American Academy of Pediatrics

Textbook of Pediatric Care

American Academy of Pediatrics

TEXTBOOK OF PEDIATRIC CARE

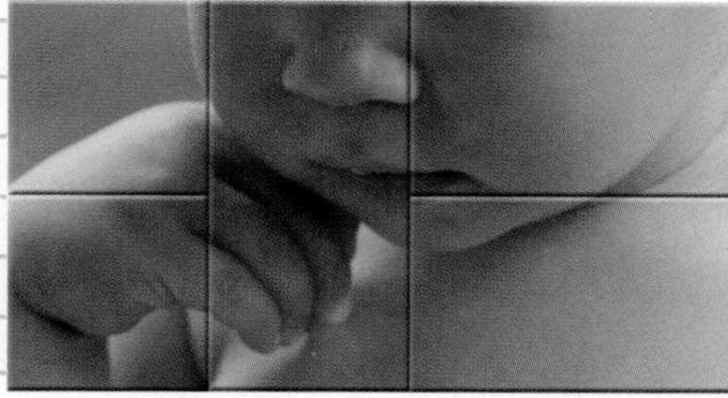

Thomas K. McInerny, MD, FAAP
Editor in Chief
Professor and Associate Chair for Clinical Affairs, Department of Pediatrics
University of Rochester School of Medicine and Dentistry
Rochester, New York

Co-editors

Henry M. Adam, MD, FAAP
Professor of Clinical Pediatrics, Albert Einstein College of Medicine
Children's Hospital at Montefiore
Bronx, New York

Deborah E. Campbell, MD, FAAP
Professor of Clinical Pediatrics, Albert Einstein College of Medicine
Director, Division of Neonatology, Children's Hospital at Montefiore
Bronx, New York

Deepak M. Kamat, MD, PhD, FAAP
Professor of Pediatrics, Wayne State University
Vice Chair of Education
Director, Institute of Medical Education, The Carman and Ann Adams Department of Pediatrics
Children's Hospital of Michigan
Detroit, Michigan

Kelly J. Kelleher, MD, MPH, FAAP
Professor of Pediatrics and Psychiatry, Colleges of Medicine and Public Health
Director, Center for Innovation in Pediatric Practice
Vice President for Health Services Research Columbus Children's Research Institute
Columbus, Ohio

Robert A. Hoekelman, MD, FAAP
ExOfficio

American Academy of Pediatrics
DEDICATED TO THE HEALTH OF ALL CHILDREN™

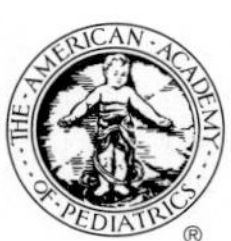

Director, Department of Marketing and Publications: **Maureen DeRosa, MPA**
Director, Division of Product Development: **Mark Grimes**
Senior Developmental Editor: **Martha Cook, MS**
Editorial Assistant: **Carrie Peters**
Director, Division of Publishing and Production Services: **Sandi King, MS**
Manager, Editorial Production: **Theresa Wiener**
Director, Division of Marketing: **Jill Ferguson**
Manager, Clinical and Professional Publications Marketing: **Linda Smessaert**
Director, Division of Sales: **Robert Herling**
Cover Design: **Linda Diamond**
Internal Designer and Project Manager: **Dana Peick, Cadmus Communications**
Production Editor: **Janice Massey, Cadmus Communications**

Library of Congress Control Number: 2007925935

ISBN-13: 978-1-58110-268-0
MA0402

The recommendations in this publication do not indicate an exclusive course of treatment or serve as a standard of medical care. Variations, taking into account individual circumstances, may be appropriate.

Every effort has been made to ensure that the drug selection and dosage set forth in this text are in accordance with the current recommendations and practice at the time of publication. It is the responsibility of the health care provider to check the package insert of each drug for any change in indications and dosage and for added warnings and precautions.

The mention of product names in this publication is for informational purposes only and does not imply endorsement by the American Academy of Pediatrics.

The publishers have made every effort to trace the copyright holders for borrowed material. If they have inadvertently overlooked any, they will be pleased to make the necessary arrangements at the first opportunity.

Printed in the United States of America.

Publisher's Cataloging-In-Publication Data
(Prepared by The Donohue Group, Inc.)

Textbook of pediatric care / Thomas K. McInerny, editor in chief; co-editors: Henry M. Adam, Deborah E. Campbell, Deepak M. Kamat, Kelly J. Kelleher.

p. : ill., charts ; cm.

Includes bibliographical references and index.
ISBN: 978-1-58110-268-0

1. Pediatrics—Textbooks. I. McInerny, Thomas K. II. Adam, Henry M. III. American Academy of Pediatrics.

RJ45 .T59 2009
618.92 2007925935

Suggested Citation: McInerny TK, Adam HM, Campbell DE, Kamat DM, Kelleher KJ, eds. *American Academy of Pediatrics Textbook of Pediatric Care.* Elk Grove Village, IL: American Academy of Pediatrics; 2009.

9-210/0908
1 2 3 4 5 6 7 8 9 10

DEDICATION

We dedicate this first edition to Robert Hoekelman, MD, whose legacy of excellence, commitment to quality health care for children, and dedication to education in pediatrics are reflected in these pages.

Foreword

The American Academy of Pediatrics (AAP) and our member pediatricians dedicate ourselves to the health, safety, and well-being of infants, children, adolescents, and young adults. An important aspect of our work is creating the educational materials necessary to provide appropriate, equitable, and high-quality pediatric care. To this end, the AAP has capitalized on its extensive knowledge and resources to create the *AAP Textbook of Pediatric Care*.

The AAP is the leading publisher in the field of pediatrics, offering more than 500 publications, both print and electronic, for pediatricians and other health professionals who care for children. This kind of leadership saves lives, improves children's health, and supports the high quality of the profession of pediatrics.

The *AAP Textbook of Pediatric Care* was created by a distinguished editorial team led by Thomas K. McInerny, MD, FAAP. Featuring contributions from experienced clinicians worldwide, this textbook addresses clinical issues faced by physicians who care for children: screening, diagnosis, treatment, and management for both common and uncommon diseases. Priorities for the 21st century, including the practice of evidence-based medicine, electronic health records, finance, and continuous quality improvement, are also addressed.

Because the practice of pediatrics is constantly changing and because we have a need for information accessible in multiple ways, we also offer this information as part of our new Web-based resource, *Pediatric Care Online*. Please see www.pediatriccareonline.org for updates to the textbook and the latest news in pediatric health care.

Renée R. Jenkins, MD, FAAP
President, American Academy of Pediatrics, 2007–2008

Introduction

Medical experts and patients alike increasingly recognize the value of the medical home and pediatric primary care. Adding to the complexity of the practice of pediatrics within the framework of the medical home is that physicians who care for children do so in various settings: community health clinics, private group practices, solo practices, and hospitals, as well as in rural, urban, and suburban communities. The *American Academy of Pediatrics Textbook of Pediatric Care* provides information for physicians who care for children no matter the setting, with an emphasis on the medical home as the ideal. This first edition, created on the basis of the fourth edition of *Primary Pediatric Care,* edited by Robert Hoekelman, MD, provides the latest evidence-based recommendations for the diagnosis and treatment of children cared for by pediatricians, family physicians, and nurse practitioners. The American Academy of Pediatrics (AAP) and its extensive resources were instrumental in ensuring the completeness and accuracy of this textbook. We particularly appreciate the efforts by the AAP committees and sections in reviewing the chapters relevant to their areas of expertise.

Some of the key topic areas of the textbook of which we are most proud include the unique section on developing well-functioning systems of care and continuous quality improvement in practice patterns. In addition, because pediatricians are increasingly on the front lines in providing mental health care, we increased the emphasis on developmental, behavioral, and psychosocial health care. The section on neonatology provides the information necessary to care for high-risk and healthy newborns in areas without ready access to tertiary care hospitals.

We include the helpful "When to Refer" and "When to Admit" guidance at the end of each chapter, and after each chapter is a summary of the most highly regarded implementation materials. These materials include links to resources for engaging patients and families, medical decision support, practice management and care coordination, and community advocacy and coordination, as well as related Web sites, AAP policy statements, and suggested readings. To make things easier for the busy physician, we created a supplement to the text, the *AAP Textbook of Pediatric Care: Tools for Practice,* which provides the reader with copies of many of the hundreds of screening questionnaires, forms, tables, and other implementation tools collected by the editors and authors. This supplement also offers a short summary of pediatric basic life support and helpful guidance with pictures of the most common procedures performed by pediatricians.

Most exciting is the delivery of the text and associated tools in an electronic format. *Pediatric Care Online* (www.pediatriccareonline.org) brings together this text and other leading pediatric resources into one integrated site. In addition to online access to the *AAP Textbook of Pediatric Care, Pediatric Care Online* includes *Red Book* content; *Bright Futures*; an interactive periodicity schedule; and a topical quick reference guide, as well as tools, patient education materials, calculators, and timely clinical updates.

Part 1, Delivering Pediatric Health Care, discusses health care delivery and finance, as well as organizational issues for pediatric practices including the use of electronic health records, Web-based resources, evidence-based medicine, and quality improvement methodologies. Chapters on child health supervision, the medical home, family-centered care (including caring for families new to the United States), and community-wide approaches to promote child health are also offered. This part concludes with a chapter on ethical and legal issues.

Part 2, Evaluation and Communication, addresses the elements of history taking, physical examination, imaging, and discussing the diagnosis with patients and families. Because the population of children in the United States is becoming increasingly more diverse and systems of medical care are evolving, chapters on cultural issues in primary pediatric care, the art of referral consultation and collaborative management, and hospital care are also provided.

Part 3, Principles of Patient Care, has been reorganized into 6 sections: Health Promotion, Disease Prevention, Screening and Case Finding, Treatment of Disease, Care of the Child With Special Health Care Needs, and Palliative and End-of-Life Care.

Because prevention is such an important part of primary pediatric care, Section Three provides the latest recommendations for screening and preventing medical, emotional, and behavioral problems, as well as anticipatory guidance. Section Four includes an extensive discussion on the management of symptoms and diseases, including some of the newer treatments using hypnosis, biofeedback, and complementary and alternative medicine. Finally, because advances in pediatric medical care have led to the survival of many children with serious chronic illnesses, Section Five provides information important to the primary care pediatrician's role in coordinating the care of children with chronic illnesses, and Section Six discusses palliative care.

Because many diseases originate during the 9 months from conception to birth, Part 4, Maternal and Fetal Perinatal Health: Effect on Pregnancy Outcomes, discusses prenatal and perinatal health issues.

Part 5, Care of the Term and Late Preterm Infant, presents information useful to the primary care pediatrician in caring for well and mild-to-moderately ill newborns. This part is divided into 4 sections: Assessment and Physical Examination of the Newborn, Routine Care Issues, Discharge Planning and Follow-up Care, and Neonatal Medical Conditions.

Part 6, Psychosocial Issues in Child Health Care, has been significantly expanded in recognition of the fact that primary care pediatricians need to provide mental health care for children with mild-to-moderate emotional disorders, as well as a medical home for all children affected by emotional disorders. Section One, Psychological and Social Development of Children, provides an overview of the theories and concepts of development and mental health and the role of early education programs in promoting mental health. Section Two, Factors Influencing the Psychosocial Health of Children, discusses many of the external and environmental influences affecting children's health such as adoption, custody, divorce, foster care, domestic violence, and abuse. Section Three, School Health, provides information regarding the all important roles that schools play in the psychosocial development of children. Section Four, Emotional and Behavioral Problems, first discusses the general approaches to managing children with emotional problems, followed by chapters with detailed information on mental health problems most commonly encountered by primary care pediatricians.

Part 7, Adolescence, discusses issues specific to teenagers, such as interviewing and counseling; adolescent sexuality including contraception, pregnancy, and abortion; and a chapter on gay, lesbian, and bisexual youth.

Part 8, Presenting Signs and Symptoms, provides extremely useful information to the primary care pediatrician in the order that illnesses are presented to clinicians, thus enabling the clinician to reach a differential diagnosis quickly.

Part 9, Specific Clinical Problems, details the common diseases of children seen in primary care settings. The latest evidence-based medicine information is used to enable the clinician to follow the recommended guidelines for diagnosis and treatment of childhood illnesses.

Part 10, Critical Situations, presents important information regarding the common life-threatening illnesses and injuries seen in children, enabling the clinician to diagnose and treat these serious conditions rapidly.

Providing the best care for children is a complex and dynamic task. We provide in this textbook the foundation of best clinical practice in this task and are pleased to refer the reader to *Pediatric Care Online* (www.pediatriccareonline.org) for an integrated, online source of information and updates.

Thomas K. McInerny
Henry M. Adam
Deborah E. Campbell
Deepak M. Kamat
Kelly J. Kelleher

Contributors List

Nahed Abdel-Haq, MD, FAAP
Department of Pediatrics
Wayne State University
Division of Infectious Diseases
Children's Hospital of Michigan
Detroit, Michigan
305: *Parasitic Infections*

Henry M. Adam, MD, FAAP
Professor of Clinical Pediatrics, Albert Einstein College of Medicine
Children's Hospital at Montefiore
Bronx, New York
53: *Physiology and Management of Fever*

Darius J. Adams, MD
Assistant Professor, Clinical Biochemical Geneticist
Albany Medical Center
Albany, New York
105: *Specific Congenital Metabolic Disorders*

Horacio Esteban Adrogué, MD
Associate Professor of Internal Medicine
Division of Nephrology and Hypertension
Medical Director of Kidney/Pancreas/Pancreatic Islet Transplantation
The University of Texas Medical Branch (UTMB)
Galveston, Texas
269: *Hemolytic-Uremic Syndrome*
272: *Henoch-Schönlein Purpura*
357: *Acute Renal Failure*

Lindsey A. Albrecht, MD
Endocrine Fellow
UC Davis Medical Center
Department of Pediatrics
Sacramento, California
286: *Intersex*

Elizabeth Meller Alderman, MD, FAAP
Clinical Professor of Pediatrics
Albert Einstein College of Medicine
Children's Hospital at Montefiore
Bronx, New York
114: *Child Custody*

C. Andrew Aligne, MD, MPH
Co-Director of Pediatric Links with the Community
Department of Pediatrics
University of Rochester School of Medicine and Dentistry
Rochester, New York
9: *Community-wide Approaches to Promoting Child Health*
35: *Prevention of Smoking*

Jorge A. Alvarez
Research Associate
Department of Pediatrics, Division of Pediatric Clinical Research
Batchelor Children's Research Institute
University of Miami Leonard M. Miller School of Medicine
Miami, Florida
32: *Preventive Cardiology*

Neil Joseph B. Alviedo, MD
Division of Neonatology
Children's Hospital of Michigan and
Hutzel Women's Hospital
Wayne State University
Detroit, Michigan
103: *Prenatal Drug Abuse and Neonatal Drug Withdrawal Syndrome*

Ahdi Amer, MD
Assistant Professor of Pediatrics, Wayne State University School of Medicine
Children's Hospital of Michigan
Detroit, Michigan
311: *Plagiocephaly*

John S. Andrews, MD, FAAP
Associate Professor of Pediatrics
Associate Head for Education, Department of Pediatrics
University of Minnesota
Minneapolis, Minnesota
199: *Limp*

Richard J. Antaya, MD, FAAP
Associate Professor of Dermatology and Pediatrics
Yale University School of Medicine
New Haven, Connecticut
314: *Psoriasis*

Jugpal S. Arneja, MD, FAAP
Assistant Professor, Surgery, Wayne State University
Children's Hospital of Michigan
Detroit, Michigan
248: *Cleft Lip and Cleft Palate*

Susan S. Aronson, MD, FAAP
Clinical Professor of Pediatrics
The Children's Hospital of Philadelphia
The University of Pennsylvania
Philadelphia, Pennsylvania
109: *Early Education and Child Care Programs*

Basim I. Asmar, MD, FAAP
Professor of Pediatrics
Wayne State University School of Medicine
Director, Division of Infectious Diseases
Children's Hospital of Michigan
Detroit, Michigan
305: *Parasitic Infections*

Andrea Gottsegen Asnes, MD, MSW, FAAP
Assistant Professor
Yale University School of Medicine
Department of Pediatrics
Associate Medical Director
Child Abuse Program
Yale-New Haven Children's Hospital
New Haven, Connecticut
122: *Sexual Abuse of Children*

William L. Atkinson, MD, MPH
Director, Immunizations Services Division
Centers for Disease Control and Prevention
Atlanta, Georgia
29: *Immunizations*

Marc A. Auerbach, MD
Fellow, Pediatric Emergency Medicine
New York University, Bellevue Hospital Center
New York, New York
355: *Poisoning*

Peter A. M. Auld, MD, FAAP
Emeritus Professor of Pediatrics
Weill Medical College of Cornell University
New York, New York
72: *Assistive Reproductive Technologies, Multiple Births, and Pregnancy Outcomes*

Jeffrey R. Avner, MD, FAAP
Professor of Clinical Pediatrics
Co-Director, Medical Student Education in Pediatrics
Albert Einstein College of Medicine
Chief, Pediatric Emergency Medicine
Children's Hospital at Montefiore
Bronx, New York
184: *Gastrointestinal Hemorrhage*
338: *Altered Mental Status*

Matthew A. Bakos, MD
Clinical Assistant Professor of Dermatology
Wright State University
Dayton, Ohio
85: *Neonatal Skin*

Felix P. Banadera, MD
Division of Neonatology
Children's Hospital of Michigan and
Hutzel Women's Hospital
Wayne State University
Detroit, Michigan
103: *Prenatal Drug Abuse and Neonatal Drug Withdrawal Syndrome*

Shireen Banerji, PharmD, DABAT
Clinical Toxicology Coordinator, Rocky Mountain Poison & Drug Center
Clinical Instructor, University of Colorado Health Science Center School of Pharmacy, Department of Clinical Pharmacy
Denver, Colorado
346: *Envenomations*

Nancy K. Barnett, MD, FAAP
Associate Staff, Dermatology
Tufts New England Medical Center
Boston, Massachusetts
160: *Alopecia and Hair Shaft Anomalies*
194: *Hyperhidrosis*
211: *Pruritus*
284: *Insect Bites and Infestations*

Stephen R. Barone, MD, FAAP
Pediatric Program Director, Schneider Children's Hospital
Associate Professor of Pediatrics, New York University School of Medicine
New York, New York
283: *Infectious Mononucleosis and Other Epstein-Barr Viral Infections*

Christine E. Barron, MD, FAAP
Assistant Professor of Pediatrics
Brown Medical School
Providence, Rhode Island
356: *Rape*

John Baum, MD
Professor of Pediatrics
Professor of Medicine Emeritus
University of Rochester School of Medicine and Dentistry
Rochester, New York
198: *Joint Pain*

Rebecca A. Baum, MD
Fellow, Developmental Behavioral Pediatrics
Nationwide Children's Hospital
Columbus, Ohio
249: *Colic*

Erawati V. Bawle, MD, FAAP
Professor, Pediatrics
Wayne State University School of Medicine
Chief, Division of Genetic and Metabolic Disorders
Children's Hospital of Michigan
Detroit, Michigan
258: *Down Syndrome: Managing the Child and Family*

William R. Beardslee, MD
Academic Chairman
Department of Psychiatry
Children's Hospital Boston
Gardner Monks Professor of Child Psychiatry
Harvard Medical School
Boston, Massachusetts
108: *Mental Health of the Young: An Overview*

Peter F. Belamarich, MD, FAAP
Associate Professor of Clinical Pediatrics
Albert Einstein College of Medicine
Children's Hospital at Montefiore
Bronx, New York
158: *Abdominal Distention*
166: *Constipation*

John P. Bent, MD
Associate Professor
Albert Einstein College of Medicine
Children's Hospital at Montefiore
Bronx, New York
222: *Stridor*

Robert J. Berkowitz, DDS
Professor and Chair, Division of Pediatric Dentistry
University of Rochester School of Medicine and Dentistry
Rochester, New York
33: *Prevention of Dental Caries*

Judy C. Bernbaum, MD, FAAP
Director, Neonatal Follow Up Program
Children's Hospital of Philadelphia
Professor of Pediatrics, University of Pennsylvania School of Medicine
Philadelphia, Pennsylvania
95: *Health and Developmental Outcomes of Infants Requiring Neonatal Intensive Care*
96: *Follow-up Care of the Graduate From the Neonatal Intensive Care Unit*

Robert J. Bidwell, MD, FAAP
Associate Professor of Pediatrics
John A. Burns School of Medicine
University of Hawaii
Honolulu, Hawaii
140: *Children With Gender-variant Behaviors and Transgender Youth*
157: *Gay, Lesbian, and Bisexual Youth*

Carol J. Blaisdell, MD, FAAP
Associate Professor of Pediatrics and Physiology
Division of Pediatric Pulmonology and Allergy
University of Maryland School of Medicine
Baltimore, Maryland
237: *Apparent Life-threatening Events*

Diane E. Bloomfield, MD, FAAP
Assistant Professor
Albert Einstein College of Medicine
Children's Hospital at Montefiore
Bronx, New York
88: *Care of the Newborn After Delivery*
230: *Weight Loss*

Lisa I. Bohra, MD
Department of Pediatric Ophthalmology
Children's Hospital of Michigan
Detroit, Michigan
301: *Ocular Trauma*

Denise A. Bothe, MD
Fellow, Developmental Behavioral Pediatrics
Case Western Reserve University
Rainbow Babies and Children's Hospital
Cleveland, Ohio
56: *Self-regulation Therapies: Hypnosis and Biofeedback*

William E. Boyle, MD, FAAP
Professor of Pediatrics and of Community and Family Medicine
Dartmouth Medical School
Hanover, New Hampshire
12: *The Pediatric History*

Michael T. Brady, MD, FAAP
Chair and Professor of Pediatrics
Nationwide Children's Hospital
The Ohio State University
Columbus, Ohio
276: *Human Immunodeficiency Virus Infection and Acquired Immunodeficiency Syndrome*

Susan L. Bratton, MD, MPH, FAAP
Professor of Pediatrics
University of Utah
Division of Critical Care Medicine
Salt Lake City, Utah
354: *Pneumothorax and Pneumomediastinum*

Nancy E. Braverman, MD, MS
Assistant Professor
Institute of Genetic Medicine and Department of Pediatrics
Johns Hopkins Medical Center
Baltimore, Maryland
48: *Recognition of Genetic-Metabolic Diseases by Clinical Diagnosis and Screening*

T. Berry Brazelton, MD, FAAP
Professor of Pediatrics Emeritus, Harvard Medical School
Children's Hospital Boston
Founder, Brazelton Touchpoints Center
Boston, Massachusetts
130: *A Developmental Approach to the Prevention of Common Behavioral Problems*

Joel S. Brenner, MD, MPH, FAAP
Associate Professor of Pediatrics
Eastern Virginia Medical School, Sports Medicine Program
Medical Director, Children's Hospital of the King's Daughters
Norfolk, Virginia
163: *Back Pain*

David A. Brent, MD
Academic Chief, Child and Adolescent Psychiatry
Western Psychiatric Institute & Clinic
University of Pittsburgh School of Medicine
Pittsburgh, Pennsylvania
143: *Mood Disorders*

Luc P. Brion, MD, FAAP
Director, Fellowship Training Program in Neonatal-Perinatal Medicine, The University of Texas Southwestern Medical Center at Dallas
Dallas, Texas
98: *Neonatal Jaundice*

David I. Bromberg, MD, FAAP
Director of the Community Practice Program
University of Maryland at Baltimore
Baltimore, Maryland
13: *Interviewing Children*

Alvin C. Bronstein, MD
Medical Director, Rocky Mountain Poison and Drug Center
Associate Professor of Surgery, University of Colorado Health Sciences Center
Denver, Colorado
346: *Envenomations*

Ann M. Buchanan, MD, MPH
Physician, Pediatric AIDS Corps
Baylor International Pediatric AIDS Initiative
Lilongwe, Malawi
Africa
293: *Meningitis*

Michael G. Burke, MD, MBA, FAAP
Assistant Professor of Pediatrics
The Johns Hopkins University School of Medicine
Saint Agnes Hospital
Baltimore, Maryland
177: *Extremity Pain*

James J. Burns, MD, FAAP
Chief, General pediatrics
Baystate Children's Hospital
Springfield, Massachusetts
Associate Professor, Pediatrics
Tufts University School of Medicine
Boston, Massachusetts
331: *Tonsillectomy and Adenoidectomy*

Eric M. Butter, PhD
Assistant Professor, Pediatrics
The Ohio State University
Children's Research Institute
Columbus, Ohio
136: *Autism*

Carol J. Buzzard, MD
Associate Professor of Pediatrics
University of Rochester School of Medicine and Dentistry
Children's Heart Center at Strong
Rochester, New York
191: *High Blood Pressure in Infants, Children, and Adolescents*

Deborah E. Campbell, MD, FAAP
Professor of Clinical Pediatrics, Albert Einstein College of Medicine
Director, Division of Neonatology, Children's Hospital at Montefiore
Bronx, New York
77: *Continuing Care of the Infant After Transfer From Neonatal Intensive Care*
78: *Discharge Planning for the High-Risk Newborn Requiring Intensive Care*
80: *Perinatal Bereavement*
82: *Maternal Medical History*
83: *Physical Examination of the Newborn*
84: *Postnatal Assessment of Common Prenatal Sonographic Findings*
87: *Prenatal Visit*
92: *Care of the Late Preterm Infant*
94: *Follow-up Care of the Healthy Newborn*
95: *Health and Developmental Outcomes of Infants Requiring Neonatal Intensive Care*
96: *Follow-up Care of the Graduate From the Neonatal Intensive Care Unit*

Mary T. Caserta, MD
Associate Professor of Pediatrics
Division of Infectious Diseases
University of Rochester School of Medicine and Dentistry
Rochester, New York
353: *Meningococcemia*

Pimpanada Chearskul, MD
Division of Infectious Diseases
Children's Hospital of Michigan
Detroit, Michigan
305: *Parasitic Infections*

Catherine Chen, MD
Clinical Research Fellow, Department of Dermatology
Eastern Virginia Medical School
Norfolk, Virginia
232: *Acne*
241: *Bacterial Skin Infections*
259: *Drug Eruptions, Erythema Multiforme, Stevens-Johnson Syndrome, and Toxic Epidermal Necrolysis*
335: *Verrucae (Warts) and Molluscum Contagiosum*

Maurice J. Chianese, MD, FAAP
Chief of Pediatrics
ProHEALTH Care Associate, LLP
Lake Success, New York
Clinical Assistant Professor of Pediatrics
New York University School of Medicine
183: *Foot and Leg Problems*

Kevin Y. Ching, MD
Fellow, Division of Pediatric Emergency Medicine
New York University/Bellevue Hospital Center
New York, New York
355: *Poisoning*

Meera Chitlur, MD
Department of Pediatric Hematology/Oncology
Children's Hospital of Michigan
Detroit, Michigan
270: *Hemoglobinopathies and Sickle Cell Disease*

Louisa Chiu, MD
General Surgery Resident
Cleveland Clinic
Cleveland, Ohio
266: *Gastrointestinal Obstruction*

Jill M. Cholette, MD
Pediatric Critical Care Fellow
University of Rochester School of Medicine and Dentistry
Rochester, New York
347: *Esophageal Caustic Injury*

Emma Ciafaloni, MD
Associate Professor of Neurology
University of Rochester School of Medicine and Dentistry
Rochester, New York
295: *Muscular Dystrophy*

Garfield A.D. Clunie, MD
Assistant Professor of Obstetrics & Gynecology and Women's Health
Albert Einstein College of Medicine
Montefiore Medical Center
Bronx, New York
70: *Prenatal Diagnosis*
71: *Fetal Interventions*

Bruce H. Cohen, MD
BrainTumor and Neuro-Oncology Section
Neurological Institute
Cleveland Clinic
Cleveland, Ohio
242: *Brain Tumors*

Judith A. Cohen, MD
Medical Director
Center for Traumatic Stress in Children & Adolescents
Allegheny General Hospital
Pittsburgh, Pennsylvania
Professor of Psychiatry
Drexel University School of Medicine
Philadelphia, Pennsylvania
146: *Posttraumatic Stress Disorder*

William I. Cohen, MD, FAAP
Developmental-Behavioral Pediatrician
Director, Down Syndrome Center of Western Pennsylvania
Children's Hospital of Pittsburgh
Professor of Pediatrics and Psychiatry
University of Pittsburgh School of Medicine
Pittsburgh, Pennsylvania
285: *Intellectual Disability*

Robert C. Cohn, MD
Chairman, Department of Pediatrics
MetroHealth Medical Center
Associate Professor of Pediatrics
Case Western Reserve University School of Medicine
Cleveland, Ohio
239: *Asthma*

Molly Cole
Family Voices of Connecticut
67: *Partnering With Families in Hospital and Community Settings*

Blaise L. Congeni, MD, FAAP
Professor of Pediatrics
Northeastern Ohio Universities College of Medicine
Director, Division of Infectious Diseases
Akron Children's Hospital
Akron, Ohio
61: *Antimicrobial Therapy*

Kelly M. Conn, MPH
Researcher
University of Rochester School of Medicine and Dentistry
Rochester, New York
18: *Adherence to Pediatric Health Care Recommendations*

Elizabeth Alvarez Connelly, MD, FAAP
Assistant Professor of Dermatology
Department of Dermatology & Cutaneous Surgery
Assistant Professor, Department of Pediatrics
Co-Director, Division of Pediatric Dermatology
University of Miami Miller School of Medicine
Miami, Florida
319: *Seborrheic Dermatitis*

Carol K. Conrad, MD
Assistant Professor of Pediatrics
Division of Pulmonary Medicine
Center of Excellence in Pulmonary Biology
Stanford University
Stanford, California
337: *Airways Obstruction*

W. Carl Cooley, MD, FAAP
Medical Director, Crotched Mountain Foundation
Medical Director, Center for Medical Home Improvement
Greenfield, New Hampshire
Associate Professor of Pediatrics, Dartmouth Medical School
Hanover, New Hampshire
110: *Family-centered Care in Pediatric Practice*

David N. Cornfield, MD, FAAP
Anne T. and Robert M. Bass Professor in Pediatric Pulmonary Medicine
Director, Center of Excellence in Pulmonary Biology
Stanford University School of Medicine
Stanford, California
Chief, Pulmonary, Allergy, and Critical Care Medicine
Lucille Packard Children's Hospital
Palo Alto, California
337: *Airways Obstruction*

Susan M. Coupey, MD, FAAP
Professor of Pediatrics and Chief, Adolescent Medicine
Albert Einstein College of Medicine
Children's Hospital at Montefiore
Bronx, New York
141: *Substance Use Disorders: Evaluation and Management*
154: *Adolescent Sexuality*

Timothy P. Culbert, MD, FAAP
Medical Director, Integrative Medicine and Cultural Care
Children's Hospitals and Clinics of Minnesota
Minneapolis, Minnesota
57: *Complementary and Alternative Medical Therapies*

Sharon S. Cummings, MPH
The University of Texas School of Public Health
Houston, Texas
125: *School Health Education*

David R. Cunningham, PhD
Professor and Director
Division of Communicative Disorders, Department of Surgery
University of Louisville School of Medicine
Louisville, Kentucky
39: *Auditory Screening*

Joseph R. Custer, MD
Attending Physician, Pediatric Critical Care Unit
Associate Professor of Pediatrics
Department of Pediatrics and Communicable Disease
University of Michigan Health Care System
University of Michigan
Ann Arbor, Michigan
358: *Shock*

Lara A. Danziger-Isakov, MD, MPH, FAAP
Assistant Professor of Pediatrics
Cleveland Clinic Lerner College of Medicine
at Case Western Reserve University
The Children's Hospital at Cleveland Clinic Foundation
Cleveland, Ohio
318: *Rocky Mountain Spotted Fever*

Viral A. Dave, MD, DCH
Neonatologist
Onsite Neonatal Partners
Norwalk Hospital
Norwalk, Connecticut
92: *Care of the Late Preterm Infant*

Philip W. Davidson, PhD
Professor of Pediatrics, Environmental Medicine and Psychiatry
University of Rochester School of Medicine and Dentistry
Rochester, New York
16: *Disclosing a Diagnosis With Parents and Patients*

Lilia C. De Jesus, MD
Neonatologist, Division of Neonatal-Perinatal Medicine
Wayne State School of Medicine
Children's Hospital of Michigan
Detroit, Michigan
103: *Prenatal Drug Abuse and Neonatal Drug Withdrawal Syndrome*

Sonia Dela Cruz-Rivera, MD
Assistant Clinical Professor of Pediatrics
Albert Einstein College of Medicine
Children's Hospital at Montefiore Medical Center
Bronx, New York
93: *Healthy Newborn Discharge*

Marcela Del Rio, MD
Assistant Professor of Pediatrics
Division of Pediatric Nephrology
Children's Hospital at Montefiore
Bronx, New York
188: *Hematuria*

Pamela K. Den Besten, DDS, MS
Professor and Chair
Division of Pediatric Dentistry, School of Dentistry
University of California at San Francisco
San Francisco, California
33: *Prevention of Dental Caries*

Joan DiMartino-Nardi, MD
Professor of Clinical Pediatrics
Children's Hospital at Montefiore Medical Center
Albert Einstein College of Medicine
Bronx, New York
192: *Hirsutism, Hypertrichosis, and Precocious Sexual Hair Development*

Linda Meyer Dinerman, MD
Private Practice
Adolescent-Young Adult Medicine
Huntsville, Alabama
171: *Dysmenorrhea*
227: *Vaginal Discharge*

Elaine A. Dinolfo, MD, MS, FAAP
Assistant Professor of Pediatrics
Albert Einstein College of Medicine
Children's Hospital at Montefiore
Bronx, New York
88: *Care of the Newborn After Delivery*
230: *Weight Loss*

Aleksandra Djukic, MD, PhD, FAAP
Assistant Professor of Neurology and Pediatrics
Montefiore Medical Center
Albert Einstein College of Medicine
Bronx, New York
106: *Neurologic Abnormalities*

Nienke P. Dosa, MD, MPH, FAAP
Assistant Professor of Pediatrics
Center for Neurodevelopmental Pediatrics
State University of New York
Syracuse, New York
68: *School-related Issues for Children With Special Needs*

M. Catherine Driscoll, MD
Children's Hospital at Montefiore
Professor of Clinical Pediatrics
Albert Einstein College of Medicine
Bronx, New York
102: *Neonatal Hematology*

George T. Drugas, MD, FACS, FAAP
Associate Professor of Surgery and Pediatrics
University of Rochester School of Medicine and Dentistry
Rochester, New York
347: *Esophageal Caustic Injury*

Howard Dubowitz, MD, MS
Professor of Pediatrics
Chief, Division of Child Protection
University of Maryland School of Medicine
Baltimore, Maryland
120: *Child Physical Abuse and Neglect*

David L. Dudgeon, MD, FAAP
Clinical Professor of Surgery
University of Arizona School of Medicine
Phoenix, Arizona
266: *Gastrointestinal Obstruction*

Paula M. Duncan, MD, FAAP
Professor of Pediatrics
University of Vermont College of Medicine
Burlington, Vermont
7: *Child Health Supervision*

Paul H. Dworkin, MD, FAAP
Professor and Chairman of Pediatrics
University of Connecticut School of Medicine
Physician-in-Chief
Connecticut Children's Medical Center
Hartford, Connecticut
36: *Screening: General Considerations*
129: *School Learning Problems and Developmental Differences*

Marian F. Earls, MD, FAAP
Medical Director
Guildford Child Health, Inc.
Associate Clinical Professor of Pediatrics
UNC School of Medicine
Greensboro Area Health Education Center
Greensboro, North Carolina
44: *Developmental Surveillance and Intervention*

Marvin S. Eiger, MD
Associate Clinical Professor, Department of Pediatrics
The Mount Sinai School of Medicine
Attending Physician, Pediatrics, The Beth Israel Medical Center
New York, New York
26: *Feeding of Infants and Children*

Mohammad F. El-Baba, MD
Division Chief, Pediatric Gastroenterology
Children's Hospital of Michigan
Assistant Professor, Department of Pediatrics
Wayne State University
Detroit, Michigan
172: *Dysphagia*

Dianne S. Elfenbein, MD, FAAP
Associate Professor of Pediatrics
University of Massachusetts Medical School
Worcester, Massachusetts
155: *Adolescent Pregnancy and Parenthood*

Jonathan Fanaroff, MD, JD, FAAP
Assistant Professor of Pediatrics
Case Western Reserve University School of Medicine
Associate Director, Rainbow Center for Pediatric Ethics
Rainbow Babies & Children's Hospital
Cleveland, Ohio
81: *Medical-Legal Considerations in the Care of Newborns*

Marianne E. Felice, MD, FAAP
Professor and Chair, Department of Pediatrics
University of Massachusetts Medical School
Physician-in-Chief, UMass Memorial Children's Medical Center
Worcester, Massachusetts
52: *The Ill Child*
155: *Adolescent Pregnancy and Parenthood*
356: *Rape*

Lauren A. Ferrara, MD
Maternal Fetal Medicine Fellow
Mount Sinai School of Medicine
New York, New York
70: *Prenatal Diagnosis*

Arthur H. Fierman, MD, FAAP
Associate Professor of Pediatrics
New York University School of Medicine
New York, New York
49: *Screening and Initial Management of Lead Poisoning*

Jeffrey S. Fine, MD, FAAP
Assistant Professor of Pediatrics and Emergency Medicine
New York University School of Medicine
New York, New York
355: *Poisoning*

Martin A. Finkel, DO, FACOP, FAAP
Professor of Pediatrics
New Jersey Child Abuse Research Education & Service Institute
University of Medicine & Dentistry of New Jersey School of Osteopathic Medicine
Stratford, New Jersey
120: *Child Physical Abuse and Neglect*

Howard Fischer, MD, FAAP
Associate Professor of Pediatrics, Wayne State University School of Medicine
Chief, Division of Ambulatory Pediatrics and Adolescent Medicine,
Children's Hospital of Michigan
Detroit, Michigan
250: *Common Cold*

Martin M. Fisher, MD, FAAP
Chief, Division of Adolescent Medicine
Schneider Children's Hospital
North Shore – Long Island Jewish Health System
New Hyde Park, New York
Professor of Pediatrics, New York University School of Medicine
New York, New York
135: *Anorexia and Bulimia Nervosa*

Randall G. Fisher, MD, FAAP
Associate Professor, Division of Pediatric Infectious Diseases
Eastern Virginia Medical School
Norfolk, Virginia
241: *Bacterial Skin Infections*

Francisco Xavier Flores, MD
Assistant Professor
Pediatric Nephrology
University of South Florida College of Medicine
Tampa, Florida
272: *Henoch-Schönlein Purpura*

Glenn Flores, MD, FAAP
Professor of Pediatrics and Public Health
Director, Division of General Pediatrics
Judith and Charles Ginsburg Chair in Pediatrics
University of Texas Southwestern Medical Center
Children's Medical Center of Dallas
Dallas, Texas
10: *Caring for Families New to the United States*

Gilbert B. Forbes, MD[†]
Professor Emeritus of Pediatrics
University of Rochester School of Medicine and Dentistry
Children's Hospital at Strong
Rochester, New York
27: *Nutritional Requirements*

Christopher B. Forrest, MD, PhD
Senior Vice President, Chief Transformation Officer, Children's Hospital of Philadelphia
Professor of Pediatrics, University of Pennsylvania School of Medicine
Philadelphia, Pennsylvania
1: *Health Care Delivery System*
2: *Pediatrician and Health Care Finance*

Rene J. Forti, MD, FAAP
Assistant Professor of Clinical Pediatrics
Albert Einstein College of Medicine
Attending Physician, Pediatric Emergency Medicine
Children's Hospital at Montefiore
Bronx, New York
338: *Altered Mental Status*

[†]Deceased

Howard R. Foye Jr, MD, FAAP
Clinical Associate Professor of Pediatrics
University of Rochester School of Medicine and Dentistry
Rochester, New York
25: *Anticipatory Guidance*

Elaine M. Frank, PhD
Associate Professor and Chair
Department of Communication Sciences and Disorders
University of South Carolina
Columbia, South Carolina
45: *Language and Speech Assessment*

Lorry R. Frankel, MD, FAAP
Professor of Pediatrics, Critical Care Medicine
Stanford University School of Medicine
Stanford, California
344: *Drowning and Near Drowning*

Gina M. French, MD, FAAP
Associate Professor of Community Pediatrics
Kapiolani Medical Center for Women and Children
University of Hawaii, John A. Burns School of Medicine
Honolulu, Hawaii
34: *Prevention of Obesity*

Katherine T. Fullerton, MD
Fellow, Pediatric Emergency Medicine
Bellevue Hospital/New York University School of Medicine
New York, New York
355: *Poisoning*

Sheila Gahagan, MD, MPH, FAAP
Professor of Clinical Pediatrics
University of Michigan Medical School
Department of Pediatrics
Ann Arbor, Michigan
299: *Obesity and Metabolic Syndrome*

Robert J. Gajarski, MD, FAAP
Associate Professor of Pediatrics, Division of Cardiology
C.S. Mott Children's Hospital, University of Michigan
Ann Arbor, Michigan
251: *Congenital and Acquired Heart Disease*

Manisha Gandhi, MD
Maternal-Fetal Medicine Fellow
Mount Sinai School of Medicine
New York, New York
71: *Fetal Interventions*

John P. Gearhart, MD, FAAP
Professor and Director of Pediatric Urology
James Buchanan Brady Urological Institute
The Johns Hopkins Hospital
Baltimore, Maryland
279: *Hypospadias, Epispadias, and Cryptorchism*

Tasha C. Geiger, PhD
Instructor of Pediatrics
Golisano Children's Hospital at Strong
University of Rochester School of Medicine and Dentistry
Rochester, New York
107: *Theories and Concepts of Development*

Paul L. Geltman, MD, MPH, FAAP
Assistant Professor of Pediatrics, Boston University School of Medicine
Department of Pediatrics, Cambridge Health Alliance
Cambridge, Massachusetts
10: *Caring for Families New to the United States*

Welton M. Gersony, MD
Alexander S. Nadas Professor of Pediatrics
Pediatric Cardiology
Morgan Stanley Children's Hospital of New York–Presbyterian
New York, New York
317: *Rheumatic Fever*

Harry L. Gewanter, MD, FAAP, FACR
Pediatric Rheumatology, Pediatric and Adolescent Health Partners
Midlothian, Virginia
288: *Juvenile Idiopathic Arthritis*

Timothy Gibson, MD, FAAP
Division Chief, Hanshaw Inpatient Hospitalist Service
UMass Memorial Children's Medical Center
Assistant Professor of Pediatrics
University of Massachusetts Medical School
Worcester, Massachusetts
52: *The Ill Child*

Melanie A. Gold, DO, FAAP
Associate Professor of Pediatrics
Division of Adolescent Medicine
Children's Hospital of Pittsburgh
University of Pittsburgh School of Medicine
Pittsburgh, Pennsylvania
118: *Gay- and Lesbian–parented Families*
153: *Interviewing Adolescents*

Johanna Goldfarb, MD, FAAP
Professor of Pediatrics, Cleveland Clinic
Lerner College of Medicine, Case Western Reserve University
Children's Hospital, Cleveland Clinic
Cleveland, Ohio
303: *Osteomyelitis*
321: *Septic Arthritis*

David L. Goldman, MD
Associate Professor of Pediatrics
Albert Einstein College of Medicine
Bronx, New York
214: *Recurrent Infections*

Stuart L. Goldstein, MD, FAAP
Associate Professor of Pediatrics
Baylor College of Medicine
Medical Director, Renal Dialysis Unit and Pheresis Service
Texas Children's Hospital
Houston, Texas
357: *Acute Renal Failure*

Ian Scott Goodman, MD
Chief Resident, Pediatrics
Baystate Children's Hospital
Springfield, Massachusetts
331: *Tonsillectomy and Adenoidectomy*

Richard Gorlick, MD, FAAP
Associate Professor of Pediatrics and Molecular Pharmacology
Albert Einstein College of Medicine
Vice Chairman
Division Chief of Hematology/Oncology
Department of Pediatrics
Children's Hospital at Montefiore
Bronx, New York
291: *Leukemias*

Rhonda M. Graves, MD, FAAP
Director, Pediatric Residency Program
New York University School of Medicine
New York, New York
115: *Children of Divorce*

Michelle A. Grenier, MD, FAAP
Assistant Professor of Pediatrics, Baylor College of Medicine
Texas Children's Hospital
Houston, Texas
40: *Cardiovascular Screening*

Lindsey K. Grossman, MD, FAAP
Professor and Associate Chair for Community and Government Affairs
University of Maryland Department of Pediatrics
Baltimore, Maryland
168: *Dental Stains*
203: *Malocclusion*
274: *Herpes Infection*

James P. Guevara, MD, MPH, FAAP
Assistant Professor of Pediatrics, University of Pennsylvania School of Medicine
Attending Physician, The Children's Hospital of Philadelphia
Philadelphia, Pennsylvania
137: *Attention-deficit/Hyperactivity Disorder*

John H. Gundy, MD, FAAP
Associate Clinical Professor of Pediatrics
Yale University School of Medicine
New Haven, Connecticut
14: *Pediatric Physical Examination*

Monika Gupta, MD
Fellow, Critical Care
Department of Pediatrics and Communicable Diseases
University of Michigan
Ann Arbor, Michigan
358: *Shock*

Bernard Guyer, MD, MPH
Zanvyl Krieger Professor of Children's Health
The Johns Hopkins Bloomberg School of Public Health
Baltimore, Maryland
28: *Morbidity and Mortality Among the Young*

Waseem Hafeez, MBBS, FAAP
Associate Professor of Clinical Pediatrics
Albert Einstein College of Medicine
Attending Physician
Division of Pediatric Emergency Medicine
Children's Hospital at Montefiore
Bronx, New York
196: *Irritability*

Joseph F. Hagan Jr, MD, FAAP
Clinical Professor in Pediatrics
University of Vermont College of Medicine
Hagan & Rinehart Pediatricians, PLLC
Burlington, Vermont
7: *Child Health Supervision*

David S. Hains, MD
Pediatric Resident, Columbus Children's Hospital
Columbus, Ohio
51: *Use of Urinalysis and Urine Culture in Screening*

Caroline Breese Hall, MD, FAAP
Professor of Pediatrics and Medicine
Division of Infectious Diseases
University of Rochester School of Medicine and Dentistry
Rochester, New York
201: *Lymphadenopathy*
243: *Bronchiolitis*
340: *Croup (Acute Laryngotracheobronchitis)*

William J. Hall, MD
Professor of Medicine
University of Rochester School of Medicine
Rochester, New York
243: *Bronchiolitis*
340: *Croup (Acute Laryngotracheobronchitis)*

Jill S. Halterman, MD, MPH
Associate Professor of Pediatrics
University of Rochester School of Medicine and Dentistry
Rochester, New York
18: *Adherence to Pediatric Health Care Recommendations*

Ada Hamosh, MD
Clinical Director, Institute of Genetic Medicine
Scientific Director, OMIM
Scutland Professor of Pediatric Genetics
The Johns Hopkins University School of Medicine
Baltimore, Maryland
48: *Recognition of Genetic-Metabolic Diseases by Clinical Diagnosis and Screening*

David C. Hanson, MD, FAAP
Assistant Professor of Pediatrics
University of Minnesota Medical School
Minneapolis, Minnesota
177: *Extremity Pain*

Winita Hardikar, MBBS, FRACP, PhD
Head of Hepatology
Royal Children's Hospital Melbourne
Associate Professor
University of Melbourne
Melbourne, Australia
273: *Hepatitis*

Christopher Harris, MD, FAAP
Monroe Carell Jr. Children's Hospital at Vanderbilt
Nashville, Tennessee
312: *Pneumonia*

J. Peter Harris, MD, FAAP
Professor of Pediatrics
University of Rochester Medical Center
Rochester, New York
164: *Cardiac Arrhythmias*

Sandra G. Hassink, MD, FAAP
Director, Childhood and Adolescent Weight Management Clinic
Alfred I. duPont Hospital for Children
Wilmington, Delaware
Assistant Professor of Pediatrics, Jefferson Medical College, Thomas Jefferson University
Philadelphia, Pennsylvania
34: *Prevention of Obesity*

Amy Heneghan, MD, FAAP
Associate Professor of Pediatrics
Case Western Reserve University School of Medicine
Cleveland, Ohio
47: *Family Screening and Assessments*

Neil E. Herendeen, MD, MBA
Associate Professor of Pediatrics
University of Rochester Medical Center
Rochester, New York
235: *Animal Bites*
255: *Cystic and Solid Masses of the Face and Neck*

Andrew D. Hershey, MD, PhD
Professor of Pediatrics and Neurology
University of Cincinnati
Director, Headache Center
Associate Director, Neurology Research
Children's Hospital Medical Center
Cincinnati, Ohio
185: *Headache*

Mel Heyman, MD, FAAP
Professor of Pediatrics
University of California
San Francisco, California
264: *Gastroesophageal Reflux Disease*

Joanne M. Hilden, MD, FAAP
Vice President of Medical Affairs
Peytoon Manning Children's Hospital at St. Vincent
Pediatric Hematologist/Oncologist
St. Vincent Children's Center for Cancer and Blood Diseases
Indianapolis, Indiana
242: *Brain Tumors*

Ginette A. Hinds, MD
Dermatology Resident
Yale University
New Haven, Connecticut
314: *Psoriasis*

Andrea S. Hinkle, MD
Associate Professor of Pediatrics
Golisano Children's Hospital at Strong
University of Rochester School of Medicine and Dentistry
Rochester, New York
244: *Cancers in Childhood*

Robert A. Hoekelman, MD, FAAP
Professor and Chairman Emeritus, Department of Pediatrics
University of Rochester School of Medicine and Dentistry
Rochester, New York
183: *Foot and Leg Problems*

Charles J. Homer, MD, MPH, FAAP
Chief Executive Officer, National Initiative for Children's Healthcare Quality
Associate Clinical Professor of Pediatrics
Harvard Medical School
Associate Professor
Harvard School of Public Health
Boston, Massachusetts
6: *Quality Improvement in Pediatric Primary Care*

Sharon G. Humiston, MD, MPH
Associate Professor of Emergency Medicine and Pediatrics
Department of Emergency Medicine
University of Rochester School of Medicine & Dentistry
Rochester, New York
29: *Immunizations*

Robert Iannone, MD
Adjunct Assistant Professor of Pediatrics
Division of Oncology
The Children's Hospital of Philadelphia
Philadelphia, Pennsylvania
253: *Contagious Exanthematous Diseases*

Sonia O. Imaizumi, MD, FAAP
Associate Professor, Pediatrics
Robert Wood Johnson Medical School
Associate Division Head, Neonatology
Children's Regional Hospital
Camden, New Jersey
65: *Home Health Care*
95: *Health and Developmental Outcomes of Infants Requiring Neonatal Intensive Care*
96: *Follow-up Care of the Graduate of the Neonatal Intensive Care Unit*

Franca M. Iorember, MD, MPH
Fellow, Pediatric Nephrology
Department of Pediatrics
Columbus Children's Hospital
The Ohio State University
Columbus, Ohio
261: *Enuresis*

Timo J. Jahnukainen, MD, PhD
Assistant Professor of Pediatrics
Department of Pediatric Nephrology and Transplantation
University of Helsinki
Helsinki, Finland
334: *Urinary Tract Infections*

Amrish Jain, MD
Fellow, Division of Pediatric Nephrology and Hypertension
Children's Hospital of Michigan
Detroit, Michigan
236: *Anuira and Oliguira*

Matthew P. Janik, MD
Dermatology Resident
Wright State University, School of Medicine
Dayton, Ohio
85: *Neonatal Skin*

Megan E. Janoff
Columbia University and New York State Psychiatric Institute
New York, New York
50: *Substance Use Disorders: Early Identification and Referral*

Sandra H. Jee, MD, MPH, FAAP
Assistant Professor of Pediatrics
Department of Pediatrics
University of Rochester School of Medicine and Dentistry
Rochester, New York
116: *Children in Foster and Kinship Care*

Michael S. Jellinek, MD, FAAP
Professor of Psychiatry and of Pediatrics
Harvard Medical School
Chief, Child Psychiatry Service
Massachusetts General Hospital
Boston, Massachusetts
46: *Psychosocial Screening*
138: *Conduct Disorders*

Jerri Ann Jenista, MD, FAAP
Pediatrician, Departments of Pediatrics and Emergency Medicine
St. Joseph Mercy Hospital
Ann Arbor, Michigan
260: *Enterovirus Infections*
275: *Human Herpesvirus-6 and Human Herpesvirus-7 Infections*

Peter S. Jensen, MD
Ruane Professor of Child and Adolescent Psychiatry
Columbia University
Director, Center for Advancement of Children's Mental Health
New York, New York
133: *Medication Management for Emotional and Behavioral Problems*

Alain Joffe, MD, MPH, FAAP
Director, Student Health and Wellness Center
The Johns Hopkins University
Associate Professor of Pediatrics
Johns Hopkins Medical Institutions
Baltimore, Maryland
161: *Amenorrhea*
171: *Dysmenorrhea*
226: *Vaginal Bleeding*
227: *Vaginal Discharge*
322: *Sexually Transmitted Infections*

Jason E. Jones, MD
Assistant Professor of Psychiatry
Division of Child and Adolescent Psychiatry
University of Maryland, School of Medicine
Baltimore, Maryland
131: *Consultation and Referral for Emotional and Behavioral Problems*

R. Joe Jopling, MD, FAAP
Wasatch Pediatrics
Salt Lake City, Utah
23: *Counseling Families on Healthy Lifestyles*

Nicholas Jospe, MD
Professor of Pediatrics
Golisano Children's Hospital at Strong
Strong Memorial Hospital
University of Rochester
Rochester, New York
278: *Hyperthyroidism*

Jeffrey M. Kaczorowski, MD, FAAP
Associate Professor of Pediatrics
University of Rochester
Rochester, New York
9: *Community-wide Approaches to Promoting Child Health*

Ronald J. Kallen, MD, FAAP
Associate Professor, Clinical
Department of Pediatrics
Feinberg School of Medicine, Northwestern University
Chicago, Illinois
316: *Renal Tubular Acidosis*

Deepak M. Kamat, MD, PhD, FAAP
Professor of Pediatrics, Wayne State University
Vice Chair of Education
Director, Institute of Medical Education
The Carman and Ann Adams Department of Pediatrics
Children's Hospital of Michigan
Detroit, Michigan
311: *Plagiocephaly*
315: *Pyloric Stenosis*

Ruth K. Kaminer, MD, FAAP
Clinical Professor of Pediatrics
Albert Einstein College of Medicine
Bronx, New York
43: *Identification of Developmental Delays and Early Intervention System*

Paul B. Kaplowitz, MD, PhD, FAAP
Chief of Endrcrinology
Children's National Medical Center
Professor of Pediatrics
George Washington University School of Medicine and Health Sciences
Washington, District of Columbia
218: *Short Stature*

Jeffrey M. Karp, DMD, MS
Assistant Professor, Division of Pediatric Dentistry
School of Medicine and Dentistry
University of Rochester
Rochester, New York
33: *Prevention of Dental Caries*

Frederick J. Kaskel, MD, PhD, FAAP
Professor and Vice-Chairman of Pediatrics
Director, Division of Pediatric Nephrology
Children's Hospital at Montefiore
Albert Einstein College of Medicine
Bronx, New York
174: *Dysuria*

Dona Rani Kathirithamby, MD
Associate Professor of Rehabilitation Medicine
Assistant Professor of Pediatrics
Albert Einstein College of Medicine
Children's Evaluation and Rehabilitation Center
Bronx, New York
66: *Pediatric Rehabilitation*

John Kattwinkel, MD, FAAP
Charles Fuller Professor of Neonatology
University of Virginia
Charlottesville, Virginia
330: *Sudden Infant Death Syndrome*

Harpreet Kaur, MD
Fellow, Division of Neonatology
Albert Einstein College of Medicine
Bronx, New York
82: *Maternal Medical History*
83: *Physical Examination of the Newborn*

Alex R. Kemper, MD, MPH, MS, FAAP
Director, Program on Pediatric Health Services Research
Duke Clinical Research Institute
Durham, North Carolina
42: *Vision Screening*

Kathi J. Kemper, MD, MPH, FAAP
Caryl J Guth Chair for Holistic and Integrative Medicine
Professor, Pediatrics and Public Health Sciences
Author, The Holistic Pediatrician
Wake Forest University School of Medicine
Winston-Salem, North Carolina
57: *Complementary and Alternative Medical Therapies*

Jonette E. Keri, MD, PhD
University of Miami Leonard M. Miller School of Medicine
Assistant Professor of Dermatology and Cutaneous Surgery
Chief, Dermatology Service, Miami VA Hospital
Miami, Florida
240: *Atopic Dermatitis*
252: *Contact Dermatitis*

Bryce A. Kerlin, MD
Assistant Professor of Clinical Pediatrics
The Ohio State University
Division of Pediatric Hematology/Oncology/BMT
Columbus Children's Hospital
Columbus, Ohio
41: *Screening for Anemia*

John A. Kerner Jr, MD
Professor of Pediatric Gastroenterology and Fellowship Director, and Director of Nutrition
Lucile Packard Children's Hospital/Stanford University Medical Center
Palo Alto, California
265: *Gastrointestinal Allergy*
268: *Gluten-sensitive Enteropathy (Celiac Sprue)*

Mohamad A. Khaled, MD, MSurg
Neurosurgery Resident
University of Virginia
Charlottesville, Virginia
277: *Hydrocephalus*

Unab I. Khan, MD
Assistant Professor of Pediatrics
Children's Hospital at Montefiore
Albert Einstein College of Medicine
Bronx, New York
154: *Adolescent Sexuality*

Diana King, MD, FAAP
Assistant Professor of Pediatrics
Albert Einstein College of Medicine
Children's Hospital at Montefiore
Bronx, New York
196: *Irritability*

Robert A. King, MD
Professor of Child Psychiatry Medical Director
Tourette's/OCD Clinic
Yale Child Study Center
Yale University School of Medicine
New Haven, Connecticut
224: *Tics*

Jonathan D. Klein, MD, MPH, FAAP
Associate Professor of Pediatrics and of Community and Preventive Medicine
University of Rochester School of Medicine and Dentistry
Rochester, New York
152: *Counseling Parents of Adolescents*

Michael D. Klein, MD, FAAP
Surgeon-in-Chief, Children's Hospital of Michigan
Arvin I. Philippart, III, MD, Chair in Pediatric Surgical Research and Professor of Surgery
Wayne State University
Detroit, Michigan
336: *Acute Surgical Abdomen*

William J. Klish, MD, FAAP
Professor of Pediatrics
Baylor College of Medicine
Houston, Texas
27: *Nutritional Requirements*

Penelope K. Knapp, MD, FAAP
Professor Emeritus, Psychiatry and Pediatrics
University of California, Davis
Davis, California
22: *Supporting Development of the Family*

Tsoline Kojaoghlanian, MD
Department of Pediatric Infectious Diseases
Department of Microbiology and Immunology
Children's Hospital at Montefiore
Albert Einstein College of Medicine
Bronx, New York
101: *The Infant With Suspected Infection*

Faye Kokotos, MD, FAAP
Assistant Professor of Pediatrics
Albert Einstein College of Medicine
Children's Hospital at Montefiore
Bronx, New York
88: *Care of the Newborn After Delivery*

E. Anders Kolb, MD
Director, Blood and Bone Marrow Transplantation
Alfred I. duPont Hospital for Children
Wilmington, Delaware
162: *Anemia and Pallor*
291: *Leukemias*

David J. Kolko, PhD
Professor of Psychiatry, Psychology, and Pediatrics
University of Pittsburgh School of Medicine
Director, Special Services Unit
Western Psychiatric Institute & Clinic
Pittsburgh, Pennsylvania
132: *Options for the Delivery of Mental Health Services*
146: *Posttraumatic Stress Disorder*

Sabine Kost-Byerly, MD, FAAP
Director, Pediatric Pain Management
Department of Anesthesiology/Critical Care Medicine
The Johns Hopkins University School of Medicine
Baltimore, Maryland
55: *Management of Chronic Pain in Children*

Richard E. Kreipe, MD, FAAP
Professor of Pediatrics
Division of Adolescent Medicine
Golisano Children's Hospital at Strong
University of Rochester School of Medicine and Dentistry
Director, Leadership Education in Adolescent Health Interdisciplinary Training Program
Rochester, New York
151: *Challenges of Health Care Delivery to Adolescents*

Leonard R. Krilov, MD, FAAP
Chief, Pediatric Infectious Diseases
Vice Chairman Department of Pediatrics
Winthrop University Hospital
Professor of Pediatrics
State University of New York Stony Brook School of Medicine
Mineola, New York
247: *Chronic Fatigue Syndrome*
283: *Infectious Mononucleosis and Other Epstein-Barr Viral Infections*

Lakshmanan Krishnamurti, MD
Associate Professor of Pediatrics
Director, Comprehensive Hemoglobinopathies Program
Division of Hematology/Oncology/Bone Marrow Transplantation
Children's Hospital of Pittsburgh of UPMC
Pittsburgh, Pennsylvania
287: *Iron-Deficiency Anemia*

Robert K. Kritzler, MD
Deputy Chief Medical Officer
Johns Hopkins Health Care
Baltimore, Maryland
212: *Puberty: Normal and Abnormal*

Daniel P. Krowchuk, MD, FAAP
Professor of Pediatrics and Dermatology
Chief, General Pediatrics and Adolescent Medicine
Wake Forest University School of Medicine
Winston-Salem, North Carolina
213: *Rash*

Zuzanna Kubicka, MD
Department of Newborn Medicine
Children's Hospital
Boston, Massachusetts
104: *Common Metabolic Disturbances in the Newborn*

Emily S. Kuschner, MA
Doctoral Student, Clinical and Social Sciences in Psychology
University of Rochester
Rochester, New York
16: *Disclosing a Diagnosis With Parents and Patients*

Erik E. Langenau, DO, FAAP, FACOP
Associate Program Director of Pediatrics
Maimonides Infants and Children's Hospital of Brooklyn
Brooklyn, New York
207: *Odor (Unusual Urine and Body)*

John D. Lantos, MD, FAAP
Professor of Pediatrics
Chief, General Pediatrics
University of Chicago
Chicago, Illinois
11: *Ethical and Legal Issues for the Primary Care Physician*

Ruth Lawrence, MD, FAAP
Professor of Pediatrics and Obstetrics/Gynecology
University of Rochester School of Medicine and Dentistry
Golisano Children's Hospital at Strong Memorial Hospital
Rochester, New York
90: *Breastfeeding: Drugs, Herbs, and Environmental Toxins*

Lori Legano, MD, FAAP
Assistant Professor of Pediatrics
New York University School of Medicine
New York, New York
115: *Children of Divorce*

Pieter le Roux, D Litt et Phil
Associate Professor of Psychiatry and Pediatrics
University of Rochester School of Medicine and Dentistry
Rochester, New York
145: *Phobias and Anxiety*

Laurel K. Leslie, MD, MPH, FAAP
Associate Professor of Medicine and Pediatrics
Tufts Medical Center
Floating Hospital for Children
Boston, Massachusetts
137: *Attention-deficit/Hyperactivily Disorder*

John M. Leventhal, MD, FAAP
Professor of Pediatrics and Child Study Center
Yale University School of Medicine
Medical Director, Child Abuse and Child Abuse Prevention Programs
Yale-New Haven Children's Hospital
New Haven, Connecticut
122: *Sexual Abuse of Children*

Terry L. Levin, MD
Clinical Professor of Radiology
Albert Einstein College of Medicine
Montefiore Medical Center
Bronx, New York
15: *Pediatric Imaging*

Sara Buchdahl Levine, MD, MPH, FAAP
Post-Doctoral Fellow, Division of Adolescent Medicine
Children's Hospital at Montefiore
Albert Einstein College of Medicine
Bronx, New York
141: *Substance Use Disorders: Evaluation and Management*

Rebecca Levin-Goodman, MPH
Senior Manager, Injury, Violence, and Poison Prevention Initiatives
Division of Safety and Health Promotion
American Academy of Pediatrics
Elk Grove Village, Illinois
30: *Injury Prevention*

Adam S. Levy, MD
Assistant Professor, Pediatrics
Albert Einstein College of Medicine
Children's Hospital at Montefiore
Bronx, New York
162: *Anemia and Pallor*
208: *Petechiae and Purpura*

Paul A. Levy, MD, FACMG
Assistant Professor of Pediatrics
Children's Hospital at Montefiore
Albert Einstein College of Medicine
Department of Pediatrics, Division of Genetics
Bronx, New York
175: *Edema*

Samuel M. Libber, MD, FAAP
Assistant Professor of Pediatrics
The Johns Hopkins University School of Medicine
Baltimore, Maryland
209: *Polyuria*

Steven E. Lipshultz, MD, FAAP
Professor and Chairman, Department of Pediatrics
Professor of Epidemiology and Public Health and Professor of Medicine (Oncology)
University of Miami Miller School of Medicine
Chief of Staff, Holtz Children's Hospital of the University of Miami-Jackson Memorial Medical Center
Director, Batchelor Children's Research Institute
Associate Director, Mailman Center for Child Development
Member, Sylvester Comprehensive Cancer Center
Miami, Florida
32: *Preventive Cardiology*
191: *High Blood Pressure in Infants, Children, and Adolescents*
349: *Heart Failure*

Gregory S. Liptak, MD, MPH, FAAP
Professor of Pediatrics, Upstate Medical University
Director, Center for Neurodevelopmental Pediatrics
Syracuse, New York
68: *School-related Issues for Children With Special Needs*
245: *Cerebral Palsy*
257: *Diaper Rash*
324: *Spina Bifida*

George A. Little, MD, FAAP
Professor of Pediatrics and of Obstetrics/Gynecology
Children's Hospital at Dartmouth
Dartmouth-Hitchcock Medical Center
Lebanon, New Hampshire
73: *Fetal Assessment*
79: *Support for Families Whose Infant Is Sick or Dying: Collaborative Decision Making*
104: *Common Metabolic Disturbances in the Newborn*

Mark N. Lobato, MD
CAPT U.S. Public Health Service
Division of Tuberculosis Elimination
Centers for Disease Control and Prevention
Atlanta, Georgia
332: *Tuberculosis and Latent Tuberculosis Infection*

Ann M. Loeffler, MD
Francis J. Curry National Tuberculosis Center
San Francisco, California
Legacy Emanuel Children's Hospital
Portland, Oregon
332: *Tuberculosis and Latent Tuberculosis Infection*

Anthony M. Loizides, MD
Assistant Professor of Pediatrics
Albert Einstein College of Medicine
Attending Physician, Division of Pediatric Gastroenterology and Nutrition,
Children's Hospital at Montefiore
Bronx, New York
159: *Abdominal Pain*

Christina M. Long, DO
Fellow, Department of Neonatology
Children's Hospital at Montefiore
Bronx, New York
78: *Discharge Planning for the High-Risk Newborn Requiring Intensive Care*
99: *Respiratory Distress and Breathing Disorders in the Newborn*

Dominique N. Long, MD
Pediatric Endocrine Fellow
Johns Hopkins Medical Institutions
Baltimore, Maryland
212: *Puberty: Normal and Abnormal*

Liana Perez Loughlin, Esq
Miami, Florida
349: *Heart Failure*

Mark G. Luciano, MD, PhD, FACS
Head, Pediatric and Congenital Neurosurgery
Department of Neurosurgery
Cleveland Clinic
Cleveland, Ohio
277: *Hydrocephalus*

Shailender Madani, MD
Assistant Professor, Carman & Ann Adams Department of Pediatrics
Wayne State University School of Medicine
Pediatric Gastroenterologist
Children's Hospital of Michigan
Director, Fellowship Program
Pediatric Gastroenterology, Hepatology & Nutrition
Children's Hospital of Michigan GME Program
Detroit, Michigan
264: *Gastroesophageal Reflux Disease*

Stephen J. Maddox Jr, MD, FAAP
Associate Director of Newborn Services
Hospital of St. Raphael
New Haven, Connecticut
49: *Screening and Initial Management of Lead Poisoning*

Prashant V. Mahajan, MD, MPH, MBA, FAAP
Vice Chief, Division of Pediatric Emergency Medicine
Associate Professor of Pediatrics and Emergency Medicine
Carman and Ann Adams Department of Pediatrics
Children's Hospital of Michigan
Detroit, Michigan
58: *Body Fluids, Electrolyte Concentration, and Acid-Base Composition*
59: *Fluids and Electrolytes in Clinical Practice*
341: *Dehydration*
348: *Head Injuries*

Shefali Mahesh, MD
Children's Hospital at Montefiore
Albert Einstein College of Medicine
Bronx, New York
210: *Proteinuria*

Michael G. Marcus, MD
Director, Pediatric Pulmonology, Allergy/Immunology
Department of Pediatrics
Maimonides Medical Center
Brooklyn, New York
167: *Cough*

Ronald V. Marino, DO, MPH, FAAP
Associate Chairman of Pediatrics, Winthrop University Hospital
Professor of Clinical Pediatrics, SUNY Medical School At Stony Brook
Stony Brook, New York
128: *School Absenteeism and School Refusal*

Robert W. Marion, MD
Professor of Pediatrics and Obstetrics and Gynecology and Women's Health
Ruth L. Gottesman Professor of Child Development
Director, Children's Evaluation and Rehabilitation Center and the Rose F. Kennedy University Center for Excellence in Developmental Disabilities
Chief, Divisions of Genetics and Developmental Medicine
Albert Einstein College of Medicine
Children's Hospital at Montefiore
Bronx, New York
86: *Common Congenital Anomalies*
178: *Facial Dysmorphism*
333: *Umbilical Anomalies*

Bruce C. Marshall, MD
Associate Professor of Medicine
The Johns Hopkins University School of Medicine
Baltimore, Maryland
254: *Cystic Fibrosis*

James E. Martin, RRT, NPS, CPFT
Clinical Specialist, Department of Pediatrics
MetroHealth Medical Center
Cleveland, Ohio
239: *Asthma*

Tej K. Mattoo, MD, DCh, FRCP(UK), FAAP
Chief, Division of Pediatric Nephrology and Hypertension
Children's Hospital of Michigan
Detroit, Michigan
236: *Anuria and Oliguria*

Lynne G. Maxwell, MD, FAAP
Associate Professor
University of Pennsylvania
Department of Anesthesiology and Critical Care
Senior Anesthesiologist
The Children's Hospital of Philadelphia
Philadelphia, Pennsylvania
62: *Preoperative Assessment*
63: *Postoperative Care*

Jay H. Mayefsky, MD, MPH, FAAP
Professor of Clinical Pediatrics and Family and Preventive Medicine
Rosalind Franklin University of Medicine and Science
North Chicago, Illinois
Senior Attending Physician, Stroger Hospital of Cook County
Chicago, Illinois
173: *Dyspnea*

Bernadette Mazurek Melnyk, PhD, RN, CPNP/NPP
Dean and Distinguished Foundation Professor in Nursing
Arizona State University College of Nursing
Tempe, Arizona
126: *Nursing Roles in School Health*

Margaret C. McBride, MD, FAAP
Professor of Pediatrics
Northeast Ohio University College of Medicine
Director, NeuroDevelopmental Center
Akron Children's Hospital
Akron, Ohio
320: *Seizure Disorders*
360: *Status Epilepticus*

Christina M. McCann, PhD
Assistant Professor, Department of Pediatrics
University of Rochester School of Medicine and Dentistry
Rochester, New York
145: *Phobias and Anxiety*

Edith A. McCarthy, MD
Assistant Professor of Pediatrics
New York University School of Medicine
New York, New York
72: *Assistive Reproductive Technologies, Multiple Births, and Pregnancy Outcomes*

Michael A. McCulloch, MD
Fellow, Department of Pediatrics, Division of Cardiology
University of Virginia Health Science Center
Charlottesville, Virginia
251: *Congenital and Acquired Heart Disease*

Hiram L. McDade, PhD
Associate Professor and Graduate Director
Department of Communication Sciences and Disorders
University of South Carolina
Columbia, South Carolina
45: *Language and Speech Assessment*

Kathleen A. McGrath, RN, MS, CPNP
Advanced Practice Nurse, Pediatric Cardiology
Golisano Children's Hospital at Strong
University of Rochester
Rochester, New York
32: *Preventive Cardiology*

Thomas K. McInerny, MD, FAAP
Professor and Associate Chair for Clinical Affairs
Department of Pediatrics
University of Rochester School of Medicine and Dentistry
Rochester, New York
2: *Pediatrician and Health Care Finance*
3: *Practice Organization*

H. Cody Meissner, MD, FAAP
Chief, Pediatric Infectious Disease
Tufts-New England Medical Center
Professor of Pediatrics
Tufts University School of Medicine
Boston, Massachusetts
292: *Lyme Disease*

Ruth J. Messinger, MSW
Associate in Pediatrics (Retired)
University of Rochester Medical Center
Rochester, New York
16: *Disclosing a Diagnosis With Parents and Patients*

Sarah E. Messiah, MPH, PhD
Research Assistant Professor and Epidemiologist, Department of Pediatrics
Division of Pediatric Clinical Research
University of Miami, Miller School of Medicine
Batchelor Children's Research Institute
Miami, Florida
191: *High Blood Pressure in Infants, Children, and Adolescents*

Ryan S. Miller, MD, FAAP
Division of Pediatric Endocrinology
The Johns Hopkins University School of Medicine
Baltimore, Maryland
209: *Polyuria*

Tracie L. Miller, MD, MS
Professor, Department of Pediatrics
Director, Division of Pediatric Clinical Research
University of Miami Leonard M. Miller School of Medicine
Miami, Florida
32: *Preventive Cardiology*
349: *Heart Failure*

Cynthia S. Minkovitz, MD, MPP, FAAP
Department of Population, Family and Reproductive Health
The Johns Hopkins Bloomberg School of Public Health
Division of General Pediatrics and Adolescent Medicine
The Johns Hopkins University
Baltimore, Maryland
28: *Morbidity and Mortality Among the Young*

Laura J. Mirkinson, MD, FAAP
Chief of Pediatrics
Blythedale Children's Hospital
Valhalla, New York
20: *Hospitalist Medicine: Communicating With Patients and Families*

Rachel Y. Moon, MD, FAAP
Goldberg Center for Community Pediatric Health
Children's National Medical Center
Associate Professor of Pediatrics
George Washington University School of Medicine and Health Sciences
Washington, District of Columbia
330: *Sudden Infant Death Syndrome*

William J. Moss, MD, MPH
Associate Professor
Departments of Epidemiology, International Health, and Molecular Microbiology and Immunology
The Johns Hopkins Bloomberg School of Public Health
Baltimore, Maryland
276: *Human Immunodeficiency Virus Infection and Acquired Immunodeficiency Syndrome*

Richard T. Moxley III, MD
Professor of Neurology, University of Rochester Medical School
University of Rochester Medical Center
Rochester, New York
295: *Muscular Dystrophy*

Daniel W. Mruzek, PhD
Assistant Professor of Pediatrics (Psychology)
University of Rochester School of Medicine and Dentistry
Strong Center for Developmental Disabilities
Rochester, New York
16: *Disclosing a Diagnosis With Parents and Patients*

James A. Mulick, PhD
Professor, Pediatrics and Psychology
The Ohio State University
Children's Research Institute
Columbus, Ohio
136: *Autism*

Upender K. Munshi, MBBS, MD(Paediatrics), FAAP
Associate Professor of Pediatrics
Albany Medical College
Albany, New York
75: *Identifying the Newborn Who Requires Specialized Care*

Philip R. Nader, MD, FAAP
Professor Emeritus of Pediatrics
University of California, San Diego
San Diego, California
124: *Overview of School Health and School Health Program Goals*

Suhas M. Nafday, MD, MRCP(Ire), DCH, FAAP
Director of Newborn Services, Children's Hospital at Montefiore
Assistant Professor of Pediatrics, Albert Einstein College of Medicine
Bronx, New York
97: *Abnormalities of Fetal Growth*
99: *Respiratory Distress and Breathing Disorders in the Newborn*

Joshua P. Needleman, MD
Division of Pediatric Pulmonology
Children's Hospital Los Angeles
Los Angeles, California
231: *Wheezing*

Robert D. Needlman, MD, FAAP
Associate Professor of Pediatrics
Case Western Reserve University School of Medicine
MetroHealth Medical Center
Cleveland, Ohio
121: *Children in Self-care*

P. Christine Nguyen, MD
Pediatric Gastroenterology, California Pacific Medical Center
San Francisco, California
Adjunct Clinical Assistant Professor, Stanford University Medical School
Palo Alto, California
265: *Gastrointestinal Allergy*

Hiep T. Nguyen, MD, FAAP
Assistant Professor in Surgery (Urology)
Harvard Medical School
Director of Robotic Surgery and Research
Department of Urology, Children's Hospital
Urological Diseases Research Center
Boston, Massachusetts
300: *Obstructive Uropathy and Vesicoureteral Reflux*

Cameron L. Nicholson, MD
Pediatric Hematology/Oncology
Cleveland Clinic Foundation
Cleveland, Ohio
242: *Brain Tumors*

Linda S. Nield, MD, FAAP
Associate Professor of Pediatrics
West Virginia University School of Medicine
Morgantown, West Virginia
240: *Atopic Dermatitis*
252: *Contact Dermatitis*
290: *Labial Adhesions*
328: *Stomatitis*

Amanda C. North, MD
Assistant Professor of Pediatric Urology
Montefiore Medical Center
Bronx, New York
279: *Hypospadias, Epispadias, and Cryptorchism*

A. Barbara Oettgen, MD, MPH, FAAP
Assistant Professor of Pediatrics
University of Virginia Health Sciences Center
Charlottesville, Virginia
309: *Phimosis*

Ikenna C. Okereke, MD
Cardiothoracic Surgery Fellow
Beth Israel Deaconess Medical Center
Boston, Massachusetts
306: *Pectus Excavatum and Pectus Carinatum*

Alex Okun, MD, FAAP
Associate Professor of Clinical Pediatrics
Department of Pediatrics
Albert Einstein College of Medicine
Children's Hospital at Montefiore
Bronx, New York
69: *Palliative, End-of-Life, and Bereavement Care*

Karen N. Olness, MD, FAAP
Professor of Pediatrics and Family Medicine and International Health
Division of Behavioral Pediatrics and Psychology
Case Western Reserve University
Rainbow Babies and Children's Hospital
Cleveland, Ohio
17: *Cultural Issues in Primary Pediatric Care*
56: *Self-regulation Therapies: Hypnosis and Biofeedback*

Craig C. Orlowski, MD
Golisano Children's Hospital at Strong
University of Rochester School of Medicine and Dentistry
Rochester, New York
280: *Hypothyroidism*

Enrique M. Ostrea Jr, MD, FAAP
Professor of Pediatrics
Wayne State University
Children's Hospital of Michigan and
Hutzel Women's Hospital
Detroit, Michigan
103: *Prenatal Drug Abuse and Neonatal Drug Withdrawal Syndrome*

Samuel T. Ostrower, MD
Otorhinolaryngology-Head and Neck Surgery
Albert Einstein College of Medicine
Montefiore Medical Center
Bronx, New York
193: *Hoarseness*

Philip O. Ozuah, MD, PhD
Professor and University Chairman
Martin S. Davis Endowed Chair
Physician-in-Chief
Children's Hospital at Montefiore
Albert Einstein College of Medicine
Bronx, New York
180: *Fatigue and Weakness*
190: *Hepatomegaly*
219: *Splenomegaly*
225: *Torticollis*

Lane S. Palmer, MD, FACS, FAAP
Chief, Pediatric Urology
Schneider Children's Hospital of the North Shore-Long Island Jewish Health System
New Hyde Park, New York
Associate Clinical Professor of Urology and Pediatrics
Albert Einstein College of Medicine
Bronx, New York
216: *Scrotal Swelling and Pain*

Debra H. Pan, MD
Assistant Professor of Pediatrics
Albert Einstein College of Medicine
Attending Physician
Division of Pediatric Gastroenterology and Nutrition
Children's Hospital at Montefiore
Bronx, New York
197: *Jaundice*

Guy S. Parcel, PhD
Dean
M. David Low Chair in Public Health
Jon P. McGovern Professor in Health Promotion
University of Texas School of Public Health
Houston, Texas
125: *School Health Education*

Sanjay R. Parikh, MD, FAAP, FACS
Chief, Division of Pediatric Otorhinolaryngology–Head and Neck Surgery
The Children's Hospital at Montefiore
Associate Professor of ORL-HNS and Pediatrics
Albert Einstein College of Medicine
Bronx, New York
193: *Hoarseness*
262: *Foreign Bodies of the Ear, Nose, Airway, and Esophagus*

Hiren P. Patel, MD, FAAP
Clinical Assistant Professor of Pediatrics
Columbus Children's Hospital
The Ohio State University College of Medicine
Columbus, Ohio
51: *Use of Urinalysis and Urine Culture in Screening*

Ian M. Paul, MD, MSc, FAAP
Assistant Professor of Pediatrics and Health Evaluation Sciences
Penn State College of Medicine
Hershey, Pennsylvania
281: *Iatrogenic Disease*
345: *Drug Overdose*

Pearl A. Payne, PhD
Department of Wellness and Therapeutic Sciences
Division of Communication Disorders
Murray State University
Murray, Kentucky
147: *Stuttering*

Robert A. Pendergrast Jr, MD, MPH, FAAP
Associate Professor of Pediatrics
Medical College of Georgia
Augusta, Georgia
163: *Back Pain*

Jack M. Percelay, MD, MPH, FAAP
ELMO Pediatrics
New York City, New York
21: *Hospital Care*

Matthew B. Perkins, MD, MBA
Child and Adolescent Psychiatry Research Fellow
Columbia University
New York, New York
133: *Medication Management for Emotional and Behavioral Problems*

Ellen C. Perrin, MD, FAAP
Director, Division of Developmental-Behavioral Pediatrics and The Center for Children with Special Needs
The Floating Hospital for Children
Tufts-New England Medical Center
Boston, Massachusetts
111: *Principles of Effective Discipline*

Deborah Persaud, MD
Associate Professor
The Johns Hopkins University School of Medicine
Pediatric Infectious Diseases
Baltimore, Maryland
276: *Human Immunodeficiency Virus Infection and Acquired Immunodeficiency Syndrome*

Louis G. Petcu, MD, MS, FACS
ENT Consultant
Baystate Children's Hospital
Springfield, Massachusetts
331: *Tonsillectomy and Adenoidectomy*

Rosemarie A. Pezzullo, MD, FAAP
St. Barnabas Hospital
Clinical Instructor of Pediatrics
Bronx, New York
119: *Homelessness and the Family*

Randall A. Phelps, MD, PhD, FAAP
Developmental and Behavioral Pediatrician
Assistant Professor of Pediatrics
Child Development and Rehabilitation Center
Oregon Health and Science University
Eugene, Oregon
285: *Intellectual Disability*

Michael E. Pichichero, MD, FAAP
Professor of Microbiology and Immunology
Professor of Pediatrics and Medicine
University of Rochester School of Medicine & Dentistry
Rochester, New York
289: *Kawasaki Disease*
327: *Staphylococcal Toxic Shock Syndrome*

Joaquim M.B. Pinheiro, MD, MPH, FAAP
Professor of Pediatrics
Albany Medical College
Albany, New York
74: *Assessment and Stabilization at Delivery*

Steven W. Pipe, MD
Associate Professor of Pediatrics
Pediatric Medical Director
Hemophilia and Coagulation Disorders Program
Medical Director, Special Coagulation Laboratory
University of Michigan
Ann Arbor, Michigan
343: *Disseminated Intravascular Coagulation*

Leslie P. Plotnick, MD
Professor of Pediatrics
Johns Hopkins Medical Institutions
Baltimore, Maryland
209: *Polyuria*
212: *Puberty: Normal and Abnormal*

Gregory A. Plotnikoff, MD, MTS
Associate Professor
Internal Medicine and Pediatrics
University of Minnesota Medical School
Minneapolis, Minnesota
Keio University Medical School
Tokyo, Japan
57: *Complementary and Alternative Medical Therapies*

Gregory E. Prazar, MD, FAAP
Pediatrician
Exeter Pediatric Associates
Exeter, New Hampshire
139: *Conversion Reactions and Hysteria*
150: *Temper Tantrums and Breath-holding Spells*

E. Rebecca Pschirrer, MD, MPH
Clerkship Director, Department of OB/GYN
Assistant Professor, Dartmouth Medical School
Director of Prenatal Diagnosis, Division of Maternal-Fetal Medicine, Department of OB/GYN
Director of Obstetric Ultrasound, Department of Radiology
Dartmouth Hitchcock Medical Center
Lebanon, New Hampshire
73: *Fetal Assessment*

Mala Puri, MD
Fellow, Department of Pediatric Endocrinology
Albert Einstein College of Medicine
Children's Hospital at Montefiore
Bronx, New York
192: *Hirsutism, Hypertrichosis, and Precocious Sexual Hair Development*

Oscar H. Purugganan, MD, MPH
Assistant Clinical Professor, Pediatrics
Albert Einstein College of Medicine
Children's Evaluation and Rehabilitation Center
Rose F. Kennedy Center
The Children's Hospital at Montefiore
Bronx, New York
202: *Macrocephaly*
204: *Microcephaly*

Andrew D. Racine, MD, PhD, FAAP
Director, Division of General Pediatrics
Children's Hospital at Montefiore
Professor of Clinical Pediatrics
Albert Einstein College of Medicine
Bronx, New York
179: *Failure to Thrive*

Eva G. Radel, MD, FAAP
Professor of Clinical Pediatrics
Albert Einstein College of Medicine
Division of Pediatric Hematology/Oncology
Children's Hospital at Montefiore
Bronx, New York
60: *Blood Products and Their Uses*
271: *Hemophilia and Other Hereditary Bleeding Disorders*

Keyvan Rafei, MD
Assistant Professor of Pediatrics
University of Maryland School of Medicine
Baltimore, Maryland
237: *Apparent Life-threatening Events*

Yaseen Rafee, MD
Pediatric Infectious Diseases Fellow
Wayne State University
Detroit Medical Center
Detroit, Michigan
305: *Parasitic Infections*

Prema Ramaswamy, MD, FAAP
Co-Director, Pediatric Cardiology
Maimonides Infants and Children's Hospital of Brooklyn
Brooklyn, New York
Assistant Professor of Pediatrics
Mount Sinai School of Medicine
New York, New York
223: *Syncope*

Cynthia M. Rand, MD, MPH, FAAP
Assistant Professor
University of Rochester School of Medicine and Dentistry
Rochester, New York
29: *Immunizations*

Rajesh C. Rao, MD
Assistant Clinical Professor
Wayne State University
Oakland University
Detroit, Michigan
301: *Ocular Trauma*

Karen Ratliff-Schaub, MD, FAAP
Assistant Professor of Pediatrics
The Ohio State University
Nationwide Children's Hospital
Columbus, Ohio
127: *School Readiness*

Jawhar Rawwas, MD
Pediatric Hematology and Oncology
Children's Hospitals and Clinics of Minnesota
Minneapolis, Minnesota
282: *Immune Thrombocytopenia Purpura*

Sushma Reddy, MD
Pediatric Cardiology Fellow
Columbia University
New York, New York
315: *Pyloric Stenosis*

Kimberly J. Reidy, MD
Fellow, Division of Pediatric Nephrology
The Children's Hospital at Montefiore
Bronx, New York
188: *Hematuria*

Horacio A. Repetto, MD
Consultant Professor of Pediatrics
Facultad de Medicina
Universidad de Buenos Aires
Buenos Aires, Argentina
South America
269: *Hemolytic-Uremic Syndrome*

Karen Teeple Reuter, MS, RN, AZCSN
Lead Nurse, Middle Schools/High Schools
School Nurse, Shadow Mountain High School
Paradise Valley Unified School District
Phoenix, Arizona
President, Arizona School Nurse Consortium
126: *Nursing Roles in School Health*

Marina Reznik, MD, MS, FAAP
Assistant Professor of Pediatrics
Albert Einstein College of Medicine
Children's Hospital at Montefiore
Bronx, New York
180: *Fatigue and Weakness*
190: *Hepatomegaly*
219: *Splenomegaly*

Abraham C. Rice, MD
Assistant Professor of Pediatrics
Contra Costa Regional Medical Center
Martinez, California
117: *Domestic Violence and the Family*

Denise M. Richardson, MD
Assistant Professor
Division of Child & Adolescent Psychiatry
Department of Psychiatry
University of Maryland, School of Medicine
Baltimore, Maryland
217: *Self-stimulating Behaviors*

Julius B. Richmond, MD, FAAP†
John D. MacArthur Professor of Health Policy Emeritus
Department of Social Medicine
Harvard Medical School
Boston, Massachusetts
108: *Mental Health of the Young: An Overview*

Angel Rios, MD, FAAP
Associate Professor of Pediatrics
The Children's Hospital at Albany Medical Center
Albany, New York
105: *Specific Congenital Metabolic Disorders*

Yolanda Rivas, MD
Assistant Professor of Pediatrics
Albert Einstein College of Medicine
Division of Pediatric Gastroenterology and Nutrition
Children's Hospital at Montefiore
Bronx, New York
197: *Jaundice*

Ruby F. Rivera, MD, FAAP
Assistant Professor of Pediatrics
Albert Einstein College of Medicine
Children's Hospital at Montefiore
Bronx, New York
170: *Dizziness and Vertigo*

Brett W. Robbins, MD, FAAP
Assistant Professor of Pediatrics and Internal Medicine
University of Rochester Medical Center
Rochester, New York
5: *Evidence-based Medicine*

Sarah M. Roddy, MD, FAAP
Associate Professor of Pediatrics and Neurology
Loma Linda University School of Medicine
Loma Linda, California
206: *Nonconvulsive Periodic Disorders*
320: *Seizure Disorders*
360: *Status Epilepticus*

Victoria Weeks Rogers, MD, FAAP
Director, Clinical Outcomes and Outreach Program at The Barbara Bush Children's Hospital at Maine Medical Center
Portland, Maine
6: *Quality Improvement in Pediatric Primary Care*

Chokechai Rongkavilit, MD
Associate Professor, Division of Pediatric Infectious Diseases
Children's Hospital of Michigan
Department of Pediatrics, Wayne State University School of Medicine
Detroit, Michigan
329: *Streptococcal Toxic Shock Syndrome*

Orna Rosen, MD, FAAP
Assistant Professor of Pediatrics
Division of Neonatology
Children's Hospital at Montefiore
Bronx, New York
86: *Common Congenital Anomalies*

Donna Andrea Rosenberg, MD, FAAP
Associate Clinical Professor
Department of Pediatrics
University of Colorado
Denver, Colorado
144: *Münchausen Syndrome by Proxy*

Maris D. Rosenberg, MD, FAAP
Associate Professor of Clinical Pediatrics
Children's Evaluation and Rehabilitation Center
Albert Einstein College of Medicine
Bronx, New York
66: *Pediatric Rehabilitation*

Lainie Friedman Ross, MD, PhD, FAAP
Associate Professor of Pediatrics
Associate Director, MacLean Center for Clinical Medical Ethics
University of Chicago
Chicago, Illinois
11: *Ethical and Legal Issues for the Primary Care Physician*

Arlene A. Rozzelle, MD, FAAP
Assistant Professor, Plastic Surgery
Wayne State University School of Medicine
Chief, Plastic Surgery
Children's Hospital of Michigan
Director, Cleft/Craniofacial Anonases Team
Detroit, Michigan
248: *Cleft Lip and Cleft Palate*

Camille Sabella, MD, FAAP
Associate Professor of Pediatrics
Cleveland Clinic Lerner College of Medicine of Case Western Reserve University
Children's Hospital, Cleveland Clinic
Cleveland, Ohio
307: *Pertussis*

†Deceased

Anca M. Safta, MD
Pediatrics Gastroenterology/Nutrition/Liver Fellow
Lucile Packard Children's Hospital, Stanford University Medical Center
Palo Alto, California
268: *Gluten-sensitive Enteropathy (Celiac Sprue)*

Olle Jane Z. Sahler, MD, FAAP
Professor of Pediatrics, Psychiatry, Medical Humanities, and Oncology
University of Rochester School of Medicine and Dentistry
Rochester, New York
107: *Theories and Concepts of Development*

A. John Sargent, III, MD
Professor of Psychiatry and Pediatrics
Baylor College of Medicine
Houston, Texas
134: *Family Interactions: Children Who Have Unexplained Physical Symptoms*

Richard M. Sarles, MD
Professor of Psychiatry and Pediatrics
University of Maryland, School of Medicine
Baltimore, Maryland
131: *Consultation and Referral for Emotional and Behavioral Problems*
205: *Nervousness*
217: *Self-stimulating Behaviors*

Sharada A. Sarnaik, MD
Professor of Pediatrics, The Carman and Ann Adams Department of Pediatrics
Wayne State University School of Medicine
Children's Hospital of Michigan
Detroit, Michigan
270: *Hemoglobinopathies and Sickle Cell Disease*

Eric A. Schaff, MD, FAAP
Clinical Assistant Professor, University at Buffalo
Medical Director, Planned Parenthood of Delaware
Wilmington, Delaware
156: *Contraception and Abortion*

Richard J. Schanler, MD, FAAP
Associate Chairman, Department of Pediatrics and Chief, Neonatal-Perinatal Medicine
Schneider Children's Hospital at North Shore
Professor, Albert Einstein College of Medicine
Bronx, New York
89: *Breastfeeding the Newborn*

Lawrence Schachner, MD
Chairman and Harvey Blank Professor of Dermatology
University of Miami Miller School of Medicine
Miami, Florida
319: *Seborrheic Dermatitis*

Miriam B. Schechter, MD, FAAP
Assistant Clinical Professor of Pediatrics
Children's Hospital at Montefiore
Bronx, New York
176: *Epistaxis*

Steven C. Schlozman, MD
Associate Director, Medical Student Education in Psychiatry, Harvard Medical School
Associate Director, Child and Adolescent Psychiatry Residency, MGH/McLean Program in Child Psychiatry
Staff Child Psychiatrist, Massachusetts General Hospital
Assistant Professor of Psychiatry, Harvard Medical School
Boston, Massachusetts
46: *Psychosocial Screening*

Barton D. Schmitt, MD, FAAP
Professor of Pediatrics
University of Colorado School of Medicine
Denver, Colorado
142: *Encopresis*

Marcie B. Schneider, MD, FAAP, FSAM
Associate Clinical Professor of Pediatrics
Department of Pediatrics
Albert Einstein College of Medicine
Bronx, New York
Associate Attending
Department of Pediatrics
Greenwich Hospital
Greenwich, Connecticut
135: *Anorexia and Bulimia Nervosa*

Cindy M. Schorzman, MD
Family Practice Physician
Group Health Cooperative
Olympia, Washington
118: *Gay- and Lesbian-parented Families*

Alan R. Schroeder, MD, FAAP
Pediatric Critical Care
Santa Clara Valley Medical Center
San Jose, California
359: *Status Asthmaticus*

Scott A. Schroeder, MD, FAAP
Professor of Pediatrics
Albany Medical College
Section Chief, Division of Pediatric Pulmonary Medicine and Cystic Fibrosis Center
Albany Medical Center
Albany, New York
165: *Chest Pain*
189: *Hemoptysis*

Andrew L. Schwaderer, MD
Assistant Professor of Pediatrics
Section of Nephrology
Columbus Children's Hospital
The Ohio State University
Columbus, Ohio
261: *Enuresis*

Cindy L. Schwartz, MD
Professor of Pediatrics
Director, Pediatric Hematology-Oncology
Hasbro Children's Hospital/Brown Medical School
Providence, Rhode Island
244: *Cancers in Childhood*

Kathleen B. Schwarz, MD
Professor of Pediatrics
The Johns Hopkins University School of Medicine
Baltimore, Maryland
273: *Hepatitis*

W. Frederick Schwenk, II, MD, FAAP
Professor of Pediatrics
Mayo Clinic
Rochester, Minnesota
256: *Diabetes Mellitus*
342: *Diabetic Ketoacidosis*

Elizabeth Secord, MD
Wayne State University
Children's Hospital of Michigan
Carman and Ann Adams Department of Pediatrics
Division of Allergy and Immunology
Detroit, Michigan
339: *Anaphylaxis*

Robert T. Seese, MD
Fellow in Pediatric Infectious Diseases
The Children's Hospital at The Cleveland Clinic
Cleveland, Ohio
318: *Rocky Mountain Spotted Fever*

Robert D. Sege, MD, PhD, FAAP
Chief of Pediatric and Adolescent Medicine
Tufts New England Medical Center
Boston, Massachusetts
31: *Violence Prevention*

George B. Segel, MD
Professor of Pediatrics and Medicine
University of Rochester School of Medicine and Dentistry
Rochester, New York
201: *Lymphadenopathy*

Henry M. Seidel, MD
Professor Emeritus of Pediatrics
School of Medicine, The Johns Hopkins University
Baltimore, Maryland
19: *Art of Referral, Consultation, and Collaborative Management*

Catherine R. Sellinger, MD, FAAP
Assistant Professor of Pediatrics
Albert Einstein College of Medicine
Children's Hospital at Montefiore
Bronx, New York
170: *Dizziness and Vertigo*

Aimee E. Seningen, MD
Adolescent Medicine Fellow
Children's Hospital of Pittsburgh
Pittsburgh, Pennsylvania
153: *Interviewing Adolescents*

M. Mohsin Shah, MD
Resident, Neurological Surgery
University of Missouri
Columbia, Missouri
352: *Increased Intracranial Pressure*

Anjali A. Sharathkumar, MD
Clinical Lecturer
Department of Pediatrics and Communicable Diseases
University of Michigan
Ann Arbor, Michigan
343: *Disseminated Intravascular Coagulation*

Tanvi S. Sharma, MD
Instructor in Medicine
Harvard Medical School
Department of Pediatrics
Division of Infectious Diseases
Children's Hospital Boston
Boston, Massachusetts
349: *Heart Failure*

Robert L. Sheridan, MD, FAAP
Chief, Burn Surgery Service, Shriners Hospital for Children
Co-Director, Sumner Redstone Adult Burn Center, Massachusetts General Hospital
Associate Professor of Surgery, Harvard Medical School
Boston, Massachusetts
361: *Thermal Injuries*

Peter G. Sherman, MD, FAAP
Director, Residency Program in Social Pediatrics
Montefiore Medical Center
Associate Professor of Clinical Pediatrics and Family and Social Medicine
Albert Einstein College of Medicine
Bronx, New York
117: *Domestic Violence and the Family*
119: *Homelessness and the Family*

Laura Jean Shipley, MD, FAAP
Clinical Associate Professor of Pediatrics
University of Rochester, Department of Pediatrics
Rochester, New York
9: *Community-wide Approaches to Promoting Child Health*

Lisa H. Shulman, MD, FAAP
Associate Clinical Professor of Pediatrics
Albert Einstein College of Medicine
Children's Evaluation and Rehabilitation Center
Rose F. Kennedy Center
Bronx, New York
66: *Pediatric Rehabilitation*

Calvin C.J. Sia, MD, FAAP
Professor of Pediatrics
University of Hawaii School of Medicine
Honolulu, Hawaii
8: *Medical Home Collaborative Care*

George K. Siberry, MD, MPH, FAAP
Assistant Professor of Pediatrics
Divisions of General Pediatrics and Pediatric Infectious Diseases
The Johns Hopkins University School of Medicine
Baltimore, Maryland
246: *Chickenpox*

Erica M. Sibinga, MD, MHS, FAAP
Assistant Professor of Pediatrics
The Johns Hopkins University School of Medicine
Baltimore, Maryland
199: *Limp*

David M. Siegel, MD, MPH, FAAP
Professor of Pediatrics and Medicine
University of Rochester School of Medicine and Dentistry
Edward H. Townsend Chief of Pediatrics
Rochester General Hospital
Rochester, New York
198: *Joint Pain*
288: *Juvenile Idiopathic Arthritis*

Edward M. Sills, MD, FAAP
Director, Pediatric Rheumatology
The Johns Hopkins Hospital and The Johns Hopkins University School of Medicine
Baltimore, Maryland
302: *Osteochondroses*
325: *Spinal Deformities*

Michael R. Simon, MD
Clinical Professor Emeritus
Departments of Internal Medicine and Pediatrics
Wayne State University School of Medicine
Detroit, Michigan
Allergy and Immunology Section
William Beaumont Hospital
Royal Oak, Michigan
339: *Anaphylaxis*

Catherine C. Skae, MD, FAAP
Assistant Professor of Pediatrics
Albert Einstein College of Medicine
Children's Hospital at Montefiore
Bronx, New York
225: *Torticollis*
262: *Foreign Bodies of the Ear, Nose, Airway, and Esophagus*

Douglas P. Sladen, PhD
Assistant Research Professor
Vanderbilt University Medical Center
Department of Hearing and Speech Sciences
Nashville, Tennessee
186: *Hearing Loss*

Eric Small, MD, FAAP
Clinical Assistant Professor of Pediatrics, Orthopedics, Rehabilitation Medicine
Mount Sinai School of Medicine
New York, New York
38: *Preparticipation Physical Examination*

Gary A. Smith, MD, DrPH, FAAP
Director, Center for Injury Research and Policy
Children's Hospital
Associate Professor of Pediatrics
The Ohio State University College of Medicine
Columbus, Ohio
30: *Injury Prevention*

Michael L. Smith, MD, FAAP
Associate Professor of Medicine and Pediatrics
Vanderbilt University Medical Center
Nashville, Tennessee
298: *Neurocutaneous Syndromes*

Shirley A. Smoyak, RN, PhD
Professor II, Rutgers, The State University of New Jersey
Continuous Education and Outreach
New Brunswick, New Jersey
112: *Changing American Families*

Matthew D. Smyth, MD, FAAP
Assistant Professor of Neurosurgery and Pediatrics
Washington University
St Louis Children's Hospital
St Louis, Missouri
352: *Increased Intracranial Pressure*

Kristin C. Sokol, MPH
Research Associate, Department of Pediatrics
Division of Pediatric Clinical Research
University of Miami, Miller School of Medicine
Batchelor Children's Research Institute
Miami, Florida
191: *High Blood Pressure in Infants, Children, and Adolescents*

Joshua Sparrow, MD
Assistant Professor of Psychiatry, Harvard Medical School
Children's Hospital Boston
Director of Special Initiatives, Brazelton Touchpoints Center, Children's Hospital Boston
Boston, Massachusetts
130: *A Developmental Approach to the Prevention of Common Behavioral Problems*

Phyllis W. Speiser, MD
Professor of Pediatrics
New York School of Medicine, Chief of Pediatric Endocrinology
Schneider Children's Hospital
New Hyde Park, New York
233: *Adrenal Dysfunction*

Mark L. Splaingard, MD
Professor of Clinical Pediatrics
Ohio State University School of Medicine
Director, Sleep Center
Nationwide Children's Hospital
Columbus, Ohio
148: *Sleep Disturbances*

Alfred J. Spiro, MD, FAAP
Professor of Neurology and Pediatrics
Albert Einstein College of Medicine
Director, MDA Muscle Disease Clinic
Bronx, New York
195: *Hypotonia*

S. Andrew Spooner, MD, MS, FAAP
Chief Medical Information Officer
Cincinnati Children's Medical Center
Cincinnati, Ohio
4: *Electronic Health Record and Web-based Resources*

Sarah H. Springer, MD, FAAP
International Adoption Health Services of Western Pennsylvania
Pediatric Alliance, P.C.
Pittsburgh, Pennsylvania
113: *Adoption*

Anthony Stallion, MD, FACS, FAAP
Staff Pediatric Surgeon
Department of Pediatric Surgery
Children's Hospital-Cleveland Clinic
Cleveland, Ohio
266: *Gastrointestinal Obstruction*
306: *Pectus Excavatum and Pectus Carinatum*

Thomas J. Starc, MD, MPH
Professor of Clinical Pediatrics
Columbia University
Division of Pediatric Cardiology
Children's Hospital of New York
New York, New York
32: *Preventive Cardiology*
317: *Rheumatic Fever*

Russell W. Steele, MD, FAAP
Division Head, Pediatric Infectious Diseases
Ochsner for Children
Ochsner Clinic Foundation
New Orleans, Louisiana
308: *Pharyngitis and Tonsillitis*

David H. Stein, MD, MPH, MSt
Johns Hopkins Dermatology
Johns Hopkins Bloomberg Public Health
Baltimore, Maryland
284: *Insect Bites and Infestations*

Ruth E.K. Stein, MD, FAAP
Professor of Pediatrics
Albert Einstein College of Medicine
Children's Hospital at Montefiore
Bronx, New York
64: *Children With Ongoing Health Conditions*

Elissa L. Stern, LCSW, MPH
Social Worker
Children's Hospital at Montefiore
Bronx, New York
66: *Pediatric Rehabilitation*

David M. Stevens, MD
Assistant Professor of Pediatrics
Albert Einstein College of Medicine
Bronx, New York
176: *Epistaxis*

R. Scott Strahlman, MD, FAAP
Instructor, Department of Pediatrics
The Johns Hopkins University School of Medicine
Baltimore, Maryland
Pediatrician, Columbia Medical Practice
Columbia, Maryland
238: *Appendicitis*
263: *Fractures and Dislocations*

Victor C. Strasburger, MD, FAAP
Professor of Pediatrics
Professor of Family & Community Medicine
Chief, Division of Adolescent Medicine
University of New Mexico School of Medicine
Albuquerque, New Mexico
123: *Children, Adolescents, and the Media*

Donna M. Strobino, PhD
Professor, Department of Population, Family, and Reproductive Health
The Johns Hopkins Bloomberg School of Public Health
Baltimore, Maryland
28: *Morbidity and Mortality Among the Young*

Dennis M. Styne, MD, FAAP
Rumsey Chair and Professor
Section Chief Pediatric Endocrinology
University of California Davis Medical Center
Department of Pediatrics
Sacramento, California
286: *Intersex*

Christina Kan Sullivan, MD, FAAP
Assistant Clinical Professor of Pediatrics
Albert Einstein College of Medicine
Children's Hospital at Montefiore Medical Center
Bronx, New York
93: *Healthy Newborn Discharge*

Katarina Supe-Markovina, MD
Assistant Professor, Department of Pediatrics
Division of Pediatric Nephrology
Montefiore Medical Center
Bronx, New York
174: *Dysuria*

Srinivasan Suresh, MD, MBA
Assistant Professor of Pediatrics and Emergency Medicine
Associate Director, Pediatric Residency Program
Children's Hospital of Michigan
Wayne State University
Detroit, Michigan
326: *Sports Injuries*
350: *Hypertensive Emergencies*
351: *Hypoglycemia*

Nicole J. Sutton, MD, FAAP
Assistant Professor of Pediatrics
Albert Einstein College of Medicine
Children's Hospital at Montefiore
Bronx, New York
100: *Evaluation of the Infant With Suspected Heart Disease*

Jack T. Swanson, MD, FAAP
Pediatrician, McFarland Clinic
Ames, Iowa
91: *Circumcision*

Sarah A. Sydlowski, AuD
Division of Communicative Disorders, Department of Surgery
University of Louisville School of Medicine
Louisville, Kentucky
39: *Auditory Screening*

Moira Szilagyi, MD, PhD, FAAP
Associate Professor of Pediatrics
University of Rochester
Medical Director, Starlight Pediatrics
Monroe County Department of Health
Rochester, New York
116: *Children in Foster and Kinship Care*

Peter G. Szilagyi, MD, MPH, FAAP
Professor of Pediatrics
Chief, General Pediatrics
University of Rochester School of Medicine and Dentistry
Rochester, New York
18: *Adherence to Pediatric Health Care Recommendations*
29: *Immunizations*
235: *Animal Bites*
255: *Cystic and Solid Masses of the Face and Neck*

Tina Q. Tan, MD, FAAP
Associate Professor of Pediatrics, Feinberg School of Medicine
Northwestern University
Infectious Diseases Attending: Co-Director, Pediatric Travel Medicine Clinic
Director, International Adoptee Clinic
Children's Memorial Hospital
Chicago, Illinois
304: *Otitis Media and Otitis Externa*
323: *Sinusitis*

Howard L. Taras, MD, FAAP
Professor of Clinical Pediatrics
Division of Community Pediatrics and School Health
University of California, San Diego
La Jolla, California
124: *Overview of School Health and School Health Program Goals*

Peter J. Tebben, MD
Assistant Professor of Medicine and Pediatrics
Division of Endocrinology, Diabetes, Metabolism, and Nutrition
Division of Pediatric Endocrinology and Metabolism
Mayo Clinic College of Medicine
Rochester, Minnesota
256: *Diabetes Mellitus*
342: *Diabetic Ketoacidosis*

Anne Marie Tharpe, PhD
Professor
Vanderbilt University Medical Center
Department of Hearing and Speech Sciences
Nashville, Tennessee
186: *Hearing Loss*

Joseph D. Tobias, MD, FAAP
Vice-Chairman, Department of Anesthesiology
Russell and Mary Shelden Chair in Pediatric Intensive Care
Chief, Division of Pediatric Anesthesiology
Professor of Pediatrics and Anesthesiology
University of Missouri
Columbia, Missouri
54: *Management of Acute Pain in Children*

Kristine Torjesen, MD, MPH
Research Assistant Professor of Pediatrics
University of North Carolina at Chapel Hill
Chapel Hill, North Carolina
17: *Cultural Issues in Primary Pediatric Care*

Christine Tracy, MD
Assistant Clinical Professor of Pediatrics
Albert Einstein College of Medicine
Attending Physician, Pediatric Cardiology
Children's Hospital at Montefiore Medical Center
Bronx, New York
187: *Heart Murmurs*

Maria Trent, MD, MPH, FAAP
Assistant Professor of Pediatrics
Departments of Pediatrics and Population, Family & Reproductive Health
The Johns Hopkins University School of Medicine & Bloomberg School of Public Health
Baltimore, Maryland
161: *Amenorrhea*
226: *Vaginal Bleeding*

Julian J. Trevino, MD
Associate Professor, Dermatology
Wright State University, School of Medicine
Dayton, Ohio
85: *Neonatal Skin*

Robert Turbow, MD, JD
Attending Neonatologist, Phoenix Children's Hospital
Phoenix, Arizona
CEO–PatientPatents, Inc.
San Luis Obispo, California
Adjunct Professor of Biology and Biomedical Engineering, California Polytechnic State University
San Luis Obispo, California
81: *Medical-Legal Considerations in the Care of Newborns*

Martin H. Ulshen, MD
Professor of Pediatrics
Chief, Division of Pediatric Gastroenterology and Nutrition
Department of Pediatrics
Duke University Medical Center
Durham, North Carolina
169: *Diarrhea and Steatorrhea*
200: *Loss of Appetite*
229: *Vomiting*

Elise W. van der Jagt, MD, MPH, FAAP
Professor of Pediatrics and Critical Care
Director, Pediatric Hospital Medicine Program
Golisano Children's Hospital at Strong
University of Rochester School of Medicine and Dentistry
Rochester, New York
181: *Fever*
182: *Fever of Unknown Origin*

Heather A. Van Mater, MD
Clinical Lecturer of Pediatrics
University of Michigan
Ann Arbor, Michigan
299: *Obesity and Metabolic Syndrome*

William S. Varade, MD
Associate Professor of Pediatrics
University of Rochester School of Medicine and Dentistry
Attending Physician, Golisano Children's Hospital at Strong
Rochester, New York
296: *Nephritis*
297: *Nephrotic Syndrome*

Abhay N. Vats, MD
Associate Professor of Pediatrics
Children's Hospital of Pittsburgh
University of Pittsburgh School of Medicine
Pittsburgh, Pennsylvania
334: *Urinary Tract Infections*

Alfin G. Vicencio, MD
Assistant Professor of Pediatrics, Division of Pediatric Respiratory and Sleep Medicine
Albert Einstein College of Medicine
Children's Hospital at Montefiore
Bronx, New York
222: *Stridor*
231: *Wheezing*

Susan J. Vig, PhD
Professor, Clinical Pediatrics
Albert Einstein College of Medicine
Bronx, New York
43: *Identification of Developmental Delays and Early Intervention System*

Joseph A. Vitterito II, MD
Division of Neonatology
Department of Pediatrics
Dartmouth Hitchcock Medical Center
Lebanon, New Hampshire
Medical Director, Rhode Island School for the Deaf
79: *Support for Families Whose Infant Is Sick or Dying: Collaborative Decision Making*

Ellen R. Wald, MD, FAAP
Professor and Chair, Department of Pediatrics
University of Wisconsin Children's Hospital
Madison, Wisconsin
313: *Preseptal and Orbital Cellulitis*

Ruth R. Walden
State Coordinator
Family Voices New York
Albany, New York
67: *Partnering With Families in Hospital and Community Settings*

Audrey M. Walker, MD
Associate Professor of Psychiatry and Pediatrics
Albert Einstein College of Medicine
Director of Training, Child and Adolescent Psychiatry
Albert Einstein College of Medicine/Montefiore Medical Center
Director of Child and Adolescent Psychiatry
Montefiore Medical Center
Bronx, New York
221: *Strange Behavior*

Christine A. Walsh, MD, FAAP
Director, Pediatric Dysrhythmia Center
Children's Hospital at Montefiore
Divisions of Pediatric Cardiology and Critical Care Medicine
Professor of Clinical Pediatrics
Albert Einstein College of Medicine
Bronx, New York
100: *Evaluation of the Infant With Suspected Heart Disease*
187: *Heart Murmurs*

Richard C. Wasserman, MD, MPH, FAAP
Professor of Pediatrics
University of Vermont College of Medicine
Burlington, Vermont
42: *Vision Screening*

Eric R. Weinberg, MD
Assistant Professor
Cornell Weill Medical College
Pediatric Emergency Department
New York Presbyterian Hospital
New York, New York
355: *Poisoning*

Geoffrey A. Weinberg, MD, FAAP, FIDSA
Professor of Pediatrics
University of Rochester School of Medicine and Dentistry
Director, Pediatric HIV Program
Golisano Children's Hospital at Strong, Strong Memorial Hospital
Rochester, New York
293: *Meningitis*

Michael L. Weitzman, MD, FAAP
Professor of Pediatrics,
The New York University School of Medicine
New York, New York
49: *Screening and Initial Management of Lead Poisoning*
115: *Children of Divorce*

John Scott Werry, MD
Emeritus Professor of Psychiatry
Department of Psychiatry
University of Auckland
Auckland, New Zealand
224: *Tics*

Barry K. Wershil, MD
Blume Biomecular Scholar
Professor of Pediatrics
Albert Einstein College of Medicine
Chief, Division of Pediatric Gastroenterology and Nutrition
The Children's Hospital at Montefiore
Bronx, New York
159: *Abdominal Pain*

Donna Beth Willey-Courand, MD
Associate Professor of Pediatrics, Pulmonary Division
University of Texas Health Science Center at San Antonio
Director, Cystic Fibrosis Center
CHRISTUS Santa Rosa Children's Hospital
San Antonio, Texas
254: *Cystic Fibrosis*

Judith V. Williams, MD, FAAP
Professor, Department of Dermatology
Eastern Virginia Medical School
Norfolk, Virginia
232: *Acne*
241: *Bacterial Skin Infections*
259: *Drug Eruptions, Erythema Multiforme, Stevens-Johnson Syndrome, and Toxic Epidermal Necrolysis*
335: *Verrucae (Warts) and Molluscum Contagiosum*

Craig M. Wilson, MD
Professor of Epidemiology, Pediatrics, and Medicine
Director, UAB Sparkman Center for Global Health
Chair, Adolescent Medicine Trials Network for HIV/AIDS Interventions (ATN)
University of Alabama at Birmingham
Birmingham, Alabama
267: *Giardiasis*
310: *Pinworm Infestations*

Jeffrey J. Wilson, MD
Assistant Professor of Clinical Psychiatry
Columbia University, College of Physicians and Surgeons
New York, New York
Private Practice of Psychiatry
Hackensack, New Jersey
50: *Substance Use Disorders: Early Identification and Referral*

Harland S. Winter, MD, FAAP
Associate Professor of Pediatrics
Harvard Medical School
Director, Pediatric Inflammatory Bowel Disease Program
MassGeneral Hospital for Children
Boston, Massachusetts
264: *Gastroesophageal Reflux Disease*

Lawrence S. Wissow, MD, MPH, FAAP
Department of Health, Behavior, and Society
The Johns Hopkins Bloomberg School of Public Health
Baltimore, Maryland
24: *Communication Strategies*

Karen S. Wood, MD, FAAP
Assistant Professor of Pediatrics, University of North Carolina
Medical Director, Pediatric Transport, Carolina Air Care
UNC Hospitals
Chapel Hill, North Carolina
76: *Care of the Sick or Premature Infant Before Transport*

Robert A. Wood, MD
Professor of Pediatrics and Director, Pediatric Allergy and Immunology
The Johns Hopkins University School of Medicine
Baltimore, Maryland
234: *Allergic Rhinitis*

Robert P. Woroniecki, MD, MS, FAAP
Assistant Professor of Pediatrics/Pediatric Nephrologist
Children's Hospital at Montefiore
Bronx, New York
210: *Proteinuria*

Kenneth W. Wright, MD, FAAP
Director, Wright Foundation for Pediatric Ophthalmology
Clinical Professor of Ophthalmology
USC Keck Medical School
Director, Pediatric Ophthalmology Research and Education
Cedars-Sinai Medical Center
Los Angeles, California
215: *Red Eye/Pink Eye*
220: *Strabismus*
228: *Visual Development, Amblyopia, and Vision Testing*

Stephanie Yee-Guardino, DO
Fellow, Pediatric Infectious Diseases
Children's Hospital, Cleveland Clinic
Cleveland, Ohio
303: *Osteomyelitis*
321: *Septic Arthritis*

Richard S.K. Young, MD, MPH, FAAP
Associate Clinical Professor of Pediatrics and Neurology
Yale University School of Medicine
Attending Neurologist and Pediatrician
Hospital of St. Raphael
New Haven, Connecticut
294: *Meningoencephalitis*

Michelle Zebrack, MD
Division of Pediatric Critical Care
Primary Children's Medical Center
University of Utah School of Medicine
Salt Lake City, Utah
354: *Pneumothorax and Pneumomediastinum*

Basil J. Zitelli, MD, FAAP
Professor of Pediatrics
University of Pittsburgh School of Medicine
Children's Hospital of Pittsburgh
Pittsburgh, Pennsylvania
37: *Physical Examination as a Screening Tool*

Aaron L. Zuckerberg, MD, FAAP
Director, Pediatric Anesthesiology Critical Care Medicine and The Children's Diagnostic Center, Sinai Hospital
North American Partners in Anesthesia
Assistant Professor, Pediatrics
University of Maryland Medical School
Baltimore, Maryland
62: *Preoperative Assessment*

Contents

Part 1
DELIVERING PEDIATRIC HEALTH CARE

1 Health Care Delivery System, 2
Christopher B. Forrest, MD, PhD

2 Pediatrician and Health Care Finance, 17
Christopher B. Forrest, MD, PhD
Thomas K. McInerny, MD

3 Practice Organization, 25
Thomas K. McInerny, MD

4 Electronic Health Record and Web-based Resources, 28
S. Andrew Spooner, MD, MS

5 Evidence-based Medicine, 38
Brett W. Robbins, MD

6 Quality Improvement in Pediatric Primary Care, 42
Charles J. Homer, MD, MPH
Victoria Weeks Rogers, MD

7 Child Health Supervision, 48
Paula M. Duncan, MD
Joseph F. Hagan Jr, MD

8 Medical Home Collaborative Care, 52
Calvin C.J. Sia, MD

9 Community-wide Approaches to Promoting Child Health, 55
C. Andrew Aligne, MD, MPH
Jeffrey M. Kaczorowski, MD
Laura Jean Shipley, MD

10 Caring for Families New to the United States, 59
Paul L. Geltman, MD, MPH
Glenn Flores, MD

11 Ethical and Legal Issues for the Primary Care Physician, 74
Lainie Friedman Ross, MD, PhD
John D. Lantos, MD

Part 2
EVALUATION AND COMMUNICATION

12 The Pediatric History, 88
William E. Boyle, MD

13 Interviewing Children, 97
David I. Bromberg, MD

14 Pediatric Physical Examination, 101
John H. Gundy, MD

15 Pediatric Imaging, 146
Terry L. Levin, MD

16 Disclosing a Diagnosis With Parents and Patients, 153
Ruth J. Messinger, MSW
Daniel W. Mruzek, PhD
Emily S. Kuschner, MA
Philip W. Davidson, PhD

17 Cultural Issues in Primary Pediatric Care, 156
Karen N. Olness, MD
Kristine Torjesen, MD, MPH

18 Adherence to Pediatric Health Care Recommendations, 161
Jill S. Halterman, MD, MPH
Kelly M. Conn, MPH
Peter G. Szilagyi, MD, MPH

19 Art of Referral, Consultation, and Collaborative Management, 165
Henry M. Seidel, MD

20 Hospitalist Medicine: Communicating With Patients and Families, 168
Laura J. Mirkinson, MD

21 Hospital Care, 171
Jack M. Percelay, MD, MPH

Part 3
PRINCIPLES OF PATIENT CARE

SECTION 1: HEALTH PROMOTION

22 Supporting Development of the Family, 179
Penelope K. Knapp, MD

23 Counseling Families on Healthy Lifestyles, 189
R. Joe Jopling, MD

24 Communication Strategies, 200
Lawrence S. Wissow, MD, MPH

25 Anticipatory Guidance, 207
Howard R. Foye Jr, MD

26 Feeding of Infants and Children, 212
Marvin S. Eiger, MD

27 Nutritional Requirements, 219
William J. Klish, MD
Gilbert B. Forbes, MD

Section 2: Disease Prevention

28 Morbidity and Mortality Among the Young, 233
Bernard Guyer, MD, MPH
Cynthia S. Minkovitz, MD, MPP
Donna M. Strobino, PhD

29 Immunizations, 244
Sharon G. Humiston, MD, MPH
William L. Atkinson, MD, MPH
Cynthia M. Rand, MD, MPH
Peter G. Szilagyi, MD, MPH

30 Injury Prevention, 266
Rebecca Levin-Goodman, MPH
Gary A. Smith, MD, DrPH

31 Violence Prevention, 272
Robert D. Sege, MD, PhD

32 Preventive Cardiology, 278
Jorge A. Alvarez
Tracie L. Miller, MD, MS
Thomas J. Starc, MD, MPH
Kathleen A. McGrath, RN, MS, CPNP
Steven E. Lipshultz, MD

33 Prevention of Dental Caries, 293
Robert J. Berkowitz, DDS
Pamela K. Den Besten, DDS, MS
Jeffrey M. Karp, DMD, MS

34 Prevention of Obesity, 297
Sandra G. Hassink, MD
Gina M. French, MD

35 Prevention of Smoking, 305
C. Andrew Aligne, MD, MPH

Section 3: Screening and Case Finding

36 Screening: General Considerations, 312
Paul H. Dworkin, MD

37 Physical Examination as a Screening Tool, 316
Basil J. Zitelli, MD

38 Preparticipation Physical Evaluation, 317
Eric Small, MD

39 Auditory Screening, 326
David R. Cunningham, PhD
Sarah A. Sydlowski, AuD

40 Cardiovascular Screening, 334
Michelle A. Grenier, MD

41 Screening for Anemia, 342
Bryce A. Kerlin, MD

42 Vision Screening, 343
Alex R. Kemper, MD, MPH, MS
Richard C. Wasserman, MD, MPH

43 Identification of Developmental Delays and Early Intervention System, 346
Ruth K. Kaminer, MD
Susan J. Vig, PhD

44 Developmental Surveillance and Intervention, 349
Marian F. Earls, MD

45 Language and Speech Assessment, 354
Hiram L. McDade, PhD
Elaine M. Frank, PhD

46 Psychosocial Screening, 358
Steven C. Schlozman, MD
Michael S. Jellinek, MD

47 Family Screening and Assessments, 364
Amy Heneghan, MD

48 Recognition of Genetic-Metabolic Diseases by Clinical Diagnosis and Screening, 373
Nancy E. Braverman, MD, MS
Ada Hamosh, MD

49 Screening and Initial Management of Lead Poisoning, 393
Stephen J. Maddox Jr, MD
Michael L. Weitzman, MD
Arthur H. Fierman, MD

50 Substance Use Disorders: Early Identification and Referral, 398
Jeffrey J. Wilson, MD
Megan E. Janoff

51 Use of Urinalysis and Urine Culture in Screening, 404
David S. Hains, MD
Hiren P. Patel, MD

Section 4: Treatment of Disease

52 The Ill Child, 409
Timothy Gibson, MD
Marianne E. Felice, MD

53 Physiology and Management of Fever, 418
Henry M. Adam, MD

54 Management of Acute Pain in Children, 423
Joseph D. Tobias, MD

55 Management of Chronic Pain in Children, 435
Sabine Kost-Byerly, MD

56 Self-regulation Therapies: Hypnosis and Biofeedback, 448
Denise A. Bothe, MD
Karen N. Olness, MD

57 Complementary and Alternative Medical Therapies, 455
Gregory A. Plotnikoff, MD, MTS
Kathi J. Kemper, MD, MPH
Timothy P. Culbert, MD

58 **Body Fluids, Electrolyte Concentration, and Acid-Base Composition,** 467
Prashant V. Mahajan, MD, MPH, MBA

59 **Fluids and Electrolytes in Clinical Practice,** 471
Prashant V. Mahajan, MD, MPH, MBA

60 **Blood Products and Their Uses,** 481
Eva G. Radel, MD

61 **Antimicrobial Therapy,** 489
Blaise L. Congeni, MD

62 **Preoperative Assessment,** 515
Aaron L. Zuckerberg, MD
Lynne G. Maxwell, MD

63 **Postoperative Care,** 552
Lynne G. Maxwell, MD

SECTION 5: CARE OF THE CHILD WITH SPECIAL HEALTH CARE NEEDS

64 **Children With Ongoing Health Conditions,** 564
Ruth E.K. Stein, MD

65 **Home Health Care,** 569
Sonia O. Imaizumi, MD

66 **Pediatric Rehabilitation,** 573
Lisa H. Shulman, MD
Dona Rani Kathirithamby, MD
Maris D. Rosenberg, MD
Elissa L. Stern, LCSW, MPH

67 **Partnering With Families in Hospital and Community Settings,** 583
Ruth R. Walden
Molly Cole

68 **School-related Issues for Children With Special Needs,** 588
Nienke P. Dosa, MD, MPH
Gregory S. Liptak, MD, MPH

SECTION 6: PALLIATIVE AND END-OF-LIFE CARE

69 **Palliative, End-of-Life, and Bereavement Care,** 593
Alex Okun, MD

Part 4

MATERNAL AND FETAL PERINATAL HEALTH: EFFECT ON PREGANCY OUTCOMES

SECTION 1: PERINATAL HEALTH

70 **Prenatal Diagnosis,** 604
Lauren A. Ferrara, MD
Garfield A.D. Clunie, MD

71 **Fetal Interventions,** 614
Manisha Gandhi, MD
Garfield A.D. Clunie, MD

72 **Assistive Reproductive Technologies, Multiple Births, and Pregnancy Outcomes,** 620
Edith A. McCarthy, MD
Peter A.M. Auld, MD

SECTION 2: PERINATAL CARE: CARING FOR THE HIGH-RISK INFANT

73 **Fetal Assessment,** 627
E. Rebecca Pschirrer, MD, MPH
George A. Little, MD

74 **Assessment and Stabilization at Delivery,** 653
Joaquim M.B. Pinheiro, MD, MPH

75 **Identifying the Newborn Who Requires Specialized Care,** 666
Upender K. Munshi, MBBS, MD(Paediatrics)

76 **Care of the Sick or Premature Infant Before Transport,** 674
Karen S. Wood, MD

77 **Continuing Care of the Infant After Transfer From Neonatal Intensive Care,** 682
Deborah E. Campbell, MD

78 **Discharge Planning for the High-Risk Newborn Requiring Intensive Care,** 709
Christina M. Long, DO
Deborah E. Campbell, MD

79 **Support for Families Whose Infant Is Sick or Dying: Collaborative Decision Making,** 729
Joseph A. Vitterito II, MD
George A. Little, MD

80 **Perinatal Bereavement,** 736
Deborah E. Campbell, MD

Part 5

CARE OF THE TERM AND LATE PRETERM INFANT

SECTION 1: ASSESSMENT AND PHYSICAL EXAMINATION OF THE NEWBORN

81 **Medical-Legal Considerations in the Care of Newborns,** 742
Jonathan Fanaroff, MD, JD
Robert Turbow, MD, JD

82 **Maternal Medical History,** 752
Harpreet Kaur, MD
Deborah E. Campbell, MD

83 **Physical Examination of the Newborn,** 757
Harpreet Kaur, MD
Deborah E. Campbell, MD

84 **Postnatal Assessment of Common Prenatal Sonographic Findings,** 774
Deborah E. Campbell, MD

85 **Neonatal Skin**, 778
Julian J. Trevino, MD
Matthew A. Bakos, MD
Matthew P. Janik, MD

86 **Common Congenital Anomalies**, 788
Orna Rosen, MD
Robert W. Marion, MD

Section 2: Routine Care Issues

87 **Prenatal Visit**, 797
Deborah E. Campbell, MD

88 **Care of the Newborn After Delivery**, 800
Diane E. Bloomfield, MD
Elaine A. Dinolfo, MD, MS
Faye Kokotos, MD

89 **Breastfeeding the Newborn**, 809
Richard J. Schanler, MD

90 **Breastfeeding: Drugs, Herbs, and Environmental Toxins**, 824
Ruth Lawrence, MD

91 **Circumcision**, 828
Jack T. Swanson, MD

92 **Care of the Late Preterm Infant**, 831
Viral A. Dave, MD, DCH
Deborah E. Campbell, MD

Section 3: Discharge Planning and Follow-up Care

93 **Healthy Newborn Discharge**, 840
Christina Kan Sullivan, MD
Sonia Dela Cruz-Rivera, MD

94 **Follow-up Care of the Healthy Newborn**, 849
Deborah E. Campbell, MD

95 **Health and Developmental Outcomes of Infants Requiring Neonatal Intensive Care**, 852
Deborah E. Campbell, MD
Sonia O. Imaizumi, MD
Judy C. Bernbaum, MD

96 **Follow-up Care of the Graduate From the Neonatal Intensive Care Unit**, 867
Judy C. Bernbaum, MD
Deborah E. Campbell, MD
Sonia O. Imaizumi, MD

Section 4: Neonatal Medical Conditions

97 **Abnormalities of Fetal Growth**, 883
Suhas M. Nafday, MD, MRCP(Ire), DCH

98 **Neonatal Jaundice**, 892
Luc P. Brion, MD

99 **Respiratory Distress and Breathing Disorders in the Newborn**, 902
Suhas M. Nafday MD, MRCP(Ire), DCH
Christina M. Long, DO

100 **Evaluation of the Infant With Suspected Heart Disease**, 916
Nicole J. Sutton, MD
Christine A. Walsh, MD

101 **The Infant With Suspected Infection**, 928
Tsoline Kojaoghlanian, MD

102 **Neonatal Hematology**, 940
M. Catherine Driscoll, MD

103 **Prenatal Drug Abuse and Neonatal Drug Withdrawal Syndrome**, 947
Enrique M. Ostrea Jr, MD
Neil Joseph B. Alviedo, MD
Felix P. Banadera, MD
Lilia C. De Jesus, MD

104 **Common Metabolic Disturbances in the Newborn**, 960
Zuzanna Kubicka, MD
George A. Little, MD

105 **Specific Congenital Metabolic Disorders**, 970
Angel Rios, MD
Darius J. Adams, MD

106 **Neurologic Abnormalities**, 988
Aleksandra Djukic, MD, PhD

Part 6
PSYCHOSOCIAL ISSUES IN CHILD HEALTH CARE

Section 1: Psychological and Social Development of Children

107 **Theories and Concepts of Development**, 997
Tasha C. Geiger, PhD
Olle Jane Z. Sahler, MD

108 **Mental Health of the Young: An Overview**, 1014
William R. Beardslee, MD
Julius B. Richmond, MD

109 **Early Education and Child Care Programs**, 1018
Susan S. Aronson, MD

110 **Family-centered Care in Pediatric Practice**, 1027
W. Carl Cooley, MD

111 **Principles of Effective Discipline**, 1029
Ellen C. Perrin, MD

Section 2: Factors Influencing the Psychosocial Health of Children

112 **Changing American Families**, 1036
Shirley A. Smoyak, RN, PhD

113 Adoption, 1042
Sarah H. Springer, MD

114 Child Custody, 1053
Elizabeth Meller Alderman, MD

115 Children of Divorce, 1056
Rhonda M. Graves, MD
Lori Legano, MD
Michael L. Weitzman, MD

116 Children in Foster and Kinship Care, 1061
Moira Szilagyi, MD, PhD
Sandra H. Jee, MD, MPH

117 Domestic Violence and the Family, 1074
Peter G. Sherman, MD
Abraham C. Rice, MD

118 Gay- and Lesbian-parented Families, 1082
Cindy M. Schorzman, MD
Melanie A. Gold, DO

119 Homelessness and the Family, 1087
Peter G. Sherman, MD
Rosemarie A. Pezzullo, MD

120 Child Physical Abuse and Neglect, 1091
Howard Dubowitz, MD, MS
Martin A. Finkel, DO

121 Children in Self-care, 1103
Robert D. Needlman, MD

122 Sexual Abuse of Children, 1106
John M. Leventhal, MD
Andrea Gottsegen Asnes, MD, MSW

123 Children, Adolescents, and the Media, 1114
Victor C. Strasburger, MD

Section 3: School Health

124 Overview of School Health and School Health Program Goals, 1122
Howard L. Taras, MD
Philip R. Nader, MD

125 School Health Education, 1131
Guy S. Parcel, PhD
Sharon S. Cummings, MPH

126 Nursing Roles in School Health, 1135
Bernadette Mazurek Melnyk, PhD, RN, CPNP/NPP
Karen Teeple Reuter, MS, RN, AZCSN

127 School Readiness, 1140
Karen Ratliff-Schaub, MD

128 School Absenteeism and School Refusal, 1145
Ronald V. Marino, DO, MPH

129 School Learning Problems and Developmental Differences, 1149
Paul H. Dworkin, MD

Section 4: Emotional and Behavioral Problems

130 A Developmental Approach to the Prevention of Common Behavioral Problems, 1156
Joshua Sparrow, MD
T. Berry Brazelton, MD

131 Consultation and Referral for Emotional and Behavioral Problems, 1163
Jason E. Jones, MD
Richard M. Sarles, MD

132 Options for the Delivery of Mental Health Services, 1168
David J. Kolko, PhD

133 Medication Management for Emotional and Behavioral Problems, 1177
Matthew B. Perkins, MD, MBA
Peter S. Jensen, MD

134 Family Interactions: Children Who Have Unexplained Physical Symptoms, 1183
A. John Sargent III, MD

135 Anorexia and Bulimia Nervosa, 1186
Marcie B. Schneider, MD
Martin M. Fisher, MD

136 Autism, 1196
Eric M. Butter, PhD
James A. Mulick, PhD

137 Attention-deficit/Hyperactivity Disorder, 1201
Laurel K. Leslie, MD, MPH
James P. Guevara, MD, MPH

138 Conduct Disorders, 1220
Michael S. Jellinek, MD

139 Conversion Reactions and Hysteria, 1226
Gregory E. Prazar, MD

140 Children With Gender-variant Behaviors and Transgender Youth, 1233
Robert J. Bidwell, MD

141 Substance Use Disorders: Evaluation and Management, 1245
Susan M. Coupey, MD
Sara Buchdahl Levine, MD, MPH

142 Encopresis, 1251
Barton D. Schmitt, MD

143 Mood Disorders, 1256
David A. Brent, MD

144 Münchausen Syndrome by Proxy, 1263
Donna Andrea Rosenberg, MD

145 Phobias and Anxiety, 1280
Pieter le Roux, D Litt et Phil
Christina M. McCann, PhD

146 Posttraumatic Stress Disorder, 1285
Judith A. Cohen, MD
David J. Kolko, PhD

147 **Stuttering,** 1291
Pearl A. Payne, PhD

148 **Sleep Disturbances,** 1294
Mark L. Splaingard, MD

149 **Suicide and Suicidal Attempts in Adolescents,** 1312
American Academy of Pediatrics Committee on Adolescence

150 **Temper Tantrums and Breath-holding Spells,** 1316
Gregory E. Prazar, MD

Part 7
ADOLESCENCE

151 **Challenges of Health Care Delivery to Adolescents,** 1322
Richard E. Kreipe, MD

152 **Counseling Parents of Adolescents,** 1328
Jonathan D. Klein, MD, MPH

153 **Interviewing Adolescents,** 1331
Melanie A. Gold, DO
Aimee E. Seningen, MD

154 **Adolescent Sexuality,** 1338
Susan M. Coupey, MD
Unab I. Khan, MD

155 **Adolescent Pregnancy and Parenthood,** 1346
Dianne S. Elfenbein, MD
Marianne E. Felice, MD

156 **Contraception and Abortion,** 1351
Eric A. Schaff, MD

157 **Gay, Lesbian, and Bisexual Youth,** 1358
Robert J. Bidwell, MD

Part 8
PRESENTING SIGNS AND SYMPTOMS

158 **Abdominal Distention,** 1369
Peter F. Belamarich, MD

159 **Abdominal Pain,** 1376
Anthony M. Loizides, MD
Barry K. Wershil, MD

160 **Alopecia and Hair Shaft Anomalies,** 1384
Nancy K. Barnett, MD

161 **Amenorrhea,** 1390
Maria Trent, MD, MPH
Alain Joffe, MD, MPH

162 **Anemia and Pallor,** 1395
E. Anders Kolb, MD
Adam S. Levy, MD

163 **Back Pain,** 1405
Joel S. Brenner, MD, MPH
Robert A. Pendergrast Jr, MD, MPH

164 **Cardiac Arrhythmias,** 1411
J. Peter Harris, MD

165 **Chest Pain,** 1420
Scott A. Schroeder, MD

166 **Constipation,** 1424
Peter F. Belamarich, MD

167 **Cough,** 1432
Michael G. Marcus, MD

168 **Dental Stains,** 1437
Lindsey K. Grossman, MD

169 **Diarrhea and Steatorrhea,** 1440
Martin H. Ulshen, MD

170 **Dizziness and Vertigo,** 1457
Ruby F. Rivera, MD
Catherine R. Sellinger, MD

171 **Dysmenorrhea,** 1461
Linda Meyer Dinerman, MD
Alain Joffe, MD, MPH

172 **Dysphagia,** 1463
Mohammad F. El-Baba, MD

173 **Dyspnea,** 1467
Jay H. Mayefsky, MD, MPH

174 **Dysuria,** 1474
Katarina Supe-Markovina, MD
Frederick F. Kaskel, MD, PhD

175 **Edema,** 1479
Paul A. Levy, MD

176 **Epistaxis,** 1482
Miriam B. Schechter, MD
David M. Stevens, MD

177 **Extremity Pain,** 1489
Michael G. Burke, MD, MBA
David C. Hanson, MD

178 **Facial Dysmorphism,** 1496
Robert W. Marion, MD

179 **Failure to Thrive,** 1501
Andrew D. Racine, MD, PhD

180 **Fatigue and Weakness,** 1509
Philip O. Ozuah, MD, PhD
Marina Reznik, MD, MS

181 **Fever,** 1515
Elise W. van der Jagt, MD, MPH

182 **Fever of Unknown Origin,** 1524
Elise W. van der Jagt, MD, MPH

183 **Foot and Leg Problems,** 1528
Robert A. Hoekelman, MD
Maurice J. Chianese, MD

184 **Gastrointestinal Hemorrhage,** 1543
Jeffrey R. Avner, MD

185 Headache, 1550
Andrew D. Hershey, MD, PhD

186 Hearing Loss, 1557
Anne Marie Tharpe, PhD
Douglas P. Sladen, PhD

187 Heart Murmurs, 1560
Christine Tracy, MD
Christine A. Walsh, MD

188 Hematuria, 1566
Kimberly J. Reidy, MD
Marcela Del Rio, MD

189 Hemoptysis, 1570
Scott A. Schroeder, MD

190 Hepatomegaly, 1575
Philip O. Ozuah, MD, PhD
Marina Reznik, MD, MS

191 High Blood Pressure in Infants, Children, and Adolescents, 1579
Kristin C. Sokol, MPH
Sarah E. Messiah, MPH, PhD
Carol J. Buzzard, MD
Steven E. Lipshultz, MD

192 Hirsutism, Hypertrichosis, and Precocious Sexual Hair Development, 1590
Joan DiMartino-Nardi, MD
Mala Puri, MD

193 Hoarseness, 1598
Samuel T. Ostrower, MD
Sanjay R. Parikh, MD

194 Hyperhidrosis, 1603
Nancy K. Barnett, MD

195 Hypotonia, 1604
Alfred J. Spiro, MD

196 Irritability, 1609
Diana King, MD
Waseem Hafeez, MBBS

197 Jaundice, 1615
Debra H. Pan, MD
Yolanda Rivas, MD

198 Joint Pain, 1625
David M. Siegel, MD, MPH
John Baum, MD

199 Limp, 1630
Erica M. Sibinga, MD, MHS
John S. Andrews, MD

200 Loss of Appetite, 1637
Martin H. Ulshen, MD

201 Lymphadenopathy, 1639
George B. Segel, MD
Caroline Breese Hall, MD

202 Macrocephaly, 1646
Oscar H. Purugganan, MD, MPH

203 Malocclusion, 1650
Lindsey K. Grossman, MD

204 Microcephaly, 1652
Oscar H. Purugganan, MD, MPH

205 Nervousness, 1656
Richard M. Sarles, MD

206 Nonconvulsive Periodic Disorders, 1657
Sarah M. Roddy, MD

207 Odor (Unusual Urine and Body), 1660
Erik E. Langenau, DO

208 Petechiae and Purpura, 1667
Adam S. Levy, MD

209 Polyuria, 1670
Ryan S. Miller, MD
Samuel M. Libber, MD
Leslie P. Plotnick, MD

210 Proteinuria, 1676
Shefali Mahesh, MD
Robert P. Woroniecki, MD, MS

211 Pruritus, 1681
Nancy K. Barnett, MD

212 Puberty: Normal and Abnormal, 1683
Dominique N. Long, MD
Robert K. Kritzler, MD
Leslie P. Plotnick, MD

213 Rash, 1688
Daniel P. Krowchuk, MD

214 Recurrent Infections, 1695
David L. Goldman, MD

215 Red Eye/Pink Eye, 1702
Kenneth W. Wright, MD

216 Scrotal Swelling and Pain, 1717
Lane S. Palmer, MD

217 Self-stimulating Behaviors, 1724
Richard M. Sarles, MD
Denise M. Richardson, MD

218 Short Stature, 1727
Paul B. Kaplowitz, MD, PhD

219 Splenomegaly, 1730
Marina Reznik, MD, MS
Philip O. Ozuah, MD, PhD

220 Strabismus, 1733
Kenneth W. Wright, MD

221 Strange Behavior, 1742
Audrey M. Walker, MD

222 Stridor, 1747
Alfin G. Vicencio, MD
John P. Bent, MD

223 Syncope, 1753
Prema Ramaswamy, MD

224 Tics, 1758
Robert A. King, MD
John Scott Werry, MD

225 Torticollis, 1764
Philip O. Ozuah, MD, PhD
Catherine C. Skae, MD

226 Vaginal Bleeding, 1766
Maria Trent, MD, MPH
Alain Joffe, MD, MPH

227 Vaginal Discharge, 1771
Linda Meyer Dinerman, MD
Alain Joffe, MD, MPH

228 Visual Development, Amblyopia, and Vision Testing, 1775
Kenneth W. Wright, MD

229 Vomiting, 1783
Martin H. Ulshen, MD

230 Weight Loss, 1786
Diane E. Bloomfield, MD
Elaine A. Dinolfo, MD, MS

231 Wheezing, 1790
Alfin G. Vicencio, MD
Joshua P. Needleman, MD

Part 9
SPECIFIC CLINICAL PROBLEMS

232 Acne, 1802
Catherine Chen, MD
Judith V. Williams, MD

233 Adrenal Dysfunction, 1808
Phyllis W. Speiser, MD

234 Allergic Rhinitis, 1818
Robert A. Wood, MD

235 Animal Bites, 1822
Neil E. Herendeen, MD, MBA
Peter G. Szilagyi, MD, MPH

236 Anuria and Oliguria, 1825
Amrish Jain, MD
Tej K. Mattoo, MD, DCh, FRCP(UK)

237 Apparent Life-threatening Events, 1829
Keyvan Rafei, MD
Carol J. Blaisdell, MD

238 Appendicitis, 1836
R. Scott Strahlman, MD

239 Asthma, 1839
Robert C. Cohn, MD
James E. Martin, RRT-NPS, CPFT

240 Atopic Dermatitis, 1850
Linda S. Nield, MD
Jonette E. Keri, MD, PhD

241 Bacterial Skin Infections, 1853
Randall G. Fisher, MD
Catherine Chen, MD
Judith V. Williams, MD

242 Brain Tumors, 1860
Cameron L. Nicholson, MD
Joanne M. Hilden, MD
Bruce H. Cohen, MD

243 Bronchiolitis, 1865
Caroline Breese Hall, MD
William J. Hall, MD

244 Cancers in Childhood, 1873
Andrea S. Hinkle, MD
Cindy L. Schwartz, MD

245 Cerebral Palsy, 1903
Gregory S. Liptak, MD, MPH

246 Chickenpox, 1911
George K. Siberry, MD, MPH

247 Chronic Fatigue Syndrome, 1919
Leonard R. Krilov, MD

248 Cleft Lip and Cleft Palate, 1923
Arlene A. Rozzelle, MD
Jugpal S. Arneja, MD

249 Colic, 1931
Rebecca A. Baum, MD

250 Common Cold, 1934
Howard Fischer, MD

251 Congenital and Acquired Heart Disease, 1937
Michael A. McCulloch, MD
Robert J. Gajarski, MD

252 Contact Dermatitis, 1973
Jonette E. Keri, MD, PhD
Linda S. Nield, MD

253 Contagious Exanthematous Diseases, 1976
Robert Iannone, MD

254 Cystic Fibrosis, 1982
Donna Beth Willey-Courand, MD
Bruce C. Marshall, MD

255 Cystic and Solid Masses of the Face and Neck, 1995
Neil E. Herendeen, MD, MBA
Peter G. Szilagyi, MD, MPH

256 Diabetes Mellitus, 1998
Peter J. Tebben, MD
W. Frederick Schwenk II, MD

257 Diaper Rash, 2010
Gregory S. Liptak, MD, MPH

258 Down Syndrome: Managing the Child and Family, 2016
Erawati V. Bawle, MD

259 **Drug Eruptions, Erythema Multiforme, Stevens-Johnson Syndrome, and Toxic Epidermal Necrolysis**, 2026
Judith V. Williams, MD
Catherine Chen, MD

260 **Enterovirus Infections**, 2032
Jerri Ann Jenista, MD

261 **Enuresis**, 2040
Franca M. Iorember, MD, MPH
Andrew L. Schwaderer, MD

262 **Foreign Bodies of the Ear, Nose, Airway, and Esophagus**, 2045
Catherine C. Skae, MD
Sanjay R. Parikh, MD

263 **Fractures and Dislocations**, 2050
R. Scott Strahlman, MD

264 **Gastroesophageal Reflux Disease**, 2054
Shailender Madani, MD
Harland S. Winter, MD
Mel Heyman, MD

265 **Gastrointestinal Allergy**, 2064
P. Christine Nguyen, MD
John A. Kerner Jr, MD

266 **Gastrointestinal Obstruction**, 2071
Louisa Chiu, MD
David L. Dudgeon, MD
Anthony Stallion, MD

267 **Giardiasis**, 2084
Craig M. Wilson, MD

268 **Gluten-sensitive Enteropathy (Celiac Sprue)**, 2088
Anca M. Safta, MD
John A. Kerner Jr, MD

269 **Hemolytic-Uremic Syndrome**, 2094
Horacio Esteban Adrogué, MD
Horacio A. Repetto, MD

270 **Hemoglobinopathies and Sickle Cell Disease**, 2098
Sharada A. Sarnaik, MD
Meera Chitlur, MD

271 **Hemophilia and Other Hereditary Bleeding Disorders**, 2105
Eva G. Radel, MD

272 **Henoch-Schönlein Purpura**, 2112
Horacio Esteban Adrogué, MD
Francisco Xavier Flores, MD

273 **Hepatitis**, 2115
Winita Hardikar, MBBS, PhD
Kathleen B. Schwarz, MD

274 **Herpes Infections**, 2129
Lindsey K. Grossman, MD

275 **Human Herpesvirus-6 and Human Herpesvirus-7 Infections**, 2134
Jerri Ann Jenista, MD

276 **Human Immunodeficiency Virus Infection and Acquired Immunodeficiency Syndrome**, 2138
William J. Moss, MD, MPH
Deborah Persaud, MD
Michael T. Brady, MD

277 **Hydrocephalus**, 2146
Mohamad A. Khaled, MD, MSurg
Mark G. Luciano, MD, PhD

278 **Hyperthyroidism**, 2154
Nicholas Jospe, MD

279 **Hypospadias, Epispadias, and Cryptorchism**, 2157
Amanda C. North, MD
John P. Gearhart, MD

280 **Hypothyroidism**, 2161
Craig C. Orlowski, MD

281 **Iatrogenic Disease**, 2167
Ian M. Paul, MD, MSc

282 **Immune Thrombocytopenia Purpura**, 2170
Jawhar Rawwas, MD

283 **Infectious Mononucleosis and Other Epstein-Barr Viral Infections**, 2175
Stephen R. Barone, MD
Leonard R. Krilov, MD

284 **Insect Bites and Infestations**, 2179
David H. Stein, MD, MPH, MSt
Nancy K. Barnett, MD

285 **Intellectual Disability**, 2184
Randall A. Phelps, MD, PhD
William I. Cohen, MD

286 **Intersex**, 2193
Lindsey A. Albrecht, MD
Dennis M. Styne, MD

287 **Iron-Deficiency Anemia**, 2201
Lakshmanan Krishnamurti, MD

288 **Juvenile Idiopathic Arthritis**, 2211
David M. Siegel, MD, MPH
Harry L. Gewanter, MD

289 **Kawasaki Disease**, 2220
Michael E. Pichichero, MD

290 **Labial Adhesions**, 2228
Linda S. Nield, MD

291 **Leukemias**, 2231
E. Anders Kolb, MD
Richard Gorlick, MD

292 Lyme Disease, 2249
H. Cody Meissner, MD

293 Meningitis, 2252
Geoffrey A. Weinberg, MD
Ann M. Buchanan, MD, MPH

294 Meningoencephalitis, 2267
Richard S.K. Young, MD, MPH

295 Muscular Dystrophy, 2273
Richard T. Moxley III, MD
Emma Ciafaloni, MD

296 Nephritis, 2286
William S. Varade, MD

297 Nephrotic Syndrome, 2296
William S. Varade, MD

298 Neurocutaneous Syndromes, 2303
Michael L. Smith, MD

299 Obesity and Metabolic Syndrome, 2320
Heather A. Van Mater, MD
Sheila Gahagan, MD, MPH

300 Obstructive Uropathy and Vesicoureteral Reflux, 2333
Hiep T. Nguyen, MD

301 Ocular Trauma, 2343
Lisa I. Bohra, MD
Rajesh C. Rao, MD

302 Osteochondroses, 2352
Edward M. Sills, MD

303 Osteomyelitis, 2355
Stephanie Yee-Guardino, DO
Johanna Goldfarb, MD

304 Otitis Media and Otitis Externa, 2360
Tina Q. Tan, MD

305 Parasitic Infections, 2366
Nahed Abdel-Haq, MD
Pimpanada Chearskul, MD
Yaseen Rafee, MD
Basim I. Asmar, MD

306 Pectus Excavatum and Pectus Carinatum, 2416
Ikenna C. Okereke, MD
Anthony Stallion, MD

307 Pertussis (Whooping Cough), 2419
Camille Sabella, MD

308 Pharyngitis and Tonsillitis, 2425
Russell W. Steele, MD

309 Phimosis, 2430
A. Barbara Oettgen, MD, MPH

310 Pinworm Infestations, 2432
Craig M. Wilson, MD

311 Plagiocephaly, 2433
Ahdi Amer, MD
Deepak M. Kamat, MD, PhD

312 Pneumonia, 2437
Christopher Harris, MD

313 Preseptal and Orbital Cellulitis, 2440
Ellen R. Wald, MD

314 Psoriasis, 2447
Ginette A. Hinds, MD
Richard J. Antaya, MD

315 Pyloric Stenosis, 2454
Sushma Reddy, MD
Deepak M. Kamat, MD, PhD

316 Renal Tubular Acidosis, 2459
Ronald J. Kallen, MD

317 Rheumatic Fever, 2475
Welton M. Gersony, MD
Thomas J. Starc, MD, MPH

318 Rocky Mountain Spotted Fever, 2481
Robert T. Seese, MD
Lara A. Danziger-Isakov, MD, MPH

319 Seborrheic Dermatitis, 2485
Elizabeth Alvarez Connelly, MD
Lawrence Schachner, MD

320 Seizure Disorders, 2488
Sarah M. Roddy, MD
Margaret C. McBride, MD

321 Septic Arthritis, 2505
Stephanie Yee-Guardino, DO
Johanna Goldfarb, MD

322 Sexually Transmitted Infections, 2509
Alain Joffe, MD, MPH

323 Sinusitis, 2534
Tina Q. Tan, MD

324 Spina Bifida, 2537
Gregory S. Liptak, MD, MPH

325 Spinal Deformities, 2545
Edward M. Sills, MD

326 Sports Injuries, 2550
Srinivasan Suresh, MD, MBA

327 Staphylococcal Toxic Shock Syndrome, 2562
Michael E. Pichichero, MD

328 Stomatitis, 2569
Linda S. Nield, MD

329 Streptococcal Toxic Shock Syndrome, 2573
Chokechai Rongkavilit, MD

330 Sudden Infant Death Syndrome, 2579
Rachel Y. Moon, MD
John Kattwinkel, MD

331 Tonsillectomy and Adenoidectomy, 2583
Louis G. Petcu, MD, MS
Ian Scott Goodman, MD
James J. Burns, MD

332 Tuberculosis and Latent Tuberculosis Infection, 2590
Ann M. Loeffler, MD
Mark N. Lobato, MD

333 Umbilical Anomalies, 2604
Robert W. Marion, MD

334 Urinary Tract Infections, 2607
Timo J. Jahnukainen, MD, PhD
Abhay N. Vats, MD

335 Verrucae (Warts) and Molluscum Contagiosum, 2615
Catherine Chen, MD
Judith V. Williams, MD

Part 10

CRITICAL SITUATIONS

336 Acute Surgical Abdomen, 2624
Michael D. Klein, MD

337 Airways Obstruction, 2630
Carol K. Conrad, MD
David N. Cornfield, MD

338 Altered Mental Status, 2638
Rene J. Forti, MD
Jeffrey R. Avner, MD

339 Anaphylaxis, 2643
Elizabeth Secord, MD
Michael R. Simon, MD

340 Croup (Acute Laryngotracheobronchitis), 2647
Caroline Breese Hall, MD
William J. Hall, MD

341 Dehydration, 2654
Prashant V. Mahajan, MD, MPH, MBA

342 Diabetic Ketoacidosis, 2662
Peter J. Tebben, MD
W. Frederick Schwenk II, MD

343 Disseminated Intravascular Coagulation, 2670
Steven W. Pipe, MD,
Anjali A. Sharathkumar, MD

344 Drowning and Near Drowning, 2676
Lorry R. Frankel, MD

345 Drug Overdose, 2682
Ian M. Paul, MD, MSc

346 Envenomations, 2686
Shireen Banerji, PharmD
Alvin C. Bronstein, MD

347 Esophageal Caustic Injury, 2705
Jill M. Cholette, MD
George T. Drugas, MD

348 Head Injuries, 2709
Prashant V. Mahajan, MD, MPH, MBA

349 Heart Failure, 2717
Tanvi S. Sharma, MD
Liana Perez Loughlin, Esq
Tracie L. Miller, MD, MS
Steven E. Lipshultz, MD

350 Hypertensive Emergencies, 2726
Srinivasan Suresh, MD, MBA

351 Hypoglycemia, 2731
Srinivasan Suresh, MD, MBA

352 Increased Intracranial Pressure, 2739
M. Mohsin Shah, MD
Matthew D. Smyth, MD

353 Meningococcemia, 2746
Mary T. Caserta, MD

354 Pneumothorax and Pneumomediastinum, 2754
Michelle Zebrack, MD
Susan L. Bratton, MD, MPH

355 Poisoning, 2762
Jeffrey S. Fine, MD
Marc A. Auerbach, MD
Kevin Y. Ching, MD
Katherine T. Fullerton, MD
Eric R. Weinberg, MD

356 Rape, 2790
Marianne E. Felice, MD
Christine E. Barron, MD

357 Acute Renal Failure, 2797
Stuart L. Goldstein, MD
Horacio Esteban Adrogué, MD

358 Shock, 2801
Monika Gupta, MD
Joseph R. Custer, MD

359 Status Asthmaticus, 2813
Alan R. Schroeder, MD

360 Status Epilepticus, 2819
Sarah M. Roddy, MD
Margaret C. McBride, MD

361 Thermal Injuries, 2821
Robert L. Sheridan, MD

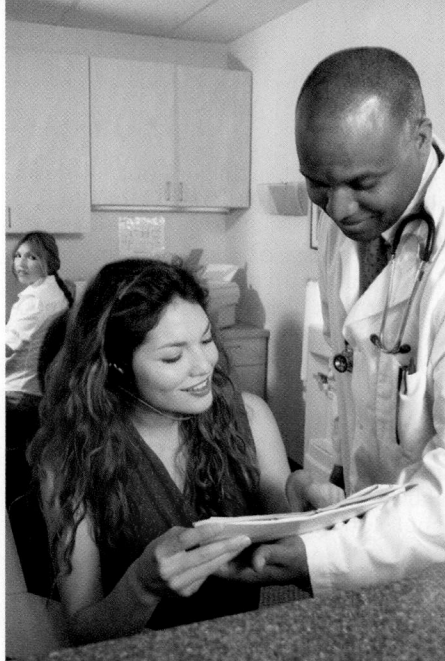

Part 1

Delivering Pediatric Health Care

1 Health Care Delivery System
2 Pediatrician and Health Care Finance
3 Practice Organization
4 Electronic Health Record and Web-based Resources
5 Evidence-based Medicine
6 Quality Improvement in Pediatric Primary Care
7 Child Health Supervision
8 Medical Home Collaborative Care
9 Community-wide Approaches to Promoting Child Health
10 Caring for Families New to the United States
11 Ethical and Legal Issues for the Primary Care Physician

Chapter 1

HEALTH CARE DELIVERY SYSTEM

Christopher B. Forrest, MD, PhD

Children's access to health care, the content and quality of services provided, and the outcomes of care all occur within the context of the health care delivery system. Understanding how health services can improve child health should begin with examining the structure of children's health care and the processes that occur once health professionals and patients interact. Findings from the relatively new scientific field of child health services research provide the pediatric care physician with a more accurate and complete picture of how health care affects child health.[1]

This chapter uses a structure-process-outcome framework to describe the health care delivery system and to analyze its effects on children.[2] Structure refers to financial and organizational arrangements of the delivery system that are present before health professionals and patients interact. Structural elements include the pediatric workforce, child health care delivery sites, financing of services, and the medical home. Assessing the process of care includes investigating the scope of pediatric practice, the content of visits, pediatricians' referrals to specialists, and the quantity of different types of services delivered to children. The chapter concludes with an examination of the connections between pediatric services and child health outcomes.

HEALTH CARE DELIVERY SYSTEM: AN OVERVIEW

Health care is purchased by government, by employers with contributions from workers, and by individual consumers. Nearly one half of all health care is financed by the federal, state, and local governments. The organization of services—that is, the arrangement of providers and suppliers within the system—is strongly determined by how they are paid. Financing is a primary driver of organization. Changes occurred in the early 1980s when the prospective payment system was instituted by the federal government in the Medicare program. Hospital payment shifted from a cost basis (payment for each service billed by the hospital) to a fixed fee that was based on the principal problem managed during the hospitalization (known as the diagnosis-related group [DRG]). This DRG-based payment system paid hospitals the same amount of money for all patients with appendicitis, regardless of how long they stayed or what services were provided. DRGs provided financial incentives to shorten lengths of stay and to shift services to the outpatient sector. The introduction of the DRG-based hospital payment system stimulated the proliferation of large outpatient specialty and surgical centers, with less emphasis on inpatient hospital bed growth. Today the United States has one of the lowest hospital admission rates throughout all developed nations, which is one of the legacies of the prospective payment system.

The delivery, or process of care, occurs when patients come into contact with providers or suppliers. The number and content of visits (utilization), the costs of these services, and the volume and types of surgical procedures are all examples of processes of care.

The degree to which health care is consistent with the best available medical evidence and linked to positive and desired health outcomes determines the level of quality of care. The end results of the health care delivery process are patient outcome, that is, changes in health, functional status, and patient well being.

STRUCTURE OF THE DELIVERY SYSTEM

Pediatric Workforce

Pediatrics and children's health care are not synonymous. A pluralistic mix of internal medicine, family medicine, pediatric specialties, and nonphysician clinicians provides services to the nation's children.[3] Individuals 17 years and younger make 23% of primary care visits to family physicians, whereas adolescents make more visits to specialists without pediatric training than to those with pediatric training. Nonetheless, pediatrics is widely viewed as the principal specialty responsible for setting child health care policy and ensuring the health of the nation's children.

Over the last several years, the increasing use of health care among older adults has been associated with pediatricians assuming responsibility for a larger share of primary care visits made by children, whereas the number of child visits to family physicians has decreased. Key trends in the pediatric workforce discussed in this chapter are (1) sustained interest in the field among graduating medical students; (2) more rapid growth in pediatricians than the population of children in the United States; (3) the dominance of women in the field; (4) the importance of international medical graduates to the pediatric workforce, especially the subspecialty workforce; and (5) a geographic maldistribution of providers.

By 2004 the total number of licensed physicians in the United States was approximately 870,000, with 8% (nearly 70,000) self-designating as pediatricians. The number of physicians has been growing steadily and at a faster rate than overall population growth. Approximately 70% of self-designated pediatricians obtain board certification from the American Board of Pediatrics (ABP), and 43,000 pediatricians are currently board certified in general pediatrics. Among certified general pediatricians, 1 in 5 obtains an additional certificate in a pediatric subspecialty.[4,5] Although hospitals and health plans use board certification as a measure of clinical competence and expertise, the benefits of board certification on the quality and outcomes of patient care are not well established. The lack of this evidence may be a result of too few research studies devoted to this topic, inadequate measures of quality of care, health metrics that are poorly sensitive to change among children, or a problem with board certification itself in that it does not truly differentiate clinical competence among practitioners.

Across all medical specialties, women constitute 27% of all physicians but a much larger share for pediatrics. Currently, 69% of pediatric trainees are women, which contrasts with only 30% in 1975.[4] The rise in the number of female pediatricians is one of the more impressive and important trends shaping the pediatric workforce. Women are more likely than men to work part time, and they spend fewer hours in direct patient care over their work lives. To maintain the same number of full-time equivalent physicians, more pediatricians may need to be trained each year in the future if the proportion of women in pediatrics remains as high as it is now or even increases[4,5]

In 2005, 202 accredited general pediatric residency training programs existed in the United States and another 16 in Canada,[4] and 10,190 pediatricians were enrolled in the US programs. When compared with 1991 figures, this growth is a 37% increase in the absolute number of pediatric residents, a rate of growth that far exceeds the proportional increase in the number of children in the country.[6] Interest in pediatrics as a career choice continues to be strong. Approximately 14% of medical school seniors select a pediatric training program.

In 1967 the ABP and the American Board of Internal Medicine agreed that individuals who had 2 years of general internal medicine and 2 years of general pediatrics were eligible for board certification in both specialties.[4] In 2005, over 90 combined med-peds residency programs in the United States offered 388 1st-year positions. However, the number of med-peds positions has been declining since 1997 when 459 1st-year slots were available. The percentage of women enrolled is less than in categorical pediatrics and has been stable over the last few years at approximately 50%. In rural communities or small towns, med-peds physicians may play a role as a consultant in the care of high-risk newborns and children who have a chronic illness or as a hospitalist for children and adults. In more competitive environments, internal medicine and pediatric practices can use the med-peds physician to attract new patients, especially adolescents and families desiring health care for everyone in the same practice. Because med-peds physicians can alter their practice according to patient demand, the amount of pediatric care that these health professionals will provide will likely decrease with the aging of the population.

Only 11% of pediatricians in the United States practice in rural communities to care for the 29% of the childhood population that live therein. By contrast, 37% of the children who live in large metropolitan areas are cared for by almost 59% of practicing pediatricians. The remaining 30% of practicing pediatricians live and practice in suburbia, serving 34% of the nation's children. Growth over the last decade in the number of child health physicians has not remedied the geographic disparities in their distribution. Except for pediatricians practicing in sparsely populated areas, which have limited hospital and technical support services and few pediatric specialists, pediatricians generally practice similarly throughout the United States. These professionals, as those in other specialties, tend to settle in areas that have a high per capita income.

On average, one certified general pediatrician can be found for every 1700 children throughout the United States.[4] This ratio is generally deemed to be an adequate supply of pediatricians, particularly given the higher growth in the number of pediatricians compared with the rate of growth of children. However, the statistic does not reflect important regional variation in the supply of pediatricians, with many rural and inner-city areas experiencing child health professional shortages. Approximately 1 in 10 children live in an area without a pediatrician. The location where residents complete their training is important determinant of job residence: States with fewer residency-training slots have lower pediatrician-to-child ratios. Interestingly, most geographic variation observed in the United States is not due to shortages of physicians, but results from substantial oversupply in particular locations.

International medical graduates (IMGs) constitute an important share of the pediatric workforce. The most common countries of citizenship for IMGs are (in rank order) the United States (ie, US citizens trained abroad), India, and Pakistan. In 1991, 33% of all 1st-year pediatric residents were IMGs, but this proportion dropped to 24% by 2005. IMGs account for a larger share of the subspecialist workforce. Nearly 1 in 3 board-certified pediatric subspecialists are IMGs. The subspecialties with the greatest proportions of IMG board-certified physicians are nephrology (41%), neonatology (40%), endocrinology (33%), and gastroenterology (33%). These data suggest that, for the foreseeable future, the pediatric workforce will require a large number of IMGs to work as both general and subspecialist pediatricians.[7]

Medical Training, Licensure, and Certification

Consumers and providers of health services differ in the priorities they place on the 3 main challenges of the health care delivery system: (1) ensuring *access* to care, (2) controlling *costs*, and (3) improving the *quality* of care. Costs of and access to medical care are of prime importance to consumers, who tend to assume that quality of care will always be good. In contrast, neither access nor cost is an important component of medical school training, which focuses almost exclusively on how to make a diagnosis; how to support this diagnosis with appropriate information from the history, physical examination, and laboratory findings; and how to institute treatment that is appropriate to the diagnosis. The nature of most educational settings (university based, research oriented, with generally a highly specialized faculty) is responsible for a medical educational process that focuses largely on the biological bases of disease. In contrast, relatively little attention is devoted to understanding the social, occupational, and environmental causes of ill health, although issues such as these are major determinants of disease and dysfunction or patients' subjective assessment of their own health. Obtaining reliable and valid children's reports of their health is now possible in research settings. Application of these methods in clinical settings is a likely direction for clinical care and will enhance the ability of health care delivery systems to monitor their effectiveness.

The medical profession has always assumed responsibility for regulating entry into its ranks and for assessing the quality of care provided. Although state boards have the legal authority to dispense licenses to practice, all states delegate this responsibility to the profession, which nominates candidates, whom the state then licenses. Individuals merely must demonstrate that they graduated from medical school and can achieve a passing grade on a cognitive examination developed by the profession itself, either in the state (state licensing examinations) or nationally (the National Board of Medical Examiners or the Federation of State Licensing Boards, ie, *Flex* examinations).

The ABP requires certification renewal every 7 years for pediatricians certified after 1987. This renewal entails successful completion of the Program for Renewal of Certification in Pediatrics (PRCP), which includes a structured home study curriculum and a supervised, open-book written, or computer-based examination. Diplomates certified before 1988 may choose to renew their certification by completing the PRCP voluntarily.

Most health care provider organizations use certification and recertification data as one means of ensuring quality of care, requiring their pediatricians to be either board certified (having passed the written examination) or board eligible (having completed 3 years of pediatric residency training in an accredited program) with certification within 5 years of completion of residency training. Pediatricians are not required to demonstrate competence under the conditions of actual practice, either when they enter practice or at any time afterward.

Although all practitioners must demonstrate at least a minimal amount of theoretic knowledge as a condition of licensure before they enter practice, the relationship between performance in tests and subsequent quality of practice has not been consistently demonstrated. Even the procedure by which physicians become certified as specialists provides dubious assurance of high quality. Board certification, apart from its relationship to longer lengths of postgraduate training, appears to have no relationship to practice quality. Continuing education requirements and periodic recertification procedures imposed by professional organizations are unlikely to improve the situation unless the model of quality of care on which the original educational and certification procedures are based is broadened to encompass assessment of the effect of services on health status.

Pediatric Specialization

In addition to general pediatrics, 16 areas of pediatric subspecialization are certifiable by the ABP (Table 1-1). A growing number of pediatricians appear to be selecting a career as a specialist. The absolute number of subspecialty trainees increased by 46% between 1996 and 2003. In 2005, 66% of 1st-time general pediatrics diplomates selected a career as a general pediatrician, 29% a career in a pediatric subspecialty, and 5% in another nonpediatric specialty. The top 5 career choices among pediatric subspecialty fields are neonatal-perinatal medicine, critical care medicine, hematology-oncology, cardiology, and emergency medicine. Women graduating from medical schools more recently are more likely than their older female counterparts to choose a subspecialty career, although male physicians still predominate within most subspecialties, particularly those that are procedure oriented (eg, cardiology, gastroenterology).

Table 1-1 Number of Board-Certified Pediatric Subspecialists Through 2005

PEDIATRIC SUBSPECIALTY	NUMBER CERTIFIED
Adolescent medicine (1994)*	505
Cardiology (1961)	1870
Critical care medicine (1987)	1287
Developmental-behavioral pediatrics (2002)	427
Emergency medicine (1992)	1291
Endocrinology (1978)	1055
Gastroenterology (1990)	872
Hematology-oncology (1974)	1874
Infectious diseases (1994)	992
Medical toxicology (1994)	30
Neonatology-perinatal medicine (1975)	4421
Nephrology (1974)	668
Neurodevelopmental disabilities (2001)	241
Pulmonology (1986)	767
Rheumatology (1992)	215
Sports medicine (1993)	108

*Year in parentheses indicates when subspecialty board was established.
From American Board of Pediatrics. Workforce Data: The American Board of Pediatrics, 2005-2006. Available at: www.abp.org/ABPWebSite/stats/wrkfrc/workforce05.pdf.

Only 59% of the certified pediatric subspecialists' time is spent in direct patient care. The remainder is spent in administration, research, and teaching, because 60% practice in academic health centers, which contrasts with fewer than 33% of internal medicine subspecialists who do so. For individuals who are not in academia, almost 50% of endocrinologists and gastroenterologists do part-time work in general pediatrics, as do 73% of those entering nephrology.

Hospitalists

The traditional American system of care in which primary care physicians have cared for their hospitalized patients is undergoing a revolutionary change in many urban and suburban areas. A recent alternative allows primary care physicians to relinquish the care of their hospitalized patients voluntarily to a new group of inpatient generalists called *hospitalists*. Estimates suggest that 8000 US physicians function as hospitalists, just 600 of whom in 2002 were pediatricians. In 2003, 40% of pediatricians were affiliated with a hospital that employed a hospitalist. This proportion is expected to grow over the next several years.[8]

Hospitalists are physicians whose main responsibility is the general medical care of hospitalized patients and whose responsibilities may also include teaching, research, and hospital care management. Patients are referred by their primary care physicians and are referred back at the time of hospital discharge. Strong emphasis is placed on communication between the 2 physicians during the patient's hospital stay. The disadvantages of this arrangement include a loss of continuity of care between the primary care physician and the patient and a decreased scope of practice among general pediatricians.

On the other hand, the use of hospitalists allows for increased productivity by the office-based pediatrician. During office hours, leaving the office with waiting patients to see a hospitalized patient is difficult for a practitioner. Other reported advantages of hospitalists include their competency in technical skills (skills easily lost to the physician who visits the hospital only occasionally), shorter patient hospital stays because of constant in-hospital supervision, and the immediate availability of urgent care. (See Chapter 21, Hospital Care, and Chapter 20, Hospitalist Medicine: Communicating With Patients and Families.)

Nonphysician Clinicians

A large body of research evidence indicates that nonphysician clinicians—nurse practitioners and physician assistants—provide health care for many health conditions that is of equal quality to physicians. Because they can be trained at lower costs to society and their salaries are lower than those of physicians, many physician organizations and health maintenance organizations employ these professionals as primary care physicians and physician extenders in specialty settings. States are giving more independence to nonphysician clinicians, a tendency that has also stimulated their growth.

Pediatric nurse practitioners (PNPs) are usually prepared at the master's degree level. They are trained in the discipline of nursing, which has a strong emphasis on patient education and methods for coping with illness. Approximately 90% practice in primary care settings. A small share may be certified in a specialty. PNPs conduct physical examinations, track medical histories, make diagnoses, treat minor illnesses and injuries, monitor chronic disease maintenance therapy, and provide an array of counseling and educational services. In many states, PNPs prescribe medications independently, admit patients to hospitals, and make hospital rounds.

Physician assistants (PAs) are health personnel who are typically trained in 2 or 3 years to render basic health services that are also performed by physicians. PAs are health care professionals licensed to practice medicine with physician supervision. Similar to nurse practitioners, PAs conduct physical examinations, diagnose and treat illnesses, order and interpret tests, and counsel on preventive health care; they may also assist in surgery and in other procedures. In 49 states, PAs can write prescriptions. Because of the close working relationship the PAs have with physicians, PAs are educated in the medical model designed to complement physician training. The demand is huge for PNPs (approximately 10,000 in the United States) and for PAs, (approximately 6000 in pediatric activity). Estimates indicate that 33% of PNPs practice in hospital clinics, 23% in private pediatric practices, 13% in community and public health settings, and 30% in schools and health maintenance organizations. In some underserved and rural areas, PNPs are the only source of primary pediatric care.

Child Health Care Delivery Sites

Children receive health care services in a large variety of inpatient and outpatient settings. Although home visits and home-based care were once commonplace in the United States, the vast majority of pediatric professionals no longer make house calls. In other countries, however, nurse home visitation, particularly for families of newborn and infant children, is a routine part of pediatric care.

Inpatient Care Facilities

Hospitals have changed dramatically over the last 20 years in response to financial pressures to reduce lengths of stay and rates of admission. Many hospitals now offer a wide range of services, including inpatient care, outpatient diagnostic procedures, surgery, and outpatient physician visits. Whereas all inpatient care occurs in hospitals, hospital care can no longer be equated with inpatient care.

Approximately 5000 hospitals exist in the United States, and 250 (5%) of these are considered children's hospitals. Children's hospitals can be categorized as free-standing (approximately 20%) children's hospitals within larger general hospitals (approximately 45%) and other specialty, orthopedic, rehabilitative, and psychiatric hospitals (approximately 35%).[9] Approximately 3 million children are hospitalized each year, and children's hospitals account for a third of these admissions. Thus the majority of children are treated in general hospitals with pediatric inpatient care units.

According to data from the Agency for Healthcare Research and Quality, 7% of Americans are hospitalized annually, but only 3% of children and adolescents have a hospital stay (8% of children younger than 6 years enter the hospital at least once per year, whereas only 2% of those 6 to 17 years of age are hospitalized during the course of a year).[10] Children residing in low-income communities are more likely to be admitted to the hospital via the emergency department compared with those from higher-income residences. This difference may be a result of poorer access to primary care physicians in low-income communities and thus greater reliance on emergency departments. The average number of days a child remains in the hospital ranges from 3 to 4, but great variation exists in length of stay according to reason for hospitalization, type of health insurance, and, to a smaller degree, the type of hospital.

Only 15% of hospitals have a for-profit tax status, whereas 58% are nonprofit, 22% are owned by state and local governments, and 5% are owned by the federal government. The not-for-profit tax status allows these institutions to forgo paying taxes to the government and to borrow money in the tax-exempt bond market. In return for these benefits, nonprofit hospitals are expected to provide services to the community, perhaps by accepting all patients regardless of ability to pay or by mounting community health programs.

Twenty percent of hospitals are teaching hospitals, which means that they are affiliated with one of the nation's 130 medical schools. Nearly one half of all US hospitals are located in rural areas, where the vast majority are small institutions with fewer than 100 beds total. In 2004, slightly less than 1 hospital bed for every 1000 children existed in the United States. Children's access to inpatient services in the United States is excellent.

Outpatient Care Facilities

Outpatient visits for children occur in a large variety of publicly and privately owned facilities, the most important of which are physician's offices, community health centers, hospital-based outpatient clinics, school-based health centers, emergency departments, urgent-care centers, and, most recently, retail-based clinics located in drug stores and stores such as Wal-Mart and Target.[11] Unfortunately, services that occur for the same patient in these varied settings are poorly coordinated and devoid of a centralized locus of information, needs assessment, or outcome evaluation. Some authors have called the child health care delivery system a *non-system of care* as a result of this lack of integration.

ACCESS TO OUTPATIENT SERVICES. Approximately 70% of children have at least 1 visit to a physician's office each year, 6% visit physicians in a hospital clinic, and 12% have 1 or more emergency department visits.[10] Many studies have documented that children make fewer than the number of visits recommended by the American Academy of Pediatrics (AAP). Barriers to accessing outpatient services are a chief cause of this underuse. The most important barrier to accessing care is financial. For example, use of dentists in the United States remains low, with just 42% of children seeing a dentist annually, a consequence of lack of insurance financing for these services. For other types of services, children's insurance may not fully cover the office visit. (Lack of coverage among insured persons for needed services is a problem that has been labeled *underinsurance*.) Additional access barriers to seeking outpatient care include geographic access problems (lack of child health care practitioners in the community or difficulty traveling to the practice site) and organizational access problems (for nonnative English speakers a lack of interpreters, limited after hours care, or long appointment waits).

One-parent families and those with 2 working parents now make up the majority of families in the United States.[12] To maintain access to services, practices have been forced to extend their office hours to provide coverage during evenings and on weekends, in addition to on-call coverage at night. This trend is a radical departure from the office hours that pediatricians traditionally provided. After-hours coverage is provided in settings that are convenient, such as using the pediatrician's own office or an examination suite at the local community hospital. Many pediatricians join with their colleagues in sharing after-hours or weekend coverage. They take turns covering the telephone and meeting patients' needs, with prompt referral back to the patient's designated physician. This approach provides efficient off-hours medical care and affords each practitioner more time for rest, relaxation, and the pursuit of personal interests. To improve geographic access, pediatricians also have embraced the concept of the satellite office as a response to the movement of young families to the suburbs. These offices offer the same complete pediatric care available in the main office but are more accessible to suburban dwellers. Satellite offices often outgrow the main office as communities change in character or demographics and establish an identity of their own.

PHYSICIAN ORGANIZATIONS. Pediatric physician organizations can be categorized into solo practice, group practice (single-specialty practices with general pediatricians only and multispecialty groups, which include general pediatrics and other types of specialties), health maintenance organizations, hospital-based practices, and free-standing emergency departments. The practice locations for office-based pediatricians in 2000 are shown in Table 1-2.[13]

Once common, solo practice is now clearly in decline. One in 10 physicians works in solo practice, but only 1 in 25 new physicians entering the workforce are choosing solo practice. Staffing an office with a single physician provides better continuity of care for patients and requires autonomous decision making on the business aspects of health care. This autonomy has been appealing to some physicians. On the other hand, physicians in solo practice have a more difficult time arranging for after-hours, weekend, and vacation coverage than their group practice peers. Pediatricians entering the medical marketplace are increasingly concerned not only with their incomes, but also with such quality of life factors as time spent in the office, vacation, and coverage flexibility. Other benefits of group practice include administrative economies of scale, more stable cash flow, stronger negotiating position with health plans, greater financial reserves, which

Table 1-2 Practice Settings for Office-Based Pediatricians, 2000

TYPE OF PRACTICE SETTING	PERCENTAGE OF PRACTICE TYPE
Self-employed solo practice	10
Two-physician group	6
Pediatrics group	26
Multiple-specialty group	12
Health maintenance organization (staff model)	5
Academic medical center	15
Nongovernment hospital	11
Government hospital or clinic	6
Other (eg, free-standing emergency department, community health center)	11

From American Academy of Pediatrics. Socio-economic Survey of Pediatricians. Available at: www.aap.org/research/periodicsurvey/ps43soci.htm.

may facilitate investments in practice improvements such as health information technology, and the possibility of physicians developing areas of special expertise, which is useful for both primary care and specialty practices. Most medical groups in this country have fewer than 10 physicians.

Community health centers are one component of the federal government's consolidated Health Center Program that also includes homeless health centers, centers in public housing, and migrant health centers. For over 30 years, the Bureau of Primary Health Care within the US Department of Health and Human Services, the Health Resources and Services Administration, has provided federal support for health center programs.[14] These resources are used to fund services for medically underserved populations, particularly uninsured children and their families, immigrant and seasonal farm workers and their families, homeless persons, public housing residents, and those needing school-based health care. Community health centers focus on providing comprehensive primary health care to persons in medically underserved areas. Approximately 4% of all primary care visits among children in the United States occur at community health centers, 8% in hospital primary care clinics, and the rest (88%) occur in physicians' offices.[15] The proportions of visits made to community health clinics and hospital clinics are much higher for the uninsured and minority racial and ethnic groups because of poorer access to physician practices for these groups.

Several other public-sector *safety-net* provider systems offer health care services for uninsured and underinsured pediatric patients. These entities include local public health departments, community and migrant health centers, public hospital systems, and school-based clinic systems. In addition, many not-for-profit organizations assist in meeting the health care needs of uninsured and underinsured children.

MEDICAL HOME. Over 90% of children identify a single practice as the place they usually go for their preventive and illness-related care. Children with a usual source of care use fewer emergency department services, are more satisfied with their care, and have shorter hospital stays than counterparts who lack such a place. Recent parlance has substituted the medical home for usual source of care, and a growing amount of policy development and quality improvement activities have addressed this concept.

Even for children who have a regular source of care, this source does not always provide all the required services, nor does it always integrate the services that the child has received elsewhere. Many children who have a physician whom they identify as their usual source of care go to other physicians when they need medical services. Primary care physicians may not be aware of these other visits, even though they may significantly influence the patient's response to subsequent care. Patients are often required to change their primary care physician when their parents' employer changes its managed health care contract.

This fragmented, uncoordinated care presents a major challenge to the profession's health care goals. If practitioners, health programs, and health institutions continue to function separately, without coordination, and if individuals continue to seek care from several sources, then duplication of services will result, with an ever-increasing cost of care without commensurate gains. In fact, effectiveness is likely to diminish because different practitioners often give patients conflicting advice and treatment. The medical home concept is an approach for rectifying these problems. Desirable attributes of the medical home have been promulgated by the AAP.[16]

The pediatric primary care medical home is important for all children, not simply those who have long-term special health care needs. In addition to providing routine preventive services, anticipatory guidance, and acute care, the medical home adds several components to the conventional examination room–based model of primary care: registries of patients with specific diseases to better facilitate ongoing chronic care management; care coordination process that link children and families to appropriate medical, social, and community services; active and integrated comanagement between primary and specialty care; and patient education, particularly for patients with chronic and psychological disorders. The medical home should be easily accessible for patients, promote continuity of care, provide a wide range of services to meet most of the needs of children, and coordinate care received in all locations. These functions—access, continuity, comprehensiveness, and coordination—are the core attributes of primary care as defined by the Institute of Medicine.[17] Research evidence demonstrates that when these functions are attained at a high level, children are less likely to be hospitalized for health problems that might be managed in outpatient settings, families report greater satisfaction with care, and health care costs are reduced.[18] (For a comprehensive discussion regarding the medical home, see Chapter 8, Medical Home Collaborative Care.)

PATIENT-CALL CENTERS OR AFTER-HOUR PROGRAMS. Pediatric call centers or after-hours programs (AHPs) have been established in all areas of the United States. Patients greatly value ready access to medical advice outside of office hours, a trend that has grown with the rise of 2 parents in the workforce because pediatricians' obligations to their patients do not cease when the office closes and because many calls are for nonurgent matters.

AHPs are staffed by trained personnel on nights, weekends, and holidays. They give advice for symptomatic care and appropriate prescription refills, make referrals to an emergency facility or to an after-hours pediatric office, or advise seeing the patient's own pediatrician during office hours. AHPs operate under professional overview, using standardized protocols provided by pediatricians who use their services. In many instances, health care systems subsidize AHPs on behalf of their network of pediatricians because of the efficiency and cost savings attributed to them.

In a large, multicenter study, 65% of parents reported no preference about speaking with a physician or nonphysician for after-hours care, but 28% indicated a preference to speak with a physician.[19] Over 80% of parents follow through with recommendations made by the call center professionals.

PROCESSES OF HEALTH CARE

The process of health care is composed of the interactions between patients and professionals. From the physician's perspective, key processes include identification of and screening for new problems; patient education; matching appropriate services to a patient's needs; diagnosis using cognitive processes, laboratory testing, and imaging studies; treatment with watchful waiting, information giving and guidance, prescribing, and therapeutic procedures; follow-up of ongoing problems; referral to specialists and community resources; and admission to hospital. From the patient and family's perspectives, the key process of health care are seeking health care and choosing to use services, disclosing health-related information and asking questions, self-management for ongoing problems, participating in the recommended care plan, and assessing treatment effectiveness.

Scope of Pediatric Practice

The time a pediatrician spends in office practice remains challenging and interesting, although it is channeled differently than it was in the past. Through much of the early and middle 20th century, the practicing general pediatrician was the daily expert, always on call in the office for families in need or making frequent house calls and hospital rounds. The practitioner provided care to premature infants, to well and sick newborns, and to well and sick children in and out of the hospital. General pediatricians diagnosed and treated rheumatic fever, glomerulonephritis, all forms of infectious illnesses, and most forms of cardiac, neurologic, and allergic diseases. In short, general pediatricians dealt with all minor and most major illnesses. Subspecialists were few, usually found only in academic medical centers. Concepts such as *primary* and *tertiary* care were unknown, and pediatric intensivists, neonatologists, and other subspecialists did not exist in community hospitals. Time for parental health education was reduced because the pediatrician had to provide definitive care in the office, the home, and the hospital for virtually all diseases affecting their patients.

Today, the office-based, primary care pediatrician deals with illnesses that are only potentially serious and spends a good bit of time promoting health and well being. The patient is almost always seen in the office, rarely in the hospital, and almost never in the home. The variety of illnesses treated by the primary care pediatrician today does not even remotely resemble those of the past. Upper respiratory tract infections, moderate lower respiratory tract problems, feeding problems, gastrointestinal upsets, and minor trauma account for 75% to 85% of illness care. A large portion of practice time is now spent giving well-child care, dealing with family dynamics, and managing the new morbidities of mental illness, obesity, and school failure. The new scope of contemporary pediatric primary care is summarized in Box 1-1.

Changes in how acute infections are managed or prevented will have important and perhaps even dramatic effects on the future scope of pediatric practice. National policy recommendations to decrease use of

BOX 1-1 Scope of Pediatric Primary Care Practice

- Prenatal counseling to families preparing for the birth of their child
- Immunization for all age groups in the practice, with prior educational advice as to the benefit, risk, and alternatives, if any
- Acute illness management, including watchful waiting, appropriate prescribing, education, and follow-up
- Injury prevention by giving advice about seat belts, smoke alarms, water safety, home safety, poison control, and bicycle helmets
- Minor injury treatment
- Coordinating services for children with complex medical needs
- Structuring the practice consistent with the principles of the medical home
- Collaborating with families to support the achievement of educational goals from infancy through adolescence
- Becoming an expert on violence prevention and abuse avoidance
- Advice and support during divorce, marital crises, or other the loss of a family member
- Counseling families on lifestyle goals, such as the need for family time and for an understanding of work-related time constraints and stresses and how the family copes with them
- Promoting good health habits through advice about a prudent diet and nutrition, exercise, and dental hygiene
- Promoting avoidance of bad health habits such as sedentary activity, excessive television watching and video game playing, and parental smoking
- Identification and management of developmental and psychosocial problems, which is composed of screening, talk therapy, medication management, referral and comanagement with behavioral health specialists, and linkage with appropriate community resources
- Encouraging community activism through knowledge and use of common resources and involvement with school boards, religious groups, school athletic programs, and community facilities
- Care of adolescents and young adults, with the twin goals of providing guidance and anticipating problems in areas such as sexuality, sexually transmitted disease avoidance, drug and alcohol abuse and teenage pregnancy prevention, and education and career goals advice
- Supporting families to ensure that all children become flourishing adults

antibiotics for viral illnesses and otitis media have led to fewer prescriptions and visits for these conditions. New vaccines will further reduce the burden of acute illnesses in pediatric practice and will free pediatricians to provide more comprehensive services to enhance child health and development; promote healthy transitions into school, adolescence, and adulthood; reduce the suffering associated with psychosocial problems; and collaborate with families to maximize the chances that all children become flourishing adults.

Between 1993 and 2000 the proportion of pediatricians working part time increased from 11% to 20%. On average, however, the way in which pediatricians spent their time was constant between these years (Figure 1-1). Office-based pediatricians work 52 hours per week, spending approximately 40 of these hours in direct patient care. Direct patient care occurs predominantly in office settings, but pediatricians also spend approximately 5 hours per week in hospitals, several hours on the telephone talking with parents, and small portions of time in the emergency department and delivery room. Full-time pediatricians work approximately 55 hours per week, whereas part-time workers spend 35 hours per week.

Referrals: Linking Primary Care With Specialty Care

Physicians providing primary pediatric health care assume responsibility for a broad spectrum of preventive and curative care and for coordinating the care their patients receive from other physicians. When primary care physicians need assistance in diagnosing and managing difficult cases, desire a specialized test or procedure (eg, endoscopy or surgery), or believe that management of their patients' health problems falls outside their scope-of-practice, they seek consultation and referral. (See Chapter 19, Art of Referral, Consultation, and Collaborative Management.) Approximately 2% of all general pediatric visits lead to a referral, and pediatricians make approximately one referral a day.[20]

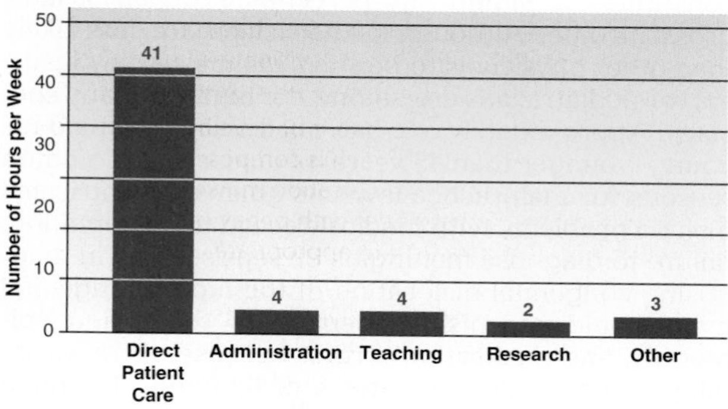

Figure 1-1 Hours per week spent in direct patient care, administration outside the practice, medical teaching, clinical or health services research, and other activities (eg, volunteer work) among pediatricians who have completed postgraduate training. *(American Academy of Pediatrics. Socio-economic Survey of Pediatricians. Available at: www.aap.org/research/periodicsurvey/ps43soci.htm.)*

Referrals are also made in telephone conversations with parents, which account for 25% of all referrals. For 75% of referrals, pediatricians anticipate sharing care with, not delegating care entirely to, the specialist; unfortunately, this practice is not often achieved.

The 15 most common health problems that general pediatricians refer to specialists and the types of specialists referred to for each problem are shown in Table 1-3. Approximately 1 in 10 referrals are made for management of otitis media. Most referrals are not for chronic diseases or for children with special health care needs but are made for time-limited musculoskeletal, skin, eye, or ear, nose, and throat problems. An important caveat is the large share of referrals comprised by psychosocial and developmental problems, which, if combined, would be the most common reason for referral. Many specialties have overlapping scopes of practice, which is reflected in Table 1-3; for example, pediatricians send patients with hernias and hydroceles to both general surgeons and urologists. Why 1 type of specialist is selected rather than another is related to a pediatrician's personal preference and the relationships the primary care physician may have with specialist colleagues.

Visits to Pediatricians

The National Center for Health Statistics reported that, in 2004, 910 million visits were made to office-based physicians, 13% of these were to pediatricians. The annual number of visits made by children and adolescents is highly related to age: 6.7 visits per person for children younger than 1 year, 2.8 visits per person for 1 to 4 year olds, and 1.9 visits per person for those between 5 and 14 years of age.

In 1993, pediatricians reported an average of 103 visits per week, whereas by 2000 the figure had decreased to 94, or approximately 19 patients per day. An average visit lasts 15 minutes, although duration of visits varies substantially according to content of the visit. Appointments made for comprehensive preventive care visits are much longer, for example, than others made for illness follow-up.

The primary reasons for pediatric visit are summarized in Table 1-4. Approximately one third of visits are for well-child care or prevention, another third is for diagnosis and treatment of physical problems, and the rest are for a variety of additional reasons. With the changing scope of pediatric practice, the share of visits devoted to acute management of physical health problems (currently approximately 30% of visits) is expected to decrease, whereas follow-up and management of psychosocial problems should increase.

Among young children, an equal proportion of visits are made to pediatric subspecialists and nonpediatric-trained specialists. By adolescence, however, a greater share of visits occurs with specialists who are not trained as pediatricians. Pediatric societies have championed the notion that the specialty care of children and adolescents should be provided by pediatric-trained medical and surgical specialists. For example, the Surgical Advisory Panel of the AAP in 2002 asserted that all children 5 years or younger who require surgical care should be referred to a pediatric surgeon.[21]

Table 1-3 The 15 Most Common Health Problems General Pediatricians Refer to Specialists and Nonphysician Clinicians With Specialized Skills.

HEALTH PROBLEM REFERRED	PERCENTAGE OF ALL REFERRALS MADE BY GENERAL PEDIATRICIANS	TWO MOST COMMON TYPES OF SPECIALISTS REFERRED TO (PERCENTAGE OF TOTAL)
Otitis media	9.2	Otolaryngologist (95.3) Audiologist (3.5)
Refractive errors	5.6	Ophthalmologist (67.3) Optometrist (32.7)
Musculoskeletal signs and symptoms	5.0	Orthopedic surgeon (71.0) Physical therapist (11.8)
Benign skin lesions	4.5	Dermatologist (80.7) Plastic surgeon (10.8)
Behavioral problems	3.5	Psychologist (58.5) Psychiatrist (18.5)
Fractures (excluding digits and hips)	2.9	Orthopedic surgeon (92.5) Otolaryngologist (7.5)
Joint disorders, trauma related	2.7	Orthopedic surgeon (87.8) Physical therapist (12.2)
Developmental delay	2.6	Neurologist (20.8) Orthopedic surgeon (12.5)
Hearing loss	2.5	Audiologist (71.3) Otolaryngologist (28.3)
Strabismus, amblyopia	2.5	Ophthalmologist (97.8) Optometrist (2.2)
Viral warts and molluscum contagiosum	2.5	Dermatologist (87.0) Podiatrist (8.7)
External abdominal hernia and hydrocele	2.3	Pediatric or general surgeon (90.7) Urologist (9.3)
Depression and anxiety	2.3	Psychiatrist (52.4) Psychologist (40.4)
Allergies	2.1	Allergist (89.5) Ophthalmologist (5.3)
Chronic pharyngitis and tonsillitis	2.0	Otolaryngologist (94.6) Speech therapist (2.7)

From Forrest CB, Glade GB, Baker A, et al. The pediatric primary-specialty care interface: how pediatricians refer children and adolescents to specialty care. *Arch Pediatr Adolesc Med.* 1999;153:705-714. Copyright © American Medical Association. Reprinted by permission.

Physician Disciplining and Medical Liability

One of the most common methods used to address poor quality is through physician disciplining programs and the medical malpractice system, even though the overall effect on quality of children's health care is low. In some countries, government agencies deal with patients' dissatisfaction and complaints. The consequences of these deliberations may be to exonerate the physician or recommend sanctions (usually financial) against the physician. The medical profession in the United States has been impotent in meaningfully disciplining its members because no way has been found to impose sanctions short of revoking a license, which is rarely done. To date, both professional and legislative bodies have failed to come to grips with this issue.

Pediatricians practice in an environment marked by skyrocketing professional liability claims, and, in some communities, insurance carriers have stopped underwriting pediatric malpractice policies.[22] Some physicians pay annual premiums as high as $25,000, which constitutes a significant percentage of physicians' gross income. Although pediatricians are less likely than other physicians to be sued, claims paid by insurers for pediatricians are among the highest of any specialty. Approximately one half of all claims are paid for young (younger than 45 years) pediatricians. Common reasons for malpractice lawsuits against pediatricians include problems with medical record documentation, failure to diagnose meningitis or sepsis, delay in diagnosing congenital dislocation of the hip or congenital hypothyroidism, mismanagement of croup and epiglottitis, and medication errors. Because of the variability among states in statutes of limitation for filing malpractice claims on behalf of minors, and because of failure to set monetary limits for malpractice awards, pediatricians are at risk not only for high awards, but also for settlement many years after the alleged malpractice occurred.

The 2001 periodic survey by the AAP revealed that, overall, no change in the frequency or nature of pediatricians' experiences had occurred with malpractice suits over the prior 15 years. On average, a pediatrician

Table 1-4 Reasons for Pediatric Visits

REASON FOR VISIT	PERCENTAGE
Well-child care or prevention	37
Physical health problems: diagnosis, treatment, or both	30
Referral or consultation	2
Follow-up for a specific health problem	15
Psychosocial health problems: diagnosis, treatment, or both	8
Ambiguous or unclear problems	6
Other	2

From American Academy of Pediatrics. Socio-economic Survey of Pediatricians. Available at: www.aap.org/research/periodicsurvey/ps43soci.htm; Forrest CB, Glade GB, Baker A, et al. The pediatric primary-specialty care interface: how pediatricians refer children and adolescents to specialty care. *Arch Pediatr Adolesc Med* 1999;153:705-714.

is sued 1.7 times. Approximately one third of claims are dropped by the plaintiff, and another third are settled out of court. Pediatricians are 3 times as likely as plaintiffs to win a case if it goes to court. Patients seen when covering another pediatrician's practice and hospitalized patients are most likely to generate malpractice suits.

To avoid malpractice suits, pediatricians should make prudent referrals, test appropriately, maintain good records, spend adequate time with patients, listen carefully to and address their concerns thoroughly, and use other techniques as listed in Box 1-2. However, no evidence has been found that either adopting these approaches or attending risk-management educational programs in reducing medical malpractice suits is effective. Defensive medicine has had an economic effect by increasing medical care expenditures. The best estimates are that it increases total health care costs in the United States by approximately 0.5% to 4%. Some of these practice changes may improve medical care; others may be unnecessary or even harmful. Because of a perceived change in physician-patient relationships resulting from the threat of liability, the pleasure of practice has lessened. Changes that are fair and equitable to both the public and the medical profession depend on societal attention to this difficult problem.

OUTCOMES OF CARE

The purpose of health care is not merely to build delivery systems or produce services. Citizens have child health care delivery systems to improve children's health, functioning, and well being. Thus the most important measures of pediatric health care effectiveness are related to the impact of services on child health, functioning, and well being.

The claim *children are healthy* is a myth with origins in the anachronistic notion of children as little adults. The key issue is the definition of *healthy*. If children are considered *little adults,* then their lower disease burden is certainly an indicator of better health. Only 10% of children have one of the long-term disorders—diabetes, cardiovascular disease, or asthma—that are typically included in disease-specific studies. The low prevalence of medical disorders calls into question the appropriateness for children of the conventional disease-oriented model of health. Certainly, a focus on children with chronic conditions merits continued attention. However, if improvement in the health of all children is the goal, then pediatric care physicians need to expand the conceptualization of child outcomes to capture the variability of health within the general population.

The dynamic developmental trajectories of childhood and the importance of the family to child outcomes are additional reasons why a child-specific outcomes framework is needed. Perspectives of health that incorporate a time dimension and the need to consider factors that threaten and promote future health are now recognized to encompass commonly accepted definitions of health. Using this comprehensive concept of health, more than 50% of children have a significant need in terms of their well being and self-esteem, symptom burden, risk behaviors, or psychosocial resilience.

The time dimension of health suggests the need to focus attention on risks—health states and behaviors that are precursors to future morbidity, injury, and illness. Although the consequences of risks may not manifest themselves until adulthood, antecedents to risk behaviors and states are molded during childhood, and many risk behaviors make their debut in adolescence. The weight-activity-nutrition complex illustrates this life-course perspective. In childhood, the antecedents to obesity—eating and activity behaviors—are formed. By late middle childhood and early adolescence, approximately 1 in 6 individuals is overweight, with a heightened risk for future disease. For most individuals, the consequences of obesity—diabetes, asthma, low back pain, hypertension, and heart disease—do not become a problem until adulthood, although they occasionally appear in adolescence and even in childhood.

Promoting child health has intrinsic merit and has benefits for adulthood. Viewing health across the life span has been called the *life course model of health*. The model suggests that health is produced across the life span, but childhood is a critical period. Unique person-environment interactions exist at each stage of development, some of which can have profound effects on future health.

In summary, a framework for assessing the effects of health delivery systems on child outcomes must be specific to the unique needs and experiences of children, developmentally sensitive, incorporate a time dimension, and rooted in a life-course model of health production. Table 1-5 provides such a framework, showing the key child outcome concepts and examples of specific metrics. Each of the 8 child outcome domains from Table 1-5 is discussed here, with special emphasis given to linkages with medical services.

Survival

The significant declines in mortality over the last century can be attributed more to improvements in public health than to specific technological advances applied to individual patients. The discovery of antibiotics is the only scientific advance applied to individual patients who are

BOX 1-2 Ways to Avoid Malpractice Suits

STANDARDS

Meet normative standards of health care delivery (ie, according to expert opinion as found in medical textbooks, articles in scientific journals, or evidence-based medicine reviews) and empirical standards (ie, according to local medical practice).

COMMUNICATION

- Use positive methods in communicating with patients and parents, showing respect, understanding, concern, and compassion.
- Train staff members to be sensitive to a patient's needs at all times.
- Train staff members to manage patient telephone calls properly and to log all incoming and outgoing telephone calls, including patient problems and instructions given.

DOCUMENTATION

- Document the care process as completely as possible.
  1. Record on the 1st page of a patient's chart drug allergies and problem list.
  2. Record for each visit the history, findings on physical examination (including pertinent negative findings), diagnostic tests ordered (including their results), and treatment prescribed in sufficient detail for purposes of recall.
  3. Record all immunizations given and all screening test results.
  4. Record all telephone calls during which medical information about the patient was received or advice given;
     include date and time.
- Document using an electronic health record or write as legibly as possible.
- Place in the patient's chart discharge summaries of hospitalizations and referral letters to and responses from consultants.
- Never alter a chart in response to a claim. If a change in the meaning of a note is warranted as a result of newer findings or recollections, then write and date a new note referring to the previous note, leaving the original untouched.

ill that has had a major impact in improving length of life. The marked improvement in life expectancy over the last century has resulted primarily from lowered infant mortality. Infant mortality began to decline long before specific medical interventions were imposed, and the decline resulted from general improvements in sanitation, maternal nutrition, hygiene, and infant feeding. Immunizations are an important, although not primary, determinant of this decline. After infancy, deaths in childhood are so relatively infrequent that they are an insensitive indicator of the value of medical interventions. Some researchers have argued that disease-specific mortality statistics, such as 5-year cancer survival, are the most compelling mortality statistics to use to assess system effectiveness because they are directly related to the adequacy of treatment.

Injury and Disease

Even though pediatricians may not be able to prevent the occurrence of most disorders, they should be expert at recognizing these problems when they occur. The application of diagnostic or therapeutic strategies requires first that problems, or potential problems, be recognized. Evidence indicates that the existence of many types of health problems is often overlooked. For example, physicians are consistently poorer at recognizing the existence of behavior problems and social factors related to illness than they are at recognizing problems that have obvious biophysiological or anatomic manifestations. However, even organic problems may be neglected. Many children, and adults as well, have health conditions that their physicians fail to identify even when information about these conditions is available. Failure to recognize the problems that patients bring to physicians is a serious shortcoming in the provision of health services.

Problem recognition also extends to prevention of disease. One type of prevention, *primary prevention,* is traditional to pediatricians. It consists of recognizing susceptibility to disease and applying interventions to prevent disease from occurring. Although immunizations are the most obvious example of primary prevention, prevention goes far beyond this measure. In some instances, only certain people are at risk of acquiring disease later in life; pediatricians must direct efforts at discovering who these people are, at keeping them under surveillance, and at trying to eliminate the situations that allow the illness to develop. This approach is known as *secondary prevention.* As social, occupational, environmental, and behavioral factors become recognized as important antecedents of many chronic illnesses, pediatricians will become more involved in activities directed toward preventing them.

Up to now, secondary prevention has not been a common feature of pediatric practice, and children who are at risk have generally been identified at the initiative of government and social agencies. Examples of such efforts include hearing and vision screening in schools, special screening programs for specific disease in special populations (sickle cell anemia, Tay-Sachs disease), and state-mandated neonatal screening for inherited metabolic disorders (eg, phenylketonuria). A major challenge for pediatricians is recognizing and dealing with occupational hazards that result in parents unknowingly exposing their children to toxic materials invisibly carried home from the workplace.

Much of health care is devoted to minimizing the effect of diseases on health. Reducing the impact of injury by limiting the duration of disability is an outcome that health care delivery systems can affect, although the provision of health services is not the only determinant of functional recovery. Similarly,

Table 1-5 Child Outcomes Framework for Assessing the Effects of Health Care Delivery Systems, Organized by 8 Domains

OUTCOME	MEASURES (EXAMPLES)
SURVIVAL	
Survival	• Infant mortality rate: number of children who die before their 1st birthday per 1000 live-born children • Life expectancy: number of years that a newborn child can expect to live • Five-year survival rates for specific diseases, such as cancer • Cause-specific mortality rate, such as mortality caused by asthma
INJURY AND DISEASE	
Injury	• Unintentional injuries • Intentional injuries • Child abuse and neglect rates • Suicide rates among youth
Development of disease	• Vaccine-preventable infections, such as measles, hepatitis B, pertussis • New cases of specific disorders, such as asthma, depression, attention deficit disorder, type 2 diabetes, seizure disorder, allergies, acne, metabolic syndrome, anxiety
Disease complications	• Severe dehydration • Suicide associated with depression • Iatrogenic complications associated with surgical interventions • Iatrogenic complications associated with medications • Consequences of untreated or inadequately treated infections, such as poststreptococcal glomerulonephritis, Lyme arthritis, pelvic inflammatory disease • School days lost resulting from illness
Disease severity	• Among patients with diabetes, glycated hemoglobin level • Among patients with asthma, forced expiratory volume in 1 second • Among children with hypertension, systolic and diastolic blood pressure levels • Cancer stage at diagnosis
GROWTH	
Growth	• Birth weight: low birth weight (<2500 g) and very low birth weight (<1500 g) • Underweight and failure to thrive: sex-specific weight for age is less than or equal to the 5th percentile • Overweight: sex-specific weight for age is greater than or equal to the 95th percentile
FUNCTIONING AND DEVELOPMENT	
Mobility	• Attainment of age-appropriate mobility developmental milestones (eg, age child walked) • Days of restricted activity • Amount and frequency of physical activity
Self-management	• Attainment of age-appropriate self care developmental milestones (eg, getting dressed independently) • Sleep habits • Nutritional intake behaviors • Dental hygiene • Adherence to medication regimens
Communication	• Attainment of age-specific receptive language capacities • Attainment of age-specific expressive language capacities
Interpersonal interactions	• Developing satisfying and fulfilling friendships • For youth and young adults, developing intimate relationships
Intellectual performance	• School readiness • Academic performance, such as grades and grade completion • Graduation from secondary school
FAMILY	
Family impact	• Parental work days lost resulting from a child's illness • Parental worry about child's health
Family connectedness	• Parental time spent with children in activities such as play, recreation, meals • Quality and frequency of child-parent discussions about the child's life • Parental monitoring of children's activities within and outside the home
RISKS	
Risk behaviors	• Tobacco smoking • Alcohol use • Drug use • Early sexual debut • Not wearing a seat belt while riding in a motor vehicle • Not using a helmet while riding a bicycle

Table 1-5 Child Outcomes Framework for Assessing the Effects of Health Care Delivery Systems, Organized by 8 Domains—cont'd

OUTCOME	MEASURES (EXAMPLES)
SYMPTOMS AND COMFORT	
Symptoms	• Physically experienced sensations, feelings, and perceptions that are the result of a disease process • Emotionally experienced sensations, feelings, and perceptions that are the result of a disease process
Comfort	• Physically experienced body sensations, feelings, and perceptions that are not associated with a known disease process • Emotionally experienced body sensations, feelings, and perceptions that are not associated with a known disease process
WELL BEING	
Well being	• Happiness • Self-worth • Life satisfaction • Flourishing: attaining a meaningful life

health care attempts to prevent or mitigate the effects of disease complications and to stabilize the disease itself so as to reduce its severity. Because managing the complexity, stability, and complications of disease are common and effective parts of pediatric practice, indicators of the adequacy of disease control are obvious candidates for outcomes for which the health care delivery system should be accountable.

The fact that many commonly applied therapeutic maneuvers are of unproved usefulness and may even be dangerous is well known. For example, several studies demonstrate that surgical rates in the United States are much higher than those in other developed countries, without any demonstrable difference in the need for surgery as defined by prevalence of disease or illness. Even within the United States, the number of hospital admissions, the length of stay in the hospital, and the rate of surgical procedures vary markedly from area to area, unrelated to differences in medical need. This potential overuse of specialized services might actually result in poorer outcomes, with more patients than necessary experiencing iatrogenic complications of interventions. Another problem is the misuse of drug therapy. For many physicians, drug manufacturers' representatives and advertisements are the primary sources of information on new drugs. Several surveys have shown a widespread lack of appreciation by physicians of the dangers of many drugs and much unwarranted use of drugs. Outcomes data will be helpful in determining the usefulness of various therapeutic maneuvers and will guide the appropriate usage of drugs.

To ensure that diagnostic procedures and instituted therapy are adequate and that problems are being resolved as expected, patients must be monitored; this approach is known as *outcomes assessment*. Medical textbooks and teaching rarely include information that helps the practitioner define appropriate intervals for reassessing particular health problems. Such information has to come from careful studies of the natural history of patients' problems, with and without intervention, and such studies are rare. Moreover, little is known about the extent to which practitioners follow up problems they treat. When the issue has been examined, research shows that failure to follow up on treated patients results in unresolved health problems; at the very least, it produces a highly inefficient health care system: Care is paid for, but no benefit is gained. At the most, outcomes assessment will ultimately lead to societal demands for greater accountability of the profession.

The likely scenario is that future physicians will be encouraged, and perhaps even required, to keep certain types of data about children in their practices. A data set for hospitals to use for each patient admitted and a similar set for ambulatory care have been accepted by the National Center for Health Statistics and recommended for wide use. This information includes registration data (patient identification number, name, address, birth date, gender, race, and marital status) and encounter data (facility identification number, provider identification number, patient identification number, source of payment, date of encounter, patient's purpose for visit, physician's diagnosis, diagnostic and management procedures, and disposition). Adoption of this or a similar system for collecting and standardizing information will facilitate the understanding of health and disease processes and the role medical care plays in influencing them. (For more details, see Chapter 6, Quality Improvement in Pediatric Primary Care.)

Growth

Monitoring children's growth is one of the cornerstones of pediatric primary care. Assessing growth requires pediatricians to examine both tails of the distribution: underweight and overweight. The ability of pediatricians to identify growth problems is well established. Whether pediatric professionals have an important effect on preventing growth problems is less clear. Today, approximately 1 in 6 children is overweight. Interventions that pediatricians can apply to prevent the problem of being overweight are lacking. Problems with inadequate weight are more easily addressed by health care; however, the degree to which a health care delivery system can affect the healthy growth of an entire population remains to be demonstrated. (See Chapter 299, Obesity and Metabolic Syndrome.)

Functioning and Development

Children's functional capacities in the areas of self-management, mobility, communication, interpersonal interactions, and intellectual capacity rapidly change and acquisition of new abilities characterizes stages of development; they are also targets of health services. Monitoring age-appropriate development of new capacities and intervening with children who have problems in each dimension is a fundamental part of well-child care.

Reducing the number of days of restricted activity, for example, due to acute illness or asthma is often a primary treatment outcome. When asked about the meaning of *being healthy,* children and youth talk about "being able to do what I want to do, play what I want to play, or see my friends." Similarly, children know that healthful self-management habits are an important part of their health status, and counseling on these topics is part of virtually every routine health visit. One of the *new morbidities* with which pediatricians have become more concerned is learning and intellectual development. For young children, pediatricians counsel parents about the importance of reading to brain development, enjoyment, and for being prepared to learn once the child starts school. Programs such as Reach Out and Read (www.reachoutandread.org/) have been developed to provide office-based practitioners with tools for promoting early childhood literacy.

As children get older, pediatricians work with them and their families in setting educational goals, monitoring children's performance in school, and, with youth, setting goals for their young adult professional lives. Perhaps the single best indicator of the health of a population of children and youth is the rate of graduation from secondary school. Healthy children finish high school and successfully transition into adulthood.

Family

Children's health outcomes are inextricably bound with their family. The family and home life are the most important contexts in the production of children's health and for promoting their development. Parenting and family involvement in a child's life are especially critical. A variety of studies have shown that accumulated childhood exposures to different types of abuse or household dysfunction directly increase the risk of psychiatric disorder and several chronic diseases that emerge later in life. Abuse appears to alter the structures and functions of a child's brain and the body's reactivity to stress. Unstable (especially rejecting) parent-child relationships produce biological changes that interact with future environmental stimuli to produce adult disease.

Child health can affect the family by influencing parental emotions and mood (eg, excessive worry about a sick child, a depressed mood in a parent who devotes a large share of time to the care of a child with a special health care need) and parents' work productivity. These family outcomes can then affect children's health in a reciprocal dynamic relationship.

Risks

When a child or youth engages in high-risk behavior, the chances of future injury or disease are increased. Not wearing a helmet while riding a bike enhances the likelihood that if the child is in a bike accident, a head injury will occur. Tobacco smoking in adolescence negatively affects pulmonary function and begins a cascade of negative effects on future cardiovascular and pulmonary structure and function. Early sexual debut heightens the chances for acquiring sexually transmitted diseases and teen pregnancy.

Routine health visits for adolescents should always address risk avoidance. Significant effects of these interventions, primarily information giving and counseling, on the incidence and frequency of risk behaviors have not been shown in research studies. This type of evidence is needed to guide risk avoidance interventions better. Until these data are made available, most professionals would not want to be held accountable for the levels of risk behavior in the population for whom they care.

Symptoms and Comfort

Feelings of discomfort can be experienced physically and emotionally, and they may or may not be linked to a disease. Almost one half of all office-based visits involve some degree of symptom management. Children who feel uncomfortable are less involved in desired activities, more likely to miss school, and more unhappy than others without the same feelings. Relieving the suffering associated with illness is a core function of health services delivery. Thus the level of comfort of a patient population or the symptom burden of a diseased subgroup is a clear outcome indicator that can be linked to health services.

Well Being

Well being has 2 components. The 1st component, simply stated, is *happiness*—the degree to which life experiences match the individual's expectations. Health care delivery systems add to the happiness of children by ensuring that the risk of injury and disease is as low as possible and the impact of disorders when injury or disease occurs is minimized by preventing unwanted symptoms and ensuring the highest level of comfort possible, by promoting growth and development, by counseling on behavior (both ways to improve health directly and ways to avoid harm), and by supporting families in the care of their children.

The 2nd component is meaning, predictability, and flourishing. Healthy children see and plan for their future. Children who have led healthy lives are more likely to become flourishing adults.

Outcomes and Health Services

Some of the outcomes in Table 1-5 are more amenable to services than others. The knowledge base linking services to outcomes is largest for the biological outcomes—survival, disease, and growth. Surprisingly, no consensus exists on the specific outcome metrics that the effectiveness of health care delivery systems on which should be evaluated. For which outcomes should health care delivery systems be held fully accountable, partially accountable, or not at all accountable? This question remains largely unanswered, which severely limits the profession's ability to use outcomes assessment to improve health care services. Future health care delivery systems for children must become more outcomes oriented. Deciding which outcomes on which to base these new delivery systems is an urgent task facing all child health care professionals and managers.

TOOLS FOR PRACTICE

Engaging Patients and Family

- *Learn More About Pediatric Subspecialists Fact Sheets* (fact sheets), American Academy of Pediatrics (www.aap.org/family/pedspecfactsheets.htm).

Medical Decision Support

- *American Board of Pediatrics* (Web page), American Board of Pediatrics (www.abp.org/abpwebsite/).
- *Subspecialty Workforce Data and Resources* (Web page), American Academy of Pediatrics (www.aap.org/workforce/copwssw.htm).
- *The Mapping Health Care Delivery for America's Children Project* (interactive tool), American Academy of Pediatrics and Dartmouth Medical School, Center for the Evaluative Clinical Sciences (www.aap.org/mapping/).
- *Women in Pediatrics* (Web page), American Academy of Pediatrics (www.aap.org/womenpeds/).

Practice Management and Care Coordination

- *Developing a Telephone Triage and Advice System for a Pediatric Office Practice* (book), American Academy of Pediatrics (www.aap.org/bookstore).
- *Pediatric Call Centers and the Practice of Telephone Triage and Advice: Critical Success Factors* (report), American Academy of Pediatrics (www.aap.org/sections/telecare/11_98.pdf).
- *Pediatric Telephone Protocols, Office Version, 11th ed* (book), American Academy of Pediatrics and Schmitt, BD (www.aap.org/bookstore).
- *Practice Management Online* (Web page), American Academy of Pediatrics (practice.aap.org/).

AAP POLICY STATEMENTS

American Academy of Pediatrics and the Medical Home Initiatives for Children With Special Needs Project Advisory Committee. The medical home. *Pediatrics.* 2002; 110(1):184-186. (aappolicy.aappublications.org/cgi/content/full/pediatrics;110/1/186).

American Academy of Pediatrics, Committee on Pediatric Workforce. Enhancing the racial and ethnic diversity of the pediatric workforce. *Pediatrics.* 2000;105(1):129-131. (aappolicy.aappublications.org/cgi/content/full/pediatrics;105/1/129).

American Academy of Pediatrics, Committee on Pediatric Workforce. Pediatrician workforce statement. *Pediatrics.* 2005;116(1):263-269. (aappolicy.aappublications.org/cgi/content/full/pediatrics;116/1/263).

American Academy of Pediatrics, Committee on Pediatric Workforce. Scope of practice issues in the delivery of pediatric health care. *Pediatrics.* 2003;111(2):426-435. (aappolicy.aappublications.org/cgi/content/full/pediatrics;111/2/426).

American Academy of Pediatrics, Committee on Pediatric Workforce. The pediatrician workforce: current status and future prospects. *Pediatrics.* 2005;116(1):e156-e173. (pediatrics.aappublications.org/cgi/content/full/116/1/e156).

REFERENCES

1. Forrest CB, Simpson L, Clancy C. Child health services research: challenges and opportunities. *JAMA.* 1997;277:1787-1793.
2. Donabedian A. The quality of care: how can it be assessed? *JAMA.* 1988;260:1743-1748.
3. Freed GL, Nahra TA, Wheeler JRC. Which physicians are providing health care to the nation's children? Trends and changes during the past 20 years. *Arch Pediatr Adolesc Med.* 2004;158:22-26.
4. Althouse LA, Stockman JA. Pediatric workforce: a look at general pediatrics data from the American Board of Pediatrics. *J Pediatr.* 2006;148:166-169.
5. American Board of Pediatrics. Workforce Data: The American Board of Pediatrics, 2005-2006. Available at: www.abp.org/ABPWebSite/stats/wrkfrc/workforce05.pdf. Accessed February 21, 2007.
6. Goodman DC and the Committee on Pediatric Workforce. The pediatrician workforce: current status and future prospects. *Pediatrics.* 2005;116:156-173.
7. Mayer ML, Preisser JS. The changing composition of the pediatric medical subspecialty workforce. *Pediatrics.* 2005;116:833-840.
8. Freed GL, Uren RL. Hospitalists in children's hospitals: what we know now and what we need to know. *J Pediatr.* 2006;148:296-299.
9. National Association of Children's Hospitals and Related Institutions. Children's Hospitals provide advanced clinical care for all children. Available at: www.nachri.org. Accessed February 21, 2007.
10. Simpson L, Owens PL, Zodet MW, et al. Health care for children and youth in the United States: annual report on patterns of coverage, utilization, quality, and expenditures by income. *Ambul Pediatr.* 2005;5:6-44.
11. American Academy of Pediatrics, Retail-Based Clinic Policy Work Group. AAP principles concerning retail-based clinics. *Pediatrics.* Dec 2006;118(6):2561-2562.
12. DeNavas-Walt C, Proctor BD, Lee CH, US Census Bureau. *Current Population Reports P60-229. Income, Poverty, and Health Insurance Coverage in the United States: 2004.* Washington, DC: US Government Printing Office; 2005.
13. American Academy of Pediatrics. Socio-economic Survey of Pediatricians. Available at: www.aap.org/research/periodicsurvey/ps43soci.htm. Accessed on February 17, 2007.
14. O'Malley AS, Forrest CB, Politzer RM, et al. Health center trends, 1994-2001: what do they portend for the federal growth initiative? *Health Aff.* 2005;24:465-472.
15. Forrest CB, Whelan EM. Primary care safety-net delivery sites in the United States: a comparison of community health centers, hospital outpatient departments, and physicians' offices. *JAMA.* 2000;284:2077-2083.
16. American Academy of Pediatrics. Medical home initiatives for children with special health care needs, policy statement, organizational principles to guide and define the child health care system and/or improve the health of all children. The medical home. *Pediatrics.* 2002;110:184.
17. Donaldson M, Yordy KD, Lohr KN, et al., eds. *Primary Care: America's Health in a New Era.* Washington, DC: National Academies Press; 1996.
18. Cooley WC. Redefining primary pediatric care for children with special health care needs: the primary care medical home. *Curr Opin Pediatr.* 2004;16:689-692.

19. Kempe A, Luberti AA, Hertz AR, et al. Delivery of pediatric after-hours care by call centers: a multicenter study of parental perceptions and compliance. *Pediatrics*. 2001;108:E111.
20. Forrest CB, Glade GB, Baker A, et al. The pediatric primary-specialty care interface: how pediatricians refer children and adolescents to specialty care. *Arch Pediatr Adolesc Med*. 1999;153:705-714.
21. American Academy of Pediatrics, Surgical Advisory Panel. Guidelines for referral to pediatric surgical specialists. *Pediatrics*. Jul 2002;110(1):187-191.
22. American Academy of Pediatrics, Committee on Medical Liability. Malpractice claim review offers mixed news for pediatricians. *AAP News*. 2001;18(4):154.

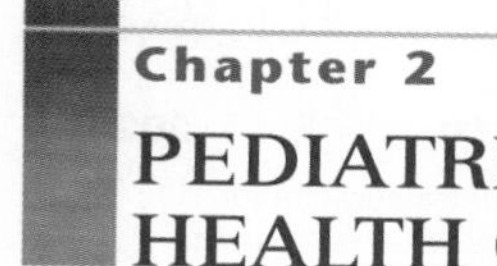

Chapter 2

PEDIATRICIAN AND HEALTH CARE FINANCE

Christopher B. Forrest, MD, PhD; Thomas K. McInerny, MD

INTRODUCTION

The vast majority of the patients in the primary care pediatrician's practice have some form of health insurance that covers a significant proportion of the charges for office visits, immunizations, laboratory tests, imaging, medications, and, of course, hospital expenses and other ancillary health care needs. Because more than 70% of US children are covered by employer-based insurance, this form of coverage is discussed first. Medicaid, the State Children's Health Insurance Program, and the problem of uninsured children are discussed later in the chapter.

EMPLOYER-BASED INSURANCE

A myriad of insurance products are available, and variations on existing products are growing at a seemingly exponential rate. Because of the rapidly rising rate of health care expenses borne by employers and federal and state governments in the last quarter of the 20th century and the first decade of the 21st century, employers and federal and state governments have been collaborating with insurers to find ways to decrease health care costs, including decisions by corporations to reduce their commitment to providing health insurance benefits to their employees and their dependents (Figure 2-1, Health Care Timeline). In effect, the market has witnessed a shift in supply-side to demand-side incentives, reflecting a shift toward more consumerism in benefit plan design and pick-up.

Initially, managed care seemed to provide the answer; but when consumers reacted to tight controls on utilization of services, and when health insurance premiums returned to double-digit annual increases, many employers moved away from health plans models that used such financial and organizational restrictions as capitated physician payment, primary care gatekeeping, and utilization review. Over the last few years, soaring health care costs have led to a shift of financial burden to families, leading to the emergence of consumer-driven health plans with high deductibles and health savings accounts.

Health plan products are tailored to meet the particular requirements of each employer, resulting in a confusing panoply of plans with different co-pays, deductibles, types of benefits and their limits, co-insurance requirements, restrictions, and authorization requirements. As a result, the primary care pediatrician often has contracts with 20 or more insurance companies for hundreds of different products. Keeping track of the rules and regulations associated with these plans is a monumental task but one that must be accomplished for pediatricians to look after the financial welfare of their patients and practices. This chapter explains the major types of plans and the implications for pediatricians in general terms. However, pediatricians must become aware of the details of the types of insurance products being used by the families in their practices. This task almost always requires the services of a professional (accountant, lawyer, financial advisor) with specific knowledge of the health insurance industry. Additionally, the American Academy of Pediatrics (AAP) provides an extensive list of resources and advice on its Web site through the Section on Administration and Practice Management (www.aap.org/sections/soapm/soapm_home.html) and the Practice Management Online Web site (www.practice.aap.org).

TRADITIONAL INDEMNITY

The oldest form of health insurance, dating back to the mid-20th century, is called *traditional indemnity* (also known as traditional fee-for-service or conventional insurance). This type of insurance was intended to cover the hospital expenses for employees with little or no coverage of outpatient expenses. Indemnity plans typically had a deductible and co-insurance (a percentage of any bills the patient incurred after reaching a deductible amount up to a maximal threshold level). Another aspect of these plans is that the patient was allowed to choose any provider without risk of the plan interfering with medical decision making. Although it has been largely replaced by managed care and other products, traditional indemnity still accounts for approximately 10% of policies. Thus most of the in-office services, including, at times, immunizations and basic preventive care, provided by primary care pediatricians for patients with indemnity insurance are not covered by the insurance plan and must be paid out of pocket by the patient. The most significant exceptions to this rule are services provided for trauma such as lacerations and fractures, which are covered by indemnity insurance. Almost all indemnity plans today would be considered managed indemnity in that they have some form of utilization review, such as prior approval for hospitalization. Although billing patients directly for provided services is relatively straightforward in this instance, collecting the payments from patients may pose some problems, particularly for patients whose financial circumstances are strained. Unfortunately, the pediatrician must use the services of a collection agency for a certain percentage of these patients and, rarely, may need to terminate care for patients who chronically are in arrears. (Pediatricians should follow the state regulations regarding termination of care closely so as to avoid abandoning patients and to limit the risk of lawsuits.) Of course, if the patient with indemnity insurance is hospitalized,

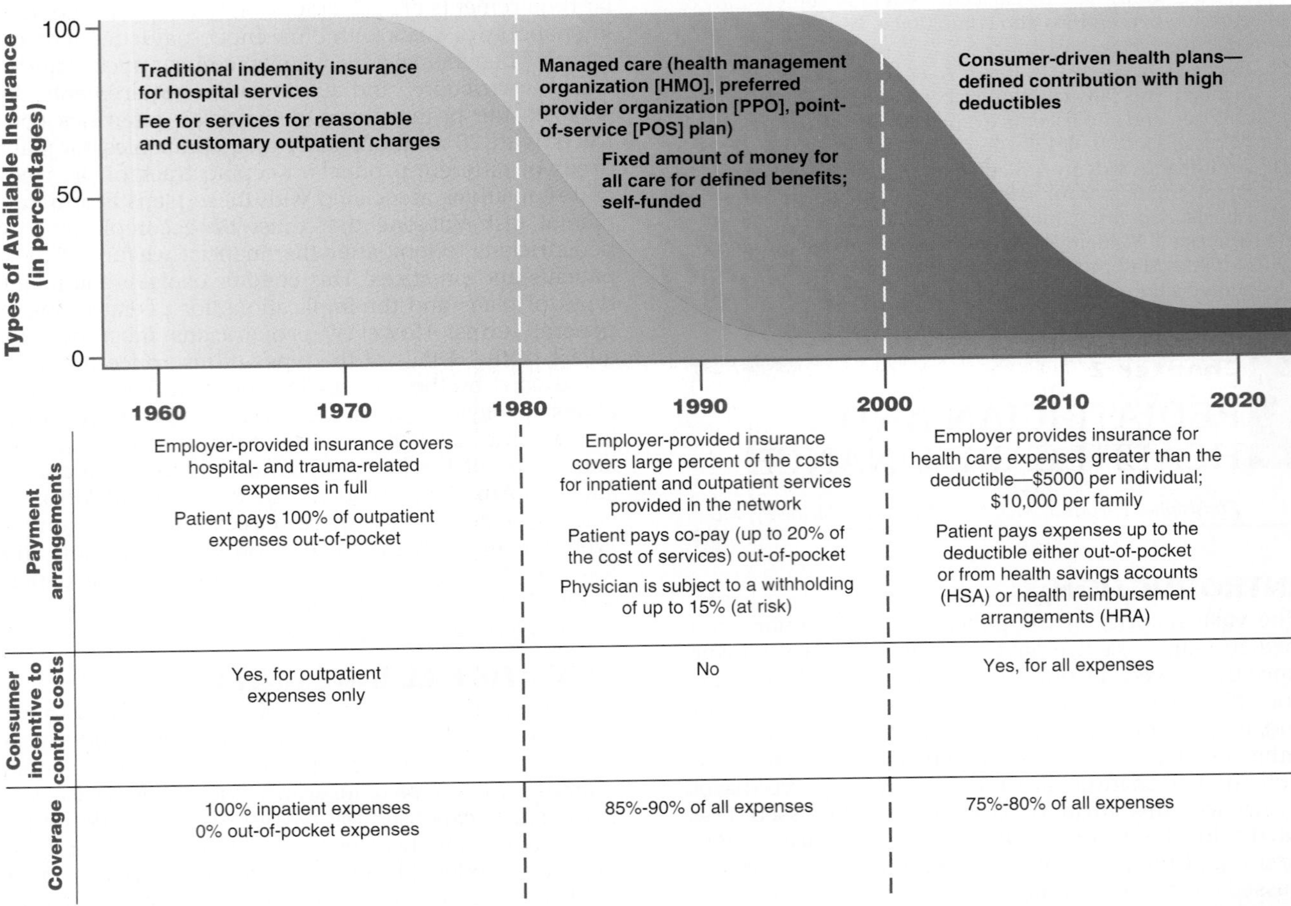

Figure 2-1 Employer-based health care financing timeline.

then the pediatrician will be paid by the insurance company for hospital services that are provided.

MANAGED CARE

As the rate of hospitalization and hospital expenses grew dramatically in the 1970s, combined with no real financial incentives to avoid hospitalization, employers grew increasingly dissatisfied with the annual premium increases imposed on them by insurers. To solve this dilemma, the insurers designed plans to reduce health care costs by managing care, or in some circles by managing costs, and by providing incentives to reduce use of health care services, particularly expensive hospital care and medical technology. The hallmark of managed care is that it combines the functions of health care financing with some aspects of health care delivery. Unfortunately, most physicians paid little attention to this rapidly growing product, were not involved in the design of the plans, and were not aware of the specifics of these plans. As a result, many physicians, including pediatricians, signed contracts with managed care organizations (MCOs) or health maintenance organizations (HMOs), otherwise known as prepaid health care, with little or no understanding of the provisions of these contracts and put themselves at considerable financial risk. Although managed care plans (HMOs and point-of-service plans) are declining in the marketplace, they still account for 25% to 50% of the products offered to employees by their employers.

Pediatricians need to understand the details of their patients' managed care plan so as to be appropriately paid for the services they provide. The following is a brief outline of the major features of managed care; for specifics, the reader is referred to *The Pediatrician's Guide to Managed Care* published by the AAP and written by the Academy's Committee on Child Health Financing. (See Tools for Practice for more information.)

To understand managed care, the pediatrician needs to learn the meanings of several consumer acronyms and the characteristics of health plans (Box 2-1, Table 2-1).

Briefly, the basic principle of managed care is that the insurance company caps the employers' expenses by assuming the risk of large health care expenses; the insurance companies then manage their risk in several ways. In the case of HMOs, the insurer passes a certain percentage of this risk to the physicians and

BOX 2-1 Consumer Health Care Plans—Acronyms and Characteristics

HMO (health maintenance organization)—a combination of an insurance company and a panel of health care providers
MCO (managed care organization)—synonymous with HMO
IPA (independent [or sometimes individual] practice organization)—a group (or panel) of health care providers that negotiates with insurers to provide care for patients insured under an HMO product at a capitated rate and that assumes risk for the loss of withhold
PHO (physician hospital organization)—a group of physicians joined with a hospital that negotiates with insurers to provide care (including hospital expenses) for a panel of patients
POS (point of service)—a type of HMO in which the primary care physician refers patients to specific specialists and hospitals
PPO (preferred provider organization)—a group of health care providers that contracts with an insurer to provide services at a discounted rate of payment

physician organizations through the mechanisms of capitation and withholds. In this model, physicians join together as medical groups or through individual practice associations (IPAs) to negotiate with the insurers to provide care for a specified number of patients for a capitated rate of a certain number of dollars per patient (member) per month. Thus the physician organization receives a fixed amount of dollars from the insurance company on a monthly basis to cover the expenses of care for the patients, or members, enrolled in that HMO. In many instances, the individual physicians are paid on a fee-for-service basis, but a certain percentage (usually 15%) is withheld from the payment from the insurance company for the services provided and placed in reserve to cover any cost overruns to the IPA. Thus physicians were presumably incentivized to reduce medical expenses so that they could be ensured of receiving 100% of the amount withheld as a return at the end of the year after all the expenses were accounted for. An important point to note is that for most primary care pediatricians practicing in a private partnership arrangement with over 50% of the gross income going to the expenses of the practice, a 15% withhold that is not returned reduces the pediatrician's own personal income by 30% or more. The effect on the use of these withhold arrangements appears to be negligible to small because most pediatricians have contracts with many health plans, only a few of which may have withhold provisions. Thus the total revenue that is at risk for any single health plan is often small.

In addition to capitation and withhold, MCOs also sought to reduce expenses by requiring preauthorization for referrals to specialists, certain procedures, diagnostic tests, and hospitalizations. More recently, as costs of drugs covered by insurers began to rise dramatically, insurance companies provided incentives for physicians and patients to prescribe lower-cost drugs by creating formularies and tiered lists of drugs. Finally, most insurers and IPAs began in the 1980s to pay the physicians and pediatricians using the resource-based relative value scale (RBRVS) system using the American Medical Association's *Current Procedural Terminology* codes and the Medicare system's RBRVS and the associated relative value units to determine fees for the types of office visits and procedures. (See Section on Provider Payment for more details on RBRVS.) The net result of all these measures was that physicians lost some control over how to care for their patients or bill for their services. Unfortunately, many pediatricians failed to review their 20- to 30-page detailed contracts with the insurers, simply signing them, often without even reading them, only to discover well into the contract year that they were suffering significant financial losses by failing to understand the terms of the contract. Thus the most important lesson to be learned is that these contracts must be read very carefully with expert advice and negotiated firmly with the MCOs, removing unfavorable terms of the contract. Indeed, in some instances, the pediatrician might be best served to avoid signing a bad contract at all. (See Tools for Practice at the end of this chapter for the Many Questions Pediatricians Should Ask Before Signing a Managed Care Contract.) Of course, the pediatrician would then be unable to care for the patients covered by that particular plan, which complicates this decision. However, occasionally, the plan providers may agree to the pediatrician's terms if the providers feel compelled to include the pediatrician's practice on their panel of physicians.

In a few areas, some plans or IPAs will capitate physicians directly for the health care expenses of their patients so that the physician assumes the full risk of expense overruns. This circumstance can be financially disastrous if the physician is not extremely aware of the costs of providing care to patients and absolutely certain that the agreed-on capitation rate will cover these costs. Generally, direct capitation is to be avoided by all but the most financially astute.

SELF-FUNDED OR SELF-INSURED PLANS

Escalating health care premiums over the last 20 years have compelled employers to look for creative solutions for controlling costs.[1] Managed care was 1 response to these rising costs; self-funded or self-insured plans are another. Nearly one half of employers participate in self-funded health plans, which are more prevalent among large employers because they can spread claims risks over a large employee population. Self-funded plans are exempt from state mandates of health benefits, and they are less expensive because of lower administrative costs than fully insured plans. Employers are able to customize the benefit structure based on the needs of the employee base, which can also achieve some costs savings if certain services are not offered. Important for pediatricians, exemptions from state benefit mandates means that they do not need to provide coverage of preventive care visits and immunizations (the so-called *ERISA* exemption, from the Employee Retirement Income Security Act of 1974).

Table 2-1 Characteristics of Insurance Policies—Managed Care

DIMENSION	INDEMNITY INSURANCE	PPO	POS	IPA OR NETWORK HMO	GROUP OR STAFF HMO
Qualified providers	Almost all	Almost all (network)	Network; out of network almost all	Network only	Network only
Payment of providers	Fee for service	Discounted fee for service	Network: similar to an HMO; out of network: fee for service	Capitation or mixed capitation-fee for service	Salary
Demand-side cost sharing	Moderate	Low in network; moderate otherwise	Low in network; very high otherwise	Low in network; high out of network	Low in network; high otherwise
Role of insurer	Pay bills	Pay bills; form network	Same as in underlying HMO	Pay bills; form network; monitor utilization	Provide care
Limits on utilization	Demand-side	Supply-side (price)	Supply-side (in network); demand-side (nonnetwork)	Supply-side (price, quantity)	Supply-side (price, quantity)

HMO, Health maintenance organization; *IPA,* independent practice association; *POS,* point of service; *PPO,* preferred provider organization.
From Newhouse JP. *Pricing the Priceless: A Health Care Conundrum.* Cambridge, MA: Massachusetts Institute of Technology Press; 2002. Used by permission.

Because employers retain control over health care reserves, they can maximize interest income, which is another benefit. In these plans, the employers took all the risk of the health care expenses for their employees rather than paying a premium to an insurer to assume this risk. Employers usually contract with health insurance companies to act as 3rd-party administrators to contract with physicians, hospitals, and other providers and process the claims, which makes the status of the plan as self-funded versus fully funded transparent to workers and their families.

PREFERRED PROVIDER ORGANIZATIONS

Preferred provider organizations (PPOs) are another form of managed care and are characterized by groups of physicians (a *network*) who agreed to provide service at a discounted fee. Employees and their families are incentivized to use the physicians in the PPOs by having only to pay a small co-pay or out-of-pocket expense to see the PPO physician and no coverage or less coverage for physicians who are not members of the PPO. One variation of this system is called the point-of-service (POS) plan in which patients have lower co-pays to visit physicians in the plan than those outside of the plan. For pediatricians, PPOs and POS plans offer the advantage of not having to deal with a withhold but have the disadvantage of needing to provide services at a discounted fee. Another important consideration for the pediatrician is whether pediatric medical and surgical subspecialists and children's hospitals are participating members of these plans. If not, then the primary care pediatrician is faced with the decision of referring the patient to a nonpediatric subspecialist or general hospital, the services of which are covered, versus to a nonparticipating pediatric subspecialist or a children's hospital, requiring the patient's family to pay some or all of the cost of care out of pocket. Clearly, primary care pediatricians should try to persuade insurers and employers to include pediatric subspecialists and children's hospitals in these plans. Once again, these contracts must be read carefully so the pediatrician has a thorough understanding of what benefits are included and excluded and how the contract provisions may affect referral patterns. In addition, many insurance companies may commit physicians to joining *silent PPOs,* that is, PPOs covered by the insurance company but not clearly stated in the contract. Some of these PPOs may have different payment rates, benefits for physicians, or physician and hospital panels, all of which can lead to significant problems. Therefore pediatricians should strive to ensure that their insurance contracts do not commit them to becoming members of these *silent PPOs.*

HEALTH SAVINGS ACCOUNTS, CONSUMER-DRIVEN HEALTH PLANS

In the early 21st century, health care costs continued to rise at what employers were characterizing as unsustainable rates, and health economists pointed out that the current systems really provided no significant incentives for employees to reduce use of unnecessary services. Employers have concluded that managed care plans in the latter part of the 20th century were ineffective cost-containment tools. The next version of health plan that has emerged effectively renders workers and their families cost-containment agents. These plans go by many names but can be broadly labeled as consumer-driven health plans (CDHPs). CDHPs combine 2 significant features designed to motivate the employees to spend their health care dollars wisely. The first feature is a high-deductible insurance plan requiring the employee to pay from $1000 to $5000 of health care expense out of pocket. This payout can be counterbalanced by a *health savings account*, funded by the employee, or a *health reimbursement account*, funded by the employer to provide a method to put tax-free dollars into a savings account to be used to pay for the out-of-pocket expenses. In theory, given that the employee is now paying for health care services out of the employee's own pocket or dipping into a savings account, the employee will seek out only necessary services at the lowest price available. In many cases, the funds dedicated to these plans are accessed through the use of health debit cards, which has implications for the pediatric office. A second and more variable feature of CDHPs is that they offer information about the prices and, when available, quality of provider services. Making consumers more cost conscious and increasing the amount of information they have about the products they are purchasing are intended to improve the competitiveness of health care.

CDHPs are indeed a major change in the financing of health care because they provide the employee with a fixed amount of dollars for health care expenses (defined contribution), rather than a listing of covered health services (defined benefit). Many people believe that these types of plans have led to the *commodification* of medicine; that is, medical care is treated exactly the same as any other commodity, such as automobiles or washing machines. In practice, many concerns exist about employees or patients acting as effective consumers of their health care.[2]

Of particular concern to the pediatrician is the fact that CDHPs, unlike managed care plans, may not cover preventive services, making health assessment visits and immunizations out-of-pocket expenses. Furthermore, parents may balk at following through with laboratory tests, procedures, or referrals to specialists as recommended by their primary care pediatrician. Given that employees are incentivized to roll over unused funds year to year, parents may be less willing to use the dollars for preventative care or other non–acute-emergency situations. Thus many experts have grave concerns that, as these plans grow in popularity, preventive health care for children, including immunization rates, will decline and children with chronic illnesses will not receive appropriate care from pediatric subspecialists. Although CDHPs account for only approximately 5% of the market share in 2006, they are expected to grow rapidly in popularity in the years to come. Therefore pediatric providers need to be proactive regarding these plans by encouraging patients, employers, and insurers to provide preventive care for children with no out-of-pocket expenses and to provide mechanisms to encourage appropriate care for chronic illnesses to avoid complications.[3]

PROVIDER PAYMENT

Physicians are paid using a variety of methods, including fee-for-service, capitation, salary, blended payment, and pay-for-performance methods (Table 2-2). Each payment method has intrinsic incentives that affect the volume of service utilization. Fee for service is payment for each service rendered. Because more revenue is generated by providing more services, fee-for-service payment provides financial incentives for providers to provide more care. The actual fee level is determined through a negotiation process with third-party payers. Patients without insurance typically pay more (paradoxically) than their insured counterparts because insurance companies negotiate discounts as a result of their group purchasing power. Fee-for-service payment is the most common method employed in the United States for paying physicians.

Very few patients ever ask about the price of a service before they obtain it. Critics of the current fee-for-service system say it is too opaque; fees should be available to a patient just as the cost of a car, DVD player, or other consumer good is provided. Without this type of cost information, health care can never be truly competitive because competition requires that purchasers compare and contrast services and products according to a subjective assessment of the amount of value to them per unit price. Other analysts contend that health care can never function as a market because (1) many health problems are unpredictable and can occur suddenly, thereby shortening the interval of decision-making deliberation, (2) individuals do not make rational decisions when considering their health, (3) data on quality of care are just as important as cost in judging value, and quality metrics are still being developed and validated, and (4) health care decision making is quite complex for many health problems requiring true collaboration among health professionals, patients, and their families.

The biggest reform to the fee-for-service payment system came in 1992 when the federal government adopted a relative value system of reimbursement to pay physicians for care of the elderly under the Medicare program. This system, the RBRVS, measures work in 4 dimensions: (1) time, (2) mental effort and judgment, (3) technical skill and physical effort, and (4) psychological stress. Higher payments are given for more complex services. Each procedure is assigned a relative value unit (RVU), which is a metric that assigns all cognitive and technical services a value on the same scale. RVUs are converted into dollar amounts by multiplying them by a conversion factor. For example, an office visit for a new patient undergoing a comprehensive evaluation yields an RVU over 3 times greater than a follow-up visit for an established patient undergoing a limited work-up. The same dollar conversion factor is applied to these RVUs to obtain the payment amount. Because RVUs are the same for all specialties, one approach to comparing costs of care among providers would be to make the RBRVS method of physician payment universal. Physician organizations need only make publicly available their conversion factors. This single number would allow patients to compare costs readily across physicians. The American Medical Association has suggested such an approach to promote the competitiveness of physician services, which account for approximately one fifth of total health care spending.

The RBRVS has had a modest effect on equalizing payment by lowering fees for technical procedures and raising fees for cognitive services. By late 2000, many pediatric RBRVS codes were developed to ensure that pediatricians would be reimbursed according to the same principles as those underlying the original

Table 2-2 Provider Payment Methods and Potential Effects on Service Use

PAYMENT METHOD	DESCRIPTION	POTENTIAL EFFECTS ON SERVICE USE
Fee for service	Payment is made for each procedure generated. Procedures can be a visit, test, or intervention such as surgery or endoscopy. Payment is retrospective—rendered after the service is provided.	Increase
Capitation	The patient is the unit of payment. The capitated payment may be for a set of services, such as primary care only. Payment is prospective (ie, given in advance of patients receiving any care).	Decrease
Salary	The unit of payment is time. Physicians are paid according to a contracted number of hours worked.	Decrease
Blended payment	Fee for service and capitation can be blended (eg, capitation for acute care but fee for service for preventive care); partial salary can be used (eg, 90% of total) with additional payments made according to productivity (number of patients seen or number of relative value units generated).	Align incentives to balance productivity and efficiency
Pay for performance	Payments, which are often given as bonuses, are made according to the degree to which quality and outcome targets are achieved.	Increase the specific set of services for which the pay-for-performance quality formula is calculated. Decrease undesirable services.

system. Many provider contracts with payers are based on an RBRVS fee schedule.

Capitated payment refers to a method whereby a lump sum is paid for each patient cared for over a period, such as a month. Physicians make more money by caring for more patients, rather than providing more services to each patient. Individual physicians usually do not receive the capitated payment unless they are in self-employed solo practice. In many instances, the payment is made to an intermediary entity such as the physician organization, which may choose to pay individuals physicians according to their contribution of total RVUs generated by the practice or some other approach. In theory, capitation should reduce medical expenses, allowing physicians to care for more patients and reduce utilization of services. However, capitation has not worked well in practice because of its complexity, and this factor is causing its decline in use.

PAY-FOR-PERFORMANCE PROGRAMS

In this country and abroad, tremendous interest exists in changing physician compensation to promote better quality and patient outcomes. The fact that fee-for-service, capitated, and salaried payment systems fall short in aligning financial incentives with clinical excellence is well recognized. More accountability for the quality of services, not just the production of services, is being demanded by purchasers of health care, primarily employers, who are concerned that rising health spending is not translating into better quality of care or improved worker health.

Pay-for-performance (PFP) programs can be defined as *use of incentives to encourage and reinforce the delivery of evidence-based practices and health care system transformation that promote better outcomes as efficiently as possible*.[4] The term *incentives* is used to denote reinforcers, which is anything that alters the chances that a desired behavior occurs, or at the organizational level, that a preferred structural change occurs.

Many hospitals now have contracts with insurance plans that include a portion of payment that is linked to attainment of specific quality of care standards, targets, improvements, or health outcomes. On a small scale, health care organizations have begun reimbursing physicians for meeting quality standards. Estimates indicate that less than 5% of physician compensation among participants in PFP programs is from incentive pay for quality. However, the number of physicians and the amount of money that will be involved in some form of PFP in the near future is likely to increase substantially, although the impact on physician income remains unclear.[5]

Both positive and negative outcomes may result from PFP programs. Aligning payment to promote quality may have important beneficial effects on outcomes. On the other hand, PFP may change the holistic, patient-oriented approach to patient care if health care is delivered by managing metrics rather than patients. Quality of care for conditions not included in the incentive system might deteriorate because of opportunity costs within a practice—that is, addressing a small set of health conditions to the detriment of care for other problems. Practice administrative costs may rise if additional funds are not provided to generate the PFP metrics.

Over the next several years, PFP will likely be one of the most common provider payment systems used in the United States. All general practitioners in the United Kingdom currently participate in a PFP program and receive a large share of their income from these bonus payments.

UNINSURED CHILDREN

In 2004, 16% of all Americans were without health insurance, but just 11% of children and adolescents lacked insurance, according to figures tabulated by the US Census Bureau.[6] The lower rate of uninsured young people is a result of 2 government-sponsored programs, Medicaid and the SCHIP, which provide coverage for a large number of children living in low-income families.

Despite its enormous wealth, the United States is the only developed nation without a national program of health insurance. Being uninsured is a problem unique to the United States among industrialized nations. A large body of research has shown that being uninsured is associated with postponing needed health care, forgoing preventive services, poorer quality of care, greater risk of avoidable hospitalization, and, among infants, a higher risk of mortality.[7]

MEDICAID AND STATE CHILDREN'S HEALTH INSURANCE PLAN

Medicaid was established in 1965 with the passage of Title XIX of the social security act. It was created to provide insurance coverage for certain categories of low-income individuals. Funding for the program comes from a blend of state and federal matching dollars.[8] The federal government sets guidelines for administration of Medicaid, but each state is given authority to administer its own program. Implementing the federal guidelines is monitored by the Centers for Medicare & Medicaid Services. States have discretion in determining certain eligibility criteria above mandated levels, how providers are paid, coverage of some optional services, and whether beneficiaries will be enrolled in managed health plans. Although children and their parents constitute 75% of beneficiaries, they account for only 36% of program expenditures. Most of the costs of Medicaid result from services consumed by disabled individuals.

SCHIP was passed in 1997 as Title XXI of the Social Security Act. It provides federal funds to states seeking to expand insurance coverage to low-income children and willing to invest state resources to do so.[9] Similar to Medicaid, SCHIP is a federal-state partnership with administration of the program left to the states with federal oversight. Today, all 50 states and the District of Columbia participate in SCHIP. The goal of SCHIP was to expand insurance coverage to the nation's children, and evaluations done over the last few years suggest that this primary goal has been successful. In 2006, over 4 million children (or 5% of all children) were enrolled in the SCHIP program nationwide. Most of these SCHIP plans are similar to commercial managed health care plans with benefits similar to those provided in employer-based plans, typically less complete than Medicaid's Early and Periodic Screening, Diagnostic, and Treatment (EPSDT) package. Thus the *working poor* families covered by SCHIP may be subject to significant out-of-pocket expenses for uncovered services. Most primary care pediatricians participate in these plans because they provide insurance for families and patients who would be otherwise uninsured. Of course, as with other managed care plans, the pediatrician needs to understand the provisions of the contracts thoroughly because they are often quite complex. Furthermore, pediatricians should encourage working poor families to enroll in these plans if they are eligible.

Twenty-two million (approximately 25%) of the nation's children are insured by Medicaid. Medicaid funds 1 in 3 births in this country. Primary care pediatricians have varying percentages of their patients covered by Medicaid, depending on practice locations. Nearly three fourths of uninsured children live in households with incomes that are less 200% of the federal poverty level (approximately $30,000 for a family of 3 in 2003), and two thirds of these children live in families with at least one full-time worker. Many of these uninsured children are eligible for either Medicaid or SCHIP.

Data compiled by the Urban Institute show that most uninsured children are eligible for publicly sponsored insurance, either Medicaid or SCHIP. If all uninsured children who were eligible for one of these programs actually participated in them, insurance coverage might be provided for nearly 98% of all children. Increasing participation in publicly sponsored insurance programs is therefore the key to reducing the rate of uninsured children. Two of the most important barriers to participation include (1) a lack of awareness that a low-income child is eligible for either Medicaid or SCHIP (the 2 main government-sponsored insurance programs), even if they do not receive welfare cash assistance, and (2) difficult and perplexing enrollment procedures.

In 2002, 51 million people were Medicaid beneficiaries; 50% were low-income children, 25% low-income parents, 16% disabled individuals, and 9% elders. Mandated covered services include inpatient and outpatient hospital services; nursing facility and home health care; physician, midwife, and certified nurse practitioner services; and laboratory, radiology, family planning, immunizations, and the EPSDT program. The EPSDT component requires states to screen Medicaid-eligible children periodically for illnesses and physically disabling conditions and to refer them for definitive treatment. In addition, with EPSDT, a federal requirement exists to provide outreach and case management services for Medicaid-eligible children.

Children eligible for Medicaid are divided into 2 groups. One group is eligible based on income and age and the other on participation in the Supplemental Security Income (SSI) program. SSI is an entitlement program under which a child who has a documented disability can receive substantially enhanced benefits such as extended eligibility for Medicaid and monthly cash allotments. Disability determination for SSI is generally made by the county social services department and can provide access to a wide array of services and benefits. Caring for SSI beneficiaries is costly because of their very high health care needs.

Together, Medicaid and SCHIP provide states with powerful policy levers for expanding coverage to uninsured low-income children. Income eligibility for Medicaid is lower than SCHIP, with the latter closing the gap between the Medicaid income criteria for each age group and 200% of the federal poverty line. For example, Medicaid offers coverage to 1- to 5-year-old children whose family's income is less than 133% of the federal poverty line, whereas, for the same age group, SCHIP covers children in the 133% to 200% of the federal poverty line for family income.

MEDICAID MANAGED CARE

Traditionally, Medicaid provides an excellent benefit package under its EPSDT requirement, which closely matches the AAP *Scope of Healthcare Benefits*. However, in many states, this benefit package is offset by extremely low payment rates to physicians for providing services to Medicaid fee-for-service (FFS) patients. More recently, the states that administer the Medicaid program have encouraged or required families to enroll in Medicaid managed health care plans in an effort to reduce expenses. In many instances, the fees provided by these Medicaid managed care plans for physician services have been higher than traditional Medicaid FFS payments. Because Medicaid managed care plans have been shown to improve preventive care and immunization rates for their enrollees, pediatricians should encourage their patients to switch from Medicaid FFS to Medicaid managed care plans. In addition, by law, Medicaid families have not been required to pay premiums or co-pays, given that studies have shown that poor families will not obtain appropriate services for their children if required to pay for these expenses. Unfortunately, in 2006, Congress passed legislation (the Deficit Reduction Act) permitting the states to change the rules regarding EPSDT, premium payments, and co-payments, threatening to reduce significantly the value of Medicaid as a safety net for health care for poor children. Therefore pediatricians need to (1) understand thoroughly the terms of their contracts to provide services for patients covered by Medicaid, and (2) advocate with state health department officials and legislators about the dangers of altering Medicaid significantly with negative consequences for the health of the nation's poor children.

Many states provide opportunities for pediatricians to advise state health department officials on how to improve the percentage of poor children who enroll in Medicaid and SCHIP and the quality of care provided. Pediatricians should take advantage of these opportunities to advocate for better children's health care.

OTHER PUBLIC PROGRAMS AND CHILDREN WITH SPECIAL HEALTH CARE NEEDS

Two sources of care are available for uninsured and underinsured children with special health care needs (CSHCN): (1) the federal Title V Maternal and Child Health Block Grant and (2) the Individuals with Disabilities Education Act (IDEA), formerly the Education for all Handicapped Children Act (PL 99-457).

In all states, Title V funds may be used for coordination of multidisciplinary health care services and for financing health care not covered by private insurance. Through their education or health systems, states provide early intervention services for infants and toddlers from birth to age 3 years who have special health care needs. Services available through Title V and IDEA are essential for uninsured and underinsured patients. Information on how these services are accessed can be obtained from the local health departments and school systems.

FOOD AND NUTRITION SUPPLEMENTATION PROGRAMS

In most communities, several programs are available that provide food and nutrition supplementation for eligible children and their families. These programs include Special Supplemental Food Programs for Women, Infants and Children; the Community Supplemental Food Program; and the Food Stamps Program. All of these programs provide either direct food allotments or coupons redeemable for retail food purchases. Many counties provide nutrition counseling as part of these services.

SUBSIDIZED PRESCHOOL AND CHILD CARE SERVICES

Although not specifically a health service, preschool and child care services can enhance the development of eligible children and improve their access to some health care services. Federally funded Head Start programs, which serve 3 and 4 year olds primarily, are available in all communities. Children also receive health screening, immunizations, and meals through these center-based developmental programs. In addition, many communities support free preschool programs through local school systems. Subsidized child care programs can often be identified by local social services departments. Some provide health screening.

IMPLICATIONS

Health care financing is extremely complex. To ensure that they can provide appropriate services at reasonable levels of reimbursement, pediatricians must thoroughly understand the details of the plans in which their patients are enrolled. In this respect, the primary care physician is a businessperson and must operate using sound business principles. First and foremost, pediatricians must comprehend the details and implications of the contracts they sign, remove or change unfavorable terms for themselves or their patients, or, in some instances, not sign bad contracts at all. Good contracting is the key to excellent pediatric care and financial survival.

Primary care pediatricians must also understand the intricacies of coding, billing, collecting, and compliance to be certain that they are neither underbilling or overbilling for their services provided. In particular, both the federal and state governments and, increasingly now, commercial insurers are auditing pediatricians' charts to determine that the services provided match the charges coded for the services. If a pattern of overcoding is determined to be present, then pediatricians may be liable for a hefty fine or, even worse, a suit for fraud and abuse. On the other hand, undercoding to avoid these problems may lead to significant financial hardships. The best way to ensure appropriate coding is through frequent self-audit and feedback using experts in coding to review the charts and charges.

Primary care pediatricians should also take a more active role in educating their patients' families on the intricacies of their health insurance plans. Unfortunately, most parents are unaware of the specific benefits, co-pay, deductible, and referral requirements of their health plans and therefore must rely on the pediatrician's office to explain these to them. Furthermore, the pediatrician should encourage families to review their health plan choices carefully, especially with regard to the preventive care benefits and availability of pediatric subspecialists and children's hospitals. Finally, pediatricians should suggest to parents that they work with their employer's human resource personnel to ensure that plans with appropriate benefits for children are available from their employer.

Pediatricians can also work directly with insurers to advocate for inclusion of appropriate services and procedures in their benefit packages, which is particularly true for new immunizations recommended by either the Centers for Disease Control and Prevention or the AAP Committee on Infectious Disease. Many AAP chapters have formed pediatric councils consisting of a handful of pediatricians and medical directors from the major insurers in that state and meet on a regular basis to discuss how to improve the quality of health services for children covered by those plans. Discussing fees is not permitted because this violates Federal Trade Commission rules regarding restraint of trade.

Finally, pediatricians need to advocate for access to and coverage of high quality health care services for children to state health department officials and legislators. Unfortunately, the health care needs of children are often overlooked at the federal and state level. In keeping with the AAP mission of ensuring the highest quality health care for infants, children, adolescents, and young adults, pediatricians must speak up for those who have no voice.

TOOLS FOR PRACTICE

Community Coordination and Advocacy

- *Insure Kids Now* (Web page), US Department of Health & Human Services (www.insurekidsnow.gov/).

Engaging Patients and Family

- American Academy of Pediatrics, Committee on Coding and Nomenclature. Brochure: 2006 RBRVS: What Is it and How Does it Affect Pediatrics? Available at: www.aap.org/visit/rbrvsbrochure.pdf.

Practice Management and Care Coordination

- *A Pediatrician's Guide to Managed Care* (book), American Academy of Pediatrics (www.aap.org/bookstore).
- *Many Questions Pediatricians Should Ask Before Signing a Managed Care Contract* (Web page), American Academy of Pediatrics (practice.aap.org/content.aspx?aid=1620&nodeID=2015).
- *Pay-for-Performance Literature Matrix* (chart), Feed GL, Uren RL, University of Michigan (www.abp.org/jpeds/p4p/p4pcurrent.pdf).
- *Contract Negotiation with Payers* (on-line course), American Academy of Pediatrics (www.pedialink.org/cme/_coursefinder/CMEdetail.cfm?aid=31177&area=liveCME).
- *Practice Management Online* (Web page), American Academy of Pediatrics (practice.aap.org/).

AAP POLICY STATEMENTS

American Academy of Pediatrics, Committee on Child Health Financing. Medicaid policy statement. *Pediatrics.* 2005;116:274-280. (aappolicy.aappublications.org/cgi/content/full/pediatrics;116/1/274).

Committee on Child Heath Financing. Scope of Health Care Benefits for Children From Birth Through Age 21. *Pediatrics.* 2006;117:979-982. (aappolicy.aappublications.org/cgi/content/full/pediatrics;117/3/979).

REFERENCES

1. Ginsburg PB. Controlling health care costs. *N Engl J Med.* 2004;351:1591-1593.
2. Rice T. *The Economics of Health Reconsidered.* 2nd ed. Washington, DC: Health Administration Press; 2003.
3. McManus MA, Berman S, McInerny TK, et al. Weighing the risks of consumer-driven health plans for families. *Pediatrics.* 2006;117(4):1420-1424.
4. Forrest CB, Villagra V, Pope J. Managing the metric versus managing the patient: the physician's view of pay-for-performance. *Am J Manag Care.* 2006;12(2):83-85.
5. Freed GL, Uren R. *Pay-for-Performance Literature Matrix.* Available at www.abp.org/jpeds/p4p/p4pcurrent.pdf. Accessed October 24, 2007.
6. DeNavas-Walt C, Proctor BD, Lee CH. *US Census Bureau. Income, Poverty, and Health Insurance Coverage in the United States: 2004.* Current Population Reports, P60-P222. Washington, DC: US Government Printing Office; 2005.
7. Fry-Johnson YW, Daniels EC, Levine R, et al. Being uninsured: impact of children's healthcare and health. *Curr Opin Pediatr.* 2004;17:753-758.
8. Vivier P. The impact of Medicaid on children's healthcare and health. *Curr Opin Pediatr.* 2004;17:759-763.
9. Shone LP, Szilagyi PG. The State Children's Health Insurance Program. *Curr Opin Pediatr.* 2004;17:764-772.

Chapter 3

PRACTICE ORGANIZATION

Thomas K. McInerny, MD

The organization of the practice is critical for the primary care physician's success in providing high-quality care and implementing and maintaining sound business principles. A study of 44 private pediatric and family medicine practices in North Carolina shows that low levels of preventive service performance and a significant percentage of bankruptcies were largely a result of poor organizational characteristics.[1] A well-organized practice can meet the demands of patients and payers for high-quality, cost-effective care by developing positive attributes in 4 major areas: (1) culture, (2) recruitment and retention, (3) achieving goals, and (4) planning.

CULTURE OF A PRACTICE

The culture of a practice is the subjective feeling of the physicians, staff, and patients about what it is like to work in and visit the practice. Is the atmosphere pleasant, friendly, caring, and supportive? Is it just the opposite, or is it somewhere in between? The culture of the practice is set by the physicians, the natural leaders of the practice. Their attitudes and beliefs are mirrored by the practice staff. Thus being aware of the images they project and ensuring that they are positive is the responsibility of the pediatricians. First and foremost, physicians in well-organized practices believe that caring for children and working with parents to achieve the best possible health outcomes for their children is a special privilege. Patient telephone calls and office visits are seen as welcome opportunities to achieve these goals. Admittedly, sometimes on particularly busy days, maintaining this positive attitude can be difficult, but doing so is most important, lest a negative attitude be projected toward patients and parents by the physicians or staff.

Another characteristic of a well-organized practice is respect for all staff by the physicians and staff members. All members of the practice must treat each other with courtesy and dignity at all times, avoiding negative remarks or comments. If someone in the practice shows a need for improvement, then this need should be discussed with the individual privately in a positive fashion. Creating a respectful atmosphere in the practice will be highly beneficial for staff performance and families' perception of the practice.

Teamwork is another extremely important cultural characteristic of a well-organized practice. Delivering high-quality care is a complex process requiring the coordinated efforts of physicians, nurses, receptionists, and administrative personnel. The activities of these individuals must be coordinated to develop a well-functioning team with clearly defined roles and responsibilities and a seamless system of transition among the staff.

Finally, notably, a well-organized practice functions in a democratic fashion rather than an authoritarian one. Decisions regarding practice policies, goals, and activities need to be reached by a thorough discussion with all members of the practice, hopefully leading to consensus so that all staff members are invested in the decisions that are made. This process requires physicians and staff to listen respectfully and with an open mind to everyone's opinions and encourage frank discussion regarding potential solutions to problems and challenges.

RECRUITMENT AND RETENTION

Recruitment of high-quality physicians, nurses, receptionists, and administrators into the pediatric practice is an important goal for a well-organized practice. However, recruitment is only one half of the equation, with retention of valued employees forming the other half. Given that orientation of new staff members to their functions within the practice is a disruptive, time-consuming, and expensive process, high turnover rates are to be avoided. Furthermore, families greatly appreciate hearing a familiar voice or seeing a familiar face in their interactions with the practice. Additionally, long-term staff members gain an understanding of family characteristics that can be particularly helpful in providing care for those families. Finally, physicians and staff develop efficient patterns of interaction with each other over time, which greatly improves the overall functioning of the practice. Thus taking the appropriate measures necessary to retain a high-quality staff is in the pediatrician's best interests. Financial rewards are obviously effective, but other techniques can be used that can be quite helpful as well. For example, frequent (daily) praise and appreciation provides employees with a sense of well being and value. In addition, letting the staff know the outcomes of patients of concern with whom they have interacted will give them a sense of true investment in the care of the patient. Other methods of rewarding staff are occasional gifts to thank them for exemplary service during particularly stressful times. Finally, including all staff members in celebrations such as achieving major practice goals, arrival of any new physician, 25th anniversaries, or retirements will let staff members know their value in the practice.

ACHIEVING THE GOALS

The 2 major goals of a well-organized practice are providing high quality care for its patients and implementing and maintaining sound business principles for financial success. Providing high-quality care requires more than well-trained physicians and staff. The practice needs to develop systems of care designed to achieve the best practice results. Both the Institute of Medicine[2] and the Institute for Healthcare Improvement[3] have called for the implementation of appropriate systems of care at all levels in the medical care spectrum. The systems of care principles are taken from those developed by the manufacturing industry and have been demonstrated to reduce variation and improve quality of product. Many of these principles are applicable to medical practice and have been shown to improve outcomes significantly. One of the most important systems of care principles is measurement. Randolph and his colleagues show that some practices that measured immunization rates found that these rates were significantly lower than the physicians' estimates.[1] The common business saying, "you can't manage what you don't measure" is applicable to pediatric practices. Pediatric practices should institute a host of measurement processes such as immunization registries, appointments kept ratios, waiting time for appointments, and time taken to answer telephone calls, among other processes. See Chapter 6, Quality Improvement in Pediatric Primary Care, for detailed information on small cycles of improvement necessary for quality improvement. As part of this process, physicians need to be aware of the latest guidelines for care as published by the American Academy of Pediatrics (AAP) and other organizations and to work to institute these guidelines as a regular part of their practice. Essential to the quality improvement process are regular meetings of the physicians and staff to determine best how to put in place systems of care necessary to ensure high-quality outcomes. Finally, a well-organized pediatric practice must assess patient satisfaction and work toward improving staff members' performance in this area that will become increasingly important as patients have more incentive to seek out high-quality care with newer health insurance products described in a later chapter. Thus listening to and acting on patient complaints and surveying patients on a regular basis to assess their satisfaction are important activities. In addition, the practice might form a *family advisory council* consisting of patients and parents that meets on a regular basis (eg, 4 to 6 times per year) with physicians, nurses, and staff members to discuss ways to improve services for patients and families.

Given that the primary care practice of pediatrics is a business, sound business principles are required for practices to perform well financially. First, physicians should employ high-quality professional consultants for advice in running the practice. Experts in medical legal matters should be employed to assist with contracts and negotiation and to provide suggestions to reduce the risk of medical malpractice suits. Accountants with specific knowledge of medical economics should review the practice's financial accounts on a regular basis and provide advice to improve financial performance. Similarly, management consultants with experience in medical practice management should be consulted for advice in the structure of the practice. For practices of 3 or more physicians, an office manager with expertise in the business aspects of running a medical practice should be employed. In many cases, someone with a master's degree in business administration will be more effective than someone with less training. Although well-trained individuals may be expensive, they will usually return their salary many times over and should therefore be considered as an investment rather than an expense. In addition to an office manager, one or more of the physicians in the practice need to serve as managing partners, often overseeing a particular aspect of practice management such as personnel, financial performance, or quality improvement. Practices also should benchmark their performance financially by comparing their revenues and expenses to the performances of best practices of similar size. The AAP Section on Administration and Practice Management has used the services of the Medical Group Management Association to survey pediatric practices and can provide the results of these surveys on its Web site, Practice Management Online. Finally, attention to detail is absolutely required to ensure that the services provided are appropriately coded and billed for and that collections are tracked carefully and maximized.

The use of computers in the well-organized pediatric practice is increasingly essential in the era of the information age. Computerized billing systems have long been the norm for pediatric practices, and their hardware and software systems should be periodically upgraded to meet the demands imposed by an increasingly complex health insurance system. Consultants are available either locally or nationally who can be of great assistance in purchasing the right computerized system for the practice. Beyond this effort, computerized or electronic medical records are becoming essential to provide high quality care (see Chapter 4, Electronic Health Record and Web-based Resources). The benefits of electronic medical records in providing reminder recall systems, improving immunization rates, and notifying patients of the recommended frequency of health assessment visits to care for children with chronic illnesses, to alert clinicians regarding patients' allergic reactions to drugs, and to prevent drug-drug interactions have been well documented. Although these systems are quite expensive, the benefit to patients and the reduction in personnel expenses for filing and transcribing justify the investment. For the latest information regarding electronic medical records, physicians should visit the AAP Council on Computers and Information Technology Web site (www.aapscot.org/).

PLANNING

Another key element in determining the success of a business is planning for the future. Thus a well-organized practice will hold annual retreats to assess past progress, survey the local and national medical environmental trends, and develop a set of goals and measurable objectives for the next year. Preparation for this retreat should include a *Strengths, Weaknesses, Opportunities, and Threats* (SWOT) analysis, with particular attention paid to anticipated changes in health care financing (eg, an increase in the number of patients moving to consumer-driven health plans), birth rates, population changes, and physician supply changes. The practice should formulate a strategic plan for the coming year and review the plan on a quarterly basis to determine progress toward the goals and objectives. Hiring a professional facilitator to assist in the retreat activities may be worth the small investment.

CONCLUSION

Clearly developing and maintaining a well-organized pediatric practice requires hard work, constant attention, and skills that are not usually taught in medical school or residency. However, physicians must devote the time, perform the hard work, and acquire the skills necessary if they are to provide high-quality care for patients and be successful financially. The AAP and other professional societies offer courses in practice management; in addition, the AAP offers practice management resources and tools on its Web site (practice.aap.org/). Running a successful practice can be challenging, but the rewards are well worth the effort.

TOOLS FOR PRACTICE

Community Coordination and Advocacy

- *Advisory Council Workplan—Getting Started* (form), Institute for Family-centered Care (www.familycenteredcare.org/advance/IFCC_Advisoryworkplan.pdf).
- *Creating Patient and Family Advisory Councils* (booklet), Institute for Family-centered Care (www.familycenteredcare.org/advance/creatingadvisroycouncil.pdf).
- *Family Consultant Feedback* (form), Center for Children with Special Health Care Needs (www.cshcn.org/).
- *FAQ Serving on Advisory Boards and Councils* (fact sheet), Family Voices (www.familyvoices.org/toolbox/FAC/VT-cshnfAQ.doc).
- *Patients and Families as Advisors—Attitude Checklist* (questionnaire), Institute for Family-centered Care (www.familycenteredcare.org/advance/IFFCC_checklist.pdf).

Medical Decision Support

- *Cost Survey for Pediatric Practices 2006* (book), Medical Group Management Association (www.aap.org/bst/showdetl.cfm?&DID=15&Product_ID=4183&CatID=133).

- *HIPAA: A How-To Guide for Your Medical Practice* (book), American Academy of Pediatrics (www.aap.org/bookstore).
- *Medical Liability for Pediatricians* (book), American Academy of Pediatrics (www.aap.org/bookstore).
- *Practice Management FAQ* (fact sheet), American Academy of Pediatrics (www.aap.org/moc/index.cfm).
- *Practice Management Online* (Web page), American Academy of Pediatrics (practice.aap.org/).

REFERENCES

1. Randolph G, Fried B, Loeding L, et al. Organizational characteristics and preventive service delivery in private practices: a peek inside the "black box" of private practices caring for children. *Pediatrics*. 2005;115(6):1704-1711.
2. Hurtado MP, Swift EK, Corrigan JM. *Crossing the Quality Chasm: A New Health System for the 21st Century*. Washington, DC: National Academy Press, Institute of Medicine; 2001.
3. Institute for Healthcare Improvement. Available at www.ihi.org/. Accessed October 10, 2007.

Chapter 4

ELECTRONIC HEALTH RECORD AND WEB-BASED RESOURCES

S. Andrew Spooner, MD, MS

INTRODUCTION

A tremendous amount of time and money is being spent on implementing electronic health record (EHR) systems. The rapid rise in the use of EHRs has been a response, in part, to the call for better information management in health care. George W. Bush, in his 2004 and 2006 State of the Union addresses, emphasized the need for electronic health records,[1-3] and legislators, as well as health care leaders, are calling for the use of EHRs.[4] Despite this widespread interest, almost 20 years may be needed for all physicians' practices in the United States to become completely paperless.[5] The reason for this prolonged course lies in the numerous barriers to implementing EHR systems, including the cost and the complexity of moving health care processes to electronic forms.[6,7] Fortunately, the EHR market is responding to the need for systems that work for child health care.

Pediatric providers face troublesome questions when facing the decision to implement an EHR, including whether they should do it, how to select a system, and how to finance it.

EHRs are not the only important application of information technology in pediatric practice. Web-based resources offer unprecedented access to medical reference information, diagnostic decision support, continuing medical education, and medical information for families.

DEFINITIONS

Electronic Health Record Versus Electronic Medical Record

The Institute of Medicine defines an EHR system:

> An EHR system includes (1) longitudinal collection of electronic health information for and about persons, where health information is defined as information pertaining to the health of an individual or health care provided to an individual; (2) immediate electronic access to person- and population-level information by authorized, and only authorized, users; (3) provision of knowledge and decision-support that enhance the quality, safety, and efficiency of patient care; and (4) support of efficient processes for health care delivery. Critical building blocks of an EHR system are the electronic health records (EHR) maintained by providers. . .and by individuals (also called personal health records).[8]

In the literature and in the popular press, the term electronic medical record (EMR) is often used interchangeably with EHR. Given the popularity of the term EMR, defining EMR as the portion of an EHR system that is maintained by a physician in a typical medical practice would be reasonable. In this chapter, however, we will use EHR to refer to the system a health care provider would use in a medical office to help implement the primary care of infants, children, and adolescents.

Electronic Heath Record System and Child Health

When the range of EHR systems is examined, a person quickly realizes that not all systems are designed for pediatric care. Although EHR systems that do not support pediatric functions are in place,[9,10] no functions of an EHR are purely pediatric. For example, drug dosing by body weight is critical in pediatrics but has enough usefulness in adult care that it would also be desirable in nonpediatric systems. Weight and height monitoring certainly have application in adult care, but it is much more important in pediatrics. Child health providers need to examine certain qualities of any system intended for use with infants, children, and adolescents (Table 4-1). To expect any system to support all functions perfectly would be unwise. Figure 4-1 provides an example of how an EHR system can present pediatric solutions in varying degrees.

Necessary Functions of an Electronic Health Record in the Pediatric Setting

Growth Monitoring

Fundamental to the practice of pediatrics is the analysis of growth, as documented by height, weight, and head circumference. In the United States, curves showing the distribution of these measurements at each age are published by the Centers for Disease Control and Prevention[11]; special curves for premature infants[12] and populations of children with specific congenital conditions such as achondroplasia,[13] Down syndrome,[14] or Turner syndrome[15] are also available. Caution must be used in applying these special charts to a given patient because, in some cases, the data on which they are based were collected before the availability of treatments that may improve growth rates. Standard practice is to plot these values on the appropriate curve at each encounter.

Table 4-1 Pediatric Functions of an Electronic Health Record With Questions to Ask About Electronic Health Record Systems

FUNCTIONAL AREA	QUESTIONS TO ASK
Growth monitoring	Does the system plot growth data (height, weight, head circumference) over time and allow simultaneous comparison to normative curves? Does the system plot body mass index against appropriate normative curves, thus providing percentile ranking? Does any indication exist for abnormal growth parameters (eg, flagging any weight below a certain percentile value as abnormal)? Does the display of growth data allow magnification *(zooming)* of the display when examination of densely packed data points is necessary? Does the system indicate corrections for prematurity on the growth plots? Can the user load normative curves other than the *standard* CDC curves, as in, for example, disease-specific normative curves? Does the system allow printouts of the growth curves for parents?
Immunization management	Does the system have any active interfaces to any state immunization registries? If so, then are they one-way or two-way interfaces? Can the system analyze a record of immunizations and recommend what immunizations are due at the time of an encounter? Can the system analyze a record of immunizations and indicate when the next immunizations are due? Will the system also alert providers whenever the patient's record is accessed? Can the system store lot numbers and *vaccine information statement* dates for automatic entry into the record for new immunizations? Can the system incorporate data indicating that a given series of immunizations is complete without having to manually enter the data on individual immunizations administered in the past? If so, then is this information on series completion incorporated appropriately into decision support functions? Can the user set up a procedure to have the computer fill out paper immunization forms for school entry based on data in the patient's record?
Medication prescribing	Does the system suggest a drug dose based on body weight? Does the system allow dosing based on a *dosing weight* rather than actual body weight? Failing to have this feature, does the system provide a drug-dosing calculator that automatically retrieves body weight for calculation purposes? Failing to have this feature, does the system display body weights in the same view in which the user is expected to create prescriptions? Does the system check drug doses for appropriateness based on dose ranges? Does the system support indication-specific dose ranges for a given medication? Does the system alert the pediatrician to drug allergies? Does the system alert the pediatrician to possible adverse drug-to-drug interactions? Will the system provide the pediatrician with a list of all patients on a certain medication? This information can be useful if the FDA issues a drug recall notice.
Data norms	Does the system display the percentile value of each height, weight, and head circumference in every place where such data are displayed? Does the system indicate abnormal blood pressure based on age and height? Can the user apply different normative ranges for laboratory results based on different ages? Does the system allow graphic plotting of laboratory values over time? Does the system allow querying of the laboratory database to find all patients with a particular abnormal laboratory value? Are physical examination findings whose normal appearance changes with age (eg, Babinski sign) shown as normal at appropriate ages?
Privacy	Does the system allow the user to label a chart for special privacy policies? If a way can be found for parents to access information from the system (as in, for example, a Web site that allows parental review of health record), does a way exist to limit this access in the case of adolescents? Does a way exist to represent complex guardianship or health care agent relationships in the system?
Terminology	In the portion of the EHR in which diagnoses are recorded, can the user specify rare congenital syndromes without resorting to free text? Can the problem list include items that are not diseases, for example, *developmental delay, immunizations up to date,* or *school avoidance?*

CDC, Centers for Disease Control and Prevention; *FDA,* US Food and Drug Administration.

Continued

Table 4-1 Pediatric Functions of an Electronic Health Record With Questions to Ask About Electronic Health Record Systems—cont'd

FUNCTIONAL AREA	QUESTIONS TO ASK
	In recording birth history, can the system distinguish specific terms that apply to the mother from those that apply to the baby? Does the system allow retrieval of all patients with a particular diagnosis, symptom, or physical finding?
Granularity	Are ages displayed in units that are appropriate to the patient's age (eg, 3 weeks of age is not shown as 0 months of age)? Can the user enter weight to the nearest gram?
Pediatric decision support	In the case in which guidelines are supported, can the system omit guidelines that are appropriate only for adults? Can the system filter reminders by age to reduce the number of inappropriate alerts? Can the system trigger reminders based on age so as to increase the relevance of alerts? Can the system trigger reminders based on age combined with other data such as diagnosis or time since last encounter?

CDC, Centers for Disease Control and Prevention; *FDA*, US Food and Drug Administration.

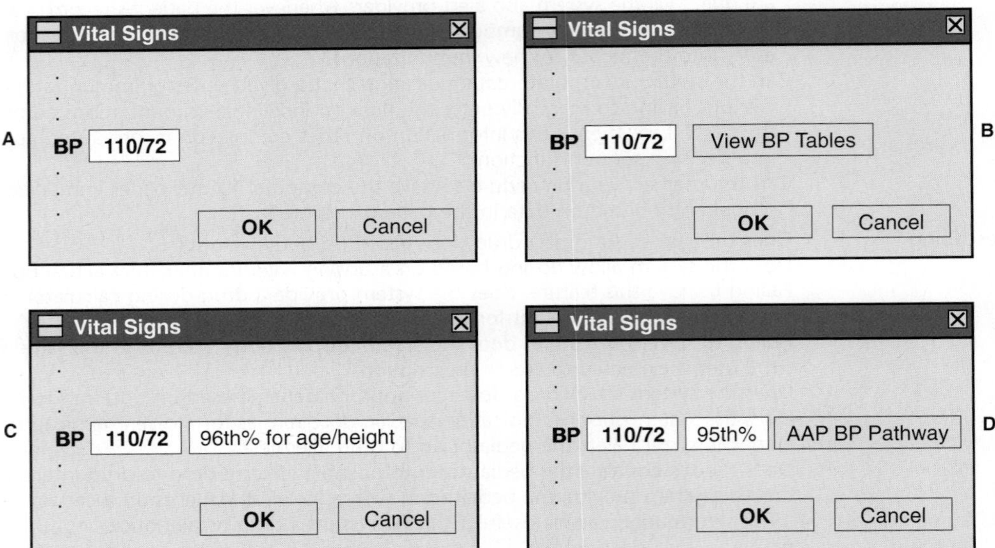

Figure 4-1 The pediatric context. The degree to which an EHR system understands cases in which pediatric care differs from adult care is a measure of its ability to present the pediatric context. Four fragments from a hypothetical user interface illustrate the different levels of pediatric context that a system can provide. **A**, Level 0: No recognition of pediatric factors. The system displays the patient's blood pressure. This behavior is expected, but it fails to reflect the pediatric complexities of blood pressure display. **B**, Level 1: Recognition of pediatric factors but no automation of special functions. The system begins to offer some pediatric context by offering the user the opportunity to look up norms for blood pressure in the same portion of the user interface that displays the blood pressure. **C**, Level 2: Recognition and basic automation. The system goes one step further by calculating the percentile value for the blood pressure (perhaps the higher of systolic or diastolic percentile values). **D**, Level 3: Recognition, automation, and integration with pediatric-specific evidence. The system calculates the percentile and offers to take the user to a pediatric-specific guideline pathway of some sort.

Although the use of growth charts in this way has not been expressly validated, it is a practically universal practice in pediatrics. Manually plotting these points is laborious and error prone. Computer systems into which these data are entered can easily display a plot of growth data over time, just as they can produce a temporal plot of other clinical data. Pediatricians expect that these plots will behave in much the same way as paper plots; with careful attention to design, computer-based growth charts can retain the analytic usefulness of the paper curves while adding functions that no paper system can hope to offer.[16] The evaluation of any EHR intended for use in the pediatric setting should include a careful examination of growth chart functions, including calculation of body mass index and body mass index percentiles by age and gender. (See Table 4-1 for specific questions to ask.)

Immunization Management

A complex, yet common, task in pediatric practice is determining which immunizations are due and when they are to be administered. The rules for indications and dosing intervals change at least every year and often more frequently as new vaccines come to market and as the epidemiologic factors of preventable diseases change.[17] Most EHR systems sold today do not offer the pediatrician any decision support for this task, and a significant minority fail to provide the ability to record immunizations.[18] Clearly, immunization management is one of the more obvious functional areas in which a computer can assist the pediatrician in working efficiently; yet the large difference in complexity between child and adult immunization management poses an often-insurmountable implementation challenge to vendors of EHR systems. The ideal system will alert providers regarding overdue immunizations whenever the patient's EHR is accessed. (See Table 4-1 for appropriate questions to ask.)

Medication Prescribing

To a much greater degree than in adult care, pediatric prescribers compute doses of medications based on a recommended dosage of drug to be used per unit of body weight. Although the fact that body surface area and ideal body weight are used in pediatrics is true, in general pediatric practice, actual body weight is the most common basis for dose calculations. Of the EHR systems that offer prescribing (most do), very few offer weight-based dosing support. This circumstance is due to many factors, including lack of standardization of dosages; although the US Food and Drug Administration (FDA)-approved labeling of drugs includes weight-based dosages for products approved for use in children, some products used in children are not FDA approved,[19] and many have recommended dosages in drug handbooks that differ from the approved product labeling. Another barrier to computerized weight-based dosing decision support is the practice of rounding to convenient doses (eg, fractions of a teaspoon), which makes calculating doses even more complex. In addition, the best systems will alert pediatricians regarding allergies to medications and possible adverse drug-drug interactions.

Data Norms

When interpreting data from children—especially numeric data—age (and sometimes gestational age, body measurements, or stage of sexual maturity) must be taken into account. For example, in adults, blood pressure is easy to interpret without referring to any of these factors; if it is above 120/80 mm Hg, then it is abnormal. In child health care, interpreting blood pressure requires either time-consuming references to tables or the assistance of an electronic information system that incorporates pediatric norms. Assistance with interpretation using gender- and age-based norms is technically easy but is often not implemented in EHRs. Pediatricians who are evaluating any clinical information system should pay particular attention to how the system assists the user with normative data (see Table 4-1).

Privacy

Pediatricians must handle certain data with special privacy considerations. The care of adolescents is the most common area in pediatric practice that requires an extra layer of protection in handling information. Some of these extra layers are the result of legislation, as in the case of parental notification laws[20] or laws governing consent to treatment.[21-23] Most of the complexity of handling adolescents' information comes from the policies of individual practices and variability of state laws. These policies are designed to encourage adolescents to seek care independently for sensitive medical issues (sexually transmitted infections, reproductive health, abuse, mental health) while striking a balance between the adolescent's autonomy and the parents' authority. With electronic systems, data are easier to locate, view, and move. EHRs might support data-access policies that take age, diagnosis, and consent status into account. For example, in the case of a visit with an adolescent that involved mental health concerns, in a practice in which the parent has agreed to allow the adolescent autonomy in seeking health care, the system might restrict display of information about that visit in situations in which the parent is likely to see it, unless the adolescent gave express permission to allow parental review. No EHR system on the market allows a privacy-protection scheme this elaborate; however, as more pediatricians use these systems, market pressure will produce greater capability in this area.

Privacy policies are also important in situations in which the identity of a child's guardian may be uncertain, as in cases of divorce, adoption, or foster care. Current EHRs cannot expressly support these complexities. The information explosion that the EHR creates[24] will make control of data access critical; we will need to insist that privacy policies that are common in pediatric care be created in EHR systems.

Terminology

Until recently, the only method for getting information into a system has been hand-typed, or free, text. Free text has limited usefulness in that it is difficult to create, is subject to typographic errors, and lends itself to colloquialisms. Given that clinical applications rely on the existence of defined sets of terms, terminology systems have been developed to eliminate these problems and add the desirable feature of semantic structure, whereby a user can start with a given term and navigate the terminology system to find related terms rapidly and unambiguously. For example, if the physician wanted to modify the diagnosis of meningitis in a problem list based on a culture result, then a quick, one-step descent into the logical hierarchy of the terminology system would list the various types of meningitides listed by causative agent. The EHR would then be able to apply pathogen-specific antibiotic selection support.

Properly constructed terminology systems have the added advantage of allowing the formation of databases by symptoms and signs, as well as diagnoses, so that the pediatrician can query the database to provide a list of all patients with a certain finding (abdominal pain or enlarged liver) or diagnosis. As new information or treatments become available, the pediatrician can then quickly find all patients for whom this information is relevant.

When terminology systems are reviewed, noticing an implicit assumption that the terms apply only to adults is common. For example, the term *premature birth* may seem to apply to a child, but in some terminology systems, this term may refer only to the obstetric history of a mother. This term might be placed into a template for a child's medical history only to find that any semantic navigation starting with this term takes the user into a set of inappropriate obstetric terms.

Evaluating the usefulness of a terminology system is extremely difficult because the effects of the adult orientation of term hierarchies are subtle. The long-term solution to this problem is for pediatricians to work with organizations that make terminologies to ensure that the pediatric perspective is represented. Pediatricians need to be aware of the limitations inherent in terminology systems in EHRs.

Granularity

Pediatrics involves smaller units of time, weight, and distance than adult health care. The scale of these measurements varies with age and with care setting. For example, age to the nearest minute is important in the delivery room, but in the newborn nursery, age to the nearest hour is usually sufficient. In the first few months of life, the patient's age should be expressed initially in days but later in weeks and then months. Body weight to the nearest gram is required in the neonatal ICU setting but is not usually necessary in the outpatient follow-up of older infants. EHRs intended for use with young infants should be able to adjust units of measure to the appropriate scale for the situation at hand. Forced rounding of weights to the nearest kilogram or tenth of a kilogram is likely to cause problems in pediatric care settings; yet this sort of scale mismatch is a common phenomenon in EHR systems. Part of the evaluation of any EHR system should include the attempt to manage basic data on very small and very young infants.

Aliases

Name changes are more common in children than in adults because of naming conventions at birth. Names associated with laboratory values obtained for a newborn may not match the name of the patient when the infant is brought to the pediatrician's office for primary care. Name changes may also occur for children as a result of divorce, remarriage, or adoption. EHRs should be able to store and allow searching for results based on an arbitrary number of aliases.

Patient and Parent Education

Most EHR systems, and many stand-alone systems, offer electronic sources of information for parents and patients. For these sources to be effective in pediatrics, this educational information needs to be available in versions that are appropriate—in both wording and reading level—for parents whose reading levels are variable. Many authorities recommend that these informational materials be written at a 4th-grade level.

Data Source

Information in adult care comes from the patient in most cases. In pediatrics, a parent provides most information, but schools, other family members, and a potentially complex system of guardians and representatives may also contribute to data on a child. EHR systems should support an indication of the source of medical history.

Managing Children With Chronic Illnesses

EHRs can be tremendously useful (if not indispensable) in assisting pediatricians in following the guidelines developed for providing optimal care for children with chronic illnesses. Good systems will alert pediatricians when patients need to be seen at recommended intervals, to have laboratory tests performed, and to refill medications, among other tasks. Appropriate disease management for children with chronic illnesses is nearly impossible with paper-based records. The proper use of EHRs should greatly improve the health outcomes of these patients.

Deciding to Implement an Electronic Health Record

Generally, the decision to implement an EHR system, the choice of vendor, and the responsibility to fund it falls to the practitioner. These decisions are complex, time consuming, and momentous. Despite the widely touted assumption that the use of EHRs improves the quality of care, this claim has never been validated for an EHR system as a whole. Although individual pieces of an EHR have been shown to improve adherence to health supervision guidelines,[25,26] documentation completeness,[27] and medication errors,[28,29] the sparse results on health outcomes has been mixed.[30] The best reason to implement an EHR in pediatric practice is to automate and control processes that serve the larger goal of providing excellent care. The EHR should give child health professionals the opportunity to spend less time on mundane tasks such as following documentation guidelines and more time doing important tasks such as talking to families.

Several methods can be used for approaching the first step, which is choosing a list of EHR systems to consider implementing:

Integration. The most important predictor of success in an EHR implementation is how well the system works with existing information systems in the environment, especially systems that are critical to the financial success of the clinical operation. Most physician groups and hospitals begin their EHR project by looking at what systems work with their practice management and administrative systems.

Peer recommendations. Another powerful influence over the product-selection process is word-of-mouth recommendations from professional peers. The American Academy of Pediatrics (AAP) Council on Clinical Information Technology supports these communications via its meetings and Web site (cocit.aap.org).

Certification. Tremendous interest lies in certifying the functions of EHR systems. A public-private collaboration known as the Certification Commission for Health Information Technology[31] is developing methods to certify that EHR systems perform functions that qualify for certain pay-for-performance incentives.[32] Other groups in the private sector are working along similar lines.[33] The effect of these certification efforts, it is hoped, is to create some national standards for how EHR systems work. To the extent pediatricians are involved in these certification efforts, pediatricians may some day be able to determine rapidly which systems work for pediatrics.

Once candidate systems have been selected, most physicians attempt to evaluate them systematically by interviewing vendors and attending demonstrations. Professional meetings, including those sponsored by the AAP, offer an efficient way of beginning this process through exhibit halls or public competitions between systems. Site visits to practices that are similar to the care provider's own are expensive but offer the most realistic information on how the system performs. The value of site visits is limited by the fact that no two practices are alike and that the user will offer a biased opinion about a system purchased and implemented at great cost.

The cost of EHR systems is the most frequent barrier cited by physicians to EHR implementation.[34] No easy answer to the question exists of how much an EHR costs. Pricing plans from vendor to vendor vary wildly, and no vendor offers a pricing plan that a health care provider can apply without a lengthy interaction with a sales representative. Published data from the American Academy of Family Physicians suggest that an EHR system costs approximately $5500 per practitioner per year and $7200 per practitioner per year for a combined EHR and practice management system that includes billing, patient scheduling, account receivable, and similar nonclinical functions.[35] Open-source EHR software[36] in which the software itself is included in the price may not be any cheaper than commercially sold software, given that the bulk of the costs of an EHR system comprises installation, set-up, and ongoing support.

A recognized factor in the success of any EHR system implementation is support among the physicians who will be using the system. Implementing an EHR system is disruptive to a practice because it changes almost all established work patterns. EHR implementation also requires physicians and staff to agree on the best procedures for a given task because computerization tends to require uniform procedures. An essential component is to have a *physician champion* who has major responsibility for the EHR implementation in the practice. This person should be a genuine leader in the practice. In addition to the physician leader (and, perhaps, leaders in other job roles), the practice needs to decide on a process for introducing the system into the work of the practice. The 2 general implementation approaches are the *big bang,* in which a given system is brought up to full operation over a very short period (say, a week), or the gentler but slower incremental approach, whereby pieces of the system are put into place gradually and used more and more over a longer period. Another technique for introducing an EHR system in a manageable fashion is to either reduce the number of patients to be seen during the rollout (not an economic possibility for most pediatricians) or use the system on only a small number of patients per day at first. The incremental approach with graduated numbers of patients is feasible but extends the period in which the practice must operate in an environment in which some information is on paper and some is in the EHR.

The full transition to an EHR system, in which no paper charts are used at all, is another challenge to EHR implementation. Obviously, information in the paper chart is useful and necessary for a long time—years in some cases. Manually entering data from the old charts is infeasible for all but the most complex patients, whose charts might benefit from manual sifting of old data. For the majority of patients, scanning of selected pieces of paper (growth charts, immunization records, latest clinic visit, latest consultant reports) is sufficient. Alternatively, the health care provider can simply continue to pull paper charts for the visits and enter new data in the EHR. This task can continue until enough time has passed that the paper charts are no longer worth having for the majority of patients. Most pediatricians will continue to maintain physical storage facilities for old paper charts because of statutory requirements, but the cost of maintaining this storage will eventually shrink because of the advancing infrequency of the need to access archival data.

The question of whether the cost of an EHR system has a financial return is legitimate. Some of the benefits of an EHR system accrue to people and organizations other than the physician. For example, if physicians are asked to provide immunization data from their EHR to update the state immunization registry, in all likelihood, the entire cost of this project will fall to the physician. This circumstance also applies to other information management tasks mandated by a health plan. Although these tasks are made possible by the EHR, the health plan is not going to subsidize the cost of the physician's EHR, although some pay-for-performance initiatives provide financial incentives for the use of EHRs.

For the pediatrician's practice, EHRs can reduce personnel costs significantly by eliminating the pulling, filing, and locating (often extremely time consuming) of paper charts for office visits, telephone calls, and prescription refills, among other duties. EHRs can also dramatically reduce the labor required to gather data for quality reporting purposes, provided the system is set up to capture the appropriate data elements.

Other cost savings from EHRs include:

- Reducing transcription costs
- Reducing medical records staff
- Reducing storage space
- Saving time in waiting for chart pulls
- Eliminating competition for the paper chart with others in the practice
- Saving time not having to deal with illegible or off-formulary prescriptions
- More efficient tracking of laboratory results and referrals

Whether a savings in time spent documenting care occurs depends on the state of the user's paper-based documentation in the first place. If the most common Medicare and Medicaid guidelines are followed for coding for evaluation and management services, then the EHR will undoubtedly perform this task faster and more accurately than any paper system. Often in pediatric practices, the paper chart system does not comply with these guidelines. Implementation of an EHR can raise the bar dramatically for documentation detail, given that Medicare compliance is a major selling point for these systems in adult care. Because the trend suggests that documentation compliance guidelines from all payers will be getting stricter, a system by which an EHR is the only way a physician can be expected to generate the detail necessary to justify payment may be a foregone conclusion, regardless of efficiency considerations.

Web-based Resources

Implementing an EHR places the pediatrician in a position to access the Web more readily for information, decision support analysis, and electronic communication with consultants and patients.

Since its inception, the Web has been a rich source of pediatric information for both professionals and patients[37]; it can also facilitate the way a pediatrician communicates with patients and stays current in the field of pediatrics. The cost of high-speed access to the Web can be more than offset by savings on paper reference materials, by time saved in communicating with families, and by savings on continuing medical education activities.

Search

To take advantage of the Web, the user must become proficient at navigating search engine sites to search for information. Even though many practitioners are familiar with search procedures for specialized medical databases such as MEDLINE (publicly accessible via pubmed.gov), the procedures for searching the Web depend on which search engine a person uses for the search. Even though these search sites may be used profitably by simply typing in some relevant text and pressing the return key, the user can do much better by learning a few search techniques.

The most popular index site for the Web is Google (www.google.com), but Yahoo (search.yahoo.com), Alta Vista (altavista.com), and MSN Search (search.msn.com), as well as a host of others, are also widely used. Each site has its own peculiarities for how to format the text the user types in the search field (the *search string*) to produce the best search. The following examples follow Google's conventions.

Google processes the search string by assuming a logical *AND* between terms. The user can override this process by explicitly using the capitalized term *OR*, as in *textbook pediatric OR surgical* to perform a search for textbooks in either area. Wildcard characters are not allowed (*p*diatric* would not work to find pediatric and podiatric) and are usually not necessary because spelling variations are usually handled behind the scenes. The user can exclude terms by prefixing a dash before the term that the user wants to exclude; *hip dysplasia -canine* would help filter out veterinary pages from the search result. The user may search within a given search results by clicking on *Search within results* button at the bottom of the page.

Google ignores the case of the text in the search string. For example, typing *Down* instead of *down* will not increase the chance of finding Web pages on Down syndrome.

To restrict the search result to a given site, the user can use the *site* modifier, as in *vaccine refrigeration site:cdc.gov*, which would be more efficient at finding CDC guidelines on vaccine storage than a search that did not include the modifier.

Google, as with other search engines, has connections to databases of information other than Web page content. Use of the *phonebook* modifier illustrates this feature in a way that is relevant to anyone who has to interpret pager numbers. If the user types a 10-digit telephone number, then Google will perform a reverse telephone number lookup in its residential telephone number database. If the user types a business name and a geographic location, then Google will return phone-book listings as part of the search results. For example, if the user were looking for a pediatric office in Tempe, AZ, the user would simply type *pediatrics tempe az* into Google.

The Google search engine does more than just search the Web. One extra function of interest to pediatricians is the conversion function, in which the user simply uses the word *in* in the search string to do unit conversions, for example, *5.6 kg in lb*, *40.5 c in f*, or *3 lb 5 oz in kg*.

Many more special features of the syntax of search strings are available in Web search index sites. None of them are strictly necessary to use, but much more efficient use of the Web can be made by spending a few minutes reading the documentation about how to enter search strings in any Web index site.

Medical Reference

The use of search engines can retrieve useful information, but textbooks and other medical literature still offer a more reliable authoritative source of information for pediatric practice. Many traditional pediatric textbooks are available on line (for a fee) via the publisher's Web site or as part of a collection of material. Virtual textbooks with plenty of pediatric content are also available on line but not in print form, such as the free eMedicine and the subscription-based *Up to Date*, both described in Table 4-2. These sources are available from the Web; some can also provide content for handheld devices for even more convenient access to reference information. Many AAP publications are also available on line, for example, the *Red Book* at www.aapredbook.org.

Diagnostic Decision Support

The use of a computer to aid in the diagnosis of children with challenging presentations has been a tantalizing possibility since the dawn of the computer age.[38,39] Diagnostic decision support systems with pediatric clinical domains have been available for years[40]; yet few pediatricians use these systems, and demand for such systems has been so low that only one commercial electronic medical record system vendor has attempted to integrate a pediatric diagnostic

Table 4-2 Web-based Medical Reference, Continuing Medical Education, and Patient Education Resources for Pediatricians

SITE	URL	DESCRIPTION	PEDIATRIC CME	PATIENT INFORMATION
Baylor University	baylorcme.org	Video and slides of presentations given at Baylor	Yes, via a test to be taken after viewing the materials; no charge to the user	No
Contemporary Pediatrics	contemporarypediatrics.com	Articles from the magazine	Yes (take test after reading article); no charge to the user; via cmeweb.com	Yes, associated with many articles
Dxplain	merckmedicus.com	Diagnostic decision support system that turns clinical findings into differential diagnoses; no charge to the user	No	No
Emedicine.com	emedicine.com	Textbook of medicine, including pediatrics; no charge to the user	Yes, via tests taken after reading articles; fee based	Yes
Isabel	isabelhealthcare.com	Diagnostic decision support with its origins in pediatric conditions; requires subscription fee	No	No
KidsHealth (Nemours Foundation)	kidshealth.org	Parent and patient information about a wide range of conditions and issues, in English and Spanish	No	Yes
MD Consult	mdconsult.com	Full text of pediatric textbooks, journals, guidelines; requires subscription fee	No (but CME found in other specialties)	Yes
Medline Plus	medlineplus.gov	An index site run by the National Library of Medicine, collecting high-quality, Web-based patient information on almost any health topic; no charge to the user	No	Yes
Medscape	medscape.com	Summaries of presentations made at national meetings; no charge to the user	Yes (take test after reading article); no charge to the user	Yes
Merck Medicus	merckmedicus.com	Electronic versions of hard-copy textbooks and journals, plus some custom content; no charge to the user	Yes (take test after reading article); no charge to the user	Yes, including some interactive features
Online Mendelian Inheritance in Man	www.ncbi.nlm.nih.gov/omim	Database of inherited disorders; allows searching by phenotypes	No	No
PediaLink	pedialink.org	A product of the American Academy of Pediatrics; basic access part of AAP membership	Yes (various methods); fee based	No
University of Nebraska	www.unmc.edu/Pediatrics/GrandRounds/	Downloadable video of grand rounds presentations; no charge to the user	Yes (take test after viewing presentation); no charge to the user	No
Up to Date	uptodate.com	Textbook of medicine, including pediatrics; requires subscription fee	Yes, via continuous, timed monitoring of system use; fee based	Yes

CME, Continuing medical eduction; *PCO,* pediatric care outline; *URL,* uniform resource locator.

decision support program into its product.[41] Furthermore, using on-line diagnostic decision support represents a break in the workflow of our paper-based systems. Perhaps when EHRs become more widespread, resurgence in interest in the use of these diagnostic aids will take place, if they can be integrated into new patterns of work. Table 4-2 includes several of these kinds of resources.[42-45]

Gathering Information About Patients

Some pediatricians are asking parents to fill out electronic screening questionnaires before the health assessment visit, either from home on line or in the pediatrician's waiting room. This technique can be a useful way to reduce the time spent gathering information and can increase the time available for discussing parental concerns. One such system is *CHADIS*.

Patient and Family Support

Health information is one of the most common searches for families who use the Web to answer questions.[46] Many physicians provide Web sites for their patients to provide basic information about the practice or even to interact with the physician or clinic staff (eg, www.medem.com). Table 4-2 includes some Web sites with excellent information for patients. These sites can be used as part of information prescriptions[47] for patients or as part of the pediatrician's printable handout library.

On-Line Continuing Medical Education

Numerous Web sites offer free or low-cost pediatric continuing medical education (CME) programs.[48] This type of on-line learning has been shown to be at least as effective as in-person seminars.[49] Table 4-2 lists some on-line CME resources with significant pediatric content. These Web sites use several different models for presenting the educational experience.

The most common model consists of presenting an article on a topic then offering some multiple-choice questions that can be answered to document that the user read and understood the article. The amount of CME credit is expressed in terms of time; each article qualifies for up to a certain number of hours of CME credit, which the user claims at the end of the exercise.

Although the article-based model is easy to set up and administer, it does require the user to set aside special time to examine a topic in depth. A more natural model of *continuous professional development* exists on some sites.[50] In this model, a computer system records the details of a physician's actual use of electronic reference material during the course of ordinary patient care. For example, if pediatricians needed to refresh their memory on the diagnosis of congenital syphilis during efforts to care for a possibly exposed neonate and they spent 10 minutes on line reading some guidelines and textbook material, then they would receive 10 minutes of CME credit. This method of attesting to a physician's ability to stay current has greater face validity than methods based on seminar attendance. More important, it tends to reinforce the habit of seeking the most current and detailed information about a patient's care. As high-speed Web access continues to rise in pediatricians' practices, this model should be seen as a productive way to fulfill the user's continuous professional development responsibility.[51] The AAP PediaLink (pedialink.org) is one method of organizing all continuous professional development in one Web site.

TOOLS FOR PRACTICE

Medical Decision Support

- *EMR Review Project* (on-line forum), American Academy of Pediatrics (www.aapcocit.org/emr/).
- *EHRs: Where's the Value—Speaker Kit* (Web page), American Academy of Pediatrics (www.aap.org/moc/index.cfm).
- *Electronic Medical Record FAQ* (fact sheet), American Academy of Pediatrics (www.aapscot.org/emrfaqs.pdf).
- *Implementing an Electronic Health Record Toolkit* (CD ROM) American Academy of Pediatrics (www.aap.org/bookstore).

AAP POLICY STATEMENTS

American Academy of Pediatrics, Task Force on Medical Informatics. Special requirements for electronic medical record systems in pediatrics. *Pediatrics.* 2007;119(3): 631-637. (aappolicy.aappublications.org/cgi/content/full/pediatrics;119/3/321).

Gerstle RS, and the American Academy of Pediatrics, Task Force on Medical Informatics. E-mail communication between pediatricians and their patients. *Pediatrics.* 2004;114:317-321. (aappolicy.aappublications.org/cgi/content/full/pediatrics;114/1/317).

SUGGESTED RESOURCES

Burt CW, Hing E. Use of computerized clinical support systems in medical settings: United States, 2001-2003. Advance data from vital and health statistics. *MMWR.* May 2005; 54(RR18):463.

Davis DA. Does CME work? An analysis of the effect of educational activities on physician performance or health care outcomes. *Int J Psychiatry Med.* 1998;28:21-39.

Davis DA et al. Changing physician performance. A systematic review of the effect of continuing medical education strategies. *JAMA.* 1995;274:700-705.

REFERENCES

1. Amatayakul M. The path to EHR. *Healthc Financ Manage.* 2004;58:98-99.
2. Bush GW. State of the union address, 2004.
3. Bush GW. State of the union address, 2006.
4. Hernandez R, Healy PD. Oddly, Hillary and, yes, Newt agree to agree. *New York Times.* May 13, 2005;A:1.
5. Ford EW, Menachemi N, Phillips MT. Predicting the adoption of electronic health records by physicians: when will health care be paperless? *J Am Med Inform Assoc.* 2006;13:106-112.
6. Johnson KB. Barriers that impede the adoption of pediatric information technology. *Arch Pediatr Adolesc Med.* 2001;155:1374-1379.
7. Gans D, Kralewski J, Hammons T, et al. Medical groups' adoption of electronic health records and information systems. Practices are encountering greater-than-expected barriers to adopting an EHR system, but the adoption rate continues to rise. *Health Aff (Millwood).* 2005;24:1323-1333.

8. The National Academic Press, Committee on Data Standards for Patient Safety. Key Capabilities of an Electronic Health Record System: *Lett Report*. 2003. Available at www.nap.edu. Accessed September 28, 2007.
9. Shiffman RN, Spooner SA, Kwiathowski K, et al. Information technology for children's health and health care: report on the Information Technology in Children's Health Care Expert Meeting, September 21-22, 2000. *J Am Med Inform Assoc*. 2001;8:546-551.
10. American Academy of Pediatrics, Task Force of Medical Informatics. Special requirements for electronic medical record systems in pediatrics. *Pediatrics*. 2997;119(3):631-637.
11. Ogden CL, Kuczmarski RJ, Flegal KM, et al. Centers for Disease Control and Prevention 2000 growth charts for the United States: improvements to the 1977 National Center for Health Statistics version. *Pediatrics*. 2002;109:45-60.
12. Fenton TR. A new growth chart for preterm babies: Babson and Benda's chart updated with recent data and a new format. *BMC Pediatrics*. 2003;3:13.
13. Trotter TL, Hall JG. Health supervision for children with achondroplasia. *Pediatrics*. 2005;116:771-783.
14. American Academy of Pediatrics: Health supervision for children with Down syndrome. *Pediatrics*. 2001;107:442-449.
15. Frias JL, Davenport ML. Health supervision for children with Turner syndrome. *Pediatrics*. 2003;111:692-702.
16. Rosenbloom ST, Qi XF, Riddle WR, et al. Implementing pediatric growth charts into an electronic health record system. *J Am Med Inform Assoc*. 2006;13(3):302-308.
17. American Academy of Pediatrics, Advisory Committee on Immunization Practices, and American Academy of Family Physicians. Recommended childhood and adolescent immunization schedule–United States, 2006. *Pediatrics*. 2006;117:239-240.
18. Kemper AR, Uren RL, Clark SJ. Electronic health records in primary care pediatric practices. *Pediatrics*. 2006 (in press).
19. American Academy of Pediatrics, Committee on Drugs. Unapproved uses of approved drugs: the physician, and the Food and Drug Administration: subject review. *Pediatrics*. 1996;98:143-145.
20. Ford C, English A, Sigman G. Confidential health care for adolescents: position paper for the society for adolescent medicine. *J Adolesc Health*. 2004;35:160-167.
21. English A, Kenney KE. *State Minor Consent Laws: A Summary*. 2nd ed. Chapel Hill, NC: Center for Adolescent Health & the Law; 2003.
22. Kuther TL. Medical decision-making and minors: issues of consent and assent. *Adolescence*. 2003; 38:343-358.
23. Vukadinovich DM. Minors' rights to consent to treatment: navigating the complexity of State laws. *J Health Law*. 2004;37:667-691.
24. Berner ES, Moss J. Informatics challenges for the impending patient information explosion. *J Am Med Inform Assoc*. 2005;12:614-617.
25. Gioia PC. Quality improvement in pediatric well care with an electronic record. *Proc AMIA Symp*. 2001; 209-213.
26. Adams WG, Mann AM, Bauchner H. Use of an electronic medical record improves the quality of urban pediatric primary care. *Pediatrics*. 2003;111: 626-632.
27. Soto CM, Kleinman KP, Simon SR. Quality and correlates of medical record documentation in the ambulatory care setting. *BMC Health Serv Res*. 2002;2:22.
28. Chamberlain JM, Slonim A, Joseph JG. Reducing errors and promoting safety in pediatric emergency care. *Ambul Pediatr*. 2004;4:55-63.
29. Kaushal R, Jaggi T, Walsh K, et al. Pediatric medication errors: What do we know? What gaps remain? *Ambulatory Pediatrics*. 2004;4:73-81.
30. Delpierre C, Cuzin L, Fillaux J, et al. A systematic review of computer-based patient record systems and quality of care: more randomized clinical trials or a broader approach? *Int J Qual Health Care*. 2004;16:407-416.
31. Hagland M. Guaranteed certified. CCHIT announces its first wave of certifications in the outpatient arena. *Healthcare Informatic*. 2006 Sep:23(9):14-16.
32. Hackbarth G, Milgate K. Using quality incentives to drive physician adoption of health information technology. *Health Aff (Millwood)*. 2005;24:1147-1149.
33. Leavitt M, O'Kane ME. Joint Statement from the National Committee for Quality Assurance and the Certification Commission for Healthcare Information Technology. Complementary nature of NCQA and CCHIT activities surrounding EHR certification, 2005. Available at: www.ncqa.org/communications/Joint%20Statement%20on%20EHR%20Cert%20Rev%203%20_2_.pdf. Accessed September 28, 2007.
34. Gans D, Kralewski J, Hammons T, et al. Medical groups' adoption of electronic health records and information systems. Practices are encountering greater-than-expected barriers to adopting an EHR system, but the adoption rate continues to rise. *Health Aff (Millwood)* 2005;24:1323-1333.
35. Kibbe DC, Waldran S. *Partners for Patients Electronic Health Record Market Survey*. Washington DC: American Academy of Family Physicians, Center for Health Information Technology; 2005.
36. California Healthcare Foundation (chcf.org) Goulde M et al. (eds). Open source software: a primer for health care leaders. California Healthcare Foundation, 2006. Open Source Software: A Primer for Health Care Leaders. iHealth Reports Series. 2006. Available at www.chcf.org/documents/ihealth/OpenSourcePrimer.pdf. Accessed September 28, 2007.
37. Spooner SA. The pediatric Internet. *Pediatrics*. 1996;98: 1185-1192.
38. Athreya BH, Athreya RB, Coriell LL. Edge-punch card as a tool in differential diagnosis. *Am J Dis Child*. 1970;119:53-56.
39. Barness LA, Tunnessen WW, Worley WE, et al. Computer-assisted diagnosis in pediatrics. *Am J Dis Child*. 1974;127:852-858.
40. Johnson KB, Feldman MJ. Medical informatics and pediatrics. Decision-support systems. *Arch Pediatr Adolesc Med*. 1995;149:1371-1380.
41. Isabel Healthcare. Isabel and NextGen: Web-based interface developed. Available at www.isabelhealthcare.com/home/emrintegration1#twob. Accessed September 28, 2007.
42. Barnett GO, Cimino JJ, Hupp JA, et al. DXplain. An evolving diagnostic decision-support system. *JAMA*. 1987;258:67-74.
43. Britto J. ISABEL at the helm. A Web-based diagnosis system speeds clinical decisions for pediatric physicians. *Health Manag Technol*. 2004;25:28-29.
44. Greenough A. Help from ISABEL for paediatric diagnoses. *Lancet*. 2002;360:1259.
45. Ramnarayan P, Tomlinson A, Rao A, et al. ISABEL. a web-based differential diagnostic aid for paediatrics: results from an initial performance evaluation. *Arch Dis Child*. 2003;88:408-413.
46. Madden M, Rainie L. *Pew Internet and American Life Project Surveys*. Washington, DC: Pew Internet & American Life Project; 2003.

47. D'Alessandro DM, Kreiter CD, Kinzer SL, et al. A randomized controlled trial of an information prescription for pediatric patient education on the Internet. *Arch Pediatr Adolesc Med.* 2004;158:857-862.
48. Sklar B. CME List: *Pediatrics.* Available at www.cmelist.com/pediatrics.htm. Accessed January 21, 2007.
49. Fordis M, King JE, Ballantyne CM, et al. Comparison of the instructional efficacy of Internet-based CME with live interactive CME workshops: a randomized controlled trial. *JAMA.* 2005;294:1043-1051.
50. Zeiger RF. Toward continuous medical education. *J Gen Intern Med.* 2005;20:91-94.
51. Sectish TC, Floriani V, Badat MC, et al. Continuous professional development: raising the bar for pediatricians. *Pediatrics.* 2002;110:152-156.

Chapter 5
EVIDENCE-BASED MEDICINE

Brett W. Robbins, MD

Evidence-based medicine (EBM) is the conscientious, explicit, and judicious use of current best evidence to solve clinical problems.[1] It requires integration of individual clinical expertise and patient preferences with the best available external clinical evidence from systematic research and consideration of available resources.[2] Pediatricians have been using the medical literature throughout their careers. However, without formal training in epidemiology or the library sciences, they have been left without guidance when using the medical literature to answer their clinical questions. EBM provides the pediatrician with an explicit process to locate, appraise, and apply clinical research reports to their patients. The 4-part process of EBM (ask, acquire, appraise, apply) provides an organized framework to facilitate bringing evidence to the point of patient care.

WHY BOTHER?

First, proliferation of the medical literature is rapid. An estimated 10,000 new randomized trials are published each month. The clinician need only look to recent advances in wart treatment[3] or the clinical diagnosis of neonatal jaundice[4] to understand that an organized approach is needed to keep up with the literature. Second, clinical practice is rich with questions. On average, for every 3 outpatients seen, clinicians have 2 questions that are pivotal to the care of these patients.[5] A similar number of questions come up for every inpatient seen.[6] Third, clinicians are at the pinnacle of their knowledge at the completion of residency training. After graduation, a significant decline occurs in medical knowledge about common medical problems.[7] Fourth, traditional continuing medical education activities do not change physician behavior or improve patient outcomes.[8] Fifth, graduates of residency programs that are robust in EBM do not experience the decline in knowledge about common medical problems.[9] In summary, EBM is worth the effort because patients deserve to be cared for by clinicians who are both good communicators with sound clinical judgment and up to date on the literature dealing with the conditions they treat.

Step 1: Ask

Formulating an answerable and searchable clinical question is the most important step of the EBM process. It focuses the busy clinician on exactly what is needed to move on with patient care. Spending 2 minutes to formulate and format a good clinical question is well worth the investment because this effort saves time later in the searching process.

The 2 types of questions in clinical medicine are background and foreground. Background questions deal with disease-specific information and the basics of a condition. An example of a background question is, "What is Kawasaki disease, and how does it usually present itself?" The answers to background questions are most often found in standard textbooks and review articles. Foreground questions deal with patient-specific information regarding the diagnosis, prognosis, or therapy of a condition. Unlike background questions, the answers to these questions are best found in the medical literature. Time is saved searching for answers to foreground questions if they are first formatted into the **p**atient, **i**ntervention, **c**omparison, **o**utcome, **t**ype of question, and **t**ype of study, also known as the PICOTT format. An example of a foreground question is, "In patients with Kawasaki disease, does intravenous immunoglobulin lead to symptomatic improvement and prevent the development of coronary artery aneurysms?" Putting this question into the PICOTT format focuses busy clinicians on exactly the answer they are interested in finding and begins the search process (Box 5-1).

Step 2: Acquire

Clinicians acquire information from the medical literature in 2 ways: (1) passively (gathering) and (2) actively (hunting). Clinicians gather information when they peruse articles that come to them, either through subscription or happenstance. Acquiring the article takes little effort, but the author of the article, not the clinician, defines the question. This process is further limited by a lack of context for the article because other data that may exist on this same question are not known. Thus, although gathering takes little energy, little is under the direct control of the clinician.

Hunting is actively pursuing an answer to a clinician-generated PICOTT question. In general, the search

BOX 5-1 Example of a Foreground Question

Patient: Child with Kawasaki disease
Intervention: Intravenous immunoglobulin
Comparison: Nothing or placebo
Outcome(s): Symptomatic improvement and prevention of coronary artery aneurysms
Type of question: Therapy
Type of study needed: Randomized controlled trial

terms are drawn directly from the PICOTT question itself. Time is best spent hunting in grounds known to have valid, preappraised, and summative evidence (Table 5-1). The best databases will do most of the work. Clinicians should search in a database where they know all the information has been systematically searched to include everything that exists on the topic. The gold-standard database, in this regard, is the *Cochrane Database of Systematic Reviews,* which is a database that is systematically searched, preappraised, and up to date. This database currently includes 2785 systematic reviews and 1625 reviews that are in progress. (Interestingly, Cochrane reviewers believe they need 10,000 systematic reviews before most of clinical medicine is covered.) The reviews are updated yearly on average. Other databases of systematic reviews such as DARE are reviews of published systematic reviews and thus are not updated regularly. *Clinical Practice Guidelines* and *Clinical Evidence* are also systematically searched and preappraised. These sources are also updated periodically. Second-tier databases include summaries of individual articles such as the *ACP Journal Club* and *InfoPOEMs.* As a last resort, the clinician can search in databases that are unfiltered for validity such as Medline (see Table 5-1 for links to these databases). If the best searching efforts are unfruitful, then asking the help of a well-trained medical librarian can be quite rewarding.

Step 3: Appraise

Once an article is located, the next step is to determine its validity. *JAMA* has published a series of 25 articles known as the Users' Guides to the Medical Literature.[2] Each article in the series describes a different type of article using principles of epidemiology. All relevant types of articles are covered, from randomized controlled trials to cost-effectiveness analyses. A clinical example is used to lead the reader through 3 tasks: (1) assessing validity, (2) quantifying results, and (3) applying the evidence to patients. Their titles are written in terms the clinician can understand, such as therapy, prognosis, and harm. However, behind these terms is a specific study design, such as the randomized controlled trial, cohort study, and case-controlled study. Table 5-2 displays the terminology of the most frequently used Users' Guides, including the common terms each guide uses to quantify the results. It also includes the most efficient method of finding each type of article in Medline.

Assessing Validity

Each Users' Guide to the Medical Literature has a list of criteria to determine if a study is valid. These criteria are based on epidemiologic principles and are explained in detail using a clinical example. The criteria roughly appear in their order of importance, but they are not intended to lead to a dichotomous decision of being valid or not valid for a study. Rather, they are intended to assist the clinician in determining the relative validity of the study and thus the relative strength of its results. If a study is not valid, then its results are in question and should not be used in the clinical decision-making process. An example of the validity criteria for therapy (randomized-controlled trial) is found in Box 5-2.

Quantifying Results

The Users' Guides provide methods to determine the magnitude of effect of an intervention in a more clinically meaningful way than is offered by P values. Each type of article has its own methods and terms, such as number needed to treat (NNT) for therapy, likelihood ratios (LR) for diagnosis, and relative risk (RR) for prognosis. For example, the NNT is calculated by dividing 100 by the absolute difference between the outcome rates of the intervention and placebo groups. The resulting number is the number of patients that need to be treated to prevent one bad outcome or to cause a good outcome. For example, in a study of 61 children with common warts,[3] of those randomized to treatment with duct tape, 15% failed to resolve. Of the patients randomized to standard cryotherapy, 40% failed to resolve. This result was statistically significant

Table 5-1 Schema for Ranking Sources of Evidence

SOURCE	SUMMATIVE	VALID	PREAPPRAISED	SYSTEMATICALLY SEARCHED
Cochrane Database of Systematic Reviews (www.cochrane.org)	+	+	+	+
Database of Abstracts of Reviews of Effects (www.york.ac.uk/inst/crd/darehp.htm)	+	+	+	+
Evidence-Based Clinical Practice Guidelines (www.guidelines.gov)	+	+	+	+
Clinical Evidence (www.clinicalevidence.com)	+	+	+	+
ACP Journal Club (www.acpjc.org)	–	+	+	+
InfoPOEMs/InfoRetriever (www.infopoems.com)	–	+	+	+
Textbooks/Up-to-Date (www.uptodate.com)	+	–	–	–
AAP Grand Rounds (aapgrandrounds.aappublications.org/)	–	–	–	+/–
Medline (www.pubmedcentral.nih.gov/)	–	–	–	–

Table 5-2 Commonly Confused Terminology in Evidence-based Medicine

STUDY TYPE	TIMELINE	LOGISTICS	STATISTICS USED	COMMENTS	HOW TO FIND ON OVID MEDLINE
Randomized controlled trial (therapy or prevention)	Prospective	Single group of patients randomized to two or more therapeutic or screening methods	Relative risk reduction Absolute risk reduction Number needed to treat	Gold standard Most powerful information	Limit to randomized control trial publication type
Cohort (prognosis)	Prospective or retrospective	Single group of patients gathered at a common point in their diseases followed forward in time	Relative risk—*predicts* outcomes	A comparison cohort may or may not exist Framingham study is good example of retrospective cohort	Combine the following MeSH heading with subject search—exp cohort studies
Case control (harm)	Retrospective	Group of patients with the disease compared with group of patients without the disease Look backward for exposure(s)	Odds ratios—*predicts* exposure(s)	Logistically the most difficult to do and control for bias when conducting	Combine the following MeSH heading with subject search—exp case-control studies
Diagnostic test (diagnosis)	Prospective (optimally)	Single group of patients thought to have a disease All get tested	Sensitivity Specificity Likelihood ratios Odds ratio	This point is where clinicians use pretest and posttest probabilities along with thresholds	Combine the following MeSH heading with subject search—exp "sensitivity and specificity"
Meta-analysis (overview)	Retrospective look at multiple studies	All relevant studies addressing the same question combined mathematically as if they were one large trial	Effect size	Can combine any of the study types, most commonly therapy and diagnosis	Limit to meta-analysis publication type

($P = .05$), with an NNT of 100/(40-15) or 4. Thus the clinician would need to treat 4 children's warts with duct tape rather than cryotherapy to prevent one from failing to resolve. The NNT is much more clinically meaningful than a simple P value and helps the clinician balance risk and benefit more explicitly. Not only is a low NNT important, it is also necessary to understand the risks and benefits of the treatment and underlying disorder to make an informed decision regarding the proposed therapy. Duct tape occlusion of a wart is nearly risk free, and the wart itself, although unsightly, does not pose a serious health risk. Thus, when the proposed treatment and the underlying disorder are low risk, an impressive NNT may not be needed to convince a clinician to employ the therapy. The NNT is difficult to interpret without its precision, or 95% confidence intervals. For our duct tape example, given that the study population is small ($N = 51$), the confidence intervals around our NNT of 4 are wide (2-111). Thus we are 95% certain that our true NNT falls somewhere between 2 and 111. Because the confidence intervals around our NNT are so wide, we are uncertain whether duct tape is significantly more effective than cryotherapy or minimally more effective based on this one study.

Step 4: Apply

After determining that an article is valid and quantifying its results, the final step is to decide whether it applies to the patient. This process has less to do with the inclusion and exclusion criteria than with the patient's underlying physiologic condition. Just because the patient would be excluded from the study does not mean the evidence cannot be applied to the patient's situation. Inclusion and exclusion criteria are written for logistic purposes of the study itself rather

BOX 5-2 Validity Criteria for a Randomized Controlled Trial

Did experimental and control groups begin the study with a similar prognosis?

- Were patients randomized?
- Was randomization concealed?
- Were patients analyzed in the groups to which they were randomized? That is, did an intention to treat exist?
- Were patients in the treatment and control groups similar with respect to known prognostic factors? That is, were baseline characteristics equal?

Did experimental and control groups retain a similar prognosis after the study started?

- Were patients aware of group allocation?
- Were clinicians aware of group allocation?
- Were outcome assessors aware of group allocation?

Was follow-up complete?

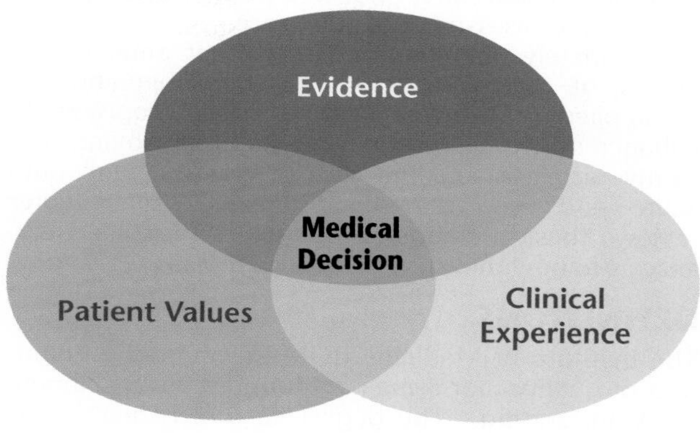

Figure 5-1 Venn diagram of clinical decisions.

than to whom the information can be applied. However, if something in the patient's underlying physiologic condition is so different from the patients in the study, then the study may not apply to this particular patient. For the duct tape and wart example, the clinician might have difficulty thinking of an example of a physiologic trait that, if so different in the patient than those in the study, would make the task of applying the evidence to the patient difficult.

The most important step in applying evidence to patients is making the clinical decision whether to use the intervention described in the study. In making this decision, clinicians must balance four factors: (1) the evidence, (2) their own clinical judgment, (3) the patient's values and preferences, and (4) the clinical state and circumstances at the time the decision needs to be made (Figure 5-1). The clinician must decide how much weight to give each of these four factors in making the decision. The process of EBM provides the validity and thus strength of the evidence. In doing so, it does not replace clinical judgment, but rather informs it. Patients have the right to refuse an effective intervention with valid evidence behind it, even if the intervention is judged to be worthwhile. Furthermore, even if an intervention is proven to be effective by valid evidence and the clinician and patient agree to use it, the intervention may not be readily available or financially viable. This fluidity of interaction of these four issues results in different decisions on different days with the same evidence, perhaps even with the same patient.

TIME

A clinician's most valuable asset is time. For EBM to be useful to the busy pediatrician, it has to be time efficient. Three suggestions might make EBM time efficient in a busy practice. First, the more clinicians use the process, the more efficient they will become. The first time medical students perform a history assessment and physical examination on a patient, they are incredibly time inefficient. With practice, however, the residents and attending physicians can perform a thorough history assessment and a physical examination in a fraction of the time required by medical students. Learning the EBM process mimics learning how to perform a history assessment and a physical examination; efficiency comes with time and practice. Second, hunting in and gathering from databases that are known to be fertile are both suggested. Medline should be avoided at nearly all costs, focusing, instead, on databases such as the *Cochrane Database, Clinical Evidence*, and guidelines.gov. In doing so, clincians can be assured that the information obtained has been thoroughly searched, assessed, and summarized. Third, hunting and gathering only those questions that are common to actual practice, are critical to an individual patient's care, or involve subjects about which clinicians are intensely curious are also suggested. Primary care pediatricians should know all the data on the treatment of otitis media but not on the treatment of acute leukemia.

GETTING STARTED

The *Users' Guides to the Medical Literature*[2] is the best resource on how to learn, practice, and teach EBM because it is complete, easy to read, and well organized; it also comes with a CD-ROM and on-line version with all the mathematics distilled to simple calculators. The next time an article from the literature is read, the *correlate chapter* feature should be used to guide the assessment of the article. Over one half of the foreground questions asked in practice deal with therapy, diagnosis, and disease management.[10] Thus, if clinicians are adept at critically appraising these types of articles, then they are well prepared to answer the majority of their clinical questions. The next time a clinical question is worth the time investment to research, the clinician should start with one of the fertile databases. If the inquiry is a common question or about a common disorder, then in all likelihood relevant evidence that is preappraised, presearched, and presummarized will be found.

CONCLUSION

Patients deserve to have physicians who make decisions regarding their care based on sound evidence. EBM provides an explicit, transparent process to track down information, assess its validity, and apply it to individual patients. It does not replace sound, seasoned clinical judgment, but rather informs it. A growing array of resources is now available that makes the process timely and thus useful to the busy primary care pediatrician.

TOOLS FOR PRACTICE

Medical Decision Support

- *BMJ Clinical Evidence* (book), British Medical Journal (www.clinicalevidence.com/ceweb/index.jsp).
- *Evidence-Based Pediatric and Child's Health*, 2nd edition (book), British Medical Journal Books (www.aap.org/bookstore).

AAP POLICY STATEMENT

American Academy of Pediatrics, Steering Committee on Quality Improvement and Management. Classifying recommendations for clinical practice guidelines. *Pediatrics*. 2004;114(3):874-877. (aappolicy.aappublications.org/cgi/content/full/pediatrics;114/3/874).

REFERENCES

1. Haynes RB, Sackett DL, Gray JM, et al. Transferring evidence from research into practice: 1. The role of clinical care research evidence in clinical decisions. *ACP J Club*. 1996;125:A14-A16.
2. Guyatt GH, Rennie D. *Users' Guides to the Medical Literature. A Manual for Evidence-Based Clinical Practice*. Chicago, Ill: JAMA Press; 2001.
3. Focht DR, Spicer C, Fairchok MP. The efficacy of duct tape vs cryotherapy in the treatment of verruca vulgaris. *Arch Paed Adolesc Med*. 2002; 156:971-974.
4. Moyer VA, Ahn C, Sneed S. Accuracy of clinical judgment in neonatal jaundice. *Arch Pediatr Adolesc Med*. 2000;154:391-394.
5. Covell DG, Uman GC, Manning PR. Information needs in office practice: are they being met? *Ann Intern Med*. 1985;103:596-599.
6. Osheroff JA, Forsythe DE, Buchanan BG, et al. Physician's information needs: analysis of questions posed during clinical teaching. *Ann Intern Med*. 1991;114(7): 576-581.
7. Sackett DL, Haynes RB, Taylor DW, et al. Clinical determinants of the decision to treat primary hypertension. *Clin Res*. 1977; 24:648.
8. Davis DA, Thomson MA, Oxman AD, et al. Changing physician performance: a systematic review of the effect of continuing medical education strategies. *JAMA*. 1997; 274:700-705.
9. Shin JH, Haynes RB, Johnston ME. Effect of problem-based, self-directed undergraduate education on lifelong learning. *CMAJ*. 1993;148(6):969-976.
10. Schilling LM, Steiner JF, Lundahl K, et al. Residents' patient specific clinical questions: opportunities for evidence-based learning, *Acad Med*. 2005;80(1): 51-56. Available at: www.cche.net/usersguides/main.asp.

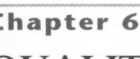

Chapter 6

QUALITY IMPROVEMENT IN PEDIATRIC PRIMARY CARE

Charles J. Homer, MD, MPH; Victoria Weeks Rogers, MD

INTRODUCTION

Quality of care has become a central theme in the delivery and management of health care. The focus on quality results from overwhelmingly consistent data that health care in the United States has a "serious and pervasive...overall quality problem," and that "the burden of harm conveyed by the collective impact of all of our health care quality problems is staggering."[1,2]

Data from both inpatient and outpatient settings in pediatrics show widespread gaps in care. A recent detailed analysis of ambulatory health care for children found that children receive recommended care less than one half of the time, and the performance of children's health care was 10% points lower than a comparable assessment of adult care.[3]

Fortunately, methods and tools that enhance the quality of care are increasingly available and can be applied in primary care settings. Programs to enhance care have been successful in improving preventive services and the care of children with both acute and long-term conditions.[4-6] This chapter reviews these methods and provides practical guidance as to how they may be applied in daily work.

DEFINITIONS

The Institute of Medicine (IOM) developed a definition of quality that remains a foundation for current thinking, stating, "The degree to which health services for individuals and populations increase the likelihood of desired health outcomes and are consistent with current professional knowledge."[7] This definition acknowledges the importance of outcomes, the key role of both individuals and the public in determining which outcomes matter, the essential role of probability (doing the right thing even if the right result does not always occur), and the constraint placed on current quality by the current state of knowledge.

The IOM refined its definition in the report entitled *Crossing the Quality Chasm*, which outlined six specific aims for the health care system, now widely viewed as the critical dimensions of quality.[1,2] These aims, as well as the explanations behind these key dimensions, are that health care be:

- *Safe:* Safety is a system property rather than a reflection of individual shortcomings; and system redesign is the necessary strategy to address shortcomings in this area.
- *Effective:* Effective care refers to the reliable delivery of care that is known to be more likely to achieve desired results, that is, care that is consistent with evidence.

- *Efficient:* Efficient care refers to the judicious and appropriate use of resources or, more specifically, not delivering care known to be ineffective (eliminating overuse).
- Patient centered: Patient centeredness is the core, central aim of health services. The fundamental definition of quality refers to outcomes desired by patients as the key aim of care. The experience of care is one dimension of patient centeredness, and satisfaction with care is one component—a subjective assessment of how these experiences compare with expectations.
- *Timely:* Timeliness refers to eliminating the abundant waits and delays that are omnipresent in health care; it is a dimension that clearly affects efficiency and patient centeredness, and it affects safety (eg, delay in providing a needed immunization as a result of scheduling) and effectiveness (waits in appointments for appropriate medical tests and therapies).
- *Equitable:* Quality applies to the care of all patients, not simply subsets of patients in the care of the physician. The IOM report, *Unequal Treatment: Confronting Racial and Ethnic Disparities in Health Care,* demonstrates that disparities of care exist throughout the health care system and calls for widespread educational and improvement efforts to eliminate them.[2]

Until recently, quality improvement efforts in primary care focused on one or, at most, two aspects of quality—such as effectiveness (eg, use of appropriate medications for asthma or rates of immunization) or patient centeredness (eg, typically, satisfaction). Nonetheless, the IOM concept of quality previously described suggests that high-quality programs that meet the needs of children and families are characterized by excellence, not simply in one or two of the six quality aims but rather by excellence in all six areas. Practices that provide the best care deliver the right care—based on evidence and associated with the best outcomes—in a manner that is respectful of family needs and values, that does not waste either resources or time, that does not cause preventable harm, and that is delivered without bias and designed to achieve equitable results across different patient populations.

Moreover, because of the nature of primary care, care must be designed to address the full spectrum of child health needs—preventive care, acute care, and the care of children with special health care needs. In most cases, care should also address community needs, addressing the particular public health concerns of the practice setting.

The fundamental concept required to address all of these issues in a practice is to view the primary care practice as a system or, in some cases, as one component of a larger system such as a medical group or hospital network.[8] When viewed as a system, the methods and tools of improving system performance can be applied to practices, as they can to hospitals and to industry.

Establishing Priorities

Given the breadth and scope of quality, as well as the substantial gaps in performance across the spectrum of quality dimensions, choosing where to begin is daunting. One strategy to set priorities is to use a monitoring tool such as a quality compass, balanced scorecard, or family of measures. Although such *dashboards* or *scorecards* are often viewed only in the context of corporate management, the concept here is to develop a set of indicators that reflect practice performance across the six dimensions of quality for a practice, as well as across dimensions practices already likely monitored, such as financial performance and staff satisfaction. Such a management tool can assist practice leadership in setting priorities. In many instances, external organizations, such as managed care plans, require measures in one or more of the quality dimensions, and national quality award programs—such as the Baldridge Award—look for such a systematic approach to priority setting and performance monitoring.

In choosing to develop and apply a monitoring tool, practices should first consider their overall purpose in establishing a measurement system. Although these tools can be used to comply with insurance requirements and identify priorities for mandated projects, a more appropriate purpose is to enable practices to provide appropriate, timely care for the child and the child's family, with the overall goal being to promote better health outcomes for children, families, and the community. Because practices need to stay organizationally vital to provide this care, a reasonable additional aim is to sustain the organization in the long term.

What should a monitoring tool measure? Individual practices or practice networks may choose different measures, but an ongoing commitment to quality includes monitoring across the full spectrum of care.

In the area of safety, practices can measure several dimensions. One critical aspect of safety in primary care is reporting and responding to critical results and high-risk tests. These areas can be assessed by identifying abnormal values from laboratory results and tracking the proportion of patients with these results who were notified appropriately or had appropriate follow-up actions documented.

The measure of timeliness in primary care is increasingly standardized. The most widely used measure is the time to the third available appointment in a practice (regardless of visit type).[9] Another measure of timeliness that assesses the performance of the broader health system is the wait for a subspecialty appointment (using the same third available construct).

Measuring the effectiveness of care should include all three aspects of care—acute, chronic, and preventive.

Acute care is a major component of pediatric primary care. Fewer firm measures of care exist in this field. Among the most widely used measures of the quality of acute care is the appropriate use of antibiotics, a measure now widely in use through the *health employer and data information set* (HEDIS), a standard set of measures used to assess quality of managed care plans developed by the National Committee on Quality Assurance. This measure tracks the rate of antibiotic prescriptions for children between 3 months and 18 years of age who were diagnosed with an upper respiratory tract infection. A second measure of the quality of acute care endorsed by the National

Committee on Quality Assurance is the appropriate management of pharyngitis, which measures the rate of children between 2 and 18 years of age who were diagnosed with pharyngitis, prescribed an antibiotic and tested for group A *Streptococcus*.[10]

Numerous metrics are available to assess the effectiveness of care for children with chronic conditions. The most widely used metrics relate to care for children with asthma, the most common chronic medical condition. These metrics include measures of care processes, such as whether severity is assessed or whether appropriate medications are prescribed, and measures of patient outcomes, such as hospitalization, emergency department visits, and days without symptoms over a specified period. Measures also exist for the care of children with attention-deficit/hyperactivity disorder (ADHD) that are broadly consistent with the guidelines of the American Academy of Pediatrics (AAP). These measures include the use of criteria established in the fourth edition of the *Diagnostic and Statistical Manual of Mental Disorders* (DSM-IV) in making the diagnosis and undertaking appropriate follow-up after the prescription of a stimulant or other medication. Measures of symptoms and function can also be collected to provide a more comprehensive assessment of care quality. More rigorous measures of effectiveness combine, or bundle, multiple measures into a single *raise-the-bar* indicator, requiring that all appropriate processes be undertaken for a specific patient (eg, assessing severity, using a written management plan, prescribing appropriate medication for a child with asthma).[11]

Because the needs and concerns of families with children with special health care needs are quite similar regardless of the specific condition, broad measures assessing the degree to which practices fulfill these needs are available. These measures assess, among other items, the extent to which practices provide coordination of care and link families to available resources. Such measures can be obtained from the "Children With Chronic Conditions Set" of the Consumer Assessment of Health Plan Survey (CAHPS).[12] These measures are based on the most effective source of information—the parent or caretaker.

Preventive care is the most often-assessed aspect of primary care for children. Typical measures of effectiveness of preventive services include immunization rates, the performance of screening tests (eg, developmental assessments), and the provision of anticipatory guidance consistent with recommendations. The recent dramatic increase in childhood obesity has led to specific emphasis on the quality of preventive care related to this condition. These measures typically include performing the body mass index percentile calculation, categorizing the obesity risk status, and providing counseling about appropriate health behaviors.

A more sophisticated approach to assessing quality of preventive services might entail assessing whether a patient specific health-risk assessment was undertaken and whether appropriate follow-up assessments and plans were developed depending on these risks. Parent-reported measures of preventive care—particularly related to promoting appropriate development—are also available (see Tools for Practice).

Measures of efficiency in primary care pediatrics are often monitored by practices themselves or by third-party payers; these measures might include productivity, use of high-cost pharmaceuticals or radiologic tests, and hospitalization or emergency department use.

Patient and family centeredness can only truly be assessed by patients and families themselves. The dimensions of these measures are typically included in patient experience-of-care surveys. These dimensions usually include:

- Perceived access
- Courtesy and respect
- Provision of information
- Involvement in decision making
- Care coordination
- The physical environment of the practice
- Overall assessment

These dimensions have been assessed on a widely available plan level measure, the Consumer Assessment of Health Plan Survey (CAHPS).[14] A medical group and practice–level CAHPS for child health has recently become available.

The measurement of equity in care is relatively simple in concept but has often been controversial in implementation. To assess equity, practices need a reliable indicator of membership in a particular group (eg, racial group, income or insurance category, language spoken). Then all the other measures in the scorecard can be stratified by the different categories (examining, for example, whether rates of prescribing appropriate medication for patients with persistent asthma vary by race or whether critical test follow-up rates differ according to language).

If practices identify improving community health as one of their aims, then broader community-based measures of health would also be appropriate, such as rates of injury caused by intentional or unintentional trauma and population-based indicators of obesity and diabetes. These data might lead to specific practice-based initiatives or prompt more active engagement in advocacy and program development within the broader community.

A comprehensive practice-measurement set combines these clinical metrics with additional performance metrics such as financial performance and measures of staff satisfaction. Practice leaders developing such scorecards for a single practice within a larger system must also realize that maximizing performance on a single unit is typically not the goal of an overall institution, and therefore care must be taken to avoid doing so in a way that harms performance elsewhere. For example, maximizing productivity in a practice by referring all complex patients to specialists may cause decreased access to that specialist for other practices.

Undertaking comprehensive monitoring and assessment is not typical of primary care practices. Indeed, the burden on an individual practice of compiling these measures on a regular basis in the absence of an effective clinical information system, such as an electronic health record and effective practice registries, is substantial. On the other hand, the ability to generate such performance data and then use the data to manage and improve quality within a system is a clear advantage of electronic health information systems and one clear argument for the potential benefit of such systems.

Measurement does not result in improvement in quality; rather, it simply documents the current status of a program. For quality to improve, measurement must be linked to (1) purpose, (2) better ideas for how to practice, and (3) a process that reliably produces change and enhanced results.[14]

UNDERTAKING AN IMPROVEMENT PROJECT

Regardless of the priority chosen, the fundamental approach used in improving quality at the practice level, is similar. The first step is chartering a team to undertake improvement. In a small practice the team might consist of the entire practice—physician, nurse, and manager. In a larger practice, improvement teams typically include part of the practice but must maintain ongoing communication with the rest of practice so that improvements can subsequently spread. If the practice has a senior partner or some other form of formal leadership, then the leadership should develop the charge for the team. The team should be multidisciplinary and in almost all cases should involve patients and families as team members.

Establishing Aims

The first task of an improvement team is establishing an aim, which may be refining the aim as laid out by leadership. Aims for improvement programs should be based on data and should be sufficiently bold to engage the energies of the project team. Similar to any research hypothesis, aims should be directional and specify magnitude. Aims should be closely aligned with the mission and vision of the organization and—whenever possible—reflect the priorities of patients and families. A hypothetical aim statement might be, "Our project aim is to increase the function of children with attention-deficit disorder cared for in our practice; we will do so by improving the care of children with ADHD so that greater than 95% receive perfect care, without disparities"; in this case, *perfect care* is precisely defined (eg, use of DSM-IV criteria for diagnosis, development of shared goals, use of evidence based treatment, follow-up consistent with AAP guideline). This example clearly indicates the interrelatedness of the six quality aims. Although ostensibly focused on effectiveness of care (giving evidence-based treatment for ADHD) the project will also necessarily involve issues of safety (monitoring for side effects and complications), efficiency (use of mental health specialists), timeliness (wait for assessment and treatment), patient and family engagement, and, given the current lower level of use of evidence-based treatments among black children who meet criteria for this diagnosis, equity.

Selecting Performance Measures

The second step in an improvement program is establishing measures to assess performance and track gains. Measuring for improvement should generally focus only on the most important elements to undertake the work. Ideally, measures should be derived from data collected routinely in the course of care, such as through an electronic health record or patient registry or through ongoing patient survey activity, but in most cases must be supplemented by project specific data collection and analysis. Importantly, data should be plotted and tracked over time using simple tools such as run charts or more sophisticated tools such as control charts rather than aggregated for evaluation-oriented before-and-after studies.[14] A typical improvement project will include four to eight measures, including measures of the processes of care (was the right thing done?), of the outcomes of care (did the right result occur?), and of potential adverse outcomes (balancing measures; did unintended harm occur?). In the example, ADHD measures of process would include whether information about child symptoms and function were assessed from a parent and one other source (eg, teacher) and whether DSM-IV criteria were used. Outcome measures might include symptom scales and measures of function. Balancing measures might include patient satisfaction and physician productivity.

Identifying Good Ideas

The third step for an improvement initiative is identifying changes, or innovations, that are likely to lead to accomplishing the desired aims. Such changes can often be found in the medical literature, with attention to the realization that medical innovations often take between 1 and 2 decades to enter widespread use after being proven effective. Changes can also be found outside of health care; safety innovations, for example, are typically imported from high-reliability industries such as aviation, nuclear power, and high-speed trains. Patients, families, and health care staff are additional valuable sources of innovation. Generic change concepts from industry are another useful source of innovation that can be customized to the health care setting.[14]

Example of a Good Idea: Care Model for Child Health in a Medical Home

An idea that is widely applicable to improving the quality of primary care—particularly preventive care and the care of children with special health care needs—is the *care model for child health in a medical home*, a modest modification of the *chronic care model* developed by Wagner and colleagues (Figure 6-1).[15,16] The *care model* asserts that primary care is best delivered not by an individual provider alone but rather by a health care team and that the team will best serve the patient if it can anticipate patient needs and act accordingly. The team can function most effectively when supportive clinical information, decision support, care delivery, and self-management support systems are in place within a practice or clinic and when larger organizational systems are also aligned in support of the overall approach. The *care model* further asserts that patients must participate in their own care as members of the care team. To accomplish this task, patients need sufficient knowledge, skills, and abilities to monitor and manage their well being. In child health, of course, a parent is the one who often serves as the patient's voice and agent. The *care model* advises that health care practices and systems draw on community resources to help patients achieve better outcomes.

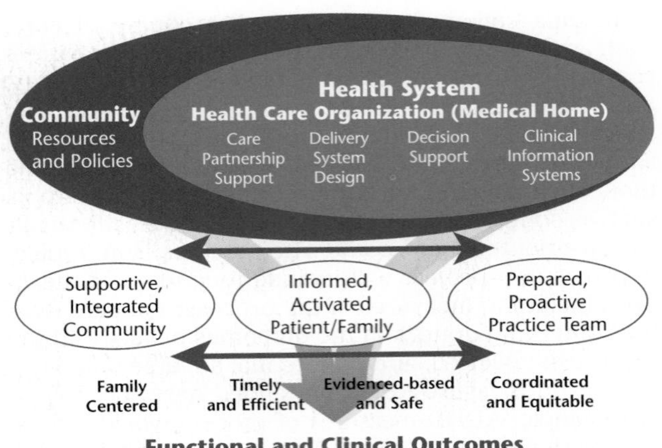

Figure 6-1 The Care Model for Child Health in a Medical Home. This diagram indicates the desired outcomes of excellent care for children; the shared contribution of the health care system and community resources to improved results; the key role of organizational policies and leadership; and the four specific elements of an effective medical home—information system, decision support, delivery system design, and care partnership support. (*Homer CJ, Cooley WC. Creating a medical home for children with special health care needs. In Sobo EJ, Kurtin PS, eds.* Optimizing care for young children with special health care needs. *Baltimore: Paul H. Brookes; 2007. Reprinted by permission.*)

Practices with appropriate clinical information systems are able to list which of their patients have specific clinical conditions (eg, asthma), the severity or complexity of these conditions (eg, severe persistent asthma), and whichever other bits of information are relevant to the patient management question at hand (eg, are all eligible children with asthma using the proper dose of antiinflammatory medication?). Information systems can also indicate which patients have received specific preventive services (eg, immunization, screenings and assessment of healthy weight) and provide reminders when they are due.[17,18]

Two aspects of the design of the delivery system merit particular notice. Interactions among health care providers, patients, and families should be designed to address issues of importance to patients and their families and to anticipate future needs. The most effective settings for such interactions are planned visits. Planned visits are routine in preventive care (well-child visits) but are less common—although essential—in the care of children with special health care needs. Because of the fragmentation of services for children, the *care model for child health* also emphasizes care coordination. A designated office staff member may provide care coordination, or care coordination functions may be distributed in explicit ways among several individuals. Finally, because children are ethnically and culturally diverse, capturing ethnic information in patient registries is important to ensure that practices can examine their care and outcomes by patient subgroups. Trained interpreters in the care partnership enable appropriate goal setting and care planning.

Chronic care itself needs to be based on evidence when evidence is available and on expert guidance when such evidence is not available or needs interpretation. Basing care on evidence requires a mechanism for practices to determine what type and degree of evidence is required to drive change, to review and obtain evidence-based recommendations, to share such information with patients and families, to embed the evidence in medical record systems so that faulty memory does not impede care, and to maintain ready access to subspecialty expertise.

The most critical component of the *care model* is providing care in such a way that promotes patients' ability to provide self-care and manage their own care. This framing acknowledges that health care professionals are facilitators and that the actions of patients are the final determinants of what happens. The core aspect of self-management support is the development of shared goals between patients and clinicians and the subsequent development of specific, mutually agreed-on plans to achieve these goals.

Because care for children includes supporting both the family's ability to provide care and the child's ability to assume self-care, practices should provide both *self-management support*—that is, support the ability of the child to manage their own health and health care—and *family-management support*—that is, promoting the ability of the family to manage that care. For example, children with diabetes or asthma need to take increasing responsibility for monitoring their own condition and for adjusting their own medical regimen as they approach adolescence. The medical home—the place where the *care model* is implemented—needs to support the child's increasing competence in managing the child's own well being and to counsel and support the family in monitoring the success of that effort while also maintaining the child's safety.

The *care model* highlights two additional areas critical to providing preventive care and care that meets the needs of persons with chronic conditions. The first area is alignment of health care provider activities with organizational aims. Secondly, practices must draw on the resources of the larger community to meet patient needs. This provision includes obtaining access to not only formal supports and entitlements such as housing services or special education, but also informal supports provided by resources such as churches and libraries.

Although not simple, the *care model for child health* is a powerful framework for the organization (and reorganization) of pediatric primary care. Combined with evidence-based guidelines, as well as an effective strategy to undertake small tests of change that will ultimately effect large changes in practice systems, it results in better care for children and families. This model provides the detail that is needed to make the medical home concept a reality.

Implementing Change

In primary care practices, fully implementing a new approach—such as the *care model* described previously—in a way that anticipates all the challenges that such change will bring is not typically possible. A more effective approach to introducing change is through the use of repeated small tests of change, sometimes referred to as the *Shewhart* cycle—after the industrial engineer who first developed the approach—or, more commonly, the *plan-do-study-act* (PDSA) cycle.[14]

The PDSA cycle starts with the question, "What is the largest meaningful test of change that we can conduct by next Tuesday?" that is, the priority for a PDSA cycle is to expeditiously try something out while doing it in a way that is planned and doing it in a way that allows learning (study) and revision (act). A typical health care PDSA cycle involves the care of one patient at one point in time by one health care provider, such as the use of a new dehydration assessment form or patient instruction diagram. A full cycle involves planning what will be done (including the questions of what, where, and when, if not why), performing the test, reflecting on what happened during the test, and modifying the test for the next cycle. Effective improvement programs conduct numerous cycles, building one on the other and addressing different dimensions of the care system with different series of tests.

This approach to improvement—the combination of aims, measures, changes, and the PDSA cycle—is known as the *model for improvement*. Developed by Associates in Process Improvement, the *model for improvement* is among the most widespread improvement frameworks in health care.[14] Different approaches use different terminology and have somewhat different emphases but in general share the use of aims, measures, and repeated tests of change.

COLLABORATIVE LEARNING

Sharing data allows individual organizations both to set priorities better and to identify practice settings that have better performance for learning (also known as *benchmarking*). The benefits of collaborative learning have formed the basis for numerous collaborative improvement programs in children's health care. Many networks initially established for clinical and health services research, including AAP Pediatric Research in Office Settings and the Continuity Research Network for academic primary care, have the potential to serve this purpose. Topic-specific learning collaboratives conducted by the National Initiative for Children's Healthcare Quality and other organizations can also serve this function. Many regional improvement programs have also been established—often involving state professional association chapters working together with public health, academic institutions, and public and private health insurance agencies. Participation in such external efforts typically accelerates learning and improvement and facilitates the pediatricians' efforts in quality improvement, which is often difficult to accomplish without external resources.

SUMMARY

Widespread deficiencies abound in health care across all six dimensions of quality (safety, timeliness, effectiveness, efficiency, equity, and patient centeredness). A systematic approach to monitoring quality can help set priorities for improvement, although the specific topics and initiatives to be undertaken must also be customized to the specific institutional environment. Use of a quality improvement approach such as the *model for improvement* increases the likelihood of making positive changes in care in outcomes. The *care model for child health* is one powerful idea that can be used to organize and improve the quality of primary care practices, particularly when combined with evidence-based recommendation such as Bright Futures. Collaboration across organizations can accelerate improvement efforts as well.

TOOLS FOR PRACTICE

Community Advocacy and Coordination

- *Quality Dividend Calculator* (interactive tool), National Committee for Quality Assurance (www.ncqacalculator.com/Index.asp).

Medical Decision Support

- *American Academy of Pediatrics Clinical Practice Guidelines* (Web page), American Academy of Pediatrics (aappolicy.aappublications.org/practice_guidelines/index.dtl).
- *Bright Futures: Guidelines for Health Supervision of Infants, Children, and Adolescents* (book), Bright Futures (brightfutures.aap.org/web/).
- *eQIPP* (online courses), American Academy of Pediatrics (www.pedialink.org/learnmore-view.cfm?show=5).

Program Management and Care Coordination

- *Child Health Care Quality Toolbox Measuring Quality in Children's Health Programs* (toolkit), Agency for Healthcare Research and Quality (www.ahrq.gov/chtoolbx/).
- *Child and Adolescent Health Measurement Initiative* (Web page), Agency for Healthcare Research and Quality (www.cahmi.org/).
- *Consumer Assessment of Healthcare Providers and Systems (CAHP)* (Web page), Agency for Healthcare Research and Quality (www.cahps.ahrq.gov/default.asp).
- *Item Set for Children With Chronic Conditions* (Web page), Agency for Healthcare Research and Quality (https://www.cahps.ahrq.gov/CAHPSkit/files/102_Children_with_Chronic_Conditions_Set.htm).
- *Quality Improvement Innovation Network (QuIIN)* (Web page), American Academy of Pediatrics (www.aap.org/moc/quiin/).
- *Safer Health Care for Kids* (Web page), American Academy of Pediatrics (www.aap.org).
- *Selected Findings on Child and Adolescent Health Care From the 2004 National Healthcare Quality and Disparities Reports* (fact sheet), Agency for Healthcare Research and Quality (www.ahrq.gov/qual/nhqrchild/nhqrchild.htm).

AAP POLICY STATEMENTS

American Academy of Pediatrics and the Steering Committee on Quality Improvement and Management. Classifying Recommendations for Clinical Practice Guidelines. *Pediatrics*. 2004;114(3):874-877. (aappolicy.aappublications.org/cgi/content/full/pediatrics;114/3/874).

American Academy of Pediatrics, the Steering Committee on Quality Improvement and Management and the Committee on Practice and Ambulatory Medicine. Principles for the Development and Use of Quality Measures. *Pediatrics*. 2008;121(2):411-418. (aappolicy.aappublications.org/cgi/content/full/pediatrics;121/2/411).

American Academy of Pediatrics and the National Initiative for Children's Health Care Quality Project Advisory Committee. Principles of Patient Safety in Pediatrics. *Pediatrics*. 2001;107(6):1473-1475. (aappolicy.aappublications.org/cgi/content/full/pediatrics;107/6/1473).

American Academy of Pediatrics Medical Home Initiatives for Children With Special Needs Project Advisory Committee. The Medical Home. *Pediatrics*. 2002;110(1):184-186. (aappolicy.aappublications.org/cgi/content/full/pediatrics;110/1/184).

SUGGESTED RESOURCES

Alliance for Pediatric Quality (www.kidsquality.org/).

American Academy of Pediatrics Quality Improvement and Management—Member Center (www.aap.org/moc/qualityimprove/qualityimp.htm).

American Academy of Pediatrics Practice Management Online—Quality Improvement (practice.aap.org/topicBrowse.aspx?nodeID=1000.1023).

Improving Chronic Illness Care (www.improvingchroniccare.org/).

Institute for Health Care Improvement (www.ihi.org/ihi).

Institute of Medicine (www.iom.edu/).

REFERENCES

1. Institute of Medicine. *Crossing the Quality Chasm: A New Health System for the Twenty-first Century*. Washington, DC: National Academies Press; 2001.
2. Institute of Medicine, Committee on Understanding and Eliminating Racial and Ethnic Disparities in Health Care. Smedley BD, Stith AY, Nelson AR, eds. *Unequal Treatment: Confronting Racial and Ethnic Disparities in Health Care*. Washington, DC: National Academies Press; 2003.
3. Mangione-Smith R, DeCristofaro AH, Setodji CM, et al. The quality of ambulatory care delivered to children in the United States. *N Engl J Med*. 2007;357(15):1515-1523.
4. Mangione-Smith R, Schonlau M, Chan KS, et al. Measuring the effectiveness of a collaborative for quality improvement in pediatric asthma care: does implementing the chronic care model improve processes and outcomes of care? *Ambul Pediatr*. 2005;5(2):75-82.
5. Young PC, Glade GB, Stoddard GJ, et al. Evaluation of a learning collaborative to improve the delivery of preventive services by pediatric practices. *Pediatrics*. 2006;117(5):1469-1476.
6. Margolis PA, Lannon CM, Stuart JM, et al. Practice-based education to improve delivery systems for prevention in primary care: a randomized trial. *BMJ*. 2004;328(7436):388.
7. Institute of Medicine, Committee to Design a Strategy for Quality Review and Assurance in Medicare. Lohr KN, ed. *Medicare: A Strategy for Quality Assurance*. Vol 1. Washington, DC: National Academies Press; 1990.
8. Randolph G, Fried B, Loeding L, et al. Organizational characteristics and preventive service delivery in private practices: a peek inside the "black box" of private practices caring for children. *Pediatrics*. 2005;115(6):1704-1711.
9. Murray M, Berwick, DM. Advanced access: reducing waits and delays in primary care. *JAMA*. 2003;289:1035-1040.
10. National Committee for Quality Assurance. NCQA Releases HEDIS® 2004, 10 New Measures Address Public Health, Service Issues. Available at: www.ncqa.org/communications/news/Hedis2004.htm. Accessed August 15, 2007.
11. Nolan T, Berwick DM. All-or-none measurement raises the bar on performance. *JAMA*. 2006;295:1168-1170.
12. US Department of Health and Human Services, Agency for Healthcare Research and Quality. Item Set for Children with Chronic Conditions. Available at: www.cahps.ahrq.gov/CAHPSkit/files/102_Children_with_Chronic_Conditions_Set.htm. Accessed August 15, 2007.
13. US Department of Health and Human Services, Agency for Healthcare Research and Quality. CAHPS® Surveys and Tools to Advance Patient-Centered Care. Available at: www.cahps.ahrq.gov/default.asp. Accessed August 15, 2007.
14. Langley GJ, Nolan KM, Nolan TW, et al. *The Improvement Guide: A Practical Approach to Enhancing Organizational Performance*. San Francisco, CA: Jossey-Bass; 1996.
15. Wagner EH, Austin BT, Von Korff M. Improving outcomes in chronic illness. *Managed Care Q*. 1996;4(2):12-25.
16. Wagner EH, Austin BT, Von Korff M. Organizing care for patients with chronic illness. *Milbank Q*. 1996;74(4):511-544.
17. Bodenheimer T, Wagner EH, Grumbach K. Improving primary care for patients with chronic illness. *JAMA*. 2002;288(14):1775-1779.
18. Bodenheimer T, Wagner, EH, Grumbach K. Improving primary care for patients with chronic illness: the chronic care model, part 2. *JAMA*. 2002;288(15):1909-1914.

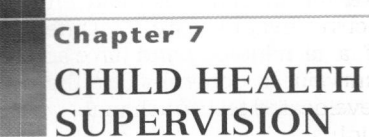

Chapter 7

CHILD HEALTH SUPERVISION

Paula M. Duncan, MD; Joseph F. Hagan Jr, MD

INTRODUCTION

According to the World Health Organization, "Health involves much more than simply the absence of disease; health involves optimal physical, mental, social, and emotional functioning and well-being."[1] In the care of American children, the health supervision visit allows health professionals to endorse and to effect this concept of health. In this preventive encounter, health promotion is addressed for all children and adolescents, including those with special health care needs.

GOALS OF THE PREVENTIVE SERVICES VISIT

For health promotion to be achieved, contemporary expert consensus defines key elements for inclusion in every preventive health care visit. Tasks of the preventive services visit include:

- Disease detection
- Disease prevention
- Health promotion
- Anticipatory guidance

In addition, preventive health care for youth occurs in the context of family. Any successful intervention will involve solicitation of family health concerns so that they might be addressed in a comprehensive fashion. Child health professionals, including pediatricians, family medicine physicians, nurse practitioners, and physician assistants, together with their nurses and other office and clinic staff, seek to provide a package of preventive services efficiently. Partnering with families enhances the relevance of services offered to the youth and family.

Disease detection is often cited as the medical impetus for health supervision activities, yet few serious disease states are found in preventive services visits. On the other hand, regularly scheduled visits are a unique opportunity to plot a child's growth and development, noting the congruence or divergence of the child's developmental trajectory when compared with norms. The growth charts of length, weight, weight for length, and head circumference for the infant and weight, height, and body mass index for the older child and adolescent are key predictors in the surveillance of physical growth. Similarly, a child's development in the motor, cognitive, and social-emotional domains should be monitored, acknowledging the importance of early brain development and its effect on long-term health.

Surveillance and screening activities are performed in each well-child visit. Surveillance is the longitudinal monitoring of growth and development or other health parameters by an experienced observer in partnership with the parent. It occurs in every health encounter and is enhanced by the opportunity for repeated visits and observations with advancing developmental stages. Effective surveillance usually relies on the experience of a skilled clinician over time. Nonetheless, clinical surveillance alone is inadequate to detect physical or developmental variation or significant deviation with high sensitivity. Screening is the more formal process using a specific screening tool for evaluating patients for conditions in the preclinical phase of disease when symptoms or signs are not obvious. Screening is appropriate when early detection is possible; when a tool with high sensitivity, specificity, and predictive value is available; when the cost of screening is reasonable; when treatments are available; and when a treatment benefit exists to early detection as compared with later detection.

Surveillance for a child's healthy development is an essential element to the child preventive health care visit. Structured developmental screening at 9, 18, and 24 or 30 months has been recommended and is a component of *The Bright Futures Guidelines,* 3rd edition.[2] Positive results at primary screening may lead to secondary screening or in depth medical evaluation. For example, the child found to have no words at the 15-month visit might appropriately receive secondary screening for autism spectrum disorders, using a specific or secondary screening instrument, such as the Modified Checklist for Autism in Toddlers (M-CHAT).[3]

Disease prevention involves guidance that is essential for all children and guidance directed at specific identified groups. Immunization is the classic disease-prevention strategy in pediatrics. "Back to Sleep" advice, associated with a reduction in the incidence of sudden infant death syndrome by 50%,[4] is information of utmost importance to all families because all children are at risk. Similarly, accurate advice regarding nutrition and the importance of physical activity is of value to all families, given the increasing problems in our culture with pediatric and adult overweight status. However, more specific and more intensive advice will be targeted for children with overweight parents or when parents have type 2 diabetes mellitus.

In situations in which behavioral change may be indicated, shared decision-making strategies are often most effective. Acknowledging and building on the parent and youth expertise about successful strategies for their situation demonstrates respect and positive expectation on the part of the clinician. Informed by the most current scientific knowledge, this individualized and collaborative problem-solving approach involving preventive planning exemplifies the unique opportunity of the preventive services visit.

Health-promotion activities are designed to optimize development and generalize the activities of specific and targeted disease prevention. Eschewing an emphasis on specific disease states, health-promotion activities are instead focused on helping children, adolescents, and families make appropriate lifestyle choices, which enhance health. Certainly, health-promotion activity will also include counseling aimed at changing unhealthy lifestyles.

The choice of health-promotion topics for a particular visit is a particular concern for the primary care physician. Where do you begin? How far do you go? Of the many topics that can be covered, which should be? Time limitations to the encounter exist for both physicians and families. Furthermore, Barkin and colleagues[5] noted that as the number of topics covered by physicians increases, family recall decreases. Consensus regarding visit content is needed, and guidelines (discussed later in this chapter) can be consulted.

Anticipatory guidance recognizes the unique relationship of the child health professional with child and family over time.[6] Knowing the tasks and demands of child and family development allows the clinician to anticipate information that will be important to the child over the upcoming months or years. Applying this knowledge to a particular child's situation allows the pediatric clinician to give family-specific advice that is cogent, coherent, and relevant to the child's developmental progress for the immediate future. Choice of anticipatory guidance topics depends on the practitioner's assessment of the child's developmental stage, the family's unique predicament and derivative needs, and the practitioner's own assessment and beliefs regarding what is the best advice for the child and family. Although experience and guidelines can direct the practitioner's choices, assessing family needs and strengths is the core element directing the guidance provided. The clinician's familiarity with the community strengths, challenges, and cultural characteristics provides a context that also affects these choices. The partnership between the medical home and local public health professionals helps provide population-based data and links to necessary community resources.

ACCOMPLISHING EFFECTIVE HEALTH SUPERVISION

Intrinsically, the 4 tasks of the health supervision visit previously mentioned are, at the same time, specific and general. Health supervision activities must meet practice and community standards. They must reproducibly reach a bar of quality in content and in practice.

This approach brings a consistency to each clinical encounter, with similar interventions with every patient. However, to be relevant to the child and family centered, every health supervision activity must be specific to the needs of the patient child and family. Repetitions are to be avoided. The experienced practitioner of pediatric health care uses the generalities of health promotion and anticipatory guidance in seeking to detect the specifics of disease detection and disease prevention. Properly constructed electronic health records may assist in health supervision activities.

Quality children's health care is effective, safe, patient centered, family centered, timely, efficient, and equitable. How can quality children's health care be achieved in any practice and replicated to meet a standard of care? How can this task be accomplished in the time available? To answer these concerns, the setting, the process, and the content of care for child and adolescent health supervision must be addressed.

SETTING: THE MEDICAL HOME

The American Academy of Pediatrics believes that every child deserves a medical home.[7] The *medical home* is a practice that is "accessible, continuous, comprehensive, family centered, coordinated, compassionate, and culturally effective.[8]

In this model, every child and family enjoys a relationship with their child's health practitioners. This relationship may be with an individual practitioner or with a group of providers. Value, depth, and breadth are added to this relationship by experienced pediatric nurses and dedicated support staff. The medical home may also include mental health services by either mental health professionals on staff or in collaborative practices. Community support personnel can assist in connecting families with additional nonmedical community services. Clearly, the broad range of services that a family may require or a practice might wish to provide is not necessarily contained in the well-child visit itself. Community collaborations will be essential to provide funding mechanisms for broader services.

PROCESS: GUIDELINES FOR CARE

Preventive service visits in the medical home are recommended for all children at certain ages or stages of development. The American Academy of Pediatrics Recommendations for Preventive Pediatric Health Care,[9] typically termed the *periodicity schedule,* directs the provision of certain services at age-specific visits.

The Periodicity Schedule is the foundation for current Federal Early Periodic Screening, Diagnosis, and Treatment (EPSDT) service requirements that direct specific aspects of care to be accomplished if Medicaid reimbursement is claimed. Similarly, the periodicity schedule has been used for public health recommendations regarding the care of children and adolescents and used to define the standard of care by 3rd-party payers.

Although the Periodicity Schedule directs specific elements of care, a large number of professional groups have developed guidelines for how this care can and should be provided. In current practice, 3 major sources provide guidelines for health supervision visits:

1. *The Bright Futures Guidelines,* from Maternal Child Health Bureau of the US Department of Health and Human Services[2]
2. The American Academy of Pediatrics' *Guidelines for Health Supervision*[9]
3. The American Medical Association's *Guidelines for Adolescent Preventive Services (GAPS)*[10]

Additionally, *GAPS* delineates a schema and system for how preventive care to adolescents might be efficiently provided. Subsequently, this *GAPS* approach has been used in other age groups.

Under the leadership of the Maternal Child Health Bureau, the 3 organizations responsible for the existing guidelines joined with representatives of the National Association of Pediatric Nurse Practitioners, the American Academy of Family Physicians, and other organizations in the development of *The Bright Futures Guidelines,* 3rd edition. "The *Bright Futures Guidelines* are a set of principles, strategies, and tools that are theory based, evidence driven, and systems oriented and can be used to improve the health and well being of all children through culturally appropriate interventions that address the current and emerging health-promotion needs at the policy, community, health systems, and family levels." Consistent with the American Academy of Pediatrics' Periodicity Schedule, Bright Futures details the content of each age-based visit and recommends interventions. These guidelines will become the primary and authoritative guidelines for use in American health care practices caring for children.

CONTENT: CRAFTING THE VISIT

For the health supervision visit to be family centered, the patient and family agenda must be identified and addressed. To be timely and efficient, a family's needs and assets must be determined. Equitable care recognizes the contributions of community and the family's connectedness to their community.

To complete the health supervision visit in the time allowed, the practitioner must be prepared to collect historical information regarding child and family health, their needs, and the family's and youth's agenda. This information will allow the practitioner and family to structure the visit so that relevant disease-prevention and health-promotion advice and services can be provided. Topics discussed are recorded to provide follow-up and avoid repetition. Relevant anticipatory guidance materials supplement the practitioner's discussion of selected topics identified by practitioner and family as important. The *Bright Futures Guidelines* outlines a schema for health supervision that is both time efficient and comprehensive. The Bright Futures toolkit provides family and patient questionnaires for each visit to assist in tailoring each visit to the child's current needs. Many pediatricians ask families to complete these questionnaires before the health supervision visit so that the valuable time available can be used to address concerns raised. Electronic health records offer promise in the important task of data collection and management.

EVIDENCE

Of the many components of a health supervision visit, those elements for which there is evidence of effectiveness must be highlighted. Interventions for which evidence of effectiveness exists take precedence over other interactions of arguable, though uncertain, value. Practitioner and family time is limited, and proven interventions must not be displaced. Nonetheless, satisfactory studies on preventive health care issues are sparse, including those that demonstrate effectiveness of components of the physical examination of the well child.

Multiple and varied services to children and families are deemed important to child health and well being as defined by professional guidelines, community protocol, or other representations of expert opinion. Here absent evidence does not demonstrate lack of usefulness. Absent evidence commonly indicates lack of study. For example, no strong evidence supporting the utility of a health supervision physical examination has been discovered. However, the physical examination, including measurements of growth, body mass index, and blood pressure, together with appropriate screening tests, may allow the detection of health problems or health risk behaviors. Evidence for management of problems detected may be available and more definitive. In situations in which evidence exists, the careful clinician will practice in a manner consistent with that evidence and embed evidence-based elements into their well-child care. Lacking evidence from randomized controlled trails, most authoritative guidelines are derived from experts' examination of the scientific data that exist to help prevent disease, detect disease and risk early, and promote health and a positive developmental trajectory. This evidence-informed approach is founded on the principle of *do no harm* and judiciously combines science and experience.

Expert opinion can provide a valuable compilation of key elements of the clinical health encounter that may be used by the practitioner to discern a standard of care and design appropriate encounters. Nonetheless, enhancing or diverging from this standard in the interest of serving the individual patient and family is reasonable and appropriate for clinical encounters. In recent studies, office-based quality-improvement strategies have been associated with the establishment of a platform of consistent preventive services delivery and decreased variability within and between practices on these important measures. Efforts have been designed to ensure that all the most important services are delivered in each practice setting (eg, immunizations, vision screening in children younger than 5 years, *Chlamydia* screening in sexually active female adolescents).

FUTURE DIRECTIONS

Health promotion has long focused on disease prevention. Health supervision content must change as health promotion evolves to include encouraging the acquisition of developmental competencies, attending to morbidities of behavioral and mental health, and addressing social needs. Schor[11] has examined opportunities for enhancing the content and the process in health supervision. As health and social mandates change, health supervision must evolve if it is to be both vibrant and valuable.

TOOLS FOR PRACTICE

Medical Decision Support

- *Bright Futures: Guidelines for Health Supervision of Infants, Children, and Adolescents* (book), Bright Futures (*brightfutures.aap.org/web/*).
- *Bright Futures Toolkit* (tool kit), Bright Futures (brightfutures.aap.org/web/).
- *Guidelines for Adolescent Preventative Services, GAPS* (guideline), American Medical Association. AAP Endorsed. (www.ama-assn.org/ama/pub/category/1980.html).
- *Modified Checklist for Autism in Toddlers (M-CHAT),* (form), Thyde Dumont-Mathieu, MD, MPH, Deborah Fein, PhD, Jamie Kleinman, BA (www.dbpeds.org/media/mchat.pdf).

AAP POLICY STATEMENTS

American Academy of Pediatrics Committee on Practice and Ambulatory Medicine. Recommendations for preventive pediatric health care. *Pediatrics.* 2000;105(3):645-646. (pediatrics.aappublications.org/cgi/content/full/105/3/645).

American Academy of Pediatrics Medical Home Initiatives for Children With Special Needs Project Advisory Committee. The medical home. *Pediatrics.* 2002;110(1): 184-186. (aappolicy.aappublications.org/cgi/content/full/pediatrics;110/1/184).

REFERENCES

1. World Health Organization. Preamble to the Constitution of the World Health Organization. New York, NY: 1946. Available at: www.searo.who.int/. Accessed February 16, 2007.
2. Hagan JF Jr, Shaw JS, Duncan PM, eds. *Bright Futures: Guidelines for Health Supervision of Infants, Children, and Adolescents.* 3rd ed. Elk Grove Village, IL: American Academy of Pediatrics; 2008.
3. Dumont-Mathieu T, Fein D, Kleinman J, American Academy of Pediatrics. Screening for autism in young children: the Modified Checklist for Autism in Toddlers (M-CHAT). Available at: www.dbpeds.org/articles/detail.cfm?textid=377. Accessed April 23, 2006.
4. American Academy of Pediatrics, Task Force on Sudden Infant Death Syndrome. The changing concept of sudden infant death syndrome: diagnostic coding shifts, controversies regarding the sleeping environment, and new variables to consider in reducing risk. *Pediatrics.* 2005; 116(5)1245-1255.
5. Barkin SL, Scheindlin B, Brown C, et al. Anticipatory guidance topics: are more better? *Ambul Pediatr.* 2005;5(6):372-376.
6. Brazelton TB. Symposium on behavioral pediatrics. Anticipatory Guidance. *Pediatr Clin North Am.* 1975; 22(3):533-544.
7. American Academy of Pediatrics and the Medical Home Initiatives for Children With Special Needs, Project Advisory Committee. The medical home. *Pediatrics.* 2002;110(1):184-186.
8. Committee on Quality of Health Care in America, Institute of Medicine. *Crossing the quality chasm: a new health system for the 21st century.* Available at: www.IOM.edu. Accessed June 4, 2007.
9. American Academy of Pediatrics, Stein MT, Wolraich, MI, Cohen GJ, et al. *Guidelines for Health Supervision III.* Elk Grove Village, IL: American Academy of Pediatrics; 2002.

10. American Medical Association. *Guidelines for Adolescent Preventive Health Services (GAPS) Recommendations*. Chicago, IL: American Medical Association; 1997. Available at www.ama-assn.org/ama/pub/category/1980.html. Accessed March 30, 2007.
11. Schor EL. Rethinking well-child care. *Pediatrics*. 2004; 114(1):210-216.

Chapter 8

MEDICAL HOME COLLABORATIVE CARE

Calvin C. J. Sia, MD

Every child deserves a medical home. The primary care physician assumes the role of a *medical home* by offering care that is accessible, coordinated, comprehensive, continuous, culturally effective, and compassionate. As the point of initial contact for child health medical services, the medical home physician is in a unique position to offer comprehensive health care through preventive, child health supervision visits, in addition to treating acute and chronic illnesses. The basic functions and role of the medical home are established when the primary care physician builds a partnership and mutual-trusting relationship with the child and family through periodic visits from infancy through young adulthood.[1]

The concept of the medical home is especially applicable to the care of children with special health care needs (CSHCN) and chronic disabling conditions. As defined by Maternal Child Health Bureau and adopted by the American Academy of Pediatrics, CSHCN are defined as those who have or who are at increased risk for a chronic physical, developmental, behavioral, or emotional condition and who also require health and related services of a type or amount generally beyond that required by most typically developing children.[2] These children include those at risk or who have conditions principally the result of biological reasons (eg, genetic conditions such as trisomy 21 or phenylketonuria), those at risk or with difficulties principally the result of their environmental or socioeconomic context (eg, prematurity, children growing up in poverty), and those who have or who are at risk for conditions caused by a combination of biological, environmental, or psychosocial factors (eg, children growing up in families affected by parental mental illness, domestic violence, or substance abuse). Chronic conditions may include asthma, diabetes mellitus, or juvenile rheumatoid arthritis.

ROLE OF THE MEDICAL HOME

Reflecting the major advances in medical care over the last century and the dramatic changes in society as a whole, child health problems have moved from the old morbidity of malnutrition and contagious diseases (1960s and into the 1970s) to the new morbidity of developmental disabilities, school dysfunction, emotional problems, violence, and injuries (1970 into the 1990s), to beyond the new morbidity, the *millennial morbidity* that include bioenvironmental interface, socioeconomic influences on health, health disparities, technological influences on health, obesity, and increasing mental health concerns (2000s).[3] Few children escape the influence of these environmental factors. The medical home is adapting pediatric practice to these changes and is assuming a new role in facing these challenges. To be an effective medical home, the primary care physician needs to incorporate the support of the family along with a specific knowledge of the community's resources to facilitate, promote, and advocate for the optimal physical, mental, and social health of the individual child and all children within a community.[4] Unfortunately, most current pediatricians have had little formal training to make them comfortable, sensitive, and facile in these areas.

The medical home physician may become (1) the primary *care coordinator* and *medical case manager* for the child in consultation with pediatric subspecialists or professionals working with the child and family as part of a specific intervention program or (2) a *co-coordinator* or *collaborative care provider* with a group of specialists or an interdisciplinary team. A clear understanding of the role of the medical home as the primary coordinator of the child's care is recommended from the onset of collaborative care. Open communication with the family and agencies or institutions involved with the child is crucial from the onset of referral and consultation and should continue on an ongoing basis. Open communication is most important in sharing periodic management goals and objectives and developing and implementing an individualized care plan for the CSHCN.

Barriers in achieving successful collaborative care include lack of communications among child health professionals and agencies, problems with understanding changing health care financing and reform (including managed care, consumer driven health plans, and appropriate payments for physician's services), lack of an integrated system of care in the community, lack of training and expertise resulting in physicians feeling uncomfortable in the role sometimes delegated to social workers, and maldistribution or limited number of pediatric subspecialists, pediatric surgical specialists, and mental health professionals in the workforce.

Fundamental to the success of the medical home is a partnership with the family in care of the CSHCN. The primary care physician and family must reconcile differences of parents' expectations for the child with current knowledge and capacity of the medical home and community's resources. Care coordination is a dynamic process that involves the physician's expertise, the concerns and needs of the family, and relationships with other medical, health, social, or educational professionals. Appropriate referrals, based on sound scientific knowledge, community standards of care or best practices, are coordinated with an interdisciplinary or interagency team's focus on the specific needs of the child and family.[5]

First Contact—Early Intervention

The medical home is often the first contact that identifies early developmental changes during well-child health supervision visits. The primary care physician observes, listens, and gathers information in each visit with the child and parents, sorting out issues and using the triage approach to identify medical and nonmedical problems that require diagnostic evaluation. Developmental screening and surveillance are crucial parts of this role. Comfort with variations in normal development is essential in this process. Proper referral for testing or professional consultants is made, and follow-up visits to integrate and interpret these studies are scheduled. A comprehensive care plan is developed with the family, outlining medical concerns, social concerns, and educational needs. The medical home may mediate any conflicts and suggest alternatives of care. The primary care physician must be nonjudgmental in his relationship with the family and culturally effective in approaching the family, providing interpretation and translation of what is known scientifically and what is still unknown or unproven in treatment. A central medical record is kept, and summaries are duplicated for the family when needed. A problem-oriented front sheet in the medical records of the medical home allows the physician a quick review and summary of current areas of concern for each visit. Increasingly, electronic health records (EHRs) containing all medical information about a patient from multiple sources are becoming the optimal method to organize the information regarding CSHCN. Ideally, parents should have access to the EHR. Additionally, the EHR can be used to track guideline recommended visits and tests, reminding and recalling patients as necessary.

Office Setting

Within the office setting, the physician or an office staff member is the care coordinator for the child and the family as a whole. Appropriate access and time for visits to the office are planned for in the routine appointments, and a care plan is developed and reviewed at these visits. Periodic evaluation and discussions with the child and parents are helpful in monitoring the child's physical growth, development, and overall management and health care. The current medical record should contain all pertinent medical information, consultations, and professional reports. The record should be accessible to the parents and appropriate staff with respect for the family's confidentiality.

Coordination and collaborative care often requires extended office time. This process may involve telephone calls or conferences with child care centers; principals, teachers, or school counselors; social workers, public health nurses; and other professionals, in addition to medical and surgical consultants. These consultations should be discussed with the parents, who are then advised as to how to proceed with follow-up care. Appropriate payment should be sought through third-party payers (health insurance carriers). The insurers may assist with financing medical case management and care coordination.

Proper use of pediatric *Current Procedural Terminology* coding for documentation of time spent on direct care and care coordination ensures appropriate payment to the medical home. Thus proper office management and documentation of time spent is a critical part of coordination and collaborative care.[6]

Transitional Plans

Because CSHCN and children with chronic diseases are living longer, transitional planning for adolescence to adulthood should begin by age 14. These plans should include discussions on what services will be needed, who will provide them, and how will they be financed. The medical home will often collaborate with the child's school in formulating transition plans. Individualized transitional plans should address educational, recreational, and vocational opportunities for adolescents as they enter into young adulthood. Transfer of care should be discussed and should occur at a mutually agreeable time for the youth, family, and current and future medical home.[7]

ROLE OF THE FAMILY

Family-centered care places the family at the center in comprehensive, coordinated, and collaborative care. The family is a source of strength and the principal caregiver. Equally important is that the parents are the experts in their child's care. The medical home respects the knowledge, skills, and experiences that parents bring to this relationship and empower the parents by offering counseling, educational materials, and referral to training programs. Varying cultural traditions, values, and diversity of families are honored and respected. Mutual understanding allows for negotiations in collaborative relationships.[8]

Federal support for parents' role in the care for CSHCN is clearly demonstrated under the Education of the Handicapped Act Amendments (Public Law 99-457) and its reauthorization under the Individuals with Disabilities Education Act (Public Law 101-476, 1990) as Part C, Zero to Three programs. Individualized family service plans are developed by Zero to Three programs with the family and medical home to provide a blueprint for provision of care for the CSHCN.[9] Ultimately the successful family recognizes its role as the primary care coordinator and child advocate and negotiates services from educational, health, social, or financial resources with support of the medical home.

ROLE OF COMMUNITY

Successful community-based care requires knowledge of community resources that support the healthy development of children and advocacy. The physician in the medical home must know the eligibility requirements for various health, education, and social-welfare programs. Without this knowledge, barriers to care coordination and interagency collaboration will be difficult to overcome.

The Maternal Child Health Bureau plays an important role through Title V in integrating the system of care for CSHCN and improving performance measures and outcomes in each state. Programs that promote the system of care include (1) Individuals with Disabilities Education Act through its early childhood programs (Zero to Three—individualized family service plans), (2) public schools through the development of an individualized educational plan, and (3) Medicaid and Early Periodic Screening Diagnosis and Treatment through periodic well-child supervision visits that include screening and surveillance. These programs provide a safety net for children, especially those growing up in poverty, and they assist parents in maximizing their child's development.[5] An appropriate measurement of quality of care provided by the medical home, family, and community is the Medical Home Index from the Center for Medical Home Improvement (www.medicalhomeimprovement.org/). This Index offers helpful guidelines for the primary care physician in becoming an effective medical home. It blends improvement strategies with progressive measurement of the *medical homeness* of the individual practice. It quantifies how well the practice partners with the family in the process of coordinating care for CSHCN.[10]

CONCLUSION

The medical home plays a vital role in support of comprehensive, coordinated, and collaborative care for children. Comprehensive care requires a detailed understanding of the medical home concept; knowledge of the physical, mental, social, and behavioral needs of children; and recognition of community resources. Care coordination calls for the medical home to:

1. Develop an anticipatory and proactive integrated plan for appropriate services for the child and family.
2. Assist the parents in accessing needed services and resources.
3. Facilitate communication among multiple professionals.
4. Avoid duplication of services and unnecessary costs.
5. Optimize the physical and emotional health and well being of the child.
6. Improve the child's and the family's quality of life.[5]

The medical home and collaborative care offers the knowledgeable, caring, and compassionate primary care physician the ability to address the needs of the whole child and family in the community and to adapt to the challenges of the 21st century's new morbidity.

TOOLS FOR PRACTICE

Community Advocacy and Coordination

- *Medical Home Mentorship Program* (Web page), American Academy of Pediatrics (www.medicalhomeinfo.org/model/index.html).
- *Medical Home Surveillance and Screening Activities* (Web page), American Academy of Pediatrics (www.medicalhomeinfo.org/screening/index.html).

Engaging Patient and Family

- *The Medical Home and Early Intervention Programs* (booklet), American Academy of Pediatrics (www.medicalhomeinfo.org/health/Downloads/ElBrochureF.pdf).

Medical Decision Support

- *Bright Futures* (Web page), Bright Futures (brightfutures.aap.org/web/).
- *Every Child Deserves a Medical Home Training Curriculum* (curriculum), American Academy of Pediatrics (www.medicalhomeinfo.org/training/index.html).
- *Maternal and Child Health Bureau* (Web page), Maternal and Child Health Bureau (mchb.hrsa.gov/).
- *Medical Home Initiatives & Resources by State* (Web page), American Academy of Pediatrics (www.medicalhomeinfo.org/states/index.html).
- *Medical Home–Tools for Providers* (Web page), American Academy of Pediatrics (www.medicalhomeinfo.org/tools/providerindex.html).
- *What is the Individualized Family Service Plan?* (fact sheet), North Bay Regional Center (www.nbrc.net/plan.html).

Practice Management and Care Coordination

- *Care Coordination Measurement Tool* (form), American Academy of Pediatrics (www.medicalhomeinfo.org/tools/Tools/Final MH CC Measurement Tool.doc).
- *Enhancing Collaboration Between Primary and Subspecialty Care Providers for Children and Youth with Special Health Care Needs* (booklet), Antonelli R, Stille C, and Freeman L, Georgetown University Center for Child and Human Development (www.medicalhomeinfo.org/publications/Downloads/Primary_Specialty_Collaboration.pdf).
- *Individuals with Disabilities Education Act (IDEA)* (Web page), US Department of Education (idea.ed.gov/).
- *Medical Home Index* (booklet), Center for Medical Home Improvement (www.medicalhomeimprovement.org/outcomes.htm).

RELATED WEB SITES

- *Center for Medical Home Improvement* (Web page), Center for Medical Home Improvement (www.medicalhome-improvement.org/default.htm).
- *Healthy and Ready to Work Center* (Web page), Healthy and Ready to Work Center (www.hrtw.org).
- *The National Center for Medical Home Initiatives for Children with Special Needs* (Web page), American Academy of Pediatrics (www.medicalhomeinfo.org/index.html).
- *Utah MedHome Portal* (Web page), Utah Collaborative Medical Home Project (medhomeportal.org/).
- *Washington State Medical Home* (Web page), Washington Department of Health and Washington State Medical Home Leadership Network (www.medicalhome.org/index.cfm).
- *Zero to Three* (Web page), Zero to Three (www.zerotothree.org/site/PageServer).

AAP POLICY STATEMENTS

American Academy of Pediatrics Committee on Fetus and Newborn, American College of Obstetricians and Gynecologists, and Committee on Obstetric Practice. The Apgar Score. *Pediatrics*. 2006;117(4):1444-1447. (aappolicy.aappublications.org/cgi/content/full/pediatrics;117/4/1447).

American Academy of Pediatrics Committee on Fetus and Newborn. Noninitiation or Withdrawal of Intensive Care for High-Risk Newborns. *Pediatrics*. 2007;119(2):401-403. (aappolicy.aappublications.org/cgi/content/full/pediatrics;119/2/401).

American Heart Association. Guidelines for Cardiopulmonary Resuscitation (CPR) and Emergency Cardiovascular Care (ECC) of Pediatric and Neonatal Patients: Pediatric Basic Life Support. *Pediatrics*. 2006;117(5):e1029-e1038. AAP endorsed.

MacDonald H and American Academy of Pediatrics Committee on Fetus and Newborn. Perinatal Care at the Threshold of Viability. *Pediatrics*. 2002;110(5):1024-1027. (aappolicy.aappublications.org/cgi/content/full/pediatrics;110/5/1024).

REFERENCES

1. Sia CCJ, Tonniges TF, Osterhus E, et al. History of medical home concept. *Pediatr Suppl.* 2004;113:1473-1478.
2. McPherson M, Arango P, Fox H, et al. A new definition of children with special health care needs. *Pediatrics.* 1998;102:137-139.
3. Palfrey JS, Tonniges T, Green M, et al. Introduction: addressing the millennial morbidity—the context of community pediatrics. *Pediatr Suppl.* 2005;115:1121-1123.
4. American Academy of Pediatrics, Medical Home Initiatives for Children with Special Needs Project Advisory Committee. The medical home. *Pediatrics.* 2002;110:184-186.
5. American Academy of Pediatrics, Council on Children with Disabilities. Care coordination in the medical home: integrating health and related systems of care for children with special health care needs. *Pediatrics.* 2005;116:1238-1241.
6. National Center of Medical Home Initiatives for Children with Special Health Care Needs Program. *Every Child Deserves a Medical Home Training Program: Practices, Policies, and Procedures.* Rev ed. Elk Grove Village, IL: American Academy of Pediatrics; 2003.
7. American Academy of Pediatrics, American Academy of Family Physicians, American College of Physicians-American Society of Internal Medicine. A consensus statement on health care transitions for young adults with special health care needs. *Pediatrics.* 2002;110:1304-1306.
8. National Center of Medical Home Initiatives for Children with Special Health Care Needs. *Every Child Deserves a Medical Home Training Program: Family-Professional Partnerships.* Rev ed. Elk Grove Village, IL: American Academy of Pediatrics; 2003.
9. National Center of Medical Home Initiatives for Children with Special Health Care Needs. *Comprehensive, Coordinated, Collaborative Care.* Rev ed. Elk Grove Village, IL: American Academy of Pediatrics; 2003. Appendix B 1-6: National Center of Medical Home Initiatives for Children with Special Health Care Needs.
10. Cooley WC, McAllister JW. Building medical homes: improvement strategies in primary care for children with special health care needs. *Pediatrics.* 2004;113:1499-1506.

Chapter 9

COMMUNITY-WIDE APPROACHES TO PROMOTING CHILD HEALTH

C. Andrew Aligne, MD, MPH; Jeffrey M. Kaczorowski, MD; Laura Jean Shipley, MD

HISTORY AND DEFINITION OF COMMUNITY PEDIATRICS

"It is especially important now for pediatricians to reexamine and reaffirm their role as professionals in the community—as community pediatricians—and prepare themselves for it, just as diligently as they prepare for traditional clinical roles."

AMERICAN ACADEMY OF PEDIATRICS[1]

Early in the 20th century, Abraham Jacobi, MD (1830-1919), *the father of American pediatrics,* had already noted that child health was influenced by community factors. In 1968, Robert J. Haggerty, MD, defined the term *community pediatrics* as "taking responsibility for all children in a community, providing preventive and curative services and understanding the determinants and consequences of child health and illness."[2] To improve the health of children, Haggerty noted that pediatricians must become partners with other child advocates and community leaders.[3,4] Now, in the early 21st century, with many new medical threats to children such as obesity and type 2 diabetes, appreciation for the importance of community-wide approaches to promoting child health is growing.[5,6]

COMMUNITY DIMENSIONS OF MEDICAL PRACTICE AND LIFE AS A PHYSICIAN

"It is more important to know what sort of patient has a disease, than to know what sort of disease a patient has."

SIR WILLIAM OSLER

A community-level perspective, which combines clinical practice and public health principles, can lead to better quality of medical care by broadening the physician's understanding of why illness occurs. A paradigm that includes environmental and social causes will often lead to the right diagnosis and treatment in a more efficient, faster, and better way than the standard biological approach. This concept is true for difficult cases, often described in the pediatric journals, in which a thorough social history would have prevented weeks of illness, hospitalization, and invasive testing. However, this notion also applies to common issues such as recurrent otitis media, in which effectively addressing passive smoking can do more good than surgery, antibiotics, or repeating standard health advice.[7] Simply knowing how to refer families for local nonmedical resources (smoking-cessation programs, battered women shelters, mental health care providers, youth activities) can be of great benefit in many cases. Furthermore, listening to families in a more comprehensive way will not only improve the quality of care, but also enhance the physician-patient relationship, helping decrease the risks and costs of malpractice litigation while making practice more enjoyable. For many individuals, medical practice has become a stressful ordeal when it can be a rewarding calling.[8] People generally choose a career in medicine because they want to help others. However, the rigors of medical education and the financial and time pressures of office practice can often dehumanize physicians and turn medicine into a mundane job.[9,10] Participation in community activities allows physicians to remember why they chose the medical profession in the first place and to feel a renewed sense of personal fulfillment.[11]

COMMUNITY DIMENSIONS OF HEALTH AND DISEASE

"Inferior doctors treat the disease of a patient. Mediocre doctors treat the patient as a person. Superior doctors treat the community as a whole."

HUANG DEE, NAI-CHANG, CHINA
(FROM THE 1ST MEDICAL TEXT, 2600 BC)

In the last century, a major shift has occurred from acute infectious diseases (especially affecting children) to chronic noninfectious diseases (affecting mainly adults). This shift is called the *epidemiologic transition*. According to Dr. Thomas McKeown, this movement represents a shift from "diseases of lack" to "diseases of excess."[12] Infectious diseases are related to lack of food, housing, sanitation, and other necessities, whereas chronic diseases are related to excesses of food, drugs, pollution, and other factors. In this paradigm, the best way to decrease sickness in the developing world is to improve supplies of necessities such as food and clean water, and the best way to decrease illness in the industrialized world is to decrease nonnecessities such as smoking and junk food. At the population level, advanced medical care does not make much of a difference when compared with the effect of social and environmental factors.[13] Modern medical care benefits individual patients, and the public health paradigm improves the health of an entire community.

Behaviors established before or during adolescence (smoking, overeating, inactivity, and violence, among other elements) are major risk factors for adult disease. In other words, improving adult health means changing behaviors in children. A person might even say, "Everything is pediatric." The average life span is much longer now than it was 200 years ago: approximately 75 years instead of approximately 40. Most of the increased average life span is due to a decrease in childhood mortality that occurred before the existence of antibiotics or other tools of modern medicine.

The health of a community is partially dependent on accessible medical services.[14] Other significant determinants of health include genetics, the physical environment, the social environment, an individual's active and passive behaviors, and public policies and interventions that influence all of these factors.[15,16] The major killer in this country—heart disease—has risk factors other than biomedical ones that affect outcome;[17] smoking, alcohol consumption, diet, and exercise are behavioral factors. Factors in the physical environment that can affect heart disease risk are exposure to pollutants (secondhand smoke) and neighborhood features that make exercising and eating healthy foods easier or harder.[18] When considering potential interventions for improving individual or public health, the pediatric primary care physician should focus on modifiable risk factors. For instance, although respiratory syncytial virus is everywhere each year, only some people, under certain conditions, will become ill as a result of exposure. The infectious disease is not caused just by the virus (agent), but also by problems with the patient (host) and the patient's life conditions (environment). Perhaps the baby was premature (host factor), or perhaps the infant is living in crowded housing (environmental factor). This combination of agent, host, and environmental factors has been termed the *epidemiologic triangle*. Once the paradigm of a single, specific cause for a specific disease is understood to be overly limiting, the fact becomes clear that respiratory syncytial virus alone does not cause clinical bronchiolitis, and other avenues for effective intervention can then be uncovered.

An example of successful large-scale application of community health concepts is the campaign to reduce the sudden infant death syndrome (SIDS) epidemic. SIDS is the major cause of death of infants between 1 month and 1 year of age. The National Institutes of Health has spent millions of dollars on animal experiments and other basic science research to uncover the cause of SIDS. However, epidemiologic research led to the discovery of prone sleeping as a risk factor and the subsequent highly successful *Back to Sleep* campaign led by the American Academy of Pediatrics (AAP) that cut United States SIDS mortality in half.[19] (See Chapter 330, Sudden Infant Death Syndrome.) Of note, prone sleeping became commonplace because of unsupported recommendations from physicians who thought it would help by decreasing gastric reflux. Many thousands of children's lives were saved by using an evidence-based epidemiologic approach instead of relying on a theory-based biomedical model. Effective prevention, including changing of health behaviors, is possible and powerful but generally requires a concentrated, population-based approach.[20,21]

APPLYING COMMUNITY HEALTH PRINCIPLES IN THE COMMUNITY

> *"There are no specific diseases. There are specific disease conditions."*
>
> FLORENCE NIGHTINGALE

The task of identifying risk and protective factors for any issue begins by studying the existing literature. One of the main barriers to physician involvement in community activities is the impression that problems are too big to tackle. This impression is based on the often-repeated reality of well-intentioned people creating and running programs that fail because they do not have an evidence base for their activities. Bloodletting, which seems insane now, was the standard of care in this country approximately 100 years ago. Practicing in the absence of evidence is similar to driving blindfolded; the driver might get to the destination safely, but the likelihood that someone would be killed is increased. The same principle is true in public health practice; evidence-based information exists to guide the implementation of public health programs proven to be of value. One health department decided to address the issue of large numbers of people drowning each year in the community. The assumption was made, quite reasonably, that people drown because they do not know how to swim. The health department launched a huge program to teach swimming. Not only did drownings not go down, they actually went up. How can such a debacle be prevented?

In 5 minutes, anyone can find out what works to decrease drowning at a population level.

- Go online to PUBMED, the free version of Medline (www.pubmed.gov).
- Search the site for *drowning/ep, pc* (for epidemiology, prevention, and control).
- Scan the article titles. For example, a recent systematic review conducted for an AAP policy statement may seem particularly relevant.
- Click on that entry for a full-text version of the article. Discover that no evidence exists for swimming lessons, which, indeed, may actually be harmful at a population level and that decent evidence exists for pool fences.

- Notice that other resources, such as a journal that recently devoted an entire issue to drowning prevention, are available.
- Click on *Related Articles* to focus the search results, if necessary.

Thus a search of the evidence-based literature reveals that fencing pools is an effective public health measure, whereas teaching more people how to swim is not. Very rarely, nothing will be known about the issue or intervention in which you are interested.

PRACTICAL COMMUNITY ACTIVITIES FOR BUSY PEDIATRICIANS

> *"Example is not the main thing in influencing others. It is the only thing."*
>
> Dr. Albert Schweitzer, Nobel Peace Prize winner

Perceived time constraints and a lack of adequate funding prevent many pediatricians from participating in community-based activities. Nevertheless, making a huge difference is often possible, even with small investments of time or money. Building a new adolescent clinic in the inner city can be a life's work for an individual. However, this same person can be on the board of directors of that particular teen clinic by going to a lunch meeting once every 3 months, and the lunch will even be free. Other examples of activities that make a difference for children but that take less than an hour a month are listed later in this chapter. Most community-based organizations (CBOs) and government agencies that work on children's health issues have no pediatricians involved at all and are generally welcoming of physician participation. Leveraging professional status and pediatric expertise by partnering with an existing CBO is a way to dramatically multiply the return on the time invested in the community.

The following 10 community pediatric activities take approximately 1 hour per month or less:

1. Vote!
2. Donate to a political campaign or a not-for-profit organization. Donating will cost money but takes no time. Donations to nonprofit groups are tax deductible.
3. Keep a resource guide of agencies in the community for referral for patients.
4. Cancel subscriptions to magazines in the waiting room that advertise cigarettes.
5. Sign up at *ListServes.com*. The easiest way to write a letter to government representatives is to have someone else write it. The document is signed and sent by clicking a button. Although evidence has shown that most elected officials do not respond, react to, or even read mass mailings of generic letters from *ListServes.com*, seen as too impersonal, their staff tabulates the numbers of such mailings and reports these numbers to the legislators. Telephone calls, letter to the editors, and face-to-face meetings are more fruitful. Such a service is easily set up by signing up for the e-mail of an organization you support. People in the organization will keep track of important issues and do much of the work. To join the AAP Federal Advocacy Action Network, see www.aap.grassroots.org.
6. Make the Web site for the local newspaper the home page on your computer's Internet account so that quick updates on events in the community can be received.
7. If any stocks are owned, then vote the proxy ballots. Mercury thermometers were recently phased out of pharmacies in part because of shareholder activism.
8. Practice passive activism. Some forms of action on behalf of kids take no time. For example, *Save the Children* bank checks can be obtained; a percentage of the money spent for checks contributes to advocacy for kids. Acquiring credit cards that donate a portion of each purchase to the AAP or other nonprofits is also possible.
9. Vote with shopping dollars. Consumer choices have social implications. What kind of car affects air pollution or increases dependence on foreign oil? The location of a house determines where property taxes go. Some clothes are made by companies that exploit children. Awareness of the political implications of purchases can offer pain-free ways of making a difference.
10. Attend once-a-year fundraising events for local charities that benefit children.

The following activities take a little more time commitment, in blocks of a few hours every now and then, but can still be done effectively in approximately 12 hours a year.

- **Visit with, write to, or call a public official.** Original letters printed on paper count more than mass e-mails. Telephone calls count even more. In-person visits are the most effective. Politicians care about getting reelected; they do not want to alienate the people who are respected by every mother in town. Pediatricians who advocate for children's health make an impression. Most people contact their representatives to advocate for themselves, not for others. Take care to differentiate between advocating for pediatricians and advocating for children.
- **Write a letter to the editor.** Letters to the editor are read carefully and tallied by politicians, and they often have more effect in your community than might be expected. A little humor or a good anecdote will help get the letter published. Given that this communication is public, avoid attacking any individuals, and focus on the positive.
- **Testify before official bodies.** Testifying before the city council or county legislature usually requires making a telephone call, having the caller's name placed on a list, and then showing up for an hour or so to talk for 2 minutes. Giving testimony does not require being a great orator or a distinguished professor. A pediatric primary care physician knows more about pediatrics than the county supervisor. A dozen physicians advocating to stop something that harms children will often be enough to block a bad policy.
- **Gain representation on boards and councils.** Many local children's nonprofit organizations would be overjoyed to have a pediatrician on the board of directors. Being on a nonprofit board

often requires simply showing up for quarterly lunch meetings.

- **Register voters.** Children's needs are often neglected because children cannot vote, and young parents often do not vote. Having a box of registration slips in the waiting room can help remedy this imbalance.
- **Serve as a media spokesperson for a CBO.** Physicians have instant credibility. One local pediatric resident became a media expert on children's nutrition just because she was a physician volunteering with a food bank. Not much time was needed for her to talk to reporters, but it was a huge boost of free publicity for her CBO's cause.

A note on public speaking: Most elements of public speaking can be practiced before standing in front of an audience. Many books, audio programs, and training seminars can be used to improve public speaking skills. Additionally, the not-for-profit group called Toastmasters can be helpful. Public speaking, as with anything, becomes easier with practice. Starting out small in a way that is comfortable and speaking briefly on a well-known and important topic is helpful. (See AAP Media training materials www.aap.org/moc/pressroom/handbook.htm [AAP member password required].)

The point of this chapter is to emphasize how small commitments of time or money can make a big difference. Obviously, larger commitments can make even bigger differences.[22] Many physicians make significant investments in their communities by volunteering, regularly working at free clinics, or starting an organization for a specific cause. For example, being a school physician or member of the school board allows a pediatrician to influence school health and nutritional policies significantly. The AAP Community Access to Child Health (CATCH) grants have been used to help develop home visiting programs, family resource centers, and other programs that promote child and family wellness. Some pediatricians even run for high office.[23] As of this writing, a pediatrician was just elected President of Chile.

CONCLUSION: EVERYTHING IS COMMUNITY PEDIATRICS

> *"What is needed is a realization that power without love is reckless and abusive, and love without power is sentimental and anemic."*
>
> MARTIN LUTHER KING, JR

Historically, community-level social and environmental characteristics have been the major determinants of child health and therefore of population health. Pediatricians who partner with CBOs on issues about which they are passionate and who follow evidence-based public health practices can leverage small investments of time into huge positive effects on children's health. If 60,000 pediatricians commit an hour or 2 a month, on average, a million hours a year of community action would be available for children.[24]

Although the *Back to Sleep* program was a success, the United States still has the highest infant mortality rate in the industrialized world.[25] The factors responsible for this statistic are modifiable but are not addressed by medical interventions alone. For their dedication to children's health to be more than *sentimental and anemic,* pediatricians need to step out of their offices and take up leadership roles in their communities.

SUGGESTED RESOURCES

Ambulatory Pediatrics Association. *Training Residents to Serve the Underserved: A Resident Education Curriculum.* McLean, VA: Ambulatory Pediatric Association; 1993.

Botash AS, Weinberger HL. Academia's role in community access to child health. *Pediatrics.* 1999;103:1424-1425.

Browner WS. *Publishing and Presenting Clinical Research.* Baltimore, MD: Williams & Wilkins; 1999.

Carnegie D. *The Quick and Easy Way to Effective Speaking.* Garden City, NY: Dale Carnegie & Associates; 1962.

Hoff R. *Do Not Go Naked into your Next Presentation: Nifty Little Nuggets to Quiet the Nerves and Please the Crowd.* Kansas City, MO: Andrews & McMeel; 1997.

Kaczorowski J, Aligne CA, Halterman JS, et al. A block rotation in community health and child advocacy: improved competency of pediatric residency graduates. *Ambul Pediatr.* 2004;4:283-288.

Lewis BA. *The Kid's Guide to Social Action: How To Solve the Social Problems You Choose—and Turn Creative Thinking Into Positive Action.* Minneapolis, MN: Free Spirit Publishing; 1998.

Nader PR, Kaczorowski J, Tonniges T, et al. Education for community pediatrics. *Clin Pediatr (Phila).* 2004;43:505-521.

Shope TR, Bradley BJ, Taras HL. A block rotation in community pediatrics. *Pediatrics.* 1999;104:143-147.

Sinetar M. *Do What You Love, The Money Will Follow.* Mahwah, NJ: Paulist Press; 1987.

Twist L. *The Soul of Money: Transforming Your Relationship With Money and Life.* New York, NY: WW Norton & Company; 2003.

TOOLS FOR PRACTICE

Community Advocacy and Coordination

- *A Pediatrician's Guide to Proposal Writing* (booklet), American Academy of Pediatrics (www.aap.org/commpeds/resources/proposalwriting.pdf).
- *AAP Advocacy Web Page* (Web page), American Academy of Pediatrics (www.aap.org/advocacy.html).
- *AAP Chapter Web sites* (Web page), American Academy of Pediatrics (www.aap.org/member/chapters/chapserv.htm).
- *AAP Communications Handbook* (booklet), American Academy of Pediatrics (www.aap.org/moc/index.cfm).
- *Toastmasters International—Become the Speaker and Leader You Want to Be* (Web page), Toastmasters International (www.toastmasters.org/).
- *Community Access To Child Health (CATCH)* (Web page), American Academy of Pediatrics (www.aap.org/catch/).
- *Community Pediatrics Bibliography* (booklet), American Academy of Pediatrics (www.aap.org/commpeds/resources/bibliography_tableofcontents.htm).
- *Community Pediatrics State Resource Page* (Web page), American Academy of Pediatrics (www.aap.org/commpeds/state_resources/index.html).
- *Community Pediatrics Training Initiative (CPTI)* (Web page), American Academy of Pediatrics (www.aap.org/commpeds/cpti/default.htm).

- *Community Resources and Tools* (Web page), American Academy of Pediatrics (www.aap.org/commpeds/resources/index.html).
- *Healthy People 2010* (Web page) US Department of Health and Human Services (www.healthypeople.gov/).
- *Healthy Tomorrows Partnership for Children Program (HTPCP)* (Web page), American Academy of Pediatrics (www.aap.org/commpeds/htpcp/overview.html).
- *Kids Count Data Book* (Web page), Anne E Casey Foundation (www.aecf.org/kidscount/sld/databook.jsp).
- *Media Center for Members* (Web page), American Academy of Pediatrics (www.aap.org/moc/index.cfm).
- *School Health Leadership Training Kit for Pediatricians* (Web page), American Medical Association (www.schoolhealth.org/trnthtrn/trainmn.html).
- *The Community Guide* (Web page), Centers for Disease Control and Prevention (www.thecommunityguide.org/).
- *The Community Toolbox* (Web page), University of Kansas (ctb.ku.edu/).
- *The Pediatric Links with the Community Program* (Web page), University of Rochester (www.plccare.org/).

Medical Decision Support

- *APA Educational Guidelines for Pediatric Residency* (Web page), Ambulatory Pediatric Association (www.ambpeds.org/egwebnew/index.cfm?cfid=985340&cftoken=36531429).
- *The Cochrane Collaboration* (Web page), The Cochrane Collaboration (www.cochrane.org/index.htm).

AAP POLICY STATEMENTS

American Academy of Pediatrics and the Medical Home Initiatives for Children With Special Needs Project Advisory Committee. The medical home. *Pediatrics*. 2002;110(1):184-186. (aappolicy.aappublications.org/cgi/content/full/pediatrics;110/1/184).

American Academy of Pediatrics, Committee on Community Health Services. The pediatrician's role in community pediatrics. *Pediatrics*. 2005;115(4):1092-1094. (aappolicy.aappublications.org/cgi/content/full/pediatrics;115/4/1092).

REFERENCES

1. American Academy of Pediatrics, Committee on Community Health Services. The pediatrician's role in community pediatrics. *Pediatrics*. 2005;115:1092-1094.
2. Haggerty RJ. Community pediatrics. *N Engl J Med*. 1968;278:15-21.
3. Haggerty RJ, Roghmann KJ. *Child Health and the Community*. 2nd ed. New Brunswick, NJ: Transaction Publishers; 1993.
4. Haggerty RJ, Aligne CA. Community pediatrics: the Rochester story. *Pediatrics*. Apr 2005;115(4):1136-1138.
5. Palfrey JS, Tonniges TF, Green M, et al. Introduction: addressing the millennial morbidity—the context of community pediatrics. *Pediatrics*. 2005;115(4:2):1121-1123.
6. Satcher D, Kaczorowski J, Topa D. The expanding role of the pediatrician in improving child health in the 21st century. *Pediatrics*. 2005;115(4:2):1124-1128.
7. Byrd RS, Hoekelman RA, Auinger P. Adherence to AAP guidelines for well-child care under managed care. *Pediatrics*. 1999;104:536-540.
8. Remen RN. *Kitchen Table Wisdom: Stories That Heal*. New York, NY: Riverhead Books; 1996.
9. Marion R. *The Intern Blues: The Private Ordeals of Three Young Doctors*. New York, NY: Faucett Crest; 1989.
10. Wear D, Bickel J, eds. *Educating for Professionalism: Creating a Culture of Humanism in Medical Education*. Iowa City, IA: University of Iowa Press; 2002.
11. Chin NP, Aligne CA, Stronczek A, et al. Evaluation of a community-based pediatrics residency rotation using narrative analysis. *Acad Med*. 2003;78:1266-1270.
12. McKeown T. *The Origins of Human Disease*. Oxford, UK: Basil Blackwell; 1988.
13. McKeown T. *The Role of Medicine: Dream, Mirage, or Nemesis?* Princeton, NJ: Princeton University Press; 1979.
14. Kindig D, Stoddard G. What is population health? *Am J Public Health*. 2003;93:380-383.
15. Marmot MG, Wilkinson RG, eds. *Social Determinants of Health*. New York, NY: Oxford University Press; 1999.
16. Aligne CA, Auinger P, Byrd RS, et al. Risk factors for pediatric asthma: contributions of poverty, race, and urban residence. *Am J Respir Crit Care Med*. 2000;162:873-877.
17. Sagan LA. *The Health of Nations: True Causes of Sickness and Well-Being*. New York, NY: Basic Books; 1987.
18. Rose G. Sick individuals and sick populations. *Int J of Epidemiol*. 1985;14:32-38.
19. Duggan A, Jarvis J, Derauf DC, et al. The essential role of research in community pediatrics. *Pediatrics*. 2005;115(4):1195-1201.
20. Sanders LM, Robinson TN, Forster LQ, et al. Evidence-based community pediatrics: building a bridge from bedside to neighborhood. *Pediatrics*. 2005;115(4:2):1142-1147.
21. Chamberlin RW. Preventing low birth weight, child abuse, and school failure: the need for comprehensive, community-wide approaches. *Pediatr Rev*. 1992;13:64-71.
22. Burton OM. Community-level child health: a decade of progress. *Pediatrics*. 2005;115(4:2):1139-1141.
23. Maier T. *Dr. Spock: An American Life*. New York, NY: Basic Books; 1998.
24. Aligne CA, Kaczorowski J. Afterword. *Pediatrics*. 2005;115(4):1212.
25. Maternal and Child Health Bureau. Child health USA 2002: Comparison of National Infant Mortality Rates. Available at: www.mchb.hrsa.gov/chusa02/main_pages/page_22.htm. Accessed September 28, 2007.

Chapter 10

CARING FOR FAMILIES NEW TO THE UNITED STATES

Paul L. Geltman, MD, MPH; Glenn Flores, MD

INTRODUCTION

The United States is a nation of immigrants. Since 1820, an estimated 69,869,450 people have immigrated to the United States.[1] Currently, 3,206,290 foreign-born children live in the United States, accounting for 1 in 23 American children.[2] This chapter provides a comprehensive approach to providing high quality health care to immigrant children. Recent detailed reviews of immigrant health care have focused on screening tests and checklists.[3,4] In addition to reviewing important medical and health-promotion topics for immigrant children, this chapter addresses basic demographics, barriers to health care, and linguistic and cultural issues for immigrant and refugee children in the United States.

DEMOGRAPHICS OF IMMIGRANTS AND REFUGEES

From 2001 to 2004, 3,780,019 immigrants entered the United States, and 160,537 more received refugee status or political asylum.[1] In 2004, 946,142 immigrants and asylees received legal status in the United States. The 5 largest countries of origin of immigrants to the United States are (in order) Mexico, India, Philippines, China, and Vietnam (Figure 10-1). Most US immigration is through family sponsorship, with 43% being immediate family members of US citizens and 23% receiving family sponsorship (Figure 10-2).

Official immigration figures, however, do not account for the large numbers of undocumented immigrants living and working in the United States. Among the estimated 12 million undocumented immigrants in the United States, 16%, or 1.8 million, are children.[5]

ACCESS TO HEALTH CARE IN THE UNITED STATES

The pediatric primary care physician should consider financial issues and insurance coverage when providing care to immigrant families. For example, more than one half (51%) of low-income noncitizen children are uninsured, compared with approximately one sixth (16%) of children in citizen families.[6] Low-income noncitizen children are approximately 3 times as likely to be uninsured as similar children in citizen families, and approximately one quarter (24%) of low-income noncitizen children participate in Medicaid or the State Children's Health Insurance Program, compared with approximately one half of citizen children (50% for citizen children in noncitizen families and 47% for citizen children in citizen families). The American Academy of Pediatrics advocates the provision of "comprehensive, coordinated, and continuous health services provided within a medical home..." for immigrants and awareness of and sensitivity to financial and other barriers that "interfere with achieving optimal health status."[7] An unfortunate start to a pediatrician's relationship with new patients who are uninsured immigrants would be to perform a large battery of screening laboratory tests, which would financially burden the family.

Studies of Latino children indicate a wide variety of other access barriers to care for immigrant children. For example, a study of a predominantly immigrant Latino population revealed that more than one quarter of parents (26%) said that language problems were the single greatest barrier to getting health care for their child (specifically, 15% of parents said that the greatest obstacle was physicians and nurses who do not speak Spanish, and 11% cited lack of interpreters).[8] A long wait at the physician's office was reported as the greatest barrier by 15%, 13% mentioned the lack of medical insurance, 7% cited difficulty paying for medical bills, and 6% identified transportation. Study parents also identified several barriers to care that had caused them not to bring their child in for medical visits in the past; transportation problems were reported most often (21%), followed by not being able to afford health care (18%), excessive waits to see the physician (17%), lack of health insurance (16%), inconvenient clinic hours (14%), difficulty making appointments (13%), and culture and language problems (11%).

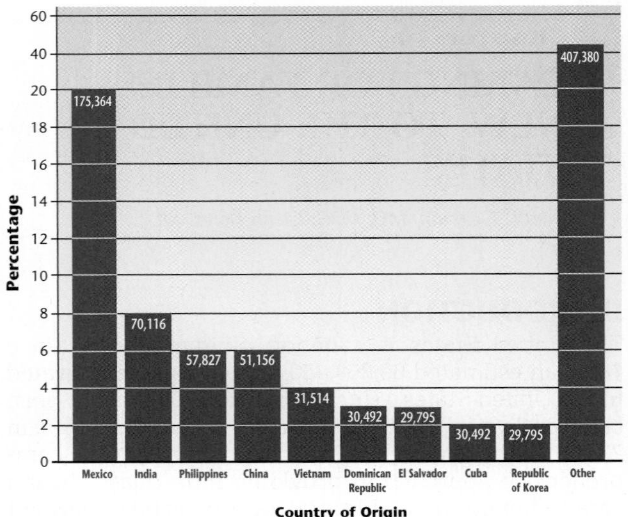

Figure 10-1 Top countries of origin of immigrants to the United States—2004

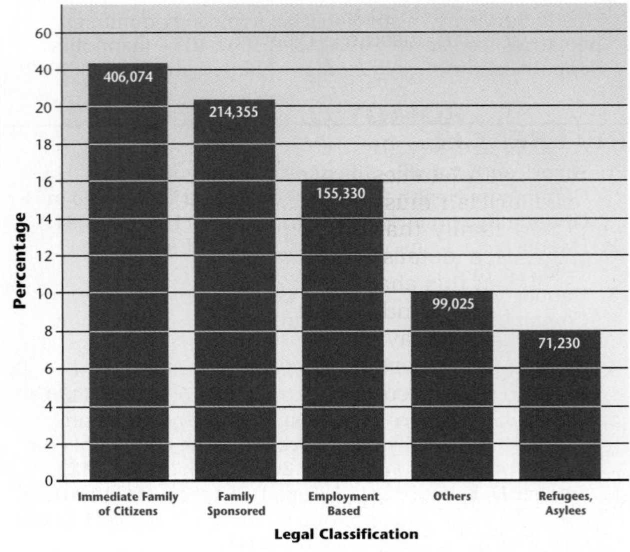

Figure 10-2 Distribution of legal classifications of immigration visa sponsorship for immigrants to the United States in 2004.

Access to primary care and other medical services can be highly variable among immigrant communities. Ethnic minorities and low-income children in the United States consistently have had significantly worse rates of having a usual source of care and other indicators.[9] In addition, specific ethnic groups have varying levels of access to and use of health care even within their own communities.[10] These differences, independent of income and educational levels, suggest a strong role for cultural and linguistic factors in determining use of care. As such, outreach to ethnic communities and assistance with clinic interpretation are important steps in facilitating initiation into care.

Other research on the largest racial/ethnic group among US immigrants, Latinos, suggests that health insurance status is a major determinant of access to and use of care.[11] A large study of Latinos in Los Angeles found that employment-linked health insurance posed a significant barrier to care for children.[12] Many Latino immigrant children live in two-parent households, with parents (particularly noncitizens) working in entry level jobs without benefits or the ability to afford health care insurance premiums. Similarly, children with working parents who were still eligible for Medicaid were less likely than others to be continuously enrolled. Children in this category also had less access to care in all measures studied.

Since these studies were done, federal welfare and immigration reform legislation in 1998 further restricted access to Medicaid for noncitizens to reduce expenditures and discourage immigrants from becoming public charges. Nonetheless, recent research documented that in the 2 years before enactment of this legislation, immigrants had substantially lower *per capita* health care expenditures (55%) than their US-born counterparts.[13] Among children, the expenditures were 74% lower among immigrants; yet rates of expenditures for emergency room services were 3 times higher. The latter finding suggests that immigrant children are going without basic primary care services and are missing out on the benefits of a medical home.

HEALTH PROMOTION

Two tasks are key for the primary care pediatrician working with families new to the United States. First, the pediatrician must establish relationships with the child and family that are linguistically and culturally effective (see details on cultural competency action steps later in this chapter). By showing interest in the families' background, culture, and community issues, the pediatrician may also gain a reputation as a sympathetic and supportive physician whom other members of that ethnic community can trust. The following section describes in more detail the issues associated with this task. An important point to remember is that postponing other aspects of medical screening is reasonable if it seems inappropriate based on cultural, linguistic, or economic reasons.

Second, the pediatrician must begin a process of health promotion and preventive medicine that may be new to the family. This process is informed by knowledge of the family's home and social circumstances with which the pediatrician can assess the level of need for environmental intervention and injury prevention. Between trying to understand the cultural expectations of immigrant patients and families and introducing concepts of health promotion and preventive medicine, the clinician will embark on a journey of communication with new Americans. This journey may be relatively straightforward and brief with patients and families who share more Western beliefs, or it may involve multiple levels of complexity that will require a fair amount of time and effort.

LANGUAGE BARRIERS TO CARE AND PROVIDING ADEQUATE LANGUAGE ACCESS

Approximately 52 million Americans speak a language other than English at home, and 23.1 million are limited English proficient (LEP), defined as a self-rated English-speaking ability of less than "very well."[14] The 2000 US Census revealed that approximately 10 million US school-aged children (5 to 17 years) speak a language other than English at home (or 19%), almost triple the number reported in 1979, and 3.5 million (7%) are LEP.[15] Between 1990 and 2005, the number of people in the United States speaking a language other than English at home increased from 31.8 million to 52 million, and the number of Americans who are LEP rose from 14 million to 23.1 million.

This marked growth in the number of Americans who speak a language other than English at home or who are LEP can be attributed to the rapid increase in the foreign-born population in the United States, which grew from 9.6 million in 1970 to 28.4 million in 2000.[16] The vast majority of LEP Americans (64%, or 13.8 million) speak Spanish; Asian and Pacific Island languages (led by Chinese) are the next most common among LEP Americans (comprising 17%, or 3.6 million), followed by other Indo-European languages (16%, or 3.4 million), and all other languages (3%, or 600,000).[17]

Language barriers have many adverse consequences in health care,[18,19] including impaired health status,[20,21] a lower likelihood of having a usual source of medical care,[18,19,22] lower rates of screening and other preventive services,[22-24] nonadherence with medications,[25] a greater likelihood of a diagnosis of more severe psychopathology and leaving the hospital against medical advice among psychiatric patients,[26,27] a lower likelihood of being given a follow-up appointment after an emergency department visit,[28] an increased risk of intubation in asthmatic children,[29] an increased risk of drug complications,[30] higher resource utilization for diagnostic testing,[31] lower patient satisfaction,[18,32,33] impaired patient understanding of diagnoses, medications, and follow-up,[34,35] fewer telephone calls to physicians offices,[36] fewer referrals to specialists,[36] and an increased risk of medical errors and injuries.[37-40] Latino parents consider the lack of interpreters and Spanish-speaking staff to be the greatest barriers to health care for their children, and 1 out of every 17 parents in one study reported not bringing their child in for needed medical care because of these language issues.[8]

To assess the language needs of patients and caregivers accurately, determining whether a child's

BOX 10-1 Key Mechanisms for Ensuring Adequate Language Access for Patients, Caregivers, and Families With Limited English Proficiency

- **A trained medical interpreter or bilingual provider should be available for each medical encounter.** Providing language services that are available throughout the encounter is especially important, including during registration, the history and physical, procedures, visits to the laboratory and radiology, and scheduling follow-up appointments.
- **Use telephone interpreter services when in-person interpreters or bilingual providers are unavailable.**
- **Ensure adequate language access *door-to-door* (ie, at all points of interaction with the health care system).** This provision includes multilingual operators, telephone trees, or both (for scheduling appointments, leaving messages and getting phone advice), multilingual signage at all key wayfaring points (parking garages, clinic entrances, registration, paths to the emergency department, laboratory, radiology, and the pharmacy), and multilingual registration clerks.
- **Routinely collect and record patient and family data on primary language spoken at home and LEP.** This provision permits efficiently meeting the language needs of the patient population and scheduling interpreters in advance for all future medical visits.
- **Use pharmacies that can print prescription labels, provide medication information packets, and communicate in non-English languages.** Failure to do so can result in documented medical errors and injuries.[37-40] Printing clinic prescription pads with checkboxes such as ☐ *Spanish* or ☐ *Chinese* is particularly helpful and a useful reminder.
- **Have patient information and anticipatory guidance pamphlets available in non-English languages common in the physician's practice.** Ideally, certified translators should be available to translate written documents for patients. Useful Web resources with materials already translated include the National Network of Libraries of Medicine Other Language Resources site (nnlm.gov/outreach/consumer/multi.html), US Department of Health and Human Services' Español-Healthfinder (www.healthfinder.gov/espanol/), CDC en Español (www.cdc.gov/spanish/), and Health Information in Chinese Uniting Patients, Physicians and the Public (library.med.nyu.edu/patient/hicup/).
- **Translate consent forms into all relevant non-English languages for your patient population.**
- **Help LEP patients and families to learn English through referrals to free or low-cost English as 2nd-language courses.** This excellent resource (www.literacydirectory.org) locates classes according to the family's zip code.
- **Increase the number of bilingual health care providers and staff.** This provision can be achieved through enhanced efforts to recruit bilingual staff, continuing professional education, intensive language courses, and bonuses for demonstrating foreign language fluency.

caregiver is LEP is essential. LEP has been shown to be superior to the primary language spoken at home as a measure of the impact of language barriers on children's health and health care.[41] The following questions, which come from the US Census,[17] are an excellent means of quickly assessing LEP and language needs and should be asked routinely of the primary caregiver during the 1st visit:

1. Does this person speak a language other than English at home?
   - Yes
   - No *[Stop here; person is considered English proficient]*
2. What is this language?
   (For example: Korean, Italian, Spanish, Vietnamese)
3. How well does this person speak English?
   - Very well
   - Well
   - Not well
   - Not at all

   [Person is LEP if reply is anything other than "Very well" and requires medical interpreter or bilingual provider.]

Although millions of Americans are LEP, many patients who need medical interpreters are not provided with interpreters. Every LEP patient should have access to a trained medical interpreter or bilingual health care provider.[42] Ample scientific evidence documents that optimal communication, patient satisfaction, and outcomes and the fewest interpreter errors occur when LEP patients have access to trained professional interpreters or bilingual providers.[18] In addition, federal guidance on Title VI of the Civil Rights Act of 1964 has established that denial or delay of medical care for LEP patients because of language barriers constitutes a form of discrimination and requires all recipients of federal funds, including Medicaid, State Children's Health Insurance Program, and Medicare, to provide adequate language assistance to LEP patients.[43] Key mechanisms for ensuring adequate language access for LEP patients and families are summarized in Box 10-1.

Detailed information on improving language access in health care is available in the Office of Minority Health's "A Patient-Centered Guide to Implementing Language Access Services in Healthcare Organizations."[44]

CULTURAL ISSUES

Cultural issues affect multiple aspects of pediatric care, including outcomes, quality, costs, satisfaction with care, and patient safety.[39,45,46] Failing to appreciate the importance of culture in pediatrics can result in a variety of adverse consequences, including difficulties with informed consent, miscommunication, inadequate understanding of diagnoses and treatment plans by families, dissatisfaction with care, preventable morbidity and mortality, unnecessary child abuse evaluations, and disparities in prescriptions, analgesia, and diagnostic evaluations.[39,45,46] On the other hand, providing culturally competent health care to children is associated with better health outcomes. For example, pediatric patients with asthma receiving care at practice sites with the highest cultural competence scores are significantly less likely to be underusing preventive asthma medications and have better parental ratings of the quality care.[47]

Because culture can profoundly affect the care of immigrant children, pediatric primary care physicians should be familiar with the most important cultural issues that affect clinical care, including (1) folk illnesses with symptoms that overlap with biomedical conditions, (2) biomedical conditions that can result from harmful folk illness remedies or parental beliefs and practices, and (3) cultural healing practices that can be confused with child abuse.[39,45,46] Tables 10-1 through 10-3 are organized so that the clinicians can immediately locate cultural information relevant to their prevalent patient populations. These 3 tables can be helpful in obtaining accurate histories and improving patient satisfaction through the use of culturally acceptable alternative treatments (see Table 10-1 on page 64), generating rapid differential diagnoses and treatment plans (see Table 10-2 on page 66), and making informed decision about child abuse (see Table 10-3 on page 69).

Cultural competency is defined as the recognition of and appropriate response to key cultural features that affect clinical care.[39,45] Providing culturally competent health care should be the goal of every clinician caring for immigrant children. Box 10-2 summarizes a model of cultural competency that can be helpful in clinical encounters with patients from any cultural group.

Helpful Web-based resources for addressing the cultural issues in pediatric care include DiversityRX (www.diversityrx.org), the Office of Minority Health's Web site (www.omhrc.gov), and the University of Michigan Health System's Program for Multicultural Health (www.med.umich.edu/multicultural/ccp/culture.htm).

GROWTH AND NUTRITION

Growth abnormalities and nutritional disorders are among the most common health problems of immigrant children, particularly refugees,[48] adoptees,[49] and immigrants from similarly deprived backgrounds. Common nutritional disorders such as iron deficiency may be seen in the majority of some populations of immigrant children, such as young refugees. Nutritional deficiencies such as in iron and calcium may also predispose immigrant and refugee children to susceptibility to environmental toxins such as lead.[50,51] Other disorders such as rickets, vitamin A deficiency,[52] and iodine deficiency and goiters may also be quite common in some populations.

With hunger and food insecurity well documented among US immigrant and refugee populations,[53] the primary care physician must assess growth and nutritional status of immigrant and refugee children. Eligible families should be referred to available programs for nutritional support, such as The Special Supplemental Nutrition Program for Women, Infants, and Children and subsidized school meals programs. A multivitamin with iron and minerals is likely to be beneficial for most immigrant children. Clinicians should closely monitor nutritionally deprived children for catch-up growth (seen even in longitudinal growth in some cases)[54] and developmental disorders, such as precocious puberty that have been associated with rapid catch-up.[55] Conversely, those at risk of overweight may be seen in some immigrant populations that reflect socioeconomic conditions and lifestyles in countries of origin that range from the formerly socialist countries of Eastern Europe[48] to the urban environments of Sub-Saharan Africa.[56]

All immigrant children should have complete blood counts performed, and those younger than 7 years should have their blood lead levels evaluated. Because a risk of acquiring elevated blood lead after arrival in the United States has been documented among refugees,[51,57] testing should be repeated after 90 days. This testing is appropriate even in parts of the United States that generally do not have significant environmental lead contamination. Regardless of the region in the United States, new American children face the unknown risk posed by the use of traditional medicines and other culturally specific practices that may expose children of many different immigrant populations to lead. These types of exposures for immigrant children have been documented repeatedly over the years in the *Morbidity and Mortality Weekly Report*. The Centers for Disease Control and Prevention's (CDC) Web site (www.cdc.gov/nceh/lead/) contains information about lead poisoning among refugee and immigrant children.

ORAL HEALTH

A high prevalence of dental caries has been documented among immigrant[58,59] and refugee children.[60] Many immigrants will lack experience with preventive oral health measures, including topical fluoride and water fluoridation, and face significant barriers to care in the United States. Research on the effect of acculturation on oral health practices among refugees and immigrants has demonstrated that the many LEP immigrants often adopt American lifestyle behaviors that are associated with poor oral health outcomes while giving up protective behaviors from their home countries.[61] However, because of LEP and partial acculturation, these immigrants do not fully adopt Western preventive oral health practices.[62,63]

The primary care physician can play an important role in promoting healthy personal oral hygiene practices and supporting traditional customs and related behaviors (eg, breastfeeding, diets low in refined sugar, use of chewing sticks with antimicrobial properties) that may provide oral health, nutritional, and other benefits to the child while also promoting proven oral hygiene practices in the United States (eg, ensuring consumption of fluoridated water or oral supplementation, use of fluoride-containing toothpaste). Other office-based practices, such as application of fluoride varnish on young immigrant children, appear promising but lack evidence to support their implementation

Table 10-1 Selected Folk Illnesses With Symptoms That Overlap With Biomedical Conditions Affecting the Health Care of Children

REGIONAL ORIGIN	FOLK ILLNESS	ETHNICITY OR NATIONALITY THAT MAY HAVE FOLK ILLNESS BELIEF	SYMPTOMS OF FOLK ILLNESS	BIOMEDICAL CONDITIONS THAT OVERLAP WITH FOLK ILLNESS
Latin America	*Empacho* (and *pega*)	Latino	Vomiting, stomach pain, headache, abdominal distention, loss of appetite, diarrhea, fever, crying	Gastroenteritis, viral infections, milk allergy, appendicitis, intussusception, anatomic obstruction
	Caida Mollera	Latino	Diarrhea, excessive crying, fever, loss of appetite, irritability, fallen fontanelle	Gastroenteritis, dehydration, sepsis, meningitis
	Susto	Latino	Drowsiness, insomnia, irritability, exaggerated startle reflex, diarrhea, anorexia, fever, nightmares	Persistent symptoms after pesticide toxicity
	Mal Ojo, Quebrante or *Olhado*	Latino Brazilian	Inconsolable crying, fever, diarrhea, vomiting, pain, gassy stomach	Gastroenteritis, dehydration
	Quebranto	Costa Rican	Irritability, crying, leg-length discrepancy	Developmental dysplasia of the hip
	Doença de Criança	Brazilian	Diarrhea, fallen fontanelle, convulsions, cyanosis, crying, vomiting (and 17 other less common symptoms)	Gastroenteritis, dehydration, malaria, bacterial meningitis, dengue, measles, pneumonia
	Ventre Caido	Brazilian	Vomiting, diarrhea, loss of appetite, fatigue, cough	Gastroenteritis, dehydration
Africa	*Nyènkènè bilènkè*	Mali	Red urine	Schistosomiasis
	Umsheko	Swaziland	Wet, loose, nongreen stools accompanied by grumbling stomach, loss of appetite, vomiting	Gastroenteritis, dehydration
	Kuhabula	Swaziland	Sunken fontanelle, loss of strength, vomiting, crying, ribs *appear to come together*	Gastroenteritis, dehydration
	Umphezulu	Swaziland	Green or yellow diarrhea, unusual crying, loss of appetite, distended stomach or navel, grumbling stomach, sunken fontanelle, blood vessels visible on stomach or forehead	Gastroenteritis, dehydration
Indian subcontinent	*Mandama*	Singhalese (Sri Lanka)	Diarrhea, abdominal distention, lethargy, *lean legs*	Gastroenteritis, dehydration
	Dud haga	Rural Bangladesh	Watery stools, crying, abdominal pain	Gastroenteritis, dehydration
	Ajirno	Rural Bangladesh	Diarrhea, abdominal distention, gripping of the stomach	Gastroenteritis, dehydration
	Amasha	Rural Bangladesh	Mucoid and sometimes bloody diarrhea	Gastroenteritis, dehydration, dysentery
	Daeria	Rural Bangladesh	Frequent stools with rice-water appearance, sunken eyes, thirst, vomiting, reduced urine output, weakness	Cholera, gastroenteritis, dehydration

Table 10-1 Selected Folk Illnesses With Symptoms That Overlap With Biomedical Conditions Affecting the Health Care of Children—cont'd

REGIONAL ORIGIN	FOLK ILLNESS	ETHNICITY OR NATIONALITY THAT MAY HAVE FOLK ILLNESS BELIEF	SYMPTOMS OF FOLK ILLNESS	BIOMEDICAL CONDITIONS THAT OVERLAP WITH FOLK ILLNESS
	Phrooey	Northern Pakistan	Green diarrhea, blisters on body, infections of the ear and eye	Gastroenteritis, dehydration
	Sarishna	Northern Pakistan	Green watery stools, burning yellow urine, weakness, eyes turned upward	Gastroenteritis, dehydration
	Loose motions	Northern Pakistan	White watery stools, fallen fontanelle	Gastroenteritis, dehydration
	Sardawan	Northern Pakistan	Frequent green watery stools, sunken eyes, weakness	Gastroenteritis, dehydration
	Maleeh	Northern Pakistan	Yellow or green watery stools	Gastroenteritis, dehydration
	Saya or *parchawan*	Northern Pakistan	Persistent green, whiter, or yellow diarrhea	Gastroenteritis, dehydration
	Nazar (evil eye)	Northern Pakistan	Green watery stools, fever, sunken eyes, dry lips, weak extremities	Gastroenteritis, dehydration
	Kand-pota (fallen fontanelle)	Northern Pakistan	Watery green stools, vomiting	Gastroenteritis, dehydration
	Sardi or *Padsa*	Marathas (India)	Cough, runny nose, congested chest, fever	Mild upper respiratory infection
	Potat ala	Marathas (India)	Labored respirations, stomach "going up and down," fever, phlegm, cough, congested chest	Moderate to severe respiratory infections, including pneumonia
	Paltha dabba	Marathas (India)	Tight or hard stomach (worse at night), cough, eyes closed, nostrils flare, fisted hands	Severe pneumonia
	Phagyra vat	Marathas (India)	Tight or hard stomach, anorexia, constipation	Moderate to severe respiratory infections, including pneumonia
Asia and Pacific Islands	*Kitsune-tsuki* (fox possession)	Japanese	Delusions, disordered thinking, auditory hallucinations, paranoia	Psychosis, schizophrenia
	Piang	The Philippines	Cough, fever	Acute respiratory infection, including pneumonia
	Naeng	Korea	Vaginal discharge, back pain, cold hands and feet, abdominal pain, vaginal itching	Vaginal candidiasis, sexually transmitted diseases

Adapted from Flores G, Rabke J, Pine W, et al. The importance of cultural and linguistic issues in the emergency care of children. *Pediatr Emerg Care.* 2002;18:271-284. Copyright © Lippincott Williams & Wilkins. Reprinted by permission.

Table 10-2 Biomedical Conditions in the Health Care of Children that Can Result from Harmful Folk Illness Remedies or Parental Beliefs and Practices

REGIONAL ORIGIN	CONDITION	ASSOCIATED FOLK ILLNESS, PARENTAL BELIEF, OR SYMPTOM	ETHNICITY OR NATIONALITY THAT MAY HAVE FOLK ILLNESS OR PARENTAL BELIEF	HARMFUL TREATMENT ASSOCIATED WITH CONDITION	CULTURALLY ACCEPTABLE ALTERNATIVE FOLK TREATMENTS
Latin America	Lead poisoning	*Empacho*	Latinos	Powders containing lead oxides *(azarcón, greta, albayalde)*	Abdominal massage with warm oil, mint tea
	Subdural hematoma	*Caida de mollera*	Latinos	Infant shaken while held upside down with head partially immersed in boiling water	Put soap foam on fontanelle Gently push up on palate
	Gonococcal conjunctivitis	Conjunctivitis	Latinos[b]	Adult urine as treatment for conjunctivitis in children	Special diet: vegetable soup and fresh fruits, carrot juice, eliminate flour tortillas, bread, soda
	Disseminated *Salmonella arizona* infections	Sinus and skin conditions, diarrhea, infections, itchy feet, AIDS, diabetes, connective tissue diseases, heart disease, cancer	Latinos	Capsules or powder containing dried ground rattlesnake, raw dried rattlesnake meat: *polvo de vibora, carne de vibora, vibora de cascabel*	Variety of harmless, disease-specific herbal preparations
	Hepatic veno-occlusive disease	Cough	Latinos	*Gordolobo yerba,* tea made from herb *Senecio longilobus,* which contains hepatotoxic pyrrolizidine alkaloids	Herbal teas using small amounts of oregano, cinnamon, or chamomile (not sweetened with honey)
Africa	Wound infection or cellulitis around infant's umbilicus	*Umphezulu* (type of diarrhea)	Swaziland (Africa)	*Traditional* vaccination *(kugata):* razor blade cuts made around infant's umbilicus rubbed with ashes	Herbal teas
	Urinary retention, dysuria, urinary tract infections, incontinence, fever, menstrual difficulties, cysts, abscesses, fistulae, obstetric complications; vaginal pain, bleeding discharge	Reasons cited by cultures for practice: tradition, group identity or norms, chastity, marital reasons, hygiene	Widespread in 33 African nations, most commonly Somalia, Djibouti, Ethiopia, Eritrea, Sudan, Sierra Leone; certain Islamic peoples in Asia, Middle East	Female circumcision, genital mutilation, *Sunna,* infibulation, Pharaonic circumcision, traditional or ritual female genital surgery	Education regarding health risks; discuss culturally-acceptable alternatives with community or religious groups; advocacy against procedure by community, religious, women's and law organizations; use of least damaging procedure

Table 10-2 Biomedical Conditions in the Health Care of Children that Can Result from Harmful Folk Illness Remedies or Parental Beliefs and Practices—cont'd

REGIONAL ORIGIN	CONDITION	ASSOCIATED FOLK ILLNESS, PARENTAL BELIEF, OR SYMPTOM	ETHNICITY OR NATIONALITY THAT MAY HAVE FOLK ILLNESS OR PARENTAL BELIEF	HARMFUL TREATMENT ASSOCIATED WITH CONDITION	CULTURALLY ACCEPTABLE ALTERNATIVE FOLK TREATMENTS
					(such as small nick/incision of prepuce) in families insisting on practice
Indian subcontinent[c]	Dehydration	*Dud haga*	Bangladesh	1. Breastfeeding discontinued because (a) breast milk considered *poisoned* by shadow, evil eye, black magic, new pregnancy, illness, diet, cold; (b) pseudoscientific laboratory *breast milk analysis* reveals pus, germs, mobile bacteria, or blood (Pakistan) 2. Reduce child's oral intake of liquid because liquid believed to worsen diarrhea or vomiting feared	Mother avoids eating green vegetables, fish, meat
		Nazar	Pakistan	Give formula until breast milk no longer considered *poisonous*	
		Eshwaha, diarrhea in general	Sri Lanka		Apply *chanted oil* (available from folk healers, Buddhist priests); Education
	Burns in circular pattern on abdomen	*Phugrya va* (respiratory illness)	India	Burning acidic seed *(biba)* in circle on abdomen	Rub ghee (clarified butter) on abdomen
	Lead poisoning (including death)	Maintenance of infant health	India	Lead-containing tonics, such as *ghasard,* with lead concentration up to 1.6%	Education; ascertain whether multivitamin drops are acceptable replacement
	Lipoid pneumonia, bronchiectasis	Cleaning airway of newborn; treatment of respiratory infections		Apply butter or oil to nostrils or oropharynx	Replace with saline drops

Adapted from Flores G, Rabke J, Pine W, et al. The importance of cultural and linguistic issues in the emergency care of children. *Pediatr Emerg Care.* 2002;18:271-284. Copyright © Lippincott Williams & Wilkins. Reprinted by permission.

[a]Biomedical condition that can result from harmful folk illness remedies or parental beliefs and practices.

[b]Ethnicity of affected children not explicitly stated in study.

[c]Certain ethnic groups from these regions may also practice female circumcision, which is described as one of the conditions in the African region.

Continued

Table 10-2 Biomedical Conditions in the Health Care of Children that Can Result from Harmful Folk Illness Remedies or Parental Beliefs and Practices—cont'd

REGIONAL ORIGIN	CONDITION	ASSOCIATED FOLK ILLNESS, PARENTAL BELIEF, OR SYMPTOM	ETHNICITY OR NATIONALITY THAT MAY HAVE FOLK ILLNESS OR PARENTAL BELIEF	HARMFUL TREATMENT ASSOCIATED WITH CONDITION	CULTURALLY ACCEPTABLE ALTERNATIVE FOLK TREATMENTS
Middle East[c]	Lead poisoning (including encephalopathy, death)	Teething Cosmetics	Saudi Arabia Kuwait Oman	Teething powders: *Saoott, Cebagin* Cosmetics: *Koh* Other: *Bint al dahab*	Teething powders or solutions without lead
	Lipoid pneumonia, bronchiectasis	Cleaning airway of newborn; treatment of respiratory infections	Saudi Arabia	Apply butter or oil to nostrils or oropharynx	Replace with saline drops
	Hypernatremia (fatal)	Healthy newborn skin	Turkey	Salting infant's skin or placing salt in swaddling material before swaddling	Education regarding health risks
Asia and Pacific Islands[c]	Lead Poisoning	Fever, rash	Hmong (Cambodia)	*Pay-loo-ah,* a red or orange powder with lead concentration of 1-80% (and occasionally arsenic)	Education regarding risks; replacement with culturally-acceptable harmless herbal preparations
	Life-threatening bradycardia; respiratory and central nervous system depression	Chinese herbal medicine used for analgesia by parents	Chinese	Unintentional poisoning due to ingestion of *Jin Bu Huan* tablets, Chinese herbal medicine used for analgesia by adults, containing L-THP (potent dopamine receptor antagonist, sedative)	Parental education regarding potential toxicity for children
	Opiate toxicity in infants	Diarrhea	Hmong	Enema made from opium seeds, unidentified capsule	Education regarding risks; culturally acceptable harmless herbal preparations

Adapted from Flores G, Rabke J, Pine W, et al. The importance of cultural and linguistic issues in the emergency care of children. *Pediatr Emerg Care.* 2002;18:271-284.

[a]Biomedical condition that can result from harmful folk illness remedies or parental beliefs and practices.

[b]Ethnicity of affected children not explicitly stated in study.

[c]Certain ethnic groups from these regions may also practice female circumcision, which is described as one of the conditions in the African region.

Table 10-3 Cultural Healing Practices That Can Be Confused With Child Abuse

REGIONAL ORIGIN	CLINICAL PRESENTATION	CULTURAL PRACTICE	ETHNICITY OR NATIONALITY ASSOCIATED WITH PRACTICE	SYMPTOMS OR ILLNESSES TREATED
Latin America	Patterned circular erythema, petechiae, occasional burns	Cupping *(ventosas):* create vacuum in cup by burning alcohol over inverted cup, place cup on affected anatomy	Latino	Pain, fever, poor appetite, congestion
Asia and Pacific Islands	Circular burns (2nd or 3rd degree) and scars	Moxibustion: moxa herb or yarn rolled into ball or cone, ignited, applied to body part and allowed to burn to point of pain	Laotian Cambodian Chinese Japanese	Fever, abdominal pain, ear infections, enuresis, temper tantrums
	Linear ecchymoses, hyperpigmentation, transient microscopic hematuria	*Cao Gio (scratch the wind),* or coin rubbing: symptomatic area covered with mentholated oil or balsam, then rubbed linearly with coin or other object until ecchymoses occurs	Vietnamese	Fever, cough, vomiting, headaches, chills, seizures, myalgias
	Linear ecchymoses	*Quat Sha (spoon scratching):* porcelain spoon used to rub skin on back (after water or saline applied) until ecchymoses appear	Chinese	Fever, headache

Adapted from Flores G, Rabke J, Pine W, et al. The importance of cultural and linguistic issues in the emergency care of children. *Pediatr Emerg Care.* 2002; 18:271-284. Copyright © Lippincott Williams & Wilkins. Reprinted by permission.

as a cost-effective measure in primary care practices.[64] In addition, the primary care physician should facilitate entry into routine dental care for children.

BEHAVIORAL HEALTH AND FUNCTIONAL HEALTH SCREENING

Mental health and behavioral problems are common among immigrant and refugee children, in part, because many such families experience traumas. In 1 large meta-analysis of studies of internationally adopted children, researchers found an elevated prevalence of behavioral problems and use of mental health services compared with nonadopted children.[65] Behavioral disorders among traumatized immigrant families may be difficult to diagnose and treat in primary care settings. Even in situations in which parents identify behavioral symptoms in their children, parents may be reluctant to have children treated for behavioral disorders because of cultural beliefs or concerns about immigration status.[66] Cultural factors may likely present similar challenges for diagnosing and treating behavioral disorders among nontraumatized children as well. Many immigrants and refugee families will visit their medical clinicians with symptoms or complaints such as headache or stomachache because of underlying behavioral or emotional problems or somatization.

Somatization is common in many cultures around the world. Studies have documented the high prevalence of somatization and its association with increased clinic visits in immigrant and refugee communities in the United States.[67,68] Caring for patients with somatization may be challenging.[69] However, the clinician's validation of the impairment from somatic symptoms and focus on functional improvement may facilitate the establishment of trust necessary for uncovering the emotional basis for the symptoms. In the setting of pediatric primary care, the clinician may find simple screening instruments such as the Pediatric Symptom Checklist (www.mgh.harvard.edu/allpsych/pediatricsymptomchecklist/psc_home.htm) or the Child Health Questionnaire (www.healthact.com) helpful in documenting functional impairment from somatization and behavioral health problems, although language and literacy barriers can be problematic with immigrant and refugee communities. Such screening may obviate the need

BOX 10-2 Model for Cultural Competency in Health Care

1. Normative cultural values
   - Identify values that affect care.
   - Accommodate for these values in clinical encounter.
2. Language issues
   - Use interpreter services unless fluent in patient's primary language.
   - Follow guidelines for effective interpreter use.
   - Encourage efforts to increase foreign language skills of staff and English skills of LEP patients
3. Folk illnesses
   - Recognize those that may affect clinical care.
   - Suggest alternatives to harmful folk remedies.
   - Accommodate nonjudgmentally into clinical encounter.
   - Integrate into biomedical treatment plan whenever possible.
4. Parent and patient beliefs
   - Identify beliefs that may affect clinical care.
   - Suggest alternatives to harmful home remedies.
   - Carefully explain etiology and treatment rationale for given biomedical condition.
5. Provider practices
   - Maintain vigilance for ethnic disparities in screening, prescriptions, procedures, and outcomes.
   - When disparities occur, determine problems source and address practices that might be responsible.

From Flores G, Abreu M, Schwartz I, et al. The importance of language and culture in pediatric care: case studies from the Latino community. *J Pediatrics.* 2000;137:842-848. Copyright © Lippincott Williams & Wilkins. Reprinted by permission.

for use of disease-specific diagnostic questionnaires that are either too lengthy for practical use or may be emotionally upsetting to patients and families. Resources and on-line training for primary care physicians wishing to work with traumatized immigrants (or any patients who are survivors of significant violence) are also available from the Harvard Program in Refugee Trauma (www.hprt-cambridge.org).

SCREENING TESTS FOR INFECTIOUS DISEASES

Parasitic Infections

Many important diseases have nearly world-wide distributions and high prevalence among immigrant and refugee populations. When considering laboratory testing, the clinician must weigh the degree of risk posed by the condition to the patient (including its level of acuity), the patient's insurance status, and the prevalence of the condition among populations from the geographic origin of the patient. For example, stool microscopy for ova and parasites will be indicated for many immigrants; however, clinicians might consider ordering only fluorescent staining for *Giardia* for patients from the formerly socialist, industrialized countries of Eastern Europe in which the risk of helminth infection is quite low. Additionally, the peripheral eosinophil count is a simple test that can give the clinician insight into the possibility of invasive parasite infections.

For patients from tropical climates in which the risk of helminths is high, empiric treatment with albendazole has been shown to be cost effective[70] and is used overseas by the CDC for refugees.[71] The CDC has also recommended empiric treatment of some African refugee populations (Southern Sudanese and Somali Bantu) for strongyloidiasis and schistosomiasis (www.cdc.gov/ncidod/dq/refugee_health.htm). Empiric treatment for helminthes, strongyloides, and schistosome can be accomplished in a single day with 1 oral dose of albendazole, 1 dose of ivermectin, and 2 doses of praziquantel. Because of a potentially life-threatening but rare side effect of ivermectin when used in patients with *Loa loa* infection, an alternate regimen for African immigrants from regions with endemic loaisis includes albendazole twice per day for 3 to 7 days and praziquantel as described previously.

Malaria

Recent literature[72,73] has documented a high prevalence of malaria among recent refugee arrivals from Africa. Among symptomatic cases, the triad of fever, splenomegaly, and thrombocytopenia were highly specific for malaria. Of note, a fairly high proportion of children with malaria were asymptomatic. In the report by Maroushek et al, 29% of children with malaria were asymptomatic. Because of the predominance of *Plasmodium falciparum* in most of Africa, individuals often will develop some immunity over time, thus reducing symptoms. Such is not the case with other forms of malaria that predominate in other parts of the world, particularly in Southeast Asia.

Primary care pediatricians should consider malaria testing of all refugees and immigrants from Sub-Saharan Africa and those from any malaria-endemic country who exhibit symptoms suggestive of malaria. Clinicians should test liberally, given that the Maroushek study found that no symptom, either alone or in combination with other symptoms, was predictive of the presence or absence of malaria. Guidelines for treatment of malaria, including criteria for determining severity level and eligibility for outpatient treatment, are available from the CDC (www.cdc.gov/malaria/diagnosis_treatment/tx_clinicians.htm). In addition, 24-hour consultation is available from the CDC at 770-488-7788 during weekday business hours and by page at 770-488-7100 after hours and on weekends and holidays.

Tuberculosis

Finally, tuberculosis infection is a major health issue for immigrant children. The foreign-born population increasingly comprises a disproportionate share of cases of active tuberculosis infection in the United States, with a case incidence closer to their country of origin for the first 5 years in the United States. Children, particularly younger children, are usually in the early stages of latent tuberculosis infection, with high likelihood of progression to active disease. All immigrant children from developing and formerly socialist countries should have tuberculin skin testing. If the child is significantly malnourished or immunocompromised, then the clinician should consider placing control tests (eg, *Candida* antigen) as well.[74]

Other highly prevalent infectious diseases that may warrant screening tests include hepatitis B, hepatitis C, HIV, syphilis (both congenital and sexually acquired), and other sexually transmitted diseases. Clinicians, again, should weight individual and geographic risk, as well as the expense and benefits for the patient, when considering such testing.

IMMUNIZATIONS AND SEROLOGIC TESTING

A safe presumption is that very few immigrant or refugee children seen as new patients in a pediatric practice will be up to date with US vaccine standards set by the CDC Advisory Committee on Immunization Practices (ACIP) (see www.cdc.gov/nip). Such is the case simply because newer vaccines used commonly in the United States are not available or used commonly in most other countries. Examples include vaccines for *Haemophilus influenzae, pneumococcus,* and *varicella*. In addition, many immigrants will not have adequate documentation of past vaccines. In some cases, documents may actually be fraudulent. Common problems include incomplete or inaccurate documentation of vaccine records, receipt of vaccines at unacceptable intervals or times, and poor immune response as a result of malnutrition. Immunization should be a priority for new immigrant children who may have school enrollment delayed pending completion of immunizations. The public health imperative for completing immunization is also illustrated by recent outbreaks of imported measles in Indiana[75] and Boston, the multistate mumps outbreak in the Midwest,[76] and congenital rubella syndrome in a refugee infant born in New Hampshire.[77] Regarding measles, mumps, and rubella, clinicians should be alert when reviewing records to receipt of vaccines with only 1 or 2 components and receipt of measles vaccine before age 1 year, as recommended by the World Health Organization for countries with endemic measles but not considered a valid dose by ACIP.

For younger children, clinicians should begin primary or catch-up immunization according to ACIP schedules. For school-aged children and adolescents who have insurance coverage, clinicians may choose a mixture of immunization and serologic testing for immunity to satisfy school and other requirements for proof of immunity. Studies of serotesting among refugees and immigrants have documented high levels of immunity to some diseases such as hepatitis B,[78] varicella, measles, and rubella.[79] In the case of varicella, serotesting before immunization is a cost-effective strategy.[80] Typically, seroprevalence will increase throughout childhood, with large increases at 1 year of age (for measles in particular) and at school age. By early adolescence, most immigrants will have either naturally acquired immunity or prior immunization for these diseases, except for hepatitis B, which will reflect the level of endemicity in the immigrant's country of origin. For hepatitis A vaccine, recommended for universal immunization by ACIP in 2006, most immigrants will have naturally acquired immunity if they lived in endemic regions until school aged.[81]

CONCLUSION

Primary care physicians caring for children new to the United States serve an important role as the gateway to the medical home. They must strike a balance between performing a screening examination function and promoting access to affordable health care that incorporates effective preventive measures. Language and cultural divides that separate clinician from patient may be bridged by providing access to language services for LEP patients and ensuring the delivery of culturally competent care. At the same time, clinicians should be attentive to the acute and chronic health issues specific to immigrant children and their families. By effectively screening for and treating these issues and promoting wellness with cultural sensitivity, the primary care physician can create strong bonds with immigrant families and communities and ensure that immigrant children receive the highest quality pediatric primary care with high levels of patient and parent satisfaction.

TOOLS FOR PRACTICE

Community Coordination and Advocacy

- *Spanish Centers for Disease Control and Prevention* (Web page), Centers for Disease Control and Prevention (www.cdc.gov/spanish/).

Medical Decision Support

- *Child Health Questionnaire* (questionnaire), Healthactchq Inc. (www.healthact.com/chq.html).
- *DiversityRX* (Web page), DiversityRX (diversityrx.org/HTML/DIVRX.htm).
- *Espanol-Healthfinder* (Web page), US Department of Health & Human Services (www.healthfinder.gov/espanol/).
- *Health Information in Chinese patient education documents,* (Web page), Health Information in Chinese Uniting Patients, Physicians, and the Public (library.med.nyu.edu/patient/hicup/).
- *Immigrant, Refugee and Migrant Health* (Web page), Centers for Disease Control and Prevention (www.cdc.gov/ncidod/dq/refugee/index.htm).
- *Lead* (Web page), Centers for Disease Control and Prevention (www.cdc.gov/lead/).
- *Malaria* (Web page), Centers for Disease Control and Prevention (www.cdc.gov/malaria/diagnosis_treatment/index.htm).
- *Measuring Trauma, Measuring Torture* (book), Harvard Program in Refugee Trauma (www.hprt-cambridge.org/).
- *Multicultural Health Generalizations* (Web page), University of Michigan Health System (www.med.umich.edu/multicultural/ccp/culture.htm).
- *National Immunization Program* (Web page), Centers for Disease Control and Prevention (www.cdc.gov/nip/default.htm-schedules).

- *Other Languages Resource* (Web page), National Network of Libraries of Medicine (nnlm.gov/outreach/consumer/multi.html).
- *Pediatric Symptom Checklist* (checklist), Michael Jellenik, M.D. and J. Michael Murphy, Ed.D. (www.mgh.harvard.edu/allpsych/PediatricSymptomChecklist/psc_home.htm).

AAP POLICY STATEMENTS

American Academy of Pediatrics, Committee on Community Health Services. Healthcare for children of immigrant familes. *Pediatrics*. 1997;100(1):153-156. (aappolicy.aappublications.org/cgi/content/full/pediatrics;100/1/153).

American Academy of Pediatrics, Medical Home Initiatives for Children with Special Needs Project Advisory Committee. The medical home. *Pediatrics*. 2002;110(1):184-186. (aappolicy.aappublications.org/cgi/content/full/pediatrics;110/1/184).

REFERENCES

1. US Department of Homeland Security. *Yearbook of Immigration Statistics: 2004*. Washington, DC: US Department of Homeland Security, Office of Immigration Statistics; 2006.
2. US Census Bureau. Detailed Tables. Available at: factfinder.census.gov/. Accessed August 7, 2006.
3. Adams KM, Gardener LD, Assefi N. Healthcare challenges from the developing world: post-immigration refugee medicine. *BMJ*. 2004;328:1548-1552.
4. Jenista JA. The immigrant, refugee, or internationally adopted child. *Pediatr Rev*. 2001;22:419-428.
5. Passel JS. *The Size and Characteristics of the Unauthorized Migrant Population in the U.S.: Estimates Based on the March 2005 Current Population Survey*. Washington, DC: Pew Hispanic Center; 2006. Available at: pewhispanic.org/files/reports/61.pdf. Accessed October 3, 2007.
6. Ku L. Report Documents Growing Disparities in Health Care Coverage Between Immigrant and Citizen Children as Congress Debates Immigrant Care Legislation. Center on Budget and Policy Priorities. Available at: www.cbpp.org/10-14-03health.htm. Accessed August 7, 2006.
7. American Academy of Pediatrics, Committee on Community Health Services. Providing care for immigrant, homeless, and migrant children. *Pediatrics*. 2005; 115:1095-1100.
8. Flores G, Abreu M, Olivar MA, et al. Access barriers to health care for Latino children. *Arch Pediatr Adolesc Med*. 1998;152:1119-1125.
9. Newacheck PW, Hughes DC, Stoddard JJ. Children's access to primary care: differences by race, income, and insurance status. *Pediatrics*. 1996;97:26-32.
10. Flores G, Bauchner H, Feinstein AR, et al. The impact of ethnicity, family income, and parental education on children's health and use of health services. *Am J Public Health*. 1999;89:1066-1071.
11. Hubell FA, Waitzkin H, Mishra SI, et al. Access to medical care for documented and undocumented Latinos in a Southern California county. *West J Med*. 1991;154:414-417.
12. Halfon N, Wood DL, Valdez RB, et al. Medicaid enrollment and health services access by Latino children in inner-city Los Angeles. *JAMA*. 1997;277:636-641.
13. Mohanty SA, Woolhandler S, Himmelstein DU, et al. Health care expenditures of immigrants in the United States: a nationally representative analysis. *Am J Public Health*. 2005;95:1431-1438.
14. US Census Bureau. US Census—2007. Selected Social Characteristics in the United States: 2005. Data Set: 2005 American Community Survey. Available at: factfinder.census.gov/. Accessed March 21, 2007.
15. US Census Bureau. Table 2. Language use, English ability, and linguistic isolation of the population 5 to 17 years by state: 2000. Available at: www.census.gov/population/cen2000/phc-t20/tab02.pdf. Accessed January 4, 2006.
16. US Census Bureau. Profile of the Foreign-Born Population in the United States: 2000. (Issued December, 2001). Available at: www.census.gov/prod/2002pubs/p23-206.pdf. Accessed June 5, 2007.
17. US Census Bureau. Language Use and English Speaking Ability: 2000. (Issued October, 2003). Available at: www.census.gov/prod/2003pubs/c2kbr-29.pdf. Accessed June 5, 2007.
18. Flores G. The impact of medical interpreter services on the quality of health care: a systematic review. *Med Care Res Rev*. 2005;62:255-299.
19. Flores G, Laws MB, Mayo SJ, et al. Errors in medical interpretation and their potential clinical consequences in pediatric encounters. *Pediatrics*. 2003;111:6-14.
20. Kirkman-Liff B, Mondragón D. Language of interview: relevance for research of southwest Hispanics. *Am J Pub Health*. 1991;81:1399-1404.
21. Hu DJ, Covell RM. Health care usage by Hispanic outpatients as a function of primary language. *West J Med*. 1986;155:490-493.
22. Weinick RM, Krauss NA. Racial/ethnic differences in children's access to care. *Am J Pub Health*. 2000;90:1771-1774.
23. Marks G, Solis J, Richardson JL, et al. Health behavior of elderly Hispanic women: does cultural assimilation make a difference? *Am J Psych Health*. 1987;77:1315.
24. Woloshin S, Schwartz L, Katz SJ, et al. Is language a barrier to the use of preventive services? *J Gen Intern Med*. 1997;12:472-477.
25. Manson A. Language concordance as a determinant of patient compliance and emergency room use in patients with asthma. *Med Care*. 1988;26:1119-1128.
26. Alpert M, Kesselman M, Marcos L, et al. The language barrier in evaluating Spanish-American patients. *Arch Gen Psychiatry*. 1973;29:655-659.
27. Baxter M, Bucci W. Studies in linguistic ambiguity and insecurity. *Urban Health*. 1981;June:36-40.
28. Sarver J, Baker DW. Effect of language barriers on follow-up appointments after an emergency department visit. *J Gen Intern Med*. 2000;15:256-264.
29. LeSon S, Gershwin ME. Risk factors for asthmatic patients requiring intubation. I. Observations in children. *J Asthma*. 1995;32:285-294.
30. Gandhi TK, Burstin HR, Cook EF, et al. Drug complications in outpatients. *J Gen Intern Med*. 2000;15:149-154.
31. Hampers LC, Cha S, Gutglass DJ, et al. Language barriers and resource utilization in a pediatric emergency department. *Pediatrics*. 1999;103:1253-1256.
32. Carrasquillo O, Orav EJ, Brennan TA, et al. Impact of language barriers on patient satisfaction in an emergency department. *J Gen Intern Med*. 1999;14:82-87.
33. Morales LS, Cunningham WE, Brown JA, et al. Are Latinos less satisfied with communication by health care providers? *J Gen Intern Med*. 1999;14:409-417.
34. Baker DW, Parker RM, Williams MV, et al. Use and effectiveness of interpreters in an emergency department. *JAMA*. 1996;275:783-788.
35. Crane JA. Patient comprehension of doctor-patient communication on discharge from the emergency department. *J Emerg Med*. 1997;15:1-7
36. Flores G, Olson L, Tomany-Korman SC. Racial and ethnic disparities in early childhood health and healthcare. *Pediatrics*. 2005;115;e183-e193.
37. Harsham P. A misinterpreted word worth $71 million. *Med Econ*. 1984;61:289-292.

38. Koren G, Barzilay Z, Greenwald M. Tenfold errors in administration of drug doses: a neglected iatrogenic disease in pediatrics. *Pediatrics*. 1986;77:848-849.
39. Flores G, Abreu M, Schwartz I, et al. The importance of language and culture in pediatric care: case studies from the Latino community. *J Pediatrics*. 2000;137:842-848.
40. Flores G. Language barrier. AHRQ WebM&M Morbidity and Mortality Rounds on the Web 2006; April. Available at: www.webmm.ahrq.gov/case.aspx?caseID=123. Accessed June 5, 2007.
41. Flores G, Abreu M, Tomany-Korman SC. Limited English proficiency, primary language spoken at home, and disparities in children's health and healthcare: how language barriers are measured matters. *Public Health Rep*. 2005;120:418-430.
42. Flores G. Language barriers to health care in the United States. *N Engl J Med*. 2006;355:229-231.
43. Hayashi D. Guidance Memorandum. January 29, 1998. Title VI Prohibition Against National Origin Discrimination—Persons with Limited-English proficiency. Available at: www.hhs.gov/ocr/lepfinal.htm. Accessed June 5, 2007.
44. American Institutes for Research. A Patient-Centered Guide to Implementing Language Access Services in Healthcare Organizations. Available at: www.omhrc.gov/assets/pdf/checked/hc-lsig.pdf. Accessed June 5, 2007.
45. Flores G. Culture and the patient-physician relationship: achieving cultural competency in health care. *J Pediatrics*. 2000;136:14-23.
46. Flores G, Rabke J, Pine W, et al. The importance of cultural and linguistic issues in the emergency care of children. *Pediatr Emerg Care*. 2002;18:271-284.
47. Lieu TA, Finkelstein JA, Lozano P, et al. Cultural competence policies and other predictors of asthma care quality for Medicaid-insured children. *Pediatrics*. 2004; 114:e102-e110.
48. Geltman PL, Radin M, Zhang Z, et al. Growth status and related medical conditions among refugee children in Massachusetts, 1995-1998. *Am J Public Health*. 2001; 91:1800-1805.
49. Albers LH, Johnson DE, Hostetter MK, et al. Health of children adopted from the former Soviet Union and Eastern Europe. Comparison with preadoptive medical records. *JAMA*. 1997;278:922-924.
50. US Department of Health and Human Services, Centers for Disease Control and Prevention. Elevated blood lead levels among internationally adopted children—United States, 1998. *MMWR*. 2000;49:97-100.
51. Geltman PL, Brown MJ, Cochran J. Lead poisoning among refugee children resettled in Massachusetts, 1995-1999. *Pediatrics*. 2001;108:158-162.
52. Seal AJ, Creke PI, Mirghani Z, et al. Iron and vitamin A deficiency in long-term African refugees. *J Nutr*. 2005; 135:808-813.
53. Kasper J, Gupta SK, Tran P, et al. Hunger in legal immigrants in California, Texas, and Illinois. *Am J Public Health*. 2000;90:1629-1633.
54. Yip R, Scanlon K, Trowbridge F. Improving growth status of Asian refugee children in the United States. *JAMA*. 1992;267:937-940.
55. De Monleon JV. Foreign adopted children growth follow-up. *Annales d Endocrinologie*. 2001;62:458-460.
56. Renzaho AMN. Fat, rich, and beautiful: changing socio-cultural paradigms associated with obesity risk, nutritional status and refugee children from sub-Saharan Africa. *Health & Place*. 2004;10:105-113.
57. US Department of Health and Human Services, Centers for Disease Control and Prevention. Elevated blood lead levels in refugee children—New Hampshire, 2003-2004. *MMWR*. 2005;54:42-45.
58. Pollick H, Rice A, Echenberg D. Dental health of recent immigrant children in the newcomer schools, San Francisco. *Am J Public Health*. 1987;77:731-732.
59. Sgan-Cohen HD, Steinberg D, Zusman SP, et al. Dental caries and its determinants among recent immigrants from rural Ethiopia. *Community Dent Oral Epidemiol*. 1992;20:338-342.
60. Cote S, Geltman P, Nunn M, et al. Dental caries of refugee children compared with U.S. children. *Pediatrics*. 2004;114:e733-e740.
61. Culhane-Pera KA, Naftali ED, Jacobson C, et al. Cultural feeding practices and child-raising philosophy contribute to iron-deficiency anemia in refugee Hmong children. *Ethn Dis*. 2002;12:199-205.
62. Cruz GD, Shore R, Le Geros RZ, et al. Effect of acculturation on objective measures of oral health in Haitian immigrants in New York City. *J Dent Res*. 2004;83:180-184.
63. Mariño R, Stuart GW, Wright FA, et al. Acculturation and dental health among Vietnamese living in Melbourne, Australia. *Community Dent Oral Epidemiol*. 2001;29:107-119.
64. Quinonez RB, Stearns SC, Talekar BS, et al. Simulating cost-effectiveness of fluoride varnish during well-child visits for Medicaid-enrolled children. *Arch Pediatr Adolesc Med*. 2006;160:164-170.
65. Juffer F, van Ijzendoorn MH. Behavior problems and mental health referrals of international adoptees. *JAMA*. 2005;293:2501-2515.
66. Geltman PL, Augustyn M, Barnett ED, et al. War trauma experience and behavioral screening of Bosnian refugee children resettled in Massachusetts. *J Dev Behav Pediatr*. 2000;21:257-263.
67. Lin EHB, Carter WB, Kleinman AM. An exploration of somatization among Asian refugees and immigrants in primary care. *Am J Public Health*. 1985;75:1080-1084.
68. Jamil H, Hakim-Larson J, Farrag M, et al. Medical complaints among Iraqi American refugees with mental disorders. *J Immigr Health*. 2005;7:145-152.
69. Perron JN, Hudelson P. How do junior doctors working in a multicultural context make sense of somatisation? *Swiss Med Wkly*. 2005;135:475-479.
70. Muennig P, Pallin D, Sell RL, et al. The cost effectiveness of strategies for the treatment of intestinal parasites in immigrants. *N Engl J Med*. 1999;340:773-779.
71. Miller JM, Boyd HA, Ostrowski SR, et al. Malaria, intestinal parasites, and schistosomiasis among Barawan Somali refugees resettling to the United States: a strategy to reduce morbidity and decrease the risk of imported infections. *Am J Trop Med Hyg*. 2000;62:115-121.
72. Maroushek SR, Aguilar EF, Stauffer W, et al. Malaria among refugee children at arrival in the United States. *Pediatr Infect Dis J*. 2005;24:450-452.
73. Ndao M, Bandyayera E, Kokoskin E, et al. Comparison of blood smear, antigen detection, and nested-PCR methods for screening refugees from regions where malaria is endemic after a malaria outbreak in Quebec, Canada. *J Clin Microbiol*. 2004;42:2694-2700.
74. US Department of Health and Human Services, Centers for Disease Control and Prevention. ATS/CDC Statement Committee on Latent Tuberculosis Infection. Targeted tuberculin testing and treatment of latent tuberculosis infection. *Am J Respir Crit Care Med*. 2000;161:S221-S247.
75. US Department of Health and Human Services, Centers for Disease Control and Prevention. Import-Associated Measles Outbreak—Indiana, May-June 2005. *MMWR*. 2005;54:1073.
76. US Department of Health and Human Services, Centers for Disease Control and Prevention. Update: multistate outbreak of mumps—United States, January 1-May 2, 2006. *MMWR*. 2006;55:1-5.

77. US Department of Health and Human Services, Centers for Disease Control and Prevention. Brief Report: Imported Case of Congenital Rubella Syndrome—New Hampshire, 2005. *MMWR*. 2005;54:1160.
78. Barnett ED, Christiansen D, Figueira M. Seroprevalence of measles, rubella, and varicella in refugees. *Clin Infect Dis*. 2002;35:403-408.
79. Hurie MB, Gennis MA, Hernandez LV, et al. Prevalence of hepatitis B markers and measles, mumps, and rubella antibodies among Jewish refugees from the former Soviet Union. *JAMA*. 1995;273:954-956.
80. Figueira M, Barnett ED, Christiansen D, et al. Cost-benefit of serotesting compared with universal immunization for varicella in refugee children from six geographic regions. *J Travel Med*. 2003;10:203-207.
81. Barnett ED, Holmes AH, Geltman PL, et al. Immunity to hepatitis A in people born and raised in endemic areas. *J Travel Med*. 2003;10:11-14.

Chapter 11

ETHICAL AND LEGAL ISSUES FOR THE PRIMARY CARE PHYSICIAN

Lainie Friedman Ross, MD, PhD; John D. Lantos, MD

The hallmark of clinical ethics in the setting of general internal medicine is its focus on the competent adult patient. In the physician-patient dyad, the patient is the decision maker and the focus is patient autonomy. If the patient becomes incompetent, the focus remains on patient autonomy because the guiding principle is to ask what the patient would have wanted (substituted judgment).[1] In contrast, the foundation of pediatric clinical ethics is a triad that includes the physician, the child, and his or her parent or parents. In the triad, the legally entitled decision maker is not the patient. Historically, parents were legally empowered to make virtually all decisions for their children. All children were presumed to be incompetent, and their opinions were not sought. The guiding principle was the *best interest of the child* standard. However, in the last 2 decades, there have been sociopolitical developments around the world to increase the child's legal authority and to give the child, particularly the older child, his or her own voice (autonomy).[2-5] Some people argue that mature children (specifically adolescents) should be allowed to make their own decisions without their parents' permission, even without their parents' awareness.[2,3] This issue is an area of tension and controversy because reasonable people disagree about the degree to which children's values and choices should direct their health care.[2,5,6]

Much of the literature of pediatric ethics focuses on the extreme cases: the premature infant who weighs 600 g, the child who has leukemia whose parents refuse chemotherapy, or the child whose sibling needs a kidney transplant. The unique issues that pediatricians in primary care practice face have not received comparable adequate scholarly attention or rigorous analysis. This circumstance may be because the ethical issues that arise in the daily practice of primary care pediatrics are usually not concerned with decisions about illnesses that are immediately life threatening. Nevertheless, pediatricians in primary care practice often face decisions that may have profound effects on a child's physical and mental health and on many emotional, spiritual, and economic elements of family life.

Societal standards about difficult moral choices in medicine have evolved through a dialogue among patients, patient advocacy groups, health care providers, bioethicists, professional societies, and the various branches of government. Legal disputes have been especially important for issues such as do-not-resuscitate orders, brain death, and treatment withdrawal. The controversies and disputes that arise in primary care seldom lead to legal actions. When they do, lower courts rather than appeals courts often decide these disputes. Lower-court decisions are seldom published and do not establish precedent. As a result, in many cases, neither statutory law nor case law is directly applicable to the issues at hand.

This chapter presents common scenarios that arise in primary care pediatrics and that raise thorny ethical issues. Some of these issues are procedural—that is, they require a decision about who should decide. Others are substantive—that is, they require consideration of what the right decision is and what constraints should apply to any decision maker. In some cases, legal constraints exist on decision making; in others, the law allows the physician wide latitude. The focus is on situations in which the law is less clear because many applicable laws vary from state to state and because these situations require that pediatricians make their own moral judgments.

CASE STUDIES AND ANALYSIS

Case 1

Alan, an 8-year-old boy, comes to your office because he has multiple warts on his hands. The school is concerned that he is contagious, and he is not allowed to participate in contact sports until his condition is treated or, at a minimum, is under treatment. You explain to Ms A, his mother, and to Alan that many therapeutic options are available, including cryotherapy in the physician's office, a salicylate-based therapy or duct tape that is to be applied nightly, or watchful waiting. Ms A requests that you give Alan the in-office treatment. Alan says that he does not want any painful treatment and will apply the ointment nightly. What do you do?

Discussion

On the surface, the case does not appear to involve an ethical issue because Alan, his mother, and the pediatrician all agree that Alan needs treatment. However, many very different treatments are available. Each approach has different benefits and burdens, and the evidence for the superiority of any one treatment is not strong. The child prefers one balance of the benefits and burdens, the parent prefers another. Their different values, when brought to play on the therapeutic options, have created a conflict between the parent and child. The pediatrician may not have a strong opinion about which option is best.

The first step in any such conflict is further discussion. Understanding why Ms A prefers the liquid nitrogen therapy would be valuable. Issues to be weighed include efficacy, cost, convenience, attendant risks, and compliance. Ms A's choice is pragmatic; she sees the liquid nitrogen as being more reliable than other treatments. Ms A is afraid, based on experience, that her child will be poorly compliant with the nightly salicylate-based treatment. She does not want to have a nightly battle. Alan has had liquid nitrogen therapy before and finds it quite painful. He promises his mother that he will comply with the nightly ointment applications.

In many such discussions, parents and children will come to an acceptable compromise. For example, Ms A may agree to a trial of home therapy during which Alan will agree to apply salicylate without parental reminders at home. If he fails to do so, then they will return for cryotherapy. In some cases, however, their positions are intractable, and the question remains, "Who should have the final word?" The American Academy of Pediatrics (AAP), Committee on Bioethics, published recommendations regarding the roles of parents and children in decision making for children.[3] The committee recommends that the resolution of conflicts between parents and children depend, in part, on the child's decision-making capacity. For children whose decision-making capacity is developed, the committee recommends that the child's decision be final. For the child whose capacity is developing, such as Alan, the committee urges the physician to try to achieve consensus. If the child and parent cannot reach consensus, then the AAP supports 3rd-party intervention.[3] Although some people may find this approach reasonable, others might find it hopelessly cumbersome. What 3rd party would be available in a busy pediatric office? Furthermore, some parents may be intolerant of 3rd-party scrutiny. These parents may find even the physician's scrutiny an inappropriate threat to their legitimate parental authority.

What are the pediatrician's options if consensus is not achieved? If pediatricians side with parents, then the protesting child will receive a painful treatment. What if children resist? Such actions convey to children the problematic message that their opinions do not matter. On the other hand, to side with children on the grounds of developing maturity places parents in an awkward position because they must now buy the medication and apply it to their children's hands nightly. What if Ms A resists and says, "OK, doctor, at what time will you come by to place the medicine on Alan's hands?" Her response demonstrates the bind that physicians have in their relationships with their patients. The challenge for professionals is to be caring without taking unnecessary control of the life of the child for whom they do not and cannot take full responsibility.[7]

In a case such as this one, it appears reasonable that parents should have ultimate decision-making authority. The risks of either treatment are low, as are the burdens of therapy, and the child is at an age during which it is unlikely that he would be capable of taking responsibility for his own medication regimen. When these conditions are met, parental authority should prevail. Still, physicians have the right, and the obligation, to involve children in the decision-making process and to explain to the child why his wishes and requests are being overridden, even if his parents complain that this action threatens their autonomy.

Case 2

Betty, a 15-year-old girl, comes into the physician's office for a yearly physical. Her examination is normal. She attends St. Mary's High School where she is on the honor roll. She is popular with her friends and tells you that she has recently fallen in love with Bob. She says that she is not sexually active yet, but she asks for birth control pills. She also asks that you not tell her parents because she knows that her sexual activity is against their moral and religious beliefs, and she fears they will prohibit her from seeing Bob.

Case 3

Vicky, a 15-year-old girl, is brought to your office by her mother, Ms V, who states that she knows that her daughter is sexually active, and she wants her to get long-term contraception to avoid pregnancy. Ms V is a single mother who became pregnant with Vicky when Ms V was 14, and she wants to protect her daughter from the hardships she faced. Vicky acknowledges that she has a boyfriend, Tom, and is sexually active. She states that he wants her to get pregnant, although she is ambivalent. She does not want contraception because she fears her boyfriend will leave her.

Discussion

Currently, more than 45% of high school girls and 48% of high school boys have had sexual intercourse.[8] Approximately 900,000 American adolescents become pregnant every year.[9] Many teens do not seek medical or gynecologic care or contraception for months or even years after they initiate sexual activity.[9,10] Most teens who become pregnant are unmarried, and most of their pregnancies are unplanned.[11] More than 60% of these girls will decide to take the pregnancy to term, and virtually all of these teenagers will take on the responsibilities of parenthood.[11] Pregnant adolescents have a higher incidence of medical complications for themselves and their fetuses than do older women.[11,12] Their children do not fare as well psychosocially as do children of adult mothers.[11] Thus one can say both that Betty is acting unusually responsibly for a 15-year-old and that Ms V's concerns are well founded.

Both of these requests should be interpreted as an opportunity for dialogue. Are Bob and Tom classmates, or are they a few years older than Betty and Vicky? If they are older, then how much older? If Bob and Tom are over 18, then concerns about abuse or legal reporting requirements arise. What would Betty do if she were to get pregnant, even though she was taking the pill? Has she discussed this concern with Bob? How will Betty's deception affect her relationship with her family? As Vicky's physician, you may want to address the issue of whether Vicky finds this three-way conversation embarrassing. You might suggest to Ms V that the best way to protect Vicky from an unwanted pregnancy might be to encourage her to talk with you confidentially. Ms V and Vicky may be receptive to this idea. This approach does not resolve whether Vicky should receive treatment that her mother requests but that Vicky rejects. However, it may give you an opportunity to discuss with Vicky the most likely outcome of adolescent pregnancy: single parenthood and its attendant responsibilities. You may try to help her see that pregnancy should be a positive decision (ie, I want to be a parent) and not a passive decision (ie, it will make my partner happy). You may want to encourage her to get counseling to help her sort out the complicated issues that she is facing.

Although parents generally have the legal right and responsibility to make medical decisions for their adolescent children, treatment related to reproductive health is an exception under the special consent statutes. These statutes vary by state, vary in their scope, and may apply differently to physicians in different practice settings, but all of these statues give adolescents the legal autonomy independently to seek and consent to the diagnosis and treatment of drug and alcohol abuse, contraceptive counseling, and the procurement of contraceptives.[13] Some states even allow minors to consent to abortions without disclosure or consent from their parents. The statutes were designed to encourage adolescents to seek health care for problems that they might deny or ignore or for which they might delay seeking treatment if they had to get parental permission. Pediatricians should know the specifics of laws in their state. Although such statutes allow physicians to provide this care, they do not compel them to do so. Thus a pediatrician facing a patient such as Betty has the legal latitude to make a moral decision. However, even a pediatrician who thinks that prescribing contraception is inappropriate for Betty should inform her that she has a right to obtain contraception and should refer her to another provider.

The purported purpose of the specialized consent statutes is laudable: to encourage early, responsible sexual health care for adolescents. The pragmatic justification is compelling. Given that adolescents can be and frequently are sexually active even when birth control and other sexual health services are relatively inaccessible, they should be given the opportunity to be responsible for their sexual activity. However, whether the pragmatic justification is sufficient to justify empowering all adolescents to consent to or refuse all types of reproductive health care is unclear. Rather, both moral and pragmatic considerations might lead one to empower Betty and to disempower Vicky. In both cases, the goal would be to minimize the chances that either girl would get pregnant.

Three moral arguments can be made in these situations that would lead to 3 different decisions. First, we might base these decisions on a pure best-interest standard. That is, we might simply judge that it is not in either Betty or Vicky's interest to get pregnant. Thus we would make the decisions that best advance these interests and prescribe contraceptives for both. This decision can be framed as a way of preserving their future autonomy; that is, granting autonomy to adolescents regarding their sexual activity when they are 15 may be autonomy-restricting over a lifetime. As with many decisions that children make, we might justify restricting a child's autonomy now to give her greater lifetime autonomy.[14] Second, one might argue that these teens have the right to make decisions for themselves in these matters. Following this view, we would confidentially prescribe contraceptives for Betty but not for Vicky. Third, one might argue that parents have a valid 3rd-party interest in their children's development and activities, even when the children become teens and achieve a significant level of competency. To act on these interests and to participate in their child's moral development, they need to have the opportunity to try to inculcate their beliefs through rational discourse.[14,15] They can accomplish this task only if they are aware of what their teens are doing. This argument acknowledges the child's decisional capacity, but it also asserts that decision-making capacity is necessary but may not be sufficient to grant an adolescent health care autonomy. In this case, one might prescribe contraception as requested by Vicky's mother but not for Betty, whose parents are not aware of their daughter's intentions.

This range of responses is consistent with both the specialized consent statutes and the AAP position on consent, permission, and assent. Teens are empowered to obtain contraception, but pediatricians are not required to provide such treatment.[16] Parents are empowered to request medical treatment that they deem to be beneficial to their child, but pediatricians are not required to provide it. Thus pediatricians must make a personal moral decision about how they will respond with 1 major caveat: When a pediatrician is not willing to provide a treatment that is a valid medical option (eg, contraception to minors), the pediatrician does have an obligation to refer the patient and family to other health care providers who are willing to do so.

Case 4

Ms C calls you the day before she is scheduled to bring in her 14-year-old son Charles for his yearly physical examination. She notes that Charles was previously an A student, but now he is getting Cs and Ds. The family is going through turmoil because Mr C moved out of the house 3 months ago to live with his pregnant girlfriend. Ms C admits to being depressed and cries easily but has not sought outside help. Charles has been withdrawn and often comes home late and refuses to tell his mother where he has been. She fears that Charles is using drugs and would like you to screen him without telling him what you are doing.

Discussion

Ms C's request is a call for help. Ms C and Charles need psychiatric treatment regardless of whether Charles is using drugs. Ideally, both of his parents need to realize how their actions and emotions are affecting their son's behavior. Charles needs parental supervision at a time when both parents are disengaged for different reasons. Each year, more than 1 million children experience the divorce of their parents.[17] The parental conflict that is often experienced around the separation is often expressed as behavioral problems in the child, and the pediatrician should be prepared to provide support or to refer for appropriate counseling.[17]

A crucial question for Ms C is, "How will the surreptitious drug testing help?" A test that comes back negative does not prove that Charles is not using drugs. False-negative tests can occur because the half-life of many drugs is less than 24 hours and because urine drug testing tests only for some of the substances more commonly abused. Serum testing is more sensitive but can only be used for specific drugs, thus you would need a list of the drugs that are suspected. If the screen comes back positive, then Ms C will need to decide how she will approach Charles. Charles is presently not trusting of adults who have betrayed him. Surreptitious testing will increase his distrust.

The preferable course of action would be to ask Ms C to give you permission to establish a confidential relationship with Charles. You might explain that this approach is likely to be much better for Charles in the long run. In our experience, most parents are willing to accept this advice. If Ms C gives you such permission, then you should arrange to meet with Charles privately and explain the confidential nature of the relationship. You should be honest about when confidentiality would be broken—specifically, in cases in which you believe that Charles is a danger to himself or others.[18]

The opportunity to speak confidentially in his physician may be what Charles needs to help him cope with the turmoil at home.[19] Charles may be willing to discuss whether he is abusing drugs and may be willing to be tested for drugs as well.[20,21] However, many other issues need to be addressed with Charles that are even more compelling. Is he suicidal? Is he engaging in any other risky behaviors (of which drug use is but one dimension)? Is he depressed? Is he willing to seek psychiatric counseling or begin antidepressant medication? Are there any adults whom he trusts?

Despite your suggestion, Ms C may still demand that you test Charles for drugs. In fact, situations occur in which the grounds for suspecting drug abuse are compelling, and teens who are using drugs may not be in a position to assess the risks and benefits of testing or treatment.[20,21] However, pragmatically, testing Charles would be difficult without his cooperation unless he was deceived about the purpose of specimen collection. Pediatricians (similar to other physicians) should not deceive their patients. Thus if Charles' mother insists on testing, then the pediatrician should insist on informing Charles of the nature of the test. Ideally, Charles should voluntarily cooperate for testing. Involuntary testing should be performed only if reason exists to doubt his competency or if information exists that strongly suggests that he is at high risk of substance abuse.[20] Even if testing is not voluntary, the disclosure that testing will be performed will help maintain trust and keep the door open for future communication. Ms C has a moral obligation to care for her son and to determine what medical information she needs to do so. However, this obligation does not give her the right to demand that you lie to him about what you are doing or to violate his right to privacy without compelling evidence that it is in his medical best interest.[20]

The physician also should use this appointment and the discussion about drug testing as an opportunity to encourage Charles and Ms C to seek counseling and to give Charles anticipatory guidance about any and all risky behaviors in which he is involved.[20,21]

Case 5

Mr and Mrs D are the proud parents of David, a well-appearing 6-week-old boy. During their first well-baby visit, you learn that Mr D had retinoblastoma as a child and had his left eye removed. You recommend genetic testing to determine if the child is at risk. Mrs D states that they were offered such testing in utero and that they refused and still refuse genetic testing.

Discussion

Retinoblastoma may be inherited as an autosomal-dominant gene, or it may develop spontaneously. Given that Mr D had retinoblastoma, David has a 50% risk for developing retinoblastoma. Before the discovery of the gene for retinoblastoma, children born into families that had a positive history for retinoblastoma underwent ophthalmologic surveillance every 3 months. The value of the genetic information is that if David tests negative for the gene, then he can avoid frequent eye examinations. If he tests positive, then he will need to undergo frequent screening to enhance the likelihood of early detection. If detected early, then the prognosis for survival and vision is improved.

Testing young children for early-onset conditions encompasses 2 very different categories of conditions: (1) conditions such as Duchenne muscular dystrophy, for which early (presymptomatic) diagnosis and treatment do not affect the course of the disease, and (2) conditions such as retinoblastoma, for which early diagnosis and treatment may improve treatment or even save lives.

In the 1st category of early-onset conditions, the value of presymptomatic diagnosis is to help avoid delay in diagnosis when early symptoms are nonspecific, to target surveillance screening more accurately, to allow parents to prepare for a child who will have special needs, and to give parents information to use in their reproductive planning.[22,23] On the other hand, early diagnosis may be detrimental in a number of ways. The *vulnerable child* syndrome has been shown to cause morbidity that may be even greater than the morbidity associated with the disease that is diagnosed. Early diagnosis may affect parent-child bonding adversely if the parents hold back on emotional investment because they fear their child will die. In older children, it may adversely affect the child's self-image and self-esteem.[22] Finally, in the United States, obtaining appropriate health insurance for the child and even for healthy siblings may cause difficulties for the parents.[23,24] Parental expectations for the future may also be limited unnecessarily.[22] In situations such as this one in which early testing has not been shown to improve morbidity or mortality, the risk-benefit balance of presymptomatic testing will depend on the values and needs of each family.[22,23] In such situations, parental choices should be respected.[25] In situations in which clear evidence exists that early testing might reduce morbidity and mortality, parental discretion may be limited by medical neglect statutes. In these cases, a pediatrician might choose to report a case to child protective services. Then, a judge would decide whether to order testing.

The value of presymptomatic testing in the second category is to prevent serious morbidity and mortality. Because articulating a compelling argument to explain why children should not be tested in these circumstances is difficult, wide consensus exists that children in families known to carry such genes should be tested.[22,23] Also assumed is that parents are the child's appropriate decision makers. The question is whether, if parents refuse testing or diagnostic work-ups, physicians should feel compelled to seek state permission to override their refusal.

In such a case, the pediatrician needs to engage Mr and Mrs D in dialogue to try to determine why they are refusing testing. They may have refused genetic testing in utero because amniocentesis entails risks of morbidity and mortality and, assuming that a positive test would not have led them to terminate the pregnancy, would not have offered any tangible benefits. However, genetic testing for the gene for retinoblastoma in a 6-week-old child is a simple blood test and the result clarifies whether the child needs frequent ophthalmologic follow-up. Mr and Mrs D may continue to refuse testing because of lack of knowledge, fear of stigma or discrimination, or fear that this procedure may interfere with obtaining insurance, particularly if either parent is looking for a new job, which may include a change in insurance.

What should be done if Mr and Mrs D continue to refuse testing? Ideally, knowing David's genetic status would be valuable, but as long as Mr and Mrs D are compliant with frequent surveillance, their decision is neither abusive nor neglectful. The eye examinations themselves are minimally invasive, although young children may require sedation. Physicians should respect this decision but realize that it adds the additional responsibility that they ensure that David does get appropriate quarterly examinations. If Mr and Mrs D refuse or fail to comply with quarterly ophthalmologic examinations, then this failure is neglectful, and they should be reported to the appropriate child protection authorities.

Case 6

Ms F delivered Frances, a healthy full-term infant, 24 hours ago. Ms F is a very well-informed parent, and she requests that Frances not receive either vitamin K or hepatitis B vaccine because she does not want to put Frances through any more discomfort than the birth process. You come to draw the newborn screen for phenylketonuria and other metabolic conditions before discharge, but she refuses. She agrees to reconsider and will take the card to her private pediatrician, whom she plans to see in 2 days. You suspect that she will again refuse newborn metabolic screening. How should you respond?

Discussion

Traditionally, the conditions screened for with the Guthrie card were rare diseases for which early treatment would reduce morbidity and mortality. In 1968 the World Health Organization enumerated 10 criteria for evaluating screening programs,[26] including (1) that the disease must represent an important health problem for which an accepted treatment exists that can prevent most or all of the morbidity or mortality associated with the condition; (2) that the screening test be simple and cheap and the follow-up confirmatory testing highly accurate; (3) that a system be in place to ensure quick communication of results to relevant parties; and (4) that the cost of case finding, diagnosis, and treatment must be economically balanced in relation to expenditures on medical care as a whole.[26] More recently, newborn screening programs are expanding in part as a result of the development of tandem mass spectrometry and advances in gene chip technology, which allows for the detection of numerous conditions, not all of which meet all of the World Health Organization criteria.

In the United States, 48 of the 50 states have mandatory universal newborn screening programs. Although states have different panels of required tests, the most common tests are those for phenylketonuria, hypothyroidism, hemoglobinopathies (including sickle cell disease), congenital adrenal hyperplasia, and galactosemia. Although screening is characterized as *mandatory*, in actual practice, parents can and occasionally do refuse testing. However, they generally are not asked for permission and therefore, to refuse, they must be informed and proactive. Most parents (and physicians) are unaware of the parents' right to refuse.

Mandated medical interventions, whether diagnostic or therapeutic, override important parental rights.[23,27] Generally, the state should not interfere in the medical decisions that parents make for their children. To do so undermines the family unit. The only exceptions to this rule are situations in which parental decisions expose their child to serious morbidity or mortality,[28] although wide interpretation may exist as to what degree or urgency, likelihood of harm, or magnitude of harm may justify overriding parental rights. Thus parents whose religious beliefs lead them to oppose blood transfusions should not be permitted to refuse blood for their child in a life-threatening situation. They may, however, refuse in situations that are less directly life threatening. Newborn screening does not meet the criteria of an imminent risk of immediate danger because the probability of harm is remote. Each of the conditions included in the newborn screen occurs in fewer than 1 in 1000 children. Some of these conditions may be diagnosable clinically; some may never manifest clinically. A parent who refuses newborn screening is taking a very small albeit serious risk. Their refusal should be respected.

Nevertheless, physicians should educate parents who refuse screening so that they understand why physicians believe that the benefits greatly outweigh the risks. Most parents will then accede to screening. In Maryland, where testing is voluntary, fewer than 1 parent in 1000 refuses testing for newborns.[29] The risk that these refusals create is much less than the risk of a false-negative test and less than the number of children not tested because of lost and improperly obtained specimens.[30]

Given the experience in Maryland, one might ask whether parental permission should be required for a universal newborn screening program. What are the arguments for seeking parental consent for newborn screening? (1) Procuring parental permission for newborn screening is a symbol of respect for the family—respect that is well placed, given that families are the primary source of childrearing and given that families, and not the state, will bear the greatest costs if diagnosis is delayed. (2) By requiring consent, parents must be educated about the purpose and limitations of screening, which may give them incentive to follow up on abnormal screening results. Knowledge of negative test results can be reassuring to parents, particularly those who have personal knowledge of any of the conditions for which their infant is being tested.

The major benefit of not requiring consent is to simplify the process of screening. Obtaining parental permission for newborn screening can be time consuming. In this day and age, physicians are more and more pressed for time. In some cases, they may not have time to seek parental consent, and newborns may suffer as a result. A related argument is that the consent process for newborn screening is perfunctory. Neither argument morally justifies circumventing the consent process, although the practicalities may make true informed consent impossible. If each condition would only require a minute of explanation, consent might take more than an hour in states with expanded screening panels. Given the public health value of many of the conditions screened for, the goal of the consent process for newborn screening should not be to fully inform parents of each condition, but rather to inform parents of the general purpose of population health screening, which is to find individuals at risk for conditions for which early intervention reduces morbidity and mortality. For most parents, this explanation will be adequate.[31] For parents who want additional information, pamphlets should be available and referrals for more extensive counseling should be possible. In rare cases, parents will choose to opt out. Given the low probability of a positive test, these parents should be counseled, but their refusals should be respected unless prohibited by state law (eg, Nebraska[32]).

Case 7

Tina is a 4-year-old new patient. Her parents are seeking to enroll her in school for the first time. You ask for Tina's immunization records, and her parents state that she has received no immunizations. They request that you write a school note excusing their daughter from vaccination based on religious beliefs. On further questioning, you discover that the parents do not really have a religious objection to immunizations but have refused immunizations because they have heard that these vaccines may cause seizures or autism.

Discussion

Childhood immunization rates are 1 of the 10 leading health indicators used to assess the health of the nation as part of the *Healthy People 2010* initiative, reflecting the high value placed on childhood immunizations. In the United States, childhood vaccinations for numerous infectious diseases are mandatory for entry into public schools and licensed child-care facilities, although some private religious schools do not require them. Despite the success, the mandatory nature of immunizations represents a tension between individual autonomy and public health. Most states recognize a religious or philosophic exemption, although the courts have found that evaluating the sincerity, strength, and religious or philosophic nature of the refusals can be legitimate.[33]

Parents refuse vaccinations for many reasons. For some parents, refusal is based on religious or philosophic beliefs; for others, it is based on fear of vaccine safety.[34] In the 1970s a report in *Archives of Disease of Childhood* suggested a connection between the whole-cell pertussis vaccine and neurologic damage in children.[35] This finding was a major impetus to developing a safer acellular pertussis vaccine. In the late 1990s, fears arose over the measles-mumps-rubella (MMR) vaccine and its relationship to autism after the *Lancet* published a report of severe developmental regression in children by Wakefield and colleagues.[36] The research team noted that the onset of symptoms occurred after MMR immunization, although they had not proved a causal link.[36] In 2003, Simon Murch, one of Wakefield's collaborators, denounced assertions of a link between MMR and autism and declared the existence of "unequivocal evidence that MMR is not a risk factor for autism."[37] In 2004, evidence revealed that Wakefield had concealed the fact that his research had been funded in part by the legal team seeking redress for parents who believed that their children had been injured by the MMR vaccine,[37] and many of the original collaborators retracted their support for a link between autism and the MMR vaccine.[38] In addition, numerous medical studies, including a large Institute of Medicine review, confirmed the lack of association between autism and the MMR vaccine.[39]

In the United States, children who are undervaccinated are demographically different from children who receive no vaccinations.[40] Risk factors for being underimmunized include minority status, poverty, living in an urban area, living in a household with more than 3 children, and low maternal education. In contrast, children who have no vaccinations tend to be white children whose parents are married, older, and wealthier or children in religious communities whose parents have a religious objection to immunization. They often live in communities of like-minded families. The clustering of these families decreases herd immunity and makes these communities more susceptible to outbreaks. In September 2005, 4 children in an Amish community in Minnesota were found to have polio infections, a disease that had not been seen in the United States since 1979.[41]

What should a pediatrician do when parents refuse recommended immunizations? Some pediatricians will discontinue care for such families.[42] They claim that they cannot care for patients who do not trust their medical recommendations. In contrast to this approach, the AAP Committee on Bioethics recommends that the pediatrician should listen carefully and respectfully to the parents' concerns and to share honestly what is known about the risks and benefits of the vaccine in question and to correct any misperceptions and misinformation.[43] They should explore the possibility that cost is a reason for refusal. Rather than dismiss the family, the AAP recommends that pediatricians take advantage of their ongoing relationship with the family and revisit the immunization discussion on subsequent visits.[43] The AAP has also developed a form to document the parents' refusal.[44]

If parents refuse immunizations for their children, then the pediatrician should document this refusal on the school form. In some states, this documentation is adequate for school entrance. In other states, parents may have to provide additional evidence as to the philosophic or religious nature of their objection.

Case 8

Mr and Ms G come to the clinic with Gary, their 5-year-old son. Gary was adopted as a newborn. Mr and Ms G have told you they plan to tell Gary about his origins, but each time you ask, they give reasons why they have not yet done so. They have kept the adoption secret from all but their immediate family.

Case 9

Mr and Ms S bring their 5-year-old child, Sam, for a well-child visit. The family has just moved from California. As you try to take a full medical history, the parents become visibly uncomfortable. Finally, Mr S takes Sam out of the room to play in the waiting room, at which time Ms S explains that they had infertility problems and used donor sperm and that Mr S is not Sam's genetic father. They have only sketchy information about the sperm donor, who was a 25-year-old healthy white medical student. They have chosen not to tell Sam about his genetic parentage.

Discussion

Adoption is a legal procedure through which a permanent family is created for a child whose birth parents are unable, are unwilling, or are legally prohibited from caring for their child. Adoption has existed throughout history, although the focus has changed. Historically, "adoption served the needs of adults. . .for the purpose of kinship, religion or the community," in contrast to our current focus on the needs and well being of the child.[45]

In the United States, formal adoptions peaked in 1970 when approximately 175,000 adoptions occurred.[46] Adoptions have decreased because of many social factors, including the decrease in the stigma of single mothers and the increased availability of abortion.[46] In 1992, the last year that adoption data were collected, almost 127,000 formal adoptions occurred.[47] Despite the large number of children and families who are directly affected by adoption, the medical literature on adoption is scant.

Before World War II, professional adoption workers advised, if not insisted, that children be told of their adopted status for the pragmatic reason that learning of adoption from parents in a loving environment rather than by well-meaning or even malicious neighbors, schoolmates, or relatives was better for the child. After World War II, the professional community argued against disclosing. By the mid-1970s the pendulum returned not only in favor of disclosing adoption, but also in openness in all aspects of adoption.[45] Nevertheless, some families still try to keep the adoption a secret.

The assisted reproductive technologies (ARTs) offer individuals another possible means to achieve parenthood (Chapter 72, Assistive Reproductive Technologies, Multiple Births, and Pregnancy Outcomes). ARTs have offered some new twists. Whereas adoption separated genetic and social parenthood, ARTs allow individuals to separate genetic, gestational, and social parenthood. For example, through in vitro fertilization, a woman can gestate a fetus who is the product of her husband's sperm and a nongenetically related egg donor whose identity is often unknown. More common are children born by the use of sperm donors, such as in the case of Sam. In the early days of donor insemination, the husband's sperm was mixed with the donor's sperm to leave open the possibility that the child was the genetic heir. Now, determination of paternity is widely available and accessible and makes this pretense obsolete. Recently, the American Society for Reproductive Medicine has issued a statement encouraging the disclosure of gamete donations,[48] although empirical studies show that the majority of families do not.[49,50]

For Gary and Sam, the clinical value of knowing their correct genetic family history is that it may allow their health care providers to perform particular diagnostic measures or to counsel them about ways to minimize their genetic susceptibilities through particular lifestyle choices. As our understanding of genetics improves, emphasis on collecting family history information increases,[51,52] and yet data suggest it may be highly inaccurate.[53] Family history is growing in importance because we understand that many illnesses have a genetic component; and yet, we are also learning that genotype frequently does not correlate with phenotype[54] and that family history may or may not provide additional data.[55,56]

However, questions also arise as to whether children have a right to know their genetic inheritance, whether parents have a right to maintain secrecy, or both. The literature about the psychologic risks of disclosure and nondisclosure is small and inconclusive. Nevertheless, today, most psychologists and psychiatrists support disclosure because of its role in health care screening, diagnosis, and treatment and the importance of genetic identity to one's self-identity. Reasons to respect nondisclosure include the potential threat that such knowledge may pose to the parent-child relationship and the integrity of the family. Which reasons are stronger depends on how one weighs the advantages and disadvantages.

Although it might be argued that knowing their biologic identity is better for children, the physician's right to interfere in interpersonal family dynamics is and should be limited to situations of clear-cut abuse or neglect; nondisclosure of biological relationships does not rise to this level. Pediatricians should encourage disclosure in a developmentally appropriate manner and should discourage parents from *waiting until the right minute*.[57] The physician should encourage disclosure on the grounds that (1) secrecy may be detrimental to a trusting relationship between parents and children; (2) later discovery by the child may have an adverse effect on self-esteem; and (3) the child otherwise may learn of the genetic discrepancy in a less secure setting (eg, accidentally overhearing a relative). Nevertheless, physicians should not disclose this information to children without the parents' permission.

Case 10

Ms H brings her 17-year-old son Harold to the clinic for a preparticipation high school basketball sports physical examination. On taking the history, you learn that Harold's father died from a heart condition last year at the age of 40. Harold's uncle died in his late 20s when playing competitive tennis. You are concerned about the possibility of a familial cause of sudden death caused by a cardiac condition known as hypertrophic obstructive cardiomyopathy (HCM). You recommend either an echocardiogram or genetic testing to see whether Harold has HCM. Harold and his mother refuse. You then write on his school physical form that he is at risk for HCM and should not participate in school sports without a cardiac work-up. Harold and his mother are quite angry. Harold is an all-state player and is being recruited heavily by many universities. The mother plans to take Harold to another physician and demands that you not inform his school or anyone else of your concerns. Harold and his mother do not disclose the family history to a colleague in a practice across town, who approves him for interscholastic athletics.

Discussion

HCM is an autosomal-dominant condition that is usually asymptomatic in pre-adolescents. It is an idiopathic cause of cardiomyopathy, and the risk of sudden death, particularly during intense athletic activity, increases with age.

Harold is at risk for a life-threatening event that is exacerbated by physical activity. This diagnosis would make him ineligible for sports and take away his opportunity for a college sports scholarship. Of course, failure to diagnose this condition may result in premature death in a high school gymnasium. Competitive sports participation is clearly risky for Harold.

You try to convince Harold and his mother to have the echocardiogram. They acknowledge that he is at risk, but Harold states that basketball is his life, and he is willing to risk his life to play.

Harold and Ms H view the issue as one of autonomy. They understand the risks and benefits of playing, given Harold's possible cardiac condition, and they believe that playing basketball is better for Harold despite the risk of sudden death. They also view the issue as one of confidentiality. They ask that you not disclose to the school the family history that you discovered when interviewing Harold and his mother.

This case is one in which the parent and child are in consensus but in disagreement with the physician. The family's position for confidentiality and nondisclosure must be weighed against the physician's belief that he or she needs to protect this child from his mother and himself. Consensus guidelines state that adolescents with HCM should not participate in sports such as basketball.[58] The physician can and must decide that the harm to patient privacy and confidentiality are outweighed by the potentially life-threatening nature of his cardiac condition. As a moral agent, the physician has an obligation to prevent a serious imminent risk of sudden death to a minor. Harold and his mother cannot relieve the physician of this obligation.

The physician also has an obligation to protect the community. Imagine the reaction if Harold were allowed to play and he did die on the basketball court in front of many classmates and their families. Such an event might cause serious psychologic trauma to the observers. How would the community respond if they knew that the physician might have prevented this event? The physician has an obligation to protect Harold and the community from such unnecessary trauma. However, Harold's mother is correct that the physician must not breach confidentiality without the permission of the patient or parent. Instead, the physician should notify child protection about this unusual form of medical neglect, although whether child protective services would find the parent medically neglectful is not clear cut. Even when Harold turns 18 years of age, the school, in loco parentis, should refuse to let him play basketball or other sports that may lead to his sudden death.[59]

Case 11

Mr K brings Kevin for his prekindergarten examination during which you notice some linear ecchymoses on his back. You ask Kevin how he got them, and he answers that his father beat him for talking back at dinner last night. Kevin's father confirms this explanation, explaining that he believes that corporal punishment is effective. He admits to using a belt because his hand "did not produce the desired effect." You inform the family that corporal punishment that leaves marks is abusive and that you plan to report your suspicions of child abuse to the department of family services. The father is irate, arguing that discipline is a family matter and that his religious faith supports his convictions of *spare the rod and spoil the child.*

Discussion

A recent AAP position statement on guidance for effective discipline begins by noting that "parents often ask pediatricians for advice about the provision of appropriate and effective discipline."[60] The most controversial aspect of this issue is the role, if any, for corporal punishment. Although a recent survey of AAP members found that approximately 85% of respondents generally or completely opposed the use of corporal punishment,[61] more than 90% of American families report having used spanking as a means of discipline at some time.[60]

Kevin's father raises the point that his actions are based on his religious beliefs. Some religious groups take a strong position in support of corporal punishment. Currently, religious exemptions to most of the child abuse and neglect statutes can be found, but the exemptions do not apply to corporal punishment, nor should they. The religious exemptions were written to protect parents who sought prayer-based therapy for their child rather than allopathic medical care; they were not meant to protect a parent from being charged with abuse for beating a child.

To examine the benefits and burdens of corporal punishment, the AAP co-sponsored a consensus conference on this topic in February 1996.[62] The conference concluded with 13 consensus statements that addressed the role of spanking and corporal punishment in parental discipline. Statement No. 6 commented on the lack of data on the effectiveness of spanking in general, and Statement No. 8 commented that the data show corporal punishment to be ineffective in older children and adolescents and "is associated with increased risk for dysfunction and aggression later in life."[62] The strongest statement against corporal punishment was Statement No. 12, which states that "concerning forms of corporal punishment more severe than spanking, the data suggest that the risk for psychological or physical harm outweigh any potential benefits."[62]

Despite common usage and acceptance of corporal punishment, the data show that, over time, spanking is a less effective strategy than noncorporal methods for reducing undesired behavior. Furthermore, this type of punishment becomes less effective with continued use.[60] The AAP recommends that parents "be encouraged and assisted in developing methods other than spanking in response to undesired behavior."[60] The AAP mentions both the *time-out* method and the removal of privileges as "two common discipline approaches that have been associated with reducing undesired behavior."[60] The AAP statement noted further that many parents go beyond spanking and use an object or other forms of unacceptable corporal punishment: "When punishment fails, parents who rely on it tend to increase the intensity of its use rather than to change strategies."[60] This action is no longer discipline but child abuse.

Pediatricians should help parents understand the facts about corporal punishment and to realize that any such punishment (beyond an occasional mild spanking) is unacceptable and will be reported.

No morally justifiable reason exists for a parent to inflict physical harm on a child. Although physical manifestations of violence are an imperfect measure of the severity of punishment, they at least define an unacceptable threshold. The marks on Kevin are a sign that his father used more physical force than is morally acceptable. Reporting to child protective services may be necessary. The physician must work with this family to modify their discipline strategy. Pediatricians can role-model alternative forms of discipline by making their office *spanking-free zones*.

Case 12

Mr and Mrs R call you to arrange a prenatal visit. They have a healthy 2-year-old daughter who was born by cesarean section (c-section) weighing 8 pounds 5 ounces. The couple explains that they were very dissatisfied with their care because they had wanted a natural childbirth but their nurse midwife "panicked" after 18 hours of labor and that they were forced into having an unwanted c-section. They have decided to have their second child at home with a lay midwife. They ask if you would be willing to be "on call" for the home birth, in case any complications arise. On further questioning, she is clearly well versed in the risks and benefits of vaginal birth after cesarean section (VBAC). She states that she lives within a 10-minute drive of a major hospital and will go there if things are "not going well." You argue that the additional time may risk her health and the health of the fetus. You tell her that VBAC is associated with uterine rupture and that this event might lead to death for both Ms R and her baby. She says she understands but is determined to proceed with the home birth.

Discussion

Currently, over 40,000 out-of-hospital births occur annually in the United States mostly in birth centers, clinics, and residences.[63] Of these births, nearly 26,000 occur at home. In 2002, Pang and colleagues reviewed outcomes of planned home births in Washington State over a 7-year period and found that planned home births had greater infant and maternal risks than did hospital births.[64] However, a more recent study of the safety of home births in North America in the year 2000 found that planned home births for low-risk women using certified professional midwives had similar intrapartum and neonatal mortality to that of low-risk hospital births but was associated with lower rates of medical intervention.[65]

VBAC is a more risky event compared with a typical vaginal delivery and is associated with more risks than a repeat c-section.[66] The risk of uterine rupture is 0.7%, and the risk of hypoxic-ischemic encephalopathy is also increased (absolute risk, 0.46 per 1000 women at term undergoing a trial of labor).[66] In 2004 the American College of Obstetrics and Gynecology (ACOG) published a practice bulletin in which it stated that good and consistent scientific evidence existed that most women with 1 previous cesarean delivery are candidates for attempting vaginal birth after cesarean delivery.[67] However, because uterine rupture may be catastrophic, ACOG recommended that VBAC be attempted only in institutions equipped to respond to emergencies.[67]

Clearly, Mrs R's decision to attempt a VBAC at home is against the ACOG recommendations and is risky for both Mrs R and her fetus. It is not what you would recommend. We believe that informing the parents that you believe that their action is placing Mrs R and the fetus at risk of harm is morally obligatory. The pediatrician should recommend in-hospital delivery both for the sake of the child and for the pregnant woman. In the end, however, Mrs R has and should have broad autonomy with respect to her obstetric decisions, and many of these are beyond the purview of the pediatrician.

At the same time, physicians have a right to refuse to participate in treatment that goes against their moral conscience. Refusing to participate in home births would be morally acceptable for physicians. The parents should be given as much information as possible about the risks of uterine rupture and the danger signs. They should be informed about appropriate medical interventions for the newborn, including vitamin K, newborn screening, and hepatitis immunizations. Alternatively, the pediatrician may decide to participate out of concern for the best interest of the newborn. Needless to say, pediatricians should carefully document all discussions about risks and their strong recommendations against home birth. Physicians may want to discuss their decisions with legal or risk management personnel before doing to.

Whether you participate in the home birth or not, Mr and Mrs R may still ask if you are willing to be the pediatrician of their children. The authors of this text encourage pediatricians to accept such families into their practices so as to be in a position to advocate for the medical needs of these children. The children will suffer if the medical community abandons them because of their parents' alternate beliefs and lifestyles. Whether pediatricians agree or do not agree with their patients' obstetric decision, the live newborn and siblings need a medical home.[68]

CONCLUSION

In the medical care of children, ethical conflicts can develop within the family and between the health care provider and the family, or the health care provider and family may be in conflict with the state. The preceding cases represent different health care scenarios that will be familiar to everyone who is involved in the primary health care of children. In each case, we propose a methodologic system for resolving conflicts. The 1st and most important step is in-depth discussion among physicians, parents, and children to try to understand why people hold the beliefs that they do. Physicians should be open minded and willing to compromise, up to a point. The 2nd important consideration is some assessment of the benefits and the burdens of the proposed treatment or action and of the available alternatives. Generally, parents have both the legal responsibility and the moral authority to make medical decisions for their children. The pediatrician's respect for the child's opinion should increase as the child grows older, acquires increased capacity to understand and make decisions, and approaches the age of legal majority. In all of the previously mentioned situations, pediatricians must balance their own assessments of what is best for the child with an understanding that children benefit from interacting with their families in an environment that is safe from 3rd-party intrusion. Pediatricians also must remember that their expertise is in deciding what is medically best for a child, whereas parental decisions need to reflect what is best for the child overall balanced by the parents' right, privilege, and responsibility to preserve their cultural, social, and moral values.

AAP POLICY STATEMENTS

American Academy of Pediatrics, Committee on Adolescence. Contraception and adolescents. *Pediatrics*. 1999; 104(5):1161-1166. (aappolicy.aappublications.org/cgi/content/full/pediatrics;104/5/1161).

American Academy of Pediatrics, Committee on Bioethics. Ethical issues with genetic testing in pediatrics. *Pediatrics*. 2001;107:1451-1455. (aappolicy.aappublications.org/cgi/content/full/pediatrics;107/6/1451).

American Academy of Pediatrics, Committee on Bioethics. Informed consent, parental permission, and assent in pediatric practice. *Pediatrics*. 1995;95:314-317. (aappolicy.aappublications.org/cgi/content/abstract/pediatrics;95/2/314).

American Academy of Pediatrics, Committee on Substance Abuse. Testing for drugs of abuse in children and adolescents. *Pediatrics*. 1996;98:305-307. (aappolicy.aappublications.org/cgi/content/abstract/pediatrics;98/2/305).

American Academy of Pediatrics, Medical Home Initiatives for Children with Special Needs Project Advisory Committee. The medical home. *Pediatrics*. 2002;110:184-186. (aappolicy.aappublications.org/cgi/content/full/pediatrics;110/1/184).

Diekema DS, American Academy of Pediatrics, Committee on Bioethics. Responding to parental refusals of immunization of children. *Pediatrics*. 2005;115:1428-1431. (aappolicy.aappublications.org/cgi/content/full/pediatrics;115/5/1428).

REFERENCES

1. Buchanan AE, Brock DW. *Deciding for Others: The Ethics of Surrogate Decision Making*. Cambridge, NY: Cambridge University Press; 1989.
2. Alderson P, Montgomery J. *Health Care Choices: Making Decisions with Children*, London, UK: Institute for Public Policy Research; 1996.
3. American Academy of Pediatrics, Committee on Bioethics. Informed consent, parental permission, and assent in pediatric practice. *Pediatrics*. 1995;95:314-317.
4. Weir RF, Peters C. Affirming the decisions adolescents make about life and death. *Hastings Center Report*. 1997;27(6):29-40.
5. Canadian Paediatric Society. Treatment decisions regarding infants, children and adolescents. *Paediatrics and Child Health*. 2004;9:99-103.
6. Ross LF. *Children, Families and Health Care Decision Making*. Oxford, UK: Oxford University Press; 1998.
7. Goldstein J, Freud A, Solnit AJ. *Before the Best Interests of the Child*. New York, NY: Free Press; 1979.
8. Grunbaum JA, Kann L, Kinchen S, et al. Youth risk behavior surveillance—United States, 2003. *MMWR Morbid Mortal Wkly Rep*. 2004;53(SS-2):1-29.
9. American Academy of Pediatrics, Committee on Adolescence. Contraception and adolescents. *Pediatrics*. 1999; 104:1161-1166.
10. Alan Guttmacher Institute. *Sex and America's Teenagers*. New York, NY: Alan Guttmacher Institute; 1994.
11. Klein JD. American Academy of Pediatrics, Committee on Adolescence. Adolescent pregnancy: current trends and issues. *Pediatrics*. 2005;116:281-286.
12. Fraser AM, Brockert JE, Ward RH. Association of young maternal age with adverse reproductive outcomes. *N Eng J Med*. 1995;332:1113-1117.
13. Tillett J. Adolescents and informed consent: ethical and legal issues. *J Perinat Neonatal Nurs*. 2005;19:112-121.
14. Ross LF. Health care decision making by children. Is it in their best interest? *Hastings Center Report*. 1997;27: 41-45.
15. Gaylin W. Competence: no longer all or none. In: Gaylin W, Macklin R, eds: *Who Speaks for the Child: The Problems of Proxy Consent*. New York, NY: Plenum Press; 1982:27-54.
16. Costello JC. If I can say yes, why can't I say no? Adolescents at risk and the right to give or withhold consent to health care. In: Humm SR, Ort BA, Anbari MM, et al, eds. *Child, Parent and State*. Philadelphia, PA: Temple University Press; 1994:490-503.
17. Cohen GJ, American Academy of Pediatrics, Committee on Psychosocial Aspects of Child and Family Health. Helping children and families deal with divorce and separation. *Pediatrics*. 2002;110:1019-1023.

18. Weddle M, Kokotailo P. Adolescent substance abuse. Confidentiality and consent. *Pediatr Clin North Am.* 2002;49:301-315.
19. Ford CA, Millstein SG, Halpern-Felsher BL, et al. Influence of physician confidentiality assurances on adolescents' willingness to disclose information and seek future health care. A randomized controlled trial. *JAMA.* 1997; 278:1029-1034.
20. American Academy of Pediatrics, Committee on Substance Abuse. Testing for drugs of abuse in children and adolescents. *Pediatrics.* 1996;98:305-307.
21. Kulig JW, American Academy of Pediatrics, Committee on Substance Abuse. Tobacco, alcohol, and other drugs: the role of the pediatrician in prevention, identification, and management of substance abuse. *Pediatrics.* 2005;115:816-821.
22. American Society of Human Genetics Board of Directors, American College of Medical Genetics Board of Directors. Points to consider: ethical, legal, and psychosocial implications of genetic testing in children and adolescents. *Am J Hum Genet.* 1995;57:1233-1241.
23. Andrews LB. *Assessing Genetic Risks: Implications for Health and Social Policy.* Washington, DC: National Academy Press; 1994.
24. Shinaman A, Bain LJ, Shoulson I. Preempting genetic discrimination and assaults on privacy: report of a symposium. *Am J Med Genet.* 2003;120:589-593.
25. Ross LF. Predictive genetic testing for conditions that present in childhood. *Kennedy Inst Ethics J.* 2002; 12:225-244.
26. Wilson JMG, Jungner G. *Principles and Practice of Screening for Disease.* Geneva, Switzerland: World Health Organization; 1968.
27. American Academy of Pediatrics, Committee on Bioethics. Ethical issues with genetic testing in pediatrics. *Pediatrics.* 2001;107:1451-1455.
28. Diekema DS. Parental refusals of medical treatment: the harm principle as threshold for state intervention. *Theor Med Bioet.* 2004;25:243-264.
29. Faden R, Chwalow AJ, Holtzman NA, et al. A survey to evaluate parental consent as public policy for neonatal screening. *Am J Pub Health.* 1982;72:1347-1352.
30. Holtzman NA, Leonard CO, Farfel MR. Issues in antenatal and neonatal screening and surveillance for hereditary and congenital disorders. *Annu Rev Public Health.* 1981;2:219-251.
31. Campbell E, Ross LF. Parental attitudes and beliefs regarding the genetic testing of children. *Community Genetics.* 2005;8:94-102.
32. Douglas Cty. v. Anaya, S-03-1446, 269 Neb. 552. Douglas County, Nebraska, appellee, v. Josue Anaya and Mary Anaya, husband and wife, as parents of Rosa Ariel Anaya, a minor child, appellants. Filed March 25, 2005. No. S-03-1446.
33. Silverman RD, May T. Private choice versus public health: religion, morality, and childhood vaccination law. *Margins (Baltimore).* 2001;1:505-521.
34. Fredrickson DD, Davis TC, Arnold CL, et al. Childhood immunization refusal: provider and parent perceptions. *Fam Med.* 2004;36:431-439.
35. Kulenkampff M, Schwartzman JS, Wilson J. Neurological complications of pertussis inoculation. *Arch Dis Child.* 1974;49:46-49.
36. Wakefield AJ, Murch SH, Anthony A, et al. Ileal-lymphoid-nodular hyperplasia, non-specific colitis, and pervasive developmental disorder in children. *Lancet.* 1998;351:637-641.
37. Colgrove J, Bayer R. Could it happen here? Vaccine risk controversies and the specter of derailment. *Health Aff (Millwood).* 2005;24:729-739.
38. Murch SH, Anthony A, Casson DH, et al. Retraction of an interpretation. *Lancet.* 2004;363:750.
39. Immunization Safety Review Committee, Board on Health Promotion and Disease Prevention, Institute of Medicine of the National Academies. *Immunization Safety Review: Vaccines and Autism.* Washington, DC: National Academies Press; 2004.
40. Smith PJ, Chu SY, Barker LE. Children who have received no vaccines: who are they and where do they live? *Pediatrics.* 2004;114:187-195.
41. Centers for Disease Control and Prevention. Poliovirus infections in four unvaccinated children—Minnesota, August-October 2005. *MMWR Morb Mortal Wkly Rep.* 2005;54:1053-1055.
42. Flanagan-Klygis EA, Sharp L. Frader JE. Dismissing the family who refuses vaccines: a study of pediatrician attitudes. *Arch Pediatr Adolesc Med.* 2005;159: 929-934.
43. Diekema DS, American Academy of Pediatrics, Committee on Bioethics. Responding to parental refusals of immunization of children. *Pediatrics.* 2005;115:1428-1431.
44. American Academy of Pediatrics. Documenting parental refusal to have their children vaccinated. Available at: www.cispimmunize.org/pro/pdf/RefusaltoVaccinate_revised%204-11-06.pdf. Accessed October 14, 2007.
45. Carp EW. *Family Matters: Secrecy and Disclosure in the History of Adoption.* Cambridge, MA: Harvard University Press; 1998.
46. Stolley KS. Statistics on adoption in the United States. *The Future of Children: ADOPTION.* 1993;3(1):26-42.
47. Evan B, Donaldson Adoption Institute. Overview of adoption in the United States. Available at: www.adoptioninstitute.org/FactOverview.html. Accessed October 14, 2007.
48. The Ethics Committee of the American Society for Reproductive Medicine. Informing offspring of their conception by gamete donation. *Fertil Steril.* 2004; 82(suppl 1):S212-S216.
49. Murray C, Golombok S. To tell or not to tell: the decision-making process of egg-donation parents. *Hum Fertil.* 2003;6:89-95.
50. Lycett E, Daniels K, Curson R, et al. School-aged children of donor insemination: a study of parents' disclosure patterns. *Hum Reprod.* 2005;20:810-819.
51. Centers for Disease Control and Prevention, National Office of Public Health Genomics. Evaluating family history for preventive medicine and public health. Available at: www.cdc.gov/genomics/activities/famhx.htm. Accessed October 14, 2007.
52. National Coalition for Health Professional Education in Genetics. Family History Working Group. Available at: www.nchpeg.org/content.asp?dbsection=working. Accessed October 14, 2007.
53. Hastrup JL, Hotchkiss AP, Johnson CA. Accuracy of knowledge of family history of cardiovascular disorders. *Health Psychol.* 1985;4(4):291-306.
54. Patch C, Roderick P, Rosenberg W. Comparison of genotypic and phenotypic strategies for population screening in hemochromatosis: assessment of anxiety, depression, and perception of health. *Genet Med.* 2005;7:550-556.
55. Steeds RP, Channer KS. How important is family history in ischaemic heart disease? *QJM.* 1997;90:427-430.
56. Nabholz CE, von Overbeck J. Gene-environment interactions and the complexity of human genetic diseases. *J Insur Med (Seattle).* 2004;36(1):47-53.
57. Borchers D, American Academy of Pediatrics, Committee on Early Childhood, Adoption, and Dependent Care. Families and adoption: the pediatrician's role in supporting communication. *Pediatrics.* 2003;112: 1437-1441.

58. Maron BJ, Ackerman MJ, Nishimura RA, et al. Task Force 4: HCM and other cardiomyopathies, mitral valve prolapse, myocarditis, and Marfan syndrome. *J Am Coll Cardiol*. 2005;45:1340-1345.
59. Mitten MJ. When is disqualification from sports justified? Medical judgment vs. patients' rights. *Phys Sports Med*. 1996;24:75-78.
60. Stein MT, Perrin EL, American Academy of Pediatrics, Committee on Psychosocial Aspects of Child and Family Health. Guidance for effective discipline. *Pediatrics*. 1998;101:723-728.
61. American Academy of Pediatrics, Division of Child Health Research. Periodic Survey #38: AAP survey on corporal punishment reveals divergent views. October 1997 through March 1998. Available at: www.aap.org/research/periodicsurvey/ps38a.htm. Accessed October 14, 2007.
62. Bauman LJ, Friedman SB. Corporal punishment. *Pediatr Clin North Am*. 1998;45:403-414.
63. Hosmer L. Home birth. *Clin Obstet Gynecol*. 2001;44:671-680.
64. Pang JW, Heffelfinger JD, Huang GJ, et al. Outcomes of planned home births in Washington State: 1989-1996. *Obstet Gynecol*. 2002;100:253-259.
65. Johnson KC, Daviss BA. Outcomes of planned home births with certified professional midwives: large prospective study in North America. *BMJ*. 2005;330:1416. Available at: www.bmj.com/cgi/reprint/330/7505/1416. Accessed October 14, 2007.
66. Landon MB, Hauth JC, Leveno KJ, et al, National Institute of Child Health and Human Development Maternal—Fetal Medicine Units Network. Maternal and perinatal outcomes associated with a trial of labor after prior cesarean delivery. *N Engl J Med*. 2004;351:2581-2589.
67. American College of Obstetricians and Gynecologists [ACOG] Committee on Practice Bulletins-Obstetrics with the assistance of Porter TF, Zelop CM. Practice bulletin no. 54. Vaginal birth after previous cesarean delivery. *Obstet Gynecol*. 2004;104:203-212.
68. American Academy of Pediatrics, Medical Home Initiatives for Children with Special Needs Project Advisory Committee. The medical home. *Pediatrics*. 2002;110:184-186.

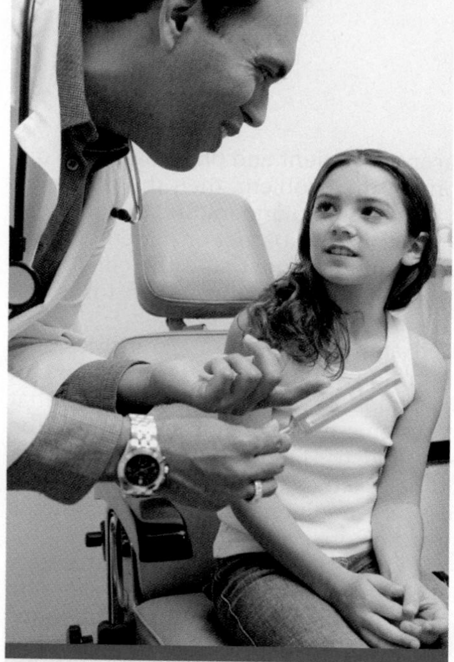

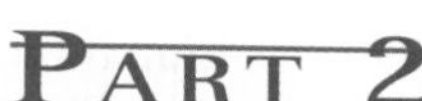

PART 2

Evaluation and Communication

12 The Pediatric History
13 Interviewing Children
14 Pediatric Physical Examination
15 Pediatric Imaging
16 Disclosing a Diagnosis With Parents and Patients
17 Cultural Issues in Primary Pediatric Care
18 Adherence to Pediatric Health Care Recommendations
19 Art of Referral, Consultation, and Collaborative Management
20 Hospitalist Medicine: Communicating With Patients and Families
21 Hospital Care

Chapter 12

THE PEDIATRIC HISTORY

William E. Boyle, MD

"A good history carefully obtained from an intelligent mother puts the physician in possession of a fund of information about the patient which is of greatest value, not only in arriving at a diagnosis in the illness for which he is consulted, but is exceedingly helpful in the future management of the child."

L. EMMETT HOLT, 1908[1]

A history is a narrative related by the patient or the patient's family. It is a unique and personal story in which are embedded the words, phrases, and clues that direct the physician to the general or specific medical problem of the patient. The patient or family brings complaints of illness, which the practitioner must translate into medical theories of disease. Care must be taken so that nothing is lost in translating this personal story into a precise disease entity. It requires the physician to pay close attention to this detailed sequence of events and, through careful direct questioning, to formulate a differential diagnosis. Parents and patients hope the physician will hear their story and interpret it correctly. This task is not easy.

Perhaps in no other medical field is a history as important as it is in pediatrics. Early detection of problems related to health—including growth, development, and nutrition—and prevention of future difficulties relies on the practitioner's thorough knowledge of the child and the family, their lifestyle, and their environment. Unlike most other areas of medicine, the pediatric history is usually given by someone other than the patient. Thus a certain amount of subjectivity and objectivity is lost. Signs and symptoms are filtered through parental perspectives before emerging as historical data, therefore these perspectives are influenced by parental hopes and fears. A pediatric history is a compilation of information gathered in a variety of ways through interviews, direct observations, questionnaires, and medical records that usually provides a concise record of the child and the family.

In the past, training in interviewing and history taking took place for an acute problem in which the concern or complaint was readily stated or easily seen. Today, however, children are seen for an increasing number of psychosocial problems, usually outside the hospital. These problems may include learning difficulties, chronic or disabling conditions, or behavioral or developmental problems, all of which require sensitive, insightful listening. The pediatrician must have a thorough knowledge of the child's health status, developmental stage, and cognitive level, as well as the family's functional characteristics, belief systems, and socioeconomic circumstances. Much of pediatrics deals with vague questions or concerns, such as "Why does she cry so much?" "Why is he so thin?" or "Is that cough serious?" These concerns must be answered and expectations managed if the encounter is to be fruitful. If the parent or patient and physician have different perceptions of the problem, then the physician must attempt to tease out and understand the patient's or the parents' concerns. The parent or patient may be worried about something tangential to the chief complaint; this situation is sometimes referred to as the *second diagnosis*.

Today's children and their families are increasingly diverse, and they bring with them a wide variety of cultural beliefs and customs. Physicians must be aware that their own belief systems may differ from those of the patient and family and try to make accommodations. Questions should be asked as to what the family thinks caused the illness or condition and what treatments have been attempted before seeing the physician.

Much transpires during the initial interview between a practitioner and a family other than the gathering of a history. The tone of all future encounters is established, and, ideally, the family begins to develop a trusting, confident relationship with the practitioner. Just as the practitioner is trying to assess the problem at hand, so too are the parents (and child) *sizing up* the clinician. A warm, friendly, nonjudgmental, courteous manner facilitates a good relationship. Taking a history requires some degree of decision making on the part of the interviewer as to what is relevant. Taking a history is not merely gathering a list of all symptoms and pertinent historical *negatives*; it involves the synthesis of various facts, attitudes, and observations. To perform this task well requires experience, tact, and a degree of intuition. The task is difficult. A history is compiled best if, for each visit, the practitioner can obtain the answers to 3 questions:

1. "Why did you come today?"
2. "What are you worried about most?"
3. "Why does that worry you?"

Answers to these questions not only direct further inquiry, but also provide clues to parent and patient concerns that need to be allayed or dealt with directly during the visit and, perhaps, thereafter. For example, a parent who brings a child to a physician because of swollen cervical lymph nodes may be worried that they have a malignancy because an aunt who died of Hodgkin's disease had the same problem. Parents, older children, and adolescents need to be told what symptoms and signs do *not* represent, as well as what they do represent, especially if the parents and patient are worried that the symptoms and signs indicate a serious or fatal illness.

SETTING AND AMBIANCE

Pediatric histories are taken in a variety of locations, and a comfortable environment enhances communication. If the practitioner is courteous, interested, and helpful, then a trusting, positive relationship is likely to develop. Patients and parents are acutely aware of what the physician thinks of them or what they perceive the physician's opinion of them to be; this perception is termed the *reflexive self-concept.* ("The doctor thinks I'm a good parent.") If the reflexive self-concept is high, then parent (or patient) satisfaction and compliance with recommendations for management are more likely to be high. Some questions to consider are:

Does the practitioner imply disinterest in the patient by cutting short the parent's description or allowing constant interruptions during the history taking?

Is privacy ensured?

Are children made comfortable?

Is there a place for clothing and belongings (other than a lap)?

Obviously, seating should be available for all, and the history taker should remain seated for the session. The practitioner should strive to maintain eye contact and not constantly view a computer screen or notes. Parents or guardians should be called by their formal names (Mrs. Williams, Mr. Adams), unless a personal relationship has been established that enables the use of first names. Children should be referred to by their first names rather than *he, she,* or *the infant.* Notes can be taken as long as doing so does not distract from the continuity or spontaneity of the interview. Most parents find coping with more than one child as being disruptive and distracting; therefore seeing more than one child at a time or having others in the room should be discouraged. Toys or books should be available to help occupy infants and toddlers, if necessary.

Clothing and appearance may affect the ease with which a relationship is established. Parents and children view a visit to the pediatrician as a special occasion and frequently dress accordingly. They hope their practitioner will view the visit in the same manner. The practitioner's dress should be appropriate and consistent with local values. Most pediatricians do not wear a white coat because it may evoke fearful memories for the child, although this notion has never been substantiated. Whatever the attire, a sense of competence must be conveyed.

TYPES OF INTERVIEWS

The initial history may be taken during an interview with the parents before their infant's birth, in the hospital after the birth, in the physician's office during the visit for whatever reason, in an emergency department at the time of an acute illness, or in a hospital room after admission for a specific illness or elective surgery. The time devoted to the initial interview and the amount of information gathered depends on the circumstances. Similarly, subsequent history taking will vary in depth and breadth, depending on the reason for the visit and the amount of time that has elapsed since the last visit.

This chapter focuses on the information to be gathered and the techniques used in obtaining the comprehensive pediatric history. Circumstances may preclude completion of this exercise during the initial visit. For example, the initial history obtained for a child who has acute otitis media and who is squeezed in during fully scheduled office hours will be brief and relate primarily to the chief complaint. The rest of the history can be obtained during a scheduled follow-up visit.

Prenatal Interview

Ideally, the parents should have their first encounter with a pediatrician before their infant is born. To many people, the idea of bringing an infant in utero to the pediatrician seems strange; but much information can be gathered at this time, and a strong, understanding relationship between the parents and the pediatrician can be fostered. Furthermore, some issues can be addressed before the postpartum period. For example, a pregnant woman with little psychosocial support may be identified and appropriate aid offered. In addition, society in the United States is mobile; most young couples live alone and are often far removed from parents and siblings, and they often turn to professionals for support and assistance.

Obstetricians traditionally care for women only throughout pregnancy and the immediate postpartum period. Pediatricians traditionally assume care of the infant at birth. Many women find difficulty in leaving someone who has supported them through a difficult psychobiological change and developing a new relationship while they learn the new role of motherhood. A prenatal interview can greatly assist in this transition.

Prenatal interviews do not need to be long or detailed; 20 to 30 minutes should suffice. In addition to gathering facts, the pediatrician should set a tone for future encounters. Husband and wife should be interviewed together, if possible, so that parental concerns can be aired, and they can be helped to support each other. Parents are anxious about their adequacy and the health of their unborn infant, and a supportive attitude and tacit acknowledgment that these fears are understandable can be helpful.

A thorough family history is a way of showing concern, not just for the child, but also for the entire family. Parents should understand the physician's interest in them as individuals and not merely as Teddy's or Sarah Jane's mother and father. The prenatal interview provides an excellent opportunity to inquire about belief systems and cultural values.

During a typical prenatal interview, plans for labor and delivery should be discussed, as well as a program of childbirth education and the type of infant feeding that is contemplated. Pointing out certain safety issues to which the parents should attend is wise at this time, before their infant comes home, such as obtaining a child safety seat and a smoke detector and setting the hot water heater at a safe temperature (see Chapter 30, Injury Prevention). Many couples will already know the sex of their unborn child through prenatal ultrasound. Circumcision should be discussed, if they know they are having a boy. If blood tests (newborn screening), immunizations (for hepatitis B virus), or vitamin K administration will be performed, then these subjects should be described and discussed.

The mother's blood type, medications taken, and rubella status (if known) should be elicited. Genetic information should be gathered about both sets of grandparents. In addition to inherited disorders and birth defects, familial tendencies such as obesity, hypertension, and short stature should be investigated. Asking what the couple's own parents were like is also wise because parenting techniques, styles, and cultural beliefs are frequently passed from one generation to the next.

After dealing with the family history, the clinician needs to gather some information about other supportive individuals. Who will help out when the infant comes home? Will the husband have a paternity leave of some sort? Grandparents traditionally visit shortly after delivery, and the pediatrician should point this out and ask if they will be helpful or a burden. The pediatrician should also inquire if transportation and a telephone are readily available. The physician should be alert at all times for evidence of undue stress, isolation, and prior psychosocial issues such as maternal depression or drug abuse because these factors are known to be predictors of poor parenting. The parents will want to know when the pediatrician will see the infant in the hospital, what the appointment schedule will be, and how the pediatrician can be reached. Fees for visits can also be discussed at this time.

The parents should be allowed to ask questions about their concerns. Supporting their instincts, rather than directing and showing the pediatrician's own personal bias, is best. The pediatrician should anticipate certain normal variations such as sleepy infants, the postpartum *blues*, and the physiologic slump that lasts from 6 to 8 weeks after birth. Parental questions may seem trivial (skin care, type of diapers), but they all revolve around the question, "Will we be good parents?" Strong reassurance that their instincts are good serves to reinforce and strengthen the couple's tendencies toward good parenting and leads to a confident beginning as parents.

At the conclusion of the interview, the practitioner should have an idea of the parents' lifestyle and coping mechanisms, and the parents should feel reassured that they have a supportive person who will help them enter parenthood.

As prenatal interviewing has become more widespread, interview requests for 2nd or subsequent pregnancies have become more common. These sessions are generally not quite so formal and can take place during the routine health maintenance visits of an older child. Parental concerns deal not only with the health and soundness of the unborn, but also with coping with another child. "Will I be able to divide myself and still survive?" The mother may find herself torn between her infant in utero and her older infant. Efforts to push the older child into relinquishing diapers, crib, stroller, or high chair should be discouraged. Separation at the time of delivery can be a problem for a child, who must be told that mommy will leave for a while and then return. This separation should occur shortly before the expected delivery. The separation will also stress the supports that the family has developed, and the clinician should review these at this time. Recounting any previous birth experience is similarly important so that conflicts or problems may be identified and thus prevented.

Comprehensive Pediatric History Interview

Traditionally, history taking has been a stepwise delineation of the events that led to the practitioner-patient encounter. Most clinicians learn this technique while dealing with hospitalized or acutely ill children, in a location where the problem frequently was visible or obvious. Fortunately, a great deal of history taking now occurs in settings other than the hospital and frequently does not involve illness and is termed the *pediatric history interview*. History taking is merely a part of the interview, which should include observation of behavior and family interactions. Essentially, a history is a story about an encounter between practitioner and parent and child that includes subjective and objective data and omits some details considered irrelevant.

Box 12-1 is a suggested outline for components of a comprehensive pediatric history. In certain settings, some of the data will have already been gathered, but a thorough knowledge of each component of the history is essential.

Usually, the interview begins with the parents stating the concerns that led to the present encounter—the *chief complaint*. The parents should be allowed, with as little interruption as possible, to relate their story as they recall it. Certain areas may be amplified and clarified, but direct or challenging questions should be avoided. After eliciting the chief complaint, the practitioner should enumerate the events associated with it in an orderly sequence *(present illness)*. In addition to facts, parental concerns and feelings about these symptoms should be elicited. The parents should be asked to speculate on what they think is causing the complaint or symptom. This information can be valuable in several respects. First, it demonstrates the level of parental concern, which may influence subsequent care and treatment. Thus parents who equate nosebleeds with leukemia, for instance, will need more than simple reassurance. Second, parental concerns about causation may color the history a great deal; for example, their concern about developmental delay can influence the information they supply about achievement of early milestones. Third, cultural bias or guilt as to causation may exist that should be addressed. Discovering how the present illness affects the rest of the family is always important. Who misses work? Who loses sleep? This information will help the physician better understand the family's concerns about and responses to a given symptom or illness and what, if any, secondary gain exists for the child.

Although the chief complaint must remain the central focus of the interview, it is frequently obvious that this complaint is not the main problem. This circumstance is especially true when dealing with very young children. Tired, anxious, or frightened parents often perceive their reactions to an infant as being abnormal in some way; they then project this perception as something being wrong with the infant, which makes seeking help acceptable. Once the practitioner recognizes this perception, an attempt should be made to create an atmosphere that allows the parents to express all their concerns. Questions such as, "Are there any other problems with Kathy you would like to discuss?" or "Is there anything else bothering you about Connor?" might facilitate communication.

After the present illness has been defined and elaborated, certain significant events should be enumerated *(medical history)*. Much of this material is factual and can be obtained by using a direct question-and-answer format. Significant events such as operations, serious injuries, and hospitalizations should be verified by obtaining and reviewing appropriate hospital records.

BOX 12-1 Comprehensive Pediatric History

The following comprehensive pediatric history is exhaustive and obviously not meant to be used in its entirety with all patients. However, depending on the patient's age and gender and the nature of the chief complaint and the present illness, the interviewer will need to explore in depth some or all of the subjects listed. In most instances, common sense must be used in deciding how much information should be gathered.

Date of interview

Identifying data: Record the date and place of birth, gender, race, religious preference, nickname (particularly for children 2 to 10 years of age), parents' first names (and last names, if different), and where the parents can be reached during work hours.

Source of and reason for referral

Source of the history: This source may be the parents, the patient, or sometimes a relative or friend. The practitioner should use judgment of the validity of the source's reporting. Other possible sources of the history are the patient's medical record or a letter from a referring physician or the school nurse.

Chief complaints: When possible, quote the parents or the patient. Clarify whether these complaints are the concerns of the parents, the patient, or both. In some instances, they are the concerns of a 3rd party, such as a teacher.

Present illness: This condition should be a clear, chronologic narrative of the problems for which the patient is seeking care. Include the onset of the problem, the setting in which it developed, its manifestations and treatments, its impact on the patient's life, and its meaning to the patient or the parents, or both. Describe the principal symptoms in terms of (1) location, (2) quality, (3) quantity or severity, (4) timing (ie, onset, duration, frequency), (5) setting, (6) factors that have aggravated or relieved these symptoms, and (7) associated manifestations. Relevant data from the patient's chart, such as laboratory reports, also belong in the *present illness* section, as do significant negatives (ie, the absence of certain symptoms that will aid in differential diagnosis). Include how each member of the family responds to the patient's symptoms, their concerns about them, and whether the patient achieves any secondary gains from them.

Medical history: General state of health as the parents or patient perceives it.

Birth history: This information is particularly important during the first 2 years of life and when dealing with neurologic and developmental problems. Review the hospital records if preliminary information from the parents indicates significant difficulties before, during, or after delivery.

Prenatal history: Determine the mother's health before and during the pregnancy, including nutritional patterns and specific illnesses related to or complicated by the pregnancy; doses and duration of all legal and illegal drugs taken during the pregnancy, including alcohol ingestion and cigarette smoking; weight gain; vaginal bleeding; duration of the pregnancy; and the parents' attitudes toward the pregnancy and parenthood in general and toward this child in particular.

Natal history: Determine the nature of the mother's labor and delivery, including degree of difficulty, analgesia used, and complications encountered; birth order, if a multiple birth; and birth weight.

Neonatal history: Determine the onset of respirations; resuscitation efforts; Apgar scores and estimation of gestational age; specific problems with feeding, respiratory distress, cyanosis, jaundice, anemia, convulsions, congenital anomalies, or infection; the mother's health after delivery; separation of the mother and infant and the reasons for the separation; the mother's initial reactions to her baby and the nature of bonding; and patterns of crying and sleeping and of urination and defecation.

Feeding history: This information is particularly important during the first 2 years of life and in dealing with problems of undernutrition and overnutrition.

Infancy:

Breastfeeding: frequency and duration of feedings, use of complementary or supplementary artificial (formula) feedings, difficulties encountered, and time and method of weaning.

Artificial (formula) feeding: type, concentration, amount, and frequency of feeds; difficulties encountered (regurgitation, colic, diarrhea); and timing and method of weaning.

Vitamin, iron, and fluoride supplements: type, amount given, frequency, and duration.

Solid foods: types and amounts of baby foods given, when introduced and infant's response, introduction of junior and table foods, start of self-foods, start of self-feeding, and the mother's and child's responses to the feeding process.

Childhood:

Eating habits: likes and dislikes, specific types and amounts of food eaten, parents' attitudes toward eating in general and toward this child's undereating or overeating, and parents' response to any feeding problems. With childhood feeding problems, the parents may need to keep a diet diary for 7 to 14 days to allow accurate assessment of the child's food intake.

Growth and development history: This history is particularly important during infancy and childhood and in dealing with problems such as delayed physical growth, psychomotor and intellectual retardation, and behavioral disturbances.

Physical growth: Determine the actual (or approximate) weight and height at birth and at 1, 2, 5, and 10 years; record any history of slow or rapid gains or losses; and note the tooth eruption and loss pattern.

Developmental milestones: Determine the ages at which the patient held head up while prone; rolled over from front to back and back to front; sat with support and alone; stood with support and alone; walked with support and alone; said first word, combinations of words, and sentences; tied own shoes; and dressed without help.

Social development:

Sleep: amount and patterns during the day and at night; bedtime routines; type and location of bed; and nightmares, terrors, and somnambulation.

Toileting: methods of training used, when bladder and bowel control were attained, occurrence of accidents or of enuresis or encopresis, parents' attitudes, and terms used in the family for urination and defecation (important to know when a young child is admitted to the hospital).

Continued

BOX 12-1 Comprehensive Pediatric History—cont'd

Speech: hesitation, stuttering, baby talk, lisping, and estimate of the number of words in the child's vocabulary.

Habits: bed-rocking; head-banging; tics; thumb-sucking; nail-biting; pica; ritualistic behavior; and use of tobacco, alcohol, or drugs.

Discipline: parents' assessment of child's temperament and response to discipline; methods used and their success or failure; negativism; temper tantrums; withdrawal episodes; and aggressive behavior.

Schooling: experience with child care, nursery school, and kindergarten; age and adjustment on entry; current level of parents' and child's satisfaction; academic achievement; and school's concerns.

Sexuality: relationships with members of the opposite gender; inquisitiveness about conception, pregnancy, and girl-boy differences; parents' responses to child's questions and what they have taught the child about masturbation, menstruation, nocturnal emissions, the development of secondary sexual characteristics, and sexual urges; and dating patterns.

Personality: degree of independence; relationships with parents, siblings, and peers; group and independent activities and interests; congeniality; special friends (real or imaginary); major assets and skills; and self-image.

Childhood illness: Determine the specific illnesses the child has had, as well as any recent exposures to communicable diseases.

Immunizations: Record the specific dates of administration of each vaccine so that a booster program can be maintained throughout childhood and adolescence; also record any untoward reactions to a vaccine. The parents should have their own written record of the child's immunizations.

Screening procedures: Record the dates and results of any screening tests. For all children, these tests should include vision, hearing, urinalysis, and hematocrit, as well as newborn screening for genetic-metabolic disorders. For certain high-risk children, additional tests may include tuberculosis, sickle cell, HIV, blood lead, cholesterol, alpha$_1$-antitrypsin deficiency, and any other screening that may be indicated.

Operations, injuries, and hospitalizations: Elicit the details of these events and the child's and the parents' reactions to them. If the child is old enough, then ask age-appropriate questions about safety and prevention of injuries.

Allergies: Pay particular attention to the allergic diseases that are more prevalent during infancy and childhood: eczema, urticaria, perennial allergic rhinitis, asthma, food intolerance, and insect venom hypersensitivity.

Current medications: Include home remedies, alternative medicines, nonprescription drugs, and medicines borrowed from family members or friends. If the patient appears to be taking one or more medications, then survey one 24-hour period in detail: "Take yesterday, for example. Starting from when he woke up, what was the first medicine Thomas took? How much? How often during the day did he take it? What is he taking it for? What other medications?"

Family history: Record the education attained, job history, emotional health, and family background of each parent or parent substitute; the family's socioeconomic circumstances, including income, type of dwelling, and neighborhood; parents' work schedules; family cohesiveness and interdependence; support available from relatives, friends, and neighbors; ethnic and cultural milieu in which the family lives; and parents' expectations of the patient and attitudes toward the child in relation to siblings. (All or part of this information can be recorded in the *present illness* section, if pertinent to it, or under *psychosocial history.*)

Also record the age and health or age and cause of death of each immediate family member, including the parents and siblings (Figure 12-1). Ascertain consanguinity of the parents by inquiring if they are related by blood.

Note the occurrence in the family of any of the following conditions: diabetes, tuberculosis, heart disease, high blood pressure, stroke, kidney disease, cancer, arthritis, anemia, headaches, mental illness, or symptoms resembling those of the patient.

Psychosocial history: This information is an outline or narrative description that captures the important and relevant information about the patient as a person: the patient's lifestyle, home situation, and significant others.

Typical day: How does the patient spend time between arising and going to bed?

Religious and health beliefs of the family: What beliefs of the family are relevant to the perceptions of wellness, illness, and treatment?

What is the patient's outlook on the future?

Review of systems:

General: Usual weight, recent weight change, weakness, fatigue, fever, pallor.

Skin: Rashes, lumps, itching, dryness, color change, changes in hair or nails.

Head: Headache, head injury.

Eyes: Vision, glasses or contact lenses, last eye examination, pain, redness, excessive tearing, double vision.

Ears: Hearing, tinnitus, vertigo, earaches, infection, discharge.

Nose and sinuses: Frequent colds, nasal stuffiness, hay fever, nosebleeds, sinus trouble.

Mouth and throat: Condition of teeth and gums, bleeding gums, last dental examination, frequent sore throats, hoarseness.

Neck: Lumps in the neck, swollen glands, goiter, pain in the neck.

Breasts: Lumps, pain, nipple discharge.

Respiratory system: Cough, sputum (color, quantity), hemoptysis, wheezing, asthma, bronchitis, pneumonia, tuberculosis, pleurisy; results of last chest roentgenogram.

Cardiac system: High blood pressure, rheumatic fever, heart murmurs; dyspnea, cyanosis, edema; chest pain, palpitations; results of past electrocardiograms or other heart tests.

Gastrointestinal tract: Trouble swallowing, loss of appetite, nausea, vomiting, hematemesis, indigestion; frequency of bowel movements, change in bowel habits, rectal bleeding or black, tarry stools, constipation, diarrhea; abdominal pain, food intolerance, excessive passing of gas; jaundice, hepatitis.

Urinary tract: Frequency of urination, polyuria, nocturia, dysuria, hematuria, urgency, hesitancy, incontinence, urinary tract infections.

Genitoreproductive system—male patients: Discharge from or sore on penis, history of venereal disease and its treatment, hernias, testicular pain or masses, frequency of intercourse, libido, sexual difficulties, sexual preference.

BOX 12-1 Comprehensive Pediatric History—cont'd

Genitoreproductive system—female patients: Age at menarche; regularity, frequency, and duration of periods; amount of bleeding, bleeding between periods, last menstrual period; dysmenorrhea; discharge, itching, venereal disease, and its treatment; number of pregnancies, number of deliveries, number of abortions (spontaneous and induced); complications of pregnancy; birth control methods; frequency of intercourse; libido; sexual difficulties; sexual preference.

Musculoskeletal system: Joint pains or stiffness, arthritis, backache; if these conditions are present, then describe location and symptoms (eg, swelling, redness, pain, stiffness, weakness, limitation of motion or activity), muscle pains, or cramps.

Neurologic system: Fainting, blackouts, seizures, paralysis, local weakness, numbness, tingling, tremors, memory loss.

Psychiatric issues: Nervousness, tension, moodiness, depression.

Endocrinologic issues: Thyroid trouble, heat or cold intolerance, excessive sweating, diabetes, and excessive thirst, hunger, or urination.

Hematologic issues: Anemia, easy bruising or bleeding, past transfusions and possible reactions to them.

Modified from Bickley LS, Hoekelman RA: Interviewing and the health history. In: Bickley LS, Hoekelman RA, eds. *Bates' Guide to Physical Examination and History Taking.* 7th ed. Philadelphia, PA: JB Lippincott; 1999. Used with permission.

When obtaining the patient's early history, the practitioner should elicit medically significant facts from conception to the onset of the present illness. All areas delineated in Box 12-1 should be touched on to some degree. The amount of information obtained may vary, but prenatal problems such as bleeding, eclampsia, or infection should be noted, and birth weight, type of delivery, and neonatal problems, if any, should be described. Information about nutrition can reveal a great deal about family dynamics and parental perceptions and expectations. "Tell me how Jennifer eats" frequently brings forth a torrent of information; but its value, nutritionally speaking, may be limited. "Good eaters" and "picky eaters" frequently weigh the same, and children who "hardly eat a thing" are often overweight.

In dealing with issues of development, asking an indirect question such as, "Tell me what Ann did during her 1st (or 2nd) year" is frequently best. This inquiry usually elicits much more information than do direct questions about motor milestones. The clinician should seek information concerning the level of skill rather than the age of achievement; for example, knowing that the child might make simple wants known at 2 years of age is more important than the age when the first word was uttered. Some information about social adaptability and temperament should be obtained (see Chapter 13, Interviewing Children, and Chapter 153, Interviewing Adolescents).

Previous health care is important, and the child's immunization status is a significant part of the early history. The practitioner should record all immunizations, skin tests, and pertinent screening information on a separate sheet that is readily accessible and retrievable. Filling out a few history forms later for camp or entry into preschool will prove the value of this record. A list of current and past medications used, including prescription, nonprescription, and homeopathic remedies, should be obtained.

Allergies and allergic reactions to medications are also an important part of the early history. Specific allergic reactions should be described in as much detail as possible. Medications that cause vomiting or diarrhea are numerous but not usually allergenic. Idiosyncratic reactions to drugs such as amoxicillin and phenothiazides should also be described.

The *family history* contains variable information but is often difficult to construct. An attempt should be made to trace back at least 2 generations on each side of the family. Figure 12-1 shows one method of recording such data. The names, birth dates, and health of the 3 generations concerned are usually listed below the pedigree (although not shown here), using a number indicating each person. As more data such as births, deaths, and disease become available, they can be added easily.

Consanguinity of parents should be investigated specifically by asking if the parents are related by blood. In addition to seeking known inherited diseases such as diabetes, hemophilia, or neuromuscular

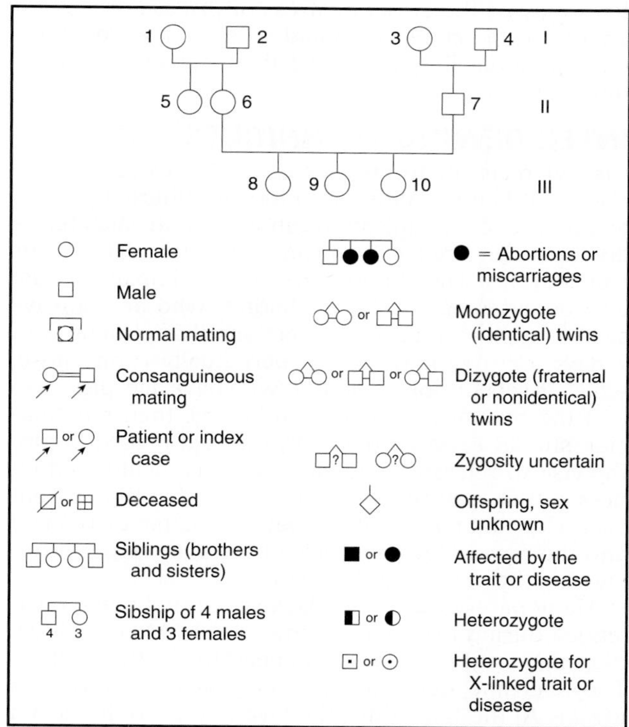

Figure 12-1 Chart and symbols used to construct a family history, or family pedigree. The Roman numerals indicate generations; the Arabic numerals indicate specific persons.

disorders, the clinician should note familial tendencies such as obesity, short stature, early heart disease, and hypertension. Inquiring about the parenting techniques of forebears is sometimes appropriate. Research has shown that abusive parents were frequently deprived or abused as children. Asking specifically about the health of the parents' brothers or sisters is also important because these individuals are often overlooked during an interview.

The *psychosocial history* describes the child in the child's present milieu and relationships with family, peers, school, and community. This history should include information about the physical setting (eg, housing), environment, and degree of isolation. Important points to determine include how children spend the day, who cares for them, what they like to do, and what their hobbies are. Inquiry should be made about the support system within the family, for example, the nature of an extended family, supportive or conflicting roles, the elements of stress that exist for this child, and how the child and family cope with them.

The psychosocial history should also touch on the parents' attitudes toward discipline and expectations about achievement. When appropriate, the practitioner should determine how the parents compare this child to the child's siblings or to other children. Asking the parents to describe the child's temperament (eg, "mellow," "feisty," "lazy"), as well as what they see as the child's strengths, is also helpful.

The *review of systems* should be detailed to obtain a baseline evaluation of all systems and their level of function. Children change over time, and various systems may be the target of stress or disease processes. Therefore the clinician should reassess all organ systems periodically and record their apparent level of function.

INTERVIEWING TECHNIQUES

Clarifying certain terms is essential. For example, *diarrhea* and *flu* mean different things to different people, and no true communication can occur until such terms are defined. *Tired* may mean sleepiness, fatigue, or true lethargy. The temporal nature of complaints must also be assessed carefully. Children who are "always sick" may have recurrent infections that clear in 5 to 7 days, or they may have a perpetually runny nose, which is seen in some children who have allergies.

If the patient has been seen before, then the clinician should review the child's medical record before the visit to refresh the memory on past health and illnesses that may relate to the reason for the current visit. Consultants should review the letter of referral and the reason for and goals of the visit before interviewing the parents and patient.

Many parents see their skills as parents being challenged during the pediatric interview: "After all, if we did things right, we wouldn't need to see the doctor." They become defensive and may answer questions *ideally*. At the same time, they want to share fears and worries with a caring, empathetic practitioner. The pediatrician must strive to develop this trusting relationship. By being facilitative, the clinician enables the parents to express fears and frustrations. Statements such as "That must have worried you" or "I bet that's upsetting" let parents know that the clinician is concerned with much more than the facts in the interview. On the other hand, statements or questions suggesting that the parents have not managed their child's illness properly such as "You should have brought Gretchen in sooner," or "It would have been better not to have fed Stephanie," or "Why did you do *that?*" should always be avoided.

The techniques used to obtain a complete and accurate history vary with the situation and the person being interviewed.

Types of Questions

In emergencies, the clinician should ask only direct (non–open-ended) questions that quickly elicit the important facts needed to make decisions regarding treatment. In nonemergencies in which time is not a factor, direct questions should be used to obtain identifying data and concerns. In nonemergent situations, having the parent or child tell the story without interruption is best. Time will dictate how much additional information is obtained.

Direct questions should be asked one at a time. Rapid-order direct questions such as "Has Karl ever had eczema, hay fever, asthma, or allergic reactions to drugs?" are logical to the questioner but are likely to confuse the respondent and lead to an overall "no" answer when a "yes" would be appropriate for one or more of the elements of the question.

Indirect (open-ended) questions are extremely useful in eliciting the present illness and psychosocial history. The answers to open-ended questions such as "How does Bonnie spend a typical day?" often provide clues to underlying, unstated problems and cues for pursuing specific elements of the patient's illness.

Direct questions are also important in eliciting the details of the present illness and the psychosocial history. For example, if a cough is mentioned as a symptom in the patient's illness, then the following sequence of direct questions is appropriate: "How long has Kathy had the cough?" "When does she have it?" "Does it wake her up at night?" "What does it sound like?" "Does she cough up any phlegm?" "How much?" and "What does it look like?" Thus open-ended questions identify the direction for further inquiry, and direct questions help determine the importance of the symptoms or signs identified.

Leading, direct questions such as "Does Jane do well in school?" should be avoided because they are more likely to result in *expected*, affirmative answers than are nonleading, direct questions such as "What kinds of grades does Jane get in school?"

Helping the Parent or Patient Communicate

Throughout the interview, the parents or patient should be assisted in several ways to relate all necessary information fully. The practitioner should use medical terminology the parents or the patient understands. Words such as *tinnitus, palpitation*, and *incontinence* may have little meaning to the parents or patient, who will often be too embarrassed to ask for a definition and may simply answer "no" when asked if these signs and symptoms are present.

The interview process is one of interaction between the clinician and the parents or patient. The person providing information should do most of the talking, and the practitioner should do most of the listening. However, the clinician can encourage the parents or patient to communicate the story by using the following 7 techniques:

1. *Facilitation.* This technique is designed to convey interest in what the parent or patient is saying. Maintaining eye contact, leaning forward, nodding in affirmation, and saying "yes," "uh huh," "I see," and similar responses all convey interest and encourage the parent or patient to continue. Additional information might be gained by giving an example, such as "In other situations like this, some parents have thought of alternative medicines. Have you thought so too?"
2. *Reflection.* Repetition of words the parent or patient has said encourages the provision of more detail, as is demonstrated in the following example:

   Parent: "Kara woke up in the middle of the night breathing hard."

   Interviewer: "Breathing hard?"

   Parent: "Yes. She seemed to be breathing fast and making a wheezing noise."

   Interviewer: "A wheezing noise?"

   Parent: "Yes, in and out—a musical wheezing sound."

   By using reflection, the interviewer was able to elicit the nature of the child's breathing difficulty without influencing its description or diverting the parent's thoughts.
3. *Clarification.* The interviewer must often clarify what the parent or patient has said, for example, "What do you mean by 'Rob wasn't acting right?'"
4. *Empathy.* Recognizing and responding to a parent's or a patient's feelings of concern, fear, or embarrassment shows understanding and acceptance and encourages continued expression of the emotion. "I can understand why that upset you" or "That must have been difficult to deal with" is an empathetic expression that tells the parent or patient that the clinician appreciates what the parent or patient has been experiencing and is sympathetic. The practitioner can also ask how the parent or patient feels or felt about a particular situation that has been related. This question displays an interest in the parent's or the patient's feelings, as well as an interest in the medical facts.
5. *Confrontation.* This technique is used to clarify what seems to be a contradiction between the parent's or the patient's feelings and actions: "You say that Alison loves school but misses a lot because she has an upset stomach most mornings." Although confrontation is used to seek clarification, it may also lead to interpretation of the meaning of the contradiction.
6. *Interpretation.* This technique is used to move beyond clarification to an inference to be made from the circumstances presented. Thus the previous example might lead to the following statement and questions by the practitioner: "Maybe there is some relationship between Alison's upset stomach and her wanting or not wanting to go to school. Do you think that's possible?"
7. *Recapitulation.* This technique is especially useful when a long and complicated history or an unusual history is presented. The physician summarizes to the parent or patient the history as the physician understands it. This task may be done at more than one point during the interview and serves to confirm the validity of the history; it also allows for possible changes.

Toward the end of the interview, asking the question, "Is there anything else you think I should know?" is sometimes helpful. This open-ended inquiry leaves parents with the sense that things were not rushed and that room still exists for discussion.

Hindrances to Communication

Although a calm, reserved, interested demeanor is important to enhance communication, the practitioner must guard against appearing casual. Constant eye contact with the parent, interrupted by glances at the child (if present), should be maintained. Evidence of boredom or impatience—looking away from the parents or patient, tapping the fingers or a pencil on a tabletop, or rushing through the interview—must be avoided. Laptop computer records of the patient should be reviewed beforehand and not during the interview. Inappropriate smiling or laughter also hinders good communication. The parents or patient always should believe that they have the practitioner's undivided attention. If time is short, then the parents or patient should be informed and another appointment made for completing the interview.

Interviewing the Child

A great deal of information can be gained by interviewing the child directly (see Chapter 13, Interviewing Children). Many children interact spontaneously with the pediatrician and answer direct questions readily. In many instances, only the child can reveal the severity of the pain or the extent of the symptoms. Approaching children indirectly, encouraging them to talk about their symptoms, is sometimes better than seeking direct answers. For example, "Tell me about your cold, Gordon" is preferable to "Do you cough?" The pediatrician should always support the child's *own story.* It should be taken seriously, and confidences should not be violated except in unusual circumstances.

With chronic problems, such as constipation or enuresis, reviewing with patients their knowledge of the complaint is helpful. A child can be asked what was discussed before coming to the physician's office, how the child feels about the visit, how the child's symptoms affect the daily routine and alter the child's lifestyle, and whether the child is able to attend school and carry out all regular activities. Asking children what they think is causing their symptoms, what they are worried about, and why it worries them is also important.

Interviewing the child provides another opportunity to assess parent-child interaction. Many parents cannot let their child speak without addition, interruption, or correction. A school-aged child who clings to a parent and cannot be coaxed to make eye contact with the practitioner or interact in any way is a concern. As adolescence approaches, parent-child conflicts become more intense. Given the chance, many adolescents will make this distressing situation obvious. Under these circumstances, separate interviews are probably preferable (see Chapter 153, Interviewing Adolescents).

Typical Day Technique

In many situations, information about a child's typical day can be helpful and informative, and most parents can relate this information readily. In addition to concrete material (eg, sleep patterns, feeding activities), much can be learned about areas of stress and harmony within a family. Parents frequently find difficulty in discussing situations without seeking approval, even if tacit, of their own actions. Mothers who are confused or unsure of themselves may frequently ask advice on a particular aspect of their child's behavior as it is presented in the description of the child's typical day; however, deferring answers until the entire day has been described is best.

Discussion can begin with an introduction, such as, "To find out more about Kim, I am going to ask you to tell me how she spends a typical day." The clinician should then begin by asking what time the child arises and what happens. Some parents will launch into vivid descriptions and will require little direction, whereas others must be encouraged. Details can be elicited by asking some simple questions such as, "What is her mood on awakening?" "Who takes care of her?" and "What does she usually eat for breakfast?" Discussion can include food likes and dislikes, skill in eating, and conduct at the table. The practitioner can also learn about the child's activities, habits, and television viewing practices. The subject of discipline might come up during this discussion, and the parents' beliefs about prohibitions and punishments can be ascertained.

Lunchtime, afternoon rest periods, and activities are reviewed in much the same way. Descriptions of trips to the market or to other stores can provide information about behavior with others and reactions to new experiences.

The evening meal is often stressful in many families, and how it proceeds can provide many clues to family dynamics. For example, the physician should find out when the parents arrive home, whether the child eats with the parents, and, if so, the types of interactions that occur. Information about the events surrounding preparation for sleep, bedtime rituals, and sleeping patterns is also important.

At the end of such an interview, assessing not only the child's style and temperament, but also the family's strengths and weaknesses should be possible. This information is essential for advising parents of children who are having developmental and maturational problems.

QUESTIONNAIRES

In certain instances, parental questionnaires may be used to supplement the history. Some questionnaires may be used as part of a general health appraisal; others are more applicable to a specific problem. Questionnaires are especially helpful for assessing school problems and developmental issues. The American Academy of Pediatrics policy statement on developmental screening lists developmental screening tools that may be incorporated into health maintenance visits.[2] The wise practitioner will be thoroughly familiar with the questionnaire format and its pitfalls before using it; all such instruments may supply additional information, but all may also be subject to observer bias and should be interpreted accordingly.

RECORDING HISTORICAL INFORMATION

Two main goals exist in recording the historical data gained in an interview: (1) documenting the patient's symptoms and medical history, which will help in formulating a diagnosis and therapeutic plan, serve as a legal record of the practitioner-patient encounter, and provide information for billing purposes; and (2) making a reasonable accounting of the patient's medical status.

The medical record should contain all the medically significant facts of the child's life. The recorded history is a synthesis of material and observations gained during the interview, compiled in a legible, retrievable form.

The present illness must be recorded clearly and concisely. Consistency is paramount, especially when dealing with time. Events must be recorded by using either of these methods: "Dick developed a cough on March 17" or "Dick developed a cough 5 days before our interview on March 23." Using terms such as *Tuesdays* and *Fridays* are difficult to identify 2 weeks after an interview.

Data obtained during an interview can be recorded in a variety of ways, such as tape-recording the entire session, a method often used by psychiatrists. Merely noting *Dx-acute otitis media; Rx amoxicillin* × *10 days* on an index card is inappropriate. Paperless records on a computer should be encouraged. Records should be legible, and much of the data should be retrievable without having to pore over volumes of paper. This process requires some foresight and planning so that different parts of the history can be separated for later use. Ideally, the historical database should be standard and uniform. However, certain problems (hip clicks, birthmarks) change with time and vary by age and gender (menstrual irregularities), by type of population served, and by geographic locale.

Questionnaires facilitate record keeping and are designed to be age appropriate. They can be filled out by the parent or by a nurse, physician's assistant, or other office personnel. However, they also present several drawbacks. First, questions tend to be answered in an idealized way because parents usually have a skewed opinion of their children. Second, all logical sequencing of information gathering is lost, and degrees of concern are not readily expressed. Third, unless the chart is updated frequently by subsequent questionnaires, much of the information soon becomes irrelevant.

The skills involved in gathering and recording a history and communicating compassionately and courteously with patients and their families are difficult to master. These skills are not innate but rather require work, insight, perseverance, and practice. The work is hard, but the rewards are great.

TOOLS FOR PRACTICE

Practice Management and Care Coordination

- *Office Visit Family "Mini"Survey (Pre-Visit)* (questionnaire), Exeter Pediatrics (www.medicalhomeinfo.org/tools/Surveys/EXETER Pre Survey.doc).

Engaging Patients and Family

- *Child Health and Development Inventory System* (CHADIS) (on-line questionnaire), Barbara J. Howard, MD (www.childhealthcare.org).
- *Child Health Record* (booklet), American Academy of Pediatrics (www.aap.org/bookstore).
- *You and Your Pediatrician* (brochure), American Academy of Pediatrics (patiented.aap.org).

Medical Decision Support

- *Bright Futures: Guidelines for Health Supervision of Infants, Children, and Adolescents Set* (book), American Academy of Pediatrics (www.aap.org/bookstore).
- *Framingham Safety Survey* (questionnaire), Injury Prevention Program (www.aap.org/family/TIPPGuide.pdf).
- *TIPP Safety Surveys: The First Year of Life* (questionnaire), American Academy of Pediatrics (www.aap.org/bookstore).
- *TIPP Safety Surveys: The First Year of Life (Spanish)* (questionnaire), American Academy of Pediatrics (www.aap.org/bookstore).

SUGGESTED RESOURCES

Bickley LS, Hoekelman RA. Interviewing and the health history. In: Bickley LS, Hoekelman, RA, eds. *Bates' Guide to Physical Examination and History Taking.* 7th ed. Philadelphia, PA: JB Lippincott; 1999.

Cassell EJ. Talking with patients. In: *Clinical Technique.* Vol 2. Cambridge, MA: MIT Press; 1985:194-196.

Feinstein AR. *Clinical Judgment.* Baltimore, MD: Williams & Wilkins; 1967.

Hagen JF, Shaw JS, Duncan PM, eds. *Bright Futures: Guidelines for Health Supervision of Infants, Children, and Adolescents.* 3rd ed. Elk Grove Village, IL: American Academy of Pediatrics; 2008.

Klaus MH, Kennell JH. *Parent-Infant Bonding.* 2nd ed. St Louis, MO: Mosby; 1982.

Thornton SM, Frankenburg WK, eds. *Child Health Care Communications. Johnson & Johnson Pediatric Round Table VIII.* New York, NY: Praeger; 1983.

Wessel MA. The prenatal pediatric visit. *Pediatrics.* 1963;32:926-930.

REFERENCES

1. Holt LE. *The diseases of infancy and childhood.* New York, NY: Appleton-Century-Crofts; 1908.
2. American Academy of Pediatrics Council on Children With Disabilities, Section on Developmental Behavioral Pediatrics, Bright Futures Steering Committee and Medical Home Initiatives for Children With Special Needs Project Advisory Committee. Policy Statement: Identifying Infants and Young Children With Developmental Disorders in the Medical Home: An Algorithm for Developmental Surveillance and Screening. *Pediatrics* 2006 118:405-420. Available at: aappolicy.aappublications.org/cgi/content/abstract/pediatrics;118/1/405. Accessed May 8, 2007.

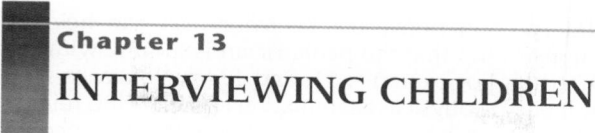

Chapter 13

INTERVIEWING CHILDREN

David I. Bromberg, MD

In assessing pediatric problems in which psychosocial and emotional factors are particularly important, the pediatrician must have a clear understanding of children and their relationship to their world. For each child, this relationship has three interrelated parts: (1) the relationship with the family, (2) the relationship with the community (mainly school), and (3) the relationship with peers. Diagnostic interviewing is the primary method of attaining this understanding (motivational interviewing is detailed in Chapter 24, Communication Strategies). A great deal of information is available from the parents (see Chapter 12, The Pediatric History) and the school (see Chapter 124, Overview of School Health and School Health Program Goals). However, a wealth of qualitatively unique information and insight can be obtained through a thorough interview with the child.

STRUCTURE OF THE INTERVIEW

The interview can be divided into three parts: (1) establishment of rapport, (2) the body of the interview (data collection), and (3) summation of the session (closure). The major goal is to collect data about the child, but other important functions are also served. For example, over the course of the interview, pediatricians can establish themselves as helping people by showing an understanding of the child's feelings and problems and a willingness to offer help rather than judgmental advice.

Establishment of Rapport

Attempting to teach a person how to establish rapport is somewhat akin to teaching someone how to ride a bike; the person has to do it to learn it. Nevertheless, several concepts are useful. Rapport is built continually throughout the interview and the ongoing relationship and is not limited to introductory remarks. Showing a sincere interest in and empathy for what the youngster has to say is essential. Verbalizing the feelings represented by a child's story can be helpful in this regard.

Patient (an 8-year-old boy being evaluated for school underachievement): I got sent to the principal's office yesterday.

Physician: Oh, really? What happened?

Patient: We had a substitute, and everyone was throwing this eraser around the room.

Physician: Then what happened?

Patient: I guess I threw it last, and she yelled at me and sent me to the office.

Physician: Sometimes it doesn't seem fair to get into trouble for something the whole class is doing.

Patient: (brightening) Yeah, but I guess I shouldn't have thrown it.

Interpreting nonverbal behavior also can help by demonstrating that the pediatrician is in tune with the youngster. For example, 11- and 12-year-olds are seen routinely for physical examinations on entering middle or junior high school. Sitting undressed and draped on an examining table, many of these youngsters appear angry or overly shy. They often avoid eye contact, scowl, and give brief answers. By saying, "I guess it's pretty embarrassing to have to undress and have a physical exam," the physician acknowledges the youngster's feelings, which can aid substantially in establishing rapport. Once rapport has been established, the examiner can watch the hostility wash away, and the subsequent interview can progress much more profitably. Reflecting feelings is generally a useful way for the health care practitioner to display caring and a desire to communicate. This process can involve responding to an unspoken message, for example, by commenting, "It sounds like you're pretty angry about that" or by summarizing the point of a story.

Patient (a 10-year-old boy being seen for behavioral problems after his parents' separation): It's just not the same since my dad left.

Physician: Really? What differences have you noticed?

Patient: Well, yesterday I had soccer practice, and my dad usually takes me, but he wasn't around to do it.

Physician: Didn't your mom take you?

Patient: Oh, yeah. She's really trying hard to do all the things; but Dad and I always talk about the practice, and Mom just doesn't know much about soccer.

Physician: So, you've really missed your dad since he moved away, but you don't want to say so to your mom.

The same message can be communicated by checking back with the child, prefaced by saying something such as, "Just to be sure we're understanding each other . . ."

When performing a behavioral assessment, the examiner should remember that the child, who is often brought to the office with little or no explanation, rarely initiates the consultation. Exploring children's fears and expectations, as well as the activities they may be missing by being in the office, can help break the ice. For younger children, this process may involve clarifying that they will not be undergoing any blood tests or receiving immunizations. The physician should discuss the format of the evaluation and the demands that will be placed on the youngster. Explicitly stating the following clearly establishes the format of the sessions: "Mary, first I will be talking with you and your family about your school difficulty, and afterwards I will be meeting just with you so that we can get to know one another better; then next week I will give you a physical examination." For older children, recognizing the difficulty of talking about themselves (or to be talked about) is worthwhile.

Physician: What concerns has the school expressed about John's behavior in the 3rd grade?

Mother: The teacher is worried that he can't stay on task and is always out of his seat. He can be very disruptive in class.

Physician: How about at home?

Mother: Well, he leaves things all over the house, and he often annoys his younger sister and brother. He tends to . . .

Patient: I do not. They always pick on me.

Physician: John, it can be pretty hard to have people talk about you, especially about things that are difficult for you. Remember, it's not that everyone is just angry at you, but we're trying to understand a problem in order to make it better.

Third-person techniques can facilitate conversation with a child. Rather than attributing feelings or characteristics to the patient, the interviewer can talk about these feelings in other youngsters. The statement "Many 9-year-olds who wet the bed are embarrassed and afraid of sleeping over at a friend's house" allows a youngster to claim these same feelings but does not confront the child directly. It also shows that the physician will not be shocked or dismayed by this information.

The interviewer must maintain a developmental perspective in relating to the patient. Complimenting a 3-year-old on climbing the steps to the examining table would be quite appropriate, whereas the same comment to an 8-year-old would be condescending.

In his book, *Childhood and Society*,[1] Erikson describes the "eight ages of man," or critical periods of development. Each age is presented as a task in development of the ego. The eight ages are summarized as the accomplishment of the following characteristics: (1) basic trust versus basic mistrust, (2) autonomy versus shame and doubt, (3) initiative versus guilt, (4) industry versus inferiority, (5) identity versus role confusion, (6) intimacy versus isolation, (7) generativity versus stagnation, and (8) ego integrity versus despair. Erikson's tasks of development provide a useful framework for both evaluating and relating to children. Commenting on issues of autonomy in the 3- to 4-year-old, issues of initiative in the 5- to 6-year-old, and issues of industry in the 7- to 9-year-old often engages the child successfully.

Physician (to an 8-year-old who is being counseled for encopresis): To review, we've discussed why you soil your pants. We've also come up with a plan for helping you stop. Do you think you would be interested in this program?

Patient: Sure. It sounds easy.

Physician: Actually, it involves a lot of hard work. In talking with you today, I think that you are a pretty hard worker, and I believe that you could do a very good job with this program. So, if you're willing, we could start this week.

Patient: Yeah. I think I'd like to do it.

Proceeding from very concrete discussions with the preschooler and early school-aged child to more abstract explanations as the child gets older is also important.

Data Collection

By the conclusion of the interview, the examiner ideally should have accumulated data covering three main areas: (1) the child's perceptions about the presenting problem; (2) information about the child's relationships with family, school, and peers; and (3) an assessment of the youngster's psychological and cognitive functioning.

Understanding the child's perception of the presenting problem is usually difficult. Denial of emotional issues is common in school-aged children. The 5- to 12-year-old frequently claims to be neither worried nor upset about the problem being evaluated. The physician must listen closely and be sensitive to nonverbal cues to understand the youngster's relationship to the presenting complaint. Using third-person techniques may be helpful.

Physician: How has school been going?

Patient: Oh, I do OK. My grades are pretty good.

Physician: Your mother had mentioned that reading and phonics are sometimes difficult for you.

Patient: Well, maybe a little bit.

Physician: Many children have told me that they feel dumb when they have trouble with reading.

Patient: Yeah, I know I do. Sometimes I just get so mad.

When a child is reluctant to discuss problems, another useful approach is to ask the child for "both sides of the coin," for example, to state what the child likes and dislikes about school. The same technique can be used to assess the child's feelings toward individuals or toward self. For example, "What are you good at doing? What things are difficult for you?" Social skills can also be evaluated in this manner: "What do your friends like about you? What things do you do that make them angry with you?"

Information about the child's relationships with family, school, and peers is obtained best by using open-ended questions, which leave the respondent a great deal of latitude in interpretation. The pediatrician will often obtain this information during routine health supervision visits. A multidisciplinary group under the auspices of the National Center for Education in Maternal and Child Health published *Bright Futures National Guidelines for Health Supervision of Infants, Children, and Adolescents*,[2] in which they outlined the preventive and health-promotion needs of youngsters. For each health supervision visit, the authors suggest *trigger questions* the pediatrician should ask the parents and the child. These questions form a valuable foundation for a semistructured interview with children. Presented here is a sample interview using these trigger questions (in italics) during a checkup for a 10-year-old girl.

Physician: How is school going?

Patient: Fine.

Physician: And how are your grades?

Patient: They're OK, straight As.

Physician: That's terrific. You should be quite proud. What do you do to have fun and with whom do you like to do it?

Patient: I'm interested in acting and am rehearsing for a play. Some of my friends are in acting with me.

Physician: Are you involved in any other after-school activities?

Patient: I wanted to play indoor soccer, but my mother doesn't want me to do it.

Physician: Why is that?

Patient: She thinks that I'm involved in too many activities.

This interview might serve as the basis for discussing a healthy lifestyle, overcommitment, and balancing of physical and sedentary activities. Other trigger questions explore safety, health-risk behaviors (including drugs, alcohol, cigarettes, sexual activity, and pressures), and body image.

The physician should attempt to be nonjudgmental and allow the youngster maximal leeway in presenting the child's own thoughts or feelings. Asking, for example, "You have lots of friends, don't you?" displays the examiner's preference for friendships and closes the subject to the child. A more effective question might be, "Do you have many friends or do you prefer doing things by yourself?" This type of question allows the child to choose either option without the physician prejudicing the choices.

Psychological functioning can be assessed by paying careful attention to both the content and the process of the interview. The assessment should include an estimate of intellectual functioning, an evaluation of the child's approach to problem solving (eg, impulsivity, frustration), and the child's fears and fantasies, self-concept, and superego functioning (conscience). A useful framework for this analysis is the mental status examination. Because a complete discussion of this examination is beyond the scope of this textbook, the interested reader is referred to Simmons' *Psychiatric Examination of Children*.[3]

Numerous assessment techniques are available for gathering important data, ranging from the very unstructured play evaluation to the very structured questionnaire. The choice of particular tools depends on the patient's age and verbal abilities and the examiner's expertise and style. For school-aged children, a semistructured interview probably is the most appropriate. This type of interview combines specific questions about the specific problem, peer relations, and related issues with the use of projective techniques. A discussion of several diagnostic techniques the pediatrician can use is included later in the section called Pediatric Psychodiagnostics.

Closure

At the end of the interview, the examiner should summarize for the child. A review of the session, highlighting the important points, is useful. An attempt should be made to offer the youngster honest, positive reinforcement and an optimistic outlook wherever possible. Plans for future meetings also should be discussed. A typical ending statement might be, "Bobby, I know you really worked very hard today, having to tell me all those things about yourself. It was especially hard to tell me how sad you were when your grandma died; but now I think we'll be able to make it easier for you to get back to school. I look forward to seeing you and your family next week."

The end of a session is typically the time that unanswered questions may be raised. The following excerpt is from an attention-deficit/hyperactivity disorder summation conference with a patient and the parents:

Physician: I am glad we had the opportunity to review attention-deficit/hyperactivity disorder today and to discuss James' medical treatment. I would like to see you again in 3 months.

Patient: (hesitatingly) Doctor, during the visit, you told my mother that I was taking stimulants. Does that mean that I take drugs?

Physician: That must have been confusing. Let's review the differences between medications and drugs.

PARENTS' ROLE

The relationship binding physician, patient, and parents is complex. Children are brought to the physician to have a problem fixed. The pediatrician must define the relationship to the child and parents, paying careful attention to the issue of confidentiality and to the patient's therapeutic needs. What format the interview should take and in what order the practitioner will see the child and parents is the initial decision. The physician must then decide how to share information among the parties.

Mature preadolescents and teenagers are often seen alone and first in the diagnostic process. The physician thereby demonstrates the primacy of the physician-teenager relationship. Although establishing a similar relationship with a latency-aged or preschool-aged patient may be equally important, these youngsters may be frightened by an initial separation from their parents. In most instances, a better approach is to see the child and parents together for the first diagnostic interview. This method allows the youngster a chance to become more comfortable with the examiner in a less-threatening setting. Parents are occasionally uncomfortable about discussing behavioral or emotional concerns with their children present. Children, however, are usually well aware of these concerns and find an honest discussion much less frightening than their fantasies about the process should they not be included. Interviewing parents and children together gives the pediatrician an opportunity to observe parent-child interactions and attitudes. After an initial joint interview, both parents and child should be seen separately.

The issue of confidentiality is a difficult one to balance. On one hand, the youngster has the right to tell the examiner specific things that should be held in confidence. On the other hand, the parents need information to play an effective role in the therapeutic process. Discussing treatment recommendations with the youngster before the final sum-up session with the family may be helpful. The parents play a crucial role in the diagnostic process and in executing the therapeutic program. The physician should plan the consultation process carefully to maximize an effective relationship with both patient and parents.

PEDIATRIC PSYCHODIAGNOSTICS

Many techniques and types of questions are available to help engage youngsters in an interview and to uncover defended emotional material. Projective techniques allow the youngster to respond to loosely structured stimuli, giving answers that reflect the child's personality. Examples include, "If a genie were to come and give you three wishes, what would you wish for?" or "If you were stranded on a desert island and could have only one person with you, who would it be?" Another area involves the child's happiest, saddest, and maddest times.

Physician: What is the happiest time that you remember?

Patient: Probably when the whole family took the vacation at the beach last summer.

Physician: How about the saddest time?

Patient: I really can't think of one.

Physician: Really, no sad times?

Patient: Well, I guess when my grandma had to go to the hospital last year.

Physician: That certainly can be frightening. Have you ever been so sad that you've thought of hurting yourself or wanting to die?

Patient: Oh, no. I've never thought about that.

Physician: How about the maddest you've been? Does your temper ever get the better of you?

The responses to these questions must be evaluated in the context of what is known about the child. Other semistructured projective techniques are described in the following sections.

Sentence Completion

The physician should tell the child that they are going to play a sentence game. The physician gives the first part of a sentence, and the child has to finish it with the first thought that comes to mind. Short sentence fragments are used, such as "Boys are...," "Girls are...," "Mothers should...," "I feel bad when I..." The answers may indicate areas of conflict or may introduce other topics of interest to the child.

Drawings

Many children find that expressing themselves through drawings is easier than through verbal communication. Several formats can be used. The pediatrician might ask a youngster to make the best drawing of a person that the child can. Standards are available in using the Draw-a-Person test to assess an IQ.[4] Kinetic family drawings are obtained by asking the child to draw a picture of the child's family doing something.[5] Family relationships and activity can be discussed by using this stimulus. Figure placement, size relationships, and use of symbols all may be useful in interpreting the drawing. Allowing a child simply to draw a picture and tell a story about it can also be helpful.

Storytelling

Stories can be useful for talking about emotions or conflicts. A storytelling format that uses fables was developed by Despert and expanded by Fine.[6] With this technique, the physician tells the child that they are going to play a storytelling game in which the child must finish stories that the physician begins. The child is then given a series of up to 20 fables that touch on many characteristic areas of conflict.

Physician: A boy and his mother go for a nice walk in the park all by themselves. They have a lot of fun together. When he comes home, the boy finds that his daddy is angry. Why is he angry?

Patient: Because the dinner wasn't ready.

Physician: What do you think the boy's father did when he got angry?

Patient: He yelled a lot at the mommy.

Physician: What does your father do when he gets angry?

The storytelling has offered several insights about this family that might have been difficult to obtain in other ways.

SUMMARY

Engaging children in a helping relationship is the core of pediatric practice. The formation of a close, empathic relationship with a patient begins with the diagnostic interview. Therefore the examiner should be alert to both the process and the content of this interview and should select diagnostic tools that will foster a trusting relationship between physician and child.

TOOLS FOR PRACTICE

Engaging Patient and Family

- *For Today's Teens: A Message From Your Pediatrician* (brochure), American Academy of Pediatrics (patiented.aap.org).

Medical Decision Support

- *Bright Futures: Guidelines for Health Supervision of Infants, Children, and Adolescents Set* (book), Bright Futures (brightfutures.aap.org).

REFERENCES

1. Erikson EH: *Childhood and Society*. 2nd ed. New York, NY: WW Norton; 1963.
2. Hagan JF Jr, Shaw JS, Duncan PM, eds. *Bright Futures: Guidelines for Health Supervision of Infants, Children, and Adolescents*. 3rd ed. Elk Grove Village, IL: American Academy of Pediatrics; 2008.
3. Simmons JE. *Psychiatric Examination of Children*. 4th ed. Philadelphia, PA: Lea & Febiger; 1987.
4. Goodenough FL: *Measurement of Intelligence by Drawings*. New York, NY: World; 1926.
5. Burns RC, Kaufman SH: *Actions, Styles, and Symbols in Kinetic Family Drawings*. New York, NY: Brunner/Mazel; 1972.
6. Fine R: Use of Despert fables (revised form) in diagnostic work with children. *J Proj Tech*. 1948;12:106.

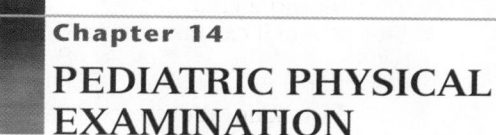

Chapter 14

PEDIATRIC PHYSICAL EXAMINATION

John H. Gundy, MD

The examination of an infant or child by a physician or nurse practitioner can accomplish several goals simultaneously. With children, as opposed to adults, the physical examination is often the first direct contact between the examiner and the patient, the history having been obtained primarily from a parent. Therefore one of the crucial outcomes of the examination is the relationship between the physician and the child. The quality and quantity of care plans and the child's future attitude in medical settings will depend in part on this relationship. This chapter emphasizes approaches to examining children of different ages that will enhance the physician-child relationship.

The physician-parent relationship, which is initiated when the history is taken, can be strengthened during the physical examination if the practitioner takes a relaxed, gentle approach toward the child and, no less important, performs a thorough examination appropriate to the setting and the chief complaint. Parents develop trust in physicians in several ways, not the least of which is the consideration the practitioner shows for the child's fears and the parents' concern about a particular symptom or sign. For each organ system discussed in this chapter, the common symptoms for which physicians are consulted are linked to a suggested level of detail in performing a physical examination.

The physician must be sensitive to the potential for iatrogenic concerns initiated by the patient's or the parent's comments during the examination and should anticipate the child's wondering, "What's wrong with me?" and the parent's worrying, "What did I do wrong?" Reactions such as these are very common. A thorough grounding in the normal stages of growth and development of the organ systems and the body as a whole allows the examining physician to respond to such questions by emphasizing the normal physical findings, as well as by interpreting abnormal findings in the context of normal developmental patterns. The description of each organ system in this chapter begins with important stages of growth and development, particularly specific steps that can be monitored by serial physical examinations. The characteristics of common physical abnormalities will be linked whenever possible to the child's age and stage of growth. The physical examination has limited value as a screening mechanism for occult disease (see Chapter 37, Physical Examination as a Screening Tool) and has proved to be much less productive in detecting problems in schoolchildren than, for instance, a comprehensive history. In general, the physical examination of children confirms abnormalities suggested by the history, as well as normal growth and development. When the child is examined in the presence of one or both parents, the physical examination can provide strong clues about the strength and characteristics of the parent-child relationship.

Each portion of the physical examination is discussed according to the special characteristics of each of five age groups: (1) newborn period, (2) infancy (1 week to 12 months), (3) early childhood (1 through 5 years), (4) late childhood (6 to 12 years), and (5) adolescence (12 to 18 years).

APPROACH TO THE PATIENT

Newborn Period

At least one examination of the newborn should be performed in the presence of one or both parents to address the parents' questions about their baby and to evaluate the parent-infant relationship. A description of the examination of a newborn is described in Chapter 83, Physical Examination of the Newborn.

In many hospitals a second more thorough examination is performed within 12 to 24 hours of birth to assess the degree of recovery from the birth process and to determine the presence or absence of signs of respiratory distress and the ability to feed. This examination can serve as a safety check before transfer of the baby from the *transition* nursery to the *routine* nursery. It should take place in a warmed environment with the baby undressed to allow thorough observation of the respiratory rate, the degree of respiratory effort, as evidenced by intercostal retractions, the color, and spontaneous activity. In many instances, quiet babies can arouse themselves with a *startle*, or Moro, response that can interfere with the examination. Giving the baby something on which to suck (rubber nipple, examiner's finger, or baby's fist) and holding the baby's arms against the baby's sides will help keep the infant as relaxed as possible; performing the examination several hours after a feeding is ideal. Although assessing the intensity and pitch of the cry is important, as many of the painless parts of the examination as possible should be performed before fully arousing the baby. Therefore, with the baby supine and after making general observations, many examiners begin by listening to the heart and lungs, then palpating the abdomen before examining the remaining systems, leaving the usually uncomfortable abduction of the hips until last.

Examination of the undressed baby with the parents present just before discharge affords the opportunity to point out normal findings, answer questions about perceived imperfections (and sometimes allow both parents a first look at their baby's entire body), discuss care of the circumcision and umbilicus, and observe the quality of the parent-infant attachment while the baby is held or fed. Holding the baby en face (the mother's face is rotated so that her eyes and those of the infant meet fully in the same vertical plane of rotation (Figure 14-1), smiling at the baby, responding to signs of hunger or satiation, and talking about the baby positively and confidently are all signs that strong parent-infant bonds are being formed and have been enhanced by the hospital experience. The neonatal behavioral assessment scale[1] was developed by T. Berry Brazelton, MD, in 1973 and is suitable for assessing the temperament, behavior, and developmental capabilities of infants up to 2 months of age. The information can be shared with parents to help them develop appropriate caregiving strategies.

Infancy

Infants between the ages of 1 and 6 months are almost always a pleasure to examine because of their responsiveness to the examiner's face and their increasing interest in environmental objects such as tongue depressors and penlights. At this age, infants can be examined successfully on the examination table, with the parent usually standing close beside the table.

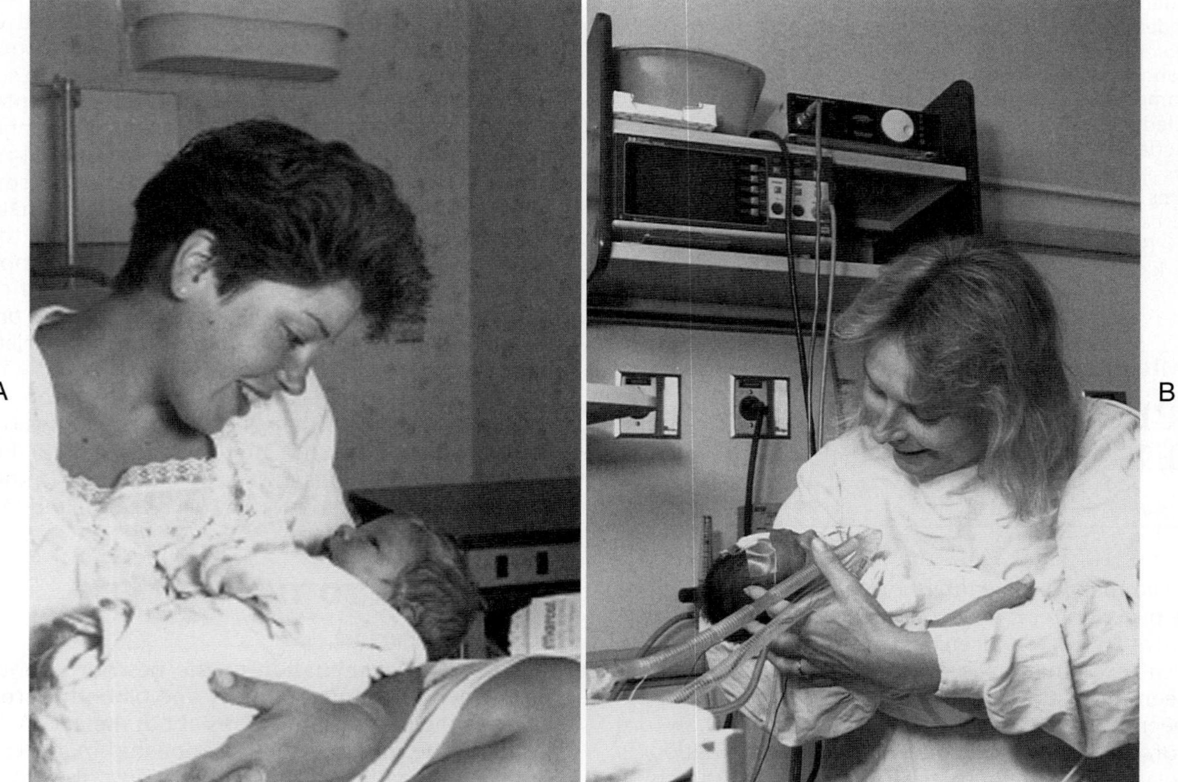

Figure 14-1 **A,** Full-term 1-day-old infant looking *en face* eye to eye with his mother. **B,** The mother of a 2-day-old, 31-week, 1400-g premature infant on a ventilator positions herself so that she can look eye to eye with her son. *(Courtesy Ruth A. Lawrence, MD.)*

With the infant unclothed except for the diaper, the practitioner should observe for spontaneous activity, state of alertness, and responsiveness to both the examiner and the parent. The order of the examination varies. If the infant is asleep in the parent's lap or held upright at the breast or shoulder, then the heart and respiratory rates can be obtained, and the heart, lungs, and even the abdomen can be examined without waking the baby. Again, the relatively uncomfortable abducting of the hips and speculum examination of the tympanic membranes are best left until last. Prolonged or painful procedures, such as deep palpation of the abdomen or a rectal examination, are best done while the baby is being fed. The infant should be examined as if physically attached to the parent, and the parent's response, especially to painful procedures, should be noted. In many clinical situations, direct observation of breastfeeding or bottle feeding is extremely useful and can help identify problems such as improper feeding techniques, weak sucking movements, and dysfunctional swallowing (see Chapter 89, Breastfeeding the Newborn). Infants 6 to 12 months of age are increasingly difficult to examine because of their normally developing anxiety about faces other than their parents' and the perceived separation from the parent. Offering interesting objects or allowing infants to sit and reach for objects or to walk or crawl around the office can help distract them. Direct eye contact with the strange face of the examiner can be especially frightening to the baby. Examination at these ages is usually easier if the baby is held in the parent's arms or on the parent's lap.

Early Childhood

With children 1 to 5 years of age, the most effective initial approach is to form a supportive relationship with the parent or an older sibling, who will hopefully become the physician's ally in the examination of the child. This alliance is aided by identifying the parent's emotional state and anxiety level during the history and then responding nonjudgmentally. For instance, if the parent appears both anxious about the child's symptoms and guilty about having had to bother the physician, then the physician might say, "I know it can be frightening to hear a baby cough like that, and I'm glad you brought him in to be examined." A parent who appears angry can sometimes be defused by a remark such as, "I know how aggravating it must be to have to bring your child in for so many ear infections."

In most situations, children in this age group are easiest to examine while they are being held by their parents, a position that is also comforting to the child when the history is initiated. A few toys and books on a low table, colorful photographs and children's drawings on the walls, and the absence of a white coat on the examiner often lead children to relax and encourage them to leave the parent and explore the office. Offering the child a piece of examining equipment such as a stethoscope or percussion hammer to handle can be helpful while the history is being taken. The examiner can often alleviate fear by showing the child the otoscope and demonstrating its use before using it on the child. Observing the child's handling of objects and interest and confidence in exploring a new environment, as well as the parent's reaction to the child's curiosity or fear, gives the examiner information important to understanding the child's developmental status and anticipating the parent's ability to cope with any problems the child may have.

In general, older children in this age group are increasingly able to communicate verbally with the examiner. A conversation that starts about the child's cat or siblings can lead to a description of what is about to be done. Continuing to describe what is being done ("I am now listening to your heart beating") can soothe even the child who starts off by screaming and kicking. With a frightened child, the parent may interpret prolonged silence on the examiner's part as disapproval or anger with the child or parent. In addition, a continuing conversation with the parent and the child during the examination signals to the child that the examiner is on the parent's side, which may increase the child's confidence that nothing too drastic will be done.

Having the child remain dressed until just before the examination is best, some of which can be accomplished by only partly removing pieces of clothing. Even before having the parent undress the child, important general observations about the child can be made, such as the activity level, gross- and fine-motor coordination, receptive and expressive language function, skin color, respiratory rate and effort, and ability to cope with a foreign environment. Some specific portions of a developmental assessment, such as throwing and catching a ball, drawing a circle, or *blowing out* the otoscope light (as a candle), can often break the ice and help the child into a gamelike atmosphere that can be continued throughout the examination.

Again, the order of the examination should be flexible; painful procedures (ears, throat) and frightening ones (anything that requires lying down) should be postponed until last. A steady pace, coupled with gentle but firm anticipatory statements ("Now I'm going to have you lie down so I can listen to your tummy"), enhances a relatively brief encounter, which, in turn, keeps the parent on the practitioner's side.

Restraining the child is often necessary, for instance, to accomplish an adequate examination of the tympanic membranes. Restraint can be accomplished in several ways, all enhanced by continuing the descriptions and discussions calmly. The parent is usually the best assistant. The child can be restrained by holding the outstretched arms against the child's head or against the child's abdomen while the examiner's body and one elbow immobilize the lower half of the child's body. The parents should be reassured that struggling is a normal response to an examination in this age group but that it can be aggravated if the parents berate or threaten the child. The examiner's goal should be to evaluate the child's health and illness while maintaining the trust and confidence of both the child and the parent. Achieving this goal requires long hours of practice, the flexibility to ask other professionals for help when the examiner's (or the parent's) patience is about to run out, and, most important, an enjoyment of the diversity, unpredictability, and spontaneity of children.

Late Childhood

Children 6 to 12 years of age are usually a pleasure to examine and rarely present any problems. A key ingredient for a successful examination is a relaxed conversation with the child about subjects such as school, hobbies, or favorite friends interspersed with brief comments about the examination itself. Occasionally a child who had an unpleasant experience with a physician as an infant will need more time for the preparatory description of the examination. School-aged children usually prefer to wear a simple drape over their underpants, and they prefer that siblings of the opposite sex be kept out of the room, particularly when the genitalia are examined. The order of the examination can be the same as for adults (vital signs, then head to foot, leaving the genitalia, perineal, and rectal [when required] until last), with care taken to anticipate any painful manipulations or procedures. As with younger children, the examiner can make the following critical observations before touching the child: activity level, ability to follow simple directions, ability to read passages of varying difficulty and to write, clarity of articulation, mood, level of neuromaturational functioning as tested by tasks such as hopping on one foot and rapidly alternating hand movements, and the relationship with the parent.

Adolescence

Most adolescents (12 to 18 years) prefer being examined without their parents in the room. They respect a straightforward, uncondescending approach, and parents respect the examiner who approaches adolescents as though they were adults. Decisions about who will be present and the issue of confidentiality should be discussed before the examination. With the parent out of the room, the examiner can review pertinent history or concerns directly with the adolescent. Some special clinics for adolescents use brief, self-administered questionnaires so that the examiner can tune in to the adolescent's present concerns more quickly. Most pubertal boys and girls have concerns about what is happening to their body, and a physical examination allows the examiner to explain and try to alleviate these concerns. While performing the examination, the examiner can reassure the pubertal child about normal developmental stages such as unilateral gynecomastia in boys, rapidly enlarging feet, the beginning of acne, and the interrelationships of the adolescent growth spurt and sexual development. The examiner's ability to approach the child's emerging sexuality factually or nonanxiously will help adolescents view themselves, at least briefly, with objectivity. Instruction in breast and testicular self-examination can help in this regard.

VITAL SIGNS AND EVALUATION OF SOMATIC GROWTH

Just as general observation of a child's behavior can give important clues about the child's general level of functioning, measuring vital signs and the characteristics of somatic growth often provides the basis for decisions about the child's overall health or illness. An abnormal vital sign or physical measurement is often the only outward indication of a problem in a child. Interpretation of vital signs and physical measurements depends on knowledge of the normal biological changes of the growing infant, child, and adolescent. One principal characteristic of human growth is that different organ systems mature at different rates and times throughout fetal life, infancy, and childhood. Figure 14-2 compares the longitudinal growth of the body as a whole with three component tissues: (1) lymphoid, (2) neural, and (3) genital.

Temperature

Body temperature is usually measured rectally in infants and in children up to 3 or 4 years of age (because rectal temperatures have been used in clinical studies to determine the significance of temperature levels in infants and young children vis a vis management of potentially life-threatening infectious illnesses) and tympanically in older children. Oral temperatures can also be taken but are less reliable. The axillary temperature is sometimes measured, especially in infants whose bottoms are excoriated or in small premature infants. This reading is generally 2°F lower than the rectal temperature. The rectal temperature is usually measured with the infant or child held prone on the parent's lap (Figure 14-3). The buttocks are separated, and the lubricated thermometer is inserted through the anal sphincter at an angle of approximately 20 degrees above the horizontal for a distance of 1½ inches. The thermometer is held in place for approximately 1 minute, either by the examiner or by the parent. Because of the relative thermal instability of newborns, especially prematurely born babies, the ambient temperature is often measured and recorded at the same time and can sometimes explain an abnormally elevated or depressed rectal temperature. Newborns' temperatures are normally higher than those of older children, averaging approximately 99.5°F (37.5°C) during the first 6 months of life. The temperature falls below 99°F (37.2°C) after age 3 and reaches 98°F (36.7°C) by age 11. A circadian rhythm of body temperature is observable by age 2 and is well developed by age 5, with increasingly higher temperatures during the daylight hours and a fall in temperature during the night (Figure 14-4). In infants and children, little relationship often exists between the degree of temperature elevation and the severity of illness. In fact, hypothermia sometimes develops in infants who have profound infection, and children can have rectal temperatures as high as 101°F (38.3°C) after vigorous activity. For children admitted to the hospital for elective procedures to have elevated temperatures initially is not uncommon, probably because of transient anxiety.

Pulse

The heart rate is measured by palpating the peripheral pulse (femoral, radial, or carotid arteries), by observing the pulsating anterior fontanelle, or by palpating or auscultating the heart directly. The pulse can be increased significantly in infants and children by anxiety, fever, and exercise before or during the examination, as well as by inflammatory illnesses, shock, and congestive heart failure. Major changes occur in the

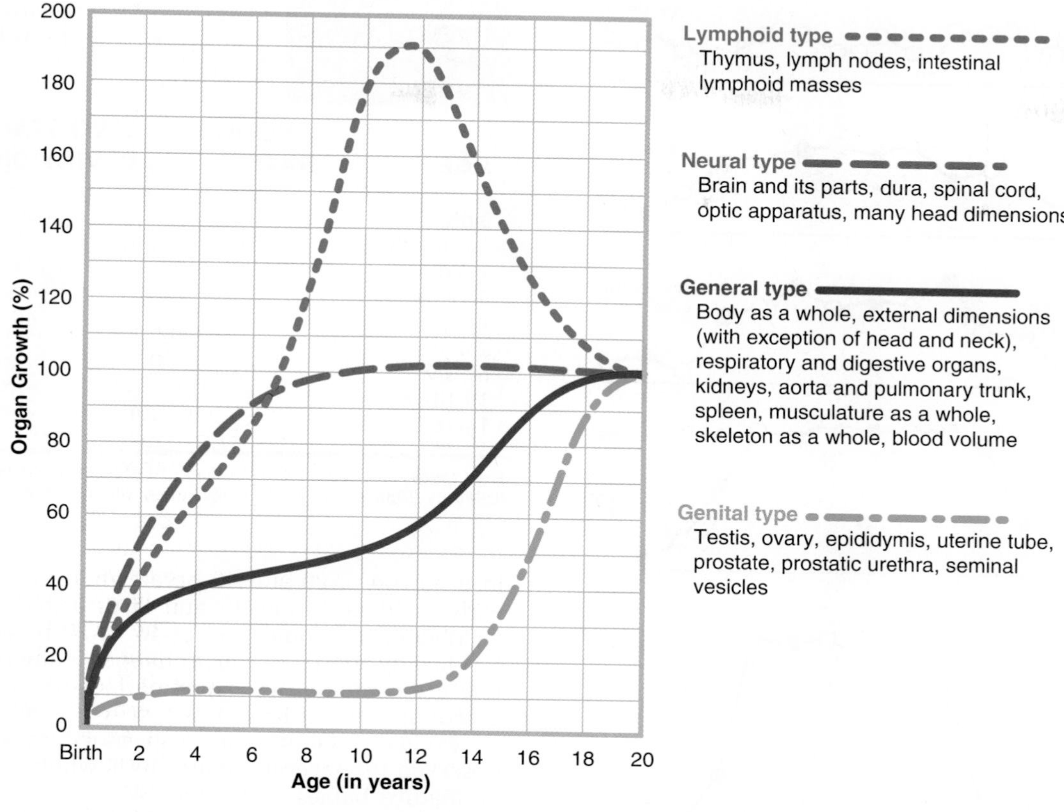

Figure 14-2 Differential organ growth curves. *(Adapted from Harris JA, et al.* The Measurement of Man. *Minneapolis, MN: University of Minnesota Press; 1930; published in Lowrey GH.* Growth and Development of Children. *8th ed. Chicago, IL: Mosby; 1986. Copyright © 1986, Elsevier, with permission.)*

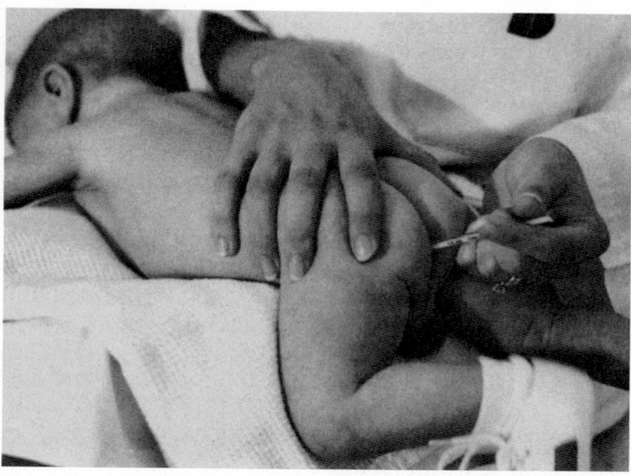

Figure 14-3 Temperature measurement in infants. *(Photograph by P. Ruben.)*

resting heart rate with increasing age, probably reflecting increasing functional control by the vagus nerve (Table 14-1). A circadian rhythm in the heart rate is observed by age 2, with a fall of 10 to 20 bpm during sleep; an absence of this rate slowing with sleep can be helpful in diagnosing acute rheumatic fever or thyrotoxicosis.

The examiner should also assess the rhythm of the heartbeat; equal spacing between consecutive beats is recorded as regular sinus rhythm. The cardiac rhythm is more commonly irregular than regular, especially in early and late childhood, reflecting sinus arrhythmia (change in the pulse rate associated with respiration) and increasing vagal control. Extrasystoles, appearing as irregularly spaced beats with or without a compensatory pause, are common in healthy children; they can usually be abolished by exercise and rarely occur as the only physical finding of underlying heart disease. Heart rates above 180 bpm (especially if rigidly regular) in infants beyond the neonatal period may indicate atrial tachycardia. Other arrhythmias in children are rare and occur mostly in those who have underlying heart disease (eg, congenital heart disease, rheumatic fever, Kawasaki disease). Tachycardia with shock in infants and children is usually associated with a weak pulse and cold, sweaty extremities. Tachycardia caused by congestive heart failure usually coexists with significant tachypnea, with or without hepatic enlargement. Heart block can occur in children who have Lyme disease with myocardial involvement.

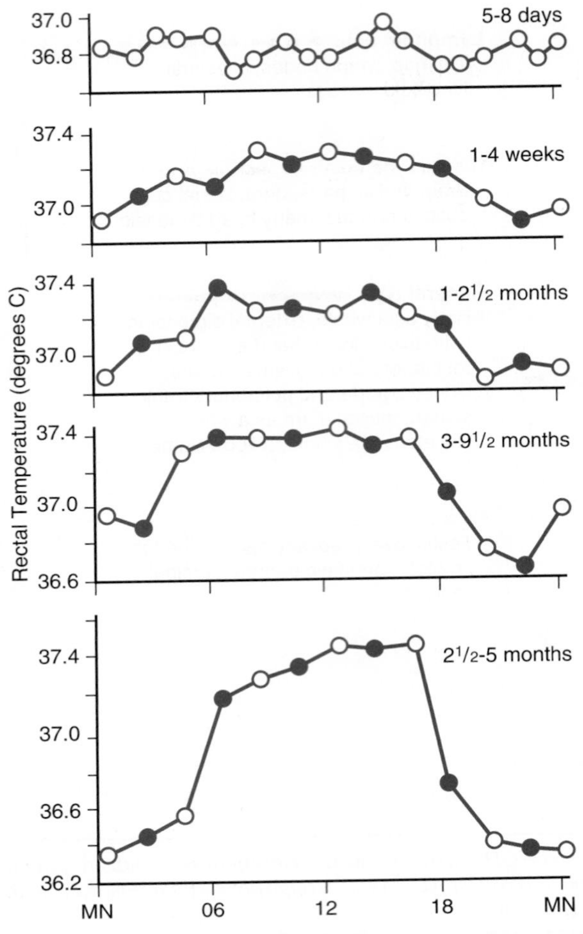

Figure 14-4 Mean rectal temperature at different hours in groups of infants at different ages. Except in the youngest group, measurements were taken every 4 hours. The hollow and solid circles represent different groups of 3 to 18 infants observed over 2 to 11 days. *MN*, Midnight. *(Adapted from Davis JA, Dobbing J.* Scientific Foundations of Pediatrics. *2nd ed. Baltimore, MD: University Park Press; 1981.)*

Respirations

Observations of the rate, depth, and respiratory effort begin at the first encounter with the child. The rate of respiration, as in the heart rate, is influenced significantly by emotion and exercise, necessitating a waiting period in some instances until a resting state is reached or to count the rate immediately if the infant or child is first encountered asleep. The rate may be counted by observing abdominal excursion in infants and thoracic excursion in children, ideally at a moment when the child is not paying attention to the examiner. In a sleeping infant, the respiratory sounds may be counted with the bell of the stethoscope held just in front of the nose. The respiratory rate varies with age, reflecting variables such as aspirated amniotic fluid in the newborn and increasing numbers of alveoli and increasing lung compliance with postnatal growth. The rate varies between 30 and 80 breaths/min in a newborn, 20 and 40 breaths/min in infancy and early childhood, and 15 and 25 breaths/min in late childhood; the adult level of 15 to 20 breaths/min is reached by age 15. Because changes in the respiratory rate are common over short periods, the rate should be counted for at least 1 minute, especially in crying or excited infants. The respiratory rate must be observed for several minutes in newborns, especially premature babies less than 2 kg and younger than 36 weeks' gestational age, to discover apneic episodes (absent respirations for 20 seconds or more) and periodic breathing (apneic periods lasting between 5 and 10 seconds). In early and late childhood, irregular respirations such as Cheyne-Stokes breathing are seen only in severely ill children, such as those who have overwhelming infection or severe head trauma.

Depth of respiration is determined subjectively and compared with norms observed for the patient's age group; deep breathing may be observed in states of metabolic acidosis and shallow breathing in severe obstructive states such as asthma. Respiratory effort is partly a subjective determination, as in estimating the degree of dyspnea, and is discussed in the section on the chest and lungs later in this chapter.

Table 14-1 Average Heart Rate for Infants and Children at Rest

AGE	AVERAGE RATE	TWO STANDARD DEVIATIONS
Birth	140	50
1st month	130	45
1-6 mo	130	45
6-12 mo	115	40
1-2 yr	110	40
2-4 yr	105	35
6-10 yr	95	30
10-14 yr	85	30
14-18 yr	82	25

From Lowery GH: *Growth and Development of Children.* 8th ed. Chicago, IL: Mosby; 1986. Copyright © 1986, Elsevier, with permission.

Blood Pressure

Because of an interest in the possibility of identifying individuals who have essential hypertension before they reach adulthood, blood pressure is determined in children and in hospitalized infants regularly. Measuring the blood pressure is essential when evaluating a child who is suspected of having congenital heart disease or chronic renal disease or who is unconscious. Blood pressure measurements in healthy ambulatory patients are compared with standard norms based on gender, age, and height (Tables 14-2 and 14-3). The auscultatory method of determining blood pressure is useful and is practiced in children older than 5 or 6 years; between ages 2 and 5, some children are cooperative, but others become agitated and anxious. A helpful point to remember is that the blood pressure of hospitalized children, especially those admitted for elective reasons, is higher during the first

Table 14-2 Blood Pressure Levels for Boys by Age and Height Percentile*

AGE (YEAR)	BP PERCENTILE ↓	SYSTOLIC BP (mm Hg) ← PERCENTILE OF HEIGHT →							DIASTOLIC BP (mm Hg) ← PERCENTILE OF HEIGHT →						
		5th	10th	25th	50th	75th	90th	95th	5th	10th	25th	50th	75th	90th	95th
1	50th	80	81	83	85	87	88	89	34	35	36	37	38	39	39
	90th	94	95	97	99	100	102	103	49	50	51	52	53	53	54
	95th	98	99	101	103	104	106	106	54	54	55	56	57	58	58
	99th	105	106	108	110	112	113	114	61	62	63	64	65	66	66
2	50th	84	85	87	88	90	92	92	39	40	41	42	43	44	44
	90th	97	99	100	102	104	105	106	54	55	56	57	58	58	59
	95th	101	102	104	106	108	109	110	59	59	60	61	62	63	63
	99th	109	110	111	113	115	117	117	66	67	68	69	70	71	71
3	50th	86	87	89	91	93	94	95	44	44	45	46	47	48	48
	90th	100	101	103	105	107	108	109	59	59	60	61	62	63	63
	95th	104	105	107	109	110	112	113	63	63	64	65	66	67	67
	99th	111	112	114	116	118	119	120	71	71	72	73	74	75	75
4	50th	88	89	91	93	95	96	97	47	48	49	50	51	51	52
	90th	102	103	105	107	109	110	111	62	63	64	65	66	66	67
	95th	106	107	109	111	112	114	115	66	67	68	69	70	71	71
	99th	113	114	116	118	120	121	122	74	75	76	77	78	78	79
5	50th	90	91	93	95	96	98	98	50	51	52	53	54	55	55
	90th	104	105	106	108	110	111	112	65	66	67	68	69	69	70
	95th	108	109	110	112	114	115	116	69	70	71	72	73	74	74
	99th	115	116	118	120	121	123	123	77	78	79	80	81	81	82
6	50th	91	92	94	96	98	99	100	53	53	54	55	56	57	57
	90th	105	106	108	110	111	113	113	68	68	69	70	71	72	72
	95th	109	110	112	114	115	117	117	72	72	73	74	75	76	76
	99th	116	117	119	121	123	124	125	80	80	81	82	83	84	84
7	50th	92	94	95	97	99	100	101	55	55	56	57	58	59	59
	90th	106	107	109	111	113	114	115	70	70	71	72	76	74	74
	95th	110	111	113	115	117	118	119	74	74	75	76	77	78	78
	99th	117	118	120	122	124	125	126	82	82	83	84	85	86	86
8	50th	94	95	97	99	100	102	102	56	57	58	59	60	60	61
	90th	107	109	110	112	114	115	116	71	72	72	73	74	75	76
	95th	111	112	114	116	118	119	120	75	76	77	78	79	79	80
	99th	119	120	122	123	125	127	127	83	84	85	86	87	87	88
9	50th	95	96	98	100	102	103	104	57	58	59	60	61	61	62
	90th	109	110	112	114	115	117	118	72	73	74	75	76	76	77
	95th	113	114	116	118	119	121	121	76	77	78	79	80	81	81
	99th	120	121	123	125	127	128	129	84	85	86	87	88	88	89
10	50th	97	98	100	102	103	105	106	58	59	60	61	61	62	63
	90th	111	112	114	115	117	119	119	73	73	74	75	76	77	78
	95th	115	116	117	119	121	122	123	77	78	79	80	81	81	82
	99th	122	123	125	127	128	130	130	85	86	86	88	88	89	90
11	50th	99	100	102	104	105	107	107	59	59	60	61	62	63	63
	90th	113	114	115	117	119	120	121	74	74	75	76	77	78	78
	95th	117	118	119	121	123	124	125	78	78	79	80	81	82	82
	99th	124	125	127	129	130	132	132	86	86	87	88	89	90	90
12	50th	101	102	104	106	108	109	110	59	60	61	62	63	63	64
	90th	115	116	118	120	121	123	123	74	75	75	76	77	78	79
	95th	119	120	122	123	125	127	127	78	79	80	81	82	82	83
	99th	126	127	129	131	133	134	135	86	87	88	89	90	90	91

BP, Blood pressure; *SD*, standard deviations.

*The 90th percentile is 1028 SD, 95th percentile is 1.645 SD, and the 99th percentile is 2.326 SD over the mean.

From US Dept of Health and Human Services, National Institutes of Health, and National Heart, Lung and Blood Institute. *The Fourth Report on the Diagnosis, Evaluation, and Treatment of High Blood Pressure in Children and Adolescents.* National Institutes of Health publication 05-5267. Bethesda, MD: US Dept of Health and Human Services, National Institute of Health; 2005.

Continued

Table 14-2 Blood Pressure Levels for Boys by Age and Height Percentile*—cont'd

AGE (YEAR)	BP PERCENTILE ↓	SYSTOLIC BP (mm Hg) ← PERCENTILE OF HEIGHT →							DIASTOLIC BP (mm Hg) ← PERCENTILE OF HEIGHT →						
		5th	10th	25th	50th	75th	90th	95th	5th	10th	25th	50th	75th	90th	95th
13	50th	104	105	106	108	110	111	112	60	60	61	62	63	64	64
	90th	117	118	120	122	124	125	126	75	75	76	77	78	78	79
	95th	121	122	124	126	128	129	130	79	79	80	81	82	83	83
	99th	128	130	131	133	135	136	137	87	87	88	89	90	91	91
14	50th	106	107	109	111	113	114	115	60	61	62	63	64	65	65
	90th	120	121	123	125	126	128	128	75	76	77	78	79	79	80
	95th	124	125	127	128	130	132	132	80	80	81	82	83	84	84
	99th	131	132	134	136	138	139	140	87	88	89	90	91	92	92
15	50th	109	110	112	113	115	117	117	61	62	63	64	65	66	66
	90th	122	124	125	127	129	130	131	76	77	78	79	80	80	81
	95th	126	127	129	131	133	134	135	81	81	82	83	84	85	85
	99th	134	135	136	138	140	142	142	88	89	90	91	92	93	93
16	50th	111	112	114	116	118	119	120	63	63	64	65	66	67	67
	90th	125	126	128	130	131	133	134	78	78	79	80	81	82	82
	95th	129	130	132	134	135	137	137	82	83	83	84	85	86	87
	99th	136	137	139	141	143	144	145	90	90	91	92	93	94	94
17	50th	114	115	116	118	120	121	122	65	66	66	67	68	69	70
	90th	127	128	130	132	134	135	136	80	80	81	82	83	84	84
	95th	131	132	134	136	138	139	140	84	85	86	87	87	88	89
	99th	139	140	141	143	145	146	147	92	93	93	94	95	96	97

BP, Blood pressure; *SD*, standard deviations.
*The 90th percentile is 1028 SD, 95th percentile is 1.645 SD, and the 99th percentile is 2.326 SD over the mean.
From US Dept of Health and Human Services, National Institutes of Health, and National Heart, Lung and Blood Institute. *The Fourth Report on the Diagnosis, Evaluation, and Treatment of High Blood Pressure in Children and Adolescents.* National Institutes of Health publication 05-5267. Bethesda, MD: US Dept of Health and Human Services, National Institute of Health; 2005.

1 or 2 days and then tends to plateau at lower levels; the blood pressure of sick, hospitalized children tends to remain constant throughout the hospitalization. Several determinations may be needed to obtain values unaffected by anxiety. Having children "watch the silver column rise" and explaining that the cuff will gently squeeze their arm usually reduces anxiety.

The size of the cuff is important because a cuff that is too small will produce falsely elevated values. The optimal cuff size is one that covers two thirds of the distance between the antecubital fossa and the acromion or between the popliteal fossa and the gluteal fold. The rubber bag inside the cuff should encircle at least 50% of the extremity. Every site where infants and children are examined should have cuffs ranging from 1 to 4 inches in width. Some obese teenagers require extra large adult cuffs.

With the auscultation method, the point at which the sounds are first heard is recorded as the systolic pressure, and the point at which the sounds disappear is recorded as the diastolic pressure. When the pulse sounds cannot be auscultated, a distal artery (radial, popliteal, or dorsalis pedis) can be palpated; the point at which the first pulsation is felt is approximately 10 mm Hg lower than the auscultated systolic pressure. The flush method can be used in infants and young children. The elevated extremity, with the uninflated cuff in place, is stroked and *milked* from the hand to the elbow. The cuff is then inflated to a point above the estimated systolic pressure, and the pressure is slowly released. A sudden flush or reddening of the extremity, compared with the color of the opposite extremity, will occur at a point approximately halfway between the systolic and diastolic pressures. Normally the systolic pressure is higher in the lower extremities, and the diastolic pressure is the same in the arms and the legs.

Somatic Growth

Assessing somatic growth is crucial in every evaluation of an infant or a child because growth is the central characteristic of healthy children and deviations from the child's norm provide an early warning of pathological processes. Several tools are available to aid in this evaluation; the most important, however, are growth charts, constructed either by longitudinal, serial measurements of a single cohort of children or by measurements of large numbers of children of different ages over a brief period. Although physical measurements of a child at a single point in time will give some useful clinical information, serial measurements over months or years provide an accurate record of the infant's or child's overall general pattern of growth, with deviations from the subject's norm

Table 14-3 Blood Pressure Levels for Girls by Age and Height Percentile*

AGE (YEAR)	BP PERCENTILE ↓	SYSTOLIC BP (mm Hg) ← PERCENTILE OF HEIGHT →							DIASTOLIC BP (mm Hg) ← PERCENTILE OF HEIGHT →						
		5th	10th	25th	50th	75th	90th	95th	5th	10th	25th	50th	75th	90th	95th
1	50th	83	84	85	86	88	89	90	38	39	39	40	41	41	42
	90th	97	97	98	100	101	102	103	52	53	53	54	55	55	56
	95th	100	101	102	104	105	106	107	56	57	57	58	59	59	60
	99th	108	108	109	111	112	113	114	64	64	65	65	66	67	67
2	50th	85	85	87	88	89	91	91	43	44	44	45	46	46	47
	90th	98	99	100	101	103	104	105	57	58	58	59	60	61	61
	95th	102	103	104	105	107	108	109	61	62	62	63	64	65	65
	99th	109	110	111	112	114	115	116	69	69	70	70	71	72	72
3	50th	86	87	88	89	91	92	93	47	48	48	49	50	50	51
	90th	100	100	102	103	104	106	106	61	62	62	63	64	64	65
	95th	104	104	105	107	108	109	110	65	66	66	67	68	68	69
	99th	111	111	113	114	115	116	117	73	73	74	74	75	76	76
4	50th	88	88	90	91	92	94	94	50	50	51	52	52	53	54
	90th	101	102	103	104	106	107	108	64	64	65	66	67	67	68
	95th	105	106	107	108	110	111	112	68	68	69	70	71	71	72
	99th	112	113	114	115	117	118	119	76	76	76	77	78	79	79
5	50th	89	90	91	93	94	95	96	52	53	53	54	55	55	56
	90th	103	103	105	106	107	109	109	66	67	67	68	69	69	70
	95th	107	107	108	110	111	112	113	70	71	71	72	73	73	74
	99th	114	114	116	117	118	120	120	78	78	79	79	80	81	81
6	50th	91	92	93	94	96	97	98	54	54	55	56	56	57	58
	90th	104	105	106	108	109	110	111	68	68	69	70	70	71	72
	95th	108	109	110	111	113	114	115	72	72	73	74	74	75	76
	99th	115	116	117	119	120	121	122	80	80	80	81	82	83	83
7	50th	93	93	95	96	97	99	99	55	56	56	57	58	58	59
	90th	106	107	108	109	111	112	113	69	70	70	71	72	72	73
	95th	110	111	112	113	115	116	116	73	74	74	75	76	76	77
	99th	117	118	119	120	122	123	124	81	81	82	82	83	84	84
8	50th	95	95	96	98	99	100	101	57	57	57	58	59	60	60
	90th	108	109	110	111	113	114	114	71	71	71	72	73	74	74
	95th	112	112	114	115	116	118	118	75	75	75	76	77	78	78
	99th	119	120	121	122	123	125	125	82	82	83	83	84	85	86
9	50th	96	97	98	100	101	102	103	58	58	58	59	60	61	61
	90th	110	110	112	113	114	116	116	72	72	72	73	74	75	75
	95th	114	114	115	117	118	119	120	76	76	76	77	78	79	79
	99th	121	121	123	124	125	127	127	83	83	84	84	85	86	87
10	50th	98	99	100	102	103	104	105	59	59	59	60	61	62	62
	90th	112	112	114	115	116	118	118	73	73	73	74	75	76	76
	95th	116	116	117	119	120	121	122	77	77	77	78	79	80	80
	99th	123	123	125	126	127	129	129	84	84	85	86	86	87	88
11	50th	100	101	102	103	105	106	107	60	60	60	61	62	63	63
	90th	114	114	116	117	118	119	120	74	74	74	75	76	77	77
	95th	118	118	119	121	122	123	124	78	78	78	79	80	81	81
	99th	125	125	126	128	129	130	131	85	85	86	87	87	88	89
12	50th	102	103	104	105	107	108	109	61	61	61	62	63	64	64
	90th	116	116	117	119	120	121	122	75	75	75	76	77	78	78
	95th	119	120	121	123	124	125	126	79	79	79	80	81	82	82
	99th	127	127	128	130	131	132	133	86	86	87	88	88	89	90

BP, Blood pressure; *SD*, standard deviations.

*The 90th percentile is 1.28 SD, 95th percentile is 1.645 SD, and the 99th percentile is 2.326 SD over the mean.

From US Dept of Health and Human Services, National Institutes of Health, and National Heart, Lung and Blood Institute. *The Fourth Report on the Diagnosis, Evaluation, and Treatment of High Blood Pressure in Children and Adolescents.* National Institutes of Health publication 05-5267. Bethesda, MD: US Dept of Health and Human Services, National Institute of Health; 2005.

Continued

Table 14-3 Blood Pressure Levels for Girls by Age and Height Percentile*—cont'd

AGE (YEAR)	BP PERCENTILE ↓	SYSTOLIC BP (mm Hg) ← PERCENTILE OF HEIGHT →							DIASTOLIC BP (mm Hg) ← PERCENTILE OF HEIGHT →						
		5th	10th	25th	50th	75th	90th	95th	5th	10th	25th	50th	75th	90th	95th
13	50th	104	105	106	107	109	110	110	62	62	62	63	64	65	65
	90th	117	118	119	121	122	123	124	76	76	76	77	78	79	79
	95th	121	122	123	124	126	127	128	80	80	80	81	82	83	83
	99th	128	129	130	132	133	134	135	87	87	88	89	89	90	91
14	50th	106	106	107	109	110	111	112	63	63	63	64	65	66	66
	90th	119	120	121	122	124	125	125	77	77	77	78	79	80	80
	95th	123	123	125	126	127	129	129	81	81	81	82	83	84	84
	99th	130	131	132	133	135	136	136	88	88	89	90	90	91	92
15	50th	107	108	109	110	111	113	113	64	64	64	65	66	67	67
	90th	120	121	122	123	125	126	127	78	78	78	79	80	81	81
	95th	124	125	126	127	129	130	131	82	82	82	83	84	85	85
	99th	131	132	133	134	136	137	138	89	89	90	91	91	92	93
16	50th	108	108	110	111	112	114	114	64	64	65	66	66	67	68
	90th	121	122	123	124	126	127	128	78	78	79	80	81	81	82
	95th	125	126	127	128	130	131	132	82	82	83	84	85	85	86
	99th	132	133	134	135	137	138	139	90	90	90	91	92	93	93
17	50th	108	109	110	111	113	114	115	64	64	65	66	67	67	68
	90th	122	122	123	125	126	127	128	78	79	79	80	81	81	82
	95th	125	126	127	129	130	131	132	82	83	83	84	85	85	86
	99th	133	133	134	136	137	138	139	90	90	91	91	92	93	93

BP, Blood pressure; *SD*, standard deviations.
*The 90th percentile is 1.28 SD, 95th percentile is 1.645 SD, and the 99th percentile is 2.326 SD over the mean.
From US Dept of Health and Human Services, National Institutes of Health, and National Heart, Lung and Blood Institute. *The Fourth Report on the Diagnosis, Evaluation, and Treatment of High Blood Pressure in Children and Adolescents.* National Institutes of Health publication 05-5267. Bethesda, MD: US Dept of Health and Human Services, National Institute of Health; 2005.

indicating some intrinsic defect or environmental insult. The physical measurements used most often in assessing children are height and weight and, in infants and young children, the head circumference, as well. The body mass index (BMI), a ratio of the weight to the square of the height, has been found to define obesity or risk of obesity accurately in children.[2] To be clinically useful, all of these measurements should be made and recorded with care and use of a consistent technique.

Of the different growth charts currently available, the ones used most often are published by the National Center for Health Statistics. These charts include length for age or stature for age, weight for age, head circumference for age (to 36 months), and weight for length or weight for stature from birth to 3 and BMI from age 3 to 18. Separate charts are available for boys and girls of 2 age groups: birth to 36 months and 2 to 20 years (Figures 14-5 through 14-12 on pages 111 through 114). The percentile lines on these charts indicate the number of healthy children expected to fall above and below the index child's measurement. For instance, a 2-year-old girl whose length is 34 inches is in the 50th percentile for length; 50% of all healthy 2-year-old girls will be expected to be taller, and will be 50% shorter.

Specialized growth charts for children with various congenital anomalies (eg, Down syndrome) are available and should be used when appropriate.

Other growth charts indicate the mean and standard deviations from the mean by chronologic age. Standard deviations (SD) are defined mathematically; for example, 1 SD above and below the mean includes approximately 67% of the measurements, and 2 SD above and below the mean includes approximately 95% of the measurements.

Velocity growth curves (Figure 14-13 on page 115) are used to measure differential rates of growth at different ages, especially among adolescents and children suspected of having endocrine disorders. These charts illustrate the two periods of rapid growth—infancy and puberty—and the differences by gender at puberty and can be helpful in children with delayed onset of puberty.

Height

Standing height can be measured fairly accurately in children older than 2 or 3 years. Some growth charts, such as the Stuart growth charts, use standing height measurements beginning at age 6 years; others, such as the National Center for Health Statistics charts, plot standing heights beginning at age 2 years. Stand-up scales with attachments for measuring height are

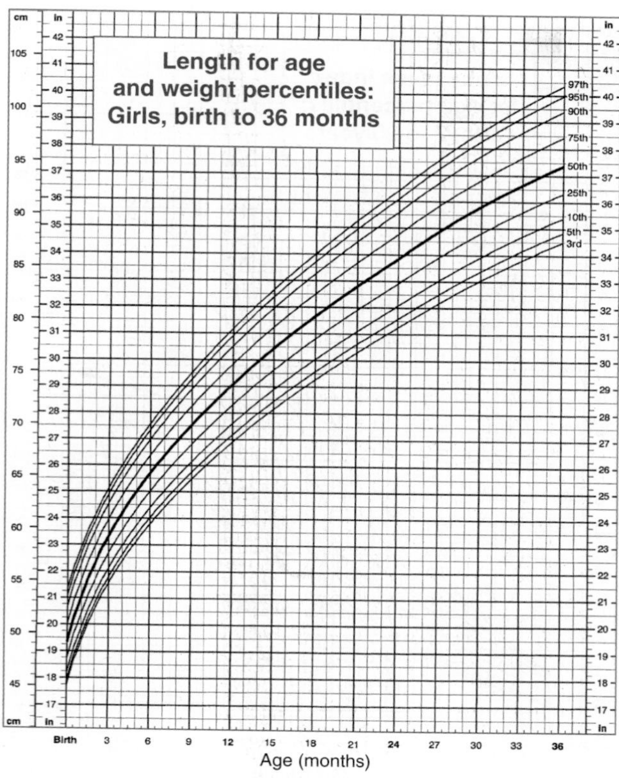

Figure 14-5 Length for age and weight percentiles, girls, birth to 36 months. *(Developed by the National Center for Health Statistics in collaboration with the National Center for Chronic Disease Prevention and Health Promotion [2000].)*

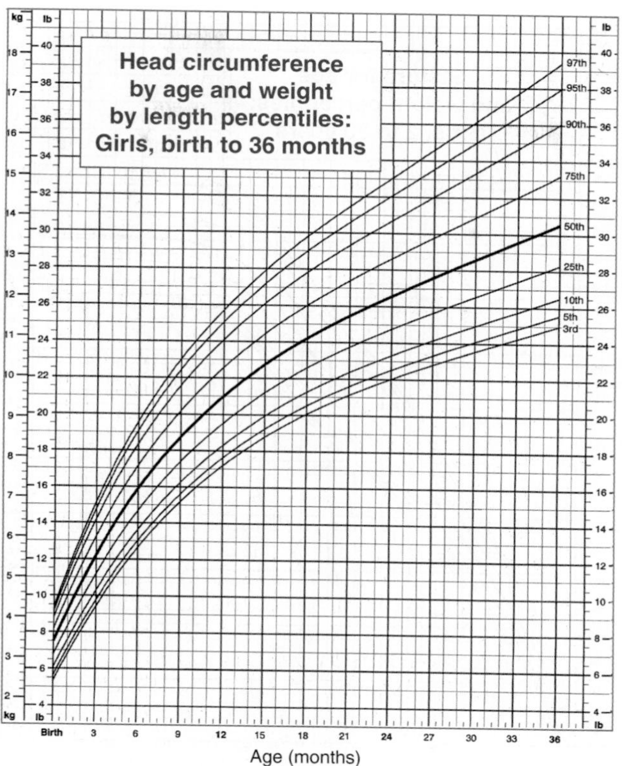

Figure 14-6 Head circumference by age and weight by length, girls from birth to 36 months. *(Developed by the National Center for Health Statistics in collaboration with the National Center for Chronic Disease Prevention and Health Promotion [2000].)*

generally inaccurate. Short of buying an expensive wall-mounted apparatus (Stadiometer), accurate measurements can be made by attaching a graduated tape or ruler to a wall and placing a flat surface or right angle on top of the head to determine the height (Figure 14-14 on page 115). This measurement should be made with the child standing in stockings or bare feet, with the heels back and shoulders just touching the wall.

Length of Infants

An infant's length is measured most accurately by using flat boards placed across and perpendicular to the examining table in contact with the vertex of the head and the soles of the feet and reading the measurement from a scale attached to the surface of the table (Figure 14-15 on page 115); care must be taken, in newborns particularly, to extend the hips and knees fully.

Weight

Infants are weighed on infant scales, with the baby clothed only in a diaper. Children old enough to stand are weighed in their underpants on stand-up scales. Stand-up scales, because of their usually wobbly base, may be frightening to children 1 to 3 years of age, and the child must sometimes be weighed by subtracting the parent's weight from the combined parent-child weight.

Ideally, serial measurements are made using the same scale. In most typically growing children, the height and weight measurements, when plotted on growth charts, fall within two standard percentile lines of each other (eg, the 3rd, 10th, 25th, 50th, 75th, 90th, and 97th percentiles). Children whose measurements are either above the 97th, below the 3rd percentile, or declining or accelerating over time (crossing percentile lines) require further evaluation, as do children whose height and weight differ by more than two percentile lines or categories.

Body Mass Index

The BMI is calculated by dividing the weight in pounds or kilograms by the square of the height in inches (or centimeters and multiplying by 703). A BMI greater than the 85th percentile is considered at risk for obesity, and greater than the 95th percentile defines obesity. The trend of BMI measurements over time can be useful in alerting parents to possible future problems. For example, increasing BMI percentiles in 4 to 10 year olds is often predictive of obesity in adolescence.

Head Circumference

The head circumference is measured and plotted on a standard growth chart during each health maintenance examination from birth to age 2 years, the

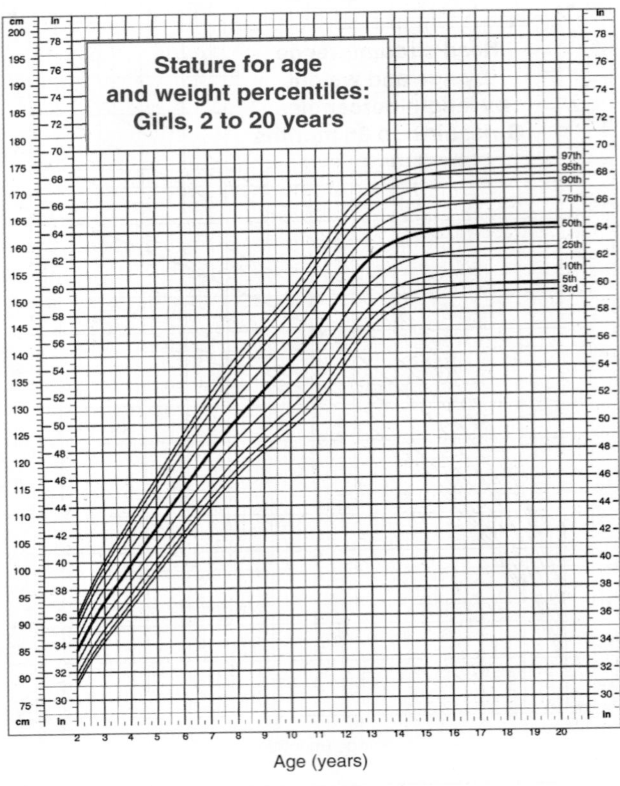

Figure 14-7 Stature for age and weight percentiles, girls, 2 to 20 years. *(Developed by the National Center for Health Statistics in collaboration with the National Center for Chronic Disease Prevention and Health Promotion [2000].)*

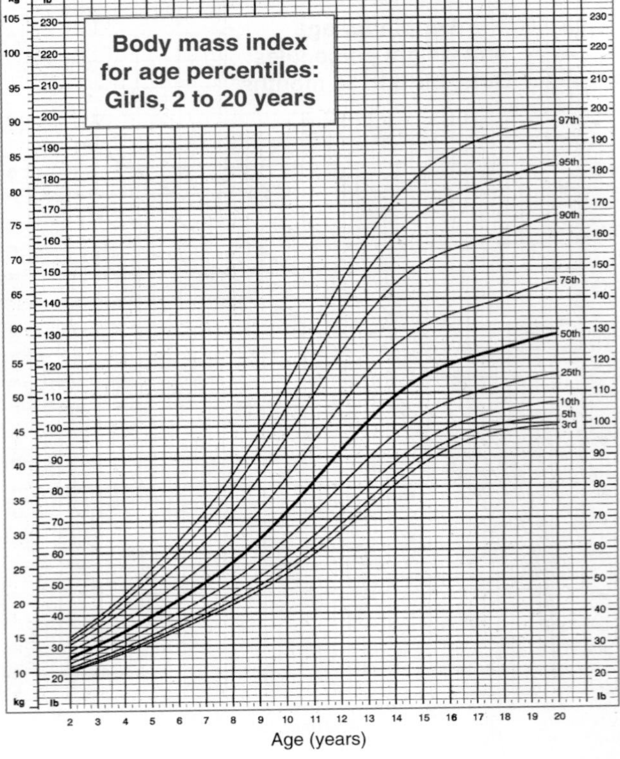

Figure 14-8 Body mass index for age percentiles, girls, 2 to 20 years. *(Developed by the National Center for Health Statistics in collaboration with the National Center for Chronic Disease Prevention and Health Promotion [2000].)*

period of maximal rate of brain growth. In children older than 2 years, head circumference measurements are obtained at the initial examination of any child and when any component of the growth curve has been abnormal, or if intellectual disability or a suspicion of fetal alcohol syndrome exists.

The measurement is made by placing a cloth tape measure around the maximal occipitofrontal circumference, taking three separate readings and selecting the largest value. When measuring the heads of infants, having the infant supine with the arms held firmly against the body by the parent or a nurse is usually necessary; with children, examiners can improve cooperation by first demonstrating the use of the measuring tape on themselves.

Chest and Other Measurements

In newborns the chest circumference is compared with the head circumference, the head having a larger circumference. The chest circumference normally equals and then exceeds the head circumference during the 1st year of life. Chest circumference is measured at the level of the nipples midway between expiration and inspiration. Another chest measurement sometimes used in monitoring children who have chronic pulmonary disease is the thoracic index, obtained by dividing the anteroposterior diameter by the transverse chest diameter. This index normally decreases from 0.85 at birth to 0.74 at age 6 years because of the more rapid growth of the transverse diameter. The transverse (side-to-side) diameter and anteroposterior (sternum-to-vertebrae spinous process) diameter are measured most accurately with special calipers at the level of the nipples. Additional somatic measurements can help in the evaluation of children whose somatic growth is abnormal. The ratio of the upper half of the body to the lower half is obtained by measuring the distance from the crown to the symphysis pubis and then from the symphysis pubis to the floor (or, with an infant, to the heel) while the child is standing. This ratio changes from 1.7:1 in the newborn to 1:1 in the adult. The arm span, normally equal to the standing height, is measured from fingertip to fingertip of the 3rd fingers with the arms outstretched. This measurement is especially important in diagnosing Marfan syndrome because the arm span is greater than the height in this condition. Norms for these measurements by age and by height are available in pediatric endocrinology textbooks. Waist circumference measurement can be helpful in predicting or diagnosing metabolic syndrome in overweight children.[3]

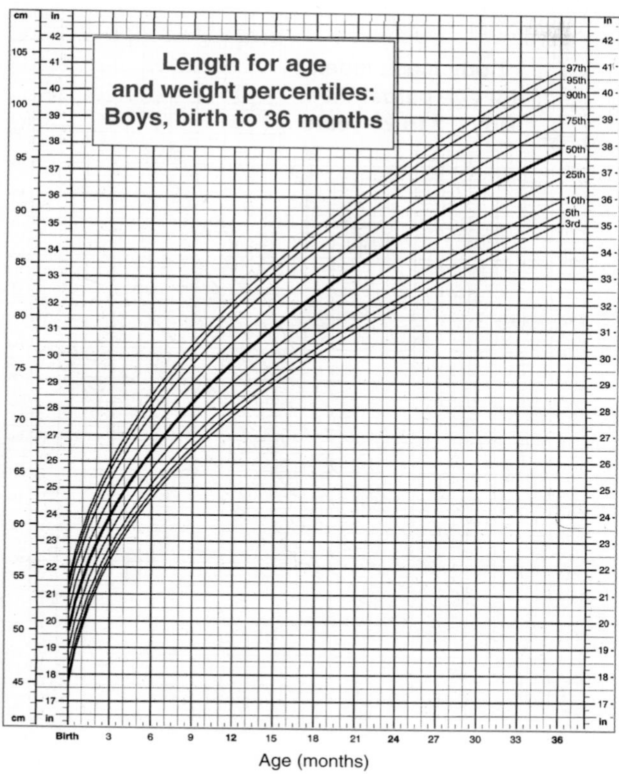

Figure 14-9 Length for age and weight percentiles, boys, birth to 36 months. *(Developed by the National Center for Health Statistics in collaboration with the National Center for Chronic Disease Prevention and Health Promotion [2000].)*

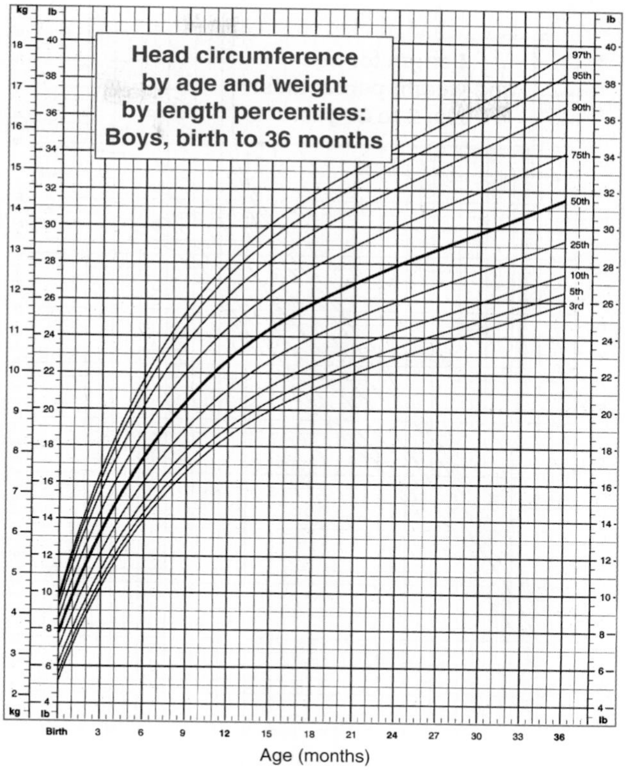

Figure 14-10 Head circumference by age and weight by length, boys from birth to 36 months. *(Developed by the National Center for Health Statistics in collaboration with the National Center for Chronic Disease Prevention and Health Promotion [2000].)*

ORGAN SYSTEMS

Skin

During the development of the fetus, neural crest cells, or melanoblasts, which have the potential for producing melanin, migrate from the dorsal region of the developing embryo. Under genetic control and mediated by tyrosinase, the melanoblasts produce varying amounts and shades of melanin, which make up the pigment of the skin, hair, and irides. Midline, ventral areas of defective pigmentation, such as piebaldism, can result from several developmental causes and are sometimes associated with defects in the development of the neural crest cells that give rise to the bipolar cells of the auditory nerve. Individuals in whom tyrosinase is absent lack pigmentation and have albinism. Localized areas of depigmentation shaped as a leaf are seen in tuberous sclerosis.

The periderm is a superficial layer of epidermis with absorption properties that normally are shed before birth; persistence of the periderm is seen in the *collodion baby* and in forms of congenital ichthyosis. Hair follicles begin developing during the 3rd fetal month, and skin keratinization first occurs at their openings. Sebaceous glands, whose secretions contribute to the formation of vernix caseosa, are active starting in the latter months of pregnancy; after birth, they are relatively inactive until puberty. Apocrine glands are formed in the fetus but are not developed fully until puberty. Sweat glands, which grow most rapidly between the 22nd and 24th fetal weeks, are inactive in the fetus. They become active in the newborn after several weeks and reach a maximal rate of activity by age 2 years. Sweat gland secretion may be under some degree of cortical control, which may explain children's tendency to sweat at all times and adults' tendency to sweat more while asleep.

Adipose tissue begins to develop during fetal life and constitutes 28% of the body weight at term. The number of fat cells increases especially rapidly during the 1st year of life, with adipose tissue constituting 40% to 70% of the body weight at 4 months of age. Cell numbers increase at a slower rate until puberty, when a second growth spurt occurs. In adults, adipose tissue constitutes 15% to 40% of body weight in men and 25% to 50% in women. The fat content of adipose tissue in a nonobese individual increases from 40% at birth to 80% in the adult.

Examination of the skin often yields important clues to both normal and pathological systemic processes. For instance, the characteristics of the newborn's skin reflect, in part, the length of gestation, and observations such as the opacity of the skin and the distribution of body hair can help determine the gestational

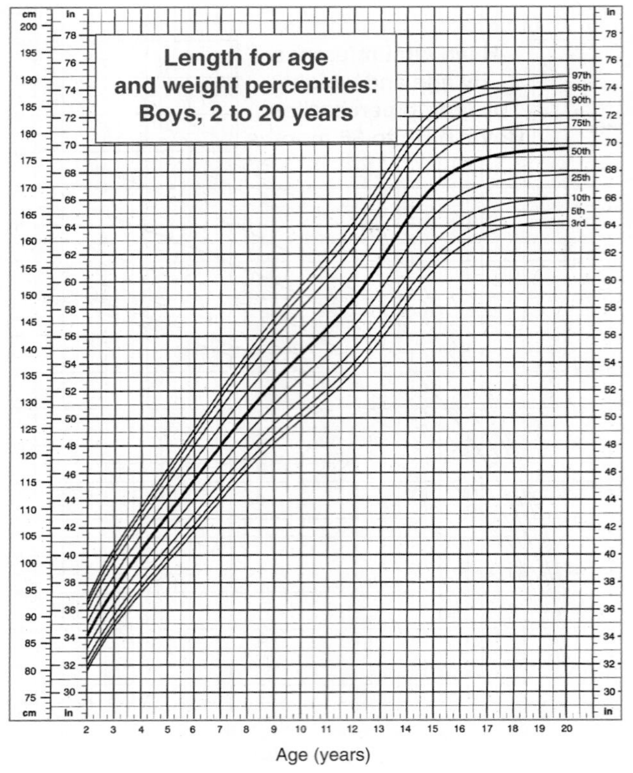

Figure 14-11 Stature for age and weight for age percentiles, boys, 2 to 20 years. *(Developed by the National Center for Health Statistics in collaboration with the National Center for Chronic Disease Prevention and Health Promotion [2000].)*

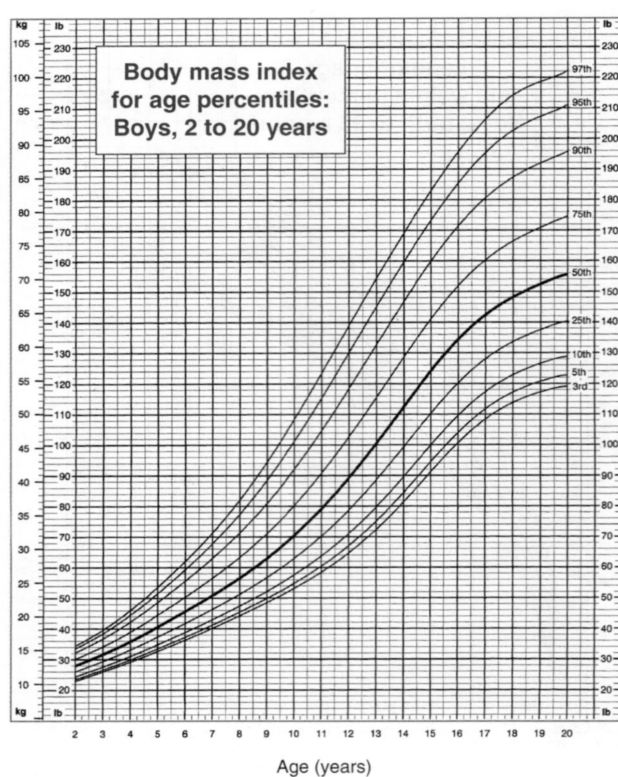

Figure 14-12 Body mass index for age percentiles, boys, 2 to 20 years. *(Developed by the National Center for Health Statistics in collaboration with the National Center for Chronic Disease Prevention and Health Promotion [2000].)*

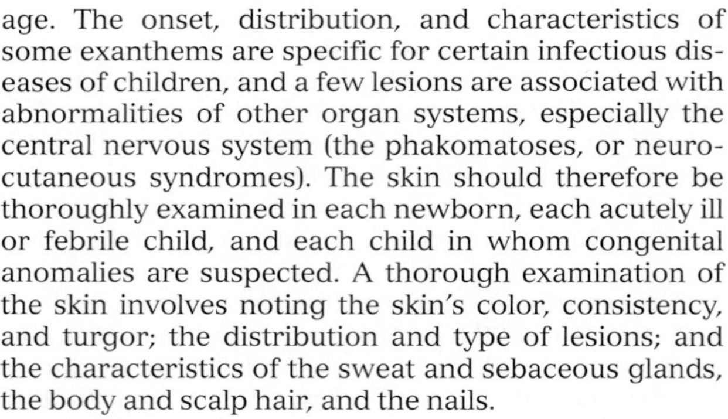

age. The onset, distribution, and characteristics of some exanthems are specific for certain infectious diseases of children, and a few lesions are associated with abnormalities of other organ systems, especially the central nervous system (the phakomatoses, or neurocutaneous syndromes). The skin should therefore be thoroughly examined in each newborn, each acutely ill or febrile child, and each child in whom congenital anomalies are suspected. A thorough examination of the skin involves noting the skin's color, consistency, and turgor; the distribution and type of lesions; and the characteristics of the sweat and sebaceous glands, the body and scalp hair, and the nails.

Newborn Period

During the 1st minutes after birth, the newborn's Apgar score is determined partly by assessment for the presence and distribution of cyanosis. A normal, nonchilled newborn usually progresses from generalized cyanosis to generalized pinkness while normal respirations are established during the first 5 to 10 minutes of extrauterine life. Acrocyanosis, especially on exposure to a cool environment, is common in newborns for several weeks after birth, as is mottling of the skin, a lattice-like pattern of pale and dark areas that appear especially on the extremities. Severe cold stress can cause generalized cyanosis. Occasionally, in newborns, transient cyanosis of an entire half of the baby (harlequin color change) or of one or more extremities is noted, presumably as the result of temporary vascular instability. Persistent generalized cyanosis is usually a sign of depression caused by maternal drugs or anesthesia, primary pulmonary disease, congenital heart disease, overwhelming infection, or hypoglycemia. Plethora in newborns may indicate high levels of hemoglobin (seen, for instance, in the twin-to-twin transfusion syndrome), and pallor in newborns may be a sign of anemia or cold stress or, less commonly, of congestive heart failure or shock.

A newborn's skin is covered by varying amounts of white, greasy, vernix caseosa, with larger amounts present in preterm babies. The newborn's skin color is determined partly by the amount of subcutaneous fat present. Premature babies have a smaller amount of subcutaneous fat and generally appear redder than full-term babies; their skin is also more transparent, and therefore subcutaneous blood vessels are more visible. Yellow staining of the vernix by meconium suggests that birth was preceded by acute fetal distress; with more prolonged fetal distress, as in the postmature baby who has placental insufficiency, the

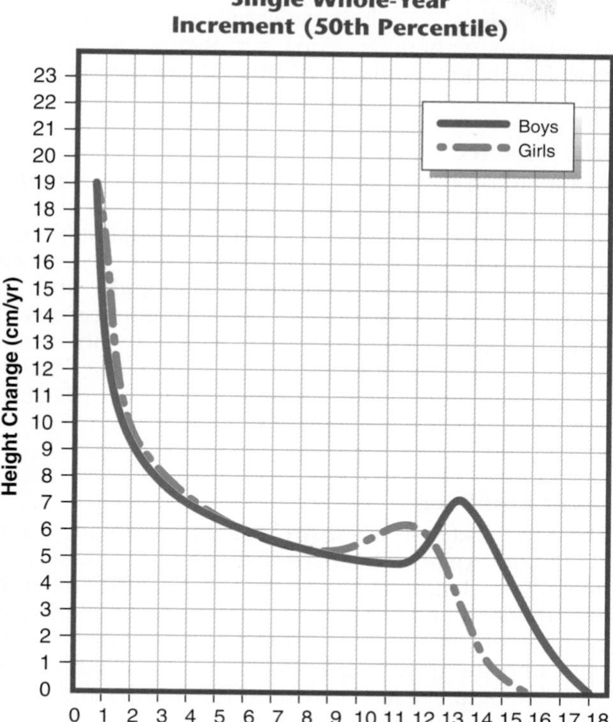

Figure 14-13 Velocity curves for length and height for boys and girls based on intervals of 1 year. *(Adapted from Lowrey GH.* Growth and Development of Children. *8th ed. Chicago, IL: Mosby; 1986. Copyright © 1986, Elsevier, with permission.)*

yellow (or yellow-green) staining can involve the umbilicus and nails. The skin tends to progress from being smooth to scaly, with varying amounts of desquamation and fissuring as the gestation progresses from preterm to postterm. This latter condition usually changes to normal, smooth skin without specific treatment within 1 to 2 weeks. Nonspecific edema, especially of the hands and feet, is less prominent as the gestational age approaches term. Generalized or localized petechiae, ecchymoses of the scalp or face, lacerations of the external ears, and diffuse or localized scalp edema all can be caused by physical trauma sustained during birth.

Jaundice can be expected to appear in at least 50% of normal-term babies and in a higher percentage of preterm babies in the 3rd or 4th day of life, usually indicating the presence of physiological jaundice. However, jaundice appearing at any time during the neonatal period may be an early sign of infection or of metabolic or primary hepatic disease. The early onset of jaundice also raises the question of blood group incompatibility and erythroblastosis. (For more information on jaundice in the newborn, see Chapter 98, Neonatal Jaundice.)

The amount of melanin in the skin varies at birth. Babies of black parents may demonstrate very little melanin as neonates. Pigmented areas over the lumbar region and buttocks, known as mongolian spots, are commonly present in black, darker-complexioned white, and Asian babies at birth. They become less prominent and eventually disappear during childhood. A number of other spots can be seen on a healthy newborn's skin, including the common telangiectasias (nevus flammeus) on the eyelids, bridge of the nose, upper lip, and nape of the neck, which usually disappear during infancy; red or purple strawberry hemangiomas or more deep-seated, cavernous hemangiomas; tiny white papules on the nose, cheeks, forehead, and occasionally the trunk caused by plugging of the sebaceous glands (milia); pinpoint vesicles

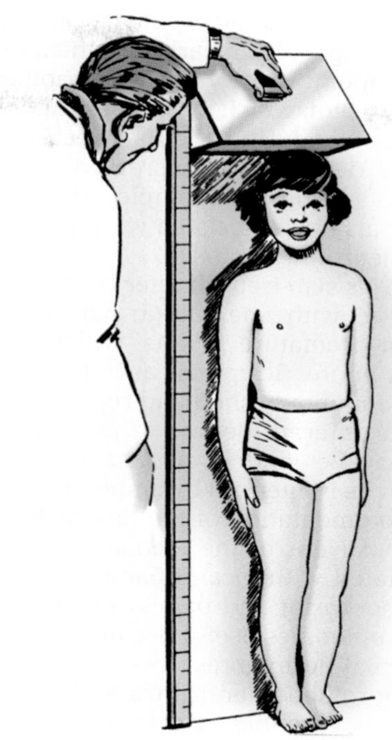

Figure 14-14 Measurement of height. *(Adapted from* Evaluation of body size and physical growth of children, *1976, Rockville, MD, the Maternal and Child Health Program, US Department of Health, Education, and Welfare.)*

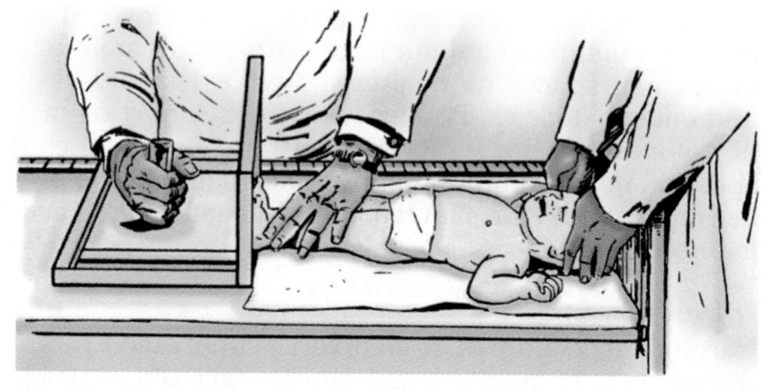

Figure 14-15 Measurement of length in the infant. *(Adapted from* Evaluation of body size and physical growth of children, *1976, Rockville, MD, the Maternal and Child Health Program, US Department of Health, Education, and Welfare.)*

with or without surrounding erythema caused by plugging of the sweat glands (miliaria); erythematous flares with central pinpoint white vesicles or papules, known as erythema toxicum, which may appear and disappear over several hours during the 1st week of life; and areas of either decreased or increased pigmentation, café au lait spots being one example, which may occur in isolation or may be associated with generalized disease, such as neurofibromatosis.

The newborn's skin (see Chapter 85, Neonatal Skin) is often covered with fine lanugo hair, more prominently seen in premature infants, which is lost after several weeks of life. Scalp hair at birth, which varies in amount, is commonly shed and replaced by permanent hair of a different degree of pigmentation. The fingernails may be long in postmature babies, and their color can be influenced by amniotic fluid staining and melanin pigmentation of the nail beds. Incurving of the lateral margins of the toenails is common and can be associated with local inflammation. Examination of the fingerprint and palmar crease patterns in newborns is sometimes useful because of the association of abnormal dermatoglyphics with certain chromosomal abnormalities and intrauterine infections.[4] Magnification is essential in determining the fingerprint pattern on the distal phalanges and the position of the axial triradius of the palm. A single transverse palmar crease (simian line) can occur in normal individuals but is more commonly associated with chromosomal abnormalities such as Down syndrome.

The newborn's skin should be checked carefully for defects and sinus tracts, especially over the entire length of the spine and the midline of the head from the nape of the neck to the bridge of the nose. Sinus tracts sometimes communicate with intracranial and intraspinal spaces or masses, as with dermoid cysts and encephaloceles. Preauricular sinuses may or may not communicate with a persistent brachial cleft space. A more common minor abnormality of the preauricular area is the skin tag, which usually has a cartilaginous core.

Infancy

Careful inspection of a completely undressed infant during health maintenance checks will often reveal minor abnormalities such as cradle cap and diaper dermatitis, the sometimes chronic lesions of infantile acne that first appear at 3 to 4 weeks of age, and less commonly, scattered ecchymoses of varying ages that can signal child abuse. Palpation of the skin, preferably over the lateral abdominal wall, allows qualitative measurement of subcutaneous adipose tissue during infancy and observation of skin turgor (the rate of return to resting position after the skin is lifted and released), which is decreased with dehydration. Observation of capillary refill can be useful in determining cardiac output.

Early and Late Childhood

For all children, evaluation of acute or chronic rashes is helped greatly by a thorough description of the rash's major characteristics (macular, papular, pustular, vesicular, petechial, ecchymotic, oozing, scaly, exfoliative, abraded, erythematous, or pigmented), location (trunk, face, extremities, or intertriginous or hairy areas), number of lesions, developmental history, and temporal association with other signs and symptoms. In fact, most infectious exanthems of children are diagnosed by certain constellations of these factors.

Adolescence

Examination of the skin of adolescents allows monitoring of important pubertal changes such as areolar pigmentation, pigmentation of the external genitalia, development of pubic and axillary hair, increased functioning of sweat and apocrine glands, and an increase in subcutaneous fat. The prominent signs of acne vulgaris on the face and trunk can be anticipated in many adolescents (see Chapter 232, Acne). Acanthosis nigricans in an obese adolescent is suggestive of the development of metabolic syndrome.

Head and Face

The rapid rate of brain growth during infancy and childhood explains the increased size of the head relative to body length in newborns and infants compared with that of adults. The facial contours and dimensions change considerably during the first 10 years of life, reflecting the downward and forward growth of the mandible and vertical growth of the maxilla and nasal bones. These changing proportions are best summarized by the proportion of cranium-to-face volumes at different ages: 8:1 at birth, 5:1 at age 2, and 2:1 by age 18. A thorough examination of the head includes measuring the head circumference and plotting the value on a standard growth chart, observing the shape and symmetry, and palpating the sutures and fontanelles; occasionally, percussion, auscultation, and transillumination are needed. The head should be examined thoroughly in clinical situations involving growth or developmental failure, suspected congenital anomaly or chromosomal defect, suspected trauma, a seizure disorder, or fever in an infant and as part of every health maintenance examination from birth to age 2 years. (See Chapter 178, Facial Dysmorphism.)

Newborn Period

The newborn's skull is composed of partly calcified, bony plates that interface with each other at predictably located suture lines. The major sutures palpable at birth are the coronal, lambdoid, sagittal, and metopic sutures (Figure 14-16). Because of overriding of one cranial bone on another after molding of the skull during the descent through the birth canal, the newborn's sutures often have the feel of ridges. The anterior fontanelle is located at the junction of the sagittal and coronal sutures and varies considerably in size in normal infants; it usually measures approximately 1 inch at its greatest diameter and is diamond shaped. The posterior fontanelle, found at the junction of the sagittal and lambdoid sutures, is only occasionally palpable at birth. Vascular pulsations, transmitted by the cerebrospinal fluid (CSF), can normally be seen over the anterior fontanelle. With normal CSF pressure and with the infant in an upright position and not crying, the anterior fontanelle is soft and flat on palpation. A bulging fontanelle is a sign of increased intracranial

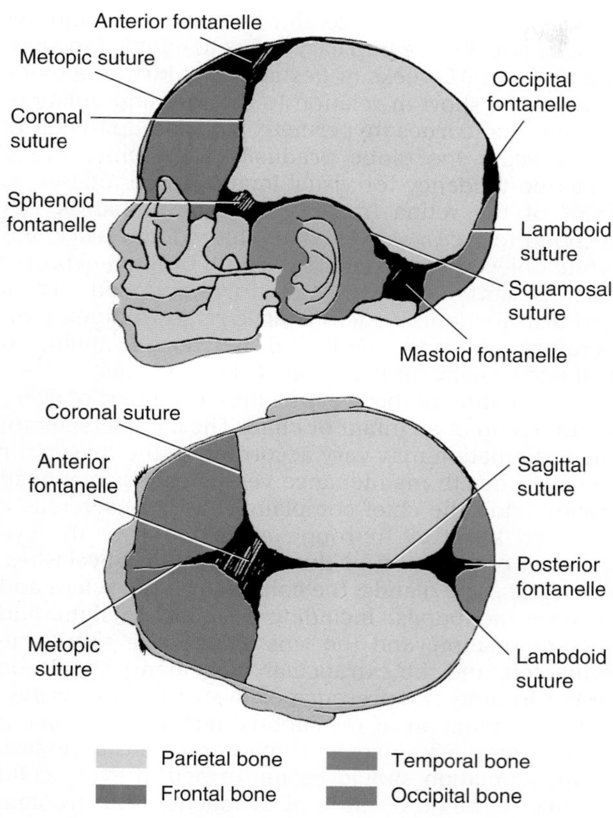

Figure 14-16 Two views of the neonatal skull showing clinically important fontanelles and sutures. *(Adapted from Scanlon JW, et al.* A System of Newborn Physical Examination. *Baltimore, MD: University Park Press; 1979.)*

pressure (see Chapter 352, Increased Intracranial Pressure); a depressed fontanelle is a sign of decreased intravascular volume, as in dehydration.

At birth, palpating localized edema over one or more areas of the head is common. A palpable swelling, particularly over the vertex, that recedes after 1 or 2 days represents subcutaneous edema and is called caput succedaneum. Swollen areas with margins that are limited to suture lines and that often require weeks to recede represent subperiosteal hemorrhage and are called cephalhematomas. These areas resolve partly by calcification, which may initially have the feel of a mass with a heaped-up bony rim and a soft center. Other commonly seen effects of the birth process include linear or curved abraded or lacerated areas, especially over the zygomatic arches and preauricular areas, resulting from use of obstetrical forceps. The infant's face may be asymmetrical at birth because of intrauterine positioning, with the chin touching one shoulder. Facial palsy, exhibited by a drooping corner of the mouth during crying, is usually caused by obstetrical forceps exerting pressure over the facial nerve in the preauricular area.

The cranial bones normally become firmer on palpation with increasing gestational age. One exception occurs when the sutural edges of the cranial bones are pliable and *springy,* a condition known as craniotabes, which is found in many healthy infants and, in rare cases, is a sign of rickets. A disproportionately large head at birth may indicate hydrocephalus or intrauterine growth retardation in which overall brain growth is often relatively normal.

Transillumination of the newborn and infant head is useful in evaluating asymmetrical or disproportionately large heads, as well as unexplained neurologic signs and symptoms. The procedure is accomplished in a completely darkened room by use of a bright light source, such as a 3-battery flashlight or a special high-intensity light. If a flashlight is used, then it should be fitted with a soft foam rubber collar and held against the head tangentially in such a way as to allow uniform intensity of illumination of the head around the full circumference of the light. Localized bright spots may indicate acquired problems, such as subdural effusions, or congenital defects, such as porencephalic cysts. The entire head will light up in the presence of hydranencephaly.

Infancy, Childhood, and Adolescence

By measuring and plotting serial occipitofrontal head circumferences, the examiner can monitor the normal growth of the brain within the normally yielding cranial bones, which are separated from each other by suture lines that remain open until brain growth is complete. A head circumference that is increasing at an abnormally slow rate may indicate either a slowly growing brain (intrinsic or acquired defect) or cranial sutures that have closed too soon (craniosynostosis). Craniosynostosis, a diagnosis that requires confirmation by roentgenography, is often associated with prominence or ridging of the involved suture line. The normally proportioned small head is called microcephaly, and a small head associated with premature suture closure is labeled according to the shape distortion caused by the suture involved: scaphocephaly (closure of the sagittal suture, resulting in restricted lateral growth of the head so that it is abnormally long and narrow); plagiocephaly (closure of coronal or lambdoidal suture, resulting in a lopsided appearance to the head so that its maximal length is on a diagonal, rather than along the midline); and acrocephaly (closure of the coronal and sagittal sutures, resulting in an upward growth of the head so that it has a pointed, or conical, shape).

A head that is growing too rapidly when compared with the rate of height and weight gain should always be evaluated for hydrocephalus and subdural effusions. In some instances, the head is merely asymmetrical, with a normally increasing head circumference; this suggests either intrauterine or extrauterine positional effects, such as the flat occiput seen in babies who are left to lie on their backs for long periods and the flattening of one occipital bone and the opposite frontal bone sometimes associated with torticollis (cranioscoliosis). Prominent frontal bone bossing, with or without associated saddle-nose deformity, may be a sign of the developing osteomyelitis associated with congenital syphilis. The anterior fontanelle is not normally palpable after 18 months of age and may disappear as early as 3 months of age.

Percussion of the head by directly tapping with the middle finger normally elicits a flat sound. A *cracked pot* sound may be heard in infants whose fontanelle is open or in infants who have increased intracranial pressure whose fontanelle is closed, as is seen with hydrocephalus. Auscultation of the head for localized bruits, indicating vascular anomalies, is included in the evaluation of children who have seizures or other neurologic abnormalities. Up to age 5 years, however, systolic or continuous bruits may be heard over the temporal areas in healthy children. Examination of the face begins with an overall impression, which occasionally yields important diagnostic clues, such as the dull, immobile face associated with hypothyroidism; the open-mouthed expression of the child who has chronic nasopharyngeal obstruction caused by hypertrophied adenoids; the multiply bruised face of the battered child; and the small nose, open mouth, and prominent epicanthal skinfolds of the child who has Down syndrome. Facial puffiness, or edema, especially involving the eyelids, can be an early sign of fluid retention caused by acute or chronic renal disease or congestive heart failure. The distance between the eyes, usually measured as the interpupillary distance, can be larger or smaller than usual in several syndromes of chromosomal origin and with other developmental anomalies.

The Chvostek sign, elicited by tapping the cheek just under the zygoma and causing unilateral facial grimacing, is sometimes a sign of hypocalcemia or hyperventilation tetany in older children; it can also be present in healthy infants and young children.

Parotid gland swelling is often difficult to distinguish from cervical adenitis. The swollen parotid gland lies mainly anterior to the angle of the mandible and often pushes the ear pinna away from the side of the head, which can be seen when the patient is viewed from behind. Swelling and tenderness below a line drawn from the angle of the mandible to the mastoid process is caused by cervical adenitis. Nonobstructive parotitis is usually viral. When acute, it is usually caused by the mumps virus but can be bacterial. When recurrent or chronic, HIV infection should be considered (see Chapter 276, Human Immunodeficiency Virus Infection and Acquired Immunodeficiency Syndrome).

Eyes

Studies of the process of mother-infant bonding during the neonatal period highlight the functional importance of an intact visual system in babies from the first minutes after birth.[5] Although examination of the eye offers clues to congenital and acquired systemic abnormalities, the overriding goal of examining the eyes of infants and children is to ascertain that normal functioning is taking place and that potentially remediable processes affecting visual acuity are detected early.

At birth the eye is almost fully grown compared with the other organs and the body. By this time the retina is completely developed except for the central foveal region, which is fully developed by 4 months of age, as is myelination of the central optic radiations and differentiation of the optic cortex. The cornea increases in diameter from 10 mm at birth to the final adult size of 11.5 mm. The lens doubles in weight between birth and age 20 and then increases another 50% by age 80. The pupillary reflex to light is functioning by 29 to 31 weeks of gestation. At birth the globe tends to be short in relation to the focusing ability of the lens and cornea (hypermetropia), and up to age 12 to 14 years the globe gradually lengthens, with a resulting tendency for visual images to be focused in front of the retina (myopia).[6] At birth, babies can respond to faces, as well as to colored and black and white objects. The fixed focal length of the newborn's eyes (20 cm), along with the aforementioned factors and distracting influences (startle reflex, hunger, temperature changes), limit the newborn's ability to respond visually for more than brief moments.

Examination of the eye is an important part of every examination of an infant or child. The completeness of the examination may vary according to the reason for the visit (health maintenance versus emergency head trauma) and the chief complaint (headaches versus a sprained knee). A thorough examination of the eye includes observation of the lids, including eyelashes, tear ducts, and glands; the conjunctiva; the sclera and cornea; the pupils, including reaction to light and accommodation; and the lens. Globe size should be estimated, and the extraocular movements should be tested to note any presence of nystagmus or strabismus. Examination of the fundus includes assessment of the optic disk, macula, retina, and central vessels; this examination should be performed in every child who is examined because of headache, head trauma, or other suspected intracranial lesion. Assessment of visual acuity should be part of every health maintenance examination.

Newborn Period

Several attempts may be required to examine a newborn's eyes completely because of transient edema of the eyelids caused by the birth process or by the conjunctivitis induced by antibiotic instillation soon after birth to prevent gonococcal and other bacterial conjunctivitis. The upper eyelid may have a midline notch from incomplete fusion of its embryonic medial and lateral portions. The eyelids are normally fused until the 8th month of gestation. The lids are often slippery with vernix caseosa and conjunctival exudate, which should be removed gently with a dry cloth, allowing separation of the lids with a finger placed on each lid. Occasionally, one or both eyelids will be everted after birth. Episcleral and subconjunctival hemorrhages, either focal or diffuse, are commonly present after birth and can be expected to recede spontaneously. Less commonly, hyphema (blood in the anterior chamber) may be present. Cloudiness of the cornea can be caused by congenital glaucoma and requires ophthalmologic consultation. Opaque particles or strands in the lens may be cataracts or remnants of the artery that supplies the lens in its early stages of development (hyaloid artery). The iris is often less pigmented at birth; its final color develops during the 1st year of life. Although a ring of white specks around the periphery of the iris (Brushfield spots) is present in some healthy infants, it is more prominent and common in children who have Down syndrome. Defects in the iris, particularly in the ventral aspect, can be associated with parallel defects in the lens and retina (colobomas) and represent incomplete closure of the embryonic optic fissure.

Thorough examination of the newborn's retina is difficult without the use of mydriatics. The appearance of a red reflex, seen when the ophthalmoscope is held 10 to 12 inches in front of the eye, ascertains that no major obstructions to light and its reflection from the retina are present between the cornea and the retina, such as corneal opacities, cataracts, and retinal tumors. Funduscopic examination of the newborn is indicated in babies in whom the red reflex is absent (leukocoria), in babies who have been given prolonged supplemental oxygen, and in babies in whom central nervous system (CNS) trauma or septicemia is suspected. In some newborn nurseries, every newborn is given a funduscopic examination. With the ophthalmoscope, the cornea can usually be seen at +20 diopters, the lens at +15 diopters, and the fundus at 0 diopters. The fundus is examined 30 minutes after instillation of a drop of 2.5% phenylephrine (Neo-Synephrine) ophthalmic solution in each eye, optimally with the assistance of another person who can offer the baby a sugar nipple. The physician notes the size and color of the optic disk and macula and any areas of hemorrhage or increased or decreased pigmentation of the retina. In newborns and infants the optic disk is paler than in older children, the peripheral retina vessels are not well developed, and the foveal light reflection is absent. Papilledema rarely occurs before age 3 years because of the ability of the fontanelles and open sutures to absorb increases in intracranial pressure.

Perhaps the most productive method for observing both the structure and function of the newborn's eyes is for the examiner to hold the infant upright, in which position the infant often opens the eyes spontaneously. Abnormalities in the size of the eyes should be noted, inasmuch as microphthalmia is a part of several rare congenital defect syndromes. Narrowing of the space between the lids may be an isolated condition, blepharophimosis, or part of Komoto syndrome, which also includes ptosis, epicanthus inversus, and telecanthus; unilateral eyelid droop associated with a constricted pupil indicates Horner syndrome. Any upward or downward slanting of the axis of the eyelids (palpebral fissures) should also be noted; upward slanting is characteristic of children who have Down syndrome. Although inner epicanthal folds can occur in healthy infants, they are common in children who have Down syndrome and in those with other chromosomal abnormalities. The setting-sun sign (a portion of the white sclera is seen between the upper lid margin and the iris) occurs in some healthy premature and full-term infants, but persistence suggests the possibility of hydrocephalus.

When the baby is held at arm's length and turned slowly in one direction (Figure 14-17), the eyes turn toward that direction. When rotation stops, the eyes turn toward the opposite direction after a few quick, unsustained, nystagmoid movements. More sustained nystagmus with this maneuver or at rest may indicate blindness or other CNS problems. When only the head is moved slowly through its full range of motion, the eyes do not move but remain in their original position (doll's eye reflex). This maneuver can demonstrate paresis of the lateral rectus muscle. Strabismus (the condition in which the visual axes of both eyes in fixing a distal point are not parallel) is commonly seen as an intermittent phenomenon in healthy newborns and may persist up to 6 months of age (see Chapter 220, Strabismus). The infant should be examined thoroughly for inward deviation of the eye, or esotropia, and outward deviation, or exotropia: whether alternating, fixed, or transient. Prominent epicanthal folds can sometimes give the erroneous impression of strabismus (pseudostrabismus). Any fixed divergence of the eyes and any transient outward divergence in the newborn require immediate neurologic and ophthalmologic consultation.

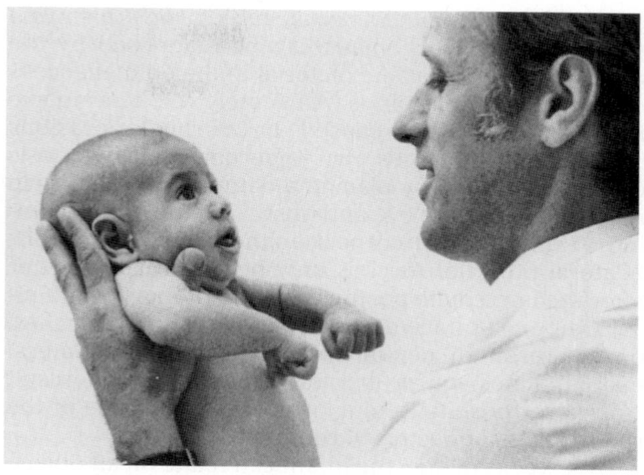

Figure 14-17 Vestibular function testing in the infant. *(Photograph by P. Ruben.)*

Visual acuity in the newborn is assessed indirectly by means of visual reflexes such as consensual pupillary constriction in response to a bright light, blinking in response to a bright light and to an object moved quickly toward the eyes, and opticokinetic nystagmus, which the healthy infant demonstrates when a cylinder that has alternating vertical black and white lines is rotated at specified distances from the eyes.

Infancy

In addition to the findings on the examination described for the newborn, a few common problems affect particularly young infants. Tears are often not present at birth but are produced by 4 months of age. The nasolacrimal duct, however, is sometimes not patent until 1 year of age, leading to a chronically tearing eye with or without purulent discharge. Pressure over the nasolacrimal sac on the medial edge of the lower eyelid will confirm the diagnosis of nasolacrimal duct obstruction by yielding mucoid or purulent fluid. In most instances, minimal or no conjunctival inflammation exists, and ophthalmologic consultation is not indicated unless the tearing and discharge persist beyond 12 months of age.

Acute conjunctival inflammation with purulent exudate in neonates can be caused by *Neisseria gonorrhoeae, Staphylococcus aureus,* or *Chlamydia trachomatis. C trachomatis* can be diagnosed by the presence of cytoplasmic material in the epithelial cells of conjunctival scrapings. An acutely red, tearing eye in infants is often caused by corneal abrasions inflicted by the infant's own fingernails; this diagnosis can be confirmed by placing a damp fluorescein strip in the corner of the eye and observing the green staining of the abraded corneal epithelium. Unilateral or bilateral ptosis of the lids may be appreciated better after the immediate postbirth period; it may be a familial trait, part of a syndrome of congenital anomalies, or the result of oculomotor nerve palsy. Unilateral exophthalmos, or protrusion of the eye, can result from a retroorbital tumor or abscess. Absence of the red reflex is suggestive of retinoblastoma.

By 4 weeks of age, the infant can fixate on an object; by 6 weeks, coordinated movements in following an object are seen. By 3 months, the infant can follow an object moving across the child's midline, and convergence of the eyes is present. Beginning at 4 to 5 months the infant can reach for and grasp colored toys and children's books and can visually circumnavigate the examiner's office.

Childhood and Adolescence

After the neonatal period and up to 3 to 5 years of age, visual acuity continues to be determined by the observations of the parents and the examiner. Standardized tests of distance visual acuity for children from 3 to 5 years use picture cards and older than 5 use letters or numbers.[7]

Infants and children who fail to perform according to the tests outlined here should be examined further for blindness or intellectual disability. Besides instances of blindness that are genetically determined or caused by perinatal insults, amblyopia (or reduced visual acuity) results from suppression of one or two unequal images in the visual cortex. Its importance is that it can be reversed only if diagnosed early enough to allow treatment of the underlying cause. The causes of amblyopia are divided into two major categories: (1) obstructive amblyopia secondary to a cataract, corneal opacity, or severe ptosis and (2) amblyopia ex anopsia secondary to uniocular squint (strabismus) or refractive (anisometropia) error. Strabismus is detected by using the corneal light reflection (Hirschberg) test and the cover-uncover test. The symmetry of the corneal light reflections is observed while the child focuses on a penlight 12 inches from the eyes; asymmetry indicates esotropia or exotropia. In the cover-uncover test, with the child focusing on the penlight, the visual axis of one eye is interrupted by the examiner's hand; any movement of the uncovered eye indicates strabismus. Similarly, when the examiner's hand is removed, the original uncovered eye moves back to its original position.

Loss of visual acuity in one eye detected during a screening evaluation is often the first indication of amblyopia. Vision is screened by using the Snellen illiterate E chart for children between the ages of 3 and 5 years and the Snellen E chart for children 5 years of age and older (see Chapter 42, Vision Screening).

The most common abnormalities of children's eyes seen in an ambulatory setting are swelling and redness of the eyelids and a red, tearing eye. Swelling and redness of the eyelids occur with obstruction of the nasolacrimal duct, blepharitis, hordeolum, and chalazion. Edema, tenderness, and warmth of the eyelid, usually indicative of periorbital cellulitis, can be caused by infection resulting from local trauma or insect bites, or they can be associated with upper respiratory tract infections and otitis media. Orbital cellulitis is characterized by marked lid edema, proptosis, chemosis, reduced vision, and decreased motility with pain on movement of the globe (see Chapter 313, Preseptal and Orbital Cellulitis). A red, tearing eye can be caused by acute conjunctivitis, subconjunctival hemorrhage, keratitis, acute iridocyclitis, and acute glaucoma. Conjunctivitis characterized by prominence of the conjunctival blood vessels is one of the signs of Kawasaki disease. Evaluation of children who have sustained head trauma or who are suspected of having an overwhelming infection requires careful, repeated testing of the extraocular movements in the six cardinal fields of gaze and of the pupillary light reflex and observation of the conjunctivae and fundi, looking for unilateral abnormalities, hemorrhage, and papilledema. For example, lateral rectus muscle palsy is often the earliest sign of increased intracranial pressure (see Chapter 352, Increased Intracranial Pressure). Retinal hemorrhages can be seen in infants who have shaken baby syndrome.

Ears

The inner ear develops early in the 1st trimester of pregnancy, and response to sound can be shown in the 26th fetal week. At birth the cochlea and vestibule are anatomically mature. Successful examination of the ears in infants and children, a skill that requires years of practice, is extremely important because of the high incidence of middle ear abnormalities in children. The student should approach the use of the otoscope and the almost universal presence of ceruminous impediments to visualization of the external auditory canal in children with patience and a willingness to ask for confirmation of findings as often as needed. The practitioner should include a thorough examination of the ears in every physical examination, noting the characteristics of the external ear, external canal, and tympanic membrane and assessing hearing acuity.

Newborn Period

The external ear is flat and shapeless until 34 weeks of gestation; once folded, it may remain so unless placed back in the flat position. Between 34 and 40 weeks of gestation, an incurving of the periphery of the pinna develops, along with an increasing ability to return spontaneously from the folded to the flat position. Minor anomalies in the shape of the external ear should be noted, including the occasional preauricular skin tags or preauricular sinuses. The position of the upper attachment of the external ears should be noted in relation to a line connecting the inner and outer canthus of the eye. Attachments that fall below this line are sometimes associated with other congenital abnormalities, including renal agenesis. Patency of the external auditory canals can be determined by direct observation after pulling the pinna away from the side of the head. The tympanic membrane is coated with vernix caseosa for several days after birth and usually cannot be visualized.

Auditory screening in neonates begins with identifying those at risk for hearing loss because of a familial hearing disorder; intrauterine viral infection; hyperbilirubinemia, with bilirubin levels above 20 mg/dL; previous treatment with an ototoxic drug (eg, gentamycin); or defects of the ear, nose, or throat. Neonates with any of these factors should be screened for hearing loss, their subsequent language development should be monitored closely, and they should be referred to an audiologist for any signs suggesting hearing loss (see Chapter 45, Language and Speech Assessment; and Chapter 39, Auditory Screening).

In some states, all newborns are screened routinely for hearing acuity using auditory brainstem response or evoked autoacoustic emissions testing.[8]

Infancy and Childhood

Several techniques can help the practitioner visualize the tympanic membrane. The infant's head should be stabilized to prevent painful jamming of the speculum into the ear canal. This task can sometimes be accomplished by having the parent or a nurse hold the infant against the chest with the infant's head on one shoulder and then the opposite shoulder. The head is usually stabilized best by laying the infant supine on the examining table and having the parent or a nurse hold the baby's arms against the body or extended on either side of the head. Providing some type of visual distraction, and verbal reassurances, while positioning the infant usually affords the examiner a brief, struggle-free period for performing the otoscopic examination. Varying amounts of resistance are almost universal; however, and a rapid examination is desirable for the infant, the parents, and the examiner. One hand is used to grasp the ear pinna and gently pull it laterally and posteriorly to straighten the lumen of the external canal. In infants the external canal tends to be perpendicular to the temporal bone, with a slight upward angle (further growth of the skull will give the canal a slightly anterior and downward direction). If the otoscope is held upside down, then the infant's head can be stabilized further by the hand holding the ear pinna and the ulnar edge of the hand holding the otoscope (Figure 14-18).

The examiner can further stabilize the infant's body by leaning across the chest and abdomen. The ear speculum then is introduced into the external canal and gently advanced to the point where the bony portion of the canal prevents further entry. Cerumen, which can be soft, firm, or flaky and varies from white to dark brown, may have to be removed. A flexible, wire-loop ear curette can remove small to moderate amounts of soft cerumen and poses less risk of abrading the canal wall or tympanic membrane than does a rigid curette. Curetting is done most safely through the otoscopic head. Larger amounts of hard, inspissated cerumen may require irrigation with warm water and sometimes before treatment with softening agents such as hydrogen peroxide. An ear canal filled with purulent exudate usually indicates acute otitis media with perforation or otitis externa (the latter is accompanied by pain when the pinna is moved); irrigation is usually unsuccessful and may be dangerous, especially with perforation of the tympanic membrane. Several sizes of specula should be tried to find the largest size that fits into the ear canal, thus allowing visualization of the largest area of tympanic membrane. The otoscope must usually be rotated to view all the important landmarks.

A normal tympanic membrane (Figure 14-19) is semitransparent, roughly cone shaped, and inclined away from the examiner. The light reflex in the anteroinferior quadrant is often the first landmark seen, with its origin at the central umbo. The examiner, moving the light superiorly from the umbo, can see the long process of the malleus through the membrane, which ends in a bony protuberance that marks the junction of the pars tensa inferiorly and the pars flaccida superiorly. Vague outlines of the incus can

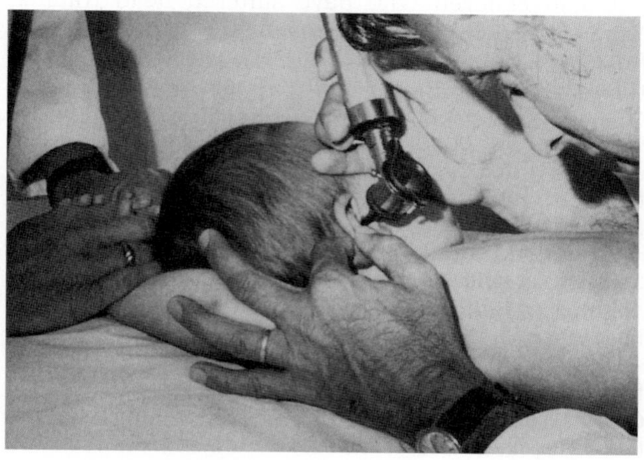

Figure 14-18 Otoscopic examination of the child. *(Photograph by P. Ruben.)*

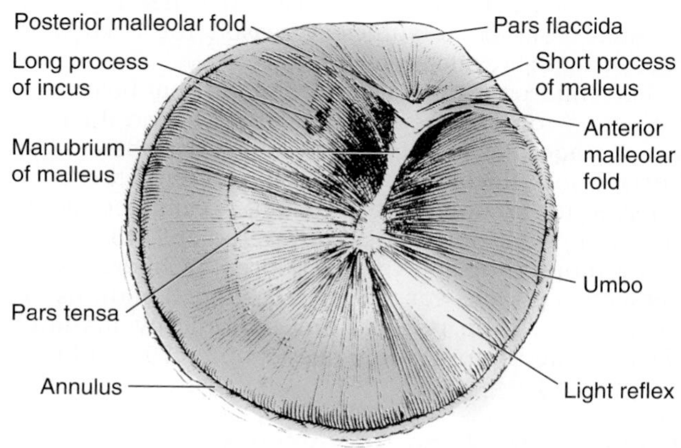

Figure 14-19 Anatomy of the tympanic membrane. *(Adapted from Strome M, ed.* Differential Diagnosis in Pediatric Otolaryngology. *Boston, MA: Little, Brown; 1975.)*

sometimes be seen in the posterosuperior quadrant. Air insufflation, by means of a diagnostic otoscopic head fitted with a small bulb, permits direct observation of the eardrum's movement as positive and then negative pressure is applied gently (pneumatoscopy).

As acute otitis media develops, the tympanic membrane becomes increasingly opaque and erythematous, usually progressing superiorly to inferiorly, with progressive outward bulging and eventual loss of the outlines of the malleus and of the light reflex. Air insufflation will demonstrate decreasing mobility and sometimes the changing menisci of fluid levels within the middle ear. As the condition heals, these changes resolve inferiorly to superiorly; final resolution of opacity, limited motion, and fluid levels sometimes requires several months.

Bullous myringitis appears as a bubble-like swelling that can almost fill the bony portion of the external ear canal. Blood behind the eardrum, either red or purple, is a sign of basilar skull fracture and should be anticipated in children who have suffered head trauma. White plaques on the eardrum are scars from old infections. A white mass in the posterosuperior quadrant may be a cholesteatoma, which is present with chronic obstructive middle ear disease. When examining acutely ill children suspected of having a middle ear infection, the mastoid process should be inspected for overlying swelling and erythema and palpated for tenderness: signs of acute mastoiditis.

All infants should have access to hearing screening using a physiological measure (otoacoustic emissions testings or auditory brainstem response testing) no later than 1 month of age. Regardless of newborn screening outcome, all infants should be monitored for age-appropriate auditory behaviors and communications skills. Typically, infants make cooing sounds (semipurposeful vocalization of vowel sounds) by 6 weeks of age, laugh out loud by 3 months, babble (repetitive sounds, such as "baabaa") by 6 months, echo sounds made in their presence by 9 months, and say their first meaningful word between 12 and 15 months. An infant who fails to progress beyond any of these developmental stages or who regresses should receive an audiologic evaluation to rule out hearing loss. Parental concern is sufficient reason for a child to receive further evaluation.[9]

For children 1 to 5 years of age, normal hearing is necessary for language development beyond the one-word stage. All infants with known risk factors for hearing loss (including caregiver concern) should be referred for an otologic evaluation. A validated global screening tool should be administered at 9, 18, and 24 to 30 months of age to all children.[9] Children with persistent middle ear effusion lasting 3 months or longer should be referred for otologic evaluation.[9] (For detailed information, see Chapter 39, Auditory Screening.)

Late Childhood and Adolescence

The tympanic membrane in older children can usually be examined without resistance with the child sitting. If the child has ear pain or has had a previous painful examination, then the supine position will make head stabilization easier. A qualitative hearing test for children in this age group can be accomplished by using tuning forks, particularly those with frequencies in the human voice range of 500 to 2000 Hz. The examiner's own acuity, presuming that it is normal, can be compared with the child's. Comparing bone and air conduction (Rinne test) and testing for lateralization of bone conduction with the handle of the tuning fork held against the midforehead (Weber test) can distinguish qualitatively between conductive and nerve hearing loss; with conductive loss, air conduction is less than bone conduction, and lateralization to the affected ear is present. Audiometric screening for this age group is routine in many schools. Some children who have chronic middle ear disease have fluctuating hearing loss that can be missed on a single pure-tone screening. In such cases, pneumatoscopy, impedance audiometry, and tympanometry can provide the definitive diagnosis.

Nose

The relative size and shape of the nose are normally influenced by the downward and forward growth of the maxillary bones and, to a lesser extent, by the increase in the bizygomatic width during childhood. The bony orbits are nearer adult size in the newborn than are the other facial bones, and the palate grows most rapidly during the 1st year of postnatal life. The paranasal sinuses are represented only by the centrally placed ethmoid sinuses at birth; the maxillary sinuses develop from birth and are usually apparent on roentgenograms by 4 years of age and the sphenoid sinuses by age 6. The frontal sinuses have usually reached the level of the roof of the orbits by age 6 to 7 years. The nose humidifies incoming air and traps bacteria and noxious materials in its continuous mucous blanket, moving them toward the pharynx by ciliary action. Olfactory function appears to be present at birth and to increase with age.

A thorough examination of the nose involves inspecting the external form, the condition of the external nares, the mucous membranes of the septum, and the turbinates and floor of the nose, as well as noting any exudate present. The nose should be examined in all newborns and in all children who have upper respiratory tract symptoms, noisy breathing, epistaxis, head trauma, headache, and fever.

Newborn Period

In examining the newborn's nose, ruling out the presence of unilateral or bilateral choanal atresia, which can produce severe respiratory distress, is important, inasmuch as most newborns are unable to breathe easily through their mouths. This examination is performed by introducing a soft No. 8 feeding tube into each external naris and advancing the catheter to the pharynx. Advancing the feeding tube farther into the stomach rules out esophageal obstructions such as atresia and allows aspiration of the amniotic fluid from the stomach. A simpler technique for testing choanal patency is to close 1 nostril and then the other nostril while holding the mouth closed. When choanal atresia is present, the infant will struggle for breath when the patent nasal airway is occluded. Obstructed nasal breathing is sometimes seen briefly after birth because of inhaled blood and amniotic debris, which can cause moderate-to-severe distress, especially in the few infants who have congenitally narrow nasal cavities. A profuse, purulent nasal discharge in the neonatal period might suggest the presence of congenital syphilis.

Infancy, Childhood, and Adolescence

By elevating the tip of the child's nose and using a nasal speculum, the practitioner can inspect the membranes covering the nasal septum, floor of the nose, and inferior, middle, and superior turbinates in the lateral nasal wall for signs of inflammation and bleeding points. The nasal septum is occasionally deviated to one side, sometimes obstructing breathing on that side. The fairly common occurrence of intranasal foreign bodies should be anticipated when examining any child who has chronic nasal discharge, with or without associated bleeding. Epithelial polyps of the nasal mucosa are rare in children and usually indicate underlying cystic fibrosis or chronic allergic rhinitis. A pale, swollen, boggy nasal mucosa indicates allergic rhinitis, whereas with viral rhinitis the nasal membranes are red and bleed easily. Sinusitis should be suspected whenever purulent exudate appears from beneath any of the three nasal turbinates, especially in a child who has a history of chronic nasal congestion, chronic tracheobronchitis, recurrent otitis media, and fever. Transillumination of the paranasal sinuses in younger children is of limited value to physicians other than otorhinolaryngologists because of the variable development of the sinuses before ages 8 and 10. After 10 years of age the frontal sinuses can be transilluminated in a darkened room by holding a bright light source (transilluminator attachment for an otoscope-ophthalmoscope handle) against the superomedial aspect of the orbit; the maxillary sinuses can be transilluminated by holding the light against the lateral aspects of the hard palate within the closed mouth. Percussion of the frontal and maxillary sinuses may be helpful in diagnosing sinusitis; the infected sinus will be tender. Percussion of the mandible can be used as a control.

Clear fluid draining from the nose after head trauma should be tested for sugar, which is present with a CSF leak. In a child who has a history of epistaxis, the anteroinferior portion of the septum is a common location of prominent blood vessels (Kiesselbach plexus) that bleed easily, especially when aggravated by local inflammation and self-inflicted abrasions.

Swelling around the bridge of the nose can be caused by a cavernous hemangioma or, less commonly, a nasal encephalocele. Erythematous swelling that involves the lateral portion of the bridge of the nose and adjacent eyelids can be a sign of orbital or periorbital cellulitis, which requires immediate intensive investigation and treatment.

Primary care physicians are often asked to examine a child who has suffered trauma to the nose. Consultation with a subspecialist should be sought immediately if the child has prolonged bleeding from the nose after an injury, if evidence exists of a septal hematoma, or if any question exists of depression of the base of the nose or of deviation from the nose's normal straight-line vertical axis.

Mouth and Pharynx

The size and shape of the mouth and pharynx change during infancy and childhood, with further growth during the 1st year of the hard palate and of the mandible, which expands on all surfaces through the 2nd year, extending downward and forward as a result of mandibular condylar growth. The most useful clinical evidence of growth around the mouth is the eruption, further growth, and shedding of the 20 primary (deciduous) teeth, with subsequent eruption of the 32 secondary (permanent) teeth. Intrauterine tooth growth begins during the 2nd fetal month. The deciduous teeth usually begin to erupt by the 6th month of extrauterine life; roughly, one new tooth erupts for each month after 6 months of age, with eruption of all deciduous teeth by 28 to 36 months of age.[10] Figure 14-20 summarizes the chronology of eruption and shedding of teeth in the growing human. Shedding of the deciduous teeth and eruption of the permanent teeth normally begins at age 5 in boys and age 5½ in girls and continues through age 14, with eruption of the permanent teeth completed by age 20. Delayed eruption of the permanent teeth may be a sign of delayed onset of puberty in adolescence or delayed bone age for other reasons.

The pharyngeal tonsils steadily increase in size during childhood and then begin to recede during puberty, a pattern of growth shared with adenoidal lymphoid tissue and peripheral lymph nodes. The mouth and pharynx should be examined carefully during all health maintenance visits and in all children who have respiratory symptoms, fever of unknown origin, and ear or facial pain. A complete examination involves inspecting and palpating the lips, buccal mucosa, gingiva, hard palate, and mandible, as well as inspecting the teeth, tongue, soft palate, tonsillar pillars, tonsils, and posterior pharyngeal wall.

Newborn Period

The newborn's mouth is often examined initially by means of the sucking reflex, with the examiner's finger inside the baby's mouth; this technique can quiet the baby and expedite other parts of the examination. The relative size of the mandible is noted (small mandibles are sometimes associated with underdevelopment of other facial bones as a result of a generalized or genetic disorder). Clefts of the upper lip may be unilateral, bilateral, or midline and may be associated with palatal clefts. A common normal variant is a prominent mucosal fold connecting the inner midline of the upper lip to the posterior portion of the upper gum, leaving a deep notch in the midline of the gum and spacing of the upper central incisors. The upper and lower gums have finely serrated borders. Occasionally, small white mucus-retention cysts (Bohn nodules), which may be mistaken for teeth, are present. White retention cysts at the midline of the posterior border of the hard palate are known as Epstein pearls. Both types of mucus-retention cysts disappear spontaneously within a few months. Filmy, patchy white membranes over the gingiva, inner lips, and buccal mucosa that cannot be removed by scraping and that sometimes overlie an erythematous base can be seen in some healthy newborns; these are characteristics of

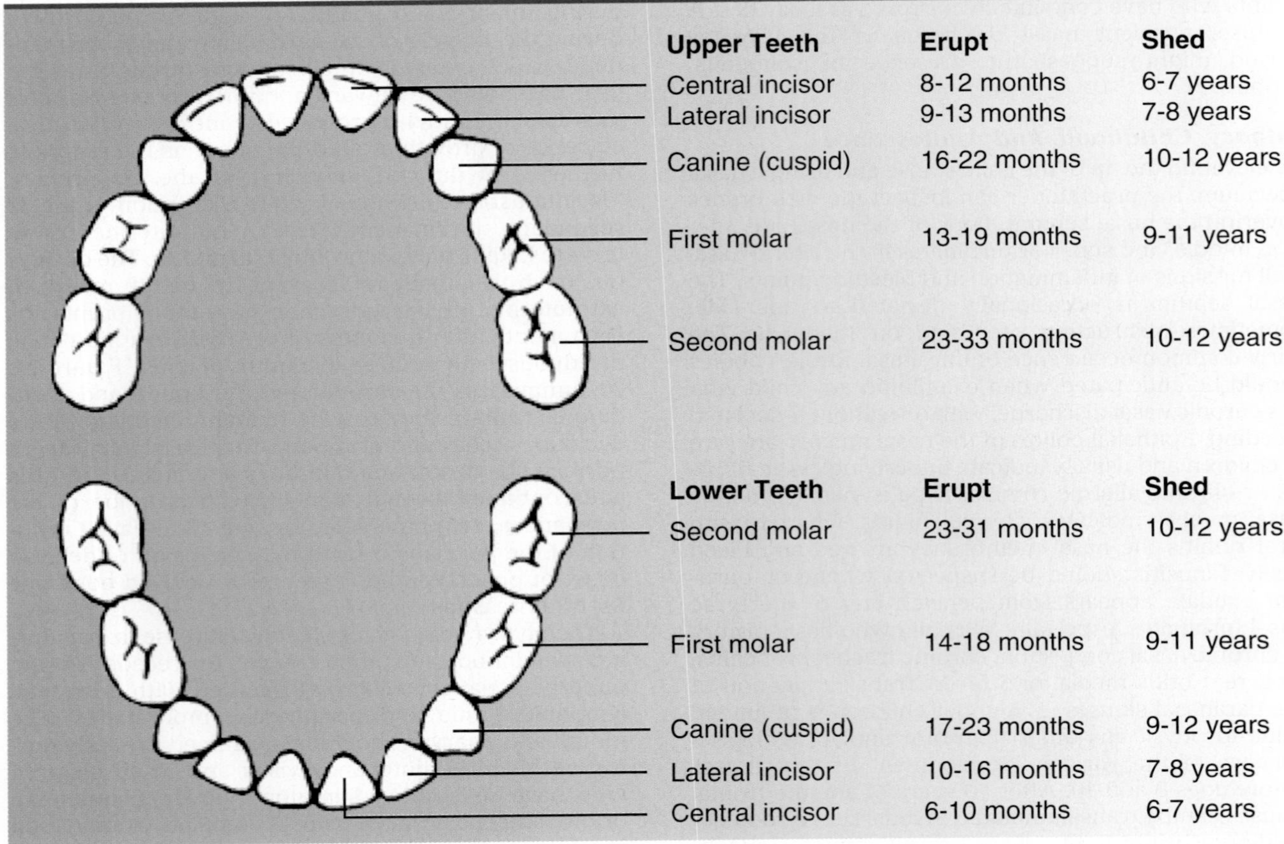

Primary Teeth

Upper Teeth	Erupt	Shed
Central incisor	8-12 months	6-7 years
Lateral incisor	9-13 months	7-8 years
Canine (cuspid)	16-22 months	10-12 years
First molar	13-19 months	9-11 years
Second molar	23-33 months	10-12 years

Lower Teeth	Erupt	Shed
Second molar	23-31 months	10-12 years
First molar	14-18 months	9-11 years
Canine (cuspid)	17-23 months	9-12 years
Lateral incisor	10-16 months	7-8 years
Central incisor	6-10 months	6-7 years

Figure 14-20 Primary teeth eruption chart. *(Copyright © American Dental Association. Reprinted with permission. Available at: www.ada.org/public/topics/tooth_eruption.asp.)*

Candida albicans stomatitis (thrush). Thorough examination of the palate should be performed to defect clefts, both complete and submucosal. In addition, a high arched palate suggests various syndromes (eg, Pierre Robin syndrome).

A prominent tongue, which may protrude from the mouth, is seen in congenital hypothyroidism and in Down syndrome. A frenulum attaches to the tongue's inferior surface and may extend almost to its tip. When this area is thickened and shortened, protrusion of the tongue is limited. Although a source of concern to parents, this *tongue tie* (ankyloglossia) does not often interfere with speech or breastfeeding and rarely requires surgical lysis. Salivation is relatively scanty in a healthy newborn; therefore excessive collection of saliva and mucus in the mouth should prompt investigation for esophageal atresia.

A newborn's pharynx is difficult to visualize except during crying because of the strong gag reflex induced by the tongue blade, which may cause the pharynx to fill with stomach contents. Tonsillar tissue is not visible in newborns.

The quality of the infant's cry should be noted. A strong, lusty cry indicates a healthy baby whose airways and lungs are functioning normally; expiratory grunting is associated with respiratory distress; inspiratory stridor is caused by several lesions obstructing upper and lower airways; a high-pitched cry suggests intracranial diseases, either congenital or acquired; a hoarse cry suggests hypocalcemic tetany or cretinism; and absence of a cry suggests severe illness or intellectual disability.

Infancy, Childhood, and Adolescence

Because examining the mouth and pharynx of preschool children is usually difficult, these attempts are best saved until the end of the examination. Some manner of restraint is usually required; one of the most effective methods is to have the child seated on the mother's lap with the child's head held stationary by the mother's hand (Figure 14-21). Some infants and toddlers will permit a brief period of "looking at the teeth," with the tongue depressor used gently to retract the lips and buccal mucosa. A crying infant usually gives the examiner struggle-free glimpses of the mouth and pharynx without the need for manipulation. While adequately restrained, a frightened child with clenched teeth can be examined by slipping the tongue depressor laterally and behind the teeth and onto the tongue. In older children, firm pressure on

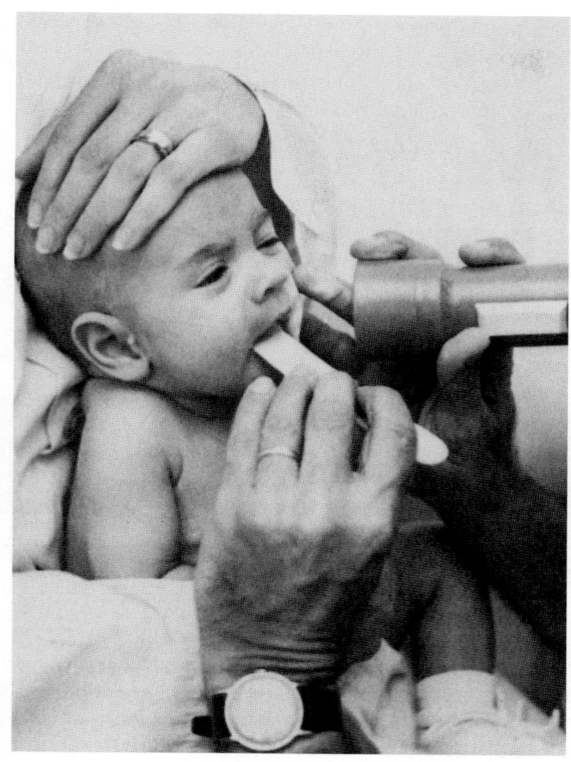

Figure 14-21 Examination of the pharynx in the infant. *(Photograph by P. Ruben.)*

the anterior half of the tongue, with the tongue not protruded, will allow adequate vision of the whole mouth and pharynx; in infants the gag reflex must usually be induced by slipping the tongue depressor onto the posterior half of the tongue. In general, sick children, including those who have respiratory tract infections, are the most reluctant to have the physician peer into their mouth. Healthy children, on the other hand, can sometimes be persuaded to stick out their tongue and say "aaah" if the practitioner demonstrates how to do so.

Salivation normally increases to full capacity during the 3rd month of life, the age when salivary drooling is first observed because of the infant's limited ability to swallow and the lack of lower front teeth to serve as a dam. Increased salivation associated with respiratory distress and fever usually suggests herpes simplex stomatitis or epiglottitis. Salivation may also increase temporarily with the eruption of new teeth. During the winter the lips can be dry and cracked, especially at the corners of the mouth. Deeper fissures at the corners of the mouth, cheilosis, occur in several states of nutritional deficiency and with severe thrush.

The gingivae should be inspected for localized or diffuse inflammatory lesions. Shallow, white-based ulcers with surrounding erythema can be seen, usually singly, on the gingivae in association with upper respiratory tract infections. Numerous gingival ulcers with concomitant involvement of the tongue and lips associated with increased salivation, fever, and pain usually result from primary herpes simplex infection, which is most common during the first years of life. Recurrent herpes simplex stomatitis, or cold sores, involving the lips can occur after the primary bout of stomatitis. Localized or diffuse gingival inflammation is most often associated with dental disease, particularly plaque buildup at the gingival borders because of inadequate tooth brushing. Dental abscesses sometimes exhibit an erythematous soft-tissue mass that exudes pus at the dental-gingival border of the involved tooth. Gingivae that bleed easily most often reflect poor mouth hygiene and irritation by bacterial plaque, but the condition can signal, albeit rarely, blood dyscrasia, a clotting deficit, or vitamin C deficiency (scurvy).

The buccal mucosa can be involved with nonspecific ulcerative processes, but it is occasionally the site of important signs of specific infectious diseases. In measles, on the 2nd or 3rd day of the illness, before the onset of the generalized rash, Koplik spots can be seen on the buccal mucosa; these are white pinpoint spots that appear at the level of the lower teeth. In parotitis, usually caused by the mumps virus but occasionally by other organisms, Stensen duct openings, found at the level of the upper molars, are red, swollen, and tender. Scattered white ulcers of varying size can appear on the buccal mucosa in chickenpox. In Kawasaki disease, several abnormalities can be seen, including cracked, fissured lips and diffuse redness of the pharynx. Chronic thrush may be an early sign of HIV infection in infants and children.

The teeth are counted with the expectation that the infant will have, on the average, one tooth for each month of age past 6 months up to 28 to 36 months of age, when the full complement of 20 primary teeth will have erupted. Delayed tooth eruption can accompany either serious chronic disease or generalized developmental delay. In infants, the individual teeth are examined for localized or generalized enamel hypoplasia, which can reflect a variety of causes, including hereditary enamel hypoplasia, intrauterine insults such as infections, and prematurity (Figure 14-22). The infant's teeth may have a permanent yellow, gray, or brown discoloration if the mother took tetracycline during her pregnancy or if the baby was treated with the drug; mottled, pitted teeth with a lusterless, opaque enamel may be the result of an excessive fluoride intake. Oral iron preparations can stain the teeth green, as can an elevated bilirubin level during the neonatal period.

The spacing of the teeth should be observed, giving special attention to teeth that are too close together or too far apart, both of which may cause spacing problems later on. Dental occlusion can be checked by having the child bite down and then observing for maxillary protrusion (overbite) or mandibular protrusion (underbite). Malocclusion has numerous causes, including chronic mouth breathing caused by nasal or nasopharyngeal obstruction, the rare instances of mandibular overgrowth secondary to temporomandibular arthritis in juvenile rheumatoid arthritis, and maxillary overgrowth in untreated hereditary hemolytic anemias, such as Cooley anemia.

The texture and appearance of the tongue may indicate specific diseases. Dryness, with or without coating, may be seen in chronic mouth breathing or in

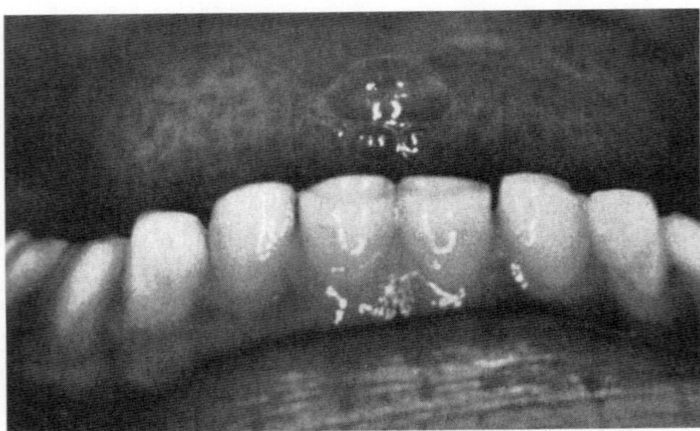

Figure 14-22 Enamel hypoplasia in a premature child. *(From McDonald RE, Avery DR.* Dentistry for the Child and Adolescent. *7th ed. St Louis, MO: Mosby; 2000. Copyright © 2000, Elsevier, with permission.)*

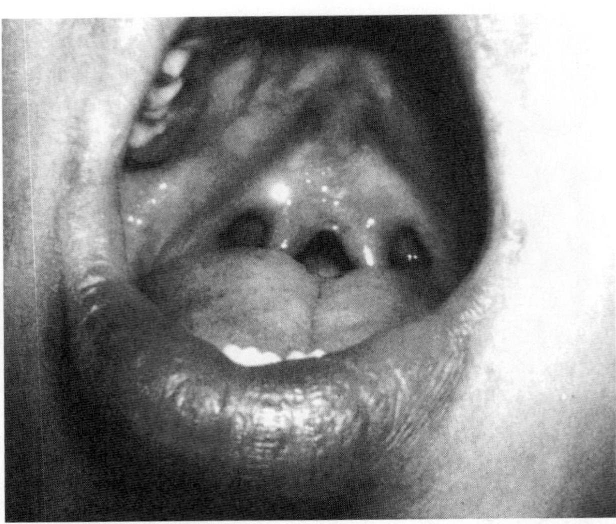

Figure 14-23 Submucosal cleft palate with bifid uvula.

states of dehydration. Strawberry tongue, a result of the prominence of the papillae, is seen during the course of scarlet fever and in Kawasaki disease. Thrush and herpes simplex, previously described, can involve the tongue. Geographic tongue, in which the surface has the appearance of a relief map, may be nonspecific or may be associated with underlying allergic disease. Deep furrows in the tongue (scrotal tongue) have no significance. Fine and gross tremor of the tongue, including fasciculations and fibrillations, can be seen in both CNS disease (eg, Sydenham chorea) and peripheral nerve and neuromuscular junction diseases (Werdnig-Hoffmann disease).

Petechiae are sometimes present on the hard and soft palates in association with pharyngitis, especially streptococcal pharyngitis. The upward motion of the uvula and soft palate should be confirmed during phonation and with the gag reflex to rule out paralysis. A bifid uvula (Figure 14-23) should be recognized because it can be associated with a submucous cleft of the soft palate. In this condition the soft palate is relatively short and does not reach the posterior pharyngeal wall. Palatal closure against the posterior pharyngeal wall, essential for normal articulation and voice resonance, can be aided in this condition by the presence of hypertrophied nasopharyngeal lymphoid tissue. Therefore, during the preoperative examination of a child scheduled for adenoidectomy, the practitioner should check for submucous cleft of the palate because it may affect the decision to operate (see Chapter 331, Tonsillectomy and Adenoidectomy).

The anterior and posterior pillars that border the tonsils are difficult to distinguish in most infants. The tonsils (palatal tonsils) are proportionately larger in preschool and school-aged children than in adults. Tonsillar size is estimated arbitrarily on a scale of 1% to 4%, 1% indicating easy visibility and 4% indicating that the tonsils meet in the midline. The tonsils normally appear more prominent during gagging or crying, and their relative size can be assessed accurately only while the infant or child is at rest. The tonsillar crypts normally contain varying amounts of desquamated cells, which appear as white spots on the surface. However, true tonsillar exudate is usually less localized to the crypts and extends over a greater portion of the surface. Some examiners try to distinguish the color of the exudate: yellow being more common with streptococcal infection, white with viral infections, and gray with diphtheria. A grayish discoloration of the tonsils (rather than an exudate) is sometimes seen with infectious mononucleosis. The only reliable way to determine cause is to obtain a throat culture, especially of the tonsillar exudate in children older than 2 to 3 years. Tonsillar erythema and edema, which should also be noted, are particularly conspicuous with streptococcal infection.

Shallow, white-based ulcers that have erythematous edges, which may involve the adjacent pillars and posterior pharynx, suggest herpangina, caused by coxsackievirus A, and can be distinguished from the more anterior location of the herpes simplex ulcers. The diphtheritic membrane may be confluent over the tonsils, pharynx, and uvula, and bleeding ensues when the membrane is scraped away with a tongue blade. In infants a diffusely red pharynx and tonsillar area, with or without exudate, most likely has a viral origin. A peritonsillar abscess is suggested by asymmetrical enlargement of the tonsils, or peritonsillar swelling (best detected by palpation) often associated with lateral displacement of the uvula toward the unaffected tonsil.

The posterior pharyngeal wall should be inspected for evidence of lymphoid hyperplasia, which has a cobblestone appearance and indicates chronic postnasal drainage, as seen in chronic allergic rhinitis or bacterial sinusitis. Postnasal drainage into the pharynx is to be expected in infants and children who have upper respiratory tract infections, and the characteristics of the mucus suggest various causes. Clear mucus is present in allergic rhinitis or in the early stages of acute rhinitis, whereas purulent mucus appears in the late stages of a viral rhinitis or with chronic bacterial sinusitis.

The presence and size of the adenoidal lymphoid tissue can be estimated indirectly by noting the amount of mouth breathing at rest, by observing the ease of breathing through the nostrils, and by noting any nasality to the voice. Direct palpation of the adenoids with a finger introduced through the mouth and around the soft palate is possible only under anesthesia. Using the nasopharyngeal mirror for visualization of the adenoids is most helpful to those who use it every day, such as otolaryngologists.

The epiglottis is sometimes visualized by chance when the throat of a child who has an upper respiratory tract infection is examined. In children who have croupy cough, especially if of sudden onset and associated with high fever, drooling, and signs of upper airway obstruction, the epiglottis must be visualized to rule out acute bacterial epiglottitis, a true emergency in children. The epiglottis may be swollen several times its usual size and is cherry red. Because of the danger of complete airway obstruction and of cardiac arrest during this examination, endotracheal tubes, a tracheotomy set, and an oxygen source should be at hand. Most primary care physicians choose to rely on a lateral neck roentgenogram initially to evaluate the size of the epiglottis and postpone direct visualization until a surgeon is present.

Neck

The neck is relatively short in infants and lengthens during childhood as a result of vertebral growth. Consequently the epiglottis descends from the level of the first cervical vertebral body at birth to the lower third of the third cervical vertebral body by adulthood. The larynx is one third the adult size at birth. It grows rapidly until age 3, becoming wider and longer, and then grows slowly until puberty, when another rapid increase in all dimensions occurs, especially in boys. The trachea at birth is approximately one third the adult length, and both the anteroposterior and lateral diameters of the trachea increase by nearly 300% from birth to puberty. The thyroid gland increases approximately 10 times in weight from birth through puberty, with most growth occurring during puberty. Cervical lymph nodes, a few of which may be palpable at birth, increase in size, monitoring the growth curve for the body's lymphatic tissues in general; those in most healthy children are less than 1 cm in diameter. The neck should be examined thoroughly from time to time in healthy infants and children and always in children who have a respiratory or febrile illness. This examination should include noting the overall neck dimensions; the resistance to passive motion; the size and location of the lymph nodes, thyroid gland, and the trachea; the status of neck vessels; and the presence of masses.

Newborn Period

The newborn's relatively short neck should be inspected for position and overall size. Torticollis, a condition in which the head is tilted to one side with the chin rotated toward the opposite shoulder, is usually associated with a palpable hematoma of the involved sternocleidomastoid muscle. Torticollis is believed to arise from a birth injury and may require physical therapy. Opisthotonos, in which the neck and back are held in extreme extension, is an ominous sign that indicates either meningeal irritation or, in an infant who has jaundice, kernicterus. In infants, frequent opisthotonic positioning associated with a relative paucity of trunk flexion movements may be an early sign of the spasticity of cerebral palsy. An unusually short neck may indicate cervical spine anomalies (Klippel Feil syndrome), and a webbed neck is seen in Turner syndrome. The newborn clavicles should be palpated routinely to rule out clavicular fractures, which usually occur at the junction of the middle and outer thirds of the bone and can occur during birth. Palpable neck masses in the newborn include the midline thyroglossal duct cyst, the supraclavicular cystic hygroma, which transilluminates, and branchial cleft cysts with or without associated skin tags and fistulas along the anterior border of the sternocleidomastoid muscle. Palpable cervical lymph nodes in healthy newborns are usually smaller than 5 mm in diameter. A crackly sensation on palpation in the supraclavicular areas usually indicates pneumomediastinum.

Infancy, Childhood, and Adolescence

When palpably enlarged lymph nodes are found, the examiner should note their location, size and number, consistency, tenderness, mobility, and attachment to other structures. Anterior cervical lymph nodes commonly enlarge in association with upper respiratory tract infections, dental infections, and stomatitis and less commonly with mycobacterial infection. Enlargement of the posterior cervical nodes is common secondary to insect bites or inflammatory lesions of the scalp. Cervical lymph nodes are enlarged generally with many viral syndromes, especially rubella, measles, and infectious mononucleosis. Lymph nodes enlarged because of an inflammation usually return to normal size days or weeks after the primary infection has subsided. One or more enlarged cervical lymph nodes, combined with other signs, are seen in Kawasaki disease. Lymph nodes that are enlarging without any signs of infection suggest Hodgkin disease and other lymphomas. Chronically enlarged lymph nodes can be seen throughout the body in HIV infection (see Chapter 276, Human Immunodeficiency Virus Infection and Acquired Immunodeficiency Syndrome).

Every infant and child who has an acute illness should be checked for nuchal rigidity, an important sign of meningeal irritation from meningitis. Ideally the infant or child should be quiet and relaxed, lying supine as the examiner cradles the infant's head with both hands and gently lifts it from the examining table, noting the degree of suppleness and any resistance to flexion. Flexion of the fully extended legs associated with neck flexion (Brudzinski sign) and flexion of one fully extended lower extremity while its opposite, flexed 90 degrees at the hip, is fully extended (Kernig sign) are present less often in infants who have meningitis than in older children and adolescents. A child who has nuchal rigidity is unable to touch the chin to the chest and assumes a tripod position when asked to sit up, that is, rests backward on extended arms while the legs are extended on the examining table.

The thyroid gland is normally difficult to palpate, if palpable at all, before puberty; it should be palpated, as should the trachea, from in front of and from behind the child. An enlarged thyroid can occur in children who have euthyroid, hypothyroid, or hyperthyroid states, and it can be caused by iodine deficiency or iodine excess (from cough medicines containing iodine), congenital or familial blockage of thyroxine synthesis, thyroiditis, diffuse or nodular hyperplasia, and, in rare cases, carcinoma. Normally the trachea is slightly deviated to the right; deviation from this norm indicates mediastinal shift, as may occur with foreign body–induced atelectasis and with pneumothorax. Neck venous pulsations and distention, usually difficult to determine in infants because of their relatively short necks, can give clues to heart disease and congestive heart failure in older children.

Children who have painful or limited neck motion should be checked for a full range of flexion, extension, lateral rotation, and lateral flexion. A fairly common cause of limited head motion is wryneck, or torticollis, which can occur after a play injury or sometimes in association with a respiratory tract infection. The head is tilted to one side, with sternocleidomastoid tenderness on the long or stretched side (as distinguished from neonatal torticollis, in which the involved sternocleidomastoid muscle is on the short side); the underlying cause of wryneck is a rotary subluxation of the first two cervical vertebrae.

Chest and Lungs

The chest wall in the fetus and newborn is round; with further growth it gradually flattens, with the lateral diameter exceeding the anteroposterior diameter. The thoracic index (transverse-anteroposterior diameter) is measured serially in some clinics that treat children who have chronic obstructive lung disease, such as cystic fibrosis, as a means of monitoring the degree of formation of a *barrel chest*. The infant's chest wall is relatively thin compared with an adult's; therefore heart and lung sounds are transmitted more clearly. Respirations are predominantly abdominal in infants, reflecting the greater role of the diaphragm in breathing; by age 6, they are predominantly thoracic, reflecting the increased role of the thoracic musculature in normal breathing.

By 16 weeks of gestation the bronchial tree is fully developed, with the adult number of segments and subsegments. Alveoli, in comparison, are just forming by the time of birth, with only 8% of the average adult number present. The number of alveoli increases until age 8, after which they primarily increase in size rather than in number until adulthood. Pulmonary blood vessels develop parallel to the developing bronchial tree and alveoli and increasing amounts of muscle appear in the walls of the more distal arterioles over time. By 28 weeks of gestation, airway and blood vessel development is usually adequate for gas transfer. By 34 to 36 weeks of gestation, sufficient amounts of a surface-active lipid are present within the alveoli to maintain them in a partly expanded position, rather than remaining collapsed at the end of each expiration. As noted previously, the respiratory rate declines with age, partly because of further postnatal development of the alveoli, with a resulting increase in lung volume.

The breasts of many healthy male and female infants are transiently hypertrophied at birth, sometimes producing small amounts of clear or white fluid, called witch's milk. This hypertrophy normally disappears by 2 to 3 months of age. Many pubertal boys have transient unilateral or bilateral firm, sometimes painful, subareolar masses that disappear within a year of onset. A girl's pubertal breast development is often asymmetrical and proceeds through several stages, starting with an increase in the areolar diameter between ages 8 and 13, and is completed between ages 12 and 19.

The chest and lungs should be examined thoroughly in every child who has any respiratory symptoms, fever, abdominal pain, or chest pain. The examiner should note size, symmetry, movement with respirations, localized tenderness or masses, and breast characteristics. The three goals of an examination of the lungs using observation, percussion, and auscultation are (1) to determine the nature of respiration, including rate, depth, and ease; (2) to establish the adequacy of gas exchange, as indicated by signs of hypoxia or hypercapnia; and (3) to localize disease. The examiner should use and become familiar with the sound characteristics of one stethoscope. Except when auscultating the chest of a small premature baby, an adult-sized stethoscope with both a bell and a diaphragm is generally effective for examining infants and children of all ages.

Newborn Period

During the few moments after birth, the adequacy of the developing lungs for gas exchange, which is influenced by factors such as maternal anesthesia, birth trauma, and the normality of the infant's central nervous and cardiovascular systems, is grossly assessed by the Apgar score (Table 14-4), which includes observations about the color and initiation of respirations. Once normal respirations have been established, the baby's chest is inspected for deformities, such as a markedly bulging sternum (pectus carinatum) or a markedly concave one (pectus excavatum); asymmetry caused by uneven chest expansion, absence of or deformed ribs, or absence of the pectoral muscle (Poland syndrome); and overall size, inasmuch as small thoracic cages are a feature of several congenital anomalies. The respiratory rate normally falls from as high as 60 breaths/min immediately after birth to 30 to 40 breaths/min by several hours of age. In a healthy newborn the auscultated breath sounds are heard easily and have a higher pitch than those in the older child and adult.

A newborn in respiratory distress from any cause exhibits some or all of the following signs: nasal flaring, tachypnea, cyanosis, expiratory grunting, intercostal retractions (subcostal, substernal, and supraclavicular retractions are also possible), and decreased air entry, as measured by decreased breath sounds. Simple auscultation of a newborn in respiratory distress should aid in the diagnosis of (1) unilateral lesions, such as aspiration pneumonia, congenital diaphragmatic hernia, congenital hypoplastic segments or emphysema, and unilateral pneumothorax and (2) congenital heart disease.

The respiratory rate of newborns, particularly premature newborns, can be quite irregular during the

Table 14-4 Apgar Score

SIGN	SCORE 0	1	2
Heart rate	Absent	<100 bpm	>100 bpm
Respiratory effort	Absent	Weak, irregular	Good, crying
Muscle tone	Flaccid	Some flexion of extremities	Well, flexed
Reflex irritability (catheter in nose)	No response	Grimace	Cough or sneeze
Color	Blue, pale	Body pink; extremities blue	Completely pink

From Klaus MH, Fanaroff AA. *Care of the High-Risk Neonate*. 4th ed. Philadelphia, PA: WB Saunders; 1993.

first few days of life and can sometimes slow to the point of apnea. Two patterns should be differentiated in premature newborns. Periodic breathing is associated with relatively brief periods of apnea lasting 5 to 10 seconds, usually without secondary bradycardia. It occurs more commonly when the baby is awake and is uncommon before 5 days of age. True apneic spells, on the other hand, last longer than 20 seconds, are associated with bradycardia, can be associated with pulmonary disease, and are more common in newborns who weigh less than 1250 g.

Infancy, Childhood, and Adolescence

In these children, auscultation and percussion, along with observation of breathing patterns, are particularly useful techniques for evaluating the chest and lungs. Auscultation is often accomplished most successfully when the infant or child is only minimally aware of being examined, for example, while asleep, being fed, or being held up to the parent's shoulder. When preschool children are asked to "take a deep breath," they often hold their breath. Starting is easier by auscultating while the child breathes at a resting level. If the child is crying, then the inspiratory phase can be thoroughly auscultated, but predominantly expiratory adventitious sounds, such as wheezes, can be missed. After the examiner listens to breath sounds at rest or during crying, a useful technique for accentuating adventitious sounds, particularly during the expiratory phase, is inducing forced expiration. The examiner may accomplish this task by holding the hands on opposing anterior and posterior sides of the chest, with the stethoscope in one hand held against the chest, and gently squeezing the hands together as expiration is ending. Breath sounds in infants and children tend to be audible during both inspiration and expiration (ie, bronchovesicular) and are heard more clearly than in adults. Secretions in any part of the respiratory tree are usually reflected by loudly audible coarse rhonchi heard throughout the chest, and the examiner should repeat the observations to rule out transmitted sounds from the nose or pharynx. The inexperienced examiners may be tempted to suspect pneumonia in most children evaluated for acute respiratory illnesses because of the fairly usual occurrence of tracheal and bronchial inflammation with common viral infections. The more or less generalized coarse rhonchi (continuous, low-pitched sounds) from bronchial secretions and the wheezes (higher pitched, predominantly expiratory) from bronchiolar secretions should be distinguished from the much less common, usually localized, crackling rales caused by alveolar fluid or exudate and heard best at the end of inspiration. Pneumonia in infants and young children is almost always accompanied by fever and tachypnea, whereas rales, bronchial breath sounds, dullness to percussion, and a productive cough are less common findings than in adults.

Several objective signs of respiratory distress can be seen in infants and children. Orthopnea occurs in children who have asthma or congestive heart failure. Maximal use of accessory muscles of respiration produces several useful physical signs, including head bobbing, seen especially in infants, with the head bobbing forward in synchrony with each inspiration, and flaring of the nasal alae, resulting from contraction of the anterior and posterior dilator naris muscles. These signs indicate increased work of breathing, or inspiratory efforts shortened by pain, as occurs in pleuritis or thoracic trauma. Intercostal retractions, an exaggerated inspiratory sinking in of intercostal and sometimes supraclavicular soft tissue, indicate increased inspiratory effort and reflect airway obstruction and lung stiffness. Bulging of the intercostal space during expiration occurs with increased expiratory effort, such as in asthma, bronchiolitis, and cystic fibrosis. Subcostal retractions, seen anteriorly at the lower costal margins, reflect flattening of the diaphragm and occur in conditions with diffuse lower airway obstruction. Substernal retractions can be seen in children who have severe upper airway obstruction and in newborns, especially premature infants, who have various pulmonary diseases. Audible wheezes usually indicate obstruction of the larger airways, and grunting can be associated with pneumonia, chest pain, and respiratory distress syndrome in neonates. A thud may be heard on inspiration in children who have a tracheal foreign body as the object moves in response to airflow.

The adequacy of gas exchange is judged primarily by seeking signs of hypoxia. Cyanosis, which results when the amount of reduced hemoglobin in the capillaries exceeds 5 g, is either peripheral (as with exposure to a cold environment) or central (seen as blue mucous membranes), the latter being of pulmonary or cardiac origin. Tachycardia, dyspnea on exertion, and

CNS depression are additional signs of hypoxia that can be critical in monitoring a child who has marginally adequate gas exchange, as in severe croup. Progressive signs of hypercapnia in acute respiratory illnesses include hot hands, small pupils, engorged fundal veins, muscular twitching, coma, and papilledema.

Localization of intrathoracic lesions in children is aided by palpating for tracheal deviation and observing for unequal respiratory movements of half of the chest, localized areas of dull or flat percussion notes, and the presence of tactile fremitus. Percussion can also be used to delineate the lower boundaries of the lungs in inspiration and expiration.

Heart

The major anatomic characteristics of the heart form long before birth, as do most congenital heart defects. In a healthy newborn's heart the right ventricle has a muscle mass equal to that of the left ventricle, reflecting the fetal circulation in which both ventricles pump blood into the systemic circulation, the left through the aorta and the right through the ductus arteriosus. After birth the left ventricle gains weight relative to the right ventricle, reaching the adult weight ratio of approximately 2:1 by age 1 year, reflecting the major changes in postnatal circulation. At birth, or shortly thereafter, the ductus arteriosus normally closes, and the flap of the foramen ovale is held closed by the rise in pressure in the left atrium. As many as one half of all newborns have transient murmurs during the first 24 to 48 hours of life, some of which are caused by a late-closing ductus arteriosus.

Congenital heart defects can be classified according to the embryonic stages of development during which an abnormality arises: position anomalies (dextrocardia with or without situs inversus), anomalous growth of the atrial chambers (atrioventricular canal, ostium primum defect, persistent foramen ovale), anomalous bulboventricular growth and septation (ventricular septal defect, tetralogy of Fallot, double outlet right ventricle, transposition of the great vessels), and maldevelopment of the truncus (truncus arteriosus, patent ductus arteriosus, coarctation of the aorta). See Chapter 251, Congenital and Acquired Heart Disease.

The significant and normal changes in pulse and blood pressure that occur with age in infants and children have been described earlier in this chapter. An important point to remember is that optimal auscultation of the heart requires use of a stethoscope with both a bell and a diaphragm, the bell picking up lower-pitched sounds and the diaphragm picking up higher-pitched ones. Proper use of the bell involves holding it lightly against the chest while the diaphragm is pressed firmly to the chest. Stethoscope tubing should be no more than 10 to 12 inches long. During auscultation, gentle traction on the earpiece end of the stethoscope enhances the audibility of heart sounds by making a tighter seal between the earpiece and the examiner's external auditory canal. Because infants have relatively rapid heart rates, detecting abnormalities in their heart sounds demands that each of the two major heart sounds be listened to in isolation, giving attention to each interval between these sounds. As in adults, the heart is auscultated initially over the 4 cardinal areas (apex, or mitral area; lower left sternal border, or tricuspid area; second left intercostal space at the sternal margin, or pulmonary area; and second right intercostal space, or aortic area). Auscultation then proceeds to the remainder of the precordium and chest, including the infraclavicular and supraclavicular area, the axillae, the back, and the neck.

A thorough examination of the heart should be part of all physical examinations of infants and children; it involves noting the heart rate and rhythm, heart size, and characteristics of the first and second heart sounds, especially in the second left interspace. With murmurs, the following information should be recorded: timing in the cardiac cycle (early, late, or pansystolic; protodiastolic, middiastolic, or presystolic), quality (blowing, harsh, rumbling, vibratory or other), grade of maximal intensity (on a scale of I to VI, with V and VI being associated with a palpable thrill), duration, point of maximal intensity, and transmission (see Chapter 187, Heart Murmurs). In all infants and children whose findings suggest congenital heart disease, palpation of peripheral pulses is especially important to determine if the pulses in the lower extremities are diminished and those in the upper extremities increased, as occurs with coarctation of the aorta. Blood pressure is measured as described earlier in this chapter.

Newborn Period and Infancy

An infant's general appearance can provide clues to underlying heart disease and may mandate a more sophisticated cardiac examination. Examples of conditions frequently associated with congenital heart disease are Down syndrome (endocardial cushion defect), Turner syndrome (coarctation of the aorta), trisomy 13, trisomy 18, and congenital rubella syndrome (patent ductus arteriosus, pulmonary stenosis). Important clinical signs of significant heart disease include cyanosis, growth failure, and lethargy. The most prominent signs of congestive heart failure in infants are tachypnea, tachycardia, and liver enlargement. Peripheral edema and pulmonary rales are late findings and are therefore not as helpful as in adults. Visible chest pulsations can indicate a hyperdynamic state caused by an increased metabolic rate or an inefficient pumping action from valvular or septal incompetency or other defect. Dextrocardia is suggested by a right-sided cardiac impulse and may be associated with abdominal situs inversus (reversal of the position of the liver, spleen, and intestines).

The apical impulse in infants is normally palpated in the 4th left interspace just outside the midclavicular line; after age 7, it is in the adult position of the 5th left interspace in the midclavicular line. The point of maximal impulse of the heart can suggest individual ventricular enlargement. An impulse at the xiphoid process or lower left sternal border suggests right-ventricular hypertrophy, whereas an impulse maximal at the apex suggests left-ventricular hypertrophy.

Infants' heart sounds are often difficult to differentiate from their breath sounds because the pitches and rates of each can be similar. Watching the abdominal excursions with respiration and palpating a peripheral pulse while auscultating the chest can aid in this differentiation. In evaluating children with suspected heart disease the examiner should be prepared to spend at least several minutes listening to the precordial area, at which time the heart and respiratory rates and rhythms can be determined. For each heart sound the intensity, point of maximal intensity, and degrees of splitting should be noted. Normally the second heart sound is louder than the first in the second left interspace and is often split (reflecting the pulmonary valve closing after the aortic valve); the split often widens with inspiration. Examples of abnormalities of the heart sounds are the loud first sound heard at the apex in mitral stenosis; the loud second sound in the pulmonary area, indicating pulmonary hypertension; and the fixed, split second sound in the pulmonary area with atrial septal defect. A 3rd heart sound can be heard at the apex of normal children and should be distinguished from the higher intensity, third-sound gallop that occurs with tachycardia and indicates congestive heart failure.

Heart murmurs are more difficult to localize in infants than in children and adolescents because, in infants, they are often so well transmitted and heard throughout the chest. Gross anatomic localization can be helpful, however, as illustrated by (1) the prominence over the back of the murmurs of coarctation of the aorta and some cases of patent ductus arteriosus, (2) the precordial systolic murmur of ventricular septal defect growing louder as the examiner descends the left sternal border to the xiphoid, and (3) the murmur or murmurs of peripheral pulmonary artery stenosis becoming louder as the examiner moves the stethoscope laterally from the precordium. On the other hand, the typical to-and-fro continuous murmur of patent ductus arteriosus described in older children may be absent in affected infants and represented only by a precordial systolic murmur.

Childhood and Adolescence

A cardiac examination in children and adolescents follows the outline already given and is different from the examination of infants largely because of the need to distinguish organic murmurs from the innocent or functional murmur, which occurs in as many as 50% of healthy children. Innocent murmurs are unassociated with any symptomatic, roentgenographic, or electrocardiographic evidence of heart disease, and the three types have several characteristics in common. They are usually low pitched and therefore heard best with the bell. Innocent murmurs are musical or vibratory (Figure 14-24), as distinguished from the more complex range of frequencies of significant murmurs. Their intensity is usually no greater than I or II/VI, and both their presence and intensity vary with change in the child's position or respiratory phase. Innocent murmurs are heard most commonly either at the second left interspace or halfway between the lower left sternal border and the apex. At these sites the murmurs are of short duration and occur early in systole. A third common location is above or below either clavicle, where the murmur is called a venous hum. This murmur is an impressive-sounding murmur and often continuous throughout systole; it is heard best with the child sitting and does not occur in the supine position.

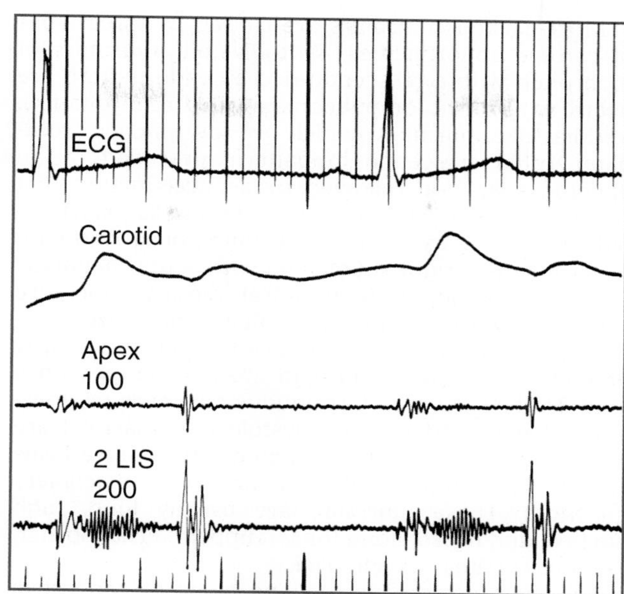

Figure 14-24 An innocent murmur: phonocardiogram. The even harmonic quality of a stringlike murmur is illustrated. *2 LIS,* Second left intercostal space. *(From Fyler DC. Nadas' Pediatric Cardiology. Chicago, IL: Mosby; 1992. Copyright © 1992, Elsevier, with permission.)*

In contrast to innocent murmurs, significant murmurs are usually, but not always, of greater intensity, are less localized, and are more likely to radiate over parts of the chest; they also do not usually change in loudness with a change in the child's position or respiratory phase. Systolic murmurs can be classified as stenotic, regurgitant, or uneven. Stenotic systolic murmurs are associated with a pressure gradient across the aortic or pulmonary valve and are of high frequency, are diamond shaped, and are transmitted to the neck. Soft systolic murmurs heard in the pulmonary area and associated not with a valvular pressure gradient but with increased flow are present with an atrial septal defect. Atrioventricular valve regurgitant murmurs begin immediately with the first sound, are either decreased or pansystolic, are blowing in character, and are best heard at the lower left sternal border or at the apex, radiating to the axilla and back. The murmur of mitral insufficiency, which is heard at the apex in a large percentage of children who have acute rheumatic fever, can be transient and soft; its discovery can be aided by auscultating over the apex with the child supine and rotated partly onto the left side. The systolic murmur along the left sternal border heard with a ventricular septal defect is usually pansystolic but has a harsher quality than the atrioventricular valve regurgitant murmurs and is transmitted less well to the axilla, neck, and back. An uneven systolic murmur is heard with patent ductus arteriosus along the upper left sternal border. Although pansystolic with or without a diastolic component, the sound of the murmur varies in pitch and intensity from beat to beat.

Most diastolic murmurs are caused by three types of cardiac abnormalities. Protodiastolic murmurs of high pitch with a crescendo-decrescendo pattern are heard with aortic or pulmonary valve regurgitation. Middiastolic murmurs, which are low pitched, rumbling, often crescendo in pattern, preceded by an opening snap and followed by an accentuated first sound, are heard with mitral (and, in rare cases, tricuspid) stenosis. Diastolic flow murmurs, occurring with all large left-to-right shunts and with acute rheumatic fever in association with mitral regurgitation, are caused by increased flow through a normal-sized atrioventricular orifice and are of low frequency, are early or middiastolic in timing, and are associated with a loud 3rd heart sound. Continuous murmurs (ie, murmurs that extend through systole into diastole) are heard most commonly with patent ductus arteriosus and are sometimes called *to-and-fro* or *machinery* murmurs. These murmurs are usually loud, high pitched, and heard along the left upper sternal border, radiating to the neck and back.

The most common presenting signs of congestive heart failure in children, as in infants, are tachypnea, orthopnea, liver enlargement, and sometimes increased sweating. Peripheral edema and pulmonary rales tend to be late findings. In children, the appearance of facial edema more commonly indicates either an allergic reaction or renal disease, such as acute glomerulonephritis. Swelling and redness of the hands and feet are features of Kawasaki disease, as is congestive heart failure (and, in a small number, myocardial infarction). Heart failure in children most often occurs with acute or chronic myocarditis (especially acute rheumatic fever), in some children with congenital heart disease, in overwhelming infections, and in hypovolemic states.

Hypertension in children is usually of renal origin, once anxiety has been ruled out. The types of underlying renal disease include acute illnesses such as acute poststreptococcal glomerulonephritis and acute pyelonephritis, end stages of various chronic renal diseases (glomerulonephropathies, chronic obstruction or infection, developmental renal anomalies), kidney tumors such as Wilms tumor, and renal vessel thrombosis and anomalies. Other causes of hypertension include those related to (1) the CNS (poliomyelitis, encephalitis, increasing intracranial pressure of many causes), (2) cardiovascular disease (coarctation of the aorta and aortic run-offs, as with patent ductus arteriosus, anemia, and thyrotoxicosis), (3) endocrine-metabolic disturbances (cortisone therapy, pheochromocytoma, Cushing disease, congenital adrenal hyperplasia, primary aldosteronism, and porphyria), (4) lead and mercury poisoning, and (5) essential hypertension, in which none of these conditions exists. Essential hypertension is more prevalent among adolescents who have a family history of hypertension. Using the standardized tables for blood pressure based on gender, age, and height is important to identify accurately those children whose blood pressure exceeds the 95th percentile and who are in need of further evaluation and treatment.

The physical findings of heart disease in infants and children only begin to define the nature of the cause of the disease. Chest roentgenography and electrocardiography, as well as echocardiography, advanced imaging techniques, and cardiac catheterization, are used to define the diagnosis further. Thus physical examination of the heart is an important step in cardiac diagnosis but is only the first of many steps that require interpretation by a qualified cardiologist.

Abdomen

The size and shape of the abdomen changes with age, reflecting, in part, changes in the intraabdominal and intrathoracic organs. During the neonatal period, the abdomen is relatively protuberant because of (1) the intrathoracic expansion of the lungs with downward movement of the diaphragm and (2) the relatively large liver caused by intrauterine extramedullary hematopoiesis. The first meconium stool is usually passed within 24 hours of birth, and intestinal gas is visible by roentgenogram throughout the normal bowel by 48 hours of age. The horizontal position of the stomach within the abdomen in infancy accounts for the increased postprandial protuberance of the epigastric area. The more vertical, adult position of the stomach is developed slowly throughout childhood. The stomach's capacity increases rapidly during the first years of life, from an average of 30 to 90 mL at birth to 210 to 360 mL at age 1 and 500 mL at age 2; it then increases slowly to the adult capacity of 750 to 900 mL. Abdominal protuberance in preschool children is caused by a transient, normal lumbar lordosis. The abdominal musculature is relatively hypotonic at birth, allowing deep palpation. Midline defects include the relatively common and usually transient diastasis recti, the fairly common umbilical hernia, and the rare omphalocele.

The abdomen should be examined thoroughly during all health maintenance examinations and in children who have gastrointestinal symptoms, fever, cough, and any other evidence of acute illness. This examination involves inspection of the abdominal contour and size; palpation for tenderness, an enlarged liver, spleen, or kidneys, and masses; percussion; and auscultation of bowel sounds. Examination of the rectum is indicated in all children who show evidence of an intraabdominal or a pelvic disorder or who have fecal elimination problems or rectal bleeding.

Newborn Period and Infancy

Absence of the normal prominence of the abdomen in a newborn should lead to further investigation for diaphragmatic hernia or high intestinal atresia. Subcutaneous abdominal wall blood vessels are easily visible in most infants because of their relatively small amount of subcutaneous fat. Abdominal movement is due to the prominent role of the diaphragm in breathing and, in addition, to intestinal peristalsis. Visible peristaltic waves can be observed over any quadrant of the abdomen, especially in premature babies, who have relatively thin abdominal walls. Prominent gastric peristaltic waves moving from left to right across the upper portion of the abdomen (best observed by lighting the abdomen from the side) are present with congenital pyloric stenosis, which usually exhibits by 4 to 6 weeks of age (see Chapter 315, Pyloric Stenosis).

The umbilical stump is inspected at birth for meconium (yellow) staining, a sign associated with chronic fetal distress. The normal umbilicus contains two ventrally placed, thick-walled, smaller arteries and one dorsally placed, thin-walled, larger vein. Infants who have a single umbilical artery may have other congenital malformations, but, more often than not, it is an isolated anomaly. The umbilical stump, if left uncovered after birth, shrinks to a relatively hard, dark-brown eschar, which normally separates from the abdomen by 1 to 2 weeks after birth. The central core area of the umbilicus is usually covered with skin no later than 3 to 4 weeks of age, a process that is sometimes delayed by growth of pink granulation tissue (umbilical granuloma). Transient spotty bleeding of the umbilical area after separation of the umbilical eschar is common and usually lasts no longer than a few days. Chronic drainage of clear fluid from the umbilicus suggests the presence of persistently patent urachus, a urachal cyst, or a communicating Meckel diverticulum or omphalomesenteric duct. Erythema of the periumbilical skin with or without purulent or foul-smelling discharge suggests omphalitis, a local infection that can spread rapidly to the bloodstream and meninges. Umbilical hernias may be associated with palpable abdominal wall defects that vary from 0.5 to 5 or 6 cm in diameter and that protrude equally as far, especially when the infant is crying or straining.

A light touch of the examining fingers against the infant's abdominal wall usually contacts the liver edge, 1 to 2 cm below the right costal margin. A spleen tip may be palpated in healthy infants at the left costal margin. Midline structures such as the enlarged pylorus of infants who have pyloric stenosis are sometimes difficult to palpate because of the contraction of the rectus muscles. Holding the infant's thighs in a flexed position and palpating while the infant is sucking will usually permit deep, midline palpation. The kidneys are accessible to palpation, especially at birth, by the technique of ballottement. One hand is held with the fingers in the costovertebral angle while the other hand presses downward from the anterior costal margin. The posterior hand then *flips* the kidney toward the anterior hand, which can usually *catch* the lower pole of the kidney. It can also be felt as it drops back against the posterior hand. In this manner, symmetry of kidney size can be determined. A unilaterally large kidney occurs with a multicystic kidney, unilateral hydronephrosis, Wilms tumor, invasive neuroblastoma, or renal-vein thrombosis. Other palpable abdominal masses include the dilated bladder secondary to urethral obstruction, the bilateral flank masses of hydronephrosis and polycystic kidney disease, duplications of the bowel, and rare primary hepatic tumors. Palpable masses associated with signs of intestinal obstruction (vomiting, abdominal distention, and failure to pass stool) include the meconium masses associated with imperforate anus, Hirschsprung disease, meconium plug syndrome, and meconium ileus; midgut volvulus associated with intestinal malrotation; and the sausage-shaped, usually right lower quadrant abdominal mass of intussusception associated with bloody or currant jelly stools. Infants who have signs of intestinal obstruction and no palpable mass require immediate further evaluation for congenital atresia or stenosis of any portion of the bowel, peritonitis, and, in premature infants, necrotizing enterocolitis. In addition, tumors of the ovary, such as teratoma, may be palpated as masses in the lower quadrants of the abdomen.

Percussion of an infant's abdomen can be helpful in determining the size of organs or masses and in outlining the relatively large area of the upper portion of the abdomen filled by the stomach. Ascites may accompany peritonitis, liver or kidney disease, and lymphangiomas of the small-bowel mesentery. Bowel sounds (peristaltic sounds) are metallic tinkling sounds heard normally every 10 to 30 seconds. They occur more frequently with intestinal obstruction or gastroenteritis and are diminished with ileus, which can accompany almost any infectious process in infants, especially pneumonitis or gastroenteritis.

A rectal examination, performed with the 5th finger, can be useful in differentiating bladder from sacral masses, in palpating the uterus, and in detecting the absence of rectal feces in some infants who have Hirschsprung disease. Some practitioners prefer to use the index finger for this examination because of its greater length, flexibility, sensitivity, and mobility.

Childhood and Adolescence

The shape of the abdomen becomes increasingly scaphoid in school-aged children, except for children who have exogenous obesity. Frightened, uncomfortable, or ticklish children can be examined successfully if the thighs are held in partial flexion and the abdomen is approached first with the stethoscope. While listening for bowel sounds, the stethoscope can be pushed gently into the abdomen, and areas of rigidity or tenderness can be noted. The examiner's hands should be warm, and in older children, deep breathing will enhance abdominal palpation. Another useful technique is placing the child's hand between the abdominal wall and the examiner's hand. Detecting rigidity or tenderness can be especially difficult in a crying or nonverbal child. The examiner can watch for facial grimacing and can attempt to catch the brief instant of relative relaxation of the abdomen at the end of expiration. The protuberant abdomen of a child whose lungs are hyperexpanded and who experiences forceful abdominal muscle contractions on expiration and sore abdominal muscles (present, for instance, in status asthmaticus) can be especially difficult to examine for intraabdominal abnormalities. Having such a child raise the head from the supine position usually lessens intraabdominal pain but increases abdominal muscle soreness.

Abdominal tenderness in children can be localized by the responses to direct palpation, by referred pain on rebound tenderness, by *shake* tenderness in which the child's pelvis is lifted gently off the examining table and gently shaken, by pain accompanying hyperextension of the hips (psoas sign) or external rotation of the hip with the knee held in flexion (obturator sign), and by abdominorectal palpation. Tenderness from an inflamed appendix is usually maximal in the right lower quadrant. Diffuse tenderness can accompany paralytic ileus secondary to extraabdominal or intraabdominal infection, as well as the more serious peritonitis or perforated viscus. Midline tenderness in the lower portion of the abdomen can be elicited by

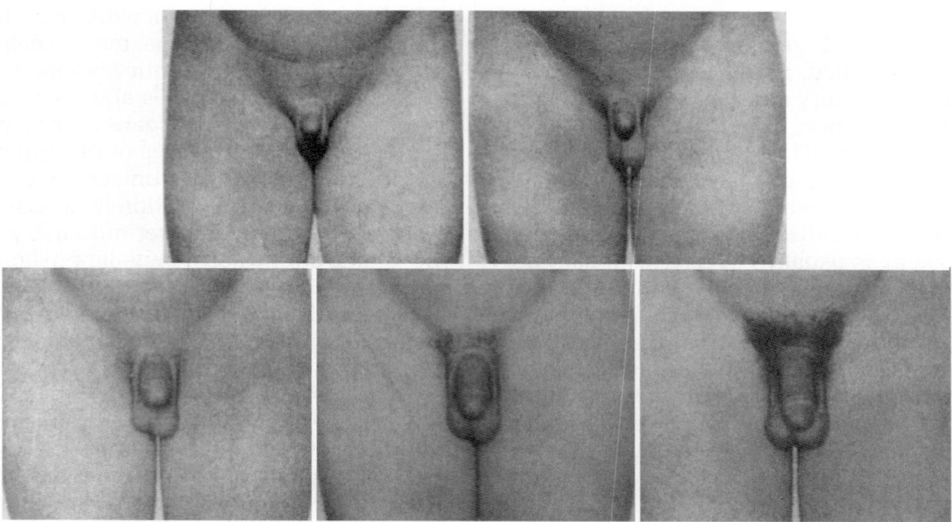

Figure 14-25 Standards for genitalia maturity ratings in boys. Shown are Tanner stages 1 through 5 of development. *(From Tanner JM.* Growth at Adolescence. *2nd ed. Oxford, UK: Blackwell; 1962. Copyright © Blackwell Publishing. Reprinted by permission.)*

palpating the abdominal aorta or a full bladder. Children with appendicitis or peritonitis often tend to change position slowly from lying, to sitting, to standing, or moving on and off the examination table. If the abdomen is soft, then the cecum and sigmoid colon can often be rolled between the examining fingers and the adjacent iliac crest. The entire colon is sometimes palpable when filled with feces in association with functional fecal retention. In healthy children, the tip of the spleen and the edge of the liver may be palpable, especially on deep inspiration. The spleen commonly enlarges in association with several acute infectious diseases and with several blood dyscrasias. The liver can enlarge as a result of heart failure, hepatitis, septicemia, a primary or metastatic tumor, blood dyscrasias, and various storage diseases. Upper quadrant direct tenderness and shock tenderness (elicited by gently pounding the lower anterior rib cage), which may be signs of liver or splenic bleeding or rupture, should be investigated in all children who have sustained trauma to the abdomen.

Genitalia

By the end of the 3rd fetal month the undifferentiated fetal gonad has developed into an ovary or, under the influence of the Y chromosome, into a testis. With production of testosterone by the fetal testis (the medulla of the fetal gonad), the wolffian duct system further develops into the epididymis, ductus deferens, and seminal vesicles; development of the müllerian duct system is inhibited by an as yet unidentified factor. The testes descend into the scrotum between the 7th and 8th months of gestation, followed by a sleeve of parietal peritoneum, the processus vaginalis, which closes off in most babies by the time of birth. At the time of birth, one or more testes are undescended in 3% to 4% of male babies. Most of these descend by 3 months of age, leaving 1% of babies by age 1 year with unilateral or bilateral undescended testes. The processus vaginalis can remain patent and retain its connection with the peritoneal cavity, causing an inguinal hernia that is usually apparent within a few months after birth. A fluid-filled segment of the processus vaginalis within the scrotum, a hydrocele, is present in 10% of male babies and can be associated with an inguinal hernia. Many hydroceles apparent at birth disappear spontaneously within the first few months of life.

In the absence of fetal testosterone and another undetermined factor, the müllerian duct system develops into the fallopian tubes, uterus, and upper vagina. After birth, as a result of withdrawal of maternal estrogen, the uterus decreases in size and then grows slowly back to its birth size by age 5 years. By age 10 years the corpus of the uterus has grown to a size equal to that of the uterine cervix. The cervix grows rapidly again in the premenarcheal years, followed by further growth of the uterine corpus. The stages of development during puberty in boys and girls are illustrated in Figures 14-25 and 14-26. Sequential recording of a given child's progress can be used both to diagnose abnormal development and to reassure a worried normal adolescent. The reader should refer to Chapter 212, Puberty: Normal and Abnormal, for details regarding pubertal changes and stages.

Thorough examination of the external genitalia is mandatory immediately after birth to allow rapid evaluation of babies whose genitalia are ambiguous (see Chapter 286, Intersex). The external genitalia are examined during all health maintenance examinations and in all children seeking medical attention for abdominal pain. The penis, testes, and external inguinal rings should be examined in boys, and the clitoris, labia majora and minora, vaginal orifice, urethral orifice, and external inguinal rings should be examined in girls. Measuring the size of the penis or clitoris and

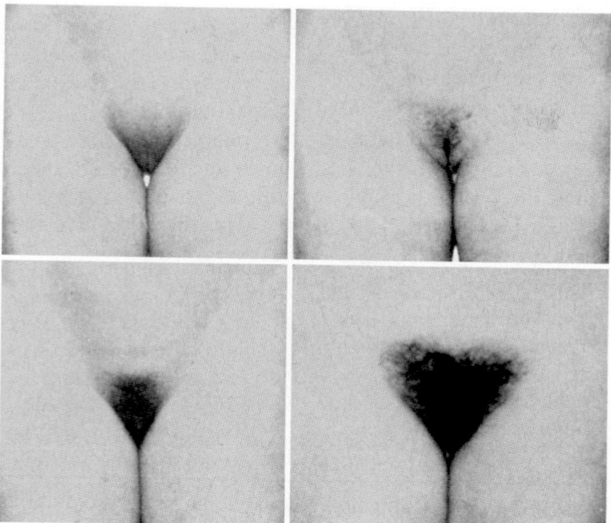

Figure 14-26 Tanner stages 2 through 5 of development of pubic hair in girls. Stage 1 is not shown because pubic hair does not exist in this stage. *(From Tanner JM.* Growth at Adolescence. *2nd ed. Oxford, UK: Blackwell; 1962. Copyright © Blackwell Publishing. Reprinted by permission.)*

comparing to standard-size norms is important when considering various endocrine disorders. Internal inspection of the vagina and cervix and bimanual abdominorectal palpation of the internal genitalia are not part of the routine examination of children; they are, however, performed in the evaluation of problems such as vaginal discharge or bleeding (see the following discussion).

When the primary care physician evaluates an infant, a child, or an adolescent for suspected sexual abuse,[10] the child and parent must be prepared with patience and with attention to their fears and concerns. (See Chapter 122, Sexual Abuse of Children.)

Newborn Period

The appearance of the external genitalia at birth provides information that is useful in assessing gestational age. In boys, the testes are undescended before the 30th week of gestation, are high in the inguinal canal between the 30th and 36th weeks, and have normally completely descended into the scrotum by 40 weeks. The scrotal rugae appear, progressing inferiorly to superiorly, between the 30th and 40th weeks. In girls, the labia majora are widely separated, and the clitoris is prominent up to the 36th week; by 40 weeks the labia majora completely cover the labia minora and clitoris.

A white vaginal discharge, occasionally mixed with blood, can be seen for several days after birth, the result of withdrawal from the relatively high levels of maternally derived estrogen. Maternal estrogen also can cause a transient hypertrophy of the labia majora. The urethral and vaginal orifices can be visualized by downward and lateral traction on each side of the perineum (Figure 14-27). The hymen varies in thickness and size, the central orifice usually measuring up to 4 mm in diameter in infants. Rarely is the hymen imperforate at birth.

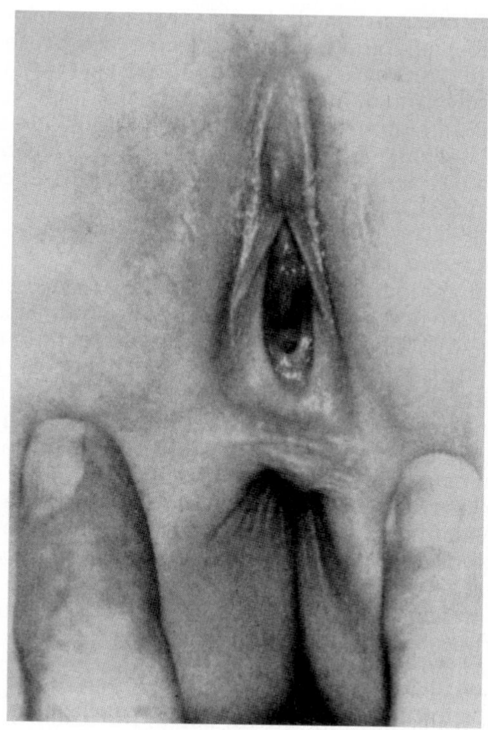

Figure 14-27 Inspection of the infant vulva.

The foreskin of the penis is usually nonretractable at birth, a condition that can persist for years. Ordinarily, sufficient retraction is possible to allow visualization of the external urethral meatus at the tip of the glans penis. The ventral surface of the penis should be inspected at birth for hypospadias (an abnormal position of the external urethral meatus located anywhere between the midline scrotum to the tip of the glans) (see Chapter 279, Hypospadias, Epispadias, and Cryptorchism) because its presence is a contraindication to circumcision. Hypospadias may be accompanied by chordee, a fixed, downward bowing of the penis. In rare cases the urethral meatus is located on the dorsal surface of the penis, a condition known as epispadias. After circumcision the glans penis and the remaining lip of foreskin are swollen and erythematous for several days.

Palpation of the testes should proceed downward from the external inguinal ring to the scrotum to counteract the active cremasteric reflex in infants. This technique is important in diagnosing the undescended testis accurately. Inguinal hernias in infants occur as unilateral or bilateral inguinal and scrotal bulges that are usually reducible and may appear only with crying or straining. Hydroceles are scrotal and sometimes inguinal masses that are often attached to the testes and are nonreducible and nontender and that transilluminate.

In rare cases the appearance of the external genitalia may make the task of determining gender difficult. For instance, a midline phallus with apparent scrotal hypospadias and partly fused scrotal-appearing skin with no palpable scrotal masses may be present. In this situation, careful inspection and, in some cases, probing of the midline of the perineum for a vaginal orifice is an important first step in diagnosing ambiguous external genitalia in a female baby, as is abdominorectal examination to palpate for the presence of a uterus (see Chapter 286, Intersex).

Infancy and Early Childhood

Several minor physical abnormalities are common during the first years of life. In boys, ammoniacal dermatitis involving the perineum (diaper rash) in either a circumcised or an uncircumcised infant can cause balanitis, an acute inflammation of the glans penis, which is sometimes associated with purulent exudate. After an episode of balanitis, the external urethral meatus may become stenotic, causing a narrow urinary stream and prolonged emptying of the bladder. Balanitis in an uncircumcised boy can leave adhesions between the glans penis and the foreskin, preventing retraction of the foreskin.

Diagnosing an undescended testis accurately is important because corrective surgery can protect the functioning of a normal, undescended testis only if performed during the first few years of life. An acutely tender testis may indicate torsion of the testis, orchitis, a complication of mumps that commonly occurs in young men, or epididymitis.

In female infants, paper-thin adhesions between the labia minora are common during the first few years of life, sometimes completely covering the vulvar vestibule, with a small opening through which urine escapes. These labial adhesions can sometimes be parted by applying gentle pressure laterally on the labia majora. They will also disappear if a cream containing estrogen is applied for several weeks.

Vulvovaginal discharge in preschool-aged girls most often is caused by vaginal foreign bodies, usually bits of toilet paper; occasionally a specific bacterial organism can be cultured, or pinworms may be discovered. Cultures that are positive for *N gonorrhoeae* and *C trachomatis* almost always indicate sexual abuse. Making these diagnoses occasionally requires vaginoscopy with a special instrument, such as the Huffman vaginoscope (Figure 14-28) or a nasal speculum, although some child abuse experts are against using any instruments when examining for possible sexual abuse. Vaginal specimens for smears and cultures can be obtained with the least pain by first instilling a small amount of sterile nutrient broth into the vagina with a medicine dropper.

Although digital examination of the vagina is not usually possible in prepubertal girls, the uterus can be palpated for size, shape, and tenderness, with one hand placed over the lower portion of the abdomen and a finger of the other hand inserted into the rectum.

During a rectal examination in a girl, the cervix is the predominant part of the uterus that is palpable; in most instances, the ovaries are not felt. Examination of the rectum in both boys and girls is usually helped by telling the child, "This will be just like having your temperature taken" and by talking with the child in a relaxed manner while performing the examination.

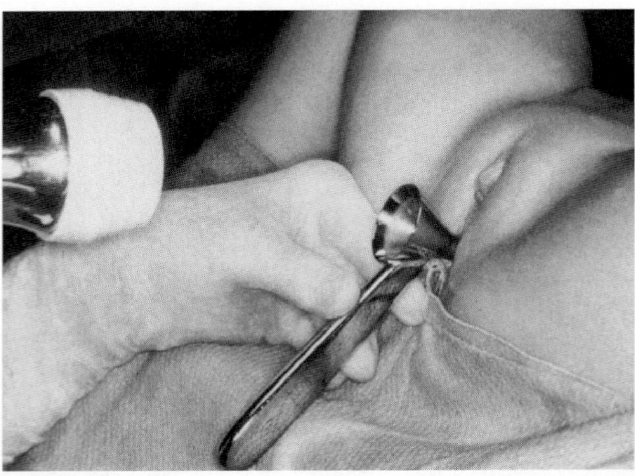

Figure 14-28 Inspection of the vagina using a children's vaginoscope and simple illumination with a flashlight.

Late Childhood

Children usually begin to have uncomfortable feelings about being undressed in front of adults by the time they reach the age of 5 or 6. Soliciting reassurance from the parent and using drapes or gowns may make the examination of school-aged children easier.

Occasionally, secondary sex characteristics begin to develop in children in this age group. Evaluation of such children must distinguish among premature thelarche, premature adrenarche, premature menarche, and precocious puberty, per se. (See Chapter 212, Puberty: Normal and Abnormal.)

One method for examining normally retractile testes is to palpate the scrotum with the boy squatting or sitting on the examining table with his legs crossed in the yoga position; the examiner begins to palpate over the inguinal areas and works downward onto the scrotum. This technique is especially helpful when examining boys with exogenous obesity, whose external genitalia may be engulfed in excess peripubic and perineal adipose tissue. By age 4, palpating for an inguinal hernia over the external inguinal ring while the boy coughs is usually possible, with the examining finger inserted into the scrotal tissue and slid upward into the inguinal canal. Tender, acute swelling of the scrotum can be caused by torsion of the testes, epididymitis, orchitis (often caused by mumps), or an incarcerated inguinal hernia.

Varicoceles are semifirm masses, sometimes of equal size to the testis, that are palpable within the spermatic vessels and may be associated with infertility unless surgically removed.

Adolescence

Examination of an adolescent's genitalia presents the practitioner with an opportunity to reassure the adolescent about the normal progression of the stages of puberty. The examiner should remember that adolescents have an excellent ability to deny real concerns and worries; therefore the physician should be especially sensitive to questions that might relate to a concern about venereal disease, pregnancy, or even cancer. Honest, direct answers to the adolescent's questions, coupled with a thorough description of the examination before it is performed, will help establish a trusting relationship.

Bimanual abdominorectal palpation of the uterus, as just described, is usually adequate when examining prepubertal and virginal pubertal girls. A complete pelvic examination is indicated for any adolescent who has vaginal discharge, dysuria, pyuria, lower abdominal pain, irregular vaginal bleeding, or amenorrhea, and for a sexually active adolescent. This examination is aided by proper instruments, including a vaginoscope or small speculum, culture media, glass slides, and a cytology fixative. The physician should be patient and gentle, minimizing painful procedures and embarrassment for the patient. After the external genitalia have been inspected and the internal organs have been examined with a speculum or vaginoscope, the uterus and ovaries are palpated using the bimanual abdominovaginal technique; normally the ovaries are not palpable. Specimens should be obtained periodically in sexually active adolescents to culture for *N gonorrhoeae* and *C trachomatis* and to evaluate cervical cytology for herpes virus effects. In male patients, the penis should be carefully examined for any lesions and the urethral meatus inspected for discharge. In addition, at all health assessment visits, the inguinal canals should be palpated for hernias, asking the patient to cough to increase intraabdominal pressure.

Musculoskeletal System

The changes in the musculoskeletal system of infants, children, and adolescents over time give the examiner the most visible evidence of human growth. If a child's sequential measurements of height fall within the norms of a standard growth curve, then evidence is strong not only that bone growth is normal, but also that the numerous factors necessary for normal growth are operating appropriately. In addition, because of its visibility, the musculoskeletal system is most often the source of questions from parents concerning possible deviations from normal, including the possible effects of trauma, a leading cause of morbidity and mortality in children.

The outward manifestations of growth of the trunk and extremities reflect primarily growth of bone, muscle, and adipose tissue. Bone grows in the fetus starting with cartilage, then from the primary centers of ossification, primarily in the long bones. Postnatally, new bone formation occurs in secondary centers of ossification at the ends of long bones and the vertebral bodies and in the membranes of the flat bones of the cranium and clavicle. In addition to longitudinal growth of long bones and vertebral bodies, internal remodeling takes place throughout infancy and childhood, resulting in less dense bone, a changing thickness of the bone cortex, and changing amounts of red marrow and fat within the diaphyses of bone. In addition to hormonal factors, mechanical forces caused by muscle attachments and gravity influence bone remodeling. Bone growth is completed with ossification of the growth cartilage and union of the epiphyses and diaphyses of long bones by age 21 years. The roentgenographic appearance of the onset, size, and shape of secondary ossification centers can be compared with established norms in determining the bone age, a measurement that can be helpful despite its variability in assessing children who are suspected of having abnormal growth.

Growth in stature predominates in the lower extremities before puberty and in the trunk during puberty. The distal extremities reach adult size before the proximal extremities, thus the common complaint of preadolescent children that their feet are too big.

Muscle growth, which results from increases in the number, size, and length of cells, proceeds throughout childhood according to the following increasing proportions of muscle mass to body weight: 1:5 to 1:4 at birth, 1:3 in early adolescence, and 2:5 in early maturity. A spurt in the increase in muscle cell numbers occurs at age 2, and maximal increase occurs between the ages of 10 and 16. Muscle cell size increases faster in girls than in boys between the ages of 3 and 10, but after age 14, boys surpass girls in both the number and size of muscle cells. The number of muscle fibers increases slowly until the 5th decade of life.

A thorough evaluation of the musculoskeletal system should be part of every newborn examination, every child health maintenance examination, and the examination of any child who has an abnormality of growth, stature, or gait. It includes an appraisal of (1) posture, position, and gross deformities; (2) skin color, temperature, and tenderness; (3) bone or joint tenderness; (4) range of joint motion; (5) muscle size, symmetry, and strength; and (6) the configuration and motility of the back.

Newborn Period

The position and appearance of the extremities at birth can reflect intrauterine position. The folded position of the lower extremities on the abdomen in the fetus results in the common appearance in newborns of externally rotated, somewhat bowed, lower extremities and inverted feet. A baby born after a breech presentation often has markedly flexed hips and extended knees. Traction on the brachial plexus during delivery can cause what usually is a temporary paresis of the proximal upper extremity muscles (Erb palsy), most often appearing as an asymmetrical Moro reflex (discussed in detail later). Another common cause of an asymmetrical Moro reflex resulting from a birth injury is a fractured clavicle, which can be confirmed by palpating an area of crepitance, usually over the distal third of the clavicle.

Gross deformities should be recognized at birth, both for early treatment and for possible clues to generalized genetic or metabolic diseases. Relatively common deformities include short or absent extremities, absence of one bone in an extremity, hypertrophy of one bone in an extremity or of an entire half of the body (hemihypertrophy), extra fingers or toes (polydactyly), webbed or fused fingers or toes (syndactyly), and annular constricting bands around a portion of an extremity with or without distal amputation or lack of development. The ratio of extremity length to body length should be noted. In a healthy newborn the ratio of the upper segment of the body to the lower segment (above and below the symphysis pubis) is approximately 1.7:1. In various types of dwarfism the extremities alone may be short, as in achondroplasia, or both extremities and trunk may be shortened, as in Morquio disease. The entire length of the vertebral column should be examined and palpated for bony defects with or without overlying skin defects such as sinus tracts, tufts of hair, sacral *dimples*, or asymmetry of the upper portion of the intragluteal crease. The joints should be tested for range of motion, noting any asymmetry, undue tightness, or contractures, as well as the muscle tone. A floppy or hypotonic baby may have CNS disease, a metabolic disturbance, primary muscle disease, or anterior horn cell disease. Limited unilateral joint motion with or without associated bone or joint tenderness and fever should be investigated extensively as a possible sign of osteomyelitis.

Perhaps the most important part of the examination of a newborn's extremities is the examination of the lower extremities, giving special attention to the hips and feet. The hips are examined particularly to rule out developmental hip dysplasia, a condition that is relatively easy to treat and with good results if treatment is started early. The examiner tests for a dislocated femoral head by abducting hip at a time and feeling over the greater trochanter for a click or clunk when the femoral head passes back into the acetabulum (Ortolani sign). This maneuver usually requires 70 to 80 degrees of hip abduction. Downward pressure over the hips transmitted through the flexed knee can be used to attempt to produce posterior dislocation of the femoral head in the Barlow test (Figure 14-29). The click or clunk of the reducing femoral head should be distinguished from the clicks felt with rotation of the hip and the click felt with simultaneous movement of the knee. After the newborn period, the hip click (Ortolani sign) heard with congenitally dislocated hips disappears, and other signs become helpful in making this diagnosis. The thigh may appear shorter on the affected side, the thigh skinfolds may be asymmetrical (although this occurs in some normal babies), and the hip will have limited abduction on the affected side. Tight hip abductors in the neonatal period are not a sign of congenital hip dislocation.

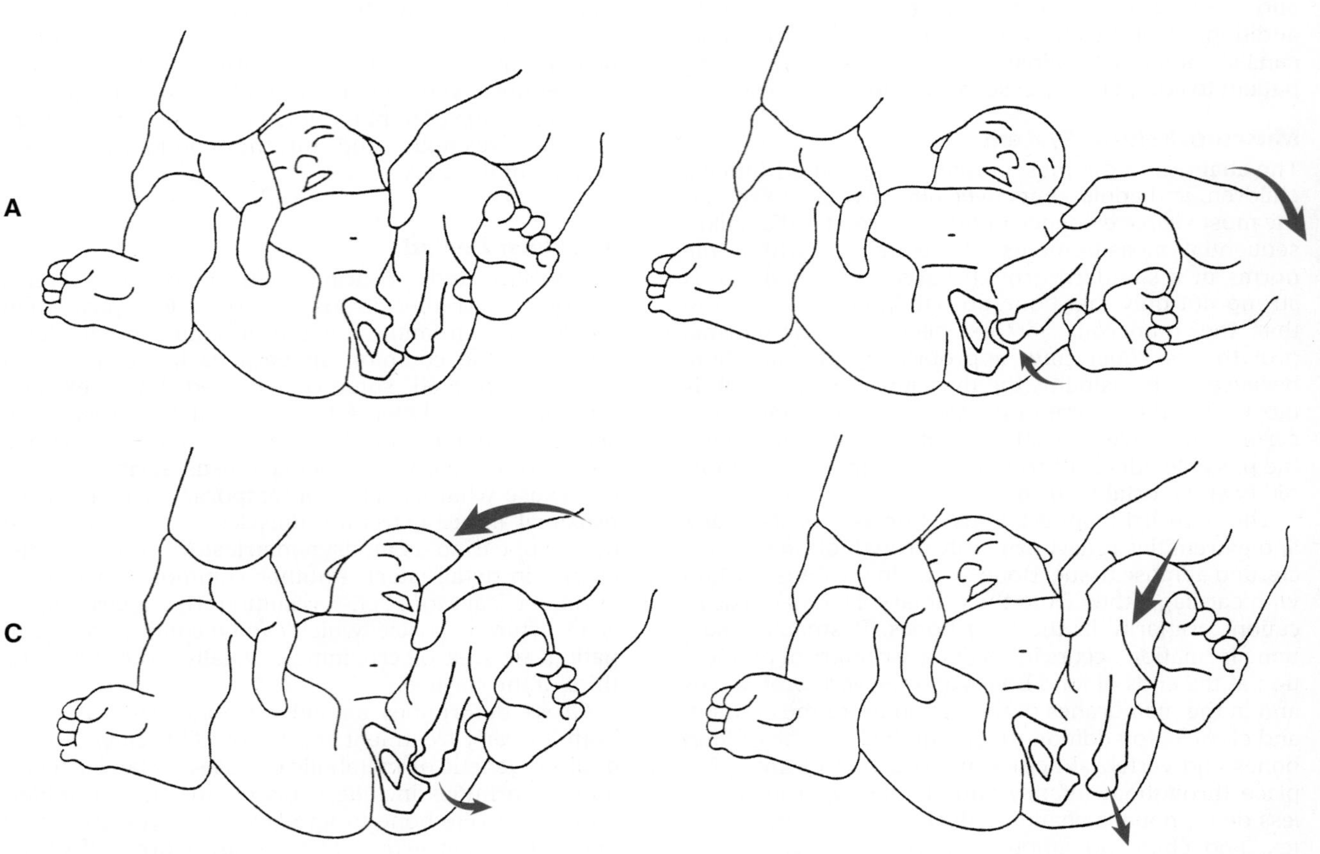

Figure 14-29 **A** and **B**, The Ortolani maneuver reduces a posteriorly dislocated hip. The affected hip is gently abducted while the femoral head is reduced with an anteriorly directed force provided by the fingers placed over the greater trochanter. **C** and **D**, The Barlow test assessing for dislocation of a located hip. This test is performed by gently adducting the examined hip, while directing a posterior force across the hip. *(From Pizzutillo PD.* Practical Orthopaedics in Primary Care. *New York, NY: McGraw-Hill; 1977. Reprinted by permission of The McGraw-Hill Companies.)*

A newborn's and an infant's feet often appear flat because of a plantar fat pad that gradually disappears during the first 1 to 2 years of life. The most severe foot deformity at birth is the talipes equinovarus deformity, or clubfoot. True clubfoot deformities cannot be corrected passively, nor do they correct with stroking of the foot's lateral side. This deformity comprises fixed forefoot adduction, fixed inversion especially of the hindfoot, equinus position, internal tibial torsion, and small calf muscles.

Viewing the sole of the resting foot (not spontaneously inverted or everted) allows observation for the normal single anteroposterior plantar axis. In metatarsus varus deformity the forefoot is adducted in relation to the hindfoot, thus describing two anteroposterior axes, and this position is not correctable by stroking the foot's lateral border. In calcaneovalgus deformity the foot is dorsiflexed and everted. (See Chapter 183, Foot and Leg Problems, for a complete discussion of developmental orthopedic variations of the lower extremities.)

Infancy and Early Childhood

An infant's lower extremities often remain bowlegged with externally rotated feet for the first 1 to 2 years of life. With ambulation, the feet gradually assume the straight-ahead position, and the knock-knee, or genu valgum, position is normally seen between the ages of 2 and 6 years or older.

Severe bowing of the legs raises the question of rickets or epiphyseal damage from inflammation or trauma (Blount disease). The infant whose toes turn in should be examined for metatarsus varus, internal tibial torsion, or femoral anteversion. Flatfeet, or feet without a longitudinal arch, are common, especially in children who have generalized ligamentous laxity.

A toddler's lower extremities are examined best by first observing the spontaneous gait with the infant undressed. The normal gait is usually wide based and somewhat unstable, with prominent lumbar lordosis. Then, especially if positional deformities are noted, a thorough examination of the hips, knees, legs, ankles, and feet with the child in the supine position can confirm the presence of any fixed deformity. A child who has a limp should be examined thoroughly for signs of trauma; localized bone or joint tenderness from fracture or infection; joint effusions with limited range of motion from trauma, infection, or noninfectious arthritis; peripheral muscle weakness; unilateral or bilateral spasticity, especially exhibited by a tight Achilles tendon; and proximal muscle weakness, particularly weakness resulting from unrecognized hip disease such as congenital dislocated hip or coxa vara. Testing for coxa vara can be performed by having the child raise one foot while standing. This action normally produces an elevation in the contralateral hip. Inability of the hip abductors to elevate the contralateral hip is considered a positive Trendelenburg sign (Figure 14-30).

Child abuse should be suspected in all cases of trauma if (1) the history of the injury is inconsistent with its severity; (2) signs exist of multiple blunt

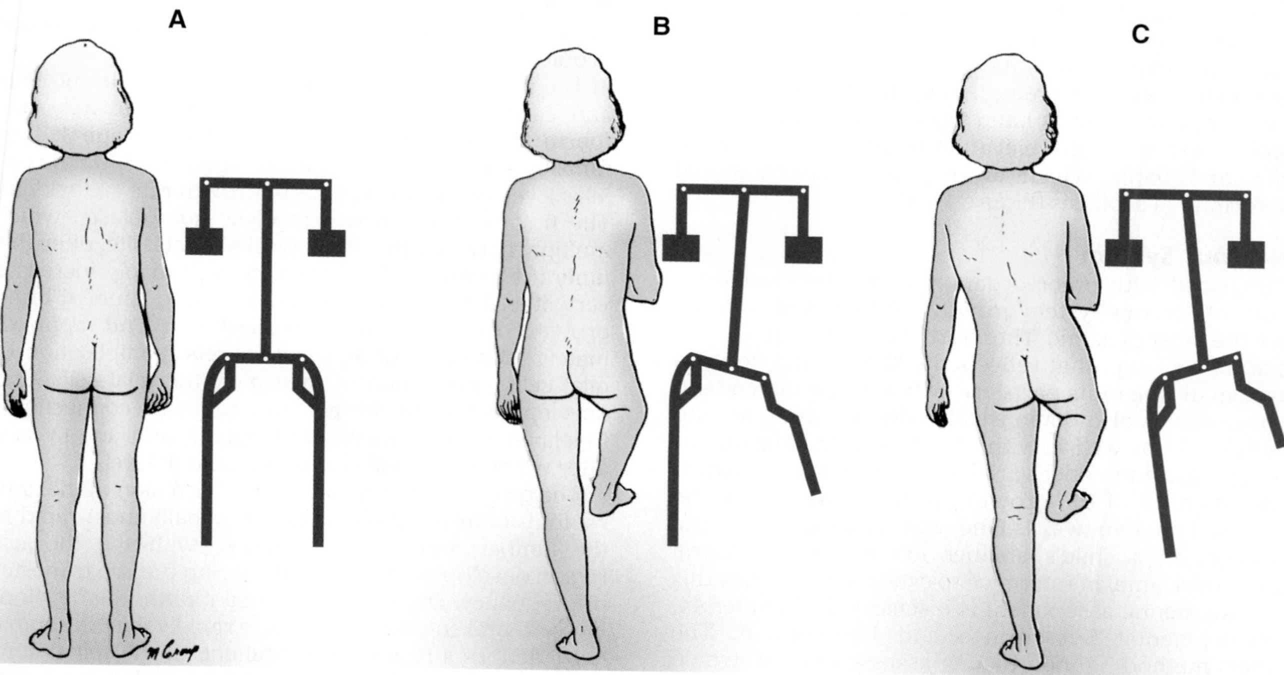

Figure 14-30 Trendelenburg sign, showing weakness of the gluteus medius muscle. **A**, Normal standing. **B**, Dropping of the pelvis of the contralateral side when standing on the affected leg. **C**, Compensation for weakness when walking by shifting the center of gravity of the trunk to elevate the pelvis on the opposite side. *(Adapted from Ferguson AM Jr. Orthopaedic Surgery in Infancy and Childhood. 5th ed. Baltimore, MD: Williams & Wilkins; 1981, with permission.)*

trauma to the extremities, trunk (especially the buttocks), and face; (3) trauma is recurrent; and (4) significant delay occurs between the episode of injury and the request for medical attention.

The child who has a tender elbow held in pronation, usually after a pulling episode (nursemaid elbow), suffers from subluxation of the radial head, which can be reduced easily by supinating the arm while applying pressure to the radial head.

Late Childhood and Adolescence

A limp in a child between the ages of 4 and 8 years, especially if accompanied by knee pain, may suggest Legg-Calve-Perthes disease. The same symptoms in a child between the ages of 9 and 12 years may be caused by a slipped femoral capital epiphysis. Tenderness over the tibial tubercle may be a sign of Osgood-Schlatter disease. Painful heels can be caused by partial evulsion of the Achilles tendon, retrocalcaneal bursitis, or plantar fasciitis.

In the examination of an injured knee, the following elements should be tested: the medial and lateral collateral ligaments, by abducting and adducting the tibia on the femur; the cruciate ligaments, by pulling the tibia forward, then pushing it backward with the knee flexed; the medial and lateral menisci, by extending the knee with the foot held in eversion and then inversion; the patella, by pushing it posteriorly against the femur; and the joint space for effusion, by pressing over the suprapatellar bursa and then attempting ballottement of the patella.

School-aged children and adolescents should be examined for scoliosis, or lateral curvature of the vertebral column. Significant spinal curvature can be seen with the child standing erect; lesser degrees of curvature can be observed by having the child bend forward approximately 50 degrees, letting the shoulders droop forward and the arms hang freely. The examiner then looks for a unilateral elevation of the lower thoracic ribs and flank, which accompanies the rotational deformity of scoliosis (Figure 14-31).

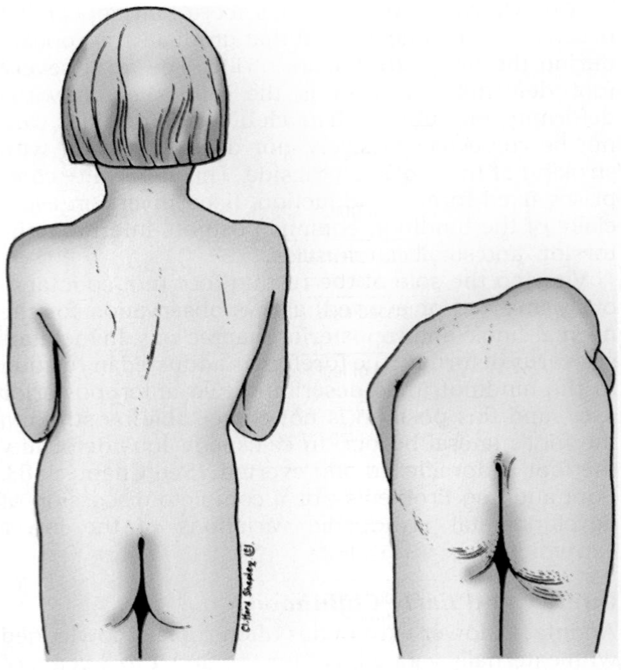

Figure 14-31 Examination for scoliosis. *(Adapted from James JIP.* Scoliosis. *Edinburgh, Scotland: E&S Livingstone; 1976.)*

Nervous System

Compared with other organ systems, the manifestations of nervous system growth in infants and children are the most dynamic. Therefore the definitions of *normal* for any sign that reflects the state of the nervous system or one of its parts are critically age dependent. These norms also demonstrate wide variation among individuals, as well as within a single individual on different days and under variable conditions. The growth and integrity of the growing nervous system can be assessed in two ways. One way is to describe the changes in a child's abilities in various behavioral areas over time, in reference to established norms; this developmental assessment is discussed in Chapter 44, Developmental Surveillance and Intervention. The other method is neurologic assessment, in which often-changing physical signs that reflect the state of subsystems of the nervous system are described over time. Although the developmental stage depends partly on the neurologic stage, it is also influenced greatly by the child's environmental experiences. The major goal of neurologic assessment in children is to monitor the maturation of the nervous system, although the methods described for localizing nervous system lesions in adults are useful in evaluating certain problems in children.

The nervous system grows most rapidly during fetal and early postnatal life, reaching approximately one fourth the adult size at birth, one half by age 1, four fifths by age 3, and nine tenths by age 7 years. At the cellular level, two distinct peaks of growth rate are evident. The first peak of growth involves neuroblasts, which multiply between 10 and 18 weeks of fetal life; after this time, the number of neuronal cells probably increases very little. The second and more striking spurt of brain growth occurs between midgestation and approximately 18 months of age and reflects multiplication of glial cells, production of myelin by the glial cells, and development of dendrites and synaptic connections. Myelination continues relatively rapidly until age 4 years, after which it gradually increases to adult levels.

The growth of the spinal cord, after fusion of the neural folds cranially and caudally, is initially most rapid in the lumbar and cervical regions, with the thoracic region developing most rapidly during the 3rd trimester of pregnancy. During the 3rd fetal month, the developing vertebral column grows more rapidly than the spinal cord, and, as a result, the cordal end of the spinal cord moves cranially from the level of the fourth lumbar vertebra in the 5th month to the adult level of the first or second lumbar vertebra by the 2nd postnatal month. Myelination of the cord precedes cephalocaudad.

Spontaneous and reflexive motor activity, reflecting developing muscular innervation and spinal reflex

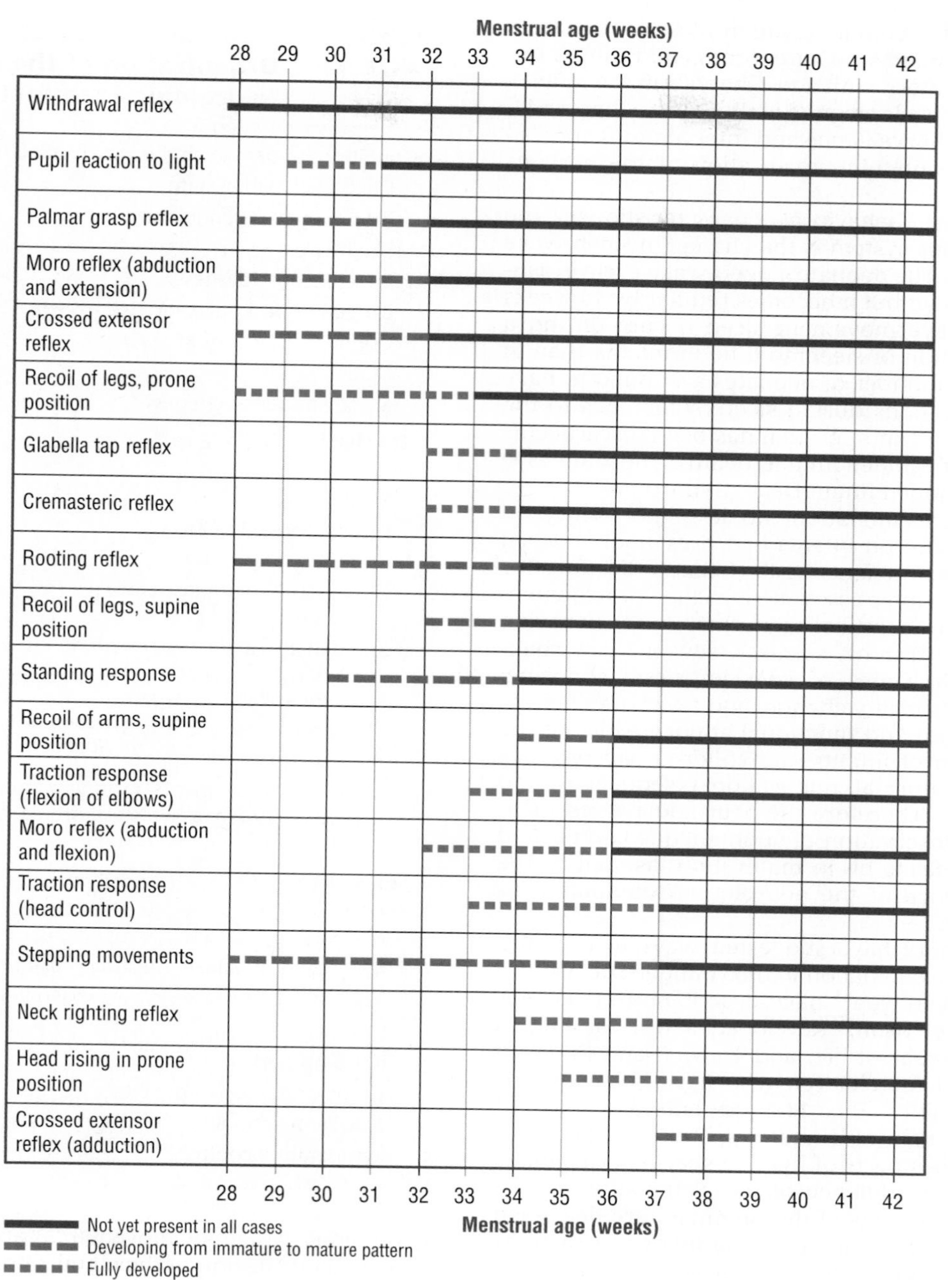

Figure 14-32 Developmental sequence of various reflexes and motor automatisms. *(Adapted from Davis JA, Dobbing J, eds.* Scientific Foundations of Paediatrics. *2nd ed. Baltimore, MD: University Park Press; 1981.)*

arcs, begins during the 10th week of fetal life. At 12 weeks of fetal age a primitive rooting and grasp response can be seen; withdrawal of the lower extremities in response to stimulation of the feet and the gastrocnemius stretch reflex are seen at 16 weeks; by 19 weeks, regular respiratory movements are seen in response to hypoxia. Tonic myotactic reflexes, responsible for the recoil of an extended extremity, are well developed in the term infant. The rhythmicity of motor neuron activity, which is responsible for jerky repetitive movements during activity (eg, the jerking jaw movements that accompany crying), increases with increasing gestational age. At term, stretch reflexes, such as the knee jerk, are diminished by sleep, whereas exteroceptive reflexes (superficial abdominal and Babinski reflexes) are not.

The normal sequence of changes in an infant's posture, muscle tone, and reflexes that occurs with increasing gestational age from 28 to 40 weeks has been described by several observers and, despite their differences, can be used in assessing a neonate's gestational (menstrual) age (Figure 14-32). Similarly, the persistence and eventual cessation of certain characteristics of the infant's posture, tone, and reflexes follow a defined pattern with age. Changes in the infant's and the child's developmental abilities (see Chapter 44, Developmental Surveillance and Intervention) are also based on the continuing maturation of the nervous system.

An additional behavioral characteristic of the maturing nervous system is the change in sleep-wake cycles with age. The neonate's sleep-wake cycle is usually quite irregular, but it becomes regular by 15 weeks of age. Rapid eye movement sleep occurs during a greater proportion of sleeping time in infants than in adults. A small number of neonates are found to have irregular respirations during sleep, sometimes to the point of apnea, a condition that has been discarded as a precursor of sudden infant death syndrome (see Chapter 330, Sudden Infant Death Syndrome).

A neurologic examination should be performed on every neonate and on infants and preschool children during health maintenance visits. Other indications for a thorough neurologic assessment include developmental delay, failure in school, abnormal social behavior, headache, head trauma, seizures, sensory disturbances, changes in states of consciousness, abnormal gait, recent personality change, and fever of unknown origin. Structural and functional abnormalities of the nervous system of infants and children can produce delays in the normal maturational sequences and localizing signs. Therefore the neurologic assessment must include observation of spontaneous and elicited activity that reflects brain maturation, as well as the ordered sequence of the neurologic examination as used for adults.

Several authors have suggested ways to organize the neurologic examination in the younger age groups. Prechtel and Beintema[11] have described a system for neonates; Amiel-Tison,[6] developed a test for infants during the 1st year of life; and Touwen and Prechtl[12] designed a test for children who have behavioral or learning disabilities. Box 14-1 presents a method of organizing the data of a neurologic examination; this scheme combines parts of the age-specific evaluations with the standard adult neurologic examination.

Various components of this summary are discussed in other chapters in this text. The following sections highlight the approach to the neurologic examination of children of different age groups, including major areas of emphasis for each group.

BOX 14-1 Organization of the Pediatric Neurologic Examination

Conditions under which the examination is conducted
- Child's behavioral state
- Environmental conditions

Mental status
- State of consciousness
- Language (receptive and expressive)
- Cognitive functioning
- Mood
- Social and self-awareness

STATION AND GATE

Head
- Skull
- Cranial nerves I to XII

Motor
- Muscle size, symmetry, contractures, tone, and strength
- Spontaneous activity when prone, supine, sitting, standing, and walking, including fine- and gross-motor abilities
- Resistance to passive stretch
- Coordination
- Involuntary movements, including fasciculations, tremor, chorea, athetosis, dystonia, and myotonic jerks

SENSORY

Reflexes
- Neonatal
- Deep-tendon reflexes, including plantar response
- Abdominal, cremasteric, and anal reflexes
- Clonus

Autonomic nervous system
- Cardiac and respiratory rate
- Bladder functioning
- Temperature control

Newborn Period and Infancy

Careful observation is the most important tool in the neurologic examination of the newborn and infant, taking into account the optimal environmental conditions previously described. Even when an infant is asleep and dressed, the examiner can note the posture, especially the degree of flexion of the extremities; any hyperextension of the neck, including overt opisthotonos; the symmetry of the position of the extremities; and the amount, quality, and symmetry of spontaneous movements, including tonic or clonic convulsions. Holding the thumb curled under the flexed fingers is a sign present with many brain abnormalities (cerebral thumb). In normal premature infants, continuous athetoid movements are common (eg, simultaneous flexion of the elbow and internal rotation of the upper portion of the arm). Athetoid postures are also common in term infants. Tremor with or without crying is seen in many healthy newborns during the first days of life. Spontaneous assumption of the tonic neck position, that is, extension of the isolateral extremities after rotation of the head to one side—the asymmetric tonic neck reflex (ATNR)—may occur in healthy infants, but an obligatory ATNR (one that is always present) is abnormal. The face is observed for expression (alert, bland, fussing, crying); symmetry of eye closure after a tap on the glabella (glabella reflex); and symmetry of position and movement of the eyes, including presence of symmetry and pupillary constriction and blinking of the eyelids in response to a hand clap approximately 12 inches from the infant's face.

With the baby undressed, resistance to passive stretch is tested in the extremities, trunk, and neck, noting particularly any symmetrical and asymmetrical increase or decrease. Many infants in whom spasticity develops later are hypotonic during the neonatal period. Symmetry of the biceps, patellar, superficial abdominal, cremasteric, and anal reflexes is noted, and eliciting ankle clonus (recording the number of beats obtained) is attempted. The palmar and plantar grasps are tested (Figure 14-33) for differences of intensity between the two sides (unilaterally decreased in Erb palsy, for instance) or bilateral absence, as with cord lesions. As shown in Figure 14-33, pressing the infant's palm from the ulnar side, with the infant's head in the midline position, is important. Babinski reflex (with a flexor response and fanning of the toes), which is expected in normal newborns, is tested for symmetry, as is the withdrawal reflex of the lower extremities.

The rooting response is elicited while the baby's hands are held against the chest (Figure 14-34). In addition to the response shown, with stimulation of the upper lip, the mouth is opened and the head is retroflexed; with stimulation of the lower lip, the mouth opens and the jaw drops. This reflex is absent in depressed infants; when the examiner's fingers are placed into the depressed infant's mouth, the sucking response is decreased in strength, frequency of sucks, and duration.

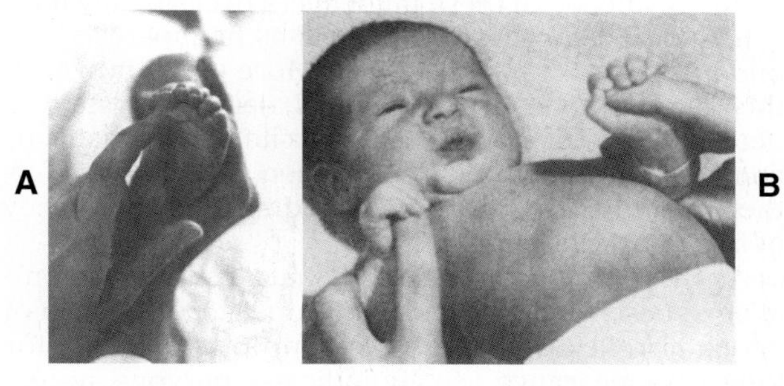

Figure 14-33 A, Plantar grasp. B, Palmar grasp. *(A from Whaley LF, Wong DL.* Nursing Care of Infants and Children. *4th ed. St Louis, MO: Mosby; 1991. B from Prechtl H.* The Neurological Examination of the Full-Term Newborn Infant. *2nd ed. London, UK: Heinemann; 1977. Reprinted by permission.)*

In the traction response test (Figure 14-35) the examiner pulls the supine infant into a sitting position and notes the degree of resistance to extension of the arms at the elbow and the degree to which the head is held upright. In a term infant, some degree of flexion of the elbow is maintained, and head control is relatively weak, with neither head flexors nor extensors predominating.

The Moro reflex is a critically important sign of an intact nervous system, particularly during the neonatal period. It is best elicited by supporting the infant's supine body in one hand then suddenly allowing the head supported by the other hand to drop a few centimeters during a moment when the head is midline and the neck muscles are relaxed. A complete Moro reflex consists of symmetrical abduction of the arms at the shoulder, extension of the forearm at the elbow, and extension of the fingers (Figure 14-36), all followed by adduction of the arms at the shoulder and crying. The Moro reflex can also be elicited by holding the supine baby in both arms and then suddenly lowering the entire body about 12 inches or by producing a sudden loud noise that startles the baby.

The prone infant is observed for spontaneous head movements (brief lifting or turning from side to side), spontaneous crawling movements, and the incurvation, or Galant, reflex (lateral curvation of the trunk after stimulation with a finger or pin along a paravertebral line from the shoulder to the buttocks approximately 3 cm from the midline). The infant is then held prone in the air with the examiner's hands around the infant's chest. The normal newborn is somewhat flaccid during this maneuver, but the hypertonic or opisthotonic baby will lift the head and extend the lower extremities to varying degrees. While holding the infant upright with the examiner's hands placed beneath the infant's axillae from behind, the placing and stepping responses are noted. In the placing response, the dorsum of one foot is allowed to brush against the undersurface of a tabletop edge and is followed normally by simultaneous flexion of the knees and hips and placement of the stimulated foot on the table. In the stepping response, the soles of the feet are allowed to touch the surface of the table, which elicits alternating stepping movements with both legs.

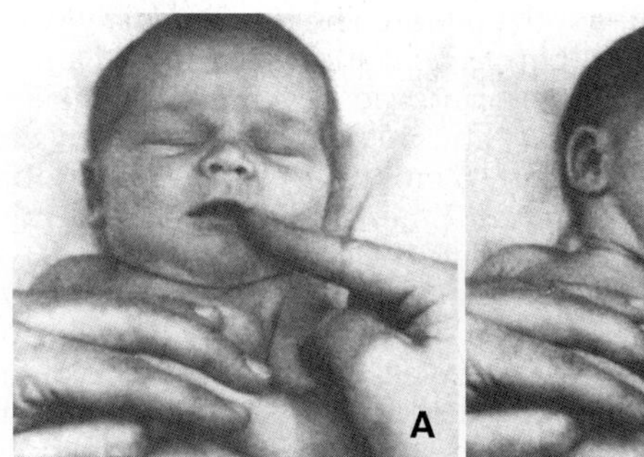

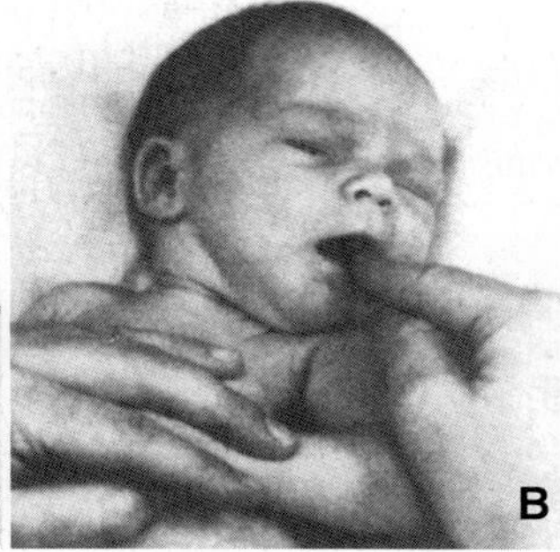

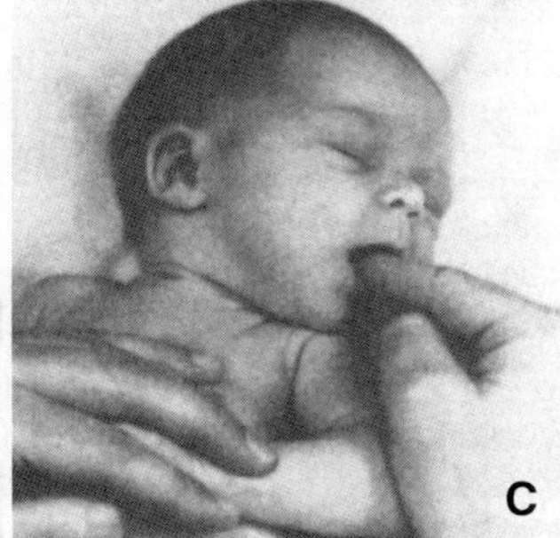

Figure 14-34 Rooting response. A, Stimulation. B, Head turning. C, Grasping with the mouth. *(From Prechtl H.* The Neurological Examination of the Full-Term Newborn Infant. *2nd ed. London, UK: Heinemann; 1977. Reprinted by permission.)*

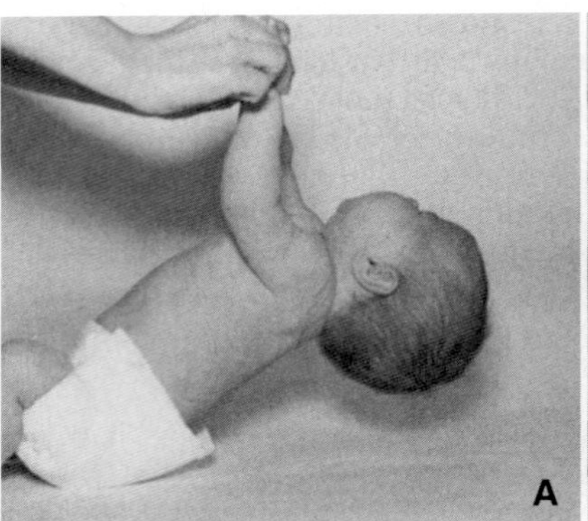

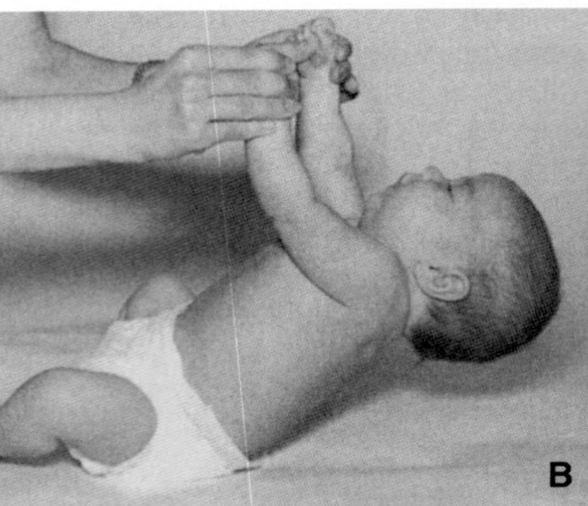

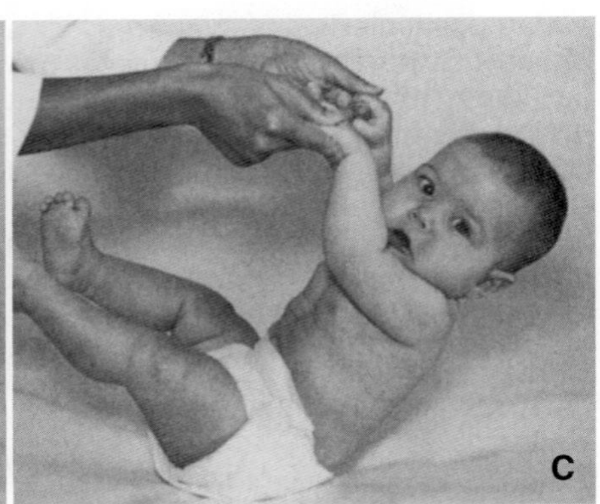

Figure 14-35 Sitting development. **A**, First 4 weeks or so: complete head lag when being pulled into sitting position. **B**, Approximately 2 months: considerable, but not complete, head lag when being pulled into sitting position. **C**, 4 months: no head lag when being pulled into sitting position. *(Whaley LF, Wong DL.* Nursing Care of Infants and Children. *4th ed. St Louis, MO: Mosby; 1991. Copyright © 1991, Elsevier, with permission.)*

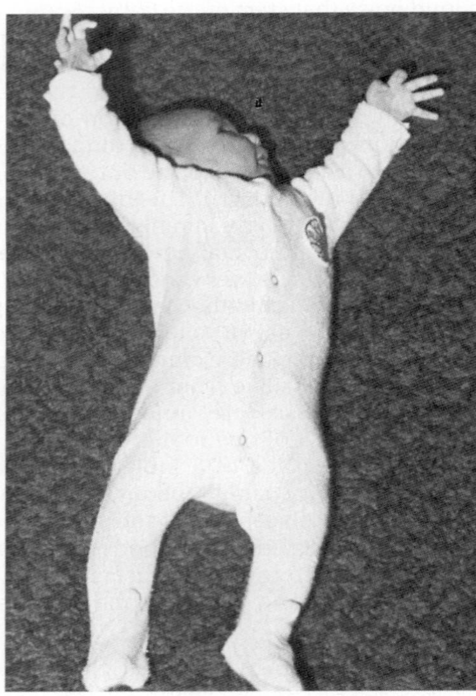

Figure 14-36 Moro reflex. *(Whaley LF, Wong DL.* Nursing Care of Infants and Children. *4th ed. St Louis, MO: Mosby; 1991. Copyright © 1991, Elsevier, with permission.)*

Throughout the neurologic examination, the practitioner should note the quality and duration of the infant's cry and should listen for the high-pitched, excessive, or weak cries that can accompany brain lesions. Cranial nerve testing is completed by testing the corneal and jaw jerk reflexes (cranial nerve V); the response during rotation of the upright infant's eyes to turning in the same direction the infant is moved while being held upright facing the examiner with the examiner's hands gripping the baby in the axillae (cranial nerve VIII); the gag reflex, symmetrical elevation of the palate and swallowing movements (cranial nerves IX and X); and by observing for non–injury-related torticollis (cranial nerve XI) and the symmetry of the tongue, including observation for fasciculations (cranial nerve XII).

The results of all these maneuvers occasionally indicate a localized brain lesion, such as hemiparesis secondary to intracranial bleeding. More often, however, the general state of the infant's nervous system is determined to be normal, hyperexcitable, apathetic, or comatose. The physician must then decide what further diagnostic tests are indicated and the frequency of follow-up examinations.

As the infant matures, the neonatal reflexes (automatisms) described previously disappear. Persistence of neonatal reflexes beyond age-appropriate norms for their disappearance usually indicates nervous system abnormality. Some of the techniques for examining neonates are continued during the 1st year to ascertain whether strength and coordination have developed further. For instance, a healthy 4-month-old infant no longer demonstrates head lag when pulled to a sitting position; a 5-month-old infant lifts the head from the supine position when about to be pulled up; and the infant sits without support between 6 and 9 months of age. The infant usually walks without support between 12 and 18 months of age.

Monitoring the development of hand coordination is important. A healthy infant can reach and grasp objects by 5 months of age, transfer objects from hand to hand by 7 months, and pick up a raisin using a pincer grasp by 10 months (Figure 14-37). After 8 months of age a healthy infant demonstrates symmetrical parachute and lateral propping reactions. The parachute reflex can be assessed using a flinging motion of the ventrally suspended infant toward the examination table, which should elicit extension of the arms. In the lateral propping reaction the sitting infant is pushed to one side, and the arms should extend to prevent falling. During these maneuvers the examiner looks for asymmetrical movements.

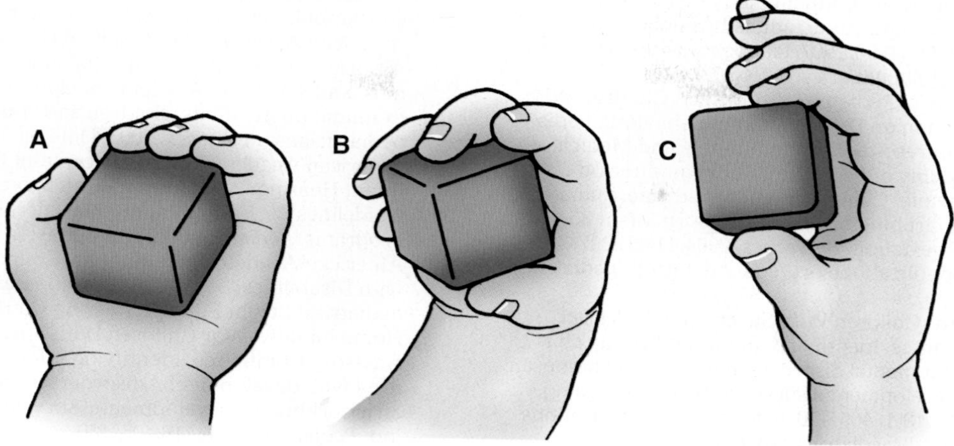

Figure 14-37 Manipulation. **A**, 6 months: immature palmar grasp of a cube. **B**, 8 months: grasp at the intermediate stage. **C**, 1 year: mature pincer grasp of a cube.

Early and Late Childhood

Further growth of the nervous system in infants and children is monitored by observing walking, the development of speech and language abilities, interaction with parents, and the ability to manipulate small objects, use pencils and crayons, climb and run, throw and catch a ball, and follow simple directions. Muscle strength in the lower extremities is best tested by observing gait, heel and toe walking, standing and hopping on one leg, and the ability to rise from the floor from a supine position. Coordination can be observed in these maneuvers, and in heel-to-shin, finger-to-nose pointing, and tandem walking. If the child's development is delayed, or if the child has a history of school failure, then further testing of neurophysiological maturation (described in Chapter 44, Developmental Surveillance and Intervention) can help define abilities and areas that need special attention.

As with infants, the neurologic examination of school-aged children who have nervous system abnormalities usually defines some degree of maturational delay. Localizing neurologic signs are less common, occurring in children most often as a result of traumatic intracranial bleeding or brain tumors or after CNS infection.

Adolescence

Although reading ability and comprehension, improved coordination, and increased strength can all be used to monitor further neuromuscular maturation in adolescents, the neurologic examination in this age group is similar to the adult examination. When evaluating a young person's mental status the examiner should remember that many healthy adolescents display variable mood swings, confused thinking, and resistance to authority. A thorough neurologic examination in adolescents includes observation of mental status, examination of cranial nerve function, extremity muscle tone and strength, sensory examination, deep-tendon reflexes, and tandem walking, finger-to-nose, and Romberg sign testing to assess cerebellar function. Any asymmetrical signs or abnormalities can be helpful in localizing CNS lesions and in suggesting appropriate laboratory tests and imaging studies.

TOOLS FOR PRACTICE

Medical Decision Support

- *A View Through the Otoscope: Distinguishing Acute Otitis Media from Otitis Media with Effusion* (video), American Academy of Pediatrics (www.aap.org/sections/infectdis/video.cfm).
- *Growth Charts—tutorials and information* (Web page), Centers for Disease Control and Prevention (www.cdc.gov/growthcharts/).
- *Growth Charts*, Centers for Disease Control and Prevention (www.cdc.gov/nchs/about/major/nhanes/growthcharts/clinical_charts.htm#Clin%201) also available at AAP bookstore (www.aap.org/bookstore) and (www.who.int/childgrowth/standards/en/index.html).
- *Primary Teeth Eruption Chart*, American Dental Association (www.ada.org/public/topics/tooth_eruption.asp).
- *The Neonatal Behavioral Assessment Scale* (scale), The Brazelton Institute (www.brazelton-institute.com/train.html).

AAP POLICY STATEMENTS

American Academy of Pediatrics, Committee on Nutrition. Prevention of pediatric overweight and obesity. *Pediatrics*. 2003;112(2):424-430. (aappolicy.aappublications.org/cgi/content/full/pediatrics;112/2/424).

American Academy of Pediatrics, Committee on Practice and Ambulatory Medicine, Section on Ophthalmology, American Association of Certified Orthoptists, American Association for Pediatric Ophthalmology and Strabismus, and

American Academy of Ophthalmology. Eye examination in infants, children and young adults by pediatricians. *Pediatrics*. 2003;111(4):902-907. (aappolicy.aappublications.org/cgi/content/full/pediatrics;111/4/902).

American Academy of Pediatrics, Council on Children With Disabilities, Section on Developmental Behavioral Pediatrics, Bright Futures Steering Committee, and Medical American Academy of Pediatrics, Subcommittee on Hyperbilirubinemia. Clinical practice guideline: management of hyperbilirubinemia in the newborn infant 35 or more weeks of gestation. *Pediatrics*. 2004;114(1):297-316. (aappolicy.aappublications.org/cgi/content/full/pediatrics;114/1/297).

Home Initiatives for Children With Special Needs Project Advisory Committee. Identifying infants and young children with developmental disorders in the medical home: an algorithm for developmental surveillance and screening. *Pediatrics*. 2006;118(1):405-420. (aappolicy.aappublications.org/cgi/content/full/pediatrics;118/1/405).

Kellogg N, American Academy of Pediatrics, Committee on Child Abuse and Neglect. Clinical report: the evaluation of sexual abuse in children. *Pediatrics*. 2005;116(2):506-512. (aappolicy.aappublications.org/cgi/content/full/pediatrics;116/2/506).

SUGGESTED RESOURCES

Davis JA, Dobbing J. *Scientific Foundations of Paediatrics*. 2nd ed. Baltimore, MD: University Park Press; 1981.

Ferguson AB. *Orthopaedic Surgery in Infancy and Childhood*. 5th ed. Baltimore, MD: Williams & Wilkins; 1981.

Fyler DC. *Nadas' Pediatric Cardiology*. St Louis, MO: Mosby-Yearbook; 1992.

James JIP. *Scoliosis*. Edinburgh, Scotland: E&S Livingstone; 1976.

Lowrey GH. *Growth and Development of Children*. 8th ed. Chicago, IL: Mosby; 1986.

McDowell F, Wolff HG. *Handbook of Neurological Diagnostic Methods*. Baltimore, MD: Williams & Wilkins; 1960.

Pizzutillo D. *Practical Orthopaedics in Primary Practice*. New York, NY: McGraw-Hill; 1997.

Smith TF, O'Day D, Wright PF. Clinical implications of preseptal (periorbital) cellulitis in childhood. *Pediatrics*. 1978;62:1006.

Sperling MA. *Pediatric Endocrinology*. Philadelphia, PA: WB Saunders; 1996.

Szilagy P. The pediatric physical examination. In: Bickley LS, ed. *Bates' Guide to Physical Examination and History Taking*. 9th ed. Philadelphia, PA: JB Lippincott; 2007.

REFERENCES

1. Brazelton TB, Nugent JK. *The Neonatal Behavioral Assessment Scale*. Cambridge, MA: Mac Keith Press; 1995.
2. American Academy of Pediatrics, Committee on Nutrition. Prevention of pediatric overweight and obesity. *Pediatrics*. 2003;112(2):424-430.
3. American Academy of Pediatrics, Subcommittee on Hyperbilirubinemia. Clinical practice guideline: management of hyperbilirubinemia in the newborn infant 35 or more weeks of gestation. *Pediatrics*. 2004:297-316. Available at: aappolicy.aappublications.org/cgi/content/abstract/pediatrics;114/1/297. Accessed May 7, 2007.
4. Jones KL. *Smith's Recognizable Patterns of Human Malformation*. Philadelphia, PA: WB Saunders; 1991.
5. Klaus MH, Kennell JH. *Bonding: the Beginnings of Parent-Infant Attachment*. St Louis, MO: Mosby; 1983.
6. Amiel-Tison C: A method for neurological evaluation within the first year of life. *Ciba Found Symb*. 1978:(59):107.
7. American Academy of Pediatrics, Committee on Practice and Ambulatory Medicine, Section on Ophthalmology, American Association of Certified Orthoptists, American Association for Pediatric Ophthalmology and Strabismus, and American Academy of Ophthalmology. Eye examination in infants, children and young adults by pediatricians. *Pediatrics*. 2003;111(4):902-907.
8. American Academy of Pediatrics, Joint Committee on Infant Hearing. 2007 Position Statement: Principles and Guidelines for Early Hearing Detection and Intervention Programs. *Pediatrics* 2007;120:898-921.
9. American Academy of Pediatrics, Council on Children with Disabilities, Section on Developmental Behavioral Pediatrics, Bright Futures Steering Committee, Medical Home Initiatives for Children With Special Needs Project Advisory Committee. Identifying infants and young children with developmental disorders in the medical home: an algorithm for developmental surveillance and screening. *Pediatrics*. 2006;118:405-420.
10. American Academy of Pediatrics, Kellogg N, and the Committee on Child Abuse and Neglect. The evaluation of sexual abuse in children. *Pediatrics*. 2005;116(2):506-512.
11. Prechtl H, Beintema D. *The Neurological Examination of the Full-Term Newborn Infant*. 2nd ed. London, UK: Heinemann; 1977.
12. Touwen BCL, Prechtl H. *The Neurological Examination of the Child With Minor Dysfunction*. London, UK: Heinemann; 1970.

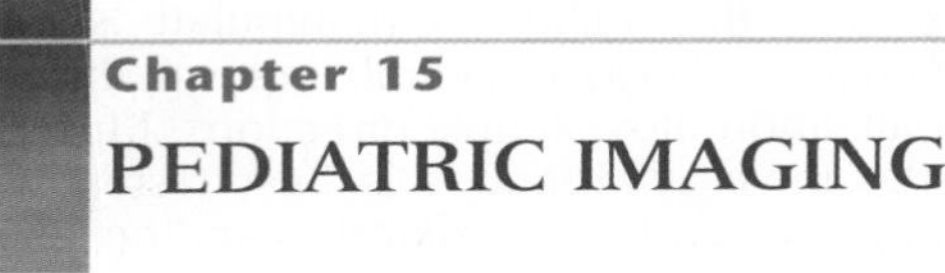

Chapter 15
PEDIATRIC IMAGING

Terry L. Levin, MD

IMAGING MODALITIES

With the advent of new technologies in radiology, the choices of imaging modalities available to the clinician have become increasingly complex. Selecting the best imaging modality is most often directed by the clinical question at hand. The more focused the question, the clearer the choice of imaging technique.

The initial evaluation of a child often begins with a plain radiograph performed in the radiology department. Technical considerations, such as patient positioning and film exposure, affect the quality of the final radiograph and are better managed in the radiology department, rather than using portable units, whenever possible. Findings on the plain radiograph will often indicate if further imaging is needed and in many cases will dictate the choice of imaging modality, whether fluoroscopy, ultrasound (US), computed tomography (CT), magnetic resonance imaging (MRI), or nuclear scintigraphy.

Fluoroscopy

Fluoroscopy provides real-time evaluation of the airway and both the gastrointestinal (GI) and the genitourinary (GU) tracts. In patients with possible tracheomalacia, dynamic changes in airway diameter can be identified. Fluoroscopic upper GI series with or without small bowel follow-through allows assessment of swallowing function, esophageal and GI motility, gastroesophageal reflux, and position of the duodenojejunal junction. The small bowel follow-through can evaluate small bowel abnormalities, particularly in children with inflammatory bowel disease. Similarly, the colon is well evaluated by fluoroscopically guided contrast enemas. Fluoroscopic voiding cystourethrography is useful in evaluating the bladder and urethra and to assess for vesicoureteral reflux in children with urinary tract infections. Videofluoroscopy allows studies to be replayed and analyzed at a later time. The length of the fluoroscopic procedure determines the radiation dose.

Ultrasound

Ultrasound (US) is the initial study of choice when evaluating solid organs in children[1]; it delivers no ionizing radiation, requires no patient sedation, and can be performed at the patient's bedside, if necessary. US is limited by body habitus and overlying bowel gas or air. Because the quality of the images depends on the skill of the US operator, the operator must be trained and experienced in working with children. In the GI tract, US is particularly useful in diagnosing pyloric stenosis, appendicitis, and intussusception. It may also be used to assess bowel-wall thickening in cases of inflammatory bowel disease. US is effective in evaluating the GU system and biliary system, as well as the neonatal brain and spine. Doppler US has proven useful in evaluating the renal arteries in children with hypertension, in evaluating vascular and nonvascular lesions, in assessing for ovarian and testicular flow abnormalities, and in determining vessel position and patency. More recently, contrast agents for US have been introduced, which consist of microbubbles and have been used in the evaluation of vesicoureteral reflux.[2,3]

Computed Tomography

CT is based on a volumetric acquisition of information. Helical CT significantly shortens image time, and coronal and sagittal reconstructed images are possible. Three-dimensional reconstructions can be obtained with multidetector CT and are effective in cardiac imaging and in evaluating the airway and skeletal system.[4] The newer-generation CT scanners allow increased speed of scanning such that motion artifact is reduced, and a single breath hold may be sufficient to image large areas. This feature is particularly helpful in young children. CT is not limited by overlying gas and provides a larger field of view than US. It is the imaging modality of choice in evaluating the lungs and is far more sensitive in detecting small lung lesions than plain chest radiographs.[5] CT is also the imaging modality of choice in cases of trauma. Newer uses of CT include CT renal angiography for evaluating for renovascular hypertension,[6] and CT urography to evaluate the renal collecting systems.[7] Neutral oral contrast agents, which distend the small bowel and provide excellent assessment of the bowel lumen and the bowel wall, are useful in patients with inflammatory bowel disease, particularly Crohn disease.[8]

CT has several limitations. Patients must be cooperative, and sedation may be required in young children. Because it is based on grey-scale analysis, intravenous or oral contrast is often required, particularly in children who have very little body fat. With the advent of newer intravenous contrast agents, the risk of adverse contrast reactions has decreased. However, such reactions may still occur, and informed consent is necessary.

A significant limitation of CT is its high radiation dose. A single abdominal CT scan is equivalent to 400 to 500 plain chest radiographs. Based on information from the atom bomb survivors in Japan, recent reports describe a statistically increased risk of malignancy in children exposed to CT imaging, particularly leukemia. From the referring physician's perspective, CT scans should be obtained when specifically indicated and not used as screening examinations. "The procedure should be restricted to cases where it is specifically indicated, and promises to convey a commensurate benefit in terms of a diagnosis that is difficult to obtain by any other means."[9]

Magnetic Resonance Imaging

MRI requires no ionizing radiation and has the advantage of providing multiplanar imaging. The patient must be cooperative, and sedation may be necessary. Examination time is longer than that with a CT scan. Noniodinated contrast agents may be used in select cases and have a low incidence of adverse reactions. MRI provides excellent evaluation of vessels, solid organs, bone marrow, and soft tissues, but it cannot assess lung disease. Cardiac MRI evaluates both cardiac anatomy and cardiac function. MRI provides excellent evaluation of the central nervous system and is the imaging modality of choice to assess the spine, spinal cord, and spinal canal. MR urography displays urograms of nondilated and dilated collecting systems,[7,10,11] and it provides information on both anatomy and function by determining renal transit time.[6] MRI has replaced conventional intravenous pyelograms. MR cholangiography is also useful as a noninvasive method of assessing the biliary and pancreatic ducts.[12,13]

Nuclear Scintigraphy

Nuclear scintigraphy has many uses in children. The diisopropyl iminodiacetic acid (DISIDA) scan can assess biliary excretion and gallbladder function, and is a useful adjunct to US, which provides only anatomic information. The scintigraphic renogram provides differential renal function that can provide information on the degree of renal parenchymal damage. Additionally, when performed after intravenous Lasix administration, it is helpful in confirming the presence or absence of renal obstruction.[14]

Scintigraphy has many applications in pediatric oncology. Positron emission tomography is useful in assessing tumor activity, particularly in cases of lymphoma. Positron emission tomography-CT combines both modalities in a fusion image. This combination provides both anatomic and functional information, and plays an important role in tumor staging, assessing of therapeutic response, and monitoring disease after completion of therapy.[15-17] In patients with neuroblastoma, meta-iodobenzylguanidine (MIBG) scanning is sensitive in detecting tumor activity in both primary and metastatic foci and is effective in evaluating patients for tumor recurrence. The use of thallium scanning (Tl-201) has been used to assess therapeutic response in patients with osteogenic sarcoma and Ewing sarcoma. Decreased tumor uptake of thallium after chemotherapy indicates a favorable response to therapy.[17]

SYSTEMS APPROACH

Chest

The initial evaluation of the chest begins with a plain radiograph. Pneumonia, atelectasis, cardiac enlargement, pleural effusion, and adenopathy can be assessed by plain radiograph. Assessment for an aspirated foreign body is best performed by inspiratory and expiratory films of the chest or bilateral decubitus views of the chest. Parenchymal and airway disease, including congenital, neoplastic, infectious, or inflammatory conditions of the lung, are best evaluated by noncontrast CT. With current software, 3-dimensional endoscopic reconstructions of the airway may be obtained.[4] Intravenous contrast-enhanced CT scans of the chest provide further information on pleural enhancement, loculation, or thickening in the setting of empyema, extent of hilar and mediastinal adenopathy in patients with neoplastic disease, and the presence of vascular anomalies. Congenital abnormalities of the aorta and its branch vessels can be evaluated by either contrast-enhanced CT or MRI (Figure 15-1). Cardiac disease is best assessed by echocardiogram or MRI.

Abdomen

Evaluation of the liver, spleen, and pancreas are best performed by US.[1] Masses, vascular abnormalities, and diffuse parenchymal abnormalities may be identified on US. Infectious processes such as abscesses may also be identified.

US is also the best method of assessing the gallbladder and biliary ductal anatomy. Gallstones not visualized on CT will be evident on US, and biliary duct dilation, stones, or masses can be identified. Findings of cholecystitis, including gallbladder distension, wall thickening, and edema, will be identified. Biliary function, however, is best evaluated with nuclear scintigraphy. Additionally, nuclear scintigraphy is the study of choice in diagnosing biliary atresia. MR cholangiography is a noninvasive method that provides excellent visualization of the biliary ducts (Figure 15-2).

Gastrointestinal Tract

Contrast studies are the study of choice in evaluating the bowel once a plain radiograph has been taken to assess the abdominal bowel gas pattern. Barium or water-soluble contrast agents are administered orally or via feeding tube. In the esophagus, intrinsic lesions such as stenoses, fistulae, rings, foreign bodies, and esophagitis are well defined. Extrinsic lesions such as vascular rings or slings have a characteristic appearance (Figure 15-3). Motility disorders and gastroesophageal reflux may also be diagnosed. Contrast studies also provide information on intrinsic or extrinsic abnormalities of the stomach, including masses and ulcer disease, and is useful in evaluating the integrity of the gastroesophageal junction in children after fundoplication.

In children with suspected possible malrotation, an upper GI series will define the location of the duodenojejunal junction and confirm or exclude proximal small bowel distension. Midgut volvulus also may be diagnosed by US. Characteristically, the normal position of the superior mesenteric artery and vein will be reversed, and a *whirlpool* sign will be demonstrated on color Doppler scanning.[18] US has replaced the upper GI series for the evaluation of the pylorus in cases of suspected pyloric stenosis. The elongated and

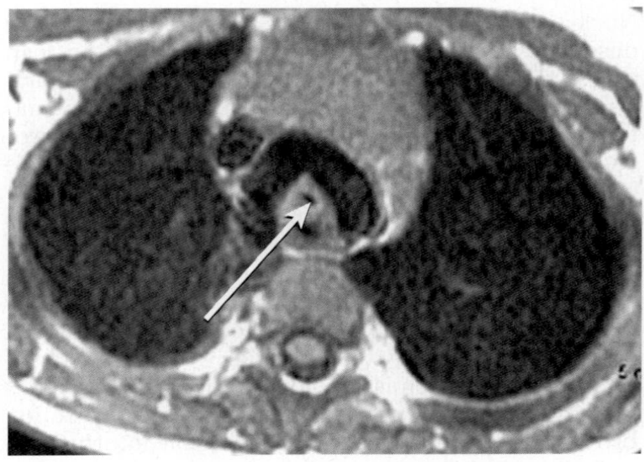

Figure 15-1 T1-weighted axial MR image clearly demonstrates a double aortic arch. Note the narrowed trachea *(arrow)*.

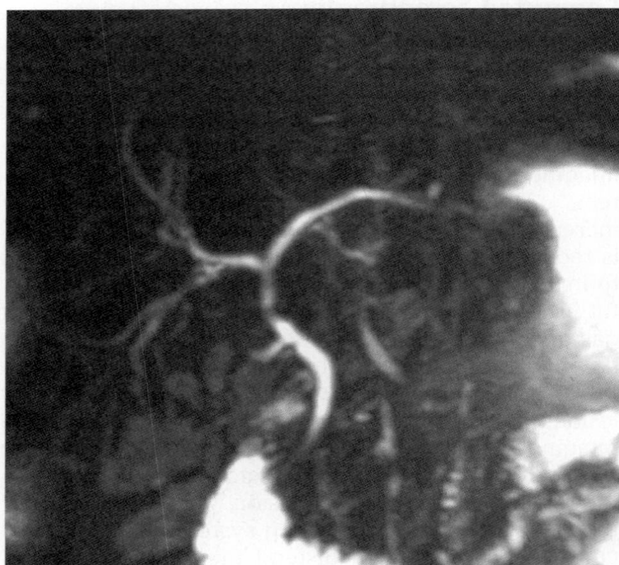

Figure 15-2 Heavily T2-weighted maximal image projection from an MR cholangiogram nicely demonstrates the normal biliary tree.

thickened pyloric muscle characteristic of pyloric stenosis is readily identifiable by US (Figure 15-4).

Small bowel disease, particularly inflammatory bowel disease, is best evaluated by upper GI series and small bowel follow-through or CT. Terminal ileal strictures, fistulae, and mesenteric infiltration can be clearly diagnosed on delayed images focused on the right lower quadrant. CT is helpful in evaluating for associated abscesses.[8] The small bowel follow-through also is effective in evaluating for small bowel polyps, although with the introduction of newer neutral oral contrast agents, the role of CT will likely increase.[8] Nuclear scintigraphy is the method of choice in diagnosing Meckel diverticulum.[19] In cases of possible intussusception, the imaging evaluation should begin with supine, prone, and decubitus views of the abdomen in an attempt to identify a filling defect in the transverse or ascending colon. If intussusception is suspected on plain radiograph, then US confirmation may be obtained. In cases in which an intussusception is present, a multilayered, masslike structure will be located in the abdomen. US has the advantage of providing further information such as the presence or absence of ascites or a lead point and presence or absence of vascularity within the intussuscipiens and intussusceptum. Air reduction enema has replaced contrast enema reduction of intussusceptions. Air is insulflated in a retrograde fashion into the rectum under fluoroscopic guidance. A pressure valve may be used to ensure that the insulflated pressure does not exceed 120 mm Hg.

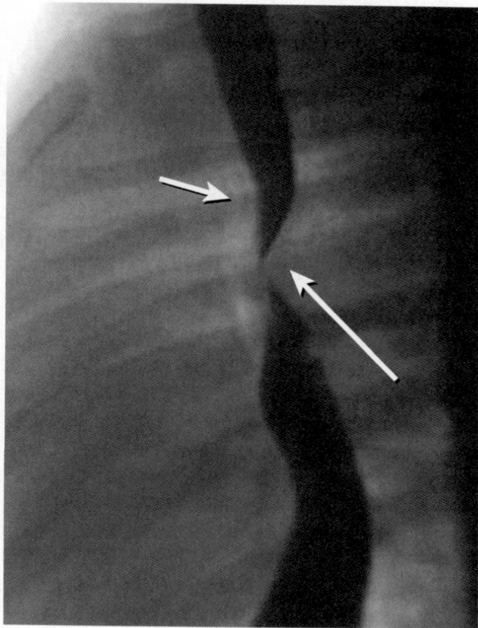

Figure 15-3 Lateral view from a barium esophagram demonstrates an extrinsic impression on the posterior aspect of the esophagus *(long arrow)* and the anterior aspect of the esophagus *(short arrow)*. The finding is consistent with a vascular ring.

The diagnosis of appendicitis can be difficult. Several imaging choices are available to aid in the diagnosis, and many opinions have been given on which modality is best. In a thin, cooperative child, US is an effective method of identifying the inflamed appendix, which will appear as a thick-walled, noncompressible structure with increased vascularity on Doppler US (Figure 15-5). US may also demonstrate the presence of an abscess or appendicolith. Lack of visualization of the appendix does not exclude appendicitis. Recent studies have found that US provides a high degree of diagnostic accuracy in patients with clinical findings suggestive of appendicitis, with a sensitivity of 86%, a specificity of 95%, a positive predictive value of 91%, a negative

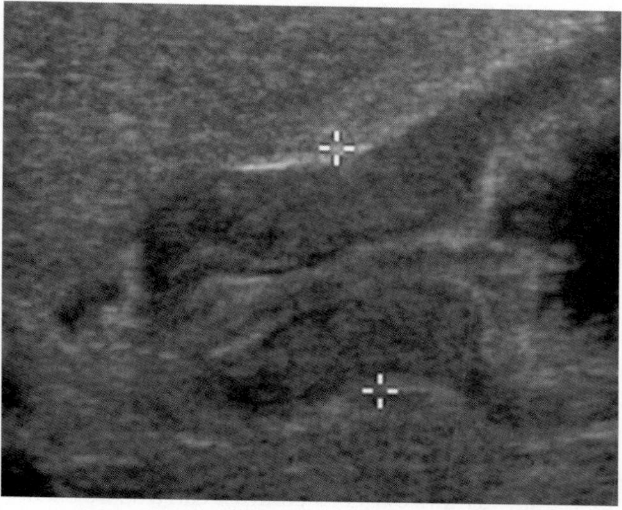

Figure 15-4 Longitudinal US image demonstrates the characteristic thickened and elongated pyloric muscle of pyloric stenosis. Calipers delineate the diameter of the pylorus.

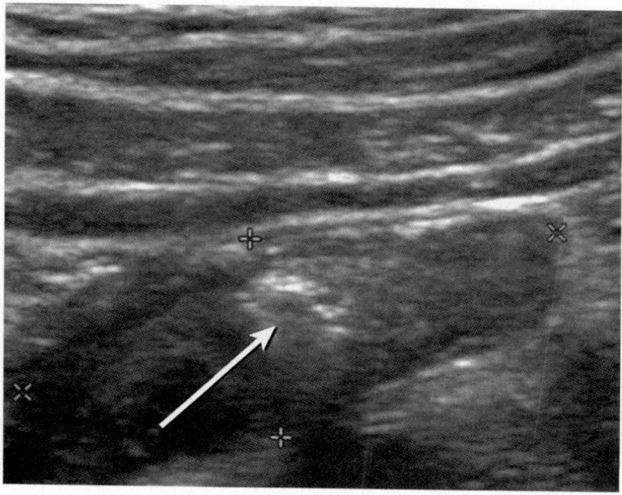

Figure 15-5 US image of an inflamed appendix. Note the appendicolith *(arrow)*. Calipers delineate the inflamed appendix.

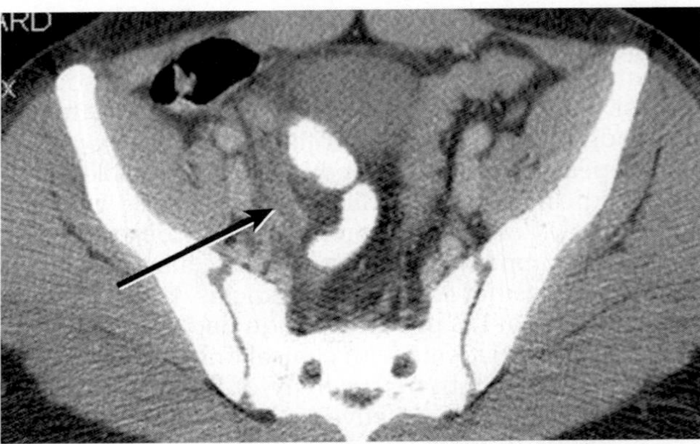

Figure 15-6 Transverse contrast-enhanced CT image of a thickened nonruptured inflamed appendix. A blind ending thickened loop of enhancing bowel is present *(arrow)*.

predictive value of 92%, and a diagnostic accuracy of 92%.[20] Many authors suggest that US be used as the primary imaging modality in evaluating for appendicitis. In cases in which US is nondiagnostic, CT can be used.[20,21] Other authors support the use of CT, with a reported sensitivity and specificity of 96.5% and 98%, respectively, as the initial imaging technique to diagnose appendicitis.[22] Some authors advocate a focused CT scan to reduce radiation exposure.[23] Contrast-enhanced CT-imaging characteristics of acute appendicitis include an enhancing blind ending structure near the cecum (Figure 15-6). Associated abscesses, periappendiceal stranding, appendicolith, and free air can also be readily identified. Rectal contrast can also be used to facilitate contrast filling of the appendix. Visualizing a normal appendix reliably excludes appendicitis.[24]

Recent articles in the surgical literature note that, currently, more than one half of patients with suggested appendicitis are imaged. In many instances, imaging findings provide little increase in diagnostic accuracy when compared with a treating surgeon's clinical examination. Even though imaging may aid in difficult cases,[25] appendicitis remains a clinical diagnosis, and imaging may contribute to delay in treatment and subsequent appendiceal rupture.[26-28]

Patients with ruptured appendicitis, recurrent fever, and possible interloop abscesses are best assessed by CT. US may also be helpful, although air-filled loops may obscure underlying pathologic anomalies.

The colon may be evaluated by contrast enema. This approach is effective in determining the cause of abdominal distension in a neonate with a distal bowel obstruction and is also useful in identifying a transition zone in older patients with Hirschsprung disease.

Genitourinary Tract

The initial assessment of the pediatric GU tract begins with US. The kidneys and bladder are well assessed for hydronephrosis, infectious processes, masses, stones, and anatomic abnormalities by US. Further evaluation for vesicoureteral reflux and structural anomalies of the urethra and upper tracts may be performed by voiding cystourography (Figure 15-7).

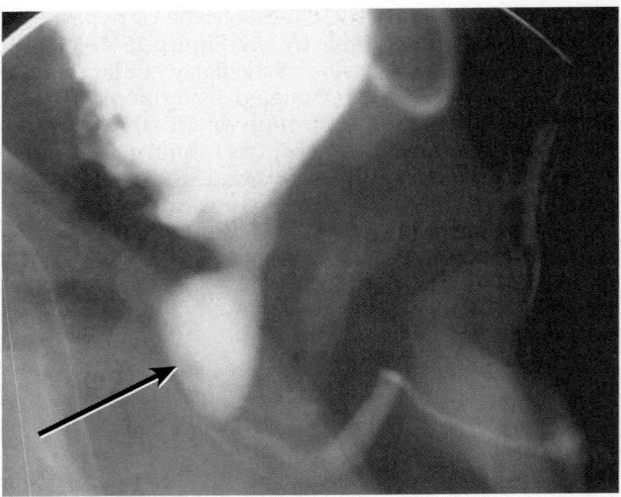

Figure 15-7 Voiding cystourethrogram reveals a trabeculated bladder and a dilated posterior urethra *(arrow)*. Findings are consistent with posterior urethral valves.

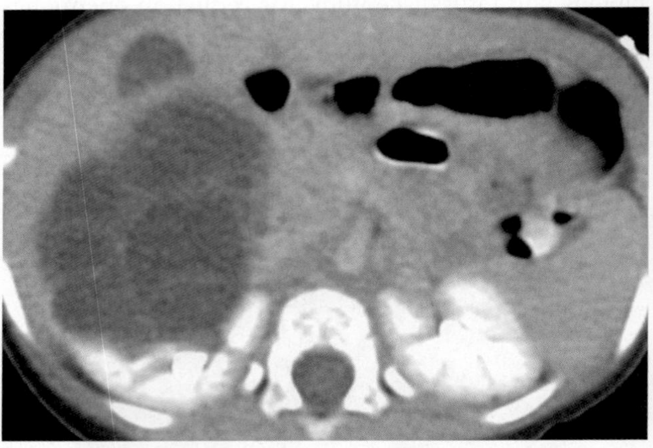

Figure 15-8 Contrast-enhanced CT image of a Wilms tumor.

In the case of a renal mass identified on US, US may assess for the presence of tumor thrombus within the ipsilateral renal vein and the presence of tumor in the contralateral kidney. CT is the study of choice to evaluate for lung metastases. Additionally, contrast-enhanced CT will provide information on tumor extent and vascularity and will also evaluate the contralateral kidney (Figure 15-8). MRI will provide similar information on tumor extent and vascularity and the status of the contralateral kidney. MRI provides superior evaluation of vascular invasion into the inferior vena cava or renal veins but is not effective in assessing for the presence of lung metastases. In the case of neuroblastoma, MRI provides superior evaluation of intraspinal extension and bone marrow involvement.

In patients with renovascular hypertension, Doppler US can detect anatomic abnormalities and provide

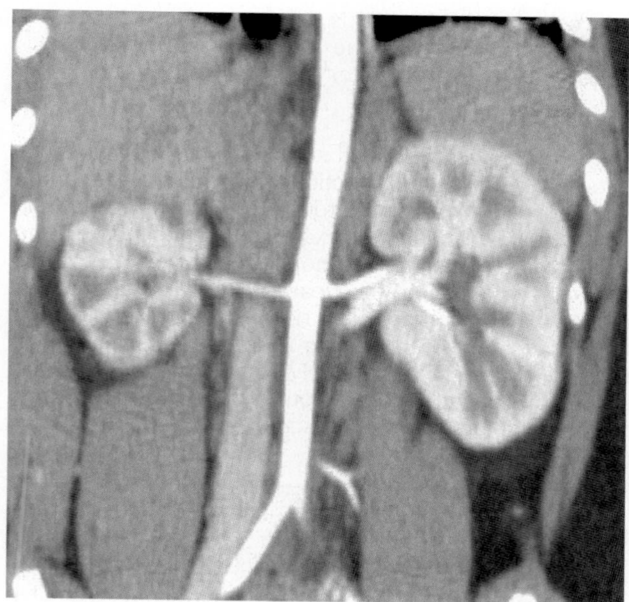

Figure 15-9 Coronal CT image from a CT renal angiogram. Note normal renal arteries.

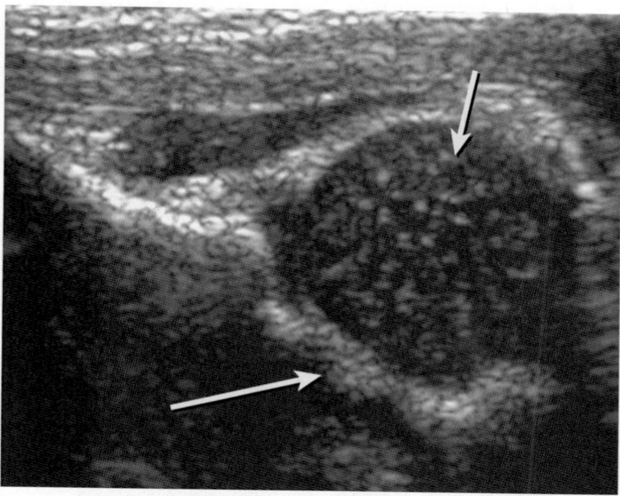

Figure 15-10 Longitudinal image from a hip US. The cartilaginous femoral head *(short arrow)* is well seated in the acetabulum *(long arrow)*.

information on flow velocities and resistive indices in the renal arteries and their branch vessels. However, the examination requires breath-holding and is difficult to perform in small children. CT renal angiography provides excellent anatomic detail of renal artery abnormalities, particularly when images are reconstructed in multiple planes (Figure 15-9). The renal arteries can also be well evaluated by MR angiography.

US may be used to evaluate for pyelonephritis. However, contrast-enhanced CT clearly demonstrates areas of decreased renal perfusion secondary to edema in patients with pyelonephritis in whom US is equivocal. Dimercaptosuccinic acid (DMSA) nuclear scintigraphy is also effective in diagnosing the parenchymal defects characteristic of pyelonephritis. Although CT will demonstrate the extension of an inflammatory process into the perirenal space, nuclear scintigraphic information is limited to abnormalities within the renal parenchyma. Upper tract stone disease is best assessed by US. Noncontrast CT imaging has the advantage of identifying ureteral stones that may not be detected on US because of overlying bowel gas. Renal function is best evaluated by nuclear scintigraphy. Recently, MR urography has been introduced and may also provide information on anatomic features and function.[6]

Bone

Evaluation of the skeletal system begins with a plain radiograph. This method is effective in defining fractures, joint effusions, gross marrow infiltration, extent of scoliosis, and healing areas of bone infarction. In children who are suspected of having nonaccidental trauma, skeletal surveys are indicated and include the evaluation of the skull, spine, ribs, pelvis, long bones, hands, and feet.[29] Skeletal surveys are also useful in evaluating patients with bone dysplasias.

Musculoskeletal US is useful in evaluating infants with developmental dysplasia of the hip (Figure 15-10), in assessing for joint effusions, and in directing the aspiration of the effusions under US guidance. US may also be used to evaluate for subperiosteal collections in cases of osteomyelitis.[30]

MRI has the advantage of being able to define marrow, cortical, and soft-tissue involvement and has become the imaging modality of choice in evaluating for skeletal lesions and osteomyelitis (Figure 15-11). MRI also has the ability to evaluate cartilage[31] and is particularly useful in the skeletally immature child.

The use of CT in assessing the pediatric musculoskeletal system is limited. In the setting of trauma, CT reconstructions may be used to determine the degree of malalignment and displacement of fracture fragments at an articular surface. Additionally, in children with developmental dysplasia of the hip after varus derotational osteotomy and casting, CT best determines the position of the femoral head relative to the acetabulum. Last, scanograms to evaluate for leg length discrepancy can now be performed with a CT scout, rather than plain radiographs.

Bone scintigraphy is useful in cases of possible osteomyelitis but can be limited by the normally increased radiotracer uptake seen in the metaphyses of growing bones, which may obscure areas of abnormally increased uptake in sites of metaphyseal osteomyelitis, a problem not encountered with MRI. Nuclear scintigraphy may be useful in cases of possible child abuse and may detect rib fractures that may not be evident on plain radiographs.[29] Nuclear scintigraphy is also helpful in cases in which multifocal bone disease is suggested, such as malignancy or multifocal osteomyelitis.

Nervous System

Central nervous system imaging is performed by US, CT, or MRI. In neonates and infants with open fontanelles, US is an excellent method of imaging the brain.

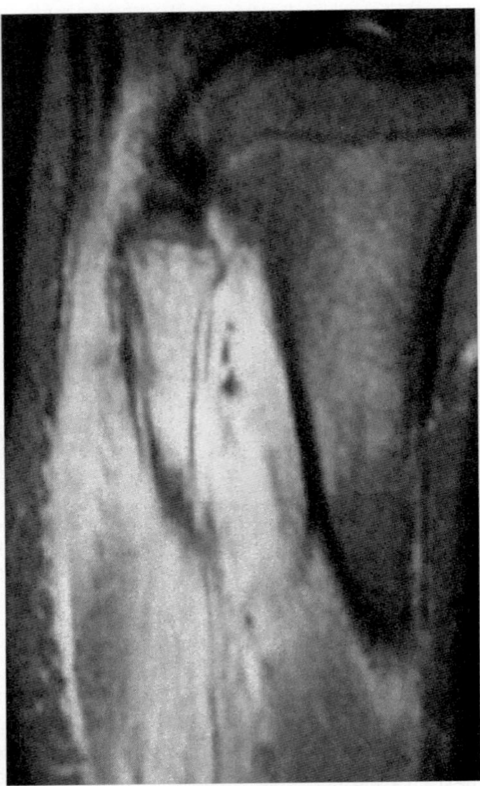

Figure 15-11 T2-weighted MR image of the leg demonstrates high signal within the fibular marrow with adjacent soft tissue changes. The findings are consistent with osteomyelitis.

Repeat US studies can be performed to follow intracranial hemorrhage and ventricular size. Areas of the brain not well visualized by US and better evaluated by CT or MRI include the brain surface and the frontal and occipital poles. In the neonate, assessment of the spinal cord can be performed with US, given that the posterior elements have not fused, and an acoustic window is present. US is effective in determining the position of the conus in the infant with a sacral dimple. It may also identify intraspinal abnormalities such as lipomas. Findings may be confirmed with MRI.[32]

The neonatal brain also may be assessed by CT or MRI. Both modalities demonstrate similar findings, with greater interobserver agreement with MRI. Additionally, MRI provides no ionizing radiation to the patient.[33] In older children, MRI has the same advantages over CT and more clearly demonstrates myelination abnormalities, edema, and infarcts. MRI is the study of choice in evaluating the spine, spinal cord, and spinal canal in children because the posterior elements have fused. Newer uses of MRI include diffusion-perfusion imaging and MR spectroscopy.[34]

Although CT imaging of the brain has been largely replaced by MRI, it remains the most sensitive modality to detect subarachnoid blood and calcifications, which may be present in congenital lesions such as TORCH (***t***oxoplasmosis, ***o***ther agents, ***r***ubella, ***c***ytomegalovirus, ***h***erpes simplex) infections and tuberous sclerosis. In addition, CT is the study of choice in evaluating the temporal bone and in assessing for fractures of the face and spine.[34]

CONCLUSION

Although newer imaging modalities now offer more detailed anatomic and functional information, the many imaging choices available to the clinician can be overwhelming. The choice of examination depends on the question that the clinician hopes to answer. The more focused the question, the clearer the choice of imaging modality. Radiation dose and risk of sedation, if required, and the ability of the child to undergo the examination must be considered. Ultimately, the pediatric radiologist should be consulted to help guide the clinician through the myriad of imaging choices.

TOOLS FOR PRACTICE

Engaging Patients and Family

- *What Is a Pediatric Radiologist?* (fact sheet), American Academy of Pediatrics (www.aap.org/family/pedspecfactsheets.htm).
- *Tests and Procedures* (sample fact sheet), Cincinnati Children's Hospital Medical Center (www.cincinnatichildrens.org/svc/alpha/r/radiology/tests.htm).
- *Radiation Dose with Computed Tomography (CT)* (fact sheet), Cincinnati Children's Hospital Medical Center (www.cincinnatichildrens.org/svc/alpha/r/radiology/radiation-cat-scans.htm).
- *Pediatric Abdominal Ultrasound*, Fact Sheet, Radiology Info, (www.radiologyinfo.org/en/info.cfm?PG=abdomus-pdi&bhcp=1).
- *Pediatric Nuclear Medicine* (fact sheet), Radiology Info (www.radiologyinfo.org/en/info.cfm?PG=nuclear-pdi).
- *Pediatric Computed Tomography (CT)* (fact sheet), Radiology Info, (www.radiologyinfo.org/en/info.cfm?PG=pedia-ct).

REFERENCES

1. Lambot K, Lougue-Sorgho LC, Gorincour G, et al. Imaging of the pediatric pancreas: state of the art [in French]. *J Radiol*. 2005;86:807-815.
2. Ascenti G, Zimbaro G, Mazziotti S, et al. Harmonic US imaging of vesicoureteral reflux in children: usefulness of a second generation US contrast agent. *Pediatr Radiol*. 2004;34(6):481-487.
3. Darge K, Moeller RT, Trusen A, et al. Diagnosis of vesicoureteric reflux with low-dose contrast-enhanced harmonic ultrasound imaging. *Pediatr Radiol*. 2005;35(1):73-78.
4. Manson D, Babyn P, Riller R, et al. Three-dimensional imaging of the pediatric trachea in congenital tracheal stenosis. *Pediatr Radiol*. 1994;24(3):175-179.
5. Meisel JA, Guthrie KA, Breslow NE, et al. Significance and management of computed tomography detected pulmonary nodules: a report from the National Wilms Tumor Study Group. *Int J Radiat Oncol Biol Phys*. 1999;44(3):579-585.
6. Jones RA, Perez-Brayfield MR, Kirsch AJ, et al. Renal transit time with MR urography in children. *Radiology*. 2004;233(1):41-50.
7. Kawashima A, Glockner JF, King BF Jr. CT urography and MR urography. *Radiol Clin*. 2003;41(5):945-961.

8. Megibow AJ, Babb JS, Hecht EM, et al. Evaluation of bowel distention and bowel wall appearance by using neutral oral contrast agent for multi-detector row CT. *Radiology*. 2006;238(1):87-95.
9. Hall EJ. Lessons we have learned from our children: cancer risks from diagnostic radiology. *Pediatr Radiol*. 2002; 32:700-706.
10. Rothpearl A, Frager D, Subramanian A. MR urography: technique and application. *Radiology*. 1995;194(1):125-130.
11. Kocaoglu M, Ilica AT, Bulakbasi N, et al. MR urography in pediatric uropathies with dilated urinary tracts. *Diagn Interv Radiol*. 2005;11(4):225-232.
12. Arcement CM, Meza MP, Arumania S, Towbin RB. MRCP in the evaluation of pancreaticobiliary disease in children. *Pediatr Radiol*. 2001;31(2):92-97.
13. Miyazaki T, Yamashita Y, Tang Y, et al. Single-shot MR cholangiopancreatography of neonates, infants and young children. *Am J Roentgenol*. 1998;170(1):33-37.
14. Piepsz A, Ham HR. Pediatric applications of renal nuclear medicine. *Semin Nucl Med*. 2006;36(1):16-35.
15. Hudson MM, Krasin MJ, Kaste SC. PET imaging in pediatric Hodgkin's lymphoma. *Pediatr Radiol*. 2004;34(3): 190-198.
16. Tatsumi M, Cohade C, Nakamoto Y, et al. Direct Comparison of FDG PET and CT findings in patients with lymphoma: initial experience. *Radiology*. 2005;237:1038-1045.
17. Jadvar H, ALavi A, Mavi A, et al. PET in pediatric diseases. *Radiol Clin North Am* 2005;43:135-152.
18. Pracros JP, Sann L, Genin G, et al. Ultrasound diagnosis of midgut volvulus: the "whirlpool" sign. *Pediatr Radiol*. 1992;22(1):18-20.
19. Kumar R, Tripathi M, Chandrashekar N, et al. Diagnosis of ectopic gastric mucosa using ^{99}Tc^{m}-pertechnetate: spectrum of scintigraphic findings. *Br J Radiol*. 2005;78(932):714-720.
20. Kaiser S, Frenckner B, Jorulf HK. Suspected appendicitis in children: US and CT—a prospective randomized study. *Radiology*. 2002;223(3):633-638.
21. Hernandez JA, Swischuk LE, Angel CA, et al. Imaging of acute appendicitis: US as the primary imaging modality. *Pediatr Radiol*. 2005;35(4):392-395.
22. Raman SS, Lu DS, Kadell BM, et al. Accuracy of nonfocused helical CT for the diagnosis of acute appendicitis: a 5-year review. *Am J Roentgenol*. 2002;178(6):1319-1325.
23. Mittal VK, Goliath J, Sabir M, et al. Advantages of focused helical computed tomographic scanning with rectal contrast only vs triple contrast in the diagnosis of clinically uncertain acute appendicitis: a prospective randomized study. *Arch Surg*. 2004;139(5):495-499.
24. Acosta R, Crain EF, Goldman HS. CT can reduce hospitalization for observation in children with suspected appendicitis. *Pediatr Radiol*. 2005;35(5):495-500.
25. Horton MD, Counter SF, Florence MG, et al. A prospective trial of computed tomography and ultrasonography for diagnosing appendicitis in the atypical patient. *Am J Surg*. 2000;179(5):379-381.
26. Karakas, SP, Guelfguat M, Leonidas JC, et al. Acute appendicitis in children: comparison of clinical diagnosis with ultrasound and CT imaging. *Pediatr Radiol*. 2000;30(2):94-98.
27. Partrick DA, Janik JE, Janik JS, et al. Increased CT scan utilization does not improve the diagnostic accuracy of appendicitis in children. *J Pediatr Surg*. 2003;38(5):659-662.
28. York D, Smith A, Phillips JD, et al. The influence of advanced radiographic imaging on the treatment of pediatric appendicitis. *J Pediatr Surg*. 2005;40(12):1908-1911.
29. Kleinman PK, Marks SC, Blackbourne B. The metaphyseal lesion in abused infants: a radiologic-histopathologic study. *Am J Roentgenol*. 1986;146(5):895-905.
30. Keller MS. Musculoskeletal sonography in the neonate and infant. *Pediatr Radiol*. 2005;35:1167-1173.
31. Jaramillo D, Shapiro F. Growth cartilage: normal appearance, variants and abnormalities. *Magn Reson Imaging Clin North Am*. 1998;6(3):455-471.
32. Fitz CR. Techniques in neuroimaging. In: Silverman FN, Kuhn JP eds. *Essentials of Caffey's Pediatric X-Ray Diagnosis*. Chicago, IL: Year Book Medical Publishers, Inc; 1990:106-174.
33. Robertson RL, Robson CD, Zurakowski D, et al. CT versus MR in neonatal brain imaging at term. *Pediatr Radiol*. 2003;33(7):442-449.
34. Grossman RI, Yousem DM. In: *Neuroradiology: The Requisites*. 2nd ed. Philadelphia, PA: Mosby; 2003.

Chapter 16

DISCLOSING A DIAGNOSIS WITH PARENTS AND PATIENTS

Ruth J. Messinger, MSW; Daniel W. Mruzek, PhD; Emily S. Kuschner, MA; Philip W. Davidson, PhD

Simplifying treatment choices and clarifying prognoses are critical goals in the disclosure of any diagnosis with parents. An important step in this process is the sharing of pertinent information with the child or with the child's parents or advocates. In most circumstances in which the illness is minor or carries an excellent prognosis, the diagnostician presents such information straightforwardly to the patient or the parents. However, in cases that involve children who are gravely ill, severely disabled, autistic, learning disabled, or emotionally disturbed or those who have an intellectual disability, the situation becomes far more complex. Parents, years after the fact, vividly remember how and when the *bad news* was related.[1] The interpretive presentation, often involving one or more specialists, must become part of a broader counseling session that deals with feelings and emotions, as well as facts, to ensure understanding of the information being shared.

This chapter focuses on the process of information sharing with parents or patient as an extension of the diagnostic process. The goal of interpreting diagnostic findings is more than merely announcing technical information. The real objective in providing this information is to establish a partnership between the primary care physician and the parents that will enhance the parents' capacity to respond appropriately to their child's condition, to comply with the recommended treatment, and to become a partner with the rest of the treatment team. This partnership between parents and professionals is even more crucial when considering that federal legislation mandates participation by parents in decisions about their children who have special needs (eg, autism, intellectual disability) and chronic conditions (eg, ventilator dependency). The Reauthorization of the Individuals with Disabilities Education Act (Public Law No. 108-446), for example, emphasizes family-centered, coordinated, case-managed care and parent-driven planning of service provision to their offspring ages 0 to 2 years who have disabilities.

No blueprint exists for building the crucial relationship between clinician and parents; however, interpretation of the physician's findings to parents without unnecessary delay is essential in case management, as is the need to attend to the family's expectations and questions initially and over time. Moreover, negative attitudes, disrespect for the parents' knowledge and beliefs, and the clinician's own biases and anxieties interfere with constructive communication about a child's diagnosis and treatment. This dialogue may be complicated further when clinicians become frustrated by their inability to cure or *save* the child, when they know that no local resources are available to deal with the child's problem, or when the parents ask questions that the clinician cannot answer.[2]

A professional-parent relationship based on the posture, "I have the information, and I know what's best for your child," represents a basic misinterpretation of the kind of relationship between parent and clinician that is necessary when information about a complex and threatening illness or disability has to be shared. Diagnosis and treatment are biomedical, but psychosocial and educational matters and their presentation to parents are decidedly nonmedical. Assuming that simply having information or knowledge about *what is best* for the child is sufficient for communicating diagnostic, therapeutic, and prognostic information to the parents is inappropriate. Parents usually know their child better than anyone else and are central as nurturers, caretakers, and guardians of their children.

To communicate effectively, clinicians must maintain a flow of information between parents and themselves; simply telling parents the facts of an evaluation does not guarantee that they will hear or understand. Considering this circumstance, disclosure should be an interactional process that is conversational in nature and demonstrates respect for the equality and individual needs of the parents.[3,4] Such communication can be described in general terms, but its effective implementation depends on careful individual planning and a reasonable investment of time. Box 16-1 outlines a method for conducting an *interpretive* conference. The format outlines four equally important steps that are essential for effective communication when the child is evaluated by the clinician (physician, nurse, psychologist, social worker, or educational specialist) alone or when several professionals have been involved as members of an interdisciplinary team in the diagnostic evaluation.

BOX 16-1 Interpretive Conference Format Outline

I. Entry pattern
   A. Review of evaluation procedures conducted
   B. Parents' and child's perceptions
   C. Restatement of parental concerns
      1. Main worry
      2. Additional concerns
II. Presentation of findings
   A. Encapsulation: brief overview
   B. Reaction by parents and patient
   C. Detailed findings
      1. Reactions to normal test results
      2. Reactions to abnormal test results
III. Recommendations—only after time has been allowed for reactions
   A. Restatement of concerns with both parents
   B. Recommendations—one at a time
   C. Reactions after each recommendation
   D. Sharing with the child
IV. Summary
   A. Repetition of findings, in varied wording if possible
   B. Restatement by parents or patient
   C. Planning for future contacts

PREPARATION FOR AN INTERPRETIVE CONFERENCE

The interpretive conference must be planned beforehand to ensure that the conference will achieve its purpose. The conference should occur as soon as possible after the examination and testing of the patient. The clinician who conducts the conference is best prepared, emotionally and cognitively, immediately after the last visit or staffing conference, and parents are anxious to hear about the outcome of the evaluation as soon as possible.

If more than one professional is involved in the conference, then the basic aim should be to establish maximal communication between parents and professionals while this expertise is available, thus ensuring that most parental questions can be answered effectively. With certain conditions, such as intellectual disability, autism, and learning or emotional disorders, the physician may not be included in the conference or may not be the primary spokesperson. In these circumstances the psychologist, special educator, or social work clinician might serve this role.

Parents sometimes view the physician as the *ultimate authority figure*, and, in these cases, the credibility of a team that does not include the physician may be impaired. On the other hand, the physician need not automatically be cast in the role of leader at an interpretive conference unless the bulk of the information to be discussed is biomedical. In no case should the interpretation of technical material to parents be left in the hands of nonprofessionals or professionals whose lack of expertise might lead to parental misunderstanding. Additionally, only professionals who participated in the diagnostic work-up should reveal the information.

Once the team members have been selected, they should meet long enough to organize the conference, following the outline in Box 16-1. This planning session should allow enough time to ensure that all the team members agree on the major information to be shared with the parents and that all terminology is understood. Because organization of the conference is the key to satisfactory communication, team members should also select a leader who will structure the conference. This selection is of paramount importance. The leader's responsibility is to control the flow of information from professionals to parents and vice versa to ensure two-way communication. *Control* implies not only organization but also a certain empathic sensitivity for the parents' feelings and reactions so that emotional highs and lows can be adequately recognized, permitted, and dealt with in ways that respect the families' cultural proscriptions and without undermining the purpose of the conference. These preparations are especially important when only one clinician is to be present at the conference. During disclosure, the lone clinician will not have the colleagues present to add omitted points or rephrase statements that remain unclear to parents.

CONDUCTING THE CONFERENCE

Entry Pattern

The beginning of the interview often sets the tone for what follows. The assumption is that planning has included specific physical requirements that create an empathic climate, privacy, and freedom from interruption and that the professional has arranged to arrive on time. Reviewing diagnostic results should be shared with a minimum of technical jargon so that parents are not intimidated when asked to discuss their main worry. During such a discussion a hidden agenda often surfaces, related either to the cause of the problem or to the problem itself. Therefore, before the information is presented to the parents, the parents' perception of the child and the child's current situation should be sought. For example, the practitioner might ask both parents, "How do you see Mary's problems and strengths today?" Even if both parents have accompanied their child throughout the evaluation, each may have different knowledge about and reactions to what is happening.[5,6] This time also is appropriate to ask what others have told them of their child's condition.

Presentation of Findings

Dwelling on technical data that do little to enhance the parents' understanding of their child's disorder accomplishes nothing and may interfere with establishing good professional-parent communication. Such data only serve to confuse, rather than clarify, the parents' concerns. When several different tests have been performed in a lengthy, technical evaluation, understanding that the data presented summarize the results of all those tests is especially helpful for parents. Some parents need a name for their child's illness or problem. If labels have not already been used by others, then they may well be in the future. Most parents want honest appraisals and will resent ambiguous assurances that border on deception. *Honesty with tact is vital.* For example, if an infant has been born having fetal alcohol syndrome, the parents should be clearly and directly informed of the diagnosis rather than their being given vague or technical terms such as *multiple craniofacial and other anomalies* to explain their child's condition. Similarly, if the determination has been made that a school-aged child has an intellectual disability, then this finding should be presented gently but directly, with avoidance of euphemisms or inaccurate terms (eg, *slow learner, learning disabled*).

The practitioner or practitioners should focus on the parents' own perceptions of their child when explaining findings, particularly as these may relate to the parent's experiences with other children. Age or grade equivalents rather than ratio scores are useful when conveying the presence of developmental delay or immaturity is necessary. For example, the clinician might say, "Susan's language development is delayed. You tell me that she, at age 2, babbles but has no words. Babbling is the typical way a 10 month old communicates." Rather than "Your son's test scores show 'scatter,' and he has a learning disability," a clearer statement would be, "Joey reads and understands written information more like a third grader than a ninth grader."

It often is said that after the parents hear the bad news, they hear very little else. For this reason the actual presentation should begin with areas of strength or normality. In fact, this presentation is as much a part of the clinician's responsibility as describing weaknesses, and doing so provides parents with the opportunity to more clearly see current ability and establish new hopes for their child's future.[7] Abnormal findings stated honestly but gently should be restated more than once and by using different words to convey the same findings. Indeed, Kaminer and Cohen[8] emphasize the relationship between empathy and honesty: "The literature documents that communication skills can be taught or at least improved. Acquiring an understanding heart seems to be more difficult." Parents should be encouraged to react to the diagnosis of the problem and to accept their feelings, including the anger that is often directed at the clinician. Professionals need to learn how to cope with parent anger and not to expect gratitude. Responses that reflect shock, guilt, bereavement, and inadequacy frequently are seen in various intensities and combinations. Parents need to be assured of the normalcy of those responses.[9,10] Communication at this level is also influenced by any sociocultural and educational differences between the professionals and the parents.

Recommendations

Specific information should be shared at a pace that can be handled emotionally and cognitively. Parents seldom feel comfortable asking for clarification; however, if they are asked to restate their main worry and other concerns, the practitioner's recommendations can become meaningful and relevant. Parents often welcome clearly written take-home materials that provide current and accurate information on the relevant diagnosis, including general descriptions of treatment and intervention options. In fact, Brogan and Knussen[4] found that the provision of written materials by clinicians was a key factor in promoting parent satisfaction with their disclosure experience. Information regarding additional resources, such as family resource rooms at some medical libraries and local family support groups, as well as reputable internet sites, give parents options for educating themselves about their child's diagnosis. Questions about complementary and alternative treatments (eg, specialized diets for autism) should be treated with compassion, respect, and honesty.[11] Finally, parents usually find it helpful to receive recommendations that include opportunities to communicate with other parents who have a child with a similar problem and referral elsewhere for help.

Recommendations are not complete until the clinician and both parents are able to decide what will be communicated to the child and who will do it. Parents' wishes and the cognitive and emotional development of the child are important considerations in this important issue. After recommendations have been shared and before the session is terminated, findings, once again, should be highlighted. One successful method for obtaining feedback is to ask parents to restate what they heard and what decisions were made. This approach provides the professional with the parents' perception and understanding of the problem and allows for further clarification, if necessary.

In many instances, more than one interpretive session is indicated. This session can be planned by arranging for parents to contact the clinician by telephone (at a specific time) after they have had time to think about and react to the information that was shared or when further questions and concerns arise. The session should be terminated only after the clinician has stated a willingness and an ability to participate in a therapeutic alliance with the parents.

SUMMARY

Discussion of diagnostic findings is a dynamic process that is an initial step in building a therapeutic milieu. The model presented here organizes a typically complex, often unwieldy, process between the professional and the parents that can easily end disastrously and decrease chances for successful therapeutic intervention with the patient. If the clinical findings, diagnosis, and prognosis are presented clearly during the conference, then two-way communication will be fostered because both the professional and the parents can identify the limits of the situation and focus on the problems that can be dealt with successfully. This method of imparting information enhances the professional-parent relationship and encourages immediate and future communication and compliance with recommendations.

REFERENCES

1. Ptacek JT, Eberhardt TL. Breaking bad news: a review of the literature. *JAMA*. 1996;276:496-502.
2. Fallowfield L, Jenkins V. Communicating sad, bad, and difficult news in medicine. *Lancet*. 2004;:312-319.
3. Sattler JM. *Assessment of Children, Behavioral and Clinical Applications*. 4th ed. San Diego, CA: Jerome M. Sattler, Publisher; 2002.
4. Brogan CA, Knussen C. The disclosure of a diagnosis of an autistic spectrum disorder. *Autism*. 2003;7:31-46.
5. Bailey D, Blasco P, Simeonsson R. Needs expressed by mothers and fathers of young children with disabilities. *Am J Ment Retard*. 1992;97:1-10.
6. Rimmerman A, Turkel L, Crossman R. Perception of child development, child-related stress and dyadic adjustment: pair analysis of married couples of young children with developmental disabilities. *J Intellectual Dev Disabil*. 2003;28:188-195.
7. Skotko B. Mothers of children with Down syndrome reflect on their postnatal support. *Pediatrics*. 2005;115: 64-77.
8. Kaminer R, Cohen H. How do you say, "your child is retarded"? *Contemp Pediatr*. 1988;5:36-49.
9. Girgis A, Sasone-Fisher R. Breaking bad news I: current best advice for clinicians. *Behav Med*. 1998;24:53-59.
10. Hasnat MJ, Graves P. Disclosure of developmental disability: a study of parent satisfaction and the determinants of satisfaction. *J Paediatr Child Health*. 2000;36: 32-35.
11. Hyman S, Levy S. Autism spectrum disorders: when traditional medicine is not enough. *Contemp Pediatr*. 2000;10:101-111.

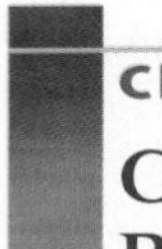

Chapter 17

CULTURAL ISSUES IN PRIMARY PEDIATRIC CARE

Karen N. Olness, MD; Kristine Torjesen, MD, MPH

Child health professionals in North America have more cross-cultural issues to consider than do child health professionals elsewhere in the world, and they receive little guidance and preparation for these issues. US child health care providers encounter cross-cultural issues when diagnosing and treating families who are newcomers to the United States or those whose cultural heritages relate to parents or grandparents who immigrated to the United States. Furthermore, US child health care providers are mobile and may themselves work in several different cultural environments during a lifetime. In the future the services of US child health experts will likely be required increasingly in less industrialized countries,[1] where 90% of the world's babies are born. Primary care practitioners encounter different types of cross-cultural situations (Boxes 17-1, 17-2, and 17-3). As they become familiar with particular beliefs, practitioners learn how to cope with these situations. However, clients may never overtly demonstrate more complex cross-cultural issues; these issues can result in poor adherence, the seeking of another physician, or misinterpretation of the diagnosis and treatment. The goal of cross-cultural medicine, now taught in many medical schools, is not to familiarize physicians with all cultural issues related to medicine but rather to sensitize physicians to different cultural beliefs that may affect expectations regarding the role of the physician and how families view diseases and treatments.

BOX 17-1 Example 1

You are working in a pediatric emergency room, and you evaluate an 11-month-old child who was born in the Middle East. He has had a fever and cold for a week. On examination, you find signs of otitis media and round, ulcerated areas on both wrists. The family explains that they were treating the child with crushed garlic cloves taped onto the child's wrists.

BOX 17-2 Example 2

You are a middle-aged pediatrician working in the outpatient department of a large county hospital. A Hmong-American child is brought in with a cold and fever. You conduct a thorough examination, including otoscopy, and diagnose otitis media. Through the translator, you prescribe amoxicillin and arrange for a follow-up appointment. Two days later the child, who is still febrile, returns in the company of 10 adult relatives and the translator. You begin an examination. However, when you reach for the otoscope, the translator says that the family requests that you not use it.

BOX 17-3 Example 3

You work in a small group practice and have many Mexican-American families as clients. One of the nurse assistants is Mexican American, and she brings her children to the practice for well-child care. She is well liked by families and colleagues within the practice. One day, she mentions that her 4-year-old son is ill, and she asks to leave early. You offer to see him, and she replies that he has *empacho*, a gastrointestinal illness, and that she is taking him to see a healer in the family because empacho cannot be cured by conventional medical treatment.

DEFINITIONS

Americans living in urban areas encounter cultural differences every day. The individual's perception of social self, as well as culture and cultural norms all play a part in the way reality is defined. *Social self* refers to the way individuals perceive or present themselves to others. It includes the degree of acceptance of the culture or subculture in which the individuals live and how they project this acceptance or rejection to those around them. *Culture* is defined as a way of life for a group of people: how they work; how they relax; their values, prejudices, and biases; and the way they interact with one another. *Cultural norms* are the ethical, moral, or traditional principles of a given society and include unwritten definitions of health, sickness, and abnormality. Social self, culture, and cultural norms change over generations of families. Persons of the same ethnic group may have very different cultures or cultural norms. Consider, for example, the different cultures of a Chinese farmer living in a rural area of Shanxi province and a fourth-generation American who is ethnically Chinese, has a doctorate in economics, and lives in a mostly white suburb of Minneapolis. Focusing on individual families as unique cultural units rather than on the cultural origins or ethnic background of the family is preferable because what is typical of a group does not necessarily predict the beliefs of an individual.[2,3] *Cultural competency* is defined as the recognition of and appropriate response to key cultural features that affect clinical care.[4]

EXPLANATIONS OF DISEASE: CULTURAL VARIATIONS

Namboze[5] noted that cultural beliefs about disease causation in Ganda society fall under the following categories: magical, supernatural, infectious, and hereditary. She notes that some of these beliefs are beneficial and can be included in health teaching. Other beliefs are harmless and best left alone by child health professionals; some cultural practices, however, are harmful. In general, these types of cultural beliefs and practices are common to all societies.

Many ethnic groups within the United States bring their ill children to both pediatricians and traditional healers within the community.[6-9] Special ceremonies, herbal remedies, chanting, and prayer are often prescribed by the latter. Sharing this information with their pediatricians is unusual for the family unless the pediatrician is of the same ethnic group, speaks the same language, or has a longstanding, trusting relationship with the family.

Notably, families from many different cultural backgrounds may purchase vitamins, minerals, and food supplements at health food stores or consult chiropractors for their children and may not inform their pediatricians about all treatments being used.[10]

A recent survey of American adults found that 34% reported using at least one unconventional therapy in the last year. A third of these adults saw practitioners of unconventional therapy, making an average of 19 visits in 1 year. The type of therapy included relaxation and imagery techniques, chiropractic and spiritual healing, commercial weight-loss programs, megavitamin therapy, homeopathy, acupuncture, and massage.[11]

CULTURAL ASSESSMENT

Appraising a family's cultural beliefs, values, and customs is an essential part of health assessment. A cultural assessment is as important as a physical or psychological assessment and can be used to understand behavior that might otherwise be interpreted as negative or noncompliant. A cultural assessment involves asking open-ended questions about the family's cultural background and beliefs and listening to the responses in a nonjudgmental way. The ability to be interculturally sensitive is desirable but difficult. Teufel[12] has noted that ethnocentricity counteracts the ability to be interculturally sensitive and describes six stages of development toward the ideal. Initially the other culture is denied, and cultural differences go unrecognized. The second stage is defensive and a person may either denigrate the other culture or claim the person's own to be superior. The third stage is that differences between cultures are trivialized, but such a perspective does not recognize the different social, physical, and spiritual environments in which worldviews are constructed. In the fourth stage the individual moves toward accepting that a cultural difference exists and that another culture is worthy of understanding. In the fifth stage, the person adapts to the difference and shifts from an ethnocentric world view to one that is ethnorelative. Finally, the ideal is that the difference is integrated. The individual attains the ability to analyze and evaluate situations from one or more cultural perspectives and is neither totally a part of nor totally apart from the person's own culture but lives on a comfortable boundary.

The practitioner should avoid stereotypical assumptions and remain sensitive to individual differences within cultural groups while gathering information concerning a particular family. For example, although alcoholism is prevalent in many Native American tribes, assuming that any Native American treated is an alcoholic would be erroneous. A tendency exists to assume that all members of a similar cultural background share commonalities, such as language, religion, and viewpoints. Developing a false sense of cultural knowledge can impede the practitioner from learning specific aspects about a particular family. An accurate understanding of several cultures would certainly take an anthropologist years of study. The best recommendation is to review the available literature and interview colleagues who are members of a specific cultural group. Observation and interview are two useful tools when assessing cultural background. Although gathering information about ethnic group affiliation, preferred language, and dietary practices may take a relatively short time, knowing about the values and beliefs, including health beliefs, of a given family may take a long time.[13]

The American Medical Association distributes a manual on providing culturally competent care to adolescents.[14] This guide lists open-ended questions to facilitate understanding of how an adolescent from another culture perceives personal health problems, for example, "Apart from me, who do you think can help you get better?"

Ethnic Group Affiliation and Racial Background

Racial background refers to specific physical and structural characteristics. These characteristics are transmitted genetically and distinguish one group from another. Some diseases are more prevalent for genetic reasons in certain racial or ethnic groups, such as sickle cell disease in blacks and Tay-Sachs disease in families of Ashkenazi Jewish origin.

Within the boundaries of one country, such as Uganda or Laos, scores of different tribes may be found that vary with respect to physical characteristics, genetically transmitted diseases, and health beliefs. On the other hand, some beliefs and lifestyles that affect health are common to ethnic groups that could not have had communication with one another. An example of this circumstance is the childrearing habit that leads to toddler malnutrition. After giving birth, the mother is isolated with the new baby for several weeks. The older toddler, who has been with the mother continually before the sibling's birth, is now rejected. This child is depressed, eats poorly, and develops malnutrition. The word *kwashiorkor*, an African tribal word, means *disease of the deposed or separated child*.

Health Beliefs and Practices

Viewpoints on health and healing vary from group to group. The basic definition of illness in North America stems from the dominant culture and is based on Western scientific thought, which views illness as a breakdown in a body part because of an infectious organism or injury.[15] Extreme effort is necessary to see illness and healing from a different perspective. The issue of pain is discussed in Zborowski's classic study.[16] Although the dominant American culture values stoicism and nonemotional expressions of pain, other cultures may express pain through screaming, moaning, and verbal complaining.[17] An understanding of these differences is essential in assessing and treating pain in children.[18] Zatzick and Dimsdale[19] reviewed 13 studies in which subjects were exposed to various noxious stimuli, and pain responses of different cultural groups were compared. None of the studies demonstrated cultural differences in the ability to discriminate painful stimuli. This finding suggests that differences in expression of pain among cultural groups do not have a neurosensory origin.

Beliefs and perceptions regarding disabilities relate to culture. Many Asian societies are concerned about the spiritual cause of a disability—for example, failure to follow a tradition. A child born with a disability may be the recipient of punishment assigned to a parent or relative.[20] These beliefs are present among Americans from Asian cultures and may affect whether rehabilitation treatment is perceived as important.

Religious Influences or Special Rituals

The dominant culture has separated church and state for so many years that separating these specific entities in health care is quite common as well. However, for many cultures, religion strongly influences beliefs concerning health and illness, death, and treatment. Assessing the role of significant religious leaders is important, especially during times of life-threatening illness. Special religious ceremonies may be comforting to the ill child and to family members. These beliefs should be integrated into the treatment.

Language Barriers and Communication Styles

Determining which language is spoken at home is essential in assessing the culture. Assessing a family's ability to read and write in English is also important. Although the family and child may speak English, their words and understanding, especially related to abstract concepts, may be limited. Significant problems may occur when translations are made of standard research consent forms.[21] A translator should accompany the primary caregiver when explaining complex topics. The translator must be culturally competent to address questions and misunderstandings.[22] Nonverbal communication may have different meanings in different cultures. Many Americans of East Asian descent nod out of respect, not necessarily out of understanding. Some nonverbal behaviors can lead to alienation and eventually withdrawal; thus their meanings are essential in keeping communication open. For example, crossing the legs in such a way as to point the sole of the foot toward a person from Southeast Asia is interpreted as an insult. In Bulgaria, a person nods the head to mean "no" and moves the head back and forth to denote "yes."

Parenting Styles and Role of Family

Understanding that parenting is neither good nor bad in any culture, simply different, is the basis of acknowledging differing cultures' attitudes toward the family. Assuming that the dominant American culture has all the answers is inaccurate when parenting is considered. Although the dominant American culture may value independence in children, another culture may value submissiveness. Attitudes toward family members vary with each culture. Culture will address how different members' advice is regarded and whether these members are involved in decisions. Culture will also affect the values held about children, family structure, and gender.[23] Parental attitudes regarding infant development and sleeping arrangements often reflect cultural values.[24]

Dietary Practices

Diet is an integral part of a person's culture. Dietary practices can include not only preferences and dislikes of particular foods, but also food preparation, consumption, frequency, time of eating, and utensils used. When a prescribed diet is part of a patient's treatment, assessing the cultural influences involved is essential. Consulting a nutritionist, a cultural informant, or colleagues of various ethnic backgrounds can be helpful. In the United States, children from underserved, ethnically diverse population groups are at increased risk for obesity, increased serum lipid levels, and dietary consumption patterns that do not meet the standards in the *Dietary Guidelines for Americans*.[25,26] However, the overall diet and eating styles in the United States represent a unique culture in the world, generally different from that of the countries of origin, and result in more than 80% of US children consuming more than recommended amounts of total fat and saturated fat. This circumstance is a good example of how facets of culture can change dramatically over a few generations.

HOW PEOPLE INTERACT: EXPECTATIONS FOR APPROPRIATE BEHAVIOR

Perhaps in a century, all people of the world will share a common culture with respect to appropriate interactions. The US population has scores of views regarding appropriate interpersonal interactions.[27] More than a common language is required to develop consensus regarding, for example, eye contact, touching, personal space or territory, appearance, gestures, use of the voice, greetings, partings, and facial expressions. Most humans tend to use the rules regarding these interactions developed from childhood cultural experiences. Complicating this tendency within the United States is that chaotic living situations for children may not provide models for appropriate interpersonal interactions. Young children who watch television a great deal and who are unable to distinguish what is real from what is acting often imitate unusual or inappropriate interpersonal interactions.

In diplomatic circles, norms can be found, some of them written, with respect to communication. Diplomats are encouraged to learn about cultural norms within their host country—for example, who can shake hands, how close to another one stands at a reception, and how much eye contact is allowed. Nonetheless, diplomats make mistakes and are therefore misinterpreted. American child health professionals who interact with peers from other cultures should study cultural norms before working with foreign colleagues, whether in this country or their own. Visitors from East Africa and Southeast Asia often complain that they find American friendliness superficial. The immediate pleasant friendliness of Americans would represent a more advanced stage of personal intimacy and friendship in their cultures, and they are offended when they discover that it does not necessarily reflect depth. They also find difficulty in accepting gifts from Americans because, in many cultures, gifts are given only in exchange for something or to acquire an advantage. Direct expression of feelings is inappropriate and considered bizarre in many cultures. In Thailand, for example, a person turns anger toward another object, either animate or inanimate, called *prachot*. This practice is performed consciously to alert the person (who is the object of the person's displeasure and annoyance) as to how the injured party feels. In Southeast Asia, avoiding confrontation is considered positive, and expressing anger, hatred, and annoyance overtly is considered negative.

Several training programs are available to increase sensitivity among people toward varying cultural norms and values. Pediatricians who plan to work in other cultures may benefit from a game *(Bafa'-bafa')* in which participants are divided into two groups and provided with values, expectations, and customs of a new culture.[28] Such training programs should be incorporated into standard training of pediatric residents in the United States.[29]

PERCEPTUAL DIFFERENCES AMONG CULTURES

Perceptual differences among various groups of humans relate not only to group beliefs, customs, and experiences, but also to differences in sensory systems that may have evolved in response to the need for individual survival or to society's needs. These differences in auditory, visual, musical, and tactile skills are well documented and may relate to differences in eye-hand coordination, information processing, and language and spatial perceptions.

Some of the differences may be genetic, but others reflect the emphasis, focus, and practice of a skill within a culture. For example, an infant's perceptual abilities are modified by listening to a particular language. Syllables, words, and sentences used in all human languages are formed from a set of speech sounds called *phones*. Only part of the phones is used in any particular language. Young infants can discriminate nearly every phonetic contrast, but this broad-based sensitivity declines by 1 year of age.[30] Adults have difficulty discriminating phonemes that do not connote meaning in their own native language and are thus handicapped when learning a new language. English-speaking natives have difficulty in perceiving the difference between two *k* phonemes (sounds) used in Thai. Japanese-speaking adults have difficulty distinguishing between the English */ra/* and */la/*. Adults who learn another language early but who do not practice the language as they mature may lose their ability to differentiate among its sounds.

Learning the language of another culture helps in understanding that culture. Dependency on translators is fraught with the likelihood of misunderstanding, especially in medicine. In some cultures, the status of the translator affects what information is provided by the patient and how it is prepared for the ears of the foreign health professional. If the patient is of *higher* status than the translator, then an awkward situation can result for the translator. If the translator has little specific knowledge about health and medical matters, then translation is less than ideal. Furthermore, abstract concepts may not translate well from English to other languages. For example, expressing abstract concepts in Norwegian or in Russian is much more difficult than in English. Many words from Western languages do not exist in Asian languages; therefore the concepts do not exist. Similarly, some Asian concepts cannot be expressed in English. The Lao language, for example, is richer in terms of words related to family relationships than is the English language.

ETHICAL ISSUES IN CROSS-CULTURAL MEDICINE

Many ethical issues operate in making transcultural diagnostic and treatment decisions. These issues relate to communication barriers, varying explanations for disease, and different expectations regarding what is honest or valuable.

Can an American pediatrician truly explain a surgical consent form to newly arrived parents of a Southeast Asian baby? When newly arrived refugees fear that they will be returned and therefore sign anything or do anything to gain favor, then is asking them to sign a consent form to have blood drawn for clinical research ethical?

Mental illness is defined very differently among cultures.[31] Is using psychotherapy considered ethical when therapist and patient are unmatched culturally?

Oppenheim and Sprung[32] have reviewed cross-cultural differences in ethical decisions related to critical care. They compare Chinese and Israeli cultures with respect to informed consent in intensive care units. For Chinese, giving all information regarding grave decisions directly and openly to the patient or to the parent of the patient is considered callous and inconsiderate. Therefore informed consent as a Western physician understands it may not be reached. Recognizing that physicians' attitudes may differ from those of the patient is important in considering ethical decisions in the intensive care unit, even when the physician and patient are from the same ethnic group.

NEED FOR EDUCATION OF HEALTH CARE PROFESSIONALS

Megatrends, such as increasing flows of refugees and immigrants, will make all pediatric practices more multicultural and multiethnic.[33] The American Academy of Pediatrics recently issued a policy statement defining culturally effective health care and its importance for pediatrics.[34,35] This statement notes that by the year 2020, approximately 40% of school-aged Americans will be minority group children. *Culturally effective pediatric health care* is defined as the delivery of care within the context of appropriate physician knowledge, understanding, and appreciation of cultural distinctions. Such understanding should take into account the beliefs, values, actions, customs, and unique health care needs of distinct population groups. The American Academy of Pediatrics believes that such knowledge and skills can be taught and acquired through educational courses. It recommends that the pediatric community develop and evaluate curricular programs in medical schools and residency programs to enhance the provision of culturally effective health care and to develop continuing medical education materials for pediatricians and nonpediatricians, with the goal of increasing culturally effective health care. In 1999 the Society for Developmental and Behavioral Pediatrics approved curricular guidelines for residency training in developmental-behavioral pediatrics.[36] These guidelines emphasize the need for pediatric residents to develop skills in working with diversity in cultural beliefs. For example, the curriculum suggests that residents, as a routine, identify the relevant racial, cultural, religious, and educational backgrounds of the patient during case presentations. Ohio State University, University of California San Francisco, and Maimonides Medical Center have all published examples of programs to help pediatric residents communicate in culturally diverse environments.[37-39]

SUMMARY

Cross-cultural issues in pediatrics affect communication, expectations, and medical explanations. Pediatricians, although enculturated by their specialty training, also have individual ethnic cultural norms that affect their beliefs and values. Therefore learning about beliefs of their colleagues and patients is helpful for child health professionals. Wherever a strong belief exists in a folk explanation for the cause of an illness, pediatricians are likely to be most successful if they acknowledge the belief and attempt to work with it. When simultaneous use of a traditional and Western medical regimen is possible and will do no harm, it is likely to enhance long-term, trusting relationships. Awareness of cultural evolution, perceptual differences related to cultural background, and implications for decision making with respect to children is essential for child health professionals.

TOOLS FOR PRACTICE

Medical Decision Support

- *Culturally Effective Pediatric Care* (Web page), American Academy of Pediatrics (www.aap.org/commpeds/cepc/index.html).
- *Delivering Culturally Effective Health Care to Adolescents* (report), American Medical Association (AMA) (www.ama-assn.org/ama1/pub/upload/mm/39/culturally effective.pdf).

AAP POLICY STATEMENT

American Academy of Pediatrics, Committee on Pediatric Workforce. Ensuring Culturally Effective Pediatric Care: Implications for Education and Health Policy. *Pediatrics*. 2004;114(6):1677-1685. (aappolicy.aappublications.org/cgi/content/full/pediatrics;114/6/1677).

REFERENCES

1. American Academy of Pediatrics. Culturally effective pediatric care: education and training issues. *Pediatrics*. 1999;103:167-170.
2. McEvoy J, Lee C, Groisman A, et al. Are there universal parenting concepts among culturally diverse families in an inner-city clinic? *J Pediatr Health Care*. 2005;19:142-150.
3. Kinsman SB, Sally M, Fox K. Multicultural issues in pediatric practice. *Pediatr Rev*. 1996;17:349-354.
4. Flores G. Language barriers to health care in the United States. *N Engl J Med*. 2006;355:229-231.
5. Namboze JM. Health and culture in an African society. *Soc Sci Med*. 1983;17:2041-2043.
6. Hufford DJ. Folk medicine and health culture in contemporary society. *Prim Care*. 1997;24:723-741.
7. Krajewski J. Folk-healing among Mexican American families as a consideration in the delivery of child welfare and child health care services. *Child Welfare*. 1991; 70:157-167.
8. Olness KN. Cultural aspects in working with Lao refugees. *Minn Med*. 1979;62:871-874.
9. Barnes LL, Plotnikoff GA, Fox K, et al. Spirituality, religion and pediatrics: intersecting worlds of healing. *Pediatrics*. 2000;103(suppl 4):899-908.
10. Carrillo JE, Green AR, Betancourt JR. Cross cultural primary care: a patient-based approach. *Ann Intern Med*. 1999:130:829-834.
11. Wolsko PM, Eisenberg DM, Davis RB, et al. Use of mind-body medical therapies. *J Gen Intern Med*. 2004;19:43-50.
12. Teufel KW. A call for dialogue: health communication interventions in the context of culture [thesis]. Antioch College, March 1999.
13. Rosales NB. Commentary: cultural effectiveness—ask and listen. *Pediatrics*. 2005;115(suppl 4):1165-1166.
14. American Medical Association. *Culturally Competent Health Care for Adolescents: A Guide for Primary Care Providers*. Chicago, IL: Department of Adolescent Health, The Association; 1994.
15. Stulc DM. The family as a bearer of culture. In: Cookfair JM, ed. *Nursing Process and Practice in the Community*. St Louis: MO: Mosby; 1991.
16. Zborowski M. Cultural components in response to pain. *J Soc Issues*. 1952;8:16-30.
17. Todd KH. Pain assessment and ethnicity. *Ann Emerg Med*. 1996;27:421-423.
18. Bernstein B, Pachter LM. Cultural considerations in children's pain. In: Schecter NL, Berde C, Yaster M, eds. *Pain in Infants, Children, and Adolescents*. Baltimore, MD: Williams & Wilkins; 1993.
19. Zatzick DF, Dimsdale JR. Cultural variations in response to painful stimuli. *Psychosom Med*. 1990;52:544-557.
20. Fitzgerald M, Armstrong J. Culture and disability in the Pacific. *International Exchange of Experts and Information in Rehabilitation Newsletter*. Jan 1993.
21. McCabe, J, Morgan F, Curley H, et al. The informed consent process in a cross cultural setting: is the process achieving the intended result? *Ethn Dis*. 2005;15: 300-304.
22. Flores G. Culture, ethnicity, and linguistic issues in pediatric care: urgent priorities and unanswered questions. *Ambul Pediatr*. 2004;4(4):276-282.
23. Harwood RLK. The influence of culturally derived values on Anglo and Puerto Rican mothers' perception of attachment behavior. *Child Dev*. 1992;63:822-839.
24. Morelli GA, Rogoff B, Oppenheim D, et al. Cultural variation in infants' sleeping arrangements: questions of independence. *Dev Psychol*. 1992;28:604-613.
25. Bronner YL. Nutritional status outcomes for children: ethnic, cultural, and environmental contexts. *J Am Diet Assoc*. 1996;96:891-903.
26. Davis SP, Northington L, Kolar K. Cultural considerations for treatment of childhood obesity. *J Cult Divers*. 2000;7(4):128-132.
27. Marsh P. *Eye to Eye: How People Interact*. Topsfield, MA: Salem House; 1988.
28. Shirts RG: *Bafa'Bafa': A Cross-Cultural Simulation*. Del Mar, CA: Simile; 1977.
29. Sidelinger DE, Meyer D, Blaschke, GS, et al. Communities as teachers: learning to deliver culturally effective care in pediatrics. *Pediatrics*. 2005;115(4): 1165-1166.
30. Werker JF. Becoming a native listener. *Am Scientist*. 1989;77:54-59.
31. Krener PG, Sabin C. Indochinese immigrant children problems in psychiatric diagnosis. *J Am Acad Child Psychiatry*. 1985;24:453-458.
32. Oppenheim A, Sprung CL. Cross-cultural ethical decision-making in critical care. *Crit Care Med*. 1998; 26(3):423-424.
33. Haggerty RJ: Child health 2000: new pediatrics in the changing environment of children's needs in the 21st century. *Pediatrics*. 1995;96:804-812.
34. American Academy of Pediatrics. Culturally effective pediatric care: education and training issues. *Pediatrics*. 1999;103:167-170.
35. Britton CV, American Academy of Pediatrics, Committee on Pediatric Workforce. Ensuring culturally effective pediatric care: implications for education and health policy. *Pediatrics*. 2004;114(6):1677-1685.
36. Coury DL, Berger SP, Stancin T, et al. Curricular guidelines for residency training in developmental-behavioral pediatrics. *J Dev Behav Pediatr*. 1999;20:S1-S38.
37. Goleman MJ. Teaching pediatrics residents to communicate with patients across differences. *Acad Med*. 2001; 76(5):515-516.
38. Altshuler L, Kachur E. A culture OSCE: teaching residents to bridge different worlds. *Acad Med*. 2001; 76(5):514.
39. Takayama JI, Chandran C, Pearl DB. A one-month cultural competency rotation for pediatrics residents. *Acad Med*. 2001;76(5):514-515.

Chapter 18

ADHERENCE TO PEDIATRIC HEALTH CARE RECOMMENDATIONS

Jill S. Halterman, MD, MPH; Kelly M. Conn, MPH; Peter G. Szilagyi, MD, MPH

Adherence, often referred to as *compliance*, is defined as the extent to which a person's health-related behaviors coincide with agreed recommendations from a health care provider.[1] Difficulties with adherence have been described since the time of Hippocrates. Nonadherence with drug therapy may reflect the failure to fill prescribed medications, delayed or forgotten doses, incorrect amounts of medication or improper dosing intervals, and failure to complete full courses of therapy. For children, the problems surrounding drug adherence are unique because the adherence of the parent and the child must be considered. This chapter focuses on adherence with medication use to illustrate the extent and consequences of nonadherence in pediatrics, determinants of nonadherence, and strategies to improve adherence within a pediatric population.

EXTENT OF NONADHERENCE

Many studies document adherence problems for pediatric patients. For example, 40% to 80% of children do not receive a complete 10-day course of treatment prescribed for otitis media or streptococcal pharyngitis.[2,3] Furthermore, for chronic conditions that require a long duration of daily therapy, lack of adherence is frequently cited as a significant problem. In 2 studies of young children with asthma, patients took only one half of their prescribed doses of antiinflammatory medications, as measured by canister weights and electronic monitoring devices.[4,5] Furthermore, adherence to penicillin prophylaxis for children who have sickle cell anemia has been determined to be only 43%, as measured by urine assay.[6] Similar problems have been described among children who have other chronic conditions, including diabetes mellitus, renal disease, cancer, rheumatic fever, and tuberculosis, in which adherence has been as low as 40%.[6-9] Because patients have been shown to over-report medication use, adherence rates are likely lower than most health care providers believe.[10]

CONSEQUENCES OF NONADHERENCE

Poor adherence or nonadherence can compromise the efficacy of a medical regimen. Certain children who have diabetes mellitus are hospitalized repeatedly for ketoacidosis and demonstrate highly elevated hemoglobin $A1_c$ levels related to nonadherence to the prescribed regimen for insulin therapy. Furthermore, nonadherence can adversely affect medical decisions, leading to inappropriate increases in dose, changes in the scheduling regimen, or additional medical tests or procedures. For infectious diseases, problems with nonadherence may cause relapses of infections or the emergence of resistant microbial strains. Finally, nonadherence interferes with the physician-parent relationship and prevents accurate evaluations of a treatment's efficacy.

DETERMINANTS OF NONADHERENCE

Physicians tend to overestimate the adherence of their patients and are unable to predict adherence by considering sociodemographic characteristics. Therefore considering factors that may influence adherence among pediatric patients would be useful. These factors include the patient or family's knowledge and recall of the treatment plan, other family factors such as perceptions of illness severity and treatment risks and benefits, interactions between the clinician and patient, and characteristics of the treatment regimen (Figure 18-1).

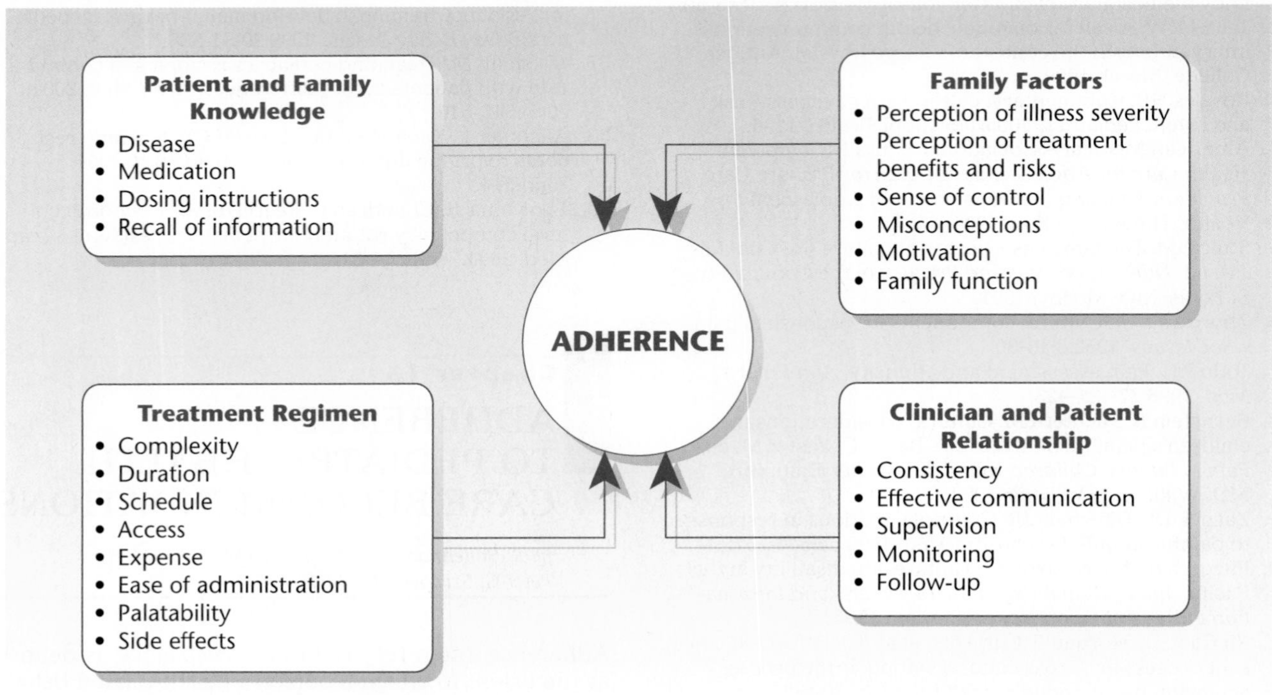

Figure 18-1 Determinants of adherence among pediatric patients.

Patient-Family Knowledge

For a patient to adhere to a therapeutic regimen, the instructions that are given must be understood. However, parents frequently do not possess all the information they need to follow a particular regimen. Confusion about the appropriate use of asthma medications has been shown to be associated with medication nonadherence, with many patients mistaking maintenance medications, which should be administered daily, for symptomatic medications used intermittently (eg, bronchodilators).[10-12] Furthermore, families often do not understand medical terms commonly used by medical personnel during visits.[13] Many individuals have difficulty with instructions involving medication dosing and mistakenly choose the incorrect dosing device for liquid medications.[14]

Patients also must be able to recall necessary information throughout the duration of therapy to comply with the recommendations. However, patients are known to forget much of what physicians tell them, and the more patients are told, the greater the proportion they will forget.[15] Patient recall declines rapidly with time. Approximately 50% of the information given to patients is forgotten within 15 minutes of a physician visit.[16,17]

Family Factors

The family's perception of the illness and treatment, and their sense of control over the illness, influences their adherence to a therapeutic regimen. Among parents of children with asthma, fears and misconceptions about preventive medications are common and negatively affect patient adherence.[11,18,19] Health belief models suggest that an individual's adherence depends on his or her degree of motivation about health-related issues, perception of susceptibility to the illness, perception of disease severity, and feelings about treatment benefits and cost.[20] Caretakers who show concern about their child's illness, perceive the illness as a threat, and believe in the accuracy of the diagnosis and the benefits of treatment are more likely to comply with a therapeutic regimen.[21] Additionally, social vulnerability in caretakers, including depression and other psychiatric illness, negatively affects families' ability to adhere to treatment plans.[22-25]

Clinician-Patient Relationship

Effective communication enhances patient adherence significantly.[26,27] Patients tend to show improved compliance when they are treated by the same practitioner consistently[8,28] and develop a long-term partnership for continued care.[29] Patient supervision, monitoring, and consistent follow-up improve adherence, particularly with chronic treatment regimens.[30-32] Support can also be found for written practitioner-patient contracts to improve adherence.[33]

Treatment Regimen

Details of the treatment regimen itself can affect patient adherence. Lower rates of adherence are associated with treatments that require long-term medications, multiple medications, complicated or inconvenient schedules, and frequent medication administration.[8,34-36] Other important issues include expense and access to appropriate therapies. In children, ease of administration, volume of medication, and palatability also must be considered.

STRATEGIES FOR IMPROVING ADHERENCE

Strategies for improving patient adherence begin with recognizing this widespread problem and considering the aforementioned components and how they may relate to patients and families (Table 18-1). Physicians

Table 18-1 Strategies for Improving Adherence

PROBLEM	POTENTIAL SOLUTION
Patient-family knowledge	Provide individualized, written information. Give clear, simple instructions. Address important features early in discussion. Provide measuring devices, calendars.
Family factors	Address fears and misconceptions. Understand cultural issues and beliefs. Enlist support from other family members. Provide families with sense of control over illness.
Clinician-patient relationship	Increase continuity of care. Set treatment goals in collaboration with family. Consider written contracts. Explain likely side effects and suggest ways these can be minimized. Provide routine supervision and monitoring. Use a health team approach.
Treatment regimen	Use simplified, short regimens. Tailor dose intervals to the patient's daily routine (preferably once or twice daily dosing). Consider palatability, volume of medication. Consider facilitated drug delivery systems. Prescribe medication with lowest co-pay.

can help improve a patient's understanding of disease and treatment by providing individualized, written information with oral instruction. Such information should contain clear, simple, understandable terms and should be relayed from patient to physician to ensure understanding. Although important details should be emphasized, an overload of information should be avoided. Furthermore, the most important details should be presented early in the discussion. Providing measuring devices and calendars may also be helpful for patients who have limited resources.

Another means by which physicians can help improve adherence is to address beliefs, fears, and potential misconceptions that the family may hold. Potential solutions may involve encouraging families to disclose worries and concerns, providing accurate information, offering other sources of information, and enlisting support from other family members with sensitivity toward their cultural beliefs. Modification of beliefs may be necessary for certain families to increase adherence. Furthermore, patients should be provided with a sense of control over their illness via accurate information in a supportive environment.

Patient-physician interactions can be improved by increasing continuity of care and increasing practitioner awareness of family concerns. Treatment goals should be set in collaboration with the child and his or her family to allow for a therapeutic framework in which the patient and provider can work together. The physician should explain likely side effects, and suggest ways that these effects can be minimized. A written contract may be helpful in some cases, particularly when long-term therapy is needed. Furthermore, routine supervision with adherence monitoring may be necessary to ensure continuation of therapies for chronic disease. This monitoring may involve follow-up appointments, telephone calls, home visits, blood level monitoring, or counting unused pills. Other members of the health care team, including nurses and social workers, can help provide support for families to improve adherence and can assist with contracts, monitoring, and education. Information and counseling from pharmacists have also been shown to be helpful.[37]

Finally, a treatment should be as simple as possible to maximize the likelihood of patient adherence. Medications should be prescribed by using the shortest regimen that is reasonable, and dosing should be tailored to the patient's daily routine. Prescriptions that recommend more than 2 doses per day should be avoided unless absolutely necessary. When possible, single agents should be prescribed and changes to a regimen introduced one at a time.[38] For pediatric doses, the most concentrated form of liquid medication is usually preferable so that smaller volumes are needed. Furthermore, being aware of the palatability of different medications when a choice can be made is helpful for physicians. In some cases, generic drugs may be preferable to reduce the cost of the treatment. Issues of access to prescribed therapies should be addressed during the original encounter. Newer drugs or drug delivery systems that include sustained-release medications and insulin pumps may improve adherence among certain patients. Finally, given that most insurance plans providing coverage for drug expenses use a 3-tiered co-pay program, the physician should prescribe the medication entailing the least out-of-pocket expense for the patient whenever possible.

SUMMARY

Successful treatment of children often depends on adherence with a therapeutic regimen; unfortunately, nonadherence is common. The issue of adherence in pediatrics includes the extent and consequences of the problem, factors related to nonadherence, and potential strategies for improving adherence. An understanding of this complicated issue requires consideration of many factors involving the patient, the family, the physician, and the regimen itself.

Pediatricians should consider nonadherence as a potential issue with all patients. The differential diagnosis in a child who is unresponsive to therapy should include an adherence history that assesses whether the child has taken the medication. Improving adherence requires a multifactorial approach that involves providing accurate, concise, and understandable information to families; addressing health-related beliefs; improving communication between physicians and families; and simplifying and individualizing the treatment. Ideally, all patients requiring sustained therapy should receive adherence monitoring, with consistent followup and support from the health care team. Barriers to adherence should be identified early in the course of therapy to allow for timely intervention and to minimize negative consequences.

TOOLS FOR PRACTICE

Engaging Patients and Family

- *Antibiotics and Your Child* (brochure), American Academy of Pediatrics (patiented.aap.org).

REFERENCES

1. Sackett DL, Haynes RB, Guyatt GH, et al. Helping patients follow the treatments you prescribe. In: *Clinical Epidemiology: A Basic Science for Clinical Medicine*. Boston, MA: Little, Brown and Co; 1991:249-281.
2. Bergman AB, Werner RJ. Failure of children to receive penicillin by mouth. *N Engl J Med*. 1963;268:1334-1338.
3. Dajani AS. Adherence to physicians' instructions as a factor in managing streptococcal pharyngitis. *Pediatrics*. 1996;97:976-980.
4. Celano M, Geller RJ, Phillips KM, et al. Treatment adherence among low-income children with asthma. *J Pediatr Psychol*. 1998;23:345-349.
5. Gibson NA, Ferguson AE, Aitchison TC, et al. Compliance with inhaled asthma medication in preschool children. *Thorax*. 1995;50:1274-1279.
6. Teach SJ, Lillis KA, Grossi M. Compliance with penicillin prophylaxis in patients with sickle cell disease. *Arch Pediatr Adolesc Med*. 1998;152:274.
7. Feinstein AR, Harrison FW, Epstein JA, et al. A controlled study of three methods of prophylaxis against streptococcal infection in a population of rheumatic children. *N Engl J Med*. 1959;260:697-702.
8. Fotheringham MJ, Sawyer MG. Adherence to recommended medical regimens in childhood and adolescence. *J Paediatr Child Health*. 1995;31:72-78.

9. Gordis L, Markowitz M, Lilienfeld AM. Studies in the epidemiology and preventability of rheumatic fever. IV. A quantitative determination of compliance in children on oral penicillin prophylaxis. *Pediatrics*. 1969;43: 173-182.
10. Bender B, Milgrom H, Rand C, et al. Psychological factors associated with medication nonadherence in asthmatic children. *J Asthma*. 1998;35:347-353.
11. Boulet L. Perception of the role and potential side effects of inhaled corticosteroids among asthmatic patients. *Chest*. 1998;113:587-592.
12. Farber HJ, Capra AM, Finkelstein JA, et al. Misunderstanding of asthma controller medications: association with nonadherence. *J Asthma*. 2003;40:17-25.
13. Korsch BM, Gozzi EK, Francis V. Gaps in doctor-patient communication. I. Doctor-patient interaction and patient satisfaction. *Pediatrics*. 1968;42:855-871.
14. Madison-Kay DJ, Mosch FS. Liquid medication dosing errors. *J Fam Pract*. 2000;49(8):741-744.
15. Cassata DM. Health communication theory and research: an overview of the communication specialist interface. In: Nimmo D, ed. *Communication Yearbook II*. New York, NY: ICA; 1978.
16. Ley P. Primacy, rated importance, and the recall of medical statements. *J Health Soc Behav*. 1972;13:311-319.
17. Ley P, Bradshaw PW, Eaves D, et al. A method for increasing patients' recall of information presented by doctors. *Psychol Med*. 1973;3:217-220.
18. Chan P, DeBruyne JA. Parental concern towards the use of inhaled therapy children with chronic asthma. *Pediatrics International*. 2000;42:547-551.
19. Conn KM, Halterman JS, Fisher SG, et al. Parental beliefs about medications and medication adherence among urban children with asthma. *Ambulatory Pediatrics*. 2005;5:305-310.
20. Janz NK, Becker MH. The health belief model: a decade later. *Health Educ Q*. 1984;11:1-47.
21. Becker MH, Drachman RH, Kirscht JP. A new approach to explaining sick-role behavior in low-income populations. *Am J Public Health*. 1974;64:205-216.
22. Bartlett SJ, Krishnan JA, Riekert KA, et al. Maternal depressive symptoms and adherence to therapy in inner-city children with asthma. *Pediatrics*. 2004;113:229-237.
23. Delambo KE, Ievers-Landis CE, Drotar D, et al. Association of observed family relationship quality and problem-solving skills with treatment adherence in older children and adolescents with cystic fibrosis. *J Pediatr Psychol*. 2004;29:343-353.
24. LeSon S, Gershwin ME. Risk factors for asthmatic patients requiring intubation. I. Observations in children. *J Asthma*. 1995;32:285-294.
25. Mellins CA, Brackis-Cott E, Dolezal C, et al. The role of psychosocial and family factors in adherence to antiretroviral treatment in human immunodeficiency virus-infected children. *Pediatr Infect Dis J*. 2004;23:1035-1041.
26. Apter AJ, Reisine ST, Affleck G, et al. Adherence with twice-daily dosing of inhaled steroids: socioeconomic and health-belief differences. *Am J Respir Crit Care Med*. 1998;157:1810-1817.
27. Hanchak NA, Patel MB, Berlin JA, et al. Patient misunderstanding of dosing instructions. *J Gen Intern Med*. 1996;11:325-328.
28. Litt IF, Cuskey WR. Compliance with medical regimen during adolescence. *Pediatr Clin North Am*. 1980;27: 3-15.
29. Legorreta AP, Christian-Herman J, O'Connor RD, et al. Compliance with national asthma management guidelines and specialty care: a health maintenance organization experience. *Arch Intern Med*. 1998;158:457-464.
30. Haynes RB. A critical review of the "determinants" of patient compliance with therapeutic regimens. In: Sackett DL, Haynes RB, eds: *Compliance with Therapeutic Regimens*. Baltimore, MD: Johns Hopkins University Press; 1976.
31. Maiman LA, Becker MH, Liptak GS, et al. Improving pediatricians' compliance-enhancing practices. A randomized trial. *Am J Dis Child*. 1988;142:773-779.
32. Rokart JF, Hofmann PB. Physician and patient behavior under different scheduling systems in a hospital outpatient department. *Med Care*. 1969;7:463-470.
33. Lewis CE, Michnich M. Contracts as a means of improving patient compliance. In: Barofsky I, ed. *Medication Compliance: A Behavioral Management Approach*, Thorofare, NJ: Charles B Slack; 1977.
34. Hussar DA. Importance of patient compliance in effective antimicrobial therapy. *Pediatr Infect Dis J*. 1987;6:971-975.
35. Rapoff MA, Barnard MU. Compliance with pediatric medical regimens. In: Cramer JA, Spilker B, eds. *Patient Compliance in Medical Practice and Clinical Trials*. New York, NY: Raven Press; 1991.
36. Thatcher Shope J. Medication compliance. *Pediatr Clin North Am*. 1981;28:5-21.
37. Canada AT. The pharmacist and drug compliance. In: Sackett DL, Haynes RB, eds. *Compliance with Therapeutic Regimens*. Baltimore, MD: Johns Hopkins University Press; 1976.
38. Dunbar JM, Stunkard AJ. Adherence to diet and drug regimen. In: Levy R, Dennis BH, Ritkino BM, eds. *Nutrition, Lipids, and Coronary Heart Disease*. New York, NY: Raven Press; 1979.

Chapter 19

ART OF REFERRAL, CONSULTATION, AND COLLABORATIVE MANAGEMENT

Henry M. Seidel, MD

Consultation, referral, and collaborative management are at the heart of patient care and rely on successful communication. The communication may be verbal or nonverbal, and it may be given in person, by telephone, or by written correspondence. The necessary skills must be second nature to physicians and evolve with the recognition that each patient is culturally and spiritually unique, with an idiosyncratic life situation blessed and beset by physical and emotional assets and limitations. The physician needs to understand the patient's and the parent's verbal and nonverbal language and search for hidden agendas—concerns not overtly expressed.

Primary care physicians (PCPs) also need to understand the language of their specialist colleagues. They, too, have vulnerabilities, assets, and limitations, as well as particular practice habits. Indeed, language and culture inconsistencies are likely because specialists have more narrow concerns. The role of the PCP is to understand both the patient's and the specialist's cultures and provide the bridge between them.

Good communication is hampered by the uncertainty that underlies patient care, the often intangible factors that influence decision-making, and the need for the patient to grasp the uncertainty. Communication is aided when the physician can:

- Listen attentively and sensitively.
- Be precise.
- Be prompt in making contact.
- Avoid rigidity.
- Avoid the use of jargon.
- Be sensitive to and comfortable with uncertainty.
- Confirm what other professionals have asserted.
- Avoid the confusion of mixed messages.
- Avoid impromptu off the cuff or corridor consultations or discussions.
- Maintain a rightful voice in decision making (respect for a patient's or a colleague's autonomy in decision making does not void responsibility).
- Maintain concise, complete records, confirming spoken communication (including telephone conversations).
- Define precisely the role of each professional involved.
- Ensure that orchestration of the entire process is delegated to 1 person, most often the primary care physician.

Also beneficial to a patient is to:

- Ensure a comfortable, private setting for conversation.
- Understand the patient's and family's perspective, worries, and goals.
- Describe the process and sequence of care in understandable, unpatronizing words.
- Gauge the family's response by reading their body language and listening carefully.
- Review the conversation and decisions and ask to hear a summation to be sure of appropriate understanding.
- Involve the patient and family in decision making.

Also important to your specialist colleague is to:

- Report any behavioral, emotional, social, and economic factors that can influence decision making.
- Define clearly individual responsibilities according to the skills, intentions, and goals of all the professionals involved.

BOX 19-1 Reasons for Consultation in Health and Medical Disciplines

1. Uncertainty in diagnosis
2. Confirmation of diagnosis
3. Specific skill required for diagnostic process, for example:
   a. Pediatric subspecialist to perform a variety of diagnostic techniques
   b. Radiologist to consider all the imaging modalities and to select them appropriately
   c. Endoscopist to see a lesion and perform a biopsy
   d. Surgeon to explore and remove a lesion, to obtain a biopsy specimen, or to correct a problem
   e. Pathologist to interpret the nature of the tissue removed
   f. Psychologist, psychiatrist, or mental health counselor to search for emotional issues affecting the patient's mental or physical health
   g. Teacher and social worker to discover aspects of patient's school environment and family life unknown to the referring physician
4. Uncertainty as to appropriate management or therapy, or both
5. Specific skill required for therapy or management, or both, for example, the variety of surgical disciplines—when *consultation* becomes *collaborative management*
6. Reassurance for the patient and family or the primary pediatrician, for example:
   a. Reassurance as to the diagnosis (even in the face of certainty)
   b. Reassurance as to a suggested course of action
7. Assistance in long-term follow-up and management of chronic illness, for example:
   a. Specialist
   b. Speech, physical, or occupational therapist
   c. Rehabilitationist
   d. School personnel

CONSULTATION

The purpose of consultation is to gain assistance in the diagnosis and management of a patient's problem and to reassure the patient and family (Box 19-1). In many instances, you will want confirmation of your impression and plan. Insecurity may sometimes make you hesitate to ask for a consultation because of fear of being thought incompetent. Omniscience is beyond anyone's capacity. Trust among you, the patient, and the family is essential and is usually reinforced, not undermined, by appropriate consultation. The PCP is most often responsible for arranging a consultation and should be sure of the consultant's education, experience, expertise, and ability to relate well with patients.

The need for a consultation often arises during the stress of an acute illness when the family and patient may react to the suggestion with increased anxiety, given that parents almost invariably fear the worst. Acknowledge their fears and put them in context. Minimizing the gravity of an illness in an effort to be protective is generally inappropriate. In this area, sensitive and careful listening and communication is most important. Problems in choosing a consultant can be forestalled if frank discussion of skills, personalities, cost, and the practice settings of the persons involved takes place. Avoiding being too specific about what the consultant might say or recommend is usually best so that leeway for flexible decision making is not compromised.

A consultation is not a referral. The physician who requests a consultation ordinarily is not intending to transfer care to another physician or even, necessarily, to share care (although doing so may often be appropriate).

Guidance for requesting a consultation include the following:

- Be precise in stating the goals for the consultation, providing all the necessary information and defining the questions you would like answered.

- Clarify the extent of the consultation; do not abdicate your role in decision making.
- Do not be so rigid that the consultant is deprived of flexibility in decision making.
- Monitor the family's level of anxiety, inform the consultant as necessary, and reassure the family appropriately.
- Keep an accurate, precise written record of telephone conversations with the consultant and family.

Although following these suggestions may be time consuming, doing so may help avoid misunderstandings that might turn out to be expensive and emotionally exhausting.

SECOND OPINIONS

Second opinions have been suggested, particularly in the event of surgery, as a means of ensuring more appropriate and, perhaps, cost-saving decision. No certainty exists, however, that a second opinion will have greater validity than the first. An obvious absurdity can result if the patient is subjected to a third expert to overcome a tie vote. Further opinions rarely are necessary when a primary physician and a consultant communicate well and keep the patient fully and appropriately informed. Recommendations made by a consultant or collaborative colleague are not binding and may be rejected by the patient, family, and primary physician. In keeping with the principles of family-centered care, everyone involved retains the privilege of contribution to the ultimate decision. In particular, should a consultant's or collaborative colleague's advice be rejected, the reasoning must be clearly documented. Finally, given that evidence-based medicine provides guidelines for more conditions, the need for second opinions should be reduced.

The consultative process can be abused. Used without clear need, it can be confusing, add to cost, and depersonalize individual care. What Peter Berczeller has characterized as "management by committee" underlies much of a resident's experience in recent years, as more and more people are involved in the continuing care for a person's problems.[1] Judicious self-reliance is no longer as often the tempering factor it must be if a clinician is to develop professional maturity. *Judicious* is an important word. The clinician must respect his or her own limits. This task can be accomplished without surrendering the responsibility to orchestrate.

REFERRAL

Referring a patient to another physician and giving up the privilege of primary care of that patient is often necessary.[2] Among other reasons, this necessity may be because the family is moving to a new community, the patient's health insurance company does not include you on its list of providers, the child's problems might be better served by others in yours or the family's judgment, or your retirement may be impending. The goal, then, is to ensure the continuity of care with a minimum of disruption. An appropriate outcome is better ensured if you:

- Are precise in stating the patient's goals
- Satisfy the need for all relevant information in hard copy (providing a front sheet that includes a problem list, current medications, and allergies is often helpful)

Ensure that the new physician involved demonstrates flexibility in decision making by referring the patient to a physician who respects the family's role in making decisions.

COLLABORATIVE MANAGEMENT

In many instances, patient care has complexities that require 2 or more health professionals to share care. The goal of collaborative management is the appropriate use of the skills of everyone involved with respectful, shared decision making that involves the patient and the family. Collaborative management increases the risk of:

- Loss of the orchestrating voice of the primary care pediatrician.
- Failure to define clearly the respective roles of the physicians involved.
- Delivery of mixed messages to the patient.
- An unsettling uncertainty that may not be expeditiously resolved for the patient.
- Some loss of the patient's trust in one or other of the professionals involved.
- Avoiding these pitfalls is everyone's responsibility; but the primary care physician should ensure that the orchestration is smooth and that the flow of information is unimpeded. The behaviors that are essential to successful communication certainly apply. Success will happen if:
  - Information is provided in parallel to all involved;
  - The patient is immediately informed and given an explanation if uncertainty exists;
  - The responsibility of care is clearly defined and truly shared, and usurpation is avoided;
  - The roles of the PCP and specialist in covering all aspects of the patient's care are clearly defined so that nothing is overlooked;
  - Casual *off-the-cuff* corridor or telephone conversations are avoided;
  - A thorough hard record is maintained and shared expeditiously;

Collaborative management often evolves from a consultation. When this need is ended, the time at which the patient returns to the PCP if, for example, a surgical procedure is involved, must be clearly defined. The consultant may need to continue some contact with the patient, and these visits may parallel primary care visits. When the relationship with the consultant ends, the PCP must be made aware and must then ensure follow-up care. Circumstances are often imposed by complex, chronic problems that mandate collaboration over years and perhaps the lifetime of the patient. The rules, however, do not vary.

NONPHYSICIAN HEALTH PROFESSIONALS

Increasingly, pediatric physicians have shared the care of children with many nonphysician health professionals, including nurses, nurse practitioners, and physician assistants; physical, occupational, and speech therapists; educational, developmental, and clinical psychologists; audiologists; social workers; and nutritionists. The PCP is responsible for understanding the resources provided by these professionals, tapping into their expertise, collaborating with them when indicated, and maintaining effective communication among everyone involved. The rules for communication are the same as those that govern consultation with another physician. The nonphysician health professional assumes the responsibilities of any consultant, including that of maintaining open and respectful communication. The PCP should assist the family in sorting through and ordering multiple recommendations from multiple therapists.

TOOLS FOR PRACTICE

Practice Management and Care Coordination

- Referral Fax Back Form, American Academy of Pediatrics, The National Center of Medical Home Initiatives for Children with Special Needs (www.medicalhomeinfo.org/tools/doc_guide.html#sample).
- Sample Referral to Emergency Room Form, Cincinnati Children's Hospital Medical Center (www.medicalhomeinfo.org/tools/doc_guide.html#sample).
- Care Coordination Measurement Tool (form), American Academy of Pediatrics, The National Center of Medical Home Initiatives for Children with Special Needs (www.medicalhomeinfo.org/tools/Toolkits.html).
- Consultation Referral Form, Cincinnati Children's Hospital Medical Center (www.cincinnatichildrens.org/NR/rdonlyres/D86E76FC-FAA6-4F21-9D9F-371D35CC365D/0/consultreferralform.pdf).
- Emergency Department Referral Form, Cincinnati Children's Hospital Medical Center (www.cincinnatichildrens.org/NR/rdonlyres/06B930C3-A7C7-4862-8654-04A83EAC6588/0/edreferfax.pdf).
- Emergency Information Form for Children with Special Needs, American Academy of Pediatrics (www.aap.org/advocacy/blankform.pdf).
- Interactive Emergency Information Form for Children with Special Needs (dynamic form), American Academy of Pediatrics (www.aap.org/advocacy/eif.doc).
- *Instructions for Parents on the Emergency Form* (fact sheet), American Academy of Pediatrics (www.aap.org/advocacy/epcparent.htm).

REFERENCES

1. Berczeller PH. The malignant consultation syndrome. *Hosp Pract*. 1991;33:15-17.
2. Howard BJ. The referral role of pediatricians. *Pediatr Clin North Am*. 1995;42:103-118.

Chapter 20

HOSPITALIST MEDICINE: COMMUNICATING WITH PATIENTS AND FAMILIES

Laura J. Mirkinson, MD

With the growth of the hospitalist movement has come a change in the organization of inpatient services. In the hospitalist model, the shift of responsibility for the patient during the inpatient stay from the primary care physician (PCP) to the hospitalist has placed a burden of responsibility on both to ensure the continuity of care for the patient[1]; research indicates that ineffective communication between the two types of providers on many levels can adversely affect patient care and safety.[2] Differences in the attitudes of community pediatricians toward hospitalist programs vary widely and include significant concerns about communication.[3] Successful communication between hospitalists and PCPs is an essential component of effective hospitalist medicine and a primary way of avoiding interruptions in patient care. The collaborative relationship between these physicians ensures a smooth transition of patient care from the inpatient to the outpatient service, and vice versa.[4] Support for the continuity of care facilitates a global understanding of the patient and assists in appropriate diagnosis and initiation of inpatient therapy and effective outpatient follow-up. This deeper understanding allows each physician to consider more effectively the impact of social, financial, and other factors that are unique to each patient's personal history.

The PCP's knowledge and insight are critical in providing the best care for the patient. Essential background information and prior therapeutic interventions can often only be provided by the patient's PCP. These factors are instrumental in preventing interruptions in care, making critical decisions such as end-of-life care, suggesting social service interventions, and recognizing the value of specialty services for patients with special health care needs. Similarly, hospitalists have a unique insight regarding repeat hospitalizations and access to information available in inpatient medical records. Hospitalists have the opportunity to use the services of many ancillary providers within the hospital system. For example, hospitalists caring for children may have access to information about social services and community resources not readily available to the PCP. Successful interaction between different care providers promotes an atmosphere of collegiality and mutual learning, and it creates an open and supportive professional and educational medical community. Communication fosters a culture of safety and may reduce medication errors and unnecessary medication use. It supports patient education, has the potential to improve the use of chronic and preventive medicines, supports the needs of patients with limited resources or without a medical home, and helps coordinate the care of chronically ill and vulnerable patients and provide greater insight in family conferences.

Box 20-1 provides guidance for communication between PCPs and hospitalists. The benefits of a partnership in patient education may help prevent unnecessary hospitalizations and may promote patient and family knowledge about chronic diseases, medications, and disease triggers. Many concerns regarding patient safety, such as medication reconciliation, follow-up of outstanding laboratory results, or the need for additional outpatient clinical tests or procedures, can be mitigated by establishing effective and collegial communication between health care providers. Everyone involved should be able to recognize easily that both the PCP and the hospitalist are advocates for the patient. Differences in approach to diagnosis and treatment should be discussed in an open and mutually respectful manner. An optimal plan is a collaborative one; however, ultimately, the attending physician of record will be responsible for making decisions about the hospital stay. Finally, effective communication and handoff supports physicians' efficiency and satisfaction in their own practices.

Transitions in patient care, such as inpatient hospitalization and discharge, when a hospitalist assumes the care of a PCP's patient, and vice versa, present opportunities to lose patient information and decrease communication. Similarly, subspecialty consultations, procedures, and therapeutic suggestions can be lost to the PCP if not adequately communicated by the hospitalist. Thus, in addition to collegial communication, continuing education for hospitalists, subspecialists, and PCPs in physician-physician communication and physician-patient communication improves rapport, a necessary component of the therapeutic relationship between the members of this triad.

BOX 20-1 Guidance for Communication Between Primary Care Physicians and Hospitalists

- Communication should, first and foremost, promote quality of care and patient safety.
- Communication should always occur at the time of admission and discharge and, depending on the patient case and physician preferences, may occur during hospitalization.
- During hospitalization, hospitalist decisions regarding specialty consultations, transfers to other institutions, and changes in level of care should be communicated to the primary care physician (PCP).
- Hospitalists, PCPs, and subspecialists should be easily accessible to each other by an established method of communication.
- PCPs should maintain communication with patients and their families who are on a hospitalist service.
- The treatment plan and follow-up suggestions are an essential part of the discharge transfer of care communication.
- Hospitalists, subspecialists, and PCPs share in the responsibility to ensure adequate follow-up after discharge, including establishing follow-up appointments, informing patients of outstanding clinical tests, and educating patients about the necessity for follow-up care.

As a particular hospitalist service evolves, the opportunities to survey both PCPs and patients can potentially generate information about the best practices for contact among hospitalists, PCPs, and patients in this setting. Methods of communication are varied and are often tailored to a particular service and patient population, although most PCPs prefer to communicate with hospitalists by telephone at admission and discharge.[5] Other options include faxes, transcribed dictation, and, under the appropriate circumstances, e-mail.[6]

Interventions that increase patient satisfaction and improve safety after discharge are essential for hospitalist services. These interventions may include identifying a specific individual from the hospitalist team to (1) contact patients after discharge, (2) identify patients who have missed follow-up appointments, and (3) track pending clinical results. For some services, providing follow-up telephone calls from a pharmacist has helped answer questions and resolve medication-related problems.[7] First and foremost, communication should promote patient safety. It should occur by a recognized method at established intervals of hospitalization, when the level of care changes significantly, or when additional services, such as a subspecialty consultation, are needed. The treatment plan must include preparations for follow-up after discharge and a method of communicating outstanding test results.

The importance of a controlled transfer of patient information after discharge cannot be overemphasized. The hospitalist and the PCP are locked into a relationship of shared responsibility and shared liability for patient care. A practice that focuses first on the best interests of the patient will ultimately benefit the physicians involved and help improve the quality of care after discharge from the hospital. The fact that a physician's legal duty is to provide follow-up care is well established. In the case of hospitalists and PCPs, this responsibility is shared. The patient must leave the hospital with these necessary tools: an understanding of the diagnosis and inpatient treatment, a recognition of the need for any ongoing medical therapy or routine follow-up care, and a follow-up care plan with an identified PCP who has timely, adequate, and accurate information about the hospitalization. A final and essential part of the discharge plan is an effective method for communicating outstanding laboratory or other clinical test results to the PCP, the patient, or both.[8]

The failure to relay information about clinical test results that are outstanding at the time of discharge is documented in the medical literature[9] and identifies an important patient safety issue. By definition, hospitalist services have a large volume of potentially actionable test results pending at the time of discharge and may not have an established system for tracking these results or providing follow-up information to PCPs or patients. Fortunately, an inherent strength of hospitalist services is their ready access to patient information through integrated hospital information systems and their ability to coordinate care for patients with other specialists. These systems need to be used to enable and promote collaboration and communication between hospitalists and community physicians.

The presence of a skilled pediatric hospitalist on an inpatient service provides a unique opportunity for teaching many members of the medical team. It is an ideal setup for direct evidence-based clinical teaching of medical students and residents, as well as providing immediate interaction with nursing and other ancillary staff. A pediatric hospitalist presence in the hospital promotes the consideration of pediatric concerns at many levels and provides a pediatric focus during administrative and peer-review hospital committee activities. In addition, the pediatric hospitalist has the opportunity to improve the quality of care provided to hospitalized children by implementing and overseeing the use of evidence-based diagnosis and treatment guidelines published by the American Academy of Pediatrics and other professional organizations. They may also conduct other quality improvement activities such as reducing nosocomial infections and adverse reactions to medications.

TOOLS FOR PRACTICE

Practice Management and Care Coordination

- *Action Care Plan* (form), Center for Medical Home Improvement (www.medicalhomeimprovement.org/assets/pdf/Working_Full.pdf).
- *Care Cordination Measurement Tool* (form), American Academy of Pediatrics, The National Center of Medial Home Initiatives for Children with Special Needs (www.medicalhomeinfo.org/tools/Toolkits.html).
- *Care Plans* (form), Hitchcock Clinic, Concord Pediatric. (www.medicalhomeinfo.org/training/materials/April2004Curriculum/PPP/PPPAppendices/HitchcockCarePlan_1.pdf).
- *Child History Fact Sheet* (form), Center for Infants and Children With Special Needs (www.medicalhomeinfo.org/tools/Documentation/CHILD HISTORY FACT SHEET mini.doc).
- *Comprehensive Care plan packet* (booklet), National Medical Home Learning Collaborative II (www.medicalhomeinfo.org/tools/CarePlans/Comprehensive CarePlanningII.pdf).
- *Consultation Referral Form* (form), Cincinnati Children's Hospital Medical Center (www.cincinnatichildrens.org/NR/rdonlyres/D86E76FC-FAA6-4F21-9D9F-371D35CC365D/0/consultreferralform.pdf).
- *Effect of Child's Disability on Family Members Interview* (questionnaire), Robert E. Nickel, MD and Larry W. Desch, MD (www.brookespublishing.com/pgforms/pdfs/03-FamilyInterview.pdf).
- *EPIC IC Medical Home Project Actionable Care Plan* (form), PA Medical Home Program—EPIC IC (www.medicalhomeinfo.org/tools/CarePlans/Actionable care plan.doc).
- *Hospital Discharge Packet* (form), Center for Infants and Children With Special Needs: Children's Hospital Medical Center of Cincinnati (www.medicalhomeinfo.org/tools/Documentation/Hospital Discharge.doc).
- *Integrated Services Care Plan* (form), PA Medical Home Program—EPIC IC. (www.medicalhomeinfo.org/tools/CarePlans/Integrated care plan DRAFT.doc).
- *Medical Home Assessment* (form), Los Angeles Medical Home Project for CSHCN (www.medicalhomeinfo.org/tools/CarePlans/Assessment form.doc).
- *Medical Summaries* (form), PA Medical Home Program—EPIC IC (www.medicalhomeinfo.org/tools/CarePlans/MEDICAL SUMMARY.doc).
- *My care plan* (form), Palmetto Pediatric (www.medicalhomeinfo.org/tools/CarePlans/Palmettocareplan.doc).
- *Primary Care Family Assessment* (form), Robert E. Nickel, MD and Larry W. Desch, MD (www.brookespublishing.com/pgforms/pdfs/03-PrimaryCareAssessment.pdf).
- *Referral Fax Back Form*, American Academy of Pediatrics (www.medicalhomeinfo.org/tools/Documentation/PA-Referral Fax Back Form.doc).
- *Sample Referral to Emergency Room Form*, Cincinnati Children's Hospital Medical Center (www.medicalhomeinfo.org/tools/doc_guide.html#sample).

Engaging Patient and Family

- *20 Tips to Prevent Medical Errors in Children* (fact sheet), AHRQ (www.aap.org/saferhealthcare/files/5907_20tipkid.pdf).

Medical Decision Support

- *Safer Health Care for Kids* (Web page), American Academy of Pediatrics (www.aap.org/saferhealthcare).

AAP POLICY STATEMENTS

American Academy of Pediatrics, Committee on Drugs and Committee on Hospital Care. Prevention of medication errors in the pediatric inpatient setting. *Pediatrics*. 2003;112(2):431-436. (aappolicy.aappublications.org/cgi/content/full/pediatrics;112/2/431).

American Academy of Pediatrics, National Initiative for Children's Health Care Quality Project Advisory Committee. Principles of patient safety in pediatrics. *Pediatrics*. 2001;107(6):1473-1475. (aappolicy.aappublications.org/cgi/content/full/pediatrics;107/6/1473).

REFERENCES

1. American Academy of Pediatrics, Section on Hospital Medicine. Guiding principles for pediatric hospitalist programs. *Pediatrics*. 2005;115:1101-1102.
2. Institute of Medicine. *Cross the Quality Chasm: A New Health System for the 21st Century*. Washington, DC: National Academy Press; 2001.
3. Srivastava R, Norlin C, James BC, et al. Community and hospital-based physicians' attitudes regarding pediatric hospitalist systems. *Pediatrics*. 2005;115:34-38.
4. Percelay J, American Academy of Pediatrics, Committee on Hospital Care. Physicians' roles in coordinating care of hospitalized children. *Pediatrics*. 2003;111:707-709.
5. Pantilat SZ, Lindenauer PK, Katz PP, et al. Primary care physician attitudes regarding communication with hospitalists. *Am J Med*. 2001;111(9B):15S-20S.
6. Bauchner H, Adams W, Burstin H. "You've got mail": issues in communication with patients and their families by e-mail. *Pediatrics*. 2002;109:954-956.

7. Dudas V, Bookwalter T, Kerr KM, et al. The impact of follow-up telephone calls to patients after hospitalization. *Am J Med.* 2001;111(9B):26S-30S.
8. Alpers A. Key legal principle for hospitalists. *Am J Med.* 2001;111(9B):5S-9S.
9. Roy CL, Poon EG, Karson AS, et al. Patient safety concerns arising from test results that return after hospital discharge. *Ann Intern Med.* 2005;143:121-128.

Chapter 21
HOSPITAL CARE

Jack M. Percelay, MD, MPH

Hospitalization of a child is a stressful and frightening event that may have negative long-term psychological consequences for child and family* alike, even when the immediate medical outcome is excellent. To make hospitalization less traumatic for children and their families, primary care physicians (PCPs) must work proactively to create integrated and efficient processes and systems for hospital admission and discharge. For each child hospitalized, PCPs must be sensitive to the child and family's individual experiences and customize the care to their needs. Only by addressing both the generic processes and the individual child and family can the optimal physical, mental, and social health and well being for children and families who require hospitalization be achieved.

HOSPITAL ADMISSION

For PCPs, the first system issue that must be addressed is where to hospitalize children in the PCPs' practice (Box 21-1). Choices may be influenced by experience, geographic proximity, insurance plans, and the hospital's physician, nursing, and other resources. More objective criteria include outcomes data, use of guidelines and pathways, and other assessments of the hospital's efforts to provide safe, high-quality care. Regardless of the decision, the hospital information should be included in a practice brochure so parents know in advance what hospital and emergency room to visit should the need arise. As the physician who has a preexisting relationship with the patient and family, the PCP's expression of confidence and trust in the institution and the individuals who will be caring for the hospitalized child is a valuable source of reassurance to the family.

Children tend to be admitted to the hospital under one of three scenarios: (1) a single planned elective admission, (2) a single unanticipated urgent or emergent admission, or (3) a repeat admission, scheduled or unanticipated, for a preexisting problem. For elective admissions, a variety of tools and resources, including hospital tours, brochures, and Web-based resources, are available to help families and children prepare for a scheduled surgical or procedural admission. The approach used should be tailored to the child's age and developmental status.

Children with underlying chronic illness or injury who have potential or planned recurrent hospitalizations may benefit from the mastery that can come from repetition and familiarity, or they may experience the fear of having a negative experience repeated. The combination of child life services, pain control, and sedation services can help make procedures and the hospital stay much less frightening. The PCP's role is to stay abreast of the child's progress, to remain a resource to the family, to support the well being of siblings, and to serve as a conduit and translator for the family to relay concerns and questions that the family may be comfortable sharing with the PCP but not directly with other subspecialty or hospital care providers. From a performance improvement standpoint, children and families who are frequently hospitalized are experts on how the hospital experience can be improved for everyone. Their feedback should be actively solicited.

The unplanned emergent or urgent admission precludes advance preparation for the individual family and thus mandates an effective system. Preparation starts with deciding on a hospital affiliation, informing parents of these relationships, and having a plan in the office to deal with the emergently ill child. The hospital pediatric department should have already determined policies and circumstances under which children may be directly admitted from the physician's office or whether all children are admitted uniformly through the emergency room. For emergent admissions, the PCP's immediate responsibility is to facilitate the process for the family. The hospital should be notified, and the admitting physician or staff member should be contacted directly. Such communications should not be delegated to the office staff. The parents should be provided with a one-page handout with directions to the hospital and instructions on where to go. Professional transport should be requested if medically indicated. A child who requires oxygen in the office should not be transported in the back seat of a parent's car.

Once the decision has been made to admit the child, the role of the PCP, as well as the roles that other physicians and health care providers will play, should be explained to the family. The parents should be informed of the times when the inpatient attending physician performs rounds to ensure that the parents can be available when the physician sees the child. Other consulting physicians caring for the child should do the same. The American Academy of Pediatrics (AAP) is a strong proponent of family-centered care, and it encourages rounds to be a shared event among physicians, nurses, patient, and family.[1] Decision making should be open and inclusive of parental input. Family-centered walk rounds are becoming the standard of care on teaching services. No longer are parents told of a decision that the attending physician and house staff made in a separate room or outside in the hallway. The family's input should be solicited as the problem, prognosis, and treatment options are explained. At the time of admission, the health care

*The term *parent* or *parents* is used in this text to reflect the child's primary adult caretakers and is often used interchangeably with the term *family.* Families and adult caretakers take many forms. The term *parent* is not meant to apply solely to a child's biological mother or father.

BOX 21-1 Advance Preparation for Hospital Admission

OFFICE PREPARATION

- Select hospital affiliation in advance.
- Include affiliated hospital information in practice brochures, with recommendations for where children should go for pediatric emergency care.
- Prepare office for medical emergencies.
- Have appropriate supplies available (eg, oxygen tank, epinephrine).
- List telephone numbers for 9-1-1, ambulance services, emergency rooms, admitting telephone numbers for hospital, subspecialists, surgeons, and hospitalists.

HOSPITAL RESOURCES FOR ELECTIVE ADMISSIONS

- Tours of surgical or procedural areas (or both), often led by child life specialists or operating room/ anesthesia personnel
- Internet or virtual tours (more common for large referral centers)
- Electronic or print orientation materials for hospital logistics
- Pictures, maps, and suggestions of what to bring to the hospital
- Visitation policies
- Dietary rules
- Electronic or print orientation materials addressing the stress of hospitalization
- Electronic or print information for specific clinical conditions and procedures
- Doll or puppet play delivered by qualified personnel

INFORMING CHILDREN ABOUT ELECTIVE ADMISSIONS

- *Infants:* Calm and prepared parents are the best preparation for infants.
- *Preschool children:* Inform children 1 to 2 days before going to the hospital. Use simple, neutral language, but be honest: "You'll get a medicine so it doesn't hurt much." "You will feel tugging." "There will be a funny feeling." "I don't know."
- *Children 5 to 6 years of age:* Inform children 3 to 5 days in advance; explain why the procedure is necessary and that it is not punishment.
- *Children 7 to 11 years of age:* Inform children 1 week in advance. Provide sufficient time to answer all their questions.
- *Children 12 years and older:* Ideally, children of this age are participants in their health care and involved with the planning from the beginning.

SPECIAL CONSIDERATIONS FOR CHILDREN WITH RECURRENT ADMISSIONS

- Repetition offers the chance to develop mastery, especially with the assistance of child life. Patients may be taught visualization and distraction techniques.
- A risk exists of increased fear and anxiety of repeating negative experiences.
- Support groups for patients, parents, and siblings may be available.
- Subspecialty team for children with chronic disease will typically provide psychosocial support.
- Patients and families who are frequently admitted to the hospital can provide useful feedback on how the hospital experience can be improved for all.

UNANTICIPATED, EMERGENT ADMISSION FROM THE OFFICE

- Depending on the child's age, the PCP may decide to tell parents separately and then inform the child with the parents present.
- Mode of urgency of admission and mode of transport (911 vs ambulance vs parents) should be determined.
- Do not overwhelm parents with detailed orientation brochures. Provide a written handout with directions to the hospital and where to go (admissions, emergency room, and floor) once in the hospital. One-page brochures from the receiving physician's practice (emergency room, subspecialist, surgeon, hospitalist) may help.
- Directly notify the receiving physician by telephone of the pending admission. Provide a copy of the most recent notes, laboratory tests, imaging studies, and current medications along with a problem list or summary of the patient's medical history. Include PCP office contact information to receive reports from hospital.
- Discuss clinical assessment and recommendations with the admitting physician.
- Discuss relevant psychosocial and cultural considerations with the admitting physician and hospital staff.

ROLE OF THE PCP IN THE HOSPITAL

- Determine the attending physician of record—PCP, a hospitalist, a subspecialist, a surgeon?
- When will the family next see or hear from the PCP? How are hospital rounds handled?
- What other physicians and health care providers will be involved in the child's care?
- Is this facility a teaching institution, and will house staff be involved? Explain different levels of training and clarify roles to the family.

PREPARING FAMILIES FOR HOSPITALIZATION

- Provide a realistic overview of expected events and time course of the hospital stay. Specifically inform the parents of any procedures planned at admission.
- Acknowledge that this time will be stressful for the entire family and that resources are available to help.
- Whenever appropriate, discuss criteria for discharge home from the hospital at the time of admission.

providers should emphasize that they and the family members are partners in the child's care. This discussion should also be held at the time of admission to set the tenor for a collaborative relationship among child, family, physicians, and other members of the health care team. Even if the PCP is not the attending physician of record, the family should still be informed that the PCP is available as a resource, especially if the family members believe they are not getting the information they need.

Admission is also a good time to acknowledge the stress of hospitalization. Recognizing these stresses and risks in advance and providing resources is crucial in helping families cope. For the affected child and family, no hospitalization is simple. The patient, siblings, and parents all experience stress. The hospital should have mental health care providers and stress-reduction resources available to patients and families, and the hospital should actively screen for families having difficulties so that intervention can occur before any problems get out of hand. The preexisting and ongoing relationship with the family puts the PCP in the special position of being able to provide important support simply through familiarity, empathy, and caring. Additionally, PCPs are in a unique position to help with the impact hospitalization commonly has on siblings. When another physician is caring for the child in the hospital, excellent communication with this individual is paramount. Use of consultants (Chapter 19, Art of Referral, Consultation, and Collaborative Management) and hospitalists (Chapter 20, Hospitalist Medicine: Communicating with Patients and Families) is discussed elsewhere in this book. In addition to discussing medical issues, the admitting physician should be provided with relevant psychosocial and cultural considerations. What are the family's strengths in coping with the stress of a hospitalized child? Where can the family benefit from assistance? Because the PCP is the only one with an established relationship and history with the family, input from the PCP is invaluable. The foreseeable hospital events should be briefly outlined to the family at the time of admission. The PCP should describe difficult or painful procedures to the parents to help prepare the patient and family; here again, the PCP serves as the bridge to a successful transfer of trust and confidence. In fact, the discharge planning process starts at the time of admission. The family should be told of the anticipated duration of the child's hospitalization and the child's likely status and disposition when the child leaves the hospital. The parents should be told about any medication, equipment, or nursing care that may be required after discharge, The parents should also know ahead of time whether the child will be fully recovered or whether the child will need to recover further at home. For children with more serious illnesses, these projections may not be possible. In the face of such uncertainty, family members may be reassured that they are not alone and that they have the continued support of their PCP.

DISCHARGE PLANNING

As is true for admission to the hospital, discharge from the hospital must be addressed as both a unique event for each individual patient and family and as a generic system process. The PCP has a responsibility to help prepare each individual patient and family according to their unique needs, strengths, and cultural beliefs to leave the hospital. Similarly, within the hospital structure, PCPs must contribute to developing robust inpatient systems with the necessary resources to promote a safe, comprehensive, effective, and efficient discharge process capable of dealing with the anticipated needs of the populations being served (Boxes 21-2 and 21-3).

Discharge planning should be addressed daily to make sure the process proceeds effectively and efficiently. A smooth discharge is the result of comprehensively delivered care and education throughout the hospitalization by all members of the health care team. Box 21-2 describes the discharge planning roles of various members of the health care team. Good planning means anticipating the usual snafus, delays, mistakes, and limitations of personnel and supplies. Requests should be submitted early. Parents should be educated about their child's care from the start. Parents who are prepared and empowered to participate in their child's care and in the decision-making processes are more informed and capable caregivers during the hospital stay and at home after discharge.

BOX 21-2 Discharge Planning Roles and Resources

Nursing: Nurses provide direct clinical care, education, and psychosocial support from the moment they meet the child and family. Their involvement in discharge planning is crucial. Home visiting nursing is usually arranged by case managers or social workers. Hospital nursing staff assists by providing a nursing care plan and indicating specific services that are needed.

Case management: Case management workers help access other health care and social resources in the community. They are particularly valuable for transfer to another institution. They can often help the family with financial access to care. Some insurance companies may offer case management services to help coordinate outpatient needs.

Social services: Social workers provide case management services in some institutions. They provide valuable psychological support to families. Together with case managers, they help when financial and legal (eg, custody, autonomy) considerations affect care.

Child life: Child life specialists are as skilled at preparing children and families for discharge as they are at preparing them for admission. Some child life programs may provide ongoing support groups for previously hospitalized children and their siblings.

Pharmacy: Pharmacists can help double-check medications and check for drug interactions. Outpatient medications are rarely provided by in hospital pharmacies because of reimbursement issues. Families should use a single pharmacy to take advantage of computerized record keeping and to monitor for potential drug interactions.

Physical, speech, respiratory, and occupational therapy: Therapists who treat children in the hospital can help link children with outpatient providers to continue services begun in the hospital.

Mental health: Psychologists, counselors, and clergy can provide mental health services on an inpatient basis and help to identify community resources.

Flow, congestion, and efficiency of the process are issues for both larger and smaller hospitals. When bed availability is limited, an efficient discharge process is particularly valuable. Some institutions schedule discharges in 30-minute appointment slots to provide a coordinated timetable for the nurses and parents and to avoid congestion and delays. Other system issues that need to be addressed include patient and family education, disposition determination, instructions, medications, equipment, nutrition, discharge instructions, follow-up plans, communication, ongoing therapy needs, and psychosocial support. These topics are addressed in Box 21-3.

Direct face-to-face, one-on-one teaching is provided by nurses, therapists, educators, and physicians as part of routine care. High-volume diagnoses, such as asthma, may warrant group classes. Most children go back home from the hospital, but others may be transferred to a different hospital or to a rehabilitation, chronic care, or other skilled nursing facility. Knowledge of local resources and experience in planning and making these transitions is crucial. When equipment is delivered early, parents can learn home care under supervision in the hospital to make sure that whatever problems are going to arise are identified and remedied while the child is still in the hospital with expert help readily available. Discharge instructions, such as medication instructions, must be clear and understandable and provided in a language that the family can understand. All too often, instructions are written in medical jargon rather than in the family's native tongue. Even for native-English speakers, instructions need to be written at a literacy level targeted to families, not physicians or nurses. The AAP has low-level literacy brochures available for common inpatient problems, but these lack the specificity required for discharge instructions. Each hospital should have plans for dealing with non-English speakers, such as local bilingual staff or a telephone-based commercial medical translation service.

For patients with long hospital stays and complex needs who either lack a PCP or whose PCP was not involved in the hospital stay, the PCP responsible for follow-up may choose to meet with the family in the hospital before discharge. Family conferences with the patient's various providers and therapists can help clarify follow-up plans for children with complex needs. The families need to know the appropriate contact (PCP, specialist, or emergency room) for different types of problems. Whenever possible, the child's subspecialty care should be centered at one institution for improved communication and convenience. Advantages include the ability to coordinate multiple physician visits with one trip; a single, unified medical record; and established

BOX 21-3 Discharge Planning Considerations

Discharge planning begins at admission. Work with other team members to assess the family's and the child's needs so that all necessary arrangements are completed once the child is medically cleared to leave the hospital.

Discharge timing should be coordinated and perhaps even scheduled with nursing to avoid bottlenecks. Notify parents and prepare discharge instructions, prescriptions, appointments, and other information 12 to 24 hours in advance.

Discharge teaching begins with patient education at admission. In addition to face-to-face teaching, provide multilingual written, electronic, video, and visual materials in layperson's terms.

Discharge instructions should be written, legible, straightforward, and in the patient's language. Preprinted, multilingual, low-literacy handouts for the hospital's most common diagnoses are helpful. For children with complex medical needs, clearly identify specific problems that should be referred to the PCP and which problems require follow-up with the (particular) subspecialist.

Discharge medications need to be double-checked, reconciled, and checked for interactions. Regimens should be simplified to maximize compliance. The medication list should be given to the PCP. Ensure that the family has the financial and logistic resources to fill prescriptions. Consider having family fill prescriptions before discharge. Specific nutritional supplies may also be required.

Durable medical equipment should be ordered once the need is recognized. Plan to have equipment in place and family instructed in its use at least 1 day before discharge. Provide troubleshooting hints and contact numbers should problems arise.

Home nursing requests should be submitted early. Resources are often limited. Whenever appropriate, teach parents to provide care in the hospital under supervision of nursing staff. This approach empowers parents and reduces the level of home nursing services required.

Therapy (physical, speech, respiratory, occupational) initiated in the hospital often needs to be continued. Develop a plan for ongoing care. Such care frequently requires transition to a different outpatient therapist.

Follow-up appointments should be clearly specified. For children with complex medical needs or families with limited resources, consider scheduling these appointments before discharge. If transportation is an issue, then ask case management or social services for help.

Discharge summaries must be timely, standardized, and complete. Communicate by telephone with other care providers on the day of discharge and provide family with a one-page summary of hospital stay, discharge medications and instructions, and pending tests.

Psychological and emotional support services need to be continued beyond discharge, just as medications and nursing care. The child, parents, siblings, and extended family may all have needs. Outpatient resources are often limited. Work with in-hospital providers, case managers, and social workers to advocate for and arrange these services.

relationships among subspecialists. However, given institutional limitations and patient preferences, multiple institutions and providers are often involved in a child's care. Thus complete written communication and record keeping is crucial for all the providers who constitute the child's medical home.

If the PCP was not the primary inpatient attending physician, then the physician caring for the child in the hospital should telephone the child's PCP on the day of discharge. Ideally, the hospital will have a transcription and fax and/or e-mail system that provides a complete discharge summary to the PCP on either the day of discharge or the next day. At a minimum, parents should go home with a legible one-page fill-in-the-blank summary that includes diagnosis, pertinent findings, hospital events, discharge medications and instructions, follow-up appointments, and a list of tests pending at discharge. Until a universal electronic medical record is developed, families of children with complex medical histories or needs will do well to maintain their own records of their child's medical history, regularly updating it with medications and any significant events. The AAP has samples for children in general[2] and specifically for children with complex needs.[3]

Finally, and in many cases most importantly, the infrastructure and resources of the hospital and the commitment of the entire staff must be directed toward the psychosocial needs of the child and family. As previously emphasized, the stress of hospitalization should have been addressed from admission. Transition out of the hospital has its own set of stressors. Just as child life specialists can help prepare children for a surgical procedure, they can help prepare children and families for discharge home. For some families, discharge from the hospital is the beginning of dealing with a chronic disease or ongoing disability. Even if a child fully recovers from an acute event, the child and family's senses of security may be shattered. Mental health needs identified during the hospital stay do not resolve with discharge. Ongoing needs should be anticipated and community resources accessed. These resources are often inadequate in the United States, and one of the responsibilities of pediatricians caring for children is to advocate for improved community mental health services for children and families.

For PCPs who practice in community hospitals with few pediatric resources, several AAP policy statements may be useful in supporting arguments for comprehensive, state-of-the-art care for children. The child life services statement[4] outlines the benefits and potential services provided by child life specialists. If the hospital does not employ a child life specialist, many useful child life materials are available through the Internet. PCPs can advocate for continuing education in this crucial area for the hospital's pediatric nursing staff, as well as staff from such areas as the emergency room, anesthesia, operating room, recovery room, radiology, and phlebotomy.

The AAP statement about physicians' roles in coordinating care of hospitalized children[5] specifically addresses responsibilities of physicians caring for children at admission and discharge, and the expected interactions with the PCP. The medical home statement further outlines the goal of comprehensive care that spans the outpatient and inpatient arenas.[6]

SUMMARY

Hospitalization can be made a less stressful experience for children and their families through advance preparation and development of systems that are designed to provide comprehensive, safe, family- and patient-centered care by health care team members who attend to the psychosocial needs of children and their families. Most problems can be anticipated and thus mitigated by preparation.

TOOLS FOR PRACTICE

Engaging Patient and Family

- *Going to the Hospital* (fact sheet), Nemours Foundation – Kids Health (www.kidshealth.org/kid/feel_better/places/hospital.html).
- *Patient Education Compendium* (package), American Academy of Pediatrics (www.aap.org/bookstore).
- *Preparing Children for Hospital Visits* (fact sheet), Johns Hopkins Children's Center (www.hopkinschildrens.org/pages/clinical/hlcc_hospital.cfm).
- *Preparing for Hospitalization* (fact sheet), Children's Hospital of Philadelphia (www.chop.edu/pat_care_fam_serv/prep_for_hosp.shtml).
- *Recommended Books: Helping Children Cope with Hospital/Doctor Visits, Surgical Procedures and Grief* (Web page), Cincinnati Children's Hospital Medical Center (www.cincinnatichildrens.org/visit/stay/books/).
- *Your Child's Hospital Stay* (booklet), UCSF Children's Hospital at UCSF Medical Center (www.ucsfhealth.org/childrens/patient_guide/services/YourChildsStay.pdf).

Practice Management and Care Coordination

- *Action Care Plan* (form), Center for Medical Home Improvement (www.medicalhomeimprovement.org/assets/pdf/Working_Full.pdf).
- *Care Coordination Measurement Tool* (form), American Academy of Pediatrics (www.medicalhomeinfo.org/tools/Tools/Final MH CC Measurement Tool.doc).
- *Care Plans (I & II)* (form), Hitchcock Clinic—Concord Pediatric (www.medicalhomeinfo.org/training/materials/April2004Curriculum/PPP/PPP Appendices/HitchcockCarePlan_1.pdf).
- *Child History Fact Sheet* (form), The Center for Infants and Children with Special Needs (www.medicalhomeinfo.org/tools/Documentation/CHILD HISTORY FACTSHEET mini.doc).
- *Comprehensive Care Plan Packet* (booklet), National Medical Home Learning Collaborative II (www.medicalhomeinfo.org/tools/CarePlans/ComprehensiveCarePlanningII.pdf).
- *Consultation Referral Form*, Cincinnati Children's Hospital Medical Center (www.cincinnatichildrens.org/NR/rdonlyres/D86E76FC-FAA6-4F21-9D9F-371D35CC365D/0/consultreferralform.pdf).

- *Documentation Forms*, American Academy of Pediatrics (www.aap.org/bookstore).
- *Emergency Information Form for Children with Special Needs*, American Academy of Pediatrics (www.aap.org/booksore).
- *EPIC-IC Medical Home Project Actionable Care Plan* (form), PA Medical Home Program—EPIC IC (www.medicalhomeinfo.org/tools/CarePlans/Actionable care plan.doc).
- *Hospital Discharge Packet* (form), The Center for Infants and Children with Special Needs: Children's Hospital Medical Center of Cincinnati (www.medicalhomeinfo.org/tools/Documentation/Hospital Discharge.doc).
- *Integrated Services Care Plan* (form), PA Medical Home Program—EPIC IC (www.medicalhomeinfo.org/tools/CarePlans/Integrated care plan DRAFT.doc).
- *Medical Summaries* (form), PA Medical Home Program—EPIC IC (www.medicalhomeinfo.org/tools/CarePlans/MEDICALSUMMARY.doc).
- *My Care Plan* (form), Palmetto Pediatric (www.medicalhomeinfo.org/tools/CarePlans/Palmettocareplan.doc).
- *Referral Fax Back Form*, American Academy of Pediatrics (www.medicalhomeinfo.org/tools/Documentation/PA-Referral Fax Back Form.doc).
- *Sample Referral to Emergency Room Form*, American Academy of Pediatrics (www.medicalhomeinfo.org/training/materials/April2004Curriculum/PPP/PPPAppendices/App R - fax form.pdf).

Other Resources

- Cincinnati Children's Hospital Medical Center. Recommended books for kids. Available at: www.cincinnatichildrens.org/visit/stay/books. Accessed February 22, 2007.
- University of California, San Francisco, Medical Center. Available at: www.ucsfhealth.org/childrens/patient_guide/services/admissions.html. Accessed December 11, 2007.
- The Children's Hospital of Philadelphia. Available at: www.chop.edu/pat_care_fam_serv/prep_for_hosp.shtml. Accessed April 15, 2008.
- Johns Hopkins Children's Center. Available at: www.hopkinschildrens.org/pages/clinical/hlcc_hospital.cfm. Accessed April 15, 2008.
- Nemours Foundation. KidsHealth. Available at: www.kidshealth.org/kid/feel_better/places/hospital.html. Accessed April 15, 2008.

AAP POLICY STATEMENTS

American Academy of Pediatrics, Child Life Council and Committee on Hospital Care. Child Life Services. *Pediatrics*. 2006;118(4):1757-1763. (aappolicy.aappublications.org/cgi/content/full/pediatrics;118/4/1757).

American Academy of Pediatrics, Committee on Hospital Care. Family-Centered Care and the Pediatrician's Role. *Pediatrics*. 2003;112(3):691-696. (aappolicy.aappublications.org/cgi/content/full/pediatrics;112/3/691).

American Academy of Pediatrics, Committee on Pediatric Emergency Medicine. Preparation for Emergencies in the Offices of Pediatricians and Pediatric Primary Care Providers. *Pediatrics*. 2007;120(1):200-212. (aappolicy.aappublications.org/cgi/content/full/pediatrics;120/1/200).

American Academy of Pediatrics, Medical Home Initiatives for Children With Special Needs Project Advisory Committee. The Medical Home. *Pediatrics*. 2002;110(1):184-186. (aappolicy.aappublications.org/cgi/content/full/pediatrics;110/1/184).

Jaimovich DG, American Academy of Pediatrics, Committee on Hospital Care, and Section on Critical Care. Admission and Discharge Guidelines for the Pediatric Patient Requiring Intermediate Care. *Pediatrics*. 2004;113(5):1430-1433. (aappolicy.aappublications.org/cgi/content/full/pediatrics;113/5/1430).

Percelay JM and American Academy of Pediatrics, Committee on Hospital Care. Physicians' Roles in Coordinating Care of Hospitalized Children. *Pediatrics*. 2003;111(3):707-709. (aappolicy.aappublications.org/cgi/content/full/pediatrics;111/3/707).

REFERENCES

1. American Academy of Pediatrics, Committee on Hospital Care. Family-centered care and the pediatrician's role. *Pediatrics*. 2003;112:691-697.
2. American Academy of Pediatrics Bookstore. Practice Management, Documentation Forms. Available at: www.aap.org/bookstore. Accessed June 7, 2007.
3. American College of Emergency Physicians and American Academy of Pediatrics. Emergency Information Form for Children With Special Needs. Available at: www.aap.org/advocacy/blankform.pdf. Accessed June 7, 2007.
4. Child Life Council and American Academy of Pediatrics, Committee on Hospital Care. Child life services. *Pediatrics*. 2006;118:1757-1763.
5. Percelay JM, American Academy of Pediatrics, Committee on Hospital Care. Physicians' roles in coordinating care of hospitalized children. *Pediatrics*. 2003;111:707-709.
6. American Academy of Pediatrics. Medical Home Initiatives for Children With Special Needs Project Advisory Committee. The medical home. *Pediatrics*. 2002;110:184-186.

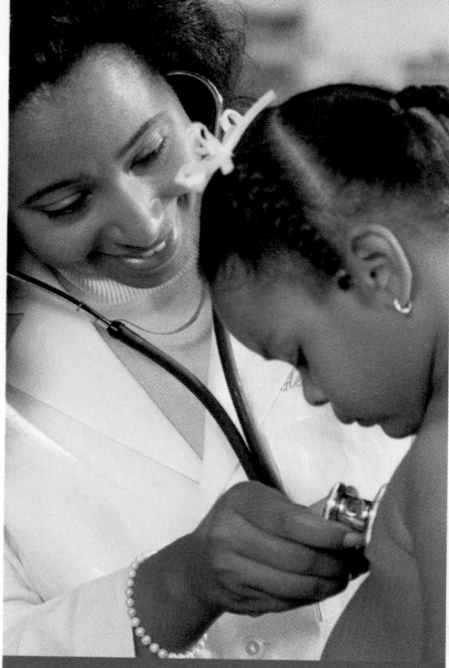

PART 3

Principles of Patient Care

Section One: Health Promotion

22 Supporting Development of the Family
23 Counseling Families on Healthy Lifestyles
24 Communication Strategies
25 Anticipatory Guidance
26 Feeding of Infants and Children
27 Nutritional Requirements

Section Two: Disease Prevention

28 Morbidity and Mortality Among the Young
29 Immunizations
30 Injury Prevention
31 Violence Prevention
32 Preventive Cardiology
33 Prevention of Dental Caries
34 Prevention of Obesity
35 Prevention of Smoking

Section Three: Screening and Case Finding

36 Screening: General Considerations
37 Physical Examination as a Screening Tool
38 Preparticipation Physical Evaluation
39 Auditory Screening
40 Cardiovascular Screening
41 Screening for Anemia
42 Vision Screening
43 Identification of Developmental Delays and Early Intervention System
44 Developmental Surveillance and Intervention
45 Language and Speech Assessment
46 Psychosocial Screening
47 Family Screening and Assessments
48 Recognition of Genetic-Metabolic Diseases by Clinical Diagnosis and Screening
49 Screening and Initial Management of Lead Poisoning
50 Substance Use Disorders: Early Identification and Referral
51 Use of Urinalysis and Urine Culture in Screening

Continued

Section Four: Treatment of Disease

52 The Ill Child
53 Physiology and Management of Fever
54 Management of Acute Pain in Children
55 Management of Chronic Pain in Children
56 Self-regulation Therapies: Hypnosis and Biofeedback
57 Complementary and Alternative Medical Therapies
58 Body Fluids, Electrolyte Concentration, and Acid-Base Composition
59 Fluids and Electrolytes in Clinical Practice
60 Blood Products and Their Uses
61 Antimicrobial Therapy
62 Preoperative Assessment
63 Postoperative Care

Section Five: Care of the Child With Special Health Care Needs

64 Children With Ongoing Health Conditions
65 Home Health Care
66 Pediatric Rehabilitation
67 Partnering With Families in Hospital and Community Settings
68 School-related Issues for Children With Special Needs

Section Six: Palliative and End-of-Life Care

69 Palliative, End-of-Life, and Bereavement Care

SECTION ONE

Health Promotion

Chapter 22

SUPPORTING DEVELOPMENT OF THE FAMILY

Penelope K. Knapp, MD

The first responsibility of parents is to provide for their children's health and safety as they grow. In turn the growth of children depends on their relationships with their parents and other family members and on how parents provide their children good experiences and protect them from bad ones. Elements that determine how parents accomplish these tasks include their own history, health, and personality, the environment in which they live and the match between their personal capacities and the age, temperament, and needs of their children.[1]

The pediatric primary care physician (PCP) plays a critical role in the support of the family, not only to maintain the child's health, but also to identify risks and to offer preventive intervention. The PCP is likely to be the first and only clinician evaluating the child, at least during infancy and early childhood. Continuing contact with the child and family allows recognition of emerging difficulties and opportunity for early interventions. This chapter focuses on supporting the family from the earliest stages of a child's developmental and social-emotional functioning—that is, the child's developing mental health. This support begins optimally during pregnancy, or at least during infancy.

The parents' own relationships with other adults nurture their relationship with the infant or child. While they are engaged in the daily and demanding project of caring for an infant or raising a child, parents rely on other supportive adults. The relationship with the PCP may be crucial, particularly if parents are vulnerable, ill-equipped, or unprepared for parenthood or lack support from others or if the child has special health care or social-emotional needs.

Parents often bring their concerns about their children's emotional and behavioral states to the PCP. Such concerns vary with the age of the child. Infants may exhibit dysregulation of physiologic functions such as fussy behavior, colic, feeding problems, or sleeping difficulties. Toddlers may display behavioral disturbances, such as aggression, defiance, impulsivity, and overactivity. Other frequently encountered early childhood concerns are constitutional factors (eg, temperament); developmental delays; processing difficulties; physiologic, sensory, or sensory-motor problems; organizational difficulties; and problems with *goodness of fit* between parent and infant or child (Tables 22-1 and 22-2).

Resiliency, or a healthy response to stress, is seen in individual family members and in families as a whole. Supporting the family well should build resiliency by increasing the parents' problem-solving abilities and knowledge. In contrast to offering the sort of support that encourages the parent to call on the PCP for any small issue, support that enhances resiliency will build on the parent's strengths. For example, an anxious young mother may possess, as strengths, a capacity for sharp observation of any small change in her baby and a library of childrearing manuals. The PCP might help her organize her observations of her infant and take the time to help her process, assess, and apply what she learns from her reading.

ATTACHMENT

Attachment is a broad concept describing the relationships that, during infancy and early childhood, support or jeopardize emotional flourishing. Attachment powerfully influences how children regulate their emotions and behaviors and how they use their capacity to deploy their intelligence in learning. It may foreordain the flourishing or constraints of later relationships.

Attachment describes a dyad, rather than a feature of the child. In North America, 65% of infants and toddlers have a secure attachment with a sensitive, responsive, available parent.[2] Securely attached children feel valued, worthwhile, and effective. They are able to explore and master new experiences, and they are able to become autonomous confidently because they know that an adult primary caregiver is available. At preschool ages, securely attached children display empathy, compliance, and positive affect, and they can regulate their own state and emotions. Thirty-five percent of children have insecure attachments. Insecure avoidant attachment patterns (20%) are found if the parent is insensitive to the child's cues, avoids contact, or rejects the child. Insecurely attached children believe that they cannot rely on adults to meet their needs or that, if they show they need closeness, they will be rejected. Therefore they do not learn to recognize their own needs for closeness and connectedness. In preschool these children display hostile, distant interactions, act tough to get their needs met, and may be defiant or aggressive; they may even victimize others. They may also seek approval through achievements by presenting a false independence.

Insecure ambivalent or resistant attachment patterns (10%) are found if the parents' care is inconsistent and unpredictable. Ambivalently attached infants heighten

Table 22-1 Primary Care Physician Queries for Primary Caregivers

PHYSICIAN'S CONSIDERATION	QUESTION FOR PRIMARY CAREGIVER
PRENATAL VISIT	
History of maternal depression*	In the last 6 months, have you felt down, sad, depressed, hopeless for more than a month? In the last 6 months, have you felt no energy to the extent that you did not want to do the things you usually do for more than a month?
Family's social supports	Who is helping you prepare for Baby?
NEWBORN VISIT	
The infant's competence and readiness to respond to her (or his) parents	Do you see how Baby brightens when she (or he) hears your voice?
The parents' capabilities, as they handle and care for the infant, to reinforce their sense of competence	Do you see how Baby likes it when you (hold or feed or talk to) her (or him)?
1-WEEK VISIT	
How mother deals with fatigue and the big project of anticipating and meeting the infant's needs	Are you finding sufficient time to take care of yourself? This ability will help you give Baby the best care.
Parent perceptions of the infant	Do you have a feeling for what kind of temperament or personality Baby has?
Social support, father's (or partner's or other family member's) roles in care of the infant	Who is helping you with caring for Baby? What are they doing to help?
Maternal mood, social support, family	See Table 22-2
1- TO 2-MONTH VISIT	
Development of a rhythm for feeding, sleep, fussiness, and soothing	Tell me how you know what Baby wants. What works best for you and Baby to feed or soothe or get Baby to sleep? Tell me what happens with you and Baby when Baby is alert and awake.
Involvement of others in assisting with the infant's care	Does Baby behave differently when she (or he) is responding to you and when she (or he) is responding to others (father, grandmother, siblings, etc.)?
Social support, family help with care of infant	Who is helping you care for Baby?
Maternal mood, social support, family	See Table 22-2
4-MONTH VISIT	
Infant's developing social repertoire	Does Baby coo and make sounds that respond to your talking to her (or him)? What do you notice makes Baby smile?
Social support, father's role is care of infant, and depression screen	Have you begun to find some ways that you can play with Baby? Tell me how Baby shows that she (or he) loves you.
Social support, family help in care of the infant	Who is helping you with caring for Baby?
Mother's return to work	How are you dealing with return to work? What have you found for child care?
Maternal mood, social support, family	See Table 22-2
6-MONTH VISIT	
Parents' response to the infant's developing mobility and strength	Tell me about how you feel when Baby begins to move (roll over, grasp things). Excited? Afraid she (or he) will get hurt?
Developing communication between parent and infant	Tell me about what new ways Baby is communicating with you. Tell me what new things Baby understands or notices.
Social support, family help in care of the infant	Who is helping you care for Baby?
Mother's return to work	How are you dealing with return to work? How is Baby doing in child care?
Maternal mood, social support, family	See Table 22-2

Table 22-1 Primary Care Physician Queries for Primary Caregivers—cont'd

PHYSICIAN'S CONSIDERATION	QUESTION FOR PRIMARY CAREGIVER
9-MONTH VISIT	
Infant's increasing communicativeness and social awareness and mobility	Tell me about how Baby is beginning to talk—with words and with movements. Tell me about how you feel when Baby begins to move (roll over, grasp things). Excited? Afraid she (or he) will get hurt?
Infant's attachment and discrimination of others	Tell me about how Baby gets along with new or unfamiliar people.
Maternal mood, social support, family	See Table 22-2

*These two questions summarize the Edinburgh Depression Scale.

Table 22-2 Probing Questions to Evaluate Maternal Mood and Support

KEY COMPONENT	WHAT TO ASK
Maternal mood state	How are your sprits?
Perception of fetus (baby)	What has Baby been telling you about himself or herself?
Marital or partner supports	How has Partner been handling all of this?
Next steps	You notice a lot. Things sound difficult. Let's help you find someone with whom to talk.

their expression of negative feelings to gain their mother's attention; they may be angrier, more aggressive, and less compliant. Their parent may be excessively close or even intrusive, then push away, a pattern seen frequently with depressed caregivers. Adaptively, such children work hard to keep the adult engaged because they never know when they will get attention. Such children may be anxious, dependent, or whiny. In preschool these children may appear inept, dependent, or clingy, and they tend to be easy victims. Disorganized-disoriented attachment patterns (5%-10%) combine features of the other patterns and are most frequently seen in abused children.

FAMILY AS A DEVELOPMENTAL CRUCIBLE

Aspects of Development for Which Family Is Essential

Brain development is most rapid in the early months of life. The earlier an infant receives optimal stimulation in a relationship with a parent, the more the infant will thrive—that is, the infant's brain will grow well. The earlier an infant is deprived of such experience or is subjected to the experience of a toxic relationship, the more lasting the effects will be on the infant's developing brain.[3] In any society, preventable damage to developing brains will incur subsequent social costs.

Research has shown that brain development depends not only on adequate nutrition,[4,5] but also on experience-dependent learning.[6] The brain is a highly evolved organ of adaptation; it will modify itself in response to experience, it will be stunted if deprived of experience,[7] it will flourish if furnished with optimal experience,[8] and its functioning will skew if the individual's experience is toxic.[9-12] The experience that is crucial for building a baby's brain is interpersonal exchange.[13]

For babies, stress includes neglect. If the balance between experiences that painfully overstimulate the infant, such as hunger, and experiences that restore the baby to a calm state, such as being fed or soothed, is frequently absent, then the baby's developing brain adapts by constructing patterns of regulation that are poorly modulated; thus so the baby may cry unappeased until exhausted or withdraw into a conserving state of reduced responsiveness.

Risks

The impact of the parent-baby environment is powerful because it affects how the intricate circuitry of the brain is wired. A parent alone can raise an infant and child, but the parent who is functionally single, including the divorced parent or the parent who lives in marital discord, is likelier to raise a child with behavioral, emotional, and academic difficulties.[14] Parents who are unable to participate fully in raising their children also lose an opportunity for their own continued personal growth.[15]

The family environment in which the infant's mother lives may either stress her or protect her from stress, and this will influence her infant's well being. Depression in mothers is associated with disruption of bonding and attachment, with the quality of their child's relationships later in life,[16,17] with later behavioral disturbances,[18] and with later depression, language delays,[19,20] and intellectual disability.

Teenaged mothers face increased challenges in parenting.[21] Other known risk factors for stressed parenting are social disadvantage, poverty, perinatal substance abuse, sexual or physical abuse, the baby's low birth weight, parental mental illness, and early childhood behavior disorder.[4,22] These risk factors tend to cluster.[23,24] Moreover, effects of early stress and neglect may be cumulative.

SUPPORTING MULTIPLE FAMILY TYPES

Culture

Cultures acculturate, meaning that children are raised according to the customs of the culture. Although many elements of child development are driven by maturation, anticipatory guidance must also take into account the cultural belief and style of the parent. Cultural expectations about nursing, nutrition, toilet training, emerging child autonomy, expression of emotion, discipline, and learning are particular to cultures. PCPs must be open to hearing the family's points of view, even if they are alien to the PCP's own culture. (See Chapter 10, Caring for Families New to the United States; and Chapter 17, Cultural Issues in Primary Pediatric Care.)

Grandparents

Grandparents powerfully influence mothers, in supportive or unsupportive ways, and this influence may be present even if the grandmother is not. A mother may have reactions to her infant that derives from her own childhood learning about nurturance, which is based on how she was treated and/or how she experienced her siblings.[25] Grandparents may have direct relationships with infants and children and participate in child rearing. The PCP should be mindful about whether the suggestions made are in line with or divergent from what the mother hears from her own mother or from other family members.

Grandparents may operate as parents. In 1990, 3.2 million children in the United States lived primarily with grandparents, an increase of 40% over previous decades.[26] This circumstance may result from illness, substance abuse, child neglect or abuse, abandonment, incarceration, military deployment, long work-related absence, or death. When supporting parenting grandparents the PCP knows that although the grandparents have their own parenting experiences on which to draw, their energy may be limited, or they may carry a burden of grief or doubt because of their own grown child's difficulties.

Mothers, Fathers, and Partners

Parenting alone is challenging. A father's or a mother's (or other partner's) emotional support of the other parent will benefit an infant's emotional development.[27] The PCP's support of the family includes optimizing the partner's participation in infant care. If possible the partner will be present at delivery, will have plenty of infant contact, and will be familiar with the newborn's developing abilities. Fathers' roles complement those of mothers in fashions that vary according to cultural expectations and that are currently changing in US culture. Fathers' experiences of diapering, feeding, and comforting their infants provide a sense of competence and involvement, and ideally such activities increase their understanding and support of the mother.

Failing to engage the father has direct and indirect adverse effects on the developing infant.[14,28] Fathers have greater impact than mothers on boys' regulatory capacities through physical play. Toddlers with less-emotionally supportive fathers were more discontented and less task oriented during problem solving.[29]

Marital strain or discord interferes with the parenting functions of each parent; it is also usually perceived as disturbing by even very young children. Routine inquiry about how the parents are getting along together in the project of rearing the child will allow the PCP to provide early intervention if troubles exist. Early recognition of domestic violence is crucial to protect the child from emotional trauma, as well as to protect a battered parent. If serious family discord is present and the issue is beyond the PCP's ability to intervene, then a mental health referral should be made.

Foster Parents

Annually, more than 250,000 children in the United States are placed in foster care because of abuse or neglect, with over 500,000 children in the foster care system at any point in time.[30] For children removed from their parents for abuse or neglect, their PCP will support the childrearing efforts of other relatives of the child or of foster parents. (See also Chapter 116, Children in Foster and Kinship Care.)

Foster children may be separated not only from their birth parents, but also from their own personal and medical histories. The PCP will assess risks to the child's health (eg, missed immunizations, undiagnosed HIV) and to the child's development (eg, unrecognized or poorly explained developmental delays). Assessment of the child's emotional well being is equally important. Risks to the child's emotional well being are obvious, beginning with the blighted attachment that led to the out-of-home placement and are exacerbated by the child's loss and uprooting. Evaluation and early intervention of the child's risk is vital to protect or restore a child's ability to form lasting relationships with caring adults.

Kinship care is the fastest-growing out-of-home placement option. Compared with foster care, kinship care may offer more placement stability and stronger family identity for the child. However, kinship caregivers are likelier to be single, older, less educated, and in poorer health than nonrelative foster parents. Moreover, their own relationships with the child's parents may complicate the child's access to and relationship with the birth parent. Although the needs of kinship caregivers may be greater and more complicated than those of foster parents, they are less likely to request needed services for the child or themselves.

Siblings

If siblings have warm and joyful relationships, then family well being increases; if they do not, then strain is inevitable. Preparing siblings for the arrival of a new baby is sensible. Presenting the sibling with a new challenge just before the new baby comes, such as giving up the pacifier, moving from crib to bed, or navigating toilet training, is unwise. Powerful feelings of jealousy and love may be expressed intensely, especially by siblings whose verbal abilities are immature. Toddlers regress when a new baby preempts their status as youngest child, whereas older siblings may feel more positive and may take pride in their ability to engage the baby and even to assist with care—for example, by amusing the baby while the mother does a chore or by fetching diapers. Older siblings also continue to desire, demand, and deserve exclusive time with their parents every day. The storms of sibling rivalry, although painful for parents to navigate, are a sign of children's attachment. Helping parents appreciate their small children's points of view will help them respond supportively while setting limits.

The parents should keep children's routines consistent, be understanding about negative feelings, and understand their coping patterns. For example, some toddlers may introduce an imaginary friend to the household after the baby comes home, and this friend may express negative feelings about the baby and relay certain special demands for treats or services. Understanding that the imaginary friend is speaking for the toddler, and that this is the toddler's way of coping, helps parents respect the older child's feelings.

TRANSITIONS AND ADAPTATIONS

Temperament

Infant temperament—that is, activity level, mood, intensity, and emotional reactivity—may challenge the goodness of fit between parent and baby, and may make it difficult for the parent to respond optimally. *Goodness of fit* is a concept that describes the ease or difficulty of parents' and infants' reactions to each other. Poor fit may be recognized during well-child visits—for example, damped-down interactions between a withdrawn baby and a passive mother or escalating distress between a high-arousal baby with an anxious or intrusive mother. The PCP will need to monitor the relationship alertly and consider early intervention if matters worsen. A temperamentally difficult, high-arousal baby expresses emotions intensely, such as crying loudly and for a long time. The parent's response may be more or less successful in helping the baby learn from this response cycle (Table 22-3).[31] Temperamental traits will influence the child's development of self-regulation, both directly and indirectly, by how it influences the parent's response.[32] The PCP may model for the mother by being present with, attentive to, and responsive to the child. Asking parents to identify their child's temperamental style and to describe what they do that works best is helpful.

Infant reactivity and infant regulation are intertwined. The PCP can help the mother understand how the infant reacts and how she reacts to the baby's reactions, as well as how to develop strategies that help the baby develop self-regulation[33] and learn the contingent responses of mother-infant mutual regulation; this ability is termed *attunement*.[16] Crucial to attunement is the mother's accuracy in recognizing her infant's emotions, and early intervention helps her accomplish this task. For example, if during a well-child visit the PCP observes that the mother seems mechanical or disengaged from her infant, then the PCP might observe, "See how she brightens up when you talk to her." Mothers' sensitive responses are timed and matched to infant's feelings. Insensitive responses are poorly timed, intrusive, or unresponsive.

Optimally the mother is sensitive to the whole range of baby's emotion, and she responds consistently. The baby expresses full emotional range because this display facilitates closeness with the mother. If the mother withdraws or is unavailable emotionally when the baby is distressed, then the baby learns to minimize negative feelings to avoid rejection. If the mother responds inconsistently, then the baby escalates emotions to increase the odds that mother will stay close, or to bring the baby close to her (see Table 22-3).

Table 22-3 Patterns of Emotional Regulation in Response to Caregiver

MOTHER	BABY
Is sensitive to whole range of baby's emotions; responds consistently	Expresses full emotional range because this facilitates closeness with mother
Withdraws or is unavailable emotionally if baby is distressed	Baby learns to minimize negative feelings to avoid rejection
Responds inconsistently	Baby escalates emotions to increase the odds that mother will stay close or to bring her close

From Cassidy J. Emotion regulation: influences of attachment relationships. *Monogr Soc Res Child Dev.* 1994;59(2-3):228-283. Copyright © Blackwell Publishing. Reprinted by permission.

In the second year of life, difficulties with attunement and infant self-regulation evolve into recognizable patterns. If the mother is inconsistent, then the infant becomes more dependent, which impedes exploration of the environment, because the child is focused on the mother's availability. (See Chapter 130, A Developmental Approach to the Prevention of Common Behavioral Problems.)

The coercive parent models aggressive ways of attaining goals and elicits negative feelings from children, which they express as defiance. If a child complies out of fear (a pattern seen in abused children), then the child's compliance may be evidence of avoidance and submission and may lead to depression and muffled hostility. By contrast, a toddler who complies because the child understands the mother's goals, may demonstrate self-regulation.

Maturation

As infants grow, their regulation of basic biological and behavioral rhythms matures. Three major periods of reorganization have been recognized.[32] At 2 to 3 months the baby becomes better organized, focuses better, remembers more with less exposure, and is able to anticipate and react to repeated patterns of interactions with caregivers.[33] Regularizing the schedule of sleep and feeding helps infants regulate their rhythms at this stage.

At 7 to 9 months, babies differentiate different emotional states and use these states to regulate their own behavior and feelings. They become aware of object permanence—the capacity to retain a mental image of someone, which underlies wariness to strangers and protests of separations. Their developing mobility may either make them feel more efficacious or less safe. They begin to use means-to-ends behaviors to maintain contact with their parents, abilities that allow recognition of their attachments as secure or insecure.[34] Supporting parents' responsiveness to the infant's social behaviors—looking, cooing, and smiling—will strengthen secure attachment.

At 18 to 20 months, toddlers' increased localization and specificity of brain function and development of language competence allow them to remember specific events and sequences, to develop working models of relationships through their interactions, and to be more aware of themselves—as shown, for example, by self-recognition in a mirror.[26]

Work

Sixty percent of mothers of children younger than 3 years work outside the home in the United States; they typically return to work 3 months after giving birth. The infants and toddlers are cared for by their fathers (27%), other relatives (27%), nannies (7%) or are in child-care centers (22%) or family-care homes (17%).[35] Parents must often share responsibility for stimulating their infants' development. Supporting them in this effort means that the PCP must guide them in selecting good-quality child care. However, the quality of one half of child care settings serving infants and toddlers is rated as poor or just fair.[36] Good child care requires consistent, responsive, affectionate caregiving by a few adults. The PCP will need to advocate with parents to press for the best child care setting, to assist them in observing their children's adaptations to child care, and to cope with the often difficult feelings aroused by having to leave the child to work. (See Chapter 109, Early Education and Child Care Programs.)

CHILDREN AT RISK AND INTERVENTIONS THAT WORK

Developmental Disorders

Estimates indicate that 5% to 10% of children have a developmental disability. PCPs regularly assess children's developmental status, but research has shown that such surveillance has poor overall sensitivity.[36] Earlier recognition of developmental delay (birth to 2 years) allows referral to developmental programs that have been shown to maximize developmental attainment. This circumstance has led to the enactment of federal laws PL 99457 (Education of Handicapped Act Amendment), the Individuals with Disabilities Education Act, and to the American Academy of Pediatrics' endorsement of early identification of developmental delay. Parents' concerns are a generally reliable indicator of children's developmental problems, and they can be efficiently ascertained by using parent-response screening tools such as Parents' Evaluation of Developmental Status (PEDS)[37] and the Ages and Stages Questionnaires (ASQ).[38,39] (See also Chapter 43, Identification of Developmental Delays and Early Intervention System; and Chapter 44, Developmental Surveillance and Intervention.)

Supporting parents of a child with developmental delay requires providing accurate information and giving the family a sense of efficacy and possibility that they can be effective in supporting their child's development by participating in early intervention.

Neglect and Abuse

The PCP, a mandated reporter of child neglect and abuse, is critically positioned to recognize abuse and neglect. Infants and young children are most vulnerable to the damaging effects on brain development and disordered self-regulation that are known to lead to emotional and behavioral disorders.[40] Ideally, early signs are recognized and families are guided to early intervention. The task of balancing between maintaining a supportive relationship with troubled parents and the obligation for mandated reporting is a difficult one. (See Chapter 120, Child Physical Abuse and Neglect.)

Children With Special Health Care Needs

The PCP provides a medical home for children with special health care needs. Supporting these children's parents requires not only addressing medical issues, but also addressing parents' distress and the burden of care.[41,42] Links to human services agencies, community resources, and early intervention services are essential in developing a network of support and care.[43] (See Chapter 64, Children With Ongoing Health Conditions; and Chapter 65, Home Health Care.)

Adolescent Mothers

Immature mothers may have particular difficulty meeting the demands of parenting, and they may be dependent on their own families for help with this task at a time when their own developmental needs propel them toward autonomy and independence. Typically, adolescent mothers lack economic resources for transportation, for completing school, and for supporting themselves. They may need more frequent health supervision visits to provide education and emotional support. Referral to parenting classes may be beneficial. Preventive intervention, beginning prenatally, with adolescent and first-time mothers who lack resources has been shown to effectively reduce later problems, such as inappropriate use of emergency room, special education, and child protective services.[44] (See Chapter 155, Adolescent Pregnancy and Parenthood.)

Maternal Depression

Risk factors for postpartum mood disorders are shown in Table 22-4. Distinguishing among postpartum blues (maternity blues), postpartum depression, and postpartum psychosis is important. Fifty percent to 80% of mothers experience postpartum blues within the first 2 days or weeks, and the blues last hours or days. Mild depression, irritability, confusion, mood instability, headache, anxiety, and fatigue are common, but if they are limited, then they are not regarded as a clinical disorder that warrants professional intervention. Nonetheless, postpartum blues are associated with increased risk for postpartum depression; therefore the PCP should monitor the mother's progression or recovery. (See Chapter 47, Family Screening and Assessments.)

Symptoms of acute depression, agitation, and inability to carry out normal daily responsibilities are warning signs of more serious depression. Postpartum depression has an incidence of 7% to 17% in adult mothers, and 26% in adolescent mothers. Its onset is generally within 6 weeks. Severity and

Table 22-4 Risk Factors for Developing Postpartum Mood Disorders

TIME	POSTPARTUM BLUES	POSTPARTUM DEPRESSION	POSTPARTUM PSYCHOSIS
Before birth	Personal history of depression Family history of depression Premenstrual depression Poor social adjustment Stressful life events Fear of labor Ambivalent feelings about pregnancy Pessimism in late pregnancy	Personal history of depression Family history of depression Premenstrual depression Poor social adjustment Marital discord Stressful life events Unwanted pregnancy Depression or anxiety during pregnancy	History of postpartum psychosis Personal history of bipolar disorder Family history of bipolar disorder
After birth	Viewing pregnancy as emotionally difficult	Infant medical problems Postpartum blues	—

Table 22-5 Symptoms of Postpartum Depression

SUBTYPE	CLINICAL FEATURES	INCIDENCE, ONSET, OR DURATION	CLINICAL SIGNIFICANCE
Postpartum blues (maternity blues)	Mild depression, irritability, confusion, mood instability, headache, anxiety, fatigue	50-80% Onset: first 2 weeks Duration: hours or days	Not regarded as a clinical disorder that warrants professional intervention Experiencing blues is associated with increased risk of postpartum depression
Postpartum depression	Major depressive disorder; may include anxiety, irritability, anhedonia, fatigue, sleep disturbance	7-17% in adult women, 26% in adolescent mothers Onset: generally within 6 weeks postpartum Duration: may vary Severity: may vary	Significantly disrupts early mothering Affects infant's development of attachment, self-regulation, and thriving
Postpartum psychosis	Most severe peripartum mood disorder Symptoms: delusions, hallucinations, impaired reality concept, rapid mood swings ranging from depression to elation, insomnia, abnormal or obsessive thoughts about the infant	1-2 in 1000 Onset: within a few days, usually within first 3 weeks Duration: may be prolonged	5% suicide, 4% infanticide Psychiatric emergency; presumptive diagnosis warrants hospitalization (although rate of hospitalization is less than for women with psychosis not precipitated by childbirth) Up to two thirds of women experience symptom relapse in subsequent pregnancies

duration vary. This major depressive disorder may include anxiety, irritability, anhedonia, fatigue, and sleep disturbance. Depression is clinically significant because it disrupts early mothering and affects the infant's development of attachment, self-regulation, and thriving. Postpartum psychosis is rare (1 to 2 per 1000) but is a true psychiatric emergency that requires hospitalization. It is the most severe peripartum mood disorder. Postpartum psychosis typically appears within 3 weeks after giving birth, and it may be prolonged. Symptoms include delusions, hallucinations, impaired reality concept, and rapid mood swings ranging from depression to elation, insomnia, and abnormal or obsessive thought. A 5% suicide rate exists with postpartum psychosis, as well as a significant risk of infanticide. Up to two thirds of women will experience relapse of symptom in subsequent pregnancies.[45,46]

Distinguishing features of maternal depression types are summarized in Table 22-5. The damage of maternal depression to a mother's emotional availability to her child is significant,[16] and intervention can be very effective.[47]

Emotional and Behavioral Disturbances

Risk factors for childhood mental health disorders are well described and include poverty, low birth weight, exposure to environmental toxins, child maltreatment or neglect, exposure to trauma or violence, the presence of mental disorder or substance abuse (or both) in a parent, and prenatal damage from substance exposure (tobacco, alcohol, drugs). Child mental disorders are prevalent, occurring in one in five children. Psychiatric symptoms in young children are not always transient.[48] One child in 10 has a severe emotional disorder that requires specialized mental health consultation or treatment. However, four of five children who need services do not receive them. Only a minority of PCPs have ready access to specialized mental health services for their patients; thus basic intervention skills must be incorporated into practice.[49] (See Chapter 131, Consultation and Referral for Emotional and Behavioral Problems.)

The next step for the PCP who is aware of risk, or who intuits an emerging social-emotional or regulation disorder, is screening. Parent-completed screening tools may facilitate a focused discussion between the PCP and the parents, and they may allow the PCP to point the parents to interventions or to refer them to mental health services. Systematic screening of parents' stresses and supports will set a baseline for planning intervention.[50] The Ages and Stages Social-Emotional screening tool has accompanying parent handouts and information for the provider.[38,39] The Parent Stress Index Short Form is another tool scored to learn whether the parent-child problem arises primarily from parental stress alone, from the fact that the child has a challenging temperament, or from a troubled parent-child relationship.[51] This approach assists the PCP in knowing whether to get help for the mother or the child or to focus on an intervention to assist their relationship. The Temperament and Behavior Scale helps characterize the child's reactivity style and points to intervention strategies.[52] The Modified Checklist for Autism in Toddlers defines emerging symptoms of autistic spectrum disorders so that early intervention, which is far more effective than later efforts, can be planned.[53]

The field of infant and early child psychiatry is quickly developing and provides a resource for the PCP for early intervention. Infant mental health has been defined as the flourishing of a baby's capacity for warm connection with baby's parents and others, of the baby's capacity to experience and gradually modulate emotions and actions, and of the development of emotional regulation.[54] In recognition that the *Diagnostic and Statistical Manual of Mental Disorders* (DSM) system offers little to describe infants and preschool children, a classification for psychiatric disorders in preschool children has been developed: the *Diagnostic Classification of Mental Health and Developmental Disorders of Infancy and Early Childhood* (DC:0-3).[55] It presents a five-axis diagnostic system, parallel to the *Diagnostic and Statistical Manual of Mental Disorders*, fourth edition (DSM-IV) except for axis 2, which describes the child's relationships, and axis 5, which describes the parent-infant relationship global assessment. Axis 1 includes a description of regulatory disorders, which require both a distinct behavioral pattern and a sensory, sensory-motor, or organizational processing difficulty. These descriptions (hypersensitive, underreactive, motorically disorganized, and impulsive) are helpful guides for PCPs to organize their observations of children. The DC:0-3 diagnosis can be converted to a DSM-IV-TR or *International Classification of Disease*, ninth edition (ICD-9) diagnosis in states that do not recognize the DC:0-3 for billing purposes.

Interventions for early childhood regulatory disorders and for attachment disorders have been described and shown to be effective. The key is to bring about a change in the response of the parent, usually the mother (or primary caregiver).[25,56] Therapeutic interventions to modify how the mother understands her attachment to her infant have been described.[25,56] Dyadic approaches, rather than an exclusive focus on maternal sensitivity, are more effective in helping the mother learn to alter an insecure attachment once it has developed.[57]

Evidence-based interventions for early childhood social-emotional disorders have been described.[58] They optimally build on and strengthen parents' capacities.[59-62] The efficacy of these interventions and their cost effectiveness over the long term have been demonstrated.[63]

TOOLS FOR PRACTICE

Engaging Patient and Family

- *A Parent's Guide to Building Resilience in Children and Teens: Giving Your Child Roots and Wings* (book), Kenneth R. Ginsburg, MD, FAAP (www.aap.org/bookstore).
- *Choosing Child Care: What's Best for Your Family?* (brochure), American Academy of Pediatrics (patiented.aap.org).
- *How Do Infants Learn?* (brochure), American Academy of Pediatrics (patiented.aap.org).
- *Parenting Your Infant* (brochure), American Academy of Pediatrics (patiented.aap.org).
- *Playing is How Toddlers Learn* (brochure), American Academy of Pediatrics (patiented.aap.org).
- *Sibling Relationships* (brochure), American Academy of Pediatrics (patiented.aap.org).
- *Welcome to the World of Parenting!* (brochure), American Academy of Pediatrics (patiented.aap.org).

Medical Decision Support

- *Ages and Stages Questionnaires (ASQ): A Parent-Completed, Child-Monitoring System* (questionnaire) Bricker D, Squires J (www.brookespublishing.com/store/books/bricker-asq/index.htm).
- *Ages and Stages Questionnaires: Social-Emotional (ASQ:SE): A Parent-Completed, Child-Monitoring System for Social-Emotional Behaviors* (questionnaire), Squires J, Bricker D, Twombly E (www.brookespublishing.com/store/books/squires-asqse/index.htm).
- *Bright Futures: Guidelines for Health Supervision of Infants, Children, and Adolescents* (book) Bright Futures (brightfutures.aap.org/web/).
- *Caring for Infants and Toddlers* (other), The Future of Children (www.futureofchildren.org/usr_doc/vol_11_no_1_no_photos.pdf).
- *Children, Families, and Foster Care* (other), The Future of Children (www.futureofchildren.org/usr_doc/vol_14_no_1_no_photos.pdf).

- *Modified Checklist for Autism in Toddlers (M-CHAT)*, Robins DL, Fein D, Barton ML, Green JA (www.utmem.edu/pediatrics/general/clinical/m-chat.pdf).
- *Parents Evaluation of Developmental Status (PEDS)* (questionnaire), Glascoe, FP (pedstest.com/index.php).
- *Parenting Stress Index Short Form (PSI-SF)* (questionnaire), Abidin, R (www3.parinc.com/products/product.aspx?Productid=PSI-SF).
- *Temperament and Atypical Behavior Scale (TABS): Early Childhood Indicators of Developmental Dysfunction* (questionnaire), Bagnato SJ, Neisworth JT, Salvia JJ, Hunt FM (www.brookespublishing.com/store/books/bagnato-tabs/index.htm).

AAP POLICY STATEMENTS

American Academy of Pediatrics, Council on Children With Disabilities, Section on Developmental Behavioral Pediatrics; Bright Futures Steering Committee and Medical Home Initiatives for Children With Special Needs Project Advisory Committee. Identifying infants and young children with developmental disorders in the medical home: an algorithm for developmental surveillance and screening. *Pediatrics*. 2006;118(1):405-420. (aappolicy.aappublications.org/cgi/content/full/pediatrics;118/1/405).

Coleman WL, Garfield C, American Academy of Pediatrics, Committee on Psychosocial Aspects of Child and Family Health. Fathers and pediatricians: enhancing men's roles in the care and development of their children. *Pediatrics*. 2004;113(5):1406-1411. (aappolicy.aappublications.org/cgi/content/full/pediatrics;113/5/1406).

REFERENCES

1. Shonkoff JP, Philips DA, eds. *From Neurons to Neighborhoods: The Science of Early Childhood Development*. Washington, DC: Institute of Medicine; 2000. Available at: books.nap.edu/books/0309069882/html/index.html. Accessed March 7, 2007.
2. Main M. The organized categories of infant, child, and adult attachment: flexible vs inflexible attention under attachment-related stress. *J Am Psychoanal Assoc*. 2000; 48:1055-1096.
3. Knapp PK. Understanding early development and temperament. In: Jensen P, Knapp PK, Mrazek D, eds. *Beyond DSM-IV: Evolutionary and Developmental Approaches to Clinical Diagnosis*. New York, NY: Guilford Press; 2006.
4. Brooks-Gunn J, McCarton CM, Casey PH, et al. Early intervention in low-birth-weight premature infants. Results through age 5 years from the Infant Health and Development Program. *JAMA*. 1994;272:1257-1262.
5. National Institute of Child Health & Development [NICHD], Early Child Care Research Network. The effects of infant child care on infant-mother attachment security: results of the NICHD Study of Early Child Care. *Child Dev*. 1997;68:860-879.
6. Huttenlocher PR. Synaptogenesis, synapse elimination and neural plasticity in human cerebral cortex. In: Nelson CA, ed. *Threats to Optimal Development: Integrating Biological, Psychological and Social Risk Factors*. Minneapolis, MN: Minnesota Symposia in Child Psychology; 1994.
7. Greenough WT. Experience and brain development. *Child Dev*. 1987;58:539-559.
8. Carlsson E, Sroufe LA. Contribution of attachment theory to developmental psychopathology. In: Cicchetti D, Cohen DJ, eds. *Developmental Psychopathology. Vol 1. Theory and Methods*. New York, NY: John Wiley & Sons; 1995.
9. Benes FM. Developmental changes in stress adaptation in relation to psychopathology. Special issue: neural plasticity, sensitive periods, and psychopathology. *Dev Psychopathol*. 1994;6:723-739.
10. Coplan JD, Andrews MW, Rosenblum LA, et al. Persistent elevations of cerebrospinal fluid concentrations of corticotropin-releasing factor in adult nonhuman primates exposed to early-life stressors: implications for the pathophysiology of mood and anxiety disorders. *Proc Natl Acad Sci U S A*. 1996;93:1619-1623.
11. Lewis MD. Trauma reverberates: psychological evaluation of the caregiving environment of young children exposed to violence and traumatic loss. In: Osofsky J, Fenichel E, eds. *Islands of Safety: Assessing and Treating Young Victims of Violence*. Arlington, VA: Zero to Three/ National Center for Infants, Toddlers, and Families; 1996.
12. Raine A, Brennan P, Mednick B, et al. High rates of violence, crime, academic problems, and behavioral problems in males with both early neuromotor deficits and unstable family environments. *Arch Gen Psychiatry*. 1996;53:544-549.
13. Courchesne E, Chisum H, Townsend J. Neural activity–dependent brain changes in development: implications for psychopathology. *Dev Psychopathol*. 1994;6:697-722.
14. Hetherington EM, Bridges M, Isabella GM. What matters? What does not? Five perspectives on the association between marital transitions and children's adjustment. *Am Psychol*. 1998;53:167-184.
15. Furstenberg FF Jr, Harris KM. When and why matter: impacts of father involvement on children of adolescent mothers. In: Lerman RI, Ooms TJ, eds. *Young Unwed Fathers: Changing Roles and Emerging Policies*. Philadelphia, PA: Temple University Press; 1993.
16. Field T. The effects of mother's physical and emotional unavailability on emotion regulation. *Monogr Soc Res Child Dev*. 1994;59:208-227.
17. Murray L. The impact of postnatal depression on infant development. *J Child Psychol Psychiatry*. 1992;33:543-561.
18. Laucht M, Esser G, Schmidt MH. Parental mental disorder and early child development. *Eur Child Adolesc Psychiatry*. 1994;3:124-137.
19. Field T. Early interactions between infants and their post-partum depressed mothers. *Infant Behav Dev*. 1984; 7:527-532.
20. Field T. Infants of depressed mothers. *Infant Behav Dev*. 1995;18:1-13.
21. Hubbs-Tait L, Pond-Hughes K, Culp AM, et al. Children of adolescent mothers: attachment representation, maternal depression, and later behavior problems. *Am J Orthopsychiatry*. 1996;66:416-426.
22. Campbell F, Ramey C. Effects of early intervention on intellectual and academic achievement: a follow-up study of children from low-income families. *Child Dev*. 1994; 65:684-698.
23. Kolvin I, Miller FJ, Scott D et al. *Continuities of Deprivation: The Newcastle 1000 Family Study*. Aldershot, UK: Avebuun/Government; 1990.
24. Lagasse LL, Seifer R, Lester BM. Interpreting research on prenatal substance exposure in the context of multiple confounding factors. *Clin Perinatol*. 1999;26:39-54.
25. Fraiberg S. *Clinical Studies in Infant Mental Health: The First Year of Life*. New York, NY: Basic Books; 1980.
26. Crockenberg S, Leerkes E. Infant social and emotional development in family context. In: Zeanah CH Jr, ed. *Handbook of Infant Mental Health*. 2nd ed. New York, NY: Guilford Press; 2000.
27. American Academy of Child and Adolescent Psychiatry. Puritt D, ed. American Academy of Child and Adolescent Psychiatry. *Your Child*. New York, NY: Harper-Collins; 1998.

28. Fivaz-Depeursinge E, Corboz-Warnery A. *The Primary Triangle*. New York, NY: Basic Books; 1999.
29. Belsky J, Rovine M, Fish M. The developing family system. In: Gunnar M, Thelen E, eds. *Minnesota Symposia on Child Psychology. Vol 22. Systems and Development*. Hillsdale, NJ: Erlbaum; 1989.
30. Bass S, Shields MK, Behrman RE. Children, Families, and Foster Care: Analysis and Recommendations. *The Future of Children: Children, Families and Foster Care*. (2004). Available at: www.futureofchildren.org/pubs-info2825/pubs-info_show.htm?doc_id=209538. Accessed August 6, 2007.
31. Cassidy J. Emotion regulation: influences of attachment relationships. *Monogr Soc Res Child Dev*. 1994;59(2-3): 228-283.
32. Crockenberg S. Are temperamental differences in babies associated with predictable differences in care giving? In: Lerner JR, Lerner RM, eds. *New Directions for Child Development Vol 31. Temperament and Social Interaction During Infancy and Childhood*. San Francisco, CA: Jossey-Bass; 1986.
33. Tronick EZ, Cohn J, Shea E. The transfer of affect between mothers and infants. In: Brazelton TB, Yogman MW, eds. *Affective Development in Infancy*. Norwood, NJ: Ablex; 1986.
34. Ainsworth MDS, Blehar M, Waters E, et al. *Patterns of Attachment*. Hillsdale, NJ: Erlbaum; 1978.
35. Larner MB, Behrman RE, Young M, et al. Caring for Infants and Toddlers: Analysis and Recommendations. *The Future of Children: Caring for Infants and Toddlers*; (2001). Available at: www.futureofchildren.org/pubs-info2825/pubs-info_show.htm?doc_id=79324. Accessed March 7, 2007.
36. Rydz D, Shevell MI, Majnemer A, et al. Developmental screening. *J Child Neurol*. 2005;20:4-21.
37. Glascoe FP. Parents' Evaluation of Developmental Status: how well do parents' concerns identify children with behavioral and emotional problems? *Clin Pediatr*. 2003; 42:133-138.
38. Bricker D, Squires J. *Ages and Stages Questionnaires: A Parent-Completed, Child-Monitoring System*. Baltimore, MD: Paul H Brooks Publishing; 1999.
39. Bricker D, Squires J. *Ages and Stages Questionnaire: Social-Emotional (ASQ)*. Baltimore, MD: Paul H Brooks Publishing; 1999.
40. Perry DB, Pollard RA, Blakley TL, et al. Childhood trauma: the neurobiology of adaptation and "use-dependent" development of the brain: how states become traits. *Infant Ment Health J*. 1995;16: 271-291.
41. Knapp PK, Harris EC. Consultation liaison psychiatry—a review of the past 10 years. I. Clinical findings. *J Am Acad Child Adolesc Psychiatry*. 1998;37: 17-25.
42. Knapp PK, Harris EC. Consultation liaison psychiatry—a review of the past 10 years. II. Research on treatment approaches and outcomes. *J Am Acad Child Adolesc Psychiatry*. 1998;37:139-146.
43. Stein REK, Westbrook LE, Bauman LJ. The questionnaire for Identifying Children With Chronic Conditions (QulCC-R), a measure based on a noncategorical approach. *Pediatrics*. 1997;99:513-521.
44. Olds D, Henderson CR Jr, Kitzman HJ, et al. *Prenatal and Infancy Home Visitation by Nurses: Recent Findings. The Future of Children*. Vol 9. Los Altos, CA: David and Lucille Packard Foundation; 1999.
45. Austin MP. Antenatal screening and early intervention for "perinatal" distress, depression and anxiety: where to from here? *Arch Women Ment Health*. 2004; 7:1-6.
46. Burt V, Henrick VC. Women's mental health. In: Hales R, Yudofsky S, eds. *Textbook of Clinical Psychiatry*. Washington, DC: American Psychiatric Press; 2003.
47. Beardslee WR. *Out of the Darkened Room: When a Parent Is Depressed: Protecting the Children and Strengthening the Family*. Boston, MA: Little, Brown and Company; 2002.
48. Lavigne JV, Arend R, Rosenbaum D, et al. Psychiatric disorders with onset in the preschool years: I. Stability of diagnoses. *J Am Acad Child Adolesc Psychiatry*. 1998;37:1246-1254.
49. American Academy of Pediatrics. Bright Futures. Available at: www.brightfutures.aap.org/. Accessed March 7, 2007.
50. Dunst C, Trivetter C, Deal A. *Enabling and Empowering Families: Principles and Guidelines for Practice*. Cambridge, MA: Brookline Books; 1988.
51. Abidin R. *Parenting Stress Index Short Form—Test Manual*. Charlottesville, VA: Pediatric Psychology Press; 1990.
52. Bagnato SJ, Neisworth JT, Salvia JJ, et al. *Temperament and Atypical Behavior Scale (TABS) Early Childhood Indicators of Developmental Dysfunction*. Baltimore, MD: Paul H Brooks Publishing; 1999.
53. Baron-Cohen S, Allen J, Gillberg C. Can autism be detected at 18 months? The needle, the haystack, and the CHAT. *Br J Psychiatry*. 1992;161:839-843.
54. Thompson RA. Emotion regulation: a theme in search of definition. *Monogr Soc Res Child Dev*. 1984;59: 250-283.
55. Zero to Three. *The Diagnostic Classification for Children Zero to Three (DC:0-3): Diagnostic Classification of Mental Health and Developmental Disorders of Infancy and Early Childhood*. Washington, DC: Zero to Three; 1994. Available at: www.zerotothree.org/. Accessed March 7, 2007.
56. Lieberman AF, Weston DR, Pawl JH. Preventive intervention and outcome with anxiously attached dyads. *Child Dev*. 1991;62:199-209.
57. Dozier M, Stovall KC, Albus KE. A transactional intervention for foster infants' caregivers. In: Chicchetti D, Toth SL, eds. *Rochester Symposium on Developmental Psychopathology. Vol 9. Developmental Approaches to Prevention and Intervention*. Rochester, NY: University of Rochester Press; 1999:195-219.
58. Hoagwood K, Burns BJ, Kiser L, et al. Evidence-based practice in child and adolescent mental health services. *Psychiatr Serv*. 2001;52:1179-1189.
59. Sanders M. Triple P—Positive Parenting Program: toward an empirically validated multilevel parenting and family support strategy for the prevention of behavioral and emotional problems in children. *Clin Child Fam Psychol Rev*. 1999;2:71-90.
60. Webster-Stratton C, Hammond M. Treating children with early-onset conduct problems: a comparison of child and parent training interventions. *J Consult Clin Psychol*. 1997;65:93-109.
61. Beauchaine TP, Webster-Stratton C, Reid MJ. Mediators, moderators, and predictors of one-year outcomes among children teated for early-onset conduct problems: a latent growth curve analysis. *Consult Clin Psychol*. 2005;73:371-388.
62. Herschell A, Calzada E, Eyberg SM, et al. Parent-child interaction therapy: new directions in research. *Cognit Behav Pract*. 2002;9:9-16.
63. Karoly LA, Greenwood PW, Everingham SS, et al. *Investing in Our Children: What We Know and Don't Know About the Costs and Benefits of Early Childhood Interventions*. Santa Monica, CA: Rand Corp; 1998.

Chapter 23

COUNSELING FAMILIES ON HEALTHY LIFESTYLES

R. Joe Jopling, MD

A healthy lifestyle is the result of ongoing and numerous decisions individuals make to maximize their genetic and environmental potential for a healthy life. These decisions include increasing physical activity, learning how to make better dietary choices on a daily basis, and learning healthy methods to deal with psychosocial stresses.[1]

Fitness is not related to athletic ability or to physical appearance; rather, it best correlates to physical activity frequency, intensity, and duration. The decline in physical activity among children, adolescents, and young adults in the United States is well documented,[2,3] and the relationship between these lifestyle choices and many preventable diseases of adulthood has been strongly suggested, if not proved.[4-9] The problem is pervasive and seems refractory to change. This chapter attempts to present a practical approach to counseling families in primary care on healthy lifestyle issues. The Centers for Disease Control and Prevention (CDC) (www.cdc.org) and the *Bright Futures: Guidelines for Health Supervision of Infants, Children, and Adolescents* (brightfutures.aap.org) will be the best 2 resources to keep up with rapid changes in this quickly evolving field.

HEALTHY LIFESTYLE PARAMETERS AND PREVENTABLE DISEASES

Cardiovascular diseases (myocardial infarction, hypertension, and stroke), obesity, type 2 diabetes, and some types of cancer (eg, lung and colon cancer) are major sources of morbidity and mortality, and they are thought to be preventable, at least in part, by lifestyle changes.[10,11] A lifestyle is learned in childhood and becomes more difficult to change with age. Therefore the younger the patient is, the more easily lifestyle changes can be made, and the more likely that these changes will help prevent or reduce the effects of the previously mentioned diseases later in life. Preventing inherently active children from becoming sedentary adults should be easier and more cost effective than trying to change unhealthy habits once adulthood has been reached.[11]

Most experts agree that the decline in fitness and physical activity correlates directly with an increase in the risk factors for cardiovascular disease such as obesity, hypertension, high serum cholesterol, type 2 diabetes, smoking, psychosocial stress, and physical inactivity.

Obesity

Sixty percent of adults in the United States are overweight, and more than 30% are obese; 16% of children are now considered overweight (body mass index [BMI] greater than the 95th percentile), a 45% increase in just 10 years.[12] (See Chapter 299, Obesity and Metabolic Syndrome.)

Hypertension

Ten percent of adults and 5% of children are considered hypertensive. This statistic, coupled with those for obesity, is particularly sobering because the risk of dying of cardiovascular disease appears to be greatest in the families of children who are obese, especially those who have persistent high blood pressure.[13]

High Serum Cholesterol

Between 10% and 20% of adults have high serum cholesterol levels, and high cholesterol is not simply a condition of adulthood; the problem begins in childhood. Atherosclerotic fatty streaks have been found in children as young as 3 years. By age 22, anywhere from 45% to 77% of individuals may have evidence of atherosclerosis.[9]

Type 2 Diabetes

Approximately 10 to 15 years ago, type 2 diabetes in children was almost nonexistent. In 2000, almost one half of all new-onset diabetes in children were type 2.[14] This increase is related to diet (fast food, soft drinks, unhealthy school lunch options, snack food, and large food portions) and inactivity (increasing options of television, video games, and computers while decreasing options of free play, physical education in school, and noncompetitive sports teams).

Smoking

Most cigarette smokers begin smoking before age 20. In the National Youth Survey of 2002 and 2004, the percentage of middle school children (grades 6 through 8) who were current users of any tobacco product was 13% of all boys and 11% of all girls. In the same survey, the percentage of high school adolescents (grades 9 through 12) who were current users of any tobacco product was 30% of all boys and 24% of all girls.[15]

Psychosocial Stress

Psychosocial problems are diagnosed more often and earlier than any time in the last 2 decades.[16] The incidences of several known risk factors such as divorce, single-parent families, gangs, and bullying are on the rise. These risk factors are thought to be associated with the increased rates of diagnosis for psychosocial problems in primary care.[17]

Physical Inactivity

An epidemiologic study reported in 1987 by the CDC has shown that physical inactivity is as strong a risk factor for coronary heart disease as are the traditional risk factors (smoking, hypertension, and high serum cholesterol).[10] Even more important, physical inactivity was shown to be 3 to 6 times more prevalent than any other risk factor. Only 20% of adults exercise adequately, and 60% do not exercise at all. In 2003, one third of high school students did not engage in the minimal recommended level of moderate or vigorous physical activity.[18] Even when offered, physical education classes often emphasize team sports rather than individual lifelong activities (ie, aerobic activities that can be done alone, such as walking, jogging, swimming, or cycling). In 2002, the CDC conducted the Youth Media Campaign Longitudinal Survey, a nationally representative

BOX 23-1 Components of a Healthy Lifestyle

CARDIORESPIRATORY ENDURANCE
Cardiorespiratory endurance is achieved by performing any one of several aerobic exercises while maintaining the heart rate at 60% to 80% of a calculated maximum for at least 30 minutes at a time, at least 3 times a week, for at least 6 consecutive months.

MUSCLE STRENGTH AND ENDURANCE
Leg muscle strength enables a person to perform aerobic exercise. Abdominal muscle strength aids in proper breathing technique and helps protect the lower back. Upper body strength is important to overall muscle balance and aids in many everyday activities.

FLEXIBILITY
Flexibility helps prevent musculoskeletal injuries and makes a person feel more spry. Without warm-up and cool-down stretching periods, an exercise program can lead to loss of flexibility.

HEALTHY DIET
A diet high in complex carbohydrates, moderate in protein, low in fat, and moderate in total calories is essential to any fitness program.

STRESS-MANAGEMENT AND COMMUNICATION SKILLS
In today's fast-paced world, techniques for managing stress and improving communication skills have become increasingly important components of good health.

Modified from Jopling RJ. Health-Related Fitness as Preventive Medicine. *Pediatr Rev.* 1988;10:141-148.

survey of children aged 9 to 13 years and their parents, which indicated that 61.5% of children aged 9 to 13 years do not participate in any organized physical activity during their nonschool hours and that 22.6% do not engage in any free-time physical activity.[19] Several factors seem to make matters worse: rural location (especially in the South), lower educational level, and lower socioeconomic status.[2]

Aggravating the problem of inactivity is that children in the United States average 25 hours a week watching television, which is compounded by having a television in a child's bedroom. Video games and computer use fall into the same category as television viewing, and all of them are often accompanied by munching some type of unhealthy snack food. (See Chapter 123, Children, Adolescents, and the Media.)

As mentioned previously, almost all experts agree that the best way to resolve these fitness problems is to change people's lifestyles. One of the best ways to accomplish this task is to develop a program for the whole family. This program should focus on cardiorespiratory endurance, strength and endurance of the large-muscle groups, flexibility, a healthful diet, stress-management techniques, and improved communication skills (Box 23-1).

Several programs can be accessed on the CDC Web site. The VERB™ campaign encourages young people aged 9 to 13 years to be physically active every day. The campaign combines paid advertising, marketing strategies, and partnership efforts to reach the distinct audiences of preteens and their parents. BAM! Body and Mind (www.bam.gov/) is an on-line destination for kids created by the CDC, an agency of the US Department of Health and Human Services. Designed for kids 9 through 13 years, BAM! Body and Mind gives them the information they need to make healthy lifestyle choices. The site focuses on topics that kids say are important to them, such as stress and physical fitness, using kid-friendly lingo, games, quizzes, and other interactive features. BAM! Body and Mind also serves as an aid to teachers, providing them with interactive, educational, and fun activities that are linked to the national education standards for science and health. The site includes aspects of physical activity, diet, peer pressure, and bullying, among other topics. Additionally, physical activity resources are available for health care professionals at the Web site www.cdc.gov/youthcampaign/.

CARDIORESPIRATORY ENDURANCE

Cardiorespiratory endurance is best achieved by performing aerobic exercise for at least 30 minutes per session while maintaining the heart rate at 60% to 80% of a calculated maximum. The minimal exercise time needed for an aerobic effect was initially thought to be 15 minutes and then 20 minutes; now the time is 30 minutes.[20]

The American College of Sports Medicine recognizes three 10-minute episodes of physical activity in a day to be as beneficial as one 30-minute episode. This recognition certainly allows for more flexibility in designing any physical activity program for all members of the family. Inactive people should start at whatever level and duration of continuous activity they can tolerate safely and gradually work up to 30 minutes.

In the adult literature, whenever a positive relationship is found between exercise and a decline in serum cholesterol, the correlate seems to be that the more vigorous and sustained the exercise is, the greater its effect will be.[21] This relationship implies that more is better with regard to intensity; however, as with duration, the recommendations for intensity level have changed. Initially, exercise physiologists proposed that a person had to reach a target heart rate to achieve an aerobic exercise threshold that led to improved aerobic fitness. Most exercise physiologists and cardiologists now believe that unless an individual is already relatively fit, even discussing target heart rates is a mistake. Initially, of more importance is to stress becoming physically active at any level and then begin to increase this level gradually.[22] Borg[23] has proposed a perceived exertion scale as an adequate measure of heart rate, a concept that has been validated more than once.[24] A common rule of thumb for finding the proper intensity is to exercise at least enough to perspire while maintaining the ability to carry on a conversation.

For people who are fit enough to use the heart rate as a guide, the recommendation is that a person who has been relatively active should aim for a target rate of approximately 60% when starting an aerobic exercise program. Exceeding 80% of the maximal heart rate is unwise at any time. People who are already active and who want more specific information should consult published guidelines for heart rates during exercise (Table 23-1). The fact that these numbers are

Table 23-1 Suggested Training Heart Rates*

AGE (YR)	HEART RATE (BEATS/MIN) MAXIMUM	80%	60%
5-9	220	176	132
10	210	168	126
11	209	167	125
12	208	166	125
13	207	165	124
14	206	165	123
15	205	164	123
16	204	163	122
17	203	162	122
18	202	162	121
19	201	161	121
20	200	160	120
22	198	158	118
24	196	157	117
26	194	155	116
28	192	154	115
30	190	152	114
32	189	151	113
34	187	150	112
36	186	149	111
38	184	147	110
40	182	146	109
45	179	143	107
50	175	140	105
55	171	137	102
60	160	128	96
65	150	120	90

*These numbers are taken from a variety of sources and are suggested guidelines initially developed for training athletes. Individuals will vary. If the target heart rate seems too hard to maintain, then a lower rate should be accepted. Conversely, if the target heart rate does not seem high enough to produce a sweat, then the individual should work harder.

From Jopling RJ. Health-Related Fitness as Preventive Medicine. *Pediatr Rev.* 1988;10:141-148.

based on suggestions for training adult athletes cannot be overemphasized, and these statistics should not be considered as hard-and-fast rules. Gradually warming up before exercising—and cooling down afterward—may help ensure a safe workout by allowing muscles, joints, and the cardiovascular system to adapt to the changes of exercise. The optimal times to stretch, and thereby to help maintain flexibility, are just after the warm-up and cool-down periods.

When discussing intensity, an important factor to consider is the possibility of overuse syndromes brought on by well-meaning adults who put undue pressure on children or overzealous adolescents who push themselves too hard. Exercising to the point of pain should be discouraged because it eventually leads to injury and can exacerbate a previous injury that was incompletely rehabilitated. *Slow but sure* is the best advice and should be emphasized when trying to make long-term changes for both children *and* their parents. Parents should consult their own medical care provider before starting any new physical activity program other than walking.

BOX 23-2 Suggestions For Fitness Activities*

Free-play time	Racquet sports
Brisk walking	Jogging
Cycling	Hiking
Swimming	Soccer
Aerobic exercise class	Jumping rope
Dancing	Strength training
Basketball	Volleyball
Tumbling	Stretching
Skating	Martial arts
Playground activities	Tag games

*Minimum of 30 minutes daily.

Note: Stretch before and after every activity. For a more balanced fitness program, include activities for stomach muscles (modified sit-ups) and upper body muscles (push-ups or pull-ups).

From the Governor's Family FUN Award Program, Utah Governor's Council on Health and Physical Fitness, Salt Lake City, Utah.

Exercising at least 3 times a week helps maintain an aerobic fitness level; exercising 5 times a week usually ensures a change in a person's aerobic fitness level. These training guidelines are well established for adults, and although less documentation exists for children, they have been applied to children as young as age 6 years. Any exercise program has the highest dropout rates in the first 6 months. Patients should strive toward slow, sustainable changes with long-term goals and should be cautioned not to expect noticeable changes in the first month. Slow changes will also help prevent overuse injuries.

Numerous activities can qualify as aerobic (Box 23-2). Brisk walking deserves special mention because it is an aerobic activity that can be done by almost everyone right from the beginning of any fitness program. Few exercises enable a family to exercise as a unit and at the same time allow all of the members to achieve an aerobic intensity level. However, walking at a brisk pace can usually be done at the same time by all, or at least by most, family members; it can be done around the neighborhood for convenience or as a hike for variation. If inclement weather is a problem, then the family can walk inside a shopping mall or a gym.[25] An alternative for indoor activity for people who already own video game players is Dance Dance Revolution™.

Jump ropes, treadmills, stationary bicycles, or stair-steppers may be reasonable investments to ensure family access to aerobic exercise day or night and year round. With a little insistence, one of these activities can replace snacking as the activity that most frequently accompanies television viewing.[25]

LARGE-MUSCLE STRENGTH AND ENDURANCE

Large-muscle strength and endurance are related to aerobic exercise in 2 ways: (1) large-muscle groups are usually the ones used in aerobic activities, and (2) repetition of the large-muscle relaxation-contraction cycle

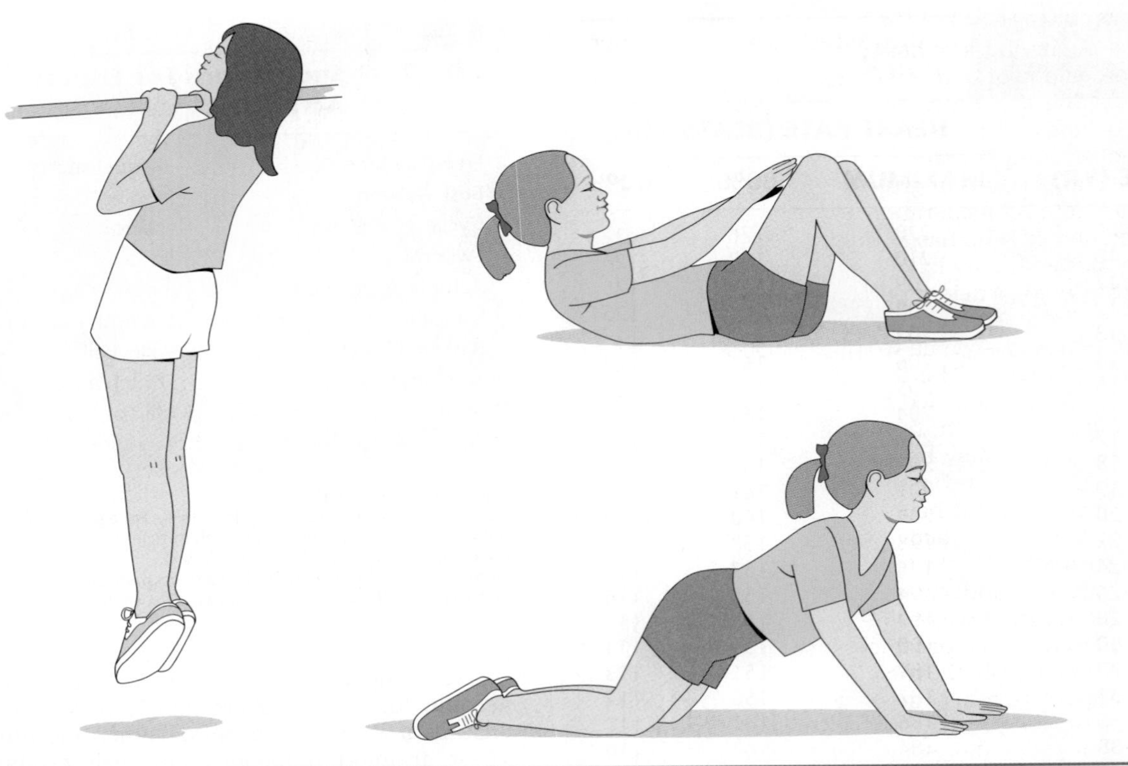

Figure 23-1 Suggested exercises to increase muscular strength. *(From "Youth Fitness," an educational handout from Ross Laboratories.)*

for a sufficient length of time increases the mitochondrial mass of the muscle tissue and thus increases the amount of aerobic enzymes per unit of tissue mass. Muscle contraction tends to occlude local circulation when the muscle is contracting at more than 30% of its maximal capacity. As muscles become stronger, they can perform more work before interfering with local circulation and therefore stay aerobic longer whether performing intense exercise or everyday activities.

Core muscles (abdominal, back, hip, gluteal) help in proper breathing and protect the lower back. Safely strengthening the core muscles involves gradually increasing their use by performing modified sit-ups or Swiss ball exercises. Traditional sit-ups increase strain to the low back and can cause injury. Modified sit-ups are done with the knees flexed and the soles of the feet on the floor or with the lower legs resting on the seat of a chair. The lumbar spine is kept in contact with the floor during the sit-up (Figure 23-1).

Upper-body strength is also important because it is helpful in everyday activities and balances the person's overall health-related fitness. Push-ups, modified push-ups, pull-ups, or flexed arm hangs are easy ways to improve upper body strength (see Figure 23-1). Weight training, as opposed to weightlifting, can be useful to help develop neuromuscular coordination in children as young as 5 years. Free weights, rubber tubing, medicine balls, and Swiss balls can be used for these exercises. If free weights are used to strengthen muscles, then low weight and 3 sets of 12 to 15 repetitions are recommended because this regimen will develop muscle endurance rather than muscle bulk. Increases in weight should be no more than 10% (typically no more than 2 to 5 pounds). Weight machines are *not* recommended for children because they are designed for adults. Children should always have supervision by an adult who has knowledge regarding weight training for kids. Knowledgeable adult supervision and maintaining proper technique are critical in preventing injuries.[26]

FLEXIBILITY

Whether flexibility helps prevent musculoskeletal injuries related to exercise is controversial. Stretching at the end of the warm-up period does not prevent injury during exercise for most children, but it may have benefits for those with previous injuries or decreased flexibility.[27] Stretching at the end of the cool-down period can help prevent muscles from tightening after exercise, which reduces flexibility and increases muscle soreness. Activities such as yoga and tai chi not only help with flexibility, but also have additional psychological benefits (see later discussion).

Static stretching involves stretching a muscle group to the point at which a sense of tightness is first felt, holding the stretch for 30 seconds, and then releasing the stretch. This routine is repeated several times for each muscle group. Any school's athletic trainer can review proper stretching (see the National Athletic Trainers' Association Web site [www.nata.org] for more information).

BODY COMPOSITION

Before beginning any health-related fitness program, the percentage of body fat or BMI is determined. Body composition is a more accurate reflection of health-related fitness than using weight or weight-to-height percentile comparisons. The weight and height percentile comparisons of growth charts do not take body habitus into consideration. A muscular or large-framed person who has a healthy to even low percentage of body fat may have a weight percentile greater than the person's height percentile.

When first starting a physical activity program, a person may actually gain weight, although the percentage of body fat will be the same or even lower. This phenomenon is explained by the higher density of muscle compared with fat; therefore, as a person starts to exercise, muscle may be added faster than fat is lost, which would make for an overall weight gain. This occurrence seems to be especially true for individuals who were not very active before starting a physical activity program.

Hydrostatic (underwater) weighing is considered the most accurate way to measure body composition; it has a 1% to 3% error factor, and it is the most inconvenient and usually the most expensive method. Using skin calipers is much more convenient and, with a skilled examiner, can approach a 3% to 5% error factor. When skin calipers are used, the more skin sites are measured, the more accurate the final determination of percentage of body fat will be. The triceps and calf are the sites that school systems most often use when mass testing is done and, for this reason, should be used if only 2 sites are selected. The proper techniques for using skin calipers can be found in many references.[28]

The BMI is based on the calculation of kilograms (weight) per meter (height) squared.[11] This number is plotted on a percentile graph based on the person's age and gender and compared with figures for others of the same age and gender. In general, the BMI is recommended when hydrostatic or skin caliper methods are not available for determining the percentage of body fat because it is dramatically more convenient and less expensive; in addition, no examiner skill is involved, thus no variation exists from one examiner to another. Whatever body composition measurement method is used, the final numbers are most helpful when comparing a person's progress over time, much as growth charts or blood pressure charts are used to follow a particular patient's trend over 6 months or longer.

SPECIAL CONSIDERATIONS IN ASSESSING PROGRESS IN ACHIEVING FITNESS

Close monitoring is required for persons with eating disorders. The population at the highest risk for eating disorders is late–grade school girls through college-aged young women. Therefore in evaluating the progress toward fitness, assessing the waking pulse rate (taken when the patient first wakes up and before getting out of bed), rather than measuring weight or body fat, is suggested for patients in this population who are considered at risk for a eating disorder by their medical provider. The waking pulse rate should decrease as the patient becomes healthier, just as other parameters should, but it allows the focus to be on the patient becoming healthier rather than losing weight or body fat. This concept is especially relevant for people who are concerned about body image. Alternately, achieving activity goals such as being able to jog or walk for a certain distance or time is a way to assess progress. Whatever method is used, the most relevant assessment is progress over time.

HEALTHY DIET

Sustaining and improving fitness is difficult if not impossible without routine physical activity and a healthy diet.[29] For the growing child or adolescent who is not obese, a safe and practical starting point for a healthy diet is to worry less about total calories and more about the types of calories. To lose weight, an individual may logically believe that a person must make sure that the total caloric intake for 1 day is less than the total caloric output for that day. In reality, however, the emphasis should be placed on the fact that crash diets and ketogenic diets are essentially starvation diets that are impossible to sustain and usually lead to overeating and poor dietary choices.

Commonly, attempts and failures occur repeatedly in a cycle called a *yo-yo diet*. Ironically, these diets also lead to loss of muscle tissue while sparing fat tissue as the body conserves the highest caloric density tissue in an effort to survive a starvation cycle. Studies have shown that even when the total number of daily calories remains unchanged, eating the largest meal of the day at breakfast instead of at night helps people lose weight. Other general dietary recommendations include increasing dietary fiber, reducing the use of salt in the diet, and increasing daily water intake.

Proper dietary recommendations in the past were fairly simple. Unfortunately, the public is inundated with a confusing array of diet and dietary information. Most primary care physicians do not consider themselves experts in this area. However, everyone would be well served if primary care physicians used a few trusted sources and individualized dietary recommendations. Fewer than 40% of children 2 to 19 years of age meet the US Department of Agriculture's recommendations for dietary intake.[30] The Web site for the US Department of Agriculture allows providers and families to develop a general plan for the family and even a personalized pyramid for each family member; it also has specific programs for kids (www.health.gov/dietaryguidelines/dga2005/document/ and www.mypyramid.gov). Simply following the proportions and servings of the updated Food Guide Pyramid is a good recommendation for most patients. Table 23-2 shows the total number of calories recommended per day in relation to age in years. Some specific suggestions for improving dietary habits are listed in Box 23-3.

Carbohydrates should be the main source of calories. The acceptable macronutrient distribution range for carbohydrates is 45% to 65% of total calories. Complex carbohydrates, which tend to have a low glycemic index, such as those found in fruits, vegetables, legumes, and whole-grain cereals, are preferable to simple carbohydrates, which tend to have a high glycemic index, and are especially preferable to the highly processed carbohydrates found in foods such as candy.[31] Although protein is an important macronutrient in the diet, most Americans are already currently consuming enough (acceptable macronutrient distribution range is 10% to 35% of calories) and do not need to increase their intake. Protein can be found in foods other than meat. When meat is part of protein consumption, fish and poultry are considered safer from a cardiovascular standpoint because they have a lower percentage of fat than many cuts of beef and pork.

For adults and for children older than 2 years, recommendations suggest that no more than 30% of total daily calories come from fats, with vegetable fats (except palm oil and coconut oil) recommended over animal fats.[32] How much fat is appropriate for the diet of a child younger than 2 years is still controversial. The American Academy of Pediatrics (AAP) currently recommends 30% to 40% of calories from fat to ensure adequate fat for myelinization of the nervous system.[29] Although most dietary recommendations apply to children older than 5 years, some experts believe that as early as 2 years of age is an appropriate time to begin to expand children's taste experience to foods lower in fat. When fat is removed from the diet, energy levels fall; therefore moderation in fat reduction is important for children. The AAP recommendation of whole milk from 1 to 2 years of age, 2% milk from 2 to 5 years of age, and skim milk after 5 years of age is enough to produce a significant decline in the amount of fat intake for most children.[30] All age groups would do well to be given low-fat luncheon meats when luncheon meat is served.[30] (For a detailed review of the role of dietary cholesterol in cardiovascular disease, refer to Kwiterovich.[5]) Recommending the counsel of a registered dietitian is critical in cases such as obesity, type 2 diabetes, familial hyperlipidemia, and hypertension.

In 1991, the Report of the Expert Panel on Blood Cholesterol Levels in Children and Adolescents[33] stated that (1) high levels of serum total cholesterol, low-density lipoprotein cholesterol, and very–low-density lipoprotein cholesterol and low levels of high-density lipoprotein cholesterol are linked to the extent of early atherosclerotic lesions in adolescents and young adults;

BOX 23-3 Suggestions for Practicing Good Nutrition

Develop a weekly meal plan.
Eat balanced meals from the 4 food groups.
Bake, boil, or broil rather than fry.
Reduce sugar intake.
Eat fruit for a snack.
Use high-fiber cereals, grains, and breads.
Use low-fat dairy products.
Eat more chicken and fish than beef and pork.
Eat low-fat meals.
Cut consumption of butter and gravies in half.
Do not add salt to food.
Do not add sugar to food.
Eat raw and fresh fruits and vegetables.

Modified from the Governor's Family FUN Award Program, Utah Governor's Council on Health and Physical Fitness, Salt Lake City, Utah.

Table 23-2 Recommended Total Daily Calories* (Moderate Activity Level)

GROUP AND AGE (YR)	WEIGHT (KG [LB])	HEIGHT (CM [IN])	ENERGY NEEDS (KCAL [RANGE])
CHILDREN			
1-3	13 (29)	90 (35)	1300 (900-1800)
4-6	20 (44)	112 (44)	1800 (1300-2300)
7-10	28 (62)	132 (52)	2000 (1650-3300)
BOYS AND MEN			
11-14	45 (99)	157 (62)	2500 (2000-3700)
15-18	66 (145)	176 (69)	3000 (2100-3900)
19-22	70 (154)	177 (70)	2900 (2500-3300)
23-50	70 (154)	178 (70)	2900 (2300-3100)
51-75	70 (154)	178 (70)	2300 (2000-2800)
76%	70 (154)	178 (70)	2050 (1650-2450)
GIRLS AND WOMEN			
11-14	46 (101)	157 (62)	2200 (1500-3000)
15-18	55 (120)	163 (64)	2200 (1200-3000)
19-22	55 (120)	163 (64)	2200 (1700-2500)
23-50	55 (120)	163 (64)	2200 (1600-2400)
51-75	55 (120)	163 (64)	1900 (1400-2200)
76%	55 (120)	163 (64)	1600 (1200-2000)

*These recommendations may vary significantly up or down for specific sports and for very active children and adolescents.
Modified from the *Food and Nutrition Board: Recommended Dietary Allowances.* 10th ed. Washington, DC: National Academy of Sciences, National Research Council; 1989.

(2) children and adolescents who have an elevated serum cholesterol, particularly low-density lipoprotein cholesterol, often come from families that have a high incidence of coronary heart disease among adult members; (3) high blood cholesterol aggregates in families as a result of shared environments and genetic factors; and (4) children and adolescents who have high cholesterol levels are more likely than the general population to have high levels as adults. The panel has recommended a strategy to lower blood cholesterol levels in children older than 2 years and adolescents by using a population approach coupled with an individual approach.

The population approach attempts to effect a change in the entire population of the country. It includes the general recommendation that the American diet be well balanced, chosen from a variety of foods, and adequate in total calories to support growth and development. It also includes the specific recommendations that saturated fatty acids be less than 10% of total calories, that total fat be less than 30% of total calories, and that total cholesterol be less than 300 mg/day. The population approach is meant to be a cooperative effort among parents, health professionals, schools, government, the food industry, and the mass media.

The individualized approach is an effort to identify and treat children and adolescents who are at greatest risk of having high serum cholesterol as adults and at subsequent risk of coronary heart disease. The panel recommends using a family history of high serum cholesterol as the basis for obtaining a serum cholesterol value for people younger than 20 years. Specifically, the panel suggests screening of children and adolescents whose parents or grandparents underwent diagnostic coronary arteriography and were found to have atherosclerosis at age 55 or younger. The panel also suggests screening a child or adolescent if (1) the parents or grandparents, at age 55 or younger, suffered a documented myocardial infarction, angina pectoris, peripheral vascular disease, cerebrovascular disease, or sudden cardiac death, and (2) one parent has had a blood cholesterol level of 240 mg/dL or higher. Finally, the panel suggests screening when the family history is unknown, particularly if other risk factors are present. For individuals older than 20 years, obtaining a baseline serum cholesterol level is recommended, followed by repeat serum cholesterol determinations every 5 years.

Potential for missing children at risk exists in this screening format,[34-36] which has led some advocates to propose mass screening, beginning as early as 2 years of age. However, mass screening also has several potential problems because it leads to high rates of children identified as at risk.[37]

1. Individuals who have high cholesterol levels have enough variation in cardiovascular outcomes to make exact prediction of risk for mortality for any one person difficult.
2. Overzealous use of low-fat diets and cholesterol-lowering drugs among at-risk children can have significant side effects.
3. Serious psychological consequences may result in children labeled at risk for an early death from cholesterol screening.
4. Labeling can affect insurability and employment opportunities.

STRESS MANAGEMENT AND COMMUNICATION SKILLS

Many of the diseases targeted for prevention are related to psychological stress. The psychological components of a healthy lifestyle are fairly familiar topics to primary care physicians, who present aspects of stress management, behavior modification, and improved communication skills when discussing anticipatory guidance topics with parents and patients. Although books and videos are available to introduce stress-management skills, the actual skills that patients or families choose must be practiced in less stressful times to be effective in truly stressful times. This concept implies a significant commitment in time and effort. Helpful to the family is to have the primary care physician prepare family members by discussing where to go for help and what kind of skills to try first.

Common examples of stress-management techniques include deep breathing, ascending muscle relaxation, body awareness, positive mental imagery, meditation, priority setting, time management, and simple body stretches. Families should be reminded that routine physical activity and a healthy diet have been proven to have independent therapeutic value in treating anxiety and depression. Yoga and tai chi have physical benefits; however, the psychological benefits are equally as important in a healthy lifestyle context. In fact, Western societies might do well to examine the Eastern philosophy of personal responsibility for quiet introspection and balance in life. Examples of family activities that can aid in stress management are listed in Box 23-4. (For more detailed information, the reader is referred to the chapters in this book on anxiety, depression, and eating disorders.)

BOX 23-4 Suggested Family Activities for Stress Management

Keep a family calendar.
Keep a family job list.
Hold a family meeting.
Have a family game night.
Attend a health fair.
Read together.
Keep a stress diary.
Get involved in service projects.
Set aside meditation and quiet time.
Prepare a meal together.
Keep a journal.
Engage in family outdoor adventures.
Have a family picnic.
Get adequate sleep.
Cut television time in half.
Discuss family budgeting.
Attend cultural events.

Modified from the Governor's Family FUN Award Program, Utah Governor's Council on Health and Physical Fitness, Salt Lake City, Utah.

SMOKING CESSATION

Evidence shows that pediatricians are the physicians most commonly in touch with adolescents and are among the most likely to be able to help convince the adolescent of the importance of smoking cessation. One of the best windows of opportunity for pediatricians to help any parent who smokes is when the child has just been diagnosed with an illness that is made worse by smoke inhalation. The best chance for success lies in a combination approach of behavior modification and pharmacotherapy. The basic classifications of over-the-counter and prescription medications include various doses of nicotine in transdermal patches, chewing gums, nasal spray, or oral inhaler and bupropion in oral tablets. This addictive habit is a difficult and recalcitrant problem. See Chapter 35, Prevention of Smoking, and the section on Important Resources later in this chapter and Tools for Practice at the end of this chapter for more detailed information.

ADHERENCE

Adherence is the basis for success or failure in any effort at prevention or intervention by medical care providers. The keys to compliance are multiple. The first key is gaining knowledge of a new concept through education by the medical provider. Next, the patient must be persuaded of the concept's importance by gaining a positive attitude toward the new concept. Implementation of the new concept begins through methods suggested by the medical provider. Finally, the motivation to adopt the new concept on a long-term basis comes through repeated reinforcement and tracking of the new behavior.[38-40] The clinician's first step is to establish rapport by listening carefully to the concerns of the patient and family. Involve the patient and parents by jointly developing a plan based on the common understanding of the issues of the visit. The plan is implemented by offering the family opportunities to learn new behaviors, develop new experiences, and modify their environment.[1] Realistic goals should be set that are achievable by incremental change. The plan is evaluated by identifying strategies for tracking the patient's progress. Teaching the patient (when possible) and the family about the problem may be motivation enough for starting a change in lifestyle. Long-term adherence, however, is more difficult. The physical and mental benefits of the program may provide a self-sustaining motivation as they become noticeable. During the gap between starting a program and reaching a point at which the benefits are tangible (as early as the 3rd month or as late as the 12th month), the dropout rate is greatest. The average dropout rate in the first 6 to 12 months of starting a fitness program is frequently 50% or higher.[41] The beneficial changes achieved through any health-related fitness program are not sustained if the program is discontinued. These issues explain why the family must comprehend the concepts needed for long-term lifestyle changes. Many factors have been studied in efforts to encourage compliance. Some of the important findings in an adult survey included scheduling of the time, accessibility to facilities, weather, time of year, and an interested friend or family member.[42] In a survey of children and adolescents with diabetes who participated in an exercise program, the most important factors in compliance were enthusiastic leadership, individual attention, and parental support.[43] Research has shown that children of physically active parents are more physically active themselves.[8] A study on the prevention of progression to severe obesity by use of family therapy showed some effectiveness when the program was started in childhood (before age 11 years).[44] Therefore the help of a motivated and involved adult is essential for children to acquire positive lifestyle habits. This role is most likely to be filled by one or both parents. If the parents are unable to fulfill this role, then other immediate or extended-family members might be willing to help. Outside of the family, possibilities include other adults who might have contact with the child (school counselors and teachers, community youth organization members, youth leaders in a house of worship).

A study of previously sedentary adults showed that those who exercised at home were more likely to achieve long-term compliance than those who attended exercise classes if both groups received the benefit of planning and encouragement from experts.[45] The convenience of home is certainly important; and many people may not stay with an exercise program because either they themselves or well-meaning trainers push too hard. The same study showed that the home-based group tended toward moderation in intensity.

By instructing the patient and family to keep a daily log of all areas of lifestyle changes and to return with the log in 1 month, the physician can provide an incentive to comply and a basis for discussion at the follow-up visit. For example, if 1 day the patient walked for 30 minutes, participated in a family meeting, and had broiled skinless chicken (instead of hamburgers) for one of the day's meals, the person might write the following on the calendar:

F (for fitness): walked 30 minutes.
U (for unity, or family stress management): had a family meeting.
N (for nutrition): ate broiled, skinless chicken.

Everyone needs motivation and encouragement to stay with any lifestyle change; and one of the keys to achieving this goal is to make the process fun. This concept is important for adults, but it is critical for children. Spelling out FUN on the calendar helps reinforce the importance of making the program enjoyable.

Use of age- and time-appropriate rewards is essential for some youth. For example, the family might go to the zoo if 1 week's goal is met; each family member might buy a desired article of clothing if 1 month's goal is met; and a family vacation to a favorite spot might be the reward if a 6- or 12-month goal is met. Family members should be allowed to help decide what reward is important for them.

Varying the selection of exercise activities makes for a more interesting exercise program and helps prevent overuse injuries, both of which will aid in adherence. For example, a person might walk twice a week, ride a stationary bike twice a week, and play games at the park as part of a family outing once a week.

For many individuals and families, lack of time to begin or maintain a fitness program is a major obstacle. A good starting point is to divide the day into

30-minute increments, then make the program a priority to be worked into one of these increments. Specific suggestions for achieving the desired exercise time include getting up 30 minutes earlier in the morning, taking 30 minutes of the lunch break, or allotting 30 minutes after dinner. Three 10-minute episodes of activity over the day may be as beneficial from a health standpoint as one 30-minute activity.[46]

OPPORTUNITIES FOR DISCUSSING HEALTH-RELATED FITNESS

One of the best times to broach the topic of health-related fitness is during a consultation for a specific problem (eg, obesity, reactive airway disease). At these times, the parent, patient, or both may be especially receptive to specific therapeutic or preventive measures.[47] Obesity is especially difficult to treat without the team approach, which is usually offered through various hospitals and private clinics. Preventive health care visits such as well-child checkups, camp physicals, and sports preparticipation physicals are some of the other physician visits that provide opportunities for discussion of this topic. Children are obese at increasingly younger ages; thus health-related fitness should be discussed from the toddler years onward. The AAP recommends encouraging free play outdoors for infants, toddlers, and preschoolers.[48,49] The *Bright Futures* approach to physical activity makes the point of using the words *physical activity* during discussion of infant and toddler developmental phases, thus planting the seed of thought about a healthy lifestyle at early preventive health care visits.

Height, weight, BMI, blood pressure, and resting pulse rate measurements can be obtained easily, recorded in the chart, and can be plotted on an age- and gender-appropriate graph before the patient sees the primary care physician on any of the previously mentioned visits. BMI can be determined with relative ease and proficiency by the nurse or examining physician using a BMI wheel. This information can then be compared with age- and gender-appropriate graphs to be used as a baseline for future reference and can serve as the basis for introducing this topic to the patient and parents.

A study done through the Pediatric Research in Office Settings network demonstrated that an upper limit of information exists that any family can successfully retain during preventive health care visits, with 5 to 8 topics being the upper limit.[50] Ultimately, the most important key to success to any intervention that a medical provider undertakes is to individualize the information presented at every visit for every patient. This approach is especially critical to something as important and as overwhelming as a discussion on a healthy lifestyle can be. The primary care physician cannot usually impart all the information needed to begin changing a family's lifestyle in the 20 or 30 minutes generally allotted for preventive health care visits. The physician should remember to introduce the topics of discussion by individualizing the major points already listed in an educational handout that the patient or parent can take home, to make specific suggestions that are the most likely to be understood and followed to get the family started, and to set up a follow-up visit for 2 to 4 weeks later. At the follow-up visit, the daily log can be reviewed, measurements can be repeated (if appropriate), and the program can be reinforced and clarified.

Can pediatricians afford to take the time that is necessary to educate their patient population, to fight for insurance reimbursement, and to encourage schools to include this topic in their curriculum? Some researchers believe that the answers await longitudinal studies, but most professionals in the areas of medicine, nutrition, and exercise believe that adopting a healthy lifestyle can enhance the quality and duration of life, surely a worthwhile effort.

TOOLS FOR PRACTICE

Community Coordination and Advocacy

- *Action for Healthy Kids* (Web page), Action For Healthy Kids (www.actionforhealthykids.org/).

Practice Management and Care Coordination

- *Obesity Coding Fact Sheet* (fact sheet), American Academy of Pediatrics (www.aap.org/obesity/codingfactsheet.PDF).

Engaging Patients and Family

- *A Parent's Guide to Childhood Obesity: A Road Map to Health* (book), American Academy of Pediatrics (www.aap.org/bst/showdetl.cfm?&DID=15&Product_ID=4176).
- *About BMI for Children and Teens* (fact sheet), Centers for Disease Control and Prevention (www.cdc.gov/nccdphp/dnpa/bmi/childrens_BMI/about_childrens_BMI.htm).
- *BAM! Body and Mind* (Web page), Centers for Disease Control and Prevention (www.bam.gov).
- *Get Fit, Stay Healthy* (brochure), American Academy of Pediatrics (patiented.aap.org).
- *Encourage Your Child to Be Physically Active* (brochure), American Academy of Pediatrics (patiented.aap.org).
- *Feeding Guide for Children, Appendix A.3, Pediatric Obesity: Prevention, Intervention, and Treatment Strategies for Primary Care* (chart), American Academy of Pediatrics.
- *Feeding Kids Right Isn't Always Easy* (brochure), American Academy of Pediatrics (patiented.aap.org).
- *Growing Up Healthy* (brochure), American Academy of Pediatrics (patiented.aap.org).
- *My Pyramid—Steps to Healthier You* (Web page), US Department of Agriculture (www.mypyramid.gov/).
- *Right From the Start: ABCs of Good Nutrition for Young Children* (brochure), American Academy of Pediatrics (patiented.aap.org).
- *Sports and Your Child* (brochure), American Academy of Pediatrics (patiented.aap.org).
- *Television and the Family* (brochure), American Academy of Pediatrics (patiented.aap.org).
- *What's to Eat? Healthy Foods for Hungry Children* (brochure), American Academy of Pediatrics (patiented.aap.org).
- *VERB* (Web page), Centers for Disease Control and Prevention (www.verbnow.com/).

Medical Decision Support

- *BMI—Body Mass Index: Child and Teen Calculator: English* (interactive tool), Centers for Disease Control and Prevention (apps.nccd.cdc.gov/dnpabmi/Calculator.aspx).
- *Bright Futures: Guidelines for Health Supervision of Infants, Children, and Adolescents* Set (book), Bright Futures (brightfutures.aap.org/web/).
- *Care of Children and Adolescents With Type 1 Diabetes: A Statement of the American Diabetes Association* (policy statement), American Diabetes Association (care.diabetes journals.org/cgi/content/full/28/1/186).
- *Environmental Assessment, Appendix A.4, Pediatric Obesity: Prevention, Intervention, and Treatment Strategies for Primary Care* (questionnaire), American Academy of Pediatrics (practice.aap.org/content.aspx?aid=2001).
- *Family History: Your Child's Genetics and Family History, Appendix A.4, Pediatric Obesity: Prevention, Intervention, and Treatment Strategies for Primary Care* (questionnaire), American Academy of Pediatrics (practice.aap.org/contentaspx?aid=2001).
- *Food Diary: What is Your Child Eating Now? Appendix A.4, Pediatric Obesity: Prevention, Intervention, and Treatment Strategies for Primary Care* (questionnaire), American Academy of Pediatrics (practice.aap.org/content.aspx?aid=2001).
- *Goal Assessment, Appendix A.4, Pediatric Obesity: Prevention, Intervention, and Treatment Strategies for Primary Care* (questionnaire), American Academy of Pediatrics (practice.aap.org/content.aspx?aid=2001).
- *Goal Achievement Plan Appendix A.4, Pediatric Obesity: Prevention, Intervention, and Treatment Strategies for Primary Care* (questionnaire), American Academy of Pediatrics (practice.aap.org/content.aspx?aid=2001).
- *Growth Charts—Tutorials and Information* (Web page), Centers for Disease Control and Prevention (www.cdc.gov/growthcharts/).
- *Growth Charts* (chart), Centers for Disease Control and Prevention, (www.cdc.gov/nchs/about/major/nhanes/growthcharts/clinical_charts.htm#Clin%201); also available at AAP bookstore (www.aap.org/bookstore).
- *Home Environment Assessment, Appendix A.4, Pediatric Obesity: Prevention, Intervention, and Treatment Strategies for Primary Care* (questionnaire), American Academy of Pediatrics (practice.aap.org/content.aspx?aid=2001).
- *Introducing Patients to Healthy Family Lifestyles* (fact sheet), R. Joe Jopling, MD (practice.aap.org/content.aspx?aid=2001).
- *Parental Concerns Assessment, Appendix A.4, Pediatric Obesity: Prevention, Intervention, and Treatment Strategies for Primary Care* (questionnaire), American Academy of Pediatrics (practice.aap.org/content.aspx?aid=2001).
- *Pediatric Obesity: Prevention, Intervention, and Treatment Strategies for Primary Care* (book), American Academy of Pediatrics (www.aap.org/bookstore).
- *Physical Activity Assessment, Appendix A.4, Pediatric Obesity: Prevention, Intervention, and Treatment Strategies for Primary Care* (questionnaire), American Academy of Pediatrics (practice.aap.org/content.aspx?aid=2001).
- *Physician Tracking Form for Pediatric Obesity, Appendix A.4, Pediatric Obesity: Prevention, Intervention, and Treatment Strategies for Primary Care* (form), American Academy of Pediatrics (practice.aap.org/content.aspx?aid=2001).
- *Set Backs Worksheet, Appendix A.4, Pediatric Obesity: Prevention, Intervention, and Treatment Strategies for Primary Care* (questionnaire), American Academy of Pediatrics (practice.aap.org/content.aspx?aid=2001).
- *Snacking Worksheet, Appendix A.4, Pediatric Obesity: Prevention, Intervention, and Treatment Strategies for Primary Care* (questionnaire), American Academy of Pediatrics (practice.aap.org/content.aspx?aid=2001).
- *VERB Campaign* (Web page), Centers for Disease Control and Prevention (www.cdc.gov/youthcampaign/index.htm).

AAP POLICY STATEMENTS

American Academy of Pediatrics, Committee on Adolescence. Identifying and Treating Eating Disorders. *Pediatrics*. 2003;111(1):204-211. (aappolicy.aappublications.org/cgi/content/full/pediatrics;111/1/204).

American Academy of Pediatrics, Committee on Communication. Children, adolescents, and advertising. *Pediatrics*. 2006;118(6):2563-2569. (aappolicy.aappublications.org/cgi/content/full/pediatrics;118/6/2563).

American Academy of Pediatrics, Committee on Early Childhood, Adoption, and Dependent Care. The pediatrician's role in family support programs. *Pediatrics*. 2001;107:195-197. (aappolicy.aappublications.org/cgi/content/full/pediatrics;107/1/195).

American Academy of Pediatrics, Committee on Environmental Health. Ambient air pollution: health hazards to children. *Pediatrics*. 2004;114(6):1699-1707. (aappolicy.aappublications.org/cgi/content/full/pediatrics;114/6/1699).

American Academy of Pediatrics, Committee on Nutrition. Prevention of pediatric overweight and obesity. *Pediatrics*. 2003;112(2):424-430. (aappolicy.aappublications.org/cgi/content/full/pediatrics;112/2/424).

American Academy of Pediatrics, Committee on Nutrition. Prevention of pediatric overweight and obesity. *Pediatrics*. 2003;112(2):424-430. (aappolicy.aappublications.org/cgi/content/full/pediatrics;112/2/424).

American Academy of Pediatrics, Committee on Nutrition. The use and misuse of fruit juice in pediatrics. *Pediatrics*. 2001;107(5):1210-1213. (aappolicy.aappublications.org/cgi/content/full/pediatrics;107/5/1210).

American Academy of Pediatrics, Committee on Public Education. Children, adolescents, and television. *Pediatrics*. 2001;107(2):423-426. (aappolicy.aappublications.org/cgi/content/full/pediatrics;107/2/423).

American Academy of Pediatrics, Committee on School Health. Soft drinks in schools. *Pediatrics*. 2004;113(1):152-154. (aappolicy.aappublications.org/cgi/content/full/pediatrics;113/1/152).

American Academy of Pediatrics, Committee on Sports Medicine and Fitness. Strength training by children and adolescents. *Pediatrics*. 2001;107(6):1470-1472. (aappolicy.aappublications.org/cgi/content/full/pediatrics;107/6/1470).

American Academy of Pediatrics, Council on Sports Medicine and Fitness and Council on School Health. Active healthy living: prevention of childhood obesity through increased physical activity. *Pediatrics*. 2006;117(5):1834-1842. (aappolicy.aappublications.org/cgi/content/full/pediatrics;117/5/1834).

American Academy of Pediatrics, Gahagan S, Silverstein J, Committee on Native American Child Health and the Section on Endocrinology. Prevention and treatment of type 2 diabetes mellitus in children, with special emphasis on American Indian and Alaska Native Children. *Pediatrics*. 2003;112(4):e328. (aappolicy.aappublications.org/cgi/content/full/pediatrics;112/4/e328).

American Academy of Pediatrics, Section on Breastfeeding. Breastfeeding and the use of human milk. *Pediatrics*. 2005;115(2):496-506. (aappolicy.aappublications.org/cgi/content/full/pediatrics;115/2/496).

American Diabetes Association. Type 2 diabetes in children and adolescents. *Diabetes Care*. 2000;23(3):381-389. AAP Endorsed.

National High Blood Pressure Education Program Working Group on High Blood Pressure in Children and Adolescents. The fourth report on the diagnosis, evaluation, and treatment of high blood pressure in children and adolescents. *Pediatrics*. 2004;114(2):555-576. AAP Endorsed.

RELEVANT ENDORSED STATEMENT

American Heart Association, Gidding SS, Dennison BA, Birch LL, et al. Dietary recommendations for children and adolescents: a guide for practitioners. *Pediatrics*. 2006;117(2):544-559. Available at: aappolicy.aappublications.org/cgi/content/full/pediatrics;117/2/544. Accessed April 12, 2006.

SUGGESTED RESOURCES

Anderson B. *Stretching*. Bolinas, CA: Shelter Publications (Random House); 1980.

Centers for Disease Control and Prevention. Nutrition. Available at: www.cdc.gov/nccdphp/dnpa/nutrition/index.htm. Accessed October 1, 2007.

American Academy of Pediatrics. Overweight and Obesity. Available at www.aap.org/obesity. Accessed October 1, 2007.

Centers for Disease Control and Prevention. Physical Activity for Everyone: Introduction. Available at: www.cdc.gov/nccdphp/dnpa/physical/everyone.html. Accessed October 1, 2007.

Hagan JF Jr, Shaw JS, Duncan PM, eds. *Bright Futures: Guidelines for Health Supervision of Infants, Children, and Adolescents*. 3rd ed., Elk Grove Village, IL: American Academy of Pediatrics; 2008.

Jellinek M, Patel BP, Froehle MC, eds. *Bright Futures in Practice: Mental Health—Volume I. Practice Guide*. Arlington, VA: National Center for Education in Maternal and Child Health; 2002.

Jopling RJ. Getting families to "eat right". *Contemp Pediatr.* 1992;9:97-118.

Patrick K, Spear B, Holt K, et al, eds. *Bright Futures in Practice: Physical Activity*. Arlington, VA: National Center for Education in Maternal and Child Health; 2001.

Rogers EM: *Diffusion of Innovations*. New York, NY: The Free Press (Simon & Schuster); 1995. Story M, Holt K, Sofka D, eds. *Bright Futures in Practice: Nutrition*. 2nd ed. Arlington, VA: National Center for Education in Maternal and Child Health; 2002.

Rowland TW. *Exercise and Children's Health*. Champaign, IL: Human Kinetics Publishers; 1990.

REFERENCES

1. Jopling RJ. Health-related fitness as preventive medicine. *Pediatr Rev*. 1988;10:141-148.
2. Centers for Disease Control and Prevention. Self-reported physical inactivity by degree of urbanization—United States, 1996. *MMWR*. 1998;47(50):1097-1100.
3. Centers for Disease Control and Prevention. Physical activity levels among children aged 9-13 years—United States, 2002. *MMWR*. 2003;52(33):785-788.
4. Consensus conference. Lowering blood cholesterol to prevent heart disease [No authors listed]. *JAMA*. 1985;253:2080-2086.
5. Kwiterovich PO Jr. Biochemical, clinical, epidemiologic, genetic, and pathologic data in the pediatric age group relevant to the cholesterol hypothesis. *Pediatrics*. 1986;78:349-362.
6. Lauer RM, Clarke WR. Childhood risk factors for high adult blood pressure: the Muscatine Study. *Pediatrics*. 1989;84:633-641.
7. US Department of Health and Human Services, National Institutes of Health. Lipid *Research Clinics Population Studies Data Book, Volume 1. The Prevalence Study*. Pub No 80-1527, Washington, DC: US Government Printing Office; 1980.
8. Moore LL, Lombardi DA, White MJ, et al. Influence of parents physical activity levels on activity levels of young children. *J Pediatr.* 1991;118:215-219.
9. Nicklas TA, Farris RP, Major C, et al. Cardiovascular risk factors from birth to 7 years of age: the Bogalusa Heart Study. *Pediatrics*. 1987;80:767-806.
10. Powell KE, Thompson PD, Caspersen CJ, et al. Physical activity and the incidence of coronary heart disease. *Annu Rev Public Health*. 1987;8:253-287.
11. Rippe JM. The health benefits of exercise. *Physician Sports Med*. 1987;15:115.
12. Centers for Disease Control and Prevention. Results from the 1999-2002 National Health and Nutrition Examination Survey (NHANES) using measured heights and weights. Available at www.cdc.gov/nchs/about/major/nhanes/nhanes01-02.htm. Accessed on February 2, 2007.
13. Burns TL, Moll PP, Lauer RM. Increased familial cardiovascular mortality in obese schoolchildren: the Muscatine Ponderosity Family Study. *Pediatrics*. 1992;89:262-268.
14. Nesmith JD. Type 2 diabetes mellitus in children and adolescents. *Pediatr Rev*. 2001;22(5):147-152.
15. Centers for Disease Control and Prevention. Corrected data tables: tobacco use, access, and exposure to tobacco in media among middle and high school students—United States, 2004. *MMWR*. 2005;54(12):297-301.
16. Gardner W, Kelleher KJ, Wasserman R, et al. Primary care treatment of pediatric psychosocial problems: a study from the Pediatric Research in Office Settings and Ambulatory Sentinel Practice Network Child Behavior Study. *Pediatrics*. 2000;106(4):e44.
17. Felitti VJ. The relationship of adult health status to childhood abuse and household dysfunction. *Am J Prevent Med*. 1998;14(4):245-258.
18. Grunbaum JA, Kann L, Kinchen S, et al. Youth risk behavior surveillance—United States, 2003. *MMWR*. 2004;53(SS12):1-13.
19. Centers for Disease Control and Prevention. Physical Activity levels children aged 9-13 years—United States 2002. *MMWR* Aug 2003;52(33):785-788.
20. Pate RR, Pratt M, Blair SN, et al. Physical activity and public health: a recommendation from the Centers for Disease Control and Prevention and the American College of Sports Medicine. *JAMA*. 1995;273: 403-407.
21. Geitmaker SL, Dietz WH. Increasing pediatric obesity in the United States. *Am J Dis Child*. 1987;141: 535-539.
22. Blair SN, Kohl HW. Physical activity or physical fitness: which is more important for health? *Med Sci Sports Exerc*. 1998;20(suppl):S8.
23. Noble BJ, Borg GA, Jacobs I, et al. A category-ratio perceived exertion scale: relationship to blood and muscle lactates and heart rate. *Med Sci Sports Exerc*. 1983;15: 523-528.
24. Dunbar CC, Robertson RJ, Baun R, et al. The validity of regulating exercise intensity by ratings of perceived exertion. *Med Sci Sports Exerc*. 1992;24:94-99.
25. Jopling RJ. Let's make fitness a family affair. *Contemp Pediatr.* 1992;4:23.
26. American Academy of Pediatrics. AAP policy statement: strength training by children and adolescents. *Pediatrics*. 2001;107(6):1470-1472. Available at aappolicy.aappublications.org/cgi/content/full/pediatrics;107/6/1470. Accessed on February 2, 2007.

27. Shrier I. Stretching before exercise does not reduce the risk of local muscle injury: a critical review of the clinical and basic science literature. *Clin J Sport Med*. 1999;9(4): 221-227.
28. Eisenmann PA, Johnson SC, Benson JE. *Coaches Guide to Nutrition and Weight Control*. Champaign, IL: Human Kinetics; 1990.
29. Brownell KD, Nelson SS. Modern methods for weight control: the physiology and psychology of dieting. *Physician Sports Med*. 1987;15:122.
30. Munoz KA, Krebs-Smith SM, Ballard-Barbash R, et al. Food intakes of US children and adolescents compared with recommendations. *Pediatrics*. 1997;100: 323-329.
31. US Department of Agriculture. Food Groups to Encourage. Dietary Guidelines for Americans 2005. Available at: www.health.gov/dietaryguidelines/dga2005/document/html/chapter5.htm. Accessed on February 2, 2007.
32. Kraus H. Unfit kids: a call to action. *Contemp Pediatr*. 1988;5:18-30.
33. US Department of Health and Human Services. National *Cholesterol Education Program: Report of the Expert Panel on Blood Cholesterol Levels in Children and Adolescents*. NIH Pub No 91-2732, Washington, DC: US Department of Health and Human Services; 1991.
34. Garcia RE, Moodie DS. A case for routine cholesterol surveillance in childhood. *Pediatrics*. 1989;84:751-755.
35. Resnicow K, Cross D. Are parents' self-reported total cholesterol levels useful in identifying children with hyperlipidemia? An examination of current guidelines. *Pediatrics*. 1993;92:347-353.
36. Wadowski SJ, Karp RJ, Murray-Bachmann R, et al. Family history of coronary artery disease and cholesterol: screening children in a disadvantaged inner city population. *Pediatrics*. 1994;93:109-113.
37. Hoekelman RA. A pediatrician's view: cholesterol mania [editorial]. *Pediatr Ann*. 1990;19:229.
38. Martin AR, Coates TJ. A clinician's guide to helping patients change behavior. *West J Med*. 1987;146: 751-753.
39. McCann DP, Blossom HJ. The physician as a patient educator: from theory to practice. *West J Med*. 1990153:44-49.
40. Rogers, EC. *Diffusion of Innovations*. 4th ed. New York, NY: Free Press; 1995.
41. Song TK, Shepard RJ, Cox M. Absenteeism, employee turnover and sustained exercise participation. *J Sports Med Phys Fitness*. 1983;22:392-399.
42. Shepard RJ. Motivation: the key to fitness compliance. *Physician Sports Med*. 1985;13:88-101.
43. Rowland TW. Motivational factors in exercise training programs for children. *Physician Sports Med*. 1988;14:122-128.
44. Flodmark CE, Ohlsson T, Rydén O, et al. Prevention of progression to severe childhood obesity in a group of obese schoolchildren treated with family therapy. *Pediatrics*. 1993;91:880-884.
45. King AC, Haskell WL, Taylor CB, et al. Group- vs home-based exercise training in healthy older men and women: a community-based clinical trial. *JAMA*. 1991;266:1535-1542.
46. American College of Sports Medicine. Exercise and Sports Science. 1998, June 1 Position Stand: The Recommended Quantity and Quality of Exercise for Developing and Maintaining Cardiorespiratory and Muscular Fitness, and Flexibility in Healthy Adults. Available at: www.acsm-msse.org/pt/pt-core/template-journal/msse/media/0698a.htm. Accessed on February 1, 2007.
47. Strong WB, Dennison BA. Pediatric preventive cardiology: atherosclerosis and coronary heart disease. *Pediatr Rev*. 1988;9:303-314.
48. American Academy of Pediatrics, Council on School Health and Council on Sports Medicine and Fitness. Active healthy living: prevention of childhood obesity through increased physical activity. *Pediatrics*. 2006; 117(5):1834-1842.
49. American Academy of Pediatrics, Committee on Public Education. Children, adolescents and television. *Pediatrics*. 2001;107:423-426.
50. Barkin SI, Scheindlin B, Brown C, et al. Anticipatory guidance topics: are more better? *Ambul Pediatr*. Nov-Dec 2005;5(6):372-376.

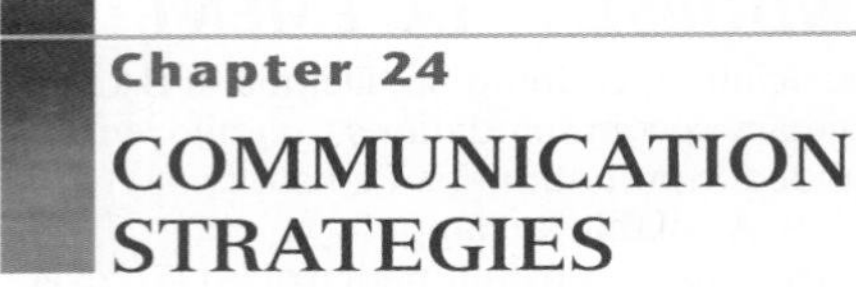

Chapter 24

COMMUNICATION STRATEGIES

Lawrence S. Wissow, MD, MPH

Approximately 15% of school-aged children and adolescents in the United States are thought to have an emotional or behavioral disorder.[1,2] Nearly two thirds of those who are depressed receive no formal mental health care, and only one half receive counseling or some other form of assistance at school.[3] Providing adequate care for this group of young people requires several strategies, including reducing stigma and financial barriers, educating young people and their families about the benefits of seeking care, and increasing the availability of effective services in accessible settings.[4]

One way of broadening access and reducing both financial and psychological barriers involves promoting the detection—and in some cases treatment—of mental health problems by primary care physicians. Primary care visits offer many potential advantages for helping families with mental health problems. Primary care's philosophy of promoting and tracking healthy development fits well with the task of preventing and monitoring for emerging mental health issues. Longitudinal relationships have the potential to build trust and willingness to share sensitive information. Long-term relationships also mean that mental health care can be delivered episodically as needed, in a familiar setting, and in the context of care for medical issues.

However, many young people (and their parents) do not disclose their emotional problems to their primary care physicians.[5] Parent and provider assessments of child mental health frequently do not agree,[6] and estimates suggest that families follow through with only approximately 40% of the mental health referrals made by primary care physicians.[7] These difficulties are not surprising when considering the challenges posed by how pediatric primary care is structured. Visits are relatively short, and many competing concerns need to be addressed. If problems are found, referral sources may be limited, and primary care physicians report low levels of confidence in managing mental health problems themselves.[8]

The skills presented in this chapter were chosen to help primary care physicians efficiently uncover and clarify mental health needs, have therapeutic encounters with people who are demoralized or angry, and give advice about mental health problems, including making referrals, that will be accepted and followed. The skills offer an approach to clinical interaction that contrasts with the style of most routine encounters. The traditional pediatric style is energetic and directive. It assumes that patients and their families come with questions and needs and that the physicians should respond with a straightforward diagnosis and plan for treatment. This approach works much of the time, especially for situations in which few emotional overlays exist. However, this approach can fail when people are ambivalent, ashamed, or anxious or if they believe that their freedom is being challenged. In these situations, patients do not always admit what really concerns them, and they may resist the advice that is offered.

An alternative style is what has been called *patient centered* or *quiet and curious.*[9,10] In this approach, clinicians provide a setting in which patient concerns can be expressed, in which patients take the lead in developing goals and the strategies to attain them, and in which information is offered when patients say they are ready to hear it. This approach can be an efficient method for helping people institute change in their lives, and it helps clinicians and patients work together during times when change is not yet possible. The techniques described here are framed in the context of emotional and behavioral concerns, but their use is not limited to visits with an explicit mental health agenda. They have wide application to situations in which families and clinicians are trying to understand each other's attitudes and develop mutually acceptable plans of action. Many of the skills will seem intuitive or already part of common practice; others may seem new. The results of many studies suggest that these sorts of skills can be learned fairly quickly; however, not surprisingly, opportunities for practice, feedback, and self-assessment lead to greater clinical impact.[11]

Some clinicians may not be able to imagine themselves using every one of these phrases or tactics. Approaches can be tailored to the individual's own style or selectively used by different clinicians sharing a practice. Effective practices structure their approach to care around the talents and interests of their staff members.[12] Helping patients with difficult emotional and behavioral problems is rarely a solo effort.

EFFICIENTLY ELICITING AN AGENDA AND SETTLING ON A TOPIC FOR THE VISIT

Many, if not most, patients never tell their physician their full list of concerns.[5,13] Physicians contribute to this avoidance by interrupting and prematurely taking over the discussion and by ignoring patients' hints that they have something to bring up.[14] Why might patients be so hesitant to speak up? People can be ambivalent about disclosing distressing situations. One aspect they may fear in particular is losing control of the situation—if they admit they have a problem, then someone will tell them what to do about it or do something themselves before the patient can object. Evidence suggests, for example, that some patients do not tell physicians about depression because they are afraid that the physician will pressure them or their child into taking medication.[15]

Many methods can be used to elicit a full range of concerns. Despite being busy, the clinician can show interest and attention through good eye contact, not fussing with the chart or other objects, and by closing the door. These efforts suggest that the clinician has time to listen (even if the physician believes time is limited). Initial greetings can be open ended: "How have things been since the last time?" or "How can I be of help?" rather than, "So I see we are here for shots today."

Once patients have begun to speak, interest can be shown by nodding, allowing a little pause that encourages them to continue, or summing up what has been said and asking for more detail. Perhaps the 2 most important techniques include not jumping in prematurely with a focused question and not ignoring hints about bigger problems. Patients can interpret focused questions asked too early as a sign of what they *should* be discussing, decreasing the chance they will spontaneously disclose key concerns or information. Similarly, hints often represent patients' desire to go beyond what they believe is the primary care physician's agenda for the visit.

Of course, the main reason clinicians do not always ask open-ended questions to elicit concerns or follow up on hints is the fear that they will lose control of time. Families may disclose far more concerns than can be discussed in a short visit, or they may ramble about things that seem only tangentially related. Sometimes it seems obvious that the multiple concerns all relate to a single underlying issue. The clinician can speculate on this possibility, check for the patient's agreement, and then ask about which aspect is the most troubling or about the issue with which the patient would like to start:

> You've raised several things related to how he is doing in school—paying attention in class, sitting still, doing his homework. Is there one of these that you see as most important at this point? Perhaps we should start by thinking about that.

If several concerns are elicited and their relationship is not clear, the clinician can play back the list and the impression of what seems to be the most important:

> You've mentioned several things, but it seems that your worry about his staying out late is what concerns you the most, is that right? Maybe that is what we should focus on today." Conversely, if a priority is not clear, "You've mentioned several concerns—which ones did you want to make sure we talked about today?

When patients ramble, the clinician can gently interrupt, summarize what has been heard so far, and ask for additional concerns:

> I'm sorry to interrupt, but so that we don't run out of time, let me see if I understand your concern(s). [The clinician can recite the list and get confirmation.] OK, good. Now, was there anything else that concerned you?

Visits frequently involve both adults and children. Children may be reluctant participants; they rarely initiate visits in which emotional or behavioral topics are likely to be brought up.[16] Connecting with them, however, is likely to be crucial to ensuring their collaboration with any treatment that results. Parents are more satisfied, children learn more, and outcomes may be improved when physicians give information to both parents and children.[17] In addition, children and parents provide contrasting information about many problems—parents report more overt behavior problems than children, but they tend to lack knowledge of children's mood problems and underestimate the extent to which children have been exposed to stresses outside the home.[18,19] Thus the clinician needs to make an effort to engage everyone who is present and make a connection with each person: a specific greeting for each and a handshake, if appropriate. While talking, the clinician should shift eye contact and body position to address everyone; the clinician should also get everyone's name if unclear and use their names when addressing them. The visit agenda should be developed from talking to all parties, not just the parent. Each person should be invited to add to the list or validate the priorities.

TIMING AND DELIVERY OF ADVICE

Even when people seem to be clearly stating a concern or even directly asking for advice, they may not always likely accept suggestions made in response. Both patients and physicians play a role in creating problems at this stage in a visit.[20] Patients may not be ready to take action, even when they are quite concerned about something. They may not see the problem as that important, they may see equally strong reasons not to act, or they may have little confidence in their ability to make a change. Even patients who are ready to change may feel cornered, challenged, shamed, or otherwise disempowered by well-intentioned clinicians whose advice seems formulaic or comes with a label that patients are not ready to assume. People are generally more likely to act when they develop their own motivation to do so, rather than when they believe that they are being pushed or actively persuaded.

Advice has to be tailored to where individuals are in their readiness to make a change, to their confidence that they can do it, and to their particular goals and values. Although providing advice this way is not nearly as complicated as it sounds (and is not necessarily any more time consuming than straightforward advice offering), it does require a few steps.

First, time should be taken to understand how people define a problem, what they see as the relative importance of addressing it now, and how confident they are that they can make a change.

> I know that this is something that you want to act on, but tell me first a little bit about what has brought you to want to act on it now. How confident do you feel that you can do something about it now? Is there anything that makes you worry that this might not be the time to act [or that you shouldn't do anything about this problem]?

Second, the clinician should find out the issues about which patients have been thinking. Most people come to a physician for advice after already having tried various things or asking family members or friends for help. Ideally, the clinician should have an opportunity to validate and reinforce something that the patient has already decided to do. In addition, learning about the patient's opinion may help avoid or be more tactful about suggesting something the patient already thinks is not likely to work.

> I am happy to give you some ideas, but first I wonder what sorts of things you have been thinking about or have heard about? Is there anything that you have already tried or anything that you feel has or hasn't worked for this?

Third, the clinician should try to present ideas as a range of choices. Even if the choices overlap or appear to be variants on the same thing, patients feel more in control if they perceive that room is available to choose. Even if they reply by asking what the clinician thinks is best, patients still have the knowledge that alternatives exist.

Fourth, the clinician should ask about potential barriers to carrying out the advice. Not uncommonly, people agree to things that they know will be difficult or impossible for them to do. The clinician can help families find telephone numbers or plan how they will get to a referral. It can be worthwhile to go back over the rationale for interventions, so that family members present at the visit can feel comfortable about explaining them to important people in their lives.[21]

Finally, the clinician should engage children as much as possible in developing and troubleshooting treatment plans. Language that children can understand should be used while filling in more details for the parent as needed. When developing a treatment plan, the clinician can ask children to walk through it to determine what part they want to play. Feedback on specific parts should be elicited, making a note of specific aspects to follow up with the child at subsequent visits.[17] For example:

> So, it seems that you and your mom agree that we should try medicine to see if it can help you do better in school. That's going to mean taking a pill every morning. How are you at taking pills? Are you good at remembering things? Do you have any ideas about how we should do that? Next time, can you tell me how that plan you had for remembering worked out?

WHEN PEOPLE SEEM AMBIVALENT ABOUT ACTING ON A PROBLEM

In some instances, ambivalence is obvious; people tell the physician that they cannot make up their mind about how they feel or what they want to do. Sometimes the clinician can only read it in their expression. These situations present 3 challenges: (1) avoiding turning ambivalence into resistance, (2) getting permission to provide information that may help resolve the ambivalence, and (3) turning ambivalence into a decision to act. The clinician hopefully communicates empathy, a willingness to provide information and support, and patience during a decision-making process that may span more than one visit.

The *elicit-provide-elicit* model[20] is a way of getting permission to give information that might help people decide, thus avoiding a lecture that can result in further ambivalence or even resistance. First, the clinician elicits a request for information:

> You mentioned that you were worried about his mood but that you were not a real fan of counselors or of medicines. Would you like to hear some thoughts about those things?

Next, the clinician provides information in a neutral way, keeping it simple and slow paced. Finally, the clinician elicits a response: "What do you make of that? Does any of that make sense to you?" The clinician should be ready to hear the response and initiate another cycle if doing so seems helpful.

Also helpful is to quantify the patient's feeling that taking action is important and the patient's confidence in the ability to act.[20] Patients can be asked to rate, on a scale of 0 to 10, the importance of an issue and their confidence in their ability to address it. These exercises have 3 goals: (1) they help elicit self-affirming statements about resolve and confidence, (2) they help people define for themselves factors that would motivate them to act, and (3) they generate numbers that can be used as benchmarks for further discussion. If the number is low but not zero (that is, low importance or confidence), the clinician should ask, "That is not a lot, but what are the things that make it not zero?" "What would have to happen to increase the importance [or confidence] up a couple of points?" If the number is relatively high (that is, high importance or confidence), then the clinician should ask, "Why is it so high?" "How could you move it up even higher?" "What stops you from moving up higher?"

Next, the clinician can examine the pros and cons.[20] In this exercise, which may develop information similar to quantifying, people are asked to consider the pros and cons (or potential benefits and costs) of leaving a problem as it is and the pros and cons of making an effort to change. The physician can jot down a 2 × 2 chart as patients talk. An important point to remember is that this exercise is not meant to induce some simple weighing of the good and bad and coming up with a decision. For example, the goal is not to have someone say that, on the whole, smoking looks good because it makes her social interactions go better, and therefore they will not attempt to quit. Rather, the goal is for the clinician to be able to empathize with the dilemma that the patient faces and at the same time to help the patient focus on what the decision really involves.

> I can see why this is a difficult decision for you; smoking makes it easier to socialize, and you are afraid that if you stop you will gain weight; but at the same time you recognize that it is not good for your health. That's a tough place to be. Does thinking about it leave you with any new ideas or questions?

WHEN PEOPLE SEEM UNAWARE OF A PROBLEM

In some instances, the clinician may think that someone has a problem, but the patient does not agree. An example might be a parent who uses physical punishment to an extent that the clinician thinks is unproductive. The goal is to help the parents identify for themselves the reasons why they might want to recognize the issue as a problem. However, the advice is likely to be heard politely and ignored, or rejected outright, if the clinician approaches it head on with a *prescription*.

One way to start a discussion is to use the *elicit-provide-elicit* model described previously.

> You mentioned that sometimes you use spanking to get her to behave. That's an area that people have a lot of thoughts about—would you like to hear some more about it?

Another way is to ask how the issue has caused a problem for the patient, the parent, or the family.[10] The question is deliberately phrased as "how" rather than "if," with the tacit assumption that problems exist. If the patient answers, then the clinician should amplify it with, "What else have you noticed?"

> So that's probably been a mixed blessing for you; it gets her to behave but everyone feels badly afterwards . . .

Answers to either of these approaches can be an opening into helping people focus on both dilemmas and discrepancies posed by their behavior. How current behaviors contrast with stated goals and values is gently and respectfully pointed out. Notably, this approach is different from warnings and negative predictions. Instead, the clinician's comments are always framed as empathetic speculations.

> I remember you telling me that you would like to be a lawyer when you grow up. I was wondering how that fits with the kind of grades you are getting now?" or "You have talked about how important it is to feel respected; it seems like your friends might not respect you when they see how you behave when you drink. Can you tell me a little more about how respect works among your friends?

Contrast these comments with:

> See, even you acknowledge that your drinking isn't consistent with your career plans or how you want your friends to see you.

WHEN ADVICE SEEMS TO BE REJECTED OVERTLY OR SUBTLY

The clinician's goal is, of course, to avoid resistance by eliciting patients' concerns and attitudes, giving advice when people are ready, and working to avoid barriers to action. However, none of these approaches works all the time. How does the clinician know that the advice is being rejected? Patients may overtly argue, become defensive, deny or minimize problems, or simply ignore what the clinician is saying.[10] Why might this circumstance happen? The traditional view of resistance is that it reflects lack of motivation, personality issues, or a lack of insight and intelligence. Although all of these factors may play some role, clinicians' behaviors also play a part. In particular, individuals may become resistant:

- As a defense against feeling ashamed of their current or past behavior
- If they believe that they are being coerced, cornered, or rushed
- If they are being urged to do something before they are ready to do it
- If they do not want to lose face in front of another family member who is in the room

A variety of ways can be used to *roll with resistance*.[10] One alternative is to reflect the thought back: "So you have heard some bad things about Ritalin." In many instances, people will then come back to the clinician with a statement that offers some kind of opening. They may go into detail about their concern, providing an opportunity to show respect for their position, provide information, and understand parameters that might form an alternative plan. They may become more conciliatory, revealing that they do, in fact, see both sides of the issue. This action also opens a possible path to a workable solution. As a second alternative, the clinician can also apologize and back up:

> I am sorry if I got ahead of where you were thinking. It is perfectly fine to put this issue aside until you feel that you have all the information that you need. Where do you think we should start?

As a 3rd alternative, the clinician can agree, but "with a twist":

> You are right—medicines certainly can be a problem if they are not used carefully. Those cases you have heard about where children had problems with medicine—do you know anything about the dose they were using or how they were checking for side effects?

WHEN PARENTS OR CHILDREN BELIEVE THEY HAVE BEEN COERCED INTO COMING

Children and teens frequently say that coming to the physician for a particular problem was not their idea. Parents sometimes have been told by an agency, school, or court that they must see the physician for counseling or medication. The clinician can often empathize with patients and families in this situation, and doing so in a way that puts down the referring source is sometimes tempting:

> The school people think every kid needs Ritalin. or The social services people seem to refer everyone whether they need it or not.

Although these statements may contain a grain of truth from your perspective, they can undermine the legitimacy of the whole therapeutic system, including the clinician's part in it. Perhaps worse, they reinforce the patient or family's role as a victim, which ultimately is not helpful. An alternative goal is to start a process through which the patient or family can again start to feel a sense of control. This process can be seen as having 3 stages: (1) acknowledging anger, (2) distancing tactfully from the coercive referral, and (3) offering choice.[20]

> I would be angry too if I felt that someone was telling me what to do that way. I know that I can't make anyone do anything they don't want to do. The schools know a lot about kids and classroom behavior, so I respect their concern; but I am your physician, and my first responsibility to you is to figure out what is right for you. Let's first take a good, broad look at the situation and decide what you think is best to do. I will be glad to talk to the school and explain to them whatever we decide.

A variant for a child or teen might be the following:

> I realize that it wasn't your idea to come, but I am really interested in hearing how you feel about this issue. Would you want to talk to me alone now or with your mother here? I guess it is doubly hard getting told you have to talk to someone and then not even having the choice of who that is. Do you think you might feel more comfortable with someone else? I can help you set that up if you would like.

HELPING PEOPLE WHO SAY THEY ARE STUCK, HOPELESS, OR HAVE TRIED EVERYTHING

Anger, low mood, and anxiety cause tunnel vision that makes seeing a way out of problems difficult; hopelessness and demoralization become vicious circles.[22] Focusing on goals for the future and how to get there can initially be more productive than a detailed analysis of how problems came about; focusing on goals is sometimes all that is needed. Solution-focused therapy grew out of a need for ways to help people in the course of brief interactions.[23,24]

Asking specifically about just how bad patients are feeling and specifically if patients feel in danger of being hurt, hurting themselves, or hurting someone else is always important. These problems need to be addressed immediately. If people report a major fall in their mood, energy, self-esteem, or interest in daily affairs, then they may be depressed, and further treatment may be warranted. For many individuals, however, more transient periods of low mood and discouragement can be helped by identifying and building on strengths and past successes, by reframing events and feelings so that negative attributions about the patient can be made positive or at least neutral, and by breaking down distant and diffuse goals into small, concrete steps that are more readily accomplished.

At least two key elements exist to solution-focused interactions. First, the patient is considered to be the expert on both desired goals and on ways to get there; the clinician is a facilitator and coach. Following from this point, the patient—often through telling the *story* of the problem—provides the outlines of the solution. Second, solution-focused interactions look at observable behavior that either leads to or is part of a desired goal. This element is in comparison to focusing on stopping an undesired behavior or focusing on having poorly observable things such as *attitude* as goals.

Solution-focused interactions often start by asking someone to tell the story of the person's problem. *Story* means the patient's understanding of how the person came to be in a particular situation. Although many people will initially say that they do not know, the clinician can prompt the parent or patient to simply describe when the problem started and how it has evolved: "I know that we could probably talk about this for hours, but in a few minutes, starting at the beginning, tell me how you got to this point."

The first, and often the only, response necessary is your ability to play the story back in a way that provides validation and empathy. To change, people need to feel understood and supported. The clinician need not agree with everything the patient did, but the difficulty of the situation and the strengths that the person has demonstrated can be supported, and how the problems make sense, given the circumstances, can be pointed out:

> So, here you are, a single parent trying to hold down two jobs, with a child who is not the easiest in the world to manage. Then on top of that, your own mother gets sick and needs you. What a tough situation.

A related technique is to look for situations that seem big to the clinician but that seem to be glossed over in the family's or patient's account. For example, a parent tells the story of progressive difficulties with a child's behavior and quickly mentions in the middle of the account the fact that the parent's own parent died during that time. In the clinician's playing back of the story, this factor is noted and speculated that it must have had an impact: "So in the middle of all these difficulties with the school, you lose your own mother. That must have made things particularly hard." The patient who makes corrections or provides more information that changes the clinician's interpretation is not a problem; this is part of the conversation. What matters in this exchange is that the patient has a chance to clarify the story in their own mind.

A 3rd technique when listening to stories is to observe and comment on "shoulds." "Shoulds" can be stated explicitly, as in "whenever he does X, I have to do Y"; as regrets, as in "I should have done ..."; or implicitly, through a pattern of behavior that recurs in a story[25]:

> So you are saying that every time he gets into trouble it is your job to bail him out. That sounds like an important rule that you are following—where did it come from?

In using this comment, the clinician is not suggesting that the rule is bad or even suggesting an alternative point of view. However, by asking someone if this procedure really is a rule that is followed and asking the patient to comment on its origin, the clinician presents an opportunity and grants permission to make a modification.

Eliciting stories usually segues into "So where do we go from here?" or "So what do you want to have happen next?" The clinician can help families set concrete, observable goals. In general, useful goals have the following characteristics:

- People develop goals for themselves.
- Goals are framed in terms of positive behaviors that are observable.
- Goals are often framed in very small steps. "What is the first change in that direction that you would like to see?"
- Goals can be counted or documented objectively; thus progress can be assessed.

When people say that they are at a loss for a goal, the clinician can ask them what they believe would be the first, small sign that things were beginning to improve—preferably so small that they feel confident they could achieve it.[24] For example, if a father's lack of participation in a child's bedtime is the focus of disagreement between parents, then a 1st achievable step might be seeing if the father would be the one to get the child a cup of water while the mother is reading the bedtime story. The clinician can also ask for a highly detailed account of the problem, look at the sequence of events that leads up to it, and identify places where a behavior or response might be changed. People can also be asked to recall exceptions—a time when the desired outcome or state actually occurred, even if only briefly. The discussion can then move on to what might have been happening then and whether these circumstances might be recreated.

WHEN PARENTS AND CHILDREN ARGUE DURING THE VISIT

Parent-child arguments during a visit can derail plans for diagnosis and treatment, and they frequently leave everyone involved feeling impotent and in a bad mood. In some instances, arguments can be avoided by taking steps at the outset of the visit to ensure that everyone gets a chance to speak. Clinicians can provide this opportunity informally by shifting their gaze and body position from parent to child and back, implying that the clinician is both listening and expecting to hear from everyone. If the parent interrupts the child or vice versa, then they can be asked to wait briefly while the other finishes.

One way to break up arguments is to interrupt them to point out areas of agreement:

> I hear you both saying that relationships in the family are important, but you [the teen] are concerned about being respected by your parents and you [the parent] are concerned about how much time he spends at home. Do you think there is a common thread to those things that we could talk about?

Arguments can also be normalized to take some of the emotion out of them:

> It's pretty common for parents and children to disagree about curfews and calling to say where you are. It's part of the whole process of learning how to be independent and responsible. How has your family been handling that?

If one or both parties seem particularly angry or are saying things that seem hurtful, several methods can be used to appeal for a calmer approach. One technique is to suggest that the argument is happening in the context of a caring relationship:

> This must be hard—it's difficult when 2 people care a lot about each other but really disagree. Is there a way you could tell X how you feel but also let him know how much you care about him?

Another technique is to point out the use of polarizing or black-and-white words and thinking. These terms tend to promote escalating insults; they also obscure concerns that might be the focus of a plan. Examples include: "He is always late—he never picks up after himself." "He is lazy—he doesn't care about anyone else in the family." Responses on your part can be:

> Ever, never, always—those words have a way of putting people on the defensive. Can you try telling her those concerns again but without using those words?"[25] "People often get upset if they feel you are labeling them—and it can really stick with kids even if they tell you they don't care. Can you tell him what he does that upsets you without using that label to explain why he does it?

CONCLUSION

Building skills in communication is an endeavor that spans a career. Endless variations in clinical situations and patient and family personalities offer the opportunity to learn new skills and analyze new experiences. As physicians mature, they develop new insights and new relational preferences that change the way they interact with their patients and families. They grow older; but, on the whole, their patients and parents stay relatively young. The growing gap both enriches the patient-physician relationship and creates hurdles to be overcome. Continuing to challenge physicians to improve their communication skills remains an important component of clinical practice.

Many of the communication techniques described in this chapter are described in detail in the books, *The Family Is the Patient: Using Family Interviews in Children's Medical Care,* and *Health Behavior Change: A Guide for Practitioners* (see Suggested Resources).

Detailed suggestions about general approaches to mental health issues in primary care and information about diagnosis and treatment for a range of commonly occurring behavioral and developmental problems may be found in *Bright Futures in Practice: Mental Health*.[26,27] A blueprint for interacting with schools including sharing responsibility for diagnosis and follow-up was developed by Drs Foy and Earls[28] and is helpful in caring for children with behavioral or developmental disorders. Conferences and training courses in effective communication and motivational enhancement techniques are available (see Related Web Sites).

Work on this chapter was supported by National Institute of Mental Health grant MH 062469.

TOOLS FOR PRACTICE

Engaging Patient and Family

- *Tips for Parents of Adolescents* (brochure), American Academy of Pediatrics (www.aap.org/bst/).

Medical Decision Support

- *American Academy on Communication in Healthcare* (Web page), American Academy on Communication in Healthcare (AACH) (www.aachonline.org/).
- *Bright Futures: Guidelines for Health Supervision of Infants, Children, and Adolescents* (book), Bright Futures (brightfutures.aap.org/web/).
- *Bright Futures Toolkit* (toolkit), Bright Futures (brightfutures.aap.org/web/).
- *Health Behavior Change: A Guide for Practitioners* (book), Rollnick S, Mason P, Butler C (intl.elsevierhealth.com/catalogue/title.cfm?ISBN=9780443058509).
- *Mid-Atlantic Addiction Technology Transfer Center* (Web page), Mid-Atlantic Addiction Technology Transfer Center (www.mid-attc.org/).
- *The Family is the Patient: Using Family Interviews in Children's Medical Care, 2nd edition* (book), Allmond BW, Tanner JL, Gofman HF.

RELATED WEB SITES

- American Academy on Communication in Healthcare (www.aachonline.org) offers a variety of conferences and training courses.
- Mid-Atlantic Addiction Technology Transfer Center (www.mid-attc.org/) provides links to courses and online materials with a focus on motivational enhancement techniques.

SUGGESTED RESOURCES

Allmond BW Jr, Tanner JL, Gofman HF. *The Family Is the Patient: Using Family Interviews in Children's Medical Care*. 2nd ed. Baltimore, MD: Williams & Wilkins; 1999.

The American Academy on Communication in Healthcare. Available at: www.aachonline.org. Accessed July 10, 2007.

Hagan JF Jr, Shaw JS, Duncan PM, eds. Bright Futures: Guidelines for Health Supervision of Infants, Children, and Adolescents. 3rd ed. Elk Grove Village, IL: American Academy of Pediatrics; 2008.

The Mid-Atlantic Addiction Technology Transfer Center. Available at: www.mid-attc.org. Accessed July 10, 2007.

Rollnick S, Mason P, Butler C. *Health Behavior Change: A Guide for Practitioners*. Edinburgh, Scotland: Churchill Livingstone; 1999.

REFERENCES

1. Lahey BB, Flagg EW, Bird HR, et al. The NIMH Methods for the Epidemiology of Child and Adolescent Mental Disorders (MECA) Study: background and methodology. *J Am Acad Child Adolesc Psychiatry*. 1996;35:855-864.
2. Costello EJ, Edelbrock C, Costello AJ, et al. Psychopathology in pediatric primary care: the new hidden morbidity. *Pediatrics*. 1988;82:415-424.
3. Wu P, Hoven CW, Bird HR, et al. Depressive and disruptive disorders and mental health service utilization in children and adolescents. *J Am Acad Child Adolesc Psychiatry*. 1999;38:1081-1090.
4. National Advisory Mental Health, Council Workgroup on Child and Adolescent Mental Health Intervention Development and Deployment. *Blueprint for Change: Research on Child and Adolescent Mental Health*. Washington, DC: National Institute of Mental Health; 2001.
5. Horwitz SM, Leaf PJ, Leventhal JM. Identification of psychosocial problems in pediatric primary care: do family attitudes make a difference? *Arch Pediatr Adolesc Med*. 1998;152:367-371.
6. Murphy JM, Kelleher K, Pagano ME, et al. The family APGAR and psychosocial problems in children: a report from ASPN and PROS. *J Fam Pract*. 1998;46:54-64.
7. Rushton J, Bruckman D, Kelleher KJ. Primary care referral of children with psychosocial problems. *Arch Pediatr Adolesc Med*. 2002;156(6):592-598.
8. Olson AL, Kelleher KJ, Kemper KJ, et al. Primary care pediatricians' roles and perceived responsibilities in the identification and management of depression in children and adolescents. *Ambul Pediatr*. 2001;1:91-98.
9. Stewart M. Patient-physician relationships over time. In: Stewart M, Brown JB, Weston WW, et al, eds. *Patient-Centered Medicine: Transforming the Clinical Method*. Thousand Oaks, CA: Sage Publications; 1995.
10. Miller WR, Rollnick S. *Motivational Interviewing: Preparing People to Change Addictive Behavior*. New York, NY: Guilford Press; 1991.
11. Gysels M, Richardson A, Higginson IJ. Communication training for health professionals who care for patients with cancer: a systematic review of training methods. *Support Care Cancer*. 2004;13;356-366.
12. Crabtree BF, Miller WL, Tallia AF, et al. Delivery of clinical preventive services in family medicine offices. *Ann Fam Med*. 2005;3:430-435.

13. Barsky AJ. Hidden reasons some patients visit doctors. *Ann Intern Med.* 1981;94(4 pt 1):492-498.
14. Levinson W, Gorawara-Bhat R, Lamb J. A study of patient clues and physician responses in primary care and surgical settings. *JAMA.* 2000;284: 1021-1027.
15. Rost K, Zhang M, Fortney J, et al. Persistently poor outcomes of undetected major depression in primary care. *Gen Hosp Psychiatry.* 1998;20:12-20.
16. van Dulmen AM. Children's contributions to pediatric outpatient encounters. *Pediatrics.* 1998; 102:563-568.
17. Lewis CC, Pantell RH, Sharp L. Increasing patient knowledge, satisfaction, and involvement: randomized trial of a communication intervention. *Pediatrics.* 1991;88:351-358.
18. MacLeod RJ, McNamee JE, Boyle MH, et al. Identification of childhood psychiatric disorder by informant: comparisons of clinic and community samples. *Can J Psychiatry.* 1999;44:144-150.
19. Richters JE, Martinez P. The NIMH Community Violence Project: I. Children as victims of and witnesses to violence. *Psychiatry.* 1993;56:7-21.
20. Rollnick S, Mason P, Butler C. Health behavior change: a guide for practitioners. Edinburgh, Scotland; Churchill-Livingston; 1999.
21. McKay MM, McCadam K, Gonzalez J. Addressing barriers to mental health services for inner-city children and their caretakers. *Comm Mental Health J.* 1996;32:353-361.
22. Elliott R, Rubinsztein JS, Sahakian BJ, et al. The neural basis of mood-congruent processing biases in depression. *Arch Gen Psychiatry.* 2002:597-604.
23. Walter J, Peller J. *Becoming Solution-Focused in Brief Therapy.* New York, NY: Brunner/Mazel; 1992.
24. Klar H, Coleman WL. Brief solution-focused strategies for behavioral pediatrics. *Pediatr Clin N Am.* 1995;42: 131-141.
25. Allmond BW Jr, Tanner JL, Gofman HF. *The Family Is the Patient: Using Family Interviews in Children's Medical Care.* 2nd ed. Baltimore, MD: Williams & Wilkins; 1999.
26. Jellinek M, Patel BP, Froehle MC, eds. *Bright Futures in Practice: Mental Health—Volume 1, Practice Guide.* Arlington, VA: National Center for Education in Maternal and Child Health; 2001.
27. Jellinek M, Patel BP, Froehle MC, eds. *Bright Futures in Practice: Mental Health—Volume 2, Tool Kit.* Arlington, VA: National Center for Education in Maternal and Child Health; 2001.
28. Foy JM, Earls MF. A process for developing community consensus regarding the diagnosis and management of attention-deficit/hyperactivity disorder. *Pediatrics.* 115(1):e97-e104; 2005.

Chapter 25
ANTICIPATORY GUIDANCE

Howard R. Foye Jr, MD

Anticipatory guidance is the key to achieving two of the primary goals of pediatric care: (1) promoting health and (2) preventing disease. Providing anticipatory guidance in primary care is challenging because of the range and complexity of appropriate issues, the enormous individual differences among normal children and their families, and the limited time in health supervision visits. Despite the time constraints, these challenges can be the greatest source of interesting variety and rewarding physician-patient interactions in the practice of primary pediatric care.

Anticipatory guidance involves three types of tasks: (1) gathering information, (2) establishing a therapeutic alliance, and (3) providing education and guidance. Many discussions of anticipatory guidance focus only on the third task. Without the first two, however, education and guidance are often misguided or ineffective.

GATHERING INFORMATION AND ESTABLISHING A THERAPEUTIC ALLIANCE

Gathering information is a prerequisite if the pediatrician is to understand and respect the unique qualities of the child and family. Effective anticipatory guidance, as with any teaching, should begin with an understanding of the patient's or family's knowledge base, preconceptions, and motivation; guidance is effective to the extent that it is targeted to the individual. A therapeutic alliance between the parents and the physician, based on mutual trust and respect, is another prerequisite for effective anticipatory guidance. In addition to enhancing the effectiveness of teaching, this alliance can be a powerful source of emotional support. By listening respectfully, sympathizing with the parents' frustrations, and reinforcing effective parenting positively, the pediatrician can help the parents gain a sense of competence and confidence in their parenting. As the child develops, establishing a therapeutic alliance directly with the child becomes increasingly important. This relationship is crucial to support anticipatory guidance as the child becomes more independent.

Box 25-1 outlines information that should be gathered before anticipatory guidance is provided. The two major categories are information about the *child* and information about the *child's environment.* Traditional pediatric health care focuses on the child, particularly on issues of promoting physical health, preventing disease, detecting and treating disorders, and monitoring for attainment of developmental milestones. More recently, pediatric health care has broadened its focus to include issues of behavior and the environment in which the child is developing. The list is imposing, particularly with the time limitations of primary care visits, but at least brief attention must be given to these areas to target anticipatory guidance appropriately. Prior knowledge of the child and family obviates the need to survey all these topics at each visit, although frequent updates are important.

The traditional method for gathering information on these diverse topics is through thorough history taking and careful observation during the medical visit. However, the majority of physicians are not able to spend sufficient time or capture all the details that may be available through other data-gathering methods. Several studies underscore the increased sensitivity of standardized tools as compared with routine medical history taking in eliciting health-risking behaviors or history.[1] In fact, patients and families are

BOX 25-1 Information Gathered Before Anticipatory Guidance is Given

A. Information about the *child*
   1. *Concerns:* expressed by parent or child
   2. *Health:* current status and follow-up of past problems
   3. *Routine care:* feeding, sleep, and elimination
   4. *Development:* evaluated by school performance or with standardized tests (eg, Denver Developmental Screening Test, Early Language Milestone Scale)
   5. *Behavior:* temperament and interaction with family, peers, and others
B. Information about the child's *environment*
   1. *Family composition* (at home)
   2. *Caregiving schedule:* who and when
   3. *Family stresses:* (eg, work, finances, illness, death, moving, marital and other relationships)
   4. *Family supports:* relatives, friends, organizations, material resources
   5. *Stimulation* in the home
   6. *Stimulation or activities* outside the home, (eg, preschool or school, peers, organizations)
   7. *Safety*

highly satisfied with the use of computerized assessments for medical history and socially challenging topics to the physician-family dialogue.[2] Bright Futures (www.brightfutures.aap.org) provides an extensive list of paper-and-pencil and electronic tools that clinicians may use in the waiting room or in examination rooms before the physician encounter to assist in collecting the information.

Regardless of the mechanism used to collect the information, fundamental principles about gathering information and establishing a therapeutic alliance for anticipatory guidance need to be highlighted:

1. The parents and child must be given the opportunity to express their concerns at the beginning of every visit; the pediatrician's agenda for the visit will not get the patient or family's attention until the physician has addressed *their* agenda.
2. Because developing a good relationship with the child, as well as the parents, is important, the pediatrician should interact warmly with the child at each visit. Even if only briefly, the physician should greet, talk, and play with the child before proceeding to more threatening procedures such as a physical examination and immunizations.
3. The pediatrician always should inquire about how things are going for the parents. Particularly in today's society of fragmented families, parenting can be lonely and demanding. To be a good nurturer, a person needs to be nurtured. The physician should take advantage of every opportunity to compliment the parents and to encourage them to save time for themselves and each other. By supporting the parents and helping them support each other, the pediatrician can indirectly help them nurture their child.

PROVIDING EDUCATION AND GUIDANCE

With the information outlined in Box 25-1, the primary care physician (PCP) is in a position to provide anticipatory guidance that is focused on the unique qualities and needs of each family. Box 25-2 outlines topics for anticipatory guidance by visit. Covering all of the issues listed at each visit is impossible. A reasonable goal at each health supervision visit would be to at least ask an open-ended question about each of the general categories (health, safety, nutrition, development and behavior, child care, and family). This exchange gives the family an opportunity to guide the discussion to specific topics of interest. Discussing a small number of salient topics is likely to be much more helpful than a rapid, rote litany of checklist items. The checklist approach to anticipatory guidance, reinforced by insurance company chart audit report cards and many authors of primary care guidelines, can interfere with the conversation between patient and practitioner that should characterize high quality anticipatory guidance. Providing anticipatory guidance at the time of taking the history about a certain issue, rather than waiting until the end of the visit, may be the most efficient use of time.

One way to expand the scope of anticipatory guidance with a very small commitment of time is to use preprinted handouts. The American Academy of Pediatrics publishes an extensive variety of patient education materials. These materials provide an efficient way to present standard information that the PCP may want to provide to all families. To avoid littering the parking lot with handouts, the PCP should introduce the material during the conversation with the family, emphasizing why the topic is important. Preprinted handouts are only a supplement, not a substitute for personal discussion with the family.

Many important topics may be overlooked if anticipatory guidance is limited to topics linked to specific ages. Topics that are among the most important at any age include:

1. *Family stresses* (eg, single parenthood, divorce, separation, moving, illness, death, unemployment)
2. *Temperament*[3,4]
3. *Hurried children*[5] (tight schedules and pressure to achieve and grow up fast)
4. *Self-esteem*[6] (development of a sense of competence)

The lists in Box 25-2 should not limit the pediatrician's scope but merely serve as examples and reminders. Much anticipatory guidance will follow from information gathered at the beginning of the visit, including new concerns of the parent or child and follow-up of old problems.

The following sections supplement information in Box 25-2 by briefly discussing the major developmental tasks of each period and related issues of anticipatory guidance. For each age, the major developmental tasks are described for three broad categories of development: (1) socioemotional development,

BOX 25-2 Topics for Anticipatory Guidance

All visits should begin by addressing the concerns of the parents (or adolescent, when applicable).

INFANCY VISITS

- Family resources (family support systems, transition home [assistance after discharge], family resources, use of community resources)
- Parental (maternal) well being (physical, mental, and oral health; nutritional status; medication use; pregnancy risks)
- Breastfeeding decision (breastfeeding plans, breastfeeding concerns [past experiences, prescription or nonprescription medications or drugs, family support of breastfeeding], breastfeeding support systems, financial resources for infant feeding)
- Safety (car safety seats, pets, alcohol or substance use [fetal effects, driving], environmental health risks [smoking, lead, mold], guns, fire or burns [water heater setting, smoke alarms], carbon monoxide detectors)
- Newborn care (introduction to the practice, illness prevention, sleep [back to sleep, crib safety, sleep location], newborn health risks [hand washing, outings])

EARLY CHILDHOOD VISITS

- Family support (adjustment to the child's developmental changes and behavior, family-work balance, and parental agreement or disagreement about child issues)
- Establishing routines (bedtime and naptimes)
- Feeding and appetite changes (self-feeding, nutritious foods, choices, and grazing)
- Establishing a dental home (first dental checkup)
- Safe environment (car safety seats, home safety, and drowning)

MIDDLE CHILDHOOD VISITS

- School readiness (established routines, after-school care and activities, parent-teacher communication, friends, bullying, maturity, management of disappointments, fears)
- Mental health (family time, routines, temper problems, social interactions)
- Nutrition and physical activity (healthy weight; appropriate well-balanced diet; increased fruit, vegetable, whole-grain consumption; adequate calcium intake; 60 minutes of physical activity per day)
- Oral health (regular visits with dentist, daily brushing and flossing, adequate fluoride)
- Safety (pedestrian safety, booster seat, safety helmets, swimming safety, child sexual abuse prevention, fire escape or drill plan and smoke alarms, firearms)

ADOLESCENCE VISITS

Including all the priority issues in every visit may not be feasible, but the goal should be to address issues important to this age group over the course of the four visits.

- Physical growth and development (physical and oral health, body image, healthy eating, physical activity)
- Social and academic competence (connectedness with family, peers, and community; interpersonal relationships; school performance)
- Emotional well being (coping, mood regulation and mental health, sexuality)
- Risk reduction (tobacco, alcohol, and other drugs; pregnancy; sexually transmitted infections)
- Violence and injury prevention (seat belt and helmet use, driving and substance abuse, suicidality, interpersonal violence [fights], bullying)

Modified from Hagan JF Jr, Shaw JS, Duncan PM, eds. *Bright Futures: Guidelines for Health Supervision of Infants, Children, and Adolescents.* 3rd ed. Elk Grove Village, IL: American Academy of Pediatrics; 2008.

(2) cognitive development, and (3) physical or motor development.

Prenatal Visit

The family's developmental tasks before delivery involve preparing for the birth and early care of the infant. The main goal of the prenatal visit is to begin a therapeutic alliance with the family. Specific objectives include learning about the family member's health and social history and discussing their plans and concerns about the remainder of the pregnancy, labor, delivery, and early child care. Other objectives include a discussion of the nature of the pediatrician's working relationship with the family and details about how the practice functions.

Newborn Visits

The major developmental tasks for newborn infants involve transitioning to the extrauterine environment. The major tasks for parents include bonding and learning to respond appropriately to the emotional and physical needs of their infant. The objectives of newborn care include assessing the infant's physical status, behavioral individuality, and caregiving environment at home; managing health problems; and promoting bonding and parenting competence and confidence.

Up to 6 Months

The major developmental tasks in the first 6 months include caregiver-infant reciprocity[7] (socioemotional development), attention to events in the external environment (cognitive development), and rapid growth and visually guided manipulation with the hands (physical or motor development).

Reciprocity describes mutually satisfying and predictable interactions between an infant and a caregiver. The development of reciprocity is influenced both by the clarity and predictability of the cues provided by the infant and by the caregiver's sensitivity, responsiveness, and predictability. Reciprocity is more difficult to achieve when the infant is irritable or unpredictable or when the caregiver's responsiveness is hindered by fatigue, depression, or distractions caused by family stress. The following anticipatory guidance may be helpful: (1) discussing the normal unpredictability of feeding and sleeping schedules and the frequency of unexplained episodes of crying in the first few months, (2) discussing parenting of infants who have various temperaments, and (3) discussing and counseling about issues that may interfere with the caregiver's ability to provide a responsive environment for the infant.

The major cognitive developmental task for the infant in this period involves a shift from activities centered on the body (eg, sucking) to a greater interest in the external environment. At first, this shift is exhibited by increasing visual and auditory attention to external events. Then, from 4 to 6 months of age, the infant's ability to guide the grasp and manipulation of objects visually progresses rapidly.

From 6 to 12 Months

The major developmental tasks of the 6- to 12-month-old infant include attachment,[8] basic trust versus mistrust[9] (socioemotional development), object permanence, early means-end relationships[10] (cognitive development), and mobility (physical or motor development).

The concepts of *attachment* and *basic trust* are similar. Basic trust develops in the first year to the extent that an infant learns that the caregiver is a predictable and reliable provider of essential physical and emotional needs. Trust in this most important aspect of the external environment—the primary caregiver—is believed to result in more confident exploration of the wider environment during the second year, when autonomy becomes the major socioemotional issue. Attachment theorists refer to this phase as *exploration from a secure base*. An infant who is insecurely attached (who mistrusts more than trusts) because of unpredictable or unreliable caregiving in the first year will more likely be inhibited in exploring the environment. The insecurely attached infant is also more likely to be clinging and demanding as a result of insecurity about the caregiver's availability. These behaviors may lead to the erroneous conclusion that the infant is too *attached* to the caregiver. An important point to remember, however, is that most infants go through a period of separation anxiety toward the end of the first year, when clinging behavior increases. Additionally, some infants who are temperamentally more timid or socially withdrawn may have an extended period of *clinginess*.

Object permanence means that the infant understands that objects continue to exist even when they are not present in the immediate physical environment. Calls for an absent primary caregiver are often the earliest evidence that the infant has developed this cognitive ability. Separation anxiety and night waking may also be manifestations of this new achievement. A budding understanding of means-end relationships is apparent in the infant's ability to remove a barrier or to use a second object to retrieve a toy that is out of reach. Another manifestation may be the infant's association of the coat closet with Mommy's departure and therefore the bitter protests that occur when the mother approaches the closet.

Increasing mobility has many implications for anticipatory guidance, particularly regarding issues of safety.

From 1 to 2 Years

The major developmental tasks of the 1 to 2 year old include autonomy versus shame and doubt[9] and ambivalence regarding dependence and independence (socioemotional development); exploration, early language, and *pretend* play (cognitive development); and ambulation and slower growth (physical or motor development).

The issue of autonomy is at the heart of the *terrible twos,* which actually start during the second year of life. This period is characterized by frustrating, dramatic behavioral shifts from stubborn independence ("I want to do it myself" and "no" to most parental requests) to infantile clinging and dependence. Parents often wish that their child were both more independent and less independent at the same time. The wild fluctuations are related to the child's newly acquired walking and climbing skills, as well as the child's eagerness to explore, which often outstrips the cognitive ability to anticipate danger or surprise. The brazen explorer can be quickly reduced to a tearful clinger.

The second year is a very exciting time for cognitive development. The developing ability to understand and to use language is a manifestation of the child's cognitive ability to use symbols for objects. By age 2, the child's play becomes a theater for imitating past events and demonstrating a budding ability to think symbolically and creatively.

A decline in the growth rate in the second year is the cause of one of the most frequent parental concerns in this period: "He eats like a bird." Explaining normal growth and intake usually reassures the parents.

Preschool: 2 to 5 Years

The major developmental tasks of the preschool period include initiative versus guilt,[9] mastery (eg, toilet training) and peer interactions with true sharing (socioemotional development); speech, deferred imitation, and imagination (cognitive development); and steady growth and increasing coordination (physical or motor development).

The initiative that characterizes this period is demonstrated in widening interactions with the physical environment and with people outside the family. Good parenting involves giving the child opportunities to exercise initiative and to experience mastery over new challenges, while ensuring close supervision to provide necessary support and encouragement and to prevent harm. An overprotective or restrictive caregiving environment may result in fear or guilt and may inhibit initiative and the developing sense of self-mastery. A caregiving environment that pushes the child too hard toward independence may not provide enough supervision and support to allow the child to master the developmental tasks of this period.

During the preschool period, language develops so remarkably that the parents may forget that the preschooler's thinking is often still illogical. It is characterized by an egocentrism that cannot comprehend a perspective other than the child's own and assumes that other people have seen and experienced exactly what the child has. It also is characterized by magical thinking (the blurring of fantasy and reality). Wishes, dreams, and actual events are not clearly distinguished. These logical limitations may help explain the common occurrence of irrational fears and exasperating misunderstandings between parent and child. A wish that a new sibling would go away may be a frightening source of guilt and self-blame when the new infant is hospitalized. The child may think that wishing made it happen. Careless comments by a parent may also be a source of anxiety for a child who cannot distinguish a threat from reality.

Middle Childhood: 5 to 10 Years

The major developmental tasks of middle childhood include industry versus inferiority[9] (socioemotional development); concrete logical thinking,[10] basic functions of mathematics, and classification of objects (cognitive development); and preadolescence (physical or motor development).

This period is when the pediatrician should increasingly engage the child directly in discussions and anticipatory guidance. By the end of this period, some physicians are already spending part of each visit alone with the child.

Middle childhood is the period when critical appraisal of a child's abilities begins in earnest. Although preschool children (and their parents) frequently compare themselves with their age mates, comparisons become much more quantitative and official in middle childhood. Tests and opportunities for public humiliation in school are unending. Even when teachers are careful to avoid overt comparisons, the children know how they measure up. After-school activities, particularly sports, are often highly competitive. The reasons why a child may develop a sense of inferiority is easy to understand, particularly in a culture that so emphasizes being number one, as if anything else is not good enough.

The socioemotional task of industry (ie, motivation to succeed through work) requires that the child experience success. Lack of success in tasks leads to a feeling of inferiority, discouragement, and defeat. This issue is important for anticipatory guidance because parents may have also accepted the notion that the child is not good at anything. Some creative thinking must be done to provide successful experiences for each child so that lack of motivation does not rob the child of potential.

Adolescence

The major developmental tasks of adolescence include identity versus role confusion[9] (socioemotional development), abstract and hypothetical thinking[10] (cognitive development), and puberty (physical or motor development).

Adolescence frequently is divided into three stages. Early adolescence (roughly 10 to 13 years of age) is the period of most rapid physical growth and sexual development. Because of the rapid changes, many children are preoccupied with their bodies and with comparing themselves with their peers. In addition, they begin to separate from their parents, frequently challenging parental authority. During middle adolescence (roughly 14 to 17 years of age), preoccupation with physical changes lessens. This period is characterized by intense involvement with peers, conflicts over independence with parents and, often, sexual exploration. Late adolescence (roughly 18 to 21 years of age) is characterized by increased concern over future plans, including college studies and career plans. Social skills are more advanced, and many adolescents are involved in committed, intimate relationships.

LITERATURE FOR PARENTS AND CHILDREN

Literature for parents and children's books are frequently valuable supplements to discussions with the pediatrician about topics of anticipatory guidance. In many instances, practitioners lack sufficient time to discuss an issue in depth in the office. One alternative is to begin a discussion in the time available and then suggest a pertinent reference. Literature references for the parents and child are listed at the end of the chapter; however, follow-up is crucial. Perhaps the next regular visit is soon enough, but inviting the family to call or making an appointment if family members wish to discuss further questions sooner would always be appropriate. Of course, a definite follow-up visit or referral should sometimes be scheduled immediately.

A note of caution is warranted about recommending books. Some parents have a tendency to overintellectualize parenting, to place too much reliance on specific *expert* advice that is not individualized to their family. Good literature for parents points out that specific advice needs to be tailored to the unique qualities of the child and the parents and to the environment in which they live. Good parenting involves more than general knowledge about children and behavior management; it also involves sensitivity and responsiveness to the special qualities of each child and self-awareness about how the parent's feelings and events in the environment influence interactions with the child. Written advice alone is therefore not sufficient. The parents must interpret and modify the advice to fit their situation. Some parents can do this themselves; many will benefit from anticipatory guidance by the pediatrician.

TOOLS FOR PRACTICE

Practice Management and Care Coordination

- *Documentation Forms* (form), American Academy of Pediatrics (www.aap.org/bookstore).

Engaging Patient and Family

- *A Parent's Guide to Building Resilience in Children and Teens* (book), American Academy of Pediatrics/Ginsburg (www.aap.org/bookstore).
- *Baby & Child Health—The Essential Guide From Birth to 11 Years* (book), American Academy of Pediatrics (www.aap.org/bookstore).
- *Caring for Your Baby and Young Child: Birth to Age 5* (book), American Academy of Pediatrics (www.aap.org/bookstore).
- *Caring for Your School-Age Child: Ages 5 to 12* (book), American Academy of Pediatrics (www.aap.org/bookstore).

- *Caring for Your Teenager* (book), American Academy of Pediatrics (www.aap.org/bookstore).
- *Food Fights: Winning the Nutritional Challenges of Parenthood Armed With Insight, Humor, and a Bottle of Ketchup* (book), American Academy of Pediatrics/Shu/Jana (www.aap.org/bookstore).
- *Heading Home With Your Newborn: From Birth to Reality* (book), American Academy of Pediatrics/Shu/Jana (www.aap.org/bookstore).
- *Immunizations & Infectious Diseases: An Informed Parent's Guide* (book), American Academy of Pediatrics (www.aap.org/bookstore).
- *Parent and Child Guides to Pediatric Visits* (fact sheet), American Academy of Pediatrics (www.aap.org/bookstore).
- *Patient Education for Children, Teens, and Parents* (book), American Academy of Pediatrics (www.aap.org/bookstore).
- *Patient Education for Children, Teens, and Parents (Spanish)* (book), American Academy of Pediatrics (www.aap.org/bookstore).
- *Patient Education Online* (other), American Academy of Pediatrics (www.aap.org/bookstore).
- *The Wonder Years* (book), American Academy of Pediatrics (www.aap.org/bookstore).
- *TIPP: The Injury Prevention Program* (fact sheet), American Academy of Pediatrics (www.aap.org/family/tippmain.htm).
- *Touchpoints Three to Six: Your Child's Emotional and Behavioral Development* (book), T. Berry Brazelton, Joshua D. Sparrow.
- *Touchpoints: Your Child's Emotional and Behavioral Development* (book), T. Berry Brazelton.
- *Your Child's Health: The Parents' Guide to Symptoms, Emergencies, Common Illnesses, Behavior, and School Problems* (book), Barton Schmitt.

Medical Decision Support

- *Bright Futures: Guidelines for Health Supervision of Infants, Children, and Adolescents* (book), Bright Futures (brightfutures.aap.org/web/).
- *Bright Futures Toolkit* (toolkit), Bright Futures (brightfutures.aap.org/web/).
- *Developmental and Behavioral Pediatrics: a Handbook for Primary Care* (book), S. Parker, B. Zuckerman, M. Augustyn.
- *Encounters with Children: Pediatric Behavior and Development* (book), S. Dixon, M. Stein.
- *Guidelines for Adolescent Preventative Services, GAPS* (guideline), American Medical Association. AAP endorsed. (www.ama-assn.org/ama/pub/category/1980.html).
- *Growth Charts* (chart), American Academy of Pediatrics (www.aap.org/bookstore).
- *Growth Charts Tutorials* (Web page), Centers for Disease Control and Prevention (www.cdc.gov/growthcharts).
- *Information Gathered Before Anticipatory Guidance is Given* (checklist), Howard R. Foye Jr, MD.
- *Pediatric Nutrition Handbook—5th Edition* (book), American Academy of Pediatrics (www.aap.org/bookstore).
- *Topics for Anticipatory Guidance* (checklist), Howard R. Foye Jr, MD.

AAP POLICY STATEMENT

American Academy of Pediatrics Committee on Practice and Ambulatory Medicine. Periodicity schedule/recommendations for preventive pediatric health care. *Pediatrics.* 2000;105(3):645-646.

REFERENCES

1. Council on Children With Disabilities; Section on Developmental Behavioral Pediatrics; Bright Futures Steering Committee; Medical Home Initiatives for Children With Special Needs Project Advisory Committee. Identifying infants and young children with developmental disorders in the medical home: an algorithm for developmental surveillance and screening. *Pediatrics.* 2006;118:405-420.
2. Hassol A, Walker JM, Kidder D, et al. Patient experiences and attitudes about access to a patient electronic health care record and linked web messaging. *J Am Med Inform Assoc.* 2004;11(6):505-513. E-publication August 6, 2004.
3. Thomas A, Chess S, Birch H. *Temperament and Behavior Disorders in Children.* New York, NY: New York University Press; 1968.
4. Carey WB. Teaching parents about infant temperament. *Pediatrics.* 1998; 102(5):1311-1316.
5. Elkind D. *The Hurried Child: Growing Up Too Fast Too Soon.* Cambridge, MA: Perseus; 2001.
6. White R. Motivation reconsidered: the concept of competence. *Psychol Rev.* 1959;66:297-333.
7. Brazelton TB, Koslowski B, Main M. The origins of reciprocity: the early mother-infant interaction. In: Lewis M, Rosenblum L, eds. *The Effect of the Infant on Its Caregiver.* New York, NY: John Wiley & Sons; 1974.
8. Bowlby J. *Attachment.* 2nd ed. New York, NY: Basic Books; 1982.
9. Erikson E. *Childhood and Society.* New York, NY: WW Norton; 1993.
10. Ginsburg H, Opper S. *Piaget's Theory of Intellectual Development.* 3rd ed. Englewood Cliffs, NJ: Prentice-Hall; 1988.

Chapter 26

FEEDING OF INFANTS AND CHILDREN

Marvin S. Eiger, MD

Most infants and children grow normally and maintain a satisfactory state of health despite variations in nutritional management. The goal of nutrition is to produce an adequately (but not overly) nourished child whose diet is readily digestible, with all the essential nutrients provided through a reasonable distribution of calories derived from protein, fat, and carbohydrate. The pattern and content of feeding in infancy strongly affects dietary habits later in life. Thus considerable care must be given to constructing the early dietary milieu.

INFANT FEEDING

Based on studies of nutritional requirements in infancy, reasonable dietary recommendations for full-term infants are 7% to 16% of calories from protein, 30% to 55% from fat, and the remainder from carbohydrate.[1] Human milk provides approximately 7% of calories from alpha-lactalbumin, a bioavailable protein that is absorbed almost entirely by the infant, 55% from mostly saturated fat containing all the essential fatty acids needed by the infant, and 38% from lactose. Recent research has shown that the high content of saturated fat of human milk is nature's method of programming the breastfed infant to metabolize fats more efficiently, thereby decreasing the risk of adult coronary disease. Most commercially prepared cow milk–based formulas in the United States are modeled after human milk and provide 9% to 15% of calories from a less bioavailable protein, beta-lactoglobulin, which is responsible for the increased gastric curd tension and the large protein loss in the stool of the artificially fed infant. Cow milk formulas contain 45% to 50% of their caloric density mostly from polyunsaturated fats and the remainder from carbohydrate, usually lactose.

With the possible exceptions of vitamin D, iron, and fluoride, the infant fed breast milk from a healthy mother receives more-than-adequate nutrition without further supplementation for at least the first 6 months of life. Thus, from a physiological and teleologic point of view, the maxims *breast is best* and *human milk is for humans, cow milk is for cows* are unchallengeable. Only in the last 50 years or so has any question been raised as to whether a mother would breastfeed her baby. With the advent of pasteurization, dependable refrigeration, and production of formulas from cow milk, alternatives have become available. Thus the decision to breastfeed depends on the customs of the community, lifestyle, the mother's personality, and the attitudes of the obstetrician, pediatrician, and family.

In 1997 the American Academy of Pediatrics (AAP), in its strongest policy statement ever, advised pediatricians and other child health clinicians of the importance and the need to recommend breastfeeding over formula feeding.[2] The AAP policy, recommending human milk as ideal nutrition and the preferred method of feeding for all infants, including premature and sick newborns, states that breastfeeding should begin within the first hour postpartum and that exclusive nursing should be continued without supplementation for approximately the first 6 months, after which solids may be added while nursing is continued through the first year and beyond by mutual consent of mother and baby. Breastfeeding, best initiated immediately after delivery by continuous rooming in and nursing on cue, should be evaluated by a trained observer within the first 24 to 48 hours. Mother and baby should be observed for proper latch-on technique and infant weight, and general health should be assessed 3 to 5 days after discharge, and both the mother and the infant should be monitored closely by the pediatrician for the first 6 weeks until breastfeeding is well established. (See Chapter 89, Breastfeeding the Newborn.) The pediatrician, while remaining sensitive to the mother's own feelings and needs, must be aware of the advantages of human milk over cow milk for infant feeding and encourage mothers to breastfeed.

Comparison of Human Milk and Cow Milk

Milk is the primary source for satisfying nutritional needs during the entire first year of life. Solid foods are unnecessary for most infants until they reach 6 to 8 months of age. Therefore the physician should be knowledgeable about the composition of human milk and cow milk. The manufacturers of infant formulas constantly modify cow milk to produce a product more comparable to human milk. Interestingly, the growth rates of the human infant and the calf are different. An infant takes two to three times longer than a calf to double its birth weight. Inasmuch as cow milk contains 3.5 g of protein per deciliter to human milk's 1.1 g, a ratio of 3:1, the symmetry of nature is satisfied. (Table 26-1 and Appendix C, Table C-13 provides further comparisons of human milk and various cow milk formulas.)

Besides the larger amount of protein in cow milk than in human milk, the proteins in the two milks have qualitative differences. The percentage of casein, as compared with whey proteins (lactalbumin and lactoglobulins), is higher in cow milk. Both proteins have high biological value, but casein causes higher curd tension in the infant's stomach and thus must be treated by homogenization, heating, and acidification for better digestion.

The fat of cow milk (butterfat) contains predominantly saturated fatty acids and is less well digested by infants than is the fat of human milk, which contains monounsaturated fatty acids, such as oleic acid, and polyunsaturated fatty acids, such as essential linoleic acid. The fat composition in human milk allows for excellent fat and calcium absorption and ensures that all essential fatty acids are provided. Human milk, in contrast to cow milk, is rich in lipase, which when added to intestinal lipase aids in the rapid splitting of free fatty acids from triglycerides to ensure quick absorption. Research has shown that free fatty acids are the most important sources of energy for the young infant, and the lipase in human milk makes these free fatty acids available rapidly, even before digestion with intestinal lipase begins.

Lactose is present in higher concentrations in human milk than in the milk of any other mammal. Lactose is split into glucose and galactose. Galactose is synthesized into galactolipid, which is an essential component of the central nervous system in mammals. In most commercial formulas, lactose is provided as the carbohydrate in a percentage similar to that found in human milk. The total ash content of human milk (0.2%) is less than one-third that of cow milk (0.7%); this amount provides an increased margin of safety for renal excretion during illness in early infancy.

Breastfeeding Versus Artificial Feeding

The protective effects of breastfeeding are summarized in Box 89-1 in Chapter 89, Breastfeeding the Newborn.

Table 26-1 Comparison of Nutrients in Formulas and Mature Human Milk

COMPONENT (PER DL)	RECOMMENDED DAILY DIETARY ALLOWANCES (0-6 MONTHS)	HUMAN MILK—VALUES VARIABLE	*HUMANIZED* FORMULAS: ENFAMIL® WITH IRON	*HUMANIZED* FORMULAS: SIMILAC® WITH IRON	*HUMANIZED* FORMULAS: SMA®	EVAPORATED MILK; 1:1 DILUTION	EVAPORATED MILK 13 OZ, WATER 19 OZ, CARBOHYDRATE 1 OZ	WHOLE MILK 3.5% FAT
Calories (kcal)	117 kcal/kg	67-75	67	68	67	69	67	66
Protein (g)	2.2g/kg	1.1	1.5	1.6	1.5	3.5	2.8	3.5
Fat, total (g)	Not listed	4.5	3.7	3.6	3.6	3.8	3.0	3.5-3.7
Saturated	—	2.2	1.2	1.4	1.6	2.4	1.9	2.2
Unsaturated	—	2.3	2.5	2.2	2.0	1.4	1.1	1.3
Cholesterol (mg)	Not listed	7-47	1.4	1.6	3.3	0-3	8-28	10-35
Carbohydrate (g)	Not listed	6.8 Lactose	7 Lactose	7.1 Lactose	7.2 Lactose	4.8 Lactose	7.0 Lactose sucrose	4.9 Lactose
Calcium (mg)	360	34	55	58	44	126	100	118
Phosphorus (mg)	240	14	46	43	33	102	81	92
Sodium (mg)	Not listed	16	28	25	16	60	48	50
Potassium (mg)	Not listed	51	69	75	56	152	122	137
Magnesium (mg)	60	4	4	4	5	12	10	12
Iron (mg)	10	0.05	1.2	1.2	1.3	0.05	0.04	0.05
Copper (Φg)	Not listed	40	60	40	50	Estimate 30	Estimate 20	30
Zinc (mg)	3	0.3-0.5	0.4	0.5	0.4	0.3-0.5	0.2-0.4	0.3-0.5
Iodine (Φg)	35	3	7	10	7	5	4	5
Vitamin A (IU)	1400	200	170	250	264	185	150	140
Thiamine (mg)	0.3	0.016	0.05	0.07	0.07	0.03	0.02	0.17
Riboflavin (mg)	0.4	0.036	0.06	0.1	0.1	0.19	0.16	0.17
Niacin (mg)	5	0.1	0.8	0.7	0.7	0.1	0.1	0.1
Pyridoxine (mg)	0.3	0.01	0.04	0.04	0.04	0.04	0.03	0.06
Folacin (mg)	0.05	0.005	0.01	0.005	0.005	0.005	0.004	0.005
Vitamin B_{12} (Φg)	0.3	0.03	0.2	0.2	0.1	0.08	0.06	0.4
Vitamin C (mg)	35	4	5	6	6	0.5	0.4	1
Vitamin D (IU)	400	2	42	40	42	Fortified 40	Fortified 32	Fortified 42
Vitamin E (IU)	4	0.2	1.3	1.5	1	0.04	0.03	0.04
Vitamin K (Φg)	Not listed	1.5	6	9	5.8	Estimate 6	Estimate 5	6

Data from Fomon SJ. *Infant Nutrition.* 2nd ed. Philadelphia, PA: WB Saunders; 1980; and the Committee on Dietary Allowances. *Recommended Dietary Allowance.* 9th ed, rev. Washington, DC: National Academy of Sciences; 1980.

An infant can digest human milk much more easily than the milk of other mammalian species. Breast milk forms softer curds in the infant's stomach than does cow milk and is assimilated more rapidly. Although human milk contains less protein than formulas made from cow milk, infants use virtually all the protein in breast milk, whereas a large amount of the protein in formula is passed in the stool. A breastfed infant rarely gets diarrhea and rarely becomes constipated because breast milk does not form hard stools in the intestinal tract.

Breast milk has no synthetic compounds, no preservatives, and no artificial ingredients. It is always available at the right temperature and the right consistency. Suckling at the breast is good for the infant's tooth and jaw development. Nursing is technically different from artificial feeding in that the bottle-fed infant does not have to exercise the jaws so energetically, inasmuch as light suckling alone produces a rapid flow of milk. Bottle-fed infants use their tongue in a manner quite opposite to that of the breastfed baby; the flow of milk through the rubber nipple is produced by a tongue-thrusting motion with each suck while the infant's lips create a negative pressure in the oral cavity, thus suctioning milk from the bottle.

Perhaps most important, although most nebulous, are the psychological benefits the infant derives from breastfeeding.[3] Factors such as the more intimate interaction between the breastfeeding mother and child and the more immediate satisfaction of the nursing baby's hunger seem to give promise to healthier mental development. The infant also gains a sense of security from the warmth and closeness of the mother's body. Breastfeeding eliminates the practice of bottle propping; the infant, out of necessity, must be drawn close at each feeding. Although the bottle-feeding mother also can show her love for her baby by holding and cuddling the baby at feeding times, in actual practice, she may do less of this action, and of course she cannot duplicate the unique skin-to-skin contact between the nursing mother and her infant. Montagu[4] states, "The breastfeeding relationship constitutes the foundation for the development of all human social relationships, and the communications the infant receives through the warmth of the mother's skin constitute the first of the socializing experiences of his life." Babies gain a sense of well being from secure handling, and mothers who nurse their infants successfully often seem more confident in managing them. Whether the woman who is sure of her maternal abilities is more likely to breastfeed—or whether the experience itself infuses her with self-confidence—is difficult to determine. Mothers who nurse may be better able to soothe their babies when they are upset, perhaps because the very act of putting them to the breast is such a comfort to them that the mother does not have to search for other methods of reassurance.

The *nursing couple*, mother and baby, forge an especially close and interdependent relationship. The baby depends on the mother for sustenance and comfort, and the mother looks forward to feeding times to gain a pleasurable sense of comfort with her infant and a period of rest and relaxation during her busy day. Because of this unique relationship, many women consider the nursing months among the most fulfilling of their lives.

A mother should not breastfeed unless she is fully convinced that she wants to do so. In most instances the wishes of the baby's father affect the decision to breastfeed inasmuch as the extended family has been replaced by the nuclear family, and the father has become the nursing mother's chief support system. For most women, nursing is accomplished easily; however, if for any reason the desire to breastfeed is lacking or poorly supported, then initiating or continuing nursing may be difficult and may produce emotional strains that might disrupt the mother-child-father relationship. Physicians should support the mother completely, whether her decision is to nurse, not to nurse, or to discontinue nursing, regardless of their personal opinions on the matter. For a working mother, breastfeeding requires a great deal of patience, development of time-saving routines, and cooperation at the workplace, where privacy for expressing milk and storage facilities should be available. Many large corporations are recognizing this need and realizing the economic and psychological advantages of enabling nursing mothers to return to work early. Lightweight, efficient, easy-to-use electric pumps can be rented inexpensively over the long term and can be left at the workplace so that milk can be expressed, refrigerated, and taken home for the infant's next-day feeding. If expressed milk is to be used within 48 hours, then it may be placed in the refrigerator; if frozen immediately after collection and kept in the freezer, then it should be used within 6 months. Although the breastfeeding routine may be more challenging for the working mother, a sympathetic family and physician and access to various support systems will help her continue nursing.[5]

If bottle feeding is chosen, or if breastfeeding is not feasible or successful, then the infant will still thrive on an artificially prepared formula. Commercially prepared formulas for typical infants are modifications of whole cow milk that approximate the composition of human milk. Thus the *humanized* formulas compare favorably with breast milk in their content of protein, carbohydrate (lactose), and saturated and unsaturated fats. Special formulas are available for milk-intolerant infants and for those who have specific malabsorptive problems.

Feeding Schedule

When bottle feeding is used, a demand schedule should be encouraged, as is the case with the breastfed infant. Bottle-fed babies should be fed only as much as they desire, although maternal pressure may subtly urge them to empty the bottle. This action should be discouraged inasmuch as overfeeding at this age may establish a pattern of eating that will eventually result in obesity. Because the gastric emptying time of bottle-fed babies is longer, they require less frequent feedings than do breastfed babies. An artificially fed infant usually shows a greater weight gain than a breastfed infant. No evidence has been found that this increased weight gain is desirable; indeed, it probably is not.

Whether breast fed or bottle fed, an infant who is fed on demand will adjust intake to needs for growth.

The following patterns, with some variations, are usually established:

BREASTFEEDING

Age (in Months)	Number of Feedings per 24 Hours
Birth-1	6-8
2-6	4-5
7-10	3-4
11-12	3

BOTTLE FEEDING

Age (in Months)	Ounces per Feeding
1	2-4
2	5
3	5-6
4	6-7
5-12	8

During the second or third month of life, most infants eliminate the night feeding.

Preparation of Formula

In the United States, most artificial feeding with cow milk is accomplished with proprietary formulas prepared commercially and supplied as *ready to feed* or *easy to mix* in presterilized bottles and cans. The ready-to-feed formulas are supplied with attached nipples in 4-, 6-, and 8-ounce disposable bottles and in 1-quart cans. Ready-to-feed formulas offer convenience to mothers who must travel with their infants and are often used as complementary and supplementary feedings for breastfed babies. However, these formulas are too expensive for most families to use every day. Easy-to-mix, concentrated formulas are supplied in 13-ounce cans of liquid, which are mixed with equal amounts of water, and in 6-ounce cans of powder, which are mixed with appropriate amounts of water, usually in a 1:2 ratio.

In some parts of the United States and the rest of the world, the cost of commercially prepared formula is too high for mothers who cannot or choose not to breastfeed, and a home-prepared formula is used.

Calculation of the ingredients needed for a home-prepared infant formula made from whole cow milk (20 cal/oz) or evaporated milk (44 cal/oz) is based on four principles: (1) All formulas should contain milk, water, and carbohydrate and have an energy content of approximately 20 cal/oz; (2) full-term infants require 110 to 120 cal/kg and 150 to 180 mL of fluid/kg each day; (3) 2 ounces of evaporated milk or 4 ounces of whole milk/kg are required each day; and (4) most infants require feeding five or six times every 24 hours. According to these principles, a 24-hour supply of formula for a 10-lb (4.5 kg) baby would consist of approximately 500 calories and 750 mL. The amount of evaporated milk required would be 10 oz (300 mL),* which would provide 440 calories. The balance of fluid required (450 mL) would be made up with water, and the balance of 60 calories would be supplied with carbohydrates (eg, table sugar, 60 cal/tbsp; Karo® syrup, 60 cal/tbsp; and Dextri-Maltose®, 30 cal/tbsp). The formula, then, would consist of 10 oz of evaporated milk, 15 oz of water, and 1 to 2 tbsp of carbohydrate (depending on the kind used). The 25 oz of formula would contain 500 calories, or 20 cal/oz, and would be divided into five or six bottles, each containing 4 to 5 oz. When larger amounts of formula are needed or when whole milk is used, the four formula principles can be met by either of the following mixtures: 13 oz of evaporated milk, 19 oz of water, and 120 calories (2 to 4 tbsp) of carbohydrates; 23 oz of whole milk, 9 oz of water, and 180 calories (3 to 6 tbsp) of carbohydrates. These formulas would meet the needs of a baby weighing 6 kg or more. A fifth principle of artificial feeding is that babies rarely require more than 1 quart of formula per 24 hours.

The method of mixing formulas described previously assumes that a full 24-hour supply will be prepared. Single 8-oz feedings (3 oz of evaporated milk, 5 oz of water, and 30 calories of carbohydrate) or fractions thereof can be mixed based on the amount the baby usually takes.

Depending on where the family lives, the mother may need to be instructed to prepare her infant's formula under aseptic conditions or to use terminal sterilization; milk is a rich culture medium, and significant contamination may result if neither of these methods is used in areas where the purity of the water supply is questionable. However, in most urban areas with safe water systems, sterilization is unnecessary. Box 26-1 presents, in instructional form, a step-by-step method of preparing and sterilizing infant formulas. This process should be followed when well water is used and when organism counts in tap water are too high. Aseptic methods of preparing single feedings or 24-hour supplies of formula also can be used under these circumstances. With these methods, the water, bottles, nipples, and utensils must be boiled beforehand. Refrigerating prepared formula reduces the number of bacteria found in contaminated bottles. Realistically, as Kendall, Vaughn, and Kusakcioglu[6] have shown, fewer than 50% of mothers can prepare a sterile formula by using either method. If a pediatrician suspects that a mother is unlikely to use aseptic or terminal sterilization techniques, then a presterilized proprietary formula or single-feeding mixture should be used. Using some form of sterile formula preparation is probably wise during the first 4 months of life.

Although most mothers warm their infant's bottle before feeding, no evidence has been found that babies prefer their milk warmed. Parents should be cautioned to avoid warming baby bottles in microwave ovens, which can result in overheating of the formula and can cause esophageal burns on ingestion. In addition, steam can form inside the bottle, causing an explosion.

Vitamin Supplements

Vitamin K

Vitamin K deficiency results in hypoprothrombinemia and hemorrhage and can occur in the young infant without supplementation. Vitamin K sufficiency depends on production by the intestinal flora. The gut of

*For ease of calculation, 1 oz is considered to contain 30 mL.

BOX 26-1 Preparation and Terminal Sterilization of Infant Formula

PREPARATION

1. Measure the prescribed number of ounces of hot water into a clean quart pitcher.
2. Stir in the carbohydrate. Measure powdered sugar with a standard-size tablespoon and level each spoonful with a table knife.
3. Add the prescribed number of ounces of milk to the formula and stir to mix well.
4. Pour the formula into clean nursing bottles.
5. Put nipples and caps on the bottles, leaving the caps loose.

STERILIZATION

1. Put the bottles of formula on a rack in the sterilizer or deep kettle. Caps should be loose, not screwed on tightly. Fill the sterilizer with approximately 3 inches of water, and cover.
2. Bring the water to a boil over moderate heat, then allow to boil gently (with the sterilizer still covered) for 25 minutes.
3. Remove the sterilizer from the heat. Leave it closed (do not even lift the lid) until the side of the sterilizer has cooled enough so that it can be touched with the palm of the hand.
4. Open the sterilizer. Then cool the bottles gradually, adding a small amount of cool water to the hot water in the sterilizer. (Gradual cooling prevents *skimming*, which frequently causes nipple clogging.)
5. Remove the cooled bottles and screw the caps tight.
6. Store the bottles of formula in the refrigerator.

the newborn is essentially sterile, and the intestinal flora of the breastfed infant produce relatively less vitamin K. The content of vitamin K in human milk is low. Therefore, to ensure vitamin sufficiency, a single intramuscular dose of vitamin K is given to all newborns at delivery.

Except for vitamin K, most infants have adequate vitamin stores from birth until rapid postnatal growth ensues at 10 to 14 days of life; vitamin supplementation should begin by that time. Most commercially prepared formulas have an adequate vitamin content; therefore, except for babies who have special needs, infants given these formulas do not need additional vitamins. Although human milk can be expected to satisfy the recommended requirements for vitamins A, C, and E and the B vitamins, providing breastfed infants a preparation containing the minimum daily requirement of vitamin D might be advisable if the mother's vitamin D intake is inadequate or if the mother's or the infant's exposure to sunlight is limited.

Vitamin D

Although vitamin D requirements can be met by sunlight exposure, defining what is adequate sunlight exposure is not possible for a given infant. Furthermore, in recent years, concern about the risk of later skin cancer has led to the recommendation against sunlight exposure even in young infants and for the use of sunscreen ointments, which also reduce cutaneous vitamin D production. An adequate intake of vitamin D for infants (400 IU/day) is not met with human milk alone. Cases of rickets in infants caused by both inadequate vitamin D intake and limited exposure to sunlight, especially in dark-pigmented infants, have been reported. Thus infants who are breastfed, without supplements of vitamin D, are at increased risk of rickets. Vitamin D supplementation is recommended. Whether maternal dietary supplementation precludes the need for infant vitamin D supplementation is questioned.

Vitamin A

Vitamin A supplementation is not needed in the breastfed infant in most areas of the world. In some developing countries, vitamin A deficiency has been found in breastfed infants and children.

Water-Soluble Vitamin Concentrations

Water-soluble vitamin concentrations in human milk may be affected by maternal diet. This circumstance becomes a problem only if the mother's diet lacks adequate intakes of water-soluble vitamins. Maternal malnutrition and alcoholism are situations in which nutritional rehabilitation should include a multivitamin supplement for the mother. Mothers who are strict vegetarians (vegans) may not receive adequate vitamin B_{12} from their diet alone, which may result in low B_{12} concentrations in their milk. Their infants may exhibit vitamin B_{12} deficiency without obvious symptoms in the mother. Therefore vegan mothers should receive a multivitamin supplement to ensure adequate availability of micronutrients. In these circumstances, water-soluble vitamin supplements do not need to be given to the infant. Infants fed home-prepared formulas should receive supplemental vitamins (A, C, and D), as well as iron and fluoride. These supplements are available commercially in a combination liquid (eg, TRI-VI-FLOR with Iron), of which 1 mL is given orally by dropper daily.

Fluoride Supplements

All children older than 6 months living in areas that lack adequate fluoridation (0.3 ppm) of the water supply should receive daily fluoride supplements of 0.25 mg/day because fluorides have been demonstrated to inhibit the development of dental caries. Maternal fluoride intake does not affect fluoride content of human milk.

Iron Supplementation in Infancy

The AAP Committee on Nutrition recommends that during the first year of life, infants should have an iron intake of 1 mg/kg/day to a maximum of 15 mg/day to prevent iron-deficiency anemia. Milk, both human and cow, is deficient in iron. Commercial formulas are supplemented with 8 to 12 mg/L of iron. Breastfed infants need not receive this amount of iron with their vitamin supplements because the small amount of iron in breast milk is almost completely bioavailable to the nursing infant; thus human milk provides sufficient iron until the sixth month of life. However, an iron preparation should be administered to the breastfed infant who has low iron stores or anemia.

Weaning

Weaning customs vary considerably around the world. In many countries, babies are routinely nursed well into the second and sometimes the third year of life. The 1997 policy statement on breastfeeding of the American Academy of Pediatrics recommends nursing ideally for at least the first year and as long thereafter as mother and child desire to continue. Both the World Health Organization and UNICEF recommend breastfeeding for at least 2 years. The emotional benefits that a mother and baby derive from breastfeeding are just as great at 9 months or at 1 year or even later. The age at which the infant is weaned from the breast should be based on a mutual decision between mother and infant. Child-led weaning is commonly practiced throughout the world; however, in the United States, various social and cultural factors, unfortunately, tend to dictate earlier weaning than in other countries. Mothers who are having a gratifying breastfeeding experience and who are made aware of the nutritional, immunologic, and emotional benefits their nursing infants enjoy throughout and even beyond the breastfeeding period will want to continue as long as possible, and the pediatrician is behooved to urge them to do so. If weaning occurs when the infant is younger than 12 months, then cow milk formula should be provided in a bottle or cup. The older infant may be weaned directly to whole milk from a bottle or cup.

The process of weaning should be gradual and should begin with substituting one breastfeeding with a bottle or cup feeding, usually at the midday meal. Once the bottle or cup is accepted, other breastfeedings are similarly eliminated and replaced gradually over a period of 1 to 4 weeks. The mother's milk supply will diminish during this time, as the stimulus of regular emptying of the breast is removed. However, many mothers are able to continue one or two daily breastfeedings over several months, should they so choose.

Occasionally, because of an illness in the mother or infant or the development of a serious complication of nursing, discontinuing breastfeeding abruptly is necessary. To diminish the mother's discomfort, she should be instructed to wear a tight breast binder, reduce her fluid intake, and apply ice packs to her breasts. The administration of 20 mg of stilbestrol orally each day for 3 days is effective in reducing her discomfort and in *drying up* her milk supply but is seldom necessary. Whenever possible, weaning should not be instituted during very warm weather because some babies will initially refuse any feeding other than breast milk for as long as 24 to 48 hours. A fruits infant can be weaned from a bottle to whole cow milk from a cup at 12 months of age.

Skim milk should not be given to infants until they reach at least 2 years of age because, at a time when milk serves as the major source of food, skim milk would provide too few calories, an excessive protein intake, and an inadequate amount of essential fatty acids.

Feeding Solid Foods

Introduction to Solid Foods

From a developmental point of view, cogent reasons exist as to why solids should not be added to the infant's diet before 4 to 6 months of age. When a solid object such as a spoon or a tongue depressor is intro[...] between the lips of a young baby, the baby purses [...] lips, raises the tongue, and pushes against the object vigorously (extrusion reflex). By 4 to 6 months, this behavior changes so that when a spoon is inserted between the lips, they part, the tongue depresses, and food placed in the mouth is drawn to the back of the pharynx and swallowed. Thus the physiologically appropriate time to begin feeding solids is some time between 4 and 6 months. Notably, once again, the 1997 policy statement of the American Academy of Pediatrics recommends that solid food not be initiated until after 6 months.[2] Somewhat later, at approximately 7 to 9 months of age, rhythmic biting movements begin, even in the absence of teeth; foods requiring some chewing may be added to the diet at this time.

Schedule for Solid Foods

An appropriate regimen for introducing solid foods begins with grains and fruits. Rice cereal appears to be the least allergenic of the cereals and thus should be offered first. Progression through vegetables, meats, and eggs can be accomplished in the following manner:

5-6 mo	Cereals and fruits
6-7 mo	Meats and vegetables
7-8 mo	Egg yolk
8-9 mo	Egg white

To ensure an adequate amount of protein, fat, and carbohydrate during the sixth to twelfth months, infants should be offered and should consume no more than an average of 28 oz of milk each day in addition to their quota of solids. An example of an infant diet in this age group follows:

Breakfast	Cereal and fruits
Midmorning snack	Cup of orange juice
Lunch	Meat, yellow or green vegetables, fruit, milk
Mid-afternoon snack	Cup of orange juice or milk
Dinner	Cottage cheese or yogurt, egg, vegetable, fruit, and milk
Bedtime	Milk

Solid foods may be prepared easily from fresh ingredients and pureed by use of a food grinder or blender, or commercially prepared baby foods may be used.

In late infancy and particularly during the toddler period (12 to 30 months), a normal physiological decline in appetite occurs, paralleling the decrease in growth rate. The parents should be made aware both of this normal decline in interest in food, particularly at meal times, and of the concomitant reduction in milk intake, which may drop to 16 oz/day by 24 to 36 months of age. By 4 to 7 years of age the appetite normally increases, as does the growth rate. The intake of *total* calories increases rapidly during the first year of life, then less rapidly to approximately age 4, and then rapidly again. The average full-term infant, by 7 to 10 days of life, will consume approximately 300 cal/day; thereafter the first-year increment is nearly 600 cal/day, the second-year increment nearly 275 cal/day, the third- and fourth-year increments nearly 100 cal/day, and the fifth- to seventh-year increments nearly 130 to 140 cal/day. Thus, despite a decrease in appetite, the actual *intake of calories* does not decrease during the preschool period, and growth patterns remain satisfactory.

PRUDENT DIET FOR THE SCHOOL-AGED CHILD AND THE ADOLESCENT

The diet of a school-aged child and an adolescent should be similar to that of an active adult; however, the extra caloric needs created by the period of rapid growth should be taken into account. Dietary habits and food preferences are closely linked with early associations and family influences. *Children will eat what they see their families eat.* Parents must be told that their infants and young toddlers, when they become older children and adults, will crave salt and sugar in their foods if they have been accustomed to eating these additives in early life. Basically, preparing foods without additives for infants and young children will ensure adequate nutrition and lay the groundwork for sound eating habits in later life.

The pediatrician is in a position to educate entire families in ways to eat more healthful foods in an attempt to prevent obesity and atherosclerosis. Physicians need to know the facts about good nutrition if they are to effect changes in the lifetime habits of families that involve consuming fewer calories and less fat, salt, and refined sugars.

The American Heart Association has endorsed a prudent diet for the child and adolescent, which in simplified form has the following requirements:

- A high-quality protein with every meal
- Milk (preferably skimmed) with vitamin D added and other low-fat dairy products
- Vegetables high in vitamin A
- Fruits for vitamin C
- Whole-grain or enriched breads or cereals
- Vegetable oils high in polyunsaturated fats
- Meat—four servings per week of 4 oz each
- Fish (a good source of polyunsaturated fats)—one to two times a week
- Poultry (low fat)—one to two times a week
- Dark green, leafy, or deep yellow vegetables—at least four times a week, preferably once a day
- Eggs—a maximum of four a week

A prudent diet thus limits the use of fatty meats, high-fat dairy products, eggs, and hydrogenated shortenings and promotes the consumption of fish and the substitution of polyunsaturated vegetable oils and margarines for butter, lard, and other saturated fats.

TOOLS FOR PRACTICE

Engaging Patient and Family

- *Juvenile Rheumatoid Arthritis* (fact sheet), American Academy of Pediatrics (www.aap.org/publiced/BKO_Arthritis.htm).

Medical Decision Support

- *Breastfeeding Handbook for Physicians* (book), American Academy of Pediatrics (www.aap.org/bookstore).
- *Eating Behaviors of the Young Child: Prenatal and Postnatal Influences for Healthy Eating* (book), Dietz W, Birch L (www.aap.org/bookstore).
- *Pediatric Nutrition Handbook* (book), American Academy of Pediatrics (www.aap.org/bookstore).

AAP POLICY STATEMENTS

American Academy of Pediatrics, Section on Breastfeeding. Breastfeeding and the use of human milk. *Pediatrics.* 2005;115(2):496-506. (aappolicy.aappublications.org/cgi/content/full/pediatrics;115/2/496).

Gartner LM, Greer FR, American Academy of Pediatrics, Section on Breastfeeding and Committee on Nutrition. Prevention of rickets and vitamin D deficiency: new guidelines for vitamin D intake. *Pediatrics.* 2003;111(4):908-910. (aappolicy.aappublications.org/cgi/content/full/pediatrics;111/4/908).

SUGGESTED RESOURCES

Auerbach KG, Riordan J. *Breastfeeding and Human Lactation.* Boston, MA: Jones & Bartlett; 1993.

Bennett I, Simon M. *The Prudent Diet.* Port Washington, NY: David White; 1973.

Briggs G, Freeman R, Yaffe S. *Drugs in Pregnancy and Lactation.* 2nd ed. Baltimore, MD: Williams & Wilkins; 1986.

Eiger MS, Olds SW. *The Complete Book of Breastfeeding.* 3rd ed. New York, NY: Workman, Bantam Books; 1999.

Eiger MS, Rausen AR, Silverio J. Breast vs. bottle-feeding. A study of morbidity in upper middle class infants. *Clin Pediatr* (Phila). 1984;23(9):492-495.

Winikoff B, Baer EC. The obstetrician's opportunity: translating "breast is best" from theory to practice. *Am J Obstet Gynecol.* 1980;138:105-117.

REFERENCES

1. Fomon SJ. *Infant Nutrition.* 2nd ed. Philadelphia, PA: WB Saunders; 1980.
2. American Academy of Pediatrics, Work Group on Breastfeeding. Breastfeeding and the use of human milk. *Pediatrics.* 1997;100:1035-1039.
3. Lozoff B, Brittenham GM, Trause MA, et al. The mother-newborn relationship: limits of adaptability. *J Pediatr.* 1977;91:1-12.
4. Montagu A. *Touching: The Human Significance of the Skin.* New York, NY: Harper & Row; 1971.
5. Olds SW. *The Working Parents' Survival Guide.* New York, NY: Bantam Books; 1983.
6. Kendall N, Vaughn VC, Kusakcioglu A. Study of preparation of infant formulas. *Am J Dis Child.* 1936;122:215.

Chapter 27

NUTRITIONAL REQUIREMENTS

William J. Klish, MD; Gilbert B. Forbes, MD

To live, to grow, and to thrive, human beings must take in nutrients from their environment. Before birth the mother supplies these nutrients; thereafter, they must be ingested. If too little is provided, then the infant or child will not grow and may become ill; too much may lead to toxicity or obesity. Nutritionists have tried for decades to define the optimal intakes for various nutrients; a few are known, yet for most the only data available are in the form of educated guesses. In an attempt to cover the maximal conceivable need (because individuals vary in size, individual differences in requirements may exist), quasi-official bodies such as the National Academy of Sciences (NAS) have recommended generous allowances of most nutrients. Although these allowances would provide for the upper extremes of need, in effect, NAS advises most of the population to eat more than they need. Dietary surveys among healthy individuals thus show that the diets of many people do not satisfy the listed recommended dietary allowances. Perhaps this fact is just as well, inasmuch as overnutrition now is a greater problem in this country than undernutrition, and concern exists over the possibility that the former may shorten the life span.

Nutritional requirements can be considered based on age, body size, growth rate, physiological losses (as in menstruation and lactation), and caloric intake. The following discussion deals primarily with the typical child; for the most part, situations that call for special nutritional advice are discussed in other chapters.

Note should be taken of the contribution of food technology to the modern nutritional scene: the pasteurization of milk, the addition of certain vitamins and minerals to some foods, alterations in milk composition to serve the needs of young infants better, hypoallergenic formulas, and the special formulas for infants who have certain inborn errors of metabolism (eg, phenylketonuria). This technology has made it possible to feed the majority of infants most satisfactorily. An undesirable consequence has been a decline in breastfeeding; this decline may be particularly disadvantageous in poor countries and in depressed areas where sanitation is inadequate and the supply of animal protein is meager. However, interest in breastfeeding has revived in recent years in all societies.

ENERGY

Energy Metabolism

The body continuously expends energy in the form of heat and work. Body temperature must be maintained, physical activity provided for, and the processes of digestion, cellular transport, and tissue synthesis supported. The unit of energy generally employed in metabolism is the kilocalorie (kcal),* usually designated simply as a *calorie* (cal). Foods have approximately the following energy equivalents when burned in the body:

- 1 gram of protein = 4 calories (protein is 16% nitrogen)
- 1 gram of carbohydrate = 4 calories
- 1 gram fat = 9 calories

That the body cannot exist on only one or even two of these sources of energy is axiomatic; thus fortunately, nature has provided a mixture of the three in many foods. Satisfactory, palatable diets for infants and children (and adults as well) provide 8% to 15% of total calories from proteins and 30% to 50% each from fats and carbohydrates.

Energy intake is placed to five broad uses:

1. *Resting metabolic rate* (RMR), also known as *resting energy expenditure* (formerly *basal metabolic rate*). This term refers to energy expenditure at rest in the fasting state. Based on body weight, the RMR is higher in infants than in adults, primarily because (1) infants' surface area/weight ratio is higher, (2) a certain amount of infants' *basal* energy is used for growth, and (3) the relative size of the viscera and brain (the most metabolically active organs in the body) is considerably greater in infants than in adults. During the first year of life the RMR is approximately 55 cal/kg/day; thereafter this value diminishes gradually to the adult level of approximately 25 to 30 cal/kg/day. Because adipose tissue has a low metabolic rate, the RMR *per kilogram of body weight* is lower in obese individuals than in thin ones and in women compared with men. However, the RMR bears a linear relationship to *lean weight* in adolescents and adults.
2. *Requirement for growth.* The synthesis of tissue obviously requires energy. The exact amount is not known, but studies of young children recovering from malnutrition and studies of intentionally overfed adults show that 4 to 8 extra calories are required for each gram of weight gain. During the first 4 months of life, one third of the total caloric intake is used for growth. By the end of the second year of life, this level has dropped to 1% to 2% of calories.
3. *Energy lost in excreta.* Some nitrogen is excreted in the urine, and feces contain both protein and fat. Estimates suggest that such losses constitute approximately 10% of the energy intake of the normal diet.
4. *Thermic effect of feeding* (formerly *specific dynamic action*). Resting metabolism rises somewhat after a meal, especially after a generous protein intake, and may not return to the baseline for several hours. The amount of energy dissipated in this manner is estimated to be 5% to 10% of total calories ingested.
5. *Requirement for physical activity.* Studies of adults show that sedentary men require approximately 2700 cal/day and very active men, 4000 cal/day; for women, these values are 2000 and 3000 cal/day, respectively. Thus very active people need 1½ times more food. Although estimates of this sort are not available for infants and children, casual observation confirms that physical activity varies from person to person. Some infants are more restless than others, and, obviously, the energy expenditure of high school athletes is different from that of their spectator friends. Because a major portion of the total energy expenditure is directly proportional to

*A kilocalorie is the amount of heat required to raise the temperature of 1 kg of water by 1° C (from 14.5° to 15.5° C); it equals 1000 small calories. Some experts would like to replace this with another unit of energy, the *joule* (equivalent to 10^7 ergs), which physical scientists commonly use. One kilojoule (kJ) equals 0.239 kcal; to convert kilocalories to kilojoules, multiply by 4.18.

Table 27-1 Calories (kcal) Expended per Hour by Adults

ACTIVITY	CALORIES MEN	WOMEN
Sleeping	65	54
Sitting quietly	83	69
Walking (3 miles/hr)	220	180
Swimming, tennis	400	300
Rowing	450+	360+

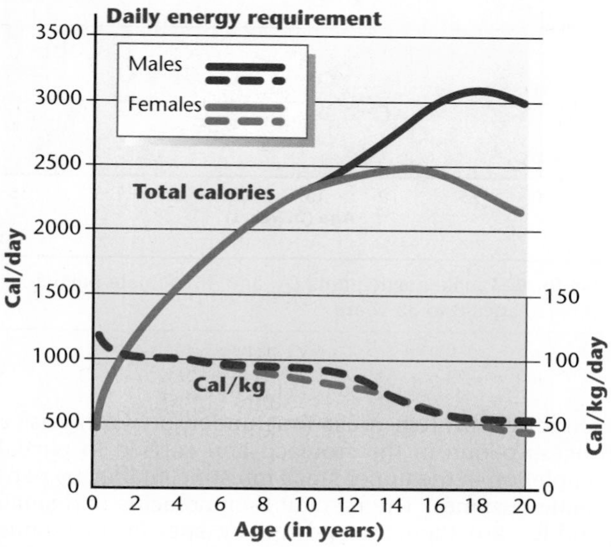

Figure 27-1 Daily energy requirement as a function of age and sex.

body weight, large persons expend more energy in a given task and at rest.

Table 27-1 lists energy expenditures for adults (these values would apply to late adolescents as well) for various activities. The total daily energy requirement as a function of age and sex is depicted in Figure 27-1. These data are based on reports by the Food and Nutrition Board of the NAS and the World Health Organization (WHO). The diagram shows the estimated average requirement. (The reader should note the sex difference both in total calories and calories per kilogram during adolescence. This difference is due to [1] boys' greater lean weight and [2] their greater physical activity. The values for individuals 19 to 20 years of age equal those for young adults.)

In this context, considering the growth of the lean body mass (LBM) is instructive inasmuch as it represents the bulk of the body's metabolically active tissue, whereas the adipose tissue component is relatively inert. The data shown in Figure 27-2 are based on total body potassium measurements.* (The reader should note that the LBM growth curve differs from that of total body weight because the latter includes a variable proportion of fat.) The adolescent growth spurt in LBM is considerably greater for boys than for girls. Obviously an adolescent boy has a greater need for calories and for many nutrients, particularly calcium and nitrogen. Indeed, in the midst of his adolescent growth spurt, a boy's need for iron to provide growth of blood volume and muscle mass may equal that of a postmenarchal girl.

Figure 27-1 shows the *average* energy requirement. Larger individuals need more calories, both for maintenance and for a given degree of physical activity; smaller people need less. This requirement amounts to 18 to 20 cal/day for each kilogram of weight difference. Under normal circumstances, appetite is a good indicator of energy need. In situations of abnormal growth, either too little or too much, this chart can help the pediatrician determine whether the stated intake of food is appropriate and thus whether food intake might be a contributing factor.

Low–birth-weight neonates need a generous intake of calories (ie, 130 to 150 cal/kg/day) to provide for catch-up growth, and their inadequate fat stores demand that feeding be started as soon after birth as possible.

One additional point is worth noting. If calories are obtained from a variety of foods, then an adequate intake of calories usually ensures an adequate intake of essential nutrients. Therefore calories should be the first item evaluated in assessing a dietary history.

Energy Needs During Pregnancy and Lactation

The large number of teenage pregnancies demands that pediatricians and child health personnel be aware of the extra energy requirements for pregnancy and lactation. Studies of chronically undernourished poverty groups have shown that providing additional calories during pregnancy can improve birth weight and the chances of infant survival; now generally known is that a weight gain of 10 to 13 kg is desirable. Weight gain during pregnancy, as well as the prepregnancy weight, influences birth weight. The extra energy cost to the mother is estimated at 150 to 300 cal/day throughout pregnancy, depending on how much she curtails her physical activity. Although based on adults, these figures should pertain equally well to the pregnant teenager.

Lactation requires even more energy. Each deciliter of milk produced contains 72 calories, and milk production is said to be 80% efficient; thus the mother must ingest 90 extra calories for each deciliter of milk produced. A total milk production of 850 mL/day therefore requires an extra 760 calories. An underweight mother should be urged to get more than this requirement, whereas the well-nourished mother

*One of the naturally occurring isotopes of potassium (^{40}K) is radioactive, and the body contains enough of this isotope to allow its measurement by specially designed scintillation counters. Because potassium is found only in lean tissue, LBM can be estimated.

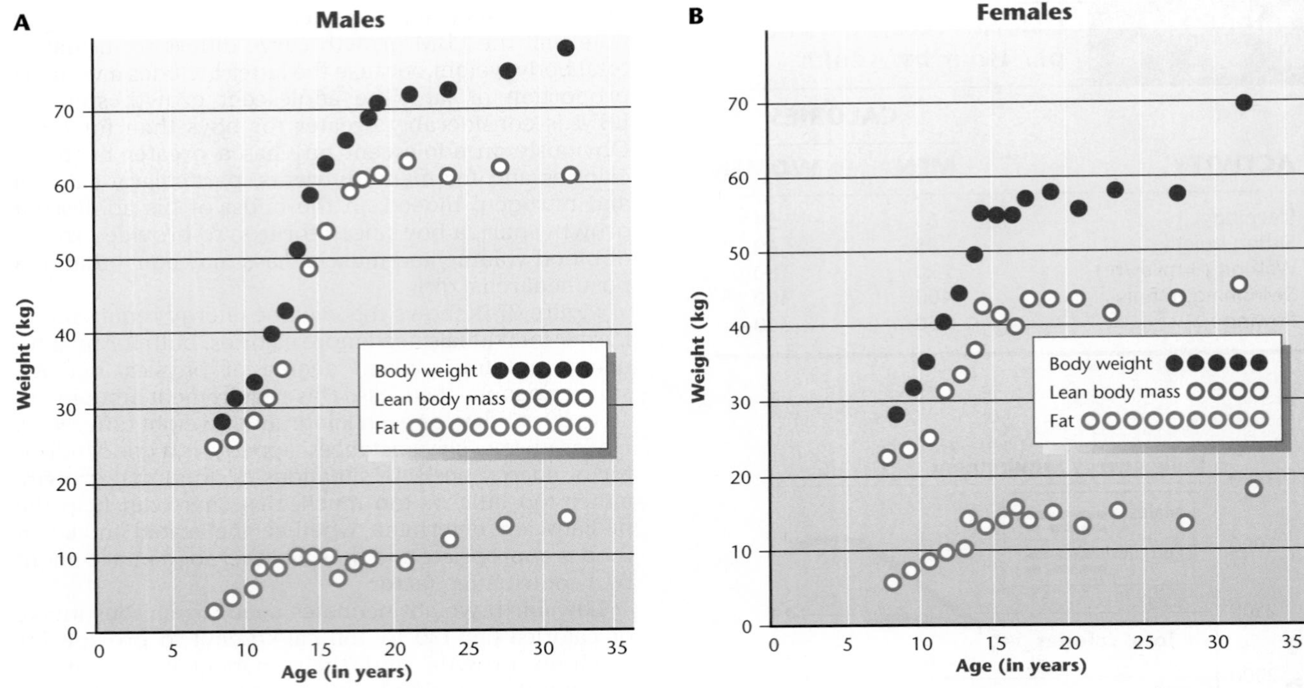

Figure 27-2 Mean body weight and estimated lean body mass *(LBM)* and fat by counting the isotopes of potassium (^{40}K) for 604 male participants *(A)* and 467 female participants *(B)* ages 8 to 35 years.

needs less—perhaps only an extra 500 cal/day—because she can draw on her generous fat stores.

PROTEIN

Proteins are high–molecular-weight polypeptides that serve many functions in the body. Enzymes are proteins, as are antibodies and some hormones; hemoglobin, plasma albumin, and the contractile elements of muscle are also proteins. All proteins are composed of approximately 20 amino acids, in varying proportions; the function of a particular protein is governed by the sequence of amino acids within the molecule. Of these amino acids, nine cannot be synthesized by the body; therefore they are known as *essential amino acids*—histidine, isoleucine, leucine, lysine, methionine, phenylalanine, threonine, tryptophan, and valine. Indications suggest that cystine and taurine may be essential for low–birth-weight infants; these essential amino acids must be supplied in food.

As with energy, the body needs a constant supply of protein; during growth, new tissue must be synthesized because *all* tissues (even bone and adipose tissue) contain protein. Even during adult life a constant turnover of protein takes place, with some nitrogen being lost in the urine even on a protein-free diet and during fasting. A protein requirement exists for growth and maintenance, and this requirement is unremitting because the body has no storage site for protein. An inadequate supply results in a slowing of growth, a compromise of many body functions, and the wasting of muscle; in severe deprivation, impaired resistance to infection, reduced mentality, and even death may result.

Ingested protein must first undergo hydrolysis, a process begun in the stomach and carried to partial completion in the upper small intestine, mainly by pancreatic enzymes. The resultant amino acids and small peptides are then transported by specific metabolic processes, which themselves involve special proteins, into the interior of the intestinal mucosal cells (the peptide bonds having been split at the brush border), and the amino acids are absorbed into the portal blood.

The end products of protein metabolism appear in the urine mainly as urea, the deaminated amino acids being either converted to carbohydrate and fat or burned to carbon dioxide and water.

Biological Quality

The variable amino acid composition of food proteins leads to variations in the efficiency with which they supply the body's needs. The methods for estimating the biological quality of a given protein include tests on animals, observation of the growth of children on differing diets, nitrogen balance studies on adult volunteers, and a chemical score based on the amino acid content. Although these methods do not always yield the same result, general consensus has been reached on the biological quality of the proteins in various food groups. In Table 27-2, the two sources with the highest quality protein (human milk and whole egg) are arbitrarily assigned a score of 100. Simply stated, a child must ingest more of a low-quality protein to achieve proper nutrition and the desired growth rate. The low quality of vegetable proteins is due to relative

Table 27-2 Relative Biological Quality of Food Protein

FOOD	SCORE
Human milk	100
Whole egg	100
Cow milk	95+
Meat	80+
Processed soy flour	80+
Vegetable proteins	50-70

Table 27-3 Safe Level of Protein Intake*

AGE GROUP OR CONDITION	INTAKE
Premature Infant	3-4 g/kg/day
TYPICAL INFANT	
<2 mo	2.2 g/kg/day
3-6 mo	1.9 g/kg/day
6-12 mo	1.5 g/kg/day
TYPICAL CHILD	
1-3 yr	1.2 g/kg/day
3-10 yr	1.0 g/kg/day
Adolescent	0.8-1.0 g/kg/day
PREGNANCY	
Second trimester	+6 g/day
Third trimester	+11 g/day
Lactation	+17 g/day

*Based on high biological quality proteins: milk, eggs, and meat. Add 20% to 50% for vegetable proteins.

deficiencies of one or more essential amino acids. For example, wheat is low in lysine, corn is low in lysine and tryptophan, rice is low in lysine and threonine, and beans are low in methionine. Commercial formulas based on processed soy flour have proved satisfactory for infants. Some vegetables are so low in protein (eg, cassava has only 0.35 g of protein per 100 cal) that it becomes impossible to eat enough to meet the protein need. However, a judicious mixture of vegetables can yield a most satisfactory result. Strict vegetarians have survived in apparent health for many years, and tests of suitable vegetable mixtures have shown good results in the treatment of protein malnutrition.

Generally speaking, wisdom dictates that some animal protein be included in the diet; even if only a third of the total protein intake comes from this source, the risk of a specific amino acid deficit becomes negligible.

Protein Requirement

Many problems exist in estimating the precise protein requirement for any age; indeed, estimates for early infancy are based on the average intake of human milk by infants who appear to be thriving. Table 27-3 represents a composite of estimates by NAS and WHO. Although protein can be limited in the diets of infants and children in poorer nations, the vast majority of

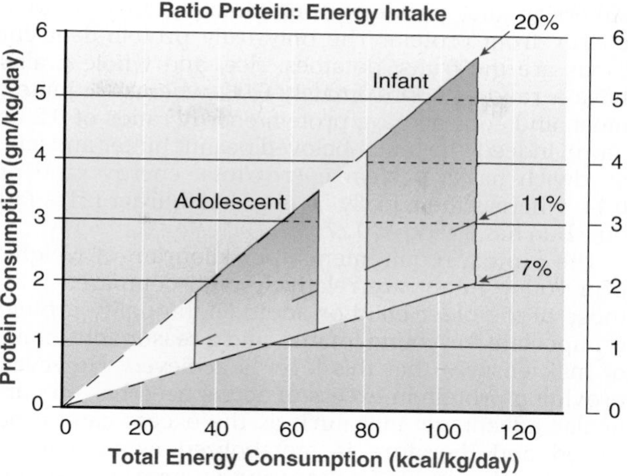

Figure 27-3 Ratio of protein intake to energy intake for normal infants and adolescents. The trapezoids define the usual range of energy intake and the stated limits for the percentage of energy from protein. The ratio represents that of calories from protein to total calories (not grams of protein to total calories). The dotted lines define protein intake per unit body weight. *(Modified from Appelbaum M, Astier-Dumas M, eds.* L' alimentation des Adolescents. *Paris, France: Maison de la Chemie, Sante' du CIDIL; 1988.)*

Americans have access to sufficient quantities of high-quality protein. Figure 27-3 illustrates the concept of the protein/energy ratio of the diet, with the two oblique lines defining the limits of this ratio, here expressed as a percentage of total calories from protein. The upper oblique line is based on cow's milk, in which 20% of the calories are supplied by protein (ie, protein energy/total energy ratio approximately 0.2); a higher ratio would probably never be needed. The lower oblique line is based on human milk, in which 7% of calories are from protein (ie, the ratio is 0.07); the fact that human infants can grow and thrive on this rather low-protein food testifies to its adequacy. If energy intake is adequate and the protein/energy ratio of the diet falls between these limits, then protein intake will be satisfactory.

A diet composed of items from each of the four basic food groups (dairy products; meat, eggs, and legumes; fruits and vegetables; and grains) that also meet the individual child's energy requirement should provide an adequate amount of protein. No evidence has been found that high-protein diets promote growth, enhance athletic performance, or improve the outcome of pregnancy. Indeed, premature infants who have a high relative growth rate thrive on milk formulas that provide 8% to 10% of their calories from protein; severely malnourished infants can also recover on similar diets. Protein quality is obviously important. The lower oblique line in Figure 27-3 is based on high-quality protein, such as that in foods such as milk, meat, and eggs. For diets that consist largely of vegetables, in which proteins are only approximately two thirds as efficient as the high-quality protein sources, the slope of this line should be increased to approximately 11%. The average

American diet provides approximately 15% of total energy from protein. The only truly protein-deficient foods are the fruits; potatoes, rice, and whole grains have a ratio of approximately 0.08, whereas legumes, meat, and eggs all have protein/energy ratios of 0.2 or more. Indeed, the much-beloved peanut butter and jelly sandwich has a protein energy/total energy ratio of 0.14, whereas the equally favored hamburger (21% fat) on a bun has a ratio of 0.27.

The protein requirements (per kilogram of weight) of a young infant are relatively high compared with those of the older child or adult. High-quality protein is important for young infants, and a reasonable intake of milk ensures that this level is achieved. However, providing protein in excess of actual need has no particular advantage, inasmuch as the excess cannot be stored and therefore is metabolized as an energy source and appears in the urine as urea and amino acids. Studies of infants recovering from severe malnutrition have shown that satisfactory recovery can be achieved at protein intakes as low as 2.5 g/kg. In fact, serious doubt exists that diets really high in protein are needed under any circumstances, save those associated with abnormal protein losses (eg, as with extensive burns or gastrointestinal disease).

Several groups require special consideration, as Table 27-3 shows. The rapid growth rate of low–birth-weight newborns demands a protein intake of 3 to 4 g/kg during the early months of life. Lactating women need an extra supply: 850 mL of human milk contains 10 g of protein; under the assumption that protein utilization is only 60% efficient, the mother should receive an extra 17 g of protein daily. The extra demand for protein during pregnancy is appreciable but not great; the body of the term newborn contains approximately 400 g of protein, to which should be added the 500 g contained in the placenta, gravid uterus, and breasts and in the expanded blood volume. Most of this increased need for protein occurs during the latter half of pregnancy.

Excessive amounts of protein (5 g/kg or more) can lead to toxicity. The concentration of blood urea nitrogen rises, the urine may contain albumin and casts and, if water intake is low, the excessive renal solute load leads to an increase in obligatory renal water excretion and to dehydration; this plus the increased thermic effect of food can result in fever, the so-called protein fever.

FAT

Fat is a constituent of all body tissues. The term *fat* is applied to a heterogeneous group of low–molecular-weight compounds that contain fatty acids and that have in common the property of being soluble in solvents such as chloroform and ether. Neutral fats, or triglycerides, are fatty acid esters of glycerol. They serve the functions of energy storage and insulation against the cold and provide a cushion for internal organs. This depot fat accounts for approximately 14% of body weight in term newborns and 10% to 30% in adults. Figure 27-2 shows that body fat content varies with age and sex. Obese individuals may have as much as 50% fat.

The high energy content of adipose tissue (composed of fat-laden adipocytes and a connective tissue stroma) is due to two factors: (1) the high caloric value of fat itself, which has the energy equivalent of gasoline; and (2) the fact that, unlike protein and carbohydrate, fat deposition is not accompanied by an increase in tissue water. This property makes for efficient energy storage; indeed, a moderately thin adult can survive fasting for at least a month, and the very obese have survived for as long as 250 days. Newborn animals (including humans) and adult hibernators have a special adipose organ—brown fat—that supplies energy quickly in response to cold. Fatty acids are classified according to the number of double bonds in the hydrocarbon chain. *Saturated fat* contains a relatively small percentage of fatty acids having double bonds, and *polyunsaturated fat* contains a high percentage of fatty acids having such bonds. Generally the former have higher melting points and thus a firmer consistency at room temperature (a comparison of lard and corn oil is an example). Fats of vegetable origin tend to be more unsaturated than those of animal origin; human milk fat is less saturated than cow milk fat. In addition to neutral fats, other fats can be found. Some fats contain phosphorus or galactose, which are essential components of tissue. Some fats—the lipoproteins—are linked to protein; these fats contribute to the stability of cell membranes and serve in combination with proteins and polysaccharides as structural components of cells (lysozymes and myelin sheaths are examples).

Except for linoleic, linolenic, and arachidonic acids, the multitude of fats found in the body can be formed from protein or carbohydrate precursors. Although symptoms and signs of essential fatty acid deficiency (dermatitis and impaired growth and lipid transport) have been observed under experimental conditions and in patients fed parenterally for long periods, the requirement is low—only 1% to 2% of total calories—thus such deficiencies have not been described under natural circumstances. Essential fatty acids are precursors of an important series of compounds, the prostaglandins, certain cytokines, and thromboxane. Cholesterol, which is a sterol and not a fat in the true sense, plays an important role in metabolism. It is a precursor of bile acids, vitamin D, adrenocortical steroids, and sex hormones. Cholesterol is synthesized in the body and thus is present in foods of animal origin, and its absorption by the intestine is facilitated by a high-fat diet. Diets high in fat and cholesterol are thought to accelerate the process of atherosclerosis. Fat digestion occurs in the upper small intestine by the action of pancreatic and intestinal lipases, which split off two fatty acids from glycerol. The 2-monoacyl-glycerol residue combines with bile salts to form micelles, which incorporate fat-soluble vitamins and cholesterol and which act to dissolve the free fatty acids and are taken up by the mucosal cells. Here the triglycerides are reconstituted and released into the lymph as chylomicrons. Short- and medium-chain fats (12-carbon chains or less) are handled differently; these can be hydrolyzed by the brush border of mucosal cells, and the resultant fatty acids released into the portal vien. Fat exists in several forms in plasma: as triglycerides, free fatty acids, lipoproteins, and phospholipids. Fatty acids are a source of energy for muscle, and they can be esterified by adipocytes to form depot fat; they also can be synthesized in liver and adipose tissue from dietary carbohydrate precursors.

Unsaturated fatty acids that have a double bond at the third carbon from the methyl terminal (alpha-linolenic acid is one such omega-3 fatty acid) are present in significant amounts in marine fish oils. These fatty acids and their derivatives reduce platelet aggregation and appear to retard the progress of atherosclerosis. Fish-eating populations have decreased atherosclerotic disease and also have slightly increased bleeding times.

CARBOHYDRATES

As the name implies, carbohydrates are a series of compounds composed of carbon, hydrogen, and oxygen. They are generally classified into three groups: (1) monosaccharides, which contain five or six carbon atoms (eg, glucose, fructose); (2) disaccharides, which have 12 carbon atoms (eg, sucrose, lactose); and (3) polysaccharides, which are high–molecular-weight polymers (eg, glycogen, starch). The main function of carbohydrates is to supply energy, although certain specialized forms are involved in antigen-antibody reactions. DNA and RNA both contain a 5-carbon sugar (deoxyribose and ribose, respectively); glucose and galactose are essential constituents of tissues such as collagen and cerebrosides; and the various glycoproteins have specialized functions.

Some tissues, such as muscle, can use fatty acids as a prime source of energy, but the brain derives most of its energy from glucose. In theory, the body can exist without dietary carbohydrate (CHO) because it can be formed from protein and fat; however, diets that are very low in CHO (less than 5% of calories) quickly lead to excessive combustion of fat, a rise in fatty acid and ketone body levels in the blood, and occasionally acidosis. Acidosis occurs when a ketogenic diet is used to treat epilepsy.

Monosaccharides require no digestion. Disaccharides are hydrolyzed in the upper small intestine by specific enzymes. Digestion of starch begins in the mouth (salivary amylase) and is carried to completion in the intestine by the action of pancreatic amylase and specific disaccharidases in the brush border of the jejunal epithelial cells. The resultant mixture of simple sugars, principally glucose, is taken into the mucosal cells and then into the portal circulation. In the liver, fructose and galactose are converted to glucose; some glucose is released to the general circulation, and some is stored as glycogen. The entry of glucose into cells of all types, save brain cells, is facilitated by the action of insulin. The level of blood glucose is maintained by the combined action of pituitary and adrenal, as well as pancreatic, hormones.

Diets very high in monosaccharides or disaccharides may cause diarrhea, and consuming these sugars (particularly sucrose) in a physical form that adheres to the teeth promotes dental caries. Generally, the proportions of protein, CHO, and fat in the diet can vary considerably without metabolic or nutritional risk. The limits are rather wide: protein, 8% to 20% of calories; CHO, 15% to 60% of calories; and fat, 25% to 60% of calories. Contrary to widespread belief, obesity is *not* the result of an abnormal distribution of calories among these three dietary components (eg, starches are no more *fattening* than fat); rather, the *total* caloric intake is at fault. Evidence suggests that high-fat diets, particularly those that provide large amounts of saturated fats and cholesterol, can be detrimental to health; however, an excess of total calories and a sedentary lifestyle are also important in this regard.

WATER

All tissues contain water (dental enamel has 1% to 2%), and for most tissues, water is the principal constituent. Most chemical reactions take place only in an aqueous medium, and the rate of water turnover in the body is relatively high. Thus the fact that most edible foods contain large amounts of this dietary essential is no accident.

Water is continuously lost from the body by several routes. An obligatory loss occurs in urine because the kidney has a limited capacity to produce concentrated urine. In children and adults this limit is approximately 1400 mOsm/L,* corresponding to a specific gravity of approximately 1.040. Thus diets high in solutes, which are largely excreted in the urine (nitrogen, sodium, phosphorus), call for a large urine volume. Notably, very young infants are able to achieve a urine concentration of only 700 mOsm/L. Water is also lost continuously from the lungs and skin in the absence of sweating, the so-called insensible water loss, the amount of which is roughly proportional to the RMR. Such losses amount to approximately 10 mL/kg/day in an adult and 30 mL/kg/day in an infant. Water loss through sweating varies with the environmental temperature and humidity and with physical activity. Under extreme conditions an adult can lose 500 mL/hour through sweating.

Daily fecal water loss amounts to approximately 150 mL in an adult and 10 mL/kg in an infant.

Besides food and drink, the body has its own source of water. The burning of fat and CHO produces carbon dioxide and water, the so-called water of oxidation (100 g of fat yields 107 mL of water, and 100 g of glucose yields 60 mL). For an adult, this production amounts to approximately 300 mL/day and for an infant, approximately 90 mL/day. Figure 27-4 depicts the overall water economy for the average infant and the average adult. The infant is at greater risk from water deprivation inasmuch as infants' water turnover is much larger—approximately 16% of total body water each day, compared with approximately 6% per day in adults. Similarly, infants are at greater risk from conditions that accelerate water loss (eg, vomiting, diarrhea), from heat stress, and from diets that provide excessive amounts of solute for urinary excretion (high protein, high salt). Not accidentally, human milk has a high ratio of water to solute.

MINERALS

The diet must provide the minerals that are essential components of body tissues. A deficiency of these

*An osmole is the molecular weight in grams of an osmotically active particle, whether it be a nonionized compound such as glucose or urea or an ion such as sodium or chlorine. A milliosmole (mOsm) is one thousandth of an osmole.

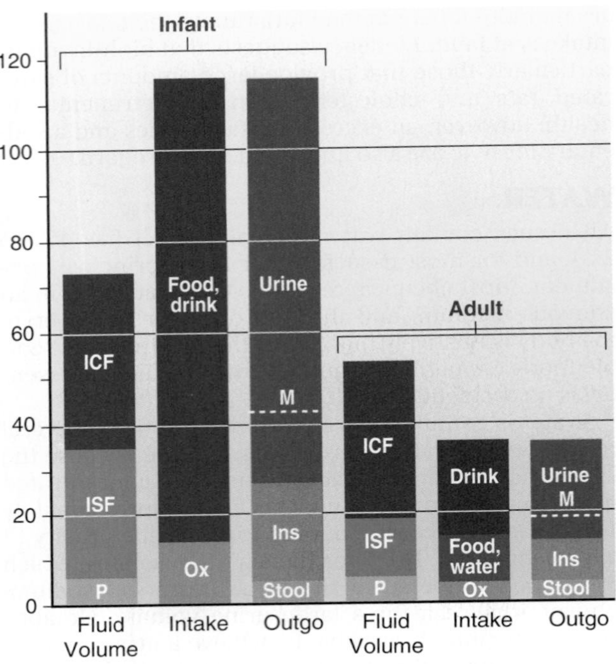

Figure 27-4 Comparisons of body fluid volumes (percentage of body weight) and daily intake and outgo of water (mL/kg) for an infant and an adult. The values shown are averages and vary somewhat with the method used and the subject's fat content. *Dashed line (M),* value for minimal water expenditure; *P,* plasma volume; *ISF,* interstitial fluid volume; *ICF,* intracellular fluid volume; *Ox,* water of oxidation; *Ins,* insensible water loss. *(Farmer T, ed.* Pediatric Neurology. *3rd ed. New York, NY: Harper & Row; 1983.)*

minerals leads to diminished growth and to disease, and excessive intakes may result in toxicity. Table 27-4 provides information on the functions, dietary sources, and requirements for minerals for which requirements have been estimated. Except for iron and fluoride, a well-balanced diet provides a satisfactory intake of minerals. Iron deficiency is now the most common nutritional deficiency in the United States. Attempts to improve this situation have been made through iron fortification of cereal products and infant formulas. Fluoride is added to the drinking water in many communities, as well as to toothpastes.

Notably, the average American diet provides a generous amount of salt to the point that some nutritionists are concerned about this level as a possible factor in the pathogenesis of hypertension.

Besides those listed in Table 27-4, several minerals are known to be essential for animals and presumably for humans. These elements are chloride, chromium, manganese, molybdenum, nickel, silicon, tin, and vanadium. Deficiencies of these minerals are unlikely except with protracted parenteral feeding or, in the case of chloride, with excessive vomiting.

VITAMINS

As the word itself implies, vitamins are necessary for proper tissue function and thus for growth. These compounds act as cofactors for several enzymes. Most vitamins cannot be synthesized in the body and therefore must be supplied in the diet. Exceptions to this rule include vitamin D (activation of skin sterols by sunlight) and vitamin K (synthesized by intestinal bacteria). Small amounts of vitamin B_{12} are manufactured by intestinal bacteria, and some niacin is produced by conversion from tryptophan but not in quantities sufficient to meet requirements. Vitamin deficiencies result in disease, and excessive intakes may lead to toxicity. The story of the discovery of the relationship of certain diseases to dietary inadequacies, of the presence of certain *vital amines* in trace amounts of food, and of the elucidation of their chemical structures and metabolic functions is a fascinating one, as well as being intimately associated with the development of modern nutritional science.

Table 27-5 lists the vitamins known to be important for humans, including the chemical name, function, estimated dietary requirement, dietary sources, and toxicity level.

Notably, certain foods are fortified with vitamins. By law, vitamin D must be added to milk, and vitamins are now added to many commercial infant formulas, to certain cereal products, to some breads, to fruit substitute drinks, and to other foods. Vitamin products are sold widely. As a result, overt vitamin deficiencies now are rare in the United States. Nevertheless, infants and children are at greater risk than adults because their requirements are proportionally greater, and thus dietary deficiency results in disease more quickly.

Claims have been made that massive intakes of vitamin C and the B complex will protect against respiratory tract infection and atherosclerosis and will ameliorate abnormal behavior and poor school performance. Such claims for *megavitamin therapy* and *orthomolecular treatment* are without merit.

A daily intake of 400 mcg of folic acid, started before conception and continued during pregnancy, has been associated with a significant decrease in the incidence of neural tube defects (see Table 27-5). For women who have borne an infant who has such a defect, a daily intake 10 times greater (ie, 4 mg), begun before conception, is recommended.[1]

NUTRITION IN THE UNITED STATES TODAY

Of the many factors that bear on today's nutritional scene, none has had a greater impact than *food technology* and *sanitation*. These modern developments have resulted from combined actions of government, industry, nutritional scientists, and physicians.

Before the turn of the century, the greatest hazards to infant health were infection and improper food. The whole history of infant nutrition is one of attempts to devise a satisfactory milk for babies who were unable to be fed at the breast. In the past, raw milk was not considered a satisfactory food for young infants. This realization led the fortunate few to employ wet nurses for their young.

The following features of raw cow milk render it less than suitable for young infants. *Bacterial contamination* arises from several sources: the cow itself

Table 27-4 Nutritionally Important Minerals

MINERAL	FUNCTION	PHYSIOLOGY	EFFECTS OF DEFICIENCY	EFFECTS OF EXCESS	DAILY REQUIREMENT	SOURCES
Calcium	Structure of bone, ion transport across cell membranes, neuromuscular excitability, blood coagulation	Absorption aided by vitamin D and parathyroid hormone (PTH), hindered by phosphate; PTH facilitates release from bone, thyrocalcitonin inhibits; gravity and muscle tension needed for skeletal stability	Osteoporosis only with severe deficiency, muscle paralysis, or malabsorption	Hypercalciuria with excessive vitamin D, and immobilization	Infants—400-600 mg; adolescents—600-700 mg; pregnancy (latter half), lactation—1000-1200 mg	Milk, cheese, green leafy vegetables, beans, canned salmon
Copper	Cofactor for certain enzymes, cross-linking of collagen	Plasma level 110 mcg/dL, mostly as ceruloplasmin; intestinal absorption hindered by excessive zinc	Anemia, osteoporosis, defective myelination	None, except with massive ingestion	0.5-2 mg	Liver, meats, grains
Fluoride	Bone and tooth structure, resistance to dental caries	Deposited in bone as fluorapatite	Tendency for dental caries	4-8 mg/day—mottled teeth; 20+ mg/day for long periods—osteosclerosis; large doses—acute poisoning	1 mg/L in drinking water	Seafoods, many municipal water supplies
Iodine	Constituent of thyroid hormone	Concentrated in thyroid gland	Simple goiter, endemic cretinism	Iodism	40-150 mcg	Seafoods, iodized salt
Iron	Constituent of hemoglobin, myoglobulin, enzymes	Absorption regulated by gastrointestinal mucosa, level of blood hemoglobin; menstrual loss averages 0.7 mg/day	Anemia: if severe, cardiac failure, poor growth, lethargy	Hemosiderosis, poisoning by medicinal iron	Infants—1 mg/kg; adolescents—10-18 mg	Liver, whole grains, eggs, legumes, meat

Table 27-5 Nutritionally Important Vitamins

VITAMIN	CHARACTERISTICS	BIOCHEMICAL ACTION	EFFECTS OF DEFICIENCY	EFFECTS OF EXCESS	DAILY REQUIREMENT	FOOD SOURCES
Vitamin A (retinol); 1 IU = 0.3 mcg retinol	Fat soluble, heat stable; bile necessary for absorption, specific binding protein in plasma; stored in liver	Component of visual purple; integrity of epithelial tissues, bone cell function	Night blindness, xerophthalmia, keratomalacia, poor growth, impaired resistance to infection	Hyperostosis, hepatomegaly, alopecia, increased cerebrospinal fluid pressure	Infants—300 mcg; adolescents—750 mcg; lactation—1200 mcg	Milk fat, eggs, liver
Provitamin A (beta-carotene); one-sixth the activity of retinol	Converted to retinol in liver, intestinal mucosa	—	—	Carotenemia	—	Dark-green vegetables, yellow fruits and vegetables, tomatoes
Biotin	Water soluble; synthesized by intestinal bacteria; deficiency with large intake of egg *white,* total parenteral nutrition	Coenzyme	Dermatitis, anorexia, muscle pain, pallor	Unknown	Unknown	Liver, egg yolk, peanuts
Cobalamin (vitamin B_{12})	Slightly soluble in water, heat stable only at neutral pH, light sensitive; absorption (ileum) dependent on gastric intrinsic factor; cobalt a part of the molecule	Coenzyme component; red blood cell maturation; CNS metabolism	Pernicious anemia, neurologic deterioration	Unknown	1-2 mcg	Animal foods only; meat, milk, eggs
Folacin (group of compounds containing pteridine ring, *p*-aminobenzoic and glutamic acids)	Slightly soluble in water, light sensitive, heat stable; some production by intestinal bacteria; ascorbic acid involved in interconversions; interference from oral contraceptives, anticonvulsants	Tetrahydrofolic acid (the active form): synthesis of purines and pyrimidines, and methylation reactions	Megaloblastic anemia	Only in patients with pernicious anemia not receiving cobalamin	Infants—60 mcg; adolescents—200 mcg; pregnancy—400 mcg	Liver, green vegetables, cereals, oranges
Niacin (nicotinic acid, nicotinamide)	Water soluble, heat and light stable; availability from corn enhanced by alkali; synthesized in the body from tryptophan (60:1), some by intestinal bacteria	Component of coenzymes I and II (NAD, NADP); many enzymatic reactions	Pellagra: dermatitis, diarrhea, dementia	Nicotinic acid (not the amide): flushing, pruritus	6.6 mg/1000 cal	Meat, fish, whole grains, green vegetables

Table 27-5 Nutritionally Important Vitamins—cont'd

VITAMIN	CHARACTERISTICS	BIOCHEMICAL ACTION	EFFECTS OF DEFICIENCY	EFFECTS OF EXCESS	DAILY REQUIREMENT	FOOD SOURCES
Pantothenic acid	Water soluble, heat stable	Component of coenzyme A; many enzymatic reactions	Observed only with use of antagonists; depression, hypotension, muscle weakness, abdominal pain	Unknown	Unknown—estimated at 5-10 mg	Most foods
Vitamin B_6 (pyridoxine, pyridoxal, pyridoxamine)	Water soluble, heat and light labile; interference from isoniazid; pyridoxal is the active form	Cofactor for many enzymes	Dermatitis, glossitis, cheilosis, peripheral neuritis; infants—irritability, convulsions, anemia	Polyneuropathy	Infants—0.2-0.3 mg; adults—1-2 mg	Liver, meat, whole grains, corn, soybeans

CNS, Central nervous system; *NAD*, nicotinamide adenine dinucleotide; *NADP*, nicotinamide adenine dinucleotide phosphate.

(tubercle bacilli, streptococci [mastitis is common in high-producing herds], and *Brucella* organisms) and the various humans who handle the milk, any one of whom may add bacteria to the milk from respiratory or cutaneous foci. Lack of suitable refrigeration in former days (or in some areas still) accentuated the problem.

Cow milk contains approximately three times as much protein as human milk, and this high-protein content (a large fraction of which is casein) accounts for the formation of tough, voluminous curds on gastric acidification and thus leads to *impaired digestibility*. According to casual observation, formula-fed infants have larger stool volumes than do breastfed babies. The sum total of solutes available for renal excretion is 2½ times higher in cow milk than in human milk, and this *high solute load* calls for a higher obligatory urine volume; thus the infant is at greater risk from hot weather. For the newborn the high phosphorus content of cow milk is one factor in the pathogenesis of neonatal hypocalcemia. Raw cow milk supplies barely enough *ascorbic acid* (21 mg/L) to prevent scurvy, and, unfortunately, the process of pasteurization destroys approximately one half the vitamin present. A few infants are *allergic* to cow milk protein and suffer gastrointestinal disturbances or eczema as a result.

Modern technology has overcome these difficulties. Pasteurization, combined with mandated refrigeration, has virtually eliminated bacterial contamination; evaporated milk and commercial infant formulas are sterile and keep well without refrigeration. Heat treatment also improves digestibility, and diluting the milk with water and adding CHO to restore the caloric content reduces the solute load.

Industry also has modified modern cow milk formulas by adding ascorbic acid, vitamin D, and iron, reducing the phosphorus content, developing hypoallergenic milks based on soybean, hydrolyzed casein or amino acids, reducing the sodium and protein content, and substituting vegetable fat for milk fat. Some commercial infant formulas contain added vitamin E and B complex and nucleotides. Recently, long-chain polyunsaturated fatty acids (docosahexaenoic acid and arachidonic acid) that are present in breast milk have been added to most infant formulas. Some, but not all, studies have shown benefits from these fatty acids on visual and neurodevelopmental outcomes. Some formulas are free of lactose (this sugar might not be tolerated by babies who have gastrointestinal disorders), and others contain partially hydrolyzed whey as a source of nitrogen, which is reported to reduce the risk of atopy similar to breast milk. This wide variety of infant formulas makes it possible to feed every baby satisfactorily by formula from nonhuman sources. Modern technology has wrought a change of unprecedented magnitude in infant welfare.

However, these technological advances have two disadvantages: (1) cost and (2) the decline in breastfeeding. Cost is a problem for poor Americans and a major stumbling block to the exportation of food technology to poverty-stricken nations. Moreover, the more advanced the technology is, the higher the cost will be. For example, a mother who nurses her 2- to

3-month-old infant needs only to drink an extra pint of pasteurized milk each day to satisfy the additional calcium and protein requirements, plus eat an extra two slices of bread and one potato (or 10 g of butter) to complete the caloric need, together with giving her baby vitamin D drops every day. Using an evaporated milk-water-Karo® syrup formula also is inexpensive (additional vitamin C is needed), whereas the cost of a commercial ready-to-feed formula complete with added vitamins is considerably greater.

The ease and convenience of formula feeding have led inevitably to a decline in breastfeeding in this society and even in some developing countries. Evidence of the benefits of breastfeeding for the mother and child make it appropriate to encourage breastfeeding. (See Chapter 89, Breastfeeding the Newborn; and Chapter 26, Feeding of Infants and Children.) An encouraging note is that many more mothers have chosen to nurse their babies in recent years. However, an important point to remember is that human milk contains very little vitamin D; thus nurslings must be given this vitamin, and mothers should be advised to eat a well-balanced diet. Governmental regulations, public health activities, food technology, and governmental assistance are of the utmost importance to the modern nutritional scene. Municipal water supplies are now pure, and pasteurization is a uniform requirement for the sale of cow milk commercially. Dairy cattle are tested for tuberculosis and brucellosis, and those that have mastitis are removed from milk production. Other measures include inspection of food handlers and meats, inspection of restaurant kitchens, codes for infant formulas shipped from one state to another, and codes for canned foods. The result is that diseases such as typhoid fever, bovine tuberculosis, trichinosis, botulism, and staphylococcal food poisoning are now rare.

Modern agricultural practices, food processing, and distribution services have resulted in the widespread availability of reasonably priced, palatable, attractively displayed, high-caloric foods, with the result that many of the citizens in this country, be they children or adults, find it easy to eat more than they need. That obesity is so prevalent is not surprising.

Many studies have shown the deleterious effects of severe infection, particularly gastroenteritis, on nutrition (vitamin turnover increases, and nitrogen balance becomes negative). The high prevalence of infantile malnutrition in developing countries is due in part to the occurrence of repeated infections. The US Food and Drug Administration was formed in 1938; this agency has the authority to regulate, among other things, food quality, food labeling, use of food additives, and vitamin fortification. The Federal Trade Commission monitors advertising claims. These measures have resulted in better, cleaner, and more wholesome food. One of the most dramatic improvements was effected by the mandatory addition of vitamin D to milk, which has led to virtual elimination of dietary-deficiency rickets in this country.

Food assistance programs are now fairly widespread. These programs include school lunch programs; the food stamp program; the program for women, infants, and children (known as the Special Supplemental Nutrition Program for Women, Infants, and Children [WIC]); and, in reality, the farm subsidy program. As a result, families that have limited financial means can augment their otherwise meager food supply. Millions of people are receiving food stamps, and approximately a half million are enrolled in the WIC program.

Finally, local, state, and federal governments play an important role in providing free or low-cost health care for poor people and salaries for school and public health nutritionists and for helping to defray the cost of special foods for children who have certain diseases, such as phenylketonuria.

The result of these efforts, both industrial and governmental, is that with but one exception (iron-deficiency anemia), overt nutritional deficiency now is uncommon in the United States, and obesity and dental caries have become the most prevalent nutritional conditions.

Two quasi-official organizations have published recommendations for nutritional allowances (*not* requirements): the Food and Nutrition Board of the NAS—National Research Council—and the Food and Agricultural Organization (FAO) of the United Nations. The former organization publishes a series of pamphlets at roughly 5-year intervals that include a listing of recommended dietary allowances for people of all ages. These recommendations are based on knowledge of actual requirements to which is added a generous safety factor to account for supposed individual variation in requirements and for variations in food quality. Except for calories, the recommended amounts all are in excess of actual need for the average individual; however, dietary surveys reveal that a sizable proportion of the population consumes less of many nutrients than the NAS recommends. The FAO recommendations are closer to actual requirements for protein, calcium, and several vitamins (see WHO *Handbook*); unfortunately, this list of nutrients is not as complete as the one published by the NAS.

POSSIBLE ROLE OF INFANT AND CHILD NUTRITION IN ADULT HEALTH

Generally, the nutritional status of infants and children today is reasonably good. Some experts say the biggest challenge is the adult, that is, whether current infant feeding practices are compromising their health and longevity.

Several facts have been established. An intake of fluoride in early life, at a time when dental enamel is forming, results in a long-term diminution of the dental caries rate. A well-known fact is that a high intake of sucrose, particularly in solid, sticky foods, predisposes a person to dental caries; thus early learning of food habits that minimize the consumption of such foods should be beneficial.* Childhood obesity tends

*Statements by manufacturers reveal a generous consumption of sucrose. For the United States, this level amounts to approximately 50 kg per capita per year, equivalent to 125 g, or 500 calories, per day. Furthermore, this figure has remained fairly constant over the last 50 years.

to persist into adult life, and this obesity shortens life span; therefore attempts to prevent childhood obesity are important. Severe malnutrition in *early life* may impair intellectual performance† and should be prevented through procedures such as early feeding of premature infants, use of intravenous alimentation in certain critical situations, and early requests for medical advice and treatment of diseases that compromise nutrition during infancy.

The most challenging question relates to atherosclerosis and its cardiac and cerebral consequences. (This discussion forgoes consideration of the inherited abnormalities of lipoprotein metabolism associated with early-onset arterial disease.) Arterial changes (the fatty streaks) appear in childhood, and by age 20 an appreciable percentage of men already have atherosclerotic plaques. The dietary components that have been considered as possible factors in initiating or intensifying this aging process are total calories, animal protein, saturated fats, and cholesterol. Cross-cultural surveys of adult autopsies reveal that any or all of these factors may be at fault; some evidence also indicates that *postcoronary* adults who limit their intake of calories, saturated fat, and cholesterol have a better prognosis. The possible preventive role of fish has been mentioned earlier; however, certain species now are contaminated with mercury and polychlorinated hydrocarbons and therefore should not be eaten.

Experiments conducted many years ago showed that rats fed (from weaning) an amount of food equal to approximately two thirds of their usual intake lived much longer and had less arterial disease and fewer tumors that those fed ad libitum. These results have been confirmed by Ross,[2] who states, "The effects of chronic restriction in food intake on laboratory animals have been so apparent that it is difficult to avoid concluding that no environmental factor so decisively reduces the rate or expression of the aging process," and, "The mechanisms through which nutrition influences the aging processes are already operative during the *youthful stage* [this chapter's authors' use of italics] of life." If dietary restriction is postponed until maturity, then the benefits are not as great.

Recent surveys show that Americans' average protein intake is at least twice the estimated requirement, that average milk consumption is approximately a pint a day, that solid food supplements are offered to infants at a very early age, and that obesity is prevalent; thus the results of the animal experiments are worth serious consideration. Berry[3] makes this cogent comment: "Throughout the world the State does not accept the responsibility to protect its individuals from overnutrition" as it does to minimize undernutrition. Interestingly, strict vegetarians are leaner and have lower levels of serum lipids and lower blood pressures than do nonvegetarians.

Some students of nutrition claim that evidence suggests that modern refined foods have a deleterious effect in that their consumption favors the incidence of diverticulosis and colonic tumors. These individuals advocate a diet that is higher in fiber, such as whole-grain cereals, bran, and raw vegetables. Others caution against an excess of dietary fiber because this may interfere with the absorption of certain minerals.

Committees of the US Senate and of the American Heart Association suggest that reducing the intake of saturated fats, refined sugar, salt, and cholesterol—while proportionally increasing the amount of complex carbohydrates—and balancing energy intake with energy expenditure would be advantageous for everyone. These *dietary goals* should apply to children (but *not* infants) and to adults as well.

WELL-BALANCED DIET

Consumption of a variety of foods is the best protection against nutritional deficiency. Except for the first few months of life when milk is the principal (if not the sole) food, the daily diet should include items from each of the following general food groups, known in nutritional circles as *the basic four*: (1) meat, fish, poultry, eggs; (2) dairy products (milk, cheese, milk products); (3) fruits and vegetables; and (4) cereals.

Today the term *junk food* is often heard in reference to prepared foods high in refined carbohydrate and low in protein and vitamins, full of so-called empty calories. These foods do supply energy, and the idea the simpler life of previous generations is brought to mind, when foods of similar composition (eg, apple pie, cake with thick frosting, jellied preserves, home-canned fruits) were consumed freely, without opprobrium, their production considered the hallmark of a successful housewife.

Vegans, strict vegetarians, should be counseled by a nutritionist because their diet is devoid of vitamin B_{12} and is likely to be low in calcium. Grains and vegetables must be chosen so as to include all the essential amino acids.

People who follow fad diets of one sort or another and those who limit their food intake voluntarily in an effort to lose weight should also receive nutritional guidance, inasmuch as such diets may lack one or more essential nutrients. Reports have been published of growth failure in adolescents who consume low-fat diets, given that such diets usually are too low in calories.

TOOLS FOR PRACTICE

Engaging Patient and Family

- *Feeding Kids Right Isn't Always Easy* (brochure), American Academy of Pediatrics (patiented.aap.org).
- *Food Fights: Winning the Nutritional Challenges of Parenthood Armed With Insight, Humor, and a Bottle of Ketchup* (book), American Academy of Pediatrics/Laura A. Jana, MD, FAAP, and Jennifer Shu, MD, FAAP (www.aap.org/bookstore).
- *Growing Up Healthy* (brochure), American Academy of Pediatrics (patiented.aap.org).

†Reasonable evidence exists of such an effect when malnutrition occurs in the early months of life and particularly when it is prolonged. In late infancy and childhood the effect has not been demonstrated clearly, probably because brain maturation is well on its way to completion. Nor has nutritional deprivation during pregnancy been shown to impair intellectual performance of the offspring. The effect of malnutrition per se is very difficult to study because it is almost always accompanied by cultural or emotional disadvantages.

- *Guide to Your Child's Nutrition* (book), American Academy of Pediatrics (www.aap.org/bookstore).
- *Right From the Start: ABCs of Good Nutrition for Young Children* (brochure), American Academy of Pediatrics (patiented.aap.org).
- *What's to Eat? Healthy Food for Hungry Children* (brochure), American Academy of Pediatrics (patiented.aap.org).

Medical Decision Support

- *Committee on Nutrition Policy Statements* (Web page), American Academy of Pediatrics (aappolicy.aappublications.org/cgi/collection/committee_on_nutrition).
- *Pediatric Nutrition Handbook, 5th Edition* (book), American Academy of Pediatrics (www.aap.org/bookstore).

RELATED WEB SITES

- *Nutrition Information* (Web page), World Health Organization (www.who.int/topics/nutrition/en/).
- *Nutrition Topics* (Web page), Centers for Disease Control and Prevention (CDC) (www.cdc.gov/nccdphp/dnpa/nutrition/index.htm).
- *USDA Food and Nutrition* (Web page), United States Department of Agriculture (www.usda.gov/wps/portal/!ut/p/_s.7_0_A/7_0_1OB?navtype=SU&navid=FOOD_NUTRITION).

SUGGESTED RESOURCES

American Psychiatric Association Task Force. *Megavitamins and Orthomolecular Therapy in Psychiatry*. Washington, DC: The Association; 1973.

Burkitt DP, Walker ARP, Painter NS. Dietary fiber and disease. *JAMA*. 1974;229:1068.

Cheatham CL, Colombo J, Carlson SE. n-3 Fatty acids and cognitive and visual acuity development: methodologic and conceptual considerations. *Am J Clin Nutr*. 2006;83:1458S-1466S.

Fomon SJ. *Infant Nutrition*. 2nd ed. Philadelphia, PA: WB Saunders; 1974.

Forbes GB. Food fads: safe feeding of children. *Pediatr Rev*. 1980;1:207.

Forbes GB. *Human Body Composition: Growth, Aging, Nutrition, and Activity*. New York, NY: Springer-Verlag; 1987.

Grand RJ, Sutphen JL, Dietz WH, eds. *Pediatric Nutrition*. Boston, MA: Butterworth; 1987.

Hytten FE, Leitch I. *Physiology of Human Pregnancy*. 2nd ed. Oxford, UK: Blackwell Scientific; 1971.

Klein PS, Forbes GB, Nader PR. Effects of starvation in infancy (pyloric stenosis) on subsequent learning abilities. *J Pediatr*. 1975;87:8-15.

Kleinman RE. ed. Pediatric Nutrition Handbook. 5th edition, Elk Grove Village, IL: American Academy of Pediatrics, 2004.

Leaf A, Weber PC. Cardiovascular effects of n-3 fatty acids. *N Engl J Med*. 1988;318:549-557.

Lechtig A, Delgado H, Lasky R, et al. Maternal nutrition and fetal growth in developing countries. *Am J Dis Child*. 1975;129:549-553.

McCann ML, Schwartz R. The effects of milk solute on urinary cast excretion in premature infants. *Pediatrics*. 1966;38:555-563.

McKigney JI, Munro HN, eds. *Nutrient Requirements in Adolescence*. Cambridge, MA: MIT Press; 1976.

Mertz W. The essential trace elements. *Science*. 1981;213:1332-1338.

National Academy of Sciences, Food and Nutrition Board. *Recommended Dietary Allowances*. 10th ed. Washington, DC: The Academy; 1989.

Pike RL, Brown ML. *Nutrition: An Integrated Approach*. 2nd ed. New York, NY: John Wiley & Sons; 1975.

Rush D, Davis H, Susser M. Antecedents of low birth weight in Harlem, New York City. *Int J Epidemiol*. 1972;1:375-387.

Sacks FM, Castelli WP, Donner A, et al. Plasma lipids and lipoproteins in vegetarians and controls. *N Engl J Med*. 1975;292:1148-1151.

Stein Z, Susser M, Saenger G, et al. *Famine and Human Development*. New York, NY: Oxford University Press; 1975.

Tsang RC, Nichols BL, eds. *Nutrition During Infancy*. Philadelphia, PA: Hanley & Belfus; 1988.

Von Berg A, Koletzko S, Grubl A, et al. Effect of hydrolyzed cow milk formula for allergy prevention the first year of life. *J Allergy Clin Immunol*. 2003;111:533-540.

Walker WA, Watkins JB, eds. *Nutrition in Pediatrics*. 2nd ed. Hamilton, Ontario: BC Dedkham; 1996.

Waterlow JC, Alleyne GAO. Protein malnutrition in children. In: Anfinsen CB Jr, Edsall JT, Richards FM, eds. *Advances in Protein Chemistry*. Vol 25. New York, NY: Academic Press; 1971.

World Health Organization. *Energy and Protein Requirements. Report of a Joint FAO/WHO/UNU Expert Consultation*. Tech Rep Series 724. Geneva, Switzerland: WHO; 1985.

REFERENCES

1. Rosenberg IH. Folic acid and neural-tube defects: time for action? *N Engl J Med*. 1992;327:1875-1877.
2. Ross MH. Nutrition and longevity in experimental animals. In: Winick M, ed. *Nutrition and Aging*. New York, NY: John Wiley & Sons; 1976.
3. Berry WTC. Nutrition in a health service. In: McLaren DS, Burman D, eds. *Textbook of Paediatric Nutrition*. New York, NY: Churchill Livingstone; 1976.

SECTION TWO

Disease Prevention

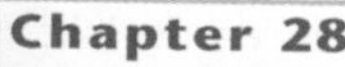

Chapter 28

MORBIDITY AND MORTALITY AMONG THE YOUNG

Bernard Guyer, MD, MPH; Cynthia S. Minkovitz, MD, MPP; Donna M. Strobino, PhD

INTRODUCTION

Today, children's health reflects the introduction of new health services technologies and the dramatic improvements in social and economic conditions of the past century. The infant mortality rate (IMR), one of the most sensitive indicators of the overall health of a population, declined to 6.8 infant deaths per 1000 live births in 2001—an all-time low; the IMR was 6.9 in 2003. Life expectancy at birth in the United States reached a new high of 77.6 years in 2003. Age-adjusted death rates continue to decline for almost all diseases and injuries.[1]

Improvement in child mortality rates, however, does not tell the whole story. Rates of morbidity and disability from some conditions—asthma, diabetes, attention-deficit disorders, and obesity—have increased in recent decades. Furthermore, indicators of health care utilization, such as immunization coverage, show that the health care system may not be serving many US children. International comparisons of key indicators, such as IMR, show the United States is lagging behind other industrialized nations that have better organized primary health care systems and universal health insurance coverage. Finally, disparities in health status among US children, according to race and socioeconomic status, reflect widening societal inequalities.

The demographic and social determinants that will shape children's health in the 21st century are changing. The United States is increasingly ethnically diverse through immigration and population growth. Children constitute an ever-smaller proportion of the population, with little political influence and limited access to public resources. Finally, the burden of personal debt and massive government deficits is being shifted to the next generation, with uncertain implications for children's health care access and health status.

Identifying the epidemiologic patterns of death, disease, and disability among children is an essential component of effective health policy for young Americans. Children have medical needs that are different from those of adults because children are dependent on adults, are on an upward developmental trajectory, and the epidemiologic mechanism of children's health conditions differs from that of adults.[2] The National Research Council[3] recommended that the definition of children's health be expanded to encompass development potential and overall well being and account for the influences of biological, physical, and social environments.

This chapter presents the current mortality, morbidity, and demographic profile of US children, highlighting the important trends in health that have occurred over the last 20 years and projections for the future. The analysis is restricted to the United States, although in some cases, international comparisons are drawn.

DEMOGRAPHIC PROFILE OF CHILDREN AND POPULATION PROJECTIONS TO THE YEAR 2020

Demographic Profile of Children in the United States

In 2003, 73 million children younger than 18 years were estimated to be living in the United States.[4] These children were roughly equally divided—between 23 and 25 million—among the three age groups: 0 to 5, 6 to 11, and 12 to 17 years.[4] The number of children in the population has fluctuated since the 1950s, primarily because of the high fertility rates during the baby-boom years, 1946 to 1964.[5] In 1950 an estimated 47 million children were younger than 18 years in the US population. This number increased markedly during the 1950s to more than 64 million in 1960 and exceeded 69 million in 1970.[6-8] The number of children in the US population is projected to reach close to 80 million in 2020.[4]

Measuring the percentage of children in the population provides an assessment of the need for investments in future populations. This percentage rose during the 1950s and 1960s from 31% in 1940 and 1950 to a peak of 36% in 1960. It did not decline much until the late 1970s, when the first half of the baby-boom cohorts reached young adult age. Children younger than 18 years constituted 26% of the US population in 1997[8] and 25% in 2003.[4]

The dependency ratio, a measure of the proportion of persons who are considered dependent (children [younger than 18 years] and the elderly adults [older than age 65]) to persons eligible to participate in the labor force (18 to 64 years of age) is a crude estimate of the extent to which the productive population must provide resources for the dependent population. The computed ratio increased dramatically from 64 dependents per 100 persons in 1950 to 82 in 1960, primarily because of a rise in the youth dependency ratio. The overall ratio remained high in 1970 but dropped to 65 in 1980 and has remained slightly below that level since then; the figure was 64 in 2003.[9] During more recent years, however, the youth dependency ratio dropped, whereas the elderly ratio increased from 13 in 1950 to 20 in 1990[6,8] and 22 in 2003.[9]

The US child population has become increasingly more diverse, racially and ethnically, since 1980 (1980 was the first year for which data on the Hispanic population were available nationally) (Figure 28-1). The percentage of children of Hispanic origin has risen faster than for other racial and ethnic groups[8] because of the higher fertility and greater proportion of women of childbearing age among Hispanics than other groups.

The rise in minority children in the population is associated with an increase in the foreign-born population over the last 3 decades, and this rise has an effect on the needs of families with children. The percentage of children with foreign-born parents was 20% in 2004, increasing from the 15% recorded 10 years earlier in 1994. Children with foreign-born parents (81%) were more likely than children with native parents (68%) to live in households with two parents present. In 2003, 19% of school-aged children spoke a language other than English at home. This percentage was particularly high among school-aged Asian (64%) and Hispanic children (68%).[4]

The size of the household of the average US family has decreased over the last 3 decades, from 3.1 to 2.6 persons.[10] Children increasingly are living in families that have only one parent. In 2003, 68% of children lived in families with two parents, 23% in families with mother only, 5% with a father only, and 4% with no parent. In 1980, 77% of children lived in two-parent families while 88% did so in 1960.[4] The decline in two-parent families is associated with an increase in mother-only families and, to a lesser extent, father-only families.[11]

The percentage of children living in two-parent families varies markedly by race and ethnicity. Although 77% of non-Hispanic white children lived in families having two parents in 2004, 65% of Hispanic black children and only 35% of non-Hispanic children did so.[4] A greater percentage of non-Hispanic black children live in mother-only families (53%) compared with non-Hispanic white children (18%) or Hispanic children (29%).[11] Children who live in female-headed households have fewer economic resources available to them than children who live in two-parent families; female-headed households (42%) were almost five times more likely in 2000 to have incomes below the poverty level than two-parent households (9%). In 2000 the median family income for married couple households ($57,245) was over two times greater than the median for female-headed households ($25,458) and 1.6 times that for male-headed households ($35,141).[12]

The percentage of children living below the US poverty level increased from 15% in 1975 to a high of 22% in 1993; it was 16% in 2000 and 17% in 2004. In 2003 a greater percentage of non-Hispanic black children (34%) and Hispanic black children (30%) lived in poverty compared with non-Hispanic white children (10%). The percentage of children living in extreme poverty, below 50% of the poverty level, was 7% in 2003,[4] comparable to the figure in 1980 but below the peak of 10% in 1993. Poverty rates for Native-American children are high; 38% lived in families with incomes below 100% of poverty in 1996.[7] The percentage of children living in

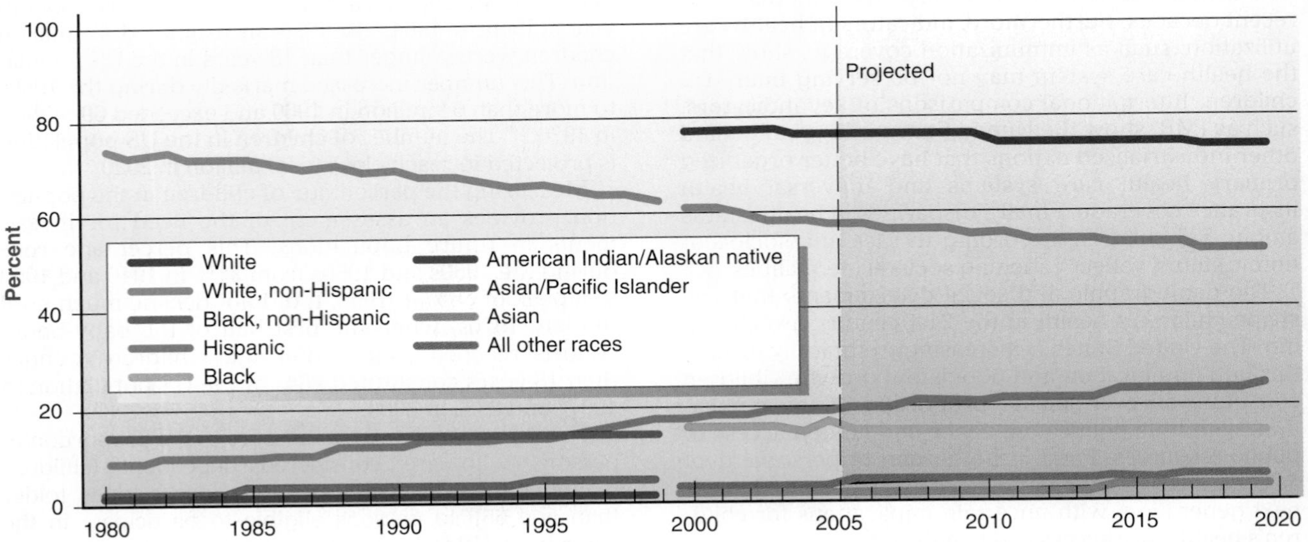

Figure 28-1 Percent of US children aged 0 to 17 years by race and Hispanic origin, 1980-2004 and projected 2005-2020. Note: Beginning in 2000, respondents were asked to choose one or more races; therefore data are not strictly comparable. With the exception of the *Two-or-More-Races* group (part of the *All Other Races* group), all race groups shown in this figure from 2000 onward refer to people who indicated only one racial identity within the racial category presented. The use of the *race-alone* population in this figure does not imply that it is the preferred method of presenting or analyzing data. Persons of Hispanic origin may be of any race. (*US Census Bureau.* Population Estimates and Projections. *Washington DC: US Government Printing Office; 1996.)*

families with very high incomes rose between 1980 and 2003 from 4% to 13%.[4]

Another change in the family environment is the dramatic rise in labor force participation of women with children, peaking at 73% in 2000; the percentage was 71% in 2004. The rise has been particularly large among women with young children. This change has been accompanied by an increased use of some form of child care among children ages 0 to 6 years who are not yet in kindergarten; the percentage in nonparental care was 61% in 2001, similar to the figure for 1995. Children in higher income families (67%), above 200% of poverty, are more likely to be in nonparental care than children in families with incomes between 100% and 200% of the poverty level (54%).[4]

Future Population Projections in the United States

The number of children in the US population is expected to increase to approximately 79 million children by 2020.[8] The composition of the population will increasingly include racial and ethnic groups other than non-Hispanic whites. Although black children were the largest minority group in 1996, Hispanic children surpassed them in numbers by 2003, and Asian children are expected to comprise 6% of the US child population by 2020.[8] These changes will occur gradually as new birth cohorts age and as those of Hispanic and Asian immigrate to the United States.[6]

The percentage of children in the total US population is projected to decline slightly over the next 15 years to approximately 24% of the population; in fact, it is never expected to be as high as it was in the 1960s. The dependency ratio is projected to remain relatively constant through 2010, although a slight decline in the youth ratio and a slight rise in the elderly ratio are anticipated. It is expected to rise rapidly, however, between 2010 and 2020, almost entirely because of a rapid increase in the elderly ratio when the first cohorts of the baby-boom generation reach age 65. By 2020 the elderly dependency ratio[9] is expected to be approximately one-third less than the youth dependency ratio (40), in contrast to 1990, when the elderly dependency ratio was less than one half (20) the youth dependency ratio (42).[6,8]

These population projections, if correct, have important implications for availability and appropriateness of child health services. The changing ethnic and racial diversity of the child population means that persons who provide health care to children will need, increasingly, not only to understand the different cultural approaches of their population to health and health care use, but also to provide culturally and linguistically-appropriate services and resources. Health education, an important component of pediatric care, increasingly will need to address this cultural and language diversity.

The rising elderly dependency ratio means that children will be increasingly less visible in the political world in which they have never been a strong constituent. Debates about allocation of scarce resources will need to achieve a delicate balance between the health and resource needs of the nation's children and those of the elderly, a debate that is likely to become more favorable to the elderly population based on numbers alone. Health care providers and public health professionals will continue to need to serve as advocates for this most vulnerable population. The future of children and subsequent generations depends on professionals' advocacy for them in the ongoing political debate.

Births

The number of births in the United States in 2004 was 4,115,590 (preliminary), an increase from the lowest number of births recorded in the United States at the end of the 1990s. The 2004 birth rate, however, was 14.0 per 1000 total population, the lowest level ever in the nation. The fertility rate, defined as the number of births per 1000 women ages 15 to 44 years, was 66.3, a slight increase over recent years (Table 28-1).[1]

Births to Teenagers

Childbearing among teenagers continued to fall dramatically, reaching 41.2 births per 1000 girls and women 15 to 19 years of age, 33% lower than the rate for 1991 (Table 28-2). The proportion of all births to teen mothers fell to 10.3%.[1] Teen birth rates have

Table 28-1 Vital Statistics of the United States, 1980-2004 (Selected Years)

	NUMBER		RATE*				
	2003	2004	1980	1990	2000	2003	2004
Live births	4,089,950	4,115,590	15.9	16.7	14.4	14.1	14.0
Fertility rate	—	—	68.4	70.9	65.9	66.1	66.3
Deaths	2,443,908	—	8.8	8.6	8.5	8.4	—
Age-adjusted rate	—	—	10.4	9.4	8.7	8.3	—
Natural increase	1,646,042	—	7.1	8.1	5.9	5.7	—
Infant mortality	28,428	—	12.6	9.2	6.9	6.9	—
Population base (in thousands)	—	—	226,546	248,710	281,422	290,810	293,655

*Rates per 1000 population, except for fertility, which is per 1000 women ages 15-44 years, and infant mortality, which is per 1000 live births.

Note: Birth data for 2004 and mortality and infant mortality data for 2003 are preliminary. Birth data for 2003, all data for 2002, and data for earlier years are final.

From Centers for Disease Control and Prevention, National Center for Health Statistics. *National Vital Statistics System, and the US Census Bureau.* Modified from Hoyert DL, Mathews TJ, Menacker F, et al. Annual summary of vital statistics—2004. *Pediatrics.* 2006;117(1):168-183.

Table 28-2 Birth Rates for Teens by Age, Race, and Hispanic Origin—United States, Final, Selected Years 1990-2003 and Preliminary 2004 (15-19 Years)

AGE AND RACE AND HISPANIC ORIGIN OF MOTHER	1990	2000	2004	PERCENTAGE CHANGE 1991-2004
All races	59.9	47.7	41.2	−33
Non-Hispanic white	42.5	32.6	26.8	−38
Non-Hispanic black	116.2	79.2	62.7	−47
Asian or Pacific Islander	26.4	20.5	17.4	−36
Native American	81.1	58.3	52.5	−38
Hispanic	100.3	87.3	82.6	−21

From Centers for Disease Control and Prevention, National Center for Health Statistics. *National Vital Statistics System. Natality (NVSS-N).* Modified from Hoyert DL, Mathews TJ, Menacker F, et al. Annual summary of vital statistics—2004. *Pediatrics.* 2006;117(1):168-183.
Note: Rates per 1000 women in specified group. People of Hispanic origin may be of any race.

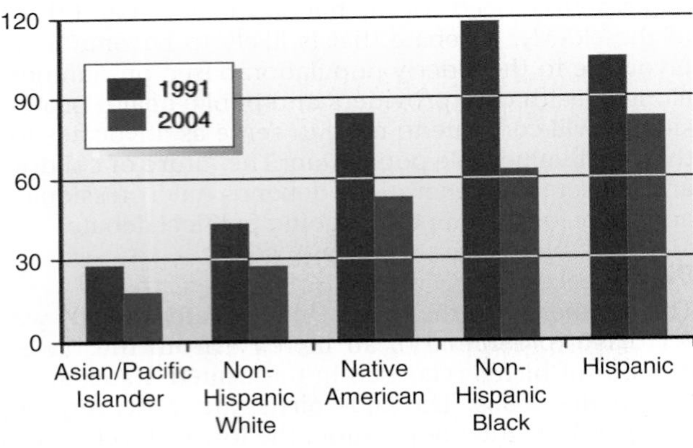

Figure 28-2 Birth rates for teens aged 15 to 19 years by race and Hispanic origin—United States, 1991 and 2004. (*Reprinted from Hoyert DL, Mathews TJ, Menacker F, et al. Annual Summary of Vital Statistics: 2004.* Pediatrics *2006; 117(1):168-183.)*

declined since 1991 for all races and Hispanic origin groups (Figure 28-2); the largest decline was seen among non-Hispanic black teens (47% since 1991). Overall, teen birth rates range from 17.4 births per 1000 girls and women 15 to 19 years of age for Asian or Pacific Islander teens to 82.6 for Hispanic teens.[1]

Unmarried Mothers

In 2004, 36% of all births occurred to unmarried women, having increased dramatically over 4 decades from 5% in 1960 (Table 28-3). The percentage of births to unmarried women was particularly high among Hispanic (46%) and black women (69%).[1]

Prenatal Care

Eighty-four percent of mothers began prenatal care in the first trimester of pregnancy in 2003 (see Table 28-3). The percentage of women who had late (beginning in the third trimester) or no care declined 41% since 1990 and was 3.6% of births in 2003.[1]

Racial disparities in timely prenatal care are declining. Since 1990 the percentage of non-Hispanic black mothers who had first-trimester care rose 24% (from 61% to 76%), whereas the comparable percentage increase for non-Hispanic white mothers was 7% (from 83% to 89%). Progress in accessing early prenatal care use has been most pronounced among Hispanic women; first-trimester care climbed 28 percentage points since 1990 (from 60% to 78%).[1]

Multiple Births

The multiple birth rate (defined as the number of births in twin, triplet, and greater deliveries per 1000 live births) was 33.4 per 1000 births in 2003 (see Table 28-3). The vast majority of multiple births are twins. Since 1980 the number of twin births has risen 67%.[1]

The higher order multiple birth rate (the number of births in triplet, quadruplet, and greater deliveries per 1000 live births) was 1.87 in 2003. The number and rate of higher-order multiple births have quadrupled since 1980. The dramatic rise in multiple births, and especially of higher-order multiple births, over the last several decades has been attributed, in part, to increases in the use of fertility-enhancing therapies and delayed childbearing (the risk of multiple birth increases with maternal age even without the use of fertility-enhancing therapies).[1]

Multiple births are much more likely than singleton births to be low birth weight or preterm (<37 completed weeks' gestation). Despite their likely survival advantage over singletons at lower birth weights and shorter gestations, multiples are at greater risk of early death. In 1996, multiple births accounted for 16% of all neonatal deaths and were seven times more likely than singletons to die within the first month of life.[13]

Birth Weight

The percentage of low–birth-weight infants (<2500 g) was 8.1% in 2004 and has risen by 21% since 1984 (Figure 28-3). The rate of increase in low–birth-weight births among singleton births, however, is substantially less at 4%. The percentage of very low–birth-weight infants (<1500 g) was 1.47% in 2004, a rise from 1.15% in 1980 (see Table 28-3).[14]

Low birth weight is a major determinant of infant health; despite improvements in survival rates among these smaller infants in recent years, the risk of early death among moderately low–birth-weight infants (1500 to 2499 g) is six times higher than heavier

Table 28-3 Percentage of Births With Selected Characteristics by Race and Hispanic Origin of Mother—United States, Final 1990, 2003, and Preliminary 2004

	ALL RACES			NON-HISPANIC WHITE			NON-HISPANIC BLACK			HISPANIC		
	2004	2003	1990	2004	2003	1990[a]	2004	2003	1990	2004	2003	1990[a]
<20 Years of age	10.3	10.3	12.8	7.4	7.5	9.6	17.3	17.4	23.2	14.3	14.3	16.8
≥40 Years of age	2.7	2.6	1.2	3.0	3.0	1.2	2.1	2.1	0.8	1.9	1.9	1.2
Unmarried[b]	35.7	34.6	28.0	24.5	23.6	16.9	69.2	68.5	66.7	46.4	45.0	36.7
Smoker[c]	—	10.7	18.4	—	14.3	21.0	—	8.3	15.9	—	2.7	6.7
First-trimester prenatal care	—	84.1	75.6	—	89.0	83.3	—	75.9	61.0	—	77.5	60.2
VLBW[d]	1.5	1.4	1.3	1.2	1.2	0.9	3.1	3.1	2.9	1.2	1.2	1.0
LBW[d]	8.1	7.9	7.0	7.2	7.0	5.6	13.7	13.6	13.3	6.8	6.7	6.1
Preterm birth[e]	12.5	12.3	10.6	11.5	11.3	8.5	17.9	17.8	18.9	12.0	11.9	11.0
Live births in twin deliveries (not percentage)	—	31.5	22.6		—	35.2	22.9	—	34.7	26.7	21.3	18.0
Live births in higher-order multiple deliveries (not percentage)	—	1.9	0.7		—	2.6	0.9	—	1.1	0.5	0.9	0.4

LBW, Low–birth weight; *VLBW*, very low–birth weight.
[a]Excludes data for New Hampshire and Oklahoma, which did not report Hispanic origin.
[b]Includes mothers 20 years of age and older. For 1990, excludes data for New York (exclusive of New York City) and Washington, which did not report educational attainment of mother.
[c]For 2003, excludes data for California, and for 1990 excludes data for California, Indiana, New York, Oklahoma, and South Dakota, which did not report tobacco use during pregnancy.
[d]VLBW is birth weight of <1500 g (3 lb, 4 oz), and LBW is birth weight of <2500 g (5 lb, 8 oz).
[e]Born before 37 completed weeks of gestation.
From Centers for Disease Control and Prevention, National Center of Health Statistics. *National Vital Statistics System. Natality (NVSS-N)*. Modified from Hoyert DL, Mathews TJ, Menacker F, et al. Annual summary of vital statistics—2004. *Pediatrics*. 2006;117(1):168-183.

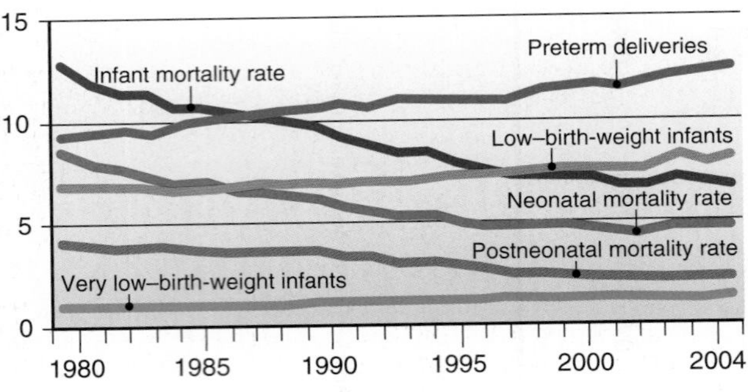

Figure 28-3 Infant mortality rate, neonatal mortality rate, postneonatal mortality rate, number of low–birth-weight infants, number of very low–birth-weight infants, and number of preterm deliveries (<37 weeks of gestation) per 1000 births in the United States, 1980-2004. (*Reprinted from Hoyert DL, Mathews TJ, Menacker F, et al. Annual Summary of Vital Statistics: 2004.* Pediatrics *2006;117(1): 168-183.)*

infants, and the risk of early death among very low–birth-weight infants is 100 times higher.[1]

The trend in increasing low birth weight over the last several decades is related to maternal race and ethnicity in an unexpected way. Since 1990 the percentage of low–birth-weight infants born to non-Hispanic white mothers has risen 29% to 7.2% in 2004; among Hispanic mothers the rate of low–birth-weight births has risen 11% to 6.8%; and among black mothers, the rate of low–birth-weight births has risen 3% to 13.7%. Some of this increase, particularly among white births, can be attributed to the rise in multiple births. The elevated risk of low birth weight for births to non-Hispanic black women is largely attributable to their higher incidence of preterm birth.

Preterm Birth

In 2004, 12.5% of births were preterm (<37 completed weeks of gestation), having steadily increased from 9.4% in 1981 to 10.6% in 1990 (see Figure 28-2). This increase in preterm births is partly explained by the concurrent increase in multiple births, which are more likely to be born preterm. Among non-Hispanic white women the percentage of preterm births rose sharply (by 35%) from 8.5% in 1990 to 11.5% in 2004. The percentage of preterm births among black mothers was 17.9% in 2004, having peaked at 19.0% in 1991. These shifting distributions have implications for primary care physicians who can expect to care for more ex-premies and low–birth-weight babies who often have complications requiring specialized medical and rehabilitative care.[15]

Deaths

Infant Mortality

The preliminary IMR in the United States in 2003 was 6.9 per 1000 live births, a slight increase from the lowest IMR ever recorded in the United States in 2001. The neonatal mortality rate (NMR; death of infants younger than 28 days) declined to 4.7, and the postneonatal mortality rate (PNMR; 28 days through 11 months) fell to 2.3. IMRs were elevated among infants whose mothers were younger than 20 years or older than 40 years, were unmarried, did not complete high school, started prenatal care after the first trimester of pregnancy, or smoked during pregnancy. IMRs are also higher for male infants, multiple births, and infants born preterm or with low birth weight.[13,16]

Infant mortality in the United States has declined by more than 40% since 1980 (see Figure 28-2). The NMR declined more rapidly during the 1980s, whereas the PNMR declined more rapidly during the 1990s.

Racial differences in the IMR remain a major national concern. Although all racial groups have experienced declines in the IMR, the relative difference in rates between black and white newborns, expressed as the ratio of black to white IMRs, increased from 2.0 in 1980 to 2.4 in 2002. The racial disparities in IMR present continued challenges for researchers and health care providers alike.

Birth Weight–Specific Infant Mortality

Birth weight is one of the most important predictors of infant mortality. The IMR for a given population can be partitioned into two key components: (1) the birth-weight distribution and (2) birth weight–specific mortality rates (the death rate for infants at a given weight). The IMR decreases when either the percentage of low–birth-rate births decreases or the birth weight–specific mortality rates decrease. All of the decline in the IMR since 1980 has been the result of declines in birth weight–specific IMR and not because of the prevention of low birth weight.[17] These declines have been attributed primarily to improvements in obstetric and neonatal care. However, the United States has been unsuccessful in reducing the proportion of preterm and low–birth-rate births, despite a variety of policy and program initiatives.

In 2003, approximately two thirds of all infant deaths occurred among the 7.0% of infants who were of low birth weight. Approximately 90% of infants with birth weights less than 500 g die within the first year of life and most die within the first few days of life. An infant's chances of survival increase rapidly thereafter with increasing birth weight. At birth weights of 1250 to 1499 g, approximately 95% of babies survive the first year. IMR is lowest for infants at birth weights of 4000 to 4499 g, with small increases thereafter among the heaviest infants.[13,16]

Leading Causes of Infant Death

More than one half of all infant deaths in 2002 were attributable to five leading causes: (1) congenital anomalies (20%); (2) disorders related to short gestation and unspecified low birth weight (17%); (3) sudden infant death syndrome (SIDS) (8%); (4) maternal complications of pregnancy (6%); and (5) complications of placenta, cord, and membranes (4%). SIDS rates have fallen by 42% since 1992, when the American Academy of Pediatrics issued a recommendation to reduce the risk of SIDS by placing infants on their backs or sides to sleep.[18]

International Comparisons of Infant Mortality

Table 28-4 shows infant mortality rates for countries that have at least a population of 2.5 million and for

Table 28-4 Infant Mortality Rate for 2000, 2001, and 2002*

COUNTRY	INFANT MORTALITY RATE†		
	2002	2001	2000
Hong Kong	2.3	2.6	3.0
Singapore	3.0	2.4	2.9
Japan	3.0	3.1	3.2
Finland	3.0	3.2	3.8
Sweden	3.3	3.7	3.4
Norway	3.5	3.9	3.8
Czech Republic	3.9	4.0	4.1
Spain	4.1‡	3.4	4.0
France	4.1†	4.5	4.4
Austria	4.1	4.8	4.8
Germany	4.2‡	4.3	4.4
Belgium	4.4‡	4.5	4.8
Denmark	4.4	4.9	5.3
Italy	4.5‡	4.7	4.5
Switzerland	4.5	5.0	4.9
Portugal	5.0	5.0	5.6
Australia	5.0	5.4	5.2
Korea	5.1	5.3	4.5
Netherlands	5.1	5.4	5.1
Greece	5.1‡	5.1	5.2
Ireland	5.1	5.8	6.2
United Kingdom	5.2	5.5	5.6
Israel	5.4	5.1	5.5
Canada	5.4	5.2	5.3
New Zealand	5.6	5.3	6.1
Cuba	6.5	6.2	7.2
United States	7.0	6.8	6.9

*For countries of more than 250,000 with infant mortality rate equal or less than the United States in 2002 and 2001.
†Infant mortality rate per 1000 live births.
‡Organization for Economic Cooperation and Development data.
From *United Nations, 2002 Demographic Yearbook.* New York, NY: United Nations; 2005. Modified from Hoyert DL, Mathews TJ, Menacker F, et al. Annual summary of vital statistics—2004. *Pediatrics.* 2006;117(1):168-183.

which the IMR was lower than the rate for the United States in both 2001 and 2002. The United States ranks 27th in infant mortality in relation to other developed countries, but quick judgments should not be made regarding the reasons for this poor ranking. Reporting of data on live births, especially for the smallest babies with the highest mortality rates, appears to differ across countries, as does the timing of when a live birth must be registered and the reporting of stillbirths.[19] Moreover, the quality of data and coverage of the birth registration systems vary by country and may also affect international comparisons. These differences in reporting, however, do not account for all of the disparity between the IMR in the United States and the other countries. A major reason for the poor ranking of the United States continues to be its persistently high rate of low birth weight relative to other developed countries.[19]

Expectation of Life

The estimated expectation of life at birth for a given year represents the average number of years that a group of infants would be expected to live if, throughout their lifetime, they were to experience the age-specific death rates prevailing during their year of birth. Based on preliminary data for 2003 the expectation of life at birth reached a new record high of 77.6 years. In 2003, life expectancy at birth was 80.5 years for white women, 76.1 years for black women, 75.4 years for white men, and 69.2 years for black men.

Deaths Among Children

In 2003 the death rate for children 1 to 4 years of age was 31.1 per 100,000 population, 14.6 per 100,000 population for 5 to 9 year olds, 19.1 for 10 to 14 year olds, and 65.3 for 15 to 19 year olds.[1] Since 1979, death rates have declined by 45% for children 1 to 4 years of age, by 41% for children 5 to 9 years, by 27% for children 10 to 14 years, and by 26% for teens 15 to 19 years of age.[20]

For children 1 to 4 years of age (Table 28-5), unintentional injury was the leading cause of death, with congenital anomalies the second and cancer the third. Unintentional injuries accounted for 34.2% of all deaths in this age group, although the rate has declined by 52% since 1979. Homicide is the fourth-leading cause of death; since 1979, death rates for homicide for this age group have declined by only 8%.[20]

For children 5 to 9 years of age (see Table 28-5), unintentional injury, cancer, congenital anomalies, and homicide were the leading causes of death. Unintentional injury accounted for 37.9% of all deaths in 2003, and cancer accounted for 17.5% of deaths in this age group. Since 1979, death rates for each of these leading causes of death have declined by at least 20%.

Unintentional injury was the leading cause of death and accounted for 36% of all deaths to children 10 to 14 years of age (see Table 28-5). The second-leading cause was cancer. The death rates caused by unintentional injuries and cancer for this age group declined by 41% and 39%, respectively, since 1979. In contrast, the death rate for suicide doubled during this period.

For teens ages 15 to 19 years (see Table 28-5), unintentional injuries, the leading cause of death, accounted for nearly 50% of all deaths in 2003, although the rate has dropped by 43% since 1979. Homicide, the second-leading cause, accounted for 14% of all deaths. The teen homicide rate increased by 24% from 1979 to 1996 but decreased 18% between 1996 and 1997. Suicide was the third-leading cause of death for this age group, accounting for 11% of all deaths. Since 1979, suicide rates increased 13% for this age group.

Despite recent declines, injuries—both unintentional and intentional (homicides and suicides)—continue to be the leading causes of mortality, morbidity, and disability in children.[21] Pediatric practice needs to keep up with the developing science of injury prevention, integrating effective interventions into clinical practice, and anticipatory guidance.[22]

Disability and Morbidity

Identifying epidemiologic trends for children who have a chronic illness is important for several reasons. First, although the vast majority of children are healthy because of advances in medical technology, increasing numbers of children are growing up with a chronic illness.[23-25] Second, children who have a chronic illness receive a disproportionate amount of

Table 28-5 Deaths and Death Rates for the Five Leading Causes of Childhood Death in Specified Age Groups in 2003—United States, Final 2002 and Preliminary 2003

AGE, CAUSES OF DEATH, AND INTERNATIONAL CLASSIFICATION OF DISEASES (10TH REVISION CODES)	RANK*	2003			2002		
		NUMBER	PERCENT	RATE†	NUMBER	PERCENT	RATE†
TOTAL: 1-19 YEARS							
All causes	—	25,216	100.0	31.0	25,820	100.0	33.5
Accidents (unintentional injuries) (V01-X59, Y85-Y86)	1	10,892	43.2	13.4	11,496	44.5	14.9
Assault (homicide) (*U01-*U02, X85-Y09, Y87.1)	2	2512	10.0	3.1	2671	10.3	3.5
Malignant neoplasms (C00-C97)	3	2118	8.4	2.6	2197	8.5	2.9
Intentional self-harm (suicide) (*U03, X60-X84, Y87.0)	4	1712	6.8	2.1	1777	6.9	2.3
Congenital malformations, deformations and chromosomal abnormalities (Q00-Q99)	5	1098	4.4	1.4	1195	4.6	1.6
All causes	—	4911	100.0	31.1	4858	100.0	31.2
Accidents (unintentional injuries) (V01-X59, Y85-Y86)	1	1679	34.2	10.6	1641	33.8	10.5
1-4 YEARS							
Congenital malformations, deformations and chromosomal abnormalities (Q00-Q99)	2	514	10.5	3.3	530	10.9	3.4
Malignant neoplasms (C00-C97)	3	383	7.8	2.4	402	8.3	2.6
Assault (homicide) (*U01-*U02, X85-Y09, Y87.1)	4	342	7.0	2.2	423	8.7	2.7
Diseases of heart (I00-I09, I11, I13, I20-I51)	5	186	3.8	1.2	165	3.4	1.1
5-9 YEARS							
All causes	—	2882	100.0	14.6	3018	100.0	15.2
Accidents (unintentional injuries) (V01-X59, Y85-Y86)	1	1091	37.9	5.5	1176	39.0	5.9
Malignant neoplasms (C00-C97)	2	504	17.5	2.6	537	17.8	2.7
Congenital malformations, deformations and chromosomal abnormalities (Q00-Q99)	3	175	6.1	0.9	199	6.6	1.0
Assault (homicide) (*U01-*U02, X85-Y09, Y87.1)	4	116	4.0	0.6	140	4.6	0.7
Diseases of heart (I00-I09, I11, I13, I20-I51)	5	97	3.4	0.5	92	3.0	0.5
10-14 YEARS							
All causes	—	4048	100.0	19.1	4132	100.0	19.5
Accidents (unintentional injuries) (V01-X59, Y85-Y86)	1	1471	36.3	6.9	1542	37.3	7.3
Malignant neoplasms (C00-C97)	2	555	13.7	2.6	535	12.9	2.5
Intentional self-harm (suicide) (*U03, X60-X84, Y87.0)	3	249	6.2	1.2	260	6.3	1.2
Congenital malformations, deformations and chromosomal abnormalities (Q00-Q99)	4	196	4.8	0.9	218	5.3	1.0
Assault (homicide) (*U01-*U02, X85-Y09, Y87.1)	5	194	4.8	0.9	216	5.2	1.0
15-19 YEARS							
All causes	—	13,375	100.0	65.3	13,812	100.0	67.8
Accidents (unintentional injuries) (V01-X59, Y85-Y86)	1	6652	49.7	32.5	7137	51.7	35.0
Assault (homicide) (*U01-*U02, X85-Y09, Y87.1)	2	1860	13.9	9.1	1892	13.7	9.3

Table 28-5 Deaths and Death Rates for the Five Leading Causes of Childhood Death in Specified Age Groups in 2003—United States, Final 2002 and Preliminary 2003—cont'd

AGE, CAUSES OF DEATH, AND INTERNATIONAL CLASSIFICATION OF DISEASES (10TH REVISION CODES)		2003			2002		
	RANK*	NUMBER	PERCENT	RATE†	NUMBER	PERCENT	RATE†
Intentional self-harm (suicide) (*U03, X60-X84, Y87.0)	3	1457	10.9	7.1	1513	11.0	7.4
Malignant neoplasms (C00-C97)	4	675	5.0	3.3	723	5.2	3.5
Diseases of heart (I00-I09, I11, I13, I20-I51)	5	374	2.8	1.8	405	2.9	2.0

*Rank based on 2003 data. Ranking is shown for five leading causes for specified age groups. For an explanation of ranking procedures, see Technical Appendix in *Vital Statistics of the United States,* Vol. II, Mortality Part A (published annually).
†Rate per 100,000 population in specified group.
From Centers for Disease Control and Prevention, National Center for Health Statistics. *National Vital Statistics System. Mortality, 2002-2003.* Modified from Hoyert DL, Mathews TJ, Menacker F, et al. Annual summary of vital statistics—2004. *Pediatrics.* 2006;117(1):168-183.

health care resources, suggesting that these children are particularly vulnerable to policies and health care reforms that limit access to particular services.[26] Third, some children with chronic illness have complex medical and other service needs that require an array of community resources for optimal functioning for them and their families. Fourth, children who have a chronic illness have needs distinct from adults with the same illness. Developing policies and allocating resources for health, educational, social services, mental health services, and other community programs requires knowledge of the characteristics of the target population.

Children With Chronic Conditions

The historical use of varying definitions of children who have one or more chronic illnesses has contributed to prevalence estimates ranging from 4% to 31%. These differences have dramatic implications for public policy and resource allocation. Applying noncategorical methods and using data from the National Health Interview Survey (NHIS) *1994 Disability Supplement,* studies have identified overall rates of children younger than 18 years who have chronic conditions to range from 15%[27] to 18%.[28] Differences in prevalence by gender, age, and socioeconomic status have been noted across many studies. In general, higher proportions of chronic illness are found among boys than girls and older rather than younger children.

In the recent National Survey of Children with Special Health Care Needs, 12.8% or 9.4 million children were reported to have special health care needs using the Maternal and Child Health Bureau definition.[29] In this survey, the prevalence of special needs was highest among Native American/Alaska Native children (16.6%), multiracial (15.1%), and non-Hispanic white children (14.2%), with the lowest prevalence noted among Hispanic (8.6%) and Asian children (4.4%).

The majority of children who have a chronic illness have a single condition rather than multiple conditions, although a small proportion have severe conditions. Using NHIS 1988 data, Newacheck and Taylor[28] reported that among the nearly 20 million children younger than 18 years who had chronic conditions, 70% had one condition, 21% had two conditions; and 9% had three or more conditions. In the same study, the authors found that 65% had mild, 29% moderate, and 6% severe conditions. Children who have multiple conditions and have severe conditions are of interest because they are at increased risk for acquiring developmental, learning, and behavioral problems; having functional limitations; experiencing more bed days and school absences; having poorer overall health status; and using more health care resources.[24] Primary care

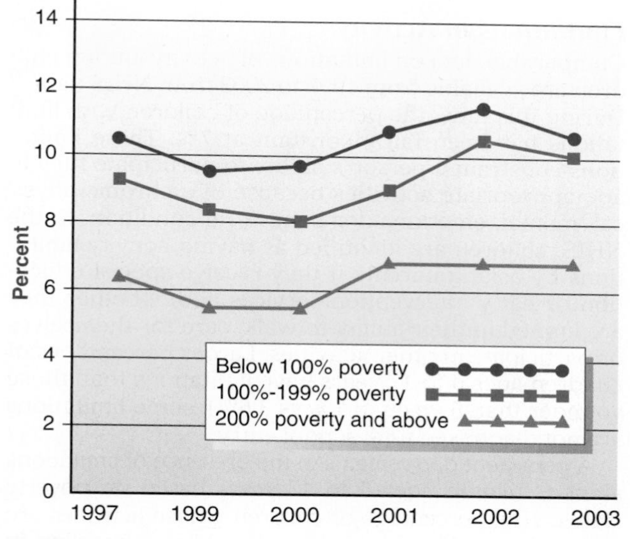

Figure 28-4 Differences in activity limitation by poverty status for children aged 5 to 17 years. (Federal Interagency Forum on Child and Family Statistics. *America's Children: Key National Indicators of Well-Being, 2005.* Federal Interagency Forum on Child and Family Statistics, Washington, DC: U.S. Government Printing Office.)

Table 28-6 Selected Chronic Conditions per 1000 Persons Causing Limitation of Activity Among Children by Age, 2002-2003

	UNDER 5 YEARS		5-11 YEARS		12-17 YEARS	
TYPE OF CHRONIC HEALTH CONDITION	RATE	SE	RATE	SE	RATE	SE
Speech problem	10.7	1.0	18.5	1.1	4.6	0.5
Asthma or breathing problem	8.2	0.9	8.4	0.7	8.3	0.8
Mental retardation or other developmental problem	7.0	0.8	10.2	0.8	9.6	0.8
Other mental, emotional, or behavioral problem	2.7	0.5	12.0	1.0	14.2	1.1
Attention-deficit/hyperactivity disorder	2.1	0.4	17.6	1.2	21.8	1.3
Learning disability	2.9	0.5	23.3	1.2	33.9	1.7

SE, Standard error.
From Centers for Disease Control and Prevention, National Center for Health Statistics. *Health, United States, 2005*.

physicians play an important role in providing a medical home and coordinating care for children with special health care needs.

Limitations in Activity

Comparable data on limitations of activity among children are available from 1997 to 2003 from NHIS data.[30] During this time, the percentage of children with limitations has been fairly constant at 7%. These limitations constrain a person's ability to participate fully in age-appropriate activities because of a chronic physical, mental, emotional, or behavioral condition. In the NHIS, children are identified as having activity limitations by asking parents if they receive special education or early intervention services and, whether they are limited in their ability to walk, care for themselves or participate in other activities. Larger percentages of children ages 5 to 17 years have limitations than those younger than 5 years (8.1% vs 3.6%); some limitations are not diagnosed until school entry.

A persistent gap remains in the presence of limitations among children ages 5 to 17 years based on poverty status.[4] The percentage of children whose activities are limited is considerably greater for children residing in families with household incomes below 200% of the poverty level than for children living in higher income families (Figure 28-4). In 2003, 10% of children ages 5 to 17 years living in the former households had activity limitations compared with 7% of children in families at or above 200% of the poverty level.[4]

Limitations in activity also vary by gender and race. In 2003, 10% of boys and 6% of girls ages 5 to 17 years were limited in activities caused by chronic health conditions. Among children of different races and ethnic backgrounds, more white non-Hispanic and black non-Hispanic children were reported to have activity limitations than Hispanic children.[4]

The major chronic health conditions causing activity limitations vary by age (Table 28-6). For preschool children, the most common causes are speech problems, asthma, and intellectual disability or other developmental problems. For school-aged children, learning disabilities are the leading cause, followed by attention-deficit/hyperactivity disorder; other mental, emotional, or behavioral problems; and intellectual disability or other developmental problems. Most children have single conditions causing limitations; one in five have multiple conditions.[30]

Specific Conditions

Although 82% of children are reported to be in excellent or very good health, the prevalence of selected conditions is high.[31] According to the 2004 NHIS, 12.2% of all children have ever been told they have asthma, and 5.5% of children are reported to have had an attack in the past year. Nearly 1 in 10 children have hay fever (9.2%) and more than 1 in 10 have respiratory allergies (11.6%), with 12.5% reported to have other allergies in the past year. Among children 3 to 17 years of age, 8% have ever been told they have learning disabilities, and 7% have attention-deficit/hyperactivity disorder. Generating particular concern has been the growing percentage of children who are overweight. These children are more likely to become overweight adults and are at risk for physical and social sequelae and chronic diseases both in childhood and as adults. Sixteen percent of youth ages 6 to 19 are overweight,[30] as defined by having a body mass index at or above the 95th percentile. This level represents a substantial increase from the 6% reported in 1980.

CONCLUSION

Children's general health has improved over the last 2 decades, in part because of prevention of serious illnesses by the development and widespread use of new vaccines. However, many opportunities are still available to reduce morbidity and mortality in children. Primary care physicians can play a significant role in this process by working directly with their patients and parents and by advocating for children with other segments of society.

TOOLS FOR PRACTICE

Community Advocacy and Coordination

- *Health, United States,* Centers for Disease Control and Prevention (www.cdc.gov/nchs.hus.htm).
- *Healthy People 2010* (Web page), US Department of Health and Human Services (www.healthypeople.gov/).

- *The National Survey of Children with Special Health Care Needs Chartbook* (other), US Department of Health and Human Services (mchb.hrsa.gov/chscn/).
- *Web-based Injury Statistics Query and Reporting System* (Web page), Centers for Disease Control and Prevention (www.cdc.gov/ncipc/wisgars/).

RELATED WEB SITES

- *Child Trends* (Web page), Child Trends (www.childtrends.org/).
- *Morbidity and Mortality Weekly Report* (MMWR) (Web page), Centers for Disease Control and Prevention (www.cdc.gov/mmwr/).
- *National Center for Health Statistics* (Web page), Centers for Disease Control and Prevention (www.cdc.gov/nchs/).
- *National Health Interview* (Web page), Centers for Disease Control and Prevention (www.cdc.gov/nchs/nhis.htm).
- *US Census Bureau* (Web page), US Census Bureau (www.census.gov/).

REFERENCES

1. Hoyert DL, Mathews TJ, Menacker F, et al. Annual summary of vital statistics—2004. *Pediatrics.* 2006;117(1):168-183.
2. Jameson EJ, Wehr E. Drafting national health care reform legislation to protect the health interests of children. *Stanford Law Policy Rev.* 1993;Fall:152-176.
3. National Research Council and Institute of Medicine, Committee on Evaluation of Children's Health, Board on Children, Youth, and Families, Division of Behavioral and Social Sciences and Education. *Children's Health, the Nation's Wealth: Assessing and Improving Child Health.* Washington, DC: The National Academies Press; 2004.
4. Federal Interagency Forum on Child and Family Statistics, Federal Interagency Forum on Child and Family Statistics. *America's Children: Key National Indicators of Well-Being, 2005.* Washington, DC, US Government Printing Office; 2005.
5. Morgan SP. Characteristic features of modern American fertility. *Pop Dev Rev.* 1996;22:19-63.
6. Campbell PR, US Bureau of the Census. *Population Projections for States, By Age, Race, and Sex: 1993 to 2020. Current Population Reports.* Washington, DC: US Government Printing Office; 1994.
7. Child Trends, Inc. *Trends in the Well-Being of America's Children and Youth. 1998 ed. Part 1: Indicators of Children's Well-Being.* Washington, DC: Office of the Assistant Secretary for Planning and Evaluation, US Department of Health and Human Services; 1999.
8. Day JC, US Bureau of the Census. *Population Projections of the United States By Age, Sex, Race, and Hispanic Origin: 1995 to 2050. Current Population Reports.* Washington, DC: US Government Printing Office; 1996.
9. US Census Bureau, Population Estimates Branch. *Estimated Population of States by Age Group and Sex, 2000-2003.* Washington, DC: US Government Printing Office; 2004.
10. Population Resource Center. A Population Perspective of the United States, 2004. Available at: www.prcdc.org Accessed July 3, 2007.
11. Child Trends, Inc. *Trends in the Well-Being of America's Children and Youth, 1997 ed.* Washington, DC: Office of the Assistant Secretary for Planning and Evaluation, US Department of Health and Human Services; 1997.
12. Legislative Commission on the Economic Status of Women. Status of Women Profile Report. Table 13a. Median Family Income By Family Type and State Listing. Compiled from Census 2000 Summary File 3 (SF3), Table PCT40. Available at: www.lcesw.leg.mn. Accessed July 3, 2007.
13. MacDorman MF, Atkinson JO. Infant mortality statistics from the 1996 period linked birth/infant death data set. *Natl Vital Stat Rep.* 1998;46(23):1-23.
14. Ventura SJ, Martin JA, Curtin SC, et al. Births: Final data for 1997. *National Vital Statistics Reports,* Vol. 47, No. 18. Hyattsville, MD: National Center for Health Statistics; 1998.
15. Behrman RE, Butler AS, eds. *Preterm Birth; Causes, Consequences, and Prevention. Report of the IOM Committee on Understanding Premature Birth and Assuring Healthy Outcomes.* Washington DC, National Academy Press; 2006.
16. Mathews TJ, Menaker F, MacDorman MF. Infant mortality Statistics from the 2002 period: linked infant birth/death data set. *Natl Vital Stat Rep.* 2004;53(10):1-32.
17. Guyer B, MacDorman MF, Martin JA, et al. Annual summary of vital statistics—1997. *Pediatrics.* 1998;102(6): 1333-1349.
18. Arias E, MacDorman MF, Strobino DM, et al. Annual summary of vital statistics—2002. *Pediatrics.* 2003;112(6 pt 1): 1215-1230.
19. Liu K, Moon M, Sulvetta M, et al. International infant mortality rankings: a look behind the numbers. *Health Care Financ Rev.* 1992;13(4):105-118.
20. Martin JA, Kochanek MS, Strobino DM, et al. Annual summary of vital statistics—2003. *Pediatrics.* 2005;115(3):619-634.
21. Bonnie RJ, Fulco CE, Liverman CT eds. *Reducing the Burden of Injury; Advancing Prevention and Treatment.* Washington, DC: National Academy Press; 1999.
22. Rivara FP. Pediatric injury control in 1999; where do we go from here? *Pediatrics.* 1999;103(4 pt 2):883-888.
23. Newacheck PW, Stoddard JJ, McManus M. Ethnocultural variations in the prevalence and impact of childhood chronic conditions. *Pediatrics.* 1993;91(5 pt 2):1031-1039.
24. McPherson M, Arango P, Fox H, et al. A new definition of children with special health care needs. *Pediatrics.* 1998;102(1 pt 1):137-140.
25. Newacheck PW, Stoddard JJ. Prevalence and impact of multiple childhood chronic illnesses. *J Pediatr.* 1994;124(1):40-48.
26. Ireys HT, Anderson GH, Shaffer TJ, et al. Expenditures for care of children with chronic illnesses enrolled in the Washington State Medicaid Program, fiscal year 1993. *Pediatrics.* 1997;100(2 pt 1):197-204.
27. Stein REK, Silver EJ. Operationalizing a conceptually based noncategorical definition: a first look at US children with chronic conditions. *Arch Pediatr Adolesc Med.* 1999;153(1):68-74.
28. Newacheck PW, Taylor WR. Childhood chronic illness: prevalence, severity and impact, *Am J Public Health.* 1992;82(3):364-371.
29. US Department of Health and Human Services, Health Resources and Services Administration, Maternal and Child Health Bureau. *The National Survey of Children with Special Health Care Needs Chartbook 2001.* Rockville, MD: Maternal and Child Health Bureau; 2004.
30. National Center for Health Statistics. *Health United States; 2005.* Hyattsville, MD: National Center for Health Statistics; 2005.
31. Bloom B, Dey AN. Summary statistics for US children: National Health Interview Survey, 2004. *Vital and Health Statistics.* Vol. 10, No. 227. Hyattsville, MD: National Center for Health Statistics; 2006.

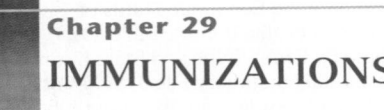

Chapter 29

IMMUNIZATIONS

Sharon G. Humiston, MD, MPH; William L. Atkinson, MD, MPH; Cynthia Rand, MD, MPH; Peter G. Szilagyi, MD, MPH

INTRODUCTION

Vaccine-preventable diseases left a legacy of suffering that must not be forgotten. We should remember our progress from a time when smallpox eradicated entire human communities to a time when humans eradicated wild smallpox. We should also remember that, although we have made marked progress in recent years, children in this country and many children elsewhere die when they lose their very personal battles with vaccine-preventable diseases.

Vaccination is one of the most important achievements in pubic health in the twentieth century.[1] The most salient feature of this achievement is decreased disease levels. Compared with prevaccination-era disease levels, the current US disease levels are from 92% to 100% lower.[2] Recent immunization successes include the first-ever interruption of indigenous measles[3] and rubella[4] transmission in the United States and the interruption of wild type polio transmission in the Western hemisphere.[5] Routine childhood vaccination is one of the few health care interventions that saves both lives and dollars; compared with a no-vaccination program, routine vaccination saves from $29 (for measles-mumps-rubella [MMR] vaccination) to $2 (for hepatitis B vaccination) for every dollar spent.

The primary reason for the record low disease incidence is record high immunization coverage levels,[6] an achievement by the health care system that was accomplished during a period of increasing complexity in the immunization schedule. These successes were due largely to major efforts by private and public health care providers. Sustaining success will require even greater effort because the process of vaccinating children is becoming increasingly complicated as the number of vaccines and vaccine combination choices increases.

The current US recommended childhood and adolescent immunization schedule is updated annually or biannually; the most current version is available on the Centers for Disease Control and Prevention (CDC) Web site.[7]

BACKGROUND INFORMATION ON VACCINES

Principles of Vaccination

For more information on the principles of vaccination, the reader is referred to the "Suggested Resources" section at the end of this chapter.[8]

Live Versus Inactivated Vaccines

Currently available vaccines are either live or inactivated. Live vaccines include:

- Those that protect against viruses (eg, MMR, varicella, rotavirus, live attenuated influenza intranasal vaccine [LAIV], yellow fever, vaccinia, oral polio vaccine)
- Those that protect against bacteria (eg, BCG, oral typhoid vaccine).

Live vaccines replicate in the body. Live injected vaccines usually induce immunity through a single dose and, unlike inactivated vaccines, are susceptible to vaccine failure caused by circulating antibodies, including residual maternal antibodies in infants.

Inactivated vaccines include:

- Inactivated viruses (eg, inactivated polio vaccine [IPV], hepatitis A, rabies)
- Inactivated subunits (eg, acellular pertussis, hepatitis B, human papillomavirus [HPV], split virus influenza, typhoid Vi)
- Toxoid (diphtheria, tetanus) agents
- Polysaccharides—either unconjugated (pneumococcal, meningococcal) or conjugated (*Haemophilus influenzae* type b [Hib], pneumococcal, meningococcal)

Inactivated vaccines do not contain infectious particles that can replicate in the body; they generally require several doses to immunize the patients completely.

Spacing and Timing

ROUTINE SCHEDULE. The routine vaccination schedules are harmonized among the American Academy of Pediatrics (AAP), the American Academy of Family Physicians (AAFP), and the CDC Advisory Committee on Immunization Practices (ACIP) (Figure 29-1). The harmonized schedules are not simple, but they do allow for office preferences by indicating acceptable ranges for routine on-time vaccination scheduling. The ranges were created so that offices might more easily accommodate routine vaccination into their well-child care schedule. To ensure timely vaccinations, vaccinating early within the acceptable age range is important.

INTERVALS BETWEEN DIFFERENT VACCINES NOT ADMINISTERED SIMULTANEOUSLY. Using all routine vaccines simultaneously is safe and effective, provided that vaccines are not combined within a single syringe. No contraindications exist to giving any 2 different routine childhood vaccines at the same visit.

Vaccines that are not administered simultaneously may be given without regard to intervals, with 1 or 2 exceptions: (1) Live vaccines not given by the oral route (ie, MMR, varicella, LAIV) that are not administered simultaneously should be separated by at least 4 weeks.[8] This *4-week separation rule* is intended to reduce the theoretical risk of interference from the first vaccine on the subsequent vaccine. If, for example, varicella vaccine is given only 1 week after an MMR, then the varicella vaccine should be repeated or serologic testing should be used to confirm seroconversion. (2) AAP guidelines specify that if the adolescent formulation (tetanus toxoid, reduced diphtheria toxoid, and acellular pertussis [TdaP], adsorbed) is not given at the same visit as meningococcal conjugate vaccine, then the 2 should be separated by at least 4 weeks.[9] ACIP guidelines do not make this stipulation.

Providers, parents, and, no doubt, children prefer fewer injections. As a consequence of the increasing

Recommended Immunization Schedule for Persons Aged 0-6 Years—UNITED STATES • 2008

For those who fall behind or start late, see the catch-up schedule

Vaccine ▼ Age ▶	Birth	1 month	2 months	4 months	6 months	12 months	15 months	18 months	19-23 months	2-3 years	4-6 years
Hepatitis B[1]	HepB	HepB		See footnote 1	HepB						
Rotavirus[2]			Rota	Rota	Rota						
Diphtheria, Tetanus, Pertussis[3]			DTaP	DTaP	DTaP	See footnote 3	DTaP				DTaP
Haemophilus influenzae type b[4]			Hib	Hib	*Hib[4]*	Hib					
Pneumococcal[5]			PCV	PCV	PCV	PCV				PPV	
Inactivated Poliovirus			IPV	IPV	IPV						IPV
Influenza[6]					Influenza (Yearly)						
Measles, Mumps, Rubella[7]						MMR					MMR
Varicella[8]						Varicella					Varicella
Hepatitis A[9]						HepA (2 doses)				HepA Series	
Meningococcal[10]										MCV4	

This schedule indicates the recommended ages for routine administration of currently licensed childhood vaccines as of December 1, 2007, for children through age 6 years. For additional information, see **www.cdc.gov/nip/recs/child-schedule.htm**. Any dose not administered at the recommended age should be administered at any subsequent visit when indicated and feasible. Additional vaccines may be licensed and recommended during the year. Licensed combination vaccines may be used whenever any components of the combination are indicated and other components of the vaccine are not contraindicated and if approved by the Food and Drug Administration for that dose of the series. Providers should consult the respective ACIP statement for detailed recommendations. Clinically significant adverse events that follow immunization should be reported to the Vaccine Adverse Event Reporting System (VAERS). Guidance about how to obtain and complete a VAERS form is available at **www.vaers.hhs.gov** or by telephone **(800) 822-7967**.

Range of recommended ages **Certain high-risk groups**

1. Hepatitis B vaccine (HepB). (Minimum age: birth)

At birth:

- Administer monovalent HepB to all newborns prior to hospital discharge.
- If mother is hepatitis surface antigen (HBsAg)-positive, administer HepB and 0.5 mL of hepatitis B immune globulin (HBIG) within 12 hours of birth.
- If mother's HBsAg status is unknown, administer HepB within 12 hours of birth. Determine the HBsAg status as soon as possible and if HBsAg-positive, administer HBIG (no later than age 1 week).
- If mother is HBsAg-negative, the birth dose can be delayed, **in rare cases,** with provider's order and a **copy of the mother's** negative HBsAg laboratory report in the infant's medical record.

After the birth dose:

- The HepB series should be completed with either monovalent HepB or a combination vaccine containing HepB. The second dose should be administered at age 1-2 months. The final dose should be administered no earlier than age 24 weeks. Infants born to HBsAg-positive mothers should be tested for HBsAg and antibody to HBsAg after completion of at least 3 doses of a licensed HepB series, at age 9-18 months (generally at the next well-child visit).

4-month dose:

- It is permissible to administer 4 doses of HepB when combination vaccines are administered after the birth dose. If monovalent HepB is used for doses after the birth dose, a dose at age 4 months is not needed.

2. Rotavirus vaccine (Rota). (Minimum age: 6 weeks)

- Administer the first dose at age 6-12 weeks.
- Do not start the series later than age 12 weeks.
- Administer the final dose in the series by 32 weeks of age. Do not administer any dose later than age 32 weeks.
- Data on safety and efficacy outside of these age ranges are insufficient.

3. Diphtheria and tetanus toxoids and acellular pertussis vaccine (DTaP). (Minimum age: 6 weeks)

- The fourth dose of DTaP may be administered as early as age 12 months, provided 6 months have elapsed since the third dose.
- Administer the final dose in the series at age 4-6 years.

4. *Haemophilus influenzae* type b conjugate vaccine (Hib). (Minimum age: 6 weeks)

- If PRP-OMP (PedvaxHIB® or ComVax® [Merck]) is administered at ages 2 and 4 months, a dose at age 6 months is not required.
- TriHiBit® (DTaP/Hib) combination products should not be used for primary immunization but can be used as boosters following any Hib vaccine in children age 12 months or older.

5. Pneumococcal vaccine. (Minimum age: 6 weeks for pneumococcal conjugate vaccine [PCV]; 2 years for pneumococcal polysaccharide vaccine [PPV])

- Administer one dose of PCV to all healthy children aged 24-59 months having any incomplete schedule and 2 doses of PCV at least 8 weeks apart to incompletely vaccinated children with underlying medical conditons.

6. Influenza vaccine. (Minimum age: 6 months for trivalent inactivated influenza vaccine [TIV]; 2 years for live, attenuated influenza vaccine [LAIV])

- Administer annually to children aged 6-59 months and to all close contacts of children aged 0-59 months.
- Administer annually to children 5 years of age and older with certain risk factors, to other persons (including household members) in close contact with persons in groups at higher risk, and to any child whose parents request vaccination.
- For healthy nonpregnant persons (those who do not have underlying medical conditions that predispose them to influenza complications) ages 2-49 years, either LAIV or TIV may be used.
- Children receiving TIV should receive 0.25 mL if age 6-35 months or 0.5 mL if age 3 years or older.
- Administer 2 doses (separated by 4 weeks or longer) to children younger than 9 years who are receiving influenza vaccine for the first time or who were vaccinated for the first time last season, but only received one dose.

7. Measles, mumps, rubella vaccine (MMR). (Minimum age: 12 months)

- Administer the second dose of MMR at age 4-6 years. MMR may be administered before age 4-6 years, provided 4 weeks or more have elapsed since the first dose, and both doses are administered at age 12 months or older.

8. Varicella vaccine. (Minimum age: 12 months)

- Administer second dose at age 4-6 years; may be administered 3 months or more after first dose.
- Don't repeat second dose if administered 28 days or more after first dose.

9. Hepatitis A vaccine (HepA). (Minimum age: 12 months)

- HepA is recommended for all children aged 1 yr (i.e., 12-23 months). The 2 doses in the series should be administered at least 6 months apart.
- Children not fully vaccinated by age 2 years can be vaccinated at subsequent visits.
- HepA is recommended for certain other groups of children, including in areas where vaccination programs target older children.

10. Meningococcasl vaccine. (Minimum age: 2 years for meningococcl conjugate vaccine [MCCV4] and for meningococcal polysaccharide vaccine [MPSV2])

- MCV4 is recommedned for children aged 2-10 years with terminal complement deficiencies or anatomic or functional asplenia and certain other high-risk groups. Use of MPSV4 is also acceptable.
- Persons who received PMSV4 and who remain at increased risk for meningococcal

The Recommended Immunization Immunization Schedules for Persons Aged 0-18 Years are approved by the Advisory Committee on Immunization Practices (www.cdc.gov/vaccines/recs/acip), the American Academy of Pediatrics (http://www.aap.org), and the American Academy of Family Physicians (http://www.aafp.org).

Department of Health and Human Service • Centers for Disease Control and Prevention • safer • healthier • people™

DEPARTMENT OF HEALTH AND HUMAN SERVICES • CENTERS FOR DISEASE CONTROL AND PREVENTION

Recommended Immunization Schedule for Persons Aged 7-18 Years—UNITED STATES • 2008

For those who fall behind or start late, see the green bars and the catch-up schedule

Vaccine ▼ / Age ▶	7-10 Years	11-12 Years	13-14 Years	15 Years	16-18 Years
Tetanus, Diphtheria, Pertussis[1]	See footnote 1	Tdap	Tdap		
Human Papillomavirus[2]	See footnote 2	HPV (3 doses)	HPV Series		
Meningococcal[3]	MCV4	MCV4	MCV4		
Pneumococcal[4]	PPV				
Influenza[5]	Influenza (Yearly)				
Hepatitis A[6]	HepA Series				
Hepatitis B[7]	HepB Series				
Inactivated Poliovirus[8]	IPV Series				
Measles, Mumps, Rubella[9]	MMR Series				
Varicella[10]	Varicella Series				

This schedule indicates the recommended ages for routine administration of currently licensed childhood vaccines as of December 1, 2007, for children aged 7-18 years. Additional information is available at **www.cdc.gov/vaccines/recs/schedules**. Any dose not administered at the recommended age should be administered at any subsequent visit, when indicated and feasible. Additional vaccines may be licensed and recommended during the year. Licensed combination vaccines may be used whenever any components of the combination are indicated and other components of the vaccine are not contraindicated and if approved by the Food and Drug Administration for that dose of the series. Providers should consult the respective Advisory Committee on Immunization Practices statement for detailed recommendations, including for high risk conditions: **www.cdc.gov/vaccines/pubs/ACIP-list.htm**. Clinically significant adverse events that follow immunization should be reported to the Vaccine Adverse Event Reporting System (VAERS). Guidance about how to obtain and complete a VAERS form is available at **www.vaers.hhs.gov** or by telephone, **(800) 822-7967**.

Range of recommended ages | Catch-up immunization | Certain high-risk groups

1. **Tetanus and diphtheria toxoids and acellular pertussis vaccine (Tdap).** *(Minimum age: 10 years for BOOSTRIX® and 11 years for ADACEL™)*
   - Administer at age 11-12 years for those who have completed the recommended childhood DTP/DTaP vaccination series and have not received a tetanus and diphtheria toxoids (Td) booster dose.
   - Adolescents aged 13-18 years who missed the 11-12 year Td/Tdap booster dose should also receive a single dose of Tdap if they have completed the recommended childhood DTP/DTaP vaccination series.
2. **Human papillomavirus vaccine (HPV).** *(Minimum age: 9 weeks)*
   - Administer the first dose of the HPV vaccine series to females at age 11-12 years.
   - Administer the second dose 2 months after the first dose and the third dose 6 months after the first dose.
   - Administer the HPV vaccine series to females at age 13-18 years if not previously vaccinated.
3. **Meningococcal vaccine.** *(Minimum age: 11 years for meningococcal conjugate vaccine [MCV4]; 2 years for meningococcal polysaccharide vaccine [MPSV4])*
   - Administer MCV4 at age 11-12 years and at age 13-18 years is not to previously vaccinated.
   - Administer MCV4 to previously unvaccinated college freshmen living in dormitories; MPSV4 is an acceptable alternative.
   - MCV4 is recommended for children aged 2-10 years with terminal complement deficiencies or anatomic or functional asplenia and certain other high-risk groups. Use of MPSV4 is also acceptable.
4. **Pneumococcal polysaccharide vaccine (PPV).**
   - Administer PPV to certain high-risk groups.
5. **Influenza vaccine.**
   - Administer annually to persons in close contact with children aged 0-59 months.
   - Administer annually to persons with certain risk factors, health-care workers, and other persons (including household members) in close contact with persons in groups at higher risk.
   - Administer 2 doses (separated by 4 weeks or longer) to children younger than 9 years who are receiving influenza vaccine for the first time or who were vaccinated for the first time last season, but only received one dose.
   - For healthy persons (those who do not have underlying medical conditions that predispose them to influenza complications) ages 2-49 years, either LAIV or TIV may be used.
6. **Hepatitis A vaccine (HepA).**
   - The 2 doses in the series should be administered at least 6 months apart.
   - HepA is recommended for certain other groups of children, including in areas where vaccination programs target older children.
7. **Hepatitis B vaccine (HepB).**
   - Administer the 3-dose series to those who were not previously vaccinated.
   - A 2-dose series of Recombivax HB® is licensed for children aged 11-15 years.
8. **Inactivated poliovirus vaccine (IPV).**
   - For children who received an all-IPV or all-oral poliovirus (OPV) series, a fourth dose is not necessary if a third dose was administered at age 4 years or older.
   - If both OPV and IPV were administered as part of a series, a total of 4 doses should be administered, regardless of the child's current age.
9. **Measles, mumps, and rubella vaccine (MMR).**
   - If not previously vaccinated, administer 2 doses of MMR during any visit, with 4 or more weeks between the doses.
10. **Varicella vaccine.**
    - Administer 2 doses of varicella vaccine to persons without evidence of immunity.
    - Administer 2 doses of varicella vaccine to persons younger than 13 years of age at least 3 months apart. Do not repeat the second dose, if administered 28 or more days following the first dose.
    - Administer 2 doses of varicella vaccine to persons aged 13 years or older at least 4 weeks apart.

The Recommended Immunization Immunization Schedules for Persons Aged 0-18 Years are approved by the Advisory Committee on Immunization Practices (www.cdc.gov/vaccines/recs/acip), the American Academy of Pediatrics (http://www.aap.org), and the American Academy of Family Physicians (http://www.aafp.org).

SAFER • HEALTHIER• PEOPLE™

Figure 29-1 A, Recommended childhood immunization schedule for ages 0 through 6 years of age. B, Recommended Adolescent immunization schedule for ages 7 through 18 years of age. *(Department of Health and Human Services; Centers for Disease Control and Prevention. Advisory Committee on Immunization Practices) (www.cdc.gov/nip/acip); American Academy of Pediatrics (www.aap.org); American Academy of Family Physicians (www.aafp.org).*

number of diseases that can be prevented through vaccination, the number of required injections increased dramatically. The number of combination vaccines available also increased.[10,11] Combination vaccines reduce the number of injections and are preferred by ACIP, AAFP, and AAP when available.[12] All vaccines for which the child is eligible should be offered whenever possible. This strategy not only keeps the child on schedule, but also prevents an additional, unnecessary office visit.

MINIMAL AGE AND INTERVALS BETWEEN DIFFERENT DOSES OF A MULTIDOSE VACCINE. Vaccine doses that are given too early in life or too soon after a previous dose may be less effective. Table 29-1 shows the earliest acceptable ages of administration of the routinely recommended childhood vaccines and the minimal spacing between their doses.[13]

Providers frequently ask whether to count a vaccine dose given at an interval shorter than the minimal interval. For example, should a child who received doses 3 and 4 of diphtheria-tetanus-acellular pertussis (DTaP) vaccines within less than 6 months be revaccinated? Was the dose valid if a child received an MMR vaccination before 12 months of age? Though state requirements for school entry vary, ACIP considers a vaccination valid if the vaccine dose was within 4 days of the minimal interval.[8] Vaccine doses, of course, are considered invalid if an incorrect amount was used. Steps should be taken to prevent these errors from occurring, and the clinician should remember that vaccination is a safe procedure, even if the child is given more than the recommended number of doses. Overvaccination with live vaccines is without consequence because the extra vaccine virus will not infect an already-immune person. Overvaccination with inactivated vaccines might cause an increase in local reactions if antibody levels are high.

Prolonged intervals between doses of a multidose vaccination series do not diminish vaccine effectiveness once the series has been completed. Series never need to be restarted because of prolonged intervals (with the exception of oral typhoid vaccine).

LATE-START OR INTERRUPTED SCHEDULE. Some children start routine vaccination late. The recommended compressed, catch-up, or accelerated immunization schedule for such children is derived from the minimal intervals for the routine vaccinations. A catch-up schedule is published annually with the routine schedule.[14]

The presentation of a new patient whose vaccination status is unknown presents a challenge. In this situation, the clinician must determine if any immunization record exists for the child and, if so, to obtain a copy of the record or a report from the previous provider. If no record can be found, then the child should be presumed to be unvaccinated, and the vaccination series should be given using the accelerated schedule. Serologic testing can be considered for some antigens (eg, MMR, hepatitis B).

INTERVALS BETWEEN LIVE INJECTED VACCINES AND ANTIBODY-CONTAINING BLOOD PRODUCTS. Live injected vaccines (eg, MMR and varicella vaccines) have to replicate in the body to induce immunity and may be compromised by circulating antibodies against the vaccine virus. Live vaccines not administered by injection (eg, LAIV, oral typhoid, live oral poliovirus vaccine [OPV]) are believed to be unaffected by circulating antibodies. Inactivated vaccines are not significantly affected by circulating antibodies and can be administered without regard to the relative timing of the administration of immune globulin–containing products.

MMR and varicella vaccine doses given more than 14 days before immune globulin–containing products are administered have time to replicate and are effective. When live injected vaccines are given after antibody-containing blood products, the situation is more complex. The specific immune globulin–containing product and its dose dictate the waiting period necessary before a valid dose of a live injected vaccine is given. MMR and varicella vaccination should be delayed from 3 months to 11 months, depending on the specific immune globulin preparation administered. Details of the appropriate waiting period can be found in the AAP *Red Book*[15] and on the CDC Web site.[16]

Vaccinations Administered in Foreign Countries

Determining the immunization status of foreign-born children or other children who have been partially or completely vaccinated in another country can be difficult. Vaccines, their abbreviations, and vaccination age criteria often differ among countries. The immunization status needs to be determined for all children and special attention paid to the rest of the family in the case of recent immigration.

The first assumption to make is that the vaccines administered in other countries were as potent as those available in the United States. Then, it becomes a matter of determining which vaccines were administered and whether the doses qualify as valid doses when considering the minimal ages of administration and the minimal time intervals between doses. Determining which vaccines were administered can be difficult because the standard abbreviations recorded in handheld vaccination records may be different from those used in the United States. Translation of foreign-language terms can be facilitated with materials from the CDC.[17] Assistance with specific questions can be obtained from your state immunization program or from the CDC National Center for Immunization and Respiratory Diseases via telephone (800-232-4636) or e-mail (nipinfo@cdc.gov). Once the vaccine types are determined, Table 29-2 can be used to determine which doses are valid and which, if any, need to be repeated. Doses given earlier than the minimal age or interval should generally by repeated.

Variation in vaccination strategies creates a problem for clinicians caring for internationally adopted children and recent immigrants. Although evidence suggests that the documented vaccination status of foreign adopted children is not always accurate, the current recommendation when interpreting the vaccination status of international adoptees is that documented vaccinations (that include the doses and dates of administration) are acceptable proof of vaccination.[8]

Contraindications and Precautions

The reader is encouraged to visit www.cdc.gov/nip/recs/contraindications.htm and check for CDC's detailed *Guide to Contraindications to Vaccinations*. Contraindications and precautions are also summarized on the *Summary of Recommendations for Childhood and Adolescent Immunization*, which is available at www.immunize.org/catg.d/rules1.pdf.

ANAPHYLACTIC ALLERGY. Anaphylactic-type allergy to a vaccine or a vaccine component, which includes even mild urticarial reactions, is a contraindication to further vaccination with the vaccine in question.

ENCEPHALOPATHY. Encephalopathy after a previous dose of a pertussis-containing vaccine is a contraindication to further vaccination with a pertussis-containing vaccine (eg, DTaP, TdaP).

MINOR, ACUTE ILLNESSES. Some children will be ill at the time of a well-child visit or will be in need of a vaccination at an illness visit. In these situations, the clinician must decide whether to recommend vaccination based on 2 questions: (1) Will vaccination be safe

Table 29-1 Recommended and Minimum Ages and Intervals Between Vaccine Doses[a]

VACCINE AND DOSE NUMBER	RECOMMENDED AGE FOR THIS DOSE	MINIMUM AGE FOR THIS DOSE	RECOMMENDED INTERVAL TO THE NEXT DOSE	MINIMUM INTERVAL TO THE NEXT DOSE
Hepatitis B-1[b]	Birth	Birth	1-4 months	4 weeks
Hepatitis B-2	1-2 months	4 weeks	2-17 months	8 weeks
Hepatitis B-3[c]	6-18 months	24 weeks		
DTaP-1[b]	2 months	6 weeks	2 months	4 weeks
DTaP-2	4 months	10 weeks	2 months	4 weeks
DTaP-3	6 months	14 weeks	6-12 months[d]	6 months[d,e]
DTaP-4	15-18 months	12 months	3 years	6 months[d]
DTaP-5	4-6 years	4 years	—	—
Haemophilus influenzae type b (Hib)-1[b,f]	2 months	6 weeks	2 months	4 weeks
Hib-2	4 months	10 weeks	2 months	4 weeks
Hib-3[g]	6 months	14 weeks	6-9 months[d]	8 weeks
Hib-4	12-15 months	12 months	—	—
Inactivated poliovirus vaccine (IPV)-1[b]	2 months	6 weeks	2 months	4 weeks
IPV-2	4 months	10 weeks	2-14 months	4 weeks
IPV-3	6-18 months	14 weeks	3-5 years	4 weeks
IPV-4	4-6 years	18 weeks	—	—
Pneumococcal conjugate vaccine (PCV)-1[f]	2 months	6 weeks	2 months	4 weeks
PCV-2	4 months	10 weeks	2 months	4 weeks
PCV-3	6 months	14 weeks	6 months	8 weeks
PCV-4	12-15 months	12 months	—	—
MMR-1[h]	12-15 months[i]	12 months	3-5 years	4 weeks
MMR-2[h]	4-6 years	13 months	—	—
Varicella (Var-1[h])	12-18 months	12 months	3-5 years	12 weeks[i]
Var-2[h]	4-6 years	15 months	—	—
Hepatitis (Hep) A-1[b]	12-23 months	12 months	6-18 months[d]	6 months[d]
Hepatitis Hep A-2b	18-41 months	18 months	—	—
Influenza inactivated vaccine (TIV)[j]	6-59 months	6 months	6 months[k]	4 weeks
Influenza live attenuated vaccine (LAIV)[j]	—	5 years	1 month	14 weeks
Meningococcal conjugate vaccine (MCV)	11-12 years	11 years	—	—
Meningococcal polysaccharide vaccine (MPSV)-1	—	2 years	5 years[l]	5 years[l]
MPSV-2[m]	—	7 years[l]	—	—
Tetanus-diphtheria (Td)	11-12 years	7 years	10 years	5 years
Tdap[n]	≥11 years	10 years	—	—
Pneumococcal polysaccharide vaccine (PPV)-1	—	2 years	5 years	5 years

Table 29-1 Recommended and Minimum Ages and Intervals Between Vaccine Doses[a]—cont'd

VACCINE AND DOSE NUMBER	RECOMMENDED AGE FOR THIS DOSE	MINIMUM AGE FOR THIS DOSE	RECOMMENDED INTERVAL TO THE NEXT DOSE	MINIMUM INTERVAL TO THE NEXT DOSE
PPV-2[o]	—	7 years	—	—
Human papillomavirus (HPV)-1[p]	11-12 years	9 years	2 months	4 weeks
HPV-2	11-12 years	109 months	4 months	12 months
HPV-3	11-12 years	112 months	—	—
Rotavirus (RV)-1[q]	2 months	6 weeks	2 months	4 weeks
RV-2	4 months	10 weeks	2 months	4 weeks
RV-3	6 months	14 weeks	—	—
Zoster[r]	60 years	60 years	—	—

DTaP, Diphtheria and tetanus toxoids and acellular pertussis vaccine; *MMR,* measles, mumps, and rubella; *TIV,* trivalent (inactivated) influenza vaccine; *LAIV,* live, attenuated (intranasal) influenza vaccine; *Td,* tetanus and reduced diphtheria toxoids; *Tdap,* tetanus toxoid, reduced diphtheria toxoid, and reduced acellular pertussis vaccine.

[a]Use of licensed combination vaccines is preferred over separate injections of their equivalent component vaccines. (CDC: Combination vaccines for childhood immunization: recommendations of the Advisory Committee on Immunization Practices [ACIP]; the American Academy of Pediatrics [AAP]; and the American Academy of Family Physicians [AAFP], *MMWR.* 1999;48[No. RR-5]). When administering combination vaccines, the minimum age for administration is the oldest age for any of the individual components; the minimum interval between doses is equal to the greatest interval of any of the individual components.

[b]Combination vaccines containing the hepatitis B component are available (HepB-Hib, DTaP-HepB-IPV, HepA-HepB). These vaccines should not be administered to infants younger than 6 weeks of age because of the other components (ie, Hib, DTaP, IPV, and HepA).

[c]HepB-3 should be administered at least 8 weeks after HepB-2 and at least 16 weeks after HepB-1, and it should not be administered before age 24 weeks.

[d]Calendar months.

[e]The minimum recommended interval between DTaP-3 and DTaP-4 is 6 months. However, DTaP-4 need not be repeated if administered at least 4 months after DTaP-3.

[f]For Hib and PCV, children receiving the first dose of vaccine at age 7 months or older require fewer doses to complete the series (CDC: Recommended childhood and adolescent immunization schedule—United States, 2006. *MMWR.* 2005; 54 [Nos. 51 and 52]:Q1-Q4).

[g]If PRP-OMP (Pedvax-Hib®, Merck Vaccine Division) was administered at 2 and 4 months of age, a dose at 6 months of age is not required.

[h]Combination measles-mumps-rubella-varicella (MMRV) vaccine can be used for children 12 months through 12 years of age. Also see footnote *i.*

[i]The minimum interval from Var-1 to Var-2 for persons beginning the series at 13 years or older is 4 weeks.

[j]Two doses of influenza vaccine are recommended for children younger than 9 years of age who are receiving the vaccine for the first time. Children younger than 9 years who have previously received influenza vaccine, and persons 9 years of age and older, require only one dose per influenza season.

[k]The minimum age for inactivated influenza vaccine varies by vaccine manufacturer. Only Fluzone (manufactured by sanofi pasteur) is approved for children 6-35 months of age. The minimum age for Fluvirin (manufactured by Novartis) is 4 years. For Fluarix and FluLaval (manufactured by GlaxoSmithKline), the minimum age is 18 years.

[l]Some experts recommend a second dose of MPSV 3 years after the first dose for people at increased risk for meningococcal disease.

[m]A second dose of meningococcal vaccine is recommended for people previously vaccinated with MPSV who remain at high risk for meningococcal disease. MCV is preferred when revaccinating persons aged 11 to 55 years, but a second dose of MPSV is acceptable. (CDC: Prevention and Control of Meningococcal Disease Recommendations of the Advisory Committee on Immunization Practices [ACIP], *MMWR.* 2005;54: No. RR-7.)

[n]Only one dose of Tdap is recommended. Subsequent doses should be administered as Td. If vaccination to prevent tetanus and/or diphtheria disease is required for children 7 through 9 years of age, Td should be administered (minimum age for Td is 7 years). For one brand of Tdap the minimum age is 11 years. The preferred interval between Tdap and a previous dose of Td is 5 years. In persons who have received a primary series of tetanus-toxoid containing vaccine, for management of a tetanus-prone wound, the minimum interval after a previous dose of any tetanus-containing vaccine is 5 years.

[o]A second dose of PPV is recommended for persons at highest risk for serious pneumococcal infection and those who are likely to have a rapid decline in pneumococcal antibody concentration. Revaccination 3 years after the previous dose can be considered for children at highest risk for severe pneumococcal infection who would be younger than 10 years of age at the time of revaluation. (CDC: Prevention of pneumococcal disease: recommendations of the Advisory Committee on Immunization Practices [ACIP]. *MMWR.* 1997;46[No. RR-8]).

[p]HPV is approved only for females at 9 to 26 years of age.

[q]The first dose of RV must be administered at 6 to 12 weeks of age. The vaccine series should not be started at 13 weeks of age or older. RV should not be administered to children 33 weeks of age or older regardless of the number of doses received between 6 and 32 weeks of age.

[r]Herpes zoster vaccine is approved as a single dose for persons 60 years and older with a history of varicella.

Source: Centers for Disease Control and Prevention. Recommended and Minimum Ages and Intervals Between Vaccine Doses. Available at: www.cdc.gov/vaccines/pubs/pinkbook/downloads/appendices/A/age-interval-table.pdf. Accessed October 1, 2007.

for this ill child, and (2) if not vaccinated at this visit, will the child be brought back for vaccination?

Minor illnesses, including upper respiratory tract infections, otitis media, and diarrheal illnesses, whether the individual is febrile or not, are not valid contraindications to vaccination. A second, perhaps more difficult, consideration is whether minor vaccine side effects such as fever will cause diagnostic confusion during the follow-up period for the illness—a problem that may be especially difficult when caring for very young infants.

Clinicians often struggle to determine the likelihood that any given child will return for a scheduled vaccination visit. Although past appointment-keeping behavior will help in the judgment, it is not completely reliable. Because vaccinating children who have minor illnesses is safe and effective, and because it may be unclear whether a child will be brought back for an appointment, vaccinating the ill child is best, especially if he or she has missed previous preventive care visits.

IMMUNOCOMPROMISE. Immunocompromised children and their close contacts require individual attention. In general, live vaccines cannot be used in immunocompromised individuals because of the potential for severe or fatal reactions from uncontrolled replication of the vaccine virus.* Because inactivated vaccines cannot replicate, they are safe for use in immunocompromised children, but these children may have a diminished immune response to inactivated vaccines.

Children who have congenital immunodeficiency, leukemia, lymphoma, or generalized malignancy should not receive live vaccines. Persons receiving treatments that cause immunosuppression (for example, alkylating agents, antimetabolites, and radiation therapy) also should not receive live vaccines. Persons receiving daily, large doses of corticosteroids (the equivalent of 2 mg/kg of prednisone per day) for 14 days or longer should not receive live virus vaccines; live vaccines should be deferred for at least 30 days after cessation of therapy or reduction in dose. Live vaccine use is not contraindicated if the corticosteroid is aerosolized (as in asthma inhalers) or topical, nor if it is given on an alternate day, short course (fewer than 14 days), or if the child is on a physiologic replacement schedule. For vaccination of bone marrow transplant patients, the clinician should consult the *Red Book*[18] or the CDC guidelines.[19]

Notably, persons who do not have evidence of severe immunosuppression—even if infected with HIV—should receive MMR and varicella vaccines. Children who have symptomatic HIV infection should not receive either of these vaccines.[20] Immunocompromised people with limited humoral immunodeficiency (eg, hypogammaglobulinemia, immunoglobulin A deficiency) may be routinely vaccinated with varicella vaccine.

Persons living with an immunocompromised household contact should be vaccinated as indicated. MMR and varicella vaccines, which are live vaccines contraindicated for use in immunocompromised people themselves, should be given to susceptible contacts of immunocompromised people. Oral polio vaccine, which is used in other countries though not in the United States, should not be given to people who are immunocompromised or who are close contacts of immunocompromised persons.

PREGNANCY. Pregnant women generally should not receive live vaccines because of the theoretical risk of fetal damage.* Women should avoid pregnancy for 4 weeks after vaccination with MMR, MMR with

Table 29-2 Recommended Immunization Schedule for Children and Adolescents Who Start Late or Who Are More Than 1 Month Behind* United States•2008

CATCH-UP SCHEDULE FOR CHILDREN AGED 4 MONTHS THROUGH 6 YEARS

VACCINE	MINIMUM AGE FOR DOSE 1	MINIMUM INTERVAL BETWEEN DOSES			
		DOSE 1 TO DOSE 2	DOSE 2 TO DOSE 3	DOSE 3 TO DOSE 4	DOSE 4 TO DOSE 5
Hepatitis B[1]	Birth	4 weeks	8 weeks (and 16 wk after 1st dose[1])	—	—
Rotavirus[2]	6 weeks	4 weeks	4 weeks	—	—
Diphtheria, tetanus, pertussis[3]	6 weeks	4 weeks	4 weeks	6 months	6 months[3]
Haemophilus influenza type b[4]	6 weeks	4 weeks (if 1st dose is given at age <12 mo) 8 weeks as the final dose (if 1st dose is given at age 12-14 mo) No further doses needed if 1st dose is given at age ≥15 mo	4 weeks[4] (if current age is <12 mo) 8 weeks as the final dose[4] (if current age is ≥12 mo and 2nd dose is given at age <15 mo) No further doses needed if previous dose is given at age ≥15 mo	8 weeks as final dose (only necessary for children aged 12 mo to 5 yr who received 3 doses before age 12 mo)	—
Pneumococcal[5]	6 weeks	4 weeks (if 1st dose is given at age <12 mo and current age is <24 mo) 8 weeks as final dose (if 1st dose is given at age ≥12 mo or current age is 24-59 mo)	8 weeks as final dose (if current age is ≥12 mo)	8 weeks as final dose (only necessary for children aged 12 mo to 5 yr who received 3 doses before age 12 mo)	

*Immunocompromise is a precaution but not a contraindication to the live, oral pentavalent rotavirus vaccine.

*An exception is yellow fever vaccination for a pregnant woman traveling to a yellow fever endemic area.

Table 29-2 Recommended Immunization Schedule for Children and Adolescents Who Start Late or Who Are More Than 1 Month Behind* United States•2008—cont'd

CATCH-UP SCHEDULE FOR CHILDREN AGED 4 MONTHS THROUGH 6 YEARS

VACCINE	MINIMUM AGE FOR DOSE 1	MINIMUM INTERVAL BETWEEN DOSES: DOSE 1 TO DOSE 2	DOSE 2 TO DOSE 3	DOSE 3 TO DOSE 4	DOSE 4 TO DOSE 5
		No further doses needed for healthy children (if 1st dose is given at age ≥24 mo	No further doses needed for healthy children (if previous dose is given at age ≥24 mo	—	—
Inactivated poliovirus[6]	6 weeks	4 weeks	4 weeks	4 weeks[6]	—
Measles, mumps, rubella[7]	12 months	4 weeks[4]	—	—	—
Varicella[8]	12 months 6 weeks	—	—	—	—
Hepatitis A[9]	12 months	6 months	—	—	—

CATCH-UP SCHEDULE FOR CHILDREN AGED 7 THROUGH 18 YEARS

VACCINE	MINIMUM AGE FOR DOSE 1	MINIMUM INTERVAL BETWEEN DOSES: DOSE 1 TO DOSE 2	DOSE 2 TO DOSE 3	DOSE 3 TO BOOSTER DOSE
Tetanus, diphtheria/ Tetanus,diphtheria, Pertussis[10]	7 years[10]	4 weeks	4 weeks if 1st dose give at <12 months 6 months if 1st dose give at ≥12 months	6 months (if 1st dose is given at age <12 months
Human papillomavirus[11]	9 years	4 weeks	12 weeks	
HepatitisA[9]	12 months	6 months		
Hepatitis B[1]	Birth	4 weeks	—	—
Inactivated poliovirus[6]	6 weeks	4 weeks		4 weeks[6]
Measles, Mumps, Rubella[7]	12 months	4 weeks	—	—
Varicella[8]	12 months	4 weeks if 1st dose give at ≥13 years 3 months if 1st dose give at <13 years	—	—

*This table provides catch-up schedules and minimum intervals between doses for children who have delayed immunizations. Restarting a vaccine series is not necessary, regardless of the time elapsed between doses. The appropriate section for the child's age should be used.

[1]HepB. Administer the 3-dose series to those who were not previously vaccinated. A 2-dose series of Recombivax HB is licensed for children 11-15 years.

[2]Rotavirus. Do not start series later than age 12 weeks. Administer final dose in the series by age 32 weeks. Do not administer a dose later than age 32 weeks.

[3]DTaP. The 5th dose is not necessary if the 4th dose was admin-istered after the 4th birthday. Not indicated for those ≥7 years.

[4]Hib. Vaccine is not generally recommended for children aged 5 years or older. If <12 months and the 1st 2 doses were PRP-OMP (Pedvax HIB or ComVax), the 3rd and final dose should be administered at age 12-15 months and at least 8 weeks after the 2nd dose.

[5]PCV. At ages 24-59 months administer 1 dose of PCV to incompletely vaccinated healthy children and 2 doses of PCV at 8 weeks apart to incompletely vaccinated children with certain high-risk conditions.

[6]IPV. For children who received an all-IPV or all-oral poliovirus (OPV) series, a 4th dose is not necessary if a 3rd dose was admin-istered at age ≥4 years. If both OPV and IPV were administered as part of a series, then a total of 4doses should be given, regardless of the child's current age. Vaccine is not generally recommended for persons aged ≥18 years.

[7]MMR. The 2nd dose of MMR is routinely recommended at age 4 to 6 years but may be administered earlier if desired. If not previously vaccinated, give 2 doses of MMR during any visit with 4 or more weeks between the doses.

[8]Varicella. The 2nd dose of varicella vaccine is recommended routinely at age 4 to 8 years but may be administered earlier if desired. Do not repeat the 2nd dose in persons younger than 13 years of age if administered 28 or more days after the 1st dose.

[9]HepatitisA. Vaccine is recommended for certain groups of children, including in areas where vaccination programs target older children. See MMWR 2006;55(No. RR-7):1-23.

[10]Td and Tdap. Tdap should be substituted for a single dose of Td in the primary catch-up series or as a booster if age appropriate; use Td for other doses. A 5-year interval from the last Td dose is encouraged when Tdap is used as a booster dose. A booster (fourth) dose is needed if any of the previous doses were administered at younger than 12 months of age. Refer to ACIP recommendations for further information. See *MMWR* 2006;55(No. RR-3).

[11]HPV. Administer the vaccine series to females at age 13-18 years if not previously vaccinated

Report adverse reactions to vaccines through the federal Vaccine Adverse Event Reporting System. For information on reporting reactions after immunization, visit mfww.vaers.hhs.gov or call the 24-hour national toil-free information line (800) 822-7967. Report suspected cases of vaccine-preventable diseases to your state or local health department. For additional information about vac-cines, including precautions and contraindications for immunization and vaccine shortages, visit the National Immunization Program Web site at www.cdc.gov/nip or contact (800) CDC-INFO ([800] 232-4636) (in English, En Espanol—24/7) varicella vaccine (MMRV), or varicella vaccines. Pregnant women generally may receive inactivated vaccines and toxoids.[21] Detailed guidelines on vaccination of pregnant women can be found on the CDC Web site.[22]

PREMATURITY. Preterm infants should be vaccinated using the routine schedule based on their chronologic age (ie, time since birth, regardless of gestational age) and the standard doses of vaccine. One exception to this rule relates to hepatitis B vaccine; to maximize vaccine efficacy, infants weighing less than 2000 g and whose mothers are documented to be hepatitis B surface antigen negative should not receive hepatitis B vaccine until they reach a body weight of 2000 g or chronologic age of 1 month.[23,24] As with full-term infants, premature infants whose mothers' hepatitis B surface antigen status is positive should receive the vaccine and hepatitis B immune globulin (HBIg). If the mother's hepatitis B surface antigen is unknown, then the hepatitis B vaccine and HBIg should be given within 12 hours of birth, regardless of birth weight, but the birth dose should not be counted as part of the vaccine series.

Vaccine Safety

Vaccine safety concerns have been based on data (eg, RotaShield® and intussusception), a biologically plausible but unsubstantiated association (eg, thimerosal in the birth dose of hepatitis B vaccine and autism), or speculation (MMR vaccine and autism). New concerns are likely to arise. Reliable sources of vaccine safety information that are regularly updated include the following:

- Immunization Action Coalition (www.immunize.org/safety/)
- National Network for Immunization Information (www.immunizationinfo.org/)
- Vaccine Education Center (www.chop.edu/consumer/)
- Vaccine Safety Institute (www.vaccinesafety.edu/)

Universal Childhood Vaccines

Diphtheria-Tetanus-Acellular Pertussis Vaccine

DTaP is the recommended form[25] of the oldest combination vaccine, DTP, which is a combination of diphtheria toxoid, tetanus toxoid, and acellular pertussis vaccine. Vaccination against tetanus and diphtheria has been highly successful. For example, the prevaccination annual incidence of diphtheria was 100,000 to 200,000 cases, but only 52 cases of diphtheria were reported in the United States between 1980 and 2002. Similarly, the US incidence of tetanus fell from 500 to 600 each year in the 1940s to 25 cases in 2002. Pertussis has been a more recalcitrant disease; after having dropped 99% from the mid-1940s to 1976, the number of cases reported in 2004 was 25,616.[26]

DTaP is licensed for all of the preschool doses. Unfortunately, two thirds of reported cases of pertussis occur in older children and adults, who represent a reservoir for the bacteria and a continuing source of infection for young children. (Please see the discussion of adolescent pertussis immunization, later in this chapter.)

STORAGE. DTaP, DTP, or DTP-Hib vaccines should arrive at the office unfrozen and should be refrigerated on arrival at a temperature of 2° to 8° C. The vaccine should not be frozen. The shelf life is up to 1 year. The vials must be shaken vigorously before withdrawing the individual doses.

ADMINISTRATION. The vaccine is administered intramuscularly using a dose of 0.5 mL. The ACIP has stated that, although completing the pertussis vaccination series using vaccine from a single manufacturer is preferred, when this is not feasible, any available licensed pertussis vaccine may be used. That is, revaccinating individuals with the same manufacturer's product is not necessary to complete the vaccination series; the series can be finished with any of the pediatric acellular vaccines.

ADVERSE REACTIONS. Adverse reactions to diphtheria and tetanus toxoids include (1) local reactions, such as redness and induration, (2) nodule at the injection site, and (3) Arthus-type hypersensitivity reactions. Mild adverse reactions to DTaP include (1) local reactions of redness, swelling, induration, and tenderness and (2) systemic reactions of drowsiness, vomiting, crying, and low-grade fever. Moderate-to-severe reactions include high fevers of 40.5° C (105° F) or higher, persistent and inconsolable crying of more than 3 hours' duration, hypotonic-hyporesponsive episodes, and febrile seizures. All of these reactions occur much less frequently with DTaP than with DTP, and all are believed to occur without permanent sequelae.

CONTRAINDICATIONS AND PRECAUTIONS. Contraindication to DTaP vaccination include (1) a history of severe (anaphylactic) allergic reaction after a prior dose of DTaP vaccine or a vaccine component and (2) encephalopathy within 7 days of a previous dose. Precautions to DTaP include a convulsion within 3 days of a previous dose; persistent, severe, inconsolable screaming or crying for 3 or more hours within 48 hours of a previous dose; collapse or shocklike state within 48 hours of a previous dose; and a temperature of 40.5° C (105° F) that is unexplained by another cause within 48 hours of a previous dose. Vaccination should be deferred in the event of a moderate to severe acute illness until the illness subsides.

Hepatitis A Virus Vaccine

In 2005, universal hepatitis A virus vaccination was recommended for all children between 12 and 23 months, with optional catch-up vaccination through the preschool years.[27] Previously, the vaccine was recommended only for children ages 2 years and older in states and communities that had a relatively high incidence of hepatitis A.[28]

In addition to the routine childhood immunization recommendation, hepatitis A vaccine is recommended for persons at increased risk of hepatitis A virus infection because they travel or work in countries of high to intermediate endemicity, have homosexual sex with men, use illegal drugs, work with hepatitis A–infected primates or laboratory specimens, or take clotting factor concentrates. The vaccine is also recommended for people with chronic liver disease.

Two manufacturers make inactivated hepatitis A vaccines, both brands given by intramuscular injection. A 2-dose schedule is used for the hepatitis A vaccine.*

*A combination hepatitis B (adult dose) and hepatitis A (pediatric dose) vaccine, Twinrix®, is available and licensed only for persons 18 years of age or older. It is given as a 3-dose series in a 0-, 1-, and 6- to 12-month schedule. Twinrix® should not be used for routine childhood immunization.

Hepatitis A vaccine has an efficacy rate of more than 90% after the 1st dose has been administered and approximately 100% after the 2nd dose.

STORAGE. The vaccine should arrive unfrozen and should be stored at temperatures between 2° and 8° C. The shelf life is up to 3 years.

CONTRAINDICATIONS AND PRECAUTIONS. Hepatitis A vaccine should not be given to individuals who have a history of severe (anaphylactic) allergy to the vaccine or its components such as alum and phenoxyethanol. Serious adverse events have not been associated with hepatitis A vaccination. The most frequent side effects are local reactions, including soreness at the injection site.

Hepatitis B Virus Vaccine

Vaccination with hepatitis B virus (HBV) vaccine prevents HBV infection and its complications, which include hepatocellular cancer. Thus hepatitis B vaccine was the 1st anticancer vaccine. In the United States before the routine use of hepatitis vaccine, an estimated 200,000 to 300,000 new HBV infections occurred annually, with 20,000 to 30,000 new chronic infections per year. Risk factors for HBV infection are lifestyles, occupations, or environments in which contact with blood or other body fluids from infected persons occurs frequently, but a large proportion of infected individuals were not known to have any risk factor.

The initial strategy of targeting hepatitis B vaccination toward high-risk persons failed to significantly reduce the incidence of HBV infection. In 1991, universal infant vaccination was recommended by ACIP,[29] AAP, and AAFP. The ACIP expanded its hepatitis B vaccination recommendations to include previously unvaccinated children ages 11 to 12 years in 1994 and in 1997 expanded them to include all unvaccinated children ages 0 to 18 years, as well as making hepatitis B vaccine available to this group through the Vaccines for Children (VFC) program.[30]

STORAGE. The vaccine should arrive at the office with a refrigerant but unfrozen. It should be refrigerated on arrival and stored at 2° to 8° C. The vaccine should not be frozen. The shelf life is up to 3 years.

ADMINISTRATION. A vaccination series started with one manufacturer's product can be completed with the other manufacturer's product. The seroconversion rate is greater than 95% for infants, children, and adolescents receiving all 3 doses. The vaccine is 80% to 100% effective at preventing infection.

A 3-dose schedule is recommended for active immunization. For routine infant immunization, the initial dose should be given to the newborn before hospital discharge. The minimal intervals between doses are[8]:

- Between the 1st and 2nd doses—4 weeks
- Between the 2nd and 3rd doses—8 weeks
- Between the 1st and 3rd doses—16 weeks

The 3rd dose should be administered no earlier than 24 weeks of age. For infants, children, and adolescents through 19 years of age, the dose is 0.5 mL of either the pediatric formulation of Recombivax HB or Engerix B.

CONTRAINDICATIONS AND PRECAUTIONS. Administration of hepatitis B vaccine is contraindicated for individuals who had a serious (anaphylactic) allergic reaction to a prior dose of hepatitis B vaccine or a vaccine component. The most common adverse event after receiving the hepatitis B vaccine is pain at the injection site. Mild systemic complaints, including fatigue, headache, and irritability, occur in fewer than 20% of children. Low-grade fever occurs in up to 6% of children. Serious systemic adverse events and allergic reactions are rare.

HIGH-RISK GROUPS FOR HEPATITIS B. High-risk groups include Alaskan Natives, American Asian and Pacific Islanders, and children of immigrants or refugee families from countries having high rates of HBV infection. Special efforts should be made to vaccinate non–US born and immigrant children, who should also be screened for hepatitis B surface antigen (HBsAg).

BABIES BORN TO HEPATITIS B SURFACE ANTIGEN–POSITIVE MOTHERS. All women should be screened for HBsAg during pregnancy, and women at high-risk of HBV infection (eg, intravenous drug users) should be screened again at the time of delivery. The results of hepatitis B testing should be available at the time of delivery so that perinatal transmission can be prevented by administration of both hepatitis B vaccine and HBIg. The regimen is approximately 95% effective in preventing infection.

All infants born to women who are HBsAg positive should receive hepatitis B vaccine and HBIg (at a different injection site) within 12 hours of birth, regardless of gestational age or birth weight. For infants weighing less than 2000 g, this birth dose should not be counted as part of the series; that is, 3 additional doses of hepatitis B vaccine should be given, the first of which should be at 1 month of age. Combination vaccines containing a hepatitis B component, COMVAX and Pediarix, cannot be given to infants before 6 weeks of age. Though these combination vaccines are not licensed for use in infants born to HBsAg-positive mothers, ACIP has recommended off-label use of COMVAX or Pediarix after 6 weeks of age to complete the hepatitis B vaccination series for these infants after a birth dose of a single-antigen hepatitis B vaccine.

After the hepatitis B immunization series is complete (preferably at 6 months of age), all infants of HBsAg-positive mothers should be tested for the presence of anti-HBs and HBsAg at 9 to 15 months of age.

Infants born to women who were not tested for HBsAg should receive an initial dose of hepatitis B vaccine within 12 hours of birth. The mother should be tested immediately, and if she tests positive, then the infant should receive HBIg within 7 days.

LOW–BIRTH-WEIGHT INFANTS. Hepatitis B vaccination should be postponed if an infant is born to an HBsAg-negative woman and weighs less than 2000 g. Low–birth-weight infants whose mother's surface antigen status is positive or unknown should receive immediate vaccination and HBIg, as previously described.

Haemophilus Influenzae *Type B Vaccine*

The near elimination of invasive Hib disease in the United States is a success story that happened within the careers of mature practicing primary care providers. In the prevaccination era, 1 in 200 children developed invasive Hib disease by the age of 5 years.[31] The most recent surveillance data show that the annual number of cases decreased by 99%.[2]

The Hib vaccines in use today are conjugated vaccines; that is, the polysaccharide component of the capsule (polyribosylribitol phosphate [PRP]) is bonded chemically to a protein carrier to enhance immunogenicity (especially in infants) and response to booster doses. Available vaccines vary by the carrier protein to which PRP is bonded. Carriers include a mutant diphtheria toxin (HbOC), tetanus toxoid (PRP-T), and a *Neisseria meningitidis* outer membrane protein complex (PRP-OMP). Hib vaccine has high efficacy—approximately 97% after 3 doses.

STORAGE. Hib vaccines should arrive in insulated containers to prevent freezing. They should arrive unfrozen and should be refrigerated immediately and stored between 2° and 8° C. Freezing reduces or destroys potency. Shelf life is up to 2 years.

ADMINISTRATION. The differences among the vaccines result in slightly different administration schedules, for example:

- PRP-T (Act-Hib) and HbOC (Hib titer) should be given as a 4-dose series at 2, 4, 6, and 12 to 15 months of age.
- PRP-OMP (COMVAX, PedvaxHIB) can be given as a 3-dose series at 2, 4, and 12 to 15 months of age. If a child receives different brands of Hib vaccine at 2 and 4 months of age, then a Hib vaccine dose should be given at 6 months—even if one of the earlier doses was PRP-OMP—and this primary series should be followed by a booster at 12 to 15 months of age.

Hib vaccine also is marketed in several combination vaccines, including separate combinations with DTaP and hepatitis B vaccines. The package insert should be consulted for product-specific dosing schedules. Notably, the DTaP-Hib combination (TriHibit) is licensed only for the 4th dose of the DTaP-Hib series. Completing the series with a different Hib product from the product used to start the Hib vaccination series is acceptable, again, with the stipulation that this would necessitate a 3-dose primary series, after which a booster is given at 12 to 15 months of age.

The number of doses needed to complete the Hib series is different for children who have a late start on Hib vaccination or who have a lapsed series.[32] Table 29-3 lists a detailed Hib vaccination schedule.

ADVERSE EVENTS. Adverse events after Hib vaccination are mild and infrequent. Between 5% and 30% will have a local reaction consisting of swelling, redness, or pain. Systemic adverse events such as fever are uncommon.

CONTRAINDICATIONS AND PRECAUTIONS. The only contraindication to Hib vaccination is a history of severe (anaphylactic) allergic reaction after a prior dose of Hib vaccine or a vaccine component. Vaccination should be deferred in the event of a moderate to severe acute illness until the patient's health improves.

Influenza Virus Vaccine

To decrease the burden of influenza disease on children,[33,34] annual influenza vaccination is recommended for all children 6 to 59 months of age and for older children who have any of the following conditions:

- Asthma and other chronic pulmonary or cardiovascular system diseases (does not include hypertension)
- Any condition that can compromise respiratory function or the handling of respiratory secretions or that can increase the risk for aspiration
- Immunosuppressive conditions, HIV infections, sickle cell disease and other hemoglobinopathies
- Chronic metabolic diseases, including diabetes mellitus, renal dysfunction, and long-term aspirin use

The vaccine is also recommended for persons who live with or care for an individual for whom the vaccine is recommended or an infant who is too young to be vaccinated (ie, younger than 6 months of age), women who will be pregnant during influenza season, and residents of nursing homes and other chronic care facilities.[35,36]

Currently, influenza immunization can be achieved using an injectable trivalent inactivated vaccine (TIV) or an LAIV. Both vaccines consist of 3 highly purified, egg-grown influenza virus subtypes. The composition is based on the viral strains expected during the winter influenza virus season. TIV consists of either purified surface antigens or viral particles prepared by disrupting the membrane; it is licensed for use in persons 6 months of age or older. LAIV is licensed only for use in healthy persons (ie, those who do not have a chronic illness) 5 to 49 years of age and who are not pregnant.

ADMINISTRATION. TIV is administered intramuscularly in an age-dependent dose and schedule as follows:

- Children 6 to 35 months of age require 2 doses the first time they receive influenza vaccine, with single annual doses thereafter (0.25 mL in each intramuscular dose).
- Children 3 to 8 years of age require 2 doses the first time they receive influenza vaccine, with single

Table 29-3 Detailed Vaccination Schedule for *Haemophilus Influenzae* Type b Conjugate Vaccines

VACCINE	AGE AT 1ST DOSE (MONTHS)	PRIMARY SERIES	BOOSTER
HbOC PRP-T (HibTITER, ActHIB)	2-6	3 doses, 2 months apart	12-15 months*
	7-11	2 doses, 2 months apart	12-15 months*
	12-14	1 dose	2 months later
	15-59	1 dose	None
PRP-OMP (PedvaxHIB)	2-6	2 doses, 2 months apart	12-15 months*
	7-11	2 doses, 2 months apart	12-15 months*
	12-14	1 dose	2 months later
	15-59	1 dose	None

*At least 2 months after previous dose.
From Detailed Vaccination Schedule for *Haemophilus influenzae* type b Conjugate Vaccine. Available at www.cdc.gov/vaccines/pubs/pinkbook/downloads/hib.pdf. Accessed October 3, 2007.

annual doses thereafter (0.50 mL in each intramuscular dose).

- Children 9 years of age or older require only 1 dose annually (0.50 mL in each intramuscular dose).

For the 2-dose regimen, the minimum interval recommendation between doses depends on the vaccine (4 weeks between doses of TIV, 6 weeks between doses of LAIV).

In 2006, TIV from 3 manufacturers were licensed for use in the United States. The vaccines have different approved age indications as shown here and should not be used outside their US Food and Drug Administration (FDA)-approved age indications.

- Fluzone (sanofi pasteur) approved for persons 6 months of age and older
- Fluvirin (Novartis) approved for persons 4 years and older
- Fluarix (GlaxoSmithKline) is approved for persons 18 years and older

STORAGE. TIV should arrive at the office unfrozen and should be refrigerated immediately on arrival. The vaccine should be stored between 2° and 8° C; shelf life is up to 18 months.

LAIV should be shipped frozen in insulated container with dry ice at 4° F (−20° C) or colder and must not have thawed in shipment. The vaccine must be maintained in a continuously frozen state at 5° F (−15° C) or colder, and no freeze-thaw cycles are permitted. To thaw before administering, the sprayer should be held, but not rolled, in palm of hand (rolling may dislodge the dose divider clip), or LAIV may be thawed in a refrigerator and stored at 35° to 46° F (2° to 8° C) for no more than 60 hours before use. Vaccine thawed in the refrigerator that is not used within 60 hours must be discarded in an impenetrable sharps container.[37]

ADVERSE EVENTS. TIV rarely causes febrile or other systemic reactions. Local reactions including soreness, redness, and induration at the site of the injection occur in fewer than 30% of vaccinees. Immediate hypersensitivity reactions, such as hives, angioedema, allergic asthma, or anaphylaxis, occur rarely after influenza vaccination. LAIV may be associated with coryza or nasal congestion, headache, fever, vomiting, abdominal pain, and myalgias; these symptoms were associated more often with the 1st dose and were self-limited.

CONTRAINDICATIONS AND PRECAUTIONS. Administration of influenza vaccine is contraindicated for individuals who had a serious (anaphylactic) allergic reaction to a prior dose of influenza vaccine or a vaccine component (eg, eggs).

For details about influenza vaccines, the reader is encouraged to consult their package inserts at the following links:

- FluMist (MedImmune): www.fda.gov/cber/label/inflmed080505LB.pdf
- Fluzone (sanofi pasteur): www.fda.gov/cber/products/inflave071405.htm
- Fluvirin (Novartis): www.fda.gov/cber/products/inflchi091405.htm
- Fluarix (GlaxoSmithKline): www.fda.gov/cber/products/inflgla083105.htm

Measles-Mumps-Rubella Vaccine

MMR vaccine is a combination of 3 live attenuated vaccines that together protect against measles, mumps, and rubella. The purpose of the measles and mumps vaccines is to protect against these specific diseases; the purpose of the rubella vaccine is to prevent congenital rubella syndrome by preventing the occurrence of rubella, which, itself, is a mild disease, in the general population, thereby preventing its spread to susceptible pregnant women. The incidence of all 3 viruses has declined more than 99% compared with the prevaccination era. As stated previously, MMR is also available combined with varicella vaccine as MMRV (ProQuad, Merck Vaccine Division).[38,39]

In the United States, only 1 strain of each vaccine virus in MMR is available. Each one is highly immunogenic, leading to seroconversion in 90% to 95% or more of recipients vaccinated at 15 months old or later.

STORAGE. MMR vaccine should arrive at the office in an insulated container at a temperature less than 10° C. It should be refrigerated on arrival and stored between 2° and 8° C (never frozen). The shelf life is up to 2 years; the expiration date is marked on the vials. On reconstitution, the vaccine should be stored in a dark place between 2° and 8° C and must be used within 8 hours.

MMRV must be shipped and stored at 4° F (−20° C) or colder at all times; it must not be stored at refrigerator temperature at any time. MMRV must be administered within 30 minutes of reconstitution.

ADMINISTRATION. The AAP and ACIP recommend administration of 2 doses of MMR vaccine for children; these doses are 0.5 mL delivered subcutaneously. The 1st dose should be given at 12 to 15 months of age and the 2nd before elementary school entry (4 to 6 years of age).[40,41] The purpose of the 2nd MMR dose is to produce immunity in the small proportion of children who fail to respond to the first. MMRV is approved only for children 12 months through 12 years of age and may be administered whenever MMR or varicella vaccines, or both, are indicated.

ADVERSE REACTIONS. Because MMR is composed of live attenuated vaccines, if side effects other than those related to allergy occur, they do so 5 to 12 days after administration. Adverse reactions include: rash—5% to 10% (measles, rubella), fever—5% to 15% (measles), thrombocytopenia—1 per 30,000 (measles), parotitis—rare (mumps); adults, but not children, often have arthralgia, and children may have transient arthritis—less than 1% of children recipients (rubella). An association between autism and MMR has been postulated but is not supported by scientific evidence.[42,43]

CONTRAINDICATIONS AND PRECAUTIONS. Contraindications to MMR vaccination include the following:

- History of a severe (anaphylactic) allergic reaction to a prior dose or a vaccine component (eg, neomycin, gelatin)
- Significant immunosuppression from any cause, including cancer or its treatment, immunodeficiency diseases, or immunosuppressive therapy. Asymptomatic HIV infection is not a contraindication to receipt of MMR (see the discussion under "Immunocompromise," earlier in this chapter)
- Pregnancy

Precautions to MMR vaccination include:

- Moderate or severe acute illness (defer vaccination until illness improves)
- Recent receipt of a blood transfusion, blood products, or immune (γ) globulin[16]

Table 29-4 Recommended Schedule for Use of 7-Valent Pneumococcal Conjugate Vaccine (PCV7)[a]

AGE AT 1ST DOSE (MONTHS)	NUMBER OF DOSES IN PRIMARY SERIES	ADDITIONAL DOSE
2-6	3 doses, 2 months apart[b]	1 dose at 12-15 months, at least 8 weeks after the primary series has been completed
7-11	2 doses, 2 months apart[b]	1 dose at 12-15 months, at least 8 weeks after the primary series has been completed
12-23	2 doses, 2 months apart[c]	None
24-59 without high-risk condition	1 dose	None
24-59 with high-risk condition[d]	2 doses, 2 months apart	None
>59	0	None

[a]Among previously unvaccinated infants and children by age at time of first vaccination
[b]For children vaccinated at age <1 year, the minimum interval between doses is 4 weeks.
[c]The minimum interval between doses is 8 weeks.
[d]High-risk conditions include sickle cell disease, asplenia, HIV infection, chronic illness, cochlear implant, and immunocompromising conditions.

- A history of thrombocytopenia or thrombocytopenia purpura

(Note that contraindications and precautions to MMRV make up those for both MMR and varicella vaccines.)

Pneumococcal Vaccine—Conjugated

Streptococcus pneumoniae (pneumococcus) has been one of major causes of serious infectious childhood diseases in the United States. Before the conjugate pneumococcal vaccine was widely used, each year in the United States, *S pneumoniae* caused 3000 cases of meningitis, 50,000 cases of bacteremia, 125,000 cases of pneumonia requiring hospitalization, a far greater number of cases of outpatient pneumonia, and 4 million cases of otitis media. Before the conjugate vaccine, a pure polysaccharide pneumococcal vaccine was licensed only for children 2 years of age and older, missing the age group of children with the highest incidence of invasive pneumococcal disease (ie, children younger than 2 years of age). The emergence of antimicrobial resistance heightened concern about pneumococcus and increased the desire for a pneumococcal vaccine for infants and toddlers.

The pneumococcal conjugate vaccine (PCV) is analogous to the Hib conjugate vaccine, in which a protein is joined to the polysaccharide. The currently licensed formulation contains 7 serotypes (thus the acronym PCV7) that accounted for most of the invasive pneumococcal diseases in children in the prevaccine era. Prelicensure studies of the conjugate vaccine indicated a high efficacy against invasive disease, 10% reductions in acute otitis media, and reductions in nasopharyngeal carriage of the bacteria. For these reasons, the AAP and ACIP recommend that all children should be routinely vaccinated with PCV7 beginning at 2 months of age.[44,45] Postlicensure studies have confirmed marked reductions in invasive pneumococcal disease, as well as possible indirect protection of other populations, such as older adults through herd immunity.

Special efforts should be made to ensure on-time vaccination of children with medical conditions that put them at increased risk of invasive pneumococcal disease, such as sickle cell disease, asplenia, HIV infection or other immunocompromising conditions, and chronic disease (eg, cardiopulmonary disease except asthma, chronic liver disease, or diabetes mellitus). Black, American Indian, and Alaska native children are also considered to be at high risk.

ADMINISTRATION. PCV7 is administered intramuscularly as a 0.5-mL dose. Administration should begin at 2 months but not earlier than 6 weeks of age. The recommended interval between the subsequent 2 doses is 2 months; the minimal interval is 4 weeks. The booster dose should be given at 12 to 15 months of age, at least 2 months after the 3rd dose.

Recommended schedules vary for children who had a delayed 1st dose or a lapse in vaccination as shown in Table 29-4[46] and Table 29-5.[47]

ADVERSE REACTIONS. Local reactions (1 in 4) and low-grade fever (1 in 3 with fever of more than 100.4° F) are common following PCV7, though fever over 102.2° F is not common (1 in 50). To date, no serious reactions have been associated with the vaccine.[48]

CONTRAINDICATIONS AND PRECAUTIONS. Contraindications to PCV7 include a severe (anaphylactic) allergic reaction following a prior dose of the vaccine or its components. Vaccination should be deferred for children with a moderate to severe acute illness until the illness improves.

Pneumococcal Vaccine—Polysaccharide

The pure polysaccharide pneumococcal vaccine (PPV) consists of purified capsular polysaccharide antigen from 23 types of the pneumococcal bacteria. The vaccine is given by intramuscular or subcutaneous injection. Unlike the conjugate pneumococcal vaccine, this vaccine does not reduce nasopharyngeal pneumococcal carriage, nor does it protect children younger than 2 years of age.

Use of the pure PPV is recommended for children older than 2 years of age who have conditions that place them at increased risk of systemic pneumococcal infection. At least 2 months should separate the last dose of PCV7 and 1st dose of PPV. For children undergoing splenectomy or chemotherapy initiation, vaccination should occur more than 2 weeks before splenectomy or the start of chemotherapy, if possible. For children, one revaccination is recommended after 3 to 5 years (not every 3 to 5 years).

Table 29-5 Recommendations for Use of 7-Valent Pneumococcal Conjugate Vaccine (PCV7)[a]

AGE AT VISIT (MONTHS)	PREVIOUS PCV7 VACCINATION HISTORY	RECOMMENDED REGIMEN
7-11	1 dose	1 dose at 7-11 mo; another ≥2 mo later at 12-15 mo
	2 doses	Same as above
12-23	1 dose before age 12 mo	2 doses ≥2 mo apart
	2 doses before age 12 mo	1 dose ≥2 mo after the most recent dose
24-59	Any incomplete schedule	1 dose[b]

[a]Among children with a lapse in vaccine administration.
[b]Children with high-risk conditions (eg, sickle cell disease, asplenia, HIV infection, chronic illness, cochlear implant, immunocompromising conditions) should receive 2 doses ≥2 mo apart.

STORAGE. Pure PPV should arrive at the office unfrozen and should be refrigerated immediately on arrival. The vaccine should be stored between 2°C and 8°C. Shelf life is up to 2 years.

ADVERSE REACTIONS. Adverse events following vaccination include mild local reactions in approximately 50% of recipients and fever or severe local reactions in less than 1%.

CONTRAINDICATIONS AND PRECAUTIONS. Contraindications to PPV include a severe (anaphylactic) allergic reaction following a prior dose of the vaccine or its components. Vaccination should be deferred for children with a moderate to severe acute illness until the illness improves.

Polio Vaccine

Polio vaccination has been so successful that the spread of wild type poliovirus has been eliminated from the Americas. The peak annual incidence of paralytic polio in the United States was 21,269 cases in 1952. Since 1979, all cases of paralytic polio acquired in the United States have been vaccine-associated paralytic polio among recipients of OPV or their close contacts. As a result of the Global Eradication Initiative, in 2006, poliovirus was endemic only in Nigeria, India, Afghanistan, and Pakistan, though importations into 8 other countries occurred.[49]

Two polio vaccines have been developed: enhanced-potency IPV and OPV. Routine polio vaccination in the United States is currently accomplished with IPV, which is administered subcutaneously (or intramuscularly) with a dose of 0.5 mL and consists of formaldehyde-killed poliovirus. OPV, in contrast, is a live attenuated vaccine that is administered orally. Though still used routinely in many countries (eg, Mexico), use of OPV was discontinued in the United States in 2000.[50,51]

STORAGE. IPV should arrive at the office unfrozen and should be refrigerated between 2° and 8° C. The shelf life is up to 18 months.

ADMINISTRATION. In many states, 4 polio vaccinations are required before school entry—3 doses in the primary series and 1 supplementary dose. If an all-IPV schedule is used and the 3rd dose is administered after the child's 4th birthday, then no supplemental dose is indicated.

ADVERSE REACTIONS. No serious adverse effects have been reported following IPV.

Rotavirus Vaccine

Rotavirus is the most common cause of severe gastroenteritis in infants and young children in the United States, and evidence shows that previously reported rates of rotavirus hospitalization actually may be underestimates.[52] The CDC estimates that rotavirus infection leads to 55,000 hospitalizations each year for acute gastroenteritis.[53]

In February 2006 an attenuated pentavalent bovine-human rotavirus vaccine (PRV) was licensed for use in the United States. PRV is expected to cover more than 80% of the strains that are currently responsible for rotavirus acute gastroenteritis worldwide.[54] In large prelicensure studies, PRV was efficacious and well tolerated.[55] The efficacy of the vaccine against rotavirus gastroenteritis caused by G1 through G4 serotypes was 74% against any severity and 98% against severe disease. Use of this vaccine was associated with a 94.5% reduction in G1 through G4 rotavirus–related hospitalizations and emergency department visits in the 1st full rotavirus season after the 3rd PRV dose.

The 1st dose should be given between 6 and 12 weeks of age. An interval of 4 to 10 weeks should pass between doses in the series. All 3 doses should be given by 32 weeks of age. Age should be calculated based on chronologic age. Premature infants can be immunized if they are clinically stable and are being or have been discharged from the hospital nursery. If a child spits out or vomits after vaccination, then the dose should not be repeated; the series should simply continue according to the recommended intervals.[56]

STORAGE. The recommended dose of PRV is 2 mL orally; this dose comes as a liquid in latex-free single-dose tubes. PRV should be transported and stored at 2° to 8° C (36° to 46° F) and protected from light.[57]

CONTRAINDICATIONS AND PRECAUTIONS. Contraindications to PRV include a severe (anaphylactic) allergic reaction after a prior dose of the vaccine or its components. Vaccination should be deferred for children with a moderate-to-severe acute illness until the illness improves. Other precautions to use include altered immunocompetence, preexisting chronic gastrointestinal disease, and history of intussusception.

ADVERSE REACTIONS. Within a week of receiving PRV, children are slightly (1% to 3%) more likely to have mild, temporary diarrhea or vomiting than unvaccinated children. Unlike a previously licensed rotavirus vaccine, no evidence has been found that PRV causes intussusception or other serious adverse events.[58]

Other live oral rotavirus vaccines are in development.

Varicella Vaccine

In the prevaccination era, almost everyone was infected with varicella, resulting in approximately 4 million cases of chickenpox per year. Varicella is not a reportable disease in all states; thus US incidence figures are not available. Estimates suggest that varicella was responsible for approximately 11,000 hospitalizations and 100 deaths per year. The majority of the hospitalizations occurred among previously healthy children and adolescents, and almost one half of the deaths occurred among children and adolescents.

The AAP[59] and ACIP[60] first recommended routine varicella vaccination in 1996. Most states now have varicella vaccination requirements for child care and school entry. The Oka/Merck strain, a live attenuated vaccine virus developed in the early 1970s in Japan, is the sole vaccine virus strain licensed in the United States today. The efficacy of the vaccine is approximately 70% for preventing any varicella disease and more than 95% for preventing severe varicella disease. Since this vaccine came into use, a 75% decrease in varicella-related hospitalizations has occurred, and a similar decrease has been seen in the number of chickenpox-related deaths. However, the number of outbreaks of varicella among immunized children (breakthrough varicella) has been growing. These cases tend to be quite mild. Some, but not all, investigators have found that a longer interval since immunization and immunization at the youngest ages, especially 12 months, are risk factors for breakthrough disease.[61] Parents should be told of the possibility of breakthrough infection and that breakthrough illness is generally very mild.

Varicella vaccine is also available combined with MMR vaccine as MMRV for use in children 12 months to 12 years of age (ProQuad, Merck) (See the "Measles-Mumps-Rubella Vaccine" section earlier in this chapter.)

ADMINISTRATION. The recommended dose is 0.5 mL injected subcutaneously. For children 12 months through 12 years of age, a single dose is recommended. For children 13 years of age or older who have neither a history of the disease nor of previous varicella vaccination, 2 doses are provisionally recommended, each separated by 4 to 8 weeks. Varicella vaccine may be given simultaneously with MMR, but, if not given on the same day, at least 28 days should elapse between the administration of the 2 doses.

Whether immunity is lifelong is unknown, and the answer to this question is complicated by persistent exposure to circulating wild type varicella virus, which boosts immunity in vaccinated children.

STORAGE. Varicella vaccine has stringent cold chain and storage requirements. The vaccine should arrive at the office frozen, having been shipped in dry ice, which should still be present in the shipping container. It must be stored in a freezer with a separate door at 5° F or colder. The shelf life of vaccine that is properly handled is 18 months. If stored at refrigerator temperatures, then varicella vaccine must be used within 72 hours, and it cannot be refrozen. Notably, MMRV must be stored frozen at all times and cannot tolerate refrigerator temperatures.

After reconstitution, varicella vaccine must be administered within 30 minutes.

CONTRAINDICATIONS AND PRECAUTIONS. Contraindications to varicella vaccination include the following:

- History of a severe (anaphylactic) allergic reaction to a prior dose or a vaccine component (eg, neomycin, gelatin)
- Substantial suppression of cellular immunity from any cause, including cancer or its treatment, immunodeficiency diseases, or immunosuppressive therapy, though persons with impaired humoral immunity may be vaccinated. Specifically, asymptomatic HIV infection and pure humoral immunodeficiencies (eg, immunoglobulin A deficiency, hypogammaglobulinemia) are not contraindications to receipt of varicella vaccine.
- Pregnancy

Precautions to varicella vaccination include:

- Moderate or severe acute illness (vaccination is deferred until illness improves)
- Receipt of a blood transfusion, blood products, or immune (γ) globulin[42]
- The manufacturer recommends discontinuing salicylates for 6 weeks after receiving varicella vaccine because of the association between aspirin use and Reye syndrome after acquiring chickenpox.

(Note that contraindications and precautions to MMRV make up those for both MMR and varicella vaccines.)

ADVERSE REACTIONS. Adverse reactions to varicella vaccine include (1) local complaints such as pain, soreness, redness, and swelling, which occur in 19% of young children and 24% to 33% of adolescents; (2) a varicella-like rash at the injection site, which occurs within 2 weeks in 3% of 1st-dose recipients; and (3) a varicella-like rash at noninjection sites, which occurs within 3 weeks in 4% to 6% of children. The incidence of zoster is less after varicella vaccination than after natural infection,[61] but zoster may be caused by varicella vaccine virus.

Routine Adolescent Immunization

A major new effort is underway to protect adolescents from vaccine-preventable diseases. Routine well-child visits should be established for adolescents to provide vaccines and other preventive care measures. Three main categories of vaccines for adolescents should be considered: (1) routinely recommended vaccines (discussed later in this chapter), (2) vaccines needed because of special high-risk conditions (eg, influenza, pneumococcal polysaccharide), and (3) vaccines that were previously missed. The last category includes, for example, vaccinating persons who have had no previous varicella vaccination (or history of disease), fewer than 2 doses of MMR, or fewer than 3 doses of hepatitis B vaccine.

Meningococcal Conjugate Vaccine

Neisseria meningitidis is a much-dreaded cause of meningitis and overwhelming sepsis. In addition to the risk of meningococcal disease in early childhood (9 in 100,000), a second peak of disease incidence occurs in adolescence and early adulthood, with the highest risk at age 18 (2 in 100,000). Overall rates of invasive meningococcal disease have increased in the last decade, with 1400 to 2800 cases each year.[62] Freshmen college students living in dormitories are at greater risk than their similarly aged peers.[63] The disease is fatal in 10% to 14% of cases, and, although infants are more likely to be infected with the disease than adolescents are, adolescents have a higher mortality rate from infection.[64] Serious consequences can result from invasive infection, including deafness, neurologic deficits, and limb loss. Since 1981, a polysaccharide meningococcal vaccine (MPSV4) was available. In 2005 the FDA approved a new meningococcal quadrivalent conjugate vaccine (MCV4), and the ACIP voted to recommend routine vaccination with MCV4 for the following adolescents (if not previously vaccinated with MCV4)[65]:

- At 11 to 12 years of age
- At high school entry (approximately 15 years of age)
- College freshmen living in dormitories

Additionally, the vaccine is recommended for groups that have an elevated risk of meningococcal disease, such as military recruits, persons who have anatomic or functional asplenia, persons with terminal complement component deficiencies, persons who travel to or reside in countries in which *N meningitidis* is hyperendemic or epidemic (particularly if contact with the local population will be prolonged), and microbiologists who are routinely exposed to isolates of *N meningitidis*.

Unlike MPSV4, MCV4 is conjugated (ie, the polysaccharide is linked to a protein); thus it offers improved duration of immunity. Whereas the older polysaccharide vaccine guarded against disease for 3 to 5 years, the new vaccine may offer protection for a decade. Additionally, conjugated vaccines are known to limit disease spread among unvaccinated persons by reducing asymptomatic bacterial carriage among those who are vaccinated. MCV4 is serogroup specific against groups A, C, Y, and W-135, similar to the polysaccharide vaccine. No vaccine is available against serogroup B disease, which causes more than 50% of meningococcal disease in young children and 30% of meningococcal disease in adolescents and young adults.[66]

MCV4 has been shown to have high immunogenicity, with significant titers in 98% of recipients after 1 dose.[67]

ADMINISTRATION. The meningococcal conjugate vaccine is licensed for ages 11 to 55. It is administered intramuscularly at a dose of 0.5 mL.

The vaccine can be given concomitantly with other vaccines, including Td or TdaP.

Common adverse effects from the vaccine include local pain (59%), headache (35%), and fatigue (30%).[68]

STORAGE. Vaccine should be stored at temperatures of 2°C to 8°C (35°F to 46°F) and should not be frozen. It is packaged in single-dose vials. Product that has been frozen should not be used.

ADVERSE REACTIONS. In the summer of 2005, five cases of Guillain Barré syndrome were reported that exhibited within 2 to 4 weeks after meningococcal conjugate vaccine administration. This incidence is not thought to be greater than that expected in the general population, but investigation is ongoing, and a history of Guillain Barré syndrome is a precaution to MCV4 use.[69]

Tetanus-Diphtheria-Acellular Pertussis Vaccine

Although the current rate of reported *Bordetella pertussis* infection is at least 50-fold less than before the DTP vaccine was introduced in the 1940s, the number of cases of pertussis reported over the last 2 decades has been increasing, with an incidence of almost 25,827 cases reported in 2004. The greatest rise in incidence has been among adolescents ages 10 to 19, although more than 90% of fatalities from the disease still occur in very young infants.[70] The upsurge is thought to represent, in some part, an increase in reporting. Over the last decade, (1) many states have expanded their investigations to find pertussis cases epidemiologically linked to another case, and (2) improved testing has become available. Specifically, in 1995, polymerase chain reaction became available for confirming bacterial presence; this test increases pertussis detection because pertussis culture has many false negatives. Despite improved abilities to identify cases, many individuals with a persistent cough have gone untested; thus reported cases largely underestimate the true pertussis disease burden.[71] Persistent *B pertussis* circulation remains problematic because the disease is communicable before it is recognizable and because immunity from childhood vaccination wanes after 5 to 10 years, leaving adolescents and young adults susceptible to disease.[72]

Vaccinating adolescents for pertussis is intended to reduce both pertussis morbidity among adolescents and the reservoir of disease. The latter effect presumably will decrease infant mortality, especially among children who are too young to have received the childhood DTaP series.

Two TdaP vaccines for adolescents are FDA approved—Adacel (for ages 11-64) and Boostrix (for ages 10 to 18). Both vaccines, which are indicated only as boosters, contain lower amounts of tetanus toxoid and pertussis antigen than the childhood vaccine (DTaP) and thus are not interchangeable with the infant formulation. Both vaccines were shown to produce significant pertussis antibody booster responses in 95% to 99% of patients and induced similar tetanus-diphtheria antibody responses to Td vaccine.[73,74]

ADMINISTRATION. The ACIP and AAP recommend that adolescents ages 11 to 12 years old be given TdaP in place of the Td booster previously given.[65,75] The Committee also recommended that TdaP be given to adolescents ages 13 to 18 who missed the early adolescent dose of Td. Adolescents ages 11 to 18 who have already been vaccinated with Td are encouraged to receive a dose of TdaP to further protect against pertussis. (A dose of TdaP is also recommended for adults younger than 65 years of age.[76]) Although the manufacturers' prescribing information recommends a 5-year interval after a Td vaccination before administering TdaP,[77,78] ACIP recommends a 2-year minimal interval based on a Canadian study that demonstrated no increase in side effects with the shorter interval.

Minimal intervals have not been prescribed before or after TdaP, and any other vaccine can be given concomitantly with it. TdaP is recommended for wound management in place of Td. If the individual has no history of receipt of the primary DTaP series, then he or she should receive 3 doses of vaccine; the 1st should be with TdaP, and the next 2 should be Td at 4 weeks and 6 months after the TdaP.

STORAGE. The dose for both brands of TdaP is 0.5 mL injected intramuscularly. Boostrix is available in 0.5-mL single-dose vials and syringes, and Adacel is available in 0.5-mL single-dose vials. Both products should be refrigerated (2° to 8° C, [35° to 46° F]) but not frozen.

ADVERSE REACTIONS. Side effects from TdaP include mild pain at the injection site (75% to 88%), redness and swelling (11% to 22%), low-grade fever, headache, and fatigue. All side effects are comparable to those from Td vaccination.

CONTRAINDICATIONS AND PRECAUTIONS. Contraindications to TdaP include a severe (anaphylactic) allergic reaction after a prior dose of the vaccine or its components, as well as a history of encephalopathy within 7 days of administration of a pertussis-containing vaccine. Vaccination should be deferred for persons with a moderate to severe acute illness until the illness improves. Contraindications and precautions are detailed on the CDC Web site at www.cdc.gov/nip/vfc/acip_resolutions/605dtap.pdf.

Human Papillomavirus Vaccine

HPV is the most common sexually transmitted infection in the United States, with an estimated 6 million infections each year, 74% of which occur in adolescents ages 15 to 24.[79] Although 32% to 46% of adolescents and young women are infected with HPV, a small percentage go on to develop cervical dysplasia and eventually cervical cancer.[80,81] Specific subtypes of HPV are considered high-risk and are associated with cervical carcinoma, whereas others are low-risk and can lead to genital or other cutaneous warts. HPV subtypes 16 and 18 are known to be present in least 70% of cervical cancers, and types 6 and 11 are the related to 90% of anogenital warts.[82,83]

The HPV DNA structure consists of an early and late functional region, which encodes 6 early (E1, E2, E4, E5, E6, E7) and 2 late (L1, L2) proteins. The L1 protein forms part of the viral capsid that can be reproduced using recombinant techniques in eukaryotic cells. The proteins self-assemble into virus-like particles (VLPs), which lack a viral DNA core and thus are not infectious. The VLPs in the vaccine can induce antibody titers 100-fold higher than natural infection.[84]

One HPV vaccine is licensed, and one candidate vaccine is undergoing clinical trials. In a study of the now-licensed quadrivalent vaccine (targeting HPV types 6, 11, 16, and 18) given at 0, 2 and 6 months of age, the incidence of HPV disease was decreased by 90% over 36-month follow-up compared with individuals receiving placebo.[85] A 2nd vaccine (targeting types 16 and 18) provided at 0, 1, and 6 months of age had a 92% to 95% efficacy against incident HPV-type specific infection.[86]

Investigators have found that vaccine efficacy, physician endorsement, cost, knowledge about HPV, and personal beliefs about vaccination are important predictors of HPV vaccine acceptability among adolescent and adult women.[87,88] The vaccine has been shown to be cost effective when combined with continued Papanicolaou testing.[89] Papanicolaou testing would continue to be recommended because not all HPV types could be included in one vaccine.

Other vaccines for sexually transmitted infections may become available within the next decade. A vaccine against herpes simplex virus (HSV) was found to have an efficacy of 74% in HSV-seronegative women but was not effective for men or HSV-1–seropositive women.[90] The potential effect of such a vaccine depends, in large part, on its ability to blunt viral shedding.[91] Several vaccines against *Chlamydia trachomatis* are in development, ranging from DNA vaccines to live attenuated vaccines. Animal studies are promising, but vaccines for adolescents are still several years away.[92]

CONCLUSION: GREAT EXPECTATIONS FOR THE FUTURE OF VACCINATION

Until the late 1980s, routine childhood vaccination had been a field marked by slow, but steady, progress. Since that time (and into the foreseeable future), routine vaccination has been anything but routine. Driven by major advances in biotechnology, the performance of childhood immunization, in terms of disease prevention, has been remarkable. However, this increased performance has come at the cost of increased complexity, including more choices among vaccines and combinations of vaccines and a more complex and rapidly changing immunization schedule. For example, combination vaccines allow prevention of diseases with fewer injections; however, the presence of nonoverlapping, noncomplementary vaccines (eg, DTaP-Hib, Hib-HBV) makes the choice of which vaccines to purchase difficult.

Advances in biotechnology will continue to bring new combination vaccines, vaccines against additional diseases, improvements in existing vaccines, and more changes in the routine vaccination schedule. At this time, more than 20 vaccines are at various stages of development and testing. More combination vaccines will lead to greater complexity in the short term, but these combinations will eventually produce protection from disease with fewer injections; they will also facilitate vaccination against newly preventable diseases by piggybacking new vaccines onto accepted and fully implemented vaccines.

Just as vaccine technology is changing, so is the US immunization delivery system. For example, a greater proportion of immunizations are now given in the private sector than was the case a decade ago. This privatization of immunization delivery is being driven by the need for efficiency, changes in the financing of vaccines, changes in the health care industry, and parental preferences. On average, health department clinics generally see a more impoverished population of children than do private practitioners. Therefore, as the health department clinics are being used less frequently for referral of children who have no insurance coverage for immunizations, the private sector will care for an increasing share of high-risk patients.

Much has been accomplished since 1796 when Edward Jenner inoculated James Phipps with cowpox, terming the procedure *vaccination* (after the word *vacca* for cow). The future is bright for children to live free of many vaccine-preventable diseases. By combining technologic advances of vaccines with aggressive delivery of immunizations by primary care clinicians and public health practitioners, the present health care system will ensure healthier lives for children.

TOOLS FOR PRACTICE

Engaging Patients and Family

- *After the Shots.... What to do if your child has discomfort* (fact sheet), Immunization Action Coalition (www.immunize.org/nslt.d/n17/p4015.htm).
- *Are you 11-19 years old?* (fact sheet), Immunization Action Coalition (www.immunize.org/catg.d/11teens8.pdf).
- *Vaccines for Adolescents* (fact sheet), Centers for Disease Control and Prevention (www.cdc.gov/nip/publications/flyers/f_imz_child.pdf).
- *Common Immunization and Vaccination Questions* (fact sheet), American Academy of Pediatrics (www.cispimmunize.org/ill/ill_main.htm).
- *Chickenpox* (fact sheet), American Academy of Pediatrics (www.cispimmunize.org/ill/ill_main.htm).
- *The Chickenpox Vaccine* (brochure), American Academy of Pediatrics (patiented.aap.org).
- *Child Health Record* (booklet), American Academy of Pediatrics (www.aap.org/bookstore).
- *Recommended Childhood and Adolescent Immunization Schedule United States-2007* (fact sheet), American Academy of Pediatrics (www.cispimmunize.org/ill/ill_main.htm).
- *Diphtheria* (fact sheet), American Academy of Pediatrics (www.cispimmunize.org/ill/ill_main.htm).
- *Haemophilus Influenzae type b* (brochure), American Academy of Pediatrics (patiented.aap.org).
- *Haemophilus Influenzae Type b* (fact sheet), American Academy of Pediatrics (www.cispimmunize.org/ill/ill_main.htm).
- *Hepatitis B* (brochure), American Academy of Pediatrics (patiented.aap.org).
- *Hepatitis B* (fact sheet), American Academy of Pediatrics (www.cispimmunize.org/ill/ill_main.htm).
- *Immunizations & Infectious Diseases: An Informed Parents Guide* (book), American Academy of Pediatrics (patiented.aap.org).
- *Immunizations for Babies: A schedule for parents* (fact sheet), Immunization Action Coalition (www.immunize.org/catg.d/p4010.htm).
- *Immunization Information on the Internet* (fact sheet), American Academy of Pediatrics (www.cispimmunize.org/ill/ill_main.htm).
- *Immunizations: What You Need to Know* (brochure), American Academy of Pediatrics (patiented.aap.org).
- *Influenza* (fact sheet), American Academy of Pediatrics (www.cispimmunize.org/ill/ill_main.htm).
- *Measles* (fact sheet), American Academy of Pediatrics (www.cispimmunize.org/ill/ill_main.htm).
- *Meningococcal Disease—Information for Teens and College Students* (brochure), American Academy of Pediatrics (patiented.aap.org).
- *MMR Vaccine and Autism* (fact sheet), Centers for Disease Control and Prevention (www.cdc.gov/nip/vacsafe/concerns/autism/autism-mmr-facts.htm).
- *Multiple Vaccines and the Immune System* (fact sheet), Centers for Disease Control and Prevention (www.cdc.gov/od/science/iso/concerns/multiplevaccines.htm).
- *Mumps* (fact sheet), American Academy of Pediatrics (www.cispimmunize.org/ill/ill_main.htm).
- *Parents Guide to Childhood Immunization* (booklet), Centers for Disease Control and Prevention (www.cispimmunize.org/mediapgs/pg_pdf.html).
- *Pertussis (Whooping Cough)* (fact sheet), American Academy of Pediatrics (www.cispimmunize.org/ill/ill_main.htm).
- *Pneumococcal Disease* (fact sheet), American Academy of Pediatrics (www.cispimmunize.org/ill/ill_main.htm).
- *Pneumococcal Infection and Vaccine* (brochure), American Academy of Pediatrics (patiented.aap.org).
- *Polio* (fact sheet), American Academy of Pediatrics (www.cispimmunize.org/ill/ill_main.htm).
- *Rubella (German Measles)* (fact sheet), American Academy of Pediatrics (www.cispimmunize.org/ill/ill_main.htm).
- *Tetanus (Lockjaw)* (fact sheet), American Academy of Pediatrics (www.cispimmunize.org/ill/ill_main.htm).
- *Vaccine Information Statements (VIS)* (fact sheet), Centers for Disease Control and Prevention (www.cdc.gov/nip/publications/VIS/default.htm).
- *Vaccine Safety FAQ #1* (fact sheet), American Academy of Pediatrics (www.cispimmunize.org/fam/facts/SafetyFAQ.pdf).
- *Vaccine Safety FAQ #2* (fact sheet), American Academy of Pediatrics (www.cispimmunize.org/fam/facts/FAQ-Vaccine%20Safety2.pdf).
- *What Parents Should Know About Measles-Mumps-Rubella (MMR) Vaccine and Autism* (fact sheet), American Academy of Pediatrics (www.cispimmunize.org/ill/ill_main.htm).
- *What Parents Should Know About Thimerosal* (fact sheet), American Academy of Pediatrics (www.cispimmunize.org/fam/autism/thimerosal.htm).
- *What Vaccines Do You Need? Adolescent and Adult* (questionnaire), Centers for Disease Control and Prevention (www2.cdc.gov/nip/adultImmSched/).
- *Immunization: What You Need to Know* (brochure), American Academy of Pediatrics (patiented.aap.org).

Medical Decision Support

- *AAP Immunization Initiatives Newsletter* (Newsletter), American Academy of Pediatrics (aappolicy.aappublications.org/cgi/content/abstract/pediatrics;115/5/1428).

- *ACIP Recommendations* (Web page), Centers for Disease Control and Prevention (www.cdc.gov/nip/publications/acip-list.htm).
- *Compare the Risks* (fact sheet), American Academy of Pediatrics (www.cispimmunize.org/).
- *Contraindications to Vaccines Chart* (chart), Centers for Disease Control and Prevention (www.cdc.gov/nip/recs/contraindications_vacc.htm).
- *GBS and Menactra Meningococcal Vaccine* (fact sheet), Centers for Disease Control and Prevention (www.cdc.gov/od/science/iso/concerns/gbsfactsheet.htm).
- *Guide to Contraindications to Vaccinations* (Web page), Centers for Disease Control and Prevention (www.cdc.gov/nip/recs/contraindications.htm).
- *Immunization Schedules as Laminated Cards* (card), Centers for Disease Control and Prevention (www.cdc.gov/nip/recs/lamincard-instruct.htm).
- *Immunization Practice Toolkit* (toolkit), Centers for Disease Control and Prevention (www2.cdc.gov/nip/isd/immtoolkit/default.htm).
- *Mercury and Vaccines (Thimerosal)* (Web page), Centers for Disease Control and Prevention (www.cdc.gov/od/science/iso/concerns/thimerosal.htm).
- *Principles of Vaccination* (booklet), Centers for Disease Control and Prevention (www.cdc.gov/nip/publications/pink/prinvac.pdf).
- *Photos of Children With Vaccine Preventable Diseases* (Web page), American Academy of Pediatrics (www.cispimmunize.org/mediapgs/photos.htm).
- *Quick Reference—Vaccine Preventable Diseases Chart* (Web page), Centers for Disease Control and Prevention (www.cdc.gov/nip/diseases/disease-chart-hcp.htm).
- *Red Book,* 27th edition (book), American Academy of Pediatrics (www.aap.org/bookstore).
- *Summary of Recommendations for Childhood and Adolescent Immunization* (fact sheet), Immunization Action Coalition (www.immunize.org/catg.d/rules1.pdf).
- *Screening Questionnaire for Child and Teen Immunization* (questionnaire), Immunization Action Coalition (www.immunize.org/catg.d/p4060scr.pdf).
- *Six Common Misconceptions about vaccination and how to respond to them* (Web page), Centers for Disease Control and Prevention (www.cdc.gov/nip/publications/6mishome.htm).
- *Vaccine Adverse Event Reporting System* (Web page), Centers for Disease Control and Prevention (vaers.hhs.gov/).
- *Vaccine Safety: The Providers Role* (fact sheet), Centers for Disease Control and Prevention (www.cdc.gov/nip/vacsafe/providers_role.htm).

Community Coordination and Advocacy

- *State Vaccine Requirements for School Entry* (other), National Network for Immunization Information (www.immunizationinfo.org/vaccineInfo/index.cfm).

Practice Management

- *The Business Case for Pricing New Vaccines* (fact sheet), American Academy of Pediatrics (www.aap.org/moc/displaytemp/BusinessCase.pdf).
- *Pediatric Council Immunization* Toolkit (Web page), American Academy of Pediatrics (www.aap.org/secure-moc/chapters/immunkit.pdf).
- *Standing Orders* (fact sheet), Immunization Action Coalition (www.immunize.org/standingorders/).
- *Vaccine Management—Recommendations for Storage and Handling of Selected Biologicals* (booklet), Centers for Disease Control and Prevention (www.cdc.gov/nip/publications/vac_mgt_book.pdf).
- *Vaccine Storage and Handling Toolkit* (Web page), Centers for Disease Control and Prevention (www2a.cdc.gov/nip/isd/shtoolkit/splash.html).

Web Sites

- *Childhood Immunization Support Program—Immunization Initiatives* (Web page), American Academy of Pediatrics (www.cispimmunize.org/).
- *The Children's Hospital of Philadelphia—Vaccine Education Center* (Web page), CHOP Vaccine Education Center (www.chop.edu/consumer/jsp/division/generic.jsp?id=75697).
- *Epidemiology & Prevention of Vaccine-Preventable Diseases* (Web page), Centers for Disease Control and Prevention (www.cdc.gov/nip/publications/pink/def_pink_full.htm).
- *Immunization Action Coalition* (Web page), Immunization Action Coalition (www.immunize.org/).
- *Institute for Vaccine Safety* (Web page), Institute for Vaccine Safety (www.vaccinesafety.edu/).
- *National Network for Immunization Information* (Web page), National Network for Immunization Information (www.immunizationinfo.org/).
- *Travelers Health—What You Need to Know About Vaccinations and Travel: A Checklist* (Web page), Centers for Disease Control and Prevention (www.cdc.gov/travel/vaccinat.htm).

AAP POLICY STATEMENTS

American Academy of Pediatrics. Age for routine administration of the second dose of measles-mumps-rubella vaccine. *Pediatrics.* 1998;101:129-133. (aappolicy.aappublications.org/cgi/content/full/pediatrics;101/1/129).

American Academy of Pediatrics. Combination vaccines for childhood immunization: recommendations of the Advisory Committee on Immunization Practices. *Pediatrics.* 1999;103:1064-1077. (aappolicy.aappublications.org/cgi/content/full/pediatrics;103/5/1064).

American Academy of Pediatrics. Immunization of preterm and low birth weight infants. *Pediatrics.* 2003;112:193-198. (aappolicy.aappublications.org/cgi/content/full/pediatrics;112/1/193).

American Academy of Pediatrics. Prevention and control of meningococcal disease: recommendations for use of meningococcal vaccines in pediatric patients. *Pediatrics.* 2005;116:496-505. (aappolicy.aappublications.org/cgi/content/full/pediatrics;116/2/496).

American Academy of Pediatrics. Prevention of pertussis among adolescents: recommendations for use of tetanus and diphtheria toxoids and acellular pertussis (Tdap) vaccines. *Pediatrics.* 2006;117(3):965-978. (aappolicy.aappublications.org/cgi/content/full/pediatrics;117/3/965).

American Academy of Pediatrics. Prevention of rotavirus disease: guidelines for use of rotavirus vaccine. *Pediatrics.* 2007;119(1):171-182.

American Academy of Pediatrics. Recommendations for influenza immunization of children. *Pediatrics.* 2008;121(4): e1016-e1031. (aappolicy.aappublications.org/cgi/content/full/pediatrics;121/4/e1016).

American Academy of Pediatrics. Recommended immunization schedules for children and adolescents—United States 2007. *Pediatrics.* 2008;121(1):219-220. (aappolicy.aappublications.org/cgi/content/full/pediatrics;121/1/219).

American Academy of Pediatrics. Reduction of the influenza burden in children. *Pediatrics.* 2002;110(6):e80. (aappolicy.aappublications.org/cgi/content/full/pediatrics;110/6/e80).

American Academy of Pediatrics. Responding to parental refusals of immunization of children—clinical report. *Pediatrics.* 2005;115(5):1428-1431. (aappolicy.aappublications.org/cgi/content/full/pediatrics;115/5/1428).

American Academy of Pediatrics, Committee on Infectious Diseases. Prevention of Varicella: Recommendations for use of varicella vaccines in children, including a recommendation for a routine 2-dose varicella immunization schedule. *Pediatrics.* 2007;120(1):221-231. (aappolicy.aappublications.org/cgi/content/full/pediatrics;120/1/221).

SUGGESTED RESOURCES

Books

Centers for Disease Control and Prevention. *Epidemiology and Prevention of Vaccine-Preventable Diseases.* Atkinson W, Hamborsky J, McIntyre L, et al, eds. 10th ed. Washington, DC: Public Health Foundation, 2007. This resource is an excellent book that discusses diseases, their epidemiology, and the vaccines. Included as appendices are key immunization resources. The book is available from the Public Health Foundation at 1-877-252-1200 or 1-800-41TRAIN. The text and accompanying slides also are available at www.cdc.gov/vaccines/pubs/pinkbook/default.htm.

American Academy of Pediatrics, Pickering LK, ed. *Red Book 2006: Report of the Committee on Infectious Diseases.* 27th ed. Elk Grove Village, IL: American Academy of Pediatrics; 2006. This book can be ordered at aapredbook.aappublications.org.

Marshall GS, Dennehy PH, Greenberg DP, et al. *The Vaccine Handbook. A Practical Guide for Clinicians.* Philadelphia, PA: Lippincott Williams & Wilkins; 2004. (This resource is also available for personal digital assistant.)

Centers for Disease Control and Prevention. *Vaccine Management: Recommendations for Handling and Storage of Selected Biologicals.* Washington, DC: US Department of Health and Human Services; 1996. Available at: www.cdc.gov/nip/publications/vac_mgt_book.pdf.

Humiston SG, Good C. *Vaccinating Your Child: Questions and Answers for the Concerned Parent.* 2nd ed. Atlanta, GA: Peachtree Publications; 2000. This resource includes a foreword by David Satcher, MD, former U.S. Surgeon General, and former director of the CDC. Available at: www.peachtree-online.com/Adults/Catalog/vaccinating.htm.

Immunization Action Coalition. *Needle Tips.* This resource is a periodical that is published every 6 months by the Immunization Action Coalition. It contains timely and extraordinarily user-friendly information of interest to all who provide immunizations. A free subscription can be obtained by writing to IAC, 1573 Selby Avenue, St. Paul, MN 55104, by calling 651-647-9009, or by visiting www.immunize.org.

Offit P, Bell L. *Vaccines: What You Should Know.* 3rd ed. New York, NY: Wiley Publications; 2003. (Also available as an e-book.) Available at: www.wiley.com/wileycda/wileytitle/productCd-0471420042,descCd-authorInfo.html.

Journal articles

Centers for Disease Control and Prevention. Vaccine-preventable diseases: improving vaccination coverage in children, adolescents, and adults: a report on recommendations of the Task Force on Community Preventive Services. *MMWR.* 1999;48(RR8):1-18.

Other resources

For more information on the principles of vaccination, please refer to *The Epidemiology and Prevention of Vaccine-Preventable Diseases.* This text is available free on the Internet at www.cdc.gov/vaccines/pubs/pinkbook/default.htm. In addition, the ACIP's *General Recommendations on Immunization* is an invaluable resource.

REFERENCES

1. Centers for Disease Control and Prevention. Ten great public health achievements—United States, 1900-1999. *MMWR.* 1999;48(50):1141. Available at www.cdc.gov/mmwr/PDF/wk/mm4850.pdf. Accessed June 19, 2006.
2. Centers for Disease Control and Prevention. Impact of Vaccines in the 20th Century. Available at: www.cdc.gov/vaccines/pubs/pinkbook/downloads/appendices/G/impact-of-vaccines.pdf. Accessed June 19, 2006.
3. Centers for Disease Control and Prevention. Measles—United States, 1996, and the interruption of indigenous transmission. *MMWR.* 1997;46(11):242-246. Available at: www.cdc.gov/mmwr/preview/mmwrhtml/00046958.htm. Accessed June 19, 2006.
4. Centers for Disease Control and Prevention. Global measles and rubella laboratory network—January 2004-June 2005. *MMWR.* 2005;54(43):1100-1104.
5. Robbins FC, de Quadros CA. Certification of the eradication of indigenous transmission of wild poliovirus in the Americas. *J Infect Dis.* 1997;175(suppl 1):S281-S285.
6. Centers for Disease Control and Prevention. National, state, and urban area vaccination coverage among children aged 19-35 months—United States, 2004. *MMWR.* 2005;54(29):717-721. Available at: www.cdc.gov/mmwr/preview/mmwrhtml/mm5429a1.htm. Accessed June 19, 2006.
7. Centers for Disease Control and Prevention. Immunization Schedules. Available at www.cdc.gov/vaccines/recs/schedules/default.htm. Accessed June 21, 2007.
8. Kroger AT, Atkinson WL, Marcuse EK, et al. General Recommendations on Immunization: Recommendations of the Advisory Committee of Immunization Practices (ACIP). *MMWR.* 2006;55(RR15):1-48. Available at: www.cdc.gov/mmwr/preview/mmwrhtml/rr5515a1.htm. Accessed June 22, 2007.
9. American Academy of Pediatrics, Committee on Infectious Diseases. Prevention of pertussis among adolescents: recommendations for use of tetanus toxoid, reduced diphtheria toxoid, and acellular pertussis (TdaP) vaccine. *Pediatrics.* 2006;117(3):965-978.
10. Centers for Disease Control and Prevention. Notice to readers: FDA licensure of diphtheria and tetanus toxoids and acellular pertussis adsorbed, hepatitis B (recombinant), and poliovirus vaccine combined, (PEDIARIX™) for use in infants. *MMWR.* 2003;52(10):203-204. Available at: www.cdc.gov/mmwr/preview/mmwrhtml/mm5210a8.htm. Accessed June 19, 2006.
11. US Department of Health and Human Services, US Food and Drug Administration. Product approval information. (Haemophilus b Conjugate [Meningococcal Protein Conjugate] and Hepatitis B [Recombinant] Vaccine, trade name COMVAX®). Available at: www.fda.gov/cber/approvltr/hbHB100296L.htm. Accessed June 19, 2006.
12. American Academy of Pediatrics. Committee on Infectious Diseases 1998-1999. Combination vaccines for childhood immunization: recommendations of the Advisory Committee on Immunization Practices, the American Academy of Pediatrics, and the American Academy of Family Physicians. *Pediatrics.* 1999;103(5):1064-1077. Available at: aappolicy.aappublications.org/cgi/content/full/pediatrics;103/5/1064. Accessed June 19, 2006.

13. Centers for Disease Control and Prevention. Recommended and Minimum Ages and Intervals between Vaccine Doses. Available at: www.cdc.gov/vaccines/pubs/pinkbook/downloads/appendices/A/age-interval-table.pdf. Accessed June 19, 2006.
14. Centers for Disease Control and Prevention. Recommended Immunization Schedule for Children and Adolescents Who Start Late or Who Are More than 1 Month Behind. Available at: www.immunize.org/cdc/child-schedule.pdf (see page 2). Accessed June 19, 2006.
15. American Academy of Pediatrics. Measles Table 2. In: Pickering LK, Baker, CJ, Long SS, et al, eds. *Red Book: 2006 Report of the Committee on Infectious Diseases.* 27th ed. Elk Grove Village, IL: American Academy of Pediatrics; 2006.
16. Centers for Disease Control and Prevention. Suggested Intervals between Administration of Immune Globulin Preparations for Different Indications and Measles-Containing Vaccine and Varicella Vaccine. Available at: www.cdc.gov/vaccines/pubs/pinkbook/downloads/appendices/A/mmr_ig.pdf. Accessed June 19, 2006.
17. Centers for Disease Control and Prevention. Translations of Foreign-Language Terms. Available at: www.cdc.gov/vaccines/pubs/pinkbook/downloads/appendices/B/foreign-products-tables.pdf. Accessed June 19, 2006.
18. American Academy of Pediatrics, Pickering LK, ed. *Red Book 2006: Report of the Committee on Infectious Diseases.* 27th ed. Elk Grove Village, IL: American Academy of Pediatrics; 2006. Available at: aapredbook.aappublications.org.
19. Centers for Disease Control and Prevention. Vaccination of Hematopoietic Stem Cell Transplant Recipients. Available at: www.cdc.gov/vaccines/pubs/downloads/hsct-recs.pdf. Accessed June 19, 2006.
20. American Academy of Pediatrics, Committee on Infectious Diseases and Committee on Pediatric AIDS. Measles immunization in HIV-infected children. *Pediatrics.* 1999;103(5):1057-1060. Available at: aappolicy.aappublications.org/cgi/content/full/pediatrics;103/5/1057. Accessed June 19, 2006.
21. National Network for Immunization Information. Immunization Issues—Vaccines for Pregnant Women. Available at: www.immunizationinfo.org/immunization_issues_detail.cfv?id=90. Accessed June 19, 2006.
22. Centers for Disease Control and Prevention. Guidelines for Vaccinating Pregnant Women. Available at: www.cdc.gov/nip/publications/preg_guide.htm. Accessed June 19, 2006.
23. Mast EE, Margolis HS, Fiore AE, et al. A comprehensive immunization strategy to eliminate transmission of hepatitis b virus infection in the United States: recommendations of the Advisory Committee on Immunization Practices, Part 1: immunization of infants, children, and adolescents. *MMWR.* 2005;54(RR16):1-23. Available at: www.cdc.gov/mmwr/preview/mmwrhtml/rr5416a1.htm. Accessed June 19, 2006.
24. Saari TN, Committee on Infectious Diseases. Immunization of preterm and low birth weight infants. *Pediatrics.* 2003;112(1):193-198. Available at: pediatrics.aappublications.org/cgi/content/full/112/1/193. Accessed June 19, 2006.
25. Centers for Disease Control and Prevention. Pertussis vaccination: use of acellular pertussis vaccines among infants and young children: recommendations of the Advisory Committee on Immunization Practices. *MMWR.* 1997;46(RR-7):1-25. Available at: www.cdc.gov/mmwr/preview/mmwrhtml/00048610.htm. Accessed June 19, 2006.
26. Centers for Disease Control and Prevention. Final 2005 reports of notifiable diseases. *MMWR.* 2006;55:880-881.
27. Fiore AE, Wasley A, Bell BP. Prevention of hepatitis A through active or passive immunization: recommendations of the Advisory Committee on Immunization Practices (ACIP). *MMWR.* 2006;55(RR07):1-23. Available at: www.cdc.gov/mmwr/preview/mmwrhtml/rr5507a1.htm. Accessed June 19, 2006.
28. Centers for Disease Control and Prevention. Prevention of hepatitis A through active or passive immunization: recommendations of the Advisory Committee on Immunization Practices (ACIP). *MMWR.* 1999;48(RR-12):1-37. Available at: www.cdc.gov/mmwr/preview/mmwrhtml/rr4812a1.htm. Accessed June 19, 2006.
29. Mast EE, Margolis HS, Fiore AE, et al. A comprehensive immunization strategy to eliminate transmission of hepatitis B virus infection in the United States: recommendations of the Advisory Committee on Immunization Practices (ACIP). Part 1: Immunization of infants, children, and adolescents. *MMWR.* 2005;54(RR16):1-23. Available at: www.cdc.gov/mmwr/preview/mmwrhtml/rr5416a1.htm?s_cid=rr5416a1_e. Accessed June 21, 2007.
30. Centers for Disease Control and Prevention. Update: recommendations to prevent hepatitis B virus transmission—United States. *MMWR.* 1999;48(2):33-34. Available at: www.cdc.gov/mmwr/preview/mmwrhtml/00056293.htm. Accessed June 19, 2006.
31. Centers for Disease Control and Prevention. Haemophilus b conjugate vaccines for prevention of Haemophilus influenzae type b disease among infants and children 2 months of age and older: recommendations of the Advisory Committee on Immunization Practices (ACIP). *MMWR.* 1991;40(RR01):1-7. Available at: www.cdc.gov/mmwr/preview/mmwrhtml/00041736.htm. Accessed June 19, 2006.
32. Centers for Disease Control and Prevention. Detailed Vaccination Schedule for Haemophilus Influenzae type b Conjugate Vaccines. (See page 9 of 13.) Available at: www.cdc.gov/vaccines/pubs/pinkbook/downloads/hib.rtf. Accessed June 19, 2006.
33. Rennels MB, Meissner HC, American Academy of Pediatrics, Committee on Infectious Diseases. Technical report: reduction of the influenza burden in children. *Pediatrics,* 2002;110(6):e80. Available at: www.pediatrics.org/cgi/content/full/110/6/e80. Accessed June 19, 2006.
34. American Academy of Pediatrics, Committee on Infectious Diseases. Reduction of the influenza burden in children. *Pediatrics.* 2002;110(6):1246-1252. Available at: aappolicy.aappublications.org/cgi/content/full/pediatrics;110/6/1246. Accessed June 19, 2006.
35. Centers for Disease Control and Prevention. Record of the Meeting of the Advisory Committee on Immunization Practices, February 21-22, 2006 (page 67 of 111).
36. Harper SA, Fukuda K, Uyeki TM, et al. Prevention and control of influenza: recommendations of the Advisory Committee on Immunization Practices (ACIP). *MMWR.* 2005;54(RR08):1-40. Available at: www.cdc.gov/mmwr/preview/mmwrhtml/rr5408a1.htm. Accessed June 19, 2006.
37. Centers for Disease Control and Prevention. Vaccine Management: Recommendations for Storage and Handling Selected Biologicals: LAIV. Available at: www.cdc.gov/nip/publications/vac_mgt_book.htm. Accessed June 19, 2006.
38. Shinefield H, Black S, Digilio L, et al. Evaluation of a quadrivalent measles, mumps, rubella and varicella vaccine in healthy children. *Pediatr Infect Dis J.* 2005;24(8):665-669.
39. US Department of Health and Human Services, US Food and Drug Administration. Product Approval Information—Licensing Action (Measles, Mumps, Rubella and Varicella Virus Vaccine Live). Available at: www.fda.gov/cber/approvltr/mmrvmer090605L.htm. Accessed June 19, 2006.

40. Centers for Disease Control and Prevention. Measles, mumps, and rubella—vaccine use and strategies for elimination of measles, rubella, and congenital rubella syndrome and control of mumps: recommendations of the Advisory Committee on Immunization Practices (ACIP). *MMWR*. 1998:47(RR-8):1-57. Available at: www.cdc.gov/mmwr/preview/mmwrhtml/00053391.htm. Accessed June 19, 2006.
41. American Academy of Pediatrics, Committee on Infectious Diseases. Policy Statement: Age for routine administration. *Pediatrics*. 1998;101(1):129-133. Available at: aappolicy.aappublications.org/cgi/content/full/pediatrics;101/1/129. Accessed June 19, 2006.
42. National Network for Immunization Information. Immunization Science. Available at: www.immunizationinfo.org/immunization_science.cfm?cat=2. Accessed June 19, 2006.
43. Institute of Medicine of the National Academies. Immunization Safety Review: Measles-Mumps-Rubella Vaccine and Autism, April 2001. Available at: www.iom.edu/CMS/3793/4705/4715.aspx. Accessed November 21, 2006.
44. Overturf GD, American Academy of Pediatrics—Committee on Infectious Diseases. Technical report: prevention of pneumococcal infections, including the use of pneumococcal conjugate and polysaccharide vaccines and antibiotic prophylaxis. *Pediatrics*. 2000;106(2):367-376. Available at: aappolicy.aappublications.org/cgi/content/full/pediatrics;106/2/367. Accessed June 19, 2006.
45. Centers for Disease Control and Prevention. Preventing pneumococcal disease among infants and young children: recommendations of the Advisory Committee on Immunization Practices (ACIP). *MMWR*. 2000;49(RR09):1-38. Available at: www.cdc.gov/mmwr/preview/mmwrhtml/rr4909a1.htm. Accessed June 19, 2006.
46. Centers for Disease Control and Prevention. Recommended Schedule for Use of 7-Valent Pneumococcal Conjugate Vaccine (PCV7) among Previously Unvaccinated Infants and Children By Age at Time of First Vaccination. (Table 10) Available at: www.cdc.gov/mmwr/preview/mmwrhtml/rr4909a1.htm#tab10. Accessed June 19, 2006.
47. Centers for Disease Control and Prevention. Recommendations for Use of 7-Valent Pneumococcal Conjugate Vaccine (PCV7) among Children with a Lapse in Vaccine Administration. (Table 11) Available at: www.cdc.gov/mmwr/preview/mmwrhtml/rr4909a1.htm#tab11. Accessed June 19, 2006.
48. Centers for Disease Control and Prevention. Pneumococcal Conjugate Vaccine Information Statement. Available at: www.immunize.org/vis/pnPCV7.pdf. Accessed June 19, 2006.
49. Global Polio Eradication Initiative. Global Case Count. Available at: www.polioeradication.org/. Accessed June 19, 2006.
50. American Academy of Pediatrics, Committee on Infectious Diseases. Policy Statement: Prevention of recommendations for use of only inactivated poliovirus vaccine for routine immunization. *Pediatrics*. 1999;104(6):1404-1406. Available at: aappolicy.aappublications.org/cgi/content/full/pediatrics;104/6/1404. Accessed June 19, 2006.
51. Centers for Disease Control and Prevention. Poliomyelitis prevention in the United States: updated recommendations of the Advisory Committee on Immunization Practices (ACIP). *MMWR*. 2000;49(RR05):1-22. Available at: www.cdc.gov/mmwr/preview/mmwrhtml/rr4905a1.htm. Accessed June 19, 2006.
52. Hsu VP, Staat MA, Roberts N, et al. Use of active surveillance to validate international classification of diseases code estimates of rotavirus hospitalizations in children. *Pediatrics*. 2005;115(1):78-82.
53. Centers for Disease Control and Prevention, National Center for Infectious Diseases, Respiratory and Enteric Viruses Branch. Rotavirus. Available at: www.cdc.gov/rotavirus. Accessed June 19, 2006.
54. Rotavirus and Rotavirus Vaccines: Proceedings of the 6th International Rotavirus Symposium. Available at: www.sabin.org. Accessed June 19, 2006.
55. Vesikari T, Matson DO, Dennehy P, et al. Safety and efficacy of a pentavalent human-bovine (WC3) reassortant rotavirus vaccine. *N Engl J Med*. 2006;354(1):23-33. Available at: content.nejm.org/cgi/content/abstract/354/1/23. Accessed June 19, 2006.
56. Centers for Disease Control and Prevention. Prevention of Rotavirus Gastroenteritis among Infants and Children: Provisional ACIP Recommendations for the Use of Rotavirus Vaccine (RV). Available at: www.cdc.gov/mmwr/preview/mmwrhtml/rr5512a1.htm. Accessed June 19, 2006.
57. US Department of Health and Human Services, US Food and Drug Administration. RotaTeq Prescribing Information. Available at: www.fda/gov/cber/label/rotateqLB.pdf. Accessed June 19, 2006.
58. Centers for Disease Control and Prevention. Rotavirus Vaccine Information Statement. Available at: www.immunize.org/vis/rota_06.pdf. Accessed June 19, 2006.
59. American Academy of Pediatrics, Committee on Infectious Diseases. Recommendations for the use of live attenuated varicella vaccine. *Pediatrics*. 1995;95:791-796.
60. Centers for Disease Control and Prevention. Prevention of varicella: recommendations of the Advisory Committee on Immunization Practices (ACIP). *MMWR*. 1996;45(RR-11):1-36.
61. Feder HM Jr, Hoss DM. Herpes zoster in otherwise healthy children. *Pediatr Infect Dis J*. 2004;23(5):451-457.
62. Bilukha OO, Rosenstein N, National Center for Infectious Diseases, Centers for Disease Control and Prevention. Prevention and control of meningococcal disease: recommendations of the Advisory Committee on Immunization Practices (ACIP). *MMWR*. 2005;54(RR-7):1-21.
63. Bruce MG, Rosenstein NE, Capparella JM, et al. Risk factors for meningococcal disease in college students. *JAMA*. 2000;286(6):688-693.
64. Harrison LH, Pass MA, Mendelsohn AB, et al. Invasive meningococcal disease in adolescents and young adults. *JAMA*. 2001;286(6):694-699.
65. American Academy of Pediatrics, Committee on Infectious Diseases. Prevention of pertussis among adolescents: recommendations for use of tetanus toxoid, reduced diphtheria toxoid, and acellular pertussis (TdaP) vaccine. *Pediatrics*. 2006;117(3):965-978.
66. Meningococcal disease and college students: recommendations of the Advisory Committee on Immunization Practices (ACIP). *MMWR Recom Rep*. 2000;49(RR-7):13-20.
67. US Department of Health and Human Services, US Food and Drug Administration. *Vaccines and Related Biological Products Advisory Committee, September 22, 2004: Briefing Information*. Rockville, MD: US Department of Health and Human Services, Food and Drug Administration; 2004. Available at: www.fda.gov/ohrms/dockets/ac/04/briefing/2004-4072b1.htm. Accessed June 19, 2006.
68. US Department of Health and Human Services, US Food and Drug Administration. Product approval information—licensing action. Rockville, MD: US Department of Health and Human Services, Food and Drug Administration, Center for Biologics Evaluation and Research; 2005. Available at: www.fda.gov/cber/products/meactra.htm. Accessed June 19, 2006.

69. Centers for Disease Control and Prevention. Guillain-Barré syndrome among recipients of Menactra meningococcal conjugate vaccine—United States, June-July 2005. *MMWR*. 2005;54(40):1023-1025.
70. Hopkins RS, Jajosky RA, Hall PA, et al, and the Centers for Disease Control and Prevention. Summary of notifiable diseases—United States, 2003. *MMWR*. 2005; 52(54):1-85.
71. Anonymous. Pertussis—United States, 1997-2000. *MMWR*. 2002;51(4):73-76.
72. Hewlett EL, Edwards KM. Clinical practice. Pertussis—not just for kids. *N Eng J Med*. 2005;352(12):1215-1222.
73. Van Damme P, Burgess M. Immunogenicity of a combined diphtheria-tetanus-acellular pertussis vaccine in adults. *Vaccine*. 2004;22(3-4):305-308.
74. Pichichero ME, Rennels MB, Edwards KM, et al. Combined tetanus, diphtheria, and 5-component pertussis vaccine for use in adolescents and adults. *JAMA*. 2005; 293(24):3003-3011.
75. Broder KR, Cortese MM, Iskander JK, et al. Preventing tetanus, diphtheria, and pertussis among adolescents: use of tetanus toxoid, reduced diphtheria toxoid and acellular pertussis vaccines: recommendations of the Advisory Committee on Immunization Practices (ACIP). *MMWR*. 2006;55(RR03):1-34. Available at: www.cdc.gov/mmwr/preview/mmwrhtml/rr5503a1.htm?s_cid=rr5503a1_e. Accessed June 21, 2007.
76. Kretsinger K, Broder KR, Cortese MM, et al. Preventing tetanus, diphtheria, and pertussis among adults: use of tetanus toxoid, reduced diphtheria toxoid and acellular pertussis: vaccine recommendations of ACIP, supported by the Healthcare Infection Control Practices Advisory Committee (HICPAC), for use of Tdap among health-care personnel. *MMWR*. 2006;55(RR17):1-33. Available at: www.cdc.gov/mmwr/preview/mmwrhtml/rr5517a1.htm. Accessed June 21, 2007.
77. GlaxoSmithKline. Boostrix prescribing information, May 2005. Available at: us.gsk.com/products/assets/us_boostrix.pdf. Accessed June 19, 2006.
78. Aventis Pasteur, Ltd. Adacel prescribing information, Sanofi Pasteur. Accessed 11/14/05. Available at: www.vaccineshoppe.com/US_PDF/ADACEL_2021114-2021543_6.05.pdf. Accessed June 19, 2006.
79. Weinstock H, Berman S, Cates W Jr. Sexually transmitted diseases among American youth: incidence and prevalence estimates, 2000. *Perspect Sex Reprod Health*. 2004;36(1):6-10.
80. Ho GY, Bierman R, Beardsley L, et al. Natural history of cervicovaginal papillomavirus infection in young women. *N Eng J Med*. 1998;338(7):423-428.
81. Winer RL, Lee SK, Hughes JP, et al. Genital human papillomavirus infection: incidence and risk factors in a cohort of female university students. *Am J Epidemiol*. 2003;157(3):218-226.
82. Munoz N, Bosch FX, de Sanjose S, et al. International Agency for Research on Cancer Multicenter Cervical Cancer Study Group. Epidemiologic classification of human papillomavirus types associated with cervical cancer. *N Engl J Med*. 2003;348(6):518-527.
83. von Krogh G. Management of anogenital warts (condylomata acuminata). *Eur J Dermatol*. 2001;11:598-604.
84. Schiller JT, Hidesheim A. Developing HPV virus-like particle vaccines to prevent cervical cancer: a progress report. *J Clin Virol*. 2000;19(1-2):67-74.
85. Villa LL, Costa RL, Petta CA, et al. Prophylactic quadrivalent human papillomavirus (types 6, 11, 16, and 18) L1 virus-like particle vaccine in young women: a randomized double-blind placebo-controlled multicentre phase II efficacy trial. *Lancet Oncol*. 2005;6(5): 271-278.
86. Harper DM, Franco EL, Wheeler C, et al. Efficacy of a bivalent L1 virus-like particle vaccine in prevention of infection with human papillomavirus types 16 and 18 in young women: a randomized controlled trial. *Lancet*. 2004;364(9447):1757-1765.
87. Zimet GD, Mays RM, Winston Y, et al. Acceptability of human papillomavirus immunization. *J Womens Health Gend Based Med*. 2000;9(1):47-50.
88. Kahn JA, Rosenthal SL, Hamann T, et al. Attitudes about human papillomavirus vaccine in young women. *Int J STD AIDS*. 2003;14(5):300-306.
89. Kulasingam SL, Myers ER. Potential health and economic impact of adding a human papillomavirus vaccine to screening programs. *JAMA*. 2003;290(6):781-789.
90. Stanberry LR, Spruance SL, Cunningham AL, et al. Glycoprotein-D-adjuvant vaccine to prevent genital herpes. *N Eng J Med*. 2002;347(21):1652-1661.
91. Garnett GP, Dubin G, Slaoui M, et al. The potential epidemiological impact of a genital herpes vaccine for women. *Sex Transm Infec*. 2004;80(1):24-29.
92. Zhang D, Yang X, Berry J, et al. DNA vaccination with the major outer-membrane protein gene induces acquired immunity to Chlamydia trachomatis (mouse pneumonitis) infection. *J Infect Dis*. 1997;176(4):1035-1040.

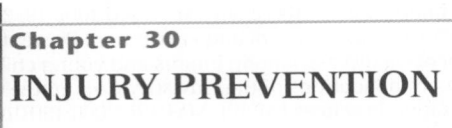

Chapter 30

INJURY PREVENTION

Rebecca Levin-Goodman, MPH; Gary A. Smith, MD, DrPH

INTRODUCTION

By many measures, injury is the most significant health problem of childhood and adolescence. Injury control includes (1) preventing events that might cause injury; (2) diminishing the likelihood or severity of injury, even though events with injury-causing potential occur; and (3) minimizing the effects of the injury, once it occurs, through state-of-the-art emergency response, medical care, and rehabilitation. This section concentrates on the first 2 parts of injury control, those classically considered as primary injury prevention, and describes the role of the pediatrician in the primary care setting in ensuring injury prevention. It highlights the critical opportunity to prevent injury by providing counseling about injury and injury prevention to children and families. Pediatricians can assume effective roles for injury prevention at many additional levels, for example, with schools, communities, local health departments, and state and national agencies and legislatures. Successful injury control demands active advocacy outside the pediatrician's office.

INCIDENCE

The number of unintentional injury deaths during childhood has been decreasing as a result, in part, of the hard work of pediatricians and public health professionals. However, injuries still cause a majority of deaths of children and adolescents aged 1 to 19 years. Although the leading causes of injury death vary by age group (Table 30-1), events involving motor vehicles, firearms, drowning, suffocation, and fires are important in every age group.

Table 30-1 Numbers and Rates of Injury Deaths by Age and Event and Percentage of All Deaths Caused by Injury, US Children and Adolescents (2004)

	AGE IN YEARS											
	<1		1-4		5-9		10-14		15-19		0-19	
EVENT	N	R	N	R	N	R	N	R	N	R	N	R
All Injury	1481	36.27	2065	12.92	1275	6.50	2069	9.79	10,637	51.33	17,527	21.50
Unintentional injury	1052	25.76	1641	10.27	1126	5.74	1540	7.29	6825	32.93	12,184	14.94
Motor vehicle traffic	139	3.40	520	3.25	584	2.98	922	4.36	5113	24.67	7278	8.93
Drowning	62	1.52	430	2.69	131	0.67	138	0.65	304	1.47	1065	1.31
Suffocation	725	17.76	125	0.78	45	0.23	68	0.32	68	0.33	1031	1.26
Poisoning	13	*	18	*	8	*	47	0.22	643	3.10	729	0.89
Fires, burns	28	0.69	228	1.43	169	0.86	87	0.41	66	0.32	578	0.71
Suicide	0	*	0	*	2	*	283	1.34	1700	8.20	1985	2.43
Homicide	325	7.96	377	2.36	122	0.62	207	0.98	1932	9.32	2963	3.63
Firearms (all intents)	7	*	51	0.32	61	0.31	239	1.13	2494	12.03	2852	3.50
Percentage of all deaths caused by injury	5%		43%		44%		52%		78%		33%†	

Data from Centers for Disease Control and Prevention, National Center for Injury Prevention and Control. Web-based Inquiry Statistics Query and Reporting System [database]. Available at: www.cdc.gov/ncipc/wisqars. Accessed May 1, 2007.

N, Number of deaths; *R*, deaths per 100,000 population.

*Rates based on 20 or fewer deaths may be unstable and are omitted.

†Sixty-three percent of deaths of persons aged 1 to 19 years are due to injury.

Although deaths may be the most often-noted injury statistic, injury results in acute morbidity, short- and long-term disability, and high medical care costs. The causes of nonfatal injury encompass those that produce fatal injury, but falls, burns, poisonings, fights, sports, and recreational activities (including play) are more prominent causes of nonfatal injury than they are of fatalities. For almost all types of injury, boys are at greater risk than girls. This increased risk has yet to be explained fully but may stem from several factors, including innate behavioral differences, societal expectations, and exposure. Children living in poverty are more likely to suffer serious and fatal injury of many types than advantaged children, and injury risk varies by geographic factors as well.

Successful injury prevention in the primary care setting is based on a clear understanding of the principles of injury prevention and on sound counseling skills.

PRINCIPLES OF INJURY CONTROL

Events leading to injury are, for the most part, predictable and preventable. They should not be considered as *accidents* because this term implies a sense of randomness and lack of preventability. In some instances, prevention is achieved through eliminating injury-producing events (eg, building divided highways to reduce motor vehicle crashes). Prevention is sometimes achieved by eliminating injury even though the event takes place (eg, protecting child passengers by restraining them in car safety seats).

When energy affects the body acutely at a damaging level, injury results. For most pediatric injuries, the energy is mechanical. However, thermal, chemical, radiation, and electrical energy are also agents of injury. To prevent injury, energy must be kept away from the child, or the energy transfer to tissue must be diffused over time or space (or both) so that it does not reach damaging levels. The former is well illustrated by building a bicycle path as an alternative to riding on streets with motor vehicles. The latter is illustrated by the protection provided by a helmet in a fall from a bicycle. The helmet absorbs and dissipates the forces of the impact over a larger area of the head so that the brain is exposed to a lower level of energy over a longer period, even though the fall has occurred.

Injury-control strategies may be categorized in several ways. Haddon's matrix places strategies in a framework according to phase (before the event, during the event, or after the event) and factor (human, vector or vehicle, physical environment, and socioeconomic environment). Comprehensive injury-prevention efforts incorporate interventions from multiple matrix cells. Table 30-2 lists examples of variables and injury prevention interventions stratified according to Haddon's matrix.

Active and Passive Injury Prevention

Prevention strategies can be active or passive. Active strategies require involvement of the child who needs protection or the child's parent every time protection is needed. Seat belts in automobiles are a good example of an active strategy. Passive (or automatic) strategies protect the individual whether the person needing protection is mindful of the need and takes

Table 30-2 Haddon's Matrix and Examples of Variables and Injury Prevention Interventions

	EPIDEMIOLOGIC DIMENSION			
PHASE	HUMAN	VECTOR OR VEHICLE	PHYSICAL ENVIRONMENT	SOCIOECONOMIC ENVIRONMENT
Preevent	Judgment Coordination	Safe storage of firearms Infant walker ban	Bicycle paths Swimming pool barriers	Speed limits Graduated driver licensing
Event	Car safety seat use Use of protective equipment	Airbags Energy-absorbing surfacing on playgrounds	Smoke alarms Highway guard rails	Helmet laws Enforcement of seat belt laws
Postevent	Age Physical condition	Activated charcoal Fuel system integrity	Time to emergency treatment Availability of rehabilitation programs	Training of emergency medical system personnel Cardiopulmonary resuscitation training

Adapted from American Academy of Pediatrics, Committee on Injury and Poison Prevention. *Injury Prevention and Control for Children and Youth*. 3rd ed. Elk Grove Village, IL: American Academy of Pediatrics; 1997; and PediaLink continuing medical education course, Moving Kids Safely: Introduction to Car Safety Seats.

appropriate action or not. Airbags are a good example. Both active and passive strategies can be quite successful when used, but passive strategies, when they exist, are usually favored over active strategies. Active strategies require compliance, and a risk always exists that they will not be fully used. Active strategies are often least likely to be adopted by the persons at greatest risk.

Education, Engineering, and Enforcement

Another framework for categorizing injury-prevention measures is the *3 Es*. Education is the approach that is most familiar to health professionals; examples include counseling during health supervision visits and public education campaigns. Engineering involves modifying a hazard or the environment to prevent injuries or reduce the severity of injuries. Enactment and enforcement of legislation and regulation can motivate people to adopt safety-promoting behaviors, require environmental modifications to reduce hazards, and facilitate changes in social norms. Injury prevention is usually most effective when all 3 approaches are incorporated. For example, bicycle helmet use can be promoted through education in schools, design of more comfortable or attractive helmets, and local laws or ordinances requiring helmet use.

Intentional Versus Unintentional Injuries

Injuries are often classified as unintentional or intentional. This dichotomy is useful in many ways; however, the intent of human behavior is not always clear cut and is better described as a continuum. For example, should injuries that result in part from inadequate parental supervision be considered unintentional or intentional resulting from child neglect? Additionally, strategies that prevent unintentional injury (eg, locking up firearms, turning down the water heater temperature) may also prevent some intentional injuries. For these reasons, and because injuries result from both, injury-control efforts often address both intentional and unintentional injury. Nevertheless, some forms of intentional injury, for example, child abuse and child and adolescent suicide and homicide, are so important as causes of pediatric morbidity and mortality that they demand focused attention. Furthermore, the causes of intentional injury are extremely complex, and violence-prevention efforts must take a multifaceted approach that includes the pediatrician. The pediatrician's important role in violence prevention is discussed in Chapter 31, Violence Prevention.

Pediatrician Roles

Pediatricians can attempt to persuade individuals to decrease their risk of injury through educational efforts with individuals or groups. Injury-control advocates have additional strategies at their disposal. Pediatricians can be involved in many of these activities, including media campaigns, legislation, regulation, litigation, environmental design, and cultural change. For most causes of injury, multiple strategies will need to be applied. The pediatrician can also become involved in research to identify risk and protective factors for injury and to evaluate prevention interventions.

ANTICIPATORY GUIDANCE

Evidence of positive outcomes after injury-prevention counseling in clinical practice was identified by a structured review of the literature.[1] The evidence for the effectiveness of injury-prevention counseling is stronger in some areas than it is in others, prompting continual calls for additional research, improvements in counseling, and investment in more passive injury-control strategies. For example, the redesign of baby walkers resulted in a dramatic decrease in injuries associated with falls down stairs in this product, demonstrating the

BOX 30-1 Topics Recommended by the American Academy of Pediatrics for Office-Based Unintentional Injury-Prevention Counseling

INFANTS

Traffic safety: Appropriate use of car safety seats rear-facing in the back seat

Burn prevention: Smoke alarms, hot water temperature no higher than 120°F

Fall prevention: Window and stairway guards and gates, avoiding walker use

Choking and strangulation prevention: Keeping small objects and balloons or plastic bags away from infants, blind and drapery cord safety

Drowning prevention: Supervising baths, emptying buckets

Safe sleep environment: Back to sleep in a crib that meets current safety standards

CPR training: Parent knowledge of infant or child CPR and local emergency medical services (911)

PRESCHOOLERS

Traffic safety: Appropriate use of car safety seats, not leaving children unsupervised in or around cars

Burn prevention: Smoke alarm batteries; keeping children away from hot objects

Fall prevention: Window and stairway guards and gates; preventing furniture tip-overs

Poison prevention: Storage of poisons; poison control phone number (1-800-222-1222)

Drowning prevention: Pool fencing; *touch supervision*

Firearm safety: Preferably keeping firearms out of the home or at least keeping firearms unloaded and locked separately from locked ammunition

SCHOOL-AGED CHILDREN

Traffic safety: Booster seat and seat belt use, avoiding riding on ATVs and in the beds of pickup trucks; safe pedestrian practices; helmets for biking

Water safety: Swimming lessons, but no swimming alone; personal flotation devices for boating

Sports safety: Safety equipment, physical conditioning, and protective equipment for rollerblading and skateboarding

Firearm safety: Preferably keeping firearms out of the home or at least keeping firearms unloaded and locked separately from locked ammunition; asking about firearms in other homes the child visits

ADOLESCENTS

Traffic safety: Seat belt use, role of alcohol in motor vehicle crashes, and minimizing distracted driving; graduated driver licensing; rules for teenage drivers; helmets for biking, motorcycling, and riding an ATV

Water safety: Role of alcohol and other drugs in water-related injuries; personal flotation devices for boating

Sports safety: Safety equipment; physical conditioning

Firearm safety: Preferably keeping any firearms out of the home or at least unloaded and locked separately from locked ammunition

ATV, All-terrain vehicle; *CPR,* cardiopulmonary resuscitation.
Modified from American Academy of Pediatrics, Committee on Injury, Violence, and Poison Prevention. Office-based counseling for unintentional injury prevention. *Pediatrics.* 2007;119:202-206.

effectiveness of the passive prevention approach after years of unsuccessful anticipatory guidance and the use of warning labels.[2]

Even though injury-prevention counseling has become a cornerstone of pediatric practice, it can be daunting, not only because of the time and expertise it requires, but also because of its breadth. Injury risk is so universal and the sources of possible injury so diverse that a pediatrician cannot counsel on all possible risks. Injury-prevention topics can be prioritized based on severity of the injury, frequency with which the injury occurs, and the availability of effective preventive strategies. Pediatricians will want to be sensitive to the individual circumstances of patients and families as well. For instance, farm families may need advice that city families do not, and vice versa. Knowing that a family has a boat or a backyard swimming pool prompts a special discussion of drowning risk. In another example of the need to customize anticipatory guidance, counseling a family that has 2 automobiles about car safety seats poses a different set of issues than does counseling a family that relies on taxis for transportation; yet child passenger safety is a high priority for both.

The American Academy of Pediatrics (AAP) recommends that parents be given advice by the pediatrician about various injury issues, depending on the age of the child (Box 30-1).[3] The AAP also provides several tools to facilitate counseling, including age-specific survey instruments to assess risk and handouts for families, as part of TIPP—The Injury Prevention Program.[4] (The counterpart AAP program for intentional injury prevention is Connected Kids: Safe, Strong, Secure, as described in Chapter 31, Violence Prevention.)

Counseling about any injury-prevention topic requires both knowledge and counseling skill. In addition to TIPP materials, several resources are listed at the end of this chapter that can provide a pediatrician with the knowledge for advising parents (and communities) about injury prevention. Counseling technique is not specific to injury prevention but can be adapted from existing methods for prompting and supporting healthy behavior change (eg, motivational interviewing). Counseling techniques that include motivational interviewing are addressed in Chapter 24, Communication Strategies.

Traffic Safety

Car Safety Seats

Because motor vehicle crashes are the leading cause of death of children and adolescents, the topic warrants frequent discussion during well-child care. Use

Table 30-3 Appropriate Car Safety Seat Selection Based on Child's Age, Height, and Weight

IF THE CHILD IS	USE THE FOLLOWING TYPE OF CAR SAFETY SEAT	AND REMEMBER THE FOLLOWING
Younger than 1 year OR under 20 lb	Rear-facing car safety seat (infant-only or convertible)	NEVER place a rear-facing car safety seat in the front seat with an airbag.
Older than 1 year AND over 20 lb	Recommended: rear-facing convertible seat to seat's height or weight (usually 30 or 35 lb) limit Then: forward-facing car safety seat (convertible, combination, or forward-facing only) to seat's height or weight limit	When switching a convertible seat from rear-facing to forward-facing, adjustments are usually needed to the harness, the angle of the seat, and the seat belt.
Too tall or heavy for a forward-facing seat with a harness (often around 4 years of age or 40 lb)	Booster seat	Booster seats must be used with lap and shoulder belts.
Big enough to fit in the adult seat belt (usually around 4′ 9″ and between 8 and 12 years of age)	None. Use the vehicle's seat belt if it fits properly (shoulder belt across chest and shoulder, lap belt low and snug on thighs, child's back against vehicle seat back and knees bent at edge of vehicle seat).	Children should sit in the back seat until they turn 13 years of age.

Adapted from American Academy of Pediatrics, Committee on Injury and Poison Prevention. Selecting and using the most appropriate car safety seats for growing children: guidelines for counseling parents. *Pediatrics.* 2002;109:550-553.

of car safety seats is a complex issue that pediatricians should not expect to master fully. Rather, pediatricians should know how to counsel parents on appropriate car safety seat selection based on developmental milestones (age, height, weight, and behavior) and where to refer parents for more information. When counseling on car safety seat selection, pediatricians should be familiar with state laws. However, recognizing that state laws often do not reflect best practice in car safety seat use is important. Table 30-3 provides information about car safety seat selection. Parents should be encouraged to read the instruction manuals for their car safety seats and vehicles to learn how to install and use car safety seats. For more information, parents can be referred to local *child passenger safety technicians*; a pediatric practice may even choose to have a staff member complete the 3- to 4-day training course to become a certified technician.

Counseling Teen Drivers

Counseling on motor vehicle safety remains important even after children have outgrown car safety seats. In fact, such counseling may be more important because motor vehicle–related death rates increase dramatically in adolescence, and novice teen drivers and their passengers are at particularly high risk. The pediatrician can play a key role in helping parents and teens negotiate their changing relationship, balancing the need to ensure the teen's safety with the teen's growing independence and increasing mobility. A state's graduated driver licensing (GDL) system may provide a good starting point for counseling, and pediatricians should be familiar with their states' laws. Under GDL, teen drivers graduate from a learner's permit to an intermediate or provisional license to a regular driver's license after spending a required amount of time and after demonstrating proficiency in a lower stage; each stage has its own restrictions. However, because many states' GDL laws are relatively weak and a few states do not have GDL laws, parents should be counseled about additional restrictions (eg, limits on the number of teenage passengers, limits on nighttime driving) that they should place on novice teen drivers. Parents and teens both should be counseled on seat belt use and the dangers of impaired driving. They should also be encouraged to have a safe ride agreement, whereby the teen promises to call the parent rather than driving while impaired or with another impaired driver and the parent agrees to provide a ride home in a nonjudgmental way. Pediatricians can consider having a family develop a parent-teen driving contract that specifies restrictions on teen drivers, when the restrictions will be relaxed, and the consequences for violating the restrictions.

Firearms

Because firearms-related injuries (unintentional and intentional) are the 2nd leading cause of death of children and adolescents, firearms are an important topic on which to provide anticipatory guidance.[5] Pediatricians are often reluctant to counsel on this topic, and parents may view such counseling as intrusive or outside the purview of pediatrics. Fortunately, strategies are available that can make counseling on firearms more palatable to both parents and pediatricians. For families with infants and toddlers, firearms can be discussed in the context of childproofing and children's natural curiosity. For parents of depressed adolescents, the association between presence of firearms in the home and higher risk of teen suicide can be discussed. Especially for parents who are receptive to firearm injury–prevention counseling, the pediatrician can introduce the concept of asking about the presence of guns in other homes where their children spend time.

TOOLS FOR PRACTICE

Community Advocacy and Coordination

- *Child Passenger Safety Issue Brief,* American Academy of Pediatrics (www.aap.org/securemoc/statelegislation/boosterseats_issuebrief.pdf).
- Injury Free Coalition for Kids (www.injuryfree.org/).
- Insurance Institute for Highway Safety (www.iihs.org/).
- *National Center for Injury Prevention and Control* (Web page), Centers for Disease Control and Prevention (www.cdc.gov/ncipc/).
- National Highway Traffic Safety Administration (hotline), 1-800-424-9393; (www.nhtsa.gov).
- National Poison Control Number (hotline), 1-800-222-1222; (www.edisonnj.gov).
- *Reducing the Burden of Injury: Advancing Prevention and Treatment* (book), Institute of Medicine (www.iom.edu/cms/3793/5627.aspx).
- Safe Kids Worldwide (www.safekids.org).
- *Safety and First Aid* (Web page), American Academy of Pediatrics (www.aap.org/healthtopics/safety.cfm).
- Seat Check (www.seatcheck.org/).
- *Teen Driving Issue Brief* (report), American Academy of Pediatrics (www.aap.org/securemoc/statelegislation/gdl_issuebrief.pdf).
- *Transportation Safety* (Web page), American Academy of Pediatrics (www.aap.org/healthtopics/carseatsafety.cfm).
- US Consumer Product Safety Commission, 800-638-2772.
- *Water Safety* (Web page), American Academy of Pediatrics (www.aap.org/healthtopics/watersafety.cfm).
- *WISQARS™,* Web-Based Injury Statistics Query and Reporting System (on-line database), Centers for Disease Control and Prevention (www.cdc.gov/ncipc/wisqars/).

Engaging Patient and Family

- *A Parent's Guide to Water Safety* (brochure), American Academy of Pediatrics (patiented.aap.org).
- *Air Bag Safety* (fact sheet), American Academy of Pediatrics (www.aap.org/bookstore).
- Asking Saves Kids Campaign (ASK) (www.paxusa.org/ask/index.html).
- *Baby Walkers* (fact sheet), American Academy of Pediatrics and National Association of Children's Hospitals and Related Institutions (www.aap.org/bookstore).
- *Car Safety Seats: A Guide for Families* 2007 (brochure), American Academy of Pediatrics (patiented.aap.org).
- *Choking Prevention and First Aid for Infants and Children* (brochure), American Academy of Pediatrics (patiented.aap.org).
- *Home Safety Checklist* (fact sheet), American Academy of Pediatrics (www.aap.org/bookstore).
- *Keep Your Family Safe: Fire Safety and Burn Prevention at Home* (brochure), American Academy of Pediatrics (patiented.aap.org).
- *Parent-Teen Driving Agreement and Fact Sheet* (fact sheet), American Academy of Pediatrics (www.aap.org/bookstore).
- *One-Minute Car Safety Seat Check-up* (fact sheet), American Academy of Pediatrics (patiented.aap.org).
- *Partners for Child Passenger Safety* (Web page), Children's Hospital of Philadelphia (www.chop.edu/consumer/jsp/division/generic.jsp?id=77971).
- *Protect Your Child From Poison* (brochure), American Academy of Pediatrics (patiented.aap.org).
- Seat Check (www.seatcheck.org).
- *The Injury Prevention Program (TIPP),* American Academy of Pediatrics (www.aap.org/family/tippmain.htm).
- *Toy Safety* (brochure), American Academy of Pediatrics (patiented.aap.org).
- *Trampolines* (fact sheet), American Academy of Pediatrics (www.aap.org/bookstore).

Medical Decision Support

- *Anticipatory Guideline Topics for Car Seat Safety* (fact sheet), American Academy of Pediatrics (pediatrics.aap.org/content.aspx?aid=2001).
- *Car Seat Selection Based on Child's Age, Height, and Weight* (fact sheet), American Academy of Pediatrics (pediatrics.aap.org/content.aspx?aid=2001).
- *TIPP—Guide to Safety Counseling in Office Practice* (booklet), American Academy of Pediatrics (www.aap.org/family/tippguide.pdf).
- *TIPP Safety Program,* American Academy of Pediatrics (www.aap.org/bookstore).
- *TIPP and Connected Kids on CD-ROM: Injury and Violence Prevention Counseling Resources* (CD-ROM), American Academy of Pediatrics (www.aap.org/bookstore).

AAP POLICY STATEMENTS

American Academy of Pediatrics, Committee on Injury and Poison Prevention. Selecting and using the most appropriate car safety seats for growing children: guidelines for counseling parents. *Pediatrics.* 2002;109(3):550-553. (aappolicy.aappublications.org/cgi/content/full/pediatrics;109/3/550).

American Academy of Pediatrics, Committee on Injury and Poison Prevention. Firearm-related injuries affecting the pediatric population. *Pediatrics.* 2000;105(4):888-895. (aappolicy.aappublications.org/cgi/content/full/pediatrics;105/4/888).

American Academy of Pediatrics, Committee on Injury, Violence, and Poison Prevention. Office-based counseling for unintentional injury prevention. *Pediatrics.* 2007;119(1):202-206. (aappolicy.aappublications.org/cgi/content/full/pediatrics;119/1/202).

American Academy of Pediatrics, Committee on Injury, Violence, and Poison Prevention, Committee on Adolescence. The teen driver. *Pediatrics.* 2006;118:2570-2581.

For a complete list of all policy statements from the American Academy of Pediatrics, Committee on Injury, Violence, and Poison Prevention visit: aappolicy.aappublications.org/cgi/collection/committee_on_injury_violence_and_poison_prevention.

REFERENCES

1. DiGuiseppi C, Roberts IG. Individual-level injury prevention strategies in the clinical setting. *The Future of Children: Unintentional Injuries in Childhood*. 2000;10:53-82. Available at www.futureofchildren.org. Accessed April 27, 2007.
2. Shields BJ, Smith GA. Success in the prevention of infant walker-related injuries: an analysis of national data, 1990-2001. *Pediatrics*. 2006;117:e452-e459.
3. American Academy of Pediatrics, Committee on Injury, Violence, and Poison Prevention. Office-based counseling for unintentional injury prevention. *Pediatrics*. 2007;119:202-206.
4. American Academy of Pediatrics, Committee on Injury, Violence, and Poison Prevention. TIPP®—The Injury Prevention Program. Elk Grove Village, IL: American Academy of Pediatrics; 1994. Available at: www.aap.org/family/tippmain.htm. Accessed April 27, 2007.
5. American Academy of Pediatrics, Committee on Injury and Poison Prevention. Firearm-related injuries affecting the pediatric population. *Pediatrics*. 2000;105:888-895.

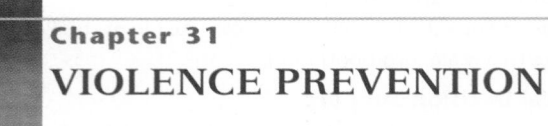

Chapter 31

VIOLENCE PREVENTION

Robert D. Sege, MD, PhD

UNDERSTANDING VIOLENCE

Most peer violence in the United States results from conflicts among friends, acquaintances, or intimate partners. Estimates of the incidence of stranger violence range from 6% to 40% of new cases among all instances of personal violence.[1,2]

Violence of all levels of severity is often a result of conflicts between persons who know each other, often quite well. Although physicians have traditionally viewed patients as the victims, the distinction between victim and perpetrator is more fluid and varied than previously thought. From a public health perspective, the conclusion from years of research is dramatically simple: Young people who fight get hurt, whether in their families or in their communities.

Primary prevention in pediatrics must extend beyond preventing a child from becoming a victim; it must help the child learn nonviolent problem-solving skills and attitudes. Developing these skills and attitudes begins in infancy. Effective, nonviolent discipline throughout childhood and adolescence is 1 key to developing resilient children who can resist being drawn into violence.[3] In addition, parents can help reduce the risk of serious violence through attention to the child's environment—both decreased exposure to media violence and domestic violence and decreased access to firearms effectively reduce serious violence. Parents can encourage a nonviolent attitude by resisting toys that promote violence, such as toy guns, violent video games, and toys that encourage racial or ethnic stereotypes.[4]

Violence Is Learned

In the 1980s, Patterson proposed a model based on an extensive review of the literature that accounted for the developmental progression of antisocial behavior.[5] These results have been confirmed by more recent longitudinal studies conducted. Aggression naturally increases during early childhood; parents serve to temper and redirect these impulses before school entry.[6] Thus the foundations of antisocial behavior begin with coercive or inadequate parenting in early childhood. Children whose parents are unable to set effective limits, particularly in households where extensive use of corporal punishment is used, develop dysfunctional behavior patterns in interactions with their peers and with adult authorities, including teachers. These children then have behavioral problems even before they enter school. In school, the children are both rejected by *normal* peers and have difficulties academically. In later childhood and adolescence, these ostracized children find each other and form peer groups that reward violence and antisocial behavior. The result of this cycle, which began in early childhood, is juvenile delinquency.

More recent descriptions of growing up in violent urban settings have reiterated the importance of peer relationships but stressed the central role that being willing to fight plays in establishing social hierarchy.[7] Boys, in particular, need to establish themselves as courageous fighters early in life, or else they fear that they will be harassed by others. Nevertheless, the majority of the young men growing up in these communities have figured out how to avoid participating in violence; they repeatedly state that they are able to walk away from potential fights. Their resilience begins early in life.

This overall trajectory model provides a focus for interventions in the pediatric office. In 1999 the American Academy of Pediatrics (AAP) Task Force on Violence endorsed a similar, far-reaching model that traces the origins of violent behavior to earliest childhood,[8] which formed the foundation of the new Connected Kids: Safe, Strong, Secure anticipatory guidance program. The Connected Kids program includes parent and patient education materials that encourage the development of resilience as a means of preventing child abuse and youth violence.[9]

Although many social and environmental factors place children at high risk for violence, countervailing resilience factors, many beginning in early childhood, help reduce the risk.

Witnessing Violence: Domestic Violence

The greatest risks of violence for infants and toddlers revolve around the family through domestic violence and child abuse. One of the goals of the pediatric provider in speaking with families of new babies can be to assess family functioning, including the risks of domestic violence. Pediatricians who are suspicious that a patient's parent has been the victim of spousal abuse should ask directly, but confidentially. The physician should have information available in the office concerning battered women's advocates or shelters, legal aid resources, and safety plans.[10] Many offices place small cards with relevant telephone numbers in the restroom so this information can be obtained discreetly.

Witnessing Violence: Television Violence

Children in the United States spend more time watching television than any other activity except sleep. While watching television, they observe an enormous amount of violence; the average child will *see* more than 10,000 deaths resulting from violence before completing high school.[11]

Television violence differs from real-life violence in quality and quantity. On television, violence is used by both heroes and villains and is therefore generally viewed as socially acceptable behavior. Although adults feel competent to separate fiction from reality, research suggests that even adults who are exposed to television violence have a more negative view of society and feel more hopeless and alienated than do less frequent viewers. Adults who rely on television as their major news source, for example, feel less safe in their homes and neighborhoods than do other adults.

Children, because they have more difficulty separating facts from fantasy, are even more likely to be affected by television violence. The American Psychological Association, in reviewing hundreds of research studies, has concluded that exposure to television violence is a major risk for children.[12] Children who view television are more likely to experience violence as victims or aggressors and are much less likely to intervene in tense situations, as bystanders, to reduce the likelihood of violence.

The AAP Committee on Communications has recommended that pediatricians counsel families to reduce the amount of television viewed by young children. Television and its influence on children are discussed further in Chapter 123, Children, Adolescents, and the Media.

Violence in Urban Minority Communities

Ethnographic research conducted in some of America's poorest urban neighborhoods has identified another pattern of violence in which fighting and the willingness to fight are key components of a broader protective strategy for coping with extremely dangerous environments. Young people have observed that individuals who are unable to defend themselves are likely prey to multiple and repeated attacks. Parents also understand this phenomenon and encourage their children to *stand up for themselves* by becoming able fighters.[7] This pattern of violence is known as the *code of the streets* or as the *sucker* phenomenon. Other parents adopt protective strategies that keep their children out of harm's way in the first place, often by enrolling them in supervised after-school programs or keeping them safely in the house, watching television, rather than risking participation in the street culture.

In counseling patients in these communities, physicians need to be aware of this logic and refrain from offering unrealistic or counterproductive advice. Nevertheless, in discussions with most young people, we need to remember that these same communities also contain nonviolent problem solvers who are well known to their classmates. Thus the reality of the code of the streets need not prevent individual children and adolescents from avoiding violent injuries through avoiding the culture of violence.

Primary Prevention: Anticipatory Guidance—Young Children

During infancy and early childhood, patterns of behavior and family interactions are established. The proper role of the pediatric provider is to ameliorate risk factors and reinforce factors that protect the child from harm. In this age group, the following topics should be addressed to the parents during anticipatory guidance: (1) reduction in exposure to violence, including both domestic violence and television violence, and (2) teaching appropriate, nonviolent methods of discipline (violence-free parenting). Because patients and families see their physicians often during this period, opportunities for brief, focused interventions are numerous. Our research has demonstrated the effectiveness of focused guidance at changing parental use of alternatives to corporal punishment and awareness of the effects of television violence during early childhood.[13]

Violence-Free Parenting: Effective Parenting Without Corporal Punishment

As children enter the second year of life, patterns of discipline become established in families. Developmentally, this age is the time when children are typically separating emotionally and cognitively from their parents, a time of potential stress in the family. Several lines of research evidence suggest that a link exists between the use of corporal punishment and the subsequent use of violence by children as they grow. The AAP issued a policy statement in 1998 advocating that pediatricians counsel families in the use of alternatives to corporal punishments.[14] This approach forms a cornerstone of the new Connected Kids: Safe, Strong, Secure program from the AAP.[15]

Many families, however, believe in the need for corporal punishment. A direct challenge to family beliefs is unlikely to lead to successful behavior change. Instead, the pediatrician may incorporate several salient observations about families who use corporal punishment. First, most of the parents who use corporal punishment do not like to hit their children. Instead, they use corporal punishment when all other methods of correcting their child's behavior seem to have failed.[16] This approach results in an erratic pattern of punishment because parents end up using threats and cajoling to avoid spanking. Second, these same parents often believe that some children "don't need to be spanked." One appropriate goal for guiding these families is to teach them effective techniques for discipline that will allow their children to be among those who do not *need* to be spanked.

Most importantly, many parents have little knowledge of other effective alternatives to corporal punishment. Faced with a choice of spanking a child or letting him or her *run wild*, many parents will opt for corporal punishment. The goal for anticipatory guidance at this age therefore is to describe and endorse specific effective behavioral techniques to help discipline children. Maintaining toddler discipline is understood best from the child's perspective; toddlers gain power over their world by being able to understand what is happening and predict what will happen next. Maintaining a schedule for children—for example, bedtimes, naptimes, mealtimes, bath time, and playtime—helps give the child this feeling of mastery.

Toddlers crave parental attention. The best kind of attention, of course, is parental praise for good behavior. In the absence of this positive reinforcement, toddlers may feel ignored and misbehave simply to grab the attention of their parents. The parental misperception that children who are praised will become self-centered and egotistical blocks the effective use of parenting and parental attention to encourage good behavior. Parents can be told very simply to tell their child, "I love it when you...."

Of course, times will occur when a child's misbehavior necessitates negative consequences. The most effective yet simple negative reinforcement technique for parents to use is *time out* from positive reinforcement. Parents can be taught that time-out periods can be used judiciously, in the background of positive reinforcement, and consistently whenever the child has certain behavior patterns that need to be stopped. Children should be placed in time-out for approximately 1 minute per year of age. Parents should explain clearly to the child why the time-out was deserved and ignore the child during the time-out. Longer explanations and discussions should be deferred until things have calmed down.

School Age

As children get older, the external influences of their behavior become more important. Television has an enormous effect at this age, and children also begin dealing with playground fights and bullying.

Bullying

Bullying prevention is an important task for school administrators. Bullying—the repeated infliction of harm on younger, smaller, or less powerful peers—is a nearly universal problem for school-age children. Severe and even lethal bullying has been described in the United Kingdom, Japan, and Scandinavia, as well as in the United States. Bullies are usually larger and stronger (among boys) or more socially powerful (among girls) than are their victims. Typically, bullies will begin the school year by trying to pick on several children. Children who become singled out as targets are weaker, physically and emotionally, and are unable to strike back, either physically or verbally. Although bullying is a problem of school-age children, the negative behaviors often happen outside of school supervision: before school, after school, or at recess. Thus classroom teachers are often unaware of the problem and are almost always unable to solve it without significant support from their administrators.

Bullying has severe adverse consequences for both bully and victim. Victims may be hurt physically, often cannot concentrate on their studies, and develop poor self-esteem. Recent news reports suggest that several perpetrators in school shootings in the United States were victims of bullies, and their lethal outbursts may have resulted from the effects of being bullied.

Children who are bullies, in contrast, often feel powerful and effective. They typically come from chaotic households, and their parents feel ineffective in controlling their child's behavior. In many instance, bullies do not experience effective limit-setting at home. In the long term, the outcome for bullies is poor: by age 30, they are more likely to be incarcerated and less likely to be employed, married, or in other stable adult relationships than their peers.

Olweus has developed an effective antibullying program in Scandinavia, where it has led to a dramatic reduction in bullying.[17] Reports in the United States suggest that this program may also be effective here. Antibullying programs begin with information gathering. Students, who are asked to complete anonymous surveys, are quite willing to report to school administrators where and when bullying usually occurs. Active efforts to control bullying occur on 3 levels: (1) in the school building and grounds, (2) in the classroom, and (3) with individual students.

School-wide interventions focus on 2 issues: (1) ensuring a safe physical environment and (2) endorsing and coordinating classroom activities. To ensure a safe physical environment, staff monitoring is improved before and after school and at lunch, and any architectural or landscaping changes needed to improve supervision are made. A school-wide assembly is convened in which the announcement is made that bullying will not be tolerated anywhere in the school environment and that all necessary steps will be taken to control it.

Classroom teachers lead discussions with their students. These discussions identify roles of bullies, victims, and bystanders and establish that bullying behavior will not be tolerated. The students themselves are helped to generate rules to prevent bullying and to prevent the social isolation of victims. The students agree to (1) report bullying behavior, and (2) resist attempts by the bullies to ostracize their victims. Successful antibullying programs work, in part, by mobilizing the large number of bystanders. In so doing, they make bullies less respected and accepted by their peers and thereby reduce the allure of bullying.

Individual measures reinforce the antibullying messages. When bullies are identified, the child receives a stern message from the principal, and the principal also speaks with the child's parents. Parents are told of the possible short- and long-term consequences for their child, and a social worker or guidance counselor is assigned to work with them on setting appropriate and enforceable behavioral limits at home.

Recently, bullying has also been identified as an important precursor to other forms of violence. The federal government has launched Stop Bullying Now, a comprehensive set of resources for parents, schools, and communities (see www.stopbullyingnow.hrsa.gov). This approach implements the approach of Olweus in the American context.

Adolescents

Violence among adolescents has long been a major concern of urban teens and their parents.[18] The recent outbreaks of school violence have led to the same concerns among many other groups. Pediatric providers have several clear roles to play in working with their adolescent patients to reduce the risk of violence: (1) screening all adolescents to identify those at high risk, (2) preventing reinjury to injured adolescents, and (3) referring high-risk or traumatized adolescents for appropriate treatment. (See also Chapter 146 Posttraumatic Stress Disorder.) In addition to screening for risk, recent research strongly supports identifying and reinforcing teen resilience factors. Attachment to school, family, community, and pro-social peer groups all exert strong protective effects, even in the face of risk factors. Programs that provide opportunities for teenagers to belong to a pro-social group and develop mastery of particular activities—ranging from academics to dance—protect young adults from health-risk behaviors, including fighting. Based on these successes, over the next few years, social programs for youth will likely move from focused risk reduction to positive youth development models.

Screening

Screening for violence risk can take either of 2 forms: (1) a specific violence history or (2) a general screen for related risk factors.

Violence History

Teenagers can be asked directly about their experiences with violence, using the acronym FISTS and asking the screening questions listed in Box 31-1.

Fighting

Teens who have been in more than 1 physical fight in the preceding 12 months are at increased risk of violence-related injury.

Injuries

A review of medical records of teens who were seriously injured or killed through violence usually reveals previous episodes of injuries that required medical attention. Multiple or serious previous injuries may indicate an increased risk of future injury.

Sexual Violence

Teen-dating violence is both a serious problem in itself and a harbinger of future domestic violence.

Threats

Previous threats with a weapon indicate that the patient is at future risk of weapons-related injury, either through the circumstances that led to the original threat or because these young people are far more likely to arm themselves than are those who have never been threatened directly.

Self-Defense

Young people who have learned to deescalate situations of conflict (or to avoid them altogether) deserve praise and encouragement. On the other hand, teens who arm themselves in self-defense are at extremely high risk, as discussed previously. (See the discussion on "Bullying," earlier in this chapter.)

Violence-Related Risk Factor Screening

A second, broader set of risk factors influences the likelihood of serious violence-related injury. Problem teen behaviors tend to cluster as a result of both intrapersonal and social factors. As shown in Figure 31-1, analysis of office-based risk factor screening results has identified three classes of risk. Young people in school who report neither drug use nor fighting to their primary care provider are at low risk of violence-related injuries.[19] Teens who are in school and are passing their courses but who report either fighting or drug use are at medium risk—approximately three times that of low-risk students. Adolescents who are failing school, already dropped out of school, or report both fighting and drug use are at approximately a 7-fold increased risk for future violence-related injury than are low-risk students. In the clinical setting, most practitioners already inquire about school performance and drug use as part of the HEADS screening; the addition of a single question, "How many fights have you been in the past 12 months?" completes the screening. Patients who are in school and deny fighting or drug use are at low risk. Patients who are in school but report either drug use or fighting are at intermediate risk. Patients who have either dropped out of school or report both drug use and fighting are at high risk and should be referred to appropriate community-based intervention services.

Finally, clinicians should be aware of the strong clustering of health risk behaviors among teens. For example, male teenagers who smoke are at increased risk for carrying weapons.

Counseling and Referral for Adolescents at Increased Risk

Intervention for patients who are identified as being at increased risk for violence-related injuries through either screening approach must be tailored to fit both the degree of risk and the individual circumstances of each child. Teens at low risk deserve acknowledgment of their success at avoiding this problem, particularly noting that courage is often needed to walk away from a fight. Teens at moderate risk need to hear that the risks are real and individual: "You are strong and healthy. However, I am worried about your telling me that you have been in several fights this year." Basic information concerning techniques for defusing particularly tense situations should be discussed. Teens who carry weapons, have left school, or are otherwise at high risk deserve intense social service or psychologic intervention. Adolescent health providers need to maintain a roster of appropriate community-based

BOX 31-1 Taking a Violence History—Adolescents and Young Adults (FISTS)

Fighting: When was your last pushing or shoving fight? How many fights have you been in the last month? In the last year?

Injuries: Have you ever been injured in a fight? Has anyone you know been injured in a fight? Has anyone you know been injured or killed?

Sexual violence: What happens when you and your boyfriend or girlfriend have an argument? Have you ever been forced to have sex against your will?

Threats: Have you ever been threatened with a knife? With a gun?

Self-defense: How do you avoid getting in fights? Do you carry a weapon for self-defense?

Alpert EJ, Sege RD, Bradshaw YS. Interpersonal violence and the education of physicians. *Acad Med* 1997;72(1 suppl):S41-S50. Used with permission from Lippincott-Williams & Wilkins.

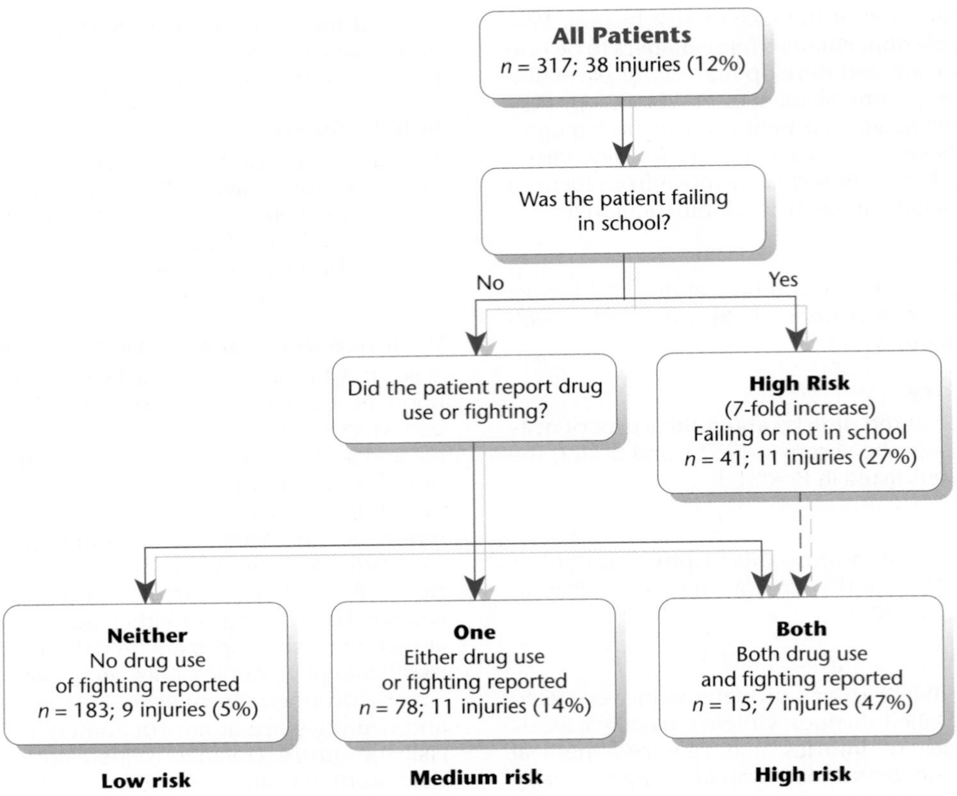

Figure 31-1 Classification of patients into high, medium, and low risk for future violence-related injury. *(Reprinted from Sege RD, Stringham P, Short S, et al. Ten years after: examination of adolescent screening questions that predict future violence-related injury.* J Adolesc Health. *1999;24:395-402. Used with permission from the Society for Adolescent Medicine.)*

referral agencies or individual counselors for these children and emphasize the importance of followup to both the patient and parents.

After a Fight (Secondary Prevention)

Patients who have been hurt in a fight are at high risk for further violence, either as the victim of another violence-related injury or by attempting to exact revenge on the assailants. The immediate need after an injury is for crisis intervention. Ask the patient: "Is the fight over? Do you feel safe leaving here? If the fight is ongoing, is there someone who can mediate?" If the situation is volatile, then the patient and family should be referred to social services or, occasionally, the police. Police intervention is warranted whenever the patient is in danger or reveals specific plans to harm another person. At a minimum, parents and patients should be advised of the risk of serious injury and that successful injury prevention involves learning how to deescalate conflicts.

After a serious injury, the following steps have been advocated:

- Have the child tell you about the problem. Allow the narrative to flow freely, avoiding judgments. This approach allows feelings of revenge to be expressed and offers an opportunity to learn of the patient's perspective before offering advice.
- Evaluate the youth's other risks: Does he or she carry a weapon? Does he or she use alcohol or other drugs? Is the youth involved in a gang?
- Discuss with the patient the known risk factors for violence, including the fact that most violent injuries occur between friends or acquaintances and often involve alcohol or drugs. Carrying weapons *increases* the risk of serious injury by encouraging the patient to take unnecessary risks and by encouraging his or her opponent to *draw first.*
- Develop a plan to stay safe after leaving the hospital or clinic. Does he or she have a relative with whom to stay who lives out of the neighborhood? Do the police need to be involved?
- Discuss conflict-avoidance strategies. This discussion can start with the particular incident involved and may need to be continued on subsequent visits. Health care professionals need to respect the patient's need not to be labeled as a *sucker* by peers.
- Refer to others, including a psychologist or social worker. For many patients, this referral may involve reaching out to church members, recreation departments, or mentoring programs.

Advocacy

As is apparent from the previous discussion, youth violence, although a serious health risk, is a complex social problem that requires broad-based public action. Pediatric providers, in addition to caring for their own patients, are often able to influence public debate in areas that affect child health. The AAP and other organizations have advocated for social policies that benefit children.

Pediatric providers who serve as school consultants have a critical role to play. School boards and principals should be advised of the importance of age-appropriate violence-prevention programs. A significant number of successful school programs are available for adaptation and use in other schools. Primary schools can focus on adequate supervision of playgrounds, teaching and modeling nonviolent problem-solving skills, and implementing effective antibullying programs. Middle schools can use proven antiviolence and conflict-resolution curricula that can be incorporated into health education programs. Successful high school programs can involve the use the school health clinics to provide services to students who have problems of violence, drug abuse, or pregnancy. Schools have successfully developed peer education programs to help reinforce these areas of concern. Peer mediation, which allows students another formal venue for resolving conflict, has been widely adopted and appears to be quite successful, both in school and in the communities in which the students live.

Media violence has recently received greater public attention, in part because of concerted efforts by pediatricians and child psychologists to call attention to the dangers of excess exposure to media violence. In addition to counseling individual families, many pediatricians have provided testimony at public hearings or endorsed community television *tune-out* weeks.

Despite a general reduction in traumatic injury and death, child and adolescent deaths caused by firearms continue to soar. Individual families can be counseled that the safest home for children is one without handguns, and that any guns present in the home should be locked and unloaded. State and federal regulations now under consideration would mandate the provision of trigger locks and prevent the marketing of certain kinds of weapons. Physician testimony and endorsement by medical professional organizations have helped push forward these initiatives.

SUMMARY

Violence is a major cause of death and disability for children in the United States. Although the problem has complex social roots and requires multifaceted solutions, pediatricians have important roles to play. Primary prevention of violence begins with anticipatory guidance for parents of infants and toddlers. Secondary prevention involves the identification, counseling, and referral of high-risk patients and should be a part of a standard care for older children and adolescents. Finally, pediatricians can advocate for school policies and state and federal legislation to reduce the risk of violence for children.

TOOLS FOR PRACTICE

Engaging Patients and Family

- TIPP and Connected Kids (CD-ROM), American Academy of Pediatrics (www.aap.org/bookstore).
- *Bullying Is Not Ok—Connected Kids* (brochure), American Academy of Pediatrics (www.aap.org/bookstore).
- *Your Child Is On the Move: Reduce the Risk of Gun Violence—Connected Kids* (brochure), American Academy of Pediatrics (www.aap.org/bookstore).
- *Teaching Good Behavior—Tips on How to Discipline—Connected Kids* (brochure), American Academy of Pediatrics (www.aap.org/bookstore).
- *Parenting Your Infant—Connected Kids* (brochure), American Academy of Pediatrics (www.aap.org/bookstore).
- *Playing Is How Toddlers Learn—Connected Kids* (brochure), American Academy of Pediatrics (www.aap.org/bookstore).
- *Young Children Learn a Lot When They Play—Connected Kids* (brochure), American Academy of Pediatrics (www.aap.org/bookstore).
- *Welcome to the World of Parenting—Connected Kids* (brochure), American Academy of Pediatrics (www.aap.org/bookstore).
- *Pulling the Plug on TV Violence—Connected Kids* (brochure), American Academy of Pediatrics (www.aap.org/bookstore).
- *How Do Infants Learn—Connected Kids* (brochure), American Academy of Pediatrics (www.aap.org/bookstore).
- *Expect Respect: Healthy Relationships—Connected Kids* (brochure), American Academy of Pediatrics (www.aap.org/bookstore).
- *Teaching the Basics of Violence Prevention* (fact sheet), American Academy of Pediatrics (www.aap.org/healthtopics/violprev.cfm).
- *Attention, Consistency, and Violence Prevention* (fact sheet), American Academy of Pediatrics (www.aap.org/healthtopics/violprev.cfm).
- Youth Violence (Web site), Centers for Disease Control and Prevention (www.cdc.gov/ncipc/factsheets/yvoverview.htm).

Medical Decision Support

- *Connected Kids Clinical Guide* (booklet), American Academy of Pediatrics (www.aap.org/ConnectedKids/ClinicalGuide.pdf).
- Connected Kids Full Training Module (PowerPoint slide set), American Academy of Pediatrics (www.aap.org/ConnectedKids/CKtrain.ppt).
- Connected Kids Introduction and Tips for Use (PowerPoint slide set), American Academy of Pediatrics (www.aap.org/ConnectedKids/CKtrain-intro.ppt).
- Connected Kids—Infancy and Early Childhood Training (PowerPoint slide set), American Academy of Pediatrics (www.aap.org/ConnectedKids/CKtrain-green.ppt).
- Connected Kids—Middle Childhood Training (PowerPoint slide set), American Academy of Pediatrics (www.aap.org/ConnectedKids/CKtrain-blue.ppt).
- Connected Kids—Adolescence Training (PowerPoint slide set), American Academy of Pediatrics (www.aap.org/ConnectedKids/CKtrain-red.ppt).

- *Youth Violence* (fact sheet), Centers for Disease Control and Prevention (www.cdc.gov/ncipc/factsheets/yvfacts.htm).
- Youth Violence (Web site), Centers for Disease Control and Prevention (www.cdc.gov/ncipc/factsheets/yvoverview.htm).

Community Coordination and Advocacy

- Stop Bullying Now (Web site), Health Resources and Services Administration (www.stopbullyingnow.hrsa.gov/index.asp).
- ASK Campaign (Web site), PAX (www.paxusa.org/ask/index.html).

AAP POLICY STATEMENTS

American Academy of Pediatrics, Committee on Injury and Poison Prevention. Firearm-related injuries affecting the pediatric population. *Pediatrics.* 2000;105(4):888-895. (aappolicy.aappublications.org/cgi/content/full/pediatrics;105/4/888).

American Academy of Pediatrics, Committee on Native American Child Health and Committee on Injury and Poison Prevention. The prevention of unintentional injury among American Indian and Alaska Native children: a subject review. *Pediatrics.* 1999;104(6):1397-1399. (aappolicy.aappublications.org/cgi/content/full/pediatrics;104/6/1397).

American Academy of Pediatrics, Committee on Public Education. Children, adolescents, and television. *Pediatrics.* 2001;107(2):423-426. (aappolicy.aappublications.org/cgi/content/full/pediatrics;107/2/423).

American Academy of Pediatrics, Committee on Public Education. Media violence. *Pediatrics.* 2001;108(5):1222-1226. (aappolicy.aappublications.org/cgi/content/full/pediatrics;108/5/1222).

American Academy of Pediatrics, Laraque D, and the Committee on Injury, Violence, and Poison Prevention. Injury risk of nonpowder guns. *Pediatrics.* 2004;114(5):1357-1362 (doi:10.1542/peds.2004-1799). (aappolicy.aappublications.org/cgi/content/full/pediatrics;114/5/1357).

American Academy of Pediatrics, Task Force on Violence. The role of the pediatrician in youth violence prevention in clinical practice and at the community level. *Pediatrics.* 1999;103(1):173-181. (aappolicy.aappublications.org/cgi/content/full/pediatrics;103/1/173.)

REFERENCES

1. Sege RD, Kharasch S, Perron C, et al. Pediatric violence-related injuries in Boston: results of a city-wide emergency department surveillance program. *Arch Pediatr Adolesc Med.* 2002;156(1):73-76.
2. Sege R, Stigol LC, Perry C, et al. Intentional injury surveillance in a primary care pediatric setting. *Arch Pediatr Adolesc Med.* 1996;150(3):277-283.
3. American Academy of Pediatrics, Committee on Psychosocial Aspects of Child and Family Health. Guidance for effective discipline. *Pediatrics.* 1998;101(4):723-728.
4. American Academy of Pediatrics, Glassy D, Romano J, and the Committee on Early Childhood, Adoption, and Dependent Care. Selecting appropriate toys for young children: the pediatrician's role. *Pediatrics.* 2003;111(4):911-913.
5. Patterson GR, DeBaryshe D, Ramsey E. A developmental perspective on antisocial behavior. *Am Psychol.* 1989;44:329-335.
6. Tremblay RE, Nagin DS, Seguin JR, et al. Physical aggression during early childhood: trajectories and predictors. *Pediatrics.* 2004;114:e43-e50. Available at: pediatrics.aappublications.org/cgi/content/full/114/1/e43. Accessed October 2, 2007.
7. Canada G. *Fist, Stick, Knife, Gun: A Personal History of Violence in America.* Boston, MA: Beacon Press; 1995.
8. American Academy of Pediatrics, Task Force on Violence. The role of the pediatrician in youth violence prevention in clinical practice and at the community level. *Pediatrics.* 1999;103:173-181.
9. Sege R, DeVos E, Hatmaker-Flanigan E, et al. American Academy of Pediatrics Connected Kids program: case study. *Am J Prev Med.* 2005;29(5 suppl):215-219.
10. Alpert EJ, Sege RD, Bradshaw YS. Interpersonal violence and the education of physicians. *Acad. Med.* 1997;72(suppl 1):S41-S50.
11. American Academy of Pediatrics, Committee on Public Education. Children, adolescents, and television. *Pediatrics.* 2001;107(2):423-426.
12. Donnerstein E, Slaby RG, Eron LD. The mass media and youth aggression. In: Eron LD, Gentry JH, Schlegel P, eds. *Reason to Hope: A Psychosocial Perspective on Violence and Youth,* Washington, DC: American Psychological Association; 1996.
13. Sege RD, Perry C, Stigol L, et al. Short-term effectiveness of anticipatory guidance to reduce early childhood risks for subsequent violence. *Arch Pediatr Adolesc Med.* 1997;151(4):392-397.
14. American Academy of Pediatrics, Committee on Psychosocial Aspects of Child and Family Health. Guidance for effective discipline. *Pediatrics.* 1998;104:723-728.
15. Sege RD, Flanigan E, Levin-Goodman R, et al, American Academy of Pediatrics. Connected Kids program case study. *Am J. Prev Med* 2005;29(5 suppl 2):215-219. Available at: www.aap.org/connectedkids.
16. Sege RD, Hatmaker-Flanigan E, DeVos E, et al. Anticipatory guidance and violence prevention: results from family and pediatrician focus groups. *Pediatrics.* 2006;117(2):455-463.
17. Olweus D. *Bullying at School,* Oxford, UK: Blackwell Publishers; 1993.
18. Centers for Disease Control and Prevention. *Mortality Trends, Causes of Death, and Related Risk Behaviors among US Adolescents.* Atlanta, GA: CDC; 1995.
19. Sege R, Stringham P, Short S, et al. Ten years after: examination of adolescent screening questions that predict future violence-related injury. *J Adolesc Health.* 1999;24:395-402.

Chapter 32

PREVENTIVE CARDIOLOGY

Jorge A. Alvarez; Tracie L. Miller, MD, MS; Thomas J. Starc, MD, MPH; Kathleen A. McGrath, RN, MS, CPNP; Steven E. Lipshultz, MD

A pediatrician must consider multiple factors when assessing a child's global risk for premature cardiovascular disease. Other chapters in this text cover general aspects of screening, the physical examination, and specific targets such as hypertension (see Chapter 191), heart failure (see Chapter 349, Heart Failure), and congenital and acquired heart disease (see Chapter 251).

Table 32-1 Schedule for Integrated Cardiovascular Health Promotion in Children

AGE (YEARS)	FAMILY HISTORY*	CHOLESTEROL	OBESITY	BLOOD PRESSURE	DIET	PHYSICAL ACTIVITY	SMOKING
0 to 2	Early heart disease[†] (age ≤55 yr) Parent's total cholesterol ≥240 mg/dL	Parental cholesterol screening	Plot height and weight on growth charts Parent obesity	Family history of hypertension	Diet history *Early foods influence future food preferences*	Parent physical activity *Discourage television and video viewing*	Parental or household smoking? If yes, counsel to quit; referral to smoking cessation
2 to 6	Update family history Early heart disease[†] (age ≤55 yr) Parent's total cholesterol ≥240 mg/dL	Fasting lipids screening Total cholesterol screening	Plot height, weight, and BMI (kg/m²) on growth charts BMI percentiles	Start routine blood pressure measures at 3 yr of age (determine if >90th or 95th percentile for sex, age, and height)	Diet history *Low-saturated-fat diet[‡] including 1% or nonfat milk* Moderate salt intake	*Encourage active child-parent play* *Limit sedentary behaviors such as television and video viewing*	Parental or household smoking? If yes, counsel to quit; referral to smoking cessation *Antismoking counseling[§]*
6 to 10	Update family history Early heart disease[†] (age ≤55 yr) Parent's total cholesterol ≥240 mg/dL	Fasting lipids screening Total cholesterol screening	Plot height, weight, and BMI (kg/m²) on growth charts BMI percentiles	Blood pressure measures Blood pressure percentiles	Diet history *Low-saturated-fat diet[‡] including 1% or nonfat milk* *Moderate salt intake*	Physical activity history *Lifestyle and family activities* *Limit sedentary behaviors such as television and video viewing*	Parental/household smoking? If yes, counsel to quit; referral to smoking cessation *Anti-smoking counseling[§]*
Older than 10	Update family history Early heart disease[†] (age ≤55 yr) Parent's total cholesterol ≥240 mg/dL	Fasting lipid screening Total cholesterol screening	Plot height, weight, and BMI (kg/m²) on growth charts BMI percentiles	Blood pressure measures Blood pressure percentiles	Diet history *Low-saturated-fat diet[‡] including 1% or nonfat milk* *Moderate salt intake*	Physical activity history *Lifestyle and family activities* *Daily moderate to vigorous activity* *Limit sedentary behaviors*	Parental or household smoking? Assess child smoking If yes, counsel to quit; referral to smoking cessation *Antismoking counseling[§]*

Assessment items are in normal typeface, counseling items are in *italics*.
*Includes parents, grandparents, and blood-related aunts and uncles.
[†]Documented myocardial infarction, coronary artery disease, angina pectoris, or sudden cardiac death at age 55 years or younger or family history not available.
[‡]The diet should average <30% (but not <20%) of calories from total fat, <10% of calories from saturated fats, <10% of calories from polyunsaturated fats; and the lesser of 300 mg/dL or 100 mg cholesterol per 1000 kcal energy intake.
[§]Includes immediate physical, social, and physiological effects of smoking, risk of addiction, counter-arguing ?techniques, and resisting social and environmental pressures to smoke.
From Williams CL, Hayman LL, Daniels SR, et al. Cardiovascular health in childhood: a statement for health professionals from the Committee on Atherosclerosis, Hypertension, and Obesity in the Young (AHOY) of the Council on Cardiovascular Disease in the Young, American Heart Association. *Circulation.* 2002;106:143-160.

This chapter addresses three major topics that should be a part of routine pediatric preventive cardiology assessment for all children and adolescents: (1) atherosclerosis, (2) obesity, and (3) smoking with a focus on atherosclerosis. The patient recommendations, screening tests, and practice guidelines needed to provide care are summarized and serve as a quick reference tool for any preventive care consultation.[1,2]

ATHEROSCLEROSIS

Atherosclerosis continues to be a leading cause of death and disability in the United States. Although myocardial infarction, stroke, and other clinical manifestations of atherosclerosis usually appear in the adult, evidence is mounting that their pathogenesis begins much earlier. Furthermore, epidemiologic studies provide overwhelming evidence that atherosclerosis is not an inevitable consequence of aging but rather, in many cases, an acquired disease with well-described risk factors.[3-5]

Although many risk factors for heart disease remain beyond the control of the individual, some factors such as hyperlipidemia and level of physical activity can be modified, and at least one factor—smoking—is completely avoidable. A goal of primary care is to prevent disease and to prevent the development of risk factors in children, ultimately reducing morbidity and mortality from atherosclerosis. Several risk factors for coronary heart disease are now easily identified during childhood, and scientifically based recommendations to begin prevention in childhood have been developed, with continuous review and enhancement. Because the process of atherosclerosis and the habits that influence the risk of heart disease begin early in life, preventive measures should be initiated during childhood[6,7] (Table 32-1).

The known risk factors for atherosclerosis include hypertension, smoking, elevated low-density lipoprotein cholesterol (LDL-C), decreased high-density lipoprotein cholesterol (HDL-C), diabetes mellitus, advancing age, male sex, a family history of premature heart disease, hypertriglyceridemia, sedentary lifestyle, and obesity.[8-10] Primary prevention in childhood should seek to eliminate or minimize these risk factors when possible. A relatively new concept, that of *primordial prevention*, also challenges health care providers to prevent risk factors by addressing the social and environmental factors that maintain them. These social and environmental changes are particularly important in addressing obesity, smoking, and sedentary lifestyle.

As an example of the importance of the early influence of environmental factors, a classic study led by Enos, Beyer, and Holmes of military personnel killed in the Korean War showed that young American soldiers had a 77% incidence of coronary arterial lesions, whereas such lesions were virtually nonexistent among young Korean soldiers. This study not only described the early initiation of the atherosclerotic process, but also suggested the role of dietary and lifestyle modifiers.[11] Similarly, findings from the Bogalusa Heart Study[3] and the Pathobiological Determinants of Atherosclerosis in Youth (PDAY) study group[12,13] showed that risk factors, such as cholesterol levels and smoking, contribute to the formation of atherosclerosis in a graded manner and that these findings are present in children and young adults long before the onset of clinical heart disease.

Hypercholesterolemia is a primary target for preventing atherosclerosis. Total cholesterol measures the cholesterol contained in several lipid particles, including LDL-C, HDL-C, and very-low-density lipoprotein cholesterol (VLDL-C). LDL-C is one of the atherogenic lipoproteins and receives the focus for screening algorithms, whereas HDL-C is considered protective against the development of coronary heart disease.[14]

Both genetic and environmental factors play a role in the development of hypercholesterolemia. Plasma cholesterol levels are influenced by the quantity and quality of dietary fat intake and by the individual's ability to synthesize and degrade cholesterol. Severe or familial hypercholesterolemia secondary to a defect in the LDL receptor occurs in approximately 1 in 500 individuals.[15] Children who have this defect commonly have LDL-C values between 200 and 300 mg/dL, which is two to three times higher than the acceptable limits of normal (Table 32-2). These children inherit the receptor defect and have a strong predilection for atherosclerotic heart disease as young adults. More than 600 different mutations of the LDL receptor have been described. Approximately 50% of men who have one of these mutations will have a myocardial infarction by age 50, and between 75% and 85% will have a myocardial infarction by age 60. Approximately 50% of women will develop ischemic heart disease by age 60. Fortunately, even in these high-risk patients, treatment can decrease the incidence of heart disease.[16]

Table 32-2 Classification of Total and LDL Cholesterol Levels in Children and Adolescents From Families With Hypercholesterolemia or Premature Cardiovascular Disease

CATEGORY	TOTAL CHOLESTEROL (mg/dL)	LDL CHOLESTEROL (mg/dL)
Acceptable	<170	<110
Borderline	170-199	110-129
High	≥200	≥130

LDL, Low-density lipoprotein.
From National Cholesterol Education Program: Report of the Expert Panel on Blood Cholesterol Levels in Children and Adolescents. *Pediatrics.* 1992:89:525.

In 1991 the National Cholesterol Education Program (NCEP) issued guidelines for preventing heart disease in children.[17] The American Academy of Pediatrics (AAP) published a revised statement in 1998 that included additional scientific justification for the emphasis on cholesterol screening and treatment.[18] In 2002 the American Heart Association (AHA) issued a scientific statement reemphasizing the NCEP's approach to both screening and treatment strategies, along with a comprehensive and easy-to-follow review of other key areas in the area of preventive cardiology.[2] The reader who is interested in a more in depth evaluation of each of the pertinent topics related to preventive cardiology is referred to the AHA scientific statement for additional information.

Although most authorities agree that preventing heart disease is laudable, the optimal methods of prevention have generated controversy on such fundamental issues as (1) what age to begin screening, (2) who actually should be screened, and (3) how ultimately to treat those individuals who have elevated cholesterol levels.[19-22] The most recent report by the United States Preventive Services Task Force found that although good evidence existed of children with dyslipidemia becoming adults with dyslipidemia, the study ultimately concluded that the evidence was insufficient to recommend for or against screening of lipid disorders in children and adolescents.[23] As has occurred with the adult guidelines, the pediatric NCEP guidelines will undoubtedly be revised as more information about treating hypercholesterolemia and long-term outcomes accrues. For now, however, pediatricians should use the basic strategy proposed by the NCEP and endorsed by the AAP and AHA.[1,18]

Table 32-3 Characteristics of the American Heart Association Step 1 and Step 2 Diet

NUTRIENT	STEP 1	STEP 2
Calories	Adequate for normal growth	Same
Total fat	≤30% of calories	Same
Saturated fat	<10% of calories	≤7%
Polyunsaturated fat	Up to 10% of calories	Same
Monounsaturated fat	Remainder of fat calories	Same
Carbohydrates	Apprx 55% of calories	Same
Protein	Apprx 15-20% of calories	Same
Cholesterol (mg/day)	<300	<200

Data from National Cholesterol Education Program. Report of the Expert Panel on Blood Cholesterol Levels in Children and Adolescents. *Pediatrics.* 1992:89:525.

BOX 32-1 American Heart Association Pediatric Dietary Strategies for Individuals Aged Over 2 Years: Recommendations to All Parents and Families

Balance dietary calories with physical activity to maintain normal growth.

Perform 60 minutes of moderate to vigorous play or physical activity daily.

Eat vegetables and fruits daily; limit juice intake.

Use vegetable oils and soft margarines low in saturated fat and trans fatty acids instead of butter or most other animal fats in the diet.

Eat whole-grain breads and cereals rather than refined grain products.

Reduce the intake of sugar-sweetened beverages and foods.

Use nonfat (skim) or low-fat milk and dairy products daily.

Eat more fish, especially oily fish, broiled or baked.

Reduce salt intake, including salt from processed foods.

From Gidding SS, Dennison BA, Birch LL, et al. Dietary recommendations for children and adolescents: a guide for practitioners: consensus statement from the American Heart Association. *Circulation.* 2005;112:2061-2075.

BOX 32-2 Tips for Parents to Implement American Heart Association Pediatric Dietary Guidelines

Reduce added sugars, including sugar-sweetened drinks and juices.

Use canola, soybean, corn oil, safflower oil, or other unsaturated oils in place of solid fats during food preparation.

Use recommended portion sizes on food labels when preparing and serving food.

Use fresh, frozen, and canned vegetables and fruits and serve at every meal; be careful with added sauces and sugar.

Introduce and regularly serve fish as an entrée.

Remove the skin from poultry before eating.

Use only lean cuts of meat and reduced-fat meat products.

Limit high-calorie sauces such as Alfredo, cream sauces, cheese sauces, and hollandaise.

Eat whole-grain breads and cereals rather than refined produces; read labels, and ensure that *whole grain* is the 1st ingredient on the food label of these products.

Eat more legumes (beans) and tofu in place of meat for some entrées.

Breads, breakfast cereals, and prepared food, including soups, may be high in salt or sugar or both; read food label for content, and choose high-fiber, low-salt, low-sugar alternatives.

From Gidding SS, Dennison BA, Birch LL, et al. Dietary recommendations for children and adolescents: a guide for practitioners: consensus statement from the American Heart Association. *Circulation.* 2005;112:2061-2075.

Recommendations for Cholesterol Screening

The NCEP suggests two separate approaches to hypercholesterolemia in children: (1) a broad, population-based approach and (2) an individualized patient approach. Universal screening of all children is not recommended despite the suggestion that cholesterol testing based only on family history would miss a substantial number of hypercholesterolemic children.[24,25]

Population Screening

The panel suggests that all children older than 2 years follow the *Step 1 Diet,* which is relatively low in fat: (1) no more than 30% of total calories should come from fat, (2) less than 10% of total calories should come from saturated fat, and (3) total cholesterol consumption should be less than 300 mg per day (Table 32-3). This diet should contain a variety of foods and should be adequate to support growth and maintain an ideal body weight for height and age. In 2005 a consensus statement issued by the AHA and endorsed by the AAP contained more detailed dietary recommendation for all children while remaining within the same general guidelines set forth by the NCEP in 1991[26] (Boxes 32-1 and 32-2). Overall, the population approach attempts to shift the distribution of exposure in a favorable direction, the classic hallmark of public

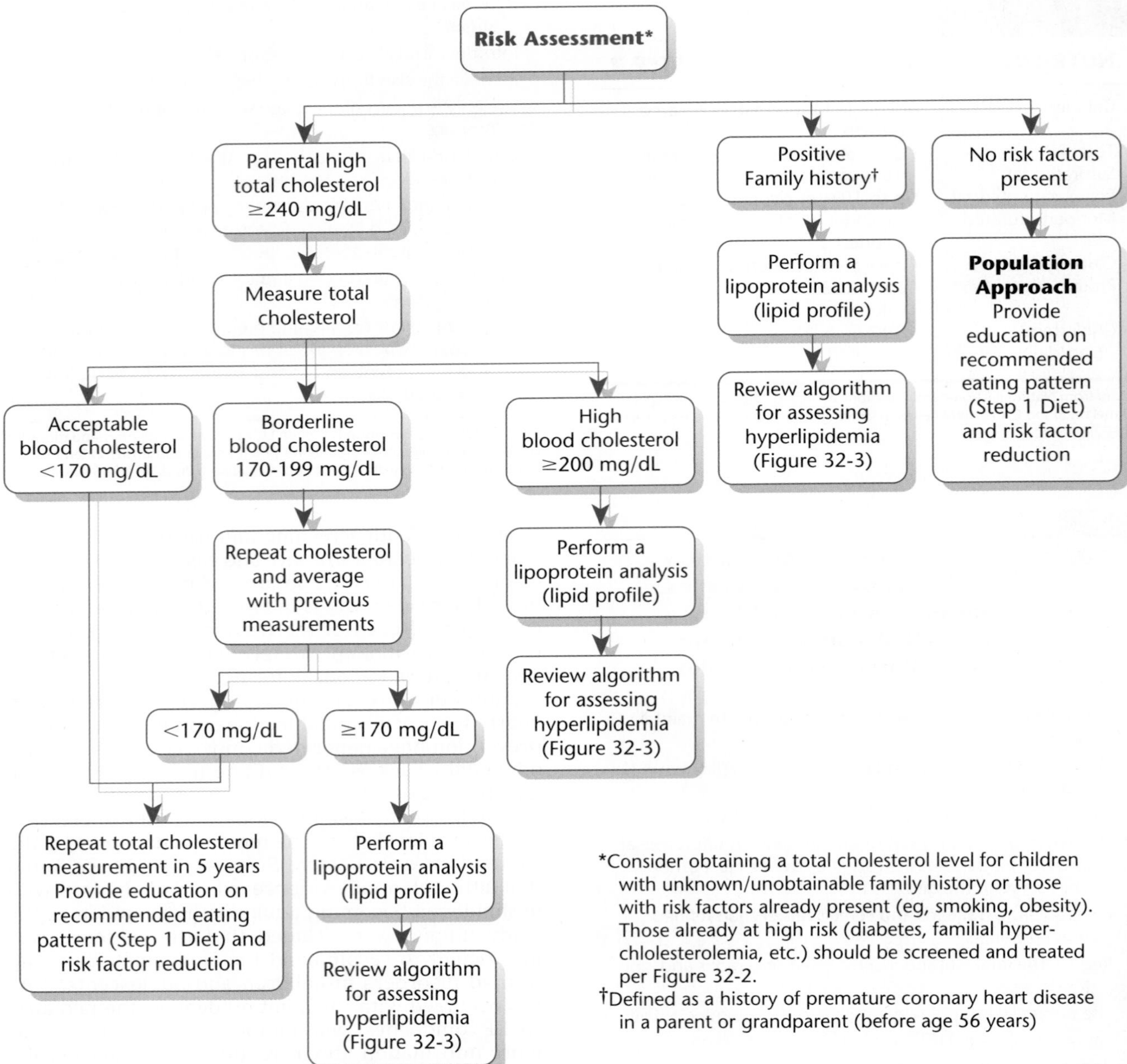

Figure 32-1 Individualized approach: algorithm for assessing initial cholesterol screening. *(Modified from National Institutes of Health.* National Cholesterol Education Program: Report of the Expert Panel on Blood Cholesterol Levels in Children and Adolescents. *NIH Pub No 91-2732. Rockville, MD: US Department of Health and Human Services; 1979.)*

health, with pediatricians taking a vital part in this effort.[27]

Individualized Screening

In addition to the population-wide diet recommendations, the NCEP guidelines suggest assessing risk and performing cholesterol testing in children older than 2 years with a positive family history, meaning children whose parent or grandparent has or had premature coronary heart disease, defined as onset of disease younger than 56 years (Figure 32-1 on page 282). Conditions that suggest heart disease include a history of documented myocardial infarction, angina pectoris, peripheral vascular disease, cerebrovascular disease, or sudden cardiac death, as well as coronary atherosclerosis as determined by angiography, or a history of balloon angioplasty or coronary artery bypass graft surgery. In addition, children who have a parent with hypercholesterolemia (total cholesterol ≥240 mg/dL) also should be screened. Children whose parental history is unknown or unobtainable, especially if they have other risk factors, may also be screened to identify those in need of nutritional advice. Parents with unknown cholesterol levels should be encouraged to obtain a full lipoprotein analysis, commonly referred to as a *lipid profile.* Cholesterol levels may also need to be determined for children at higher risk for coronary heart disease independent of family history: for example, those who smoke, are obese, consume diets rich in saturated fats and cholesterol, or have diabetes mellitus.

For children who have a family history of premature heart disease, the NCEP guidelines suggest obtaining a fasting lipid profile that includes total cholesterol, LDL-C, HDL-C, and triglycerides. For children with a family history of hypercholesterolemia and no history of early heart disease, the NCEP suggests initial screening by measuring total cholesterol only (see Figure 32-1).

The AHA and AAP have recently proposed a risk stratification and treatment algorithm for children who are at increased risk for premature coronary heart disease. It identifies children with homozygous or heterozygous familial hypercholesterolemia, diabetes mellitus (type 1 or 2), chronic kidney disease or end-stage renal disease, Kawasaki disease, congenital heart disease, chronic inflammatory disease, and post–cardiac transplant or cancer treatment survivors as needing special consideration for more careful attention to cardiovascular risk factors. Children with these conditions are categorized into two tiers (Table 32-4). An algorithm for screening with tier-specific test value cutoffs (Figure 32-2 on page 284) is provided. Also included are therapeutic goals for all strata (Box 32-3 on page 285), as well as condition-specific recommendations for the highest risk group (Box 32-4 on page 286).[2,28]

Recommendations for Treatment

Most of the information regarding the risk of heart disease in adults is based on fasting LDL-C values; therefore recommendations in children are also based on fasting LDL-C values. Because cholesterol standards vary by age, treatment values are based on percentile ranks of children in the United States that exceed the upper *norms.* A total cholesterol level greater than 200 mg/dL and LDL-C greater than 130 mg/dL represent values above the 95th percentile for children and are designated as *high.* A total cholesterol level less than 170 mg/dL and LDL-C less than 110 mg/dL represent values below the 75th percentile and are *acceptable.* Values between these limits are considered *borderline* (see Box 32-4).

Table 32-4 High-Risk Stratification: Tier I Condition-Specific Treatment Recommendations

RISK CATEGORY	RATIONALE	DISEASE PROCESS OR CONDITION
Tier I: high risk	Manifest CAD <30 years of age; clinical evidence	Homozygous familial hypercholesterolemia Diabetes mellitus, type 1 Chronic kidney disease or end-stage renal disease Post–orthotopic heart transplantation Kawasaki disease with current coronary aneurysms
Tier II: moderate risk	Accelerated atherosclerosis: pathophysiological evidence	Heterozygous familial hypercholesterolemia Kawasaki disease with regressed coronary aneurysms Diabetes mellitus, type 2 Chronic inflammatory disease
Tier III: at risk	High-risk setting for accelerated atherosclerosis: epidemiological evidence	Post–cancer-treatment survivor Congenital heart disease Kawasaki disease without detected coronary involvement

CAD, Coronary artery disease.
From Kavey R-EW, Allada V, Daniels SR, et al. Cardiovascular risk reduction in high-risk pediatric patients: a scientific statement from the American Heart Association Expert Panel on Population and Prevention Science; the Councils on Cardiovascular Disease in the Young, Epidemiology and Prevention, Nutrition, Physical Activity and Metabolism, High Blood Pressure Research, Cardiovascular Nursing, and the Kidney in Heart Disease; and the Interdisciplinary Working Group on Quality of Care and Outcomes Research: Endorsed by the American Academy of Pediatrics. *Circulation.* 2006;114(24):2710-2738.

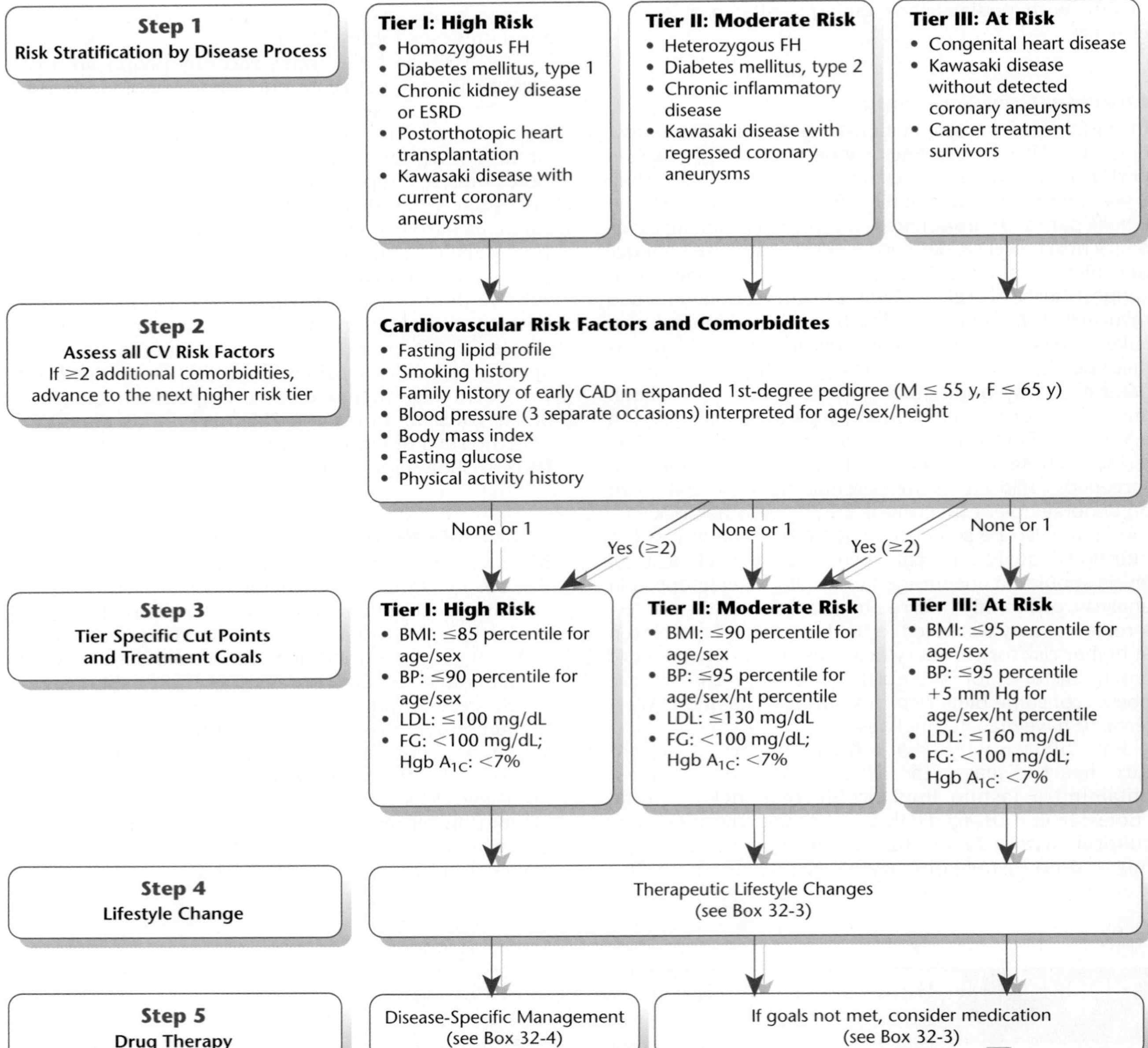

Figure 32-2 High-risk pediatric populations: risk stratification and treatment algorithm. Directions: Step 1: Risk stratification by disease process (see Table 32-4). Step 2: Assess all cardiovascular risk factors. If two or more comorbidities exist, then assign patient to the next higher risk tier for subsequent management. Step 3: Tier-specific intervention cut points or treatment goals defined. Step 4: Initial therapy: for tier I, initial management is therapeutic lifestyle change (see Box 32-3) plus disease-specific management (see Box 32-4). For tiers II and III, initial management is therapeutic lifestyle change (see Box 32-3). Step 5: for tiers II and III, if goals are not met after initial management, consider medication as outlined in Box 32-3. *BP,* Blood pressure; *CAD,* coronary artery disease; *CV,* cardiovascular; *ESRD,* end-stage renal disease; *FG,* fasting glucose; *FH,* familial hypercholesterolemia; *HgbA$_{1C}$,* hemoglobin A_{1C}; *ht,* height; *LDL,* low-density lipoprotein. *(Modified from Kavey R-EW, Allada V, Daniels SR, et al. Cardiovascular risk reduction in high-risk pediatric patients: a scientific statement from the American Heart Association Expert Panel on Population and Prevention Science; the Councils on Cardiovascular Disease in the Young, Epidemiology and Prevention, Nutrition, Physical Activity and Metabolism, High Blood Pressure Research, Cardiovascular Nursing, and the Kidney in Heart Disease; and the Interdisciplinary Working Group on Quality of Care and Outcomes Research: endorsed by the American Academy of Pediatrics.* Circulation. *2006;114[24]:2710-2738.)*

BOX 32-3 High-Risk Stratification: Tiers I, II, and III Treatment Recommendations

Growth and diet

- Nutritionist evaluation, diet education for all, see Step 1 Diet recommendations (see Table 32-3)
- Calculate BMI percentile for sex and height.[a]
  - If initial BMI >95th percentile:
    - Step 1:
      - □ Age-appropriate reduced-calorie training for child and family
      - □ Specific diet and weight follow-up every 2 to 4 weeks for 6 months; repeat BMI calculation at 6 months
      - □ Activity counseling (see below)
  - If follow-up BMI >85th percentile for tier I, >90th percentile for tier II, or >95th percentile for tier III:
    - Step 2:
      - □ Weight-loss program referral plus exercise training program appropriate for cardiac status

Blood pressure (tiers I, II, and III)

- BP measurement or interpretation for age, sex, and height
  - If SBP or DBP = 90th to 95th percentile or BP >120/80 mm Hg (3 separate occasions within 1 month):
    - Step 1: Recommend decreased calorie intake, increased activity for 6 months.
  - If initial SBP or DBP >95th percentile (confirmed within 1 week) or 6-month follow-up SBP or DBP >95th percentile:
    - Step 2: Initiate pharmacologic therapy per Fourth Task Force recommendations.

Lipids

- LDL-C (tiers II and III)
- See Box 32-4 for recommendations for LDL-C for tier I.
- If initial LDL-C ≥130 mg/dL (tier II) or >160 mg/dL (tier III):
  - Step 1: nutritionist training for Step 2 Diet (see Table 32-3) along with avoidance of trans fats for 6 months
- If repeat LDL-C ≥130 mg/dL in tier II or >160 mg/dL in tier III and child 10 years of age:
  - Step 2: Initiate statin therapy with LDL-C goal of 130 mg/dL.

Triglycerides

- If initial TG >150 to 400 mg/dL:
  - Step 1:
    - Nutritionist training for low simple carbohydrate, low-fat diet
    - If elevated TGs are associated with excess weight, nutritionist referral for weight loss management: energy balance training plus activity recommendations (see below)
- If TG >700 to 1000 mg/dL, initial or F/U:
  - Step 2:
    - Consider fibrate or niacin if >10 years of age.[b]
    - Weight loss recommended when TG elevation is associated with overweight or obesity.

Glucose (tiers I, II, and III, except for patients with diabetes mellitus)

- If fasting glucose = 100 to 126 mg/dL:
  - Step 1: Recommend reduced-calorie diet, increased activity aimed at 5% to 10% decrease in weight over 6 months.
- If repeat fasting glucose = 100 to 126 mg/dL:
  - Step 2: Recommend insulin-sensitizing medication as per endocrinologist.
- Casual glucose >200 mg/dL or fasting glucose >126 mg/dL = diabetes mellitus ⇒ endocrine referral for evaluation and management
- Maintain HbA_{1C} <7%

Smoking (tiers I, II, and III)

- Step 1: Obtain parental smoking history at every visit; child smoking history beginning at age 10. Provide active antismoking counseling for all; smoke-free home strongly recommended at each encounter.
- Step 2: Provide smoking cessation referral for any history of cigarette smoking.

Activity (tiers I, II and III)

- For children in all tiers, participation in activity is at the discretion of the physician or physicians directing care. For specific cardiac diagnoses such as Kawasaki disease and congenital heart disease, activity guidelines are referenced.
  - Step 1: Obtain specific activity history for each child, focusing on time spent in active play and screen time (television + computer + video games). Goal is ≥1 hour of active play per day; screen time limited to ≤2 hours/day.
- Encourage activity at every encounter.
  - Step 2: After 6 months, if goals not met, consider referral for exercise testing, recommendations from exercise specialist.

Specific treatment goals for each risk factor and each tier are given in the algorithm (see Figure 32-2).

BMI, Body mass index; *BP,* blood pressure; *DBP,* diastolic blood pressure; *F/U,* follow-up; *HbA1C,* hemoglobin A_{1C}; *LDL-C,* low-density lipoprotein cholesterol; *SBP,* systolic blood pressure; *TG,* triglycerides.

[a]Normal BMI values for age and sex are available at www.cdc.gov/growthcharts

[b]Elevation of triglycerides to ≥1000 mg/dL is associated with significant risk for acute pancreatitis. A fasting TG of 700 mg/dL is likely to rise to >1000 mg/dL postprandially. Treatment recommendation is congruent with guidelines for management of dyslipidemia in diabetic children.

From Kavey R-EW, Allada V, Daniels SR, et al. Cardiovascular risk reduction in high-risk pediatric patients: a scientific statement from the American Heart Association Expert Panel on Population and Prevention Science; the Councils on Cardiovascular Disease in the Young, Epidemiology and Prevention, Nutrition, Physical Activity and Metabolism, High Blood Pressure Research, Cardiovascular Nursing, and the Kidney in Heart Disease; and the Interdisciplinary Working Group on Quality of Care and Outcomes Research: endorsed by the American Academy of Pediatrics. *Circulation.* 2006;114(24):2710-2738.

All of these cutoff values were agreed on by consensus of the NCEP Expert Panel on Blood Cholestrol Levels in Children and Adolescents and are based on data published in 1980 from the Lipid Research Clinics Prevalence Study from children of varied ages (1 to 19 years of age for total cholesterol and 5 to 19 years of age for LDL-C). However, the most recent report using data from the National Health and Nutrition

BOX 32-4 High-Risk Stratification: Tiers I Conditions Specific Treatment Recommendations

- Rigorous age-appropriate education in diet, activity, and smoking cessation for all
- Specific therapy as needed to achieve BP, LDL-C, glucose, and Hb_{A1C} goals as indicated for each tier, as outlined in algorithm; timing individualized for each patient and diagnosis. Step 1 and step 2 therapy for all outlined in Box 32-3.

Homozygous FH

- LDL management: scheduled apheresis every 1 to 2 weeks beginning at diagnosis to maximally lower LDL-C, plus statin and cholesterol absorption inhibitor
- Rx per cardiologist or lipid specialist. (Specific therapeutic goals for LDL-C are not meaningful with this diagnosis.)
- Assess BMI, BP, and FG: step 1 management for 6 months
- If tier I goals not achieved, proceed to step 2.

Diabetes mellitus, type 1

- Intensive glucose management per endocrinologist, with frequent glucose monitoring or insulin titration to maintain PG <200 mg/dL, Hb_{A1C} <7%
- Assess BMI, fasting lipids: step 1 management of weight, lipids for 6 months
- If goals not achieved, proceed to step 2; statin Rx if >10 years of age to achieve tier I treatment goals
- Initial BP >90th percentile: step 1 management plus no added salt, increased activity for 6 months
- BP consistently >95th percentile for age, sex, and height: initiate ACE inhibitor therapy with BP goal <90th percentile or <130/80 mm Hg, whichever is lower.

CKD or end-stage renal disease

- Optimization of renal failure management with dialysis or transplantation as per nephrologist.
- Assess BMI, BP, lipids, FG: step 1 management for 6 months
- If goals not achieved, proceed to step 2; statin Rx if >10 years of age to achieve tier I treatment goals.

After heart transplantation

- Optimization of antirejection therapy, treatment for CMV, routine evaluation by angiography or perfusion imaging per transplant physician
- Assess BMI, BP, lipids, FG: initiate step 2 therapy, including statins, immediately in all patients >1 year of age to achieve tier I treatment goals

Kawasaki disease with coronary aneurysms

- Antithrombotic therapy, activity restriction, ongoing myocardial perfusion evaluation as per cardiologist
- Assess BMI, BP, lipids, FG: step 1 management for 6 months
- If goals not achieved, proceed to step 2; statin Rx if >10 years of age to achieve tier I treatment goals

ACE, Angiotensin-converting enzyme; *BP*, blood pressure; *CKD*, chronic kidney disease; *CMV*, cytomegalovirus; *FG*, fasting glucose; *FH*, familial hypercholesterolemia; *HbA_{1C}*, hemoglobin A_{1C}; *LDL-C*, low-density lipoprotein cholesterol; *PG*, plasma glucose; *Rx*, prescription/treatment.
From Kavey R-EW, Allada V, Daniels SR, et al. Cardiovascular risk reduction in high-risk pediatric patients: a scientific statement from the American Heart Association Expert Panel on Population and Prevention Science; the Councils on Cardiovascular Disease in the Young, Epidemiology and Prevention, Nutrition, Physical Activity and Metabolism, High Blood Pressure Research, Cardiovascular Nursing, and the Kidney in Heart Disease; and the Interdisciplinary Working Group on Quality of Care and Outcomes Research: endorsed by the American Academy of Pediatrics. *Circulation.* 2006;114(24):2710-2738.

Examination Survey (NHANES) III (1988-1994) showed modest increases in the values at both the 75th and 95th percentiles for total cholesterol (to 181 and 216 mg/dL, respectively) and for the 95th percentile for LDL-C (to 152 mg/dL) but not for the 75th percentile, which remained relatively stable at 109 mg/dL. Analyzing more recent NHANES data, independent researchers estimated new age- and sex-specific cutoffs based on the changes in population-level cholesterol distribution.[29] This estimation has prompted discussion in changing the recommended cutoffs, and the reader who is interested in further investigation is referred to a recent commentary on the study and its implications.[30] At the time of writing, however, no change has been made in the guidelines issued by the NCEP. In the remainder of this chapter the 1991 NCEP guidelines accepted by the AAP and other organizations are used.[31]

If the initial fasting total cholesterol level is high or, after an initial borderline value, the average of the first and second test values is greater than 170 mg/dL, then lipid profile, including an assessment of LDL-C, should be ordered (see Figure 32-1). The final evaluation should be based on the average of at least two LDL-C measurements, and treatment should follow the general strategy described later in this chapter and in Figure 32-3:

Acceptable (LDL-C <110 mg/dL): Repeat cholesterol testing in 5 years, and advise the family to follow the Step 1 Diet.

Borderline (LDL-C 110 to 129 mg/dL): Advise the family to follow the Step 1 Diet, provide advice regarding other risk factors, and reevaluate the child in 1 year.

High (LDL-C ≥130 mg/dL): Before recommending dietary or medical treatment, obtain a history detailing the use of drugs such as isotretinoin (Accutane), steroids, and alcohol to identify any secondary cause of hypercholesterolemia. In addition, screen for other secondary causes of elevated cholesterol such as liver, thyroid, and renal disease (Box 32-5).

The initial dietary treatment is to follow a Step 1 Diet (see Table 32-3). This diet is safe and efficacious for managing children with borderline to high LDL-C levels.[32] However, the child must consume adequate calories while decreasing fat intake. Current dietary guidelines

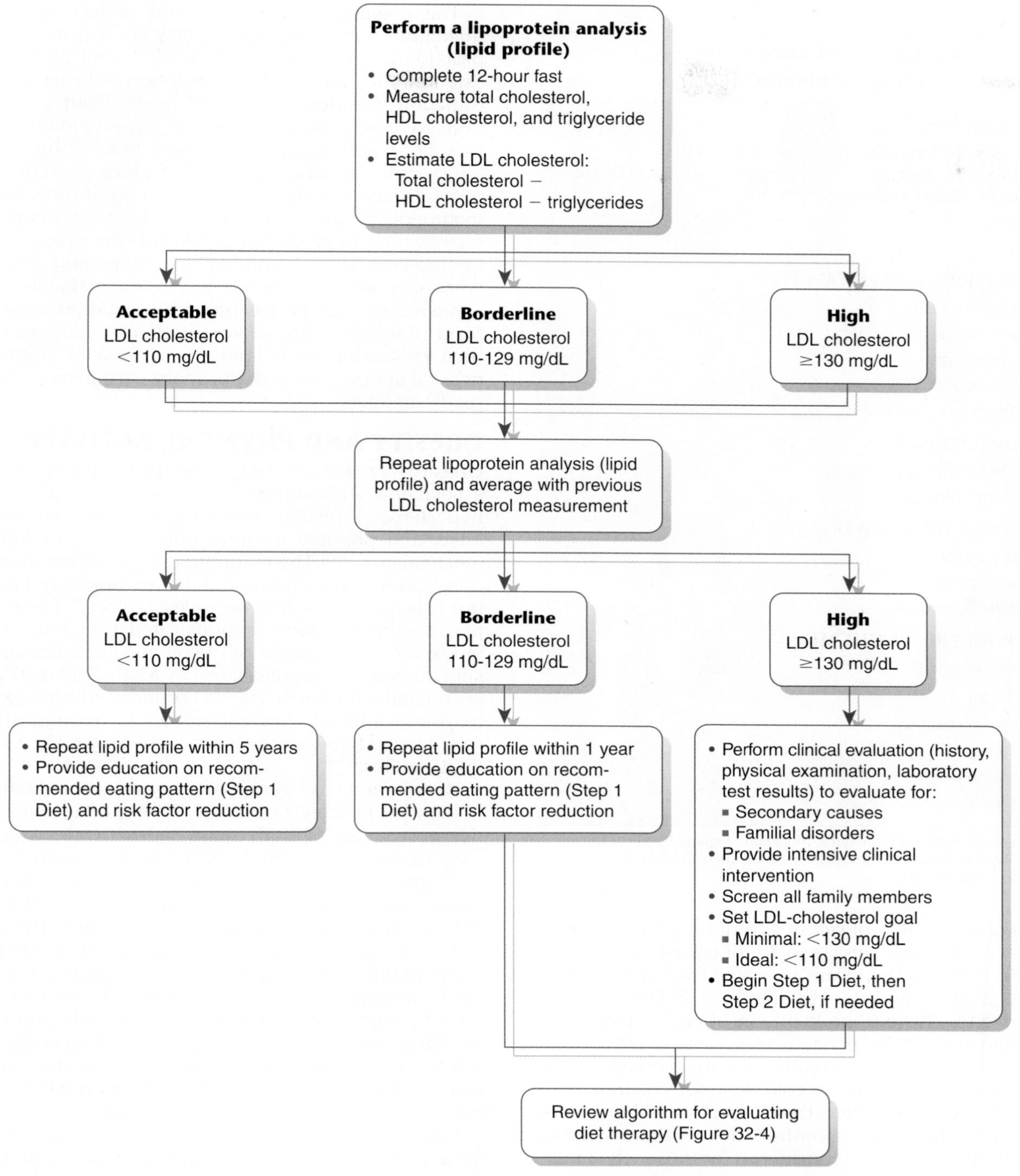

Figure 32-3 Individualized approach: algorithm for assessing and managing hyperlipidemia based on LDL cholesterol. *(Modified from National Institutes of Health. National Cholesterol Education Program:* Report of the expert panel on blood cholesterol levels in children and adolescents. *NIH Pub No 91-2732. Rockville, MD: US Department of Health and Human Services; 1979.)*

suggest that all children should consume enough calories to reach or maintain desirable weight. With the increase in the prevalence of overweight and obesity in children, weight reduction in these children is often helpful in correcting cholesterol profiles. However, in contrast to adults, some children with hypercholesterolemia are not overweight, and in children who are not overweight, caloric restriction is not the primary treatment for hypercholesterolemia, as it is often for adults.

For children whose LDL-C remains above 130 mg/dL after at least 3 months of careful adherence to the Step 1 Diet, the Step 2 Diet (Figure 32-4), with no more than

BOX 32-5 Causes of Secondary Hypercholesterolemia

EXOGENOUS

Drugs: corticosteroids, isotretinoin (Accutane), thiazides, anticonvulsants, beta-blockers, anabolic steroids, certain oral contraceptives

Alcohol

Obesity

ENDOCRINE AND METABOLIC

Hypothyroidism

Diabetes mellitus

Lipodystrophy

Pregnancy

Idiopathic hypercalcemia

STORAGE DISEASES

Glycogen storage diseases

Sphingolipidoses

OBSTRUCTIVE LIVER DISEASES

Biliary atresia

Biliary cirrhosis

Alagille syndrome

CHRONIC RENAL DISEASES

Nephrotic syndrome

OTHERS

Anorexia nervosa

Progeria

Collagen disease

Klinefelter syndrome

Modified from National Cholesterol Education Program: Report of the Expert Panel on Blood Cholesterol Levels in Children and Adolescents. *Pediatrics*. 1992;89:525.

approximately 30% of calories from total fat (similar to the Step 1 Diet) and less than 7% of calories (compared to 10% in Step 1 Diet) from saturated fat, is advised (see Table 32-3). Adherence to the Step 2 Diet is often improved by having the family meet with a registered dietician trained in managing hyperlipidemia in children.[33] Consider drug treatment with binding resins, such as cholestyramine or colestipol, for children older than 10 years whose LDL-C level remains above 190 mg/dL after 6 to 12 months of dietary therapy. Drug therapy should also be considered for those who maintain a level of LDL-C above 160 mg/dL *and* who have a family history of premature cardiovascular disease (see Figure 32-4). Commercially available dietary products, such as special margarines with plant sterols and stanols to reduce LDL-C absorption, are available in supermarkets; however, the 2005 AHA/AAP Dietary Recommendations caution against using these spreads given the possible decrease in absorption of fat-soluble vitamins and beta-carotene.[26] Other medications such as 3-hydroxy-3-methylglutaryl coenzyme A reductase inhibitors (HMG CoA-reductase inhibitors, or statins) are not recommended routinely for children, except in consultation with a lipid specialist.[21]

The cholesterol screening and dietary treatment guidelines can be initiated safely by a primary care practitioner (see Figures 32-1, 32-2, and 32-3) interested in nutrition and the prevention of heart disease. Initiation includes a review of family history, evaluation for secondary causes of hyperlipidemia (see Box 32-5), and dietary counseling. In addition, identifying children who have risk factors for coronary heart disease should lead to screening of other family members, including the parents, because many risk factors tend to cluster in families. If the primary care pediatrician is not comfortable managing children who have severe hypercholesterolemia that is unresponsive to dietary treatment or children who are from families with early onset of heart disease, then evaluation by a lipid specialist with continued general support from the primary care pediatrician is recommended.

OBESITY AND PHYSICAL ACTIVITY

Obesity increases the risk for heart disease through its association with abnormalities such as dyslipidemia, hypertension, insulin resistance, and glucose intolerance, and possibly through other, as yet undefined, mechanisms.[34,35] The magnitude of the effect of childhood obesity on cardiac risk is not precisely known, but it is an area of intense investigation.[36] For example, the PDAY study demonstrated that body mass index and the thickness of the panniculus adiposus (ie, subcutaneous fat as measured by a skin-fold test) were correlated with the degree of coronary atherosclerosis in young adults.[12] Several studies have suggested a relationship between the level of obesity and abnormal lipid profiles.[37,38]

A common and reasonable approach in defining obesity in children is based on the use of age and gender percentiles of body mass index (BMI), which is easy to calculate (BMI=kg/m^2). Children who have a BMI greater than the 95th percentile are considered *obese*, and those with a BMI between the 85th and 95th percentile are considered *overweight*. The Centers for Disease Control and Prevention (CDC) in 2000 adopted different terms to avoid the negative labeling of children; namely, *risk of overweight* is used for children between the 85th and 95th percentile and *overweight* is used for those above the 95th percentile. The terms *overweight* and *obesity* are often used interchangeably, and attention should be paid when reading the scientific literature for definitions.

Charting materials for BMI by age and gender should be a part of every primary care physician's practice. Free templates can be found online from the CDC.[39] Although adiposity in childhood is strongly associated with adiposity in adulthood, and although BMI is considered an appropriate measure of obesity, the United States Preventive Services Task Force concluded that evidence was insufficient to recommend for or against screening of overweight in children and adolescents.[40] Current recommendations from the AHA[1] and AAP[41] suggest that pediatricians should feel more confident in assessing and charting BMI, beginning at 2 years of age, and in counseling parents to address the at-risk child's eating and activity patterns. (See Chapter 34, Prevention of Obesity.)

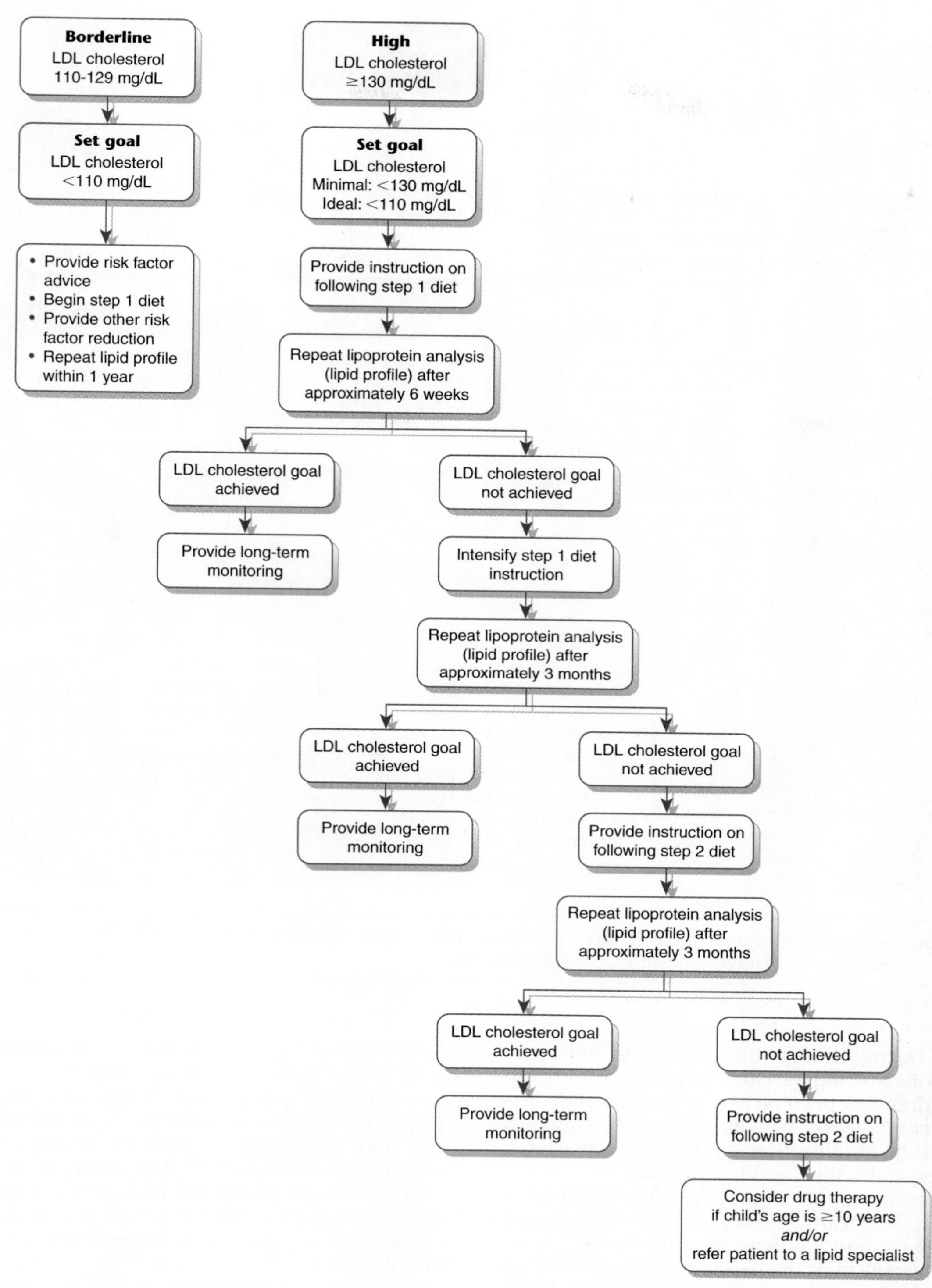

Figure 32-4 Individualized approach: algorithm for evaluating diet therapy in children with borderline or high screening LDL-cholesterol levels. *(Modified from National Institutes of Health. National Cholesterol Education Program:* Report of the expert panel on blood cholesterol levels in children and adolescents. *NIH Pub No 91-2732. Rockville, MD: US Department of Health and Human Services; 1979.)*

BMI can be easily calculated and charted for all children (see Table 32-1); and overweight children (BMI >95th percentile) should be further screened for hypertension, orthopedic complaints, hypoventilation, and abnormalities of lipids and glucose metabolism.[7,41,42] Figure 32-5 provides an algorithm to assist in screening. Additional specialty evaluations should be recommended in individual situations, with the

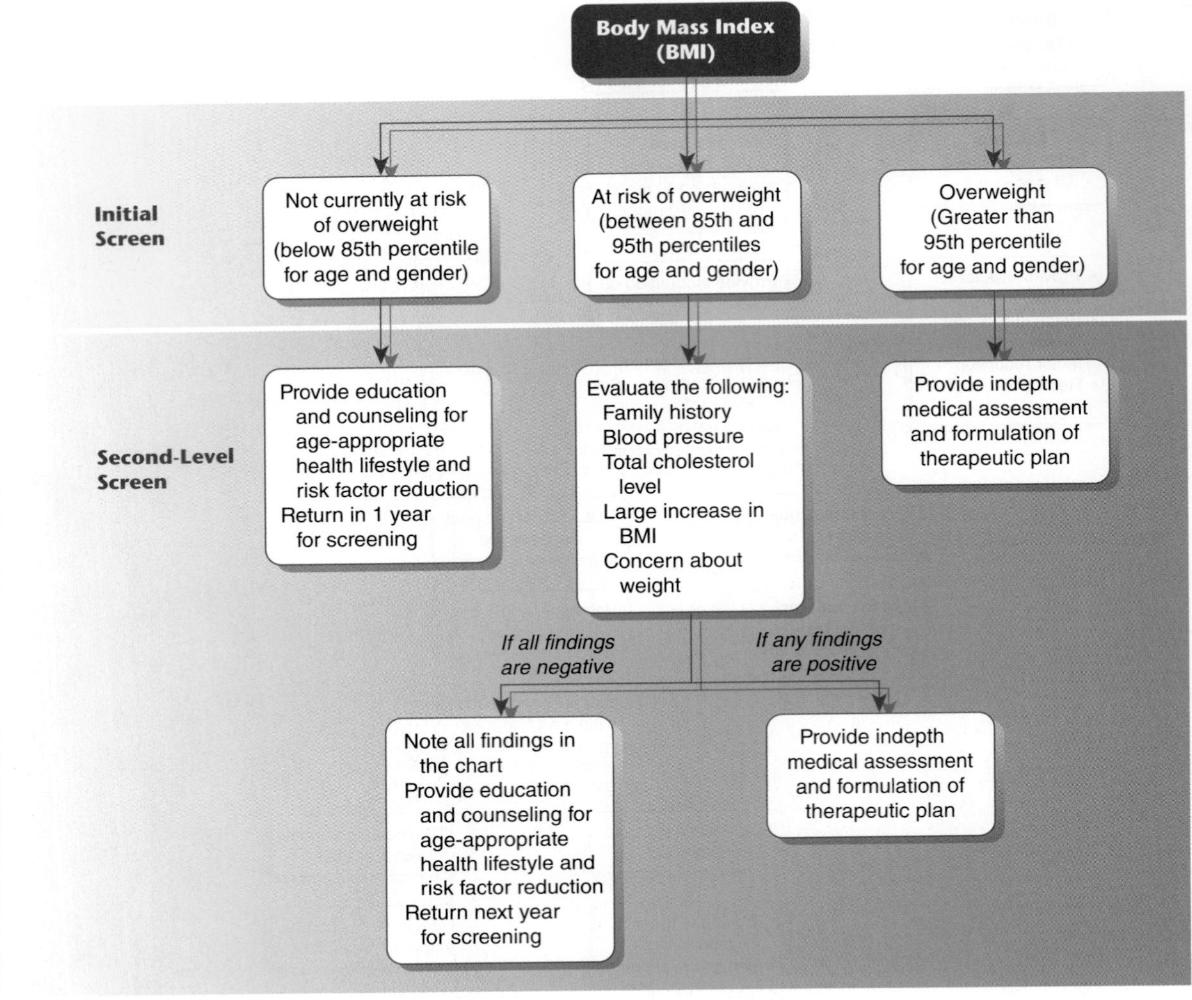

Figure 32-5 Evaluation of overweight in children. *(Modified from Barlow SE, Dietz WH. Obesity Evaluation and Treatment: Expert Committee Recommendations.* Pediatrics. *1998;102[3]:e29.)*

magnitude of the abnormalities being an important consideration. No single treatment program for overweight children has been proven to be uniformly successful. A combination of diet and exercise therapy with behavioral modification and family counseling is often needed and is the first-line approach.

The importance of physical activity in preventing or ameliorating other cardiac risk factors such as obesity, hyperlipidemia, and hypertension has been recognized increasingly over the last several years.[26,42] Furthermore, in adults, higher levels of physical activity have been associated with decreased rates of heart disease, above and beyond those associated with changes in known cardiac risk factors.[43,44]

Health care professionals should encourage children to make physical activity a part of their daily routine (Box 32-6).[37,45] A *Cochrane Review* found that although many diet and exercise interventions to prevent obesity in children are not effective in preventing weight gain, they improve eating behaviors and physical activity levels.[46] Children and their families should be encouraged to be physically active, and studies suggest that children are more likely to be physically active if their parents are active (see Table 32-1).[47] Recent recommendations by the AHA and endorsed by the AAP stress the importance of physical activity appropriate for age.[1,26,42] For example, school-aged children should participate in regular physical activity most days of the week for at least 1 hour per day and should limit television and computer time to less than 2 hours per day.[26,42]

SMOKING

The evidence that cigarette smoking is a risk factor for cardiovascular disease is overwhelming. Studies as early as 1940 documented a relationship between tobacco use and coronary artery disease.[48] In 1964 the Surgeon General first reported the link between smoking and heart disease. In 1979 the Surgeon General addressed the growing problem of children who smoked or were exposed to smoke and, in 1994, addressed the need for smoking prevention in young

BOX 32-6 Counseling Guidelines for Healthy Physical Activity

- Regular walking, bicycling, and outdoor play; use of playgrounds and gymnasiums; interaction with other children
- Participation in regular household chores
- Emphasis on play rather than exercise
- Fewer than 2 hours per day watching television, videos, and computer activities
- Weekly participation in age-appropriate organized sports, lessons, clubs, games
- Daily school or child care physical education that includes 20 minutes of coordinated large muscle exercise
- Access to school buildings and community facilities that enable safe participation in physical activity
- Extracurricular programs in schools and community recreation centers to meet needs and interests of specific populations such as racial and ethnic minority groups, girls, persons who have disabilities, and low-income groups
- Opportunities for physical activity that are fun, increase confidence, and involve friends and peers
- Regular family outings that involve walking, cycling, swimming, and other recreation
- Positive role modeling for a physically active lifestyle by parents, other caretakers, physicians, and school personnel

Data from Anderson AJ, Sobocinski KA, Freedman DS, et al. Body fat distribution, plasma lipids, and lipoproteins. *Arteriosclerosis.* 1988;8:88-94.

people.[49-51] A 1996 AHA task force presented more evidence that tobacco use increases the risk of cardiovascular disease.[52] Tobacco use adversely affects lipid levels and is associated with decreased exercise capacity, increased platelet aggregation, increased incidence of respiratory illness, increased incidence of low–birth-weight deliveries, and increased infant mortality. In addition, exposure to passive smoking is linked with changes in risk factors for coronary artery disease in children.[53] Passive smoking is associated with reduced HDL-C in nonsmoking children,[54] as well as those with high-risk lipid profiles.[55] In 2006 the Surgeon General issued an update on findings and recommendations to eliminate secondhand or passive smoke exposure for children.[56]

Adolescents are more likely to smoke or use tobacco than any other age group. In 2002 the National Youth Tobacco Survey estimated that 13% of middle school and 28% of high school students were current users of tobacco products.[57] In 2003 the National Youth Risk Behavior Survey showed a decline in reported current tobacco use among high school students; however, the estimate was still 22%.[58] The risk of smoking initiation increases from ages 12 to 16 years, with most initiating and becoming addicted during this critical period.[59] Although most youth do not become nicotine dependent until after 2 to 3 years of smoking, addiction can occur after smoking as few as 100 cigarettes.[60]

Children whose parents or siblings smoke are at an increased risk of beginning to smoke. Other factors that may predict smoking include peer influence, less-educated parents, independence and rebelliousness, and decreased concerns about the health risks associated with smoking. Identifying these factors and addressing them openly is helpful in counseling. Primary care physicians should advise smoking parents about the risks and refer them to a smoking cessation program. Pediatricians should actively participate in and support school and community antismoking campaigns. Although the current decline in the prevalence of smoking among children is a positive change, the potential for addiction brings smoking prevention into the realm of pediatric practice. The risks of smoking should be a part of routine preventive care discussions (see Table 32-1). For further reading on smoking prevention, including age-specific strategies, please refer to Chapter 35, Prevention of Smoking.

CONCLUSION

Given the prevailing evidence from adults with atherosclerotic cardiovascular disease and the emerging risk factors in children, the pediatric primary care physician should start to identify and treat these potential atherosclerotic cardiac risk factors in children. Even more important, the pediatric primary care physician can educate children and families on preventive strategies that obviate the development of these risk factors and their progression into adulthood. The long-term hope is that these early interventions will ultimately decrease the burden of atherosclerotic heart disease in adult life.

TOOLS FOR PRACTICE

Engaging Patient and Family

- *Exercise (Physical Activity) and Children* (fact sheet), American Heart Association (www.americanheart.org/presenter.jhtml?identifier=4596).

Medical Decision Support

- *American Heart Association Guidelines for Primary Prevention of Atherosclerotic Cardiovascular Disease Beginning in Childhood* (guidelines), American Heart Association (www.circ.ahajournals.org/cgi/content/full/107/11/1562).
- *Cardiovascular Health in Childhood: A Statement for Health for Health Professionals From the Committee on Atherosclerosis, Hypertension, and Obesity in the Young (AHOY) of the Council on Cardiovascular Disease in the Young, American Heart Association* (policy statement), American Heart Association (www.circ.ahajournals.org/cgi/content/full/106/1/143?ck=nck).
- Growth Charts—tutorials and information (Web page), Centers for Disease Control and Prevention (www.cdc.gov/growthcharts/).
- *Growth Charts* (chart), Centers for Disease Control and Prevention, (www.cdc.gov/nchs/about/major/nhanes/growthcharts/clinical_charts.htm#Clin%201). Also available at AAP bookstore: www.aap.org/bookstore.

- *Pediatric Obesity: Prevention, Intervention, and Treatment Strategies for Primary Care* (book), American Academy of Pediatrics (www.aap.org/bookstore).
- *Understanding Obesity in Youth. A Statement for Healthcare Professionals From the Committee on Atherosclerosis and Hypertension in the Young of the Council on Cardiovascular Disease in the Young and the Nutrition Committee, American Heart Association* (policy statement), American Heart Association (www.circ.ahajournals.org/cgi/content/full/94/12/3383).

AAP POLICY STATEMENTS

American Academy of Pediatrics Committee on Nutrition. Cholesterol in childhood. *Pediatrics*. 1998;101(1):141-147. (aappolicy.aappublications.org/cgi/content/full/pediatrics;101/1/141).

American Heart Association. Dietary recommendations for children and adolescents: a guide for practitioners: consensus statement from the American Heart Association. *Circulation*. 2005;112(13):2061-2075. AAP endorsed.

Kavey R-EW, Allada V, Daniels SR, et al. Cardiovascular risk reduction in high-risk pediatric populations. *Circulation*. 2006;114(24);2710-2738. AAP endorsed.

REFERENCES

1. Williams CL, Hayman LL, Daniels SR, et al. Cardiovascular health in childhood: a statement for health professionals from the Committee on Atherosclerosis, Hypertension, and Obesity in the Young (AHOY) of the Council on Cardiovascular Disease in the Young, American Heart Association. *Circulation*. 2002;106(1):143-160.
2. American Academy of Pediatrics. Cardiovascular risk reduction in high-risk pediatric populations. *Pediatrics*. 2007;119(3):618-621.
3. Berenson GS, Srinivasan SR, Bao W, et al. Association between multiple cardiovascular risk factors and atherosclerosis in children and young adults. The Bogalusa Heart Study. *N Engl J Med*. 1998;338(23):1650-1656.
4. Juonala M, Jarvisalo MJ, Maki-Torkko N, et al. Risk factors identified in childhood and decreased carotid artery elasticity in adulthood. The Cardiovascular Risk in Young Finns Study. *Circulation*. 2005;112(10):1486-1493.
5. Kavey R-EW, Daniels SR, Lauer RM, et al. American Heart Association guidelines for primary prevention of atherosclerotic cardiovascular disease beginning in childhood. *Circulation*. 2003;107(11):1562-1566.
6. Williams C. Prevention of coronary artery disease. In: Gewitz MH, ed. *Primary Pediatric Cardiology*. Armonk, NY: Futura Publishing; 1995.
7. Gidding SS. Preventive pediatric cardiology. Tobacco, cholesterol, obesity, and physical activity. *Pediatr Clin North Am*. 1999;46(2):253-262.
8. Stamler J, Dyer AR, Shekelle RB, et al. Relationship of baseline major risk factors to coronary and all-cause mortality, and to longevity: findings from long-term follow-up of Chicago cohorts. *Cardiology*. 1993;82(2-3):191-222.
9. Pasternak RC, Grundy SM, Levy D, et al. 27th Bethesda Conference: matching the intensity of risk factor management with the hazard for coronary disease events. Task Force 3. Spectrum of risk factors for coronary heart disease. *J Am Coll Cardiol*. 1996;27(5):978-990.
10. Expert Panel on Detection Evaluation and Treatment of High Blood Cholesterol in Adults. Executive summary of the third report of the National Cholesterol Education Program (NCEP) Expert Panel on Detection, Evaluation, and Treatment of High Blood Cholesterol in Adults (Adult Treatment Panel III). *JAMA*. 2001;285(19):2486-2497.
11. Enos WF, Beyer JC, Holmes RH. Pathogenesis of coronary artery disease in American soldiers killed in Korea. *JAMA*. 1953;158:912-914.
12. McGill HC Jr, McMahan CA, Malcom GT, et al. Relation of glycohemoglobin and adiposity to atherosclerosis in youth. Pathobiological Determinants of Atherosclerosis in Youth (PDAY) Research Group. *Arterioscler Thromb Vasc Biol*. 1995;15(4):431-440.
13. McGill HC Jr, McMahan CA, Zieske AW, et al. Association of coronary heart disease risk factors with microscopic qualities of coronary atherosclerosis in youth. *Circulation*. 2000;102(4):374-379.
14. Gordon DJ, Rifkind BM. High-density lipoprotein—the clinical implications of recent studies. *N Engl J Med*. 1989;321(19):1311-1316.
15. Brown MS, Goldstein JL. A receptor-mediated pathway for cholesterol homeostasis. *Science*. 1986;232(4746):34-47.
16. Scientific Steering Committee on behalf of the Simon Broome Register Group. Mortality in treated heterozygous familial hypercholesterolaemia: implications for clinical management. *Atherosclerosis*. 1999;142(1):105-112.
17. National Cholesterol Education Program. Report of the Expert Panel on Blood Cholesterol Levels in Children and Adolescents. *Pediatrics*. 1992;89(3 pt 2):525-584.
18. American Academy of Pediatrics, Committee on Nutrition. Cholesterol in childhood. *Pediatrics*. 1998; 101(1 Pt 1):141-147.
19. Newman TB, Browner WS, Hulley SB. The case against childhood cholesterol screening. *JAMA*. 1990;264(23): 3039-3043.
20. Garber AM. Cholesterol screening should be targeted. *Am J Med*. 1997;102(2A):26-30.
21. Gidding SS. Controlling cholesterol in children. *Contemp Pediatr*. 2001;18:77-78, 83-100.
22. O'Loughlin J, Lauzon B, Paradis G, et al. Usefulness of the American Academy of Pediatrics recommendations for identifying youths with hypercholesterolemia. *Pediatrics*. 2004;113(6):1723-1727.
23. US Preventive Services Task Force. Screening for lipid disorders in children: recommendation statement. *Pediatrics*. 2007;120(1):e215-e219.
24. Dennison BA, Kikuchi DA, Srinivasan SR, et al. Parental history of cardiovascular disease as an indication for screening for lipoprotein abnormalities in children. *J Pediatr*. 1989;115(2):186-194.
25. Starc TJ, Belamarich PF, Shea S, et al. Family history fails to identify many children with severe hypercholesterolemia. *Am J Dis Child*. 1991;145(1):61-64.
26. Gidding SS, Dennison BA, Birch LL, et al. Dietary recommendations for children and adolescents: a guide for practitioners: consensus statement from the American Heart Association. *Circulation*. 2005;112(13):2061-2075.
27. Rose G. Sick individuals and sick populations. *Int J Epidemiol*. 1985;14(1):32-38.
28. Kavey R-EW, Allada V, Daniels SR, et al. Cardiovascular risk reduction in high-risk pediatric patients: a scientific statement from the American Heart Association Expert Panel on Population and Prevention Science; the Councils on Cardiovascular Disease in the Young, Epidemiology and Prevention, Nutrition, Physical Activity and Metabolism, High Blood Pressure Research, Cardiovascular Nursing, and the Kidney in Heart Disease; and the Interdisciplinary Working Group on Quality of Care and Outcomes Research: endorsed by the American Academy of Pediatrics. *Circulation*. 2006;114(24): 2710-2738
29. Jolliffe CJ, Janssen I. Distribution of lipoproteins by age and gender in adolescents. *Circulation*. 2006;114(10):1056-1062.
30. Gidding SS. New cholesterol guidelines for children? *Circulation*. 2006;114(10):989-991.

31. Hickman TB, Briefel RR, Carroll MD, et al. Distributions and trends of serum lipid levels among United States children and adolescents ages 4-19 years: data from the Third National Health and Nutrition Examination Survey. *Prev Med.* 1998;27(6):879-890.
32. Writing Group for the DISC Collaborative Research Group. Efficacy and safety of lowering dietary intake of fat and cholesterol in children with elevated low-density lipoprotein cholesterol. The Dietary Intervention Study in Children (DISC). *JAMA.* 1995;273(18): 1429-1435.
33. Kaistha A, Deckelbaum RJ, Starc TJ, et al. Overrestriction of dietary fat intake before formal nutritional counseling in children with hyperlipidemia. *Arch Pediatr Adolesc Med.* 2001;155(11):1225-1230.
34. Kaplan NM. The deadly quartet. Upper-body obesity, glucose intolerance, hypertriglyceridemia, and hypertension. *Arch Intern Med.* 1989;149(7):1514-1520.
35. Gidding SS, Leibel RL, Daniels S, et al. Understanding obesity in youth. A statement for healthcare professionals from the Committee on Atherosclerosis and Hypertension in the Young of the Council on Cardiovascular Disease in the Young and the Nutrition Committee, American Heart Association. Writing Group. *Circulation.* 1996;94(12):3383-3387.
36. Must A, Jacques PF, Dallal GE, et al. Long-term morbidity and mortality of overweight adolescents. A follow-up of the Harvard Growth Study of 1922 to 1935. *N Engl J Med.* 1992;327(19):1350-1355.
37. Anderson AJ, Sobocinski KA, Freedman DS, et al. Body fat distribution, plasma lipids, and lipoproteins. *Arteriosclerosis.* 1988;8(1):88-94.
38. Barakat HA, Burton DS, Carpenter JW, et al. Body fat distribution, plasma lipoproteins and the risk of coronary heart disease of male subjects. *Int J Obes.* 1988;12(5):473-480.
39. Centers for Disease Control and Prevention. Clinical Growth Charts. Available at: www.cdc.gov/nchs/about/major/nhanes/growthcharts/clinical_charts.htm. Accessed 20 February 2006.
40. US Preventive Services Task Force. Screening and interventions for overweight in children and adolescents: recommendation statement. *Pediatrics.* 2005;116(1):205-209.
41. Barlow SE, Dietz WH. Obesity evaluation and treatment: expert committee recommendations. *Pediatrics.* 1998;102(3):e29.
42. Daniels SR, Arnett DK, Eckel RH, et al. Overweight in children and adolescents: pathophysiology, consequences, prevention, and treatment. *Circulation.* 2005;111(15): 1999-2012.
43. Blair SN, Kampert JB, Kohl HW, et al. Influences of cardiorespiratory fitness and other precursors on cardiovascular disease and all-cause mortality in men and women. *JAMA.* 1996;276(3):205-210.
44. Paffenbarger RS Jr, Hyde RT, Wing AL, et al. The association of changes in physical-activity level and other lifestyle characteristics with mortality among men. *N Engl J Med.* 1993;328(8):538-545.
45. American Heart Association. Scientific Position: Exercise (Physical Activity) and Children. Available at: www.americanheart.org/presenter.jhtml?identifier=4596. Accessed February 2, 2006.
46. Summerbell CD, Waters E, Edmunds LD, et al. Interventions for preventing obesity in children. In: *The Cochrane Library.* Issue 1. Oxford, UK: Update Software; 2006.
47. Moore LL, Lombardi DA, White MJ, et al. Influence of parents' physical activity levels on activity levels of young children. *J Pediatr.* 1991;118(2):215-219.
48. English JP, Willus FA, Berkson J. Tobacco and coronary disease. *JAMA.* 1940;115(16):1327-1329.
49. United States Surgeon General's Advisory Committee on Smoking and Health. *Smoking and Health: Report of the Advisory Committee to the Surgeon General of the Public Health Service.* Washington, DC: US Dept. of Health, Education, and Welfare, Public Health Service; 1964.
50. Public Health Service, Office of the Surgeon General, United States Office on Smoking and Health, United States Surgeon General's Advisory Committee on Smoking and Health. *Smoking and Health: A Report of the Surgeon General.* Rockville, MD: US Department of Health, Education, and Welfare, Public Health Service, Office of the Assistant Secretary for Health; 1979.
51. United States Office on Smoking and Health, United States Public Health Service, Office of the Surgeon General. *Preventing Tobacco Use Among Young people: A Report of the Surgeon General.* Washington, DC: US Department of Health and Human Services, Public Health Service, Centers for Disease Control and Prevention, National Center for Chronic Disease Prevention and Health Promotion; 1994.
52. Ockene IS, Miller NH. Cigarette smoking, cardiovascular disease, and stroke: a statement for healthcare professionals from the American Heart Association. American Heart Association Task Force on Risk Reduction. *Circulation.* 1997;96(9):3243-3247.
53. Gidding SS, Schydlower M. Active and passive tobacco exposure: a serious pediatric health problem. *Pediatrics.* 1994;94(5):750-751.
54. Feldman J, Shenker IR, Etzel RA, et al. Passive smoking alters lipid profiles in adolescents. *Pediatrics.* 1991;88(2):259-264.
55. Neufeld EJ, Mietus-Snyder M, Beiser AS, et al. Passive cigarette smoking and reduced HDL cholesterol levels in children with high-risk lipid profiles. *Circulation.* 1997;96(5):1403-1407.
56. Public Health Service, Office of the Surgeon General. *The Health Consequences of Involuntary Exposure to Tobacco Smoke: A Report of the Surgeon General.* Rockville, MD: US Department of Health and Human Services, Public Health Service, Office of the Surgeon General; 2006.
57. Centers for Disease Control and Prevention. Tobacco use among middle and high school students—United States, 2002. *MMWR Morb Mortal Wkly Rep.* 2003;52(RR-45): 1096-1098.
58. Centers for Disease Control and Prevention. Cigarette use among high school students—United States, 1991-2003. *MMWR Morb Mortal Wkly Rep.* 2004;53(RR-23): 499-502.
59. Giovino GA. Epidemiology of tobacco use in the United States. *Oncogene.* 2002;21(48):7326-7340.
60. American Academy of Pediatrics, Committee on Substance Abuse. Tobacco's toll: implications for the pediatrician. *Pediatrics.* 2001;107(4):794-798.

Chapter 33

PREVENTION OF DENTAL CARIES

Robert J. Berkowitz, DDS; Pamela K. Den Besten, DDS, MS; Jeffrey M. Karp, DMD, MS

Dental caries is one of the most common bacterial infections afflicting children and adolescents. The disease is a localized, progressive destruction of tooth structure by bacterial activity. The occurrence of dental caries is related to critical interrelationships among the tooth, dietary carbohydrate, saliva, and specific oral bacteria. The decay process is initiated by demineralization of the outer tooth surface as a result of organic acids formed during bacterial fermentation of dietary carbohydrates. Simultaneously, saliva functions as a remineralizing and buffering solution to counter the effect of demineralization. Should bacterial-derived demineralization exceed saliva's remineralization and buffering capacity, carious lesions form. Incipient lesions first appear as opaque white spots; with progressive loss of tooth mineral, cavitation occurs.

ETIOLOGY

Microbial Factors

Mutans streptococci are a primary etiologic agent in human dental caries.[1] Therefore an important approach toward preventing dental caries is to reduce intraoral levels of mutans streptococci. Many studies focusing on epidemiologic, chemotherapeutic, and immunologic strategies are currently under way.

Salivary Factors

Observations in desalivated experimental animals and xerostomic humans clearly indicate that saliva is the primary host defense against dental caries. Salivary hypofunction may be a consequence of a variety of factors, including (in part) the following: radiotherapy when the salivary glands are within the radiation ports, chronic administration of anticholinergic or parasympatholytic drugs, and salivary gland disease (eg, Sjögren syndrome). Accordingly, such patients should be referred to pediatric dentists for aggressive dental caries preventive measures. The relationship between salivary gland hypofunction and dental caries is related to several factors. First, the physical flow of saliva augmented by the activity of the oral musculature removes a large number of bacteria from the teeth. Second, salivary proteins and enzymes (lysozyme, lactoferrin, and lactoperoxidase) work with other salivary components to kill bacteria, interfere with bacterial replication, or interfere with the acidogenic potential of cariogenic bacteria. Third, saliva can also interfere with bacterial attachment through molecular interactions. Finally, saliva has properties that directly protect the tooth surface from demineralization. Salivary bicarbonate, phosphate, and histidine-rich peptides diffuse into plaque biofilm and act directly as buffers. In addition to helping to counter plaque biofilm acidity, saliva remineralizes teeth. The presence of fluoride in trace quantities reduces enamel crystal solubility, allowing remineralization. Given that remineralization is promoted by the frequent introduction of a low concentration of fluoride into the mouth, the small amount of fluoride in fluoridated drinking water is sufficient to promote remineralization.[2]

Dietary Factors

Most dietary sugars, carbohydrates, and starches are readily metabolized to organic acids by mutans streptococci and are termed *cariogenic substrates*. Multiple investigations in humans and laboratory animals demonstrate that frequent and prolonged oral exposure to sugars, carbohydrates, and starches facilitates dental caries activity.[3] Stated differently, it is not how much sugar a person eats but how a person eats sugar that determines the sugar's relative cariogenic potential. For example, the cariogenic potential of apple juice contained in a nursing bottle that is sampled throughout the night or naptimes, or both, is quite different from that of the same volume of apple juice consumed at a single meal. Similarly, sugars contained in food products retained orally for a long time are more cariogenic than those in food products retained orally for short times (eg, the sugar in a liquid that is immediately swallowed versus the sugar in a sticky raisin or caramel that can stick to teeth).

PREVENTION

Fluoride

Water Fluoridation

The relationships among natural water fluoride concentrations, dental caries prevalence, and enamel fluorosis were determined in studies by H. Trendley Dean in the 1930s and 1940s. The recommendation for an optimal level of water fluoridation was refined to a range of 0.7 to 1.2 ppm fluoride, depending on the amount of water intake. Fluoridation of public water supplies has proven to be the most effective, convenient, and economical measure available to prevent dental caries.[4]

Fluoride Supplements

The dramatic reduction in dental caries in populations drinking fluoridated water led to recommendations to administer fluoride as a dietary supplement for people who did not receive it in their drinking water. Fluoride was assumed to have a systemic mode of action resulting in the formation of a more dental caries–resistant enamel structure, leading to the conclusion that fluoride supplements should mimic previous estimates of dietary fluoride intake. Fluoride supplements were therefore proposed for the period during which teeth were developing. However, fluoride acts topically to prevent dental caries through salivary remineralization of demineralized enamel. This action works best by frequent exposure to relatively low levels of fluoride, as occurs with drinking fluoridated water.[1] The realization that systemic fluoride ingestion is not the major mechanism of action of fluoride in dental caries prevention and reports on increased dental fluorosis (see Dental Fluorosis) have led to new fluoride supplementation recommendations (Table 33-1). Because the risk of fluorosis increases with increased exposure to fluoride, pediatricians should assess a child's exposure to other fluoride sources such as toothpaste and fluoridated commercial beverages before prescribing fluoride supplements. If supplements are given, then they should be sucked or chewed to enhance the topical action of the fluoride in the supplements.

Dental Fluorosis

Dental fluorosis is a hypomineralization of enamel that occurs when higher than optimal levels of fluoride are ingested during the period of enamel formation. Fluorosis may vary from very mild to severe. Very mild to mild cases appear as chalky whitening of the enamel; severe fluorosis exhibits as mottled enamel

Table 33-1 Daily Fluoride Supplement Dose Schedule*

AGE	CONCENTRATION OF FLUORIDE IN DRINKING WATER (ppmF)		
	<0.3	0.3-0.6	>0.6
Birth-6 mo	0	0	0
6 mo-3 yr	0.25 mg	0	0
3-6 yr	0.5 mg	0.25 mg	0
6-16 yr	1.0 mg	0.5 mg	0

ppmF, Parts per million fluoride (1 mg of fluoride per liter of water = 1 ppmF).
*Fluoride dose regimen accepted by the American Academy of Pediatrics, the American Academy of Pediatric Dentistry, and the American Dental Association (1994).

that is pitted and brown in color. Recent reports have shown a trend toward a higher prevalence of dental fluorosis relative to historical data from earlier studies. This increase in the prevalence of fluorosis was found to correlate with the ingestion of fluoride from sources other than drinking water, including fluoride supplements, fluoridated toothpaste, and commercial beverages containing fluoridated water.[5,6]

Accordingly, the Council on Dental Therapeutics of the American Dental Association has endorsed a new fluoride supplementation schedule (see Table 33-1). Fluoride supplements are not recommended prenatally or during the first 6 months of life. In addition, breastfed infants residing in optimally fluoridated communities should not receive fluoride supplements. As indicated in Table 33-1, the dose level is based on the patient's age and fluoride content of the water supply. The recommended supplement dose should be considered a maximum, and other sources of ingested fluoride, such as from toothpastes and commercial beverages, should also be taken into account. The fluoride level of a water supply can usually be obtained by calling the local water board. Should the patient use a private water supply, then a fluoride analysis is indicated. The patient's parent should be instructed to use a plastic container for the water specimen (a glass container may impair the accuracy of the fluoride assay) and send to an appropriate laboratory. When providing supplements, no fluoride prescription should be written for more than 120 mg of fluoride. Even if a child ingested the entire supply, probably only mild gastric upset would ensue. However, in such an event, a poison control center should be contacted immediately.

Toothpaste can also provide a topical form of fluoride supplement for children who swallow the toothpaste after brushing. For children who are not able to spit, a maximal recommended fluoride dose may be ingested simply by brushing a child's teeth once or twice a day. To reduce the risk of dental fluorosis from toothpaste ingestion, a small amount of toothpaste (pea size) should be used in brushing a young child's teeth, and the parent should dispense the toothpaste. Young children should not have access to toothpaste.

Fluoride Dentifrice (Toothpaste)

Fluoride-containing dentifrices are highly effective in preventing dental decay. Toothbrushing with a pea-size amount of dentifrice on a toothbrush should be encouraged as soon as teeth begin to erupt. Before the age 6 years, children tend to swallow rather than expectorate dentifrice, and nearly all of the ingested fluoride is absorbed, primarily from the small intestine. Therefore, although the use of a fluoride-containing dentifrice should be encouraged, the amount used for young children should be limited.

Fluoride Rinses

Fluoride rinses containing 0.05% fluoride are highly effective in reducing dental decay. These products are available without a prescription and should be recommended for children older than 6 years who are at risk for dental decay because of conditions such as compromised salivary flow rates, orthodontic therapy, and a high dental caries experience. They are not recommended for children younger than 6 years because of their inability to expectorate properly, resulting in excessive fluoride ingestion.

Fluoride Varnish

Fluoride varnishes that can be painted on the teeth are now available in the United States. Fluoride varnishes contain high concentrations of fluoride (up to 22,600 ppm) suspended in a viscous delivery medium. They can be applied to the teeth of high-risk children by trained personnel in various settings, including the medical office.[7] Fluoride varnishes, unlike foams, rinses, and gels, do not require trays or oral suction equipment.

Oral Hygiene

Thorough daily brushing and flossing of the teeth helps prevent dental caries and periodontal disease. Teeth are mechanically cleansed to disturb the attachment of dental plaque biofilm to the tooth surface. Parents should verify that the child's teeth are clean before bedtime because the buffering capacity and antimicrobial action of saliva decreases during sleep with diminished secretion of saliva. Parents should receive professional instruction regarding oral hygiene techniques for children. Information regarding performing oral hygiene can be obtained from the American Dental Association at its Web site (www.ada.org). Clinical studies demonstrate that most children 8 years and younger do not have the hand-eye coordination required for adequate oral hygiene; accordingly, parents must assume responsibility for oral hygiene. The degree of parental involvement should reflect the child's level of competency.

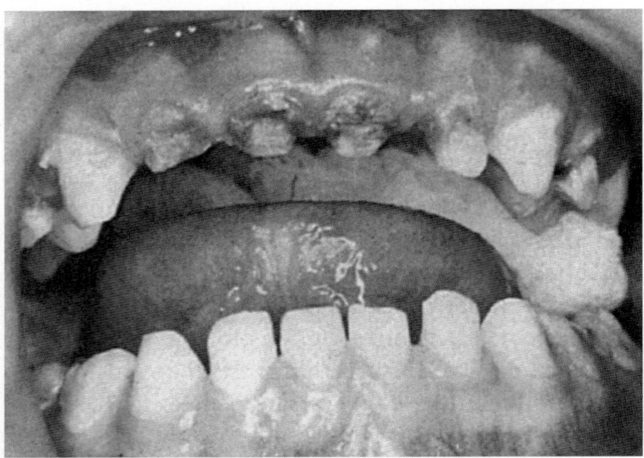

Figure 33-1 Nursing bottle dental caries in a child aged 2½ years.

Sealants

Excellent oral hygiene and optimal fluoride exposure have minimal effect in preventing dental caries in the pits and fissures on the occlusal (biting) surfaces of the posterior teeth. The use of sealants has been shown to be effective in preventing pit and fissure caries.[7] Sealants are plastic coatings that are applied professionally to the occlusal surfaces of the posterior teeth. A survey conducted by the National Institute of Dental Research indicated that relatively few schoolchildren in the United States have sealants on their teeth.[8] Unfortunately, although efficacious, the use of sealants is not routine in the prevention of dental caries.[9]

Diet

Decreasing the frequency of cariogenic substrate ingestion prevents dental caries. Parents and children should be encouraged to avoid eating between-meal snacks that contain cariogenic substrates. The use of gum, candy, and soft drinks containing sugar substitutes (mannitol, sorbitol, xylitol, and aspartame [with precautions]) is an effective approach for the child who has a sweet tooth. Chewing sugarless gum has been proven clinically to enhance salivary flow rate and, in turn, neutralize plaque biofilm pH. In addition, infants should be weaned from the bottle by 1 year of age to eliminate their risk for early childhood dental caries (also known as nursing bottle dental caries) (Figure 33-1). Otherwise, bedtime and naptime nursing bottles should contain only water. Finally, sweetened elixirs of medications used on a chronic basis result in an increase in oral exposure to cariogenic substrates, thereby increasing dental caries risk. Patients exposed to this risk factor should be referred to a pediatric dentist for aggressive dental caries preventive measures.

ROLE OF THE PEDIATRICIAN

The pediatrician has an important role in the prevention and early diagnosis of dental caries.[10] Pediatricians should routinely question parents about feeding behaviors and make recommendations that promote dental health. In addition, examination of the dentition should be performed on every child as part of a routine physical examination. The required equipment consists of an intraoral light and pediatric tongue blade. The examiner should begin with the distal maxillary molar and continue with the inspection of each tooth from right to left. The procedure should be repeated from the patient's left to right in the mandibular arch. Dental caries, which frequently appear as a darker stained area, usually begins in the pits and fissures on the biting surfaces of the molar teeth. The 2nd most frequent sites for dental caries development are the contact surfaces between the molar teeth. These areas are difficult to examine, even by the dentist, who usually depends on intraoral radiographs. Carious lesions may also be detected on the front surface of the primary incisor teeth near the gingiva. These types of lesions are routinely found in the child with severe early childhood dental caries. Retracting the lips is necessary to inspect adequately the entire surface of primary incisor teeth. Any child with evidence of cavitation, stained fissures, or areas of enamel decalcification should be referred to a dentist immediately. Every child should be evaluated by a dentist by 12 months of age.[10]

TOOLS FOR PRACTICE

Community Advocacy and Coordination

- *Preventing Dental Caries with Community Programs* (fact sheet), Centers for Disease Control and Prevention (www.cdc.gov/oralhealth/factsheets/dental_caries.htm).

Engaging Patients and Family

- *A Guide to Children's Dental Health* (brochure), American Academy of Pediatrics (patiented.aap.org).
- *How to Prevent Tooth Decay in Your Baby's Teeth* (fact sheet), American Academy of Pediatrics (www.aap.org/bookstore).
- *Brush Up on Healthy Teeth—A Quiz for Parents* (fact sheet), Centers for Disease Control and Prevention (www.cdc.gov/oralhealth/pdfs/brushupquiz.pdf).
- *Brush Up on Healthy Teeth—Simple Steps for Kids' Smiles* (fact sheet), Centers for Disease Control and Prevention (www.cdc.gov/oralhealth/pdfs/brushuptips.pdf).
- *Brushing Up on Oral Health: Never Too Early to Start* (brochure), American Academy of Pediatrics (www.aap.org/family/healthychildren/07winter/oralhealth.pdf).
- *Dental Sealants FAQ* (fact sheet), Centers for Disease Control and Prevention (www.cdc.gov/oralhealth/factsheets/sealants-faq.htm).
- *Teething and Dental Hygiene* (fact sheet), American Academy of Pediatrics (www.aap.org).
- *Tooth Development* (fact sheet), American Academy of Pediatrics (www.aap.org).
- *What is a Pediatric Dentist?* (fact sheet), American Academy of Pediatrics (www.aap.org/sections/peddentist/pediatricdentist_eng.pdf).
- *Your School-Age Child's Teeth* (fact sheet), American Academy of Pediatrics (www.aap.org).

Medical Decision Support

- *Oral Health Resources* (Web page), Centers for Disease Control and Prevention (www.cdc.gov/oralhealth/).
- *Oral Health Risk Assessment Training for Pediatricians and Other Child Health Professionals* (Web page), American Academy of Pediatrics (www.aap.org/commpeds/dochs/oralhealth/screening.cfm).

- *Surveillance for Dental Caries, Dental Sealants, Tooth Retention, Edentulism and Enamel Fluorosis—United States, 1988-1994 and 1999-2002* (fact sheet), Centers for Disease Control and Prevention (www.cdc.gov/oralhealth/factsheets/nhanes_findings.htm).
- *The Children's Oral Health Electronic Newsletter* (newsletter), American Academy of Pediatrics (www.aap.org/commpeds/dochs/oralhealth/enews.cfm).

AAP POLICY STATEMENTS

American Academy of Pediatrics, Section on Breastfeeding. Breastfeeding and the use of human milk. *Pediatrics*. 2005; 115(2):496-506. (aappolicy.aappublications.org/cgi/content/full/pediatrics;115/2/496).

American Academy of Pediatrics, Section on Pediatric Dentistry. Oral health risk assessment timing and establishment of the dental home. *Pediatrics*. 2003;111(5):1113-1116. (aappolicy.aappublications.org/cgi/content/full/pediatrics;111/5/1113).

REFERENCES

1. Loesche WJ. Role of Streptococcus mutans in human dental decay. *Microbiol Rev*. 1986;50:353-380.
2. Mandel ID. The functions of saliva. *J Dent Res*. 1987; 66:623-627.
3. Bibby B. Influence of diet on the bacterial composition of plaques. In: Stiles HM, Loesche WJ, O'Brien TC, eds. *Microbiol Aspects of Dental Caries*. Vol II. London, UK: Information Retrieval; 1976.
4. Newbrun E. Effectiveness of water fluoridation. *J Pub Health Dent*. 1989;49(5):279-289.
5. Beltran ED, Burt BA. The pre- and posteruptive effects of fluoride in the caries decline. *J Pub Health Dent*. 1988; 48:233-240.
6. Pendrys DG. Dental fluorosis in perspective. *J Am Dent Assoc*. 1991;122:63-66.
7. Rozier RG, Sutton BK, Bawden JW, et al. Prevention of early childhood caries in North Carolina medical practices: implications for research and practice. *J Dent Educ*. 2003;67:876-885.
8. American Dental Association. Sealant use low. *Am Dent Assoc News*. Apr 1989;20:24.
9. Ripa LW. The current status of pit and fissure sealants. A review. *J Can Dent Assoc*. 1985;51:367-375, 377-380.
10. American Academy of Pediatrics, Section on Pediatric Dentistry. Oral health risk assessment timing and establishment of the dental home. *Pediatrics*. 2003;5: 1113-1116.

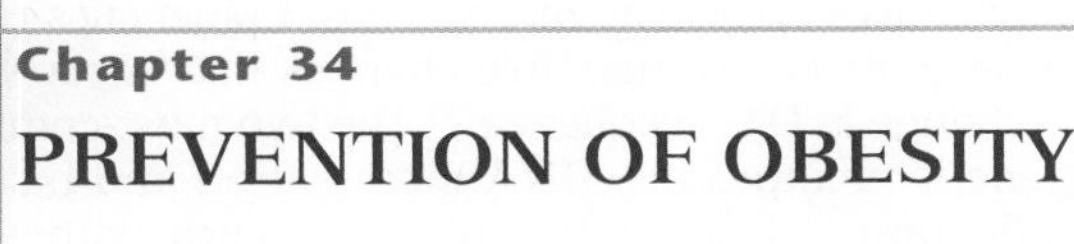

Chapter 34

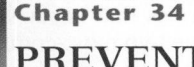

PREVENTION OF OBESITY

Sandra G. Hassink, MD; Gina M. French, MD

Childhood obesity has emerged as a major health problem that increases the risk for chronic illnesses in children. Obesity comorbidities include dyslipidemia, type 2 diabetes, nonalcoholic steatohepatitis, polycystic ovarian syndrome, slipped capital epiphysis, Blount disease, and sleep apnea. These illnesses along with depression and self-esteem issues are occurring in children with increasing frequency and mandate that obesity prevention, intervention, and treatment become part of the pediatrician's repertoire.

INCIDENCE OF OBESITY

The incidence of obesity has increased dramatically in the United States and the world in the last 2 decades (Figure 34-1). The number of children who are overweight has increased as well, rising from 4% in 1962 to 16% in 2002[1] (Figure 34-2 on page 299). Body mass index (BMI, calculated as wt/ht^2) is a measure that correlates with body fat,[2] and this index has been used to screen populations for obesity and to categorize individuals to target obesity prevention, intervention, or treatment. In adults a BMI of 25 or greater is considered overweight, and a BMI of 30 or greater is obese. Increased BMI in adults is correlated with increases in obesity-related comorbidities.[3] In children, body fat changes throughout development, and therefore BMI percentile must be used. (See BMI charts in Chapter 14, Pediatric Physical Examination.) The recommendations of the Institute of Medicine[4] and the American Medical Association Expert Committee Recommendations[5] for children classify BMI between 85% and 94% as overweight and BMI greater than the 95% as obese (Box 34-1 on page 299).

Calculation of BMI (and classification of weight status at least once a year) is considered an essential part of pediatric well care.[5] BMI of greater than 99% has been associated with a very high risk of cardiovascular risk factors (high blood pressure, elevated insulin and lipid abnormalities) and severe adult obesity.[6]

Obesity is rapidly overtaking smoking as the largest preventable cause of disease in the United States.[7] It has the potential to make the current generation of US children the first to have a shorter life expectancy than their parents.[8]

EFFECTS OF OBESITY

Pediatricians must be prepared to prevent, identify, and treat obesity, as well as obesity-related comorbidities. These comorbidities include diseases that have traditionally been considered as adult diseases: sleep apnea, type 2 diabetes, hypertension, dyslipidemia, polycystic ovarian syndrome, and nonalcoholic steatohepatitis. The uniquely pediatric comorbidities of slipped capital femoral epiphysis and Blount disease occur as a result of injury to open growth plates in the hip and knee. Depression and low self-esteem have also been associated with childhood obesity. Box 34-2 on page 300 provides a summary of screening and treatment measures for obesity-related comorbid diseases. Pediatricians also need to be prepared to deal with obesity-related emergencies, such as hyperosmolar hyperglycemia, pseudo tumor cerebri, pulmonary emboli, and cardiomyopathy, which occur in obese children. These comorbidities of obesity add to the burden of chronic disease in children and the health care system. Annual hospital costs (in 2001 dollars) for childhood obesity more than tripled between 1981 and 1999 to $127 million per year. Discharge diagnoses of diabetes, obesity-related sleep apnea, and gallbladder disease increased by 15% to 74%.[9]

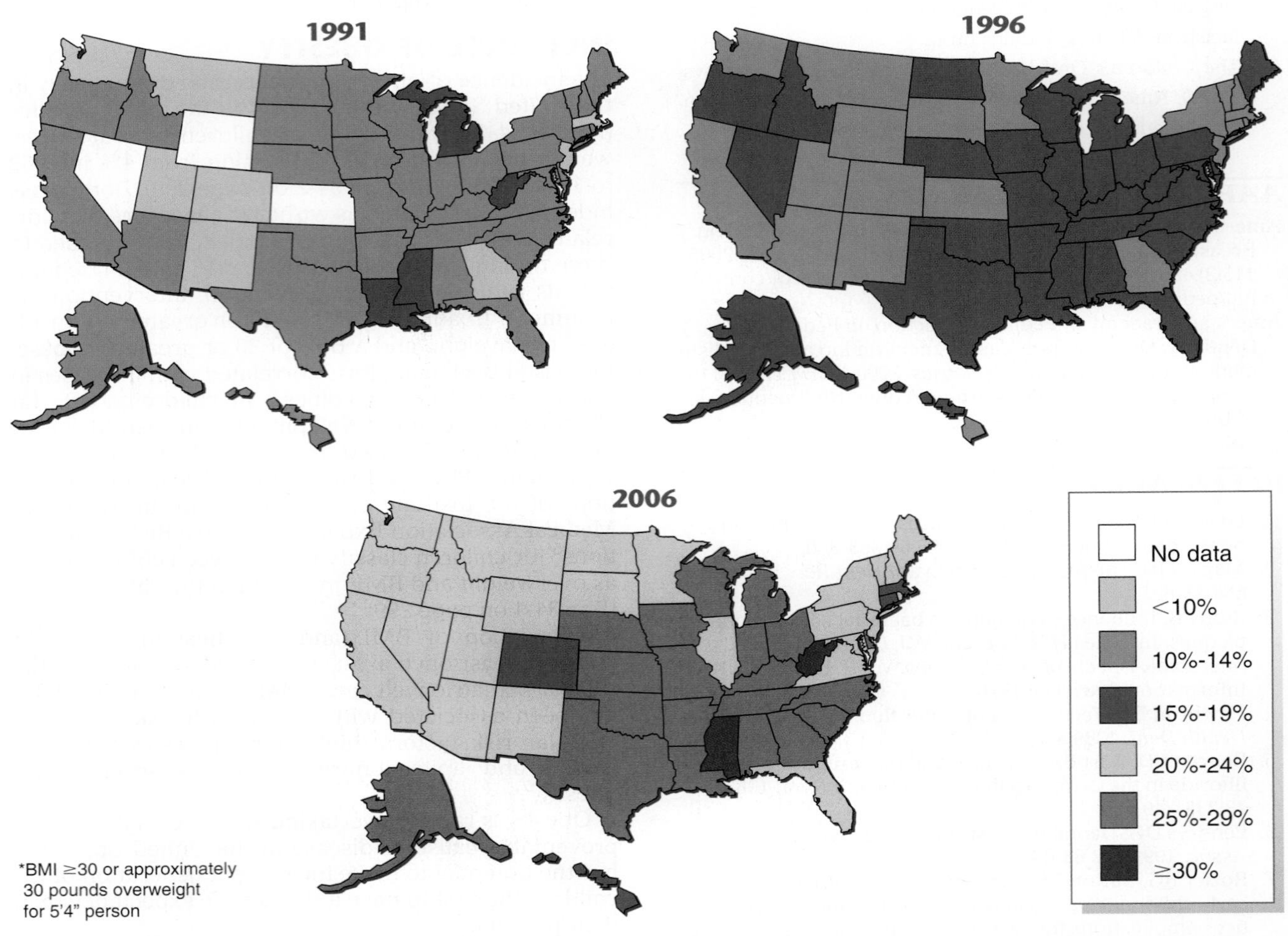

Figure 34-1 Obesity trends among US adults (Behavioral Risk Factor Surveillance System [BRFSS] for 1991, 1996, and 2006). *(Adapted from Behavioral Risk Factor Surveillance System, CDC.)*

FACTORS ASSOCIATED WITH OBESITY

The cause of the obesity epidemic is multifactorial and complex. Genetic predisposition, the environment, and nutrition and activity behavior each play a role in the development of obesity. These factors play out at the individual, family, community, and population level, accounting for the global shift in obesity demographics.

Genetic Effects

The contribution of genetics to obesity has been studied in twins and shows that BMI is highly correlated with genetic factors.[10] BMI measures of identical twins reared apart correlate strongly with the BMI of their biological parents rather than their adoptive parents, indicating a strong genetic predisposition toward weight gain.[11] Parental obesity also increases the risk of a child becoming an obese adult,[12] allowing for early identification of obesity risk.

Infants of mothers who are obese or have diabetes during pregnancy have an increased risk for childhood and adult obesity.[13] The explanation of gene environment interaction involves *epigenetic mechanisms*. Epigenetics refers to "a set of reversible heritable changes that occur without a change in DNA sequence"[14] The two most-common epigenetic changes are DNA methylation and histone modification.[15] Epigenetic change occurs with environmental interaction with the genome. Studies have shown that epigenetic changes in monozygotic twins cause increasing genetic divergence over time.[16] Environmental factors can act during intrauterine development via epigenetic modification of gene expression without altering DNA sequences[17] to increase the risk of obesity, type 2 diabetes, and cardiovascular disease.[18]

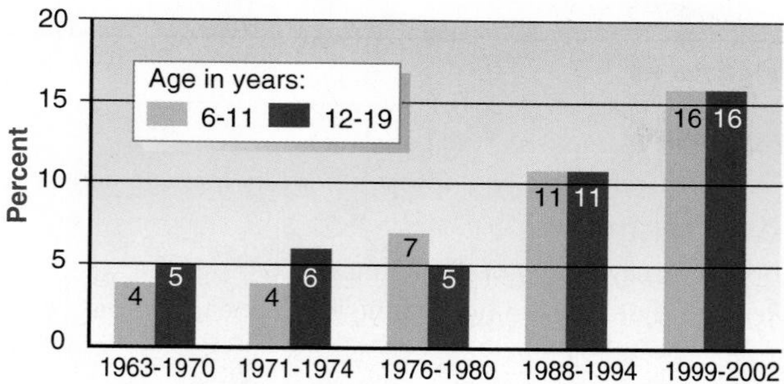

Note: Excludes pregnant women starting with 1971 to 1974. Pregnancy status is not available for 1963 through 1965 and 1966 through 1970. Data for 1963 through 1965 are for children 6 to 11 years of age; data for 1966 through 1970 are for adolescents 12 through 17 years of age, not 12 through 19 years.

Figure 34-2 Prevalence of overweight among children and adolescents, ages 6 to 19 years of age: United States, 1999-2002. *(Adapted from the Centers for Disease Control and Prevention/National Center for Health Statistics (CDC/NCHS), the National Household Education Surveys (NHES), and the 1999-2002 National Health and Nutrition Examination Survey (NHANES). Available at: www.cdc.gov/nchs/products/pubs/pubd/hestats/overwght99.htm. Accessed August 29, 2007.)*

BOX 34-1 Classification of Children by Body Mass Index (BMI) Percentage

BMI <5%: underweight
BMI 5%-84%: healthy or normal weight
BMI 85%-95%: overweight
BMI >95%: obese

Environmental Effects

Early infant weight gain is independently associated with being overweight in childhood. Infants who gain excess weight in the first 4 months of life are likely to be overweight at the age of 7 years.[19] In addition, weight increase between birth and 12 months of age as a ratio of birth weight is independently associated with becoming overweight at 6 years of age. When combined with protein intake at 9 to 12 months of age this early weight gain was able to explain 50% of the variance in boys' BMIs at 6 years.[20]

Prolonged breastfeeding (6-12 months) has been associated with a reduced risk of becoming overweight among non-Hispanic white children.[21] In an evidence-based review of breastfeeding studies, breastfeeding was associated with reduction in the risk of obesity and type 2 diabetes in the children and a reduction in type 2 diabetes in mothers.[22]

The shifting nutrition and activity environment plays a role in both population risk and individual risk of obesity. The concept of the *thrifty genotype* has been used to describe the transition of a population that evolved under conditions of periodic food scarcity to a state of abundant food and increased inactivity.[23] This concept may partially explain the differential susceptibility of ethnic populations such as Native Americans. Populations in underdeveloped countries who are transitioning to a Western lifestyle are also experiencing a rapid rise of childhood obesity.[24] Minority and disadvantaged children are disproportionately affected by obesity,[25] possibly reflecting a greater exposure to obesity-promoting environments. For example, children from low-income groups, blacks, and Hispanics watch more television than white children.[26] Lower physical activity levels have been associated with low family income, time spent indoors, higher crime areas, and maternal education level,[27] factors that differentially affect disadvantaged populations.

Changes in the secular environment have increased calories available to children and families. Portion sizes of commercially available foods began to increase above recommended dietary guidelines in the 1970s and have increased steadily since, with the average chocolate chip cookie over 700% larger than its counterpart at the onset of the obesity epidemic.[28] Studies in adults[29] and children[30] show that people eat more as portion sizes increase.

The availability and consumption of snack foods can also lead to excess calorie consumption. One extra serving of potato chips in excess of daily calorie needs would have resulted in a weight gain of 13 pounds per year in 1977 and 23 pounds per year in 1994.[24]

Eating out has been cited as one of the factors important in the development of the obesity epidemic. Between 1977 and 1996 the proportion of foods that children consumed from restaurants and fast-food outlets increased by nearly 300%.[31] Fast-food consumption is a significant risk factor for obesity.[32] In one study, children who consumed fast food took in an average 187 kcal/day more than children who did not consume fast food. In the same study, 30% of children ate fast food on any given day.[33]

Obesity correlates with the number of hours of television viewing.[34] After-school time is a particularly vulnerable time for children in terms of television exposure.[35] Food advertising may play a role in increases in high-energy food. Children are the targets of significant advertising of foods with high caloric density. They see an average of one food commercial per 5 minutes of television time and may see 3 hours of food commercials per week.[36] Food advertising ranges from product placement in movies and television shows to vending machines in schools and includes the use of sports heroes to sell soda and the use of highly advertised collectable toys to sell fast-food meals. Exposure to such advertisements affect children's food choices even in preschool.[37]

Consumption of more than one soda per day by children as young as 2 years was correlated with obesity.[38] Soda consumption was also associated with excess weight gain in children studied from age 7 through preadolescence.[39]

Inactivity has also been associated with obesity. In a 30-year longitudinal twin study, twins in the pair who were inactive over the course of the study had significantly more weight gain and waist circumference than the active twin.[40] In a review of obesity prevention trials, moderate to vigorous physical activity was significantly correlated with obesity prevention in children.[41] Nutrition- and activity-related behaviors act at the

BOX 34-2 Summary of Screening and Treatment Measures

TYPE 2 DIABETES

History: maternal diabetes during pregnancy, small for gestational age, intrauterine growth restriction, family history of diabetes

Review of systems: polyuria; polydipsia, nocturia; recurrent vaginal, bladder, or other infections; recent weight loss

Physical examination: acanthosis nigricans

Laboratory assessments: elevated fasting glucose, glycosuria, positive glucose tolerance test, hyperinsulinemia

NONALCOHOLIC STEATOHEPATITIS

History: no specific history; some cases have other family members affected

Review of systems: possible nausea and right upper quadrant discomfort

Physical examination: hepatomegaly

Laboratory and imaging assessments: elevated serum aminotransferases, echogenicity of liver on ultrasound

Treatment: referral to pediatric gastroenterologist for evaluation and definitive diagnosis; weight loss

HYPERTENSION

History: family history of hypertension or other obesity-related comorbidity

Review of systems: usually asymptomatic

Physical examination: elevated systolic or diastolic blood pressure

Laboratory assessments: evaluation for other causes of hypertension as indicated

Treatment: referral to pediatric hypertension specialist, dietary treatment, pharmacologic treatment

DYSLIPIDEMIA

History: family history of lipid disorders, cardiovascular disease

Review of systems: asymptomatic; other obesity comorbidities, particularly signs of metabolic syndrome

Physical examination: no specific signs; acanthosis nigricans may indicate metabolic syndrome

Laboratory assessment: lipid panel

Treatment: referral to lipid specialist; dietary management

SLEEP APNEA

History: family history of sleep apnea

Review of systems: snoring, snoring with apnea, daytime tiredness, napping, poor concentration in school, enuresis

Physical examination: large tonsils or adenoids

Imaging assessment: nighttime polysomnography

Treatment: referral to pediatric pulmonologist, weight loss

SLIPPED CAPITAL FEMORAL EPIPHYSIS

History: knee or hip pain

Review of systems: knee or hip pain, limp

Physical examination: limp, pain in knee or hip

Imaging: hip and knee films

Treatment: immediate referral to pediatric orthopedist

BLOUNT DISEASE

History: bowing

Review of systems: bowing (tibia vera), knee pain, limp

Physical examination: bowing, knee pain, limp

Imaging: knee films

Treatment: referral to pediatric orthopedist

DEPRESSION

History: family history of depression, history of abuse, psychological trauma, teasing, low self-esteem

Review of systems: loss of interest, anger, irritability, sadness, suicidal ideation

Physical examination: no signs; may have sad, irritable appearance with lack of self-care

Laboratory or imaging assessments: none

Treatment: mental health referral for counseling or pharmacologic treatment

From Hassink S, ed. *Pediatric Obesity Prevention, Intervention and Treatment Strategies for Primary Care.* Elk Grove Village, IL: American Academy of Pediatrics; 2007.

interface between the individual and family and the environment. The primary care physician can counsel parents and patients on lifestyle issues that affect children's nutrition and activity. Table 34-1 provides age-appropriate obesity prevention information. (See also Chapter 23, Counseling Families on Healthy Lifestyles.)

Obesity prevention and treatment are family based. Children's eating habits and preferences can be predicted by their mother's behaviors. Maternal preferences predict child preferences for milk type and amount and predict the intake of calcium and cholesterol in the child's diet.[42] Early parental behavior influences a child's eating behavior through at least five mechanisms: (1) availability and accessibility of foods, (2) meal structure, (3) adult food modeling, (4) food socialization practices, and (5) food-related parenting styles.[43]

Parental modeling appears to be consistently correlated with child eating behaviors and attitudes. Attempts by parents to control what their children eat or to use food to control other behaviors has much less consistent effects, sometimes having the opposite effect from that which is desired.[44] The authoritative parenting style that sets limits in a supportive rather than punitive way has been linked with improved health outcomes, including preventing obesity.[45]

Engaging parents and families to partner in obesity prevention and treatment is a core skill for pediatricians. Techniques such as motivational interviewing show promise as feasible office-based interventions.[46] (See Chapter 24, Communication Strategies, for a description of motivational interviewing and other techniques for communicating with children and families.)

Table 34-1 Age-Appropriate Obesity-Prevention Guidance

AGE OF CHILD	NUTRITION INFORMATION	APPROPRIATE ACTIVITY
Newborn or infant	Promote breastfeeding. Teach parents to recognize hunger and satiety cues. Assess family's eating habits and nutrition environment. Limit juice.	Encourage face-to-face play time, with infant to lay groundwork for shared activity. Take daily walk in stroller to establish outdoor time. Use safe toys. Limit television viewing.
Toddler	Remind parents of appropriate portion sizes. "Parents provide (correct portions), child decides (what to eat)". Encourage structured meals and snack time with family. Model desired eating behavior. Address *picky eating, food refusal, and grazing* if problematic. Discuss safe eating to prevent choking. No sugar-sweetened beverages.	Encourage *free play* in safe indoor and outdoor environment. Spare use of strollers. Limit television and computer time. No television or computer in the bedroom. Review age-appropriate motor-skill development.
Preschool	Parents, not children, should be deciding on food choices. Limit eating out. Review growth charts with goal to *keep on the chart.* Help parents identify and assess all the different nutritional environments in their child's day (ie, child care, school, extended family, friends). No sugar-sweetened beverages. Be aware of food marketing that targets children. Help parents maintain structured meals and snacks. Help parents address child's behavior around demands for food if a problem.	Encourage free play. Encourage outdoor play. Encourage participation not competition. No more than 2 hr/day television or computer time. Encourage family time that is physically active.
School age	Check nutritional choices at school, after-school care, extracurricular activities; may need to pack food from home. Advocate for change if necessary. Address weekend, vacation, and summer nutritional challenges. Minimize *junk food.* No sugared beverages. *Nutrition decisions are health decisions.* Do not bring food into the house that you do not want your child to eat. Monitor after-school eating.	Balance free play and entry-level sport participation (fundamental skill development with minimal competition and flexible rules). Focus on fun activities. Limit television and computer time. No television or computer in bedroom, Do not mix television watching and eating. Help child find other indoor activity options.
Early adolescent	Encourage family meals. Discuss the importance of breakfast (breakfast skipping is common at this age). Help child and family with healthy after-school snack. Help child make decisions around social eating. No sugar-sweetened beverages.	Help schedule physical activity around homework and social demands. Encourage extracurricular activities to avoid sedentary time after school. Limit television and computer time. Social-skill building if needed can help encourage participation in peer activities.
Middle adolescent	Review growth chart with adolescent. Help teen self-assessment eating and nutritional choices. Encourage breakfast. Discourage meal skipping. Discuss social eating, healthy choices. Limit fast food. No sugared beverages.	Find ways to help teen keep participating in physical activity. Encourage lifestyle activities. Limit television and computer time; find alternatives such as volunteering, hobbies, clubs.
Late adolescent and young adult	Encourage self-monitoring. Discuss structure and time management of meals, activity, and sleep. Go over health priorities. Provide nutrition information on fast food. Screen for binge eating.	Maintain activity of daily living. Limit television and computer time. Encourage lifestyle sports and activities. Take advantage of community and school recreation facilities.

OBESITY ASSESSMENT, PREVENTION, AND TREATMENT

The most current methods for preventing childhood obesity are recommended by an expert panel and endorsed by the American Academy of Pediatrics.[5]

Assessment

All children should have BMI measured at least yearly and weight status classified (see Box 34-1). Children with a BMI in the 99th percentile should be identified to allow for additional study.

Well Visit

At each well-child visit for all children the physician should:

1. Measure height and weight and calculate and classify BMI.
2. Assess self-efficacy readiness to change lifestyle behaviors.
3. Assess diet, including attention to the following behaviors that may be targets for change:
   - Frequency of eating outside the home
   - Excessive consumption of sweetened beverages, including juice
   - Consumption of excess portion sizes
   - Frequency of breakfast
   - Excessive snack-food consumption
   - Low fruit and vegetable consumption
   - Meal frequency and snack patterns and portions
4. Assess activity, including the following:
   - Environmental support and barriers to physical activity
   - Whether child is meeting a recommendation of 60 minutes of moderate exercise every day
   - Level of sedentary behavior, including television and computer time of less than 2 hours a day in children older than 2 years
5. Take a focused family history for obesity, type 2 diabetes, and cardiovascular disease, including hypertension and early deaths from cardiovascular disease or stroke.
6. Assess risk for current or future obesity-related comorbidities.
7. Perform a complete physical examination that includes pulse and blood pressure, as well as signs of obesity-related comorbidities.
8. Order the following laboratory tests:
   - Lipid profile for children with BMI of 85% to 94% with no risk factors
   - Aspartate aminotransferase, alanine aminotransferase, fasting glucose for children with BMI of 85% to 94% with risk factors for obesity-related conditions
   - Fasting lipid profile, aspartate aminotransferase, alanine aminotransferase, fasting glucose, blood urea and nitrogen with creatinine for children with BMI greater than 95%

Prevention of Obesity

For children ages 2 to 18 years with a BMI greater than 5% and less than 84% the physician should counsel as follows:

1. Diet:
   - Limit sugar-sweetened beverages.
   - Encourage recommended fruits and vegetables.
2. Activity:
   - Limit television and computer time to 1 to 2 hours per day.
   - Allow no television or computer in bedroom.
   - Engage in moderate physical activity daily.
3. Behavior:
   - Eat breakfast daily.
   - Limit eating out.
   - Encourage family meals; limit portion sizes.
4. Actively engage families with parental obesity or maternal diabetes because of increased risk of child developing obesity.
5. Encourage authoritative parenting style, discouraging restrictive parenting style.
6. Encourage parents to model healthy diets and portion sizes, physical activity, and limited television time.
7. Encourage a diet rich in calcium, high in fiber, and balanced macronutrients; and limit consumption of energy-dense foods.
8. Ask parents and children about physical activity at school and child care.

Treatment of Obesity

Children who have a BMI greater than 85% should be treated appropriately. Treatment consists of four stages depending on the status of the child and includes all guidance found in the prevention section presented previously and the following points. This state is *stage 1,* also known as *prevention plus.*

The *prevention plus* stage involves the following areas:

Nutrition:

1. Five or more servings of fruits and vegetables per day
2. A maximum of 2 hours of television or computer time per day, and no television in the bedroom
3. One hour or more of physical activity daily
4. No sugar sweetened beverages

Behavior:

1. Eat breakfast daily.
2. Limit eating out.
3. Eat family meals 5 to 6 days a week.
4. Allow children to self-regulate eating at meals, and avoid overly restrictive behavior.

The goal of prevention plus is weight maintenance and should include monthly follow-up appointments. If no improvement is seen after 3 to 6 months, then the physician should move to the next stage, *stage 2, structured weight management protocol:*

In stage 2 the primary care physician should stress the following areas:

1. Developing a plan for use of a low-energy, dense, balanced macronutrient diet
2. Increased structured daily meals and snacks
3. Supervised active play at least 60 minutes a day
4. Television and computer time less than 1 hour per day
5. Increased monitoring of these behaviors, encouraging parents to do so as well

The goal of stage 2, the structured weight-management protocol, is weight maintenance that results in decreasing BMI as height increases. Weight loss is not to exceed 1 pound per month in children 2 to 11 years or 2 pounds per week in children older than 11 years.

If no improvement is seen in BMI or weight after 3 to 6 months, then the primary care physician should advance to *stage 3,* which is a multidisciplinary intervention by an obesity care team. If this stage is not successful, then the patient is referred to *stage 4,* a tertiary-care intervention.

TOOLS FOR PRACTICE

Community Coordination and Advocacy

- Action for Healthy Kids (Web page), Action For Healthy Kids (www.actionforhealthykids.org/).

Practice Management

- *Obesity Coding Fact Sheet* (fact sheet), American Academy of Pediatrics (www.aap.org/obesity/codingfactsheet.PDF).

Engaging Patients and Family

- *A Parent's Guide to Childhood Obesity: A Road Map to Health* (book), American Academy of Pediatrics (www.aap.org/bookstore).
- *About BMI for Children and Teens* (fact sheet), Centers for Disease Control and Prevention (www.cdc.gov/nccdphp/dnpa/bmi/childrens_BMI/about_childrens_BMI.htm).
- *BAM* (Web page), Centers for Disease Control and Prevention (www.bam.gov).
- *Better Health and Fitness Through Physical Activity* (brochure), American Academy of Pediatrics (patiented.aap.org).
- *Encourage Your Child to Be Physically Active* (brochure), American Academy of Pediatrics (patiented.aap.org).
- *Feeding Guide for Children, Appendix A.3, Pediatric Obesity: Prevention, Intervention, and Treatment Strategies for Primary Care* (chart), American Academy of Pediatrics.
- *Feeding Kids Right Isn't Always Easy* (brochure), American Academy of Pediatrics (patiented.aap.org).
- *Growing Up Healthy* (brochure), American Academy of Pediatrics (patiented.aap.org).
- My pyramid—steps to healthier you (Web page), US Department of Agriculture (www.mypyramid.gov/).
- *Right From the Start: ABCs of Good Nutrition for Young Children* (brochure), American Academy of Pediatrics (patiented.aap.org).
- *Sports and Your Child* (brochure), American Academy of Pediatrics (patiented.aap.org).
- *Television and the Family* (brochure), American Academy of Pediatrics (patiented.aap.org).
- *What's to Eat? Healthy Foods for Hungry Children* (brochure), American Academy of Pediatrics (patiented.aap.org).
- *VERB* (Web page), Centers for Disease Control and Prevention (www.verbnow.com/).

Medical Decision Support

- *BMI—Body Mass Index: Child and Teen Calculator: English* (interactive tool), Centers for Disease Control and Prevention (apps.nccd.cdc.gov/dnpabmi/Calculator.aspx).
- *Bright Futures: Guidelines for Health Supervision of Infants, Children, and Adolescents* (book), Bright Futures (brightfutures.aap.org/web/).
- *Care of children and adolescents with type 1 diabetes: a statement of the American Diabetes Association* (policy statement) American Diabetes Association (care.diabetesjournals.org/cgi/content/full/28/1/186).
- *Environmental Assessment, Appendix A.4, Pediatric Obesity: Prevention, Intervention, and Treatment Strategies for Primary Care* (questionnaire), American Academy of Pediatrics (practice.aap.org/content.aspx?aid=2001).
- *Family History: your child's genetics and family history, Appendix A.4, Pediatric Obesity: Prevention, Intervention, and Treatment Strategies for Primary* (practice.aap.org/content.aspx?aid=2001).
- *Care* (questionnaire), American Academy of Pediatrics (practice.aap.org/content.aspx?aid=2001).
- *Food diary: what is your child eating now? Appendix a.4, pediatric obesity: prevention, intervention, and treatment strategies for primary Care* (questionnaire), American Academy of Pediatrics (practice.aap.org/content.aspx?aid=2001).
- *Goal Assessment, Appendix A.4, Pediatric Obesity: Prevention, Intervention, and Treatment Strategies for Primary Care* (questionnaire), American Academy of Pediatrics (practice.aap.org/content.aspx?aid=2001).
- *Goal Achievement Plan Appendix A.4, Pediatric Obesity: Prevention, Intervention, and Treatment Strategies for Primary Care* (questionnaire), American Academy of Pediatrics (practice.aap.org/content.aspx?aid=2001).
- *Growth Charts—tutorials and information* (Web page), Centers for Disease Control and Prevention (www.cdc.gov/growthcharts/).
- *Growth Charts* (chart), Centers for Disease Control and Prevention (www.cdc.gov/nchs/about/major/nhanes/growthcharts/clinical_charts.htm#Clin%201) also available at AAP bookstore (www.aap.org/bst).
- *Home Environment Assessment, Appendix A.4, Pediatric Obesity: Prevention, Intervention, and Treatment Strategies for Primary Care* (questionnaire), American Academy of Pediatrics (practice.aap.org/content.aspx?aid=2001).
- *Introducing Patients to Healthy Family Lifestyles* (fact sheet), Jopling RJ (practice.aap.org/content.aspx?aid=2001).
- *Parental Concerns Assessment, Appendix A.4, Pediatric Obesity: Prevention, Intervention, and Treatment Strategies for Primary Care* (questionnaire), American Academy of Pediatrics (practice.aap.org/content.aspx?aid=2001).
- *Pediatric Obesity* (on-line course), American Academy of Pediatrics (www.pedialink.org).
- *Pediatric Obesity Clinical Decision Support Chart* (chart), Maine Center for Public Health and the Maine Chapter of the American Academy of Pediatrics (www.aap.org/bookstore).

- *Pediatric Obesity: Prevention, Intervention, and Treatment Strategies for Primary Care* (book), American Academy of Pediatrics (www.aap.org/bookstore).
- *Physical Activity Assessment, Appendix A.4, Pediatric Obesity: Prevention, Intervention, and Treatment Strategies for Primary Care* (questionnaire), American Academy of Pediatrics (practice.aap.org/content.aspx?aid=2001).
- *Physician Tracking Form for Pediatric Obesity, Appendix A.4, Pediatric Obesity: Prevention, Intervention, and Treatment Strategies for Primary Care* (form), American Academy of Pediatrics (practice.aap.org/content.aspx?aid=2001).
- *Set Backs Worksheet, Appendix A.4, Pediatric Obesity: Prevention, Intervention, and Treatment Strategies for Primary Care* (questionnaire), American Academy of Pediatrics (practice.aap.org/content.aspx?aid=2001).
- *Snacking Worksheet, Appendix A.4, Pediatric Obesity: Prevention, Intervention, and Treatment Strategies for Primary Care* (questionnaire), American Academy of Pediatrics (practice.aap.org/content.aspx?aid=2001).
- *VERB Campaign* (Web page), Centers for Disease Control and Prevention (www.cdc.gov/youthcampaign/index.htm).

RELATED WEB SITES

- Childhood Obesity, National Initiative for Healthcare Quality (www.nichq.org/NICHQ/Topics/PreventiveCare/Obesity).
- Nutrition, Centers for Disease Control and Prevention (www.cdc.gov/nccdphp/dnpa/nutrition/index.htm).
- Overweight and Obesity: Home, Centers for Disease Control and Prevention (www.aap.org/obesity).
- Physical Activity for Everyone: Introduction, Centers for Disease Control and Prevention (www.cdc.gov/nccdphp/dnpa/physical/index.htm).

AAP POLICY STATEMENTS

American Academy of Pediatrics, Gahagan S, Silverstein J, Committee on Native American Child Health and the Section on Endocrinology. Prevention and treatment of type 2 diabetes mellitus in children, with special emphasis on American Indian and Alaska Native children. *Pediatrics.* 2003;112(4):e328. (aappolicy.aappublications.org/cgi/content/full/pediatrics;112/4/e328).

American Academy of Pediatrics, Committee on Adolescence. Identifying and treating eating disorders. *Pediatrics.* 2003;111(1):204-211. (aappolicy.aappublications.org/cgi/content/full/pediatrics;111/1/204).

American Academy of Pediatrics, Committee on Communication. Children, adolescents, and advertising. *Pediatrics.* 2006;118(6):2563-2569. (aappolicy.aappublications.org/cgi/content/full/pediatrics;118/6/2563).

American Academy of Pediatrics, Committee on Nutrition. Prevention of pediatric overweight and obesity. *Pediatrics.* 2003;112(2):424-430. (aappolicy.aappublications.org/cgi/content/full/pediatrics;112/2/424).

American Academy of Pediatrics, Committee on Nutrition. The use and misuse of fruit juice in pediatrics. *Pediatrics.* 2001;107(5):1210-1213. (aappolicy.aappublications.org/cgi/content/full/pediatrics;107/5/1210).

American Academy of Pediatrics, Committee on Public Education. Children, adolescents, and television. *Pediatrics.* 2001;107(2):423-426. (aappolicy.aappublications.org/cgi/content/full/pediatrics;107/2/423).

American Academy of Pediatrics, Committee on School Health. Soft drinks in schools. *Pediatrics.* 2004;113(1):152-154. (aappolicy.aappublications.org/cgi/content/full/pediatrics;113/1/152).

American Academy of Pediatrics, Committee on Sports Medicine and Fitness. Strength training by children and adolescents. *Pediatrics.* 2001;107(6):1470-1472. (aappolicy.aappublications.org/cgi/content/full/pediatrics;107/6/1470).

American Academy of Pediatrics, Committee on Sports Medicine and Fitness and Council on School Health. Active healthy living: prevention of childhood obesity through increased physical activity. *Pediatrics.* 2006;117(5):1834-1842. (aappolicy.aappublications.org/cgi/content/full/pediatrics;117/5/1834).

American Academy of Pediatrics, Section on Breastfeeding. Breastfeeding and the use of human milk. *Pediatrics.* 2005;115(2):496-506. (aappolicy.aappublications.org/cgi/content/full/pediatrics;115/2/496).

American Diabetes Association. Type 2 diabetes in children and adolescents. *Diabetes Care.* 2000;23(3):381-389. AAP endorsed.

National High Blood Pressure Education Program Working Group on High Blood Pressure in Children and Adolescents. The fourth report on the diagnosis, evaluation, and treatment of high blood pressure in children and adolescents. *Pediatrics.* 2004;114(2):555-576. AAP endorsed.

REFERENCES

1. US Department of Health and Human Services, Centers for Disease Control and Prevention, National Center for Health Statistics. Prevalence of Overweight Among Children and Adolescents—United States, 1999-2002. Available at: www.cdc.gov/nchs/products/pubs/pubd/hestats/overwght99.htm. Accessed August 14, 2007.
2. Chan YL, Leung SS, Lam WW, et al. Body fat estimation in children by magnetic resonance imaging, bioelectrical impedance, skinfold and body mass index: a pilot study. *J Paediatr Child Health.* 1998;34(1):22-28.
3. Sturm R. Increases in morbid obesity in the USA: 2000-2005. *Public Health.* 2007:121(7):492-496.
4. Koplan JP, Liverman CT, Kraak VA, eds, and the Committee on Prevention of Obesity in Children and Youth. *Preventing Childhood Obesity: Health In The Balance.* Washington, DC: National Academies Press; 2005.
5. American Medical Association. Appendix: Expert Committee Recommendations on the Assessment, Prevention, and Treatment of Child and Adolescent Overweight and Obesity. American Medical Association. Available at: www.ama-assn.org/ama1/pub/upload/mm/433/ped_obesity_recs.pdf. Accessed August 14, 2007.
6. Freedman DS, Mei Z, Srinivasan SR, et al. Cardiovascular risk factors and excess adiposity among overweight children and adolescents; the Bogalusa Heart Study. *J Pediatr.* 2007;150(1):12-17.
7. Mokdad AH, Marks JS, Stroup DF, et al. Actual causes of death in the United States, 2000. *JAMA.* 2004;291(10):1238-1245.
8. Olshansky SJ, Passaro DJ, Hershow RC, et al. A potential decline in life expectancy in the United States in the 21st century. *N Engl J Med.* 2005;352(11):1138-1145.
9. Wang G, Dietz WH. Economic burden of obesity in youths aged 6 to 17 years: 1979-1999. *Pediatrics.* 2002;109(5):E81-E81.
10. Stunkard AJ, Foch TT, Hrubec Z. A twin study of human obesity. *JAMA.* 1986;256(1):51-54.
11. Stunkard AJ, Sorensen TI, Hanis C, et al. An adoption study of human obesity. *N Engl J Med.* 1986;314(4):193-195.
12. Whitaker RC, Wright JA, Pepe MS, et al. Predicting obesity in young adulthood from childhood and parental obesity. *N Engl J Med.* 1997;337(13):869-873.
13. Whitaker RC, Dietz WH. Role of prenatal environment in the development of obesity. *J Pediatr.* 1998;132(5):768-776.
14. Choi JK, Kim SC. Environmental effects on gene expression phenotype have regional biases in the human genome. *Genetics.* 2007;175(4):1607-1613.

15. Jaenisch R, Bird A. Epigenetic regulation of gene expression: how the genome integrates intrinsic and environmental signals. *Nat Genet.* 2003;33(suppl):245-254.
16. Fraga MF, Ballestar E, Paz MF, et al. Epigenetic differences arise during the lifetime of monozygotic twins. *Proc Natl Acad Sci USA.* 2005;102(30):10604-10609.
17. Godfrey KM, Lillycrop KA, Burdge GC, et al. Epigenetic mechanisms and the mismatch concept of the developmental origins of health and disease. *Pediatr Res.* 2007; 61(5 pt 2):5R-10R.
18. McMillen IC, Robinson JS. Developmental origins of the metabolic syndrome: prediction, plasticity, and programming. *Physiol Rev.* 2005;85(2):571-633.
19. Stettler N, Zemel BS, Kumanyika S, et al. Infant weight gain and childhood overweight status in a multicenter, cohort study. *Pediatrics.* 2002;109(2):194-199.
20. Gunnarsdottir I, Thorsdottir I. Relationship between growth and feeding in infancy and body mass index at the age of 6 years. *Int J Obes Relat Metab Disord.* 2003; 27(12):1523-1527.
21. Grummer-Strawn LM, Mei Z, Centers for Disease Control and Prevention, Pediatric Nutrition Surveillance System. Does breastfeeding protect against pediatric overweight? Analysis of longitudinal data from the Centers for Disease Control and Prevention Pediatric Nutrition Surveillance System. *Pediatrics.* 2004;113(2):e81-e86.
22. Ip S, Chung M, Raman G, et al. Breastfeeding and maternal and infant health outcomes in developed countries. *Evid Rep Technol Assess* (Full Rep). 2007;(153):1-186.
23. Neel JV. Diabetes mellitus: a "thrifty" genotype rendered detrimental by "progress"? *Am J Hum Genet.* 1962;14; 353-362.
24. Hassink SG. *Clinical Guide to Pediatric Weight Management and Obesity.* Philadelphia, PA: Lippincott Williams & Wilkins; 2007.
25. Centers for Disease Control and Prevention, National Center for Health Statistics. *National Health Examination and Nutrition Survey, Hispanic Health and Nutrition Survey (1982-1984) and National Health Examination Survey (1963-1965 and 1966-1970).* Hyattsville, MD: National Center for Health Statistics; 2004.
26. Kumanyika S, Grier S. Targeting interventions for ethnic minority and low-income populations. *The Future of Children: Childhood Obesity.* 2006;16(1):187-207.
27. Ferreira I, van der Horst K, Wendel-Vos W, et al. Environmental correlates of physical activity in youth—a review and update. *Obes Rev.* 2007;8(2):129-154.
28. Young LR, Nestle M. The contribution of expanding portion sizes to the US obesity epidemic. *Am J Public Health.* 2002;92(2):246-249.
29. Rolls BJ, Roe LS, Meengs JS, et al. Increasing the portion size of a sandwich increases energy intake. *J Am Diet Assoc.* 2004;104(3):367-372.
30. Fisher J, Rolls BJ, Birch LL. Children's bite size and intake of an entrée are greater with large portions than with age-appropriate or self-selected portions. *Am J Clin Nutr.* 2003;77(5):1164-1170.
31. St-Onge MP, Keller KL, Heymsfield SB. Changes in childhood food consumption patterns; a cause for concern in light of increasing body weights. *Am J Clin Nutr.* 2003; 78(6):1068-1073.
32. Agras WS, Mascola AJ. Risk factors for childhood overweight. *Curr Opin Pediatr.* 2005;17(5):648-652.
33. Bowman SA, Gortmaker SL, Ebbeling CB, et al. Effects of fast-food consumption on energy intake and diet quality among children in a national household survey. *Pediatrics.* 2004;113(1 pt 1):112-118.
34. Robinson TN. Television viewing and childhood obesity. *Pediatr Clin North Am.* 2001;48(4):1017-1025.
35. O'Brien M, Nader PR, Houts RM, et al. The ecology of childhood overweight: a 12-year longitudinal analysis. *Int J Obes (Lond).* 2007;3. [E-publication ahead of print.]
36. Story M, French S. Food advertising and marketing directed at children and adolescents in the US. *Int J Behav Nutr Phys Act.* 2004;1(1):3.
37. Borzekowski DL, Robinson TN. The 30-second effect: an experiment revealing the impact of television commercials on food preferences of preschoolers. *J Am Diet Assoc.* 2001;101(1):42-46.
38. Warner ML, Harley K, Bradman A, et al. Soda consumption and overweight status of 2-year-old Mexican-American children in California. *Obesity (Silver Spring).* 2006;149(11):1966-1974.
39. Tam CS, Garnett SP, Cowell CT, et al. Soft drink consumption and excess weight gain in Australian school students; results from the Nepean study. *Int J Obes (Lond).* 2006;30(7):1091-1093.
40. Waller K, Kaprio J, Kujala UM. Associations between long-term physical activity, waist circumference and weight gain: a 30-year longitudinal twin study. *Int J Obes (Lond).* 2007;24. [E-publication ahead of print.]
41. Connelly JB, Duaso MJ, Butler G. A systematic review of controlled trials of interventions to prevent childhood obesity and overweight: a realistic synthesis of the evidence. *Public Health.* 2007;121(7):510-517.
42. Oliveria SA, Ellison RC, Moore LL, et al. Parent-child relationships in nutrient intake: the Framingham Children's Study. *Am J Clin Nutr.* 1992;56(3):593-598.
43. Nicklas TA, Morales M, Linares A, et al. Children's meal patterns have changed over a 21-year period: the Bogalusa Heart Study. *J Am Diet Assoc.* 2004;104(5):753-761.
44. Brown R, Ogden J. Children's eating attitudes and behavior: a study of the modeling and control theories of parental influence. *Health Educ Res.* 2004;19(3):261-271.
45. Rhee KE, Lumeng JC, Appugliese DP, et al. Parenting styles and overweight status in first grade. *Pediatrics.* 2006;117(6):2047-2054.
46. Schwartz RP, Hamre R, Dietz WH, et al. Office-based motivational interviewing to prevent childhood obesity: a feasibility study. *Arch Pediatr Adolesc Med.* 2007; 161(5):495-501.

Chapter 35

PREVENTION OF SMOKING

C. Andrew Aligne, MD, MPH

INTRODUCTION

Smoking is the number one preventable cause of death in the United States and a growing problem in the developing world.[1,2] Tobacco smoke is a poisonous mixture that includes known carcinogens and toxins such as benzene and carbon monoxide. The link between active smoking and adult disease (lung cancer, stroke, heart attacks, and other conditions) is perhaps the most thoroughly investigated disease association in history and is now universally accepted, even by the tobacco companies.[3,4] Nevertheless, considerable public confusion remains about the dangers of passive smoking because of disinformation from the tobacco companies about a supposed scientific controversy in this area.[5] Despite its public denials, even the tobacco industry's research shows that passive smoking is harmful.[1,6] The evidence that passive smoking is a cause of death, disease, and disability comes from many types of studies, performed over many years, in nations all over the world; passive smoking harms children.[7] Reducing smoking prevalence, youth smoking, and childhood exposure to passive smoke is a national health priority.[8]

MORTALITY

The harmful effects of tobacco begin at the earliest ages. Absorption of tobacco smoke by children is a function of the number of cigarettes smoked around the child and the proximity of the smokers, and a dose-response relationship has been noted between exposure and health effects.[9] Thus, although studies show that maternal smoking (as opposed to smoking by fathers and other caretakers) is most strongly associated with pediatric morbidity, the risk of disease increases with increasing total exposure from all sources (even prenatally).[10] Maternal smoking during pregnancy is associated with increased risk of fetal loss, prematurity, low birth weight, and perinatal death.[10] Passive smoking is also a significant underlying risk factor for deaths caused by sudden infant death syndrome, respiratory syncytial virus bronchiolitis, asthma, and fire injuries.[10] As a result, estimates suggest that more children under the age of 5 are killed by parental smoking than by motor vehicle crashes, poisonings, drownings, gunshots, and all other unintentional injuries combined.[11]

MORBIDITY

Passive smoking, also known as environmental tobacco smoke (ETS), is associated with an increased risk of many pediatric health problems, including respiratory disease ranging from the common cold to pneumonia and cystic fibrosis exacerbations, acute and chronic otitis media, difficulty with breastfeeding, atopic eczema, skin infections, meningitis, birth defects, decrease in linear growth of 1 to 2 cm, cataracts, colic, febrile seizures, and dental caries.[7,12,13]

WHAT SHOULD PEDIATRICIANS DO ABOUT CIGARETTE SMOKING? STANDARD RECOMMENDATIONS

Parental smoking increases the risk that a child will become an adult active smoker. Most smokers start the habit before adulthood, so that (adult) smoking is, in fact, a *pediatric* disease[14] (Figure 35-1). Pediatricians and family physicians are the only health care professionals who routinely come into contact with nonsmokers who are at high risk of becoming smokers (ie, preadolescents). They may also be the only medical professionals in routine contact with parents of young children, given that young men and women rarely visit physicians for check-ups. Thus, because of their regular contact with young children and their families, pediatricians and family physicians have a unique opportunity to intervene against both active and passive smoking. The American Academy of Pediatrics has recommended numerous steps that physicians can take. Among these measures are the following: do not smoke, promote a smoke-free environment, do not display magazines that advertise tobacco, and support community antismoking programs.[15,16]

The 1st step in any clinical effort to reduce smoking is simply to ask about it.[17] Studies of parents' attitudes reveal approximately 90% of parents expect pediatricians to discuss passive smoking.[18] Inquiries should be nonaccusatory. For communication techniques such as motivational interviewing, see Chapter 24, Communication Strategies. Any discussions of smoking should communicate that smoking is an addictive behavior that harms the smoker and those around the

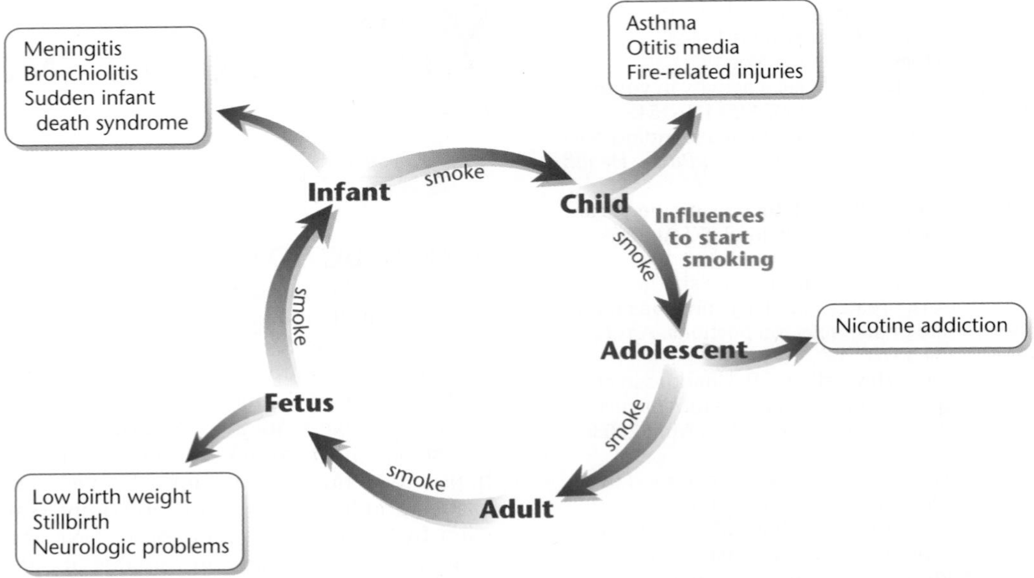

Figure 35-1 The life cycle of the effects of smoking on health. *(Adapted from Aligne CA, Stoddard JJ. Tobacco and children: an economic evaluation of the medical effects of parental smoking.* Arch Pediatr Adolesc Med. *1997;151: 648-653. Copyright © 1997 American Medical Association. Used by permission.)*

smoker and that encouragement and help to stop this habit is being offered. Informational brochures and smoking-cessation programs should be made available. The physician should consider recommending nicotine replacement therapy. Physicians who wish to increase their skills in smoking-cessation counseling can obtain additional information and training from the National Cancer Institute (www.cancer.gov). Nonsmokers, including quitters, should be congratulated. Smoking status should be recorded routinely, similar to a vital sign and in the problem list, starting with the prenatal visit. In addition, certain medical complaints represent red flags and teachable moments that should prompt the pediatrician to bring up passive smoking.[19] For example, visits for recurrent otitis or hospitalizations for asthma constitute opportunities to reinforce the link between smoking and illness in the child. Preteens who are at particularly high risk to become smokers are those who are poor, white girls and with relatives or friends who smoke; thus focusing on preadolescent girls for prevention may be the best place to break the cycle of both active and passive smoking.[20]

For smoking parents who are unwilling or unable to quit, efforts must be directed toward reducing exposure of children to ETS.[21] This task can be accomplished best by not allowing smoking inside the home or other places that the child spends significant amounts of time (including automobiles); however, this mandate is not easily accomplished, especially in areas with harsh winters. If a family member insists on smoking indoors, then this person should smoke as far away from the child as possible, perhaps going under a kitchen exhaust fan or by an open window. Reduction of ETS exposure even without cessation does improve the health of children with asthma.[22]

BARRIERS TO IMPLEMENTING STANDARD RECOMMENDATIONS

Efficacy of Counseling Parents

Despite considerable interest and effort, smoking cessation in the pediatric office setting has not been demonstrated to be an effective and practical intervention. Even in well-funded, intensive clinical trials, counseling of smoking mothers to quit in pediatric practices had no significant long-term effect.[23] The Cochrane review on the effectiveness of interventions aimed at reducing exposure of children to ETS concluded the following:

> Brief counseling interventions cannot be extrapolated to adults in the setting of child health. There is limited support for more intensive counseling interventions. There is no clear evidence for differences between the respiratory, non-respiratory ill child, well child and peripartum settings as contexts for reduction of children's ETS exposure.[24]

Preventing Smoking in Children

A randomized trial of counseling parents and preteens to prevent smoking showed that prevention efforts had no effect.[25] Although bupropion and nicotine-replacement therapy (gum, patch, lozenge, spray, among other measures) with motivated adult quitters leads to a significant increase in quit rates, pharmacotherapy for adolescent smokers has not demonstrated effectiveness overall.[26,27] A need exists for well-designed randomized controlled trials for this population of smokers and studies specifically designed for adolescents. Given that the 1st rule of pediatrics is that children (including teens) are not simply little adults, this special designation should not be surprising. However, the fact that interventions that are effective in adult care settings have not worked in pediatric settings is disheartening. The US Preventive Services Task Force found limited evidence that screening and counseling children and adolescents in the primary care setting are effective in either preventing initiation or promoting cessation of tobacco use. The US Preventive Services Task Force concluded that the evidence is insufficient to recommend for or against routine screening for tobacco use or interventions to prevent and treat tobacco use and dependence among children or adolescents.[28]

Reasons for Failure of Intervention

Most studies of pediatric office–based parental smoking cessation have focused on postpartum women who stopped smoking during pregnancy, and the intervention consisted of brief advice delivered by the pediatrician. Participating pediatricians were required to spend extra time with every mother of a newborn to ascertain the complete smoking history and then to follow up at subsequent visits. Poor compliance was noted on the part of the physicians, perhaps because of the length of time added to visits that are already hectic. Another problem with approaches used is that they were based on the *health beliefs* model (physician advice will change patient behavior) and on the hypothesis that women who have quit for up to 9 months during pregnancy will just need a little help after delivery to remain abstinent. However, this concept does not accurately correspond with the reality of maternal smoking behavior. DiClemente et al have suggested that pregnant smokers do not really quit and then relapse postpartum; rather, they suspend smoking temporarily during pregnancy with the intention of starting again as soon as the baby is born.[29] The *stages of change* model classifies smokers in 5 stages of quitting: (1) precontemplation, (2) contemplation, (3) preparation, (4) action, and (5) maintenance.[30] The suspenders' psychological stage of change is actually more like contemplation than action; therefore postpartum relapse rates are very high (often 80% or more).[31] Meanwhile, the teens may be in a *precontemplation* stage of cessation because they often do not identify themselves as nicotine addicts.

One possibility explaining why interventions are not successful is because they are incomplete, lacking either pharmacotherapy or else the right type of counseling.[32-34] Although benefits to being more intensive and comprehensive are obvious, the feasibility of implementing a cessation intervention at the individual client level decreases as the complexity of doing so increases.[35] In addition, pediatricians often lack formal training in cessation counseling and may not be comfortable with the process.[36-38] Another major barrier is the lack of reimbursement for cessation in the pediatric setting and the complexities of a pediatrician recommending pharmaceuticals (over the counter) for a parent as opposed to a patient, even though the patient is suffering from passive smoking, the treatment of which involves parental cessation.[39,40]

FUTURE DIRECTIONS FOR PEDIATRIC OFFICE–BASED INTERVENTIONS TO REDUCE SMOKING

Further research is needed to demonstrate evidence of real-world effectiveness before recommending implementation of any new clinical interventions. Based on the lack of proven success to date, shifting the paradigm of how people think about behavior change in patients and physicians looking for broad system changes in the delivery of pediatric cessation services may be wise.[41] The lessons from past failures suggest that future clinical efforts should involve a focus on motivated quitters, the availability of cessation experts, and reimbursement from medical insurance for comprehensive nicotine addiction treatment including brief motivational counseling, which addresses individual psychosocial barriers to successful abstinence, and pharmacotherapy such as nicotine replacement therapy for the physiological effects of nicotine withdrawal. An approach that is effective, quick, easy, familiar, and emotionally satisfying for caring but busy professionals is more likely to be adopted. For example, referral of interested parents or teens by the pediatrician to a qualified cessation expert or a quit line would not add any significant amount of time to the average routine office visit.[42] Used in combination with community-level interventions, for example, mass media messages encouraging use of a quit line, such an approach could be successful in overcoming barriers for both smokers and physicians.

RECOMMENDATIONS FROM EVIDENCE-BASED GUIDELINES: COMMUNITY-LEVEL TOBACCO CONTROL

Given the difficulties associated with smoking intervention in the pediatric office, fortunately, many effective community-level tobacco control interventions are available. The *Guide to Community Preventive Services*, a systematic review of published studies, conducted on behalf of the Task Force on Community Preventive Services examined the question, What strategies are most effective in reducing the number of people who start using tobacco and increasing the number who stop? The task force found that interventions to increase the unit price for tobacco products are effective both in reducing the number of people who start using tobacco and in increasing the number who quit. Mass media campaigns are effective in reducing initiation of tobacco use when combined with other actions (eg, increasing the excise tax). Mass media campaigns may also decrease consumption of tobacco products and increase tobacco use cessation. Providing counseling and support to patients by telephone, when included as one component of a multicomponent strategy to help smokers quit, is effective in increasing the number of adult smokers who succeed.[43]

In fact, population-level interventions are so effective that considerable progress has been made in tobacco control in the last decade despite the lack of effect from office-based activities. Although most young children still are regularly exposed to tobacco smoke, only 23% of high school seniors are active smokers—down from 35% in 1996.[44,45] This dramatic decrease is due, in large part, to the activities of tobacco-control advocates. Certain kinds of cigarette advertising that targeted children (eg, Joe Camel) have been stopped. The *master settlement agreement* between the states' attorneys general and the tobacco companies helped to raise the price of cigarettes and to fund effective antismoking advertising campaigns. In addition, numerous states and localities have banned indoor smoking and raised cigarette taxes.[46,47] Remaining vigilant, though, is important because the recent decline has begun leveling off, and the tobacco companies have continued marketing to minors even after the master settlement agreement.[48] Pediatricians can help with community-level efforts to decrease smoking by connecting with their local tobacco-control coalitions. (See Chapter 9, Community-wide Approaches to Promoting Child Health.)

CONCLUSIONS

Cigarette smoking is the number 1 cause of premature death in the United States, and it generally starts before adulthood; it is a pediatric disease. Children are innocent victims of passive smoking, which contributes to a wide variety of health problems. Passive smoking is perhaps the major preventable cause of death in infants and young children. Systematic policy and practice changes are needed to allow comprehensive smoking-cessation interventions to be implemented fully in the pediatric clinical setting, and further effectiveness research is needed in this area to refine practical solutions. On the other hand, existing community-level tobacco-control interventions have already proven to be effective. If pediatricians are interested in combating the scourges of active and passive smoking, then they must energetically support public health efforts to promote a tobacco-free environment for all children.

TOOLS FOR PRACTICE

Community Advocacy and Coordination

- *Campaign for Tobacco-Free Kids* (Web page), Tobacco-Free Kids (www.tobaccofreekids.org/).
- *Coverage For Tobacco Use Cessation Treatments* (fact sheet), Centers for Disease Control and Prevention (www.cdc.gov/tobacco/quit_smoking/cessation/coverage/page1.htm).
- *Environmental Tobacco Smoke and Other Indoor Air Pollution Problems Affecting Children* (slide set), American Academy of Pediatrics (www.aap.org/moc/displaytemp/etsspeech.doc).
- *Targeting Tobacco Use Nations Leading Cause of Death 2007* (fact sheet), Centers for Disease Control and Prevention (www.cdc.gov/tobacco/basic_information/00_pdfs/aagtobacco2007.pdf).
- *Tobacco Control Resource Center* (Web page), Public Health Advocacy Institute (tobacco.neu.edu/).
- *Youth Tobacco Cessation: A Guide for Making Informed Decisions* (book), Centers for Disease Control and Prevention (www.cdc.gov/tobacco/quit_smoking/cessation/youthtobacco.htm).

Engaging Patients and Family

- *Dangers of Secondhand Smoke* (brochure), American Academy of Pediatrics (patiented.aap.org).
- *Second Hand Smoke* (fact sheet), Centers for Disease Control and Prevention (www.cdc.gov/tobacco/data_statistics/factsheets/secondhandsmoke.htm).
- *Secondhand Smoke Causes Sudden Infant Death Syndrome* (fact sheet), Centers for Disease Control and Prevention (www.cdc.gov/tobacco/data_statistics/factsheets/sids.htm).
- *The Risks of Tobacco Use: A Message to Parents and Teens* (brochure), American Academy of Pediatrics (patiented.aap.org).
- *Tobacco, Drugs and Adolescents* (fact sheet), American Academy of Pediatrics (patiented.aap.org).
- *Tobacco: Straight Talk for Teens* (brochure), American Academy of Pediatrics (patiented.aap.org).
- *What Is Environmental Tobacco Smoke* (fact sheet), American Academy of Pediatrics (www.medem.com/medlb/article_detaillb.cfm?article_id=zzz1ubhwq7c&sub_cat=29).
- *Youth and Tobacco* (fact sheet), Centers for Disease Control and Prevention (www.cdc.gov/tobacco/youth/information_sheets/yuthfax1.htm).

Medical Decision Support

- *ETS Exposure Risk—3 Question Screen* (questionnaire), Groner, et al. (practice.aap.org/content.aspx?aid=2001).
- *Pediatric Environmental Health, 2nd ed* (book), American Academy of Pediatrics (www.aap.org/bookstore).
- *Smoking and Tobacco Use* (Web page), Centers for Disease Control and Prevention (www.cdc.gov/tobacco/index.htm).
- *Smoking Assessment Questionnaire* (questionnaire), Seifert, et al. (practice.aap.org/content.aspx?aid=2001).
- *Tobacco Fast Facts* (fact sheet), Centers for Disease Control and Prevention (www.cdc.gov/tobacco/basic_information/fastfacts.htm).
- *Treating Tobacco Use and Dependence—A How-To Guide For Implementing the Public Health Service Clinical Practice Guideline* (guideline), US Department of Health and Human Services, Public Health Service (www.surgeongeneral.gov/tobacco/clinpack.html).
- *Youth and Tobacco Use: Current Estimates* (fact sheet), Centers for Disease Control and Prevention (www.cdc.gov/tobacco/data_statistics/factsheets/youth_tobacco.htm).

Internet Resources

American Cancer Society (www.cancer.org/docroot/home/index.asp).

American Heart Association (www.americanheart.org/presenter.jhtml?identifier=1200000).

American Lung Association (www.lungusa.org/site/pp.asp?c=dvluk9o0e&b=22542).

National Cancer Institute, US National Institutes of Health (www.cancer.gov/).

Robert Wood Johnson Foundation Smoke Free Families (www.smokefreefamilies.org/).

Smoke Free Homes, Children's National Medical Center (www.kidslivesmokefree.org/).

AAP POLICY STATEMENTS

American Academy of Pediatrics, Committee on Drugs. The transfer of drugs and other chemicals into human milk. *Pediatrics.* 2001;108:776-789. (aappolicy.aappublications.org/cgi/content/abstract/pediatrics;108/3/776).

American Academy of Pediatrics, Committee on Environmental Health. Environmental tobacco smoke: a hazard to children. *Pediatrics.* 1997;99:639-642. (aappolicy.aappublications.org/cgi/content/abstract/pediatrics;99/4/639).

American Academy of Pediatrics, Committee on Infectious Diseases and Committee on Fetus and Newborn. Revised indications for the use of palivizumab and respiratory syncytial virus immune globulin intravenous for the prevention of respiratory syncytial virus infections. *Pediatrics.* 2003;112:1442-1446. (aappolicy.aappublications.org/cgi/content/abstract/pediatrics;112/6/1442).

American Academy of Pediatrics, Committee on Substance Abuse. Indications for management and referral of patients involved in substance abuse. *Pediatrics.* 2000;106:143-148. (aappolicy.aappublications.org/cgi/content/abstract/pediatrics;106/1/143).

American Academy of Pediatrics, Committee on Substance Abuse. Marijuana: a continuing concern for pediatricians. *Pediatrics.* 1999;104:982-985. (aappolicy.aappublications.org/cgi/content/abstract/pediatrics;104/4/982).

American Academy of Pediatrics, Committee on Substance Abuse. Tobacco, alcohol, and other drugs: the role of the pediatrician in prevention, identification, and management of substance abuse. *Pediatrics.* 2005;115(3):816-821. (aappolicy.aappublications.org/cgi/content/full/pediatrics;115/3/816).

American Academy of Pediatrics, Committee on Substance Abuse. Tobacco's toll: implications for the pediatrician. *Pediatrics.* 2001;107:794-798. (aappolicy.aappublications.org/cgi/content/abstract/pediatrics;107/4/794).

American Academy of Pediatrics, Task Force on Sudden Infant Death Syndrome. The changing concept of sudden infant death syndrome: diagnostic coding shifts, controversies regarding the sleeping environment, and new variables to consider in reducing risk. *Pediatrics.* 2005;116:1245-1255. (aappolicy.aappublications.org/cgi/content/abstract/pediatrics;116/5/1245).

REFERENCES

1. US Department of Health and Human Services. The Health Consequences of Smoking: A Report of the Surgeon General. 2004. Available at: www.hhs.gov/surgeongeneral/library/smokingconsequences/. Accessed on March 8, 2007.
2. Bartecchi CE, MacKenzie TD, Schrier RW. The global tobacco epidemic. *Sci Am.* 1995;272:44.
3. Bartecchi CE, MacKenzie TD, Schrier RW. The human costs of tobacco use (1). *N Engl J Med.* 1994;330:907-912.
4. Phillip Morris. Risks of Smoking. Available at: www.philipmorrisusa.com/en/health_issues/default.asp. Accessed March 8, 2007.
5. Frieden TR, Blakeman DE. The dirty dozen: 12 myths that undermine tobacco control. *Am J Public Health.* 2005;95:1500-1505.
6. Barnes DE, Hanauer P, Slade J, et al. Environmental tobacco smoke. The Brown and Williamson documents. *JAMA.* 1995;274:248-253.

7. DiFranza J, Aligne CA, Weitzman M. Prenatal and environmental tobacco smoke exposure and children's health. *Pediatrics*. Apr 2004;113(4):1007-1015.
8. US Department of Health and Human Services: *Healthy People 2000: National Health Promotion and Disease Prevention Objectives*. DHHS Pub No PHS 91-50213. Washington, DC: US Department of Health and Human Services; 1991.
9. Chilmonczyk BA, Salmun LM, Megathlin KN, et al. Association between exposure to environmental tobacco smoke and exacerbations of asthma in children. *N Engl J Med*. 1993;328(23):1665-1669.
10. Klonoff-Cohen HS, Edelstein SL, Lefkowitz ES, et al. The effect of passive smoking and tobacco exposure through breast milk on sudden infant death syndrome. *JAMA*. 1995;273(10):795-798.
11. Aligne CA, Stoddard JJ. Tobacco and children: an economic evaluation of the medical effects of parental smoking. *Arch Ped Adolesc Med*. 1997;151:648-653.
12. Aligne CA, Moss M, Auinger P, et al. Association of pediatric dental caries with passive smoking. *JAMA*. 2003;289:1258-1264.
13. US Department of Health and Human Services. The Health Consequences of Involuntary Exposure to Tobacco Smoke: A Report of the Surgeon General. June 27, 2006. Available at: www.surgeongeneral.gov/library/secondhandsmoke/report/. Accessed on March 8, 2007.
14. Kessler DA. Nicotine addiction in young people. *N Eng J Med*. 1995;333:186.
15. American Academy of Pediatrics, Committee on Substance Abuse Policy Statement. Tobacco-free environment: an imperative for the health of children and adolescents. *Pediatrics*. 1994;93:866-868.
16. Aligne CA, Christy C, Jain S. Inadvertent tobacco advertising in physicians' offices. *JAMA*. 2000;285:43-44.
17. Centers for Disease Control and Prevention. Quick Reference Guide for Clinicians. Treating Tobacco Use and Dependence. Available at www.surgeongeneral.gov/tobacco/tobaqrg.htm. Accessed March 8, 2007.
18. Kahn RS, Wise PH, Finkelstein JA, et al. The scope of unmet maternal health needs in pediatric settings. *Pediatrics*. 1999;103:576-581.
19. Fiore MC, Jorenby DE, Schensky AE, et al. Smoking status as the new vital sign: effect on assessment and intervention in patients who smoke. *Mayo Clin Proc*. 1995;70:209.
20. Beeber SJ. Parental smoking and childhood asthma. *J Pediatr Health Care*. 1996;10(2):58-62.
21. Tucker JS, Ellickson PL, RAND Corporation Santa Monica, CA. A Discrete Time Hazards Model of Smoking Initiation Among West Coast Youth from Age 5 to 23 Maria Orlando. Available at: www.rand.org/pubs/working_papers/2006/rand_wr395.pdf. Accessed March 8, 2007.
22. Murray AB, Morrison BJ. The decrease in severity of asthma in children of parents who smoke since the parents have been exposing them to less cigarette smoke. *J Allergy Clin Immunol*. 1993;91:102-110.
23. Severson HH, Andrews JA, Lichtenstein E, et al. Reducing maternal smoking and relapse: long-term evaluation of a pediatric intervention. *Prevent Med*. 1997;26:120-130.
24. Roseby R, Waters E, Polnay A, et al. Family and career smoking control programmes for reducing children's exposure to environmental tobacco smoke. *Cochrane Database System Rev*. 2003;3:CD001746.
25. Curry SJ, Hollis J, Bush T, et al. A randomized trial of a family-based smoking prevention intervention in managed care. *Prevent Med*. 2003;37:617-626.
26. Hurt RD, Croghan GA, Beede SD, et al. Nicotine patch therapy in 101 adolescent smokers: efficacy, withdrawal symptom relief, and carbon monoxide and plasma cotinine levels. *Arch Pediatr Adolesc Med*. Jan 2000; 154(1):31-37.
27. Grimshaw GM, Stanton A. Tobacco cessation interventions for young people. *Cochrane Database System Rev*. 2006. Available at: www.cochrane.org/reviews/en/ab003289.html. Accessed March 8, 2007.
28. US Preventive Services Task Force (AHRQ). Counseling to Prevent Tobacco Use. Available at: www.ahrq.gov/clinic/uspstf/uspstbac.htm. Accessed March 8, 2007.
29. DiClemente CC, Dolan-Mullen P, Windsor RA. The process of pregnancy smoking cessation: implications for interventions. *Tob Control*. 2000;9:16-21.
30. Prochaska JO, DiClemente CC, Norcross JC. In search of how people change: applications to addictive behaviors. *Am Psychol*. 1992;47:1102-1114.
31. Ockene JK. Smoking among women across the life span: prevalence, interventions, and implications for cessation research. *Ann Behav Med*. 1993;15:135-148.
32. Winickoff JP, Berkowitz AB, Brooks K, et al, the Tobacco Consortium, and the Center for Child Health Research of the American Academy of Pediatrics. State-of-the-art interventions for office-based parental tobacco control. *Pediatrics*. Mar 2005;115(3):750-760.
33. Emmons KM, Rollnick S. Motivational interviewing in health care settings opportunities and limitations. *Am J Prev Med*. 2001;20:68-74.
34. Fiscella K, Franks P. Cost-effectiveness of the transdermal nicotine patch as an adjunct to physicians' smoking cessation counseling. *JAMA*. 1996;275:1247-1251.
35. Windsor RA, Whiteside HP Jr, Solomon LJ, et al. A process evaluation model for patient education programs for pregnant smokers. *Tob Control*. 2000;9:29-35.
36. Perez-Stable EJ, Juarez-Reyes M, Kaplan C, et al. Counseling smoking parents of young children: comparison of pediatricians and family physicians. *Arch Pediatr Adolesc Med*. 2001;55:25-31.
37. Cabana MD, Rand CS, Becher OJ, et al. Reasons for pediatrician nonadherence to asthma guidelines. *Arch Pediatr Adolesc Med*. Sep 2001;155(9):1057-1062.
38. Oncken CA, Pbert L, Ockene JK, et al. Nicotine replacement prescription practices of obstetric and pediatric clinicians. *Obstet Gynecol*. 2000;96:261-265.
39. Ibrahim JK, Schauffler HH, Barker DC, et al. Coverage of tobacco dependence treatments for pregnant women and for children and their parents. *Am J Public Health*. 2002;92:1940-1942.
40. American Academy of Pediatrics, Committee on Child Health Financing and Committee on Substance Abuse. Policy statement: improving substance abuse prevention, assessment, and treatment financing for children and adolescents. *Pediatrics*. Oct 2001;108(4):1025-1029.
41. Fiore MC, Croyle RT, Curry SJ, et al. Preventing 3 million premature deaths and helping 5 million smokers quit: a national action plan for tobacco cessation. *Am J Public Health*. 2004;94(2):205-210.
42. Perry RJ, Keller PA, Fraser D, et al. Fax to quit: a model for delivery of tobacco cessation services to Wisconsin residents. *WMJ*. 2005;104(4):37-40.
43. Centers for Disease Control and Prevention. Guide to Community Preventive Services. Tobacco. Available at: www.thecommunityguide.org/tobacco/default.htm. Accessed March 8, 2007.
44. Centers for Disease Control and Prevention. Third National Report on Human Exposure to Environmental Chemicals. 2005. Available at: www.cdc.gov/exposurereport/report.htm. Accessed March 8, 2007.

45. Johnston LD, O'Malley PM, Bachman JG, et al. *Teen Drug Use Down But Progress Halts Among Youngest Teens.* Ann Arbor, MI: University of Michigan News and Information Services; 2005. Available at: monitoringthefuture.org/pressreleases/05cigpr.pdf. Accessed March 8, 2007.
46. Breslow L, Johnson M. California's Proposition 99 on tobacco, and its impact. *Ann Rev Public Health.* 1993;14:585-604.
47. American Lung Association. Tobacco Control Laws in Your State. Available at: lungaction.org/reports/tobacco-control05.html. Accessed March 8, 2007.
48. Farrelly MC, Healton CG, Davis KC, et al. Getting to the truth: evaluating national tobacco countermarketing campaigns. *Am J Public Health.* 2002;92(6):901-907.

SECTION THREE

Screening and Case Finding

Chapter 36

SCREENING: GENERAL CONSIDERATIONS

Paul H. Dworkin, MD

Primary care physicians are well positioned to participate in the early detection of childhood problems and conditions because of their access to young children and families. Universal screening refers to the process of testing all children at certain ages to detect those at high risk for significant deviations from normal. The emphasis is on distinguishing between children at high and low risk for certain problems, rather than on diagnosing such conditions. This screening typically involves the application of rapidly administered tests, examinations, or other procedures. Screening tools or instruments may also be used for validating history or physical findings after concerns are raised; however, this process is different and has been referred to as *second-stage screening*.

The number of conditions for which screening is currently recommended or mandated continues to increase. Research has better delineated the adverse effects of certain childhood conditions, such as the neurobehavioral and intellectual deficits associated with moderate lead poisoning and iron-deficiency anemia. Technological advances, such as automated equipment to measure auditory brainstem response to detect hearing loss in young infants and of tandem mass spectrometry to measure metabolic analytes for newborn screening, allow effective testing after an abnormal screening test. Changing morbidity within pediatric practice has emphasized the importance of identifying behavioral, developmental, and psychosocial problems early and suggests the need for revised screening policies for certain conditions such as tuberculosis. Societal changes have influenced the scope and content of screening programs. These changes include demands for confidentiality of test results, concerns with the stigma associated with certain diagnoses, and legislative mandates requiring early intervention for children who have developmental problems and other chronic conditions. The continuing debate over health care reform, with its emphasis on primary prevention and cost containment, has contributed to an increased scrutiny of screening practices.

Despite the time-honored tradition of performing screening tests during child health supervision visits, the effectiveness of many such practices is uncertain. The United States Congress Office of Technology Assessment, in a critical review of the value of child health supervision services, concluded that the only cost-effective and cost-saving screening procedure is newborn testing for metabolic disorders.[1] Because recommendations for screening practices have typically been determined by a combination of limited scientific data, empiricism, and good intentions, they have often provoked considerable debate. Recent examples of such recommendations include the following:

- The 1993 recommendation of the US Department of Health and Human Services that all infants be screened for sickle cell disease regardless of race or ethnic background[2]
- The 1993 National Institutes of Health Consensus Statement, which recommended screening of all infants for hearing impairment within the first 3 months of life and preferably before discharge from the hospital newborn nursery[3]
- The 1997 recommendation by the Centers for Disease Control and Prevention that universal screening for elevated blood lead levels be limited to areas with at least 27% of housing built before 1950 and to populations in which the percentage of 1- and 2-year-old children who have elevated blood lead levels is at least 12%[4]

The goal of this chapter is to review the criteria by which conditions are judged appropriate for screening and tests are selected for use in screening programs. Examples of screening recommendations that have generated debate and controversy illustrate the extent to which conditions and tests fulfill such criteria. Examples of evidence-based recommendations illustrate the limitations of research data to guide public policy. In addition, screening is compared with other approaches to early detection during child health supervision services.

TRADITIONAL CRITERIA FOR CONDITIONS TO BE SCREENED

Traditionally, disease conditions have been judged appropriate for screening if they fulfill certain well-accepted criteria:

1. The condition must have significant morbidity or mortality, with serious consequences if not detected and remediated early. For example, the adverse effects of early sensorineural hearing loss on language development and subsequent academic achievement and on social and emotional development are cited to

support recommendations for universal screening for hearing impairment among infants.

2. The condition must be sufficiently prevalent to justify the cost of screening programs. However, determining the true prevalence of certain conditions is difficult. For example, recommendations for universal lead screening were influenced by data indicating that 17% of all American preschool children have blood lead (BPb) levels greater than 15 mcg/dL. However, subsequent surveys from various parts of the country found that only 2% to 10% of children have BPb levels greater than 10 mcg/dL.[5]
3. The screening program must include the entire population, especially those at particular risk for the condition. Screening programs are optimally implemented within a comprehensive system of preventive child health care directed at the entire population. The lack of access of many young children and families to child health supervision services and a medical home is well recognized. Disadvantaged children at increased risk for conditions such as iron-deficiency anemia, lead poisoning, and tuberculosis are less likely to receive recommended screening tests because of their limited access to health care.
4. Diagnostic tests must allow affected individuals to be distinguished from nonaffected persons or those who are borderline. Screening should be performed only for conditions that can be diagnosed with certainty. In the example of universal screening for hearing impairment in infants, some authorities have criticized the test that measures evoked otoacoustic emissions (EOAEs) because the results may be affected by fluid or debris in the middle or external ear. In the past, the alternative auditory brainstem response (ABR) equipment available in hospitals was considered difficult to operate and time consuming, and test results were difficult to interpret.[6]
5. The condition, after detection, must be treatable or controllable. Developmental screening is based on the premise that screening positives will result in an intervention that will benefit the child. Although the benefits of early intervention for children who have physical handicaps (eg, sensory impairment, Down syndrome, cerebral palsy) or delayed speech or language are well established, more modest evidence supports the benefits of early identification and intervention for young children who have learning disabilities and mild intellectual disability.
6. Detection and treatment during the asymptomatic stage must improve prognosis, and early treatment must have significant advantage. Newborn screening for phenylketonuria is clearly beneficial because early treatment prevents later brain damage and neurologic impairment. Similarly, prophylactic penicillin has been shown clearly to reduce both morbidity and mortality from pneumococcal infections in infants who have sickle cell anemia. Screening for cystic fibrosis has been supported by evidence that treatment before the development of severe pulmonary disease will increase the chance and duration of survival.
7. Adequate resources must be available for the definitive diagnosis and treatment of disorders identified by screening. A major criticism of the Early Periodic Screening, Diagnosis and Treatment component of Medicaid has been the failure to ensure that all children whose findings on screening are suspect receive appropriate diagnostic and treatment services. The lack of adequate diagnostic and therapeutic resources for developmental, behavioral, and psychosocial problems hampers efforts at early identification. This lack of resources has raised concerns about the ethics of screening for developmental, behavioral, and psychosocial problems.[7] Universal screening for hearing impairment in infants is problematic for some individuals because follow-up diagnostic testing and treatment of hearing loss are difficult to carry out in rural or remote areas.
8. The cost of screening must be outweighed by the savings in suffering and alternative expenditure that would occur if the condition were not diagnosed until the symptomatic stage. Costs of screening programs must include not only the direct cost of the procedures themselves, but also the cost of diagnostic evaluation, monitoring, and intervention as a consequence of screening, as well as the costs of false-positive and false-negative results. For example, the cost of universal screening for hearing impairment in infants has been estimated to be $200 million per year.[6] In contrast, the lifetime economic cost of a single case of congenital deafness is estimated to exceed $1 million.[8] Screening for developmental delay defies simple cost-benefit analysis, and the cost of screening has yet to be justified by either the savings in alternative expenditures, such as special educational programs or services, or a quantifiable lessening of anxiety or suffering. Furthermore, such screening is not without risks, such as the dangers of labeling and creating a self-fulfilling prophecy.

CRITERIA FOR SCREENING TESTS

Once the decision has been made to screen for a particular disorder, judging which tests are appropriate to use in screening programs is based on widely accepted criteria:

1. Tests must be simple, practical, convenient, and safe. The relative ease and simplicity of performing EOAE testing facilitates universal screening for hearing impairment in infants. However, the decrease in specificity of this test during the first 24 hours of life poses logistical problems in that early discharge may necessitate a second screening on an outpatient basis.[9]
2. Tests must be acceptable to patients and families, with assurance of informed parental consent and confidentiality of findings. Children should not be subjected to screening procedures without parental approval. Informed parental consent includes a discussion of potential false-positive and false-negative findings, the possible need for time-consuming and often expensive follow-up evaluations, and the anxiety generated by positive screening results. Confidentiality of screening results must be maintained because positive findings for disorders such as HIV

infection and sickle cell disease may be socially stigmatizing and result in discrimination by insurance companies and potential employers.

3. Tests must be accurate and reliable. Although anodic stripping voltimetry and graphite furnace atomic absorption spectroscopy may yield blood lead (BPb) results having a ±4 mcg/dL accuracy, 10% to 20% of clinical laboratories do not meet proficiency standards.[5] Furthermore, capillary screening may include skin contamination that falsely elevates BPb.

Although a wide variety of developmental screening tests are proposed for use in health programs during infancy and early childhood, all tests have varying degrees of reliability and validity and lack well-established norms. The validity of screening tests consists of two components: (1) sensitivity, the proportion of individuals who have a disorder whose test result is positive; and (2) specificity, the proportion of individuals who do not have the disorder whose test is negative. Of particular clinical importance is the probability of an individual having the disorder when the test is positive—the test's positive predictive value—as well as the probability of not having the disorder when the test is negative—negative predictive value. The predictive value of a test depends greatly on the prevalence of the disorder in the population being tested. The low prevalence of hearing impairment (approximately 1 to 3 of every 1000 otherwise healthy newborns) contributes to the reported low specificity of EOAE testing alone and favors a two-step screening system with EOAE combined with ABR testing.[9]

4. Tests should be economical. The costs of newborn screening for metabolic disorders such as congenital hypothyroidism, galactosemia, and maple syrup urine disease are minimal because such tests are incorporated within established screening programs for phenylketonuria. The cost of screening for such rare disorders in isolation would be prohibitive.
5. Test results should lend themselves to easy interpretation. Screening test results may be complex. For example, reports of screening for sickle cell disease should include the hemoglobin phenotype and the diagnostic possibilities associated with the phenotype. The screening program must ensure the availability of appropriate education and genetic counseling for parents.

SCREENING AS A PUBLIC HEALTH SERVICE

In recent years, the criteria for screening have evolved to include a broader definition of benefits to the affected child and the child's family, including the prevention or optimization of all outcomes and negative consequences.[10] A greater emphasis on more moderate and parent-centered benefits, including a reduction in recurrence risks through genetic counseling and the avoidance of *diagnostic odysseys* associated with unrecognized conditions such as uncommon inborn errors of metabolism, have implications for policy deliberations. For example, the Centers for Disease Control and Prevention has concluded that newborn screening for cystic fibrosis is justified based on such outcomes as nutritional benefits, cognitive benefits for children at nutritional risk, reduction in diagnostic delays, the avoidance of hospitalization, and the recognition of carriers.[11]

EVIDENCE-BASED ASSESSMENTS

Recommendations for selecting disorders for population-based screening should include the systematic assessment of evidence of effectiveness using standardized methods. The US Preventive Services Task Force (USPSTF) develops recommendations for screening based on systematic reviews of evaluations of interventions, including the strength of research designs.[12] The USPSTF grades its recommendations according to one of five classifications:

A. The USPSTF strongly recommends the service based on good evidence of improved health outcomes and the conclusion that benefits substantially outweigh harms.
B. The USPSTF recommends the service based on at least fair evidence of important health outcomes and the conclusion that benefits outweigh harms.
C. The USPSTF makes no recommendation for or against the service based on at least fair evidence of improved health outcomes and the conclusion that the balance of benefits and harms is too close to justify a general recommendation.
D. The USPSTF recommends against routinely providing the service based on at least fair evidence of ineffectiveness or the conclusion that harms outweighs benefits.
I. The USPSTF makes no recommendation for or against the service based on insufficient evidence of effectiveness and the inability to determine the balance of benefits and harms.

EVIDENCE-BASED RECOMMENDATIONS

The USPSTF publishes its recommendations for pediatric prevention and screening in its *Guide to Clinical Preventive Services* (www.preventiveservices.ahrq.gov). Examples of evidence-based recommendations for screening and their classification include the following:

- Evidence is insufficient to recommend for or against routine risk assessment of preschool children by primary care clinicians for the prevention of dental disease (I).
- Evidence is sufficient to recommend against the routine screening of asymptomatic adolescents for idiopathic scoliosis (D).
- Evidence is insufficient to recommend for or against routine screening of newborns for hearing loss during postpartum hospitalization (I).
- Evidence is sufficient to recommend screening to detect amblyopia, strabismus, and defects in visual acuity in children younger than age 5 years (B).
- Evidence is insufficient to recommend routine screening for developmental dysplasia of the hip in infants (I).
- Evidence is insufficient to recommend for or against routine use of brief, formal screening instruments in primary care to detect speech and language delay in children up to 5 years of age (I).

In addition to the USPSTF, other important organizations provide evidence-based recommendations for screening procedures. Examples include the American Academy of Pediatrics (AAP) (aappolicy.aappublications.org), the Canadian Task Force on Preventive Care (www.ctfphc.org), and the American College of Medical Genetics. The AAP in collaboration with the Maternal and Child Health Bureau has incorporated its recommendations for screening within preventive care in *Bright Futures: Guidelines for Health Supervision of Infants, Children, and Adolescents.*

ALTERNATIVE APPROACHES TO EARLY DETECTION

Early detection is considered desirable for certain conditions that do not fulfill traditional criteria for screening. For example, neither the types of developmental delays for which screening is performed nor the screening tests themselves fulfill standard criteria for acceptance.[13] Nonetheless, early identification of and intervention for developmental delays are goals of child health supervision. Alternative approaches to early detection should be considered for such conditions.

SELECTIVE OR HIGH-RISK SCREENING?

Selective as opposed to universal screening may be performed for certain conditions. For example, reported differences in BPb levels between children living in urban and suburban areas have been cited to support a strategy of geographic targeting.[5] A multistage approach to more selective BPb screening is the use of a five-item questionnaire for all patients as an initial screen to identify children who are at increased risk and should therefore receive BPb testing.[4]

Selective screening programs may target a specific racial or ethnic group that has an increased prevalence of a particular disorder. For example, screening programs for Tay-Sachs disease target Ashkenazi Jews. However, selective screening will undoubtedly fail to identify certain affected individuals. For example, selective screening programs targeting a specific racial or ethnic group will not identify all infants who have sickle cell disease because defining an individual's racial or ethnic background reliably by surname, self-report, or physical characteristics is not possible. Because prophylactic administration of penicillin has been demonstrated to reduce morbidity and mortality in children who have sickle cell anemia, universal screening of all newborns is recommended, regardless of race or ethnic background.[2]

HIGH-RISK REGISTER

Before 1994 the Joint Committee on Infant Hearing favored the use of a register instead of screening to identify infants at risk for hearing impairment. The registry listed specific conditions that place a newborn at increased risk for hearing loss, for example, a family history of hearing loss, anomalies of the head and neck, and a birthweight less than 1500 g. Listing these high-risk factors in the form of a screening questionnaire and asking parents to complete the form after delivery was followed by selective ABR testing for infants considered at risk. Because risk-factor screening identifies only 50% of infants who have significant hearing loss, the Joint Committee recommended in 1994 the option of universal screening or evaluating all infants before discharge from the newborn nursery.[14] Subsequently, the AAP Task Force on Newborn Hearing endorsed the implementation of universal newborn hearing screening.[15]

PRESCREENING AND SCREENING QUESTIONNAIRES

Questionnaires as initial screens have been developed to aid in the early detection of children's behavioral, emotional, and psychosocial problems. Parents may be asked to complete these brief questionnaires before meeting with the pediatric physician. Examples include the Pediatric Symptom Checklist (PSC), designed for screening the emotional well being of school-aged children in pediatric practice,[15] and a self-administered questionnaire for structured psychosocial screening.[16] Results from small-scale validation studies have been encouraging and suggest that such questionnaires deserve further study to assess their value in pediatric office practice.

SURVEILLANCE

The approach currently practiced by primary care physicians for the early detection of developmental problems is most consistent with the process termed *developmental surveillance*. Surveillance is a flexible, continuous process whereby knowledgeable professionals observe children repeatedly during the provision of child health supervision over time.[13] The components of developmental surveillance include eliciting and attending to parents' concerns, obtaining a relevant developmental history, observing children accurately and informatively, and sharing opinions and concerns with other relevant professionals, such as preschool teachers. Parent-completed developmental questionnaires, such as the Parents' Evaluation of Developmental Status (PEDS) and the Ages and Stages Questionnaire (ASQ), also may be used to involve parents in the monitoring of their infants' and children's development.[17,18] To improve the accuracy of surveillance, pediatric primary care physicians may supplement their subjective impressions occasionally by administering a test such as the Brigance Screens-II, or they may selectively use such a professionally administered test as a *second-stage* screening instrument or validation tool when suspicions arise.[19] The AAP now recommends that surveillance be strengthened through the administration of developmental screening tests at the 9-, 18-, and 30- (or 24-) month visits.[20] (See Chapter 44, Developmental Surveillance and Intervention.)

SUGGESTED RESOURCES

Briss PA, Brownson RC, Fielding JE, et al. Developing and using the Guide to Community Preventive Services: lessons learned about evidence-based public health. *Annu Rev Public Health.* 2004;25:281-302.

Dworkin PH. Detection of behavioral, developmental, and psychosocial problems in pediatric primary care practice. *Curr Opin Pediatr.* 1993;5:531-536.

Hagan JF Jr, Shaw JS, Duncan PM, eds. *Bright Futures: Guidelines for Health Supervision of Infants, Children, and Adolescents.* 3rd ed. Elk Grove Village, IL: American Academy of Pediatrics; 2007.

Kohatsu ND, Robinson JG, Torner JC. Evidence-based public health: an evolving concept. *Am J Prev Med.* 2004;27: 417-421.

Meisels SJ, Provence S. *Screening Assessment: Guidelines for Identifying Young Disabled and Developmentally Vulnerable Children and Their Families.* Washington, DC: Zero to Three/National Center for Clinical Infant Programs; 1989.

Whitby LG. Screening for disease: definition and criteria. *Lancet.* 1974;11:819-822.

REFERENCES

1. United States Congress, Office of Technology Assessment. *Healthy Children: Investing in the Future.* Publication No. OTA-H-345. Washington, DC: US Government Printing Office; 1988.
2. US Department of Health and Human Services, Sickle Cell Disease Guideline Panel. *Sickle Cell Disease: Screening, Diagnosis, Management, and Counseling in Newborns and Infants. Clinical Practice Guideline No. 6.* Rockville, MD: US Department of Health and Human Services, Public Health Service, Agency for Health Care Policy and Research; 1993.
3. National Institutes of Health. Early identification of hearing impairment in infants and young children. *NIH Consens Statement.* 1993;11(1):1-24.
4. Centers for Disease Control and Prevention. *Screening Young Children for Lead Poisoning. Guidance for State and Local Public Health Officials.* Atlanta, GA: US Department of Health and Human Services, Public Health Service, Centers for Disease Control and Prevention; 1997.
5. Harvey B. Should blood level screening recommendations be revised? *Pediatrics.* 1994;93:201-204.
6. Bess FM, Paradise JL. Universal screening for infant hearing impairment: not simple, not risk-free, not necessarily beneficial, and not presently justified. *Pediatrics.* 1994;93:330-334.
7. Perrin EC. Ethical questions about screening. *J Dev Behav Pediatr.* 1998;19:350-352.
8. Northern JL, Downs MP. *Hearing in Children.* Baltimore, MD: Williams & Wilkins; 1991.
9. American Academy of Pediatrics, Task Force on Newborn and Infant Hearing. Newborn and infant hearing loss: detection and intervention. *Pediatrics.* 1999;103:527-530.
10. Grosse SD, Boyle CA, Kenneson A, et al. From public health emergency to public health service: the implications of evolving criteria for newborn screening panels. *Pediatrics.* 2006;117:923-929.
11. Grosse SD, Boyle CA, Botkin JR, et al. Newborn screening for cystic fibrosis: evaluation of benefits and risks and recommendations for state newborn screening programs. *MMWR Recomm Rep.* 2004;53(RR-13):1-36.
12. Harris RP, Helfand M, Woolf SH, et al. Current methods of the US Preventive Services Task Force: a review of the process. *Am J Prev Med.* 2001;20(3 suppl):21-35.
13. Dworkin PH. British and American recommendations for developmental monitoring: the role of surveillance. *Pediatrics.* 1989;84:1000-1010.
14. American Academy of Pediatrics, Joint Committee on Infant Hearing. *1994 Position Statement.* Elk Grove Village, IL: American Academy of Pediatrics; 1994.
15. Jellinek MS, Murphy JM. The recognition of psychosocial disorders in pediatric office practice: the current status of the pediatric symptom checklist. *J Dev Behav Pediatr.* 1990;11:273-278.
16. Kemper KJ. Self-administered questionnaire for structured psychosocial screening in pediatrics. *Pediatrics.* 1992;89:433-436.
17. Glascoe FP. *Collaborating With Parents. Using Parents' Evaluations of Developmental Status To Detect and Address Developmental and Behavioral Problems.* Nashville, TN: Ellsworth & Vandermeer Press; 1998.
18. Squires JK, Nickel R, Eisert D. Early detection of developmental problems: strategies for monitoring young children in the practice setting. *J Dev Behav Pediatr.* 1996;17:420-427.
19. Frankenburg WK, Dodds J, Archer P, et al: The Denver II: a major revision and restandardization of the Denver Developmental Screening Test. *Pediatrics.* 1992;89:91-97.
20. Council on Children With Disabilities, Section on Developmental Behavioral Pediatrics, Bright Futures Steering Committee, and Medical Home Initiatives for Children With Special Needs Project Advisory Committee. Identifying infants and young children with developmental disorders in the medical home: an algorithm for developmental surveillance and screening. *Pediatrics.* 2006;118: 405-420.

Chapter 37

PHYSICAL EXAMINATION AS A SCREENING TOOL

Basil J. Zitelli, MD

The clinical examination is relatively inexpensive and requires little equipment. The two components of the clinical examination—the history and physical examination—can be completed almost anywhere, and repeated examinations can be done easily.[1] The evaluation of clinical disorders emphasizes the importance of the history and physical examination as the most important diagnostic tools the clinician has available.[2-5] A diagnosis can often be made with the clinical examination without further laboratory testing. If necessary a directed laboratory investigation can be made based on information gathered in the history and physical examination. The history and physical examination should be used to formulate a diagnosis with appropriately guided laboratory evaluation used to verify the diagnosis.[6]

A good pediatric physical examination requires great observation skills, flexibility, and attention to detail. The examination begins as soon as the physician enters the room and gains a snapshot of the child. Immediate impressions of activity, color, mental status, respiratory distress, and interactions with the family and environment begin the overall assessment. During the history, observations can be made concerning developmental level and parent-child interactions. Examination of the child should be in a well-lighted and warm room so that the child is not uncomfortable without clothing. For comfort, the infant or toddler should be examined while being held in the parent's lap. The physical examination begins by direct observation of the cranial nerves, tone, movement, response to environment, color, and respiratory pattern, as well as the presence of rashes, birthmarks, and dysmorphic features. Least invasive examinations should be accomplished first, such as examination of the heart and lungs. Flexibility in the order of the examination is important to maximize comfort of the child, moving to different parts of the examination if the child shows fear or discomfort, and returning later to complete the examination. The toddler may frequently be frightened by direct eye contact during the examination. A gentle, progressive approach while avoiding direct eye contact may be more successful. Having the parent aid in the examination may reassure and calm the fearful child. Observing the child play, draw, or participate in games often gives the examiner information about cognitive skills, fine- and gross-motor function and coordination. The examiner must often be creative in producing an environment where parent and child are at ease and maximal information can be obtained. On occasion, subsequent and serial examinations are necessary to elucidate the clinical problem.

Particular attention should be paid to vital signs and growth parameters, especially plotting serial growth points on appropriate growth curves. Vital signs are a screening tool, giving information at a single point in time and serving as a frame of reference for subsequent clinical changes. Plotting growth data is important for monitoring long-term growth patterns and observing deviations from normal growth velocity. Specific growth charts should be used for individual clinical indications such as Down syndrome, Turner syndrome, and other disorders. These ongoing data-collection points constitute the surveillance that is critical for detecting subtle developmental, growth, and medical problems at early stages. In fact, a physical examination uninformed by history or such indicators has an otherwise low yield.

Listening to the patient's concerns, as William Osler declared, is unspoken caring.[7] Gentle touching with the examination enhances bonding between physician and patient. Thorough, unrushed explanation of findings of the clinical evaluation reassures and comforts the family. If further evaluation is necessary, then explanation of the process based on the clinician's evaluation provides a foundation of confidence and trust.

The clinical examination of the child demands skill, patience, gentleness, and compassion. It is the beginning not only of the patient's evaluation, but also more importantly of the physician-patient relationship. It is the cornerstone of clinical medicine.

REFERENCES

1. Jauhar S. The demise of the physical exam. *N Engl J Med.* 2006;354:548-551.
2. Peterson MC, Holbrook JH, Von Hales D, et al. Contributions of the history, physical examination, and laboratory investigation in making medical diagnoses. *West J Med.* 1992;156:163-165.
3. Sills H. Failure to thrive. The role of clinical and laboratory evaluation. *Am J Dis Child.* 1978;132:967-969.
4. Fireman P. Diagnosis of sinusitis in children: emphasis on the history and physical examination. *J Allergy Clin Immunol.* 1992;90:433-436.
5. Bohner H, Yang Q, Franke C, et al. Simple data from history and physical examination help to exclude bowel obstruction and to avoid radiographic studies in patients with acute abdominal pain. *Eur J Surg.* 1998;164:777-784.
6. Fred HL. The tyranny of technology. *Hosp Prac (Off Ed).* 1997;32:17-8, 21.
7. Osler W. A Way of Life. An address delivered to Yale students on the evening, April 20th, 1913. Springfield, IL., C. C. Thomas, 1919.

Chapter 38

PREPARTICIPATION PHYSICAL EVALUATION

Eric Small, MD

Over 6 million high school students participate in sports each year. With this many participants, the preparticipation physical evaluation (PPE) is one of the most commonly performed examinations. Over the last decade, the PPE has evolved to allow physicians to provide consistent, high-quality examinations nationwide. In the

BOX 38-1 Common Questions Parents Have About the Preparticipation Physical Evaluation (PPE)

My son had a physical examination for participation in football last year. Does he still need to see his physician this year?

Although the PPE is comprehensive, it was never designed to take the place of a regular physician visit. The setting or time allocation for the PPE is often not conducive to discussions of health issues that are of primary importance during the adolescent years, such as drug and alcohol use, smoking, sexual activity education, safety issues, and diagnosis of depression.

When should my child have a PPE relative to the beginning of an athletic season?

The best time for the PPE is approximately 4 to 6 weeks before the beginning of the athletic season. This period allows enough time for thorough evaluations, consultations, and rehabilitation of any identified musculoskeletal injuries.

Do I need to attend the PPE with my child?

Although you may not be asked to attend the PPE with your child, you should review the accuracy and completeness of the medical history and family history that are given. Your child may not know or remember some of the history. Most of the important information obtained in the PPE is obtained from the history.

How often will my son or daughter need a PPE?

The frequency of required evaluations varies by state. Most commonly, a physical evaluation is required every year. To determine the requirements of your state, check with the school district or the state high school athletic association.

Will my child need to undergo any laboratory or radiographic studies at the PPE?

Routine laboratory studies and radiographs are not generally performed. Based on information obtained during the history and physical examination, however, your physician may think that further studies are indicated.

early 1990s the American Academy of Family Physicians, the American Academy of Pediatrics, the American Medical Society for Sports Medicine, the American Orthopaedic Society for Sports Medicine, and the American Osteopathic Academy of Sports Medicine formed the Preparticipation Examination Task Force to standardize the conduct and content of these examinations. In 1992 the Task Force published recommendations for the PPE based on the consensus of the current literature. These guidelines were updated in 1997, 2002, and 2004 and serve as the basis for the current PPE.[1]

GOALS OF THE PREPARTICIPATION PHYSICAL EVALUATION

The purpose of the PPE is not to disqualify athletes; less than 2% are actually disqualified based on an evaluation's results. Rather, the primary goals of the PPE are to detect conditions that might predispose the athlete to injury, to detect conditions that might be life-threatening or disabling, and to meet legal or insurance requirements. The secondary goals are to determine general health, to counsel athletes on health-related issues, and to assess fitness level.

Identifying athletes who may need further diagnostic testing, counseling, or rehabilitation is the primary goal of the PPE, but many other expectations exist. Parents sometimes expect the PPE to be a comprehensive evaluation of the athlete's health, including areas that may be considered unrelated to sports participation, such as teenage sexuality, substance abuse, and immunizations, among others. Parents frequently think of the PPE as the only medical evaluation their child or adolescent needs, and they expect it to be comprehensive.[2] In contrast, many physicians view the PPE as a cursory examination that is only intended to detect conditions that might limit or impair athletic endeavors. Common questions parents have about the PPE, and their answers, are provided in Box 38-1.

Table 38-1 Medical History Questions

QUESTION	REASON
1. Injury or illness since last check-up?	Targets potential physical examination concerns
2. Chronic illnesses, hospitalizations, or surgeries?	Identifies potential counseling or rehabilitation issues
3. Any medications or supplements of any type?	Identifies drugs that may inhibit or interfere with sports participation
4. Allergies to medications, insects, or food?	Alerts physicians and trainers for potential allergic reactions
5. Dizziness, passed out, chest pain with exercise; history of sudden death in a close relative <50 years of age?	Identifies potential causes of sudden death caused by cardiovascular problems
6. Have you ever passed out or nearly passed out during exercise? Have you ever passed out or nearly passed out after exercise? Have you ever had discomfort, pain, or pressure in your chest during exercise? Does your heart race or skip beats during exercise? Does anyone in your family have Marfan syndrome?	Targets cardiovascular concerns
7. Ever been restricted from sports by physician?	Identifies potential disqualifying problems
8. Any skin problems?	Identifies potential transmittable disease during contact
9. Concussion, knocked out, unconsciousness, memory loss, seizure, or severe or frequent headache?	Targets neurologic concerns
10. Stinger, burner, pinched nerve, numbness or tingling in extremities?	Targets neurologic concerns
11. Problems while exercising in the heat?	Targets heat illness concerns
12. Asthma, allergies, wheezing, difficulty breathing, or chest pain?	Identifies potential for exercise-induced asthma
13. Special equipment or devices not usually used in your sport?	Identifies potential concerns for physician follow-up
14. Glasses, contacts, or vision or eye problems?	Identifies ophthalmologic concerns
15. Strain, sprain, fracture, joint pain, or swelling?	Identifies potential musculoskeletal problems
16. Concerns about weight: Do you lose weight regularly for your sport?	Identifies potential disordered eating
17. Feel stressed out?	Clue to ask follow-up questions regarding drug use, eating problems, sexuality, and home and school problems
18. Recent immunizations (tetanus, measles, hepatitis B, chickenpox)?	Health maintenance issues
19. Girls only: menstrual history?	Identifies oligomenorrhea and amenorrhea and potential risk for poor nutrition, stress fractures
20. Do you wear protective braces, splints?	Identifies injuries that have not been fully rehabilitated

Because parents and physicians view the evaluation differently, parents must be advised about the intent of the PPE, and the PPE's scope and purpose must be made clear to them. The most recent PPE guidelines suggest creating a medical home for all athletes (see Chapter 8, Medical Home Collaborative Care.)

CONDUCTING THE PREPARTICIPATION PHYSICAL EVALUATION

Methods

The PPE is typically conducted in one of three ways: (1) the locker-room method, (2) the station method, or (3) the office-based method.

In the locker-room method, athletes traditionally line up single file, and the physician examines each athlete individually. One benefit of this method is that it requires few personnel and can be performed with little preparation. However, this method affords little privacy for the athlete, it is usually so noisy that the physician has a hard time auscultating the heart and lungs, and it is often too brief.

The station method divides the examination into several components, with physicians, nurses, athletic trainers, and coaches each assigned to a single task. This method is ideally suited for screening large numbers of athletes. Two benefits of this method are (1) its relative efficiency and (2) its good ability to identify abnormalities. However, this method affords less rapport with athletes, and, similar to the locker-room method, a lack of privacy exists. Athletes have little opportunity to ask questions of the physicians regarding their own health or other medical or personal issues.

The individual office-based method has the advantage of an established physician-patient relationship in which the medical history is known and continuity of care is fostered. Disadvantages include a lack of consistency among physicians, potential unfamiliarity with the sport and its disqualifying conditions by the physician, and its lack of cost effectiveness.

Timing

Ideally, the PPE is performed early enough before the sport's season begins to ensure that athletes who have medical problems can be thoroughly evaluated and treated but not so early that intervening injuries are likely to occur. The best time for the evaluation to take place is 4 to 6 weeks before the first scheduled practice.

Although the current guidelines of the American Academy of Pediatrics (AAP) suggest that the PPE should be performed every year, other sources suggest that the PPE be conducted before the beginning of each new level of competition (ie, middle school or junior high, high school, college), with annual updates of the history and targeted physical examinations of areas of concern. However, most state high school athletic associations require annual evaluations. A recent survey of all 50 states and the District of Columbia found that 65% of states require annual examination of all athletes competing in high school sports.

EVALUATION

History

As with any health evaluation, the history identifies most potential problems for young athletes.[2-4] Most experts agree that despite the best screening of athletes to prevent sudden death, only a few who die would have been detected through history and physical examination. The key to identifying these problems is the questionnaire that systematically screens for conditions that frequently cause problems in athletes or that might lead to sudden death during athletic activity. Table 38-1 lists some of the most important questions to ask during the examination. The PPE forms provided by state high school athletic associations often do not incorporate all of the screening questions recommended by the Preparticipation Examination Task Force. The form that should be used can be accessed on the AAP Web site (see end of chapter materials.)

Athletes typically complete their history forms without input from their parents. One study showed that only 40% of PPE forms matched when filled out independently by parent and child. The athlete and the parents should therefore complete the form together to obtain a thorough and accurate history. Although the PPE forms should be completed by parent and patient, some issues may arise (particularly for those patients for whom the practice is the medical home) in

Table 38-2 Cardiovascular Screening in Athletes

CONDITION	CARDIOVASCULAR EXAMINATION	ABNORMALITY
Hypertension	Blood pressure	Varies with age—general guideline is >135/85 mm Hg in adolescents
Coarctation of aorta	Femoral pulses	Decreased intensity of pulse
Hypertrophic cardiomyopathy	Auscultation with provocative maneuvers (standing, supine, Valsalva maneuver)	Systolic ejection murmur that intensifies with standing or Valsalva maneuver
Marfan syndrome	Auscultation	Aortic (decrescendo diastolic murmur) or mitral insufficiency (holosystolic murmur)

Adapted from Maron BJ, Thompson PO, Puffer JC. Cardiovascular preparticipation screening of competitive athletes: a statement from the Sudden Death Committee [clinical cardiology] and Congenital Cardiac Defects Committee [cardiovascular disease in the young] American Heart Association. *Circulation.* 1996;94:850-856. Reprinted by permission of Lippincott Williams & Wilkins.

which adolescent privacy on certain topics, such as sexuality and substance abuse should be respected.

Physical Examination

Two key components of the physical examination (cardiovascular and musculoskeletal) identify most athletes who warrant further evaluation or disqualification. The updated medical evaluation form recommended by the Preparticipation Examination Task Force can be accessed on the AAP Web site (see end of chapter materials.)

Cardiovascular Examination

The cardiovascular examination should include evaluation of peripheral pulses, murmurs, and blood pressure. Table 38-2 summarizes important aspects of the cardiovascular examination screening. All diastolic murmurs and grade 3/6 systolic murmurs warrant further evaluation. Hypertrophic cardiomyopathy, one of the most important conditions to detect, may produce a systolic murmur that cannot be distinguished from an innocent murmur. The murmur of hypertrophic cardiomyopathy increases in intensity with a Valsalva maneuver (decreased ventricular filling, increased obstruction) and decreases with squatting (increased ventricular filling, decreased obstruction); it will also increase in intensity when the athlete moves from a squatting to standing position.

Blood pressures obtained during the PPE are often high. These readings are sometimes the result of using a blood pressure cuff that is too small, particularly in large adolescents. However, sometimes the athlete's blood pressure is truly high when an age-based table of norms is consulted. Hypertension is rarely severe enough to disqualify an athlete from participation, but it needs to be identified and monitored by the athlete's regular physician. Weight-training activities should be restricted in patients who have severe hypertension. Recent cardiovascular research showed that screening for sudden cardiac death that included a standardized history, physical examination, and electrocardiogram may have helped prevent sudden death caused by cardiomyopathy.[5]

Although sudden cardiac death in young athletes is rare, a history of syncope, chest pain with exercise, or a family history of sudden death under age 50 should be evaluated.

Musculoskeletal Examination

The musculoskeletal examination is particularly important because it typically accounts for 50% of the abnormal physical findings identified on the PPE. The examination should focus on previously injured or symptomatic areas. Ninety-two percent of orthopedic injuries are detected by history alone.[6]

Some authorities suggest a sport-specific approach to the physical examination.[7] This method emphasizes

BOX 38-2 Special Considerations for the Examination of Injured or Symptomatic Joints

- Inspect for visual deformity, muscle mass, asymmetry, and swelling.
- Palpate for localized areas of tenderness, warmth, and effusion.
- Assess range of motion (eg, an athlete with hip pain should be tested for loss of internal rotation and abduction, which can be seen in slipped capital femoral epiphysis and Legg-Calvé-Perthes disease).
- Test neurovascular status by evaluating muscle strength, sensation, reflexes, and pulses of the involved limb (eg, an athlete with a history of burners should undergo complete neurovascular testing of the neck and upper extremities).
- Test joint stability (eg, an athlete with knee pain should undergo tests for valgus and varus stress, Lachman test, and posterior drawer test).

BOX 38-3 Sport Classification by Contact

CONTACT OR COLLISION
Basketball
Boxing
Diving
Field hockey
Football (flag, tackle)
Ice hockey
Lacrosse
Martial arts
Rodeo
Rugby
Ski jumping
Soccer
Team handball
Water polo
Wrestling

LIMITED CONTACT
Baseball
Bicycling
Cheerleading
Canoeing and kayaking (white water)
Fencing
Field events (high jump, pole vault)
Floor hockey
Gymnastics
Handball
Horseback riding
Racquetball
Skating (ice, in-line, roller)
Skiing (downhill, water)
Softball
Squash
Ultimate frisbee
Volleyball
Windsurfing and surfing

NONCONTACT
Archery
Badminton
Bodybuilding
Canoeing and kayaking (flat water)
Crew rowing
Curling
Dancing
Field events (discus, javelin, shot put)
Golf
Orienteering
Power lifting
Race walking
Riflery
Rope jumping
Running
Sailing
Scuba diving
Strength training
Swimming
Table tennis
Tennis
Track
Weight lifting

Adapted from American Academy of Pediatrics, Committee on Sports Medicine and Fitness. Medical conditions affecting sports participation. *Pediatrics.* 2008;121(4):841-848.

Table 38-3 Sports Classification by Intensity

HIGH-TO-MODERATE INTENSITY; HIGH-TO-MODERATE DYNAMIC; HIGH-TO-MODERATE STATIC DEMANDS	HIGH-TO-MODERATE INTENSITY; HIGH-TO-MODERATE DYNAMIC; LOW STATIC DEMANDS	HIGH-TO-MODERATE INTENSITY; HIGH-TO-MODERATE STATIC; LOW DYNAMIC DEMANDS	LOW INTENSITY; LOW DYNAMIC; LOW STATIC DEMANDS
Boxing	Badminton	Archery	Bowling
Crew rowing	Baseball	Auto racing	Cricket
Cross-country skiing	Basketball	Diving	Curling
Cycling	Field hockey	Equestrian	Golf
Downhill skiing	Lacrosse	Field events (jumping, throwing)	Rifle shooting
Fencing	Orienteering	Gymnastics	
Football	Table tennis	Karate or judo	
Ice hockey	Race walking	Motorcycling	
Rugby	Racquetball	Rodeo	
Running (sprint)	Soccer	Sailing	
Speed skating	Squash	Ski jumping	
Water polo	Swimming	Water skiing	
Wrestling	Tennis	Weight lifting	
	Volleyball		

Adapted from American Academy of Pediatrics Committee on Sports Medicine and Fitness. Medical conditions affecting sports participation. *Pediatrics.* 2008;121(4):841-848.

the areas that are most commonly affected or injured in each specific sport. For example, a swimmer's examination would focus on the shoulders and ears (otitis externa), whereas a football player's examination would include evaluation of neurologic conditions and musculoskeletal injuries.

Box 38-2 lists special considerations for the examination of injured or symptomatic joints.

Laboratory Studies

Laboratory studies have not been shown to be cost effective or warranted in young asymptomatic athletes. Routine urinalysis and hematocrit for all athletes have been largely abandoned because these tests do not identify athletes who require disqualification, and they have a high rate of false-positive results. Similarly, electrocardiogram, echocardiogram, and stress testing are not suggested as screening tests in asymptomatic individuals because of the high rate of false-positive findings and their high cost.

SPORTS CLASSIFICATION

Sports are classified based on the likelihood of collision injury and the strenuousness of the exercise. These classifications are used to guide physicians on the risk of injury and the degree of cardiopulmonary fitness required to engage in the sport successfully. The AAP has established classification guidelines by the level of contact and intensity (Box 38-3 and Table 38-3).

CLEARANCE TO PLAY

Few athletes are disqualified from activity based on conditions identified during the PPE. Table 38-4, which is designed to be understood by both medical and nonmedical personnel, lists the most current recommendations regarding medical conditions and contraindications to participation. Working with athletes to find safe, enjoyable sports in which they can participate is important. If possible, and depending on the condition that is detected, sports participation should not be eliminated altogether. Figure 38-1 provides a sample clearance or return-to-play form.

Occasionally, an athlete or parent will disagree with a physician's recommendation for restricting participation in a particular sport. In these cases, the important steps are to explain fully the reasons for the recommendation and to consider having the athlete and parent sign a document acknowledging that this discussion occurred and that they were informed of the risks. Athletes who request a second opinion should be encouraged to do so. Ultimately, the team physician is responsible for ensuring that athletes are able to participate safely and without undue risk of injury.

SPECIAL CONSIDERATIONS

Nutritional Supplements

Sports supplements have become a billion-dollar industry. Athletes as young as age 11 are taking performance-enhancing supplements. Sports supplements contain impurities, and when taken inappropriately, they may result in adverse side effects. Side effects can include muscle cramps, dehydration, abdominal bloating, tachycardia, arrhythmia, and even death. Supplement use should be discouraged. If a young athlete is taking them, then this person should be told about their possible ill effects. The PPE is an ideal time to question athletes briefly about supplement use.

Table 38-4 Medical Conditions and Sports Participation

CONDITION	PARTICIPATE?	EXPLANATION
Atlantoaxial instability (instability of the joint between cervical vertebrae 1 and 2)	Qualified yes	Athlete needs evaluation* to assess risk of spinal cord injury during sports participation.
Bleeding disorder	Qualified yes	Athlete needs evaluation.
Carditis (inflammation of the heart)	No	Carditis may result in sudden death with exertion.
Hypertension (high blood pressure)	Qualified yes	Persons with significant essential (unexplained) hypertension should avoid weight and power lifting, bodybuilding, and strength training. Those with secondary hypertension (hypertension caused by a previously identified disease) or severe essential hypertension need evaluation.
Congenital heart disease (structural heart defects present at birth)	Qualified yes	Persons with mild forms may participate fully; those with moderate or severe forms or who have undergone surgery need evaluation.
Dysrhythmia (irregular heart rhythm)	Qualified yes	Athlete needs evaluation because some types require therapy or make certain sports dangerous, or both.
Mitral valve prolapse (abnormal heart valve)	Qualified yes	Persons with symptoms (chest pain, symptoms of possible dysrhythmia) or evidence of mitral regurgitation (leaking) on physical examination need evaluation. All others may participate fully.
Heart murmur	Qualified yes	If the murmur is innocent (does not indicate heart disease), then full participation is permitted; otherwise the athlete needs evaluation (see "Congenital heart disease" and "Mitral valve prolapse" above).
Cerebral palsy	Qualified yes	Athlete needs evaluation.
Diabetes mellitus	Yes	All sports can be played with proper attention to diet, hydration, and insulin therapy. Particular attention is needed for activities that last 30 minutes or more.
Diarrhea	Qualified no	Unless disease is mild, no participation is permitted, because diarrhea may increase the risk of dehydration and heat illness. See "Fever" below.
Eating disorders, anorexia nervosa, bulimia nervosa	Qualified yes	These patients need both medical and psychiatric assessment before participation.
Eyes: functionally one-eyed athlete, loss of an eye, detached retina, previous eye surgery or serious eye injury	Qualified yes	A functionally one-eyed athlete has a best-corrected visual acuity of <20/40 in the worse eye. These athletes would experience significant disability if the better eye were seriously injured, as would those with loss of an eye. Some athletes who have previously undergone eye surgery or had a serious eye injury may have an increased risk of injury because of weakened eye tissue. Availability of eye guards approved by the American Society of Testing Materials and other protective equipment may allow participation in most sports, but this determination must be judged on an individual basis.
Fever	No	Fever can increase cardiopulmonary effort, reduce maximal exercise capacity, make heat illness more likely, and increase orthostatic hypotension during exercise. Fever may rarely accompany myocarditis or other infections that may make exercise dangerous.
History of heat illness	Qualified yes	Because of the increased likelihood of recurrence, the athlete needs individual assessment to determine the presence of predisposing conditions and to arrange a prevention strategy.
HIV infection	Yes	Because of the apparent minimal risk to others, all sports may be played that the state of health allows. In all athletes, skin lesions should be properly covered, and athletic personnel should use universal precautions when handling blood or body fluids with visible blood.
Kidney: absence of one	Qualified yes	Athlete needs individual assessment for contact or collision and limited contact sports.

Table 38-4 Medical Conditions and Sports Participation—cont'd

CONDITION	PARTICIPATE?	EXPLANATION
Liver: enlarged	Qualified yes	If the liver is acutely enlarged, then participation should be avoided because of risk of rupture. If the liver is chronically enlarged, then individual assessment is needed before collision or contact or limited contact sports are played.
Malignancy	Qualified yes	Athlete needs individual assessment.
Musculoskeletal disorders	Qualified yes	Athlete needs individual assessment.
History of serious head or spine trauma, severe or repeated, concussions, or craniotomy	Qualified yes	Athlete needs individual assessment for collision or contact or limited contact sports and for noncontact sports if deficits exist in judgment or cognition. Recent research supports a conservative approach to management of concussions.
Convulsive disorder (well controlled)	Yes	Risk of convulsion during participation is minimal.
Convulsive disorder (poorly controlled)	Qualified yes	Athlete needs individual assessment for collision or contact or limited-contact sports. Avoid the following noncontact sports: archery, rifle shooting, swimming, weight or power lifting, strength training, or sports involving heights. In these sports, occurrence of a convulsion may be a risk to self or others.
Obesity	Qualified yes	Because of the risk of heat illness, obese persons need careful acclimatization and hydration.
Organ transplant recipient	Qualified yes	Athlete needs individual assessment.
Ovary: absence	Yes	Risk of severe injury to the remaining ovary is minimal.
Respiratory, pulmonary compromise (including cystic fibrosis)	Qualified yes	Athlete needs individual assessment, but generally, all sports may be played if oxygenation remains satisfactory during a graded exercise test. Patients with cystic fibrosis need acclimatization and good hydration to reduce the risk of heat illness.
Asthma	Yes	With proper medication and education, only athletes with the most severe asthma will have to modify their participation.
Acute upper respiratory infection	Qualified yes	Upper respiratory obstruction may affect pulmonary function. Athlete needs individual assessment for all but mild diseases. See "Fever" previously listed.
Sickle cell disease	Qualified yes	Athlete needs individual assessment. In general, if status of the illness permits, then all but high-exertion, collision or contact sports may be played. Overheating, dehydration, and chilling must be prevented.
Sickle cell trait	Yes	Individuals with sickle cell trait do not likely have an increased risk of sudden death or other medical problems during athletic participation except under the most extreme condition of heat and humidity and possibly high altitude. These individuals, as with all athletes, should be carefully conditioned, acclimatized, and hydrated to reduce any possible risk.
Skin: boils, herpes simplex, impetigo, scabies, molluscum contagiosum	Qualified yes	Because the patient is contagious, participation in gymnastics with mats, martial arts, wrestling, or other collision or contact or limited-contact sports is not allowed. Herpes simplex virus is probably not transmitted via mats.
Spleen: enlarged	Qualified yes	Persons with acutely enlarged spleens should avoid all sports because of risk of rupture. Those with chronically enlarged spleens need individual assessment before playing collision or contact or limited contact sports.
Testicle: absent or undescended	Yes	Certain sports may require a protective cup.

[*] Needs evaluation means that a physician with appropriate knowledge and experience should assess the safety of a given sport for an athlete with the listed medical condition. Unless otherwise noted, this term is used because of the variability of the severity of the disease, the risk of injury among the specific sport, or both.
Adapted from American Academy of Pediatrics, Committee on Sports Medicine and Fitness. Medical conditions affecting sports participation. *Pediatrics.* 2008;121(4):841-848.

Clearance for Return to Play

Name ______________________ Sex ________ Age ________ DOB ________

☐ Cleared without restriction

☐ Cleared with recommendations for further evaluation or treatment:

____

____

____

____

☐ Not cleared for:

☐ All sports. Reason ______________________

☐ Certain sports. Reason ______________________

Recommendations: ______________________

____

EMERGENCY INFORMATION

Allergies: ______________________

Other information: ______________________

Immunizations (eg, tetanus/diphtheria; measles, mumps, rubella; hepatitis A, B; influenza; poliomyelitis; pneumococcal; meningococcal; varicella)

☐ Up to date *(see attachment documentation)*

☐ Not up to date. Specify: ______________________

____

Name of physician *(print or type)* ______________________ Date ________

Figure 38-1 Sample clearance for return to play. *(Adapted from the American Academy of Family Physicians, American Academy of Pediatrics, American College of Sports Medicine, American Medical Society for Sports Medicine, American Orthopaedic Society for Sports Medicine, and American Osteopathic Academy of Sports Medicine. Copyright ©2004.)*

Obesity

Childhood obesity has reached epidemic proportions. Up to 30% of children are obese, and many of these youngsters are seeking to participate in sports. Obesity is not a contraindication to sports participation unless a comorbid finding such as severe hypertension is found. Obese children are at increased risk of heat injury and should be counseled accordingly. Sports participation with emphasis on activities that improve fitness should be encouraged for the obese child.

Concussion

A history of previous concussions should be addressed during the PPE. Consensus about concussion has been updated from the former three grades of severity to two: simple and complicated. Complicated concussion includes amnesia, loss of consciousness, seizure, or prolonged symptoms. Neuropsychological testing is suggested with repeat concussion or complicated concussion. Patients must meet three criteria to return to play: (1) asymptomatic at rest, (2) asymptomatic with exercise, and (3) no neurocognitive deficits (memory loss, concentration problems, fatigue, fogginess, confusion).

Medical Home

The most underserved population in health care today is adolescents. In many instances, their only contact with the medical system is the PPE. However, referring all young athletes to a pediatric primary care physician for routine care and for follow-up of any ongoing medical conditions is important.

SUMMARY POINTS

- A PPE is performed to prevent injury and assess medical conditions; it is not performed primarily to disqualify an athlete.
- An entire PPE should ideally be performed by one physician, even if a mass screening is taking place.
- Sudden cardiac death in young athletes is a rare event, but a history of syncope or chest pain with exercise or a family history of sudden death under age 50 should be evaluated.
- The musculoskeletal history and physical examination are the best ways to discover orthopedic problems.
- Concussion, heat injury, and use of nutritional supplements are topics that need to be discussed and emphasized during the PPE.

TOOLS FOR PRACTICE

Engaging Patient and Family

- *Sports and Your Child* (brochure), American Academy of Pediatrics (patiented.aap.org).
- *Sports Success Rx! Your Child's Prescription for the Best Experience: How to Maximize Potential and Minimize Pressure* (book), American Academy of Pediatrics (www.aap.org/bookstore).

Medical Decision Support

- *Care of the Young Athlete* (book), American Academy of Pediatrics and American Academy of Orthopaedic Surgeons (www.aap.org/bookstore).
- *Preparticipation Physical Evaluation, 3rd edition* (book), American Academy of Family Physicians, American Academy of Pediatrics, American College of Sports Medicine, American Medical Society for Sports Medicine, American Orthopaedic Society for Sports Medicine, and American Osteopathic Academy of Sports Medicine (www.aap.org/bookstore).
- *Preparticipation Physical Evaluation* (form), American Academy of Family Physicians, American Academy of Pediatrics, American College of Sports Medicine, American Medical Society for Sports Medicine, American Orthopaedic Society for Sports Medicine, and American Osteopathic Academy of Sports Medicine (www.aap.org/bookstore).

AAP POLICY STATEMENT

American Academy of Pediatrics, Committee on Sports Medicine. Medical conditions affecting sports participation. *Pediatrics*. 2008;121(4):841-848. (aappolicy.aappublications.org/cgi/content/full/pediatrics;121/4/841).

SUGGESTED RESOURCES

American Academy of Family Physicians, American Academy of Pediatrics, American College of Sports Medicine, American Medical Society for Sports Medicine, American Orthopaedic Society for Sports Medicine, American Osteopathic Academy of Sports Medicine. *The Preparticipation Physical Evaluation*. 3rd ed. Minneapolis, MN: McGraw-Hill; 2005.

American Academy of Pediatrics, Committee on Sports Medicine and Fitness. Medical conditions affecting sports participation. *Pediatrics*. 2001;107:1205-1209.

26th Bethesda Conference. Recommendations for determining eligibility for competition in athletes with cardiovascular abnormalities. January 6-7, 1994. *Med Sci Sports Exerc*. 1994;26(10 suppl):S223-S283.

Corrado D, Basso C, Pavei A, et al. Trends in sudden cardiovascular death in young competitive athletes after implementation of a preparticipation screening program. *JAMA*. 2006;296:1593-1601.

Fahrenbach MC, Thompson PD. The preparticipation sports examination: cardiovascular considerations for screening. *Cardiol Clin*. 1992;10:319-328.

Glover DW, Maron BJ. Profile of preparticipation cardiovascular screening for high school athletes. *JAMA*. 1998;279:1817-1819.

Grafe MW, Paul GR, Foster TE. The preparticipation sports examination for high school and college athletes. *Clin Sports Med*. 1997;16:569-591.

Maron BJ, Mitchell JH. Revised eligibility recommendations for competitive athletes with cardiovascular abnormalities. *J Am Coll Cardiol*. 1994;24:848-850.

McCrory P, Johnston K, Meeuwisse W, et al. Summary and agreement statement of the 2nd International Conference on Concussion in Sport, Prague 2004. *Br J Sports Med*. 2005;39:196-204.

Mitten MJ, Maron BJ, Zipes DP. Task Force 12: legal aspects of the 36th Bethesda Conference Recommendations. *J Am Coll Cardiol*. 2005;45:1373-1375.

Smith DM, Kovan JR, Rich BSE, et al, eds. *Preparticipation Physical Evaluation*. 2nd ed. Minneapolis, MN: McGraw-Hill; 1997.

Wingfield K, Matheson GO, Meeuwisse WH. Preparticipation evaluation: an evidence-based review. *Clin J Sport Med*. 2004;14:109-122.

REFERENCES

1. American Academy of Family Physicians, American Academy of Pediatrics, American College of Sports Medicine, American Medical Society for Sports Medicine, American Orthopaedic Society for Sports Medicine, American Osteopathic Academy of Sports Medicine. *Preparticipation Physical Examination*. 3rd ed. Minneapolis, MN: McGraw-Hill Healthcare Information; 2005.
2. Krowchuk DP, Krowchuk HV, Hunter M, et al. Parents' knowledge of the purposes and content of preparticipation physical examination. *Arch Pediatr Adolesc Med*. 1995;149(6):653-657.

3. Koester MC, Amundson CL. Preparticipation screening of high school athletes: are recommendations enough? *Phys Sportsmed*. 2003;31(3):35-38.
4. Carek PJ, Futrell M. Athletes' view of the preparticipation physical examination. *Arch Fam Med*. 1999;8(4):307-312.
5. Corrado D, Basso C. Schiavon, M, et al. Screening for hypertrophic cardiomyopathy in young athletes. *N Engl J Med*. 1998;339(6):364-369.
6. National High Blood Pressure Education Working Group on Hypertension Control in Children and Adolescents. Update on the 1987 task force report on high blood pressure in children and adolescents: a working group report on the National High Blood Pressure Education Program. *Pediatrics*. 1996;98(4 pt 1):649-658.
7. Smith J, Laskowski ER. The preparticipation physical examination: Mayo Clinic experience with 2,739 examinations. *Mayo Clin Proc*. 1998;73(5):419-429.

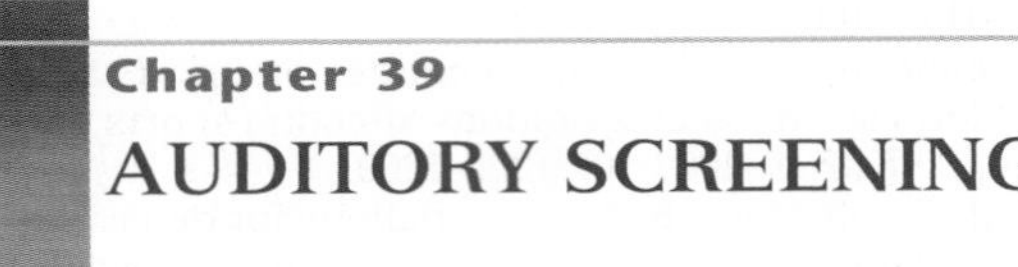

Chapter 39

AUDITORY SCREENING

David R. Cunningham, PhD; Sarah A. Sydlowski, AuD

JUSTIFICATION FOR SCREENING

Hearing loss, the most common congenital abnormality in newborns, is 20 times more prevalent than phenylketonuria and occurs twice as often as hypothyroidism, galactosemia, phenylketonuria, and sickle cell disease combined.[1] Routine screening for hearing loss is a justifiable procedure based on the prevalence of the disorder in the general pediatric population and at-risk groups along with the availability of effective interventions. Between 1 and 6 per 1000 babies without risk factors and approximately 13.3 per 1000 babies with high-risk factors are born with hearing loss greater than 40 dB.[2,3] However, these estimates fail to account for babies who have mild (<40 dB) sensorineural hearing losses. Add to this number children with progressive hearing losses and acquired childhood hearing losses and the importance of infant and childhood hearing screening is undeniable.

Approximately 14.9% of all children in the United States have a hearing loss with thresholds of at least 16 dB hearing level.[4] Any hearing loss, including a minimal degree of loss (15-25 dB), may cause speech and language delay and difficulty in social and educational environments. (See Chapter 45, Language and Speech Assessment.) The consequences are profound; approximately 37% of children with a mild sensorineural hearing loss will fail at least one grade in school.[5] Late-identified children with bilateral permanent hearing loss leave the educational system at the age of 18 years having achieved an average sixth-grade reading level and an average language-age equivalent of 12 years.[6] These developmental delays have been found to result in reduced educational and employment levels in adulthood.[7]

To maximize communicative competence and literacy in children who are hard of hearing or deaf, the Joint Committee on Infant Hearing (JCIH) published a position statement (endorsed by the National Institutes of Health [NIH] and the American Academy of Pediatrics [AAP])[8] recommending an agenda of early hearing detection and intervention.[7] The Committee endorsed the goal of testing children by 1 month of age, identifying those with hearing loss by 3 months of age, and treating hearing-impaired children by 6 months of age, as suggested in the landmark 1998 study by Yoshinaga-Itano et al.[9] Despite the evidence that early identification and intervention are critical to the overall communicative, cognitive, educational, and emotional development of children with hearing loss, the average age of identifying early-onset hearing loss in the United States was between 12 and 25 months but may be improving.[1] Early intervention in the form of audiologic management, otologic treatment, amplification, parental counseling, and special education is important not only because of the seriousness of the medical sequelae of active otopathologic conditions, but also because of the negative consequences that even a mild hearing loss has for language growth, academic success, and behavioral development.

GOALS OF SCREENING

The goal of hearing screening programs in general is to identify children with a moderate-to-severe hearing loss as early as possible to prevent the detrimental effects that late diagnosis has on language and speech development.[10]

Approximately 40% to 50% of infants with hearing loss would remain unidentified if *high-risk* indicators were used as a screening method instead of direct testing of all children.[6] In 1993 the NIH Consensus Development Conference recommended that all babies be screened for hearing loss before being discharged from the hospital.[7] As of 2005, all 50 states and the District of Columbia had mandatory universal newborn hearing screening (UNHS) programs in place,[11] the goal of which is to detect moderate to severe hearing loss. (State-specific information is available at www.infanthearing.org/states/index.html.)

NEONATAL AND EARLY INFANT PERIOD

Empirical evidence suggests that the best solution for the detection and subsequent intervention for hearing loss in the neonatal and early infant period is the implementation of a UNHS program[6,7,12-16] (Box 39-1 and Figure 39-1). Regardless of prior screening outcomes, all infants who are at risk for delayed-onset or progressive hearing loss should receive audiologic monitoring every 6 months for the first 3 years of life. (Box 39-2 summarizes the risk factors for hearing loss.) Additionally, all infants with or without risk factors should receive ongoing surveillance of communicative development beginning at 2 months of age during well-child visits.[7]

Based on data suggesting the long-term developmental consequences of hearing loss in infants, the JCIH defines the targeted hearing loss for UNHS programs as permanent bilateral or unilateral, sensory, or conductive hearing loss averaging 40 dB in the frequency region that is important for speech recognition

BOX 39-1 Principles That Provide the Foundation for Effective Early Hearing Detection and Intervention (EHDI) Systems

1. All infants should have access to hearing screening using a physiological measure no later than 1 month of age.
2. All infants who do not pass the initial hearing screening and the subsequent screening should have appropriate audiologic and medical evaluations to confirm the presence of hearing loss no later than 3 months of age.
3. All infants with confirmed permanent hearing loss should receive early intervention services as soon as possible after diagnosis but no later than 6 months of age. A simplified, single point of entry into an intervention system appropriate for children with hearing loss is optimal.
4. The EHDI system should be family centered with infant and family rights and privacy guaranteed through informed choice, shared decision making, and parental consent in accordance with state and federal guidelines. Families should have access to information about all intervention and treatment options and counseling regarding hearing loss.
5. The child and family should have immediate access to high-quality technology, including hearing aids, cochlear implants, and other assistive devices when appropriate.
6. All infants and children should be monitored for hearing loss in the medical home. Continued assessment of communication development should be provided by appropriate professionals to all children with or without risk indicators for hearing loss.
7. Appropriate interdisciplinary intervention programs for infants with hearing loss and their families should be provided by professionals knowledgeable about childhood hearing loss. Intervention programs should recognize and build on strengths, informed choices, traditions, and cultural beliefs of the families.
8. Information systems should be designed and implemented to interface with electronic health records and should be used to measure outcomes and report the effectiveness of EHDI services at the patient, practice, community, state, and federal levels.

From Joint Committee on Infant Hearing, American Academy of Audiology, American Academy of Pediatrics, American Speech-Language-Hearing Association, Directors of Speech and Hearing Programs in State and Welfare Agencies. Year 2007 position statement: principles and guidelines for early hearing detection and intervention programs. *Pediatrics*. 2007;120:898-921.

(approximately 500-4000 Hz).[7] This guideline generally eliminates from identification children with transient conductive hearing losses and mild sensory or conductive hearing impairments, as well as those with hearing loss related to auditory neuropathy or neural conduction disorders, which makes audiologic monitoring and routine screening later in life even more important. This issue will be discussed in more detail in later sections of this chapter. Objective physiological measures must be used to identify newborns and young infants with hearing loss. Although different programs use different screening criteria and a conclusive recommendation has yet to be reached, the literature suggests that otoacoustic emissions (OAEs) and auditory brainstem response (ABR) measures used together provide much more accurate information than either test alone and that both are necessary for a comprehensive screening program.[16-18] Northern and Hayes report that using a two-stage OAE-ABR screening protocol will result in only 1.7 infants with normal hearing being referred for a complete diagnostic evaluation for every baby who has hearing loss (based on a prevalence rate of two to three hearing-impaired infants per 1000 births).[19-21] In other words the two screening technologies are complementary when used in a two-stage screening protocol. Regardless of the protocol used, studies indicate that the best time frame for UNHS programs is approximately 3 to 4 days after birth, provided social or financial reasons do not suggest an earlier discharge from the hospital.[19-22] Korres et al reported that the highest referral rates occur within the first 24 hours of life.[19-21] The 2007 JCIH position statement recommends different protocols for the neonatal intensive care unit and well-baby nurseries. Screening of neonatal intensive care unit babies admitted for more than 5 days should always include ABR testing. Additionally, any baby readmitted to the hospital within the first month of life who also has risk factors for hearing loss should have a repeat hearing screening before discharge.[7]

Both OAEs and ABRs are noninvasive recordings of the physiological activity that underlies normal auditory function. Both tests are easily recorded in neonates, although environmental noise and the presence of birth fluids in the ear canal may influence test results. OAEs and ABR testing examines different levels of audition. OAEs are rapidly recorded and provide information regarding the presence or absence of hearing loss but cannot distinguish the degree or type of hearing loss.[23] OAEs are also generally absent in the presence of sensory hearing loss greater than or equal to 40-dB hearing level. However, OAEs are also sensitive to ear canal obstruction and middle ear effusion and may therefore cause a failed test result in the presence of normal cochlear function.[23] Because OAEs examine the integrity of the cochlea, neural dysfunction such as auditory neuropathy or neural conduction disorders without overlaying sensory loss will not be detected. In comparison, ABR testing reflects the activity of the cochlea, the auditory nerve, and the central auditory pathway up to the level of the brainstem. The test may also be affected by the presence of environmental noise or fluid in the external auditory canal. ABR reflects conductive hearing loss, sensory hearing loss, and neural conduction disorders such as auditory dyssynchrony and neuropathy.

Despite the sensitivity of a two-step screening protocol, some infants with hearing loss will still be missed. According to the JCIH, some examples of hearing loss types and configurations that are typically missed by current standards include isolated low-frequency (ie, <1000 Hz) hearing loss or steeply sloping high-frequency (ie, >2000 Hz) hearing loss. ABR

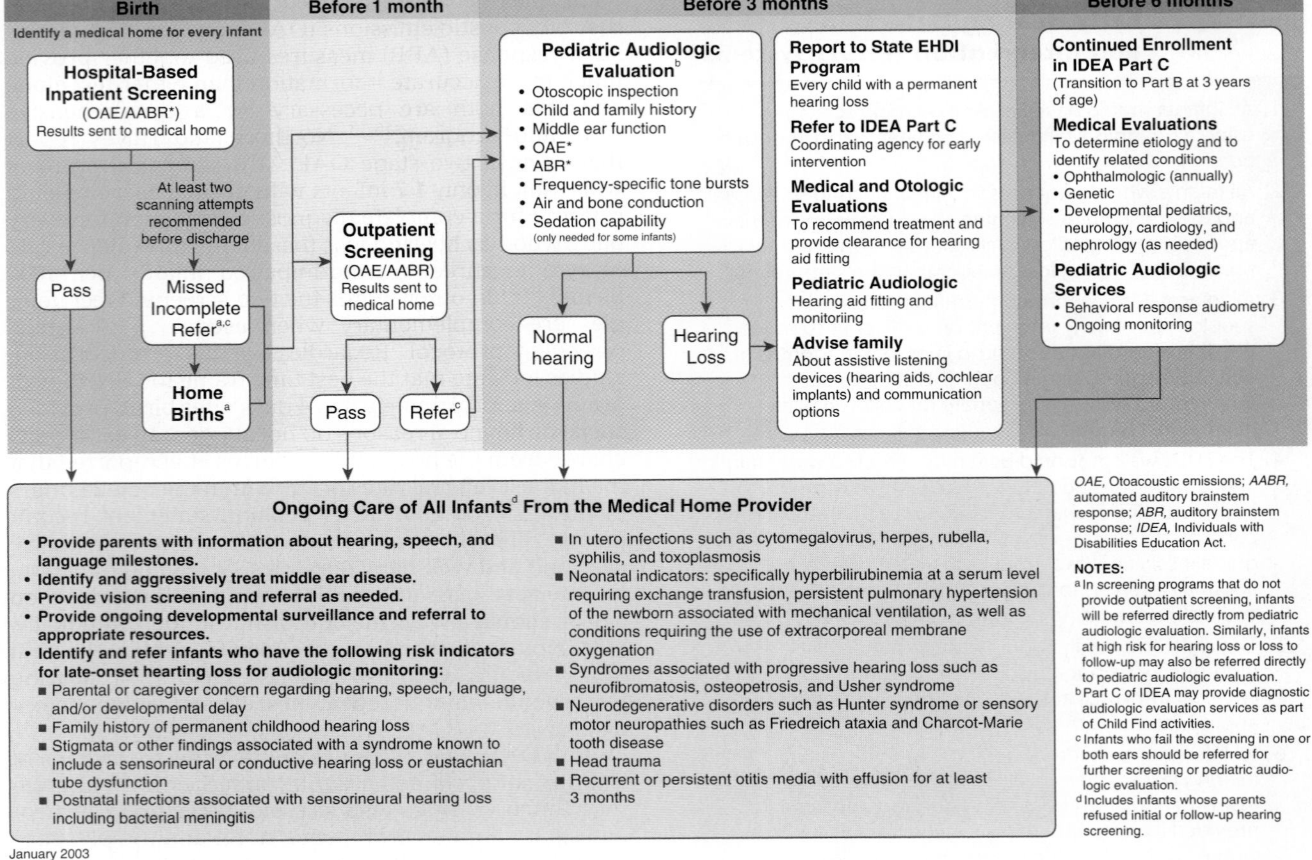

Figure 39-1 Universal Newborn Hearing Screening, Diagnosis, and Intervention—Guidelines for Pediatric Medical Home Providers. *(Adapted from the American Academy of Pediatrics. The National Center of Medical Home Initiatives for Children with Special Needs. Available at: www.medicalhomeinfo.org/screening/Screen%20Materials/Algorithm.pdf. Accessed August 3, 2007.)*

testing can also suggest normal hearing in the presence of mid-frequency (500-2000 Hz) hearing loss. Acquired or progressive hearing loss will also be unidentified in the neonatal population. Other factors that may result in a false-negative outcome include the performance and recording characteristics of the test technology, the pass-refer criteria, and excessive retesting using the same technology.[7,24] In 2000 the JCIH and the AAP revised their goals for UNHS protocols to achieve a screening population capture rate of 95%, follow-up rate of 95%, a referral rate of less than 4%, and a false-positive rate less than 3%, all confirmed by 3 months of age and with intervention occurring by 6 months of age.[2,7] If 95% of babies born are screened for hearing loss, as the JCIH recommends, then technology and protocols to screen for hearing loss at birth can detect approximately 90% of those with hearing loss.[24] The primary factor contributing to the effectiveness of hearing screening is appropriate follow-up.

TODDLER AND PRESCHOOL PERIOD (2 TO 5 YEARS)

In the toddler and preschool periods the screening protocol is modified to include the identification of otopathologic abnormalities (especially otitis media with effusion), mild conductive hearing loss, and previously undiagnosed, acquired, or progressive sensorineural hearing impairment. Routine periodic screening of school-aged children is recommended to ensure hearing that is optimal for educational participation. Although the method of screening children in these age groups has not changed significantly, awareness of and sensitivity to the effects of hearing loss on skill development and educational achievement is far greater.

The primary goal of screening in the 2- to 5-year-old period is the detection of medically remediable otopathologic abnormalities, progressive hearing loss, or late-onset acquired hearing loss. Furthermore, parents and pediatricians should recognize that children with

BOX 39-2 Risk Indicators Associated With Permanent Congenital, Delayed-Onset, or Progressive Hearing Loss in Childhood*

1. Caregiver concern† regarding hearing, speech, language, or developmental delay
2. Family history† of permanent childhood hearing loss
3. Neonatal intensive care of more than 5 days or any of the following regardless of length of stay: ECMO,† assisted ventilation, exposure to otoxic medications (gentamycin and tobramycin) or loop diuretics (furosemide, lasix), and hyperbilirubinemia requiring exchange transfusion
4. In-utero infections, such as CMV,† herpes, rubella, syphilis, and toxoplasmosis
5. Craniofacial anomalies, including those involving the pinna, ear canal, ear tags, ear pits, and temporal bone anomalies
6. Physical findings, such as white forelock, associated with a syndrome known to include a sensorineural or permanent conductive hearing loss
7. Syndromes associated with hearing loss or progressive or late-onset hearing loss,† such as neurofibromatosis, osteopetrosis, and Usher syndrome; other frequently identified syndromes such as Waardenburg, Alport, Pendred, and Jervell and Lange-Nielson
8. Neurodegenerative disorders,† such as Hunter syndrome, or sensory motor neuropathies, such as Friedreich ataxia and Charcot-Marie-Tooth syndrome
9. Culture-positive postnatal infections associated with sensorineural hearing loss,† including confirmed bacterial and viral (especially herpes virus and varicella) meningitis
10. Head trauma, especially basal skull or temporal bone fracture† requiring hospitalization
11. Chemotherapy†

CMV, Cytomegalovirus; *ECMO*, extracorporeal membrane oxygenation.
*All infants with a risk indicator for hearing loss should be referred for an audiologic assessment at least once by 24 to 30 months of age. Children with risk indicators highly associated with delayed-onset hearing loss, such as having received ECMO or having CMV infection, should have more frequent audiologic assessments.
†Risk indicators that are of greater concern for delayed-onset hearing loss.
From Committee on Infant Hearing, American Academy of Audiology, American Academy of Pediatrics, American Speech-anguage-earing Association, Directors of Speech and Hearing Programs in State and Welfare Agencies. Year 2007 position statement: principles and guidelines for early hearing detection and intervention programs. *Pediatrics.* 2007; 120:898-921.

mild hearing loss are typically missed by UNHS programs.[24] Screening procedures for young children are performed with the assumption that the more severe sensorineural hearing losses will have been identified by 2 years. However, 20% to 30% of hearing loss in children up to age 18 is acquired or progressive hearing loss,[1,16] and 75% of children will have at least one episode of otitis media by their third birthday.[25] Even though this age group is particularly difficult to screen, obtaining accurate results is nonetheless important in this population. The principal cause of hearing loss in this age range is otitis media, a pathologic abnormality capable of producing subtle, but significant, auditory learning disorders and permanent middle-ear damage.[26] Additionally, many conditions place children at risk for late-onset or progressive hearing loss (see Box 39-2), thus these conditions also must be considered when screening this population.

Children in this age group are usually screened for hearing loss at well-baby clinics, pediatricians' offices, Head Start programs, and preschool programs. Although the screening procedures may differ from site to site depending on the availability of equipment and trained personnel and on the level of background noise in the screening environment, the ideal protocol would include the following elements:

1. Physical examination
2. A detailed family history
3. Acoustic immittance testing (tympanometry)
4. Otoscopic inspection of the ear canal
5. Behavioral testing (or evoked OAEs in the case of children who cannot condition to behavioral testing)
6. An elicitation of parental or caregiver concern about the child's hearing and speech and language development.[26,27] The importance of this element should not be underestimated. According to the NIH, 70% of children with acquired hearing impairments are initially identified by parents.[16] Parents are typically as much as 12 months ahead of physicians in identifying their child's hearing loss.[3] Thus the NIH stresses that parental concern regarding hearing is sufficient reason to initiate prompt, formal, comprehensive hearing evaluation.[16]
7. Failure to attain appropriate language milestones should result in prompt referral for further hearing evaluation.[16]

Although behavioral responses are the gold standard of hearing screening for this age group, for children who are unable to participate in behavioral procedures, screening with OAEs is acceptable, although even a mild conductive component may obscure results. Screening stimuli that lack frequency-specificity or behavioral observation techniques based on noncalibrated signals, such as rattles, music boxes, noisemakers, whisper tests, and finger-rub tests, among others, are neither recommended nor acceptable.[26] Behavioral testing for children up to 36 months of age can be conducted using visual reinforcement audiometry, whereas children older than 36 months should be able to participate in conditioned play audiometry. Both tests should be performed at a level of 30 dB in a sound booth. Any child who does not respond at this level at any one frequency should be referred for a comprehensive evaluation by a licensed audiologist. A more in-depth discussion of appropriate screening procedures for this age group can be found in the American Speech-Language-Hearing Association *Audiologic Assessment Panel's Guidelines for Audiologic Screening*.[10] Parents, particularly those with a child who is at risk for progressive or acquired hearing loss, should also be counseled regarding auditory and communicative milestones for their child (Box 39-3) so that they may monitor their child's development.

BOX 39-3 Checklist of Selected Speech-Language-Auditory Milestones Achieved By Infants and Children Who Have Intact Cognition and Hearing*

BIRTH TO 3 MONTHS
Startles to loud noise
Awakens to sounds
Blinks or widens eyes in response to new sounds

3 TO 4 MONTHS
Quiets to mother's voice
Stops playing; listens to new sounds
Looks for source of new sounds not in sight

6 TO 9 MONTHS
Enjoys musical toys
Coos and gurgles with inflection
Says "mama"

12 TO 15 MONTHS
Responds to the baby's own name and "no"
Follows simple requests
Uses expressive vocabulary of three to five words
Imitates some sounds

18 TO 24 MONTHS
Knows body parts
Uses expressive vocabulary (two-word phrases, minimum of 20-50 words)
50% of speech intelligible to strangers

BY 36 MONTHS
Uses expressive vocabulary of four- to five-word sentences (approximately 500 words)
Uses speech that is 80% intelligible to strangers
Understands some verbs

*Failure to achieve these milestones by expected age ranges might relate to hearing loss that necessitates audiologic testing.
From Cunningham M, Cox EO, Committee on Practice and Ambulatory Medicine, Section on Otolaryngology and Bronchoesophagology. Hearing assessment in infants and children: recommendations beyond neonatal screening. *Pediatrics.* 2003;111:436-440.

SCHOOL-AGE PERIOD (5 TO 18 YEARS)

The primary goal of hearing screenings in this age group is identical to that of the toddler-preschool period, with the addition of the maintenance of educationally optimal hearing. Typically these children are screened in the school setting by trained professionals and are referred to the physician only if they fail the screening. School-aged children should be screened on initial entry into school, annually in kindergarten through third grade, in seventh and eleventh grades, and as needed, requested, or mandated by regulation.[10] In this age group the most likely cause of hearing abnormality is an otopathologic abnormality; however, some children are still at risk for acquired or progressive hearing loss. At-risk children should be routinely monitored for hearing loss (see Box 39-2). Additionally, during this period, central auditory processing disorders typically become apparent. Children as young as 7 years may be diagnosed with a central auditory processing disorder by an audiologist. Parent and teacher reports are particularly important during this period and should be regarded seriously.

The ideal protocol would include the following elements:

1. Otoscopic inspection of the ear canal
2. Acoustic immittance testing (tympanometry)
3. Behavioral testing under headphones or with insert phones
4. Elicitation of parental or caregiver concern about the child's hearing and speech and language development and educational performance

Behavioral testing should be performed in the traditional method of hand-raising in response to frequency-specific tones (1000, 2000, and 4000 Hz) presented under headphones at 20 dB. Failure to respond at even one frequency in one ear should result in referral for complete audiometric evaluation by a licensed audiologist. Should failure of acoustic immittance testing occur at both initial testing and retesting 6 weeks later, then referral will be made to the primary care physician for evaluation of middle-ear disorder. A more in-depth discussion of appropriate screening procedures for this age group can be found in the American Speech-Language-Hearing Association *Audiologic Assessment Panel's Guidelines for Audiologic Screening.*[10]

FOLLOW-UP CARE AND BENEFITS OF TREATMENT

The most critical aspect of an effective screening program is the subsequent follow-up care and treatment of children identified with hearing loss, those who fail their newborn hearing screening, or those labeled as at risk for progressive, late-onset, or acquired hearing loss. If no meaningful intervention and management occurs after hearing screening, or if children with a proclivity to acquired hearing loss are not screened frequently and appropriately, then the program has failed in its primary purpose: initiating a process of timely habilitation. Timely, consistent follow-up is one of the greatest challenges to hearing screening programs. In the year 2000, approximately 50% of children who were referred for a follow-up examination failed to return for one.[7] A combination of administrative error and lack of parental education appear to be to blame. Inadequate data systems, inconsistent reporting requirements, and lack of communication among medical professionals have all been cited as reasons for the poor follow-up rate.[12] In a 2004 study of medical care after school hearing screening, one of the most common barriers to follow-up was that 33% of parents surveyed did not suspect a hearing problem or doubted the screening test accuracy, or both.[28] The importance of parental education cannot be overemphasized. A study conducted by Wittman-Price and Pope in 2002 found that although 97% of parents rated UNHS programs as *very important* on a survey and left the hospital with a scheduled follow-up appointment, only 77%

returned their infant for follow-up testing.[12] However, in an intervention group which received a 20-minute educational session on UNHS programs at a prenatal class and received educational literature, 100% of parents of referred infants returned for follow-up testing.[12] Consistent, coordinated medical reporting and management combined with parental education are critical to the success of UNHS and early hearing detection and intervention programs. The AAP developed a checklist and flow chart to assist in the tracking of patients by their medical team (Figure 39-2; see also Figure 39-1).[29] Simple systems such as these are an asset to primary care physicians and other members of the team.

The initial follow-up evaluation for an infant or child who fails a hearing screen or who is at risk for acquired or progressive hearing loss must include a comprehensive audiologic evaluation by a licensed audiologist, the purpose of which is to assess the integrity of the auditory system, to estimate hearing sensitivity, and to identify all intervention options.[7] At least one ABR test is also recommended as part of the complete diagnostic assessment of children younger than age 3 years before a permanent hearing loss can be confirmed. Once a hearing loss or the presence of middle-ear dysfunction has been confirmed by the audiologist, the child should be referred for otologic and medical consultation to determine the cause of the hearing loss, to identify related physical conditions, and to provide recommendations for medical treatment, if appropriate, as well as referrals for other services.[7] Approximately 40% of children with hearing

Universal Newborn Hearing Screening, Diagnosis, and Intervention

Patient Checklist for Pediatric Medical Home Providers

Patient Name: ______________________

Date of Birth: ____/____/____

Birth	**Hospital-Based Inpatient Screening Results (OAE/AABR)** (also home births) **Left ear:** o Missed o Incomplete o Refer[a,c] o Pass **Right ear:** o Missed o Incomplete o Refer[a,c] o Pass	Date: ___/___/___
Before 1 month	**Outpatient Screening Results (OAE/AABR)** **Left ear:** o Incomplete o Refer[a,c] o Pass **Right ear:** o Incomplete o Refer[a,c] o Pass	Date: ___/___/___
Before 3 months	o **Pediatric Audiologic Evaluation**[b] o Hearing loss o Normal hearing	Date: ___/___/___
	Documented Child and Family Auditory History	Date: ___/___/___
	o **Report to State EHDI Program** (results of diagnostic evaluation)	Date: ___/___/___
	o **Refer to Early Intervention** (IDEA, Part C)	Date: ___/___/___
	o **Medical and Otologic Evaluations** (to recommend treatment and provide clearance for hearing aid fitting)	Date: ___/___/___
	o **Pediatric Audiologic** (hearing aid fitting and monitoring)	Date: ___/___/___
	o **Advise family** (about assistive listening devices [hearing aids, cochlear implants] and communication options)	Date: ___/___/___
Before 6 months	o **Enrollment in Early Intervention (IDEA, Part C)** (transition to Part B at 3 years of age)	Date: ___/___/___
	Medical Evaluations (to determine etiology and identify related conditions)	
	o Ophthalmologic (annually)	Date: ___/___/___
	o Genetic	Date: ___/___/___
	o Development pediatrics, neurology, cardiology, and nephrology (as needed)	Date: ___/___/___
	o **Ongoing Pediatric Audiologic Services**	

Ongoing Care of All Infants[d]

- o Provide parents with information about hearing, speech, and language milestones.
- o Identify and aggressively treat middle ear disease.
- o Conduct vision screening and provide referral as needed.
- o Provide ongoing developmental surveillance and referral.
- o Provide referrals to otolaryngology and genetics as needed.
- o Identify risk indicators for late-onset hearing loss:

____

(Refer for audiologic monitoring.)

Service Provider Contact Information

Pediatric Audiologist:
Early Intervention Provider:
Other:
Other:
Other:

[a]In screening programs that do not provide Outpatient Screening infants will be referred directly from inpatient screening to pediatric audiologic evaluation. Similarly, infants at high risk for hearing loss or loss to follow-up may also be referred directly to pediatric audiologic evaluation.
[b]Early intervention (IDEA, Part C) may provide diagnostic audiologic evaluation services as part of Child Find activities.
[c]Infants who fail the screening in one or both ears should be referred for further screening or pediatric audiologic evaluation.
[d]Includes infants whose parents refused initial or follow-up hearing screening.

OAE, Otoacoustic emissions; *AABR*, automated auditory brainstem response; *ABR*, auditory brainstem response; *IDEA*, Individuals with Disabilities Education Act; *EHDI*, early hearing detection and intervention.

This project is funded by an educational grant from the Maternal and Child Health Bureau, Health Resources and Services Administration, US Department of Health and Human Services.

March 2004

Figure 39-2 Universal Newborn Hearing Screening, Diagnosis, and Intervention—Patient Checklist for Pediatric Medical Home Providers. *(Adapted from American Academy of Pediatrics. The National Center of Medical Home Initiatives for Children with Special Needs. Available at: www.medicalhomeinfo.org/screening/EHDI/EHDI%20info%20for%20providers/Checklistbw.pdf. Accessed August 3, 2007.)*

loss have other disabilities. These evaluations should typically include the following elements:

1. Complete patient and family history to identify risk factors for hearing loss
2. Physical examination, and possibly laboratory and radiologic tests, to identify malformations or abnormalities of anatomic structures
3. Monitoring of developmental milestones
4. Referral for genetic evaluation and counseling by medical geneticist
5. Referral to an ophthalmologist to test for visual acuity[7]
6. Other specialty referrals, such as a speech and language evaluation, may also be suggested once etiology and developmental concerns have been identified[7]

After these comprehensive evaluations, audiologic intervention is usually recommended. Many treatment options are available, depending on the type and degree of the child's hearing loss. Kemper et al noted that specific treatment was recommended for 51% of children who had follow-up appointments after a failed school screening.[28] This number is even higher for those identified after UNHS evaluation. For children with conductive hearing loss, medical and surgical options are often available. In the case of a child with atresia or a similar anatomic condition that precludes medical or surgical treatment, the fitting of a bone-conduction or bone-anchored hearing aid by an audiologist is typically the treatment of choice. Amplification or the use of assistive listening devices are typically recommended for children with sensorineural hearing loss. Children as young as 4 weeks of age may be fit with hearing aids if appropriate physiological test results have been obtained. Once diagnosed with a permanent hearing loss, children should be fit with hearing aids within 1 month.[7] Cochlear implantation is often considered for a child with severe to profound hearing loss (Box 39-4 summarizes the criteria).[30] The US Food and Drug Administration currently approved cochlear implantation in children as young as 12 months. Children with auditory neuropathy also benefit from treatment; however, at the time of publication, conclusive evidence regarding the most effective treatment for this population does not exist. Audiologic management should be supervised by a licensed audiologist. For all of these children, speech and language assessment and therapy is essential to development and to the attainment of the goal of intelligible speech by the time the child enters kindergarten.[31]

Financial concerns should not limit a child's access to intervention services for hearing loss. The Individuals with Disabilities Education Act (IDEA) ensures that children who have hearing loss receive appropriate, family-centered, multidisciplinary intervention services at no charge to the family from birth through the school years.[32] In addition, a variety of options are available to cover the cost of amplification for a child with permanent hearing loss, including private insurance, Medicaid, and the early intervention services provided by IDEA.[32] Specifics vary by state; however, assisting patients in familiarizing themselves with the options they have available is worthwhile. (State-specific information is available at www.infanthearing.org.)

BOX 39-4 Candidacy Criteria for Cochlear Implantation*

12 TO 24 MONTHS

- Profound sensorineural hearing loss (SNHL) in both ears
- Lack of progress in development of auditory skills with appropriate binaural hearing aids
- High motivation and realistic expectations from the family
- Other medical conditions, if present, do not interfere with cochlear implant procedure

25 MONTHS TO 17 YEARS 11 MONTHS

- Severe-to-profound SNHL in both ears
- Receives little or no benefit from hearing aids (speech scores of 30% or less in best-aided condition)
- Lack of progress in development of auditory skills
- High motivation and realistic expectations from family
- No medical contraindications

*Data based on recommendations for Cochlear Freedom™ system.
From Cochlear Americas. Candidacy Criteria. Available at: www.cochlearamericas.com/americas/378.asp. Accessed August 3, 2007, with permission.

ROLE OF THE PRIMARY CARE PHYSICIAN

According to the JCIH, the AAP, and the NIH, all infants, regardless of newborn hearing screening outcome, should receive ongoing monitoring for the development of age-appropriate auditory behaviors and communication skills. Any infant who demonstrates an auditory or communicative delay should undergo comprehensive audiologic evaluation by a licensed audiologist.[7] Additionally, any child who is at risk for hearing loss should undergo a complete audiologic evaluation at least once by 24 to 30 months of age. Being coordinator, caretaker, and advocate for the patient is the responsibility of the primary care physician. Additionally, because 30% to 40% of children with confirmed hearing loss will demonstrate developmental delays or other disabilities, the pediatrician should monitor developmental milestones and initiate referrals related to suspected disabilities.[7] The pediatrician should strive for consistent medical management of all patients with hearing loss. Most importantly, the primary care physician should be a part of a medical team who, in collaboration with parents, the audiologist, and other health professionals, provides accessible, family-centered, continuous, comprehensive, coordinated, compassionate, and culturally appropriate health care.[1,7]

CONCLUSION

Hearing is crucial for the development of speech and language skills in children, and the presence of hearing loss has a negative impact on social, emotional, and educational development. For this reason, hearing screening is a critical component of medical care for infants and children. Efficient screening methods combined with appropriate and timely follow-up and intervention are necessary to achieve the goal of testing by 1 month of age, identifying hearing loss by 3 months of age, and intervening by 6 months of age, which is important to provide optimal access to sounds during the most critical periods of development. The implementation of UNHS programs has decreased the average age of identification dramatically. However, taking the lead in the management and coordination of their patients' care is the responsibility of pediatricians and primary care physicians. Routinely referring children who fail their hearing screenings to a licensed audiologist for appropriate follow-up and management of their hearing is particularly important. Without adequate tracking and follow-up, coordinated by a team approach, maximal benefit cannot be achieved.

TOOLS FOR PRACTICE

Community Advocacy and Coordination

- *50 State Summary of Newborn Hearing Screening Laws* (other), National Conference of State Legislatures (www.ncsl.org/programs/health/hear50.htm).

Engaging Patient and Family

- *Causes of Hearing Loss in Children* (fact sheet), American Speech-Language Hearing Association (www.asha.org/public/hearing/disorders/causes.htm?print=1).
- *Children and Hearing Aids* (fact sheet), American Speech-Language Hearing Association (www.asha.org/public/hearing/treatment/child_aids.html).
- *Just in Time So Your Baby's Care Is Right on Time: Early Hearing Detection and Intervention* (other), Centers for Disease Control and Prevention (www.cdc.gov/ncbddd/ehdi/documents/justintime/136poster.pdf).
- *Newborn Hearing Screening and Your Baby* (brochure), American Academy of Pediatrics (www.aap.org/bst).

Medical Decision and Support

- *Bright Futures: Guidelines for Health Supervision of Infants, Children, and Adolescents* (book), Bright Futures (brightfutures.aap.org/web/).
- *PediaLink–Childhood Hearing* (interactive tool), American Academy of Pediatrics (www.pedialink.org/cme/_coursefinder/CMEdetail.cfm?aid=22410&area=liveCME).
- *The "State" of Early Hearing Detection and Intervention in the United States* (other), National Center for Hearing Assessment and Management, Utah State University (www.infanthearing.org/states/index.html).
- *Universal Newborn Hearing Screening: Current Testing Techniques* Gorga M, Eiten L, Boys Town National Research Hospital (www.infanthearing.org/physicianeducation/UNHSFactSheet_Boystown.pdf).
- *Universal Newborn Hearing, Screening, Diagnosis, and Intervention: Patient Checklist for Pediatric Medical Home Providers* (checklist), American Academy of Pediatrics and National Center for Hearing Assessment and Management, Utah State University (www.medicalhomeinfo.org/screening/EHDI/EHDI%20info%20for%20providers/Checklistbw.pdf).
- *Universal Newborn Hearing, Screening, Diagnosis, and Intervention: Guidelines for Pediatric Medical Home Providers* (guideline), American Academy of Pediatrics (www.medicalhomeinfo.org/screening/Screen%20Materials/Algorithm.pdf).

AAP POLICY STATEMENTS

American Academy of Pediatrics, Committee on Environmental Health. Noise: a hazard for the fetus and newborn. *Pediatrics*. 1997;100:724-727. (aappolicy.aappublications.org/cgi/content/full/pediatrics;100/4/724).

American Academy of Pediatrics, Cunningham M, Cox EO, Committee on Practice and Ambulatory Medicine, Section on Otolaryngology and Bronchoesophagology. Hearing assessment in infants and children: recommendations beyond neonatal screening. *Pediatrics*. 2003;111:436-440. (aappolicy.aappublications.org/cgi/content/full/pediatrics;111/2/436).

American Academy of Pediatrics, Task Force on Newborn and Infant Hearing. Newborn and infant hearing loss: detection and intervention. *Pediatrics*. 1999;103:527-530. (aappolicy.aappublications.org/cgi/content/full/pediatrics;103/2/527).

Joint Committee on Infant Hearing, American Academy of Audiology, American Academy of Pediatrics, American Speech-Language-Hearing Association, Directors of Speech and Hearing Programs in State Health and Welfare Agencies. Year 2000 position statement: principles and guidelines for early hearing detection and intervention programs. *Pediatrics*. 2000;106:798-817. (aappolicy.aappublications.org/cgi/content/full/pediatrics;106/4/798).

SUGGESTED RESOURCES

American Academy of Pediatrics. *Bright Futures: Guidelines for Health Supervision of Infants, Children, and Adolescents*. 3rd ed. Elk Grove Village, IL: American Academy of Pediatrics; 2004.

Brookhouser P, Worthington D, Kelly W. Fluctuating and/or progressive sensorineural hearing loss in children. *Laryngoscope*. 1994;104:958-964.

Joint Committee on Infant Hearing. Year 2007 position statement: principles and guidelines for early hearing detection and intervention programs. *Pediatrics*. 2007; in press.

Nance WE. The genetics of deafness. *Mental Retard Dev Disabil Res Rev*. 2003;9:109-119.

RELATED WEB SITES

- Centers for Disease Control and Prevention, Early Hearing Detection and Intervention Program (Web page), Centers for Disease Control and Prevention Early Hearing Detection and Intervention Program (www.cdc.gov/ncbddd/ehdi/).
- National Center for Hearing Assessment and Management Utah State University (Web page), National Center for Hearing Assessment and Management (NCHAM), Utah State University (www.infanthearing.org/index.html).
- National Center of Medical Home Initiatives for Children with Special Needs: Newborn and Infant Hearing

Screening Activities (Web page), American Academy of Pediatrics (www.medicalhomeinfo.org/screening/hearing.html).

- National Institute on Deafness and Other Communication Disorders (Web page), National Institute on Deafness and Other Communication Disorders (www.nidcd.nih.gov/health).

REFERENCES

1. Campbell D. The role of the primary-care provider in the hearing health of children. *Hear J*. 2000;53(11):40-44.
2. Connolly JL, Carron JD, Roark SD. Universal newborn hearing screening: are we achieving the Joint Committee on Infant Hearing (JCIH) objectives? *Laryngoscope*. 2005;115(2):232-236.
3. Cunningham M, Cox EO, and the Committee on Practice and Ambulatory Medicine, the Section on Otolaryngology and Bronchoesophagology. Hearing assessment in infants and children: recommendations beyond neonatal screening. *Pediatrics*. 2003;111(2):436-440.
4. Krueger WW, Ferguson L. A comparison of screening methods in school-aged children. *Otolaryngol Head Neck Surg*. 2002;127(6):516-519.
5. Bess FH, Dodd-Murphy J, Parker RA. Children with minimal sensorineural hearing loss: prevalence, educational performance, and functional status. *Ear Hear*. 1998;19(5): 339-354.
6. Yoshinaga-Itano C, Gravel JS. The evidence for universal newborn hearing screening. *Am J Audiol*. 2001;10(2): 62-64.
7. American Academy of Pediatrics: Joint Committee on Infant Hearing. Year 2007 position statement: principles and guidelines for early hearing detection and intervention programs. *Pediatrics*. 2007;120:898-921.
8. Moeller MP. Early intervention and language development in children who are deaf and hard of hearing. *Pediatrics*. 2000;106(3):43-52.
9. Yoshinaga-Itano C, Sedey AL, Coulter DK, et al. Language of early- and later-identified children with hearing loss. *Pediatrics*. 1998;102(5):1161-1171.
10. American Speech-Language-Hearing Association, Audiologic Assessment Panel. *Guidelines for Audiologic Screening*. Rockville, MD: American Speech-Language-Hearing Association; 1997.
11. National Conference of State Legislatures. 50 State Summary of Newborn Hearing Screening Laws. Available at: www.ncsl.org/programs/health/hear50.htm. Accessed August 3, 2007.
12. Baroch KA. Universal newborn hearing screening: fine-tuning the process. *Curr Opin Otolaryngol Head Neck Surg*. 2003;11(6):424-427.
13. Keren R, Helfand M, Homer C, et al. Projected cost-effectiveness of statewide universal newborn hearing screening. *Pediatrics*. 2002;110(5):855-864.
14. Downs MP. The quest for early identification and intervention. *Semin Hear*. 2000;21(4):285-294.
15. Erenberg A, Lemons J, Sia C, and the Task Force on Newborn and Infant Hearing. Newborn and infant hearing loss: detection and intervention. *Pediatrics*. 1999; 103(2):527-530.
16. National Institutes of Health. Early identification of hearing impairment in infants and young children. *NIH Consens Statement*. 1993;11(1):1-24.
17. Hall JW, Smith SD, Popelka GR. Newborn hearing screening with combined otoacoustic emissions and auditory brainstem responses. *J Am Acad Audiol*. 2004;15(6):414-425.
18. Northern JL, Hayes D. Universal screening for infant hearing impairment: necessary, beneficial and justifiable. *Audiology Today*. 1994;6(3):10-13.
19. National Center for Hearing Assessment and Management, Utah State University. Available at: www.infanthearing.org/. Accessed on August 3, 2007.
20. Centers for Disease Control and Prevention. Early Hearing Detection & Intervention (EHDI) Program. Available at: www.cdc.gov/ncbddd/ehdi/. Accessed on August 3, 2007.
21. National Institute on Deafness and Other Communication Disorders. Health Information. Available at: www.nidcd.nih.gov/health/. Accessed on August 3, 2007.
22. Hall JW. *Handbook of Otoacoustic Emissions*. San Diego, CA: Singular Thomson Learning; 2000.
23. Hood LJ. *Clinical Application of the Auditory Brainstem Response*. San Diego, CA: Singular; 1998.
24. Prieve BA. What newborn screening doesn't tell us. *Hear J*. 2000; 53(11): 36-39.
25. American Speech-Language-Hearing Association. Causes of Hearing Loss in Children. Available at: www.asha.org/public/hearing/disorders/causes.htm?print=1. Accessed August 3, 2007.
26. Northern JL, Downs MP. *Hearing in Children*. 4th ed. Baltimore, MD: Williams & Wilkins; 1991.
27. Niskar AS, Kieszak SM, Holmes A, et al. Prevalence of hearing loss among children 6 to 19 years of age: the Third National Health and Nutrition Examination Survey. *JAMA*. 1998;279:1071-1075.
28. Kemper AR, Fant KE, Bruckman D, et al. Hearing and vision screening program for school-aged children. *Am J Prev Med*. 2004;26:141-146.
29. American Academy of Pediatrics. The National Center of Medical Home Initiatives for Children with Special Needs. Newborn and Infant Hearing Screening Activities. Available at: www.medicalhomeinfo.org/screening/hearing.html. Accessed August 3, 2007.
30. Cochlear Americas. Candidacy Criteria. Available at: www.cochlearamericas.com/americas/378.asp. Accessed August 3, 2007.
31. Yoshinaga-Itano C. Early identification: an opportunity and challenge for Audiology. *Semin Hear*. 1999;20(4): 317-331.
32. American Speech-Language-Hearing Association. Children and Hearing Aids. Available at: www.asha.org/public/hearing/treatment/child_aids.html. Accessed August 3, 2007.

Chapter 40

CARDIOVASCULAR SCREENING

Michelle A. Grenier, MD

Congenital and acquired heart diseases are among the most common of pediatric chronic disorders. Because of the severe consequences of undetected disease, screening may be indicated in some situations. This chapter reviews the types of conditions and the indications and methods for screening for cardiovascular disease.

BURDEN OF DISEASE

Pediatric heart diseases are a heterogeneous group of conditions. Individually, they are not common, but as a group, pediatric heart diseases are frequent enough to raise questions about the need for universal screening. Congenital structural lesions occur in 0.8% to 1% of all births.[1,2] Detection and, more importantly, treatment have improved for these conditions, making early detection essential. Interest has been growing in screening for lesions that are associated with sudden death. Improved screening strategies suggest that the incidence of cardiomyopathies may be higher than expected, with 1.13 new cases per 100,000 births,[3] with hypertrophic cardiomyopathy (HCM) remaining the most common cause of sudden cardiac death in healthy, often athletic adolescents.[4] Rhythm disturbances of concern are long QT syndrome (LQTS), an inherited disorder of cardiac ion channels, and the more recently described Brugada syndrome. Both syndromes predispose affected individuals to sudden death from ventricular tachycardia. The cost of sudden and unexpected death in a seemingly healthy young individual is well known. In addition to the myopathies or arrhythmias, some conditions include aspects of both rhythm abnormalities and cardiomyopathy. One such condition is arrhythmogenic right-ventricular cardiomyopathy (ARVC). Among cases of sudden death in North America, ARVC accounts for 5%.[5] A mandated preparticipation screening of Italian athletes in a national program may have reduced the incidence of sudden cardiac death in athletes in Italy.[6]

In addition to these congenital causes of heart disease, acquired conditions can also be severe and lead to sudden death or heart failure. Acquired conditions may be infectious (myocarditis, vasculitis, pericarditis, endocarditis), toxic (Adriamycin, thalassemias, medications), or vascular (atherosclerosis) in origin.

The incidence of sudden cardiac death from all of these cardiac diseases is approximately one death in 200,000 high school athletes participating in competitive sports per year or one in 70,000 over a 3-year period. At least as important as these numbers is the devastating effect on the public when a young person in the prime of life dies unexpectedly. In addition, an even larger number of youth with these conditions will be disabled by heart failure.

SCREENING FOR HEART DISEASE

The devastating consequences, hidden nature of the disease, relatively common occurrence of the different cardiovascular conditions, and often prolonged asymptomatic periods have led numerous authors to recommend widescale screening for cardiovascular disease in childhood. Unfortunately, to identify the many types of cardiac conditions, echocardiograms and electrocardiograms (ECGs) would be necessary for all children and adolescents. The costs of such a dragnet approach would be prohibitive. Moreover, a large number of false positives might be generated by the ECGs. Thus comprehensive assessments such as these are probably not indicated.

Although echocardiograms and ECGs are not indicated for the entire population, clinicians should maintain a high level of alert for these potential killers by conducting a thorough history, physical examination, and laboratory evaluation. The necessary screening tools are readily available to all practitioners (Box 40-1). Most of the tools should be readily available to all practitioners in all settings and should provide sufficient clues to heart disease to prompt referrals to a pediatric heart specialist.

These tools and a high index of suspicion will be useful in identifying some cases of occult cardiovascular disease in children and adolescents. However, some subpopulations may be particularly vulnerable or require additional consideration. Therefore the evidence

BOX 40-1 Office Tools for Evaluating Cardiovascular Health in Children

- Positive communication skills that help forge a relationship with families
- Growth curves and documentation of normal developmental milestones
- Accurate scales and a stadiometer for height (or a tape measure)
- Tape measure for head circumference and *wing span*
- Accurate blood pressure cuffs with a range of appropriate size cuffs. An oscillometric cuff is easier to use on infants and small children than it is on older children and adolescents. However, aneroid cuffs are portable and may by more reliable, particularly in older children who may be hypertensive.
- A reliable pulse oximeter or the ability to identify cyanosis readily
- A calculator to calculate BMI, as well as the Centers for Disease Control and Prevention guidelines for the normal range of BMI by gender and age. If these figures are not readily available to the practitioner, then the formula for calculating BMI is weight (in kilograms) divided by height (in meters) squared.[a] Printed tables may be obtained from the Centers for Disease Control and Prevention.
- Clinical examination by observation, palpation, and auscultation
- Access to radiographs, electrocardiography, and echocardiography
- Blood biomarkers. When combined with the total clinical picture, biomarkers may be useful in distinguishing heart diseases from other causes of distress.[b] These tools may not be available to the primary care physician, and the interpretation of results may require discussion with the subspecialist who uses these tests with greater frequency.
- In some tertiary care centers, thorough clinical screening may allow the identification of the affected individual and genotype; genetic testing of individual family members may follow.

[a]Discher CL, Klein D, Pierce L, et al. Heart failure disease and management: impact on hospital care, length of stay, and reimursement. *Congest Heart Fail.* 2003;9:77-83.

[b]Vasan RS, Benjamin EJ, Larson MG, et al. Plasma natriuretic peptides for community screening for left ventricular hypertrophy and systolic dysfunction: the Framingham Heart Study. *JAMA.* 2002;288:1252-1259.

around fetal screening, infant screening, hypertension screening, and screening of young athletes is reviewed here.

Fetal Screening

A fetal diagnosis of complex congenital heart disease may prompt delivery at a tertiary care center. However, the cost/benefit ratio is unknown. Advance knowledge of an infant's cardiac defect may allow the family more time to process the disease emotionally, but the emotional effect of this advance knowledge is difficult to assess.

Indications for fetal echocardiogram include:

- Obvious structural abnormality visualized on routine fetal sonogram
- Perceived rhythm abnormality
- Sibling with congenital heart defect or cardiomyopathy
- Known fetal chromosomal abnormality
- Family history of syndromes or heart disease
- Maternal lupus or phospholipid antibodies
- Maternal diabetes
- Maternal exposure to infectious diseases
- Multiple spontaneous abortions
- Known teratogens and toxins[7]

Neonatal and Infant Screening

Most neonates have not been screened by fetal echocardiography because screening all fetuses is presently not cost effective. Current screening efforts rely on standard pediatric tools (see Box 40-1) in making the diagnosis of significant heart disease in neonates with appropriate referral to the pediatric heart specialist.

Pediatricians screen most infants in the immediate newborn period, in the first 2 weeks and again at 2 months of life. Detecting lesions that are dependent on the ductus arteriosus, such as critical coarctation, pulmonary atresia, and hypoplastic and left heart syndrome, among others, is critical early postnatally because the consequences of ductal closure in this cohort are devastating. The presentation is often nonspecific. Coarctation may occur surreptitiously with a cranky infant who is mildly tachypneic and diaphoretic. Frequently, these infants appear septic. Other ductal-dependent lesions lend themselves to cyanosis, which may be readily apparent, although less so in the darker-skinned infant and anemic infant. The 2-month screening (see next section) is particularly important in detecting left-to-right shunts because the patient's pulmonary vascular resistance drops maximally at that point.

A detailed family history may provide important clues. In a busy pediatric practice, asking all of these questions may not be feasible. The medical and family history process may be facilitated by using a written intake questionnaire, which may be mailed to the individual or given at the initial visit. Allowing the individual family member privacy and some time to think may produce a more thorough family and medical history. This approach is a relatively inexpensive and useful tool for screening. Screening questions include the following:

1. Was the pregnancy normal?
2. Does anyone in the family have known heart disease that began before the person turned 50 years of age?
3. Did anyone require cardiac intervention or subacute bacterial endocarditis prophylaxis for a heart murmur?
4. Does the family have any history of sudden infant death?
5. Did anyone die abruptly under the age of 50 years? (The screen should ask whether automobile accidents or swimming deaths had occurred, considering that these may give clues that a family history of LQTS or Brugada syndrome exists.)
6. Was anyone in the family born deaf? (An association exists with the Jervell and Lange-Nielsen form of LQTS and abnormalities of ion flux the organ of Corti.)
7. Does anyone in family have seizures? (Seizures are possibly caused by ventricular tachycardia.)
8. Does anyone have known potassium abnormalities? (Postassium abnormalities are also associated with LQTS.)
9. Do any family members have known developmental delays, physical handicaps, or syndromes?
10. Does anyone have diabetes?
11. Does anyone have thyroid disease, lupus, rheumatoid arthritis? (May have associations with pericarditis, cardiomyopathies, and atrioventricular block.)
12. Does anyone have an enlarged heart? (Indicates cardiomyopathy.)
13. Does anyone have a pacemaker or take antiarrhythmic drugs?
14. Are any people in the family tall? (May indicate connective tissue disease.)
15. Did anyone in the family die of an aneurysm? (Indicates connective tissue disease and familial aortic aneurysm.)
16. Is anyone in your family overweight?
17. Has anyone in the family had kidney disease or a kidney transplant? (Applicable when screening for systemic hypertension.)

Screening Infants Using the Medical History and Review of Systems

During the initial encounter with a new patient, a cardiovascular screening should thoroughly probe the medical history and review of systems. A poor Apgar score, tachypnea, or cyanosis at birth, although nonspecific, are signs of a possible cardiac lesion.

In the review of systems, any indications of poor or lengthy feeding, tachypnea, dyspnea, or diaphoresis with feeding can be indications that cardiac disease and congestive heart failure (CHF) are present.

Although reflux is common in infants, persistent reflux with sweating and pallor or cyanosis may be an indication that a heart lesion is present with associated CHF caused by diminished gut perfusion, hepatosplenomegaly, or both.

A cranky, colicky infant who is also pale, tachypneic, or is not growing well may have CHF or intermittent arrhythmia.

Frequent upper respiratory symptoms such as dyspnea, tachypnea, and wheezing are often an indication of pulmonary edema caused by CHF or congenital heart disease associated with immune deficiency.

The clinician should ask how well the patient sleeps; an infant with heart failure or arrhythmia may sleep restlessly.

Screening Infants Using the Physical Examination

Vital signs are crucial. If the numbers are outside the normal range, then assessment should be repeated in the examining room. If an infant appears cyanotic or dusky, then a pulse oximetry reading is indicated.

The physical examination must include palpation of upper and lower extremity pulses, including femoral pulses, to assess for coarctation. Although previously thought to be useful in identifying infants with coarctation, four-extremity blood pressures are less sensitive and specific than previously thought.[8] Assessing for blood pressure elevation in the upper extremity then comparing upper and lower extremity pulses simultaneously during the physical examination may increase accuracy. Despite this approach, and because coarctation is the most frequently missed cardiac lesion, having four-extremity blood pressure performed at least once on all infants is still good practice.

A horizontal or negative growth curve may indicate failure to thrive, which is frequently associated with CHF. The clinician should remember that infants and children with cyanotic and valvular heart disease may continue to grow along a normal curve, if not severely compromised by their defects.

The physical examination of infants with heart disease should include the following areas.

HEAD, EARS, EYES, NOSE, AND THROAT. Any jugular venous distention, brisk carotid upstroke, or cranial bruit should be cause for a referral to a pediatric cardiologist. Neck webbing prompts suspicion of Noonan or Turner syndrome. A bifid uvula prompts thoughts of Loeys-Dietz syndrome with predilection toward bicommissural aortic valves, aortic root dilatation and, ultimately, dissection.

CHEST. A precordial bulge is quite concerning for cardiomegaly. Pectus excavatum and carinatum may signal the presence of a connective tissue disorder such as Marfan syndrome.

LUNGS. Persistent, recalcitrant wheezing and frequent respiratory symptoms are suspect for pulmonary edema.

CARDIAC SYSTEM. Many children have innocent murmurs, which are soft or musical and systolic in nature; some of these murmurs are even continuous and extinguish on having the child lie supine. Murmurs, which are present in diastole or continuously, require referral, as do harsh and loud, persistent systolic murmurs, clicks, snaps, rubs, and 3rd and 4th heart sound gallop rhythms.

ABDOMEN. Organomegaly is suspect for CHF and storage diseases, which are associated with cardiomyopathy.

EXTREMITIES. Clubbing is a sequela of cyanotic disease. Arachnodactyly causes suspicion of Marfan syndrome. Polydactyly, clinodactyly, absent radii lend suspicion of genetic syndromes.

Appearance as a Screening Tool

The following questions about appearance should be asked:

- Is the child dysmorphic?
- Does the child have similarities in appearance to mom or dad?

The clinician should not use this *look alike* phenomenon to exclude syndromes. Parents may not realize they have a syndrome if they have never been diagnosed. A parent with bad acne may in fact have tuberous sclerosis.

If the child is dysmorphic, and if a syndrome is suspected, then the clinician should consider heart disease as an associated issue. A very strong association exists between structural heart abnormalities or cardiomyopathies and syndromes or chromosomal abnormalities.

Screening With Noninvasive Tools

Most screening tools for heart disease that do not involve direct imaging provide supportive rather than definitive evidence of heart disease. The key is to have a high index of suspicion for possible heart disease when interpreting noninvasive tests, even if performed for noncardiac disease.

CHEST RADIOGRAPH. The chest radiograph may be useful if a clinical suspicion of cardiopulmonary disease exists. It allows assessment of visceral situs, pulmonary blood flow patterns, and the shape and size of the cardiac silhouette. Although some cardiologists have abandoned the chest radiograph, preferring the echocardiogram, indicators of heart disease should not be missed on radiography even if it is being performed for noncardiac indications. Dextrocardia or situs inversus indicates some form of cardiac disease, as do increased cardiopulmonary blood flow and cardiomegaly. Cardiomegaly may be caused by volume or pressure overload lesions, cardiomyopathies or myocarditis, Ebstein anomaly, and pericardial effusions.

The side of the aortic arch may be inferred. A right-sided aortic arch is seen in 10% of the population but is more common with conotruncal defects such as tetralogy of Fallot. A right-sided arch may also be seen in persons with a double aortic arch, which produces a vascular ring. The thymic sail should be obvious in newborns and neonates. Its absence should cause the pediatric physician to consider thoughts of DiGeorge syndrome and conotruncal defects. The pulmonary blood flow pattern is important because Kerly B lines may confirm the suspicion of pulmonary edema consistent with shunt lesions or cardiomyopathy or myocarditis. Chronic lesions may produce hyperinflation and flattened diaphragms, indicating cardiac asthma.

BARIUM ESOPHAGOGRAM. The barium esophagram (barium swallow) is still readily accessible, does not require sedation, and remains a great screening tool for vascular rings and slings. It is less expensive than magnetic resonance imaging, the interpretation of which is most crucial. Indentation of the esophagus indicates abnormal vasculature, which requires further investigation by a pediatric cardiologist. This test is indicated in stridorous infants, in those with reflux, and in any infant in whom the suspicion of right-sided aortic arch is raised. However, direct imaging techniques are required to make a definitive diagnosis.

ELECTROCARDIOGRAM. The ECG is a relatively insensitive, nonspecific screening tool for structural heart defects but is an important screening tool for rhythm disturbances. It is inexpensive, readily accessible, and provides baseline information regarding heart lesions.[9]

Use of the ECG as a routine screening tool in newborns (to identify cardiac abnormalities that may predispose the child to sudden infant death syndrome)[10] and in athletes as part of preparticipation screening in competitive sports is not universally established but has been adopted in some parts of Europe.

In newborns suspected of having heart disease, particular attention must be paid to the QRS axis and the T wave morphology. A superior axis may suggest the presence of major cardiac defects such as atrioventricular septal defect, tricuspid atresia, or some forms of double-outlet right ventricle. The persistence of an upright T wave in V1 beyond the first week of life usually indicates significant right-ventricular hypertrophy in the context of cardiac or pulmonary disease. If the heart rhythm is not sinus, then heart disease should be considered. Additionally, if degrees of atrioventricular block are found, then maternal systemic lupus must be considered.

Greatly elevated (sinus) heart rates may be present in patients with CHF. Extremely low heart rates (not sinus) may be consistent with atrioventricular block.

The configuration of the P waves and QRS complexes is important. Ventricular preexcitation patterns, such as those seen with Wolf-Parkinson-White (WPW) syndrome may be present within families but may also be an indication of Ebstein anomaly. WPW syndrome is also seen with left-ventricular noncompaction-type cardiomyopathy (LVNC).

The diagnosis of Brugada syndrome depends on the appropriate analysis of the QRS complex, including ST segment elevation in the right precordial leads.

An rSR′ pattern may be a normal variant, evidence of right-ventricular hypertrophy or the initial sign of an atrial septal defect. More pronounced right bundle branch block patterns, which are not surgically induced, may be present in some of the mitochondrial dystrophies (Kearns-Sayre syndrome), arrhythmogenic right-ventricular dysplasia (ARVD), Beckwith-Weideman syndrome, and some septal defects but may also be present in familial right bundle branch block, which is generally benign.

Ventricular hypertrophy as indicated by ECG has long been a signal that an echocardiogram is necessary. Although right- and left-ventricular hypertrophy may be signs of cardiomyopathy, shunt, or pressure overload lesions, voltage is not uniformly accurate in predicting disease.[11] If increased voltage is combined with a strain pattern, then cardiac disease is likely. In fact, certain ECGs are considered pathognomonic for disease, for example, the massively increased voltage, strain pattern, and shortened PR interval seen with Pompe disease. Many patients who are severely affected with LVNC exhibit a similar pattern of severe ventricular hypertrophy by ECG, which is pathognomonic for this disease, and of strain, with or without evidence of preexcitation. QT interval will be further discussed in the screening for arrhythmia section.

SERUM MARKERS OF HEART DISEASE. Although cardiac enzymes and B-type natriuretic peptide (BNP) levels are routinely used in screening a symptomatic adult for cardiac ischemia or heart failure, their use as screening tools is not established for diagnosing heart disease in children. Instead, they serve as secondary tools that aid in defining the severity of the disease.

Troponin I and troponin T are components of the cardiomyocyte that may be released during myocyte degradation. These markers have been useful in identifying adults with ischemic heart disease. The use of troponin analysis in children is less clear. However, when attempting to distinguish between dilated cardiomyopathy and myocarditis, the active release of troponins may be more consistent with acute myocarditis than chronic dilated cardiomyopathy.

BNP is released from the ventricle during times of cardiac stress and appears to correlate well with heart failure in adults and children. A linear correlation of BNP appears to exist with degree of heart failure.[12] Additionally, the specific level of BNP may be predictive of adverse cardiac events in children.[13]

Other biomarkers are presently being investigated as possible indications of heart disease. More conventional markers of disease, including C-reactive protein, sedimentation rate, blood chemistry, and complete blood cell counts, are nonspecific and not very useful in screening for heart disease.

ECHOCARDIOGRAM. Echocardiogram is expensive and time consuming; thus screening every newborn with this test is not cost effective. Indiscriminate performance of echocardiograms may create more anxiety than comfort among practitioners and parents. The finding of a tiny patent ductus arteriosus or patent foramen ovale on a routine echocardiogram often results in unnecessary follow-up that increases parental anxiety and drives up medical expenditure.

However, appropriate echocardiogram screening of children with heart murmurs appreciated by a thorough clinical examination performed by general pediatricians is reported to be 80% sensitive in identifying pathological heart disease. This number increases to 96% sensitivity when a pediatric cardiologist performs the examination.[14]

A screening echocardiogram may be warranted in neonates with siblings with complex congenital heart disease (although it is of low yield with a normal cardiac examination). A screening echocardiogram is warranted in any syndromic neonate, particularly when Down syndrome is suspected. If maternal exposure to toxins or potential teratogens is suspected, then a screening echocardiogram may be warranted. Some cardiologists consider echocardiogram for infants born to mothers with gestational diabetes.

If the history and physical examination are completely within normal limits, then the likelihood of pathological heart disease is low.

Screening for Cardiovascular Diseases in Children and Adolescents

In the United States, the diagnosis of structural heart disease is frequently made early in life because of the frequency of recommended pediatric visits within the first 2 years of life. Still, some occult cardiac defects and cardiomyopathies may not come to light until children grow and their physiological features change. Examples of such defects include bicuspid aortic valve, HCM, atrial septal defects, partial anomalous pulmonary veins, and coronary artery anomalies.

History

The history of present illness, family history, medical history, and review of systems is crucial. A history of multiple family members with diabetes may indicate a predisposition for acquired heart disease or metabolic or mitochondrial cardiomyopathy. If a patient is hospitalized yearly for respiratory infections (a frequent presentation of atrial septal defects, pulmonary vein anomalies, and dilated cardiomyopathies), or if the patient prefers a more sedentary lifestyle, then it may be because the patient does not have the energy to play because of an underlying heart defect. Symptoms of chest pain and palpitations are often nonspecific in growing children and adolescents but warrant evaluation for heart disease in appropriate cases. Presyncope should be thoroughly evaluated by the primary care physician. A history of syncope warrants screening for cardiovascular disease. In a child with a heart murmur, the clinician should ask if this murmur is new. The answer may help differentiate between innocent versus pathological murmurs. Coarctation of the aorta may sometimes occur beyond infancy, and physical examination should include palpation of femoral pulses and measurement of upper and lower extremity blood pressure in suspected cases.

In addition to the history, questions to ask of children and adolescents include the following:

- What grade are you in, and how are you doing in school? (Chronically ill children tend to have more difficulty concentrating on school activities.)
- Do you participate in activities outside of school? What type? (Some children do not have the energy to participate in activities.)
- How well do you sleep at night? How many pillows do you use for sleeping? Has anyone ever told you that you snore? Are you sleepy during the day? Do you nap? (These questions are useful in identifying sleep apnea, which has been linked with systemic hypertension, severe sinus bradycardia with obstruction, and cor pulmonale.)
- How often and how much do you eat? (This question may be difficult for some children and adolescents to answer; the question may be further refined by asking what the patient has had to eat today. A chronically ill child may have high caloric needs; a patient with organomegaly caused by CHF, storage disease, or both may have early satiety and abdominal pain.)

Screening for Systemic Hypertension, Obesity, and Metabolic Syndrome as Precursors to Cardiovascular Diseases

Cardiac risk factors such as systemic hypertension, obesity with or without metabolic syndrome, and obstructive sleep apnea caused by obesity are additive risk factors for future cardiac disease.[15-17] The American Academy of Pediatrics has endorsed guidelines for diagnosing systemic hypertension.[18]

BLOOD PRESSURE SCREENING. Mass screening such as those performed at high school as part of athletic examinations may produce a variety of false positives. However, they do allow referral to the primary care physician for further assessment.

A written questionnaire may be given to the patient or family member to complete while waiting to see the practitioner. In addition to the previously asked questions, the following questions might be added:

1. How and when were you diagnosed with high blood pressure?
2. Have you had any tests for your high blood pressure?
3. Have you gained or lost weight recently? How much and over what period?
4. What are your favorite foods? How often do you eat out?
5. What are your favorite drinks? How much water do you drink in a day?
6. What medicines (prescription and over the counter) are you taking?
7. Do you take any dietary supplements such as creatine, protein shakes, or MetRx? (Anabolic steroids will cause acne and blood pressure elevation.)
8. How active are you? Is your exercise limited? By what?
9. Do other people in your family have high blood pressure? Does anyone have kidney dialysis, transplants, or diabetes?
10. How do you sleep at night? Do you snore? How many pillows do you use under your head when sleeping?
11. Do you ever have trouble with palpitations, breathing difficulties, fainting, or dizziness? (If the initial blood pressure is taken in an outer room and it is elevated, then the patient should be allowed to lie down in the examining room for at least 5 minutes. Then, the blood pressure assessment is repeated. The readings are compared with those recently established by the Task Force for Systemic Hypertension in Children, using gender, height, and weight percentiles.[18] If three readings on different visits are consistently greater than the 97th percentile, then the patient should be referred to a subspecialist [either a pediatric cardiologist or nephrologist] for further assessment.)

OBESITY AND COMORBIDITIES. Childhood obesity has become increasingly prevalent. (See Chapter 299, Obesity and Metabolic Syndrome). Once an individual has been identified as obese by body mass index (BMI) the associated comorbidities should be assessed by history and physical examination. Appropriate referrals can be made to nutritionists, behavioral modification specialists, physical therapists, exercise or rehabilitative programs, pulmonology or sleep specialists, and an endocrinologist.

Electrocardiography. Although ECGs should be obtained in obese children with systemic hypertension, in those with obstructive sleep apnea, in those with hyperlipidemia, and in any obese child who is seeking exercise clearance, the presence of obesity may preclude a reliable ECG. The layer of adipose may provide voltage insulation, arbitrarily decreasing the total voltage. However, the presence of right-ventricular hypertrophy, which may be seen with cor pulmonale caused by obstructive sleep apnea, left-ventricular hypertrophy, bundle branch blocks, and ischemic changes, would all prompt further cardiologic investigation.

Echocardiography. Children with systemic hypertension and obstructive sleep apnea should have an echocardiogram. The echocardiogram is technically challenging in obese individuals, given that resolution is often poor. Although some studies have reported increased left-ventricle mass in obese individuals, obese children have not been thoroughly assessed. The lack of increased left-ventricle mass or left-ventricle hypertrophy by echocardiogram should not be a measure of comfort.

Given that obesity may first occur as an endothelial disease, the newer noninvasive imaging modalities may be in order. Possibly, carotid or intimal thickening and vascular reactivity studies might move into the realm of early identification of cardiovascular diseases in obese children and adolescents in the not-so-distant future.

Serum Markers. Individuals with obesity or systemic hypertension should have blood tests conducted, including:

- Metabolic profile (including liver function tests)
- Complete blood cell count with differential
- Thyroid function tests
- Aldosterone, uric acid testing renin (if systemic hypertension or as a baseline marker)
- Insulin level testing (likely to be elevated)
- Glycated hemoglobin test
- Glucose tolerance testing if suspicion of diabetes exists
- C-reactive protein testing as a nonspecific marker for cardiac inflammatory disease
- Fasting lipid profile
- Brain natriuretic peptide assessment. This test is often performed at baseline and serial follow-up in patients with suspected or proven cardiomyopathy; obese individuals have been documented to have lower BNP levels.[19] Therefore a false-negative result may occur.

Athletic Screening: Ruling Out Sudden Death

Genetic diseases such as HCM, Marfan syndrome, and ARVD may be suspected in individuals based on family history, medical history, and current illness history. However, many of the diseases that cause sudden cardiac death are relatively silent, and the history and physical examination alone do not possess the power to guarantee the identification of many critical cardiovascular abnormalities that may occur in young athletes.[20] One retrospective analysis of 134 young athletes who died suddenly showed that 3% of those screened were suspected of having heart disease, with less than 1% receiving accurate diagnoses.[21] Even with the addition of noninvasive screening (echocardiograms and ECGs performed in populations of 250 to 2000 athletes, followed up over 1 year), very few definitive examples of lethal cardiovascular abnormalities have been detected.[22] Given the expense, time, and labor intensiveness of genetic molecular screening for the widely heterogeneous cardiovascular diseases, screening blood testing for mutations is untenable.

Detection of the most common cause of sudden cardiovascular death in young athletes, HCM, is possible by the use of echocardiography. Unexplained left-ventricular hypertrophy in the absence of a hemodynamic cause is defined as HCM. Other relevant abnormalities associated with sudden cardiac death, such as valvar heart disease (mitral valve prolapse and aortic valve stenosis), aortic root dilatation, and left-ventricular dysfunction (myocarditis or dilated cardiomyopathy), may be identified. However, some relevant diseases such as coronary anomalies, early coronary diseases, and ARVD may occasionally be missed even with echocardiographic assessment.

Cost efficiency is an important consideration in mass screening. The cost of an echocardiogram ranges from $600 to $2000.[6] If the occurrence of HCM in an athletic population is assumed to be 1 in 500, even at $500 per study, the cost would be $250,000 to identify a person previously undiagnosed case using echocardiogram as a primary screening tool.[23] Institutions cannot be expected to bear the expense of these screening programs. Additional emotional, financial, and medical burdens exist of false-negative and false-positive echocardiographic results.

The ECG is a more practical and cost-efficient alternative to routine echocardiography for population-based screening.[24] In most cases, an ECG is abnormal in 75% to 95% of patients with HCM[11] and will usually assist in identifying LQTS and Brugada syndrome. Not all affected relatives within a family with LQTS will exhibit an ECG abnormality, and some patients with coronary anomalies have entirely normal ECG. Therefore the ECG does not have the power of the echocardiogram as a preliminary screening tool, and it has a relatively low specificity because of the frequency with which ECG alterations may occur in normal athletic physiological circumstances. False-positive ECG results complicate its use as a primary screening tool, anticipating that 20% to 25% of all athletes will exhibit these abnormalities, prompting further echocardiographic study.[23] In fact, elite athletes without structural cardiac abnormalities are likely to exhibit ECG abnormalities most consistent with HCM and ARVD.[25]

If an abnormality is identified, then the patient deserves full evaluation by a pediatric cardiologist, who may refer to the 27th Bethesda Conference recommendations predicated on the likelihood that intense athletic training will increase the risk of disease progression, sudden death, or both. Quantifying these risks is not presently possible.[26]

Cardiovascular screening depends on a high index of suspicion of disease in young children; those who appear healthy and fit, with normal clinical examinations, are the most difficult to refer for further assessment. The risk of sudden cardiac death associated with many of the clinically relevant cardiac diseases is not known.

TOOLS FOR PRACTICE

Engaging Patient and Family

- *Chest X-ray* (fact sheet), American Heart Association (www.americanheart.org/presenter.jhtml?identifier=3005143).

- *Echocardiography (Ultrasound of the Heart)* (fact sheet), American Heart Association (www.americanheart.org/presenter.jhtml?identifier=3005161).
- *Electrocardiogram (EKG or ECG)* (fact sheet), American Heart Association (www.americanheart.org/presenter.jhtml?identifier=3005172).

Medical Decision Support

- *Cardiovascular Screening: Patient History Form* (form), American Academy of Pediatrics (practice.aap.org/content.aspx?aid=2001).
- *Preparticipation Physical Evaluation* (book), American Academy of Pediatrics, American Academy of Family Physicians, American College of Sports Medicine, American Medical Society for Sports Medicine, American Orthopaedic Society for Sports Medicine, and American Osteopathic Academy of Sports Medicine (www.aap.org/bookstore).
- *Preparticipation Physical Evaluation Form* (form), American Academy of Pediatrics, American Academy of Family Physicians, American College of Sports Medicine, American Medical Society for Sports Medicine, American Orthopaedic Society for Sports Medicine, and American Osteopathic Academy of Sports Medicine (www.aap.org/bookstore).
- *Sudden Cardiac Death Sports Short* (fact sheet), American Academy of Pediatrics (www.aap.org/family/SportsShorts_09.pdf).

AAP POLICY STATEMENT

National High Blood Pressure Education Program Working Group on High Blood Pressure in Children and Adolescents. The Fourth Report on the Diagnosis, Evaluation, and Treatment of High Blood Pressure in Children and Adolescents. *Pediatrics*. 2004;114(2):555-576. AAP endorsed.

REFERENCES

1. Ferencz C, Rubin JD, Brenner JI, et al. Congenital heart disease: prevalence at livebirth. The Baltimore-Washington Infant Study. *Am J Epidemiol*. 1985;121:31-36.
2. Wilson PD, Correa-Villasenor A, Loffredo CA, et al. Temporal trends in the prevalence of cardiovascular malformations in Maryland and the District of Columbia, 1988. The Baltimore-Washington Infant Study Group. *Epidemiology*. 1993;4:259-265.
3. Lipshultz SE, Sleeper LA, Towbin JA, et al. The incidence of pediatric cardiomyopathy in two regions of the United States. *N Engl J Med*. 2003;348:1647-1655.
4. Maron BJ, Shirani J, Poliac LC, et al. Sudden death in young competitive athletes: clinical, demographic and pathological profiles. *JAMA*. 1996;276:199-204.
5. Liberthson RR. Sudden death from cardiac causes in children and young adults. *N Engl J Med*. 1996;334:1039-1044.
6. Corrado D, Basso C, Schiavon M, et al. Screening for hypertrophic cardiomyopathy in young athletes. *N Engl J Med*. 1998;339:364-369.
7. Rychik J, Ayres N, Cuneo B, et al. American Society of Echocardiography guidelines and standards for performance of the fetal echocardiogram. *J Am Soc Echocardiogr*. 2004;17:803-810.
8. Crossland DS, Furness JC, Abu-Harb M, et al. Variability of four extremity blood pressure in normal neonates. *Arch Dis Child Fetal Neonatal Ed*. 2004;89:F325-F327.
9. Ashley EA, Raxwal V, Froelicher V. An evidence-based review of the resting electrocardiogram as a screening technique for heart disease. *Prog Cardiovasc Dis*. 2001;44:55-67.
10. Quaglini S, Rognoni C, Spazzolini C, et al. Cost-effectiveness of neonatal ECG screening for the long QT syndrome. *Eur Heart J*. 2006;27(15):1824-1832.
11. Maron BJ. The electrocardiogram as a diagnostic tool for hypertrophic cardiomyopathy: revisited [editorial]. *Ann Noninvas Electrocardiol*. 2001;:277-279.
12. Vasan RS, Benjamin EJ, Larson MG, et al. Plasma natriuretic peptides for community screening for left ventricular hypertrophy and systolic dysfunction: the Framingham Heart Study. *JAMA*. 2002;288:1252-1259.
13. Price J, Thomas AK, Grenier MA, et al. B-type natriuretic peptide levels in pediatric outpatients with chronic left ventricular dysfunction. *Pediatr Cardiol*. 2005;26:497.
14. Yi MS, Kimball TR, Tsevat J, et al. Evaluation of heart murmurs in children: cost-effectiveness and practical implications. *J Pediatr*. 2002;141:504-511.
15. Kavey RE, Daniels SR, Lauer RM, et al. American Heart Association guidelines for primary prevention of atherosclerotic cardiovascular disease beginning in childhood. *Circulation*. 2003;107:1562-1566.
16. Stamler J, Stamler R, Neaton JD, et al. Low risk-factor profile and long-term cardiovascular and noncardiovascular mortality and life expectancy: findings for 5 large cohorts of young adult and middle-aged men and women. *JAMA*. 1999;282:2012-2018.
17. Daviglus ML, Stamler J, Pirzada A, et al. Favorable cardiovascular risk profile in young women and long-term risk of cardiovascular and all-cause mortality. *JAMA*. 2004;292:1588-1592.
18. National High Blood Pressure Education Program Working Group on High Blood Pressure in Children and Adolescents. The fourth report on the diagnosis, evaluation, and treatment of high blood pressure in children and adolescents. *Pediatrics*. 2004;114:555-576.
19. Horwich TB, Hamilton MA, Fonarow GC. B-type natriuretic peptide levels in obese patients with advanced heart failure. *J Am Coll Cardiol*. 2006;47:85-90.
20. Pfister GC, Puffer JC, Maron BJ. Preparticipation cardiovascular screening for US collegiate student-athletes. *JAMA*. 2000;283:1597-1599.
21. Lewis JF, Maron BJ, Diggs JA, et al. Preparticipation echocardiographic screening for cardiovascular disease in a large, predominantly black population of collegiate athletes. *Am J Cardiol*. 1989;64:1029-1033.
22. Maron BJ, Bodison SA, Wesley YE, et al. Results of screening a large group of intercollegiate competitive athletes for cardiovascular disease. *J Am Coll Cardiol*. 1987;10:1214-1221.
23. Maron BJ, Gardin JM, Flack JM, et al. Assessment of the prevalence of hypertrophic cardiomyopathy in a general population of young adults: echocardiographic analysis of 4111 subjects in the CARDIA study. *Circulation*. 1995;92:785-789.
24. Corrado D, Basso C, Schiavon M, et al. Identification of athletes with hypertrophic cardiomyopathy at risk for sudden death: cost-effectiveness of screening strategies [abstract]. *Circulation*. 2002;106(suppl II):II-701.
25. Pellicia A, Maron BJ, Culasso F, et al. Clinical significance of abnormal electrocardiographic patterns in trained athletes. *Circulation*. 2000;102:278-284.
26. Maron BJ, Mitchell JH. 26th Bethesda Conference. Recommendations for determining eligibility for competition in athletes with cardiovascular abnormalities. *J Am Coll Cardiol*. 1994;24:845-899.

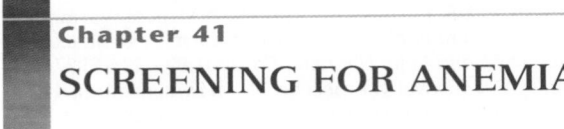

Chapter 41

SCREENING FOR ANEMIA

Bryce A. Kerlin, MD

Anemia is a symptom with many possible causes and should be investigated for the appropriate diagnosis. Anemia may be defined by laboratory values (low hemoglobin) or by physiologic consequences (inadequate oxygen-carrying capacity); both are equally important. This chapter focuses on the former because screening programs are directed primarily at detecting disease in otherwise asymptomatic children (see Chapter 162, Anemia and Pallor).

REASONS TO SCREEN FOR ANEMIA

Anemia is a public health issue. Screening for anemia is the most reliable and cost-effective method for detecting occult iron deficiency, the most common cause of anemia. Anemia is only 1 manifestation of iron deficiency; adequate iron stores are critical for normal neurocognitive development, and inadequate levels should be detected and treated as early as possible. Thus iron deficiency is the major impetus behind public health recommendations for anemia-screening programs.[1]

PREVALENCE OF ANEMIA

The prevalence of iron deficiency varies depending on the diagnostic criteria applied but may be as high as 2.9% in some settings. Although the prevalence has been decreasing over the last several decades because of improved dietary recommendations and the use of iron-fortified formulas, continued vigilance is required.[2] Additionally, the early detection of sickle cell anemia (affects approximately 1 of every 600 African American children), through either newborn screening or pediatric screening, with rapid institution of penicillin prophylaxis has dramatically reduced the incidence of fatal pneumococcal sepsis in this population.[3]

SCREENING PROGRAMS

Screening for anemia in infants and young children begins shortly after birth via the newborn screening programs.[4] All 50 states and the District of Columbia now require screening for sickle cell anemia through these programs; many states also report variant hemoglobins identified incidentally during the screening process. Many of the variant hemoglobins are benign, particularly when heterozygous; a search engine provided by the Globin Gene Server (globin.cse.psu.edu/) can be used to guide the pediatrician regarding their clinical relevance. Although newborn screening improves the sensitivity of detection for α-thalassemia, some forms of β-thalassemia may not be detectable until after hemoglobin switching from fetal forms has been completed around 6 to 12 months of age. Therefore the American Academy of Pediatrics recommends screening at 9 to 12 months, again between 15 months and 5 years for children at risk (Box 41-1), and at least once during adolescence for males and annually for menstruating females to detect the more common congenital anemias (infants) and occult iron deficiency (older children and adolescents).[5]

BOX 41-1 Children at Risk

1. Preterm or low–birth-weight infants
2. Infants receiving unfortified formula
3. Infants receiving cow's milk before age 12 months
4. Breastfed infants not getting iron supplementation after age 6 months
5. Children consuming >24 oz cow's milk per day
6. Children with special health care needs

LABORATORY EVALUATION

Screening for anemia generally is accomplished by determining the whole-blood hemoglobin concentration using blood obtained by skin puncture of the finger or heel. The sample may be analyzed in the primary care office setting using a small portable spectrophotometer or one of the many bench-top particle counters now available. By either method, the procedure is quick and reliable, with minimal quality control and maintenance required. The hemoglobin concentration determined by this method is compared with reference values for age-matched normal children. Hemoglobin levels that are less than the lower reference limit (2 standard deviations below the mean) are defined as anemic.

Positive screening tests for anemia must be confirmed and correlated with the clinical presentation. Important information that is relevant to the anemic patient is a history of neonatal jaundice, ethnicity, dietary intake, and family history of splenectomy, cholecystectomy, iron therapy, or blood transfusions. Further information about the morphologic characteristics of the patient's red blood cells should also be obtained to guide further diagnostic evaluation. Confirmation is usually performed by submitting a venous blood sample anticoagulated with ethylenediaminetetraacetic acid (EDTA) to the hematology laboratory for a complete blood count and microscopic examination of a Wright stained peripheral blood smear.

In the absence of an underlying inflammatory illness, serum ferritin is the most reliable indicator of iron status. Other studies that may be helpful in determining iron status include serum iron and iron-binding capacity; however, these findings may be misleading if the patient has recently partaken in an iron-rich meal and are best obtained in the fasting state. A lead level should be considered, particularly for younger children with iron deficiency because they may be more prone to lead intoxication secondary to the pica associated with iron deficiency.

DIFFERENTIAL DIAGNOSES

Iron deficiency anemia will generally have microcytic-hypochromic indices (low mean corpuscular volume

[MCV] and mean corpuscular hemoglobin concentration [MCHC], a high red-cell distribution width [RDW]), and it may be associated with thrombocytosis, although thrombocytopenia may be observed in severe iron deficiency. Other types of anemia that should be included in the differential diagnosis of microcytic anemia include thalassemia, sickle-thalassemia syndromes, some hemoglobinopathies (C and E), hereditary pyropoikilocytosis, severe lead intoxication, and the anemia of chronic disease. The differential diagnoses for normocytic and macrocytic anemias are considered in Chapter 162, Anemia and Pallor.

RECOMMENDATIONS

For mild microcytic anemia (ie, hemoglobin ≥8 to 10 g/dL), empiric treatment with iron supplementation (3 to 4 mg elemental iron/kg/day) is appropriate. The reticulocyte count should increase within 1 week of beginning iron therapy, and the hemoglobin should rise by at least 1 g/dL within a month.[2] Treatment should continue in patients who respond for an additional 2 months to ensure adequate replacement of iron stores. For patients who fail to respond, additional laboratory evaluation is indicated, and referral to a hematologist should be considered. Appropriate dietary counseling is important to prevent recurrence. An evaluation should be undertaken to identify sources of occult blood loss that may be contributing to the iron deficiency, particularly in older children who are not consuming inordinate amounts of cow's milk. If the anemia is more severe, then confirmatory laboratory evaluation should be obtained at the time empiric iron therapy is begun.

Iron requirements are highest for infants and adolescents because of the increased growth velocity at these stages of development. Therefore these children are at greatest risk of occult iron deficiency, and particular attention to appropriate dietary recommendations and indications for iron supplementation is essential. A comprehensive, up-to-date discussion of suitable dietary and supplementation recommendations is maintained by the Centers for Disease Control and Prevention's *Morbidity and Mortality Weekly Report Recommendations and Reports* (www.cdc.gov/mmwr/preview/mmwrhtml/00051880.htm).[6]

TOOLS FOR PRACTICE

Engaging Patients and Family

- Symptoms of Anemia (fact sheet), American Academy of Pediatrics (www.aap.org/pubed/ZZZ6G06JL5C.htm?&sub_cat=107).
- Understanding Anemia (fact sheet), American Academy of Pediatrics (www.aap.org/pubed/ZZZ9S6QUA7C.htm?&sub_cat=107).
- *Anemia and Your Young Child* (brochure), American Academy of Pediatrics (www.aap.org/bst/showdetl.cfm?&DID=15&Product_ID=2339).

Medical Decision Support

- Globin Gene Server (Web site), Penn State University (globin.cse.psu.edu/).

REFERENCES

1. Hagan JF, Shaw JS, Duncan PM, eds. *Bright Futures: Guidelines for Health Supervision of Infants, Children, and Adolescents*. 3rd ed., Elk Grove, IL: American Academy of Pediatrics, 2008.
2. Oski FA. Iron deficiency in infancy and childhood. *N Engl J Med*. 1993;329(3):190-193.
3. Embury SH. *Sickle Cell Disease: Basic Principles and Clinical Practice*. Philadelphia, PA: Lippincott-Raven; 1996.
4. Williams D. National Newborn Screening and Genetics Resource Center. National Newborn Screening Status Report. Available at: genes-r-us.uthscsa.edu/index.htm. Accessed February 4, 2006.
5. Committee on Practice and Ambulatory Medicine. Recommendations for preventive pediatric health care. *Pediatrics*. Mar 2000;105(3):645-646.
6. Centers for Disease Control and Prevention. Recommendations to prevent and control iron deficiency in the United States. *MMWR Recomm. Rep*. 1998;47(RR-3):1-36.

Chapter 42

VISION SCREENING

Alex R. Kemper, MD, MPH, MS; Richard C. Wasserman, MD, MPH

BURDEN OF ILLNESS

Amblyopia, a permanent uncorrectable vision loss, is a major threat to vision that is preventable when detected in early childhood.[1] During development, the visual cortex must receive focused images from both eyes to learn how to see. Conditions that interfere with the normal visual image during this time, such as strabismus, certain refractive errors, or cataracts, can lead to amblyopia if not identified and corrected. Approximately 5% of preschool-aged children have amblyopia, and up to 10% have vision problems, such as refractive error. The prevalence of refractive error increases with age and affects over 20% of high school–aged children.[1,2]

BENEFITS OF SCREENING AND EARLY IDENTIFICATION

The likelihood of successfully treating amblyopia decreases with age. The goal is to detect amblyogenic conditions before 5 years of age. The earlier these conditions are identified and treated, the more likely and the more easily amblyopia can be prevented.

From a public health standpoint, screening for vision problems is readily justified on the following counts:

- Vision problems are common.
- Vision problems pose a threat to children's current and future well being.
- Vision problems are likely to go undetected without screening.
- Screening tests are available that can identify children who have or are at risk for vision problems.
- Efficacious treatments for vision problems are readily available.

- Early diagnosis and treatment confer significant advantages in outcome for many vision problems (eg, congenital cataracts, strabismus, amblyopia).

TOOLS

The goals of vision screening are (1) to identify deficits in vision or conditions that might ultimately threaten vision before they otherwise would be discovered and (2) to ensure that appropriate diagnostic and therapeutic referrals are made so that conditions threatening vision are ameliorated. To achieve the first goal, the practitioner and staff must learn the appropriate vision screening techniques and procedures and then apply them systematically in their practice. To achieve the second goal, the practitioner must structure the primary care encounter so that screening results are communicated accurately to parents, appropriate referrals are made (when indicated), and proper follow-up is achieved.

Appropriate vision screening techniques and procedures vary to some degree for infants and toddlers (younger than 3 years), preschool children (3 to 5 years), and school-aged children and adolescents.[3,4] The practitioner's physical examination provides some of the elements of vision screening, especially in infants and toddlers, but vision is tested more efficiently by ancillary personnel and apart from the physical examination. Children who have developmental disabilities are often at increased risk for vision problems and may require special expertise for assessment. Criteria for referral are discussed in the next sections.

INFANTS AND TODDLERS

Physical Examination

The eyes are first examined as part of the newborn examination and should be assessed subsequently at each health supervision visit. As part of the examination, the eyes should be inspected for any structural abnormalities. The red reflex is evaluated for abnormality or asymmetrical appearance through an ophthalmoscope. After an infant can fixate on an object, generally by 3 months of age, the corneal light reflections should be tested by using a penlight held in midline 12 inches in front of the eye (Hirschberg test). Asymmetry of the light's reflection on the two corneas suggests strabismus. The examiner should assess ocular motility by having the child follow a brightly colored object or toy. Information from the cover-uncover test is sometimes difficult for the unskilled to interpret. This test detects movement of each eye when the other is covered and then uncovered. Such movement suggests either a unilateral visual defect or an ocular muscle weakness in the eye that moves. (See Chapters 220, Strabismus; and 228, Visual Development, Amblyopia, and Vision Testing for more detailed discussions of the physical examination of the eyes.)

Formal Screening

New technology, such as photorefractive screening *(photoscreening)* and autorefraction, are now available for screening young children. However, the validity and reliability of these devices in the primary care setting are unknown.[5]

Special Circumstances

Infants whose circumstances or family history place them at special risk for visual problems, such as preterm infants at risk for retinopathy of prematurity, those who have a family history of congenital eye problems, or those who have genetic (eg, trisomy 21) or acquired problems (eg, cerebral palsy) that place their eyes at risk, should be evaluated by an ophthalmologist.

Parents sometimes give a history of asymmetry of the child's eyes when none can be demonstrated at the visit. Because some problems of muscle imbalance occur only when the child is fatigued, the examiner would be wise to pay attention to such a history and refer the patient to a specialist if these complaints are persistent. A family history of amblyopia, a *lazy eye*, or *crossed eyes* confers a higher risk of problems and should prompt consideration of referral.

PRESCHOOL CHILDREN

Physical Examination

Inspection, bilateral red reflex, corneal light reflection, and ocular motility, should be performed at each health supervision visit.

Formal Screening

Testing for visual acuity should be attempted beginning at age 3 years, and an interpretable result should be achieved by age 4 years. Having a child who is uncooperative or inconsistent in responses return for a repeat test is reasonable. Repeated failure to achieve an interpretable test result may be an indication of a visual problem.

At this age, the simpler tests of acuity that do not rely on knowledge of letters are the most acceptable. The Lea chart has become popular because children may have an easier time identifying the four symbols (apple, circle, square, and house) on this test than some of the other tests.[6] In general, these tests are available for testing from a distance of 10 and of 20 feet. At 10 feet, children are less likely to become distracted by other activities in the immediate environment.

Testing for binocular vision (stereoacuity) is not a substitute for assessing visual acuity, but it is a useful adjunct and will sometimes identify a child whose vision problems have been missed on physical examination and acuity testing. Acceptable tests for this age group include the Random Dot E Test and the Stereo Fly Test.[7]

Special Circumstances

Children at high risk for poor vision, as discussed previously, should be referred if satisfactory results cannot be obtained on screening.

SCHOOL-AGED CHILDREN AND ADOLESCENTS

Physical Examination

Eyes should be inspected and the bilateral red reflex, corneal light reflex, and ocular motility tests should be performed at each health supervision visit.

Formal Screening

Once a child knows the alphabet, the Snellen letters on a wall chart are appropriate for visual acuity screening. For school-aged children and adolescents, vision testing machines that combine acuity testing with tests of binocular vision are readily accepted and require less office space.

Special Circumstances

School difficulties may be a presenting symptom of visual problems, and all children who have such troubles should have their vision evaluated if not done recently. Although the prevention of amblyopia becomes less of a concern with increasing age, the overall prevalence of vision problems increases steadily over time; therefore children should continue to be tested at health supervision visits.

PERSONNEL AND EQUIPMENT

Nonprofessional personnel who have a high school education can be trained to administer all of these formal tests. The equipment necessary for most of these tests is readily available from medical supply houses and is inexpensive. Vision not tested with testing machines requires a well-lighted environment with at least 10 feet of available space. Vision testing machines require less space but are expensive.

REFERRAL

When strabismus or amblyopia is suspected, the child should be referred to an eye care specialist who is skilled in working with young children.

A child who has a structural abnormality of the eye or its movements, any asymmetry or abnormality of the red reflex, any asymmetry of the corneal reflections, aversion to the occlusion of one eye, or any movement of the eyes on the cover-uncover test should be referred.

Preschool children failing to pass a visual acuity test in either or both eyes at the 20/40 level or who display a two-line discrepancy between the eyes (eg, 20/20 and 20/40) should be referred. In addition, any child who cannot be tested successfully by age 4 years after repeated attempts should be referred. School-aged children and adolescents who fail to pass at the 20/30 level in either or both eyes should be referred. In addition, children who have developmental disabilities who cannot be tested successfully should be referred.

Children of any age who fail a test of binocular vision should be referred.

IMPROVING VISION SCREENING AND ITS OUTCOMES

The primary care practice and clinic settings, because they provide continuity of care, remain ideal places to carry out vision screening. Practitioners need to screen systematically all of the children whom they see for health supervision visits. They should record and communicate the results of the screening to parents and make sure that follow-up and referral appointments are made and kept. Rates of screening are suboptimal, and many children whose visual testing is abnormal never receive evaluation by an eye care specialist.[3,6,8,9]

Few data are available about the accuracy of vision screening in the primary care setting. As in any screening program, a proportion of children will fail vision screening but have a normal ophthalmologic evaluation. False-positive tests are a feature of all screening programs and should not discourage practitioners from screening. Vision screening examinations will detect the overwhelming proportion of children who have treatable vision problems; practitioners must ensure that these cases are detected and treated properly.

TOOLS FOR PRACTICE

Engaging Patient and Family

- *Eyeglasses for Infants and Children* (fact sheet), American Academy of Ophthalmology (www.medem.com/medlb/article_detaillb_for_printer.cfm?article_ID=ZZZSOWVEH4C&sub_cat=117).
- *How do I know if my child has a vision problem?* (fact sheet), American Academy of Pediatrics (www.aap.org/publiced/BR_Eyes.htm).
- *What is a Pediatric Ophthalmologist?* (fact sheet), American Academy of Pediatrics (www.aap.org/sections/he3006.pdf).
- *When to See an Eye MD* (fact sheet), American Academy of Pediatrics (www.medem.com/search/article_display.cfm?path=\\TANQUERAY\M_ContentItem&mstr=/M_ContentItem/ZZZS1ZGZY9C.html&soc=AAO&srch_typ=NAV_SERCH).

Medical Decision Support

- *Eye Examination in Infants, Children, and Young Adults by Pediatricians* (fact sheet), American Academy of Pediatrics (aappolicy.aappublications.org).
- *Pediatric Ophthalmology for Primary Care, 3rd edition* (book), Wright KW (www.aap.org/bookstore).
- *See Red Cards (Red Reflux Testing)* (fact sheet), American Academy of Pediatrics. (www.aap.org/sforms/seered.htm).
- *Visual Impairment in children ages 0-5: screening* (report), US Preventive Services Task Force (www.ahrq.gov/clinic/uspstf/uspsvsch.htm).
- *Wright Eye Chart* (chart), Kenneth W. Wright, MD, FAAP, (www.aap.org/bookstore).

AAP POLICY STATEMENTS

American Academy of Pediatrics, Committee on Practice and Ambulatory Medicine and Section on Ophthalmology. Use of photoscreening for children's vision screening. *Pediatrics.* 2002;109(3):524-525. (aappolicy.aappublications.org/cgi/content/full/pediatrics;109/3/524).

American Academy of Pediatrics, Committee on Practice and Ambulatory Medicine and Section on Ophthalmology, American Association of Certified Orthoptists, American Association for Pediatric Ophthalmology and Strabismus, and American Academy of Ophthalmology. Eye examination in infants, children, and young adults by pediatricians. *Pediatrics.* 2003;111:902-907. (aappolicy.aappublications.org/cgi/content/full/pediatrics;111/4/902).

SUGGESTED RESOURCES

American Academy of Pediatrics, Committee on Practice and Ambulatory Medicine, Section on Ophthalmology. Eye examination and vision screening in infants, children, and young adults. *Pediatrics*. 1996;98:153-157.

Hartmann EE, Sobson V, Hainline L, et al. Preschool vision screening: summary of a task force report. *Pediatrics*. 2000;106:1105-1116.

REFERENCES

1. Epelbaum M, Milleret C, Buisseret P, et al. The sensitive period for strabismic amblyopia in humans. *Ophthalmology*. 1993;100:323-327.
2. Angle J, Wissmann DA. The epidemiology of myopia. *Am J Epidemiol*. 1980;111:220-228.
3. American Academy of Pediatrics, Committee on Practice and Ambulatory Medicine, Section on Ophthalmology. Eye examination and vision screening in infants, children, and young adults. *Pediatrics*. 1996;98:153-157.
4. Hartmann EE, Sobson V, Hainline L, et al. Preschool vision screening: summary of a task force report. *Pediatrics*. 2000;106:1105-1116.
5. American Academy of Pediatrics, Committee on Practice and Ambulatory Medicine, Section on Ophthalmology. Use of photoscreening for children's vision screening. *Pediatrics*. 2002;109:524-525.
6. Hered RW, Murphy S, Clancy M. Comparison of the HOTV and Lea Symbols charts for preschool vision screening, *J Pediatr Ophthalmol Strabismus*. 1997;34:24-28.
7. Simons K. Amblyopia characterization, treatment, and prophylaxis. *Surv Ophthalmol*. 2005;50:123-166.
8. Campbell LR, Charney E. Factors associated with delay in diagnosis of childhood amblyopia. *Pediatrics*. 1991;87:178-185.
9. Wasserman RC, Croft CA, Brotherton SE. Preschool vision screening in pediatric practice: a study from the pediatric research in office settings (PROS) network. *Pediatrics*. 1992;89(5 pt 1):834-838.

Chapter 43

IDENTIFICATION OF DEVELOPMENTAL DELAYS AND EARLY INTERVENTION SYSTEM

Ruth K. Kaminer, MD; Susan J. Vig, PhD

When a primary care physician (PCP) identifies a child who has delayed development, every effort should be made to connect the child to the early intervention system quickly. The importance of early intervention as a national concern has been reflected in federal legislation. The Amendments to the Education of the Handicapped Act (PL 99-457 Part H), enacted by Congress in 1986 and subsequently incorporated into the Individuals with Disabilities Education Act (IDEA) of 1989, gave states the option of participating in the early intervention system, and all 50 states chose to do so. The legislation requires participating states to develop a coordinated, comprehensive, multidisciplinary system of early intervention services for young children (birth to 3 years) and their families. The 1997 Amendments to IDEA (PL 105-17 Part C) have prioritized the provision of services in natural environments. This amendment means that services should be offered, when possible, in home and community settings, such as child care facilities, in which children who have no disabilities participate.

Key components of the legislation include a definition of developmental delay; a comprehensive system of identifying and referring children, called "Child Find"; a public awareness program; policy regarding personnel standards; and procedural safeguards to ensure protection of confidentiality and the rights of families to due process. In each state, a lead agency is designated to administer, supervise, and monitor early intervention programs and activities. Most states have assigned these roles to the department of education or the department of health. Early intervention legislation requires a comprehensive, multidisciplinary evaluation to determine the needs of children and families. After evaluation, family members and professionals work together to develop an *individualized family service plan* that describes the services, supports, and coordination of services to be provided for the child and family.

PROVIDING EARLY INTERVENTION

PCPs play an important role in this process by identifying and serving children who have developmental delays. Good pediatric practice embodies the principles on which the IDEA legislation is based: a family orientation and an awareness of the need to support a child's future independent functioning. PCPs have learned that any factor affecting a child's functioning affects the parents and family, regardless of the cause of such limitations.

The PCP's role in identifying and serving children who have known developmental delays may be interpreted narrowly or broadly, depending on the physician's training, interest, and level of comfort (see Chapter 44, Developmental Surveillance and Intervention). However, minimal expectations include screening for developmental delays by routinely asking the parents during health maintenance visits about their concerns, using appropriate, validated screening instruments, and referring children whose development is questionable or delayed for evaluation and services. The developmental surveillance questions and developmental milestones outlined in the Bright Futures guidelines are effective tools for accomplishing this task.[1] More detail on developmental screening is provided in Chapter 44, Developmental Surveillance and Intervention. Routine screening of vision and hearing in preschoolers as described in Chapter 42, Vision Screening; and Chapter 39, Auditory Screening, is an accepted part of health maintenance.

PCPs with a special interest in the care of patients with developmental disabilities may participate with other professionals in multidisciplinary evaluations of the child's delay, help the parents understand the child's strengths and weaknesses, interpret medical information for early intervention providers, and monitor the outcomes of intervention. Parents need and value the support of their PCP in dealing with the possibility or reality of developmental delay in their child.[2]

MONITORING EARLY INTERVENTION

Once children have entered the early intervention system, the PCP's role shifts from identifying delays to monitoring the child's progress and giving parents guidance. Parents often have the unstated expectation that the intervention will correct the developmental delay. Although this correction may sometimes occur, it is not universally true. After dealing with the stress of identifying the delay, parents often need the period of optimism that starting intervention provides. However, some developmental problems will persist and will require different kinds of intervention at different ages, and the PCP must be aware of and help parents understand this issue. Box 43-1 offers an outline for monitoring progress in a child with known developmental delay.

The PCP's role in monitoring the progress of children receiving early intervention services includes asking parents for an update on the child's functioning, identifying what progress has been achieved, and learning what the current intervention goals are. Changes in the child's functioning may require a change in types of intervention. For example, in the first year of life, infants born prematurely frequently have abnormalities of tone and asymmetries in motor function for which physical and occupational therapy are provided. These problems tend to improve by 1 year of age, only to be replaced by newly identified delays in language or cognition, which require speech and language therapy or special education services. Ongoing contact with the family about the child enables the PCP to determine that some delays have resolved and to identify others that have emerged. Sharing this information with parents helps them obtain and understand modifications in the child's intervention program.

With the increased publicity about early diagnosis of autism spectrum disorder and its prompt treatment, parents are turning to their PCPs for advice on diagnosis and treatment of this condition. Many therapeutic interventions, both biomedical and psychosocial, are being promoted by various advocacy or professional groups, but only a few of these have been scientifically studied. For parents seeking guidance from their PCP on treatment, the American Academy of Pediatrics Committee on Children with Disabilities Statement on Complementary and Alternative Medicine is a useful resource.[3]

BOX 43-1 Follow-Up of Children With Developmental Delay

- Developmental diagnosis
- Current parental concerns
- Current intervention
- Progress reported by parent with or without a preschool or school report
- Observed functioning
- Newly identified needs of child or family
- Plan for evaluation, coordination, and service provision
- Follow-up

BARRIERS TO CARE

Although many PCPs are involved in identifying, evaluating, referring, and managing children who have developmental delays, the following barriers may prevent some PCPs from getting involved in these roles.

Reluctance to Identify Developmental Delays

PCPs may be reluctant to identify developmental delays because the parents have to be confronted with the possibility of these delays. Just as PCPs share the parents' enjoyment of their children's developmental progress, they share their distress when the adequacy of that progress is questioned. Some parents wait for the PCP to voice the concerns they have begun to feel, and they interpret the physician's silence as an indication that no problem exists. By routinely questioning parents about development and behavior at all contacts and observing the child's development along with the parent, the PCP creates a comfortable atmosphere for discussing concerns identified either by the parents or the PCP.

Questions About the Efficacy of Early Intervention

A PCP who is convinced that early intervention will help a child and family is more likely to identify children who need this service. The efficacy of early intervention in improving children's developmental outcomes is documented in well-designed studies. The Infant Health and Development Program, an extensive eight-site clinical trial for low–birth-weight infants, demonstrated such an impact. Children who had participated for 3 years with their families in this comprehensive early intervention program, which provided health, developmental, and family services, had higher IQs and fewer maternally reported problems at corrected age 36 months than did controls.[4] Follow-up studies at 8 years of age showed intervention-related advantages in cognitive, receptive language and academic skills for the heavier low–birth-weight premature children.[5] In addition, follow-up studies of economically disadvantaged children have shown that daily participation in intensive, center-based early intervention is associated with a higher IQ, stronger school achievement, fewer failing grades at age 12, and less grade retention and special education placement at age 15.[6] In general, the best developmental outcomes have been associated with early intervention programs that are comprehensive, involve both the family and the child, and focus on strengthening the parent-child relationship.[7] The two groups that appear to benefit most are (1) children who have biological risk factors and who are growing up in adverse circumstances and (2) all children who have mild degrees of developmental delay.[6]

Concerns About Overidentifying Delays

PCPs often have concerns about overidentifying delays, upsetting the family, and subjecting the child to unnecessary evaluations. However, sensitive exploration of possible delays harms neither the parents nor the child, whereas avoiding the issue may be detrimental. Evaluation is a way of gaining a better understanding of the child, and a diagnosis of developmental delay is often required to enter the system of developmental services. The evaluation process itself becomes a useful intervention by educating the parent, supporting the parent in observing and interpreting the child's behavior, and exploring new ways of interacting with the child.[8]

Time Pressures

The increasing pressure to see more patients in less time and the limitations on the number of health care maintenance visits by some managed care systems make identifying developmental issues hard for the PCP. Eliciting the child's current developmental function by parent interview or observation takes time, and talking to the parent about delays or deviations and achieving consensus on a plan of action also take time. These tasks are uniquely a PCP's role because no other professional whose opinions carry the same authority is involved in the lives of children. Several strategies may enable a busy PCP to address developmental issues. These strategies include using short questionnaires for parents who are literate, such as the Child Development Review,[9] or training an office nurse or another staff member to perform developmental screening. The most effective method is scheduling a separate appointment for developmental screening by the PCP when developmental concerns are identified on regular visits. Some early intervention systems will reimburse participating PCPs for performing developmental screenings. These strategies are reviewed in Chapter 44, Developmental Surveillance and Intervention.

Lack of Familiarity With Resources

PCPs may not have the time to be involved in the early intervention system. However, they must learn how to connect patients and families to this system so that children may obtain services to which they are entitled. Literature for patients can be obtained from state or county health departments that describe early intervention programs, and such literature should be available in the PCP's office. Most medical school–affiliated pediatric departments have specialists in developmental disabilities who are a useful resource for evaluation and referral to publicly funded services.

CONCLUSION

Hearing from parents that the PCP reassured them about the child's delay by saying, "He'll outgrow it" is painfully common for specialty clinicians who evaluate children with developmental disabilities. Although children may outgrow various problems, a physician should always investigate the parents' concerns thoroughly before reassuring them. Without careful screening and monitoring, only children who have more severe delays are likely to be identified. However, evidence suggests that early intervention may make a critical difference in the development, behavior, and success of children with mild delays. The PCP is ideally situated to provide ongoing support to families who must navigate the early intervention system, regardless of the severity of the developmental delay.

TOOLS FOR PRACTICE

Medical Decision Support

- *Bright Futures* (Web page), American Academy of Pediatrics/Bright Futures (www.brightfutures.aap.org/web/).
- *Coding Conundrums—Consultation Codes* (fact sheet), Lynn Wegner, MD, FAAP, and Michelle Macias, MD (www.dbpeds.org/articles/detail.cfm?TextID=120).
- *First Signs* (Web page), First Signs (www.firstsigns.org/index.html).
- *Learn the Signs. Act Early.* (Web page), Centers for Disease Control and Prevention (www.cdc.gov/ncbddd/autism/actearly/).
- *The Medical Home and Early Intervention Program* (booklet), American Academy of Pediatrics (www.medicalhomeinfo.org/health/Downloads/ElbrochureF.pdf).

Practice Management and Care Coordination

- *Individuals with Disabilities Education Act (IDEA)* (Web page), US Department of Education (www.idea.ed.gov/).
- *National and State Resources* (Web page), National Early Childhood Technical Assistance Center (www.nectac.org/contact/contact.asp).
- *State Resource Sheets* (fact sheet), National Dissemination Center for Children With Disabilities (www.nichcy.org/states.htm).

AAP POLICY STATEMENTS

American Academy of Pediatrics, Committee on Children With Disabilities. Role of the pediatrician in family-centered early intervention services. *Pediatrics*. 2001; 107(5):1155-1157. (aappolicy.aappublications.org/cgi/content/full/pediatrics;107/5/1155).

American Academy of Pediatrics, Committee on Children With Disabilities. The pediatrician's role in development and implementation of an individual education plan (IEP) and/or an individual family services plan (IFSP). *Pediatrics*. 1999;104(1):124-127. (aappolicy.aappublications.org/cgi/content/full/pediatrics;104/1/124).

American Academy of Pediatrics, Council on Children With Disabilities, Section on Developmental Behavioral Pediatrics, Bright Futures Steering Committee, and Medical Home Initiatives for Children With Special Needs Project Advisory Committee. Identifying infants and young children with developmental disorders in the medical home: an algorithm for developmental surveillance and screening. *Pediatrics*. 2006;118(1):405-420. (aappolicy.aappublications.org/cgi/content/full/pediatrics;118/1/405).

REFERENCES

1. Green M, Palfrey JS, eds. *Bright Futures: Guidelines for Health Supervision of Infants, Children, and Adolescents*. 2nd ed. Arlington, VA: National Center for Education in Maternal and Child Health; 2000.
2. American Academy of Pediatrics, Committee on Children with Disabilities. Pediatrician's role in the development and implementation of an individualized education plan (IEP) and/or an individualized family service plan (IFSP). *Pediatrics*. 1999;104(1):124-127.
3. American Academy of Pediatrics, Committee on Children with Disabilities. Counseling families who choose complementary and alternative medicine for their child with chronic illness or disability. *Pediatrics*. 2001;107(3):598-601. Available at aappolicy.aappublications.org/cgi/content/full/pediatrics;107/3/598. Accessed June 26, 2007.

4. The Infant Health and Development Program. Enhancing the outcomes of low-birth-weight, premature infants. A multisite, randomized trial. *JAMA*. 1990;263(22): 3035-3042.
5. McCarton CM, Brooks-Gunn J, Wallace IF, et al. Results at age 8 years of early intervention for low-birth-weight premature infants. The Infant Health and Development Program. *JAMA* 1997;277(2):126-132.
6. Ramey CT, Campbell FA, Burchinal M, et al. Persistent effects of early childhood education on high-risk children and their mothers. In: Feldman MA, ed. *Early Intervention*. Malden, MA: Blackwell Science; 2004.
7. Bennett FC, Guralnick MJ. Effectiveness of developmental intervention in the first five years of life. *Pediatr Clin North Am*. 1991;38(6):1513-1528.
8. Vig S, Kaminer R. Comprehensive interdisciplinary evaluation as intervention for young children. *Infants Young Child*. 2003;16(4):342-353.
9. Ireton HR. *Child Development Reviews*. Minneapolis, MN: Behavior Science Systems; 1990.

Chapter 44
DEVELOPMENTAL SURVEILLANCE AND INTERVENTION

Marian F. Earls, MD

Individuals who provide primary health care for children have long recognized the importance of developmental screening and surveillance in helping families optimize their children's acquisition of skills, understand behavior, and facilitate learning. For children who have developmental differences or delays, universal or focused screening provides the opportunity for early identification and referral for intervention.

Pediatricians know from brain research that experience affects brain development, both prenatally and postnatally. For example, infants living in a neglectful environment have changes in neurogenesis and synapse pruning. The implications for prevention and intervention are profound because growth, development, and behavior are inextricably linked. Therefore screening needs to consider the whole child, including social and emotional development in the context of family and community.

Approximately 16% of children have developmental or behavioral disabilities, including speech and language delays, intellectual disability, learning disabilities, and emotional problems.[1] Even at preschool age, 13% of children have mental health problems.[2] In 2005 the Centers for Disease Control and Prevention reported that 5% of 4 to 17 year olds in the United States (2.7 million children) were described by their parents as having severe emotional or behavioral difficulties in the National Health Interview Survey.[3] These rates increase with the co-occurrence of risk factors such as poverty, maternal depression, substance abuse, domestic violence, and foster care placement. In 2005, approximately 38% of children in the United States lived in low-income families. This number has been increasing since 2000, after a decade of decline. These children have an increased risk for language, learning, and behavioral problems. An infant living with a depressed mother can show disordered attachment as early as 2 months of age and can have poor performance on the Bayley Scales of Infant Development at 1 year of age. As an older child and adolescent, the prognosis is poor because of the increased likelihood of conduct disorder. Many premature infants, especially those of extremely low birth weight (<1000 g) are at risk for visual and hearing impairment, language delays and learning problems, and problems with motor development. In addition, for an infant who has had a prolonged neonatal intensive care unit course, bonding can be a challenge, particularly if ongoing medical or feeding issues exist.

Despite the medical community's knowledge of prevalence and risk, detection of developmental and behavioral problems before school age is very poor (approximately 30%).[4] This circumstance completely eliminates the possibility of early intervention. By contrast, 70% to 80% of children with developmental disabilities are correctly identified when standardized screening tests are used.[5] The primary medical home provides the perfect setting for screening and surveillance, improving prevention and early identification.

Discussing assets and promoting connections for support needs to be part of early conversations with families, along with open discussion regarding risk factors.[6] When psychosocial screenings reveal risk, the office is the source for initial discussion and referral to community resources. This role assumes previous networking by the practice with community partners and a working knowledge and connection to community providers such as counselors, agencies, early intervention programs, child care, Head Start, and schools.

Psychosocial screening includes asking about family relationships, maternal depression, domestic violence, and substance abuse.[7] Brief screening tools regarding these individual issues are available, as well as general tools that address all of these topics. Other important questions regarding stable housing, financial resources, and insurance coverage are also pertinent. The practice can assist families with contacting community agencies. In a family-centered practice, financial issues need to be considered for each family for a plan of care to be realistic and possible (eg, for cost of medication or transportation to a referral).

Developmental and behavioral screening, completed by the parents and reviewed by the physician, allows early identification of potential problems or delays. Of equal importance, screening also reviews appropriate expectations at a given developmental age, facilitating understanding regarding the child's behavior and potentially facilitating appropriate discipline use by parents. A conversation about the screening identifies the child's strengths and weaknesses, gives a template for anticipatory guidance, and elicits and respects parental concerns. In this way, parental self-efficacy and confidence is promoted. Encouraging sharing age-appropriate books together from an early age has benefits for the relationship, developing language skills and success for early reading skills. For children with at-risk scores, referral to early intervention services occurs. For a parent whose child has a medical condition or developmental problem, a connection to a family support network can provide parent-to-parent support. Early empowerment for parenting has implications for long-term outcomes, including readiness to learn, school success, and social success.

BENEFITS OF EARLY IDENTIFICATION AND INTERVENTION

Early identification allows for referral and for early intervention even for children with significant developmental diagnoses that cannot be cured or completely remediated. Early intervention improves function for the child and family. Early intervention can also save up to $100,000 per student in special-education costs over the course of the child's education.[8]

Waiting until a problem is observable to screen is pointless. If a problem is already observable, then a screen is unnecessary, and time for intervention has been lost. Informal checklists, in use by many primary care physicians, have no validated criteria for referral and result in missed referral opportunities.

SCREENING TOOLS FOR THE PRIMARY CARE PRACTICE

Developmental screening tools are of different types and include direct elicitation, interview, and parent questionnaires. Effective screens have sensitivity and specificity of at least 70% to 80%. Screens included in this group are the Ages and Stages Questionnaire (ASQ), the Parents' Evaluation of Developmental Status (PEDS), PEDS Developmental Milestones (PEDS DM), the Infant Developmental Inventory (IDI), the Bayley Infant Neurodevelopmental Screener (BINS), and the BRIGANCE Screens and Inventories. For a complete description of tools with information on forms, content, sensitivity and specificity, and for ordering, the reader is referred to the screening section of www.dbpeds.org. Excluded tests as a result of poor validation or sensitivity and specificity are the Prescreening Developmental Questionnaire, the Denver Developmental Screening Test II, Developmental Indicators for the Assessment of Learning III, and Gesell Developmental Observation Test.

For family psychosocial screening, a variety of tools are available, ranging from very brief to multiple-item screens. Most of these tools screen for maternal depression, domestic violence, and substance abuse. (See Chapter 47, Family Screening and Assessments.)

Screening rates for development and behavior, maternal depression, and family risk or protective factors are poor in primary care practice. The American Academy of Pediatrics Survey of Fellows No. 53 in 2002 revealed that 71% of fellows used only clinical observation without a screening instrument to identify children with a developmental delay. Only 23% reported using a standardized tool. Reasons given for not screening include (1) screening takes too long, (2) tools are difficult to administer, (3) children may not cooperate, and (4) reimbursement is limited. Perceived barriers are time, cost, and staff required. For tools completed by a parent, an inclusive reading level must also be considered, although the best tools have been developed with an eye to readability. Language availability is an important consideration in some practices. Concerns about practicality are especially important. Many practices have found that the use of the most familiar and common tool, the Denver Developmental Screening Test, is untenable in a busy practice because of demands on the physician's time. A parent-completed tool can solve concerns with time and efficiency. A comparison of tools by time, cost, staff, reading level, and language availability is shown in Table 44-1. A similar comparison of social emotional screening tools is listed in Table 44-2.

Several advantages exist to using a parent questionnaire, not the least of which is that it is a family-centered process, recognizing the parent as the expert on the child. The parent is engaged as a partner in the care of the child. A parent tool does not require administration by staff and can be completed while the parent is in the waiting room or examination room so that it does not impinge on visit time or office flow. It also removes the problem of trying to elicit skills from a toddler or preschooler by a virtual stranger and in a setting that is not the child's natural environment.

Parents give accurate and good quality information, and they are good reporters of what their child can do. Parents' concerns are accurate indicators of true problems, particularly for speech and language, fine-motor, hearing, and general function. When asked how old their child acts compared with other children, parent estimations correlate well with developmental quotients for cognitive, motor, self-help, and academic skills. Recall (eg, milestones) is unreliable, however.[9] If parental reading skills are a concern, then parents can be asked if they would like to complete the screen independently or have someone go through it with them.

OFFICE PROCESS

Integrating screening and surveillance into the office process and flow is crucial for successful implementation of screening programs.

Steps include:

1. Assess protocols for developmental screening already in use in the practice.
2. Map the workflow. This process needs to include the physician, nursing staff, and the office manager and should be tailored to the practice. For example, the nurse can give the screening tool to the parent at intake to be completed in the examination room so as to be ready for the physician to review and score after coming into the room.
3. Select tool or tools.
4. Identify system supports for parent education, referral, and community services.
   a. Meet with key partners. Inviting community partners to a lunch meeting at the practice to share screening plans and align goals is a good idea.
   b. Establish a process for referral and communication.
5. Orient all staff members to new procedures.

The primary care physician does not need to become an expert at diagnosing and managing

Table 44-1 Developmental and Behavioral Screening Tools

	ASQ	BINS	PEDS	PEDS DM	IDI	BRIGANCE
Type	Parent questionnaire	Direct elicitation	Parent questionnaire	Parent questionnaire	Parent questionnaire	Direct elicitation
Ages	4 mo-5 yr	3-24 mo	0-8 yr	0-7 to 11 yr	3-18 mo	0-23 mo 2-2.5 yr 3-4 yr
Staff required	Paraprofessional	Master's or equivalent	Paraprofessional	Paraprofessional	Paraprofessional	Professional
Cost	$199.00/kit	$195.00/kit	$69.95 manual $30.00 kit	$275.00/starter kit Extra: laminated questionnaire book $110.00 each	$14.00/pad (25 sheets)	For each age range: $110.00/manual $148.00/120 data sheets
Refills, copies	Ok to copy	Refills: score sheet	Refills: $30.00/ 50 sheets	Refills: record form $32/100 sheets	Refills: $14.00	Refills: $148.00/ 120 sheets
Time	3 min to score	20-30 min to administer 10 min to score	5 min to score	5-10 min to score	10 min to score	10-15 min to administer
Languages	English, Spanish, French, Korean	English	English, Spanish, Vietnamese, Hmong, Somali	English, Spanish (7/07)	English, Spanish	English, Spanish
Reading level	4th-6th grade	NA	5th grade	3rd to 4th grade	Unknown (not in descriptive material)	NA

ASQ, Ages and Stages Questionnaire; *BINS,* Bayley Infant Neurodevelopmental Screener; *IDI,* Infant Developmental Inventory; *PEDS,* Parent's Evaluation of Developmental Status; *PEDS DM,* Parent's Evaluation of Developmental Status—Developmental Milestones.

Table 44-2 Social-Emotional Screening Tools

	ASQ SE	TABS	BITSEA	EYBERG	PSC
Type	Parent questionnaire or interview	Parent questionnaire or interview	Parent questionnaire or interview	Parent questionnaire or interview	Parent questionnaire or interview
Ages	6-60 mo	11-71 mo	12-36 mo	2-16 yr	4-18 yr
Cost	$125/kit	$85/kit	$99.00/kit	$147/kit	Free, downloadable
Refills, copies	Free to copy	$25 for pad of 50 sheets	$35 for 25 sheets	$29 for pad of 25 sheets	Free to copy
Time	10 min	5 min	7-10 min	5 min	5 min
Languages	English, Spanish	English, Spanish	English, Spanish, French, Dutch, Hebrew	English	English, Spanish, Chinese
Reading level	4th-6th grade	3rd grade	—	6th grade	—

ASQ SE, Ages and Stages Questionnaire (social-emotional); *BITSEA,* Brief Infant Toddler Social Emotional Assessment; *Eyberg,* Eyberg Child Behavior Inventory; *PSC,* Pediatric Symptom Checklist; *TABS,* Temperament and Atypical Behavior Scale.

Table 44-3 The Longitudinal Relationship with Children and Families

VISIT	PRIMARY SCREEN	PERTINENT ISSUES	PARENTING	SECONDARY SCREEN
1 week and 1 mo	Psychosocial	Support, housing, transportation, peak crying in 2nd mo	Newborn care, feeding, sleep, reading cues, soothing strategies	—
2 mo	Maternal depression (Edinburgh Postnatal Depression Scale)	Socioeconomic, family relationships, attachment	Sleep, reading cues	—
4 mo	Maternal depression	Same as 2 mo, reaching, rolling, social smile	Sleep, reading cues	—
6 mo	Psychosocial: MH, SA, DV	Emergent motor and social skills mobility	Sleep, book sharing, age-appropriate expectations	ASQ SE, if indicated
9 mo	ASQ, PEDS	Emerging stranger anxiety, mobility, feeding self	Sleep, book sharing, discipline	—
12 mo	ASQ, PEDS (if not at 9 months)	Emerging language, joint attention, mobility	Sleep, book sharing, discipline, toilet training	ASQ SE, TABS, or BITSEA, if indicated
15 mo	Psychosocial MH, SA, DV	Language, home environment	Same as above	—
18 mo	ASQ, PEDS	Language, independence	Sleep, book sharing, discipline, toilet training	ASQ SE, TABS or BITSEA; MCHAT, if indicated
24 mo (or 30 mo)	ASQ/PEDS (if not at 30 months) Psychosocial	Language, independence	Interaction with peers, discipline, toilet training, book sharing	ASQ SE, TABS, BITSEA, Eyberg (if indicated), MCHAT
30 mo (or 36 mo)	ASQ, PEDS (if not at 30 mo)	Communication, social skills	Book sharing	ASQ SE, etc., if indicated
48 mo	ASQ, PEDS	School readiness, communication, social skills, early graphomotor	Book sharing	ASQ SE, TABS, Eyberg, PSC, if indicated
60 mo	ASQ, PEDS	Same as above	Same as above	Same as above
6 to 18 yr	PSC	Learning, peers, self-esteem	Building self-esteem, making good choices	ADHD, depression, anxiety screens

ADHD, Attention-deficit/hyperactivity disorder; *ASQ,* Ages and Stages Questionnaire; *BINS,* Bayley Infant Neurodevelopmental Scale; *BITSEA,* Brief Infant Toddler Social Emotional Assessment; *DV,* domestic violence; *IDI,* Infant Developmental Inventory; *MCHAT,* Modified Checklist for Autism in Toddlers; *MH,* mental health; *PEDS,* Parents' Evaluation of Developmental Status; *PSC,* Pediatric Symptom Checklist; *SA,* substance abuse; *SE,* social-emotional; *TABS,* Temperament and Atypical Behavior Scale.

developmental and behavioral disorders. However, the physician is a resource for referrals for further assessment and interventions, a partner in finding information, a sounding board, and a facilitator to negotiate the system. If a screen returns an at-risk score, then the primary care physician refers for more detailed assessment to confirm or rule out a diagnosis. The assessment is generally performed outside the practice (developmental and behavioral pediatrician, infant-toddler specialist, psychologist, speech and language pathologist, physical therapist). The primary care physician screens periodically, which is surveillance. Surveillance increases the sensitivity and accuracy of the assessment of the child's skills and progress.

The physician should review and discuss the screen with the parents at the time of the visit. The screen provides a template for anticipatory guidance, facilitates patient flow (by reducing *doorknob concerns* as the physician leaves the examination room), and improves patient and physician satisfaction.

Primary developmental and behavioral screens and psychosocial screening can be interwoven into the schedule of well-child visits and into the growing relationship with the family. One such schedule is highlighted in Table 44-3. Screens are included at times in the schedule in anticipation of critical turning points. However, these screens are meant to be flexible to respond to individual family concerns. For children who have been born prematurely, screens should be used according to adjusted age until age 2 years. In the schedule in Table 44-3, family psychosocial screening is performed at the 1st visit with the family and is really part of the history-taking process. It can then take place with any updating of history at later visits. Psychosocial screening can be interwoven into registration material when a family first comes to the practice, at visits when developmental screening questionnaires are not being used, and into the conversations between the physician and parents at any visit. Screening should be routine for all families, not targeted because of assumptions about risk. Parent-completed screens can be performed in the examination room while waiting for the physician or in the waiting room. Depending on the technology used by the practice and the resources of its families, some tools are available in an on-line version and can be completed by the family before the visit.

For children who screen at risk for social-emotional problems, effective social-emotional secondary screens are available to help the primary care physician in the medical home make decisions about referrals and types of interventions. The primary care practice may opt not to do secondary screening and to refer for further assessment when the primary screen indicates an at-risk area. Alternately, a secondary screen can be performed at a follow-up visit with the primary physician, by a care manager, or by a social worker in the practice. As an example, the Modified Checklist for Autism in Toddlers (MCHAT)[10] screens for risk of autism spectrum disorders and can be used if a child has indicators of risk on the communication portion of the primary screen.

Billing issues are an important aspect of screening. For screening tools, the American Medical Association *Current Procedural Terminology* code is 96110. It can be billed with a well-visit code or an evaluation and management code, and it has 0.36 relative value units.

CONCLUSIONS

Screening and surveillance need to be a regular part of well-child care because growth, development, and behavior are inextricably linked. Parent-completed tools include parents as experts; and when used from the beginning of the family-practice relationship, these tools provide the basis for the establishment of the medical home for the child and family. Creating collaborative relationships that link the family, the practice, and the community constitutes best practice.

TOOLS FOR PRACTICE

Community Coordination and Advocacy

- *Improving Developmental Screening Through Public Policy* (fact sheet), Margaret Dunkle (www.dbpeds.org).
- *Zero to Three* (Web page), Zero to Three (www.zerotothree.org/site/PageServer?pagename=homepage).

Practice Management and Care Coordination

- *Developmental Screening/Testing Coding Fact Sheet for Primary Care Pediatricians* (fact sheet), American Academy of Pediatrics (www.medicalhomeinfo.org/tools/Coding/Developmental Screening-Testing Coding Fact Sheet.doc).
- *Screening Implementation Worksheet* (questionnaire), ABCD project of the Commonwealth Fund (www.dbpeds.org).

Engaging Patient and Family

- *Developmental Screening* (fact sheet), Centers for Disease Control and Prevention (www.cdc.gov/ncbddd/autism/actearly/screening.html).
- *Interactive Developmental Checklists for Parents* (interactive tool), Centers for Disease Control and Prevention (www.cdc.gov/ncbddd/autism/actearly/interactive/index.html).
- *Is Your One-Year-Old Communicating with You?* (brochure), American Academy of Pediatrics (www.aap.org/bst/showdetl.cfm?&DID=15&Product_ID=4054).
- *Learn the Signs. Act Early. Materials for Waiting Room/Office* (other), Centers for Disease Control and Prevention (www.cdc.gov/ncbddd/autism/ActEarly/downloads_hcp.html).
- *The Wonder Years* (book), American Academy of Pediatrics (www.aap.org/bookstore).
- *Your Child's Growth: Developmental Milestones* (brochure), American Academy of Pediatrics (patiented.aap.org).

Medical Decision Support

- *Ages & Stages Questionnaire (ASQ)* (questionnaire), Diane Bricker, Ph.D., and Jane Squires, Ph.D., with assistance from Linda Mounts, M.A., LaWanda Potter, M.S., Robert Nickel, M.D., Elizabeth Twombly, M.S., and Jane Farrell, M.S. (www.brookespublishing.com/store/books/bricker-asq/index.htm).

- *Bayley Infant Neurodevelopmental Screener (BINS)* (questionnaire), The Psychological Corporation (harcourtassessment.com/HAIWEB/Cultures/en-us/Productdetail.htm?Pid=015-8028-708&Mode=summary).
- *Brigance* (questionnaire), Brigance A. N. Billerica (www.curriculumassociates.com/products/detail.asp?title=BrigScreensOverview&Type=SCH&CustId=9368528118006291612073).
- *Bright Futures: Guidelines for Health Supervision of Infants, Children, and Adolescents* (book), Bright Futures (brightfutures.aap.org/web/).
- *Bright Futures Toolkit* (toolkit), Bright Futures (brightfutures.aap.org/web/).
- *Commonly used screening tools* (fact sheet), Frances P. Glascoe, PhD (www.dbpeds.org).
- *Developmental and Behavioral Pediatrics Online* (Web page), American Academy of Pediatrics (www.dbpeds.org/).
- *Developmental Milestones* (fact sheet), Cynthia Dedrick, PhD (www.dbpeds.org).
- *First Signs* (Web page), First Signs (www.firstsigns.org/index.html).
- *From Neurons to Neighborhoods: The Science of Early Childhood Development,* (book), Shonkoff J, Phillips D, editors; National Research Council, Institute of Medicine, National Academy Press (www.nap.edu/books/0309069882/html).
- *Infant Developmental Inventory* (questionnaire), Harold Ireton (www.childdevelopmentreview.com/Samples/idi1-1.pdf).
- *Learn the Signs. Act Early* (Web page), Centers for Disease Control and Prevention (www.cdc.gov/ncbddd/autism/actearly).
- *Parent's Evaluation of Developmental Status (PEDS)* (questionnaire), Ellsworth & Vandermeer Press (pedstest.com/content.php?content=peds-intro.html).

RELATED WEB SITES

Commonwealth Fund (www.cmwf.org/).
National Academy for State Health Policy (www.nashp.org/_catdisp_page.cfm?LID=124).
National Center for Children in Poverty (www.nccp.org/).

SUPPLEMENTAL MATERIALS

Screening

American Academy of Pediatrics. Developmental Behavioral Pediatrics Online (www.dbpeds.org).
National Center for Infants, Toddlers and Families. Zero To Three® (www.zerotothree.org).
Centers for Disease Control and Prevention, National Center on Birth Defects and Developmental Disabilities. Learn the Signs. Act Early (www.cdc.gov/actearly).
National Center for Education in Maternal and Child Health and Georgetown University. Bright Futures (www.brightfutures.org).

Screening and Autism

First Signs, Inc. A Parent's Guide to the First Signs and Next Steps (www.firstsigns.org).

Successful Implementation

The Commonwealth Fund (www.cmwf.org).
National Academy for State Health Policy (www.nashp.org).

Children in Poverty

National Center for Children in Poverty (NCCP) (www.nccp.org).

SUGGESTED RESOURCES

Earls M, Hay S. Setting the stage for success: implementation of developmental and behavioral screening and surveillance in primary care practice, the North Carolina Assuring Better Child Health and Development (ABCD) Project. *Pediatrics*. 2006;118(1):e183-e188.
Shonkoff J, Phillips D, eds. *From Neurons to Neighborhoods: The Science of Early Childhood Development.* Washington, DC: National Research Council, Institute of Medicine, National Academy Press; 2000.

REFERENCES

1. Boyle CA, Decoufle P, Yeargin-Allsop MY. Prevalence and health impact of developmental disabilities. *Pediatrics.* 1994;93:863-865.
2. Squires J, Nickel R. Never too soon: identifying social emotional problems in infants and toddlers. *Contemp Pediatr.* 2003;3:117.
3. National Center for Health Statistics. QuickStats from the National Center for Health Statistics. *MMWR.* 2005;54(RR-34):852-853.
4. Palfrey JS, Singer JD, Walker DK, et al. Early identification of children's special needs: a study in five metropolitan communities. *J Pediatr.* 1987;111(5):651-659.
5. Squires J, Nickel RE, Eisert D. Early detection of developmental problems: strategies for monitoring young children in the practice setting. *J Dev Behav Pediatr.* 1996;17(6):420-427.
6. Search Institute. Available at: www.search-institute.org. Accessed April 10, 2007.
7. Kemper KJ, Kelleher KJ. Family psychosocial screening: instruments and techniques. *Ambul Child Health.* 1996;1:325-339.
8. Glascoe F. Early detection of developmental and behavioral problems. *Pediatr Rev.* 2000;21(8):272-279.
9. Glascoe FP, Dworkin PH. The role of parents in the detection of developmental and behavioral problems. *Pediatrics.* 1995;95(6):829-836.
10. Robins D, Fein D, Barton M, et al. The modified checklist for autism in toddlers: an initial study investigating the early detection of autism and pervasive developmental disorders. *J Autism Dev Disord.* 2001;31(2):131-144.

Chapter 45

LANGUAGE AND SPEECH ASSESSMENT

Hiram L. McDade, PhD; Elaine M. Frank, PhD

Each child who enters school is assumed to possess a well-developed system of spoken language skills. It is upon this system the foundation for social interaction and higher levels of communication is built. It is not uncommon for children who are slow to develop spoken words, whose speech is unintelligible at age 3 years, or who exhibit word-finding difficulties to be later identified in second or third grade as needing special assistance in reading, spelling, writing, and math. Actually, Johnny, who still was not talking at 2 years of age, or Billy, whose speech could not be understood at age 4 years of age, never outgrew their problems. They simply became manifested in other channels of language learning. The literature is compelling regarding the relationship between failure in reading and writing in the primary grades and a history of earlier communication difficulties. Children with early language problems are at an increased risk for later reading problems.[1-7] In a 5-year follow-up study of 3-year-old children, as many as 50% of those diagnosed as having preschool articulation or phonologic disorders were receiving some type of special education by the third grade.[8]

Because the age at which typical children achieve spoken language milestones varies the fundamental question confronting the health professional is this: "Is the child I am examining, who appears to be slow in speech or language development, simply at the low end of the normal continuum (and presumably will catch up without professional assistance), or is this a child who is at risk for later learning difficulties?" Speech-language pathologists, occupational therapists, and other early interventionists see these children only after problems are suspected and referrals are made. Nurses and primary care physicians, through regular well-baby checkups, immunizations, booster shots, and acute illnesses, are often the only trained professionals who monitor young children on a regular basis before school entry. Consequently this accessibility to young children carries with it a responsibility: making early and appropriate referrals to specific specialists trained to perform comprehensive evaluations.

SPEECH AND LANGUAGE DEVELOPMENT

Because the emergence of certain critical speech and language abilities follows a relatively stable timetable a child's communication competency may be assessed using a validated screener. The purpose of such screenings is not to diagnose but rather to identify children in need of further testing. Children who are identified as having a concern, either by parent report or by using a validated screener, should be referred for evaluation by a developmental specialist or a speech-language pathologist. Such a referral provides two benefits: (1) children found to be deficient in speech and language abilities are assured early intervention, and (2) children whose developmental status remains uncertain may be reassessed at appropriate intervals. For the latter group the evaluation provides objective baseline data that allow the examiner to measure the child's rate of progress over time. Delayed onset of language may be the first indication of more global developmental delays.

PRESPEECH DEVELOPMENT

Children develop communication skills long before the onset of first words. They wave *good-bye* months before saying "bye-bye," raise their hands to be held before saying "up," and shake their head before saying "no," among other developing skills. Within the first year of life the normally developing infant progresses from a purely reflexive newborn to a purposeful communicator. During this time, several preverbal *red flags* may be indicative of potential developmental problems. Examples include:

- Failure to smile or show joyful expressions by 6 months
- No reciprocal turn taking with sounds and facial expressions by 9 months
- No pointing or reaching to communicate by 12 months

Two valuable resources that provide guidance for evaluating preverbal infants include the American Academy of Pediatrics brochure, entitled "Is Your One-Year-Old Communicating With You?"[9] and the Firstsigns.org Web site,[10] which provides information on screening and referral processes.

LATE TALKERS

As a group, the terms *late talker* and *slow expressive language development* refers to children who have fewer than 50 spoken words and no word combinations by 24 months of age, with otherwise-normal receptive language, cognitive and social-emotional development, and adaptive behavior.[11-13] To date the research appears inconclusive regarding the longtem outcomes for late talkers, although some of the literature suggests that 40% to 50% of these children continue to exhibit expressive language delays throughout the preschool years, with 25% exhibiting problems well into elementary school.[14-17] Positive predictors of children who will outgrow their delayed speech are (1) age-appropriate development in receptive language, cognitive, and self-help skills; (2) no oral-motor concerns; (3) no social or interactive concerns; (4) appropriate play skills; and (5) no family history of speech-language disorders or learning disabilities.[18]

The emergence of two-word phrases is a significant milestone in language learning. During this stage the rudimentary rules of grammar are first evidenced. Normally developing children, as young as 18 months, begin producing two-word combinations. A child who has failed to achieve this milestone by 24 months of age is at risk for later language-based difficulties and should be referred for further testing.[5] To many parents the child's productions of *hot dog, choo-choo,* and *merry-go-round* represent word combinations when they are, in fact, simply learned labels of objects and thus considered single words. Asking, "Can you give me an example of some of your child's word combinations?" helps parents give a clearer picture of the child's language abilities (eg, common early two-word combinations include *no juice, what that, my cup,* and *look, kitty*).

PRESCHOOL SPEECH AND LANGUAGE DEVELOPMENT

By age 3 years, most children have a spoken vocabulary of more than 500 words. In addition, their grammatical skills have developed to the point at which they routinely speak in three- and four-word sentences. At this age, some of the basic rules of grammar are finely tuned. Plural, possessive, and past tense forms of words are emerging, and use of pronouns such as *I, me, you,* and *mine* is common. Three year olds demonstrate an appropriate understanding of *why?* questions, indicating an appreciation of cause and effect. Most important, the speech of a 3 year old is highly intelligible, and despite frequent mispronunciations, parents and most strangers have little difficulty understanding the child. In short, 3 year olds have the capacity to carry on a reasonable conversation with an adult.

The language of 4 year olds approaches adult competency with respect to grammatical skills. Unlike 2 and 3 year olds, 4 year olds speak in complete sentences. Rarely are words omitted from the four- and five-word sentences that these children typically produce. Although 4 year olds do not have as many different ways to say the same things as do older children, they usually have at least one way to express all thoughts and desires. The vocabulary of a 4 year old is also quite extensive. By this age, most children can recognize and name several colors, count to 10 by rote, understand the prepositions *in, on, under, beside, in front,* and *in back* (but not *behind* until age 5), and answer complex questions such as *how much? how long?* and *what if . . . ?* Three and 4 year olds are beginning to formulate questions using mature constructions, such as *is it broken?* By age 5, children have developed most of the language-based concepts that are important for schooling. They can sort and classify objects by category, name all the basic colors, and understand the concept of time, which allows them to answer *when* questions, and the concept of numbers up to 10 integers. The acquisition of individual speech sounds (with the exception of *th*) should be fully developed by age 5 years. Occasional mispronunciations may be heard, but these are usually restricted to sound blends (eg, *truck* and *sprinkle*) and difficult-to-pronounce, multisyllabic words.

INTELLIGIBILITY OF SPEECH

In the course of normal development, children commonly mispronounce certain sounds or have problems producing particular words that involve difficult sound combinations. The mastery of speech sounds is a gradual process that takes place over a period of 6 to 7 years. As children master various sounds and sound combinations, their speech becomes more adult like. An important point to keep in mind, however, is that regardless of the frequent errors in pronunciation the speech of young, normally developing children is easily understood by their caregivers. Parents who complain they cannot understand their child's speech suggests that the pattern of mispronunciation is so unusual and so unpredictable that it is not characteristic of normal mispronunciations. A related, but perhaps equally important, concern regarding speech intelligibility is the reaction of the child. Many children with unintelligible speech become so frustrated by their inability to communicate effectively with those around them that they cease talking and resort to gestures and pantomime to fulfill their communicative needs. Children with childhood apraxia of speech (CAS) often exhibit this complaint. CAS refers to the inability to program voluntary movements of the articulators in absence of paralysis, paresis, or incoordination.[7] Such children have often mastered only one or two speech sounds, exhibit groping while attempting to search for the correct tongue placement, and have great difficulty imitating simple words. Because of their frequent nonverbal nature, children with CAS are often misdiagnosed as having an expressive language disorder.

HEARING ASSESSMENT

Because normal speech and language development requires an intact auditory system, hearing screening is an integral part of any developmental evaluation. The Joint Committee on Infant Hearing has endorsed early detection of hearing loss and early intervention through a national program of universal newborn hearing screening.[19] This program, which has been adopted in many states, provides the opportunity for infants with significant hearing impairment early identification and intervention. Children who fail the neonatal hearing screening are given additional in-depth assessment, allowing intervention to begin in the first 3 to 4 months. Among toddlers and preschoolers, parental concern was identified by the National Institutes of Health Consensus Conference on Early Identification of Hearing Impairment (1993) as a significant factor in the identification of hearing impairment in 70% of children with hearing impairment.[20] Toddlers younger than age 3 may be difficult to screen and should be tested using physiological testing such as brainstem audiometry and tympanometry, Screening stimuli that do not have calibrated levels or frequency information or that rely on behavioral observation are not recommended (ie, rattles, music toys, other noisemakers). For children ages 3 to 5, play audiometry and tympanometry may be helpful. In the play audiometry technique, children are trained to provide an operant response to a sound that establishes an estimate of hearing acuity. Among school-aged children, the American Speech-Language-Hearing Association *Guidelines for Audiology Screening* (1997) recommend hearing screening on the initial entry into school (kindergarten) and annually through the third grade, with repeat testing in the seventh and eleventh grades. These screening tests should be completed at 20 dB for 1000, 2000, and 4000 Hz under earphones.[21]

Any child with a speech and language delay should have a hearing screening using the age-appropriate method, tympanometry, and an otolgic evaluation. Sensorineural hearing losses in children should be identified as early as possible to reduce the effect of hearing loss on speech and language development. An important study on language development in hearing-impaired children concluded that those who received appropriate amplification and intervention before 6 months of age had significantly better language scores than those receiving intervention after 6 months.[22] For the mild and moderately hearing-impaired infant, traditional hearing amplification and aural habilitation is provided by audiologists and speech-language pathologists. Options for severely impaired infants and children may include referral for consideration of cochlear implant surgery and specialized aural habilitation postoperatively. Families who strongly identify with deaf culture may rightfully not choose this option for their infants and young children.

ACQUIRED SPEECH AND LANGUAGE DISORDERS IN CHILDREN

Acquired communication disorders can be secondary to stroke, seizure disorder, meningitis, or other diseases, but the majority of childhood-acquired speech and language disorders are a result of brain trauma. The incidence of hospitalization from trauma is between 150,000 and 200,000 children each year.[23] Causes of injury are falls, bicycle accidents, child abuse, and motor-vehicle accidents. Open-head injuries from gunshot wounds have increased among children and adolescents.[24] Among children who have a traumatic brain injury (TBI), studies have reported a high rate of risk-taking behavior, limited judgment, and learning problems. Factors influencing the recovery pattern of cognition and language in children include the severity, volume, and location of the injury and the age of the child at the time of injury.[24] A brain injury often interferes with acquisition of new knowledge and skills; therefore older children have the advantage of greater knowledge acquired before the brain injury, whereas younger children must gain more new knowledge and skills with a brain developing with injured areas.[23]

TBI can result in a focal or, more often, a diffuse brain injury. The TBI sequelae often include speech, language, communication disorders, and swallowing problems. The language problems may include:

- Disorganized, tangential, wandering discourse
- Imprecise language
- Word-retrieval difficulties
- Disinhibited, socially inappropriate language, with ineffective use of contextual cues
- Restricted output and lack of initiation
- Difficulty comprehending extended language in spoken or written form and detecting main ideas
- Difficulty understanding abstract language, including indirect or implied meaning
- Inefficient verbal learning caused by reduced memory ability

Because these problems are different from the grammatical difficulties typical of children who have developmental problems, they are frequently misunderstood and not seen as being symptomatic of a language disorder. Speech disturbances can include apraxic speech, characterized by difficulty initiating and programming speech, or dysarthric speech resulting from paralysis or paresis of oral or pharyngeal musculature. This muscle weakness may contribute to a secondary swallowing or dysphagic disorder.

Standardized testing may not be sensitive to the social communication and language effects of TBI. Insightful clinical evaluation of speech and language function is essential in determining the need for rehabilitative or specialized educational intervention. Although a positive correlation between initial indices of severity (including the Glasgow coma scale and the length of coma) and the long-term outcome is relatively strong, individual outcomes may vary. Children who have a mild head injury and only a short-term loss of consciousness may require minimal medical intervention but may still experience interruption in normal cognitive functioning. Behavioral changes, including easy fatigability, inconsistent performance, and slow processing, are often evident. Children who have a more severe head injury may require intensive speech and language inpatient rehabilitation and outpatient follow-up. The pediatrician or school personnel should refer these children for an individual education program through the school district. Because the consequences of speech, language, and related cognitive function are often difficult to identify through screening procedures, children with a TBI should be referred for a speech-language-cognitive assessment if any memory, learning, comprehension, or attention problems are reported.

Therapeutic intervention goals may be rehabilitative or compensatory. Rehabilitation of attention, awareness, perception, memory, learning, organization, social cognition, problem solving, and general executive system functioning are necessary for cognitive processing and language functioning. Compensatory techniques may include memory devices, organizational patterning, or referent cues. Stimulating speech programming and muscular strengthening may improve oral communication, or compensatory techniques may be required in the form of augmentative communicative devices (eg, communication boards, computerized speech). Successful educational reentry for children who have a TBI should include assistance in school programming and in-service for family, teachers, other school personnel, and the child's peers. Children whose TBI is significant will need continued monitoring through successive developmental stages to achieve maximal functional ability and academic success.

WHEN TO REFER

- No smile or joyful expression by 6 months
- No reciprocal turn taking, with sounds and facial expressions by 9 months
- No babbling, pointing, or gestures by 12 months
- No spoken words by 15 months
- No two-word combinations by 24 months
- Inability of parents to understand their child's speech at 30 months
- Continued poor intelligibility at 36 months of age
- Difficulty answering *wh* questions by 48 months of age
- Poor ability to associate letters with their sounds by the end of kindergarten
- Parents voice concern about their child's hearing, speech, or language
- Any regression in speech, language, or social skills at any age

TOOLS FOR PRACTICE

Engaging Patient and Family

- *Building Speech and Language Skills* (fact sheet), Kathleen E. Mahn MS, CCC-SLP (www.dbpeds.org/articles/detail.cfm?TextID=%20275).
- *Is Your One-Year-Old Communicating with You?* (brochure), American Academy of Pediatrics (patiented.aap.org/).

AAP POLICY STATEMENTS

American Academy of Pediatrics, Council on Children With Disabilities, Section on Developmental Behavioral Pediatrics; Bright Futures Steering Committee and Medical Home Initiatives for Children With Special Needs Project Advisory Committee. Identifying infants and young children with developmental disorders in the medical home: an algorithm for developmental surveillance and screening. *Pediatrics*. 2006;118(1):405-420. (aappolicy.aappublications.org/cgi/content/full/pediatrics;118/1/405).

American Academy of Pediatrics, Joint Committee on Infant Hearing. Year 2007 position statement. Principles and guidelines for early hearing detection and intervention programs. *Pediatrics*. 2007;120(4):898-921. (aappolicy.aappublications.org/cgi/content/full/pediatrics;120/4/898).

RELATED WEB SITES

American Speech-Language-Hearing Association (www.asha.org/default.htm).

First Signs (firstsigns.org).

REFERENCES

1. Aram DM, Ekelman BL, Nation JE. Preschoolers with language disorders: 10 years later. *J Speech Hear Res*. 1984;27:232-244.
2. Silva P, Williams S, McGee R. A longitudinal study of children with developmental language delay at age three: later intelligence, reading and behavior problems. *Dev Med Child Neurol*. 1987;29:630-640.
3. Botting N, Simkin Z, Conti-Ramsden G. Associated reading skills in children with a history of specific language impairment (SLI). *Reading Writing*. 2006;19:77-98.
4. Catts HW. Speech production deficits and reading disabilities. *J Speech Hear Disord*. 1989;54:422-428.
5. Catts HW, Fey MD, Zhang X, et al. Language bases of reading and reading disabilities: evidence from a longitudinal investigation. *Scientific Studies of Reading*. 1999;3:331-362.
6. Stothard SE, Snowling MJ, Bishop DVM, et al. Language-impaired preschoolers: a follow-up into adolescence. *J Speech Language Hear Res*. 1998:41:407-418.
7. Snowling MJ, Bishop DVM, Stothard SE. Is preschool language impairment a risk factor for dyslexia in adolescence? *J Child Psychol Psychiatry*. 2000;41:587-600.
8. Zimmerman D, McDade H, Montgomery A. The relationship between preschool speech problems and later school performance. *ASHA Leader*. 1998;3:108.
9. American Academy of Pediatrics. Is your one year old communicating with you? Available at: patiented.aap.org. Accessed August 15, 2007.
10. First Signs, Inc. Red Flags. Available at: www.firstsigns.org/concerns/flags.htm. Accessed August 15, 2007.
11. Agin MC, Geng L, Nichol M. *The Late Talker*. New York, NY: St Martin's Press; 2003.
12. Agin MC. The "late talker"—when silence isn't golden. *Contemp Pediatr*. 2004;21:22-32.
13. Paul R. Clinical implications of the natural history of slow expressive language development. *Am J Speech-Language Pathol*. 1996;5:5-22.
14. Scarborough HS. Very early language deficits in dyslexic children. *Child Dev*. 1990;61:1728-1743.
15. Berko Gleason J. *The Development of Language*. 6th ed. Boston, MA: Allyn & Bacon; 2004.
16. Rescorla L, Roberts J, Dahlsgaard K. Late talkers at two: outcome at age 3. *J Speech Hear Res*. 1997;40:556-566.
17. Rescorla L. Do late-talking toddlers turn out to have reading difficulties a decade later? *Ann Dyslexia*. 2000; 50:87-102.
18. Paul R. Profiles of toddlers with slow expressive language development. *Top Language Dev*. 1991;11:1-13.
19. American Academy of Pediatrics, Joint Committee on Infant Hearing. Year 2000 position statement: principles and guidelines for early hearing detection and intervention program. *Audiology Today*. 2000;12(special issue): 7-27.
20. National Institute on Deafness and Other Communication Disorders. *National Institutes of Health Consensus Statement. Early Identification of Hearing Impairment in Infants and Young Children*. Rockville, MD: National Institute of Health; 1993.
21. American Speech-Language-Hearing Association. *Guidelines for Audiologic Screening: Panel on Audiologic Assessment*. Rockville, MD: American Speech-Language-Hearing Association; 1997.
22. Yoshinaga-Itano C, Sedey AL, Coulter DK, et al. Language of early- and later-identified children with hearing loss. *Pediatrics*. 1998;102:1161-1171.
23. Sohlberg MM, Mateer CA. *Cognitive Rehabilitation: An Integrative Neuropsychological Approach*. New York, NY: Guilford Press; 2001.
24. Murdoch BE, Theodoros DG, eds. *Traumatic Brain Injury: Associated Speech, Language, and Swallowing Disorders*. San Diego, CA: Singular Thomson Learning; 2001.

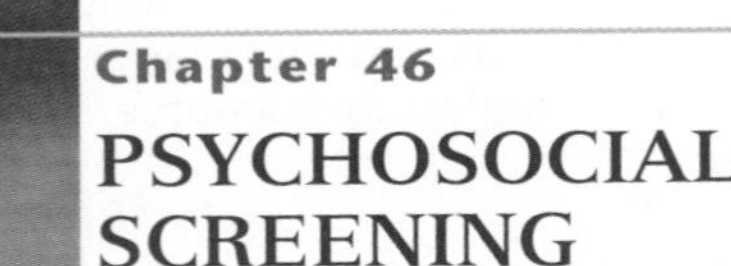

Chapter 46

PSYCHOSOCIAL SCREENING

Steven C. Schlozman, MD; Michael S. Jellinek, MD

NEED FOR PSYCHOSOCIAL SCREENING

Prevalence of Psychosocial Dysfunction

Between 5% and 20% of American children[1-3] suffer from psychosocial difficulties that include significant functional impairments and psychiatric disorders defined by the fourth edition of the *Diagnostic Statistical Manual of Mental Disorders* (DSM-IV) and the text revision edition (DSM-IV-TR). In addition a significant number of children and adolescents consider suicide. Childhood psychiatric disorders are estimated to increase by 50% by the year 2020.[4]

Psychiatric diagnoses do not always take into account important developmental and functional assessments. For example, family discord may lead to school phobia or oppositionality in young children and to depression and substance abuse in adolescents. A more holistic nosologic discussion is available through the *Diagnostic and Statistical Manual of*

Mental Disorders, Primary Care Version (DSM-IV-PC), a manual defining psychosocial issues within a developmental context.[5]

The DSM-IV-PC discusses a broad range of problems, some of which are consistent with formal psychiatric diagnoses and many issues that are clinically relevant in spite of not meeting full DSM-IV criteria. Dysfunction is grouped into three main categories: (1) normal variation, (2) problems, and (3) disorders. Normal variation allows for different temperaments, personalities, and developmental paths among healthy children. Problems refer to a broad range of issues that may not meet formal criteria for a discrete psychiatric disorder. For example, the DSM-IV-PC recognizes that although a child's anxious reaction to divorce may be a normal and expected developmental response the child might still be in need of support and services during this difficult time. Finally, disorders refer to specific conditions that meet the DSM-IV criteria for a psychiatric disorder.

Secondary Consequences of Psychosocial Issues

Beyond mental health concerns, psychosocial issues in primary care have multiple secondary consequences. Psychosocial dysfunction is a major risk factor for unintentional injuries, the most common cause of death in children. Fires, falls from windows, drowning, and motor-vehicle accidents are more common among children who have higher rates of psychosocial stressors.[6-8] Detection of these broader stressors is challenging, given that DSM-IV diagnoses generally do not take into account developmental expectations and corresponding functional assessments. Thus the pediatrician is served best by broadly screening for psychosocial dysfunction rather than focusing exclusively on psychiatric diagnoses.

Barriers to Detecting Psychosocial Difficulties

Despite a high prevalence of psychosocial difficulties encountered by children and adolescents the majority of these problems are not detected by primary care physicians.[9-14] Possible reasons for this lack of recognition include time limitations, hesitancy among practitioners to attach possibly stigmatizing labels to children, the absence of widely available and easily implemented screening procedures, lack of adequate training regarding psychosocial issues, and limited resources for referral and treatment. Additionally, some evidence suggests that primary care physicians may offer discouraging reactions to the presentation of psychosocial difficulties in their practice.[15] The theoretical benefits of managed care with its preventive focus and consistent quality-assurance activities to improve care processes are being overshadowed by pressures of productivity that have decreased the number of minutes per patient and by barriers to referral. In many communities the medical referral relationship between primary care and pediatric subspecialists does not extend to mental health clinicians because of insurance barriers. However, in principle, managed care should encourage referral by emphasizing screening and quality and, perhaps, lower costs over time.

Reasons to Screen for Psychosocial Dysfunction

The clear epidemiologic burden of psychosocial challenges facing children and adolescents in the context of limited specialty care demands that primary care physicians play an active role in the detection and treatment of this multidimensional issue. The nature of pediatric practice has changed with the decreasing burden of infectious disease and the growing need to address psychosocial issues ranging from psychiatric disorders to psychosocial impact of chronic illnesses and injury prevention. Because psychosocial challenges are heterogeneous in nature, and because the average primary care visit includes limited time and increasing psychosocial demands, screening practices routinely with structured instruments hold the most promise for accurate detection of significant difficulties in the primary care setting.

Goals of Psychosocial Screening

Obtaining a comprehensive psychosocial history is time consuming and inefficient. Some children's psychosocial issues are recognized because of parental complaints of overt behavioral problems or because of school referral. Less obvious problems, such as dysfunction stemming from divorce or depression, are often identified in the primary care setting. The goal of psychosocial screening is to provide screening methods in harmony with pediatric primary care for early, efficient, and effective recognition of developing psychosocial problems.

STRATEGIES TO INCREASE RECOGNITION OF PSYCHOSOCIAL DYSFUNCTION

Interviewing

Careful attention to developmental aspects of the child's life, such as the child's family, friends, school, play, and mood, will help the pediatrician assess the child's overall function.[16] Despite the obvious time involved, face-to-face interviewing, in which high-risk issues are discussed with the patient and parents, offers many advantages. The physician can address key issues directly, communicating to the family the importance of psychosocial issues, thus increasing the likelihood that the family will consider these issues appropriate to bring to the physician's attention.

Raising questions face to face builds trust; examples of clinically relevant questions are available through the American Academy of Pediatrics *Guidelines for Health Supervision* and the *Bright Futures* manuals and are easily accessible on line at brightfutures.aap.org/.[17] Topics mentioned in both documents include instructions such as the following:

- At intake, ask all parents for a family history of psychiatric disorder (eg, depression, substance use). A family history of depression, anxiety, substance use, and attention-deficit/hyperactivity disorder (ADHD) places the child at high risk.

- At annual visits, ask about parental discord and marital stability.
- For newborns, assess parental coping, family support, and maternal depression. A depressed mother has a profound emotional and cognitive impact on an infant, and given the very good response to treatment the pediatrician can do a real service to the family and the baby by early intervention.
- For toddlers, ask about the child's autonomy and the ability to *separate*.
- For early school-aged children, ask about social functioning.
- For adolescents, ask parents about their child's autonomy, and ask the adolescent about mood and substance use.

Screening Tools

Parent Questionnaires

Because of the time constraints inherent in a face-to-face approach, alternative strategies have been developed to screen more efficiently for psychosocial difficulties. Ideally these tools are used to supplement face-to-face time. The Achenbach Child Behavior Checklist (CBCL) is the most-studied and best-validated behavioral screening device available for children ages 4 to 16 years.[18] The Achenbach CBCL is completed by the child's parents and is divided into two distinct item groups: (1) behavior problems and (2) school competency. Although the results of the Achenbach CBCL are reliable and valid the main drawbacks to the use of this instrument include length of administration (more than 100 items requiring approximately 20 minutes of the parents' time) and some complexity in methods for scoring and interpreting the results of the questionnaire.

A possible and less cumbersome alternative to the Achenbach CBCL is the Pediatric Symptom Checklist (PSC), a 35-item survey also given to the parents and requiring only a few minutes to complete.[16,19] In addition, the results of the PSC can be scored quickly, with 2 points assigned to each question answered "often," 1 point assigned to each answered "sometimes," and 0 points assigned to each answered "never." Administration and scoring commonly take 3 to 5 minutes. A score greater than 28 suggests a 70% likelihood that the child has significant psychosocial difficulties; scores less than 28 suggest a greater than 95% likelihood that the child has no substantial psychosocial problems. Thus, if the parents complete the PSC in the waiting room and have it scored by a receptionist or clinical assistant, then the pediatrician can quickly recognize and more closely evaluate significant psychosocial issues.

However, although the PSC works well in adolescent populations, it is somewhat hampered in this age group by the parents' limitations in correctly assessing, through a questionnaire, their child's intrapsychic state. Specifically, some parents will not know that their child is depressed because the child appears to be in reasonable spirits and functioning well; thus the PSC will, in this circumstance, yield a false-negative result. Despite this difficulty, because the PSC primarily assesses function, it still yields efficient and important information that can direct further inquiry.[20]

A relatively new screening device is the Strength and Difficulties Questionnaire.[21,22] This instrument includes 25 items that assess specifically for emotional difficulties; problems with conduct, hyperactivity, and inattention; peer relationship indicators; and prosocial behavior. This screening tool is completed by parents and teachers of children ages 4 to 16 years, and additional versions exist for assessing younger children. The Strength and Difficulties Questionnaire is similar to the PSC but is perhaps slightly more complicated to score.

Patient Questionnaires

For young children the Human Figure Drawing Screening Device has been found useful in elucidating occult anxiety and depression in some children.[23]

The issue of identifying the adequately functioning but depressed teenager can be addressed in several ways. Columbia University has started a nationwide program called Teenscreen.[24] This program helps schools and health care providers construct different means by which adolescents can be screened for depression, as well as suicidality. Interestingly, some political opposition exists to this program, with several political groups suggesting that not all Americans are in favor of screening children for psychiatric difficulties. A more traditional approach involves use of the Beck Depression Inventory, completed by the adolescent at the time of the primary care visit. Twenty percent or more of teenagers have scores that raise concerns using this screening instrument.[25,26]

Specific Screening

Some pediatric practices have gone beyond general psychosocial and depression screening to help identify children with Asperger syndrome or autism, using the Modified Checklist for Autism in Toddlers (M-CHAT),[27,28] the Parents Evaluation of Developmental Status[29,30] (PEDS), and screening for adolescent substance use.[31,32] Offering critiques or endorsements of every screening device available is not the goal of this chapter. All of the methods discussed have utility, and clinicians must choose an instrument that best addresses their practice, level of interest, and their patient population.

Assessing Severity of Psychosocial Dysfunction

When psychosocial issues are identified through screening or clinical interview, patients should be assessed for the severity of the impairment in functioning. Although conditions such as psychosis or serious suicidal ideation are clearly severe, other problems, such as depression or anxiety, are quite variable in their severity. Not all cases of depression, for example, need specialized treatment, although some depressed children require an aggressive and multimodal approach and even hospitalization.

An assessment of severity includes the following three items[33]:

1. *Symptoms:* number, frequency, duration, and places where the symptoms are experienced
2. *Functioning:* developmental impact on functioning in key areas such as family, friends, school, activities, and self-esteem

3. *Burden of suffering:* intensity of suffering, duration, limitations on family activities, danger to self and others, and intrusion into developmental tasks or daily activities

FACTORS AFFECTING PSYCHOSOCIAL HEALTH

In the process of screening and assessment for psychosocial health, understanding risk factors that may be associated with future problems is also important. Several biological and environmental factors may be protective against the risk of adversity leading to serious psychosocial problems. Table 46-1 outlines both protective and risk factors for psychosocial difficulties.[33] The number of moderate risk factors can have a cumulative effect on a child's dysfunction, greater than any one severe risk factor. Children facing three or more risk factors have a very high likelihood of psychosocial problems.[16] Individual risk factors that have special significance include single-parent households and poverty.[16]

In fact the issue of poverty deserves special mention. Although numerous studies have connected low social-economic status with increased risk of psychosocial dysfunction,[28,34-37] research suggests that pediatricians tend to address a larger proportion of psychosocial concerns in highly educated families than in less-educated families. One potential explanation for this discrepancy is that more-educated parents might feel more comfortable bringing psychosocial issues to their pediatrician's attention, whereas less-educated parents might not realize that the pediatrician's office is appropriate for psychosocial inquiries. In addition, some studies have shown that middle- to upper-class parents tend to overreport their children's psychosocial problems, whereas lower-class parents tend to underreport. A recently posited alternative explanation for why poverty is a risk factor includes the possibility that some mothers are more likely to ask the community for support with their child's psychosocial difficulties. This practice may be more prevalent in lower-income families.[38] All of these findings demonstrate the need for a thorough and systematic review of psychosocial issues in all patients within a pediatric practice.

BRIEF EVALUATION

Many psychosocial problems will be elucidated through focused interviewing or using different screening instruments. For best results, clinicians should be relatively consistent with their screening instruments, familiarizing themselves with one instrument with which they and their colleagues are most comfortable. In addition, patients might have a definite psychosocial complaint, often mentioned by parents or school personnel. At this point the clinician should attempt to elaborate the symptoms, further defining the nature of the complaint. Risk factors and developmental concerns should be considered, and the child's daily functioning should be examined. Several guidelines will be helpful in this process.[33]

1. For younger children, observe them while directing questions to the parents.
2. For school-aged children, use confirmatory questions, if possible, without parents being present.
3. For adolescents, perform a separate interview with the patient alone. Assess important issues such as substance use and depression. Inquire about sexual activity. Consider parental functioning, especially abuse, depression, and substance use.

Table 46-1 Children's Well Being: Risk and Protective Factors

CATEGORY	PROTECTIVE FACTORS THAT DECREASE THE IMPACT OF STRESS	RISK FACTORS THAT INCREASE THE IMPACT OF STRESS
Health	Good health	Chronic disease, ill health
Temperament	Example, pleasant mood	Example, negative mood, irritable
Cognitive status	Normal IQ (particularly verbal)	Learning disability or low IQ
Emotional health	Good mental health function	Preexisting emotional disorder
Sociability	Good peer relations	Poor peer relations
Child reaction to stress	Perceives stress as limited; does not blame self	Perceives continued threat; blames self
Quality of attachment	High quality, high continuity; securely attached	Low quality, discontinuous; ambivalent, insecurely attached
Parent competence	Competent	Incompetent
Family resources	Adequate economic resources	Poverty or discrimination
Quality, stability, safety of environment	Adequate, stable, safe	Inadequate, unstable, unsafe
Family relationships	Good communication; little conflict	Poor communication; excessive conflict
Emotional and physical health of caregivers	Caregivers in good emotional and physical health	Mental illness or physical illness in caregivers
Availability or access to community resources	High access	Low access

4. Review relevant risk factors and potentially protective factors.
5. Assess safety, paying special attention to potential accidents, suicidal ideation, and risk-taking behaviors.
6. Complete a severity estimate using the Achenbach CBCL and the PSC formats, ranking the current issue as mild, moderate, or severe.

Once information is gathered the presenting complaint should be categorized as either a normal variation that requires no further action or a problem that requires special consideration. Many issues can be addressed at the primary care level, often with co-management by mental health professionals or school personnel. Other more serious problems require outside referral for evaluation by a specialist and, possibly, ongoing treatment. The most severe cases often require emergency referral.

THE FUTURE IS NOT QUITE HERE

The future of psychosocial screening is ripe with promise. Perhaps the most exciting aspect concerns the possible use of genetic screening to subtype risk factors for psychosocial difficulties and to predict treatment response. For example, Caspi[39,40] and colleagues reported an autosomal recessive genotype of the serotonin transporter gene that is strongly correlated with the propensity to develop depression after a negative life event. Patients who were heterozygous or autosomal dominant appeared significantly less at risk for psychosocial difficulties after difficult events. Importantly, however, the technology and the understanding of these and similar findings are not yet applicable to routine practice; rather, they represent important directions of future inquiries. Similarly, numerous organizations suggest that sophisticated neuroimaging assays and the use of electroencephalographic evaluations have the capacity to predict the onset of psychosocial problems. The current standard of care and the state of the research concerning these techniques suggest that the information gleaned from these evaluations is no better than a careful clinical evaluation. For this reason, at this point little practical stock can be placed in these tests, but they do hold great promise for the future.

CHANGING PRACTICE ENVIRONMENT AND NEXT STEPS

Although the epidemiology of pediatric practice has shifted dramatically from infectious disease to immunologic and psychosocial concerns, the changes in reimbursement secondary to managed care constraints have made psychosocial screening and referral for appropriate treatment increasingly difficult. For the majority of children in the United States, mental health services are carved out of pediatric care, with financial incentives that discourage referral and comprehensive treatment.[41] These carved-out companies limit the role of psychiatrists primarily to medication management, creating an environment increasingly overemphasizing psychotropic medication at the expense of both comprehensive and alternative treatments.[1,30,41,42] Furthermore, capitation may be an additional disincentive to referral to specialty services.

However, innovative practices may be able to provide more children with adequate treatment in spite of the current health care insurance climate.

General psychosocial screening usually results in a substantial increase in recognition and an increase in referral rate from the 1% to 2% range to 4%. Many practices in the not-too-distant future will set up electronic questionnaires on tablets in the waiting room or from home through the Internet. Built-in screening tests can be determined by the child's age and risk factors. For example, a family history of ADHD or a cluster of positive answers to school dysfunction questions may elicit, through internal logic, an ADHD screening questionnaire. Given the prevalence of disorders, some pediatricians already have mental health professionals in their practices to provide follow-up to screening, consultation, and ongoing services. The idea of the office social worker being at the hub of referral services, providing individual family and group treatment in the pediatric office setting, can be easily imagined. These groups might include preventive efforts regarding recent divorce, ongoing support for parents raising children with ADHD, or treatment for adolescents using substances or dealing with depression. Depending on the local reimbursement climate, screening, evaluation, and in-office services may be covered and self-sustaining.

Addressing a child psychosocial development and dysfunction is among the highest priorities for parents who experience their child's emotional suffering on a daily basis. To this end the primary care pediatric office, with adequate reimbursement, is in an ideal setting to provide crucial screening and to initiate important treatments.

TOOLS FOR PRACTICE

- *Achenbach Child Behavior Checklist* (checklist), Achenbach T (www.aseba.org/products/forms.html).
- *Bright Futures: Guidelines for Health Supervision of Infants, Children, and Adolescents* (book), Bright Futures (brightfutures.aap.org/web/).
- *CRAFFT: A Brief Screening Test for Adolescent Substance Abuse* (questionnaire), Knight JR and associates, Children's Hospital Boston (www.slp3d2.com/rwj_1027/webcast/docs/screentest.html).
- *Modified Checklist for Autism in Toddlers (M-CHAT)* (checklist), Robins DL, Fein D, Barton ML, Green JA (www.utmem.edu/pediatrics/general/clinical/m-chat.pdf).
- *Parents Evaluation of Developmental Status (PEDS)* (questionnaire) Glascoe FP (pedstest.com/index.php).
- *Pediatric Symptom Checklist* (checklist), Jellinek M, Murphy JM (psc.partners.org/psc_home.htm).
- *Strength and Difficulties Questionnaire* (questionnaire), Goodman R (www.sdqinfo.com/).
- *Surgeon General's Conference on Children's Mental Health* (www.hhs.gov/surgeongeneral/topics/cmh/childreport.htm).

- *TeenScreen Program*, Columbia University (www.teenscreen.org/).
- *The Classification of Child and Adolescent Mental Diagnoses in Primary Care* (book), Wolraich ML and The Task Force on Coding for Mental Health in Children (www.aap.org/bookstore).

SUGGESTED RESOURCES

Hagan JF, Shaw JS, Duncan PM, eds. *Bright Futures: Guidelines for Health Supervision of Infants, Children, and Adolescents*, 3rd ed. Elk Grove Village, IL: American Academy of Pediatrics; 2008.

Jellinek M, Little M. Supporting child psychiatric services using current managed care approaches: you can't get there from here. *Arch Pediatr Adolesc Med.* 1998;152:321-326.

Jellinek M, Patel BP, Froehle MC, eds. *Bright Futures in Practice: Mental Health—Volume 1, Practice Guide*. Arlington, VA: National Center for Education in Maternal and Child Health; 2001.

Jellinek M, Patel BP, Froehle MC, eds. *Bright Futures in Practice: Mental Health—Volume 2, Tool Kit*. Arlington, VA: National Center for Education in Maternal and Child Health; 2001.

Jellinek MS. Approach to the behavioral problems in children and adolescents. In: Stern TA, Herman JB, Slavin PL, eds. *The MGH Guide to Psychiatry in Primary Care*. New York, NY: McGraw-Hill; 1997.

Massachusetts General Hospital: *The Pediatric Symptom Checklist (PSC)* (Web site), psc.partners.org. Accessed September 28, 2007.

Murphy JM, Arett HL, Bishop SJ, et al. Screening for psychosocial dysfunction in pediatric practice: a naturalistic study of the Pediatric Symptom Checklist. *Clin Pediatr.* 1992;31:660-667.

US Department of Health and Human Services, Office of the Surgeon General. *Report of the Surgeon General's Conference on Children's Mental Health*. Washington, DC: US Goverment Printing Office; 1999.

REFERENCES

1. Office of Technology Assessment. *Children's Mental Health: Problems and Services: A Background Paper.* Washington, DC: Office of Technology Assessment; 1986. Available at: www.wws.princeton.edu/ota/ns20/alpha_f.html. Accessed August 2, 2007.
2. Pincus HA, Tanielian TL, Marcus SC, et al. Prescribing trends in psychotropic medications: primary care, psychiatry, and other medical specialties. *JAMA.* 1998;279:526-531.
3. Gould MS, Wunsch-Hitzig R, Dobrenwend B. Estimating the prevalence of childhood psychopathology: a critical review. *J Am Acad Child Psychiatry.* 1991;20:526-531.
4. US Department of Health and Human Services, Office of the Surgeon General. *Report of the Surgeon General's Conference on Children's Mental Health*. Washington, DC: US Goverment Printing Office; 1999. Available at: www.surgeongeneral.gov/topics/cmh/childreport.htm#vis. Accessed August 2, 2007.
5. Woiraich ML, ed. *The Classification of Child and Adolescent Mental Diagnoses in Primary Care: Diagnostic and Statistical Manual for Primary Care (DSM-IV-PC) Child and Adolescent Version*. Elk Grove Village, IL: American Academy of Pediatrics; 1996.
6. Bijur PE, Stewart-Brown S, Butler N. Child behavior and accidental injury in 11,966 preschool children. *Am J Dis Child.* 1986;140:487-492.
7. Kemp A, Silbert J. Childhood accidents: epidemiology, trends and prevention, *J Accident Emerg Med.* 1997;14:316-320.
8. Larrison JO, Aurelius G. Accidents in childhood: relation to psychosocial conditions and mental development. *Acta Paediatr.* 1996;85:285-291.
9. Bishop SJ, Murphy JM, Jellinek MS, et al. Psychosocial screening in pediatric practice: a survey of interested physicians. *Clin Pediatr* (Phila). 1991;30:142-147.
10. Costello EJ. Primary care pediatrics and child psychopathology: a review of diagnostic, treatment, and referral practices, *Pediatrics.* 1986;78:1044-1051.
11. Glascoe FP, Toward A. Model for and evidence-based approach to developmental/behavioral surveillance. Promotion and patient education. *Ambul Child Health.* 1999;5:197-208.
12. Costello EJ, Janiszewski S. Who gets treated? Factors associated with referral in children with psychiatric disorders. *Acta Psychiatr Scand.* 1990;18:523-529.
13. Sharp L, Pantell RH, Murphy LO, et al. Psychosocial problems during child health supervision visits: eliciting, then what? *Pediatrics.* 1992;89:619-623.
14. Starfield B. Behavioral pediatrics and primary health care. *Pediatr Clin North Am.* 1982;29:377-390.
15. Wissow LS, Larsen S, Anderson J, et al. Pediatric responses that discourage discussion of psychosocial problems in primary care. *Pediatrics.* 2005;115:1569-1578.
16. Jellinek M, Little M, Murphy JM, et al. The Pediatric Symptom Checklist: support for a role in a managed care environment. *Arch Pediatr Adolesc Med.* 1995;149:740-746.
17. Hagan JF, Shaw JS, Duncan PM, eds. *Bright Futures: Guidelines for Health Supervision of Infants, Children, and Adolescents,* Third Edition. Elk Grove Village, IL: American Academy of Pediatrics; 2008.
18. Achenbach TM. *Manual for the Child Behavior Checklist/4-18 and 1991 Profile*. Burlington, VT: University of Vermont Department of Psychiatry; 1991.
19. Jellinek MS, Murphy JM, Pagano ME, et al. Use of the Pediatric Symptom Checklist to screen for psychosocial problems in pediatric primary care: a national feasibility study. *Arch Pediatr Adolesc Med.* 1999;153:254-260.
20. Duke N, Ireland M, Borowsky IW. Identifying psychosocial problems among youth: factors associated with youth agreement on a positive parent-completed PSC-17. *Child Care Health Dev.* 2005;31:563-573.
21. Goodman R. The Strengths and Difficulties Questionnaire: a research note. *J Child Psychol Psychiatry.* 1997;38:581-586.
22. Goodman R. The extended version of the Strengths and Difficulties Questionnaire as a guide to child psychiatric caseness and consequent burden. *J Child Psychol Psychiatry.* 1999;40:791-799.
23. Tielsch AH, Allen PJ. Listen to the draw: screening children in primary care through the use of human figure drawings. *Pediatr Nurs.* 2005;31:320-327.
24. Columbia University. TeenScreen© Program. Available at: teenscreen.org/. Accessed August 2, 2007.
25. Beck AT, Ward CH, Mendelson M, et al. An inventory for measuring depression. *Arch Gen Psychiatry.* 1961;45:561-571.
26. Kashani JH, Sherman DD, Parker DR, et al. Utility of the Beck Depression Inventory with clinic-referred adolescents. *J Am Acad Child Adolesc Psychiatry.* 1990;29:278-282.
27. Dumont-Mathieu T, Fein D. Screening for autism in young children: the Modified Checklist for Autism in Toddlers (M-CHAT) and other measures. *Ment Retard Dev Disabil Res Rev.* 2005;11:253-262.

28. Robins D, Fein D, Barton M, et al. Modified Checklist for Autism in Toddlers (M-CHAT). Available at: www.utmem.edu/pediatrics/general/clinical/m-chat.pdf. Accessed August 2, 2007.
29. Parent's Evaluation of Developmental Status. Available at: www.pedstest.com/index.php. Accessed August 2, 2007.
30. Murphy JM, Arnett HL, Bishop SJ, et al. Screening for psychosocial dysfunction in pediatric practice: a naturalistic study of the Pediatric Symptom Checklist. *Clin Pediatr* (Phila). 1992;31:660-667.
31. Knight JR, Sherritt L, Shrier LA, et al. Validity of the CRAFFT substance abuse screening test among adolescent clinic patients. *Arch Pediatr Adolesc Med.* 2002;156: 607-614.
32. The Center for Adolescent Substance Abuse Research. The CRAFFT Questions. Available at: www.slp3d2.com/rwj_1027/webcast/docs/screentest.html. Accessed August 2, 2007.
33. Jellinek MS. Approach to the behavioral problems in children and adolescents. In: Stern TA, Herman JB, Slavin PL, eds. *The MGH Guide to Psychiatry in Primary Care.* New York, NY: McGraw-Hill; 1997.
34. Jellinek M. The present status of child psychiatry in pediatrics. *N Engl J Med.* 1982;306:1227-1230.
35. Hack S, Jellinek MS. Historical clues to the diagnosis of the dysfunctional child and other psychiatric disorders in children. *Pediatr Clin North Am.* 1998;45:25-48.
36. Kleinman RE, Murphy JM, Little M, et al. Hunger in children in the United States: potential behavioral and emotional correlates. *Pediatrics.* 1998;101:E3.
37. Lipman EL, Offord DR, Boyle MH. Relation between economic disadvantage and psychosocial morbidity in children. *CMAJ.* 1994;151:431-437.
38. Barlow M, Wildman B, Stancin T. Mothers' helpseeking for pediatric psychosocial problems. *Clin Pediatr.* 2005; 44:161-167.
39. Caspi A, Sugden K, Moffitt TE, et al. Influence of life stress on depression: moderation by a polymorphism in the 5-HTT gene. *Science.* 2003;301(5631):386-389.
40. Caspi A, McClay J, Moffitt TE, et al. Role of genotype in the cycle of violence in maltreated children. *Science.* 2002;297(5582):851-854.
41. Jellinek M, Little M. Supporting child psychiatric services using current managed care approaches: you can't get there from here. *Arch Pediatr Adolesc Med.* 1998;152: 321-326.
42. Schreter RK. Coping with the crisis in psychiatric training. *Psychiatry.* 1997;60:51-59.

Chapter 47

FAMILY SCREENING AND ASSESSMENTS

Amy Heneghan, MD

Parents are encouraged to promote their child's growth and development and to foster a loving, consistent, and well-balanced relationship with their child. Parents who are struggling with depression, poverty, addiction, and violence face immense challenges in meeting their child's needs. Primary care physicians can and should partner with parents, offering them information and resources.

RATIONALE FOR FAMILY PSYCHOSOCIAL SCREENING AND ASSESSMENT

Much evidence supports family psychological screening.[1] The American Academy of Pediatrics (AAP) Task Force on the Family advocates for family-oriented pediatric care to improve family outcomes.[2] The Task Force specifically stated that the "health and well-being of children is inextricably linked to their parents' physical, emotional, and social health."[3] The recent National Academy of Sciences report, *From Neurons to Neighborhoods,* highlights the scientific evidence of how the quality of the child's environment, especially the quality of caregiving relationships, influences the development of young children and their long-term outcomes.[4] *Bright Futures: Guidelines for Health Supervision* encourages pediatricians to support families as part of providing primary health care for children.[5] *Bright Futures in Practice: Mental Health* recommends that during health supervision visits, pediatricians "ask parents about any new experiences or stresses in their own lives."[6] Because primary care physicians develop on-going relationships with families, they are uniquely poised to discuss, and have been urged to screen for, a variety of family stresses that may negatively affect children.[7-13]

Given the evidence-based guidelines to address family psychosocial issues in caring for children, the question remains, Will parents be willing to discuss such issues? Several studies suggest this circumstance is indeed the case.[14-16] A nationally representative sample of parents surveyed stated that most parents believe clinicians should address family and community influences on child health and development.[17] Kahn et al found that almost 90% of parents would welcome discussion of such issues as maternal depression, family stresses, and smoking cessation.[16]

How can pediatric providers incorporate family psychosocial screening in pediatric primary care? Barriers to discussing family stresses include lack of time, lack of training or expertise, and perceived or real lack of available resources.[15,18,19] Barriers may be community specific, and some may be more difficult to rectify than others. The AAP is addressing 1 stated barrier: education. The Future of Pediatrics Education (FOPE) II residency education guidelines have specifically called for educating pediatric residents about family health and maternal depression in particular.[20] Practicing pediatricians would also be more likely to address both parent and child problems more readily if they used tool kits such as that from *Bright Futures in Practice: Mental Health.*[21] Information technology and resource coordination also support screening efforts when done properly.

Screening for specific issues includes maternal depression, intimate partner violence, and smoking. In 1996, Kemper et al advocated for family psychosocial screening.[22] Six particular factors were identified that place children at risk for morbidity, that are readily assessed, and that have the potential for intervention in the pediatric primary care setting. These conditions included parental depression, domestic violence, parental substance abuse, housing instability, and social support.[22] This chapter addresses the psychosocial issues that the AAP has specifically addressed as essential components of primary care and that are supported by evidence regarding identification and effective treatments. These issues are maternal depression, intimate partner violence, and parental smoking. Although these 3 important factors affecting children's health and well being will be highlighted, attention to all facets of a child's family environment is important.

MATERNAL DEPRESSION

Depression and depressive symptoms in mothers with children are prevalent and represent a significant public health concern. Rates of maternal depressive symptoms in pediatric primary care settings range from 12% to 42%.[10,23-25] For women ages 15 to 44, depression is the leading disease burden worldwide.[26] Maternal depressive symptoms are ubiquitous within all social and economic groups; nonetheless, women at highest risk are those with a personal or family history of depression, previous episode of postpartum depression, low income, low level of education, poor maternal health status, or other stressful life events.[27-29]

Etiology and Definitions

The cause of depression in women is unclear but likely involves a complex interaction of biochemical, interpersonal, and social factors.[30,31] A spectrum of diseases and disease severities exist, including postpartum blues, postpartum depression, postpartum psychosis, and maternal depression. Postpartum blues occurs in approximately 70% of women, lasts approximately 10 days, and typically does not interfere with a woman's ability to function. Postpartum depression is more persistent and debilitating than postpartum blues. It occurs in approximately 15% of women, may develop insidiously over the initial 3 postpartum months or more acutely, and lasts an average of 7 months if left untreated. Of the 4 million births annually, depression affects 500,000 women, making it the most common complication of childbearing. This condition is well described in the American Psychiatric Association *Diagnostic and Statistical Manual of Mental Disorders,* 4th edition,[32] and includes signs and symptoms that are clinically indistinguishable from major depression that occurs in women at other times (Box 47-1). Postpartum depression can interfere with a mother's ability to care for herself or her child. Maternal depression is a term often used to describe chronic or acutely depressed women with dependent children and is "more like asthma than appendicitis"[33] in that it recurs and relapses. Finally, a serious, but rare mental health problem, postpartum psychosis, occurs in 1 to 2 of every 1000 births, occurs within the initial 2 weeks of delivery, and is characterized by the acute onset of major disturbances in thinking and behavior, hallucinations, and delusions. Postpartum psychosis is a psychiatric emergency requiring immediate action because of risk of suicide and infanticide.

Rationale for Screening for Maternal Depression

Healthy People 2010 identifies depression as 1 of the 10 most important health concerns in the Unites States.[34]

BOX 47-1 Signs and Symptoms of Maternal Depression

- Sadness or low mood
- Feeling down
- Feeling worthless
- Loss of interest or pleasure (anhedonia)
- Anxiety
- Guilt
- Loss of energy
- Anger
- Increased or decreased sleep
- Increased or decreased appetite
- Delusions or paranoia
- Thoughts of death (their own or their child's)
- Suicidal ideation

The *President's New Freedom Commission on Mental Health Report* confirms that "mental illnesses rank 1st among illnesses that cause disability in the United States, Canada, and Western Europe" and pose "a serious public health challenge that is under-recognized as a public health burden."[35] After an extensive review of the research evidence, the Agency for Healthcare Research and Quality concluded that "good evidence" can be found to recommend screening for depression in primary care settings.[36] The US Preventive Services Task Force similarly finds "sufficient evidence" to screen routinely for depression in primary care settings.[37,38]

Despite this evidence, pediatricians are reluctant to discuss maternal mental health in routine pediatric primary care. Pediatricians recognize only 25% of mothers with depressive symptoms.[13] In a national sample, Olson and colleagues described pediatricians' perceived roles, management practices, and barriers encountered in addressing maternal depression.[18] Fifty-seven percent believed that recognizing maternal depression was their responsibility, and 7% believed that they were responsible for treatment. Two thirds of pediatricians surveyed provided mothers with a referral to a mental health professional, primary care provider, or support group. Time constraints and incomplete training were barriers to addressing maternal depression most often raised by the pediatricians surveyed. Despite these known barriers, screening for maternal depression is necessary when viewed in the context of the effects on children.

Maternal Depression: Effects on Children

Maternal depression has significant potential to negatively affect children (Box 47-2). Numerous studies over the last 2 decades confirm negative consequences for children across all ages in behavior, attachment, emotional and cognitive development, and children's mental health.[39-44]

Maternal depression has also been associated with diminished practices of child safety,[45] improper sleep positioning,[46] delayed immunizations,[46] increased use of acute health services,[47] increased food instability,[48] and fewer optimal parenting practices, such as prolonged breastfeeding, reading, or playing.[11] The

BOX 47-2 Maternal Depression: Effects on Children*

INFANT BEHAVIORS

Limited play and exploratory behaviors
Less responsive to facial expressions
More emotionally labile (ie, fussy)
Increased drowsiness
Less sociable with strangers
Difficulties with emotion regulation

MATERNAL-CHILD INTERACTIONS

Decreased reciprocity in interaction of the infant
Decreased enjoyment of the infant by mother
Lack of patience to soothe the infant
Less active interactions with the infant

CHILDREN'S MENTAL AND EMOTIONAL HEALTH

Hyperactivity
Defiance and disrespect
Higher rates of depression
Increased substance abuse in adolescent years

CHILDREN'S COGNITIVE DEVELOPMENT

Delayed cognitive development
Lower scores on the McCarthy Scale of Children's Abilities in infants
Poor school performance in later years

PREVENTIVE HEALTH AND PARENTING PRACTICES

Shorter duration of breastfeeding
Less play and reading
Less use of safety items (ie, outlet covers)
Higher use of acute health services
Lower rate of up-to-date immunizations

*This list is not exhaustive and is meant as a sample of effects.

literature is vast and growing: Maternal depression affects children. Treating maternal depression can, in fact, have a positive effect on both mothers and their children and can reduce psychopathologic conditions in children.[49] This fact alone supports the necessity for early identification and treatment of maternal depression.

Screening for Maternal Depression

Mothers at risk for depression may not seek health care from their own primary care physicians, yet they do see their child's pediatrician many times during the postpartum period and beyond. Every well-child visit presents the opportunity to ask a mother if she is feeling overwhelmed, stressed, anxious, or depressed. Some simple steps can be taken that may open windows of communication that will encourage a mother to discuss her feelings. Although many mothers initially may be hesitant to discuss their feelings because of fear of judgment and recrimination, consistent attention to maternal emotional needs in the context of primary care for children is key. Mothers will be open to help if a consistent, trusting relationship exists and if concerns about maternal depression become an expected component of each pediatric visit.[50]

Screening Strategies

- Note the mother-child interaction. By noting mother-child interaction, the pediatrician can assess attachment and bonding. This assessment is the most rudimentary but is already an inherent component of a primary care visit.
- Ask questions. Simply asking, "How are you doing?" is not advisable. Ask specific questions about feelings of sadness, levels of energy, sleep, anxiety, and appetite, and offer specific suggestions for questions. Some examples include, "How are you feeling about being a mother?" "How is your energy level?" "Have you had any periods of sadness? Feeling blue? Crying?" "Are you feeling overly worried about your infant?" "How have you been eating? Sleeping?" "Do you have any worries about your overall mood?"
- Ask about resources mothers have to assist them (eg, family members, child care, financial assistance).
- Ask about other stressors that may have a negative impact on children (eg, marital problems, substance abuse, housing instability).
- Ask about history of depression. Be specific.
- Ask about suicidal ideation. Make appropriate emergency referrals as needed.
- Listen. Mothers will talk about their concerns if they believe you are listening without judging them.
- Consider using a standardized screening tool to assess a mother's symptoms.

Screening Tools for Depression

Several depression screening tools are available for use in primary care settings. The Edinburgh Postpartum Depression Scale (EPDS) is the most commonly used screening tool for mothers of very young children. The EPDS is a 10-item questionnaire that is easy to use and can be scored immediately. In 2 large community-based studies of women up to 12 weeks postpartum, the EPDS had a sensitivity of 93% to 100% and a specificity of 83% to 90% for major depression when compared with structured diagnostic interviews.[51-53] The questionnaire is available at the end of this chapter, on line, and in multiple languages that can be obtained at www.mhcs.health.nsw.gov.au/health-public-affairs/mhcs/publications/7005.html. Other depression screening tools include the Center for Epidemiologic Studies Depression scale (CES-D),[54] the Beck Depression Inventory (BDI),[55] and the Patient Health Questionnaire (PHQ-9).[56]

Brief screening tools are also useful and have been shown to have good validity and ease of use in practice. The PHQ-2 consists of 2 questions that are comparable to the PHQ-9. These screening questions are shown in Box 47-3.[57] The US Preventive Task Force has advocated that the following 2 questions be asked of the mother at every primary care visit:

1. During the past 2 weeks, have you ever felt down, depressed, or hopeless?
2. During the past 2 weeks, have you felt little interest or pleasure in doing things?

If a mother reveals that she is depressed or scores above a cutoff on a screening tool, then discussing

BOX 47-3 Screening Questions

SCREENING FOR DEPRESSION

US Preventive Services Task Force

1. During the past 2 weeks, have you ever felt down, depressed, or hopeless? ☐ Yes ☐ No
2. During the past 2 weeks, have you felt little interest or pleasure in doing things? ☐ Yes ☐ No

The answer of *Yes* to either question is considered a positive score.

Patient Health Questionnaire (PHQ-2)

Over the past 2 weeks, how often have you been bothered by any of the following problems?

1. Little interest or pleasure in doing things ______ ______
2. Feeling down, depressed, or hopeless. ______ ______

Answers 0-3

0 = Not at all, 1 = Several days, 2 = More than one half the days, 3 = Nearly every day

Score of 3 or more points is considered positive.

SCREENING FOR INTIMATE PARTNER VIOLENCE

HITS (Hurt, Insulted, Threatened with harm, and Screamed at them)

How often does your partner?

1. Physically hurt you ______ ______
2. Insult or talk down to you ______ ______
3. Threaten you with harm ______ ______
4. Scream or curse at you ______ ______

Answers: 1 = Never, 2 = Rarely, 3 = Sometimes, 4 = Fairly often, or 5 = Frequent

Each item is scored from 1-5. Thus scores for this inventory range from 4-20. A score of greater than 10 is considered positive.

Partner Violence Screen (PVS)

1. Have you been hit, kicked, punched, or otherwise hurt by someone within the past year? If so, by whom? ☐ Yes ☐ No
2. Do you feel safe in your current relationship? ☐ Yes ☐ No
3. Is there a partner from a previous relationship who is making you feel unsafe? ☐ Yes ☐ No

A *Yes* response on any question is considered positive for partner violence.

SCREENING FOR SMOKING

Smoking Assessment Questionnaire

1. Does "_________'s" mother currently smoke? ☐ Yes ☐ No
2. In the home? ☐ Yes ☐ No
3. Does "_________'s" father currently smoke? ☐ Yes ☐ No
4. In the home? ☐ Yes ☐ No
5. Is your child exposed to cigarette smoke on a regular basis (any exposure at least 1 time a week) from anyone other than the parents (eg, stepparents, day care providers, grandparents, siblings, friends)? ☐ Yes ☐ No

Edinburgh Postnatal Depression Scale (EPDS)

The EPDS was developed for screening postpartum women in outpatient, home-visiting settings or at the 6- to 8-week postpartum examination. It has been used for numerous populations, including US women and Spanish-speaking women in other countries. The EPDS consists of 10 questions. The questionnaire can usually be completed in less than 5 minutes. Responses are scored 0, 1, 2, or 3 according to increased severity of the symptom. Items marked with an asterisk (*) are reverse scored (ie, 3, 2, 1, and 0). The total score is determined by adding together the scores for each of the 10 items. Validation studies have used various threshold scores in determining which women were positive and in need of referral. Cutoff scores ranged from 9 to 13 points. Therefore to err on safety's side, a woman scoring 9 or more points or indicating any suicidal ideation—that is, she scores 1 or higher on question #10—should be referred immediately for follow-up. Even if a woman scores less than 9, if the clinician believes that the client is suffering from depression, then an appropriate referral should be made. The EPDS is only a screening tool. It does not diagnose depression; that is done by appropriately licensed health care personnel. ©1987 The Royal College of Psychiatrists. The Edinburgh Postnatal Depression Scale may be photocopied by individual researchers or clinicians for their own use without seeking permission from the publishers. The scale must be copied in full, and all copies must acknowledge the following source: Cox JL, Holden JM, Sagovsky R. Detection of postnatal depression. Development of the 10-item Edinburgh Postnatal Depression Scale. *Br J Psychiatr* 1987;150:782-786. Written permission must be obtained from the Royal College of Psychiatrists for copying and distribution to others or for republication (in print, online, or by any other medium).

Translations of the scale and guidance as to its use may be found in Cox JL, Holden J. *Perinatal mental health: a guide to the Edinburgh Postnatal Depression Scale.* London: Gaskell; 2003.

Continued

BOX 47-3 Screening Questions—cont'd

INSTRUCTIONS FOR USERS

1. The mother is asked to indicate 1 of 4 possible responses that comes the closest to how she has been feeling the previous 7 days.
2. All 10 items must be completed.
3. Care should be taken to avoid the possibility of the mother discussing her answers with others.
4. The mother should complete the scale herself, unless she has limited English or has difficulty with reading.

Name: ______________________

Baby's Age: ____________ Date: ____________

Given that you have recently had a baby, we would like to know how you are feeling. Please check the box next to the answer that comes closest to how you have felt IN THE PAST 7 DAYS, not just how you feel today.

Example: I have felt happy:
- ☐ Yes, all the time
- ☐ Yes, most of the time
- ☐ No, not very often
- ☐ Not at all

Checking Box #2 would mean: "I have felt happy most of the time" during the past week. Please complete the following questions in the same way.

In the past 7 days:

1. I have been able to laugh and see the funny side of things
   - ☐ 0 As much as I always could
   - ☐ 1 Not quite so much now
   - ☐ 2 Definitely not so much now
   - ☐ 3 Not at all
2. I have looked forward with enjoyment to things
   - ☐ 0 As much as I ever did
   - ☐ 1 Rather less than I used to
   - ☐ 2 Definitely less than I used to
   - ☐ 3 Hardly at all

*3. I have blamed myself unnecessarily when things went wrong
   - ☐ 3 Yes, most of the time
   - ☐ 2 Yes, some of the time
   - ☐ 1 Not very often
   - ☐ 0 No, never

4. I have been anxious or worried for no good reason
   - ☐ 0 No, not at all
   - ☐ 1 Hardly ever
   - ☐ 2 Yes, sometimes
   - ☐ 3 Yes, very often

*5. I have felt scared or panicky for no very good reason
   - ☐ 3 Yes, quite a lot
   - ☐ 2 Yes, sometimes
   - ☐ 1 No, not much
   - ☐ 0 No, not at all

*6. Things have been getting to me
   - ☐ 3 Yes, most of the time I haven't been able to cope
   - ☐ 2 Yes, I haven't been coping as well as usual
   - ☐ 1 No, most of the time, I have coped quite well
   - ☐ 0 No, I have been coping as well as ever

*7. I have been so unhappy that I have had difficulty sleeping
   - ☐ 3 Yes, most of the time
   - ☐ 2 Yes, sometimes
   - ☐ 1 Not very often
   - ☐ 0 No, not at all

*8. I have felt sad or miserable
   - ☐ 3 Yes, most of the time
   - ☐ 2 Yes, quite often
   - ☐ 1 Not very often
   - ☐ 0 No, not at all

*9. I have been so unhappy that I have been crying
   - ☐ 3 Yes, most of the time
   - ☐ 2 Yes, quite often
   - ☐ 1 Only occasionally
   - ☐ 0 No, never

*10. The thought of harming myself has occurred to me
   - ☐ 3 Yes, quite often
   - ☐ 2 Sometimes
   - ☐ 1 Hardly ever
   - ☐ 0 Never

US Preventive Services Task Force, © Agency for Healthcare Research and Quality; Patient Health Questionnaire (PHQ-2), © Pfizer, Inc.; Sherin KM, Sinacore JM, Li XQ, et al. HITS: a short domestic violence screening tool for use in a family practice setting. *Fam Med.* 1998;30(7):508-512; Feldhaus KM, Koziol-McLain J, Amsbury HL, et al. Accuracy of 3 brief screening questions for detecting partner violence in the emergency department. *JAMA.* 1997;277(17);1357-1361; Seifert JA, Ross CA, Norris JM. Validation of a five-question survey to assess a child's exposure to environmental tobacco smoke. *Ann Epidemiol.* 2002;12:273-277. Holden JM, Sagovsky R. Edinburgh Postnatal Depression Scale (EPDS). *Br J Psychiatr.* 1987;150:782-786. These screens are reproduced with permission.

the results and formulating a follow-up plan is important.

- Point out that she is not alone and that many mothers experience similar feeling. Encourage mothers to get the help they might need and to be the best mother they can be.
- Assure mothers that support is available if they need it and that you are a partner that can help.
- Stress that depression is treatable.
- Help mothers meet other mothers and learn about other community resources (eg, support groups).
- Provide a list of print and on-line resources that might be helpful to the mother at risk.
- Ask if the mother has a primary care physician of her own and gain permission to initiate a conversation with that professional.
- Offer to initiate a referral to a mental health professional, support group, or other therapeutic agency.
- Ask to speak with other family members who might be supportive to the mother.
- Initiate an emergency behavioral evaluation by a specialist if the mother shows severe impairment, psychosis, or suicidal ideation, or if you believe that the child is at imminent physical risk. If any concern for child safety exists, then strongly consider contacting child protective services.

- Schedule frequent office visits to follow-up with the mother and her child or children.
- Be prepared for a mother to deny her symptoms and initially be unwilling to seek further treatment. A strong therapeutic alliance and close follow-up can help encourage mothers to address depressive symptoms.

PARENTAL SMOKING

A 1994 survey estimates that 43% of children aged 2 months to 11 years live in homes with at least 1 smoker.[58] In 2006, the Surgeon General's office noted that 60% of children in the United States between 3 and 11 years of age, approximately 22 million children, are exposed to second-hand smoke.[59]

Among adults in the United States, approximately 45 million adults smoked cigarettes in 2004.[60] Exposure to environmental tobacco smoke (ETS) poses a significant public health risk to children. The AAP issued a policy statement with strong recommendations for pediatricians to inform parents about the health hazards of passive smoking and to provide guidance on smoking cessation during primary care visits.[61] Risks include increased rates of lower respiratory infections, middle ear effusions, asthma exacerbations, and sudden infant death syndrome.[62-64] Children exposed to ETS are also at increased risk of cancer as adults, especially lymphoma and leukemia.[65,66] The consequences of ETS on children pose such immediate health risks and long-term health concerns that routine screening of children's exposure to ETS is warranted.

Exposure to second-hand smoke primarily comes from parental tobacco use. Despite recommendations from *Bright Futures,* pediatricians infrequently assess and advise parents to quit smoking.[62] Lack of training or knowledge about treatment may interfere with treatment recommendations. Simple, validated tools that assess ETS exposure have also been lacking. Nevertheless, pediatricians can address children's exposure to ETS by asking a few simple questions.

SCREENING FOR ENVIRONMENTAL TOBACCO SMOKE

Children's exposure to ETS can be assessed by measuring the biochemical marker cotinine or by a more practical method of parental report. Groner et al compared hair cotinine samples with 3 simple questions to create a validated measure of ETS exposure risk.[67] These 3 questions are:

1. Does the child's mother smoke?
2. Do others smoke?
3. Do others smoke inside?

Seifert et al created a 5-item screen (see Box 47-3) that also asks about others who smoke and who might regularly interact with the child.[68] Both screening tools can be readily used in even the busiest practices and can help guide pediatricians in counseling parents about smoking.

Smoking is a highly addictive behavior, but treatment is effective and strongly recommended to reduce the negative effects of smoking, for parents and their children. However, few pediatric providers and family practitioners routinely screen or counsel patients about smoking.[69] Pediatricians should familiarize themselves with treatment options that are available, not only to help their adolescent patients who smoke, but also to assist the parents of their youngest patients. A list of helpful Web sites and resources are provided in Tools for Practice.

INTIMATE PARTNER VIOLENCE

Intimate partner violence has been identified by the AAP as a significant problem for women and children.[70,71] In 1998 the AAP issued a policy statement proclaiming that "pediatricians are in a position to recognize abused women in pediatric settings and that intervening is an active form of child abuse prevention."[68] As many as 2 million women will experience intimate partner violence each year.[72] Yearly, over 3 million children witness interparental violence.[73] Such children are at risk for developmental delay, sleep disorders, school failure, oppositional defiant disorder, and depression.[74,75] Many children are victims of abuse themselves.[76,77]

Bright Futures in Mental Health recommends that women be asked about intimate partner violence and suggests specific interventions.[6] Nonetheless, asking mothers about intimate partner violence during a pediatric visit is often difficult, especially when older children are present.[78,79] Pediatricians may be unprepared to raise questions with mothers, yet this area of inquiry is critical and has been recommended by numerous advisory boards.[80]

SCREENING FOR INTIMATE PARTNER VIOLENCE

During every pediatric visit, pediatricians can ask mothers a few simple questions. The AAP[70] states that the following questions are helpful: "We all have disagreements at home. What happens when you and your partner disagree?" "Does shouting, pushing, or shoving occur?" "Does anyone get hurt?" "Has your partner ever threatened to hurt you or your children?" "Do you ever feel afraid of your partner?" "Has anyone forced you to have sex in the last few years?"

The American Medical Association has suggested 3 questions[81]:

1. Are you in a relationship now or have you ever been in a relationship in which you have been harmed or felt afraid of your partner?
2. Has your partner ever hurt any of your children?
3. Are you afraid of your current partner?

Several easy-to-use, validated measures have been used successfully in primary care practices. The Woman Abuse Screening Tool (WAST),[82] the HITS questions (Hurt, Insulted, Threatened with harm, and Screamed at them),[83] and the Abuse Assessment Screen (AAS)[84,85] have all been studied. They are all brief and focused, which makes them easy to implement in primary care and may alleviate some of the discomfort about addressing a topic that is too often neglected and may have threatening consequences for children or their parents.

SUMMARY

Although the evidence is clear that early identification and treatment of maternal depression, smoking, and intimate partner violence are beneficial to children, routine screening for these family factors will not occur without a pragmatic approach that considers the issues of time, communication skills and core knowledge, and parental willingness. Most important, effective treatments and resources must be available to assist families. Screening for family issues without confidence in the ability to communicate effectively with a family, knowledge about the treatment options available to assist a family in need, and a clear system of care to provide ongoing help for an identified need is problematic and even unethical.[86]

A paradigm shift is underway in primary care pediatrics. Considering the child in the context of the child's family is imperative, and new approaches to family assessments are needed. Strategies that incorporate theories of behavioral health counseling, such as the 5 *A*'s (Ask, Advise, Assess, Assist, Arrange) that have been used to counsel patients about smoking[87,88] are readily transportable to other family issues, such as maternal depression, parental smoking, and intimate partner violence. Preventing adverse outcomes and maximizing each child's potential is the essence of primary care pediatrics; family well being is critically important in achieving this lofty goal.

TOOLS FOR PRACTICE

Community Coordination and Advocacy

- *Environmental Tobacco Smoke and Other Indoor Air Pollution Problems Affecting Children* (slide set), American Academy of Pediatrics (www.aap.org/moc/displaytemp/etsspeech.doc).
- *Why Is Health Insurance Coverage for Tobacco Use Treatments So Important* (fact sheet), Centers for Disease Control and Prevention (www.cdc.gov/tobacco/educational_materials/cessation/index.html).

Engaging Patients and Family

- *Dangers of Secondhand Smoke* (brochure), American Academy of Pediatrics (patiented.aap.org).
- *Family—Well-Functioning* (fact sheet), American Academy of Pediatrics (www.aap.org/).
- *Expect Respect: Healthy Relationships* (brochure), American Academy of Pediatrics (patiented.aap.org).
- *Family—Dealing with Conflicts* (fact sheet), American Academy of Pediatrics (www.aap.org/).
- *Secondhand Smoke* (fact sheet), Center for Disease Control and Prevention (www.cdc.gov/tobacco/factsheets/secondhand_smoke_factsheet.htm).
- *Secondhand Smoke Causes Sudden Infant Death Syndrome* (fact sheet), Centers for Disease Control and Prevention (www.cdc.gov/tobacco/factsheets/sids_factsheet.htm).
- *What is Environmental Tobacco Smoke* (fact sheet), American Academy of Pediatrics (www.medem.com/).

Medical Decision Support

- *AAP Intimate Partner Violence questions* (form), American Academy of Pediatrics (practice.aap.org/content.aspx?aid=2001).
- *Abuse Assessment Screen (AAS)* (questionnaire), Centers for Disease Control and Prevention (www.ispub.com/ostia/index.php?xmlFilePath=journals/ijapa/vol4n1/violence.xml).
- *AMA Intimate Partner Violence Screening questions* (form), American Medical Association (practice.aap.org/content.aspx?aid=2001).
- *Beck Depression Inventory (BDI)* (questionnaire), Harcourt Assessment, Inc. (harcourtassessment.com).
- *Center for Epidemiological Studies Depression Scale* (questionnaire), National Institute for Mental Health (www.hepfi.org/nnac/pdf/sample_cesd.pdf).
- *Edinburgh Postnatal Depression Scale (EPDS)* (questionnaire), British Journal of Psychiatry (www.dbpeds.org/media/edinburghscale.pdf).
- *Environmental Tobacco Smoke exposure risk—3-question screen* (questionnaire), Groner JA, et al. (practice.aap.org/content.aspx?aid=2001).
- *HITS: A Short Domestic Violence Screening Tool* (questionnaire), Sherin K. (practice.aap.org/content.aspx?aid=2001).
- *Intimate Partner Violence* (fact sheet), Centers for Disease Control and Prevention (www.cdc.gov/ncipc/factsheets/ipvfacts.htm).
- *Patient Health Questionnaire (PHQ-2)* (questionnaire), Pfizer Inc. (www.nyc.gov/html/doh/downloads/pdf/csi/depressionkit-clin-sticker.pdf).
- *Patient Health Questionnaire (PHQ-9)* (questionnaire), Pfizer Inc. (www.phqscreeners.com).
- *Pediatric Environmental Health, Second Edition* (book), American Academy of Pediatrics (www.aap.org/bst/showdetl.cfm?&DID=15&Product_ID=1697&CatID=132).
- *Woman Abuse Screening Tool* (questionnaire), Brown (www.hotpeachpages.net/canada/air/medbook/13.html).

Practice Management

- *Screening Implementation Worksheet* (questionnaire), ABCD project of the Commonwealth Fund (www.dbpeds.org/articles/detail.cfm?TextID=343).

AAP POLICY STATEMENTS

American Academy of Pediatrics, Committee on Environmental Health. Environmental tobacco smoke: a hazard to children. *Pediatrics*. 1997;99(4):639-642. (aappolicy.aappublications.org/cgi/content/full/pediatrics;99/4/639).

American Academy of Pediatrics, Committee on Child Abuse and Neglect. The role of the pediatrician in recognizing and intervening on behalf of abused women. *Pediatrics*. 1998;101(6):1091-1092. (aappolicy.aappublications.org/cgi/content/full/pediatrics;101/6/1091).

SUGGESTED RESOURCES

Depression

Bennett SS, Indman P. *Beyond the Blues*. San Jose, CA. Moodswings Press; 2003.

Honikman J. *I'm Listening: A Guide to Supporting Postpartum Families. A Guide to Understanding and Treating Prenatal and Postpartum Depression*. Proceedings of the 2nd World Congress on Women's Mental Health, Washington, DC, March 17-20, 2004.

Beardslee WR. *Out of the Darkened Room: When a Parent is Depressed: Protecting the Children and Strengthening the Family.* Self-published; 2002.

Henry AD, Clayfield JC, Phillips JN, eds. *Parenting Well When You're Depressed: A Complete Resource For Maintaining a Healthy Family.* Oakland, CA, New Harbinger Publications; 2001.

Goodman SH, Gotlib IH. *Children of Depressed Parents: Mechanisms of Risk and Implications for Treatment.* Washington, DC: American Psychological Association; 2001.

Smoking

Glynn TJ. *How to Help Your Patients Stop Smoking: A Manual for Physicians.* National Cancer Institute. Bethesda, MD: Dept. of Health and Human Services, Public Health Service, National Institutes of Health; 1998.

Intimate partner violence

Berry DB. *Domestic Violence Sourcebook.* Los Angeles, CA: RGA Publishing Groups, Inc; 1995.

Brewster S. *To Be An Anchor in the Storm: A Guide for Families and Friends of Abused Women.* Seattle, WA, Seal Press; 2000.

Children's Safety Network. *Domestic Violence: A Directory of Protocols for Health Care Providers* [booklet]. Newton, MA: Children's Safety Network, Education Development Center, Inc; 1994.

Brownmiller S. *Against Our Will: Men, Women, and Rape.* New York, NY: Random House; 1993.

Davies J, Lyon E, Monti-Catania D. *Safety Planning With Battered Women: Complex Lives/Difficult Choices.* New York, NY: Random House; 1993.

Edelson J, Jaffe P. *Ending the Cycle of Violence: Community Responses to Children of Battered Women.* Thousand Oaks, CA: Sage Publications; 1994.

REFERENCES

1. Haggerty R, Roghmann K, Pless I. *Child Health and the Community.* New York, NY: John Wiley & Sons; 1975.
2. American Academy of Pediatrics. Family pediatrics: report of the Task Force on the Family. *Pediatrics.* 2003;111(6):1541-1571.
3. Wertlieb D. Converging trends in family research and pediatrics: recent findings for the American Academy of Pediatrics Task Force on the Family. *Pediatrics.* 2003;111(6 pt 2):1572-1587.
4. Shonkoff J, Philips D. *From Neurons to Neighborhoods. The Science of Early Childhood Development.* Washington, DC: National Academy Press; 2000.
5. Green M, Palfrey J, eds. *Bright Futures: Guidelines for Health Supervision of Infants, Children, and Adolescents.* 2nd ed, rev. Arlington, VA: National Center for Education in Maternal and Child Health; 2002.
6. Jellinek M, Patel B, Froehle M, eds. *Bright Futures in Practice: Mental Health Practice Guide.* Arlington, VA: National Center for Education in Maternal and Child Health; 2002.
7. Cheng T, Perrin E, DeWitt T, et al. Use of checklists in pediatrics practice. *Arch Pediatr Adolesc Med.* 1996;150:768-769.
8. Simonian SJ, Tarnowski KJ, Stancin T, et al. Disadvantaged children and families in pediatric primary care settings: II. Screening for behavior disturbance. *J Clin Child Psychol.* 1991;20(4):360-371.
9. Kemper K, Babonis T. Screening for maternal depression in pediatric clinics. *ADJC.* 1992;146:876-878.
10. Olson A, Dietrich A, Prazar G, et al. Two approaches to maternal depression screening during well child visits. *J Dev Behav Pediatr.* 2005;26(3):169-176.
11. McLearn K, Minkovitz C, Strobino D, et al. Maternal depressive symptoms at 2-4 months post partum and early parenting practices. *Arch Pediatr Adolesc Med.* Mar 2006;160:279-284.
12. Elwy A. All parents need family pediatrics. *Pediatrics.* 2006;117(1):218-219.
13. Heneghan A, Silver E, Bauman L, et al. Do pediatricians recognize mothers with depressive symptoms? *Pediatrics.* 2000;106(6):1367-1373.
14. Burklow K, Vaughn L, Valerius K, et al. Parental expectations regarding discussions on psychosocial topics during pediatric office visits. *Clin Pediatr.* Oct 2001;40: 555-562.
15. Heneghan A, Morton S, DeLeone N. Paediatricians' attitudes about discussing maternal depression during a paediatric primary care visit. *Child Care Health Dev.* 2007;33:333-339.
16. Kahn R, Wise P, Finkelstein J, et al. The scope of unmet maternal health needs in pediatric settings. *Pediatrics.* 1999;103:576-581.
17. Kogan M, Schuster M, Yu SM, et al. Routine assessment of family and community health risks: parent views and what they receive. *Pediatrics.* 2004;113(6):1934-1943.
18. Olson A, Kemper K, Kelleher K, et al. Primary care pediatricians' roles and perceived responsibilities in the identification and management of maternal depression. *Pediatrics.* 2002;110(6):1169-1176.
19. Horwitz S, Kelleher K, Stein R, et al. Barriers to the identification and management of psychosocial issues in children and maternal depression. *Pediatrics.* Under review.
20. Pascoe J. Letter: maternal depression and the pediatrician. *Pediatrics.* 2004;113(2):424.
21. Jellinek M, Patel B, Froehle M, eds. *Bright Futures in Practice: Mental Health Tool Kit.* No. 2. Arlington, VA: National Center for Education in Maternal and Child Health; 2002.
22. Kemper K, Kelleher K. Rationale for family psychosocial screening. *Ambulatory Child Health.* 1996;1:311-324.
23. Orr ST, James S. Maternal depression in an urban pediatric practice: implications for health care delivery. *AJPH.* 1984;74(4):363-365.
24. Heneghan A, Silver E, Bauman L, et al. Depressive symptoms in inner-city mothers of young children: who is at risk? *Pediatrics.* 1998;102:1394-1400.
25. Chaudron L, Szilagyi P, Kitzman H, et al. Detection of postpartum depressive symptoms by screening at well-child visits. *Pediatrics.* 2004;113(3):551-558.
26. Murray C, Lopez A. *The Global Burden of Disease.* Cambridge MA: Harvard University Press; 1996.
27. Fleming A, Klein E, Corter C. The effects of social support group on depression, maternal attitudes and behavior in new mothers. *J Child Psychol Psychiatr.* 1992;33(4): 685-698.
28. Field T. Early intervention for infants of depressed mothers. *Pediatrics.* 1998;102(5 suppl):1305-1310.
29. Brown G, Harris T, Bridge L, et al. Life stress, chronic subclinical symptoms and vulnerability to clinical depression. *J Affect Disord.* 1986;11:1-19.
30. Wisner K, Parry B, Pointek C. Postpartum depression. *N Engl J Med.* 2002;347:194-199.
31. Nicolson P. Understanding postnatal depression: a mother-centered approach. *J Adv Nurs.* 1990;15:689-695.
32. Diagnostic Interview Schedule. The Diagnostic Interview Schedule for DSM-IV. Washington University in St. Louis. Available at: epi.wustl.edu/DIS/dishisto.htm. Accessed December 27, 2006.
33. Klinkman M, Schwenk T, Coyne J. Depression in primary care—more like asthma than appendicitis: The Michigan Depression Project. *Can J Psychiatr.* 1997;42:966-973.

34. President's New Freedom Commission on Mental Health. *Achieving the Promise: Transforming Mental Health Care in America Final Report*. Rockville, MD: The Commission; 2003.
35. United States Institute of Medicine. *Crossing the Quality Chasm: A New Health System for the 21st Century*. Washington, DC: National Academy Press; 2000.
36. Gaynes B, Gavin N, Meltzer-Brody S, et al. Perinatal Depression: Prevalence, Screening Accuracy, and Screening Outcomes. Evidence Report/Technology Assessment No. 119. Available at: www.ahrq.gov/clinic/epcsums/peridepsum.htm.
37. Pignone M, Gaynes B, Rushton J, et al. Screening for depression in adults: a summary of the evidence for the U.S. Preventive Services Task Force. *Ann Intern Med.* 2002;136(10):765-776.
38. US Preventive Services Task Force. Screening for depression: recommendations and rationale. *Ann Intern Med.* 2002;136(10):760-764.
39. Beck C. The effects of postpartum depression on child development: a meta-analysis. *Arch Psychiatr Nurs.* 1998;12:12-20.
40. Goodman S, Gotlib I, eds. *Children of Depressed Parents: Mechanisms of Risk and Implications for Treatment.* Washington, DC: American Psychological Association; 2002.
41. McLennan J, Offord D. Should postpartum depression be targeted to improve child mental health? *J Am Acad Child Adolesc Psychiatry.* 2002;41(1):28-35.
42. Beardslee W. Children of parents with affective disorder. *Pediatr Rev.* 1989;10(10):313-319.
43. Downey G, Coyne J. Children of depressed parents: an integrative review. *Psychol Bull.* 1990;108:50-76.
44. Zuckerman BS, Beardslee WR. Maternal depression: a concern for pediatricians. *Pediatrics.* 1987;79:110-117.
45. McLennan JD, Kotelchuck M. Parental prevention practices for young children in the context of maternal depression. *Pediatrics.* 2000;105(5):1090-1095.
46. Chung E, McCollum K, Elo I, et al. Maternal depressive symptoms and infant health practices among low-income women. *Pediatrics.* 2004;113:e523-e529.
47. Minkovitz C, Strobino D, Scharfstein D, et al. Maternal depressive symptoms and children's receipt of health care in the first 3 years of life. *Pediatrics.* 2005;115(2):306-314.
48. Casey P, Goolsby S, Berkowitz C, et al. Maternal depression, changing public assistance, food security, and child health status. *Pediatrics.* 2004;113(2):298-304.
49. Weissman M, Pilowsky D, Wickamaratne P, et al. Remissions in maternal depression and child psychopathology: a STAR*D-child report. *JAMA.* 2006;295(12):1389-1398.
50. Heneghan A, Mercer M, DeLeone N. Will mothers discuss parenting stress and depressive symptoms with their child's pediatrician? *Pediatrics.* 2004;113:400-467.
51. Shakespeare J, Blake F, Garcia J. A qualitative study of the acceptability of routine screening of postnatal women using the Edinburgh Postnatal Depression Scale. *Br J Gen Pract.* 2003;53(493):614-619.
52. Jadresic E, Araya R, Jara C. Validation of the Edinburgh postnatal depression scale (EPDS) in Chilean postpartum women. *J Psychosom Obstet Gynecol.* 1995;16:187-191.
53. Cox J, Chapman G, Murray D, et al. Validation of the Edinburgh postnatal depression scale (EPDS) in non-postnatal women. *J Affect Dis.* 1996;39:185-189.
54. Radloff LS. The CES-D scale: a self-report depression scale for research in the general population. *Appl Psychol Meas.* 1977;1(3):385-401.
55. Beck A, Ward C, Mendelson M, et al. An inventory for measuring depression. *Arch Gen Psychiatr.* 1961;4:561-571.
56. Kroenke K, Spitzer R, Williams J. The PHQ-9: validity of a brief depression severity measure. *J Gen Inter Med.* 2001;16:6006-6013.
57. Lowe B, Kroenke K, Grafe K. Detecting and monitoring depression with a two-item questionnaire (PHQ-2). *J Psychosom Res.* 2005;58:163-171.
58. Pirkle J, Flagal K, Bernert J, et al. Exposure of the US population to environmental tobacco smoke: the Third National Health and Nutrition Examination Survey, 1988 to 1991. *JAMA.* 1996;275(16):1233-1240.
59. US Department of Health and Human Services. *The Health Consequences of Involuntary Exposure to Tobacco Smoke: A Report of the Surgeon General.* Rockville, MD: Public Health Service, Office of Surgeon General; 2006.
60. American Cancer Society. Questions About Smoking, Tobacco and Health. Available at: www.cancer.org/docroot/PED/content/PED_10_2x_Questions_About_Smoking_Tobacco_and_Health.asp. Accessed December 27, 2006.
61. American Academy of Pediatrics, Committee on Environmental Health. Environmental tobacco smoke: a hazard to children. *Pediatrics.* 1997;99(4):639-642.
62. Zapka J, Fletcher K, Pbert L, et al. The perceptions and practices of pediatricians: tobacco intervention. *Pediatrics.* 1999;103:e65.
63. Klerman L. Protecting children: reducing their environmental tobacco smoke exposure. *Nicotine Tob Res.* 2004;6(suppl 2):S239-S253.
64. American Academy of Pediatrics, Committee on Environmental Health. Environmental tobacco smoke: a hazard to children. *Pediatrics.* 1997;99(4):639-642.
65. Sandler D, Wilcox A, Everson R. Cumulative effects of lifetime passive smoking on cancer risk. *Lancet.* 1985;1:312-315.
66. Sandler D, Everson R, Wilcox A, et al. Cancer risk in adulthood from early life exposure to parents' smoking. *Am J Public Health.* 1985;75:487-492.
67. Groner J, Hoshaw-Woodard S, Koren G, et al. Screening for children's exposure to environmental tobacco smoke in a pediatric primary care setting. *Arch Ped Adolesc Med.* 2005;159:450-455.
68. Seifert J, Ross C, Norris J. Validation of a five-question survey to assess a child's exposure to environmental tobacco smoke. *Ann Epidemiol.* 2002;12:273-277.
69. Winickoff JP, Tanski SE, Mcmillen RC, et al. Addressing parental smoking in pediatrics and family practice: a national survey of parents. *Pediatrics.* 2003;112(5):1146-1151.
70. American Academy of Pediatrics, Committee on Child Abuse and Neglect. The role of the pediatrician in recognizing and intervening on behalf of abused women. *Pediatrics.* 1998;101:1091-1092.
71. Thompson RS, Krugman R. Screening mothers for intimate partner abuse at well-baby care visits. *JAMA.* 2001;285(12):1628-1630.
72. American Medical Association, Council on Scientific Affairs. Violence against women: relevance for medical practitioners. *JAMA.* 1992;267:3184-3189.
73. Kerker B, Horwitz S, Leventhal J, et al. Identification of violence in the home: pediatric and parental reports. *Arch Pediatr Adolesc Med.* 2000;154(5):457-462.
74. Wolfe D, Korsch B. Witnessing domestic violence during childhood and adolescence, implication for pediatric practice. *Pediatrics.* 1994;94:594-599.
75. Gleason W. Children of battered women: developmental delays and behavioral dysfunction. *Violence Vict.* 1995;10:153-160.
76. Ross S. Risk of physical abuse to children of spouse abusing parents. *Child Abuse Negl.* 1996;20:589-598.

77. Christian C, Scribano P, Seidl T, et al. Pediatric injury resulting from family violence. *Pediatrics*. 1997;99(2):E8.
78. Zink T, Jacobson J. Screening for intimate partner violence when children are present. *J Interpers Violence*. Aug 2003;18:872-890.
79. Erickson M, Hill T, Siegel R. Barriers to domestic violence screening in the pediatric setting. *Pediatrics*. 2005;115:1569-1578.
80. Nygren P, Nelson H, Klein D. Screening children for family violence: a review of the evidence for the US Preventive Service Task Force. *Ann Fam Med*. 2004;2(2):161-169.
81. Siegel RM, Hill TD, Henderson VA, et al. Diagnostic and treatment guidelines on domestic violence. *Pediatrics*. 1999;104(4);874-877.
82. Brown J, Lent B, Schmidt G, et al. Application of the Women Abuse Screening Tool (WAST) and WAST-Short in the family practice setting. *Fam Pract*. 2000;49:896-903.
83. Sherin K, Sinacore J, Li X, et al. HITS: a short domestic violence screening tool for use in a family practice setting. *Fam Med*. 1998;30(7):508-512.
84. Norton L, Peipert J, Zierler S, et al. Battering in pregnancy: an assessment of two screening methods. *Obst Gynecol*. 1995;85:321-325.
85. Nelson H, Nygren P, Mclnerney Y, et al. Screening women and elderly adults for family and intimate partner violence: a review of the evidence of the U.S. Preventive Services Task Force. *Ann Intern Med*. 2004;140(5): 387-396.
86. Perrin EC. Ethical question about screening. *J Dev Behav Pediatr*. 1998;19(5):350-352.
87. Fiore M, Bailey W, Cohen S, et al. *Treating Tobacco Use and Dependence: A Clinical Practice Guideline*. Rockville, MD: US Dept Health and Human Services, Agency for Healthcare Research and Quality; 2000.
88. Prochaska J, Velicer W, Rossi J, et al. Stages of change and decisional balance for 12 problem behaviors. *Health Psychol*. 1994;13(1):39-46.

Chapter 48

RECOGNITION OF GENETIC-METABOLIC DISEASES BY CLINICAL DIAGNOSIS AND SCREENING

Nancy E. Braverman, MD, MS; Ada Hamosh, MD

This is a time of rapid progress in the identification of human genes, including genes in which mutations cause disease or a predisposition to it. Consequently, genetic tests are currently available for an increasing number of disorders. Many of these tests will be used only when clinical suspicion is aroused. Prompt diagnosis of genetic disease is important for two reasons. First, therapeutic interventions are now available for some genetic disorders. Early therapy may result in a better outcome for a significant number of conditions. Second, diagnosis is followed by genetic counseling, which informs parents about recurrence risk and future reproductive options.

In the first part of this section, early clinical manifestations of inherited metabolic disorders are considered and how they should be evaluated by primary care clinicians. In the second part, population-wide screening is considered—that is, testing without regard to occurrence in a family. With the advent of expanded newborn screening, infants with selected genetic-metabolic diseases will be recognized with less severe symptoms, providing a unique opportunity to reduce the early mortality and morbidity associated with these disorders. However, clinicians should not rely on newborn screening alone; practitioners will continue to suspect and diagnose metabolic disease throughout the lifetime of their patients. The outcome of newborn screening programs will highlight a wide clinical spectrum in these disorders from the severely affected to the functionally benign, educating the practitioner regarding the natural history of disease and its unforeseen complications and encouraging critical appraisal of current and novel management interventions.

SUSPECTING METABOLIC DISEASE

Although inborn errors of metabolism individually are rare, their collective incidence is approximately 1 in 1000 live births. Approximately one in five sick full-term newborns who have no risk factors for infection and 1 in 100 children who have a serious medical problem will have a metabolic disease as the origin of their symptoms. Thus, over the course of practice, a primary care physician can expect to see several patients who have these disorders. Primary care physicians will often be the first person to evaluate these children, and they should be familiar with the clinical presentations and how to proceed with the initial laboratory evaluation. Formal diagnosis and treatment are usually done in consultation with a specialist.

The first disorders of metabolism to be identified were specific enzyme defects in intermediary catabolic or biosynthetic pathways in cells. Their symptoms result from the buildup of toxic precursors or the inability to produce a necessary product, or both. With advances in understanding cellular processes, some defects in transport proteins,[1,2] membrane proteins,[3] organelle assembly,[4] intracellular processing and trafficking,[5] and many other biological processes that result in biochemical disturbances with clinical expression can now be recognized. A scheme for classifying these disorders according to metabolite and organelle affected is presented in Table 48-1. Over 300 diseases caused by inborn errors of metabolism exist, and more will likely be identified in the future.[6] Relevant textbooks and Web site portals with details on these diseases provide more information.[7-16]

Diagnostic suspicion that a patient has a metabolic disorder does not require comprehensive knowledge of the various biochemical pathways involved. These disorders have typical clinical presentations, specific historical clues, and pertinent findings on clinical examination that should lead to their consideration. Furthermore, some of the laboratory tests that are obtained routinely in ill children can help determine the presence of metabolic disease.

Characteristic Presentation

Many common pediatric illnesses produce similar signs and symptoms. Such high-risk scenarios are

Table 48-1 Classification of Genetic-Metabolic Disorders*

METABOLITE AFFECTED	BIOCHEMICAL PATHWAY	CLINICAL EXAMPLES
Amino acids	Amino acid catabolism	Phenylketonuria, homocystinuria, tyrosinemia type 1, maple syrup urine disease, nonketotic hyperglycinemia
	Urea cycle disorders	Ornithine transcarbamylase deficiency (X-linked), citrullinemia, arginosuccinic aciduria, carbamoylphosphate synthase deficiency
	Amino acid transport	Lysinuric protein intolerance, cystinuria hyperornithinemia-hyperammonemia-homocitrullinuria syndrome
	Synthesis of creatine, and neurotransmitters	Creatine deficiency disorders, disorders of GABA metabolism and monoamine synthesis
Organic acids	Organic acid metabolism	Propionic acidemia, methylmalonic acidemia, isovaleric acidemia, glutaric acidemia type 1, holocarboxylase synthetase deficiency
Fatty acids	Fatty acid oxidation	Short chain, median chain and very long–chain acyl-CoA dehydrogenase deficiency, long chain 3-hydroxyacyl-CoA hydrogenase deficiency, carnitine uptake defect, carnitine palmitoyl transferase deficiencies (CPT 1 and CPT 2)
	Cholesterol synthesis	Mevalonic acidemia, Smith-Lemli-Opitz syndrome, Conradi-Hünermann-Happle syndrome (X-linked)
Carbohydrates	Carbohydrate intolerances	Galactosemia, hereditary fructose intolerance
	Glycogen breakdown (glycogen storage disorders)	*Hepatic forms:* glucose-6-phosphatase deficiency (GSD 1), debrancher enzyme deficiency (GSD 3) *Muscle forms:* muscle glycogen phosphorylase deficiency (GSD 5) *Lysosomal form:* Pompe disease (GSD 2)
	Glucose catabolism (glycolysis) and synthesis (gluconeogenesis)	Pyruvate dehydrogenase deficiency, pyruvate carboxylase deficiency, fructose diphosphatase deficiency
Vitamins, minerals, and cofactors	Activation, transport, recycling	Biotinidase deficiency; molybdenum cofactor deficiency; biopterin, cobalamin, and copper disorders

ORGANELLES AFFECTED	SUBGROUPS	CLINICAL EXAMPLES
Peroxisome	Peroxisome biogenesis	Zellweger syndrome, neonatal adrenoleukodystrophy, infantile Refsum disease, rhizomelic chondrodysplasia punctata
	Single peroxisome enzyme or protein deficiencies	X-linked adrenoleukodystrophy, adult Refsum disease, hyperoxaluria type 1
Lysosome	Lysosomal storage disorders	*Mucopolysaccharidoses:* Hurler-Scheie syndrome (MPS 1), Hunter syndrome (MPS 2, X-linked), Sanfilippo syndrome (MPS 3A-D) *Sphingolipidoses:* Tay-Sachs disease; Krabbe disease; metachromatic leukodystrophy; Niemann-Pick, Gaucher, Fabry diseases (X-linked) *Glycoprotein degradation:* mannosidosis, fucosidosis
	Lysosomal enzyme transport	*Mucolipidoses:* I-cell disease (ML 2, ML 3), cystinosis, sialic acid storage disease
Mitochondria	Respiratory chain complexes	Leigh syndrome, multiple acyl-CoA dehydrogenase deficiency (glutaric acidemia type 2), MELAS, MERRF, NARP (maternal inheritance, mitochondrial DNA encoded defects)
ER, Golgi	Intracellular protein processing and trafficking	*Glycosylation*: congenital disorders of glycosylation

*Many of the clinical examples provided refer to groups of disorders and do not distinguish specific enzymatic defects; for example, homocystinuria can result from several different enzyme deficiencies. All disorders are autosomal recessive unless otherwise noted.

ER, Endoplasmic reticulum; *GABA,* γ-aminobutyric acid; *MELAS,* mitochondrial encephalomyopathy, lactic acidosis, and stroke syndrome; *MERRF,* mitochondrial encephalomyopathy and ragged red fibers; *NARP,* neuropathy, ataxia, and retinitis pigmentosa.

Table 48-2 High-Risk Scenarios for Consideration of Metabolic Disorders

CLINICAL PICTURE	DISORDERS TO CONSIDER
Acute illness in a previously healthy newborn	Aminoacidopathies, organic acidemias, urea cycle defects, galactosemia
Neonatal seizure disorder	Pyridoxine-dependent seizures, nonketotic hyperglycinemia, sulfite oxidase deficiency, Zellweger syndrome
Recurrent episodes of illness (lethargy, vomiting, ataxia, encephalopathy, strokelike episodes, myopathy)	Aminoacidopathies, organic acidemias, urea cycle defects, defects in fatty acid metabolism, disorders of carbohydrate metabolism, mitochondrial disorders
Near-miss sudden infant death syndrome	Fatty acid oxidation defects
Neurologic regression	Lysosomal storage disorders, X-linked adrenoleukodystrophy
Chronic, progressive symptomology (poor feeding, poor growth, slow development, neurologic and other organ system dysfunction)	Aminoacidopathies, organic acidemias, disorders of carbohydrate metabolism, mitochondrial and peroxisomal diseases
Cardiomyopathy	Pompe disease, mitochondrial disorders, fatty acid oxidation defects, congenital disorders of glycosylation
Hepatopathy	Tyrosinemia type 1, galactosemia, mitochondrial disorders, bile acid defects
Maternal HELLP syndrome	Fatty acid oxidation disorders

HELLP, Hemolysis, elevated liver enzymes, low platelets.

considered by symptom complex and age in this section and in Table 48-2. Serious acute illness in a previously well newborn or recurrent episodes of illness in a child are classic presentations of metabolic disease. Unfortunately, metabolic disease is often not considered until other disorders are excluded. Diagnostic delay is particularly common for metabolic disorders that have a nonacute presentation, especially when slow development is the major initial finding. For the best outcomes, metabolic disease should be included in the earliest differential diagnoses.

Neonatal Presentation

Sudden deterioration of a full-term normal neonate within the first few days of life is a hallmark of metabolic disease. Many infants remain free of symptoms for the first 24 hours of life. When feeding begins, toxic metabolites accumulate, vomiting may occur, and the infant becomes increasingly lethargic. Neurologic abnormalities, respiratory distress, and shock highlight the progression of many severe illnesses in a neonate who has a limited repertoire of responses. The differential diagnosis includes sepsis, congenital heart disease, neurologic insults, gastrointestinal obstruction, and metabolic disease.

The clinician should pay particular attention to the possibility of metabolic disease when risk factors for infection are absent or when the infant deteriorates in spite of antibiotic therapy. The documentation of infection, cardiomyopathy, or brain abnormalities does not exclude underlying metabolic disease. Serious infection occurs in metabolically debilitated patients; for example, untreated infants who have galactosemia are at increased risk for developing *Escherichia coli* sepsis.[17] Cardiomyopathies develop in several categories of metabolic disease, including disorders of fatty acid oxidation, and may occur during infancy.[18] Metabolic crisis may result in diffuse cerebral swelling and stroke. Seizure activity predominates in certain disorders; others are associated with developmental brain abnormalities.

Some disorders (peroxisomal defects, disorders of pyruvate metabolism, and respiratory chain defects) occur within the first 24 hours of life. They may be associated with dysmorphic features and congenital abnormalities. Hydrops is an unusual presentation of some lysosomal storage diseases.[19]

The infant who has a metabolic disorder may also demonstrate less fulminantly within the first few months of life with poor feeding, recurrent vomiting, and generalized hypotonia. Infants who have tyrosinemia type I experience liver dysfunction, and their status can deteriorate rapidly.[20] In one third of patients who have inborn errors of metabolism, disease does not become clinically apparent until childhood or even later.

Late-Onset Presentation

Late-onset presentation of disease is more variable than neonatal presentation and frequently involves precipitating factors such as diet and illness. In some instances, mutations in the responsible genes encode a protein with more residual activity than in patients with neonatal presentations who may have none. Associated findings of poor growth, developmental delay, or other underlying chronic abnormalities are often found; however, illness resulting from a metabolic disorder can also occur acutely in a previously well individual. Toddlers who have medium-chain acyl-coenzyme A (CoA) dehydrogenase deficiency typically exhibit the condition acutely.[21,22] Some patients who have urea cycle defects have late-onset presentations.[23] Such presentations may involve neurologic symptoms and include encephalopathy, psychiatric symptoms, ataxia, and stroke-like episodes. Recovery may be slow, with permanent or transient neurologic dysfunction. Nongenetic diagnoses usually considered include Reye syndrome, ingestion of toxic substances, and encephalitis. In children with recurrent vomiting, lethargy, and dehydration that resembles a viral illness, each episode is protracted, and improvement often requires parenteral fluids. Patients who have methylmalonic academia, isovaleric acidemia, and maple syrup urine disease (MSUD) can exhibit symptoms later on in this fashion. Recurrent crises of fever, vomiting, and diarrhea associated with dysmorphic features are found in mevalonic aciduria.[24] The recurrence of similar episodes of illness is characteristic of metabolic disease. Abdominal pain, vomiting, and evidence of pancreatitis (eg, increased serum amylase) occur in approximately 8% of patients who have organic acidemia and may be the first findings. Organic acidemias constitute a high proportion of otherwise-unexplained pancreatitis in children.[25] Postpartum coma may lead to the diagnosis of an underlying urea cycle defect. Overall, late-onset presentations are instructive examples of genetic and environmental interactions because of their variability.

Neuropsychological Regression

Neuropsychological regression is a characteristic feature of lysosomal storage disorders. Typically a child demonstrates either normal or slow developmental progress and then fails to reach developmental milestones. Progressive deterioration occurs at variable ages and rates. Certain associated physical findings can narrow the differential diagnosis in this group.

Chronic, Progressive Symptoms

Metabolic disease can affect any of the major organ systems chronically and progressively without episodes of acute illness.

EVALUATION

History

Dietary History

For disorders in which protein catabolism is defective (amino acid and organic acid disorders), high protein intake precipitates symptoms such as vomiting, lethargy, and coma. An infant who vomits, who improves on glucose feeding, and in whom vomiting recurs within a few days of reinstitution of milk feeding might have a metabolic disease. The history may reveal the onset of illness on weaning from breast milk, which has a lower protein content than commercial formulas, or the association of illness with high-protein meals. Some older patients are found to avoid protein by limiting their protein intake. Carbohydrate intolerances occur with the introduction of fructose (fruit juices) in hereditary fructose intolerance[26] or lactose (human or cow milk) in galactosemia.

Response to Infection, Fever, and Fasting

Obtaining a history of unusual lethargy during mild illness or intolerance of fasting is an important clue for diagnosing metabolic disease. Infections, fever, and fasting result in an overall catabolic state.[27] Under these conditions, disorders involving impaired glucose production and fatty acid catabolism are exacerbated, and endogenous protein catabolism may precipitate expression of amino acid and organic acid disorders. Glycogen storage disease may occur within the first few months of life, when time between feedings is lengthened. Disorders of fatty acid oxidation classically occur during an episode of intercurrent illness with prolonged fasting. Immunizations, which may produce mild illness in normal children, can cause metabolic decompensation in children who have inborn errors of metabolism. Immunization should not be avoided in these children; rather, patients with metabolic disorders should be monitored carefully after immunization. Influenza vaccines are recommended yearly.[28]

Adverse Reactions to Anesthesia and Surgery

Other situations that stress metabolic systems, such as general anesthesia and surgery, can precipitate illness in patients who have metabolic disease. Patients who have homocystinuria are prone to thromboembolism on administration of high-osmolar contrast dyes and during surgery.[29] Some patients who have myopathy are at risk of developing malignant hyperthermia when halothane is administered.[30]

Family History

Obtaining a complete family history for all patients suspected of having metabolic disease is essential. Most of these disorders are inherited in an autosomal-recessive fashion. Parental consanguinity, similarly affected siblings, or early death of a sibling increases the likelihood of autosomal-recessive disease. However, consanguinity is uncommon in the United States, and nuclear families are small. Thus a negative family history does not exclude the possibility of a metabolic disorder. Some autosomal-recessive metabolic disorders are found at higher frequency in certain ethnic groups. The finding of similarly affected male relatives on the maternal side is consistent with X-linked disorders. Disorders of the mitochondrial genome show an exclusively maternal pattern of inheritance.

Physical Examination

Metabolic disease affects multiple organ systems and produces a variety of physical findings. Box 48-1 lists common signs, including classic radiologic findings. Some general themes exist. In disorders that occur along with episodic illness, significant findings may be present or exacerbated only during the acute phase. Neurologic abnormalities and vomiting predominate in episodic presentations, but hepatomegaly, cardiomyopathy, and muscle weakness may also be present, as in disorders of fatty acid oxidation. Tachypnea and hyperpnea are often overlooked as signs of metabolic acidosis or respiratory alkalosis.

Other disorders feature a characteristic pattern of findings that develop over time. Coarse facial features, corneal clouding, hepatosplenomegaly, macrocephaly, and skeletal changes suggest mucopolysaccharidoses, disorders of glycoprotein degradation, and mucolipidoses.[31] The constellation of alopecia, chronic dermatitis, ataxia, and seizures is seen with biotinidase deficiency.[32] Lens dislocation, long extremities, and vascular occlusion caused by thrombosis are found in homocystinuria.[29] When physical examination reveals

BOX 48-1 Pertinent Clinical Findings in Genetic-Metabolic Disorders

NEUROLOGIC
- Encephalopathy
- Strokelike episode
- Macrocephaly or microcephaly
- Developmental delay
- Ataxia
- Choreoathetosis
- Dystonia
- Peripheral neuropathy
- Hypotonia or hypertonia
- Seizures
- Myoclonus
- Deafness
- Brain malformation
- Cerebral calcification

OPHTHALMOLOGIC
- Cataracts
- Lens dislocation
- Corneal opacity
- Macular cherry-red spot
- Macular degeneration
- Retinal pigment change
- Optic atrophy

RESPIRATORY
- Tachypnea
- Hyperpnea

CARDIOVASCULAR
- Cardiomyopathy
- Pericardial effusion
- Rhythm disturbance
- Thrombosis
- Bleeding diathesis
- Anemia

ABDOMINAL
- Hepatomegaly
- Cirrhosis
- Jaundice
- Splenomegaly
- Nephrolithiasis
- Renal Fanconi syndrome
- Renal cyst
- Pancreatitis

MUSCULAR
- Hypertrophy
- Myopathy
- Myalgias
- Recurrent myoglobinuria

SKIN
- Eczematous rash
- Ichthyosis
- Photosensitivity
- Angiokeratomas
- Xanthomas

HAIR
- Sparse
- Brittle, dry, coarse

SKELETAL
- Scoliosis
- Kyphosis
- Joint contractures
- Dysostosis multiplex
- Epiphyseal calcifications

OTHER
- Dysmorphic features
- Coarse facial features

abnormalities in more than one organ system, metabolic disease should be suspected.

Laboratory Evaluation

Routine laboratory investigations can provide useful diagnostic clues. The key laboratory abnormalities in many of these disorders are metabolic acidosis, hypoglycemia with or without ketosis, and hyperammonemia. The particular combination can help predict which biochemical pathway is affected and thus which group of disorders to consider. Metabolic acidosis is routinely assessed by reviewing serum electrolytes for bicarbonate level and blood gas for pH. If the serum bicarbonate level is low, then the anion gap is calculated by the sodium content minus the sum of bicarbonate and chloride ($Na - [HCO_3 + Cl]$). An increased anion gap (>16) with a normal chloride concentration reflects the presence of unmeasured anions, such as organic acids, lactate, and ketones.[33] These compounds accumulate in amino acid and organic acid disorders. Accumulation of lactic acid predominates as a result of defects of the mitochondrial respiratory chain, multiple carboxylase deficiency, and disorders of carbohydrate metabolism. A nongenetic cause of lactic acidosis is severe tissue hypoxia. A normal anion gap with an increased chloride concentration reflects bicarbonate wasting that results from intestinal dysfunction or renal tubular defects. An important point to note is that a normal blood pH does not rule out a mild metabolic acidosis because neutrality is maintained by various buffer systems. Low serum sodium concentration with normal or high serum potassium suggests the salt-losing form of congenital adrenal hyperplasia (CAH).

Hypoglycemia occurs either because of a primary defect in the generation of glucose (disorders of glycogen breakdown and gluconeogenic pathways) or because of toxic interference with these pathways (organic acidemias). Carbohydrate depletion or impaired glucose metabolism stimulates lipid catabolism, providing ketones as an alternative fuel and resulting in ketosis. Hypoglycemia without significant ketosis is the hallmark for disorders of fatty acid oxidation in which the pathway is blocked before the formation of ketones or for excessive insulin secretion. Hyperglycemia is occasionally seen in organic acidemias.

Ammonia is produced normally from protein catabolism and detoxified in the liver through the urea cycle. Ammonia levels are increased primarily in urea cycle disorders and as secondary phenomena in organic acidemias, disorders of fatty acid oxidation, and liver disease. Hyperammonemia induces central hyperventilation, resulting in respiratory alkalosis.[23]

Low uric acid levels, which often escape attention, are consistently present in molybdenum cofactor deficiency and disorders of purine catabolism but may also be the result of renal tubular defects.[34] (See Chapter 316, Renal Tubule Acidosis.) Leukopenia and thrombocytopenia have been found in patients who have organic acidemias. Patients who have methylmalonic acidemia develop evidence of renal dysfunction.[35]

A primary laboratory evaluation is listed in Table 48-3. When the results suggest a metabolic disorder, more specific testing is performed. These secondary tests are often available on site or through an experienced reference laboratory; they are listed in Table 48-4. In disorders that have episodic symptoms, laboratory values may be abnormal only at the time of acute illness. Furthermore, partial treatment with intravenous fluids, transfusions, or dietary changes can mask abnormalities. Drug metabolites can result in false-positive findings.[36] By testing for metabolic disease early in the course of illness, diagnostic results are more likely to be obtained. A practical approach consists of collecting specimens (urine, heparinized plasma, spinal fluid) early, storing them frozen, and sending them later for analysis, if warranted.

TREATMENT

Treatment of metabolic disease can be divided into two categories: (1) acute therapy and (2) chronic management.

Table 48-3 Initial Blood and Urine Tests for Suspected Genetic-Metabolic Disorders

TEST	ABNORMAL FINDING	DISEASE
BLOOD		
Blood gases, electrolytes	Metabolic acidosis, increased anion gap	Organic acidemias, maple syrup urine disease, disorders of carbohydrate metabolism, mitochondrial defects
	Respiratory alkalosis	Urea cycle defects
Glucose	Low with ketosis	Disorders of carbohydrate metabolism, organic acidemias
	Low without ketosis	Fatty acid oxidation defects
Ammonia	High	Urea cycle defects, organic acidemias, fatty acid oxidation defects
Lactate, pyruvate	High	Disorders of carbohydrate metabolism, respiratory chain defects
Uric acid	High	Glycogen storage disorders, fatty acid oxidation defects, organic acidemias
	Low	Molybdenum cofactor deficiency
Urea nitrogen	Low	Urea cycle disorders
Liver transaminases	High	Tyrosinemia, galactosemia, hereditary fructose intolerance, fatty acid oxidation defects
Phosphate	Low	Hereditary fructose intolerance, fructose 1,6 diphosphatase deficiency
Creatine kinase	High	Fatty acid oxidation disorders, mitochondrial myopathies, muscular dystrophies
Blood count	Neutropenia, thrombocytopenia	Organic acidemias
URINE		
Odor*	Sweaty feet, musty, tomcat urine, maple syrup odor	Organic acidemias, aminoacidopathies
Ketones†	Positive	Organic acidemias, maple syrup urine disease, disorders of carbohydrate metabolism
Reducing substances‡	Positive with glucose, galactose, fructose	Galactosemia, hereditary fructose intolerance

*Assess by opening a closed container left at room temperature for 3 hours.
†Essential test whenever hypoglycemia is documented.
‡Requires urine glucose determination for interpretation.

Table 48-4 Specific Laboratory Tests for Genetic-Metabolic Disorders*

SUBSTANCE TESTED	TYPE	DISEASE
Blood	Quantitative plasma amino acids	Aminoacidopathies, organic acidemias, disorders of carbohydrate metabolism
	Carnitine levels (total, free, and esterified), acylcarnitine profile	Disorders of fatty acid metabolism
	Very long–chain fatty acids, plasmalogens, phytanic acid	Peroxisomal disorders
Urine	Quantitative amino acids	Specific amino acid transport defects
	Organic acids	Organic acidemias
	Oligosaccharide thin layer chromatography	Lysosomal disorders of glycoprotein degradation
	Screens (ferric chloride, dinitrophenylhydrazine, sulfite mucopolysaccharide spot)	Aminoacidopathies, organic acidemias, sulfite oxidase deficiency mucopolysaccharidoses (frequent false positives and false negatives)
Cerebrospinal fluid	Amino acids, glucose, neurotransmitters, lactate	Nonketotic hyperglycinemia (requires simultaneous plasma amino acids), disorders of neurotransmitters, mitochondrial disorders
Blood, skin, or other tissue	Enzyme assays	Lysosomal enzymes, definitive diagnosis of most metabolic disorders

*In the event that the child dies before a definitive diagnosis is made, a small piece of muscle and liver should be flash frozen and held at −80° C; a skin sample to culture fibroblasts should be obtained by biopsy before death for enzyme studies. Heparinized plasma and urine should be frozen for metabolic studies. EDTA-anticoagulated blood should be obtained for DNA studies.

Acute Therapy

In treatment of episodes of metabolic decompensation (before or after the diagnosis has been established) the ill child is approached as usual, with particular attention paid to respiratory, cardiovascular, fluid, and neurologic status. Intake of all potentially offending compounds (protein, lactose, fructose) is stopped, and further catabolism is inhibited by providing high caloric intake. Caloric supplements should include at least 60 calories/kg/day from glucose to prevent proteolysis. These calculations generally conform to an hourly rate of D10 (with appropriate electrolytes) at twice maintenance, or 8 to 10 mg/kg/min of glucose. Insulin, starting at a low dose, may be required to maintain euglycemia and promote anabolism. Bicarbonate is useful in cases of severe acidosis. If a vitamin-responsive disorder is suspected, then a trial of vitamin cofactors (hydroxocobalamin, biotin, thiamin, riboflavin, pyridoxine, folate) can be instituted. Carnitine may be added in organic acidurias to promote excretion of toxic metabolites. In disorders of fatty acid oxidation, carnitine should be used judiciously and only to restore normal levels of free carnitine. Hyperammonemia is treated with intravenous phenylacetate, sodium benzoate, and arginine, which help detoxify and remove ammonia.[23] Progressive hyperammonemia, unresponsive to these medications, or comatose states that result from hyperammonemia or other toxic metabolites require prompt institution of hemodialysis.[37] For patients with MSUD, acute crises are best managed with the use of nasogastric branched-chain amino acid–free synthetic feeds.[38] Acute therapy and chronic treatment should be managed in consultation with a physician skilled in treating metabolic diseases. Careful monitoring of laboratory parameters and clinical status is required, with attention being given to complications that may occur as a result of the biochemical abnormalities and therapy.

Chronic Management

Long-term therapy is disease specific and involves several strategies. To reduce the accumulation of toxic metabolites the intake of offending compounds is limited to the smallest amount needed for growth and development. This approach often requires an artificial diet that includes special formulas and caloric supplementation. Regular monitoring of amino acids and other laboratory values is required so that adjustments can be made to optimize the diet for each individual patient. For some disorders the offending compound is nonessential and can be eliminated entirely from the diet. When the enzyme defect involves binding of a cofactor (usually a vitamin) or defective synthesis of the cofactor itself, therapy centers on dietary supplementation of the cofactor. Other strategies include the stimulation of alternative biochemical pathways to detoxify and remove the offending substance.[39] In tyrosinemia type I, treatment with the drug nitisinone blocks the formation of succinylacetone, a toxic compound. Administration of cysteamine, an aminothiol, to patients who have cystinosis reduces their lysosomal storage of cystine.[24] In disorders that are accompanied by fasting intolerance, treatment consists of frequent meals, which may require the administration of complex carbohydrates, such as cornstarch, between meals to allow prolonged absorption of glucose and nocturnal nasogastric feeding.[40]

Other therapeutic approaches directly provide the missing product. Mannose supplements are given to children who have some forms of congenital disorders of glycosylation,[41] and cholesterol is provided to patients who have Smith-Lemli-Opitz syndrome.[42] None of these interventions constitutes a cure, and most are only partially successful in alleviating clinical symptoms.[43-45] With a better understanding of the pathophysiological nature of these disorders, better therapies will become available. Chaperone therapy to optimize residual enzymatic activities have been proposed.[46] Liver and bone marrow transplantations have been performed in several disorders, with mixed results.[47-51] Enzyme replacement therapies have been developed for some of the lysosomal storage disorders, and others are in the pipeline.[52] Gene therapies and in utero therapies continue to be explored.[52,53] On a community level the daily care of these patients can be extensive and requires a team approach that includes education of ancillary caretakers, school systems, and the general public. As in other chronic diseases, psychosocial and financial consequences to the patient and family exist.[54]

ILLUSTRATIVE CASES

The following cases are included to illustrate some of the principles discussed in the previous sections.

Case 1

Description

A baby boy was the full-term product of a normal pregnancy and delivery. His birth weight was 3.2 kg. The infant was started on a cow milk formula and discharged on day 2 of life without incident. From days 2 to 8, anorexia, lethargy, and vomiting became progressively worse. The formula was changed to a soy base, without clinical improvement. On day 8 the mother noted respiratory difficulties. No history of fever was present. Examination revealed a dehydrated, hypothermic infant who had a weak suck and cry. Tachypnea and tachycardia were present. Perfusion was decreased in the distal extremities, but blood pressure was normal. Oxygen saturation ($Sa{O_2}$) was 98% by pulse oximetry. The abdomen was soft, without apparent hepatosplenomegaly or renal enlargement. The remainder of the examination revealed nothing abnormal. The infant had two healthy sisters, and the family had no history of early infant deaths or parental consanguinity. The initial clinical impression was of a septic infant. Intravenous fluids and antibiotics were provided, and the infant was warmed. Initial laboratory evaluation revealed the following: white blood cell count 3500/mm^3; platelets 192,000/mm^3; venous blood gases pH 7.03, carbon dioxide saturation ($Sa{CO_2}$) 31%, $Sa{O_2}$ 98%; electrolytes, Na 146 mEq/L, potassium (K) 4.4 mEq/L, Cl 103 mEq/L, HCO_3 5 mEq/L (anion gap 38); glucose 25 mg/dL; urine (obtained after rehydration) pH 5; and ketones 2%. Analysis of spinal fluid revealed normal chemistries and cell counts, and chest radiograph indicated the presence of right upper lobe pneumonia.

The primary diagnosis was sepsis with aspiration pneumonia. All cultures were negative, but this finding was thought to be the result of antibiotic administration just before obtaining the samples for culture. The hospital course was protracted, requiring several days for the acidosis to improve on intravenous fluids containing bicarbonate. Persistent vomiting and severe acidosis recurred when formula feeding was reintroduced. A barium swallow test did not reveal gastrointestinal obstruction. On day 14 of life the infant became increasingly lethargic, and laboratory investigation showed the following: white blood cell count 4300/mm^3; platelets 7800/mm^3; arterial blood gases pH 7.1; $Saco_2$ 33%; Sao_2 97%; electrolytes, Na 141 mEq/L, Cl 103 mEq/L, HCO_3 9 mEq/L (anion gap 29); glucose 80 mg/dL; ammonia 191 mcmol/L; urine pH 5.0; and urine ketones 4%.

The infant was transferred to a tertiary-care hospital for diagnosis and management of suspected metabolic disease. Plasma amino acids showed increased glycine, and measurement of urine organic acids revealed increased levels of propionic acid and methylcitrate. These findings suggested propionic acidemia.[48] This disorder is inherited in an autosomal-recessive manner. The defective enzyme is propionyl CoA carboxylase, a biotin-dependent enzyme. The enzyme defect was confirmed later in a fibroblast culture. The patient responded to intravenous fluids with appropriate amounts of glucose provided through a central line. He was not responsive to a trial of biotin. With clinical and laboratory improvement, oral feedings were instituted, first with a glucose polymer solution and then to a restricted protein diet supplemented with a special formula deficient in the precursors of propionic acid: valine, isoleucine, methionine, threonine, and odd-chain fatty acids. If the patient had not improved quickly or had continued to deteriorate, hemodialysis would have been indicated for urgent removal of toxic metabolites.

Discussion

A history of acute illness in a healthy newborn represents a typical high-risk scenario for the consideration of metabolic disease. The initial laboratory findings provide further evidence that points to metabolic disease: metabolic acidosis with an increased anion gap, hypoglycemia, and ketosis. Ketosis, an unusual finding in a neonate, indicates metabolic disease in this age group. Recurrence of symptoms when milk feedings are resumed is also characteristic. The increased ammonia level finally led to the suspicion of an underlying metabolic disorder. Poor response to therapy should have prompted an investigation for metabolic disease. Most cases of propionic academia can now be detected in expanded newborn screening programs by increases in C3 acylcarnitine species.

Case 2

Description

This infant weighed 2900 g at term. Although his development was normal and he was generally healthy, his appetite was poor, and his growth parameters fell below the 5th percentile after 6 months of age. He had four siblings who were all healthy. At age 2 years, he was noted to have mild anemia that did not improve with iron therapy, a borderline low serum albumin level, and an enlarged liver. These findings prompted further investigation, during which time he was hospitalized and received a high-calorie and high-protein formula by nasogastric tube. However, he became progressively lethargic, and on the third day of feeding, he was found unresponsive, with sluggishly reactive pupils. No seizures had been observed, and no evidence of toxic ingestion was found. Studies included neurologic, cardiac, and septic evaluations, and these results were normal. His mental status improved on intravenous fluid therapy, and additional investigations were initiated.

At examination, he was a small, proportionate child without dysmorphic features. He had sparse, dry hair that was hypopigmented over portions of his scalp. His skin was dry, and he had reduced subcutaneous fat. His liver measured 3.5 cm below the costal margin, and the tip of his spleen was palpable. Skeletal x-ray films revealed osteopenia. The following chemistries were pertinent: venous blood gas pH 7.48; $Saco_2$ 34% (respiratory alkalosis); ammonia 244 mcmol/L; lactate 1.2 mmol/L; electrolytes, Na 137 mEq/L, Cl 100 mEq/L, bicarbonate 23 mEq/L (no anion gap); blood urea nitrogen 8 mg/dL; creatinine 0.1 mg/dL; glucose 61 mg/dL. Liver function tests revealed alanine aminotransferase 115 U/L, aspartate aminotransferase 83 U/L, total protein 5.6 g/dL, albumin 2.1 g/dL, bilirubin normal. Blood counts revealed the following: white blood cell count 2700/mm^3, hematocrit 23.2%, platelets 137,000/mm^3. Urine organic acids showed large excretion of orotic acid. Plasma amino acids showed increased glutamine with low levels of ornithine, arginine, and lysine. Urine amino acids showed marked increases of these dibasic amino acids.

The biochemical profile suggested lysinuric protein intolerance, an autosomal-recessive disorder resulting from an inactive transporter for dibasic amino acids. The diagnosis was confirmed by identifying mutations in the gene encoding this transporter, *SLC7A7*. The transporter defect results in the loss of these amino acids in the urine, their reduced absorption from the intestine, and consequent low plasma concentrations. Hyperammonemia develops from a deficiency of the urea cycle intermediates, ornithine and arginine, compromising urea cycle function. Symptoms of lysinuric protein intolerance typically emerge when a breastfed infant is weaned and begins to receive higher-protein formulas and foods. Nausea and vomiting occur, and aversion to protein-rich food develops. The patients fail to thrive and have symptoms of protein malnutrition. The liver and spleen are moderately enlarged. Without treatment, marked osteoporosis, pancytopenia, interstitial lung disease, and renal glomerular disease can develop.

The initial management included intravenous fluids, citrulline supplementation, and protein restriction. On this regimen, ammonia levels normalized. Refeeding was monitored, and his protein intake was gradually increased to 1.5 g/kg, which he was able to tolerate. Citrulline, a neutral amino acid, does not require this transporter and thus can replenish urea cycle intermediates. His clinical condition and growth improved.

He is currently in the third grade and is doing well. Interestingly, his hair color darkened on protein repletion.

Discussion

The child was 2 years of age before a genetic-metabolic disorder was considered, although a complete history revealed his protein avoidance. The finding of poor growth and hepatosplenomegaly should lead to the consideration of metabolic disease. The laboratory findings of hyperammonemia combined with increases in glutamine and orotic acid indicate a functional urea cycle defect.

Case 3

Description

The child is a 6-year-old girl who was completely well until 10 days before admission, when she developed a papular rash. Although she remained afebrile, she developed progressive abdominal pain, lethargy, and dysarthria, and she had an unsteady gait. She was adopted; her biological mother has three other children, two boys and one girl, whom she reported were well. Examination of the patient revealed normal growth parameters and no dysmorphic features. Skin examination revealed only a single papule. Her neck was supple, her chest was clear, her cardiovascular examination was normal, and no hepatosplenomegaly was present. She was sleepy, with slurred speech, but arousable, and she was able to follow commands. Her reflexes were 2 to 3+ and symmetric, and no clonus was elicited.

A viral infection was suspected, and she was evaluated for her altered mental status under this assumption. Laboratory values revealed normal electrolytes. Venous blood gas indicated respiratory alkalosis. Her tests indicated the following: liver function tests, aspartate aminotransferase 635 U/L, alanine aminotransferase 899 U/L; viral titers, normal; ammonia, 235 mcmol/L. Computed tomographic scan of the head revealed nothing abnormal. Plasma amino acids showed increased glutamine with low urea cycle intermediates, ornithine, arginine, and citrulline. Urine organic acids showed an increase in orotic acid. These laboratory results are consistent with ornithine transcarbamylase (OTC) deficiency. Although this condition is an X-linked disorder, girls can be symptomatic depending on their pattern of X inactivation. Because symptomatic girls usually retain some residual enzymatic activity, they are considered to have partial OTC deficiency. For confirmation of this diagnosis, mutation analysis of the *OTC* gene was performed. Although no clinical suspicion existed that the child might have a *45, XO* karyotype, this was also evaluated because it is another reason for expression of X-linked recessive disorders in girls.

The patient responded to intravenous fluids, which provided caloric supplementation, and to sodium phenylbutyrate and arginine hydrochloride, which are ammonia-scavenging drugs. Once the ammonia level was normal, a low-protein diet was begun, and she was placed on oral phenylbutyrate and citrulline to provide a cushion against further episodes of hyperammonemia. Increased liver function tests are not typically seen with OTC deficiency, but they can occur, or they might have been related to the intercurrent illness.

Discussion

This case is an example of an apparently normal child with sudden deterioration during an illness. As with many genetic-metabolic disorders, she is at risk for additional episodes with intercurrent illness, fasting, or stress. Patients with urea cycle disorders who do not respond to ammonia-scavenging drugs are candidates for hemodialysis. If unrecognized or treatment is delayed, then cerebral edema and irreversible brain damage might occur.

Case 4

Description

This 13 year old was referred to the genetics clinic to determine the cause of his skeletal dysplasia. He had short stature and an abnormality of his wrist that resembled Madelung deformity or anterior subluxation. The diagnosis of Leri-Weill dyschondrosteosis was considered but could not be confirmed. In addition, he had high-frequency hearing loss, sleep apnea for which he had undergone removal of his tonsils and adenoids, and repairs of umbilical and inguinal hernias. He was the product of a normal full-term delivery, and no concerns were raised about his health until he was 6 years of age, when short stature was recognized. He had low levels of insulin-like growth factor 1, and growth hormone therapy was initiated. Magnetic resonance imaging of the head showed a normal pituitary but increased Virchow-Robin spaces. Analysis of a skin lesion on his back indicated dermal mucinosis. His intellect was normal. Review of the family history revealed no other members with similar findings.

At examination the boy had small stature with macrocephaly. His hair was coarse in texture, and he had mild coarsening of facial features. No corneal clouding was noted. He had a thoracic kyphosis, a prominent ribcage, and restricted extension in his elbows, wrists, phalanges, knees, and hips. Lungs were clear to auscultation, but cardiac examination revealed the presence of a murmur. His abdomen was slightly protuberant, his liver was 3 to 4 cm below the costal margin with a total span of 13 cm, and his spleen was not enlarged. Skin examination revealed unusual elevated, pebbly regions on his back. His neurologic examination revealed nothing abnormal. A radiologic survey of his skeleton showed splaying of rib ends and anterior beaking of several vertebrae. A cardiac echo showed thickened aortic and mitral valves with moderate regurgitation. He also had mild left-ventricular dilation, as well as mild dilation of the aortic root and ascending aorta. The findings on history and examination indicated a mucopolysaccharide storage disorder. A urine mucopolysaccharide spot test was positive, and enzymatic testing of leukocytes showed decreased activity of iduronate sulfatase, which is diagnostic of Hunter syndrome. This disorder is inherited in an X-linked recessive fashion, and the mother was shown to be a carrier by mutation analysis of her iduronate sulfatase gene.

Discussion

This case is an example of a slowly progressive genetic-metabolic disease that can be diagnosed by the pattern of clinical findings. Virtually all of the physical findings are characteristic of mucopolysaccharide storage disorders: macrocephaly, coarse features, joint restrictions, hernias, sleep apnea (caused by enlarged adenoids), deafness, dysostosis multiplex, cardiac valve thickening, and enlarged cerebral Virchow-Robin spaces. The pebbly or nodular skin lesions are a distinguishing feature of Hunter syndrome. This disease is characterized by a broad spectrum of clinical severity, and in the milder form, mental development and life span can be normal. The diagnosis in this adolescent was especially timely because enzyme replacement therapy is now available for this disease.

SCREENING FOR GENETIC AND METABOLIC DISORDERS

Certain disorders for which treatment is effective are asymptomatic until it is too late for effective intervention. Such is the case, for instance, for phenylketonuria (PKU); although nonspecific signs occasionally appear early in infancy (such as eczema), by the time that developmental delay is apparent, irreversible damage has occurred. For other disorders, such as galactosemia and MSUD, symptoms appear early, but the diagnosis is often delayed. Such is also the case in some infants who have congenital hypothyroidism (CH). Newborn screening can accelerate the diagnosis, provided that specimens are analyzed quickly and abnormal results are reported promptly. A *sine qua non* of newborn screening is that the prognosis can be improved by the prompt institution of therapy. Accumulated experience with screening has demonstrated that the outcome is not always as good as anticipated, and for some disorders a few infants may receive therapy unnecessarily.

A few single-gene conditions occur only after exposure to environmental agents that are not harmful to most people in the doses encountered. Screening for such susceptibilities might result in treatment that ameliorates the harmful effects or warns people at risk to avoid exposure. Among people who develop cancer (retinoblastoma and breast and colon cancer have been studied the most thoroughly) a small proportion (<10%) have inherited alleles at single loci that greatly increase their susceptibility to malignant transformation as a result of spontaneous or environmentally induced mutations of other genes. The benefits of screening the entire population for these genetic susceptibilities remain to be established. Claims of inherited risk factors for complex disorders such as Alzheimer disease need thorough assessment before population screening is even considered. Genetics plays a role in adult-onset coronary artery disease. Cholesterol screening is discussed in another part of this chapter.

Most single-gene disorders are not treatable, but persons at risk for them, as well as heterozygous carriers, can be detected by genetic tests. Carrier testing before pregnancy provides couples the option of preventing conception of children who have severe untreatable, inherited disorders, such as Tay-Sachs disease or thalassemia. They can choose to have children by adoption, artificial insemination of donor sperm, or, in the case of X-linked disorders, ovum donation or surrogacy. Carrier testing early in pregnancy by chorionic villi sampling or amniocentesis provides couples the option of preventing the birth (by selective abortion) of a similarly affected child. Prenatal cytogenetic and biochemical testing can avoid, respectively, the birth of children who have aneuploidy or neural tube defects.

Primary health care clinicians will be increasingly involved with neonatal, carrier, and prenatal screening and presymptomatic testing for adult-onset disorders. In some cases the clinician will inform patients about the availability of tests, will counsel them about having the test, and, when they decide to be tested, about the meaning of the results.

FALSE-POSITIVE AND FALSE-NEGATIVE FINDINGS

Few people being screened, whether newborns, nonpregnant women, or pregnant women, will be at risk of disease in themselves or their offspring. Except for DNA tests, many of the techniques used in screening yield positive results in the absence of the condition of interest, especially when the conditions are rare. These false-positive findings frequently occur more often than the condition of interest in the population being screened. The immunoreactive trypsinogen (IRT) test used in a few states to screen newborns for cystic fibrosis (CF) yields over five times as many false-positive as true-positive results. Because the blood phenylalanine concentration may exceed normal levels only minimally in infants who have PKU during the first few days of life the cutoff for phenylalanine level (and other metabolites) must be set lower than the minimal phenylalanine concentration needed to establish a diagnosis of PKU. Consequently, false-positive results will often exceed truly positive results.

On average, by using current methods, more than 50 false-positive findings are identified for every confirmed case.[55] For CAH, more than 200 false-positive findings occur for every true case.[55] When the screening test entails enzyme assays, as for one type of testing for galactosemia and for biotinidase deficiency, heat denaturation (by a long mailing time in hot weather or by letting samples dry on a radiator) greatly increases the percentage of false-positive results. When DNA tests are performed appropriately for single-gene disorders, false-positive results are seldom encountered. For multifactorial disorders, however (eg, colon cancer, Alzheimer disease), in which a single-gene mutation increases the risk of disease but is insufficient to cause it, positive DNA test results do not always mean that disease will occur. Other factors, mostly unknown, also play a role.

False-negative results are a problem with both DNA tests and more traditional tests. In the case of DNA tests, they occur when the test does not detect all of the different mutations capable of causing disease.

Early discharge of healthy newborns before 24 hours of age increases the number of infants who have false-negative and false-positive test results. Infants who have PKU have near-normal levels of phenylalanine in cord blood, and adequate exposure to exogenous protein is required to develop a high phenylalanine level. Similarly, when quantitation of blood galactose is used to screen for galactosemia, infants with galactosemia must have consumed sufficient amounts of galactose-containing human milk or cow milk formula to accumulate galactose. Approximately 10% of infants who have CH will have normal thyroxine (T_4) levels when screened early, and most of these infants also have normal thyroid-stimulating hormone (TSH) levels. When TSH is used as the initial screening test (common in European countries but not in the United States), as many as 25% of infants discharged early may have increased levels.[56] In screening for CAH, samples collected before 36 hours of age are much more likely to yield false-positive increases in 17-hydroxyprogesterone than are samples collected after 48 hours.[57]

Although the chance of misclassification is higher the earlier an infant is screened, most, but not all, infants who have the disorders for which screening usually is provided will be detected when tested after 24 hours of age. In view of difficulties of guaranteeing that a screening test will be performed soon after discharge, no infant should be discharged from the newborn nursery, even if younger than 24 hours, without first being screened. Raising the threshold value to reduce the number of false-positive results or lowering it to reduce the number of false-negative results for infants screened before 48 hours has the problem of increasing, respectively, the number of false-negative and false results. The use of a different value for infants screened early or late requires the laboratory to treat the two groups of infants separately. The best solution to prevent these errors is not to discharge infants until they are at least 48 hours of age.

False-positive and false-negative test results are both dangerous and costly. Parents of infants who have false-positive test results may become anxious until the result is proven to be false; even then, anxiety may linger in a small number of parents, particularly if their infants had low Apgar scores.[58] The parent-child relationship might be influenced as a result of this stress in the neonatal period.

With a high false-positive rate, more infants require follow-up testing, which adds to the cost of screening. The affected infants missed by screening suffer severely, usually at great cost to their families and society. Primary care clinicians have been found financially liable for infants missed by screening. No clinician should ever assume that an infant who has symptoms of a disorder for which screening was performed might not have that disorder.

Screening tests can give erroneous results because of the presence of other substances that interfere with the analysis. Most important for DNA-based screening is the presence of a donor's blood products as the result of recent transfusion. Certain antibiotics can interfere with the bacterial inhibition assays used in some newborn screening.

In the absence of rigorous quality-control programs, laboratory error is probably the most common cause of false-positive and false-negative newborn screening test results. Errors include misidentification of specimens and failure to transmit the results properly, as well as erroneous assays.

NEWBORN SCREENING

Newborn screening in the United States is mandated by each state. For many years, most states screened only for PKU and hypothyroidism. With the advent of newer methods and a concerted effort by the American College of Medical Genetics, the Health Resources Services Administration, and the March of Dimes, a much broader panel of disorders has been recommended.[55] The paradigm has shifted from only screening for disorders that lead to irreversible damage without screening and for which an effective treatment exists to a broader scope when the hope is that early recognition will ameliorate outcome. The National Newborn Screening and Genetics Resource Center (genes-r-us.uthscsa.edu/) maintains current information on which states screen for which disorders.

All states and the District of Columbia routinely screen newborns for PKU (1 in 14,000 live births), CH (1 in 3300 live births), galactosemia (approximately 1 in 59,000 live births), and sickle cell anemia (>1 in 400 live births of black infants).[57] All states but Florida screen for other hemoglobinopathies.[57] Forty-six states screen for MSUD (<1 in 100,000 live births),[55] 45 for homocystinuria (<1 in 100,000 live births),[57] 44 for biotinidase deficiency (approximately 1 in 80,000 live births),[55] 48 for CAH (1 in 20,000 live births),[57] 46 for medium-chain acyl-CoA dehydrogenase deficiency (1 in 15,000 live births),[55] and 24 for CF (1 in 3200 white live births).[59] Because states differ in the tests that are required, health care practitioners must be familiar with the policies of their own state, even though their states may not notify them when new tests are introduced. Whether this circumstance contributes to the failure of a few of them to act when notified of a positive test result is unknown, but their failure to act might have resulted in an infant's death.[60] Physicians should document screening test results and any follow-up on the child's medical record.

Because screening tests can be falsely negative, practitioners should not place undue faith in a negative result. A repeat test, or a more definitive one, should be obtained for infants whose findings arouse suspicion. Because of the problem of false-positive test results, treatment should not be started based merely on a single positive screening test result. Consultation with someone experienced in the evaluation of metabolic disorders should be initiated. When treatment is indicated the response may vary; careful monitoring and expert evaluation are needed. Furthermore, consultation is reassuring to the family.

Some infants may escape screening. The largest group is composed of infants born at home. They should be screened at their first visit for pediatric care. Sick infants transferred from one hospital to another fall through the cracks when each hospital believes that the other performed the screening. If any doubt exists, then the receiving hospital should rescreen the baby.

Screening for PKU and CH is cost effective. The addition of other tests from which infants will benefit usually involves only marginal cost increments. Centralization of laboratories and more stringent regulations for quality control reduce laboratory error, increase cost effectiveness, and reduce the cost to the patient.

Phenylketonuria

Infants who have PKU show few signs until they develop intellectual disability, which may not be appreciated until the second year of life and is irreversible. Screening early in infancy, followed by prompt administration of a diet low in phenylalanine, is the only way to improve the outcome of infants born with the condition. Evidence shows that intellectual performance correlates with the age at which dietary treatment is started and with the success of dietary control.[6] Studies to confirm positive test results should be performed quickly to permit the initiation of the low-phenylalanine diet as soon as possible and no later than the third week of life.

The American Academy of Pediatrics recommends that every infant in the United States be screened before discharge from the nursery but that infants initially screened before 24 hours of age should be rescreened before the third week of life. Premature and sick infants should be screened by the seventh day of life.[3] A few states recommend that all infants undergo a second screening between 2 and 4 weeks of age; and a few infants who have PKU with a negative first test have been detected by the repeat screening. The second screening costs much more per infant who has PKU detected than the first screening.

In addition to the predominant phenylalanine hydroxylase deficiency, defects in the synthesis or regeneration of biopterin cofactors for the conversion of phenylalanine to tyrosine also result in positive screening test results and clinical disease. Dietary restriction of phenylalanine is insufficient to prevent mental deterioration and seizures in these infants. The use of biopterin or neurotransmitter precursors offers some hope of improving the outcome. Infants who have these disorders will be identified by neonatal screening for PKU; they represent less than 3% of all infants who have hyperphenylalaninemia. Tests for these variant forms should be performed in any infant who persistently has high blood phenylalanine levels, even in the moderate range of 10 to 20 mg/dL, while on a normal diet.

Congenital Hypothyroidism

The cause of CH is multiple and complex, including transplacental passage of maternal antibodies that interfere with fetal thyroid development or thyroid function.[56] Maternal antibodies also can cause transient hypothyroidism. Mothers receiving antithyroid medication (propylthiouracil) may have babies who have transient hypothyroidism. Genetic factors are suggested in families that have more than one affected infant, although such findings do not rule out environmental or maternally acquired causes. For unknown reasons, girls are twice as likely to have CH as boys, and the birth prevalence is somewhat higher in Hispanics and Native Americans than in whites or Asians, in whom it is higher than in blacks.[61] (See also Chapter 280, Hypothyroidism.)

Infants who have the most profound deficiencies of T_4, usually as a result of thyroid agenesis, are more likely to have symptoms in the neonatal period, of which persistent jaundice, difficulty feeding, and lethargy are most frequent.[56,62] Nevertheless, even infants who have agenesis may be asymptomatic when they are examined as part of the evaluation of their abnormal screening test result. Placental transfer of T_4 and some fetal production of triiodothyronine in the brain may explain this circumstance. The 10% of infants who have CH that is found by a second screening (in states that screen twice) are less often symptomatic and have lower increases of TSH. Even if newborn test results are negative, hypothyroidism may still develop in infancy or childhood. The incidence of CH detected by neonatal screening is higher than that detected by clinical diagnosis in the prescreening era. This increased incidence suggests either that infants who have milder disease escaped diagnosis or that some infants being diagnosed today do not really have CH. Because of this latter possibility, the need to ensure that CH persists in equivocal cases, as discussed later, is important.

In most laboratories in the United States, T_4 is measured on the screening specimen, and if it is low, then TSH is measured on the same specimen. If the TSH is high and the findings are confirmed by another specimen, then treatment with T_4 is initiated. Most infants who persistently have low T_4 levels but who have normal TSH levels will prove on further study to have normal free T_4 concentrations and thyroid-binding globulin deficiency; they do not require treatment. A few infants who have low T_4 and normal TSH levels have pituitary gland failure, but it is encountered much less frequently than thyroid-binding globulin deficiency. Occasionally an infant who has initial low T_4 and normal TSH levels will have a delayed increase in TSH level and symptoms of hypothyroidism. If an infant has an initial low T_4 level and a normal TSH level, then TSH should be retested if symptoms appear.

The motor and cognitive development of infants who have CH at 7½ years of age correlates with the age at which T_4 treatment is started.[63] Although most infants who receive early treatment have IQ scores in the normal range,[56] many of them are at the low end compared with matched controls,[63] with approximately a 5- to 10-point loss in IQ. Patients with CH have persistent deficits in visuospatial abilities, memory, and attention, which correlate with severity of early hypothyroidism.[64,65]

The need for long-term thyroid replacement can be assumed if scans or other studies reveal absent or ectopic thyroid or goiter caused by an enzyme defect. In the absence of these findings, but when low T_4 and increased TSH levels indicate the need for early treatment, a test of continued need for thyroid replacement therapy should wait until the child is between 3 and 4 years of age. Thyroid-replacement therapy should then be discontinued for 30 days, or until signs and symptoms of CH appear. At that time, serum should be obtained for T_4 and TSH assays. If the results are normal, no further treatment is needed. Such transient cases are usually those in which the TSH level was increased only moderately (20 to 100 mU/mL) in the newborn period.

Sickle Cell Anemia

States have added sickle cell to their newborn screening programs.[57,66,67] Before screening was initiated, approximately 10% of infants in the United States who had sickle cell disease died by 10 years of age, most from pneumococcal sepsis.[68] The effectiveness of screening in reducing morbidity and mortality depends on ensuring that infants detected by screening are referred to a continuing source of care from which they can receive prophylactic penicillin and their parents can learn how to manage situations that increase the chance of sickle cell crises. As yet, no specific treatment is available for sickle cell anemia.

Many of the tests used for screening (eg, hemoglobin electrophoresis, isoelectric focusing, high-performance liquid chromatography) will reveal hemoglobinopathies in addition to sickle cell anemia, not all of which are symptomatic. Specific sickle cell anemia DNA testing will not identify other hemoglobinopathies. All forms of sickle cell testing also identify infants who have sickle cell trait who will remain healthy. However, parents of an infant who has sickle cell trait may be at risk for having an infant who has sickle cell anemia if both partners are carriers of the sickle cell gene. A screening program will have 40 times more carriers to notify than parents of infants who have sickle cell anemia. The purpose of notifying the parents of a trait is to determine, by offering to have them both tested, whether they are both carriers and consequently are at 25% risk of having affected offspring with each subsequent pregnancy. They can then be offered prenatal diagnosis in any future pregnancies. The infant who has this trait who triggers the investigative process has nothing to gain from it. Moreover, in most couples that have an infant with trait, only one partner is a carrier. Parents should be informed that newborn screening might provide information about their future risks of having a child with a serious hemoglobinopathy, and they should be given the opportunity to request the results.[69] Thalassemias are not directly screened for in the United States but will be detected when general hemoglobin electrophoresis is performed. (See Chapter 270, Hemoglobinopathies and Sickle Cell Disease, for more information.)

Galactosemia

In contrast to PKU, serious manifestations of classic galactosemia occur soon after milk feedings are started. Consequently the diagnosis can be, and often is, made clinically before screening test results are reported. The prompt administration of a lactose-free diet in newborns will save the lives of patients who have this disorder, but it may not prevent intellectual disability or other developmental problems, including a high incidence of ovarian failure. The age of starting the galactose-free diet is not significantly associated with the magnitude of developmental delay, physical growth, or speech problems.[70,71]

Whether infants who have galactosemia found by screening would have developed symptoms had they not been started on a lactose-free diet is uncertain. Some infants discovered by screening have variant forms of galactosemia, in which residual amounts of galactosyl-1-phosphate uridylyltransferase, the enzyme that is absent in classic cases, are found. Although infants who have some of these variants have acute neonatal symptoms, such symptoms are generally milder than those in the classic cases. Other infants exhibit no symptoms. Whether they are less likely to have long-term manifestations, such as developmental delay, is not clear.

Much remains to be learned about the pathogenesis of galactosemia and the development of effective therapy. Until more is known the value of neonatal screening for galactosemia is questionable, although classical galactosemia will result in death if it remains untreated. The principal goal is to ensure prompt intervention in individuals who have early onset of symptoms and whose lives are threatened. These infants can be diagnosed clinically.

Maple Syrup Urine Disease

Infants who have the classic form of MSUD usually show signs within 2 weeks of birth. The course can be fulminant and rapidly fatal, but early treatment can prevent or ameliorate the acute symptoms. If the special diet (low in branched-chain amino acids) is started early, then the long-term outcome can be good. One of the problems with routine screening is the inherent delay in obtaining results. A specimen collected on day 2 may not be reported until day 10. By that time, most infants who have the classic form will be severely ill or dead. Starting the special diet will usually save infants who are still alive at this point, but infants who survive will often have intellectual disability and neurologic problems.

Confirmation of a diagnosis of MSUD in sick infants can sometimes be hastened by contacting the laboratory responsible for performing newborn screening; a positive result may have been obtained already. In many instances the laboratory will process the specimen more quickly when it receives a special request. Infants known to be at risk because of a previously affected family member or because they are of North American Mennonite descent should undergo definitive testing (quantitative plasma amino acids) in the second day of life, with immediate initiation of a special diet for affected individuals to ensure the best possible outcome. Lapse into coma is associated with a drop of up to 40 IQ points with this condition.

The enzyme that is defective in MSUD is complex,[72] and many different mutations have been characterized. Except in a North American Mennonite community, in which a single mutation accounts for a high prevalence of the condition, several different mutations have been found.[73] Many patients are compound heterozygotes. As a result of screening and the immediate institution of the special diet, establishing genotype-phenotype relations has been difficult. Some infants started on the diet may have forms of the disorder that would have appeared only later in infancy or childhood with episodes of ataxia, failure to thrive, and mild ketoacidosis, particularly after infection or high protein ingestion.

Congenital Adrenal Hyperplasia

In 21-hydroxylase deficiency, which accounts for more than 90% of patients who have CAH, and in 11-hydroxylase deficiency, accounting for approximately 5% of cases, cortisol production is impaired. As a result of the deficiency, feedback inhibition of adrenocorticotrophic hormone is lacking, and cortisol precursors, including those that have androgenic activity, are overproduced. In girls, ambiguous genitalia should permit clinical diagnosis in the neonatal period. Because the diagnosis is not always made, however, screening might increase recognition of girls, permitting them to be raised as girls. The diagnosis is much more difficult to establish in newborn boys. Approximately two thirds of infants who have 21-hydroxylase deficiency lose salt; they may experience severe dehydration and vascular collapse accompanied by hyponatremia during the first 3 weeks of life. Unscreened boys who have salt-losing CAH are diagnosed at a median age of 26 days, versus 12 days for screened boys.[74] Boys who have simple virilizing CAH are detected only by screening.[74] Several different mutations in the gene for 21-hydroxylase have been found. The presence of salt losing depends on the particular mutation, but a complete genotype-phenotype correlation has not been established.[75]

By hastening the diagnosis and promptly instituting mineralocorticoid therapy, screening can prevent life-threatening episodes in both boys and girls. Salt-losing crises, however, can often occur before the results of screening are known. Screening also offers an advantage to affected boys who do not lose salt; corticosteroid therapy will prevent virilization, rapid early growth, and premature closure of the epiphyses with resultant short adult stature.

The observation of more living female subjects than male subjects who have this autosomal-recessive disorder suggests that boys may die in the neonatal period before they are diagnosed.[75] Through screening, an almost equal number of boys and girls are detected, and the birth prevalence with screening is considerably higher than by clinical diagnosis.[75]

17-Hydroxyprogesterone is increased in the blood in both 21- and 11-hydroxylase deficiency and is measured by the screening test. Laboratory or administrative error has accounted for the handful of false-negative results. When these results are excluded the test detects more than 98% of infants who have CAH.[75] Approximately 30 false-positive results occur for every infant who has a true-positive result. In girls the presence of ambiguous genitalia establishes a true-positive finding, but in the absence of such findings and in most boys, additional studies are needed. Measuring serum electrolytes is the most important immediate follow-up to determine the presence of salt loss, which should prompt immediate mineralocorticoid treatment.

Symptom-free adults who have genetic variant forms of 21-hydroxylase deficiency have been identified.[76] The possibility arises therefore that clinical problems will not develop in all symptom-free infants who have a confirmed deficiency, unambiguous genitalia, and no salt losing.

Prenatal diagnosis in high-risk girls is possible. Prenatal administration of dexamethasone orally to the mother at or before 10 weeks' gestation prevents or reduces intrauterine virilization in most infants. Dexamethasone is safe for both the mother and the fetus.[77]

Biotinidase Deficiency

Biotin is a cofactor of several carboxylases. Its availability through recycling is reduced in inherited deficiencies of biotinidase. The manifestations and age at onset of biotinidase deficiency vary, possibly because of differences in the degree of enzyme deficiency and the amount of biotin available to the infant. Symptoms usually appear between 2 weeks and 3 years. Ataxia, alopecia, hearing loss, decreased vision, optic atrophy, and seizures have been observed. Not yet known is whether some infants who have the disorder remain free of symptoms and consequently how many of the infants detected by screening would develop symptoms if left untreated. Because infants found by screening have higher levels of residual biotinidase than those diagnosed clinically,[78] the possibility exists that not all infants discovered by screening will ever develop symptoms. Nevertheless, the treatment—providing supplemental biotin—is simple and inexpensive. Although biotin reverses some of the symptoms after they appear, this is not always true for the hearing and visual impairments and developmental delay.[79] Moreover, whether clinical diagnosis will always be made expeditiously is by no means clear. Infants treated as a result of screening have so far remained free of symptoms.

Cystic Fibrosis

IRT is increased in the blood of most newborns who have CF.[80] Twenty-four states currently perform this test. Those that mandate two screenings, including Colorado and Maryland, use this method alone. Other states perform one IRT followed by second-tier DNA testing for common CF transmembrane conductance regulator (CFTR) mutations in infants who have high IRT levels. Some states screen only for the *F508del* mutation, which is present in 70% of CF alleles worldwide. Other states require a broader panel, especially California, which is enriched for black and Hispanic mutations. This method decreases the rate of false-positive findings identified by IRT screening alone, but it may miss up to 10% of patients with CF who do not carry a common mutation on either allele. Neonates with CF and meconium ileus usually have false-negative results. The Centers for Disease Control and Prevention issued a report that concluded that screening newborns for CF was justified based on improved long-term nutritional outcome in children identified by screening compared with those identified clinically.[81,82] In addition, newborn screening may improve childhood survival.[82] No treatment is yet available that prevents the clinical manifestations, but earlier therapy appears to ameliorate the condition.

Homocystinuria

Although vitamin B_6-dependent forms of homocystinuria are treated easily and effectively and account for approximately 50% of cases, newborn screening will not detect all affected infants.[83] The detection rate after the first week of life by tests that measure blood or urine homocystine will be higher than that of neonatal screening, which detects hypermethioninemia. In view of this circumstance, as well as the rarity of the disorder, newborn screening by bacterial inhibition assay is hard to justify. Some experts have suggested lowering the blood methionine cutoff to 1 mg/dL to decrease the false-negative rate.[84] The argument has been obviated by the institution of tandem mass spectrometry (MS/MS) for newborn screening because the results are quantitative; MS/MS is currently being used to some extent in all but six states.

Tandem Mass Spectrometry

Tandem mass spectrometry (MS/MS) is able to quantitate accurately multiple amino acids, organic acids, and metabolites of fatty acid oxidation from dried blood on filter paper.[55,57] The advent of this technique has broadened the scope of newborn screening while dramatically decreasing (by two orders of magnitude) some false-positive rates.[85] It also decreases the false-negative rates for homocystinuria.[86] MS/MS is used to screen for PKU, MSUD, homocystinuria, tyrosinemia, citrullinemia, and argininosuccinic acidemia, the last two by detecting increased citrulline. MS/MS cannot detect OTC or carbamoylphosphate synthetase deficiencies because it cannot reliably detect a low citrulline. MS/MS can detect a broad array of organic acids and metabolites of fatty acid oxidation. Newborn screening for medium-chain acyl-CoA dehydrogenase deficiency, which is common and easily treated, makes sense according to the old paradigm. For many of the other disorders that can be identified by MS/MS, no fully effective treatment exists, and early intervention may not affect outcome. However, undiagnosed infant deaths would decrease, and the availability of prenatal diagnosis in subsequent pregnancies for at-risk families would increase. The American College of Medical Genetics and March of Dimes concurred on a core panel of disorders and secondary target conditions that can be detected by MS/MS.[55]

Medium-Chain Acyl-CoA Dehydrogenase Deficiency

Medium-chain acyl-CoA dehydrogenase deficiency has an incidence of 1 in 10,000 to 14,000 in the white population and a 25% to 50% initial decompensation fatality rate. However, it is easily treated by avoiding fasting and catabolism and by instituting carnitine supplementation and intravenous glucose early in the course of intercurrent illness. Unscreened infants are usually discovered between 6 and 18 months of age. After decreased caloric intake usually associated with intercurrent illness the child first develops hypoketotic hypoglycemia, followed by hepatic encephalopathy, and ultimately death if untreated. This whole progression can occur during the 12 hours of nighttime sleep and accounted for a small percentage of deaths caused by sudden infant death syndrome in the prescreening era.[57]

NEW TECHNIQUES IN NEWBORN SCREENING

Enzyme replacement therapy has been developed to treat infant-onset Pompe disease. For the best outcome, treatment should be initiated before 6 months of age. A dried-blood spot filter paper assay has been developed. Many experts are advocating for adding this condition to the newborn screening panel. The treatment is variably effective; in some patients, it affords complete resolution of heart and muscle disease, but in others, it converts a lethal disorder to a severe chronic illness, resulting in numerous hospitalizations and slow deterioration. Cord blood stem cell transplantation can cure Krabbe disease if undertaken in the first month of life. One state has already added this condition to its newborn screening panel. New tests are being developed to screen for severe combined immunodeficiency and adrenoleukodystrophy. Much research and interest exists in this area.

Genetic Susceptibilities

In a few genetic conditions, disease is likely to appear only in certain environments. Screening of infants or young children provides warning that certain exposures will be harmful and should be avoided. If harmful exposures occur, then awareness of the genetic susceptibility might speed appropriate management. In the United States, no state currently screens newborns for such genetic susceptibilities. This circumstance may reflect a lack of confidence in the ability of the health care system or parents to ensure that the harmful exposures will be avoided. Screening workers or prospective employees for genetic susceptibilities (including the two conditions discussed later), in which the harmful agent may be encountered on the job, is of interest to some employers.[87]

Glucose-6-Phosphate Dehydrogenase Deficiency

A significant number of different alleles result in this X-linked genetic susceptibility. The usual manifestations are hemolytic anemia accompanied by jaundice and hemoglobinuria. Approximately 10% of black boys inherit the mild A form. Except for some sulfur compounds (eg, sulfamethoxazole) the drugs that trigger reactions are seldom used in the United States (eg, primaquine), although some may develop hemolysis after heavy exposure to naphthalene (mothballs). In the more severe Mediterranean variant (but only occasionally in the A variant), hemolytic anemia (favism) is encountered after ingestion of fava beans, a staple of diets in many Mediterranean countries. The initiation of a newborn screening program for glucose-6-phosphate dehydrogenase deficiency in Sardinia, together with more education about the deficiency, was associated with a marked decline in the occurrence of favism and the need for blood transfusions.[88]

$Alpha_1$-Antitrypsin Deficiency

Individuals who have severe $alpha_1$-antitrypsin (α_1-AT) deficiency, usually the result of inheriting Z alleles from both parents, are at increased risk of chronic obstructive pulmonary disease (COPD), although in population-based surveys, many people who have severe deficiency remain asymptomatic throughout life.[89] Individuals who have the deficiency and who smoke are likely to encounter pulmonary problems between 20 and 40 years of age, approximately 15 years earlier than nonsmokers.[90] Not all nonsmokers who have α_1-AT deficiency get COPD. Severe α_1-AT deficiency accounts for approximately 1% of all COPD cases. Presymptomatic screening might alert individuals who have α_1-AT deficiency to the especially harmful consequences of smoking. Treatment of α_1-AT–deficient adults with emphysema with human α_1-AT increased their serum and lung α_1-AT levels but did not improve their pulmonary function.[91] Whether such treatment would prevent COPD remains to be established. Because adolescents who have α_1-AT deficiency have normal pulmonary function,[92] screening of newborns or young children is of questionable value in improving outcome.[93]

Approximately 10% of infants who have α_1-AT deficiency develop cholestasis, and 2% to 3% later develop cirrhosis. No specific treatment or known means of preventing the liver manifestations is available, although human milk may be protective.[94] Consequently, newborn screening would not be expected to alter the prognosis. α_1-AT deficiency should be included in the differential diagnosis of persistent jaundice in young infants. Screening adolescents or young adults might be of benefit.

Carrier Screening

Carrier screening is undertaken for severe untreatable inherited disorders to provide persons identified as carriers with options for preventing the conception or birth of affected children. Carrier screening for Tay-Sachs disease has resulted in a significant decrease in the disease in many Jewish communities.[95] Carrier screening for thalassemia in Sardinia[96] and elsewhere in the Mediterranean Basin has lowered its incidence. Most American couples found by carrier screening to be at risk of having a child who has sickle cell anemia decide not to terminate the pregnancy.[97] With nondirective counseling, they may not view the disorder as severe as do those at risk of having children who have Tay-Sachs disease or thalassemia.

School-based screening programs for sickle cell and Tay-Sachs disease carriers probably recruit a much higher proportion of the at-risk population than do community programs or office or clinic screening programs. However, they may lead to the stigmatization of students identified as carriers unless all those being screened understand the reasons for the screening and the significance of the results. Nor is it clear that adolescents whose carrier status is identified will retain this information or act on it when they consider having children.[98] If prenatal diagnosis of a condition is available and abortion of an affected fetus is acceptable, then less reason exists to offer screening before pregnancy. Couples might be screened before the woman becomes pregnant or early in pregnancy, although the latter may require more expensive testing and preclude certain options, such as artificial insemination of sperm from a donor who is not a carrier.

Since 2001 the American College of Obstetrics and Gynecology has recommended offering carrier testing for CF for all pregnant white women. In 2005, it altered its recommended panel of 25 mutations.[99] Uptake of screening approached 25% of pregnancies in 2004.

Screening young women to determine whether they are carriers of X-linked disorders, such as fragile X syndrome, hemophilia, and Duchenne muscular dystrophy, is technically feasible with DNA analysis. Because of new mutations, not all births of infants who have these disorders might potentially be avoided. Such testing is not routinely offered at this time.

Prenatal Screening

Practitioners who provide care to the young do not usually have primary responsibility for managing pregnancies; however, they often will have prior contact with the mother and the father and can contribute to the parents' understanding of the indications for screening in pregnancy. They may also be contacted by obstetricians to assist in counseling or in anticipation of high-risk newborns. A review of prenatal genetic diagnosis for primary care physicians has been published.[100] Only prenatal screening tests are discussed in this chapter.

Neural Tube Defects

Folate supplementation of bread products was initiated in January 1998 when circumstances became apparent that women of childbearing age did not recognize the need for periconceptional folate supplementation, and the incidence of neural tube defects have declined.[101] Maternal serum screening of alpha-fetoprotein (AFP) between the fifteenth and twenty-first weeks of pregnancy provides women an opportunity to prevent the birth of most infants who have anencephaly and open spina bifida by prenatal diagnosis and abortion or, if they chose to carry to term, to possibly improve the outcome. Identifying fetuses affected with open spina bifida before delivery permits prelabor cesarean section, which may improve the infant's sensorimotor function.[102]

The maternal serum AFP test is capable of detecting 90% of fetuses that have anencephaly and approximately 80% of those that have open spina bifida.[103] For every true-positive result, however, approximately 30 women who do not have affected fetuses will have false-positive results. In women who have high maternal serum AFP, sonographic examination is needed to determine the accuracy of the estimate of gestational age; the normal maternal serum AFP concentration is highly dependent on gestational age. If sonography confirms the gestational age, then amniotic fluid is obtained by amniocentesis. If the amniotic fluid AFP is high, then the likelihood of an open neural tube defect exceeds 90%. Further assurance that a defect is present is obtained by performing acetylcholinesterase determinations[104] and high-detail (level 2) ultrasound. Although high-level ultrasound performed by expert sonographers detects most fetuses that have open spina bifida, it should not replace AFP screening.

Down Syndrome

Prenatal diagnosis for Down syndrome is rapidly evolving. Definitive testing requires chorionic villi sampling or amniocentesis, both of which are costly and invasive. These tests are routinely offered to women older than 35 years of age. For younger women and women older than 35 years from whom the risks of amniocentesis or chorionic villi sampling are unacceptable, several forms of biochemical marker screening tests are now available.[105] Second-trimester triple screening (free beta human chorionic gonadotropin [ß-hCG], maternal serum AFP, and estriol) detects approximately 60% of fetuses with Down syndrome. Addition of inhibin A to form a quadruple screening increases the sensitivity to approximately 70% with a 5% false-negative rate. New first-trimester screening, which includes testing for pregnancy-associated plasma protein A and free ß-hCG, is capable of detecting 70% of fetuses with Down syndrome. When coupled with first-trimester nuchal translucency testing by ultrasound, which is technically challenging and not yet widely available, the sensitivity increases to 86%, with only a 5% false-negative rate. Sequential screening (first-trimester screening, followed by second-trimester quadruple screening for persons not at high risk by first-trimester screening) can detect up to 95% of affected pregnancies, with only an overall false-positive rate of 5%. First-trimester screening for Down syndrome does not obviate the need for second-trimester screening for neural tube defects.

AVAILABILITY OF SCREENING TESTS

Health departments can usually provide information about newborn screening and hemoglobinopathy screening. Community groups for sickle cell anemia, thalassemia, Tay-Sachs disease, and CF often know where carrier screening for these conditions can be obtained. The Alliance of Genetic Support Groups (www.geneticalliance.org/) can also provide information. GeneTests (www.genetests.org/), which operates out of the University of Washington in Seattle, maintains an up-to-date list of laboratories providing DNA tests and some biochemical tests.

ETHICAL AND LEGAL ISSUES IN SCREENING

In view of the reproductive implications of most genetic screening tests, as well as respect for the autonomy of individuals, agreement is widespread that genetic screening, with the possible exception of newborn screening, requires informed consent.[106] The disclosure should include the nature of the disease; the probability that the condition will occur; the nature, benefits, and risks of the interventions should the result be positive (including pregnancy termination in the case of prenatal screening); the probability of test error; and other possible deleterious effects.

Some researchers have argued that newborn screening for incurable disorders (eg, Duchenne muscular dystrophy, fragile X syndrome) is appropriate because a prompt diagnosis affords parents the opportunity of preventing the birth of another affected child. Others have argued that the infant found to be affected by newborn screening derives no benefit from the test and may even be harmed—perhaps, for instance, by interference with parental bonding.[53] With current DNA testing technology, some persons at high risk of having affected children can be identified by carrier screening either before or early in pregnancy. Couples at risk then have the opportunity of preventing the conception or birth of any affected offspring, whereas only second or additional affected children can be avoided by newborn screening.

Third parties, such as insurers and employers, may have an interest in learning the results of genetic tests. Such third parties may use the information to deny employment or health insurance coverage to persons who have positive results. The wide consensus is that test results should not be released to such third parties without explaining to the person being screened (or the infant's parents in the case of newborn screening) the implications of obtaining consent and releasing the results. Except in unusual circumstances, health care practitioners are not obliged to notify relatives of a patient who has a positive test result but who refuses to inform relatives that they are at risk.[106]

One reason for screening newborns in hospitals is that they are a captive population. Unless screening confers a benefit not otherwise attainable, such a reason is ethically suspect. For conditions that occur in early childhood, newborn screening confers a benefit not otherwise attainable for those disorders for which treatment is effective only before symptoms appear. Such is not the case for conditions that occur later in childhood, or not until adulthood, and for which intervention in infancy or childhood is of no proven benefit. This issue is likely to emerge if and when screening for genetic predispositions to cancer and other mainly adult-onset disorders becomes possible. Telling parents and children that they are at risk for a late-onset condition for which no childhood intervention exists might alter child-rearing patterns and generate considerable anxiety. In some cases, parents and their children might differ on wanting to have the child screened. Older children should be informed of such screening and should agree to it.

FUTURE OF GENETIC SCREENING

The Human Genome Project continues to increase the identification of genes that play a role in disease. The major advances of DNA technology allow testing a small specimen containing nucleated cells for genetic variants that increase the risk of many different disorders. The ethical and legal challenges to this multiplex testing may prove more difficult than the technological hurdles. The different disorders that might be included in multiplex testing will be markedly different in their age at onset, their severity, and in the interventions available to treat, ameliorate, or prevent their occurrence. How will prospective subjects of testing, or their parents, be able to decide whether they want any or all of the tests available?

The discovery of genes that play a role in complex (polygenic or multifactorial) disorders holds great appeal; but much needs to be learned of the role of alleles at these loci in the general population, as well as in high-risk families, before screening is even considered.

Many mutations of a single gene are capable of causing or predisposing to disease. One drawback of current DNA technology is the inability to detect all of these mutations or to distinguish mutations that result in disease from those that do not. Advances in DNA technology may overcome these problems. In addition, examining gene products in readily accessible cells will be possible by amplifying the protein synthesized by the gene of interest and examining its structure or function. Alterations in structure or function are likely to indicate the presence of more disease-causing or susceptibility-conferring mutations than might DNA analysis.

Intensive efforts are being made to isolate fetal cells from maternal circulation in an effort to perform prenatal diagnosis without placing the fetus at risk.[107] If feasible, then fluorescent DNA probes will be used to determine the presence of extra chromosomes (as in Down syndrome) in the fetal cells, as well as to perform DNA analysis for disease-causing mutations. Within a few years, this technique might make the screening of every fetus for several congenital and hereditary disorders feasible. Once again the ethical and legal issues may be more difficult to solve than the technical issues.

The expansion of genetic testing and screening has increased commercial interest in manufacturing test reagents and providing genetic testing services. Health care clinicians can expect pressures from companies offering tests to provide these services. Unfortunately, tests can be made available without adequate assessment of their safety and effectiveness. Practitioners would do well to go beyond material in the lay press and in company-sponsored brochures before offering these tests to their patients.

TOOLS FOR PRACTICE

Engaging Patient and Family

- *Newborn Screening Disorders—What Parents Want to Know about Newborn Screening Disorders* (brochure), Academy of Pediatrics and The Health Resources and Services Administration, Department of Health and Human Services (test.medicalhomeinfo.org/screening/Screen Materials/Newborn screening disorders.pdf).
- *Newborn Screening Tests—These tests could save your babies life* (brochure), American Academy of Pediatrics and Health Resources and Services Administration, US Department of Health and Human Services (test.medicalhomeinfo.org/screening/Screen%20Materials/Newborn%20screening%20tests.pdf).
- *What is cystic fibrosis?* (fact sheet), American Academy of Pediatrics (www.aap.org/publiced/BK0_CysticFibrosis.htm)
- *What is Spina Bifida?* (fact sheet), American Academy of Pediatrics (www.aap.org/publiced/BK0_SpinaBifida.htm).

Medical Decision Support

- *Newborn Screening Act Sheets and Confirmatory Algorithms* (algorithm), American Academy of Pediatrics (www.acmg.net/resources/policies/ACT/condition-analyte-links.htm).
- *Newborn Screening and Related Conditions* (Web page), Centers for Disease Control and Prevention (www.cdc.gov/ncbddd/bd/genetics_screen.htm).

RELATED WEB SITES

- American College of Medical Genetics (www.acmg.net).
- Birth Defects, Centers for Disease Control and Prevention (www.cdc.gov/ncbddd/bd/default.htm).
- Gene Test (www.genetests.org/).
- Genetic Alliance (www.geneticalliance.org/).
- Infogenetics, Maternal and Child Health (DHHS) and Children's Hospital of The King's Daughters Health System Norfolk, Virginia (www.infogenetics.org/).
- March of Dimes (www.marchofdimes.com/).
- National Newborn Screening and Genetics Resource Center (genes-r-us.uthscsa.edu/).
- Newborn Screening—The National Center of Medical Home Initiatives, American Academy of Pediatrics (www.medicalhomeinfo.org/screening/newborn.html).
- Online Mendelian Inheritance in Man, Johns Hopkins University (www.ncbi.nlm.nih.gov/sites/entrez?db=OMIM).

AAP POLICY STATEMENTS

American Academy of Pediatrics, Committee on Bioethics. Ethical issues with genetic testing in pediatrics. *Pediatrics*. 2001;107(6):1451-1455. (aappolicy.aappublications.org/cgi/content/full/pediatrics;107/6/1451).

American Academy of Pediatrics, Committee on Genetics. Folic acid for the prevention of neural tube defects. *Pediatrics*. 1999;104(2):325-327. (aappolicy.aappublications.org/cgi/content/full/pediatrics;104/3/325).

American Academy of Pediatrics, Committee on Genetics. Health supervision for children with Down syndrome. *Pediatrics*. 2001;107(2):442-449. (aappolicy.aappublications.org/cgi/content/full/pediatrics;107/2/442).

American Academy of Pediatrics, Committee on Genetics. Maternal phenylketonuria. *Pediatrics*. 2001;107(2):427-428. (aappolicy.aappublications.org/cgi/content/full/pediatrics;107/2/427).

American Academy of Pediatrics, Committee on Genetics. Molecular genetic testing in pediatric practice: a subject review. *Pediatrics*. 2000;106(6):1494-1497. (aappolicy.aappublications.org/cgi/content/full/pediatrics;106/6/1494).

American Academy of Pediatrics, Rose SR, and the Section on Endocrinology and Committee on Genetics; American Thyroid Association, Brown RS, and the Public Health Committee; Lawson Wilkins Pediatric Endocrine Society. Update of newborn screening and therapy for congenital hypothyroidism. *Pediatrics*. 2006;117(6):2290-2303. (aappolicy.aappublications.org/cgi/content/full/pediatrics;117/6/2290).

Cunniff C, American Academy of Pediatrics, Committee on Genetics. Prenatal screening and diagnosis for pediatricians. *Pediatrics*. 2004;114(3):889-894. (aappolicy.aappublications.org/cgi/content/full/pediatrics;114/3/889).

Kaye CI, American Academy of Pediatrics, Committee on Genetics. Introduction to the newborn screening fact sheets. *Pediatrics*. 2006;118(3):1304-1312. (pediatrics.aappublications.org/).

Kaye CI, American Academy of Pediatrics, Committee on Genetics. Newborn screening fact sheets. *Pediatrics*. 2006;118(3):e934-e963. (pediatrics.aappublications.org/).

REFERENCES

1. Mancini GM, Havelaar AC, Verheijen FW. Lysosomal transport disorders. *J Inherit Metab Dis.* 2000;23:278-292.
2. Pascual JM, Wang D, Lecumberri B, et al. GLUT1 deficiency and other glucose transporter diseases. *Eur J Endocrinol.* 2004;150:627-633.
3. Vanier MT, Millat G. Niemann-Pick disease type C. *Clin Genet.* 2003;64:269-281.

4. Raymond G, Moser H. Clinical diagnosis and therapy of peroxisomal diseases. In: Applegarth DA, Dimmick JE, Hall JG, eds. *Organelle Diseases: Clinical Features, Diagnosis, Pathogenesis and Management.* London, UK: Chapman and Hall; 1997.
5. Jaeken J. Congenital disorders of glycosylation (CDG): It's all in it! *J Inher Metab Dis.* 2006;26:99-118.
6. Saudubray JM, Charpentier C. Clinical phenotypes: diagnosis/algorithms. In: Scriver CR, Beaudet AL, Sly WS, et al, eds. *Metabolic and Molecular Basis of Inherited Disease.* New York, NY: McGraw-Hill; 2001.
7. Online Mendelian Inheritance in Man. Available at: www.ncbi.nlm.nih.gov/entrez/query.fcgi?db=OMIM. Accessed August 14, 2007.
8. National Organization for Rare Disorders. Available at: www.rarediseases.org/. Accessed August 14, 2007.
9. Genetic Alliance. Available at: www.geneticalliance.org/. Accessed August 14, 2007.
10. Scriver CR, Beaudet AL, Sly WS, et al, eds. *Metabolic and Molecular Basis of Inherited Disease.* New York, NY: McGraw-Hill; 2001.
11. Fernandes J, Saudubray J-M, Van den Berghe G, eds. *Inborn Metabolic Diseases: Diagnosis and Treatment.* Heidelberg, Germany: Springer-Verlag; 2000.
12. Clarke JTR. *A Clinical Guide to Inherited Metabolic Diseases.* Cambridge, MA: Cambridge University Press; 2005.
13. Blau N, Hoffmann GF, Leonard J, et al, eds. *Physician's Guide to the Treatment and Follow-up of Metabolic Diseases.* New York, NY: Springer; 2005.
14. Nyhan WL, Ozand PT. *Atlas of Metabolic Diseases.* London, UK: Chapman & Hall; 1998.
15. Hoffman GF, Nyhan WL, Zschocke J, et al. *Inherited Metabolic Diseases.* Philadelphia, PA: Lippincott Williams & Wilkins; 2002.
16. GeneTests. Available at: www.genetests.org/. Accessed August 14, 2007.
17. Levy HL, Sepe SJ, Shih VE, et al. Sepsis due to Escherichia coli in neonates with galactosemia. *N Engl J Med.* 1977;297:823-825.
18. Servidei S, Bertini E, DiMauro S. Hereditary metabolic cardiomyopathies. *Adv Pediatr.* 1994;41:1-32.
19. Burin MG, Scholz AP, Gus R, et al. Investigation of lysosomal storage diseases in nonimmune hydrops fetalis. *Prenat Diagn.* 2004;24:653-657.
20. Scott CR. The genetic tyrosinemias. *Am J Med Genet C Semin Med Genet.* 2006;142:121-126.
21. Hale DE, Bennett MJ. Fatty acid oxidation disorders: a new class of metabolic diseases. *J Pediatr.* 1992;121:1-11.
22. Touma EH, Charpentier C. Medium chain acyl-CoA dehydrogenase deficiency. *Arch Dis Child.* 1992;67:142-145.
23. Brusilow SW, Maestri NE. Urea cycle disorders: diagnosis, pathophysiology, and therapy. *Adv Pediatr.* 1996;43:127-170.
24. Prietsch V, Mayatepek E, Krastel H, et al. Mevalonate kinase deficiency: enlarging the clinical and biochemical spectrum. *Pediatrics.* 2003;111:258-261.
25. Kahler SG, Sherwood WG, Woolf D, et al. Pancreatitis in patients with organic acidemias. *J Pediatr.* 1994;124:239-243.
26. Van den Berghe G. Inborn errors of fructose metabolism. *Annu Rev Nutr.* 1994;14:41-58.
27. Dixon MA, Leonard JV. Intercurrent illness in inborn errors of intermediary metabolism. *Arch Dis Child.* 1992;67:1387-1391.
28. American Academy of Pediatrics, Committee on Infectious Diseases. Policy statement: recommendations for influenza immunization of children. *Pediatrics.* 2004;113(4):1441-1447. Available at: aappolicy.aappublications.org/cgi/content/full/pediatrics;113/5/1441. Accessed August 15, 2007.
29. Mudd SH, Skovby F, Levy HL, et al. The natural history of homocystinuria due to cystathionine beta-synthase deficiency. *Am J Hum Genet.* 1985;37:1-31.
30. Johnson C, Edleman KJ. Malignant hyperthermia: a review. *J Perinatol.* 1992;12:61-71.
31. Gieselmann V. Lysosomal storage diseases. *Biochim Biophys Acta.* 1995;1270:103-136.
32. Wolf B, Heard GS. Biotinidase deficiency. *Adv Pediatr.* 1991;38:1-21.
33. Foreman J. Acid-base physiology in health and disease. In: Cohn RM, Roth KS, eds. *Metabolic Disease: A Guide to Early Recognition.* Philadelphia, PA: WB Saunders; 1983.
34. Arnold GL, Greene CL, Stout JP, et al. Molybdenum cofactor deficiency. *J Pediatr.* 1993;123:595-598.
35. Baumgarter ER, Viardot C. Long-term follow-up of 77 patients with isolated methylmalonic acidaemia. *J Inherit Metab Dis.* 1995;18:138-142.
36. Bachmann C, Boulat O, Meyrat BJ, et al. Pitfalls in amino acid and organic acid analysis: 3-hydroxypropionic aciduria. *Eur J Pediatr.* 1994;153(7 suppl 1):S23-S26.
37. Rutledge SL, Havens PL, Haymond MW, et al. Neonatal hemodialysis: effective therapy for the encephalopathy of inborn errors of metabolism. *J Pediatr.* 1990;116:125-128.
38. Morton DH, Strauss KA, Robinson DL, et al. Diagnosis and treatment of maple syrup disease: a study of 36 patients. *Pediatrics.* 2002;109:999-1008.
39. Levy H. Nutritional therapy in inborn errors of metabolism. In: Desnick RJ, ed. *Treatment of Genetic Diseases.* New York, NY: Churchill Livingstone; 1991.
40. Wolfsdorf JI, Weinstein DA. Glycogen storage diseases. *Rev Endocr Metab Disord.* 2003;4:95-102.
41. Harms HK, Zimmer KP, Kurnik K, et al. Oral mannose therapy persistently corrects the severe clinical symptoms and biochemical abnormalities of phosphomannose isomerase deficiency. *Acta Paediatr.* 2002;91:1065-1072.
42. Sikora DM, Ruggiero M, Petit-Kekel K, et al. Cholesterol supplementation does not improve developmental progress in Smith-Lemli-Opitz syndrome. *J Pediatr.* 2004;144:783-791.
43. Ridel KR, Leslie ND, Gilbert DL. An updated review of the long-term neurological effects of galactosemia. *Pediatr Neurol.* 2005;33:153-161.
44. Rubio-Gozalbo ME, Panis B, Zimmermann LJ, et al. The endocrine system in treated patients with classical galactosemia. *Mol Genet Metab.* 2006;89:316-322.
45. Sass JO, Hofmann M, Skladal D, et al. Propionic acidemia revisited: a workshop report. *Clin Pediatr (Phila).* 2004;43:837-843.
46. Sawkar AR, D'Haeze W, Kelly JW. Therapeutic strategies to ameliorate lysosomal storage disorders—a focus on Gaucher disease. *Cell Mol Life Sci.* 2006;63:1179-1192.
47. Meyburg J, Hoffmann GF. Liver transplantation for inborn errors of metabolism. *Transplantation.* 2005;80(1 suppl):S135-S137.
48. Sokal EM. Introduction: liver and liver cell transplantation for inborn errors of liver metabolism. *Acta Gastroenterol Belg.* 2005;68:451-452.
49. Kelly DA. Organ transplantation for inherited metabolic disease. *Arch Dis Child.* 1994;71:181-183.
50. Boelens JJ. Trends in haematopoietic cell transplantation for inborn errors of metabolism. *J Inherit Metab Dis.* 2006;29:413-420.
51. Moser HW. Therapy of X-linked adrenoleukodystrophy. *NeuroRx.* 2006;3:246-253.
52. Brady RO. Enzyme replacement for lysosomal diseases. *Annu Rev Med.* 2006;57:283-296.

53. Sands MS, Davidson BL. Gene therapy for lysosomal storage diseases. *Mol Ther.* 2006;13:839-849.
54. Bhat M, Haase C, Lee PJ. Social outcome in treated individuals with inherited metabolic disorders: UK study. *J Inherit Metab Dis.* 2005;28:825-830.
55. American College of Medical Genetics, Newborn Screening Expert Group. Newborn screening: toward a uniform screening panel and system. *Genet Med.* 2006; 8:1S-252S.
56. Dussault JH. Neonatal screening for congenital hypothyroidism. *Clin Lab Med.* 1993;13(3):645-652.
57. American Academy of Pediatrics, Kaye CI and the Committee on Genetics. Introduction to the newborn screening fact sheets. *Pediatrics.* 2006;118(3): 1304-1312.
58. Tluczek A, Mischler EH, Farrell PM, et al. Parents' knowledge of neonatal screening and response to false-positive cystic fibrosis testing. *J Dev Behav Pediatr.* 1992;13(3):181-186.
59. Hamosh A, FitzSimmons SC, Macek M Jr, et al. Comparison of the clinical manifestation of cystic fibrosis in black and white patients. *J Pediatr.* 1998;132(2): 255-259.
60. Listernick R, Frisone L, Silverman BL. Delayed diagnosis of infants with abnormal neonatal screens. *JAMA.* 1992;267(8):1095-1099.
61. Holtzman NA, Kronmal RA, van Doorninck W, et al. Effect of age at loss of dietary control on intellectual performance and behavior of children with phenylketonuria. *N Engl J Med.* 1986;314(10):593-598.
62. Lorey FW, Cunningham GC. Birth prevalence of primary congenital hypothyroidism by sex and ethnicity. *Hum Biol.* 1992;64(4):531-538.
63. Grant DB, Smith I, Fuggle PW, et al. Congenital hypothyroidism detected by neonatal screening: relationship between biochemical severity and early clinical features. *Arch Dis Child.* 1992;67:87-90.
64. Kooistra LLaane C, Vulsma T, Schellekens JM, et al. Motor and cognitive development in children with congenital hypothyroidism: a long-term evaluation of the effects of neonatal treatment. *J Pediatr.* 1994;124(6): 903-909.
65. Rovet JF. Congenital hypothyroidism: long-term outcome. *Thyroid.* 1999;9(7):741-748.
66. Simons WF, Fuggle PW, Grant DB, et al. Educational progress, behaviour, and motor skills at 10 years in early treated congenital hypothyroidism. *Arch Dis Child.* 1997;77(3):219-222.
67. Gaston MH, Verter JI, Woods G, et al. Prophylaxis with oral penicillin in children with sickle cell anemia: a randomized trial. *N Engl J Med.* 1986;314(25):1593-1599.
68. Agency for Health Care Policy and Research, Sickle Cell Disease Guideline Panel. *Sickle Cell Disease: Screening, Diagnosis, Management, and Counseling in Newborns and Infants.* Rockville, MD: US Department of Health and Human Services; 1993.
69. Lane PA, Eckman JR. Cost-effectiveness of neonatal screening for sickle cell disease. *J Pediatr.* 1992;120(1): 162-163.
70. Andrews LB, Fullarton JE, Holtzman NA, et al, eds, Institute of Medicine, Committee on Assessing Genetic Risks. *Assessing Genetic Risks: Implications for Health and Social Policy.* Washington, DC: National Academy of Sciences Press; 1994.
71. Donnell GN. Clinical aspects and historical perspectives of galactosemia. In: Donnell GN, de la Cruz F, Koch R, et al, eds. *Galactosemia: New Frontiers in Research.* Washington, DC: US Department of Health and Human Services; 1993.
72. Waggoner DD, Donnell GN, Buist NRM. Long-term prognosis in galactosemia: results of a survey of 350 cases. In: Donnell GN, de la Cruz F, Koch R, et al, eds. *Galactosemia: New Frontiers in Research.* Washington, DC: US Department of Health and Human Services; 1993.
73. Peinemann F, Danner DJ. Maple syrup urine disease 1954 to 1993. *J Inherit Metab Dis.* 1994;17(1): 3-15.
74. Nobukuni Y, Mitsubuchi H, Hayashida Y, et al. Heterogeneity of mutations in maple syrup urine disease (MSUD): Screening and identification of affected E1 alpha and E1 beta subunits of the branched-chain alpha-keto-acid dehydrogenase multienzyme complex. *Biochim Biophys Acta.* 1994;1225(1):64-70.
75. Brosnan PG, Brosnan CA, Kemp SF, et al. Effect of newborn screening for congenital adrenal hyperplasia. *Arch Pediatr Adolesc Med.* 1999;153(12):1272-1278.
76. Pang S, Clark A. Congenital adrenal hyperplasia due to 21-hydroxylase deficiency: newborn screening and its relationship to the diagnosis and treatment of the disorder. *Screening.* 1993;2:105-139.
77. Thompson R, Seargeant L, Winter J. Screening for congenital adrenal hyperplasia: distribution of 17 alpha-hydroxyprogesterone concentrations in neonatal blood spot specimens. *J Pediatr.* 1989;114(3):400-404.
78. Carlson AD, Obeid JS, Kanellopoulou N, et al. Congenital adrenal hyperplasia: update on prenatal diagnosis and treatment. *J Steroid Biochem Mol Biol.* 1999;69(1-6): 19-29.
79. Hart PS, Barnstein BO, Secor McVoy JR, et al. Comparison of profound biotinidase deficiency in children ascertained clinically and by newborn screening using a simple method of accurately determining residual biotinidase activity. *Biochem Med Metabol Biol.* 1992;48(1): 41-45.
80. Wolf B, Heard GS. Biotinidase deficiency. *Adv Pediatr.* 1991;38:1-21.
81. Hammond KB, Abman SH, Sokol RJ, et al. Efficacy of statewide neonatal screening for cystic fibrosis by assay of trypsinogen concentrations. *N Engl J Med.* 1991; 325(11):769-774.
82. Grosse SD, Scott D, Boyle CA, et al. Newborn screening for cystic fibrosis: evaluation of benefits and risks and recommendations for state newborn screening programs. *MMWR Morb Mortal Wky Rep.* 2004;53(RR13): 1-36.
83. Grosse SD, Rosenfeld M, Devine OJ, et al. Potential impact of newborn screening for cystic fibrosis on child survival: a systematic review and analysis. *J Pediatr.* 2006;149(3):362-366.
84. Pyeritz RE. Homocystinuria. In: Beighton P, ed. *McKusik's Heritable Disorders of Connective Tissue.* St Louis, MO: Mosby; 1993.
85. Peterschmitt MJ, Simmons JR, Levy HL. Reduction of false negative results in screening of newborns for homocystinuria. *N Engl J Med.* 1999;341(21): 1572-1576.
86. Schulze A, Kohlmueller D, Mayatepek E. Sensitivity of electrospray-tandem mass spectrometry using the phenylalanine/tyrosine-ratio for differential diagnosis of hyperphenylalaninemia in neonates. *Clin Chim Acta.* 1999;283(1-2):15-20.
87. Chace DH, Hillman SL, Millington DS, et al. Rapid diagnosis of homocystinuria and other hypermethioninemias from newborns' blood spots by tandem mass spectrometry. *Clin Chem.* 1996;42(3):349-355.
88. Holtzman NA. *Proceed With Caution: Predicting Genetic Risks in the Recombinant DNA Era.* Baltimore, MD: Johns Hopkins University Press; 1989.

89. Meloni T, Forteleoni G, Meloni GF. Marked decline of favism after neonatal glucose-6-phosphate dehydrogenase screening and health education: the Northern Sardinian experience. *Acta Haematol.* 1992;87(1-2):29-31.
90. Silverman EK, Pierce JA, Province MA, et al. Variability of pulmonary function in alpha-1-antitrypsin deficiency: clinical correlates. *Ann Intern Med.* 1989;111(12): 982-991.
91. Wulfsberg EA, Hoffmann DE, Cohen MM. Alpha 1-antitrypsin deficiency: impact of genetic discovery on medicine and society. *JAMA.* 1994;271(3):217-222.
92. Hubbard RC, Sellers S, Czerski D, et al. Biochemical efficacy and safety of monthly augmentation therapy for alpha 1-antitrypsin deficiency. *JAMA.* 1988;260(9): 1259-1264.
93. Wall M, Moe E, Eisenberg J, et al. Long-term follow-up of a cohort of children with alpha-1-antitrypsin deficiency. *J Pediatr.* 1990;116(2):248-251.
94. McNeil TF, Sveger T, Thelin T. Psychosocial effects of screening for somatic risk: the Swedish alpha 1 antitrypsin experience. *Thorax.* 1988;43:505-507.
95. Udall JN, Dixon M, Newman AP, et al. Liver disease in alpha 1-antitrypsin deficiency: a retrospective analysis of the influence of early breast- vs bottle-feeding. *JAMA.* 1985;253(18):2679-2682.
96. Kaback M, Lim-Steele J, Dabholkar D, et al. Tay-Sachs disease: carrier screening, prenatal diagnosis, and the molecular era: an international perspective, 1970-1993. *JAMA.* 1993;270(19):2307-2315.
97. Cao A, Rosatelli C, Pirastu M, et al. Thalassemias in Sardinia: molecular pathology, phenotype-genotype correlation, and prevention. *Am J Pediatr Hemat-Oncol.* 1991;13(2):179-188.
98. Loader S, Sutera CJ, Segelman SG, et al. Prenatal hemoglobinopathy screening. IV. Follow-up of women at risk for a child with a clinically significant hemoglobinopathy. *Am J Hum Genet.* 1991;49(6):1292-1299.
99. Zeesman S, Clow CL, Cartier L, et al. A private view of heterozygosity: 8-year follow-up study on carriers of the Tay-Sachs gene detected by high school screening in Montreal. *Am J Med Genet.* 1984;18(4):769-778.
100. American College of Obstetrics and Gynecology, Committee on Genetics. ACOG Committee Opinion. Number 325, December 2005. Update on carrier screening for cystic fibrosis. *Obstet Gynecol.* 2005;106(6): 1465-1468.
101. Cuniff C and the American Academy of Pediatrics, Committee on Genetics. Prenatal screening and diagnosis for pediatricians. *Pediatrics.* 2004;114(3):889-894.
102. Centers for Disease Control and Prevention. Knowledge and use of folic acid by women of childbearing age—United States, 1995 and 1998. *MMWR Morb Mortal Wkly Rep.* 1999;48(16):325-327.
103. Luthy DA, Wardinsky T, Shurtleff DB, et al. Cesarean section before the onset of labor and subsequent motor function in infants with meningomyelocele diagnosed antenatally. *N Engl J Med.* 1991;324(10):662-666.
104. Wald NJ, Cuckle HS. Open neural-tube defects. In: Wald J, ed. *Antenatal and Neonatal Screening.* New York, NY: Oxford University Press; 1984.
105. Rosen T, D'Alton ME. Down syndrome screening in the first and second trimesters: what do the data show? *Semin Perinatol.* 2005;29(6):367-375.
106. Andrews LB, Fullarton JE, Holtzman NA. *Assessing Genetic Risks: Implications for Health and Social Policy.* Washington, DC: National Academy of Sciences Press; 1994.
107. Bianchi DW, Wataganara T, Lapaire O. Fetal nucleic acids in maternal body fluids: an update. *Ann NY Acad Sci.* 2006;1075:63-73.

Chapter 49

SCREENING AND INITIAL MANAGEMENT OF LEAD POISONING

Stephen J. Maddox Jr, MD; Michael L. Weitzman, MD; Arthur H. Fierman, MD

Childhood lead poisoning represents one of the great pediatric public health success stories in the United States. For a child to suffer from acute lead encephalopathy is now rare. Virtually no children in the United States die from this disease, and most pediatricians have never seen a child who has overt symptoms resulting from this condition. Despite these successes, a large number of children continue to have levels of exposure that affect their health negatively, and unfortunately severe toxicity and even deaths do still occur, as evidenced by reports of accidental ingestion of lead-containing necklaces[1] and metallic charms.[2] More commonly, children who are exposed to lead are exposed at low levels previously thought to be harmless but now recognized to have adverse effects on cognition and behavior. Thus continued efforts in the areas of screening, public education, and removal of sources of lead are still needed.

EPIDEMIOLOGIC FEATURES OF CHILDHOOD LEAD POISONING

Blood lead levels of children in the United States have declined dramatically, as measured in the National Health and Nutrition Examination Surveys. The geometric mean blood lead level of children 1 to 5 years of age has declined from 15 mcg/dL in the 1976 to 1980 survey, to 2.7 mcg/dL in 1991 to 1994, and most recently to 1.9 mcg/dL in 1999 to 2002.[3] These changes were accompanied by corresponding declines in the prevalence of 1- to 5-year-old children with elevated blood levels (defined as $\geq$10 mcg/dL), from 77.8% (1976 to 1980) to 4.4% (1991 to 1994), to 1.6% (1999 to 2002).[4] Based on the prevalence in the 1999 to 2002 survey, an estimated 310,000 children aged 1 to 5 years in the United States have elevated blood lead levels.[3]

Although individuals of all ages may develop lead poisoning, blood lead levels tend to peak between 1 and 3 years of age. Levels vary inversely with family income. Because living in impoverished homes is linked so closely to increased exposure to lead, Medicaid enrollment is an excellent marker for elevated blood lead levels: 60% of children whose blood lead levels are at least 10 mcg/dL and 83% of those whose levels are at least 20 mcg/dL are enrolled in Medicaid. As a result, all children enrolled in Medicaid are required by federal regulation to be tested for elevated blood lead levels at 1 and 2 years of age.[5]

SOURCES OF LEAD

For most children, lead-contaminated interior and exterior household paint that has chipped, peeled, or chalked in their primary residences or in the homes of relatives, babysitters, or child care providers remains the most common and the most concentrated source of exposure. As detailed in a survey report by the US Department of Housing and Urban Development, the older the house is, the more likely it is to contain lead-based paint; the less affluent the family is, the more likely this paint is to be in disrepair.[6] Housing built before 1950 poses the greatest danger of exposure. Nationwide, the number of pre-1950 housing units has decreased from 27.5 million in 1990 to 25.7 million in 2000. Although at-risk housing can be found throughout the United States, 50% of the houses built before 1950 are located in only seven states: California, Illinois, Massachusetts, Missouri, New York, Ohio, and Pennsylvania.[4]

Other sources of lead exposure exist. Children may be exposed to lead in water, food, soil, toys, or ceramics. Parents whose clothing becomes contaminated with lead at work may inadvertently bring lead into the home. Occupations at high risk for take-home exposures include those involving battery production or repair, the making of pottery, smelting, printing, paint contracting, and working on a firing range, in a brass foundry, or on the demolition or renovation of outdoor structures. In addition, a significant number of hobbies can place children at risk, such as making lead fishing sinkers or bullets, collecting lead figurines, spending time at indoor firing ranges, and making ceramic pottery. In certain cultures, such as several from Latin America and Southeast Asia, many home remedies such as azarcon or greta can serve as sources of lead poisoning. Certain cosmetics such as Kohl, an eye makeup from the Middle East and South Asia, can contain over 80% lead.[7] Lead-glazed ceramic dishes and containers also can cause lead poisoning, especially if acidic foods such as salad dressings or citric acid juices are served on or stored in them. These sources should be considered when children who are recent immigrants are poisoned. Lead plumbing also remains an important source, especially in areas with older water supplies. This contamination was evidenced in 2003 to 2004 by the elevated lead concentrations found in Washington, DC, after changes in water disinfection procedures caused leaching of lead out of water service pipes.[8]

ADVERSE HEALTH EFFECTS

Exposure to lead has numerous adverse health consequences. Most pediatricians' concern, however, has focused on the adverse neurocognitive effects of lead toxicity. A well-established fact is that, beginning at levels of 10 mcg/dL, each 10-mcg/dL increase in blood lead results in a loss of 2 to 3 points in IQ. Lead has also been shown to have adverse effects on other aspects of children's functioning, including attention, vigilance, language development, the transfer of information from short-term to long-term memory, aggression, and antisocial or delinquent behaviors. An impressive array of studies has identified subtle but potentially serious alterations of children's neurocognitive functioning associated with lead exposure at levels previously believed to be innocuous.[9-12] No apparent threshold exists for the toxic effects of lead; that is, negative cognitive effects appear to occur at levels even lower than 10 mcg/dL. Credible research has suggested that in the 0- to 10-mcg/dL range for blood lead, the decrement in IQ associated with each unit increase in blood lead may be larger than the IQ decrement per unit increase in blood lead in the 10- to 20-mcg/dL range.[13-15] Although negative effects on behavior have been shown at levels greater than 10 mcg/dL, lower levels may also produce negative effects.[16] Prenatal lead exposure has also been studied and has been negatively associated with intellectual development of school age children.[17]

SCREENING FOR ELEVATED BLOOD LEAD LEVELS

Primary prevention has certainly proven to be the most effective means of eliminating lead poisoning in the United States, and even more intensive large-scale primary preventive measures, such as more aggressive housing rehabilitation, have been advocated.[18] However, to identify children who need individual interventions to reduce their blood lead levels, screening of blood samples remains an essential tool in the prevention of childhood lead poisoning. Guidance from the Centers for Disease Control and Prevention (CDC) has been pivotal in defining national standards for screening programs. Since 1991, the CDC has recommended the use of venous or capillary blood lead level as the laboratory examination of choice and the use of 10 mcg/dL as the cutoff point for defining an elevated lead level.[19]

Although capillary blood samples collected by finger stick are acceptable, the potential for contamination by lead deposits on the skin dictates that capillary specimens with values at or above 10 mcg/dL be confirmed with a venous sample. An important point to recognize is that the allowable error established by the Clinical Laboratory Improvement Amendments for lead testing is ±4 mcg/dL or 10% of value, whichever is greater.[20] At low levels of blood lead, allowable laboratory error can result in misclassification that might affect management recommendations for an individual child.

CDC guidelines advise state health officials to develop universal or targeted screening programs (or both) based on the risk characteristics of their local communities.[21] Within the state or the locale for which recommendations are made, the CDC advises that child health care professionals use blood lead tests to screen 1- and 2-year-olds (and 3- to 6-year-olds who have not been screened previously) who meet one or more of the criteria in Box 49-1. Of particular continued importance is the recommendation to screen all Medicaid-eligible children at 1 and 2 years of age (even if no other risk factors are present).

Screening by questionnaire to evaluate risk remains part of the guidelines suggested by the CDC, but substantial variability in the sensitivity and specificity of screening questionnaires limits the usefulness of this screening strategy. Screening questions are still used by some states and localities as one component of an overall lead-screening strategy, often with modifications in the specific questions used based on the locale. State- and locale-specific screening strategies

BOX 49-1 Recommendations for Lead Screening in Children At Risk

Child resides in a zip code area in which at least 27% of housing stock was built before 1950 or 12% or more of children have blood lead levels at or above 10 mcg/dL.

Child receives services from public assistance programs for the poor, such as Medicaid or the Supplemental Food Program for Women, Infants, and Children (WIC).

See CDC Web site for the latest and most accurate screening questions for your region. Available at: www.cdc.gov/nceh/lead/guide/1997/pdf/chapter3.pdf.

Data from Centers for Disease Control and Prevention. *Screening Young Children for Lead Poisoning: Guidance for State and Local Public Health Officials,* Atlanta, GA: US Department of Health and Human Services; 1997.

are available on the CDC Web site at www.cdc.gov/nceh/lead/grants/contacts/clppp%20map.htm.

In addition to following state- or local-level guidelines, health care professionals are encouraged to go beyond these recommendations by remaining vigilant in identifying children who should be screened because of exposure to less-usual sources of lead, such as those resulting from various parental occupations or hobbies.[21] Similarly, if parents or health care professionals have suspicion of lead exposure, then prompt performance of a blood lead test should be undertaken, regardless of patient age, general health department recommendations, or responses to screening questionnaires.

Of course, to be optimally effective, a screening policy is not enough; health care providers must participate and comply with the recommended program. In a 1994 survey, almost 50% of practicing pediatricians reported being out of compliance with the CDC lead-screening recommendations.[22] Even more disturbing was a 1998 government report showing that 81% of children receiving Medicaid, a group with a 3-fold increase risk of having elevated lead levels, had never been screened for lead.[5] Similarly, an analysis of children receiving Medicaid in Michigan in 2002 showed that only 19.6% of children under age 5 years in the cohort had ever had a blood lead test.[23]

Healthy People 2010 calls for the elimination by the year 2010 of all lead levels over 10 mcg/dL in children. Although most physicians agree that lead poisoning remains a major problem, concern is growing about the cost benefit of using blood lead level as a screening tool in an era of declining prevalence. This concern is addressed in a recent policy statement from the American Academy of Pediatrics, which reviews a cost-benefit analysis of lead screening.[8] Although the cost of lead screening is not trivial, the projected loss of income among individuals who suffered IQ decrements caused by lead poisoning in childhood is in the hundreds of billions of dollars.

Table 49-1 Recommended Schedule for Obtaining a Confirmatory Venous Sample

SCREENING TEST RESULT (mcg/dL)	PERFORM A CONFIRMATION TEST WITHIN
10-19	3 mo
20-44	1 wk-1 mo
45-59	48 hr
60-69	24 hr
>70	Immediately as an emergency laboratory test

The higher the blood lead level on the screening test is, the more urgent will be the need for confirmatory testing.

Adapted from Centers for Disease Control and Prevention. *Screening Young Children for Lead Poisoning: Guidance for State and Local Public Health Officials.* Atlanta, GA: US Department of Health and Human Services; 1997.

Follow-Up of Positive Screening Tests

In communities where universal screening is recommended, children whose blood lead screening test result at age 1 year is less than 10 mcg/dL should be rescreened at age 2 years.

If at the 2-year screen the blood lead level is again less than 10 mcg/dL and the child's potential exposures have not increased, then the child need not be subjected to subsequent screening.

The CDC has recommended a schedule of follow-up testing based on the initial screening result (Table 49-1).

Children with blood lead values of 10 to 19 mcg/dL. If a venous sample confirms that the child does have an elevated blood lead level, then parents are counseled on ways to diminish ongoing exposure (Box 49-2). Children whose blood lead levels are between 10 and 14 mcg/dL should be retested every 3 months; those whose levels are between 15 and 19 mcg/dL should be retested every 2 months. In an increasing number of locales, blood lead values greater than 10 mcg/dL may prompt a home inspection (see the next section on "Children with blood lead values of 20 to 44 mcg/dL").

Children with blood lead values of 20 to 44 mcg/dL. Children whose blood lead levels are in this range are described as having moderately elevated blood lead levels; they require both medical and environmental intervention. If the confirmatory venous lead level is 20 mcg/dL or greater, then the child should have (1) a medical evaluation, consisting of a detailed medical, nutritional, developmental, and environmental history, and a complete physical examination; (2) a laboratory evaluation of iron status, including a hematocrit and mean corpuscular volume and either a ferritin level or iron and iron binding capacity levels; (3) an environmental inspection and, when indicated, environmental intervention to diminish or curtail further exposure to lead; and (4) case management to ensure that the needed counseling and medical, nutritional, and

BOX 49-2 Avoiding Lead Hazards in the Home

Cover leaded paint that is chipping or peeling.
Move cribs, playpens, furniture, and play areas away from chipping or peeling paint.
Wet-mop floors and wet-clean windowsills and window wells with a high-phosphate detergent.
Avoid dry dusting or sweeping.
Wash children's hands, toys, and pacifiers regularly.
Use cold water for cooking; run tap water for 2 to 3 minutes every morning before using.
Repair deteriorated windowpanes in house and on porches.
Replace old windows.
Remove paint in old homes (only by trained contractors).
Families must be out of their homes during paint removal.
Postabatement cleanup, preferably by professional house-cleaners, is essential.
Relocate the family to lead-safe housing.

Data from Centers for Disease Control and Prevention: *Preventing Lead Poisoning in Young Children: A Statement by the Centers for Disease Control.* Atlanta, GA: US Department of Health and Human Services; 1991.

environmental interventions are provided quickly and effectively.

The medical evaluation should focus on identifying signs and symptoms of lead poisoning (although these are very unusual at these blood levels). A developmental assessment is conducted to determine the need for early intervention services, although blood lead levels in this range would not likely result in demonstrable delays. Concerns about inattention and hyperactivity should prompt referral for early intervention services.

Nutritional assessment is conducted to identify eating patterns that may result in increased absorption of lead from the gastrointestinal tract, such as iron deficiency, low calcium intake, or infrequent meals. Many children whose blood lead levels are in this range are eligible for support from the Special Supplemental Nutrition Program for Women, Infants, and Children and should be referred. If the child is iron deficient, then iron supplements should be prescribed. The protective effect of increased calcium intake is not proven but is generally recommended, especially when calcium intake is low. Increasing meal frequency may decrease lead absorption, but this action should be prescribed in the context of a diet that is not excessive in caloric content.

Children with lead levels of 20 to 44 mcg/dL require home inspections, usually performed by local public health departments, to identify sources of lead exposure. Although often a lengthy process, abatement of lead-based hazards and subsequent dust control are cornerstones of treatment for children whose blood lead levels are in this range.

Families should be counseled to (1) have lead-based paint abatements performed by a properly licensed contractor and, if possible, with supervision of the local health department; (2) relocate children and pregnant women to another site while abatement is being performed; and (3) have a thorough cleanup of dust before allowing children to reinhabit the home. The use of chelating agents for children whose blood lead levels are less than 25 mcg/dL is not indicated. Recent research suggests that chelation therapy may also be ineffective in treating children with levels between 25 and 44 mcg/dL. A prospective study randomized 2-year-old children with lead levels between 25 and 44 mcg/dL to receive succimer (dimercaptosuccinic acid) or placebo, with up to 3 treatment courses of 26 days each, over 6 months. The authors found no appreciable difference in lead levels and no significant differences on measures of cognition or behavior between the succimer-treated and placebo groups at follow-up at age 7 years.[24] The effects of succimer when used in more prolonged or more repeated treatment courses would require further study.

According to CDC guidelines, children whose blood lead levels are in this range should have blood lead tests repeated weekly to monthly so as to identify promptly children with lead levels that continue to rise (the higher the blood lead levels, the more frequently the child should be retested). Testing should continue until levels decline into the 10- to 19-mcg/dL range or lower. The frequency of this testing should be based on the pattern of past tests, confidence in the child's safe environment, the child's risk from his behaviors and iron status, and overall clinical judgment.

Children with blood lead values of 45 mcg/dL or higher. The clearest management strategies exist for children in this category. Children whose blood lead screens are 45 to 59 mcg/dL should be retested with venous blood within 48 hours, those whose are 60 to 69 mcg/dL should be retested within 24 hours, and those whose are at least 70 mcg/dL should have a venous blood lead level conducted on an emergency basis (see Table 49-1). Broad consensus exists that such children must be removed from sources of lead in their environments and receive chelation therapy, as described in Chapter 355, Poisoning.

TOOLS FOR PRACTICE

Community Coordination and Advocacy

- *Screening Young Children for Lead Poisoning: Guidance for State and Local Public Health Officials,* (report), Centers for Disease Control and Prevention (www.cdc.gov/nceh/lead/guide/guide97.htm).

Engaging Patient and Family

- *Lead* (Web page), Centers for Disease Control and Prevention (www.cdc.gov/lead/).
- *Lead Poisoning* (Web page), Centers for Disease Control and Prevention (www.cdc.gov/nceh/lead/CaseManagement/caseManage_main.htm).

- *Lead Screening for Children* (brochure), American Academy of Pediatrics (patiented.aap.org).

Medical Decision Support

- *Eliminating Childhood Lead Poisoning: A Federal Strategy Targeting Lead Paint Hazards* (report), President's Task Force on Environmental Health Risks and Safety Risks to Children (yosemite.epa.gov/ochp/ochpweb.nsf/content/leadhaz.htm/$file/leadhaz.pdf).
- *Managing Elevated Blood Lead Levels Among Young Children: Recommendations from the Advisory Committee on Childhood Lead Poisoning Prevention* (report), Centers for Disease Control and Prevention (www.cdc.gov/nceh/lead/CaseManagement/caseManage_main.htm).
- *Pediatric Environmental Health, 2nd edition* (book), American Academy of Pediatrics (www.aap.org/bookstore).
- *Preventing Lead Poisoning in Young Children* (report), Centers for Disease Control and Prevention (www.cdc.gov/nceh/lead/publications/PrevLeadPoisoning.pdf).
- *Recommendations for Blood Lead Screening of Young Children Enrolled in Medicaid: Targeting a Group at High Risk,* (report), Centers for Disease Control and Prevention (www.cdc.gov/mmwr/preview/mmwrhtml/rr4914a1.htm).

AAP POLICY STATEMENTS

American Academy of Pediatrics, Committee on Environmental Health. Lead exposure in children: Prevention, detection, and management. *Pediatrics*. 2005;116(4):1036-1046 (aappolicy.aappublications.org/cgi/content/full/pediatrics;116/4/1036).

Centers for Disease Control and Prevention. *Preventing Lead Poisoning in Young Children*. Atlanta, GA: Centers for Disease Control and Prevention; 2005.

REFERENCES

1. Centers for Disease Control and Prevention. Lead poisoning from ingestion of a toy necklace—Oregon, 2003. *MMWR*. 2004;53:509-511.
2. Centers for Disease Control and Prevention. Death of a child after ingestion of a metallic charm—Minnesota, 2006. *MMWR*. 2006;55;1-2.
3. Centers for Disease Control and Prevention. Blood lead levels—United States, 1999-2002. *MMWR*. 2005;54(20):513-516.
4. Meyer P, Pivetz T, Dignam TA, et al, and the Centers for Disease Control and Prevention. Surveillance of elevated blood lead levels among children—United States 1997-2001. *MMWR*. 2003;52(10):1-21.
5. Centers for Disease Control and Prevention, Advisory Committee on Childhood Lead Poisoning Prevention. Recommendations for blood lead screening of young children enrolled in Medicaid: targeting a group at high risk. *MMWR*. 2000;49(14):1-13.
6. Clickner RP, Marker D, Viet SM, et al. *Lead-Based Paint Hazards in Housing. National Survey of Lead and Allergens in Housing. Volume I: Analysis of Lead Hazards*. Rev 6.0. Rockville, MD: US Department of Housing and Urban Development, Office of Lead Hazard Control; 2001.
7. Centers for Disease Control and Prevention, Advisory Committee on Childhood Lead Poisoning. Managing Elevated Blood Lead Levels in Children: Recommendations from the Advisory Committee on Childhood Lead Poisoning Prevention. March 2002. Available at: www.cdc.gov/nceh/lead/CaseManagement/caseManage_main.htm. Accessed March 2006.
8. American Academy of Pediatrics. Lead exposure in children: prevention, detection, and management. American Academy of Pediatrics policy statement. *Pediatrics*. 2005;116(4):1036-1046.
9. Centers for Disease Control and Prevention. *The Nature and Extent of Lead Poisoning in Children in the United States: A Report to Congress*. Atlanta, GA: US Department of Health and Human Services, Agency for Toxic Substances and Disease Registry; 1988.
10. National Research Council. *Measuring Lead Exposure in Infants, Children, and Other Sensitive Populations*. Washington, DC: National Academy Press; 1993.
11. Needleman HL, Gatsonis CA. Low-level lead exposure and the IQ of children. *JAMA*. 1990;263:673-678.
12. Schwartz J. Low-level lead exposure and children's IQ: a meta-analysis and search for a threshold. *Environ Res*. 1994;65:42-55.
13. Lanphear BP, Homung R, Khoury J, et al. Low level environmental lead exposure and children's intellectual function: an international pooled analysis. *Environ Health Perspect*. 2005;113(7):894-899.
14. Canfield RL, Henderson CR, Cory-Slechta DA, et al. Intellectual impairment in children with blood lead concentrations below 10 mcg per deciliter. *N Engl J Med*. 2003;348:1517-1526.
15. Centers for Disease Control and Prevention. Preventing lead poisoning in young children. Atlanta, GA: US Department of Health and Human Services; 2005.
16. Mendelsohn A, Dreyer BP, Fierman AH, et al. Low-level lead exposure and behavior in early childhood. *Pediatrics*. 1998;101(3):e10.
17. Schnaas L, Rothenberg SJ, Flores MF, et al. Reduced intellectual development in children with prenatal lead exposure. *Environ Health Perspect*. 2006;114(5):791-797.
18. President's Task Force on Environmental Health Risks and Safety Risks to Children. Eliminating Childhood Lead Poisoning: A Federal Strategy Targeting Lead Paint Hazards. February 2000. Available at: www.cdc.gov/nceh/lead/about/fedstrategy2000.pdf. Accessed November 29, 2007.
19. Centers for Disease Control and Prevention. *Preventing Lead Poisoning in Young Children: A Statement by the Centers for Disease Control*. Atlanta, GA: US Department of Health and Human Services; 1991.
20. Centers for Disease Control and Prevention. CLIA Regulations 2004 Codifications. Subpart I, Section 493.937. Available at: www.phppo.cdc.gov/clia/regs/subpart_i.aspx#493.937 Accessed March 12, 2007.
21. Centers for Disease Control and Prevention. *Screening Young Children for Lead Poisoning: Guidance for State and Local Public Health Officials*. Atlanta, GA: US Department of Health and Human Services; 1997.
22. Campbell JR, Schaffer SJ, Szilagyi PG, et al. Blood lead screening practices among US pediatricians. *Pediatrics*. 1996;98(3):372-377.
23. Kemper AR, Cohn LM, Fant KE, et al. Blood lead testing among Medicaid-enrolled children in Michigan. *Arch Pediatr Adolesc Med*. 2005;159:646-650.
24. Dietrich KN, Ware JH, Salganik M, et al, and the Treatment of Lead-Exposed Children Clinical Trial Group. Effect of chelation therapy on the neuropsychological and behavioral development of lead-exposed children after school entry. *Pediatrics*. 2004;114:19-26.

Chapter 50

SUBSTANCE USE DISORDERS: EARLY IDENTIFICATION AND REFERRAL

Jeffrey J. Wilson, MD; Megan E. Janoff

DEFINITION OF TERMS

Adolescent substance abuse is a major public health problem and contributes to potentially preventable morbidity and mortality in this population. However, in primary care settings the screening for and prevalence of adolescent substance abuse is often overlooked. Estimates suggest that as many as 1 in 10 adolescents should receive a diagnostic evaluation for substance abuse, and at least one half of these adolescents are likely to require treatment.[1] Literature discussing substance abuse among adults in primary care settings suggests that substance abuse may be commonly overlooked and underdiagnosed. For example, Saitz et al[2] reported that of 1440 patients, less than one half (45%) reported that the physician who cared for them was aware of their substance abuse. Earlier identification of substance use disorders, before the development of serious complications, can prevent the many adverse consequences of these highly prevalent disorders among young people.[3]

Substance abuse among adolescents can be a matter of life and death. The effects of substance abuse or dependence are pervasive and adversely affect judgment, placing youth at significant risk. For example, in youth 15 to 24 years of age, 38% of all deaths are secondary to motor-vehicle accidents, the number one killer among adolescents. One half of these motor-vehicle accidents are alcohol related.[4] Although cigarette smoking and other forms of nicotine dependence have been declining in the general population, such is not the case among adolescents. In addition, 75% of adolescents who smoke will become lifetime smokers and thus face a longer exposure to nicotine toxicity.[5] Nicotine alone accounts for more substance-related deaths than all other drugs (including alcohol) together. Furthermore, adolescents who abuse nicotine and alcohol are more likely to abuse marijuana and a variety of other illicit substances. These very high-risk children (who abuse nicotine, alcohol, marijuana, and other substances) are even more likely to suffer from a variety of negative outcomes, including school failure, sexually transmitted diseases such as HIV, teenage pregnancy, and delinquency; they are also at greater risk for suicide and homicide.[6]

Epidemiologic Factors of Use

Many more youth use nicotine, alcohol, or other substances than abuse or become dependent on them. Figure 50-1 presents the 30-day prevalence rates of nicotine and alcohol use, as reported from the *Monitoring the Future* study at the University of Michigan sponsored by the National Institute of Drug Abuse. Ten percent of all 8th graders report having smoked cigarettes in the previous 30 days, and one half this number (5%) smoked cigarettes daily. Regarding alcohol, 19.5% of 8th graders used alcohol in the previous 30 days, and 6.7% had been drunk in the previous 30 days. Among 12th graders, these numbers increase to over 26.7% smoking cigarettes in the previous 30 days and over 16.9% smoking daily. Nearly 50% of high school seniors have used alcohol in the previous 30 days, whereas 30.3% have been drunk in this period. Just under 5% (3.9%) of seniors report being drunk on a daily basis.[7] Figure 50-2 presents the 30-day prevalence rates of marijuana and other drug use. Of note, 21.3% of high school seniors have smoked marijuana in the previous 30 days, whereas only 6% smoked marijuana daily. Specific other drug use is rather uncommon, in total, 11.3% of high school seniors report using some type of other illicit drug.

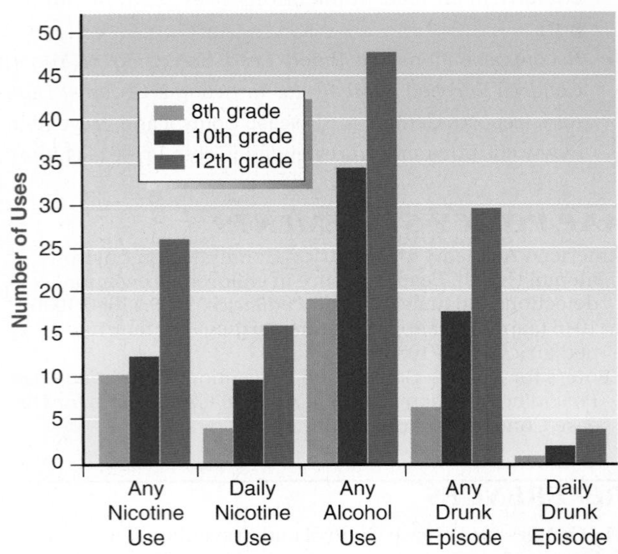

Figure 50-1 Current (previous 30-day) nicotine and alcohol use.

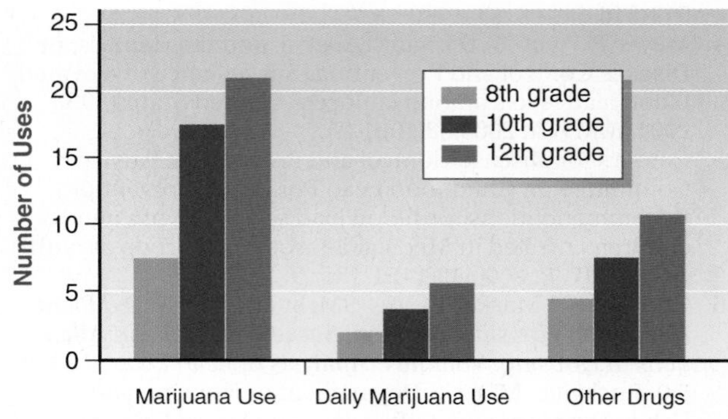

Figure 50-2 Current (previous 30-day) drug use.

Epidemiologic Factors of Substance Abuse or Dependence

Excluding nicotine, 7% of adolescents (12-17 years of age) are estimated to have a substance use disorder.[8] The highest age-specific prevalence occurs during adolescence, and rates of current dependence on alcohol and other drugs peak between ages 16 and 19 years.[9] Alcohol and marijuana are the most common substances of abuse among adolescents. Among adolescents with substance use disorders, an estimated 41% have an alcohol use disorder, 11% have an alcohol or marijuana use disorder, 5% have an alcohol use disorder with another substance use disorder (other than marijuana), 3% smoke marijuana only, and another 3% have a marijuana use disorder with another substance use disorder (other than alcohol).[8]

Gateway Hypothesis

The *gateway hypothesis* is an attempt to explain the progression of substance use (eg, from cigarettes and alcohol to marijuana or from marijuana to cocaine and possibly heroin). In general the earlier the age of onset is and the more severe the earlier stage of use is, the more likely an adolescent is to progress to problem use or substance use disorder. Marijuana is often called a *gateway drug*. For example, only 12.8% of persons who have smoked marijuana once or twice have tried cocaine; however, of those who have smoked more than 300 times, over 71% have tried cocaine. An important point to recognize is that this hypothesis is based on cross-sectional data; that is, the type of drugs of use may be one of several factors that predict transition through stages of problem use. The extent to which nicotine use predisposes a person to marijuana use, or the extent to which marijuana use predisposes a person to cocaine use, is unclear, although compelling associations exist. The age of onset of substance use is also associated with transition between stages. For example, heroin users typically report first smoking cigarettes at 12.6 years, whereas cocaine users report beginning cigarettes at 14 years, marijuana users report beginning cigarettes at 14.6 years, and alcohol-only users report beginning at 15.8 years. Regardless of the etiology of the relationship between stages of substance use, these patterns of use and the prevalence of use at different ages provide valuable clinical information for the assessment of risk related to adolescent substance abuse. For example, early-onset nicotine use can be seen as a marker for potential abuse and dependence to nicotine and other substances of abuse.[10]

Early- Versus Late-Onset Substance Use Disorders

The earlier the age of onset is, the more likely substance use is to develop into a lifetime disorder. Early-onset or adolescent substance use disorders appear to differ from substance use disorders that develop later in life. Youth who develop substance use disorders tend to have an increased degree of disruptive behaviors or delinquency. These youth also tend to have an increased degree of novelty or sensation seeking and a decreased dependence on external incentives (eg, doing well in school, performing a job well).[11] Later-onset substance use disorders tend to be associated with a decreased degree of antisocial behavior and an increased degree of reward dependence. These differences have been shown in both adolescent and adult samples. As a result the majority of adolescent substance use disorders are often accompanied by some other problem behaviors that can include school failure or truancy, depression or suicidal thoughts, early-onset sexual behavior, sexually transmitted disease, pregnancy, and legal problems, among others.[12,13] As the list of problems mount, identifying the existence of a substance use disorder as a contributor to these problems becomes easier and easier for family members and health care professionals. Because of the nature of the illness, adolescents rarely spontaneously seek help; more commonly, they are referred by a parent, other caring adults, or the justice system.

Etiology of Early-Onset Substance Use Disorders

Most of the time, substance abuse develops within a context of behavioral impulsivity, conduct problems, and difficulties in functioning that arise *before* the first use of a substance. At times, this behavioral impulsivity is accompanied by aggression, which develops during the preschool or early school-age period. Early-onset aggression is more highly associated with oppositional defiant disorder, which, in turn, is highly associated with the development of early-onset conduct disorder.[12] Disruptive behavior disorders such as conduct disorder strongly predict the transition from substance use to abuse. Untreated attention-deficit/hyperactivity disorder also appears to increase the risk of substance use by approximately two times the general risk. Attention-deficit/hyperactivity disorder that is comorbid with conduct disorder increases the risk developing a substance use disorder by up to four times the general risk.[14,15] Social factors are also important. For example, low levels of parental monitoring, parental substance abuse, and peers who also use substances all play significant roles in the development of a substance use disorder. Poverty and neglect also play an important role.[16]

DIFFERENTIAL DIAGNOSIS

The physician should realize that substance use alone does not imply a substance use disorder, and infrequent substance use may, in fact, be a normative part of adolescent development. Nevertheless, when substance use is detected or suspected, determining whether a substance use disorder is present is the responsibility of the primary care physician. Youth who exhibit substance use but not a substance use disorder should be monitored closely to determine if a substance use disorder does occur.

Substance use disorders include substance abuse and substance dependence.[17] Substance abuse is *a maladaptive pattern of substance use leading to clinically significant impairment or distress*. The specific symptoms that indicate this diagnosis can be found in Box 50-1. As an individual loses control over the use, and as the substance-related problems mount, substance dependence develops. Substance dependence

BOX 50-1 DSM-IV-TR Criteria for Substance Abuse

A. A maladaptive pattern of substance use leading to clinically significant impairment or distress, as demonstrated by one (or more) of the following, occurring within a 12-month period:
   1. Recurrent substance use resulting in a failure to fulfill major role obligations at work, school, or home (eg, repeated absences or poor work performance related to substance use; substance-related absences, suspensions or expulsions from school; neglect of children or household)
   2. Recurrent substance use in situations in which it is physically hazardous (eg, driving an automobile, operating a machine when impaired by substance use)
   3. Recurrent substance-related legal problems (eg, arrests for substance-related disorderly conduct)
   4. Continued substance use despite having persistent or recurrent social or interpersonal problems caused or exacerbated by the effects of a substance (eg, arguments with spouse about consequences of intoxication, physical fights)

B. The symptoms have never met the criteria for substance dependence for this class of substance.

From American Psychiatric Association. *Diagnostic and Statistical Manual of Mental Disorders,* 4th ed, text revision. Arlington, VA: American Psychiatric Association; 2000. Reprinted by permission.

BOX 50-2 DSM-IV-TR Criteria for Substance Dependence

A maladaptive pattern of substance use, leading to clinically significant impairment or distress, as demonstrated by three (or more) of the following, occurring at any time in the same 12-month period:

1. Tolerance, as defined by either of the following:
   a. A need for markedly increased amounts of the substance to achieve intoxication or desired effect
   b. Markedly diminished effect with continued use of the same amount of substance
2. Withdrawal, as demonstrated by either of the following:
   a. The characteristic withdrawal syndrome for the substance
   b. The same (or closely related) substance is taken to relieve or avoid withdrawal symptoms
3. The substance was taken in larger amounts or for a longer period than expected
4. A persistent desire or unsuccessful effort exists to cut down or control substance use
5. A great deal of time is spent in activities necessary to obtain the substance (eg, visiting multiple physicians, driving long distances), use the substance (eg, chain smoking), or recover from its effects.
6. Important social, occupational, or recreational activities are given up for or reduced because of substance use.
7. The substance use is continued despite knowledge of having a persistent or recurrent physical or psychological problem that is likely to have been caused or exacerbated by the substance (eg, current cocaine use despite recognition of cocaine-induced depression, continued drinking despite recognition that an ulcer was made worse by alcohol consumption).

From American Psychiatric Association. *Diagnostic and Statistical Manual of Mental Disorders,* 4th ed, text revision. Arlington, VA: American Psychiatric Association; 2000. Reprinted by permission.

is a maladaptive pattern of use, defined as *a constellation of symptoms indicating tolerance or withdrawal or loss of function as a result of substance use*. These symptoms are specified in Box 50-2. An important point to note is that these criteria were primarily created for adults, and authorities have suggested that they are not as useful in delineating the severity of adolescent substance use disorders. Given that the patterns of use of adolescents differ from those of adults (eg, availability, freedom, supervision), the validity of these criteria have been questioned. Some youth can meet one or two criteria of substance dependence but no criteria for abuse. These *diagnostic orphans* appear similar to youth with substance abuse diagnoses and make up approximately a third of youth who use alcohol regularly.[18] Because of the high prevalence of these diagnostic orphans, most experts in adolescent substance abuse recommend asking youth about both lists of symptoms, allowing the diagnosis of disorder to depend largely on the maladaptive significance of this substance use.

EVALUATION

Clinical Presentation

Accurately assessing substance use in an adolescent can be a complex undertaking. In the short amount of time that many clinicians have to evaluate patients, identifying adolescent substance abuse or dependence can be a challenge. Nonetheless, a pediatrician or family physician can have a tremendous impact on whether a youth or the youth's family seeks treatment. Many times the adolescent is not the one who is concerned about the problem; the parent is often the one who mentions this problem to the physician. A substance use disorder can often be identified by the surrounding behaviors rather than explicit knowledge of a child's substance abuse. Paying attention to these subtle clues is more important than many parents or guardians realize. Problems proximal to drug use, as listed previously, include disruptive or defiant behavior, school failure or truancy, depression or suicidal thoughts, early-onset sexual behavior, sexually transmitted disease, pregnancy, and legal problems. Encouraging parents to remain involved in their adolescents' lives will increase the likelihood that parents may identify and seek help for these problem behaviors. In addition, one of the most important protective factors in reducing the development of substance abuse is increased parental monitoring and involvement.

Clinical Interview

Creating an environment in which an adolescent is able to talk about alcohol or drug use is a critical aspect of assessment. An adolescent's self-report of substance-related problems is key to accurate diagnosis and treatment. Providing an environment conducive to self-disclosure involves careful definition of adolescent confidentiality. The usual definition of confidentiality involves a safety exclusion; that is, only information that indicates that an adolescent is a danger to self or others will be revealed to a parent or guardian. Some clinicians may include any substance use in this exclusion to confidentiality. However, the risk of this approach is creating a therapeutic relationship in which *any* talk of drug use will be muted because of fear of parental knowledge. The authors believe that a therapeutic relationship with an adolescent should accommodate the developing individuation of an adolescent from the family, and normative substance experimentation should not be so readily divulged to caretakers. Wherever a clinician feels most comfortable in setting the limits of confidentiality, these limits should be made clear with the adolescent at the beginning of treatment. Otherwise, youth may lose their trust in confiding in anyone, especially the clinician. However, when substance use places youth in dangerous situations (eg, driving under the influence) or when symptoms are sufficient to warrant a substance use disorder diagnosis or other serious impairment, parental involvement is almost always indicated. Clinicians should include the dangerousness of the substance use in this decision. If an adolescent is using substances that are highly dangerous (eg, inhalants, heroin), then this use may increase the risk/benefit ratio of maintaining confidentiality. Deciding each case based on the particular risks involved is best, keeping in mind that helping an adolescent self-identify the adolescent's own substance-related problems is usually the best-case scenario, though family intervention is usually required for treatment to be effective. An adolescent's functioning is best assessed through a variety of viewpoints; hence the clinician needs to obtain information from parents, other health care providers, and the school, if possible.

Standardized Instruments

A variety of standardized instruments can be informative for clinical practice. Types of structured instruments that can be used to assess substance use disorder include screening instruments and more comprehensive structured interviews of substance use or substance-related problems. Generally speaking the most sensitive screening instruments not only ask about substance use, but also ask about substance-related problems. For example, the Substance Abuse Subtle Screening Inventory (SASSI) is a self-report that concentrates to a larger degree on substance-related problems, that is, the adaptive significance of substance use symptoms.[19,20] Additional examples include the Personal Experience Inventory, the Problem Oriented Screening Instrument for Teenagers, and the Rutgers Alcohol Problem Index.[21] Two examples of well-designed structured interviews that more comprehensively assess the relationship between substance use and other domains of functioning include the Comprehensive Addiction Severity Index[22] and the Global Appraisal of Individual Needs.[23] Both of these tools give diagnoses of substance abuse according to *Diagnostic and Statistical Manual of Mental Disorders* and assess a variety of domains of functioning, including substance use, substance-related problems, family relationships, peer relationships, legal status, psychiatric problems, and leisure activities.[21]

The CRAFFT screening tool has been validated for adolescents and consists of six items aimed at identifying adolescents with problematic substance use. Positive answers to two or more items suggest that intervention is necessary (see Tools for Practice).

Urine Drug Screens

The meaning of a positive urine drug screen varies greatly on the context in which it is obtained. For example, an adolescent who is admitted to the hospital for a medical problem may have a urine drug screen that is positive for marijuana. Statistically, this screen more likely indicates use rather than abuse. However, use or abuse can be determined only after a clinical interview with the adolescent, the parent, a teacher or other representative from the adolescent's school, or any combination. A random positive finding from a urine drug screen for cocaine or heroin, however, would increase suspicion of a substance use disorder. When the urine drug screen is obtained in the context of a high index of suspicion of substance abuse (eg, with a youth who has been truant, verbally aggressive toward the parents, not fulfilling obligations at home, staying out late), the presence of any substance would fit with the hypothesis that the youth has a substance use disorder. The process of obtaining the urine drug screen is also informative. Youth who refuse to give urine samples or who claim they cannot urinate are often fearful of giving urine because of the consequences and are likely to be hiding their substance use. One strategy for determining the severity of use is to warn the adolescent in advance of the urine drug screen. If substance use is in fact infrequent, then the adolescent should be able to produce a clean urine. Thus a drug screen that comes back positive after advance warning is indicative of a more severe problem. Although the gold standard is supervised urine collection, in practice this method can be complicated and overly invasive. A sufficient degree of monitoring may also be obtained by the use of a plastic thermometer, which indicates the urine's temperature. The urine may also be tested for creatinine level. Youth may hydrate themselves or use diuretic substances to reduce the concentration of drugs in their urine.[19] Thus, if the urine creatinine is low, then significant substance use should be suspected. Notably, urine drugs screens for different substances vary in their sensitivity. Whereas the drug in marijuana may last from 7 to 28 days, depending on the frequency of its use, alcohol lasts only 12 hours in the urine and is difficult to detect or monitor with this method. Alcohol breathalyzers are generally more sensitive than urine tests and can be used readily. Cocaine and heroin generally last up to 48 and 72 hours, respectively. Tests for substances not included on regular drug panels can be costly; this group would include methylenedioxymethamphetamine (MDMA; *ecstasy*), lysergic acid diethylamide

(LSD; *acid*), ketamine (*special K*), and phencyclidine (PCP; *angel dust*), among others.

In most cases a combination of a sequence of urine drug screens and clinical interviewing of parents and youth are necessary to diagnose adolescent substance abuse accurately. In some cases the way a clinician uses the urine drug screen and the patient's response to the screen are the most informative aspects of the test. By manipulating the context to obtain a more specific result, or through observing the response of a belligerent adolescent, a clinician can enhance the assessment of a substance use disorder.[24]

MANAGEMENT

Referral

Clinicians may vary in the amount of time that they are able or willing to devote to the accurate assessment of adolescent substance abuse. In addition, most primary care physicians are not equipped to manage adolescent substance use disorders on their own. Thus, when a substance use disorder is diagnosed or suspected, making an appropriate referral will generally be necessary. To whom a clinician refers a patient should depend on the severity of the use problem. For example, if the youth was just arrested for driving under the influence, then a substance abuse treatment center is usually indicated. On the other hand, if the extent to which a youth is abusing alcohol or drugs is unclear, then a private mental health practitioner may seem less foreboding and less invasive. Adherence to any referral will usually vary as a function of the adolescent's relationship with the referring clinician, as well as the relationship between the clinician and the adolescent's parents or guardian. Promoting these relationships depends largely on the extent to which an adolescent and the adolescent's parents or guardian feel understood. A referral without the development of some understanding, however brief the evaluation is, has a reduced chance of occurring.

Motivational Interviewing

Using motivational interviewing techniques with adolescents can be helpful in promoting adherence to referrals. Motivational interviewing is designed to foster an increased awareness of the substance-related problems in a patient's life. This interviewing technique emphasizes supporting personal-change goals with a nonjudgmental attitude regarding an adolescent's substance use. Through focusing on developing empathy with an adolescent the clinician enters into an alliance with the adolescent that is less confrontational than most other approaches. Motivational interviewing effects change through promoting contemplation of the dissonance or discrepancy between an adolescent's personal goals and an adolescent's actions (ie, substance use). Although this approach has more evidence basis in adults, it holds great promise for use in adolescents because of its emphasis on personal choice and supporting an adolescent's developing autonomy.[25-27] A detailed discussion of the use of motivational interviewing among adolescents is found in Chapter 24, Communication Strategies, and is provided by Baer and Peterson.[28]

Outpatient Treatments

Although more is known about adult treatments for substance use disorders, significant advances have been made in the last decade in adolescent substance abuse treatment research.[11] Evidence-based treatments for substance use disorder that are found in the community include family therapy, behavioral therapy, cognitive-behavioral therapy, and 12-step facilitation therapies. Twelve-step groups are the most common available treatments in most areas, but they arguably have the least empirical support. However, these programs may integrate aspects of the evidence-based treatments. Cognitive-behavioral group approaches have both short- and long-term benefits for adolescents with substance use disorder. Differences between various group therapy modalities are minimal, and interactional group therapy has also been demonstrated to be effective. Behavioral therapy (eg, role playing, response rehearsal, homework assignments, diary keeping) is effective in reducing substance use (measured by urine drug screen, adolescent self-reports, and collateral reports), when compared with supportive therapy. When assessing different therapies, an important component of treatment is family involvement. Family therapies that include the adolescent have the most empirical support. The target of these interventions is to reduce familial contributions to the development or maintenance of adolescent substance abuse behaviors. Many parents have difficulty negotiating a relationship with their child at a developmental period when the child is usually pulling away. Experienced family therapists can usually help families find the right kind of professional guidance for the problem. Empirically validated family therapies include functional family therapy—which includes positive relabeling, consistently clear communication, and the development of a supportive recovery environment—and family system therapy. Self-reports of reduced substance use as a result of these therapies have been noted, as have increased levels of abstinence. The referring clinician should always be aware of the success rates and the evidence base for the treatment programs to which patients are referred. For a detailed review of evidence-based treatments for adolescent substance use disorders, see Deas and Thomas.[29]

Inpatient or Residential Treatments

In some instances the most available family and the best possible use of outpatient treatment resources fail to produce reduction in substance use. Inpatient detoxification can stop the vicious cycle of substance abuse, particularly when negative reinforcement (eg, withdrawal from opiates or alcohol or, to a lesser extent, marijuana) maintains dependence. Residential treatment can range from a few weeks to a year or more (eg, the traditional therapeutic community). Residential treatments can help establish alternative reinforcers to substance use that may generalize to the outside world. Adolescents who stay in such residences demonstrate long-term benefits in behavior, including reductions in substance use and criminal recidivism and increased adaptive functioning. Importantly, very high levels of attrition exist (30% to 40% within the first month; up to 80% within the first year). Nonetheless, a direct relationship appears to exist between length of treatment and outcome, and clinical observations of improved self-regulation are evident in such settings.[14] Substance abuse treatment can be effective even when mandated. Mandated community support groups have been shown to be effective in reducing criminal recidivism among incarcerated delinquents with drug-related crimes.[15]

CONCLUSION

Based on studies of substance abuse in primary care, adolescent substance abuse may be underdiagnosed in primary care settings. Evidence-based clinical techniques used for identification and referral of adolescents who are abusing substances may be adapted to primary care settings.

WHEN TO REFER

- Ongoing substance use despite monitoring prior parent or authority attempts to get the patient to abstain from or control substance use
- Progression of substance use to substances of greater risk (eg, alcohol to cocaine)
- When the patient meets any one of the criteria for substance abuse or dependence (either by parent, adolescent, or teacher or other authority figure's report)
- High index of suspicion resulting from unexplained adaptive impairment or unexplained decline in adaptive function
- Patient substance use and high index of suspicion because of parent, sibling, or peer substance use disorder
- Patient substance use and high index of suspicion because of patient psychiatric comorbidity or delinquent behaviors
- Patient with substance use is engaging in dangerous behavior (eg, self-mutilation, suicidal thoughts, driving under the influence)

TOOLS FOR PRACTICE

Engaging Patient and Family

- *Alcohol: Your Child and Drugs* (brochure), American Academy of Pediatrics (patiented.aap.org).
- *Inhalant Abuse: Your Child and Drugs* (brochure), American Academy of Pediatrics (patiented.aap.org).
- *Substance Abuse Prevention: What Every Parent Needs To Know* (brochure), American Academy of Pediatrics (patiented.aap.org).
- *Testing Your Teen for Illicit Drugs: Information for Parents* (brochure), American Academy of Pediatrics (patiented.aap.org).
- *Tobacco: Straight Talk for Teens* (brochure), American Academy of Pediatrics (patiented.aap.org).

Medical Decision Support

- *Addiction Severity Index* (questionnaire), McLellan, T (www.tresearch.org/ASI.htm).
- *CRAFFT: A Brief Screening Test for Adolescent Substance Abuse* (questionnaire), Knight JR and associates at Children's Hospital Boston (www.slp3d2.com/rwj_1027/webcast/docs/screentest.html).
- *Global Appraisal of Individual Needs (GAIN)* (questionnaire), Chestnut Health Systems (Dennis ML) (www.chestnut.org/LI/gain/index.html#Summary%20Description).
- *Personal Experience Inventory (PEI)* (questionnaire), Winters K, Henly G (www.portal.wpspublish.com/portal/page?_pageid=53,102631&_dad=portal&_schema=PORTAL).
- *Rutgers Alcohol Problem Index* (questionnaire), White HR, Labouvie E (alcoholstudies.rutgers.edu/etiology/rapi.html).
- *Substance Abuse: A Guide for Health Professionals* (book), American Academy of Pediatrics (www.aap.org/bst).
- *Substance Abuse Subtle Screening Inventory (SASSI)* (questionnaire), Substance Abuse Subtle Screening Inventory (SASSI) Institute (www.sassi.com/sassi/index.shtml).

SUGGESTED RESOURCES

Baer JS, Peterson PL. *Motivational Interviewing with Adolescents and Young Adults*. 2nd ed. New York, NY: Guilford Press; 2002.

Deas D, Thomas SE. An overview of controlled studies of adolescent substance abuse treatment. *Am J Addict*. 2001; 10(2):178-189.

Dryfoos JG. *Making it Through Adolescence in a Risky Society*. New York, NY: Oxford University Press; 1998.

Galanter M, Kleber H. *Textbook of Substance Abuse Treatment*. Washington, DC: American Psychiatric Press; 1999.

Kandel DB. *Adolescent Substance Use*. New York, NY: Cambridge University Press; 1998.

Kandel DB. *Stages and Pathways of Drug Involvement: Examining the Gateway Hypothesis*. New York, NY: Cambridge University Press; 2002.

REFERENCES

1. Ungemack JA, Hartwell SW, Babor TF. Alcohol and drug abuse among Connecticut youth: implications for adolescent medicine and public health. *Conn Med*. 1997;61(9): 577-585.
2. Saitz R, Mulvey KP, Plough A, et al. Physician unawareness of serious substance abuse. *Am J Drug Alcohol Abuse*. 1997;23(3):343-354.
3. Haverkos HW, Stein MD. Identifying substance abuse in primary care. *Am Fam Physician*. 1995;52(7):2029-2035.
4. Centers for Disease Control and Prevention. *CDC Fact Book 2000/2001*. Atlanta, GA: US Department of Health and Human Services, Centers for Disease Control and Prevention; 2000.
5. Moolchan ET, Ernst M, Henningfield JE. A review of tobacco smoking in adolescents: treatment implications. *J Am Acad Child Adolesc Psychiatry*. 2000;39(6): 682-693.
6. Dryfoos JG. *Making it Through Adolescence In a Risky Society*. New York, NY: Oxford University Press; 1998.
7. National Institute of Drug Abuse. *National Survey Results on Drug Use from the Monitoring the Future Study*. Washington, DC: US Government Printing Office; 2002.
8. Kilpatrick DG, Acierno R, Saunders B, et al. Risk factors for adolescent substance abuse and dependence: data from a national sample. *J Consult Clin Psychol*. 2000; 68(1):19-30.

9. Kandel DB. *Adolescent Substance Use*. New York, NY: Cambridge University Press; 1998.
10. Kandel DB. *Stages and Pathways of Drug Involvement: Examining the Gateway Hypothesis*. New York, NY: Cambridge University Press; 2002.
11. Galanter M, Kleber H. *Textbook of Substance Abuse Treatment*. Washington, DC: American Psychiatric Press; 1999.
12. Tarter R, Vanyukov M, Giancoila P, et al. Etiology of early age onset substance use disorder: a maturational perspective. *Dev Psychopathol*. 1999;11:657-683.
13. Clark DB, Parker AM, Lynch KG. Psychopathology and substance-related problems during early adolescence: a survival analysis. *J Clin Child Psychol*. 1999;28(3):333-341.
14. Wilens TE, Biederman J, Spencer TJ. *Attention Deficit-Hyperactivity Disorder in Youth*. Washington, DC: Cambridge University Press; 1999.
15. Wilson JJ, Steiner H. Conduct problems, substance use and social anxiety: a developmental study of recovery and adaptation. *Clin Child Psychol Psychiatry*. 2002;7(2):235-247.
16. Luthar SS, Cushing G, McMahon TJ. *Interdisciplinary Interface: Developmental Principles Brought to Substance Abuse Research*. New York, NY: Cambridge University Press; 1997.
17. Mannuzza S, Klein RG, Bessler A, et al. Adult outcome of hyperactive boys. Educational achievement, occupational rank, and psychiatric status. *Arch Gen Psychiatry*. 1993;50(7):565-576.
18. Pollock NK, Martin CS. Diagnostic orphans: adolescents with alcohol symptom who do not qualify for DSM-IV abuse or dependence diagnoses. *Am J Psychiatry*. 1999;156(6):897-901.
19. Wilson JJ, Rojas N, Haapanen R, et al. Substance abuse and criminal recidivism: a prospective study of adolescents. *Child Psychiatry Hum Dev*. 2001;31(4):297-312.
20. Feldstein SW, Miller WR. Does subtle screening for substance abuse work? A review of the Substance Abuse Subtle Screening Inventory (SASSI). *Addiction*. 2007; 102(1):41-50.
21. Winters KC, Latimer WW, Stinchfield R. Clinical issues in the assessment of adolescent alcohol and other drug use. *Behav Res Ther*. 2002;40(12):1443-1456.
22. Meyers K, McLellan AT, Jaeger JL, et al. The development of the Comprehensive Addiction Severity Index for Adolescents (CASI-A). An interview for assessing multiple problems of adolescents. *J Subst Abuse Treat*. 1995; 12(3):181-193.
23. Dennis ML, Funk R, Godley SH, et al. Cross-validation of the alcohol and cannabis use measure in the Global Appraisal of Individual Needs (GAIN) and Timeline Followback (TLDB; Form 90) among adolescents in substance abuse treatment. *Addiction*. 2004;99(suppl 2):120-128.
24. Riggs PD, Whitmore EA. *Substance Use Disorders and Disruptive Behavior Disorders*. Washington, DC: American Psychiatric Press; 1999.
25. Monti PM, Colby SM, Barnett NP, et al. Brief intervention for harm reduction with alcohol-positive older adolescents in a hospital emergency department. *J Consult Clin Psychol*. 1999;67(6):989-994.
26. Dennis M, Godley SH, Diamond G, et al. The Cannabis Youth Treatment (CYT) Study: main findings from two randomized trials. *J Subst Abuse Treat*. 2004;27(3):197-213.
27. Colby SM, Monti PM, Barnett NP, et al. Brief motivational interviewing in a hospital setting for adolescent smoking: a preliminary study. *J Consult Clin Psychol*. 1998;66(3):574-578.
28. Baer JS, Peterson PL. *Motivational Interviewing with Adolescents and Young Adults*. 2nd ed. New York, NY: Guilford Press; 2002.
29. Deas D, Thomas SE. An overview of controlled studies of adolescent substance abuse treatment. *Am J Addict*. 2001;10(2):178-189.

Chapter 51

USE OF URINALYSIS AND URINE CULTURE IN SCREENING

David S. Hains, MD; Hiren P. Patel, MD

Examination of the urine is a simple and efficient office procedure that may detect or evaluate for renal, urinary tract, and systemic disorders. A first-morning, midstream, clean-catch specimen is most reliable for this purpose. Urine examination is usually warranted only in symptomatic children to aid in diagnosis. The presence of heavy proteinuria (nephrotic syndrome or other significant renal disease), hematuria (glomerulonephritis), glucosuria (diabetes mellitus), or leukocyte esterase or nitrites (urinary tract infection) can help the pediatrician diagnose and manage the pathologic condition. Urinalysis is an important tool in evaluating the child who has renal symptoms and should also be considered in patients who have vague signs and symptoms, such as failure to thrive or malaise, because some renal disorders may exhibit in such nonspecific ways. Urinalysis is less useful as a screening procedure in asymptomatic patients than it is in patients who have symptoms.

Several principles need to be considered in screening for abnormalities in the urine.[1] First, a screening test should be reliable and accurate. Second, screening should be done for conditions that can be diagnosed with certainty and benefit from early diagnosis and treatment. Finally, a screening test should be cost effective for the individual and the general population. The cost effectiveness of mass urine screening depends on the total monetary cost and psychological cost (false positives can lead to invasive testing and anxiety) of performing the screening test compared with the cost of disease management for those diagnosed at a later time without screening.

Although the early discovery of a symptom-free child who has renal disease may prove to be beneficial, the cost effectiveness to society of mass screening in young children remains unproven. Several studies reveal rather high rates (up to 6%) of abnormalities on an initial urinalysis screen, but 80% to 90% of these abnormalities are transient.[2-4] Current data from England do not support the current practice of routine screening urinalysis.[5] Such findings reflect the high degree of sensitivity and the lack of specificity (ability to minimize false-positive results) of current urine tests in detecting significant renal or urinary tract disease in symptom-free children. The relatively low prevalence of end-stage renal disease in children limits the positive predictive value of screening for hematuria or proteinuria.

Recommendations for urine screening have evolved over time. Although a majority of pediatricians conduct screening urinalyses frequently,[6] both the American Academy of Pediatrics (AAP) and *Bright Futures Practice Guidelines* recommend that a complete urinalysis be performed once at 5 years of age (and then repeated annually for sexually active adolescents).[7,8] *Bright Futures* also recommends that a complete urinalysis be performed at least once during adolescence even if the individual is not sexually active. This policy is currently under review by the AAP and may be changed in the near future (S. Wassner, MD, and J. Flynn, MD, personal communication).

PROTEINURIA

Proteinuria is detected most easily by the dipstick method. The presence of protein causes a change in indicator color from yellow to blue-green that is proportional to the amount of protein present; albumin causes the indicator to change color more readily than do other proteins. This method does not usually detect the small quantity of protein that healthy persons normally excrete. Depending on the study, the sensitivity of detecting proteinuria with a urine dipstick ranges from 83.9% to 95.1%. The specificity ranges from 93.8% to 95.5%.[9] False-positive findings can occur in alkaline urine (pH greater than 6.5) or in urine contaminated by skin antiseptics such as chlorhexidine or benzalkonium chloride. Furthermore, the urine concentration also affects dipstick results and should be taken into consideration (see Suggested Resources for link to an interpretation algorithm for proteinuria in the context of urine specific gravity).

Proteinuria is considered to be persistent if the dipstick is positive (1+ or greater) for at least 2 of 3 random urine specimens collected at least 1 week apart.[10] Because accurately obtaining a 24-hour urine collection in children can be difficult, quantifying proteinuria using the protein-to-creatine ratio on a random urine sample is recommended.[11] A ratio greater than 0.2 mg protein per mg creatinine is considered abnormal for children older than 2 years.[12]

The prevalence rate for proteinuria in the symptom-free pediatric population depends on the definition of proteinuria used. The prevalence increases with age and is greater in girls than it is in boys. Using less stringent criteria, the prevalence of proteinuria can range from less than 1% in 6-year-old boys to as high as 6% in adolescent girls. If a more strict criteria is used (2+ on each dipstick with at least 2 performed), then the prevalence decreases considerably, with rates ranging from 0.2% to 0.45% in boys and 1% to 1.6% in girls.[2,3,13,14]

Because more than 50% to 75% of symptom-free patients found to have protein in a single urinalysis will have normal urine on repeat testing, the value of this screening as part of well-child health care has been questioned. Furthermore, of those having several positive random urinalysis results, at least 60% will have orthostatic proteinuria, a diagnosis that is not considered to be a harbinger of clinically significant renal disease.[2] In a 20-year follow-up study of young men who had persistent orthostatic proteinuria, none developed renal insufficiency, including those who had nonspecific glomerular abnormalities on renal biopsy.[15] Excluding individuals with orthostatic proteinuria, regular followup, however, remains important for these children so that changes in the pattern of protein excretion or the appearance of hematuria can be detected and appropriately investigated. Follow-up care of children determined by screening tests to have proteinuria has shown spontaneous resolution in more than 40% of cases within 4 years and an incidence of identifiable renal disease in 1 child per 1000 children screened.[16] If hematuria is excluded, then asymptomatic children who have proteinuria are not likely to have overt renal disease. Vehaskari and Rapola biopsied 28 children who had the highest protein excretion rates after identifying them from 8954 classmates by school screening; no definite morphologic renal disease was identified.[17] Topham and colleagues did find that 100% of their patients with hematuria *and* proteinuria (only 1% of original cohort of 3808) did have significant parenchymal renal disease. The patients who had only hematuria *or* proteinuria did not have any significant renal disease.[5]

On the other hand, isolated cases of significant renal disease can sometimes exhibit solely with proteinuria in the asymptomatic child. In contrast to the generally benign prognosis of isolated proteinuria, Yoshikawa and colleagues reported 53 children who were examined retrospectively after being biopsied for asymptomatic, fixed, isolated proteinuria.[18] They found that 47% had significant glomerular changes (focal segmental glomerulosclerosis, immunoglobulin A [IgA] nephropathy, mesangial proliferative glomerulonephritis, and membranous glomerulonephritis), which appeared to progress with time to chronic renal impairment. In Silverberg's studies, approximately 9% of children screened to have isolated proteinuria had evidence of pyelonephritic scarring.[13,14] Although some children who have proteinuria may have an abnormality that requires no additional management (eg, a hypoplastic kidney), others may have diseases that may improve with treatment (eg, focal glomerulosclerosis, IgA nephropathy). However, most children who have significant renal disease will have other signs and symptoms (eg, edema, poor weight gain, hypertension) that cause them to seek medical care and thus can be identified even in the absence of screening programs.

The high sensitivity and low specificity of screening for proteinuria in asymptomatic children can produce undue anxiety in patients and parents and can direct the practitioner to perform more invasive testing, which often provides no new information. Such screening may not only detract from the overall well being of the population but may be costly as well. Kaplan and colleagues estimated that approximately $200 is spent to evaluate proteinuria before referral to a pediatric nephrologist.[19] Currently, less enthusiasm can be found for mass screening for proteinuria in symptom-free children. Many researchers agree that a satisfactory compromise for the health of children is to screen a first morning urine at 5 years of age.[16,19,20] The use of the first morning urine avoids the identification of children who have orthostatic proteinuria. In the case of persistent proteinuria, a meticulous examination of fresh urinary sediment should precede any additional laboratory evaluation[16,20] (see Chapter 210, Proteinuria).

HEMATURIA

Not all discolored urine indicates hematuria. Urine can be discolored by many substances[21]; therefore the presence of blood should be confirmed by dipstick for complaints of gross hematuria. The dipstick is highly sensitive, reacting to hemoglobin levels as low as 0.015 to 0.062 mg/dL.[22] Depending on the degree of hematuria, the sensitivity of the dipstick for blood is 85% to 100%, and the specificity is 86.3% to 99.3%.[23,24] False-positive tests for blood in the urine may result from the presence of oxidizing cleansing agents (eg, povidone-iodine or hypochlorite) or microbial peroxidases. False-negative tests result from the presence of large amounts of a reducing agent such as ascorbic acid.

A positive dipstick result for blood does not discriminate between hemoglobin and myoglobin from muscle; differentiation requires spectrophotometric analysis. Furthermore, the dipstick test does not differentiate hemoglobinuria from hematuria or whether the blood originates from the upper or lower urinary tracts. For these questions, the microscopic examination of the centrifuged urine sediment is essential. Dipstick positive, red, or cola-colored urine without red blood cells (RBCs) on microscopic examination is diagnostic of free hemoglobin or myoglobin within the urine. Glomerular bleeding (upper tract) is suggested by the presence of RBC casts, proteinuria, brown or tea-colored urine, and dysmorphic RBCs. Conversely, red or pink urine or clots usually indicates lower urinary tract bleeding.

The prevalence of microscopic hematuria in an ambulatory setting ranges from 2% to 6% when a single urinalysis is abnormal to approximately 1% when more than 1 urinalysis is positive. However, the hematuria persists longer than 6 months in fewer than 0.5% of these cases.[2,25] The annual incidence of new cases (defined as at least 5 RBCs/hpf) is 0.4%. No consistent trends exist for the age, gender, and race dependence of hematuria.

Few children whose hematuria was detected in screening programs are found to have significant renal or urologic disease.[26] On the other hand, hematuria persisting for longer than 6 months is more likely to be associated with renal disease if the patient has had at least 1 episode of gross hematuria or proteinuria or has a family history of hematuria in a first-degree relative.[27,28] The most likely diagnoses in these cases are IgA nephropathy thin basement membrane disease, and Alport syndrome (hereditary nephritis). In a review of studies of screened, symptomless microhematuria, IgA nephropathy was found in 2% to 21% of biopsies, and other glomerular lesions were much less frequent.[29] The most common nonglomerular finding was asymptomatic urinary tract infection (4.8% to 6.0%), and less common were ureteropelvic junction obstruction and reflux nephropathy. In more recent follow-up studies of children referred for isolated hematuria, the most common underlying diagnosis (11% to 16%) found was hypercalciuria.[27,30]

Although screening for hematuria is limited by low specificity, potential value exists in identifying patients at risk for renal disease in patients with symptoms, gross hematuria (especially if recurrent), proteinuria or a positive family history. An examination of the first morning urine at age 5 years is recommended.[16,19,20] In the case of persistent isolated microscopic hematuria, a careful examination of fresh urinary sediment and microscopic analysis should precede any additional laboratory evaluation for asymptomatic children.[16,20] The great majority of these children will not have clinically significant disease, and current practice guidelines suggest that continued observation without workup is appropriate (see Chapter 188, Hematuria).

GLUCOSURIA

Urine glucose can be detected by glucose oxidase-impregnated dipsticks. Normally, all of the filtered glucose is reabsorbed by the proximal tubules, and glucose is not detectable in the urine when the plasma glucose is less than 180 mg/dL. Glucosuria is seen most commonly when the filtered load of glucose is increased as a result of hyperglycemia in diabetes mellitus. Less often, a defect can be found in proximal tubular reabsorption that may be selective, as in renal glucosuria, or may be part of a more generalized proximal tubular dysfunction, as in Fanconi syndrome. Measurement of blood glucose will help differentiate among these conditions. Glucosuria is also observed in the latter stages of tubular destruction seen in a variety of chronic kidney diseases. In these conditions, the urinalysis usually also shows proteinuria and the urinary sediment may contain renal tubular cells and casts.

Urine screening reveals a prevalence of glycosuria that is less than 0.1%.[3,13,14] Although up to 10 to 50 previously undetected cases of diabetes mellitus per 100,000 children could be identified, new-onset diabetes mellitus is much more likely to produce classic symptoms of polyuria and polydipsia. Rarely cases of renal glucosuria, Fanconi syndrome, and other tubular dysfunction may be identified. Therefore the cost effectiveness of screening asymptomatic patients for glucosuria is rather low and not recommended for routine visits.

BACTERIURIA

Asymptomatic bacteriuria is defined as growth of >100,000 cfu/ml in at least 2 consecutive urine specimens in a child who has no other symptoms of infection at a regular checkup. The prevalence of asymptomatic bacteriuria in school-age children is 1% to 2% in girls and 0% to 0.1% in boys.[13,14,31,32]

In a child with symptoms consistent with a urinary tract infection (UTI), the presence of leukocyte esterase or nitrites generated by gram-negative organisms from nitrates will increase suspicion for bacteriuria. Nitrites are extremely specific to bacteriuria with a specificity of 98% but a sensitivity of only 50%. Leukocyte esterase is much more sensitive (84%) compared with nitrite, but it has a lower specificity of only 78%. When either leukocyte esterase *or* nitrite is positive, the sensitivity is 88%, and the specificity is 93%. When both leukocyte esterase *and* nitrites are positive, the sensitivity is 72%, and the specificity is 96%.[33]

Dipstick detection of leukocyte esterase or nitrites is variable depending on the method of collection and the age of the patient. McGillivray and colleagues found that the sensitivity for bag-collected urine was 85%, in contrast to catheter-collected urine samples having a sensitivity of 71% in non–toilet-trained children. The specificity of bag-collected urine was 62%

versus 97% specificity of catheter-collected urine. The sensitivities of the 2 methods are decreased by approximately 20% in infants younger than 90 days.[34]

When investigating a possible UTI with a urinalysis, the AAP has provided guidelines on the use of bagged urine specimens for analysis. A negative result can be trusted, and no further invasive collection of urine is needed. On the other hand, a bagged urine sample that has either positive leukocyte esterase or nitrites, a positive Gram stain, or more than 5 white blood cells per high power field requires the physician to obtain another urine sample for urine culture via more invasive measures such as catheterization or suprapubic aspiration before starting antibiotics.[35]

Extensive investigations of asymptomatic or covert bacteriuria in school girls have shown that nontreatment does not influence the episodes of symptomatic UTI, renal growth, or renal function in normal or scarred kidneys.[36-38] Furthermore, treatment of asymptomatic bacteriuria may be associated with a greater risk for pyelonephritis because of the development of more pathogenic and resistant organisms.[31] In addition, antibiotic treatment does not prevent further renal scarring once it has occurred or restore poor renal growth.[32,36]

For a child with signs and symptoms consistent with UTI, the physician should have a low threshold for obtaining a diagnostic urinalysis. Positive results should be confirmed by urine culture and treated. Screening of asymptomatic patients for asymptomatic bacteriuria is not recommended. If asymptomatic bacteriuria is discovered, then it should not be treated. Persistent bacteriuria should be pursued with a careful history for renal and urinary tract symptoms, examination of growth and blood pressure, and possibly a renal ultrasound to determine persons who are at risk for progressive renal disease (see Chapter 334 Urinary Tract Infections).

WHEN TO REFER

- Persistent proteinuria (first morning void)
- Gross hematuria of unknown cause
- Persistent hematuria associated with proteinuria or hypertension
- Hematuria suggested to be of lower urinary tract origin accompanied by elevated serum glucose level
- Physician discomfort with diagnosis and management
- Family reassurance

TOOLS FOR PRACTICE

Engaging Patients and Family

- *What You Need to Know About Urinalysis* (brochure), National Kidney Foundation (www.kidney.org/atoz/pdf/urinalysis.pdf).

Medical Decision Support

- Pathologic Proteinuria Calculator (interactive tool), Metro Health (www.metrohealthresearch.org/schelling/).
- Practice Parameter: The Diagnosis, Treatment, and Evaluation of the Initial Urinary Tract Infection in Febrile Infants and Young Children (guideline), American Academy of Pediatrics (pediatrics.aappublications.org/cgi/reprint/103/4/843).

AAP POLICY STATEMENT

Hogg RJ, Portman RJ, Milliner D, Lemley KV, Eddy A, Ingelfinger J. Evaluation and management of proteinuria and nephrotic syndrome in children: recommendations from a pediatric nephrology panel established at the National Kidney Foundation Conference on Proteinuria, Albuminuria, Risk, Assessment, Detection, and Elimination (PARADE). *Pediatrics*. 2000;105(6):1242-1249 (doi:10.1542/peds.105.6.1242. (www.pediatrics.org/cgi/content/full/105/6/1242).

SUGGESTED RESOURCE

Pathologic Proteinuria Calculator. A program in which the urine dipstick protein can be interpreted in the context of urine specific gravity. Although the data and recommendations given are based on adult data, it can be useful for interpreting the potential significance of urine dipsticks positive for protein. Available at: www.metrohealthresearch.org/schelling/.

REFERENCES

1. Hoekelman RA. Is screening urinalysis worthwhile in asymptomatic pediatric patients? *Pediatr Ann.* 1994;23:459-460.
2. Dodge WF, West EF, Smith EH, et al. Proteinuria and hematuria in schoolchildren: epidemiology and early natural history. *J Pediatr* 1976;88:327-347.
3. Gutgesell M. Practicality of screening urinalyses in asymptomatic children in a primary care setting. *Pediatrics*. 1978;62:103-105.
4. US Renal Data System. USRDS 2005 annual data report, Chapter VIII: Pediatric End-Stage Renal Disease. *Am J Kidney Dis.* 2006;47(suppl 1):s99.
5. Topham PS, Jethwa A, Watkins M, et al. The value of urine screening in a young adult population. *Fam Pract.* 2004;21:18-21.
6. Sox CM, Christakis DA. Pediatricians' screening urinalysis practices. *J Pediatr.* 2005;147:362-365.
7. American Academy of Pediatrics, Committee on Practice and Ambulatory Medicine. Recommendations for preventive pediatric health care. *Pediatrics.* 2000;105:645-646.
8. Hagan JF Jr, Shaw JS, Duncan PM, eds. Bright Futures: Guidelines for Health Supervision of Infants, Children, and Adolescents, 3rd ed. Elk Grove, IL: American Academy of Pediatrics; 2008.
9. Pugia MJ, Lott JA, Kajima J, et al. Screening school children for albuminuria, proteinuria and occult blood with dipsticks. *Clin Chem Lab Med.* 1999;37:149-157.
10. Norman ME. An office approach to hematuria and proteinuria. *Pediatr Clin North Am.* 1987;34:545-560.
11. Hogg RJ, Portman RJ, Milliner D, et al. Evaluation and management of proteinuria and nephrotic syndrome in children: recommendations from a pediatric nephrology panel established at the National Kidney Foundation conference on proteinuria, albuminuria, risk, assessment, detection, and elimination (PARADE). *Pediatrics.* 2000;105:1242-1249. Available at: pediatrics.aappublications.org/cgi/reprint/105/6/1242.

12. Ettenger RB. The evaluation of the child with proteinuria. *Pediatr Ann.* 1994;23:486-494.
13. Silverberg DS. City-wide screening for urinary abnormalities in schoolboys. *Can Med Assoc J.* 1974;111:410-412.
14. Silverberg DS, Allard MJ, Ulan RA, et al. City-wide screening for urinary abnormalities in schoolgirls. *CMAJ.* 1973;109:981-985.
15. Springberg PD, Garrett LE Jr, Thompson AL Jr, et al. Fixed and reproducible orthostatic proteinuria: results of a 20-year follow-up study. *Ann Intern Med.* 1982;97:516-519.
16. Arant BS Jr. Screening for urinary abnormalities: worth doing and worth doing well. *Lancet.* 1998;351:307-308.
17. Vehaskari VM, Rapola J. Isolated proteinuria: analysis of a school-age population. *J Pediatr.* 1982;101:661-668.
18. Yoshikawa N, Kitagawa K, Ohta K, et al. Asymptomatic constant isolated proteinuria in children. *J Pediatr.* 1991;119:375-379.
19. Kaplan RE, Springate JE, Feld LG. Screening dipstick urinalysis: a time to change. *Pediatrics.* 1997;100:919-921.
20. Linshaw MA, Gruskin AB. The routine urinalysis: to keep or not to keep; that is the question. *Pediatrics.* 1997;100: 1031-1032.
21. Yadin O. Hematuria in children. *Pediatr Ann.* 1994;23: 474-478, 481-485.
22. American College of Physicians, Physicians' Information and Education Resource. *The Physicians' Information and Education Resource.* American College of Physicians, Philadelphia, PA; 2005.
23. Gleeson MJ, Connolly J, Grainger R, et al. Comparison of reagent strip (dipstick) and microscopic haematuria in urological out-patients. *Br J Urol.* 1993;72:594-596.
24. Moore GP, Robinson M. Do urine dipsticks reliably predict microhematuria? The bloody truth! *Ann Emerg Med.* 1988;17:257-260.
25. Vehaskari VM, Rapola J, Koskimies O, et al. Microscopic hematuria in school children: epidemiology and clinicopathologic evaluation. *J Pediatr.* 1979;95:676-684.
26. Murakami M, Yamamoto H, Ueda Y, et al. Urinary screening of elementary and junior high-school children over a 13-year period in Tokyo. *Pediatr Nephrol.* 1991; 5:50-53.
27. Bergstein J, Leiser J, Andreoli S. The clinical significance of asymptomatic gross and microscopic hematuria in children. *Arch Pediatr Adolesc Med.* 2005;159: 353-355.
28. Turi S, Visy M, Vissy A, et al. Long-term follow up of chronic recurrent isolated hematuria. *Orv Hetil.* 1989; 130:1363-1366.
29. Benbassat J, Gergawi M, Offringa M, et al. Symptomless microhaematuria in schoolchildren: causes for variable management strategies. *QJM.* 1996;89:845-854.
30. Feld LG, Meyers KE, Kaplan BS, et al. Limited evaluation of microscopic hematuria in pediatrics. *Pediatrics.* 1998; 102:E42.
31. Kemper KJ, Avner ED. The case against screening urinalyses for asymptomatic bacteriuria in children. *Am J Dis Child.* 1992;146:343-346.
32. Savage DC. Natural history of covert bacteriuria in schoolgirls. *Kidney Int.* 1975;4:S90-S95.
33. Gorelick MH, Shaw KN. Screening tests for urinary tract infection in children: a meta-analysis. *Pediatrics.* 1999; 104:e54.
34. McGillivray D, Mok E, Mulrooney E, et al. A head-to-head comparison: "clean-void" bag versus catheter urinalysis in the diagnosis of urinary tract infection in young children. *J Pediatr.* 2005;147:451-456.
35. American Academy of Pediatrics, Committee on Quality Improvement, Subcommittee on Urinary Tract Infection. Practice parameter: the diagnosis, treatment, and evaluation of the initial urinary tract infection in febrile infants and young children. *Pediatrics.* 1999;103:843-852. Available at: pediatrics.aappublications.org/cgi/reprint/103/4/843
36. Newcastle Covert Bacteriuria Research Group. Covert bacteriuria in schoolgirls in Newcastle Upon Tyne: a 5-year follow-up. *Arch Dis Child.* 1981;56:585.
37. Hansson S, Jodal U, Noren L, et al. Untreated bacteriuria in asymptomatic girls with renal scarring. *Pediatrics.* 1989;84:964-968.
38. Verrier Jones K, Asscher AW, Verrier Jones ER, et al. Glomerular filtration rate in schoolgirls with covert bacteriuria. *Br Med J.* 1982;285:1307-1310.

SECTION FOUR

Treatment of Disease

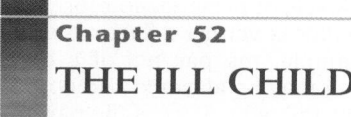

Chapter 52

THE ILL CHILD

Timothy Gibson, MD; Marianne E. Felice, MD

INTRODUCTION

To address the topic of the ill child, the primary care physician (PCP) must consider the nature, the severity, and the cause of the health concern voiced by the child or the parents. These concerns vary tremendously, from the mildest symptoms of an upper respiratory tract infection to the most severe presentation of frank shock, for example, in meningococcal sepsis. Injuries also account for a large number of medical visits, and, increasingly, psychosocial complaints such as difficulties at school or depression are brought to the attention of the pediatrician. For any health concern, the need for involving a health care professional varies immensely. Most mild complaints can be, and are, managed at home, with minimal or no contact with the medical team. Today, parents have an unprecedented array of resources available to them from which to seek medical advice. In past generations, many parents, particularly young parents, sought advice from their own parents, family members, or neighbors. Although this circumstance is still true for some families, many parents turn to other resources, including the Internet.[1] Other parents seek counsel from a clinician whenever their child is ill either by telephone or an office visit. Options vary widely as to who this clinician is (pediatrician, family medicine physician, nurse practitioner, and others) and in what setting (office visit, clinic setting, urgent care center, and others). Finally, a small number of patients will require a higher level of care, such as the emergency department, hospitalization, or an intensive care unit. This chapter addresses the anatomy of the ill child (Figure 52-1) with a discussion of the issues that are important at each level of care. The chapter ends with a discussion of how caring for the ill child has changed over the last decade and how care is likely to change further in the future.

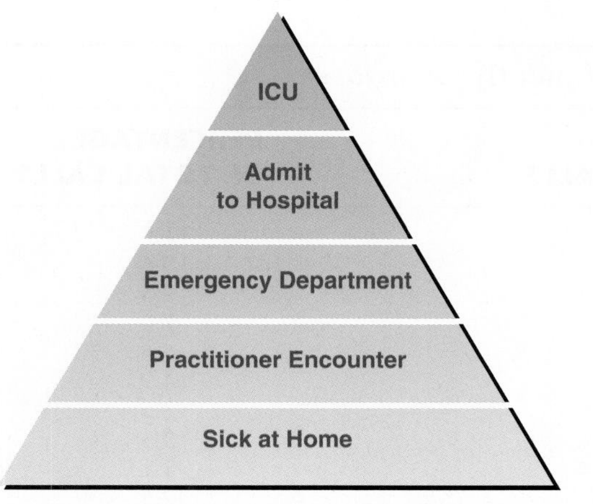

Figure 52-1 Levels of care of the ill child.

SICK CHILD AT HOME

Most children with mild medical complaints can be managed at home by attentive, competent caregivers who know them well. However, several factors exist that determine whether a parent is capable of caring for a sick child at home: Does the parent know the signs and symptoms of a serious problem compared with a mild problem? Does the parent have experience with previous children, or is this child the first child? Does the parent know whom to call or where to go if the child's condition worsens? Does the parent have a support person to whom the parent can turn for help if needed? How far away does the parent live from a health care provider? Does the parent have transportation? Is the parent comfortable with illness, or does the parent feel the need for reassurance from medical personnel for each complaint?[2] Many office visits to PCPs result in large doses of reassurance.

The parents of the mildly ill child at home have more resources at their fingertips than ever before. Increasingly, media have focused on educating consumers regarding health care advances, with the conclusions of articles published in respected medical journals being reported on television, radio, and in newspapers, long before their findings have stood the test of time. Using the Internet as a resource for medical information has increased dramatically. Many reputable medical Web sites exist. The most reliable sites (but not always the most user friendly) are those that are sponsored by large physician organizations, for example www.aap.org as the official Web site of the American Academy of Pediatrics. Some of the most popular sites are those that advertise, such as WebMD and drkoop.com, and these are also fairly trustworthy sources. However, parents who randomly search the Internet for medical information must use extreme caution. The World Wide Web is unregulated and flush with medical disinformation. Parents may turn to any number of Web sites to research their child's complaint or symptom, resulting in several possible outcomes.[3] They may visit a legitimate Web site and be reassured by what they find. They may visit a legitimate site and learn that their child's illness does, in fact, require an office or emergency department (ED) visit. They may encounter private Web sites and be unnecessarily alarmed by fantastic claims focused on rare occurrences, for instance, mild cough as the presenting symptom of a rare fatal malignancy compressing a bronchus. Pediatricians must be acutely aware of these issues and counsel patients to use caution when interpreting what they see and read.

Many over-the-counter medications are available for parents who opt to treat their children at home.[4] Pain relievers, antipyretics, gastric acid reducers, constipation remedies, and multiple classes of cold medicines are the most commonly used medications at home. Most of these medications are quite safe, but every one has potential side effects. Because these medications are obtained without a prescription, they are the most common medicines to have in the home, and thus they are some of the most common drugs encountered in overdoses in children, both intentional and accidental (Table 52-1).[5] Dosing of over-the-counter medications can be confusing to parents, with multiple trade names, formulations, and concentrations of the same drug often present and similar sounding names for very different drugs. Because most pediatric illnesses are mild and short lived, managing symptoms will often be sufficient until the natural history of the illness puts the child on the road to recovery; over-the-counter medications play a large role here. The physician should not forget that most herbal remedies do not require a prescription and are commonly used by pediatric patients.[6] To add to the confusion, many parents do not consider these substances to be medications and may omit them when asked, "Does the child take any medicines?"

Even for the mildest complaints, parents must monitor their child closely for signs of deterioration. They must have some basic medical knowledge about what is serious and what is not serious. Some of this information can be taught during well-child visits, for example, stressing to parents of newborns that fever is an emergency in very young infants and requires immediate medical attention, whereas fever in older children is often not as worrisome. If children are in the care of someone other than the parent (family member, child care provider), then parents must communicate to these caregivers the disease course to date and parameters for which the caregiver must take the next step. Different levels of parental comfort may be present for an acute illness versus a flare-up of an existing illness. For example, the parents of a child with new-onset wheezing may be alarmed and appropriately insist on being examined, whereas the parents of a child with longstanding asthma may feel much more comfortable initiating treatment on their own, sometimes even managing mild distress at home without a physician visit.

ACCESSING THE HEALTH CARE SYSTEM

The 1st foray into accessing the health care system is often a telephone call, usually to the PCP, if one is available. For as many practice models that exist, an equal number of telephone triage models are available that can be used. Smaller primary care groups may opt to not have a nurse in the office, and a secretary sends all calls directly to be answered by the physician, who may need to return telephone messages in between patient visits. Medium-sized groups may have a nurse, nurse practitioner, or physician's assistant who handles telephone calls and gives advice over the telephone. Larger multispecialty groups often have a battery of office help, from the secretary who can schedule appointments, to the medical billing specialist who answers financial questions and arranges referrals, to the medical staff who field questions and help with triage decisions based on reported signs and symptoms. Standardized protocols exist, and many excellent resources are available to the office triage staff, whatever their medical qualifications may be.[7] For example, for the chief complaint of cough,

Table 52-1 Substances on Which Children Frequently Overdose*

CATEGORY	NUMBER OF CALLS	PERCENTAGE OF TOTAL CALLS
Cosmetic or personal care products	648,187	11.7
Cleaning substances (household)	589,820	10.6
Analgesics	418,265	7.5
Plants	387,906	7.0
Cold and cough preparations	366,549	6.6
Topical preparations	273,170	4.9
Antimicrobials	194,462	3.5
Vitamins	182,458	3.3
Gastrointestinal preparations	173,473	3.1
Insecticides or pesticides	141,379	2.5

*The most commonly reported toxic exposure classes in children aged younger than 6 years from 1993 to 1997 as reported by the Association of Poison Control Centers Toxic Exposure Surveillance System.
From McGuigan MA. Common culprits in childhood poisoning. *Pediatric Drugs*. Oct-Dec 1999;1(4):313-324.

protocols may recommend reassurance and home treatment for the child who has little or no fever and has no respiratory distress. These same protocols would trigger more aggressive intervention if the triage staff elicits positive answers to questions about cough after a choking episode, as in a foreign-body aspiration or a cough that is paroxysmal and associated with cyanosis, as in pertussis. Telephone triage can be a source of anxiety for the practitioner because recommendations are given without the benefit of a physical examination and depend exclusively on trusting what the caller is reporting. The protocols themselves are subject to interpretation.[8] As a way to mitigate potential legal consequences, most triage references recommend ending any telephone encounter between a practitioner and caller by stating, "We can see you if you are not comfortable." Many pediatric practices make use of nurse-staffed night-call services after regular office hours have ended as a way to limit the number of telephone calls the on-call physician must handle, and differences can exist in the way patients perceive and act on advice given by different levels of practitioners.[9,10] These services are often run from a regional or even national center, hence the medical staff member fielding the telephone call has no direct experience with the patient. Regardless of who handles telephone calls from caregivers, clearly, telephone interactions with families are intensely time consuming and, except for a handful of experimental experiences, are not paid by insurers.

E-mail correspondence with physicians is increasingly desired by patients and has many of the same pitfalls encountered with telephone triage. Advancing technology may make electronic interactions with patients more useful, for instance the ability to e-mail an audio file of a patient with croup or a brief video clip of a patient with a seizure. Use of e-mail, though offering significant advantages, has also raised important questions, including privacy and discoverability.[11] However, e-mail correspondence can be successful only if the e-mails are checked regularly and if a systematic mechanism is in place for answering them. Unlike telephone calls, the person reading the e-mail does not have the added advantage of hearing the tone of voice of the questioner or the hesitancy in answering certain questions. For this reason, many physicians currently choose to use e-mail correspondence for nonacute questions only. This situation may change in future years.

The telephone triage system can result in several steps after the call is made (Figure 52-2). The caregiver may be reassured, with no treatment recommended. Home treatment options may be suggested without requiring a face-to-face physician encounter. An acute office visit may be recommended either immediately (eg, a child with sore throat who is not eating or

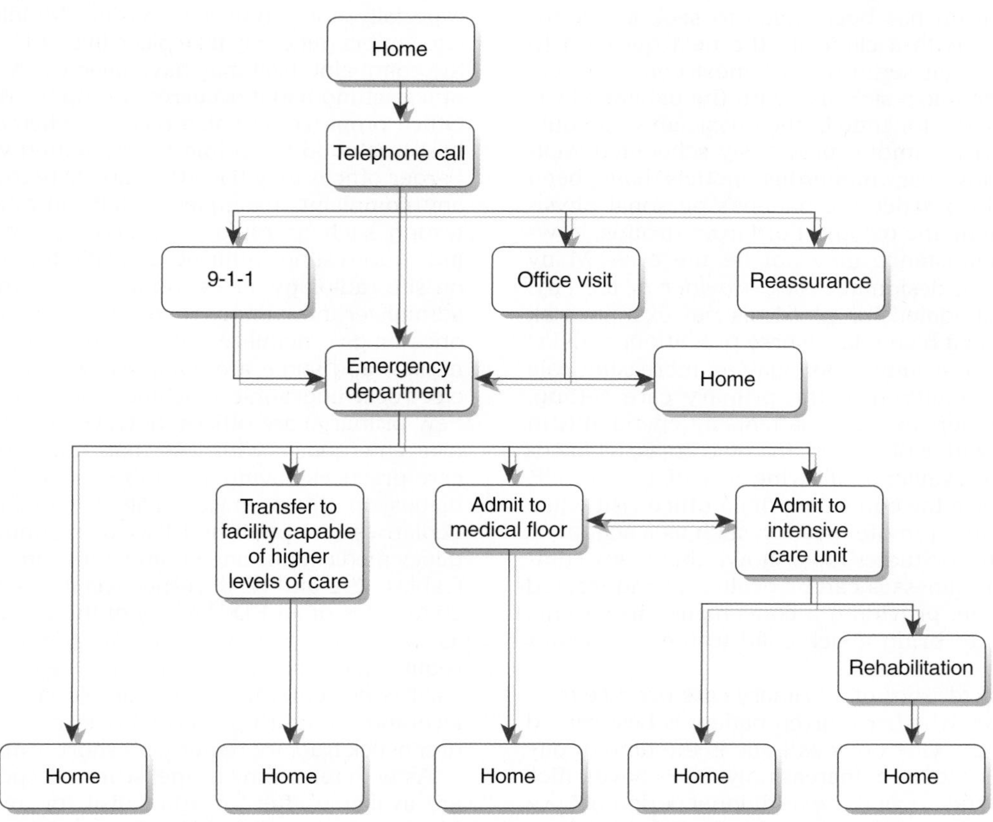

Figure 52-2 Telephone care flow chart.

drinking) or within a specified period for less urgent complaints (eg, tinea capitis, acne); an ED visit may be requested; and, finally, for truly emergent needs, the triage staff member may recommend that a patient or caregiver call their local emergency number or 9-1-1.

In addition to all the medical issues that are present, many nonmedical issues exist that must be considered when deciding how to triage a parental telephone call. Does the patient actually have a home? An intact, financially secure family can often handle a child at home with mild dehydration, but what if the family is homeless and has no immediate access to fluids or even running water? Does the caller understand the instructions given, or is understanding lacking as a result of either intellectual or language limitations? Do cultural barriers exist that may prevent recommendations from being followed? Does the family have access to an automobile for transport to a medical visit in the case of deterioration? Does the family have continual access to a telephone in case of worsening symptoms? Triage personnel must consider issues of contagion. For instance, scheduling an office visit for a patient who is likely to infect others is probably not best, the classic example being varicella. Whatever the disposition, excellent documentation of all telephone calls should be the rule, and parents should be given specific instructions on when to call again, for example, for deterioration. Plans for follow-up should be made, either again by telephone or by subsequent office visit.

Table 52-2 Office Emergency Drugs

DRUGS	PRIORITY*
Oxygen	E
Albuterol for inhalation†	E
Epinephrine (1:1000)	E
Activated charcoal	S
Antibiotics	S
Anticonvulsants (diazepam, lorazepam)	S
Corticosteroids (parenteral or oral)	S
Dextrose (25%)	S
Diphenhydramine (parenteral, 50 mg/mL)	S
Epinephrine (1:10,000)	S
Atropine sulfate (0.1 mg/mL)	S
Naloxone (0.4 mg/mL)	S
Sodium bicarbonate (4.2%)	S
FLUIDS	
Normal saline solution or lactated Ringer's solution (500-mL bags)	S
5% Dextrose, 0.45 normal saline (500-mL bags)	S

**E*, Essential; *S*, strongly suggested (essential if emergency medical services response time is >10 minutes).
†Metered-dose inhaler with spacer or mask may be substituted.
Adapted from: American Academy of Pediatrics, Committee on Pediatric Emergency Medicine, Singer J, Ludwig S, eds. *Emergency Medical Services for Children: The Role of the Primary Care Provider*. Elk Grove Village, IL: American Academy of Pediatrics; 1992.

Practitioner-Patient Encounter

Once the decision has been made to seek a face-to-face encounter with a clinician, the next question to answer is "In what setting?" The most common scenario is to schedule a sick visit with the patient's PCP. Most offices allow for time in the physician's schedule to fit in sick visits among previously scheduled well-child visits; however, numerous models have been used. In a solo practice the patient's personal physician will examine the patient. For larger groups, however, this circumstance may not be the case. Many practices have a designated *sick provider of the day,* who is not scheduled for physicals but examines all sick children on a given day. Nurse practitioners (NPs) and physician assistants (PAs) play an increasing role in the care of children in the primary care setting. These practitioners examine patients independently in collaboration with a physician. In some areas, telemedicine visits are available, allowing a pediatrician, NP, or PA to perform the equivalent of an office visit while the patient is in a remote location such as a school or child care setting. Studies have shown that many common childhood illnesses can be evaluated and treated via telemedicine, providing a convenience to parents of not having to bring a sick child to the physician's office.[12]

Many characteristics of a primary care practice exist that determines whether a given patient is best served by an office visit. One obvious issue is the time of day that the visit is required. Increasingly, PCPs have office hours that extend beyond the traditional period of 9 AM to 5 PM to include nights and weekends. School obligations and daytime parental employment obligations make these nontraditional office hours more amenable, especially for nonurgent visits. Middle-of-the-night encounters generally take place in an ED setting, even if the complaint itself may have been easily handled in an office setting had it occurred during the daytime hours. Office preparedness also dictates whether a patient is best treated in the primary care setting versus the ED. Larger offices may have the capability to handle nearly any complaint. Examples include in-office laboratory testing such as rapid streptococcal antigen or rapid influenza testing, suturing and splinting capability, and on-site radiology suites. Some offices are prepared to administer intravenous fluids and intramuscular antibiotics or give nebulized medications for respiratory illnesses, and some are equipped with pulse oximeters, electrocardiographic machines, or even defibrillators. Few primary care offices, however, are prepared for a true emergency, with less than one third of primary care practices having an Ambu bag with oxygen capabilities on the premises. The American Academy of Pediatrics has published lists of recommended emergency medications and equipment suggested for offices (Tables 52-2 and 52-3, respectively), even those within 20 minutes of an ED.[13] Many of the offices that are not as well equipped will need to triage patients who require these services to an ED, even if the complaint itself is not emergent, for example, a small superficial laceration requiring Dermabond or a nondisplaced greenstick fracture requiring a short-arm splint.

As with telephone triage, several disposition options are available after an office visit for an acute illness. Most patients will be sent home with either reassurance or treatment advice to include medications, prescription or over the counter. Occasionally, the PCP

Table 52-3 Office Emergency Equipment and Supplies

ITEM	PRIORITY*
AIRWAY MANAGEMENT	
Oxygen-delivery system	E
Bag-valve-mask (450 and 1000 mL)	E
Clear oxygen masks, breather and nonrebreather, with reservoirs (infant, child, adult)	E
Suction device, tonsil tip, bulb syringe	E
Nebulizer (or metered-dose inhaler with spacer or mask)	E
Oropharyngeal airways (sizes 00-5)	E
Pulse oximeter	E
Nasopharyngeal airways (sizes 12-30F)	S
Magill forceps (pediatric, adult)	S
Suction catheters (sizes 5-16F) and Yankauer suction tip	S
Nasogastric tubes (sizes 6-14F)	S
Laryngoscope handle (pediatric, adult) with extra batteries, bulbs	S
Laryngoscope blades (straight 0-2, curved 2-3)	S
Endotracheal tubes (uncuffed 2.5-5.5, cuffed 6.0-8.0)	S
Stylets (pediatric, adult)	S
Esophageal intubation detector or end-tidal carbon dioxide detector	S
VASCULAR ACCESS AND FLUID MANAGEMENT	
Butterfly needles (19-25 gauge)	S
Catheter-over-needle device (14-24 gauge)	S
Arm boards, tape, tourniquet	S
Intraosseous needles (16, 18 gauge)	S
Intravenous tubing, microdrip	S
MISCELLANEOUS EQUIPMENT AND SUPPLIES	
Color-coded tape or preprinted drug doses	E
Cardiac arrest board or backboard	E
Sphygmomanometer (infant, child, adult sizes; thigh cuffs)	E
Splints, sterile dressings	E
Automated external defibrillator with pediatric capabilities	E
Spot glucose test	S
Stiff neck collars (small or large)	S
Heating source (overhead warmer or infrared lamp)	S

**E, Essential; S, strongly suggested (essential if emergency medical services response time is >10 minutes).*
Adapted from: American Academy of Pediatrics, Committee on Pediatric Emergency Medicine, Singer J, Ludwig S, eds. *Emergency Medical Services for Children: The Role of the Primary Care Provider.* Elk Grove Village, IL: American Academy of Pediatrics; 1992.

will refer the child to a subspecialist for consultation, and this referral can happen immediately, for example, an otolaryngology referral for suspected peritonsillar abscess or, less urgently, for example, an orthopedic consult for leg length discrepancy or scoliosis. The PCP always has the option to send the moderate to severely ill child for immediate and further evaluation in a higher-acuity setting, namely the ED. Parents of children who are sick but stable can be recommended to drive their children to the appropriate ED, for example, the child suspected to have early appendicitis. In rare instances, a PCP may call for ambulance transport, for example, for an infant with bronchiolitis in severe respiratory distress. For the patient who is not a diagnostic dilemma but requires hospitalization, the PCP may send the patient directly for inpatient admission, bypassing the ED.

Parents may choose to bypass the primary care setting and bring the child directly to an urgent care center or ED. In many cases, this decision is appropriate by parents and may have been made with the guidance of medical personnel affiliated with their PCP. At other times, an ED visit is not appropriate, which can be a dilemma for hospitals and their administrators, given that overcrowding and long wait times often plague EDs, especially during the peak of the winter respiratory viral season. This overcrowding is frequently the result of inappropriate use of the ED for nonemergent matters, such as an uncomplicated upper respiratory tract infection or otalgia or even for pure primary care matters, such as prescription refills.[14,15] Unfortunately, many patients without insurance have nowhere else to turn for their medical care except for the ED. This circumstance, in turn, places a financial strain on the medical delivery system as a whole, with emergency care being much more costly than a less acute, but more medically appropriate, setting. Some insurers have offered financial incentives to physicians to teach patients the appropriate use of less costly acute settings when appropriate.

Once in the ED, children can receive a wide range of care, depending on the type of hospital visited and the training of the practitioner who attends to the patient.[16] Many ED visits occur at community hospitals that are not staffed by physicians who have formal pediatric emergency fellowship training. Nonetheless, in this modern era, formally trained emergency medicine physicians all receive some training in the care of children. Hence most community hospital EDs are comfortable treating all but the most complicated pediatric illnesses. Certainly the subspecialty services that are the most frequently consulted from the ED (orthopedics, surgery, otolaryngology) are accustomed to evaluating children, especially teenagers. EDs are equipped with laboratory and radiologic capabilities, and ED physicians themselves have more extensive training and experience with procedures, whether simple suturing or intubation. Because some children may be brought to EDs with very serious illness, having the capability for immediate consultation between ED physicians and pediatric subspecialists is important for all emergency departments that treat children. Most EDs are affiliated with tertiary care children's hospitals with pediatric emergency physicians available for consultation at any hour. Technology allows for *consultation from afar*, with the ability to send electrocardiograms, x-ray films, or computed tomographic scans electronically over fax lines or the Internet for pediatric specialists to review.[17]

Regardless of the patient's complaint, the ED physician's role is similar to the in-office physician, that is, to treat and discharge when appropriate or to triage the patient to a higher level of care if deemed appropriate. As with office visits, most patients seen in an ED setting are discharged home with either reassurance or a home treatment plan. A small percentage of patients will be sick enough to warrant hospitalization (see the following discussion). Transfer to another facility with pediatric capabilities is also an option open to the ED physician. For example, most general surgeons at community hospitals competently manage uncomplicated appendicitis in teenagers,[18] but most would not feel comfortable treating the 18 month old with evolving intussusception. In these cases, transfer to a tertiary care pediatric center is appropriate.

Hospitalized Patient

Just as a small percentage of acutely ill children in the office need to be sent to the ED, only a small percentage of sick children seen in the ED require hospitalization (see Figure 52-1). This circumstance is in contrast to the pattern observed 20 years ago when a lower threshold to admit sick children to the hospital existed. Seasoned pediatricians have noted that, in the current environment, children with life-threatening illnesses are now admitted to pediatric intensive care units and often do quite well; children with severe illnesses who used to be admitted to these special units are now admitted to regular pediatric inpatient units; and children with moderate illnesses who used to be admitted to pediatric inpatient units are now treated as outpatients. Furthermore, hospital stays are much shorter now than they were in past years, which means that hospitalized children today have a higher severity of illness than children hospitalized 20 years ago.[19]

Children may be admitted to a small community hospital with a pediatric service for minor illnesses, but many community hospitals are choosing to close their pediatric beds because so few patients need them. Children with complex illnesses are usually admitted to a tertiary care children's hospital or medical center where services are more comprehensive.

Classically, the patient's PCP would see patients in-house, making traditional rounds, usually once daily, and directing the child's care often with the assistance of experienced nurses or house officers. As with all aspects of pediatrics, however, inpatient care has become more specialized, giving rise to a new class of pediatricians: pediatric hospitalists.[20] Hospitalists have been used in internal medicine for more than a decade; they are now becoming more common in pediatrics as well, both in the community and tertiary or academic setting. Despite the obvious downside of not having had a longitudinal relationship with the hospitalized patient, evidence suggests that patient care is improved, patient and family satisfaction is increased, and lengths of stay are decreased.[21] In addition to being able to focus their continuing education on inpatient issues, pediatric hospitalists have the advantage of being in-house, thus able to reexamine patients multiple times daily and to respond quickly if patients should deteriorate. (See Chapter 20, Hospitalist Medicine: Communicating With Patients and Families; and Chapter 21, Hospital Care.)

Regardless of whether the PCP or a specialist is the inpatient-attending physician, a team approach is paramount to the effective treatment of the hospitalized child. Besides interacting with the attending physician and multiple members of the nursing staff during their stay, children and parents are also likely to encounter an increasing number of ancillary staff members, particularly in tertiary care settings. Medical students, house officers, and fellows will care for children who are admitted to teaching hospitals. Many children will benefit from the input of pediatric dietitians who specialize in the nutritional needs of children, including both enteral and parenteral nourishment. The injured child may benefit from the involvement of physical and occupational therapists during their inpatient stay. They not only start the process of rehabilitation, but are also invaluable partners in assessing readiness for the home environment or recognizing the need for a formal rehabilitation placement. Pediatric-trained social workers also play an important role in the overall care of a hospitalized child. Because the treatment of the hospitalized child rarely ends by the time of discharge, the competence of the caregiver and stability and safety of the home environment, wherever that may be, must be ensured. Social workers have the knowledge and skills to work with state and local child welfare agencies to ensure that these conditions are met. Formal *discharge planners* also assist in this role, arranging for home services that may be required after leaving the hospital (delivering a home nebulizer machine to a patient with asthma or arranging home nursing visits and antibiotics for a patient with osteomyelitis).

Hospital admission itself can be a trying experience for patients and their families. To deal with the physical and emotional stress of the hospitalization, most children's hospitals employ *child life* specialists.[22] Typically possessing a bachelor's or master's degree in child life, these individuals work with children both to prepare and to guide the child through each step of the inpatient stay. The teenager with cellulitis may simply need

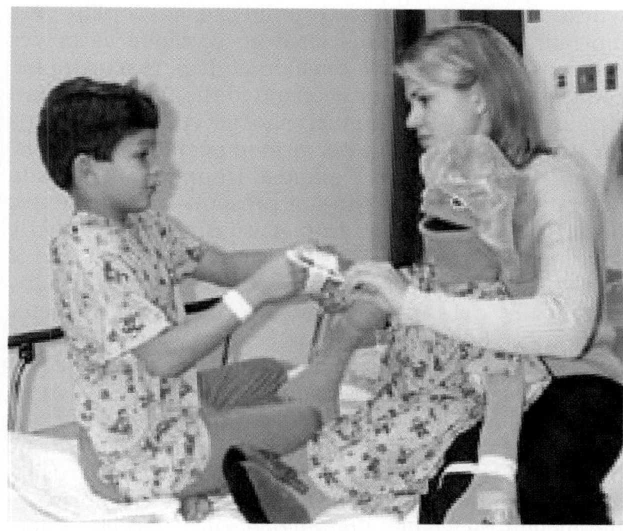

Figure 52-3 A child life worker modeling a painful procedure for a patient.

a partner with whom to play board games to help pass the time. However, the toddler with leukemia who will have multiple admissions for chemotherapy and painful procedures will probably interact with the child life team more intensely. The child life team can prepare the child before any invasive procedure, such as lumbar puncture or bone marrow biopsy, using anatomically correct dolls (Figure 52-3), or by assisting the medical team during the procedure itself with distraction methods. The child life service is an invaluable asset to both the child and the clinician.

Although the goal of any inpatient stay is to diagnose and treat the patient's underlying abnormality, recognizing and treating the symptoms of disease is equally important. To parents, pain control is likely to be just as important an issue as addressing the pathophysiological factors of an illness. Increasingly, the literature supports early and aggressive treatment of pediatric pain, even in illnesses such as appendicitis in which pain medicines were previously thought to mask the symptoms.[23] Hospitals are encouraged to use pediatric pain scales to assess the nonverbal cues that the child in pain gives. New topical anesthetics should optimally be used before venipuncture or incision. In addition, moderate or deep sedation should be used for significantly painful procedures.

Most patients will undergo an imaging study at some time during their inpatient stay. The study most commonly used remains the plain-film radiograph, relatively unchanged over many decades. Plain films are typically the 1st step in imaging the lung fields for pneumonia, the heart size for cardiomegaly, the skeleton for fractures, or the bowel gas pattern for signs of obstruction. Newer imaging techniques that have found an ever-widening role include computed tomography, magnetic resonance imaging, ultrasonography, and nuclear medicine studies. Interventional radiologists have carved a niche performing radiology-guided procedures, such as deep-abscess drainage or percutaneous biopsy.[24,25] (See Chapter 15, Pediatric Imaging.)

Pediatric subspecialists are often consulted during a patient's hospitalization. Because of the advances in pediatric health care, patients with serious illnesses are living longer, which has led to increased involvement of fellowship-trained pediatric subspecialists. For example, the improved survival of very premature infants weighing less than 1000 grams has a domino effect on the future use of health care resources.[26] Many former *preemies* have chronic pulmonary disease and are cared for by pediatric pulmonologists, or they have seizure disorders and are cared for by pediatric neurologists.

Occasionally, a child is ill enough to require admission to an intensive care setting, either directly from an ED or transferred from a lower acuity setting. Nurse-to-patient ratios are such that each child is given greater attention and closer monitoring. Technologic advances have changed intensive care medicine perhaps more than any other facet of pediatrics.[27] Patients and their physiologic status can be monitored extremely closely, including directly monitoring intracranial pressure, central venous pressure, or arterial blood pressure with indwelling catheters. Failing cardiovascular and respiratory systems can be assisted by intravenous blood pressure medications and mechanical ventilation, respectively. Novel surgical approaches have greatly decreased both morbidity and mortality, examples of which include cerebral hemispherectomy for intractable seizures or the multistep Glenn procedure for infants born with certain cyanotic heart lesions. Clearly, with the ability to provide highly specialized care comes the obligation to discuss the risks and benefits of any given intervention with patients and their families. The intensive care unit is often the setting for *do-not-resuscitate* discussions, clearly much more difficult when discussing children than adults. Although the pediatric intensivist has occasion to lead these discussions, in many instances, the patient's PCP can offer a unique perspective and should be invited to participate in the process. Along with the potential for dramatic recovery comes the realization that, despite heroic efforts, occasionally a child cannot recover from the injury or illness. End-of-life decisions must often be made in the intensive care setting. In many hospitals, ethics committees are available to assist in these determinations. Child life specialists and social workers play an important role in the coping process. Chaplains or other religious figures may be of support to some families. In many cases, approaching the family of the dying child to inquire about organ donations is appropriate; personnel specifically trained for this purpose should conduct this conversation in a sensitive manner.

Disposition

Because family-centered care has been shown to improve outcomes, the parents of hospitalized children should be involved in all major care decisions, including discharge criteria.[28] The hospitalized patient is rarely asymptomatic on discharge. The healing process, and often the diagnostic work-up, may continue after discharge. Close follow-up should be arranged for the discharged patient. Effective communication between the inpatient attending and the PCP is essential. The PCP should be informed of any unresolved medical issues, the names and dosing schedules of any discharge medications, and any arrangements for follow-up appointments with consultants. Some patients will require follow-up studies, and the PCP should be made aware of these requirements.[29] Most children's hospitals will fax a discharge summary with recommended treatments, procedures, and follow-up visits to the PCP within 24 hours of the patient's discharge. The patient will occasionally require the hands-on involvement of medical personnel at home after discharge. These patients benefit from the involvement of visiting nurses or home health nurses who can administer medications, take vitals signs, and draw blood for follow-up laboratory studies, among other tasks. Home physical or occupational therapy can be arranged for appropriate patients as well.

Infrequently, the hospitalized patient will require transfer to a rehabilitation facility after discharge. Injuries account for the majority of these patients, especially patients who have suffered a traumatic brain or spinal cord injury.[30] Any patient, however, who has been hospitalized for an extended period may suffer from muscle wasting and deconditioning, and these patients also frequently require a rehabilitation placement. Regardless of the reason, great care should be taken to ensure that the proposed facility has adequate experience with children. Some children may require long-term care in a skilled nursing facility, perhaps requiring permanent enteral nutrition through a gastrostomy tube or permanent ventilation via a tracheostomy. A previously healthy child may suffer a massive central nervous system insult, such as overwhelming meningitis, and permanently lose the ability to perform activities of daily living. The decision to have a child be cared for in a nursing facility can be emotionally devastating for families. Fortunately, with highly skilled visiting nurse services, caring for technologically dependent children at home may be possible for families. As with discussions regarding end-of-life issues, family decisions regarding long-term care should be made with the input of appropriate subspecialists, such as intensivists, neurologists, or neurosurgeons. Families must weigh not only whether they are willing to provide the necessary care, but also whether they are capable of providing this care with respect to both the skill and the time commitment required. The PCP can assist families in this decision and in arranging home nursing services. Increasingly, children with terminal illness are discharged home for palliative care with the assistance of hospice services, because this setting can be far more satisfying for the patient and family than remaining in the hospital. Again, the PCP can be helpful to families in coordinating hospice services.

CHILD WITH SPECIAL HEALTH CARE NEEDS—PROSPECTS FOR THE FUTURE

The health of children certainly has improved dramatically over the last several decades and will likely continue to do so. Vaccinations have nearly wiped out several infectious diseases, at least in the developed world, that once caused immense morbidity and mortality.[31] This trend is likely to continue as newer vaccines continue to be developed. Laparoscopic procedures have significantly changed the field of pediatric surgery,[32] allowing much shorter recovery periods for the most commonly performed pediatric surgeries. Prenatal screening has expanded from initial efforts to detect phenylketonuria to the present ability to detect dozens of inborn errors of metabolism, allowing early treatment of many of these diseases. The science of genomics holds great promise for the cure of many genetically determined illnesses, including diabetes and cancer. Public health initiatives are likely to become a backbone of the approach to treating certain diseases in children, such as obesity, type II diabetes, and depression, designated the *millennial morbidity*.

The future of the care of the ill child is likely to be marked by new challenges, however. Increasing resistance to antibiotics has already resulted in the rise of methicillin-resistant *Staphylococcus aureus* infections,[33] and other pathogenic organisms are likely to follow suit. As violence in the media and video games becomes more common, the incidence of aggressive and antisocial behavior may also increase. The very technology that has dramatically decreased mortality may also lead to increased morbidity. Neonatologists now routinely resuscitate infants born at 24 weeks' gestation,[34] and advances in care allow many of these infants to survive and leave the newborn intensive care unit. Such patients will require ongoing care that is intensive, specialized, and costly. In this realm, society as a whole must also grapple with the high cost of technologically advanced medical care. The United States spends more per capita on health care than any other nation,[35] yet vital statistics suggest that the country lags behind other industrialized countries on certain specific outcomes, such as infant mortality. As advances continue to be made in the science of medicine, and as the cost of these advances skyrocket, the emphasis on value, as well as a focus on evidence-based medicine combined with outcomes data (Figure 52-4), will clearly play a large role. As always,

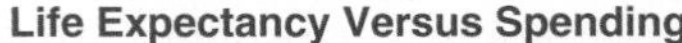

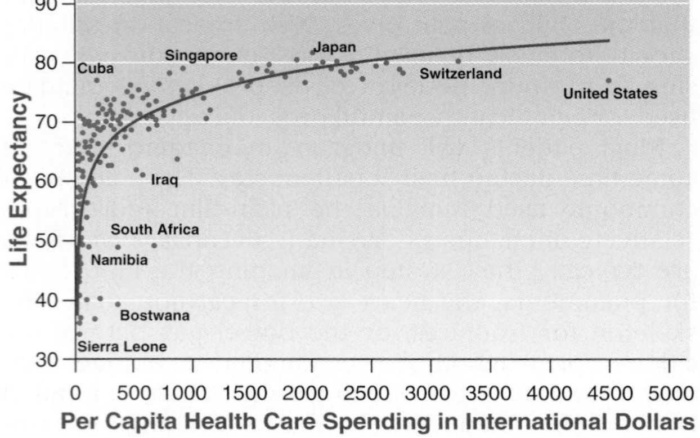

Figure 52-4 Health care spending versus life expectancy.

preventing disease is far more cost effective than treatment. The PCP will continue to play an important role in disease prevention through direct care of patients and via advocacy for increased governmental and community preventive measures.

TOOLS FOR PRACTICE

Engaging Patient and Family

- *Medicine and the Media: How to Make Sense of the Messages* (brochure), American Academy of Pediatrics (patiented.aap.org).
- *PsoriasisNet* (Web page), American Academy of Dermatology (www.skincarephysicians.com/psoriasisnet/index.html).
- *What Is a Pediatric Hospitalist?* (fact sheet), American Academy of Pediatrics (www.aap.org/sections/hospcare/whatishospitalist.pdf).

Practice Management and Care Coordination

- *Pediatric Telephone Protocols: Office Version, 11th Edition* (book), Barton Schmitt, MD (www.aap.org/bookstore).

AAP POLICY STATEMENTS

American Academy of Pediatrics, Child Life Council and Committee on Hospital Care. Child Life Services. *Pediatrics.* 2006;118(4):1757-1763. (aappolicy.aappublications.org/cgi/content/full/pediatrics;118/4/1757).

American Academy of Pediatrics, Committee on Hospital Care. Family Centered Care and the Pediatrician's Role. *Pediatrics.* 2003;112(3):691-696. (aappolicy.aappublications.org/cgi/content/full/pediatrics;112/3/691).

American Academy of Pediatrics, Committee on Pediatric Emergency Medicine. Pediatric Care Recommendations for Freestanding Urgent Care Facilities. *Pediatrics.* 2005;116(1):258-260. (aappolicy.aappublications.org/cgi/content/full/pediatrics;116/1/258).

American Academy of Pediatrics Committee on Pediatric Emergency Medicine. Preparation for Emergencies in the Offices of Pediatricians and Pediatric Primary Care Providers. *Pediatrics.* 2007;120(1):200-212. (aappolicy.aappublications.org/cgi/content/full/pediatrics;120/1/200).

American Academy of Pediatrics Committee on Pediatric Emergency Medicine. The Role of the Pediatrician in Rural Emergency Medical Services for Children. *Pediatrics.* 2005;116(6):1553-1556. (aappolicy.aappublications.org/cgi/content/full/pediatrics;116/6/1553).

Gerstle RS, and the American Academy of Pediatrics Task Force on Medical Informatics. Clinical Report: E-mail Communication Between Pediatricians and Their Patients. *Pediatrics.* 2004;114(1):317-321. (aappolicy.aappublications.org/cgi/content/full/pediatrics;114/1/317).

REFERENCES

1. Spitzer AR. The Internet—a new medical problem or invaluable ally? *Pediatrics.* 2004;114:817-819.
2. Wagner PJ, Phillips W, Radford M, et al. Frequent use of medical services: patient reports of intentions to seek care. *Arch Fam Med.* 1995;4(7):594-599.
3. Pandolfini C, Impicciatore P, Bonati M. Parents on the Web: risks for quality management of cough in children. *Pediatrics.* 2000;105(1):e1.
4. Kogan MD, Pappas G, Yu SM, et al. Over-the-counter medication use among US preschool-age children. *JAMA.* 1994;272(13):1025-1030.
5. McGuigan MA. Common culprits in childhood poisoning: epidemiology, treatment and parental advice for prevention. *Paediatr Drugs.* 1999;1(4):313-324.
6. Woolf AD. Herbal remedies and children: do they work? Are they harmful? *Pediatrics.* 2003;112(1 pt 2):240-246.
7. Schmitt BD. *Pediatric Telephone Protocols: Office Version.* 11th ed. Elk Grove Village, IL: American Academy of Pediatrics; 2006.
8. Wachter DA, Brillman JC, Lewis J, et al. Pediatric telephone triage protocols: standardized decisionmaking or a false sense of security? *Ann Emerg Med.* 1999;33(4):388-394.
9. Lee TJ, Baraff LJ, Wall SP, et al. Parental compliance with after hours telephone triage advice: nurse advice service versus on-call pediatricians. *Clin Pediatr.* 2003;42(7):613-619.
10. Lee TJ, Baraff LJ, Guzy J, et al. Does telephone triage delay significant medical treatment? Advice nurse service vs on-call pediatricians. *Arch Pediatr Adolesc Med.* 2003:157(7):635-641.
11. Gerstle RS, American Academy of Pediatrics, Task Force on Medical Informatics. E-mail communication between pediatricians and their patients. *Pediatrics.* 2004;114(1):317-321.
12. McConnochie KM, Wood NE, Kitzman HJ, et al. Telemedicine reduces absences due to illness in urban children: evaluation of an innovation. *Pediatrics.* 2005;115:1273-1282.
13. American Academy of Pediatrics, Committee on Pediatric Emergency Medicine. Pediatric care recommendations for freestanding urgent care facilities. *Pediatrics.* 2005;116(1):258-260.
14. Weir R, Rideout E, Crook J. Pediatric use of emergency departments. *J Pediatr Health Care.* 1989;3(4): 204-210.
15. Halfon N, Newacheck PW, Wood DL, et al. Routine emergency department use for sick care by children in the United States. *Pediatrics.* 1996;98(1):28-34.
16. Hampers LC, Faries SG. Practice variation in the emergency management of croup. *Pediatrics.* 2002;109(3):505-508.
17. Callahan CW, Malone F, Estroff D, et al. Effectiveness of an Internet-based store-and-forward telemedicine system for pediatric subspecialty consultation. *Arch Pediatr Adolesc Med.* 2005;159(4):389-393.
18. Alexander F, Magnuson D, DiFiore J, et al. Specialty versus generalist care of children with appendicitis: an outcome comparison. *J Pediatr Surg.* 2001;36(10):1510-1513.
19. Dougherty G. When should a child be in the hospital? A. Frederick North, Jr, MD, revisited. *Pediatrics.* 1998;101(1 pt 1):19-24.
20. Narang AS, Ey J. The emerging role of pediatric hospitalists. *Clin Pediatr.* 2003;42(4):295-297.
21. Bellet PS, Whitaker RC. Evaluation of a pediatric hospitalist service: impact on length of stay and hospital charges. *Pediatrics.* 2000;105(3 pt 1):478-484.
22. American Academy of Pediatrics, Committee on Hospital Care. Child life services. *Pediatrics.* 2000;106(5):1156-1159.
23. Green R, Bulloch B, Kabani A, et al. Early analgesia for children with acute abdominal pain. *Pediatrics.* 2005;116(4):978-983.
24. Kaye RD, Sane SS, Towbin RB. Pediatric intervention: an update. Part I. *J Vasc Interv Radiol.* 2000;11(6):683-697.
25. Kaye R, Sane SS, Towbin RB. Pediatric intervention: an update. Part II. *J Vasc Interv Radiol.* 2000;11(7):807-822.
26. Slonim AD, Patel KM, Ruttimann UE, et al. The impact of prematurity: a perspective of pediatric intensive care units. *Crit Care Med.* 2000;28(3):848-853.

27. Irazuzta J. Monitoring in pediatric intensive care. *Indian J Pediatr.* 1993;60(1):55-65.
28. American Academy of Pediatrics, Committee on Hospital Care. Family-centered care and the pediatrician's role. *Pediatrics.* 2003;112(3 pt 1):691-697.
29. Pantilat SZ, Lindenauer PK, Katz PP, et al. Primary care physician attitudes regarding communication with hospitalists. *Am J Med.* 2001;111(9B):15S-20S.
30. Ylvisaker M, Adelson PD, Braga LW, et al. Rehabilitation and ongoing support after pediatric TBI: twenty years of progress. *J Head Trauma Rehab.* 2005;20(1):95-109.
31. Centers for Disease Control and Prevention. Impact of vaccines universally recommended for children—United States, 1990-1998. *MMWR Morb Mortal Wkly Rep* 1999; 48:243-247.
32. Schrag S, Gorwitz R, Fultz-Butts K, et al. Prevention of perinatal group B streptococcal disease. Revised guidelines from CDC. *MMWR Recomm Rep.* 2002;51(RR-11): 1-22.
33. Zetola N, Francis JS, Nuermberger EL, et al. Community-acquired methicillin-resistant Staphylococcus aureus: an emerging threat. *Lancet Infect Dis.* 2005;5(5):275-286.
34. Louis JM, Ehrenberg HM, Collin MF, et al. Perinatal intervention and neonatal outcomes near the limit of viability. *Am J Obstet Gynecol.* 2004;191(4):1398-1402.
35. Anderson GF, Hussey PS, Frogner BK, et al. Health spending in the United States and the rest of the industrialized world. *Health Aff.* 200;24(4):903-914.

Chapter 53

PHYSIOLOGY AND MANAGEMENT OF FEVER

Henry M. Adam, MD

Viewing fever both as a response to illness and as a disease in itself has a long history, at least in Western cultures. Hippocrates perceived fever as a defense mounted by the body against an underlying disorder; the Galenic and medieval traditions understood fever to be a means of restoring balance among the humors by burning off an excess of phlegm (water) with yellow bile (fire).[1] On the other hand, the writers of the Gospels saw fever itself as the disease that Jesus "rebuked," miraculously curing Simon's mother-in-law.[2,3]

This *double vision* regarding fever has persisted despite our relatively sophisticated understanding of the physiologic mechanisms of temperature control, blurring how we as physicians and as parents see the child who is febrile. Although our science teaches us that fever, as part of the inflammatory response, is only a sign or symptom of the real pathologic process, we have the need to *treat* fever with a drug and a sponge, as if it were the noxious culprit itself. Fever, as opposed to hyperthermia, rarely poses a threat to a child's well being; in fact, the argument has been made that as an energy-expensive phenomenon, fever is not likely to have weathered evolution without conferring some survival benefit.[4] Considering that fever is the most common signal of illness in children, serving as the chief complaint for as many as one third of all pediatric office visits, we would do well to clarify our approach to its management that is distinct from the illnesses that cause it.

FEVER AND THERMOREGULATION

Fever is a regulated elevation of body temperature, mediated by the anterior hypothalamus, that occurs in response to any insult that stimulates the body's inflammatory defenses.[5] Similar to a thermostat, the hypothalamic set point controls the temperature that the body tries to maintain. Some provocation, most commonly a viral infection in children, induces macrophages to release low–molecular-weight proteins called cytokines, among them interleukin-1 and interleukin-6 and probably tumor necrosis factor, that function as endogenous pyrogens. They circulate to the anterior hypothalamus, where by increasing local levels of prostaglandin E_2 they induce a rise in the set point.[4,6] With the body's thermostat now up-regulated, several mechanisms come into play to bring the core temperature (defined as the temperature of blood within the pulmonary artery[7]) up to the new set point. Because the core temperature, even as it begins to elevate, is lower than the thermostat setting, a person developing fever feels chilled. Physiologically, the body's response is to generate more internal heat, setting skeletal muscles to shivering and stimulating cellular metabolism while minimizing heat loss to the environment by vasoconstricting the skin and turning off sweat glands. The one strategy is analogous to heating up the furnace, the other to closing the windows.

Hyperthermia, on the contrary, is an unregulated rise in core temperature to a level above the hypothalamic set point, either from overproduction of heat (thyroid storm), a reduced ability to dissipate heat (a bundled-up baby), or as with heat stroke from overexertion on a hot and humid day, a combination of the two.[8] The body's response to hyperthermia is the opposite of its response when a fever is induced; instead of an initial chill, intense flushing ensues as blood vessels in the skin vasodilate and sweat glands activate in an attempt to lose as much heat as possible to the outside. The furnace is burning out of control; the only strategy is to try to open the windows wide.

Whereas hyperthermia may raise body temperature to dangerous, even deadly, levels, fever appears to be a homeostatic process, physiologically regulated within benign limits. DuBois[9] first noted how unusual it was, even for patients who had an untreated serious infection, to have fever exceeding 106° F (41.1° C). Two studies, one retrospective[10] and the other prospective[11] that examined large numbers of children who came to emergency departments were consistent in finding that in only 0.05% of visits did the child have a temperature of 106° F or higher. Although the pediatric literature conflicts about whether a temperature greater than 106° F (frequently called hyperpyrexia) is a marker for particular risk for serious underlying infection,[10-14] no study suggests that the elevated temperature itself poses a threat to an otherwise healthy child except in the extraordinarily rare event that fever exceeds 107° F (41.7° C). A child who has a temperature greater than 106° F is likely to have an element of hyperthermia, such as dehydration, in addition to fever. Evidence is accumulating that as an intrinsic feature of the febrile response, the body releases *endogenous cryogens*, peptides that counterbalance pyrogens and modulate how high the hypothalamus sets its thermostat.[4] Vasopressin and melanocyte-stimulating hormone, as well as some of the cytokines that also may act as pyrogens, appear to help limit the height fever can reach.[4]

As a centrally regulated response to an inflammatory insult, fever may well serve as a helpful component of the body's acute phase reaction and is an adaptive response widely present in the animal kingdom among cold-blooded and warm-blooded species.[4,14-16] At least some species of fish and lizards, when infected, move to a warmer part of their environment, thus raising their body temperatures. This behaviorally induced fever has demonstrable survival benefit, which can be negated with antipyretic agents that lower temperature and increase mortality.[15-17] Fever can retard the growth and reproduction of many invasive pathogenic microorganisms, both bacterial and viral, and it appears to lower the amount of iron that is available to invading bacteria, many of which have a greater iron requirement at higher temperatures.[18] Among its other effects on human physiology, fever enhances neutrophil migration and the production of superoxides; it promotes T-cell proliferation and increases the release and activity of interferon.[4,19] Interestingly, some of fever's apparently beneficial stimulation of immunologic function may be reversed at very high temperatures, in the hyperpyretic range.[20]

Unfortunately, no conclusive experimental information is available to prove that fever benefits humans clinically in the course of an infection, and some data suggest that, at least within the context of endotoxemia, the metabolic cost of fever contributes to mortality. However, in a teleologic sense, its metabolic cost argues for fever playing some protective role in the infected host. A process that results in a 7% to 10% increase in energy expenditure for every 1° C rise in temperature is not likely to have persisted so widely in nature, among invertebrates, fish, amphibians, and reptiles, as well as among birds and mammals, for millions of years without conferring some survival advantage.[4,21]

FEVER PHOBIA

If, then, fever itself only rarely poses a threat to a child and may even be of benefit, then why are parents and pediatricians so generally aggressive about treating it? Schmitt[22] coined the phrase *fever phobia* when he described the prevalence of misunderstanding about fever among parents bringing their children to an inner city clinic. He found that 58% of parents defined fevers below 102° F (39° C) as *high*, and 16% actually believed that, if left untreated, fever might rise to 110° F (43.3° C) or higher. Almost every parent thought fever could cause harmful side effects, with 46% fearing permanent brain damage. Given these responses, not surprisingly, 63% of all the parents worried "lots" about the harm fever might cause their children and that 56% gave an antipyretic agent for a temperature within the normal range. For temperatures below 102° F (38.9° C), 85% of parents treated with a drug and 62% with sponging. Twenty years later, a study in Baltimore revisiting fever phobia in 2 urban hospital-based clinics documented the enduring persistence of the misconceptions and fears Schmitt had first identified.[23]

The population Schmitt described consisted mainly of medically indigent, poorly educated families. Kramer, Naimark, and Leduc[24] essentially repeated Schmitt's study in a private practice with middle-class parents. Almost 50% defined temperatures in the normal range as fever; 43% thought that temperatures below 104° F (40° C) could be dangerous, and 15% believed that untreated fevers could rise above 107.6° F (42° C). Death, brain damage, and stroke were among the complications of fever these educated parents feared, with 20% believing that such complications might occur at temperatures below 104° F and 95% believing that they might occur at levels below 107.6° F. One in 5 of these parents would treat normal temperatures, and virtually all (97%) would treat a temperature below 104° F.

The fact that the use of medication to treat fever is so widespread is not surprising. The English, for example, administer an estimated 68 million child-days of antipyretic drugs each year.[25] Fifty percent of the parents in Schmitt's study[22] stated that physicians or nurses were their most important source of information about fever. This claim was given credence by a survey of members of the American Academy of Pediatrics in Massachusetts[26] in which 2 of 3 believed fever itself can pose a danger to children, and 25% of the responding physicians cited death and brain damage as potential complications of fever as low as 104° F (40° C). Almost three fourths of the pediatricians always or often recommended treatment for fever, two thirds of them for temperatures under 102° F (38.9° C). The children may be the ones who swallow the medicine, but the therapy seems aimed more at the anxiety of their parents and physicians than at any real danger that fever holds for them.

DEFINITION AND MEASUREMENT

As would be expected with any physiological parameter, no single normal value represents the gold standard for body temperature. Rather, a range of normal values must take into account variations from person to person, fluctuations that reflect both a circadian pattern and age-related differences and disparities arising from the method and site of temperature measurement. A reading of 98.6° F (37° C) has traditionally been considered the *norm;* however, the average mean daily oral temperature, measured every 6 hours for 41 to 108 days, of 9 healthy young adult volunteers was 97.9° F (36.61° C), with a range of 97.5°F to 98.4° F (36.41°C to 36.9° C).[7] Young children tend to have higher normal body temperatures than older children or adults; yet infants in the first 1 or 2 months of life are less likely than older children to develop fever with an infectious illness. Normally, body temperature is higher in the late afternoon and early evening than it is late at night or early in the morning, with a swing of as much as 3° F (1.7° C).[20,26-28] Probably the temperature cited most frequently as defining fever is 100.4° F (38° C), measured rectally. However, given all the variables that affect a particular person's body temperature, any specific number used to define fever is arbitrary. The measurement of fever is discussed fully in Chapter 181, Fever.

MANAGEMENT

The management of fever rightly begins well before a child becomes febrile. As a first step, we primary care providers must recognize the part we have played in creating *fever phobia* in our patients' parents. Our almost ritualistic dependence on measuring a child's temperature, even at routine encounters in which illness is not an issue, as well as our readiness to recommend antipyretic therapy for any elevation of temperature, must certainly confuse parents when we tell them not to worry about fever itself. Offering counseling about fever when a child is already ill is not as likely to be as effective as introducing the subject routinely in the course of a health maintenance visit.[29,30] We need to explain that fever is one of the body's natural responses and is not a threat in itself and that temperature will not spiral out of control to dangerous heights without treatment other than sensible care (eg, maintaining hydration and not overbundling).[31] In identifying the underlying illness as the possible danger to the child, we would do well to educate parents about the symptoms and behaviors that should alert them to trouble and signal the need for medical attention.

Treating fever is a question of judgment. If the source of the fever poses a threat, then obviously it must be addressed specifically. However, intervening against fever per se should be a decision that is individualized to each child who is febrile. By far the most common reason for treating fever is that it makes the child uncomfortable. Although on an evolutionary scale, fever surely must be beneficial, its benefit during the course of an acute illness is not so well proven as to override concern for the child's comfort. The decision to treat for comfort's sake should not be based on any particular temperature threshold, but rather on how the child looks and behaves; many children tolerate fevers to 104° F (40° C) without apparent ill effect, whereas others become cranky and restless with a temperature barely above 100.4° F (38° C). In some cases, concern for a child's comfort may have to be balanced against the usefulness of a fever's pattern or persistence when making a diagnosis. At least one study[32] has even suggested that acetaminophen's efficacy in improving a febrile child's comfort is more presumption than fact. In a randomized, double-blind, placebo-controlled trial of 225 children 6 months to 6 years who had acute fever, those treated with acetaminophen were somewhat more active and alert than the control group but were no different in mood, comfort, appetite, or fluid intake. The acetaminophen group's fever and other symptoms lasted as long, and at the end of the trial, parents were unable to tell with any reliability whether their child had received the drug or the placebo.

Hyperthermia

Hyperthermia is different from fever, posing a real and immediate threat to any child suffering from heat illness. Successful treatment depends on restoring the core temperature to normal as rapidly as possible. Antipyretic agents, which work by lowering the hypothalamic set point, are not helpful because the set point is already below a rising body temperature that has escaped regulation; physical cooling is the mainstay of therapy.[8]

Treating for Pain Relief

Particularly when comfort is the issue for an infant in the first few months of life, 2 factors weigh against routine use of medication for fever. The half-lives of all available antipyretics are significantly prolonged early in infancy, making inadvertent overdose more of a problem. With their larger surface area relative to volume, infants are also more responsive to physical interventions that reduce body heat, such as removing clothing and blankets, keeping the room temperature moderate, and improving air circulation.

Some researchers also believe that reducing fever with a dose of antipyretic can distinguish children who appear ill only because they are febrile from children who have a seriously threatening infection. In fact, neither the magnitude of fever reduction nor a child's clinical appearance after receiving antipyretic medication can reliably distinguish serious from trivial infectious disease.[33,34]

Treating the Compromised Child

Although fever itself is benign in an otherwise healthy child who has a self-limited viral illness, the metabolic stress it entails may be more than an already compromised child can tolerate. Increased oxygen consumption and insensible water loss, along with tachycardia and tachypnea, can further threaten a child who is significantly anemic, septic, or in shock, as well as a child rendered vulnerable by cardiac, pulmonary, renal, or any other systemic disease that strains homeostasis. Fever may also exacerbate an acute brain injury, either infectious or traumatic, and its effect on the sensorium may be confounding in a child who has a neurologic disorder.

Seizures

More troublesome is defining the role of antipyretic medication in preventing febrile seizures. Children who are most at risk for febrile seizures (those 3 months to 3 years of age) are also the children who most frequently have self-limited viral illnesses. Urging parents to treat their young children's fever with an antipyretic agent will likely promote fever phobia, as well as an unwarranted fear of the risk that a febrile seizure poses. Undeniably, a convulsive episode in a young child is terribly frightening, but only very rarely is it dangerous.[35] Aggressive attention to the possibility of a seizure with any fever will only magnify the anxiety parents already feel about both—and without any convincing evidence the strategy will work. The relationship between fever and seizures is neither clear nor predictable. The convulsive activity in a febrile seizure can, in fact, precede the fever, making causality at best uncertain. Parents are often not aware that their child has a fever until after the seizure has occurred. Some children *seize* with low-grade fever and not again when their temperature is high. The lower the child's temperature is with the first seizure, the greater the risk; this circumstance makes having a sense of control more difficult for parents because lower-grade fevers are hard to detect. Parents overcall fever when they use palpation,[37] which may lead either to excessive dosing with an antipyretic drug or confirmatory rectal probes that become part of too many children's routine. Last, whether around-the-clock administration of acetaminophen or ibuprofen can prevent recurrence of febrile seizures has even been questioned.[38,39] Although no approach seems perfect, a reasonable compromise might be to use antipyretics prophylactically only for the approximately 3% of children who have had a first febrile convulsion, in which the risk for recurrence is 1 in 3.[36] Even then, parents deserve reassurance that another seizure is neither their fault nor a real threat to their child's well being. In fact, the threat may come from the treatment if prophylaxis becomes too aggressive. The use of alternating antipyretics, given every 2 hours, has worked its way into practice without real evidence to give it support but certainly with the potential to generate toxic reactions.

Medical Management

If a fever is to be treated beyond routine attention to hydration and ambient conditions, then the most sensible approach follows from understanding how the brain controls the body's temperature. When the hypothalamic set point rises, fever follows. Acetaminophen and nonsteroidal antiinflammatory drugs (NSAIDs), particularly aspirin and ibuprofen, are all effective antipyretic agents because they lower the hypothalamic set point back toward normal by inhibiting the synthesis of prostaglandin E_2.

In most circumstances, aspirin should not be the drug of choice for children because of its reported association with Reye syndrome.[40,41] Whether this association is unique to aspirin or generic to NSAIDs, which all have similar modes of action, remains unclear. When reducing fever is the principal concern, acetaminophen has the advantage of a long record of safety; it has almost no side effects, other than allergic reactions, unless ingested in toxic amounts (more than 140 mg/kg), which is at least 10-fold greater than its therapeutic dose (10 to 15 mg/kg).[42] Children younger than 6 years, the group most frequently febrile, are significantly less susceptible than older children and adults to liver destruction, the major toxicity of acetaminophen poisoning.

At its optimal dose (10 mg/kg), ibuprofen reduces fever as effectively as acetaminophen, and because its duration of action is moderately longer, it can be given every 6 hours rather than every 4 hours.[43,44] However, ibuprofen's less-frequent dosing has a cost; typically of antiinflammatory agents, it can cause gastritis and gastrointestinal bleeding, and it inhibits platelet function. The clinical situation determines whether ibuprofen's suppression of inflammation is a benefit or potentially an undesirable side effect. In a child who is febrile with rheumatoid disease, ibuprofen offers relief that acetaminophen cannot; a child whose fever arises from infection may well do better with the inflammatory response left intact. Other NSAIDs, with properties and side effects similar to those of ibuprofen, are coming on the market. Naproxen is available in a pediatric suspension; because of its relatively long half-life, it can be given twice daily, at a dose of 5 mg/kg.

Physical Cooling

As an alternative to medication, physical cooling can lower the body temperature of a child who is febrile, but the physiologic mechanism of fever explains why the result may paradoxically make the child feel worse. With fever, the hypothalamic thermostat is set above normal, dictating that the body generate heat. Whereas acetaminophen or NSAIDs push the thermostat back down, damping the impulse to produce heat, physical measures such as sponging work the opposite way; in effect, they open the windows to let heat escape without adjusting the thermostat at all. As cooling begins, the hypothalamus senses wider divergence between its own set point and the body's actual temperature; to close the gap, it sends out the directive to generate still more heat, with muscular shivering and a rise in the general metabolic rate. Aside from how uncomfortable the child may feel, with the set point remaining high once the sponging is finished, the temperature is likely to renew its climb.

Of course, under some circumstances, physical cooling has a place. Some fevers that warrant intervention clinically may not respond to antipyretic drugs, as in a neurologically impaired child whose temperature control is aberrant. If an underlying illness gives special urgency to reducing the metabolic stress that comes with a fever, then the combination of an antipyretic medication and cooling not only works more quickly than either alone,[45] but it also makes physiological sense; while cooling physically draws heat off, the drug lowers the set point to avert a rebound temperature rise. The same holds for the rare fever high enough to be a concern itself or for a fever that is complicated by some element of hyperthermia. When sponging a child, tepid water (approximately 90° F [32° C]) is probably best. It sets a moderate but effective gradient down from body temperature, rather than the precipitous decline colder water would induce, and it is less likely to distress the child who has a shivering response. Alcohol solutions have no place at all in the management of a febrile child because alcohol can be absorbed through the skin.

Hippocrates saw it right when, without the insights of our science, he somehow appreciated fever as part of the body's natural defense. We often do best to let nature have its way.

TOOLS FOR PRACTICE

Engaging Patients and Family

- *Understanding Fever* (fact sheet), American Academy of Pediatrics (www.aap.org/publiced/BR_Fever.htm).
- *Understanding Febrile Seizures* (fact sheet), American Academy of Pediatrics (www.aap.org/publiced/BR_FebrileSeizures.htm).
- *Fever and Your Child* (brochure), American Academy of Pediatrics (patiented.aap.org).

AAP POLICY STATEMENT

American Academy of Pediatrics, Committee on Quality Improvement, Subcommittee on Urinary Tract Infection. Practice parameter: the diagnosis, treatment, and evaluation of the initial urinary tract infection in febrile infants and young children. *Pediatrics*. 1999;103(4):843-852. (aappolicy.aappublications.org/cgi/content/abstract/pediatrics;103/4/843).

SUGGESTED READINGS

Kluger MJ. Fever revisited. *Pediatrics*. 1992;90:846-850

Mackowiak PA. Concepts of fever. *Arch Intern Med*. 1998; 158:1870-1881.

May A, Bauchner H. Fever phobia: the pediatrician's contribution. *Pediatrics*. 1992;90:851-854.

Schmitt BD. Fever phobia: misconceptions of parents about fevers. *Am J Dis Child*. 1980;134:176-181.

Simon HB: Hyperthermia. *N Engl J Med*. 1993;329:483-487.

REFERENCES

1. Richards DW. Hippocrates and history: the arrogance of humanism. In: Bulger RJ, ed. *Hippocrates Revisited*. New York, NY: Medcom Press; 1973.
2. Luke, 4:38-39.
3. Matthew, 8:14-15.
4. Kluger MJ. Fever revisited. *Pediatrics*. 1992;90:846-850.
5. Mackowiak PA. Concepts of fever. *Arch Intern Med*. 1998;158:1870-1881.
6. Ushikubi F, Segi E, Sugimoto Y, et al. Impaired febrile response in mice lacking the prostaglandin E receptor subtype EP3. *Nature*. 1998;395:281-284.
7. Lorin MI. Measurement of body temperature. *Semin Pediatr Infect Dis*. 1993;4:4-8.
8. Simon HB. Hyperthermia. *N Engl J Med*. 1993;329: 483-487.
9. DuBois EF. Why are fever temperatures over 106°F rare? *Am J Med Sci*. 1949;217:361-368.
10. McCarthy PL, Dolan TF Jr. Hyperpyrexia in children. Eight-year emergency room experience. *Am J Dis Child*. 1976;130:849-851.
11. Press C, Fawcett NP. Association of temperature greater than 41.1°C (106°F) with serious illness, *Clin Pediatr*. 1985;24:21-25.
12. Alpert G, Hibbert E, Fleisher GR. Case-control study of hyperpyrexia in children. *Pediatr Infect Dis J*. 1990;9: 161-163.
13. Bonadio WA, McElroy K, Jacoby PL, et al. Relationship of fever magnitude to rate of serious bacterial infections in infants aged 4-8 weeks. *Clin Pediatr (Phila)*. 1991;30: 478-480.
14. Surpure JS. Hyperpyrexia in children: clinical implications. *Pediatr Emerg Care*. 1987;3:10-12.
15. Bernheim HA, Kluger MJ. Fever effect of drug-induced antipyresis on survival. *Science*. 1976;193: 237-239.
16. Covert JB, Reynolds WW. Survival value of fever in fish. *Nature*. 1977;267:43-45.
17. Vaughn LK, Bernheim HA, Kluger MJ. Fever in the lizard Dipsosaurus dorsalis. *Nature*. 1974;252:473-474.
18. Kluger MJ, Rothenberg BA. Fever and reduced iron: their interaction as a host defense response to bacterial infection. *Science*. 1979;203:374-376.
19. Roberts NJ Jr. Impact of temperature elevation on immunologic defenses. *Rev Infect Dis*. 1991;13: 462-472.
20. Lorin MI. Rational, symptomatic therapy for fever. *Semin Pediatr Infect Dis*. 1993;4:9.
21. Kluger MJ. Fever. *Pediatrics*. 1980;66:720-724.
22. Schmitt BD. Fever phobia: misconceptions of parents about fevers. *Am J Dis Child*. 1980;134:176-181.
23. Crocetti M, Moghbeli N, Serwint J. Fever phobia revisited: have parental misconceptions about fever changed in 20 years? *Pediatrics*. 2001;107:1241-1246.
24. Kramer MS, Naimark L, Leduc DG. Parental fever phobia and its correlates. *Pediatrics*. 1985;75:1110-1113.
25. Rylance GW, Woods CG, Cullen RE, et al. Use of drugs by children. *BMJ* 1988;297:445-447.
26. May A, Bauchner H. Fever phobia: the pediatrician's contribution. *Pediatrics*. 1992;90:851-854.
27. Dinarello CA, Wolff SM. Pathogenesis of fever in man. *N Engl J Med*. 1978;298:607-612.
28. McCarthy PL: Fever in infants and children. In: Machowiak PA, ed. *Fever: Basic Mechanisms and Management*, New York, NY: Raven Press; 1991.
29. Casey R, McMahon F, McCormick MC, et al. Fever therapy: an educational intervention for parents. *Pediatrics*. 1984;73:600-605.
30. Robinson JS, Schwartz ML, Magwene KS, et al. The impact of fever health education on clinic utilization. *Am J Dis Child*. 1989;143:698-704.
31. Fruthaler GJ. Fever in children: phobia vs facts. *Hosp Pract (Off/Ed)*. 1985;20(11A):49-53.
32. Kramer MS, Naimark LE, Roberts-Brauer R, et al. Risks and benefits of paracetamol antipyresis in young children with fever of presumed viral origin. *Lancet*. 1991; 337:591-594.
33. Baker RC, Tiller T, Bausher JC. Severity of disease correlated with fever reduction in febrile infants. *Pediatrics*. 1989;83:1016-1019.
34. Torrey SB, Henretig F, Fleisher G. Temperature response to antipyretic therapy in children: relationship to occult bacteremia. *Am J Emerg Med*. 1985;3:190-192.
35. Maytal J, Shinnar S. Febrile status epilepticus. *Pediatrics*. 1990;86:611-616.
36. Berg AT, Shinnar S, Hauser WA. A prospective study of recurrent febrile seizures. *N Engl J Med*. 1992;327:1122-1127.
37. Banco L, Veltri D. Ability of mothers to subjectively assess the presence of fever in their children. *Am J Dis Child*. 1984;138:976-978.
38. Schnaiderman D, Lahat E, Sheefer T, et al. Antipyretic effectiveness of acetaminophen in febrile seizures: ongoing prophylaxis versus sporadic usage. *Eur J Pediatr*. 1993;152:747-749.
39. van Stuijvenberg M, Derksen-Lubsen G, Steyerberg EW, et al. Randomized, controlled trial of ibuprofen syrup administered during febrile illnesses to prevent febrile seizure recurrences. *Pediatrics*. 1998;102:1-7.
40. American Academy of Pediatrics, Committee on Infectious Diseases. Special report: aspirin and Reye syndrome. *Pediatrics*. 1982;69:810-812.
41. Centers for Disease Control and Prevention. Surgeon General's advisory on the use of salicylates and Reye syndrome. *MMWR Morb Mortal Wkly Rep*. 1982;31:289-290.
42. Temple AR. Pediatric dosing of acetaminophen, *Pediatr Pharmacol (New York)*. 1983;3:321-327.
43. Kauffman RE, Sawyer LA, Scheinbaum ML. Antipyretic efficacy of ibuprofen vs acetaminophen. *Am J Dis Child*. 1992;146:622-625.
44. Walson PD, Galletta G, Chomilo F, et al. Comparison of multidose ibuprofen and acetaminophen therapy in febrile children. *Am J Dis Child*. 1992;146:626-632.
45. Steele RW, Tanaka PT, Lara RP, et al. Evaluation of sponging and of oral antipyretic therapy to reduce fever. *J Pediatr*. 1970;77:824-829.

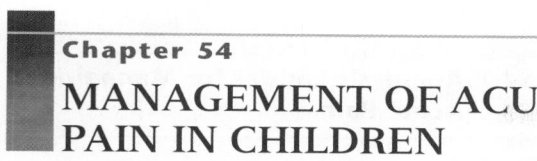

Chapter 54

MANAGEMENT OF ACUTE PAIN IN CHILDREN

Joseph D. Tobias, MD

INTRODUCTION

Major changes in pediatric pain management began with the rejection of previously held beliefs that neonates, infants, and children do not feel, experience, or react to pain as adults do because of the immaturity of their peripheral and central nervous systems. These misconceptions, compounded by fears of addiction and adverse effects, led to the undertreatment of pain in both the outpatient and the hospital settings. Clinical studies have demonstrated that infants and children experience a similar severity of postoperative pain as adults and that even preterm infants demonstrate alterations in physiological and biochemical markers of stress after painful stimuli.[1-5] Aside from the obvious humanitarian concerns, the inadequate treatment of pain during infancy may have long-lasting consequences, including the development of chronic pain syndromes or a heightened sensitivity to subsequent painful stimuli that may persist throughout childhood.[3-5] Despite the ongoing emphasis on the need to treat acute pain, pain management in the hospital, emergency room, and the outpatient setting is less than optimal, reflecting the need for ongoing education and scientific evaluations to determine the optimal methods of acute pain management.[6-8]

In addition to the wide variations in ages of the pediatric patient, several variables exist in the acute pain process that may affect treatment options and decisions. Causes of acute pain include trauma, acute medical illnesses, and surgical procedures. Pain treatment may occur in the hospital or the outpatient setting, in a tertiary care center or in a community hospital. The patient's underlying status may range from a healthy patient free of systemic disease to a compromised host with several co-morbid features.

MEASURING ACUTE PAIN

The first step in the treatment of acute pain is assessing its severity, which may be used to guide therapy, and assessing the response to therapy. Although older children can identify when they hurt and how bad the pain is, the evaluation of preverbal children or those with cognitive impairment is difficult and can complicate the issues of pain management. Although generalized irritability and agitation may be related to pain, it may also be related to other factors, including absence of parents or hunger. To overcome such problems, various pain scales and assessment tools have been created. These tools range from simple, bedside checklists with four to five components that require only 5 to 10 seconds to lengthy surveys that are cumbersome and time consuming. Regardless of the clinical scenario, the patient's response to the analgesic therapy must be evaluated. Pain cannot be identified if it is not assessed.

One method of evaluating children for pain is to consider the pain score to be the 5th vital sign and encourage the nursing staff to assign a pain score for all hospitalized patients whenever the other vital signs are checked. The pain score is checked to identify untreated pain even if the patient is not receiving analgesics. Pain is a frequent accompaniment of many of the diseases that lead to the hospitalization of infants and children. Compliance with the use of pain scales is mandated by various hospital credentialing boards and by auditing agencies that frequently evaluate pain management protocols as a benchmark criterion.

Pain assessment tools can be categorized into self-report, observational, and physiological scales. Many of the more involved scoring systems use components from two or all three of these types of scales. Pain assessment in the verbal patient is relatively straightforward using a self-reported, visual analogue score such as asking the patient to identify where the pain falls on a straight line from 0 (no pain) to 10 (worst imaginable pain). These techniques rely on patients' ability to assess and report their own pain. Variations of the scales aimed at being more user friendly and applicable in younger children (5 to 7 years of age) include the use of poker chips, a ladder, colored crayons, or pictures of children in varying degrees of distress. With the poker chip scale, the child expresses pain as a certain number of red poker chips (1 to 4).[9] Mild pain would be 1 poker chip, whereas 4 poker chips are the most hurt the child could have. The pain ladder is a picture of a ladder with 9 steps or rungs. At the bottom of the ladder is no hurt, and at the top of the ladder is hurt as bad as it could be. The children are then asked to point at the appropriate place on the ladder that may indicate the amount of pain that they are experiencing. The severity of pain can also be expressed by selecting a colored crayon, with red indicating severe pain and blue indicating little or no pain. The use of colors to express pain has been shown to have some variability among various ethnic groups as the association of blue with calm or no pain and red with pain does not cross all ethnic groups.

Alternatively, the child can use a *faces* scale.[10] This scale uses actual photographs of children in various degrees of distress and are available in various ethnic groups. The faces scale is meant to be used as a self-report type of scoring system. However, some centers have modified its use and used the faces scale as an observational tool. Primary care physicians assess the child and select the face and hence the degree of pain that they think the patient is feeling. Another self-report score developed by Beyer and Wells uses simple drawings instead of photographs of 6 faces with the eyes, nose, and a mouth in various positions from a smile to a frown. These faces are placed beside a corresponding 100-point vertical scale.[11] A more involved assessment tool that combines both observational and self-report tools is the Children's Hospital of Eastern Ontario pain score (CHEOPS).[12] Given its complexity, CHEOPS is used more commonly for clinical research than in actual clinical practice. The scale assigns a score of 0 to 2 for 6 categories, including cry, facial expression, verbal complaints of pain, position of the torso, whether the child is touching the wound, and position of the legs.

In many children, such as the preverbal child or those with cognitive impairment, the assessment of pain is more difficult because the patient is unable to express the severity of the pain. The tools used in these scenarios are limited to those using observational scoring, physiological factors, or a combination of both. Observational tools may include an assessment of the patient's facial features, body positioning, and the presence or absence of crying. Physiological parameters commonly used in pain scales include heart rate, blood pressure, respiratory rate, and oxygen saturation. Although not practical for everyday bedside use, clinical research of pediatric pain may also include physiological parameters, including neurohumoral changes such as the alterations in the plasma concentration of stress hormones.

Because many patients' conditions or age preclude the use of self-report scales, several observational tools have been described and validated for neonates,[13,14] preterm infants,[15] and patients with cognitive impairment.[16] For patients with cognitive impairment, different options can be used that may be helpful in the assessment of their pain, including the noncommunicative children's pain checklist—postoperative version (NCCPC-PV).[17] NCCPC-PV includes the grading of several specific behaviors such as vocalization, socialization, facial expression, activity, body and limb positioning, and physiological signs that have been shown to indicate pain in children with cognitive impairment.[16] Alternatively, scales such as the face, legs, activity, cry, and consolability (FLACC) scoring system, which is used for preverbal children, can be modified for cognitively impaired children by adding specific descriptors and parent-identified behaviors for each individual patient.[18] These tools have been shown to have excellent interobserver reliability and are quick and easy to use even in a busy clinical practice.

Effective pain management first identifies patients in pain and includes an ongoing assessment of the response to the therapy. The chosen tool used is not as crucial as the standard use of the tool in all hospitalized children.

PHARMACOLOGIC MANAGEMENT OF ACUTE PAIN

Treatment regimens should incorporate a graded approach (Box 54-1) similar to what has been used for the treatment of cancer-related pain, regardless of the cause of pain.[19] Although a primary assessment of the severity of pain is made to guide initial therapy, if effective analgesia is not achieved with the approach rung of the ladder, then the physician must consider moving up to the next step. Selecting an analgesic also depends on the setting in which the pain is treated. Outpatient management requires nonintravenous routes, including oral administration, whereas the inpatient setting provides an appropriate scenario for the administration of parenteral opioids. Treatment with a nonopioid analgesic agent such as a prostaglandin synthesis inhibitor (acetaminophen, acetylsalicylic acid, or a nonsteroidal anti-inflammatory drug [NSAID] such as ibuprofen) is used for mild pain such as that after a soft-tissue surgical procedure or that caused by a mild medical illness such as pharyngitis or otitis media. Moderate pain such as that after a bony orthopedic procedure or a fracture can usually be controlled with a combination of a prostaglandin synthesis inhibitor and a weak opioid (eg, an acetaminophen with codeine preparation) for the outpatient. More severe pain such as sickle cell vasoocclusive crisis, major burn, or the pain after a major surgical procedure (thoracotomy or an exploratory laparotomy) generally requires either a regional anesthetic technique or parenteral opioids.

BOX 54-1 Analgesic Ladder for Managing Acute Pain

MILD PAIN

NSAIDs, acetaminophen, or salicylates

MODERATE PAIN

1. NSAIDs or acetaminophen with weak opioid (oxycodone, hydrocodone, codeine)
2. Intravenous opioids (with addition of fixed-interval NSAID or acetaminophen)
   a. Intravenous opioid by PCA
   b. Continuous infusion of opioid with as-needed rescue does of opioid
   c. Fixed, interval dosing of opioid
3. Regional anesthetic techniques

SEVERE PAIN

1. Continue fixed interval dosing of NSAID or acetaminophen
2. Intravenous opioid by PCA
3. Regional anesthetic techniques

NSAID, Nonsteroidal anti-inflammatory drug; *PCA*, patient-controlled analgesia.

Mild-to-Moderate Pain in the Outpatient Setting (Prostaglandin Synthesis Inhibitors and Weak Opioids)

With tissue disruption, fatty acids are released from cell membranes and are metabolized to prostaglandins, which result in local inflammation and pain by stimulating the free nerve endings of C and A fibers. NSAIDs, acetaminophen, and salicylates inhibit the enzyme cyclooxygenase, thereby blocking prostaglandin formation. In distinction to opioids, the prostaglandin synthesis inhibitors demonstrate a ceiling effect such that, once a specific plasma concentration is achieved, increasing the dose provides no further analgesia. Although the majority of these agents are available as over-the-counter medications, they represent an effective and relatively safe means of controlling mild-to-moderate pain. The prostaglandin synthesis inhibitors include para-aminophenol derivatives (acetaminophen), NSAIDs (ibuprofen), and salicylates (acetylsalicylic acid and choline magnesium trisalicylate).[20]

Role of Prostaglandin Synthesis Inhibitors

The role of the prostaglandin synthesis inhibitors to treat acute pain includes their use as the sole agent for

Table 54-1 Potency and Half-Life of Opioids

OPIOID AGONISTS	POTENCY (RATIO COMPARED WITH MORPHINE)	HALF-LIFE	ACTIVE METABOLITES
Morphine	1	2-3 hr	Yes
Meperidine	0.1	2-3 hr	Yes
Hydromorphone	5-8	2-3 hr	No
Oxymorphone	10	1-4 hr	No
Methadone	1	12-24 hr	No
Fentanyl	100	20-30 min	No
Sufentanil	1000	20-30 min	No
Alfentanil	20	10-15 min	No
Remifentanil	100	5-8 min	No
AGONIST-ANTAGONISTS			
Butorphanol	5	2-4 hr	No
Nalbuphine	1	4-5 hr	No
Pentazocine	0.3-0.4	2-3 hr	No

minor pain, their combination with weak opioids for oral administration to control moderate pain, and their addition to parenteral opioids and regional anesthetic techniques for severe pain. In the last situation, their use does not replace opioids, but rather provides adjunctive analgesia, thereby lowering the total amount of opioid required. Because the majority of opioid-related adverse effects are dose related, decreasing total opioid consumption play a significant role in decreasing or preventing opioid-associated adverse effects.

Route of Administration of Prostaglandin Synthesis Inhibitors

Although oral administration is used most frequently, with this route, obstacles to effective analgesia may exist, including a delay in the onset, decreased bioavailability when compared with parenteral administration, refusal to take the medication, vomiting, and an inability to give enteral medications caused by ileus or abdominal complaints. When considering the actual agent to be used, acetaminophen and ibuprofen are the most commonly prescribed medications of this class. Both of these medications are available in several preparations, including chewable tablets, elixirs, and infant drops. Acetaminophen is also available in suppository form and sustained-release tablets. Intravenous acetaminophen products (the prodrug propacetamol and a newer pure acetaminophen form) are available outside of the United States.

Specific Uses of Prostaglandin Synthesis Inhibitors

Acetaminophen, a para-aminophenol derivative, has a significant role in the management of acute pain, whereas phenacetin is no longer used because of its toxicity profile and the risk of renal papillary necrosis. The association of Reye syndrome with salicylates combined with the diverse array of NSAIDs released onto the market has markedly reduced the use of aspirin products. Despite the limited use of salicylates, the role for choline magnesium trisalicylate remains, which combines the analgesic advantages of a salicylate with limited effects on platelet function. It is an effective choice in patients with qualitative and quantitative platelet issues. Table 54-1 outlines the more commonly prescribed prostaglandin synthesis inhibitors for children. In the perioperative setting, the oral premedication (midazolam) can be combined with either acetaminophen (15 mg/kg) or ibuprofen elixir (10 mg/kg).[21] This technique allows the patient analgesia on awakening and masks the taste of the midazolam premedication. If preoperative administration is not chosen, then an acetaminophen suppository (40 mg/kg) can be placed after anesthetic induction. With rectal administration, a larger dose of acetaminophen is required to achieve analgesic plasma concentrations of 10 to 20 mcg/mL.[22] Suggested doses for acetaminophen in neonates and infants were derived from six pediatric acetaminophen dosing studies.[23]

Another possibility for perioperative pain management is the postoperative administration of either ibuprofen or acetaminophen when the child complains of pain in the recovery room. This approach is valued in the outpatient setting when the practitioner is confronted with a patient in acute pain. Waiting until the child complains is less desirable in the perioperative setting because the onset of activity of any of these agents after oral or rectal administration is 20 to 30 minutes. If intravenous access is established, then a small dose of an intravenous opioid (fentanyl 0.5 mcg/kg, morphine 0.02 mg/kg, or nalbuphine 0.02 to 0.04 mg/kg) can be used to provide immediate analgesia while waiting for the onset of the oral or rectal acetaminophen or ibuprofen. When the patient is ready for discharge home, ongoing analgesia can be provided with either acetaminophen or ibuprofen. Although administering these agents on an as-needed basis is common, fixed-interval dosing may provide more effective analgesia. Fixed-interval dosing is the administration of the medication around the clock for the first 24 to 48 hours without waiting for the child to complain of pain. For this purpose, acetaminophen (10 to 15 mg/kg) every 4 hours or ibuprofen (10 mg/kg) every 6 hours can be used. If the patient is receiving acetaminophen as a fixed-interval dose and has breakthrough pain, then a supplemental dose of ibuprofen can be administered, and vice-versa. Fixed-interval dosing is also recommended when opioids are used in the treatment of severe pain (see discussion later in this chapter). By maintaining a plasma concentration of the prostaglandin synthesis inhibitor, a synergistic effect is achieved, and pain can be managed with a decreased total dose of opioid.

When fixed-interval acetaminophen is administered, the primary care physician must ensure that the infant or child is not receiving acetaminophen in other forms, such as cold medicines. Additionally, given that several different acetaminophen preparations are available from numerous manufacturers, ensuring that the parents and the primary care physician know the concentration of acetaminophen or ibuprofen in the specific product is equally important. The most common cause of acetaminophen toxicity in patients younger than 10 years remains inadvertent overdosing by parents.[24]

Role of Weak Opioids

Aspirin or acetaminophen can be combined with a weak opioid such as codeine, tramadol, oxycodone, or hydrocodone for the outpatient treatment of moderate pain or when NSAIDs alone fail to control mild pain. A hepatic microsomal enzyme metabolizes codeine to morphine for a significant part of its analgesic effect. In a cohort of 96 children, 47% had genotypes associated with low activity of the enzymes necessary for the conversion of codeine to morphine, and in 36% of the patients, neither morphine nor its metabolites were detected.[25] The authors concluded that the reduced ability to metabolize codeine may be more common than previously reported and that codeine analgesia is less reliable than morphine. Although health care practitioners may choose codeine because of a misconception that it has less sedative or respiratory depressant effects, opioids when used in equipotent doses result in equivalent degrees of sedation and respiratory depression. Given the issues with codeine and its variable pharmacodynamics, agents such as oxycodone or hydrocodone are preferable.

Several of these preparations are available in both liquid and tablet formulations. The use of a liquid or tablet is determined by the patient's age and preference. For younger patients, acetaminophen with codeine elixir containing 120 mg of acetaminophen and 12 mg of codeine per 5 mL is a frequently chosen option, with dosing based on the codeine component (0.5 to 1.0 mg/kg every 4 to 6 hours). Tablet preparations contain 325 mg of acetaminophen with 15 mg codeine (Tylenol 2), 30 mg codeine (Tylenol 3), or 60 mg codeine (Tylenol 4). Codeine is also available as a parenteral formulation for subcutaneous administration; however, its use via this route is not recommended. Although this formulation has also been used for intravenous administration, this practice is not suggested because of the potential for allergic and anaphylactoid reactions. Oxycodone and hydrocodone are also available in both liquid and tablet forms in combination with either acetaminophen or acetylsalicylic acid. Hydrocodone (7.5 mg) is also available as a tablet combined with 200 mg ibuprofen (Vicoprofen). The dose should be based on the oxycodone or hydrocodone component, starting at 0.1 to 0.15 mg/kg (maximal starting dose 5 mg) every 4 to 6 hours. Regardless of the preparation used, with dose escalation, the amount of acetaminophen may exceed the maximal recommended dose of 60 to 90 mg/kg/day. When higher doses of the opioid component are needed, switching to preparations that contain codeine, oxycodone, or hydrocodone without the acetaminophen or aspirin is best to prevent the possibility of toxicity. A sustained-release formulation of oxycodone (OxyContin) is also available. Its sustained-release action provides an analgesic plasma concentration that can be maintained with a dosing interval of every 8 to 12 hours. Although used occasionally to achieve a baseline steady-state plasma concentration of opioid to provide analgesia after major operative procedures, given its abuse potential, potential for diversion for illegal use, and a lack of data regarding its pharmacokinetics in children, the risk-benefit ratio of such regimens must be considered.

Tramadol (Ultram)[26-29] is a unique analgesic agent in that it has a dual mechanism of action, including agonism at the μ-opioid receptor and inhibition of norepinephrine and serotonin reuptake in the central nervous system. Although initially thought to have limited abuse potential, clinical experience has demonstrated an abuse potential that may be similar to that of other weak opioids. Tramadol's potency is roughly equivalent to that of meperidine.

An intravenous intraoperative dose of tramadol (2 mg/kg) decreases the need for rescue opioid analgesia in the recovery room in patients receiving tramadol.[27] Tramadol is well tolerated and provides effective pain relief. Tramadol analgesia is rated as very good or excellent by 69% of parents and 70% of patients. Adverse events are mild or moderate and similar in incidence to that seen with other oral opioids.[27-29]

Tramadol has a longer half-life (6 to 7 hours) than other oral agents and an active metabolite with a half-life of 10 to 11 hours. The active metabolite is renally excreted and can accumulate in patients with renal insufficiency or failure, making it a poor choice in this setting. Despite its longer half-life, tramadol fails to decrease analgesic needs after discharge when compared with placebo.[27] The adverse effect profile of tramadol is similar to that of other opioids (see later discussion); however, as with meperidine, a unique adverse effect generally seen only with large doses or in patients with renal failure is seizure activity.[30] Respiratory depression may be less with equipotent doses of tramadol when compared with other weak opioids.[30,31]

Tramadol is available in injectable solution, suppository, liquid, and tablet formulations. A tablet containing 50 mg of tramadol and the combination of 37.5 mg of tramadol with 325 mg of acetaminophen in a tablet (Ultracet) are the only two preparations available in the United States. The 50-mg tablet is scored and can be cut in half, allowing its administration to smaller children. The manufacturer's recommendations for dosing include 0.5 to 1.0 mg/kg (initial maximal dose of 50 mg) every 3 to 4 hours as needed. However, doses up to 2 mg/kg have been used in some pediatric trials.[28,29]

Moderate-to-Severe Pain, Inpatient Setting (Prostaglandin Synthesis Inhibitors)

In the inpatient setting, the options for controlling acute pain are more diverse, including the option for the use of parenteral prostaglandin synthesis inhibitors and opioids. Even when the choice is made to use parenteral opioids, the prostaglandin synthesis inhibitors have a role in controlling pain in that they can be used to decrease the total postoperative opioid requirements and thereby opioid-related adverse effects.

Although a significant amount of literature exists regarding the use of the parenteral agent ketorolac (Toradol), less-expensive alternatives including oral ibuprofen and acetaminophen may also be beneficial. In patients receiving opioids, the addition of either ibuprofen (10 mg/kg orally every 6 hours) or acetaminophen (15 mg/kg orally or rectally every 4 hours) on a fixed-interval schedule is suggested. Children receiving rectal ibuprofen (40 mg/kg/day) after inpatient surgery have lower pain scores and decreased opioid requirements in the recovery room, during the day of operation, and during the first 72 hours after the procedure.[32] Additionally, the incidence of opioid-related adverse effects is lower in patients receiving ibuprofen. Although rectal preparations of ibuprofen are not available in the United States, similar results have been reported in both children and adults with the use of rectal indomethacin or acetaminophen.[33]

When oral or rectal administration is not feasible, intravenous administration is possible using the parenteral NSAID ketorolac. Although preliminary clinical trials suggested that ketorolac was as effective as opioids in treating acute pain, its more applicable clinical role is similar to that of other NSAIDs as an adjunct to opioid analgesia during the postoperative perioed.[34] Ketorolac may also be effective in acute pain of other causes, including inflammatory and musculoskeletal pain, such as patients with pleuritic pain or vasoocclusive crisis caused by sickle cell disease.

In patients ranging in age from 1 to 16 years, ketorolac (0.5 mg/kg) demonstrated similar pharmacokinetic properties as that reported in adults and a plasma concentration in the adult therapeutic range will be maintained for 6 hours in the majority of patients.[35]

Although after its initial release (recommendations for ketorolac dosing included 1 mg/kg up to 60 mg), newer information has resulted in a decrease in dosing regimens down to 0.5 mg/kg. More recently, in the adult population, a ceiling effect has been reported such that no further analgesia was noted with doses greater than 7.5 to 10 mg.[36] Although no comparable studies in children have been conducted, current practice includes dosing at 0.5 mg/kg up to a maximum of 10 mg every 6 hours. Once the patient is able to tolerate oral medications, the switch is made to an oral NSAID or acetaminophen.

To date, data regarding ketorolac in patients younger than 1 year of age are limited.[37,38] In 1 study, daily morphine requirements (0.04 ± 0.05 versus 0.15 ± 0.06 mg/kg/day, $p < 0.01$) were significantly decreased in 10 infants who received ketorolac. No differences in pain scores were noted between the two groups, and no adverse effects related to ketorolac were noted.[37] Another study reported no adverse renal or hematologic effects in their retrospective review of ketorolac use in 53 children younger than 6 months of age who received at least 1 dose of ketorolac after cardiac surgery.[38] The greatest increase in serum creatinine from baseline was 0.3 mg/dL. Four patients had minor episodes of bleeding while receiving ketorolac. Contraindications to the use of ketorolac include patients with bleeding dyscrasias or settings in which acute hemorrhage is a concern (ie, patients with abnormal coagulation function, the trauma patient, patients after intracranial or otolaryngologic surgery). Foster and Williams reported two patients who developed bradycardia that was temporally related to the administration of ketorolac.[39]

Adverse effects of NSAIDs and acetylsalicylic acid generally result from the inhibition of prostaglandins distant from the sites of inflammation (Box 54-2). Acetaminophen or magnesium choline trisalicylate should be considered instead of NSAIDs in patients with qualitative or quantitative platelet disorders because neither agent alters platelet function. Alterations in glomerular filtration rate with NSAIDs are uncommon, except in patients with preexisting renal dysfunction, with the concomitant administration of other nephrotoxic agents, in the presence of hypovolemia, or with prolonged administration. An additional concern with NSAIDs is the inhibition of new bone formation and in some centers, use of these agents is restricted in patients undergoing spinal fusion and other procedures in which bone grafts are used.[40]

Recent efforts to maintain analgesia while diminishing the incidence of adverse effects of NSAIDs have focused on the use of specific isomers of the NSAIDs or agents that selectively inhibit cyclooxygenase (COX) type 2 versus type 1. Although NSAID isomers are still in the investigational phase, experience with other medications has demonstrated the potential for decreasing adverse effects while maintaining efficacy by separation of the two enantiomers of a chiral

BOX 54-2 Adverse Effects of Nonsteroidal Anti-inflammatory Drugs

- Central nervous system effects, including headache, dizziness, drowsiness
- Nausea and vomiting
- Peptic ulcer formation
- Gastrointestinal bleeding
- Decreased glomerular filtration rate, renal insufficiency or failure
- Platelet dysfunction
- Bronchospasm
- Interaction with other medications (this effect varies from 1 NSAID to another)

NSAID, Nonsteroidal anti-inflammatory drug.

compound. Ibuprofen is a chiral mixture of its two optical isomers, and animal data suggest that the S(+)-isomer may provide analgesia while having limited effects on the homeostatic COX (see discussion later in this chapter), thereby limiting its adverse effect profile.[41]

COX type I, referred to as the homeostatic COX, controls renal blood flow, protects the gastric mucosa, and maintains normal platelet function. COX type II, referred to as inducible COX, is responsible for the inflammatory process. Celecoxib (Celebrex), valdecoxib (Bextra), and rofecoxib (Vioxx) were the first COX-2 inhibitors introduced into clinical use. As with nonspecific NSAIDs and acetaminophen, when used as an adjunct to opioid analgesia, these medications were effective in decreasing opioid requirements and opioid-related adverse effects.[42] However, the enthusiasm for these agents and their clinical use has decreased dramatically after several investigations demonstrating their association with an increased risk of cardiovascular events, including myocardial infarctions.[43-45]

Strong Opioids

Several options are available when considering the use of strong opioids for the treatment of moderate-to-severe pain in infants and children. The most clinically relevant differences between the opioids are their potency, duration of action, and their metabolic fate, including the presence or absence of active metabolites (Table 54-2). The opioids exhibit their end-organ effects through the interaction with specific opioid receptors (μ or κ) in the peripheral and central nervous system. Opioids may act as either pure agonists (bind and activate μ- and κ-receptors) or agonists-antagonists (bind and activate κ-receptors while binding to, but not activating, μ-receptors). The agonist-antagonists, including nalbuphine (Nubain), butorphanol (Stadol), and pentazocine (Talwin), should not be administered to patients who have been chronically receiving opioids because they can precipitate withdrawal symptoms. Although these agents have a decreased potential to cause repression depression, a ceiling effect also exists for their analgesia. With dose escalation for increasing or persistent pain, a limit or ceiling exists to the analgesia achieved. Although the potency and efficacy of agonists-antagonist for severe pain is less than that of pure agonists, they are useful for mild-to-moderate pain when oral administration of other agents, such as acetaminophen with codeine, is not feasible or when a more rapid onset of action is desired. One option to treat moderate pain postanesthesia is to administer a single intravenous dose of an agonist-antagonist opioid followed by a switch to an oral agent when the patient is discharged home. For this purpose, nalbuphine is a good option. An additional benefit of nalbuphine is that it clinically provides more sedation than other opioids because of its effects on the κ-opioid receptor and therefore, in addition to providing analgesia, may provide sedation for the agitated postoperative patient. The agonist-antagonists should also be considered when supplemental intravenous analgesia is required in patients who are receiving or have received neuraxial (epidural or intrathecal) opioids within the last 24 hours. The potential for respiratory depression that can occur with the combination of intravenous and neuraxial opioids is less if an agonist-antagonist is used rather than a pure agonist such as morphine.

When opioids are chosen for postoperative analgesia, three choices must be made, including (1) the opioid to be used, (2) the mode of administration, and (3) the route of administration. Information to help decide which opioid is best for postoperative analgesia is relatively limited. Several acceptable alternatives are available, any of which will provide equivalent analgesia provided that equipotent doses are administered. The potential for respiratory depression is present with all of the pure opioid agonists and is not more likely with any specific opioid provided that equipotent doses are administered.

Choosing the Appropriate Opioid

In the acutely ill patient, in the presence of co-morbid diseases, such as a compromised cardiovascular status,

Table 54-2 Salicylate and Nonsteroidal Anti-inflammatory Drug Preparations Commonly Used in Acute Pain Management

MEDICATION	PREPARATION	DOSE FORMS
Ibuprofen	Oral suspension	100 mg/5 mL
	Infant drops	50 mg/1.25 mL
	Chewable tablets	50 and 100 mg
	Children's caplets	100 mg
	Tablets	200, 400, 600, and 800 mg
Choline magnesium trisalicylate	Liquid	500 mg/5 mL
	Tablets	500, 750, and 1000 mg
Naproxen	Suspension	125 mg/5 mL
	Delayed-release tablets	275 and 500 mg
	Tablets	250, 275, 375, 500, and 550 mg
Tolmetin	Tablets	200 and 600 mg
	Capsules	400 mg
Acetylsalicylic acid	Several different preparations available	—

or when a risk for pulmonary hypertension exists, the synthetic opioids (fentanyl, sufentanil, alfentanil, remifentanil) with their cardiovascular stability, beneficial effects on pulmonary vascular resistance, and their ability to blunt the sympathetic stress response may be advantageous. Because the synthetic opioids have short plasma half-lives (less than 30 minutes), they are generally administered by a continuous infusion to maintain a plasma concentration adequate to provide analgesia. No inherent advantage appears to exist in regards to any of the currently available synthetic opioids, except that fentanyl is the least expensive. Remifentanil, metabolized by plasma esterases, has the shortest half-life of any of the synthetic opioids (approximately 10 minutes). Unlike the other opioids that are dependent on hepatic metabolism, no difference exists in the clearance of remifentanil across the age ranges; thus its half-life is consistent even in neonates. Given these properties, remifentanil has become a popular agent for intraoperative use with limited applications outside of the operating room. The synthetic opioids are also used in critically ill infants and children in the intensive care unit as a means of providing sedation and analgesia during mechanical ventilation.

Although the synthetic opioids maintain a stable hemodynamic pattern in patients with compromised cardiovascular function, alternatives such as morphine are acceptable in patients with normal cardiovascular function. For the majority of patients, morphine is generally the first-line agent. The dose depends on the mode of administration that is chosen (Box 54-3). Because of decreased hepatic metabolism and increased permeability of the blood-brain barrier with an increased risk of respiratory depression, dosing with any opioid should start at 50% of the listed dose in infants younger than 3 months. Furthermore, monitoring of respiratory function with continuous pulse oximetry is recommended when opioids are used in this age group or in patients with compromised cardiorespiratory status. Morphine can cause venodilation and may decrease blood pressure, especially in patients with hypovolemia. Additionally, histamine release from morphine may lead to pruritus, an adverse effect that tends to be particularly common in adolescents and young adults. Morphine is metabolized in the liver to morphine-6-glucuronide (M6G), which is significantly more potent that the parent compound. Given that it is water soluble, M6G penetrates the central nervous system poorly and, in most circumstances, is of little consequence. However, because M6G is cleared by the kidneys and can accumulate in patients with renal failure or insufficiency and lead to respiratory depression, alternative opioids such as hydromorphone (see discussion later in this chapter), which has no active metabolites, should be considered.

Other opioids that have been used in the treatment of acute pain include hydromorphone (Dilaudid), meperidine (Demerol), and methadone (Dolobid). Hydromorphone may be advantageous when adverse effects related to histamine release such as pruritus occur with morphine. Given that pruritus tends to be more common in adolescents and young adults, this author's practice is to use hydromorphone as the opioid of choice for control of severe pain in this population. Hydromorphone's potency is 5 to 8 times that of morphine and therefore one fifth to one seventh of the morphine dose is used. Patient-controlled analgesia (PCA) solutions are prepared such that an equipotent amount of the opioid is present in each milliliter of the solution (1 mg/mL for morphine, 1 mg/mL for nalbuphine, 0.15 mg/mL for hydromorphone, and 10 mg/mL for meperidine).

Meperidine (pethidine in Europe and the United Kingdom) is approximately one tenth as potent as morphine and is associated with a relatively high incidence of adverse central nervous system effects, including dysphoria, agitation, and seizures. Meperidine's central nervous system toxicity, including its epileptogenic potential, results from the accumulation of normeperidine, a metabolite produced by the hepatic N-methylation of the parent compound. Normeperidine has a long half-life (15 to 20 hours) and is dependent on renal clearance. High or toxic levels occur more commonly in the setting of renal failure or insufficiency with the coadministration of drugs such as phenobarbital that stimulate hepatic microsomal enzymes and with large doses (greater than 2 g/day in an adult). Because meperidine offers no particular advantage over other opioids and may in fact be less efficacious than morphine in controlling acute pain,[46] morphine or hydromorphone is preferred.

Methadone has a potency similar to that of morphine; however, the plasma half-life is 12 to 24 hours. Its long plasma half-life provides a continuous steady-state serum concentration after a single-bolus administration, thereby providing prolonged analgesia without the need for a continuous infusion or the use of a PCA device. Intraoperatively, a single intravenous dose of 0.2 mg/kg has been shown to result in lower pain scores and a decreased need for supplemental opioid analgesic agents during the initial 36 postoperative hours.[47] The longer duration of action offers analgesic advantages over the intermittent administration of agents with shorter half-lives and may be useful in situations in which PCA devices or continuous

BOX 54-3 Morphine Dosing*

Initial intravenous titration for acute, moderate-to-severe pain:
- 0.01 to 0.02 mg/kg every 5 min; titrate to effective analgesia

As-needed or fixed-interval dosing:
- 0.05 mg/kg every 3 hr

Continuous infusion:
- 0.01 to 0.03 mg/kg/hr

Patient-controlled analgesia:
- Bolus: 0.02 mg/kg every 10 min
- Infusion: 0.004-0.005 mg/kg/hr

*The doses listed are for initial doses in patients who have not previously been receiving opioids. These doses should be adjusted up or down as necessary to achieve the desired level of analgesia while limiting adverse effects. When opioids are used in infants younger than 6 months or in patients with severe systemic illnesses or other comorbid diseases that place them at risk for opioid-related adverse effects, the starting dose should be 50% of the above-listed doses. Cardiorespiratory function monitoring is suggested.

infusions are not available. However, the use of intravenous methadone in the acute pain setting remains somewhat investigational and is therefore limited to institutions involved in ongoing clinical trials or in the hands of investigators with significant experience with its use. Additionally, the intravenous preparation may not be readily available in many institutions.

Deciding Mode of Administration

INTRAVENOUS ADMINISTRATION. After deciding which opioid to prescribe, the second decision to be made is the mode of administration. Intravenous options include on-demand (as-needed) dosing, fixed-interval administration, continuous infusion, or PCA. To provide optimal analgesia, opioids should be administered in a manner that maintains a steady-state serum concentration. For moderate-to-severe pain, as-needed or on-demand administration generally does not provide adequate analgesia. A significant delay can occur from the time that the child is recognized as being in pain until the medication is drawn up, administered, and has time to take effect. The optimal mode for the delivery of opioids to provide analgesia remains PCA, which allows the patient to administer a preset amount of opioid at specific intervals. These devices may be used in children as young as 5 to 6 years.[48]

Appropriate education is required before instituting a pediatric PCA program to avoid potential adverse effects and ineffective use of this technique. Decisions regarding PCA include the opioid to be used, the bolus dose, the lockout interval (the time that must elapse between doses), whether a continuous or basal infusion will be used in addition to the intermittent bolus doses, and the maximal total hourly dose. Although any opioid can be used with PCA, the majority of experience is with morphine. A common starting pointing for the bolus dose is 0.02 mg/kg every 10 minutes as needed; however, this level may need to be adjusted based on the patient's previous exposure to opioids or co-morbid disease processes. Before starting PCA for acute pain, effective analgesia must be obtained. To accomplish this task, an opioid is titrated in incremental intravenous bolus doses (morphine 0.02 mg/kg every 5 minutes) until the desired level of analgesia is obtained. Once this level is reached, the PCA device is started. A frequent problem is that patients are provided adequate analgesia in the recovery room after a surgical procedure and are then discharged to the floor only to have a significant amount of time expire until the PCA pump arrives. When this circumstance happens, the patients will need to repeatedly push the PCA button to reestablish an analgesic plasma concentration of the opioid. Making arrangements for the PCA pump to be delivered to the recovery room and started before the patient is discharged to the floor is ideal.

One of the relatively controversial issues regarding PCA is whether to include a low basal infusion rate in addition to the patient-administered bolus doses. The use of a basal infusion rate is thought by some experts to contradict the inherent safety factor of PCA; with the basal infusion rate, opioid is infused regardless of the patient's demands. Different results have been reported in children depending on the dose used for the basal infusion rate. When comparing PCA with and without a basal infusion rate of 0.02 mg/kg/hour, the pain scores showed no difference, and adverse effects were increased, including nausea, sedation, and hypoxemia in the patients that received the basal infusion rate.[49] In a follow-up study, a low basal infusion of 0.004 mg/kg/hour (4 mcg/kg/hr) improved the sleep pattern when compared with no basal infusion rate.[50]

When used in its classic sense, PCA requires an awake, cooperative patient who is able to comprehend its purpose and is able to push the button. Therefore its use may be limited in certain patients because of underlying illness or diminished cognitive capabilities. An additional controversy regarding PCA is whether to allow the use of nurse- or family-controlled analgesia in these patient populations. When used in this fashion, the PCA device eliminates the delay in opioid administration that may occur as the nurse signs out the medication and draws it up. Equivalent levels of analgesia and equivalent opioid consumption are observed when comparing PCA with nurse-controlled analgesia,[51] although the inherent safety factor of PCA is lost.

NONINTRAVENOUS ADMINISTRATION OF OPIOIDS. Although most moderate-to-severe acute pain is treated with intravenous opioids, certain situations limit or preclude intravenous administration. Nonintravenous routes include subcutaneous, oral, transdermal, and transmucosal (sublingual, buccal, intranasal, rectal, and inhaled) administration.[52] Many of these techniques are considered investigational and are therefore likely to have a limited role in the day-to-day management of acute pain in children. The intramuscular route is strictly avoided because variability in uptake and absorption leads to erratic serum levels and ineffective analgesia. Additionally, children will deny pain to avoid a shot.

The simplest and cheapest of the nonintravenous routes remains oral administration. Although this route is frequently chosen for outpatients, its use remains limited in hospitalized patients. The oral administration of the weak opioids, including codeine and oxycodone, is a viable option even in hospitalized patients provided that the pain is considered mild to moderate. Other opioids such as morphine, hydromorphone, and methadone can be administered orally. Decreased oral bioavailability necessitates the use of larger doses. Regardless of the opioid chosen, problems that arise with oral administration include a delay in onset of action, the need for larger doses because of decreased bioavailability, and underlying medical or surgical problems that preclude the use of the gastrointestinal tract. Although the use of these opioids via the oral route is common practice for controlling cancer-related pain in the outpatient setting, information regarding this technique for controlling moderate-to-severe pain in the inpatient setting is limited. A novel technique termed *oral PCA* (hydromorphone or morphine) has been used to treat acute pain related to medical illnesses.[53]

Subcutaneous administration has generally been reserved for the patient with terminal cancer. However, studies suggest its efficacy for controlling acute postoperative pain.[54,55] Subcutaneous administration is associated with significantly fewer hypoxemic events (oxygen saturation less than 90%) than intravenous administeration.[54] When compared with intermittent intramuscular administration of opioids, 95% of the nurses preferred the subcutaneous route and 74% stated that they would give morphine more readily via the subcutaneous route compared with intramuscular administration.[55] For subcutaneous administration, a butterfly needle or a standard intravenous catheter is inserted into the subcutaneous tissue of the thigh, abdominal wall, subclavicular area, or deltoid. Dosing regimens such as basal infusions, continuous infusions, and boluses are the same as for intravenous administration. Although the plasma concentration of the opioid during subcutaneous administration are equivalent to those achieved with intravenous administration, the peak plasma concentration is not achieved as rapidly after subcutaneous administration when compared with intravenous bolus dosing. The fluid volume used to deliver the opioid should be restricted to a maximum of 1 to 3 mL/hour. The site should be changed at 7 day intervals or sooner if erythema or local tissue reaction is noted. Several different opioids can be administered subcutaneously, including morphine, hydromorphone, and fentanyl.[56] Methadone can cause significant tissue reaction with erythema and is not recommended for subcutaneous administration.

Adverse Effects of Opioids

Several adverse effects may occur with opioids that interfere with the delivery of effective analgesia (Table 54-3). Respiratory depression is directly related to potency and occurs with all opioids; equi-analgesic doses of opioids produce equivalent degrees of respiratory depression. Factors that may predispose patients to respiratory depression include extremes of age, severe underlying systemic diseases, preexisting altered mental status, and the addition of other medications that potentiate the central respiratory depressant effects of opioids (Box 54-4). The presence of these comorbid problems does not preclude the use of opioids; however, initial doses should start at approximately 50% of the usual regimens, and monitoring of cardiorespiratory function is suggested to help provide the early identification of cardiovascular and respiratory compromise.

Respiratory depression may also occur in the setting of renal failure in patients receiving morphine. Whereas morphine undergoes primarily hepatic metabolism, the metabolite M6G is dependent on renal excretion. M6G possesses respiratory depressant activity and analgesic activity several times that of the parent compound. In patients with altered renal function, an opioid such as hydromorphone, which does not have active metabolites, may be a safer alternative.

In patients who develop respiratory depression, the first priority remains airway management with provision of supplemental oxygen or bag-mask ventilation as needed followed by the incremental administration of naloxone. Because several different dilutions of naloxone are available, particular attention must be paid to the individual ampule. Standard pediatric ampules contain either 0.4 or 1.0 mg/mL. Naloxone should be administered in incremental doses of 1 to 2 mcg/kg, repeated every 3 minutes as needed, up to a total dose of 10 mcg/kg. The administration of small incremental doses is suggested because reversing respiratory depression is possible without reversing analgesia. Using the doses recommended in many reference texts (10 to 15 mcg/kg) will result in a precipitous reversal of all analgesia, which may lead to agonizing consequences for the patient. These large doses are used only for reversing opioid effects in the setting of an acute overdose. Once respiratory depression is reversed, continued monitoring of the patient is important because the half-life of naloxone is only 20 to 30 minutes compared

Table 54-3 Adverse Effects of Opioids and Treatment Strategies*

ADVERSE EFFECT	TREATMENT STRATEGY
Respiratory depression	Stop opioid Airway management as needed Naloxone 1 mcg/kg every 3 minutes up to 10 mcg/kg; consider use of infusion for longer acting opioids
Constipation or ileus	Stool softeners Cathartic agents Motility agent (metoclopramide)
Nausea or vomiting	Phenothiazine (promethazine 0.25 mg/kg up to 12.5 mg)* 5-HT_3 antagonist: ondansetron (0.1 mg/kg up to 4 mg)
Pruritus	Diphenhydramine (0.5 mg/kg up to 12.5 mg) Change opioid

*Monitoring respiratory status is suggested when opioids are used with phenothiazines because of the possible potentiation of opioid-induced respiratory depression.

BOX 54-4 Patients At Risk for Opioid-Related Adverse Effects*

1. Infants younger than 6 months
2. Patients with severe underlying systemic illness:
   Cardiorespiratory dysfunction
   Hepatic insufficiency
   Renal insufficiency
   Altered mental status
   Airway obstruction
   Central or obstructive apnea
3. Concomitant use of other medications:
   Barbiturates
   Phenothiazines
   Benzodiazepines

*The presence of the problems mentioned does not preclude opioid administration. When opioids are used in these patients, 50% of the usual dose is recommended in addition to continuous monitoring of cardiorespiratory function.

with 2 to 3 hours or longer for many opioids, including morphine, meperidine, or hydromorphone. Although 2 longer-acting opioid antagonists (naltrexone and nalmefene) are available, information regarding their use in children is limited.

Although the life-threatening effects of opioids such as respiratory depression are most worrisome, more commonly, the non–life-threatening problems interfere with the delivery of effective analgesia. Inadequate analgesia may occur in younger children and infants because of physicians' unfounded fears of addiction. The incidence of addiction in patients receiving opioids for acute pain management is exceedingly rare. Physical dependence follows the prolonged administration (more than 5 to 7 days) of opioids and sedative agents. These problems should not limit the use of opioids, but rather emphasizes the need to have protocols in place that outline the options for preventing and treating of such problems.[57]

Additional adverse effects of opioids include sedation, constipation, pruritus, nausea, and vomiting. Stool softeners given concurrently with opioid therapy may help prevent constipation. Although tolerance to some of the other adverse effects of opioids such as sedation may develop, tolerance to the opioids' effects on gastrointestinal motility does not occur. Cathartic or osmotic agents (Milk of Magnesia, 70% sorbitol) may be needed for refractory cases or when constipation has already developed. Preventing constipation with a daily dose of Milk of Magnesia during outpatient opioid therapy is easier than treating the problem once it has occurred. Patients receiving opioids for acute pain are frequently inactive and may have less than normal fluid intake, which only serves to aggravate the problem of constipation. New opioid antagonists that do not cross the blood brain barrier may soon be available. These agents may be effective in eliminating the effects of opioids on gastrointestinal motility while preserving their analgesic activity. These agents may be available in the near future for both oral and intravenous administration.

Nausea and vomiting are probably the most bothersome of the non–life-threatening adverse effects of opioids. Three different mechanisms may be involved: (1) a direct stimulation of the central chemoreceptor trigger zone of the medulla, (2) decreased gastrointestinal motility and increased pyloric tone, and (3) sensitization of the vestibular apparatus. Regardless of the mechanisms involved, treatment is primarily symptomatic and may include phenothiazines, metoclopramide, 5-HT_3 antagonists such as ondansetron, or a new class of drug, the neurokinin-1 receptor antagonists, aprepitant, which has recently been introduced for clinical use. Phenothiazines such as promethazine are available in a preparation for rectal administration, and ondansetron has recently been released in a wafer that dissolves in the mouth. Although most experience is with the phenothiazines, adverse effects may occur with these agents, including dystonic reactions, lowering of the seizure threshold, alteration of cardiac repolarization, and potentiation of opioid-induced respiratory depression. When the phenothiazines are used to treat nausea in patients receiving PCA, stopping the PCA for 30 minutes before and after the dose may be appropriate because phenothiazines potentiate of opioid-induced respiratory depression. Other options to treat nausea and vomiting include metoclopramide (0.1 mg/kg up to 10 mg) or one of the serotonin antagonists (ondansetron, dolasetron, or granisetron). Ondansetron is administered intravenously in a dose of 0.15 mg/kg (maximum of 4 mg) intravenously every 6 hours as needed. Unlike the phenothiazines, ondansetron, dolasetron, and granisetron do not cause sedation or potentiate the respiratory depressant effects of opioids. If nausea or vomiting persists despite symptomatic treatment, then changing opioids may be helpful. No particular opioid appears to cause a higher incidence of nausea and vomiting.

Pruritus may occur as an isolated symptom or in association with urticaria. The mechanisms of opioid-induced pruritus are multifactorial and include a direct central effect, as well as histamine release. Strategies to control pruritus include the administering of antihistamines such as diphenhydramine (0.5 mg/kg up to 12.5 mg) or changing to another opioid. The sedative properties of diphenhydramine may also potentiate opioid-induced sedation. When pruritus is not controlled with antihistamines, changing to another opioid with less histamine-releasing properties may be helpful. For intravenous use, these substances include hydromorphone, oxymorphone, and the synthetic agent fentanyl. Given the higher incidence of pruritus in some patient populations (adolescents, patients with sickle cell disease), initiating PCA with hydromorphone in these patients is suggested. Patients with severe skin diseases such as cutaneous involvement of graft-versus-host disease may be particularly likely to develop opioid-induced pruritus. In this group of patients, using fentanyl may be necessary to provide analgesia and prevent pruritus.[58] In such circumstances, the physician should consult with the anesthesiology department or pain service for dosing guidance.

Regional Anesthetic Techniques

Regional anesthetic techniques such as neuraxial blockade (epidural or spinal-intrathecal analgesia) or peripheral nerve blockade can be continued into the postoperative period to provide effective analgesia while preventing the potential adverse effects associated with parenteral opioid therapy. The administration of local anesthetic agents into the epidural or intrathecal space provides profound analgesia; however, undesirable side effects of the use of high concentrations of local anesthetics include blockade of the sympathetic nervous system with hypotension, urinary retention, and blockade of motor function. Epidural and intrathecal opioids can provide intense, segmental, localized analgesia without sensory, motor, or sympathetic nervous system effects. However, adverse effects of neuraxial opioids may include respiratory depression, nausea, pruritus, sedation, and urinary retention. As a result, a combination of low-dose epidural local anesthetics and opioids are commonly used to take advantage of their synergistic effects and limit the side effects of each. Fentanyl and morphine are commonly used opioids, and bupivacaine is the usual local anesthetic of choice. The lipid solubility of the opioid predicts its clinical behavior. Fentanyl is very lipid soluble, penetrating the dura and rapidly binding to spinal cord opioid receptors, producing a fast onset of action but a short duration of action. Significant vascular absorption of fentanyl also occurs, decreasing its epidural effect and reducing its advantage over parenteral administration. Morphine is lipid insoluble and has a slower onset of action but a much longer duration of action. However, given its hydrophilic nature, morphine remains in the cerebrospinal fluid for a longer period with cephalad spread and the risks of delayed respiratory depression for up to 24 hours after neuraxial administration, thereby mandating ongoing monitoring of respiratory function during this time. Other methods of postoperative analgesia include the use of long-acting local anesthetic agents for either wound infiltration or peripheral nerve blockade. Examples of peripheral nerve blockade include brachial plexus blocks for upper extremity pain, femoral nerve blocks for femur and knee surgeries, sciatic nerve blocks for analgesia below the knee, and intercostal nerve blocks for thoracic and abdominal surgeries. Options include the placement of a catheter to allow for continuous infusion during the postoperative period and to provide long-term analgesia for up to 3 to 5 days. Although these regional anesthetic techniques are used most commonly for the control of acute postoperative pain, they may also have applications in the treatment of acute pain of other causes.[59]

SUMMARY

Ongoing evidence continues to demonstrate the deleterious physiological effects of pain and the beneficial results of effective postoperative analgesia. A graded, 3-step approach is recommended with the initial therapy based on an assessment of the severity of pain. This strategy uses a combination of NSAIDs or acetaminophen, the weak opioids (codeine, oxycodone, hydrocodone), and intravenous opioids. In the setting of moderate-to-severe pain, acetaminophen or an NSAID should be continued on a fixed-interval basis as a means of decreasing total opioid consumption and thereby opioid-related adverse effects. Decisions regarding opioid use include the choice of opioid, its route of administration, and its mode of administration. For severe pain in the hospitalized patient, PCA is the preferred mode of administration. Although the intravenous administration of opioids remains the primary route of administration for moderate and severe pain in the hospital setting, future formulations and developments may allow for the increased use of nonparenteral routes. Regional anesthetic techniques are frequently used to control acute postoperative pain, although these techniques may also be applicable to treat acute pain of other causes. In addition to the appropriate choice of medications, an integral aspect of pain management is the assessment of the patient's pain, of the response to therapy, and of the need to increase or decrease the level of analgesia.

TOOLS FOR PRACTICE

Engaging Patient and Family

- *Anesthesia and Your Child* (brochure), American Academy of Pediatrics (patiented.aap.org).

Medical Decision Support

- *Children's Hospital Eastern Ontario Pain Scale (CHEOPS)*, Children's Hospital Eastern Ontario (www.anes.ucla.edu/pain/assessment_tool-cheops.htm).
- *Face Legs Activity Cry and Consolability (FLACC) scoring system*, University of Michigan (Merkel, Voepel-Lewis, and Malviya) (www.resourcenurse.com/Referencemtls/Other_Reference_Materialby_Specialty/Pain_Mgt/FLACCPAINSCALE.doc).
- *Non-communicating Children's Pain Checklist—Postoperative Version* (NCCPC PV), Lyn Breau, Patrick McGrath, Allen Finley, Carol Camfield (216.239.51.104/search?q=cache:Wy_cQl8CkL8J:aboutkidshealth.ca/PDF/AKH_Breau_post-op.pdf+NCCPC-PV&hl=en&ct=clnk&cd=3&gl=us).
- *Pediatric Pain Management for Primary Care—2nd Edition* (book), American Academy of Pediatrics (www.aap.org/bookstore).
- *Poker Chip Scale* (www.ama-cmeonline.com/pain_mgmt/module06/03pain/03_01.htm#).
- *The Oucher* (scale), Judith Beyer, PhD, RN; Antonia M Villaruel; Mary J Denyes (www.oucher.org/differences.html).
- *Visual Analog Scale*, AHRQ and Texas Cancer Council (www.partnersagainstpain.com/printouts/A7012AS1.pdf).
- *Wong-Baker FACES Pain Rating Scale (questionnaire)*, Wong DL, Baker CM (www.mosbysdrugconsult.com/WOW/faces.html).

AAP POLICY STATEMENTS

American Academy of Pediatrics Committee on Fetus and Newborn and Section on Surgery, Canadian Paediatric Society and Fetus and Newborn Committee. Prevention and Management of Pain in the Neonate: An Update. *Pediatrics*. 2006;118(5):2231-2241. (doi:10.1542/peds.2006-2277). (aappolicy.aappublications.org/cgi/content/full/pediatrics;118/5/2231).

American Academy of Pediatrics Committee on Psychosocial Aspects of Child and Family Health and Task Force on Pain in Infants, Children, and Adolescents. The Assessment and Management of Acute Pain in Infants, Children, and Adolescents. *Pediatrics*. 2001;108(3):793-797. (aappolicy.aappublications.org/cgi/content/full/pediatrics;108/3/793).

Zempsky WT, Cravero JP, and the American Academy of Pediatrics Committee on Pediatric Emergency Medicine and Section on Anesthesiology and Pain Medicine. Relief of Pain and Anxiety in Pediatric Patients in Emergency Medical Systems. *Pediatrics*. 2004;114(5):1348-1356. (aappolicy.aappublications.org/cgi/content/full/pediatrics;114/5/1348).

REFERENCES

1. Mather L, Mackie J. The incidence of postoperative pain in children. *Pain*. 1983;271-282.
2. Anand KJ, Hickey PR. Halothane-morphine compared with high-dose sufentanil for anesthesia and postoperative analgesia in neonatal cardiac surgery. *New Engl J Med*. 1992;32:1-9.
3. Peters JW, Schouw R, Anand KJ, et al. Does neonatal surgery lead to increased pain sensitivity in later childhood? *Pain*. 2005;114:444-454.

4. Bartocci M, Bergqvist LL, Lagercrantz H, et al. Pain activates cortical areas in the preterm newborn brain. *Pain*. 2006;122:109-117.
5. Anand KJ, Runeson B, Jacobson B. Gastric suction at birth associated with long-term risk for functional intestinal disorders in later life. *J Pediatr*. 2004;144:449-454.
6. Beyer JD, DeGood DE, Ashley LC, et al. Patterns of postoperative analgesic use with adults and children following cardiac surgery. *Pain*. 1983;17:71-81.
7. Kim MK, Galustyan S, Sato TT, et al. Analgesia for children with acute abdominal pain: a survey of pediatric emergency room physicians and pediatric surgeons. *Pediatrics*. 2003;112:1122-1126.
8. Petrack EM, Christopher NC, Kriwinsky J. Pain management in the emergency department: patterns of analgesic utilization. *Pediatrics*. 1997;99:711-714.
9. Hester NO, Foster R, Kristensen K. Measurement of pain in children: generalizability and validity of the pain ladder and the poker chip tool. In: Tyler DC, Krane EJ, eds. *Advances in Pain Research and Therapy*. New York, NY: Raven Press; 1990.
10. Bieri D, Reeve RA, Champion GD, et al. The faces pain scale for the self-assessment of the severity of pain experience by children: development, initial validation, and preliminary investigation for ratio scale properties. *Pain*. 1990;41:139-150.
11. Beyer JE, Wells N. The assessment of pain in children. *Pediatr Clin North Am*. 1989;36:837-854.
12. McGrath PJ, Johnson G, Goodman JT, et al. CHEOPS: a behavioral scale for rating postoperative pain in children. In: Fields HL, Dubner R, Cewero F, eds. *Advances in Pain Research and Therapy*. New York, NY: Raven Press; 1985.
13. Taddio A, Nulman I, Koren BS, et al. A revised measure of acute pain in infants. *J Pain Symptom Manage*. 1995;10:456-463.
14. Krechel SW, Bildner J. CRIES: a new neonatal postoperative pain measurement score. Initial testing of validity and reliability. *Paediatr Anaesth*. 1995;5:53-61.
15. Stevens B, Johnson C, Petryshen P, et al. Premature infant pain profile: development and initial validation. *Clin J Pain*. 1996;12:13-22.
16. Breau LM, Finley GA, McGrath PJ, et al. Validation of the non-communicating children's pain checklist—postoperative version. *Anesthesiology*. 2002;96:528-535.
17. McGrath PJ, Rosmus C, Camfield C, et al. Behaviors caregivers use to determine pain in non-verbal, cognitively impaired individuals. *Dev Med Child Neurol*. 1998;40:340-343.
18. Malviya S, Voepel-Lewis T, Burke C, et al. The revised FLACC observational pain tool: improved reliability and validity for pain assessment in children with cognitive impairment. *Paediatr Anaesth*. 2006;16:258-265.
19. Schug SA, Zech D, Dorr U. Cancer pain management according to WHO analgesic guidelines. *J Pain Symptom Manage*. 1990;5:27-32.
20. Tobias JD. Weak analgesics and nonsteroidal anti-inflammatory agents in the management of children with acute pain. *Pediatr Clin North Am*. 2000;47:527-543.
21. Tobias JD, Lowe S, Hersey S, et al. Analgesia after bilateral myringotomy and placement of pressure equalization tubes in children: acetaminophen versus acetaminophen with codeine. *Anesth Analg*. 1995;81:496-500.
22. Birmingham PK, Tobin MJ, Henthorn TK, et al. 24-hour pharmacokinetics of rectal acetaminophen in children. *Anesthesiology*. 1997;87:244-248.
23. Anderson BJ, van Lingen RA, Hansen TG, et al. Acetaminophen developmental pharmacokinetics in premature neonates and infants: a pooled population analysis. *Anesthesiology*. 2002;96:1336-1345.
24. Rivera-Peneera T, Gugig R, Davis J, et al. Outcome of acetaminophen overdose in pediatric patients and factors contributing to hepatotoxicity. *J Pediatr*. 1997;130:300-304.
25. Williams DG, Patel A, Howard RF. Pharmacogenetics of codeine metabolism in an urban population of children and its implications for analgesic reliability. *Br J Anaesth*. 2002;89:839-845.
26. Tobias JD. Tramadol for postoperative analgesia in adolescents following orthopedic surgery in a third world country. *Am J Pain Manage*. 1996;6:51-53.
27. Viitanen H, Annila P. Analgesic efficacy of tramadol 2 mg/kg for paediatric day-case adenoidectomy. *Br J Anaesth*. 2001;86:572-575.
28. Finkel JC, Rose JB, Schmitz ML, et al. An evaluation of the efficacy and tolerability of oral tramadol hydrochloride tablets for the treatment of postsurgical pain in children. *Anesth Analg*. 2002;94:1469-1473.
29. Rose JB, Finkel JC, Arquedas-Mohs D, et al. Oral tramadol for the treatment of pain of 7-30 days' duration in children. *Anesth Analg*. 2003;96:78-81.
30. Tobias JD. Seizure after overdose of tramadol. *South Med J*. 1997;90:826-827.
31. Bosenberg AT, Ratcliffe S. The respiratory effects of tramadol in children under halothane anaesthesia. *Anaesthesia*. 1998;53:960-964.
32. Maunuksela EL, Ryhanen P, Janhunen L. Efficacy of rectal ibuprofen in controlling postoperative pain in children. *Can J Anaesth*. 1992;39:226-230.
33. Sims C, Johnson CM, Bergesio R, et al. Rectal indomethacin for analgesia after appendectomy in children. *Anaesth Intens Care*. 1994;22:272-275.
34. Vetter TR, Heiner EJ. Intravenous ketorolac as an adjuvant to pediatric patient-controlled analgesia with morphine. *J Clin Anesth*. 1994;6:110-113.
35. Dsida RM, Wheeler M, Birmingham PK, et al. Age-stratified pharmacokinetics of ketorolac tromethamine in pediatric surgical patients. *Anesth Analg*. 2002;94:266-270.
36. Reuben SS, Connelly NR, Lucie S, et al. Dose-response of ketorolac as an adjunct to patient-controlled analgesia with morphine in patients after spinal fusion surgery. *Anesth Analg*. 1998;87:98-101.
37. Burd RS, Tobias JD. Ketorolac for pain management after abdominal surgical procedures in infants. *South Med J*. 2002;95:331-333.
38. Moffett BS, Wann TI, Carberry KE, et al. Safety of ketorolac in neonates and infants after cardiac surgery. *Pediatr Anesth*. 2006;16:424-428.
39. Foster PN, Williams JG. Bradycardia following intravenous ketorolac in children. *Eur J Anesth*. 1997;14:307-309.
40. Glassman SD, Rose SM, Dimar JR, et al. The effect of postoperative nonsteroidal anti-inflammatory drug administration on spinal fusion. *Spine*. 1998;23:834-838.
41. Bonabello A, Galmozzi MR, Canaparo R, et al. Dexibuprofen [S(+)-isomer ibuprofen] reduces gastric damage and improves analgesic and anti-inflammatory effects in rodents. *Anesth Analg*. 2003;97:402-408.
42. Joshi W, Connelly NR, Reuben SS, et al. An evaluation of the safety and efficacy of administering rofecoxib for postoperative pain management. *Anesth Analg*. 2003;97:35-38.
43. Howard PA, Delafontaine P. Nonsteroidal anti-inflammatory drugs and cardiovascular risk. *J Am Coll Cardiol*. 2004;43:519-525.
44. Konstam MA, Weir MR, Reicin A, et al. Cardiovascular thrombotic events in controlled, clinical trials of rofecoxib. *Circulation*. 2001;104:2280-2288.

45. Solomon DH, Glynn RJ, Levin R, et al. Nonsteroidal antiinflammatory drug use and acute myocardial infarction. *Arch Intern Med.* 2002;162:1099-1104.
46. Vetter TR. Pediatric patient-controlled analgesia with morphine versus meperidine. *J Pain Symptom Manage.* 1992;7:204-208.
47. Berde CB, Beyer JE, Bournaki MC, et al. Comparison of morphine and methadone for prevention of postoperative pain in children. *J Pediatr.* 1991;119:136-141.
48. Berde CB, Lehn BM, Yee JD, et al. Patient-controlled analgesia in children and adolescents: a randomized, prospective comparison with intramuscular administration of morphine for postoperative analgesia. *J Pediatr.* 1991;118:460-466.
49. Doyle E, Robinson D, Morton NS. Comparison of patient-controlled analgesia with and without a background infusion after lower abdominal surgery in children. *Br J Anaesth.* 1993;71:670-673.
50. Doyle E, Harper I, Morton NS. Patient-controlled analgesia with low dose background infusions after lower abdominal surgery in children. *Br J Anaesth.* 1993;71: 818-822.
51. Murphy DF, Graziotti P, Chaldiadis G, et al. Patient-controlled analgesia: a comparison with nurse-controlled intravenous opioid infusion. *Anaesth Intens Care.* 1994; 22:589-592.
52. Tobias JD. The non-intravenous administration of opioids in children. *Am J Anesthesiol.* 1997;24:254-263.
53. Litman RS, Shapiro BS. Oral patient-controlled analgesia in adolescents. *J Pain Symptom Manage.* 1992;7:78-81.
54. Doyle E, Morton NS, McNicol LR. Comparison of patient-controlled analgesia in children by i.v. and s.c. routes of administration. *Br J Anaesth.* 1994;72:533-536.
55. Lamacraft G, Cooper MG, Cavalletto BP. Subcutaneous cannulae for morphine boluses in children. *J Pain Symptom Manage.* 1997;13:43-49.
56. Dietrich CC, Tobias JD. Subcutaneous fentanyl infusions in the pediatric population. *Am J Pain Manage.* 2003;13:146-150.
57. Tobias JD. Tolerance, withdrawal, and abstinence syndromes following long-term sedation and analgesia of children in the pediatric ICU. *Crit Care Med.* 2000;28: 2122-2132.
58. Tobias JD. Patient-controlled analgesia using fentanyl in pediatric patients with sickle cell vaso-occlusive crisis. *Am J Pain Manage.* 2000;10:149-153.
59. Tobias JD. Epidural anesthesia: indications and applications in a pediatric population outside of the perioperative period. *Clin Pediatr.* 1993;32:81-85.

Chapter 55
MANAGEMENT OF CHRONIC PAIN IN CHILDREN

Sabine Kost-Byerly, MD

DEFINITIONS AND PATHOPHYSIOLOGICAL MECHANISMS

The International Association for the Study of Pain defines pain as an "unpleasant and emotional experience with actual or potential tissue damage, or described in terms of such damage."[1] The experience requires a complex interaction of all parts of the nervous system: *transduction, transmission, modulation,* and *perception.* The conversion of a noxious stimulus (mechanical, chemical, or thermal) into electrical energy by a peripheral nociceptor (free afferent nerve ending) is called *transduction.* Tissue inflammation with the release of prostaglandins, bradykinin, and a variety of other mediators can augment the receptiveness of the peripheral nerve endings. Nonsteroidal antiinflammatory drugs (NSAIDs), opioids, and local anesthetics can reduce or inhibit the response of the nervous system at this level. The next phase of nociception is characterized by the *transmission* of information through the peripheral nervous system to the dorsal horn of the spinal cord. Initial sharp pain is propagated via fast A-δ fibers, whereas dull, throbbing pain is transmitted via slower C fibers. Another set of fibers, A-β (tactile) fibers, have a low threshold of stimulation. Local anesthetics and α-2 agonists can effectively interrupt transmission. From the dorsal horn of the spinal cord and along the spinothalamic tract, excitatory neuropeptides such as glutamate (at the N-methyl-D-aspartate [NMDA] receptor) and substance P (at the neurokinin-1 receptor) can modulate the message such that it is facilitated or augmented. Simultaneously, endogenous descending analgesic systems dampen or completely obliterate the nociceptive response. Local anesthetics, α-2 agonists, opioids, NSAIDs, tricyclic antidepressants (TCAs), selective serotonin reuptake inhibitors (SSRIs), and NMDA receptor antagonists can interfere with the nociceptive response at the level of modulation. Finally, when reaching the central nervous system, pain is *perceived* as an individualized unpleasant and emotional experience. Hypnotics, sedatives, anxiolytics, opioids, and α-2 agonists can interrupt perception.

Any pain that persists for longer than 3 months is considered chronic pain. Chronic pain can be continuous or episodic and recurrent, as in migraine headaches. Pain may last for hours, days, or even weeks but then resolve completely, only to recur at a later date. Many patients with chronic pain can have adequate pain relief with their daily management but may still experience breakthrough pain. Episodes of breakthrough pain should be assessed to identify certain patterns (eg, during physical therapy, before the next dose is due). Appropriate interventions and adjustments in medication will prevent patient frustration and possible noncompliance.

TYPES OF PAIN

Two types of pain have been identified: (1) nociceptive and (2) neuropathic. After an injury, the painful stimulus is transmitted via the normal physiological pathways, from the peripheral nerve ending to the central nervous system. It can originate in the musculoskeletal system as somatic pain or in the internal organs as visceral pain. Examples of somatic pain are osteoarthritis and rheumatoid arthritis, which is often described as constant and achy. Pain caused by pancreatitis or bladder spasms is typical of visceral pain. Patients likely complain about cramping and sharp pain in these conditions.

Neuropathic pain is initiated by a primary lesion or dysfunction in the nervous system. It has a central origin when it results from an injury to the central nervous system at the level of the spinal cord or above. A typical example is pain developing after a stroke. Neuropathic pain of peripheral origin involves neural structures distal to the spinal cord. These neuropathies are caused by a multitude of conditions, such as metabolic derangements (diabetes mellitus, vitamin deficiencies), viral illnesses (herpes zoster), or toxins (chemotherapeutic agents). Independent of the origin, patients typically complain of persistent, deep aching pain, constant burning sensations, and paroxysmal cramping or lancinating pain.

Neuropathic pain is associated with peripheral and central sensitization. Peripheral sensitization refers to tissue inflammation augmenting the receptiveness of the peripheral nerve, leading to a heightened response to a painful stimulus (primary hyperalgesia). Central sensitization is due to an increase in the excitability of spinal neurons. The combination of peripheral and central sensitization leads to an increase in the magnitude and duration of pain. In the affected area, patients might experience pain caused by a normally innocuous stimulus (allodynia), an exaggerated response to a normally mildly painful stimulus (hyperesthesia), and pain in neighboring areas not originally affected by injury (secondary hyperalgesia). Proposed mechanisms to explain the characteristics of neuropathic pain include a decreased threshold of the peripheral nociceptor caused by an abnormal accumulation of sodium channels, neurogenic inflammation, and ectopic discharges in C and A-β nerve fibers. An increased responsiveness to norepinephrine might contribute to the localized autonomic dysregulation observed in some chronic pain syndromes. In the central nervous system, hyperexcitability mediated by the NMDA receptor in the dorsal horn of the spinal cord, altered modulatory responses to a stimulus, and changes in the somatosensory cortical map of the affected body area are believed to contribute to the neuropathic pain experience.

In children, the primary care physician will encounter neuropathic pain after trauma and surgery for neurologic injury. Symptoms range from continued sensitivity at the site of an incision to phantom pain after amputation. In children with cancer, peripheral neuropathic pain is common after treatment with chemotherapeutic agents such as vincristine, although not always persistent. Neuropathic pain can also be caused by direct nerve compression by a tumor or extensive lymphadenopathy. Complex regional pain syndrome (CRPS) types 1 and 2 (formerly known as reflex sympathetic dystrophy and causalgia), once thought to be rare in children, have been described in more than 1000 children in the literature. Particularly challenging to treat is neuropathic pain caused by a neurodegenerative disorder or after central nervous system injury because communication with the patient and therefore assessment are often limited.

PREVALENCE

Chronic or frequent recurrent pain complaints have become apparent in large numbers of adolescent girls. In the United States, almost 30% of adolescent girls have reported headaches, 21% stomachaches, and 24% back pain more than once a week, with 53% of these girls experiencing pain in more than 1 location.[2] Heavy abuse of nicotine, caffeine, and alcohol was associated with these symptoms, whereas parent and teacher support was found to be protective. Approximately 25% of Dutch girls have reported chronic pain when defined as chronic pain or recurrent pain present for longer than 3 months,[3] with musculoskeletal pain in an extremity, headaches, and abdominal pain the most common complaints. Girls report both more frequent and more intense pain than boys. The prevalence of migraine headaches has been estimated at 10% in children[4] and up to 28% in adolescents.[5]

Experience of chronic pain does not always lead to health care use. Approximately 50% of children and adolescents with back pain, limb pain, and abdominal pain seek medical advice, whereas only 30% do so for headaches.[6] Medication use, on the other hand, is much more common for headaches than for other pains. Increasing age, greater intensity of pain, and longer duration of pain but not the frequency of pain are associated with greater use of health care services. Clearly, chronic or recurrent pain is common in children. Better assessment and treatment will have implications for the individual patient and public health in general.

EFFECT ON PATIENT AND FAMILY

Surgery and acute pain not only affect the immediate well being of children, but they also have other implications. The child might miss a few days of school, parents might have to request leave from work, or friends and relatives might be asked to provide supervision for siblings at home. In the same way, chronic pain can affect the child, the child's daily life, and other members of the family and social environment. Following the World Health Organization's model of impact of disease, the experience of chronic pain can be divided into 4 areas: (1) *disease* or *disorder,* (2) *impairment,* (3) *disability,* and (4) *handicap*. *Impairment* is assessed by taking a history and performing a physical examination. Reported symptoms such as pain, edema, or joint tenderness are a measure of the severity of the *impairment*. The *disability* caused by the disease can be evaluated by asking how the child's activities in home, school, and community are affected. Restricted involvement or inability to participate in sports or to attend school is a sign of the degree of *disability*. School absence has been found to be a common indicator for disability in children with a variety of conditions associated with chronic pain. Disability can be influenced not only by the child's severity of pain and emotional status, but also by parental coping style and expectations of teachers and school administrators. Parents who are protective and discourage active coping behavior in their children can unwittingly promote a withdrawal from life at school.[7] Large schools with several thousand children can be difficult to navigate for children on crutches or in wheelchairs. Hearing from parents that school administrators advise home teaching is not unusual because accommodating the child is too time consuming. Unfortunately, removal from school can lead to *handicap,* the restriction of social roles and interactions available to the child. Children who attend school, at least on a part-time basis, even just for 1 class a week, are generally easier to rehabilitate than those who have completely withdrawn from school. In these cases, the primary care physician might have to become an advocate for the child.

EVALUATION

Pain is a subjective experience. Only patients know where, when, and how much pain they are experiencing. In infants, toddlers, and children with significant cognitive impairments, pain and discomfort after a painful stimulus are assessed indirectly by measuring changes in physiological parameters, such as facial expressions, body movement, and intensity of crying. Validated and reliable instruments have been developed to assess acute pain in children older than 3 years.[8] These *self-report measures* use numbers, pictures, or words to assess pain in a graded fashion from mild to severe. The most commonly used scale for the preschool age is the Wong-Baker faces scale,[9] which uses a cartoon smiling face that shows gradual changes in 5 steps to a crying face. Because of their limited vocabulary, younger children are usually unable to describe the particular qualities associated with chronic pain. Comparative expressions such as *crushing, burning, stabbing,* or *dull* are beyond the comprehension and lifetime experiences of younger children. For older children, the primary care physician can offer a list of descriptive adjectives associated with pain and ask the child to pick several terms most representative of the pain. Location of the pain can be assessed with the help of a doll or action figure. Older school-aged children and adolescents can be asked to draw an outline of the body, front and back, and point out the most painful areas. Because chronic pain varies from day to day and with different activities, asking the older child to keep a pain journal is also useful. Entries into the journal should be as timely as possible because recall of intensity and frequency of pain at a later date is unreliable.

History and Physical Examination

A thorough history and physical examination are helpful in establishing the correct diagnosis and appropriate treatment plan. A complete pain history should be taken that addresses the following questions:

When was pain first noted?
Was the onset sudden or gradual?
Did an injury precede the pain?
Was pain limited to 1 area of the body, or did it migrate?
How often was the child in pain?
Was the pain worse in the morning or at night?
Is sleep affected by pain?
How is the child's mood?

Exacerbating factors should be explored because they can point to activities that should be modulated or avoided. Alleviating factors are just as important because these can be integrated into a treatment protocol. Children whose pain improves when taking a hot bath might be amenable to exploring aqua therapy as a complementary therapy.

If the child has seen previous practitioners for the same pain complaint, then every effort should be made to document which previous interventions have been used, the quality and efficacy of these interventions, and how the child responded. Medication doses in previous therapies should be closely evaluated for adequate dosing. Finding that use of adjuvant medications such as antidepressants or anticonvulsants have been stopped at too low a dose to represent an adequate trial of the medication is not unusual. This circumstance only contributes to long lists of medications that the patient deems to be *not* working. On the other hand, reintroducing a previously unsuccessful treatment is not only time consuming and costly, but it also increases the family's frustration with the health care system.

A detailed past surgical and medical history should be included. Medical and psychological comorbidities need to be identified. The behavioral and physical development of the child in comparison to siblings and peers might provide clues to the diagnoses of chronic pain conditions. Children with diffuse musculoskeletal pain, eventually diagnosed as having benign hypermobility syndrome, have significant motor development issues already present in early childhood, including poor coordination, general *clumsiness,* and difficulties with handwriting.[10]

Family history and social history needs to be reviewed. Certain pain syndromes, such as migraines, have long been known to aggregate in families. Children with disabilities have been recognized as being at increased risk for abuse and neglect.[11]

A thorough physical examination from head to toe is invaluable in reaching a diagnosis and designing a treatment plan. The primary care physician will already have gained information during the history phase of the evaluation by paying close attention to facial expressions, body position, protective behaviors, movement, and gait. Palpation of the head in patients with chronic or recurrent headaches might reveal tender areas. Most practitioners are familiar with facial headaches caused by chronic or recurrent sinusitis. These headaches can have a neuropathic component because of irritation of the superior and inferior orbital nerves. Tenderness at the facial foramina of the nerves can be exquisite. A similar irritation of the occipital nerves may be seen after posterior fossa surgeries such as a cervico-medullary decompression. Patients may suffer from headaches preoperatively and may be concerned that the procedure was unsuccessful. Tenderness at the foraminal opening should be sought. Treating neuropathic pain with TCAs or anticonvulsants and referring to a pain specialist for injection of the area with local anesthetics and steroids should be considered. A patient exhibiting intolerable pain a few days after an injury such as a sprained ankle might also have hypersensitivity of the skin to even the lightest touch and an erythematous, edematous, and warm extremity. Though the practitioner will have to consider cellulitis, the pain might also be a presentation of CRPS. On the other hand, the same syndrome may be present if the patient instead had a painful, cold, and lividly discolored extremity—with deep-vein thrombosis as the differential diagnosis. The findings on the physical examination will guide further studies. A patient whose pain is initially confined to the hand or elbow may protect the arm by positioning it close to the body; the shoulder is slightly elevated, the trapezius muscle is tightened, and the head might be cocked to the side. This unnatural position leads to secondary musculoskeletal pain in the shoulder and neck region, potentially requiring a different intervention than the primary pain. Children with cognitive impairments are especially difficult to evaluate but are at risk for chronic pain syndromes caused by spasticity, scoliosis, or chronic hip dislocations. A gentle, nonthreatening examination paying close attention to changes in facial expressions or muscle tone might bring the practitioner closer to a diagnosis. For children who have supportive equipment such as splints and wheelchairs, the clinician should to take a look at the child while using the equipment. A growth spurt may turn the perfectly fitting wheelchair with chest wall supports for upright sitting into a compression device. Chest wall pain, back pain, or even femoral nerve and brachial plexus compression syndromes may be found on examination.

Laboratory Evaluation

Laboratory, radiographic, and scintigraphic studies are used in children with chronic pain of unclear origin to further define a differential diagnosis. Laboratory screening tests might suggest an inflammatory or infectious process, which can help in the decision-making process and determine which specialists, if any, should be consulted. Three-phase bone scans can show increased or decreased uptake of the radioactive tracer. Unfortunately, these findings are only of limited diagnostic value. No consistent pattern of tracer uptake has been found to be diagnostic of a specific chronic pain condition. Nerve conduction studies and electromyography can help distinguish more diffuse cases of neuropathic pain from a localized nerve injury or a nerve entrapment. Quantitative sensory testing and autonomic testing are offered by a variety of pain centers. The sensitivity and specificity of the results of these studies are unclear at this point.

Consultation

For patients with significant disability caused by their painful condition and prolonged school absences, the primary care physician should consult with a psychologist or psychiatrist. The child's functional limitations and disabilities can be better assessed and documented, a possible learning disability and school avoidance might become apparent, or presence of comorbid depression interfering with successful pain management might be diagnosed.

Once the assessment is complete, an individualized treatment plan is implemented. Age-appropriate short-term goals should be combined with long-term ones, such as walking along the shallow end of a pool without a brace, participating in a summer day camp, or obtaining a driver's license.

MANAGEMENT

The goal of effective chronic pain management is a reduction of the child's pain, improvement in daily functioning, and return to age-appropriate activities. Before initiating any therapy, the primary care physician should ask the child and family members what their expectations are. Expectations of no pain or complete pain relief might be unrealistic and will lead to disappointment and frustration even if the child's condition significantly improves. Instead of a simple pharmacologic intervention, multimodal therapy is usually needed. Multimodal therapy can include referrals to a physical therapist, psychologist, orthopedist, rheumatologist, or other health care specialist. The primary care physician has a vital role in the process of care coordination, in concert with the family.[12] Care coordination has been shown to improve family satisfaction and reduce health care costs.[13,14] As medical home professionals, primary care physicians should also assess each child's specific needs for special educational services or early intervention services. To this effect, primary care physicians should be aware of local resources and federal, state, and local requirements.[15]

All therapies need to be weighed for their risks and benefits, particularly more aggressive interventional or surgical modalities. Many pharmacologic therapies have not been specifically evaluated in children. Level-1 evidence for chronic pain therapy is virtually nonexistent in children. Benefits and potential adverse effects should be discussed in detail with the parents and child, taking the child's developmental stage into consideration.

In general, the approach to treatment of chronic pain in children is more conservative. Far fewer interventional procedures are performed in children than adults. The need for sedation or anesthesia to perform interventions safely such as a sympathetic nerve block is at least partly responsible for the more conservative treatment. Primary care physicians can successfully integrate many of the therapies into their practice.

Once treatment has been initiated, continually assessing and documenting pain control and changes in function is important. These assessments need to be made over a long period because many patients will have days when their pain will temporarily increase. Any positive patient and family behavior and contributions should be welcome and reinforced. Figure 55-1 highlights a possible algorithm for managing chronic pain.

Nonpharmacologic Therapies

Ideally, nonpharmacologic therapies are fully integrated into a multimodal approach to chronic pain management in children. They should be viewed as neither something to try before "we have to get the heavy guns out" nor the last resort because "everything else we've tried has failed." Many nonpharmacologic therapies emphasize self-management skills and can improve patients' confidence in their abilities. Primary care physicians can familiarize themselves with these therapies during introductory workshops or seminars currently offered at many professional meetings.

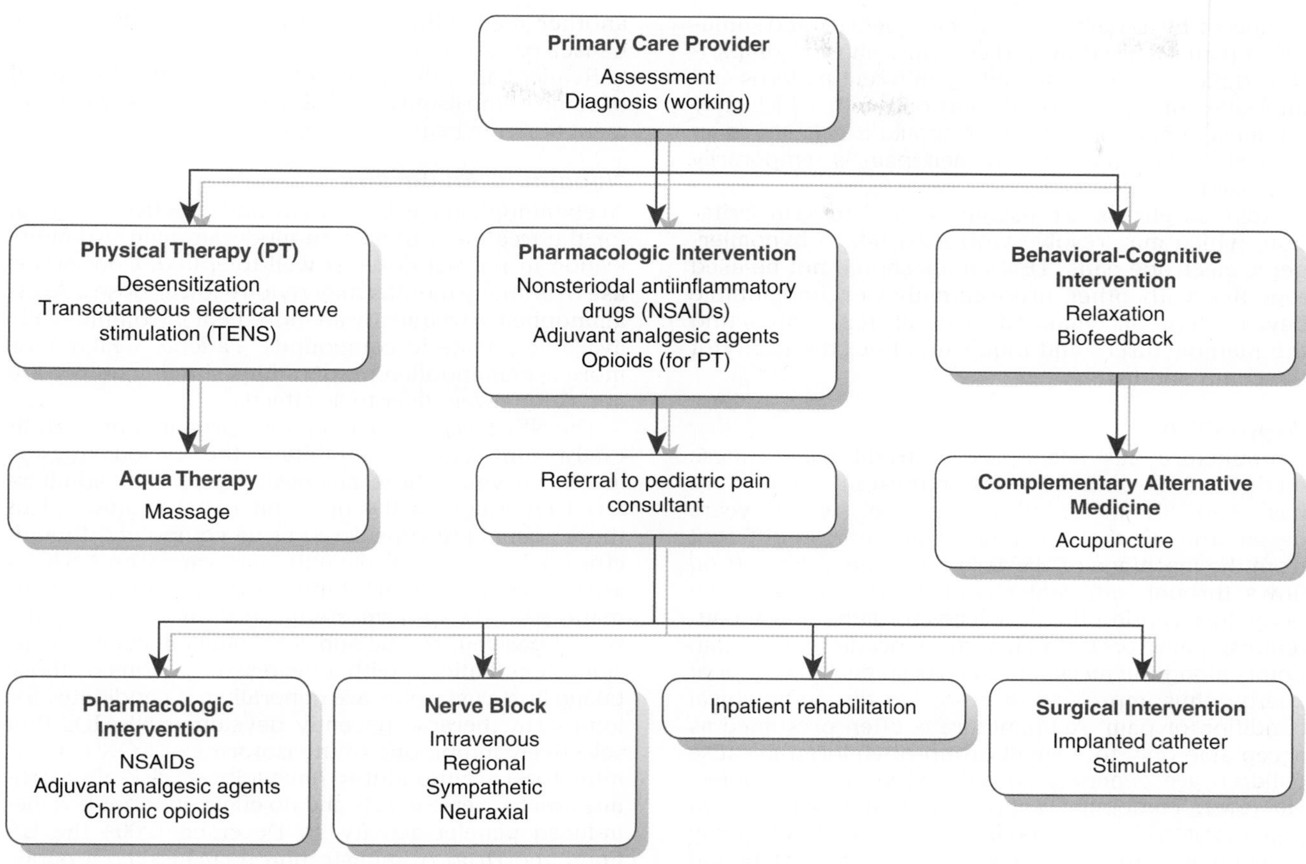

Figure 55-1 Algorithm for approach to chronic (neuropathic) pain. The primary care provider can initiate therapy. If no improvement is noted, then the patient may be referred to the pediatric pain specialist who will continue effective modalities and add more aggressive therapy.

Cognitive-Behavioral Interventions

Cognitive-behavioral interventions rely on providing age-appropriate information to the child and on the child's natural interest in imaginative play. Simple *comfort measures* such as swaddling, massage, or soft music are commonly used for infants; but even older children like to have their favorite stuffed animal or blanket with them in times of distress. *Distraction* with kaleidoscopes, bubbles, movies, or videos are helpful for many children, even those with limited communication skills. *Suggestion* requires greater participation by the child. A *magic* item, such as a blanket, is used to lessen the pain in 1 area or of 1 procedure. The child has to be willing to be enveloped into this *magic* story.

A variety of relaxation exercises have been evaluated in children though mostly for acute or procedure-related pain. Because many children with chronic pain experience acute exacerbation of pain, learning some of these techniques may be useful. *Breathing techniques* with deep-chest, rhythmic, or patterned breathing can be learned without professional help. Trained child-life specialists, occupational therapists, or psychologists are usually needed to explore *guided imagery, progressive muscle relaxation, biofeedback,* and *hypnosis*. Hypnosis has been found to be more effective than distraction and breathing for procedural distress in children undergoing oncologic procedures.[16] Hypnosis and guided imagery have also been shown to improve analgesia and shorten length of stay after surgery in children.[17]

Transcutaneous Electrical Nerve Stimulation

Transcutaneous electrical nerve stimulation (TENS) consists of a battery-powered unit delivering electrical impulses to skin electrodes placed in the vicinity of the painful area. Two main theories exist to explain the effects of TENS. The gate control theory stipulates that nonnoxious impulses from TENS are transmitted via large diameter afferent fibers. Simultaneous painful stimuli, traveling along small diameter afferent fibers, will be suppressed at various *gates* within the spinal cord. TENS has also been suggested to activate inhibitory, descending pathways in the central nervous system because it has been associated with an increase of endogenous opioids in the serum and spinal fluid.

A variety of amplitudes, frequencies, and stimulation patterns can be programmed; low-intensity stimulation remains sensory, higher intensity will result in muscle contraction. Research evaluating the efficacy of TENS for acute and chronic pain management has been hampered by the large variety of frequencies and stimulation patterns used in studies, which makes comparisons difficult. Patients should try different patterns and intensities of stimulation to find one with which they are most comfortable. Patients should use TENS as an adjunct for the times when their pain is temporarily increased.

Adverse effects are usually limited to skin irritation, which may resolve with a switch to hypoallergenic electrode pads. TENS units should not be used together with other programmable or implantable devices (eg, pacemakers) without first contacting the manufacturers and inquiring about the safety of the combination.

Acupuncture

Acupuncture has been part of traditional Chinese medicine for over 5000 years. Interest in acupuncture has gradually increased during the last 30 years despite the fact that the underlying theory is different from the teachings of Western medicine: Energy *(Chi)* flows through different channels *(meridians)* in the body. Interrupting the flow leads to pathological conditions, pain, or both. Inserting needles at certain points along the meridians can reestablish the flow of energy, thus improving or resolving the pathological condition or pain. Acupuncture is often presumed as acceptable only to a small group of children because children are generally considered as needle phobic. However, combining acupuncture and hypnosis in patients with chronic pain has been found to be highly acceptable, with a decline in anticipatory anxiety and significant improvements in pain after treatment.[18] Further studies are necessary to assess the efficacy of acupuncture in different painful conditions.

The use of complementary and alternative medicine to treat chronic illness or disability is increasing in the United States. The primary care physician may be asked to provide balanced advice concerning therapeutic options, though, at this point, only limited recommendations have been published regarding the use of complementary and alternative medicine in the care of children with chronic illness or disability.[19]

Pharmacotherapy

Pharmacotherapy for chronic pain includes nonopioid, opioid, and adjuvant medications. Whereas in the past, therapy progressed gradually from nonopioids to *weak* opioids (disregarding the fact that at equianalgesic doses all opioids have the same potency) and finally to *strong opioids,* multimodal analgesic therapy is currently preferred. The goal of such therapy is an augmentation of analgesia and a simultaneous reduction in adverse effects. Patients should continue to take their nonopioid analgesic with opioids because this combination may decrease the required dose of opioids and the incidence of opioid-related adverse effects.

Some adverse effects, such as sedation or dizziness, may be more apparent at the beginning of therapy. Initiating therapy at a low dose and titrating the dose carefully is therefore prudent. For children who attend school, weekends may be a good time to begin or augment therapy. Occasionally, an otherwise effective analgesic may require the addition of another medication to treat adverse effects such as nausea or pruritus.

Readers are referred to a more in-depth discussion of some of the listed analgesics in Chapter 54, Management of Acute Pain in Children.

Nonopioid Analgesics

Acetaminophen has been a safe and effective analgesic for the treatment of mild-to-moderate pain. Administration in normal doses is well tolerated. Continuous use over many months may require lower doses. Acetaminophen is frequently an ingredient in commercially available analgesic compounds. Patients taking 1 or more acetaminophen preparations simultaneously are at risk for severe liver toxic effects.

The NSAIDs provide pain relief primarily by peripherally and centrally inhibiting the cyclooxygenase (COX) enzyme. These analgesic agents are administered enterally via the oral and rectal routes. All of these agents are considered to be equipotent, though efficacy in individual patients may vary. The NSAIDs are particularly useful for inflammatory, bony, or rheumatic pain. Long-term administration must take the risk of gastrointestinal and renal side effects into consideration. Patients with a history of gastritis or those taking corticosteroids are generally not candidates for long-term therapy. Recently developed NSAIDs that selectively inhibit one of the isoforms of COX (COX-2 inhibitors) are thought to have a lower risk of gastrointestinal adverse effects and no effect on thromboxane-induced platelet activity. In December 2004 the US Food and Drug Administration (FDA) issued a public health advisory that indicated that some COX-2 inhibitors may be associated with an increased risk of thromboembolic phenomena (myocardial infarction, stroke). At this point, how this risk would affect children is unclear.

Whereas aspirin has largely been abandoned in pediatric practice because of its association with Reye syndrome, 1 aspirin-like compound with no effect on platelet function, choline-magnesium trisalicylate, has remained attractive in chronic pain management. Patients with cancer who are experiencing bony pain and decreased platelet function are the main treatment group. The drug is available in both liquid and tablet form and is administered twice a day. As in acute pain management, the most commonly used NSAID is ibuprofen. The limited duration of action of this drug with a required administration of 3 to 4 times a day may necessitate a switch to the longer-acting naproxen, which is administered twice a day. Dosing strategies for the most commonly prescribed nonopioid analgesics are listed in Table 55-1.

Opioid Analgesics

Opioid analgesics are neurotransmitters that interact with several distinct receptors in the peripheral and central nervous system. The 4 major receptors are designated mu, delta, kappa, and sigma. Most currently used opioid analgesics primarily attach to the mu receptor. Morphine is 50 to 100 times stronger at this receptor than at the delta receptor. The mu receptor and its subspecies and the delta receptor are known as being related to analgesia, respiratory depression,

Table 55-1 Dosing Strategies for Frequently Used Oral Nonsteroidal Anti-inflammatory Drugs

GENERIC NAME	PEDIATRIC ORAL DOSE AND FREQUENCY	MAXIMUM ADULT ORAL DAILY DOSE	INDICATIONS	COMMENTS
Acetaminophen	10-15 mg/kg q4h	4000 mg	Mild-to-moderate pain, fever	Lacks antiinflammatory activity
Ibuprofen	6-10 mg/kg q6-8h	2400 mg	Mild-to-moderate pain, fever, RA, OA	Oral suspension available
Naproxen	5-10 mg/kg q12h	1000 mg	OA, RA, other rheumatic or bony pain	Oral suspension available
Salicylates (aspirin)	10-15 mg/kg q4h	4000 mg	Mild-to-moderate pain, fever	Inhibits platelet aggregation, causes gastrointestinal irritability, Reye syndrome
Choline magnesium trisalicylate	8-10 mg/kg q6h	3000 mg	Mild-to-moderate pain, fever	Aspirin compound that does not affect platelets

OA, Osteoarthritis; *RA*, rheumatoid arthritis.

euphoria, and physical dependence. Butorphanol attaches at a ratio of 1:4:25 at the mu to delta to kappa receptors.

All opioid analgesics can be classed into agonist, antagonist, and mixed agonist-antagonist based on their receptor-binding capacities. Agonist attachment to a receptor leads to a cascade of intracellular activity, whereas antagonist attachment at the receptor does not have this response. Antagonists, such as naloxone, can competitively remove an agonist from the receptor and stop the action of the agonist. Butorphanol, a mixed agonist-antagonist, functions as an antagonist at the mu receptor and as an agonist at the kappa receptor. Therefore butorphanol, as with naloxone, can lead to withdrawal symptoms when it is used indiscriminately in patients taking mu opioids for a longer time. The most commonly used drugs are listed in Table 55-2.

Opioids need to be titrated to effect because response to specific opioids will vary. Though mu receptor opioids are known to produce similar degrees of adverse effects such as respiratory depression, sedation, euphoria, nausea, biliary tract spasm, and constipation, the response of particular patients will vary. If adverse effects become too cumbersome and outweigh the benefits of an opioid, then the patient may be prescribed a different one, a process known as *opioid rotation*. Ideally, the primary care physician has explained this possibility to the patient and family before initiating therapy, which will decrease frustration and maintain trust.

Most opioids for chronic pain management are administered orally. They are available as liquids of various concentrations, immediate-release tablets, and sustained-release preparations. Even for chronic pain, opioids do not always have to be administered around the clock. Providing the patient with a single dose of an opioid before physical therapy might be sufficient and might result in much better therapy. When multiple doses of a short-acting opioid are needed throughout the day, switching to sustained-release opioids is more effective—and more convenient—because they prevent peaks and troughs in the serum and provide a better steady state. The patient's daily opioid requirement should be well known before initiating any long-acting opioids. Asking the patient and the parents to keep a journal in which they document how often a short-acting opioid was required can be helpful. This information can then be evaluated with the following questions in mind:

Do they wake up in the middle of the night because of pain?

Do they need medication in the middle of the school day?

Many manufacturers of sustained-release opioids provide conversion tables, but starting at lower doses than suggested and gradually titrating over several days is advisable. Immediate-release opioids can be supplemented during this period, which will avoid oversedation and drowsiness.

Methadone is currently the only long-acting opioid in liquid form. Opioids in pill form need to be swallowed whole because chewing the pill can lead to a rapid release of the active drug and a potential overdose. Transdermal administration of the opioid is another possibility if the oral route is not available. The recent introduction of a fentanyl patch has increased this option for children, although studies with opioids lasting for up 24 hours in children are lacking. Currently available long-acting opioids are listed in Table 55-3.

Long-acting opioids may be used in combination with short-acting ones. A child who is receiving opioids on a daily basis with generally good results might still experience an occasional escalation of pain or even daily short-lived pain, which is known as breakthrough pain. In these situations, adding a short-acting opioid to the long-acting form might be

Table 55-2 Dosing Strategies for Frequently Used Oral Immediate-Release Opioid Analgesics

GENERIC NAME	PEDIATRIC ORAL DOSE AND FREQUENCY	INITIAL ADULT ORAL DOSE AND FREQUENCY	INDICATIONS	COMMENTS
Codeine	1.2 mg/kg q4-6h	15 mg q4-6h	Mild-to-moderate pain	By mouth only Usually prescribed with acetaminophen
Oxycodone—immediate release	0.1 mg/kg q4-6h	5 mg q4-6h	Moderate-to-severe pain	By mouth only Less nauseating than codeine Usually prescribed with acetaminophen in adults
Morphine—immediate release	0.3 mg/kg q4-6h	5-15 mg q4-6h	Moderate-to-severe pain	May cause seizures in high doses Causes histamine release, vasodilatation; avoid in patients with asthma
Hydromorphone		2-4 mg q4-6h	Moderate-to-severe pain	
Methadone	0.1 mg/kg q6-24h	2.5-10 mg q6-24h	Severe chronic pain when opioids are needed for a prolonged period Pain refractory to other opioids	QT prolongation possible in susceptible patients Toxicity caused by accumulation within 3-5 days Do not increase more often than every 5-7 days Use only in opioid-tolerant patients
Oral transmucosal fentanyl citrate		200 mcg; 200- to 1600-mcg lozenge units	Breakthrough pain in opioid-tolerant patients	Should only be used in opioid-tolerant patients

Table 55-3 Dosing Strategies for Frequently Used Sustained-Release Opioid Analgesics

GENERIC NAME	PEDIATRIC DOSE AND FREQUENCY	INITIAL ADULT DOSE RANGE AND FREQUENCY	INDICATIONS	COMMENTS
Morphine—sustained release	No specific pediatric dosing has been established, follow adult dosing	Dose dependent on previous opioid requirement; lowest dose: 15 mg q12h Interval: Ms Contin and Oramorph q8-12h	Moderate-to-severe pain when opioids are needed for a prolonged period	Patient needs to be able to swallow whole pill Fatal overdose possible if chewed
Oxycodone—sustained release	No specific pediatric dosing has been established, follow adult dosing	Dose dependent on previous opioid requirement; lowest dose: 10 mg q12h	Moderate-to-severe pain when opioids are needed for a prolonged period	Patient needs to be able to swallow whole pill Fatal overdose possible if chewed
Fentanyl transdermal system (Duragesic)	No specific pediatric dosing has been established, follow adult dosing	Dose dependent on previous opioid requirement Lowest dose: 12 mcg/hr Patch needs to be changed q72h	Moderate-to-severe pain when opioids are needed for a prolonged period	Initial dose should not exceed 25 mcg/hr Unauthorized simultaneous use of multiple patches can lead to fatal overdose

indicated, particularly when other nonpharmacologic or nonopioid measures have failed. Frequent need for a short-acting opioid in addition to the long-acting form should lead to a reassessment: Is the dose of the long-acting opioid too low? Is the patient more active than before therapy started? Does the patient feel only the short-acting opioid *really works?* As the serum blood level changes rapidly with the short-acting opioid, patients might experience a higher degree of euphoria and decide that only the short-acting drug helps. A frank and honest discussion of these effects can prevent unnecessary changes by primary care physicians.

Though usually reserved for oncologic and palliative-care patients, long-acting opioids can be combined with intravenous patient-controlled analgesia (PCA). The PCA device is programmed without a continuous rate because the long-acting opioid provides baseline analgesia throughout the day. Intermittent patient-initiated doses will relieve episodic pain. Occasionally, when no other intravenous fluids are administered, a low continuous rate is required to maintain the patency of the venous access.

Adverse effects generally associated with opioid administration, such as sedation, drowsiness, nausea, and vomiting, can be apparent the 1st few days when opioids are initiated but often resolve in patients taking opioids in the long-term. Increases in dose may be accompanied by a temporary recurrence of adverse effects. Reaction time can be slowed even when the patient does not subjectively feel drowsy or sleepy. Teenaged drivers and their parents have to be advised of this effect. Bowel motility will be affected even after a prolonged administration of opioids, and constipation is a common complaint. Therefore combining opioid therapy with a bowel regimen is wise. Adolescent patients taking opioids for years may experience delayed puberty because testosterone and estrogen levels can be decreased. Hormonal supplements might be necessary.

Once patients have received opioids on a regular basis for more than a week to 10 days, they cannot simply stop using these drugs; they need to be weaned off of them. The body has developed a physical tolerance, receptors have changed in response to the long-term administration, and immediate discontinuation of drug therapy would lead to withdrawal symptoms. Decreasing the total dose by 10% every day to every other day is a common approach to weaning opioids, although this area is one of continuing research.[20] For children who have received opioids for months, this approach might be too aggressive. Weaning just once or twice a week might be more adequate, especially in an outpatient setting where symptoms of withdrawal might be missed. Parents should be informed that signs of withdrawal include subtle ones, such as yawning, lacrimation, rhinorrhea, nasal stuffiness, or insomnia, as well the more commonly associated, extreme ones of restlessness, chills, tachycardia, hypertension, nausea and vomiting, crampy abdominal pains, and diarrhea. When the parent reports subtle signs of withdrawal, stopping the weaning process for a few days before resuming it at a slower rate is best. More severe signs of withdrawal require a return to a higher dose, stabilization at the higher dose for a few days, and then again a slower rate of continued weaning.

Controlled Substances, Patient Care, and the Law

The use of opioids for chronic pain has been controversial. Some authors have argued that opioids should never be used for chronic, nonmalignant pain. Their use would only lead to dependency, tolerance, and dose escalations. Clearly, daily use of opioids always result in physical dependence, though not psychological addiction, tolerance, and a potential need for a higher dose. The use of opioids may be justified when it can be demonstrated that the pain has been reduced and the patient's function has significantly improved. When initiating opioid therapy, the status of the patient should be clearly documented, and therapy should be objectively assessed later. The clinician is advised to sign a contract with the family that details who can write prescriptions for opioids, where these prescriptions can be filled, whom to contact when the prescribed doses are inadequate, and what happens if patients run out of medications early or loses their medications. The individual patient's and the family's risk for abuse and diversion of medications needs to be reviewed carefully. State medical boards and the US Drug Enforcement Administration provide further information on their respective Web sites.[21,22]

Adjuvant Analgesics

Adjuvant analgesics are most commonly used in the treatment of chronic neuropathic pain. Few randomized controlled studies have examined the efficacy of these analgesics in chronic pain management, although they have been used for at least 20 years. Experiences in adults have been extrapolated to administration in children because no comparable studies in children have been conducted. The practitioners accustomed to the efficacy of NSAIDs or opioids in acute pain management are often surprised by how little improvement these medications seem to provide (for every 100 patients taking antidepressants for chronic pain, only 30 experience at least a 50% reduction in pain[23]).

None of these medications have been specifically approved for the treatment of chronic pain in children. Several of them have an FDA indication for particular neuropathic pain syndromes in adult patients, such as postherpetic neuralgia or diabetic peripheral neuropathy. Most of the current use is off label. The child and the family need to be advised that the treatment often involves trial and error. Medications will need to be gradually titrated to effect, but adverse effects might limit this approach.

ANTICONVULSANTS. Anticonvulsants suppress neural hyperexcitability, which might explain their effectiveness in chronic pain management. Gabapentin has been indicated for the adjunctive treatment of partial seizure in children as young as 3 years. Therefore the experience in children with this particular drug is more extensive than with others in this class. Gabapentin is currently the most widely used adjunctive analgesic for children and is usually well tolerated. The most common adverse effects are dizziness, somnolence, ataxia, fatigue, and weight gain. Weight gain can be particularly concerning when treatment for lower extremity pain is required because added weight does not help in the rehabilitation process. Therapy is usually initiated on a once-a-day basis and advanced up to 3 doses a day if necessary. Doses can be increased every 2 to 5 days. Many physicians begin with nighttime dosing and also increase the nighttime dose first so that potential sedation and dizziness may be less apparent. If patients experience an improvement in pain relief, doses can be raised as long as no significant adverse effects occur. The patient and family should be told that these medications do not work immediately; a week might pass before patients note any improvement at all. Pregabalin was approved in 2004 for treatment of pain caused by peripheral neuropathy and postherpetic neuralgia. Pregabalin is commonly used off label for other neuropathic pain disorders in adults, but no experience in children is available at this point. Other anticonvulsants have not been studied as closely as gabapentin. Adverse effects and toxicity have limited their use. Lamotrigine has been associated with Stevens-Johnson syndrome, tiagabine with seizures, and topiramate with hyperthermia. Older anticonvulsants such as phenytoin, carbamazepine, and valproate require periodic monitoring for potential end-organ toxic effects.

ANTIDEPRESSANTS. Evidence of the efficacy of antidepressants in chronic pain management has been best for agents that have a local anesthetic-like effect on neural sodium channels and interfere with the reuptake of norepinephrine. These drugs include TCAs such as nortriptyline and amitriptyline. SSRIs seem to be less effective but are helpful when associated depression, sleep disturbance, and anxiety are present.

In October 2004 the FDA directed manufacturers of all antidepressant drugs to revise the labeling for their products to include a boxed warning and expanded warning statements that alert health care providers to an increased risk of suicidality (suicidal thinking and behavior) in children and adolescents being treated with these agents. When initiating antidepressant therapy, the FDA advises health care providers to evaluate children and adolescents every week for the first 4 weeks, then every other week for the next 4 weeks, and again at 12 weeks to assess for potential mood changes.[24]

Other side effects of TCAs include dry mouth, constipation, urinary retention, sedation, and cardiovascular effects such as hypotension and disturbances of conduction. Rare reports have surfaced of sudden death associated with TCA therapy. A baseline electrocardiogram should be obtained to identify children with a preexisting conduction defect, and a subsequent electrocardiogram should be performed if higher doses are required. The side effect profile varies between the drugs: Nortriptyline has fewer anticholinergic side effects than amitriptyline, whereas amitriptyline is the more sedating. Sedation can be turned into a therapeutic advantage when treating patients who complain of nighttime awakenings caused by pain. Patients should be advised to avoid high-caloric drinks to relieve the sensation of dry mouth because they can contribute to undesirable weight gain.

With anticonvulsants, pain relief is delayed and cannot be expected for at least a week or more. No established correlation exists between plasma concentration of TCAs and analgesic efficacy. Routine measurement of plasma drug levels is rarely indicated. If use of the drug needs to be discontinued, then the dosing should be tapered over 1 to 2 weeks to avoid irritability and agitation.

MEMBRANE STABILIZERS. Membrane stabilizers are drugs that interfere with the ionic fluxes required for the initiation and conduction in peripheral and central neurons. These medications are available in a variety of applications: intravenous lidocaine, oral mexiletine, and transdermal lidocaine patches. All of these drugs are thought to be particularly helpful in the treatment of neuropathic pain. Intravenous lidocaine and oral mexiletine are 2nd-line therapy usually reserved for patients who show insufficient improvement after therapy with other adjuvants such as anticonvulsants or antidepressants. A positive response to an infusion of lidocaine is thought to be predictive of successful therapy with mexiletine. Adverse effects include nausea, vomiting, sedation, and ataxia, which limit the usefulness of this therapy. Initiation of this therapy will most frequently occur after consultation with a pediatric pain specialist; however, the relatively new application of transdermal lidocaine might be considered by the primary care physician. As with many therapies, these patches have not been specifically evaluated in children. Their indication, at this point, is solely for postherpetic neuralgia, but they have been found to be useful in a variety of other localized neuropathic pain conditions. The patches can be cut to size and are applied to the area for 12 continuous hours a day. Adverse effects are usually limited to local irritation because the systemic absorption of lidocaine through intact skin is low. Parents should be warned, though, to keep the patches out of reach of small children because overdose can occur when the patches are chewed or swallowed. At least 95% or 665 mg of lidocaine will still be present in the patch after 12 hours of application.

ALPHA AGONISTS. Drugs such as clonidine are centrally and peripherally sympathoplegic. They stimulate α-adrenoreceptors in the brain stem, resulting in reduced sympathetic outflow from the central nervous system, and they stimulate prejunctional receptors on peripheral neurons, reducing norepinephrine release. Epidural use of clonidine has been found to be effective for neuropathic pain syndromes. Transdermal clonidine prophylaxis has also been evaluated as an adjunct preventing withdrawal symptoms in children who were sedated in the intensive care units for a prolonged period.[25] Adverse effects may include sedation, bradycardia, and hypotension. A list of the most frequently used adjuvant analgesics can be found in Table 55-4.

Interventional Therapy

If the patient's condition does not improve after a period of several weeks despite a multidisciplinary approach, including psychological and pharmacologic

Table 55-4 Dosing Strategies for Frequently Used Adjuvant Analgesics

GENERIC NAME	PEDIATRIC DOSE AND FREQUENCY	INITIAL ADULT DOSE RANGE AND FREQUENCY	INDICATIONS	COMMENTS
Gabapentin	5-60 mg/kg divided into 2 to 3 daily doses Start at 5 mg/kg for <20 kg, 100 mg for <50 kg, 300 mg for >50 kg Titrate q1-3d as needed	300 mg Titrate 300 mg/day q1-3d, up to 3600 mg divided 3 times daily	Postherpetic neuralgia Neuropathic pain, migraine prophylaxis	CNS effects (somnolence, dizziness, etc) Do not stop abruptly—risk of seizure in susceptible patients
Pregabalin	No specific pediatric dosing established	50 mg; 50 mg tid or 75 mg bid Titrate up to 300 mg/day in 1 wk as needed	Postherpetic neuralgia, diabetic neuropathy, neuropathic pain	CNS effects (somnolence, dizziness, etc) Do not stop abruptly—risk of seizure in susceptible patients
Topiramate	No specific pediatric dosing established	25 mg Titrate to 50 mg q12h in 4 wks as needed	Migraine prophylaxis	Risk of metabolic acidosis, oligohidrosis, hyperthermia
Amitriptyline	10-25 mg qhs Titrate up to 2-3 mg/kg (max. 150 mg), every qhs or twice-daily dosing	25-50 mg qhs Titrate up to 150 mg/day	Neuropathic pain, chronic pain	Sedation, anticholinergic and cardiac effects
Nortriptyline	10-25 mg qhs Titrate up to 1-3 mg/kg (max. 150 mg), every qhs or twice-daily dosing	25-50 mg qhs Titrate up to 150 mg/day	Neuropathic pain, chronic pain	Anticholinergic and cardiac effects
Doxepin	12.5 mg/kg qhs Titrate up to 100 mg/day in 1-3 doses	75 mg, divided in 1-3 doses Titrate up to 150 mg/day	Neuropathic pain, chronic pain	Do not use in children <12 years of age
Trazodone	No specific pediatric dosing established	50 mg qhs Titrate up to 200 mg qhs or 400 mg/day in divided doses	Chronic pain	Risk of priapism—avoid in male patients

CNS, Central nervous system.

interventions and physical therapy, the pain specialist might consider a regional anesthetic. A regional anesthetic may be particularly helpful if the painful condition is limited to a single extremity as is often the case in CRPS type 1. Interventional therapy may be limited to the injection of a single peripheral nerve with local anesthetics and steroids or extend to the intravenous regional block of a whole extremity. It may comprise a block of the sympathetic nervous system or a neuraxial block via an epidural injection. Most young children will require sedation for these procedures; thus primary care physicians should refer the patient to a pain management facility that is capable of providing this kind of care.

Intravenous Regional Block (Bier Block)

Intravenous regional anesthesia is indicated for painful conditions of the arm below the elbow or the leg blow the knee. An intravenous cannula is inserted in a distal vein in the limb, and a tourniquet is applied to the upper arm or thigh. Before inflation of the tourniquet, the limb may be exsanguinated (blood removed) by wrapping the distal part of the limb with an elastic bandage. This procedure can increase the efficacy of the block but may be poorly tolerated in patients with chronic pain. Local anesthetic and ketorolac infusion have been found to be efficacious in some children with CRPS type 1.[26] Complications, though rare, can occur if the tourniquet suddenly deflates soon after the local anesthetic has been injected. The sudden increase in serum level of the local anesthetic will lead to the well-known neurologic adverse effect of an overdose: dizziness, tinnitus, loss of consciousness, and convulsions. Serious cardiac adverse effects are rare but can occur if bupivacaine is the local anesthetic or if convulsions are inadequately treated.

Sympathetic Blocks

Sympathetic blocks are injections of local anesthetic into a particular area of the ganglionic chain of the sympathetic nervous system: at the stellate ganglion for the upper extremity and at the lumbar sympathetic plexus for the lower extremity. The pain specialist may use ultrasound, fluoroscopy, or computed tomography for guidance in the placement of the block. Indications for this intervention are chronic pain syndromes such as CRPS type 1, in which the sympathetic nervous system may contribute to the painful condition. After the block, the patient experiences a warming in the extremity, and the practitioner can register a measurable increase in temperature in the extremity, which helps in assessing the efficacy of the block in multiple ways. If temperature is increased and the patient reports pain relief, then the pain is considered as sympathetically maintained. If the pain relief lasts beyond the expected duration of the local anesthetic block, then the injection will be considered not only diagnostic, but also therapeutic. Depending on the duration of pain relief, the block can be repeated. Repeated injections might provide progressively longer periods of pain relief. If the injection resulted in an increase in temperature but no improvement in pain occurred, then the condition has to be considered as sympathetically independent. Repeating the block has no benefit. If the injection did not result in a temperature change in the extremity the block was technically inadequate. Even in this condition, the patient might report an improvement in pain, a so-called placebo response, a situation the specialist will have to contemplate when deciding on further interventions.

At this point, no controlled studies have been performed in children or adolescents evaluating the efficacy of sympathetic blocks. Adverse effects include typical findings of Horner syndrome in case of a stellate ganglion block: drooping of the eyelid, conjunctival injection, and stuffy nose on the injected side. Hoarseness can also occur. These effects will persist only for the duration of action of the injected local anesthetic. Other adverse effects include local anesthetic overdose after unintentional intravascular injection or injury to adjoining structures such as a pneumothorax. If a sympathetic nerve block has repeatedly provided good analgesia but was of insufficient duration, then a surgical sympathectomy may be considered.

Implanted Devices

In children, therapeutic interventions will only occasionally progress to the invasiveness of an implanted device. Primary care physicians are already familiar with these forms of therapy as an advanced mode in the management of spasticity in a child with cerebral palsy. An intrathecal catheter is surgically implanted at the lumbar level of the spinal cord. It is then tunneled to a reservoir device, which is usually placed in a subcutaneous pocket in the lower abdomen. The reservoir can be filled with local anesthetic, opioids, and clonidine. Because the drugs are delivered directly into the spinal fluid, drug doses can be much smaller than is the case with enteral or parenteral delivery. Patients have to return to the pain management center every 4 to 8 weeks for a refill. The device is programmable via telemetry. Program modes can range from a simple continuous infusion to more complex modes with additional boluses at particular times of the day when increased pain can be anticipated.

In the case of spinal cord stimulation, electrodes are surgically placed in the epidural space and connected to an implanted controller. Multiple parameters of the repetitive electrical impulses such as duration, intensity, and pulse width can be manipulated. Patient cooperation during implantation is paramount to achieve an optimal result. Therefore this device is reserved for the occasional older adolescent with severe, unrelenting pain. Discussions of adverse effects for these therapies have to include not only possible immediate surgical complications, but also the need for long-term maintenance.

Referral to a Pediatric Pain Specialist

Patients with complex disease processes and significant disability and impairment in function will challenge the primary care physician. Patients who have uncontrolled pain or loss of function despite therapy, significant comorbid diseases, a need for more invasive testing or treatment, or a family who is looking for another opinion should be referred to a pain specialist. The primary care physician has 2 options in this case: either (1) remain the primary coordinator of the multimodal treatment team with the pain specialist as one of the providers, or (2) allow the pain specialist to become the coordinator of the team. Which option is right will depend not only on the complexity of the patient's problem, but also on the distance the family will have to travel to see the specialist. Ideally, the primary care physician, who is familiar with the patient, the family, and the local resources, will work in close consultation with the pain specialist.

Discontinuing Treatment

Periodically, all treatment modalities should be assessed to see whether they are still effective or even necessary. A change in function may no longer be dependent on a particular therapy because the overall physical status of the patient has improved. Discontinuing therapy can be a challenge because many patients and families fear that the painful condition will recur. A gradual *weaning* of therapy is an option even when no clear pharmacologic necessity exists.

Palliative Care

Insufficient relief of pain is one of the most common patient complains in the management of progressive cancer or other terminal conditions. All therapeutic interventions that have been discussed in this chapter should be considered in the management of a patient with a potentially life-threatening disease. Waiting until the child has only days to live to consider more invasive therapy will lead to needless, avoidable suffering. The American Academy of Pediatrics therefore recommends offering components of palliative care at the diagnosis and throughout a potentially life-threatening disease.[27] For placement of an implantable device, the child should have a life expectancy of approximately 6 months. If the life expectancy is less than 6 months, then a tunneled catheter connected to a conventional infusion pump or a PCA device is an option. Neurolytic blocks can provide the patient and family with valuable pain-free or painless time.[28]

CONCLUSION

The prevalence and significance of chronic pain in children and adolescents have only recently been recognized.

Chronic pain can limit the functional abilities of the child, prevent normal age-appropriate development, and have a significant impact on other members of the family. A multidisciplinary approach is preferred when assessing the patient and providing therapy. A team comprising the primary care physician, who has an established rapport with the family, and specialists, such as a physical therapist, psychologist, and pain management consultant, may be most effective in providing care even for the challenging patient.

TOOLS FOR PRACTICE

Medical Decision Support

- *Pediatric Chronic Pain* (policy statement), American Pain Society (www.ampainsoc.org/advocacy/pediatric.htm).
- *Pediatric Pain Management for Primary Care, 2nd Edition* (book), American Academy of Pediatrics (www.aap.org/bookstore).
- *Questions to ask parents to evaluate pain* Sabine Kost-Byerly (practice.aap.org/content.aspx?aid=2001).
- *Wong-Baker FACES Pain Rating Scale (questionnaire)*, Wong DL, Baker CM (www.mosbysdrugconsult.com/WOW/faces.html).

AAP POLICY STATEMENTS

American Academy of Pediatrics, Committee on Children with Disabilities. Counseling families who choose complementary and alternative medicine for their child with chronic illness or disability. *Pediatrics.* 2001;107(3):598-601. (aappolicy.aappublications.org/cgi/content/full/pediatrics;107/3/598).

American Academy of Pediatrics, Committee on Bioethics and Committee on Hospital Care. Palliative care for children. *Pediatrics.* 2000;106(2):351-357. (aappolicy.aappublications.org/cgi/content/full/pediatrics;106/2/351).

American Academy of Pediatrics, Committee on the Psychosocial Aspects of Child and Family Health and the Task Force on Pain in Infants, Children, and Adolescents. The assessment and management of acute pain in infants, children, and adolescents. *Pediatrics.* 2001;108(3):793-797. (aappolicy.aappublications.org/cgi/content/full/pediatrics;108/3/793).

REFERENCES

1. Pain terms: a list with definitions and notes on usage. Recommended by the IASP Subcommittee on Taxonomy. *Pain.* 1979;6:249-252.
2. Ghandour RM, Overpeck MD, Huang ZJ, et al. Headache, stomachache, backache, and morning fatigue among adolescent girls in the United States. *Arch Pediatr Adolesc Med.* 2004;158:797-803.
3. Perquin CW, Haseboek-Kampschroeur AA, Hunfeld JA, et al. Pain in children and adolescents: a common experience. *Pain.* 2000;87:51-58.
4. Abu-Arefeh I, Russell G. Prevalence of headaches and migraines in schoolchildren. *BMJ.* 1994;309:765-769.
5. Split W, Neuman W. Epidemiology of migraine among students from randomly selected secondary schools in Lodz. *Headache.* 1999;39:494-501.
6. Roth-Isigkeit A, Thysen U, Stoven H, et al. Pain among children and adolescent: restrictions in daily living and triggering factors. *Pediatrics.* 2005;115:e152-e162.
7. Dunn-Geier BJ, McGrath PJ, Rourke BP, et al. Adolescent chronic pain: the ability to cope. *Pain.* 1986;26:23-32.
8. Beyer JE, Wells N. The assessment of pain in children. *Pediatr Clin North Am.* 1989;36(4):837-854.
9. Wong DL, Baker CM. Pain in children: comparison of assessment scales. *Pediatr Nurs.* 1988;14:9-17.
10. Adib N, Davis K, Grahame R, et al. Joint hypermobility syndrome in childhood. A not so benign multisystem disorder? *Rheumatology.* 2005;44:744-750.
11. American Academy of Pediatrics, Committee on Child Abuse and Neglect and Committee on Children With Disabilities. Assessment of maltreatment of children with disabilities. *Pediatrics.* 2001;108:508-512.
12. American Academy of Pediatrics and the Council on Children with Disabilities. Coordination in the medical home: integrating health and related systems of care for children with special health care needs. *Pediatrics.* 2005;116:1238-1244.
13. Liptak GS, Burns CM, Davidson PW, et al. Effects of providing comprehensive ambulatory services to children with chronic conditions. *Arch Pediatr Adolesc Med.* 1998;152:1003-1008.
14. Criscione T, Walsh KK, Kastner TA. An evaluation of care coordination in controlling inpatient hospital utilization of people with disabilities. *Ment Retard.* 1995;33:364-373.
15. American Academy of Pediatrics, Committee on Children with Disabilities. The pediatrician's role in development and implementation of an individual education plan (IEP) and/or an individual family service plan (IFSP). *Pediatrics.* 1999;104:124-127.
16. Zeltzer L, LeBaron S. Hypnosis and nonhypnotic technique for reduction of pain and anxiety during painful procedures in children and adolescents with cancer. *J Pediatr.* 1982;101:1032-1035.
17. Lambert SA. The effects of hypnosis/guided imagery on the post-operative course of children. *Dev Behav Pediatr.* 1996;17:307-310.
18. Zeltzer LK, Tsao JC, Stelling C, et al. A phase I study on the feasibility and acceptability of an acupuncture/hypnosis intervention for chronic pediatric pain. *J Pain Symptom Manage.* 2002;24:437-446.
19. American Academy of Pediatrics, Committee on Children with Disabilities. Counseling families who choose complementary and alternative medicine for their child with chronic illness or disability. *Pediatrics.* 2001;107:598-601.
20. Berens RJ, Meyer MT, Mikhailov TA, et al. A prospective evaluation of opioid weaning in opioid-dependent pediatric critical care patients. *Anesth Analg.* 2006;102:1045-1050.
21. Federation of the State Medical Boards of the United States, Inc., University of Wisconsin Pain and Policy Studies Group. Model Guidelines for the Use of Controlled Substances for the Treatment of Pain. Available at: www.medsch.wisc.edu/painpolicy/domestic/model.htm. Accessed January 5, 2007.
22. US Department of Justice Drug Enforcement Administration, Office of Diversion Control. Prescription Pain Medications: Frequently Asked Questions and Answers for Health Care Professional and Law Enforcement Personnel. Available at: www.deadiversion.usdoj.gov. Accessed January 5, 2007.
23. McQuay HJ, Tramer M, Nye BA, et al. A systematic review of antidepressants in neuropathic pain. *Pain.* 1996;68:217-227.
24. US Food and Drug Administration. Antidepressant Use in Children, Adolescents, and Adults. Drug Information Web site. Available at: www.fda.gov/cder/drug/antidepressants. Accessed January 5, 2007.

25. Deutsch ES, Nadkarni VM. Clonidine prophylaxis for narcotic and sedative withdrawal syndrome following laryngotracheal reconstruction. *Arch Otolaryngol Head Neck Surg*. 1996;122:1234-1238.
26. Suresh S, Wheeler M, Patel A. Case series: IV regional anesthesia with ketorolac and lidocaine: is it effective for the management of complex regional pain syndrome 1 in children and adolescents? *Anesth Analg*. 2003;96:694-695.
27. American Academy of Pediatrics, Committee on Bioethics and Committee on Hospital Care. Palliative care for children. *Pediatrics*. 2000;106:351-357.
28. Staats PS, Kost-Byerly S. Celiac plexus blockade in a 7-year-old child with neuroblastoma. *J Pain Symptom Manage*. 1995;10:321-324.

Chapter 56

SELF-REGULATION THERAPIES: HYPNOSIS AND BIOFEEDBACK

Denise A. Bothe, MD; Karen N. Olness, MD

Children learn self-hypnosis easily and can apply it to help solve problems such as acute and chronic pain, undesirable habits, anxiety associated with chronic illnesses such as hemophilia or cancer, performance anxiety, and enuresis. The teaching and application of self-hypnosis is enhanced by the addition of biofeedback, which provides proof to the child that changes in thinking result in changes in body responses. Training in hypnosis has been used for many years by athletes and other performers. Children, adolescents, and their families can gain an increased sense of control and participation in their treatment by learning effective coping strategies, such as those available through self-hypnosis, with or without biofeedback.

HISTORY

Hypnosis techniques have been used since the late 18th century. The Franklin Commission, which investigated the claims of Franz Mesmer, included experiments involving children. In the 1840s, two British surgeons, John Elliotson and James Braid, both reported surgical procedures on children during which hypnosis was the sole anesthesia method.[1,2] In the late 19th century, European clinicians reported successfully treating negative habits and pain in children with hypnosis.[3] The first research studies in children using hypnosis were in the 1960s and assessed hypnotizability.[4] Since then, researchers have recognized that children generally learn hypnosis more quickly and easily than do adults. The first use of biofeedback with children was reported in the 1970s, and since the 1970s, increasing research documents the ability of children to use hypnosis, with or without biofeedback, to treat many clinical conditions.[5-7]

Three-day training workshops on hypnosis with children were first taught in 1976 and have been available annually since then. (See Suggested Resources section for workshops offered.)

DEFINITIONS

Hypnosis is defined as a focused state of awareness, sometimes involving relaxation, during which the individual has enhanced ability to facilitate specific physiologic and behavioral outcomes. *Hypnotherapy* is defined as a treatment modality that uses hypnosis by integrating that focused state of awareness into treatment.

Many terms have been used to describe the process of Hypnosis (Box 56-1). *Mesmerism* was the original term used to describe the clinical work of Franz Mesmer. James Braid, an English surgeon, first coined the term *hypnosis*. This designation was unfortunate because *hypnos* came from the Latin root for sleep, implying that the person in hypnosis is asleep. Although such is not the case, hypnosis remains misunderstood. Since then, many other terms (see Box 56-1) such as *self-regulation* and *mind-body skills training* have been used. (*Cyberphysiology* is another term coined in the 1980s to describe these same techniques. The prefix *cyber* is derived from the Greek *kybernan*, which means to steer or take the helm; thus cyberphysiology refers to a person's ability to steer or regulate a physiological or behavioral response.)

Some of the more common misconceptions about hypnosis include the following:

- Hypnotists exert mind control over passive subjects.
- Hypnosis is magic.
- When under hypnosis the person is sleeping.
- Only a few people are able to be hypnotized.

None of these statements is true. The person is fully awake during hypnosis and aware of the environment. The mind and mental imagery of the person using these mind-body skills causes the physiological changes. Although some people find these skills easier to do than other people, anyone can learn self-hypnosis.

Biofeedback is a term coined in 1969 to describe the procedure of using a physiologic response measure, or signal from the body, to give feedback to the person. This feedback increases the awareness of the body and how it is functioning. Biofeedback is a useful tool in training individuals to strengthen their

BOX 56-1 Terms Used to Describe Self-regulation Techniques Involving Hypnosis

Self-hypnosis	Relaxation
Mind-body skills training	Progressive relaxation
Self-regulation	Meditation
Biofeedback	Visual imagery
Diaphragmatic breathing	Guided imagery
	Cyberphysiology

mind-body connection and learn self-regulation skills. Although biofeedback is a useful adjunct, training in biofeedback requires self-hypnosis instructions, which lead to the desired physiological changes.

Measure of physiologic response include skin temperature, galvanic skin resistance (GSR) or electrodermal activity, electroencephalographic (EEG) data, breathing, heart rate, and heart rate variability. Simple skin-temperature monitors make a cheap and effective biofeedback tool. Nocturnal enuresis alarms are essentially biofeedback tools. The Mind Body Computer Game is specifically designed for children, and it uses appealing images on the computer screen to direct children to change the image by changing their thinking. A sensor connected to the computer measures GSR, and these changes are reflected in computer image changes. For example, a computer-generated animal will smile as the child becomes more relaxed.

Another computer program that was originally designed for adults and has also been successful with children is the Freeze Framer program (www.heartmath.com) (Figure 56-1). A finger sensor connected to the computer measures the heart rate variability. As the person relaxes, the image on the computer screen gives positive feedback. For example, a hot-air balloon floats up and across a field as the player relaxes. This program calculates heart rate variability and shows the patient and practitioner how well the patient was able to relax. This feedback can then be compared with other sessions from the same patient to determine progress.

COMMON GROUND

Health professionals use many terms such as *imagery, relaxation imagery, progressive relaxation,* and *meditation,* among others, all of which refer to the same process by which hypnosis is induced. Although great confusion and disagreement exists in the definitions of the variety of terms used, common ground can be found among terms. For example, hypnosis often uses relaxation and imagery techniques, and biofeedback can be used to augment a person's body-physiological awareness during hypnosis. In addition, imagery and relaxation techniques, which are hypnosis methods, are used in biofeedback to help increase the person's focus and awareness. Culbert and colleagues describe current thoughts on the biofeedback-hypnosis interface and the rationale for integrating these self-regulation or cyberphysiologic techniques with children and adolescents.[8] These skills all foster empowerment, mastery, and self-control. Many athletes use these skills to improve performance, and many patients have used them to improve their health and body functions.

GUIDELINES FOR LEARNING AND TEACHING SELF-HYPNOSIS

Before training a child in self-regulation skills, the child health professional should prepare the child and family (Box 56-2). The choice of strategies for teaching self-hypnosis to children varies, depending on the child's age and developmental stage, the preferred type of mental imagery (ie, visual, auditory, kinesthetic, olfactory), learning style, preferred activities, dislikes, and personality. The child health professional who provides coaching or teaching of hypnosis should emphasize that the child is in control and can choose when and where to use self-hypnosis. The child health professional should be knowledgeable about the basic problem of the child before embarking on a hypnotherapeutic intervention. For example, a general pediatrician should be able to assess whether all necessary diagnostic tests have been completed for the presenting problems of headache or enuresis before offering training in self-hypnosis. A general pediatrician would not teach self-hypnosis to a child with posttraumatic stress

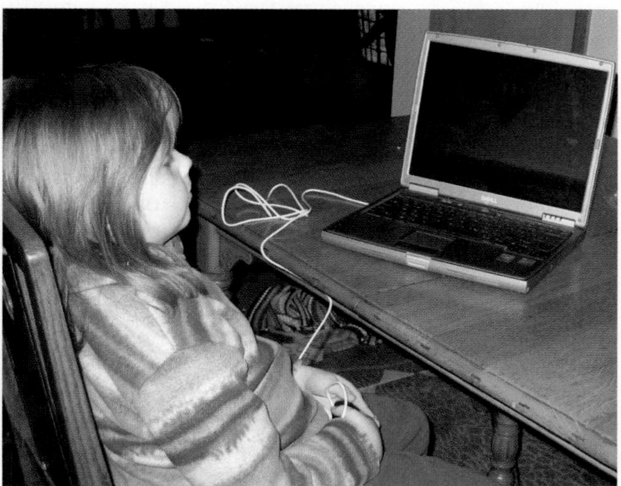

Figure 56-1 Biofeedback program measures heart rate variability through a finger sensor connected to the child's finger.

BOX 56-2 When Teaching a Child Self-regulation Techniques

1. Understand the problem with a thorough diagnostic evaluation, as well as the limitations of the problem on the child and the significance of symptoms for the family.
2. Understand the child by learning about the child's personality, interests, likes, dislikes, developmental stage, and about any learning disabilities.
3. Emphasize the need for practice by explaining that becoming proficient in self-hypnosis requires practice as learning, for example, a sport or music skill.
4. Emphasize that the child is the client, not the parent; thus parents should not remind their child to practice.
5. Throughout the process, emphasize the child's control because the child learning that the *child being in control* is the principle key to success.

From Kohen DP, Olness KN. Self-regulation therapy: helping children help themselves. *Ambul Child Health.* 1996;2:43-58. Used by permission of Blackwell Publishing Ltd.

BOX 56-3 Techniques to Help a Child Focus and Relax

Learning may include:

- Deep breathing
- Relaxation (eg, progressive muscle relaxation)
- Mental imagery
- Guided imagery
- Therapeutic suggestions
- Adjunct biofeedback

disorder (PTSD) unless the clinician were working closely with a child psychiatrist or psychologist who was experienced in assessment and treatment of PTSD.

Training in self-hypnosis is helpful to a clinician interested in using these skills to help children. Much can be learned about language used to promote mind-body control and self-confidence in a child. The language used should be permissive, allowing the child to feel a sense of control. However, many techniques that use mind-body or hypnosis methods can be used in a primary care setting without formal training. Understanding a child's needs, increasing the child's understanding of mind-body control, and helping the child feel comfortable will promote a sense of control and will increase the child's ability to regulate his or her body and behavior. Techniques that help a child focus and relax may be taught as part of hypnosis (Box 56-3). Deep breathing, often called diaphragmatic breathing, or *belly breathing,* is a powerful way to focus the person's attention and start the relaxation process. Progressive muscle relaxation is useful for older children who understand the instructions. Young children may respond better to *becoming floppy* as they relax. An article written by Leora Kuttner[9] describes strategies for working with preschool children in pediatric practice.

Imagery techniques work best when the clinician has an understanding of the child's developmental stage, likes, dislikes, and fears. The clinician should help children choose relaxation and imagery methods that suits them. The child should practice 10 minutes twice daily for 1 month then once daily for the second month. Because biofeedback and hypnosis are designed to promote self-control, the parents should not remind their child to practice; children should develop their own reminder system (eg, a ribbon around the neck of a favorite stuffed animal). Adding a biofeedback measure (eg, to monitor pulse and heart rate variability or peripheral temperature or GSR) may help the child improve. An audiotape may also be an effective reinforcer.

CLINICAL APPLICATIONS

Mind-body interventions constitute a major portion of the overall use of complementary and alternative medicine by the public. In 2002, five relaxation techniques and imagery, biofeedback, and hypnosis, taken together, were used by more than 30% of the adult US population.[10]

BOX 56-4 Clinical Applications of Child Hypnosis

- Pain:
  - Acute (eg, injury, illness, procedural)
  - Chronic or recurrent (eg, chronic illness, disability, trauma, recurrent procedures)
- Habit problems and disorders (eg, thumb sucking, nail biting, hair pulling [trichotillomania], habit coughs, tics)
- Behavioral problems (eg, attention problems, anger management)
- Medical-biobehavioral disorders (eg, asthma, migraine, Tourette syndrome, inflammatory bowel disease, warts, pruritus)
- Anxiety (eg, performance [examinations, stage fright, sports], anxiety disorders, PTSD, phobias)
- Psychophysiologic problems (eg, enuresis, encopresis, conditioned nausea and vomiting, irritable bowel syndrome, sleep disorders)
- Chronic disease, multisystem disease, terminal illness (eg, cancer, hemophilia, AIDS, cystic fibrosis, diabetes, chronic renal disease)

From Kohen DP, Olness KN. Self-regulation therapy: helping children help themselves. *Ambul Child Health.* 1996;2:43-58. Used by permission of Blackwell Publishing Ltd.

Hypnosis and biofeedback are generally categorized in the mind-body aspects of complementary and alternative medicine; however, increasingly, medical institutions are considering hypnosis and biofeedback as part of mainstream medicine. Pediatricians and other health care professionals see many children who exhibit symptoms of high stress levels, including such symptoms as anxiety, depression, headaches, abdominal pain, and school avoidance. Children and parents often feel out of control, with busy lives, worries, or chronic health problems. Children and adolescents may attempt to cope in self-injurious ways, such as with the use of alcohol, nicotine, and drugs.

A thorough medical evaluation should precede hypnosis, with or without biofeedback treatment. Children referred for integrative treatment may not have had adequate diagnostic evaluations. In a study that reviewed 200 cases of children referred specifically for treatment with hypnosis, biofeedback, or both, 25% had unrecognized biologic bases for symptoms such as enuresis, headache, anxiety, and recurrent abdominal pain.[11] Some of the children referred for hypnosis to control headaches proved to have sinusitis, food allergies, brain tumor, and carbon monoxide poisoning.

Children have been taught self-hypnosis for a wide range of problems (Box 56-4). The mind-body skills learned with hypnosis can give a child the capacity to change attitudes, emotions, and behavior, habits, autonomic reactivity, and biological functions. This self-regulation offers techniques that facilitate a their ability to:

- Direct their behavior.
- Modulate physiological changes in desired directions.

- Control their thoughts for the purpose of symptom control.
- Attain and maintain health and wellness.
- Improve function or enhance performance.

PAIN MANAGEMENT

Pain is a subjective experience, and children exhibit different tolerance levels. Hypnosis techniques can be used for pain control, for example, in emergency rooms[12] or for children with cancer who are undergoing procedures.[13] When in acute pain, children are in a more focused state of awareness and are highly motivated to feel better. Because of this motivation, they may be more likely to respond to suggestions that increase their sense of control, which they can then use to decrease their sensation of pain. Helping children *dissociate* by imagining that they are in a favorite place can have a calming effect. In some situations, such as a first time migraine headache, it can be difficult to work with a child who is acutely miserable. While not always possible, it is preferable overall to teach children these techniques when they are well, allowing them to prepare themselves for the possible acute episode. Some of these effective self-regulatory techniques are described in the literature.[14]

Chronic pain and recurrent pain are more difficult to manage than acute pain. A child who experiences pain over a long period or learns to expect the pain to return again and again may become increasingly anxious and develop feelings of hopelessness. Teaching self-regulation is more complicated in these situations because of the need to address the severity and the negative expectancy that accompanies chronic pain. It has been shown[15] that children will benefit more and require less training if they are offered training very early, ideally within a few days, after diagnosis of a chronic or life threatening disease. "No Fears No Tears"[16] and "No Fears No Tears 13 Years Later,"[17] are two video productions that illustrate the use of self regulation strategies with children who have cancer.

If the self-regulatory techniques seem ineffective for the child with chronic or recurrent pain, then the clinician should reevaluate the situation. The pain may be serving a protective psychological purpose. Significant mental health issues, such as PTSD, depression, or abuse may exist, and psychotherapeutic evaluation and intervention may be needed. (See Case Report, Box 56-5.)

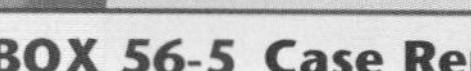

BOX 56-5 Case Report

Sarah, a 6-year-old girl, was brought to the pediatrician by her mother because of severe abdominal pain of 2 months' duration. The pains started suddenly 1 day in the morning after breakfast and before school. They occurred many mornings of the week and lasted for 1 to 2 hours. Sarah would clutch her stomach and double over with pain. She did not have vomiting or diarrhea or fever. After the pain resolved, each day she appeared healthy. She had no history of constipation. Medical work-up was negative for any medical causes of her pain.

A complete history revealed that Sarah did not want to go to school. She was afraid because a classmate on her school bus was saying things to scare her. The abdominal pain kept her home and protected her from the child who was scaring her.

Sarah's pediatrician spoke with her mother about addressing this issue with school officials and then asked Sarah if she wanted to learn a way to help herself prevent the pain from arising and decrease the intensity when it did occur. Sarah was interested. She liked dolls and stuffed animals; thus she was asked if she had one that was very soft and squishy, and she did. Sarah was taught to take slow deep breaths "into her belly," and then advised to "make her belly very soft" as her squishy stuffed animal. This exercise would help her belly work better and prevent the pain from coming. Sarah demonstrated in the office that she was able to perform this task. She was then advised to practice this deep breathing and making her belly soft at home. (This teaching took approximately 5 minutes of the office visit.)

One month later, Sarah's mother brought her back for a well-child check. Sarah had only one more episode of abdominal pain after learning how to relax herself and her abdomen. She has not had similar recurrent abdominal pains since. Sarah's mother also addressed the issue of the child who was scaring her by talking to the principal, teacher, and bus driver. Sarah now enjoys going to school and does well with her friends and schoolwork.

HABIT DISORDERS

Habit problems are common in children. Habit problems such as thumb sucking, nail biting, hair pulling (trichtillomania), or habitual cough are potentially responsive to hypnotherapy. In a retrospective study, a significant number of children with habit cough responded well to hypnosis with resolution of their symptoms of cough.[18]

Some types of habits, such as tics or hair pulling, often begin during a stressful experience and initially carry with them emotional significance. In most instances, the emotional significance disappears, yet the habit remains. Habits such as habitual cough may begin with an upper respiratory infection but persist long after the infection is gone; others such as thumb sucking may have begun as a comfort measure in young childhood and have became habitual. As long as no motivation exists behind the habit (eg, if the habit helps the child avoid school) and the child is motivated to change (not just the parent), hypnosis techniques are effective in extinguishing the habit. Emphasizing the child's control in mastering the problem is crucial to success in eliminating the problem.

ENURESIS

Before considering hypnotherapy for enuresis, the clinician should distinguish whether the enuresis is primary or secondary and whether the enuresis occurs day and night or night only. (See Chapter 261, Enuresis.) Organic causes such as urinary tract infection, diabetes, or constipation must be ruled out. Primary enuresis may be considered a maturational issue, whereas secondary enuresis, after a period of dryness, may be associated with a significant stressor in the child's life. Enuresis that has no organic cause is expected to resolve spontaneously over time. Depending on the age of the child, enuresis can be quite

BOX 56-6 Case Report

Dan, age 16, was referred to learn self-hypnosis for control of test anxiety. He had been an excellent student during all his school years until a year earlier when he began to perform poorly on examinations. No changes occurred in his studying habits. He did very well on homework. No family changes had occurred. He got along well with two older siblings, both of whom are now in college. Dan had a girlfriend, a classmate, who was also a good student and was looking forward to college.

Dan's mother described him as having always been *perfectionistic.* She said that he began expressing worry about examinations when his older brother was taking student aptitude tests. Dan said that he studied and felt that he knew the material but that he froze during the examinations and was unable to think clearly. He also said that he slept poorly on the night before examinations.

Dan said that he enjoyed reading, drawing, playing computer games, swimming, and soccer. He said that his dream was to become an architect. He said that he had been afraid of dogs when a young child but this was no longer so. Dan also said he got approximately 6 hours of sleep a night on school nights and slept 10 to 12 hours a night on weekends.

The pediatrician explained to Dan that she was able to teach him self-hypnosis to reduce test anxiety and that his daily practice would be required. She described the use of self-hypnosis by Olympic athletes and the type of practice that was required. The pediatrician emphasized that Dan's parents were not allowed to remind him to practice. Dan said that he wished to learn and was willing to practice.

The pediatrician taught Dan a self-hypnosis method involving progressive relaxation and focus on a winning soccer game. She asked that he practice this method twice daily and return in a week. When Dan returned, he said he had been practicing regularly. At this visit, Dan was hooked to a temperature sensor and was able to watch a screen that demonstrated the increase in his peripheral temperature as he relaxed and achieved self-hypnosis. The pediatrician then taught him specific suggestions to use before his examinations, including suggestions related to sleeping well, and to include future programming of pleasant events associated with successful examinations.

Dan continued to practice daily and was followed up by telephone every 2 weeks for 2 months. At that time, Dan had no further test anxiety, was achieving high scores on tests, and had good grades.

frustrating and interfere with activities, such as sleep-overs. Children with nocturnal enuresis often feel shame or guilt. Various methods have been used for children and parents who wish to stop enuresis, such as motivational behavior management (including the child in cleanup of the wet bed, bedwetting alarms) and medications such as imiprimine and desmopressin. Hypnotherapy is helpful for many children with enuresis. In a study that compared two groups of children treated with hypnotherapy versus imiprimine, comparable results were seen with each group. At long-term follow-up, the group treated with hypnotherapy had a significantly larger positive response.[19] Drugs such as imipramine can have significant side effects and can be life threatening. Desmopressin has negligible known side effects, but some parents are reluctant to give their child medication. The bedwetting alarm is a type of conditioning device and is quite effective, although some children find the alarm to be aversive. Hypnosis as a treatment is at least equivalent, has longer duration, and is not potentially life threatening. When considering choice of treatment for enuresis, self-regulation therapy or hypnosis is the least invasive, and many children respond favorably.

BEHAVIORAL AND ATTENTION DISORDERS

Self-regulation has value as an adjunct in management of behavioral problems. In addition to therapeutic interventions, such as counseling and behavioral modification, teaching self-regulation techniques to a child can be a constructive way to build self-esteem and more effectively control the maladaptive behaviors. Attention-deficit/hyperactivity disorder is one of the most common behavioral problems encountered in children. Recommended management usually involves behavioral modification and primarily stimulant medication. Recent studies with biofeedback and hypnosis techniques have demonstrated beneficial effects of EEG biofeedback on measures of intelligence, on behavioral rating scales assessing the frequency of core symptoms of attention-deficit/hyperactivity disorder, on computerized tests of attention (eg, the Test of Variables of Attention [TOVA]), and on quantitative EEG measures of cortical arousal.[20] This training may prove to be as effective as stimulant medication for the treatment of attentional problems in children.

STRESS MANAGEMENT AND ANXIETY

Self-regulation skills are an excellent way to manage stress. Relaxation and hypnosis are useful for helping children and adolescents with anxiety. (See Case Report, Box 56-6.)

With children who have an anxiety disorder, such as general anxiety, separation anxiety, or selective mutism, hypnosis techniques can be a useful adjunct along with therapeutic counseling.

MEDICAL PROBLEMS

Some diseases respond well to self-regulation techniques. One group of diseases can be classified into biobehavioral disorders in that they have clear pathophysiological origins, as well as significant

BOX 56-7 Case Report—Migraine Headache

Anne, an 11-year-old girl, had a history of migraine headaches for 3 years. Her mother also had migraines since childhood. Anne was evaluated by a child neurologist who, at various times, had prescribed propranolol, Periactin, and Elavil. He also suggested regular sleep and avoidance of certain foods.

Anne did well in school and had many friends. She enjoyed music and played the piano. She had two younger siblings, ages 8 and 6. She said that she was afraid of thunder.

At the initial visit, Anne was having a migraine episode at least once a week. Most episodes were preceded by a visual aura, and they lasted approximately 12 hours. They were accompanied by nausea and sometimes vomiting. Anne said that she would sleep as soon as possible after a migraine began and would usually awaken without the pain with a shaky feeling for several hours thereafter.

Anne was interested in learning self-hypnosis for control of her migraines. Anne chose to focus on music for her hypnotic induction. She imagined favorite music as she gradually relaxed all of her muscles. She did well during the 1st practice.

At her second visit, Anne's finger temperature was monitored during her examination. Her peripheral temperature increased 4°F during this practice, proof that she was relaxing. She learned about pain signals and was offered options for turning the signals off if she should develop a migraine episode.

The third visit took place 3 weeks later. Anne had one migraine during that period, a significant decrease. Subsequently, she was followed up by telephone. In the 6-month follow-up period, she had two migraine episodes, both associated with sleep deprivation.

BOX 56-8 Case Report—Warts

Warts are another common condition seen in primary care pediatrics. Warts are reported to respond to many interventions and often resolve by themselves. In many intances, children will undergo numerous topical treatments without success or with recurrence. Many case studies of successful wart treatment using hypnotherapy have been conducted.*

David, age 7, had warts on his hands and legs for 2 years. He had been treated by a dermatologist with topical treatments and freezing the warts. Each time, the warts recurred. David had three warts on his left leg, three on the right leg, two on the left hand, and five on the right hand.

David was in second grade. He enjoys school and has friends in both school and the neighborhood. He likes bicycle riding, playing soccer, and ice skating.

David has an older sister and a younger brother. He said he wanted to get rid of the warts because he did not like the way they looked and because the previous treatments hurt.

David was told that many children had eliminated warts by doing a relaxation exercise and giving a message to themselves to stop feeding the warts. He was told about practice at home and about the need for a good reminder system for the practice; his mother was told not to remind him to practice.

David imagined himself playing soccer as a hypnotic induction and was asked to imagine playing until the game was won. Then, he should tell himself to stop feeding each of the 13 warts.

David returned in 2 weeks. At this point, David had seven warts and was very pleased. He continued practice for another month, and 12 of the warts were gone. No new warts appeared. After 3 months, all the warts were gone.

*Felt BT, Hall H, Olness K, et al. Wart regression in children: comparison of relaxation imagery to topical treatment and equal time interventions. *Am J Clin Hypn.* Oct 1998;41(2):130-137.

psychoemotional components. Examples of these conditions include asthma, migraine, and irritable bowel syndrome. Relaxation and self-hypnosis with these problems help promote a sense of self-control and a reduction of symptoms.

Children and adolescents with asthma can learn self-hypnosis to reduce wheezing in acute episodes. Research using hypnosis, both with and without biofeedback, has demonstrated decreased functional morbidity, with fewer emergency room visits, fewer missed school days, and a better sense of control in children who were taught to use these techniques.[21]

Children with migraine headaches have been shown to respond well, with a significant decrease in frequency of their headaches after self-regulation training, when compared with propranolol and placebo.[22] (See Case Reports, Boxes 56-7 and 56-8.)

DIABETES

A child with diabetes must cope with frequent blood tests, a special diet, and daily injections. When a child with diabetes feels out of control, compliance with diet and medicines can prove inadequate. Hypnotherapy can provide a child with a way to learn to cope and gain a sense of mastery, both of which may help reduce anxiety and improve compliance.

MEDICAL PROCEDURES

Medical procedures are usually a source of anxiety for children and are often painful. These procedures include routine immunization injections, venipuncture, and pelvic examinations. Reductions in anxiety and pain have been noted in children who were taught skills using hypnosis techniques.[23] A randomized controlled study assessing the effects of hypnosis on distress of children undergoing a voiding cystourethrogram procedure found significant reductions in distress for the group of children that received hypnosis.[24]

HYPNOSIS IN THE ROUTINE PEDIATRIC OFFICE VISIT

Integrating self-regulation techniques into primary care practice[25] offers the opportunity for child health professionals to facilitate a sense of mastery and competency in the children under their care. Although many clinicians may not realize it, they have long been applying some of the hypnotic principles and using some of the sensitive language in their clinical work with children. In an introductory course on hypnosis, clinicians become aware of the importance of carefully selecting their language and monitoring the timing and pacing with which to introduce new words in their encounters with children. Clinicians often realize that integrating these techniques will be easier and faster than they may have originally believed.[26]

Brief self-regulation interventions can be integrated into primary care practice. Following are some examples of simple techniques that can be used to make a child more comfortable during routine office procedures, such as receiving shots, or throat cultures, or just being examined by a *stranger.*

- Having a child *blow away* pain by using a pinwheel, bubbles, or a pretend candle is an effective tool for decreasing a child's experience of pain during injections or venipuncture.
- Bubbles can also be used to get the attention of the young child who starts screaming as soon as the clinician walks into the room and to help the child to feel more comfortable.
- A stuffed animal or doll can be used as an example before examining a child. By pointing out how the doll or stuffed animal is comfortable being examined, the child is often more comfortable when being examined.
- Slow deep breaths while focusing on a pleasant thought may help the child who needs a throat culture to keep still with the child's mouth open.
- Favorite music can also be a nice way to help the child focus and relax during procedures.

How can the child health practitioner learn to use hypnosis in the practice?

1. *Take a basic 3-day hypnosis-training workshop.* See Suggested Resources section.
2. *Identify and stay in touch with a mentor after the first workshop.* Most of the workshops will offer mentoring assistance to encourage the new learner and provide advice regarding clinical situations. Workshops also have an active list-serve resource for child health professionals who share knowledge about hypnosis with children.
3. *Take follow-up workshops, to read textbooks and hypnosis journals, and attend annual hypnosis scientific meetings.*
4. *Take board-certified examination in hypnosis.* Tests from the American Boards of Medical Hypnosis, Hypnosis in Psychology, Hypnosis in Dentistry, and Hypnosis in Social Work are available. Information can be obtained from the American Society of Clinical Hypnosis or the Society for Clinical and Experimental Hypnosis.

RESEARCH IN CHILD HYPNOSIS

Active research in child hypnosis has taken place over the last 40 years. Initial research work studied measures of child hypnotic susceptibility, such as the Stanford Children's Hypnotic Susceptibility Scale.[27] Most subsequent research has been clinical research that documents the efficacy of hypnosis with children in areas such as pain management, habit problems, wart reduction, and performance anxiety. The variability in preferences, learning styles, and developmental stages complicates the design of research protocols, which study hypnosis with children. These protocols are often written to describe identical hypnotic inductions, often recorded, to be used at prescribed times. Measured variables do not include whether a child likes the induction, listens to the tape, or whether the child focuses on entirely different mental imagery of the child's own choosing. Furthermore, learning disabilities are often subtle and may not be recognized without detailed testing that is not usually done before research studies involving child hypnosis. Learning disabilities, such as auditory processing handicaps, may interfere with the ability of children to learn and remember self-hypnosis training. Each of these variables complicates efforts to perform meta-analyses on hypnosis and related interventions. Interventions called *relaxation imagery, imagery, visual imagery,* or *progressive relaxation* each lead to a hypnotic state. The proper analysis of studies on efficacy of hypnosis in children should be to combine all studies that describe strategies that induce hypnosis in children.

Some research studies are defined as controlled but mix therapeutic interventions. For example, Scharff, Marcus, and Masek[28] reported on "A controlled study of minimal contact thermal biofeedback treatment in children with migraine." Children were randomly assigned to thermal biofeedback, attention, or wait-list control groups. The hand-warming biofeedback group received four sessions of cognitive behavioral stress management training, thermal biofeedback, progressive muscle relaxation, imagery training of warm places, and deep-breathing techniques. Thus children were also being taught self-hypnosis.

Several controlled laboratory studies have demonstrated that an association exists between learning self-hypnosis and changes in humoral or cellular immunity (or both) in children. In one study, Karen Olness and colleagues[29] examined the self-regulation of salivary immunoglobulin A by children, which demonstrates that self hypnosis can facilitate some immunomodulation in children. This work was the basis for a clinical trial by Hewson-Bower, who demonstrated that training in self hypnosis for children with frequent upper respiratory infections resulted in a reduction of infectious episodes and fewer illness days if upper respiratory infections did occur.[30]

The International Society of Hypnosis is currently sponsoring Cochrane reviews of hypnotherapeutic interventions, including those with children.

TOOLS FOR PRACTICE

Medical Decision Support

- *Imaginative Medicine: Hypnosis in Pediatric Practice* (video), Laurence Sugarman, MD, FAAP (www.laurencesugarman.com/doc/order.php).
- *No Fears, No Tears* (video), Leora Kuttner, PhD (www.fanlight.com/catalog/films/286_nfnt.php).
- *No Fears, No Tears—13 Years Later* (video), Leora Kuttner, PhD (www.fanlight.com/catalog/films/277_nfnt.php).

- *Provisional Section on Complementary, Holistic, and Integrative Medicine Mind-Body articles* (Web page), American Academy of Pediatrics (www.aap.org/sections/chim/P&R-Mind.htm).

RELATED WEB SITES

- *American Society of Clinical Hypnosis* (Web page), American Society of Clinical Hypnosis (www.asch.net/).
- *Hypnosis Workshop* (Web page), Society for Developmental and Behavioral Pediatrics (www.sdbp.org/).
- *International Society of Hypnosis* (Web page), International Society of Hypnosis (www.ish-web.org/page.php).

SUGGESTED RESOURCES

Training Organizations

Society for Developmental and Behavioral Pediatrics, www.sdbp.org.

Society for Clinical and Experimental Hypnosis. www.sceh.us/.

American Society of Clinical Hypnosis (training workshops bimonthly), www.asch.net.

REFERENCES

1. Elliotson J. *Numerous Cases of Surgical Operations Without Pain in the Mesmeric State*. Philadelphia, PA: Lea and Blanchard; 1843.
2. Braid J. *Neurypnology, or the Rationale of Nervous Sleep*. New York, NY: Julian Press; 1960 (original publication 1843).
3. Bramwell JM. *Hypnotism: Its history, Practice, and Theory*. New York, NY: Julian Press; 1903 (reissued with new introduction 1956).
4. London P. *Children's Hypnotic Susceptibility Scale*. Palo Alto, CA: Consulting Psychologists Press; 1963.
5. Miller NE. Learning of visceral and glandular responses. *Science*. 1969;163:434-445.
6. Brown B. *New Mind, New Body*. New York, NY: Harper and Row; 1974.
7. Dikel W, Olness K. Self-hypnosis, biofeedback, ad voluntary peripheral temperature control in children. *Pediatrics*. 1980;66:335-340.
8. Culbert TP, Reaney JB, Kohen DP. "Cyberphysiologic" strategies for children: the clinical hypnosis/biofeedback interface. *Int J Clin Exp Hypn*. 1994 Apr;42(2):97-117.
9. Kuttner L. Helpful strategies in working with pre-school children in pediatric practice. *Pediatr Ann*. 1991;20(3): 120-127.
10. Wolsko PM, Eisenberg DM, Davis RB, et al. Use of mind-body medical therapies. *J Gen Intern Med*. 2004;19(1):43-50.
11. Olness K, Libbey P. Unrecognized biological basis of behavioral symptoms in pediatric patients referred for hypnotherapy. *Am J Clin Hypn*. 1987;30:1.
12. Kohen DP. Applications of relaxation mental imagery (self-hypnosis) in pediatric emergencies. *Int J Clin Exp Hypn*. 1986;34:283-294.
13. LeBaron S, Hilgard JR. *Hypnotherapy of Pain in Children with Cancer*. Los Altos, CA: William Kaufman; 1984.
14. Kuttner L. *A Child in Pain: How to Help, What to Do*. Point Roberts, WA: Hartley and Marks; 1996.
15. Olness KN, Kohen DP. Hypnosis and Hypnotherapy with Children. 3rd ed. New York, NY: Guilford Press; 1996.
16. Kuttner L. *No Fears, No Tears: Children with Cancer Coping with Pain* [30 minute video and manual]. Vancouver, British Columbia, Canada: Canadian Cancer Society; 1986.
17. Kuttner L. *No Fears No Tears 13 Years Later*. Vancouver, British Columbia, Canada: Canadian Cancer Society; 1999.
18. Anbar RD, Hall HR. Childhood habit cough treated with self-hypnosis. *J Pediatr*. Feb 2004;144(2):213-217.
19. Banjeree S, Srivastav A, Palan B. Hypnosis and self-hypnosis in the management of nocturnal enuresis: a comparative study with imipramine therapy. *Am J Clin Hypn*. 1993;36(2):113-119.
20. Monastra VJ, Lynn S, Linden M, et al. Electroencephalographic biofeedback in the treatment of attention-deficit/hyperactivity disorder. *Appl Psychophysiol Biofeedback*. 2005;30(2):95-113.
21. Kohen DP. Relaxation/mental imagery (self-hypnosis) for childhood asthma: behavioral outcomes in a prospective controlled study. HYPNOS. *Swed J Hypn Psychother Psychosom Med*. 1995;22:133-144.
22. Olness KN, MacDonald JT, Uden DL. Comparison of self-hypnosis and propranolol in the treatment of juvenile classic migraine. *Pediatrics*. 1987;79:593-597.
23. Olness KN, Kohen DP. *Hypnosis and Hypnotherapy with Children*. 3rd ed. New York, NY: Guilford Press; 1996.
24. Butler LD, Symons BK, Henderson SL, et al. Hypnosis reduces distress and duration of an invasive medical procedure for children. *Pediatrics*. 2005;115:77-85.
25. Sugarman LI. Hypnosis in a primary care practice: developing skills for the new morbidities. *J Dev Behav Pediatr*. 1996;17:300-306.
26. Kohen DP, Olness KN. Self-regulation therapy: helping children help themselves. *Ambul Child Health*. 1996;2: 43-58.
27. London P. *Children's Hypnotic Susceptibility Scale*. Palo Alto, CA: Consulting Psychologists Press; 1963.
28. Scharff L, Marcus D, Masek B. A controlled study of minimal-contact thermal biofeedback treatment in children with migraine. *J Pediatr Psychol*. 2002;27(2): 109-119.
29. Olness KN, Culbert T, Uden D. Self regulation of salivary immunoglobulin A by children. *Pediatrics*. 1989;83:66-71.
30. Hewson-Bower B. *Psychological Treatment Decreases Colds and Flu in Children by Increasing Salivary IgA* [thesis]. Murdoch University, Perth, Western Australia: 1995.

Chapter 57

COMPLEMENTARY AND ALTERNATIVE MEDICAL THERAPIES

Gregory A. Plotnikoff, MD, MTS; Kathi J. Kemper, MD, MPH; Timothy P. Culbert, MD

Interest in complementary and alternative medicine (CAM) has redefined modern Western medicine. Formerly unconventional therapies such as acupuncture, biofeedback, guided imagery, and hypnotherapy have been integrated into pediatric care in many clinics and hospitals (see Chapter 56, Self-Regulation Therapies: Hypnosis and Biofeedback). Other nonpharmaceutical therapies such as herbs, dietary supplements, massage, and chiropractic care are widely used by the public and are increasingly available at conventional hospitals. Formal definitions of health care quality now acknowledge the importance of respecting spirituality and culturally based healing traditions in daily practice.

In the 2001 American Academy of Pediatrics periodic survey of fellows, most pediatricians reported that they have limited knowledge of CAM and desired to know more. Seventy percent of pediatricians reported having patients who use complementary and alternative therapies. Fifty-one percent reported that they were concerned that CAM use by patients might delay standard medical care, and 36% were concerned that CAM use occasionally impairs physician-patient communication. However, fewer than 20% of pediatricians routinely ask about the use of CAM therapies. Most (83%) wanted to learn more about complementary and alternative therapies so they might appropriately counsel families interested in them.[1]

Similarly, most parents report the desire to discuss CAM with their pediatrician. This group includes more than 80% of those who use CAM for their children. However, fewer than one half of these parents report having done so.[2] Lack of communication may compromise the quality of pediatric care.

Pediatricians do not need to be content experts on CAM, nor do they need to reject their training in biomedicine or critical thinking. However, the tremendous growth in demand for CAM plus parental use of the Internet and mass media for health information suggests the necessity for new competencies in pediatric care. These disciplines include the capacity to:

- Inquire regarding CAM use
- Counsel on CAM from an evidence-based perspective
- Partner with and refer appropriately to CAM practitioners

This chapter defines CAM and describes how to inquire, how to counsel, and how to partner and refer. For physicians who seek further skills development, this chapter also cites additional physician training opportunities.

WHAT IS COMPLEMENTARY AND ALTERNATIVE MEDICINE?

CAM includes all health care systems, therapies, and products that are not considered part of conventional medicine as practiced in the United States. These therapies can be used to supplement conventional care, thus the term *complementary*, or used in place of conventional care, hence the term *alternative*.

Integrative medicine is the preferred term because it incorporates both conventional medicine and complementary and alternative therapies for which sufficient evidence of safety and efficacy exist. The Consortium of Academic Health Centers for Integrative Medicine, which consists of 36 prominent medical schools, further defines integrative medicine as

> ... the practice of medicine that reaffirms the importance of the relationship between practitioner and patient, focuses on the whole person, is informed by evidence, and makes use of all appropriate therapeutic approaches, health care professionals and disciplines to achieve optimal health and healing.[3]

More so than with conventional medicine, this understanding emphasizes the centrality of the therapeutic relationship, the importance of prevention, and the healing power of nature. Integrative medicine seeks to use the best of scientifically based medical therapies whenever appropriate but provide compassion and attention to the patient's spiritual and emotional needs, as well as appropriate complementary and alternative approaches when they enhance conventional medicine.[4]

The National Institutes of Health's 2001 survey of 31,044 adults assessed and ranked the use of 5 categories of CAM. In order of prevalence of use by adults, these categories are (1) mind-body medicine, (2) biologically based therapies, (3) manipulative and body-based methods, (4) alternative medical systems, and (5) energy therapies.

Mind-Body Medicine

Mind-body medicine includes all therapies that activate emotional, mental, social, spiritual, and behavioral factors to modulate positively physiological mechanisms, including immune and endocrinologic function.[5] Over 35 years ago, Green, Green, and Walters stated that

> ... every change in the physiologic state is accompanied by an appropriate change in the mental-emotional state, conscious or unconscious, and every change in the mental-emotional state is accompanied by an appropriate change in the physiologic state.[6]

The bidirectional influences of mind on body and body on mind can have significant mediating effects, both positive and negative, on health outcomes for children. Broadly considered, mind-body therapies include relaxation, stress management, yoga, hypnosis, guided imagery, biofeedback, prayer, meditation, music therapy, support groups, and psychological therapies such as cognitive behavioral therapy. In the last 20 years, mind-body therapies have become recognized as safe and effective for many pediatric conditions, including headaches, asthma, enuresis, sleep problems, pain, and stress-related symptoms.[7-13]

According to the National Institutes of Health, spiritual and religious practices such as prayer represent the most prevalent complementary therapies in the United States. More than twice as many US adults use prayer for health and healing than use herbal medicines.[14] Nearly 80% of US adults believe that religion, to a large extent, helps patients and families cope with illness.[15] Nearly 75% of the public believes that praying for someone else can help cure that person's illness, and 56% of adults state that faith has helped them recover from illness, injury, or disease.[16] Spirituality may or may not involve formal religion. Spiritual concerns arise in clinical settings when important connections with self, with others, with nature, and with a higher power are threatened or disrupted. Spiritual beliefs are frequently important in medical decisions.[17] Spiritual well being is closely linked to successful coping,[18] faster recovery,[19] and higher quality of life.[20] Many patients may want help with meaning, hope, or overcoming fears[21]; and unmet spiritual needs are associated with despair[22] and increased mortality.[23] Parents often have significant spiritual needs around the life-threatening illness or death of a child.[24]

Music and music therapy—the intentional use of melody, rhythm, harmony, timbre, form, and style for healing—are important nonpharmaceutical regulators of physiological, social, and psychological well being. In premature infants, music therapy has been shown to increase oxygen saturation and weight gain and decrease salivary cortisol and distress behaviors.[25-27] In postsurgical patients, intraoperative and postoperative music reduces both pain and pharmaceutical requirements, including use of both sedatives and analgesics.[28,29] In pediatric oncology patients, music therapy can reduce pain and suffering and improve both mood and attitude.[30-33] In intensive care units, music reduces patient anxiety and depression[34-37]; and for dying patients, music therapy has been shown to improve the quality of life.[38,39]

Nonphysician providers of mind-body therapies include psychologists, nurses, social workers, chaplains, and music therapists. Frequently, master's level and higher levels of education in these fields include training in 1 or more mind-body therapies. Formal graduate-level training is required for both chaplaincy and music therapy certification. Advanced training and certification in hospital chaplaincy is available through the Association for Clinical Pastoral Education.

Biologically Based Therapies

Biologically based therapies includes all therapies that use natural products such as herbs, vitamins, and other supplements to modulate physiological function. Approximately 20% of the US adult population has used or uses herbal medicines for therapeutic purposes. Use is substantially higher among patient populations, including children suffering from chronic or recurrent illnesses.[40-48] The most recent data show that 46.2% of 1280 interviewed adolescents had used dietary supplements in their life, with 29.1% having used a supplement in the previous month. Nearly 10% of adolescents report using supplements with prescription medications in the previous month.[49]

The numerous Internet, mass media, and multilevel marketing campaigns for herbs and dietary supplements overwhelm most parents. The most frequently used natural products among children include chamomile, Echinacea, and St. John's wort. However, the most frequently used supplements are multivitamins, single vitamins, and mineral supplements (eg, vitamin C, zinc, calcium) and other supplements such as omega-3 fatty acids, fish oils, and melatonin. In adolescents, use of weight-loss supplements and creatine are closely linked to attempts to change body shape.[50]

Since the passage of the Dietary Supplement Health and Education Act of 1994 (DSHEA), supplements have been available over the counter as dietary supplements. The dietary supplements industry now generates at least $18.7 billion dollars a year. Though neither food nor drug, these substances are still regulated by the US Food and Drug Administration (FDA) but with less stringent requirements more akin to foods than drugs. Good Manufacturing Practice (GMP) regulations are identical to those for food. Unlike food and drugs, dietary supplements can be sold without premarket approval and do not require a specific post-marketing study. Supplements can be sold based on evidence of safety in the possession of the manufacturer. Supplements can only be removed from the market if the FDA can prove them to be unsafe under ordinary conditions of use. This ban recently occurred with the sympathomimetic herb ephedra (*Ephedra sinica* and related plants), which had been widely marketed for weight reduction. The FDA ruling was later overturned in a court ruling.

Under DSHEA, herbal medicines can be sold for *stimulating, maintaining, supporting, regulating,* and *promoting health* rather than for treating disease. As dietary supplements rather than drugs, herbal medicines may not claim to restore normal or to correct abnormal function. Additionally, herbs may not claim to *diagnose, treat, prevent, cure,* or *mitigate*. For example, herbal medicine companies can assert that their product supports cardiovascular health but not that it lowers cholesterol. To do so would suggest that the product is for treating a disease (hypercholesterolemia) and is therefore subject to FDA pharmaceutical regulations. However, most herbs are used by the public for the treatment of a disease or symptoms of a disease (Table 57-1). Only functional foods (eg, oat bran, soy, cranberries, certain processed butter-like spreads) can claim specific health benefits. Such approvals require significant supporting clinical data and FDA approval.

Nonspecialist recommendations for herbal medicine use abound in the mass media and in numerous local and national stores. Licensed practitioners who promote herbal medicine use include naturopaths and chiropractors for whom advanced training often exists as part of their degree programs. Not all naturopaths, however, are graduates of accredited naturopathic medical schools. International Board Certified Lactation Consultants frequently prescribe herbs to nursing mothers; examples of such drugs include galactagogues to stimulate milk production. At present, no national certification exists for the specific provision of complementary and alternative biologically based therapies.

Manipulative and Body-Based Methods

Manipulative and body-based methods include all therapies that focus on manipulation and movement of 1 or more parts of the body. The best-known examples are chiropractic, osteopathy, and massage. All examples incorporate touch, an essential human need with therapeutic, interpersonal, and cultural dimensions. Massage is one of the oldest health care practices and was used in ancient times in India, China, Arabia, Egypt, and Greece. Experience at one of the largest pediatric CAM programs at a children's hospital in the Midwest suggests that massage and other forms of bodywork are among the most popular options—inpatient or outpatient—as selected by children and teens.[50-55] Similar observations have been documented in pediatric oncology patients[56] and adolescents.[57] Massage may be provided most often by parents or other family members. The appropriate amount of massage has not yet been measured, but family members frequently appreciate the chance to

Table 57-1 Commonly Used Herbal Therapies

COMMON NAME (LATIN NAME)	COMMON USES
Aloe *(Aloe vera)*	Burns, minor wounds, skin irritations, aphthous stomatitis, constipation, gastric and duodenal ulcers
Astragalus (*Astragalus* species)	Immune booster
Calendula *(Calendula officinalis)*	Skin soother
Cascara *(Rhamnus purshiana)*	Constipation
Cayenne *(Capsicum frutescens)*	Topical treatment for pain, postherpetic neuralgia, nasal spray for migraines and cluster headaches
Chamomile *(Matricaria recutita)*	Sedative, colic, antiinflammatory, antispasmodic
Clove oil *(Syzygium aromaticum)*	Teething pain
Coffee (*Coffea* species)	Stimulant, attention-deficit/hyperactivity disorder, bronchodilator
Dandelion *(Taraxacum officinale)*	Mild diuretic, liver tonic
Dill *(Anethum graveolens)*	Antispasmodic, provides colic relief, decreases flatulence
Echinacea (*Echinacea* species)	Immune stimulation, antiinflammatory
Ephedra (ma huang) (*Ephedra* species)	Vasoconstriction; allergy, upper respiratory infection; asthma; appetite suppressant
Evening primrose oil *(Oenothera biennis)*	Eczema, premenstrual syndrome
Feverfew *(Tanacetum parthenium)*	Migraine headaches, rheumatoid arthritis
Garlic *(Allium sativum)*	Antimicrobial, cholesterol lowering
Ginger *(Zingiber officinale)*	Antiemetic, antinausea
Ginkgo *(Ginkgo biloba)*	Enhances blood flow past clogged arteries; prevents memory loss; marketed to treat attention-deficit/hyperactivity disorder
Ginseng (*Panax* species)	Stimulant, adaptogen; enhances endurance and performance
Hawthorn *(Crataegus oxycantha)*	Cardiac stimulant; enhances cardiac contractility
Hops *(Humulus lupulus)*	Sedative
Kava kava *(Piper methysticum)*	Anxiolytic
Lavender (*Lavendula* species)	Sedative
Licorice (*Glycyrrhiza* species)	Antiinflammatory, antiviral, demulcent
Milk thistle *(Silybum marianum)*	Hepatoprotection against cirrhosis, hepatitis
Oats *(Avena sativa)*	Antipruritic; eczema, varicella
Pine bark extract (*Pinus* species)	Antioxidant promoted to treat attention-deficit/hyperactivity disorder
Rhubarb root *(Rheum officinale)*	Constipation, chronic renal failure
Saint John's wort *(Hypericum perforatum)*	Depression, antiviral
Skullcap (*Scutellaria* species)	Sedative
Slippery elm bark *(Ulmus fulva)*	Demulcent; pharyngitis
Tea tree oil *(Melaleuca alternifolia)*	Topical antimicrobial; treats acne, minor skin infections, including fungal and yeast infections
Thyme *(Thymus vulgaris)*	Antimicrobial, expectorant; treats colds, sore throats, cough
Valerian *(Valeriana officinalis)*	Sedative
Witch hazel *(Hamamelis virginiana)*	Topical antiseptic, antiinflammatory

learn a skill that can contribute to the comfort and well being of the patient. Massage can also include many different techniques and forms that require more significant training, including structural integration (rolfing), movement integration (Feldenkreis technique, Alexander technique), pressure point techniques (shiatsu, acupressure), cranial sacral therapy, reflexology, and many others.

The manipulation, compression, and stretching of the skin, muscles, and joints activates a variety of mechanisms that support and promote health, including:

- Mechanical—enhances blood flow to the muscles and soft tissues and enhances lymphatic flow[58]
- Immunologic—enhances specific immune cell functions such as natural killer cell activity[59]
- Neurologic—triggers relaxation response and lowers sympathetic nervous system arousal, reduces serum cortisol, enhances endogenous serotonin and dopamine levels,[60] and modulates pain perception[61]
- Energetic—by traditional thought, certain massage practices can provide balance and improve the flow of life force energy or *chi*

The massage experience may be enhanced through the use of clinical aromatherapy—the therapeutic application of essential oils distilled from plants. Topical oils that enhance blood flow and engender a sense of warmth (called rubefacients) are often added and include lemongrass and black pepper oil. Specific scents can have application to specific symptoms, such as lavender or chamomile for relaxation, ginger or spearmint for nausea, and peppermint or lemon for fatigue.

Chiropractors and osteopaths are licensed in all 50 states, and their services are widely covered by insurance, including Medicaid. Doctors of osteopathy are considered mainstream physician practitioners, and graduates of osteopathic medical schools can enter pediatric residency programs. Most chiropractic schools now offer courses in pediatric care. Chiropractors tend to take few radiographs of children, to use lighter force when making adjustments, and to often use a device called an activator to make adjustments. Chiropractors also use special pediatric tables or treat the children in their parents' laps. Massage therapists are also licensed in all 50 states, but training and licensure requirements are quite variable. The largest professional national organization of bodyworkers is the American Massage Therapy Association. Membership requires training in an accredited school and completion of 500 hours of training.

Alternative Medical Systems

Alternative medical systems are based on comprehensive theories found outside of conventional Western biomedicine. These systems are frequently culturally based healing traditions, the theories and unique physical examinations of which are the basis for specific recommendations on lifestyle, diet, exercise, herbal medicines, and spiritual practices to restore balance in body and mind. The best-known examples in the West are Ayurveda from the Indian subcontinent and Traditional Asian Medicine from ancient China. However, in the West, the cultural and metaphysical foundations of Eastern traditions are frequently removed or hidden. Thus from the very broad field of Traditional Asian Medicine comes the therapy of acupuncture, which can be practiced with no reference to the ancient 5-element theory on which treatments are based. The best-known modern alternative medical system is homeopathy.

Among major teaching hospitals that have a pediatric pain service, 33% offer acupuncture therapy to treat chronic pain.[62] This therapy is one component of traditional Asian medicine systems in which vital energy, chi (qi), is believed to circulate through the body in channels called meridians. When the circulation of this vital energy is blocked or disrupted, disease is present; when the flow is balanced, harmonized, and restored, the patient returns to health. Acupuncture, which is the inserting of needles into key points on known meridians, is one means of restoring flow of chi.

Acupuncture point stimulation can be an effective and well-accepted intervention with children and teens, but care must be taken to present it in a nonthreatening light.[63] Thus use of the term *acupoint stimulation* avoids eliciting fear of needles. Acupoint stimulation can be achieved by massage, comfortable electrical stimulation, stickers with beads, or very thin (>30 gauge) nonhollow acupuncture needles. Acupoint stimulation can be taught to and performed by parents and children for home treatments. In many instances, after gradually establishing comfort and trust with a noninvasive approach, children and teens will agree to needle insertion. Acupuncture, when done correctly, is virtually painless and well tolerated for older children. Immediate benefits are rarely seen; thus acupuncturists often ask patients to commit to 4 to 6 visits before deciding to stop treatment.

Homeopathy is a system of medical treatment invented in the early 1800s by a German physician, Samuel Hahnemann, for whom Hahnemann Medical School was named. Homeopathy was frequently taught and practiced in US medical schools until rigorously criticized in the Flexner Report (1910). Currently, homeopathy is popular in Europe, Russia, India, and South America.

Homeopathy is based on 2 principles: (1) the *Law of Similars* or *like cures like* and (2) the *Law of Dilutions*. The Law of Similars means that a remedy that would cause a symptom in a healthy person is used to treat the same symptom in a sick person. For example, a treatment, termed remedy, made from the poison ivy plant *(Rhus toxicum)* might be used to treat a child suffering from eczema. Although pediatricians might reasonably be concerned about dangerous-sounding homeopathic medications such as *belladonna*, serious side effects from homeopathic treatment are exceedingly rare, far less common than side effects from standard over-the-counter and prescription medications.

This safety profile is attributable to its 2nd principle, the Law of Dilutions, which states that the more a remedy is diluted, the more powerful it becomes. This Law is counter-intuitive because, for most medicines, the larger the dose is, the more powerful the effects will be. However, in homeopathy, the most powerful remedies are the ones that have been diluted hundreds, thousands, or even millions of times. Dilutions of 1 to 10 are designated by the Roman numeral X (1X = 1/10, 3X = 1/1000, 6X = 1/1,000,000). Similarly, dilutions of 1 to 100 are designated by the Roman numeral C (1C = 1/100, 3C = 1/1,000,000, and so on). Most remedies today range from 6X to 30X, but some products are as dilute as 200C. Dilutions beyond 12X or 24C contain none of the original molecules.

Homeopaths believe that these highly dilute solutions contain an energy, or information, that the patient uses to heal symptoms. They report that the right remedy may worsen symptoms briefly before they improve. Many physicians believe that the remedies are nothing more than placebos that trigger the patient's psychoneuroimmunologic healing systems. Randomized-controlled trials suggest activity exists for remedies for diarrhea[64] and otitis media[65] but no activity for attention-deficit disorder.[66] Common over-the-counter remedies include combination products for teething, colic, allergies, and bedwetting.

An estimated 12,000 homeopaths practice in the United States; of these, approximately 50% are lay practitioners, 35% are chiropractors, and approximately 10% are physicians. The remaining 5% are other health professionals. Almost 2 million visits were made to homeopathic practitioners in the United States in 1997. Retail sales of homeopathic remedies were estimated at $250 million in the late 1990s.[67]

Most states allow certified health professionals such as physicians, osteopaths, dentists, veterinarians, and, in some cases, chiropractors and nurses to practice acupuncture or homeopathy. Specific training programs exist in acupuncture and homeopathy to supplement standard educational programs for each discipline. Insurance reimbursement is sometimes available to physicians. For laypersons to be certified practitioners in Traditional Asian Medicine or acupuncture, they can enroll in schools accredited by the Accreditation Commission in Acupuncture and Oriental Medicine (NCCAOM), which is recognized by the US Department of Education. Certification in acupuncture or traditional Chinese herbal medicine is obtained after testing by NCCAOM.

The private, nonprofit Council for Homeopathy Education reviews homeopathic programs. Certification in homeopathy is given after testing by the Council. Certification boards exist for health care professionals including medical physicians and doctors of osteopathy (American Institute of Homeopathy), chiropractors (National Board of Homeopathic Education), and naturopaths (Naturopathic Academy of Homeopathic Physicians). Persons who are not health care professionals are registered with the North American Society of Homeopaths.

Energy Therapies

Energy therapy includes all therapies that affect physiological function by the modulation of hypothesized energy fields, defined in different cultures as spirit or chi or energy or life force. Examples include Therapeutic Touch, Healing Touch, and Reiki. Practitioners transmit bioenergetic healing energy through their hands to foster healing. Actual touching the patient does not always take place. This category also includes therapies that use measurable electromagnetic fields such as magnet therapies to relieve the underlying causes of unexplained pain.

Therapeutic Touch was invented in the 1970s by a New York University nursing professor, Dolores Krieger, and a lay healer, Dora Kunz. Based on their observations of numerous religious healers, they distilled the process into 5 steps that practitioners might bring to healing outside of a specific religious faith or belief. These steps are:

1. Having a clear and conscious intent to be helpful and heal
2. Being centered in a peaceful state of mind
3. Using hands to assess the patient's energy (typically moving the hands 1 to 3 inches away from the body in a slow downward sweep from the head to the toes)
4. Using hands to help restore the patient's energy to a balanced, harmonious, peaceful state
5. Releasing the patient to complete the healing process while the healer returns to the healer's own centered, peaceful state of mind

Nurses and other health professionals in more than 80 countries have received training in Therapeutic Touch from its founders. It is currently taught in nursing schools across the United States. Nursing practice in many hospitals, including children's hospitals, includes policies and procedures for performing Therapeutic Touch.

Reiki is a similar practice that comes from a Japanese tradition. Practitioners are trained by a Reiki master through apprenticeship and spiritual and energetic initiation. Neither Therapeutic Touch nor Reiki have national certifying examinations or state licensure. Therapeutic Touch and Healing Touch are typically provided by nurses in both inpatient and outpatient settings. Reiki is typically provided by lay practitioners outside of medical settings. No reports of side effects have been documented from such treatments. The primary clinical benefits of Therapeutic Touch are increased relaxation, diminished anxiety, diminished pain, and enhanced sense of well being.[68-71]

TALKING WITH PATIENTS ABOUT COMPLEMENTARY AND ALTERNATIVE MEDICINE

Although many physicians are concerned that families who use CAM may be dissatisfied with mainstream medical care and fear they may abandon effective therapies in favor of unproved alternatives, data do not support these concerns. Fifty-five percent of all surveyed adults believed that use of complementary and alternative medicines would support health when used with conventional medical treatments.[72] For the most part, families seek therapies that are consistent with their values, worldview, and culture, and they seek care from therapists who respect them as individuals and who offer them time and attention.[73,74] Families continue to value highly the care they receive from compassionate, comprehensive primary care pediatricians; and they seek additional information on healthy lifestyles, dietary supplements, and environmental therapies over which they may exert some control.[75] They also seek care from complementary and alternative medical therapists who offer personal attention, hope, time, and therapies that are consistent with their culture and values. Families who seek out complementary and alternative medical therapies rarely abandon their pediatrician, but they may not feel comfortable discussing these therapies if they perceive the pediatrician to be antagonistic or judgmental toward them.

To provide the best care, pediatricians should ask all patients about CAM use. This task is best accomplished in a seamless, structured, and nonjudgmental manner during the medical interview. To set a positive tone, the care provider can begin new patient interviews with questions about the number of meals eaten together as a family, fun things the family does together, hopes and dreams for the child, and aspects of the child of which they are most proud. At each return visit, a helpful question would be to also ask, "Since the last visit, which other health professionals has your child visited?" As with all good interviewing, listening for understanding rather than agreement or disagreement enhances the therapeutic alliance.

Social History

During the social history, the care provider should inquire about:

- Diet, exercise, and environment to provide insight about risks and actions taken to promote health
- Illness care at home
- Any special foods, teas, rubs, prayers, or rituals that are helpful for the patient's family
- Any mind-body therapies to manage stress, reduce chronic symptoms, or promote well being

One such question might be, "When you are stressed, what is most helpful for you? Which of your activities do you find is best for your health?" To assess psychological wellness, stress and time-management, self-esteem, and self-concept, a thorough academic history and questions about learning style, friends, hobbies, and extracurricular activities should be included.

Questions regarding spirituality can be inserted at this point in the inquiry, as appropriate. Multiple mnemonics exist to guide physicians in their interviews to understand the patient's and family's source of meaning, purpose, richness, and direction (Box 57-1). Conscious choices expressed in the social history represent strengths that can be used for achieving health goals. Clearly, ethical boundaries exist around faith and spirituality. The physician's role is not to provide answers but to support the search for answers.

BOX 57-1 Spiritual Assessment Tools

FICA

F: Faith or belief—What is your faith or belief?

I: Importance and influence—Is faith important in your life? How?

C: Community—Are you part of a religious community?

A: Awareness and addressing—What would you want me as your physician to be aware of? How would you like me to address these issues in your care?

HOPE

H: Hope—What are your sources of hope, meaning, strength, peace, love, and connectedness?

O: Organization—Do you consider yourself part of an organized religion?

P: Personal spirituality and practices—What aspects of your spirituality or spiritual practices do you find most helpful?

E: Effects—How do your beliefs affect the kind of medical care you would like me to provide?

SPIRIT

S: Spiritual belief system—What is your formal religious affiliation?

P: Personal spirituality—Describe the beliefs and practices of your religion or spiritual system that you personally accept or do not accept.

I: Integration within a spiritual community—Do you belong to a spiritual or religious group or community? What importance does this group have for you?

R: Ritualized practices and Restrictions—Are there specific practices that you carry out as part of your religion/spirituality (eg, prayer or meditation)?

I: Implications for medical care—Would you like to discuss religious or spiritual implications of health care?

T: Terminal events planning—As we plan for your care near the end of life, how does your faith affect your decisions? Are there particular aspects of care that you wish to forgo or have withheld because of your faith?

Adapted from Puchalski CM, Romer AL. Taking a spiritual history allows clinicians to understand patients more fully. *J Pall Med.* 2000;3:129-137; Anandarajah G, Hight E. Spirituality and medical practice: using the HOPE questions as a practical tool for spiritual assessment. *Am Fam Physician.* 2001;63:81-88; and Maugans TA. The SPIRITual history. *Arch Fam Med.* 1996;5:11-16.

This point of the inquiry is also the time for assessing all potential environmental factors contributing to health and illness in children.[76] A useful mnemonic for an environmental history is ACHHOO, with each letter representing a potential exposure site to known toxins such as lead, mercury, second-hand tobacco smoke, pesticides, and other contaminants:

*A*ctivities
*C*ommunity
*H*ousehold
*H*obbies
*O*ccupation
*O*ral behaviors

Allergies and Current and Past Medications

When documenting current and past medication use, additional questions to include in routine practice consist of the following:

1. Do you use multivitamins, for example, Poly-Vi-Sol or Flintstones chewable vitamins?
2. Do you use over-the-counter medications, for example, any medications for colds, pain or constipation?
3. Do you use herbal medicines, for example, any herbs such as *Echinacea* or chamomile?
4. Do you take specific vitamins and minerals, for example, any vitamins such as vitamin C, D, or E? Do you take any mineral supplements such as calcium, iron, magnesium, or selenium?
5. Do you take dietary supplements, for example, any supplements such as fish oils?

   Follow-up questions include:
   - What brand?
   - What dose?
   - How often?
   - What directions are you following?
   - What goals are you hoping to achieve by taking it?
   - Are you using any other remedies now?

Understanding the supplements used and the patient and family's source of information for making treatment decisions can be quite helpful for comprehending what is important to the family.

Interviewing for herbal medicine use is crucial for identifying patients who are at risk for interactions with prescription medications or for excessive bleeding in surgery. Too frequently, professionals and patients follow a *don't ask, don't tell* policy. *Ask, then ask again* is a practice policy that is foundational to safe and effective patient care. Patients should be asked to bring all remedies with them to every visit so that the chart can be updated and usage monitored. Patients with special risks of drug interactions include those who take the following pharmaceutical agents: anticoagulants, hypoglycemics, antidepressants, sedative-hypnotics, antihypertensives, and medications with narrow therapeutic windows such as digoxin and theophylline.

Medical History

In addition to immunizations, surgeries, and hospitalizations, the interview for the medical history is a good time to ask about use of complementary and alternative therapies that often require multiple visits, such as chiropractic, other body work, and acupuncture. Understanding what worked or did not work for the patient provides further insights into what is important for the patient and family. Additionally, questioning during this portion of the inquiry can help identify health issues that may be important to address in the context of a holistic approach to health.

COUNSELING FAMILIES ABOUT COMPLEMENTARY AND ALTERNATIVE MEDICINE

The goal of counseling about CAM is to strengthen the physician-patient relationship through honest dialogue that is clinically responsible, ethically appropriate, and legally defensible. Parental inclusion of complementary and alternative therapies for their children, in itself, does not constitute child neglect.[77] Similarly, physician provision of complementary and alternative therapies does not, in itself, represent professional misconduct.

Increasingly, pediatricians will find themselves sharing patients with massage therapists, chiropractors, acupuncturists, and others. Pediatric patient advocacy requires assessing for safety and efficacy, as well as respecting the autonomy of the parent-child relationship. When patients or families report seeing other health professionals and describe current CAM use, physicians should follow 3 steps in response to the answers provided:

Step 1. Determine if the complementary and alternative therapy represents a rejection of standard care for a serious or life-threatening disease for which a reasonable chance exists of cure or if use of the complementary and alternative therapy will delay proven treatment. In such cases, the 1st step is to protect the child while understanding the parents' goals. Reporting requirements for abuse and neglect may apply. (See Chapter 120, Child Physical Abuse and Neglect.)

Step 2. Determine if the complementary and alternative therapies used are known to be unsafe, ineffective, or both. Excellent Web-based and other resources are noted at the end of this chapter to guide this assessment. Frequently used resources include the National Library of Medicine's PubMed or TOXLINE, the Natural Medicines Comprehensive Database, and the National Institute's of Health National Center for Complementary and Alternative Medicine, Office of Dietary Supplements, and the National Cancer Institute.

In the event of use of a known toxic agent or an ineffective agent with possible harm, the physician's responsibility is to counsel from the documented evidence that the therapy should be stopped. Resistance to such advice may place the parents at risk for charges of negligence or abuse.

In the absence of data on toxicity or efficacy, the pediatrician's role is to monitor as clinically appropriate. This role can include scheduling telephone follow-up or office visits. In both cases, document the following in the medical record:

- Therapy used and the goal of the therapy
- Patient or family preferences and expectations regarding the therapy
- Provider of the therapy, location, and treatment plan (as known by the family). This information should include names, telephone numbers, any other contact information, and specialties.
- Review of the safety and efficacy issues of the therapy from the medical literature
- Results of counseling including the pediatrician's treatment plan for monitoring the treatment and its results
- Advice provided or resources recommended for further information

Step 3. Ensure that the patient and family's decision to use a complementary and alternative therapy is based on a fully-informed judgment and that their verbal consent was obtained and documented. This documentation includes what options have been discussed, offered, tried, or refused. (General guidelines for counseling are found in Box 57-2.) Counseling on spiritual concerns requires special consideration for clinical and ethical reasons. Although not classically part of medical training, adults in the United States consistently report that physicians talking with patients about spirituality is appropriate.[78,79] Recently,

BOX 57-2 How to Talk With Patients About Complementary and Alternative Therapies

1. DO talk about the different kinds of therapies families may have tried to help their child.
2. Do NOT wait for families to bring it up.
3. Ask in an open-minded, nonjudgmental fashion. Avoid using potentially pejorative terms such as *unproved, unconventional,* or *alternative*.
4. Elicit further information with questions about specific therapies. For example, have you tried any HERBAL therapies, such as Echinacea or ginkgo? Have you tried any DIETARY therapies, such as avoiding wheat or milk? Have you sought care from any OTHER HEALTH PROFESSIONALS such as acupuncturists or chiropractors?
5. Elicit the values, beliefs, and influences that led parents to these therapies. For example, were these suggested by family members? Were they consistent with their religious, spiritual, or cultural beliefs? What is the value of natural or organic approaches? Do you have a fear of side effects of mainstream treatments?
6. Whenever possible, join with the parents and support their decision to pursue avenues that may help their child. Be an ally rather than a tyrant.
7. Ask how well the family thinks the therapies worked or did not work *before* offering your opinion.
8. Offer to talk with other therapists involved in the child's care to maintain coordinated, comprehensive care.
9. Offer to learn more to help answer the family's questions.
10. Offer families additional information and resources to address their questions about alternative and complementary therapies.

83% of 921 primary care patients surveyed in Ohio reported that they wanted physicians to ask about spiritual beliefs in certain circumstances, such as with serious illness or the loss of loved ones.[80] In response to the accumulating data on the importance of spirituality and health, even the Joint Commission for the Accreditation of Health Care Organizations now requires that patient spirituality be addressed as part of routine inpatient care.[81]

Spirituality may be understood as connection with the sources of ultimate meaning. Spirituality may or may not include formal religion. Spiritual concerns arise with threatened losses or disruptions of such connections. These issues can include key relationships with parents, other family members, and friends or what the child believes God to be. For efficient and effective clinical care when spiritual issues are present, the following guidelines should be kept in mind:

1. Anticipate the presence of spiritual concerns with every illness. These concerns can include those of the patient, the family, and care team member, and as well as one's own.
2. Comprehend how the patient's and the family's faith or spirituality can be a resource during illness.
3. Seek to understand how the patient's or the family's cultural and spiritual worldview influence understanding of the disease, the appropriate treatment, and the recovery process.
4. Determine what effect, positive or negative, the patient's or the family's spiritual orientation or interpretation has on perceived needs.
5. Partner with, and refer to, chaplains or the patient's or the family's preferred spiritual care provider for assistance with significant spiritual concerns.

To achieve these goals, open-ended questions are always helpful. The physician should create a safe environment in which patients and families can articulate their questions. In contrast to the role of physicians in routine medical care, for spiritual concerns, solving problems and providing answers are rarely helpful. For spiritual concerns, the best answers are found rather than given. The physician's role is to support the search for answers.

HOW TO PARTNER WITH AND REFER TO COMPLEMENTARY AND ALTERNATIVE MEDICINE PRACTITIONERS

Because of increasing interest and evidence of safety and efficacy, pediatricians will increasingly want to partner with and refer to CAM practitioners. This task is quite easy when credentialed practitioners exist in conventional settings such as hospital-based integrative pediatric clinics or consultation services. However, when a pediatrician provides the therapy or refers to practitioners in the community, the State Medical Board Guidelines for Physician Use of Complementary and Alternative Medical Therapies apply.[82] Key points include documenting the following in the medical record:

1. Parity of evaluation (medical history and physical examination as thorough as for conventional care)
2. Informed consent (review of diagnosis, all medical options for that diagnosis, discussion of risks and benefits of the recommended treatment, including potential interference with ongoing conventional care, and any applicable financial interests)
3. Treatment plan objectives and goals (expected favorable outcomes and monitoring plan for duration of treatment)

Physicians who refer to CAM practitioners should do so only to licensed or otherwise state-regulated health care practitioners with the requisite training and skills to use the complementary and alternative therapy being recommended. Physicians are expected to not sell, rent, or lease health-related products or engage in personal branding. Physicians must also be able to demonstrate a basic understanding of the medical scientific knowledge connected with any complementary and alternative therapy.

Physicians are not liable for any negligence on the part of a CAM provider unless (1) the referral delayed necessary conventional treatment, (2) the physician knew the provider was not competent to provide the therapy, or, (3) the physician hired the CAM provider or provided joint treatment with the provider.[82]

When making referrals for children with complex chronic illness or chronic pain, pediatricians must carefully prioritize and schedule necessary conventional therapies. They must also coordinate care with all subspecialists. Equally important, however, pediatricians must consider the effect on time and expenses of families who are vulnerable as they seek any available therapies for children. The pediatrician should set appropriate expectations, support appropriate hope, and avoid overscheduling and overtreating children.

CONCLUSION

Increasingly, the public expects pediatricians to provide wise counsel on CAM and to make appropriate referrals for complementary and alternative therapies. Pediatricians may also seek additional training in CAM to enhance their clinical practice. (See Related Web Sites.)

TOOLS FOR PRACTICE

Engaging Patients and Family

- *Are You Considering Using CAM?* (fact sheet), American Academy of Pediatrics (nccam.nih.gov/health/decisions/index.htm).

Medical Decision Support

- *Social and Environmental CAM history* (questionnaire), American Academy of Pediatrics (practice.aap.org/content.aspx?aid=2001).

RELATED WEB SITES

Complementary and Alternative Medical Training for Physicians

Mind-Body Medicine: Hypnosis and Biofeedback

- Society for Developmental and Behavioral Pediatrics (www.sdbp.org).
- American Society for Clinical Hypnosis (www.asch.net).

- Association for Applied Psychophysiology and Biofeedback (www.aapb.org).
- Biofeedback Certification Institute of America (www.bcia.com).
- Center for Mind-Body Medicine (www.cmbm.org).
- Mind-Body Medical Institute (www.mbmi.org).

Mind-Body Medicine: Spiritual Care

- Massachusetts General Hospital/Kenneth B. Schwartz Center (www.theschwartzcenter.org/programs.asp#pastoral).
- Association for Clinical Pastoral Education (www.acpe.edu).

Biologically Based Therapies

- University of Arizona Program in Integrative Medicine (on-line and residential programs) (integrativemedicine.arizona.edu/online_courses/).
- North Carolina Northwest Area Health Education Center and Wake Forest University (on line) (northwestahec.wfubmc.edu/learn/herbs_ce/index.cfm).
- Keio University Medical School (on line; Kampo and traditional Asian herbal medicine). (web.sc.itc.keio.ac.jp/kampo/vc/index.html).
- Center for Mind-Body Medicine (clinical nutrition) (www.cmbm.org).

Manipulative and Body-Based Therapies

- American Massage Therapy Association (www.amtamassage.org).
- American Massage Therapy Foundation (www.massagetherapyfoundation.org).

Alternative Medical Systems: Medical Acupuncture

- Stanford University/University of California-Los Angeles/Helms Medical Institute (www.hmieducation.com).
- American Academy of Medical Acupuncture (www.medicalacupuncture.org).
- New York Medical College (www.nymc.edu/cpm).
- Harvard University Medical School (cme.hms.harvard.edu/index.asp).

Energy Therapies

- Healing Touch International (www.healingtouch.net).
- Therapeutic Touch (www.therapeutic-touch.org).

Resources for Selecting a Complementary and Alternative Medical Practitioner

- National Center for Complementary and Alternative Medicine, National Institutes of Health, US Department of Health and Human Services. NIH guidelines for selecting a CAM practitioner. (nccam.nih.gov/health/practitioner/index.htm).
- Cohen MH, Kemper KJ, Stevens L, et al. Pediatric use of complementary therapies: ethical and policy choices. *Pediatrics*. 2005;116:e568-e575.
- Cohen MH, Kemper KJ. Complementary therapies in pediatrics: a legal perspective. *Pediatrics*. 2005;115: 774-780.
- Cohen MH, Hrbek A, Davis RB, et al. Emerging credentialing practices, malpractice liability policies, and guidelines governing complementary and alternative medical practices and dietary supplement recommendations: a descriptive study of 19 integrative health care centers in the United States. *Arch Intern Med.* 2005; 165:289-295.

Counseling Resources

General

- Informational topics and handouts from National Institutes of Health, National Center for Complementary and Alternative Medicine (NCCAM):
  - Backgrounder Information Clearinghouse (nccam.nih.gov/health/backgrounds).
  - Treatment Information Clearinghouse (nccam.nih.gov/health/bytreatment.htm).
  - Making CAM Decisions (nccam.nih.gov/health/decisions/index.htm).
- Children's Hospitals and Clinics of Minnesota. Colorful, informational monographs for children, plus videos of children and CAM therapies (www.childrensintegrativemed.org).
- American Academy of Pediatrics, Section on Complementary Health and Integrative Medicine (www.aap.org/sections/chim/).
- AAP guidance: American Academy of Pediatrics, Committee on Children with Disabilities. Counseling families who choose complementary and alternative medicine for their child with chronic illness or disability. *Pediatrics* 2001;107(3):598-601.
- Therapeutic guidance: Kemper KJ. *The Holistic Pediatrician: A Pediatrician's Guide to Safe and Effective Therapies for the 25 Most Common Ailments of Infants, Children and Adolescents*. 2nd ed. New York, NY: Harper Paperbacks; 2002.
- Environmental health: Pediatric Environmental Health Specialty Units (www.aoec.org).
- Academic Consortium on Integrative Medicine (www.imconsortium.org).
- American Holistic Medical Association (www.holisticmedicine.org).
- Cochrane Collaboration Database. Specific therapies including herbs and dietary supplements (www.cochrane.org).
- Micromedex Alternative Medicine Database (www.library.ucsf.edu/db/micromedex.html).
- Natural Medicines Comprehensive Database (www.naturaldatabase.com).
- American Botanical Council (www.herbalgram.org).
- Medicinal and Poisonous Plant Database (www.biologie.uni-hamburg.de/b-online/ibc99/poison/).
- Society for Medicinal Plant Research (www.ga-online.org).
- US Pharmacopeia (www.usp.org).
- InteliHealth (Harvard Medical School) (www.intelihealth.com).
- National Cancer Institute (www.cancer.gov/cancertopics/treatment/cam).
- University of Texas, M.D. Anderson Cancer Center (www.mdanderson.org/departments/cimer/).
- Columbia University/Children's Hospital New York-Presbyterian Herbert Irving Child and Adolescent Cancer Center Integrative Therapies Program for Children with Cancer (www.integrativetherapiesprogram.org/links/index.php).

Spirituality

- Meert KL, Thurston CS, Briller SH. The spiritual needs of parents at the time of their child's death in the pediatric intensive care unit and during bereavement: a qualitative study. *Pediatr Crit Care Med.* 2005;6:420-427.
- Barnes LL, Plotnikoff GA, Fox K, et al. Spirituality, religion and pediatrics: intersecting worlds of healing. *Pediatrics.* 2000;106(4 suppl):899-908.
- Lo B, Ruston D, Kates LW, et al for the Working Group on Religious and Spiritual Issues at the End of Life. Discussing religious and spiritual issues at the end of life. *JAMA.* 2002;287:749-754.
- Center for Spirituality, Theology and Health (www.dukespiritualityandhealth.org).
- George Washington Institute on Spirituality and Health (www.gwish.org).
- The Health Care Chaplaincy (www.healthcarechaplaincy.org).
- Institute for Public Health & Faith Collaborations. Interfaith health program at Emory University (www.ihpnet.org).
- University of Minnesota Center for Spirituality and Healing (www.csh.umn.edu).
- Wayne E. Oates Institute (www.oates.org).

AAP POLICY STATEMENTS

American Academy of Pediatrics, Committee on Children with Disabilities. Counseling families who choose complementary and alternative medicine for their child with chronic illness or disability. *Pediatrics.* 2001;107:598-601. (aappolicy.aappublications.org/cgi/content/full/pediatrics;107/3/598).

American Academy of Pediatrics, Committee on Pediatric Workforce. Scope of practice issues in the delivery of pediatric health care. *Pediatrics.* 2003;111(2):426-435. (aappolicy.aappublications.org/cgi/content/full/pediatrics;111/2/426).

REFERENCES

1. Kemper KJ, O'Connor KG. Pediatricians' recommendations for complementary and alternative medical (CAM) therapies. *Ambul Pediatr.* 2004;4:482-487.
2. Sibinga EM, Ottolini MC, Duggan AK, et al. Parent-pediatrician communication about complementary and alternative medicine use for children. *Clin Pediatr (Phila).* 2004;43:367-373.
3. Consortium of Academic Health Centers for Integrative Medicine. Available at: www.imconsortium.org/. Accessed February 1, 2006.
4. Snyderman R, Weil AT. Integrative medicine: bringing medicine back to its roots. *Arch Intern Med.* 2002;162:395-397.
5. Astin JA, Forys K. Psychological determinants of health and illness: integrating mind, body and spirit. *Adv Mind Body Med.* 2004;20:14-21.
6. Green E, Green A, Walters E. Voluntary control of internal states: psychological and physiological. *J Transpersonal Psych.* 1970;2:1-26.
7. Sussman D, Culbert T. Pediatric self-regulation. In: Levine MD, Carey WB, Crocker AC, eds. *Developmental-Behavioral Pediatrics.* 3rd ed. Philadelphia, PA: WB Saunders; 1999.
8. Astin JA, Shapiro SL, Eisenberg DM, et al. Mind-body medicine: state of the science, implications for practice. *J Am Board Fam Pract.* 2003;16:131-147.
9. Morgenthaler TI, Owens J, Alessi C, et al, and the American Academy of Sleep Medicine. Practice parameters for the psychological and behavior treatment of insomnia: an update. *Sleep.* 2006;29(11):1415-1419.
10. Andrasik F, Schwartz M. Behavioral assessment and treatment of pediatric headache. *Behav Modif.* 2006;30:93-113.
11. Tsao J, Zeltzer L. Complementary and alternative medicine approaches for pediatric pain: a review of the state-of-the-science. *ECAM.* 2005;2:1149-1159.
12. Mellon M, McGrath M. Empirically supported treatments in pediatric psychology: nocturnal enuresis. *J Pediatr Psychol.* 2000;25(4):219-224.
13. Lehrer PM, Vaschillo E, Vaschillo B, et al. Biofeedback treatment for asthma. *Chest.* 2004;126(2):352-361.
14. Barnes PM, Powell-Griner E, McFann K, et al. Complementary and alternative medicine use among adults in the United States, 2002. *Adv Data.* 2004;343:1-19.
15. Dujardin RC. Faith in medicine. *Detroit Free Press.* December 26, 1996:7D.
16. McNichol T. When religion and medicine meet: The new faith in medicine. *USA Weekend.* April 7, 1996:4.
17. Silverstri GA, Knittig S, Zoller JS, et al. Importance of faith on medical decisions regarding cancer care. *J Clin Oncol.* 2003;21:1379-1382.
18. Koenig HG, Cohen HJ, Blazer DG, et al. Religious coping and depression among elderly, hospitalized medically ill men. *Am J Psychiatry.* 1992;149:1693-1700.
19. Koenig HG, George LK, Peterson BL. Religiosity and remission of depression in medically ill older patients. *Am J Psychiatry.* 1998;155:536-542.
20. Fisch MJ, Titzer ML, Kristeller JL, et al. Assessment of quality of life in outpatients with advanced cancer: the accuracy of clinician estimations and the relevance of spiritual well-being—a Hoosier Oncology Group Study. *J Clin Oncol.* 2003;21:2754-2759.
21. Moadel A, Morgan C, Fatone A, et al. Seeking meaning and hope: self-reported spiritual and existential needs among an ethnically-diverse cancer population. *Psychooncology.* 1999;8:378-385.
22. McClain CS, Rosenfield B, Breitbart W. Effect of spiritual well-being on end-of-life despair in terminally-ill cancer patients. *Lancet.* 2003;361:1603-1607.
23. Pargament KI, Koenig HG, Tarakeshwar N, et al. Religious struggle as a predictor of mortality among medically ill elderly patients: a two-year longitudinal study. *Arch Intern Med.* 2001;161:1881-1885.
24. Meert KL, Thurston CS, Briller SH. The spiritual needs of parents at the time of their child's death in the pediatric intensive care unit and during bereavement: a qualitative study. *Pediatr Crit Care Med.* 2005;6:420-427.
25. Standley JM. A meta-analysis of the efficacy of music therapy for pre-mature infants. *J Pediatr Nurs.* 2002;17(2):107-113.
26. Standley JM, Moore RS. Therapeutic effects of music and mother's voice on premature infants. *Pediatr Nurs.* 1995;21(6):509-512, 574.
27. Block S, Jennings D, David L. Live harp music decreases salivary cortisol levels in convalescent preterm infants. *Pediatr Res.* 2003;53(4, part 2):469a.
28. Koch ME, Kain ZN, Ayoub C, et al. The sedative and analgesic sparing effect of music. *Anesthesiology.* 1998;89(2):300-306.
29. Nilsson U, Rawal N, Unosson M. A comparison of intra-operative or postoperative exposure to music—a controlled trial of the effects on postoperative pain. *Anesthesia.* 2003;58(7):699-703.
30. Barrerra ME, Rykov MH, Doyle SL. The effects of interactive music therapy on hospitalized children with cancer: a pilot study. *Psychooncology.* 2002;11(5):379-388.
31. Magill L. The use of music therapy to address the suffering in advanced cancer pain. *J Palliat Care.* 2002;17(3):167-172.
32. Beck SL. The therapeutic use of music for cancer-related pain. *Oncol Nurs Forum.* 1991;18(8):1327-1337.

33. Standley JM, Hanser SB. Music therapy research and applications in pediatric oncology treatment. *J Pediatr Oncol Nurs*. 1995;12(1):3-10.
34. Guzzetta CE. Effects of relaxation and music therapy on patients in a coronary care unit with presumptive acute myocardial infarction. *Heart Lung*. 1989;18(6):609-616.
35. Evans D. The effectiveness of music as an intervention for hospital patients: a systematic review. *J Adv Nurs*. 2002;37(1):8-18.
36. Vickers AJ, Cassileth BR. Unconventional therapies for cancer and cancer-related symptoms. *Lancet Oncol*. 2001;2(4):226-232.
37. Chlan L. Effectiveness of a music therapy intervention on relaxation and anxiety for patients receiving ventilatory assistance. *Heart Lung*. 1998;27(3):169-176.
38. Halstead MT, Roscoe ST. Restoring the spirit at the end of life: music as an intervention for oncology nurses. *Clin J Oncol Nurs*. 2002;6(6):332-336.
39. Hilliard RE. The effects of music therapy on the quality and length of life of people diagnosed with terminal cancer. *J Music Ther*. 2003;40(2):113-137.
40. Pitetti R, Singh S, Hornyak D, et al. Complementary and alternative medicine use in children. *Pediatr Emerg Care*. 2001;17(3):165-169.
41. Breuner CC, Barry PJ, Kemper KJ. Alternative medicine use by homeless youth. *Arch Pediatr Adolesc Med*. 1998;152:1071-1075.
42. Lanski SL, Greenwald M, Perkins A, et al. Herbal therapy use in a pediatric emergency department population: expect the unexpected. *Pediatrics*. 2003;111(5 Pt 1):981-985.
43. Sawni-Sikand A, Schubiner H, Thomas RL. Use of complementary/alternative therapies among children in primary care pediatrics. *Ambul Pediatr*. 2002;2(2):99-103.
44. Sanders H, Davis MF, Duncan B, et al. Use of complementary and alternative medical therapies among children with special health care needs in southern Arizona. *Pediatrics*. 2003;111(3):584-587.
45. Hagen LE, Schneider R, Stephens D, et al. Use of complementary and alternative medicine by pediatric rheumatology patients. *Arthritis Rheum*. 2003;49(1):3-6.
46. Heuschkel R, Afzal N, Wuerth A, et al. Complementary medicine use in children and young adults with inflammatory bowel disease. *Am J Gastroenterol*. 2002;97(2):382-388.
47. Kelly KM, Jacobson JS, Kennedy DD, et al. Use of unconventional therapies by children with cancer at an urban medical center. *J Pediatr Hematol Oncol*. 2000;22(5):412-416.
48. Reznik M, Ozuah PO, Franco K, et al. Use of complementary therapy by adolescents with asthma. *Arch Pediatr Adolesc Med*. 2002;156(10):1042-1044.
49. Wilson KM, Klein JD, Sesselberg TS, et al. Use of complementary medicine and dietary supplements among US adolescents. *J Adolesc Health*. 2006;38(4):385-394.
50. Culbert T. Children's Hospitals and Clinics of Minnesota. Integrative Medicine Program Data, 2005-2006. Personal communication, 2006.
51. Field T. Massage therapy for skin conditions in young children. *Dermatol Clin*. 2005;23(4):717-721.
52. Khilnani S, Field T, Hernandez-Reif M, et al. Massage therapy improves mood and behavior of students with attention-deficit/hyperactivity disorder. *Adolescence*. 2003;38(152):623-638.
53. Diego MA, Field T, Hernandez-Reif MA, et al. Aggressive adolescents benefit from massage therapy. *Adolescence*. 2002;37(147):597-607.
54. Field T. Preterm infant massage therapy studies: an American approach. *Semin Neonatol*. 2002;7(6):487-497.
55. Field T. Massage therapy. *Med Clin North Am*. 2002;86(1):163-171.
56. McCurdy EA, Spangler JG, Wofford MM, et al. Religiosity is associated with the use of complementary and alternative medicine. *J Pediatr Hematol Oncol*. 2003;25(2):125-129.
57. Wilson KM, Klein JD. Adolescents' use of complementary and alternative medicine. *Ambul Pediatr*. 2002;2(2);104-110.
58. Hansen TI, Kristensen JH. Effect of massage, shortwave diathermy and ultrasound on ^{133}Xe disappearance rate from muscle and subcutaneous tissue in human calf. *Scand J Rehabil Med*. 1973;5:179-182.
59. Ironson G, Field T, Scafidi F, et al. Massage therapy is associated with enhancement of the immune system's cytotoxic capacity. *Int J Neurosci*. 1996;84:205-217.
60. Field T, Hernandez-Reif M, Diego M, et al. Cortisol decreases and serotonin and dopamine increase following massage therapy. *Int J Neurosci*. 2005;115: 1397-1413.
61. Lund I, Ge Y, Yu LC, et al. Repeated massage-like stimulation induces long-term effects on nociception: contribution of oxytocinergic mechanisms. *Eur J Neurosci*. 2005;22:1553-1554.
62. Lin YC, Lee AC, Kemper KJ, et al. Use of complementary and alternative medicine in pediatric pain management service: a survey. *Pain Med*. 2005;6:452-458.
63. Kemper KJ, Highfield ES. When should you consider acupuncture for pediatric patients? *Contemp Pediatr*. 2002;19(12):31-46.
64. Jacobs J, Jonas WB, Jimenez-Perez M, et al. Homeopathy for childhood diarrhea: combined results and meta-analysis from three randomized, controlled clinical trials. *Pediatr Infect Dis J*. 2003;22:229-234.
65. Jacobs J, Springer DA, Crothers D. Homeopathic treatment of acute otitis media in children: a preliminary randomized placebo-controlled trial. *Pediatr Infect Dis J*. 200;20:177-183.
66. Jacobs J, Williams AL, Girard C, et al. Homeopathy for attention-deficit/hyperactivity disorder: a pilot randomized-controlled trial. *J Altern Complement Med*. 2005;11:799-806.
67. Ullman D. Homeopathy and managed care: manageable or unmanageable. *J Altern Complement Med* 1999;5:65-73.
68. Kemper KJ, Kelly EA. Treating children with therapeutic and healing touch. *Pediatr Ann*. 2004;33(4): 248-252.
69. Giasson M, Bouchard L. Effect of therapeutic touch on the well-being of persons with terminal cancer. *J Holist Nurs*. 1998;16(3):383-398.
70. Wilkinson DS, Knox PL, Chatman JE, et al. The clinical effectiveness of healing touch. *J Altern Complement Med*. 2002;8(1):33-47.
71. Lafreniere KD, Mutus B, Cameron S, et al. Effects of therapeutic touch on biochemical and mood indicators in women. *J Altern Complement Med*. 1999;5(4):367-370.
72. Barnes P, Powell-Griner E, McFann K, et al. Complementary and alternative medicine use among adults: United States, 2002. *CDC Adv Data Report #343* May 2004.
73. Astin JA. Why patients use alternative medicine: results of a national study. *JAMA*. 1998;279:1548.
74. Neuberger J. Primary care: core values. Patients' priorities. *BMJ*. 1998;317:260.
75. Kaptchuk TJ, Eisenberg DM. The persuasive appeal of alternative medicine, *Ann Intern Med*. 1998;129:1061-1065.
76. American Academy of Pediatrics, Committee on Environmental Health and Etzel RA, ed. *Pediatric Environmental Health*. 2nd ed. Elk Grove Village, IL: American Academy of Pediatrics; 2003.
77. Cohen MH, Kemper KJ. Complementary therapies in pediatrics: a legal perspective. *Pediatrics*. 2005;115:774-780.
78. King DE, Bushwick B. Beliefs and attitudes of hospital inpatients about faith healing and prayer. *J Fam Pract*. 1994;3:349-352.
79. Ehman JW, Ott BB, Short TH, et al. Do patients want physicians to inquire about their spiritual or religious beliefs if they become gravely ill? *Arch Intern Med*. 1999;159:1803-1806.
80. McCord G, Gilchrist VJ, Grossman SD, et al. Discussing spirituality with patients: a rational and ethical approach. *Ann Fam Med*. 2004;2:356-361.
81. Joint Commission for the Accreditation of Health Care Organizations. *Comprehensive Accreditation Manual for Hospitals*. Oakbrook Terrace, IL: Joint Commission for the Accreditation of Health Care Organizations; 2003. Available at: www.jcrinc.com/13519/. Accessed October 1, 2007.
82. Cohen MH, Kemper KJ. Complementary therapies in pediatrics: a legal perspective. *Pediatrics*. 2005;115:774-780.

Chapter 58

BODY FLUIDS, ELECTROLYTE CONCENTRATION, AND ACID-BASE COMPOSITION

Prashant V. Mahajan, MD, MPH, MBA

Evaluating and managing fluid and electrolyte disorders in children requires an understanding of the composition of the human body and the regulatory mechanisms that maintain homeostasis. The primary care physician will encounter the issue of managing fluids and electrolytes in a large number of patients. Selecting the optimal fluid and electrolyte solution will vary depending on the age of the patient, cause of the disease, severity of the condition, and the presence of a coexisting morbidity in the patient. Normal homeostasis is maintained by a complex interaction among the solutes, body water, hormonal influence, and the hypothalamic-pituitary-renal axis. Guiding the approach to fluid therapy in any child are a few basic principles of human physiology, including the regulation of body water, electrolytes, and acid-base equilibrium.

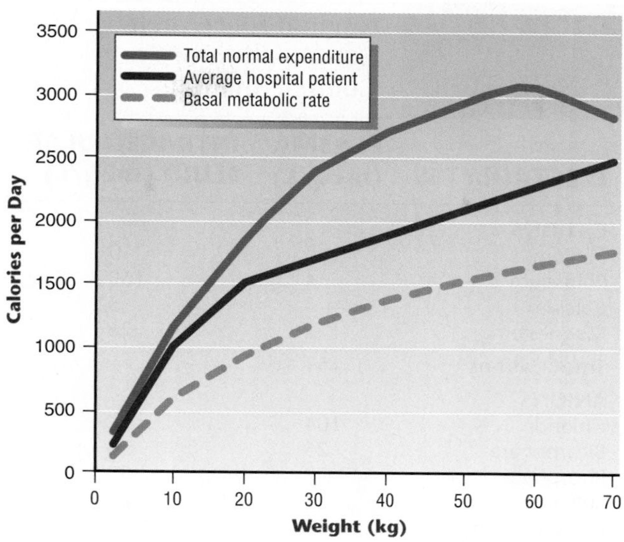

Figure 58-1 Metabolic requirements of the average hospitalized patient. The center line represents calculated caloric requirements for average hospitalized patients. See text for explanation of the three sections of the curve. (*Adapted from Holliday MA, Segar WE. The Maintenance Need for Water in Parenteral Fluid Therapy. Pediatrics. 1957;19(5):823-832.*)

BODY FLUID COMPARTMENTS

The entire body mass is composed of total body water (TBW) and body solids (fat, skeletal muscle, and cellular solids). TBW, which is 55% to 75% of body mass, varies with sex, age, and fat content.[1] Traditionally, TBW has been viewed as a composite of intracellar fluid (ICF) and extracellular fluid (ECF).[2] ECF is composed of intravascular fluid (plasma) and interstitial fluid (Figure 58-1).

TOTAL BODY WATER

Water is the most plentiful constituent of the human body. The size of the body's fluid compartments changes significantly in the 1st year of life. TBW comprises approximately 75% of an infant's mass and approximates the adult figure of 60% by 1 year of age. TBW varies inversely with the fat content of the body. TBW decreases in dehydration and thus is a smaller percentage of body weight.[2]

FLUID COMPARTMENTS—EXTRACELLULAR FLUID AND INTRACELLULAR FLUID

The ECF is divided into plasma water (5% of body weight) and interstitial fluid (15% of body weight). The term *effective circulating volume* refers to the blood volume that is perfusing the tissues of the body and is in contact with and stimulating the volume and pressor receptors.[3,4] The delicate balance between intravascular fluid and interstitial fluid is maintained by hydrostatic pressures (the result of the pumping action of the heart), as well as osmotic pressures and oncotic pressures (the result of the presence of proteins, mainly albumin). Pathological conditions such as nephrotic syndrome reduce the plasma oncotic pressure and tend to increase the interstitial fluid volume at the expense of intravascular fluid volume, whereas states of dehydration cause a decrease in both interstitial and intravascular volume.

ELECTROLYTE COMPOSITION

In plasma, sodium is the major cationic particle, with smaller concentrations of calcium, magnesium, and potassium present. Electroneutrality is maintained by an equal number of anionic particles, primarily chloride, bicarbonate, and protein. In addition to these particles are the unmeasured anions that are not part of the laboratory profile (the anion gap), namely phosphate, sulfate, and various organic acids.

The composition of ICF is different from that of plasma (Table 58-1). Potassium is the most abundant intracellular cation, followed by magnesium and a relatively small amount of sodium. The major intracellular anions are organic phosphates and proteins, with smaller concentrations of bicarbonate and sulfate.

The large concentration gradient of electrically charged particles between ECF and ICF is critical to maintaining various cellular functions, such as nerve conductance, muscle movement, and secretory processes. This gradient is maintained by active transport mechanisms found in cell membranes.

The laboratory measurement of serum concentration of electrolytes does not always reflect total body

Table 58-1 Normal Electrolyte Composition of Fluid Compartments

ELECTROLYTES	PLASMA (mEq/L)	INTRACELLULAR FLUID (mEq/L)
CATIONS		
Sodium	140	±10
Potassium	4	160
Calcium	5	3.3
Magnesium	2	26
Total Cations	**151**	—
ANIONS		
Chloride	104	±2
Bicarbonate	25	±8
Phosphate	2	95
Sulfate	1	20
Organic acids	6	—
Protein	13	55
Total Anions	**151**	—

content, and care must be taken when interpreting these results. For example, a shift of intracellular potassium into the intravascular space may lead to a normal serum level while masking a significant decrease in total body content of potassium.

OSMOLALITY AND OSMOTIC PRESSURE

The ICF and ECF are separated from each other by cell membranes that are highly water permeable but selectively impermeable to solutes. The movement of water across the cell membrane is responsible for maintaining osmotic equilibrium. Water will flow along an osmotic gradient from areas of low osmolality to areas of high osmolality, thus maintaining osmotic equilibrium between the ECF and the ICF. Osmolality is a measure of the amount of dissolved solids in the various fluid compartments and is determined by the number of molecules in solution, independent of their size.

By far the most substantial contribution to normal plasma osmolality is made by sodium and its associated anions. Under most circumstances the plasma osmolality is approximately equivalent to twice the concentration of plasma sodium. However, under unusual circumstances, or for precision, the osmolality can be calculated using the following formula:

$$2[\text{Na}]\text{mEq/L} + \frac{\text{glucose mg/dL}}{18} + \frac{\text{BUN mg/dL}}{2.8}$$

Changes in the ECF content of sodium or glucose will cause significant fluid shifts between the ECF and ICF. This shift has important clinical implications, especially in diabetic ketoacidosis, in which hyperglycemia causes a shift of water from the ICF to the ECF and dilutes the plasma sodium (hyponatremia) in spite of an elevated osmolality. In this case, the plasma sodium needs to be corrected for hyperglycemia. The formula for correction is:

$$\text{measured Na} + 1.6 \times \frac{\text{measured glucose mg/dL} - 100\text{ mg/dL}}{100}$$

Normally a difference of 10 mOsm/kg exists between the measured and calculated osmolality. This osmolar gap (the result of unmeasured osmoles) should be calculated because it may reflect the presence of unmeasured osmoles such as ethanol, ethylene glycol, methanol, mannitol, and others, especially when a clinical suspicion of poisoning exists.

REGULATING TOTAL BODY WATER AND OSMOLALITY

Homeostasis is maintained by independent systems for (1) water balance, which determines osmolality, and (2) sodium balance, which determines volume status. Although the most important determinant of plasma osmolality is sodium, the body maintains normal osmolality not by the regulation of sodium but by the regulation of TBW. Maintaining intravascular fluid volume takes precedence over maintaining osmolality.

Regulating Osmolality

Normal plasma osmolality is maintained between 285 and 290 mOsm/kg by modification of water intake and excretion. Although some water is produced in the body during oxidation and some water is lost from the lungs, skin, and gastrointestinal tract, only water intake and urinary losses are regulated. The osmolality in plasma is detected by osmoreceptors in the hypothalamus, which regulates the secretion of antidiuretic hormone (ADH). Thus, during states of elevated plasma osmolality, secretion of ADH is increased, which increases the permeability of the renal collecting ducts to water and maintains normal osmolality by reducing urinary free-water losses. At the same time, a different set of osmoreceptors stimulate the cerebral cortex to facilitate water intake by increasing the sensation of thirst. Healthy adults begin to experience thirst at plasma osmolality levels of 290 mOsm/kg, with profoundly increasing intensity as the osmolality reaches 300 to 305 mOsm/kg. At this point the person consumes large amounts of water (assuming free access, which is not the case with infants and young children) until plasma osmolality is brought back below the thirst-threshold level. Secretion of ADH occurs at a lower threshold than that for thirst and is initiated (thus inhibiting renal water loss) at a plasma osmolality level above 280 mOsm/kg. Similarly a reduction in plasma osmolality leads to suppression of ADH, increased urinary water loss, and simultaneous suppression of the thirst mechanism.

Regulating Volume

Plasma sodium is the single most important determinant of intravascular volume. Sodium homeostasis depends on the ability of the kidneys to alter its excretion in the urine, which occurs in response to change in effective circulating volume and circulating levels of plasma sodium. This mechanism will be further discussed under Sodium and Sodium Homeostasis.

Sodium and Sodium Homeostasis

Sodium is the major osmotically active cation in plasma. The total body content of sodium approximates 60 mEq/kg, but almost 43% of this content is contained in bone, most of which plays almost no role in daily regulation of sodium concentration. Most of the remainder is concentrated in the interstitial and plasma fractions, with only a small amount in the intracellular space.

Sodium homeostasis results from the balance of sodium intake and excretion. Intake is controlled by dietary habits, and although some central regulation for sodium intake may be higher given that thirst is present (many patients who lose salt seem to develop a craving for sodium), it appears to be poorly developed and has not yet been localized. The typical American adult's diet contains 100 to 170 mEq of sodium per day; the amount of sodium in the infant's diet varies according to the amount of formula or human milk the infant receives. Most of the dietary sodium is absorbed actively in the jejunum. Aldosterone secretion increases gastrointestinal sodium absorption.

Sodium excretion is controlled primarily by the kidneys but also by the gastrointestinal tract and skin. Although a large amount of sodium is presented to the kidneys during glomerular filtration, almost 99% of it is resorbed in the kidney tubules. In conditions of severe sodium depletion, volume depletion, or both, the amount resorbed may increase to nearly 100%; in cases of sodium and water overload, it may decrease to approximately 90%. The renin-angiotensin-aldosterone system, when stimulated by decreased renal blood flow, facilitates a greater degree of sodium resorption in the distal convoluted tubules and collecting ducts through the action of aldosterone at these sites.

Hypernatremia (serum sodium greater than 145 mEq/L) may follow dehydration if a greater loss of water than sodium occurs. These losses may occur through the lungs, skin, stool, or urine (especially in the presence of diabetes insipidus). Another important, although infrequent, cause of hypernatremia in young children is the overuse of commercial enema preparations containing high concentrations of phosphate and sodium. Elevated sodium content of human milk has been implicated as a cause of hypernatremia in breastfed infants.[5]

Signs and symptoms of hypernatremic dehydration may be difficult to interpret accurately, and the severity of dehydration may not be apparent based on physical examination alone. ECF volume remains relatively well preserved because of the shift of water from the ICF caused by a change in plasma osmolality; therefore clinical signs of dehydration are often absent. Hypernatremia results in marked changes in central nervous system function, especially if the electrolyte disturbance occurs rapidly (within a few hours), which is common in small children. Affected infants exhibit marked irritability alternating with severe lethargy. Seizures may occur and may be followed by coma if the condition is not diagnosed and adequate therapy is not initiated. Brain hemorrhage can occur because of the movement of water from the brain cells and tearing of the intracerebral veins. If the state of hypernatremia persists, then the brain cells react by increasing their intracellular concentrations of osmotically active solutes (previously referred as idiogenic osmoles). This action reduces neuronal dehydration and has important clinical implications. Rapid correction (ie, reduction of plasma sodium) leads to a shift of free water to the ICF (mainly neurons), leading to cerebral edema, which produces seizures and coma. Thus lowering the serum sodium level slowly over a period of 24 to 48 hours with frequent monitoring is important. In addition, elevation of the serum sodium concentration may lead to skeletal muscle rigidity and hyperactive deep-tendon reflexes.

Hyponatremia (serum sodium $<$ 130 mEq/L) occurs whenever body sodium stores are diluted or depleted. It is more often related to failure to excrete adequate amounts of water than to simple overhydration; however, in small infants the intake of hypotonic formulas or human milk low in sodium may lower the plasma sodium concentration substantially. Hyponatremic dehydration is less common in children with acute diarrhea and is most often encountered because large stool losses are replaced with solutions containing little or no sodium. Any situation that increases the secretion of ADH may be associated with low serum sodium concentrations. This circumstance is seen in patients who have the syndrome of inappropriate ADH secretion resulting from central nervous system disease, pneumonia,[6] or meningitis.[7] Addison disease and congenital adrenal hyperplasia are associated with excessive loss of sodium in the urine and with retention of potassium. Children who have obstructive uropathy and progressive renal failure are less able to resorb sodium from their renal tubules; therefore they sustain large sodium losses and may exhibit mild dehydration with a borderline or low serum sodium concentration. Children treated with vasopressin or 1-deamino-8-D-arginine vasopressin may develop iatrogenic hyponatremia,[8,9] as may children receiving diuretic therapy. The administration of enemas low in saline concentration also may result in hyponatremia. An excessive loss of sodium and water occurs in individuals suffering from heat-related illnesses. The serum sodium concentration reported by the laboratory may be artificially low in the presence of marked hyperlipidemia and hyperproteinemia (pseudohyponatremia). Highly elevated concentrations of blood glucose (as in diabetic ketoacidosis) are associated with real and factitious hyponatremia.

Signs and symptoms of hyponatremia are related to the duration of the lowered serum sodium concentration, the rate of decrease in serum sodium, and to the plasma volume status. Most signs and symptoms are due to ICF shifts especially related to cerebral edema. These patients will have more manifestations of signs of dehydration as a result of a reduction in effective circulating volume. Hyponatremia associated with diminished plasma volume results in anorexia, muscle cramps, lethargy, and shortness of breath on exertion. With further decreases in sodium concentration, nausea, emesis, and muscle weakness ensue, which may proceed to delirium and seizures.[6,10] Hyponatremia associated with acute water intoxication is more likely to result in seizures and coma than in conditions in which the plasma volume remains unchanged.

Potassium

Potassium is the major intracellular cation. The total potassium content is approximately 50 mEq/kg of body weight, with concentrations of intracellular and extracellular potassium of 145 mEq/L and 4 to 5 mEq/L, respectively.[2]

The kidney is the primary organ involved in potassium homeostasis. Potassium is filtered by the glomerulus and is resorbed and secreted by the tubule. Most potassium absorption occurs in the proximal portions of the gastrointestinal tract where it is excreted in the colon in exchange for sodium. Thus disorders of kidney and altered absorption in the gastrointestinal tract are associated with significant abnormalities in serum potassium levels. Aldosterone is intimately involved in regulating potassium by increasing its excretion from the gastrointestinal tract, the skin (losses here are relatively minimal), and the kidneys. Urinary excretion of potassium results from tubular secretion rather than glomerular filtration. Aldosterone acts at the level of the distal tubule to foster sodium resorption and potassium secretion. Thus sustained hypovolemic states result in enhanced renal potassium losses. Potassium frequently shifts between the intracellular and extracellular spaces, mediated mostly by alterations in the serum acid-base status. An increase in extracellular potassium concentration occurs with systemic acidosis, and alkalosis leads to movement of potassium into the cell.

Increased potassium levels, though infrequent in children, can be life threatening because of its effect on membrane potential, especially in cardiac muscle. The earliest sign of cardiac toxicity are in the form of tall, peaked T waves (with normal or short QT interval and short PR interval). They are seen at serum concentrations of 5.5 to 6.5 mEq/L. A widened QRS complex with prolonged PR interval is seen at levels between 6.5 and 7.5 mEq/L. Subsequent increases in serum potassium levels are associated with broad P waves, QT prolongation (7.0 to 8.0 mEq/L), and absent P waves with markedly widened QRS (sine wave pattern) at levels above 8.0 mEq/L. Most patients with hypokalemia are asymptomatic, particularly if the disorder is mild (3.0 to 3.5 mEq/L). Most frequently the clinical findings in hypokalemia include muscle weakness and ileus. Cardiac effects may also be exhibited on the electrocardiogram by low voltage, flattening of the T waves, depression of ST segments, prominence of U waves, arrhythmias, and asystole. However, these effects are usually not seen until the serum potassium concentration falls below 2.0 mEq/L. When levels fall below 2.0 mEq/L, an ascending paralysis can develop, with eventual respiratory muscle paralysis. The likelihood of symptoms caused by hypokalemia depend on the rapidity of decrease and presence of underlying heart disease; these children should be treated promptly (especially children who are receiving digitalis derivatives).

Other Ions

Concentrations of chloride, calcium, magnesium, and phosphorous are also critical to maintenance of cellular function, but their role in typical fluid disturbances is relatively minor and will not be discussed here. The remaining ion of interest is bicarbonate, which is crucial in the acid-base buffering system in plasma that is responsible for the close maintenance of a normal pH in the setting of widely varying conditions. Control of the concentration of bicarbonate is the result of interactions between its plasma concentration and those of carbon dioxide and water. The concentrations of these components, and thus control and maintenance of pH, are affected by the function of the kidneys and the lungs. In metabolic acidosis, when plasma pH falls in the setting of poor tissue perfusion or increased acid production, the kidney retains bicarbonate ion, whereas the lungs increase their elimination of carbon dioxide by increasing minute ventilation, driving the system toward higher pH. In respiratory acidosis, usually induced by excessive carbon dioxide production or inadequate elimination by the lungs, the kidney responds by retaining bicarbonate ion. Conversely, with respiratory alkalosis, in the case of increased minute ventilation and excessive carbon dioxide losses, the kidney excretes increased amounts of bicarbonate ion, lowering plasma pH.

In most situations requiring fluid therapy, a metabolic acidosis prevails as a result of diminished tissue perfusion. Attention to the pH and buffering characteristics of fluids administered is important, but more important is administering sufficient amounts of isotonic fluids that will result in rapid reexpansion of the ECF. The resulting enhanced tissue perfusion, elimination of tissue acids, and restoration of end-organ function will stop the acidosis.

REFERENCES

1. Perkin RM, Novotny WE, Harris GD, et al. Common electrolyte problems in pediatric patients presenting to the ED. *Pediatr Emerg Med Rep*. Nov 2001;6(11): 113-116.
2. Greenbaum LA. Pathophysiology of body fluids and fluid therapy. In: Berhman RE, ed. *Nelson Textbook of Pediatrics*. 17th ed. Philadelphia, PA: Elsevier; 2006: 191-223.
3. Hill LL. Body composition, normal electrolyte concentrations, and the maintenance of normal volume, tonicity, and acid-base metabolism. *Pediatr Clin North Am*. Apr 1990; 37(2):241-256.
4. Saxton CR, Seldin DW. Clinical interpretation of laboratory values. In: Kokko JP, Tannen RL, eds. *Fluids and Electrolytes*. Philadelphia, PA: WB Saunders; 1986.
5. Peters JM. Hypernatremia in breast-fed infants due to elevated breast milk sodium, *J Am Osteopath Assoc*. 1989;89:1165.
6. Cheng JC, Zikos D, Peterson DR, et al. Symptomatic hyponatremia: pathophysiology and management. *Acute Care*. 1988;14-15, 1989;270-292.
7. Shann F, Germer S. Hyponatremia associated with pneumonia or bacterial meningitis. *Arch Dis Child*. 1985; 60:963.
8. Beach PS, Beach RE, Smith LR. Hyponatremic seizures in a child treated with desmopressin to control enuresis: a rational approach to fluid intake. *Clin Pediatr*. 1992;31: 566.

9. Smith TJ, Gill JC, Ambroso DR, et al. Hyponatremia and seizures in young children given DDAVP. *Am J Hematol.* 1989;31:199-202.
10. Wattad A, Chiang ML, Hill LL. Hyponatremia in hospitalized children. *Clin Pediatr.* 1992;31:153.

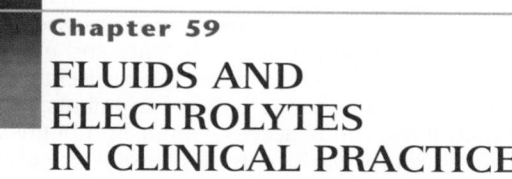

Chapter 59

FLUIDS AND ELECTROLYTES IN CLINICAL PRACTICE

Prashant V. Mahajan, MD, MPH, MBA

MAINTENANCE REQUIREMENTS

Estimating parenteral fluid requirements relies on a knowledge of the losses of water and electrolytes that occur under normal conditions. In clinical practice, maintenance fluids and electrolytes must be replaced, and deficits caused by ongoing losses, if any, must be corrected. The key to understanding maintenance fluid and electrolyte requirements is recognizing that they stem from basal metabolism.[1] Metabolism creates two by-products—heat and solute—that need to be eliminated to maintain homeostasis. Heat is lost through insensible evaporation of water from the skin (accounting for two thirds of insensible water loss; approximately 30 mL/100 kcal) and from the respiratory system (accounting for one third of insensible water loss; approximately 15 mL/100 kcal). Sensible water losses occur primarily through urine output (55 mL/100 kcal), which is needed by the body to excrete the daily solute by-products from metabolism. Obligate urine output, the minimal amount of urine needed to eliminate daily solute by-products, is approximately 25 mL/100 kcal.

Water

Daily water needs are based on insensible losses from the respiratory tract and skin and sensible losses from the urine and stool. Traditionally, water requirements have been calculated by 1 of 3 methods: (1) body weight, (2) body surface area, or (3) metabolic rate. Water need per unit of body weight changes dramatically with age and size and therefore is not very useful. Body surface area was once thought to correlate well with both metabolic expenditure and fluid needs, but this has been subsequently shown not to be the case, especially in neonates and in children between 6 months and 3 years of age. Additionally, surface area is determined by comparing height and weight with a nomogram, which is cumbersome and depends on accurate measurements (height is notoriously difficult to measure in young children and infants). Use of the metabolic rate to calculate fluid requirements is attractive because it is based on physiological principles and is a constant number; approximately 100 mL (1 dL) of water is needed for every 100 calories consumed.[2] Using an average child who has a metabolic rate midway between normal activity and basal metabolic rate as a standard, a fluid requirement can be derived based on calorie expenditure that is quite simple and can be calculated from body weight (Figure 59-1). This value results in a maintenance water requirement of 100 mL/kg/day for each of the first 10 kg, 50 mL/kg/day for each additional kilogram from 11 to 20, and 20 mL/kg/day for each subsequent kilogram. When converting to an hourly fluid rate the simplest approximation is 4 mL/kg/hr for the first 10 kg, 2 mL/kg/hr for the next 10, and 1 mL/kg/hr for each additional kilogram. This value results, for example, in an hourly maintenance rate of 32 mL/hr for an 8-kg infant (4 mL/kg × 8 kg), 50 mL/hr for a 15-kg toddler (4 mL/kg × 10 kg = 40 mL, plus 2 mL/kg × 5 kg = 10 mL), and 70 mL/hr for a 30-kg child (4 mL/kg × 10 kg = 40 mL, plus 2 mL/kg × 10 kg = 20 mL, plus 1 mL/kg × 10 kg = 10 mL) (Table 59-1). This simple approach will meet maintenance fluid requirements for most children and should be adjusted up or down depending on factors such as rate of insensible fluid losses (tachypnea, burns) or decreased fluid excretion (renal failure).

Electrolytes

The maintenance requirement of sodium for the average infant is between 2 and 3 mEq/100 cal; and potassium is closer to 2 mEq/100 cal. Because sodium and potassium are supplied routinely in the form of chloride salt, the infant or child receives between 4 and 5 mEq/100 cal of chloride ion, although the absolute chloride requirement probably is very small. An important point to remember is that the amount of water and electrolytes for maintenance needs are based on the metabolic rate and not body weight. This point is important especially while calculating electrolyte needs in an older child and adolescent.

Calories

The nutritional component of maintenance therapy should provide substrate for metabolism. Although optimal nutritional therapy provides an equal number of calories for those expended, for short-term administration of parenteral fluids, little consideration is

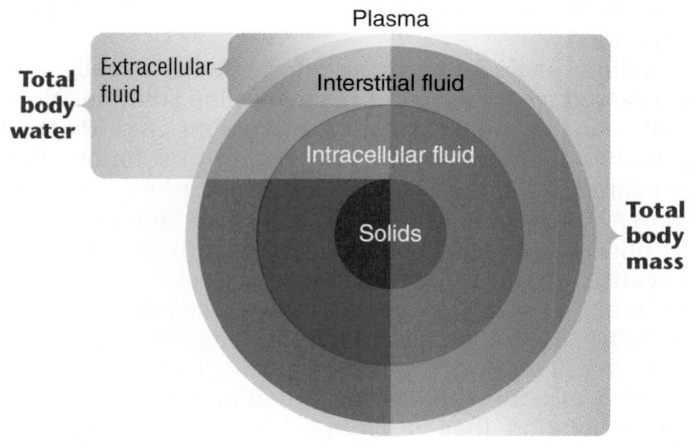

Figure 59-1 Fluid compartments of the body.

Table 59-1 Holliday-Segar Formula for Determining Daily Maintenance Fluid Requirements

WEIGHT (kg)	KCAL/DAY OR ML/DAY	KCAL/HR OR ML/HR
0-10	100 kg/day	4 mL/kg/hr
11-20	1000 + (50/kg/day)*	40 + (2 kg/hr)
>20	1500 + (20/kg/day)†	60 + (1 kg/hr)

*For each kg > 10.
†For each kg > 20.
From Holliday MA, Segar WE. The Maintenance Need for Water in Parenteral Fluid Therapy. *Pediatrics.* 1957;19(5):823-832.

usually given to replacing caloric expenditure calorie per calorie. Rather, the reason for adding calories in the form of dextrose to parenteral fluids is to prevent ketosis and the breakdown of endogenous protein. In the average hospitalized patient this process requires that approximately 25% of caloric expenditure be provided with an intravenous solution that contains glucose; therefore the aim should be 25 cal/100 cal expended energy. Because each gram of dextrose provides 4 calories, 5 g of dextrose per 100 calories expended provides sufficient energy. For infants and small children the absolute glucose requirement to prevent ketosis and overt hypoglycemia is between 4 and 6 mg/kg/minute.

COMPOSITION OF MAINTENANCE FLUID FOR PARENTERAL USE

The composition of the parenteral fluid that can be administered under normal circumstances to a hospitalized patient for a short period (up to several days) is figured based on 1 dL water, 2 to 3 mEq sodium, 2 mEq potassium, and 5 g glucose for every 100 calories expended. Because prepared intravenous fluids are formulated on a per-liter basis the composition of a suitable fluid for maintenance therapy would be 20 to 30 mEq sodium, 20 mEq potassium, and 50 g glucose (values expressed per liter) for every 100 calories expended.

Values of sodium in parenteral fluids usually are expressed as a fraction of normal saline solution. Normal saline is a 0.9% solution of sodium chloride that provides 154 mEq of sodium per liter of solution. The prepared solutions available most commonly contain either half-normal saline (77 mEq of sodium per liter) or quarter-normal saline (38 mEq of sodium per liter). Because of the body's ability to excrete any excess sodium, a solution containing quarter-normal (or 0.225%) saline is an acceptable preparation. This solution is usually formulated with 5% glucose (50 g/L); 20 mEq of potassium can be added to each liter, yielding a solution that is slightly hypertonic (compared with plasma), with an osmolarity of 386 mOsm/L. This solution is, however, hypotonic with respect to sodium.

ADMINISTRATION

Once the appropriate concentration of each solute in the parenteral fluid has been determined the solution is administered at a rate of 100 mL/100 cal of expected energy expenditure through a peripheral vein. Procedures for gaining vascular access in children are described in Appendix B, Special Procedures. Although not a new method, the technique of administering fluids and medications into the bone marrow (intraosseous infusion) has been demonstrated to be safe and effective in providing volume replacement and resuscitation drugs in an emergency. It may be used in infants and children when intravenous access cannot be obtained rapidly. Techniques for performing this procedure also are found in Appendix B. Any solution that can be given intravenously may be given via the intraosseous route.

WHEN MAINTENANCE IS NOT ADEQUATE

In the preceding sections a rational approach is outlined for supplying children with maintenance fluids. Based on the physiologic mechanism of the illness the needs of any given child may differ considerably from these maintenance requirements. However, the calculations presented remain valid over a wide range of situations if used as a basis on which unusual losses are added. Any and all of the organs normally involved in water homeostasis may be sought as sources or reasons for water loss: water lost through the gastrointestinal (GI) tract in the form of diarrhea or vomiting; massive renal excretion of water in diabetes mellitus or diabetes insipidus or after administration of osmotic or other diuretics; excessive sweating caused by autonomic instability, fever, or high ambient temperature; and an increased loss of lung water with hyperpnea from any cause, including hyperpyrexia. Processes that do not normally contribute to water loss also may be involved, such as losses through a nasogastric tube and acute blood loss. In addition, increased demands for fluids exist in various conditions of elevated metabolic rate (eg, thyrotoxicosis), in situations that create large shifts in the body's fluid compartments (usually of the vascular space), and in many perioperative conditions (third spacing) that if uncorrected may produce shock. Persistence of any of these abnormal conditions in the absence of adequate fluid intake leads to water or electrolyte deficits or both. The purpose of replacement fluid therapy is to determine a rational approach to body water and electrolyte restoration. Additionally, the fluid administration scheme has to take into consideration the ongoing losses that persist beyond the institution of parenteral fluid therapy and provide appropriate replacement of these lost fluids.

Fluids sometimes need to be supplied in amounts below those estimated for the average hospitalized patient. Any child who has a diminished urine output because of renal failure does not require as much free water as the child's healthy counterpart. Children who are placed in mist tents or maintained on ventilators lose less water through their lungs and should have a lower estimate made of insensible water loss. Children whose activity levels are below those predicted for most

Table 59-2 Signs and Symptoms Related to Degree of Dehydration*

PARAMETER	DEGREE OF DEHYDRATION		
	MILD	MODERATE	SEVERE
Weight loss in child <1 yr	3-5	10	15
Weight loss in patient >1 yr (%)	2-3	6-9	>10
Skin color	Pale	Gray	Mottled
Skin turgor	May be normal	Decreased	Tenting
Mucous membranes	Slightly dry	Dry	Dry, parched, collapse of sublingual veins
Eyes	Probably normal	Decreased tears	Sunken, absence of tears, soft globes
Central nervous system	Normal	Irritable	Lethargic
PULSE			
Quality	Strong	Somewhat decreased	Distal pulse not palpable
Rate	Probably normal	Somewhat increased (orthostatic changes)	Markedly tachycardic
OTHER PARAMETERS			
Capillary refill	Normal (<2 seconds)	2-4 seconds	>4 seconds
Blood pressure	No change	Orthostatic decrease	Decreased while supine
Urine	Probably normal or slightly decreased volume	Elevated specific gravity, decreased volume	Less than 0.5 mL/kg/hr over the previous 12-24 hr; may be anuric

*Table is most useful for situations involving isotonic dehydration. (See text for adjustments needed for other forms of dehydration.)

bedridden patients (eg, those in coma or who are paralyzed) expend fewer calories and therefore require less water (see Figure 59-1).

ESTIMATING AND CORRECTING DEFICITS AND ONGOING LOSSES

The best way to estimate fluid and electrolyte deficits is to determine how much fluid has been lost from each body compartment, the electrolyte concentration of the lost fluid, and the period over which such losses have occurred. In most situations, however, therapy must be initiated before these data can be collected. In addition, volumes of diarrheal or emetic losses may be extremely difficult to measure.

The first step in evaluating a child who has a fluid and electrolyte deficit is to determine the degree of total body volume that has been lost. Although fluids and electrolytes are lost from all body compartments the intravascular volume status is the most immediately relevant. Children who have sustained severe losses of intravascular (circulating) fluid volume are at risk for shock, which may result in irreversible organ system damage and death if not addressed promptly.

Table 59-2 contains a systematic approach to estimating fluid losses. Typically, a child may be categorized as mildly, moderately, or severely dehydrated according to clinical findings (the term *dehydration* is used here in its most common sense, meaning losses of fluid volume. Technically, dehydration refers only to pure water losses, a condition almost never seen clinically). Attention should be given to the immediate replacement of the estimated fluid losses via the oral, intravenous, or intraosseous routes, depending on the child's overall clinical status. Even before a formal calculation is made, an initial fluid bolus of 20 mL/kg over 20 to 30 minutes should be given to any child who appears to be severely dehydrated or in shock.

When calculating the final amount of fluid to be replaced, either a recent-normal weight should be used, if available, or the deficit may be calculated based on an average (50th percentile) weight for the child's age. Formerly, fluid replacements were administered over a 24-hour period, with the aim of restoring one half of the deficit in the first 8 hours of therapy and the second half in the subsequent 16 hours. It is apparent that faster rates of fluid repletion are both more effective and simpler and that complicated formulas for calculating fluid and electrolyte replacements are not necessary. In most cases, dehydration of a mild to moderate degree may be managed on an outpatient basis, often without the use of intravenous therapy at all. In general, the aim should be to replace the entire calculated deficit in the initial 4 to 6 hours of treatment.[3] This more rapid treatment hastens the restoration of circulating fluid volume, speeds the excretion of tissue acids and ketones that are the result of diminished end-organ perfusion, and contributes to the more rapid resolution of compensatory mechanisms such as renal sodium retention and potassium losses.

In the vast majority of cases, electrolyte determinations do not add useful information to management.[4-6] The exceptions to this rule include a child who has a severely abnormal mental status (irritable or lethargic), seizures, or clinical signs of hyponatremia or hypernatremia. Furthermore, normal saline should be the initial fluid of choice in virtually all instances, until a specific electrolyte abnormality is detected that mandates a more hypertonic or hypotonic solution. An important point to remember is that regardless of measured serum sodium concentration a child who is significantly dehydrated usually has a net deficit of *total body sodium;* thus even a hypernatremic child (as determined by the serum concentration of sodium) will benefit from the initial administration of normal saline.

Fluid volume for initial rehydration should be based on calculated or estimated healthy weight. After an initial bolus administration of 20 mL/kg over 20 to 30 minutes the child should be reevaluated. If evidence of shock persists, then repeated boluses should be administered, with reevaluation after each bolus. When heart rate and capillary refill time have returned to normal the rate of fluid administration may be reduced to an amount calculated to replace the remaining deficit over 4 to 6 hours. In a healthy child who has normal kidneys this task may usually be accomplished safely by administering half-normal saline (77 mEq of sodium per liter).

THERAPEUTIC APPROACH TO SPECIAL SITUATIONS

Shock

Severe plasma volume deficit, with actual or impending cardiovascular collapse, is a life-threatening pediatric emergency requiring *immediate* action; initial therapy replaces the intravascular volume depletion with normal (0.9%) saline. (See Chapter 358, Shock.) Hemorrhagic shock, which must be considered with any history of trauma or any possible internal source of bleeding (eg, a known peptic ulcer or other GI disease that might lead to acute blood loss), must be treated with administration of packed red blood cells. This treatment is required because administering additional electrolyte solutions to a patient who has an already diminished hematocrit decreases oxygen-carrying capacity further and may result in irreversible damage to vital organs (especially the heart and brain). Therefore most hospital blood banks keep a fairly ready supply of type O blood, which should be infused as rapidly as possible once the diagnosis of hemorrhagic shock has been considered. A sample of the patient's blood (obtained before transfusion) should be sent to the blood bank so that a properly matched unit of donor blood can be obtained without delay in case it is needed for further therapy. In addition, if the patient's blood type is known, then type-specific non–cross-matched blood, which carries less risk than the use of type O non–cross-matched blood, may be administered. While awaiting the arrival of blood from the blood bank, normal saline solution should be given. The use of colloid-containing plasma expanders such as albumin or dextran remains controversial and probably provides no benefit over the use of a crystalloid solution unless the shock is the result of protein loss. Additionally, if the shock is cardiogenic, then administration of albumin may worsen pulmonary edema. In sepsis, in which volume depletion is caused by leaky capillaries and exudation of plasma into extravascular spaces, fresh-frozen plasma may be useful (because it also replaces many clotting factors) and is sometimes used in combination with other fluids. Shock in babies and small children is associated almost invariably with depletion of glycogen stores. Thus hypoglycemia often may be present. Administration of 2 to 4 mL/kg of a 25% dextrose solution will correct hypoglycemia and improve the results of further resuscitation efforts. For this reason, rapid bedside determination of blood glucose concentration should always be part of the initial evaluation of the infant or child in shock (current or impending).

Serious Electrolyte Abnormalities

Although most patients who are dehydrated may be managed with the empirical administration of normal saline, and without measurement of serum electrolytes, special situations exist in which more attention must be given to electrolyte status. Clinically, these situations will become apparent if a child demonstrates signs associated with hypernatermia or hyponatremia (see later discussion) or if signs of dehydration do not resolve in response to standard management. This section examines specific electrolyte abnormalities.

Sodium

The pediatric electrolyte aberrations encountered most commonly relate to sodium balance, and they ordinarily occur with dehydration. The clinical conditions of hyponatremia and hypernatremia, which involve abnormalities of both the patient's volume status and the plasma osmolality, are discussed in the section. When significant electrolyte disturbances are evident, efforts must be made to determine the cause of the disturbance, as well as any factors that may tend to perpetuate it, so that they can be addressed in the treatment plan.

HYPONATREMIA. Hyponatremia is usually associated with hypotonicity. When it is not, the clinician must suspect either artifactual lowering of the serum sodium, such as with hyperlipidemia and hyperproteinemia, or the presence of an osmotically active substance such as glucose or mannitol.[7] These compounds cause a shift of intracellular water into the extracellular space to restore osmotic neutrality, thereby lowering effective serum sodium by 1.6 mEq/L for every 100-mg/dL rise in serum glucose or mannitol concentration. Such situations are associated almost universally with preservation of intravascular volume (except in some extreme cases of diabetic ketoacidosis) and are often apparent from the history, physical examination, or a few simple laboratory tests. Table 59-3 summarizes the causes of hyponatremia. The clinical manifestations of hyponatremia are primarily neurologic and related to cerebral edema caused by hypo-osmolality. These manifestations occur in the form of headaches, nausea, vomiting, and weakness. As the cerebral edema worsens, patients develop behavioral changes and impaired response to verbal and tactile stimuli.[8]

The most common clinical situation leading to hyponatremia is volume loss, usually caused by diarrhea, in which the child has lost fluid with a sodium concentration higher than that of the serum. If ongoing diarrheal losses are replaced with hypotonic fluids, then

Table 59-3 Causes of Hyponatremia

TYPE	CAUSE
Pseudohyponatremia (Hyperosmolality)	Hyperglycemia Mannitol
Hypovolemic hyponatremia	Gastrointestinal losses (vomiting, diarrhea) Excessive sweating Renal losses (diuretics, urinary obstruction, etc)
Euvolemic hyponatremia	Syndrome of inappropriate secretion of antidiuretic hormone Glucocorticoid deficiency Water intoxication (excessive hypotonic intravenous fluids) Child abuse, tap water enemas, psychogenic polydipsia
Hypervolemic hyponatremia	Congestive cardiac failure Cirrhosis Nephrotic syndrome

hyponatremia will develop, even if the volume deficit is not great. Sodium-rich fluid is also lost from the intravascular space when ascites or other abnormal accumulations of fluid occupy a body cavity. This phenomenon is known as *third spacing*.

When volume status is normal the clinician must consider situations that lead to a combination of sodium loss with water intake sufficient to maintain usual hydration. Such a negative sodium balance can result from severe restriction of sodium intake or profound loss of sodium through the skin, GI tract, or kidneys (salt-losing nephropathy or diuretic use).

Mild hyponatremia (serum sodium 128 to 134 mEq/dL) with normovolemia or hypovolemia is usually undetectable clinically and can be managed by providing isotonic sodium solutions with adequate fluid administration, thereby allowing excretion of water at an appropriate rate. When simultaneous large deficits of both water and saline solution occur, both must be replaced effectively; the usual normal saline solution is sufficient at the outset.

Severe total body potassium depletion, sometimes overlooked, may lead to persistent hyponatremia. Because potassium is the major intracellular cation, sodium ions enter the cells to replace potassium ions to provide electroneutrality; therefore the concentration of sodium in the extracellular space may fall. Potassium then must be supplied to allow the restoration of normal sodium balance.

More rapid correction of the sodium deficit may be necessary with serious symptoms (seizures), which may accompany a large or precipitous decline in serum sodium concentration. Rapid correction can be achieved through the administration of 3% saline solution (containing 500 mEq of sodium per liter), which allows rapid replacement of sodium without infusing a large volume of water.[9] Administration of 10 to 12 mL/kg of 3% saline over 1 hour will provide rapid and temporary relief of signs of severe hyponatremia by elevating the serum sodium level rapidly. Osmotic equilibrium is established rapidly once intravascular tonicity is restored because sodium is distributed quickly throughout all body fluid compartments. Intravenous administration of hypertonic sodium-chloride solutions is not without risk to the patient, however, especially a patient who has cardiac or renal disease. Such infusions cause a rapid shift of water into the intravascular space and may lead to acute volume overload. This therapy must therefore be reserved for potentially life-threatening situations, and the child must be monitored closely throughout the infusion. Demyelination syndromes have been noted in adults because of rapid reversal (a rise of more than 12 mEq/L in 24 hours) of long-standing or chronic hyponatremia.[10] When hyponatremia exists with *expanded* vascular volume the most likely cause is excessive secretion of antidiuretic hormone (ADH), which may occur because of increased intracranial pressure, severe pneumonia, or the stress of certain surgical procedures. Syndrome of inappropriate secretion of ADH is diagnosed based on laboratory and physical examination data and requires the presence of hyponatremia with normal or increased intravascular volume. Sodium excretion in the urine is variable but is usually higher than expected for the level of serum sodium concentration. Treatment of this disorder, whatever the cause, consists of fluid restriction and no sodium administration, unless the patient is convulsing. Some authors have urged the simultaneous use of a potent diuretic such as furosemide, which is expected to induce the loss of more water than sodium.[11] In most cases, however, fluid restriction remains the safest and most efficacious mode of therapy. Once the sodium concentration returns to near normal, moderate fluid restriction (generally to two thirds of maintenance requirements) may need to be continued, usually for at least 24 hours but sometimes for as long as the underlying disorder persists.

HYPERNATREMIA. As with decreased serum sodium concentration, hypernatremia may occur with overhydration, dehydration, or normal hydration. However, unlike hyponatremia, an elevated serum sodium level is *always* associated with hypertonicity. Table 59-4 summarizes the causes of hypernatremia.

Hypernatremia associated with overhydration is generally an iatrogenic problem created by (1) administering intravenous or oral solutions with high salt content and (2) failing to provide the requisite free water. Patients treated with large amounts of sodium bicarbonate for metabolic acidosis are also at risk of developing marked hypernatremia (approximately 1 mEq of sodium is administered for every milliliter of bicarbonate solution). Occasionally, when infant formulas are being mixed, mistakes occur that result in markedly hypertonic solutions that may induce particularly severe hypernatremias. These patients are at risk of developing obvious signs of plasma volume overload, including hypertension, congestive heart failure, and pulmonary edema. Under such circumstances, administering additional fluid is risky and may prove fatal. The

Table 59-4 Causes of Hypernatremia

MECHANISM	CAUSE
Excessive sodium	Improperly mixed formula
	Intentional (Munchausen syndrome by proxy)
	Hyperaldosteronism
Water deficit	Nephrogenic diabetes insipidus
	Central diabetes insipidus
	Increased insensible losses (prematurity, phototherapy)
Water and sodium deficits	Gastrointestinal losses (diarrhea, nasogastric suction)
	Skin losses (burns, excessive sweating)
	Renal losses (osmotic diuretics, diabetes mellitus)

most rational approach is to limit sodium and water input and to attempt to induce sodium loss to a greater extent than water. This task may be accomplished by using a potent loop diuretic such as furosemide, which will induce a net sodium loss if the child's renal function is adequate. Concurrently, the clinician must watch closely for the development of dehydration because predicting precisely how much water and sodium will be lost is impossible. Generally, some portion of the induced urine output (50%-75%) should be replaced with intravenous fluid that is slightly hypotonic (ie, 66% or 75% normal saline solution) until normal hydration and tonicity have been achieved. In patients who have severe hypernatremia (ordinarily considered as a serum sodium value greater than 160 mEq/L), serious complications may occur if the sodium concentration falls too rapidly. This action produces marked shifts of extracellular water to the intracellular space and results in cellular swelling. This swelling is most worrisome in the central nervous system because cerebral edema may occur, which may lead to seizures, coma, or death. Therefore when the serum sodium value is high and is accompanied by overhydration the preferred therapeutic approach is to restrict sodium and water, thus permitting a spontaneous diuresis to occur. Serum electrolyte values must be monitored every few hours. If the patient has substantially decreased renal function, then hemodialysis or peritoneal dialysis should be considered, especially in the presence of hypertension or pulmonary edema.

Hypernatremia associated with decreased plasma volume is encountered frequently in pediatric practice. It is caused most commonly by acute gastroenteritis that induces relatively larger losses of water than sodium. Although these children may have severe hypernatremia, their total body sodium content is usually depleted; they therefore present quite a therapeutic challenge.

Patients who have this condition need to be evaluated carefully. The physician must consider all the aspects of dehydration previously discussed but must remember that because extracellular fluid volume is relatively well preserved, the severity of the plasma volume loss may be seriously underestimated. Even with significant fluid losses, these children rarely have signs of incipient vascular collapse. When using the signs and symptoms of dehydration shown in Table 59-2 to determine the degree of dehydration, if the serum sodium concentration is greater than 155 mEq/L, then another 3% to 5% should be added to the weight loss in predicting the degree of dehydration.

Fluid therapy of hypernatremic dehydration is not nearly as straightforward as for other types of dehydration because the risk of creating major fluid shifts and cerebral edema is great. The clinician cannot simply try to remove sodium because a decrease in the plasma tonicity without an increase in plasma water may induce circulatory collapse. Therefore a cautious rehydration scheme must be developed.

Instead of being rehydrated over a short period, as with isonatremic or hyponatremic dehydration, the child who has a serum sodium greater than 155 mEq/L should have the fluid deficit replaced over 48 to 72 hours. Calculating the actual amount of sodium lost is *not* possible. The physician should estimate the water deficit (based on weight and clinical signs) and plan to replace this volume evenly over 48 to 72 hours. The solution used should be slightly hyponatremic (containing 100 to 120 mEq of sodium per liter). Glucose should be added so that the solution is not hypotonic. As soon as the urine output is judged to be adequate, potassium should be added to the intravenous solution to correct the potassium deficit and to preserve the intracellular osmolality, thus helping to prevent intracellular edema. Particularly important is to monitor serum electrolyte concentrations, serum osmolality, and urine output and osmolality as frequently as possible. Although the clinician needs to avoid a persistent elevation of the serum sodium concentration, ensuring a slow, steady decline in the serum sodium and osmolality levels is also important.[12] Decreases in serum tonicity should be limited to a rate of 5 mOsm/hr. Serum sodium concentration should fall at a rate no more rapid than 0.5 mEq/L/hr. In many cases, adding up to 40 mEq of potassium per liter to the infused solution and reducing its sodium concentration to 50 mEq/L is feasible.

Sometimes, no matter how carefully hypernatremia is handled, seizures ensue during the rehydration period. They can usually be managed successfully by infusing a solution slightly more hypertonic than the one being given (ie, normal saline or lactated Ringer's solution). If the seizures are particularly severe, or evidence exists of brain herniation, then a hypertonic agent such as mannitol may be required. Unfortunately, the diuresis induced by mannitol may worsen the dehydration substantially. In addition, mannitol should not be used if urine output has not been established.

A relatively uncommon cause of hypernatremia is diabetes insipidus, which usually leads to hypernatremia with a normal plasma volume. This circumstance presupposes an intact thirst mechanism and that the patient has access to the large volume of water required to replace renal losses. Such is not the case for small babies and certain other patients who have diabetes insipidus and hypernatremic dehydration.

Large renal losses of free water may occur because of deficient ADH (central or pituitary diabetes insipidus) or impairment of the normal renal response to the hormone (nephrogenic diabetes insipidus).

In infants and children the most common cause of central diabetes insipidus is a brain tumor, such as a craniopharyngioma. The syndrome also may follow intracranial surgical procedures or trauma. Other causes include central nervous system diseases of vascular, infectious, or granulomatous origin or histiocytosis. The most common cause of central diabetes insipidus in children and young adults is idiopathic.[13]

Nephrogenic diabetes insipidus may be evident as a congenital disorder, but it is more commonly caused by renal failure (particularly that caused by obstructive uropathy) or to electrolyte disorders, drug ingestions, or sickle cell disease. Laboratory findings in diabetes insipidus usually include a moderate to marked hypernatremia (depending on how adequately the lost fluid volume has been replaced) and dilute urine, usually produced in large volumes. Clinically, these patients exhibit a tremendous thirst (often craving ice-cold water) and usually show signs of normal hydration. The laboratory differentiation between central and nephrogenic diabetes insipidus is unnecessary when the cause is apparent (eg, after surgical removal of a craniopharyngioma) but in other situations is essential to help guide the therapeutic approach. This differentiation is generally determined by performing a water deprivation test.

Potassium

HYPOKALEMIA. A low serum potassium concentration seldom represents an emergency unless cardiac effects are seen, which do not typically occur until the serum potassium level is less than 2 mEq/L. (For symptoms of hypokalemia, see later discussion.) In patients receiving digitalis preparations, however, a combined cardiac toxicity may ensue, and the typical T-wave changes and arrhythmias of hypokalemia may occur at serum potassium levels closer to normal. Other patients at risk of exhibiting an exaggerated response to mild hypokalemia include those who have an acid-base disturbance or other ionic aberration that may create a cardiac conduction disturbance by substantially altering the flux of ions between the intracellular and extracellular spaces. At particular risk of developing such alterations are children receiving long-term diuretic therapy. Hypokalemia may occur after large losses of potassium from the kidneys in children with diabetic ketoacidosis and as a manifestation of hyperaldosteronism. (Table 59-5 lists the causes of hypokalemia.)

When emergency therapy for hypokalemia is necessary (usually in the form of intravenous potassium at a dose of 0.5 to 1.0 mEq/kg usually given over 1 hour and in the preoperative patient who has a serum potassium concentration less than 3.5 mEq/L), intravenous potassium repletion should be implemented. This task is accomplished either by increasing the concentration of potassium ion in the fluids given intravenously (maximum of 80 mEq/L) or by administering a bolus of potassium into a central vein. The maximal amount of potassium that may be given is 1 mEq/kg over a 1-hour period (with the physician at the bedside and continuous electrocardiographic monitoring), but it is generally safer to deliver only 20% or 25% of this amount and to repeat the dose as necessary to raise the concentration to a safe level. In nonemergent circumstances, enteral potassium supplementation is safer and very effective.

Table 59-5 Causes of Hypokalemia

MECHANISM	CAUSES
1. Spurious	High white cell counts
2. Transcellular shifts	Alkalosis Insulin Beta-agonists (albuterol), toxins (theophylline) Hypokalemic periodic paralysis
3. Decreased intake	—
4. Extrarenal losses	Diarrhea, sweating, laxative abuse
5. Renal losses	With metabolic acidosis (renal tubular acidosis) Without acid-base imbalance (interstitial nephritis) With metabolic alkalosis (cystic fibrosis, Bartter syndrome) With high blood pressure (licorice ingestion, Cushing syndrome)

HYPERKALEMIA. Substantial elevations of serum potassium concentration are encountered most frequently with renal failure or systemic acidosis, combined with an increased intake of potassium or a rapid breakdown of tissue or blood products. Table 59-6 summarizes the causes of hyperkalemia.

When the potassium concentration reaches 8 mEq/L or more, or if characteristic electrocardiographic abnormalities are noted at any potassium concentration, then the child is in grave danger of cardiac toxicity. Such a patient should have continuous electrocardiographic monitoring, and immediate steps should be taken to protect the heart from the effects of severe hyperkalemia. The first priority is the infusion of intravenous calcium, 0.2 mL/kg of 10% calcium chloride given over 2 to 5 minutes.[14] This infusion should be followed by the administration of sodium bicarbonate (2 to 3 mEq/kg given within a 30-minute period) to raise the serum pH level and help move the potassium into cells, thereby decreasing (transiently) the intravascular potassium concentration. Simultaneously or immediately after the previously described steps, a mixture of glucose and insulin should be infused, which also induces movement of potassium ions from the extracellular to the intracellular spaces. This mixture accelerates the usual process by which glucose moves into the cells and is converted to glycogen. A dose of 2 mL/kg of a 25% glucose solution is given along with 1 U/kg of regular insulin. This solution

Table 59-6 Causes of Hyperkalemia

MECHANISM	CAUSES
1. Spurious laboratory values	Hemolysis, leukocytosis, faulty blood draw techniques
2. Increased intake	Oral or intravenous, blood transfusion
3. Transcellular shifts	Acidosis Rhabdomyolysis, tissue necrosis, tumor lysis syndrome Drug toxicity (β-blockers, digitalis) Hyperkalemic periodic paralysis
4. Decreased excretion	Renal failure Adrenal (Addison disease, congenital adrenal hyperplasia) Kidney transplant, lupus nephritis Renal tubular acidosis (pseudohypoaldosteronism) Medications (angiotensin-converting enzyme inhibitors)

may be administered over 30 minutes and repeated as necessary. Serum glucose concentration must be monitored closely during and following therapy.

Salbutamol, a selective beta-2 agonist, has been used successfully to reduce temporarily serum potassium levels in neonates[15,16] and children.[17] It may be administered intravenously or by nebulization. The parenteral form is not yet available commercially in the United States.

Once lifesaving measures have been instituted, attention must be given to removing potassium from the body. One of the most effective means of accomplishing this task is with hemodialysis or peritoneal dialysis. One or the other should be initiated without delay in patients who have hyperkalemia accompanied by congestive heart failure and volume overload. The other mechanism used commonly for removing potassium from the body is to bind potassium in the GI tract by using an exchange resin such as sodium polystyrene sulfonate (Kayexalate).[18,19] This exchange resin is usually introduced through a retention enema that contains sorbitol. The clinician can expect a decline in serum potassium of 1 mEq/L for each g/kg of resin introduced. The dose is calculated based on the severity of the hyperkalemia, with a maximal adult dose of 60 g. Caution should be used in patients who have renal failure because sodium is absorbed as potassium is excreted, and each gram of resin contains 4.1 mEq of sodium; hypernatremia and hypervolemia may result. Additionally, the patient must be monitored for the development of hypocalcemia and hypomagnesemia. Metabolic alkalosis may result from repeated polystyrene sulfonate enemas. When hyperkalemia becomes a chronic but not life-threatening problem the best approach is to restrict dietary potassium and administer potassium-losing diuretics concomitantly.

SPECIAL SITUATIONS REQUIRING FLUID THERAPY

Fluid Therapy of the Neonate

Adequate provision of fluid replacement therapy for newborn infants depends on perinatal alterations in body composition and the infant's size and gestational age. Hydration of sick premature babies who weigh less than 1500 g is found in Chapter 76, Care of the Sick or Premature Infant Before Transport.

Total body water content decreases progressively throughout gestation and the first year of postnatal life. This decrease is accompanied by increases in the body's content of protein and fat. Shrinkage of the extracellular fluid compartment accounts largely for the decrease in total body water. In the first few days of extrauterine life, both term and premature babies normally lose up to 10% of their body weight. Although this loss is considered a physiological reduction, failure to replace such losses may lead to substantial dehydration.

All newborns show a progressive increase in their metabolic rate. The metabolic rate for full-term infants approximates 32 cal/kg/day at birth and reaches close to 43 cal/kg/day within 3 days. After this progressive increase is a slow, steady increase over the first 2 weeks of life. Premature infants maintain a higher metabolic rate than full-term babies, even when they achieve a similar weight.

In addition to the baseline metabolic expenditure of calories, newborns use energy with cold, stress, and muscular activity. The growth rate is rapid during this period, and the average newborn requires between 100 and 125 cal/kg/day.

Water requirements are governed by losses through the skin, respiratory tract, and kidneys. Evaporative losses through the skin generally average 20 to 30 mL/kg/day; respiratory losses account for approximately 15 mL/kg/day. Both parameters are affected by ambient humidity, and respiratory losses may actually be reduced by 50% with provision of high humidity to the baby's immediate environment.

The newborn's kidneys are limited in their ability to concentrate urine because of the relative shortness of the loops of Henle and the absence of a notable concentration gradient. Thus they are able at best to excrete urine with an osmolality that approaches 300 mOsm/kg. As the solute load increases the free water requirement rises; thus, for a formula-fed infant, urinary water loss may be as high as 120 mL/kg/day. However, the average range probably is closer to 60 to 75 mL/kg/day.

Electrolyte requirements for infants have not been fully established, but they seem to tolerate a fairly wide range of electrolyte provisions. Fluids that have been used successfully yield between 1 and 3 mEq of sodium per 100 calories per day; this has become the recommended starting range for maintenance fluid therapy.

When preparing a maintenance parenteral fluid formula for newborns the clinician needs to ensure adequate monitoring, which will indicate whether fluid estimates have been adequate. Also important,

Table 59-7 Summary of Treatment Based on Degree of Dehydration

DEGREE OF DEHYDRATION	REHYDRATION THERAPY	REPLACEMENT OF LOSSES	NUTRITION
Minimal or no dehydration	Not applicable	<10 kg body weight: 60-120 mL oral rehydration solution (ORS) for each diarrheal stool or vomiting episode >10 kg body weight: 120-240 mL ORS for each diarrheal stool or vomiting episode	Continue breastfeeding, or resume age-appropriate normal diet after initial hydration, including adequate caloric intake for maintenance*
Mild to moderate dehydration	ORS, 50-100 mL/kg body weight over 3-4 hr	Same	Same
Severe dehydration	Lactated Ringer's solution or normal saline in 20 mL/kg body weight intravenous amounts until perfusion and mental status improve; then administer 100 mL/kg body weight ORS over 4 hr or 5% dextrose half-normal saline intravenously at twice maintenance fluid rates	Same; if unable to drink, administer through nasogastric tube or administer 5% dextrose quarter-normal saline with 20 mEq/L potassium chloride intravenously	Same

*Overly restricted diets should be avoided during acute diarrheal episodes. Breastfed infants should continue to nurse ad libitum even during acute rehydration. Infants too weak to eat can be given breast milk or formula through a nasogastric tube. Lactose-containing formulas are usually well tolerated. If lactose malabsorption appears clinically substantial, then lactose-free formulas can be used. Complex carbohydrates, fresh fruits, lean meats, yogurt, and vegetables are all recommended. Carbonated drinks or commercial juices with a high concentration of simple carbohydrates should be avoided.

From Centers for Disease Control and Prevention, Managing acute gastroenteritis among children: oral rehydration, maintenance, and nutritional therapy for the Centers for Disease Control and Prevention. *MMWR Recomm Rep.* 2003;52:1-16.

especially with the sick neonate, is to record weights once or twice a day and to record intake, output, vital signs, urinary osmolality, electrolyte concentrations, and other indications of optimum cardiac and respiratory homeostasis frequently. Frequent changes may be needed; therefore the physician must never become locked into a particular formula but rather must apply the basic rules of fluid therapy to the situation logically and be ready to compensate for failing systems or increasing losses when necessary.

Fluid Therapy for Burns

See Chapter 361, Thermal Injuries, for fluid management of children with burns.

Hydration of the Ambulatory Patient: Alternatives to Parenteral Fluid Therapy

A fairly common practice for pediatricians in the United States is to recommend oral fluids for young patients who have mild diarrhea or vomiting. Such therapy has been suggested for many years on totally empirical grounds, and most physicians have urged the use of a dilute solution that contains sodium and potassium in concentrations of 30 and 20 mEq/L, respectively, and 5% to 7% glucose. When diarrhea leads to moderate or severe dehydration, or if substantial emesis accompanies the illness, then the standard teaching had dictated hospitalization of such children and resting the GI tract with the use of parenteral therapy, as outlined in previous sections.

Sodium absorption in the small intestine depends on the presence of glucose or small neutral amino acids such as glycine or alanine. Similarly, the absorption of glucose is enhanced by the presence of sodium salts, and this mechanism of coupled transport is responsible for the efficacy of the oral rehydration solution (ORS).[4] Movement of salt and glucose across the mucosal border is accompanied by an influx of water and other electrolyte concentrations. Maximal rates of absorption are achieved when (1) sodium and glucose are present in a 1:1 to 1:2 molecular ratio, (2) glucose concentration is between 110 and 140 mmol (2% to 2.5% solution), and (3) sodium concentration is not substantially less than that of normal jejunal fluid (usually 12 mEq/L). The World Health Organization (WHO) has derived a formula for use with all patients who have diarrheal illness regardless of its cause. It contains 90 mmol of sodium, 20 mmol of potassium, 30 mmol of bicarbonate, 80 mmol of chloride, and 111 mmol of glucose per liter. This formulation provides a solution that has an osmolality of 331 mOsm/L. When given ad lib to patients who have diarrhea, this formula corrects dehydration rapidly and can return electrolyte concentrations to the normal range regardless of the presence of hyponatremia or hypernatremia on initial evaluation. Large field studies have documented its successful use in patients who have ongoing emesis. No evidence has been found to suggest that the use of such fluid prolongs the duration of diarrhea; just the reverse appears to be the case. In addition, children given this oral rehydration therapy seem to tolerate resumption of a regular diet earlier than those treated solely with intravenous fluids. Use of a solution that has lower osmolality (224 mOsm/L) has been shown to result in superior water absorption and patient weight gain.[20]

The guidelines for managing mild, moderate, or severe dehydration as recommended by the Centers for Disease Control and Prevention, American Academy of Pediatrics (AAP), and WHO are summarized in Table 59-7.[4,21,22]

Preparations that meet WHO and AAP guidelines, as indicated previously, are available commercially. Because such preparations are available ready to use, the bicarbonate found in the WHO powder has been replaced with citrate.[23] Studies have documented equivalent efficacy of the two bases in correcting the mild acidosis that accompanies mild to moderate diarrhea. Most of the large-scale evaluations that have been performed in developed countries have excluded the use of ORS in patients in shock who are treated initially with intravenous fluids.[24,25] Despite considerable efforts to develop a super ORS, most evidence suggests that the standard WHO solution, accompanied by early return to normal diet and sufficient access to free water, is still the best overall therapy. Treatment consists of two phases: rehydration and maintenance. In the rehydration phase, fluid deficit is replaced quickly, whereas in the maintenance phase, calories are added along with fluids. The intent of this therapy is to restore age-appropriate diet as soon as possible while preventing GI rest.

In summary, oral rehydration therapy provides a cost-efficient approach to the problem of childhood diarrhea for the patient who is able to drink, is not in shock, and has a relative or other responsible person who can understand the instructions for using the oral rehydration therapy formula. Such a therapeutic approach avoids the hospitalization of a child and the consequent disruption in the lives of the family members. This treatment approach eliminates the potential complications of intravenous therapy. (See also Chapter 169, Diarrhea and Steatorrhea; and Chapter 341, Dehydration.)

WHEN TO REFER

- Abnormal electrolytes refractory to fluid therapy
- Seizure or encephalopathy
- Inability to rehydrate by chosen means (oral or intravenous)

WHEN TO ADMIT

- Failure to rehydrate completely in 6 hours
- Persistent abnormal mental status
- Inability of parent to maintain hydration at home

AAP POLICY STATEMENT

Centers for Disease Control and Prevention. Managing Acute Gastroenteritis Among Children: Oral Rehydration, Maintenance, and Nutritional Therapy. *Pediatrics*. 2004;114(2):507. AAP endorsed.

REFERENCES

1. Roberts KB. Fluid and electrolytes: parenteral fluid therapy. *Pediatr Rev*. 2001;22(11):380-387.
2. Simmons CF, Ichikawa I. External balance of water and electrolytes. In: Ichikawa I, ed. *Pediatric Textbook of Fluids and Electrolytes*. Baltimore, MD: Williams & Wilkins; 1990.
3. Hirschhorn N. The treatment of acute diarrhea in children: an historical and physiological perspective. *Am J Clin Nutr*. 1980;33:637.
4. Centers for Disease Control and Prevention. Managing acute gastroenteritis among children: oral rehydration, maintenance, and nutritional therapy from the Centers for Disease Control and Prevention. *MMWR Recomm Rep*. 2003;52(RR-16):1-16. Available at: www.cdc.gov/mmwr/pdf/rr/rr5216.pdf. Access June 7, 2007.
5. Liebelt EL. Clinical and laboratory evaluation and management of children with vomiting, diarrhea, and dehydration. *Curr Opin Pediatr*. 1998;10:461-469.
6. Nager AL, Wang VJ. Comparison of nasogastric and intravenous methods of rehydration in pediatric patients with acute dehydration. *Pediatrics*. 2002;109:566-572.
7. Weisburg LS. Pseudohyponatremia: a reappraisal. *Am J Med*. 1989;86:315.
8. Moritz ML, Ayus JC. Disorders of water metabolism in children: hyponatremia and hypernatremia. *Pediatr Rev*. 2002;23(11):371-379.
9. Sarnaik AP, Meert K, Hackbarth R, et al. Management of hyponatremic seizures in children with hypertonic saline: a safe and effective strategy. *Crit Care Med*. 1991;19:758.
10. Cheng JC, Zikos, D, Peterson DR, et al. Symptomatic hyponatremia: pathophysiology and management. *Acute Care*. 1989;14/15:270.
11. Rossi NF, Cadnapaphornchai P. Disordered water metabolism: hyponatremia. *Crit Care Clin*. 1987;5:759.
12. Jacobson J, Bohn D. Severe hypernatremic dehydration and hypokalemia in an infant with gastroenteritis secondary to rotavirus. *Ann Emerg Med*. 1993;22:1630.
13. Maghnie M, Cosi G, Genovese E, et al. Central diabetes insipidus in children and young adults. *N Engl J Med*. 2000;343:998-1007.
14. Hill LL. Body composition, normal electrolyte concentrations, and the maintenance of normal volume, tonicity, and acid-base metabolism. *Pediatr Clin North Am*. 1990;37(2):241-256.
15. Greenough A, Emery EF, Brooker R, et al. Salbutamol infusion to treat neonatal hyperkalemia. *J Perinat Med*. 1992;20:437.
16. Mauer AM, Dweck HS, Finberg L, et al. American Academy of Pediatrics Committee on Nutrition: use of oral fluid therapy and posttreatment feeding following enteritis in children in a developed country. *Pediatrics*. 1985;75:358-361.
17. McClure RJ, Prasad VK, Brocklebank JT. Treatment of hyperkalemia using intravenous and nebulised salbutamol. *Arch Dis Child*. 1994;70:126.

18. Meyer I. Sodium polystyrene sulfonate: a cation exchange resin used in treating hyperkalemia. *Med Rev ANNA*. 1993;20:93.
19. Noerr B. Sodium polystyrene sulfonate (Kayexalate). *Neonatal Netw*. 1993;12:77-79.
20. Rautanen T, Salo E, Verkasalo M, et al. Randomised double-blind trial of hypotonic oral rehydration solutions with and without citrate. *Arch Dis Child*. 1994;70:44.
21. American Academy of Pediatrics, Provisional Committee on Quality Improvement, Subcommittee on Acute Gastroenteritis. Practice parameter: the management of acute gastroenteritis in young children. *Pediatrics*. 1996; 97:424-435.
22. World Health Organization. *The Treatment of Diarrhea: A Manual for Physicians and Other Senior Health Workers*. Geneva, Switzerland: World Health Organization; 1995. Available at: www.who.int/child-adolescent-health/New_Publications/CHILD_HEALTH/ISBN_92_4_159318_0.pdf. Accessed June 7, 2007.
23. Salazar-Lindo E, Sack RB, Chea-Woo E, et al. Bicarbonate versus citrate in oral rehydration therapy in infants with watery diarrhea: a controlled clinical trial. *J Pediatr*. 1986;108:55.
24. Rautanen T, el-Radhi S, Vesikari T. Clinical experience with a hypotonic oral rehydration solution in acute diarrhea. *Acta Paediatr*. 1993;82:52-54.
25. Tamer AM, Friedman LB, Maxwell SRW, et al. Oral rehydration of infants in a large urban US medical center. *J Pediatr*. 1985;107:14.

Chapter 60

BLOOD PRODUCTS AND THEIR USES

Eva G. Radel, MD

The ability to separate blood into its components, store them appropriately, and administer them as needed has resulted in significantly improved supportive care, particularly in the areas of oncology and neonatology. However, the unfortunate occurrence of blood-transmitted acquired immunodeficiency syndrome (AIDS) has made the medical profession and the public aware of the hazards of blood products and, in some cases, has led to excessive fear of transfusion. As a result, the indications for transfusion have been reassessed, transfusion policies have become more conservative, and more effort is being devoted to a search for alternatives to the use of blood products.

GENERAL INDICATIONS FOR BLOOD TRANSFUSION

The general indications for transfusion of blood or blood products are (1) restoring blood volume when it has been acutely depleted, (2) restoring oxygen-carrying capacity, (3) restoring a particular blood component (cellular or humoral) to a level allowing adequate function, (4) replacing or supplementing an abnormally functioning component with a normal one, and (5) removing and replacing large amounts of plasma or blood cells (exchange transfusion or apheresis).

The circulating amount of a blood component almost never has to be restored to the normal range; instead, the goal should be a level that will correct pathological processes and allow normal physiological functioning for the patient's current condition. In deciding whether component replacement is necessary, physicians should ask themselves 2 questions: (1) Is it essential to correct the particular deficit immediately through replacement, and (2) does another method exist that would restore an adequate physiological state? The necessary component should be administered selectively, if possible. In some situations, nonblood-product medications such as erythropoietin, granulocyte colony-stimulating factor (filgrastim), recombinant coagulation factors, and desmopressin (1-desamino-8d-arginine vasopressin) may decrease or prevent the need for transfusion of blood products. Clinical trials are in progress for red cell substitutes.[1]

BLOOD DONORS AND HANDLING OF BLOOD PRODUCTS

In recent years, public demand has been high for directed donations from family members and friends; this demand allows an individual to avoid receiving blood from routine donors who are unknown and therefore considered potentially unsafe by some individuals. However, extra time is required for testing of the donor, and a higher incidence of high-risk activity and transmissible disease has actually been found among 1st-time directed donors than among volunteer donors.[2,3] In addition, a risk of graft-versus-host disease (GVHD) is present in immunocompetent blood recipients who have been transfused with blood products from relatives who are homozygous for one of the patient's human leukocyte antigen (HLA) haplotypes. The risk is greatest for donors who are 1st-degree relatives. This problem can be prevented by irradiating all blood products from blood relatives.[4] In some situations, however, such as for small patients who require repeated transfusions or multiple blood components, the exclusive use of 1 or 2 dedicated apheresis donors may help prevent sensitization.[5]

All possible precautions must be taken to prevent clerical errors when drawing and labeling blood specimens to be used for cross-matching blood and when starting transfusions. Mislabeling tubes and administering blood to the wrong patient are the most common causes of severe hemolytic transfusion reactions. Blood products must also be stored and handled properly. Once blood has been taken out of the blood bank, it should be used promptly and not refrigerated. If administration will be delayed, then the blood should be returned to the blood bank immediately. Improper refrigeration can cause blood to freeze, resulting in lysis of the red cells, hemoglobinuria, and poor response to transfusion. Before and after transfusion, the tubing should be flushed with normal saline solution. Blood should not have contact with solutions containing dextrose or calcium, and drugs should never be added to a blood component.

RED BLOOD CELL TRANSFUSIONS

In some situations (eg, exchange transfusions, massive bleeding), use of whole blood is desirable. However, most blood banks no longer store whole blood and have only packed red blood cells (PRBCs) available. These PRBCs can be reconstituted, if indicated, with saline, albumin (or another colloid), or fresh-frozen plasma (FFP). FFP rarely is needed in these situations, and using it exposes the recipient to some of the same risks as receiving another unit of blood. RBC preparations are described in Table 60-1.

Acute Blood Loss

Acute loss of up to 15% of the blood volume can usually be managed by volume replacement with crystalloid fluids. Larger losses may require colloid replacement, and loss of more than 30% usually requires transfusion of PRBCs.[6] If the patient is actively bleeding, then rapid administration may be necessary. Massive bleeding involving the loss and replacement of more than 1 blood volume (8% to 9% of ideal body weight in a child, 7% in an adult) in 24 hours can give rise to some unique problems.[7] The mortality in this situation has been approximately 40%. A bleeding tendency may develop partly as a result of dilution but, more importantly, as a result of a consumption coagulopathy that is related, at least in part, to the presence of shock. Acidosis and hypothermia also can contribute to increased bleeding. In an extreme emergency, non–cross-matched group O Rh negative blood may be used initially, but type-specific and subsequently fully cross-matched blood should be used as soon as it is available. Platelet transfusions should be given if the platelet count is below 50,000/mcL, and FFP is indicated if the prothrombin time or partial thromboplastin time is more than 1.5 times normal. Occasionally, cryoprecipitate can be helpful in replacing fibrinogen. An evaluation for disseminated intravascular coagulation should be done.

Restoration of Oxygen-Carrying Capacity

Transfusion is often recommended for a variety of indications to improve oxygen delivery in patients with anemia, but, in many instances, no evidence exists to support such recommendations. The patient's general clinical condition is important when determining the need to correct mild degrees of anemia. Children with chronic anemia (eg, sickle cell anemia) can sometimes tolerate hemoglobin levels of less than 6 g/dL without difficulty under baseline conditions, although superimposed acute illness or surgery may result in decompensation. Transfusions are often given to small premature newborns or to older children who are critically ill and have cardiovascular compromise. The indications in these situations are controversial, but some guidelines have been published and are shown in Boxes 60-1 and 60-2.[8,9] Careful consideration must be given to the risks of transfusion versus those of a low hemoglobin concentration. In many situations, treating the underlying cause of the anemia can avert the need for transfusion.

The volume of PRBCs given for anemia is usually in the range of 10 to 15 mL/kg (15 to 20 mL/kg in the premature infant), which can be given at a rate of approximately 5 mL/kg per hour to a patient who is clinically stable.[9] A single unit of blood should be given within 4 hours to prevent bacterial contamination. With very severe chronic anemia (hemoglobin less than 5 g/dL), the risk of congestive heart failure from transfusion may be greater than the risk of withholding

Table 60-1 Red Blood Cell Preparations

PRODUCT	PREPARATION	HEMATOCRIT (%) OR CELL COUNT	VOLUME/ UNIT (mL)	INDICATIONS OR COMMENTS
Whole blood	450 mL blood, plus anticoagulant	40%	500	Massive bleeding, exchange transfusion
Packed RBCs	Centrifuged or sedimented to remove about two thirds of plasma	55-80%	250-350	Most RBC transfusions
Prestorage leuko-reduced RBCs	Filtration at the time of collection	Contains $<5 \times 10^6$ WBCs/unit	250-300	Chronic transfusions, potential transplant recipients, febrile transfusion reactions, CMV-positive donor for patient at risk
Washed RBCs	Several manual and automated techniques available to remove plasma; must be used within 24 hr	90% Contains <1% of original plasma, <10% of WBCs	200	Repeated febrile and allergic reactions
Frozen RBCs	Frozen in glycerol, thawed, and washed; must be used within 24 hr of thawing; 10-15% loss of original RBCs	Contains <0.025% of original plasma, 1%-5% of original WBCs and platelets	200	Rare blood types, multiple severe febrile or allergic reactions, IgA deficiency, autologous blood donations

CMV, Cytomegalovirus; *IgA*, immunoglobulin A; *RBCs*, red blood cells; *WBCs*, white blood cells.

BOX 60-1 Guidelines for Transfusion of RBCs in Children Older than 4 Months

1. Emergency surgery in patient with significant preoperative anemia (Hct <24%)
2. Preoperative anemia when other corrective therapy is not available*
3. Intraoperative blood loss >15% of total blood volume
4. Hct <24%:
   a. In perioperative period, with signs and symptoms of anemia
   b. While on chemotherapy or radiation therapy†
   c. Chronic congenital or acquired symptomatic anemia
5. Acute blood loss with hypovolemia not responsive to other therapy
6. Hct <40% with:
   a. Severe pulmonary disease
   b. On extracorporeal membrane oxygenation
7. Chronic hypertransfusion programs for disorders of RBC production or complications of sickle cell disease (eg, cerebrovascular accident)

Hct, Hematocrit; *RBC,* red blood cell.
*For preoperative transfusion in sickle cell disease, see guidelines for surgery in text.
†Many radiation therapists prefer Hct >30% for radiation to have maximal effect
Adapted from Roseff SD, Luban NLC, Manno CS. Guidelines for assessing appropriateness of pediatric transfusion. *Transfusion.* 2002;42: 1398-1413. Reprinted by permission of Blackwell Publishing Ltd.

BOX 60-2 Guidelines for Transfusion of Red Blood Cells in Infants Younger Than 4 Months*

1. Hct <20% with low reticulocyte count and signs of anemia (eg, tachycardia, tachypnea, poor feeding)
2. Hct <30% in an infant:
   a. On <35% O_2 by hood
   b. On O_2 by nasal cannula
   c. On continuous positive airway pressure (CPAP) or intermittent mandatory ventilation (or both) with mean airway pressure <6 cm H_2O
   d. With significant apnea or bradycardia
   e. With significant tachycardia or tachypnea
   f. With low weight gain
3. Hct <35% in an infant:
   a. On >35% O_2 by hood
   b. On CPAP or intermittent mandatory ventilation with mean airway pressure >6-8 cm H_2O
4. Hct <45% in an infant:
   a. On extracorporeal membrane oxygenation
   b. With congenital cyanotic heart disease

H_2O, Water; *Hct,* hematocrit; *O_2,* oxygen.
*Guidelines may vary in different institutions.
Adapted from Roseff SD, Luban NLC, Manno CS. Guidelines for assessing appropriateness of pediatric transfusion. *Transfusion.* 2002;42: 1398-1413. Reprinted by permission of Blackwell Publishing Ltd.

transfusion and treating the patient medically if possible. A common example is severe iron-deficiency anemia in a patient who is clinically stable. If transfusion is necessary in such a situation, the volume given should be no more than 4 to 5 mL/kg given over 4 hours, and a diuretic may be needed. If the anemia must be corrected rapidly (eg, for emergency surgery), then a partial exchange transfusion can be done.

Chronic Transfusion

A child who is likely to undergo repeated and prolonged transfusion therapy requires several precautions that are not relevant to a patient receiving short-term transfusions:

1. Red cell phenotyping. For black patients, typing for several common red cell antigens should be done to prevent transfusion of blood containing antigens against which the recipient is likely to form antibodies. This circumstance has been a particular problem for patients who have sickle cell disease.[10] Although practice has varied in different institutions, typing for and avoiding blood that is incompatible for at least C, E, and Kell is frequently recommended.[11] Such typing has also been recommended for children with thalassemia.
2. Leukocyte depletion. Because most minor transfusion reactions are caused by leukocytes or plasma proteins, patients who are transfused frequently should receive leukocyte-reduced red cells. Leukoreduction also decreases the incidence of alloimmunization to platelets and is therefore recommended for patients who require repeated platelet transfusions, such as those with malignancy or aplastic anemia. It also significantly reduces the transmission of cytomegalovirus (CMV).[12] Although bedside filters are available, leukocytes are usually removed at the blood collection centers in the process of preparing PRBCs; at the time of this writing, this procedure is performed routinely in many countries but only selectively in the United States.
3. Hemosiderosis. Serum ferritin should be monitored, and chelation therapy may be required.
4. Hepatitis. Although routine donor screening significantly reduces the incidence of hepatitis transmission, hepatitis B vaccine should be given to individuals likely to receive repeated transfusions. Hepatitis A vaccine is also advisable.

Surgery

Individuals who have significant anemia develop more complications from surgery and anesthesia. In the past, a hematocrit of 30% (10.2 g/dL hemoglobin) was recommended as the minimal requirement for patients undergoing anesthesia. However, more recent guidelines suggest transfusion only for a hematocrit less than 24% with signs and symptoms of anemia in the perioperative period or blood loss of more than 15% of the blood volume.[9] The extent of surgery, the likelihood of massive blood loss, and coexisting factors such as impaired pulmonary function or inadequate cardiac output must be considered when deciding about the need for transfusion. The combination of anemia and hypovolemia must be prevented.

Children with sickle cell disease who require anesthesia have fewer complications if they are transfused to a hemoglobin level of more than 10 g/dL before surgery. For patients with hemoglobin sickle cell disease or others with high hemoglobin levels, this procedure may have to be performed by exchange transfusion or erythrocytapheresis.[13] (See Hemoglobinopathy and Exchange Transfusion sections later in this chapter.)

The tendency to decrease the amount of exogenous blood transfusion for elective surgery has been increasing.[14,15] Autologous blood donations have been used successfully in adolescents, children, and even in infants as young as 3 months, although the collection is technically difficult in children weighing less than 25 kg. The largest experience has been in orthopedic procedures that are associated with significant blood loss, in cardiac surgery, and in prospective bone marrow donors. Several phlebotomies can be performed over a period of a few weeks just before surgery, or the process can be conducted over a longer period, and the blood can be frozen and stored. Another approach to blood conservation during surgery is normovolemic hemodilution. Whole blood is removed and anticoagulated, volume is replaced with lactated Ringer's solution or other fluid to lower the hematocrit to 20% to 25%, and the blood is reinfused if the hematocrit drops to less than 15% or at the end of the procedure. Salvaging blood intraoperatively and postoperatively, collecting it with special equipment, and reinfusing it is an additional technique used to reduce the use of banked donor blood. These procedures can be combined with added efficacy. The use of erythropoietin and iron supplementation for several weeks before surgery may be a helpful adjunct with or without the previously described techniques and has been shown to allow repair of craniosynostosis in young infants without the need for exogenous blood.[16,17] However, at the time of this writing, the US Food and Drug Administration has issued a warning that an increased risk of cardiovascular and thromboembolic events exists with the use of erythropoietin if the hemoglobin level is allowed to increase above 12 g/dL or by more than 1 g/dL within a 2-week period.

Special Circumstances in Red Blood Cell Transfusion

Infants Younger Than 4 Months

Maternal blood is used, if possible, to cross-match blood for the infant's transfusion. However, the blood used should be ABO specific for the infant or type O with a low titer of isoagglutinins. With ABO incompatibility, the blood should be type O. If the infant is Rh-negative, then the blood should be Rh-negative as well. It should not contain any red cell antigen to which the mother has antibodies. Infants whose mothers are seronegative for CMV should receive only leukoreduced or CMV-negative blood.[8,18]

With a small premature infant who is transfused frequently, performing a cross-match procedure for each transfusion is no longer considered necessary unless plasma, platelets, or granulocytes have been administered. Many blood banks now designate certain blood units that are drawn into 4 small bags to be used for repeated transfusions for specific neonates to limit the number of donor exposures. Stored blood has been shown to be as safe and effective as fresh blood in most situations.[8,18]

Blood for very small premature infants and for all exchange transfusions should be irradiated to prevent GVHD (if this is possible without causing significant delay).[4,18]

Hemoglobinopathy

Patients who have sickle cell disease are often transfused to replace cells capable of sickling in the circulation with cells that are more deformable and will not participate in a vasoocclusive process. The blood used should be from sickle-negative donors. These patients have a high incidence of developing red cell antibodies; this incidence can be decreased by matching for specific antigens, as noted previously. Some investigators have advocated erythrocytapheresis instead of simple transfusion for patients who require chronic transfusions to limit hemosiderosis.[19] The disadvantages of this approach are increased exposure to donor units and increased cost. It has been recommended that patients with sickle cell disease not be transfused acutely to a hemoglobin above 11 g/dL to prevent hyperviscosity resulting in increased sickling.[13] Children with sickle cell disease or thalassemia may be candidates for stem cell transplantation (see the discussion in the next section).

Potential Stem Cell Transplant Recipients

Children who may be candidates for stem cell transplantation should not be given blood products from genetically related family members because it may lead to sensitization to HLA antigens and subsequent stem cell rejection. In addition, CMV infection must be prevented (see discussion on Immunosuppressed Patients in the next section).

Immunosuppressed Patients

Patients who are immunosuppressed include (1) patients being treated for a malignancy, (2) bone marrow or organ transplant recipients, (3) premature infants weighing fewer than 1250 g and other severely ill neonates, (4) fetuses receiving intrauterine transfusions, and (5) children who have severe congenital immunodeficiency disorders. These children are susceptible to GVHD because of their failure to eliminate viable lymphocytes from the transfused blood. Leukodepletion does not prevent this complication. Irradiation of all blood products with a minimum of 25 Gy is recommended for these children.[4]

CMV infection is also a risk in neonates and potential stem cell transplant recipients. If the child (or the mother of a newborn) does not already have antibodies to CMV (indicating preexisting infection), then blood products that are leukoreduced (see previous discussion) or from CMV-seronegative donors should be given. CMV-negative blood should also be given to pregnant women who are seronegative.

PLATELET TRANSFUSION

Platelet transfusions are useful primarily in situations in which production of platelets by the bone marrow is deficient. If thrombocytopenia is due to peripheral destruction, then transfusion is unlikely to raise the platelet count significantly. Platelet transfusions are contraindicated in patients with thrombotic thrombocytopenic purpura or hemolytic-uremic syndrome. Spontaneous hemorrhage does not usually occur with a platelet count above 10,000/mcL, although, in the past, maintaining the count above 20,000/mcL was often standard procedure. Patients who have chronically low platelet counts are less likely to bleed spontaneously than are those whose platelets are diminishing rapidly. Coexistent fever or a coagulation disorder may predispose patients to bleeding at somewhat higher platelet counts. Traumatic or surgical bleeding may require platelet counts above 50,000/mcL, and neurosurgical or ophthalmologic procedures may warrant platelet counts above 100,000/mcL. For small premature infants, many neonatologists prefer to maintain platelet counts above 50,000/mcL if the infant is stable and above 100,000/mcL if ill.[9] Dysfunctional platelets (eg, those that may result from a congenital platelet disorder, after extracorporeal perfusion, after administration of drugs that cause platelet dysfunction, or after massive blood replacement) also may result in bleeding at somewhat higher platelet count levels. Some guidelines for platelet transfusions are given in Box 60-3.

The half-life of transfused platelets is approximately 24 hours under normal circumstances; but survival may be shortened by fever or infection, platelet antibodies, splenomegaly, massive bleeding, or any condition that results in peripheral destruction or consumption of platelets. Platelets are not cross-matched for transfusion, but ABO-compatible platelets should be used when possible. If Rh-positive platelets must be given to an Rh-negative individual, then Rh immune globulin should be administered to prevent sensitization of the body's immune system by contaminating RBCs. For patients who need a single transfusion or a brief period of platelet transfusions, random donor platelets are satisfactory. For patients who have a malignancy or aplastic anemia and who will likely require repeated platelet transfusions, many centers prefer single-donor (apheresed) platelets (Table 60-2), although the incidence of alloimmunization and refractoriness to platelets has not been shown to be different with random pooled or pheresed platelets as long as they are leukodepleted or ultraviolet B irradiated.[20] Patients who have aplastic anemia and require frequent platelet transfusions have a high incidence of alloimmunization and may benefit from having a limited number of designated unrelated platelet donors who are apheresed regularly. For patients who have malignancies or are immunosuppressed, the precautions previously recommended for RBC transfusions should be followed. Patients who have become refractory to random donor platelets and who are not candidates for stem cell transplantation may benefit from receiving platelets from family members who are at least partly HLA matched. Unrelated but HLA-matched donors also may be good platelet donors for such individuals.

BOX 60-3 Guidelines for Prophylactic Transfusion of Platelets in Children and Infants With Reduced Platelet Production

1. Platelet count <10,000/mcL
2. Platelet count <20,000/mcL and:
   a. Severe mucositis
   b. Disseminated intravascular coagulation (DIC)
   c. Anticoagulant therapy
   d. Platelets likely to fall to <10,000/mcL in the next few days before next evaluation
   e. Risk of bleeding due to a local tumor infiltration
3. Platelet count <50,000/mcL and:
   a. Active brain tumor
   b. DIC in association with induction therapy for leukemia
   c. Extreme hyperleukocytosis
   d. Before surgery, lumbar puncture, or central venous line insertion
4. In neonates with:
   a. Platelet count <20,000/mcL if stable and not bleeding
   b. Platelet count <30,000/mcL if sick and not bleeding
   c. Platelet count <50,000/mcL if stable and:
      i. Active bleeding
      ii. Invasive procedure
   d. Platelet count <100 000/mcL if sick and:
      i. Active bleeding
      ii. Invasive procedure
      iii. DIC
5. Normal platelet count
   a. Active bleeding in association with a qualitative platelet defect
   b. Unexplained excessive bleeding in patient undergoing cardiopulmonary bypass
   c. Patient undergoing extracorporeal membrane oxygenation:
      i. Platelet count <100 000/mcL
      ii. Platelet count >100 000/mcL and active bleeding

From British for Standards in Haematology Transfusion Task Force. Transfusion guidelines for neonates and older children. *Br J Haematol.* 2004;124:433; Roseff SD, Luban NLC, Manno CS. Guidelines for assessing appropriateness of pediatric transfusion. *Transfusion.* 2002;42:1398.

GRANULOCYTE TRANSFUSIONS

White blood cells are the most difficult blood cellular components to transfuse because of problems with yield, recovery, and complications. The use of granulocyte transfusions has been controversial; some centers use them regularly and others rarely. Studies have shown conflicting results and have been difficult to compare and interpret, both in neonatology and oncology. Bacterial sepsis that is unresponsive to appropriate antibiotic therapy in a severely neutropenic patient who is not expected to recover within a week has been the major indication.[21] Some centers have also advocated granulocyte transfusions for newborns who have sepsis and neutropenia. However, recent reviews of studies of granulocyte transfusions in both of these settings did not find conclusive evidence to either support or refute their use.[22,23] Febrile reactions and pulmonary infiltrates are often seen with granulocyte transfusion and may be associated with alloimmunization to both HLA antigens and granulocyte-specific antigens. Simultaneous administration of granulocytes and amphotericin has been implicated in severe pulmonary decompensation with intraalveolar hemorrhage and should be avoided.[24]

Table 60-2 White Cell, Platelet, and Whole Plasma Preparations*

PRODUCT	PREPARATION	CELL COUNT OR CONTENT	VOLUME/UNIT (mL)	INDICATIONS AND COMMENTS
Random donor platelets	Separated from single whole-blood units	5 to 7×10^{10} platelets/unit	40 to 50	Infants, short-term need 1 unit/10 kg increases platelet count by 50,000
Single-donor platelets	Collected by apheresis	Equivalent to 6 to 8 random units	200 to 400 may be divided in 2 bags	Patients who require multiple transfusions
Apheresed granulocyte concentrates	Varying techniques to increase donor neutrophil count and yield	0.5 to 3×10^{10}/unit	500	Contains RBCs, must be ABO-compatible; must be used within 24 hr of collection
Fresh-frozen plasma	Whole plasma	1 unit of coagulation factors/mL	200 to 220 or 600 (pheresed)	Multiple factor deficiency; DIC: reversal of warfarin effect; HUS or TTP; unknown coagulation defect; deficiency of factors II, V, X, XI, or XIII. Contains all plasma factors; not virus-inactivated

*For plasma products used to treat coagulation deficiencies, see Chapter 271, Hemophilia and Other Hereditary Bleeding Disorders (Table 271-1).
Virus attenuation processes may not inactivate parvovirus, hepatitis A, and possibly other viruses.
DIC, Disseminated intravascular coagulation; *F,* factor; *HUS,* hemolytic-uremic syndrome; *RBCs,* red blood cells; *TTP,* thrombotic thrombocytopenic purpura.

CMV transmission is a risk (see discussion in the section "Special Circumstances in Red Blood Cell Transfusion").

EXCHANGE TRANSFUSION AND THERAPEUTIC APHERESIS

One unit of whole blood is equivalent to approximately twice the blood volume of a full-term neonate (ie, a double volume exchange) and will replace approximately 85% of the infant's RBCs. PRBCs can be reconstituted with FFP. The blood used should be fewer than 3 to 5 days old, and the recommendations for transfusion of newborns (see section "Special Circumstances in Red Blood Cell Transfusion") should be followed. Although manual exchange transfusion is often performed in older children for a variety of indications, this process can be difficult and time consuming. Automated cell separators simplify the process, and some can be adapted for use in young children. Whole blood is removed; plasma, platelets, leukocytes, and red cells are separated; and the desired component is removed. Except with erythrocytapheresis, the red cells are returned to the patient. Volume can be replaced with saline, albumin, or FFP.[25]

Erythrocytapheresis (partial exchange transfusion) may be performed for symptomatic polycythemia in neonates or in older children who have cyanotic heart disease by using volume replacement with saline or albumin. The volume of exchange can be calculated as follows:

Volume exchanged = (Total blood volume × [Observed hematocrit – Desired hematocrit]) ÷ Observed hematocrit

See the sample calculation in Figure 60-1.

In sickle cell disease, red cells may be removed and replaced with normal ones. An exchange of 1 red cell volume (70 mL/kg × hematocrit) will reduce the hemoglobin S (Hb S) to approximately 35%. The RBCs should be reconstituted with albumin or FFP, and an additional RBC infusion can reduce the Hb S level further. The final hematocrit should not be more than 30% to 35%. Leukocytapheresis may be performed for patients who have leukemia and very high white blood cell counts to reduce viscosity and leukostasis until chemotherapy takes effect. Plasma exchange can be done for thrombotic thrombocytopenic purpura by using FFP for replacement. Many autoimmune disorders and other related conditions have also been treated with plasmapheresis using albumin for replacement.[25]

Weight = 2.1 kg

Venous hematocrit = 70%

Blood volume = (100 mL/kg × 2.1 kg) = 210 mL

Desired hematocrit = 50%

Volume to be exchanged = (210 × [70 − 50]) ÷ 70 = 210 × (20 ÷ 70) = 60 mL

Aliquots of 10 mL can be removed and replaced by normal saline or other crystalline or colloid fluid.

Figure 60-1 Sample calculation of exchange transfusion for a polycythemic newborn.

PLASMA PRODUCTS

Plasma products used to treat coagulation disorders are described in Chapter 271, Hemophilia and Other Hereditary Bleeding Disorders. Recombinant, genetically engineered, non–plasma-derived factor concentrates are gradually replacing the blood-derived factors. Factors VIII, IX, and VIIa are currently available in the United States. However, commercial lyophilized coagulant concentrates, which are assayed such that the physician knows exactly how much of a desired factor is being administered, are still available and are less expensive. Several effective methods for inactivating viruses have made such concentrates much safer in recent years, although some viral agents such as parvovirus and hepatitis A still cause concern.

Indications for FFP administration include (1) active bleeding or prophylaxis for an invasive procedure in patients who have a congenital or acquired coagulation defect for which no specific concentrate is available or, in an emergency, until the specific defect is identified, (2) massive transfusion, (3) urgent reversal of warfarin, (4) hypercoagulable state resulting from deficiency of a plasma protein factor when rapid correction is necessary, and (5) plasma exchange for thrombotic thrombocytopenic purpura.

Albumin

Albumin is available as a 5% or 25% solution, the latter for patients who have hypoproteinemia and need large amounts of albumin and who would get a much larger sodium load with the larger volume if the less concentrated product is used. Albumin is fractionated from pooled plasma and is pasteurized to inactivate viruses.

Immune Globulin

Different immune globulin preparations are available for intramuscular (IM) administration, for intravenous (IV) use, and for subcutaneous infusion. Special products prepared from individuals who have high titers for specific infectious agents (varicella-zoster, hepatitis, and tetanus) are also available for IM administration. IM anti-Rh γ globulin (Rhogam) is given to nonsensitized Rh-negative women during pregnancy, and after delivery, abortion, amniocentesis, or chorionic villus biopsy to prevent sensitization.[26] It should also be given to Rh-negative patients who, in an emergency, require transfusion with Rh-positive platelets.[27] Intravenous γ globulin is used to treat hypogammaglobulinemia, idiopathic thrombocytopenic purpura, Kawasaki disease, and a variety of immune disorders. IV anti-D γ globulin (WinRho) is also used to treat idiopathic thrombocytopenic purpura in Rh-positive patients.[28] A rare complication of intravenous γ globulin has been renal failure.[29,30] Anti-D globulin may also result in severe hemolytic anemia.[30]

Anticoagulants

Children who have thrombotic disease are more likely than adults to have a congenital deficiency of one of the natural anticoagulants (antithrombin III, protein C, or protein S) or an abnormal coagulant protein (factor V Leiden or prothrombin 20210). Antithrombin III concentrate is available. Protein C has been approved by the US Food and Drug Administration for adults with severe sepsis but has not yet not been approved for children or for patients with congenital deficiency and thrombosis.

COMPLICATIONS OF TRANSFUSION

Acute Hemolytic Transfusion Reaction

Severe, immediate hemolytic transfusion reactions are almost always related to ABO incompatibility and clerical errors, such as incorrect labeling of a blood specimen tube sent to the laboratory for cross-matching or administering another patient's unit of blood. An acute onset of fever and chills may be accompanied by nausea, abdominal and lower back pain, dyspnea, and hypotension. Renal failure, disseminated intravascular coagulation (DIC), and shock may rapidly ensue. If such a reaction is suspected, then the transfusion must be stopped at once. Blood from the patient should be sent to the blood bank immediately, together with the remainder of the unit of donor blood or the empty bag and any attached blood tubing. A rapid screening test can be performed by obtaining a blood specimen (with care taken to prevent artificial hemolysis) and centrifuging it; pink, red, or brown plasma indicates intravascular hemolysis. At the same time, a urine sample should be checked for the presence of hemoglobin. If evidence of a hemolytic reaction is present, then adequate venous access should be established and the patient transferred to an intensive care unit for close monitoring, aggressive fluid administration, and supportive care. Treatment of DIC and renal dialysis may be needed, and blood components should be given as indicated.[31]

Delayed Hemolytic Transfusion Reaction

Delayed reactions may develop 3 to 21 days after transfusion in patients who may have had prior sensitization to red cell antigens with titers too low to be detected before the recent transfusion. An anamnestic reaction may increase antibody production so that hemolysis ensues, and the patient becomes anemic, with or without hyperbilirubinemia and hemoglobinuria. Usually, no specific therapy is required, but an additional transfusion may be needed. Severe hemolysis has been described in patients with sickle cell disease, often without detectable antibodies, with concomitant destruction of the patient's own red cells, and with associated reticulocytopenia; hemolysis may be exacerbated by further transfusion, which should be avoided if possible. Steroids have sometimes been advocated for treatment.[32]

Febrile Transfusion Reaction

Fever is the most common transfusion reaction, occurring most often in patients who receive multiple transfusions and those who receive platelet transfusions. The fever is usually associated with leukocyte-derived cytokines or with antibodies directed against leukocytes; its incidence and severity may be significantly reduced by using leukodepleted blood products.[33] The onset usually occurs 30 minutes to 2 hours after the transfusion is begun, and the patient may also have chills. If the reaction is mild and the patient has been transfused multiple times and has had previous febrile reactions, then stopping the transfusion is unnecessary, but it should be slowed. In more severe reactions, temporary interruption or discontinuation of the transfusion is indicated, with an evaluation for a hemolytic reaction. If chills and back or abdominal pain accompany the reaction, then the transfusion must be stopped immediately and precautions for a hemolytic transfusion reaction taken. Treatment with acetaminophen and, for more severe reactions, corticosteroids is helpful; for future transfusions, pretreatment may prevent such reactions.

Allergic Reactions

The cause of urticarial reactions is usually unclear, although they may be associated with antigens in donor plasma. The plasmas of allergic donors may also result in an allergic reaction if the recipient is exposed to the corresponding antigen. Individuals who have congenital immunoglobulin A (IgA) deficiency have a 20% to 25% incidence of antibodies directed against IgA. These patients may develop severe anaphylactic reactions to any blood product containing plasma proteins.[34] Anti-IgA antibodies may also develop in normal individuals and result in urticarial or anaphylactic reactions. People who have repeated minor allergic reactions should be pretreated with an antihistamine; corticosteroids may be used if more severe reactions have occurred. Frozen washed RBCs may be effective and may be available from IgA-deficient donors. Urticarial reactions cannot be prevented by leukodepletion.

Although common practice in many centers is to give prophylactic acetaminophen or diphenhydramine before blood transfusion to prevent febrile and allergic reactions, a recent study of children with cancer or after stem cell transplantation has shown that these medications are not necessary or effective when leukoreduced, irradiated blood products are given.[35]

Transfusion-Transmitted Infections

Routine screening of donors for antibodies to HIV has been in effect in the United States since 1985, when 27 per 100,000 donations were found to be HIV positive. With current screening tests for donors, the risk has been reduced to approximately 1 in 2 million.[36,37] Groups at risk for CMV infection are discussed in the section Immunosuppressed Patients. Individuals who have been infected carry the virus in their leukocytes indefinitely. In a healthy recipient, infection is asymptomatic or associated with a mild, mononucleosis-like illness 3 to 4 weeks after transfusion. Epstein-Barr virus can also be transmitted by transfusion but has less clinical significance than CMV.

Routine screening of blood donors for hepatitis B has reduced the incidence to approximately 1 in 200,000 units. In the United States, donor blood has been tested for antibody to hepatitis C virus since 1990. This agent was previously the major cause (90%) of non-A, non-B transfusion–associated hepatitis but is now estimated to have a transmission risk of approximately 1 in 800,000 units.[36,37] Other viruses that may be transmitted by transfusion include hepatitis G (not known to cause disease), hepatitis A, parvovirus, and human T-cell leukemia virus I and II. Donors are now screened for the last 2 viruses and West Nile virus.[36]

Much concern has surfaced in recent years about the possible transmission of new variant Creutzfeldt-Jakob disease and other prion-induced diseases by blood transfusion. As of the time of this writing, 3 cases in the United Kingdom, but none in the United States, have been associated with blood transfusion. In the United States, donors who have spent varying periods of time in the United Kingdom or Europe are deferred.[37]

Because of the significant decrease in transmission of viral disease by transfusion and increased use of platelet transfusions, bacterial contamination is now a more common complication. It is estimated to occur in approximately 1:2000 units of transfused platelets because platelets are stored at room temperature rather than under refrigeration, as are RBCs.[1,37] The American Association of Blood Banks currently requires testing of platelet units for bacterial contamination to reduce the risk to recipients but does not specify a method.

Malaria and babesiosis also can be transmitted by contaminated blood. The latter resembles malaria and is a problem only for patients who have undergone a splenectomy or who are immunocompromised.

Transfusion-Related Acute Lung Injury

Transfusion-related acute lung injury is a rare but very serious complication of transfusion, occurring most often after transfusion of FFP, but also after other blood products. It has been estimated to occur in 1:5000 transfusions and, with a 5% mortality, is the leading cause of transfusion-related death. Patients develop acute respiratory distress caused by noncardiogenic pulmonary edema during or up to 4 hours after transfusion and may require mechanical ventilation. It is thought to be caused primarily by antibodies (either HLA- or neutrophil-directed antibodies) in the donor's plasma, with resultant sequestration of neutrophils in the lung. The treatment is supportive.[38]

TOOLS FOR PRACTICE

Engaging Patients and Family

- *Safety of Blood Transfusions* (brochure), American Academy of Pediatrics (patiented.aap.org).

AAP POLICY STATEMENT

American Academy of Pediatrics, Section on Hematology/Oncology, Section on Allergy/Immunology. Cord blood banking for potential future transplantation. *Pediatrics*. 2007;119(1):165-170. (aappolicy.aappublications.org/cgi/content/full/pediatrics;119/1/165).

SUGGESTED RESOURCES

Goodnough LT, Shander A, Brecher ME. Transfusion medicine: looking to the future. *Lancet*. 2003; 361:161.

Roseff SD, Luban NLC, Manno CS. Guidelines for assessing appropriateness of pediatric transfusion. *Transfusion*. 2002; 42:1398-1413.

Schroeder ML. Transfusion-associated graft-versus-host disease. *Br J Haematol*. 2002;117:275.

Stainsby D, Russell J, Cohen H, et al. Reducing adverse events in blood transfusion. *Br J Haematol*. 2005;131:8.

Wales PW, Lau W, Kim PCW. Directed blood donation in pediatric general surgery: is it worth it? *J Pediatr Surg*. 2001;36:722.

REFERENCES

1. Goodnough LT, Shander A, Brecher ME. Transfusion medicine: looking to the future. *Lancet*. 2003;361:161-169.
2. Starkey JM, MacPherson JL, Bolgiano DC, et al. Markers for transfusion-transmitted disease in different groups of blood donors. *JAMA*. 1989;262:3452-3454.
3. Wales PW, Lau W, Kim PCW. Directed blood donation in pediatric general surgery: is it worth it? *J Pediatr Surg*. 2001;36:722-725.
4. Schroeder ML. Transfusion-associated graft-versus-host disease. *Br J Haematol*. 2002;117:275-287.
5. Silvergleid AJ. Autologous and designated donor programs. In: Petz LD, Swisher SN, Kleinman S, et al, eds. *Clinical Practice of Transfusion Medicine*. New York, NY: Churchill Livingstone; 1996.
6. Waltzman ML, Mooney DP. Major trauma. In: Fleisher GR, Ludwig S, Henretig FM, eds. *Textbook of Pediatric Emergency Medicine*. Philadelphia, PA: Lippincott Williams & Wilkins; 2006.
7. Stainsby D, MacLennan S, Hamilton PJ. Management of massive blood loss: a template guideline. *Br J Anaesth*. 2000;85:487-491.
8. British Committee for Standards in Haematology Transfusion Task Force. Transfusion guidelines for neonates and older children. *Br J Haematol*. 2004;124:433-453.
9. Roseff SD, Luban NLC, Manno CS. Guidelines for assessing appropriateness of pediatric transfusion. *Transfusion*. 2002;42:1398-1413.
10. Tahhan HR, Holbrook CT, Braddy LR, et al. Antigen-matched donor blood in the transfusion management of patients with SC disease. *Transfusion*. 1994;34:562-569.
11. Vichinsky EP. Current issues with blood transfusion in sickle cell disease. *Semin Hematol*. 2001;38(1):14-22.
12. Bowden RA, Slichter SJ, Sayers M, et al. A comparison of filtered leukocyte-reduced and cytomegalovirus (CMV) seronegative blood products for the prevention of transfusion-associated CMV infection after marrow transplant. *Blood*. 1995;86:3598-3603.
13. Wanko SO, Telen MJ. Transfusion management in sickle cell disease. *Hematol Oncol Clin North Am*. 2005;19: 803-826.
14. Thompson HW, Luban NL. Autologous blood transfusion in the pediatric patient. *J Pediatr Surg*. 1995;30:1406-1411.
15. Goodnough LT, Brecher ME, Kanter MH, et al. Transfusion medicine. Second of two parts: blood conservation. *N Engl J Med*. 1999;340:525-533.
16. Meneghini L, Zadra N, Aneloni V, et al. Erythropoietin therapy and acute preoperative normovolaemic haemodilution in infants undergoing craniosynostosis surgery. *Paediatr Anaesth*. 2003;13:392-396.
17. Fearon JA, Weinthal J. The use of recombinant erythropoietin in the reduction of blood transfusion rates in craniosynostosis repair in infants and children. *Plast Reconstr Surg*. 2003;109:2190-2196.
18. Strauss RG. Data-driven blood banking procedures for neonatal RBC transfusions. *Transfusion*. 2000;40:1528-1540.
19. Eckman JR. Techniques for blood administration in sickle cell patients. *Semin Hematol*. 2001;38(1):23-29.
20. The Trial to Reduce Alloimmunization to Platelet Study Group. Leukocyte reduction and ultraviolet B irradiation of platelets to prevent alloimmunization and refractoriness to platelet transfusions. *N Engl J Med*. 1997;337: 1861-1869.
21. Bishton M, Chopra R. The role of granulocyte transfusions in neutropenic patients. *Br J Haematol*. 2004;127: 501-508.
22. Mohan P, Brocklehurst P. Granulocyte transfusions for neonates with confirmed or suspected sepsis and neutropaenia. *Cochrane Database Syst Rev*. 2003;4:CD003956.
23. Stanworth SJ, Massey E, Hyde C, et al. Granulocyte transfusions for treating infections in patients with neutropenia or neutrophil dysfunction. *Cochrane Database Syst Rev*. 2005;3:CD00533.
24. Chanock SJ, Gorlin JB. Granulocyte transfusions: time for a second look. *Infect Dis Clin North Am*. 1996;10: 327-343.
25. Gorlin JB. Therapeutic plasma exchange and cytapheresis in pediatric patients. *Transfus Sci*. 1999;21:21-39.
26. Fung Kee Fung K, Eason E, Crane J, et al. Prevention of Rh alloimmunization. *J Obstet Gynaecol Can*. 2003;25: 765-773.
27. Ewing CA, Rumsey DH, Langberg AF, et al. Immunoprophylaxis using intravenous Rh immune globulin should be standard practice when selected D-negative patients are transfused with D-positive random donor platelets. *Immunohematol*. 1998;14:133-137.
28. Tarantino MD, Madden RM, Fennewald DL, et al. Treatment of childhood acute immune thrombocytopenic purpura with anti-D immune globulin or pooled immune globulin. *J Pediatr*. 1999;134:21-26.
29. Ahsan N. Intravenous immunoglobulin induced-nephropathy: a complication of IVIG therapy. *J Nephrol*. 1998;11:157-161.
30. Kees-Folts D, Abt AB, Domen RE, et al. Renal failure after anti-D globulin treatment of idiopathic thrombocytopenic purpura. *Pediatr Nephrol*. 2002;17:91-96.
31. Capon SM, Goldfinger D. Acute hemolytic transfusion reaction, a paradigm of the systemic inflammatory response: new insights into pathophysiology and treatment. *Transfusion*. 1995;35:513-520.
32. Garratty G. Severe reactions associated with transfusion of patients with sickle cell disease. *Transfusion*. 1997;37: 357-361.
33. Heddle NM. Universal leukoreduction and acute transfusion reactions: putting the puzzle together. *Transfusion*. 2004;44:1-4.
34. Sandler SG, Mallory D, Malamut D, et al. IgA anaphylactic transfusion reactions. *Transfus Med Rev*. 1995;9:1-8.
35. Sanders RP, Maddirala SD, Geiger TL, et al. Premedication with acetaminophen or diphenhydramine for transfusion with leucoreduced blood products in children. *Br J Haematol*. 2005;130:781-787.
36. Stramer SL. Viral diagnostics in the arena of blood donor screening. *Vox Sang*. 2004;2:S180-S183.
37. Goodnough LT. Risks of blood transfusion. *Crit Care Med*. 2003;31:S678-S686.
38. Sanchez R, Toy P. Transfusion related acute lung injury: a pediatric perspective. *Pediatr Blood Cancer*. 2005;45:248-255

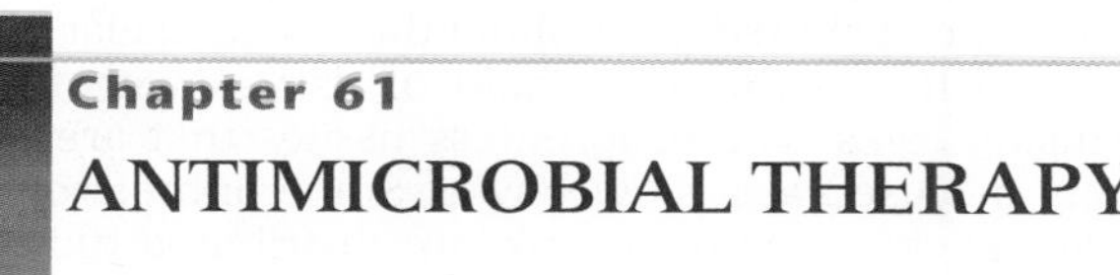

Chapter 61

ANTIMICROBIAL THERAPY

Blaise L. Congeni, MD

The use of antimicrobial agents to treat diseases caused by bacteria is part of the day-to-day practice of pediatrics. Antimicrobial therapy continuously evolves; even experts in infectious diseases have trouble staying abreast of new agents and their pharmacologic properties and pharmacodynamics. The practitioner should know how to use a limited number of antimicrobial agents well rather than having a meager knowledge of many.

APPROACH TO ANTIMICROBIAL THERAPY

Three important questions should be answered before antimicrobial therapy is initiated: (1) where is the infection (anatomic site), (2) what pathogens usually cause infections at this site, and (3) which antimicrobial agents, given by what route of administration, will achieve effective concentrations at this site? The answers to the two initial questions are usually addressed critically by the practitioner. However, selection of an antimicrobial agent is more likely to be based on a *bug-drug* relationship than on knowledge about a drug's ability to achieve an effective concentration at the site of infection.

The anatomic site of most bacterial infections can be identified by a combination of historical information and findings on physical examination. When the site of infection is more obscure, diagnostic studies such as radiographs, radionucleotide scans, computed tomography scans, magnetic resonance imaging, and ultrasound evaluation are often helpful.

The pediatrician can usually develop a list of potential bacterial pathogens based on the site of infection and the patient's age, habitat, history of exposures, and clinical signs and symptoms. The site of infection and possible causative agents help the clinician decide what (if any) specimens should be cultured for bacteria and whether the laboratory should be alerted to use special culture media or techniques. Selecting an antimicrobial agent based on its ability to achieve effective concentrations at the site of infection requires a working concept of effective concentration. To define an effective concentration, the clinician must first review some of the basic pharmacodynamics of antimicrobial agents.

PHARMACODYNAMICS AND PHARMACOKINETICS

Pharmacodynamics describes the relationship between the serum concentration of the drug and its pharmacologic and toxicologic effects. Pharmacokinetics, on the other hand, describes the absorption, distribution, and elimination of drugs. Clinicians are most often interested in the relationship between drug concentration and the antimicrobial effect, the interrelationship between pharmacokinetics and pharmacodynamics. Once administered, an antimicrobial agent is initially distributed throughout the intravascular volume and the extracellular fluid of tissues with high perfusion rates. The drug enters tissues that are not highly perfused at a slower rate. Some antimicrobial agents, such as the β-lactams, are distributed only in extracellular fluid, whereas others distribute intracellularly as well[1](rifampin, trimethoprim-sulfamethoxazole [TMP-SMX]).

Correlation of Drug Concentration and Clinical Effect

Antibiotics can be divided into 2 different groups based on their pattern of bactericidal activity.[2] The first group of agents exhibits a greater rate and extent of bactericidal activity the higher the drug concentration. These agents exhibit concentration-dependent killing. Aminoglycosides, fluoroquinolones, metronidazole, and perhaps macrolides exhibit this type of bactericidal activity.

In contrast, other antibiotics demonstrate bactericidal activity that is independent of drug concentration as long as the concentration exceeds the minimal inhibitory concentration (MIC) for a certain portion of the dosing interval. These agents demonstrate minimal concentration-dependent killing, but instead, their bactericidal activity depends on the time of exposure. Time-dependent agents include the β-lactam antibiotics, vancomycin, and clindamycin.[2]

Postantibiotic Effect

For some antibiotics, continued suppression of bacterial growth occurs even after concentrations of the agent have declined below levels that are sufficient to inhibit growth. This circumstance is termed postantibiotic effect (PAE). All antimicrobial agents exhibit PAEs in vitro against susceptible Gram-positive bacteria. Prolonged PAEs for Gram-negative bacteria are observed only after exposure to antibiotics that inhibit protein synthesis or nucleic acid synthesis.[2] A notable exception is the carbapenems, which produce prolonged PAEs with strains of *Pseudomonas aeruginosa*.

Relationship of Pharmacokinetic and Pharmacodynamic Parameters and Efficacy

When a time-dependent agent is used, organisms begin to regrow once the serum concentration of the antimicrobial agent has fallen below the MIC. Consequently, the most effective treatment regimens will allow for drug concentrations at the site of infection to be above the MIC for as large a part of the dosing interval as possible. For example, a cure of 85% to 100% can be anticipated when the drug concentration exceeds the MIC for at least 40% of the dosing interval for time-dependent agents such as β-lactams.

Some investigators have suggested that infections such as endocarditis or osteomyelitis may require more time above the MIC for clinical cure. Serum bactericidal activity typically has been measured to monitor children who have acute hematogenous osteomyelitis. Peak levels have been traditionally used, but at least 1 group of investigators has suggested that serum bactericidal activity at trough concentrations may correlate better with cure.[2] In other words, a trough serum bactericidal concentration may be a more accurate reflection of the portion of the dosing interval during which the drug concentration was above the MIC.

Infrequent dosing of concentration-dependent agents such as aminoglycosides and fluoroquinolones is effective. During the 1990s, several studies have reported equal or superior clinical efficacy when the entire aminoglycoside dose is given as a single daily dose.[3,4] This approach allows for a single peak concentration at least 10-fold higher than the MIC. Although considerable debate continues, toxicity does not appear to be increased; some investigators have suggested that toxicity depends on the length of time the drug is present in drug-sensitive tissues (eg, the kidney, the inner ear) rather than on the highest concentration attained in the serum at any point.

Minimal Inhibitory and Minimal Bactericidal Concentrations

An antimicrobial agent's activity against specific bacteria in vitro is expressed as the agent's MIC or minimal bactericidal concentration (MBC). To determine the MIC, bacteria are grown in broth to a concentration of 100,000 (10^5) microorganisms per milliliter. The broth containing the bacteria, which is clear to the naked eye, is then placed in a series of test tubes, and a decreasing amount of antimicrobial agent is added to each test tube. The broth containing the bacteria and antimicrobial agent is incubated overnight and then examined for visible turbidity. (Turbidity represents bacterial growth.) The test tube with the smallest concentration of antimicrobial agent that remains clear to the naked eye represents the MIC. To determine if the antibiotic is bactericidal, the tubes that remained clear are quantitatively subcultured onto agar plates. After overnight incubation, bacterial colonies are counted. Each colony represents 1 bacterium that survived, or 1 colony-forming unit (CFU). The smallest amount of antibiotic that results in the death of 99,900 (99.9%) of the original 100,000 microorganisms per milliliter inoculum (a 1000-fold reduction) is the MBC. MIC and MBC results are reported in micrograms of antimicrobial agent per milliliter of broth required to inhibit or kill the microorganism, respectively.

Serum Inhibitory and Bactericidal Titers

Antimicrobial activity in vivo can be approximated by determining the inhibitory or bactericidal titers. Although the test is usually performed using serum, it can be done with most body fluids that are clear, except urine. The test is performed by growing organisms to 10^5 CFU/mL of broth, as in determining the MIC. However, instead of adding known concentrations of antimicrobial agent to each test tube, serial 2-fold dilutions of serum (or other body fluids) are added to sequential tubes (undiluted serum is added to the 1st tube, serum diluted 1:2 to the 2nd tube, 1:4 to the 3rd, and so on). After incubation overnight, the tubes are examined for visible turbidity; the most dilute sample that has no visible turbidity is the serum inhibitory titer. To determine if the bacteria are being killed, the broth is cultured quantitatively as for the MBC, and the most dilute specimen that results in the death of 99.9% of the original inoculum is the serum bactericidal titer. Formerly, serum bactericidal levels were used to monitor adequacy of therapy when patients being treated for osteomyelitis or sometimes endocarditis were switched from parenteral to oral therapy. Unfortunately, few laboratories are able to offer this test any longer.

Tolerance

Tolerance to an antibiotic occurs when organisms are inhibited by the typical concentration of a bactericidal agent but require a higher concentration of the agent to achieve a bactericidal effect. The clinical significance of tolerance is still controversial, but this phenomenon may apparently be important with infections that require bactericidal activity to effect a cure.[5]

Bacteriostatic Versus Bactericidal Agents

Most infections in children do not require a bactericidal antimicrobial agent. In general, bactericidal agents are needed for optimal treatment of bacterial endocarditis, meningitis, and osteomyelitis. The effectiveness of bacteriostatic agents depends on the host's ability to opsonize and phagocytize bacteria that have been inhibited; thus bactericidal agents are usually necessary to treat bacterial infections in a neutropenic host.

Role of the Laboratory in Antimicrobial Therapy

Laboratory testing is usually unnecessary to choose antimicrobial agents for the vast majority of bacterial infections treated in the ambulatory setting. For example, otitis media is the most common infection of children that is treated with antimicrobial agents in the ambulatory setting. The site of infection is identified by physical examination. The bacterial pathogens that cause otitis media have been well established, and several antimicrobial agents have been shown to produce a clinical and microbiologic cure when given orally. Only if empirical therapy fails might performing a tympanocentesis become necessary to obtain a specimen for isolating the bacteria and performing antibiotic susceptibility tests. The practitioner can manage common infections such as impetigo, cellulitis, cervical adenitis, local abscesses, and conjunctivitis without obtaining specimens for culture simply by knowing the usual pathogens and their susceptibility to antimicrobial agents.

Culture and Susceptibility

When therapy fails, when the patient is seriously ill or is immunocompromised, or when the clinical situation is unusual, the 1st step in choosing antimicrobial therapy is to obtain appropriate specimens for culture. When bacterial pathogens are isolated from a normally sterile specimen, antimicrobial susceptibility is tested. Susceptibility is tested by either determining the MIC as described previously or by using the disk diffusion method.

In the disk diffusion method of susceptibility testing, a culture plate is inoculated with the bacteria to be tested, and paper disks containing standardized concentrations of antimicrobial agents are placed on the surface of the culture medium. The culture plates are incubated, and the moisture from the medium allows the antimicrobial agents to diffuse out of the paper disks. The farther from the disk the diffusion reaches, the lower will be the concentration of antimicrobial agent. If the bacteria are inhibited by the antibiotic, then a zone around the disk forms in which the bacteria do not grow. The zone of inhibition is measured after overnight incubation and, based on its diameter, the organism is determined to be *susceptible* or *resistant* to the antimicrobial agent. A report of *intermediate* or *indeterminant* should be interpreted to mean that the microorganism is resistant or that the MIC should be determined. The diameter of the zone of inhibition has been correlated to MIC determinations such that *susceptible* actually means that the MIC will be equal to or less than a certain concentration of the antimicrobial agent.

An organism that is reported to be susceptible by disk means that 95% of the strains of these bacteria are inhibited by serum concentrations of the antimicrobial agent if the antimicrobial agent is given at the usual dose by the usual route of administration for an infection with that organism. This concentration is called the MIC_{95}. The MIC_{95} of selected antimicrobial agents for bacteria reported as susceptible by disk are listed in Table 61-1. Clearly, the site of infection, the proposed antibiotic's activity against the pathogen, and the concentration of the antibiotic that can be achieved at the site of infection must all be considered.

Susceptible to ampicillin has very different meanings, depending on the organism being tested. Gram-negative organisms or enterococci that are reported as being susceptible to ampicillin (see Table 61-1) means that 95% of these organisms are inhibited by serum concentrations of 8 mcg/mL or less of ampicillin.[6] For Gram-positive cocci, susceptible means that 95% are inhibited by serum concentrations of 0.2 mcg/mL or less or 40 times less ampicillin than is required to inhibit Gram-negative enterics.[6] For *Haemophilus influenzae,* susceptible means that serum concentrations of 2 mcg/mL or less are required to inhibit 95% of all strains.[6] Unless the MIC has been determined for the individual isolate, the clinician must assume that MIC_{95} must be achieved at the site of infection to inhibit the isolate.

Two modifications of the disk diffusion method provide additional information when selecting an antibiotic for certain infections. The *e test* uses a strip instead of a disk. An antibiotic gradient is applied, and the zone of inhibition enables the laboratory to determine an approximated MIC by observing where growth occurs on the gradient. This test is most often used to determine MICs for different antimicrobics for *Streptococcus pneumoniae*.

The *D test* is used to determine if inducible resistance for clindamycin is likely for the offending staphylococcal isolate. The clindamycin disk is placed adjacent to the erythromycin disk. The zone of inhibition between the clindamycin and erythromycin disks is blunted, hence the appearance of a zone that resembles a *D*. Despite the presence of a large zone of inhibition, the staphylococcal isolate is considered resistant to clindamycin (Figure 61-1).

PROPERTIES OF CLASSES OF ANTIBACTERIAL AGENTS

Because of the large number of antimicrobial agents currently available, usually, several are equally effective for a given infection. The antimicrobial agents preferred by a practitioner reflect the drugs' cost, availability, physician's training, and local practices. In general, knowing how to use a small number of antimicrobial agents well is far better than knowing all of the possible alternatives. The most frequently prescribed antimicrobial agents and their selected pharmacologic and pharmacodynamic information are listed in Table 61-1. This table is an example of the information a practitioner should have at hand when using microbial agents.

Penicillins

Mechanism of Action

Although the general mechanism of action of penicillins is to inhibit cell wall synthesis, precisely how they do this is unknown. Current evidence, however, points to inhibition of transpeptidation. Most bacteria have penicillin-binding proteins (PBPs) in their cell membranes. Several PBPs can be found, and the number and type vary from bacteria to bacteria. The activity of penicillins generally correlates with the number of high-affinity PBPs the organism has.

Bacterial Resistance

Bacterial resistance to penicillins can be based on 3 principal mechanisms: (1) enzymatic degradation, (2) reduced penetration of the agent to the target site, and (3) alteration in the PBP.[7] Inactivation of the penicillin as a result of degradation caused by a penicillinase produced by the bacteria has been the most common mechanism of resistance for this class of agents. Beta-lactamase enzymes hydrolyze the β-lactam ring. A variety of β-lactamases have been identified and are classified based on substrate preference. Both Gram-positive and Gram-negative organisms can produce β-lactamases, and production of these enzymes is mediated by either plasmid or chromosomal mechanisms.

Occasionally, resistance is mediated by failure of the penicillin to reach the site of infection. Some bacteria are resistant because, as a result of shape or electric charge, penicillin cannot reach the binding site.

During the last decade, alteration in PBPs has become an important mechanism of resistance. This mechanism of resistance is responsible for methicillin resistance seen with *Staphylococcus aureus*. Alteration of PBP also is responsible for the reduced susceptibility of *S pneumoniae* to β-lactams, drug-resistant *S pneumoniae,* (DRSP). Use of β-lactamase T stable agents under these circumstances is not effective.

Infections in children caused by DRSP appear to be decreasing as a result of widespread use of the conjugate pneumococcal vaccine. Community associated infections with methicillin-resistant *S aureus* (MRSA), have increased dramatically, however. Infections caused by MRSA may require treatment with antimicrobics that do not inhibit cell wall synthesis by binding to PBPs. Agents frequently used for such infections include vancomycin, linezolid, trimethoprim-sulfamethoxazole, and clindamycin. Tetracyclines and fluoroquinolones may also be used when the age of the patient permits. When selecting a specific antistaphylococcal agent, the physician should be guided by the severity of the infection, as well as by local susceptibility patterns. For example, in life-threatening infections, vancomycin is usually used as a 1st-line therapy.

Classification

Based on their specific antibacterial activity, penicillins can be classified loosely as (1) natural, (2) penicillinase resistant, (3) amino, (4) antipseudomonal, and (5) extended spectrum. The practitioner should be well versed in the use of 1 penicillin from each class.

Pharmacologic Properties

Penicillins vary greatly in absorption after oral administration, with penicillin V, amoxicillin, cloxacillin, and

Table 61-1 Dosage, Peak Serum Concentrations, and MIC_{95} for Selected Antimicrobial Agents

		Age					
Antimicrobial Agent	**Route of Administration**	**<1 Wk* (<2000 g) mg/kg/Dose/ Interval**	**1 Wk-1 Mo* (<2000 g) mg/kg/Dose/ Interval**	**>1 Mo mg/kg/Dose/ Interval**	**Adult Dose† g/Dose/ Interval**	**Peak Serum Concentration (mcg/mL)**	**Susceptibility (MIC_{95}) (mcg/mL)‡**
Penicillin G	IV	50,000 U q8h (50,000 U 66 q12h)	50,000 U q6h (50,000 U q8h)	25,000-50,000 U q4-6h	25,000-50,000 U/kg q4-6h	400	≤0.01 *L. monocytogenes* ≤2
Procaine penicillin	IM	50,000 U q24h (50,000 U q24h)	50,000 U q24h (50,000 U q24h)	25,000-50,000 U q12-24h	25,000-50,000 U/kg q12-24h	5-6	≤0.1
Benzathine I penicillin	IM	50,000 U; 1 dose (50,000 U; 1 dose)	50,000 U; 1 dose (50,000 U; 1 dose)	50,000 U; 1 dose	2.4 × 10^6 U; 1 dose	0.2	≤0.1
Penicillin V	PO	Not recommended	Not recommended	6.25-12.5 q6h	0.25-0.5 q6h	3-5	≤0.1
Ampicillin	IV	25-50 q8h	25-50 q6h	25-75 q4-6h	1-2 q4-6h	40	Gram-negative ≤8
	IM	(25-50 q12h)	(25-50 q8h)			8	Streptococci ≤0.1 *H influenzae* ≤2
Amoxicillin	PO	Not recommended	Not recommended	10-15 q8h	0.25-0.5 q8h	4.7-7.5	As for ampicillin
Nafcillin	IV	20 q8h (25 q12h)	37.5 q6h (25 q8h)	25-50 q6h	0.5-1.5 q4-6h	11	≤1
Methicillin[§]	IV	25-50 q8h (25-50 q12h)	25-50 q6h (25-50 q8h)	—	—	—	—
Dicloxacillin	PO	Not recommended	Not recommended	3-6.25	0.25-0.5 q6h	15-18	≤1
Mezlocillin	IV	75 q12h	75 q8h	50-75 q4-6h	3-4 q4-6h	200-300	≤64
	IM	(75 q12h)	(75 q8h)			15	
Cefazolin	IV	20 q12h	20 q8h	8.3-25 q6-8h	0.5-1.5 q6-8h	188	≤8
	IM	(20 q12h)	(20 q12h)				
Cephalexin	PO	Not recommended	Not recommended	6.25-12.5 q6h	0.25-1 q6h	8-40	≤8
Cefoxitin	IV	Not recommended	Not recommended	20-26.6 q4-6h	1-2 q4-6h or 3 q8h	110-125	≤8
	IM						
Cefotaxime	IV	50 q12h (50 q12h)	50 q8h (50 q8h)	25-50 q6h	1-2 q4-12h	1 g 40 2 g 80-90	≤8
Ceftriaxone	IV	50 q24h	50-80 q24h	50 q24h	0.5-2 q24h	1 g 150	≤8
	IM	(50 q24h)	(50 q24h)	CNS: 80 q24h		1 g 50	
Ceftazidime	IV	30 q8h	50 q8h	25-50 q6h	0.5-2 q8-12h	1 g 85	≤8
	IM	(50 q12h)	(50 q8h)			1 g 34	
Amikacin	IV	10 q12h	10 q8h	5 q8h or 7.5 q12h	5 **mg/kg** q8h or 7.5 **mg/kg** q12/h	20-40	≤16
	IM	(7.5 q12h)	(7.5 q8h)			(20)	

*Doses and intervals shown in parentheses are for infants with a birth weight <2000 g; doses and intervals shown without parentheses are for infants with a birth weight >2000 g.
†Maximal recommended dose (units other than grams are in **boldface**).
‡mcg/mL of the antimicrobial required to inhibit isolate reported to be susceptible to disk diffusion method.
§Methicillin is preferred for newborns when kernicterus is a concern.

Continued

Table 61-1 Dosage, Peak Serum Concentrations, and MIC_{95} for Selected Antimicrobial Agents—cont'd

Antimicrobial Agent	Route of Administration	Age: <1 Wk* (<2000 g) mg/kg/Dose/Interval	Age: 1 Wk-1 Mo* (<2000 g) mg/kg/Dose/Interval	Age: >1 Mo mg/kg/Dose/Interval	Adult Dose† g/Dose/Interval	Peak Serum Concentration (mcg/mL)	Susceptibility (MIC_{95}) (mcg/mL)‡
Gentamicin	IV IM	2.5 q12h (2.5 q12h)	2.5 q8h (2.5 q8h)	1-2.5 q8h	1-1.7 mg/kg q8h	4-10 (7)	≤4
Tobramycin	IV IM	2 q12h (2 q12h)	2 q8h (2 q8h)	1-2 q8h	1-1.7 mg/kg q8h	4-14 (4)	≤4
Trimethoprim-sulfamethoxazole (TMP-SMX)	PO IV	Not recommended	Not recommended	3-6 TMP/15-30 SMX q12h 5 TMP/25 SMX q6h for pneumocystosis	0.16 TMP/0.8 SMX q12h	2-4/80-100	≤2/38
Sulfisoxazole	PO	Not recommended	Not recommended	30-37.5 q6h	0.5-1 q6h	40-50	≤100 (urinary tract infection only)
Erythromycin estolate	PO	10 q12h (10 q12h)	10-12.5 q8h (10 q8h)	10 q8h or 15 q12h	0.25-0.5 q6h	4.2	≤0.5
Erythromycin ethylsuccinate	PO	10 q12h (10 q12h)	10 q8h (10 q8h)	10 q6h	0.25-0.5 q6h	1.5	≤0.5
Clindamycin	PO IV	5 q8h (5 q12h)	5 q6h (5 q8h)	2.5-7.5 q6h	0.15-0.45 q6h	2.5-3.6	≤0.5
Chloramphenicol	IV PO	25 q24h (25 q24h)	25 q24h (25 q24h)	12.5-18.75 q6h 18.7-25 q6h (meningitis)	12.5-25 mg/kg q6h	19 (25)	*H influenzae* ≤4 Others ≤12.5
Tetracycline	IV PO	Not recommended	Not recommended	Children >8 yr 6.25-12.5 q6h	0.25-0.5 q6h	8 (4)	≤4
Vancomycin	IV	15 q12h (10 q12h)	10 q8h (10 q8h)	10-15 q6h	15 mg/kg q12h or 6.5-8 mg/kg q6h	30-40	≤5
Metronidazole	PO IV	7.5 q12h (7.5 q12h)	15 q12h (7.5 q12h)	5-12 q8h (7.5 q6h)	7.5 mg/kg q6h	11.5 (20-25)	≤4
Rifampin	PO	Not recommended	Not recommended	10-20 q24h	0.6 q24h	7	≤1

*Doses and intervals shown in parentheses are for infants with a birth weight <2000 g; doses and intervals shown without parentheses are for infants with a birth weight >2000 g.
†Maximal recommended dose (units other than grams are in **boldface**).
‡mcg/mL of the antimicrobial required to inhibit isolate reported to be susceptible to disk diffusion method.
§Methicillin is preferred for newborns when kernicterus is a concern.

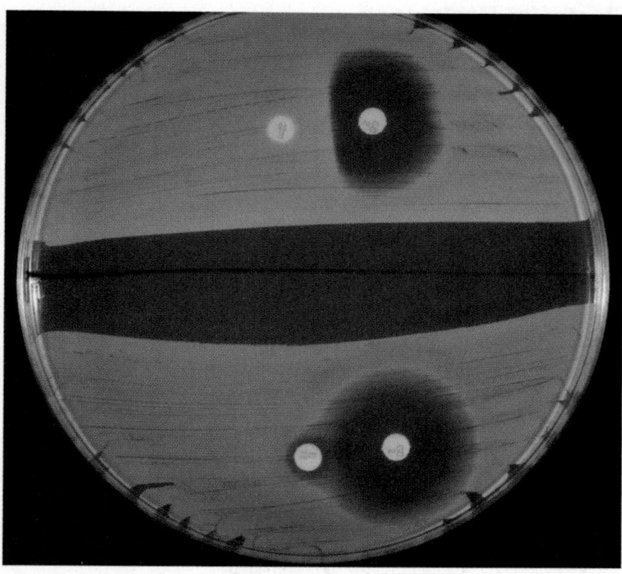

Figure 61-1 Positive D test. Petri plate with zone of inhibition surrounding disks.

dicloxacillin having the greatest absorption. Food reduces the absorption of oxacillin and dicloxacillin but not of penicillin V or amoxicillin. Procaine penicillin G and benzathine penicillin G are absorbed slowly after intramuscular injection and are given every 12 to 24 hours and every 15 to 20 days, respectively. Penicillins are excreted by renal tubular cells and have a very short half-life, ranging from less than 30 minutes to slightly more than 1 hour. Penicillins are distributed to most areas of the body if inflammation is present. However, they are poorly lipid soluble and do not enter the central nervous system (CNS) well, even if inflammation is present. Penicillins do not enter cells well. Passage of penicillins from the serum of a pregnant woman to her fetus depends on the degree of protein binding present; little of highly protein-bound penicillins reaches the fetus.

Side Effects

The most important adverse reactions to penicillins are caused by hypersensitivity; they range from skin rashes to anaphylaxis. Anaphylactic reactions to penicillin are IgE-mediated and occur in approximately 1 of every 500 courses of treatment (0.2%); approximately 1 of every 100,000 courses results in a fatality (0.001%).[8] The morbilliform rashes seen during therapy with penicillins probably are IgM-mediated and often disappear even when therapy is continued. Less common reactions include serum sickness, exfoliative dermatitis, and Stevens-Johnson syndrome.

Penicillin Desensitization

At times, administering penicillin to a penicillin-sensitive patient may be necessary, for example a patient with meningococcal meningitis who is allergic to cephalosporins and penicillins. When penicillin is administered to a patient who may have an anaphylactic reaction, immunotolerance to penicillin can be achieved by starting with very small doses. An effective protocol is to administer 5 U of penicillin G intracutaneously, in the forearm, and then, at 60- to 90-minute intervals, increase the dose to 10, 100, 1000, 10,000, and 50,000 U. If the intradermal doses are tolerated, intravenous penicillin can be instituted.

Use of Selected Penicillins

The natural penicillins listed in Table 61-1 are penicillin G (aqueous, procaine, and benzathine) and penicillin V. These antimicrobial agents are most active against both aerobic and anaerobic Gram-positive cocci, *Neisseria meningitidis, N gonorrhoeae, Fusobacterium* species, *Eikenella* species, *Listeria monocytogenes,* and *Borrelia burgdorferi*. Penicillins are still the mainstay of treatment for infections caused by group A β-hemolytic streptococci, group B streptococci, *S pneumoniae, N meningitidis,* and *L monocytogenes*. Penicillin is also the drug of choice for acute infections with *B burgdorferi* (Lyme disease) in children and for infections caused by anaerobes normally found in the mouth.

The potassium salt of penicillin G is usually used and is almost exclusively given intravenously. Either procaine or benzathine preparations are used for intramuscular administration. When given intramuscularly, aqueous penicillin G is excreted very rapidly; when given by mouth, it is poorly absorbed, and very low serum concentrations are achieved with these preparations; they can be used only for exquisitely sensitive organisms and generally should not be used to treat CNS infections. Procaine penicillin can be used in a newborn to treat neurosyphilis. Penicillin V is well absorbed from the gastrointestinal tract and is therefore preferred for oral administration. Peak serum concentrations and MIC_{95} equivalents for susceptibility by disk are listed for individual penicillins in Table 61-1.

Ampicillin has the same general activity as penicillin, but it also is active against *Escherichia coli, Proteus mirabilis, Salmonella* species, and *Shigella* species and is more active against group D streptococci and *L monocytogenes*. Amoxicillin differs from ampicillin in molecular composition only by the presence of a hydroxyl group. Because amoxicillin is absorbed much better than ampicillin, peak serum concentrations of amoxicillin after oral administration are equal to those achieved with an equivalent dose of ampicillin given intramuscularly. The antimicrobial activity of amoxicillin is virtually identical to that of ampicillin, except that it is not useful in the treatment of shigellosis; because of the increased absorption of amoxicillin, less drug is available in the intestinal tract.

Several fixed combination β-lactam–β-lactamase inhibitors are available. Beta-lactamase inhibitors include clavulanic acid, sulbactam, and tazobactam. Four agents are currently available: amoxicillin-clavulanate (Augmentin), ampicillin-sulbactam (Unasyn), ticarcillin-clavulanate (Timentin), and piperacillin-tazobactam (Zosyn). Piperacillin-tazobactam does not have a pediatric indication for its use. The β-lactamase inhibitor extends the activity of the β-lactam to include some organisms that produce β-lactamase. Amoxicillin-clavulanate, for example, is active against β-lactamase—producing

S aureus, H influenzae, N gonorrhoeae, and *Moraxella catarrhalis* that otherwise would be resistant to amoxicillin. The MIC for *E coli, Klebsiella* species, *Proteus* species, and *Bacteroides fragilis* ranges from 8 to 16 mcg/mL. This combination is no more active than amoxicillin for *S pneumoniae* strains that are resistant to penicillin. Ampicillin in a fixed combination with sulbactam is marketed as Unasyn for intravenous use only. The activity of ampicillin-sulbactam is similar to that of ampicillin-clavulanate, and this agent is frequently used in adults and children for respiratory infections and infections in which anaerobes are likely to be pathogens, such as intraabdominal or intraoral infections. Safety and efficacy for intraabdominal infections in children have not been established. Ticarcillin-clavulanate (Timentin) and piperacillin-tazobactam (Zosyn) use a β-lactam that is an extended-spectrum penicillin with antipseudomonal activity, thereby extending the spectrum of these fixed combinations further. These agents would be more appropriate for infections in which Gram-negative organisms, including *Pseudomonas,* are thought to be pathogens.

Nafcillin is one of several penicillinase-resistant penicillins used primarily to treat infections caused by *S aureus,* excluding MRSA. Most strains of *S aureus* are inhibited by concentrations of 2 to 3 mcg/mL. Because nafcillin is highly protein bound, methicillin is preferred for newborns when the possibility of kernicterus is a concern, because the amount of albumin available for binding bilirubin will be diminished. Absorption of nafcillin from the gastrointestinal (GI) tract is erratic; it should not be given orally. Dicloxacillin is absorbed from the GI tract more consistently and is a good oral agent for treating *S aureus* infections. The oral suspension of dicloxacillin has a very bitter taste, which can create problems with compliance.

Several antipseudomonad and extended-spectrum penicillins are currently available. In general, *Pseudomonas* infections should be treated with a combination of one of these agents plus an aminoglycoside, both for synergy and for reducing the emergence of resistant bacteria. A possible exception to this rule is for the treatment of a urinary tract infection caused by *Pseudomonas aeruginosa*. Mezlocillin has the antipseudomonad activity of carbenicillin and ticarcillin; it is also more active against enterococci, *Klebsiella* species, *H influenzae,* and *B fragilis*. An important point to remember is that a report of *susceptible to mezlocillin* means that concentrations as high as 64 mcg/mL will be needed to inhibit 95% of the strains tested; this circumstance is compensated for by the high serum concentrations achieved when the drug is given intravenously (the peak serum concentration is 300 mcg/mL after an intravenous dose of 4 g).

Cephalosporins

Mechanism of Action

Similar to penicillins, cephalosporins are β-lactam antibiotics that interfere with cell wall synthesis. However, the precise mechanism is not known, and the effects of cephalosporins on bacteria range from lysing the organism to producing bacteria that have unusual forms.

Bacterial Resistance

Bacterial resistance to cephalosporins can arise if the cephalosporin is inactivated by β-lactamase, if it is unable to reach antibiotic-binding proteins, if the bacteria does not have appropriate binding sites, or if tolerance develops (see the previous discussion of penicillins).

Classification

In the 1970s and 1980s, more new cephalosporins were introduced for general use than any other type of antimicrobial agent.[9] Currently, ceftriaxone and cefotaxime are 2 of the agents most commonly used for the empirical therapy of the febrile infant. The usual classification system for cephalosporins is based on antibacterial activity and is divided into 1st, 2nd, and 3rd generations (Box 61-1). Some experts have recently added a 4th generation. This classification system appears more useful for parenteral agents and may result in very dissimilar agents being grouped together. In general, the 1st-generation cephalosporins have good activity against Gram-positive cocci except enterococci, coagulase-negative staphylococcal species, and MRSA; they have limited activity against Gram-negative organisms except *E coli, Klebsiella pneumoniae,* and *P mirabilis*. Activity of these agents against Enterobacteriaceae is unpredictable; the clinician should be guided by in vitro susceptibility testing. Organisms susceptible to one cephalosporin of this class are generally susceptible to all. The 2nd-generation cephalosporins have the general activity of the 1st generation but are somewhat more active against Gram-negative organisms, including *H influenzae*. Third-generation cephalosporins are more active than 2nd-generation drugs against Gram-negative organisms but are less active against some

BOX 61-1 Cephalosporins

FIRST GENERATION
Cefadroxil*
Cefazolin
Cephalexin*
Cephalothin
Cephapirin
Cephradine†

SECOND GENERATION
Cefaclor*
Cefamandole
Cefmetazole
Cefonicid
Cefotetan
Cefotiam
Cefoxitin
Cefprozil*
Cefuroxime
Cefuroxime axetil*

THIRD GENERATION
Cefepime
Cefixime*
Cefmenoxime
Cefoperazone
Cefotaxime
Cefpiramide
Cefpodoxime proxetil*
Ceftazidime
Ceftibuten*
Ceftizoxime
Ceftriaxone
Moxalactam

*Oral.
†Oral and parenteral.
All others are parenteral.

Gram-positive organisms, especially *S aureus,* than are the 1st-generation drugs.

Cefepime is a 4th-generation cephalosporin with activity similar to cefotaxime, but it additionally demonstrates better activity against some Gram-negative organisms such as *P aeruginosa*.

Pharmacologic Properties

Because of the number of cephalosporins and the wide variations in pharmacology, each drug should be considered individually.

Side Effects

The side effects seen with cephalosporins are generally the same as those seen with penicillins. Hypersensitivity reactions are the most common side effects. Although immunologic studies have shown a substantial cross-reactivity between penicillins and cephalosporins,[10] in practice, only 5% to 10% of persons who have hypersensitivity reactions to penicillins have them with cephalosporins. In general, if a patient has had only a nonurticarial rash as the manifestation of penicillin hypersensitivity, then using cephalosporins is safe. For patients who have had urticaria or an anaphylactic reaction in response to penicillins, cephalosporins should be used with great caution. Recent studies have suggested that the frequency of cross-sensitivity between penicillins and cephalosporins is substantially less than the figures cited previously.[11] Allergy to cephalosporins in patients truly allergic to penicillins is more common with 1st-generation cephalosporins and is seen with agents with identical side chains. The fact that both the penicillins and the cephalosporins share an identical β-lactam ring seems much less important relative to predicting cross-sensitivity than previously thought. Less common side effects with cephalosporins are nephrotoxicity, diarrhea, alcohol intolerance, and bleeding.

Use of Selected Cephalosporins

FIRST-GENERATION CEPHALOSPORINS. First-generation cephalosporins are used to treat infections caused by Gram-positive cocci when penicillin cannot be used, to treat infections caused by methicillin-sensitive *S aureus,* and to provide coverage against *E coli, K pneumoniae,* and *P mirabilis.* Cefazolin is preferable to cephalothin because it has greater activity against *E coli* and *Klebsiella* species, achieves higher peak serum concentrations, and has a longer half-life. The peak serum concentration of cefazolin after a dose of 1 g given intravenously is 188 mcg/mL; the serum half-life is 1½ to 2 hours. Susceptible by disk means that 95% of the bacteria tested are inhibited by 8 mcg/mL or less. The longer half-life compared with antistaphylococcal penicillins, nafcillin, or cephalothin makes cefazolin a particularly attractive agent for patients who are not hospitalized. Cefazolin can be given 3 times a day compared with the other agents, which require dosing 4 times a day. Cephalexin (Keflex) is a 1st-generation cephalosporin that can be given orally. A peak serum concentration of 16 mcg/mL can be achieved with a dose of 0.5 g. The antibacterial activity of cephalexin is similar to that of cefazolin. Cefadroxil achieves peak serum concentrations and has antimicrobial activity similar to that of cephalexin but is excreted more slowly, allowing administration at 12- to 24-hour intervals.

SECOND-GENERATION CEPHALOSPORINS. Based on activity, 2nd-generation cephalosporins should be divided further into 2 separate groups. The true cephalosporins of the 2nd generation include cefuroxime and cefamandole.

Cefuroxime was used widely in children for the treatment of infection when Gram-positive cocci such as *S aureus* and *H influenzae* were considered likely pathogens. Many of these infections are now treated with the 3rd-generation cephalosporins, ceftriaxone, or cefotaxime because of improved penetration into the cerebrospinal fluid and because of the possibility of *S pneumoniae* as a pathogen in these circumstances. Cefuroxime is the only 2nd-generation cephalosporin that achieves therapeutic concentrations in cerebrospinal fluid (CSF). For a time, cefuroxime was advocated as single-drug therapy for bacterial meningitis in infants and children older than 2 months. However, cefuroxime does not sterilize the CSF as rapidly as does ampicillin plus chloramphenicol or selected 3rd-generation cephalosporins and should not be used to treat meningitis. Cefuroxime can be used when parenteral coverage for both *S aureus* and *H influenzae* is desirable in a patient who has no CNS infection.

The 2nd-generation cephamycins include cefoxitin, cefotetan, and cefmetazole. These agents are rarely used in children because more suitable agents are available. Cefoxitin is highly resistant to β-lactamases and is more active against anaerobes, especially *B fragilis,* than other cephalosporins. It is not as active as other 2nd-generation cephalosporins against *H influenzae* and Enterobacteriaceae, nor is it as active against Gram-positive cocci as 1st-generation cephalosporins. Cefotetan is more active against aerobic Gram-negative bacilli than cefoxitin but is less active against aerobic Gram-positive cocci. Cefmetazole appears to be more active against *S aureus* than either cefoxitin or cefotetan but is less active than cefotetan against Enterobacteriaceae and less active than cefoxitin against *B fragilis.*[12] Because of its activity against anaerobes plus some Gram-positive and Gram-negative aerobes, cefoxitin has proved useful in the treatment of pelvic inflammatory disease and lung abscesses. The peak serum concentration after a dose of 1 g given intravenously is approximately 22 mcg/mL; and the serum half-life is approximately 50 minutes. Susceptible by disk means that the MIC_{95} for the organism is 8 mcg/mL or less. Use of cefoxitin declined dramatically in the 1990s because of the development of safer, more effective agents. Fixed-combination β-lactam–β-lactamase inhibitors including Unasyn are more active against anaerobes and have better activity against Gram-positive cocci, including *S aureus.* Metronidazole and carbapenems are also more active against anaerobes than cefoxitin. Consequently, these agents are preferred in clinical situations in which cefoxitin may have been used in the past.

Second-generation cephalosporins available for oral administration include cefaclor (Ceclor), cefuroxime axetil (Ceftin), cefprozil (Cefzil), and loracarbef (Lorabid). Loracarbef is technically a carbacephem rather than a cephalosporin.[13] These agents are used primarily as the 2nd- or 3rd-line agents to treat upper respiratory infections (eg, otitis media, sinusitis) in patients who have failed less expensive 1st-line agents such as amoxicillin. The structure and spectrum of activity of loracarbef are very similar to those of cefaclor.

THIRD-GENERATION CEPHALOSPORINS. The 3rd-generation cephalosporins are more active than even the 1st- or 2nd-generation drugs against Gram-negative organisms, but these agents are less active against *S aureus*. Cefotaxime and ceftriaxone are the most active of the cephalosporins against *S pneumoniae* and other streptococci, including many strains that are resistant to penicillin.

Third-generation cephalosporins can be thought of as those that have a role in treating *Pseudomonas* infections and those that do not. Cefotaxime and ceftriaxone do not have activity against *P aeruginosa*. Cefotaxime, the initial 3rd-generation cephalosporin to be used widely in the United States, is still useful clinically. Ceftriaxone is very similar to cefotaxime in antibacterial activity but has a much longer half-life. Both cefotaxime and ceftriaxone are active against most Gram-positive aerobes except enterococci and *L monocytogenes*. Neither one is active against MRSA or coagulase-negative staphylococci. Both are active against most Gram-negative aerobic bacteria, except for *Pseudomonas* species. The diacetyl breakdown product of cefotaxime also has a broad range of activity, but specific activity is less than that of cefotaxime itself. The peak serum concentration after intravenous administration of 1 g of cefotaxime is approximately 40 mcg/mL, compared with 150 mcg/mL for ceftriaxone. The serum half-life of cefotaxime is approximately 1 hour, compared with 8 hours for ceftriaxone. Because ceftriaxone is excreted slowly, a peak serum concentration of 50 mcg/mL is achieved in adults after a dose of 0.5 g is given intramuscularly. Susceptible by disk means that the MIC95 of either drug for the bacteria tested is 8 mcg/mL or less.

The subsequent 2nd-generation cephalosporins that have good antipseudomonad activity are cefoperazone and ceftazidime. Ceftazidime is more active than cefoperazone against *Pseudomonas* in vitro but is less active than cefotaxime against Gram-positive organisms. Whether ceftazidime should be used as a single agent to treat *Pseudomonas* infections is still controversial. In adults, the peak serum concentration of ceftazidime after 1 g is given intravenously is 85 mcg/mL; the serum half-life is approximately 1 hour and 48 minutes. Approximately 90% of *Pseudomonas* isolates are inhibited by 8 mcg/mL or less of ceftazidime.

Four 3rd-generation cephalosporins are currently available for oral use; they are cefixime (Suprax), cefpodoxime proxetil (Vantin), ceftibuten (Cedax), and cefdinir (Omnicef).[13] Cefixime and ceftibuten have a similar spectrum; consequently, they are grouped together. They have limited activity against some Gram-positive cocci such as *S pneumoniae* and no activity against *S aureus*. Both are active against the Gram-negative bacilli responsible for most urinary tract infections. Because *S pneumoniae* coverage is incomplete, these agents are recommended only as 2nd-line agents for the treatment of otitis media and only if treatment with an antimicrobial that has good antipneumococcal activity fails when used alone. Both of these agents are active against *Streptococcus pyogenes* and can be used for pharyngitis. The usual dose of cefixime is 8 mg/kg/day given as a single dose; the usual dose of ceftibuten is 9 mg/kg/day given once daily or divided into 2 equal doses.

Cefpodoxime proxetil and cefdinir have a spectrum of activity for Gram-negative microorganisms that is similar to those of other oral 3rd-generation cephalosporins. These agents, however, have good activity against Gram-positive cocci, including *S pneumoniae*, *S pyogenes*, and *S aureus*, methicillin-sensitive strains. Cefpodoxime achieves higher tissue concentrations in the lungs and tonsils than do other cephalosporins. The usual dosage is 5 mg/kg every 12 hours, with a maximal dose of 400 mg/day for otitis media and 200 mg/day for pharyngitis or tonsillitis. The dosage of cefdinir for children 6 months to 12 years of age is 14 mg/kg/day in 1 or 2 divided doses. Although the oral 3rd-generation cephalosporins are effective in treating bacterial pneumonia, otitis media, tonsillitis, and pharyngitis, equally effective and less expensive alternatives are available.

FOURTH-GENERATION CEPHALOSPORINS. Currently, cefepime (Maxipime) is available for use in individuals older than 2 months. This agent has been tentatively classified as a 4th-generation cephalosporin. Available only for parenteral use, it is unique compared with other cephalosporins because of its broad spectrum of activity against both Gram-positive cocci, including methicillin sensitive *S aureus*, *S pneumoniae*, and *S pyogenes*, as well as most aerobic Gram-negative bacilli, including *P aeruginosa*. This agent has a half-life of 2 hours, which permits dosing twice daily at 100 mg/kg/day. It has been used primarily in adults for the treatment of pneumonia and febrile neutropenia. Although it appears to penetrate into the cerebrospinal fluid, it does not have an indication for the treatment of meningitis.

Other Beta-Lactam Antibiotics

Three other β-lactam antibiotics—imipenem, meropenem, ertapenem (carbapenems), and aztreonam (monobactam)—have a limited role in the treatment of bacterial infections in children. Imipenem and meropenem have an extremely broad range of activity that covers most Gram-positive organisms, including enterococci, *Listeria* species, and methicillin-susceptible staphylococci, which includes coagulase-negative staphylococci. Strains of *S pneumoniae* that demonstrate intermediate or high levels of resistance to penicillin are frequently susceptible to these agents. Imipenem and meropenem also inhibit most Enterobacteriaceae, *P aeruginosa*, and *Pseudomonas maltophilia*, as well as most anaerobic bacteria. Ertapenem has a longer half-life compared with the other available carbepenems, permitting less frequent dosing. It is not as reliably active against Gram-negative aerobes when compared with imipenem or meropenem.

Because imipenem is rapidly destroyed by a renal peptidase, it is supplied in a fixed combination with a dehydropeptidase inhibitor called cilastatin. In adults, 500 mg of imipenem with cilastatin given intravenously produces an average peak serum concentration of 33 mcg/mL; the serum half- life is approximately 1 hour. The MIC_{95} of bacteria susceptible by disk is 4 mcg/mL;

or less. Imipenem's broad spectrum of antimicrobial activity is seldom required in clinical practice.

The major risk factor that has somewhat limited the usefulness of the carbapenems is seizure activity. The risk of seizures appears to be somewhat lower with meropenem compared with imipenem. Consequently, carbapenems should be used with caution in patients who have associated risk factors that may increase the likelihood of seizures, such as renal failure and CNS conditions, including meningitis.

Imipenem recently has been licensed for use in patients as young as 1 week. Meropenem, however, does not have an indication for use in children younger than 12 years. Ertapenem does not have an indication for use in children younger than 3 months, and no indication has been found for patients with meningitis. Given the broad spectrum of activity, these agents are occasionally useful in resistant infections with *S pneumoniae,* mixed infections, including those caused by anaerobes, and in patients with febrile neutropenia.

Aztreonam, a monobactam, has little activity against Gram-positive or anaerobic bacteria because these bacteria have little PBP 3, which is the primary binding site for aztreonam. On the other hand, aztreonam is very active against Enterobacteriaceae (MIC, $\leq$0.5 mcg/mL) and moderately active against *P aeruginosa* (MIC, $\leq$16 mcg/mL). In adults, 1 g of aztreonam given intravenously results in a peak serum concentration of approximately 125 mcg/mL; the serum half-life is 1 hour and 42 minutes. Susceptible by disk means that the MIC_{95} will be 8 mcg/mL or less. The use of aztreonam in children is scant.

Aminoglycosides

Mechanisms of Action

Aminoglycosides inhibit bacterial protein synthesis by interfering with bacterial ribosomes at the interface between the smaller and larger ribosome subunits. A 2nd mechanism, not yet known, is necessary to fully explain bacterial killing.

Bacterial Resistance

Three known mechanisms of bacterial resistance to aminoglycosides have been found. Ribosomal resistance occurs when alteration in the smaller ribosomal subunit results in its inability to bind streptomycin. The most common mechanism of resistance is the production of bacterial enzymes that inactivate aminoglycosides. Because aminoglycosides are similar in structure, certain enzymes can inactivate more than 1 aminoglycoside. The capacity to produce aminoglycoside-inactivating enzymes is inherent among Gram-negative aerobic bacteria and seldom occurs by induction. The number and types of enzymes vary among places and populations. As an aminoglycoside becomes used more widely, bacteria that produce inactivating enzymes become more prevalent. The ability to produce inactivating enzymes is carried by plasmids and transferred among Gram-negative bacteria. Amikacin appears to be an unsuitable substrate for many of these inactivating enzymes; consequently, amikacin may be active against some organisms resistant to other aminoglycosides, including gentamicin and tobramycin.

The 3rd mechanism of resistance to aminoglycosides is bacterial impermeability to aminoglycosides. Permeability mutants are generally not very virulent. When an organism is susceptible to tobramycin or gentamicin (or both) but is resistant to amikacin, the amikacin resistance must be based on amikacin's inability to enter the organism. This property must be the reason because the only enzyme produced by Gram-negative organisms that inhibits amikacin also inhibits tobramycin and gentamicin.

Pharmacologic Properties

Aminoglycosides are absorbed poorly or not at all after oral administration. Absorption after intramuscular administration is excellent, with the peak serum concentration occurring 30 to 90 minutes after administration. The serum concentration after intravenous administration over 20 to 30 minutes is approximately the same as after intramuscular administration. Aminoglycosides do not cross cell membranes well and therefore achieve poor concentrations inside most cells except renal tubular cells, which actively transport these agents. In general, only low concentrations of aminoglycosides are achieved in the CNS, eyes, biliary tract, or prostatic fluid. Aminoglycosides do enter synovial fluid well.

Because aminoglycosides are excreted by glomerular filtration, care must be taken to adjust the dose for patients who have renal failure. After filtration, some of the aminoglycoside dose is reabsorbed by the proximal renal tubular cells; this reabsorption probably plays a role in nephrotoxicity caused by these drugs. By convention, the drug is infused over a 30-minute period, and the peak serum concentration is measured 30 minutes after the infusion is completed. With intramuscular administration, the peak serum concentration is measured 1 hour later. Because the therapeutic-to-toxic index is very low for aminoglycosides, the serum concentration should be monitored closely.

Side Effects

The two most common side effects of aminoglycosides are ototoxicity and nephrotoxicity. Ototoxicity is generally considered to be reversible and is caused by destruction of the outer hair cells in the organ of Corti and is possibly related to the concentration of aminoglycoside in the endolymph or perilymph that bathes these cells. The relationship between serum concentrations and the development of ototoxicity remains unclear.[7] Some investigators have suggested that elevated trough concentrations predispose a patient to ototoxicity. Others have recently postulated that once-daily dosing of aminoglycosides may actually reduce the likelihood of ototoxicity by reducing drug accumulation in the inner ear.

Hearing loss generally begins at higher frequencies than those commonly used for conversation. Consequently, routine screening of hearing may be useful in patients at risk for auditory ototoxicity such as those who have cystic fibrosis and are receiving repeated courses of aminoglycosides. Vestibular toxicity is another manifestation of ototoxicity that is thought to be irreversible and can be very disabling. Transient elevations in aminoglycoside concentrations probably do not affect hearing.

Nephrotoxicity is exhibited as a decrease in the glomerular filtration rate. As with ototoxicity, the relationship between serum concentrations and the development of nephrotoxicity is not completely understood. Nephrotoxicity is generally mild and reversible. Associated risk factors frequently are found in patients who have nephrotoxicity, including concurrent medications and illnesses. Some investigators have suggested that the risk of nephrotoxicity is reduced by administering the entire daily aminoglycoside dose once a day. Both ototoxicity and nephrotoxicity seem to occur less often in children than in adults. Nonetheless, monitoring the serum concentration is important to make sure it is both safe and therapeutic, especially when dosed 2 or 3 times daily.

Aminoglycosides can also cause neuromuscular paralysis, particularly when given along with curare-like drugs, in the presence of botulin toxin, and in patients who have myasthenia gravis. Neuromuscular paralysis does not usually occur if aminoglycosides are given intramuscularly. Neuromuscular paralysis can be treated by administering calcium.

Use

Streptomycin, the 1st aminoglycoside used clinically, is used almost exclusively to treat tuberculosis, but it is also used to treat tularemia, plague, and brucellosis. Neomycin is used primarily to reduce the number of bacteria in the large bowel. It is given by mouth, and very little reaches the bloodstream.

Three aminoglycosides—gentamicin, tobramycin, and amikacin—are currently used systemically to treat serious infections caused by Gram-negative aerobic bacteria. In general, no evidence has been uncovered that one of these aminoglycosides is clinically superior to another in the treatment of susceptible bacteria. Tobramycin is more active against *P aeruginosa* than gentamicin or amikacin, but differences in its clinical effectiveness have not been observed. Tobramycin and amikacin are somewhat less nephrotoxic than gentamicin. Amikacin is susceptible to inactivation by 1 aminoglycoside-inactivating enzyme, whereas tobramycin and gentamicin are inactivated by at least 6 enzymes. Thus organisms are less likely to be resistant to amikacin than to either tobramycin or gentamicin. Because amikacin is less toxic on a weight basis, a larger dose is given and a higher peak serum concentration is achieved. With a dose of 7.5 mg/kg of amikacin given intravenously, the peak serum concentration averages 38 mcg/mL. At a dose of 2 mg/kg of tobramycin or gentamicin, the peak serum concentration ranges from 3 to 12 mcg/mL. All 3 drugs have a serum half-life of 2 to 2½ hours. The MIC_{95} of amikacin for bacteria reported susceptible by disk is 16 mcg/mL or less; the MIC_{95} of gentamicin or tobramycin is 4 mcg/mL or less.

Once-daily dosing of aminoglycosides has been found to have several advantages over dosing every 8 to 12 hours. The pharmacodynamic model presented earlier suggests that because aminoglycosides kill in a concentration-dependent manner, once-daily dosing should offer more rapid and effective killing of bacteria.[2] Once-daily dosing results in a higher peak serum concentration, an acceptably low trough concentration, and possibly a lower incidence of nephrotoxicity and ototoxicity. Dosing once daily also facilitates more convenient administration and reduces costs. Gentamicin and tobramycin are dosed at 4 to 7 mg/kg/day, producing a peak serum concentration that ranges from 10 to 20 mcg/mL and a trough concentration below 2 mcg/mL. Actually, the serum concentration will be below the MIC for a substantial portion of the dosing interval. Amikacin is dosed at 15 mg/kg/day, with a resulting peak serum concentration of 54 mcg/mL and a trough concentration below 5 mcg/mL. Monitoring serum concentrations in patients receiving once-daily dosing is generally accomplished by obtaining a single serum sample 6 hours after the dose. A nomogram is available that then enables the physician to decide whether that dose is administered most appropriately once a day, every 36 hours, or once every other day.[14] Despite studies showing an efficacy equivalent to divided daily doses, once-daily administration of aminoglycosides has not become widespread in pediatrics. Apparently, a majority of adult patients, however, are treated using a single daily dose. Some investigators have cautioned that once-daily dosing should not be used for patients who have enterococcal endocarditis, who are newborns, or who are febrile and neutropenic.

Sulfonamides and Trimethoprim

Mechanisms of Action

Sulfonamides inhibit bacterial growth by reducing bacterial synthesis of folic acid, resulting in a decrease in bacterial nucleotides. Trimethoprim inhibits bacterial dihydrofolate reductase, which is the step in folic acid synthesis that follows the step inhibited by sulfonamides. The combination of trimethoprim and sulfamethoxazole results in a synergistic, sequential blockage of folic acid.

Bacterial Resistance

Resistance to sulfonamides can be based on overproduction of substrate by the bacteria or a change in enzyme structure to one that has diminished sulfonamide binding. Trimethoprim resistance also may be caused by a decline in the bacteria's capacity to bind the drug or to a change in dihydrofolate reductase. Resistance to both drugs can result if an organism develops decreased permeability to the drugs. Resistance occurs less often when the combination TMP-SMX is used.

Pharmacologic Properties

The sulfonamides currently used in the United States, either alone or in combination with trimethoprim, are sulfisoxazole (Gantrisin), sulfamethoxazole, and sulfadiazine. Sulfonamides are usually given orally, but intravenous preparations of sulfadiazine and sulfisoxazole are available. These sulfonamides are quickly and completely absorbed from the stomach and small intestine. Sulfonamides are distributed throughout the body, including the CSF. They readily cross the placenta and are found in fetal blood. Sulfonamides are partially metabolized in the liver, and free drug metabolites are excreted by glomerular filtration.

Trimethoprim is also usually given orally and is readily absorbed. It is well distributed throughout the body, with the CSF concentration reaching approximately 40% of the serum concentration. Excretion is primarily by renal tubular secretion.

Side Effects

A wide variety of toxicities are associated with sulfonamides, ranging from GI upset, headache, and rash to serum sickness and hepatic necrosis. Severe hypersensitivity reactions can occur, such as toxic epidermal necrolysis, Stevens-Johnson syndrome, erythema nodosum, vasculitis, and anaphylaxis. Blood cell disorders, including aplastic anemia, granulocytopenia, thrombo cytopenia, and leukopenia, have been attributed to sulfonamides. Patients who have glucose-6-phosphate dehydrogenase (G6PD) deficiency are at heightened risk for aplastic anemia. Sulfonamides should not be taken during the last month of pregnancy because they cross the placenta and compete for bilirubin-binding sites, increasing the risk for kernicterus. All of the side effects associated with sulfonamides can occur with trimethoprim as well, the most common being GI upset and hypersensitivity reactions. With prolonged use, trimethoprim can interfere with folate metabolism, resulting in a megaloblastic anemia. This condition can be prevented by administering folinic acid.

Use of Trimethoprim-Sulfamethoxazole and Selected Sulfonamides

The combination of trimethoprim and sulfamethoxazole was introduced initially to treat urinary tract infections. However, because of its wide range of antibacterial activity, it has proved useful in several bacterial infections. Gram-positive organisms susceptible to TMP-SMX include both coagulase-positive and coagulase-negative staphylococci, *S pneumoniae*, enterococci, and *Listeria* species. Currently, over 95% of MRSA strains that are community associated are susceptible to TMP-SMX. Hospital associated strains are not as likely to be susceptible. TMP-SMX also is inhibitory for a wide range of Gram-negative aerobic organisms, including *E coli, Klebsiella* species, *Salmonella* species, *Shigella* species, *H influenzae*, and *N meningitidis*.

Until recently, TMP-SMX was used primarily in the treatment of acute urinary tract infections and for long-term bacterial suppression in patients who have chronic or recurrent urinary tract infections. Currently, however, TMP-SMX is a preferred agent for the treatment of mild-to-moderate infections caused by community associated MRSA. Respiratory tract infections, otitis media, sinusitis, prostatitis, orchitis, and epididymitis are also treated on occasion with TMP-SMX. TMP-SMX remains the drug of choice for treating *Pneumocystis jiroveci* (formerly *carinii*) infections and has proved effective in preventing *P jiroveci* infection in children who have malignancies. Many adults infected with HIV do not tolerate TMP-SMX well. To date, however, this situation has not been a major problem in HIV-infected infants. The peak serum concentrations for both drugs, reached approximately 2 hours after an oral dose, average 2 mcg/mL for trimethoprim and 60 mcg/mL for sulfamethoxazole. After repeated doses, the peak serum concentration of trimethoprim approaches 9 mcg/mL. The MIC_{95} for bacteria susceptible to the combination is 2 mcg/mL or less for trimethoprim and 38 mcg/mL or less for sulfamethoxazole. However, the combination usually is synergistic in vivo.

Sulfisoxazole is used primarily to treat acute urinary tract infections or to effect long-term suppression in patients who have chronic or recurrent urinary tract infections. Sulfadiazine is effective prophylaxis for close contacts of patients who have *N meningitidis* infections if the strain is known to be susceptible (see Chapter 353, Meningococcemia). The peak serum concentrations after an oral dose of 2 g range from 30 to 60 mcg/mL for sulfadiazine, 40 to 50 mcg/mL for sulfisoxazole, and 80 to 100 mcg/mL for sulfamethoxazole.

Topical sulfonamides are used primarily in 2 settings. Ophthalmic preparations of sulfacetamide are used to treat acute conjunctivitis and as adjunctive therapy in the treatment of trachoma. Silver sulfadiazine is used in the topical treatment of burns. In this combination, the sulfadiazine serves principally as a vehicle for the release of silver ions, which have an antibacterial effect.

Macrolides and Azalides: Erythromycin, Clarithromycin, and Azithromycin

Mechanism of Action

Macrolides inhibit RNA-dependent protein synthesis at the step of chain elongation.

Bacterial Resistance

Bacteria that lack the appropriate ribosomal binding site are resistant to erythromycin, as are bacteria that are less permeable to the drug. The presence of an efflux pump results in low level resistance for streptococcal strains and this is the most common mechanism of resistance seen in the United States.

Erythromycin

Pharmacologic Properties

Several erythromycin preparations are available for oral administration. Erythromycin base is destroyed by gastric acid and is therefore useful only when given as an enteric-coated tablet. Pediatric preparations use the ester or ester salt derivatives of erythromycin because they are acid stable, soluble, and tasteless. Preparations vary in their rate and degree of absorption from the GI tract. The best absorbed is the estolate ester, which results in a peak serum concentration of approximately 4 mcg/mL. The ethylsuccinate and stearate preparations produce peak serum concentrations that range from 0.4 to 1.9 mcg/mL when given at a dose equivalent to the ester. Erythromycin is distributed throughout the body and persists in tissue longer than in the blood. Therapeutic concentrations are reached in middle ear fluid, paranasal sinuses, tonsils, and pleural fluid but not the CSF, even when the meninges are inflamed. Limited data suggest that entry into synovial fluid is poor.

Erythromycin's route of elimination is not clear. A small percentage of a dose of erythromycin can be found in the urine, and erythromycin is known to be concentrated in and excreted with bile. However, most of an administered dose cannot be recovered.

Side Effects

The most common side effect of erythromycin is GI upset characterized by abdominal pain, nausea, vomiting, or diarrhea. Erythromycin is actually used primarily to promote gastrointestinal motility in some adults. Allergic reactions occur but are relatively uncommon. Cholestatic hepatitis occurs after treatment with the estolate ester but can be seen with any of the preparations. This side effect has been seen primarily in adults. The better absorption characteristics of the estolate preparation of erythromycin probably outweigh the slight risk of cholestatic hepatitis in children.

Use

Erythromycin has a broad range of antibacterial activity and is the drug of choice for infections caused by *Mycoplasma pneumoniae, Legionella* species, *Corynebacterium diphtheriae, Bordetella pertussis, Chlamydia trachomatis,* and *Campylobacter jejuni*. Erythromycin is an alternative drug for the treatment of streptococcal and staphylococcal infections and as prophylaxis for syphilis, urinary tract infections, rheumatic fever, and bacterial endocarditis. Macrolide-resistant *S pyogenes* have been reported recently in the United States.[15] However, exactly how this discovery may affect the use of this class of drugs for the penicillin allergic individuals with streptococcal pharyngitis is unknown.

The MIC_{95} of erythromycin required to inhibit bacteria reported as susceptible by disk is 0.5 mcg/mL or less. Lactobionate and gluceptate preparations are available for parenteral administration but are not used often. The peak serum concentration after intravenous administration is approximately equal to that achieved when estolate is given by mouth.

Clarithromycin

Pharmacologic Properties

Clarithromycin is stable in gastric acid and is well absorbed from the GI tract; furthermore, its bioavailability is not affected by food.[16,17] A peak serum concentration of 4 to 5 mcg/mL is reached in 2½ to 3 hours, and concentrations in middle ear fluid and lung tissue exceed serum concentrations. The major route of excretion is in bile, but approximately one third of an administered dose can be recovered in the urine. A metabolite of clarithromycin, 14-hydroxyclarithromycin, achieves a serum concentration that is approximately 60% that of clarithromycin and is approximately twice as active against *H influenzae*.

Side Effects

Clarithromycin causes much less gastric upset than erythromycin, but diarrhea (6% of cases), vomiting (6%), abdominal pain (3%), and nausea (1%) are the most common side effects. Children frequently complain that the suspension is unpalatable and leaves an unpleasant aftertaste.

Use

Clinical trials have demonstrated the efficacy of clarithromycin in the treatment of otitis media, pharyngitis, skin and soft-tissue infections, *Mycobacterium avium* complex (MAC) infections, and *Helicobacter pylori* infections. In general, clarithromycin can be used for infections traditionally treated with erythromycin. Because of the activity of its 14-hydroxyclarithromycin-breakdown product, clarithromycin may prove useful in *H influenzae* infections.

Azithromycin

Azithromycin differs structurally from erythromycin and clarithromycin by having a 15-member rather than a 14-member ring.[16,18] Because of its unique structure, azithromycin has a much larger volume of distribution, a longer half-life, and greater penetration at the cellular level than erythromycin and clarithromycin. In vitro studies show equivalent antimicrobial activity for Gram-positive cocci and atypical pathogens, including *Mycoplasma*. Azithromycin is more effective against *H influenzae* than erythromycin or clarithromycin. Because of its volume of distribution and longer half-life, once-daily dosing is appropriate, and short-course therapy for streptococcal pharyngitis (ie, 5 days) is recommended. Given its prolonged tissue half-life, and concentration-dependent killing, azithromycin has been used with shorter courses and less frequent dosing. Newer preparations such as Tri-pak or Zmax use higher doses, given for 3 days or as a single dose, respectively. These preparations are not available for use in children.

The macrolide antibiotics may interact with other drugs by inducing cytochrome P-450. Commonly used drugs that may interact include theophylline, zidovudine, cimetidine, and most anticonvulsants. Because azithromycin does not induce formation of cytochrome P-450, drug-to-drug interactions do not occur with this formulation.

Clindamycin

Mechanism of Action

Clindamycin shares binding sites with erythromycin and chloramphenicol on the 50S ribosomal subunit and interferes with protein synthesis by inhibiting the transpeptidation reaction.

Mechanisms of Resistance

The mechanisms of bacterial resistance are the same as for erythromycin.

Pharmacologic Properties

Clindamycin is usually given orally, but preparations for intramuscular and intravenous administration are available. Approximately 90% of a dose of clindamycin is absorbed after oral administration, and peak serum concentrations are reached in 1 hour and are dose dependent. Clindamycin palmitate (oral suspension) and clindamycin phosphate (preparation for intravenous administration) are inactive but are hydrolyzed rapidly in vivo to the active free base. Clindamycin is well distributed throughout the body except for the CSF. Clindamycin is one of the few antimicrobial agents that is concentrated in polymorphonuclear neutrophils. The serum half-life of clindamycin is approximately 2 hours and 24 minutes. Most clindamycin is metabolized in the liver to products that have variable antibacterial activity. Antibacterial activity in the bile and GI tract is very high and results in a dramatic decline in sensitive bowel flora.

Side Effects

The most highly publicized complication of clindamycin is colitis caused by the toxin of *Clostridium difficile* (pseudomembranous colitis). This complication has now been associated with many other antimicrobial agents and seems to occur less often in children than in adults. Side effects of clindamycin include allergic reactions, rashes, and minor elevations in transaminase concentrations.

Use

Clindamycin is highly active against most Gram-positive aerobic bacteria and most anaerobic bacteria. The major clinical use of clindamycin is the treatment of anaerobic infections. Clindamycin is used routinely when fecal material spills into the abdomen, and it is also used to treat anaerobic bronchopulmonary infections. When used for the treatment of intraabdominal infections, it is generally given along with an aminoglycoside. Clindamycin is also used as alternate therapy for groups A and B streptococcal infections. Group A streptococci that are resistant to macrolides are almost invariably susceptible to clindamycin. It has also been used as oral therapy to complete a course of antibiotics for *S aureus* osteomyelitis. Under these circumstances, clindamycin is an especially attractive alternative in patients who are allergic to β-lactams. In the United States, many strains of penicillin-resistant *S pneumoniae* remain susceptible to clindamycin. Clindamycin is a preferred agent for the treatment of mild-to-moderate community-associated MRSA infections. However, resistance to clindamycin for this indication is rapidly increasing and varies from location to location. In contrast to TMP-SMX, clindamycin will provide coverage for both staphylococci and streptococci. Providing such coverage may be necessary before culture and sensitivity data are available. Clindamycin does not enter the CSF in useful concentrations. A peak serum concentration of 2.5 to 3.6 mcg/mL is achieved approximately 1 hour after oral administration, and a concentration of 6 to 9 mcg/mL can be reached after intravenous infusion. The MIC_{95} of clindamycin for bacteria reported as susceptible by disk is 0.5 mcg/mL or less.

Chloramphenicol

Mechanism of Action

Similar to erythromycin and clindamycin, chloramphenicol binds to the 50S ribosomal subunit and inhibits protein synthesis.

Bacterial Resistance

Mechanisms of resistance include (1) bacterial production of an acetyltransferase that inactivates chloramphenicol and (2) inability of chloramphenicol to enter bacteria.

Pharmacologic Properties

Chloramphenicol can be given orally as the free base or as chloramphenicol palmitate, which is hydrolyzed in the intestine to free base. Because chloramphenicol is extremely bitter, oral palmitate suspension is given to patients who cannot take capsules containing free base. The intravenous preparation is chloramphenicol succinate, which is also hydrolyzed to free base. Because the palmitate is hydrolyzed more completely than the succinate, its peak serum concentration is generally higher after oral administration. Chloramphenicol distributes well throughout the body, including the brain and CSF. Chloramphenicol is conjugated by the liver and excreted in an inactive form in urine.

Side Effects

The major side effects of chloramphenicol are dose-related bone marrow suppression, which is reversible; aplastic anemia, which is idiosyncratic and usually fatal; and gray-infant syndrome. Gray-infant syndrome was first described and occurs most commonly in infants, but it has been reported in all age groups. The syndrome, which is characterized by cyanosis, circulatory collapse, and death, occurs when the chloramphenicol concentration becomes very high.

Use

The importance of chloramphenicol in the treatment of infectious diseases has waxed and waned since its introduction in the late 1940s. Because of its side effects, practitioners have tended to use alternate antimicrobial agents whenever possible. However, because of its antibacterial and pharmacologic properties, it must be often included to optimize treatment. With the introduction of the 3rd-generation cephalosporins, use of chloramphenicol in the United States has declined sharply. Formerly, chloramphenicol frequently was considered the drug of choice to treat brain abscesses, bacterial meningitis in infants and children older than 2 months, typhoid fever, and salmonellosis. Currently, metronidazole frequently is selected for anaerobic coverage in brain abscesses, ceftriaxone or cefotaxime for bacterial meningitis, and either TMP-SMX or ceftriaxone to treat typhoid fever and salmonellosis. Although chloramphenicol, rather than tetracycline, is considered by many to be the drug of choice for rickettsial infections in children younger than 8 years, some experts continue to consider tetracyclines to be the drug of choice for children who have rickettsial disease or ehrlichiosis regardless of their age. Chloramphenicol frequently is active against vancomycin-resistant enterococci and is frequently included in regimens to treat such infections.

When chloramphenicol must be used, the peak serum concentration should be measured after 4 or 5 doses to ensure that the concentration is safe and therapeutic and that the drug is not accumulating in the patient. A complete blood count and differential count should be done twice a week while the patient is receiving chloramphenicol to check for dose-related bone marrow suppression. The peak serum concentration is reached 1 to 2 hours after oral or intravenous administration and averages 25 mcg/mL (orally) and 19 mcg/mL intravenously.[6] The serum half-life of chloramphenicol is approximately 4 hours. The MIC_{95} of chloramphenicol for bacteria reported as susceptible by disk is 4 mcg/mL or less for *H influenzae* and 12.5 mcg/mL or less for other organisms. Although chloramphenicol is bactericidal for *H influenzae, S pneumoniae,* and *N meningitidis,* it is bacteriostatic for most other bacteria. When used with a β-lactam to treat organisms inhibited only by chloramphenicol, antagonism may occur.[19]

Tetracycline

Mechanism of Action

Tetracycline binds to the 30S ribosomal subunit and blocks aminoacyl-tRNA binding to the receptor site; this action inhibits protein synthesis.

Bacterial Resistance

The entry of tetracycline into bacterial cells is energy dependent; resistance is usually based on interference with entry into the cell. In general, tetracycline is not altered by resistant bacteria.

Pharmacologic Properties

Several analogs of tetracycline have been produced, but the range of antibacterial activity is similar for each. The semisynthetic analogs, minocycline and doxycycline, are the most active tetracyclines but are used less often than other tetracyclines because they are considerably more expensive.

Tetracycline has a broad spectrum of activity that includes inhibition of *Streptococcus* species, *S aureus* including many MRSA, *Neisseria* species, *E coli*, and many common anaerobic bacteria. Tetracyclines are well absorbed from the intestinal tract, and the peak serum concentration is achieved 1 to 3 hours after oral administration. Tetracycline distributes in varying concentrations throughout most of the body, with concentrations in synovial fluid, urine, and the maxillary sinuses approaching the serum concentration, whereas the CSF concentration reaches only 10% to 20% of the serum concentration.

Side Effects

The side effects of tetracycline essentially preclude its use in children younger than 8 years and in pregnant women. Tetracycline causes a permanent gray-brown to yellowish discoloration of the teeth and can be associated with hypoplasia of the enamel. Skeletal growth can be depressed when the drug is given to premature infants. Although bone and tooth defects are associated with the total dose of tetracycline given and occur more often after repeated courses, avoiding use of the drug during pregnancy and in young children is prudent. Although these side effects generally preclude the use of tetracycline in children younger than 8 years, for rickettsial diseases and ehrlichiosis, some experts continue to consider doxycycline the drug of choice because the usual duration of therapy is only 7 to 10 days, and staining of teeth is related to the total dose received.[19] Doxycycline is less likely to stain teeth than other tetracyclines. In addition, tetracyclines are effective against rickettsial diseases and ehrlichiosis, but chloramphenicol may not be. Other side effects of tetracycline are allergic reactions and skin toxicity.

Use

For individuals older than 8 years, tetracycline is considered the drug of choice for brucellosis, chlamydial infections, lymphogranuloma venereum, epididymitis, granuloma inguinale, infections with spirochetes (Lyme disease, relapsing fever, leptospirosis), pelvic inflammatory disease, plague, prostatitis, and rickettsial infections. Tetracycline is also an effective alternate drug for many other infectious diseases.

In adults, the peak serum concentrations after oral administration of 500 mg of tetracycline or 200 mg of doxycycline or minocycline are 4 mcg/mL, 2.5 mcg/mL, and 2.5 mcg/mL, respectively. The peak serum concentration is reached 1 to 3 hours after administration. The serum half-life of tetracycline is 8 hours, compared with 16 hours for minocycline and 18 hours for doxycycline. Intravenous administration of tetracycline results in a peak serum concentration about twice that achieved when the same dose is given by mouth. The MIC_{95} of tetracycline for bacteria reported as susceptible by disk is 4 mcg/mL or less.

Vancomycin

Mechanism of Action

Vancomycin inhibits cell wall synthesis during the 2nd stage by inhibiting formation of peptidoglycan. This action is in contrast to β-lactams that inhibit cell wall synthesis during the final stage by binding to the PBPs, which are enzymes that are crucial to the formation of the cell wall.

Bacterial Resistance

Currently, vancomycin demonstrates good activity against most Gram-positive cocci. However, vancomycin-resistant enterococci have become more common. In addition, vancomycin failures caused by infections with staphylococcal strains demonstrating in vitro susceptibility and the emergence of strains with reduced susceptibility to vancomycin has been a source of concern.

Until safer, more rapidly bactericidal agents are available for use in children, several principles must be considered to ensure appropriate use of vancomycin with regard to concerns of emerging resistance. First, although monitoring vancomycin levels has been reserved exclusively for selected patients such as those with altered renal function,[20] now, monitoring levels may apparently be the best predictor of clinical outcome. Maintaining trough concentrations in excess of 10 mcg/mL, or even higher, are necessary especially in patients with endocarditis or bacteremia. Second, the clinician must be aware that current disk diffusion methods may not adequately recognize vancomycin intermediate *S aureus,* heteroresistant vancomycin intermediate strains, or even *vancomycin-resistant S aureus.*

Pharmacologic Properties

Vancomycin is absorbed minimally after oral administration and is given orally only to treat pseudomembranous colitis caused by the toxin of *C difficile*. Most experts prefer to use metronidazole for this indication because increased use of vancomycin has been associated with a marked increase in resistance of commonly encountered Gram-positive organisms. After intravenous administration, vancomycin is distributed throughout the body, except for the aqueous humor of the eye and the CSF when the meninges are not inflamed. A bactericidal concentration can be achieved in the CSF in cases of meningitis caused by susceptible organisms. Sometimes, vancomycin must be administered intraventricularly to adequately treat meningitis with or without ventriculitis. Vancomycin is excreted unchanged in the urine by glomerular filtration. Therefore monitoring the serum concentration and adjusting the dose based on renal function is important in certain circumstances. (See Side Effects.)

Side Effects

When vancomycin initially became available for clinical use, commercial preparations contained as much as 20% of another substance, and its use was limited because of its toxicity. Currently available preparations are more highly purified and less toxic. The most common side effects are fever, chills, and pain at the injection site or, less often, flushing and tingling of the face, neck, and thorax (red neck syndrome). These side effects can be prevented largely by infusing vancomycin slowly in a large volume of fluid and by pretreating the patient with an antihistamine before the 1st dose. Reports of ototoxicity and nephrotoxicity caused solely by vancomycin have been difficult to confirm. Furthermore, the relationship of toxicity to serum concentrations remains controversial. In children, ototoxicity and nephrotoxicity are apparently uncommon, and no clear correlation between serum concentrations and toxicity has been proven.

Use

In recent years, infections caused by MRSA, coagulase-negative staphylococci (eg, *Staphylococcus epidermidis*), and ampicillin-resistant enterococci have become major indications for the use of vancomycin as the drug of choice. Vancomycin is active against most aerobic Gram-positive cocci, including most *Streptococcus* species and *L monocytogenes* and, in combination with streptomycin or gentamicin, is synergistic against enterococci. Many anaerobic streptococci also are susceptible to vancomycin, whereas most Gram-negative bacteria are resistant. Some methicillin-resistant staphylococci have demonstrated tolerance to vancomycin killing, and rifampin or TMP-SMX must be added to kill bacteria. Vancomycin is the drug of choice to treat serious infections with methicillin-resistant staphylococci or coagulase-negative staphylococci and to treat enterococcal endocarditis in patients allergic to penicillin. Patients who have staphylococcal infections that are methicillin susceptible might be treated with an antistaphylococcal penicillin. Patients who have bacterial endocarditis caused by *S aureus* cleared their bacteremia slowly when treated with vancomycin compared with using an antistaphylococcal penicillin in patients whose strain was methicillin sensitive.[21]

The initial dose of vancomycin should be a full therapeutic dose, even in patients in renal failure. Subsequent doses and intervals should be adjusted to achieve a peak serum concentration of 30 to 40 mcg/mL. The MIC_{95} of vancomycin for bacteria reported as susceptible by disk is 5 mcg/mL or less.

A concentration of 20 mcg/mL of vancomycin in a heparin flush or hyperalimentation solution has been shown to prevent line-related infections in premature infants[22] and children who have cancer in whom tunneled central venous catheters have been placed.[23]

Metronidazole

Mechanism of Action

After being taken up by bacteria, metronidazole is reduced to intermediate products that are toxic to the bacteria; the organism then releases inactive end-products.

Bacterial Resistance

Resistance to metronidazole develops infrequently and has been associated with decreased entry of the drug into bacteria and a decreased rate of reduction once in their cells.

Pharmacologic Properties

Metronidazole is active against most anaerobic bacteria, *Treponema pallidum, H pylori, Campylobacter fetus, Gardnerella vaginalis, Actinobacillus* species, *Actinomycetem comitans, Capnocytophaga* species, and *Trichomonas vaginalis,* as well as certain parasites. After oral administration, metronidazole is absorbed rapidly and completely, with the peak serum concentration being proportional to the dose administered. Metronidazole is distributed well throughout the body, including the CNS and the aqueous humor of the eyes. The serum half-life is approximately 8 hours. After being metabolized, metronidazole is excreted primarily in the urine.

Side Effects

The most common side effect of metronidazole is GI upset. Metronidazole also has been associated with CNS dysfunction (seizures, encephalopathy, ataxia) and peripheral neuropathy, and it can potentiate the effects of warfarin and cause a disulfiram reaction when alcohol is consumed. A major concern with the use of metronidazole has been its carcinogenic potential. Although rats and mice that have received metronidazole for a long period have shown an increase in neoplasms, mutagenicity for human cells has not been demonstrated in vitro, and follow-up studies on women who received metronidazole for trichomonal infections have shown that they did not have an increased frequency of tumors up to 10 years later.

Use

Originally introduced to treat *T vaginalis,* metronidazole also has proved to be effective in the treatment of amebiasis and giardiasis. More recently, it has gained widespread use in the treatment of anaerobic bacterial infections; it is not effective in treating actinomycosis or *Propionibacterium acnes* infections. Metronidazole also is not optimally effective in the treatment of anaerobic lower respiratory tract infections, perhaps because of the presence of aerobic bacteria; the outcome generally is good if penicillin or ampicillin is given concomitantly.

The peak serum concentration achieved in adults after 0.5 g of metronidazole is given orally averages 11.5 mcg/mL; after an intravenous dose of 0.5 g, the serum concentration ranges from 20 to 25 mcg/mL. The MIC_{95} of metronidazole for susceptible bacteria usually is 4 mcg/mL or less. Most diagnostic microbiology laboratories do not test anaerobic bacteria routinely for susceptibility.

Rifampin

Mechanism of Action

Rifampin works by inhibiting DNA-dependent RNA polymerase at the β subunit, preventing chain initiation but not elongation.

Bacterial Resistance

Bacterial resistance to rifampin develops rapidly by mutation of the DNA-dependent RNA polymerase. The rates of mutation are so high that they preclude use of rifampin as monotherapy except for very short courses of prophylaxis.

Pharmacologic Properties

Rifampin is usually administered orally and is completely and rapidly absorbed, with the peak serum concentration achieved 1 to 4 hours after ingestion. An intravenous form of rifampin is also available. Rifampin is distributed throughout the body, deacetylated by the liver, and excreted in the bile. The serum half-life is 2 to 5 hours early in therapy, but it declines over time because of increased biliary excretion. Rifampin also can enter phagocytes and kill viable intracellular organisms, which may explain why rifampin is better able to enter and sterilize abscesses than are other antimicrobial agents.

Side Effects

When rifampin is given daily, the most common side effects are a mild, self-limited rash and mild GI complaints. When rifampin is used intermittently at high individual doses, an influenza-like syndrome with fever, aches, and chills develops in up to 20% of patients. Because rifampin crosses the placenta and teratogenic effects have been observed in rodents, it should not be used during pregnancy except in severe cases of tuberculosis. Patients or parents should be warned that urine, feces, saliva, and tears may turn a red-orange color while they are taking the drug. The patient should not wear contact lenses while on

Table 61-2 Initial Empirical Therapy for Selected Infections*

CLINICAL DIAGNOSIS	MOST LIKELY OFFENDING ORGANISMS	ANTIMICROBIAL AGENTS
Meningitis	Neonate: group B streptococci, *E coli, L monocytogenes*	Ampicillin and cefotaxime (or ceftriaxone)
	Child: *S pneumoniae, N meningitidis, H influenzae* type b	Ceftriaxone or cefotaxime (plus vancomycin if *S pneumoniae* is suggested)
Brain abscess	Streptococcal species, anaerobes, *S aureus*	Penicillin and metronidazole (plus nafcillin† if *S aureus* is suggested [plus cefotaxime or ceftriaxone if Gram-negative bacilli are suggested])
Orbital cellulitis	Streptococcal species, *S aureus, H influenzae* type b	Ceftriaxone or cefotaxime plus clindamycin or nafcillin*
Epiglottitis	*H. influenzae* type b	Ceftriaxone or cefotaxime
Pneumonia (lobar or segmental)	Neonate: group B streptococci, *S aureus,* Gram-negative organisms	Ampicillin plus an aminoglycoside
	Child: *S pneumoniae, H influenzae* type b, *S aureus, S pyogenes, M pneumoniae*	Penicillin, nafcillin,† or erythromycin
Infective endocarditis	*Streptococcus viridans, S aureus*	Nafcillin† and an aminoglycoside
Acute diarrhea (fecal WBC present)	*Salmonella, Shigella* species	If patient is systemically ill, very young, or immunocompromised, cefotaxime or ceftriaxone
Abdominal sepsis	Anaerobes, aerobic enterics, enterococci	Clindamycin, aminoglycoside, and ampicillin (Unasyn and Timentin are suitable alternatives)
Urinary tract infection	Acute: *E coli, Klebsiella* species	Gentamicin or trimethoprim-sulfamethoxazole (TMP-SMX)
	Chronic: *E coli, Proteus* species, *Pseudomonas* species	Await culture and sensitivity results
Osteomyelitis	Neonate: group B streptococci, *S aureus, S pyogenes, S pneumoniae*	Nafcillin† and an aminoglycoside
	Child: *S aureus, S pyogenes*	Nafcillin†
Pyogenic arthritis	Neonate: group B streptococci, *S aureus, S pyogenes, N gonorrhoeae*	Nafcillin† and an aminoglycoside (or cefotaxime)
	Child: *H influenzae* type b (<5 yr), *S aureus, S pyogenes, N gonorrhoeae*	Ceftriaxone or cefotaxime (test MIC for *S aureus*) plus nafcillin†
Suggested sepsis	Neonate: group B streptococci, *L monocytogenes,* Gram-negative enteric organisms	Ampicillin and an aminoglycoside (or cefotaxime)
	Infant (1-6 wk): as for neonate plus as for child	Ampicillin and ceftriaxone
	Child: *S pneumoniae, H influenzae* type b, *N meningitidis*	Ceftriaxone
COMPROMISED HOST		
Fever only	*S aureus, E coli, Pseudomonas* species	Cefotaxime or aminopenicillin
Shock (sepsis without source)	Neonate: group B streptococci, enterics	Ampicillin and an aminoglycoside
	Child: *N meningitidis, S pneumoniae*	Ceftriaxone or cefotaxime

*For most clinical diagnoses, an acceptable alternative choice of antibiotics might be proposed.
†If local prevalence of methicillin-resistant *Staphylococcus aureus* is high, then vancomycin will be empirical drug of choice.

Table 61-3 Recommendations for Preoperative Antimicrobial Prophylaxis[1]

OPERATION	LIKELY PATHOGENS	RECOMMENDED DRUGS	PREOPERATIVE DOSE
Neonatal (<72 hr of age)—all major procedures	Group B streptococci, enteric Gram-negative bacilli, enterococci	Ampicillin plus gentamicin	50 mg/kg 2.5-3 mg/kg
Cardiac (prosthetic valve or pacemaker)	*Staphylococcus epidermidis, Staphylococcus aureus, Corynebacterium* species, enteric Gram-negative bacilli	Cefazolin *OR* Vancomycin, if MRSA or MRSE is likely	25 mg/kg 10 mg/kg
GASTROINTESTINAL			
Esophageal and gastroduodenal	Enteric Gram-negative bacilli, Gram-positive cocci	Cefazolin (high risk only[2])	25 mg/kg
Biliary tract	Enteric Gram-negative bacilli, enterococci, clostridia[3]	Cefazolin	25 mg/kg
Colorectal or appendectomy (nonperforated)	Enteric Gram-negative bacilli, enterococci, anaerobes	Cefoxitin *OR* Cefotetan[4] If at high risk, gentamicin and clindamycin, plus or minus ampicillin	40 mg/kg 40 mg/kg 2 mg/kg 10 mg/kg 50 mg/kg
Ruptured viscus	Enteric Gram-negative bacilli, anaerobes, enterococci	Cefoxitin *OR* Cefotetan[4] plus or minus gentamicin *OR* Gentamicin plus clindamycin	40 mg/kg 2 mg/kg 2 mg/kg 2 mg/kg 10 mg/kg
Genitourinary	Enteric Gram-negative bacilli, enterococci	Ampicillin plus gentamicin	50 mg/kg 2 mg/kg
Head and neck surgery (incision through oral or pharyngeal mucosa)	Anaerobes, enteric Gram-negative bacilli, *S aureus*	Gentamicin plus clindamycin *OR* Cefazolin	2 mg/kg 10 mg/kg 25 mg/kg
Neurosurgery (craniotomy)	*S epidermidis, S aureus*	Cefazolin *OR* Vancomycin, if MRSA or MRSE is likely	25 mg/kg 10 mg/kg
Ophthalmic	*S epidermidis, S aureus,* streptococci, enteric Gram-negative bacilli, *Pseudomonas* species	Gentamicin, ciprofloxacin, ofloxacin, tobramycin *OR* Neomycin-gramicidin-polymyxin B or cefazolin	Multiple drops topically for 2-24 hr before procedure 100 mg subconjunctivally
Orthopedic (internal fixation of fractures or prosthetic joints)	*S epidermidis, S aureus*	Cefazolin *OR* Vancomycin, if MRSA or MRSE is likely	25 mg/kg 10 mg/kg
Thoracic (noncardiac)	*S epidermidis, S aureus,* streptococci, Gram-negative enteric bacilli	Cefazolin *OR* Vancomycin, if MRSA or MRSE is likely	25 mg/kg 10 mg/kg
Traumatic wound (nonbites)	*S aureus,* group A streptococci, *Clostridium* species	Cefazolin	25 mg/kg

MRSA, Methicillin-resistant *Staphylococcus aureus; MRSE.* methicillin-resistant *S epidermidis.*
[1]Antimicrobial prophylaxis in surgery. Treatment guidelines from the Medical Letter. *Med Lett Drugs Ther.* 2004;20:-32
[2]Esophageal obstruction, decreased gastric acidity or gastrointestinal motility, morbid obesity.
[3]Safety and effectiveness of cefotetan have not been established in children.
From American Academy of Pediatrics. Antimicrobial Prophylaxis. In: Pickering LK, Baker CJ, Long SS, McMillan JA, eds. *Red Book: 2006 Report of the Committee on Infectious Diseases.* 27th ed. Elk Grove Village, IL: American Academy of Pediatrics; 2006.

rifampin therapy because the lenses can become permanently discolored.

Use

Rifampin is extremely active against a wide range of organisms. Most strains of *S aureus* and coagulase-negative staphylococci are exquisitely sensitive to rifampin, which is also active against most other Gram-positive cocci. *H influenzae, N meningitidis,* and *N gonorrhoeae* are exquisitely susceptible to rifampin, but other aerobic Gram-negative pathogens are less so. Rifampin also is active against *Legionella* species and *Mycobacterium tuberculosis.*

Despite its widespread use for treating tuberculosis and as prophylaxis for *N meningitidis* and *H influenzae,* no pediatric preparation of rifampin is available. Instructions for preparing a suspension for pediatric use are detailed in the *Physicians' Desk Reference.*[24] Internationally, rifampin is used most commonly to treat tuberculosis and leprosy. Rifampin also is recommended for prophylaxis of close contacts of patients who have meningococcal disease and for household contacts of children who have systemic *H influenzae* type b disease. When rifampin is used for the last 4 days along with a 10-day course of penicillin-amoxicillin for the treatment of group A β-hemolytic streptococcal infections, the microbiologic failure rate falls to almost zero. Rifampin in combination with other antistaphylococcal agents has been used to treat severe staphylococcal infections such as *S aureus* endocarditis, osteomyelitis, and CSF shunt infections caused by coagulase-negative staphylococci.

The peak serum concentration of rifampin after oral administration of 600 mg to an adult or 10 mg/kg to a child averages 7 mcg/mL. Because of the long half-life of rifampin, the peak serum concentration and bioavailability are better if the drug is given once a day. The MIC_{95} of bacteria reported as susceptible by disk to rifampin is 1 mcg/mL or less.

INITIAL THERAPY OF SELECTED ACUTE INFECTIONS

In most clinical situations, the physician must decide which antimicrobial agent or agents to use before the offending organism has been positively identified through culture results, serologic tests, or microscopic examination of material obtained from the infected site. The practitioner should consider the following points before starting treatment:

- Patient's age and immune status
- Whether concomitant disease is a factor
- Patient's history of exposure to infectious agents
- Current or recent administration of antimicrobial agents
- Findings on physical examination

Appropriate specimens for bacterial and viral cultures and specimens for serologic tests and microscopic examinations should be obtained before antimicrobial therapy is started, and specific adjunctive, supportive therapy should be instituted concomitantly. Table 61-2 lists the most likely offending organisms and the antimicrobial agent or agents that might be used empirically for various diagnoses under these circumstances. Local susceptibility patterns and other special circumstances always should be considered.

PROPHYLAXIS

Antimicrobial agents can be given to prevent colonization, to eradicate carriage, to prevent bacteria that colonize 1 body site from causing disease at a usually sterile site, or to prevent bacteria that have been introduced into a usually sterile site from causing disease. In general, an antimicrobial agent that has the narrowest spectrum that is effective against the most likely pathogen or pathogens should be used at the lowest dose and for the shortest period that will prevent infection. Prophylaxis also should be restricted to situations in which it is known to be effective and

Table 61-4 Dental Procedures and Endocarditis Prophylaxis

RECOMMENDED[1]	NOT RECOMMENDED
Dental extractions	Restorative dentistry[2] (operative and prosthodontic) with or without retraction cord[3]
Periodontal procedures, including surgery, scaling and root planing, probing, and routine maintenance	Local anesthetic injections (nonintraligamentary)
Dental implant placement and reimplantation of avulsed teeth	Intracanal endodontic treatment; postplacement and buildup
Endodontic (root canal) instrumentation or surgery only beyond the apex	Placement of rubber dams
Subgingival placement of antimicrobial fibers or strips	Postoperative suture removal
Initial placement of orthodontic bands but not brackets	Placement of removable prosthodontic or orthodontic appliances
Intraligamentary local anesthetic injections	Taking of oral impressions
Prophylactic cleaning of teeth or implants during which bleeding is anticipated	Fluoride treatments
	Taking of oral radiographs
	Orthodontic appliance adjustment
	Shedding of primary teeth

[1]Prophylaxis is recommended for patients with high- and moderate-risk cardiac conditions.
[2]This includes restoration of decayed teeth (filling cavities) and replacement of missing teeth.
[3]Clinical judgment may indicate antimicrobial use in some circumstances that may create significant bleeding.
From American Academy of Pediatrics. Antimicrobial Prophylaxis. In: Pickering LK, Baker CJ, Long SS, McMillan JA, eds. *Red Book: 2006 Report of the Committee on Infectious Diseases.* 27th ed. Elk Grove Village, IL: American Academy of Pediatrics; 2006.

in which the risk of infection exceeds the potential risks of the antimicrobial agent or the emergence of resistant bacteria. Recommendations for preoperative antimicrobial prophylaxis are listed in Table 61-3, and clinical situations in which prophylactic antimicrobial agents might be effective and the recommended regimens for prophylaxis are listed in Tables 61-4, 61-5, and 61-6. The *Red Book: Report of the Committee on Infectious Diseases,* American Academy of Pediatrics) has triannually updated dose recommendations for specific antimicrobials in specific situations.[19]

ANTIMICROBIAL THERAPY FOR VIRAL, FUNGAL, AND PARASITIC INFECTIONS

Currently, only a limited number of agents and a limited number of indications are available for systemic treatment of viral, fungal, and parasitic infections in the United States; thus most primary care pediatricians are unlikely to be familiar with the use of these agents. Therefore the pediatrician should consult a specialist in pediatric infectious diseases before treating a patient with these drugs. The antiviral drugs available currently, along with their indications and dosages, are presented in Table 61-7; antifungal drugs

Table 61-5 Other Procedures and Endocarditis Prophylaxis

	RECOMMENDED[1]	NOT RECOMMENDED
Respiratory tract	Tonsillectomy, adenoidectomy, or both Surgical operations that involve respiratory mucosa Nasotracheal intubation Bronchoscopy with a rigid bronchoscope	Endotracheal intubation Bronchoscopy with a flexible bronchoscope, with or without biopsy[2] Tympanostomy tube insertion
Gastrointestinal tract[3]	No prophylaxis recommended	
Genitourinary tract	No prophylaxis recommended	
Other	—	Cardiac catheterization, including balloon angioplasty Implanted cardiac pacemakers, implanted defibrillators, and coronary stents Incision or biopsy of surgically scrubbed skin Circumcision

[1]Prophylaxis is recommended for high- and moderate-risk cardiac conditions.
[2]Prophylaxis is optional for high-risk patients.
[3]Prophylaxis is recommended for high-risk patients; optional for medium-risk patients.
From American Academy of Pediatrics. Antimicrobial Prophylaxis. In: Pickering LK, Baker CJ, Long SS, McMillan JA, eds. *Red Book: 2006 Report of the Committee on Infectious Diseases.* 27th ed. Elk Grove Village, IL: American Academy of Pediatrics; 2006.

Table 61-6 Prophylactic Regimens for Dental, Oral, Respiratory Tract, or Esophageal Procedures

SITUATION	AGENT	REGIMEN
Standard general prophylaxis	Amoxicillin	50 mg/kg orally 1 hr before procedure (maximum 2 g)
Unable to take oral medications	Ampicillin *OR*	50 mg/kg IM or IV within 30 min before procedure (maximum 1 g)
	Cefazolin or ceftriaxone	50 mg/kg IM or IV within 30 min before procedure (maximum 1 g)
Allergic to penicillins or ampicillin—oral	Clindamycin *OR*	20 mg/kg orally 1 hr before procedure (maximum 600 mg)
	Cephalexin[ab] *OR*	50 mg/kg orally 1 hr before procedure (maximum 2 g)
	Azithromycin or clarithromycin	15 mg/kg orally 1 hr before procedure (maximum 500 mg)
Allergic to penicillin and unable to take oral medications	Clindamycin *OR*	20 mg/kg IV within 30 min before procedure (maximum 600 mg)
	Cefazolin or ceftriaxone[a]	25 mg/kg IM or IV within 30 min before procedure (maximum 1 g)

IM, Intramuscularly; *IV,* intravenously.
[a]Or other first- or second-generation oral cephalosporin in equivalent dose.
[b]Cephalosporins should not be used in an individual with a history of anaphylaxis, angioedema, or urticaria with peniclins or ampicillin.
Adapted from American Academy of Pediatrics. Antimicrobial prophylaxis. In Pickering LK, Baker CJ, Long SS, et al, eds. *Red Book: 2006 Report of the Committee on Infectious Diseases.* 27th ed. Elk Grove Village, IL: American Academy of Pediatrics; 2006.

Table 61-7 Antiviral Drugs

GENERIC (TRADE NAME)	INDICATION	ROUTE	AGE	USUALLY RECOMMENDED DOSAGE
Acyclovir[1,2,3] (Zovirax)	Neonatal herpes simplex virus (HSV) infection	IV	Birth-3 mo	60 mg/kg per day in 3 divided doses for 14-21 days
	HSV encephalitis	IV	≥3 mo-12 yr	60 mg/kg per day in 3 divided doses for 14-21 days
		IV	≥12 yr	30 mg/kg per day in 3 divided doses for 14-21 days
	Varicella in immunocompetent host[4]	Oral	≥2 yr	80 mg/kg per day in 4 divided doses for 5 days; maximum dose, 3200 mg/day
	Varicella in immunocompetent host	IV	≥2 yr	30 mg/kg per day for 7-10 days or 1500 mg/m² per day in 3 doses for 7-10 days
	Varicella in immunocompromised host	IV	<1 yr	30 mg/kg per day in 3 divided doses for 7-10 days
		IV	≥1 yr	1500 mg/m² of body surface area per day in 3 divided doses for 7-10 days; some experts recommend the 30-mg/kg per day dose
	Zoster in immunocompetent host	IV	All ages	Same as for varicella in immunocompromised host
		Oral	≥12 yr	4000 mg/day in 5 divided doses for 5-7 days
	Herpes-zoster in immunocompromised host	IV	<12 yr	60 mg/kg per day, every 8 hr, for 7-10 days
			≥12 yr	30 mg/kg per day, every 8 hr, for 7 days
	HSV infection in immunocompromised hose (localized, progressive, or disseminated)	IV	<12 yr	30 mg/kg per day in 3 divided doses for 7-14 days
		IV	≥12 yr	15 mg/kg per day in 3 divided doses for 7-14 days
		Oral	≥2 yr	1000 mg/day in 3-5 divided doses for 7-14 days
	Prophylaxis of HSV in immunocompromised host	Oral	≥2 yr	600-1000 mg/day in 3-5 divided doses during period of risk
	HSV-seropositive patients	IV	All ages	15 mg/kg in 3 divided doses during period of risk
	Genital HSV infection; 1st episode	Oral	≥12 yr	1000-1200 mg/day in 3-5 divided doses for 7-10 days. Oral pediatric dose: 40-80 mg/kg per day divided in 3-4 doses for 5-10 days (maximum 1.0 g/day)
		IV	≥12 yr	15 mg/kg per day in 3 divided doses for 5-7 days
	Genital HSV infection: recurrence	Oral	≥12 yr	1000-1200 mg/day in 3 divided doses for 3-5 days
	Chronic suppressive therapy for recurrent genital and cutaneous (ocular) HSV episodes	Oral	≥12 yr	800-1200 mg/day in 2 divided doses for as long as 12 continuous mo
Adefovir (Hepsera)	Chronic hepatitis B	Oral	≥18 yr	10 mg once daily for 1-3 y; optimal duration of therapy unknown
Amantadine (Symmetrel)	Influenza A: treatment and prophylaxis	Oral	1-9 yr	Treatment or prophylaxis: 5 mg/kg per day, maximum 150 mg/day, in 2 divided doses
		Oral	≥10 yr	Treatment or prophylaxis: <40 kg: 5 mg/kg per day, in 2 divided doses; ≥40 kg: 200 mg/day in 2 divided doses
		Oral	Dose by weight, not age	Alternative prophylactic dose for children >20 kg and adults: 100 mg/day
Cidofovir (Vistide)	Cytomegalovirus (CMV) retinitis	IV	Adult dose[5]	Induction: 5 mg/kg once weekly × 2 doses with probenecid with hydration Maintenance: 5 mg/kg once every 2 weeks with probenecid and hydration

Table 61-7 Antiviral Drugs—cont'd

GENERIC (TRADE NAME)	INDICATION	ROUTE	AGE	USUALLY RECOMMENDED DOSAGE
Famciclovir (Famvir)	Genital HSV infection; 1st episode	Oral	Adult dose[5]	750 mg/day in 3 divided doses for 7-10 days
	Episodic recurrent genital HSV infection	Oral	Adult dose[5]	250 mg/day in 2 divided doses for 3-5 days
	Daily suppressive therapy	Oral	Adult dose[5]	500 mg/day in 2 divided doses for 1 yr, then reassess for recurrence of HSV infection
Fomivirsen (Vitravene)	CMV retinitis	IO	Adult dose[5]	1 vial (330 mcg) injected into the vitreous, first 2 doses 2 weeks apart then every 4 wk
Foscarnet[1] (Foscavir)	CMV retinitis in patients with acquired immuno-deficiency syndrome	IV	Adult dose[5]	180 mg/kg per day in 2 divided doses for 14-21 days, then 90-120 mg/kg once a day as maintenance dose
	HSV infection resistant to acyclovir in immuno-compromised host	IV	Adult dose[5]	80-120 mg/kg per day in 2-3 divided doses until infection resolves
Ganciclovir[1] (Cytovene)	Acquired CMV retinitis in immunocompromised host[6]	IV	Adult dose[5]	10 mg/kg per day in 2 divided doses for 14-21 days; for long-term suppression, 5 mg/kg per day for 7 days/wk or 6 mg/kg per day for 5 days/wk
	Prophylaxis of CMV in high-risk host	IV	Adult dose[5]	10 mg/kg per day in 2 divided doses for 1 wk, then 5 mg/kg per day in 1 dose for 100 days or 6 mg/kg per day for 5 days/wk
		Oral	Adult dose[5]	1 g, orally, 3 times/day (not to be used as induction)
Lamivudine (Epivir-HBV)	Treatment of chronic hepatitis B	Oral	≥2 yr	3 mg/kg per day (maximum 100 mg/day) (children coinfected with HIV and hepatitis B should use the approved dose for HIV)
Oseltamivir (Tamiflu)	Influenza A and B: treatment and prophylaxis	Oral[7]	1-12 yr	Treatment for people 1-12 yr of age (once daily for prophylaxis): <15 kg: 30 mg, twice daily; >15-23 kg: 45 mg, twice daily; >23-40 kg: 60 mg, twice daily; >40 kg: 75 mg, twice daily
		Oral	≥13 yr	75 mg, twice daily for treatment; once daily for prophylaxis
Ribavirin (Virazole)	Treatment of respiratory syncytial virus infection	Aerosol	Newborn infants and older	Given by a small-particle generator, in a solution of 6 g in 300 mL sterile water (20 mg/mL), delivered for 18 hr per day for 3-7 days or 6 g in 100 mL of sterile water for 2 hr, 3 times/day; longer treatment may be necessary in some patients
Ribavirin (Rebetol)	Treatment of hepatitis C in combination with interferon	Oral/capsule	Dose by weight	Fixed dose by weight is suggested: 25-36 kg: 200 mg AM and PM; >36-49 kg: 200 mg AM and 400 mg PM; >49-61 kg: 400 mg AM and PM; >61-75 kg: 400 mg AM and 600 mg PM; >75 kg: 600 mg AM and PM
		Oral/solution	≥3 yr	15 mg/kg per day in 2 divided doses
Rimantadine (Flumadine)	Influenza A: treatment	Oral	≥13 yr	200 mg/day in 2 divided doses
	Influenza A: prophylaxis	Oral	≥1 yr	1-9 yr of age: 5 mg/kg per day, maximum 150 mg/day, once daily ≥10 yr of age, <40 kg: 5 mg/kg per day, in 2 divided doses; ≥40 kg: 200 mg/day in 2 divided doses

IV, Intravenous; *IO*, intraocular.
[1]Dose should be decreased in patients with impaired renal function.
[2]Oral dosage of acyclovir in children should not exceed 80 mg/kg per day.
[3]Acyclovir doses listed in this table are based on clinical trials and clinical experience and may not be identical to doses approved by the US Food and Drug Administration.
[4]Selective indications; see Varicella-Zoster Infections (Chapter 246, Chickenpox).
From American Academy of Pediatrics. Antimicrobial Agents and Related Therapy. In: Pickering LK, Baker CJ, Long SS, McMillan JA, eds. *Red Book: 2006 Report of the Committee on Infectious Diseases*. 27th ed. Elk Grove Village, IL: American Academy of Pediatrics; 2006.

Continued

Table 61-7 Antiviral Drugs—cont'd

GENERIC (TRADE NAME)	INDICATION	ROUTE	AGE	USUALLY RECOMMENDED DOSAGE
Valacyclovir (Valtrex)	Genital HSV infection	Oral	Adolescents	2 g/day in 2 divided doses for 10 days
	Episodic recurrent genital HSV infection	Oral	Adolescents	1 g/day in 2 divided doses for 3 days
	Daily suppressive therapy for HSV infection	Oral	Adolescents	500-1000 mg, once daily for 1 year, then reassess for recurrences
Zanamivir (Relenza)	Influenza A and B: treatment	Inhalation	≥7 yr	10 mg, twice daily for 5 days. Not licensed for prophylaxis

IV, Intravenous; *IO*, intraocular.
[1]Dose should be decreased in patients with impaired renal function.
[2]Oral dosage of acyclovir in children should not exceed 80 mg/kg per day.
[3]Acyclovir doses listed in this table are based on clinical trials and clinical experience and may not be identical to doses approved by the US Food and Drug Administration.
[4]Selective indications; see Varicella-Zoster Infections (Chapter 246, Chickenpox).
From American Academy of Pediatrics. Antimicrobial Agents and Related Therapy. In: Pickering LK, Baker CJ, Long SS, McMillan JA, eds. *Red Book: 2006 Report of the Committee on Infectious Diseases.* 27th ed. Elk Grove Village, IL: American Academy of Pediatrics; 2006.

Table 61-8 Recommended Doses of Parenteral and Oral Antifungal Drugs

DRUG	ROUTE[1]	DOSE (PER DAY)	ADVERSE REACTIONS[2,3]
Amphotericin B deoxycholate	IV	0.25-0.5 mg/kg initially, increase as tolerated to 0.5-1.5 mg/kg; infuse as single dose over 2 hr; 0.5-1.0 mg/kg weekly for suppressive therapy	Fever, chills, gastrointestinal tract symptoms, headache, hypotension, renal dysfunction, hypokalemia, anemia, cardiac arrhythmias, neurotoxicity, anaphylaxis
	IT	0.025 mg, increase to 0.5 mg, twice a week	Headache, gastrointestinal tract symptoms, arachnoiditis/radiculitis
Amphotericin B lipid complex (Abelcet)[4,5]	IV	5 mg/kg, infused over 2 hr	Fever, chills, other reactions associated with amphotericin B, but less nephrotoxicity; hepatotoxicity has been reported
Amphotericin B cholesteryl sulfate complex (Amphotec)[4,5]	IV	3-6 mg/kg, infused at a rate of 1 mg/kg/hr	Fever, chills, other reactions associated with amphotericin B, but less nephrotoxicity; hepatotoxicity has been reported
Liposomal amphotericin B (AmBisome)[4,5]	IV	3-5 mg/kg, infused over 1-2 hr	Fever, chills, other reactions associated with amphotericin B, but less nephrotoxicity; hepatotoxicity has been reported
Caspofungin[4,5]	IV	Adults: 70-mg loading dose, then 50 mg once daily	Fever, rash, pruritus, phlebitis, headache, gastrointestinal tract symptoms, anemia. Concomitant use with cyclosporine is not recommended unless potential benefits outweigh potential risks.
Clotrimazole	PO	10-mg tablet 5 times per day (dissolved slowly in mouth)	Gastrointestinal tract symptoms, hepatotoxicity
Fluconazole[3,5]	IV	Children: 3-6 mg/kg/day, single dose (up to 12 mg/kg/day has been used for serious infections)	Rash, gastrointestinal tract symptoms, hepatotoxicity, Stevens-Johnson syndrome, anaphylaxis

Table 61-8 Recommended Doses of Parenteral and Oral Antifungal Drugs—cont'd

DRUG	ROUTE[1]	DOSE (PER DAY)	ADVERSE REACTIONS[2,3]
	PO	Children: 6 mg/kg once, then 3 mg/kg/day for oropharyngeal or esophageal candidiasis; 6-12 mg/kg/day for invasive fungal infections; 6 mg/kg/day for suppressive therapy in HIV-infected children with cryptococcal meningitis Adults: 200 mg once, followed by 100 mg/day for oropharyngeal or esophageal candidiasis; 400-800 mg/day for other invasive fungal infections; 200 mg/day for suppressive therapy in HIV-infected patients with cryptococcal meningitis	
Flucytosine	PO	50-150 mg/kg/day in 4 doses at 6-hr intervals (adjust dose if renal dysfunction)	Bone marrow suppression, renal dysfunction, gastrointestinal tract symptoms, rash, neuropathy, hepatotoxicity, confusion, hallucinations
Griseofulvin	PO	Ultramicrosize: 5-15 mg/kg, single dose; maximum dose, 750 mg Microsize: 10-20 mg/kg/day divided in 2 doses; maximum dose, 1000 mg	Rash, paresthesias, leukopenia, gastrointestinal tract symptoms, proteinuria, hepatotoxicity, mental confusion, headache
Itraconazole[3,5]	IV, PO	Children: 5-10 mg/kg per day as a single dose or divided into 2 doses Adults: 200-400 mg/day once or twice a day; 200 mg once a day for suppressive therapy in HIV-infected patients with histoplasmosis	Gastrointestinal tract symptoms, rash, edema, headache, hypokalemia, hepatotoxicity, thrombocytopenia, leukopenia; cardiac toxicity is possible in patients also taking terfenadine or astemizole
Ketoconazole[3,5]	PO	Children[6]: 3.3-6.6 mg/kg/day, single dose Adults: 200 mg, twice a day for 4 doses, then 200 mg, once a day	Hepatotoxicity, gastrointestinal tract symptoms, rash, anaphylaxis, thrombocytopenia, hemolytic anemia, gynecomastia, adrenal insufficiency; cardiac toxicity is possible in patients also taking terfenadine or astemizole
Micafungin[4,5]	IV	Adults: 50-150 mg daily	Fever, headache, nausea, vomiting, diarrhea, leukopenia, hepatic enzyme elevations, and phlebitis
Nystatin	PO	Infants: 200,000 U, 4 times a day, after meals Children and adults: 400,000-600,000 U, 3 times a day, after meals	Gastrointestinal tract symptoms, rash
Terbinafine[4]	PO	Adults: 250 mg, once a day Children: <20 kg: 67.5 mg/day; 20-40 kg: 125 mg/day; >40 kg: 250 mg/day	Gastrointestinal tract symptoms, rash, taste abnormalities, cholestatic hepatitis
Voriconazole	IV	Children: 6-8 mg/kg every 12 hr for 1 day, then 6 mg/kg every 12 hr Adults: 6 mg/kg every 12 hr for 1 day (loading dose), then 4 mg/kg every 12 hr	Visual disturbance, rash, increased liver function tests
	PO	Children: 8 mg/kg every 12 hr for 1 day, then 6 mg/kg every 12 hr Adults: <40 kg: 200 mg every 12 hr on 1 day, then 100 mg every 12 hr; >40 kg: 400 mg every 12 hr for 1 day, then 200 mg every 12 hr	

[1] *IV*, Intravenous; *IT*, intrathecal; *PO*, oral; *HIV*, human immunodeficiency virus.
[2] See package insert or listing in current edition of the *Physicians' Desk Reference* or www.pdr.net (for registered users only).
[3] Interactions with other drugs are common. Consult the *Physicians' Desk Reference*, a drug interaction reference or database, or a pharmacist before prescribing these medications.
[4] Experience with drug in children is limited.
[5] Limited or no information about use in newborn infants is available.
[6] For children 2 years of age and younger, the daily dose has not been established.
From American Academy of Pediatrics. Antimicrobial Prophylaxis. In: Pickering LK, Baker CJ, Long SS, McMillan JA, eds. *Red Book: 2006 Report of the Committee on Infectious Diseases.* 27th ed. Elk Grove Village, IL: American Academy of Pediatrics; 2006.

(their route of administration, dosages, and adverse reactions) are listed in Table 61-8. Treatment of parasitic infections is discussed in Chapter 305, Parasitic Infections, and in the AAP *Red Book 2006*, in the *Nelson's Pocket Book of Pediatric Antimicrobial Therapy*,[25] and in *The Medical Letter Handbook of Antimicrobial Therapy*.[26]

TOOLS FOR PRACTICE

Community Coordination and Advocacy

- *Day Care Letter* (template letter), Centers for Disease Control and Prevention (www.cdc.gov/drugresistance/community/campaign_materials/Color/ChildcareLetter(color).pdf).

Engaging Patients and Family

- *A veces, el remedio es peor que la enfermedad* (brochure), Centers for Disease Control and Prevention (www.cdc.gov/drugresistance/community/campaign_materials/Color/Brochure-Spanish(color).pdf).
- *Antibiotics and Your Child* (brochure), American Academy of Pediatrics (patiented.aap.org).
- *Snort, Sniffle, Sneeze. No Antibiotics Please Poster African American* (poster), Centers for Disease Control and Prevention (www.cdc.gov/drugresistance/community/campaign_materials/Color/Poster-AfricanAmerican(color).pdf).
- *Snort, Sniffle, Sneeze. No Antibiotics Please Poster Caucasian* (poster), Centers for Disease Control and Prevention (www.cdc.gov/drugresistance/community/campaign_materials/Color/Poster-Caucasian(color).pdf).
- *Snort, Sniffle, Sneeze. No Antibiotics Please* (brochure), Centers for Disease Control and Prevention (www.cdc.gov/drugresistance/community/campaign_materials/Color/Brochure-Parent(color).pdf).
- *Virus vs. Bacteria Chart* (fact sheet), Centers for Disease Control and Prevention (www.cdc.gov/drugresistance/community/campaign_materials/Black-White/VirusBacteriaChart(BW).pdf).

Medical Decision Support

- *Antibiotics and Resistance: Physician Information Sheet* (fact sheet), Centers for Disease Control and Prevention (www.cdc.gov/drugresistance/community/files/ads/resis_an.pdf).
- *Appropriate Treatment Summary: Physician Information Sheet* (fact sheet), Centers for Disease Control and Prevention (www.cdc.gov/drugresistance/community/files/ads/appropriate_treatment.pdf).
- *Cough Illness/Bronchitis: Physician Information Sheet* (fact sheet), Centers for Disease Control and Prevention (www.cdc.gov/drugresistance/community/files/ads/cough.pdf).
- *Get Smart: Know when antibiotics work* (Web page), Centers for Disease Control and Prevention (www.cdc.gov/drugresistance/community/index.htm).
- *Otitis Media: Physician Information Sheet* (algorithm), Centers for Disease Control and Prevention (www.cdc.gov/drugresistance/community/files/ads/otitis_media.pdf).
- *Pharyngitis: Treat Only Proven GAS: Physician Information Sheet* (fact sheet), Centers for Disease Control and Prevention (www.cdc.gov/drugresistance/community/files/ads/pharyn_children.pdf).
- *Practice Tips: Careful Antibiotics Use* (fact sheet), Centers for Disease Control and Prevention (www.cdc.gov/drugresistance/community/files/ads/practice_tips.pdf).
- *Red Book 2006*, American Academy of Pediatrics (www.aap.org/bst/showdetl.cfm?&DID=15&Product_ID=4143&CatID=132).
- *The Common Cold: Rhinitis Vs. Sinusitis: Physician Information Sheet* (fact sheet), Centers for Disease Control and Prevention (www.cdc.gov/drugresistance/community/files/ads/rhini_vs_sinus.pdf).

REFERENCES

1. Moellering RC Jr, ed. Proceedings of symposium, tissue-directed antibiotic therapy. *Am J Med.* 1991;91(suppl 3A):1S.
2. Craig WA.Pharmacokinetic/pharmacodynamic parameters: rationale for antibacterial dosing of mice and men. *Clin Infect Dis.* 1998;26:1-12.
3. Powell SH, Thompson WL, Luthe MA, et al. Once-daily vs continuous aminoglycoside dosing: efficacy and toxicity in animal and clinical studies of gentamicin netilmicin, and tobramycin. *J Infect Dis.* 1983;147(5):918-932.
4. Gilbert D. Once-daily aminoglycoside therapy. *Antimicrob Agents Chemother.* 1991; 35(3): 399-405.
5. Kim KS. Clinical perspectives on penicillin tolerance. *J Pediatr.* 1988;112:509-514.
6. National Committee for Clinical Laboratory Standards. *Performance Standards for Antimicrobial Disk Susceptibility Tests.* 3rd ed. Wayne, PA: NCCLC; 1984.
7. Yu VL, Merigan TC, Barriere SL, eds. *Antimicrobial Therapy and Vaccines.* Baltimore, MD: Williams and Wilkins; 1999.
8. Idsoe O, Guthe T, Willcox RR, et al. Nature and extent of penicillin side reactions with particular reference to fatalities from anaphylactic shock. *Bull World Health Organ.* 1998;38:159-188.
9. Molavi A.Cephalosporins: rationale for clinical use. *Am Fam Physician.* 1991;43:937-948.
10. Pichichero M. A review of evidence supporting the American Academy of Pediatrics recommendation for prescribing cephalosporin antibiotics for penicillin-allergic patients. *Pediatrics.* 2005;115(4):1048-1057.
11. Dash CH. Penicillin allergy and cephalosporins. *J Antimicrob Chemother.* 1975;1:107-118.
12. Karam GH, Sanders CV, Aldridge KE. Role of newer antimicrobial agents in the treatment of mixed aerobic and anaerobic infections. *Surg Gynecol Obstet.* 1990; 172(suppl):57-64.
13. Stamos JK, Yogev R. Oral cephalosporins: the newest of the new. *Contemp Pediatr.* 1993;3:298-305.
14. Nicolau DP, Freeman CD, Belliveau PP, et al. Experience with a once-daily aminoglycoside program administered to 2184 patients. *Antimicrob Agents Chemother.* 1995; 39(3):650-655.
15. Martin JM, Green M, Barbadora KA, et al. Erythromycin-resistant group A streptococci in schoolchildren in Pittsburgh. *N Engl J Med.* 2002; 346:1200-1206.
16. Klein JO. Clarithromycin: where do we go from here? *Pediatr Infect Dis J.* 1993;12:S148-S151.
17. Neu HC. The development of macrolides: clarithromycin in perspective. *J Antimicrob Chemother.* 1991;27 (suppl A):A1-A9.

18. Whitman MS, Tunkel AR. Azithromycin and clarithromycin: overview and comparison with erythromycin. *Infect Control Hosp Epidemiol*. 1992;13:357-368.
19. The American Academy of Pediatrics. Rickettsial diseases. In: Pickering LK, Baker CJ, Long SS, et al, eds: *Red Book 2006: Report of the Committee on Infectious Diseases*, 27th ed. Elk Grove Village, IL: The American Academy of Pediatrics;2006.
20. Thomas MP, Steele RW. Monitoring serum vancomycin concentrations in children: is it necessary?*Pediatr Infect Dis J*. 1998;17:351-352.
21. Levine DP. Fromm BS. Reddy BR. Slow response to vancomycin or vancomycin plus rifampin in methicillin-resistant Staphylococcus aureus endocarditis. *Ann Intern Med*. 1991;115:674.
22. Spafford PS, Sinkin RA, Cox C, et al. Prevention of central venous catheter-related coagulase negative staphylococcal sepsis in neonates. *J Pediatr*. 1994;125:259-263.
23. Schwartz C, Henrickson KJ, Roghmann K, et al. Prevention of bacteremia attributed to luminal colonization of tunneled central venous catheters with vancomycin-susceptible organisms. *J Clin Oncol*.1990;8:1591-1597.
24. Medical Economics. *Physicians' Desk Reference*. 54th ed. Montvale, NJ: Medical Economics; 2000.
25. Bradley JS, Nelson JD. *Nelson's Pocket Book of Pediatric Antimicrobial Therapy*. 16th ed. Buenos Aires, Argentina: Alliance for World Wide Editing; 2006.
26. Abramowicz M, ed. Drugs for parasitic infections. *Med Lett*. 2004; 46: 1-12.

Chapter 62

PREOPERATIVE ASSESSMENT

Aaron L. Zuckerberg, MD; Lynne G. Maxwell, MD

INTRODUCTION

Ambulatory or same-day surgery provides significant medical, psychological, and economic benefits to children and their families.[1,2] Much of the preoperative and postoperative patient care that in the past was provided in the hospital by the surgeon and anesthesiologist is now being performed by the child's primary care physician (PCP). Indeed, the PCP is often asked to *clear* children for surgery, with little, if any, guidance as to what this term means. Although outpatient procedures are generally considered to be minor and usually performed on healthy children, the anesthetics used in these procedures are not without risk. An unappreciated acute illness or undiagnosed underlying disease can increase the risk of the anesthetic beyond that of the procedure for children so affected. This chapter reviews the effects of anesthesia on children and highlights specific aspects of the child's history and physical examination that are of particular importance to the anesthesiologist and surgeon.

Although this chapter is devoted to discussion of *perioperative* issues, the reality is that the scope of pediatric anesthesia has changed greatly during the last decade. No longer is anesthesia an activity confined to the operating room, requiring the presence of an anesthesia machine. Today, with a syringe, a monitor, and the appropriate backup equipment, a child can be anesthetized in virtually any location. More than 4 million children in the United States receive anesthesia or deep sedation both in and out of operating rooms each year.[3] The forces driving these changes in children's anesthesia are many: cost containment, efficiency, increased use of sophisticated diagnostic tools, and the continued efforts to minimize the periprocedure trauma that a child experiences. More than 60% of elective pediatric surgery is now being performed on an ambulatory, or same-day, basis.* Cost concerns have shifted more pediatric surgical procedures to freestanding surgical facilities.[4] The use of diagnostic imaging (magnetic resonance imaging [MRI], computed tomography [CT], and positron emission tomography), which requires immobility, has increased greatly in children, in part, because of the ability to provide safe anesthesia in these complex environments outside the operating room. Examples of surgical and diagnostic procedures that are now routinely performed on children in an outpatient setting are listed in Box 62-1. Although the discussion is framed with reference to *preoperative* evaluation, the guidelines and principles reviewed apply equally to preprocedural and presedation assessment and preparation.

BOX 62-1 Common Outpatient Surgical Procedures

GENERAL SURGERY
- Femoral, inguinal, and umbilical herniorrhaphies
- Lymph node and other diagnostic biopsies
- Central line insertion
- Fistulotomy

GENITOURINARY SURGERY
- Orchiopexy, hydrocele
- Circumcision
- Hypospadias repair

OTORHINOLARYNGEAL SURGERY
- Myringotomy and tube placement
- Adenoidectomy (children >2 yr)
- Tonsillectomy (children >3 yr)
- Bronchoscopy
- Tympanomastoidectomy
- Tympanoplasty
- Endoscopic sinus surgery
- Cochlear implant

OPHTHALMOLOGIC SURGERY
- Strabismus
- Examination under anesthesia
- Cataract
- Eyelid repair for ptosis

ORTHOPEDIC SURGERY
- Tendon lengthening
- Cast changes
- Fracture reductions
- Arthroscopy

PLASTIC SURGERY
- Cleft lip repair
- Hand surgery
- Rhinoplasty

*Data from the Children's Hospital of Philadelphia study on 22,000 cases in the fiscal years of 2002 and 2006 with 63.5% and 62.7% of surgical or nonsurgical procedures performed with anesthesia being performed on an ambulatory basis; and from COMPARE database kept by the Child Health Corporation of America.

PREOPERATIVE (PREANESTHETIC) ASSESSMENT AND PREPARATION

The goal of this section is to familiarize the PCP with many of the key aspects of a child's preoperative evaluation, clarifying what the anesthesiologist needs to know to make the most accurate risk, benefit, and consequence calculation for an individual child. Common coexisting conditions that affect the child's perianesthetic course are discussed, and preparative regimens that ameliorate the risk of these conditions are provided. Such preparation may minimize the possibility of procedural delay or postponement, which, if it occurs, may add to the family's stress surrounding the procedure. In addition, conditions that require delay of surgery for the best interests and safety of the child are discussed.

Preoperative Evaluation: *Not* Pediatric Clearance for Surgery

Because most of the anesthetics that children receive are given on an outpatient basis, the preoperative evaluation and decisions about medical interventions to minimize the perioperative risks are being performed by the PCP. Efficiency considerations have also minimized the opportunity for hospital-based psychological preparation of the child and the family. This circumstance is problematic in that parental anxiety, which may be ameliorated by such preparation, has a negative effect on the psychological responses of the child.[5,6] The PCP has the most complete knowledge of the child's medical history and an established relationship with the entire family. As such, the PCP is in the best position to determine whether the child is in the best possible state of health given underlying medical issues and to help the family prepare psychologically for the procedure. After preoperative evaluation of the child by the PCP, the child is then reevaluated by the anesthesia and surgical teams on the morning of the procedure to determine whether an acute illness has developed. Compliance with preoperative medication administration and *nil per os* (NPO) status is determined as well. Although this process has streamlined the approach to the child on the day of the procedure, and although most of the risk factors for adverse events have been addressed, the time for adequate psychological preparation of the child and parent has been minimized. Because parental anxiety has a negative effect on the psychological reactions of the child, adequate family preparation must be accomplished through alternative means, including preprocedure telephone calls, movies, and PCP involvement. These opportunities for the PCP to affect positively both the safety and the psychological aspects of the procedure through thorough assessment and preparation (with communication of important risk factors to the anesthesia team) emphasize the importance of the preoperative visit beyond the concept of *clear for surgery*.

Preanesthetic Evaluation

The goal of the preanesthetic evaluation is to determine what the risk of anesthetizing a particular child for a specific procedure. Factors that should be taken into consideration include the probability of an adverse event and its associated estimated risk, the benefits of the procedure, and the consequences associated with proceeding with or delaying the procedure. For example, a child with an exacerbation of reactive airways disease who has acute appendicitis has a significant risk of adverse pulmonary events in the perioperative period. However, this risk is far outweighed by the anticipated benefits of the appendectomy *and* the unacceptable consequences of postponing the appendectomy until the child's asthma is better controlled. Contrast this situation with the same child undergoing elective dental restoration. The risks of the procedure are unchanged from the first example. The benefits of the procedure are obvious: improved appearance, better feedings, and elimination of pain and a possible source of infection. However, the consequences of delaying the procedure are modest and limited primarily to inconvenience. In the latter situation, the risks of proceeding far outweigh the benefits and consequences of delaying the procedure.

Based on this decision process, clearance for surgery is obviously an antiquated concept. The 3 variables—risk, benefit, and consequence—must all be considered in the decision to administer an anesthetic. The decision is a dynamic one predicated on optimization of a child's underlying disease, as well as consideration of the effect of any intercurrent processes on her overall physiology. Key in this process is an appreciation of the risk of adverse perianesthetic events common in children.

EFFECTS OF GENERAL ANESTHESIA

The components of a general anesthetic abolish the sensation of pain (analgesia); produce muscle paralysis, amnesia, and a loss of consciousness; and inhibit the adrenal-stress response to pain and surgery. Although the drugs that produce general anesthesia have narrow therapeutic indices, modern anesthetic practice produces few, if any, perioperative complications. Nevertheless, children and their parents dread the entire surgical experience. Young children are afraid of separation from their parents, older children fear potential mutilation and death, and teenagers fear all of this plus loss of control.[7] Young children will frequently struggle, scream, and cry either when separated from their parent or parents or when anesthesia is being induced, particularly if the induction technique is via mask induction of potent volatile vapors such as halothane or sevoflurane. This struggle often leads to a stormy induction of anesthesia and significantly increases the risks of airway compromise (laryngospasm, coughing, breath holding, with associated hypoxemia), anesthetic overdose (hypotension), and arrhythmias. Furthermore, memories of this struggle or of the separation from the child's parents may be long lasting, indeed, even longer lasting than the experience of surgery itself.[8] Fortunately, the emergence of new drugs for the premedication of children such as midazolam (Versed®), parental presence during the induction of anesthesia, and improved, faster, and better-tolerated volatile anesthetic gases for mask induction (sevoflurane) have lessened the incidence of such terrorizing experiences.

Parents fear for their child's life and safety as well. This sense of terror and foreboding is compounded by a sense of inadequacy and guilt. Rather than protecting their child from pain and suffering, they feel responsible for *causing* it or *allowing* it to happen.

RISKS OF ANESTHESIA

Are fear and foreboding necessary, and can they be allayed? Ultimately, the answer depends on how safe anesthesia is. In a study reviewing the risks of anesthesia in an American hospital from 1969 to 1983, the overall mortality rate was 0.9 per 10,000 anesthetics, with an incidence of cardiac arrest of 1.7 per 10,000 anesthetics.[9] In this study, children younger than 12 years had a 3-fold higher incidence of cardiac arrest (4.7 per 10,000) compared with adult patients (1.4 per 10,000).[9] Mortality risk in infants younger than 1 year is 43 per 10,000 anesthetics, decreasing to 5 per 10,000 anesthetics in the second year of life.[10] Complications leading to cardiac arrest are largely due to adverse events during airway management (laryngospasm, difficult intubation, and pulmonary aspiration of gastric contents) or halothane overdose (hypotension, arrhythmia, or both). Infants younger than 1 month have the greatest risk of serious intraoperative complications (cardiac arrest) and the highest perioperative death rates because they are more likely to be having major surgery (intrathoracic or intraabdominal) than are older children and are sicker (a greater percentage are American Society of Anesthesiologists physical status 3 to 5). A review of closed anesthesia malpractice claims revealed that complications in children were related to respiratory events with a greater frequency than in adult cases (43% versus 30%), and the mortality rate of the events documented in the cases was greater in children (50% versus 35%).[11]

American Society of Anesthesiologists Physical Status Classification

The American Society of Anesthesiologists physical status (ASA PS) classification (Table 62-1) provides a convenient method of summarizing the patient's physical condition and may provide a means of assessing the relative risk of anesthesia. ASA PS 1 patients are healthy and have no underlying disease, whereas ASA PS 4 patients are significantly incapacitated by their underlying disease. Other factors associated with increased preoperative risk are multiple coexisting diseases and the need for emergent surgery. The anesthetic mortality rate in healthy ASA PS 1 children requiring elective surgery is probably less than 1 in 50,000.

Children who are candidates for outpatient surgery are generally in the ASA PS 1 and 2 groups. Among these children who require elective surgery, factors that might impose any additional perioperative risk (eg, upper respiratory infection, recent meal) are considered unacceptable. Children (especially infants) have a higher incidence of respiratory events (laryngospasm and bronchospasm) than do adults. The risk of perioperative respiratory adverse events decreases by 8% with each increasing year of age.[12] In children younger than 9 years, the incidence of laryngospasm is 17.4 per 1000, but this rate increased more than 5-fold in children with active upper respiratory tract infections (URTI), and more than 3-fold in children with reactive airways disease.[13] The relative risks of anesthesia in children are presented in Figure 62-1.

One of the sequelae of laryngospasm occurring at the time of induction or emergence from anesthesia is negative-pressure pulmonary edema. This phenomenon occurs because of forced inspiratory effort against a closed glottis, with high negative pressure pulling fluid into the alveolar spaces.[14] Low oxygen saturation is observed. Once recognized, resolution of the child's increased oxygen requirement usually occurs in 4 to 8 hours when treated with 100% oxygen by mask and a single dose of furosemide. These patients require overnight monitoring in a high-observation unit. Subsequent intubation is rarely necessary.

Although the initial intent was to confine outpatient surgery to patients of ASA PS 1 and 2, ASA PS 3 and even ASA PS 4 patients are increasingly undergoing outpatient surgery because of pressure from payers, who deny payment for inpatient care. Unfortunately, whether this circumstance is safe or desirable is irrelevant. Because of the increased risk to these children,

Table 62-1 Physical Status Classification of the American Society of Anesthesiologists and Suitability for Outpatient Surgery

CLASS	DESCRIPTION	EXAMPLE	SUITABILITY
1	Normal healthy person	No medical condition	Excellent
2	Mild systemic disease without functional limitations	Mild asthma, anemia, controlled seizures Controlled diabetes mellitus	Generally good
3	Severe systemic disease	Moderate to severe asthma, poorly controlled seizures, pneumonia, tracheostomy without ventilatory support, poorly controlled diabetes, moderate obesity, h/o prematurity, cancer, stable organ dysfunction (moderate renal or liver insufficiency)	Intermediate Consider risks versus benefits
4	Severe systemic disease that is a constant threat to life	Severe BPD, sepsis, advanced organ insufficiency: cardiac, pulmonary (eg, tracheostomy with ventilatory support), hepatic, renal, adrenal. Morbid obesity	Poor risk
5	Moribund patient Unexpected to survive without procedure	Septic shock Severe organ failure Severe trauma	Extremely poor

BPD, Bronchopulmonary dysplasia; *h/o*, history of.

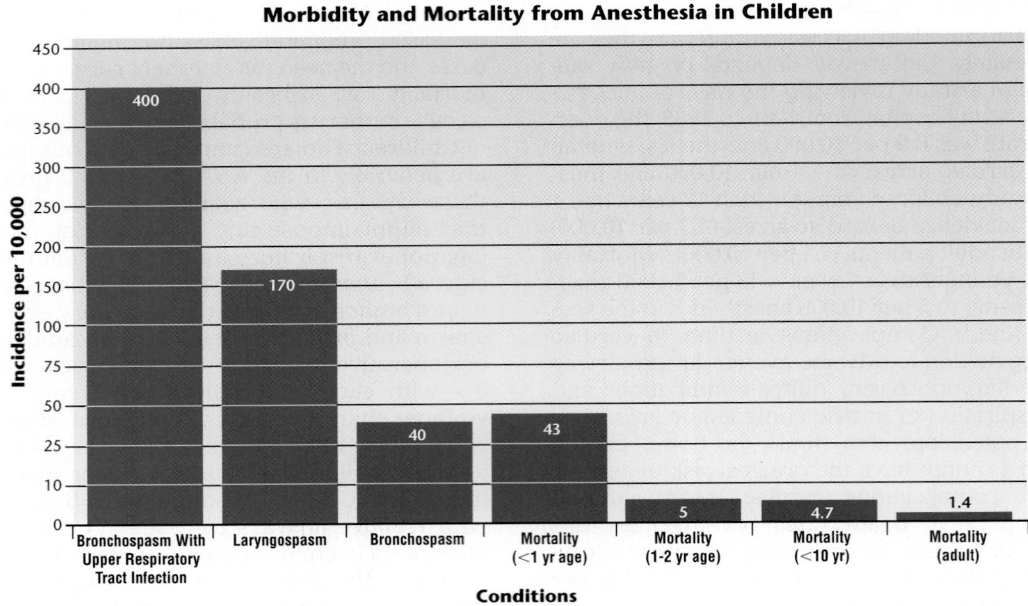

Figure 62-1 Morbidity and mortality of anesthesia in children. *(Adapted from Olsson GL, Hallen B: Laryngospasm during anesthesia: a computer-aided incidence study of 136,929 patients.* Acta Anaesthesiol Scand. *1984;28:567-575; and Morray JP, Geiduschek JM, Ramanmoorthy C, et al. Anesthesia-related cardiac arrest in children.* Anesthesiology. *2000;93:6-14.)*

Table 62-2 Relationship of Age to American Society of Anesthesiologists Physical Status and Mortality[a]

	ALL AGES	<1 MONTH	1-5 MONTHS	6-12 MONTHS	>12 MONTHS	MORTALITY BY ASA STATUS
++ DATA FROM PEDIATRIC PERIOPERATIVE CARDIAC ARREST REGISTRY						
Number of cases[b]	262	65	64	32	101	—
ASA PS 1-2	50	6	11	9	24	3 (6%)
ASA PS 3	76	5	23	12	36	20 (26%)
ASA PS 4-5	136	54	30	11	41	99 (73%)
Mortality By Age[c]	122 (47%)	43 (66%)[d]	25 (39%)[e]	12 (38%)[e]	42 (42%)[e]	

ASA PS, American Society of Anesthesiologists physical status.
[a]Data from Pediatric Perioperative Cardiac Arrest (POCA) Registry.
[b]Number of cases of cardiac arrest submitted to the POCA Registry.
[c]Number reported (or percentage of deaths reported) for age group.
[d]Fewer than expected by chance alone ($p < 0.01$ by Chi square).
[e]More than expected by chance alone ($p < 0.01$ by Chi square).
From ASA Newsletter 1998;62. Available at: www.asahq.org/Newsletters/1998/06_98/Registry_0698.html. Accessed April 17, 2007.

direct communication between the PCP and the anesthesiologist is advised well in advance of the planned surgical procedure. Better resources, in addition to this text, are now available to help PCPs educate themselves and their patients' families about the perioperative experience, from preoperative evaluation to postoperative pain management.[15]

Pediatric Perioperative Cardiac Arrest Registry

The Pediatric Perioperative Cardiac Arrest (POCA) Registry, started in 1994, is an ongoing effort to identify trends in adverse events that occur in children receiving anesthetics and provides the medical community with more contemporary data on perioperative risk. Regarding mortality, the POCA Registry continues to confirm that infants and those with severe systemic disease are at highest risk for perianesthetic mortality (Table 62-2).[16,17]

In the last decade, of cases submitted to the registry, respiratory events were responsible for 25% of all pediatric perioperative cardiac arrests, a decrease from 43% in the previous 10-year period. The most

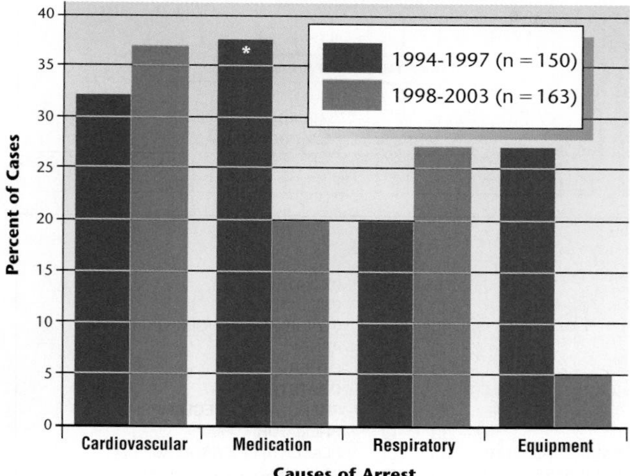

Figure 62-2 Causes of arrest from the Pediatric Perioperative Cardiac Arrest Registry. *(Morray JP, Bhananker SM. Recent Findings from the Pediatric Perioperative Cardiac Arrest [POCA] Registry.* ASA Newsletter. *2005;69[6]:10-12. Reprinted by permission of the American Society of Anesthesiologists.)*

common causes of cardiovascular causes of arrest were hemorrhagic hypovolemia and the metabolic consequences of massive blood transfusions. Medication-related causes of arrest have decreased markedly, primarily as a result of a practice change in the choice of inhalational anesthetics from halothane (hypotension, arrhythmias) to sevoflurane.[18] The newest inhalational anesthetic, sevoflurane, has replaced halothane for mask induction of anesthesia in children because it has a more pleasant odor. Sevoflurane also produces fewer cardiovascular adverse effects such as bradycardia, hypotension, and ventricular arrhythmias as a result of lesser effects on myocardial contractility and the conducting system. These trends continue when the data are subdivided into the first and last 5 years of the last decade (Figure 62-2).

Pediatric Anesthesia Malpractice Closed Claims Registry

Another outcome measure available to evaluate risk of adverse perioperative events is the closed pediatric anesthesia malpractice claims registry. In this registry, 75% of pediatric claims were made in ASA PS 1 and 2 children. The procedures most commonly cited were dental, ear, nose, throat, and maxillofacial procedures (36%) followed by abdominal procedures (17%). Although these results may be skewed by the frequency of cases performed (ASA PS 1 and 2 children are the most frequently anesthetized, and these are the most common procedures for which children are anesthetized), they suggest that procedures related to the airway are associated with increased risk. Most of the claims involving airway obstruction occurred in the dental, ear, nose, throat, and maxillofacial group.[19]

The incidence of adverse events has been cited as 75 per 1000 anesthetics, with the most common adverse events resulting from respiratory causes during the procedure and vomiting during the recovery period, although younger children experience respiratory adverse events in the recovery period as well.[20] Factors that increase the risk of a respiratory adverse perioperative event include young age, otolaryngology procedure, and the presence of a respiratory tract infection.[21]

Psychological stress and behavioral complications are additional adverse outcomes in the periprocedure experience of the child. The principal risk factors are inadequate family preparation and the lack of preprocedure anxiolysis. Parents who have not been adequately prepared exhibit significant anxiety, which has been demonstrated to be transmitted to the child; this anxiety may contribute to a stormy anesthetic induction.[22] Preprocedural sedation, usually by an oral or rectal route, is often effective in modulating a child's anxiety. Omitting a premedication in an anxious child will also result in a traumatic induction.[23] Children who experience stressful anesthetic inductions exhibit postoperative maladaptive behaviors, including enuresis, night terrors, and violent behavior.[24-27]

Children requiring repeated invasive procedures can develop a posttraumatic stress–like syndrome.[2]

Preanesthetic History and Physical Examination

The preanesthetic evaluation should focus on specific elements of the patient's medical history and physical examination that may have physiological consequences during use of an anesthetic. Fundamental elements are the pulmonary (including airway anatomy), cardiovascular, endocrine, hematologic, and neuromuscular systems. Important areas of attention when applicable include premature birth and neonatal course, oncologic disease and exposure to chemotherapeutic agents, history of corticosteroid use, history of congenital anomalies and their corrective procedures, and the presence of autism and other behavioral-communicative disorders. This last category will significantly affect the pediatric anesthesiologist's psychological approach to the child. Many departments of anesthesiology will provide the PCP with a history and physical examination form on which to report the preoperative evaluation (Figure 62-3). When not provided with such a form, the PCP should provide a history and physical examination with all abnormalities identified. The airway examination is especially important. Even when the airway is normal, the PCP should make specific note of adequacy of mouth opening, neck mobility, and the presence of loose teeth. Normal mouth opening, mandibular size, and neck mobility are fundamental to the success of intubation using the most common technique, direct laryngoscopy. Congenital (micrognathia) or acquired (jaw immobility caused by infection, trauma, or irradiation) abnormalities in these parameters can lead to great difficulty with intubation, which, if unexpected, can lead to adverse airway events and imperil the life of the patient. Alerting the anesthesiologist to these abnormalities is essential to allow for appropriate advanced preparation for special techniques to secure

Preoperative Evaluation/History and Physical

DATE ________ TIME ________ AGE ____ SEX ____ RACE ____

PROCEDURE ________

DIAGNOSIS ________

MEDICATIONS ________

ALLERGIES ________

STAMP PATIENT'S IDENTIFICATION OR PRINT CLEARLY

NURSING UNIT/CLINIC

HOSPITAL HISTORY NUMBER

PATIENT'S NAME (LAST, FIRST, MI)

Medical History and Review of Systems

YES	NO	CARDIOVASCULAR
☐	☐	MYOCARDIAL INFARCTION
☐	☐	HYPERTENSION
☐	☐	ARRHYTHMIA
☐	☐	ANGINA
☐	☐	CONGESTIVE HEART FAILURE
☐	☐	VALVULAR DISEASE
☐	☐	PERIPHERAL VASCULAR DISEASE
☐	☐	PAST CARDIAC SURGERY
☐	☐	OTHER
		PULMONARY
☐	☐	HISTORY OF SMOKING
☐	☐	ASTHMA
☐	☐	CHRONIC OBSTRUCTIVE PULMONARY DISEASE; EMPHYSEMA; BRONCHOPULMONARY DYSPLASIA
☐	☐	OTHER
		RENAL
☐	☐	RENAL FAILURE
☐	☐	OTHER
		HEPATIC
☐	☐	HEPATITIS
☐	☐	OTHER

YES	NO	ENDOCRINE
☐	☐	DIABETES
☐	☐	OTHER
		INFECTIOUS
☐	☐	SEPSIS
☐	☐	OTHER
		NEUROLOGIC
☐	☐	SEIZURE
☐	☐	ELEVATED INTRACRANIAL PRESSURE
☐	☐	CEREBROVASCULAR DISEASE
☐	☐	NEUROMUSCULAR DISORDER
☐	☐	OTHER
		GASTROINTESTINAL
☐	☐	GASTROESOPHAGEAL REFLUX; HIATAL HERNIA
☐	☐	BOWEL OBSTRUCTION
☐	☐	OTHER
		HEMATOLOGIC
☐	☐	SICKLE CELL
☐	☐	COAGULOPATHY
☐	☐	PREGNANCY; TRANSFUSION WITHIN THE LAST 3 MONTHS Y/N
☐	☐	OTHER

YES	NO	PEDIATRICS
☐	☐	PREMATURITY
☐	☐	CONGENITAL ABNORMALITY
☐	☐	APNEA
☐	☐	OTHER
		OBSTETRICS
☐	☐	PREECLAMPSIA; ECLAMPSIA
☐	☐	PREMATURITY
☐	☐	PLACENTA PREVIA; ABRUPTIO
☐	☐	LAST MENSTRUAL PERIOD ________
☐	☐	OTHER
		ANESTHETIC DIFFICULTIES
☐	☐	DIFFICULT INTUBATION
☐	☐	FAMILY HISTORY
☐	☐	OTHER
		DRUG USE
☐	☐	ETHANOL
☐	☐	OTHER

☐ HISTORY UNKNOWN EXCEPT AS NOTED ABOVE

Explanation of Positive Data ________

Physical Examination BP (RANGE): ________ P ________ R ________ T ________ WT ________ (lbs/kg)

Labs: ________

H&P PERFORMED BY ________

ECG FINDINGS: ________

RISK FACTORS:

HEMODYNAMIC COMPROMISE ________ OTHER ________

CRITICAL AIRWAY ________

FULL STOMACH ________ LAST PO ________

Impression: ASA Status | 1 | 2 | 3 | 4 | 5 | E | ________

REVIEWED BY: ________ DATE: ________ TIME: ________

CHART COPY

Figure 62-3 Example of form for submitting preoperative evaluation. *(Johns Hopkins Hospital, Department of Anesthesiology and Critical Care Medicine, 1988. Reprinted by permission.)*

BOX 62-2 Critical Information Frequently Omitted in Pediatric Primary Physician Preanesthetic History and Physical Examinations

- Weight
- Blood pressure
- Room-air oxygen saturation or saturation with baseline oxygen supplementation
- Allergies (drugs and latex)
- Cardiac murmur history
- Previous subspecialty encounters: findings, recommendations, and interventions
- Medications
- Extent of neuromuscular disease (eg, hypotonia)

BOX 62-3 Risk Factors for Adverse Perianesthetic Respiratory Events Occurring During Acute and Recent Upper Respiratory Infection

- Age younger than 5 yr
- Copious secretions
- Plan for endotracheal intubation required for procedure
- History of reactive airway disease
- History of prematurity
- Parental smoking history
- Upper respiratory infection within the previous 4 weeks
- *Wet* cough
- Wheezing

Adapted from Tait AR, Malviya S, Voepel-Lewis T, et al. Risk factors for perioperative adverse respiratory events in children with upper respiratory tract infections. *Anesthesiology.* 2001;95:299-306.

the airway. Under no circumstances should the words *cleared for surgery* be written on a prescription form after a completion of a preoperative history and physical examination. Critical information that is frequently missing from preoperative evaluations in institutions is included in Box 62-2.

The remainder of this chapter discusses pertinent issues of the preoperative assessment in a systematic fashion, identifying critical factors that would be of interest to the anesthesiologist caring for children.

AIRWAY AND PULMONARY FUNCTION

General anesthesia alters respiratory function significantly at virtually every level. Early effects result from excitation of airway reflexes (laryngospasm, increased secretions, and bronchospasm) during the inhalational induction of general anesthesia before the achievement of a depth of anesthesia appropriate for surgery. The effects of anesthesia include decreased contractility of respiratory muscles, depressed ciliary clearance, depression of the central respiratory response to hypoxia and hypercapnia, decreased lung volume, and increased intrapulmonary shunting. These effects can result in serious and potentially life-threatening consequences, including upper airway obstruction, hypoventilation or apnea, and hypoxemia. The presence of underlying conditions (eg, prematurity) or respiratory or airway diseases (eg, asthma, bronchopulmonary dysplasia) compounds the risks of anesthesia greatly for the child. Therefore detailed information about preexisting respiratory disease should be available for the anesthesiologist.

Upper Respiratory Tract Infections

No greater difference in perspective exists between the PCP and the pediatric anesthesiologist than in the diagnosis of a URTI. To the PCP, the diagnosis is usually one of reassurance: "it's just a cold." To the pediatric anesthesiologist, a URTI is a diagnosis that mandates a careful risk, benefit, and consequence analysis.

The pediatric anesthesiologist is frequently challenged to determine the appropriate management of children who are undergoing an elective procedure and who have an acute or recent URTI, which may put them at increased risk for adverse events. Children with an active or recent URTI are more likely to have episodes of laryngospasm, oxygen desaturation, bronchospasm, severe coughing, and breath holding during anesthetic induction and emergence.[28] Independent risk factors for adverse perioperative respiratory events in the setting of an active or recent URTI are summarized in Box 62-3.[29]

The incidence of perioperative respiratory events is increased 7 times in children with URTI and 11 times if the child is intubated.[30] The risk of airway complications remains high for up to 6 weeks after a URTI, probably as a result of altered airway reactivity.[31-33] Children with URTIs undergoing elective cardiac surgery have a 4-fold increased incidence of airway complications at induction of anesthesia, a 2-fold increased incidence of postoperative respiratory complications, and a 5-fold increase in postoperative bacterial infections, as well as an extended stay in the intensive care unit.[34] Mortality during or after administration of an anesthetic in a child with a URTI has rarely been reported.[35] However, airway events were responsible for almost 30% of all pediatric anesthetic deaths in the most recent summary of pediatric perioperative cardiac arrest registry data. The most common events leading to cardiac arrest in this category are laryngospasm, airway obstruction, inadequate oxygenation, inadvertent extubation, difficult intubation, and bronchospasm, some of which might be related to URTI.[18]

The adverse respiratory events that are associated with a mild to moderate URTI are frequently managed with additional oxygen supplementation, increased postanesthesia care unit stay, inhaled beta-agonists, and corticosteroids. A small percentage of patients require unplanned hospitalization for stridor, pneumonia, or other complications.[20,36]

Interestingly, several studies have found no significant increase in respiratory complications among children anesthetized *during* an acute URTI,[31] which has led some researchers to advocate *not* canceling surgery for these children. The physiological, psychological, and financial implications of delays in surgery must be weighed against the risks of increased perioperative complications of anesthetizing a child who has a URTI. Patients who have systemic manifestations, such as temperature greater than 101.3°F (38.5°C), purulent nasal discharge, and lower respiratory symptoms such as productive cough, crackles, wheezes, or positive chest radiograph findings, should have the surgical procedure delayed for 4 to 6 weeks after the resolution of symptoms.[37,38] Surgery and anesthesia can usually be performed safely in children who have none of these symptoms, particularly if they do not require endotracheal intubation (Figure 62-4).[28] Even in the absence of these symptoms in children with a history of recent URTI, adverse events are still possible; parents should be informed of this possibility and that intra- or postoperative treatment (eg, nebulization of beta-agonist for wheezing) may be required.

The child's room-air oxygen saturation may be an additional discriminating tool. If a child with a URTI has a room-air oxygen saturation of less than 96% at sea level, in the absence of chronic lung disease, then the case will be rescheduled. Parents should also be told that increased adverse perioperative respiratory events occur in children exposed to cigarette smoke at home.[39]

Asthma

Asthma is one of the most common and serious underlying medical conditions that can affect patients undergoing general anesthesia.[40-42] The incidence of reactive airway disease has increased markedly in the general pediatric population and is now approximately 25% of the pediatric surgical population. Many procedures performed routinely during anesthetic management, most notably laryngoscopy and intubation, are potent and intense stimuli that produce bronchospasm in the child with reactive airways. Intraoperative bronchospasm is frightening, is challenging to treat, and can be catastrophic. Ventilation is difficult, if not impossible, and may result in hypercapnia, acidosis, hypoxia, cardiovascular collapse, and death. Fortunately, these adverse events need not and should not happen. Maximal preoperative optimization of a patient's medical management may prevent, or at the least limit, all of the perioperative complications of asthma. In general, asthma medical therapy must be escalated preoperatively even in asymptomatic patients or patients with well-controlled asthma to limit or prevent intraoperative bronchospasm. Short courses of corticosteroids in particular are extremely effective in preventing perioperative wheezing, even in patients who have severe asthma.[43] Thus children who take asthma medications only as needed should begin use of their inhaled beta-agonists or oral medications 3 to 5 days preoperatively.[44] Children taking medications on a long-term basis (oral or inhaled) should have steroids added in doses that are normally used for an acute exacerbation. Finally, the *difficult* asthmatic child who takes bronchodilators and steroids regularly requires intensification in the frequency of nebulizer treatments, added bronchodilators, increased steroids, or, on occasion, all of these measures. Under no circumstances should asthma therapy be deescalated or stopped before surgery. Because the condition of most children with reactive airway disease is tracked using peak flow rate, optimization of the child's condition should be documented by achieving maximal peak flow rate for that child. Although theophylline therapy for reactive airway disease is much less common than in the past, children taking theophylline should have serum levels measured preoperatively to optimize drug administration and avoid possible toxic effects, which may include arrhythmias in the setting of local or general anesthetic, or catecholamine administration (topical or infiltration administration of epinephrine or cocaine). Despite fasting regimens, all oral medications may be taken with small amounts of water on the morning of surgery.

Children with asthma are not candidates for procedures performed at freestanding facilities if these children have been hospitalized for asthma within the previous 3 months, had an exacerbation in the previous month, or have a room-air oxygen saturation of 96% or less. *Elective* surgery should never be performed in a child who is wheezing actively or who has had a recent asthma attack. Decreased peak expiratory flow and forced expiratory volume in the first second of expiration (FEV_1) occur in adults and children for up to 6 weeks after an acute asthma attack, and airways are more reactive and prone to bronchospasm in this period.

Postoperative Apnea and Prematurity

Infants born prematurely (<37 weeks' gestation) are at significant risk for the development of apnea after exposure to sedative drugs and anesthetic agents.[45] Their central and peripheral chemoreceptors are immature and limit effective responses to hypoxia and hypercapnia, even without the additional burden of drug-induced depression.[46] Furthermore, anesthetic agents decrease muscle tone in the airways, chest wall, and diaphragm, thereby depressing the ventilatory response to hypoxia and hypercapnia further.[47]

This risk of apnea affects the postanesthetic care of infants born prematurely, mandating that those at risk be admitted for postprocedure monitoring. Nonanemic infants who had been born prematurely and who have attained a postconceptual age (gestational age added to age after birth) of greater than 56 weeks have a less than 1% risk of developing postoperative apnea (Figure 62-5).[48] A hemoglobin concentration of less than 10 g/dL increases the risk to greater than the mean for infants of all postconceptual ages.

Postanesthetic apnea is usually central in origin and brief and frequently resolves either spontaneously or with minor stimulation. Nevertheless, postoperative apnea is considered a serious event because cerebral arterial desaturation has been documented after only 5 seconds of apnea in these premature infants.[49] Although most apneic episodes occur within the first 2 hours after an anesthetic, apnea can be seen for up to 12 hours. Infants undergoing procedures with regional anesthesia (caudal, spinal) with *no* concomitant sedation have much less postoperative oxygen desaturation and bradycardia.[50,51] Infants who had been born prematurely and who had spinal anesthesia have demonstrated a decrease in cerebral blood flow velocity

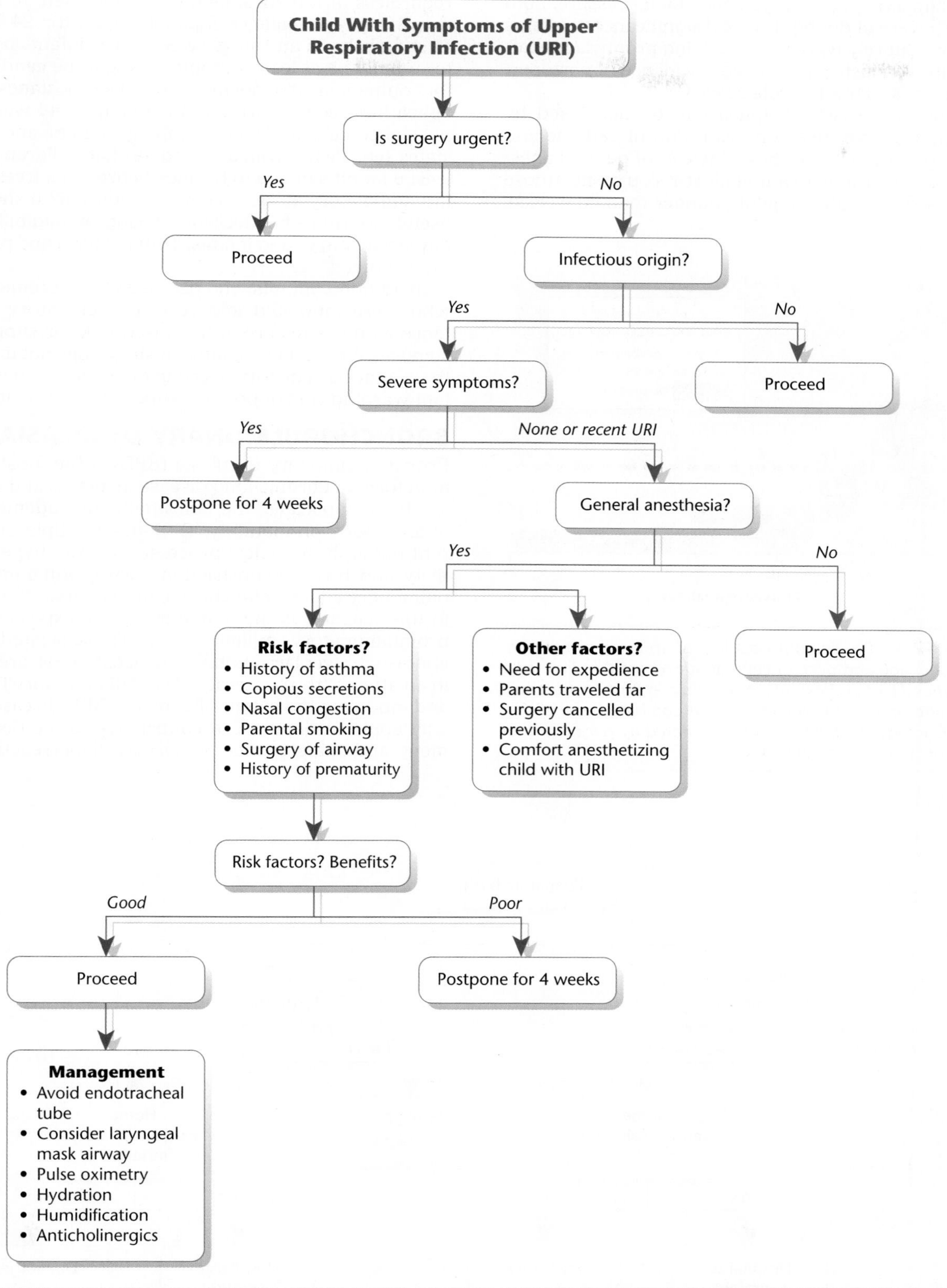

Figure 62-4 Preoperative decision making in children with upper respiratory infection symptoms. *(From Tait AR, Malviya S. Anesthesia for the child with an upper respiratory infection: still a dilemma?* Anesth Analg. *2005;100:59-65. Reprinted by permission of Lippincott Williams & Wilkins.)*

paralleling a decrease in systemic blood pressure, both of which were of doubtful clinical significance.[52] Infants born prematurely who were receiving prophylactic caffeine intravenously have a lower incidence of postoperative apnea and bradycardia as well.[53,54]

Although the risk of apnea can be decreased by both the perioperative administration of caffeine and the use of regional anesthesia instead of general anesthesia, it is advisable to admit all at-risk patients (those with a postconceptual age of younger than 60 weeks), regardless of the anesthetic technique used, to monitored, high-surveillance inpatient units for 24 hours after anesthesia and surgery. Similarly, infants born at term must be at least 1 month of age to be candidates for outpatient management because postanesthetic apnea has been reported in infants up to 44 weeks of postconceptual age.[55] Finally, many centers, and some states (eg, Pennsylvania) mandate that children be at least 6 months of age to be anesthetized in a freestanding ambulatory surgery center.[56] Figure 62-6 shows a useful algorithm for decision making on eligibility for day surgery in young infants, both full term and prematurely born.[57]

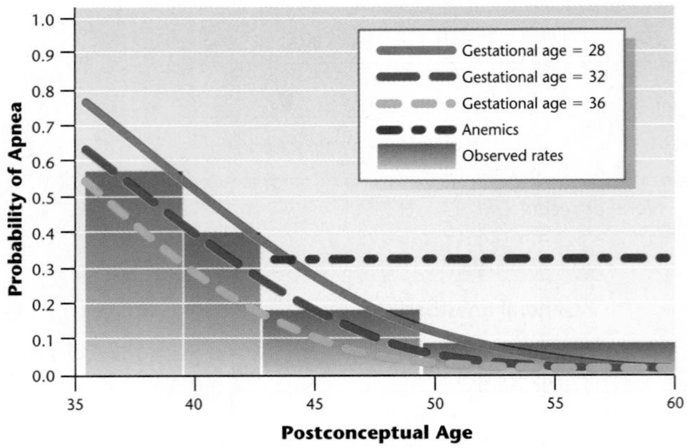

Figure 62-5 Predicted probability of apnea in relation to gestational age and postconceptual age. *(Cote CJ, Zaslavsky A, Downes JJ, et al. Postoperative apnea in former preterm infants after inguinal herniorrhaphy. A combined analysis.* Anesthesiology. *1995:82:809-822. Reprinted by permission of Lippincott Williams & Wilkins.)*

In addition, infants who had been born prematurely who were intubated and received ventilatory assistance as neonates are at increased risk for subglottic stenosis. Although a negative history does not exclude the diagnosis, a history of croup or stridor is an important warning sign of possible subglottic narrowing.

BRONCHOPULMONARY DYSPLASIA

Bronchopulmonary dysplasia (BPD) is the most common form of chronic lung disease in infants and significantly complicates the anesthetic management of infants born prematurely. BPD has multiple concurrent pathophysiological processes: airway hyperreactivity and bronchoconstriction, airway inflammation, pulmonary edema, and chronic lung injury.[58,59] Pivotal in this scenario is the immature lungs' exposure to a proinflammatory milieu, which is associated with abnormal alveolarization.[60] Corticosteroids are used in an attempt to counteract these inflammatory factors and modulate the extent of evolving BPD disease. Airway epithelial injury also contributes to the development and maintenance of airway hyperreactivity.[61]

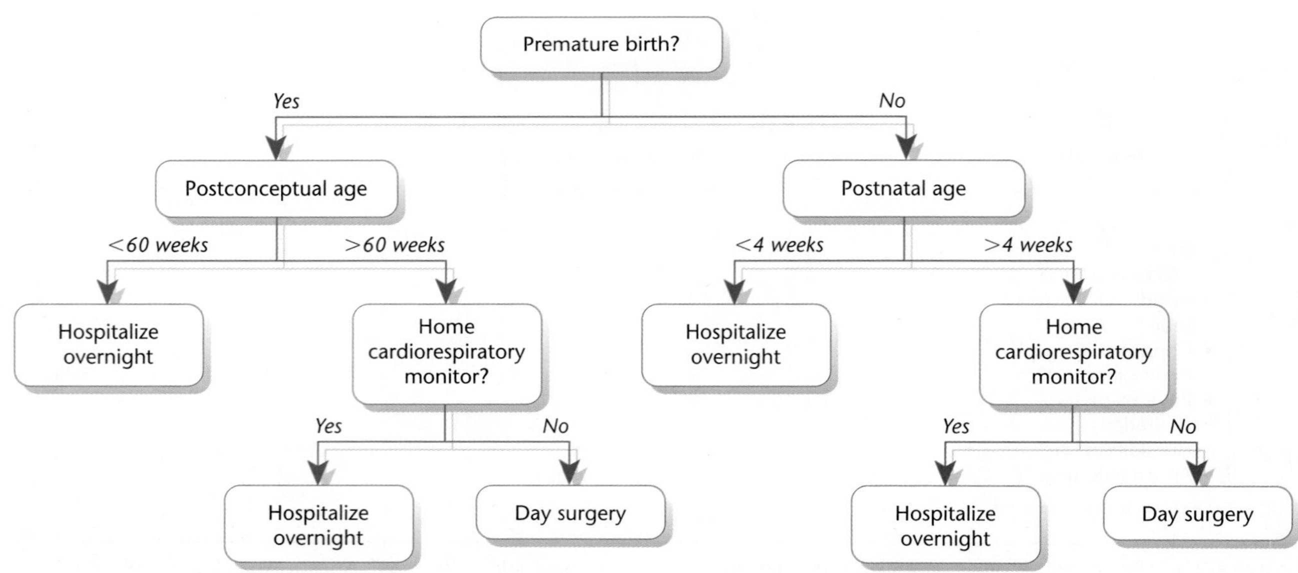

Figure 62-6 Algorithm for decision making about outpatient surgery versus overnight admission in ex-premature infants. *(Galinkin JL, Kurth CD. Neonatal and pediatric apnea syndromes.* Problems Anesth. *1998;10:444-454.)*

Many infants with BPD also have pulmonary hypertension resulting from decreased vascular development during the disease.[62]

Several effects of anesthesia, together or separately, may produce life-threatening consequences. Pulmonary vasoconstriction after anesthetic induction can aggravate ventilation-perfusion mismatch and lead to profound hypoxemia. Anesthetic effects on myocardial contractility can result in impaired right-ventricular function, reduced cardiac output, pulmonary hypoperfusion, and profound cardiovascular compromise with hypoxemia resembling acute cor pulmonale. Increased airway reactivity during induction of or emergence from anesthesia can result in a severe exacerbation of BPD, with an increased ventilation-perfusion mismatch. Increased oral and bronchial secretions induced by the anesthetic can compromise airflow and lead to airway or endotracheal tube plugging. Because of diminished respiratory reserves in these patients, such plugging can quickly cause profound hypoxia and acute right-sided heart strain, arrhythmias, and possibly death. These children may also have a degree of increased airway reactivity and tracheomalacia. Intraoperative bronchospasm or airway collapse poses a serious intraoperative risk. Finally, infections of the respiratory tract occur frequently in children who have BPD, and the presence of pneumonia can complicate the perioperative course significantly.

The pulmonary status of these children must be evaluated and their conditions optimized before anesthesia and surgery to minimize their perioperative risks of bronchospasm, atelectasis, pneumonia, respiratory, and possibly cardiac failure. Bronchodilators, antibiotics, diuretics, nutritional support, and corticosteroid therapy all may benefit these children. Respiratory infections or bronchospasm in children who have BPD must be treated thoroughly before elective surgery. For children who have severe BPD and bronchospasm, preoperative treatment with increased inspired oxygen tension may decrease pulmonary vasoreactivity and improve cardiovascular function. The possibility of associated right-ventricular dysfunction should always be considered and, when indicated, evaluated with electrocardiogram (ECG) and echocardiography. Many children take diuretics such as furosemide and spironolactone on a long-term basis, which may result in electrolyte abnormalities. These patients require a preoperative measurement of their serum electrolytes. Many infants with BPD receive frequent courses of corticosteroids, and perioperative steroid coverage may be required.

Because infants with BPD are at major risk for perioperative morbidity and mortality, these issues should be reviewed with the parents before the anesthetic is administered to their child. Frequently, children with BPD may require continuous postoperative monitoring and ventilatory assistance for an extended period (24 to 48 hours). Risks of general anesthesia and intubation in these children can sometimes be avoided with the judicious use of either a laryngeal mask airway or a regional anesthetic.[63] Parents must be cautioned, however, that either approach might be unsuccessful and that intubation might still be required.

OBSTRUCTIVE SLEEP APNEA SYNDROME

Upper airways obstruction is a consequence of abnormal upper airways anatomy, upper airways dysfunction, or both. Abnormal airways anatomy can be congenital, as in Pierre Robin syndrome, or acquired as in adenotonsillar hypertrophy. Adenotonsillar hypertrophy is the primary cause of obstructive sleep apnea syndrome (OSAS) in children age 2 to 6 years. Obesity, with increased airway soft tissue, is frequently responsible for OSAS in teenagers. Airways dysfunction may be the result of central nervous system dysfunction, neuromuscular diseases, or hypotonia. Children with OSAS commonly have a combination of obstructive and central components. Decreased upper airway muscle tone and an inadequate ventilatory response to hypercarbia and hypoxemia are responsible for this central component. The acute airways inflammation that accompanies URTI in addition to residual amounts of inhaled anesthetic agents can significantly aggravate a child's baseline level of airways obstruction.[64]

The hypoxemia and hypercarbia of chronic upper airways obstruction may lead to the development of pulmonary hypertension and right-ventricular dysfunction in these patients. Hypoxemia and hypercarbia are potent systemic and pulmonary vasoconstrictors, which, over time, induce a structural remodeling of the pulmonary vascular bed, producing systemic and pulmonary hypertension. As a result of this increase in right-ventricle pressure work, right-ventricle hypertrophy develops. Progressively, tricuspid regurgitation and paradoxical movement of the intraventricular septum produces left-ventricular outflow tract obstruction. This left-ventricular dysfunction in combination with the large negative intrathoracic pressures generated during inspiration to overcome an extrathoracic obstruction favors formation of pulmonary edema, which only serves to worsen the patient's hypoxemia and work of breathing.

Children with OSAS undergoing adenotonsillectomy have a 10% to 30% incidence of perioperative complications.[65] These complications include laryngospasm, pulmonary edema, postoperative airway obstruction, and respiratory arrest. Risk factors for these complications include the following: age younger than 3 years, severe OSAS on polysomnography, infants born prematurely, right-ventricle hypertrophy, pulmonary hypertension, recent URTI, signs of respiratory distress, trisomy 21, craniofacial anomalies, neuromuscular disease, failure to thrive, and obesity.[66,67] An oxygen saturation nadir of less than 80% during the sleep study has been noted to increase a child's probability of postoperative complications to 50%.[68] Children undergoing urgent, as opposed to elective, tonsillectomy have a 2-fold increase risk of postoperative complications.[69] Many studies have shown that children younger than 3 years have a high rate of postadenotonsillectomy airways obstruction and respiratory complications[70-72] and therefore should be admitted overnight for observation and monitoring, including cardiorespiratory monitor and continuous pulse oximetry.

The goal of the perioperative evaluation of children with OSAS is to determine whether these risk factors for postoperative morbidity exist. Significant upper airways obstruction may lead to snoring, failure to thrive, cyanosis during sleep, daytime somnolence, or any combination. Because many children who snore do not have OSAS, snoring cannot be used as a predictor of morbidity.[66] Right-ventricular dysfunction can cause jugular venous distention, hepatomegaly, peripheral edema, and failure to thrive. Preoperatively, these children should have laboratory testing, including electrolytes (looking for high bicarbonate as a metabolic response to chronic hypercarbia), baseline room-air oxygen saturation (pulse oximetry), and a hematocrit (looking for elevation as a response to chronic hypoxia). Most surgeons also request prothrombin time, partial thromboplastin time, and international normalized ratio to identify patients at increased risk of perioperative bleeding. Although a chest radiographic, ECG, and echocardiographic evaluation may be performed, only the findings of a high-velocity tricuspid regurgitant jet or abnormal intraventricular septal motion have a positive predictive value for the presence of pulmonary hypertension.[62] The presence and severity of right-ventricular dysfunction and pulmonary hypertension have profound implications on the anesthetic approach to these patients. Finally, the details of the sleep study, if performed, should be reviewed. Because of the expense of sleep studies and the unavailability of facilities and scarcity of pediatric sleep centers, many children undergoing adenotonsillectomy have the diagnosis of OSAS made on clinical grounds.[66]

Postoperatively, these high-risk children, especially those younger than 3 years, should be admitted to the pediatric intensive care unit or other highly monitored locations because the incidence of obstructive events and pulmonary complications may increase during the first 24 hours after surgery because of narrowing of the airway caused by edema, secretions, or both.[70]

CYSTIC FIBROSIS

Cystic fibrosis (CF) is a progressive pulmonary disease associated with pancreatic dysfunction, growth failure, gastroesophageal reflux, coagulopathy, and electrolyte imbalances. Children and adolescents with CF most commonly require anesthetics for otolaryngology procedures (eg, sinus surgery), central line placement, bronchoscopy, and esophagoscopy, as well as laparotomy for intestinal obstruction and the placement of enteral feeding devices.[73] Patients with CF have an incidence of postoperative complications of 10% to 22% and a perioperative mortality of 1% to 5%.[74] Most of the complications are pulmonary, and some evidence suggests that general anesthesia may have at least short-term deleterious effects on the already severely impaired pulmonary function of these patients.[75]

The primary focus in the perioperative evaluation of the child with cystic fibrosis is to determine the severity of their pulmonary disease and use all methods possible to optimize it in consultation with the pediatric pulmonologist. Pulmonary function tests will demonstrate whether the patient has hyperinflation, has lower airways obstruction, and is responsive to bronchodilators. Chest radiographs and chest CT studies document the degree of disease heterogeneity and may be useful in determining the risk of pneumothorax during positive pressure ventilation. Preoperative room air pulse oximetry further helps to quantify the degree of underlying pulmonary dysfunction. Patients with CF who are chronically hypoxemic are at risk for pulmonary hypertension and cor pulmonale. An echocardiographic evaluation should be performed in this subset of patients.

Patients with CF commonly have acute pulmonary infections superimposed on chronic colonization. A recent sputum culture will help determine whether the patient should be prescribed preoperative antibiotics or may require contact precautions. Chest physiotherapy and mucolytics are useful in improving sputum clearance. Adolescents with severe pulmonary dysfunction are at risk for massive hemoptysis; 25% of patients with CF will experience recurrent massive hemoptysis.[76]

Other aspects of the CF patient's pathophysiology should be addressed as well, in concert with other pediatric subspecialists. Preoperative nutritional support and optimization of pancreatic enzyme supplementation will help mitigate the effects of growth failure and hypoalbuminemia that affect anesthetic pharmacodynamics. Correction of electrolyte and coagulation abnormalities with oral agents is useful in decreasing the need for acute interventions on the day of the procedure.

CARDIOVASCULAR DISEASE

All anesthetic agents can affect the normal cardiovascular system profoundly and adversely. The sinus node, conduction system, and myocardial contractility all can be depressed by general anesthetics. Moreover, these drugs alter both preload and afterload by relaxing vascular smooth-muscle tone. General anesthetics also attenuate hypoxic pulmonary vasoconstriction and thereby impair ventilation perfusion matching. The combination of vasodilatation and impaired myocardial contractility often causes some degree of hypotension, especially in children who are relatively hypovolemic because of a prolonged fast or excessive fluid loss (eg, diarrhea, vomiting, hemorrhage). Because the presence of underlying heart disease increases the inherent risks of anesthesia, the preanesthetic cardiac evaluation should identify whether cardiac dysfunction, structural heart disease, or hypertension is present and whether subacute bacterial endocarditis (SBE) prophylaxis is needed.

Heart Murmur

Many children will have heart murmurs noted during their preanesthetic evaluation. Does a child with a heart murmur need a cardiology evaluation? Given the high prevalence (75% to 90%) of innocent murmurs through childhood, most children will have an audible murmur at some point; however, most of these children will not require a cardiology consultation.[77] Innocent murmurs are frequently episodic in appearance and are associated with a normally split second heart sound, normal exercise tolerance, and a normal

Table 62-3 Innocent Murmurs

	LOCATION	QUALITY	INCREASED BY	DECREASED BY
Still's murmur	LLSB without radiation	Low pitch vibratory	Exercise	Standing
Pulmonary murmur	LUSB	Blowing midsystolic	Expiration	Standing
Supraclavicular bruit	R supraclavicular fossa	Harsh systolic ejection	Pressure	Shoulder extension

LLSB, Left lower sternal border; *LUSB*, left upper sternal border.

electrocardiogram. The 3 most common murmurs are the Still's murmur, the innocent pulmonary murmur, and the arterial supraclavicular bruit. The defining characteristics of the innocent murmurs are summarized in Table 62-3.

Still's murmur is most frequent in late preschool and is exacerbated by fever, exercise, and anemia.[78] Still's murmur is low pitched and decreases with standing, which distinguishes it from a small ventricular septal defect and hypertrophic obstructive cardiomyopathy.[79] The innocent pulmonary murmur is most common during middle to late childhood and can appear during febrile illnesses, anemia, and pregnancy. A normal split second heart sound differentiates the innocent pulmonary murmur from an atrial septal defect, as well as pulmonary valvular disease.[80]

Alternatively, cardiac murmurs can be indicative of either intracardiac shunts or valvular heart disease. Because anesthetic agents have varying degrees of effects on pulmonary and systemic vascular resistance, heart rate, and contractility, an inappropriate choice of anesthetic agent can severely disturb a previously balanced pathophysiological state. For this reason, all murmurs of questionable status should be evaluated by a pediatric cardiologist, and all pathologic findings should be communicated directly to the pediatric anesthesiologist.

A newly diagnosed murmur can represent underlying congenital heart disease with intracardiac shunts or unappreciated valvular heart disease, both of which may require SBE prophylaxis. Cardiology consultation is warranted when this new murmur does not appear to be innocent or is associated with changes in exercise tolerance, respiratory status, or perfusion.

Children with congenital heart disease (whether repaired or not) should have a cardiac evaluation within 1 year before surgery, even if asymptomatic. Current use of cardiac medications, prolonged QT syndrome and residual cardiac disease all disqualify a child from having procedures performed at freestanding ambulatory surgical facilities.

Williams Syndrome

Williams syndrome is a constellation of dysmorphic facies, intellectual disability, growth deficiency, neonatal hypercalcemia, genitourinary anomalies, and congenital heart disease.[81] The principal cardiac manifestation is supravalvular aortic stenosis, which is often progressive. Other end-organ manifestations of Williams syndrome include epilepsy, persistent hypercalcemia, hypothyroidism, renovascular hypertension, and proteinuria.[82] The locus for the deletion responsible for this syndrome is in the *ELN* gene on chromosome 7, which codes for elastin.[83]

A reduced amount of elastin in the media of the aorta is thought to produce aortic narrowing at the sinotubular junction producing the supravalvular aortic stenosis; a similar process can occur in any artery.[84] Pulmonary arterial obstruction is seen in 80% of cases.[85] Sudden death is estimated to occur in at least 3% of patients with Williams syndrome; many deaths occur during the perioperative period.[86] At postmortem examination, coronary artery stenosis, and biventricular outflow tract obstruction have been identified and are thought to contribute to myocardial ischemia, decreased cardiac output, and ventricular dysrhythmias. The coronary artery stenosis may be caused by ostia obstruction from the distorted aortic valve or by abnormalities in elastin production. Retrospectively, many of these patients had evidence of myocardial ischemia on preoperative electrocardiogram or Holter monitor.[87]

Patients with Williams syndrome should be considered at high risk for perioperative complications. Given that their cardiac disease appears to be dynamic, a thorough history looking for a change in exercise tolerance, dyspnea, angina, and syncope should be sought. A complete cardiologic evaluation, including an echocardiogram, should be performed before the administration of each anesthetic, looking for evidence of outflow tract obstruction, coronary artery anomalies, and segmental wall motion abnormalities, suggestive of myocardial ischemia. Anesthetic induction must be performed with great care, avoiding extremes in heart rate and blood pressure.

Prolonged QT Syndrome

Prolonged (or long) QT syndrome (LQTS) is the perturbation of ion channels impairing ventricular repolarization, which puts patients at increased risk for Torsades de pointes, a polymorphic ventricular tachycardia. Prolongation of the QT segment results from either congenital genetic mutations or the effects of drugs or metabolic abnormalities on the ion channels responsible for repolarization (Table 62-4). Congenital LQTS can occur in children at any age. The prevalence is 1 in 5000 persons.[88,89] Most of the genetic mutations are inherited in an autosomal-dominant manner. Far less common is the autosomal-recessive LQTS and sensorineural deafness, affecting 1 in 1 million people.[90] These patients present with syncope, seizures, or sudden cardiac death after an increase in sympathetic activity, commonly in the form of exercise, an auditory stimulus, or emotional stress.

Table 62-4 Drugs That Prolong the QT Interval or Induce Torsades de Pointes

GENERIC NAME	BRAND NAME	CATEGORY*
Albuterol	Ventolin, Proventil	3
Amantadine	Symmetrel	2
Amiodarone	Pacerone, Cordarone	1
Amphetamine/dextroamphetamine	*Adderall*	3
Atomoxetine	*Strattera*	3
Azithromycin	Zithromax	2
Chloral hydrate	Noctec	2
Chloroquine	Arelan	1
Chlorpromazine	Thorazine	1
Clarithromycin	Biaxin	1
Clozapine	Clozaril	2
Dextroamphetamine	Dexadrine	3
Disopyramide	Norpace	1
Dobutamine	Dobutrex	3
Dolasetron	Anzemet	2
Dopamine	Intropin	3
Droperidol	Inapsine	1
Ephedrine	Rumatuss	3
Epinephrine	Primatene, Bronkaid	3
Erythromycin	*Erythrocin, EES*	1
Felbamate	*Felbatrol*	2
Flecainide	Tambocor	2
Foscarnet	Foscavir	2
Fosphenytoin	*Cerebyx*	2
Gemifloxacin	Factive	2
Granisetron	*Kytril*	2
Halofantrine	Halfan	1
Haloperidol	Haldol	1
Isoproterenol	Isupres, Medihaler-Iso	3
Isradipine	Dynacirc	2
Levalbuterol	*Xopenex*	3
Levofloxacin	Levaquin	2
Lithium	Lithobid, Eskalith	2
Metaproterenol	Alupent, Metaprel	3
Methadone	Dolophine, Methadose	1
Methylphenidate	*Ritalin, Concerta*	3
Milodrine	ProAmantine	3
Moxifloxacin	Avelox	2
Nicardipine	Cardene	2
Norepinephrine	Levophed	3
Octreotide	Sandostatin	2
Ofloxacin	Floxin	2
Ondansetron	*Zofran*	2
Pentamidine	Pentam, NebuPent	1
Phenylephrine	Neosynephrine	3
Pimozide	Orap	1
Procainamide	Pronestyl	1
Pseudoephedrine	PediaCare, Sudafed	3
Quetiapine	Seroquel	2
Quinidine	Quinaglute, Cardioquin	1
Risperidone	*Risperdal*	2
Salmeterol	Serevent	3
Sotalol	Betapace	1
Tacrolimus	Prograf	2
Telithromycin	Ketek	2
Terbutaline	Brethine	3
Thioridazine	Mellaril	1
Tizanidine	Zanaflex	2
Venlafaxine	Effexor	2
Ziprasidone	Geodon	2

Drugs in **bold** type are commonly used in perioperative period.
Drugs in *italics* type are commonly used in children.
*Category 1: Drugs that are generally accepted by authorities to have a risk of prolonging the QT interval and causing Torsades de pointes.
Category 2: Drugs that *may* prolong the QT interval but at this time lack substantial evidence for causing Torsades de pointes.
Category 3: Drugs to be avoided for use in patients with diagnosed or suspected congenital long QT syndrome (in addition to drugs in categories 1 and 2).
A continuously updated and complete list of drugs that prolong QT, as well a list of drugs which do not prolong QT and are therefore safe in patients with long QT, may be found at www.torsades.org/medical-pros/drug-lists/drug-lists.htm#. (Accessed July 21, 2006.)

A preoperative electrocardiographic evaluation should be performed on children with a history of any these manifestations, who have a family history of sudden death, or who are receiving long-term administration of one of the drugs listed in Table 62-4, looking for a QT_c greater than 470 ms in male patients and 480 ms in female patients. Only 60% of patients are symptomatic at the time of recognition.[91] Children with LQTS should have electrolytes measured to ensure that serum levels of potassium, calcium, and magnesium are normal. Patients with a risk of congenital LQTS should avoid all of the drugs listed in Table 62-4, if possible. Potent anesthetic vapors have effects on the cardiac conduction system and should be used in these patients with great care.[92]

SUBACUTE BACTERIAL ENDOCARDITIS PROPHYLAXIS

Antibiotic prophylaxis to prevent bacterial endocarditis has long been recommended for children who have congenital heart disease and are undergoing any procedure in which the patient is at risk for transient bacteremia (eg, dental, sinus, airway, genitourinary, gastrointestinal) or when the surgical site, though normally sterile, is contaminated. In 2006 a workgroup of the American Heart Association published new recommendations for antibiotic prophylaxis that are substantially different from those promulgated for the previous 50 years. Specifically, genitourinary and gastrointestinal procedures have been eliminated from those requiring prophylaxis and restricting prophylaxis for dental and respiratory tract procedures to patients in the categories listed in Box 62-4. Oral endotracheal intubation by itself is not an indication for SBE prophylaxis, but nasotracheal intubation requires it. Patients with hemodynamically insignificant lesions such as bicuspid aortic valve or mitral valve prolapse no longer require prophylaxis for any procedure. Patients with congenital heart disease repaired with prosthetic material require prophylaxis only for the first 6 months after repair, after which endothelialization has occurred. Such is the case for VSD as well as ASD repairs as long as no residual defect is present. Patients with prosthetic valves or those palliated with shunts or conduits require prophylaxis. The antibiotic regimen outlined in Table 62-5 should be followed.[93] In most circumstances, prophylactic antibiotics can be administered orally 1 hour before the procedure, with a minimal amount of water. When necessary, give the antibiotic intravenously when the intravenous administration is started after induction of anesthesia, because the interval between the start of the intravenous catheter and the incision generally is long enough (5 minutes) to achieve adequate blood levels. Starting an intravenous catheter in an awake child is unnecessary solely to administer antibiotics for SBE prophylaxis.

BOX 62-4 Cardiac Conditions for Which Prophylaxis with Dental or Respiratory Tract Procedures is Recommended

- Congenital heart disease (CHD)*
- Unrepaired cyanotic CHD, including palliative shunts and conduits
- Completely repaired congenital heart defect with prosthetic material or device, whether placed by surgery or by catheter intervention, during the first 6 months after the procedure†
- Repaired CHD with residual defects at the site or adjacent to the site of a prosthetic patch or prosthetic device (which inhibit endothelialization)
- Cardiac transplantation recipients who develop cardiac valvopathy
- Prosthetic cardiac valves
- Previous infective endocarditis

*Except for the conditions listed above, antibiotic prophylaxis is no longer recommended for any other form of CHD.
†Prophylaxis is recommended because endothelialization of prosthetic material occurs within 6 months of the procedure.
Adapted from Wilson W, Taubert KA, Gewitz M et al. Prevention of infective endocarditis. Guidelines from the American Heart Association Rheumatic Fever, Endocarditis, and Kawasaki Disease Committee, Council on Cardiovascular disease in the Young, and the Council on Clinical Cardiology, Council on Cardiovascular Surgery and Anesthesia, and Quality of Care and Outcomes Research Interdisciplinary Working Group. *Circulation.* 2007;116: 1736-1754. Reprinted by permission of Lippincott Williams & Wilkins.

ENDOCRINE DISEASES

Diabetes Mellitus

The perioperative management of children with diabetes mellitus has changed; no longer is avoidance of hypoglycemia sufficient. Diabetic patients are at significant risk for postoperative complications, many of which can be related to perioperative hyperglycemia.[94] Hyperglycemia is associated with increases in perioperative morbidity and mortality, delayed wound healing, white blood cell dysfunction, and increased infectious complications,. as well as an increase in morbidity and mortality in critically ill patients.[95-101] Not only is immediate perioperative glucose control important, adult patients with elevated glycosylated hemoglobin (HbA_{1C}) levels, indicative of inadequate long-term glucose control, have been shown to be at a higher risk for perioperative infectious complications as well,[102] although this risk has not been demonstrated in children.

Maintenance of glucose homeostasis in the diabetic patient in the perioperative period is complicated by the anesthetic and surgical stimulation of a stress response. This stress response produces a hyperglycemic state in the *nondiabetic* patient as a result of the increased secretion of counter-regulatory hormones: catecholamines, glucagon, cortisol, and growth hormone with a concomitant relative insulin deficiency. This insulin deficiency arises from a combination of reduced insulin secretion and insulin resistance. The change in resistance is due to the alteration of post receptor insulin binding by the counterregulatory hormones.[103] In the diabetic patient, glucose homeostasis is further deranged by their lack of insulin. Significant hyperglycemia occurs, with its attendant osmotic diuresis, electrolyte imbalance, and intracellular dehydration, and intraoperative diabetic ketoacidosis with its associated cerebral edema can develop.[104]

Table 62-5 Prophylactic Regimens for Dental, Oral, Respiratory Tract, or Esophageal Procedures

SITUATION	AGENT	REGIMEN
Standard general prophylaxis	Amoxicillin	50 mg/kg orally 1 hr before procedure (maximum 2 g)
Unable to take oral medications	Ampicillin *OR*	50 mg/kg IM or IV within 30 min before procedure (maximum 1 g)
	Cefazolin or ceftriaxone	50 mg/kg IM or IV within 30 min before procedure (maximum 1 g)
Allergic to penicillins or ampicillin—oral	Clindamycin *OR*	20 mg/kg orally 1 hr before procedure (maximum 600 mg)
	Cephalexin[ab] *OR*	50 mg/kg orally 1 hr before procedure (maximum 2 g)
	Azithromycin or clarithromycin	15 mg/kg orally 1 hr before procedure (maximum 500 mg)
Allergic to penicillin and unable to take oral medications	Clindamycin *OR*	20 mg/kg IV within 30 min before procedure (maximum 600 mg)
	Cefazolin or ceftriaxone[a]	25 mg/kg IM or IV within 30 min before procedure (maximum 1 g)

IM, Intramuscularly; *IV,* intravenously.
[a]Or other first- or second-generation oral cephalosporin in equivalent dose.
[b]Cephalosporins should not be used in an individual with a history of anaphylaxis, angioedema, or urticaria with peniclllins or ampicillin.
Adapted from American Academy of Pediatrics. Antimicrobial prophylaxis. In Pickering LK, Baker CJ, Long SS, et al, eds. *Red Book: 2006 Report of the Committee on Infectious Diseases.* 27th ed. Elk Grove Village, IL: American Academy of Pediatrics; 2006.

Table 62-6 Insulin Regimen for Procedures Lasting Less Than 2 Hours

INSULIN	DAY BEFORE PROCEDURE	DAY OF PROCEDURE
Mixed insulin	Usual intermediate or long acting	50% intermediate or long
Short acting	Usual short acting	No short acting
Glargine (Lantus)	Take usual dose the night before OR	Take no insulin
	Take none night before	Full daily dose
Insulin pump	Normal rate	Normal rate

Perioperative evaluation of diabetic patients includes determination of their insulin regimen and an assessment of the adequacy of their metabolic control. Electrolyte levels should be normal, no evidence of ketonuria should be seen, and the patient's HbA_{1C} level should be within the endocrinologist's acceptable range. The HbA_{1C} level is a dynamic reflection of mean blood glucose level during the previous 8 to 12 weeks.

Perioperative evaluation of the diabetic patient should be directed to determine whether the child is experiencing any end-organ dysfunction. Many systemic manifestations of diabetes mellitus exist, including renal microangiopathy, coronary artery disease, hypertension, retinopathy, peripheral neuropathies, delayed gastric emptying, and limited joint mobility. Limited joint mobility is the result of abnormal cross-linkage of collagen by nonenzymatic glycosylation in the presence of chronic hyperglycemia. Involvement of the cervical spine and temporomandibular joints can result in difficulties with laryngoscopy and intubation of diabetic patients.[105] Many of these complications appear as cumulative effects of diabetes, often associated with poor glucose control and only rarely seen in childhood.[102,106] A notable exception is delayed gastric emptying in diabetic children. More than 50% of children have delayed gastric emptying; elevated HbA_{1C} levels and hyperglycemia are risk factors.[107] Diabetic children require careful preoperative evaluation and planning, which may require input from the child's PCP and endocrinologist to the anesthesia and surgery teams.[108]

Preoperative Insulin Regimen

The regimen for managing diabetes during the preoperative period should be established in consultation with the child's endocrinologist and should aim toward maintaining blood glucose levels between 100 and 200 mg/dL. Most diabetic patients can undergo minor surgical procedures with insulin administered subcutaneously, as outlined in Table 62-6.

Diabetic patients should be the first case of the day, and blood glucose levels should be measured on patients' arrival to the preoperative preparation area. If the blood glucose level is greater than 250 mg/dL, then subcutaneous regular insulin or an insulin pump bolus should be administered according to a sliding scale to decrease the glucose level to 150 mg/dL.

Management Recommendations for Diabetic Children on Insulin Injections for Procedures Requiring NO Insulin Infusion

Consider for any short procedure that will cause minimal change in oral feeding postoperatively

Patient Name: ______________________________ DOB: ____________

Date: __________ Expected Date of Surgery: __________ (Patient should be scheduled as first case.)

1. Recommendations for family for **insulin dosing the day before and the morning of surgery:**
   AM ______________ Dinner ______________
   *Children taking Lantus/Levemir should reduce evening dose by 10%.
   PM ______________ Morning of surgery ______________
2. Recommendations for family for **oral agents** day before and morning of surgery.
   Please Note: Metformin (Glucophage) must be discontinued 48 hours before surgery and any procedures using contrast dye.
3. The patient should follow preoperative feeding instructions provided by surgical staff.
4. Obtain blood glucose on arrival.
   If hyperglycemic, consider administering Humalog/Novolog insulin to correct hyperglycemia. Usual subcutaneous correction factor for this patient: 1 unit Humalog/Novolog corrects blood sugar ___ mg/dL
   Consider canceling or postponing surgery if blood glucose is over 400 mg/dL **AND ketones are in urine.**
5. Check blood sugars hourly perioperatively.
   If blood sugar is over 300 mg/dL: Consider touching up with Humalog/Novolog.
   If blood sugar is below 80 mg dL: Consider 2 cc/kg D10W (if NPO) or 15 g of carbohydrate (by mouth).
6. Dip all urine for ketones.
7. Call Endocrine Fellow in case of ketones, vomiting, or persistent low blood sugars (<80 mg/dL).
8. Allow child to ingest fluids or food postoperatively per surgical protocol. When child is tolerating oral foods and liquids, the family may resume home insulin regimen. Begin subcutaneous insulin at mealtime if possible.
9. Additional instructions:
   ____
   ____
   ____

Signature of Diabetes APN ______________________________

Signature of Endocrine Attending ______________________________

Forward copy of completed form with last clinic letter to:

1. Endocrine Fellows
2. Surgical department attention
3. Preanesthesia testing

GIVE 1 COPY TO FAMILY

Figure 62-7 Insulin regimen for short procedures used at The Children's Hospital of Philadelphia. *(Used by permission of The Children's Hospital of Philadelphia.)*

For major procedures, or if the child has brittle diabetes, a continuous infusion of insulin, along with an infusion of glucose to maintain a blood glucose level between 150 and 200 mg/dL is suggested. Many institutions prohibit use of the patient's insulin pump intraoperatively with conversion to a continuous intravenous infusion. Hourly blood glucose measurements are performed throughout the procedure, and additional glucose or insulin is titrated as appropriate. Examples of perioperative insulin regimens used at the Children's Hospital of Philadelphia are shown in Figures 62-7 and 62-8.

Congenital Adrenal Hyperplasia

Congenital adrenal hyperplasia (CAH) is the consequence of numerous autosomal-recessive enzymatic deficiencies that result in inadequate cortisol production. The most common form of CAH is 21-hydroxylase deficiency in which excess amounts of progesterone and 17-hydroxyprogesterone are produced. Peripherally, these hormones are converted to the androgens testosterone and dihydrotestosterone. Mineralocorticoid production is affected in 75% of these patients, the salt-wasters. Adrenal medullary secretion of catecholamines is deficient as well. If mineralocorticoid is not given, then salt-wasters lose sodium through the kidney, colon, and sweat glands and develop a hyponatremic dehydration, which rapidly progresses to shock, exacerbated by an inadequate catecholamine response to stress.[109]

Children with CAH require lifelong hormonal replacement. Hydrocortisone at 10 to 20 mg/m^2 in 3 divided doses is administered to provide physiological glucocorticoid coverage and to suppress adrenocorticotropic hormone–mediated androgen production. 17-Hydroxyprogesterone levels are monitored to ensure sufficient androgen suppression. Salt-wasting patients require fludrocortisone (Florinef) and sodium chloride supplementation. Plasma rennin activity may be monitored to determine the adequacy of these supplements.[110]

The focus on the preoperative evaluation of the patient with CAH is to characterize the exact nature of the enzymatic deficiency to know whether both the glucocorticoid and the mineralocorticoid arms of steroidogenesis are involved. State of hydration, blood pressure, and electrolytes are evaluated to determine the adequacy of baseline supplementation. The usual maintenance hydrocortisone dose is inadequate to cover physiological stresses such as a febrile illness or surgery. Febrile patients with CAH are usually given 2 to 3 times their routine dose of hydrocortisone in 3 divided doses. Patients scheduled for major surgery are given 100 mg/m^2 hydrocortisone in 4 divided intravenous doses for the first 24 hours and then tapered slowly. Some endocrinologists prefer to administer a continuous infusion of hydrocortisone during surgery.

Secondary Adrenal Insufficiency

Adrenal suppression is decreased adrenal function resulting from exposure to exogenous steroids. A patient who is adrenally suppressed may become adrenally insufficient and hypotensive when exposed to the stress of anesthesia and surgery. The hypotension of secondary adrenal insufficiency is the result of glucocorticoid deficiency, not mineralocorticoid deficiency. Glucocorticoids enhance the vasculature's response to catecholamines, in part, by inhibiting endothelial cell production of the vasodilator prostaglandin I2. Aldosterone secretion is regulated through the renin-angiotensin system and thus is unperturbed during secondary adrenal insufficiency.[111]

Many children scheduled for anesthetics have received corticosteroids in the recent past. Who of these patients are at risk for developing an adrenal crisis in the perioperative period and therefore should be considered candidates for perioperative steroid replacement? Asthmatic children who received a single 5-day course of high-dose systemic steroids have normal adrenal function by 10 days after treatment.[112] Children who have received at least 3 courses of high-dose burst (5 days) systemic steroids within the previous year in addition to their maintenance inhaled steroids have no evidence of adrenal dysfunction 30 days after the last burst.[113] Patients receiving prolonged therapy for more than 3 weeks, evening doses, and continuous dosing (versus alternate-day dosing) are more likely to have adrenal insufficiency, which may take more up to a year to resolve.[114]

Inhaled corticosteroids also affect the hypothalamic-pituitary-adrenal axis.[115] Fluticasone appears to be the most potent of the inhaled steroids,[116] with children receiving high-dose inhaled fluticasone at greater than 400 mcg/day at risk for the development of spontaneous adrenal crisis.[117] Fluticasone at doses greater than 500 mcg/day causes adrenal suppression in 20% of children.[118] Although children receiving high doses of fluticasone may undergo a cosyntropin stimulation test to determine their risk for adrenal suppression,[119] if they do not, the best course is to administer *stress-dose* steroid perioperatively to cover this possibility. Intranasal steroids can also cause adrenal suppression in children.[120]

Even though the incidence of perioperative adrenal insufficiency of any cause is low, it remains a significant hazard for a small population of children. Box 62-5 lists the situations in which patients should receive perioperative steroids, and suggested doses are listed in Table 62-7.

Thyroid Disease

Hypothyroidism

Hypothyroidism in children is either congenital or acquired. Developmental defects of the thyroid are the most common cause of congenital hypothyroidism. Hashimoto thyroiditis is the most common noniatrogenic cause of hypothyroidism. Children with Hashimoto thyroiditis may have other autoimmune mediated disease, including primary adrenal insufficiency.

Patients with undertreated hypothyroidism have multisystem disease that can have profound anesthetic implications, the most important of which is cardiovascular dysfunction (Box 62-6). Deficiency in thyroid hormone depresses myocyte adenosine triphosphatase (ATPase) activity, and decreases the rate of calcium uptake, and decreases expression of sodium-potassium-ATPase (Na^+-K^+-ATPase) and β-adrenergic receptors.[121,122] Peripheral vascular resistance is also increased because of the absence of the vasodilatory

Management Recommendations for Diabetic Children on Insulin Injections for Procedures Requiring Insulin Infusion

Consider for any procedure that is long in duration or may interfere with oral feeding after surgery

Patient Name: ______________________ DOB: ______________

Date: ______________ Expected Date of Surgery: ______________

1. Recommendations for family for **insulin dosing** day before and morning of surgery:
   AM ____________ Dinner ________ *Children on Lantus should reduce the evening dose by 10%.
   PM ____________ Morning of surgery **HOLD MORNING INSULIN**
2. Recommendations to family for **oral agents** day before and morning of surgery.
   PLEASE NOTE: Metformin (Glucophage) must be discontinued 48 hours before surgery and any procedures using contrast dye.
3. The patient should follow preoperative feeding instructions provided by surgery.
4. Obtain blood glucose on arrival.
   Consider canceling or postponing surgery if blood glucose is over 400 mg/dL **AND any ketones are in urine.**
5. Begin insulin infusion and D10W by intravenous route simultaneously. Insulin infusion should be started before 8 AM, and at least 2 hours prior to beginning of the surgical procedure.
6. Initial intravenous insulin infusion recommendations for this patient:
   10% dextrose with electrolytes at maintenance levels
   - Regular insulin at 0.02-0.05 units/kg/hr as detailed below:
     - Select 0.02 units/kg/hr if blood sugar is 80-200 mg/dL at beginning of infusion.
     - Select 0.02 units/kg/hr if child received Lantus insulin the night before.
     - Select 0.03 units/kg/hr if blood sugar is 200-300 mg/dL.
     - Select 0.04 units/kg/hr if blood sugar is 300-400 mg/dL.
     - Select 0.05 units/kg/hr if blood sugar is >400 mg/dL at beginning of infusion.
7. Check blood sugars hourly while on insulin infusion. Titrate infusion (by increments of 0.01 units/kg/hr) and intravenous fluids to keep blood glucose levels 80-180 mg/dL.
8. Dip all urine for ketones.
9. Call Endocrine Fellow if you have questions regarding insulin infusion. Call Endocrine Fellow in case of ketones, vomiting, or persistent low blood sugars (<80 mg/dL).
10. Additional instructions:
    ____
    ____
    ____

Signature of Diabetes APN ______________________________

Signature of Endocrine Attending ______________________________

Forward copy of completed form with last clinic letter to:
1. Endocrine Fellows
2. Surgical department attention
3. Preanesthesia testing

GIVE 1 COPY TO FAMILY

Figure 62-8 Insulin regimen for longer procedures used at The Children's Hospital of Philadelphia. *(Used by permission of The Children's Hospital of Philadelphia.)*

BOX 62-5 Situations in Which *Stress-Dose* Steroid Coverage is Necessary

- Less than 10 days after a burst (5 days) of steroids
- Less than 30 days after completion of the last of multiple short courses of steroids
- Less than 1 year after completing a prolonged course of steroids (>3 mo)
- Previously treated with fluticasone over 500 mcg/dL
- Daily parenteral or enteral steroids for more than 3 weeks
- Evening doses of steroids
- Impaired response to cosyntropin stimulation test

Table 62-7 Stress-Dose Steroid Recommendations

DEGREE OF SURGICAL STRESS	DOSE
Minor: <1 hr (eg, hernia)	Hydrocortisone 25 mg/m^2 IV Methylprednisolone 5 mg/ m^2 IV
Moderate: extremity surgery	Hydrocortisone 50 mg/m^2 IV Methylprednisolone 10 mg/m^2 IV Or usual oral dose and reduced parenteral dose
Major: laparotomy	Hydrocortisone 25 mg/m^2 IV every 6 hr* Methylprednisolone 5 mg/m^2 IV 6 hr* Wean over 1-3 days

*At start of surgery through the operative day. May return to maintenance steroid administration on the first postoperative day if the patient is stable.
IV, Intravenous.

effect of triiodothyronine (T3). Although the cardiovascular profile of a patient with hypothyroidism would suggest a depressed adrenergic tone, catecholamine levels are elevated but ineffective because of the down regulation of the β-adrenergic receptors.[123]

The primary objective in the preoperative patient with a history of hypothyroidism is to confirm that the patient is euthyroid. If the thyroxine (T4) level is low and the thyroid-stimulating hormone level is elevated, *elective* surgical procedures should be postponed for at least 2 weeks to allow for adequate thyroxine supplementation. Children recently diagnosed as having hypothyroidism and those who have an unexpected bradycardia should undergo a cardiologic evaluation to determine the extent of their myocardial involvement. T4 supplementation in the perioperative period should be managed in collaboration with a pediatric endocrinologist. Measurement of an 8-AM cortisol level is useful in establishing whether the child has occult adrenal dysfunction. Although levothyroxine has a half-life of 6 to 7 days, the practice of the authors is to have children take their medication on the morning of surgery.[124]

BOX 62-6 Organ System Dysfunction Caused by Hypothyroidism

CARDIAC
- Myocardial depression
- Bradycardia, Torsades de pointes
- Hypotension 2nd-degree baroreceptor dysfunction
- Decreased intravascular volume

RESPIRATORY
- Blunted ventilatory response to hypoxia and hypercapnia

PHARMACOLOGIC
- Increased sensitivity to depressant effects of anesthetic agents
- Hypothermia
- Reduced metabolic rate
- Adrenal insufficiency
- Delayed gastric emptying

Hyperthyroidism

The most common causes of hyperthyroidism in children are the transient neonatal congenital form and Graves disease. Transient neonatal hyperthyroidism results from transplacental transfer of thyroid-stimulating immunoglobulins from the mother. The infant's hyperthyroid state resolves with clearance of maternal immunoglobulins. These infants can have congestive heart failure with profound respiratory distress. Graves disease is an autoimmune disease that commonly occurs in adolescents, with only modest cardiovascular manifestations.

Hyperthyroidism produces a hypermetabolic state that exhibits as hyperthermia, tachycardia, systolic hypertension, palpitations, and dysrhythmias. During the perioperative period, undertreated patients with hyperthyroidism can have thyroid storm with malignant hyperthermia-like symptoms. Adrenal reserve may be limited in patients with hyperthyroidism as well. Corticosteroids, because of their ability to block peripheral conversion of T4 to T3, have been shown to improve outcomes in patients with thyroid storm.[125] In addition to antithyroid medications and potassium iodide, ß-blockers are useful in the management of these children. Not only do they attenuate the cardiovascular effects of excess T3, but they also block the peripheral conversion of T4 to T3. ß-Blockers should be titrated to restore the child's heart rate to age appropriate norms.

Children with hyperthyroidism should have clinical and chemical evidence of a euthyroid state before elective procedures. Elective procedures may need to be delayed until a euthyroid state is established. Children with goiters should undergo sufficient imaging to delineate the extent of airway compromise.

HEMATOLOGIC DISEASES

Hematologic conditions that may complicate perioperative management include anemia, sickle cell disease, and the presence of a bleeding diathesis (eg, factor deficiency syndromes, long-term aspirin therapy).

Anemia is associated with a reduction in the oxygen-carrying capacity and a secondary increase in cardiac output. Anemia is often well tolerated; unfortunately, many perioperative events (eg, blood loss, anesthesia-induced myocardial depression) can subject the child whose cardiac function is intact and compensated to cellular hypoxia and cardiovascular collapse when the stresses of anesthesia and surgery overwhelm the anemic patient's delicate balance of oxygen demand and supply. Furthermore, an anemic child is more likely to need blood transfusions perioperatively if significant bleeding occurs, whereas even in the setting of moderate amounts of blood loss, avoidance of administering blood products to children who have normal preoperative hemoglobin levels is common. Although the hemoglobin value at which individual anesthesiologists choose to transfuse varies greatly, most anesthesiologists allow a normal child's hemoglobin to decline to 7 to 8 g/dL before transfusing blood.

A child who has a previously undiagnosed anemia may have a serious underlying disorder such as sickle cell anemia or a blood dyscrasia that requires additional evaluation before surgery. Thus the cause of any significant anemia (hemoglobin <9 g/dL) should be determined preoperatively. Nutritional causes (eg, iron deficiency) often require relatively brief periods of therapy to improve the child's anemia. The presence of a mild anemia should not delay urgent surgery. For elective surgery, consultation with the anesthesia and surgical teams may be required.

Sickle Cell Disease

Hemoglobin (Hgb) is a tetramer protein consisting of 2 α-globins and 2 β-globins. The hemoglobinopathies occur as a result of various mutations of the α- and β-genes. Sickle cell anemia results from a single base mutation in the β-globin gene, which substitutes valine for glutamine in position 6 of the β-chain, and places a highly reactive hydroxyl group on the globin's surface. As a result, under conditions of hypoxia, acidosis and cold temperature, Hgb S can polymerize. When one β-chain gene is inherited, the patient has sickle cell trait. When 2 β-chain genes are inherited, the patient has sickle cell anemia; a smaller number of patients can have mixed hemoglobinopathies in which a β-chain gene coexists with other mutations of the β chain, such as Hgb SC and Hgb S-β thalassemia. Clinically, 30% of patients with Hgb SS have a rapidly progressive course, leading to early end-organ failure and death, 60% have a less catastrophic course, and 10% are relatively well for most of their lives.[126,127]

Physiological Features

The physiological consequences of sickle cell anemia are chronic hemolysis, recurrent episodes of vaso-occlusion and severe pain, chronic inflammation, and progressive end-organ damage, leading to premature death. The instability of Hgb S contributes to rapid breakdown of the hydrophobic globin pocket, and oxidation of the iron (Fe^{2+}) heme to the Fe^{3+} of methemoglobin. This autooxidation generates destructive oxidative free radicals, which, along with free Fe^{+}, accumulate in the membrane structures of the sickled red blood cell.[128] Increased cell membrane iron disrupts membrane ion transport channels, contributing to intracellular dehydration, which is essential for sickling.[129] The injured red cell membrane adheres more avidly to the vascular endothelium, exposing the endothelial cell to increased oxidative stress and shearing forces, ultimately resulting in a state of chronic vascular inflammation, with important perturbations of vascular tone, coagulation, and fibrinolysis.[130] The cumulative damage to the red cell membrane of the patient with Hgb SS increases its fragility, producing a state of chronic hemolysis. Not only is anemia the consequence of this hemolysis, but also cell free Hgb scavenges and inactivates nitric oxide, and thus decreased bioavailability of nitric oxide results in inability to modulate ongoing vascular inflammation and endothelial cell dysfunction.

Vasoocclusion

Vasoocclusion, the clinical hallmark of sickle cell disease, is likely to be the result of acute changes in endothelial cell function on a foundation of chronic inflammation. Triggered by infection, surgical stress, or poor perfusion, adhesion molecules are expressed by the endothelial cells, which bind neutrophils to the vascular endothelium, with resultant proteolytic damage. Platelets are activated and aggregate at the sites of endothelial cell damage, initiating the hemostatic cascade. Thrombus formation and increased expression of adhesion molecules accentuate red cell adhesion and slow erythrocyte transit time to enable microvascular sickling to occur.[131] Perceived pain is probably the integrated response to the inflammation, ischemia, and infarction of vasoocclusion. The average rate of vasoocclusive crises is 0.8 per patient year. Although 39% of sickle cell patients have no crises, 1% have more than 6 episodes per year.[126]

Complications

Sickle cell disease is also characterized by progressive end-organ dysfunction. Pulmonary and neurologic diseases are the leading cause of morbidity and mortality.[126] Acute pulmonary complications of sickle cell anemia include reactive airway disease, pulmonary thromboembolism, and acute chest syndrome. The acute chest syndrome (ACS), an acute multifactorial process, is characterized by a new pulmonary infiltrate on chest radiograph, often associated with an increased oxygen requirement, respirophasic pain, fever, tachypnea, cough, and wheezing. Common causes include infection (*Chlamydia pneumoniae, Mycoplasma pneumoniae,* and respiratory syncytial virus), pulmonary infarction, bone marrow or fat embolism, and surgical procedures.[132] At the level of the pulmonary endothelial cell, an imbalance between adhesive forces and nitric oxide is created, favoring intrapulmonary sickle cell adhesion.[133] Compared with Hgb SS, the incidence of ACS is 33% in patients with Hgb S-β^0 thalassemia, 50% in patients with Hgb SC, and 25% or less in patients with Hgb S-β^+ thalassemia.[134] Up to 20% of children in the perioperative period will have an episode of ACS, with the highest risk being the age group between 2 and 4 years.[132,135] ACS usually develops 48 to 72 hours after the surgical procedure and may not be immediately obvious. ACS is the second most common complication of sickle cell disease, with a rate of 12.8 cases per 100 patient years, and is the leading cause of death, being responsible for up to 25% of sickle cell deaths.[136] The mortality rate in children is 1.1% and 3% overall.[126]

Sickle cell disease's chronic inflammatory state contributes to an obstructive reactive airway disease, as well as progressive pulmonary fibrosis, restrictive lung disease, and ultimately cor pulmonale and severe hypoxemia. Children with sickle cell disease are twice as likely to have reactive airway disease as their peers with normal Hgb levels. Both atopy and asthma are more common in children with Hgb SS who have had multiple ACS episodes than in those who have had a single or no episode.[137,138] The progression from sickle cell reactive airway disease in childhood to chronic restrictive pulmonary disease in adulthood is common; 10% of adolescents have pulmonary hypertension, 15% of adults have irreversible chronic lung disease, and 40% have secondary pulmonary hypertension.[139-141] Intravascular hemolysis, by scavenging nitric oxide and causing endothelial cell dysfunction, may play a role in the development of pulmonary hypertension. Patients who develop sickle cell chronic lung disease have a history of recurrent ACS episodes.[142] The 2-year mortality rate of sickle cell pulmonary hypertension is 50% compared with 2% in patients without pulmonary hypertension.[143] Echocardiographic demonstration of a high-velocity tricuspid regurgitant jet is useful in identifying patients with pulmonary hypertension.[144] Obstructive sleep apnea and nocturnal hypoxemia are common in children with sickle cell disease. Proposed mechanisms for nocturnal hypoxemia include OSAS caused by adenotonsillar hypertrophy and the chronic pulmonary disease of sickle cell disease.[145] Adenotonsillectomy results in the reduction of nocturnal hypoxemia and a decrease in the frequency of vasoocclusive crises.[146]

Patients with thalassemias and other hemoglobinopathies are also predisposed to the development of pulmonary hypertension. Up to 40% of patients with thalassemia intermedia and 75% of patients with thalassemia major have echocardiographic evidence of pulmonary hypertension.[147,148]

Sickle cell disease is the main cause of stroke in children. As a result of abnormalities on the red cell surface and activation of the coagulation system, up to 10% of children with sickle cell disease will experience a stroke, at a median age of 6 years.[149] A history of ACS, but specifically 1 episode within the previous 2 weeks, is an important risk factor, as is infantile dactylitis.[141,150] As many as 20% of children will have MRI evidence of clinically silent cerebral vascular infarctions, which are predictive of an increased risk for further strokes.[151,152] The transcranial Doppler (TCD) ultrasound measurement of increased flow velocity in the internal carotid and middle cerebral arteries is a useful screening test to determine who is at risk for stroke. Patients with the highest TCD velocities are more likely to have silent MRI lesions. The stroke risk for children with high TCD velocities is decreased from 10% to less than 1% per year with regular transfusion therapy.[153] Nocturnal oxygen saturations of less than 96% is also a risk factor for a cerebrovascular event.[154]

In the perioperative period, children with sickle cell disease are at high risk for vasoocclusive crises, ACS, transfusion associated events, stroke, and priapism. Because these perioperative complications specific to sickle cell disease are common, ranging from 15% to 20%, the preoperative assessment of the child with sickle cell disease must include a thorough investigation of end-organ damage, which puts the child at increased risk for these complications. The following variables must be evaluated: the planned procedure, the patient's age, current disease activity, cumulative disease severity (eg, hospitalizations, exchange transfusions), history of ACS episodes, abnormal chest radiograph, abnormal TCD velocity, abnormal MRI, preexisting infections, and pregnancy.

Procedures and Hospitalizations

Surgical procedures are stratified by the risk of these perioperative complications for the patient with sickle cell disease. In the nonpregnant patient, extremity procedures and hernia repairs are considered low risk. Intermediate risk procedures include tonsillectomy and adenoidectomy, hip surgery, and intraabdominal surgery. Complications occur in 15% of children undergoing tonsillectomy and adenoidectomy. Sickle cell patients undergoing myringotomy had a disproportionate incidence of postoperative complications compared with the general population.[155] Evidence is evolving that patients undergoing laparoscopic procedures may have a lower incidence of ACS when compared with those undergoing open procedures.[156,157] Intraocular, intrathoracic, and intracranial procedures are considered high risk.

The child's current disease activity is easily assessed by review of recent hospitalizations. An increase in the number of hospitalizations in the year preceding surgery is an independent predictor of perioperative vasoocclusive crisis.[158] A history of pulmonary disease is a significant independent predictor of perioperative complications.[159] Early onset of dactylitis is an early indicator of severe disease.[160] Increased age is also independently associated with an increased perioperative incidence of pain crises and ACS episodes, presumably the result of cumulative end-organ damage. Coexisting urinary or respiratory tract infections are associated with an increase in perioperative ACS.[131] A clustering of ACS episodes proximate to a surgical procedure is indicative of progressive pulmonary disease. An abnormal chest radiograph, a change in exercise tolerance, or work of breathing indicate the need for pulmonary function tests to determine the severity of the patient's underlying disease and whether preoperative bronchodilators might help optimize their underlying pulmonary disease. The importance of a history of pulmonary disease is seen in the 3-fold increase risk of perioperative complications in sickle cell patients undergoing tonsillectomy and adenoidectomy.[155] Unfortunately, patients with sickle cell disease may have silent progression of their pulmonary disease that only comes to clinical attention in a notable fashion in the perioperative period.

Limited data are available on the perioperative complications of the other hemoglobinopathies. Apparently, patients with Hgb SC are at slightly increased risk for vasoocclusive crises and at a much higher risk for ACS. Patients with Hgb S-β^+ thalassemia and Hgb S-β^0 thalassemia appear to be at a somewhat lower risk for perioperative vasoocclusive crises and ACS.[161]

Preoperative Preparation

Historically, many patients with sickle cell disease had preoperative double volume exchange transfusions or simple red cell transfusions in an effort to dilute the population of sickle cells and therefore decrease the incidence of perioperative sickle cell disease complications. However, these transfusions are not without their own risk. The risks of perioperative complications in patients with sickle cell disease should be balanced with the risks of simple and exchange transfusions. No differences have been found between a preoperative simple transfusion regimen (goal Hgb >10 g/dL) and an aggressive transfusion regimen (exchange or serial transfusions goal Hgb S, 30%). However, the incidence of transfusion related complications has been found to be twice as high in the aggressive transfusion group.[159] In patients undergoing cholecystectomy, no differences have been found between those receiving aggressive transfusions compared with those receiving conservative transfusions, although the perioperative complication rate is almost twice as high in patients who do not receive transfusions.[158] In addition, no differences in the incidence of perioperative complications has been found among patients undergoing orthopedic procedures who were randomized to aggressive transfusion, conservative transfusion, or no transfusion, with the exception of ACS occurrence. ACS occurs 3 times more in both the aggressively transfused and the nontransfused groups compared with the conservatively transfused group.[162] No prospective studies have examined varying transfusion practices in patients with sickle cell disease undergoing intrathoracic or intracranial procedures. Data are also limited for the other hemoglobinopathies; thus recommendations for preoperative preparation of these patients are less evidence based. In patients with Hgb SC disease undergoing a variety of surgical procedures, 35% of patient who did not receive preoperative transfusions suffered preoperative sickle cell–related complications, including 2 deaths; no sickle cell–related complications were noted in the transfused group.[163]

At this point, the number of randomized studies is insufficient to establish evidence-based guidelines for blood transfusions in the perioperative period.[164] As such, a suggested approach to the individual child with sickle cell disease focuses on the child's specific risk factors, in close collaboration with the pediatric hematologist and other pediatric subspecialists. Children undergoing minor elective surgical procedures may not require a preoperative transfusion, based on their risk profile. Patients at higher risk for adverse perioperative events are listed in Box 62-7.

BOX 62-7 High-Risk Patients With Sickle Cell

Sickle cell chronic lung disease
Frequent acute chest syndrome
Reactive airway disease
Abnormal chest radiograph
Abnormal pulmonary function test
History of stroke
High transcranial Doppler velocity
On chronic transfusion protocols

A patient meeting any of these criteria will usually receive some form of perioperative transfusion. Both simple transfusions to achieve an Hgb level greater than 10 g/dL and exchange transfusions to reduce the Hgb S level to less than 30% may be used; the more concerning the child's risk profile is, the more appropriate it is to choose a double-volume exchange transfusion. Children who are already on a long-term transfusion program should have their transfusions scheduled within 1 week of the planned procedure. Patients with a history of recurrent ACS are given preoperative bronchodilators and corticosteroids as well.

Inherited Coagulopathies

von Willebrand disease (vWD) is the most common of the congenital bleeding disorders. Most patients with vWD have type 1 disease, which is a quantitative deficiency of von Willebrand factor (vWF). Ninety percent of patients with type 1 vWD will respond to DDAVP with a 2- to 3-fold increase in vWF.[165] These patients can undergo minor surgical procedures with preoperative DDAVP administered intravenously 30 minutes before the procedure. Because 10% of patients with type 1 vWD do not respond to DDAVP, advance determination of the quality of the response is fundamental to the preoperative evaluation of a patient with vWD.[166] Type 1 nonresponders, as well as patients with type 2 and type 3 vWD, require preoperative administration of plasma derived, human factor VIII concentrate (Humate-P), which has a high concentration of vWF.[167] *All* patients with vWD undergoing major surgical procedures require factor replacement preoperatively.

Hemophilia A, B, and C are cross-linked inherited deficiencies of factors VIII, IX, and XI, respectively. Perioperative management of these patients depends on the planned procedures. Patients undergoing major surgical procedures require factor VIII and factor IX levels that approximate 100% of normal from 30 minutes before the procedure, through the first postoperative week. Patients undergoing minor procedures can be covered with factor levels that are 50% of normal after the second postoperative day. Some patients with mild hemophilia A have a sufficient response to DDAVP to provide adequate protection for minor procedures. The bleeding diathesis of patients with hemophilia C is not directly correlated to factor levels. The need for fresh-frozen plasma transfusion in these patients should be determined by a pediatric hematologist.

Platelet Abnormalities

Children with congenital thrombocytopenias, such as Wiskott-Aldrich syndrome, Diamond-Blackfan syndrome, and thrombocytopenia absent radii, as well as the inherited thrombocytopathies, Glanzmann thrombasthenia, and Bernard-Soulier syndrome, usually require perioperative platelet transfusions.

ONCOLOGIC DISEASE

Children treated for malignancy frequently receive medications that have the potential to cause profound perianesthetic complications. Many of these children receive prolonged doses of corticosteroids as part of their chemotherapy, which puts them at risk for adrenal suppression. The anthracycline drugs—doxorubicin and daunomycin—can cause myocardial dysfunction, whereas mithramycin and bleomycin may cause pulmonary dysfunction. Many of the children's oncologic protocols include serial echocardiographic evaluations. The most recent echocardiographic report should be included in preoperative evaluation of these children.

CEREBRAL PALSY

Cerebral palsy (CP) is a polymorphic set of motor disorders with a wide spectrum of severity. Children with CP frequently require anesthesia for the neurologic, gastrointestinal, pulmonary, and orthopedic consequences of their neurologic deficits. Many children with CP have a dysfunctional swallow, increased salivation, gastroesophageal reflux, and chronic pulmonary aspiration of both oral and gastric contents. These processes, along with an ineffective gag and poor cough commonly result in the development of reactive airway disease and recurrent pneumonias. Up to one third of patients have a seizure disorder. Communication regarding medications to the anesthesiologist is essential for the optimal perioperative care of these patients.

The preoperative evaluation of these children should include assessment of room-air oxygen saturation and the degree of underlying reactive airway disease, as well as the presence of snoring and other obstructive symptoms suggestive of inadequate airway tone. Scheduling elective procedures between episodic exacerbations of reactive airway disease and aspiration pneumonia is challenging in the most severely affected patients. Given that many of these children have a continuous condition of heightened airway reactivity, the preoperative evaluation and preparative regimen is often directed toward ensuring that the child's pulmonary status is optimal. Chest radiographs may be helpful in the child who has had previous episodes of significant pulmonary consolidation. Patients with CP are not at increased risk for malignant hyperthermia.

GENETIC DISEASES

Patients with genetic diseases frequently pose significant challenges in the perianesthetic period.[167] Children with previously considered lethal genetic diseases are living well beyond the neonatal period and are undergoing increasingly complex diagnostic studies and therapeutic procedures to modulate the consequences of their underlying genotype.

In addition to their characteristic phenotypes, these children commonly have significant airway, pulmonary, cardiac, neuromuscular, liver, and renal diseases. Airway obstruction and hypoxemia are the most preeminent concerns resulting from abnormalities of the upper airway and trachea, altered chest wall mechanics and respiratory drive, and reduction in the pulmonary bed from either hypoplasia or destruction as the result of gastroesophageal reflux. Hypertension and dysrhythmias, cardiomyopathies, and structural heart disease are commonly seen in this group of patients and affect management in this period as well. Approximately 60% of the reported 10,000 genetic diseases have central or peripheral nervous system abnormalities.[164] The presence of neuromuscular diseases will often dictate specific drug use and technique for airway management.

DOWN SYNDROME

The perioperative evaluation of the child with Down syndrome (DS) focuses on the numerous associated anomalies that have perianesthetic implications. Craniofacial and upper airway anomalies affect airway patency and management. Airways obstruction often persists after adenotonsillectomy in these patients because of mid-face hypoplasia.[169] As a result of a smaller tracheal diameter than their peers, patients with DS usually require an endotracheal tube that is 1 to 2 sizes smaller.[170] Between 40% and 50% of patients with DS have associated congenital heart disease, often requiring surgical correction, with postoperative conduction defects or valvular dysfunction (or both), as well as the need for SBE prophylaxis. Pulmonary hypertension and pulmonary vascular disease results from these cardiac lesions, as well as upper airways obstruction and endothelial cell dysfunction.[171] Children with DS are at much higher risk for the development of pulmonary hypertension in the setting of chronic upper airways obstruction than children without DS.[64,67] Perioperative complications occur in 8% to 10% of patients with DS undergoing noncardiac surgery. These complications include severe bradycardia, airways obstruction, difficult intubation, postintubation croup, and bronchospasm.[172] Patients with DS have an incidence of OSAS as high as 57%, leading some investigators to suggest that all patients with DS should be screened with polysomnography for OSAS at the age of 3 to 4 years.[173]

Cervical spine instability can lead to catastrophic neurologic injuries in the perianesthetic period. Atlantoaxial instability is a unique characteristic of DS. As a result of laxity of the ligament that holds the odontoid process of 2nd cervical vertebra (C2) against the posterior aspect of the arch of C1, C1 subluxes anteriorly compressing the spinal cord (Figure 62-9). The prevalence of atlantoaxial instability in patients with DS is approximately 15%.[174-176] Atlantoaxial instability is screened with lateral flexion and extension views of the cervical spine, odontoid views, and measurements of the neural canal width.[177,178] An atlantoaxial distance interval of greater than 4 to 5 mm in any lateral view is abnormal (Figure 62-10).[179]

Controversy surrounds the concept of routine screening. Many maintain that plain-film radiographs are not reliable in predicting cervical cord compression and therefore do not advise routine preoperative screening of these children.[180] However, the American Academy of Pediatrics and the Special Olympics Medical Committee continue to recommend routine screening for all patients with DS between 3 and 5 years of age and those desiring to participate in Special Olympics events, respectively.[181]

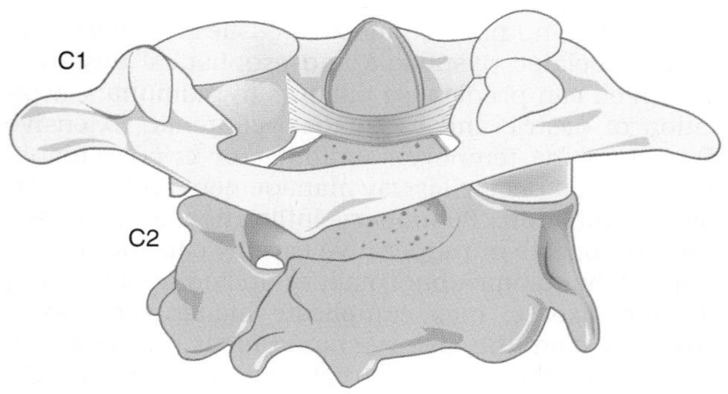

Figure 62-9 Relationship of the arch of C1 and odontoid process of C2. *(Hata T, Todd MM. Cervical spine considerations when anesthetizing patients with Down syndrome.* Anesthesiology. *2005;102:680-685. Reprinted by permission of Lippincott Williams & Wilkins.)*

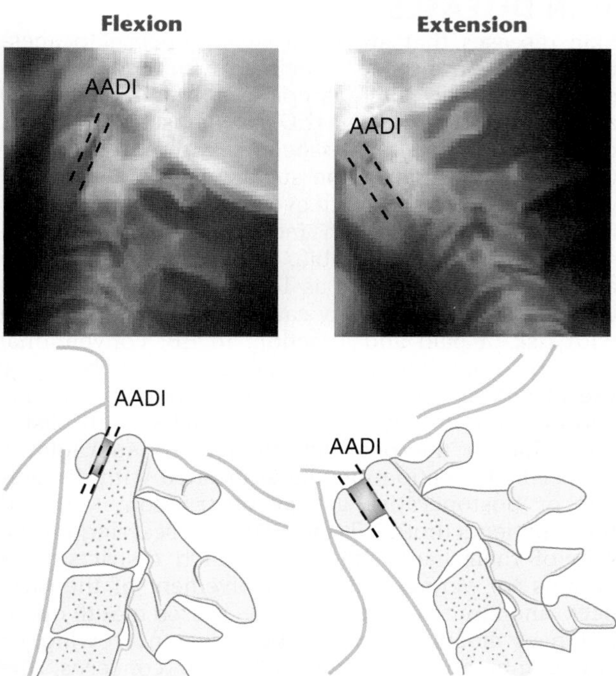

Figure 62-10 Increased distance (subluxation) between C1 and odontoid in Down syndrome. *(Hata T, Todd MM. Cervical spine considerations when anesthetizing patients with Down syndrome.* Anesthesiology. *2005; 102:680-685. Reprinted by permission of Lippincott Williams & Wilkins.)*

Parents should be asked questions concerning any recent changes in the child's neuromuscular functions, which might be indicative of cord impingement, such as loss of bowel or bladder control, sensory deficits, or motor changes. Even in the absence of symptoms, children who have DS and are 3 years or older should have lateral flexion and extension radiographs of the cervical spine before anesthesia is given so that patients at risk for subluxation can be identified. If radiographs reveal an atlantodens interval of greater than 5 mm (usually maximal in the flexion view), then the child should be referred for orthopedic or neurosurgical consultation before elective surgery.

Children younger than 3 years may be at risk, but neck radiographs will not be helpful in the diagnosis because of the lack of ossification of the structures. The anesthesiologist should use neck-protection strategies in this group of young patients.

MALIGNANT HYPERTHERMIA

First recognized as a cluster of anesthetic deaths in a family, malignant hyperthermia (MH) is an inherited disorder of skeletal muscle calcium channels, which is triggered in affected individuals by exposure to inhalational anesthetic agents, succinylcholine, or both.[182] The result is a MH crisis, which is a cascade of hypermetabolism, electrolyte derangements, arrhythmias, skeletal muscle damage, and hyperthermia, which progresses to death if untreated. The incidence of MH crisis is 1 in 15,000 general anesthetics in children.[183] The incidence increases if succinylcholine is given in addition to volatile anesthetics.[184] Appropriately treated, the mortality from a MH crisis is now estimated to be less than 10%.[185]

In the past when a patient had postoperative fever and rhabdomyolysis, MH was said to have occurred; however, other muscle abnormalities can occur in a similar fashion.[186] These other conditions are associated with abnormal increases in intracellular calcium, and these patients can have MH-like events.[187] Conditions that predispose patients to MH, rhabdomyolysis, or hyperkalemia are listed in Box 62-8. Many of these

BOX 62-8 Myopathies That Produce Malignant Hyperthermia–Like Symptoms

- Central core disease
- Duchenne muscular dystrophy
- Becker muscular dystrophy
- Myotonic dystrophy type 1
- Mitochondriopathy
- Brody myopathy
- Carnitinepalmityltransferase deficiency
- Evans syndrome
- King-Denborough syndrome

BOX 62-9 Mnemonic for Suggested Therapy for Malignant Hyperthermia

Some **H**ot **D**ude **B**etter **G**ive **I**ced **F**luids **F**ast

S Stop all trigger agents, administer 100% oxygen
H Hyperventilate: treat hypercarbia
D Dantrolene 2.5 mg/kg immediately
B Bicarbonate: treat acidosis: 1 mEq/kg
G Glucose and insulin: treat hyperkalemia: 0.5 g/kg glucose, 0.15 U/kg insulin
I Iced intravenous fluids, cooling blanket
F Fluids: ensure adequate urine output: furosemide, mannitol as needed
F Fast tachycardia: be prepared to treat ventricular tachycardia

From Zuckerberg AL. A hot mnemonic for the treatment of malignant hyperthermia. *Anesth Analg.* 1993;77:1077. Reprinted by permission of Lippincott Williams & Wilkins.

patients who in the past had been classified as having MH indeed had Duchenne muscular dystrophy instead.[188]

Most patients who are MH susceptible have normal history and physical examinations. Although some association has been found with cleft palate, ptosis, clubfoot, scoliosis, strabismus, and cryptorchidism, no evidence shows that these musculoskeletal abnormalities are related to a susceptibility to malignant hyperthermia.[189] Fifty percent of patients with MH have undergone a prior general anesthetic without complication.

The standard test to screen for MH susceptibility is the in vitro caffeine-halothane contracture test, which uses a muscle biopsy specimen. The indications for performing this test are a documented episode of hyperthermia, acidosis, and rhabdomyolysis induced by a triggering agent; an episode of masseter muscle spasm after exposure to a triggering agent; and availability of testable relatives of an MH-susceptible patient. However, this test has its limitations because it requires that the patient be at least 5 years of age and weigh 20 kg. Genetic screening, using the *RYR1* gene, has been reported. Relatives of patients who had a positive contracture test and a known causative mutation of *RYR1* were screened. The familial mutation was found in 50% of family members, characteristic of its autosomal dominance.[190] First- and second- degree family members of an MH-susceptible patient have a 50% and 25% risk, respectively, of being MH susceptible.[191]

Dantrolene, a muscle relaxant that reduces the release of calcium from muscle sarcoplasmic reticulum, has significantly improved patient outcomes. Current suggested therapy can be summarized by the mnemonic given in Box 62-9.[192]

CONNECTIVE TISSUE DISORDERS

Children who have connective tissue disorders may have multiple organ system involvement. These patients are often treated with aspirin or other nonsteroidal antiinflammatory drugs, which may complicate their perioperative management further by causing a bleeding diathesis resulting from platelet dysfunction. The effect of aspirin and nonsteroidal antiinflammatory drugs on platelet function is long lived, and their administration should be stopped 1 week preoperatively. If these drugs cannot be stopped, then a bleeding time may be performed to evaluate the extent of platelet impairment. Determination of prothrombin and partial thromboplastin times will not reflect this abnormality.

Patients who have connective tissue disorders may have associated dysphagia and esophageal dysmotility, which can predispose patients to pulmonary aspiration of gastric and esophageal contents. Extensive fibrosis of the temporomandibular or cricoarytenoid joint can complicate airway management and endotracheal intubation. Pulmonary infiltration and fibrosis may complicate intraoperative care by causing hypoxemia. Hematologic abnormalities, including anemia of chronic disease, may complicate management even further. Again, the history should focus on the extent of disease, the type of treatment, and the child's response to therapy. Laboratory assessment may include an ECG and a chest radiograph; electrolytes, blood urea nitrogen, creatinine, hemoglobin, hematocrit, and platelet levels; and evaluation of the peripheral blood smear. A patient who has quiescent disease and who has regular follow-up may need nothing other than hematocrit determination.

SKIN DISEASES

Skin diseases that are of greatest concern to anesthesiologists are those associated with increased fragility of the skin, such as epidermolysis bullosa (EB) and ectodermal dysplasia (ED). The most severe forms of these conditions are associated with blister formation and sloughing of the surface layers of the skin and oral mucosa (EB) with even minor trauma such as may be associated with moving the patient from stretcher to operating table. Use of all forms of tape and even dressings such as Tegaderm may be forbidden because removal may cause denuding of the skin with risk of pain and infection. In EB, conventional methods of intubation such as direct laryngoscopy or use of airway adjuncts, such as laryngeal mask airways or oral airways may be associated with blister formation in the pharynx, tongue, or supraglottic area. This formation may be associated with discomfort or postoperative airway obstruction. Many of these patients (both EB and ED) have scarring on the skin of their hands and feet, which restricts their options for venous access. Involvement of the face, neck, and mouth may result in decreased mouth opening, neck mobility, supraglottic airway narrowing, or any combination. Because of these concerns, the anesthesia team should have advanced notice of these patients' scheduling to afford the opportunity for complete face-to-face preoperative evaluation that will allow for appropriate consultation with the patient's dermatologist and PCP, followed by discussion with the family of risks and methods for skin protection and airway management.

MEDICATIONS

Children receive medications regularly for many illnesses. The dosage should be adjusted to ensure adequate therapeutic levels perioperatively. Administration of medications is ordinarily continued at usual doses up to and including the day of surgery. The 2 current exceptions to this practice are the use of monoamine oxidase (MAO) inhibitors and tricyclic antidepressants (TCAs). The MAO inhibitors are encountered infrequently in younger children and adolescents; however, TCAs, such as imipramine and its analogs, are used commonly in the treatment of enuresis. For children receiving MAO inhibitors, the administration of meperidine (Demerol) or pancuronium (Pavulon) can have profound, catastrophic consequences, for example, malignant hypertension and tachycardia.[193] The TCAs can produce significant conduction abnormalities undetected by electrocardiography; moreover, when combined with the volatile anesthetic halothane, TCAs have resulted in life-threatening arrhythmias in the perioperative period. Therefore discontinuing use of these agents 2 to 3 weeks before the scheduled operation is best. If discontinuation cannot be done without risk to the patient, then preoperative consultation with the anesthesiologist is necessary.

An increasing number of children are being treated for behavioral and depressive disorders with selective serotonin reuptake inhibitors such as fluoxetine (Prozac). Withdrawal can precipitate anxiety, agitation, and diaphoresis, and therefore the use of antidepressants should not be stopped to prepare for surgery.[194] Most of these drugs have such long elimination half-times that unless prolonged NPO periods are contemplated, withdrawal is unlikely perioperatively if only the preoperative dose is omitted. The anesthesiologist must be informed that patients are taking such drugs because interactions with other drugs administered perioperatively can lead to unexpected adverse effects. Fluoxetine, similar to other selective serotonin reuptake inhibitors, is a potent inhibitor of the hepatic cytochrome P-450 enzymes and therefore may result in elevated blood levels of these other drugs, which depend on these enzymes for metabolism.[195] A review of psychotropic drugs in the perioperative period advises discontinuation of use of lithium, MAO inhibitors, TCAs (eg, amitriptyline), and clozapine because of known drug-drug interactions.[196] Given that discontinued use of these medications may precipitate withdrawal or worsening of the underlying psychiatric disorder, such cessation of medications requires involvement of the patient's mental health professional.

An increasing number of children are taking newly introduced drugs for attention-deficit/hyperactivity disorder, such as Strattera, Concerta, and Adderall. At present, no evidence exists that these drugs adversely interact with anesthetics and sedatives, and therefore their use may be continued in the preoperative period. Reports of tachycardia and arrhythmias associated with the use of these drugs mandate vigilance for these events under anesthesia.

In addition, an increasing number of children, as are their parents, are taking herbal or homeopathic medications, which may lead to unexpected reactions to anesthetic drugs[197,198] (Table 62-8). Use of these substances should be disclosed to the anesthesiologist. Many anesthesiologists advise stopping use of all herbal supplements 2 weeks before a surgical procedure. Other investigators advise a more individualized approach, with different times for discontinuation of use of herbal medications, depending on their duration of action.[199] Web resources for information about herbal and homeopathic medications include the National Center for Complementary and Alternative Medicine (National Institutes of Health) (nccam.nih.gov), National Institutes of Health, Office of Dietary Supplements (dietary-supplements.info.nih.gov), and other Web sites (www.herbmed/org).

RELEVANT ASPECTS OF THE PHYSICAL EXAMINATION

The physical examination should determine the patient's general state of health with the aim of specifically discovering any conditions that might complicate anesthesia. The cardiovascular and respiratory systems demand close attention and documentation. Neurologic status should be evaluated and preexisting deficits specifically documented. Recording of all abnormalities will assist the anesthesiologist in developing an appropriate plan for the anesthesia to be administered.

The PCP should note the general body habitus, height, weight (in kg), and percentiles. An obese or cushingoid child can have significant hypoventilation or airways obstruction in the supine position and under anesthesia and is at increased risk for aspiration pneumonitis. A thorough examination of the head and neck is essential. A short neck, large tongue, and a small mandible all constitute sources of airway obstruction and may lead to delay or impossibility in intubating the trachea because of the difficulty in seeing the glottic opening (Figure 62-11). Midfacial or maxillary hypoplasia may present similar problems. In addition to difficulty with intubation, such patients may have airways obstruction on induction of anesthesia and difficulty with ventilation. Many congenital syndromes are associated with anatomic abnormalities that may cause difficulty with intubation. Some of the most common syndromes are listed in Table 62-9. Advance knowledge of patients with these conditions allows the anesthesia team to have required equipment for difficult airway management, such as fiberoptic bronchoscope, laryngeal mask airway, and light wands.[200]

In addition to having the aforementioned airway concerns, because of a large tongue and a relatively hypoplastic midface, patients who have DS may have atlantoaxial instability. This condition may exhibit only under general anesthesia and neuromuscular blockade and can result in damage to the cervical spinal cord.[176,180] Parents should be questioned about any neurologic symptoms such as long-tract signs (hyperreflexia, positive Babinski response, and clonus), hand weakness, or bladder and bowel dysfunction. History of torticollis or neck pain should be elicited.

Some *dwarfing* syndromes can be associated with airway and cardiorespiratory abnormalities that can present significant problems perioperatively. In all children, the presence of loose or fractured teeth must be documented to guard against potential aspiration

Table 62-8 Clinically Important Effects and Perioperative Concerns of Selected Herbal Medications With Recommendations for Preoperative Discontinuation

HERB: COMMON NAME(S)	RELEVANT PHARMACOLOGICAL EFFECTS	PERIOPERATIVE CONCERNS	PREOPERATIVE DISCONTINUATION
Echinacea: purple coneflower root	Activation of cell-mediated immunity	Allergic reactions; decreased effectiveness of immunosuppressants; potential for immunosuppression with long-term use	No data
Ephedra: ma huang	Increased heart rate and blood pressure through direct and indirect sympathomimetic effects	Risk of myocardial ischemia and stroke from tachycardia and hypertension; ventricular arrhythmias with halothane; long-term use depletes endogenous catecholamines and may cause intraoperative hemodynamic instability; life-threatening interaction with monoamine oxidase inhibitors	At least 24 hours before surgery
Garlic: ajo	inhibition of platelet aggregation (may be irreversible); increased fibrinolysis; equivocal antihypertensive activity	Potential to increase risk of bleeding, especially when combined with other medications that inhibit platelet aggregation	At least 7 days before surgery
Ginkgo: duck foot tree, maidenhair tree, silver apricot	inhibition of platelet-activating factor	Potential to increase risk of bleeding, especially when combined with other medications that inhibit platelet aggregation	At least 36 hours before surgery
Ginseng: American ginseng, Asian ginseng, Chinese ginseng, Korean ginseng	Lowers blood glucose; inhibition of platelet aggregation (may be irreversible); increased PT-PTT in animals; many other diverse effects	Hypoglycemia; potential to increase risk of bleeding; potential to decrease anticoagulation effect of warfarin	At least 7 days before surgery
Kava: awa, intoxicating pepper, kawa	Sedation, anxiolysis	Potential to increase sedative effect of anesthetics; potential for addiction, tolerance, and withdrawal after abstinence unstudied	At least 24 hours before surgery
St John's wort: amber, goat weed, hardhay, Hypericum, klamatheweed	Inhibition of neurotransmitter reuptake, monoamine oxidase inhibition is unlikely	Induction of cytochrome P450 enzymes, affecting cyclosporine, warfarin, steroids, protease inhibitors, and possible benzodiazepines, calcium channel blockers, and many other drugs; decreased serum digoxin levels	At least 5 days before surgery
Valerian: all heal garden heliotroper, vandal toot	Sedation	Potential to increase sedative effect of anesthetics; benzodiazepine-like acute withdrawal; potential to increase anesthetic requirements with long-term use	No data

PT-PTT, Indicates prothrombin time-partial thromboplastin time.

From Ang-Lee MK, Moss J, Yuan C. Herbal medicines and perioperative care. *JAMA.* 2001;286:208-216. Reprinted by permission of the American Medical Association.

Mallampati Signs as Indicators of Difficult Intubation

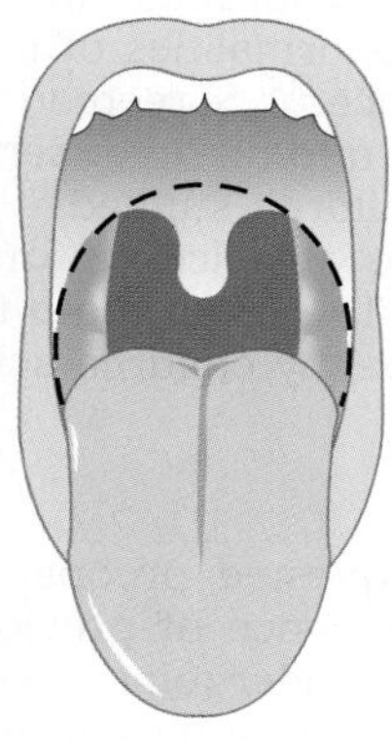

Class I
No difficulty
Soft palate, uvula, fauces and pillars visible

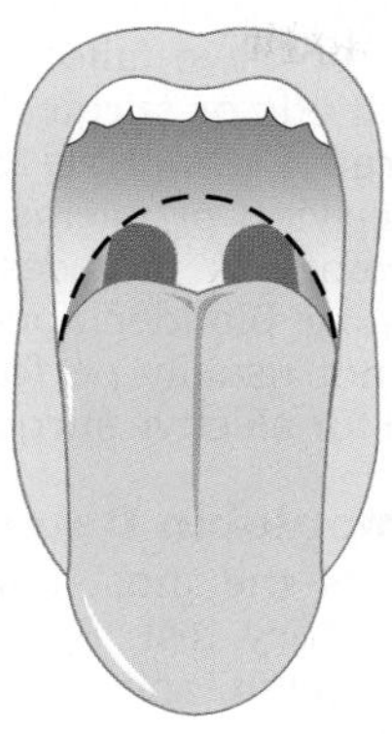

Class II
No difficulty
Soft palate, uvula, fauces visible

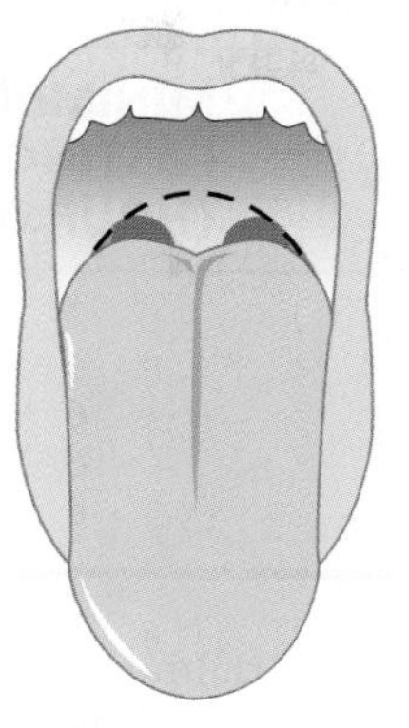

Class III
Moderate difficulty
Soft palate, base of uvula visible

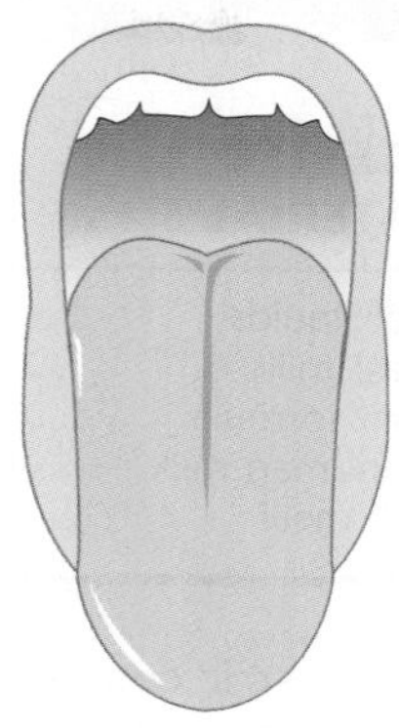

Class IV
Severe difficulty
Only hard palate visible

Figure 62-11 Mallampati airway classification. *(Modified from Euliano TY. Mallampati Classification, 2002. Available at: www.anesth.ufl.edu/at/case1/mallampati.hmtl.)*

Table 62-9 Examples of Syndromes Associated With Anatomic Abnormalities Which May Cause Difficult Intubation

SYNDROME	RELEVANT CLINICAL CHARACTERISTICS
Beckwith-Wiedemann	Macroglossia
Down (trisomy 21)	Macroglossia, midface hypoplasia, tracheal narrowing
Pierre Robin sequence	Micrognathia, cleft palate, glossoptosis
Treacher Collins	Hypoplasia of the maxilla and mandible
Hemifacial microsomia (Goldenhar)	Unilateral or bilateral mandibular hypoplasia, macrostomia
Apert	Craniosynostosis, midface hypoplasia
Freeman-Sheldon *(whistling face)*	Microstomia, facial anomalies
Mucopolysaccharidoses	Redundant facial, pharyngeal, and supraglottic soft tissue; neck immobility
Klippel Feil	Cervical vertebral fusion, neck immobility
Crouzon	Craniosynostosis, midface hypoplasia
Stickler	Mandibular hypoplasia, joint stiffness
Pfeiffer	Craniosynostosis, mid-face hypoplasia

Adapted from Litman RS. The difficult pediatric airway. In: Litman RS, ed. *Pediatric Anesthesia: The Requisites in Anesthesiology.* Philadelphia, PA: Mosby;2004. Copyright Elsevier 2004. Reprinted by permission.

because the teeth and oral mucosa may be subject to trauma during airway manipulation.

Preoperative vital signs, including weight (in kg), temperature, respiratory rate, heart rate, and blood pressure, should be recorded. Accurate weight measurement is essential because anesthetic drug dosing is calculated by weight. Preoperative recognition of any cardiovascular compromise may prevent significant perioperative problems. For example, patients who have significant chest wall or thoracic deformities (eg, severe scoliosis, dwarfism) can have marked cardiorespiratory compromise exhibited as decreased lung volumes and pulmonary function and can have myocardial strain evident on ECG or echocardiogram. Such patients are at risk for intraoperative complications and prolonged postoperative mechanical ventilation. Therefore they need preoperative pulmonary function studies and their myocardial function should be evaluated to enable the anesthesiologist to design the optimal anesthetic plan.

NOTHING BY MOUTH: THE PREOPERATIVE FAST

The most poorly understood and therefore the most emotional and contentious issue in the anesthesia-family-surgical interface is the "sacred caveat of preoperative fasting."[201] Patients with large volumes of

Table 62-10 Suggested Fasting Times for Oral Intake

INGESTED MATERIAL	MINIMUM FASTING (HOURS)
Clear liquids	2
Breast milk	4
Infant formula	6
Nonhuman milk	6
Light meal	6

acidic gastric contents are at risk for pulmonary aspiration and significant morbidity. Because this risk of pulmonary aspiration in healthy children is less than 0.05%, the practice of *NPO after midnight* has been abandoned; the American Society of Anesthesiology has revised the preoperative fasting guidelines (Table 62-10).[202]

Children are encouraged to drink clear liquids to minimize the anxiety, hypovolemia, and possible hypoglycemia that may result from a prolonged preoperative fast.[203] Long-term medications are administered with clear fluids on the morning of surgery. Healthy children are allowed to drink clear fluids until 2 hours preoperatively; breastfed infants can feed until 4 hours preoperatively; nonhuman milk and formula can be consumed until 6 hours before the scheduled procedure.[204] Despite the suggestion of the acceptability of a 6-hour fast after a *light meal,* most solid food meals have a high fat content, which delays gastric emptying. Because of these factors, many pediatric anesthesiologists require a fast of 8 hours after solid food for elective surgery. Gum chewing increases gastric fluid volume at least 2 fold, without clinically significant important buffering of the pH of the gastric fluid and therefore is generally proscribed in the preoperative period.[205] To avoid confusion, institutions' pediatric anesthesiology division should be consulted to determine their specific practice protocols.

The practice of a preoperative fast has come under intense attack by many nonanesthesiologists who are providing deep sedation or actual anesthesia using potent sedative or hypnotic medications such as propofol. Numerous studies of sedation in nonfasted children have been performed, with no reports of pediatric aspiration. Given the rarity of a severe aspiration complication, rather than encouraging the conclusion that this practice is a safe one, the impression of the authors is that this literature only leads us to a classic type II error. Until a sufficiently powered study is available, a preanesthetic fast, tempered with the liberal administration of clear fluids as outlined in Table 62-10 is suggested.

PREOPERATIVE LABORATORY EVALUATION

Laboratory studies are performed to detect significant physiological or metabolic abnormalities that may increase risk to the child in the perioperative period. In an otherwise healthy child scheduled for outpatient surgery, routine laboratory tests are rarely indicated. Routine preoperative chest radiographs in well children have failed to detect abnormalities of major anesthetic or surgical consequence.[206] Screening preoperative urinalysis also has failed to discover serious underlying problems in most children studied[207] and therefore is unnecessary in the absence of known renal or bladder abnormalities. Therefore these tests are not usually performed in healthy children scheduled for elective surgery.

Hemoglobin Determination

Hgb is the most commonly requested preoperative laboratory test. Because the incidence of previously undetected anemia in children undergoing elective surgery is extremely low (0.29%),[208] *routine determination of hematocrit and Hgb is not necessary* if the results of studies performed previously as part of well-child care have been normal. A selective Hgb determination should be used in children with chronic medical illnesses and those about to undergo procedures with the potential for significant blood loss.[209] Infants younger than 6 months should have their preoperative Hgb level measured because the physiological nadir of red blood cell production may cause the Hgb level to decrease as low as 7 g/dL. In addition, in ex-premature infants, Hgb levels of less than 10 g/dL have been associated with an increased incidence of postoperative apnea. Children of African or African-American ethnicity who have not had a Hgb and hematocrit determination after 6 months of age should have Hgb or hematocrit measurements and a sickle cell screening test performed. Most surgeons require preoperative determination of coagulation status (prothrombin time, partial thromboplastin time, and platelet count) in children undergoing procedures with an increased risk of intra- or postoperative bleeding (eg, tonsillectomy or adenoidectomy, intracranial procedures), even when no history of a bleeding disorder in the patient or the patient's family exists.

Electrolyte Abnormalities

Electrolyte abnormalities of any consequence are extremely rare in healthy children; preoperative screening for such deviations is usually unhelpful and does not alter the anesthetic management. Even for hospitalized patients who might be expected to have an incidence of laboratory abnormalities higher than that found in *healthy outpatients,* routine preoperative testing is not indicated.

Pregnancy Testing

Routine pregnancy screening of all menarcheal adolescents is performed in many institutions. The incidence of a positive pregnancy test result in the preoperative adolescent population ranges from 0.5% to 1.2%.[210-213] Many authors question the cost effectiveness of such a screening practice given the uncertainty about the adverse effects of a single anesthetic exposure on the fetus and mother and the difficulties that arise when a positive human chorionic gonadotropin result is found. In the spirit of *primum non nocere,* the institutions of the authors mandate pregnancy testing, which is performed on the day of surgery using point-of-care urine testing. When a positive result is obtained the procedure is canceled, the patient is notified, and a pediatric social worker is consulted to help the young woman begin to address the ramifications of the positive test result.

Preoperative Testing

Although the healthy child needs almost no preoperative laboratory tests, the situation is entirely different for children who have a history of or the presence of an abnormality. For example, obtaining a chest radiograph is helpful in a patient who has a history of chronic aspiration or lower airway disease. Knowing the Hgb level is important in the child who has sickle cell disease or cardiac disease. A child who has cardiovascular disease and is undergoing digoxin therapy should have the serum sodium, potassium, and digoxin levels measured. An ECG is warranted in a child who has OSAS, BPD, congenital heart disease, or severe scoliosis. Serum electrolytes should be evaluated in children with an underlying condition such as renal insufficiency or in those who are taking diuretics, angiotensin-converting enzyme inhibitors, or other medications that increase the likelihood of an abnormal result. Electrolytes should also be determined in children whose feeding is limited to enteral (nasogastric or gastrostomy tube) feedings or parenteral nutrition. Children being treated with anticonvulsants should have serum levels of these medications checked to ensure that they are in the therapeutic range. In these and similar circumstances, preoperative testing is aimed at detecting and quantifying underlying abnormalities associated with known disease that can lead to life-threatening complications during anesthesia.

Pulmonary Function Tests

Pulmonary function tests are often used to assess the response to bronchodilator therapy in patients whose bronchospasm is reversible. Although they are rarely necessary preoperatively in patients with uncomplicated asthma, these tests may be useful in predicting whether children who have pulmonary or thoracic cage abnormalities such as scoliosis are at increased risk for anesthetic complications and postoperative respiratory insufficiency. The studies used most commonly are pulse oximetry, forced vital capacity (FVC), and FEV_1. The absolute values obtained and the ratios of the 2 measurements (FEV_1/FVC) are useful predictors of the need for postoperative mechanical ventilation among patients at risk (eg, kyphoscoliosis). In adults, an FEV_1/FVC less than 50%, an FEV_1 less than 35% predicted, or an absolute FVC less than 25 mL/kg is associated with inadequate postoperative ventilation and usually results in prolonged mechanical ventilation. However, the accurate measurement of FEV_1 and FVC requires patient cooperation; therefore obtaining reliable results in children younger than 6 years is usually not possible.

MISCELLANEOUS ISSUES

Surgical Procedures

Who should be anesthetized as an outpatient? PCPs are frequently asked whether a child is an appropriate candidate for an outpatient surgical procedure. Surgical procedures suitable for an outpatient setting are those performed quickly, those that have a low likelihood of surgical or anesthetic complications, those that involve minimal physiological derangements, and those that are associated with easily controlled postoperative pain.[55] These procedures must be performed on appropriate patients. Pediatric adenotonsillectomy illustrates the importance of patient selection. Post-adenotonsillectomy respiratory compromise is seen in children younger than 3 years and in those who have neuromuscular disorders, chromosomal abnormalities, loud snoring with apnea, or a respiratory tract infection with 4 weeks of surgery.[214] Children undergoing procedures at freestanding facilities should have no risk factors for postprocedure hospital admission. Thus patients with OSAS or recent URTI should be performed in a hospital-based setting because of the small chance of overnight admissions.

The authors' patient selection for outpatient surgical procedures begins with assigning an ASA PS classification to the child. ASA PS 1 and 2 children are usually appropriate for outpatient anesthesia. PS 3 children may be outpatient candidates if their systemic disease is well controlled and unlikely to be significantly perturbed by the anesthetic and proposed procedure.

Transfusions

Questions are frequently raised by parents regarding transfusion practices. Parents are anxious about the infectious risks of transfusion, and some may have religious objections. Elimination of paid donors, evolution of methods of donor screening, and increasingly sophisticated testing of donated blood have led to a significant decrease in the incidence of infection transmitted by transfusion. The biggest remaining threat to safety of the blood supply is donation by someone who is seronegative in the window of time between infection and seroconversion. The incidence of transfusion-associated hepatitis B is 1:63,000.[215] The risk of transfusion-transmitted hepatitis C is 1:103,000.[215] Hepatitis A, in which a carrier state is rare, is not usually transmitted by transfusion.

Most cases of non-A, non-B, non-C hepatitis are due to an as yet undiscovered viral agent or are of nonviral origin.[216] Testing for HIV-I antibody was implemented in 1985, in 1992 for HIV-II, and most recently in 1996 for HIV-I p24 antigen. The risk of transfusion-transmitted HIV is now estimated to be between 1:450,000 and 1:600,000.[215,217,218] Cytomegalovirus can be transmitted by transfusion, but disease occurs rarely in immunocompetent recipients. Infection can occur and may be devastating in immunocompromised children, such as premature infants, cancer or transplant patients, and those who have congenital immunodeficiency. Testing of donated units for cytomegalovirus is essential for these immunocompromised patients.

Aside from infectious risks, reactions to transfusion include hemolytic reactions resulting from ABO incompatibility, allergic or anaphylactic reactions, febrile nonhemolytic reactions, and transfusion-associated graft-versus-host disease (TA-GVHD). Proper cross-matching and careful checking of units before administration should eliminate most risk of hemolytic reactions, but they still occur in 1:33,000 transfusions, with 1:300,000 to 1:700,000 being fatal (usually the result of massive hemolysis and renal failure caused by hemoglobinuria).[219,220] Febrile nonhemolytic reactions are immunologically mediated and occur most commonly in patients who have received transfusions previously. TA-GVHD may also occur in immunocompromised patients. To avoid the risk of TA-GVHD in patients in whom severe combined immunodeficiency syndrome is identified later in infancy, infants younger than 6 months should receive transfusions only with irradiated blood products.[221]

Parents should be realistically informed about the risks of excessive blood loss in the operation their child faces. A child who weighs as little as 40 kg who has a normal hematocrit may donate autologous blood in advance of an elective procedure. This option should be discussed with the surgeon and arranged through the hospital blood bank. Some blood banks will allow *directed* donation (allogeneic or homologous blood), in which a family member who has the same blood type as the patient donates blood for a specific family member; however, even if the institution allows this practice, up to a week may be required to prepare such a unit of blood. An important point to remember is that some blood banks do not screen directed donor units for HIV or hepatitis and that these units may represent a greater risk of infection than the regular blood supply. Therefore no actual benefit and a greater risk associated with the administration of directed donor units may exist if these units are not screened.

SUMMARY

Preoperative evaluation and preparation are directed toward minimizing the intrinsic risks of anesthesia and surgery by having the child in the healthiest possible condition before surgery. The PCP can contribute to reaching this goal by understanding the effects of general anesthesia on the physiology of children. This knowledge allows an appreciation of the anesthesiologist's concerns regarding underlying diseases, which may appear *stable* (and therefore of little present concern to the PCP) but which may have grave consequences during anesthesia. The preoperative evaluation is designed to ensure that the child's perioperative needs can be met by providing the anesthesiologist both qualitative and quantitative information regarding the child's state of health and disease. The relationship among the child, parents, and PCP places the PCP in an ideal position to prepare families for their children's surgical experience.

TOOLS FOR PRACTICE

Engaging Patient and Family

- *Anesthesia and Your Child* (brochure), American Academy of Pediatrics (patiented.aap.org).

Medical Decision Support

- *National Center for Complementary and Alternative Medicine* (Web page), National Institutes of Health (nccam.nih.gov/).
- *Office of Dietary Supplements* (Web page), National Institutes of Health (dietary-supplements.info.nih.gov/).
- *Pediatric Perioperative Cardiac Arrest (POCA) Registry, Overview* (Web page), POCA Registry (depts.washington.edu/asaccp/POCA/).
- *Preoperative Evaluation History and Physical Form* (form), Johns Hopkins Hospital (practice.aap.org/content.aspx?aid-2001).
- *What is a Pediatric Anesthesiologist?* (brochure), American Academy of Pediatrics (www.aap.org/sections/sap/he3003.pdf).

RELATED WEB SITE

- American Academy of Anesthesiologists (www.asahq.org/).

AAP POLICY STATEMENTS

American Academy of Pediatrics, Section on Anesthesiology and Section on Anesthesiology Bridges Committee. Evaluation and preparation of pediatric patients undergoing anesthesia. *Pediatrics*. 1996;98(3 Pt 1):502-508. (aappolicy.aappublications.org/cgi/content/abstract/pediatrics;98/3/502).

American Academy of Pediatrics, Section on Anesthesiology. Guidelines for the pediatric perioperative anesthesia environment. *Pediatrics*. 1999;103(2):512-515. (aappolicy.aappublications.org/cgi/content/full/pediatrics;103/2/512).

American Academy of Pediatrics, Surgery Advisory Panel. Guidelines for referral to pediatric surgical specialists. *Pediatrics*. 2002;110(1):187-191. (aappolicy.aappublications.org/cgi/content/full/pediatrics;110/1/187).

REFERENCES

1. Hughes JM. Parents' experiences of caring for their child following day case surgery: a diary study. *J Child Health Care*. 2004;8:47-58.
2. Letts M, Davidson D, Splinter W, et al. Analysis of the efficacy of pediatric day surgery. *Can J Surg*. 2001;44:193-198.
3. Centers for Disease Control and Prevention, National Center for Health Statistics. Vital and Health Statistics: Ambulatory and Inpatient Procedures in the United States, 1996. Available at: www.cdc.gov/nchs/data/series/sr_13/sr13_139.pdf. Accessed May 19, 2006.
4. Shapiro NL, Seid AB, Pransky SM, et al. Adenotonsillectomy in the very young patient: cost analysis of two methods of postoperative care. *Int J Pediatr Otorhinolaryngol*. 1999;48:109-115.
5. Kain ZN, Caldwell-Andrews AA. Preoperative psychological preparation of the child for surgery: an update. *Anesthesiol Clin North Am*. 2005;23:597-614.
6. Bevan JC, Johnston C, Haig MJ, et al. Preoperative parental anxiety predicts behavioural and emotional responses to induction of anaesthesia in children. *Can J Anaesth*. 1990;37:177-182.
7. Zuckerberg AL. Perioperative approach to children. *Pediatr Clin North Am*. 1994;41:15-29.
8. Moynihan R, Kurker C. The perioperative environment and the pediatric patient. In: Ferrari LR, ed. *Anesthesia and Pain Management for the Pediatrician*. Baltimore, MD: Johns Hopkins University Press; 1999.
9. Keenan RL, Boyan CP. Cardiac arrest due to anesthesia: a study of incidence and causes. *JAMA*. 1985;253:2373-2377.
10. Tiret L, Nivoche Y, Hatton F, et al. Complications related to anaesthesia in infants and children: a prospective survey of 40,240 anaesthetics. *Br J Anaesth*. 1988;61:263-269.

11. Morray JP, Geiduschek JM, Caplan RA, et al. A comparison of pediatric and adult anesthesia closed malpractice claims. *Anesthesiology*. 1993;78:461-467.
12. Mamie C, Habre W, Delhumeau C, et al. Incidence and risk factors of perioperative respiratory adverse events in children undergoing elective surgery. *Pediatr Anesth*. 2004;14:218-224.
13. Olsson GL, Hallen B. Laryngospasm during anesthesia: a computer-aided incidence study of 136,929 patients. *Acta Anaesthesiol Scand*. 1984;28:567-575.
14. Oudjhane K, Bowen A, Oh KS, et al. Pulmonary edema complicating upper airway obstruction in infants and children. *Can Assoc Radiol J*. 1992;43:278-282.
15. Ferrari LR. Do children need a preoperative assessment that is different from adults? *Int Anesthesiol Clin*. 2002; 40:167-186.
16. Geiduschek JM. Registry offers insight on preventing cardiac arrests in children. *ASA Newsletter* 1998;62(6): 16-18.
17. Morray JP, Geiduschek JM, Ramanmoorthy C, et al. Anesthesia-related cardiac arrest in children. *Anesthesiology*. 2000;93:6-14.
18. Morray JP, Bhananker SM. Recent findings from the Pediatric Perioperative Cardiac Arrest (POCA) Registry. *ASA Newsletter*. 2005;69(6):10-12.
19. Jimenez N. Trends in pediatric anesthesia malpractice claims over the last three decades. *ASA Newsletter*. 2005;69(6):8-9, 12.
20. Murat I, Constant I, Maud'huy H. Perioperative anaesthetic morbidity in children: a database of 24,165 anaesthetics over a 30-month period. *Pediatr Anesth*. 2004;14: 158-166.
21. Bordet F, Allaouchiche B, Lansiaux S, et al. Risk factors for airway complications during general anaesthesia in paediatric patients. *Paediatr Anaesth*. 2002;12:762-769.
22. Kain ZN, Caldwell-Andrews AA, Maranets I, et al. Predicting which child-parent pair will benefit from parental presence during induction of anesthesia: a decision-making approach. *Anesth Analg*. 2006;102: 81-84.
23. Kain ZN, Mayes LC, Wang SM, et al. Parental presence during induction of anesthesia versus sedative premedication: which intervention is more effective? *Anesthesiology*. 1998;89:1147-1156.
24. Kotiniemi LH, Ryhanen PT, Moilanen IK. Behavioural changes in children following day-case surgery: a 4-week follow-up of 551 children. *Anaesthesia*. 1997;52: 970-976.
25. Kain ZN, Wang SM, Mayes LC, et al. Distress during the induction of anesthesia and postoperative behavioral outcomes. *Anesth Analg*. 1999;88:1042-1047.
26. Stargatt R, Davidson AJ, Huang GH, et al. A cohort study of the incidence and risk factors for negative behavior changes in children after general anesthesia. *Pediatr Anesth*. 2006;16:846-859.
27. Rennick JE, Johnston CC, Dougherty G, et al. Children's psychological responses after critical illness and exposure to invasive technology. *J Dev Behav Pediatr*. 2002;23:133-144.
28. Tait AR, Malviya S. Anesthesia for the child with an upper respiratory tract infection: still a dilemma? *Anesth Analg*. 2005;100(1):59-65.
29. Tait AR, Malviya S, Voepel-Lewis T, et al. Risk factors for perioperative adverse respiratory events in children with upper respiratory tract infections. *Anesthesiology*. 2001;95:299-306.
30. Cohen MM, Cameron CB. Should you cancel the operation when a child has an upper respiratory tract infection? *Anesth Analg*. 1991;72:282-288.
31. Skolnick ET, Vomvolakis MA, Buck KA. A prospective evaluation of children with upper respiratory infections undergoing a standardized anesthetic and the incidence of respiratory events (abstract). *Anesthesiology*. 1998; 89:A1309.
32. Aquilina AT, Hall WJ, Douglas RG, et al. Airway reactivity in subjects with viral respiratory infections: the effects of exercise and cold air. *Am Rev Respir Dis*. 1980;122:3-10
33. Empey DW. Effect of airway infections on bronchial reactivity. *Eur J Resp Dis*. 1983;128(suppl):366-368.
34. Malviya S, Voepel-Lewis T, Siewert M, et al. Risk factors for adverse postoperative outcomes in children presenting for cardiac surgery with upper respiratory tract infections. *Anesthesiology*. 2003;98:628-632.
35. Coté CJ. The upper respiratory tract infection dilemma: fear of a complication or litigation. *Anesthesiology*. 2001;95:283-285.
36. Parnis SJ, Barker DS, Van Der, et al. Clinical predictors of anaesthetic complications in children with respiratory tract infections. *Paediatr Anaesth*. 2001;11: 29-40.
37. Folkerts G, Busse WW, Nijkamp FP, et al. Virus-induced airway hyperresponsivemenss and asthma. *Am J Respir Crit Care Med*. 1998;157:1708-1720.
38. Larsen GL, Colasurdo G. Neural control mechanisms within airways: disruption by respiratory syncytial virus. *J Pediatr*. 1999;135:S21-S27.
39. Jones DT, Bhattacharyya N. Passive smoke exposure as a risk factor for airway complications during outpatient pediatric procedures. *Otolaryngol-Head and Neck Surg*. 2006;135:12-16.
40. Kuehni CE, Davis A, Brooke AM, et al. Are all wheezing disorders in very young (preschool) children increasing in prevalence? *Lancet*. 2001;357:1821-1825.
41. Toelle BG, Ng K, Belousova E, et al. Prevalence of asthma and allergy in schoolchildren in Belmont, Australia: three cross sectional surveys over 20 years. *BMJ*. 2004;328:386-387.
42. Doherty GM, Chisakuta A, Crean P, et al. Anesthesia and the child with asthma. *Pediatr Anesth*. 2005;15: 446-454.
43. Silvanus M-T, Groeben H, Peters J. Corticosteroids and inhaled salbutamol in patients with reversible airway obstruction markedly decrease the incidence of bronchospasm after tracheal intubation. *Anesthesiology*. 2004;100:1052-1057.
44. Zachary CY, Evans R. Perioperative management for childhood asthma. *Ann Allergy Asthma Immunol*. 1996;77:468-472.
45. Welborn LG, Greenspun JC. Anesthesia and apnea: perioperative considerations in the former preterm infant. *Ped Clin N Am*. 1994;41:181-198.
46. Katz-Salamon M. Delayed chemoreceptor responses in infants with apnea. *Arch Dis Child*. 2004;89:261-266.
47. Isono S. Developmental changes of pharyngeal airway patency: implications for pediatric anesthesia. *Pediatr Anesth*. 2006;16:109-122.
48. Coté CJ, Zaslavsky A, Downes JJ, et al. Postoperative apnea in former preterm infants after inguinal herniorrhaphy. A combined analysis. *Anesthesiology*. 1995;82: 809-822.
49. Shah AR, Kurth CD, Gwiazdowski SG, et al. Fluctuations in cerebral oxygenation and blood volume during endotracheal suctioning in premature infants. *J Pediatr*. 1993;120:769-774.
50. Krane EJ, Haberkern CM, Jacobson LE. Postoperative apnea, bradycardia, and oxygen desaturation in formerly premature infants: prospective comparison of spinal and general anesthesia. *Anesth Analg*. 1995;80:7-13.

51. Williams RK, Adams DC, Aladjem EV, et al. The safety and efficacy of spinal anesthesia for surgery in infants: the Vermont infant spinal registry. *Anesth Analg.* 2006;102:67-71.
52. Bonnet MP, Larousse E, Asehnoune K, et al. Spinal anesthesia with bupivacaine decreased cerebral blood flow in former preterm infants. *Anesth Analg.* 2004;98:1280-1283.
53. Henderson-Smart D, Steer PA. Prophylactic caffeine to prevent postoperative apnea following general anesthesia in preterm infants. *Cochrane Database Sys Rev.* 2001;4:CD000048.
54. McNamara DG, Nixon GM, Anderson BJ. Methylxanthines for the treatment of apnea associated with bronchiolitis and anesthesia. *Pediatr Anesth.* 2004;14:541-550.
55. Noseworthy J, Duran C, Khine HH. Postoperative apnea in a full-term infant. *Anesthesiology.* 1989;70:879-880.
56. Fishkin S, Litman RS. Current issues in pediatric ambulatory anesthesia. *Anesth Clin North Am.* 2003;21:305-311.
57. Galinkin JL, Kurth CD. Neonatal and pediatric apnea syndromes. *Prob Anesth.* 1998;10:444-454.
58. Groneck P, Gotze-Speer B, Oppermann M, et al. Association of pulmonary inflammation and increased microvascular permeability during the development of bronchopulmonary dysplasia: a sequential analysis of inflammatory mediators in respiratory fluids of high-risk preterm neonates. *Pediatrics.* 1994;93:712-718.
59. Jobe AH. Glucocorticoids, inflammation and the perinatal lung. *Semin Neonatol.* 2001;6:331-342.
60. Jobe AH, Bancalari E. Bronchopulmonary dysplasia. *Am J Respir Crit Care Med.* 2001;6:331-342.
61. Shaffer TH, Wolfson MR, Panitch HB. Airway structure, function and development in health and disease. *Pediatr Anesth.* 2004;14:3-14.
62. Abman S. Pulmonary hypertension in chronic lung disease in infancy; pathogenesis, pathophysiology and treatment. In: Bland R, Coalson J, eds. *Chronic Lung Disease of Early Infancy.* New York, NY: Marcel Dekker; 1999.
63. Ferrari LR, Goudsouzian NG. The use of the laryngeal mask airway in children with bronchopulmonary dysplasia. *Anesth Analg.* 1995;81:310-313.
64. Blum RH, McGowan FX. Chronic upper airway obstruction and cardiac dysfunction: anatomy, pathophysiology, and anesthetic implications. *Pediatr Anesth.* 2004;14:75-83.
65. Rosen GM, Muckle RP, Mahowald MW, et al. Postoperative respiratory compromise in children with obstructive sleep apnea syndrome: can it be anticipated? *Pediatrics.* 1994;93:784-788.
66. American Academy of Pediatrics, Subcommittee on Obstructive Sleep Apnea Syndrome, Section on Pediatric Pulmonology. Clinical practice guideline: diagnosis and management of childhood obstructive sleep apnea syndrome. *Pediatrics.* 2002;109:704-712.
67. Ayeri TI, Roper HP. Pulmonary hypertension resulting from upper airways obstruction in Down's syndrome. *J R Soc Med.* 1998;91:321-322.
68. Wilson K, Lakheeram I, Morielli A, et al. Can assessment of obstructive sleep apnea help predict postadenotonsillectomy respiratory complications. *Anesthesiology.* 2002;96:313-322.
69. Brown KA, Morin I, Hickey C, et al. Urgent tonsillectomy: an analysis of risk factors associate with postoperative morbidity. *Anesthesiology.* 2003;99:586-595.
70. Statham MM, Elluru RG, Buncher R, et al. Adenotonsillectomy for obstructive sleep apnea syndrome in young children. *Arch Otolaryngol Head Neck Surg.* 2006;132:476-480.
71. Biavati MJ, Manning SC, Phillips DL. Predictive factors for respiratory complications tonsillectomy and adenoidectomy in children. *Arch Otolaryngol Head Neck Surg.* 1997;123:517-521.
72. McColley SA, April MM, Carroll JL, et al. Respiratory compromise after adenotonsillectomy in children with obstructive sleep apnea. *Arch Otolaryngol Head Neck Surg.* 1992;118:940-943.
73. Rocca GD. Anaesthesia in patients with cystic fibrosis. *Curr Opin Anaesthesiol.* 2002;15:95-101.
74. Saltzman DA, Johnson EM, Feltis BA, et al. Surgical experience in patients with cystic fibrosis: a 25-year perspective. *Pediatr Pulmonol.* 2002;33:106-110.
75. Richardson VF, Robertson CF, Mowat AP, et al. Deterioration in lung function after general anaesthesia in patients with cystic fibrosis. *Acta Pediatr Scand.* 1984;73:75-79.
76. Flume PA, Yankaskas JR, Ebeling M, et al. Massive hemoptysis in cystic fibrosis. *Chest.* 2005;128:729-738.
77. Harvey WP. Innocent vs. significant murmurs. *Curr Probl Cardiol.* 1976;1:1-51.
78. Klewer SE, Donnerstein RJ, Goldberg ST. Still's innocent murmur can be produced by increasing aortic velocity to a threshold value. *Am J Cardiol.* 1991;68:810-812.
79. DeMonchy C. Studies on functional heart murmurs in children: 1. The external carotid tracing of children with a precordial vibratory murmur. *Ann Paediatr.* 1966;206:356-362.
80. Danford DA, McNamara DG. Innocent murmurs and heart sounds. In: Garson A, Bricker JT, Fisher DJ, et al, eds. *The science and practice of pediatric cardiology.* 2nd ed. Baltimore, MD: William and Wilkins; 1998.
81. American Academy of Pediatrics, Committee on Genetics. Healthcare supervision for children with Williams syndrome. *Pediatrics.* 2001;107:1192-1204.
82. Medley J, Russo P, Tobias JD. Perioperative care of the patient with Williams syndrome. *Pediatr Anesth.* 2005;15:243-247.
83. Ewart AK, Morris CA, Atkinson DL, et al. Hemizygosity at the elastin locus in a developmental disorder, Williams syndrome. *Nat Genet.* 1993;5:11-16.
84. Ewart AK, Morris CA, Ensing GJ, et al. A human vascular disorder, supravalvular aortic stenosis, maps to chromosome 7. *Proc Natl Acad Sci USA.* 1993;90:3226-3230.
85. Wessel A, Pankau R, Kececioglu D, et al. Three decades of follow-up of aortic and pulmonary vascular lesions in the Williams-Beuren syndrome. *Am J Med Genet.* 1994;52:297-301.
86. Kececioglu D, Kotthoff S, Vogt J. Williams-Beuren syndrome: a 30 year follow-up of natural and postoperative course. *Eur Heart J.* 1993;14:1458-1464.
87. Bird LM, Billman GF, Lacro RV, et al. Sudden death in Williams syndrome: report of ten cases. *J Pediatr.* 1996;129:926-931.
88. Fukushige T, Yoshinaga M, Shimago A, et al. Effect of age and overweight on the QT interval and the prevalence of long QT syndrome in children. *Am J Cardiol.* 2002;89:395-398.
89. Yang P, Kanki H, Drolet B, et al. Allelic variants in long-QT disease genes in patients with drug-associated torsades de pointes. *Circulation.* 2002;105:1943-1948.
90. Kies SJ, Pabelick CM, Hurley HA, et al. Anesthesia for patients with congenital long QT syndrome. *Anesthesiology.* 2005;102:204-210.
91. Ackerman MJ. The long QT syndrome: Ion channel diseases of the heart. *Mayo Clin Proc.* 1998;73:250-269.

92. Saussine M, Massad I, Raczka F, et al. Torsades de pointes during sevoflurane anesthesia in a child with congenital long QT syndrome. *Pediatr Anesth.* 2006; 16:63-65.
93. Wilson W, Taubert KA, Gewitz M, et al. Prevention of infective endocarditis. Guidelines from the American Heart Association Rheumatic Fever, Endocarditis, and Kawasaki Disease Committee, Council on Cardiovascular Disease in the Young, and the Council on Clinical Cardiology, Council on Cardiovascular Surgery and Anesthesia, and Quality of Care and Outcomes Research Interdisciplinary Working Group. *Circulation.* 2007;116:1736-1754. Available at: circ.ahajournals.org/cgi/content/full/116/15/1736. Accessed August 24, 2007.
94. McAnulty GR, Robertshaw HJ, Hall GM. Anaesthetic management of patients with diabetes mellitus. *Br J Anaes.* 2000;85:80-90.
95. Furnary AP, Wu YX, Bookin SP. Effect of hyperglycemia and continuous intravenous insulin infusions on outcomes of cardiac surgical procedures: The Portland Diabetic Project. *Endocrine Practice.* 2004; 10:S21-S33.
96. Pierre EJ, Barrow RE, Hawkings HK, et al. Effects of insulin on wound healing. *J Trauma.* 1998;44:342-345.
97. Delamaire M, Maugendre D, Moreno M, et al. Impaired leucocyte functions in diabetic patients. *Diabet Med.* 1997;14:29-34.
98. Marhoffer W, Stein M, Maeser E, et al. Impairment of polymorphonuclear leukocyte function and metabolic control of diabetes. *Diabetes Care.* 1992;15:256-260.
99. Golden SH, Peart-Vigilance CP, Kao WH, et al. Perioperative glycemic control and the risk of infectious complications in a cohort of adults with diabetes. *Diabetes Care.* 1999;22:1408-1414.
100. Van den Berghe G, Wouters P, Weekers F, et al. Intensive insulin in the critically ill patients. *N Engl J Med.* 2001;345:1359-1367.
101. Van den Berghe G, Wilmer A, Hermans G, et al. Intensive insulin therapy in the medical ICU. *N Engl J Med.* 2006;354:449-461.
102. Dronge AS, Perkal MF, Kancir S, et al. Long-term glycemic control and postoperative infectious complications. *Arch Surg.* 2006;141:375-380.
103. Thorell A, Nygren J, Hirshman MF, et al. Surgery-induced insulin resistance in human patients: relation to glucose transport and utilization. *Am J Physiol.* 1999; 276:E754-E761.
104. Chadwick V, Wilkinson KA. Diabetes mellitus and the pediatric anesthetist. *Pediatr Anesth.* 2004;14:716-723.
105. Warner ME, Contreras MG, Warner MA, et al. Diabetes mellitus and difficult laryngoscopy in renal and pancreatic transplant patients. *Anesth Analg.* 1998;86:516-619.
106. Gallego PH, Bulsara MK, Frazer F, et al. Prevalence and risk factors for microalbuminiuria in a population-based sample of children and adolescents with T1DM in Western Australia. *Pediatr Diabetes.* 2006;7:165-172.
107. Horowitz M, O'Donovan D, Jones KL, et al. Gastric emptying in diabetes: clinical significance and treatment. *Diabet Med.* 2002;19:177-194.
108. Rhodes ET, Ferrari LR, Wolfsdorf JI. Perioperative management of pediatric surgical patients with diabetes mellitus. *Anesth Analg.* 2005;101:986-999.
109. Merke DP, Chrousos GP, Eisenhofer G, et al. Adrenomedullary dysplasia and hypofunction in patients with classic 21-hydroxylase deficiency. *N Engl J Med.* 2000;343:1362-1368.
110. Speiser PW, Brenner D. Congenital adrenal hyperplasia resulting from 21-hydroxylase deficiency. *The Endocrinologist.* 2003;13:334-340.
111. Axelrod L. Perioperative management of patients treated with glucocorticoids. *Endocrinol Metab Clin North Am.* 2003;32:367-383.
112. Zora JA, Zimmerman D, Carely TL, et al. Hypothalamic-pituitary-adrenal axis suppression after short-term high-dose glucocorticoid therapy in children with asthma. *J Allergy Clin Immunol.* 1986;77:9-13.
113. Ducharme FM, Chabot G, Polychronakos C, et al. Safety profile of frequent short courses of oral glucocorticoids in acute pediatric asthma: impact on bone metabolism, bone density, and adrenal function. *Pediatrics.* 2003; 111:376-383.
114. Doherty GM, Chisakuta A, Crean P, et al. Anesthesia and the child with asthma. *Pediatr Anesth.* 2005;15: 446-454.
115. Dahl R. Systemic side effects of inhaled corticosteroids in patients with asthma. *Resp Med.* 2006;100:1307-1317.
116. Adams N, Bestall JM. Lasserson TJ, et al. Inhaled fluticasone versus inhaled beclamethasone or inhaled budesonide for chronic asthma. *Cochrane Database Sys Rev.* 2004;2:CD002310.
117. Todd GRG, Acrini CL, Foss-Russell R, et al. Survey of adrenal crisis associated with inhaled corticosteroids in the United Kingdom. *Arch Dis Child.* 2002;87:457-461.
118. Kanniston S, Korppi M, Remes K, et al. Adrenal suppression, evaluated by a low dose adrenocorticotropin test, and growth in asthmatic children treated with inhaled steroids. *J Clin Endocrinol Metab.* 2000;85: 652-657.
119. Wilson JW, Robertson CF. Inhaled steroids-too much of a good thing? *Med J Aust.* 2002;177:288-289.
120. Gulliver T, Eid N. Effects of glucocorticoids on the hypothalamic-pituitary-adrenal axis in children and adults. *Immunol Allergy Clin North Am.* 2005;25: 5451-5455.
121. Suko J. The calcium pump of the cardiac sarcoplasmic reticulum: functional alterations at different levels of thyroid state in rabbits. *J Physiol.* 1973;228:563-582.
122. Ojamaa K, Sabet A, Kenessey A, et al. Regulation of cardiac Kv1.5 gene expression by thyroid hormone is rapid and chamber specific. *Endocrinology.* 1999;140: 3170-3176.
123. Keon TP, Templeton JJ. Diseases of the endocrine system. In: Katz J, Steward DJ, eds. *Anesthesia and Uncommon Pediatric Diseases.* 2nd ed. Philadelphia, PA: WB Saunders; 1993.
124. Spell NO 3rd. Stopping and starting medications in the perioperative period. *Med Clin North Am.* 2001;85: 1117-1128.
125. Schiff RL, Welsh GA. Perioperative evaluation and management of the patient with endocrine dysfunction. *Med Clin North Am.* 2003;87:175-192.
126. Platt OS, Brambilla DJ, Rosse WF, et al. Mortality in sickle cell disease. Life expectancy and risk factors for early death. *N Engl J Med.* 1994;330: 1639-1644.
127. Powars D, Chan LS, Schroeder WA. The variable expression of sickle cell disease is genetically determined. *Semin Hematol.* 1990;27:360-376.
128. Aslan M, Thornley-Brown D, Freeman B. Reactive species in sickle cell disease. *Ann NY Acad Sci.* 2000;899:375-391.
129. Hebbel RP. Beyond hemoglobin polymerization: the red blood cell membrane and sickle disease pathophysiology. *Blood.* 1991;77:214-237.
130. Lancaster JR Jr. Reaping of nitric oxide by sickle cell disease. *Proc Natl Acad Sci USA.* 2002;99:552-553.
131. Firth PG, Head CA. Sickle cell disease and anesthesia. *Anesthesiology.* 2004;101:766-785.

132. Vichinsky EP, Neumayr LD, Earles AN, et al. Causes and outcomes of the acute chest syndrome in sickle cell disease. National Acute Chest Syndrome Group. *N Engl J Med.* 2000;342:1855-1865.
133. Stuart MJ, Setty BN. Sickle cell acute chest syndrome: pathogenesis and rationale for treatment. *Blood.* 1999;94:1555-1560.
134. Castro O, Brambilla DJ, Thorington B, et al. The acute chest syndrome in sickle cell disease: incidence and risk factors. *Blood.* 1994;84:643-649.
135. Delatte SJ, Hebra A, Tagge EP, et al. Acute chest syndrome in the postoperative sickle cell patient. *J Ped Surg.* 1999;34:188-192.
136. Vichinsky EP, Styles LA, Colangelo LH, et al. Acute chest syndrome in sickle cell disease: clinical presentation and course. Cooperative Study of Sickle Cell Disease. *Blood.* 1997;89:1787-1792.
137. Knight-Madden JM, Forrester TS, Lewis NA, et al. Asthma in children with sickle cell disease and its association with acute chest syndrome. *Thorax.* 2005;60: 206-210.
138. Koumbourlis AC, Hurlet-Jensen A, Bye MR. Lung function in infants with sickle cell disease. *Pediatr Pulmonol.* 1997;24:277-281.
139. Minter KR, Gladwin MT. Pulmonary complications of sickle cell anemia: a need for increased recognition, treatment, and research. *Am J Respir Crit Care Med.* 2001;164:2016-2019.
140. Koumbourlis AC, Zar HJ, Jurlet-Jensen A, et al. Prevalence and reversibility of lower airway obstruction in children with sickle cell diseases. *J Pediatr.* 2001;138: 188-192.
141. Powars DR, Chan LS, Hiti A, et al. Outcome of sickle cell anemia: a 4-decade observational study of 1056 patients. *Medicine.* 2005;84:363-376.
142. Powars D, Weidman JA, Odom-Maryon T, et al. Sickle cell chronic lung disease: prior morbidity and the risk of pulmonary failure. *Medicine (Baltimore).* 1988;67:66-76.
143. De Castro LM, Jonassaint JC, Graham FL, et al. Pulmonary hypertension in SS, SC, and S-beta thalassemia: prevalence, associated clinical syndromes, and mortality. *Blood.* 2004;104:462a.
144. Gladwin MT, Sachdev V, Jison ML, et al. Pulmonary hypertension as a risk factor in patients with sickle cell disease. *N Engl J Med.* 2004;350:886-895.
145. Needleman JP, Franco ME, Varlotta L, et al. Mechanisms of nocturnal oxyhemoglobin desaturation in children and adolescents with sickle cell disease. *Pediatr Pulmonol.* 1999;28:418-422.
146. Bandla H, Splaingard M. Sleep problems in children with common medical disorders. *Pediatr Clin North Am.* 2004;51:203-227.
147. Aessopos A, Farmakis D, Deftereos S, et al. Thalassemia heart disease: a comparative evaluation of thalassemia major and thalassemia intermedia. *Chest.* 2005;127: 1223-1530.
148. Derchi G, Fonti A, Forni GL, et al. Pulmonary hypertension in patients with thalassemia major. *Am Heart J.* 1999;138:384.
149. Serjeant GR. Historical review: the emerging understanding of sickle cell disease. *Br J Haematol.* 2001;112: 3-18.
150. Ohene-Frempong K, Wiener SJ, Sleeper LA, et al. Cerebrovascular accidents in sickle cell disease: rates and risk factors. *Blood.* 1998;91:288-294.
151. Moser FG, Miller ST, Bello JA, et al. The spectrum of central nervous system abnormalities in sickle cell disease as defined by magnetic resonance imaging: a report from the Cooperative Study of Sickle Cell Disease. *A J N R.* 1996;17:965-972.
152. Miller ST, Macklin EA, Pegelow CH, et al. Silent infarction as a risk factor for overt stroke in children with sickle cell anemia. *J Pediatr.* 2001;139:385-390.
153. Adams RJ, McKie VC, Hsu L, et al. Prevention of a first stroke by transfusions in children with sickle cell anemia and abnormal result on transcranial Doppler ultrasonography. *N Engl J Med.* 1998;339:5-11.
154. Kirkham FJ, Hewes DKM, Prengler M, et al. Nocturnal hypoxaemia and central nervous system events in sickle cell disease. *Lancet.* 2001;357:1656-1659.
155. Waldron P, Pegelow C, Neumayr L, et al. Tonsillectomy, adenoidectomy, and myringotomy in sickle cell disease: perioperative morbidity. *J Pediatr Hematol Oncol.* 1999;21:129-135.
156. Kokoska ER, West KW, Carney DE, et al. Risk factors for acute chest syndrome in children with sickle cell disease undergoing abdominal surgery. *J Pediatr Surg.* 2004;39:848-850.
157. Wales PW, Carver E, Crawford MW, et al. Acute chest syndrome after abdominal surgery in children with sickle cell disease: is a laparoscopic approach better? *J Pediatr Surg.* 2001;36:718-721.
158. Haberkern CM, Neumayr LD, Orringer EP, et al. Cholecystectomy in sickle cell anemia patients: perioperative outcome of 364 cases from the National Preoperative Transfusion Study. Preoperative Transfusion in Sickle Cell Disease Study Group. *Blood.* 1997;89:1533-1542.
159. Vichinsky EP, Haberkern CM, Neumayr L, et al. A comparison of conservative and aggressive transfusion regimens in the perioperative management of sickle cell disease. The Preoperative Transfusion in Sickle Cell Disease Study Group. *N Engl J Med.* 1995;333:206-213.
160. Miller ST, Sleeper LA, Pegelow CH, et al. Prediction of adverse outcomes in children with sickle cell disease. *N Engl J Med.* 2000;342:83-89.
161. Koshy M, Weiner SJ, Miller ST, et al. Surgery and anesthesia in sickle cell disease. Cooperative Study of Sickle Cell Diseases. *Blood.* 1995;86:3676-3684.
162. Vichinsky EF, Neumayr LD, Haberkern C, et al. The perioperative complication rate of orthopedic surgery in sickle cell disease: report of the National Sickle Cell Surgery Study Group. *Am J Hematol.* 1999; 62:129-138.
163. Neumayr L, Koshy M, Haberkern C, et al. Surgery in patients with hemoglobin SC disease. Preoperative Transfusion in Sickle Cell Disease Study Group. *Am J Hematol.* 1998;57:101-108.
164. Riddington C, Williamson L. Preoperative blood transfusions for sickle cell disease. *Cochrane Database Sys Rev.* 2001;3:CD003149.
165. Mannucci PM. Desmopressin (DDAVP) in the treatment of bleeding disorders. The first 20 years. *Blood.* 1997;90: 2515-2521.
166. Nolan B, White B, Smith J, et al. Desmopressin: therapeutic limitations in children and adults with inherited coagulation disorders. *Br J Haematol.* 2000;109:865-869.
167. Federici AB, Baudo F, Caracciolo C, et al. Clinical efficacy of highly purified doubly virus-inactivated factor VIII/von Willebrand factor concentrate (Fandhdi) in the treatment of von Willebrand disease: a retrospective clinical study. *Haemophilia.* 2002;8:761-767.
168. Butler MG, Hayes BG, Hathaway MM, et al. Specific genetic diseases at risk for sedation/anesthesia complications. *Anesth Analg.* 2000;91:837-855.
169. Shott SR, Donnelly LF. Cine magnetic resonance imaging: evaluation of persistent airway obstruction after tonsil and adenoidectomy in children with Down syndrome. *Laryngoscope.* 2004;114:1724-1729.
170. Shott SR. Down syndrome: analysis of airway size and a guide for appropriate intubation. *Laryngoscope.* 2000;110:585-592.

171. Cappelli-Bigazzi M, Santoro G, Battaglia C, et al. Endothelial cell dysfunction in patients with Down's syndrome. *Am J Cardiol.* 2004;94:392-395.
172. Borland LM, Colligan J, Brandom BW. Frequency of anesthesia-related complications in children with Down syndrome under general anesthesia for noncardiac procedures. *Pediatr Anesth.* 2004;14:733-738.
173. Shott SR, Amin R, Chini B, et al. Obstructive sleep apnea. Should all children with Down syndrome be tested? *Arch Otolaryngol Head Neck Surg.* 2006;132: 432-436.
174. Selby KA, Newton RW, Gupta S, et al. Clinical predictors and radiological reliability in atlantoaxial subluxation in Down's syndrome. *Arch Dis Child.* 1991;66:876-878.
175. Cremers MJ, Ramos L, Bol E, et al. Radiological assessment of the atlantoaxial distance in Down's syndrome. *Arch Dis Child.* 1993;69:347-350.
176. Pueschel SM, Scola FH: Atlantoaxial instability in individuals with Down syndrome: epidemiologic, radiographic, and clinical studies. *Pediatrics.* 1987;80: 555-560.
177. Wang JC, Nuccion SL, Feighan JE, et al. Growth and development of the pediatric cervical spine documented radiographically. *J Bone Joint Surg Am.* 2001;83-A: 1212-1218.
178. Hata T, Todd MM. Cervical spine considerations when anesthetizing patients with Down syndrome. *Anesthesiology.* 2005;102:680-685.
179. White KS, Ball WS, Prenger EC, et al. Evaluation of the craniocervical junction in Down syndrome: correlation of measurements obtained with radiography and MR imaging. *Radiology.* 1993;186:377-382.
180. Litman RS, Zerngast BA, Perkins FM. Preoperative evaluation of the cervical spine in children with trisomy-21: results of a questionnaire study. *Pediatr Anaesth.* 1995;5:355-361.
181. American Academy of Pediatrics, Committee on Genetics. Health supervision for children with Down syndrome. *Pediatrics.* 2001;107:442-449.
182. Denborough MA, Forster JFA, Lovell RRH. Anaesthetic deaths in a family. *Br J Anaesth.* 1962;34:395.
183. Finsterer J. Current concepts in malignant hyperthermia. *J Clin Neuromusc Dis.* 202;4:64-74.
184. Wappler F. Malignant hyperthermia. *Eur J Anesthesiol.* 2001;18:632-652.
185. Denborough M. Malignant hyperthermia. *Lancet.* 1998; 352:1131-1136.
186. Brandom BW. The genetics of malignant hyperthermia. *Anesth Clin North Am.* 2005;23:615-619.
187. Jurkat-Rott K, McCarthy T, Lehmann-Horn F. Genetics and pathogenesis of malignant hyperthermia. *Muscle Nerve.* 2000;23;4-17.
188. Larach MG, Rosenberg H, Gronert GA, et al. Hyperkalemic cardiac arrest during anesthesia in infants and children with occult myopathies. *Clin Pediatr (Phila).* 1997;36:9-16.
189. Davis M, Brown R, Dickson A, et al. Malignant hyperthermia associated with exercise-induced rhabdomyolysis or congenital abnormalities and a novel RYRI mutation in New Zealand and Australian pedigrees. *Br J Anaesth.* 2002;88:808-815.
190. Girard T, Treves S, Voronkov E, et al. Molecular genetic testing for malignant hyperthermia susceptibility. *Anesthesiology.* 2004;100:1076-1080.
191. Malignant Hyperthermia Association of the United States. MH Susceptible Patient FAQs. Available at: www.mhaus.org/. Accessed July 9, 2006.
192. Zuckerberg AL. A hot mnemonic for the treatment of malignant hyperthermia. *Anesth Analg.* 1993;77: 1077.
193. Evans-Prosser CD. The use of pethidine and morphine in the presence of monoamine oxidase inhibitors. *Br J Anaesth.* 1968;40:279-282.
194. Kudoh A, Katagai H, Takazawa T. Antidepressant treatment for chronic depressed patients should not be discontinued prior to anesthesia. *Can J Anesth.* 2002;49: 132-136.
195. Stoelting RJ. *Pharmacology and Physiology in Anesthetic Practice.* 3rd ed. Philadelphia, PA: Lippincott Raven; 1999.
196. Huyse FJ, Touw DJ, van Schijndel RS, et al. Psychotropic drugs and the perioperative period: a proposal for a guideline in elective surgery. *Psychosomatics.* 2006;47:8-22.
197. Lerman J. Herbal medicine in children: caveat medicus. *Pediatr Anesth.* 2005;15:443-445.
198. Everett LL, Birmingham PK, Williams GD, et al. Herbal and homeopathic medication use in pediatric surgical patients. *Pediatr Anesth.* 2005;15:455-460.
199. Ang-Lee MK, Moss J, Yuan C. Herbal medicines and perioperative care. *JAMA.* 2001;286:208-216.
200. Litman RS. The difficult pediatric airway. In: Litman RS, ed. *Pediatric Anesthesia: The Requisites in Anesthesiology.* Philadelphia, PA: Elsevier Mosby; 2004.
201. Coté CJ: NPO after midnight for children—a reappraisal. *Anesthesiology.* 1990;72:589-592.
202. Warner MA, Caplan RA, Epstein BS, et al. Practice guidelines for preoperative fasting and the use of pharmacologic agents to reduce the risk of pulmonary aspiration: application to healthy patients undergoing elective procedures: a report by the American Society of Anesthesiologists Task Force on Preoperative Fasting. *Anesthesiology.* 1999;90:896-905.
203. Sandhar B, Goresky GV, Maltby JR, et al. Effects of oral liquids and ranitidine on gastric fluid volume and pH in children undergoing outpatient surgery. *Anesthesiology.* 1989;71:327-330.
204. Practice guidelines for preoperative fasting and the use of pharmacologic agents to reduce the risk of pulmonary aspiration: application to healthy patients undergoing elective procedures. *Anesthesiology.* 1999;90:896-905.
205. Schoenfielder RC, Ponnamma CM, Freyle D, et al. Residual gastric fluid volume and chewing gum before surgery. *Anesth Analg.* 2006;102:415-417.
206. Farnsworth PB, Steiner E, Kleiner RM, et al. The value of routine preoperative chest roentgenograms in infants and children. *JAMA.* 1980;244:582-583.
207. O'Connor ME, Drasner K. Preoperative laboratory testing of children undergoing elective surgery. *Anesth Analg.* 1990;70:176-180.
208. Hackmann T, Steward DJ, Sheps SB. Anemia in pediatric day-surgery patients: prevalence and detection. *Anesthesiology.* 1991;75:27-31.
209. Patel RI, DeWitt L, Hannallah RS. Preoperative laboratory testing in children undergoing elective surgery: analysis of current practice. *J Clin Anesth.* 1997;9:569-575.
210. Wheeler M, Cote CJ. Preoperative pregnancy testing in a tertiary care children's hospital: a medico-legal conundrum. *J Clin Anesth.* 1999;11:56-63.
211. Azzam FJ, Padda GS, DeBoard JW, et al. Preoperative pregnancy testing in adolescents. *Anesth Analg.* 1996; 82:4-7.
212. Hennrikus WL, Shaw BA, Gerardi JA. Prevalence of positive preoperative pregnancy testing in teenagers scheduled for orthopedic surgery. *J Pediatr Ortho.* 2001;21:677-679.
213. Pierre N, Moy LK, Redd S, et al. Evaluation of a pregnancy-testing protocol in adolescents undergoing surgery. *J Pediatr Adolesc Gynecol.* 1998;11:139-141.

214. Gerber ME, O'Connor DM, Adler E, et al. Selected risk factors in pediatric adenotonsillectomy. *Arch Otolaryngol Head Neck Surg.* 1996;122:811-814.
215. Schreiber GB, Busch MP, Kleinman SH, et al. The risk of transfusion-transmitted virus infections. The Retrovirus Epidemiology Donor Study. *N Engl J Med.* 1996;334: 1685-1690.
216. Alter HJ, Nakatsuji Y, Melpolder J, et al. The incidence of transfusion-associated hepatitis G virus infection and its relation to liver disease. *N Engl J Med.* 1997;336: 747-754.
217. Centers for Disease Control and Prevention. US Public Health Service guidelines for testing and counseling blood and plasma donors for human immunodeficiency virus type 1 antigen. *MMWR.* 1996;45(RR-2):1-9.
218. Lackritz EM, Satten GA, Aberle-Grasse J, et al. Estimated risk of transmission of the human immunodeficiency virus by screened blood in the United States. *N Engl J Med.* 1995;333:1721-1725.
219. Linden JV, Kaplan HS. Transfusion errors: cause and effects. *Trans Med Rev.* 1994;8:169-183.
220. Linden JV, Tourault MA, Scribner CL. Decrease in frequency of transfusion fatalities. *Transfusion.* 1997;37: 243-244.
221. Luban NC. Irradiation for neonatal and pediatric transfusions. In: Herman JH, Manno CS, eds. *Pediatric Transfusion Therapy.* Bethesda, MD: AABB Press; 2002.

Chapter 63

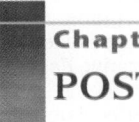

POSTOPERATIVE CARE

Lynne G. Maxwell, MD

INTRODUCTION

During the last 25 years, outpatient (ambulatory) anesthesia and surgery have revolutionized the way surgery and anesthesia are practiced in North America.[1] Safe, reliable, inexpensive, and convenient outpatient surgery is an attractive option for parents, children, their health care providers, and, perhaps most importantly, their insurers. Surgical procedures that routinely required 1 or 2 days of preadmission hospitalization and 1 to 7 days of postoperative recuperation are now commonly performed without any inpatient hospitalization at all. The cost savings are substantial; the average cost of 1 day in an American hospital is approaching $2000.[2] Government and private health care insurers are demanding increased use of ambulatory surgery services and will pay for even fewer inpatient procedures. Besides cost savings, outpatient surgery has additional advantages. Ambulatory anesthesia and surgery reduce the psychological trauma of hospitalization and family separation, cause fewer nosocomial infections, and hasten recovery.[1] Examples of surgical procedures that now are routinely performed in children on an outpatient basis are listed in Box 63-1.

BOX 63-1 Common Outpatient Surgical Procedures by Specialty

GENERAL SURGERY
Femoral, inguinal, and umbilical herniorrhaphies
Lymph node and other diagnostic biopsies
Central line insertion
Fistulotomy

GENITOURINARY SURGERY
Orchiopexy, hydrocele
Circumcision
Hypospadias repair

OTORHINOLARYNGEAL SURGERY
Myringotomy and tube placement
Adenoidectomy
Tonsillectomy
Bronchoscopy

OPHTHALMOLOGIC SURGERY
Strabismus
Examination under anesthesia

ORTHOPEDIC SURGERY
Tendon lengthening
Spica changes
Fracture reductions

COMPLICATIONS

Although the incidence of serious postoperative complications in healthy children undergoing ambulatory surgery is relatively low (<1%), some minor postoperative problems occur commonly.[1,3] These common anesthetic and surgical postoperative problems can be classified into early and late, depending on their time of onset. In many instances, the family will call on the primary care physician, rather than the surgeon or anesthesiologist, to diagnose and treat these problems. The primary care physician must therefore be aware of the existence of and recommended treatment for these complications.

SELECTION OF PATIENTS

Guidelines to select appropriate procedures and patients for outpatient surgery and anesthesia are continually evolving and are discussed in greater detail in Chapter 62, Preoperative Assessment.[4,5] In general, the procedure itself should not involve excessive bleeding or open entry into a major body cavity. Additionally, the patient should not require any special postoperative nursing care and must have a responsible adult at home who will be available to provide care until recovery is complete.

EARLY POSTOPERATIVE ANESTHETIC PROBLEMS

The most frequent complications of general anesthesia are postoperative nausea and vomiting (PONV).[6,7] These adverse effects are the most common cause of delayed discharge from the postanesthesia care unit (PACU, formerly called the recovery room) and unanticipated hospitalization after outpatient surgery.[6] The cause of these adverse effects is multifactorial, with factors such as predisposition (previous history of postoperative

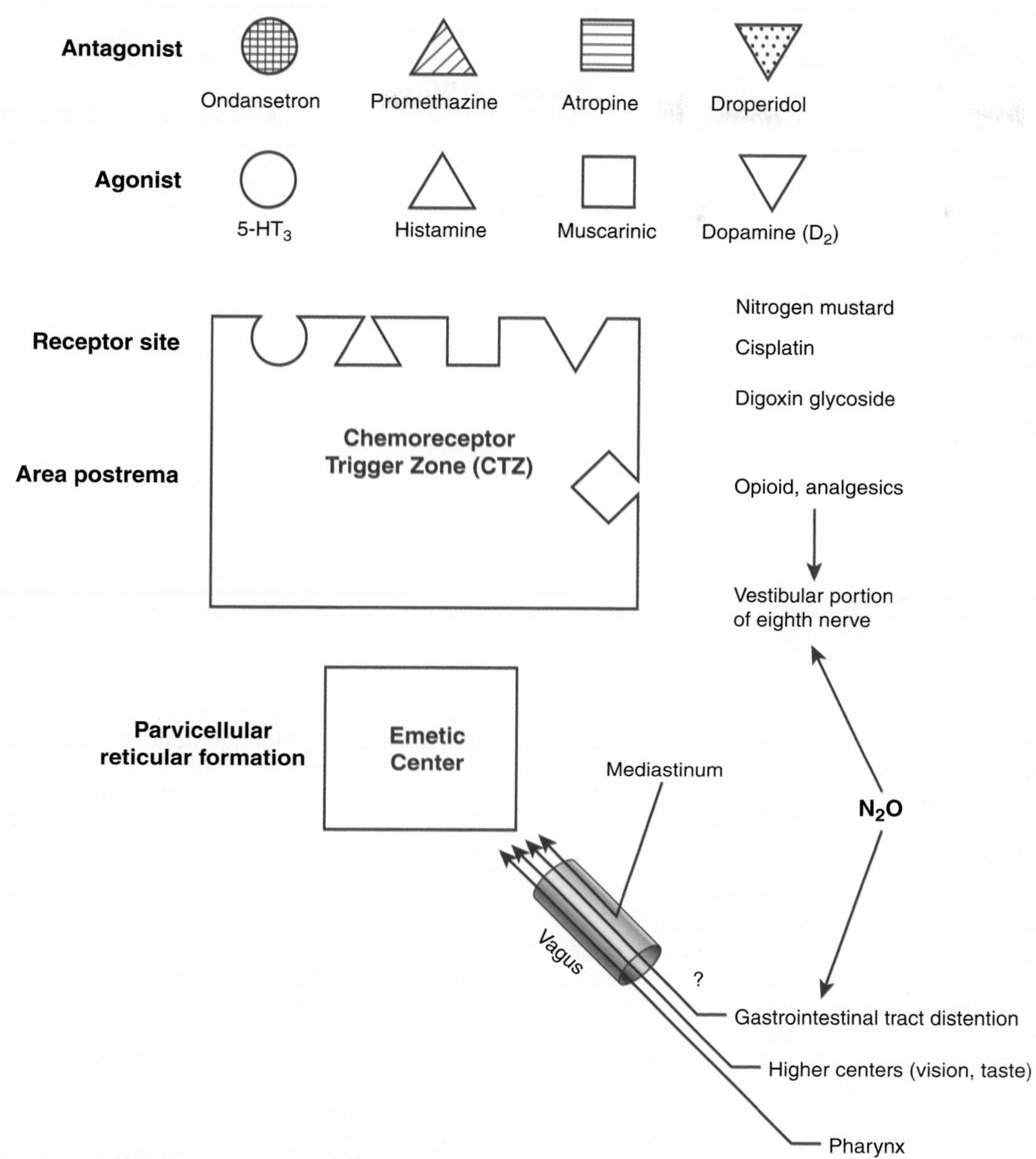

Figure 63-1 The chemoreceptor trigger zone and the emetic center with the agonist and antagonist sites of action of various anesthetic-related agents and stimuli. *(Watcha MF, White PF. Postoperative nausea and vomiting. Its etiology, treatment, and prevention.* Anesthesiology *1992;77:162-184. Reprinted with permission from Lippincott Williams & Wilkins.)*

vomiting, susceptibility to motion sickness), the anesthetic drugs or techniques used, the procedure being performed, the skill of the anesthesiologist providing the anesthetic, and motion playing an important role. Certain surgical procedures, such as strabismus surgery, middle ear surgery, orchiopexy, and umbilical hernia repair, are associated with a greater than 50% incidence of postoperative vomiting. Similarly, the perioperative use of *any* opioid is associated with a high incidence of postoperative nausea and vomiting even when general anesthetic drugs associated with a lower incidence of nausea, such as propofol, are used.[8]

The complex act of vomiting involves coordination of the respiratory, gastrointestinal, and abdominal musculature and is controlled by the emetic center. Stimuli from several areas within the central nervous system can affect the emetic center. These stimuli include afferents from the pharynx, gastrointestinal tract, and mediastinum, as well as afferents from the higher cortical centers (including the visual center and the vestibular portion of the eighth nerve) and the chemoreceptor trigger zone in the area postrema of the ventral lateral nucleus. The area postrema of the brain is rich in dopamine, opioid, and serotonin receptors.[9] Therefore blockade of these receptors is an important mechanism of action of the most commonly used antiemetics (Figure 63-1 and Table 63-1). Several techniques are available to treat or prevent postoperative nausea

Table 63-1 Receptor Site Affinity of Antiemetic Drugs

PHARMACOLOGICAL GROUP DRUG	DOPAMINE	MUSCARINIC CHOLINERGIC	HISTAMINE	SEROTONIN
PHENOTHIAZINES				
Chlorpromazine	++++	++	++++	+
Prochlorperazine	+++	+	++++	+
BUTYROPHENONES				
Droperidol	+++	—	+	+
Haloperidol	+++	—	+	—
ANTIHISTAMINES				
Promethazine	++	+++	++++	—
Diphenhydramine	+	++	++++	—
BENZAMIDES				
Metoclopramide	++	—	+	++
ANTICHOLINERGICS				
Scopolamine	+	++++	+	—
ANTISEROTONIN				
Ondansetron	—	—	—	++++

From Altman DF. Drugs used in gastrointestinal diseases. In Katzung BG, ed. *Basic and Clinical Pharmacology*. New York, NY: Lange Medical Books/McGraw-Hill; 2001. Reprinted with permission by The McGraw-Hill Companies, Inc.

and vomiting, including altering the anesthetic technique (eg, avoiding the perioperative use of opioids), using antiemetics perioperatively either prophylactically or as treatment (eg, droperidol, phenothiazines, ondansetron, or antihistamines; Table 63-2), and limiting oral intake postoperatively.[7,10,11]

Contribution of Anesthetic Technique to Postoperative Nausea and Vomiting

Certain anesthetic agents and techniques produce more vomiting than others. The effects of the general anesthetic inhalational agents sevoflurane, isoflurane, and nitrous oxide on vomiting are controversial.[12,13] Some studies report significantly more vomiting when these anesthetics are used, whereas others do not. Although some newer inhalation agents, such as desflurane, have been touted to be associated with less PONV than previous agents, gas anesthetics have repeatedly been shown to cause more PONV than intravenous anesthetic techniques. A new intravenous general anesthetic agent, propofol, produces significantly less vomiting and nausea than others, if opioids are not given concomitantly.[14] Indeed, opioids, including morphine, meperidine, fentanyl, codeine, oxycodone, or hydromorphone, have been consistently shown to cause nausea and vomiting.[15,16] Individual patients may find 1 opioid drug more nauseating than another; sometimes changing from 1 drug to another may decrease the amount of nausea and vomiting. Finally, although regional anesthetic techniques that use local anesthetics either centrally (eg, epidural) or peripherally (peripheral nerve block) produce less vomiting than general anesthetic techniques, using these techniques is rarely possible without concomitant general anesthesia in children.[17]

Avoiding opioids perioperatively may solve only part of the puzzle. Obviously, pain control is essential in children who undergo surgery, and opioids are the most common analgesic drugs used for this purpose (see Chapter 54, Management of Acute Pain in Children). An alternative may be ketorolac, a powerful nonsteroidal antiinflammatory drug (NSAID), which is almost as potent as morphine as an analgesic but does not produce nausea, vomiting, or respiratory depression.[18-20] Because NSAIDs affect platelet aggregation and adhesiveness, their use is limited in many patients who are at risk for postoperative bleeding, particularly children who have undergone tonsillectomy.[18,21] In addition, many orthopedic surgeons forbid the use of NSAIDs during and after operations in which new bone formation is important (fractures, spine fusions) because NSAIDs have been shown to impair osteoblastic activity.[22] The extent to which this effect is clinically important is controversial.[23]

Contribution of Postoperative Oral Intake to Postoperative Nausea and Vomiting

Many anesthesiologists prefer to restrict patients from taking anything by mouth until they are ready and willing to drink and eat, even if this restriction means that the child leaves the hospital while still fasting.[10,11,24] Basically, children must say that they are thirsty, or better still hungry, and must specifically ask for something to drink or eat before any food or liquid is offered. Even in the youngest patients, the risk of dehydration is low, particularly if intravenous fluids were appropriately administered perioperatively. In current anesthetic practice, virtually all children undergoing surgery and anesthesia receive intravenous fluids that contain salt and sugar in the operating room and PACU. If fluids sufficient to supply maintenance and replacement requirements were given during this period, a postoperative fast will be readily tolerated. Thus, just as anesthesiologists are abandoning stringent, prolonged preoperative fasts, they are increasingly appreciating their benefits postoperatively.[10]

Table 63-2 Dosage Guidance for Commonly Used Antiemetics

PHARMACOLOGICAL GROUP (GENERIC)	BRAND NAME	DOSAGE (mg/kg)	ADVERSE EFFECTS
PHENOTHIAZINES			
Chlorpromazine Prochlorperazine	Thorazine Compazine	IV, PO: 0.5-1.0 every 6-8 hr PO, PR: 0.1 every 6-8 hr (maximum dose 10 mg)	Drowsiness, hypotension, arrhythmias, extrapyramidal symptoms; potentiates effects of opioids, sedatives
BUTYROPHENONES			
Droperidol Haloperidol	Inapsine Haldol	IV: 0.01-0.03 every 6-8 hr IV: 0.01 every 8-12 hr	Drowsiness, hypotension, arrhythmias; droperidol has black box warning: prolongs QT interval, extrapyramidal symptoms; lowers seizure threshold; potentiates effects of opioids, sedatives
ANTIHISTAMINES			
Promethazine Diphenhydramine	Phenergan Benadryl	IV: 0.25-0.5 every 6 hr 0.5-1.0 every 4-6 hr (maximum dose 50 mg)	Drowsiness, hypotension, arrhythmias; contraindicated in patients taking MAO inhibitors; Phenergan contraindicated in children <2 years old because of cases of fatal respiratory depression*
BENZAMIDES			
Metoclopramide	Reglan	IV, PO: 0.05-0.1 every 6 hr	Adverse effects include extrapyramidal symptoms
ANTICHOLINERGIC			
Scopolamine	Hyoscine transdermal scopolamine	IV, PO: 0.005 every 4-6 hr apply behind ear 4 hr before needed; lasts 72 hr	Adverse effects include dry mouth, blurred vision, fever, tachycardia, constipation, urinary retention, drowsiness, amnesia
ANTISEROTONIN			
Ondansetron	Zofran, Zofran ODT	IV, PO: 0.15 every 8 hr, (maximum dose 4 mg)	Adverse effects include bronchospasm, tachycardia, headaches, lightheadedness, may prolong QT interval

MAO, Monoamine oxidase; *ODT*, oral dissolving tablet.
*FDA MedWatch, www.fda.gov/medWatch/SAFETY/2005/safety05.htm#phenergan (accessed 4/19/2007).

Unfortunately, many institutions continue to require that patients drink and ambulate before they can be discharged from the hospital or same-day care unit. This restriction almost certainly contributes to the incidence of unanticipated admission to the hospital after outpatient surgery because of vomiting.

Treatment of Postoperative Nausea and Vomiting

The treatment of PONV is the same as that used for viral gastroenteritis. A cooling-off period of 2 to 4 hours is followed by sips of clear fluids that contain sugar and salt (eg, oral rehydration solution, Pedialyte® [see Chapter 341, Dehydration]). Each sip is separated by several minutes. Giving fluids or solids prematurely only aggravates the problem. Finally, antiemetics can be used either prophylactically or to treat the problem once it develops. The most common antiemetics are those that block receptors within the vomiting center. Four major neurotransmitter systems play a role in mediating the emetic response: dopaminergic, histaminic, cholinergic, and serotonergic. Antiemetic drugs may act at more than 1 receptor, but they tend to have a more prominent action at 1 or 2 receptors.[9] The most commonly used antiemetics, in order of use, include benzamides (metoclopramide, trimethobenzamide hydrochloride), serotonin antagonists (ondansetron, dolasetron), phenothiazines (prochlorperazine and promethazine [Phenergan]), butyrophenones (droperidol, haloperidol), antihistamines (hydroxyzine, diphenhydramine), and anticholinergics (scopolamine, atropine).[25,26] Unfortunately, most of these antiemetic classes, with the exception of the serotonin antagonists, produce sedation, which can interfere with rapid return to baseline function and therefore hospital discharge. In addition, promethazine has been identified as a contributing cause in a significant number of deaths in children younger than 2 years to whom it had been administered for vomiting that occurred either in the postoperative period after hospital discharge or because of gastroenteritis. For this reason, in 2004, the US Food and Drug Administration mandated a black box warning. The original warning seemed to apply only to brand name suppository formulations[27]; the warning was clarified in 2006 to make sure that both health care professionals and parents understood that the warning applies to all formulations:

> Medications containing promethazine hydrochloride (HCl) should not be used for children less than 2 years of age because of the potential for fatal respiratory depression. This includes promethazine HCl in any form: syrup, suppository, tablet, or injectable. Cases of respiratory depression including fatalities have been reported with use of promethazine HCl in children less than 2 years of age. Caution should also be exercised when administering promethazine HCl in any form to pediatric patients 2 years of age and older.[28]

This warning is especially germane in children postoperatively because they may be receiving opioids for analgesia, which may cause respiratory depression.

Pharmacology of Commonly Used Antiemetic Drugs

Site of action, dose, and route of administration of the most commonly used antiemetics are listed in Table 63-1 and Table 63-2. Recently, a new dose form of ondansetron, the oral dissolving tablet, has been found to be an effective and acceptable formulation in children undergoing adenotonsillectomy,[29] as well as in infants and children with gastroenteritis treated in an emergency department.[30] This drug, as with all serotonin antagonists, is much more expensive than older antiemetics, but it has the advantage of oral dosing and lack of side effects, such as sedation or extrapyramidal reactions seen with metoclopramide. The effective dose and therefore cost of serotonin antagonists can be reduced by the coadministration of intravenous dexamethasone (Decadron) in the perioperative period, which has also been shown to prolong the duration of the antiemetic effect of these drugs.[31]

Prolonged Nausea and Vomiting

Nausea and vomiting that persists beyond 12 to 24 hours is unusual and requires evaluation to determine the state of hydration and possible necessity of intravenous rehydration and to rule out alternative conditions. In rare instances, excessive air swallowing in the postoperative period may lead to acute gastric dilation in young children. Recognition of the characteristic distended abdomen and gastric splash, if present, should be followed by nasogastric decompression.

Effect of Postoperative Vomiting on Concomitant Medications

Postoperative vomiting may interfere with the resumption of long-term oral medication regimens. With few exceptions (monoamine oxidase inhibitors, oral hypoglycemics, and diuretics), all long-term administered oral medications should be taken on the morning of surgery.[4] Indeed, the question of whether patients should take oral medications on the morning of surgery has become moot because of the liberalization of preoperative fasting guidelines. This ability of patients to take their medications preoperatively has greatly reduced the stress associated with deciding when the use of oral medications can be restarted postoperatively. Most drugs administered in the long term, such as anticonvulsants, bronchodilators, and digitalis, have half-lives of elimination that are long (>12 hours), which means that missing a dose of these drugs for 1 or 2 half-lives (12 to 24 hours) will have minimal, if any, effect on blood levels. Of course, this situation assumes that therapeutic blood levels existed before surgery began. If vomiting persists beyond 24 hours, then parenteral drug administration may be required.

POSTOPERATIVE PAIN MANAGEMENT

The treatment and alleviation of pain is fundamental to medical care.[16,32] The physician's obligation to manage pain and relieve patient suffering is a crucial element of the professional commitment to patient care. This concept is not merely a lofty ideal; effective pain management produces a myriad of patient benefits, including reduced morbidity and mortality, early mobilization, and more rapid recovery, and return to work, school, and play. (A detailed discussion of pain management can be found in Chapter 54, Management of Acute Pain in Children.)

EMERGENCE PHENOMENA AFTER GENERAL ANESTHESIA

Emergence from general anesthesia in healthy patients is often accompanied by transient symmetrical neurologic changes that, under other circumstances, are considered pathological reflexes. These otherwise pathological reflexes include sustained and nonsustained ankle clonus, bilateral hyperreflexia, the Babinski reflex, and decerebrate posturing. These reflexes can often be detected within minutes of discontinuing a general anesthetic and may persist for hours, the reason for which is unknown. However, the discovery of *focal* neurologic deficits in a postoperative patient is never normal. Such neurologic deficits should point to a possible central or peripheral nervous system injury and requires investigation.

Children are prone to disorientation, hallucinations, and, at times, uncontrollable physical activity during emergence from general anesthesia. This hyperexcitable, hyperactive state is sometimes referred to as *emergence delirium* and occurs most commonly if a patient awakens in pain after receiving a potent vapor anesthetic (eg, halothane, sevoflurane, isoflurane, desflurane).[33] Other causes include sensory deprivation (eye bandages, eye lubricant); residual anesthetic; awakening in a strange environment (the PACU); and the perioperative use of ketamine.[34] Regardless of cause, before discharge from the PACU, most of the disorientation, hyperactivity, excitability, and hallucinatory visual disturbances should be completely resolved. PACU treatment for these phenomena may include small doses of analgesics (eg, fentanyl) or flumazenil, if midazolam was administered. In some instances, atropine may be responsible for this reaction, in which case it will be accompanied by other features of anticholinergic syndrome (flushed cheeks, mydriasis, and low-grade fever). This reaction may be treated by administration of physostigmine, an anticholinesterase that crosses the blood-brain barrier and reverses the central nervous system effects of atropine by potentiating the action of acetylcholine at nerve terminals. The prevalence of such anticholinergic reactions has been reduced since the replacement of halothane with sevoflurane as the primary gas for mask anesthetic induction in children. Sevoflurane does not cause the bradycardia seen with halothane, making routine use of atropine unnecessary in pediatric anesthetic practice, except that used to counteract the muscarinic effects of anticholinesterase administration for reversal of nondepolarizing muscle relaxant.

Occasionally, some lingering evidence of these behavioral perturbations may persist for 12 to 24 hours. Thus some children who have undergone general anesthesia and surgery may experience sleep disturbances, nightmares (terrors), separation anxiety, aggression toward authority, and even loss of nighttime bladder control on the night after surgery. Indeed, children who are extremely anxious during the induction of anesthesia are more at risk of developing postoperative negative behavioral changes compared with children who appear calm during the induction process.[35] These children clearly benefit from premedication with a benzodiazepine (midazolam) before the induction of anesthesia. In fact, Kain et al[36,37] have clearly demonstrated that oral premedication with midazolam is more effective than either parental presence or extensive preoperative behavioral programs at reducing preoperative anxiety and postoperative, delayed alterations in behavior. Ketamine, in particular, is associated with sleep disturbances after its administration.[34,35] Although the incidence of nightmares after ketamine administration is less in children than adults, it has been reported to occur in 5% to 10% of patients who receive it. However, the incidence is mitigated by the concomitant administration of benzodiazepine, usually midazolam. Fortunately, regardless of the cause, sleep disturbance is time limited and rarely persists beyond 48 hours after surgery and general anesthesia. If sleep disturbances become overwhelming, they can then be treated with oral diazepam. In most cases, 1 dose given at bedtime cures the problem completely.

INTUBATION-RELATED COMPLICATIONS

On awakening from a general anesthetic, many children who have been endotracheally intubated or who have experienced either airway manipulation or instrumentation (laryngeal mask airway) will complain of a sore throat. This discomfort can be alleviated with fruit-flavored ice pops, ice chips, or common throat lozenges or sprays once cough, gag, and swallowing reflexes have returned to baseline. Analgesics are rarely required, but if they are, then acetaminophen will usually suffice.

POSTINTUBATION CROUP

Postintubation croup, or postextubation subglottic edema, has been a well-recognized entity since airways were first secured by intubation. Children are more prone to develop croup after intubation than are adults because of differences in their airway anatomy. Children have narrower laryngeal and tracheal lumens that are more easily compromised by mucosal edema. Additionally, the narrowest portion of the younger child's airway is at the level of cricoid cartilage and not at the level of the larynx. Given that an endotracheal tube can easily pass through the vocal cords and become wedged in the subglottic area, internal tracheal mucosal injury can occur. Other contributing factors to the development of croup are traumatic or repeated intubations, coughing *(bucking)* on the tube, changing the patient's position after intubation, and providing general anesthesia to children who have a current or recent upper respiratory tract infection.[38,39]

The incidence of postintubation croup has been lowered from 6% to 1% of all endotracheally intubated children.[40] This reduction has occurred through the use of sterile, implant-tested endotracheal tubes and the routine intraoperative use of humidification of the administered gases and, in children younger than 5 years, by using appropriately sized (air leak pressure of less than 30 cm of water), uncuffed endotracheal tubes.[40] Children who have Down syndrome may be at increased risk for this complication because of the increased incidence of occult subglottic narrowing.

The treatment of postintubation croup is the same as for viral laryngotracheitis. Humidification is effective in most cases. Nebulized racemic epinephrine therapy is rarely necessary. If it is, then these patients should not be discharged from the PACU to their homes. Rather, they must be admitted to the hospital for overnight observation because of the potential for rebound edema formation. The efficacy of corticosteroids in treating postintubation croup has been controversial, although most studies have shown it to be effective.[41,42] Most anesthesiologists will prescribe dexamethasone for this problem, even though no controlled, prospective trials have validated its use for this purpose.

SUCCINYLCHOLINE-INDUCED MYALGIA

In the past, many anesthesiologists commonly used succinylcholine, a short-acting, depolarizing muscle relaxant, to facilitate intubation of the trachea in children. Because of the risk of fatal hyperkalemia in children with undiagnosed Duchenne muscular dystrophy, when succinylcholine is administered, it is used less frequently.[43] Because of these risks, and because alternatives are available, the use of succinylcholine by anesthesiologists caring for children has declined in favor of relatively fast-onset, nondepolarizing muscle relaxants such as rocuronium. Use of succinylcholine is now reserved for patients who have no known risk of malignant hyperthermia or hyperkalemia and who need true rapid sequence intubation because of intestinal obstruction or increased gastric contents from a recent meal. Succinylcholine administration in all children normally will result in some damage to the muscle cell, with leakage of intracellular potassium. In fact, myalgia and increased blood levels of creatinine phosphokinase and myoglobin are expected complications of succinylcholine administration.[44,45] To some degree, the magnitude of these perturbations can be avoided by pretreating the patient with small doses of a nondepolarizing muscle relaxant or calcium. The myalgia is intense and as debilitating as the myalgia produced by an influenza infection. Treatment is supportive, and the pain usually resolves over several days.

EARLY POSTOPERATIVE SURGICAL PROBLEMS

Fever

Postoperative fever has several possible causes, which can be remembered as the 4 Ws: wind, wound, water, and walker (Table 63-3).[46] Pyrexia (rectal temperature greater than 101.2°F [38.5°C]) within 24 hours of operation and general anesthesia is common and usually caused by atelectasis. Postoperative atelectasis has many causes. Endotracheal intubation, inhalational general anesthetics, and the use of nonhumidified gases all depress ciliary motion within the tracheal-bronchial tree and thereby interfere with normal pulmonary clearance mechanisms. When these factors are combined with small tidal volume breathing, somnolence, splinting cause by pain, and cough suppression caused by pain or opioid analgesics, atelectasis occurs. Early ambulation, deep breathing, and coughing can be extremely helpful in alleviating or preventing atelectasis and postoperative fever. Indeed, this feature may be one of the important medical advantages of ambulatory surgery because patients are more likely to be up and about when they are at home rather than in the hospital.

Other causes of postoperative pyrexia are rare. Yeung, Buck, and Filler, in a retrospective analysis of the postoperative course of 256 febrile children at the Hospital for Sick Children in Toronto, Canada, found that only 4 had infections that required treatment.[46] Interestingly, all 4 of these children had significant and obvious associated signs of infection (local tenderness, crepitance, or erythema at the incision site, tachypnea, cough, dysuria, and headache). Most patients with low-grade postoperative fevers require only a physical examination to differentiate between a septic and nonseptic process. Extensive (and expensive) diagnostic workups are rarely indicated. Indeed, in most patients, fever in the early postoperative period is so common that it can be regarded as a normal response to operative trauma and general anesthesia. Other unusual causes of postoperative fever include urinary tract infections, dehydration, infected intravenous access sites, thyroid storm, pheochromocytoma, and malignant hyperthermia. Urinary tract infections do not usually produce symptoms in the immediate postoperative period. Rather, they are a cause of late postoperative fever, usually occurring 3 to 5 days after operation. These children generally are symptomatic and complain of dysuria. Infants may have hematuria. The fever associated with malignant hyperthermia usually starts intraoperatively. Malignant hyperthermia is discussed in more detail in Chapter 62, Preoperative Assessment.

Wound infection as a cause of fever is rare.[46] The postoperative day on which a given wound infection becomes apparent and the local signs of sepsis produced by the infection vary according to the organism and the concomitant use of antibiotics (Table 63-4). As a general rule, the earlier the onset of wound sepsis is, the more destructive and life-threatening the infection will be. Most wound infections do not usually become apparent until the 5th to 10th postoperative day. The rare exceptions are beta-streptococcal, *Clostridium difficile*, and *Clostridium perfringens (welchii)* infections. These organisms produce wound infections that can become apparent within 24 to 48 hours of surgery. *Clostridium* and streptococcal wound infections are life threatening. In most instances, children with these infections develop high, spiking fevers (temperatures of 102.2° to 105.8°F [39°C to 41°C]), become irrational, and may even develop jaundice. The surgical incision site is red, warm, and intensely painful on palpation. Additionally, vesicle formation, wound crepitance, and an exudate may be present. Obviously, patients who develop this type of wound infection require immediate hospitalization and treatment.

Table 63-3 Common Causes of Postoperative Fever

SITE	ETIOLOGY	TIME	INCIDENCE	SIGN SYMPTOMS	DIAGNOSIS	THERAPY
Wind (lungs)	Atelectasis	24-48 hr	Very common	Cough, shortness of breath, retractions	Examination, chest x-ray	Cough, deep breathing, incentive spirometer
Wound (operative site)	Infection	<24 hr-7 days	Rare	Pain, erythema, induration	Examination wound cultures	Antibiotics, open wound
Water (urinary tract)	Urinary tract infection	3-5 days	Very rare	Dysuria, hematuria	Examination urinalysis, culture	Remove indwelling catheter, antibiotics
Walker (legs)	Deep-vein thrombosis	>3 days	Extremely rare	Swelling, heaviness of lower extremities, superficial venous congestion, palpable cord	Examination, duplex Doppler, venogram	Bed rest, elevation, heparin (Coumadin), thrombolytics

Drainage

A small amount of serosanguineous drainage in the postoperative dressing is normal and should not be a cause for alarm. Only persistent bleeding requires immediate surgical attention.

Serosanguineous discharge from the operative site 2 to 3 days after the operation may be due to a superficial hematoma just below the incision site. A hematoma can be recognized by its characteristic ecchymoses and fluctuance. Small hematomas directly below a wound, umbilicus, or scrotum usually spontaneously drain or resorb. If the hematoma progressively expands, it may then require operative exploration to evacuate the clot and control any ongoing bleeding. In general, a nonexpanding hematoma will usually resolve within 4 to 6 weeks after surgery. If the wound hematoma is associated with pain, then the child should be examined by the operating surgeon.

Serous drainage from a wound may be caused by creation of a large dead space during the operative procedure or by liquefaction of adipose tissue. In general, seromas caused by dead space usually drain 4 to 7 days after surgery, whereas liquefaction of adipose tissue, characterized by yellow drainage, occurs 2 to 3 weeks after surgery.

Regardless of size, hematomas and seromas are excellent culture media for bacteria and increase the likelihood of wound infection.[46] Both of these postoperative problems should be closely watched for and are usually characterized by the triad of pain, wound dehiscence, and persistent drainage.

Postoperative Bleeding

Persistent bleeding is defined as bleeding and bloody ooze that continues for more than 6 to 8 hours after the operation or a need to change a blood-soaked wound dressing more than twice in the first 6 to 8 hours after surgery. It almost always indicates inadequate hemostasis and is usually due to a superficial skin arterial bleeding site, although coagulopathy might also be responsible. Until the bleeding site is investigated and controlled by the operating surgeon or the surgeon's designee, direct digital pressure applied to the wound will slow or stop the flow of blood.

Posttonsillectomy Hemorrhage

The incidence of posttonsillectomy hemorrhage is estimated to be 5% to 10%, with 1% to 3% of patients who have tonsillectomy requiring additional operation.[47,48] Bleeding that occurs after tonsillectomy may

Table 63-4 Postoperative Wound Infections

ONSET (POSTOPERATIVE DAY)	USUAL PATHOGENS	WOUND APPEARANCE	OTHER SIGNS
1-3	*Clostridium welchii*	Brawny, hemorrhagic, cool	High standard fever (temperatures of 39°C-40°C)
		Occasional gaseous crepitance	Irrational behavior
		Putrid *dishwasher* exudate	Leukocytosis (white blood cell count >15,000/mL)
		Intense local pain	Occasional jaundice
2-3	*Streptococcus*	Erythematous, warm, tender	High, spiking fever (temperatures of 39°C-40°C)
		Occasionally, hemorrhagic with blebs	Irrational at times
		Serous exudate	Leukocytosis (white blood cell count >15,000 mL)
			Rare jaundice
3-5	*Staphylococcus*	Erythematous, warm, tender	High, spiking fever (temperatures of 38°C-40°C)
		Purulent exudate	Irrational behavior at times
			Leukocytosis (white blood cell count 12,000-20,000/mL)
>5	Gram-negative rods	Erythematous, warm, tender	Sustained low-grade to moderate fever (temperatures of 38°C-40°C)
		Purulent exudate	Rational behavior
			Leukocytosis (white blood cell count 10,000-16,000/mL)
>5	Symbiotic (usually anaerobes plus gram-negative rods)	Erythematous, warm, tender	Moderate to high fever (temperatures of 38°C-40°C)
		Focal necrosis	Leukocytosis (white blood cell count >15,000/mL)
		Purulent, putrid exudate	Occasional jaundice
			Mentation variable

occur early (in the first 24 hours, but usually after hospital discharge) or late (5 to 14 days after surgery). Early bleeding is due to failure of hemostasis and may be due to coagulopathy, whereas late bleeding results from dislodgement of the scab from the operative bed. Either form may be severe and life-threatening and requires immediate emergency evaluation. Rehydration with isotonic fluid is always required because hemorrhage is frequently associated with history of poor postoperative fluid intake and volume contraction resulting from blood loss. Transfusion, although unlikely, may be required even if a subsequent operation is performed and control of bleeding is achieved.

MISCELLANEOUS EARLY POSTOPERATIVE PROBLEMS

Urinary Retention

In contrast to adults, urinary retention is rare in pediatric surgical outpatients. Most children who undergo surgery through the inguinal canal void within 8 hours of the operation, regardless of their intraoperative anesthetic technique or their postoperative analgesic regimen, which included parenteral and enteral opioids or regional anesthesia (caudal epidural blockade or ilioinguinal-iliohypogastric nerve blocks) or both.[49] This finding is significant because, theoretically, opioids and regional anesthetics, particularly caudal epidural blockade, may interfere with the neural mechanisms responsible for emptying of the bladder. In fact, many investigators who argued against the routine use of caudal anesthesia or opioids (or both) for the treatment of postoperative surgical pain based their opinions on the theoretical risk of urinary retention. Many surgeons, anesthesiologists, and ambulatory care administrators have insisted that children void before discharge after outpatient procedures that require anesthesia. However, many patients simply cannot void on command, particularly in the strange setting of a PACU or hospital. The knowledge that all patients void within 24 hours of operation and virtually all spontaneously void within 10 hours of a procedure strongly suggests that voiding before discharge is unnecessary.

To minimize bladder distention, children and adolescents should be encouraged to urinate immediately before coming to the operating room and as soon as possible postoperatively. In some practices, primary care physicians do not routinely require patients to void before postoperative discharge from the PACU. Exceptions to this rule include patients who complain of lower abdominal distention and discomfort. These patients are initially treated with ambulation, in the case of the older child or adolescent, or gentle pressure on the lower abdomen, in the case of infants. If these measures do not lead to voiding and amelioration of symptoms, then bladder catheterization should be performed. Patients requiring bladder catheterization should then be observed for their ability to urinate spontaneously. If bladder function does not return, then the patient should be admitted to the hospital, a specimen of urine should be sent for urinalysis and culture, and the patient's surgeon should decided whether a bladder catheter should be reinserted. Nevertheless, the need for bladder catheterization is rare. In the experience of some practitioners, urination after outpatient surgery requires a *less is more* attitude; that is, the more attention the physician pays to this issue, the more problems are created.

Scrotal Swelling

Scrotal swelling and concomitant discoloration of the scrotum commonly occur after inguinal herniorrhaphy or hydrocelectomy, or both. Initially, this process can produce swelling alone and may progress to bluish discoloration as bleeding and clot lysis occur. In general, the problem is usually the result of bleeding from the cut edge of the peritoneal sac derived from either a hernia or hydrocele. The swelling and color change should resolve in 4 to 6 weeks. However, if fever, erythema, tenderness, and progressive enlargement of the hemiscrotum occur, then an urgent consultation with the patient's surgeon is needed. In many instances, such patients require additional exploratory surgery and operative evacuation of the hematoma via a suprainguinal or transscrotal approach.

LATE POSTOPERATIVE SURGICAL PROBLEMS

Pyrexia (rectal temperature greater than 101.2°F [38.5°C]) 48 hours or more after outpatient surgery is unusual and may indicate a serious wound infection (see Table 63-3 and Table 63-4).[46] This circumstance requires evaluation and examination by the patient's primary care physician or surgeon. The wound is examined for signs of inflammation, such as heat, pain, redness, and swelling. If any of these signs or symptoms is present, then the operating surgeon should be informed. If the wound appears to be the source of the fever and infection, then the wound can be probed with a sterile swab (Q-Tip) and a Gram stain and culture obtained. If pus is present, the wound should be opened, copiously irrigated, and debrided. Regardless of the presence of pus, a culture swab should always be sent for Gram stain and culture.

Gram-positive infections are the most common causes of wound infection. Wound infections caused by *Staphylococcus aureus* or *S epidermidis* are usually characterized by a milky white, purulent drainage and usually occur 3 to 5 days after surgery (see Table 63-4). Staphylococcal infections usually produce high, spiking fevers (temperatures of 102.2°F to 104°F [39°C to 40°C]) and leukocytosis (white blood cell count of >12,000/mL). After Gram stain and culture, the patient is treated with a penicillinase-resistant antibiotic such as oxacillin. Enteric, encapsulated, gram-negative organisms such as *Escherichia coli* are usually associated with significant erythema, tenderness, and, possibly, purulent discharge and usually occur more than 5 days after surgery (see Table 63-4). Enteric organisms such as *E coli* are sensitive to penicillin, cephalosporins, and aminoglycosides.

Finally, in patients who develop fevers more than 5 days after a surgical procedure, primary care physicians should suspect an anaerobic infection or a mixed (symbiotic) infection of anaerobic and gram-negative rods. The skin surrounding the wound should be examined closely for the presence of crepitus and vesicle formation, purulent and putrid discharge, and focal necrosis. All of these conditions indicate the development of gas gangrene or necrotizing fasciitis. These anaerobic types of infections can be caused by the gram-positive cocci, *Clostridium perfringens* or the gram-negative rods of the *Bacteroides* species (usually *B fragilis*). *C perfringens* infection causes exquisite pain, brown discoloration, and a wound that is crepitant to palpation. Gas may be seen in the subcutaneous tissues on a plain radiograph. Wound infections caused by *Bacteroides* are usually purulent and malodorous. Both of these anaerobic infections are life threatening and require immediate hospitalization, resuscitation, and operational evaluation and intervention.

The treatment of a serious wound infection is straightforward and consists of inpatient hospitalization, opening the wound along its entire length, drainage, wide debridement of necrotic tissue, high-dose intravenous antibiotics (penicillin, clindamycin, metronidazole, cefotetan), and, in selected cases, hyperbaric oxygen therapy. These wounds are not closed but rather are allowed to close spontaneously by contracture. If only cellulitis is detected, then the wound should not be opened; however, the patient should be given intravenous antibiotic therapy. Lymphangitis, characterized by its characteristic red streaks and tender regional adenopathy, should also be treated with intravenous antibiotics in the hospital.

If the surgical incision site does not appear to be responsible for the development of fever, then a thorough history and physical examination should be performed. Particular attention should be devoted to the lungs and intravenous administration sites. As stated previously, atelectasis often follows general anesthesia and surgery. Infected intravenous insertion sites, phlebitis, or thrombophlebitis, especially in the female adolescent taking birth control pills, also can occur. Additionally, routine causes of pyrexia in children can occur in the postoperative patient and include upper respiratory tract infections, gastroenteritis, and otitis media.

VENOUS THROMBOEMBOLISM

Although not as common as in adults, venous thromboembolism (VTE) occurs in children in the postoperative period, with the incidence increasing in adolescence.[50,51] The primary care physician should be alert to symptoms of VTE, such as extremity pain, swelling, and discoloration, which may indicate deep-vein thrombosis and should be referred for immediate evaluation. Patients at highest risk are those who are immobilized after surgery and have at least 1 other risk factor. Risk factors for VTE are listed in Box 63-2. Patients who develop VTE are at risk for pulmonary embolism, which has a mortality rate as high as 20%.[52] Symptoms of pulmonary embolism include dyspnea, chest pain, cough, hemoptysis, and fever. Patients at risk for VTE should receive prophylactic measures, which may include compression stockings or pneumatic sequential compression devices (or both) until ambulatory. Patients with 3 or more risk factors may be treated with pharmacologic prophylaxis: subcutaneous heparin or low–molecular-weight heparin.

BOX 63-2 Risk Factors for Venous Thromboembolism (VTE) in the Postoperative Period

- Immobility
- Major lower extremity orthopedic surgery
- Spinal cord injury
- Major trauma or trauma to the lower extremities
- Previous history of deep-vein thrombosis or VTE or pulmonary embolism
- Pregnancy
- Oral contraceptive use
- Inflammatory bowel disease
- Nephrotic syndrome
- Burns
- Obesity
- Central venous catheter in the lower extremity
- Known acquired or inherited thrombophilia
- Acute infection

PRACTICAL ASPECTS OF THE POSTSURGICAL WOUND

Wound healing represents a highly dynamic, integrated series of cellular physiological and biochemical events. The morphological events that make up the healing of closed wounds include the following: inflammation, epithelialization, cellular influx, and fibroplasia. The inflammatory phase begins immediately. During its early stages, white blood cells migrate into the wound and engulf and remove cellular debris and tissue fragments. This phase sets the stage for subsequent events in the healing process.

After dead material is removed, the epidermis and dermis immediately adjacent to the wound edges begin to thicken within 24 hours after injury. Within 48 hours, the entire wound surface is reepithelialized. During this critical period, the wound should be kept dressed and dry. Thus wound dressings are not required after 48 hours. Wound contamination with stool and urine should be cleansed with water or saline, and the overlying dressing should be replaced. Detergent soaps and peroxide should be avoided.

Between days 2 and 3, an influx of fibroblasts into the wound occurs deep in the epithelium. By the 4th or 5th day, the fibroblasts begin to lay down collagen fibers, which continues for several months. However, remodeling of collagen takes place for more than 1 year. Practically speaking, by postoperative day 4, the wound may be washed with warm water and a bland soap (eg, Ivory, Dove, Neutrogena).

From the surgeon's point of view, all of the morphological events of wound healing lead to a single important conclusion: wounds become stronger with time. Closing the wound with suture material only serves to hasten the process. Normally, a simple wound will attain 50% of the strength of surrounding uninjured tissue by 28 days. Most wounds are closed using absorbable suture material, which maintains tensile strength for 60 to 90 days, supplies an appreciable amount of wound strength to allow for the normal healing process to take place, and does not require suture removal. Closing wounds with absorbable suture material allows the child to return to activity at an earlier time. For instance, adolescents with uncomplicated inguinal hernia repair may return to nonstrenuous activity 7 to 10 days postoperatively and may return to full activity by 4 to 6 weeks. Whenever possible, toddlers are kept off tricycles and bicycles for 7 to 10 days. Infants should be treated as if no operation was performed (ie, full bath by the 4th postoperative day and no restrictions for carrying the infant).

SCAR FORMATION

Black and white people of Mediterranean descent are predisposed to hypertrophic scars and keloid formation. Keloids are tumors characterized by massive formation of scar tissue in and beneath the skin after any trauma, including surgery. The keloid grows well beyond the borders of the incision, which is what differentiates it from hypertrophic scar formation. Furthermore, a hypertrophic scar tends to resolve with time and, as a rule, is not associated with prolonged itchiness. Keloids tend to recur after excision. Children have a greater tendency to form and re-form keloids than adults do. A thorough family history may be a predictor of this pathological process. An abnormal scar should be observed for a minimum of 6 months postoperatively. If it does not resolve, then a trial excision should be attempted, staying within the confines of the lesion to see what response is obtained. If it recurs, then it should be reexcised and 1% triamcinolone injected beneath the scar, which will produce some keloid resolution. A hypertrophic scar, on the other hand, should be treated with pressure. Overall, the management of the abnormal scar should be determined by the anatomic position of the wound, the age of the patient, and any underlying associated diseases.

Finally, all skin wounds and surgical skin incision sites will scar regardless of the expertise of the surgeon or the use of plastic surgical techniques in closing the skin. Indeed, the notion that plastic surgery is scarless is a myth. Furthermore, the scar tissue will permanently pigment (it will usually become red to dark brown-black) when exposed to intense sunlight during the first 6 months of its formation. Thus patients and their families should be advised that when going outdoors and exposing the surgical incision site to the sun, the incision site should be completely covered or protected with zinc oxide or a sunblock with an sun-protection factor number higher than 30 for 6 months after surgery.

The authors acknowledge the work of Drs Myron Yaster and Charles Paidas in previous editions of this book.

TOOLS FOR PRACTICE

Engaging Patients and Family

- *Anesthesia and Your Child* (brochure), American Academy of Pediatrics (patiented.aap.org).

Medical Decision Support

- *Pediatric Pain Management* (book), Tobias JD, Deshpande JK, American Academy of Pediatrics (www.aap.org/bookstore).

REFERENCES

1. Yaster M, Sola JE, Pegoli W Jr, et al. The night after surgery: postoperative management of the pediatric outpatient: surgical and anesthetic aspects. *Pediatr Clin North Am.* 1994;41:199-220.
2. Reinhardt UE, Hussey PS, Anderson GF. Cross-national comparisons of health systems using OECD data, 1999. *Health Affairs.* 2002;21:169-181.
3. Hannallah RS. Pediatric outpatient anesthesia. *Urol Clin North Am.* 1987;14:51-62.
4. Fisher QA, Feldman MA, Wilson MD. Pediatric responsibilities for preoperative evaluation. *J Pediatr.* 1994;125:675-685.
5. Maxwell LG, Deshpande JK, Wetzel RC. Preoperative evaluation of children. *Pediatr Clin North Am.* 1994;41:93-110.
6. Patel RI, Hannallah RS. Anesthetic complications following pediatric ambulatory surgery: a 3-year study. *Anesthesiology.* 1988;69:1009-1012.
7. Watcha MF, White PF. Postoperative nausea and vomiting: its etiology, treatment, and prevention. *Anesthesiology.* 1992;77:162-184.
8. Weir PM, Munro HM, Reynolds PI, et al. Propofol infusion and the incidence of emesis in pediatric outpatient strabismus surgery. *Anesth Analg.* 1993;76:760-764.
9. Scholz J, Steinfath M, Tonner PH. Antiemetics. In Evers AS, Maze M, eds. *Anesthetic Pharmacology: Physiologic Principles and Clinical Practice.* Philadelphia, PA: Churchill Livingstone; 2004.
10. Schreiner MS. Preoperative and postoperative fasting in children. *Pediatr Clin North Am.* 1994;41:111-120.
11. Schreiner MS, Nicolson SC, Martin T, et al. Should children drink before discharge from day surgery? *Anesthesiology.* 1992;76:528-533.
12. Divatia JV, Vaidya JS, Badwe RA, et al. Omission of nitrous oxide during anesthesia reduces the incidence of postoperative nausea and vomiting: a meta-analysis. *Anesthesiology.* 1996;85:1055-1062.
13. Muir JJ, Warner MA, Offord KP, et al. Role of nitrous oxide and other factors in postoperative nausea and vomiting: a randomized and blinded prospective study. *Anesthesiology.* 1987;66:513-518.
14. Watcha MF, Simeon RM, White PF, et al. Effect of propofol on the incidence of postoperative vomiting after strabismus surgery in pediatric outpatients. *Anesthesiology.* 1991;75:204-209.
15. Mendel HG, Guarnieri KM, Sundt LM, et al. The effects of ketorolac and fentanyl on postoperative vomiting and analgesic requirements in children undergoing strabismus surgery. *Anesth Analg.* 1995;80:1129-1133.
16. Schechter NL, Berde CB, Yaster M. *Pain in Infants, Children, and Adolescents.* Baltimore, MD: Williams and Wilkins; 1993.
17. Yaster M, Maxwell LG. Pediatric regional anesthesia. *Anesthesiology.* 1989;70:324-338.
18. Forrest JB, Heitlinger EL, Revell S. Ketorolac for postoperative pain management in children. *Drug Saf.* 1997;16:309-329.

19. Gillis JC, Brogden RN. Ketorolac: a reappraisal of its pharmacodynamic and pharmacokinetic properties and therapeutic use in pain management. *Drugs*. 1997;53: 139-188.
20. Yaster M. Non-steroidal anti-inflammatory drugs. In Yaster M, Cote CJ, Krane EJ, Kaplan RF, eds. *Pediatric Pain Management and Sedation Handbook*. St Louis, MO: Mosby Year Book; 1997.
21. Rusy LM, Houck CS, Sullivan LJ, et al. A double-blind evaluation of ketorolac tromethamine versus acetaminophen in pediatric tonsillectomy: analgesia and bleeding. *Anesth Analg*. 1995;80:226-229.
22. Chang JK, Wang GJ, Tsai ST, et al. Nonsteroidal anti-inflammatory drug effects on osteoblastic cell cycle, cytotoxicity, and cell death. *Connect Tissue Res*. 2005; 46:200-210.
23. Reuben SS, Ablett D, Kaye R. High dose nonsteroidal anti-inflammatory drugs compromise spinal fusion. *Can J Anesth*. 2005;52:506-512.
24. Splinter WM, Schreiner MS. Preoperative fasting in children. *Anesth Analg*. 1999;89:80.
25. Habib AS, Gan TJ. Evidence-based management of postoperative nausea and vomiting: a review. *Can J Anesth*. 2004;51:326-341.
26. Watcha MF, Bras PJ, Cieslak GD, et al. The dose-response relationship of ondansetron in preventing postoperative emesis in pediatric patients undergoing ambulatory surgery. *Anesthesiology*. 1995;82:47-52.
27. National Drug Association. Drug Description and Precautions. Wyeth. 1-10. Available at: www.fda.gov/medwatch/SAFETY/2004/nov_PI/Phenergan_PI.pdf. Accessed January 10, 2008.
28. US Food and Drug Administration. Promethazine HCl (marketed as Phenergan) Information. FDA Alert. Available at: www.fda.gov/cder/drug/infopage/promethazine/default.htm. Accessed January 10, 2008.
29. Cohen IT, Joffe D, Hummer K, et al. Ondansetron oral disintegrating tablets: acceptability and efficacy in children undergoing adenotonsillectomy. *Anesth Analg*. 2005;101:59-63.
30. Freedman SB, Adler M, Seshadri R, et al. Oral ondansetron for gastroenteritis in a pediatric emergency department. *N Engl J Med*. 2006;354:1698-1705.
31. Splinter WM, Rhine EJ. Low-dose ondansetron with dexamethasone more effectively decreases vomiting after strabismus surgery in children than does high-dose ondansetron. *Anesthesiology*. 1998;88:72-75.
32. Yaster M, Krane EJ, Cote CJ, et al. *Pediatric Pain Management and Sedation Handbook*. St Louis, MO: Mosby Year Book; 1997.
33. Davis PJ, Greenberg JA, Gendelman M, et al. Recovery characteristics of sevoflurane and halothane in preschool-aged children undergoing bilateral myringotomy and pressure equalization tube insertion. *Anesth Analg*. 1999;88:34-38.
34. White PF, Way WL, Trevor AJ. Ketamine: its pharmacology and therapeutic uses. *Anesthesiology*. 1982;56: 119-136.
35. Kain ZN, Wang SM, Mayes LC, et al. Distress during the induction of anesthesia and postoperative behavioral outcomes. *Anesth Analg*. 1999;88:1042-1047.
36. Kain ZN, Mayes LC, Wang SM, et al. Parental presence during induction of anesthesia versus sedative premedication: which intervention is more effective? *Anesthesiology*. 1998;89:1147-1156.
37. Kain ZN, Caramico LA, Mayes LC, et al. Preoperative preparation programs in children: a comparative examination. *Anesth Analg*. 1998;87:1249-1255.
38. Koka BV, Jeon IS, Andre JM, et al. Postintubation croup in children. *Anesth Analg*. 1977;56:501-505.
39. Schreiner MS, O'Hara I, Markakis DA, et al. Do children who experience laryngospasm have an increased risk of upper respiratory tract infection? *Anesthesiology*. 1996;85: 475-480.
40. Khine HH, Corddry DH, Kettrick RG, et al. Comparison of cuffed and uncuffed endotracheal tubes in young children during general anesthesia. *Anesthesiology*. 1997; 86:627-631.
41. Ausejo M, Saenz A, Pham B, et al. The effectiveness of glucocorticoids in treating croup: meta-analysis. *BMJ*. 1999;319:595-600.
42. Kairys SW, Olmstead EM, O'Connor GT. Steroid treatment of laryngotracheitis: a meta-analysis of the evidence from randomized trials. *Pediatrics*. 1989;83: 683-693.
43. Sullivan M, Thompson WK, Hill GD. Succinylcholine-induced cardiac arrest in children with undiagnosed myopathy. *Can J Anaesth*. 1994;41:497-501.
44. Laurence AS. Serum myoglobin release following suxamethonium administration to children. *Eur J Anaesthesiol*. 1988;5:31-38.
45. McLoughlin C, Leslie K, Caldwell JE. Influence of dose on suxamethonium-induced muscle damage. *Br J Anaesth*. 1994;73:194-198.
46. Yeung RS, Buck JR, Filler RM. The significance of fever following operations in children. *J Pediatr Surg*. 1982;17: 347-349.
47. Rakover Y, Almog R, Rosen G. The risk of postoperative haemorrhage in tonsillectomy as an outpatient procedure in children. *Int J Pediatr Otorhinolaryngol*. 1997;41: 29-36.
48. Randall DA, Hoffer ME. Complications of tonsillectomy and adenoidectomy. *Otolaryngol Head Neck Surg*. 1998;118:61-68.
49. Fisher QA, McComiskey CM, Hill JL, et al. Postoperative voiding interval and duration of analgesia following peripheral or caudal nerve blocks in children. *Anesth Analg*. 1993;76:173-177.
50. Chalmers EA. Epidemiology of venous thromboembolism in neonates and children. *Thromb Res*. 2006; 118:3-12.
51. Stein PD, Kayali F, Olson RE. Incidence of venous thromboembolism in infants and children: data from the national hospital discharge survey. *J Pediatr*. 145:563-565.
52. Van Ommen CH, Peters M. Acute pulmonary embolism in childhood. *Thromb Res*. 2006;118:12-25.

Section Five

Care of the Child With Special Health Care Needs

Chapter 64

CHILDREN WITH ONGOING HEALTH CONDITIONS

Ruth E. K. Stein, MD

All children experience minor illnesses and injuries while they are growing. Although most children have no ongoing consequences from these episodes, some children have more serious or recurrent impairments or disruptions of their health with which they live for prolonged periods. These conditions, and the children who have them, have been given many names over the past decades. Some authorities have referred to them as having chronic illness, but some of these children are not ill. Other authors have referred to them as having disabilities or handicaps, but many children do not exhibit these features. The term in vogue most recently has been to refer to these children as having special health care needs. *Children with special health care needs* (CSHCN) was a term originally coined as a euphemism for the other terms.[1] More recently the term CSHCN has been defined to include children who are not currently having any condition or impairment but who are at risk for them, such as foster children.[2] Because no agreement exists on which children to include in the at-risk category, they are referred to in this chapter as children with ongoing or chronic conditions, though many others refer to them as CSHCN and count only those with identified impairments or service needs.

DEFINITION

Identifying children with ongoing or chronic conditions requires a definition. In fact, many current definitions are quite similar. One useful definition has three key components: (1) the presence of a condition, (2) a duration or expected duration of at least 1 year, and (3) a consequence for the child.[3] This classification recognizes three main types of consequences: (1) having a functional limitation—that is, something that prevents the child from participating in the normal range of age-appropriate activities; (2) increased use of health care services beyond those used by age mates, and (3) reliance on compensatory mechanisms (medication, special treatments, assistive devices or personal assistance) to function.

The definition adopted by the Maternal and Child Health Bureau combines the latter two categories of consequences and considers *at-risk* children as well: "Those children who have or are at increased risk for a chronic physical, developmental, behavioral, or emotional condition and who also require health and related services of a type or amount beyond that required by children generally."[2] Because no validated method currently exists for fully operationalizing the Maternal and Child Health Bureau definition, and because the concept of compensatory mechanisms is conceptually and critically distinct from receipt of services, the definition with three key components is used here. Compensatory mechanisms are especially important as medical care finds new ways to minimize functional limitations and allows children to carry on with their normal activities. For example, a child with a pacemaker or one who is on insulin, inhaled steroids, or overnight infusions may only be able to *pass* and function as a healthy child because of those treatments and may have few, if any, other consequences of his underlying condition. Unless these special aspects of care are considered, children whose compensatory mechanisms are successful may be counted as healthy children, and thus the success of treatments and the need to sustain them will be underappreciated, undercounted, and underfunded.

The use of an umbrella definition that considers children regardless of their diagnosis is important because of the epidemiologic mechanism of ongoing conditions in children and adolescents includes a few common conditions, such as asthma, developmental delay, or diabetes, and far more uncommon conditions, such as birth defects and inborn errors of metabolism, malignancies, and a wide range of acquired injuries and illnesses. Even though the names of many of these conditions are known, an all-inclusive list would be extremely long, and many children would still not find their diagnoses on the list. Because of this circumstance, thinking of these children as sharing some common characteristics of duration and consequences without necessarily naming the condition is far more convenient for many purposes other than biomedical treatment. However, the specific diagnosis is extremely important to understand so as to provide the appropriate specific treatments for the condition. Many of the specific conditions and their treatment are described elsewhere in this text.

PREVALENCE

Depending on how the definition is operationalized, estimates suggest that between 15% and 20% of children have some impairment or underlying condition that qualifies them as children with special health care needs. Some of the children have only minor, if any, difficulties from their conditions; but others are severely affected. Among children who meet the definition, between one half and two thirds of these children experience a functional limitation, either with or without other types of consequences. Only approximately 10% of these children experience consequences in all three categories and these are often the children with the most severe conditions.[4]

Two factors will likely lead to an increase in numbers of children with ongoing conditions. The first factor is improvements in early detection and diagnosis as a result of molecular genetics, and the second factor is the use of preventive interventions that postpone the onset of the full manifestations of some conditions to which children are genetically vulnerable. Such interventions and earlier detection will increase the numbers of children who qualify under the definitions and thus will likely lead to an expansion of the number of children over time.

EFFECT OF THE CONDITIONS

Ongoing conditions vary in their severity from very mild ones that the health care system may regard as background noise to extremely debilitating ones that affect every aspect of the child and family's lives. However, all ongoing conditions have some implications for the children's long-range health and service needs and in many cases for their longevity as well. Additionally, all conditions affect how families view their children and their vulnerability and how parents deal with the health care and other systems. Research has demonstrated that a correlation between the pediatrician's sense of the severity of the condition and the family's perception of its impact or influence on their child and their lives cannot always be found.

Ongoing conditions affect children and their family in many and often profound ways. Children with any type of functional limitation tend to experience fewer of the usual activities and opportunities for socialization that are important for normal development. Depending on the age of the child, as well as the level of functional limitations, these effects vary considerably. The lack of exploratory opportunities can range from minor to major and therefore can influence the child's developmental trajectory. Even children who do not have limitations are sometimes overprotected by their parents, and this overprotection can result in unnecessary restrictions of opportunity for developing important social skills and psychological well being. When parents perceive that their child needs to be protected in ways that are not medically indicated or worry about their child in an exaggerated way, this circumstance is referred to as *the vulnerable child syndrome*.

Parents face a great deal of physical, emotional, and financial strain, and in many cases the entire family experiences significant social isolation. All of these stresses place additional burdens and demands on the family members. Some studies suggest that parents who assume major caretaking responsibilities for children with severe conditions are at increased risk for physical and mental health problems and divorce.

Siblings and the children themselves are often stigmatized when conditions are visible. In addition, many siblings are subjected to a situation in which they are forced to function more independently than usual because parental attention may be focused on the child with a condition. They may feel jealous, abandoned, and sad, or they may alternately assume increased adult responsibilities. Sometimes these children become caretakers for their sibling with an ongoing condition or take on the care of younger, healthy siblings.

Conditions that are invisible can also be particularly challenging emotionally because children and families face issues of disclosure and have to navigate between the world of the well and the world of their illnesses or conditions. Lack of visibility is one aspect of uncertainty, and any type of uncertainty is particularly challenging.[5] Most people seem to have the greatest difficulty with conditions that fluctuate, even when most of the time the children are relatively well. The emotional toll of these conditions is sometimes worse than a stable level of greater dysfunction.

Transition times are especially stressful. Transition times include stages and events such as becoming ambulatory, entering school or child care, moving from one school or community to another, or moving into latency or adolescence or into adulthood. When healthy children move from one major stage to another the family of a child with an ongoing condition is often confronted with the ways in which their own child is different or with the need to make special accommodations to ensure that the medical safety or special needs are managed. Pediatricians can anticipate that these times are when families may need extra help and support.

SPECIAL CARE CONSIDERATIONS

The physician caring for the child needs to be aware of multiple special aspects of care of the child with an ongoing health condition and how they may modify usual practices. These aspects of care include the provision of health care maintenance and management of acute illness.

Provision of Health Care Maintenance

Because many children with ongoing conditions have more contact with the health care system than other children, their parents often assume that they are receiving a full package of services, but this assumption is not often true. The actual number of visits that focus on issues of health care maintenance for children with ongoing conditions is much lower than for the general population. Many subspecialists assume that these services are being provided elsewhere. However, studies show that many children with ongoing conditions do not receive the routine screenings that are a part of recommended health care maintenance for all children; many are underimmunized as well. In most cases this situation represents a failure of care rather than a reflection of recommendations for modification of the immunization schedule because of the child's condition or its treatment. Pediatricians should be aware of special recommendations concerning live vaccines, especially for immunocompromised patients, and document when vaccines are being modified for that reason. If vaccination is postponed, then the clinician should have a mechanism for remembering to provide appropriate alternate protection or later immunization, if possible.

The usual anticipatory guidance should also be provided, although in the case of children with developmental impairments, anticipatory guidance should be adjusted to the appropriate developmental stage. This process may be complex because children with ongoing conditions may develop normally or even be precocious in some areas while lagging in others.

In addition to following the usual health care maintenance schedule for age-appropriate screening, specific recommendations exist for many children with ongoing conditions to have additional screening for specific vulnerabilities caused by their primary diseases or by the medications that they take. When sharing responsibility for the care of such patients with subspecialists the clinician must establish who is providing the routine screening, immunizations, and anticipatory guidance and who is monitoring these special risks so as to prevent failures or duplications of care. If a division of services exists, then the family must know this and the reasons that they need to make regular visits to both providers.

Management of Acute Illness

Children with ongoing conditions experience the same minor illnesses that affect others in the community. However, every evaluation of a seemingly minor chief complaint requires the primary care physician or emergency room physician to consider whether the symptoms are complications of the underlying disease process, side effects related to medication taken to treat the condition, or a normal intercurrent event. Even when the child has an ordinary minor illness or injury, clinicians also should consider whether the condition or its treatment requires the child to receive any special care or medication adjustment. For example, a child with diabetes who experiences an episode of gastroenteritis is likely to need adjustment to the insulin regimen. A child who is being weaned from steroids or who is on permanent physiologic levels of exogenous steroid may need extra coverage during the illness. A child with vomiting caused by gastroenteritis might require an alternate mode of administration of an essential medication or special monitoring or titration of the dose.

In evaluating the patient and the management plan for the acute minor illness the practitioner must check with the parents and older child about whether they have any special concerns or questions. This responsibility is most essential in an encounter in which the treating practitioner does not know the family, given that the family is often able to distinguish between the child's current and baseline condition in ways that may not be immediately obvious to someone who does not know the patient well. In many instances the patient or parents will raise practical issues in daily management that may not have occurred to the physician. This circumstance is particularly true when they have experienced similar circumstances in the past. Box 64-1 lists some of the questions to consider in the management of acute illness or injury.

BOX 64-1 Assessing Acute Conditions in Children With Ongoing Health Conditions

Can the chief complaint and associated symptoms be explained by the child's underlying condition?

Can the chief complaint and associated symptoms be explained by the current or recent medications or other treatments?

Might the chief complaint and associated symptoms represent a complication of the child's underlying condition or a special vulnerability caused by the underlying condition?

If so, what special evaluations should be performed?

How do the child's current physical and laboratory findings differ from the child's baseline?

Has the child skipped, vomited, or failed to absorb recent medications, and might this circumstance be causing a problem?

What features of the child's condition are of most concern to the family or patient?

What do they think the problem is?

Can these features be explained by the presumptive diagnosis of the acute condition?

What events or circumstances worry the family or patient most? Is this worry a realistic concern, and can something be done to reassure the family?

In light of the acute diagnosis, does the child need a modification of usual care or medication? Can this modification or medication be handled at home? If the situation can be handled at home, then what is the plan for follow-up, and should it be modified in light of the child's underlying condition?

Management of the Ongoing Condition

Each health condition requires special biomedical management in terms of treatments and monitoring. Regardless of the specific type of condition each child may have, stages of management, common goals of treatment, and issues that confront families across the full range of conditions can be found. Ideally the child receives care in the medical home. (See Chapter 8, Medical Home Collaborative Care.)

DIAGNOSIS

The detection and confirmation of a condition herald the first stage of management. The treatment plan may be developed by the pediatrician, or it may be a shared responsibility with a subspecialist or the staff of a referral hospital. In the latter situation the practitioner must work out a pattern of communication in which the various responsibilities of each of the parties are delineated. The practitioner needs to determine regular mechanisms for communication, ascertain key issues that need to be monitored, and determine how these responsibilities will be divided between the pediatrician and the consultant. In the case of very rare conditions, especially when the primary expertise is far from the patient's home, the pediatrician should make sure the delegated responsibilities with the specialist is reviewed and that special issues to monitor and the indications for further consultation are understood.

Confirming a diagnosis and discussing its implications with parents and the child is an ongoing process that is never accomplished in a single informing conference. Parents should be encouraged to ask questions on a regular basis, given that they are usually unable to absorb a great deal of information at the time of confirmation of the diagnosis. The practitioner should suggest to them that they write down their own and other people's questions and advice and check them out at the next visit. Providing this mechanism and a socially acceptable way to ask naive or awkward questions can be helpful in enabling family members to address issues that they may find embarrassing or difficult.

Some pediatricians are uncomfortable in sharing their uncertainty about answers to questions posed by family members. In most instances the key questions that the parents want answered are related to what will happen to their specific child. This question is one that even the most expert pediatricians cannot answer except in a probabilistic way. Parents repeatedly state that a cornerstone to working well with pediatricians over time is honesty in dealing with them, including sharing uncertainty or seeking additional information when the physician does not have ready answers.

When the information provided is especially distressing (see Chapter 16, Disclosing a Diagnosis With Parents and Patients), the parents should be advised to seek a second opinion, and the physician should recommend places where this task can be accomplished responsibly. Many parents consider seeking a second opinion, and being open to the idea is far preferable than going behind the back of the original physician. For some families, just the offer of opening the results to scrutiny is reassuring; for others who wish to follow through on the offer, it avoids the need for repeated tests and the awkwardness of their worrying about raising the issue with the physician or finding a way to discuss and reconcile conflicting recommendations.

Grief is a normal reaction to the confirmation of a diagnosis and to the loss of the idealized perfect child. Parents normally go through a series of reactions at the time of diagnosis. These reactions may include shock, denial, anger, sadness, and anxiety. Dealing with denial and anger are challenging even for a pediatrician skilled in caring for a child with a complex or serious condition, especially when the anger is directed at the pediatricians. Care must be taken to recognize the misplaced anger and to avoid letting it affect the physician-patient relationship negatively. All parents feel guilty about real or imagined things that might have prevented the condition, and addressing this guilt as universal, as well as unfounded, is important because even abusive parents or those who transmit a recognized genetic disorder do not actively want to hurt their child.

Eventually, somewhat of a normalization of emotional well being, or what has been called *reorganization,* occurs; but every condition-related event or exacerbation is likely to resurface a cascade of emotional reactions. Parents may go through these reactions at different rates from one another, and this circumstance can affect their communication with and relationship to the pediatrician. In addition, when these feelings are projected on to the child or pediatrician, the situation can become difficult. The physician should avoid overreacting to parents' behavior and should maintain a professional relationship.

DEVELOPING AND PROMOTING PARTNERSHIPS WITH FAMILIES

Unlike acute conditions, in which life quickly returns to normal, by their very nature, ongoing conditions persist, and many times the disruption that they cause continues or ameliorates slowly. Therefore families bear the brunt of the care responsibilities, and they need to be full partners in care. (See Chapter 67, Partnering With Families in Hospital and Community Settings.)

At times the traditional medical approach becomes a central barrier to the formation of partnerships with families. Two aspects are particularly problematic. The first problem is the paternalistic and hierarchical nature or medicine, which is often associated with entirely prescriptive decision making. Effective management of a chronic condition or impairment requires the pediatrician to understand that the parents are the experts in raising their child. Within a short time, parents will know more, especially about rare conditions, than the average health care practitioner, and their expertise should be valued and respected. Even at the beginning, the importance of the parents' role with and expertise about their own child necessitates active involvement and sharing of responsibility that may run counter to the traditional hierarchical paternalism of the health care system. This shared decision-making process leads to better health outcomes for the child.[6]

The second problem with a traditional medical approach is the emphasis on the deficit model, which focuses entirely on what is *wrong* with the patient rather than seeing the strengths and assets, as well as the impairments. Clinicians are trained to focus on the problem and fix it. For the most part, chronic conditions cannot be fixed entirely, and the challenge for both the family and the pediatrician is to live with it and to make it as undisruptive and unobtrusive in the child's life as possible while still maximizing the child's longer-term future health and potential. To accomplish this task, focus must be placed on the whole child, and the assets, as well as impairments, must be assessed and actively recognized.

When communications and mutual respect are established among the partners, a care plan can be developed that includes the priorities of all parties, is medically and culturally acceptable, and has a far better chance of being implemented and of being successful than one that does not recognize the parents' expertise.

GOALS OF CARE

Regardless of the nature of the condition the primary goal is to contain or minimize the impact of the condition and to provide maximal opportunity for the child to function and develop physically, socially, cognitively, and emotionally. This process involves providing optimal specific care for the biomedical treatment of the condition and helping the family *normalize* the child's and the family members' own life experiences to the fullest extent possible. To accomplish this task the pediatricians should place as few restrictions on the child's activities as possible, limiting only specific activities that are absolutely necessary to avoid. Additionally, the care should plan be implemented in a way that minimizes the burden on the family as much as possible. Sometimes this objective requires a great deal of information about the child and family that is perceived by pediatricians as prying. However, knowing something about the family's daily and weekly routines may be extremely useful in helping to normalize family life as much as possible. For example, information about the family's routines and preferences may help in suggesting minor modifications in the type or timing of medication administration or procedures that will make the child's care less disruptive. Family members may not know on their own whether and when they can safely modify schedules and when they cannot. Tailoring care to the individual family also requires a longitudinal and developmental framework in which the management strategies and responsibilities shift over time in a manner that is appropriate for the parents' increasing comfort with management of the condition and with the child's developmental progress.

INVOLVING AND PREPARING THE CHILD

Beginning with the young child the practitioner must provide developmentally appropriate information about the condition and the treatments that the child receives. The child should also be involved in the timing, nature of, and assent for special procedures, especially when real choices exist. As the child matures, communicating directly with the child, rather that exclusively through the parents, is important. Explanations that may have been given to the parents, or to a young child, require expansion and revision as the child matures. Daily care routines are optimally shifted to the child as early as possible, and well before adolescence. Being cognizant of these needs helps prepare the child for the time when the child will become independent and responsible for self-care and self-management. Just as with other childhood responsibilities, special care for the condition starts out being the parents' duty and must end up being the child's responsibility. To facilitate this transition, pediatricians need to be cognizant of the need for inclusion of age-appropriate explanations of the condition with the child and for graduated responsibility for care. The pediatrician will also need to start preparing adolescents with ongoing health conditions for transitioning their care to physicians trained to care for adults. Although the actual transfer of care will usually take place by the patients twenty-first birthday, discussions regarding this transition should start years earlier. In many instances, patients *age out* of federal- or state-funded special services at different ages, depending on the state and the nature of the service, requiring the arrangement of alternative services. Increasingly, pediatricians have been referring their young adults with special health care needs to medical-pediatrics–trained physicians, given that these professionals are experts in caring for both adults and children and are knowledgeable about childhood chronic illnesses. However, in many places, finding such individuals with such expertise and finding the appropriate professional to provide ongoing care can be a challenge.

COORDINATION OF CARE

Families often need assistance with learning about how to use different parts of the health care system and health-related services. Dealing with multiple systems, each of which has its own requirements and regulations, can be daunting for many families. The pediatrician is often the one who knows about other resources in the community that can be helpful.

Coordination of care includes two major aspects: (1) coordination within the parts of the health care system and (2) coordination with other community agencies and resources in the educational, recreational, and human services sectors. Family coalitions that range from disease-specific organizations to more general groups of parents of children with ongoing conditions, such as Family Voices (www.familyvoices.org/) or Federation of Children with Special Health Care Needs (www.fcsn.org/) may provide critical advice and networking. Other families in the practice who have struggled with finding resources may also be willing to be introduced to parents of a child with the same or another condition. In some instances, opportunities for care coordinators can be found through private agencies, insurance companies, or Title V programs. Familiarity with these programs and resources can be extremely helpful.

PERIODIC REASSESSMENT

At each stage in the care of a child with ongoing conditions, making sure that the family (including both parents, whenever possible, and the older patient) and the clinicians providing care agree on the priorities and on the plan is important. If possible a written plan should be developed that outlines the next phase of care and builds on the mutual priorities. Although this step may be time consuming initially, it saves time in the long run and is much more likely to result in adherence with therapy than presumptive decisions that are made quickly and unilaterally.

Children with ongoing conditions and their family members often experience more stress and difficulty in adjusting to the demands of their lives than other families. As a result, families with children with ongoing conditions are more likely than others in a physician's practice to need assistance from mental health services. Periodically providing a time for them to deal with the stresses and helping them understand that all families of children with ongoing conditions face these issues may help prevent serious mental health concerns.

SUMMARY

Although taking care of children with a range of special health care needs can be challenging, it is an increasingly important part of pediatric practice. This circumstance is a result of the enormous successes that have occurred in enhancing survival of children with a wide range of conditions. Now the vast majority of children who develop serious ongoing conditions survive into adolescence and adulthood, and the challenge is to help prepare them for and to lead maximally independent and fulfilling lives. Given that so many of these children have conditions with which the individual practitioner may have little cumulative experience the primary care physician should remember the principles that apply across diagnoses and apply the lessons learned from caring for other children with ongoing conditions. Doing so can make pediatric practice all the more rewarding.

RELATED WEB SITES

- Maternal and Child Health Bureau, The Health Resources and Services Administration, Department of Health and Human Services (mchb.hrsa.gov/).
- Medical Home and Transitions—The National Center of Medical Home Initiatives for Children with Special Needs, American Academy of Pediatrics (www.medicalhomeinfo.org/health/trans.html).
- National Center of Medical Home Initiatives for Children with Special Needs, American Academy of Pediatrics (www.medicalhomeinfo.org/index.html).

AAP POLICY STATEMENTS

American Academy of Pediatrics, Medical Home Initiatives for Children With Special Needs Project Advisory Committee. The medical home. *Pediatrics.* 2002;110(1):184-186. (aappolicy.aappublications.org/cgi/content/full/pediatrics;110/1/184).

American Academy of Pediatrics, American Academy of Family Physicians, American College of Physicians, American Society of Internal Medicine. A consensus statement on health care transitions for young adults with special health care needs. *Pediatrics.* 2002;110:1304-1306. (aappolicy.aappublications.org/cgi/content/full/pediatrics;110/6/1304).

REFERENCES

1. Nelson R, Stein REK. Children with special needs: recommendations and rationale. In Klerman L, ed. *Research Priorities in Maternal and Child Health.* Washington, DC: Office for Maternal and Child Health, Health Services Administration, Public Health Service, US Department of Health and Human Services; 1982.
2. McPherson M, Arango P, Fox H, et al. A new definition of children with special health care needs. *Pediatrics.* 1998; 102:137-140.
3. Stein REK, Bauman LJ, Westbrook LE, et al. Framework for identifying children who have chronic conditions: the case for a new definition. *J Pediatr.* 1993;122:342-347.
4. Stein REK, Sliver EJ. Operationalizing a conceptually-based noncategorical definition: a first look at US children with chronic conditions. *Arch Pediatr Adolesc Med.* 1999; 153:68-74.
5. Jessop DJ, Stein REK. Uncertainty and its relation to psychological and social correlates of chronic illness in children. *Social Sci Med.* 1985;20:993-997.
6. Sobo EJ, Kurtin PS. *Optimizing Care for Young Children With Special Health Care Needs: Knowledge and Strategies for Navigating the System.* Baltimore, MD; Paul H Brookes Publishing; 2007.

Chapter 65

HOME HEALTH CARE

Sonia O. Imaizumi, MD

Medical advances that occurred in the last decades of the 20th century have saved and extended the lives of an increasing number of infants and children. These same advances have also allowed these children to be cared for at home, where their social and developmental needs are better met. These children may or may not depend on assistive technology, and their health care needs may vary in intensity and duration.

The rapid growth of pediatric home health services in the 1980s and 1990s has been attributed to the increased survival of children with complex medical problems. It is also a result of pressures from third-party payers to decrease lengths of stay in institutional settings and to lower the high costs associated with intensive care. Current home health services span the entire spectrum of health care services, from a single home visit for family support or outreach to the ongoing care of the ventilator-dependent child.

No easily accessible statistics exist regarding the exact number of children receiving home health care services because they are a widely diverse group, although authorities have concluded that dependence on technology is a common occurrence among children discharged from a children's hospital. Despite this circumstance, home health care services are planned for only a small percentage of cases.[1] Lack of consistency in discharge planning and lack of clear evidence-based clinical guidelines for children needing home health care services further complicate the matter. The 3 major diagnoses of children receiving home health care are (1) cerebral palsy, (2) lack of expected physiologic development, and (3) prematurity and its associated sequelae (eg, problems with breathing, eating, growth, and development).[2]

This chapter reviews issues relevant to the delivery of home health services but will not address specific clinical guidelines relevant to particular disease processes or age groups.

FAMILY-CENTERED CARE

The principles of family-centered care place the patient and family at the center of decision making. Its philosophy is based on *mutual beneficial partnerships between families and health care providers* and were first articulated by Shelton, Jeppson, and Johnson.[3] It also recognizes each family's strengths, regardless of the family's circumstances, and how these strengths can add positively to the family's health care experiences.

The principles of family-centered care are listed in Box 65-1.[4,5] These principles offer an opportunity for families and home health care providers to negotiate their respective roles and responsibilities. This fosters open communication and respect, thus decreasing the

BOX 65-1 Principles of Family-Centered Care

Respecting child and family regardless of the family's social circumstances.

Identifying and building on family strengths and identifying areas in which a given family may need support, taking into account their goals, priorities, and values.

Exploring choices. In this era of cost cutting by insurers (private or public), the dialogue between the family and the health care team becomes even more important when parents decide that the best place for their child is at home.

Coordinating care. Most payers provide a case manager to work with the family. The primary care physician is the most important link between the family and the case manager. Good communication among all health care providers is crucial to ensure that unnecessary barriers are not added to the care of the child at home.

Providing flexible service. Home health care providers and agencies need to be aware and willing to accommodate the potential problems of interrupting normal family routines, loss of privacy, and the family's perceived loss of control of their daily lives.

Communicating. Families need to be informed so as to collaborate in their child's care and in planning this care. Home health care providers need to recognize the importance of this relationship-based care and that sharing of information is an essential part of it. This process includes documentation that takes into account the principles of family-centered care, as well as the family's literacy level and language. This documentation will enhance the child's care by facilitating handoff procedures and overall communication among all the involved care providers, thus contributing to improved continuity of care.

Providing ongoing emotional and practical support for families. This support is needed not only to help the family come to terms with the responsibility they have acquired, which may grow beyond the skills that they successfully learned when the child arrived at home as the child's trajectory progresses, but also to ensure that the child's developmental and educational needs are completely met.

Providing family-to-family support. To prevent a family from feeling isolated and alone, opportunities for families to network with others whose child is at home under similar circumstances must be facilitated. This model can also serve as a source of potential respite.

Providing respite care, which is needed to prevent burnout and child neglect.

Source: Johnson BH, Schlucter J. Family-centered care. In: McConnell MS, Imaizumi SO, eds. *Guidelines for Pediatric Home Health Care*. Elk Grove Village, IL: American Academy of Pediatrics; 2002; Ahmann E. *Home for the High Risk Infant: A Family Centered Approach*. Gaithersburg, MD: Aspen Publishers;1996.

stress generated by the loss of privacy for the families and the lack of direct professional and supervisory guidance for the home health care providers, which is always available in an inpatient setting.

The plan of care should take into consideration a frank dialogue with the parents so that they can truly understand the issues that they will encounter once the child is home, including arrangements for respite care and ways to incorporate the child's care into the family's activities with minimal interruptions. A transition plan for discontinuation of home services needs to be an ongoing process as the child's condition progresses and medical needs evolve. This termination of home health care services typically occurs because of insurer coverage limits or when such services are no longer clinically necessary.

FAMILY-DIRECTED HOME HEALTH CARE

Several factors contribute to the growing importance of family-directed home health care. In an attempt to control costs, payers frequently reduce or limit benefits, which is compounded by a shortage of nurses and other personnel trained to work with children.[6] In the family-directed model of home health care, the case manager for the child strives to become a proxy for the parents or other primary caregivers in directing the roles of professional health care and support providers but without supplanting these roles.

Reasons for a child to be placed in family-directed care include unavailability of professional care,[6] lack of support in the community as a result of the child's complex medical needs, rehospitalization for nonmedical reasons, serious illness of the professional caregiver, and family need, often in an effort to save health insurance resources.

For family-directed home health to succeed, a team approach is essential. A detailed home health care plan must be developed, with the parents, physicians, health care team, and home health care providers all working together. This type of home health care must provide some ancillary services and ongoing maintenance, just as in nurse-directed home health care programs. In this model, one of the essential roles of the primary care physician is to address the caregiver's needs, abilities, and capacities. The physician must also be willing to play an active role in dealing with the social dynamics in the home and making sure that the home health care plan is being followed and is meeting its goals. A definitive respite care plan needs to be determined ahead of time. These arrangements can include other family members, community-based respite care, personal care attendants, and out-of-home medical day care. In some instances, and as a last resort, the child may have to be rehospitalized. The latter should occur only when the family can no longer safely care for the child.

For this model to succeed, a true parent-payer-provider relationship should be developed,[6] with the identification of a willing primary care physician being a crucial first step. Other issues that need to be addressed include defining roles and responsibilities, creating an ongoing communication plan, evaluating available community resources, identifying educational resources, and obtaining reimbursements by payers.

A complete home health care plan specific for the patient needs to be created. This plan should contain all the information required for the care of the child—medical and otherwise—including filling out the emergency information form for children with special needs.[7]

The ongoing monitoring of the home health care program should include monthly status reports and regular team meetings.

WHO ARE PEDIATRIC HOME HEALTH CARE PROVIDERS?

The following main professionals deliver care in the home.[8]

Nurses

Pediatric home health care nurses should have at least 1 year's acute care experience and have basic pediatric nursing skills. They should also be familiar with the agency's policies, procedures, and charting requirements. Nurses are usually the assigned individuals for all care coordination and management in the home. They are, for the most part, the eyes and the ears of the primary care physician, and ongoing communication between these 2 professionals is essential. A clear plan needs to be in place that addresses how to handle emergency situations and coverage to ensure continuity of care during off hours. Sometimes a licensed practical nurse or home health aide can be employed for certain tasks.

Physical Therapists

Physical therapists should be graduates of an accredited therapy program and should have at least 1 year's experience working with children in an acute care setting. Home-based physical therapy is indicated for homebound patients with physical therapy needs or for children who qualify for early intervention.

The physical therapist is responsible for determining short- and long-term goals, for continually assessing the child, and for providing the family with an individualized home therapy program.

The primary care physician or the subspecialist is responsible for the medical treatment of the patient and for developing the plan of treatment with the therapist. Community resources should be used whenever possible.

Occupational Therapists

Occupational therapists should be graduates of an accredited program and should have at least 1 year's experience with children in an acute care setting. As with physical therapy, occupational therapy is indicated for homebound patients or children who qualify for early intervention. In some states, a physical therapist or registered nurse must initiate the admission to home health care, and if occupational therapy is indicated, then the care will then be taken over by the occupational therapist.

Suggestions for treatment, its frequency, and its duration are made in the initial assessment and then approved and ordered by a physician. The goals of the therapy program need to be shared with the family and reviewed on an ongoing basis with the health care team and the family.

Speech Therapists

Speech therapists should have a master's degree in speech-language pathology or audiology and a certificate of clinical competency in speech from the American Speech-Language-Hearing Association. Speech therapists should have at least 1 year's experience in an acute care setting.

Speech therapy is indicated for homebound patients who are speech and hearing impaired, who have undergone tracheostomy, and who have feeding issues. Feeding therapy can also be undertaken by appropriately trained occupational therapists (specialized knowledge and skills, feeding, aiding, and swallowing using guidelines for occupational therapy practice).[9] An individualized program with short- and long-term goals under the direction of a physician should be initiated and started with the family.

Social Workers

A home health care medical social worker should have a master's degree in social work from an accredited program and should have completed a 2-year internship. Payers do not always allow social worker intervention as part of a patient's home care benefits.[10]

Medical social workers are invaluable in providing families with support, helping the parents navigate through a fragmented and complicated health care and educational system, and connecting the parents with community resources. The medical social worker needs to communicate regularly with the primary physician.[8]

Physicians

Physicians do have a limited role in home health care. Ideally the primary care pediatrician should be the one monitoring the quality of care provided in the home, coordinating the child's medical care, and making referrals to subspecialists and early intervention programs, as well as being responsible for the development of an *individualized health care plan*. The child's individual developmental needs should be integrated with the child's health care needs. The communication of the primary care physician regarding the child's health care and developmental needs to the local early intervention and special education programs should be part of providing high-quality health care.

PAYING FOR PEDIATRIC HOME HEALTH CARE

Public Funding

Pediatric home health care could not be provided today without the existence of public funding.[11,12] Private insurance varies greatly in type and amount of coverage. For children who need long-term care, insurance benefits are quickly exhausted, and the parents must seek other resources. One such resource is Medicaid. Eligibility for Medicaid is determined by each state and is based on family income levels. The 1990s showed an increase in the income eligibility for children to qualify for Medicaid under the State

Children's Health Insurance Program—up to 180% of the federal poverty line for some states. Primary care physicians need to familiarize themselves with the eligibility criteria of the state in which they practice. In 1981, through an executive order from President Ronald Reagan, certain Medicaid eligibility requirements were waived so that every technologically dependent child was able to be cared for at home. This executive order became known as the *Katie Beckett Waiver*. After this historical waiver, states were allowed to develop other waiver programs. Pediatricians should be familiar with their local and state waiver programs.[13]

Supplemental Security Income

Supplemental security income is a cash benefit for people with disabilities and is administered by the Social Security Administration. The determination of eligibility takes into consideration financial and disability criteria. For a child, the criteria are based on the child's ability to engage in age-appropriate activities. Supplemental security income is another way of becoming eligible for Medicaid, depending on the family's circumstances and income.

Early and Periodic Screening, Diagnosis, and Treatment

The Early and Periodic Screening, Diagnosis, and Treatment (EPSDT) program is a mandated Medicaid service limited to children under 18, and it ensures comprehensive pediatric health services, with an emphasis on prevention. It requires that all diagnostic and treatment services be available to an EPSDT recipient, which means that under this program, even specific services not included under a state's Medicaid plan must be made available to an EPSDT recipient.[11,12]

Mandatory Services Covered by Medicaid and the Early and Periodic Screening, Diagnosis, and Treatment Program

Medicaid benefits are described in each state's plan, which has to be approved by the Centers for Medicare and Medicaid Services. Home health care is one of the mandatory services covered by Medicaid. However, private-duty nursing is an optional service that is not mandated, and its availability may vary from state to state.

Medicaid Managed Care Organizations

Managed care organizations receive contracts from Medicaid. To obtain these contracts, these organizations must demonstrate an adequate network of health care providers and provide a vast array of services. This system is based on providing primary care for the beneficiaries. The child's primary care physician coordinates the necessary care and makes all the needed referrals, including referral for home health care services.[11,12]

This system has built-in disincentives and barriers, and the requirements vary from state to state. Patients may be automatically moved from one plan to another without being aware of it, necessitating a change in primary care physicians. This movement among plans may interrupt continuity of care for these patients.

Medical Day Treatment Programs

In the late 1980s, *prescribed pediatric extended-care centers* were established in Florida.[13,14] These centers are prescribed by physicians and qualify for reimbursement by both public and private insurers. This model was modified and updated, leading to *prescribed pediatric centers*, which are now becoming available in other states. These centers provide skilled nursing services and allied health services, including early intervention and developmentally appropriate education.

In the late 1990s, Respite House, Inc., now known as Coach Care Center, Inc., was opened in Illinois to provide respite for families of children dependent on life-sustaining technology. In addition to providing respite services for various lengths of time, it also provides transition training for parents of children being discharged from the hospital, as well as child life and educational services. More centers following this model need to be developed around the country.

Such programs are becoming more and more necessary, not only to provide much-needed respite for parents and siblings, but also for low-income families whose parents are mandated back to work as a result of the changes in welfare laws.

As in all home health care programs, a written individual health plan needs to be developed, and the communication between all members of the health care team continues to be an essential ingredient.

CONCLUSION

Pediatric home health care has been the fastest-growing expenditure of health care in the United States, motivated by the increased survival of fragile infants and children and by managed care pressures. Despite this trend, research and studies about pediatric home health care from the primary care physician's perspective have lagged. More outcome studies are needed not only to develop evidence-based clinical guidelines, but also to learn how to address family issues such as barriers, access, stress levels, psychological problems, financial consequences, job absenteeism, and family satisfaction.

TOOLS FOR PRACTICE

Community Advocacy and Coordination

- *Caring for Our Children: National Health and Safety Performance Standards for Out-of-Home Child Care* (book), American Public Health Association and American Academy of Pediatrics (www.aap.org/bookstore).
- *The National Home and Hospice Care Survey* (Web page), Centers for Disease Control and Prevention (www.cdc.gov/nchs/about/major/nhhcsd/nhhcsdes.htm).

Medical Decision Support

- *Guidelines for Pediatric Home Health Care Manual* (book), Callarman D, Lazzari L, Family-directed home health care. In: McConnell MS, Imaizumi SO, eds (www.aap.org/bookstore).
- *The National Center of Medical Home Initiatives for Children With Special Needs* (Web page), American Academy of Pediatrics (www.medicalhomeinfo.org.index.html).

Practice Management and Care Coordination

- *Access to Care, Medicaid, and the State Children's Health Insurance Program (SCHIP)* (Web page), American Academy of Pediatrics (www.aap.org/advocacy/staccess.htm).
- *Emergency Information Form for Children With Special Needs* (form), American College of Emergency Physicians and American Academy of Pediatrics (www.aap.org/advocacy/blankform.pdf).

RELATED WEB SITES

- American Academy of Home Care Physicians (www.aacp.org).
- Centers for Medicare & Medicaid Services (www.cms.hhs.gov).
- Centers for Medicare & Medicaid Services: State Children's Health Insurance Program (www.cms.hhs.gov/home/schip.asp).
- Home Healthcare Nurses Association (HHNA) (www.hhna.org).
- National Association for Home Care & Hospice) (www.nahc.org).
- Social Security Administration: Supplemental Security Income (SSI) (www.ssa.gov/ssi/).
- US Department of Health and Human Services: The Early Periodic Screening Diagnosis, and Treatment (EPSDT) Program (www.hrsa.gov/epsdt/).

AAP POLICY STATEMENTS

American Academy of Pediatrics Committee on Child Health Financing and Section on Home Care. Financing of Pediatric Home Health Care. *Pediatrics*. 2006;118(2):834-838. (aappolicy.aappublications.org/cgi/content/full/pediatrics;118/2/834).

American Academy of Pediatrics Council on Children With Disabilities. Care Coordination in the Medical Home: Integrating Health and Related Systems of Care for Children With Special Health Care Needs. *Pediatrics*. 2005;116(5):1238-1244. (aappolicy.aappublications.org/cgi/content/full/pediatrics;116/5/1238).

Johnson CP, Kostner TA, American Academy of Pediatrics Committee/Section on Children With Disabilities. Helping Families Raise Children With Special Health Care Needs at Home. *Pediatrics*. 2005;115(2):507-511. (aappolicy.aappublications.org/cgi/content/full/pediatrics;115/2/507).

Kastner TA and American Academy of Pediatrics Committee on Children With Disabilities. Managed Care and Children With Special Health Care Needs. *Pediatrics*. 2004;114(6):1693-1698. (aappolicy.aappublications.org/cgi/content/full/pediatrics;114/6/1693).

REFERENCES

1. Feudtner C, Villareale NL, Morray B, et al. Technology-dependency among patients discharged from a children's hospital: a retrospective cohort study. *BMC Pediatrics*. 2005;5:8:1-8.
2. Zafar H, Nash D. Present and future of pediatric home care. In: McConnell MS, Imaizumi SO, eds. *Guidelines for Pediatric Home Health Care*. Elk Grove Village, IL: American Academy of Pediatrics; 2000.
3. Shelton TL, Jeppson ES, Johnson BH. *Family Centered Care for Children with Special Health Care Needs*. Washington, DC: Association for the Care of Children's Health; 1987.
4. Johnson BH, Schlucter J. Family-centered care. In: McConnell MS, Imaizumi SO, eds. *Guidelines for Pediatric Home Health Care*. Elk Grove Village, IL: American Academy of Pediatrics; 2002.
5. Ahmann E. *Home Care for the High Risk Infant: A Family Centered Approach*. Gaithersburg, MD: Aspen Publishers; 1996.
6. Callarman D, Lazzari L. Family-directed home health care. In: McConnell MS, Imaizumi SO, eds. *Guidelines for Pediatric Home Health Care*. Elk Grove Village, IL: American Academy of Pediatrics; 2002.
7. American College of Emergency Physicians and American Academy of Pediatrics. Emergency Information Form for Children With Special Needs. Available at: transition.mchtraining.
8. Townsend M, Pasek F, Prophet C, et al. Pediatric home nursing and ancillary programs in guidelines for pediatric home health care. In: McConnell MS, Imaizumi SO, eds. *Guidelines for Pediatric Home Health Care*. Elk Grove Village, IL: American Academy of Pediatrics; 2002.
9. Clark GF, Avery-Smith W, Wolf LS, et al, Eating and Feeding Task Force, Commission on Practice. Specialized knowledge and skills in eating and feeding for occupational therapy practice. *Am J Occup Therapy*. 2003;57(6):660-678.
10. Assistance to States for the Education of Children with Disabilities and Preschool Grants for Children with Disabilities, Final Rule, 71 Fed. Reg. 46539-46845 #4 CFR Parts 300 and 301. August 12, 2006.
11. Buzdygan D. Pediatric home health care: public funding. In: McConnell MS, Imaizumi SO, eds. *Guidelines for Pediatric Home Health Care*. Elk Grove Village, IL: American Academy of Pediatrics; 2002.
12. American Academy of Pediatrics, Committee on Child Health Financing, Nelson RP, Minon, M, eds. *A Pediatrician's Guide to Managed Care*. Elk Grove Village, IL: American Academy of Pediatrics; 2001.
13. Ruppert E, Host N. Out of home child care and medical day treatment programs. In: McConnell MS, Imaizumi SO, eds. *Guidelines for Pediatric Home Health Care*. Elk Grove Village, IL: American Academy of Pediatrics; 2002.
14. American Public Health Association and American Academy of Pediatrics. *Caring for Our Children: National Health and Safety Performance Standards: Guidelines for Out-of-Home Child Care Programs*. 2nd ed. Washington, DC: American Public Health Association; 2002.

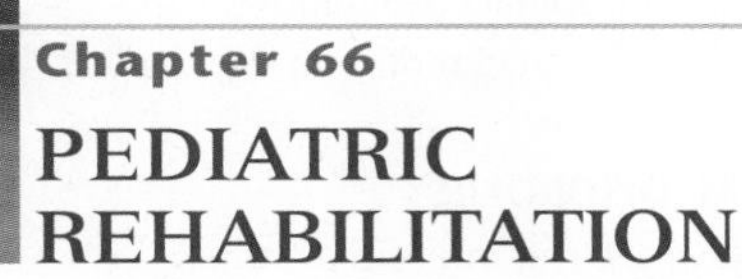

Chapter 66

PEDIATRIC REHABILITATION

Lisa Shulman, MD; Dona Rani Kathirithamby, MD; Maris D. Rosenberg, MD; Elissa L. Stern, LCSW, MPH

Rehabilitation typically refers to a return to a previous level of functioning. It is the process of restoring a person with a disability to the fullest physical, mental, social, vocational, and economic usefulness of which the person is capable. Rehabilitation is an approach for individuals who experience neurologic, neuromuscular, and musculoskeletal injuries caused by acquired disease processes (eg, stroke, tumors) or trauma (eg, traumatic brain and spinal cord injuries).[1,2]

Habilitation is the process of developing a skill to be able to function in an environment. It may be defined as the process by which various professional services are used to help a disabled person make maximal use of the person's capacities to function more effectively.[1] The term is also used to refer to various medical, therapeutic, and educational interventions that children with developmental disabilities receive.[1] *Habilitation*, by definition, would be the appropriate term to use in discussing therapeutic planning for children with congenital disorders such as cerebral palsy, spina bifida, or developmental delay. However, using the term *rehabilitation* to refer to both rehabilitative and habilitative services is common practice, given that both processes have the same ultimate goal of optimizing the functioning of the child with a disability.

Other definitions of importance to frame a discussion of childhood disabilities and their rehabilitation include those put forth by the World Health Organization.[3] *Impairment* is defined as any loss or abnormality of psychological, physiological, or anatomic structure or function. *Disability* is any restriction or lack (resulting from an impairment) of ability to perform an activity in the manner or within the range considered normal. *Handicap* is the disadvantage for an individual resulting from an impairment or disability that limits or prevents the fulfillment of a role that is normally appropriate for that individual (depending on age, sex, and social and cultural factors). Suggested modifications for this model have included incorporating the impact of environmental factors and society in limiting opportunities or facilitating them for individuals with disabilities.[4] For example, in this framework, a child with cerebral palsy would have an *impairment* in terms of motor function, a *disability* related to difficulty with ambulation, and a *handicap* relating to difficulty gaining access to buildings that are not wheelchair accessible. This handicap, however, can be eliminated by society through environmental modifications such as installing ramps.

The number of specific disorders resulting in childhood disabilities is vast. Box 66-1 lists a variety of conditions associated with childhood disabilities that are treated with interventions that fall within the realm of pediatric rehabilitation.

Pediatric rehabilitation is also used to treat children with chronic illnesses such as sickle cell anemia, HIV, pediatric tumors and malignancies, diabetes, asthma and chronic pulmonary disease, renal disease, and cardiac disease. The following areas are common to all approaches for both habilitation and rehabilitation for all childhood disabilities in all settings: evaluation and management by an interdisciplinary team; identification of areas of functional impairment; development of an intervention plan; and implementation of the intervention plan.

INTERDISCIPLINARY TEAM

Children with disabilities and their families have multiple, complex needs. Typically, no single professional can manage all of the issues. The care of the child with a disability is best handled by a team of professionals. An interdisciplinary team is made up of professionals from multiple disciplines who collaborate in a climate of mutual respect. The team addresses the full spectrum of the complex needs of the child with a disability by using a family-centered approach. Members of the

BOX 66-1 Disorders Treated With Pediatric Rehabilitation and Habilitation

NEUROMUSCULAR DISORDERS (CONGENITAL AND ACQUIRED)

- Cerebral palsy
- Spina bifida
- Myopathies and muscular dystrophies
- Neuropathies (congenital or hereditary, inflammatory, infectious, metabolic) and peripheral nerve injuries
- Congenital and traumatic spinal cord injuries
- Traumatic brain injuries (eg, accidents, stroke, shaken baby syndrome)

MUSCULOSKELETAL DISORDERS

- Arthropathies (eg, juvenile rheumatoid arthritis)
- Congenital and acquired limb deficiencies
- Congenital and traumatic orthopedic deformities
- Burns

DEVELOPMENTAL DISORDERS

- Genetic syndromes
- Developmental delay, intellectual disability
- Developmental language disorders, autism
- Learning disabilities, attention-deficit/hyperactivity disorder

BOX 66-2 Disciplines Typically Included in an Interdisciplinary Team for Children With Physical Disabilities

- Developmental pediatrician
- Primary health care physician
- Physiatrist (pediatric rehabilitation specialist)
- Orthopedist
- Neurologist
- Geneticist
- Otorhinolaryngologist
- Ophthalmologist
- Neurosurgeon
- Urologist
- Nurse practitioner and other nurses
- Dentist
- Physical therapist
- Occupational therapist
- Speech and language pathologist
- Feeding therapist
- Psychologist
- Special education professional
- Social worker
- Adaptive technology specialist
- Audiologist
- Nutritionist
- Orthotist

team dynamically bring together their differing expertise and perspectives to complete a diagnostic workup, create a plan for intervention, and resolve ongoing management issues. The family is a vital member of the team, able to provide information about the settings in which the child spends time, insight into the child's functioning and motivating factors, and clarification of family priorities.

A single member of the team is delegated as the primary clinician or case manager to serve as the main contact for the family regarding management issues and to bring the family's priorities and concerns to the team. Interdisciplinary teams vary in terms of the professionals involved, depending on the setting and the mission of the team. Interdisciplinary teams function in a range of settings, including acute-care hospitals, transitional-care units, rehabilitation hospitals, outpatient rehabilitation facilities, clinics, and home-based programs. Specialty or regional centers may have funding to create larger, more comprehensive teams. In individual communities, a team of a few professionals at different sites may work together, collaborating to create an ad hoc team to assist children and families. Box 66-2 lists common members of the team for children with physical disabilities.

IDENTIFYING SPECIFIC AREAS OF FUNCTIONAL IMPAIRMENT

Once the interdisciplinary team has clarified the diagnoses and impairments for a child with a disability, the analysis of function takes center stage. The diagnostic evaluation should address all of the areas of impairment, including the child's general health, sensory impairments, and cognitive impairments because each factor separately affects a child's functioning, and the impairments collectively affect overall functioning. Functional evaluation by the interdisciplinary team is essential for establishing the goals of treatment. Such assessments are typically performed by physicians (eg, developmental pediatricians and pediatric rehabilitation specialists, known as *physiatrists*), as well as by physical and occupational therapists. Physical therapists are the experts in interventions to address impairments in gross-motor functioning and mobility, and occupational therapists are the experts in interventions to address impairments in fine-motor and adaptive functioning and self-care skills.

The evaluation of gross-motor functioning involves assessing muscle tone, muscle strength, reflexes, sensation, movement patterns, postural status, motor coordination, gait, joint ranges, and documenting deformities. This information provides the basis for clarifying impairments and skill level relative to peers. Functional analysis examines the effect of the set of impairments on the child's functioning. In the gross-motor domain, the functions of interest include attaining gross-motor skills relating to stability and mobility (sitting, crawling, pulling to stand, ambulating) and transitions from one position to another.

Evaluating fine-motor and adaptive functioning typically involves a detailed history. Children should participate in providing the history as they are able. The functional assessment should involve assessing the child's ability for self-care: feeding, grooming, toileting, hygiene, and dressing. Functional histories should include information regarding areas of competence, as well as impairment. Parents are in a unique position to provide details to the team regarding how and where the child currently carries out adaptive tasks, highlighting strengths and strategies that may prove useful in planning interventions.

Many assessment tools can be used to examine motor and adaptive skill attainment. Norm-referenced, standardized tests are primarily diagnostic; they document a set of delays relative to norms, thereby justifying the need for intervention. Functional or qualitative assessments are criterion referenced; they assess how a child performs a task from a functional perspective. Such instruments are useful for intervention planning and follow-up to assess improvement from intervention and ultimately in establishing evidence-based outcomes research. Table 66-1 lists some of the frequently used functional outcome measures.

DEVELOPING AN INTERVENTION PLAN

When planning an effective rehabilitation program for a child with a disability, many factors need to be considered. These factors include severity of motor impairment; anticipated functional potential; age,

Table 66-1 Functional Outcome Measures in the Assessment of Motor Disability*

ASSESSMENT TOOL	AGE GROUP	AREAS OF MEASUREMENT
Pediatric Evaluation of Disability Inventory (PEDI)[a]	6 mo-7 yr	Gross-motor, adaptive function
Functional Independence Measure for Children (WeeFIM)[b]	0-18 yr	Gross-motor, fine-motor, adaptive function
Peabody Developmental Motor Scales[c]	0-9 yr	Gross-motor, fine-motor, adaptive function
Gross Motor Function Measure (GMFM)[d]	15 mo-16 yr	Gross-motor function
Motor Assessment of Infants (MAI)[e]	0-12 mo	Gross-motor, reflex function

*Adapted from: Deitz Curry JE. Promoting functional mobility. In: Dormans JP, Pellegrino L, eds. *Caring for Children With Cerebral Palsy.* Baltimore, MD: Paul H. Brookes Publishing; 1998. Reprinted by permission.

[a]Coster WJ, Haley SM. Conceptualization and measurement of disablement in infants and young children. *Infants Young Child.* 1992:4:11-12.

[b]Msall ME, DiGaudio KM, Duffy LC. Use of functional assessment on children with developmental disabilities. *Phys Med Rehabil Clin North Am.* 1993;4:517-527.

[c]Folio M, Fewell R. *Peabody Developmental Motor Scales.* Hingham, MA: DLM; 1983.

[d]Russell DJ, Rosenbaum PL, Cadman DJ, et al. The gross motor functional measure: a means to evaluate the effect of physical therapy. *Dev Med Child Neurol.* 1989;31:341-356.

[e]Chandler L, Andrews M, Swanson M. *The Movement Assessment of Infants.* Rolling Bay, WA: Rolling Bay Press; 1980.

mental capacity, and developmental status; home and family environment; and ethnic and cultural factors.

Realistic goals should be established based on these factors and the lifelong nature of physical disability. The multisystem nature of disabilities often requires an interdisciplinary approach to treatment with a team of therapists, each therapist using a variety of techniques. The interdisciplinary approach should address the following components:

- Medical management
- Therapeutic management
- Durable medical equipment, orthotics, and prosthetics
- Sports and recreation
- Psychosocial support to the family, caregiver, and patient
- Education and vocational planning
- Transitional and long-term planning

MEDICAL MANAGEMENT

Medical management of the child with a disability involves the diagnosis and treatment of associated medical issues, pain management, management of spasticity, and management of complications of tonal abnormalities.

The diagnosis and treatment of associated medical issues is an important component of the care of the child with a disability; many common conditions can greatly affect functioning. Common medical issues in children with disabilities relate to growth, feeding and nutrition, vision and hearing, seizures, pulmonary disease (eg, asthma, chronic lung disease), gastrointestinal functioning (eg, gastroesophageal reflux, oral-motor dysfunction, constipation), and dentition.

Managing pain is also an important part of the intervention plan for a child with a disability. Pain can be related to spasticity in neuromuscular disorders such as traumatic brain injury and cerebral palsy, it can be the result of joint inflammation in juvenile rheumatoid arthritis, or it can be caused by sickle crises in sickle cell disease. Pain management is also an integral part of the treatment of burns.

Medical management involves managing tonal abnormalities that affect function. This area includes the management of spasticity. Assessing spasticity should include identifying treatable conditions that can contribute to spasticity, such as urinary tract infection, decubitus ulcers, fecal impaction, and constipation. Spasticity should not be treated for its own sake but rather when it hinders functioning or causes pain. In many instances, spasticity is beneficial. For example, a child with spinal cord injury may use spasticity in standing. A patient with cerebral palsy may be able to use spasticity to walk.

The spectrum of intervention for managing spasticity includes the use of medication and surgery. Treatment differs depending on whether the spasticity is diffuse or localized. Oral medications such as diazepam, dantrolene sodium, and baclofen have been used for diffuse spasticity, although the functional improvement reported has been small. Baclofen, which is administered intrathecally via a programmable pump, achieves higher levels in the cerebrospinal fluid and thus can be effective in managing spasticity of central origin.[5] Botulinum toxin A injection is indicated for more localized spasticity, especially in younger patients without fixed contractures.[6,7] Reduction of spasticity is temporary, lasting between 3 and 8 months. Surgical treatment, in the form of selective dorsal rhizotomy, interrupts the afferent limb of the reflex arc, reducing spasticity without causing motor paralysis. Improved range of motion and muscle strength have been reported.[8]

Orthopedic interventions are indicated when medication, splints, casts, and physical therapy have failed to deter the progression of deformities and when spasticity interferes with functioning. Release or lengthening of muscles and tendons can reduce the restricted joint motion or malalignment. Orthopedic interventions should also be considered when fixed contractures interfere with function or when they hinder the provision of nursing care.

Orthopedic management also addresses the complications of tonal abnormalities. Spasticity in hip adductors and hip flexors can cause subluxation of hips progressing to hip dislocation or dislocation with degenerative changes of the femoral head with pain. Progressive bony deformities can cause pelvic obliquity and scoliosis of the spine. When hip subluxation is detected, soft-tissue release or lengthening can be performed. Comprehensive hip reconstruction may be performed in severely affected children. Orthopedic surgical procedures should be followed by physical therapy and orthotics management to maintain range of motion, strengthen weak muscles, and prevent recurrence of deformities.

THERAPEUTIC MANAGEMENT

The primary goals of intervention are to maximize functional skills, foster independence, and prevent or minimize complications. The emphasis must be on improved function rather than on improvement in the impairment. No single therapeutic method is suitable for all children; thus the therapeutic regimen must be individualized to the child.

Components of therapeutic management include physical therapy, occupational therapy, functional activity training, speech and communication therapy, and feeding therapy for oral motor dysfunction.

Physical and Occupational Therapy and Functional Activity Training

Children with disabilities often have decreased or limited exercise capacity relative to their able-bodied peers. This incapacity may result from the specific pathological features of their disability, deconditioning, or decreased muscle strength and endurance. In therapeutic management of children, physical and occupational therapists use traditional exercises and specific treatment techniques (both traditional and nontraditional), as well as adaptive equipment and assistive devices to improve muscle strength, endurance, flexibility, and range.

Traditional exercises are often not applicable in the treatment of infants and young children because very young children are unable to cooperate and participate in progressive resistive, isokinetic, and isometric exercises. Therefore using age-appropriate games, toys, and play activities to engage young children is important in improving strength, flexibility, and posture.

Maintaining passive range of motion, flexibility, and mobility of joints and preventing soft-tissue tightness is especially important in children with muscle tone abnormalities. Limitation in joint mobility interferes with normal movement and activities. Therapy to elicit active movements in infants is done by handling the child or by inducing spontaneous interaction. Normal movement patterns are facilitated by using developmentally appropriate, colorful toys and equipment. Parents are encouraged to be actively involved, and exercise programs must carry over to the home.

In preschool- and school-aged children, coordination of therapy with education is increasingly used. Participation of therapists in classroom consultation can enhance the child's education potential. Occupational therapists can assist teachers in improving graphomotor skills, activities of daily living (ADL), and fine-motor adaptive skills. Physical therapists can assist the child in achieving optimal positioning, trunk alignment, and mobility.

In treating adolescents with disabilities, therapeutic programs are geared toward preventing contractures; maintaining strength, flexibility, and endurance; improving postural alignment; and facilitating mobility. Improving functional skills and independence should be emphasized within the limits of the disability.

In addition to strength training and improvement in range of motion, physical and occupational therapists use specific therapeutic techniques. They rarely use a single approach; rather, therapists combine a variety of approaches to develop a program suitable for a particular child's needs. Many of these treatment approaches have little reliable clinical or scientific evidence to indicate efficacy of one method over another. The outcomes of various treatments have not been well studied, and assessment tools do not separate the effects of treatment from developmental progress as a result of maturation. Functional assessment measures and an emphasis on functional outcomes of interventions will soon lead to evidence-based data for various treatment modalities in children with disabilities.

Primary care physicians are often called on to prescribe therapeutic services for children. Prescribing physicians should have contact with the treating therapists, and physicians should be familiar with the goals of the therapeutic program and the techniques that will be used to achieve these goals. If such information is lacking, then the physician should consult with a physiatrist or a developmental pediatrician.

Table 66-2 lists current physical and occupational therapeutic techniques, the populations appropriate to receive these therapies, and the availability of data to support them. Many of these therapy techniques were originally used in adults and have been modified for children.

Physical and occupational therapists use various modalities in conjunction with therapeutic exercises, such as electrical stimulation, biofeedback, therapeutic cold and heat, hydrotherapy, and dry heat therapy. Electrical stimulation[9] can be used to treat muscle spasms and for functional improvement such as gait training or upper extremity use. Biofeedback,[10] with and without electromyography feedback, can help patients learn ways to gain control over motor function. Therapeutic cold decreases the muscle stretch reflex excitability and clonus and improves range of motion. It can be used to decrease spasticity temporarily and to allow mobility of extremities during therapy. In children with arthropathies such as juvenile rheumatoid arthritis, hydrotherapy, hot packs, and dry heat therapy can relieve the joint stiffness and pain and allow active range of motion of involved joints.

Hyperbaric oxygen therapy, intensive suit therapy, and magnetic therapy are nontraditional therapy techniques used in many children with neurologic disease that lack evidence-based support.[11,12]

Functional activities training is a critical component of the therapy program, especially for older children and adolescents. The training focuses on age-appropriate ADL, such as dressing, feeding, brushing teeth, and personal hygiene. Actual training goes on during therapy sessions. Adaptive equipment such as long-handled hairbrushes, modified toothbrushes, and special utensils should be provided. Carryover to home and practice are critical. Bicycling, stair climbing, and treadmill walking to improve mobility, endurance, and strength should also be included.[13]

Speech and Communication Therapy

The indications for speech and language therapy in children include congenital language delays such as those associated with intellectual disability, autism, and hearing impairment; acquired language disorders caused by neurologic disorders such as traumatic brain injury, stroke, brain tumor, or encephalopathy; and speech disorders resulting from neuromuscular processes that involve respiration, phonation, articulation, structure, and function, such as in cerebral palsy, myopathies, tracheostomy, ventilator dependency, and high spinal cord injuries.

Oral-Motor and Feeding Therapy

These same populations should be assessed for oral-motor dysfunction, which affects feeding and swallowing. Oral-motor dysfunction can be temporary (debilitative illness) or long term (neuromuscular disorder). Successful feeding involves the coordinated action of multiple systems. Normal feeding requires anatomic integrity of the oropharyngeal cavity, neuromotor control and coordination, sensory perception, adequate gastrointestinal function, sufficient cardiorespiratory support, intact autonomic nervous system, and integration of normal behavioral responses. Therefore assessment and intervention in feeding disorders require an interdisciplinary approach. The team of specialists with expertise in feeding may include speech and language pathologists, occupational therapists, nutritionists, radiologists, physiatrists, and developmental pediatricians.

Warning signs for the primary care physician regarding the possibility of a feeding disorder include the following:

- History of frequent respiratory infections
- Difficulty handling oral secretions and drooling

Table 66-2 Specific Physical and Occupational Therapy Treatment Techniques

TYPE	AGE AND DISABILITY	EMPIRICAL SUPPORT
Passive stretching	All ages All neurologic conditions	Few studies Conflicting results[a]
Neurodevelopmental Treatment[b]	All ages All neurologic conditions	Few studies Conflicting results
Sensory motor[c]	All ages All neurologic conditions	Very few studies Conflicting results
Brunnstrom method[d]	All ages All neurologic conditions	Very few studies Conflicting results
Proprioceptive neuromuscular facilitation[e]	Adolescent and young adults All neurologic conditions	Very few studies
Sensory integration[f]	Children with cerebral palsy, MR, autism, developmental delay, ADHD, LD	Many studies Conflicting results in school-aged children; positive results for infants with tactile, vestibular input
Vojta method (reflex locomotion)[g]	All ages cerebral palsy	Few studies Conflicting results
Conductive education[h]	Preschool to school age cerebral palsy, spina bifida, neurologic disorders	Many studies
Reflex patterning	All ages Neurologic conditions	No evidence[i]
Constraint-induced therapy	Adults and children cerebral palsy, hemiplegia, stroke hemiplegia	Evidence based[j-l]
Craniosacral techniques,[m] myofascial release,[n] Feldenkrais[o]	Originally used for adults, now used in children with cerebral palsy	

ADHD, Attention-deficit/hyperactivity disorder; *LD,* learning disability; *MR,* mental retardation.
[a]Pin T, Dyke P, Chan M. The effectiveness of passive stretching in children with cerebral palsy. *Dev Med Child Neurol.* 2006;48:855-862.
[b]Bobath K, Bobath B. The neuro-developmental treatment. In: Scrutton D, ed. *Management of Motor Disorders in Children with Cerebral Palsy.* Philadelphia, PA: JB Lippincott; 1984.
[c]Rood MS. Neurophysiological mechanisms utilized in the treatment of neuromuscular dysfunction. *Am J Occup Ther.* 1956;10:4.
[d]Brunnstrom S. Walking preparation for adult patients with hemiplegia. *J Am Phys Assoc.* 1965;65:17-29.
[e]Knott M, Voss DE. *Patterns and Techniques.* New York, NY: Harper & Row; 1968.
[f]Ayers AJ. *Sensory Integration and Learning Disabilities.* Los Angeles, CA: Western Psychological Services; 1972.
[g]Molnar GE, Alexander MA, eds. *Pediatric Rehabilitation.* 3rd ed. Philadelphia, PA: Hanley & Belfus; 1999.
[h]Bairstow P, Cochrane R, Rusk I. Selection of children with cerebral palsy for conductive education and the characteristics of children judged suitable and unsuitable. *Dev Med Child Neurol.* 1991;33:984-992.
[i]Cohen HJ, Birch HG, Taft LT. Some considerations for evaluating the Doman-Delacato "patterning" method. *Pediatrics.* 1970;45:302-314.
[j]Taub E, Landesman Ramey S, DeLuca S, et al. Efficacy of constraint-induced movement therapy for children with cerebral palsy with asymmetric motor impairment. *Pediatrics.* 2004;113:305-312.
[k]Naylor CE, Bower E. Modified constraint-induced movement therapy for young children with hemiplegic cerebral palsy: a pilot study. *Dev Med Child Neurol.* 2005;47:365-369.
[l]Eliasson AC, Krumlinde-Sundholm L, Shaw K, et al. Effects of constraint-induced movement therapy in young children with hemiplegic cerebral palsy: an adapted model. *Dev Med Child Neurol.* 2005;47:266-275.
[m]Upledger J, Vrevevoogd J. *Craniosacral Therapy.* Seattle, WA: Eastland Press; 1983.
[n]Manheim C, Levett D. *The Myofascial Release Manual.* Thorofare, NJ: Slack; 1989.
[o]Feldenkrais M. *Awareness Through Movement.* New York, NY: Harper & Row; 1977.
Based on Taggart P, Aguilar C. Therapeutic Exercise. In: Molnar GE, Alexander MA, eds. *Pediatric Rehabilitation.* 3rd ed. Philadelphia, PA: Hanley & Belfus; 1999.

- Coughing and choking
- Multiple swallows to process a bolus of food
- Noisy breathing
- Food refusal

Assessment of oral-motor function includes a detailed feeding history, specifically feeding behavior, feeding skill level, and nutritional status. The oral-motor structures should be examined for specific anatomic abnormalities of the oral cavity and for functional abnormalities of the lips, tongue, and jaw. Such abnormalities may be caused by the presence or absence of normal or abnormal oral reflexes necessary for coordinated feeding (eg, tongue thrust), weakness or incoordination (eg, poor lip seal), or pain (eg, temporomandibular joint syndrome). The evaluation may require assessment of oropharyngeal structure and function with video fluoroscopy to assess for structural abnormalities or evidence of aspiration. This information is often required before feeding therapy can safely be initiated. The child should be evaluated for the ability to manage oral and pharyngeal phases of swallow, as well as the ability to swallow foods of different consistencies.

Poor motor control of head, trunk, and extremities can also interfere with feeding. Muscle tone abnormalities, opisthotonic posturing, obligatory primitive reflexes, and abnormal movements can all interfere with proper positioning. Sensory abnormalities such as hypersensitivity or hyposensitivity to food texture, utensils used for feeding, or inability to tolerate being handled or held can also interfere with successful feeding. Medical factors such as gastroesophageal reflux disorder, seizures, swallowing dysfunction, or respiratory distress can cause pain, lethargy, and agitation, all leading to food refusal. When feeding difficulties are long standing as a result of any of the previously mentioned abnormalities, behavioral feeding problems can result, including refusal to participate in oral feeding therapy or selective or restricted intake, leading to inadequate nutrition.

Treatment includes an initial decision regarding the ability to eat safely and effectively. If significant obstacles to safe oral feeding are identified, then enteral feeding may be indicated. Feeding competency can be encouraged through the use of adaptive positioning chairs with head and trunk supports for positioning of children with poor head control and impaired trunk balance; the use of specialized nipples, bottles, feeders, or adaptive shallow spoons; the use of special cups to improve lip closure and sucking movements; and the use of brushes for oral stimulation to diminish hypersensitivity.

The inability to feed and swallow is a difficult experience for children and families, and it can have far-reaching consequences. It can interfere with parent-child interaction and attachment, especially in infants. In older children, it can result in isolation owing to an inability to share social experiences at mealtimes with friends and family.

DURABLE MEDICAL EQUIPMENT

Assistive technology or *durable medical equipment* refers to equipment designed to enhance the independence of children with chronic illnesses and disabilities, thus improving their quality of life. Assistive devices can be subcategorized into 5 categories of function: (1) positioning, (2) mobility, (3) ADL, (4) recreation, and (5) communication.[14]

Positioning devices promote optimal posture and alignment of joints in children who have not achieved adequate head or trunk control. They prevent contractures and decubiti formation by decreasing pressure on bony prominences. Devices such as positioning chairs serve as an alternative to beds or wheelchairs, and they allow the child to be optimally positioned while interacting with others during mealtime or other family activities. Standers provide supported passive standing for children who cannot independently bear their own weight.

Mobility devices can be subcategorized into ambulatory aids, transfer aids, and wheeled mobility aids. Ambulatory aids such as walkers help children improve balance and posture, provide support during walking, and decrease energy expenditure. Forward or anterior walkers promote trunk flexion; reverse or posterior walkers facilitate more erect posture and trunk extension. Crutches and canes are mobility aids that can be used by children who have better trunk control. Before children use ambulatory aids at home, they should be trained by a physical therapist. The devices must be checked and adjusted regularly to accommodate the growth of the child.

Transfer aids are used to assist children in changing their position on one surface or in transferring from one surface to another, such as a trapeze bar over a bed.

Wheeled mobility devices, such as wheelchairs, scooters, and strollers, are designed to meet the diverse needs of children with differing levels of physical disabilities, cognitive limitations, and recreational interests.

Proper selection of a wheelchair is essential. Manual and powered wheelchairs share the same basic components: frame, seat, wheels and tires, armrests and footrests, brakes, and seat belts. Powered wheelchairs should be considered for children with adequate cognition (a developmental level of at least 24 months) whose upper body strength or endurance is insufficient to propel a manual chair effectively. The child must be able to understand the concept of cause and effect, be able to follow one-step commands, have adequate visual skills, and have at least one reliable movement for activating a switch to operate the powered chair. Powered chairs can be operated with joysticks, jaw control, and sip-and-puff mechanisms.

ADL devices help patients during feeding, bathing, grooming, and toileting. Occupational therapy evaluation determines the need for such devices, which are used in conjunction with a therapeutic program appropriate for the child's age and functional level. Parents should be involved in the therapeutic program to provide implementation assistance and supervision of these activities.

Communication devices use augmentative and alternative communication strategies when a child's ability to speak is impaired. Taking into account the child's cognitive ability, these devices range from simple to complex and should allow expansion should the child's communication abilities improve.

Orthoses are externally applied devices that are used to modify structural and functional characteristics of the neuromuscular and skeletal system of the body. In clinical practice, orthoses generally take the form of braces, splints, or casts. Common aims in prescribing orthoses are to provide optimal positioning and maintain correct alignment of an extremity, prevent deformities by restricting abnormal joint motion, correct joint contracture, relieve discomfort, and assist in function and stability. An orthosis may be rigid and support an affected extremity in one position (static), or it may allow movement in a controlled manner (dynamic). Orthoses can be used for both upper extremities (eg, finger-thumb adductor splints, elbow extension orthoses, shoulder stabilization orthoses) and lower extremities (eg, supramalleolar orthoses, ankle-foot orthoses).

Casts are made of plaster or fiberglass and are applied to an extremity for a short period, between 2 and 6 weeks. Serial casting involves removal and reapplication to increase the range of stretch when a change in muscle tightening occurs.

Splints are commonly made of low-temperature thermoplastic materials that are heated and molded directly onto an extremity. They are not very strong or durable. Splints are generally used for upper and lower extremities in infants and young children and for upper extremities in older children. They can be easily modified and adjusted to accommodate rapid growth. Braces are usually custom made from high-temperature plastic materials cast from a plaster mold, metal joints, and leather or canvas straps with buckles or Velcro. Braces are durable, but they cannot be easily altered to accommodate growth; therefore they need to be replaced after a growth spurt or a change in neuromuscular or functional status.

With the assistance of the treating therapist, physicians provide justification and prescription for orthoses. Orthoses are fabricated either by an orthotist or by qualified and experienced physical and occupational therapists. Comfortable fit will improve acceptance. Cotton socks or stockings should be worn under the orthosis to absorb perspiration. A realistic wearing schedule must be outlined with gradually increased periods of use, from a few minutes to the desired number of hours. Skin should be examined for evidence of increased pressure (especially over bony prominences), edema, or other inflammatory responses.

Unbiased clinical research regarding the effectiveness of orthoses or even the spectrum of their application has been sparse. In children with cerebral palsy, a short-term effect on passive range of movement and diminished toe walking have been reported, but the long-term clinical significance is unclear.[15,16]

SPORTS AND RECREATION PROGRAMS

Physical benefits of exercise in adults with disabilities (adult paraplegia) have been observed. Individuals with disabilities who are involved in exercise programs have fewer decubitus ulcers, decreased incidence of urinary tract infections, and fewer hospitalizations. Improved strength, endurance, range of motion, and flexibility have been described in patients with cerebral palsy, as have increased socialization and higher self-esteem.[17]

Less information is available regarding effects of sports and recreation activities on children with disabilities. Children with disabilities are found to generally watch more television and to have a greater level of dependency than their peers.[18] Encouraging data show that self-concept scores of young disabled athletes were similar to their able-bodied peers.[19] Sports can be a significant part of an active lifestyle of children with disabilities. Adapted sports are activities that have been modified to meet the needs of children with disabilities. Adapted physical education was developed as a result of the Individuals with Disabilities Education Act of 1973, which includes instruction in physical education as a part of the child's individualized education program.

Sports for disabled youth are available in many communities through community centers, summer camps, and after-school programs and through adapted physical education programs. Such activities can be therapeutic, recreational, or competitive.

Training is provided for teachers, therapeutic and recreational specialists, and physical and occupational therapists in identifying needs, developing curricula, and providing direct instruction in adapted sports. Physical education teachers provide early exposure to sports and recreational activities for children with special needs, and they encourage participation in local, regional, and national levels as the children mature.

Therapeutic sports include hippotherapy (horseback riding for the disabled), aquatic therapy, dance therapy, yoga, tai chi, and karate. Hippotherapy has been popular in Europe since the 1950s and has been used in the United States since the 1970s for children with cerebral palsy. The concept behind the intervention is that the movement of the horse induces a pattern of movement in the rider similar to human walking. Reported benefits include improvement in muscle tone, posture, balance, and strength,[20,21] as well as improved concentration, language skills, self-confidence, and peer relations. Aquatic therapy uses water therapeutically. The increased buoyancy of water diminishes the effect of gravity; thus less effort is required to move. The temperature of the water can therapeutically relax muscles. Increased range of motion, improvement in coordination, cardiorespiratory endurance, and muscle tone have been noted.[22,23]

Many children with disabilities participate in organized athletic events. The National Wheelchair Athletic Association, National Wheelchair Basketball Association, American Athletic Association of the Deaf, and United Cerebral Palsy Athletic Association have established junior-level participation and programs for disabled athletes 6 to 18 years of age.

With the expansion of the range of competitive sports for disabled athletes, sports classification systems have been developed to allow for competition among athletes with various disabilities. Early classification was based on medical diagnoses. The current classifications are based on functional skills; therefore, athletes with different disabilities complete in a single system.

Children with disabilities face many challenges when participating in adapted sports as a result of their medical conditions, varying functional skill levels, and sometimes the need for sophisticated and expensive individualized equipment. For example, a child with spina bifida or a spinal cord injury can have decreased or absent sensation, which may result in pressure ulcers or skin breakdown as a result of minor stresses. An athlete with cerebral palsy may be predisposed to developing muscle strains and injuries as a result of abnormal stresses on spastic muscles and joints with decreased range of motion. A child with mobility impairment may require a racing or sports wheelchair, adapted skis, special balls, or safety devices for participation in the child's chosen activity.

Athletes must first be evaluated to assess their muscle strength and coordination and then to assess their ability to participate in the specific competitive sport. As with able-bodied athletes, children with disabilities should have a preprogram participation history taken and a physical examination performed. Medical issues, disability specific concerns, and developmental and behavioral issues should be addressed. General health, conditions limiting participation, and predisposing factors to injury should also be assessed.[24]

PSYCHOSOCIAL SUPPORT TO THE FAMILY AND PATIENT

The family is an important member of the interdisciplinary team. Although family members are experts on their child and the priorities and concerns of the family, they are often students—at least initially—in the diagnostic and treatment aspects of rehabilitation. Psychosocial support is needed to address parents' thoughts, feelings, questions, and concerns during the process. The patient, depending on age and developmental capacity, should also be included in the psychosocial support plan. The individual learning styles and educational levels of the caregivers and the patient need to be taken into account when working with families, and education should include presentation of materials through different modalities. Because of anxiety and stress during the course of treatment, remembering complicated information may be hard for a caregiver; therefore staff members should teach skills gradually and repeatedly.[25] Families are most satisfied when care is offered in a respectful and supportive manner.[26]

Providing psychosocial support to the family and child is an integral part of the rehabilitation plan. Support must be flexible and individualized to meet the family's changing needs. The times of greatest need are typically at the initial diagnosis and at points of transition. When a child is newly diagnosed with muscular dystrophy or has experienced traumatic brain injury, the family may cope with guilt, anger, and the loss of what might have been.[27] Transitions from one setting of care to another, such as the discharge of a premature infant from the neonatal intensive care unit or the transition from the hospital setting to the home, a rehabilitation facility, or a transitional care unit after traumatic brain injury, are points of particular stress for families. Parents may feel anxiety or stress as a result of changes in their child's level of care. They may feel unprepared for the new setting, time of discharge, or management of their child's new medical and equipment needs.[28]

To provide support to the family most effectively, family members should be engaged in the planning process early on to ensure coordination and continuity of care from one setting to another. Proper support to families includes an effective and collaborative discharge plan. This plan includes the identification of the patient's primary caregivers and an understanding of family beliefs, attitudes, motivations, competency, social supports, and biopsychosocial stressors in the home environment. In addition, an assessment of the home environment, home equipment and service needs, and provision of appropriate home care and community support services (eg, nursing services, home-based therapies, durable medical equipment, school accommodations, backup care in the community) will facilitate a smoother transition process for the patient and family.[29] Alternative therapeutic plans may need to be explored with the family and interdisciplinary team when barriers preclude a safe and agreed-on treatment plan.

In-hospital supportive counseling, parent-to-parent groups, counseling, home modifications, and training in equipment use and rehabilitation needs are essential to continue to support, strengthen, involve, and encourage the family's ability to care for the child at home or as they transition from the acute-care setting to a transitional or rehabilitation unit. A trial home visit from a rehabilitation facility may build the family's confidence and self-determination in preparation for discharge, with the availability of the interdisciplinary team to provide support and further education to the patient and family as needed.

EDUCATIONAL AND VOCATIONAL PLANNING

When transitioning a child to the home, additional support in the community must extend to the academic setting to ensure proper placement, related services, and accommodations as needed. State agencies such as Vocational and Educational Services for Individuals with Disabilities provide vocational training to prepare the child for suitable jobs. (See Chapter 65, Home Health Care; and Chapter 68, School-Related Issues for Children With Special Needs.)

IMPLEMENTATION OF THE THERAPEUTIC PLAN

Beginning in the neonatal intensive care unit and continuing through adulthood, entitlements exist that families can access so as to obtain therapeutic services for their children with disabilities and to fund these services. Early Intervention, Part C, of the Individuals With Disabilities Education Act (PL 99-457) funds follow-up of at-risk infants, evaluation of children from birth to 3 years for developmental disabilities, designation of a service coordinator, and provision of a wide range of therapeutic services for the eligible child and the child's family. Typically, children who are between 2 and 3 years of age and show continuing impairment may enter a therapeutic nursery setting and receive therapies at that site. PL 99-457 ensures that rehabilitation services continue into elementary school and through 21 years of age. Although these entitlements can provide an array of therapies to children with disabilities, they only address a portion of the necessary intervention plan for the child with a disability as described in this chapter. Meeting the needs of the child with a disability requires an interdisciplinary team that is able to integrate health care and therapeutic services in a coordinated fashion. This task is best accomplished through care coordination centered in the medical home.[30]

Nonetheless, many obstacles hinder families attempting to obtain care for children with special health care needs. The American Academy of Pediatrics policy statement on "Care Coordination in the Medical Home: Integrating Health and Related Systems of Care for Children With Special Health Care Needs" cites multiple barriers to effective care coordination, including:

- Lack of knowledge and information about the chronic condition
- Lack of community resources and a coordination process on the part of the primary care physician
- Primary care physicians who feel unprepared to be involved in equipment decisions for physically impaired children in their care
- Lack of communication between health care providers and other organizations involved in the child's care
- Lack of clearly defined roles for each team member, leading to redundancy of efforts and gaps in care

- Inadequate time and reimbursement for the administrative tasks associated with care coordination
- Language and cultural barriers between health care providers and families.[31]

Obstacles to accessing services can also be related to the family of a child with a disability. Although families who are knowledgeable about their child's condition can often effectively coordinate care, some families require more assistance with this task as a result of language barriers, educational level, economic situations, lack of insurance, and living far from sites of available specialty medical care. An effective, coordinated system of care must address these obstacles.

TOOLS FOR PRACTICE

Medical Decision Support

- *Guidelines for Pediatric Home Health Care* (book), American Academy of Pediatrics (www.aap.org/bookstore).

RELATED WEB SITES

- American Academy for Cerebral Palsy and Developmental Medicine (AACPDM) (aacpdm.org).
- American Brain Tumor Association (www.abta.org).
- American Physical Therapy Association (www.apta.org).
- American Speech-Language-Hearing Association (ASHA) (www.asha.org/default.htm).
- Brain Injury Association of America (www.biausa.org/).
- Centers for Disease Control and Prevention (www.cdc.gov/).
- Family Voices (www.familyvoices.org/).
- Internet Resource for Special Children (www.irsc.org/).
- Kids-Health-Nemours Foundation (kidshealth.org).
- March of Dimes (marchofdimes.com/).
- American Academy of Pediatrics: Medical Home Initiatives for Children With Special Needs (medicalhomeinfo.org/).
- Muscular Dystrophy Association (mdausa.org/).
- National Center on Physical Activity and Disability (ncpad.org/).
- National Dissemination Center for Children with Disabilities (www.nichcy.org/).
- National Institute of Neurological Disorders and Stroke (ninds.nih.gov/disorders/tbi/tbi.htm).
- Spina Bifida Association of America (www.sbaa.org).
- United Cerebral Palsy (UCP) (www.ucp.org/).

AAP POLICY STATEMENTS

American Academy of Pediatrics, Council on Children With Disabilities. Care coordination in the medical home: integrating health and related systems of care for children with special health care needs. *Pediatrics*. 2005;116(5):1238-1244. (aappolicy.aappublications.org/cgi/content/full/pediatrics;116/5/1238).

American Academy of Pediatrics, Medical Home Initiatives for Children With Special Needs Project Advisory Committee. The medical home. *Pediatrics*. 2002;110(1):184-186. (aappolicy.aappublications.org/cgi/content/full/pediatrics;110/1/184).

REFERENCES

1. Pellegrino L, Meyer G. Interdisciplinary care of the child with cerebral palsy. In: Dormans JP, Pellegrino L, eds. *Caring for Children With Cerebral Palsy*. Baltimore, MD: Paul H. Brookes Publishing; 1998.
2. Medline Plus, National Library of Medicine, National Institutes of Health. Rehabilitation. Available at: www.nlm.nih.gov/medlineplus/rehabilitation.html. Accessed June 21, 2007.
3. World Health Organization. *International Classification of Impairments, Disabilities and Handicap*. Geneva, Switzerland: World Health Organization; 1980.
4. National Institutes of Health. *Research Plan for the National Center for Medical Rehabilitation Research*. Bethesda, MD: National Institutes of Health; 1993. NIH Publication No. 93-3509.
5. Van Schnaeybroeck P, Nuttin B, Lagae L, et al. Intrathecal baclofen for intractable cerebral spasticity: a prospective placebo-controlled, double-blind study. *Neurosurgery*. 2000;46:603-609.
6. Speth LA, Leffers P, Janssen-Potten YJ, et al. Botulinum toxin A and upper limb functional skills in hemiparetic cerebral palsy: a randomized trial in children receiving intensive therapy. *Dev Med Child Neurol*. 2005;47:468-473.
7. Bottos M, Benedetti MG, Salucci P, et al. Botulinum toxin with and without casting in ambulant children with spastic diplegia: a clinical and functional assessment. *Dev Med Child Neurol*. 2003;45:758-762.
8. Abbott R. Sensory rhizotomy in the treatment of childhood spasticity. *J Child Neurol*. 1996;11(suppl 1):S36-S42.
9. Hazelwood ME, Brown JK, Rowe PJ, et al. The therapeutic use of electrical stimulation in the treatment of hemiplegic cerebral palsy. *Dev Med Child Neurol*. 1994;36;661-673.
10. Basmajian JV. Biofeedback in rehabilitation: a review of principles and practices. *Arch Phys Med Rehabil*. 1981;62(10):469-475.
11. Collet JP, Vanesse M, Marois P. Hyperbaric oxygen for children with cerebral palsy: a randomized multicentre trial. HBO-CP Research Group. *Lancet*. 2001;357:582-586.
12. Liptak GS. Complementary and alternative therapies for cerebral palsy. *Ment Retard Dev Disabil Res Rev*. 2005;11:156-163.
13. Schindl MR, Forstner C, Kern H, et al. Treadmill training with partial body weight support in non-ambulatory patients with cerebral palsy. *Arch Phys Med Rehabil*. 2000;81:301-306.
14. American Academy of Pediatrics. Assistive technology in the home care setting. In: *Guidelines for Pediatric Home Health Care*. Elk Grove Village, IL: American Academy of Pediatrics; 2002.
15. Morris C. A review of the efficacy of lower limb orthoses used for cerebral palsy. *Dev Med Child Neurol*. 2002;44:205-211.
16. Autti-Ramos I, Suovanta J, Anttila H, et al. Effectiveness of upper and lower limb casting and orthosis in children with cerebral palsy: an overview of review articles. *Am J Phys Med Rehabil*. 2006;85:80-103.
17. Stotts KM. Health maintenance: paraplegic athletes and nonathletes. *Arch Phys Med Rehabil*. 1986;67:109-114.
18. Brown M, Gordon WA. Impact of impairment on activity patterns of children. *Arch Phys Med Rehabil*. 1987;68:828-832.
19. Sherrill C, Hinson M, Gench B, et al. Self-concepts of disabled youth athletes. *Percept Motor Skills*. 1990;70:1093.
20. Depauw KP. Horseback riding for individuals with disabilities: programs, philosophy, and research. *Adapted Phys Ther Q*. 1986;3:226.

21. Bertoti DB. Effect of therapeutic horseback riding on posture in children with cerebral palsy. *Phys Ther.* 1988; 68:1512.
22. Broach E, Dattilo J. Aquatic therapy: therapeutic recreation intervention. *Ther Recreation J.* 1996;30:213-222.
23. Thorpe DE, Reilly MA. The effect of aquatic resistive exercise on lower extremity strength, energy expenditure, functional mobility, balance and self-perception in an adult with cerebral palsy: a retrospective case study. *J Aquat Phys Ther.* 2000;8:18-24.
24. Wilson PE. Exercise and sports for children who have disabilities. *Phys Med Rehabil Clin North Am.* 2002;13: 907-923.
25. Sheikh L, O'Brien M, McCluskey-Fawcett K. Parent preparation for the NICU-to-home transition: staff and parent perceptions. *Child Health Care.* 1993;22:227-239.
26. King G, Cathers T, King S, et al. Major elements of parents' satisfaction and dissatisfaction with pediatric rehabilitation services. *Child Health Care.* 2001;30: 111-134.
27. Bruce EJ, Schultz CL, Smyrnios KX. A longitudinal study of the grief of mothers and fathers of children with intellectual disability. *Br J Med Psychol.* 1996;69:33-45.
28. Coleman EA, Berenson RA. Lost in transition: challenges and opportunities for improving the quality of transitional care. *Ann Intern Med.* 2004:140:533-536.
29. American Academy of Pediatrics, Committee on Children With Disabilities. Transition of severely disabled children from hospital or chronic care facilities to the community. *Pediatrics.* 1986;78:531-534.
30. American Academy of Pediatrics, Medical Home Initiatives for Children With Special Needs Project Advisory Committee. The medical home. *Pediatrics.* 2002;110:184-186.
31. American Academy of Pediatrics, Council on Children with Disabilities. Policy statement. Care coordination in the medical home: integrating health and related systems of care for children with special health care needs. *Pediatrics.* 2005;116:1238-1244.

Chapter 67

PARTNERING WITH FAMILIES IN HOSPITAL AND COMMUNITY SETTINGS

Ruth R. Walden; Molly Cole

> *"In a world where few people share their experiences, parents look to professionals for understanding as well as practical help. Under favorable conditions a professional can reach out to parents and children, making them feel understood.... We love this man who told us our child was going to die. How is this possible? There was never a limit to the amount of time he would spend with us ..."*
>
> HELEN FEATHERSTONE
> (*A DIFFERENCE IN THE FAMILY*, PENGUIN, 1980)

Parenting a child with special health care needs (CSHCN) and disabilities can be challenging and rewarding. Parents are faced with accessing needs from multiple health care specialists; allied health services such as occupational, speech, and physical therapy; multiple public and private payment sources; and services from early intervention school programs and family-support programs. Success at this time hinges on the critical ability of parents to partner with their primary care professional in developing and implementing a care plan that addresses the unique needs of their children. The collaboration of the physician and the family promotes optimal health for the CSHCN.

FIRST CONTACT: SHARING UNEXPECTED NEWS

For a pediatrician, sharing the news with patients that their child has a special health care need may be a difficult and complex process. (For detailed guidance, please see Chapter 16, Disclosing a Diagnosis With Parents and Patients.) However, for the parents, this process is even more complicated. Physicians' choice of words, willingness to listen and answer questions, and their empathy and support at this time is a critical foundation to building a lasting and trusting relationship with families who may need ongoing and more specialized care within the practice. Just as the job of the primary care physician for this child's unique needs is only just beginning, when the parents receive this information, their job is only beginning as well. A parent's 1st challenge is sharing the information with other family members, including other siblings, the spouse, extended family, and with friends in the community. Having complete information in a way that family members can understand it and share it becomes critical for them. Even more challenging, parents must then incorporate their child's unique health care needs into the context of their family's hopes, dreams, strengths, and challenges. They must make tough decisions based on their family's priorities and goals. Providing the family with adequate information to make these decisions and respecting choices that families make are important factors, provided the child's life is not at risk.

To assist parents through the journey in caring for their child, the focus of the pediatrician needs to be on building a strong partnership with the family. Creating a trusting relationship, built on mutual respect and valuing the parents' knowledge about their child, takes time and requires an initial meeting that is calm, focused, and free from distractions in a safe and supportive environment. Interruptions should be limited, and the primary care physician must make sure that the location is private and comfortable. The family should be given some warning of difficult news so that they have time to bring in other family members or other supports. Many parents will state that hearing the news is not the most difficult experience for them, but rather being faced with the task of sharing it with their children and other family members and trying to answer their questions. If only one caregiver is present, then a time should be arranged to speak by telephone to the other family members. The primary care physician should help both parents think about ways to explain this situation to other children and, if possible, should talk to these other siblings as well. Brothers and sisters of the CSHCN often report that they felt left out of the care of their sibling. Their questions should be answered and suggestions should be given on how to be involved.

In many instances, when difficult news is shared with families, they only hear the first few words, becoming so distracted or anxious that they miss much of what is said. For the health professional, listening is a critical part of this exchange. The primary care physician must ensure that the family member's questions are answered, and enough patience must be used to answer them repeatedly. The ability of the primary care physician to be available to answer calls from the family, to check back with family members, and to see how they are doing is important. Parents may appear to be in denial because they have not fully absorbed the complexity of the problem.

Once a family has had time to absorb the information, to share it with other family members, and to ask questions, the time comes to make referrals for other community supports, such as early intervention, family-support groups, or other evaluations and treatments. These referrals should be part of a care coordination plan, developed with the family, to ensure that it addresses the family's concerns and answers all questions. In this partnership, the care coordination plan will be the tool to ensure that the pediatrician's priorities and the family's priorities are addressed. The referrals outlined in this plan are a mechanism to make sure that all the needs of this parent-professional partnership are addressed. During follow-up visits, parents can report what is happening in their early intervention program, school program, or family-support program, and they hear results of the pediatrician's examination, tests, and other medical referrals. Thus the basis of the partnership—mutual respect for the knowledge, skills, and experience of both the parent and the physician—is in place.

Supporting the family through even relatively simple decisions may be necessary. Specialist referrals are a decision point that should be reached in partnership with the family. The primary care physician should listen carefully to the parents as they explain their needs or concerns and address them in a sensitive and caring manner. Although parents may be overwhelmed, their concern for their child drives all that they do. Unless the family's choices will have a negative outcome, the pediatricians must try to empathize, putting themselves in the family's place before reacting.

OFFICE VISIT

Scheduling an office visit for a CSCHN can be a pleasant experience for the child and caregiver if a few accommodations are made. The child's record should be flagged to indicate that the child needs extended time for the appointment or that the child may need to be seen immediately on arrival to accommodate any special needs. The appointment should be scheduled at a time of day that will be easiest on the child, such as the first thing in the morning, at the end of the day, or right before or after lunch. Although many people request these times, definite legitimacy exists for a CSHCN to visit at a time that is best for the child. Family centeredness is important. (See Chapter 110, Family-Centered Care in Pediatric Practice.) Allowing for cultural differences is essential to ensure an optimal visit. (See Chapter 17, Cultural Issues in Primary Pediatric Care.)

The office visit should not consist of only milestones and physical examination, but rather to allow for dialogue to learn about the child. Getting to know the child and observing how the child interacts are important tasks. Having the family report on how the child plays and relates to the environment and how the child is doing socially is important because these interactions may be different from those of the typical child. The parents should be engaged in full partnership because they are the experts on their child. They know the child's likes, dislikes, behaviors, and abilities intimately. Family members may need additional time for questions to be answered and concerns to be addressed. If possible, the child should be engaged in the discussion about the child's own health and asked about any concerns or questions that the child may have. Writing out instructions for changes in routine or new medications and how they are to be taken is helpful. The primary care physician should check to be sure that the family understands the recommendations and that questions are answered before leaving the office. The nurse, social worker, or health educator may be able to provide the explanations for the families. Translation may be needed for family members who speak a different language. The need to assess the emotional status of the family, including the siblings, should be emphasized during the visit. Parents should be referred to the Directory of State Title V CSHCN Programs at their state's department of health, to Family Voices, Inc. (www.familyvoices.org), and to the local MUMS National Parent-to-Parent Network (www.netnet.net/mums/) to provide avenues for exploring funding of services and sources of emotional support and advocacy. These programs can also provide matching with families whose children have the same diagnosis.

The CSHCN often needs emergency services from the office or the hospital. The primary care physician should check with the family to see if they have an emergency plan in place. The American Academy of Pediatrics and the American College of Emergency Physicians have developed an emergency form that can be completed and updated by the physician. Copies should be kept with the parents, with child care provider, on the child's car seat or diaper bag, and in school. This information will prepare the emergency providers and hospital staff to best meet the needs of the child because it will provide baseline information. This sheet is used in collaboration with a MedicAlert bracelet or tag. Parents should be urged to contact their local ambulance company to introduce their child and to help avoid misunderstandings when an emergency arises. Also important is knowing if the local community hospital is equipped to handle an emergency for the child or if the tertiary care hospital is best suited to deal with the child's condition. The parents should also be advised whether they should contact the office in an emergency or on arrival at the hospital. The parents, if they choose, should be permitted to stay with their child during emergency procedures, including resuscitation. The primary care physician may be able to influence the hospital staff to support the family's choice. Parents may need support and care coordination during and after the emergency situation.

Many children with special needs require home care. Discharge planners may initially plan for the home care, but the primary care physician must follow up, complete the paperwork, and direct and coordinate the care. (See Chapter 65, Home Health Care.) Families should be assisted throughout the process. The primary care physician should periodically check with the family to ensure consistency and quality of care. Home care agencies are often understaffed and cannot provide consistent care for the child. Parents should be trained to care for their children at home but not to be drained by the task. The primary care physician should note that having outsiders who come into the home and intrude on family life is a burden on the entire family. Supporting the family members through this process and referring them for some training on how to deal with the home health caregiver can be helpful. If the parents needs financial assistance to access the home care, then referral to the Katie Beckett waiver program or other public financing programs in their state should be made. Parents can contact the Title V Program their state, which is prepared to direct them to the agency directing the waiver program for their state.

The office visit is a good time to prepare for the child's future. Early intervention, preschool, and school services are huge milestones for the CSHCN. Parents often know the type of setting they want for their child; they understand their child's learning style and have a feeling for the type of experience that will work to make the child's formative years most productive. The physician may be asked to partner with the family to find the most appropriate placement. School placement decisions should include benefits for the CSHCN and the class as a whole. Inclusion in the regular classroom will bring many benefits. Modifications and the services of a special education teacher can lead to positive outcomes not just for the CSHCN, but also for the other children in the class who learn to accept people who are different. However, if parents choose a less-inclusive setting in a special class, then honoring this choice is important as well.

Information as to the child's clinical needs will help in the development of the best program to meet the needs the child has, regardless of the placement choice. Forms for specific services (occupational, physical, and speech therapies among others) will be required. If possible, attending or participating by telephone in the school placement process is desired. Parents should be asked to envision what they see the child doing in 18 years. Transition to adult living, earning, and learning should take place from birth through adulthood, understanding that the child may go through many changes within that time. The physician is a role model for the family for advocating and championing the needs of the child. As an equal partner with the family, the primary care physician may be required to advocate with other physicians, insurance companies, and the educational system.

SUPPORT DURING HOSPITALIZATION

Hospitalizations, whether planned or in an emergency, are stressful times for families who have a child with special health care needs. In the emergency department, the hospital staff must engage the parents as partners in addressing the crisis at hand. The emergency plan developed with the family will assist the hospital staff in providing a smooth emergency department experience. When contacted by the emergency department physician, the child's health professional can assist in this process by providing the staff with insight into the parents' ability to report on their child's needs accurately and encouraging the staff to use the parents' input during their emergency department stay.

For a planned hospital admission, the parents must have a clear understanding of the usual information: the purpose of the admission and what is expected to happen during the time the child is hospitalized, potential challenges, and anticipated discharge. However, with the CSHCN, other considerations must also be addressed: special beds, seating, diets, and feeding needs, specialized activities with the child life department or volunteers, communication problems, and behavior concerns. Parents should be encouraged to develop a list of their child's unique care needs and bring the list with them so that these points can be easily incorporated into the care plan with hospital staff.

Many parents who have a CSHCN prefer to stay in the hospital to ensure that their child's unique needs can be met. Other parents cannot be available for long periods because of other commitments. In either case, the primary care physician is critical to the development of a strong working partnership between the family and the hospital staff. Parents have unique insight and understanding about their child's care needs, and the staff should be encouraged to seek their input during the hospital stay. The primary care physician should encourage the staff to schedule times to meet with caregivers, whether they stay at the hospital or not. Parents must be allowed to be present during procedures. The staff should be encouraged to work with the parents and to incorporate the parents' knowledge about their child's unique care needs into the hospital care plan.

Teaching hospitals pose opportunities and challenges for the CSHCN. Parents should be encouraged to be present during rounds and should be treated as a critical component of the child's hospital care team. Not only will this practice enhance outcomes for the child, but it can also be a good teaching tool for residents and other students in teaching hospitals. The primary care physician should model this partnership.

One of the usual learning opportunities in a teaching hospital is the practice of taking the child's history. Parents who have a child with frequent hospitalizations may find that this process of medical history taking, although a valuable teaching tool, is painful and stressful. Recalling traumatic and difficult events in their child's medical history at a time when their child is again being hospitalized is something that some parents will resist, and they may need support when they decline to participate in this process, if it is not critical to the treatment.

Parents often anxiously await the arrival of the primary care physician at the hospital each day. The primary care physician is their partner in their child's care, and they look for insight, support, and information each day. Let family members know when you will be in the hospital so they can talk to you. If you miss the parents, check in with them by telephone later in the day so that any of their questions can be answered and so they can be updated on their child's status.

Parents must be involved in discharge planning—from a discussion of wellness and stability to the types of supports they may need at discharge. If their child's care needs have changed as a result of this hospitalization, then the team needs to ensure that they are trained in the care and have adequate support and equipment at home. The primary care physician should assist the team, including the family members, in the discharge process. Issues such as school, accessibility, nursing, equipment, medications, and follow-up with the primary care physician and other specialists are part of the process. Additionally, the care coordination plan developed by the primary care physician and the family may need to be modified.

On the day of discharge, the discharge planner or other hospital staff members usually meet with the family to review the discharge plan. The primary care physician should review the discharge plan either on the day of discharge or at an office visit after discharge. The parents should be comfortable with the treatments, needs, and follow-up appointments, especially if any changes in care have occurred as a result of this hospitalization.

TRANSITIONS

Early intervention provides a nurturing and supportive staff and an environment for the CSHCN and the family. Services are focused on the child and family, with family centeredness at the core of all that they do. Programs are much less supportive when the child moves to the early childhood program within the child's school district. Services may be fewer than they were in early intervention; family supports may end completely or become less family centered. For many children, this move will also mean the transition from home-based to center-based services. Parents should be made aware of these differences and be supported during this potentially difficult transition. Referrals for other services through the Title V Program in their state and community agencies may become necessary to supplement the Individuals with Disabilities Education Act, Part B, 3 to 5 Preschool Services. The primary care physician may need to check with the parents to ascertain their needs more often than usual during this transition.

The transition from the smaller setting of the early childhood program to the elementary school program can be frightening for families and the CSHCN. How will the child be accepted? How will the staff meet the child's needs? Are the allied services going to continue to support progress? Is the child placed with the best teacher to meet the child's learning style? These questions are a few that the parents may have as they approach the beginning of school. During the school physical, the primary care physician may need to reassure the family. The primary care physician may agree or disagree with the placement, but the support will help the family approach the beginning or continuation of the program with less apprehension. Understanding and empathy will help the family.

Transition from elementary to middle and then from middle to high school may bring placement changes and insecurity to the child and family. Friends who have surrounded the child up to this point may not be available to support the child; teachers and staff will be new and perhaps less supportive and understanding of the child's needs. Providing clinical information and clearly and concisely explaining the needs of the child may be necessary. The primary care physician should check with the parents to determine their needs and to see how smoothly the transition is proceeding.

Transitions occur at other junctures as well. An illness may result in changes in the child's ability to attend school. A child with a terminal illness may deteriorate for long periods, and the school personnel may not understand the need to adjust their demands of the student. This circumstance may be more characteristic of middle and high schools because of the expectations of the curricula. The primary care physician's support of the family and staff within school will help increase understanding, reduce demands and expectations, and support the child or young adult through the illness. If the illness is one that results in physical or cognitive deterioration, then preparing the family and, if the parents wish, the educational program, for the changes is important. These transitions can be sources of great stress not only for the parents, but also the siblings and extended family members. Helplessly watching as the child's ability diminishes over time is difficult. Gently providing support and referrals for emotional and family support and services is critical.

The transition to adult health care takes planning and time for the primary care physician, the adolescent, and the family. Preparing the adolescent for an adult health care provider who may be less family centered requires advocating, sharing of information, mentoring the adolescent, and relying on the trust of the family. Choosing an adult health care provider should be an informed decision of the partnership: adolescent, parents, and primary care physician. Preparing the new care provider is the responsibility of the physician and parents. Adolescents should be empowered to speak on their own behalf, to describe their condition, to share how it affects them daily, and to seek care for themselves. The mentoring should begin early and continue until such time as the primary care physician discharges the adolescent from care.

FINANCIAL CONSIDERATION

The parents may face significant unpaid bills, difficulties with getting insurance to pay for services, insurance company reversing decisions, and seeking services that may be difficult to find locally. Referrals to the state insurance program, Medicaid for children, or Medicaid waiver programs if the family does not have insurance may assist families. If the primary care physician's office does not accept these sources of payment, then helping the family identify a practice that does will also be helpful if the parents are not able to afford the associated out-of-pocket expenses. Displaying brochures about the state insurance program and Medicaid within the primary care physician's office will draw the attention of parents needing these services.

END-OF-LIFE PLANNING

When dealing with a child who has a terminal diagnosis, the primary care physician must have discussions with the family at a time other than when the child is in crisis. The primary care physician should schedule a time in the office to discuss these issues. Included in this meeting should be a frank discussion of the family's wishes regarding do not resuscitate orders. (See Chapter 69, Palliative, End-of-life, and Bereavement Care.)

GUIDE TO COLLABORATING WITH FAMILIES

1. Respect the parents for their knowledge and understanding about their child and their ability to relate to their child.
2. Accept the parents, and later the youth, as full and equal partners in the care of their child. The primary care physician and both parents, all working together, will be powerful champions to obtain the best results.
3. Always take the time to listen to parents. Their words and actions will measure their emotional status and provide an opportunity to learn what their wants, desires, and hopes are for their CSHCN.
4. Learning about the meaning of the child's illness or condition is important to the parents because this information will explain their actions, reactions, and goals for their child and responses to changes in their child's condition or treatment recommendations.
5. Keep the CSHCN as the center of focus.
6. If care coordination cannot be provided in the primary care physician's practice, then the parents should be referred to outside sources of support. (See Suggested Resources.)
7. Early in the relationship with the family, discuss the fact that disagreements will occur. Make an arrangement to respect each other's judgment and to agree to disagree.

CONCLUSION

Parents are seeking physicians who are able to treat them as equals in the care of their children. They are looking for someone who will be nonjudgmental, as long as the child is safe, well cared for, and treated with respect. Parents will respect the primary care physician who admits to not knowing but will seek out the answer or the specialist who does. Parents will respect the primary care physician who can provide sensitive, nurturing, and supportive care.

> *"... Families are visionaries. Their dreams are not tied to bureaucratic limitations.*
>
> *Their ideas and hopes for their children, their families, and their communities provide challenge, inspiration, and guidance."*
>
> (Elizabeth S. Jeppson and Josie Thomas, *Essential Allies: Families as Advisors,* Institute for Family Centered Care, 1995)

TOOLS FOR PRACTICE

Community Coordination and Advocacy

- *Advisory Council Workplan—Getting Started* (form), Institute for Family-Centered Care (www.familycenteredcare.org/advance/creatingadvisorycouncil.pdf).
- *Creating Patient and Family Advisory Councils* (booklet), Institute for Family-Centered Care (www.familycenteredcare.org/advance/creatingadvisorycouncil.pdf).
- *Family Consultant Feedback* (form), Center for Children with Special Health Care Needs (www.cshcn.org/).
- *FAQ serving on Advisory Boards and Councils* (fact sheet), Family Voices (www.familyvoices.org/toolbox/FAC/VT-cshnFAQ.doc).

Practice Management and Care Coordination

- *2006 Care Coordination Toolkit* (toolkit), Center for Infants and Children with Special Needs at Cincinnati Children's Hospital Medical Center and The National Center of Medical Home initiatives for Children with Special Needs (www.medicalhomeinfo.org/tools/Coding.html).
- *Action Care Plan* (form), Center for Medical Home Improvement (www.medicalhomeimprovement.org/assets/pdf/Working_Full.pdf).
- *Actionable Care Plan EPIC IC Medical Home Project* (form), PA Medical Home Program—EPIC IC (www.medicalhomeinfo.org/tools/CarePlans/Actionable care plan.doc).
- *Care Coordination Measurement Tool* (form), American Academy of Pediatrics (www.medicalhomeinfo.org/tools/FinalMHCCMeasurementTool.doc).
- *Care Plans (I & II)* (form), Hitchcock Clinic—Concord Pediatric Care Plan Part I (www.medicalhomeinfo.org/tools/assess/htm).
- *Child History Fact Sheet*, Center for Infants and Children with Special Needs (www.medicalhomeinfo.org/tools/Documentation/CHILD HISTORY FACTSHEET mini.doc).
- *Consultation Referral Form*, Cincinnati Children's Hospital Medical Center (www.cincinnatichildrens.org/NR/rdonlyres/D86E76FC-FAA6-4F21-9D9F-371D35CC365D/0/consultreferralform.pdf).
- *Comprehensive Care plan packet* (booklet), National Medical Home Learning Collaborative II (www.medicalhomeinfo.org/tools/CarePlans/ComprehensiveCarePlanningII.pdf).
- *ED Referral Form*, Cincinnati Children's Hospital Medical Center (www.cincinnatichildrens.org/NR/rdonlyres/06B930C3-A7C7-4862-8654-04A83EAC6588/0/edreferfax.pdf).
- *Effect of Child's Disability on Family Members Interview* (questionnaire), Robert E. Nickel, MD; Larry W, Desch, MD (www.brookespublishing.com/pgforms/pdfs/03-FamilyInterview.pdf).
- *Emergency Information Form*, American Academy of Pediatrics (www.aap.org/advocacy/blankform.pdf).
- *Hospital Discharge Packet* (form), Center for Infants and Children with Special Needs: Children's Hospital Medical Center of Cincinnati (www.medicalhomeinfo.org/tools/Documentation/HospitalDischarge.doc).

- *Index of CPT Codes for Medical Home* (fact sheet), American Academy of Pediatrics (www.pafp.com/MMS/coding/medical-home-code-index.doc).
- *Integrated Services Care Plan,* PA Medical Home Program—EPIC IC (www.medicalhomeinfo.org/tools/CarePlans/IntegratedcareplanDRAFT.doc).
- *Interactive Emergency Information Form,* American Academy of Pediatrics (www.aap.org/advocacy/eif.doc).
- *Instructions for Parents on the Emergency Form* (fact sheet), American Academy of Pediatrics (www.aap.org/advocacy/epcparent.htm).
- *Medical Home Assessment,* Los Angeles Medical Home Project for CSHCN (www.medicalhomeinfo.org/tools/CarePlans/Assessmentform.doc).
- *Medical Summaries,* PA Medical Home Program—EPIC IC (www.medicalhomeinfo.org/tools/CarePlans/MEDICALSUMMARY.doc).
- *My Care Plan,* Palmetto Pediatric and Adolescent Clinic, P.A. (www.medicalhomeinfo.org/tools/CarePlans/Palmettocareplan.doc).
- *Physician Management Billing Form,* American Academy of Pediatrics (www.medicalhomeinfo.org/tools/Coding/PCMBilling.doc).
- *Primary Care Family Assessment,* Robert E. Nickel, MD; Larry W. Desch, MD (www.brookespublishing.com/pgforms/pdfs/03-PrimaryCareAssessment.pdf).
- *Referral Fax Back Form,* American Academy of Pediatrics (www.medicalhomeinfo.org/tools/referr.html).

AAP POLICY STATEMENTS

American Academy of Pediatrics, Committee on Children With Disabilities. Role of the pediatrician in family-centered early intervention services. *Pediatrics.* 2001;107(5):1155-1157. (aappolicy.aappublications.org/cgi/content/full/pediatrics;120/5/1153).

American Academy of Pediatrics, Committee on Hospital Care. Family-centered care and pediatrician's role. *Pediatrics.* 2003;112(3):691-696. (aappolicy.aappublications.org/cgi/content/full/pediatrics;112/3/691).

SUGGESTED RESOURCES

American Academy of Pediatrics. Health Topics on Children with Special Health Care Needs. Available at: www.aap.org/healthtopics/specialneeds.cfm. Accessed December 6, 2007.

American Academy of Pediatrics, National Center of Medical Home Initiatives for Children with Special Health Care Needs. What is a medical home? Available at: www.medicalhomeinfo.org/. Accessed December 6, 2007.

Family Voices, Inc. Family Voices . . . speaking on behalf of children and youth with special health care need. Available at: www.familyvoices.org. Accessed December 6, 2007.

Federation of Families for Children's Mental Health. Helping children with mental health needs and their families achieve a better quality of life. Available at: www.ffcmh.org/. Accessed December 6, 2007.

Institute for Child Health Policy. Healthy & Ready To Work. [Initiative that presents a comprehensive system of family-centered, culturally competent, community-based care for children with special health care needs who are approaching adulthood.] Available at: www.hrtw.org. Accessed December 6, 2007.

Institute for Family-Centered Care. Resources. Available at: www.familycenteredcare.org/resources/index.html. Accessed December 6, 2007.

National Dissemination Center for Children with Disabilities, State Pages, NICHCY. Available at: www.nichcy.org. Accessed December 6, 2007.

The Family Village. A Global Community of Disability-Related Resources. Available at: www.familyvillage.wisc.edu. Accessed December 6, 2007.

US Department of Health and Human Services, Maternal and Child Health Bureau, Administration on Developmental Disabilities. Kids As Self Advocates (KASA): Youth as Leaders Manual. Teens and young adults with special health care needs speaking on our own behalf. Available at: www.fvkasa.org/. Accessed December 6, 2007.

Chapter 68

SCHOOL-RELATED ISSUES FOR CHILDREN WITH SPECIAL NEEDS

Nienke P. Dosa, MD, MPH; Gregory S. Liptak, MD, MPH

Approximately 8% of children entering kindergarten and 16% of adolescents entering high school have a chronic physical, developmental, behavioral, or emotional condition that requires health and related services of a type or amount beyond that generally required by children.[1] At all grade levels, boys are one and one-half times more likely than girls to have a special health care need. This likelihood may be related to the higher proportion of boys who are diagnosed with behavioral disorders.[2] Although children with special health care needs have the same basic educational and developmental needs as their healthy peers, a significant minority have a range of problems that may interfere with their academic performance or require special medical services in school. Collaborative efforts among school personnel, health professionals, and families enhance the health, education, and development of these children and should be the basis for addressing their needs in school.

In the past, children with special health care needs were often isolated from healthy children in schools or were taught at home; thus they were deprived of crucial social contacts and a broad educational experience. Several laws now ensure that all children have access to education in the least restrictive environment.

- Public Law 94-142, the Education for All Children Act of 1975, ensures a free and appropriate public education for preschool (ages 3-5 years) and school-aged children who have disabilities. The law was amended in 1990 by Public Law 101-476 and renamed the Individuals with Disabilities Education Act (IDEA). Under IDEA, children and parents are entitled to therapeutic and related services such as occupational, physical, vision, and hearing therapy; family support; social services; mental health services; educational intervention; and case management services, even if the child is not receiving special education, as long as these services relate to a child's education. Changes made to IDEA with the Individuals with Disabilities Education Improvement Act (IDEIA) of 2004 and subsequent regulations and judicial rulings have altered IDEA. Children may now be identified as having a learning disability by their response to instruction (RTI). Establishing a discrepancy between a child's ability and achievement (ie, *wait to fail*) is no longer necessary to initiate psychoeducational evaluation and services. However, when conflict exists regarding what constitutes a *free and appropriate education,* the burden of proof lies with the party bringing suit (usually the parents) rather than the school district.

- Section 504 of the Rehabilitation Act of 1973, appended through 1998, requires school districts to eliminate barriers that exclude children with special needs from full participation. These barriers can be either physical (buildings that are not wheelchair accessible) or programmatic (keeping children with hepatitis segregated from other children). Section 504 is, in essence, an antidiscrimination law. The definition of disability is broader under Section 504 than it is under IDEA, but fewer services are provided under 504 plans than under IDEIA. Section 504 gives students access to programs such as adaptive physical education and accommodations such as extra time for test taking. However, federal funding for remediation and school-based services such as physical therapy is only made available if a student is in special education (IDEIA). Another important distinction is that federal funding is not provided to schools under Section 504.

Under both laws, children are required to have a written plan with educational goals. This plan is called an Individual Education Plan (IEP) under IDEA and a 504 Plan under Section 504. When a child turns 16, the IEP must include transition goals. These are appropriate, measurable post-secondary goals related to training, education, employment, and independent living skills, where appropriate. Involvement in formulating them is an opportunity for the pediatrician to coordinate a child's educational program with a medical treatment plan and to help families and children review beneficial services to which they are entitled.[3] An up-to-date overview of relevant public laws is available on the Wright's Law Web site, www.wrightslaw.com.[4]

SCHOOL ISSUES FOR CHILDREN WHO HAVE CHRONIC HEALTH CONDITIONS

School provides a child with academic skills and multiple experiences critical to emotional and social development. The school-related problems and concerns that all children have can be exacerbated for a child who has special health care needs. The child's chronic condition may require frequent and, occasionally, long absences; illness and medications may affect cognitive functioning; and physical limitations may restrict participation in school activities. These obstacles, when combined with inappropriate expectations of teachers and parents and altered interactions with peers, can provide formidable impediments to academic achievement, psychosocial development, and vocational placement.

Medical Issues

The primary school-related goal for the pediatrician who cares for children who have chronic conditions is to ensure a safe environment. Specific issues such as transportation, special equipment, backup, and emergency plans need to be identified. Additional issues such as notification of the parents if the child's health status changes in school, responsibility for monitoring the child's health in school, and the role of the physician need to be determined. For children who have severe or complex conditions, especially those who require technology-assisted care, a formal process of entry into school should be followed, including early notification of the school and discussion with school administrators of the child's condition and needs.[5] The physician helps develop and approve a formal health care plan, created in collaboration with the family and the child, school administration, and other health care personnel. The physician can also make recommendations regarding the program, placement, and staffing and can participate in the training of school personnel. Excellent guides for the training of school personnel who care for children who have chronic conditions are available. Box 68-1 lists the components of an emergency plan; Box 68-2 lists specific guidance for a child who has a chronic condition in school.

School Achievement

Approximately 10% to 15% of school-aged children repeat or fail a grade in school. Children with special health care needs are nearly 3 times as likely to repeat at least one grade as children who have no disabilities.[6] This risk may be present in the earliest school years; children with special needs are significantly more likely than their healthy peers to repeat kindergarten or first grade.[7] The pediatrician can help prevent school failure by promoting school readiness at health supervision visits, advocating for psychoeducational support, and by identifying health behaviors or psychosocial factors that negatively affect school performance.

BOX 68-1 Components of an Emergency Plan for a Child Who Has a Chronic Condition in School

1. Names, addresses, and telephone numbers of family and caretakers
2. Emergency telephone numbers:
   - Ambulance
   - Home care company
   - Utility companies
   - Hospital
   - Emergency department
   - Primary care physician
   - Specialists
3. Child-specific emergency plan
4. Other school personnel to contact

BOX 68-2 Components of Child-Specific Guidance

1. Important personnel
2. Background information:
   - Conditions
   - Medical history
   - Special health care needs
   - Baseline status
   - Medications
   - Diet
   - Technological aids
   - Transportation needs
3. Procedures required
4. Equipment
5. Child-specific techniques
6. Special considerations and precautions (eg, latex allergy)
7. List of possible problems for observation, reason, action
8. Daily log

In some cases, school difficulties are caused by neurocognitive, visual, or auditory impairments. Medical treatment, such as intrathecal chemotherapy and cranial irradiation, and certain medications, such as anticonvulsants, may impair cognitive functioning. Fatigue, caused by medication or underlying conditions, should also be considered. Physicians can help identify the cause of fatigue and may be able to treat the problem by adjusting medication schedules, such as with anticonvulsants, by treating the underlying condition (eg, depression, obstructive sleep apnea), or by suggesting that a rest period be incorporated into the school day.

For the majority of children who have chronic health conditions, however, these concerns are not significant. Many children face academic adversity because of the social and psychological consequences of their condition. "Chains of adversity"[8] can occur when the individual's physical impairments initiate a sequence of disadvantageous outcomes. Diminished expectations and lower self-esteem, fatigue, pain, and preoccupation with symptoms that often accompany chronic conditions can be associated with a decreased self-efficacy that may develop into a learned helplessness that results in diminished expectations and efforts. This situation may be complicated by altered parental expectations that involve many aspects of the *vulnerable child syndrome* (see Chapter 128, School Absenteeism and School Refusal). Failure to understand these psychosocial complications can lead to expectations that are unreasonably high or detrimentally low.

Children who have special health care needs often have increased school absences, which may lead to significant educational disadvantage (see Chapter 128, School Absenteeism and School Refusal). Homebound teaching often becomes available only when a child misses 2 to 4 weeks of school, yet most children who have chronic conditions have frequent, intermittent absences. Pediatricians can encourage parents and teachers to help children disadvantaged by absences from falling behind in school work and can advocate that a child be made eligible for homebound teaching without the usual waiting period. Homebound teaching has significant limitations, however, and school attendance should be encouraged whenever possible. Medical appointments should be scheduled during nonschool hours whenever possible.

Job Achievement and Independent Living

For the majority of children who have special health care needs, expectations for participation in the work force as adults should be no different from the expectations for their healthy peers. Nonetheless, many children, particularly those with developmental disabilities, fail to participate fully in society once they become young adults. High school graduation rates for students who have disabilities are lower than for those who have no disabilities, and of those who graduate, fewer go on to college. Vocational rehabilitation, a federally funded, state-operated program, is an important funding stream for adolescents with disabilities seeking postsecondary education, adaptive driving skills, or employment. Because most vocational services do not become available until candidates are 18 years of age, prevocational skills, including social skills training and independent living planning, should be included in a child's IEP or 504 Plan during the high school years.

Schools must provide opportunities for youths to be active participants in preemployment and employment activities from the earliest stages of the child's academic experience. Unfortunately, many youths with special health care needs enter the workforce later than their nondisabled peers. Nationwide, nearly 85% of high school seniors have held a regular job before graduation. In contrast, the employment rate for high school seniors with learning disabilities, emotional disturbances, or speech impairments is only 50%. Only 30% of blind youths, 25% of youths with multiple disabilities or orthopedic impairments, and 15% of youths with autism have job experience before high school graduation.[9] Participation in peer-appropriate activities at every stage of schooling is essential to successful transition to adulthood.[10] Parental support and adult role models are also important.[11]

COLLABORATION OF SCHOOL STAFF AND HEALTH PROFESSIONALS

Collaboration among school-based educational and health personnel, community-based providers, and parents is essential in caring for the chronically ill child in school. Only through well-coordinated efforts do educators become aware of the child's medical needs and do health care providers become aware of the child's learning needs.

Primary care physicians provide direct medical care and guidance about medical issues and play a vital role as advocates for their patients who have chronic conditions. As the professional who knows the child medically and psychosocially, the pediatrician can encourage academic achievement and socialization and help anticipate major transitions in a child's educational career. Familiarity with a child's IEP is a prerequisite for effective primary care of the child who has a chronic health condition. One example of the primary care physician's role would be physician guidance in the development of an adaptive physical education program for children with special needs. The National Center on Physical Activity and Disability is a clearinghouse for guidelines for physical activity that can be used for planning an adaptive physical education program for a wide variety of pediatric conditions, such as autism and spina bifida (www.ncpad.org/disability/).[12]

Teachers and parents need to know the implications of the child's medical condition for school performance. Lack of such information can result in misunderstanding of the child's medical condition, which can lead to denial of services, misinterpretation of behaviors, or undue restrictions or unrealistic expectations. With adequate information, teachers and parents can foster not only academic achievement, but also social competence. An excellent resource on the Internet that provides information for teachers and other nonmedical providers on a wide variety of pediatric conditions is the Family Village Library (www.familyvillage.wisc.edu/library.htm).[13] Teachers can implement recommendations and provide ongoing evaluation of a child's progress. Their input is central to the IEP and invaluable to comprehensive medical management.

The school nurse usually coordinates health services in the school. In most school districts the nurse is responsible for contacting physicians and parents about a child's medical needs. Nurses also often develop and implement care plans[14] and emergency plans[15] in collaboration with the school pediatrician, the primary care pediatrician, or pediatric subspecialists. Federal standards for school nurses set forth in the Healthy People 2010 initiative include a nurse-to-student ratio of 1:750. Many school districts fall short of this goal, and some schools do not have a nurse on site. School nurse practice acts currently define the scope of nursing service on a state-by-state basis. School nurses are increasingly involved with public health measures such as obesity prevention and mental health screening. In addition, the number of school-based health care clinics is growing rapidly, especially in medically underserved areas. Most of these clinics have a multidisciplinary staff (eg, a physician, nurse practitioner, social worker, health educator); their potential contribution to the care of children with special health care needs should not be overlooked. The role of the school nurse and models of school health services are discussed in greater detail in Chapter 125, School Health Education.

TOOLS FOR PRACTICE

Community Advocacy and Coordination

- *School Forms & Resources National Center of Medical Initiatives* (Web page), American Academy of Pediatrics (www.medicalhomeinfo.org/tools/school.html).
- *Transition Tools National Center for Medical Home Initiatives* (Web page), American Academy of Pediatrics (www.medicalhomeinfo.org/tools/trans.html).

Engaging Patient and Family

- *A Parent's Guide: Developing Your Child's IEP* (Web page), National Dissemination Center for Children with Disabilities (www.nichcy.org/pubs/parent/pa12txt.htm).
- *A Parent's Guide to Finding Help for Young Children with a Disability* (booklet), National Dissemination Center for Children with Disabilities (www.nichcy.org/pubs/parent/pa2.pdf).
- *Family Village* (Web page) (www.familyvillage.wisc.edu/).
- *The Paper Chase: Managing Your Child's Documents* (article), Wrightslaw (www.wrightslaw.com/info/advo.paperchase.crabtree.htm).
- *When Your Child with Special Needs Goes to School* (form), Center for Children With Special Needs, Children's Hospital and Regional Center (www.cshcn.org/forms/ReturntoSchoolFlyer_English.pdf).

Practice Management and Care Coordination

- *Emergency Information Form*, American Academy of Pediatrics (www.aap.org/advocacy/blankform.pdf).
- *Frequently Asked Questions About Section 504 and the Education of Children With Disabilities* (fact sheet), US Department of Education (www.ed.gov/about/offices/list/ocr/504faq.html).
- *Individuals with Disabilities Education Act (IDEA)* (Web page), US Department of Education (idea.ed.gov/).
- *Instructions for Parents on the Emergency Form* (fact sheet), American Academy of Pediatrics (www.aap.org/advocacy/epcparent.htm).
- *Interactive Emergency Information Form*, American Academy of Pediatrics (www.aap.org/advocacy/eif.doc).

RELATED WEB SITES

- National Center on Physical Activity and Disability: Disabilities and Conditions (www.ncpad.org/disability/).
- Wrightslaw (www.wrightslaw.com/).

AAP POLICY STATEMENTS

American Academy of Pediatrics, Committee on School Health and Committee on Bioethics. Do not resuscitate orders in schools. *Pediatrics*. 2000;105:878-879. (aappolicy.aappublications.org/cgi/content/full/pediatrics;105/4/878).

American Academy of Pediatrics, Committee on Children With Disabilities. Provision of educationally related services for children and adolescents with chronic diseases and disabling conditions. *Pediatrics*. 2007;119(6):1218-1223. (aappolicy.aappublications.org/cgi/content/full/pediatrics;119/6/1218).

American Academy of Pediatrics, Committee on Children With Disabilities. The pediatrician's role in development and implementation of an individual education plan (IEP) and/or an individual family service plan (IFSP). *Pediatrics*. 1999;104:124-127. (aappolicy.aappublications.org/cgi/content/full/pediatrics;104/1/124).

American Academy of Pediatrics, Committee on Children With Disabilities. The role of the pediatrician in transitioning children and adolescents with developmental disabilities and chronic illnesses from school to work or college. *Pediatrics*. 2000;106:854-856. (aappolicy.aappublications.org/cgi/content/full/pediatrics;106/4/854).

American Academy of Pediatrics, Committee on Injury and Poison Prevention. School bus transportation of children with special health care needs. *Pediatrics*. 2001;108:516-518.

American Academy of Pediatrics, Committee on Pediatric AIDS. Education of children with human immunodeficiency virus infection. *Pediatrics*. 2000;105:1358-1360. (aappolicy.aappublications.org/cgi/content/abstract/pediatrics;88/3/645).

American Academy of Pediatrics, Committee on Pediatric Emergency Medicine. Emergency preparedness for children with special health care needs. *Pediatrics*. 1999;104: e53. (aappolicy.aappublications.org/cgi/content/full/pediatrics;104/4/e53).

American Academy of Pediatrics, Committee on School Health. Guidelines for the administration of medication in school. *Pediatrics*. 2003;112:697-699. (aappolicy.aappublications.org/cgi/content/full/pediatrics;113/2/697).

American Academy of Pediatrics, Committee on School Health. The role of the school nurse in providing school health services. *Pediatrics*. 2001;108:1231-1232. (aappolicy.aappublications.org/cgi/content/full/pediatrics;108/5/1231).

American Academy of Pediatrics, Committee on Sports Medicine and Fitness. Human immunodeficiency virus and other blood-borne viral pathogens in the athletic setting. *Pediatrics*. 1999;104:1400-1403. (aappolicy.aappublications.org/cgi/content/full/pediatrics;104/6/1400).

American Academy of Pediatrics, Committee on Sports Medicine and Fitness. Medical conditions affecting sports participation *Pediatrics*. 2001;107:1205-1209. (aappolicy.aappublications.org/cgi/content/full/pediatrics;107/5/1205).

REFERENCES

1. US Department of Health and Human Services, Health Resources and Services Administration, Maternal and Child Health Bureau. *The National Survey of Children with Special Health Care Needs Chartbook 2001*. Rockville, MD: US Department of Health and Human Services; 2004.
2. Scahill L, Schwab-Stone M. Epidemiology of ADHD in school-age children. *Child Adolesc Psychiatr Clin North Am*. Jul 2000;9(3):541-555, vii.
3. American Academy of Pediatrics, Committee on Children with Disabilities. The pediatrician's role in the development and implementation of an Individual Education Plan (IEP) and/or an Individual Family Service Plan (IFSP). *Pediatrics*. 1999;104:124-127.
4. Wight's Law. Available at: www.wrightslaw.com/. Accessed June 7, 2007.
5. Schwab NC, Gelfman MHB, eds. *Legal Issues in School Health Services: A Resource for School Administrators, School Attorneys, and School Nurses*. North Branch, MN: Sunrise River Press; 2001.
6. Byrd RS. School failure: assessment, intervention, and prevention in pediatric primary care. *Pediatr Rev*. 2005; 26:233-243.
7. Byrd RS, Weitzman M. Predictors of early grade retention among children in the United States. *Pediatrics*. 1994;93:481-487.
8. Rutter M. Pathways from childhood to adult life. *J Child Psychol Psychiatry*. 1989;30:23-51.
9. Cameto R, Marder C, Wagner M, et al. Youth Employment [electronic version]. Reports from the National Longitudinal Transition Study, NLTS2 Data Brief Vol. 2, Issue 2. Available at: www.ncset.org/publications/printresource.asp?id=1310. Accessed June 7, 2007.
10. Buran CF, Sawin KJ, Brei TJ, et al. Adolescents with myelomeningocele: activities, beliefs, expectations, and perceptions. *Dev Med Child Neurol*. 2004;46:244-252.
11. Holmbeck GN. A developmental perspective on adolescent health and illness: an introduction to the special issues. *J Pediatr Psychol*. 2002;27:409-416.
12. National Center for Physical Activity and Disability [NCPAD]. Physical Activity Guidelines. Available at: www.ncpad.org/disability/. Accessed June 7, 2007.
13. The Family Village. Waisman Center, University of Wisconsin-Madison. Available at: www.familyvillage.wisc.edu/Specific.htm. Accessed June 7, 2007.
14. Silkworth CK, Arnold MJ, Harrigan JF, et al, eds. *Individualized Healthcare Plans for the School Nurse*. North Branch, MN: Sunrise River Press; 2005.
15. American Academy of Pediatrics. Emergency Information Form for Children with Special Health Needs. Available at: www.aap.org/advocacy/emergprep.htm. Accessed June 7, 2007.

SECTION SIX

Palliative and End-of-Life Care

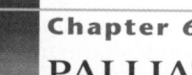

Chapter 69

PALLIATIVE, END-OF-LIFE, AND BEREAVEMENT CARE

Alex Okun, MD

Most physicians caring for children have not pursued the study of handling death as diligently as they have pursued the treatment of the diseases which cause it.

VERNICK AND KARON[1] (1965)

Depending on the involvement in the care of children with complex chronic conditions and the size of the practice, a primary care physician based in an industrialized country might work with dying children and their families as seldom as once or twice a decade or as often as once or twice a month. In developing countries and areas of the world affected by war and famine, childhood death rates are far higher than in more affluent regions. This chapter is intended as a guide to practitioners involved anywhere in palliative, end-of-life, and bereavement care of children. It is written at a time of increased attention to the need for improved services for dying children and their families.

CHILDREN INVOLVED

Each year in the United States, between 50,000 and 55,000 children die before their twentieth birthday. Another 17,000 to 20,000 young adults aged 20 to 24 years die each year. Thirty-eight percent of deaths of people younger than age 25 occur in first year of life, with two thirds of these occurring in the first 28 days. Accidents and injuries are the primary causes of death after the first year of life; malignancy, organ system disease, and congenital anomalies[2] are also main causes of death (Table 69-1). Black children aged 1 to 4 years in the United States are twice as likely to die as white children from accidents, congenital anomalies, homicide, and other causes.[3]

Childhood death in developing countries is more common and has different causes compared with those in developed countries. Between 2000 and 2003, worldwide death rates for children aged 1 month to 5 years living outside low-mortality regions in North America, Europe, and the Western Pacific were 17 times higher than the rates within these regions. Seventy-three percent of deaths in developing countries among all children under age 5 years, including neonates, were linked to six causes: (1) neonatal illness (38% overall), (2) pneumonia (19%), (3) diarrhea (18%), (4) malaria (8%), (5) measles (4%), and (6) HIV/AIDS (3%)[4] (Box 69-1). In over one half of these cases, malnutrition played a role.[5] Death rates for children younger than 5 years approached rates 50 to 100 times those in low-mortality regions over the same period in embattled areas in Africa, where millions of families are refugees.[6]

Palliative care is appropriate for children with a broad range of illnesses, prognoses, and potential for cure. The four main classes of life-limiting diseases affecting children whose treatment should incorporate principles of palliative care are as follows: (1) diseases such as cancer in which attempts at cure may fail;

Table 69-1 Deaths, Birth to 24 Years of Age, United States, 2003

BY AGE GROUP

AGE	PERCENTAGE OF TOTAL
Birth to 28 days (neonatal)	25.7
1-12 mo (postneonatal)	12.4
1-4 yr	6.8
5-9 yr	3.9
10-14 yr	5.5
15-19 yr	18.5
20-24 yr	27.2

BY MAJOR CAUSES

CAUSE	PERCENTAGE OF TOTAL
Assorted conditions present at birth*	29.0
Unintentional injuries	28.0
Homicide and suicide	14.5
Cancer	4.3
Heart disease	3.5
Sudden infant death syndrome	3.0
Other	17.7

*Assorted conditions present at birth, comprising 29% of childhood deaths overall, were coded in the following manner: congenital anomalies and malformations (20% of infant deaths); short gestation or low birth weight (17%); maternal complications of pregnancy (6%); complications of placenta, cord, or membranes (4%); respiratory distress and sepsis (6%); and other (47%).

From Hoyert DL, Heron MP, Murphy SC, et al. Deaths: final data for 2003. *Natl Vital Stat Rep.* 2006;54:1-120.

BOX 69-1 Deaths in Children Aged 1 Month to 5 Years, 2000-2003, for Countries With Low Mortality Versus All Others

Countries with low mortality:

Between the years 2000 and 2003, countries with the lowest mortality rates for children aged 1 month to 5 years were located in North America, Europe, and the Western Pacific Region. A typical community in one of these countries with a population of 100,000 children between 1 month and 5 years of age could expect, on average, 68 of those children to die in 1 year:

- 15 caused by accidents and injuries
- 53 resulting from other causes:
  21 from malignancy
  10 from congenital heart disease
  22 from congenital anomalies and other causes

All others:

Mortality rates were substantially higher in other countries located in the Americas, Europe, Africa, Southeast Asia, and the Eastern Mediterranean and Western Pacific regions. A typical community in one of these countries with a population of 100,000 children between 1 month and 5 years of age could expect, on average, 1179 of those children to have died between 2000 and 2003:

- 54 caused by accidents and injuries
- 955 resulting from infectious causes:
  361 from pneumonia
  314 from diarrhea
  152 from malaria
  57 from HIV/AIDS
  71 from measles
  170 from other causes

From World Health Organization. The World Health Report 2005: Making Every Mother and Child Count. Statistical Annex. Available at: www.who.int/whr/2005/en/. Accessed June 8, 2007. Reprinted by permission.

(2) diseases that will, if untreated, result in death but that have life-extending treatments, such as cystic fibrosis and HIV/AIDS; (3) progressive diseases for which treatment can only be palliative, such as Batten disease; and (4) nonprogressive conditions of neurologic disability that result in vulnerability that may result in death, such as cerebral palsy.[7]

DEFINITION OF TERMS

Palliative Care

Contemporary practice of palliative care embraces a broad scope of services from a point early in the illness, ideally close to the time of diagnosis of a life-threatening condition.[8-11] Palliative care seeks to "prevent or relieve the physical and emotional distress produced by a life-threatening medical condition or its treatment; help patients with such conditions and their families live as normally as possible; and provide them with timely and accurate information and support in decision-making."[9] Palliative care enhances quality of life in the event of life-limiting illness.[8,12,13] It should not be limited to children destined to die from their underlying conditions because it can also benefit those who survive in the long term or who are even cured.

End-of-Life Care

End-of-life care is a type of palliative care that is focused on aggressive control of symptoms, maintenance of comfort, and psychological and spiritual support in the relatively brief period before an anticipated death. Its orientation and organization share many features of palliative care, but it is intended for individuals whose death will come soon.

Hospice

The term *hospice* refers to a combined philosophy of care, program of care, and site of care (ie, an independent facility devoted to care for patients in the last stages of life).[9] Hospice care shares the priorities of end-of-life care but has traditionally been restricted to patients willing to forgo all resuscitative measures and most or all life-sustaining treatments. Among children dying of cancer in the United States, referrals to hospice tend to be made late in the course of illness.[14] In contrast, most admissions to hospices in the United Kingdom last a few days, are for respite care, and are followed by discharge home.[15,16]

Grief, Bereavement, and Mourning

Grief refers to feelings and behaviors in response to loss.[9] *Anticipatory grief* occurs in advance of the loss.[17,18] *Bereavement* refers to grief and other feelings and experiences that occur as a result of loss through death. *Mourning* refers specifically to social rituals and expressions that take place in the course of bereavement. The cluster of diagnoses referred to as *complicated grief*, which includes delayed grief, inhibited grief, and chronic grief, describes responses that are timed atypically or experienced more intensely or for longer than usual.[19-21]

Throughout this chapter, the term *practitioner* will be used to refer to the pediatrician, general practitioner, family practitioner, nurse practitioner, or other health professional acting as the primary care physician. The term *caregiver* will be used to refer to the child's parents or family members providing the bulk of care.

COMPONENTS OF PALLIATIVE, END-OF-LIFE, AND BEREAVEMENT CARE

Palliative and end-of-life care are "designed to fit each child's physical, cognitive, emotional and spiritual level of development."[9] They demand respect for the child as an individual[22,23] as one whose "suffering is utterly unique."[24] The child should be included in all aspects of care planning, as appropriate to the child's developmental level.[25,26] Together with bereavement care, palliative and end-of-life care view the family as "a functional unit with unique physical, psychological and spiritual needs."[23]

Palliative and end-of-life care share with curative care a focus on quality of life for the child.[9,11] They strive

BOX 69-2 Components of Pediatric Palliative and End-of-Life Care

PALLIATIVE CARE

Information and support with decision making
Detailed symptom assessment and monitoring
Helping children and families with practical needs
Spiritual and psychosocial support for children and families
Planning the site of ongoing and future care
Ensuring smooth transitions across the continuum of care

END-OF-LIFE CARE

All of the components of palliative care
Advance care planning
Information about the dying process
Support through the dying process
Help anticipating the nature and site of death
Planning for arrangements after death

Adapted from Himmelstein BP, Hilden JM, Boldt AM, et al. Pediatric palliative care. *N Engl J Med.* 2004;350:1752-1762.

to maximize physical and emotional comfort, enable as normal a life as possible for the child and family, facilitate optimal family function, respect and support the child's and the family's cultural and spiritual values, and help them prepare for the child's death[9] (Box 69-2).

Planning how and where the child will die requires that the family learn about some common manifestations of active dying. These manifestations may include the cessation of eating and drinking, slowing or cessation of voiding and stooling, cognitive clouding, social withdrawal, cooling or mottling of skin and extremities, and various patterns of respiratory irregularities. Practitioners, caregivers, and children facing end-of-life care need to discuss the forgoing of specific life-prolonging measures such as mechanical ventilation and pressors.

When a child is expected to die at home, arrangements with a funeral home or cremation service can be made in advance.[27] Just after the death, the family may wish to bathe the child or save an additional memento, such as a lock of hair, a handprint, or footprint. A set of helpful steps for pronouncing a child's death in the hospital room is provided in Box 69-3.[28]

Bereavement care requires a sustained relationship between the practitioner and the surviving family after the child's death. It begins with acknowledgment of the child's death and continues through attention to parental grief, the experience of surviving siblings, and to stressors that may intensify the grief. Bereavement care is appropriate for families that have lost a child suddenly to accident or injury or otherwise unexpectedly, such as to stillbirth or sudden infant death syndrome.

Palliative and end-of-life care for children commonly integrate treatments traditionally associated with an orientation toward cure. Transfusions of blood products, intravenous hydration, parenteral antibiotics, chemotherapy, and radiation treatment can lessen the symptoms and suffering of many dying children. Practitioners and caregivers need not make an either-or choice between palliative or end-of-life care and cure-oriented therapies.[29]

BOX 69-3 Helpful Steps for Pronouncing a Child's Death in the Hospital Room

1. Before entering the room:
   - Know the circumstances of the death.
   - Ask professional staff members which persons are present in the room and which ones are aware of the death.
   - Inquire as to the child's condition.
2. On entering the room:
   - Calm yourself.
   - Assess the family's condition.
   - Perform a brief examination: check for pulse and respiratory effort, and listen for a heartbeat.
   - Say that the child has died and offer condolence.
3. While remaining in the room:
   - Expect an acute grief reaction.
   - Listen to persons present.
   - Do not say too much.
   - Console the family as you believe is appropriate.
   - Give family time before asking for consent to autopsy.
   - Offer help notifying others.
4. Before leaving the room:
   - Say good-bye to the child.
   - Offer family time to spend together before moving the child's body to the morgue.

Adapted from Hallenbeck J. Palliative care in the final days of life: "They were expecting it at any time." *JAMA.* 2005;293:2265-2271. Reprinted by permission of the American Medical Association.

Palliative, end-of-life, and bereavement care are delivered in an ethnocultural context that demands special awareness, sensitivity, and skills on the part of the practitioner and the entire health system. Families that have experienced discrimination or that come from traditionally underserved populations may suspect that efforts to limit the extent of cure-oriented care arise from competing motives.[3] Practitioners must attend carefully to their use of language, understand how decisions are made for the child, and become familiar with each family's religious and cultural beliefs. Foreign-language interpreters should be used whenever they would be helpful. Talks with community and religious leaders and extended family members are a rich source of insight.

ETHICAL ISSUES

The imperative to provide effective and timely palliative and end-of-life care is grounded in the obligation to promote the best interests of the child and to prevent all avoidable harm.[12,26,30,31] In addition to saving lives, "the physician also must assume responsibility for incurring injury and suffering."[32] Respect honors children's autonomy and that of their caregivers and serves as the impetus for collaborative decision making.[26] It creates an obligation, called *veracity*, for the practitioner to be truthful and to inform children about their health status as fully and sensitively as possible.

Benevolent deception poses a threat to the special relationship between patients and physician and should not be practiced.[33] Partial or avoided disclosure of details about a child's condition can prevent the child who knows or suspects the diagnosis from needed reassurance that comes from discussion with the family: "lack of communication leads to a wall of secrecy and a belief that the illness is too dreadful to talk about."[34]

Decisions about withholding or withdrawing (together called *forgoing*) life-sustaining medical or surgical treatments are best made through examining the balance of potential benefit and harm or distress resulting from the pursuit of each line of treatment.[8,12,35] According to the American Academy of Pediatrics Committee on Bioethics,[13] "physicians should offer more than a 'menu' of choices—they should recommend what they believe is the best option for the patient under the circumstances" and give their reasons. The forgoing of care for critically ill or extremely premature newborns has received much legislative attention in the United States.[32,36,37]

Although withholding and withdrawing specific treatments are considered to be morally and legally equivalent, they are experienced differently by many health professionals.[9] Practitioners and caregivers unsure of the benefits of specific interventions near the end of life can plan time-limited trials of these treatments; if, after a suitable period, the burdens of a particular intervention seem to outweigh its benefits, then it can be withdrawn.

Some treatments intended to relieve pain and suffering may appear to hasten death. Treatment of severe pain with high doses of opiate analgesics often raises concerns of respiratory depression. Even when doses are carefully titrated in response to the patient's pain, opiates may have a foreseeable and unintended effect to diminish respiratory drive. Under the so-called double-effect rule, the unintended side effect is ethically permissible on the condition that only the beneficial effect of the treatment is intended.[38] The notion that death is the mechanism ... of the drug is unacceptable. Most physicians and nurses in pediatric intensive care think that hastening death may be an "acceptable, unintended side effect of terminal care."[39]

Critics of this justification question how to account for practitioners' intent; moral beings often have more than one intent for a given action.[38,40] Society holds physicians and other professionals, from home contractors to airplane pilots, accountable for other foreseeable consequences of risk-laden decisions.

Euthanasia and physician-assisted suicide are not endorsed by any advisory or governing body of physicians treating children in the North America, although other countries may permit these measures under certain circumstances.[41] Nonetheless, when palliative and end-of-life care are not successful, "physicians need to ask themselves what they hope to accomplish by insisting on the prolongation of suffering they cannot relieve."[42]

TALKING WITH CHILDREN AND FAMILIES

Parents want their children's practitioners to discuss prognosis and to help them incorporate the principles of palliative care into treatment.[43] These conversations should be centered on the patient and "focused on empathy, openness and reassurance."[44] Effective and compassionate communication with children and their parents is central to high-quality end-of-life care.[45] Practitioners may realize that children in their care are beyond hope for cure long before parents do.[43] Parents of children with life-threatening conditions value professionals who offer clear, compassionate, informative explanations; tolerate denial and expression of emotion; remain accessible and committed to follow-up; demonstrate interest in family members; and work to preserve the parent-child relationship.[46,47]

Practitioners feel anxious and inexperienced when the time comes to initiate discussions about end-of-life care with families.[48-50] During these discussions, practitioners must accept differences of opinion between caregivers, tolerate negative responses from them, and remain comfortable with nonacceptance.[51] They should try to identify which views about the care plan parents share and on which details they differ.[52] When counseling families about the prognosis for children without hope for cure, expressing the time left as a range is better than giving a specific prediction.[28] The best communication methods use clear, simple language; facilitate understanding with drawings and other memory aids; and provide frequent opportunity for review and clarification.

Children's awareness that they are dying becomes more focused and pronounced during the terminal phase of their illness.[18] Some children feel preoccupied with their own safety and security. Although more open communication with children has been generally embraced,[53] conflicts persist about the timing of disclosure. Discussing prognosis allows concerns to be voiced, elicits support, reassures unwarranted worries, permits practical assurance with immediate issues, helps prevent depression, and helps reduce isolation.[54] Children and their parents are ready to talk about limiting further life-sustaining interventions when they feel supported by trusting staff, wish to avoid further suffering, and want their time left together to be of good quality.[55]

Parents do not regret discussions they have with their children about dying.[56] Discussions about dying need to be targeted to the child's developmental level and understanding of death.[21,57] At the same time, professionals must respect the fact that such discussion is taboo in many cultures.[3,58]

Care of the dying adolescent calls for additional considerations and specialized skills in communication.[59] Life-threatening illness interferes with the attainment of independence, social skills, peer acceptance, and a healthy self-image. For an adolescent with appropriate mental capacity, practitioners should ensure that sufficient information is provided and that the adolescent is as free as possible from the controlling influence of others to make choices about treatment.[59,60] The adolescent's autonomy should be respected in all care decisions, including those at the end of life. Even in instances when adolescents "don't have the last word"[59] in treatment decisions, their thoughts and feelings deserve serious respect and consideration. When a patient asks for help in dying, the request does not necessarily indicate a psychiatric disorder.[61] The child may be exhausted from medical therapies, have unrecognized or undertreated physical symptoms, be experiencing emergent psychosocial problems, or be experiencing spiritual or religious crisis. The practitioner should assess for clinical depression, "listen and learn from the patient before responding,"[61] and seek advice from an expert. Learning to talk with families in the context of palliative, end-of-life, and bereavement care is a lifelong process.[62-64]

SYMPTOM MANAGEMENT

In-depth attention to the assessment and management of pain and other symptoms is central to palliative and end-of-life care. Great suffering is often present, especially in children with cancer, who may experience pain and dyspnea that cannot be managed by drugs. This suffering is a shortcoming in the care of dying children.[65-67]

Recognition and Treatment of Pain

Practitioners should follow an approach to analgesic use that is organized by the ladder—by the clock, by the child, and by mouth[68] (Box 69-4). A three-step ladder of analgesics of escalating potency and onset of action is promoted, in which acetaminophen or a nonsteroidal antiinflammatory drug (NSAID) such as ibuprofen is used for mild pain; weak-acting opiates are added for moderate pain; and stronger opiates, given parenterally, are chosen for severe pain. Analgesic medicines should be ordered on a standing basis *(by the clock)*, according to the chosen analgesic and route of administration, rather than on an as-needed basis. When analgesics are provided only if the patient requests them, pain escalates between doses, the cumulative amount of analgesic administered is higher, and the potential for adverse effects is increased compared with when they are provided by the clock.

Opiate doses that provide adequate analgesia vary widely among individual children. The proper dose to use *(by the child)* is the one that works without causing intolerable adverse effects. Opiates have no ceiling effect,[31] a dose beyond which escalation fails to yield greater therapeutic benefit. Adjunctive analgesic medications such as acetaminophen and NSAIDs should always be continued unless their toxicities indicate otherwise. Whenever possible, the oral route is preferred *(by mouth)* to parenteral or other routes.

Unwarranted fears of addiction and confusion about the nature of opiate tolerance and dependence inhibit some practitioners from ordering opiate analgesics optimally and some families from agreeing to their use.[31,69] Tolerance to the analgesic effects of opiates will develop after as little as 1 week, but usually

BOX 69-4 Principles of Pain Management in Children

1. By the ladder

Step	Pain Severity	Treatment
1	Mild	Oral acetaminophen or nonsteroidal antiinflammatory drugs (NSAIDs)
2	Moderate	Oral opiate analgesics; continue acetaminophen or NSAIDs
3	Severe	Parenteral opiate analgesics; continue acetaminophen or NSAIDs

2. By the clock
   Analgesic treatment around the clock, rather than on a purely as-needed basis, results in:
   - Less frequent breakthrough pain
   - Improved pain relief overall
   - Fewer peaks and troughs of analgesic levels
   - Less sedation
3. By the child
   Maximal suggested doses for acetaminophen and NSAIDs are based on the child's weight. In contrast, opiate analgesics have no ceiling effect. The appropriate dose of an opiate is that which relieves pain without unacceptable adverse effects.
4. By mouth
   Analgesic medication should be given by mouth, whenever possible, for mild to moderate pain. The parenteral route offers no advantages over the oral route other than more rapid onset of action.

Adapted from World Health Organization. *Cancer Pain Relief and Palliative Care in Children.* Geneva, Switzerland: World Health Organization; 1998. Reprinted by permission.

2 or 3 weeks, of continuous use. Symptoms of dependence may appear if the drug is abruptly withdrawn after as little as 1 to 2 weeks. The complex psychosocial dysfunction and self-destructive pursuits that characterize addiction do not appear more frequently in children with life-limiting illnesses than in others.

Tolerance develops not only to the analgesic effects of opiates, but also to most of the adverse effects. Sedation lessens after 1 to 3 days of consistent dosing. Pruritus may take longer to abate. Tolerance to the constipating effects rarely, if ever, develops. If doses of opiates are increased and unacceptable adverse effects persist, then an alternative drug can be substituted. Opiate drugs used in such a rotation can be initiated at less-than-equianalgesic doses.

Appropriate pain control begins with proper assessment. Several validated scales for the appraisal of pain are readily available.[70] These scales must be used consistently and correctly.[8,12] Observation of behavior is necessary for preverbal or nonverbal children. Self-report scales may be used for verbal children older than 4 years that use colors, poker chips, or cartoon faces to help children indicate the severity of their pain. Scales incorporating numeric ratings or visual analogs may be used in children older than 7 years who understand order.[71]

Anticipating and preventing procedural and incident pain is essential.[72] Environmental and behavioral measures, such as infant swaddling and cuddling, holding a cherished blanket or toy, and minimizing loud noises and bright lights are particularly important for young children.[8,12,71] Transcutaneous electric nerve stimulation may help relieve chronic pain.[72] Cognitive-behavioral methods such as distraction, guided imagery, biofeedback, and art and music therapy provided by child-life specialists have powerful effects.[71,72] Many practitioners and families will wish to explore modalities such as aromatherapy, herbal supplementation, or therapeutic massage.

The advice of a pain specialist should be sought when analgesic regimens pose challenges. For children who quickly develop tolerance to the analgesic effects of opiates, who experience neuropathic pain, or who experience pain that might be amenable to regional epidural or nerve block, an expert should be a part of the care team.

Recognition and Management of Other Symptoms

Dyspnea can occur as the result of several processes related to the child's underlying condition, complications of treatment, and unrelated comorbidities. In addition to treating the underlying cause or causes of the dyspnea, an approach that prioritizes symptom assessment and palliation may lead to even greater relief. Oxygen can relieve dyspnea through actions other than raising the arterial oxygen content.[28] Opiate doses effective at relieving shortness of breath are usually smaller than those used for analgesia[73] and likely work through mechanisms other than respiratory depression. Simple environmental measures can be helpful, such as introducing fresh air and using fans to circulate air.

Anorexia is a subjective experience expected toward the end of life. By its nature, anorexia is unassociated with hunger. Traditional assessments of nutrition and hydration in these instances need not lead to medically provided interventions, such as intravenous fluids or nasogastric feeding. Forced hydration may lead to edema, dyspnea, and skin breakdown. Mouth care with moistening swabs, ice chips, and gentle hygiene is sufficient for many children with advanced disease.

Fatigue is a prevalent and bothersome symptom near the end of life. It can be lessened by planned naps, limited interruptions during hospitalization, and efforts on the child's part to conserve energy. When excessive sedation is a persistent complication of narcotic analgesics required for pain control, opiate rotation or the addition of a stimulant such as caffeine can be considered.

As is the case with dyspnea, pruritus may arise from the effects of the underlying disease, its treatment, and unrelated comorbidities. Environmental alterations, soothing baths and compresses, oral antihistamines, and topical corticosteroids and moisturizers, chosen as appropriate, can improve quality of life.

The most successful management of constipation is anticipatory and may be multimodal. It includes the use of softeners and laxatives, the incorporation of higher-fiber foods, and encouraging physical activity as much as possible.

Nausea and vomiting can be lessened with antiemetic medication and by dietary and environmental modifications. Some cognitive-behavioral methods and complementary and alternative treatments may be beneficial. Seizures are distressing to observe and may or may not warrant treatment, depending on frequency, intensity, and desire on the caregivers' part to minimize sedation.

Anxiety is common in all children receiving treatment for serious illness. Interventions and support aimed at the cause are central. Delirium may be caused by metabolic abnormalities, infections, or adverse effects of drugs. Consultation should be sought if the administration of sedatives and antipsychotic medications is being considered to treat these specific symptoms. Depressive symptoms are nearly universal among children with advanced illness, yet criteria for major depressive disorder are not commonly met. Much of this suffering is an expected response to progressive disease as part of anticipatory grieving. Adverse effects of disease treatment may worsen depressive symptoms. Many children will welcome discussion of their feelings. Intense or prolonged symptoms may be improved with antidepressant medication, which should be used in consultation with a specialist.[54]

SPIRITUAL AND PSYCHOSOCIAL SUPPORT

Palliative and end-of-life care share with bereavement care a foundation in psychosocial and spiritual support for families. The classic stages of an individual's reaction to anticipatory loss and grief, popularized by Kubler-Ross[74] in 1964, may not occur sequentially, may recur, and may be experienced discordantly by members of the family and the child.[75]

Psychosocial and spiritual assessment in end-of-life care involves exploring what meaning the illness has to the child and family, understanding how they have coped, and identifying concomitant stressors in their lives.[76] Knowledge of the family's social support network, their spiritual resources, and individual emotional and psychiatric vulnerabilities will help the practitioner offer advice on strategies and steps that can be taken to minimize emotional distress. Support groups are valuable at all stages of the family's experience. The practitioner should not be reluctant to refer the family for further mental health evaluation and treatment. The practitioner should ensure personal support for the family after the child's death.[9]

Dying children often worry that they will be forgotten. Many worry about their parents' pain and sadness after they are gone. Some children feel preoccupied with their own safety and security. They may wish to put their affairs in order and to assist in planning their own funeral and burial.[77] For some children, the main goal of living during the terminal stage is to find "new meaning in life and to live in a new mindset."[78]

For the benefit of the sick child and the child's siblings, families should maintain as normal and usual a scheme of discipline and routines as possible.[75] Siblings should be as involved as they can in the care of the sick child; this will be easiest when the child is

BOX 69-5 Advice for Families That May Help Siblings Anticipating Loss or Grieving After Death

- Spend plenty of time with the children.
- Encourage children to express their feelings and thoughts in their own ways.
- Explain what happened, and be prepared to answer questions again and again.
- Appreciate children's understanding of death at different developmental levels.
- Facilitate children's involvement with friends and activities.
- Continue the usual routine of family responsibilities and discipline.
- Let children know that adults also experience anger, sadness, and fright and may express it.
- Share your own feelings and memories.
- Allow time for fun and laughter.
- Tell children how much the sick or deceased sibling loves or loved them.
- Avoid comparisons between survivors and the deceased.
- Let children know they will be cared for and loved by a consistent adult.

Adapted from Davies B, Wordon JR, Orloff SF, et al. Bereavement. In: Carter BS, Levetown M, eds. *Palliative Care for Infants, Children and Adolescents: A Practical Handbook.* Baltimore, MD: Johns Hopkins University Press; 2004; and American Academy of Pediatrics, Committee on Psychosocial Aspects of Child and Family Health. The pediatrician and childhood bereavement. *Pediatrics* 2000;105:445-447.

home.[16] Advice for helping grieving siblings is listed in Box 69-5.

Child-life specialists can help caregivers create mementos through photography, art, crafts, and music that are difficult to gather together at emotionally stressful times but will be treasured later. They can facilitate the child and siblings' expression of questions, worries, and fears.[77] Social workers can provide emotional and psychosocial support, share resources with families, and assist with referrals to community-based agencies that can enable a smooth transition to home or hospice.

Spiritual needs of children and families involved in palliative, end-of-life, and bereavement care are based in traditional religions, unique religious affiliations, and interpretations and nonreligious paradigms, all of which give meaning to the individuals' lives. The decline in health of a child can be one of the greatest spiritual and existential crises for a parent, yet it is possibly the spiritual domain in which the least training is provided to providers. Addressing children and families' spiritual needs requires exploration and understanding in the domains of professionalism and humanism that are disquieting and profound. Membership in the same religious group or sect as the family or belief in God is not required for professionals to be able to offer spiritual support. Collaboration with the family's religious leaders or hospital- or community-based chaplains may enrich support.

A practitioner should try to attend the wake, funeral, or memorial service for a child who has died under the practitioner's care.[79] Families are moved that their child meant so much to health care professionals who attend such events.[80] Attendance at the service "honor[s] the struggle of the family and the value and courage of the child."[81] Many hospitals and hospices organize memorial services or other annual events for children who have died while in care there, and families are similarly honored by the practitioner's presence. The practitioner may send a letter of condolence.[82] Sending notes or telephoning to acknowledge the child's birthday or anniversary of death is often comforting to the family, and practitioners should consider maintaining a calendar of these dates.

The practitioner has an essential role in providing practical and emotional support after death.[75,83,84] Surviving siblings who receive care from the same practitioner will be returning for visits that provide an opportunity for all to remember the child who died. The practitioner may want to create a pretext, such as a well-child visit, to bring the family back in for care so the practitioner can assess how the siblings, parents, and extended family are coping.[79]

Surviving parents commonly experience conflict, anger, discordant coping, and incongruent grieving. These experiences can lead to compounding breakdown in communication, avoidance, misunderstanding, and low intimacy. Rather than recovering from the loss of the child or experiencing resolution of the intense pain, many families prefer to conceive of successful bereavement as one of reconciliation and reconstitution.[19]

Parental grief may remain intense for years longer after the death of a child than in other instances of bereavement.[58] Mothers and fathers likely grieve in different ways[85]; helping normalize some of these differences can be reassuring to couples.[54] Facilitating communication about the most stressful aspects of the loss or those that promote the greatest degree of anxiety enables mutual help and support.[54] Connecting families to others who have lost a child or to organizations such as Compassionate Friends,[86] Candlelighters,[87] and Mothers in Sympathy and Support[88] can make additional support available to them.

Families can be helped to anticipate the surprising effect of predictable events, such as birthdays, holidays, and anniversaries, that serve as secondary stressors and traumatic reminders.[89] The practitioner is often in a sensitive position to know what factors in the family personal and social history may pertain.

CONCLUSIONS

Improvements in palliative and end-of-life care for children have begun in the United States, decades after improved survival and disease-combating therapeutic successes. Practitioners must learn to recognize children's need for palliative care, assess and manage their pain and symptoms, assess their emotional and spiritual needs and those of their families, facilitate advance-care planning, provide bereavement care to families, and recognize the indications for referral to a specialist.[21] All health professionals who work with children should have relevant basic competence in palliative, end-of-life, and bereavement care, and specialists, subspecialists, and others should have advanced competence.[9]

For the time being, the state of the art in palliative and end-of-life care for children remains simply that: an art. As evidence for effective interventions in the field emerges from well-designed empiric studies, practitioners can look forward to helpful guidelines to improve care. Professionals who offer care in this manner need to find ways to account for the extensive amount of unreimbursed time it requires and the personal toll it can take as a result of its intensity and sadness.

Individuals involved in providing care to seriously ill children require support in processing their own experiences of loss.[90,91] For some people, the rewards of working with devoted members of other disciplines and of the extreme closeness that can develop with children and their families make providing this care the best work they can imagine. With detailed attention to symptom recognition and management, and with the provision of psychological and spiritual support in an ethical, biologic, and ethnocultural context of care for the child with the illness, the interested professional will vastly improve care and caring for some of the sickest children and their families.

TOOLS FOR PRACTICE

Community Advocacy and Coordination

- *A Call for Change: Recommendations to Improve the Care of Children Living with Life-Threatening Conditions*, National Hospice and Palliative Care Organization (www.nhpco.org/files/public/ChIPPSCallforChange.pdf).

Engaging Patient and Family

- *Approaching Grief* (brochure), Children's Hospice International (www.medicalhomeinfo.org/publications/Downloads/Palliative/approaching_grief.pdf).

Medical Decision Support

- *Palliative Care Publication for Providers* (Web page), American Academy of Pediatrics (www.medicalhomeinfo.org/publications/palliative_pro.html).
- *When Children Die: Improving Palliative Care and End-of-Life Care for Children and Their Families* (book), Marilyn Field and Richard Behrman, editors (books.nap.edu/catalog.php?record_id=10390).

RELATED WEB SITES

- *American Academy of Hospice and Palliative Care* (Web page), (www.aahpm.org/).
- *Candlelighters Childhood Cancer Foundation* (Web page), (candlelighters.org/).
- *Mothers in Sympathy and Support (MISS) Foundation* (Web page), (missfoundation.org/).
- *The Compassionate Friends* (Web page), (compassionatefriends.org/).

AAP POLICY STATEMENTS

American Academy of Pediatrics Committee on Bioethics and Committee on Hospital Care. Palliative Care for Children. *Pediatrics*. 2000;106(2):351-357. (aappolicy.aappublications.org/cgi/content/full/pediatrics;106/2/351).

American Academy of Pediatrics Committee on Bioethics. Ethics and the Care of Critically Ill Infants and Children. *Pediatrics*. 1996;98(1):149-152. (aappolicy.aappublications.org/cgi/content/abstract/pediatrics;98/1/149).

American Academy of Pediatrics Committee on Bioethics. Guidelines on Forgoing Life-Sustaining Medical Treatment. *Pediatrics*. 1994;93:532-536. Reaffirmed 2004; 114(4):1126. (aappolicy.aappublications.org/cgi/content/abstract/pediatrics;93/3/532).

American Academy of Pediatrics Committee on Fetus and Newborn. Noninitiation or Withdrawal of Intensive Care for High-Risk Newborns. *Pediatrics*. 2007;119(2):401-403. (aappolicy.aappublications.org/cgi/content/full/pediatrics;119/2/401).

American Academy of Pediatrics Committee on Hospital Care. Family-Centered Care and the Pediatrician's Role. *Pediatrics*. 2003;112(3):691-696. (aappolicy.aappublications.org/cgi/content/full/pediatrics;112/3/691).

American Academy of Pediatrics Committee on Psychosocial Aspects of Child and Family Health. The Pediatrician and Childhood Bereavement. *Pediatrics*. 2000;105(2):445-447. (aappolicy.aappublications.org/cgi/content/full/pediatrics;102/2/445).

REFERENCES

1. Vernick J, Karon M. Who's afraid of death on a leukemia ward? *Am J Dis Child*. 1965;109:393-397.
2. Hoyert DL, Heron MP, Murphy SC, et al. Deaths: final data for 2003. *Natl Vital Stat Rep*. 2006;54:1-120.
3. Koenig BA, Davies E. Cultural dimensions of care at life's end for children and their families. In: Field MJ, Behrman RE, eds, and the Institute of Medicine of the National Academies Committee on Palliative and End-of-Life Care for Children and Their Families. *When Children Die: Improving Palliative and End-of-Life Care for Children and Their Families*. Washington, DC: National Academies Press; 2003.
4. World Health Organization. *The World Health Report 2005: Making Every Mother and Child Count*. Statistical annex. Available at: www.who.int/whr/2005/en/. Accessed June 8, 2007.
5. Bryce J, Boschi-Pinto C, Shibuya K, et al, and the WHO Child Health Epidemiology Reference Group. WHO estimates the causes of death in children. *Lancet*. 2005; 365:1147-1152.
6. World Health Organization. *Health and Mortality Survey Among Internally Displaced Persons in Gulu, Kitgum and Pader Districts, Northern Uganda*. Geneva, Switzerland: World Health Organization; 2005. Available at www.who.int/hac/crises/uga/sitreps/Ugandamortsurvey.pdf. Accessed June 8, 2007.
7. Association for Children With Life Threatening or Terminal Conditions and Their Families [ACT], Royal College of Paediatrics and Child. *Health Guide to the Development of Children's Palliative Care Services*. Bristol, UK: ACT; 1997.
8. American Academy of Pediatrics, Committee on Bioethics and Committee on Hospital Care. Palliative care for children. *Pediatrics*. 2000;106:351-357.
9. Institute of Medicine of the National Academies, Committee on Palliative and End-of-Life Care for Children and Their Families, Field MJ, Behrman RE, eds. *When Children Die: Improving Palliative and End-of-Life Care for Children and Their Families*. Washington, DC: National Academies Press; 2003.
10. Frager G. Pediatric palliative care: building the model, bridging the gaps. *J Palliat Care*. 1996;12:9-12.
11. Frager G. Palliative care and terminal care of children. *Child Adolesc Psychiatr Clin North Am*. 1997;6:889-909.

12. Canadian Paediatric Society Bioethics Committee. Treatment decisions regarding infants, children and adolescents. *Paediatr Child Health*. 2004;9:99-103.
13. American Academy of Pediatrics, Committee on Bioethics. Guidelines on forgoing life-sustaining medical treatment. *Pediatrics*. 1994;93:532-536.
14. Fowler K, Poeling K, Billheimer D, et al. Hospice referral practices for children with cancer: a survey of pediatric oncologists. *J Clin Oncol*. 2006;24:1099-1104.
15. McQuillan R, Finlay I. Facilitating the care of terminally ill children. *J Pain Symptom Manage*. 1996;12:320-324.
16. Children's International Project on Palliative/Hospice Services (ChIPPS) Administrative/Policy Workgroup of the National Hospice and Palliative Care Organization. *A Call for Change: Recommendations to Improve the Care of Children Living With Life-Threatening Conditions*. Alexandria, VA: National Hospice and Palliative Care Organization; October 2001.
17. Lindemann E. Symptomatology and management of acute grief. *Am J Psychiatry*. 1944;101:141-148.
18. Sourkes B. The broken heart: anticipatory grief in the child facing death. *J Palliat Care*. 1996;12:56-59.
19. Christ GH, Bonanno G, Malkinson R, et al. Bereavement experiences after the death of a child. In: Field MJ, Behrman RE, eds, and the Institute of Medicine of the National Academies Committee on Palliative and End-of-Life Care for Children and Their Families. *When Children Die: Improving Palliative and End-of-Life Care for Children and Their Families*. Washington, DC: National Academies Press; 2003.
20. Watson MA. Bereavement in the elderly. *AORN J*. 1994; 59:1079-1084.
21. Himmelstein BP, Hilden JM, Boldt AM, et al. Pediatric palliative care. *N Engl J Med*. 2004;350:1752-1762.
22. International Work Group on Death, Dying and Bereavement. Palliative care for children. *Death Stud*. 1993;17: 277-280.
23. Kane JR, Primono M. Alleviating the suffering of seriously ill children. *Am J Hospice Palliat Care*. 2001;118:161-169.
24. Wolfe J. Suffering in children at the end of life: recognizing an ethical duty to palliate. *J Clin Ethics*. 1999;11:157-163.
25. American Academy of Pediatrics, Committee on Hospital Care, Institute for Family-Centered Care. Family-centered care and the pediatrician's role. *Pediatrics*. 2003;112:691-696.
26. Fleischman AR, Nolan K, Dubler NN, et al. Caring for gravely ill children. *Pediatrics*. 1994;94:433-439.
27. Davies B, Wordon JR, Orloff SF, et al. Bereavement. In: Carter BS, Levetown M, eds. *Palliative Care for Infants, Children and Adolescents: A Practical Handbook*. Baltimore, MD: Johns Hopkins University Press; 2004.
28. Hallenbeck J. Palliative care in the final days of life: "They were expecting it at any time." *JAMA*. 2005;293:2265-2271.
29. Masri C, Farrell CA, Lacroix J. Decision making and end-of-life care in critically ill children. *J Palliat Care*. 2000;16: S45-S52.
30. American Academy of Pediatrics, Committee on Fetus and Newborn. The initiation or withdrawal of treatment for high-risk newborns. *Pediatrics*. 1995;96:362-363.
31. Liben S. Pediatric palliative medicine: obstacles to overcome. *J Palliat Care*. 1996;12:24-28.
32. Levetown M, Carter MA. Child-centered care in a terminal illness: an ethical framework. In: Doyle D, Hanks GWC, MacDonald N, eds. *Oxford Textbook of Palliative Medicine*. 2nd ed. New York, NY: Oxford University Press; 2002.
33. Hays RM, Haynes G, Geyer JR, et al. Communication at the end of life. In: Carter BS, Levetown M, eds. *Palliative Care for Infants, Children and Adolescents: A Practical Handbook*. Baltimore, MD: Johns Hopkins University Press; 2004.
34. Troup SB, Greene WZ, eds. *The Patient, Death and the Family*. New York, NY: Charles Scribner's Sons; 1974.
35. American Academy of Pediatrics, Committee on Bioethics. Ethics and the care of critically ill infants and children. *Pediatrics*. 1996;98:149-152.
36. Lantos J. Baby Doe five years later: implications for child health. *N Engl J Med*. 1987;317:444-447.
37. Sayeed SA. Baby Doe redux? The Department of Health and Human Services and the Born-Alive Infants Protection Act of 2002: a cautionary note on normative neonatal practice. *Pediatrics*. 2005;116:576-585.
38. Lo B, Rubenfeld G. Palliative sedation in dying patients: "We turn to it when everything else hasn't worked." *JAMA*. 2005;294:1810-1816.
39. Burns JP, Mitchell C, Outwater KM, et al. End-of-life care in the pediatric intensive care unit after the forgoing of life-sustaining treatment. *Crit Care Med*. 2000;28: 3060-3066.
40. Quill TE, Dresser R, Brock DW. The rule of double effect: a critique of its role in end-of-life decision making. *N Engl J Med*. 1997;337:1768-1771.
41. Verhagen AAE, Sauer PJJ. End-of-life decisions in newborns: an approach from the Netherlands. *Pediatrics*. 2005;116:736-739.
42. Frader JE. Surveying euthanasia practices: methods and morality. *J Pediatr*. 2005;146:584-585.
43. Wolfe J, Klar N, Grier HE, et al. Understanding of prognosis among parents of children who died of cancer: impact on treatment goals and integration of palliative care. *JAMA*. 2000;284:2469-2475.
44. Morrison RS, Meier DE. Palliative care. *N Engl J Med*. 2004;350:2582-2590.
45. Hurwitz CA, Duncal J, Wolfe J. Caring for the child with cancer at the close of life: "There are people who make it, and I'm hoping I'm one of them." *JAMA*. 2004;292: 2141-2149.
46. Mack JW, Hilden JM, Watterson J, et al. Parent and physician perspectives on quality of care at the end of life in children with cancer. *J Clin Oncol*. 2005;23:9155-9161.
47. Meyer EC, Ritholz MD, Burns JP, et al. Improving the quality of end-of-life care in the pediatric intensive care unit: parents' priorities and recommendations. *Pediatrics*. 2006;117:649-657.
48. Hilden JM, Emanuel EJ, Fairclough DL, et al. Attitudes and practices among pediatric oncologists regarding end-of-life care: results of the 1998 American Society of Clinical Oncology survey. *J Clin Oncol*. 2001;19: 205-212.
49. Contro N, Larson J, Scofield S, et al. Family perspectives on the quality of pediatric palliative care. *Arch Pediatr Adolesc Med*. 2002;156:14-19.
50. Andresen EM, Seecharan GA, Toce SS. Provider perceptions of child deaths. *Arch Pediatr Adolesc Med*. 2004; 158:430-435.
51. Kang T, Hoehn S, Licht DJ, et al. Pediatric palliative, end-of-life and bereavement care. *Pediatr Clin North Am*. 2005;52:1029-1046.
52. Jellinek MS, Catlin EA, Todres ID, et al. Facing tragic decisions with parents in the neonatal intensive care unit: clinical perspectives. *Pediatrics*. 1992;89:119-122.
53. Nitschke R, Humphrey GB, Sexauer CL, et al. Therapeutic choices made by patients with end-stage cancer. *J Pediatr*. 1982;101:471-476.
54. Stuber ML, Bursch B. Psychiatric care of the terminally ill child. In: Chochinov HM, Breitbart W, eds. *Handbook of Psychiatry in Palliative Medicine*. New York, NY: Oxford University Press; 2000.
55. Hinds PS, Drew D, Oakes LL, et al. End-of-life care preferences of pediatric patients with cancer. *J Clin Oncol*. 2005;23:9146-9154.

56. Kreicbergs U, Valdimarsdottir U, Onelov E, et al. Talking about death with children who have severe malignant disease. *N Engl J Med*. 2004;351:1175-1186.
57. Tellerman K, Chernoff R, Grossman L, et al. When a parent dies. *Contemp Pediatr*. 1998;15:145-153.
58. Collins JJ. Palliative care and the child with cancer. *Hematol Oncol Clin North Am*. 2002;16:657-670.
59. Freyer DR. Care of the dying adolescent: special considerations. *Pediatrics*. 2004;113-388.
60. Levetown M. Ethical aspects of pediatric palliative care. *J Palliat Care*. 1996;12:35-39.
61. Quill TE. Doctor, I want to die. Will you help me? *JAMA*. 1993;270:870-873.
62. Levy MM. End-of-life care in the intensive care unit: can we do better? *Crit Care Med*. 2001;29:N56-N61.
63. Fallowfield L. Giving sad and bad news. *Lancet*. 193;341: 476-478.
64. Sharp MC, Strauss RP, Lorch SC. Communicating medical bad news: parents' experiences and preferences. *J Pediatr*. 1992;121:539-546.
65. Wolfe J, Grier HE, Klar N, et al. Symptoms and suffering at the end of life in children with cancer. *N Engl J Med*. 2000;342:326-333.
66. Drake R, Frost J, Collins JJ. The symptoms of dying children. *J Pain Symptom Manage*. 2003;26:594-603.
67. Nelson JE, Danis M. End-of-life care in the intensive care unit: where are we now? *Crit Care Med*. 2001;29: N2-N9.
68. World Health Organization. *Cancer Pain Relief and Palliative Care in Children*. Geneva, Switzerland: World Health Organization; 1998.
69. Chaffee S. Palliative care. *Primary Care Clin Office Pract*. 2001;28:365-390.
70. Huff S, Joshi P. Pain and symptom management. In: Armstrong-Daily A, Zarbock S, eds. *Hospice Care for Children*. 2nd ed. New York, NY: Oxford University Press; 2001.
71. Jacox A, Carr DB, Payne R, et al. *Management of Cancer Pain. Clinical Practice Guideline 9*. AHCPR Publication 94-0592. Rockville, MD: Agency for Health Care Policy and Research, US Department of Health and Human Services, Public Health Service; March 1994.
72. Stevens MM, Pozza LD, Cavalletto B, et al. Pain and symptom control in paediatric palliative care. *Cancer Surv*. 1994;21:211-231.
73. Robinson WM, Ravilly S, Berde C, et al. End-of-life care in cystic fibrosis. *Pediatrics*. 1997;100:205-209.
74. Kubler-Ross E. *On Death and Dying*. New York, NY: Macmillan; 1964.
75. Barakat LP, Sills R, LaBagnara S. Management of fatal illness and death in children or their parents. *Pediatr Rev*. 1995;16:419-423.
76. Block SD. Psychological considerations, growth and transcendence at the end of life: the art of the possible. *JAMA*. 2001;285:2898-2905.
77. International Work Group on Death, Dying and Bereavement, Work Group on Palliative Care for Children. Children, adolescents and death: myths, realities and challenges. *Death Stud*. 1999;23:443-463.
78. Nitschke R, Meyer WH, Sexauer CL, et al. Care of terminally ill children with cancer. *Med Pediatr Oncol*. 2000; 34:268-270.
79. Lewis L, Brechner M, Rearman GH, et al. How you can help meet the needs of dying children. *Contemp Pediatr*. 2002;19:147-159.
80. Irvine P. The attending at the funeral. *N Engl J Med*. 1985; 312:1704-1705.
81. Wolfe L. Should parents speak with a dying child about impending death? *N Engl J Med*. 2004;351:1251-1253.
82. Bedell SE, Cadenhead K, Graboys TB. The doctor's letter of condolence. *N Engl J Med*. 2001;344:1162-1164.
83. Hynson JL, Sawyer SM. Paediatric palliative care: distinctive needs and emerging issues. *J Paediatr Child Health*. 2001;37:323-325.
84. Sandler I, Kennedy C. Parental grief and palliative care require attention. *Arch Pediatr Adolesc Med*. 2004;158: 590-591.
85. Black D. Coping with loss: the dying child. *BMJ*. 1998; 316:1376-1378.
86. Compassionate Friends. Available at: www.compassionatefriends.org/. Accessed June 7, 2007.
87. Candlelighters Childhood Cancer Foundation. Available at: www.candlelighters.org/. Accessed June 7, 2007.
88. The MISS Foundation. Available at: www.missfoundation.org/. Accessed June 7, 2007.
89. Christ GH. *Healing Children's Grief: Surviving a Parent's Death from Cancer*. New York, NY: Oxford University Press; 2000.
90. Serwint J. Physicians must address emotional toll of patient's death. *AAP News*. August 2004:81.
91. Baverstock A, Finlay F. Specialist registrants' emotional responses to a patient's death. *Arch Dis Child*. 2006;91:774-776.

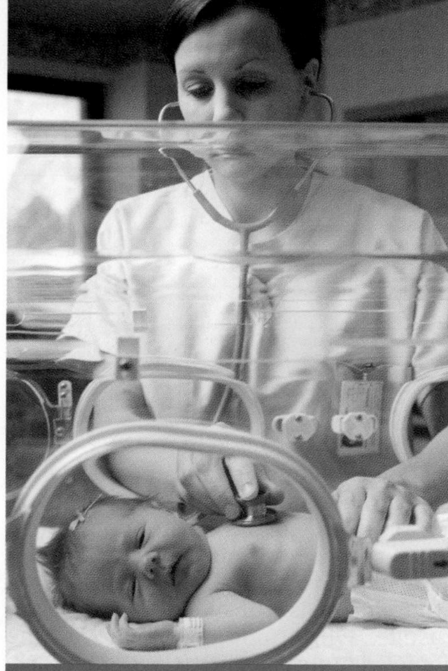

Part 4

Maternal and Fetal Perinatal Health: Effect on Pregnancy Outcomes

Section One: Perinatal Health

70 Prenatal Diagnosis
71 Fetal Interventions
72 Assistive Reproductive Technologies, Multiple Births, and Pregnancy Outcomes

Section Two: Perinatal Care: Caring for the High-Risk Infant

73 Fetal Assessment
74 Assessment and Stabilization at Delivery
75 Identifying the Newborn Who Requires Specialized Care
76 Care of the Sick or Premature Infant Before Transport
77 Continuing Care of the Infant After Transfer From Neonatal Intensive Care
78 Discharge Planning for the High-Risk Newborn Requiring Intensive Care
79 Support for Families Whose Infant Is Sick or Dying: Collaborative Decision Making
80 Perinatal Bereavement

Care of the newborn begins well before conception and has lifelong consequences affecting the health, well-being, and functional abilities of the adult. The fetal origins of disease are the focus of great interest and research as the importance of the early intrauterine environment on long-term health is increasingly recognized. The prenatal and early childhood periods are critical developmental stages especially vulnerable to the effects of various exogenous stimuli or insults that induce lasting changes in organ development or function. These effects may be further moderated by lifestyle factors such as healthy dietary habits, smoking cessation, physical activity, socioeconomic status, environmental exposures, and occupation. The association between low birth weight and an increased risk of cardiovascular disease (coronary heart disease and stroke) and type 2 diabetes during adulthood is an example. Extremes of growth that occur as adaptive responses to aberrant intrauterine environments are discussed in great detail in Part 5, Chapter 97, Abnormalities of Fetal Growth. During embryonic life, organ development and susceptibility to later disease are genetically determined. These developmental patterns are additional contributors to various high prevalence conditions that develop later in childhood and adulthood. The focus of this portion of the text encompasses facets of prenatal and pregnancy care, fetal assessment and intervention, and evaluation and care of the high risk neonate. Because these extensive topics cannot be completely reviewed here, the reader is referred to the additional readings and resources at the end of these chapters for additional information.

SECTION ONE

Perinatal Health

Chapter 70
PRENATAL DIAGNOSIS

Lauren A. Ferrara, MD; Garfield A. D. Clunie, MD

Fifty percent of early pregnancy losses and 6% to 11% of still births and neonatal deaths are attributed to chromosomal abnormalities.[1,2] The abnormalities that are nonlethal can cause significant morbidity and occur in 0.7% of newborns.[3] Although detecting all abnormalities may not be possible prenatally, some screening and diagnostic tests are available.

GENETIC SCREENING: SERUM TESTING AND FIRST-TRIMESTER ULTRASOUND

Prenatal screening first became available more than 20 years ago and has been evolving ever since. Initially, maternal age and history was the only screening available. This practice changed in the mid 1980s when Cuckle[4] demonstrated that combining maternal age with maternal serum alpha-fetoprotein increased the detection rate for aneuploidy substantially. This maternal serum screening evolved into what is known as the *quadruple screen* typically performed at 15 to 18 weeks' gestation. Four serum markers, (1) maternal serum alpha-fetoprotein, (2) human chorionic gonadotropin (hCG), (3) estriol, and (4) inhibin, are measured, yielding a 75% detection rate and a 5% false-positive rate.

In the early 1990s, Nicolaides[5] reported an association between thickened nuchal translucency (NT) and aneuploidy. NT is a sonographic finding examining the subcutaneous tissue at the back of the fetal neck. The NT is a collection of fluid that appears as an echolucent line. Combining NT with maternal age can provide early detection of these pregnancies in women at higher risk for aneuploidy, with 80% detection rate.[6]

In 1996, Wald et al[7] found 2 markers—pregnancy-associated plasma protein A (PAPP-A) and free β-hCG—that stood out as being discriminatory for Down syndrome–affected pregnancies. PAPP-A values were found to be low and free β-hCG values high in affected pregnancies. Using both analytes in combination with age provided a 62% detection rate at an earlier gestational age.

The combination of measuring NT and testing for serum markers is more effective than either of these measurements alone.[8] At 11 weeks' gestation, the detection rate for Down syndrome is 70% using NT alone. This rate increases to 87% when PAPP-A and free β-hCG are added. A fully integrated model of screening in which serum metabolites from the second trimester are measured and the risk is not completely calculated until after this second trimester screen yields the best detection rate at 96%. The major disadvantage is that the patient is not made aware of the first-trimester results, which not only removes the option of chorionic villus sampling (CVS) for early diagnosis, but also affects management option for the patient if the decision is made not to continue the pregnancy. Stepwise sequential testing allows for calculation of risk after the first trimester. If the screening is negative, then the patient would then undergo the quadruple screen, with a new risk calculated. If the first-trimester screen is positive, then the patient can have a CVS for further assessment if so desired. Even with the positive screen the patient can choose to forego CVS, and the clinician should have the quadruple screen with a new risk calculated. The patient can then undergo amniocentesis for further determination. The detection rate for the stepwise sequential testing is 95%.

Genetic Diseases Specific to Ancestry

Carrier screening for specific genetic diseases is often determined by the individual's ancestry. For example, certain autosomal-recessive diseases are more prevalent in the Ashkenazi Jewish population. These diseases include Tay-Sachs disease, Canavan disease, cystic fibrosis, familial dysautonomia, Fanconi anemia, Niemann-Pick disease, mucolipidosis type IV, Bloom syndrome, and Gaucher disease. Many of these conditions are lethal in childhood and are associated with significant morbidity. As another example, some hematologic disorders are more prevalent in some populations than in others (ie, sickle cell disease in blacks, α-thalassemia in Southeast Asians, β-thalassemia in patients from surrounding Mediterranean countries).

Carrier screening should be offered to couples either preconceptually or in early pregnancy so that prenatal diagnostic testing is an option for the couple.

Invasive Testing

If a woman is of advanced maternal age and the first- or second-trimester screening is positive for aneuploidy, or if a couple is at risk for a specific genetic disease, then the patient has the option of invasive testing. These options include 1 of 2 ultrasound-guided procedures, CVS performed between 10 and 13 6/7 weeks' gestation or amniocentesis done from 15 weeks' gestation onward. CVS is performed by inserting a needle into placental tissue and abstracting villi. An amniocentesis is performed by inserting a needle into the amniotic sac and withdrawing amniotic fluid. In experienced hands, the procedure-related loss rate for CVS is approximately 0.5% to 1%. Traditionally the procedure-related loss rate was similar to that of amniocentesis, but newer literature has shown that the loss rate with amniocentesis may be as low as 1 per 1000. More current studies are underway to assess for loss rates with CVS as a direct comparison with amniocentesis.

SECOND- AND THIRD-TRIMESTER ULTRASOUND

Ultrasound has been the best method for imaging the fetus since the 1950s. With the advent of real-time sonography, higher-frequency transducers, and Doppler sonography, the ability to provide accurate prenatal diagnoses has greatly improved. Most pregnant women in the United States will undergo an ultrasound examination, although the role of routine ultrasound has been a focus of controversy. The American College of Obstetrics and Gynecology has specific recommendations for the role of ultrasound in each trimester of pregnancy. The focus of this chapter is on the diagnosis and evaluation of major fetal anomalies.

Central Nervous System

Neural Tube Defects

Neural tube defects (NTDs) are congenital structural abnormalities of the brain and vertebral column. These abnormalities can occur as an isolated event, with other malformations, or as part of a genetic syndrome. With an incidence of 1 to 2 per 1000 live births, NTDs are the second-most common major congenital anomaly.[9]

Embryologically the neural plate appears during the third week of gestation and gives rise to neural folds that fuse in the midline to form the neural tube. Closure of the neural tube is usually complete by the end of the sixth gestational week. Failure of this process leads to the defect. The cause is a result of genetic, environmental, and dietary influences. Folic acid plays an important role in the proper formation of the neural tube,[10] which is mediated via the enzyme methylenetetrahydrofolate reductase (MTHFR). Deficiency in folic acid has been implicated in part of the mechanism for the formation of NTDs. Such is the case not only in terms of dietary deficiency, but also as a result of the mechanism of teratogenic effects of certain medications, such as antiepileptic drugs. Supplementation has been shown to decrease the incidence and recurrence.[11]

NTDs can be separated into 2 categories: cranial and spinal. Cranial defects include anencephaly, exencephaly, encephalocele, and iniencephaly. These defects occur in the skull, scalp, and brain tissue and result in death. Defects in the caudal region are more commonly known as spina bifida. These defects are malformations of the spinal cord, meninges, and vertebrae and are compatible with life. Caudal-region defects that are confined to the spine are further differentiated as open (neural tissue exposed), usually involving the spine or cranium, or closed (neural tissue not exposed).

Maternal serum screening is routinely offered to all pregnant women. Alfa-fetoprotein (AFP) is the maternal serum marker that is used as a screening tool.[12] AFP is measured at 15 to 20 weeks and is expressed as multiples of the median. A value above 2.0 to 2.5 multiples of the median is considered abnormal and necessitates further evaluation, such as a repeat test, ultrasound examination, and possibly amniocentesis. Other factors can affect interpretation, such as knowledge of proper gestational age, maternal weight, multiples of the median, and the presence of other anomalies.

Ultrasound is effective for detecting NTDs as well.[13] In experienced hands, ultrasound can be 97% sensitive and 100% specific. Detection of the NTD is by irregularities of the bony spine or a bulging of the contour of the fetal back. The posterior fossa of the fetal brain may also provide clues that an NTD is present. The banana and lemon signs may occur in the early second trimester. The banana sign refers to the shape the cerebellum makes as a result of the herniation of the spinal tissue. The lemon sign refers to the flattened frontal contour of the fetal calvarium. Other findings may include ventriculomegaly and clubbed feet. At the time of diagnosis, an amniocentesis should be performed. This test can provide information regarding the karyotype, particularly if other anomalies are detected; it also serves as a confirmatory test. AFP levels will be increased in amniotic fluid, which can also be tested for acetylcholinesterase (AChE). AChE is an enzyme found in blood cells, muscle tissue, and nerve tissue. An increase in AChE levels suggests an open NTD with 96% accuracy.

Prognosis depends on the type and location of the lesion. As stated previously, lesions involving the brain and skull are lethal; those involving the spine are usually compatible with life. An important point to note is the existence of indications regarding ambulatory, urologic, and bowel function, which is important when counseling parents regarding further interventions or parents considering termination of the pregnancy. In utero intervention is available for this anomaly (see Chapter 71, Fetal Interventions).

Ventriculomegaly and Hydrocephalus

Ventriculomegaly is defined as an increased diameter of the fetal lateral ventricles of more than 10 mm. Hydrocephalus is defined as a pathologic increase in intracranial cerebrospinal fluid (CSF). These terms are often used interchangeably in prenatal diagnosis, though technically, hydrocephalus refers to intracranial pressure, which cannot be measured in the prenatal setting.

CSF is produced within the ventricular system, with one half from the choroid plexus cysts and the other half from the cerebral capillaries. Circulation is unidirectional and moves from the lateral ventricles through the foramen of Monroe to the third ventricle. It then travels to the fourth ventricle after passing through the aqueduct of Sylvius and ends up in the spinal subarachnoid space or basal cisterns. It is then reabsorbed in the venous sinuses. In the event of either production of CSF that exceeds absorption or mechanical obstruction of flow, ventriculomegaly can result. Ventriculomegaly can be an isolated finding, with an incidence of 1.4 to 20 per 1000 live births, or it may be an indicator of other underlying central nervous system (CNS) anomalies (ie, aqueductal stenosis) or associated extra-CNS anomalies (ie, NTDs).[14,15]

The lateral ventricles can be readily assessed with ultrasound. The atria of the lateral ventricles measure, on average, 7 mm; the upper limit of normal is 10 mm. Once the diagnosis has been made, a thorough ultrasound examination should permit the operator to assess for any other associated anomalies. Amniocentesis for karyotyping should be offered because a 4% to 14% association has been reported with aneuploidy, which may also provide additional information if an NTD is suspected. Family history should be carefully reviewed because of the association with some X-linked conditions. Limitations of ultrasound evaluation exist, particularly for cortical malformations. Fetal magnetic resonance imaging (MRI) is becoming the standard of care when a CNS anomaly is diagnosed, which has been shown to alter diagnosis and management in up to 40% of cases.

Prognosis depends on the presence of other anomalies. Termination of the pregnancy, if desired, can be offered before 24 weeks' gestation. In patients continuing the pregnancy, surveillance of the ventriculomegaly is performed with serial ultrasounds. Although in utero treatment has been attempted, no improvement in outcome has resulted. Most fetuses will have normal head circumference; therefore cesarean section should be considered only for routine obstetric reasons.

Choroid Plexus Cysts

Choroid plexus cysts (CPCs) are thought to be neuroepithelial folds that fill with CSF and cellular debris. A CPC is a common ultrasound finding in healthy fetuses in the second trimester and has an incidence of 0.2% to 3.6%.[16] The choroid plexus is a major source of CSF. Development begins at 6 to 7 weeks' gestation. They grow rapidly, filling 75% of the lateral ventricles by 9 weeks' gestation and reaching full size by 20 weeks' gestation.

The typical appearance on ultrasound is a sonolucent structure with well-defined borders. CPCs are generally small (<10 mm) and can be unilateral or bilateral. The concern with this finding is its association with aneuploidy, particularly trisomy 18.[17] When determining the actual risk for trisomy 18 with isolated CPCs, the clinician must take into consideration maternal age and adjust it according to the maternal serum screen risk, if available. The risk does not depend on the age at diagnosis, but rather on the size or laterality of the cysts.[18]

Once noted on ultrasound, a detailed ultrasound should be performed to determine the presence of other anomalies, particularly those associated with trisomy 18 (ie, congenital heart defects, rocker-bottom feet). In up to 75% of fetuses with trisomy 18, additional abnormalities will be detected. Once the risk of aneuploidy is determined, amniocentesis can be offered. Many physicians suggest invasive testing only in the setting of other anomalies or if the mother is older than 35 years. In the setting of an isolated CPC, the prognosis is good, and most CPCs will resolve by the third trimester; those that do persist are usually benign. However, resolution does not change the small risk of aneuploidy.

Craniofacial Defects

The orofacial cleft is the most common craniofacial malformation found in the newborn. Clefting can be of the lip or palate in isolation or together. Of all cases, 60% to 75% will involve the lip with or without the palate, and 25% to 40% will involve the palate alone. Up to 80% of cases are unilateral; left-side involvement is twice as common as the right side. The overall incidence is population dependent. In the white population, incidence is 1 per 1000 live births; in the black population, incidence is 1 per 2273 live births. The incidence among Asians is higher, with reported rates of 1 per 500 live births.

Craniofacial development involves migration, proliferation, and differentiation of facial mesenchyme derived from neural crest cells. Many genes are involved in the regulation of this process. Normally, fusion of 3 mesodermal processes occur, which is complete by 7 weeks' gestation. Failure of this process leads to clefting involving the lip, whether it is in isolation or involves the palate. Cleft palate in isolation is different; although fusion must also take place, the formation of a cleft palate also involves other processes, particularly proper movement of palatal shelves and the tongue.

The cause is genetic, as well as environmental. The genes involved, *Dlx* and *sonic hedgehog*, influence cell programming and cell differentiation.[19] Environmental factors are the result of teratogenic effects. Medications, including antiepileptic drugs and steroids, have been implicated. Cigarette smoking, alcohol consumption, and folic acid deficiency have also been found to have an association.[20,21]

Orofacial clefting can be detected on ultrasound, but only after 14 weeks, because this is the time that the fetal face assumes its normal form. Isolated cleft palate can be extremely difficult to diagnose prenatally. Once detected, a thorough ultrasound examination should be performed to assess for other anomalies, particularly of the CNS and cardiac systems. If another anomaly is detected, then chromosomal abnormalities can be seen is as many as 60% of these fetuses. Cleft lip or palate in isolation is not associated with aneuploidy. However, amniocentesis can be offered, and it may be helpful in finding other anomalies.

No prenatal interventions are available. Management of the pregnancy should otherwise be routine. Parents should meet with the craniofacial surgeons to discuss the steps involved in postnatal surgical management.

Neck

Cystic Hygroma

Cystic hygroma is a lymphatic malformation or lymphangioma located at the level of the neck. Lymphatic fluid collects in the jugular system because of a blockage to flow. The overall prevalence in the first trimester is 1 per 100 live births.

Cystic hygromas can be large single or multiloculated fluid-filled cavities. They are easily identifiable on ultrasound examination in the first trimester. Cystic hygromas tend to be largest in the nuchal region but can extend the full length of the fetus. Once detected, a thorough ultrasound examination should be performed. The skull and spine should be examined to differentiate cystic hygroma from an NTD. The clinician should thoroughly assess for other signs consistent with hydrops fetalis (skin edema, ascites, pericardial or pleural effusions). A 50% chance of aneuploidy exists when diagnosis is made in the first trimester. The most common aneuploidy is Downs syndrome (trisomy 21), but it can also be seen with trisomy 13 and 18, as well as Turner syndrome *(45XO)*. Therefore amniocentesis or cardiovascular surgery should be performed. A fetal echocardiogram should also be performed to determine the presence of any cardiac defects. No fetal intervention is available. Serial sonograms should be performed to assess for polyhydramnios resulting from fetal inability to swallow, which can lead to uterine irritability and even preterm labor.

This finding is associated with significant mortality because of the high incidence of coexisting chromosomal abnormalities and other malformations. In the small group of fetuses in which this disorder is found in isolation with normal karyotype, the prognosis can be excellent. The major concern is the ability to maintain the airway at the time of delivery, which may require an *ex* utero *i*ntrapartum *t*reatment (EXIT) procedure during which uteroplacental blood flow and gas exchange is maintained while the fetal malformation is surgically treated. (See Chapter 71, Fetal Interventions.)

Goiter

Fetal goiter, also known as thyromegaly, is an enlargement of the fetal thyroid gland. It can occur in the maternal hyperthyroid, euthyroid, or, most commonly, hypothyroid state. When fetal goiter occurs in the hypothyroid state, it may result from transplacental passage of antithyroid medication, antithyroid antibodies, iodine deficiency, or congenital thyroid metabolic disorders. A fetal goiter that occurs in the hyperthyroid state is most commonly due to transplacental passage of thyroid-stimulating antibody levels, as in maternal Graves disease. Overall, this finding is rare. The fetal thyroid becomes fully responsive to thyroid-stimulating substances only in the second trimester; therefore diagnosis before 20 weeks is unlikely.

A fetal goiter can be seen on ultrasound examination as a homogenous anterior neck mass. In severe cases, the neck is in a persistent state of hyperextension. Polyhydramnios may also occur as a result of fetal impairment of swallowing. Other abnormal ultrasound findings include fetal tachycardia, intrauterine growth restriction (IUGR), and hydrops. Signs of fetal hypothyroidism include cardiomegaly and fetal heart block. Even with these findings, accurately predicting fetal status may be difficult.

Given the difficulty in accurately determining fetal status with ultrasound alone, periumbilical cord blood sampling should be considered to evaluate thyroid hormone levels in fetal serum.[22] The fetus can then be treated through administration of the proper medication to the mother. If the mother is euthyroid, then she may need supplementation to maintain her thyroid function. In addition, the fetus should be monitored with serial ultrasounds to assess amniotic fluid, signs of hydrops, and growth.

At delivery, the neonatologists should be present and aware of the diagnosis and therapy that have been instituted. Fetal airway needs to be maintained; thus tracheostomy or bronchoscopy may need to be performed.

Thoracic Defects

Bronchopulmonary Sequestration

Bronchopulmonary sequestration (BPS) is a rare congenital malformation of the lower respiratory tract. It is made up of a cystic mass of nonfunctional pulmonary tissue. No communication occurs with the normal bronchopulmonary tree, and it derives its blood supply from anomalous vessels. BPS is thought to comprise 0.1% to 6% of all congenital pulmonary lesions.[23]

BPS is thought to originate from a supernumerary lung bud that develops caudally to the normal lung buds and then migrates with the esophagus. Two forms have been described: intralobar and extralobar. Intralobar is more common (75%) than extralobar; it is located in the lobe and lacks its own visceral pleura. Extralobar is seen in the rest of the cases; it is located outside the normal lung and has its own visceral pleura. Extralobar lesions can be intrathoracic or subdiaphragmatic.

On ultrasound examination, BPS is a solid echogenic mass characterized by its location, vascular supply, and association with other abnormalities. Most lesions are located in the lower lobes, but they can be anywhere in the thorax or subdiaphragmatic. They have their own blood supply, which tends to arise from the thoracic aorta. Demonstration of the aberrant blood supply by Doppler sonography usually confirms the diagnosis. Other sonographic findings may be pleural effusion, mediastinal shift, and hydrops. Cardiac and vertebral anomalies may also be present. Amniocentesis should be offered if other anomalies are present. A fetal echocardiogram should be performed because of the disorder's association with cardiac anomalies.

The natural history of BPS tends to be variable. Some lesions regress; others can lead to hydrops, usually from vascular compression. The prognosis depends on the other associated findings. Fetuses with pleural effusion or polyhydramnios have a 22% and 30% survival rate, respectively; those with hydrops can be fatal. For fetuses that develop hydrops before 30 weeks' gestation, intervention can be considered via shunting. If it develops after 30 weeks, then early delivery should be considered.[23-25]

Cystic Adenomatoid Malformation

Congenital cystic adenomatoid malformation (CCAM) is also a rare lesion of the lower respiratory tract. It is composed of multicystic masses of pulmonary tissue, is unilobar in 80% to 95% of cases, and can affect any lobe of the lung. The incidence has been reported as being 1 per 10,000 to 1 per 35,000 live births.[26]

CCAM arises from an abnormality in branching and maturation of bronchiolar structures, which begins around 5 to 6 weeks' gestation. Three types of CCAMs have been identified and are thought to originate at different levels of the respiratory tract at different times during development.[27] Type I is the most common and accounts for 50% of these lesions. Lesions are characterized by either single or multiple large cysts (3-10 cm). The cysts are lined by ciliated pseudostratified columnar epithelium; these lesions are thought to be distal in origin because they have well-differentiated tissue. Type II is the second-most common type and accounts for 40% of CCAM cases. These lesions are made up of smaller cysts (<1 cm) lined with ciliated cuboidal or columnar epithelium. This type of malformation has a high association (60%) with other anomalies, including genitourinary, cardiac, and skeletal anomalies, because the disorder likely occurs earlier in development. Type III is the least common (10%). It is characterized by large homogeneous microcystic masses (<0.5 cm). A mixture of solid and cystic tissue is found from adenomatoid proliferation of the distal airways and spaces. Lesions tend to be large and lack differentiation. This insult is thought to occur at 26 to 28 days' gestation.

The tumor can be visualized by ultrasound. Types I and II can appear as cystic or echolucent structures, and type III appears as a hyperechogenic mass. Mediastinal shift can occur with types I and III. A detailed Doppler ultrasound examination should be performed to differentiate these lesions from other ones, such as congenital diaphragmatic hernia (CDH) or BPS, as well as to assess for other associated anomalies, particularly if a type-II lesion is suspected. A fetal echocardiogram should be performed to rule out cardiac anomalies, particularly in the setting of hydrops. Fetal karyotyping should be offered in the setting of other anomalies because CCAM alone has a less than 1% association with aneuploidy,[28] although karyotyping should be performed if plans are in place for in utero intervention because an abnormal result may affect the decision to do so. Serial sonography should be performed to look for signs of hydrops. These lesions can occasionally regress.

Prognosis for these lesions depends on the type of CCAM present. Fetuses with type I tend to do well; fetuses with type III disorder have a poorer prognosis. The prognosis for type II depends on the severity of other lesions, if present. In utero treatment with decompression and possible shunt placement may be reasonable when hydrops is present before 32 weeks. An EXIT procedure should be considered at the time of delivery if concern for the airway exists.

Congenital Diaphragmatic Hernia

CDH occurs when a defect develops in the diaphragm that allows the abdominal viscera to herniate into the fetal thorax. Most CDHs are unilateral (98%), with the left side being the most common.[29] The incidence is 1 per 2200 live births.[30]

The defect occurs either as failure of closure of the pleuroperitoneal folds or as a defect in migration of muscle fibers during the development of the diaphragm at 9 to 10 weeks' gestation. When the defect is present, it allows herniation to occur. Because this defect happens so early in lung development, the number of bronchial branches becomes reduced, leading to pulmonary hypoplasia. These changes are more pronounced on the side of the herniation, but the contralateral lung can be affected by compression of a shifted mediastinum.

On ultrasound examination, one of the key clues to diagnosing CDH is the location of the stomach bubble. When viewing the fetal chest, the stomach bubble is seen in the same plane as the heart in cases of CDH. Peristalsis of the bowel in the thorax may also be noted. Determination of potential liver herniation is important for prognosis and the possibility for intervention. Magnetic resonance imaging may be suitable for this purpose.[31] Fifty percent of CDHs are associated with other anomalies, including cardiac, genitourinary, and gastrointestinal anomalies. A fetal echocardiogram should be performed to assess for cardiac defects. Chromosomal abnormalities can be seen in 10% to 20% of cases; therefore amniocentesis should be offered, particularly if in utero intervention is being considered.

Prognosis depends on such factors as karyotype, liver herniation, associated anomalies, and ratio of lung area to head circumference.[30] This ratio estimates the contralateral lung size and mediastinal shift at the level of the atria. Originally thought to predict survival, this ratio is more useful in assessing morbidity than mortality. Up to 30% of these fetuses can be stillborn; therefore close surveillance in the third trimester is warranted. Serial ultrasounds may also be performed to assess growth and amniotic fluid volume. In utero intervention may play a role, which is discussed elsewhere (see Chapter 71, Fetal Interventions). Delivery should be at an appropriate tertiary-care center.

Cardiovascular Defects

Cardiac anomalies are the most common congenital lesion, with an incidence of 5 to 8 per 1000 live births. Thus review of cardiac anatomy is an integral part of the basic fetal anatomic survey.[32] Most cardiac lesions are detected in low-risk populations[33]; however, several risk factors call for more detailed evaluation, such as a fetal echocardiogram. These risk factors can be divided into 3 general categories: (1) familial, (2) maternal, and (3) fetal. Familial risk factors include parental congenital heart disease, a previous affected child, or a family history of a syndrome associated with heart disease (eg, Noonan syndrome). Maternal risks include diabetes, lupus, teratogen exposure (eg, lithium), and infection (eg, rubella). Fetal risks include detection of another anomaly, suspicion of aneuploidy, arrhythmia, and evidence of hydrops. A strong association exists between cardiac anomalies and aneuploidy[34]; therefore amniocentesis should be performed. Patients should meet with pediatric cardiologists or a pediatric cardiothoracic surgeon (or both) to discuss prognosis and postnatal treatment, including surgery. The following section will provide a brief review of some of the most common cardiac anomalies.

Atrioventricular Canal Defect

Atrioventricular (AV) canal defects consist of atrial septal defect (ASD) and ventricular septal defect (VSD) and a single common AV valve. It is also known as endocardial cushion defect. AV canal defects account for 1% to 5% of all cases of congenital heart disease.

On ultrasound examination, a large defect is noted when looking at the 4-chamber view of the heart, representing the defects in the inferior portion of the atrial septum and the superior portion of the ventricular septum. The normal conduction of the heart is affected by the large defect, often leading to bradyarrhythmia. Additional cardiac malformations may be present, including tetralogy of Fallot, coarctation, and pulmonary stenosis. The prognosis depends on the presence of other associated anomalies, including hydrops and aneuploidy.

Truncus Arteriosus

Truncus arteriosus occurs when a single large ventricular outflow tract arises from both the left and right ventricles. It is rare, accounting for only 1.5% of heat defects, with an incidence estimated at 3 per 100,000 live births. Four subtypes were originally described. Type I has a single pulmonary trunk that then divides into right and left pulmonary arteries. Type II has 2 pulmonary arteries arising from the posterior of the truncus. Type III has 2 pulmonary arteries from the lateral aspects of the truncus. In type IV, the pulmonary arteries are absent, but collaterals arise from the descending aorta.

When visualizing the outflow tracts using ultrasound, a single large ventricular outflow tract is seen. The right-ventricular outflow tract is not seen. Abnormalities of the aortic arch may also be seen, as well as the presence of hydrops.

Hypoplastic Left and Right Ventricles

Hypoplastic left ventricle, also known as hypoplastic left heart syndrome, occurs when hypoplasia of the left ventricle, atresia of the aortic and mitral valves, and hypoplasia of the aortic arch are present. Each of these components can occur at varying degrees. Hypoplastic left heart syndrome accounts for 9% of all congenital heart defects, with an incidence of 1 per 10,000 live births.

Hypoplastic right heart syndrome, also known as pulmonary atresia with intact ventricular septum, occurs when hypoplasia of the right ventricle, pulmonary atresia, and occasionally tricuspid atresia are present. This lesion accounts for less than 3% of congenital heart defects, with an incidence of 1 per 144,000 live births.

Both lesions are usually easy to detect on ultrasound examination. When looking at the 4-chamber view of the heart, an inequality of the ventricles can be seen. The affected side will appear as a small remnant and will appear hypocontractile. Both lesions may not be as clear on second-trimester ultrasound but will evolve over time. Careful anatomic survey should be performed to assess for other cardiac and extracardiac anomalies.

Tetralogy of Fallot

Tetralogy of Fallot is a malformation that consists of VSD, right-ventricular outflow obstruction, the aorta overriding the ventricular septum, and right-ventricular hypertrophy. Tetralogy of Fallot is thought to occur as a result of misalignment during embryogenesis. It accounts for 5% to 10% of congenital heart defects and has an incidence of 2 per 10,000 live births.

On ultrasound examination, an overriding aorta is the key feature for diagnosis. Color Doppler sonography may be helpful in detecting the VSD. Detailed sonogram should be performed to assess for extracardiac malformations.

Transposition of the Great Vessels

In transposition of the great vessels, the aorta connects with the right ventricle, and the pulmonary artery connects with the left ventricle. Two types have been identified, complete and corrected. Complete transposition of the great vessels, also known as D-transposition, is the more common of the 2 forms. In this form, the aorta comes off the right ventricle, and the pulmonary artery comes off the left ventricle. ASD and VSD defects are also commonly seen. It usually causes no hemodynamic compromise in utero. The corrected type of transposition of the great vessels, also known as L-transposition, refers to a connection of the right atrium to the morphologic left ventricle that connects to the pulmonary artery, whereas the left atrium connects to the morphologic right ventricle and then to the aorta. It is an abnormality in conotruncal development at 4 to 5 weeks' gestation and accounts for 4% to 6% of congenital heart defects.

The diagnosis is made on ultrasound examination when the aorta is identified as originating from the right ventricle. Demonstrating the vessels supplying the head and neck helps identify the aorta. The normal crossing over of the pulmonary artery and aorta is not seen. The outflow tracts appear to run in parallel, which is of importance, particularly in L-transposition, which can be difficult to diagnose. A detailed ultrasound examination should be performed to assess for other cardiac anomalies, such as pulmonic stenosis and coarctation, as well as extracardiac anomalies.

Atrial and Ventricular Septal Defects

ASD is a malformation in the development of the interatrial septum. Three different types are possible, depending on location. An inlet ASD is located near the entrance of the superior vena cava. A primum or outlet ASD is located in the body of the septum. Secundum ASDs occur because of an absence of the foramen ovale flap. These lesions are usually of no concern in utero because of normal right-to-left shunting. ASDs comprise 7.5% of all congenital heart defects.

A VSD is a malformation in the development of the interventricular septum. It is the most common congenital heart defect. VSDs can occur in the muscular or membranous portions of the septum. Muscular VSDs are bordered on all sides by muscle and may be further categorized as inlet, trabecular, or infundibular. Subvalvular VSDs may also occur, which are directly related to the AV and semilunar valves.

Prenatal diagnosis of ASD is difficult because of the normal presence of the foramen ovale. VSDs can also be problematic, particularly if the lesion is small. Color Doppler sonography may be useful in demonstrating flow across the septum. A detailed ultrasound examination should be performed to assess cardiac anatomy further. Serial ultrasounds should be performed to assess growth and to monitor for signs of fetal hydrops.

Arrhythmias

The normal fetal heart rate ranges from 120 to 160 beats/min. In bradycardia, the rate is sustained below 120 beats/min; in tachycardia, the sustained rate exceeds 160 beats/min. Bradyarrhythmias are caused by congenital heart block and are most commonly associated with structural anomalies such as transposition and AV canal defects. Bradyarrhythmia can also be found in a structurally normal heart when transplacental passage of certain maternal antibodies occurs in mothers with connective tissue disorders (ie, anti-Ro and anti-La in patients with systemic lupus erythematosus). First-, second-, or third-degree heart block can exist, with the last of these 3 blocks being the most common. Echocardiography should be performed to assess for cardiac anomalies. Serial ultrasounds should be performed to assess fetal growth. Bradycardia is generally well tolerated but can lead to hydrops in up to 25% of fetuses. If evidence exists of fetal compromise after 30 weeks' gestation, then delivery should be induced. Medical treatments have been proposed and are divided into those that suppress maternal immune response, such as corticosteroids, and those that increase fetal ventricular rate, such as β-mimetics.

Tachyarrhythmias are irregular cardiac rhythms caused by extrasystoles, supraventricular tachycardia, atrial flutter, or fibrillation. Extrasystoles may originate in the atria, AV node, or ventricles and usually resolve spontaneously. The most common is supraventricular tachycardia, many of which are reentry dysrhythmias. Atrial flutter is from a single reentry circuit within the atria with varying degrees of block at the AV node. Atrial fibrillation is from multiple small intraatrial reentry circuits, and organized atrial contraction is absent. These dysrhythmias have the potential for serious sequelae leading to hydrops. Complete cardiac survey should be performed to assess for cardiac anomalies. In utero treatment by administration of antiarrhythmics to the mother can convert the aberrant rhythm. Serial sonograms should be performed to assess fetal growth and to assess for signs of hydrops.

Abdominal Wall Defects

Gastroschisis

Gastroschisis is a full-thickness defect of the abdominal wall that leads to evisceration of the abdominal contents. The defect is thought to be the result of vascular compromise of either the umbilical vein or the omphalomesenteric artery. It typically arises to the right of the umbilicus. The incidence is reported as 1 per 4000 live births.[35]

Increased levels of AFP in maternal serum will be present with gastroschisis and other wall defects. Midgut herniation is normal up until 11 weeks' gestation. Herniation noted on ultrasound examination beyond this time is abnormal. Protruding bowel can be easily seen. Color Doppler sonography can be used to demonstrate the insertion of the umbilical cord medial to the defect. A thorough ultrasound evaluation should be performed to assess for other anomalies. Gastroschisis is not associated with chromosomal abnormalities. Amniocentesis should be offered if other anomalies are detected. Serial sonograms are performed to monitor growth and bowel integrity.

The prognosis with gastroschisis is generally good. No fetal intervention is available. Mode of delivery is for obstetrical indications. Parents should meet with a pediatric surgeon to discuss postnatal surgical treatment.

Omphalocele

An omphalocele is a defect of the ventral abdominal wall characterized by the lack of abdominal muscles, fascia, and skin. Protrusion of the intraabdominal contents occurs with a covering membrane that consists of peritoneum and amnion. In contrast to gastroschisis, the umbilical cord inserts into the membrane.

During development, the embryo undergoes a series of cranial, caudal, and lateral folding events. When failure of lateral folding occurs at the third to fourth week of gestation, omphaloceles can occur. The incidence is 1 per 4000 live births.[35] Maternal serum screening can be helpful making this diagnosis.

On ultrasound examination, bowel herniation can be noted. The membranous covering confirms the diagnosis of omphalocele. The presence or absence of liver herniation should be noted because this finding is important for determining prognosis. Color Doppler sonography can demonstrate the umbilical cord entering into the sac. Omphalocele is strongly associated with other anomalies and with chromosomal abnormalities. Therefore a thorough ultrasound evaluation should be performed, as well as amniocentesis. Serial sonograms should be performed to assess fetal growth.

The prognosis depends on finding other congenital anomalies and on chromosome evaluation.[36] Mortality may be as high as 20% to 30%. Large lesions have limited potential for closure. Patients should meet with pediatric surgeons to discuss postnatal surgical treatment.

Gastrointestinal Defects

Duodenal Atresia

Duodenal atresia is characterized by complete obliteration of the duodenal lumen. It is the most common type of congenital small-bowel atresia. The incidence is 1 per 10,000 live births.

At 5 weeks' gestation, the lumen of the duodenum is obliterated by proliferating epithelium. Normally, recanalization occurs, and the lumen is restored by 11 weeks. Failure of the recanalization process results in duodenal atresia or stenosis. Three types are described. Type I is membranous mucosal atresia with an intact muscular wall. The proximal duodenum is ballooned out, and the distal duodenum is narrowed. Type II duodenal atresia is rare. It has a short fibrous cord connecting the 2 ends of the duodenum. Type III has a complete separation between the duodenal ends and can be associated with gallbladder anomalies.

The majority of cases can be diagnosed by ultrasound but generally not until the third trimester. The duodenum is persistently dilated and the stomach is filled with fluid, leading to the classic *double-bubble* appearance. Significant polyhydramnios is usually present because of the fetal inability to swallow,[37] which can lead to uterine irritability and preterm labor and may often be the reason why a mother requests an ultrasound evaluation. Thirty percent of fetuses with duodenal atresia will have Down syndrome; therefore amniocentesis should be performed. A thorough cardiac evaluation should be conducted because an association exists with heart malformations.

The prognosis is related to associated malformations and karyotype.[38] The risk of preterm labor and its associated morbidity and mortality is increased. Successful surgical repair is usually possible.

Echogenic Bowel

Echogenic bowel is a sonographic finding in which the bowel appears to have the same echogenicity as the surrounding bone. The incidence ranges from 0.2% to 2%. Echogenic bowel can be a normal variant; it can also be associated with chromosomal abnormalities, fetal cystic fibrosis, cytomegalovirus infection, IUGR, intraamniotic bleeding, and intestinal abnormalities.[39] Once the echogenic bowel is detected, an amniocentesis should be offered, which enables testing for karyotype, cystic fibrosis, and infection studies. No fetal intervention is available. Prognosis depends on the cause.

Genitourinary Defects

Ambiguous Genitalia

Sexual differentiation does not occur until 6 to 7 weeks' gestation, even though phenotype is determined at the time of conception. Before 6 to 7 weeks' gestation, the gonads are undifferentiated. The presence of particular hormones and the expression of specific genes aid in the differentiation process. Masculinization is induced by the activity of dihydrotestosterone, which is formed from testosterone. Absence of or insensitivity to this hormone leads to the formation of female genitalia. Disruption in this pathway can lead to ambiguous genitalia. The overall incidence is 1 per 5000 live births.

Abnormalities of sex differentiation are chromosomal, gonadal, or phenotypical. Three categories are described. The true hermaphrodite has both ovarian and testicular tissue present. Female pseudohermaphrodites are overmasculinized females. Male pseudohermaphrodites are undermasculinized males. Many methods have been described to determine sex on ultrasound examination. (See Chapter 286, Intersex.)

Amniocentesis should be performed to determine genotype. Testing for inborn errors of metabolism should be performed. A complete maternal history and physical examination should be performed to assess for signs of androgen excess, hormone ingestion, or family history of similar findings.

Hydronephrosis

Hydronephrosis is dilatation of the renal pelvises and calyces. It is one of the most commonly reported ultrasound findings and comprises 75% of diagnosed renal abnormalities. The severity can range from mild to severe and depends on gestational age. Hydronephrosis may be physiologic or pathologic. Distinguishing the 2 entities requires thorough ultrasound evaluation and close follow-up.[40] The incidence of mild hydronephrosis is reported as 1 per 100 live births; for severe hydronephrosis, as in ureteropelvic junction obstruction, the incidence 1 per 100,000 live births. The finding may be unilateral or bilateral.

When visualizing the kidneys on ultrasound evaluation, the renal pelvises are dilated when measured. The absolute measurement depends on gestational age because normal dilatation exists with advancing gestational age. A thorough ultrasound evaluation should be performed to assess for any other abnormalities. Amniocentesis should be performed because of the increased risk of aneuploidy in severe cases. In unilateral cases, fetal intervention is not available. If severe bilateral hydronephrosis is present and evidence exists of dysplastic kidney or renal agenesis, and if the fetus is older than 30 weeks' gestation, then delivery should be considered after administering corticosteroid therapy to promote fetal lung maturation. Before 30 weeks, intervention by shunting can be considered after the normal kidney has been identified by sampling fetal urine.[41] Parents should meet with a pediatric urologist for prenatal consultation.

Ureterocele

Ureterocele is a cystic dilation of the intravesicular portion of the ureter—that is, the distal end at the junction of the bladder. Ureteroceles can be classified as simple or ectopic. Simple ureteroceles are at the normal location of the ureteral orifice in the trigone of the bladder. These are more commonly found in adults and may be associated with a varying degree of obstruction. In ectopic ureteroceles, the ureteral orifice is in an ectopic position, usually distal to the trigone. It can be associated with a duplex collecting system (75%). Ectopic ureteroceles tend to be unilateral, but it is bilateral in 10% to 20% of cases. The incidence is 1 per 5000 live births.

Unilateral hydronephrosis is often noted first on ultrasound examination, with the key feature being a dilated upper pole of the kidney with a normal lower pole. A crescent-shaped line may be seen at the base of the bladder, demonstrating the prolapsing ureterocele. The ureterocele itself is of no consequence unless it is causing bladder outlet obstruction. If obstruction is noted, then bladder decompression via needle aspiration may be indicated. Parents should meet with a pediatric urologist.

Multicystic Dysplastic Kidney

Multicystic dysplastic kidney is an extreme form of dysplasia of the kidney characterized by large dilatations of the collecting tubules with an atretic ureter. The kidney essentially consists of a group of cysts containing some connective tissue, with no real renal tissue present. Up to 80% of cases are unilateral. The incidence is reported as between 1 per 1000 to 1 per 4500 live births.[42] Multicystic dysplastic kidney is thought to arise from an early error in the development of the mesonephric blastema leading to an early obstructive uropathy.

On ultrasound examination, a cystic paraspinal flank mass is noted. Multiple cysts of varied size exist at the periphery of the kidney. They start out small but will usually get bigger over time. The overall kidney size may either be large or small. If unilateral, hypertrophy of the contralateral kidney may then be noted as a compensatory mechanism. A thorough ultrasound examination should be performed to assess for associated genitourinary and nongenitourinary anomalies. Amniocentesis should be performed because of this disorder's association with chromosomal abnormalities.

The prognosis depends on the presence of other anomalies, particularly in cases of unilateral dysplasia. If no other anomalies are present and the contralateral kidney is normal, then the prognosis is excellent. Bilateral severe cysts result in fetal death. If partial dysplastic involvement of both kidneys is found, then renal impairment may eventually occur.

Renal Agenesis

Renal agenesis is the congenital absence of either one or both kidneys. At 4 to 6 weeks' gestation, the metanephros fails to develop, which leads to the complete absence of the kidney. The incidence of unilateral agenesis is 1 per 1000 live births and of bilateral agenesis is 12 per 100,000 live births.[43,44]

The diagnosis of bilateral renal agenesis is made when severe oligohydramnios or oligohydramnios is noted after 14 weeks' gestation, along with the inability visualize the fetal bladder or kidneys. Visualization can be difficult in the absence of amniotic fluid. Amnioinfusion may be considered, in which sterile saline is infused into the uterus by using the same method as amniocentesis.[45] This procedure is helpful to rule out ruptured membranes, and it aids in the anatomic survey.

No available fetal intervention is available. Up to 40% of fetuses with bilateral renal agenesis are stillborn; the remaining fetuses die shortly after birth from respiratory or renal complications. Unilateral agenesis may be asymptomatic and consistent with life. Girls should eventually undergo pelvic ultrasound to assess for müllerian abnormalities.

Umbilical Cord

The umbilical cord normally has 2 arteries and 1 vein. In the case of a single umbilical artery, also known as a 2-vessel cord, one of the arteries is congenitally absent. Its incidence is 0.5% to 0.9%.[46]

The umbilical arteries develop from the allantois, which is a diverticulum of the yolk sac. Single umbilical artery occurs as a result of either primary agenesis of one of the umbilical arteries, secondary atresia of one of the arteries, or persistence of the common allantoic or umbilical artery.

A detailed ultrasound evaluation is necessary to assess for other anomalies, and if they are present, then amniocentesis should be performed because the risk of aneuploidy is increased. If the work-up is normal, then serial sonograms should be performed for the remainder of the pregnancy because this disorder is associated with IUGR.[47]

Skeletal Defects

Achondroplasia

Achondroplasia is a form of short-limbed dwarfism and is the most common form of nonlethal skeletal dysplasia. It is characterized by rhizomelic limb shortening with macrocephaly. Endochondral ossification is decreased. Bones that are initially formed from cartilage, such as long bones, are affected. The incidence is 1 per 26,000 live births.

On ultrasound examination, all the long bones are noted to be shortened (less than the 3rd percentile), particularly the femur. This finding is first notable at 21 to 27 weeks' gestation. The overall shape of the bones is normal. Additional findings include a large head (macrocrania), an abnormal profile caused by frontal bossing, and a protruding abdomen. Development of mild polyhydramnios may also occur in the third trimester. Once achondroplasia is detected, echocardiography and karyotyping should be performed to rule out other conditions. Finding the *FGFR3* mutation on amniocytes can confirm the diagnosis. A fetus with macrocrania near term may require delivery by cesarean; therefore serial sonograms should also be performed.

Intelligence and life span are normal. Neurologic sequelae remain a risk because of spinal cord compression. Homozygosity for achondroplasia is lethal, resulting in stillbirth or neonatal death from respiratory failure.

Osteogenesis Imperfecta

Osteogenesis imperfecta (OI) is a heterogeneous group of brittle bone disorders and is characterized by a tendency to fractures, both before and after birth. Most individuals are heterozygotes, and most types of OI are due to type-I collagen abnormalities. Approximately 25% of cases of OI are due to a spontaneous dominant mutation.[48]

OI is divided into 4 distinct categories. Type I, the classic form, is autosomal dominant and is the most common form and mildest type of OI. Affected patients have distinctly blue sclera and will develop fractures and various degrees of hearing loss. Patients with type-I OI have underproduction of normal collagen rather than abnormal (defective) collagen fibers as seen in the other forms of OI. All patients with type-I OI are able to walk independently. Affected patients have progressive loss of height resulting from kyphosis. Unlike infants with types-II, -III or -IV OI, babies with type I typically develop their first factures after birth. Type II is the severe form that results in neonatal death at or shortly after birth caused by lung hypoplasia; multiple prenatal fractures and severe bone deformity will be present. Type III is rare and is a progressively deforming disorder. Fractures are often present at birth with evidence of healed fractures that occurred in utero. Blue sclerae may be present at birth but then may fade. Hearing impairment is rare. A tendency exists toward severe disability by middle age. Type IV is autosomal dominant; long bones are variably deformed, and sclerae are normal. The incidence ranges from 1 per 28,500 to 1 per 69,000 live births. Recent investigations have also characterized 2 subgroups within type-IV OI, children with distinct bone histology that is not the result of mutation in type-I collagen genes.

On ultrasound examination, fractures and callus formation may be noted, which can result in long-bone deformity and shortening. The family history will provide clues about diagnosis. If OI is suspected prenatally and no known family history is found, then type II must be considered. Confirmation of diagnosis can be made by biochemical and histological testing. For the nonlethal forms, cesarean delivery may be of benefit to decrease the risk of fracture.

Extremities

Arthrogryposis

Arthrogryposis is a term to describe a group of disorders that are characterized by congenital nonprogressive joint contractures at multiple sites. The muscles in the affected areas are replaced with fat and fibrous tissue. The incidence is 1 per 3000 live births.

Four major causes of contractures have been identified. The first is an abnormality in muscle tissue. The second is abnormal nerve function or innervation. The third is an abnormality of connective tissue. The fourth is a mechanical limitation of movement. Clinical features include joint rigidity, short and tight muscles, and joint dislocation.

On ultrasound examination the diagnosis is made by observation of malposition of the fetal limbs. The bones are morphologically normal, but the range of motion is limited. A detailed ultrasound evaluation should be performed to rule out other associated anomalies and to delineate further the case into possible syndrome categories. Karyotyping should be offered to rule out chromosomal abnormalities.

Clubfoot

Clubfoot is a term used to describe an abnormal positioning of the foot and is characterized by equinus and inversion of the foot with associated abnormalities in the musculature of the lower leg. The incidence is 1 per 1000 live births.[47]

The fetal lower limb begins movement between 9 and 11 weeks' gestation. If neurologic or muscular abnormalities are present, then limb movements may be impaired, and joints will eventually become stiff and even contracted.

On ultrasound examination, the 2 long bones of the lower leg can be seen at the same time as the lateral aspect of the feet; it is fixed in position. Most cases of clubfoot are isolated and idiopathic. If other anomalies are associated, then a syndrome may be present. Although offering amniocentesis is controversial when the finding is isolated, it should be performed if other anomalies are suspected.[49] Parents should consult a pediatric orthopedic surgeon.

Twins

In a twin, gestation ultrasound examination is extremely important in determining chorionicity, which is important because twin-twin transfusion and the morbidity associated with it is unique to monochorionic twins. The membrane is visualized at the insertion into the placenta. In a dichorionic gestation, the membrane is thick (>2 mm) and is described as a lambda sign or a so-called *twin peak*. In a monochorionic gestation, the membrane is thin and appears as a T sign.

Intrauterine Growth Restriction

IUGR is a condition defined as birth weight below the 10th percentile at a given gestational age. The causes of IUGR are fetal, maternal, or placental. At the time of diagnosis, a detailed ultrasound examination is performed to determine whether any anomalies are present. Echocardiography is useful because cardiac anomalies are significantly associated with IUGR. Amniocentesis should be offered, particularly if IUGR is diagnosed early in gestation, because aneuploidy is also strongly associated with IUGR. Infection studies (TORCH [*t*oxoplasmosis, *o*ther agents, *r*ubella, *c*ytomegalovirus, *h*erpes simplex]) can be requested at the time of amniocentesis. Amniotic fluid volume is also assessed as a determination of placental function. Doppler ultrasound may also be performed to ensure fetal well being. Fetuses are assessed by serial sonograms because the diagnosis of IUGR carries an increased risk of fetal death.

TOOLS FOR PRACTICE

Medical Decision Support

- *Spina Bifida and Anencephaly Before and After Folic Acid Mandate* (report), Centers for Disease Control and Prevention (www.cdc.gov/mmwr/preview/mmwrhtml/mm5317a3.htm).

SUGGESTED RESOURCES

Bianchi D. *Fetology: Diagnosis & Management of the Fetal Patient*. New York, NY: McGraw-Hill; 2000.

Callen P. *Ultrasonography in Obstetrics and Gynecology*. 4th ed. Philadelphia, PA: WB Saunders; 2000.

Creasy R. *Maternal Fetal Medicine*. 5th ed. Philadelphia, PA: WB Saunders; 2004.

Van de Hof MC, Wilson RW. Fetal soft markers in obstetric ultrasound. Society of Obstetrics and Gynaecology of Canada Clinical Practice Guidelines. *J Obstetr Gynaecol Can*. 2005;27(6):592-612.

REFERENCES

1. Gardner RJM, Sutherland GR. Pregnancy loss and infertility. In: *Chromosome Abnormalities and Genetic Counseling*. 2nd ed. New York, NY: Oxford University Press; 1996. Oxford Monographs on Medical Genetics No. 29.
2. Alberman ED, Creasy MR. Frequency of chromosomal abnormalities in miscarriages and perinatal deaths. *J Med Genet*. 1977;14:313-315.
3. Milunsky A, Milunsky J. Genetic counseling, preconception, prenatal and perinatal. In: Milunsky A, ed. *Genetic Disorders and the Fetus: Diagnosis, Prevention, and Treatment*. 4th ed. Baltimore, MD: The Johns Hopkins University Press; 1998.
4. Cuckle HS, Wald NJ, Thompson SG. Estimating a woman's risk of having a pregnancy associated with Down's syndrome using her age and alpha fetal protein level. *Br J Obstet Gynecol*. 1987;94(5):387-402.
5. Nicolaides KH, Azar G, Byrne D, et al. Fetal nuchal translucency: ultrasound screening for chromosomal defects in the first trimester of pregnancy. *BMJ*. 1992; 304:867-869.
6. Snijders RL, Noble P, Sebire N, et al. UK multicenter project on assessment of risk of trisomy 21 by maternal age and fetal nuchal translucency thickness at 10-14 weeks of gestation. *Lancet*. 1998;352:343-346.
7. Wald NJ, George L, Smith D, et al. Serum screening for Down's syndrome between 8 and 14 weeks of pregnancy. *Br J Obstet Gynecol*. 1996;103:407-412.
8. Malone FD, Canick JA, Ball RH, et al. First trimester or second trimester, or both, for Down's syndrome. *N Engl J Med*. 2005;353(19):2001-2011.

9. Centers for Disease Control and Prevention. Spina bifida and anencephaly before and after folic acid mandate—United States, 1995-1996 and 1999-2000. *MMWR Morb Mortal Wkly Rep*. 2004;53(17):362-365.
10. Tmamura T, Picciano MF. Folate and human reproduction. *Am J Clin Nutr*. 2006;83:993-1016.
11. Mitchell LE, Adzick NS, Malchiome J, et al. Spina bifida. *Lancet*. 2004;364:1885-1895.
12. American College of Obstetrics and Gynecology. ACOG practice bulletin. Clinical management guidelines for obstetrician-gynecologists. Number 44, July 2003. (Replaces Committee Opinion Number 252, March 2001). *Obstet Gynecol*. 2003;102:203.
13. Norem CT, Schoen EJ, Walton DL, et al. Routine ultrasonography compared with maternal serum alpha-fetoprotein for neural tube defect screening. *Obstet Gynecol*. 2005;106(4):747-752.
14. Jorde LB, ed. *Medical Genetics*. St Louis, MO: Mosby; 2000.
15. Valsky DV, Ben-Sira L, Porat S, et al. The role of magnetic resonance imaging in the evaluation of isolated mild ventriculomegaly. *J Ultrasound Med*. 2004;23(4):519-523.
16. Nadel AS, Bromley BS, Frigoletto FD Jr, et al. Isolated choroids plexus cysts in the second trimester fetus: is amniocentisis really indicated? *Radiology*. 1992;185(2):545-548.
17. Fitzsimmons J, Wilson D, Pascoe-Mason J, et al. Choroid plexus cysts in fetuses with trisomy 18. *Obstet Gynecol*. 1989;73(2):257-260.
18. Hertzberg BS, Kay HH, Bowie JD. Fetal choroid plexus lesions. Realtionship of antenatal sonographic appearance to clinical outcome. *J Ultrasound Med*. 1989:8(2):77-82.
19. Young DL, Schneider RA, Hu D, et al. Genetic and teratogenic approaches to craniofacial development. *Crit Rev Oral Bio Med*. 2000;11(3):304-317.
20. Shaw GM, Wasserman CR, Lammer EJ, et al. Orofacial clefts, cigarette smoking and transforming growth factor-alpha gene variants. *Am J Hum Genet*. 1996;58(3):551-561.
21. Munger RG, Romitti PA, Daack-Hirsch S, et al. Maternal alcohol use and risk of orofacial cleft birth defects. *Teratology*. 1996;54(1):27-33.
22. Kilpatrick S. Umbilical blood sampling in women with thyroid disease in pregnancy: is it necessary? *Am J Obstet Gynecol*. 2003;189:1.
23. Van Raemdonck D, De Boeck K, Devlieger H, et al. Pulmonary sequestration: a comparison between pediatric and adult patients. *Eur J Cardiothorac Surg*. 2001;19(4):388-395.
24. Zach MS, Eber E. Adult outcome of congential lower respiratory tract malformations. *Thorax*. 2001;56(1):65-72.
25. Louie HW, Martin SM, Mulder DG. Pulmonary sequestration: 17-year experience at UCLA. *Am Surg*. 1993;59(12):801-805.
26. Laberge JM, Flageole H, Pugash D, et al. Outcome of the prenatally diagnosed congenital cystic adenomatoid lung malformation: a Canadian experience. *Fetal Diagn Ther*. 2001;16(3):178-186.
27. Stocker JT, Madewell JE, Drake RM. Congenital cystic adenomatoid malformation of the lung. *Human Pathol*. 1977;8:155-171.
28. Adzick NS, Harrison MR, Crobleholme TM. Fetal lung lesions: management and outcome. *Am J Obstet Gyecol*. 1998;179:884-889.
29. Adzick NS, Harrison MR, Glick PL, et al. Diaphragmatic hernia in the fetus: prenatal diagnosis and outcome in 94 cases. *J Pediatr Surg*. 1985;20:357-361.
30. Graham G, Devine PC. Antenatal diagnosis of congential diaphragmatic hernia. *Semin Perinatol*. 2005;29(2):69-76.
31. Hubbard AM, Crombleholme TM, Adzick NS, et al. Prenatal MRI evaluation of congenital diaphragmatic hernia. *Am J Perinatol*. 1999;16(8):407-413.
32. France R. A Review of fetal circulation and the segmental approach in fetal echocardiography. *J Diagn Med Sonogr*. 2006;22:29-39.
33. Sharland G. Routine fetal cardiac screening: what are we doing and what should we do? *Prenat Diagn*. 2004;24(13):1123-1129.
34. Wimalasundera RC, Gardiner HM. Congenital heart disease and aneuploidy. *Prenat Diagn*. 2004;24(13):1116-1122.
35. Martin RW. Screening for fetal abdominal wall defects. *Obstet Gynecol Clin North Am*. 1998;25(3):517-526.
36. Hughes MD, Nyberg DA, Mack LA, et al. Fetal omphalocele: prenatal US detection of concurrent anomalies and other predictors of outcome. *Radiology*. 1989;173(2):371-376.
37. Brantberg A, Blaas HG, Salvesen KA, et al. Fetal duodenal obstructions: increased risk of prenatal sudden death. *Ultrasound Obstet Gynecol*. 2002;20(5):439-446.
38. Escobar MA, Ladd AP, Grosfeld JL, et al. Duodenal atresia and stenosis; long-term follow-up over 30 years. *J Pediatr Surg*. 2004;39(6):867-871.
39. Al-Kouatly HB, Chasen ST, Streltzoff J, et al. The clinical significance of fetal echogenic bowel. *Am J Obstet Gynecol*. 2001;185(5):1035-1038.
40. Lee RS, Cendron M, Kinnamon DD, et al. Antenatal hydronephrosis as a predictor of postnatal outcome: a meta-analysis. *Pediatrics*. 2006;118:586-593.
41. Cheng AM, Phan V, Geary DF, et al. Outcome of isolated antenatal hydronephrosis. *Arch Pediatr Adolesc Med*. 2004;158:38-40.
42. Gough DC, Postlethwaite RJ, Lewis MA, et al. Mulitcystic renal dysplasia diagnosed in the antenatal period: a note of caution. *Br J Urol*. 1995;76(2):244-248.
43. Cardwell MS. Bilateral renal agenesis: clinical implications. *South Med J*. 1988;81(3):327-328.
44. Cascio S, Paran S, Puri P. Associated urological anomalies in children with unilateral renal agenesis. *J Urol*. 1999;162(3 pt 2):1081-1083.
45. Fisk NM, Ronderos-Dumit D, Soliani A, et al. Diagnostic and therapeutic transabdominal amnioinfusion in oligohydramnios. *Obstet Gynecol*. 1991;78(2):270-278.
46. Gornall AS, Kurinczuk JJ, Konje JC. Antenatal detection of a single umbilical artery: does it matter? *Prenat Diagn*. 2003;23(2):117-123.
47. Wynne-Davis R. Genetic and environmental factors in the etiology of talipes equinovarus. *Clin Orthop*. 1972;84:9.
48. Marini JC. Osteogenesis imperfecta: comprehensive managment. *Adv Pediatr*. 1988;35:391-426.
49. Treadwell MC, Stanitski CL, King M. Prenatal sonographic diagnosis of clubfoot: implications for patient counseling. *J Ped Orthop*. 1999;19(1):8-10.

Chapter 71

FETAL INTERVENTIONS

Manisha Gandhi, MD; Garfield A. D. Clunie, MD

In the past, parents have been offered 2 options after learning their unborn child has an abnormality: (1) pregnancy termination if the diagnosis is made before 24 weeks' gestation (some states allow termination after 24 weeks for fetal anomalies) or (2) continuing the pregnancy and dealing with the medical issues after birth. Continuing a pregnancy with a major fetal abnormality can lead to serious physiological consequences before birth, followed by subsequent irreversible organ failure and postnatal death. However, since the advent of sonography, and more recently with the addition of fetal magnetic resonance imaging, a third option may be considered: fetal intervention. Close follow-up with ultrasound has afforded clinicians the ability to define the natural history of many fetal anomalies, determine the clinical features that affect outcome, and plan management strategies to improve prognosis (see Chapter 70, Prenatal Diagnosis). Observing the natural history of an abnormality diagnosed in utero also leads to a better understanding of the pathophysiological processes that take place in the developing fetus. Treatment for Rh isoimmunization was the first successful example of medical intervention in the fetus and occurred in the early 1960s. Over the last 40 years, the field of fetal intervention has greatly progressed, and it has led to the creation of more alternatives for pregnancy management when a fetus is found to have an abnormality.

TYPES OF FETAL INTERVENTIONS

Although many of the prenatally diagnosed fetal malformations are best treated after birth, patients with pregnancies that are complicated by certain fetal abnormalities known to result in devastating consequences can be offered fetal intervention. Open fetal surgery frequently involves administration of inhalation anesthetics and tocolytics to the mother. A hysterotomy is performed, and the fetal malformation is repaired. This type of surgery often results in preterm labor and preterm premature rupture of membranes. The mother usually needs to be hospitalized for several days for recovery and tocolytic treatment. With the advent of minimally invasive techniques such as fetal endoscopy and ultrasound-guided fetal surgery, maternal recovery time and preterm labor rate have decreased. Fetal endoscopy, also known as fetoscopy, is based on preserving fetal homeostasis by protecting the intrauterine environment. The surgery is performed by introducing a 3- to 5-mm trocar into the uterine cavity to allow for placement of endoscopes or fetoscopic instruments. Ultrasound-guided fetal surgery (fetal image-guided surgery) is the least invasive and can be performed under local anesthesia. This type of intervention was first used for amniocentesis and percutaneous umbilical blood sampling and is now also used to place a catheter in the fetal bladder, abdomen, or chest; and to provide radiofrequency ablation for monochorionic multiple gestations.

ETHICAL CONSIDERATIONS IN MATERNAL-FETAL INTERVENTIONS

The need to balance risks to the mother and fetus against potential benefits to the fetus forms the basis for the fundamental ethical conflict when considering fetal surgery.[1] Correcting a fetal malformation with open surgery, fetoscopy, or ultrasound-guided procedures can be risky to both fetus and mother. In addition, considerations exist related to psychosocial risks to the mother and family of losing the pregnancy or, in the event of iatrogenic injury to the fetus, living with the burden of a child with further damage. Residual risks to future pregnancies also exist. Criteria have been set for considering fetal intervention and include the following: (1) prenatal diagnosis techniques should identify the malformation and almost certainly exclude any abnormalities that will result in death; (2) the defect should have a defined natural history and cause progressive injury to the fetus that is irreversible after delivery; (3) repair of the defect should be feasible and should reverse or prevent the injury process; and (4) the surgical risk must not entail excessive risk for the mother or her future fertility.[2]

Meeting these prerequisites is extremely important because most fetal malformations do not directly threaten the mother's health. The investigational nature of these interventions offered at a limited number of centers of excellence under research protocols involves the need for a rigorous nondirective informed consent process that emphasizes the experimental basis for these interventions. In addition, several of these procedures involve a multidisciplinary team, including perinatologists, neonatologists, radiologists, pediatric surgeons, anesthesiologists, residents, fellows, nurses, scrub technicians, and audiovisual technicians. Despite the investigational nature of fetal surgery, costs for certain fetal surgeries are covered by many insurers. The majority of insurance companies will pay for *medically necessary* interventions, such as the treatment for twin-twin transfusion syndrome, the placement of in utero shunts (vesicoamniotic and thoracoamniotic). They will also consider covering the cost for treatment of congenital cystic adenomatoid malformation (CCAM), extralobar pulmonary sequestration, and sacrococcygeal teratomas when complicated by hydrops in a previable fetus. In contrast, many insurers consider in utero fetal surgeries for the repair of neural tube defects and congenital diaphragmatic hernia, stem cell transplantation, and gene therapy as experimental or investigational therapies that are not medically necessary. As therapies advance, public policy and insurance practices will likely continue to evolve. Centers performing fetal surgery have established *fetal oversight committees* that serve as a multidisciplinary advisory council, which ensures continuous monitoring of quality and function.

This chapter describes the most common surgical interventions available to treat fetal abnormalities (Table 71-1).

FETAL ABNORMALITIES

Obstructive Uropathy

Obstructive uropathy is known to affect from 1 in 200 to 1 in 1000 births and can be the result of ureteropelvic junction obstruction or urethral obstruction.[3] In male fetuses, this obstruction can be seen with posterior urethral valves. Lower urinary tract lesions appear to have a higher association with morbidity than upper urinary tract lesions.[4] This abnormality can lead to decreased fetal urine output and oligohydramnios. When this occurs in the second trimester, pulmonary hypoplasia may result. Initially, affected fetuses are monitored with serial ultrasounds and reassessed

Table 71-1 Fetal Interventions

TYPE OF INTERVENTION	DESCRIPTION	CLINICAL INDICATIONS
Open surgery	Hysterotomy under general anesthesia; requires 3-7 days postoperative hospitalization; obligates cesarean delivery; preterm labor and preterm delivery are associated risks	Congenital cystic adenomatoid malformation (CCAM) Sacrococcygeal and cervical teratomas Myelomeningocele repair EXIT procedure Tracheal occlusion Neck tumors Congenital diaphragmatic hernia (CDH) (EXIT to ECMO) CCAM (EXIT lobectomy)
Fetendo fetal surgery	Fetoscopic surgery using small endoscopes; performed either percutaneously or via a small laparotomy incision; preterm labor is a risk but less so than with open surgery	Balloon occlusion trachea (CDH) Laser ablation vessels (TTTS) Cord ligation or division Cystoscopic ablation posterior urethral valves Amniotic bands division
Fetal image-guided surgery	Sonographic-guided endoscopic surgery performed through a percutaneous or small laparotomy incision; performed under regional (epidural, spinal) or local anesthesia; least invasive though a risk of preterm labor exists	Amnioreduction or amnioinfusion Fetal blood sampling Twin-reversed arterial perfusion (acardiac or acephalic twin) Vesicoamniotic shunts for obstructive uropathy Pleuro (thoraco)-amniotic shunts for pleural effusions or hydrothorax Cord monopolar cautery Balloon dilation aortic stenosis

ECMO, Extracorporeal membrane oxygenation; *EXIT*, ex utero intrapartum treatment; *TTTS*, twin-twin transfusion syndrome.

after birth. If both kidneys are noted to be affected, then surgical intervention can be considered. Before surgical intervention, an intensive work-up is performed to determine whether the patient is an appropriate surgical candidate. Fetal karyotype must be determined. Ultrasound is used to attempt to differentiate between normal and abnormal tissue. Poor prognostic indicators include echogenic kidneys and kidneys with multiple cysts. Finally, fetal urine must be sampled for electrolytes. Healthy fetuses usually produce hypotonic urine, whereas renal damage is associated with salt wasting and can lead to isotonic urine.[5] The fetal urine is sampled by draining the fetal bladder in a method similar to amniocentesis. A needle is introduced into the fetal bladder, and the bladder is completely drained. This procedure is repeated twice more, 48 to 72 hours apart. The third sample provides the most accurate assessment of the fetus' renal capabilities. Fetuses with evidence of isotonic urine are not good surgical candidates because this is evidence of minimal kidney function.[5]

The purpose of surgical intervention is to allow the fetus to produce urine again so that amniotic fluid may accumulate and the lungs and kidneys can continue to develop. The first case of an obstructive uropathy treated in utero by vesicoamniotic shunting was reported in 1982 by Golbus et al.[6] In open fetal surgery a vesicostomy is made by creating an opening in the lower fetal abdomen so urine can exit and drain into the amniotic cavity. As previously noted, open fetal surgery is frequently associated with preterm labor. Ultrasound-guided placement of a catheter for vesicoamniotic shunting involves placement of a tube into the fetal bladder so that urine can flow from the bladder into the amniotic fluid. The most common complication of this procedure is a blocked or dislodged catheter, which can lead to a cessation in shunt functioning with further worsening of the obstructive uropathy.[7]

A technique that is only available for male fetuses has been developed that involves introducing a 3-mm fetoscope into the fetal bladder for disrupting posterior urethral valves to relieve the obstruction. After birth, these neonates will require follow-up with renal ultrasound, and voiding cystourethrograms to determine if further intervention is necessary.[8]

Congenital Diaphragmatic Hernia

Congenital diaphragmatic hernia results from a muscular defect in the diaphragm that allows abdominal contents to herniate into the hemothorax. The majority of these hernias occur on the left side, and the disorder occurs in approximately 1 in 2200 births.[9] The herniated abdominal contents can cause compression in the hemithorax and can lead to pulmonary hypoplasia because the pulmonary tissue no longer has room to develop and expand. This situation can be reversible if fetal repair is performed early. Evaluation of these fetuses requires a detailed ultrasound (to rule out other defects), a fetal echocardiogram, and fetal karyotype. A poor prognosis is associated with diagnosis at less than

25 weeks' gestation and liver herniation into the hemithorax. Liver herniated into the hemithorax is associated with a postnatal survival of less than 50%.[10] If the liver is in its normal abdominal position, then these fetuses are not surgical candidates because this is already associated with a 90% survival rate.[10]

The goal of fetal intervention is to assist with the development of the lungs so that these neonates can breathe after birth. The first attempted congenital diaphragmatic hernia repair was in 1986.[11] Since then, minimally invasive fetoscopic techniques have been developed to occlude the fetal trachea in utero. This is only considered for fetuses with very severe CDH in which the liver is herniated into the chest cavity. With blockage of the trachea, the fluid that the fetal lung makes remains in the lungs and allows accelerated maturation of the lungs. This accelerated maturation leads to increased intrathoracic pressure, which can push the abdominal contents back into the abdominal cavity.[8]

Various methods have been described for tracheal occlusion, including fetoscopic neck dissection with attachment of obstructing clips to the trachea, although this method is complicated because of the fine dissection required to bring the trachea into view. The technique was modified to allow for endoscopic placement of a detachable balloon in the trachea with deflation after delivery.[4] After delivery, the infant has to be monitored in the intensive care unit and carefully followed by neonatologists and pediatric surgeons. Some of these neonates may need extracorporeal membrane oxygenation, which is a heart-lung machine that provides oxygen to the baby when the lungs are unable to do so.

Congenital Cystic Adenomatoid Malformation

CCAM is a fetal intrathoracic tumor that is most commonly diagnosed by prenatal ultrasound, but its incidence is only approximately 1 in 25,000 to 35,000 pregnancies.[4] CCAM is a congenital cystic lesion that occupies space in the lung field. It is usually unilateral or lobar, and it can decrease in size, remain stable, or increase in size. CCAM may lead to fetal hydrops by causing a mediastinal shift and compromising venous return to the heart. Affected fetuses can have associated polyhydramnios as a result of increasing intrathoracic mass size, leading to esophageal compression and decreased swallowing.[12] Two types of CCAM have been identified: (1) microcystic and (2) macrocystic. The microcystic lesions have a worse prognosis than macrocystic lesions. The period of fastest growth is from 20 to 28 weeks; therefore this time is when the most vigilance is needed.[11]

Before surgical intervention, fetal echocardiograms should be obtained. If the fetus develops hydrops, then the perinatologist can intervene with repeated thoracocenteses to decompress the cysts; this is most effective with macrocystic CCAM. Fetal surgical resection of the CCAM via open fetal surgery can also be offered. If the fetus has large lesions, then a specialized ex utero intrapartum treatment procedure may be required at delivery. This procedure involves the baby being delivered and remaining attached to the placenta while the CCAM is surgically resected or until support with extracorporeal membrane oxygenation is provided.[8]

Sacrococcygeal Teratoma

Sacrococcygeal teratoma (SCT) is the most common tumor of the fetus and neonate and affects approximately 1 in 40,000 births.[13] Arteriovenous shunting through the tumor can lead to high-output cardiac failure and fetal hydrops.[14] In addition, fetal hydrops and associated placentomegaly appears to cause a *maternal mirror* syndrome, which can lead to severe preeclampsia and requires immediate delivery.[15] SCTs are derived from totipotent somatic cells from the Henson node of the caudal cell mass.[4] Affected fetuses need detailed serial ultrasounds and echocardiograms to assess growth. Solid SCTs are highly vascularized, increasing the risk for development of hydrops in utero. In addition, rapid growth of these tumors is associated with a worse prognosis.[9]

Although open fetal surgery can be performed if the fetus develops hydrops before 32 weeks, this type of surgery does not have a good prognosis, and preterm labor remains a common complication. Minimally invasive methods have been developed that involve inserting a needle into the blood vessels that feed into the tumor and applying radiofrequency waves to ablate the vessels so that the high-velocity blood flow is stopped and the fetal hydrops can be reversed.[8] However, most fetuses can be managed expectantly.

Gastroschisis and Omphalocele

Gastroschisis and omphalocele are ventral wall defects. In gastroschisis, fetal bowel extends freely into the amniotic cavity through a small opening adjacent to the right side of the umbilicus. It is associated with an increase in maternal serum alfa-fetoprotein (AFP) levels. Because the bowel is unprotected, damage can occur from constant exposure to the amniotic fluid. Gastroschisis has an incidence of approximately 1 in 5000 and is not associated with chromosomal defects.[16] Omphalocele differs from gastroschisis because the defect is at the level of the umbilicus and the bowel that extends through the amniotic wall is protected by a membrane. Omphalocele has a high association with aneuploidy.

Both anomalies should be monitored closely with ultrasounds and fetal surveillance in the third trimester because of their effects on fetal growth, amniotic fluid, and fetal bowel.

Affected fetuses are usually treated after delivery. The surgery in the neonatal period involves returning extraabdominal contents into the abdominal cavity via a primary abdominal wall closure or via staged approach with a silo. The infant usually receives parenteral nutrition during this period, followed by feeds via a nasogastric tube until feeding by mouth can be tolerated.[16]

Neural Tube Defects

Neural tube defects (NTDs) are characterized by midline vertebral defects and are usually associated with the dorsal portion of the lumbosacral spine. NTDs develop when the neural tube fails to completely close. When the meningeal sac protrudes through the defect, it is called a meningocele, and when the sac has nerve roots, the NTD is called a myelomeningocele. Myelomeningocele affects 1 in 2000 infants worldwide.[9] Exposure of the spinal elements to the intrauterine environment can lead to progressive damage. Knowing the progression of the neurologic damage associated with these lesions in utero is difficult because distinguishing between active and passive movement of the lower extremities on ultrasound can be difficult.[9] Most of these lesions are associated with an increased maternal serum AFP level.[17] On ultrasound, a notable *lemon sign* can be noted, which is seen with the caving in of the frontal bones of the calvarium. A *banana sign* can also be seen and is associated with herniation of the cerebellum.[18] Fetal repair can provide some improvement by releasing the pressure on the posterior fossa and preventing postnatal hydrocephalus; this repair also decreases the need for ventricular shunting after birth. However, associated improvement in neurologic function is unlikely.[9] NTDs are known to be associated with paralysis, hydrocephalus, intellectual disability, and loss of control of bowel and bladder function. No benefit of surgical intervention has been proven, although trials are underway. The current treatment involves early postnatal closure, shunting for hydrocephalus, and extensive rehabilitation.[8]

Hydrocephalus

Cerebrospinal fluid pathways can become obstructed or obliterated in utero as a result of developmental or acquired abnormalities and can lead to the accumulation of cerebrospinal fluid in the ventricular system. The increase in pressure can lead to dilation of the ventricles, which is known as hydrocephalus. Hydrocephalus occurs in 0.3 to 2.5 of 1000 live births.[8] Frequently, the obstruction is at the aqueduct of Sylvius and can be associated with other congenital malformations such as Chiari type II deformity or Dandy Walker syndrome. The diagnosis is usually made by ultrasound, confirmed by magnetic resonance imaging, and followed up by serial ultrasounds.[8] For isolated, rapidly progressive ventriculomegaly, fetal ventriculoamniotic shunting has been investigated. Results of this procedure have not resulted in improved outcomes, and a moratorium has been imposed on percutaneous shunting for fetal hydrocephalus.[19] In response to poor outcomes after early shunting and delivery, treatment before 32 week's gestation is not recommended. Any fetus with hydrocephalus should undergo amniocentesis for karyotype, amniotic fluid AFP, and culture for viruses to rule out infectious processes.

Twin-Twin Transfusion Syndrome

Twin-twin transfusion syndrome (TTTS) occurs at a rate of 0.1 to 0.9 per 1000 live births,[19] and the syndrome complicates approximately 10% to 20% of monochorionic pregnancies.[9] The etiology of TTTS is based on the vascular anastomoses running across the single placenta between the 2 fetuses and the unequal sharing of blood flow. These anastomoses can lead to the shunting of blood from one fetus to the other via arteriovenous anastomoses, leading to intrauterine growth restriction in the donor fetus and to fetal hydrops in the recipient fetus.[7] The number of vascular anastomoses and the type of anastomoses within the single placenta determine whether TTTS develops because all monochorionic twins share a blood supply.[19] The syndrome is diagnosed in monochorionic twins when a marked difference is found in amniotic fluid volume between the 2 sacs, leading to polyhydramnios in one sac and oligohydramnios in the other. Significant size discordance can also develop between the twins, with the larger twin in the sac with polyhydramnios and the smaller twin in the sac with oligohydramnios.[20] The latter twin is also referred to as the *stuck twin* because of its inability to move. The increase in blood volume in the recipient twin from the shunting of blood flow can lead to strain on this fetus's heart, leading to heart failure and fetal hydrops from the chronic volume overload. If left untreated, then fetal death will result, usually of the donor twin. The surviving twin has an increased risk of neurologic ischemic events that are due to the vascular changes that can occur after its co-twin's demise.[21]

Several minimally invasive techniques can be performed to treat TTTS. Serial amnioreduction can be used to help prolong gestation by improving uteroplacental blood flow and easing maternal discomfort. In this procedure, a significant amount of amniotic fluid is removed in the twin with polyhydramnios. Care has to be taken to not remove too much fluid because placental abruption might occur from the decrease in intraamniotic pressure. An amniotic septostomy can also be made in the dividing membrane between the 2 fetuses to allow amniotic fluid to flow in between the 2 sacs. However, this can create monoamniotic twins.

For the pregnancies that develop TTTS early in gestation, fetoscopic laser coagulation can be offered. In these pregnancies, both fetuses must have a normal karyotype, a fetal echocardiogram, a detailed ultrasound, and TORCH (*t*oxoplasmosis, *o*ther agents, *r*ubella, *c*ytomegalovirus, *h*erpes simplex) laboratory work-up to rule out possible infectious causes.[19] Fetoscopic laser coagulation is considered in early-onset TTTS after failure of amnioreduction. An attempt is made to map all intertwined communicating vessels, followed by laser ablation of these vessels. A thin fiberoptic endoscope is introduced through the wall of the uterus and into the amniotic cavity of the recipient twin. The surfaces of the placental vessels are examined directly, and the abnormal vascular connections are eliminated with a laser. By eliminating the anastomoses, significant shunting of blood flow between the twins is stopped.[9] The efficacy of amnioreduction versus laser ablation is currently being studied.

Twin Reversed Arterial Perfusion Syndrome

Twin reversed arterial perfusion syndrome (TRAP) affects approximately 1 in 35,000 live births.[7] It is usually seen in a twin gestation with one acardiac twin. This twin has acephalic and acardia morphology. Acardia is lethal to the affected twin. The unaffected twin may experience significant associated morbidity and mortality. This twin must sustain the affected twin's cardiovascular system, which can lead to added circulatory burden. As in TTTS, twin reversed arterial perfusion syndrome can lead to in utero cardiac failure of the normal twin and eventual fetal death. Large-volume amnioreduction can be offered as the initial treatment, followed by ultrasound-guided radiofrequency ablation of the malformed fetus at the area of umbilical cord insertion. Laser ablation and cord coagulation can also be used to terminate the twin with acardia.[7]

Fetal Anemia

Rh sensitization has become increasingly rare since the advent of Rho(D) immune globulin (RhoGAM), but cases of Rh isoimmunization that require fetal intervention can still be found. Rh isoimmunization can develop when an Rh-negative mother is pregnant with an Rh-positive fetus. If the mother has been exposed to Rh-positive cells in the past, then she has antibodies to the Rh antigen, and these antibodies rapidly increase in number when exposed to the Rh-positive fetus. These antibodies attack the fetal red blood cells, leading to fetal anemia, which can further progress to heart failure and hydrops.[22] Currently, all pregnant women receiving prenatal care are tested for their Rh type at the beginning of pregnancy and treated with RhoGAM when necessary. If an Rh-negative woman has Rh antibodies, she is followed with antibody titers. If the titer is greater than or equal to 1:16, the fetus is monitored more closely for anemia.[22] Middle cerebral artery peak systolic velocity is monitored via pulsed-wave Doppler ultrasound.

Amniocentesis can also be performed to check the optical density of the amniotic fluid based on the heme pigment produced by hemolysis. This value, known as the ΔOD_{450} value, is plotted on a Liley curve. However, Doppler measurement of the middle cerebral artery peak systolic velocity is now the standard of care. For severe anemia, the current practice for treatment involves a fetal blood transfusion via percutaneous umbilical blood sampling (PUBS). PUBS is performed by introducing a needle into the fetal umbilical cord at the site of the cord insertion into the fetal abdomen. A small amount of blood is withdrawn, and a Coulter counter determines the fetal hematocrit. Based on this initial value, a calculation is made to determine the amount of blood that should be transfused to the fetus. Irradiated, leukodepleted, cytomegalovirus-negative, O-negative red blood cells are transfused to the fetus. This procedure may need to be repeated several times during a pregnancy until the fetus is delivered. The risks of PUBS include fetal distress, spontaneous rupture of membranes, preterm labor, and intrauterine infection.

THE FUTURE

In utero transplantation with hematopoietic stem cells can possibly treat fetuses with various congenital disorders. Gene therapy has not yet been performed in human fetuses, but experiments have been conducted with animal models. Today, many treatable inherited diseases have to be treated after birth with bone marrow transplantation, which can be complicated by lack of donor stem cells, irreversible damage in the neonate, or rejection of the donor cells. The idea of transplantation in utero is based on the theory that the fetal immune system is immature and will be more likely to overcome these problems.[23] This treatment is novel and unproven. In utero transplantation will be considered for hemoglobinopathies, immunodeficiency diseases, inborn errors of metabolism, mucolipidoses, and more. Currently, most fetal interventions are used in situations in which the fetus would die without the intervention, as in Rh isoimmunization or TTTS.

As technology advances and physicians become more proficient with these techniques, ethical considerations will arise, because interventions may exist that can be offered to correct non–life-threatening defects in utero, such as cleft lips and palates. Society will then need to weigh the cost of treating these defects in utero against the complications that can occur.

RELATED WEB SITES

- Birthplace of Fetal Surgery (fetus.ucsfmedicalcenter.org).
- Children's Hospital of Philadelphia (CHOP): Center for Fetal Diagnosis and Treatment (www.chop.edu/consumer/jsp/division/service.jsp?id=27703).
- Fetal Care Center of Cincinnati (www.fetalcarecenter.org/default.htm).

REFERENCES

1. Chervenak FA, McCullough LB, Birnbach DJ. Ethical issues in fetal surgery research. *Best Pract Res Clin Anesthesiol.* 2004;18(2):221-230.
2. Harrison MR, Globus MS, Filly RA, et al. Fetal surgical treatment. *Pediatr Ann.* 1982;22:896.
3. Harrison MR, Filly RA, Parer JT, et al. Management of the fetus with a urinary tract malformation. *JAMA.* 1982; 246(6):635.
4. Cortes RA, Farmer DL. Recent advances in fetal surgery. *Semin Perinatol.* 2004;8(3);199-211.
5. Lipitz S, Ryan G, Samuell C, et al. Fetal urine analysis for the assessment of renal function in obstructive uropathy. *Am J Obstet Gynecol.* 1993;168(1 pt 1):174.
6. Golbus MS, Harrison MR, Filly RA, et al. In utero treatment of urinary tract obstruction. *Am J Obstet Gynecol.* 1982;142:383-388.
7. Danzer E, Sydorak RM, Harrison MR, et al. Minimal access fetal surgery. *Eur J Obstet Gynecol Reprod Biol.* 2003;108:3-13.
8. University of California at San Francisco, USCF Children's Hospital. Fetal Treatment Center: The Birthplace of Fetal Surgery. Available at: fetus.ucsfmedicalcenter.org/. Accessed July 13, 2007.
9. Callen P. *Ultrasonography in Obstetrics and Gynecology.* 4th ed. Philadelphia, PA: WB Saunders; 2000.
10. Albanese CT, Lopoo J, Goldstein RB, et al. Fetal liver position and perinatal outcome for congenital diaphragmatic hernia. *J Pediatr Surg.* 1997;32(11):1634.
11. Evans MI, Harrison MR, Flake AW, et al. Fetal therapy. *Best Pract Res Clin Obstet Gynaecol.* 2002;16:671-683.
12. Adzick NS, Harrison MR, Glick PL, et al. Fetal cystic adenomatoid malformation: prenatal diagnosis and natural history. *J Pediatr Surg.* 1985;20(5):483.
13. Dillard BM, Mayer JH, McAlister WH, et al. Sacrococcygeal teratoma in children. *J Pediatr Surg.* 1970;5(1):53.
14. Bond SJ, Harrison MR, Schmidt KG, et al. Death due to high-output cardiac failure in fetal sacrococcygeal teratoma. *J Pediatr Surg.* 1990;33(2):177.
15. Langer JC, Harrison MR, Schmidt KG, et al. Fetal hydrops and death from sacrococcygeal teratoma: rationale for fetal surgery. *Am J Obstet Gynecol.* 1989; 160(5 pt 1):1145.

16. Children's Hospital of Philadelphia. The Center for Fetal Diagnosis and Treatment. Available at: www.chop.edu/consumer/jsp/division/service.jsp?id=27703. Accessed March 9, 2007.
17. Brock DJ, Barron L, Raab GM. The potential of mid-trimester maternal plasma serum alpha-fetoprotein measurement in predicting infants of low birth weight. *Br J Obstet Gynaecol.* 1980;87(7):582.
18. Nicolaides KH, Campbell S, Gabbe SG, et al. Ultrasound screening for spina bifida: cranial and cerebellar signs. *Lancet.* 1986;2(8498):72.
19. Bianchi D. *Fetology: Diagnosis and Management of the Fetal Patient.* New York, NY: McGraw-Hill; 2000.
20. Wittman BK, Baldwin VJ, Nichol F. Antenatal diagnosis of twin-twin transfusion syndrome. *Am J Obstet Gynecol.* 1981;58:123-127.
21. Fusi L, Gordon H. Multiple pregnancy complicated by single intrauterine death: problems and outcome with conservative management. *Br J Obstetr Gynaecol.* 1990;97:511-516.
22. Creasy R. *Maternal Fetal Medicine.* 5th ed. Philadelphia, PA: WB Saunders; 2004.
23. Blackman M, Kappler J, Marrack P. The role of the T-cell receptor in positive and negative selection of developing T-cells. *Science.* 1990;248:1335.

Chapter 72

ASSISTIVE REPRODUCTIVE TECHNOLOGIES, MULTIPLE BIRTHS, AND PREGNANCY OUTCOMES

Edith A. McCarthy, MD; Peter A. M. Auld, MD

INTRODUCTION

The decision to bring a child into the world is a momentous one. For some people, reproductive medicine may be necessary to realize this goal. Infertility rates in industrialized countries have risen for 3 decades, mostly as a result of couples delaying childbirth. In the United States from 1988 to 1995 the number of American women of childbearing age with fertility problems increased by 25%, from 4.9 million to 6.1 million. The Centers for Disease Control and Prevention (CDC) reports that approximately 2% of women of reproductive age (ie, 1.2 million) have had an infertility-related medical visit within the previous year, and an additional 10% have received infertility services at some time in their lives.[1] The 122,872 cycles of assisted reproductive technologies (ART) performed at reporting clinics in 2003 resulted in 35,785 live births (deliveries of 1 or more living infants) and 48,756 infants. In fact, the CDC estimates that ART accounts for slightly more than 1% of total US births.[1]

When taking a child's history, the health professional should include the history of the perinatal course, whether a history of infertility exists, and if any assistive measures were used to achieve this or previous pregnancies. In the instances when a multifetal pregnancy occurred, the discussion should include whether any associated fetal or neonatal losses occurred. Given that this issue is sensitive for many parents, such information may not be divulged spontaneously. Furthermore, many parents may have kept this information secret from close family and friends. Consequently, the health professional will need to probe gently, but thoroughly, to elicit any salient information.

The increase in infertility has been accompanied by astounding advances in the field of reproductive medicine. Since 1978, when the world's first successful human pregnancy after in vitro fertilization (IVF) was achieved, the clinical management of infertility has been completely transformed by the array of new medicines and ART, including intrauterine insemination (IUI), with or without ovulation induction, using oral clomiphene (Clomid) or injectable gonadotropins, egg donation, surrogacy, frozen embryo transfer, intracytoplasmic sperm injection (ICSI), preimplantation genetic diagnosis, assisted hatching, and cryopreservation of oocytes (eggs), embryos, and sperm. Box 72-1 provides a list of common abbreviations.

BOX 72-1 Glossary of Assisted Reproductive Treatments (ART)

THE A-B-Cs OF ART
AI: artificial insemination
AID: artificial insemination with donor sperm
COH: controlled ovarian hyperstimulation
DET: dual embryo transfer
FET: frozen embryo transfer
FTEPS: frozen-thawed epididymal spermatozoa
FTTS: frozen-thawed testicular spermatozoa
GIFT: gamete intrafallopian transfer
ICSI: intracytoplasmic sperm injection
IUI: intrauterine insemination
IVF: in vitro fertilization
MESA: microsurgical epididymal aspiration
TESE: testicular sperm extraction
ZIFT: zygote intrafallopian transfer

TREATMENT OF INFERTILITY

The following discussion is a summary of various types of assisted reproductive techniques. (Box 72-2 provides an overview of assisted conception techniques.)

Artificial Insemination With Donor Sperm and Intrauterine Insemination

Artificial insemination (AI) represents the oldest form of assisted reproduction, with attempts dating back to Princess Joana of Portugal, wife of King Henry IV of Castile, circa 1455. Efforts to develop practical methods for AI were started in Russia in 1899. IUI, a technique involving the injection of collected sperm-containing semen from a man into a woman to cause pregnancy, is used in cases of infertility or impotence or as a means by which an unmarried woman may become pregnant. Approximately 80,000 procedures using donor sperm are performed each year, resulting in the births of 30,000 babies. For many years, artificial insemination with donor sperm (AID) was the only available treatment for male factor

BOX 72-2 Overview of Assisted Conception Techniques

1. GIFT is a procedure in which eggs and sperm are placed laparoscopically in the fallopian tube where fertilization takes place.
2. ZIFT, also called tubal embryo transfer, combines IVF and GIFT. Retrieved eggs are fertilized in the laboratory and placed in the fallopian tubes rather than the uterus.
3. GIFT and ZIFT in comparison with conventional IVF:
    a. Comparable clinical pregnancy rates to the natural fecundity of the population at large.
    b. Pregnancy rates in IVF are generally lower.
    c. Disadvantage to these procedures: two successive invasive operations are required.
4. Oocyte retrieval and tubal replacement of either oocytes plus spermatozoa, two pronuclear oocytes, or cleaved embryos
5. Tubal replacement: carried out by direct access to the oviducts via the uterine cervix
6. Embryo freezing (cryopreservation): enables patients to use excess eggs and embryo
7. Donor eggs: help achieve pregnancy in women who have absent or inappropriate eggs and increase the chance of conception in women older than 40 years
8. Micromanipulation of sperm and eggs: enables fertilization and conception when sperm are defective in quantity or quality
9. Preimplantation genetic diagnosis (PGD): sampling of cells in early embryos; may be used in selecting chromosomally normal embryos for IVF procedures or in couples at risk for recessive genetic disease

GIFT, Gamete intrafallopian transfer; *IVF,* in vitro fertilization; *ZIFT,* zygote intrafallopian transfer.

infertility. Today, IUI is indicated also for idiopathic or unexplained infertility, to bypass cervical abnormalities, and to offer lesbian couples the option of childbirth. When IUI is combined with ovarian hyperstimulation, the chance of achieving a pregnancy is increased compared with IUI alone.

In Vitro Fertilization and Related Assisted Reproductive Technologies

IVF accounts for 99% of ART procedures performed by fertility clinics in the United States. IVF is an outpatient procedure that uses ovulation induction, ultrasound-guided oocyte retrieval techniques followed by IVF using sperm from the male partner or another donor, and transcervical embryo transfer 2 to 3 days after fertilization of the retrieved eggs. The procedure can be performed under sedation without the need for general anesthesia. Although IVF was originally developed to treat women who had absent or irreparable fallopian tubes, use of this procedure has since expanded widely to treat many other causes of infertility, including tubal obstruction, pelvic adhesions, endometriosis, male factor infertility, and immunologic or idiopathic infertility.

A woman's age is the single most important variable affecting success rates after IVF. Pregnancy rates drop precipitously and miscarriage rates rise in women older than 40 years because of a lack of ovarian reserve (declining number of eggs in the aging female ovary). Low ovarian reserve decreases a woman's chances for conception. To optimize success rates, many IVF programs in the United States still transfer relatively high numbers of embryos with the hope that at least one will result in a pregnancy. In fact, the 2000 National Summary and Fertility Clinic Reports of the CDC showed that 68% of ART cycles involved the transfer of three or more embryos, 34% of cycles involved the transfer of four or more, and 12% involved the transfer of five or more embryos.[2] The result has been an unprecedented increase in the incidence of multiple births. In the United States, the number of twin births has risen more than 50% over the last 2 decades since the advent of IVF, from approximately 68,000 to approximately 104,000 in 1997; furthermore, the incidence of higher-order multiple pregnancies (triplets or greater) has increased 100-fold. Detailed information regarding the current status of ART is reviewed annually in the CDC publication, *Mortality and Morbidity Weekly Review Surveillance Summaries.*[3]

Ovulation Induction

Ovulation induction, which uses ovary-stimulating drugs, has been used traditionally for women who have anovulation and oligoovulation, for whom ovulation induction improves the chance for conception each month by increasing the number of eggs that will ovulate. More recently, ovulation induction has been used in IVF cycles before IUI to enhance the number of embryos for transfer.

Intracytoplasmic Sperm Injection

ICSI represents a true revolution in assisted reproduction. ICSI involves the insertion of a single spermatozoon, selected by a trained embryologist based on its morphology and motility, into the cytoplasm of an oocyte, thereby bypassing all of the inherent obstacles for penetrating the oocyte, such as the zona pellucida.

ICSI is currently the treatment of choice for male factor infertility and for couples who have experienced previous IVF failures or low yield of eggs at egg retrieval. Male factor infertility accounts for nearly one third of all infertile couples and is caused by low sperm count, poor sperm motility, or poor sperm morphology.

PREGNANCY RATES AFTER IN VITRO FERTILIZATION

Approximately 20% of IVF pregnancies are lost, most as 1st-trimester spontaneous abortions; this number exceeds 50% in women older than 40 years.[4] The rate of loss after IVF exceeds that for spontaneous conceptions for several reasons, including the adverse effect of high ratios of estradiol to progesterone on the endometrium, an increased incidence of genetically abnormal oocytes and embryos after ovulation induction in an inherently higher-risk population, and a higher risk for ectopic pregnancy.

Table 72-1 Causes of Infertility

CAUSES OF INFERTILITY	PERCENT
Male factor	18.8
Multiple factors, women and men	17.9
Tubal factor	12.3
Multiple factors, women only	12.3
Unexplained cause	11.6
Diminished ovarian reserve	6.7
Endometriosis	6.6
Other cause	6.4
Ovulatory dysfunction	6.0

Adapted from US Department of Health and Human Services, Centers for Disease Control and Prevention. Assisted Reproductive Technology Success Rates: National Summary and Fertility Clinic Reports. Available at: www.cdc.gov/ART/ART2003/index.htm.

MAKING THE DIAGNOSIS OF INFERTILITY

A couple is considered infertile only after unprotected, well-timed intercourse for more than 12 months has failed to result in pregnancy. This rule does not apply to couples when the female is older than 35 years or when either partner has a history of fertility-related problems. *Primary infertility* (30% of infertile women) indicates that the female partner has never achieved a pregnancy; *secondary infertility* (70% of infertile women) means a previous pregnancy was achieved, regardless of outcome. Infertility, or a reduced potential for pregnancy, is distinguished from sterility, in which no chance for pregnancy exists. Most childless couples younger than 43 years who are having problems conceiving are infertile but not sterile.

Reproductive endocrinologists determine the cause of infertility and counsel the infertile couple about realistic expectations and their prognosis for future fertility. Oversimplification of success stories of ART as reported by mass media has raised patient expectations to new, and occasionally insurmountable, heights.

The most common causes of infertility are listed in Table 72-1. The cause of infertility is determined by performing a basic infertility evaluation, which includes taking a history and performing a physical examination, semen analysis, and blood tests that include follicle-stimulating hormone, luteinizing hormone, prolactin, testosterone, estradiol, progesterone, 17-OH progesterone, thyroxine, thyroid-stimulating hormone, lupus anticoagulant, anticardiolipin, and complete blood count.[5] Hysterosalpingogram and laparoscopy are indicated only if necessary to evaluate the anatomy of the endometrial cavity of the uterus and the fallopian tubes.

PERINATAL OUTCOMES AND NEONATAL ISSUES ASSOCIATED WITH ASSISTED REPRODUCTIVE TECHNOLOGIES

Although dramatic advances in reproductive technologies have offered new hope to childless couples and new opportunities to those who want to postpone childbearing, they also have raised concerns about the ultimate outcomes for infants conceived after fertility treatments such as IVF or ICSI. Parents who conceive after fertility treatments want to know if their children are at excess health risks compared with children who were conceived naturally. The 1st child conceived through the use of IVF is now 28 years of age. (Box 72-3 lists milestones in fertility medicine.) Since then, numerous scientific papers have been published on various aspects of IVF, but very few reports address perinatal complications, with even fewer studies characterizing the long-term follow-up of IVF children. Identified risks include an increased risk for preterm or low birth weight, multiple gestation, major malformations, growth delay, developmental delay (psychomotor and cognitive), infant mortality, and postnatal health problems. Concerns

BOX 72-3 Milestones in Fertility Medicine

1978: Louise Brown, the first *test tube baby*, is born in Britain.[a]

1984: The first infant created from a donor egg is born in the United States; the first infant from a frozen embryo is born in Australia.[b]

1986: A surrogate mother in New Jersey, Mary Beth Whitehead, sues to keep the baby. In a landmark case, she loses the battle for custody but wins visitation rights.

1993: The only living sextuplets in the United States are born.

1994: A postmenopausal woman in Italy uses donor eggs and her husband's sperm to give birth at age 62.

1997: The world's first living septuplets are born, 4 boys and 3 girls, after the mother received fertility drugs.[c]

1998: The world's first set of octuplets are born alive but premature, again owing to fertility agents; 1 infant died in the newborn period.

1999: A woman in New York who underwent IVF gives birth to 2 boys, 1 black and 1 white, as a result of an embryo mix-up.[d]

1999: In California, an infant is born after sperm was harvested from the deceased father and used to fertilize the egg of the mother via IVF, raising ethical questions over whether a man must consent to be a father.[e]

2006: Children who are born to mothers who conceived via artificial insemination with sperm from the same anonymous donor discover they have half-brothers and half-sisters they never knew.[f]

IVF, In vitro fertilization.

[a]Wright VC, Chang J, Jeng G, Macaluso M. Assisted reproductive technology surveillance—United States 2003. *MMWR Surveill Summ.* 2006;55(SS-4):2-22.

[b]US Department of Health and Human Services, Centers for Disease Control and Prevention, American Society for Reproductive Medicine, and Society for Assisted Reproductive Technology. *2000 Assisted Reproductive Technology Success Rates: National Summary and Fertility Clinic Reports*. December 2002. Available at: www.cdc.gov/ART/index.htm. Accessed March 7, 2007.

[c]Davis OK, Rosenwaks Z. In vitro fertilization. In: Adashi EY, Rock JA, Rosenwaks Z, eds. *Reproductive Endocrinology, Surgery, and Technology.* Philadelphia, PA: Lippincott-Raven; 1996.

[d]Yardley J. Health officials investigating to determine how woman got the embryo of another. *New York Times*. March 31, 1999.

[e]Joint Society Obstetrics and Gynaecology of Canada. Canadian Fertility and Andrology Society guideline. Pregnancy outcomes after assisted reproductive technology. *J Obstetr Gynaecol Can.* 2006;28(3):220-233.

[f]Wendy Cramer, CBS "60 Minutes". Sperm Donor Siblings Find Family Ties, March 19, 2006.

have also been raised regarding associated increased risks of genetic imprinting disorders, such as Beckwith-Weidemann syndrome and childhood cancer.

Although many studies have reported reassuring data, because of faults in methods used, study results are considered insufficient to conclude that IVF has no detrimental effect on the growth or the motor and psychological development of the children conceived with this technique. Some investigators have not found increased risks for structural abnormalities in offspring from ART pregnancies, whereas others document increased rates of adverse infant outcomes, including higher rates of birth defects. Several recent systematic reviews and meta-analyses of published studies on the outcomes of ART-assisted pregnancies are limited by the quality of the studies available for analyses. The nature of ART, however, is such that studies typically categorized as the highest quality (level I evidence)—randomized controlled clinical trials that compare one treatment strategy with another—have not been considered feasible or appropriate under current clinical practice standards. Consequently, most studies on which meta-analyses and systematic reviews have been based evaluate studies that fall within level II-1 to II-3 (controlled trial without randomization and prospective cohort or case-control studies) and level III (descriptive studies) evidence categories (Box 72-4).[6]

Congenital Malformations and Chromosomal Anomalies

Concerns regarding the risk for birth defects among infants born as the result of ART are continuing. A recent systematic review and meta-analysis identified a 30% to 40% increase in the risk of having a major birth defect resulting in the need for medical or surgical intervention.[7] Although the studies used in this analysis all had some limitation, the analysis does provide some perspective on the increased potential for a significant birth defect among infants of ART pregnancies.

Significant concerns have been raised over the possibility of adverse effects resulting from the ICSI technique, such as chromosomal abnormalities, congenital malformations, and intellectual disability. A recent study in *Pediatrics*[8] is reassuring for parents who conceived through ICSI or IVF. The findings indicate that the motor and cognitive development of children conceived through these methods is similar to that of naturally conceived children.[9] Furthermore, a recent Canadian study of the last 28 years found that the smallest surviving premature babies, many of whom were conceived via IVF, eventually attained levels of education, employment, and independence that were almost indistinguishable from those of normal-weight babies. Another recent meta-analysis conducted by Lie et al assessed the limited data comparing outcomes from ICSI pregnancies compared with conventional IVF. The authors did not find additional risks of major birth defects with ICSI.[5]

Multiple Births

The most frequent complication of IVF is multiple gestation. Since the 1970s, the national twin-birth rates have increased worldwide because of ART.[10] Approximately 35% of births after IVF in the United States in 2002 were multiple births; 4% were triplets or higher.[11] Multifetal gestation may occur resulting from ovarian hyperstimulation from ovulation induction or the implantation of multiple embryos. Ovarian stimulation alone also increases the twinning rate from a spontaneous rate of 1.2% to 5.9%. Rates of identical twinning

BOX 72-4 Effect of Assisted Reproductive Technologies on Perinatal Outcomes

1. Possible higher risk exists of obstetrical complications and perinatal mortality among untreated women with histories of infertility who conceive spontaneously (II-2).
2. Genetic counseling should be offered to couples when a history of male infertility related to sperm abnormalities is present (II-2A, II-3B).
3. Pregnancies achieved by ovulation induction and intrauterine insemination are at higher risk for perinatal complications (II-2A).

   Whether these greater risks are related to the underlying infertility itself, characteristics of the couple, or attributable to assisted reproductive techniques is unclear.
4. Pregnancies achieved by IVF with or without ICSI are at higher risk for both obstetrical and perinatal complications than spontaneous pregnancies. Similar uncertainty exists in terms of the underlying pathogenesis of these sequelae (II-2A).

   IVF-ICSI for male factor infertility should be informed about the increased risk of de novo chromosomal anomalies, primarily sex chromosome anomalies (II-2A).
5. Singleton pregnancies achieved by ART are at higher risk for adverse perinatal outcomes in comparison with spontaneous pregnancies (II-2A).
   - Perinatal mortality
   - Preterm birth
   - Low birth weight
6. Multiple gestation is a significant risk of ART, particularly gonadotropin use (II-2A).
   - Dichorionic twins are the most common.
   - Increased risk exists for monochorionic twinning.
   - Risks in assisted twin conception appears lower than in spontaneous twinning.
7. Multifetal reduction is offered for higher order multiple pregnancies (II-2A).
   - Families who have chosen this option need ongoing psychosocial support and should have counseling available to assist them with ongoing grief or loss issues.
   - Fetal growth may be compromised after multifetal reduction; consequently, careful surveillance is warranted.
8. The exact risks of ART-associated genetic imprinting and childhood cancer are unclear (III-B).

ART, Assisted reproductive technologies; *ICSI*, intracytoplasmic sperm injection; *IVF*, in vitro fertilization.

From Allen VM, Wilson RD, Cheung A, Genetics Committee of the Society of Obstetricians and Gynaecologists of Canada, et al. Pregnancy outcomes after assisted reproductive technology. *J Obstet Gynaecol Can.* 2006;28(3): 220-250. Reprinted by permission of the Society of Obstetricians and Gynaecologists of Canada.

and triplet gestation are also increased. Voluntary guidelines regarding number of IVF embryos implanted may explain the higher rates of multiple births in the United States as compared with other countries such as Britain, Finland, and Sweden.

Multifetal pregnancies are at increased risk for preterm delivery or miscarriage and have the potential for significant sequelae in the offspring, including *in utero* fetal death, low birth weight, and disability among survivors. Apparently, major morbidity—defined in this study as neonatal intensive care admission, surgical intervention, special needs, and delayed speech development—was related to multiple gestation as opposed to ART itself.[12] The risk for perinatal mortality and morbidity is 5-fold and 7-fold higher for twins and triplets, respectively. The average duration of a multifetal gestation decreases by approximately 3 weeks for each additional fetus: 37 weeks for twins, 33.5 weeks for triplets, and 31.5 weeks for quadruplets (CDC National Center for Health Statistics, 2004). This decrease has resulted in a significant debate within the reproductive medicine communities in North America and Europe about the appropriate number of embryos to implant and the role of multifetal reduction.

Multifetal pregnancy reduction (MFPR) offers an alternative to couples who have high-order multiple gestations but poses ethical and religious dilemmas for many couples. Data are limited regarding outcomes of multiple gestations with or without fetal or embryo reduction. However, reports have surfaced that outcomes for both the mother and infant after MFPR are improved.[13] Reports comparing obstetrical outcome data from quintuplets or quadruplets reduced to twins and nonreduced multiple births suggest that the obstetrical outcome of pregnancies after reduction is improved compared with the data from nonreduced pregnancies.[14] The data regarding reduction from triplet to twin gestation are less clear, with reports of both improved outcomes and no difference in outcome. In theory, reduction from triplet to twin decreases the chance of a very early prematurity and short-term morbidity. However, MFPR is itself associated with a risk for preterm delivery and fetal loss, particularly if performed after 15 weeks' gestation.[15]

The risk for multiple gestation may also be reduced by limiting the number of eggs or embryos transferred to two or one when egg or embryo quality is high. Unfortunately, many clinics continue to implant more than the recommended number of embryos in their patients in an effort to meet patient demands and achieve high success rates. Britain, Germany, Sweden, Switzerland, and other European countries have banned putting more than three embryos in women who are undergoing IVF for fear of multiple pregnancies. In the United States, the American Society for Reproductive Medicine[16] has published guidelines to assist ART programs and prospective patients in determining the appropriate number of cleavage stage (2- to 3-day embryos) that should be implanted. These guidelines specify that women under age 35 with a good prognosis should consider only one embryo and that no more than two should be transferred in this age group except under extraordinary circumstances. Women between ages 35 and 37 should receive two embryos, unless they have a poor prognosis, in which case three embryos should be the maximum implanted.

Equally important are the risks of adverse pregnancy outcome that result in maternal morbidity, with the potential for serious impact on fetal and neonatal health. The National Institutes of Health–sponsored FASTER Research Consortium has reported on the outcomes for over 36,000 pregnancies among its participating centers nationwide, noting that ovulation induction is associated with significantly increased risks for placental abruption, fetal loss after 24 weeks, and gestational diabetes. Women who are undergoing IVF experience significant increases in rates of gestational hypertension and preeclampsia, placental abnormalities (abruption, placenta previa), and cesarean delivery.[17]

Growth and Development

The long-term outcomes of children born using IVF appear similar to naturally conceived children when assessing scholastic performance, congenital malformations, and neurologic and psychomotor development.[18-22] The growth of IVF children may lag behind that of naturally conceived children during the first 3 years of life; they may also have an increased incidence of respiratory diseases and diarrhea in the neonatal period.[23] Developmental outcomes of IVF children compared with naturally conceived children are conflicting.[21,22] The most recent reports of the neurodevelopmental well being of children conceived through ICSI conclude that verbal, performance, and full-scale IQ at 5 and 8 years of age are comparable among a group of children conceived by ICSI and IVF and those conceived spontaneously.[9,24] Data on outcomes of pregnancies achieved using frozen-thawed and cryopreserved embryos suggest a slightly lower developmental index with frozen-thawed embryos, but the results were not adjusted for prematurity.[25] Long-term outcomes for children conceived by ICSI using fresh or frozen-thawed surgically retrieved spermatozoa are not known. However, both sources of sperm are equally efficacious in achieving conception.[26]

Psychosocial Effect and Family Functioning

An integral component of infertility care is the provision of counseling during the evaluation and treatment cycles. Although the body of literature regarding the mental health issues experienced by couples undergoing infertility treatment and their transition to parenthood is small and primarily women focused, the work continues to grow. In addition, interest has grown in the psychological outcomes for children who are products of reproductive technology related to parent-child relationships and parenting skills in IVF pregnancies and the potential effects of nongenetic parenting when pregnancy is achieved through the use of donor eggs or sperm. The existing literature is limited in that it tends to focus on the parenting relationships with healthy children. Little is known about the mental health issues and burdens faced by parents who have undergone fertility treatments, achieved a pregnancy, but had a sick or disabled child or experienced a fetal or neonatal loss of one or more babies in a multifetal pregnancy. Recent reports in the psychological literature suggest that stresses associated with infertility and infertility treatments may contribute to dysfunctional parenting patterns and increased susceptibility to the *vulnerable child syndrome*. Parents who make the difficult choice to reduce a multifetal pregnancy either because of a fetal abnormality in one or more babies or to improve the chances for a healthier pregnancy outcome for the mother and the remaining baby or babies experience tremendous grief, anxiety, emotional distress, and guilt. Parents must cope with conflicting feelings of joy in their surviving infant or infants and sadness and grief associated with their remembrances of the babies who died. Recognizing that mothers and fathers often use different coping mechanisms that may influence their perceptions and responses is important.[27] Golombok[28] and Hahn[29] have reviewed recent studies that suggest that ART does not appear to influence parenting and child development unduly. Two recent studies provide additional confirmation that successful ART does not predict mental health problems for parents as they transition to parenthood[30,31]

ETHICAL AND LEGAL CONSIDERATIONS

Although new techniques offer multiple reproductive choices for couples and individuals, they also have created complex ethical and legal issues.[32] For example, in ICSI, the male factor infertility that necessitated ICSI in the first place may be caused by a genetic defect, which the father may then pass unknowingly to his son. Another sensitive issue is that of posthumous reproduction. Widows can now request sperm collection and insemination with a dead husband's sperm without his prior consent or prior knowledge.[33] This capability raises ethical, practical, and legal questions concerning legitimacy, inheritance, and rights of the donor, the gestating woman, prospective rearing parent or parents, and any children who may result. Another controversial issue is that of egg freezing. When clinics freeze embryos for later use, what happens if that use never takes place? If the parents divorce or die, who gets custody of the embryos? What happens to embryos? In the United States, clinics request that parents specify how they want unused embryos handled. Some parents will donate them to other infertile couples or to scientists for research; others have them destroyed for fear of creating offspring they will never know. However, many individuals and religious institutions consider these embryos to be human beings and their disposal equivalent to murder.

Egg freezing has allowed women who are nearing menopause to freeze their own eggs for later use. This advent has increased the number of older women who have chosen to give birth beyond the typical childbearing years. In the United States, 100 women who are 50 years and older have borne children. Some ethicists believe that this circumstance is not fair to the child, and, in the words of Fr John Paris, Professor of Bioethics, "We're designing orphans by choice."[33] For this reason, few fertility clinics in the United States will treat women older than 49 years. The ethics committee of the American Society for Reproductive Medicine has issued guidelines stating, "Infertility should remain the natural characteristic of menopause."[33] However, these guidelines are voluntary, and no law prevents physicians from treating any woman who requests it. Assisted reproduction is among the least regulated medical specialties in the United States. Licensing is not required of fertility clinics in the United States.

In most of the world, IVF is covered by national health insurance. Private insurers in the United States, by contrast, often refuse to pay for it. Because each attempt costs $8000 to $10,000, patients often risk multiple births to avoid having to pay for a second visit. Although 8 states now mandate IVF coverage, in most of the United States, high-quality assisted reproductive care is available only to people who have the financial means. Although a few states have enacted legislation requiring health insurance providers to offer or provide infertility benefits, such coverage is often limited or absent altogether because of regulatory loopholes. The high cost of infertility treatment, especially the advanced ART such as IVF, has resulted in reluctance on the part of most insurance companies to provide benefits for infertility and therefore has rendered such medical intervention financially inaccessible to the general infertile population. For many women then, ovulation induction is the primary method feasible to achieve pregnancy, despite the risk of ovulation hyperstimulation and consequent multiple gestation.

CONCLUSION

ART has allowed many couples who were once considered barren or beyond childbearing age to now experience the miracle of childbirth. Furthermore, same-sex couples and single mothers or single fathers now have the option of procreating using their own genetic material through assisted reproduction often involving surrogacy. Unfortunately, technological advances often come with uncertain and often imperfect outcomes; in the case of ART, these would include multiple births, prematurity, and low birth weight. Nonetheless, evidence-based medicine points to an overwhelmingly positive result of the advances in reproductive medicine, provided physicians are responsible and follow reasonable voluntary guidelines. Primary care physicians can be instrumental in guiding families through the information-gathering and decision-making process that is necessary when faced with the obstacle of infertility.

TOOLS FOR PRACTICE

Engaging Patients and Family

- *Early Arrival: Information for Parents of Premature Infants* (booklet), American Academy of Pediatrics (www.aap.org/bookstore).

Medical Decision Support

- *2003 Assisted Reproductive Technology (ART) Report*, Centers for Disease Control and Prevention (www.cdc.gov/art/art2003/).

SUGGESTED RESOURCES

Baude P, Rowell P. Assisted conception: II. In vitro fertilisation and intracytoplasmic sperm injection. *BMJ*. 2003;327: 852-855.

Baude P, Rowell P. Assisted conception: III. Problems with assisted conception. *BMJ*. 2003;327:920-923.

Nguyen RHN, Wilcox AJ. Terms in reproductive and perinatal epidemiology: I. Reproductive terms. *J Epidem Comm Health*. 2005;59(11):916-919.

Nguyen RHN, Wilcox AJ. Terms in reproductive and perinatal epidemiology: II. Perinatal terms. *J Epidem Comm Health*. 2005;59(12):1019-1021.

Pickering S, Baude P. Further advances and uses of assisted conception technology. *BMJ*. 2003;327:1156-1158.

Rowell P, Baude P. Assisted conception: I. General principles. *BMJ*. 2003;327:799-801.

REFERENCES

1. US Department of Health and Human Services, Centers for Disease Control and Prevention. *Assisted Reproductive Technology Success Rates: National Summary and Fertility Clinic Reports*. December 2003. Available at: www.cdc.gov/ART/ART2003/index.htm. Accessed March 7, 2007.
2. US Department of Health and Human Services, Centers for Disease Control and Prevention, American Society for Reproductive Medicine, and Society for Assisted Reproductive Technology. *2000 Assisted Reproductive Technology Success Rates: National Summary and Fertility Clinic Reports*. December 2002. Available at: www.cdc.gov/ART/index.htm. Accessed March 7, 2007.
3. Wright VC, Chang J, Jeng G, et al. Assisted reproductive technology surveillance—United States 2003. *MMWR Surveill Summ*. May 2006;55(SS-4):2-22.
4. Davis OK,Rosenwaks Z. In vitro fertilization. In: Adashi EY, Rock JA, Rosenwaks Z, eds. *Reproductive Endocrinology, Surgery, and Technology*. Philadelphia, PA: Lippincott-Raven; 1996.
5. Lie RT, Lyngstadaas A, Orstavik KH, et al. Birth defects in children conceived by ICSI compared with children conceived by other IVF-methods: a meta-analysis. *Int J Epidemiol*. 2005;34:696-701.
6. Joint Society Obstetrics and Gynaecology of Canada. Canadian Fertility and Andrology Society guideline. Pregnancy outcomes after assisted reproductive technology. *J Obstetr Gynaecol Can*. 2006;28(3):220-233.
7. Hansen M, Bower C, Milne E, et al. Assisted reproductive technologies and the risk of birth defects—a systematic review. *Human Reprod*. 2005;20(2):328-338.
8. Kristoffersen P, Sutcliffe AG, Bonduelle M, et al. International collaborative study of intracytoplasmic sperm injection-conceived, in vitro fertilization-conceived, and naturally conceived 5-year-old child outcomes: cognitive and motor assessments. *Pediatrics*. 2005;15(3):e283-e289.
9. Leunens L, Celestin-Westreich S, Bonduelle M, et al. Cognitive and motor development of 8 year-old children born after ICSI compared to spontaneously conceived children. *Human Reproduct*. 2006;21(11):2922-2929.
10. Pinborg A. IVF/ICSI twin pregnancies: risks and prevention. *Human Reprod Update*. 2005;11(6):575-593.
11. Centers for Disease Control and Prevention. 2002 Assisted Reproductive Technology Report (ART). Available at: www.cdc.gov/ART/ART02/index.htm. Accessed March 7, 2007.
12. Pinborg A, Loft A, Schmidt L, et al. Morbidity I a Danish national cohort of 472 IVF/ICSI twins, 1132 non-IVF/ICSI twins and 634 IVF/ICSI singletons: health-related and social implications for the children and their families. *Human Reprod*. 2003;18(6):1234-1243.
13. Souter I, Goodwin M. Decision making in multifetal pregnancy reduction for triplets. *Am J Perinatol*. 1998; 15:63-71.
14. Berkowitz RL, Stone J, Alvarez M. The current status or multifetal pregnancy reduction. *Am J Obstet Gynecol*. 1996;174:1265-1272.
15. Antsaklis A, Souka AP, Daskalakis G, et al. Pregnancy outcome after multifetal pregnancy reduction. *J Matern Fetal Neonat Med*. 2004;16(1):27-31.
16. American Society of Reproductive Medicine, Practice Committee of the Society for Assisted Reproductive Technology. Guidelines on the number of embryos transferred. *Fertil Steril*. 2004;82(3):773-774.
17. Shevell T, Malone FD, Vidaver J, et al. Assisted reproductive technology and pregnancy outcome. *Obstet Gynecol*. 2005;106:1039-1045.
18. Mushlin DN, Spensley A, Hanson BM. Children of IVF. *J Clin Obstet*. 1985;12:865.
19. Morin N, Wirth FBL, Johnson DH, et al. Congenital malformations and psychological development in children conceived by IVF. *J Pediatr*. 1989;115:222.
20. Brandes JM, Itzkovits J, Scher A, et al. Growth and development of children conceived by IVF. *Pediatrics*. 1992;90:424.
21. Saunders K, Spensley J, Munro J, et al. Growth and physical outcome of children conceived by in vitro fertilization. *Pediatrics*. 1996;98:688.
22. Oliviennes F, Kerbrat V, Rufat P, et al. Follow up of a cohort of 422 children aged 6 to 13 years conceived by in vitro fertilization. *Fertil Steril*. 1997;67:284.
23. Koivurova S, Hartikainen AL, Sovio U, et al. Growth, psychomotor development and morbidity up to 3 years of age in children born after IVF. *Hum Reprod*. 2003; 18(11):2328-2336.
24. Ponjaert-Kristoffersen I, Bonduelle M, Barnes J, et al. International collaborative study of intracytoplasmic sperm injection-conceived, in vitro fertilization-conceived, and naturally conceived 5-year old child outcomes: cognitive and motor assessments. *Pediatrics*. 2005;115(3):e283-e289.
25. Sutcliffe AG, D'Souza SW, Cadman J, et al. Outcome in children from cryopreserved embryos. *Arch Dis Child*. 1995;72:290.
26. Ulug U, Bener F, Karagenc L, et al. Outcomes in couples undergoing ICSI: comparison between fresh and frozen-thawed surgically retrieved spermatozoa. *Int J Androl*. 2005;28:343-349.
27. Peterson BD, Newton CR, Rosen KH, et al. Gender differences in how men and women who are referred for IVF cope with infertility stress. *Human Reprod*. 2006;21(9): 2443-2449.
28. Golombok S, MacCallum F. Practitioner review: outcomes for parents and children following non-traditional conception: what clinicians need to know. *J Child Psychol Psychiatry*. 2003;44(3):303-315.
29. Hahn CS. Review: psychosocial well-being of parents and their children born after assisted reproduction. *J Pediatr Psychol*. 2001;26(8):525-538.
30. Golombok S, Murray C, Jadva V, et al. Non-genetic and non-gestational parenthood: consequences for parent-child relationships and the psychological well-being of mothers, fathers and children at age 3. *Human Reprod*. 2006;21(7):1918-1924.
31. Repokari L, Punamaki RL, Poikkeus P, et al. The impact of successful assisted reproduction treatment on female and male mental health during transition to parenthood: a prospective controlled study. *Hum Reprod*. 2005; 20(11):3238-3247.
32. Soini S, Ibaretta D, Anastasiadon V, et al. The interface between medically assisted reproduction and genetics: technical, social, ethical and legal issues. *European Society of Human Reproduction and Embryology Monographs*. 2006;1:2-51.
33. American Society for Reproductive Medicine, Ethics Committee. Ethical considerations of assisted reproductive technologies. *Fertil. Steril*. 1998;82:4-7.

Perinatal Care: Caring for the High-Risk Infant

Chapter 73

FETAL ASSESSMENT

E. Rebecca Pschirrer, MD, MPH; George A. Little, MD

Pediatricians, as primary care physicians and as subspecialist neonatologists, consult and work collaboratively with obstetric providers in preconception counseling, fetal risk identification, and peripartum decisions. They assume primary responsibility for resuscitation, stabilization, and ongoing care of the neonate from the moment of birth. Years ago, pediatricians first saw their newborn patients in the nursery, but only after the events of pregnancy and delivery.

Knowledge of fetal health includes appreciation of the interaction of the fetus with the mother, father, health professionals, and society. Now, many examples exist of the ability of fetal medicine, as part of preconception and prenatal care, to prevent or treat problems and to improve outcomes.

Parents and professionals have good reason to be concerned about the immediate and long-term effects of agents or processes on the fetus. Infections such as rubella can result in the loss of the fetus or in multisystem disease. The magnitude and seriousness of manifestations of maternal alcohol consumption, tobacco use, or substance abuse during pregnancy may be evident in the infant's physical appearance or behavior in the neonatal period and throughout the infant's life span. Furthermore, problems may not appear until a subsequent generation. The effects of diethylstilbestrol, once given to mothers for threatened abortion, did not present until the appearance of clear cell carcinoma of the vagina in female offspring 10 to 20 years later.[1]

Growth and development are as much a key to fetal medicine as they are to pediatrics, of which study of the fetus is merely the first installment. Human growth and development must be regarded as a continuum that begins with conception (Figure 73-1). This chapter outlines some of the normal physical and interactive aspects of fetal existence, then discusses selected pathophysiological states that may adversely affect that existence.

MATERNAL CONDITIONS THAT AFFECT THE FETUS AND NEWBORN

Many authorities have pointed to socioeconomic status and social environment as causes of fetal risk. Delineation of specific influences is difficult, but poverty is undoubtedly important, as are nutrition and hygiene. Intrauterine infection is more frequent in mothers of lower socioeconomic status. Emotional influences on fetal wastage have been discussed; in addition, the possibility that medical or socioeconomic deprivation contributes cannot be discounted.

Maternal Nutrition

Maternal nutritional disorders represent a definite risk to the fetus, including situations in which gross deprivation is not apparent. The supply of substrate to the fetus for growth originates with the maternal circulation and passes through an interface with fetal tissue at the placenta. Placental insufficiency can result in intrauterine growth restriction (IUGR) that is not of maternal origin. The relationship between maternal and fetal nutrition is complex. Maternal dietary changes usually do not directly or rapidly influence fetal well being; thus the positive or negative effects of changes in maternal nutrition are not easily recognized. Maternal weight is an important but not overriding concern.

Traditionally, two types of nutritional deficiency have been conceptualized: (1) general caloric or energy-related deficiency states and (2) specific deficiencies. Deprivation of maternal caloric intake to the point at which fetal growth is markedly impaired also may be associated with specific deficiencies. If maternal caloric deprivation is severe, then fertility is decreased.

Women whose prepregnancy weight is below standard for height tend to have babies whose weight is less than expected. Women who are obese tend to have heavier babies. Problems such as hyperemesis gravidarum can be sufficient to result in fetal caloric deprivation. The mother's expression of eating disorders that often start during late childhood and adolescence is a possible fetal risk.

Specific deficiencies are well recognized; their risk to the fetus can be reduced through public health and individual clinical interventions. Vitamin deficiencies are of interest, and problems such as congenital beriberi (lack of thiamin) and infant calcium disorders (lack of maternal vitamin D) are of historic interest and

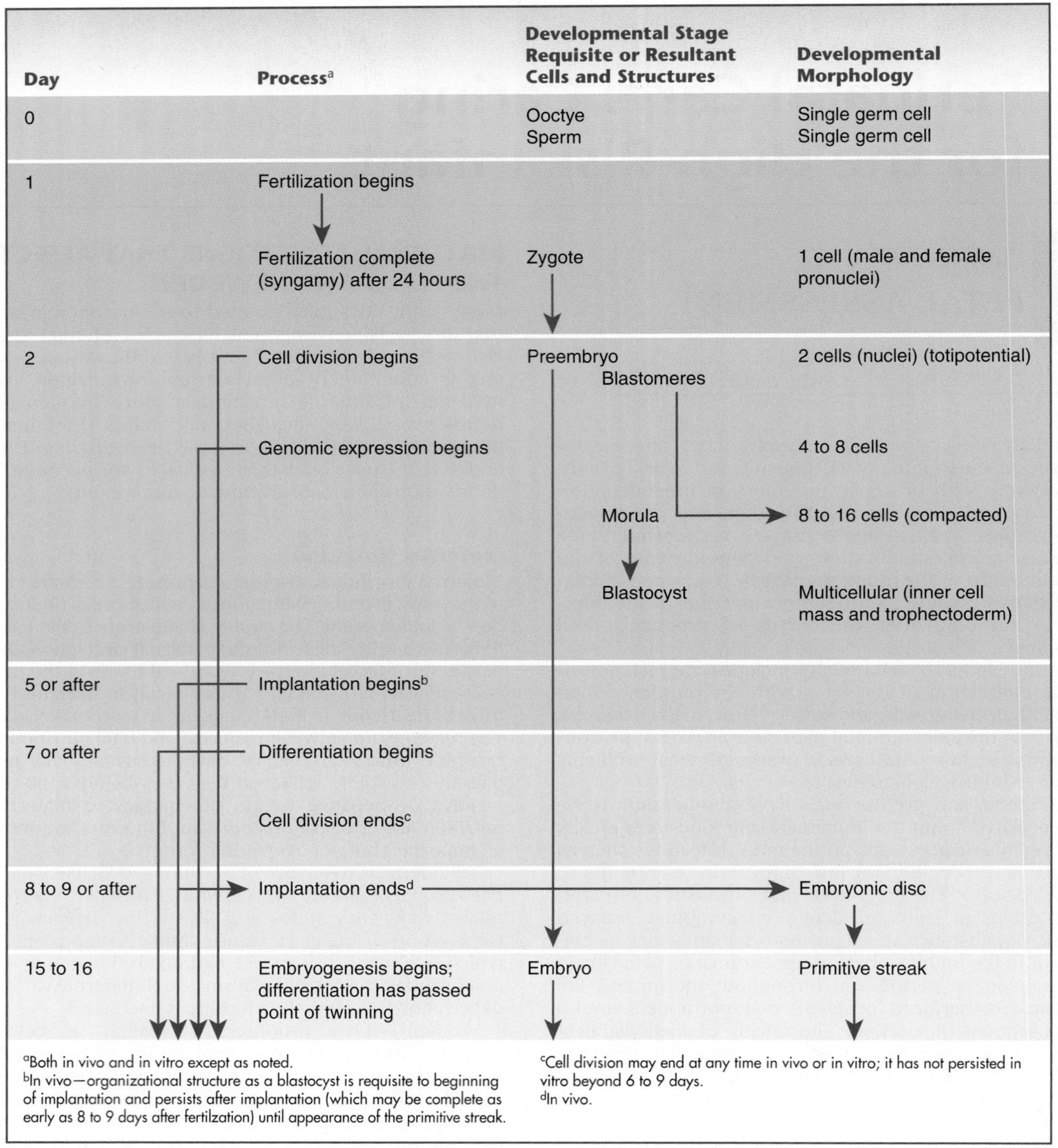

Early In Vivo and In Vitro Human Development Process

Day	Process[a]	Developmental Stage Requisite or Resultant Cells and Structures	Developmental Morphology
0		Ooctye Sperm	Single germ cell Single germ cell
1	Fertilization begins Fertilization complete (syngamy) after 24 hours	Zygote	1 cell (male and female pronuclei)
2	Cell division begins Genomic expression begins	Preembryo Blastomeres Morula Blastocyst	2 cells (nuclei) (totipotential) 4 to 8 cells 8 to 16 cells (compacted) Multicellular (inner cell mass and trophectoderm)
5 or after	Implantation begins[b]		
7 or after	Differentiation begins Cell division ends[c]		
8 to 9 or after	Implantation ends[d]		Embryonic disc
15 to 16	Embryogenesis begins; differentiation has passed point of twinning	Embryo	Primitive streak

[a]Both in vivo and in vitro except as noted.
[b]In vivo—organizational structure as a blastocyst is requisite to beginning of implantation and persists after implantation (which may be complete as early as 8 to 9 days after fertilzation) until appearance of the primitive streak.
[c]Cell division may end at any time in vivo or in vitro; it has not persisted in vitro beyond 6 to 9 days.
[d]In vivo.

Figure 73-1 Fetal and child development begins with fertilization and is similar in vivo and in vitro for 6 to 9 days. (Reprinted from Using preimplantation embryos for research. ACOG Committee Opinion No. 347. American College of Obstetricians and Gynecologists. Obstet Gynecol 2006;108:1305-1317. Used by permission.)

decreasing incidence. Studies have confirmed that neural tube defects can be reduced by consuming folic acid, with the best protection being achieved when 0.4 mg is ingested from at least 1 month before conception through the first month of pregnancy.[2]

Minerals are a major concern in pregnancy. Iodine deficiency is said to be the most common cause of preventable mental deficiency in the world; treatment during pregnancy protects the fetal brain, with later treatment being much less beneficial to neurologic status.[3] Zinc deficiency may also be associated with anomalies. Maternal anemia caused by reduced availability of iron is well known; the fetus and infant, as a result, can have low iron stores, making the infant susceptible to iron deficiency if intake after birth is inadequate.

Environmental factors, such as radiation, chemicals, and drugs, affect people of all socioeconomic classes. Radiation exposure in mammals causes fetal death, growth retardation, and congenital malformation, with the central nervous system (CNS) commonly affected. The relationship between embryonic or fetal irradiation and carcinogenesis is unclear. Effects are both dose and rate related. Death during the preimplantation period, malformation during early organogenesis, and cell deletion and hypoplasia during fetal life form a general pattern in animal studies. Guidelines exist for limiting radiation to the embryo and fetus during occupational exposure or elective diagnostic techniques; however, dilemmas often arise as a result of lack of foreknowledge about pregnancy, nonelective medical evaluations, and emotional factors. When necessary, a radiation physicist should be consulted.

Chemicals in the environment are of natural and synthetic origin, with the latter being of greater concern. Certain substances, such as pesticides and mercury, have received publicity, although more study of other potential environmental toxins is needed. Many agents are potentially more toxic to the embryo, fetus, and neonate than to older children and adults.

Mercury exposure is a major issue in environmental health, in large part because of its toxicity to the brain, especially the more susceptible fetal brain. Mercury is common in the environment in small amounts and occurs in three forms: (1) the metallic element, (2) inorganic salts, and (3) organic compounds. Exposure to predatory fish is the primary exposure, and local fish advisory bans are available from the US Environmental Protection Agency.[4] Women planning pregnancy, women who are pregnant or breastfeeding, and children younger than 15 years have been advised to avoid eating swordfish or shark and to limit the amount of tuna eaten. Updates on information regarding the safety of fish and shellfish, as well as resources for local health departments, may be found through the US Environmental Protection Agency.[4] *Consumer Reports* found variable amounts of mercury during testing of different brands of tuna.[5] Thimerosal, a mercury-containing preservative used in some vaccines, has been the subject of concern and controversy, resulting in its no longer being used in vaccines despite the lack of evidence of causality.[6] (See Chapter 29, Immunizations.)

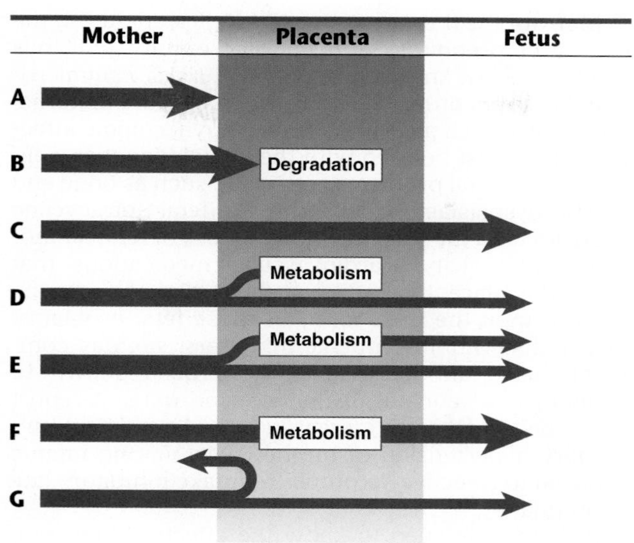

Figure 73-2 Maternal-fetal transport patterns and the role of the placenta, a fetal organ with active metabolic activity. **A,** Placental barrier with minimal uptake or transfer (eg, succinylcholine, highly charged quaternary compounds). **B,** Active placental uptake and degradation without transfer as seen with insulin. **C,** Placental uptake and transfer without significant change as with bilirubin. **D,** Placenta actively involved in uptake, partial use, and transfer (oxygen, glucose, amino acids, free fatty acids). **E,** Uptake, partial metabolism, and transfer (cyclosporine). **F,** Placenta actively modifies during transfer (25-hydroxyvitamin D_3). **G,** Carrier-coupled uptake occurs with release of ligand to the fetus and regeneration of carrier on the maternal side (transferrin-iron). *(Adapted from Pridjian G. Feto-maternal interactions: placental physiology and its role as a go-between. In: Avery GB, Fletcher MA, MacDonald MG, eds.* Avery's Neonatology: Pathophysiology and Management in the Newborn. *5th ed. Philadelphia, PA: Lippincott Williams & Wilkins;1999. Reprinted by permission.)*

Drugs and Other Substances

Drug use during pregnancy is epidemic and may be on the rise. All physicians must be concerned about all types of drug use: legitimate (nonprescription and prescription), social, illegal, and abusive. All health care professionals, especially the primary care physician, should recognize that the concept of the placenta as an effective toxic-substance barrier between maternal and fetal circulation has been discarded.

The maternal-fetal pharmacologic mechanism is complex, with the placenta serving as an organ of exchange (Figure 73-2). Placental diffusing capability or permeability of the simple variety operates for many substances; energy-utilizing transport is also important. Virtually all drugs in the maternal circulation should be assumed to cross the placenta, and all should be considered potentially teratogenic. The risk to the fetus depends on several factors, including concentration of the substance, length of exposure, and when exposure occurs during gestation.

Therapeutic agents, both prescribed and nonprescribed, may be taken before pregnancy is recognized, thereby placing the products of conception at risk during the period of organogenesis in early gestation. An important benefit of preconception or interconception care is the opportunity to identify medication uses that are necessary, such as anticonvulsants, or desirable, such as nonnarcotic analgesics, and monitor or modify exposure. Examples of problems include fetal hydantoin syndrome and the potential effects on the mother and fetus of aspirin, including clotting abnormalities and disruption of prostaglandin synthesis.

Many of the therapeutic agents indicated during the course of pregnancy and delivery require judicious use because of known and potential risks. Antimicrobial therapy is often necessary when treating maternal conditions, such as urinary tract or gynecologic infections, but must be used with the knowledge that well-recognized fetal problems can result, such as bone and dental dysplasias associated with fetal tetracycline exposure and the potential hearing loss of fetal aminoglycoside toxicity. Cardiovascular medications that cross the placenta readily, such as digitalis, can be used to treat the fetus and can cause fetal problems. Selected serotonin reuptake inhibitors, such as commonly used antidepressants, have been shown to result in mild neonatal abstinence syndrome.[7] A report has been issued of an increased rate of persistent pulmonary hypertension of the newborn among infants exposed to selective serotonin reuptake inhibitors late in pregnancy.[8]

Pediatricians need to know the effects of obstetric drugs on the fetus, including narcotics, oxytocin, and magnesium sulfate, which can cause depressed respiration, hyperbilirubinemia, and hypotonia, respectively. Socially used and abused drugs are very well known to pediatricians for their deleterious effect on the fetus, newborn, child, and adult. Mothers who smoke have babies who are smaller than those of nonsmokers by an average of 200 g. Varied active agents in smoke, such as carbon monoxide and nicotine, have physiological effects. Evidence suggests that antenatal exposure to environmental tobacco smoke affects early childhood cognitive development. Infants exposed to tobacco smoke pre- and postnatally are at increased risk for childhood asthma, respiratory infections, otitis media, and sudden infant death syndrome, as well as later behavioral problems and increased rates of adolescent smoking.[9,10] The clear medical consensus is that smoking is a health hazard for the fetus and newborn. Maternal alcohol consumption is associated with fetal alcohol syndrome and should be discouraged during pregnancy in all trimesters, although demonstrating deleterious effects is difficult from small amounts consumed.

Addictive drug use during pregnancy creates major medical and societal problems of seemingly increasing and endlessly complex proportions. Many, if not most, users have lifestyles that include factors such as poor nutrition or lack of prenatal care that present significant background risk regardless of the addictive agent. Heroin is known to reach the fetus soon after maternal use, with intrauterine dependency and withdrawal recognized. Treatment programs that use methadone or buprenorphine are recognized as preferable alternatives to continued illicit opioid abuse, although neonatal withdrawal is still a concern.[11] Outcomes of women and infants in treatment programs are significantly better than for those women not enrolled in treatment.[12]

Cocaine is considered to be responsible, directly or indirectly, for many admissions to neonatal intensive care units. Cocaine use can result in problems such as placental abruption that compromise the fetal and neonatal cardiovascular and neurologic systems. Investigative efforts to characterize and quantify long-term neurodevelopmental effects are ongoing. (See Chapter 103, Prenatal Drug Abuse and Neonatal Drug Withdrawal Syndrome.)

Identification of environmental and lifestyle risks relies largely on the maternal medical history. When specific factors such as radiation or chemical exposure are detected, assessment of fetal well being, especially its growth and morphology, may be helpful. In many situations, however, decisions to continue or terminate pregnancy are made based on nebulous possible fetal effects, may involve parental emotions and values, and may require compassionate, nondirective counseling in addition to the presentation of available scientific knowledge.

Dental Health

Women with periodontal disease are at increased risk of preterm birth[13] compared with women without periodontal disease. The increasing popularity of oral jewelry, including lip and tongue piercing, has been associated with higher incidence of periodontal disease.[14] A study that directly relates oral piercing to increased preterm delivery has yet to be accomplished; however, clearly, women who are planning a pregnancy should pursue regular dental care, with treatment of poor dentition and gingivitis, and should be encouraged to avoid oral piercing.[15]

Maternal Reproductive Capability and Health

Certain maternal factors result in fetal risk. Pregnancy can produce physiological changes in the mother that may complicate preexisting maternal conditions, thereby jeopardizing the fetus. For example, mothers who have asymptomatic cardiac disease may decompensate when they become pregnant.

Maternal biological factors such as age, weight, height, race, parity, and previous obstetric history directly affect fetal risk. Perinatal mortality increases at the extremes of maternal age; the relative risk of stillbirth increases with maternal age, regardless of medical comorbidity, parity, or race and ethnicity.[16] One large observational study determined the lowest risk to be in the 16- to 19-year range.[17] However, such observations should not be taken to encourage adolescent pregnancies; pregnancy in those younger than age 16 has definite associated risks, and pregnancy throughout the teenage years is associated with medical and social morbidity.[18] Newborn weight and height are related to maternal nutrition, socioeconomic status, and other variables, which may jeopardize the fetus by increasing the incidence of prematurity or intrapartum complications. Race is a complex factor that includes socioeconomic considerations; some congenital anomalies and medical conditions may be racially predisposed. Congenital maternal reproductive tract abnormalities are frequently associated with spontaneous abortion and with prematurity. Cervical insufficiency occurs in 1 in 500 to 600 pregnancies and can result in premature delivery. The interval between pregnancies is an important contributor to the risk of low birth weights.

Maternal medical disorders carry a significant risk to both fetus and mother. Cyanotic congenital heart disease in a mother is clearly related to fetal problems, including IUGR and prematurity. Elective abortion should be considered if maternal cardiac decompensation later in the pregnancy is anticipated. Asthma can threaten mother and fetus but is commonly well controlled with medication. Tuberculosis demands aggressive management of maternal disease with attention to potential fetal exposure to drugs. Pregnancy in women who have cystic fibrosis presents the fetus with a variety of medications, maternal pulmonary insufficiency, and possible nutritional deficiency.

Preexisting and new-onset renal disease can complicate pregnancy. Fetal risk increases markedly in the presence of maternal proteinuria, impaired renal function, and hypertension. Hypertension can result in placental changes leading to IUGR. Adverse fetal outcome from urinary tract infection relates primarily to the risk of premature birth. Successful pregnancy is possible in women with kidney transplants, with the best outcomes seen among women who have stable renal function, time since transplantation of at least 2 years, and no evidence of rejection. Some risks are associated with exposure to immunosuppressants, such as corticosteroids, but they do not prohibit a good outcome.

Maternal hematologic problems are very common. In developing countries, anemia has been demonstrated to correlate with low birth weight; the effect of moderate maternal iron deficiency on the fetus is unclear. Some hemoglobinopathies can profoundly increase fetal mortality and morbidity, either as a result of maternal health status or of fetal disease. Pregnant patients who have sickle cell disease require close attention. Immune sensitization problems (Rh, ABO) are discussed later and in Chapter 82, Maternal Medical History.

Maternal metabolic disorders can be significant for the fetus. The interaction of mother and fetus seems limitless; compounds are metabolized actively on both sides of the placenta; fetal organogenesis and development may be affected; and fetal end organs may respond to maternal abnormalities. Two conditions, diabetes and thyroid disorder, deserve special mention.

Diabetes in pregnancy causes a myriad of fetal complications, including stillbirth, increased frequency of congenital anomalies, macrosomia (a large-for-gestational-age state characterized by an increase in fat but not in total body water), and conversely, growth restriction in a small number of infants. Evidence suggests that fetal pulmonary and neurologic maturity may be delayed in these pregnancies. In addition, obstetric problems, including preeclampsia, hydramnios, and intrapartum complications, resulting from excessive size, increase risk further. Glucose is a primary metabolite of the fetus. Pregnancies complicated by diabetes may cause fluctuations in maternal-fetal glucose, with resultant fetal hyperinsulinism and hypoglycemia. These fetuses have an increase in pancreatic islet tissue, leading to fetal hyperinsulinism, which may be associated with a growth hormone effect that results in macrosomia. Severe maternal diabetes, especially when complicated by prepregnancy vascular disease, may result in small fetuses rather than macrosomia because of placental insufficiency and fetal nutritional deficit. Close control of maternal diabetes results in a better overall perinatal outcome.[19]

Maternal thyroid disease is much less common than diabetes but also has profound fetal effects. Fetal thyroid function appears by 12 weeks' gestation; thyroxine and triiodothyronine can cross the placenta in small amounts in either direction. Classic cretinism, a reflection of maternal and fetal hypothyroidism, includes obvious fetal neurodevelopmental problems and is a result of endemic iodine deficiency or autoimmune maternal thyroiditis. Evidence is accumulating that maternal hypothyroidism, even when subclinical, interferes with normal fetal brain development and may be prevented by maternal screening and treatment.[20] Spontaneous loss, stillbirths, anomalies, and prematurity can be associated with hypothyroidism. Increases in maternal thyroid replacement hormone are generally necessary during pregnancy. Hyperthyroidism, when untreated, increases fetal wastage. Its treatment, however, carries a definite risk to the fetus because antithyroid drugs may affect the fetal thyroid, and surgical intervention carries an operative risk to fetus and mother. Postoperative treatment with thyroid replacement therapy may minimize fetal complications.

Although seizure disorders are common, their course during pregnancy is difficult to predict with certainty. The status of approximately one half of those affected is unchanged, and of the remaining number, one half improve and one half become worse. Status epilepticus is an emergency for the mother and fetus. Some anticonvulsants, such as trimethadione and valproic acid, are clearly teratogenic. Carbamazepine is associated with an increased risk of neural tube defect. Phenytoin has been linked with a fetal hydantoin syndrome, although the actual incidence is much debated. Phenobarbital, carbamazepine, phenytoin, and other medications have a broad-based impact on fetal enzymatic systems; they are associated with vitamin K–dependent coagulation factor deficiency in neonates. Many perinatologists suggest additional supplementation of vitamin K in the last month of pregnancy. Women who have epilepsy have an approximately 1 in 40 chance that their children will develop the same condition.

Seizures that appear de novo in pregnancy must be thoroughly evaluated. Eclampsia usually produces other signs and symptoms and is associated with a high incidence of fetal and neonatal complications.

Maternal emotional status presents too complex a relationship with physical and familial status to be used as a specific fetal risk factor in most situations. Whether maternal emotional illness not related to pregnancy can affect the fetus directly is unclear. Pregnancy-caused or pregnancy-aggravated crises leading to abortion, drug abuse, or poor maternal nutrition generate obvious fetal consequences.

Placenta and Membrane Disorders

The placenta and associated membranes are tissues on which the fetus depends for respiration, nutrition, protection, and other functions. Manifestations of placental disease are diverse and severe and include fetal death, distress, hypoxia, shock, anemia, polycythemia, infection, congenital anomalies, and neoplasia.

The implantation site is normally in the upper uterus but may be in the lower segment, in the tubes, or, rarely, in the abdominal cavity. Maternal anatomic factors may contribute to abnormal implantations. Abdominal and tubal (ectopic) pregnancies are potential disasters for both mother and fetus; except for a rare surviving abdominal fetus, fetal wastage is nearly uniform, and maternal mortality and morbidity are common.

Placenta previa is associated with multiparity and places the fetus at risk in the event of hemorrhage; premature delivery, usually by cesarean section, is necessary. Abruption of the placenta often is associated with maternal problems, including preeclampsia, hypertension, renal disease, and multiparity. Sudden fetal death may occur after an extensive placental separation; lesser degrees of separation can result in hypoxia and acute fetal stress. Bleeding from placenta previa and abruption is usually maternal but can be fetal and sufficient to cause fetal hypovolemia and anemia.

Cord abnormalities are unusual but may have severe consequences. A short umbilical cord may be complicated by abruption. True knots are unusual, but they do occur and can cause fetal stress. Vasa previa and velamentous cord insertion are difficult to identify before labor but can result in nonreassuring fetal status or fetal exsanguination. A circumvallate placenta is associated with fetal growth restriction. Vascular abnormalities within the main placental structure occur rarely; fetal risk in monochorionic multiple pregnancies includes the possibility of twin-to-twin transfusion syndrome, in which arteriovenous vascular anastomoses result in blood flow between the fetuses and in severe circulatory problems for recipient, donor, or both.

A vascular abnormality of the cord observed in 1% of pregnancies is a two-vessel cord with a single umbilical artery, rather than the normal two. Current evidence suggests that anomalies may be associated with a two-vessel cord.[21,22] The risk of associated abnormalities, including fetal growth restriction, renal abnormalities, and aneuploidy, is approximately 7%.

Premature rupture of membranes (PROM) is a major contributor to perinatal mortality and morbidity. It is defined as rupture that occurs before the onset of labor and is usually spontaneous. Artificial rupture of membranes may be accidental during an examination or may be used to augment labor. Regardless of classification the prenatal care team must be aware that an inevitable process of increased fetal risk begins soon after rupture and that prospective treatment protocols are desirable. Most protocols stipulate evaluation and treatment in relation to the time since rupture. Prolonged rupture of membranes, which most authorities consider to be 18 hours after rupture, is the beginning of increased risk.

The primary cause of fetal and maternal morbidity and mortality in prolonged rupture of membranes is sepsis. At term, labor occurs within 24 hours of rupture in 80% of pregnancies; in preterm pregnancies, labor begins within 24 hours in less than 50%. The cause of preterm PROM is often not clear, and except for entities such as an incompetent cervix or history of a preterm delivery, no statistical correlation has been found with prior risk factors.

The frequency and degree of inflammation of membranes, cord, or fetus vary directly with time and onset of labor. Infection apparently ascends to the fetus through the cervix, with labor accelerating the process. Antibiotics given before delivery are of uncertain value in providing effective maternal treatment, but they do prevent some cases of sepsis in the fetus and newborn. Such is particularly the case of chemoprophylaxis for prevention of group B streptococcal (GBS) infection. Current practice recommendations include culture of all pregnant women for GBS infection between 35 and 37 weeks' estimated gestational age, with treatment at the time of labor with intravenous antibiotics for those found to be positive.[23] Women with GBS urinary colonization or women who have previously had an infant with invasive GBS disease should receive intrapartum chemoprophylaxis; prenatal culture screening is not necessary.[24]

A dilemma in fetal risk management occurs in the PROM pregnancy that is significantly preterm. The fetus in this situation is at risk not only from infection, but also from premature birth and its complications, especially respiratory distress syndrome. The clinician has available prepartum agents (corticosteroids) that seem to accelerate pulmonary maturity and improve postpartum status overall in certain populations. A 2000 National Institutes of Health Consensus Development Conference reiterates the previous recommendation for antenatal treatment with corticosteroids for fetuses between 24 and 32 weeks that have preterm PROM.[25] The consensus statement also clarifies the recommendation that only one course of corticosteroids should be provided during any given pregnancy.

There may be an increased risk of neurologic sequelae among babies born prematurely after PROM. An increased incidence of periventricular leukomalacia and cerebral palsy seems to be at least associated with, if not caused by, intraamniotic infection. Whether immediate induced vaginal delivery or cesarean section delivery with preterm PROM will decrease these risks is unknown at present.

Maternal-Fetal Unit

Fetal risk and poor perinatal outcomes are frequently associated with pathophysiological processes in which both mother and fetus play an integral role. Causality in some situations is well understood, as in, for example, alloimmunization, but causality for other situations such as preeclampsia is not yet clear.

Premature Birth

Prematurity and its complications are the prime contributors to perinatal mortality and morbidity. The problems of prematurity and low birth weight are similar but not identical.

The prevention and management of premature birth has been and remains the primary objective of perinatal care providers. Prematurity is multifactorial in origin, and its causes will likely remain unclear for the foreseeable future, inasmuch as the precise mechanisms that cause normal labor have yet to be elucidated. Many factors that contribute to fetal risk precipitate adverse outcomes directly or indirectly through premature birth.[26]

Pharmacologic Intervention

Tocolysis, or inhibition of uterine activity, is therapy directed at preventing premature birth once labor has begun. Pharmacologic agents have been used with this intent for years with minimal success.

The theoretical basis for the use of ß-mimetic drugs as tocolytics is their inhibitory effect on uterine contractions through activation of ß-adrenergic receptors. ß-Adrenergic receptors are subdivided into ß-1 and ß-2 groups, with the latter dominant in blood vessels and the uterus. Isoxsuprine hydrochloride (a derivative of catecholamine), ritodrine hydrochloride, and terbutaline sulfate have been used and are believed to be effective in depressing uterine contractions. A ß-mimetic that has a narrow impact on only the uterus has yet to emerge. Thus maternal and fetal or neonatal side effects do occur, with cardiovascular, pulmonary, and metabolic complications documented. For example, neonatal hypoglycemia is a recognized complication of isoxsuprine therapy.

Calcium antagonists such as nifedipine are now used as an adjunct for tocolysis. Magnesium sulfate is no more effective than other agents but is commonly used because of a better maternal side effect profile than the ß-adrenergic agents. Prostaglandin synthetase inhibitors may have a future role, but their use is limited because of their potential vasoactive effect on the fetus, especially on the ductus arteriosus.

Tocolytic therapy can be beneficial between 26 and 33 weeks' gestation. Then a relatively short delay of preterm delivery through tocolysis or other interventions is long enough (24-48 hours) to allow administration of corticosteroids for the enhancement of fetal lung maturity and maternal antibiotics for GBS sepsis prophylaxis.

Prevention of Prematurity

Prevention of preterm birth continues to be an area of ongoing research. Evaluation of lifestyle factors associated with preterm delivery and the subsequent modification of identified risk factors has yielded mixed results. More recent efforts have focused on cervical insufficiency, subclinical infection, and hormonal effects.[27]

For patients who have had previous idiopathic preterm birth, screening for bacterial vaginosis in early pregnancy and treatment with oral antibiotics has been associated with a significant decrease in risk of subsequent preterm birth. Theoretically, bacterial vaginosis promotes upper genital tract colonization, which triggers early parturition. The use of weekly progesterone to decrease the risk of recurrent preterm birth in subsequent pregnancy appears promising because the biggest risk factor for preterm delivery is a history of previous preterm delivery.[28]

Health professionals can play a major role in such preventive programs because they ensure that the need for intervention is documented and that intervention occurs. In addition to management of specific medical problems, alterations in lifestyle, work environment, and behavior patterns may be necessary. Good prenatal care and early work leave may be very important. Countries where such policies exist, such as Sweden, have low prematurity rates, but whether this circumstance is an association or a contributing relationship is unknown at present.

Multiple Gestation

The incidence of multiple gestation has recently and remarkably increased because of the application of newer reproductive technologies to treat infertility, although as reproductive technology is refined the incidence of higher-order multiple gestation is decreasing.

Spontaneously occurring multiple gestation is also relatively common (twins occur naturally in approximately 1 in 88 births). Regardless of the source of multiple gestation, fetal risk is increased. These risks range from those that are placental in origin, such as twin-to-twin transfusion, to rare fetal malformations, as in conjoined twins, to the much more frequent problems of prematurity and obstetric complications. Multiple gestation is one of the three most common causes of prematurity. Complications of labor and delivery increase the risk of hypoxia or trauma, with the second-born twin being more susceptible to damage than the first.

Obstetric Complications

Obstetric complications jeopardize the fetus, the most dire manifestation being intrapartum fetal death. Even the most ideally healthy fetus is at increased risk during labor and delivery. Stress to the fetus may be documented retrospectively by low Apgar scores, poor recovery after birth, and subsequent complications. A fetus chronically compromised by adverse factors, such as diabetes in pregnancy, may be compromised further by obstetric problems.

Abnormal presentations, such as breech and transverse lie, greatly increase fetal risk, as does cephalopelvic disproportion (a mismatch between the maternal pelvis and the fetal head). Malproportion can be predominantly fetal, as in congenital hydrocephalus, or maternal when congenital pelvic bone abnormalities exist.

Abnormal Growth and Gestation

Discrepancies between fetal growth and gestation are often manifestations of an underlying disease process but may occur without apparent cause. Regardless of cause, discrepancies in growth and gestation can often result in such severe risk to the fetus as to be more worrisome than the underlying problem. Postmaturity occurs much less frequently than prematurity, but it presents increased risk to the fetus. Continued growth in utero increases the risk of macrosomia and birth trauma. Placental insufficiency may result in the development of hypoxia and acidosis before or during labor that is characterized by nonreassuring fetal heart rate, poor Apgar scores, and perinatal hypoxic encephalopathy. Meconium passage is common and poses a risk of meconium aspiration syndrome; it may also signal peripartum infection.[29]

Deviations of growth and gestation can be cumulative for fetal risk. The premature infant also affected by IUGR tolerates intrauterine stress poorly, may exhibit respiratory distress syndrome or apnea after birth, and is at risk for the development of hypoglycemia. New information is emerging about the long-term effects of fetal growth restriction. Fetal nutritional adaptations to placental insufficiency may persist through adulthood because the risk of coronary artery disease and chronic hypertension is increased among adults who were born with IUGR.[30] The clinician should appreciate that evaluation of the fetus or newborn by birth weight and gestational age can provide specific information that facilitates diagnosis and treatment.

Alloimmunization

Alloimmunization is a disease of the maternal-fetal unit that has decreased in incidence because of successful efforts to prevent Rh disease with Rh-globulin (RhoGAM). Passage into the maternal circulation of fetal red cells, which possess antigens not present in the mother, stimulates production of antibodies. Maternal antibodies of the immunoglobulin (Ig) G class cross the placenta, resulting in a hemolytic process in the fetus that can be severe. The initial alloimmunization can occur with blood transfusions, with spontaneous or induced abortion, or with the first or subsequent pregnancy. Small amounts of red cell antigen contained in blood measuring 1 mL or less (especially if repeated) can cause an antibody response even in normal pregnancies. Sensitization risk is increased by complications such as preeclampsia or cesarean section.

Rh incompatibility is associated with a variable but often severe sensitization that can cause stillbirth, massive fetal erythropoiesis or erythroblastosis, anemia, hydrops fetalis, and other systemic manifestations. Hyperbilirubinemia occurs in the newborn and to a lesser degree in utero, whereas the maternal liver clears bilirubin.

The incidence of fetal Rh disease varies with the prevalence of Rh negativity. This genetically determined state is not often documented in Asians and Native Americans; however, it occurs in 15% of whites, resulting in the possibility of approximately 9% of their pregnancies involving an Rh-negative woman carrying an Rh-positive fetus. Despite prophylaxis with RhoGAM for the D antigen, alloimmunization still occurs in response to several other red cell antigens, including c, C, e, E, Kell, Kidd, and Duffy. These *minor* antigens can cause very serious hemolysis. Some patients acquire more than one hemolytic antibody.

Since the delineation of the cause of Rh sensitization, a wide range of diagnostic and therapeutic methods has become available that make Rh incompatibility treatment a paradigm for intensive perinatal care. Today's routine procedures for the disease include initial screening for the presence of alloimmunization and for Rh-negative women who are still candidates for prevention with RhoGAM. If hemolytic antibody is detected, then maternal serum levels and amniotic fluid analysis can assess the possibility of severe fetal illness. Amniotic fluid can be analyzed by polymerase chain reaction (PCR) DNA analysis to determine fetal blood type and the risk of hemolytic disease. Noninvasive methods of diagnosis of fetal anemia have been developed, which use ultrasound assessment of fetal cerebral blood flow in the middle cerebral artery. Peak systolic velocity in the middle cerebral artery increases as anemia worsens. This noninvasive option for monitoring decreases the risk accrued with serial amniocentesis, which can include infection, worsened sensitization, and loss of pregnancy.[31,32] When a high hemolytic risk is detected, by either ultrasound or amniocentesis, fetal blood sampling via the percutaneous umbilical route can be performed so that an accurate assessment can be made and so that in utero blood transfusion may be administered. The timing of delivery includes consideration of fetal health, the possibility of in utero transfusion, and the degree of prematurity. Immediate, aggressive neonatal intensive care, including exchange transfusion and cardiopulmonary support, may be indicated.

Incompatibilities of the ABO system result from the presence of maternal anti-A or anti-B antibodies when the fetus' blood type is group A or B and the mother's is group O. Severe hemolysis is much less common, even though ABO incompatibility is potentially present in approximately 20% of pregnancies. Fetal erythrocytes appear to have fewer antigenic loci, and maternal antibody appears in IgA, IgM, and IgG forms, with only the latter crossing the placenta. These facts may explain why ABO alloimmunization is usually of greater concern in the newborn than in the fetus. Stillbirths and hydrops fetalis are rare, but prolonged neonatal hyperbilirubinemia occurs frequently.

Gestational Hypertension

Hypertension of pregnancy is a major contributor to fetal risk. A group of diseases seen only in pregnancy and presenting with acute and chronic manifestations of hypertension, edema, and proteinuria may be lumped together in this category. *Preeclampsia* is another term for the basic process, which can be severe; when convulsions or coma occurs, *eclampsia* is present. Chronic hypertensive vascular disease with pregnancy is believed by many to be a separate disease state that can have superimposed preeclamptic manifestations.

Spontaneous premature labor of uncertain etiology occurs frequently in all hypertensive gestations. Premature birth is increased further in incidence because early delivery is frequently elected on maternal or fetal indication. As the severity of the disease increases, and particularly when eclampsia develops, stillbirth and maternal death become much more frequent. IUGR is seen in a third of perinatal deaths associated with preeclampsia. For the fetus, this disease process presents a bleak perspective; fetal stress is significant, and labor and delivery are often premature and timed for maternal treatment rather than for fetal well being. Neonatal complications are many and severe.

Successful perinatal management of maternal hypertension relies heavily on early detection during prenatal care. When the process is discovered, intensive perinatal care may be necessary, with seizure prophylaxis with magnesium sulfate a mainstay of therapy. Severe preeclampsia is a significant maternal threat and may require a decision to deliver a premature baby. Careful maternal and fetal surveillance, including assessment of fetal well being by nonstress testing, biophysical profile, amniotic fluid volume determinations, Doppler studies of umbilical blood flow, and ultrasound studies of fetal growth are all part of proper expectant management.

Intrauterine Infections

The medical community's understanding of the scope of the problem of intrauterine infections and its fetal effects has broadened considerably but is probably far from complete. Expression ranges from fetal loss from spontaneous abortion and stillbirth through severely debilitating congenital anomalies resulting from teratogenic effects, to subtle systemic manifestations, including those of the CNS, not detected until later in childhood when problems with higher cerebral function and behavior become apparent.

The important infectious agents include viruses, bacteria, spirochetes, and protozoa. The route for infection varies with the agent and can be transplacental, ascending through the cervix, with or without the rupture of membranes, which provide an imperfect protective cover, as well as through direct contact with the fetus during passage through the birth canal.

The pediatric practitioner needs to have a basic appreciation for the variety of intrauterine infectious agents and the pathophysiological processes and clinical problems they invoke. Table 73-1 is a modification of the TORCH acronym that has served well for several decades. Since it was originally derived, however, knowledge has emerged including the intrauterine manifestations of *Parvovirus* B-19 infection (fetal hydrops and death) and the complexities of HIV.

Human Immunodeficiency Virus

Fetal, intrauterine, and peripartum considerations are but a small part of the story of HIV; a complete discussion appears in Chapter 276, Human Immunodeficiency Virus Infection and Acquired Immunodeficiency Syndrome. Given the magnitude of the HIV/AIDS problem and that of the three predominant modes of transmission in the United States (sexual contact, percutaneous contact with contaminated sharps, and fetal or infant contact with an infected mother), two of which involve reproduction, the pediatrician must know the specifics of transmission and intervention. The newly developed ability to decrease vertical transmission from mother to fetus makes universal screening of pregnant women for HIV imperative, despite complaints regarding invasion of privacy. The fetus can be infected in utero, although the exact timing is uncertain; other possibilities for transmission include transplacental or peripartum, as well as postpartum (through breastfeeding). The timing of the expression of disease in children is variable and is thought to be determined by whether the infection was acquired before delivery or during parturition. Without antiviral therapy, approximately 25% of babies born to HIV-infected women will become infected themselves. The use of antepartum, intrapartum, and postpartum zidovudine decreases the risk of congenital infection to 8%. Even further decreases in transmission may be associated with multiple-agent antiretroviral therapy and by cesarean section delivery or vaginal delivery within 4 hours after rupture of membranes.[33] Whether cesarean section delivery is protective for fetuses of women who have very low or undetectable viral loads is uncertain.[34] Newborns discovered to be at risk should be continued on antiretroviral agents until their infective status becomes clarified. In the United States, where safe artificial milk is available, breastfeeding is contraindicated in HIV-infected women.[35]

Rubella

Rubella virus is recognized as a potent teratogen. Infections during the first trimester result in approximately 20% of fetuses being severely damaged or malformed, with second-trimester involvement damaging

Table 73-1 Maternal-Fetal Infections: The TORCH Acronym

INFECTION	AGENT	COMMENT
T—Toxoplasmosis	Protozoa	Transplacental passage; mild maternal illness, variable fetal or neonatal manifestations; maternal antibody test available
O—Other	Virus, bacteria, parasite	HIV, *Listeria*, syphilis, gonococcus, group B streptococcus, varicella-zoster, malaria
R—Rubella	Virus	Prototype for transplacental viral infections; severe and chronic fetal or neonatal disease; antibody test and immunization available
C—Cytomegalovirus	Virus	Transplacental passage, ubiquitous agent; broad spectrum of fetal or infant manifestations
H—Herpes simplex	Virus	Rare transplacental passage, usual intrapartum transmission from maternal genitalia; severe neonatal disease; antiviral treatment available

From Nahmias AJ. Torch complex. *Hosp Pract.* 1974;9(5):65-72.

10%. Third-trimester infection has presented few clinical problems. The expression of rubella syndrome is variable. Manifestations of first-trimester fetal disease can be severe (eg, abortion, stillbirth, severe rubella syndrome). Severe rubella syndrome includes growth restriction, eye defects (cataracts and microphthalmia), congenital cardiac defects, deafness, thrombocytopenic purpura, hepatosplenomegaly, bone lesions, pneumonitis, and cerebral defects (microcephaly, encephalitis, intellectual disability, and spastic quadriplegia). Infections in the second trimester are variable and tend to be less severe.

The high fetal risk and potentially devastating consequences of intrauterine rubella have stimulated aggressive efforts to prevent maternal rubella. Congenital rubella is a reportable disease. Vaccination of children between the ages of 1 and 12 years is routine. Administration of vaccine to women of childbearing age has been controversial because of concern of possible vaccine effects on the developing fetus. However, a registry of cases in which women received vaccine within 3 months of conception has found no cases of congenital rubella syndrome. Vaccine virus was cultured from fetal and placental tissue, but teratogenic effects were not seen. Preconception counseling should include rubella serotesting to determine the need for vaccination before conception occurs.

Cytomegalovirus Infections

The cytomegaloviruses may be the most common cause of congenital infections, occurring in somewhat less than 1% of births. This group of viruses is widespread and produces various apparent and inapparent infections in the general population: 3% to 5% of pregnant women have this virus in their cervical canal or urine. Fetal infection usually occurs through the placenta.

The fetal disease has been called *cytomegalic inclusion disease* because of the large inclusion-bearing cells found in urine and many organs. Severe cytomegalic inclusion disease includes hepatosplenomegaly, microcephaly, cerebral calcifications, mental and motor manifestations, and chorioretinitis. Reviews suggest that expression of intrauterine infections is variable and that full recognition of incidence is yet to come. Serologic tests for cytomegalovirus (CMV) are available and can provide presumptive evidence for infection; however, reliability is not as good as with rubella titers, and a vaccine is not available. Urine CMV culture is a good indicator of recent or active infection.

Herpes Simplex Virus Infections

Herpes simplex virus (HSV) infections in humans result from two strains, types 1 and 2, each with distinct serotypes yet some cross-reactivity. Perinatal disease is usually associated with type 2, although type 1 is more common in the general population. Type 2 HSV produces genital lesions and in most instances is transmitted sexually. Herpetic disease in the fetus or newborn is relatively rare but can be devastating. Transmission occurs by direct contact at birth or by ascending transcervical infection after rupture of the membranes. Transplacental infection early in pregnancy with fetal manifestations similar to those of CMV infection has been documented but is rare. Prophylaxis against recurrent HSV outbreak is suggested late in the third trimester through delivery.[36]

Newborn manifestations of intrapartum contact are well known. They range from vesicular lesions of the skin to encephalitis and severe systemic disease, with a mortality of more than 90% without treatment and severe CNS morbidity in those who survive. Expression is probably linked to primary versus recurrent maternal disease, being more intense in the former.

A major recent development is the success of antiviral agents in the treatment of systemic herpes infection, in particular encephalitis. Early diagnosis and treatment are essential. Prevention is desirable and possible. (See the discussion of herpes infections in Chapter 275, Human Herpesvirus-6 and Human Herpesvirus-7 Infections.) Current suggested management for a pregnant mother who has genital lesions is a cesarean birth to prevent fetal inoculation by passage through the birth canal.

Toxoplasmosis

Toxoplasmosis is caused by an intracellular protozoan parasite, *Toxoplasma gondii.* Infection is widespread, is congenital or acquired, and varies in expression from almost asymptomatic to generalized and fatal. The fetus is at risk for death when the infection occurs early in pregnancy or may be born with fully developed disease indicative of a long intrauterine course. Chorioretinitis, cerebral calcification, hydrocephalus or microcephaly, hepatosplenomegaly, and a host of systemic manifestations are observed. Long-term sequelae, especially involving the CNS, are present in most of the infants who have severe infection and who survive.

Pregnant women are believed to become infected through consumption of raw or undercooked meat or by ingestion of oocysts from soil or contaminated food. They may also become infected by exposure to cat feces. Prevention of toxoplasmosis in pregnancy is possible by careful handwashing after changing cat litter, gardening, or handling raw meat. The incidence of the perinatal disease is higher in certain locales.

Detection of *Toxoplasma* antibody by a reference laboratory can document the onset of infection, if IgM antibody appears, coupled with a rise of IgG antibody in paired samples over at least 2 weeks. Antibody levels can remain high for years; unchanging elevated levels indicate old infection. Infection before pregnancy appears to prevent congenital disease; however, maternal coinfection with HIV may result in reactivated maternal parasitemia and congenital infection.[37] If toxoplasmosis is suspected by serologic testing, then amniotic fluid or fetal blood can be tested by PCR for *Toxoplasma* DNA. Treatment with pyrimethamine and sulfadiazine is effective in decreasing the severity of congenital infection. Congenital toxoplasmosis may be inapparent at birth and not recognized until later in infancy or early childhood. (See Chapter 305, Parasitic Infections.)

Other Intrauterine Infections

Fetal syphilis is caused by transplacental passage of *Treponema pallidum.* Fetal infection has been thought not to occur before the eighteenth week of gestation, but this assumption is disputed. Pregnancy in a woman who has primary- or secondary-stage disease may result in stillbirth. Other manifestations vary from presentation in the newborn to those appearing in the first 2 years of life or later. In general, the earlier the onset of infection is, the more severe the lesions will be. Severe fetal infection manifests in early infancy by osteochondritis and periostitis, rhinitis (snuffles), rash, and mucosal fissures or patches. Premarital and prenatal screening for syphilis, in conjunction with antibiotic treatment, has effectively decreased the incidence of intrauterine disease, especially the more severe or classic manifestations. Unfortunately a resurgence occurred in the late 1990s. Recently trained clinicians have not had the experience in recognizing congenital syphilis that many of their older colleagues have had, which sometimes results in a delayed diagnosis. Detection of disease during pregnancy and treatment with penicillin will arrest development of the fetal disease. Penicillin remains the treatment of choice for syphilis during pregnancy, even if desensitization for penicillin allergy is required. (See Chapter 322, Sexually Transmitted Infections.)

Listeria monocytogenes is a gram-positive bacillus that probably plays an important role in overall fetal wastage. Incidence varies widely; infection is associated with ingestion of contaminated ready-to-eat food products.[38] Fetal death may occur after a relatively mild systemic maternal disease. *Listeria* chorioamnionitis can be diagnosed by amniocentesis, and successful antibiotic treatment is possible. Neonatal manifestations include systemic disease at birth or a delayed appearance as meningitis in the second to fifth week of life, with a characteristic monocellular cerebrospinal fluid.

GBS disease has many similarities in presentation to that of *Listeria* and is a more common problem. (See Chapter 99, Respiratory Distress and Breathing Disorders in the Newborn.) Infection is acquired by exposure to organisms during parturition. Maternal immune status and bacterial subtype are important determinants of virulence. The Centers for Disease Control and Prevention, the American College of Obstetrics and Gynecology, and the American Academy of Pediatrics recommend assessing colonization status at 36 weeks' gestation by culture and treating all colonized women as labor commences. If GBS status is unknown at the onset of labor, then women who have risk factors such as prolonged rupture of membranes, preterm labor, fever or systemic manifestations, or a previous child who had GBS disease should be treated.[24]

All neonatal services should have a structured approach to identifying and treating patients at risk for or having GBS disease in its two dominant modes of presentation: (1) a fulminant hemorrhagic pneumonitis in the first hours after birth or (2) neonatal meningitis that appears a few days or weeks after birth.

Other known intrauterine infections include agents of all known classes; undoubtedly, many others are yet to be discovered. Many viruses can cause fetal infection, including varicella, coxsackievirus, mumps, rubeola, echovirus, and hepatitis. *Mycoplasma pneumoniae* also is an important perinatal agent, and malaria is a significant fetal threat in many areas of the world.

FETAL ASSESSMENT

Clinicians use menstrual dating when describing the course of human pregnancy, beginning with the first day of the last menstrual period. Others use conceptual dating and a timeline that begins with conception or approximately 2 weeks after the last menstrual period. Occasional confusion arises when the differences between these two conventions are not appreciated. Furthermore, clinicians discuss pregnancy in terms of portions of weeks, such as 36 0/7, or the beginning of the thirty-sixth week. By use of menstrual dating, a pregnancy is thus in the thirty-seventh week (37 0/7), when it is considered to be at term. This concept is similar to a child not being 1 year of age until the child's first birthday, on the 366th day of life.

The typical human pregnancy lasts 36 to 40 weeks from fertilization or 38 to 42 weeks from the last menstrual period (by menstrual dating). Fetal development begins at fertilization, when a sperm combines with an oocyte to form a zygote. The fetal life span is defined here in the broad sense to include the entire gestational interval (Figure 73-3). The human product of conception technically becomes a fetus at the end of the eighth week after fertilization and remains so until birth.

Development proceeds from conception to birth in three stages: (1) the ovum, zygote, and blastocyst; (2) the embryo; and (3) the fetus. The *conceptus,* or product of conception, comprises all the structures that develop from the zygote, both embryonic (the embryo or fetus) and extraembryonic (the membranes and the placenta).

The stage of the ovum, zygote, and blastocyst, illustrated in Figures 73-1, begins with fertilization, wherein a single haploid sperm (23 chromosomes) enters the oocyte (haploid female ovum with 23 chromosomes). This stage usually takes place within the ampulla of the fallopian tube. The fertilization process is complicated and takes up to 24 hours before the genetic material from the two haploid cells fuses to form a diploid cell, the *zygote,* with a full complement of genetic material (called the *stage of syngamy*).

The *preembryo* consists of the developing cells, produced by division of the zygote, and lasts until the formation of the *primitive streak,* approximately 14 days after the beginning of fertilization. The preembryonic stage has been of special interest clinically and ethically because sustaining human preembryos in vitro is possible for up to 6 to 9 days after fertilization.

Preembryo development, during the interval before implantation in the uterine lining, includes a series of morphologic changes. Progression proceeds from blastomeres, or individual cells, to a tightly compacted group of cells called the *morula*. The blastocyst, a mass of cells with a fluid-filled inner cavity, appears at approximately 4 days after syngamy. Early mitotic divisions lead to totipotential cells that are able to produce all the products of conception. During this time, twinning becomes possible; by approximately day 7, differentiation leads to cells becoming individualized. The multicellular blastocyst with a trophectoderm and an inner cell mass initially attaches to the maternal

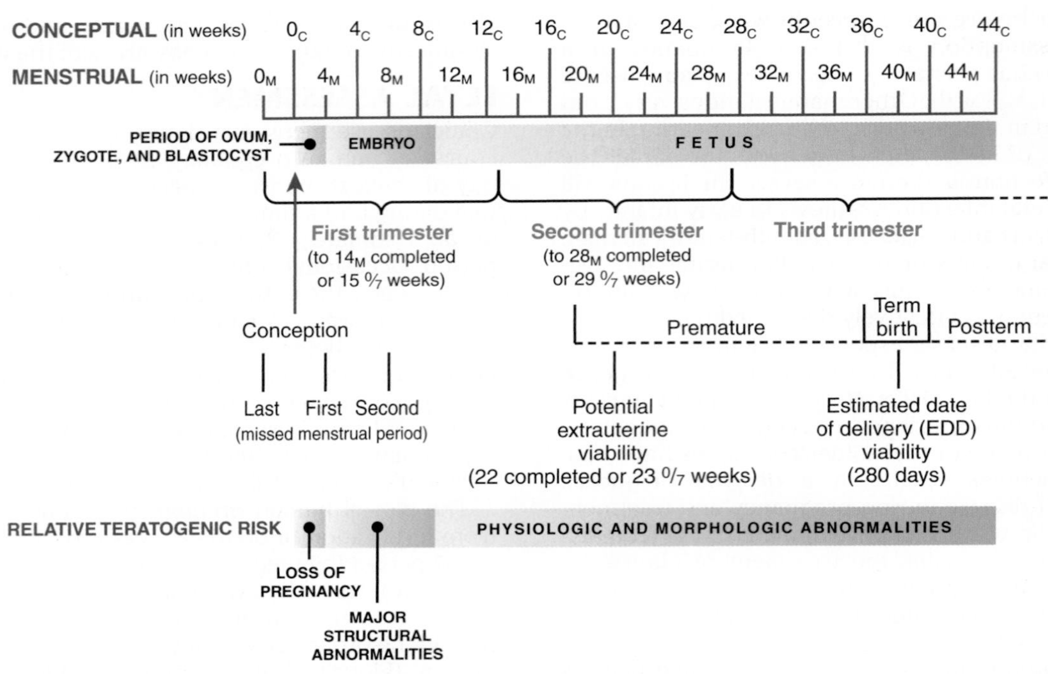

Figure 73-3 Fetal life span by conceptual and menstrual dating. Note timing of important events and relative teratogenic risk.

endometrial lining at day 8 or 9, and over the next several days, it becomes embedded, thereby completing the process of implantation.

By the time of the first missed menstrual period (see Figure 73-3) the primitive streak has been formed in the embryonic disk, embryogenesis is beginning, and a critical time has passed during which up to 50% or more of fertilizations do not complete preembryonic development and implantation successfully. Thus this stage is a period when the product of conception is at very high risk.

The *embryonic* period encompasses approximately weeks 3 to 8 and is characterized by the differentiation of all major organs that will be present in the fetus, the newborn, and the adult. Near the beginning of this interval, the woman usually becomes aware of cessation of menstruation, and laboratory tests can confirm pregnancy.

During the preembryonic period, adverse conditions may cause the death of the products of conception. This event often occurs around the time when a menstrual period would have been expected, and fertilization may not be recognized. Adverse influences during the embryonic period can cause severe interruptions in the pattern of system development, resulting in major congenital anomalies in a surviving fetus. The embryo is recognizable as humanoid toward the end of this period; malformations, such as neural tube defects, resulting, for example, from maternal ingestion of carbamazepine, may be identified.

The *fetal* stage, the longest of the three stages of the fetal life span, ends with delivery. Growth in size is the most apparent change during this interval, but maturation of organ systems and bodily processes is equally important. The high incidence and problems of premature birth make the degree of organ and enzyme system maturation of compelling interest to the pediatrician. The development of pulmonary surfactant is probably the single most important maturational process directly affecting survival in premature infants.

The late fetal stage has become the focus of increasingly sophisticated diagnostic techniques. Ultrasonography not only provides images of the fetus but also facilitates invasive procedures, such as amniocentesis to obtain amniotic fluid, and fetal blood sampling. Magnetic resonance imaging can be used in selective cases to provide further diagnostic information.[39] The pediatrician needs to keep pace with developments in this period because intrauterine treatment of the fetus appears destined to expand someday to include the addition or modification of genetic material.

Intrauterine Growth and Nutrition

The physician dealing with the newborn must have a firm conceptual framework of intrauterine growth to evaluate and treat the healthy newborn and the atypical newborn effectively. In particular the common clinical problem of prematurity can be managed more appropriately if growth patterns as they relate to gestational age are appreciated.

The growth rate of the fetus is especially rapid from 12 to 16 weeks of gestation and again during its final months. Both of these rapid-growth phases are associated with events of immediate concern to the practitioner. By the end of the sixteenth week after fertilization, the size and activity of the fetus have reached the point that many multiparous and some primiparous women are able to feel fetal motion *(quickening)*. This event can be a valuable marker when assessing fetal age and well being. The late-growth phase can be monitored by several means, especially physical examination, including the measurement of the height of the fundus above the maternal symphysis pubis and ultrasound measurements.

The period from 8 to 12 weeks after fertilization begins with a fetus whose head makes up almost one half of the total length. By 12 weeks the total length has doubled, but the head represents a smaller proportion. The 12- to 16-week interval is characterized by extremely rapid growth in length. In the 17- to 20-week interval, growth slows somewhat, but extremities assume their relative proportions. The 21- to 25-week interval after fertilization is characterized by significant gains in both length and weight.

Twenty-one weeks after fertilization, or 23 weeks from the last menstrual period, represents an extremely important milestone because the threshold for extrauterine viability is currently recognized as occurring at approximately 22 to 25 weeks (menstrual dating), with neonatal intensive care necessary to sustain that potential.[40] An important point to note is that at the threshold of viability, cognitive and neurologic impairment is common when the child has reached school age, and that the level of impairment is greater than previously recognized with the use of standardized norms.[41,42]

Many studies have attempted to quantify fetal growth through the use of postnatal data. Such growth curves, derived from measuring infants born at varying gestational ages, can give an approximation of intrauterine growth, but they have shortcomings. The baseline population is, by definition, atypical because the babies were born before term. In addition, the population of premature live births is very difficult to standardize for factors such as race, parity, socioeconomic status, maternal smoking, and maternal disease states.

Despite all this circumstance, intrauterine growth curves derived from postnatal data can be of great clinical assistance. The Colorado Intrauterine Growth Charts (Figure 73-4) are among the better known. They provide percentiles of intrauterine growth for weight, length, and head circumference. In addition, a weight-to-length ratio is shown. From weight and length data a ponderal index can be derived to depict proportionality. The growth curves in Figure 73-4 were derived from a population of hospital-born and non–hospital-born infants who had mixed racial backgrounds and were living at an altitude of approximately 5000 feet. Intrauterine growth curves derived from live births in other populations show significantly different values, particularly at some of the higher percentiles. However, the basic sigmoid shape of the curve persists. A few investigators have questioned the sigmoid shape of the growth curve as artifactual because it is based on the inaccuracies of menstrual dating. They suggest that when ultrasound dating is used the curves become linear. With the use of growth curves and ultrasound, fewer pregnancies now are delivered at 43 and 44 weeks' gestation.[43]

Intrauterine growth curves for the last trimester of pregnancy can be very helpful in both fetal and neonatal medicine. That intrauterine growth is a steady process cannot be assumed without reservation; growth might occur in bursts of undetermined length. Monitoring individual fetuses for growth against the baseline of an intrauterine growth scale can be helpful.

Fetal nutrition can be conceptualized in basic parameters that are familiar to the pediatrician. As with the child, two basic processes are under way: (1) accretion of substance for growth of new tissues and (2) oxidation or energy production for metabolism. Growth and development occur as a continuum from fetal to extrauterine existence, but the physiological mechanism of nutrition for that continuum changes abruptly at birth when the principal fetal organ for respiration and nutrition (the placenta) gives way to other organs and systems.

Glucose is a primary nutrient for the fetus, with its transplacental passage providing material for energy and for contributions to the fetal carbon pool. Initially, tissue growth is the main location for carbon and other constituents, with the 20-week fetus having little or no fat and approximately 90% water in its body composition. By term, fetal body water has decreased to approximately 76%, a figure high by adult standards; fat, a material of high carbon content, comprises approximately 16% of the fetus. These observations, coupled with the instability of neonatal glucose metabolism, when the baby is stressed by infection or other problems, should reinforce the importance of glucose metabolism in the perinatal period and particular respect for the relatively depleted stores of energy in the small premature or growth-restricted infant.

Amino acids, both essential and nonessential, are important as the building blocks of fetal protein synthesis. The uptake of essential amino acids through the placenta seemingly serves as a basic requirement for growth. Maternal nutritional state and placental function are crucial to fetal well being and growth, whereas in the neonate, amino acids and nitrogen originate with digestion of milk and uptake through the portal venous route.[44]

The clinician dealing with the newborn must consider the prior fetal nutritional state. Fortunately, when the digestive system of the neonate is unable to function at a level sufficient to provide energy and growth, physicians have the knowledge and technology available to approximate the fetal nutritional state. Total parenteral nutrition effectively returns the baby to the fetal state, in which all necessary nutrients, including essential and trace substances, enter directly into the circulation. Although this state can be maintained for reasonable intervals, such therapy does have complications, including infection and liver disease, making very long-term parenteral nutrition of the child much more problematic than it is for the fetus.

Identification and Management of Fetal and Maternal Risk

Any factor that increases the possibility of adverse pregnancy outcomes contributes to risk. Medical risk includes physiological, nutritional, obstetric, and genetic factors. Psychosocial risk includes psychological, social, environmental, and behavioral factors and

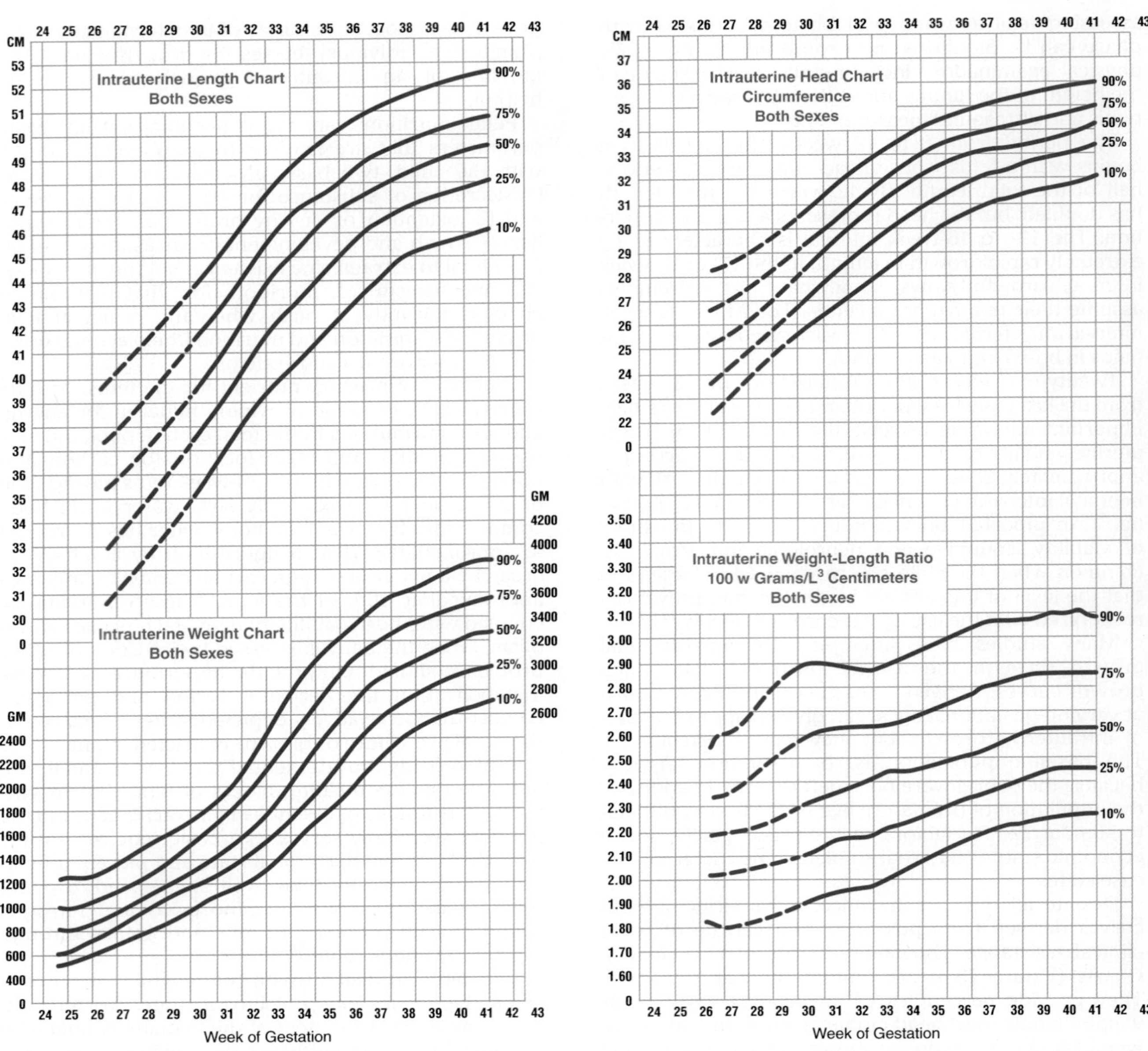

Figure 73-4 Colorado intrauterine growth charts. These charts were developed from measurements of babies after birth. They remain useful as a means for determining relative growth status of a baby compared with a reference population. *(Adapted from Lubchenco LO, Hansman C, Boyd E. Intrauterine growth in length and head circumference as estimated from live births at gestational ages from 26 to 42 weeks.* Pediatrics. *1966;37:403-408.)*

personal habits. These two broad categories of risk often act concurrently, and individual risks may overlap, accompany, or follow each other. The relationship between risk factors and adverse outcomes may be obvious, as with a specific toxic agent such as mercury; more often, however, risk is both subtle and cumulative.

Preconception Care

Health before pregnancy has become increasingly recognized as an important determinant of pregnancy outcome. Preparation for pregnancy should begin before conception, including assessment of risk and preventive or therapeutic intervention, including change of behavior. Box 73-1 illustrates the general categories and some specific problems that should be addressed in preconception care.

The concept of care before conception is related to, but not the same as, family planning; much more is involved than merely spacing of pregnancies. Wider acceptance of this concept within society may have a major effect on the outcome of pregnancy in such specific populations as adolescents. The role of the pediatrician in preconception and interconception care is vital.[45]

The importance of preconception care was emphasized in 2006 by the Centers for Disease Control and

BOX 73-1 Preconception Care Inventory

MEDICAL HISTORY

- Reproductive
- Family
- Genetic
- Current medications
- Substance use, including alcohol, tobacco, and illicit drugs
- Abuse, physical and emotional
- Environmental exposures
- General physical examination
- Immunization when indicated (rubella, hepatitis B, varicella)

SCREENING

- Sexually transmissible infections, depending on risk assessment
- Genetic disorders based on racial and ethnic back ground and family history (sickle hemoglobin pathologies, β-thalassemia, α-thalassemia, Tay-Sachs disease, cystic fibrosis, fragile X syndrome, Duchenne muscular dystrophy)

COUNSELING

- HIV prevention and testing
- Abstention from tobacco and alcohol
- Folic acid supplementation when attempting pregnancy and during first trimester
- Good control of preexisting medical conditions such as diabetes, hypertension

Modified from American Academy of Pediatrics. *Guidelines for Perinatal Care.* 4th ed. Elk Grove Village, IL: American Academy of Pediatrics and American College of Obstetrics and Gynecology.

Prevention, which convened a summit to discuss preconception care programs, research, and policy. The recommendations are specific to the implementation of health behavior, access to health care, consumer demand, research and surveillance for monitoring, and improving the health of women, children, and families.[46] Box 73-2 summarizes the primary objectives of the panel recommendations of the Centers for Disease Control and Prevention.

Prenatal Care

A report entitled *Caring for Our Future: The Content of Prenatal Care,* published by the US Department of Health and Human Services in 1989,[47] defines the three basic components of prenatal care as (1) early and continuing risk assessment, (2) health promotion, and (3) medical and psychosocial interventions and follow-up.[48] The most recent data indicate that 84% of women receive prenatal care in the first trimester, and 3.5% receive no or late prenatal care.[49]

Previous discussion has emphasized that during the prenatal period the fetus is undergoing rapid and continuous growth and development. Anything that jeopardizes this process must be recognized as a fetal risk factor and assessed. Major contributors to fetal risk are listed in Box 73-3.

BOX 73-2 Recommendations to Improve Preconception Health and Health Care

1. Improve the knowledge and attitudes and behaviors of men and women related to preconception health.
2. Ensure that all women of childbearing age in the United states receive preconception care services that will enable them to enter pregnancy in optimal health.
3. Reduce risks indicated by a previous adverse pregnancy outcome through interventions during the interconception period, which can prevent of minimize health problems for a mother and her future children.
4. Reduce the disparities in adverse pregnancy outcomes.

From Centers for Disease Control and Prevention. Recommendations to improve preconception health and health care—United States: a report of the CDC/ATSDR Preconception Care Work Group and the Select Panel on Preconception Care. *MMWR Recomm Rep.* 2006;55(RR06);1-23.

Little doubt exists that prenatal care is associated with healthier babies and mothers. Much of the original interest in and emphasis on prenatal care involved pregnancy-induced hypertension and the use of periodic blood pressure determinations. Standardized schedules (with details such as number and timing of visits, procedures, and studies) are available. In addition, the US Department of Health and Human Services offers suggestions, including the addition of preconception care, to traditional prenatal care.[47] The tests available for fetal assessment are provided in Box 73-4.

Assessing Fetal Status Before Labor

The clinician is obligated to make every effort to identify risk and practice expectant fetal medicine. Pediatricians must be familiar with the basic principles of techniques used to gather information. Family and reproductive history, fetal structure and growth, heart rate, and amniotic fluid and fetal blood analyses provide the basis for the majority of these methods. Some of these measurements are noninvasive, have been part of obstetric practice for years, and provide statistically valid information—for example, taking a history and measuring the size of the uterus. They are used to assess the need for other investigative techniques.

Fetal Activity

The duration, amplitude, and frequency of fetal movement after quickening and in the third trimester can provide important information about fetal well being. An inactive fetus may be chronically compromised, and the rapid onset of inactivity in a previously active fetus can be ominous. Daily assessment of fetal movement has some value as a test of fetal well being. Obstetricians often ask women to report if they perceive fewer than 10 fetal movements in a 2-hour period of close observation (*kick counts*[50]). Change in fetal activity does not predict specific fetal abnormalities but warrants follow-up with more standardized tests of fetal well being.

BOX 73-3 Major Contributors to Fetal Risk

GENETIC

- Chromosome abnormalities
- Inherited traits

MATERNAL-FAMILIAL ENVIRONMENT AND LIFESTYLE

- Socioeconomic status
- Social environment
- Physical environment
- Radiation
- Teratogens
- Nutrition
- Smoking or secondary exposure to smoke
- Drugs or alcohol abuse
- Lack of prenatal care

MATERNAL REPRODUCTIVE CAPABILITY AND HEALTH

- Age, weight, height
- Reproductive tract abnormalities
- Maternal medical disorders
- Cardiac
- Respiratory
- Renal
- Hematologic disorders (eg, sickle cell disease)
- Metabolic disorders (eg, diabetes, thyroid disorders, phenylketonuria)
- Epilepsy
- Emotional status

PLACENTA AND MEMBRANE DISORDERS

- Implantation (abdominal, tubal, previa)
- Vessel and cord complications
- Abruption
- Premature rupture of membranes and infection

MATERNAL-FETAL UNIT

- Multiple gestation
- Obstetric complications
- Malposition and malpresentation
- Cephalopelvic disproportion
- Abnormal fetal growth and gestation
- Alloimmunization (erythroblastosis fetalis)
- Intrauterine infections
- Pregnancy-induced hypertension

BOX 73-4 Fetal Assessment*

ANEUPLOIDY SCREENING

First-trimester screening
Second-trimester screening
  Quadruple marker screening
  Genetic sonogram
Integrated screening
Sequential screening

DIAGNOSTIC PROCEDURES

Chorionic villus sampling
Amniocentesis
Percutaneous umbilical blood sampling

FETAL WELL BEING ASSESSMENT

Fetal kick counts
Nonstress test
Biophysical profile
Modified biophysical profile: nonstress test plus amniotic fluid index
Contraction stress test
Umbilical artery Doppler velocimetry
Middle cerebral artery Doppler velocimetry

*Fetal assessment modalities available at most regional centers. See text for more information.

Fetal Heart Rate

The normal fetal heart rate (FHR) settles in the range of 110 to 160 beats/min by the final trimester and is easily monitored by a Doppler device (after 10 weeks), a fetoscope (after 20 weeks), and a stethoscope (after 28 weeks). During labor, continuous electronic fetal monitoring is used widely but has not been conclusively shown to be better than intermittent auscultation, despite many large studies.

FHR decelerations, especially fewer than 100 beats/min, is of concern because of an association with acute or chronic distress. Explanation for its presence must be sought. The list of possible causes is long and includes many that have a poor outcome, such as placental insufficiency. An intrinsic fetal cause, heart block, is not as ominous. Tachycardia usually occurs as an autonomic response to stimulation and can indicate fetal normality; it also may be associated with a maternal condition, such as pyrexia. Intrinsic fetal arrhythmias, such as supraventricular tachycardia, can result in secondary manifestations, including fetal hydrops.

Nonstress and Contraction Stress Tests

Tests that record FHR and the presence, absence, or temporal sequence of uterine contractions are used extensively. The FHR is driven by neurogenic reflex mechanisms similar to those seen in newborns.

The nonstress test (NST) observes FHR patterns by continuous fetal monitoring before the onset of labor. The interrelationship between FHR and fetal movement or spontaneous uterine contractions is observed. Such testing can begin at 26 to 28 weeks but is usually performed closer to term. NST is indicated for patients at risk for uteroplacental insufficiency and fetal death. It is repeated once or twice weekly. A normal or *reactive* NST is defined by a normal baseline heart rate (110-160 beats/min), moderate variability (5-20 beats/min), two or more accelerations of at least 15 seconds' duration, and a 15-beats/min peak above baseline in a 20-minute period.[51] A nonreactive or abnormal NST is defined as one that does not meet these standardized criteria and may actually show decelerations. The test has a false-positive rate for prediction of adverse fetal outcome of approximately 80%.

The contraction stress test (CST), or oxytocin challenge test, uses oxytocin-stimulated uterine contractions and records the FHR response. The NST is used more commonly; the CST is used by some physicians only after a nonreactive (abnormal) NST result. The presence of repeated late decelerations is considered problematic. Interpretations can be difficult, and relative and absolute contraindications exist for performing CST, in addition to a false-positive rate of approximately 50%. Interpretation requires experience. Nipple stimulation rather than oxytocin challenge is used by some practitioners to induce uterine contractions.

Fetal Biophysical Profile

Fetal well being can be assessed through the use of multiple parameters identified on ultrasound. Items such as muscle tone, body movement, breathing movement, amniotic fluid volume, and results of the NST can be identified and a score derived in a fashion similar to that for determining an Apgar score.

The biophysical profile probably has a lower false-positive rate than the CST and has been found to have a reasonable correlation with fetal blood gas scores. Some investigators have found the combination of amniotic fluid volume assessment and NST to have equivalent performance as a biophysical profile.

Uterine Size

The uterus and the products of conception are monitored closely at each prenatal visit. Measurements of fundal height above the symphysis are obtained and plotted; the umbilicus is reached by 20 to 22 weeks. Deviations from the expected curve may indicate a significant number of abnormal and high-risk states.

Fundal height at a level greater than expected may be the result of a miscalculation of dates, with the pregnancy being further along than anticipated. Another relatively straightforward cause of unexpectedly large uterine size is multiple pregnancy. Conversely, fetal causes of smaller than expected uterine size include pregnancy less advanced than anticipated and many problems that lead to IUGR.

The amniotic fluid volume deviations, oligohydramnios or hydramnios, may initially be detected by abnormal uterine size or fundal height. Confirmation and further study by ultrasonography should follow because imaging by ultrasound can more precisely estimate the volume of fluid present and assess fetal structures.

The pediatrician also needs to be alert to particular fetal situations in preterm pregnancies in which oligohydramnios occurs, inasmuch as this may be associated with a large number of disease processes, including IUGR and renal abnormalities with severely compromised urinary excretion. Under normal circumstances, amniotic fluid volume increases until 36 weeks and then decreases. Oligohydramnios thus can be associated with both postterm and postmature pregnancies. Renal agenesis (Potter syndrome) or dysplasia and structural and functional renal problems may not become evident until after birth.

Hydramnios may result from maternal problems, such as diabetes, or from fetal causes, such as tracheoesophageal fistula or diaphragmatic hernia. The pediatrician should immediately suspect fetal and neonatal abnormalities of the upper gastrointestinal tract because the normal circulation of amniotic fluid is interrupted on the absorptive side of the loop in these conditions. The baby will require special attention at birth and may require surgical intervention. CNS and neuromuscular abnormalities, such as myotonic dystrophy, impair fetal swallowing and cause hydramnios.

Ultrasonography

Clinical ultrasound has had a profound effect on all aspects of perinatal medicine. A transducer, acoustically linked to the skin surface by a gel, transmits ultrasonic vibrations, and the returning sound echoes are processed electronically to produce a two-dimensional image. New technology is now allowing production of three-dimensional images, but two-dimensional imaging remains the standard of care of diagnostic ultrasound imaging in obstetrics. Three-dimensional imaging technology may be seen as an adjunct technology.[52]

Two-dimensional images are used to evaluate fetal size and morphology. Doppler ultrasound is used to measure velocity of blood flow in fetal and maternal blood vessels. Color Doppler depicts local flow by color encoding an estimate of the mean Doppler frequency shift at a particular position, thereby demonstrating direction and velocity of blood flow. This tool is useful in evaluating fetal heart structure on echocardiogram and may be used as an adjunct in antenatal monitoring in the setting of IUGR or maternal alloimmunization.[31,53] Power Doppler ultrasound is a technique that encodes the amount of blood flow in color. Its usefulness includes evaluation of fetal vasculature and placental abnormalities.[54]

Although no clinically untoward effects of clinical ultrasound have been documented in humans, potential structural and functional biological effects have been hypothesized. Doppler ultrasound theoretically has greater potential for harm because of the continuous, rather than pulsed, wave and the amount of time in use. The US Food and Drug Administration, together with the American Institute of Ultrasound in Medicine and other organizations, has developed standards for safe information display.[55]

Controversy continues about the usefulness of and indications for routine prenatal ultrasound examination; several large clinical studies provide conflicting results. An American College of Obstetrics and Gynecology *Practice Pattern Review* developed the following conclusions: Specificity of ultrasound fetal anomaly survey is high (99%), sensitivity varies widely and depends on clinical setting and professional skill, ultrasound is safe when used appropriately, specific indications should serve as the basis for the use of ultrasound in pregnancy, and the optimal time for a single ultrasound during pregnancy is between 16 and 20 weeks gestation. The use of casual ultrasound without a medical indication should be avoided, and patients must be counseled about the limits of ultrasonography for prenatal diagnosis.[56]

A National Institutes of Health consensus development conference in 1984 concluded that when an accepted medical indication exists, ultrasound improves pregnancy outcome, and the consensus committee listed many specific risk situations. Routine screening, identification of fetal sex, and parental desire to see their fetus were not considered appropriate because of possible risk and ethical concerns. Estimates indicate that approximately 67% of pregnancies undergo ultrasound examination.[49]

Ultrasound evaluations are an important part of evaluation of fetal well being. Measurements of fetal growth pattern and distribution and amniotic fluid volume are important observations. A fetus for which biometric parameters are concordant and within acceptable range for gestational age and for which amniotic fluid volume is normal has a low risk of adverse outcome, such as stillbirth. Although the sensitivity varies with the type of birth defect and the skill of the operator, ultrasound can detect many birth defects. Ultrasound also is being used as a noninvasive tool to detect minor markers of trisomy 21.

Fetal Surgery

Fetal surgery is a controversial intervention that has attracted considerable medical and public interest. Pediatric care practitioners should be aware of the general level of activity in this field because they may be consulted by families in their practices. The media and increasingly the World Wide Web serve as informants about possible interventions, often without adequate attention to status of investigation and outcomes.

Fetal risk identification through accurate and timely prenatal diagnosis by ultrasound in conjunction with fetal sampling techniques and technical ability to intervene surgically though endoscopic or open techniques has resulted in attempts to correct fetal lesions that interfere with normal development. Fetal problems, theoretically amenable to surgical correction with resultant continued development in utero, include diaphragmatic hernia, cystic adenomatoid malformation, urinary obstruction (urethral valves), twin-twin transfusion syndrome resulting from placental vascular abnormalities, aqueductal stenosis, and myelomeningocele. Select situations such as congenital diaphragmatic hernia without liver herniation and neural tube defect have been subject to randomized controlled studies of intervention and outcome evaluation. Risks and benefit evaluation of fetal surgery should include the mother as well as the fetus.[57]

Risk Assessment and Diagnostic Testing

An increasingly valuable technique of perinatal risk assessment involves maternal serum screening for markers that correlate with risk of specific outcomes. Essentially all pregnant women in the United States should be offered testing for detection of neural tube defects and trisomy 18 and 21. Second-trimester (15-21 weeks) risk assessment includes analysis of alpha-fetoprotein, unconjugated estriol, inhibin A, and human chorionic gonadotrophin (hCG), the quadruple screen, or *quad,* screen. The sensitivity of detection of spina bifida is approximately 80%, with a 3% to 5% false-positive rate. Ultrasound sensitivity for open neural tube defect is up to 95%. Women who have unexplained elevated serum alpha-fetoprotein are at risk for adverse pregnancy outcomes other than neural tube defects, including intrauterine growth retardation and stillbirth. The sensitivity of a quad marker study panel for trisomy 21 is 79%, with a false-positive rate of 5%. First-trimester screening uses two serum analytes, β-hCG and pregnancy-associated plasma protein A, as well ultrasound measurement of the fetal nuchal translucency, allows risk assessment at 11 to 13 + 6 weeks' gestation, with a similar detection rate and false-positive rate.[58] Ultrasound in the second trimester can be used to modify the risk assessed on either a quad screen or a first-trimester screen; the screen is based on the presence or absence of markers: subtle changes in fetal anatomy which are more likely to be associated with aneuploidy, such as hypoplastic nasal bone or thickening of the nuchal fold.[59] Women whose screening results are positive are offered diagnostic testing, such as amniocentesis, and they often accept the procedural risk to achieve a definitive diagnosis.

Amniocentesis

Amniotic fluid bathes and is swallowed by the fetus, and it contains fetal cells, urine, and other substances, including pulmonary surfactant. The technique for obtaining a specimen of this fluid by percutaneous aspiration has been made more successful by the use of ultrasonography.

Diagnostic amniocentesis at 15 to 18 weeks' gestation, in conjunction with ultrasonography, confirms placental localization, fetal size, and gestational age, in addition to providing information obtained from fluid analysis. Evaluation of fetal cells through karyotyping can detect chromosomal abnormalities before potential extrauterine viability so that termination can be considered. Fluorescent in situ hybridization studies are available, which produce results for some aneuploidies within 48 hours, as opposed to the 10- to 14-day requirement for standard metaphase karyotype analysis. Molecular genetic studies on DNA extracted from fetal cells are expanding so rapidly that the pediatrician is advised to contact a prenatal diagnostic center to determine whether prenatal testing has become available for a specific disorder.[60]

Chorionic Villus Sampling

Chorionic villus sampling (CVS) involves ultrasound-directed aspiration of trophoblastic tissue surrounding the gestational sac during the first trimester. The approach can be transcervical or abdominal. CVS is usually performed at 10 to 12 completed gestational weeks, thereby providing information earlier than amniocentesis.

Studies of the safety and efficacy of CVS have found a higher rate of pregnancy loss and procedure failure than midtrimester amniocentesis. Some centers have higher rates of loss with transcervical than with transabdominal CVS. That CVS requires more professional experience than does amniocentesis is generally accepted. The advantage of CVS is more rapid and earlier diagnostic information, which allows more time for consultation and intervention, including abortion. The disadvantages of CVS include the slightly higher loss rate, lack of information about neural tube defect, and the possible need for later amniocentesis to clarify CVS results or to diagnose neural tube defect. Controversy has existed concerning possible limb reduction defects associated with CVS. The procedure is usually not performed before 10 weeks in an effort to minimize this risk.

Percutaneous Umbilical Blood Sampling (Cordocentesis)

Direct aspiration of fetal blood by means of a needle placed transabdominally through maternal skin and into a fetal blood vessel, or percutaneous umbilical blood sampling (PUBS), is another technique facilitated by ultrasound that has improved fetal diagnosis and therapy significantly. Sampling is possible from approximately 17 weeks to term, with greater apparent safety than with other techniques. Fetoscopy has a complication rate of 4% to 5%, fetal scalp sampling requires labor and cervical dilation, and placental aspiration results in contamination with maternal blood in more than 50% of attempts.

Common diagnostic indications for PUBS are the need for rapid fetal karyotype and evaluation of fetal alloimmune hemolytic disease. The main treatment is transfusion for fetal anemia. The PUBS technique is useful because it provides immediate fetal blood specimens for study of hemoglobin, platelets, blood gases, blood typing, and other parameters in the same fashion as studies in the neonate. Risk is a concern, with fetal loss a possibility. Currently, this technique requires sophisticated technology and expertise.

Fetal System Formation and Malformation

Pediatricians and other health care providers must be prepared to discuss normal fetal development, as well as fetal malformation, with parents; this discussion increasingly includes management during pregnancy and the peripartum period. *Teratology* is the study of the causes, development, structure, and classification of fetal abnormalities. Modern prenatal diagnosis provides information about the presence of structural abnormalities in a large portion of cases well before birth.

Most major malformations and disruptions of system function can be categorized as being caused by genetic or intrauterine factors, maternal conditions, and drugs or other agents. Genetic factors have their origin in parental cell lines or in aberrations of initial cellular division after fertilization and are discussed in Chapter 86, Common Congenital Anomalies. Evaluation of risk for genetic disease has advanced rapidly as the techniques for prenatal diagnosis (including fetal cell and tissue sampling) have become increasingly sophisticated. Intrauterine factors include problems such as uterine abnormalities, amniotic bands, and umbilical cord or placental abnormalities. Mechanical pressure from uterine constraint (as in severe oligohydramnios) causes morphologic changes categorized as a deformation sequence. If otherwise normally developing tissue is disrupted, as with the damage caused by amniotic bands from early amnion rupture, then the resulting damage is categorized as a *disruption sequence*.[61] Maternal medical conditions that produce metabolic imbalance, such as diabetes mellitus and phenylketonuria, are teratogenic. The effect of maternal nutrition is of major concern, especially because the relationship between folic acid deficiency and neural tube defects now is well recognized.[62] Drugs and other agents are a major concern because of the recognition that practically any drug is potentially teratogenic and because of the observation that chemical, radiation, or infectious agents may vary in degree of expression, depending on genetic predisposition or gestational age at the time of insult.

The major systems are discussed in the following sections, with attention drawn to the gestational time of origin of the major types of abnormalities.

Central Nervous System

The CNS starts from an ectodermal origin at about day 18 of gestation; development continues through delivery and long after birth. It is susceptible to teratogenic agents throughout the embryonic and fetal periods and is most susceptible during the first half to two thirds of the embryonic period.

The original neural plate develops into a neural tube that has cranial and caudal ends. The neural tube walls develop to become the brain and spinal cord; the inner part evolves into the ventricles of the brain and the central canal of the spinal cord. Brain development is complex and passes through stages of a forebrain, midbrain, and hindbrain, with subsequent development of the cerebrum, midbrain structures, pons, and cerebellum. Cells that were originally separated from the neural plate and became the neural crest develop into cranial, spinal, and autonomic ganglia, as well as the autonomic nervous system and chromaffin tissue, especially the adrenal medulla.

Malformations of the CNS confront the clinician prenatally and postnatally through imaging studies, which may prompt pediatric and neurosurgic consultation. Some of these defects are among the most profound, such as the anencephalic baby or infants who have very large encephaloceles. Application of life-supportive technology, in the form of assisted ventilation and nutrition, to babies who have such problems has been the subject of much public debate, as has the issue of organ donation.[63] Other anomalies, such as microcephaly, may be compatible with life for variable lengths of time but carry extremely bleak prognoses. Congenital malformations of the spinal column, especially those that have defects in overlying tissue, also pose major moral and ethical dilemmas to parents and health professionals, when potentially treatable complications are superimposed on a fundamentally poor prognosis. Some CNS lesions are of known origin, but others, such as meningomyelocele, may be the result of interactions between genetic predisposition and extrinsic factors. Preconception supplementation with folic acid will decrease the risk of neural tube defect.

Of major concern is the evidence that intrauterine exposure of the developing nervous system to substances such as cocaine or alcohol results in permanent functional morbidity, as well as structural changes. Although morphologic and behavioral changes often appear together, thus inviting the postulation of cause and effect, no reason exists to think that the two are always related. Pediatricians should be familiar with resources available for management of neonatal abstinence syndrome.[64]

The developing fetal brain is now known to acquire lesions that are clinically important to the infant and child. Spontaneous hemorrhagic lesions have been seen in the presence of alloimmune thrombocytopenia and cocaine exposure. Evidence is increasing of a link among intrauterine infection, preterm PROM, an increased risk of periventricular leukomalacia, and subsequent cerebral palsy.[65]

Cardiovascular System

The cardiovascular system is the first to function, with a rudimentary blood circulation beginning in the third week. Initially, two tubes fuse to form a single tube that evolves into the four-chambered heart and great vessels. By the end of the fourth or fifth week, partitioning of the chambers is complete, with two atria and two ventricles. Equally complex is the initial formation of a truncus arteriosus, aortic sac, and aortic arches, which evolve by the eighth week into a fetal circulatory pattern. This system undergoes changes in flow patterns during adjustment to extrauterine existence.

Schematic representations of the process whereby the initial pair of tubes forms a single tube with subsequent twisting and formation of chambers and very complex vascular structures (some of which become atretic, whereas others become dominant) can help in understanding spatial relationships and the reasons specific lesions develop. The lymphatic system, which develops in a similar timeline, is seen initially somewhat later than the cardiovascular system. The lymphatics have connections with the venous side of the developing cardiovascular system. Malformations of the cardiovascular system occur in approximately 7.5 in 1000 live births. The critical period for teratogenic effects ends relatively early in the intrauterine period, but the process of formation is so complex that a multitude of possibilities for maldevelopment exists. The degree of severity varies considerably.

Some structural malformations, such as the patent foramen ovale type of atrial septal defect, may be functional only when another pathological condition exists. The patent ductus arteriosus as a pathological entity occurs when closure fails after birth; in the fetal state, the patent ductus arteriosus is normal. Use of nonsteroidal antiinflammatory agents by pregnant women in the third trimester can cause premature closure of the ductus arteriosus and cardiac failure. Early malrotation of the fused cardiac tubes can result in dextrocardia, which can occur with an otherwise-normal heart and great vessel structures and may not be a clinical problem if complete situs inversus of the viscera also is present. Dextrocardia without situs inversus is often a major problem because of a tendency for associated complex intrinsic abnormalities.

Intracardiac malformations, such as septal defects, are very common, especially in the ventricle. Complex problems, with formation of the great vessels evolving from an inappropriate partitioning of the truncus arteriosus, are also fairly common. Coarctation of the aortic arch is an example of a malformation that may be some distance from the heart itself. Manifestations of malformations can occur in utero and are believed in some instances to result in infants who are large for gestational age. In severe and relatively rare instances, they can produce a form of nonimmune hydrops fetalis.

The physiological aspects of cardiac function in the fetus is basically different from that in the infant, child, and adult. The fetal circulation has several parallel circuits, rather than the series (or sequential) circuitry that is established after the closure of physiological shunts during or shortly after birth (Figure 73-5). The fetal heart has lower myocardial compliance and ventricular ability to increase stroke work. Increases in heart rate or filling pressure cause little increase in cardiac output.[66]

The pediatrician, pediatric cardiologist, and neonatologist are increasingly becoming involved with cardiac dysfunction before birth. The evaluation of fetal well-being includes that of cardiac status, with the result that problems such as cardiac arrhythmia or cardiac failure can be detected in utero. Fetal echocardiography can detect specific structural defects, with the interval from 18 to 24 weeks optimal for such an evaluation. Pregnant women who are themselves healthy are admitted to hospitals for treatment of fetal cardiovascular disease; use of antiarrhythmic drugs in the pregnant woman to treat fetal cardiac arrhythmias is an example of fetal treatment via the maternal and placental circulations. Medications used to treat fetal arrhythmias in utero may include digoxin, propranolol, flecainide, sotalol, or amiodarone.[67]

Musculoskeletal System

Formation of the musculoskeletal structures becomes apparent in the embryo by at least the fourth week, when limb buds (first the upper and then the lower) become obvious. Muscle structures originate from mesoderm, much of which arises directly from the somites. Bone evolves from mesoderm that undergoes a process of chondrification. Cardiac muscle and other smooth muscles have a different origin in the splanchnic mesoderm of the primitive gastrointestinal tract. The origin of some muscles, such as those of the iris and extrinsic eye, is unclear. The limb buds elongate while forming bone and large-muscle masses. A process of rotation and growth, in which upper and lower extremities rotate in different directions, results in the muscle groupings and dermatome patterns of the child and adult.

Malformations of the limbs are relatively common; otherwise, skeletal and muscular abnormalities are rare. The health professional providing newborn care is often struck by the significant attention paid by parents to the extremities, particularly the hands, of newborns. For this reason, relatively minor defects can have major emotional significance. Polydactyly or syndactyly are among the more common human malformations.

Many limb abnormalities are genetic in origin, but some malformations result from genetic predisposition interacting with environmental factors. The thalidomide deformities were a specific and perhaps relatively isolated example of limb teratogenesis. Sirenomelia, or caudal regression syndrome, is pathognomonic for poorly controlled maternal diabetes.

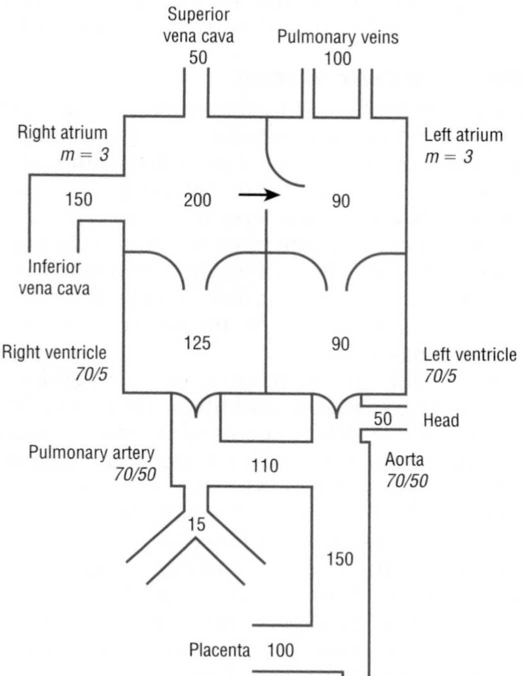

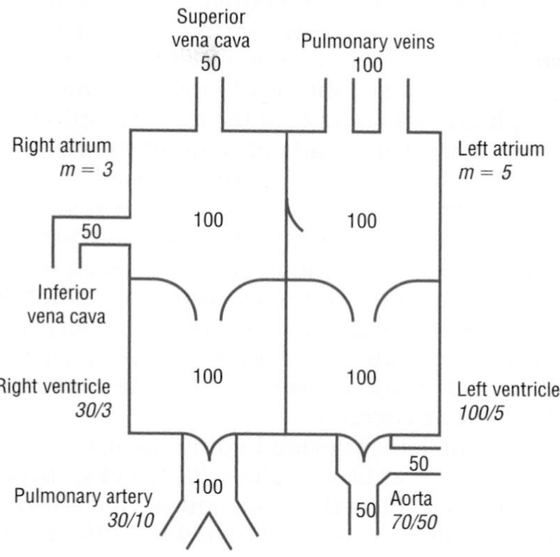

Figure 73-5 In the fetus, blood follows several routes, with a small portion going to the lungs. Oxygenated and nonoxygenated blood is admixed in the fetus, and the placenta serves as the fetal organ of respiration. The risk of expression of cardiovascular disease differs before and after birth because of changes in structure and flow. The numbers inside the diagram represent blood flow (rate), and numbers in italics represent pressure. *(Adapted from Flanagan MF, Yeager SB, Weindling SN. Cardiac disease. In: Avery GB, Fletcher MA, MacDonald MG, eds.* Avery's Neonatology: Pathophysiology and Management in the Newborn. *5th ed. Philadelphia, PA: Lippincott Williams & Wilkins; 1999. Reprinted by permission.)*

Gastrointestinal System

The alimentary tract, developing from a primitive anlage seen initially at the fourth week, has three main divisions: (1) foregut, (2) midgut, and (3) hindgut. Each of these divisions has its own specific blood supply in the celiac, superior mesenteric, and inferior mesenteric arteries. Because development of each tract can be traced, abnormalities of the individual divisions are seen. The foregut, from the pharynx to the insertion of the common bile duct, develops into various structures, including the intestine and the liver and pancreas. Midgut structures include all the small intestines (except for the duodenum proximal to the insertion of the common bile duct) plus the cecum, appendix, ascending colon, and approximately two thirds of the proximal transverse colon. The midgut structures go through a complex rotation during development, whereby an initial loop develops outside the fetal abdomen and rotates approximately 90 degrees at that time. At approximately the tenth week these midgut intestinal structures return to the abdomen and go through a further complex rotation of 180 degrees, leading to the final anatomic relationships of the intestine. Hindgut structures include the transverse, descending, and sigmoid colon and rectum through the final portion of the anal canal, which develops from an anal pit. The cloaca (the early expanded end of the hindgut) and tissues of other origin form the perineal structures.

Alimentary tract malformations are fairly common and often are associated with other anomalies. The foregut has an initial tracheoesophageal common origin, with subsequent separation. Tracheoesophageal fistulas resulting from errors in formation of the tracheoesophageal septum occur in four basic patterns; early detection is important to prevent extensive aspiration pneumonitis. Errors of midgut development and malrotation lead to many problems, the most spectacular of which is the lack of return of the bowel to the abdominal cavity, with a resultant omphalocele. Other malrotation presentations include acute intestinal obstruction and ischemia in utero or at varying lengths of time after birth, often after initial feedings. Malformations of the intestinal tube in the form of stenosis, duplication, or atresia are of unclear origin but may result from problems with recanalization or a compromised mesenteric vascular supply. Hindgut malformation occurs most commonly at the most distal portion, resulting in atresia, stenosis, membranous obstruction, or imperforate anus. Many other intestinal malformations can be seen. Of special interest is Meckel diverticulum (an outpouching in the ileum), representing the remnant of the yolk stalk.

Respiratory System

Respiratory system formation begins at approximately 26 days and goes on long after birth. Initial cell lines arise on the floor of the primitive pharynx and produce a laryngotracheal tube. Endoderm of this tube becomes the lining and glands of the lower respiratory system; connective tissue and cartilage of the respiratory system arise from splanchnic mesoderm.

Further growth of the endotracheal tube results in two lung buds that divide further into two sections on the left and three on the right; these correspond to the adult lobes. Branching continues after this point to form the pulmonary segments. At approximately 5 to 7 weeks after fertilization a pseudoglandular period exists during which major growth of the bronchi and terminal bronchioles occurs.

During the canalicular period beginning at 13 weeks and continuing to approximately 25 weeks, bronchioles and alveolar ducts develop, and significant vascularization occurs. From 24 weeks until birth, terminal sacs arise and become alveoli. These sacs are initially lined by a cuboidal epithelium, which changes to a squamous form at approximately 26 weeks' gestation. Alveolar development continues through early childhood. The association of the development with the threshold of extrauterine viability is obvious.

Surfactant is not produced until alveoli are formed. Complex cell types lining the alveoli have been described. A vacuolated cell, the type 2 pneumocyte, appears to have a secretory function and to be involved in alveolar stabilization through the elaboration of surfactant.

Anatomic malformations of the pulmonary parenchyma are unusual but include many dysplastic and cystic abnormalities. Because of the nature of fetal respiration, in which gas exchange is not occurring in the lung, these abnormalities are usually not problematic until after birth. Abnormalities of the diaphragm, the most common of which is diaphragmatic hernia, are most common on the left and often are associated with severe restriction of lung development on one or both sides. Some infants who have diaphragmatic hernia exhibit persistent pulmonary hypertension, a complication that includes increased vascular resistance similar to that seen in the fetus.

The pediatrician confronts respiratory problems closely related to the formative and maturational status of the lung. For example, at 22 to 25 weeks' gestation, alveolar formation may not be advanced to the point of being able to support life, even when exogenous surfactant, mechanical ventilation, and other interventions of present-day neonatal intensive care are used. This situation is encountered in the extremely low–birth-weight infant, or *micropremie,* and is basically a problem of pulmonary immaturity rather than prematurity. Whether respiratory distress syndrome is present after the birth of a premature baby depends largely on the functional cellular maturity of the infant's lungs. Antenatal treatment includes the use of corticosteroids to enhance fetal pulmonary maturity in pregnancies at risk for preterm delivery. Administration of a single course of corticosteroids is recommended for the pregnant woman at risk of preterm delivery, between 24 and 34 weeks' gestation.[25] Postnatal treatment includes administration of exogenous surfactant until endogenous production occurs. (See Chapter 99, Respiratory Distress and Breathing Disorders in the Newborn.)

Hematopoietic System

Initial red blood cell formation is seen as early as day 14 after conception, when cells containing embryonic hemoglobin arise from the endothelium of primitive vessels of the yolk sac. Hematopoiesis within the embryo begins in the liver at approximately the sixth week and remains the most active site during the early part of the fetal life span. The bone marrow assumes the primary role at approximately the sixth month, and other sites, especially the spleen and lymph nodes, play a contributory role.

Fetal hemoglobin (HbF) predominates for much of intrauterine existence and under normal circumstances is seen to a small degree in early infancy. Beginning at approximately the third month, some hemoglobin A (HbA) is present (5% to 10%), and the proportion of HbA to HbF increases rapidly from approximately 35 weeks to term, when blood is approximately 50% to 65% HbF. HbF has an increased oxygen affinity compared with HbA, which is probably the result of a differing action of 2,3-diphosphoglycerate, which facilitates oxygen saturation in the intrauterine environment. Blood group antigens are familial in their determination and can be identified as early as the second month of fetal life. Platelets also are seen at approximately the second month. The presence of hematopoietic abnormalities is important for the clinician to recognize. Certain hemoglobinopathies may result in intrauterine disease. α-Thalassemia results in hemoglobin Bart (tetrameric gamma chains), which has a very high oxygen affinity, resulting in intrauterine distress from tissue hypoxia and nonimmune hydrops fetalis. Several other significant hemoglobinopathies (eg, homozygous and heterozygous β-thalassemia) and structurally abnormal hemoglobins have been identified, such as HbS and HbC. PCR analysis of DNA from samples obtained by amniocentesis is possible. Hemolytic anemia that results from maternal-fetal blood group incompatibilities and transplacental passage of antibody is an immune disease; however, it has a marked effect on hematopoiesis, resulting in erythroblastosis fetalis and extensive proliferation of hematopoietic tissue. Fetal thrombocytopenia may be primarily of fetal origin, or it may be associated with some form of extrinsic agent or process, such as immune antibody of maternal origin or intrauterine infection. Many fetal intrauterine hematologic manifestations are part of disease processes involving other systems.

Middle cerebral artery Doppler velocimetry, amniocentesis, and PUBS are clinically useful in fetal hematologic disorders. Middle cerebral artery velocimetry is used to noninvasively diagnose fetal anemia, as seen, for example, with alloimmunization. PUBS can be used to diagnose thrombocytopenia and for platelet transfusions or exchange transfusions in the fetus with severe anemia caused by blood group alloimmunization.

Immune System

Immune system components function very early in fetal life, with some parts present as early as the eighth week and with a total rudimentary system capability by the twelfth week. The cellular immune system originates in liver or spleen stem cells that migrate to the thymus at approximately the eighth week. These T cells enter the bloodstream and are distributed to the body, mainly to the lymph nodes and spleen. The antibody immune system generates IgM in lymphoid tissues as early as the eleventh week and IgG at approximately the twelfth week. IgA, IgD, and IgE are seen in the fetus in small amounts toward the end of pregnancy. Current thinking suggests that specific immunoglobulin synthesis occurs in stem cells or B cells. Passive transfer of maternal antibody has been demonstrated very early in fetal life. Maternal IgG is detectable as early as the fortieth day, and practically all cord IgG is maternal in origin, arising from both passive and active enzymatic transplacental passage. IgM is not transferred passively. The complement system has some fractions present during the embryonic period at the eighth week, and by 12 to 14 weeks' gestation a considerable complement fraction is present. Malformations of the fetal immune system, either of familial or developmental origin, have been described and have contributed to an understanding of the adult system.

Abnormalities are believed to exist in all parts of the immune system, and clinicians should understand the basic possibilities because of the fetal and neonatal diseases that result. Fetal graft-versus-host reactions have been documented after intrauterine transfusions. Congenital infections activate the immune system, with an increased cord IgM level possibly being evidence of such infections. Fetal IgM is usually not present until the third trimester. At term, IgM and IgA are detectable but at levels much less than in the adult. Transplacental antibody passage with effects on the fetus, as seen in alloimmunization (erythroblastosis fetalis), is the classic clinical example of fetal disease resulting from activation of a maternal immune system response.[68]

Urogenital System

A close interrelationship exists between the development of two basic systems: (1) the urinary (or excretory) system and (2) the genital (or reproductive) system. The human embryo has three separate excretory organs: (1) the pronephros, (2) the mesonephros, and (3) the metanephros. The metanephros appears at approximately the fifth week after fertilization, functions 2 to 3 weeks later, and remains as the permanent kidneys. The other two systems involute, with the mesonephros remaining as a few ducts in the male genital tract and as a vestigial remnant in the female genital tract. The final excretory system has two main divisions. The entire collecting system from the kidney to the bladder originates from the ureteric bud; nephrons arise from the mesodermic-metanephric mass. The kidney tissue appears originally in the early pelvic region and ascends into the abdomen. The bladder develops from the urogenital sinus and splanchnic mesenchyme. Excretory system function is present by approximately the ninth week; theoretically, contributions to amniotic fluid are possible at this time and become the major component later in gestation.

The prospective phenotype of the genital system is determined at fertilization. However, an indifferent stage of genital development exists, ending at approximately the seventh week, with the gonads showing specific sexual characteristics. By the twelfth week after fertilization, the genitals are distinctly male or female. The Y chromosome appears to be responsible for the differentiation of testes. Masculinizing hormones from the testes stimulate development of mesonephric ducts into genital components and result in the external genitals forming a penis and scrotum. Feminization of the external genitalia seemingly occurs in the absence of androgens. Gonadal tissue has its origin in the lateral abdominal wall, with the testes descending into the scrotum late in fetal life.

Malformations of the urogenital system are relatively common and result in a myriad of morphologic and microscopic manifestations. Some entities, such as renal agenesis, result in intrauterine manifestations, including oligohydramnios, and in morphological changes in the fetus. Other problems may occur in the immediate neonatal period. For example, renal abnormalities that result in cystic lesions of the kidneys initially may be detected in the newborn period as abdominal masses found at physical examination or as abnormalities in renal function. Malformations in the vascular supply to the kidneys or the collecting system result in congenital problems such as obstructive uropathy that predispose the person to renal disease, occurring in infancy and childhood. Ultrasound evaluation of the fetal collecting system may demonstrate findings consistent with dilation that does not persist. Fetal observations should be evaluated after birth. Malformations arising from problems of formation of the urogenital sinus and urachus may be severe, as in extrophy of the bladder or, less obviously, as in fistulae between perineal structures.

Abnormalities of kidney function can develop in utero. Maternal exposure to angiotensin-converting enzyme inhibitors in the second and third trimester can cause renal failure and severe oligohydramnios without structural abnormalities.

Malformations of the genitals also can be complex in origin; those resulting from errors in the sex-determining mechanism can result in hermaphrodites but are rare. Errors in sexual differentiation, producing pseudohermaphrodites, are somewhat more common. The presence of neonatal ambiguous genitalia is a true medical emergency, requiring immediate evaluation. Congenital adrenal hyperplasia, which is characterized by fetal androgen excess and masculinization of the female fetus, is accompanied by a deficiency of cortisol, leading to salt wasting and shock, is one possible cause. (See Chapter 59, Fluids and Electrolytes in Clinical Practice; and Chapter 286, Intersex.)

Special Considerations

Certain situations of fetal formation and malformation deserve special mention. The special senses, specifically those of the eyes and ears, are very sensitive to teratogenic activity and result in profound effects on the developing infant and child. Eye formation begins at the fourth week and proceeds very rapidly, especially through the sixth week. Malformations of the eye and ear may be associated with errors in genetic material;

some syndromic conditions have readily identifiable eye and ear malformation patterns. Intrauterine infections, particularly rubella, can affect the eye and inner ear. CMV is a common cause of congenital deafness.[69] Errors in position or morphology of the external ear often are associated with other malformations.

Malformations of the face and palate are of major concern. These malformations have their origin in the embryonic branchial apparatus from which the face, pharynx, and attendant structures develop. Cleft lip often is associated with cleft palate but arises from distinctly different origins. Cleft lip is often recognizable on second trimester ultrasound, but prenatal diagnosis of cleft palate remains elusive. Three-dimensional ultrasound holds promise for the diagnosis of cleft palate. Difficulties in these areas are probably of mixed genetic and environmental cause. The branchial arch merging in the formation of palate structures is most susceptible to teratogenic factors between 6 and 10 weeks' gestation.

Fetus, Mother, and Family

The fetus influences the mother and family physically and emotionally. Although expectations regarding conception and childbearing vary, the most positive situation is one of physical reproductive readiness and an anticipated pregnancy. Psychological factors involved in the decision to become pregnant are extremely complex and heavily influenced by societal mores and values. More than 50% of all pregnancies in the United States, and a much higher portion of pregnancies in teenagers and unmarried women, are unanticipated, but not necessarily unwanted, at conception.[70] Psychosocial situations that detract from optimal health before conception should be interpreted as the beginning of potential fetal risk.

Many maternal and familial situations of unfortunate familiarity to the physician provide a bad start for the pregnancy; a common example is pregnancy in the younger adolescent, who is both physically and emotionally immature and who may well not have a stable interpersonal relationship with her male partner. Postconceptual factors interact once fertilization occurs, with a progression of biochemical, physical, and emotional changes that influence the mother, father, and family. Poverty has a profound impact on the physical, emotional, and cognitive well being of children, adolescents, and adults. These effects can be mitigated by health and social programs such as Medicaid and the Special Supplemental Nutrition Program for Women, Infants, and Children.[71]

These postconceptual changes, some subtle and some not, permanently alter the parents' lifestyle. New situations demand behavioral adaptations and a process of coping. If the coping process is successful, then major developmental progress has been made, especially by the mother; such is usually true to a lesser extent in the father and to varying degrees in people further removed. However, if attitudes and the coping process are unsatisfactory, then adoption or abortion may be considered.

The first missed menstrual period, an overt sign of change to many women, does not occur until after the stage of the dividing zygote is essentially complete. By the time of the second missed menstrual period, the embryonic stage is one half over (see Figure 73-3). Although the zygotic stage is relatively unaffected by teratogens, the embryonic stage is one of very high risk. Maternal and familial habits potentially injurious to the fetus are difficult to alter under any circumstances, and of course altering circumstances is impossible when the mother does not yet know that she is pregnant. Pregnancy is often not confirmed in the present medical system until after the second missed menstrual period.

The customary use of trimesters as a means of dividing pregnancy into three intervals of equal length of particular personal or medical significance is considered imprecise by obstetricians and is discouraged for clinical situations. Nonetheless, the trimester concept remains in common usage in discussions of the progression of pregnancy and its influence.

The first trimester may be the most important phase of adjustment to the fetal presence. Many women experience physical symptoms such as fatigue, nausea, and headache, as well as changes in emotional status. The second trimester is usually marked by less overt signs of physical and emotional adjustment and discomfort. System development in the fetus is basically complete, and major growth is occurring. This development leads to the phenomenon of *quickening*, when a woman feels fetal movements for the first time at approximately week 18 to 20 in the primigravida; in the multigravida, such movement may be felt 1 to 2 weeks earlier. Quickening undoubtedly represents a major milestone in the relationship between a woman and her fetus. This sign is the first overt or direct sign of independent fetal activity. Awareness of fetal movement can provide some information about gestational age. For some women, it also serves as a milestone after which abortion is an even more difficult choice.

The third trimester is marked by an acceleration of the fetal alteration of lifestyle. Maternal physical activity, previously undertaken easily, may become increasingly difficult. Sexual activity between parents may be subject to changes or even cessation. Preparation for delivery becomes more of a part of everyday life; childbirth education, financial planning, and other aspects of preparation and emotional adjustment should be in progress. Ideally, a first appointment with the pediatrician would occur at this time.

Fetus, Health Professional, and Society

Great concern over the influence of factors such as smoking, alcohol consumption, radiation, and pesticides on the fetus is supported by many studies, and research continues to expand the database. Societies that advocate preconception care and the introduction of employment, nutritional, and lifestyle changes for women as soon as they miss a period (or preferably before conception), are surely enlightened in their advocacy of improved fetal and pregnancy outcomes.

Amniocentesis, chorionic villus sampling, and percutaneous umbilical cord sampling represent procedures of major interest to individuals and society because they enable physicians to detect conditions incompatible with what is considered normal human existence. These procedures allow families to prepare for the birth of an infant who may have special needs or requirements or to make the difficult and personal decision to terminate a pregnancy. Moral and ethical concerns over these procedures are related to those associated with abortion generally. The debate over legalized abortion has brought to the fore concerns about the legal and interpersonal status of the fetus. Health professionals are embroiled in this debate, especially over whether a practitioner of perinatal medicine can personally oppose abortion and therefore not mention all alternatives to patients.

Viability, or the capability of a fetus to assume an independent extrauterine existence, is a concept that demands attention and thought. Research shows that 23 weeks from the last menstrual period is the time at which some fetuses, if born into an environment in which neonatal intensive care is available, can survive. The role of the family in decision making, especially with regard to the extent of intervention for a baby born at the threshold of viability, is a matter of great interest. In particular, the frequency of somber modes of survival need to be presented sensitively. Parents and pediatricians have advocated that for premature infants born between 23 and 25 weeks' gestation, parental wishes should be recognized and followed.

The clinician must be aware of the close approximation of potential viability and gestation limits on legal abortion in the context of significant variations in clinical estimates of fetal age. The Supreme Court decision *(Roe v Wade)* has been interpreted to support legal abortion, although state laws vary with respect to gestational age limits. Menstrual dating by history and physical examination is only accurate within a range of 2 to 4 weeks. Confirmation of pregnancy dating by ultrasound examination improves the precision of dating to approximately 10%, so that a variation of 10 to 14 days is still possible in the second trimester. Ultrasound dating in the first trimester is associated with the smallest margin of error.

TOOLS FOR PRACTICE

Engaging Patient and Family

- *Fish Advisories* (Web page), United States Environmental Protection Agency (epa.gov/waterscience/fish/).

Medical Decision Support

- *3-D Technology,* American Institute of Ultrasound in Medicine (www.aium.org/publications/statements/_statementSelected.asp?statement=23).
- *Guidelines for Perinatal Care, 6th edition* (book), American Academy of Pediatrics and American College of Obstetricians and Gynecologists (www.aap.org/bookstore).
- *Prevention of Perinatal Group B Streptococcal Disease* (guideline), Centers for Disease Control and Prevention (www.cdc.gov/mmwr/preview/mmwrhtml/rr5111a1.htm).
- *Recommendations to Improve Preconception Health and Health Care—United States: A Report of the CDC/ATSDR Preconception Care Work Group and the Select Panel on Preconception Care* (other), Centers for Disease Control and Prevention (www.cdc.gov/mmwr/preview/mmwrhtml/rr5506a1.htm).
- *Red Book: 2006 Report of the Committee on Infectious Diseases, 27th edition,* American Academy of Pediatrics (www.aap.org/bookstore).

RELATED WEB SITE

- *March of Dimes* (Web page), March of Dimes (www.marchofdimes.com).

AAP POLICY STATEMENTS

American Academy of Pediatrics and United States Public Health Service. Joint statement of American Academy of Pediatrics and United States Public Health Service. *Pediatrics.* 1999;104(3):568-569. (aappolicy.aappublications.org/cgi/content/full/pediatrics;104/3/568).

Cunniff C, American Academy of Pediatrics, Committee on Genetics. Prenatal screening and diagnosis for pediatricians. *Pediatrics.* 2004;114(3):889-894. (aappolicy.aappublications.org/cgi/content/full/pediatrics;114/3/889).

MacDonald H, American Academy of Pediatrics, Committee on Fetus and Newborn. Perinatal care at the threshold of viability. *Pediatrics.* 2002;110(5):1024-1027. (aappolicy.aappublications.org/cgi/content/full/pediatrics;110/5/1024).

SUGGESTED RESOURCES

American Academy of Pediatrics. Available at: www.aap.org/.

American College of Obstetricians and Gynecologist. Available at: www.acog.org/.

American College of Obstetricians and Gynecologists Preembryo Research. *History, Scientific Background, and Ethical Considerations.* ACOG Committee Opinion 136. Washington, DC: American College of Obstetricians and Gynecologists; 1994.

Beckman DA, Brent RL. Mechanisms of known environmental teratogens: drugs and chemicals. *Clin Perinatol.* 1986:13:649.

Centers for Disease Control and Prevention, National Immunization Program. Available at: www.cdc.gov/nip/.

Centers for Disease Control and Prevention. Available at: www.cdc.gov/.

Chalmers I, Enkin M, Keirse M, eds. *Effective Care in Pregnancy and Childbirth.* Oxford, UK: Oxford University Press; 1989.

Dorris M. *The Broken Cord.* New York, NY: Harper & Row; 1989.

Hauth JC, Merenstein GB. *Guidelines for Perinatal Care.* 3rd ed. Washington, DC: American Academy of Pediatrics, American College of Obstetricians and Gynecologists; 1997.

Hetzel BS. Iodine deficiency and fetal brain damage. *N Engl J Med.* 1994;331:1770.

Institute of Medicine. *Fetal Research and Applications: A Conference Summary.* Washington, DC: National Academy Press; 1994.

Moore KL, Persaud TVN. *The Developing Human: Clinically Oriented Embryology.* 5th ed. Philadelphia, PA: WB Saunders; 1993.

National Institutes of Health Consensus Development Program. Available at: consensus.nih.gov/.

National Institutes of Health. *Report of the Human Embryo Research Panel.* Bethesda, MD: National Institutes of Health; 1994.

United States Environmental Protection Agency. Fish Advisories. Available at: www.epa.gov/waterscience/fish/.

REFERENCES

1. Mittendorf R, Herbst AL. DES exposure: an update. *Contemp Pediatr.* 1994;11:59.
2. American College of Obstetrics and Gynecology. *Committee Opinion: The Importance of Preconception Care in the Continuum of Women's Health Care.* Washington, DC: American College of Obstetrics and Gynecology; 2005.
3. Cao XY, Jiang XM, Dou ZH, et al. Timing of vulnerability of the brain to iodine deficiency in endemic cretinism. *N Engl J Med.* 1994;331(26):1739-1744.

4. US Environmental Protection Agency. Fish Advisories. Available at: www.epa.gov/waterscience/fish. Accessed August 23, 2007.
5. Mercury in tuna: New safety concerns. *Consum Rep.* 2006;71:20.
6. American Academy of Pediatrics. Joint statement of the American Academy of Pediatrics (AAP) and the United States Public Health Service (USPHS). *Pediatrics.* 1999; 104(3 pt 1):568-569.
7. Sanz EJ, De-las-Cuevas C, Kiuru A, et al. Selective serotonin reuptake inhibitors in pregnant women and neonatal withdrawal syndrome: a database analysis. *Lancet.* 2005;365(9458):482-487.
8. Chambers CD, Hearnandez-Diaz S, Van Marter LJ, et al. Selective serotonin-reuptake inhibitors and risk of persistent pulmonary hypertension of the newborn. *N Engl J Med.* 2006;354(6):579-587.
9. DiFranza JR, Aligne CA, Weitzman M. Prenatal and postnatal environmental tobacco smoke exposure and children's health. *Pediatrics.* 2004;113(4 suppl):1007-1015.
10. Perer FP, Rauh V, Whyatt RM, et al. A summary of recent findings on birth outcomes and developmental effects of prenatal ETS, PAH and pesticide exposures. *Neurotoxicology.* 2005;26(4):573-587.
11. Jones HE, Johnson RE, Jasinski DR, et al. Buprenorphine versus methadone in the treatment of pregnant opioid-dependent patients: effects on the neonatal abstinence syndrome. *Drug Alcohol Depend.* 2005;79:1-10.
12. El-Mohandes A, Herman AA, Nabil El-Khorazaty M, et al. Prenatal care reduces the impact of illicit drug use on perinatal outcomes. *J Perinatol.* 2003;23:354-360.
13. Lopez NJ, Smith PC, Gutierrez J. Higher risk of preterm birth and low birth weight in women with periodontal disease. *J Dent Res.* 2002;81:58-63.
14. Levin L, Zadik Y, Becker T. Oral and dental complications of intra-oral piercing. *Dent Traumatol.* 2005;21:341-343.
15. Lopez NJ, DaSilva I, Ipinza J, et al. Periodontal therapy reduces the rate of preterm low birth weight in women with pregnancy-associated gingivitis. *J Periodontol.* 2005;76(11 suppl):2144-2153.
16. Reddy UM, Ko CW, Willinger M. Maternal age and the risk of stillbirth throughout pregnancy in the United States. *Am J Obstet Gynecol.* 2006;195:764-770.
17. Amini SB, Catalano PM, Dierker LJ, et al. Births to teenagers: trends and obstetric outcomes. *Obstet Gynecol.* 1996;87(5 pt 1):668-674.
18. Rosengard C, Pollock L, Weitzen S, et al. Concepts of the advantages and disadvantages of teenage childbearing among pregnant adolescents: a qualitative analysis. *Pediatrics.* 2006;118:503-510.
19. Hawthorne G. Preconception care in diabetes [review]. *Semin Fetal Neonatal Med.* 2005;10:325-332.
20. Haddow JE, Palomaki GE, Allan WC, et al. Maternal thyroid deficiency during pregnancy and subsequent neuropsychological development of the child. *N Engl J Med.* 1999;341:549-555.
21. Thummala MR, Raju TN, Langenberg P. Isolated single umbilical artery anomaly and the risk for congenital malformations: a meta-analysis. *J Pediatr Surg.* 1998;33(4):580-585.
22. Chow JS, Benson CB, Doubilet PM. Frequency and nature of structural abnormalities with single umbilical arteries. *J Ultrasound Med.* 1998;17:765-768.
23. American College of Obstetrics and Gynecology. *Committee Opinion: Prevention of Early Onset Group B Streptococcal Disease in Newborns.* Washington, DC: American College of Obstetrics and Gynecology; 2002.
24. Centers for Disease Control and Prevention. Prevention of perinatal group B streptococcal disease. Revised guidelines from CDC. *MMWR Recomm Rep.* 2002;51 (RR-11):1-22.
25. National Institutes of Health Consensus Development Panel. Antenatal corticosteroids revisited: repeat courses—National Institutes of Health Consensus Development Conference Statement, August 17-18, 2000. *Obstet Gynecol.* 2001;98(1):144-150.
26. Goldenberg RL, Rouse DJ. Prevention of preterm birth. *N Engl J Med.* 1998;339:313-320.
27. Viadeff AC, Ramin SM. From concept to practice: the recent history of preterm delivery prevention. Part 1: cervical competence [review]. *Am J Perinatol.* 2006;23:3-13.
28. Meis PJ, Klebanoff M, Thom E, et al, for the National Institute of Child Health and Human Development Maternal-Fetal Medicine Units Network. Prevention of recurrent preterm delivery by 17 alpha-hydroxyprogesterone caproate. *N Engl J Med.* 2003;348:2379-2385.
29. Tran SH, Caughey AB, Musci TJ. Meconium-stained amniotic fluid is associated with puerperal infections. *Am J Obstet Gynecol.* 2003;189(3):746-750.
30. Osmond C, Barker DJ. Fetal, infant, and childhood growth are predictors of coronary heart disease, diabetes, and hypertension in adult men and women [review]. *Environ Health Perspect.* 2000;108(suppl 3):545-553.
31. Mari G, Deter RL, Carpenter RL, et al. Noninvasive diagnosis by Doppler ultrasonography of fetal anemia due to maternal red-cell alloimmunization. *N Engl J Med.* 2000; 342(1):9-14.
32. Oepkes D, Seaward PG, Vandenbussche FP, et al. Doppler ultrasonography versus amniocentesis to predict fetal anemia. *N Engl J Med.* 2006;355(2):156-164.
33. Sperling RS, Shapiro DE, Coombs RW, et al. Maternal viral load, zidovudine treatment, and the risk of transmission of human immunodeficiency virus type 1 from mother to infant. Pediatric AIDS Clinical Trials Group Protocol 076 Study Group. *N Engl J Med.* 1996;335(22): 1621-1629.
34. Hawkins D, Blott M, Clayden P, et al. Guidelines for the management of HIV infection in pregnant women and the prevention of mother-to-child transmission of HIV. *HIV Med.* 2005;6(suppl 2):107-148.
35. American Academy of Pediatrics. Human immunodeficiency virus infection. In: Pickering LK, Baker CJ, Long SS, et al, eds. *Red Book: 2006 Report of the Committee on Infectious Diseases.* 27th ed. Elk Grove Village, IL: American Academy of Pediatrics; 2006.
36. Sheffield JS, Hill JB, Hollier LM, et al. Valacyclovir prophylaxis to prevent recurrent herpes at delivery: a randomized clinical trial. *Obstet Gynecol.* 2006;108: 141-147.
37. American Academy of Pediatrics. Toxoplasma gondii infections. In: Pickering LK, Baker CJ, Long SS, et al, eds. *Red Book: 2006 Report of the Committee on Infectious Diseases.* 27th ed. Elk Grove Village, IL: American Academy of Pediatrics; 2006.
38. Hitchins AD, Whiting RC. Food-borne Listeria monocytogenes risk assessment. *Food Addit Contam.* 2001;18: 1108-1117.
39. Levine D. *Atlas of Fetal MRI.* Boston, MA: Taylor & Francis; 2005.
40. American College of Obstetrics and Gynecology. Practice bulletin: clinical management guidelines for obstetrician-gynecologists. No. 38, September 2002. Perinatal care at the threshold of viability. *Obstet Gynecol.* 2002;100:617-624.
41. American Academy of Pediatrics. *Clinical Report: Perinatal Care at the Threshold of Viability.* Elk Grove Village, IL: American Academy of Pediatrics; 2002.
42. Marlow N, Wolke D, Bracewell MA, et al. Neurologic and developmental disability at six years of age after extremely preterm birth. *N Engl J Med.* 2005;352(1): 9-19.

43. Savitz DA, Terry JW, Dole N, et al. Comparison of pregnancy dating by last menstrual period, ultrasound and their combination. *Am J Obstet Gynecol.* 2002;187:1660.
44. Battaglia F, Meschia G. *An Introduction to Fetal Physiology.* Orlando, FL: Academic Press; 1986.
45. Klerman LV, Reynolds DW. Interconception care: a new role for the pediatrician. *Pediatrics.* 1994;93(2):327-329.
46. Centers for Disease Control and Prevention. Recommendations to improve preconception health and health care—United States: a report of the CDC/ATSDR Preconception Care Work Group and the Select Panel on Preconception Care. *MMWR Recomm Rep.* 2006;55(RR06):1-23.
47. US Department of Health and Human Services. *Caring for Our Future: The Content of Prenatal Care.* Washington, DC: US Department of Health and Human Services; 1989.
48. Rosen MG, Merkatz IR, Hill JG. Caring for our future: a report by the expert panel on the content of prenatal care. *Obstet Gynecol.* 1991;77:782-787.
49. Martin JA, Hamilton BE, Sutton PD, et al. *Births: Final Data for 2003 National Vital Statistics Report 54.* Washington, DC: US Department of Health and Human Services; 2005.
50. Velazquez MD, Rayburn WF. Antenatal evaluation of the fetus using fetal movement monitoring. *Clin Obstet Gynecol.* 2002;45:993-1004.
51. National Institute of Child Health and Human Development Research Planning Workshop. Electronic fetal heart rate monitoring: research guidelines for interpretation. *Am J Obstet Gynecol.* 1997;177(6):1385-1390.
52. American Institute of Ultrasound in Medicine. Official Statement, 3-D Technology. 2005. Available at: www.aium.org/publications/statements/_statementSelected.asp?statement=23. Accessed August 23, 2007.
53. Cosmi E, Ambrosini G, D'Antona D, et al. Doppler, cardiotocography and biophysical profile changes in growth-restricted fetuses. *Obstet Gynecol.* 2005;106(6):1240-1245.
54. Martinoli C, Pretolesi F, Crespi G, et al. Power Doppler sonography: clinical applications. *Eur J Radiol.* 1998;27(suppl 2):S133-S140.
55. American Institute of Ultrasound in Medicine. *Acoustic Output Measurement Standards for Diagnostic Ultrasound Equipment.* Laurel, MD: American Institute of Ultrasound in Medicine; 1998.
56. American College of Obstetrics and Gynecology. *Ultrasonography in Pregnancy: ACOG Practice Pattern 58.* Washington, DC: American College of Obstetrics and Gynecology; 2004.
57. Coleman BG, Adzick NS, Crombleholme TM, et al. Fetal therapy: state of the art. *J Ultrasound Med.* 2002;21(11):1257-1288.
58. Malone FD, Canick JA, Ball RH, et al. First trimester or second trimester screening, or both, for Down syndrome. *N Engl J Med.* 2005;353(19):2001-2011.
59. Shipp TD, Benacerraf BR. Second trimester ultrasound screening for chromosome abnormalities. *Prenat Diagn.* 2002;22(4):296-307.
60. Cunniff C, American Academy of Pediatrics, Committee on Genetics. Prenatal screening and diagnosis for pediatricians. *Pediatrics.* 2004;114(3):889-894.
61. Jones KL. *Smith's Recognizable Patterns of Human Malformation.* 5th ed. Philadelphia, PA: WB Saunders; 1997.
62. Czeizel AE, Dudás I. Prevention of the first occurrence of neural-tube defects by periconceptional vitamin supplementation. *N Engl J Med.* 1992;327(26):1832-1835.
63. The Medical Task Force on Anencephaly. The infant with anencephaly. *N Engl J Med.* 1990;322(10):669-674.
64. Welch-Carre E. The neurodevelopmental consequences of prenatal alcohol exposure. *Adv Neonatal Care.* 2005;5(4):217-229.
65. Bracci R, Buonocore G. Chorioamnionitis: a risk factor for fetal and neonatal morbidity. *Biol Neonate.* 2003;83(2):85-96.
66. Fineman JR, Clyman RI, Heymann MA. Fetal cardiovascular physiology. In: Creasy RK, Resnik R, Iams JD, eds. *Maternal-Fetal Medicine: Principles and Practice.* 5th ed. Philadelphia, PA: WB Saunders; 2004.
67. Kleinman CS, Nehgme RA. Cardiac arrhythmia in the human fetus. *Pediatr Cardiol.* 2004;25(3):234-251.
68. Zusman I, Gurevich P, Ben-Hur H. Two secretory immune systems (mucosal and barrier) in human intrauterine development, normal and pathological. *Int J Mol Med.* 2005;16:127-133.
69. Nance WE, Lim BG, Dodson KM. Importance of congenital cytomegalovirus infection as a cause of pre-lingual hearing loss. *J Clin Virol.* 2006;35:222-225.
70. Brown SS, Eisenberg L, eds, Institute of Medicine, Committee on Unintended Pregnancy. *The Best Intentions: Unintended Pregnancy and the Well-Being of Children and Families.* Washington, DC: National Academy Press; 1995.
71. Black RM, Cutts DB, Frank DA, et al. Special supplemental nutrition programs for women, infants, and children participation and infant's growth and health: a multisite surveillance study. *Pediatrics.* 2004;114:169.

Chapter 74

ASSESSMENT AND STABILIZATION AT DELIVERY

Joaquim M. B. Pinheiro, MD, MPH

Labor and transition to extrauterine function are physiological challenges that most humans overcome successfully. However, birth is the riskiest stage of life because failure of postnatal adaptation can result in immediate physiological instability, end-organ dysfunction, and death or disability. Approximately 10% of neonates require some resuscitative assistance during transition in the delivery room. In subgroups such as very low–birth-weight newborns (<1500 g), 90% receive immediate respiratory support; although most of these neonates need only oxygen, approximately 6% reportedly require advanced resuscitation, including chest compressions.

Prenatal history and intrapartum evaluation allow clinicians to anticipate most newborns who will need resuscitation after delivery; still, unexpected complications are common. Immediate assistance aimed at ensuring stabilization and appropriate transition of the neonate must be available and effectively established, usually in the first few minutes of life. Thus the American Academy of Pediatrics and American College of Obstetrics and Gynecology, in their *Guidelines for Perinatal Care,* recommend that "At every delivery, there should be at least one person whose primary responsibility is the neonate and who is capable of initiating resuscitation. Either that person or someone else who is immediately available should have the skills required to perform a complete resuscitation.... It is not sufficient to have someone 'on call' (either at home or in another area of the hospital)."[1]

A skilled resuscitator does not suffice to ensure an effective resuscitation. An integrated approach involving all perinatal staff is needed for immediate recognition of distressed neonates, communication among care providers, and rapid implementation of accepted resuscitation procedures. The Neonatal Resuscitation Program (NRP) (www.aap.org/nrp/), jointly sponsored by the American Heart Association and the American Academy of Pediatrics,[2] provides evidence-based guidelines and expert opinion on neonatal resuscitation. The guidelines include a curriculum for training and evaluating neonatal primary care providers, individually and in teams, and practical tools to guide resuscitation. Because the NRP curriculum is now used to train most care providers of neonatal resuscitation in the United States (and in some other countries), hospitals base their neonatal resuscitation procedures on principles espoused by the NRP, adapted to local resources. As a result, this chapter suggests practices closely aligned with those published by the NRP.

This chapter, intended for primary care physicians and other providers of neonatal primary care who may practice at hospitals without a tertiary care perinatal center and focuses on practical evaluation and management of neonates who need assistance during transition in the delivery room setting. After briefly reviewing the physiological basis of neonatal resuscitation, the necessary physical infrastructure, provider roles, and procedures for routine and contingency resuscitations are outlined. Routine care of neonates and evaluation of sick newborns after the delivery room transition are addressed in Chapter 75, Identifying the Infant Who Requires Specialized Care; and Chapter 96, Follow-Up Care of the Graduate of the Neonatal Intensive Care Unit.

ANTICIPATING HIGH-RISK DELIVERIES

Prenatal anticipation of the need for neonatal resuscitation allows time for adequate preparation. Significant resuscitative interventions in the delivery room can be expected in very premature newborns (with gestational age <32 weeks) and those with major congenital malformations.

Gestational age should be assessed before birth because obstetric criteria are more accurate for this purpose than a postnatal physical examination that uses a method such as the New Ballard Score (www.ballardscore.com/). An accurate approximation of gestational age is particularly crucial in deliveries around the edge of viability, between 21 and 25 weeks of gestation. Because no official algorithm exists to ensure uniform determinations of gestational age by obstetricians, finding discrepant gestational ages on a maternal record is common. Primary care physicians should verify the obstetrically estimated gestational age, which is optimally based on the first day of the mother's last menstrual period and confirmed by an early prenatal ultrasound. Proper advanced planning, which ranges from withholding resuscitation to advanced notification of a transport team, is contingent on obtaining reliable gestational age estimates.

Congenital malformations recognized prenatally, whether necessitating neonatal surgery or potentially interfering with cardiorespiratory transition at birth, may require specialized resuscitative interventions in the delivery room.

Common intrapartum exposures such as maternal magnesium sulfate therapy and chorioamnionitis are generally identified well in advance of the delivery. However, meconium staining of the amniotic fluid and significant decelerations of the fetal heart rate are most often noted just before delivery. Review of the obstetric history is useful to identify these and other factors (Box 74-1) that may affect the newborn's need for resuscitation and early postnatal care.

A continuum of risks is anticipated at delivery. Each institution should establish specific criteria determining which deliveries require the presence of a separate team to care for the neonate, as well as the composition of such team, according to level of risk. The traditional practice of calling a neonatal team to every cesarean delivery, initially justified by the use of general anesthesia in the mother and the frequent presence of fetal distress as the indication for urgent surgical delivery, is no longer sensible. Rates of cesarean section delivery now approach 30% in the United States, and an increasing trend exists in medically and socially elective surgical deliveries, prompted by prior cesarean deliveries or simple maternal choice. Given that the need for pediatrician attendance at low risk, elective cesarean deliveries is controversial, individual hospital obstetric and newborn service providers should consult with their risk-management department to develop policies and programs that best serve their unique circumstances.

ESSENTIAL TRANSITIONAL CARDIORESPIRATORY PHYSIOLOGY

The successful establishment of cardiorespiratory function in the newborn requires adequately grown and unobstructed conducting airways, gas-exchanging airways with sufficient surfactant and matching pulmonary vasculature, removal of fetal lung fluid, sustained breathing, and a rapid increase in pulmonary blood flow. Anatomic or functional derangements in one or more of these areas can result in cardiorespiratory insufficiency in the newborn. Although these functions may be approached by following the ABC (airway, breathing, circulation) sequence commonly taught for resuscitation, each requires integration of respiratory, hemodynamic, neurologic, and other inputs.

A functional airway must be anatomically normal, externally straight and uncompressed, and unobstructed by intrinsic structures such as the tongue or vocal cords; its lumen must also be clear of extraneous matter (eg, amniotic fluid, meconium, blood, secretions). The initial postnatal breaths clear lung fluid from the airways and establish a gaseous functional respiratory capacity; normal tone of pharyngeal and laryngeal muscles sustains a patent upper airway. Thus any condition that causes apnea, generalized hypotonia, or laryngospasm at birth will compromise the airway.

Box 74-2 lists common or typical causes of symptomatic airway obstruction in the immediate postnatal

BOX 74-1 Factors That Increase the Likelihood of Neonatal Resuscitation

PREPARTUM PRESENTATION

- Planned preterm delivery*
- Magnesium sulfate*
- Maternal infection*
- Oligohydramnios*
- Hydrops fetalis*
- Major fetal malformations*
- Multiple gestation*
- Size-date discrepancy*
- Lung immaturity
- Premature rupture of membranes
- Postterm gestation
- Diminished fetal activity
- Polyhydramnios
- Fetal anemia
- Maternal hypertension
- Maternal diabetes
- Maternal drug abuse
- Acute maternal illnesses
- Recent vaginal bleeding
- Maternal adrenergic blockade
- No prenatal care

INTRAPARTUM PRESENTATION

- Preterm delivery*
- Chorioamnionitis*
- Meconium-stained amniotic fluid*
- Abnormal fetal heart rate*
- Emergency cesarean delivery*
- Placental abruption*
- Cord prolapse*
- Maternal narcotics <4 hours before delivery
- Abnormal presentation (breech, transverse)
- Placenta previa
- Cord compression
- Precipitous labor
- Prolonged labor
- Prolonged second stage of labor >2 hours
- Shoulder dystocia
- Uterine tetany
- Ruptured membranes >18 hours
- General anesthesia
- Maternal hypotension
- Forceps- or vacuum-aided delivery

POSTPARTUM PRESENTATION

- Severe respiratory distress*
- Drug-induced depression*
- Central nervous system injury*
- Central nervous system anomalies
- Spinal cord injury
- Airway obstruction
- Sepsis or infection
- Diaphragmatic hernia
- Pneumothorax
- Deformities
- Abdominal anomalies

*Most common and significant conditions.

period. They are categorized according to whether they are extrinsic to the airway, related to intrinsic airway structures, or the result of removable luminal fluids or particulates. The actual incidence of these conditions is unknown, and they may coexist (eg, mild laryngomalacia, nasal secretions, nasal mucosal edema). Iatrogenic causes are emphasized because they are common and mostly preventable. For example, airway obstruction can easily occur during bag-mask ventilation, through mandibular pressure from the mask or from impingement of the resuscitator's fourth and fifth fingers on submandibular tissue. Laryngospasm can be readily induced by mechanical stimulation of the hypopharynx or larynx with a suction catheter or laryngoscope.

In the newborn, initial breaths inflate and aerate the lungs and promote gas exchange. Each of these elements has independent and synergistic physiological effects. Lung inflation decreases vagal tone, directly diminishing the apneic and bradycardic effects of vagal activity. Lung inflation and aeration each decrease pulmonary vascular resistance, allowing the postnatal increase in pulmonary blood flow necessary for gas exchange; the latter is optimized by the inflation-induced stimulation of surfactant secretion. The subsequent increase in systemic oxygenation has additional vagolytic effects.

Significant intrapartum hypoxia and exposure to common medications such as magnesium sulfate and narcotics depress respiratory drive, producing hypopnea or apnea in the newly born. Common and archetypal causes of apnea in the delivery room are listed in Box 74-3. In most instances, the neonate exhibits primary apnea, which is induced by respiratory reflexes and is thus readily reversed. Secondary apnea is much less common because it reflects significant hypoxia-ischemia, with resulting metabolic dysfunction of the central respiratory apparatus. Protracted depression of the respiratory drive can also be the result of transplacental transfer of maternal medications with neuroinhibitory effect.

Hypoventilation may occur despite unobstructed conducting airways and normal or increased respiratory effort. Common or typical conditions causing hyperpneic respiratory failure include severe lung immaturity (respiratory distress syndrome), lung hypoplasia (diaphragmatic hernia, oligohydramnios), and external impediments to lung inflation (tension pneumothorax, large pleural effusions, thoracic hypoplasia).

BOX 74-2 Common or Prototypical Causes of Airway Obstruction in the Newly Born

EXTRINSIC
- Mandibular pressure from facemask*
- Submandibular pressure from resuscitator's fingers
- Kinked upper airway (flexed or hyperextended)
- Masses (eg, epulis)
- Vascular ring

INTRINSIC (PARIETAL)
- Hypotonic pharyngeal muscles, tongue
- Laryngospasm
- Nasal trauma, edema
- Airway malformations (Pierre Robin sequence, choanal atresia)
- Laryngomalacia
- Vocal cord paralysis

INTRALUMINAL
- Pharyngeal secretions (with or without meconium, blood)
- Nasal secretions
- Residual lung fluid
- Aspiration of upper airway fluid and suspended particles

*Most common and significant conditions.

Circulatory adequacy depends on heart rate and stroke volume. Thus cardiac output is compromised by bradycardia, acute hypovolemia, or both. In addition, functional circulatory insufficiency can reflect an inadequate increase in pulmonary blood flow at birth, with consequent hypoxemia. Rare anatomic defects such as transposition of the great vessels with intact ventricular septum can produce severe, persistent hypoxemia from birth. However, cardiovascular lesions that depend on patency of the ductus arteriosus for maintenance of pulmonary or systemic blood flow would not become symptomatic in the delivery room.

BOX 74-3 Common or Prototypical Causes of Apnea or Hypopnea in the Newly Born

Hypoxemia
Reflexes elicited by trigeminal or ocular pressure, laryngeal stimulation
Deflated lungs
Airway obstruction
Magnesium sulfate
Recent intrapartum narcotics
General anesthesia (rare)
Hypoxia-ischemia

BOX 74-4 Common or Prototypical Causes of Inadequate Circulatory Transition in the Newly Born

Acute hypovolemia (nuchal cord, fetoplacental or fetomaternal transfusion, placental abruption, cord accidents)
Prolonged fetal bradycardia
Persistent pulmonary hypertension (lung hypoplasia, fetal distress, meconium aspiration, asphyxia)
Hypothermia
Polycythemia
Hydrops fetalis
Transposition of the great vessels (with intact ventricular septum)
Cardiomyopathy
Pneumopericardium
Tension pneumothorax

Common causes and clinical correlates of inadequate transition from fetal to newborn circulation are listed in Box 74-4. Acute hypovolemia is particularly difficult to diagnose because pallor and peripheral vasoconstriction commonly result from the catecholamine surge induced by fetal or neonatal distress (or both) and acidosis. However, when these symptoms occur in the setting of a tight nuchal cord, hypovolemia caused by significant fetoplacental transfusion should be suspected; this condition is likely underdiagnosed and occurs in approximately 3% of deliveries at term.

Another typical transitional disorder is persistent pulmonary hypertension, with right-to-left shunt at the level of the foramen ovale and ductus arteriosus and with consequent systemic hypoxemia. The persistently increased pulmonary vascular resistance may result from a combination of inadequate lung inflation, alveolar hypoxia, hypoventilation, and acidosis; these complications may be superimposed on hypoplastic or hyperreactive pulmonary vasculature, and they may be exacerbated by hypothermia developing during resuscitation.

Thermoregulation is a fundamental but easily overlooked aspect of transition in neonates requiring cardiopulmonary resuscitation. Hypothermia can develop within minutes, and it may adversely affect circulatory transition because it induces pulmonary vasoconstriction and increases oxygen consumption. Thus efforts to maintain a neutral thermal environment and minimize convective heat loss should precede resuscitation and be sustained while performing other interventions (in mnemonic terms, T-ABC[D] [temperature, airway, breathing, circulation, drugs]).

ACUTE FETAL HYPOXIA AND ASPHYXIA

Despite the myriad causes of cardiorespiratory insufficiency in the neonate, acute hypoxia that develops during or immediately after birth is a central feature of most transitional disorders. Sustained hypoxemia and ischemia result in asphyxia and ultimately death. Intermittent fetal hypoxia occurs normally with uterine contractions as a result of decreased uterine blood flow, umbilical cord compression, or both. Pathological intrapartum hypoxia likely develops most often in susceptible human fetuses by repetitive cord compression and incomplete recovery between contractions.

Much of the understanding of the physiology of asphyxia is extrapolated from Dawes' experiments with acute total asphyxia in a normal newborn rhesus monkey model.[3] Figure 74-1 illustrates the progression of cardiorespiratory and neurologic dysfunction during acute asphyxia, which is produced by delivering the animal's head into a saline-filled bag and clamping the umbilical cord. The initial response to hypoxia is reflex (primary) apnea and bradycardia.

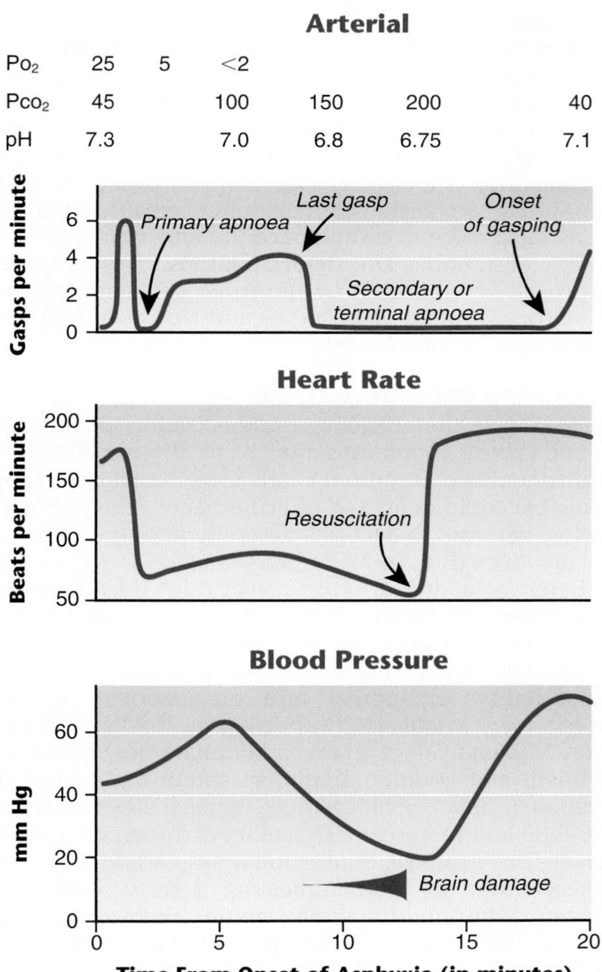

Figure 74-1 Sequence of cardiorespiratory and neurologic abnormalities during total acute asphyxia followed by positive pressure ventilation in newborn rhesus monkeys. *(From Dawes GS.* Fetal and Neonatal Physiology. *Chicago, IL: Year Book Medical Publishers, Inc; 1968:149. Copyright 2008 Elsevier Ltd. Reprinted by permission.)*

Progressive mixed acidosis ensues and induces gasping, which ceases as the respiratory centers develop severe metabolic dysfunction; this stage is the phase of secondary (or terminal) apnea and bradycardia, during which neurologic responsiveness has been lost, and only artificial resuscitation can avert death. Permanent brain injury may develop during this stage. Resuscitation with positive pressure ventilation (PPV) results in immediate recovery of the heart rate, return of blood pressure, and, finally, the reappearance of gasping respirations.

The importance of reflex mechanisms in determining immediate cardiorespiratory responses in the newly born cannot be overemphasized. Natural and iatrogenic stimuli including hypoxia, acidosis, lung deflation, trigeminal pressure, and secretions or mechanical irritation in the periglottic region act synergistically to induce laryngeal closure, central apnea, and bradycardia. These reflex responses are mediated through arterial chemoreceptors and vagal and somatosensory afferents. Conversely, simple lung inflation stimulates pulmonary stretch receptors, producing an immediate vagolytic effect while desensitizing laryngeal and carotid body reflexes and inducing further deep inspirations through the Head paradoxical reflex. Adequate lung inflation, whether spontaneous or assisted, is therefore paramount in restoring spontaneous cardiorespiratory and neurologic function in the depressed newborn.

Cardiorespiratory depression in a newborn thus results from cardiorespiratory reflexes superimposed on and interacting with a continuum of hypoxia-ischemia. Rapid assessment of the severity of physiological dysfunction in the individual baby is essential to apply appropriate resuscitative measures. In the clinical setting, practical evaluation methods must be used in place of invasive physiological measurements. The Apgar scores were traditionally devised for this purpose, but they are no longer recommended as a guide to resuscitation, partly because evaluation of heart rate, respirations, tone, reflex irritability, and color cannot be done rapidly, reliably, and unobtrusively in emergency conditions. The NRP recommends repeated assessment of the triad of respirations, heart rate, and color to guide further interventions in the delivery room. Nevertheless, Apgar scores are still routinely obtained to assess the condition of the newly born.[4] Both the Apgar scoring system and the abbreviated NRP evaluation method can be fundamentally understood from the continuum of perinatal depression studied by Geoffrey Dawes in animal models and observed by Virginia Apgar in human newborns.

As shown in Figure 74-2, the 5 clinical signs in the Apgar scoring system can be considered as sequential steps in a cycle of oxygen transport and utilization. Individual signs are further linked through reflex mechanisms. Conditions that depress fetal cardiorespiratory or neurologic function in the immediate perinatal period will produce primary apnea and hypoventilation in the newly born. Failure of lung inflation, aeration, and oxygenation triggers a sequence of progressive dysfunction. The increased vagal tone causes reflex *(primary)* apnea and bradycardia. Consequent progressive hypoxia produces cyanosis and promotes gradual

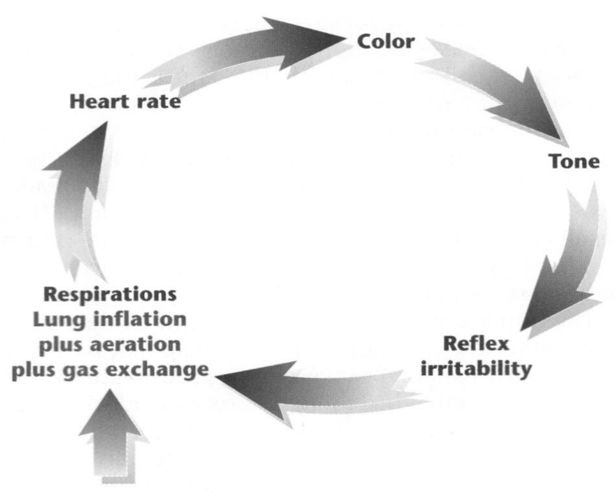

Figure 74-2 Recovery of clinical signs within the Apgar scoring system in response to assisted ventilation. Immediate responses are reflexive in nature; the cycle is sustained by oxygen transport and metabolism.

loss of neuromuscular function. Progressive hypoxia results in metabolic dysfunction in the muscular and central neurologic systems, culminating in secondary apnea and concurrent unresponsiveness to stimuli. Asystole follows prolonged, severe hypoxia.

Figure 74-2 depicts the sequence of recovery of functions when effective resuscitation with PPV is applied before the onset of asystole. The vagolytic effect of lung inflation immediately increases heart rate. Peripheral oxygenation then visibly improves, and neuromuscular function gradually recovers, ultimately producing sustained respirations.

Understanding these intrinsic relationships within the Apgar system facilitates the assessment of depressed newborns independently of the attribution of numerical scores. The abbreviated evaluation scheme suggested by the NRP includes initial muscle tone followed by repeated rapid assessment of respirations, heart rate, and color. The NRP method effectively uses the same basic functions as the Apgar system without the obtrusive scoring. Given the interdependence of the 5 clinical signs, isolated abnormalities in any measure should suggest specific causes directly affecting that sign and unrelated to hypoxia (eg, sustained bradycardia in a pink, vigorous newborn might indicate congenital heart block).

RESUSCITATION IN THE DELIVERY ROOM

Withholding, Limiting, or Withdrawing Resuscitation

Resuscitation of the newborn is a medical intervention with variable effectiveness, benefits, and risks, which largely depend on the baby's underlying conditions. In keeping with ethical principles, resuscitation should not be applied indiscriminately to all newborns with cardiorespiratory depression, particularly when the prognosis for survival is poor or survival will likely be burdensome to the child. Because most delivery room resuscitations are expected, time is usually available to discuss the expected outcomes with the family. An evidence-based, family-centered valuation of the outcomes of resuscitation should guide clinical decision making in the delivery room.[5] Ideally, the obstetric and pediatric clinicians and the parents would reach a common understanding of the goals of resuscitation before the time of birth. Only then can the extent of interventions be tailored to the individual mother and baby—including the options of withholding or limiting resuscitation of the newborn.

Resuscitation is not indicated in babies with poor prognoses that entail early death or major morbidities in the rare long-term survivor. Newborns meeting these criteria include those of confirmed gestational age less than 23 weeks or birth weight below 400 g, those with anencephaly, and those with confirmed trisomy-13 or -18 or other known lethal anomaly. Comfort care and support of the family are always indicated.

Noninitiation of resuscitation is also appropriate at the parents' request for infants with uncertain prognosis, including those with high probability of death or extreme morbidity. Newborns at 23 to 24 weeks' gestation typify a situation in which the parents' wishes for resuscitation should be ascertained, respected, and supported by clinicians. As discussed previously, clinicians must attempt to minimize the uncertainty inherent in gestational age determinations. This practice approach is supported by the American Academy of Pediatrics Committee on Fetus and Newborn and the Canadian Pediatric Society.[5-7]

Preparing for Resuscitation

To maximize the efficiency of stabilization during the initial, crucial 10 minutes after birth, the resuscitation team should be organized in advance, familiar with the available equipment, and informed about the prenatal factors relevant to accurate assessment of the individual newborn (Box 74-5).

Before or at arrival at the delivery site, the resuscitation team can rapidly assess the fetal condition by ascertaining gestational age, other major underlying diagnoses, and evidence of fetal distress. Next, the resuscitation equipment and medications can be checked systematically by applying the T-ABC(D) mnemonic. Team leadership and additional roles should be defined, and additional support should be sought if needed. If time permits, a more detailed assessment of the fetal and maternal risk factors can then be undertaken. The pediatric team should assess and plan the resuscitation by communicating clearly with the obstetric staff and the family, among themselves, and with a tertiary-care center if neonatal transport is anticipated.

By directly observing the last few minutes of the delivery, rather than waiting by the resuscitation table, the team leader can obtain useful information that is often not verbally communicated. This information may include the fetal heart rate pattern during the last contractions, presence or absence of meconium or blood in the mouth, a tight nuchal cord, the baby's facial response to suctioning or handling, and the tone

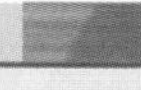

BOX 74-5 Domains of Preparation for Delivery Room Resuscitation

ASSESSMENT OF THE FETUS

- Gestational age
- Anticipated fetal pathological abnormality
- Signs of fetal distress
- Fetal heart rate tracing
- Meconium
- Pregnancy history
- Course of labor
- Intrapartum medications
- Risk factors for infection
- Other (eg, major bleeding)

RESUSCITATION EQUIPMENT

Thermoregulation

- Warmer, towels, plastic wrap

Airway

- Suction (bulb syringe and wall), catheters, meconium aspirator
- Intubation equipment (functioning laryngoscope; endotracheal tubes)

Breathing

- Ventilation equipment, tubing, oxygen supply and monitor, carbon dioxide detector

Circulation

- Location of medications, catheters

Drugs

- Other medications, if needed (eg, surfactant)

PERSONNEL ROLES

- Airway manager
- Assistant to monitor heart rate
- Other assistants as needed

immediately after expulsion. Awareness of these factors allows the resuscitator to stay one step ahead and quickly identify the hypovolemic baby after a fetoplacental transfusion or question the reported absence of heart rate in the newborn who had some flexor tone after expulsion, 40 seconds prior.

INITIAL POSTNATAL EVALUATION AND INTERVENTION

The general flow of neonatal resuscitation, as recommended by the NRP, is shown in Figure 74-3.

Cycles of assessment and consequent appropriate intervention are repeated at approximately 30-second intervals, following the ABC(D) sequence; thermoregulation is maintained throughout. Subsequent care, from routine to postresuscitation stabilization, depends on the level of intervention needed during the initial resuscitation. This algorithm may be used to perform a quick initial assessment of a newborn. Four essential questions are asked, as listed in Box 74-6. The first 2 questions can generally be answered before delivery, and the last 2 within seconds after birth. For most newborns, the answer to these 4 questions is *yes*, and such newborns require only thermoregulatory support (warmth and drying), maintenance of an open and clear airway, and assessment of color to verify respiratory and circulatory efficacy. Such babies can remain with their mothers. The subsequent discussion applies to the few newborns who need assistance with transition.

Very premature newborns (<28 weeks' gestation) lose heat rapidly, and they often develop hypothermia despite standard thermoregulatory care. Prewarmed, dry blankets diminish conductive heat losses. Most importantly, convective losses should be minimized by immediately covering the baby with a plastic barrier. This goal can be achieved by placing the baby in a clean, food-grade polyethylene bag. Alternatively, 2 sheets of nonadhesive Saran wrap (or another brand of polyvinylidene chloride film) can be used to wrap the head and the body below the neck, respectively. In some settings, increasing the temperature of the delivery room and using a warmed incubator for transfer to the neonatal unit may also be helpful.

If the amniotic fluid contains meconium, blood, or infected matter, or if the newborn infant is not breathing or exhibits hypotonia, then immediate airway management is needed while supporting thermoregulation.

The airway can be approached by external positioning and internal suctioning, in that order (see Box 74-2). External patency is ensured by positioning the head so the neck is slightly extended, in the sniffing posture; the mandible should be lifted anteriorly. Internal airway patency is achieved by suctioning to remove obstructing matter (meconium, bloody or infected secretions) from the mouth first and then the nose.

Meconium or pus in the amniotic fluid is not an exception to the *airway before breathing* rule. Failure to follow this principle in these conditions is especially risky because of the consequences of aspirating meconium or infected fluid. Because meconium-stained babies who are vigorous (as evidenced by strong respirations, normal muscle tone, and heart rate >100 beats/min) have already established an airway and effective breathing, they need only assistance in clearing the mouth and nose of any additional secretions. However, meconium-stained babies who are not vigorous (ie, they have suboptimal respirations, muscle tone, or heart rate) should receive tracheal intubation and direct suctioning, in addition to clearing of the oropharyngeal airway. Assistance with breathing, whether by stimulation or PPV, should not be given until suctioning has been performed. Suctioning of the airway before delivery of the head does not improve meconium aspiration syndrome or related outcomes in meconium-stained babies. Therefore routine intrapartum suctioning of such babies is no longer recommended. Guidelines for subsequent care of the newly born are not affected by this change in obstetrical management. Previous practices, such as judging the thickness of the meconium and visualizing the cords to decide whether to intubate, are not supported by evidence.

Approximately 30 seconds after birth, most newborns have been provided with a patent airway, as well as some tactile stimulation through drying. Recurrent

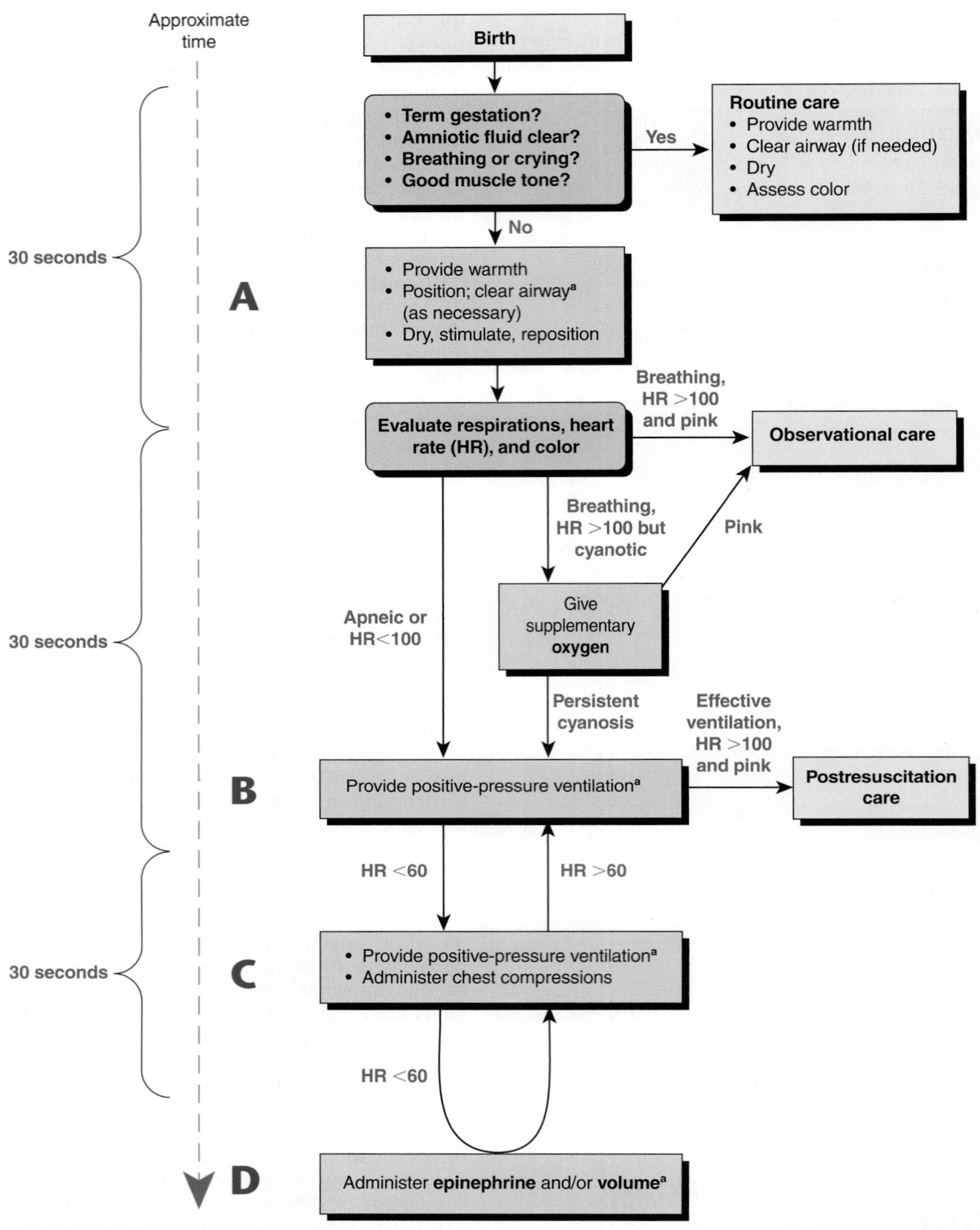

Figure 74-3 Chart describing general flow of neonatal resuscitation. resuscitation. [a]Endotracheal intubation may be considered at several steps. *(Reprinted from American Heart Association, American Academy of Pediatrics. 2005 American Heart Association [AHA] guidelines for cardiopulmonary resuscitation (CPR) and emergency cardiovascular care [ECC] of pediatric and neonatal patients: neonatal resuscitation guidelines.* Pediatrics. *2006;117:e1029-e1038. Available at: pediatrics.aappublications.org/cgi/content/full/117/5/e1029. Accessed June 12, 2007.)*

evaluation of the triad of respirations, heart rate, and color is then needed to decide whether resuscitative support should be escalated or abated, in a stepwise manner, at approximately 30-second intervals.

A newborn who is breathing and has a normal heart rate, but who is cyanotic, may need only free-flow oxygen. If cyanosis persists after 30 seconds of blow-by oxygen, then PPV should be added.

Indications for immediate institution of PPV include apnea, gasping, or bradycardia (heart rate <100 beats/min). Adequate inflation and ventilation of the lungs is by far the most essential aspect of resuscitation in the depressed newly born.

Breathing support requires equipment to deliver and monitor oxygen (Table 74-1), as well as devices to assist and monitor ventilation. Free-flow oxygen can be administered through oxygen tubing or mask or through a flow-inflating bag and mask but not through a self-inflating bag.

Assisted ventilation necessitates both a positive pressure generator such as a bag or T-piece ventilator and a mechanism to connect this device to the newborn's airway (eg, facemask, endotracheal tube) (Table 74-2). An additional team member will be needed and should be called for when beginning PPV.

Bag-mask ventilation, a critical skill in resuscitation, is often performed suboptimally. A tight seal between the mask and face is necessary to operate a flow-inflating bag or T-piece resuscitator. However, obstructing the airway by depressing the mandible with the facemask or inadvertently pressing with the free fingers on the submandibular area (see Box 74-2) must be avoided. Deliberately placing the middle and fourth fingers under the chin and the angle of the mandible, respectively, provides a jaw lift and keeps the airway open during ventilation (Figure 74-4).

Effective ventilation is indicated by a slight rise of the chest with each assisted breath, with a consequent rapid increase in heart rate; other signs include improvement in color over 30 seconds, gradual return of muscle tone, and spontaneous breathing. Assisted breaths should be given at a rate of 40 to 60 per minute, at the minimal peak inflation pressure necessary to effect a slight chest movement (most often 20-30 cm water). The NRP recommends using a fraction of inspired oxygen (FiO_2) of 100% with PPV while acknowledging preliminary evidence that suggests a lower initial FiO_2 may also be appropriate.

If bag-mask ventilation is ineffective in achieving the desired physiologic endpoints, then the airway (external or internal)-breathing sequence should be reassessed. The clinician should reposition the baby's head, lift the jaw, and reapply the facemask, check for secretions and suction as needed, increase inflation pressure, check the bag, and ensure that 100% oxygen is being administered if the baby remains depressed 90 seconds after birth.

Persistent evidence of ineffective ventilation should prompt intubation to establish a more reliable airway, followed by ventilation and reassessment.

BOX 74-6 Key Questions in Determining the Need for Resuscitation

Was the baby born after full-term gestation?

Is the amniotic fluid clear of meconium and infected matter?

Is the baby breathing or crying?

Does the baby have good muscle tone?

Table 74-1 Equipment for Oxygen Delivery and Monitoring

FUNCTION	DEVICE	COMMENT
Oxygen source	Wall outlet, tank	—
Air source*	Wall outlet, tank*	In very preterm neonates (<32 weeks), avoid hyperoxia
Adjustable FiO_2*	Oxygen blender*	
Oxygen conduit	Tubing, mask, with or without bag	Cannot be delivered through a self-inflating bag and mask
Oxygenation monitoring*	Pulse oximeter*	In very preterm neonates, avoid SpO_2 >95%

FiO_2, Fraction of inspired oxygen; *SpO_2*, oxygen saturation by pulse oximetry.
*Equipment that should be available for very preterm babies but is otherwise optional.

Table 74-2 Equipment for Assisting and Monitoring Ventilation

FUNCTION	DEVICE	COMMENTS
Pressure generator	Flow-inflating* or self-inflating bags, T-piece ventilators	Capable of function without a gas source; others need compressed gas (wall outlet, tank)
Pressure conduit into airway	Face mask, endotracheal tube, laryngeal mask airway	Assess appropriate size (and tube depth) before use
Ventilation monitoring*	Carbon dioxide detector; pressure manometer	—

*Equipment that should be available for very preterm babies but is otherwise optional.

Modifying this sequence of interventions may be appropriate in some circumstances. For example, some very premature infants may benefit from prophylactic surfactant and early use of continuous positive airway pressure; special measures to avoid hyperoxia are also necessary (Table 74-3).

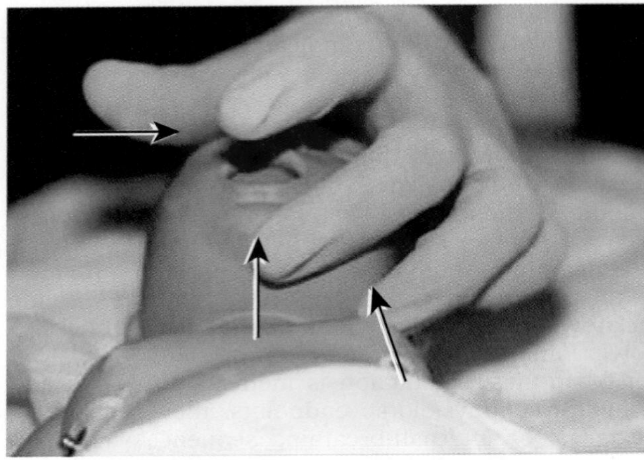

Figure 74-4 Positioning of hand to maintain open airway during bag-mask ventilation. The middle and fourth fingers are placed under the chin and the angle of the mandible, respectively, which lifts the jaw. Keeping these fingers on bony landmarks prevents inadvertent compression of submandibular tissue and airway obstruction. The first 2 fingers naturally accommodate the face mask.

Persistent bradycardia (heart rate <60 beats/min) after 30 seconds of effective PPV is an indication to initiate chest compressions. Chest compressions are preferably performed with the 2-thumb technique, with hands encircling the chest. Ventilation (with 100% oxygen) must remain adequate during chest compressions. The latter can be achieved by 2-second cycles of 3 compressions followed by one breath, coordinated as the compressor verbalizes "1-and-2-and-3-and-breathe-and..."; this technique results in 90 compressions and 30 breaths per minute. If the heart rate remains below 60 beats/min after 30 seconds of coordinated ventilation and chest compressions, then epinephrine is indicated.

Extensive or Complicated Resuscitation

Because persistent cardiorespiratory depression most often results from ineffective resuscitative efforts, the mechanics of each basic step should be reassessed before further intervention.

The physician should recheck the airway (endotracheal tube position) (Table 74-4), the effectiveness of ventilation (chest movement, breath sounds), chest compressions, and epinephrine delivery and then consider the possibility of hypovolemia.

If the baby is poorly responsive to resuscitation and blood loss is suspected (eg, pallor, hypoperfusion, history of abruption placenta, tight nuchal cord), then hypovolemia is likely. This circumstance is an indication for volume expansion with normal saline or lactated Ringer's solution. Unmatched O-negative blood may be used immediately if anemia is suspected.

Table 74-3 Medications for Neonatal Resuscitation in the Delivery Room*

MEDICATION	DOSE	ROUTE	INDICATION
Epinephrine (1:10,000)	0.1 to 0.3 mL/kg	IV preferred (first dose may be endotracheal)	Bradycardia persisting after adequate ventilation and chest compressions
Volume expander (normal saline, lactated Ringer solution, or blood)	10 mL/kg	IV, slow	Poor response to resuscitation, and suspected blood loss, shock, pallor, hypoperfusion
Sodium bicarbonate (0.5 mEq/mL)*	2 mEq/kg	IV, slow	Prolonged CPR unresponsive to adequate ventilation and other therapies
Naloxone*	0.1 mg/kg	IV or IM only (not endotracheal)	After resuscitation (ie, heart rate and color normal), for intrapartum narcotic-induced respiratory depression

CPR, Cardiopulmonary resuscitation; *IM*, intramuscular; *IV*, intravenous.
*Limited role in neonatal resuscitation.

Table 74-4 Endotracheal Tube Size and Depth for Neonates

GESTATIONAL AGE, wk	WEIGHT, g	TUBE INNER DIAMETER, mm	DEPTH OF INSERTION FROM UPPER LIP, cm
<28	<1000	2.5	6.5-7
28-34	1000-2000	3	7-8
34-38	2000-3000	3.5	8-9
>38	>3000	3.5-4.0	>9

The efficacy and safety of sodium bicarbonate in neonatal resuscitation are uncertain, and its use during brief resuscitations is discouraged.

The initial dose may be administered via the endotracheal tube, but absorption is erratic, and the preferred route for subsequent doses, if needed, is intravenous, through a shallow umbilical venous catheter, inserted to a depth of 3 cm.

Naloxone should not be administered during the primary steps of resuscitation. Intrapartum exposure to narcotics causes central apnea, not direct cardiac and neuromuscular dysfunction. Thus naloxone is indicated only after PPV has restored a normal heart rate and color, if respiratory depression continues, and a history intrapartum narcotic administration within 4 hours of birth exists.

Continued failure of effective ventilation despite appropriate endotracheal tube placement should raise consideration of airway malformations (see Box 74-2) or inability to inflate the lungs as a result of pneumothorax or diaphragmatic hernia; obvious asymmetry of breath sounds and shifted or muffled cardiac sounds suggest the latter diagnoses. Poor response to resuscitation despite adequate ventilation may indicate primary circulatory insufficiency (see Box 74-4).

Suspected tension pneumothorax, or hydrothorax, in a newborn who responds poorly to resuscitation is an indication for emergency thoracentesis. An 18- or 20-gauge angiocatheter, rather than a butterfly needle, is safe for this purpose. The catheter should be inserted at the fourth intercostal space, anterior axillary line, to drain gas, or at the midaxillary line to drain a hydrothorax.

Newborns Unresponsive to Resuscitation

Asystole persisting after 10 minutes of adequate resuscitation, which may be beyond 10 minutes of life, indicates a very low probability of intact survival. Therefore discontinuing resuscitation and instituting comfort care centered on the family's needs may be appropriate. Persistent bradycardia unresponsive to adequate resuscitation in a newborn with obvious conditions associated with lung hypoplasia (eg, oligohydramnios sequence, Potter syndrome) would also justify discontinuing resuscitation efforts.

Technical Considerations of Endotracheal Intubation

Intubation should not be viewed as a step in resuscitation but rather as a method that may be applied during any of the basic steps for distinct indications. It may be used to suction debris from the airway; to establish an artificial airway and enhance ventilation when bag-mask ventilation is ineffective, prolonged, or unadvisable (eg, diaphragmatic hernia, gastroschisis); or to administer drugs such as epinephrine or surfactant.

Experts suggest that a clinician capable of performing endotracheal intubation be available at every delivery. Assuming that such individuals are experienced with handling a laryngoscope, choosing a No. 0 blade for a preterm newborn and a No. 1 blade for term newborns and recognizing the vocal cords, the following tips are intended to improve efficacy and safety of intubation.

Intubation of a mainstem bronchus is a frequent event that can result in ineffective ventilation and other serious complications. Thus the clinician should explicitly designate both endotracheal tube size and intended depth of insertion before attempting intubation. These values can be estimated from actual or expected weight, as noted in Table 74-4. Alternatively, Tochen's rule, (6 + weight in kg = tip-to-lip depth in cm) is easy to memorize. Appropriate endotracheal tube insertion depth should first be guided by visually placing the vocal cord mark on the tube at the level of the vocal cords; external depth at the lip should then be verified before assisted ventilation is initiated. At ventilation, confirmation of endotracheal tube placement in the trachea should rely primarily on finding an increasing heart rate and exhaled carbon dioxide by using an appropriate carbon dioxide detector. Other useful methods of verifying endotracheal tube placement, such as observing chest rise, condensation in the tube, skin color, or auscultation of breath sounds, are considered less reliable. If the endotracheal tube is to remain in place after resuscitation, then an x-ray should be obtained to verify tube position.

The NRP now recognizes the laryngeal mask airway as an alternative device to assist ventilation in larger newborns who cannot be effectively managed by bag-mask ventilated or endotracheal intubation. These methods are simple to use in principle, but experience with their application is still limited in newborns.

Special Considerations for Premature Newborns

Premature babies, especially those who are very premature (less than 28 weeks' gestation), have special needs during and after resuscitation, as detailed previously and summarized in Table 74-5.

Physicians will note the new NRP emphasis on more strict management of oxygenation during neonatal resuscitation, particularly in preterm newborns. This action was prompted by preliminary clinical and laboratory evidence suggesting deleterious effects of even brief exposures to hyperoxia and equivalent effectiveness and resuscitation with room air or 100% oxygen. Because existing evidence is limited, present guidelines do not indicate a specific initial FiO_2 for assisting ventilation in very premature newborns (<32 weeks). Instead, experts suggest that an oxygen blender and pulse oximeter be used during resuscitation so that the clinician can titrate FiO_2 to increase oxyhemoglobin concentrations gradually toward 90% over several minutes. FiO_2 should be decreased as oxygen saturations exceed 95%. In the presence of bradycardia, appropriate ventilation with 100% oxygen is indicated.

For full-term newborns, the NRP guidelines recommend administering 100% oxygen for cyanosis or with PPV, without the need for pulse oximetry monitoring. However, experts recognize that alternative approaches may be reasonable.

POSTRESUSCITATION ASSESSMENT AND STABILIZATION

After initial stabilization, a more detailed assessment of the baby's condition and evaluation of relevant risk factors in the prenatal history (see Box 74-1) should be undertaken to guide further care.

Table 74-5 Special Needs of Preterm Newborns During Resuscitation

SPECIAL FEATURE OF PRETERM NEWBORNS	ADJUSTMENT TO RESUSCITATION PROCEDURES
Thermoregulation: rapid heat loss	Avoid convective losses. Use plastic wrap at <28 weeks' gestation.
Fragile skin, particularly at <25 weeks' gestation	Avoid rubbing. Use protective barriers when taping or otherwise securing devices onto skin.
Diminished respiratory drive	Low threshold for supporting ventilation. Need clinician skilled at intubation.
Likely surfactant deficiency	May benefit from prophylactic surfactant.
Lungs susceptible to immediate ventilatory injury	Provide continuous positive airway pressure or the minimal inflation pressures needed to support adequate ventilation and oxygenation.
Tissue vulnerability to hyperoxic injury	Use oxygen blender, pulse oximetry to keep SpO_2 between 85% and 95%. Consider starting resuscitation with an oxygen concentration <100%.
Susceptibility to brain hemorrhage and/or ischemia	Avoid hyperventilation, hypocapnia, and rapid infusion of fluid boluses or hypertonic solutions.
Metabolic susceptibility to hypoglycemia	Monitor for hypoglycemia.
Susceptibility to infection	Assess risk of infection. Most preterm newborns <35 weeks need an evaluation for sepsis immediately after birth, and empirical antibiotic therapy, pending diagnostic tests.

SpO_2, Oxygen saturation by pulse oximetry.

Acute postresuscitation derangements in cardiorespiratory, neurologic, and metabolic function should be sought. Reexamining the ABCs is a simple strategy to ensure sustained adequate ventilation and perfusion in addition to thermoregulation. A malpositioned endotracheal tube, large pneumothorax, or acute hypovolemia after fetoplacental transfusion can cause further physiological derangements. Frequent monitoring of vital signs is useful. However, blood pressure may remain normal despite insufficient systemic or pulmonary blood flow, which would be evident as peripheral hypoperfusion and hypoxemia, respectively. Newborns who were significantly depressed need to be evaluated for acute metabolic complications such as hypoglycemia or severe acidosis.

Preexisting conditions, such as maternal diabetes, fetal growth restriction, significant dysmorphisms found by obstetric ultrasound or during physical examination, and risk factors for sepsis, require specific diagnostic and therapeutic interventions shortly after birth.

Some congenital malformations require specific attention during stabilization. For example, relief of airway obstruction caused by Pierre Robin sequence can be accomplished by prone positioning and a nasopharyngeal airway.

Anomalies characterized by exposed internal organs, such as gastroschisis, meningomyelocele or other neural tube defects, and cloacal exstrophy, necessitate protection from heat and fluid loss, contamination by environmental microorganisms, and traumatic or ischemic injury. Immediate enclosure in a sterile plastic bag safeguards tissues from evaporation and infection. Generally, the newborn should be positioned so as to optimize blood flow to the structures. This goal can be achieved by keeping pressure off the anomaly and by keeping arterial and venous supply to the lesion unobstructed; a newborn with a gastroschisis, for example, would best be stabilized in the right lateral decubitus position. Finally, the newborn should be protected from excessive, unnecessary examinations, and appropriate pain management should be provided if needed.

UMBILICAL CORD BLOOD GAS ANALYSIS

Identifying newborns at risk for complications from intrapartum asphyxia is an issue of significant concern to obstetric and pediatric primary care physicians. Investigations into the use of arterial umbilical cord acid-base status to define the degree of fetal acidemia that correlates with a high risk for neonatal complications have been the focus of ongoing research efforts. Umbilical arterial or venous blood gases or an early neonatal arterial base deficit (before administration of bicarbonate) have been studied for their utility in delineating the degree of acidosis at the time of delivery. Umbilical arterial cord blood gas analysis provides the best information regarding fetal status, whereas umbilical venous cord blood reflects placental functioning most directly. When extensive delivery room resuscitation is necessary, an umbilical venous blood gas analysis can also be obtained from the newborn immediately on insertion of the umbilical venous catheter.

Neonatal complications are associated with fetal metabolic acidosis, rather than respiratory acidosis; even brief cord compression will produce significant hypercarbia. Therefore interpretation of umbilical cord

BOX 74-7 Causes of Acidosis in Neonates

Respiratory distress*
Sepsis
Hypovolemia*
Hypothermia*
Severe anemia*
Low cardiac output (hypotension) with poor tissue perfusion
Cardiac failure
Perinatal asphyxia*
Inborn errors of metabolism
Renal bicarbonate losses

*These conditions are relevant during delivery room resuscitation.

pH should include consideration of both respiratory and metabolic components. Although umbilical arterial pH identifies an infant at potential risk for short-term neonatal morbidity, it does not distinguish the infant at risk for a poor long-term outcome. Among infants exhibiting severe hypoxic-ischemic encephalopathy, fetal hypoxemia is found to be the cause in less than 25% of cases studied.[8] Umbilical arterial pH is normal in 80% of infants experiencing perinatal depression.[9] Box 74-7 lists the causes of acidosis in infants.

At delivery the mean umbilical arterial base deficit is 4 to 5 mmol/L (if *base excess* is reported the respective values are −4 to −5 mmol/L). Lackman et al have reported on umbilical cord blood gases in relation to birth size (appropriateness of growth for gestational age) from a population of nearly 30,000 term infants born over a 10-year period (1990-1999) in Canada. The investigators found that the mean pH was 7.26 ± 0.07 and the mean base deficit was 4.7 ± 2.9 mmol/L in umbilical arterial cord blood specimens. Among infants with intrauterine growth restriction the base deficit was 5.3 ± 3.1, whereas large-for-gestational-age babies exhibited base deficits of 4.4 ± 2.8 mmol/L.[10]

The degree of metabolic acidosis that determines the threshold for injury is defined as greater than 2 standard deviations from the mean (10-12 mmol/L) and is accepted as greater than 12 mmol/L.[11] Base deficit levels exceeding 12 mmol/L occur in less than 2% of a normal obstetric population.[11-13] Also important to note is that the majority of newborns with a base deficit greater than 12 mmol/L do not demonstrate neurologic injury. Among infants experiencing severe metabolic acidosis with base deficits greater than 16 mmol/L, the majority either die or are normal if they survive. In contrast to the symptomatic infant who requires resuscitation and has evidence of a significant metabolic acidosis, the approach to the baby who appears to be transitioning without difficulty but is found to have a base deficit greater than 12 mmol/L is less clear. At a minimum, in addition to a thorough physical assessment for signs of illness or transitional delay, a blood gas analysis should be obtained from the infant to ascertain the presence of persistent metabolic acidosis or other abnormality necessitating further evaluation or intervention. In the absence of significant hypoxemia or hypothermia, metabolic acidosis that is present at birth and persists is likely caused by circulatory insufficiency resulting most likely from hypovolemia.

The availability of umbilical cord blood gases will depend on the individual hospital policy. Although experts have argued that umbilical cord blood acid-base determination does not add to the evaluation of the vigorous term infant who is assessed to have normal Apgar scores, the medical-legal climate is such that some obstetric societies and hospitals in North America and Europe are recommending the routine surveillance of umbilical cord blood gases for all births.

DISPOSITION

Depending on the level of support provided to a newborn during resuscitation (see Figure 74-3), subsequent care may be routine or observational (more frequent evaluation in the delivery room or designated observation area), or it may involve postresuscitation care in a special care nursery.

The management of newborns with significant perinatal depression and those whose underlying conditions impart a risk of physiological instability should be discussed with a neonatologist, and referral to a neonatal intensive care unit may be necessary. Technically challenging or controversial interventions such as surfactant administration in the delivery room or therapeutic hypothermia should be planned in conjunction with the regional center.

COMMUNICATION AND DOCUMENTATION

After resuscitation interventions, assessment of the newborn and development of a postresuscitation plan of care, findings, and plans should be discussed with the parents, nursing staff, and obstetrician.

Documentation of these activities is essential. This task is facilitated by the use of structured forms that help guide the flow of resuscitation while rapidly recording evaluations and interventions at appropriate time intervals and even the corresponding orders. Attribution of Apgar scores, whether performed concurrently by an observer or in retrospect, is more meaningful if the signs assessed are recorded together with concurrent interventions. An expanded Apgar score form has been proposed for this purpose.[4]

EVALUATION AND QUALITY IMPROVEMENT IN NEONATAL RESUSCITATION

Neonatal resuscitation is a critical activity amenable to perinatal quality assurance and quality improvement. Measures related to both the resuscitation process and immediate outcomes may be useful in characterizing the effectiveness, efficiency, and timeliness of resuscitative interventions, even if only in high-risk subgroups (eg, very low–birth-weight newborns, meconium staining). The variables to be tracked should depend on the specific questions to be answered about each institution's neonatal stabilization procedures. However, a few measures reflect efficacy and safety in core processes; they may be particularly useful if they are easy to collect and if published benchmark data are available—for example, in very low–birthweight or extremely low–birth-weight newborns, the proportion of babies given chest compression, epinephrine, or both, time to first surfactant dose, and admission temperature; and in all newborns, the number of intubation attempts and proportion of endotracheal tubes misplaced should be recorded.

Maintaining a highly effective recording system for neonatal resuscitation requires not only maintenance of infrastructure and recurrent training and updating of personnel, but also a planned, systematic evaluation of procedures in high-risk cases and in sentinel events. Both intramural evaluations and external benchmarking in conjunction with the regional perinatal center are necessary elements of this process.

TOOLS FOR PRACTICE

Medical Decision Support

- *Guidelines for Perinatal Care, 6th edition,* American Academy of Pediatrics and American College of Obstetrics and Gynecology (www.aap.org/bookstore).
- *Neonatal Resuscitation Program,* American Academy of Pediatrics (www.aap.org/nrp/about/aboutnrp_index.html).
- *NRP Code Cart Chart* (poster) American Academy of Pediatrics (www.aap.org/bookstore).
- *NRP Pocket Card* (card), American Academy of Pediatrics (www.aap.org/bst).
- *NRP Slide Presentation Kit on CD-ROM, 5th edition* (CD-ROM), American Academy of Pediatrics (www.aap.org/bookstore).
- *NRP Video on DVD: Cases in Neonatal Resuscitation, 5th edition* (DVD), American Academy of Pediatrics (www.aap.org/bookstore).
- *NRP Wall Chart* (Poster), American Academy of Pediatrics (www.aap.org/bst).
- *Textbook of Neonatal Resuscitation, 5th edition,* American Academy of Pediatrics (www.aap.org/bookstore).

AAP POLICY STATEMENT

Schrag S, Gorwitz R, Fultz-Butts K, et al. Prevention of perinatal group B streptococcal disease. Revised guidelines from CDC. *MMWR Recomm Rep.* 2002;51:1-22. AAP Endorsed.

SUGGESTED READING

American Academy of Pediatrics. NRP: Neonatal Resuscitation Program. Available at: www.aap.org/nrp/. Accessed February 17, 2007.

American Heart Association, American Academy of Pediatrics. 2005 American Heart Association (AHA) guidelines for cardiopulmonary resuscitation (CPR) and emergency cardiovascular care (ECC) of pediatric and neonatal patients: neonatal resuscitation guidelines. *Pediatrics.* 2006;117:e1029-e1038. Available at: pediatrics.aappublications.org/cgi/content/full/117/5/e1029. Accessed February 13, 2007.

American Heart Association. 2005 American Heart Association guidelines for cardiopulmonary resuscitation and emergency cardiovascular care. Part 13: neonatal resuscitation guidelines. *Circulation.* 2005;112;IV-188-IV-195. Available at: circ.ahajournals.org/cgi/content/full/112/24_suppl/IV-188. Accessed February 13, 2007.

Bloom RS. Delivery room resuscitation of the newborn. In: Fanaroff AA, Martin RJ, eds. *Neonatal-Perinatal Medicine: Diseases of the Fetus and Infant.* 7th ed. St Louis, MO: CV Mosby; 2002.

REFERENCES

1. American Academy of Pediatrics, American College of Obstetricians and Gynecologists. *Guidelines for Perinatal Care.* 5th ed. Washington, DC: AAP and ACOG; 2002.
2. Kattwinkel J, ed. *Textbook of Neonatal Resuscitation.* 5th ed. Elk Grove Village, IL. American Heart Association, American Academy of Pediatrics; 2006.
3. Dawes GS. *Fetal and Neonatal Physiology.* Chicago, IL: Year Book Medical Publishers Inc; 1968.
4. American Academy of Pediatrics, Committee on Fetus and Newborn, American College of Obstetricians and Gynecologists, Committee on Obstetric Practice. The Apgar score. *Pediatrics.* 2006;117:1444-1447.
5. American Academy of Pediatrics, Committee on Fetus and Newborn. Noninitiation or withdrawal of intensive care for high risk newborns. *Pediatrics.* 2007;119:401-403.
6. Canadian Paediatric Society, Fetus and Newborn Committee, Society of Obstetricians and Gynaecologists of Canada, Maternal-Fetal Medicine Committee. Management of the woman with threatened birth of an infant of extremely low gestational age. *Can Med Assoc J.* 1994; 151:547-551, 553.
7. American Academy of Pediatrics, Committee on Fetus and Newborn, MacDonald H. Perinatal care at the threshold of viability. *Pediatrics.* 2002;110:1024-1027.
8. Low JA, Galbraith RS, Muir DW, et al. The relationship between perinatal hypoxia and newborn encephalopathy. *Am J Obstet Gynecol.* 1985;152:256-260.
9. Thorp JA, Dildy GA, Yeomans ER, et al. Umbilical cord blood gas analysis at delivery. *Am J Obstet Gynecol.* 1996;175:517-522.
10. Lackman F, Capewell V, Gagnon R, et al. Fetal umbilical cord oxygen values and birth to placental weight ratio in relation to size at birth. *Am J Obstet Gynecol.* 2001;185: 674-682.
11. Helwig JT, Parer JT, Kilpatrick SJ, et al. Umbilical cord blood acid-base state: what is normal? *Am J Obstet Gynecol.* 1996;174:1807-1812.
12. Low JA. Intrapatrum fetal asphyxia: definition, diagnosis and classification. *Am J Obstet Gynecol.* 1997;176:957-959.
13. Arikan GM, Scholz HS, Haeusler MC, et al. Low fetal oxygen saturation at birth and acidosis. *Obstet Gynecol.* 2000;95:565-571.

Chapter 75

IDENTIFYING THE NEWBORN WHO REQUIRES SPECIALIZED CARE

Upender K. Munshi, MBBS, MD (Paediatrics)

Full-term neonates born after a normal spontaneous vaginal delivery are usually assessed by the delivery room nurse, who may notify the primary care physician (PCP) if any abnormality of cardiorespiratory adaptations or any external malformations are observed. A PCP or nurse practitioner may be in attendance for high-risk deliveries, and this person will assess the baby soon after delivery. In either case, after this initial assessment, a decision is made whether the baby is stable enough to be cared for in a regular well-baby nursery or in the room with the mother or, if concern exists about the condition of the baby, to consider transfer to a neonatal intensive care unit (NICU).

NEWBORNS IN THE NEONATAL INTENSIVE CARE UNIT

Most newborns who are referred to an NICU fall into one of 3 broad categories: (1) those who have a clear need for NICU care, (2) those with a possible need for NICU care, and (3) well-seeming newborns with no apparent need for NICU care on initial assessment (Box 75-1). Newborns who appear to be fine but who have been flagged as possessing a warning sign that requires further assessment fall into the last group.

Clear Need for Neonatal Intensive Care Unit Care

Critically ill newborns include those with moderate to severe respiratory distress needing ventilatory support, infants with compromised cardiovascular function and manifestations of poor perfusion, very premature newborns, low–birth-weight infants, and infants with an obvious major system malformation that requires early medical or surgical intervention. The decision-making process for referral to a higher level of care is straightforward in this group. Referral to the NICU should be initiated immediately while the initial diagnostic and therapeutic measures commence.

BOX 75-1 Broad Categories of Newborns for Neonatal Intensive Care Unit (NICU) Referral

Group 1: Clear need for NICU

Call NICU early; arrange prompt transfer.

- Very low–birth-weight and premature infants
- Moderate to severe respiratory distress
- Compromised cardiovascular function, poor perfusion
- Life-threatening malformations such as gastroschisis, diaphragmatic hernia

Group 2: Possible need for NICU

Communicate and discuss with regional NICU team.

- Borderline maturity and birth weight
- Mild to moderate respiratory distress

Group 3: No need for NICU

Review history, physical examination and laboratory results. Watch for any warning signs; if present, then call NICU.

- Full-term appropriate or large weight
- No apparent illness at initial assessment

Possible Need for Neonatal Intensive Care Unit Care

For newborns who have near-normal birth weight and maturation criteria, mildly abnormal physical findings, or borderline laboratory results, making the decision for referral to NICU is difficult. In addition, some newborns exhibit grunting, flaring, and chest wall retractions within minutes after birth, which results in an early transfer to NICU. However, these respiratory symptoms frequently subside quickly, often during the transport itself, making such admissions unnecessary and adding to the space crunch and paperwork burden on the busy NICU staff. These transfers cause needless parental anxiety and interruption in the newborn-parent bonding, particularly when it involves transfer to another hospital. Watchful observation in consultation with the accepting NICU attending physician[1] and communication of clinical or laboratory parameters for a reasonable amount of time is appropriate.

Well-Seeming Infants and Neonatal Intensive Care Unit Care

For the majority of infants who are vigorous and healthy looking, no higher-level care will be required. However, occasionally a baby in this group may have warning signs in the prenatal or postnatal history, subtle findings in the physical examination, or concerning laboratory results that need to be addressed.

REFERRAL TO NEONATAL INTENSIVE CARE UNIT CARE

The objective of this chapter is to present a systematic approach for the PCP to identify newborns in the last 2 categories who may require admission to NICU for close monitoring and management. This chapter also identifies warning signs that may imply an underlying problem in an apparently well newborn. Early recognition of these conditions may prevent delay in referrals and resulting complications. In addition, factors other than the actual medical condition of the newborn may come into play while referrals of the newborn to other hospitals are made, although these factors will not be discussed in this chapter. Such factors may include training and competence in the field of newborn medicine for the PCP, experience of an adverse outcome in a previous case, unavailability of around-the-clock in-hospital physician coverage in some community hospitals, time crunches and financial implications caused by the commitment to ambulatory patient care, adequacy and comfort level of the nursing staff, and third-party payer characteristics.[2]

To assess a newborn properly, the PCP must possess the basic elements of the mother's care, including her history of pregnancy (including results of her screening laboratory tests and ultrasounds) and that of events around and at delivery. Any newborn showing signs of illness should have an initial basic work-up (Box 75-2), which may help with early recognition

BOX 75-2 Initial Work-Up of an Ill-Appearing Newborn

- Pulse oximeter saturation of oxygen (Sao_2)
- Rapid blood glucose strip test (Dextrostix)
- Blood cell counts: hematocrit and hemoglobin, white cells with differential, platelets
- Basic metabolic panel: serum glucose, electrolytes, urea, creatinine
- Blood gas and chest radiograph, deferring if no respiratory distress
- Blood culture, deferring if no risk of infection
- If Sao_2 or arterial pressure of oxygen in room air is low, then observe the response to 100% oxygen (hyperoxia test)

If an inborn error of metabolism is suspected, then send blood for lactate, pyruvate, ammonia, plasma amino-acid profile, carnitine, and acylcarnitine. Test urine for organic acids and reducing substance. Keep extra samples of blood and urine for specific genetic tests and store at −20°C (68°F).

of any problems and with referral of the baby to the NICU.

GROWTH AND MATURITY

Every state health care system has arbitrarily classified the newborn care facilities into levels of care in a process of providing regionalized perinatal care.[3,4] A hospital providing basic neonatal care to full-term, healthy babies would be designated as level 1. This level includes most community hospitals with obstetric services. Hospitals with resources to take care of mild to moderate problems (eg, needing incubator care, short-term ventilatory support, intravenous antibiotics, oral or nasogastric tube feeding) may qualify as level 2. Centers caring for very low–birth-weight babies and other complex problems of newborns (eg, need for full ventilatory support, parenteral nutrition, and medical and surgical subspecialty support) are classified level 3 and above.

In general, newborns born before 35 weeks' gestation or newborns weighing less than 2000 g should be cared for at a higher level than a level-1 nursery. They invariably experience problems in feeding and maintaining their body temperature. Although birth-weight measurement is objective, gestation assessment is not, the result of inaccuracies in dating the last menstrual period or of late prenatal ultrasounds. Every effort should be made to gather information that documents reliable gestational dates and to perform a proper assessment of the newborn to arrive at a plausible gestational age.

For very small and premature babies (eg, <32 weeks' gestation or birth weight <1500 g) born at a level-1 hospital, referral to higher level is straightforward. Decision making can become tricky at 32 to 36 weeks' gestation because of variability of fetal growth. Infants born to mothers with diabetes at 32 to 33 weeks' gestation may weigh far more than 2000 g, but they will need to be admitted to a NICU because they are at a high risk of respiratory distress syndrome, hypoglycemia, polycythemia, hyperbilirubinemia, hypocalcemia, and poor feeding, whereas growth-restricted babies born at 35 to 37 weeks' gestation may weigh less than 2000 g but may be feeding well and are comfortable breathing room air.

Resources at level-2 nurseries are so variable that each hospital should develop its own guidelines for gestation and birth-weight cutoffs (conforming to their respective state health department guidelines and their own available resources), below which it must refer the newborns to a higher level of care. This indication for admission comprises the bulk of referrals to higher levels of care.

SIGNS OF RESPIRATORY DISTRESS

Common causes of respiratory distress within the first few hours of life are provided in Figure 75-1. Increased frequency and work of breathing, as characterized by breathing rates of more than 60 breaths per minute, grunting, nasal flaring, and chest wall retractions, are the findings that draw the most attention of the baby's caregivers. If these signs are accompanied by central cyanosis or the need for supplemental oxygen to maintain normal color or pulse oximeter saturations, then it may indicate an underlying disorder that requires immediate diagnostic and therapeutic intervention. Presence of these signs in a preterm newborn suggests respiratory distress syndrome caused by surfactant deficiency.[5] Similar manifestation in a term or late preterm newborn may be the result of transient tachypnea of newborn (TTN) if the amniotic fluid is clear and the delivery is by cesarean.[6] Respiratory distress that improves with each hour and resolves in approximately 24 hours is due to TTN, whereas persisting or worsening respiratory distress beyond 24 hours rule out this diagnosis. Respiratory distress with presence of thick, meconium-stained fluid points toward meconium aspiration syndrome. Meconium aspiration syndrome is especially common in postterm infants who require resuscitation at delivery. These infants usually have meconium staining of nails and umbilical cord.[7] Meconium aspiration syndrome is invariably associated with persistent pulmonary hypertension of newborn, which makes the respiratory failure worse and difficult to manage.

Newborns with suspected TTN are usually stabilized by increasing the inspired oxygen concentration and providing noninvasive ventilatory support. If they start showing improvement in their respiratory status within the first few hours, then these newborns may be closely observed for further resolution within the first 12 to 24 hours of life in consultation with the accepting attending physician at the referral center.

All other categories of respiratory distress needing ventilatory support should result in transfer to a higher level of care.[8]

SEPSIS SYNDROME

Sepsis mimics most of the neonatal systemic disorders that affect newborns of all gestational ages, and its

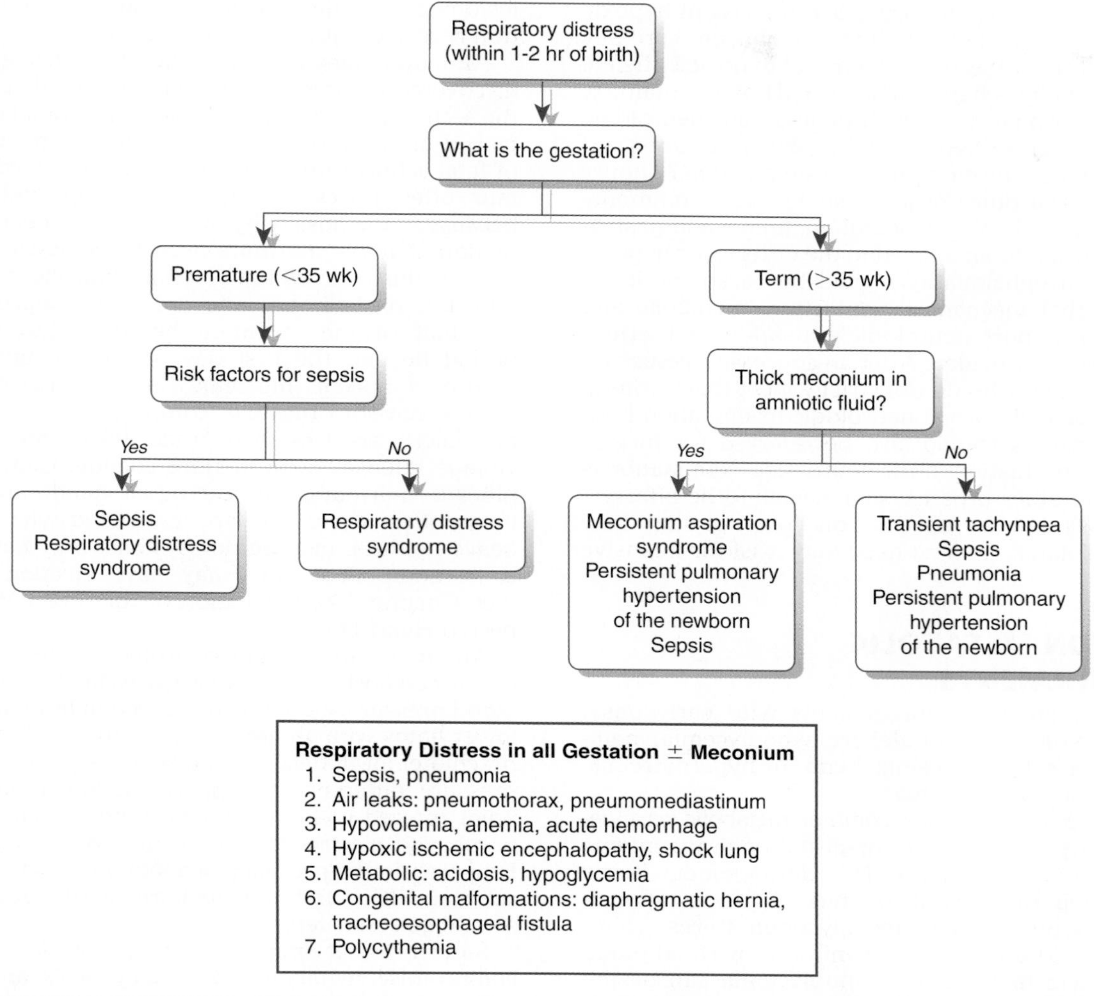

Figure 75-1 Respiratory distress within the first few hours of life.

onset can span from the delivery room to anytime thereafter. Risk factors for neonatal sepsis, such as maternal fever, chorioamnionitis, prolonged rupture of membranes, urinary tract infections, group B *Streptococcus* colonization, or a history of genital herpes, should be sought in the maternal history. In the delivery room, sepsis syndrome occurs mostly in the form of respiratory distress and cardiovascular instability in form of tachycardia; pale, mottled skin; delayed capillary refill; and hypotension. Later onset is demonstrated by a change in the baby's baseline behavior, such as poor feeding, irritability, and lethargy, as well as temperature instability in a baby who had apparently normal activity and feeding pattern.[9,10] Skin or mucous membrane lesions should be examined for the possibility of neonatal herpes; negative maternal history of genital herpes does not rule out neonatal infection.[11] (See Chapter 101, The Infant With Suspected Infection.)

The clinician needs to recognize these changes early enough to initiate diagnostic (fluid cultures) and therapeutic interventions (intravenous antibiotics) quickly. Diagnostic and therapeutic interventions should occur at the same time that the diagnosis of suspected sepsis is being entertained and that arrangements for referral to a higher level of care unit are being considered. Blood cell counts are often checked to find evidence for or against the diagnosis of neonatal sepsis; however, these results should be interpreted judiciously and not relied on as the sole factor for decision making.[12] Neutropenia in the absence of pregnancy-induced hypertension or preeclampsia syndrome is worrisome and so is a marked left shift with ratio of immature neutrophils (band forms) to total neutrophils (bands plus segmented neutrophils) of 0.3 or more.

Peripartum Events, Hypoxic Ischemic Encephalopathy, and Multiorgan Involvement

Newborns with severe cardiorespiratory compromise at birth that requires sustained aggressive resuscitation, including positive pressure ventilation, chest compressions, or epinephrine, are at a risk of hypoxic ischemic encephalopathy and should be carefully monitored. The objective evidence of hypoxic ischemic encephalopathy is based on a cord pH of less than 7.0, a 5-minute Apgar score of 3 or less, and neurologic findings (hyper- or hypotonia, irritability, seizures) and involvement of one more organ system within 72 hours of birth.[13] The other organ systems most commonly involved are kidneys, myocardium, lungs, and gastrointestinal tract. Infants meeting the criteria for hypoxic ischemic encephalopathy should be cared for in an NICU so that mechanical ventilation, metabolic and nutritional support, neurologic evaluation, and seizure control can be provided. After an aggressive resuscitation, newborns who do not strictly meet these criteria but who have abnormal neurologic examination findings or seizures should also be referred for further neurologic evaluation. If the neurologic examination is normal, no other organ system seems to be affected, and a close 24-hour observation does not show any change in status, then no need may exist for intensive care.

COMMON METABOLIC DERANGEMENTS

Common metabolic derangements with early onset (within the day 1 or 2 of life) are hypoglycemia, metabolic acidosis, hypocalcemia, hypo- or hypernatremia, and hypo- or hyperkalemia.

Hypoglycemia is the most common metabolic derangement mostly seen in large-for-gestational-age infants of mothers with diabetes. This derangement is the result of hyperinsulinemia or, in small-for-gestational-age babies, due to depleted glycogen stores. These babies should be routinely monitored by rapid blood glucose strip test. Rarely, hypoglycemia can be the result of inborn error of carbohydrate metabolism (see Chapter 351, Hypoglycemia; and Chapter 105, Specific Congenital Metabolic Disorders). Hypocalcemia is a common problem sometimes seen in infants of diabetic mothers or in situations in which maternal hypercalcemia is present causing transient suppression of fetal parathyroid function. Occasionally, early persistent hypocalcemia may be a clue to DiGeorge syndrome. Early hyponatremia may reflect maternal fluid overload or neonatal fluid overload particularly after administering electrolyte-free, intravenous dextrose solution to newborns beyond the first day of life.

Cardiovascular Malformations

Very few cardiac malformations manifest clinically in the delivery room, such as the transposition of great vessels with intact septum. The most common manifestation of serious cardiac malformations coincides with the closure of the ducts arteriosus (duct-dependent lesions), which occurs at the first 24 hours of life to the end of the first week of life; the remaining lesions appear later, when pulmonary resistance declines further (at 2-12 weeks). A normal physical examination and absence of murmur on the first day of life does not rule out cardiac malformation; approximately one half of confirmed duct-dependent lesions are in infants whose initial physical examination revealed nothing abnormal.[14,15]

Although many congenital heart malformations are discovered by prenatal fetal ultrasounds that examine the 4-chamber view of the fetal heart, not all cases are picked up because of the technically demanding skill of fetal echocardiography. Presence of a cardiac murmur often raises anxiety in the staff and parents because of the possibility of a congenital heart malformation. Audible murmurs need to be assessed: Does it have the characteristics of a clinically significant murmur, or is it an innocent one? Approximately one half of the murmurs heard in the newborn period beyond the first day of life are innocent in nature. Innocent murmurs are short systolic in nature, have no diastolic component, have no ejection clicks, are less than grade 3/6 in intensity, and change intensity with posture change. Clinically significant murmurs, on the other hand, are louder (more than grade 3/6), are associated with palpable heave or thrill, may be holosystolic, may have a diastolic component, and may have ejection clicks.[16] (See Chapter 100, Evaluation of the Infant With Suspected Heart Disease.)

An effort should be made to feel the femoral pulse on all newborns. If this pulse is difficult to feel, then blood pressure should be measured in both upper and lower limbs with an appropriate cuff size. Presence of brachiofemoral delay in pulse or significant blood pressure difference in upper and lower limbs may point toward coarctation syndromes. A chest radiograph and electrocardiogram may be of some help. However, in the presence of a significant murmur, the referral NICU and the pediatric cardiology service should be contacted.

Sudden onset of poor feeding, cardiorespiratory compromise, metabolic acidosis, cyanosis, and no significant improvement in oxygenation while breathing 100% oxygen in a newborn beyond the first day of life should arouse suspicion of a duct-dependent cardiac malformation. Examples of duct-dependent lesions are hypoplastic left heart syndrome, left outflow tract obstruction, coarctation of aorta, transposition of great vessels, tricuspid atresia, pulmonary stenosis, and atresia. Prostaglandin infusion may be initiated in consultation with the pediatric cardiology service as soon as possible.[17-19] Other important differential diagnoses, such as sepsis or inborn error of metabolism, should be also kept in mind (Box 75-3).

Neurologic Problems

A neonatal seizure is the most common neurologic cause of referral to the NICU. Treatment should be based on reliable history from parents or from witness accounts by medical personnel. Seizures may need immediate attention for control then clinical and diagnostic evaluation to find the cause. Neonatal seizures may be caused by perinatal hypoxia or ischemia, metabolic disturbances, intracranial hemorrhage or infarction, sepsis, withdrawal syndrome, or they may be of the benign familial type. In the management of a clinical seizure, an important feature is to look for hypoglycemia before providing anticonvulsant therapy. Hypoglycemia should be assessed by a rapid blood

BOX 75-3 Healthy-Appearing Newborn With a Serious Underlying Disorder

Neonatal sepsis (group B *Streptococcus* infection, *Escherichia coli* infection, herpes simplex virus infection) during incubation period
Ductal-dependent cardiovascular malformation (before ductus arteriosus starts closing)
Gastrointestinal (small-bowel obstruction, malrotation, Hirschsprung disease) before feeding and abdominal distension
Inborn errors of metabolism (before feeding and accumulation of offending metabolites)
Congenital adrenal hyperplasia, particularly in boys (before any physiological stress)
Congenital clotting disorders, particularly in boys (before circumcision)

glucose strip test, and, if present, the infant is treated with an intravenous glucose bolus first; if absent, then a loading dose of anticonvulsant is given. Other therapy will depend on the causative factor for the seizure. After the seizure is controlled, transfer should be initiated in consultation with the accepting NICU as further evaluation for the cause of seizure continues. (See Chapter 320, Seizure Disorders.)

Other neurologic causes for referral may include unexplained hypotonia *(floppy infant)*, poor feeding, hypertonia, and exaggerated reflexes. The NICU team and pediatric neurology service should be consulted regarding whether the baby requires intensive care or whether the infant is feeding and stable enough to be followed up in the outpatient department.

Prenatal Conditions

Life-threatening malformations that require early medical or surgical intervention, such as gastroschisis, omphalocele, and diaphragmatic hernia, diagnosed by prenatal ultrasound, should preferably be delivered at a hospital with an NICU with the required specialty support. Presence of polyhydramnios or oligohydramnios on prenatal ultrasounds should alert the PCP to assess for malformations in the newborn baby associated with these conditions. Polyhydramnios is associated with tracheoesophageal fistula and open neural tube defects, whereas oligohydramnios is associated with renal dysplasia, obstructive uropathy, and pulmonary hypoplasia. Occasionally, these infants are born in a community hospital without a prenatal diagnosis, or the mother experiences an unexpectedly rapid progression of labor before reaching a perinatal regional referral center. The PCP should contact the regional NICU team to optimize the pretransport stabilization.

Dysmorphology

The most common dysmorphologies are trisomy 21, 18, and 13 phenotypes and their association with major organ system malformations. Other group associations include VACTERL (vertebral anomalies, anal atresia, cardiac defects, tracheoesophageal fistula, renal anomalies, and limb anomalies) and CHARGE (coloboma, heart disease, atresia choanae, retardation of growth or development, genitourinary tract anomalies, and ear anomalies), in which the presence of one feature leads to the discovery of another. Facial dysmorphic features (eg, frontal prominence, depressed nasal bridge, palpebral fissure slants, micrognathia, ear anomalies) may be present as isolated findings, but a combination of these findings along with others found by systemic examination should be discussed with the NICU or a genetic service (or both) for diagnosis and management. These infants may or may not require NICU care, depending on the presence or absence of any associated serious systemic malformations.

Hematologic Problems

Acute hemorrhage, hypovolemia, and anemia may be life threatening and should be addressed promptly. Although volume resuscitation and blood transfusion are contemplated, the referral process to the NICU should be initiated. Early-onset jaundice and pallor (within 24 hours of life) signifying hemolysis should be assessed promptly, and the infant should be referred after consultation with the accepting NICU. A ruddy-appearing baby might have polycythemia, which is defined as a venous hematocrit level of 65% or more. It is commonly associated with infants of mothers with diabetes, small-for-gestational-age babies, Down syndrome, delayed clamping, and milking of the umbilical cord and should be discussed with the NICU team.[20] Thrombocytopenia caused by maternally acquired antibodies may occasionally be severe enough to cause life-threatening bleeding in newborns, and referral should be decided with the NICU team and in consultation with pediatric hematology service.

Neonatal hyperbilirubinemia: Jaundice within the first 24 hours after birth, particularly when associated with significant anemia, is a cause for concern and should be discussed with the regional referral hospital NICU team. Exaggerated physiological jaundice and breastfeeding jaundice is a common cause of neonatal readmission to hospital and can be managed at level-1 or level-2 facilities. (See Chapter 98 for information on the management of neonatal jaundice.)

Inborn Errors of Metabolism

Inborn errors of metabolism (IEM) are rare disorders but when considered together comprise 1 in 1500 births by some estimates. Carbohydrate metabolism related disorders (eg, galactosemia) will produce hypoglycemia, hepatic dysfunction, and acidosis. Aminoacidopathies (phenylketonuria, tyrosinemia, maple syrup disease) produce acidosis, encephalopathy, and hepatic dysfunction. Lipid metabolism disorders are errors with fatty acids and organic acidemias, medium-chain acyl-coenzyme A dehydrogenase deficiency, propionic academia, urea cycle disorders, and primary lactic acidosis. (See Chapter 104, Common Metabolic Disturbances in the Newborn; and Chapter 105, Specific Congenital Metabolic Disorders.)

In a stable baby, IEM are diagnosed either as part of the state screening program or as prenatal or postnatal diagnostic work-up in response to a positive family history of a genetic disorder. In either case the PCP should contact the designated screening program or the genetics service for guidance.[21] In an ill-appearing newborn in whom IEM are suspected (sudden deterioration after 1 or 2 days or of feeding and unexplained severe acidosis and or hypoglycemia), a few general screening tests may be performed to arrive at a diagnosis pending the results of the genetic testing (see Box 75-2).

Endocrinal problems: The most common endocrine derangement is neonatal hypoglycemia caused by increased fetal insulin in infants of diabetic mothers. Congenital hypothyroidism, generally discovered by newborn screening, is the next most common disorder.[22] Congenital adrenal hyperplasia is usually detected in newborn girls because virilization leads to ambiguous genitalia; boys with the same condition are not discovered unless the state newborn screening tests detect increased levels of 17-hydroxyprogesterone. Transient hypoparathyroidism may produce hypocalcemia, but it may occasionally be the earliest clue to DiGeorge syndrome.

Drug withdrawal: Drug withdrawal syndromes may be severe enough to cause seizures and need closer observation. Maternal history and results of drug screening tests are helpful.

ASSESSMENT OF WELL-APPEARING INFANTS

Some clinical clue always exists that leads to suspicion or diagnosis of a problem and that helps decision making about referral of an infant to the NICU. Few situations occur in which the newborn appears apparently well only to show signs of a serious disorder later (Box 75-4; see also Box 75-3). The 2 most common

BOX 75-4 Common Diagnostic Categories for an Ill-Appearing Newborn (Beyond 12-24 Hours After Birth)

Neonatal sepsis

Cardiac malformation: duct-dependent cardiac lesion

Common metabolic derangements: hypoglycemia, hypocalcemia

Inborn errors of metabolism: unexplained severe persistent acidosis or hypoglycemia

Neurologic problems: neonatal seizures, hypertonia, hypotonia

Surgical conditions: diaphragmatic hernia, gastroschisis, omphalocele, esophageal atresia with tracheoesophageal fistula, ileal atresia, malrotation, volvulus, intussusception, Hirschsprung disease, meconium ileus, hypertrophic pyloric stenosis

Endocrinal: ambiguous genitalia (congenital adrenal hyperplasia)

Hematologic problems (hyperbilirubinemia, anemia , polycythemia, severe alloimmune thrombocytopenia, congenital clotting disorders)

Genitourinary problems (renal dysplasia, moderate to severe hydronephrosis demonstrated as urinary tract infection or severe hypertension)

BOX 75-5 Warning Signs in an Apparently Well-Appearing Term Baby

SEPSIS

- Increased difference of central to peripheral skin temperature of more than 1° C in a thermo-neutral environment
- Presence of skin or mucous membrane vesicles with inflamed base
- Complete blood cell count performed for risk factors shows neutropenia with left shift

CONGENITAL HEART DISEASE

- Dysmorphic features: trisomy 21, 13, 18 syndromes, Turner syndrome
- Significant cardiac murmur
- Difference in femoral and brachial pulses or low blood pressure in lower limbs as compared with upper limbs
- Sudden onset of cardiorespiratory compromise in a previously well baby beyond the first day of life and no improvement in oxygenation while breathing 100% oxygen

INBORN ERRORS OF METABOLISM

- Poor feeding after 1 or 2 days of initial normal feeding
- Unexplained metabolic acidosis, hypoglycemia
- Respiratory alkalosis, hyperammonemia
- Family history of inborn errors of metabolism or unexplained neonatal deaths

ENDOCRINE PROBLEMS

- Hypoglycemia: hyperinsulinism in large-for-date infants of diabetic mothers
- Hypoglycemia with microphallus: hypopituitarism, growth hormone deficiency
- Hypoglycemia, hypothermia in holoprosencephaly: panhypopiturism
- Hypocalcemia and hyperphosphatemia: hypoparathyroidism
- Hyponatremia and hyperkalemia: ambiguous genitalia: congenital adrenal hyperplasia, adrenal insufficiency
- Hyperbilirubinemia, constipation, slow feeder: hypothyroidism
- Unexplained tachycardia with maternal history of Graves disease: hyperthyroidism

HEMATOLOGIC PROBLEMS

- Polycythemia: large ruddy-looking infant of diabetic mother or small-for-date chronically stressed baby caused by placental insufficiency, twin-twin transfusion
- Excessive bleeding from circumcision: clotting disorder, immune thrombocytopenia
- Jaundice within 24 hours with pallor: hemolytic disease

OTHER PROBLEMS

- Esophageal atresia or proximal bowel obstruction
- Prenatal history of polyhydramnios
- Inability to pass oro- or nasogastric tube

conditions that start as an apparently well newborn at birth who remains stable for a few days before rapidly becoming symptomatic are (1) neonatal sepsis and (2) duct-dependent congenital heart malformation.

For sepsis, risk factors for infection need to be diligently sought. Such factors include a history of maternal fever, chorioamnionitis, prolonged rupture of membranes, urinary tract infections, group B *Streptococcus* colonization, and genital herpes. Whenever indicated, laboratory tests such as blood cell counts and differential white blood cell count should be performed. Early symptoms may include a change in activity or feeding pattern and temperature instability.

Cardiac malformations might be suspected at prenatal ultrasound when assessing for a 4-chamber heart, but aortic arch defects can be subtle. At physical examination, finding weak or absent femoral pulse and a diastolic or a loud systolic murmur may provide early clues for cardiac evaluation. Rapidly developing pallor and metabolic acidosis with desaturation at pulse oximetry and poor response to 100% inspired oxygen implies congenital cardiac malformation with closing ductus arteriosus. Initiation of prostaglandin infusion after a telephone consultation with a pediatric cardiologist may be lifesaving before the transport team arrives.

After initial assessment and consideration of the conditions listed in Box 75-4 and based on the available resources at the primary care facility, a decision-making process is initiated to determine the feasibility of transfer of the newborn to a hospital that can provide a higher level of care. The first consideration is to provide the measures needed to stabilize the newborn immediately and to start the initial diagnostic work-up according to the findings of the assessment while getting in touch with the accepting NICU. The accepting neonatologist may have important suggestions and guidelines useful for pretransport stabilization and work-up for the baby. At the same time, PCPs should explain to the parents the details of and reasons for transfer of their baby to a higher level of care, and the parents should continue to be periodically updated as the clinical picture begins to unfold.

SUMMARY

History of maternal gestation, prenatal maternal laboratory results, ultrasound results, and complete physical examination of an ill-appearing newborn are essential to arrive at a provisional diagnosis. An initial basic work-up adds to the process of diagnosis and decision making (see Box 75-2). Occasionally an apparently well-appearing newborn may have a serious underlying condition, although in most cases a warning sign will be present in the history, physical examination, or in the laboratory results that may provide a clue and reason to pursue further evaluation (Box 75-5). Communication with the accepting NICU attending physician and with the baby's parents is crucial to this entire process.

TOOLS FOR PRACTICE

Medical Decision Support

- *Guidelines for Perinatal Care, 6th edition,* American Academy of Pediatrics (www.aap.org/bookstore).

AAP POLICY STATEMENT

American Academy of Pediatrics, Committee on Fetus and Newborn. Levels of neonatal care. *Pediatrics.* 2004;114(5):1341-1347. (aappolicy.aappublications.org/cgi/content/full/pediatrics;114/5/1341).

REFERENCES

1. Perlstein PH, Edwards NK, Sutherland JM. Neonatal hotline telephone network. *Pediatrics.* 1979;64:419-424.
2. Phung H, Bauman A, Tran M, et al. Factors that influence special care nursery admissions to a district hospital in South-western Sydney. *J Paediatr Child Health.* 2005;41:119-124.
3. American Academy of Pediatrics, Committee on Fetus and Newborn. Level of neonatal care. *Pediatrics.* 2004;114:1341-1347.
4. Hein HA. Regionalized perinatal care in North America. *Semin Neonatol.* 2004;9:111-116.
5. Rodriguez RJ. Management of respiratory distress syndrome: an update. *Respir Care.* 2003;48(3):279-286.
6. Jain L, Dudell GG. Respiratory transition in infants delivered by cesarean section. *Semin Perinatol.* 2006;30:296-304.
7. Munshi UK, Clark DA. Meconium aspiration syndrome. *Contemp Clin Gynecol Obstet.* 2002;2:247-257.
8. Buckmaster AG, Wright IMR, Arnolda G, et al. Practice variation in initial management and transfer thresholds for infants with respiratory distress in Australia hospitals. *J Paediatr Child Health.* 2007;43:469-475.
9. Short MA. Guide to a systemic physical assessment in infant with suspected infection and or sepsis. *Adv Neonat Care.* 2004;4(3):141-153.
10. Fischer JE. Physicians' ability to diagnose sepsis in newborns and critically ill children. *Pediatr Crit Care Med.* 2005;6(suppl):S120-S125.
11. Kimberlin DW. Herpes simplex infections of the newborn. *Semin Perinatol.* 2007;31:19-25.
12. Jackson GL, Engle WD, Sendelbach DM, et al. Are complete blood cell counts useful in the evaluation of asymptomatic neonates exposed to suspected chorioamnionitis? *Pediatrics.* 2004;113:1173-1180.
13. The American College of Obstetrics and Gynecology [ACOG]. *Neonatal Encephalopathy and Cerebral Palsy: Defining the Pathogenesis and Pathophysiology.* Washington, DC: ACOG; 2003.
14. Driscoll D, Allen HD, Atkins DL, et al. Guidelines for evaluation and management of common congenital cardiac problems in infants. American Heart Association. *Circulation.* 1994;90:2180-2188.
15. Ainsworth SB, Wyllie JP, Wren C. Prevalence and clinical significance of cardiac murmurs in neonates. *Arch Dis Child Fetal Neonatal Ed.* 1999;80:F43-F45.
16. Norman M. Detecting heart defects in newborn infant—innocent murmurs mixed with silent dangers. *Acta Paediatr.* 2006;95:391-393.
17. Richmond S, Wren C. Early diagnosis of congenital heart disease. *Semin Neonatol.* 2001;6:27-35.
18. Moss AJ. Clues in diagnosing congenital heart disease. *West J Med.* 1992;156:392-398.
19. Onuzo OC. How effectively can clinical examination pick up congenital heart disease at birth? *Arch Dis Child Fetal Neonatal Ed.* 2006;91:F236-F237.
20. Kates EH, Kates J. Anemia and polycythemia in the newborn. *Pediatr Rev.* Jan 2007;28(1):33-34.
21. Enns GM, Packman S. Diagnosing inborn errors of metabolism in the newborn: laboratory investigations. *NeoReviews.* 2001;2(8):e192-e199.
22. Vliet VG, Czernichow P. Screening for neonatal endocrinopathies: rationale, methods and results. *Semin Neonatol.* 2004;9:75-85.

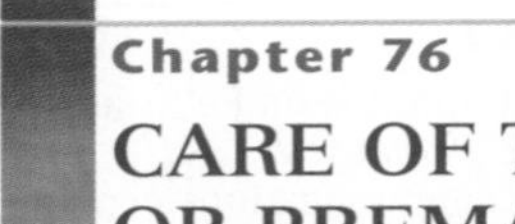

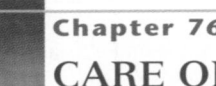

Chapter 76

CARE OF THE SICK OR PREMATURE INFANT BEFORE TRANSPORT

Karen S. Wood, MD

Organized neonatal transport programs emerged in the late 1970s when perinatal care shifted to regional centers. Regionalization of care promoted maternal-fetal transport and reduced the number of newborns requiring postnatal transport. In addition, regionalization resulted in improvements in perinatal mortality[1] and neonatal morbidity[2] as the percentage of very low–birth weight infants delivered outside of tertiary care centers decreased. Sick or premature infants, however, continue to be born at institutions that are unable to provide all of their medical needs. In some areas, organized regional perinatal care services have deteriorated. In all regions of the country, very low–birth weight infants and term infants with known congenital anomalies are born in hospitals that are not designed to provide specialized care. Some term infants will fail to transition or have unpredicted medical needs and require transport to a tertiary care center.

STABILIZING INFANTS

Stabilizing a sick or premature infant before interfacility transport means first ensuring an adequate airway and then optimizing ventilation. The next most critical issue is evaluating and obtaining an effective blood circulating volume. After the airway, breathing, and circulation (ABCs) have been established, several other parameters that are crucial to maintaining neonatal stability should be addressed, including thermoregulation, glucose homeostasis, evaluation for sepsis and the efficacy of ongoing therapies, and family crisis support. Because dealing with a sick neonate is an infrequent occurrence for people working outside of neonatal intensive care units, the S.T.A.B.L.E mnemonic was created by the developers of the S.T.A.B.L.E. course[3] to (www.stableprogram.org) to aid recall of these steps for managing the infant before transport. The mnemonic is as follows:

S = SUGAR and SAFE care
T = TEMPERATURE
A = AIRWAY
B = BLOOD PRESSURE
L = LABORATORY EVALUATION
E = EMOTIONAL SUPPORT

The remainder of this chapter will both summarize the STABLE Program Learner manual content[3] and review each of these issues, in mnemonic order, as it applies to pretransport management.

Sugar

Because the newborn infant is at risk for hypoglycemia,[4,5] checking serum glucose is imperative. Newborns, and particularly premature infants, have limited glycogen stores because most glycogen is produced and stored during the 3rd trimester. The sick newborn will have increased glucose utilization, and hyperinsulinemia may be present in the infant who is large for gestational age or the infant of a mother with diabetes. Other causes of increased glucose utilization include perinatal distress, respiratory distress, hypoxia, shock, hypothermia, sepsis, and cardiac disease. In conditions of normoxia, infants rely on aerobic metabolism, which is efficient in producing energy from glucose. However, during hypoxia, anaerobic metabolism occurs, which uses additional glucose to produce the same amount of energy. Inadequate glucose production occurs in premature infants and those who are small for gestational age. Some maternal medications potentiate infant hypoglycemia, including β-sympathomimetics, β-blockers, benzthiazide diuretics, chlorpropamide, and tricyclic antidepressants.[6] Infants with polycythemia or congenital hypopituitarism are also at risk for hypoglycemia.

The goal range for serum glucose is 50 to 110 mg/dL (2.8-6.0 mmol/L).[7] Hypoglycemia is traditionally defined as a serum glucose concentration of less than 40 mg/dL[8]; however, to provide a buffer, 50 mg/dL is designated as the concentration at which to intervene for patients undergoing transport. In most instances, sick infants are not stable enough for oral feedings, and glucose administration will require placement of a peripheral intravenous catheter or umbilical venous catheter. The initial glucose infusion rate (GIR) should be 4 to 6 mg/kg/min and can be delivered with 10% dextrose in water D10W at 80 mL/kg/day or in extremely low–birth weight (<1000 g) infants with D5W at 120 mL/kg/day. If the initial measured serum glucose concentration is less than 50 mg/dL, then a peripheral intravenous line should be started, with a GIR of 4 to 6 mg/kg/min and a 2 mL/kg D10W (200 mg/kg) glucose bolus given. Higher-concentration glucose boluses are discouraged because of the rebound hypoglycemia that can follow. A repeat serum glucose measurement should be performed 15 to 30 minutes after the bolus. If subsequent glucose measurements continue to be less than 50 mg/dL, then the clinician must ensure that the intravenous line is functioning, that a GIR of 4 to 6 mg/kg/min is being delivered, and then an additional 2-mL/kg D10W bolus should be given intravenously. As needed, 2 glucose boluses may be given before increasing the GIR, which should be done in increments of 2 mg/kg/min. The clinician should continue to repeat the serum glucose measurements until 2 successive measurements are more than 50 mg/dL. Infants with hyperinsulinemia may need a GIR twice the initial starting rate[9] and may require an increased fluid rate or a central line to achieve this goal. The steps for managing serum glucose are outlined in Box 76-1.

Temperature

A neutral thermal environment has an important effect on the well being of a newborn. Although the sentinel work by Silverman demonstrated increased survival in a neutral thermal environment for premature infants

BOX 76-1 Serum Glucose Management

Step 1: Make sure the neonate receives nothing by mouth.
Step 2: Start IV glucose infusion at 4-6 mg/kg/min
Step 3: Check serum glucose (step 3 may precede step 2)
Step 4: If serum glucose is less than 50 mg/dL then:
  a. Check IV infusion rate.
  b. Administer a bolus of 2 mL/kg D10W.
  c. Recheck serum glucose in 15-30 minutes.
  d. May proceed through step 4 twice.
Step 5: If serum glucose is less than 50 mg/dL after 2 boluses, then:
  a. Increase glucose infusion by 2 mg/kg/min.
  b. Recheck serum glucose in 15-30 minutes.
  c. Repeat step 5 as needed.
Step 6: If serum glucose is more than 50 mg/dL, then recheck serum glucose in 30-60 minutes.
Step 7: If serum glucose is more than 50 mg/dL on 2 serial checks, then space glucose measurements to 1-3 hr.

D10W, 10% dextrose in water; *IV,* intravenous.

only,[10] in practice, this principal is used for all newborns. Oxygen consumption increases at temperatures above and below the neutral thermal range. Hypothermia is a significant predictor of neonatal morbidity[11] and mortality,[12] particularly in the transport literature. Recent studies have demonstrated that head cooling[13] or whole-body hypothermia[14] may have advantages for neurologic outcome in a subset of neonates who have suffered an hypoxic insult at birth. However, for the general neonatal population, normothermia is the goal. The normal core temperature range for an infant is 36.5°C to 37.5°C (97.7°F to 99.5°F).[15] Every effort should be made to prevent heat loss in the neonate because rewarming an infant who has become hypothermic can be difficult.

All infants are at risk for hypothermia. Groups at high risk include premature infants, particularly those weighing less than 1500 g, infants who are small for gestational age; infants with hypoxia or infants who require a prolonged resuscitation; acutely ill infants with infectious, cardiac, endocrine, neurologic, or surgical issues (abdominal wall and neural tube defects); infants who are sedated or paralyzed; and infants with hypoglycemia. During the transition to extrauterine life, an infant can lose heat at rates up to 1.0°C per minute.[16] The recommended delivery room temperature range therefore is 25°C to 28°C (77°F to 82.4°F).[17]

Heat can be lost by a variety of mechanisms; however, by the law of thermodynamics, heat always flows from warm to cold.[18] Conductive heat loss occurs when the infant comes in contact with a cooler object such as a mattress, scale, stethoscope, blanket, or care provider. Warming objects (not to exceed 40°C) that the infant contacts and providing insulators, such as hats, are good ways to avoid conductive heat loss. Convective heat loss occurs from the skin surface to the surrounding air and is increased when the environmental air temperature is colder or when the air currents are higher. Careful attention to the environmental temperature, including use of a prewarmed isolette or nonobstruction of the overhead heat source on a radiant warmer, and avoiding drafts, including cold oxygen currents, can help eliminate convective heat loss. Infants weighing less than 1500 g should be covered with polyethylene plastic from neck to feet to reduce convective heat loss. Radiant heat loss occurs between solid surfaces not in contact with each other. The heat sink is usually a cold wall or window, although a cold radiant warmer or isolette can have the same effect. The infant should not be located close to a cold solid object, and thermal shades and covers should be used. Finally, heat can be lost through the mechanism of evaporation, which is a particular concern in the delivery room. Evaporative losses occur when moisture on the skin surface or in the respiratory tract is converted into vapor, with a concurrent cooling effect. This type of heat loss can be minimized by drying the infant after delivery or bathing. No infant should be bathed until a normal core temperature has been established and the infant is otherwise stable. Oxygen should be heated and humidified as soon as possible. Polyethylene plastic wrap also reduces evaporative heat loss.

Term infants have adaptive mechanisms in response to cold stress, including peripheral vasoconstriction, increased muscle activity and flexion, and brown adipose metabolism. These mechanisms require oxygen and glucose. Peripheral vasoconstriction prevents blood flow to and heat loss from the skin surface. Infants cannot shiver; however, muscle activity generates some heat, and flexion conserves the surface area from which heat can be lost. Brown adipose is metabolized in response to cold stress with norepinephrine release, creating nonshivering thermogenesis.[19] Brown adipose is accumulated throughout gestation, predominantly during the 3rd trimester, and has a unique capability for extraordinary energy production and subsequent heat production. Pulmonary vasoconstriction occurs in addition to peripheral vasoconstriction in response to norepinephrine release and can lead to persistent pulmonary hypertension. The cascade of problems that occur with hypothermia is demonstrated in Figure 76-1.[20]

In the event of heat loss, rewarming must occur, though rapidly rewarming the patient can result in vasodilation and hypotension. Unfortunately, no studies exist to define rewarming rates that are too fast or too slow. If the infant is rewarming in an isolette, then the air temperature should be set to 1.0°C to 1.5°C above the infant's core temperature; after equilibration, the air temperature should be increased by an additional 1.0°C to 1.5°C until the infant's core temperature is within the normal range. If the infant is being rewarmed with a radiant warmer, then overly aggressive rewarming should be avoided. The servo control should not be set to greater than or equal to 36.5°C unless the infant's temperature is within 1.5°C of this value. The neonate's response to rewarming should be

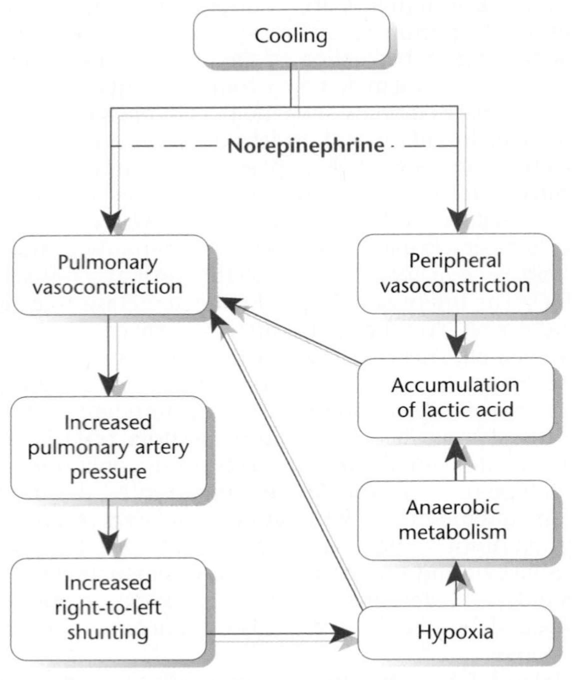

Figure 76-1 Cardiovascular response to hypothermia. *(From Baumgart S. Incubation of the human newborn infant. In: Pomerance JJ, Richardson CJ, eds.* Neonatology for the Clinician. *Norwalk, CT: Appleton & Lange, 1993. Used with permission.)*

monitored, and the speed of rewarming, depending on tolerance, should be adjusted.

Airway

Stabilizing the airway usually represents the most critical management dilemma in a pretransport newborn. The most common diagnosis requiring transport to a neonatal intensive care unit is respiratory distress. Respiratory failure can occur quickly but may be thwarted by early respiratory support, including correct airway positioning, supplemental oxygen therapy via hood or nasal cannula, continuous positive airway pressure (CPAP) via high-flow nasal cannula or CPAP device, or assisted ventilation through an endotracheal tube.[21] The amount of support needed may change during the pretransport period, necessitating constant reevaluation of the patient's respiratory requirements. An important point to remember is that if the infant is not ventilated, then other management strategies, including medications, will not be effective.

The normal respiratory rate for a newborn is 30 to 60 breaths per minute.[22] Respiratory distress may manifest as apnea, poor air entry on auscultation, cyanosis, or increased work of breathing, such as tachypnea, retractions, grunting, or flaring. The newborn can endure hypoxia for only a brief period during which the infant relies on anaerobic metabolism, metabolizes large amounts of glucose, and produces significant quantities of lactic acid. If hypoxia continues, then profound metabolic acidosis causes cellular dysfunction and cell death with organ injury.[23] A postductal saturation measurement provides an estimation of oxygenation and is useful for continuous monitoring; however, an arterial blood gas test is the gold standard for assessing oxygenation, ventilation, and acid-base balance and can guide further management. A low partial pressure of carbon dioxide in arterial blood with tachypnea typically represents a nonpulmonary cause of respiratory distress, such as congenital heart disease, metabolic acidosis, or central nervous system dysfunction. A high partial pressure of carbon dioxide with tachypnea typically represents a pulmonary cause, such as pneumonia, meconium or amniotic fluid aspiration, airway obstruction, chest mass, congenital diaphragmatic hernia, pneumothorax, or respiratory distress syndrome. A chest radiograph should be obtained to help diagnose the cause of respiratory distress and define the extent of disease. (See Chapter 99, Respiratory Distress and Breathing Disorders in the Newborn.)

Rarely does a term newborn require CPAP; therefore using the oxygen hood is usually the best technique to supply oxygen to these nonventilated newborns. Unlike the nasal cannula, the hood allows measuring the amount of oxygen being supplied to the nares. In term infants, the use of high oxygen concentrations (fraction of inspired oxygen = 1.0) in the time frame for stabilization is not considered to be toxic. Using a nasal cannula to provide oxygen therapy is common practice; however, this method also provides unnecessary CPAP, which increases the risk for air leak and is therefore not the best choice for term patients. If an insufficient amount of oxygen is being delivered via the hood or the patient's respiratory status is deteriorating, then the infant should be intubated and placed on assisted ventilation. The endotracheal tube size and placement depth is dictated by the infant's weight (Table 76-1).[24] The initial ventilator settings should consider the patient's gestational age, weight, and disease process (Figure 76-2).[25]

In contrast, in preterm infants, judicious use of oxygen therapy must occur because of the known retinal and pulmonary toxicities of oxygen.[26] Premature infants frequently need CPAP but little supplemental oxygen; therefore the best initial device for them is CPAP or a nasal cannula with a flow meter and blender to deliver the minimal necessary oxygen concentration. Given that CPAP devices are not universally available, increasing flow rates with the nasal cannula can create CPAP. For infants requiring more support, intubation and assisted ventilation should be provided (see Table 76-1 and Figure 76-2).

Respiratory distress can result from parenchymal lung disease but can also be caused by airway obstruction. Obstruction can occur at any point in the airway: nose, mouth, jaw, larynx, trachea, or bronchi. Upper airway obstruction can produce the aforementioned signs of respiratory distress, as well as stridor. The character of the stridor can suggest the level of obstruction because supraglottic lesions tend to result in inspiratory stridor, tracheal lesions result in expiratory stridor, and

Table 76-1 Endotracheal Tube Size and Placement Depth

WEIGHT (G)	TUBE SIZE (MM)	TUBE INSERTION DEPTH (CM)
<1000	2.5	6.5-7.0
1000-2000	3.0	7-8
2000-3000	3.5	8-9
>3000	3.5-4.0	>9

Adapted from Kattwinkel J. *Textbook of Neonatal Resuscitation.* 5th ed. Elk Grove Village, IL: American Academy of Pediatrics and American Heart Association; 2006.

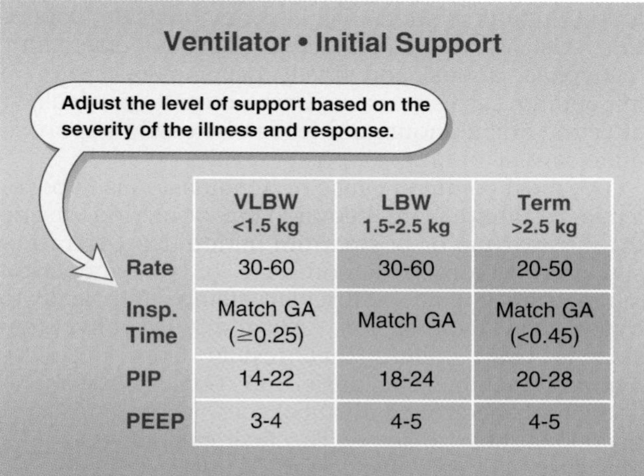

	VLBW <1.5 kg	LBW 1.5-2.5 kg	Term >2.5 kg
Rate	30-60	30-60	20-50
Insp. Time	Match GA (≥0.25)	Match GA	Match GA (<0.45)
PIP	14-22	18-24	20-28
PEEP	3-4	4-5	4-5

Figure 76-2 Proposed initial ventilator settings. *VLBW,* Very low–birth weight; *LBW,* low birth weight; *GA,* gestational age; *PIP,* peak inspiratory pressure; *PEEP,* positive end-expiratory pressure. *(Adapted from Karlsen KA.* The S.T.A.B.L.E. Program: Post-resuscitation/Pre-transport Stabilization Care of Sick Infants. Guidelines for Neonatal Healthcare Providers: Learner Manual. *5th ed. Salt Lake City, UT: S.T.A.B.L.E. Program, 2006. Used with permission.)*

glottic and subglottic problems lead to biphasic stridor.[27] (See Chapter 222, Stridor.) The diagnosis of choanal atresia can be excluded by the ability to pass a catheter through each nare. Patients with choanal atresia often only need an oral airway but may need intubation to bypass the obstruction. Nasal cannula and CPAP devices are completely ineffective in choanal obstruction. Infants with Pierre Robin sequence have micrognathia, cleft palate, and airway obstruction from the posterior position of the tongue.[28] These infants often improve with prone positioning, allowing the tongue to fall forward with gravity. If this measure fails, then an endotracheal tube can be passed through the nares to the pharynx and be used to supply humidified oxygen or CPAP. An oral airway or a laryngeal mask airway, if available, may be effective. If these mechanisms are ineffective, then endotracheal intubation should be performed. However, endotracheal intubation can be technically difficult because of the micrognathia.

Persistent pulmonary hypertension (PPHN) can occur with sustained elevation of pulmonary vascular resistance after birth and persistence of fetal circulation. Given that blood follows the path of least resistance, it is shunted from right to left, away from the lungs, through the ductus arteriosus or foramen ovale, resulting in hypoxemia. Idiopathic PPHN can occur, and PPHN can accompany hypothermia, sepsis, congenital heart disease, or birth depression. However, most cases of PPHN occur with a parenchymal lung disorder such as meconium aspiration, pulmonary hypoplasia, pneumonia, or respiratory distress syndrome. With prompt recognition and early management of PPHN, infants typically need far less support than infants with delayed diagnosis.

PPHN should be considered in any infant with respiratory distress. Infants with PPHN will have tachypnea, cyanosis, and lability in oxygen saturations. The presence of PPHN is suggested by a preductal-to-postductal oxygen saturation difference greater than or equal to 10%. Some infants with PPHN will shunt only at the atrial level and will not display this preductal-to-postductal saturation difference but will have lower-than-normal oxygen saturations. The chest radiograph in infants with PPHN may demonstrate parenchymal lung disease or decreased vascular markings, as in idiopathic PPHN, as well as a heart size that is normal or slightly enlarged. PPHN is also suggested by a low partial pressure of oxygen on an arterial blood gas sample; however, congenital heart disease needs to be ruled out in these patients. Providing adequate oxygen and eliminating acidosis may significantly improve the partial pressure of oxygen in patients with PPHN but not in patients with congenital heart disease. Comparison of an arterial blood gas test in room air and a 2nd arterial blood gas test after 30 minutes of 100% oxygen (fraction of inspired oxygen = 1.0) exposure is known as the hyperoxic challenge test. Echocardiography is the gold standard for diagnosing congenital heart disease but is often unavailable in the pretransport setting. Therapy for PPHN includes adequate ventilation and oxygenation (may require intubation), correction of acidosis or mild alkalosis,[29] provision of sedation and analgesia, maintenance of adequate cardiac output via volume and inotropic support, elimination of hypothermia, correction of polycythemia but maintenance of a normal hematocrit, and correction of metabolic abnormalities, including hypoglycemia and hypocalcemia. After all of these therapies have been optimized, inhaled nitric oxide[30] can be considered; extracorporeal membrane oxygenation[31] should be contemplated only as a last therapeutic option.

Pneumothorax occurs frequently in neonates. In fact, based on radiographic surveys, spontaneous pneumothoraces occur in 1% of all live births[32] and are a consequence of the high negative intrapleural pressures (40 to 100 cm of water[33]) seen with initial respirations in a newborn. Despite a high frequency of occurrence, the majority of pneumothoraces are asymptomatic. Parenchymal lung disease, resuscitation at birth with positive pressure ventilation, or assisted ventilation in the neonatal period increases the risk for a symptomatic pneumothorax. Surfactant replacement and ventilation using lower peak airway pressures (gentle ventilation) have decreased the incidence of air leaks, particularly in the preterm population.

Pneumothorax can be the primary cause of respiratory distress, or it can arise as a complication of lung disease. Air accumulating in the pleural space can compress the lung, affect ventilation, and, in severe cases, restrict cardiac output. A pneumothorax should be suspected in any infant who undergoes a rapid deterioration of respiratory status, especially if an associated cardiovascular collapse occurs. However, smaller air leaks can produce an insidious change in vital signs. A pneumothorax can usually be diagnosed by an anterior-posterior view chest radiograph, although a lateral view is occasionally needed. With an unstable infant, as seen with a tension pneumothorax, there may not be time to wait for the radiograph, and in these cases, transillumination of the chest can be used to diagnose the pneumothorax.[34] Transillumination indicates a pneumothorax if the fiber-optic light on the chest wall demonstrates a degree of lucency in excess of the usual 2- to 3-cm halo around the probe tip.[35] Some expanded lung tissue must be available against which to transilluminate; thus a completely collapsed lung can demonstrate a false-negative transillumination. The room should be dark, and the transilluminator light source needs to be bright. False-positive transillumination can occur with chest wall edema, subcutaneous air, pneumomediastinum, and severe pulmonary interstitial emphysema.

Asymptomatic infants with a small pneumothorax require only close observation. Infants with respiratory distress may benefit from oxygen therapy (nitrogen washout) best delivered without positive pressure via an oxygen hood. Unstable infants will require evacuation of the pneumothorax with needle decompression or thoracostomy tube placement. The presence of parenchymal lung disease or ongoing positive pressure ventilation substantially increases the need for evacuation. Needle decompression is performed in the 2nd intercostal space in the mid-clavicular line.[36] The thoracostomy tube should be placed in the 5th intercostal space in the anterior axillary line for a posterior tube and at the midpoint of the anterior axillary to mid-axillary line for an anterior tube.[37] If size 10 or 12 French thoracostomy tubes are not available and a chest tube is necessary, then a 23-gauge butterfly needle can be placed, as in needle decompression, and the end of the tubing submerged in sterile water for temporary drainage.

Blood Pressure

Hypotension results in inadequate oxygen delivery to the tissues. In newborns, hypotension occurs secondary to hypovolemia, heart failure, sepsis, or a combination of these conditions. In the extremely low–birth weight infant, adrenal insufficiency may be an isolated cause for hypotension.[38,39] Delaying treatment of shock can lead to multisystem organ failure and death; therefore early identification is essential.

The normal range for blood pressure varies by gestational age,[40] and the exact normal range remains controversial. As a rule of thumb, the mean blood pressure should approximate gestational age. Given that low blood pressure is a late finding in cardiac collapse, early signs of compromise must be identified. The physical examination findings of hypotension include weak peripheral pulses, cyanosis, poor perfusion (represented as a capillary refill time more than 3 seconds), pallor, and mottled and cool skin. Cardiac output is a product of stroke volume and heart rate. Although older patients increase cardiac output by increasing stroke volume, the infant has a poorly compliant myocardium and therefore relies on increased heart rate to increase cardiac output.[41] Infants with hypotension will initially demonstrate tachycardia but progress to bradycardia before arrest. Infants in shock will also demonstrate respiratory distress with increased work of breathing, tachypnea, apnea, and finally gasping as a sign of impending cardiac arrest. Urine output, particularly after the first 24 hours of life, can be used to approximate cardiac output.

The most common cause of hypotension is hypovolemia resulting from hemorrhage occurring during the intrapartum or postpartum period. However, sepsis, dehydration, pneumothorax, or pneumoperitoneum can impair ventricular filling and lead to hypovolemic hypotension. A second cause of hypotension is heart failure that results from asphyxia, hypoxia, metabolic acidosis, infection, severe metabolic and electrolyte disturbances, arrhythmias, or congenital heart disease. The final category of hypotension is caused by sepsis, which typically produces distributive shock with the loss of vascular tone and accompanying capillary leak. Infants can have hypotension from one or a combination of these different causes, and each will have its own management plan.

Treatment for the infant in hypovolemic shock relies on volume resuscitation. Initially, volume expansion should use lactated Ringer's solution or normal saline at 10 mL/kg. If the patient is anemic, then ideally, cross-matched packed red cells should be given. Infants should be reassessed for further volume replacement. Cardiogenic failure is best treated with inotropic agents, dopamine or dobutamine.[42] Initially, inotrope at a dose of 5 mcg/kg/min should be started and titrated to the desired mean blood pressure or effect. In septic shock, capillary leak and the ongoing 3rd-space losses will require volume replacement, and the cardiac effects will require inotropic support. Requiring large amounts of volume replacement is not uncommon for infants in septic shock. Patients with cardiogenic and septic hypotension can have significant metabolic acidosis; however, the use of sodium bicarbonate is controversial[43] and reserved for term infants who are well ventilated and have a pH of less than 7.15. The most effective therapy for these infants is to identify and treat the cause of the metabolic acidosis. Also important in the face of hypotension is maintaining adequate glucose, calcium, sodium, and potassium for optimal cardiac function.[44] (See also Chapter 358, Shock.)

Laboratory Evaluation

Before transport, the 4 laboratory specimens that are helpful to obtain are designated by the S.T.A.B.L.E. Program as the 4 Bs[45]:

Blood glucose
Blood gas
Blood count
Blood culture

Blood Glucose

The reader is referred to the discussion under "Sugar" earlier in this chapter.

Blood Gas

A blood gas test is essential because the majority of patients referred to higher-level centers will have respiratory symptoms, and the acid-base balance gives valuable diagnostic information. An arterial blood gas test is preferred if the distinction between a cardiac disorder and a respiratory disease remains in question; however, a capillary blood gas level is often easier to obtain and is acceptable to assess pH and ventilation. The blood gas analysis helps define the infant's status and can be communicated to the consultant at the referral center to determine further management and urgency of transport.

Blood Count and Blood Culture

The complete blood count and the blood culture are the essential components of an initial sepsis evaluation in a neonate. Because all neonates are immunodeficient, and because failure to treat a septic infant can be fatal, performing a sepsis evaluation in a symptomatic infant is critically important. The risk factors for neonatal sepsis include premature rupture of membranes, rupture of membranes more than 18 hours, maternal fever, recent maternal infection or illness, maternal urinary tract infection, maternal chorioamnionitis, maternal group B streptococcal colonization, fetal distress, perinatal asphyxia, low birth weight, male gender, and intrapartum or postpartum instrumentation.[46] Clinical signs of sepsis can be subtle or dramatic and include respiratory distress, temperature instability, abnormal skin perfusion, abnormal heart rate, abnormal blood pressure, feeding disturbance, and neurologic dysfunction. Given the wide spectrum of presentation for sepsis and the fact that considerable overlap exists with other diagnoses, obtaining blood work and initiating antibiotic therapy until infection is ruled out is imperative.

Causative agents for neonatal sepsis are not always bacterial. However, bacterial infections are more common in the neonate than patients at any other stage in life[47] and are the agents to which therapy should be targeted in the pretransport period. The most common infecting organisms include group B *Streptococcus, Escherichia coli, Staphylococcus aureus, Staphylococcus epidermidis,* and, less commonly, *Enterococcus, Klebsiella pneumoniae, Neisseria meningitidis, Streptococcus pneumoniae, Listeria monocytogenes, Pseudomonas aeruginosa, Serratia marcescens, Enterobacter,* and group A *Streptococcus.*[48] A blood culture, preferably 1 mL in volume, obtained from a carefully prepped site can identify the infectious agent. Obtaining the blood culture should precede antibiotic administration; however, antibiotic delivery should not be delayed if a culture cannot be obtained.

The complete blood count and differential may suggest sepsis if it reveals neutropenia, neutrophilia, immature neutrophils, or thrombocytopenia. Neutrophils are the critical component of defense against bacterial infections, and elevation of neutrophil counts can signal sepsis, although a diminished neutrophil count is much more ominous for neonatal sepsis.[49] When neutrophils are depleted, the bone marrow produces more immature neutrophils. When the percentage of immature-to-mature neutrophils exceeds 20%, the diagnosis of sepsis should be entertained.[50] Thrombocytopenia may indicate sepsis. The normal range for the platelet count of a term infant is 310,000 (+/−68,000) per mcL.[51] Thrombocytopenia is defined as a platelet count less than 150,000/mcL although counts of less than 100,000/mcL typically receive more attention. For term infants, the risk of bleeding is low until platelet counts drop below 30,000/mcL, and therefore platelet transfusions are rarely necessary in the pretransport period. An essential point to note is that the complete blood count is not diagnostic for sepsis. An infant with sepsis can have normal values in the complete blood count, and an infant without sepsis can have an abnormal complete blood count.

The suggested therapy for presumed early-onset neonatal sepsis consists of ampicillin and gentamicin. The ampicillin dose is 100 mg/kg/dose every 12 hours intravenously. This higher dose is used because meningitis is not excluded with an initial neonatal sepsis evaluation. Gentamicin should be dosed in accordance with the Neofax guidelines,[52] with dose ranges from 4 to 5 mg/kg/dose every 24 to 48 hours depending on gestational age. The antibiotic regimen is continued until sepsis is satisfactorily ruled out; this typically requires monitoring of the blood culture for a minimum of 48 hours.

Early-onset group B streptococcal (GBS) infection can occur in the 1st week of life as sepsis, pneumonia, meningitis, or any combination. The incidence of this infection has decreased in recent years with the implementation of maternal carrier screening and peripartum antibiotics.[53,54] The drug of choice for intrapartum prophylaxis of mothers is penicillin G. Neonates who demonstrate signs of sepsis at birth should have a blood culture, and they should be started on antibiotics. Given that premature infants have a 10-fold increased risk of early-onset GBS disease compared with term infants,[55] and because distinguishing GBS disease from respiratory distress syndrome is often difficult, these preterm infants more frequently deserve an initial septic evaluation. For asymptomatic infants who received appropriate intrapartum prophylaxis, a 24- to 48-hour observation period is required.[55]

Emotional Support

An ill newborn requiring transfer to another hospital represents a significant and unexpected crisis for most parents. Parent support group evaluations reveal that during the pretransport and posttransport periods, the needs of the neonate are being met, whereas the needs of the parents are frequently not. Parents should be informed of the assessment and plan for their infant. This information often needs to be repeated because families may be in shock and not fully assimilate the information that is provided.

Families receiving catastrophic news undergo the stages of grief as outlined by Elisabeth Kübler-Ross in her book, *On Death and Dying*: shock, denial, anger, bargaining, depression, testing, and acceptance.[56] During the pretransport period, it is typical for families to be in the earliest stages, expressing shock and denial, finding it incomprehensible that what was supposed to be a happy, uncomplicated event has gone awry. However, individual family members transition through these stages at different speeds and sometimes in different orders.[56] Consequently, the caretaking team needs to be capable of managing families in all stages of grief. A designated hospital staff member, usually the physician or a staff nurse, must be responsible for communicating directly with the family during the stabilization period and after departure of the infant. The parents should be encouraged to write questions down for the physician or transport team because forgetting questions is easy when under stress.

The caretakers communicating with the family should identify the infant as personally as possible. Family members should be encouraged to touch their infant, take pictures, and obtain mementos such as footprints or a lock of hair. Any additional sources of support such as family members, friends, or members of the clergy should be identified and contacted. The assigned communicator should accompany the transport team to the mother's room and stay to hear the discussion with the family because questions will inevitably arise once the team leaves. Once the transport team departs with the neonate, the caretaking team should switch its focus from taking care of the infant to taking care of the parents. A helpful measure would be to review with the family the information communicated by the transport team, such as the new caretakers for the infant, the plan of care at the receiving hospital, and directions to the receiving hospital. Also important is assessing the parent's response and coping mechanisms when the infant departs. Inquiring into the mother's plan to breastfeed and obtaining a breast pump (many insurance plans will provide mothers with a hospital grade electric breast pump if the infant is hospitalized and unable to nurse) and encouraging her to proceed with breast milk expression can be useful. In addition, offering to help the parents make subsequent contact with the center caring for their infant is appropriate. Calling the parents on arrival at the receiving hospital to update them on the status of their infant is common practice for transport personnel.

Few parents anticipate that their term newborn will be sick, and families having preterm infants are ill prepared for birth, much less for coping with an infant requiring critical care. Providing families with information, an opportunity to talk and grieve, support in their time of crisis, and close personal follow-up is an essential and often overlooked portion of providing care in the pretransport stabilization period.

The author wishes to thank Diane Marshall and Kristine Karlsen whose contributions were instrumental in the preparation of this manuscript.

TOOLS FOR PRACTICE

Engaging Patients and Family

- *What is a Neonatologist?* (fact sheet), American Academy of Pediatrics (www.aap.org/sections/perinatal/WhatisNeonatologist.pdf).

Medical Decision Support

- *Guidelines for Air and Ground Transport of Neonatal and Pediatric Patients* (book), American Academy of Pediatrics (www.aap.org/bookstore).
- *The S.T.A.B.L.E. Program: Student Manual,* 5th edition (book), Kristine A. Karlsen, MSN, RNC, NNP (www.aap.org/bookstore).
- *The S.T.A.B.L.E. Program: Learner Course Slides on CD-ROM,* 5th edition (CD-ROM), Kristine A. Karlsen, MSN, RNC, NNP (www.aap.org/bookstore).
- *The S.T.A.B.L.E. Program: Physical Exam and Gestational Age Assessment Slide Program* (CD-ROM), Kristine A. Karlsen, MSN, RNC, NNP (www.aap.org/bookstore).
- *The S.T.A.B.L.E. Program: Quick Reference Bedside Card Set,* 3rd edition (cards), Kristine A. Karlsen, MSN, RNC, NNP (www.aap.org/bookstore).
- *The S.T.A.B.L.E. Program: Blood Gas Interpretation Chart,* 2nd edition (chart), Kristine A. Karlsen, MSN, RNC, NNP (www.aap.org/bookstore).

REFERENCES

1. Cifuentes J, Bronstein J, Phibbs CS, et al. Mortality in low birth weight infants according to level of neonatal care at hospital of birth. *Pediatrics*. 2002;109(5): 745-751.
2. Hohlagschwandtner M, Husslein P, Klebermass K. Perinatal mortality and morbidity: comparison between maternal transport, neonatal transport and inpatient antenatal treatment. *Arch Gynecol Obstet*. 2001;265: 113-118.
3. Karlsen KA. *The S.T.A.B.L.E. Program: Post-resuscitation/Pre-transport Stabilization Care of Sick Infants*. 5th ed. Salt Lake City, UT: S.T.A.B.L.E. Program; 2006:8. (www.stableprogram.org)
4. Cornblath M, Schwartz R. Hypoglycemia in the neonate. *J Pediatr Endocrinol*. 1993;6(2):113-129.
5. deLonlay P, Giurgea I, Touati G, et al. Neonatal hypoglycaemia: aetiologies. *Semin Neonatol*. 2004;9:49-58.
6. Kalhan SC, Parimi PS. Disorders of carbohydrate metabolism. In: Martin RJ, Fanaroff AA, Walsh MC, eds. *Neonatal-Perinatal Medicine*. 8th ed. Philadelphia, PA: Mosby Elsevier; 2006:1472.
7. Karlsen KA. *The S.T.A.B.L.E. Program: Post-resuscitation/Pre-transport Stabilization Care of Sick Infants,*. 5th ed. Salt Lake City, UT: S.T.A.B.L.E. Program; 2006:20.
8. Cornblath M, Hawdon JM, Williams AF, et al. Controversies regarding definition of neonatal hypoglycemia: suggested operational thresholds. *Pediatrics*. 2000;105(5): 1141-1145.
9. Cowett RM, Farrag HM. Selected principles of perinatal-neonatal glucose metabolism. *Semin Neonatol*. 2004;9: 37-47.

10. Silverman WA, Fertig JW, Berger AP. The influence of the neutral thermal environment upon the survival of newly born premature infants. *Pediatrics*. 1958;22(5): 876-886.
11. Beeram M, Kolawole S. Morbidity and mortality of infants born before arrival at the hospital. *Clin Pediatr.* 1995;34(5):313-316.
12. Hood JL, Cross A, Hulka B, et al. Effectiveness of the neonatal transport team. *Crit Care Med*. 1983;11(6): 419-423.
13. Gluckman PD, Wyatt JS, Azzopardi D, et al. Selective head cooling with mild systemic hypothermia after neonatal encephalopathy: multicentre randomised trial. *Lancet*. 2005;365(9460):663-670.
14. Shankaran S, Laptook AR, Ehrenkranz RA, et al. Whole-body hypothermia for neonates with hypoxic-ischemic encephalopathy. *N Engl J Med*. 2005;353(15): 1574-1584.
15. Riesenfeld T, Hammerlund K, Sedin G. The effect of a warm environment on respiratory water loss in full term newborn infants on their first day after birth. *Acta Pediatr Scand*. 1990;79:889-893.
16. Friedman M, Baumgart S. Thermal regulation. In: MacDonald MG Mullett MD, Seshia MMK, eds. *Avery's Neonatology Pathophysiology and Management of the Newborn*. 6th ed. Philadelphia, PA: Lippincott–Williams & Wilkins; 2005:446.
17. World Health Organization, Department of Reproductive Health and Research. *Thermal Protection of the Newborn: A Practical Guide*. Geneva, Switzerland: World Health Organization; 1997.
18. Lavenda BH. Thermodynamics of an ideal generalized gas: I. Thermodynamic laws. *Naturwissenschaften*. 2005; 92(11):516-522.
19. Nedergaard J, Cannon B. Brown adipose tissue: development and function. In: Polin RA, Fox WW, Abman SH, eds. *Fetal and Neonatal Physiology*. 3rd ed. Philadelphia, PA: WB Saunders; 2004:405.
20. Baumgart S. Incubation of the human newborn infant. In: Pomerance JJ, Richardson CJ, eds. *Neonatology for the Clinician*. Norwalk, CT: Appleton and Lange; 1993:139.
21. Ambalavanan N, Schelonka RL, Carlo W. Ventilatory strategies. In: Goldsmith JP, Karotkin EH, eds. *Assisted Ventilation of the Neonate*. 4th ed. Philadelphia, PA: WB Saunders; 2003:249.
22. American Academy of Pediatrics, Committee on Fetus and Newborn, and American College of Obstetricians and Gynecologists, Committee on Obstetric Practice. *Guidelines for Perinatal Care*. 5th ed. Evanston, IL: American Academy of Pediatrics and American College of Obstetricians and Gynecologists; 2002:212.
23. Calvert JW, Zhang JH. Pathophysiology of a hypoxic-ischemic insult during the perinatal period. *Neurol Res*. 2005;27(3):246-260.
24. Kattwinkel J. *Textbook of Neonatal Resuscitation*. 5th ed. Elk Grove Village, IL: American Academy of Pediatrics and American Heart Association; 2006: Tables 5-1, 5-3.
25. Karlsen KA. *The S.T.A.B.L.E. Program: Post-resuscitation/Pre-transport Stabilization Care of Sick Infants. Guidelines for Neonatal Healthcare Providers: Learner Manual*. 5th ed. Salt Lake City, UT: S.T.A.B.L.E. Program; 2006:101.
26. Weinberger B, Laskin DL, Heck DE, et al. Oxygen toxicity in premature infants. *Toxicol Appl Pharmacol*. 2002; 181(1):60-67.
27. Sprecher RC, Arnold JE. Upper airway lesions. In: Martin RJ, Fanaroff AA, Walsh MC, eds. *Neonatal-Perinatal Medicine*. 8th ed. Philadelphia, PA: Mosby Elsevier; 2006:1150.
28. Jones KL. *Smith's Recognizable Patterns of Human Malformation*. 6th ed. Philadelphia, PA: WB Saunders Elsevier; 2006:262.
29. Ammari AN, Schulze KF. Uses and abuses of sodium bicarbonate in the neonatal intensive care unit. *Curr Opin Pediatr.* 2002;14:151-156.
30. Abman SH, Kinsella JP. Inhaled nitric oxide for persistent pulmonary hypertension of the newborn: the physiology matters! *Pediatrics*. 1995;96(6):1153-1155.
31. Farrow FN, Fliman P, Steinhorn RH. The diseases treated with ECMO: focus on PPHN. *Semin Perinatol*. 2005;29(1): 8-14.
32. Miller MJ, Fanaroff AA, Martin RJ. Respiratory disorders in preterm and term infants. In: Martin RJ, Fanaroff AA, Walsh MC, eds. *Neonatal-Perinatal Medicine*. 8th ed. Philadelphia, PA: Mosby Elsevier; 2006:1128.
33. Vyas H, Milner AD, Hopkins IE. Intrathoracic pressure and volume changes during the spontaneous onset of respiration in babies born by cesarean section and by vaginal delivery. *J Pediatr.* 1981;99(5):787-791.
34. Kuhns LR, Bednarek FJ, Wyman ML, et al. Diagnosis of pneumothorax or pneumomediastinum in the neonate by transillumination. *Pediatrics*. 1975;56(3):355.
35. Donn SM. Transillumination. In: Donn SM, Sinha SK, eds. *Neonatal Respiratory Care*. 2nd ed. Philadelphia, PA: Mosby; 2006:163.
36. Grady M. Procedures. In: Gunn VL, Nechyba C, eds. *The Harriet Lane Handbook: A Manual for Pediatric House Officers*. 16th ed. Philadelphia, PA: Mosby; 2002:65.
37. Rais-Bahrami K, Eichelberger MR. Thoracostomy tubes. In: MacDonald MG, Ramasethu J, eds. *Atlas of Procedures in Neonatology*. 3rd ed. Philadelphia, PA: Lippincott–Williams & Wilkins; 2002:281.
38. Efird MM, Heerens AT, Gordon PV, et al. A randomized-controlled trial of prophylactic hydrocortisone supplementation for the prevention of hypotension in extremely low birth weight infants. *J Perinatol*. 2005;25(2):119-124.
39. Jett PL, Samuels MH, McDaniel PA, et al. Variability of plasma cortisol levels in extremely low birth weight infants. *J Clin Endocrinol Metab*. 1997;82(9):2921-2925.
40. Kim MS, Herrin JT. Renal conditions. In: Cloherty JP, Eichenwald EC, Stark AR, eds. *Manual of Neonatal Care*. 5th ed. Philadelphia, PA: Lippincott–Williams & Wilkins; 2004:634.
41. Zahka KG. Principles of neonatal cardiovascular hemodynamics. In: Martin RJ, Fanaroff AA, Walsh MC, eds. *Neonatal-Perinatal Medicine*. 8th ed. Philadelphia, PA: Mosby Elsevier; 2006:1211.
42. Noori S, Friedlich P, Seri I. The use of dobutamine in the treatment of neonatal cardiovascular compromise. *NeoReviews*. 2004;5(1):e22-e26.
43. Ammari AN, Schulze KF. Uses and abuses of sodium bicarbonate in the neonatal intensive care unit. *Curr Opin Pediatr.* 2002;14:151-156.
44. Teitel DF, Hoffman JIE. Ventricular function. In: Gluckman PD, Heymann MA, eds. *Pediatrics and Perinatology the Scientific Basis*. 2nd ed. London, UK: Arnold; 1996:737.
45. Karlsen KA. *The S.T.A.B.L.E. Program: Post-resuscitation/Pre-transport Stabilization Care of Sick Infants. Guidelines for Neonatal Healthcare Providers: Learner Manual*. 5th ed. Salt Lake City, UT: S.T.A.B.L.E. Program; 2006:154.
46. Saez-Llorens X, McCracken GH. Perinatal bacterial diseases. In: Feigin RD, Cherry JD, eds. *Textbook of Pediatric Infectious Diseases*. 4th ed. Philadelphia, PA: WB Saunders; 1998:897.
47. Saez-Llorens X, McCracken GH. Perinatal bacterial diseases. In: Feigin RD, Cherry JD, eds. *Textbook of Pediatric Infectious Diseases*. 4th ed. Philadelphia, PA: WB Saunders; 1998:898.

48. Edwards MS. Postnatal bacterial infections. In: Martin RJ, Fanaroff AA, Walsh MC, eds. *Neonatal-Perinatal Medicine*. 8th ed. Philadelphia, PA: Mosby Elsevier; 2006:791.
49. Papoff P. Use of hematologic data to evaluate infections in neonates. In: Christensen RD, ed. *Hematologic Problems of the Neonate*. Philadelphia, PA: WB Saunders; 2000:389.
50. Steele RW, ed. *The Clinical Handbook of Pediatric Infectious Disease*. 2nd ed. New York, NY: Parthenon; 2000:25.
51. Christensen RD. Expected hematologic values for term and preterm neonates. In: Christensen RD, ed. *Hematologic Problems of the Neonate*. Philadelphia, PA: WB Saunders; 2000:132.
52. Young TE, Mangum B. *Neofax*. 18th ed. Raleigh, NC: Acorn; 2005:36.
53. Schrag SJ, Zywicki S, Farley MM, et al. Group B streptococcal disease in the era of intrapartum antibiotic prophylaxis. *N Engl J Med*. 2000; 342:15-20.
54. Lin FYC, Brenner RA, Johnson YR, et al. The effectiveness of risk-based intrapartum chemoprophylaxis for the prevention of early-onset neonatal group B streptococcal disease. *Am J Obstet Gyn*. 2001;184:1204-1210.
55. Centers for Disease Control and Prevention. Prevention of perinatal group B streptococcal disease: revised guidelines from the Centers for Disease Control. *MMWR Recomm Rep*. 2002;51(RR-11):1-22.
56. Kübler-Ross E. *On Death and Dying*. New York, NY: Simon and Schuster/Touchstone; 1997:51-165.

Chapter 77

CONTINUING CARE OF THE INFANT AFTER TRANSFER FROM NEONATAL INTENSIVE CARE

Deborah E. Campbell, MD

The elements of care for the infant returned to a community hospital after transfer to tertiary care center *(back transfer)* vary based on the child's underlying medical problems and health needs. In addition to maintaining bed availability within level III neonatal intensive care units (NICUs), an important aspect of care for the infant who is back transferred is to foster development of the parent-infant relationship and bonding. A well-known fact is that the separation imposed by the need to transport a sick newborn often long distances for tertiary care creates tremendous hardships for families. Parents' active involvement in their child's in-hospital care, preparation for their baby's discharge home, and post-hospital care are critical to facilitating the transition from hospital to home. Back transport to a community intermediate (level II) or primary (level I) care nursery can facilitate linking the child and family with follow-up systems within the community in which the child resides. (Box 77-1 describes levels of neonatal care.) Costs for care are often less than at the regional perinatal center or community level III NICU; it also promotes a reciprocal relationship between the community hospital and tertiary center that fosters communication and collaboration.

The hospital to which the infant is returned and the timing of the return transfer depend on the individual patient health care needs and capability of the receiving hospital. Under certain circumstances within some integrated health care delivery networks or regionalized perinatal care networks, an infant may be transferred to a facility with a lower level of care that was not the birth hospital to complete treatment and preparation for discharge home. Infants transferred to level II units include extremely low–birth-weight infants needing convalescent care, infants with chronic lung disease of infancy, infants with feeding problems, infants receiving antibiotic therapy, and infants with nonacute surgical, neurosurgical, and subspecialty medical issues. Some infants may have stable or regressing retinopathy of prematurity (ROP) or apnea of prematurity (AOP) requiring infrequent or no stimulation. Infants with life-limiting conditions may be transferred to a community hospital nearer to their homes and families for hospice (comfort) care. Box 77-2 provides a summary of the benefits of and requirements for return transfer.

The continuing care needs of the infant who is transferred back to a community primary or intermediate care unit will be determined by the infant's underlying medical condition and the child's clinical course while in intensive care. As the infant progresses through the convalescence period, the primary care physician will need to identify the child's ongoing medical care needs to determine the infant's readiness for discharge home or if a need exists for transitional (rehabilitation) or chronic care. The decision whether the baby is able to be discharged home or whether the infant will need chronic care once intermediate care is no longer needed is based on multiple factors, including the infant's ability to feed and demonstrate adequate weight gain, the need for home oxygen therapy and multiple medications, the need for intensive rehabilitation, the parents' ability to care for the infant safely at home, and the availability of home health care services and public health nurse services within the community in which the child will reside. Key to all phases in this process is communication among the treating physicians and staff at the tertiary care center, the receiving primary care physician and the intermediate or primary care nursery staff, and the parents. The receiving physician should speak directly with a member of the treating medical personnel in addition to reviewing a detailed written summary about the infant's medical problems and hospital course. Box 77-3 provides information that should be contained in the transfer summary.

Common medical issues in the continuing care of infants returned to community care after a stay at a level III NICU are discussed in the following sections.

ANEMIA

Anemia unrelated to underlying hemolytic anemias and congenital red cell disorders is a common medical condition seen in premature and sick neonates related to blood loss and decreased red blood cell production

BOX 77-1 Levels of Neonatal Care

Level I (basic): hospital nursery organized with the personnel and equipment to:
- Perform neonatal resuscitation and evaluate and provide postnatal care of healthy newborn infants.
- Stabilize and provide care for infants born at 35 to 37 weeks' gestation who remain physiologically stable.
- Stabilize newborn infants born at less than 35 weeks' gestational age or ill until transfer to a facility that can provide the appropriate level of neonatal care.

Level II (specialty): hospital special care nursery organized with the personnel and equipment to provide care to:
- Infants born at more than 32 weeks' gestation and weighing more than 1500 g who have physiologic immaturity such as apnea of prematurity, inability to maintain body temperature, or inability to take oral feedings
- Infants who are moderately ill with problems that are expected to resolve rapidly and are not anticipated to need subspecialty services on an urgent basis
- Infants who are convalescing from intensive care
- Level II care is subdivided into two categories:
  - Level IIA does not provide mechanical ventilation or continuous positive airway pressure (CPAP)
  - Level IIB has the capability to provide mechanical ventilation for brief durations (<24 hr) or CPAP

Level III (subspecialty): hospital neonatal intensive care unit (NICU) organized with personnel and equipment to:
- Provide continuous life support and comprehensive care for extremely high-risk newborn infants and those with complex and critical illness
- Level III is subdivided into three levels differentiated by the capability to provide advanced medical and surgical care
- Level IIIA units can provide:
  - Care for infants with birth weight of more than 1000 g and gestational age of more than 28 weeks
  - Continuous life support can be provided but is limited to conventional mechanical ventilation
- Level IIIB units can provide:
  - Comprehensive care for extremely low–birth-weight infants (1000 g birth weight or less and 28 or less weeks' gestation)
  - Advanced respiratory care such as high frequency ventilation and inhaled nitric oxide
  - Prompt and on-site access to a full range of pediatric medical subspecialists
  - Advanced imaging with interpretation on an urgent basis, including computed tomography, magnetic resonance imaging, and echocardiography
  - Pediatric surgical specialists and pediatric anesthesiologists on site or at a closely related institution to perform major surgery
- Level IIIC units have the capabilities of a level IIIB NICU and are located within institutions that can provide extracorporeal membrane oxygenation and surgical repair of serious congenital cardiac malformations that require cardiopulmonary bypass

From American Academy of Pediatrics, Committee on Fetus and Newborn. Levels of neonatal care. *Pediatrics.* 2004;114:1341-1347.

(ineffective erythropoiesis). (See Chapter 102, Neonatal Hematology, for a detailed discussion of neonatal anemia.) Blood losses may be acute or chronic resulting from repeated blood sampling, hemorrhage, and procedure-associated loss. Nutritional deficiencies of protein, iron, folic acid, or vitamin B_{12} lead to decreased erythropoiesis. Vitamin E deficiency, common in preterm infants, may lead to increased red blood cell destruction, particularly in infants receiving supplemental iron. Acquired (bacterial or viral sepsis) and congenital (TORCH infections [toxoplasmosis, other agents, rubella, cytomegalovirus, herpes simplex], parvovirus, HIV, and malaria) infection may lead to decreased erythrocyte production or increased red cell destruction.

Anemia of prematurity typically occurs in infants younger than 32 weeks' gestation and occurs between 2 and 4 months of age. It is the result of low red blood cell mass, shorter red blood cell survival, and increased requirements resulting from growth. Premature infants also exhibit more rapid and greater reduction in their hemoglobin levels than do full-term neonates, typically 7 to 8 g/dL. Nearly one half of preterm infants younger than 32 weeks' gestation will exhibit symptoms from anemia of prematurity. Among very low–birth-weight infants, 60% to 80% will receive at least one transfusion during their hospitalization, the majority within the first 2 to 4 weeks of life. The decision regarding the need for transfusion is often based on the infant's underlying health problems and the presence of signs (changes in cardiovascular and respiratory status, increased oxygen or ventilatory support requirements, deterioration in feeding efficiency, and declining weight gain). Box 77-4 lists the signs of anemia of prematurity.

Transfusion

Controversy exists in the approach to treating anemia in preterm infants, including deciding on a threshold for transfusion, defining symptomatic anemia and the role of erythropoietin in the treatment of anemia of prematurity, and reducing the need for transfusion (Table 77-1). Guidelines from the American College of Pathologists detail thresholds for transfusion based on severity of illness and the degree of technologic support needed by the infant.[1] The use of recombinant human erythropoietin (rHuEPO) to promote erythropoiesis remains controversial because studies

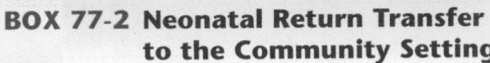

BOX 77-2 Neonatal Return Transfer to the Community Setting

BENEFITS:

- Provides continuing and convalescent care in the child's home community
- Increases availability of tertiary care beds for other critically ill infants
- Increased opportunities for parent involvement in their infant's care, facilitates parent education, and fosters parent-infant interaction
- May lessen financial burden for the family and reduce health care costs overall
- Promotes communication and collaboration between community health care providers and tertiary care providers

REQUIREMENTS:

- Infant is stable.
- Appropriate level of care is available closer to the infant's home.
- Individual patient care needs determine the level of continuing care required and the timing of the return transfer.
- Telephone consultation between the receiving health care professional and the perinatal center or community neonatal intensive care unit staff to initiate the transfer process, prepare the receiving hospital regarding the infant's current medical needs, and develop a treatment plan for the infant.
- The referring center medical staff maintains responsibility for the infant during the transport.
- Parental consent authorizing transfer, treatment, and admission to the receiving center are typically obtained by the referring hospital staff.
- The parents should be encouraged to visit the receiving intermediate or primary care nursery.
- The transport team should communicate with the receiving center regarding the estimated time of arrival.
- On arrival at the receiving hospital the transport team should discuss with the receiving staff the infant's medical history, events during the transport, and the baby's current status.
- A discharge summary from the sending hospital should accompany the infant.
- Periodic communication should be maintained between the referring and receiving hospital personnel.

have not demonstrated a significant reduction in the transfusion requirements during the first 2 weeks of life, when the majority of transfusions occur in sick neonates. The use of poly packs to split a unit of packed red blood cells into multiple aliquots has also reduced the number of donors to which a neonate is exposed. Therefore use of rHuEPO is individualized to selected cases (eg, infants with intrinsic renal disease from Jehovah's Witness or Rastafarian families

BOX 77-3 Information That Should Be Contained in the Transfer Summary

Summary of infant's clinical course in the tertiary care unit that reviews each of the infant's medical problems and complications, the treatments received, and ongoing health conditions

Current medications, nutrition needs, and feeding regimen

Results of completed diagnostic tests

Pending test results

Necessary follow-up testing, including retinopathy of prematurity checks, newborn metabolic and hearing screening, and neuroimaging

Immunizations received, immunizations due

Eligibility for and timing of palivizumab (Synagis) administration

Needed subspecialty consultations

Family assessment:

- Parents' understanding of their infant's health issues
- Parents' emotional responses and coping style in response to their infant's illness and ongoing health needs
- Financial and social support resources

Goals of continued hospital care

BOX 77-4 Symptoms of Anemia of Prematurity

Tachypnea	Decreased activity
Tachycardia	Pallor
Apnea	Flow murmurs
Poor weight gain, feeding difficulties	Metabolic acidosis

and families who refuse blood products for their infants).

Reducing iatrogenic blood losses that are the result of blood sampling for laboratory testing is important to minimize the infant's transfusion needs. Point-of-care testing devices, validated for use with neonatal blood samples, are valuable tools in reducing blood loss. Unnecessary blood sampling should be avoided as well. Use of noninvasive monitoring (transcutaneous arterial oxygen saturation [Sao_2]) is an additional tool that reduces the need for blood sampling. Experts no longer recommend that transfusions be performed to replace phlebotomy losses alone.

If a blood transfusion is required, then the volume of packed red blood cells infused is typically 10 to 15 mL/kg administered via a peripheral intravenous catheter over 2 to 3 hours. The American Association

Table 77-1 Suggested Guidelines for Packed Red Blood Cell Transfusion in Neonates*

HEMATOCRIT, HEMOGLOBIN LEVEL	AMERICAN COLLEGE OF PATHOLOGY RECOMMENDATIONS	CRITERIA OF STRATEGY (STRAUSS, 2000)†
Hematocrit (Hct) <0.4 (40%)	Acute blood loss with shock	Severe cardiopulmonary disease
Hct ≤0.35 (35%) or hemoglobin (Hg) ≤12 g/dL (≤7.44 mmol/L)	Severe RDS requiring mechanical ventilation (airway pressure [P_{aw}] >8 cm H_2O) + Fio_2 >0.5 OR Severe congenital heart disease with cyanosis or heart failure	Severe cardiopulmonary disease
Hct ≤0.3 (≤30%) or Hg ≤10 g/dL (≤6.2 mmol/L)	Moderate RDS + Fio_2 >0.35, or nasal cannula oxygen or ventilation with IMV and P_{aw} 6-8 cm H_2O	Moderate cardiopulmonary disease or major surgery
Hct ≤0.25 (≤25%) or Hg ≤8 g/dL (≤4.96 mmol/L)	Any of the following conditions: 1. Apnea and bradycardia ≥10 episodes/24 hr or ≥2 episodes requiring bag-mask ventilation 2. Sustained tachycardia >180 beats/min or sustained tachypnea >80 breaths/min over 24-hr period 3. Inadequate weight gain for 4 days with 100 kcal/kg/day (420 kj/kg/day) caloric intake 4. Mild RDS with: a. Fio_2 0.25-0.3 b. Nasal cannula 125-250 mL/min c. IMV or NCPAP with P_{aw} <6 cm H_2O	Symptomatic anemia: 1. Unexplained breathing disorders 2. Unexplained abnormal vital signs 3. Unexplained poor growth 4. Unexplained decreased activity
Hct ≤0.2 (≤20%) or Hg ≤7 g/dL (≤4.34 mmol/L) and reticulocyte count <4% (absolute reticulocyte count <100,000/mcL)	Irrespective of the presence or absence of symptoms	Irrespective of the presence or absence of symptoms

*Hematocrit and hemoglobin level and clinical symptom criteria on which to base the transfusion decision.
Fio_2, Fraction of inspired oxygen; IMV, intermittent mandatory ventilation; *NCPAP,* nasal continuous positive airway pressure; *RDS,* respiratory distress syndrome.
†Strauss RG. Transfusion approach to neonatal anemia. *NeoReviews.* 2000;1(4):e74-e80.

of Blood Banks *Standards for Blood Banks and Transfusion Services,* 23rd edition, published in 2004, specifies the testing required for blood donated in the United States.

Iron Supplementation

Infants, whether full-term or preterm, require iron supplementation during the first year of life to prevent nutritional anemia. Iron supplementation should provide 2 to 3 mg/kg/day of elemental iron for breastfed infants and babies whose formula intake does not provide the required daily iron intake. Preterm infants need supplementation in the range of 4 to 4.5 mg/kg/day of elemental iron to prevent iron deficiency anemia. During the infant's hospitalization, iron supplementation will frequently be initiated when the enteral intake is at least 100 mL/kg/day (between 2 and 4 weeks of age). Infants who have required multiple transfusions may receive a significant iron load from the transfused blood.[2,3] Monitoring of ferritin levels to determine the appropriate time to start iron therapy may be prudent in this circumstance. Vitamins providing nutritional doses of vitamin E (25 IU/day), folate, and vitamin B_{12} should also be given daily to high-risk infants.

APNEA, BRADYCARDIA, AND DESATURATION

Apnea, bradycardia, and desaturations are common problems encountered in neonatal units. (Box 77-5 provides a list of definitions.) These symptoms may occur in isolation or together. The incidence and severity of apnea increases with decreasing gestational age. The need to treat neonatal apnea varies with gestational age and symptoms. AOP is experienced by more than 50% of premature infants and nearly 100% of babies weighing less than 1000 g at birth.[4] The relationship among apnea, bradycardia, and desaturation is complex and is further complicated by the occurrence of one or more of these symptoms in relation to feeding or choking episodes. The criteria used to define *clinically significant* apnea, bradycardia, and desaturation are controversial, presenting a challenge to the clinician caring for preterm infants who exhibit these symptoms. Apnea in the larger preterm infant typically resolves by

BOX 77-5 Definitions

Apnea: Absence of breathing for ≥20 s or >10 s if associated with bradycardia (heart rate <80 bpm) or oxygen desaturation (<80%-85%)

Apnea classification:

- Central: cessation of chest wall movement (inspiration) caused by lack of central nervous system neural input (10%-25%)
- Obstructive: respiratory effort without nasal airflow (10%-20%)
- Mixed: combination of central and obstructive apneas (50%-70%)

Bradycardia: Age-related norms have been defined for infants based on postmenstrual and postnatal age.

Significant bradycardia in infants less than 44 weeks' postconceptual age: <80 bpm for >15 s or <60 bpm for >5 s

Desaturation: Oxygen saturation <80%-85% on pulse oximetry for >4 s (normal range for full-term and preterm infants from birth to 28 days of age: 93%-100%; mean oxygen pressure 70-76 mm Hg during postnatal days of life 2 to 7)

- May accompany periodic breathing (respiratory pauses)
- May or may not occur in association with bradycardia

Periodic breathing: Episode of three or more successive respiratory pauses of ≥3 s in duration, each separated by ≤20 s of normal respiration

Periodic breathing is considered significant if it occurs during more than 5% of the quiet sleep time.

*Finer NN, Higgins R, Kattwinkel J, et al. Summary proceedings from the Apnea of Prematurity Group. *Pediatrics.* 2006;117(3):547-551.
†Ramanathan R, Corwin MJ, Hunt CE, et al, and the Collaboration Home Infant Monitoring Evaluation (CHIME) Study Group. *JAMA.* 2001;285(17) 2199-2207.

34 to 36 weeks' postmenstrual age, with over 90% of infants being apnea free by 37 weeks' postmenstrual age. Among extremely low–birth-weight infants less than 28 weeks' gestation, apnea duration is longer, often not resolving until 40 to 43 weeks' postmenstrual age.[5] Despite numerous studies, consensus as to the optimal Sa_{O_2} range has not been achieved. Study outcomes for infants born less than 27 weeks' gestation have demonstrated improved survival rates and reduced morbidity (chronic lung disease, ROP) without an increase in cerebral palsy among infants who are maintained with Sa_{O_2} in the range of 84% to 94%.[6]

Preterm infants with lung disease frequently have Sa_{O_2} measurements less than 90% lasting less than 20 seconds. These episodes often occur during feedings and during periods of wakefulness and sleep and are not associated with apnea, bradycardia, or cyanosis. Infants with chronic lung disease are more likely to have severe desaturations less the 80%.[7] Episodes of prolonged desaturation (SpO_2 less than or equal to 80%) for more than 4 seconds are most frequently seen during periodic breathing or hypoventilation.[8] Experts suggest that infants less than 34 weeks' gestation receive cardiorespiratory monitoring and pulse oximetry for apnea and bradycardia during their hospitalization. Desaturations or bradycardia occurring without apnea suggest airway obstruction (obstructive apnea).

Evaluation of Apnea, Bradycardia, or Desaturation

Evaluation of the infant with apnea, bradycardia, or desaturations will vary with the frequency and severity of the infant's symptoms. Although primarily related to the infant's underlying prematurity, other causes must be considered, including infection, anemia, hyperthermia (environmental overheating), seizures, necrotizing enterocolitis, metabolic abnormalities (hypoglycemia, acidosis, hyponatremia, hypocalcemia, inborn errors of metabolism), and patent ductus arteriosus or heart failure. Excessive neck flexion may also trigger apneic or bradycardic episodes. The use of sedation, analgesia, and other medications may contribute to respiratory depression and apneic episodes. Acute stress such as that experienced by preterm infants undergoing an eye examination for ROP or after multiple procedures occurring on the same day may contribute to fatigue and an increase in feeding intolerance or apnea, bradycardia, or desaturations in the hours after the procedure. Increased symptoms may be exhibited irrespective of whether the infant receives sedation before the procedure. Gastroesophageal reflux, another common condition among preterm infants, is also believed to contribute to AOP. Although the two conditions often occur coincidentally, recent studies have failed to demonstrate a link between these two conditions in premature infants.[9,10]

Treatment of Apnea, Bradycardia, and Desaturation

Treatment of apnea, bradycardia, and desaturation will depend on the underlying cause or causes. In addition to diagnosing and treating precipitating conditions, therapy may include the use of tactile stimulation, nasal cannula with air-oxygen flow, nasal continuous positive airway pressure (CPAP), methylxanthines, or mechanical ventilation alone or in combination.

Medications

Aminophylline, theophylline, and caffeine are the methylxanthines most frequently used in the treatment of significant AOP (Box 77-6). Caffeine is considerably less toxic than theophylline and is the drug of choice for treating neonatal apnea. Treatment is deemed effective if the reduction in episodes of apnea is 50% or greater. Signs of toxicity include tachycardia, gastrointestinal intolerance, and jitteriness or agitation. Medications can usually be discontinued when the preterm infant reaches 32 to 34 weeks' postmenstrual age and has been apnea free for 7 to 10 days. Infants treated with caffeine require monitoring for 7 days because of caffeine's long half-life. The period of observation after discontinuation of theophylline is somewhat shorter, at 4 to 5 days.

Continuous Positive Airway Pressure

CPAP is a frequently used respiratory support modality in the care of neonates with transitional difficulties and premature infants with respiratory distress syndrome, chronic lung disease, and AOP. CPAP is provided through short binasal prongs (NCPAP), nasopharyngeal tube (NP-CPAP), or infant nasal mask (NM-CPAP) that are used in conjunction with a

BOX 77-6 Methylxanthines Used to Treat Apnea of Prematurity

CAFFEINE:

- Loading dose: 10 mg/kg IV or PO (20 mg/kg caffeine citrate)
- Maintenance dose: 2.5 mg/kg every 24 hr
- Therapeutic plasma level 8 to 20 mg/L
- Mean half-life is approximately 100 hr and remains prolonged until 37 to 38 weeks' postmenstrual age; caffeine half-life decreases with maturity and postnatal age
- Infants with cholestasis have longer caffeine half-life caused by impaired hepatic metabolism
- Long-term administration associated with increased oxygen consumption and reduced weight gain

AMINOPHYLLINE OR THEOPHYLLINE:

- Aminophylline is metabolized to theophylline (80% theophylline)
- Loading dose: 4 to 6 mg/kg IV or PO
- Maintenance dose: 6 mg/kg/day divided every 6, 8 or 12 hr IV or PO
- Therapeutic plasma level: 6 to 11 mg/L (theophylline)
- Plasma half-life 12 to 64 hr

IV, Intravenous; *PO,* by mouth.

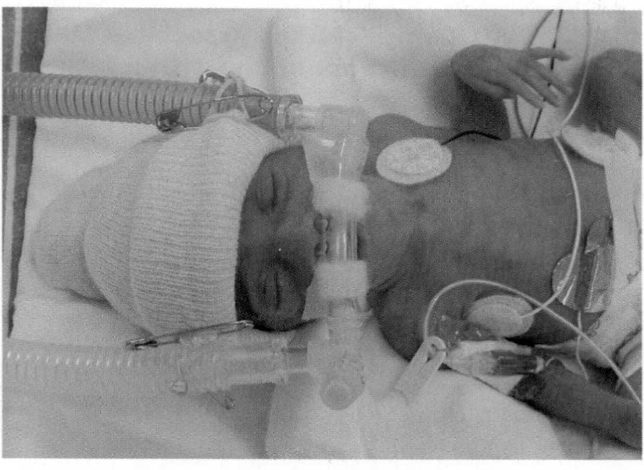

Figure 77-1 Premature infant on nasal continuous positive airway pressure.

continuous flow source (underwater seal), an infant or multipurpose ventilator equipped with a CPAP mode (Figure 77-1). These CPAP devices provide heated and humidified continuous or variable flow so as to increase an infant's functional residual capacity, improve lung compliance, and decrease airway resistance. The resultant increase in tidal volume reduces the infant's work of breathing and stabilizes minute ventilation. In addition, CPAP reduces pharyngeal and airway collapse, stabilizes chest wall musculature, and

BOX 77-7 Continuous Positive Airway Pressure Indications

Increased work of breathing; respiratory rate 30% above the normal for age

Retractions, grunting, and nasal flaring

Presence of cyanosis, pallor, and respiratory distress

Inadequate arterial blood gas values; inability to maintain partial pressure of oxygen >50 mm Hg with an Fio_2 <0.60 and adequate ventilation with a pH >7.25 and partial pressure of carbon dioxide <60 mm Hg

Fio_2, Fraction of inspired oxygen.

BOX 77-8 Conditions Benefiting From Continuous Positive Airway Pressure

Apnea of prematurity

Atelectasis

Pulmonary edema

Respiratory distress syndrome

Recent extubation

Tracheomalacia or similar lower airway abnormality

Transient tachypnea of the newborn

decreases chest wall inhibitory reflexes. CPAP is effective in mixed and obstructive apnea. Indications for CPAP use in infants include the presence of abnormalities on physical examination, inadequate arterial blood gases, poor lung expansion on chest radiograph, and conditions that are known to benefit from CPAP (Boxes 77-7 and 77-8). The duration of CPAP therapy, typically applying 4- to 6-cm water (H_2O) pressure will depend on the reason for its use and the infant's stability as the CPAP is weaned to physiologic levels (3 cm H_2O).

Complications associated with CPAP use include nasal irritation, abdominal distension, and feeding intolerance. Barotrauma and air leaks may also result if excessive pressure is applied or if an inappropriate CPAP device is used. Overdistension of alveoli will impair ventilation-perfusion ratios and lead to decreased oxygenation and carbon dioxide retention and may also reduce cardiac output and cause an air leak. Insufficient gas flow through the CPAP device creates a fluctuating baseline pressure that can increase the infant's work of breathing. Nasal prong obstruction may occur from accumulated secretions or bleeding after traumatic suctioning or nasal irritation. Humidification and gentle suctioning are important aspects of care for infants requiring CPAP to prevent nasal mucosal damage. Proper positioning of the CPAP prongs and correct nasal prong size are additional factors important to ensuring effective

CPAP therapy. The infant's head position is also important because excessive head rotation or neck extension can lead to altered effective CPAP pressure. Maintaining a closed-mouth position is also important to ensuring that the infant is receiving the prescribed positive airway pressure and oxygen concentration. Studies have demonstrated that a 2.2-cm H_2O drop in CPAP pressure occurs from the CPAP prongs to the pharynx with the mouth closed. This pressure loss increased to 3.2 cm H_2O when the infant's mouth was open.[11-13] Gastric and abdominal distension are common complications of CPAP therapy and may contribute to feeding tolerance problems or aspiration.

BRONCHOPULMONARY DYSPLASIA (CHRONIC LUNG DISEASE)

Bronchopulmonary dysplasia (BPD) develops in one third of very low–birth-weight infants (rates of BPD vary with NICU care practices[14,15] and approaches to ventilatory support) and is most common among infants less than 32 week's gestation. In addition to higher mortality rates, infants with BPD experience greater morbidity. Changes in clinical practice, particularly restriction in postnatal steroid usage caused by concerns about higher rates of cerebral palsy among infants receiving early postnatal corticosteroids, has resulted in increased numbers of very low–birth-weight infants surviving with BPD.[16] (For detailed information on BPD, see Chapter 99, Respiratory Distress and Breathing Disorders in the Newborn.)

BPD is defined by oxygen dependence at specific periods after birth (28 days' postnatal age or 36 weeks' postmenstrual age) among infants with persistent lung disease and characteristic radiographic findings (Box 77-9). Characteristic BPD findings have changed over time as the disease, originally described in larger preterm infants with severe respiratory distress syndrome (RDS) who required treatment with mechanical ventilation with high pressures (tidal volumes) and high oxygen concentrations has evolved to include more immature infants with mild to moderate lung disease who exhibit prolonged oxygen requirements.[17] Currently, classic BPD, the form of chronic lung disease resulting from severe RDS and leading to atelectasis, edema, fibrosis, smooth muscle disease, right-ventricular hypertrophy, and the need for prolonged ventilation, involves less than 25% of babies with BPD. Most infants with BPD exhibit milder RDS signs of hazy lungs, minimal airway lesions, pulmonary edema, disruption of lung growth, and alveolarization and require prolonged oxygen, CPAP therapy, or both. Complications associated with BPD are listed in Box 77-10.

BOX 77-9 Definitions of Bronchopulmonary Dysplasia (BPD)

- Oxygen (O_2) requirement at 28 days of age
- O_2 requirement at 36 weeks' postmenstrual age (PMA)
- O_2 or positive airway pressure at 36 weeks' PMA
- O_2 requirement at 36 weeks' PMA and more than 28 days of oxygen duration
- National Institutes of Health (2001) has subcategorized BPD as follows:

Mild: Supplemental oxygen for infants $\geq$28 days' PMA and on room air at 36 weeks' PMA or at discharge (for infants <32 weeks' PMA at birth) or at 56 days or at discharge (for infants $\geq$32 weeks' PMA at birth)

Moderate: Supplemental oxygen for infants $\geq$28 days' PMA with a need for supplemental oxygen <30% at 36 weeks' PMA or at discharge (for infants <32 weeks' PMA at birth) or at 56 days or at discharge (for infants $\geq$32 weeks' PMA at birth)

Severe: Supplemental oxygen for infants $\geq$28 days' PMA with a need for supplemental oxygen $\geq$30% or on nasal CPAP or mechanical ventilation at 36 weeks' PMA or at discharge (for infants <32 weeks' PMA at birth) or at 56 days or at discharge (for infants $\geq$32 weeks' PMA at birth)

BOX 77-10 Complications Associated With Bronchopulmonary Dysplasia

ApneaReactive airway disease
Infection
Feeding difficulties
Gastroesophageal reflux
Poor growth
Poor bone mineralization (osteopenia, nutritional rickets)
Electrolyte abnormalities
Nephrocalcinosis
Impaired cardiac function: pulmonary hypertension, cor pulmonale, left ventricular hypertrophy
Systemic hypertension
Poor cognitive and motor outcomes
Retinopathy of prematurity

Oxygen Therapy

Oxygen therapy is an important component of BPD management. Oxygen may be delivered to convalescing infants through various devices: oxygen hood, nasal cannulae, CPAP devices, or conventional ventilators. Precise measurement of the oxygen concentration delivered to the infant is not as easily determined when a baby is on a nasal cannula or CPAP. The actual oxygen concentration received by the infant reflects a blend of the nasally inspired oxygen and ambient (room) air inhaled through the nose and mouth. The infant's minute ventilation and ratio of nose-to-mouth breathing also alter the effective fraction of inspired oxygen (FiO_2) received.[18] This consideration is important during the process of weaning an infant from supplemental oxygen therapy and in determining whether a need exists for home oxygen use. Approximately two thirds of convalescing infants can be successfully weaned from supplemental oxygen when the infant's Sao_2 is greater than 96% and the Fio_2 is less than or equal to 0.23. A simplified formula for calculating the oxygen level delivered to the infant's hypopharynx has been devised that uses the infant's weight, nasal cannula flow, and Fio_2: 0.21 + (flow + weight) × (F_{NCO2} − 0.21), where F_{NCO2} is the Fio_2 set to be delivered via the nasal cannula.[19]

Care must be taken when providing flow through a nasal cannula because positive distending pressure has been demonstrated in premature infants weighing less than 2000 g when nasal cannula flow rates of 1 to 2 L/min are used.[20] Nasal cannula prong diameter is another factor in the delivery of positive distending pressure because a 0.3-cm nasal cannula has been shown to deliver increased pressure as a function of the flow rate used.[21]

Oxygen Saturation

Maintaining the arterial pressure of oxygen levels above 55 torr (mm Hg) is important in infants with BPD. Infants with BPD may exhibit increased oxygen requirements during nipple feeding and sleep if significant desaturations (saturation percentage of oxygen [Spo_2] <80%-85%; Spo_2 obtained by pulse oximetry) occur. The issue of Spo_2 limits (oxygen targeting) is the focus of debate and ongoing study. Spo_2 and its role in developmental outcome, as well as the incidence and severity of ROP and BPD in extremely premature babies, continue to be elucidated. The conundrum is that optimal oxygen thresholds to protect the developing eye may be harmful to the cardiovascular and respiratory function of the infant with BPD. Hypoxemia is detrimental to the baby with BPD because it leads to increased pulmonary vascular resistance, pulmonary vasoconstriction, impaired right-ventricular performance, and peripheral oxygen delivery. Further chronic hypoxemia affects brain growth and weight gain.

When caring for a premature infant with BPD who is less than 35 weeks' postmenstrual age, the Spo_2 range should be maintained between 90% and 94%. Tighter Spo_2 limits in the range of 92% to 94% is recommended but has been shown to be difficult for many nurseries to attain. An Spo_2 of 92% to 96% for infants with BPD who are more than 35 weeks' postmenstrual age is recommended. During sleep the Spo_2 should be kept above 93% because this level has been shown to improve sleep architecture.[22] In the STOP-ROP study evaluating the efficacy of two supplemental oxygen strategies to prevent the development of threshold ROP in preterm infants with BPD, maintaining Spo_2 levels above 96% was shown to increase the risk for adverse pulmonary and cardiovascular outcomes and resulted in a longer duration of oxygen treatment, medication use (diuretics, methylxanthines, and steroids) and hospitalization.[23] However, the infant with BPD and pulmonary hypertension requires adequate oxygen to reduce the pulmonary vascular resistance and avoid death. Current recommendations for these infants are to avoid Spo_2 less than 92% and maintain saturation pressure levels above 94% to 96%.

Monitoring

In addition to impairing right-ventricular heart function, BPD is associated with other cardiovascular abnormalities: left-ventricular hypertrophy, systemic hypertension, and the development of bronchial and other systemic-pulmonary collateral vessels. Postnatal steroid use may also contribute to the development of transient left-ventricular hypertrophy. Pulse oximetry is an important tool used in the routine monitoring for infants with chronic lung disease while they remain in the hospital. Monitoring should occur through all of the infant's activities of daily living—while awake, during bathing and feeding, and during active and quiet sleep. Blood pressures should be monitored at least weekly, and periodic electrocardiograms should be obtained to assess the infant for right-ventricular hypertrophy. Infants requiring prolonged ventilation and oxygen therapy or who have evidence of pulmonary hypertension should have serial echocardiography performed every 2 to 3 months.[24]

Medications

Medications used in the treatment of BPD include aerosolized beta-agonists, inhaled steroids, and diuretics (Box 77-11). The duration of medication use is predicated on the infant's clinical symptoms, tolerance of fluid volumes and growth, and continued dependence on oxygen or respiratory support. The effectiveness of bronchodilator therapy in preterm infants is unclear. Studies have demonstrated short-term improvement in respiratory function with treatment. However, long-term benefits in the treatment of BPD have not been conclusively demonstrated in randomized, controlled studies. For infants with worsening respiratory symptoms such as wheezing, increasing airway resistance, or worsening lung compliance, the clinician should consider a closely monitored trial of albuterol and ipratropium. The preferred mode of drug delivery is by use of an metered-dose inhaler plus

BOX 77-11 Medications

Hydrochlorothiazide: 20 to 40 mg/kg/day in 2 divided doses q 12 hr

Spironolactone: 2 to 4 mg/kg/day in 2 divided doses q 12 hr

Furosemide: 2 to 4 mg/kg/dose every 12-24 hr

Potassium chloride: 1 to 4 mEq/kg/day in 2-4 doses q 6-12 hr

Bronchodilators:

- Albuterol (Proventil, Ventolin): 0.5 cc by nebulizer or inhaler every 6-12 hr
- Ipratropium (Atrovent): 0.5 cc by nebulizer or inhaler every 12 hr
- Levalbuterol (Xopenex): 0.62 mg respule by nebulizer

Antiinflammatory and inflammatory drugs:

- Cromolyn (Intal): inhaler or nebulizer; takes 2 to 4 weeks for adequate trial
- Inhaled steroids:
  - Budesonide (Pulmicort): 0.25 to 0.5 mg respule every 12-24 hr
  - Fluticasone (Flovent): 0.125 mg (1 puff) every 12 hr
  - Betamethasone valerate
- Oral prednisone for serious exacerbations

spacer rather than nebulizer or via hand-bag ventilation. Consultation with a neonatologist or pediatric pulmonary specialist can assist in implementing and monitoring the efficacy of respiratory management strategies.

NUTRITION AND GROWTH

Premature Infant

Continuing care of the recovering infant or growing premature baby includes optimizing the infant's growth and nutrition. Increased calories, protein, and mineral intake are needed to promote better linear growth and mineral accretion. The recommended caloric intake will vary with the infant's underlying medical issues and degree of prematurity. Caloric requirements for most infants will range from 100 to 120 kcal/kg/day to achieve an average daily weight gain of 20 to 30 g. For the preterm baby, weight gains of 15 to 25 g/day are more typical between 28 and 32 weeks of gestation. As infants recover, more of their caloric intake is available for tissue growth and weight gain. However, during periods of increased energy expenditure, such as when the infant is weaning from CPAP or oxygen, transitioning from isolette-bassinette conditions, learning to nipple feed, or experiencing an intercurrent illness, growth may either slow or the infant may lose weight. Energy requirements for infants with chronic lung disease have been shown to be 25% higher than preterm infants without BPD. Consequently, infants with chronic lung disease require 120 to 160 kcal/kg/day. The caloric density of the feeding will depend on the infant's growth velocity, feeding efficiency, evidence of feeding fatigue, and ability to handle fluid volume.

The rate of weight gain and adequacy of growth are a significant concern in the care of the preterm infant because suboptimal growth will affect brain growth and cognitive outcomes; however, excessively rapid growth has the potential to predispose the infant to cardiovascular problems in adulthood. A common practice involves restricting the feeding volume until a weight plateau occurs before increasing the feeds. This factor is important in the growth delay experienced by many preterm infants. Common patterns of growth in preterm infants are listed in Box 77-12.

Achieving optimal postnatal growth is a challenge as growth lags considerably after birth among most very low–birth-weight infants. Figure 77-2 depicts an aggressive nutritional approach to prevent poor postnatal growth in very low–birth-weight infants. Nutrient intakes that meet current recommended daily intakes are difficult to achieve during early postnatal life. By the end of the first week, significant cumulative energy and protein deficits occur in preterm infants, irrespective of gestational age. Among the smallest infants, weight loss often exceeds 15% of their birth weight. Energy and protein deficits persist at 5 weeks of age; infants of 30 weeks' gestation or younger exhibit mean energy deficits of 813 kcal/kg and protein deficits of 23 g/kg. Among infants older than 30 weeks' gestation, comparable energy and protein deficits are evident at the end of the first week of life, although by 5 weeks of age these infants' energy and protein deficits are 382 kcal/kg and 13 g/kg, respectively.[25]

BOX 77-12 Convalescing Preterm Infant Growth Patterns

- Appropriate-for-gestational-age (AGA) infant at birth who at discharge has a body weight that is appropriate for the postmenstrual age (corrected age)
- AGA preterm infant at birth whose discharge weight is below the reference for the postmenstrual age (postnatal or extrauterine growth restriction)
- Small-for-gestational-age (SGA) infant who remains below the 10th percentile for postmenstrual age at the time of discharge
- SGA infant who exhibits early postnatal catch up growth and whose weight at discharge is appropriate for postmenstrual age

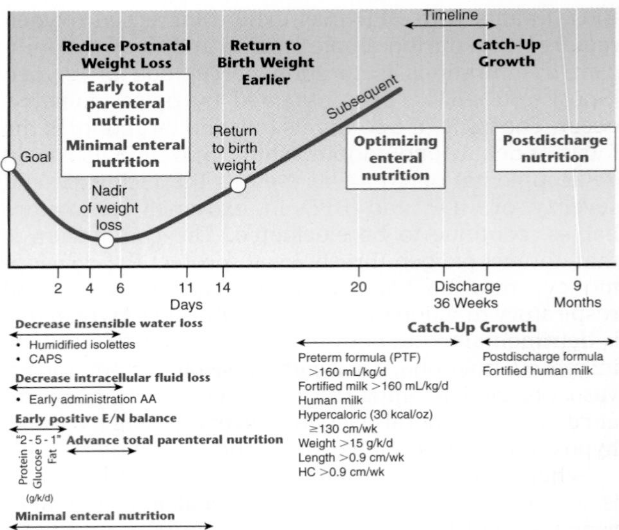

Figure 77-2 Aggressive nutrition to prevent extrauterine growth restriction. *Adamkin DH. Nutrition management of the very low-birthweight infant I. Total parenteral nutrition and minimal enteral nutrition.* Neoreviews. *2006;7:e602-e607.)*

Evidence is increasing of long-term consequences for these children who remain shorter, weigh less, and have a greater risk of neurodevelopmental impairment than their normal–birth-weight full-term counterparts. As gestational age decreases, an incremental lag occurs in weight gain and growth velocity (Figures 77-3 and 77-6). Infants with subnormal head circumferences at 8 months corrected age have an increased risk of neurologic impairment, lower IQ, and poorer academic performance. Male infants are more likely at greatest risk for extrauterine growth restriction, they require mechanical ventilation during the first day of life, need respiratory support at 28 days of age, develop necrotizing enterocolitis, and receive postnatal steroids.[26]

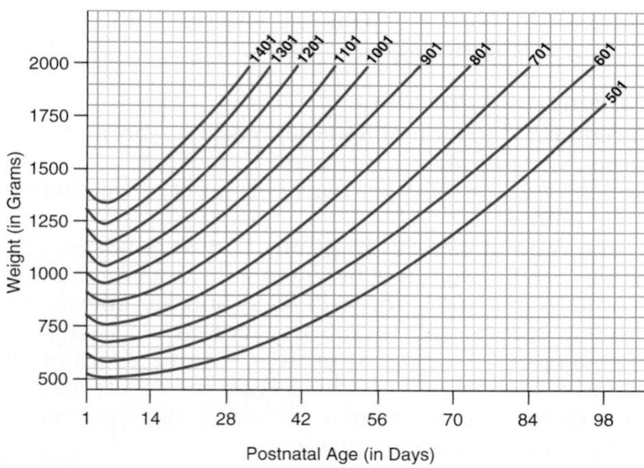

Figure 77-3 Longitudinal growth of hospitalized very low–birth-weight infants. *Ehrenkranz RA, Younes N, Lemons JA, et al. Longitudinal growth of hospitalized very low birth weight infants.* Pediatrics. *1999;104:280-289.)*

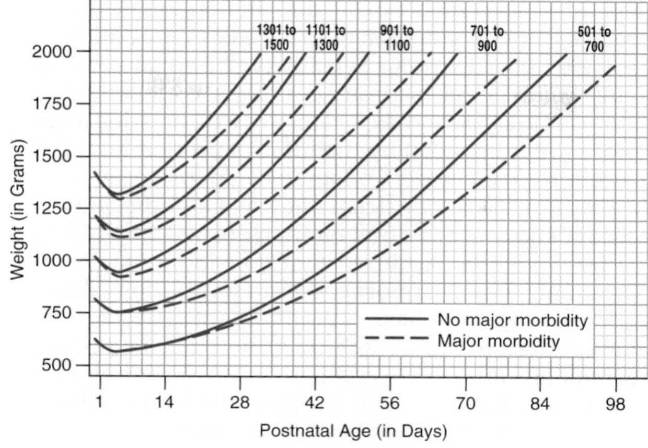

Figure 77-5 Growth curves of infants with and without major morbidity versus postnatal age in days. *Ehrenkranz RA, Younes H, Lemons JA, et al. Longitudinal growth of hospitalized very low birth weight infants.* Pediatrics. *1999;104:280-289.)*

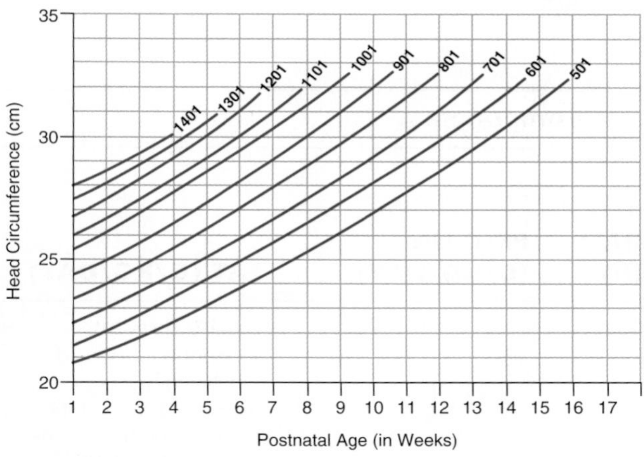

Figure 77-4 Average weekly head circumference versus postnatal age in weeks. *Ehrenkranz RA, Younes H, Lemons JA, et al. Longitudinal growth of hospitalized very low birth weight infants.* Pediatrics. *1999;104:280-289.)*

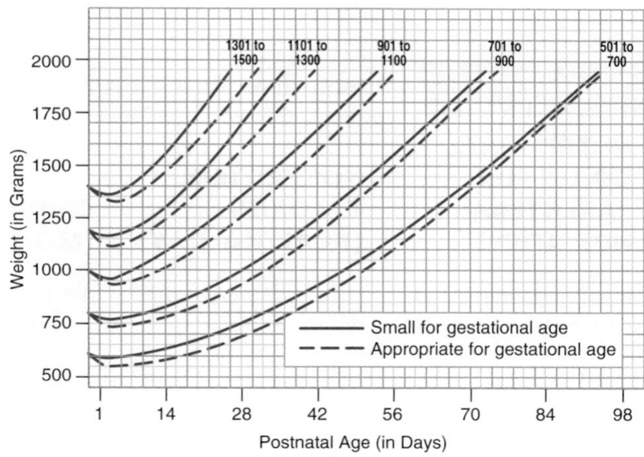

Figure 77-6 Growth curves of appropriate-for-gestational-age and small-for-gestational-age very low–birth-weight infants verus postnatal age (days). *Ehrenkranz RA, Younes H, Lemons JA, et al. Longitudinal growth of hospitalized very low birth weight infants.* Pediatrics. *1999; 104:280-289.)*

The length of time required to regain birth weight is an important predictor of the overall rate of weight gain and of the likelihood that an infant will be below the 10th percentile at the time of hospital discharge. Early initiation of parenteral nutritional support and enteral feeding is critical. Trophic and minimal enteral feedings promote intestinal motility and bile secretion and induce lactase activity, reducing sepsis and cholestasis. Early aggressive nutrition regimens limit the degree of extrauterine growth restriction and improve the postnatal metabolic and nutritional status of the infant. Daily volume increments of 10 to 35 cc/kg/day have been shown to be safe. More rapid advancement of feedings (25 to 35 cc/kg/day) results in a shorter time to regain birth weight without an increase in the rate of necrotizing enterocolitis.[27] After regaining birth weight, the weight gain goal for a preterm infant is 15 to 20 g/kg/day.

Just as inadequate growth is detrimental, excessive weight gain and growth patterns that alter the body's composition have harmful long-term cardiovascular and metabolic effects. The postnatal environment, nutrient energy sources, hormones, and factors that influence growth during the postnatal period differ from the intrauterine condition. After birth, fat becomes the primary fuel source for the neonate, in contrast to fetal dependence on glucose, lactate, and amino acids. Very preterm infants younger than 32 weeks' gestation also have decreased insulin sensitivity.[28] The rate of postnatal weight gain in preterm infants is dependent on caloric intake, whereas brain growth and increasing length are influenced by the infant's protein intake. Fat accretion is increased postnatally in preterm infants who at term-postmenstrual age have a higher body fat content and more visceral fat than normal–birth-weight full-term infants. An important consideration in planning a nutritional support program for the convalescing and growing low–birth-weight infant is recognizing that a pattern of rapid catch-up growth during the first 2 years of life, and an observed increase in central fat distribution at 5 years of age in these children predispose them to cardiovascular disease in later life.[29]

Infants who are returned to community neonatal units for continuing and convalescent care will vary in their nutritional needs, as well as their mode of nutritional intake at the time of back transfer. Some infants may be on full enteral feeding, whereas others may be transitioning from parenteral nutrition to enteral feedings. The infant's specific nutrient requirements will be influenced by the child's underlying medical problems and degree of prematurity and whether the nutrient sources are from parenteral fluids, breast milk, or infant formula.

Parenteral Nutrition

Parenteral nutrition (PN) solutions may be administered via peripheral or central intravenous lines. Tables 77-2 and 77-3 list considerations in calculating PN solutions.

The ratio of calories to grams of nitrogen is important to promote optimal nitrogen utilization for protein synthesis and tissue growth. The optimal energy-to-protein ratio is 150 to 200 nonprotein cal to 1 g of nitrogen, or 22 kcal/g of protein. The total grams of amino acids per day are divided by the factor 6.25 to yield the grams of nitrogen per day: ratio = nonnitrogen calories ÷ grams of nitrogen.

Increased calories are needed during episodes of metabolic stress. Table 77-4 lists the effects of certain diseases on specific nutrient requirements. In brief, nutritional requirements are altered as follows:

- + 12% for every degree fever
- + 20% to 30% for infants requiring surgery
- + 40% to 50% for septic infants
- + 50% to 100% for infants with long-term growth failure

Table 77-2 Parenteral Nutrition Macronutrient Components

NUTRITIONAL GOALS FOR PARENTERAL NUTRITION	NONPROTEIN CALORIES (KCAL/KG/DAY)	CARBOHYDRATE (MG/KG/MIN)	PROTEIN (G/KG/DAY)	FAT (G/KG/DAY)
Basal metabolic need (prevents catabolism)	50-60	4-6 (glucose infusion rate)	1.0-1.5	0.6-1.0 (prevents essential fatty acid deficiency; 4-5% total fat calories should be from linoleic acid and 1% from linolenic acid)
Positive balance (promotes growth)	80-100	8-10; gradually advance to max 12-13	2.7-3.5	3.0-3.5 (30-55% of the total calories from fat)

Table 77-3 Daily Total Parenteral Nutrition Intake

NUTRIENT	PRETERM INFANT	BIRTH TO 12 MONTHS
Fluid volume (cc/kg)	60-200	120-150
Protein (g/kg)	2.5-3.5	2.5-3.0
Energy (kcal/kg)	80-100	80-120
Carbohydrate (g/kg)	12-25	12-25
Lipid (g/kg)	0.5-3.0	0.5-3.0
Sodium (mEq/kg)	2-5	2-4
Potassium (mEq/kg)	2-3	2-3
Chlorine (mEq/kg)	2-5	2-4
Calcium (mg/kg) [mEq/kg]	50-90 [3-4]	40-60 [2-3]
Phosphate (mg/kg) [mmol/kg]	35-70 [1-2]	30-50 [1-2]
Magnesium (mEq/kg)	0.2-0.6	0.5-1.0

Table 77-4 Effects of Neonatal Disease on Specific Nutrient Requirements

NUTRIENT	RESPIRATORY DISTRESS SYNDROME	BRONCHO-PULMONARY DYSPLASIA	CYANOTIC CONGENITAL HEART DISEASE	CONGESTIVE HEART FAILURE	SEPSIS	INTRAUTERINE GROWTH RESTRICTION
Free water	⇓	⇓	⇔	⇓	⇔	⇑
Energy	⇑	⇑⇑	⇑	⇑⇑	⇑	⇑
Fat	⇔	⇑	⇑	⇑	⇔	⇑
Carbohydrate	⇑	⇓	⇑	⇑	⇑	⇑
Protein	⇔	⇑	⇑	⇑	⇑⇑	⇑
Calcium	⇔	⇑*‡	⇑*†	⇑*†‡	⇔	⇑
Iron	⇔	⇑*	⇑	⇔	⇓	⇑
Vitamin A	⇑*	⇑*	⇔	⇔	⇔	⇔
Vitamin E	⇔	⇑	⇔	⇔	⇔	⇔

*<1500 g; †postoperative; ‡calciuric diuretics.
From Huysman WA, de Ridder M, de Bruin N C, et al. Growth and body composition in preterm infants with bronchopulmonary dysplasia. *Arch Dis Child Fetal Neonat Ed.* 2003;88:46-51. Reprinted by permission of BMJ Publishing Group Ltd.

Peripheral parenteral solutions cannot exceed 12.5% dextrose or 3.5% amino acid; maximal calcium concentrations are also limited because of the risk of severe tissue injury in the event of extravasation. Each gram of protein provides 4 kcal. Potential risks associated with protein administration include acidosis, elevated blood urea nitrogen, hyperammonemia, and cholestasis. Taurine and cysteine are considered conditional essential amino acids for neonates and should be added to PN solutions. Dextrose yields 3.4 kcal/g and may be advanced to provide a maximal glucose infusion rate of 12 to 14 mg/kg/min. Complications associated with dextrose infusions include hyper or hypoglycemia, glycosuria and possible osmotic diuresis, and cholestasis or steatosis (or both) as a result of long-term high-caloric intake. Intravenous lipid solutions provide 10 kcal/g. A 20% soybean emulsion is commonly used because it is more efficiently cleared than the 10% solution and provides 2 kcal/mL. Lipid infusions are administered over a 20- to 24-hour period at rate of 0.12 to 0.15 g/kg/hour and should not exceed 60% of the total caloric intake. Triglyceride levels should be measured periodically and should be less than 200 mg/dL. Potential adverse effects from lipid infusions include hyperlipidemia, bilirubin displacement from albumin-binding sites by free fatty acids, potential to interfere with pulmonary clearance in infants with chronic lung disease, lipid overload resulting in hepatic failure, and coagulopathy. The ratio of calcium to phosphorous in PN solutions is 1.3 to 1.7:1 by weight.

Additional additives to PN solutions include trace elements and vitamins. Trace elements contain zinc, manganese, copper, and chromium and are typically initiated 2 to 3 weeks after birth if the infant does not have renal or liver dysfunction. During the first 2 weeks of life, zinc should be provided in a dose of 0.15 mL/kg/day (150 mcg/kg/day; 1-mg/mL concentration). Thereafter, preterm infants require an additional 300 mcg/kg/day, and full-term infants should receive 200 mcg/kg/day of zinc. Selenium is also essential for both preterm and full-term infants and should be given in a dose of 2 mcg/kg/day. Trace elements are discontinued from the PN solution if the infant develops cholestasis. Trace element requirements are adjusted to provide a total daily intake of 400 mcg/kg/day of zinc for the preterm infant (100 to 350 mcg/kg/day for full-term infants), 0.2 mcg/kg/day of chromium, and 2 mcg/kg/day of selenium. Pediatric vitamins, 2 mL/kg/day, are also added to PN solutions up to a maximum of 5 mL/day. Heparin is often added to PN solutions to be administered through a central line.

Biochemical monitoring for infants on established (maintenance) PN regimens typically includes evaluation of blood electrolytes, blood urea nitrogen, creatinine, and calcium one to three times per week. Liver function studies (albumin, total and direct bilirubin, alanine aminotransferase, γ-glutamyltransferase, alkaline phosphatase), phosphorus, magnesium, triglyceride level, and complete blood count, including differential and platelet count, are monitored weekly to biweekly while the infant is receiving parenteral nutrition. Growth should be assessed weekly, plotting the occipitofrontal circumference, weight, and length on standard postnatal growth charts (Figure 77-7).

The baby is weaned from PN as advancing enteral feeding intake is tolerated. Once the daily enteral intake exceeds 50 mL/kg/day the lipid infusion can be discontinued. Thereafter, PN can be stopped when the infant's intake is 100 to 120 mL/kg/day. Infants who develop cholestasis and continue to require prolonged PN therapy benefit from *cycling,* intermittent infusion, of the PN solution. Intermittent PN infusion promotes a feeding-fasting cycle that decreases the severity of cholestasis. If this strategy is used, then close monitoring of the infant's glucose is necessary to avoid hypoglycemia.

Enteral Nutrition

Enteral feeding regimens typically begin with expressed breast milk or formula. Infants may be nipple fed if they are clinically stable, with respiratory rates less than 60 to 70 breaths/min and they are 34 weeks' gestation or older. Infants between 32 and 34 weeks' gestation

Fetal-Infant Growth Chart for Preterm Infants

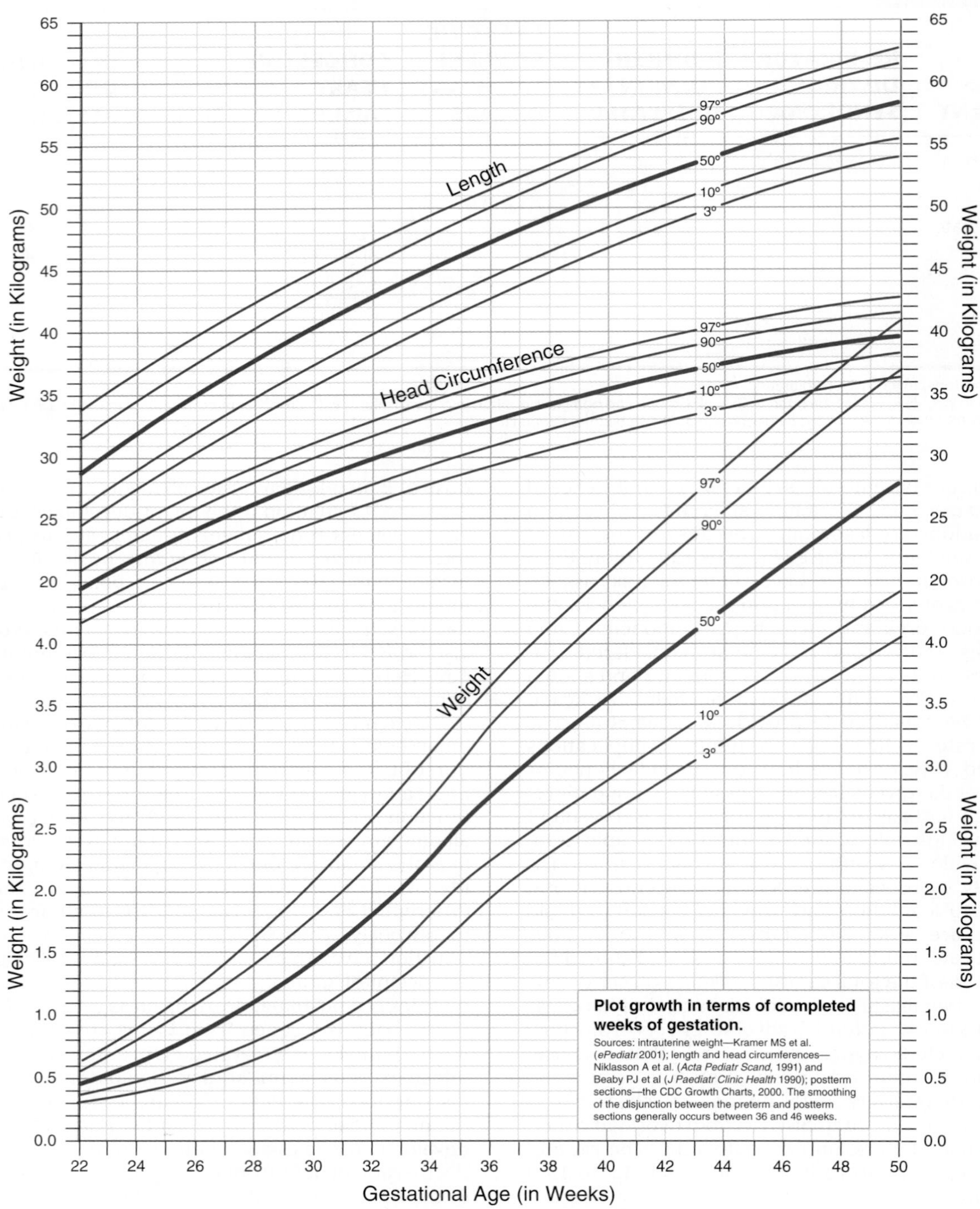

Figure 77-7 Fetal-infant growth chart for preterm infant. *(Fenton TR. A new growth chart for preterm babies: Babson and Benda's chart updated with recent data and a new format.* BMC Pediatr. *2003;3[1]:13. © 2003 Fenton; licensee BioMed Central Ltd. (www.biomedcentral.com/1471-2431/3/13).*

may be able to nipple feed but should be assessed to document their oromotor skills, state regulation, and evidence of a coordinated suck-swallow-breathing pattern. Bolus feeding rather that continuous feeding is preferred for the recovering neonate.

Feeding Intolerance

A frequent concern arises related to the significance of gastric residual volumes and the risk for necrotizing enterocolitis. The color or volume (or both) of aspirated gastric residuals are factors frequently considered in the decision whether to continue enteral feeding.[30] Investigators have shown that the color of the gastric residual did not predict the risk for developing necrotizing enterocolitis. Maximal residual volumes of more than 3.5 mL or 33% of the feed volume is suggested as the threshold for concern. However, an important point to note is that gastric residuals must be considered in the context of the infant's clinical status, vital signs, abdominal examination, stool character, and stooling pattern.

Premature infants are predisposed to feeding intolerance because of functional dysmotility and immaturity of the gastrointestinal tract, particularly after prolonged periods of no oral intake. Lack of early enteral feeding disrupts the intestine's barrier functions, which leads to gut atrophy, loss of intestinal villi and malabsorption, bacterial translocation, and impaired immune function. The initiation of early small volume minimal enteral or trophic feedings is beneficial in maintaining intestinal integrity and promoting gastrointestinal motility.

Erythromycin has been recommended for infants who are unable to establish full enteral feeding within 2 to 3 weeks of age. It has prokinetic properties as a motilin agonist that stimulates gastric emptying and proximal small intestinal contractility. Data from several randomized clinical trials have been published with conflicting results about the efficacy of erythromycin in improving feeding tolerance. Comparison of these studies is difficult because each one employed a different erythromycin dose (low vs antimicrobial), route (enteral vs intravenous), and mode (prophylactic or rescue) of treatment. Given concerns regarding erythromycin-induced hypertrophic pyloric stenosis and cardiac arrest, prophylactic treatment of preterm infants is not recommended. If a trial of erythromycin is used to promote intestinal motility, then the oral route is preferred because of the risk of significant morbidity and mortality with intravenous administration. The optimal and safest dose of erythromycin is not known. However, exposure to antimicrobial doses for more than 14 days has been associated with the development of hypertrophic pyloric stenosis. Gestational age may also be a factor in the erythromycin's proposed efficacy.[31] A recent review by Patole et al[32] summarizes the current understanding of the physiological gastrointestinal function and feeding intolerance in premature infants and the gastrointestinal effects of erythromycin. Currently, erythromycin can only be recommended for a select subset of premature infants with a protracted course of feeding intolerance.

Human Milk and Preterm Infant Formula Use

Human milk is the choice for feeding full-term and preterm infants.[33] However, for the very low–birth-weight premature infant, human milk requires fortification to provide nutrient intakes comparable to intrauterine accretion rates. Human-milk feeding has been shown to result in improved neurodevelopmental and cognitive outcomes and visual acuity among human milk–fed premature infants in comparison with their formula-fed counterparts. Fresh milk is preferred when available. (See Chapter 89, Breastfeeding the Newborn.) Routine screening cultures for evidence of bacterial contamination or heat treatment of the mother's own milk has not been shown to be necessary or cost effective.[34] If a mother's own milk is not immediately available, then use of pasteurized donor human milk, if available, may be considered. Pasteurized donor human milk maintains most of the properties of fresh human milk (immunoglobulins, growth and developmental hormones, enzymes, antiinflammatory factors) is sterile, and reduces necrotizing enterocolitis while improving feeding tolerance.[35-37] Studies have shown that healthy preterm infants born less than 30 weeks' gestation are able to tolerate milk volumes of 150 to 200 mL/kg/day without adverse effects.[38] Human milk–fed, extremely low–birth-weight infants require approximately 180 mL/kg/day to achieve adequate growth, nutrient retention, and nutritional status.

The nutrient composition of human milk varies because of the individual properties of expressed milk and changes that occur during collection, storage, and use. The energy and protein content of expressed human milk varies, as does the fat content. Human milk is not homogeneous; as the milk stands the fat content separates. Much of the variation in the energy content of milk used is the result of differences in or losses of fat in unfortified milk. Although concentrations of protein, sodium, and zinc decline during the period of lactation, the nutrient needs of premature infants remain higher than those of full-term infants, even after the preterm infant reaches term-postmenstrual age. This circumstance results in the need to fortify expressed human milk to compensate for the inadequate nutrient supply. Mineral content of calcium and phosphorus varies less during lactation but remains too low with respect to the premature infant's nutrient needs. Low calcium and phosphorus intake causes physiological changes that result in poor bone mineralization that may have long-term effects on the preterm child's height. Nutrient availability of vitamin C, vitamin A, and riboflavin declines during collection, storage, and administration of expressed milk.

Human-milk fortification is typically started when the intake reaches 50 to 80 mL/kg/day. Fortifiers such as Enfamil human milk fortifier (Mead Johnson Nutritional Division of Bristol-Myers Squibb) provides 4 kcal/packet and is typically added to 25 mL of breast milk to achieve a caloric density of 80 kcal/dL (24 kcal/oz). Similac human milk fortifier and Natural Care human milk fortifier (Ross Nutritionals, a Division of Abbott Laboratories) can be used similarly to increase the caloric and mineral content of human milk. Additional calories may be required because of poor weight gain (<10 to 15 g/kg/day) or the need for fluid restriction, (<140 mL/kg/day). Under these circumstances, one packet of fortifier may be added to 15 mL of expressed human milk to achieve 27 kcal/oz. Biochemical (alkaline phosphatase >600 to 800 IU/L) and radiographic evidence of metabolic bone disease require increased calcium and phosphorus intake. Infants receiving more than 120 mL/kg/day of fortified human milk are at a greater risk for hypercalcemia and hyperphosphatemia and thus require closer monitoring of calcium and phosphorus levels. Preterm liquid formula may also be added to human milk to increase the caloric and nutrient intake.

Premature infant formulas are typically recommended for preterm infants weighing less than 1800 grams at birth or who are less than 34 weeks' gestation. Preterm formulas are cow milk–based, whey-predominant formulas that provide between 2.7 and 3.0 grams of protein per 100 kcal. Fat calories are derived from long- and medium-chain triglycerides. Formulas designed for preterm infants (Table 77-5) should be used instead of protein hydrolysate (Alimentum, Pregestimil, Nutramigen) or elemental (Neocate) formulas that are designed for full-term infants, unless a specific indication exists for use of one of these formulas (cholestasis, malabsorption or short-bowel syndrome). Soy protein–based formulas are not recommended for preterm infants who weigh less than 1800 g[39] because its use results in reduced serum phosphorus levels, increased alkaline phosphatase levels, and reduced bone mineralization. In addition, use of soy protein–based formulas leads to poorer growth (weight and length) and lower serum albumin levels and poses the potential for aluminum toxicity.

Routine iron supplementation should begin at 2 months' postnatal age providing 2 to 4 mg/kg/day of iron. Infants with iron deficiency anemia require a higher iron intake of 4 to 6 mg/kg/day. Oral vitamin supplements are initiated after 2 weeks of age typically once the preterm neonate is able to tolerate full enteral feedings. A summary of nutrient recommendations for preterm and term infants is found in Table 77-5.

Infants With Chronic Lung Disease

Nutrition management of infants with chronic lung disease includes providing appropriate nutrient intake and calories to meet the infant's increased energy needs and decreased nutrient intake. Babies with chronic lung disease have reduced fat accretion, fat mass, growth, and muscle mass. Infants with bronchopulmonary dysplasia continue to exhibit decreased growth throughout the first year of life.[40] Medication use can alter energy requirements because methylxanthines will increase energy expenditure, and dexamethasone therapy has been associated with decreased weight gain. Infants with BPD require 15% to 25% more calories per day (140 to 150 kcal/kg/day) during the acute phases of their disease compared with their healthy peers. Protein intakes of 3.5 to 4.0 g/kg/day are considered adequate to meet the anabolic and tissue growth requirements. Diuretic use is common in the management of infants with BPD, with resultant increased urinary losses of sodium, potassium, chloride, and calcium. Replacement of excess salt and mineral losses is often required. Close monitoring of the electrolyte and mineral balance is important to prevent complications related to nutrient depletion and poor growth. Inadequate mineral intake combined with diuretic use increases the risk for osteopenia and metabolic bone disease (nutritional rickets). This risk may be further increased by using hydrolyzed, elemental formulas or preterm formulas that are modified by the addition of carbohydrate or fat but contain insufficient calcium and phosphorus for bone mineralization.

Infants With Complex Congenital Heart Disease

Similar to infants with chronic lung disease, the caloric requirements for infants with complex congenital heart disease may be as high as 150 mL/kg/day. Adequate weight gain and growth may be impeded by episodes of hypoxemia, tachypnea, and feeding fatigue that limit intake and increase energy expenditure. Gastroesophageal reflux and delayed gastric emptying further complicate appropriate nutritional management. Poor nutrition contributes to delayed wound healing, impaired immunity. and an increased risk for infection. Swallowing difficulties are a frequent complication after cardiac surgery in children. Prolonged intubation and injury to the recurrent laryngeal nerve resulting in vocal cord paralysis also contribute to feeding difficulty. Fiberoptic endoscopic evaluation of swallowing is a useful adjunct in the assessment of feeding in these babies in order to construct an appropriate feeding regimen (gavage vs nipple) and plan for oral-motor therapy.

GASTROESOPHAGEAL REFLUX AND GASTROESOPHAGEAL REFLUX DISEASE

Gastroesophageal reflux (GER), defined as the retrograde passage of gastric contents into the esophagus, occurs in approximately 50% of all young infants. Babies who exhibit symptoms or complications of GER (vomiting, poor weight gain, difficulty feeding, hematemesis, and airway symptoms such as chronic lung disease and airway inflammation, apnea, aspiration, and recurrent pneumonia) are classified as having gastroesophageal reflux disease (GERD), requiring evaluation and treatment. Therapy is empiric with little evidence for efficacy of current treatment modalities. Pediatric clinical practice guidelines published in 2001 by the North American Society for Pediatric Gastroenterology, Hepatology, and Nutrition (NASPGHAN) and endorsed by the American Academy of Pediatrics (AAP)[41] list the following points:

- A time-limited trial of medical therapy for infants with symptomatic GER should be provided.
- A 1- to 2-week trial of a hypoallergenic formula in infants with vomiting should be considered.
- Thickened feedings reduce visible vomiting but does not improve reflux.
- Antireflux formulas are not appropriate for preterm infants.
- Ensure adequate caloric intake, increase caloric density if necessary.
- Prone positioning may be beneficial for select infants with significant symptoms; however, supine sleep position is associated with the lowest risk of sudden infant death syndrome, and is the position of preference while the infant is convalescing in the neonatal unit and after discharge home.
- Infants who are maintained in the prone position require continuous monitoring.

An important caveat is that the NASPGHAN guidelines are not intended for the management of neonates in the first 3 days of life, premature babies, or infants with neurologic impairment or structural

Table 77-5 Preterm Infant Formula, Fortifier, and Supplement Information

FORTIFIER, FORMULA, SUPPLEMENT	MANUFACTURER	MEASURING	PRECAUTIONS, COMMENTS
FORTIFIER			
Human milk fortifier (provides increased protein, carbohydrate, fat, vitamins, minerals and calories for the preterm infant. Infants are rarely discharged on human milk fortifier.)	—	—	Not for use in preterm infants born more than 34 weeks' gestation, once a very low–birth-weight infant weighs >2500 g, or if the infant has an intake of more than 500 mL/day, given that human milk fortifier supplementation may exceed renal solute load Prolonged use associated with vitamin D toxicity and may supply several times RDA for vitamin A at intakes >500 mL/day. Not for postdischarge use with full-term infants or in cases of failure to thrive.
Similac human milk fortifier (powder)	Ross Labs	For 22 kcal/oz, use 1 packet and 50 mL of human milk. For 24 kcal/oz, use 1 packet and 25 mL of human milk. Measure human milk first and add powder.	Infants are rarely discharged on human milk fortifier Discontinue once the infant weighs 2000 g (4.5 lb)
Enfamil human milk fortifier (powder)	Mead Johnson	For 22 kcal/oz, use 1 packet and 50 mL of human milk. For 24 kcal/oz, use 1 packet and 25 mL of human milk. Measure human milk first and add powder.	Infants are rarely discharged on human milk fortifier Discontinue once the infant weighs 2000 g (4.5 lb)
Similac Natural Care, Advance (liquid and ready-to-feed)	Ross Labs	Provides 24 kcal/30 mL (0.8 kcal/mL); use in equal amounts with human milk for 22 kcal/oz.	Discontinue once the infant weighs 2000 g (4.5 lb) if used as human milk fortifier May be continued to a weight of 3600 g (8 lb) in preterm infants with inadequate weight gain
FORMULAS			
(provides increased protein, calcium, phosphorus, vitamins A and D. Can supplement or fortify human milk.)	—	—	Contributes to improved growth and bone mineralization compared with preterm infants fed standard infant formulas. Current recommendation is to use transitional formula until 9 mo corrected age; some infants may benefit from continued use until 12 months corrected age. Infants exhibiting rapid catch-up growth whose weight exceeds the 50% may be transitioned to standard infant formula or exclusive breastfeeding sooner.
Similac Neosure Advance (powder and ready-to-feed)	Ross Labs	*Formula:* For 22 kcal/oz (standard dilution) use, 1 packed, level scoop and 60 mL water.	Should not be used for calorie enhancement in growth restricted infants whose gestational age is >34 weeks.

Adapted from Nutrition Practice Care Guidelines for Preterm Infants in the Community (Revised August 2006) Child Development and Rehabilitation Center, Nutrition Services, Oregon Department of Human Services, Nutrition & Health Screening—WIC Program Oregon Pediatric Nutrition Practice Group.
RDA, Recommended daily allowance.

Continued

Table 77-5 Preterm Infant Formula, Fortifier, and Supplement Information—cont'd

FORTIFIER, FORMULA, SUPPLEMENT	MANUFACTURER	MEASURING	PRECAUTIONS, COMMENTS
		For 24 kcal/oz, use 3 packed, level scoops and 165 mL of water. For 27 kcal/oz, use 5 packed, level scoops and 240 mL. *Fortifier:* For 22 kcal/oz, use 1 tsp in 180 mL. For 24 kcal/oz, use 1 tsp in 90 mL. For 27 kcal/oz, use 2 tsp in 90 mL. Measure water or human milk first then add powder.	
Enfamil EnfaCare Lipil (powder)	Mead Johnson	Same as for Similac Neosure above.	Should not be used for calorie enhancement in growth restricted infants whose gestational age is > 34 weeks.
SUPPLEMENTS			
MCT Oil	Mead Johnson/ Novartis	Provides 8.8 kcal/mL; add 0.5 mL/oz of breast milk or formula.	Can cause loose stools, steatorrhea; does not provide essential fatty acids
Safflower oil	—	Provides 8 kcal/mL	—
Microlipid emulsified safflower oil	Mead Johnson	Provides 4.5 kcal/mL	Contains long-chain fatty acids
Polycose glucose polymer (liquid or powder)	Ross Labs	½ tsp of powder provides 4 kcal; 1 mL of liquid provides 2 kcal; 23 kcal/tbsp; add ½ tsp/oz of formula.	Can cause diarrhea
Moducal	Mead Johnson	30 kcal/tbsp	
Specialized formulas not recommended for routine use	—	—	—
Soy-based formulas			Not recommended for infants with birth weights <1800 g. Suboptimal carbohydrate and mineral absorption; results in less weight gain and linear growth, lower serum albumin and phosphorus levels, and higher alkaline phosphorus levels indicative of poorer bone mineralization
Enfamil AR (standard infant formula with added rice starch recommended for infant feeding of babies with gastroesophageal reflux) An alternative practice is to thicken infant formula or breast milk with rice cereal.	Mead Johnson		No data to support the use of thickened formula in preterm infants with reflux after discharge. Thickening feedings is a common practice but is controversial. Does not contain necessary vitamin and mineral content for the growing preterm infant. Some evidence that thickened feeds increase the duration of reflux episodes. For infants with feeding difficulties, thickened feedings may further exacerbate preexisting feeding difficulties.

Adapted from Nutrition Practice Care Guidelines for Preterm Infants in the Community (Revised August 2006) Child Development and Rehabilitation Center, Nutrition Services, Oregon Department of Human Services, Nutrition & Health Screening—WIC Program Oregon Pediatric Nutrition Practice Group.
RDA, Recommended daily allowance.

abnormalities of the upper gastrointestinal tract. An additional consideration is discontinuation of methylxanthines therapy because caffeine and theophylline will exacerbate reflux symptoms.

GER is common among preterm infants who may exhibit three to five episodes of reflux per hour and is related to physiological transient lower esophageal sphincter relaxation (TLESR). These episodes of TLESR occur in both asymptomatic and symptomatic infants and may be elicited by gastric distension that accompanies feeding and abdominothoracic straining that accompanies movement. Episodes of acid GER have been shown to occur frequently in healthy preterm infants and resolve in most preterm babies as they reach term postmenstrual age. Use of gavage feeding tubes is also associated with increased reflux symptoms. Clinical concerns about feeding intolerance and recurrent episodes of apnea, bradycardia, and desaturation lead to the frequent use of prokinetic agents and acid suppressant drugs.

The frequency of feeding in young infants results in relatively brief periods of gastric pH less than 4; consequently pH probe measurements may not be helpful in diagnosing significant reflux in the preterm infant. Although a common concern is that GER may contribute to apnea, numerous studies have failed to document a link between the two events.[42] Impedance studies have demonstrated retrograde reflux of air and fluid into the esophagus occurring in addition to episodes of acid reflux.[43] Approximately 25% of reflux events are strongly acidic, with total esophageal exposure time to acid estimated to be 5%.[9] Recent studies have not confirmed a temporal link between acid-based GER and AOP.[44] As a result, medication use to treat reflux is not recommended as part of the management of episodic apnea, bradycardia, and desaturation in preterm infants. Other pharmacologic and medical approaches may be necessary to optimize growth, nutrition, and respiratory function.[45] The challenge that arises in management of GER in the preterm infant is the lack of data on the efficacy of antireflux measures. Although metoclopramide has been shown to reduce reflux symptoms, its use is associated with adverse effects such as irritability, dystonic reactions, drowsiness, emesis, apnea, and involuntary muscle movements, as well as oculogyric crisis (involuntary upward conjugate gaze).[46] Metoclopramide's action as a dopamine-receptor antagonist accounts for its promotility effects in the intestine and blockade of dopamine receptors in the brain, resulting in the central nervous system effects. Therefore metoclopramide should be used with caution in the management of reflux in preterm and young infants.

Symptomatic preterm infants with GERD will exhibit significant vomiting more than three to four times per day of more than 50% of the fed volume in conjunction with:

- Recurrent episodes of apnea, bradycardia, and desaturations associated with feeding
- Signs of discomfort or distress during feeds (arching, crying)
- Difficulty advancing feeding volume
- Poor weight gain

Management strategies include:

- Infant positioning in prone with slight elevation of the head of the bed (requires continuous monitoring)
- Infant transitioned to supine sleep position 1 to 2 weeks before anticipated discharge home to lessen the risk for sudden infant death syndrome
- Consideration of discontinuation methylxanthines (caffeine or theophylline)
- If a medication trial is considered appropriate: metoclopramide started at 0.1 to 0.2 mg/kg/dose every 6 to 8 hours for 4 to 7 days

If clinical improvement occurs, then the medication can be continued and the infant reassessed every 2 weeks to determine the continued need for treatment.

The infant should be closely monitored for central nervous system changes and other adverse effects. Acid suppression therapy,[47] although not well studied in the preterm infant, may be considered: histamine-2 (H_2) blockers (ranitidine [Zantac, 1 mg/kg/dose every 12 hr], famotidine [Pepcid, 1 mg/kg/day divided every 12 hr]) or proton pump inhibitors ([Prilosec, 1.0 mg/kg/day given once daily or divided every 12 hr] or lansoprazole [Prevacid, 1.5 mg/kg/day given once daily or divided every 12 hr]).

Care must be taken if H_2-blockers are used because therapy has been associated with higher rates of necrotizing enterocolitis in very low–birth-weight infants.[48]

If a family history of allergy exists, then the clinician should consider having the mother eliminate dairy from her diet if she is expressing breast milk or initiate a trial of an elemental (casein-hydrolyzate) formula such as Pregestimil, Alimentum, or Nutramigen, Neocate, or Elecare (amino acid–based formulas) may be used for infants with severe milk intolerance. (For a full discussion of the management of GERD, see Chapter 264.)

CHOLESTASIS

Cholestasis is a complication seen among infants who have enteral feedings withheld for extended periods. At greatest risk are infants with intestinal immaturity or intrinsic gastrointestinal disease, sepsis, and hypoxemia and babies who require prolonged PN. Toxicity has been associated with amino acids such as methionine; trace elements such as copper, chromium, and manganese; and excessive energy and dextrose intakes. Medications and nutrient deficiencies of taurine, choline, fatty acids, and trace minerals have been associated with an increased incidence of cholestasis. Biochemical abnormalities include elevations in serum alkaline phosphatase, direct bilirubin, and transaminases. Direct bilirubin levels above 2 to 3 mg/dL warrant evaluation and intervention. Treatment strategies include small amounts of enteral feedings, especially for infants who require long-term PN because feedings enhance gastric motility and bile flow. Trace minerals (copper and manganese) can be eliminated from PN once enteral feeding is initiated. Cycling of PN is also suggested for infants who may require long-term PN. Choleretics such as chenodeoxycholate (Ursodiol or Actigall) are also used to treat cholestasis and are considered to be more efficacious than phenobarbital. Discontinuation of PN and progression of enteral feedings result in a gradual improvement of cholestasis over weeks to months.

OSTEOPENIA

Osteomalacia (rickets), also referred to as osteopenia of prematurity (OOP) or metabolic bone disease of prematurity, occurs frequently in very low–birth-weight infants who are at risk for poor bone mineralization caused by inadequate mineral intake, prolonged PN, and chronic diuretic therapy. Infants with ostomies may also exhibit increased electrolyte and mineral losses from high ostomy output. Medications commonly used in premature babies that result in calcium excretion and increase mineral needs include furosemide, xanthines, and dexamethasone. Anticonvulsants such as hydantoin and phenobarbital increase the turnover of vitamin D, leading to decreased serum levels of calcium and magnesium. Use of chronic thiazide diuretic also contributes to bone demineralization. Renal or liver disease increases the risk for osteopenia.

Mineral deficiencies are reported to occur in 30% to 50% of preterm infants who are fed either unfortified human milk or formulas designed for full-term infants. Infants born with very low birth weight or 28 weeks' gestation or less are at highest risk for OOP primarily as a result of inadequate phosphorus intake. Growing preterm infants who are fed human milk exclusively will not achieve bone mineral contents comparable to that attained through in utero accretion. Radiographs of the wrist and long bones reveal evidence of poor bone mineralization, with widening and cupping at the metaphyseal ends of the bones. Healing fractures may also be noted on routine radiographs involving the ribs and long bones. The risk for fractures is greatest between 6 and 12 weeks' postnatal age and when alkaline phosphorus levels exceed 1000 IU/L. Given that vitamin D deficiency is not a primary factor in OOP, supplemental vitamin D beyond nutritional requirements, 200 to 400 IU daily, is not needed. However, infants with cholestasis require additional vitamin D supplementation. Human milk should be fortified or the appropriate premature formula used. In the United States, fortification of human milk is recommended for very low–birth-weight preterm infants until a weight of 1800 to 2000 g is reached.

Routine monitoring of serum alkaline phosphatase, phosphorus, and calcium is helpful in detecting signs of metabolic bone disease. Generally, alkaline phosphatase levels will be elevated, and serum phosphorus levels will be lower in babies with osteopenia. Serum calcium levels are typically maintained within a normal range during osteopenia at the expense of bone mineralization. Serum alkaline phosphatase levels greater than 600 to 800 IU/L in conjunction with a serum phosphorus concentration less than 4.5 mg/dL warrant radiographic evaluation of the wrist or knee for evidence of rickets or severe bone loss. Physical activity in the form of passive range of motion exercise has been shown to reduce bone mineral losses, increase bone strength, and promote growth in preterm infants.[49,50]

TRANSITION TO ORAL FEEDING

Feeding disorders are common among infants, particularly babies who have been ill or are premature. The ability to nipple feed is an important developmental task that requires neurologic maturation, self-regulation, motor strength, and physiological stability. Successful nipple feeding requires coordination of sucking, swallowing, and breathing and is a process that matures with age, increasing physiological stability and self-regulation. Coordination of the tongue, pharynx, and upper trunk movements are necessary for an infant to swallow safely. The infant must also learn to protect the airway during feeding. In preterm infants this process is complicated by the occurrence in *deglutition apnea* episodes in which the infant stops breathing during successive swallows while feeding. This occurrence diminishes as the infant matures and as feeding skill improves.

More coordinated suck-swallow-breathe patterns and longer sucking bursts are noted by 37 weeks' postmenstrual age. Infants who are less mature at birth, who experience complex medical courses with significant respiratory illness, or who require prolonged ventilation or oxygen therapy have greater difficulty establishing nipple feeds and take longer to master coordination of sucking, swallowing, and breathing than their healthy counterparts. Infants who have difficulty coordinating sucking, swallowing, and breathing quickly fatigue and lose motor tone. This situation contributes to desaturation, apnea, and bradycardia while feeding. For many of these infants, feeding difficulties continue after discharge from the neonatal unit and throughout infancy. These feeding behaviors lead to the development of feeding refusal in some infants. Techniques helpful in supporting the development of oral feeding skills are listed in Box 77-13.

The first attempts at oral feeding usually occur between 32 and 33 weeks' gestational or postmenstrual age or when the infant weighs between 1600 and 1700 g and exhibits a stable respiratory status. Infants are deemed to be successfully nipple feeding when they are able to complete feedings within 20 minutes. This goal may or may not be fully achieved by the time of the infant's discharge home. The choice of nipple used may facilitate or impede feeding efficiency. Some infants benefit from use of low- or variable-flow nipples to aid pacing during the feeding. Infants who are unable to achieve full nipple feeding may require a specialized program of intensive feeding therapy. A gastrostomy may also need to be placed if the infant is unable to gain adequate weight until sufficient oral feeding is attained. Signs that an infant may not be developmentally ready to initiate nipple feeding include falling asleep, not latching on, or exhibiting respiratory irregularity and loss of muscle tone when a bottle is placed in the mouth.

Assessing an infant's oral feeding ability requires evaluating multiple considerations (Box 77-14). The physician plays a critical role in promoting breastfeeding of the hospitalized infant (Boxes 77-15 and 77-16).

HEALTH MAINTENANCE

Newborn Screening of the Critically Ill or Premature Infant

Newborn screening is an important component of acute and continuing care for the sick or preterm infant. Most neonatal units have established protocols that specify the timing when newborn metabolic screening is conducted for babies requiring specialized

BOX 77-13 Techniques to Support Development of Oral Feeding Skills

Nonnutritive sucking: offering the infant a pacifier or the infant's fingers to suck and orally explore:
- Accelerates transition from tube to oral feedings
- Enhances weight gain and increases gastrointestinal motility
- Improves the infant's behavioral state and organization
- Does not fully reflect the oral feeding experience because swallowing is less and rhythmic sucking and breathing can more easily occur

Provide tastes of breast milk or formula on the pacifier or infant's fingers; provides sensory stimulation before the introduction of nipple feeding

Kangaroo care allowing the infant to nuzzle, lick, and suck at the mother's breast

Use of slower or low flow nipples to support the infant's swallowing; bolus size will increase as the infant's feeding skills mature and coordination improves

Jaw support and proper positioning to sustain postural control

Pacing:
- Useful for infants who are not yet able to self-regulate their feeding or control successive swallows
- Pacing is done by shifting the infant slightly forward every 3 to 5 sucks or the bottle tilted down to allow the milk to drain from the nipple and giving the infant a chance to breathe

Some infants will require supplemental oxygen during nipple feeding to maintain adequate oxygenation and prevent desaturations and bradycardic episodes

Assessment and monitoring of the infant's coordination of the suck-swallow-breathing sequence is necessary for timely identification of feeding difficulties

neonatal or intensive care or transfer to another hospital. State health department newborn screening policies guide individual hospital practices. The timing of the first newborn screen is typically between 24 and 48 hours of age after the infant has established milk (human milk or formula) feeding. The infant who requires transfer to another facility, needs a blood transfusion, or is critically ill should have a newborn screening test obtained on the first day of life. A second screening test should be obtained between 1 and 2 weeks of age. If an infant is transfused before obtaining the initial newborn screening test, then a third specimen is necessary 2 to 3 months posttransfusion or when the blood cells tested are presumed to be the infant's and not reflect those of the donor. Earlier retesting may reflect donor hemoglobins and invalidate testing for galactosemia (red blood cells assayed for galactose-1-phosphate uridyltransferase). Infants receiving PN, particularly preterm infants, may have elevated amino acids (eg, phenylalanine) resulting in positive screening results.

BOX 77-14 Assessment of an Infant's Oral Feeding Ability

Assessment of an infant's oral feeding ability encompasses the following:

1. Infant's state regulation and response to tactile stimulation
2. Feeding position
3. Oral motor control
4. Physiological response to feeding episode
5. Coordination of suck-swallow-breathing sequence
   a. Consider feeding evaluation by a speech pathologist or feeding therapist.
   b. Consider airway and feeding efficiency assessment with a modified barium swallow and fiberoptic endoscopic swallowing study to evaluate the vocal cords and swallowing and assess for evidence of aspiration.
6. Caregiver-infant feeding interactions

BOX 77-15 Promotion of Breastfeeding in the Hospitalized Infant

Discuss feeding options for the infant and the benefits of providing colostrum or human milk.

Provide mother with information or handouts on human milk expression and storage.

Work with nursery and postpartum staff to ensure that human milk expression is initiated in the first 24 hours after delivery

Provide referral to lactation consultant (hospital or community-based).

Facilitate arrangements to rent or purchase a hospital-grade electric breast pump to support mother's goal of providing expressed human milk for her infant.

Most state Medicaid departments and WIC programs have guidelines that authorize payment for hospital-grade electric breast pumps for infants with the following conditions:
- Prematurity
- Neurologic disorders
- Genetic abnormalities (Down syndrome)
- Anatomic and mechanical malformations (cleft lip and palate)
- Congenital malformations requiring surgery
- Prolonged infant hospitalization
- Conditions that prevent normal breastfeeding (respiratory compromise)

Many insurers will include among subscriber benefits (these are plan specific) recommendations for electric breast pump authorization, such as prematurity, feeding difficulty caused by abnormal infant suck, or a hospitalized mother or infant

WIC, Special Supplemental Nutrition Program for Women, Infants, and Children.

BOX 77-16 Transition to Breastfeeding

Criteria to initiate nonnutritive *time at the breast*
- Begin at approximately 32 weeks' gestation.
- Infant demonstrates ability to swallow own secretions.
- Stable outside incubator for more than 10 to 15 minutes.
- Able to tolerate kangaroo care (skin-to-skin contact)
- Infant responses:
- Mouth is at the breast; may or may not latch on or suck.
- May swallow once or twice.
- May fall asleep at the breast.
- Coordinate nonnutritive nursing attempts with infant hunger cues.

Reinforce importance of expressing milk every 3 hr (100 min/day)

Initiation of nutritive sucking:
- Infant displays consistent latch-on ability.
- Infant is able to feed for approximately 5 min.
- Supplementation with expressed human milk or formula after nursing episode:
- Breastfeeds <5 min: gavage full enteral feeding volume
- Breastfeeds 5 to 10 min: gavage one half enteral feeding volume
- Breastfeeds >10 min: supplementation is not needed unless inadequate weight gain or signs dehydration exhibited

Mother should continue to pump between and after feedings.

Current newborn screening recommendations include testing for cystic fibrosis. Testing algorithms rely on immunoreactive trypsinogen (IRT) or screening for cystic fibrosis transmembrane conductance regulator mutations. Newborn infants with meconium ileus are at risk for cystic fibrosis but may have low initial IRT test results (false negative). Consequently, all babies with meconium ileus require follow-up sweat tests. Infants experiencing severe perinatal distress or have low Apgar scores may exhibit elevated IRT levels on testing (false positive). Follow-up testing is needed.

Premature infants often have abnormal newborn screening test results that are not the result of an underlying metabolic disorder. Preterm infants frequently have elevated 17-hydroxyprogesterone (17-OHP) and low thyroxine levels. The typically higher 17-OHP level in premature infants presents a difficulty in diagnosing congenital adrenal hyperplasia among this group of babies. Many states use weight-adjusted cutoff values to reduce the high false-positive rates that result with standard testing. Antenatal corticosteroid treatment does not appear to suppress 17-OHP levels. Transient hypothyroxinemia, with low thyroxine and normal thyroid-stimulating hormone levels, is common among sick preterm babies and is most often self-limited. Acute illness may further depress thyroid function and increase adrenal steroid production, contributing to persistent abnormalities on retesting. Preterm infants need to be monitored until normal test results are achieved. Infants with persistent abnormalities require assessment of thyroid function and may need treatment to reduce the risk of poor neurocognitive outcome related to hypothyroidism. Serial screening tests or diagnostic evaluation may be required based on local state health department requirements. Infants with physical or metabolic signs suggestive of the condition should undergo an immediate evaluation for the suspected disorder.

Cranial Ultrasonography Screening

Limited cerebral autoregulation in association with vascular, cellular, and anatomic features of the developing brain result in a preterm infant's vulnerability to hemorrhage and ischemic brain injury. Hemorrhagic lesions involve the germinal matrix (GM), may extend into the ventricular system, and may be found in brain parenchyma. The GM involutes during the third trimester, by 34 to 36 weeks' postmenstrual age. Ischemic injury within the periventricular area is related to hypoperfusion and ischemia occurring along the end-zone regions of the long penetrating arteries that arise from the anterior, middle, and posterior cerebral arteries. Both hemorrhage and ischemic injury may occur coincidentally. White matter injury may lead to nonhemorrhagic cerebral infarction, periventricular leukomalacia (PVL), or porencephaly. Ventriculomegaly (VM) may also occur because of loss of cerebral white matter in the absence of an intraventricular hemorrhage (IVH). Most IVH is evident by 3 days of age, although 50% of hemorrhages occur within the initial hours following birth.

The American Academy of Neurology practice parameter on *Neuroimaging of the Neonate* recommends routine screening cranial ultrasonography in preterm infants between 7 and 14 days of age on all infants younger than 30 weeks' gestation. The initial study identifies IVH. The presence of cystic PVL within the first 2 weeks of age indicates an antenatal insult. A repeat study should be obtained between 36 and 40 weeks' postmenstrual age to detect the presence of PVL and low-pressure VM. These two timeframes have been chosen as the most useful in terms of predicting long-term neurodevelopmental outcomes. However, from a clinical care perspective, diagnosing the GM hemorrhage or IVH early is often important. The Canadian Paediatric Society statement on routine screening cranial ultrasonography suggests that an earlier neurosonogram should be performed by the third day of life in infants with multiple early complications.

Follow-up studies should be obtained as clinically indicated. Because of the inverse relationship between brain injury and gestational age, an alternate approach has been suggested by Perlman and Rollins who recommend an initial cranial sonogram between days 3 to 5 with three follow-up studies at 10 to 14 days of age, 28 days of age, and before discharge for babies weighing less than 1000 g birth weight. The initial study at 3 to 5 days will identify 75% of hemorrhages in the extremely low–birth-weight preterm infant. The second ultrasound at 10 to 14 days of age will identify 84% of hemorrhages and detect early hydrocephalus and cyst formation. The 28-day scan identifies the presence of periventricular echogenicity and VM. The yield of these studies performed in more mature preterm infants decreases with increasing gestational age. Consequently the recommended periodicity for cranial ultrasonography screening in larger preterm infants is consistent with American Academy of Neurology and the Canadian Paediatric Society guidelines. Although American Academy of Neurology did not find sufficient evidence to recommend inclusion of conventional magnetic resonance imaging (MRI) of the brain at term-postmenstrual age in addition to cranial sonography to assist in the prediction of neurodevelopmental outcome, recent research has increased understanding of the utility of this imaging technique in outcome prediction.

For full-term infants who exhibit neonatal encephalopathy with a history of birth trauma, low hematocrit, or coagulopathy, recommendations call for a noncontrast computer tomographic (CT) scan to be performed. Infants whose CT scan is nonconclusive should have an MRI performed between days 2 and 8 of age to assess the location and extent of the injury, information important in diagnosis and prognosis for the infant.[51-56]

Retinopathy of Prematurity

ROP affects primarily premature infants weighing less than 1500 g or who are born before 31 weeks' gestation. The incidence of ROP is inversely related to gestational age. ROP typically involves both eyes, is one of the most common causes of visual loss in childhood, and can lead to lifelong vision impairment and blindness. ROP is classified according to the severity of the changes in the developing blood vessels and the region of the retina into which these abnormal vessels have grown. The severity is referred to as the *stage* and the retinal regions as *zones* (Figure 77-8). Fifty percent of infants weighing 1500 g or less at birth will develop some degree of ROP. For most preterm infants, ROP will regress as the infant matures. Approximately 10% of infants with ROP require medical treatment. Approximately 400 to 600 infants with ROP are classified as legally blind each year in the United States. Early treatment of severe ROP is important, producing significant reductions in unfavorable outcomes (retinal detachment, blindness, poor visual acuity).

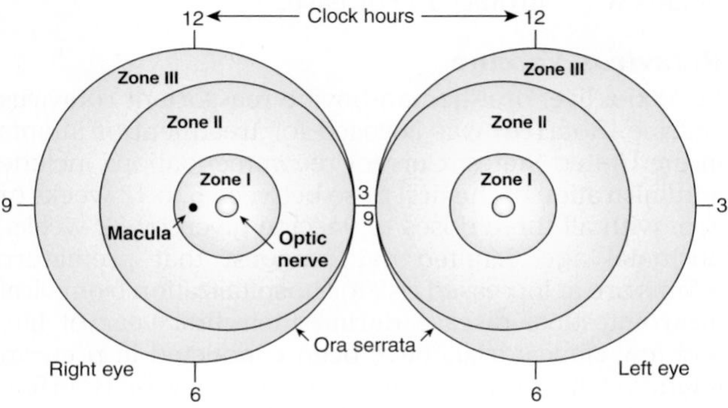

Figure 77-8 Retinopathy of prematurity is described by the examining ophthalmologist in terms of zones and stages, whereby the zone is the location of the retinopathy and the stage is the severity.

Infants who are transferred back to the community hospital setting have been shown to be more likely to miss follow-up ophthalmologic care than infants remaining in tertiary care facilities. Infants not screened for ROP during their NICU hospitalization were more likely to miss follow-up care than infants assessed before hospital discharge. This tendency reinforces the need for communication between medical care providers and written recommendations in transfer summaries detailing findings on the initial examinations (stage of ROP if present and zone to which the retina is vascularized) and specifying the timing for subsequent follow-up evaluations.

The joint statement from the AAP, American Academy of Ophthalmology, and American Association for Pediatric Ophthalmology and Strabismus entitled "Screening Examination of Premature Infants for Retinopathy of Prematurity" provides guidelines for the timing of the initial and follow-up eye examinations and offers criteria to determine the need for treatment.[57–58] Who should be screened?

- Infants with a birth weight less than 1500 g or who are 30 weeks' gestation or younger
- Selected infants with a birth weight between 1500 and 2000 g or gestational age greater than 30 weeks who have experienced an unstable clinical course, including the need for cardiorespiratory support or who are believed to be at high risk

Table 77-6 provides the appropriate timing of the first eye examination in these infants. The following schedule of follow-up examinations is recommended based on the examining ophthalmologist's findings:

- 1-week or less follow-up for:
  - Stage 1 or 2 ROP: zone I
  - Stage 3 ROP: zone II
- 1- to 2-week follow-up for:
  - Immature vascularization: zone I; no ROP
  - Stage 2 ROP: zone II
  - Regressing ROP: zone I
- 2-week follow-up for:
  - Stage 1 ROP: zone II
  - Regressing ROP: zone II
- 2- to 3-week follow-up for:
  - Immature vascularization: zone II; no ROP
  - Stage 1 or 2 ROP: zone III
  - Regressing ROP: zone III

The presence of plus disease (dilated, tortuous posterior retinal blood vessels) in zones I or II suggests that peripheral ablation, rather than observation, is necessary. Treatment may also be initiated for any of the following retinal findings:

- Zone I ROP; any stage with plus disease
- Zone I ROP: stage 3 with no plus disease
- Zone II: stage 2 or 3 with plus disease

Treatment should generally be accomplished, when possible, within 72 hours of determination of treatable disease to minimize the risk of retinal detachment. The conclusion of acute retinal screening examinations should be based on age and retinal ophthalmoscopic findings (see Figure 77-8).

Table 77-6 Timing of First Eye Examination Based on Gestational Age at Birth

GESTATIONAL AGE AT BIRTH (IN WEEKS)	AGE AT INITIAL EXAMINATION (IN WEEKS)	
	POSTMENSTRUAL	CHRONOLOGIC
22*	31	9
23*	31	8
24	31	7
25	31	6
26	31	5
27	31	4
28	32	4
29	33	4
30	34	4
31†	35	4
32†	36	4

*Guideline should be considered tentative rather than evidence-based for infants with a gestational age of 22 to 23 weeks.
†If necessary.
From American Academy of Pediatrics, Section on Ophthalmology, American Academy of Ophthalmology, American Association for Pediatrics Ophthalmology and Strabismus. Policy Statement: Screening examination of premature infants for retinopathy of Prematurity. *Pediatrics.* 2006;117:572-576.

The following medications are used to dilate the infant's eyes: amethocaine 1% (or benoxinate 0.4%), cyclopentolate 0.5% (Cyclogyl), and phenylephrine 2.5%. One drop of each preparation is instilled in each eye 30 minutes before the ophthalmologist's arrival (ie, 0800 hr for a 0830-hr starting time) and repeated 10 minutes later. The eye drops are effective for up to 2 hours from the last installation. Infants with a darker iris may require a longer time and repeat drops for their pupils to dilate. A sucrose nipple can also be used for analgesia during the eye examination.[57,58]

Immunizations

Diphtheria-tetanus-acellular pertussis (DTaP), inactivated polio vaccine (IPV), *Haemophilus influenza* type b conjugate (HiB), and pneumococcal conjugate vaccines are recommended. Current AAP recommendations include immunization of clinically stable premature and low–birth-weight infants at 2 months' postnatal age. Vaccines should be preferentially administered in the anterolateral area of the thigh using a small needle. The immune responses in preterm infants to diphtheria, pertussis, and polio antigens are similar to those seen with full-term babies. In contrast, the immunogenicity of HiB vaccine varies and is believed to be altered by the choice of conjugate protein, use of combination vaccine, and the infant's underlying medical condition. Antibody responses to vaccines in low–birth-weight and preterm infants are frequently less than those in term infants, though protective antibody levels are achieved. Reports of adverse side effects after immunization of sick preterm infants have noted an increase in the incidence of apnea and cardiorespiratory events after the first vaccinations. These events are most common among infants with preexisting apneas, bradycardias, and desaturations at the time of DTaP-IPV-HiB immunization, some of whom may require intervention. However, concerns about potential cardiorespiratory events should not preclude timely immunization. Infants at risk should be appropriately monitored after vaccination.

Hepatitis B Vaccine

The timing of the initial hepatitis B vaccine administration in preterm and low–birth-weight infants is based on birth weight and maternal hepatitis B surface antigen (HBsAg) status, given that immunogenicity is poor in newborns weighing less than 2000 g when hepatitis B vaccine is given at birth. Infants born weighing less than 2000 g to HBsAg-negative mothers should receive hepatitis B vaccine at 30 days of age or at the time of hospital discharge if this occurs before 30 days. If the mother's hepatitis B status is not known at the time of delivery, then hepatitis B vaccine should be given within 12 hours of birth. Hepatitis B immune globulin should also be administered within 12 hours for newborns weighing less than 2000 g and within 7 days if the newborn is greater than 2000 g and the mother is confirmed HBsAg positive.

Influenza Vaccine

Rarely, a chronically ill infant may require continued hospitalization at 6 months of age. The first of two doses of inactive influenza vaccine should be administered at 6 months' postnatal age, particularly for infants with chronic lung disease.[59-62]

Rotavirus Vaccine

In 2006 a live, oral human-bovine reassortant rotavirus vaccine (RotaTeq) was licensed for treatment of infants in the United States. Current recommendations include administration of the first dose between 6 to 12 weeks of age, with all three doses of vaccine given by 32 weeks' postnatal age. Limited data suggest that premature infants are at increased risk for hospitalization from viral gastrointestinal disease during their first year of life, and few clinical trials have been conducted in preterm infants evaluating the safety and efficacy of RotaTeq. Lower levels of maternal antibody to rotaviruses in very low–birth-weight premature infants pose a theoretical risk for adverse reactions among this group of babies. However, the Centers for Disease Control and Prevention Advisory Committee on Immunization Practices believes that the benefits of rotavirus vaccine in premature infants outweighs the potential risks and supports vaccination of premature infants who are at least 6 weeks postnatal age, are clinically stable and ready for hospital discharge, or have already been discharged from the hospital.[63]

In-Hospital Respiratory Syncytial Virus Prophylaxis With Palivizumab

Respiratory syncytial virus (RSV) is responsible for a significant percentage of lower respiratory tract infections (bronchiolitis and pneumonia) in young children. Immune prophylaxis is recommended for high-risk very preterm infants and babies with chronic lung disease or hemodynamically significant heart disease. The clinician should be familiar with local and regional variations in the onset and duration of RSV activity because these variations will guide when RSV immune prophylaxis should be initiated. Data from the Centers for Disease Control and Prevention National Respiratory and Enteric Virus Surveillance System (www.cdc.gov/ncidod/dvrd/revb/nrevss/index.htm) suggest that the annual seasonal peak for RSV infection begins in July in Florida, in the remainder of the South in October, and in the Northeast during November. Highest RSV activity is in October, late December, and early January in Florida, the remainder of the South, and in the Northeast, respectively.

Family-centered care is integral to the functioning of most neonatal units nationwide. Siblings, parents, and grandparents, as well as various health professionals, are in contact with vulnerable infants, thus posing frequent potential infectious exposures including to RSV. Consequently, some physicians have advocated RSV immune prophylaxis with palivizumab in preterm infants hospitalized during RSV season. Studies have demonstrated that extremely preterm infants young than 29 weeks' postmenstrual age are able to mount a protective immune response to 15 mg/kg of palivizumab. Seventy percent of infants studied were able to maintain protective palivizumab concentrations 2 weeks after the initial dose. Less than 25% of infants maintained protective concentrations at 4 weeks after administration. Midpoint concentrations (2 weeks after prophylaxis) were higher after second and third palivizumab doses among the hospitalized cohort of infants. These findings have been confirmed by other investigators. The decision to begin RSV immune prophylaxis of high-risk infants while hospitalized will need to be guided by local infection rates and considerations regarding infant risk.[64]

Positional Plagiocephaly

Positional or deformational plagiocephaly is common among sick and preterm infants or may result from positioning in a restrictive uterine environment. The calvarial bones of the cranium are more malleable in the preterm infant than their healthy peers, increasing the infant's susceptibility to external molding forces. This circumstance results in unilateral flattening in the parietooccipital region, with associated anterior advancement of the ipsilateral ear and anterior displacement (bossing) of the ipsilateral forehead. The head shape resembles a parallelogram. The weight of the infant's head and the child's overall decreased tone and strength are contributing factors as well. Preterm and sick infants, particularly those who require prolonged ventilatory support or who experience neurologic compromise, more often spend extended time with their heads in fixed positions that promote development of a long, narrow scaphocephalic-shaped head.[65] For a full discussion of plagiocephaly, see Chapter 311.

ASSESSMENT AND MANAGEMENT OF PAIN

Early repetitive pain experiences result in permanent changes in pain processing, neuroendocrine function, and development that contribute to abnormal pain thresholds, increased anxiety and stress disorders, and atypical behaviors that include exaggerated startle responses and hypervigilance. Attention should be paid to providing appropriate analgesia to alleviate procedural and postoperative pain. Several measures are available to facilitate assessment of neonatal pain. Among the commonly used measures are the Premature Infant Pain Profile (PIPP), Neonatal Infant Pain Score (NIPS), Neonatal Facial Coding System (NFCS), Neonatal Pain, Agitation and Sedation Scale (N-PASS), Cry, Requires Oxygen, Increased Vital Signs, Expression, Sleeplessness (CRIES), and COMFORT Scale.[66-69]

DEVELOPMENTALLY SUPPORTIVE CARE

Preterm and sick infants experience repetitive painful stimuli and prolonged stress, which has both short- and long-term physiological effects on the child. A developmentally supportive neonatal care environment that integrates noise and bright-light reduction, cycling of light exposure to mimic physiological diurnal variations, and grouping of care activities has demonstrated efficacy in supporting the neurodevelopment and self-regulation abilities of the sick and preterm infant. Benefits attributed to developmentally appropriate care include enhanced growth and behavioral outcomes, decreased need for respiratory support, and decreased length of hospitalization. Environmental modifications include flexed positioning, use of containment to promote state regulation, gel and shape-retaining pillows to provide head support and reduce positional plagiocephaly, adjustable ambient lighting with the use of procedure lights, and incubator covers, limiting decibel levels for continuous and transient sounds to less than 50 dB (maximum of 70 dB for transient sounds), and modifying handling and touch in synchrony with the infant's sleep-wake cycles and behavioral responses (cues). For comparison purposes, 45 dB corresponds to noise levels of normal living, talking, or background radio sound; 70 dB is equivalent to average roadway traffic or a vacuum cleaner or a quiet hair dryer 1 meter away from the ear.

Infants who are most sensitive to stimulation, particularly tactile contacts, are babies who are more immature (<32 weeks postmenstrual age), have chronic cardiorespiratory illness (BPD, cardiac disease), and those infants who demonstrate physiological and behavioral disorganization. Parents should be encouraged to touch and hold their infant, providing tactile experiences appropriate to the baby's ability to tolerate stimulation. Forms of stimulation beneficial to preterm infants include nonnutritive sucking, kangaroo care, and infant massage. Nonnutritive suck provides comfort, promotes physiological organization, and enhances growth and development. Kangaroo care promotes physiologic stability with reductions in apnea and bradycardia, improves sleep patterns and activity levels, reduces infections, decreases length of hospitalization, and promotes breastfeeding and lactation. Massage therapy also has benefits, although the infant's ability to handle stimulation needs to be assessed before massage is integrated into the infant's care regimen.[70-73]

TOOLS FOR PRACTICE

Engaging Patient and Family

- *Early Arrival: Information for Parents of Premature Infants* (brochure), American Academy of Pediatrics (patiented.aap.org).

Medical Decision Support

- *COMFORT Pain Scale* (www.cincinnatichildrens.org/NR/rdonlyres/45D6BDEA-9842-457E-9CF4-A799F11C34CF/0/comfortpainscale.pdf).
- *Cry, Requires Oxygen, Increased Vital Signs, Expression, Sleeplessness (CRIES) Instrument* (scale), Bildner J (www.cityofhope.org/prc/pdf/CRIES.pdf).
- *Guidelines for Perinatal Care, 6th edition* (book), American Academy of Pediatrics (www.aap.org/bookstore).
- *National Respiratory and Enteric Virus Surveillance System (NREVSS)*, Centers for Disease Control and Prevention (www.cdc.gov/ncidod/dvrd/revb/nrevss/index.htm).
- *Neonatal Facial Coding System* (www.cebp.nl/vault_public/filesystem/?ID=1425).
- *Neonatal Infant Pain Score (NIPS)* (scale) (www.cincinnatichildrens.org/NR/rdonlyres/3F2871BE-B165-435F-B6C8-7A2B3C9E45A5/0/neonatalinfantpainscale.pdf).
- *Neonatal Pain, Agitation and Sedation Scale (N-PASS)*, Hummel P, Puchalski M, Loyola University Health System, Loyola University Chicago (www.n-pass.com/assessment_tables.html).
- *Newborn Screening ACT Sheets and Confirmatory Algorithms*, American Academy of Pediatrics and American College of Medical Genetics (www.acmg.net/resources/policies/ACT/condition-analyte-links.htm).
- *Nutritional Support of the Very Low Birth Weight Infant: Part I* (tool kit), California Perinatal Quality Care Collaborative (www.cpqcc.org/NutritionToolkit.html).
- *Nutritional Support of the Very Low Birth Weight Infant: Part II* (tool kit), California Perinatal Quality Care Collaborative (www.cpqcc.org/NutritionIIToolkit2.htm).
- *Premature Infant Pain Profile (PIPP)*, Johnston SB (www.cebp.nl/media/m347.pdf).
- *Transitioning the Breastfeeding/Breastmilk-fed Premature Infant from the Neonatal Intensive Care Unit to Home* (scale), The Academy of Breastfeeding Medicine (www.bfmed.org/ace-files/protocol/NicuGradProtocol.pdf).

AAP POLICY STATEMENTS

American Academy of Pediatrics, Committee on Practice and Ambulatory Medicine and Committee on Fetus and Newborn. The role of the primary care pediatrician in the management of high-risk newborn infants. *Pediatrics*. 1996; 98(4):786-788. (aappolicy.aappublications.org/cgi/content/absctract/pediatrics;98/4/786).

American Academy of Pediatrics, Committee on Psychosocial Aspects of Childhood and Family Health and Task Force on Pain in Infants, Children, and Adolescents. The assessment and management of acute pain in infants, children, and adolescents. *Pediatrics*. 2001;108(3):793-797. (aappolicy.aappublications.org/cgi/content/full/pediatrics;108/3/793).

American Academy of Pediatrics, Section on Ophthalmology, American Academy of Ophthalmology, and American Association for Pediatric Ophthalmology and Strabismus. Screening examination of premature infants for retinopathy of prematurity. *Pediatrics*. 2006;117(2): 572-576. (aappolicy.aappublications.org/cgi/content/full/pediatrics;447/2/572).

American Academy of Pediatrics, Section on Transport Medicine. *Guidelines for Air and Ground Transport of Neonatal and Pediatric Patients*. Elk Grove Village, IL: American Academy of Pediatrics; 2006.

Kaye CL, American Academy of Pediatrics, Committee on Genetics. Introduction to newborn screening fact sheets. *Pediatrics*. 2006;118(3):1304-1312. (pediatrics.aappublications.org/cgi/content/full/118/3/1304).

Kaye CL, American Academy of Pediatrics, Committee on Genetics. Newborn screening fact sheets. *Pediatrics*. 2006;118(3):e934-e936. (pediatrics.aappublications.org/cgi/content/full/118/3/e934).

Saari TN, American Academy of Pediatrics, Committee on Infectious Diseases. Immunization of preterm and low birth weight infants. *Pediatrics*. 2003;112(1):193-198. (aappolicy.aappublications.org/cgi/content/full/pediatrics;112/1/193).

SUGGESTED RESOURCES

Abrams SA. In utero physiology: role in nutrient delivery and fetal development for calcium, phosphorus and vitamin D. *Am J Clin Nutr*. 2007;85(suppl):604S-607S.

Arvedson JC, GI Motility Online. Swallowing and Feeding in Infants and Young Children. Available at: www.nature.com/gimo/contents/pt1/full/gimo17.html. Accessed January 28, 2007.

Comeau AM, Accurso FJ, White TB, et al. Guidelines for implementation of cystic fibrosis screening programs. Cystic Fibrosis Foundation Workshop Report. *Pediatrics*. 2007;119:e495-e518. Available at: pediatrics.aappublications.org/cgi/content/abstract/119/2/e495. Accessed January 10, 2008.

Cincinnati Children's Hospital Medical Center. *Evidence-Based Clinical Practice Guidelines: Postoperative Feeding of Neonates With Complex Congenital Heart Disease*. [Guideline 30.] Cincinnati, OH: Cincinnati Children's Hospital Medical Center; 2002.

Cox J, ed. *Nutrition Manual for At-Risk Infants and Toddlers*. Chicago, IL: Precept Press; 1997.

Groh-Wargo S, Thompson M, Cox JH, eds. *Nutritional Care for High to Risk Newborns*. 3rd ed. Chicago, IL: Precept Press; 2000.

King JL, Naber JM, Hopkin RJ, et al. Antenatal corticosteroids and newborn screening for congenital adrenal hyperplasia. *Arch Pediatr Adolesc Med*. 2001;155: 1038-1042.

Klein CJ. Nutrient Requirements for preterm infant formulas. *J Nutr*. Jun 2002;132(6 suppl 1):1395S-1577S.

Lau C. Oral Feeding in the Preterm Infant. *NeoReviews*. 2006; 7(1)e19. Available at: www.neoreviews.org.

Linder N, Davidovitch N, Kogan A, et al. Longitudinal measurements of 17α-hydroxyprogesterone in premature infants during the first three months of life. *Arch Dis Child Fetal Neonatal Ed.* 1999;81:F175-F178.

National Academy of Sciences, Institute of Medicine. Dietary Reference Intakes, 2002. Available at: www.iom.edu.

Olgemöller B, Roscher AA, Liebel B, et al. Screening for congenital adrenal hyperplasia: adjustment for 17-hydroxyprogesterone cut-off values to both age and birth weight markedly improves the predictive value. *J Clin Endocrinol Metab.* 2003;88:5790-5794.

Rauch F, Schoenau E. Skeletal development in premature infants: a review of bone physiology beyond nutritional aspects. *Arch Dis Child Fetal Neonatal Ed.* 2002;86:F82-F85.

Reuss ML, Leviton A, Paneth N, et al. Thyroxine values from newborn screening of 919 infants born before 29 weeks' gestation. *Am J Public Health.* 1997;87:1693-1697.

Strauss RG. Transfusion approach to neonatal anemia. *NeoReviews.* 2000;1(4):e74-e80.

Tsang R, Uauy R, Koletzko B, et al. *Nutrition of the Preterm Infant.* 2nd ed. Cincinnati, OH: Digital Educational Publishing; 2005.

Widness JA. Pathophysiology, diagnosis and prevention of neonatal anemia. *NeoReviews.* 2000;1(4):e61-e68.

Wolf LS, Glass RP, eds. *Feeding and Swallowing Disorders in Infancy: Assessment and Management.* San Antonio, TX: Therapy Skill Builders; 1992.

REFERENCES

1. Simon TL, Alversen DC, AuBuchon J, et al. Practice parameter for the use of red blood cell transfusions. *Arch Pathol Lab Med.* 1998;122:130-138.
2. Cooke RWI, Drury JA, Yokall CW, et al. Blood transfusions and chronic lung disease in premature infants. *Euro J Pediatrics.* 1996;156(1):47-50.
3. Arad I, Konijn AM, Linder N, et al. Serum ferritin levels in preterm infants after multiple transfusions. *Am J Perinatol.* 1988;5(1):40-43.
4. Finer NN, Higgins R, Kattwinkel J, et al. Summary proceedings from the Apnea of Prematurity Group. *Pediatrics.* 2006;117(3):S47-S51.
5. Eichenwald EC, Aina A, Stark AR. Apnea frequently persists beyond term gestation in infants delivered at 24 to 28 weeks. *Pediatrics.* 1997;100:354-359.
6. Chow W, Milligan DW, Pennefather P, et al. Pulse oximetry, severe retinopathy and outcome at one year in babies less than 28 weeks' gestation. *Arch Dis Child Fetal Neonat Ed.* 2001;84:F106-F110.
7. Garg M, Kurner SI, Bautista DB, et al. Clinically unsuspected hypoxia during sleep and feeding in infants with bronchopulmonary dysplasia. *Pediatrics.* 1988;81: 635-642.
8. Razi NM, DeLauter M, Pandit PB. Periodic breathing and desaturation in preterm infants at discharge. *J Perinatol.* 2002;22:442-444.
9. Lopez-Alonso M, Moya M, Cabo JA, et al. Twenty-four hour esophageal impedance to pH monitoring in healthy preterm neonates: rate and characteristics of acid, weakly acidic and weakly alkaline gastroesophageal reflux. *Pediatrics.* 2006;118(2):e299-e308. Available at: pediatrics.aappublications.org/cgi/content/full/118/2/e299. Accessed January 19, 2008.
10. DiFore JM, Arko M, Whitehouse M, et al. Apnea is not prolonged by acid gastroesophageal reflux in preterm infants. *Pediatrics.* 2005;116:1059-1063.
11. De Paoli AG, Lau R, Davis PG, et al. Pharyngeal pressure in preterm infants receiving nasal continuous positive airway pressure. *Arch Dis Child Fetal Neonatal Ed.* 2005; 90:F79-F81.
12. Myers TR, American Association for Respiratory Care. AARC clinical practice guideline: selection of an oxygen delivery device for neonatal and pediatric patients—2002 revision and update. *Respir Care.* 2002;47(6):707-716.
13. American Association for Respiratory Care. AARC clinical practice guideline: Application of continuous positive airway pressure to neonates via nasal prongs, nasopharyngeal tube or nasal mask—2004 revision and update. *Respir Care* 2004;49(9):1100-1108.
14. Payne NR, LaCorte M, Sun S, et al. Evaluation and development of potentially better practices to reduce bronchopulmonary dysplasia in very low birth weigh infants. *Pediatrics.* 2006;118(suppl 2):S65-S72.
15. Payne NR, LaCorte M, Karna P, et al. Reduction of bronchopulmonary dysplasia after participation in the Breathsavers Group of the Vermont Oxford Network Neonatal Intensive Care Quality Improvement Collaborative. *Pediatrics.* 2006;118(suppl 2):S73-S77.
16. Barrington KJ. The adverse neuro-developmental effects of postnatal steroids in the preterm infant: a systematic review of RCTs. *BMC Pediatrics.* 2001;1:1. Available at www.biomedcentral.com/1471-2431/1/1. Accessed June 12, 2007.
17. Vaucher Y. Bronchopulmonary dysplasia: an enduring challenge. *Pediatr Rev.* 2002;23(10):349-358.
18. Walsh M, Engle W, Laptook A, et al. Oxygen delivery through nasal cannulae to preterm infants: can practice be improved? *Pediatrics.* 2005;116(4):865-861.
19. Jackson JK, Ford SP, Meinert KA, et al. Standardizing nasal cannula oxygen administration in the neonatal intensive care unit. *Pediatrics.* 2006;118(suppl 2): S187-S196.
20. Sreenan C, Lemke RP, Hudson-Mason A, et al. High-flow nasal cannulae in the management of apnea of prematurity: a comparison with conventional nasal continuous positive airway pressure. *Pediatrics.* 2001;107:1081-1083.
21. Locke RG, Wolfson MR, Shaffer TH, et al. Inadvertent administration of positive end-distending pressure during nasal cannula flow. *Pediatrics.* 1993;91(1):135-138.
22. Fitzgerald D, Van Asperen P, Leslie G, et al. Higher SaO2 in chronic neonatal lung disease: does it improve sleep? *Ped Pulmonol.* 1998;26:235-240.
23. The STOP-ROP Multicenter Study Group. Supplemental therapeutic oxygen for prethreshold retinopathy of prematurity (STOP-ROP), a randomized, controlled trial. I: primary outcomes. *Pediatrics.* 2000;105:295-310.
24. Abman SH. Monitoring cardiovascular function in infants with chronic lung disease of prematurity. *Arch Dis Child Fetal Neonatal Ed.* 2002;87:F15-F18.
25. Embleton NE, Pang N, Cooke RJ. Postnatal malnutrition and growth retardation: an inevitable consequence of current recommendations in preterm infants? *Pediatrics.* 2001;107(2):270-273.
26. Clark R, Thomas P, Peabody J. Extrauterine growth restriction remains a serious problem in prematurely born neonates. *Pediatrics.* 2003;111(5):986-990.
27. Rayyis SF, Ambalavanan N, Wright L, et al. Randomized trial of "slow" versus "fast" feed advancements on the incidence of necrotizing enterocolitis in very low birth weight infants. *J Pediatr.* 1999;134:293-297.
28. Hofman PL, Regan F, Jackson WE, et al. Premature birth and later insulin resistance. *N Engl J Med.* 2004;351: 2179-2186.
29. Ong KK, Ahmed ML, Emmett PM, et al. Association between postnatal catch up growth and obesity in childhood: prospective cohort study. *BMJ.* 2000;320:967-971.
30. Mihatsch WA, von Schoenaich P, Fahnenstich H, et al. The significance of gastric residuals in the early enteral advancement of extremely low birth weight infants. *Pediatrics.* 2002;109:457-459.

31. Aly H, Abdel-Hady H, Khashaba M, et al. Erythromycin and feeding intolerance in premature infants: a randomized trial. *J Perinataol.* 2007;27(1):39-43.
32. Patole S, Rao S, Doherty D. Erythromycin as a prokinetic agent in preterm neonates a systematic review. *Arch Dis Child Fetal Neonatal Ed.* 2005;90:F301-F306.
33. Schanler RJ, Gartner LM, Krebs NF, et al, eds. *Breastfeeding Handbook for Physicians.* Elk Grove Village, IL: American Academy of Pediatrics; 2005.
34. American Academy of Pediatrics. Human milk. In: Pickering LK, Baker CF, Long SS, et al, eds. *2006 Red Book: Report of the Committee on Infectious Diseases.* 27th ed. Elk Grove Village, IL: American Academy of Pediatrics; 2006.
35. Lucas A, Cole TJ. Breast milk and neonatal necrotizing enteral colitis. *Lancet.* 1990;336:1519-1523.
36. Arnold LDW. Donor human milk banking. In: Riordan J, ed. *Breastfeeding and Human Lactation.* 3rd ed. Sudbury, MA: Jones & Bartlett Publishers; 2004.
37. Ziegler EE, Thureen PJ, Carlson SJ. Aggressive nutrition of the very low birthweight infant. *Clin Perinatol.* 2002; 29:1-20.
38. Kuschel CA, Evans N, Askie L, et al. A randomized trial of enteral feeding volumes in infants born before 30 weeks' gestation. *J Paediatr Child Health.* 2000;36(6):581-586.
39. American Academy of Pediatrics, Committee of Nutrition. AAP policy statement: soy protein-based formulas: recommendations for use in infant feeding. *Pediatrics.* 1998;101(1):148-153.
40. Huysman WA, de Ridder M, de Bruin NC, et al. Growth and body composition in preterm infants with bronchopulmonary dysplasia. *Arch Dis Child Fetal Neonatal Ed.* 2003;88:F46-F51.
41. North American Society for Pediatric Gastroenterology, Hepatology, and Nutrition (NASPGHN), American Academy of Pediatrics. Clinical practice guidelines. *J Pediatr Gastroenterol Nutr.* 2001;32(suppl 2):S1-S31.
42. Poets CF. Gastroesophageal reflux: acritical review of its role in preterm infants. *Pediatrics.* 2004;113:e128-e132, Available at: www.pediatrics.org/cgi/content/full/113/2/e128. Accessed June 12, 2007.
43. Vandenplas Y, Goyvaverts H, Helven R, et al. Gastroesophageal reflux, as measured by 24-hour pH monitoring in 509 healthy infants screened for risk of sudden infant death syndrome. *Pediatrics.* 1999;88:834-840.
44. Di Fiore JM, Arko M, Whitehouse M, et al. Apnea is not prolonged by acid gastroesophageal reflux in preterm infants. *Pediatrics.* 2005;116(5):1059-1063.
45. Martin RJ, Hibbs AM. Diagnosing gastroesophageal reflux in preterm infants. *Pediatrics.* 2006;118:793-794.
46. Hibbs AM, Lorch SA. Metoclopramide for the treatment of gastroesophageal reflux disease in infants: a systematic review. *Pediatrics.* 2006;118:746-752. Available at: www.pediatrics.org/cgi/doi/10.1542/peds.2005-2664. Accessed June 12, 2007.
47. Patel AS, Pohl JF, Easley DJ. Proton pump inhibitors and pediatrics. *Pediatr Rev.* 2003;24(1):12-15.
48. Guillet R, Stoll BJ, Cotton CM, et al. Association of H-2 blocker therapy and higher incidence of necrotizing enterocolitis in very low birth weight infants. *Pediatrics.* 2006;117(2):e1-e6. Available at: www.pediatrics.org/cgi/content/full/peds.205-1543v1. Accessed June 12, 2007.
49. Moyer-Mileur LJ, Brunstetter V, McNaught TP, et al. Daily physical activity program increases bone mineralization and growth in preterm very low birth weight infants. *Pediatrics.* 2000;106:1088-1092.
50. Litmanovitz I, Dolfin T, Frieldand O, et al. Early physical activity intervention prevents decrease of bone strength in very low birth weight infants. *Pediatrics.* 2003;112: 15-19.
51. American Academy of Neurology. Practice parameter: neuroimaging of the neonate. Report of the Quality Standards Subcommittee of the American Academy of Neurology and the Practice Committee of the Child Neurology Society. *Neurology.* 2002;58:1726-1738.
52. Canadian Paediatric Society. Statement FN2001-01: routine screening cranial ultrasound examinations for the prediction of long term neurodevelopmental outcomes in preterm infants. *Paediatr Child Health.* 2001;6:39-43.
53. Perlman JM, Rollins N. Surveillance protocol for the detection of intracranial abnormalities in premature neonates. *Arch Pediatr Adolesc Med.* 2000;154:822-826.
54. Mirmiran M, Barnes PD, Keller K, et al. Neonatal brain magnetic resonance imaging before discharge is better than serial cranial ultrasound in predicting cerebral palsy in very low birth weight infants. *Pediatrics.* 2004;114: 992-998.
55. Robertson NJ, Wyatt JS. The magnetic resonance revolution in brain imaging: impact on neonatal care. *Arch Dis Child Fetal Neonatal Ed.* 2004;89:F193-F197.
56. Woodward LJ, Anderson PJ, Austin NC, et al. Neonatal MRI to predict neurodevelopmental outcomes in preterm infants. *N Engl J Med.* 2006;355:685-694.
57. American Academy of Pediatrics, Section on Ophthalmology, American Academy of Ophthalmology, American Association for Pediatric Ophthalmology and Strabismus. Policy statement: screening examination of premature infants for retinopathy of prematurity. *Pediatrics.* 2006;117:572-576.
58. Attar MA, Gates MR, Iatrow AM, et al. Barriers to screening infants for retinopathy of prematurity after discharge or transfer from a neonatal intensive care unit. *J Perinatol.* 2005;25:36-40.
59. Pfister RE, Afschbach V, Niksic-Stuber V, et al. Safety of DtaP-based combined immunization in very low birth weight premature infants: frequent but mostly benign cardiorespiratory events. *J Pediatr.* 2004;145:58-66.
60. Saari N, American Academy of Pediatrics, Committee on Infectious Disease. Immunization of the premature and low birth weight infant. *Pediatrics.* 2003;112:193-198.
61. Sen S, Cloete Y, Hassan K, et al. Adverse events following vaccination in premature infants. *Acta Paediatr.* 2001;90:916-920.
62. D'Angio CT. Active immunization of premature and low birth weight infants: a review of immunogenicity, efficacy and tolerability. *Pediatr Drugs.* 2007;9:17-32.
63. Prashar U, Alexander J, Glass R. Prevention of rotavirus gastroenteritis among infants and children: recommendations of the Advisory Committee on Immunization Practices (ACIP). *MMWR Mort Morb Weekly Rep.* 2006; 55(RR12):1-13.
64. Wu S-Y, Bonaparte J, Pyati S. Palivizumab use in very premature infants in the neonatal intensive care unit. *Pediatrics.* 2004;114:e554-e556.
65. Littlefield TR, Reiff JL, Rekate HL. Diagnosis and management of deformational plagiocephaly. *BNI Q.* 2001; 17:1-8.
66. American Academy of Pediatrics, Committee on Fetus and Newborn, Section on Surgery, and Canadian Paediatric Society Fetus and Newborn Committee. Prevention and management of pain in the neonate: an update. *Pediatrics.* 2006;118:2231-2241. Available at: www.pedia trics.org/cgi/doi/10.1542/peds.2006-2277 Accessed June 12, 2007.
67. Anand KJS, Aranda JV, Berde CB, et al. Summary proceedings from the Neonatal Pain-Control Group. *Pediatrics.* 2006;117:S9-S22. Available at: www.pediatrics.org/cgi/doi/10.1542/peds.2005-0620C. Accessed June 12, 2007.

68. Anand KJS, Hall RW. Pharmacological therapy for analgesia and sedation in the newborn. *Arch Dis Child Fetal Neonatal Ed.* 2006;91:F448-F453.
69. Stevens B, Johnston C, Gibbins S. Pain assessment in neonates In: Anand KJ, Stevens BJ, McGrath P, eds. *Pain in Neonates.* 2nd ed. Philadelphia, PA: Elsevier; 2000.
70. Sizun J, Westrup B, ESF Network Coordination Committee. Early developmental care for preterm neonates: a call for more research. *Arch Dis Child Fetal Neonatal Ed.* 2004;89:F384-F389.
71. Field TM. Stimulation of preterm infants. *Pediatr Rev.* 2003;24(1):4-11.
72. Westrup B. Newborn Individualized Developmental Care and Assessment Program (NIDCAP). Family-centered developmentally supportive care. *NeoReviews.* 2005;6(3): e115-e122.
73. Feldman R, Eidelman AI. Skin-to-skin contact (kangaroo care) accelerates autonomic and neurobehavioral maturation in preterm infants. *Dev Med Child Neurol.* 2003;45: 274-281.

Chapter 78

DISCHARGE PLANNING FOR THE HIGH-RISK NEWBORN REQUIRING INTENSIVE CARE

Christina M. Long, DO; Deborah E. Campbell, MD

INTRODUCTION

One of the most important aspects of caring for a premature or sick infant is the preparation for the infant's discharge from the hospital. The most medically complex infants have often spent weeks or months in a neonatal intensive care unit (NICU) and require a broad array of medical and other services for their postdischarge health care, including primary pediatric care, subspecialty follow-up, home or public health nursing care, early intervention services, extensive care coordination, and family support.

Comprehensive discharge planning is as important as the medical care that the infant received in the NICU; it requires a team approach that includes the neonatologist, pediatric specialists, the infant's primary care physician, hospital nurses, social worker, lactation consultant, therapists, and most important, the infant's family. The family is central to the discharge planning process and pivotal to its success. Discharge planning is necessary not only for infants who will be discharged home with their families, but also for infants who may be transferred to a transitional or chronic-care facility, such as a children's rehabilitation center.

The transition from the NICU to home can be stressful for the neonate and the infant's family. Preparing the family for a coordinated discharge, with adequate opportunities for parents to assimilate the staff's teaching and to ensure availability of the appropriate resources, can help alleviate many of the fears parents may have about taking their premature or medically fragile infant home. The infant's primary care physician is an integral member of the team, given that the role as the infant's primary medical caregiver and coordinator of the child's medical home is also key.[1-3] The hospital-based medical team is responsible for engaging the primary care physician and ensuring complete disclosure of the infant's medical information and the scope of required follow-up care services. The neonatal team also needs to ensure that the pediatric physician is fully informed about the family's material resources, as well as psychosocial and other support needs, so that the parents may properly care for and nurture their infant at home and handle their other family responsibilities.

Every neonatal or special care unit has basic criteria that must be met for the infant to be discharged from the acute-care setting. Most units require that an infant demonstrate a sustained pattern of weight gain with effective oral feeding by breast or bottle, be able to maintain a normal body temperature under ambient (thermoneutral) conditions, and maintain a stable cardiorespiratory status with resolution of apnea, bradycardia, and desaturations. Additional criteria for discharge are evidence of active parental involvement and demonstrated parental ability to comply with the child's prescribed care. Arranging for timely, appropriate medical follow-up after the infant's hospital discharge is another important aspect of the discharge planning process. Families in rural and other underserved communities may face particular challenges in accessing the needed specialized follow-up care their infants require, placing an additional burden on the family, discharging hospital, and primary care physician.

FEEDING AND NUTRITION

Discharge Criteria

Despite advances in nutritional support with attention to early aggressive nutrition, many low–birth-weight or chronically ill infants exhibit slow or inadequate postnatal growth; and among the smallest, least-mature infants, universal growth failure is evident at discharge.[4] The goal of postdischarge nutrition is to provide the necessary nutrients to optimize growth and bone mineralization and promote a pattern of weight gain and head growth that supports appropriate catch-up growth yet prevents excessive or inappropriate weight-gain patterns that may predispose the infant to adverse health consequences, such as metabolic syndrome later in life.[5,6] Infants at risk for poor growth include preterm, low–birth-weight, and severely growth-restricted infants, as well as babies born with anatomic abnormalities or neurologic disorders that interfere with effective oral feeding, limit nutrient utilization, or increase metabolic requirements that are not easily met through typical feeding regimens. Infants with complex nutritional needs include those with chronic lung disease, short bowel syndrome, cholestasis, and cardiac disease.

Individual hospitals and health systems have established criteria regarding the specific weight an infant must attain before discharge; many units aim for a weight of 1800 to 2000 grams. Significant variation exists in the actual discharge weights of NICU infants, given that the infant's comorbidities often determine the timing of discharge, as does the availability of community resources to support the infant with continuing feeding issues and the infant's mode of enteral intake at discharge—oral or via a feeding tube (nasogastric or gastrostomy). Insurance coverage for the infant's post–hospital care may support an earlier discharge for the infant with home nursing care.

For infants who experience feeding difficulties, the neonatal team, in collaboration with a speech pathologist with feeding expertise, nutritionist, or lactation consultant, must devise a feeding plan with the parents that will support the infant's nutrition and weight gain and that is feasible for the family to implement. A feeding plan should include the type of feeding, amount of feeding, frequency and method of feeding, and any special instructions necessary. For example, some infants may require special formulas that require special preparation. The parents and primary care physician should understand the feeding regimen, the nutrition and weight-gain goals, and the parents' need to demonstrate their ability to feed their infant appropriately.

During the course of the infant's hospitalization the baby's weight and other growth parameters, length, and head circumference should have been plotted on a standardized infant growth curve, such as the Fenton (Babson-Benda intrauterine and postnatal growth chart) or Ehrenkrantz postnatal growth charts that track growth of preterm infants from 22 to 50 weeks' gestation or the 2000 standard growth curves from the Centers for Disease Control and Prevention. The weight-gain goal at discharge and during the transition home is typically 20 to 30 g/day, with an intake of 100 to 120 kcal/kg/day and a volume intake of at least 180 mL/kg/day, unless a particular reason exists that an infant requires fluid restriction. Experts have recently recommended that a more appropriate weight-gain target to promote optimal growth should be 16 to 17 g/kg/day.[7] Many recovering preterm infants without feeding or cardiorespiratory problems who are fed ad libitum (on demand, without volume restriction) have daily intakes that range between 170 and 220 mL/kg/day. Preterm infants who are receiving exclusively expressed milk may exhibit a reduced weight-gain pattern. However, if the infant is consuming more than 170 to 180 mL/kg/day of human milk, then growth patterns comparable to formula-fed preterm infants are seen. Acceptable weight gain for an infant receiving only human milk should also be 20 to 30 g/day. Gastroesophageal reflux is a common problem among preterm and some term infants and may limit feeding volume and weight gain.

The following aspects of the hospital feeding plan assessment help develop a discharge feeding plan[8]:

1. Type of feeding—unfortified or fortified human milk, formula, or a combination
   - Human milk fortifier is frequently discontinued when the infant reaches a weight of approximately 1800 grams.
   - 24 cal/oz premature formula (Similac Special Care Formula or Enfamil Premature Formula) may be continued until the infant attains a weight of 1850 to 2400 grams (4.0-5.5 lb).
   - Some states' Special Supplemental Nutrition Program for Women, Infants, and Children (WIC programs) will provide these formulas postdischarge until the infant reaches 3 to 4 months' postnatal age (approximately term-corrected age).
   - 22 cal/oz transitional or postdischarge formula (Enfamil Enfacare or Similac Neosure) is started when the preterm infant achieves a weight of 1850 to 2400 grams and is continued until optimal growth is achieved, nutritional deficiencies are corrected, or the infant reaches 6 to 9 months' corrected age.
     - Sick preterm infants with birth weights between 1500 and 1850 grams who have required parenteral nutrition and diuretics and are exhibiting suboptimal growth may also benefit from transitional or postdischarge formula if breastfeeding is not the chosen feeding method.
2. Volume of feedings—milk intake (in mL/kg/day) and volume per feeding if bottle fed
   - Goal is an intake of approximately 180 mL/kg/day.
   - Intakes of less than 160 mL/kg/day are suboptimal.
3. Method of feeding—breast, bottle, lactation aid, cup, tube feeding (oro- or nasogastric tube or gastrostomy tube) or a combination of methods
   - Feeding is suboptimal if the infant cannot consume all feeds orally because of fatigue or poor coordination.
   - Assess the adequacy of the infant's latch if breastfeeding.
4. Adequacy of growth—average daily weight gain and weekly rate of linear and head growth
   - Growth is deemed adequate when weight (>20 g/day), length (>1 cm/week), and head circumference (>0.5 cm/week) are within normal for corrected age or improving.
   - Growth is inadequate if the weight gain is less than 20 g/day or length gain is less than 0.5 cm/week
5. Adequacy of nutrition—biochemical monitoring of nutritional status (blood urea nitrogen, phosphorus, and alkaline phosphatase)
   - Oral multivitamin supplementation may be required for the infant who is breastfeeding or ingesting less than 32 oz of formula per day.
   - Until the infant is taking in at least 500 mL/day of formula, vitamin D in a dose of 200 IU/day should be provided.
   - Preterm infants who are exclusively breastfeeding should begin elemental iron supplementation at 2 months of age at a dose of 2 to 4 mg/kg/day.
   - Formula-feeding, preterm infants should receive an iron-fortified formula.

Mothers who have been expressing milk during their infant's hospitalization should be assisted in transitioning to breastfeeding in advance of the infant's discharge. Clinical guidelines are available that offer information for use by both clinicians and mothers.[8-11] High-risk infants who have been receiving fortified feeds should be monitored at least 1 week on unfortified human milk to assess properly the adequacy of growth and nutrient intake. Infants with signs of persistent inadequate growth and nutritional deficiencies (low serum albumin, blood urea nitrogen levels, and elevated serum alkaline phosphatase) and infants who have difficulty completing their feedings will benefit from continued nutritional supplementation after discharge. Determining whether the infant can be fed on demand or needs to continue on a schedule is another important factor to ensure that infants with poor state regulation, chronic conditions, feeding difficulties, and feeding fatigue achieve the desired intakes.

Optimally the goal is for the infant to breastfeed rather than for the mother to continue to express breast milk for administration by bottle. A common parental concern relates to the adequacy of the infant's intake once the mother is no longer able to monitor the baby's oral intake visually. Information and guidance are necessary to foster maternal confidence in her ability to nourish her infant adequately without benefit of a volume measure.[12-14] The mother should be counseled to continue expressing or pumping milk at least three times daily to build her milk supply. Iron and multivitamin supplementation should be started once the infant is receiving unfortified human milk.

Mothers who are expressing milk must often contend with a decreasing milk supply during the infant's extended hospitalization. Some women use pharmacologic and herbal products to boost their milk supply. Metoclopramide (Reglan) is effective in increasing and maintaining milk production in some women. Metoclopramide increases prolactin secretion and is prescribed in a dose of 10-mg tablet taken orally, three to four times per day for 1 week, followed by a 1-week period during which the medication is tapered.[15] (Continuing kangaroo care after discharge is another technique that can improve milk production and encourage a faster transition to breastfeeding.[16]) Some breastfeeding women prefer to use herbal products or natural foods to increase their milk supply. Herbs commonly used include fenugreek, goat's rue, milk thistle, anise, basil, blessed thistle, fennel seeds, and marshmallow.[17] No standard dosing, preparation, or combinations of these substances exist, and they are not approved by the US Food and Drug Administration (FDA). Fenugreek, a member of the pea family listed as generally safe by the FDA, may be consumed in capsules or as a tea; side effects are rare, but it can cause hypoglycemia. Goat's rue is recommended in several European countries; used alone, no side effects have been reported. Milk thistle is an herb that, according the American Herbal Products Association, may be safely consumed during lactation.[18] (Mother's milk tea is a blend of plants used in increased milk supply; it is promoted as having no caffeine, and none of the ingredients have pharmacologic actions. Other herbal teas considered safe during lactation include chicory, orange spice, peppermint, raspberry, red bush tea, and rose hips.[18]) Although the FDA does not approve the use of herbal medicines for lactation purposes, many have been proven safe. However, many herbs are contraindicated in lactation, including aloe, buckthorn bark, buckthorn berry, cascara sagrada bark, coltsfoot leaf, senna leaf, peppermint oil, caraway oil, kava kava, petasites root, Indian snakeroot, rhubarb root, senna leaf, and uva ursi.[19]

Special Considerations

If the infant does not gain appropriate weight with unfortified human milk, then two to three feedings of an enriched transitional formula (Neosure or Enfacare) or postdischarge formula (22 kcal/oz) should be added to the infant's feeding regimen (Table 78-1 provides formula modifications). The infant should be monitored in the hospital for improved growth. Human milk fortifier and preterm formulas typically used during the NICU hospitalization are not usually recommended at discharge because the nutrient content is greater than the infant's needs and because the preparation can be difficult. Human milk fortifier is typically discontinued when an infant reaches approximately 36 weeks' postmenstrual age and weighs 1800 to 2000 grams. If suboptimal weight gain or growth continues, then additional supplementation should be provided, with an increase in the caloric density to 24 to 30 kcal/oz.

A similar process of feeding method assessment and formula adjustment should be performed for the formula-feeding preterm infant.

During the hospital course, infants with cardiac, renal, pulmonary, and gastrointestinal disease may have a requirement for increased calories. This requirement for special nutrition often continues after discharge. These infants must be discharged home on the correct formula, which will provide adequate nutrition for an infant's needs. For example, patients with renal disease many require a formula with a low solute load and low phosphorous content (Similac PM 60:40). Infants with a cleft lip and palate require a comprehensive feeding assessment to determine the extent of feeding difficulties and whether special nipples or an obturator are needed to facilitate oral feeding. Babies born with a cleft lip or palate can successfully breastfeed, although the infant may require an obturator if the cleft palate is large.

Eligibility for the Special Supplemental Nutrition Program for Women, Infants, and Children

An important resource for neonates ready for discharge from the NICU is the WIC program. WIC is a federal-grant program administered by federal and state agencies in each of the 50 states, the District of Columbia, Native-American tribal organizations, and five territories that include Northern Mariana, American Samoa, Guam, Puerto Rico, and the Virgin Islands. The WIC program targets the low-income population with infants and children who are at nutritional risk. The program provides supplemental nutritious foods, nutrition education, screening, and referrals to other health, welfare, and social service centers. Applicants must meet all of the eligibility requirements, including categorical, residential, income, and nutritional risks. Categorically eligibility includes pregnant women (during pregnancy and up to 6 weeks after birth), postpartum women (up to 6 months after the birth of the infant or the end of pregnancy), breastfeeding women

Table 78-1 Formula Adjustments

FORMULA	CALORIES DESIRED	MIXING INSTRUCTIONS (WATER)	FORMULA POWDER	FINAL VOLUME
Standard 20 cal/oz	22	5.5 oz	3 scoops	6 oz
	24	5 oz	3 scoops	10 oz
	26	3 oz	2 scoops	3.5 oz
	27	8.5 oz	6 scoops	10 oz
Neosure 22 cal/oz	20	4.5 oz	2 scoops	5 oz
	24	5.5 oz	3 scoops	6 oz
	26	5 oz	3 scoops	5¾ oz
	27	8 oz	5 scoops	9 oz
Enfamil EnfaCare Lipil 22 cal/oz	20	4.5 oz	2 scoops	5 oz
	24	5.5 oz	3 scoops	6 oz
	26	5 oz	3 scoops	5.5 oz
	27	8 oz	5 scoops	9 oz
Neocatev 20 cal/oz	20	3.5 oz	4 scoops	4 oz
	22	4 oz	4.5 scoops	4.5 oz
	24	5 oz	7 scoops	6 oz
Pregestimil or Nutramigen 20 cal/oz	22	5.5 oz	3 scoops	6 oz
	24	5 oz	3 scoops	5.5 oz
	26	3 oz	2 scoops	3.5 oz
	27	7 oz	5 scoops	8 oz
Nutramigen with liquid concentrate	22	11 oz	1 can concentrate	24 oz
	24	9 oz	1 can concentrate	22 oz
	26	7 oz	1 can concentrate	20 oz
	27	6 oz	1 can concentrate	19 oz
Human milk fortified with standard formula	22	4 oz HM	¾ Tsp	—
	24	3 oz HM	1 Tsp	
	26	6 oz HM	1 scoop	
	27	5.5 oz HM	1 scoop	
Human milk fortified with Neosure	22	6 oz HM	1¼ Tsp	—
	24	6 oz HM	2½ Tsp	
	26	5 oz HM	1 Tbsp	
	27	6 oz HM	1 scoop	
Human milk fortified with Enfacare	22	6 oz HM	1 Tsp	—
	24	4 oz HM	1¼ Tsp	
	26	5 oz HM	1 Tbsp	
	27	3 oz HM	2 Tsp	

HM, Human milk.

(up to the infant's first birthday), infants (up to 1 year of age), and children (up to 5 years of age). Applicants must live in the state in which they apply and have an income at or below an income level or standard set by the state agency to which they apply. Applicants must be seen by a health professional who determines if the applicant meets nutritional risk criteria.[20] WIC-eligible patients should be referred for enrollment before hospital discharge.

TEMPERATURE REGULATION

An infant's ability to maintain a normal body temperature is another necessary criterion in determining readiness for discharge from the hospital. This factor is of particular importance for the low–birth-weight infant and babies who have exhibited poor growth caused by a prolonged illness, feeding difficulties, or feeding restrictions that limit fluid and caloric intake. Infants who have underlying neurologic dysfunction may also exhibit difficulty with body temperature regulation. The infant who is ready for discharge should be able to maintain thermoneutrality when dressed in infant clothing and covered with a blanket. A normal body temperature in the range of 36.5°C to 37.5°C[21] (with the infant in an open bassinette should be maintained for at least 24 hours). If any evidence of temperature instability exists, then the infant should not be discharged. Infants at less than 34 weeks' gestation are least likely to be able to maintain body temperature in an open bassinette, although more mature infants may also exhibit difficulty with temperature regulation because they are recovering from serious illness, have limited adipose stores, or have high energy expenditure associated with learning to feed or ongoing cardiorespiratory disease. Infants who are unable to maintain their body temperature under routine ambient environmental conditions should continue to be cared for in a heated isolette. An additional important factor to consider relates to the infant who exhibits a change in the ability to maintain body temperature without a change in the environmental conditions. Temperature instability is a nonspecific, though frequently present, sign suggestive of infection.

RESPIRATORY

Home Oxygen Therapy and Pulse Oximetry

Some infants discharged from neonatal units will have residual lung disease requiring supplemental oxygen therapy at home. The decision regarding an infant's need for home oxygen therapy is often based on a combination of objective and subjective criteria. The infant's clinical care needs must be balanced with the parents' caregiving responsibilities at home and an assessment of the parents' ability or desire to have their infant home on oxygen. Some parents will prefer having their infant transition to a chronic-care or rehabilitative facility until their infant no longer requires oxygen. Other parents will undertake the challenge of combining parenting with medical caregiving to bring their baby home sooner. Additional considerations include availability of home health care support, local equipment vendors, and the expertise of the child's primary care physician who will be managing the infant's continuing respiratory care needs at home. Individual hospital policies delineate the specific criteria for home oxygen therapy (Box 78-1).

Preterm infants with lung disease frequently have brief arterial oxygen saturations less than 90% during feedings, periods of wakefulness, and sleep that are not associated with apnea, bradycardia, or cyanosis. Infants with chronic lung disease are also more likely to have severe oxygen desaturations less than 80%.[22] (Improved survival rates and reduced morbidity [chronic lung disease, retinopathy of prematurity] without an increase in cerebral palsy have been observed among infants born less than 27 weeks' gestation who are maintained with oxygen saturations in the range of 84% to 94%.[23]) Desaturations or bradycardia that occur without apnea suggest airways obstruction (obstructive apnea). Although most neonatal units will not discharge a preterm infant until at least 34 weeks' postmenstrual age, if the decision is made to send such an infant home, then the option of a brief period of home monitoring should be considered, given that episodes of prolonged desaturation greater than 4 seconds occur frequently during periodic breathing or hypoventilation.[24] Infants who continue to exhibit cardiorespiratory instability with recurrent episodes of desaturation, apnea, or bradycardia requiring intervention should not be discharged from the hospital. The frequency of these episodes and the interventions required may be useful in determining the feasibility of the infant transitioning to a chronic-care facility versus remaining in an acute-care hospital.

Controversy exists regarding specific guidelines for discharging infants on home oxygen therapy. The concentration of oxygen to be used, its duration, the need for cardiorespiratory monitoring versus pulse oximetry, and strategies for weaning the infant from oxygen are areas of debate. Consultation with pediatric pulmonary specialists who will participate in the infant's postdischarge medical care is an additional important aspect of discharge planning for these infants (see Box 78-1).

BOX 78-1 Discharge Criteria for Home Oxygen Therapy

- Maintains oxygen saturations above 92%-93%
- Can cope with short periods without oxygen if the nasal cannula is removed or dislodged
- No apneic events for a predetermined period
- Immunizations up to date, and palivizumab prophylaxis as appropriate to the time of year of respiratory syncytial virus activity for the region where the child resides
- Parents and caregivers capable of caring for infant on home oxygen therapy
- Satisfactory home environment with a functioning telephone
- Satisfactory home environment with functioning electricity and adequate electrical outlets
- Home care visit completed (before discharge)
- Parents and caregivers trained on use of oxygen, equipment, and cardiopulmonary resuscitation
- Advice given for smoking cessation
- Advice given regarding avoidance of open-flame use in the presence of oxygen
- Parents or caregivers advised to travel with cylinders and inform their home and vehicle insurance companies
- Appropriate resources for parental help in place and emergency contact telephone numbers given to parents
- Communication with the primary care pediatrician completed (before discharge)

Adapted from Balfour-Lynn I, Primhak R, Shaw B, Home oxygen therapy for children: who, how and when? *Thorax*. 2005;60:76-81. Reprinted by permission of BMJ Publishing Group Ltd.

Experts recommend that infants with residual lung disease and infants at risk for developing pulmonary hypertension be discharged on home oxygen therapy if they are unable to maintain their oxygen saturation above 93%. Infants with chronic lung disease whose oxygen saturation is maintained above 93% on home oxygen with low-flow oxygen have been shown to have a reduced risk of sudden infant death, improved weight gain, lower pulmonary artery pressure and airway resistance, and fewer hypoxemic episodes.[25] The goal for oxygen therapy is to maintain the oxygen saturation equal to or greater than 95%. Oxygen, however, is not benign. Oxygen toxicity can occur in premature infants and contribute to ongoing lung injury, in addition to inhibiting lung healing.[26] Infants with documented persistent apnea also require home monitoring.[27,28] Some infants with persistent feeding difficulties may have increased oxygen or air-flow requirements to prevent desaturations during feeding. These infants typically have poor oromotor coordination and may have associated posterior pharyngeal dysfunction causing airway collapse. Provision of low-flow

BOX 78-2 Equipment Required for Home Oxygen Therapy

Oxygen concentrators are preferred with a back-up cylinder and portable cylinder for use during travel.

Oxygen concentrators require two outlets.

Low-flow meters must provide the appropriate flow range for infants and young children (many require less than 1-L/min of flow).

Humidification system required for some specific flow rates.

Appropriately sized nasal prongs required, with facemask and extension tubing.

Lightweight ambulatory equipment required.

Families must have functioning electricity and must be provided with documentation for the local electric company to prevent electricity disruption.

An assessment should be made regarding the need for an emergency generator as a back up electricity source.

Adapted from Balfour-Lynn I, Primhak R, Shaw B, Home oxygen therapy for children: who, how and when? *Thorax.* 2005;60:76-81. Reprinted by permission of BMJ Publishing Group Ltd.

air or low concentrations of oxygen may be beneficial in preventing episodes of desaturations or bradycardia during feeding. A feeding assessment by a qualified speech pathologist with infant feeding expertise will facilitate making this diagnosis and deciding the need for supplemental flow or oxygen during feeding.

After requirements for discharge are met, the required equipment (Box 78-2) is delivered, and the parents and other caregivers are properly trained, the type of monitoring required at home must be determined—a cardiorespiratory monitor or a pulse oximeter. Pulse oximetry is a method of measuring and monitoring arterial blood oxygenation. It provides a simple, noninvasive technique for measuring arterial oxygenation saturation. However, no evidence has been found that pulse oximetry improves the outcome of babies on home oxygen therapy. Pulse oximetry is notable for frequent false alarms, especially when the infant is active. In addition, oxygen saturation is only one measurement of an infant's respiratory status. A sick infant may still maintain normal oxygen saturation while receiving oxygen despite changes in other physiological parameters. Therefore the issue of discharging an infant with pulse oximetry remains controversial, although it is helpful in the periodic assessment of the infant's status with measurement of the infant's oxygenation during activity (bathing, crying), sleep, feeding, and while in a vehicle safety seat or infant seat.

Most third-party insurers have policies guiding their approval process for home oxygen therapy and home monitoring for high-risk groups of infants. The hospital caregivers will coordinate the initial insurance company approvals, but the pediatric primary care physician will need to become familiar with the specific insurer's guidelines regarding periods of coverage and authorizations required for continued therapy at home. The neonatal team in consultation with the pulmonary specialist typically determines the concentration of inspired oxygen and equipment required by the infant and provides the home health care company, equipment vendor, and the family with specific instructions for the equipment set-up and use. The equipment vendors typically provide the family with detailed instruction on the equipment set-up and use and provide 24-hour access for technical support and equipment replacement in the event a problem arises. No consensus exists about the optimal alarm settings required for home oxygen saturation monitoring, although, in general, typical alarm settings are heart rate greater than 200 beats per minute and less than 80 beats per minutes and oxygen saturation less than 80%.

An infant who is discharged on home oxygen therapy requires close medical follow-up. The infant should also have a follow-up visit with a pulmonary specialist, if feasible. In communities where appointments for subspecialty care are not easily accessible for families, the pediatric primary care physician will need to have an identified pulmonary specialist with whom to possibly consult on management issues.

Supplemental Oxygen Requirements During Air-Flight

An important, though infrequent, consideration is the potential need for supplemental oxygen during air flight for infants who families plan air travel after discharge. Commercial air travel has been shown to decrease oxygenation in children.[29,30] Experts recommend that children, particularly infants with residual lung disease, undergo a preflight assessment of their response to a hypoxemic challenge to determine their need for in-flight oxygen therapy. If the pulse oximeter saturation decreases below 85% during the hypoxic challenge test, then supplemental in-flight oxygen is necessary. For infants with a history of respiratory disease, experts recommend that supplemental oxygen be provided if the pulse oximeter saturation is less than 90%.[31,32] The majority of formerly preterm infants who are younger than 12 months' corrected age at the time of the proposed air travel and not requiring oxygen supplementation in room air are at risk for hypoxemia during air flight.[33] Infants at highest risk are younger than 3 months' corrected age, irrespective of whether the infant has chronic lung disease. This factor suggests that young infants with a history of neonatal respiratory disease should not undertake air travel without supplemental oxygen unless preflight hypoxia testing is performed.

Home Ventilation

Improving survival rates among very medically complex infants with severe cardiorespiratory disease, craniofacial anomalies, and neurologic abnormalities affecting respiratory control have resulted in a group of infants who require long-term ventilatory support and home ventilation. The discharge planning and care coordination of infants needing ventilator assistance at home requires extensive preparation and the coordination before the child and family can safely move to a community setting. Before considering home ventilation, the infant must be medically stable with stable ventilator settings for at least 1 week and require a fractional inspired oxygen concentration less than or equal to 0.4 (40% oxygen), have stable blood gases within the normal range for the infant's diagnosis, and have a secure airway with a mature tracheostomy that is healed (at least 1 week postoperative). The infant should not require intensive care (one-on-one) nursing or invasive monitoring.

The infant's parents must be committed to home ventilation, and adequate home health care personnel must be available, including the parent and at least one other person (parent or other family member or a registered or licensed practical nurse). If other children or individuals with developmental disabilities are in the home, then an intensive assessment should occur as to the feasibility, safety, and appropriateness of the infant's discharge to the home. Infants who are being discharged on home ventilation should have professional home nursing for at least 16 hours per day to support the safe transition of the infant from the hospital and ensure the parents' ongoing education and technical skills in managing the respiratory equipment.

The home environment needs to be evaluated by the equipment vendor and the home health care agency to ensure adequate space, electricity, and other utilities and a safe home environment. The respiratory equipment vendor must ensure 24-hour access and in-home support. The local community emergency medical services providers (fire department and emergency medical system) should be made aware of the infant's home ventilation need. Local utility companies, including telephone and electric companies, need to be made aware of the child's technology dependence to ensure that services are not interrupted. Arrangements for routine and emergency transport of the infant for primary, specialty, and emergency care visits must be clearly detailed. Community resources must also be identified and linkages established to ensure that the infant and family receive appropriate medical, psychosocial, and early intervention services. Parent and other home caregiver education must include tracheostomy care and changing, airway suctioning, medication administration, manual ventilation and resuscitation, and recognition of changes in the infant's status—lethargy or agitation, cyanosis, respiratory distress, temperature instability (hyperthermia or hypothermia), and dehydration.

Apnea, Bradycardia, and Desaturations

Apnea, bradycardia, and desaturation commonly occur in premature infants. A detailed discussion about the underlying pathophysiological mechanism is provided in Chapter 77, Continuing Care of the Infant After Transfer From Neonatal Intensive Care. The timing of discharge for a preterm infant with a history of apnea, bradycardia, and desaturation is controversial, as is the definition of when the infant can be deemed *medically stable* for discharge. Treatment of apnea, bradycardia, and desaturation depends on its underlying cause. The etiology of these signs further influences the decision regarding the appropriate time for discharge of an infant experiencing apnea, bradycardia, and desaturation. The standard practice is to delay the discharge of premature infants until they have achieved a set duration of days without any apnea, bradycardia, or desaturations.

No standard or universally accepted guidelines exist regarding the duration of this observation period or the effectiveness of delaying discharge. However, among the most immature infants, a period of observation that is too short may predispose a subset of infants to apparent life-threatening events at home. Apnea in the larger preterm infant resolves in the majority of affected infants by 34 to 36 weeks' postmenstrual age, with more than 90% of infants being apnea free by 37 weeks' postmenstrual age. The duration of apnea is extended, often not resolving until 40 to 43 weeks' postmenstrual age, among extremely low–birth-weight infants born at less than 28 weeks' gestation.[34] Premature infants may also exhibit apnea as a developmental process; however, persistent apnea may also occur because of other factors, such as sepsis, temperature instability, sedation, gastroesophageal reflux, and physiological instability in response to positioning and handling. Each infant needs to be evaluated individually when determining the cause of the apnea and the possibility of discharge. Infants requiring treatment with methylxanthines for apnea of prematurity should have medications discontinued when the preterm infant reaches 32 to 34 weeks' postmenstrual age and be apnea free for 7 to 10 days before discharge if home monitoring is not planned. Infants treated with caffeine require an extended period of observation for 7 days because of caffeine's long half-life; the period of observation after discontinuation of theophylline is somewhat shorter at 4 to 5 days.

Recommendations for the period of symptom-free days before hospital discharge for the infant who does not require home monitoring range from 3 to 8 days. Evidence suggests that continuing hospital care for preterm infants with significant apnea until cessation of apnea for a predetermined duration is a reasonable clinical practice.[35,36] Infants who have been apnea free for 8 days or more are unlikely to have another apneic episode, unless other associated complications exist.[37] In a survey of neonatal units, the margin of safety for infants with gestational age greater than or equal to 30 weeks between the last documented episode of apnea and hospital discharge was 5 to 7 days.[38] Zupancic et al explored the economic implications of monitoring for resolution of apnea of prematurity for a fixed number of days before discharge home. Results of the economic modeling performed demonstrated a sharp decline in the utility or *value* for the cost of continuing hospital care as the duration of monitoring increased and decreasing cost effectiveness for infants who were born at higher gestational ages. Currently, no studies have established either the efficacy or the cost effectiveness of the various durations of monitoring.[39]

Predischarge Polysomnography (Event Monitoring)

Predischarge monitoring of infants with a history of apnea of prematurity using 12- to 24-hour pneumocardiogram recordings are a routine aspect of discharge planning in some hospitals. A pneumocardiogram is a diagnostic test that provides a continuous recording of heart rate and respirations that can detect periods of central apnea and periodic breathing. A four-channel device also employs a nasal thermistor to detect airflow and a pulse oximeter to measure oxygen saturation through the activities occurring during the period of monitoring. The thermistor can help distinguish between central and obstructive apnea. Pneumocardiograms may be used as screening tests to determine which infants are at risk for life-threatening apnea; however, no evidence exists to support predischarge monitoring as predictive of life-threatening apnea or sudden infant death syndrome. In addition, although such studies may reveal ongoing episodes of apnea, bradycardia, or desaturation, they reflect the events over a limited time frame and may not identify all infants at continuing risk. The infant being tested may not exhibit signs during the examination. Therefore no current guidelines have been formulated to recommend the routine use of pneumograms in infants with apnea; however, distinguishing the type of apnea that an infant experiences may be useful clinically.

Home Apnea Monitoring

Apnea monitors were first introduced in the 1960s for managing apnea of prematurity in hospital settings.[40] Subsequently, home cardiorespiratory monitoring became widely used, with the hypothesis that sudden infant death syndrome (SIDS) might be prevented by monitoring for apnea. No scientific evidence has been found to support the premise that cardiorespiratory monitoring at home reduces the incidence of SIDS or that apnea is a precursor to SIDS.[27] Apnea of prematurity does not predispose an infant to SIDS, although prematurity, itself, is a risk factor for SIDS. The efficacy of home cardiorespiratory monitoring for siblings of infants who died of SIDS has also not been proven. Given the lack of evidence that home cardiorespiratory monitoring has any impact on SIDS, prevention of SIDS is not an acceptable indication for home cardiorespiratory monitoring. Di Fiore et al concluded that infants referred for apnea monitoring studies because of persistent bedside monitor alarms had very infrequent apnea of at least 20 seconds' duration. A high frequency of desaturation and bradycardia was noted in response to short respiratory pauses when compared with infants with no persistent bedside monitor alarms.[41] Some premature infants continue to experience recurrent apneic episodes despite evidence that they are otherwise ready for discharge because they have achieved full oral feeding and demonstrate appropriate temperature regulation. The decision to discharge a premature infant on home apnea monitoring is typically based on the infant experiencing *clinically significant cardiorespiratory events.* These events are defined as apnea greater than 20 seconds' duration, apnea of less than 20 seconds that is associated with bradycardia (heart rate [HR] less than 80 beats/min), a 33% drop in HR below the resting HR or a decline in the oxygen saturation below 85%, bradycardia with an HR less than 80 beats/min, or oxygen desaturation less than 80% for more than 5 seconds. Infants who have experienced apparent life-threatening events associated with apnea, color change, marked change in muscle tone with hypotonia or flacidity, and choking and gagging should also be considered for home apnea monitoring. Home monitoring until 43 to 45 weeks' postmenstrual age may offer an acceptable alternative to continued hospitalization if the parents are in agreement and if close coordination and follow-up care is provided by the pediatric primary care physician.[27]

Home monitoring may be also medically necessary and justified for other infants with significant medical conditions. Infants who are technology dependent requiring home ventilation (continuous positive airway pressure or nasal bilevel positive airway pressure), who have a tracheostomy or require home oxygen therapy, or who have neurologic or craniofacial abnormalities that affect respiratory control or function are typically discharged with home monitoring. The American Academy of Pediatrics offers specific recommendations for home cardiorespiratory monitoring (Box 78-3). Parents and caregivers must learn that home cardiorespiratory monitoring does not guarantee avoidance of sudden death from an underlying cause.

If home monitoring is prescribed, then the parents and other caregivers must be trained in the correct application and operation of the monitor and in infant cardiopulmonary resuscitation (see Tools for Practice). The family should have 24-hour access to an equipment specialist from the home care supply vendor, as well as medical support, should questions or problems arise with the equipment or its use. Most insurers have detailed policies that delineate eligibility requirements for the use of apnea monitors. Confirming with individual carriers whether the patient meets the criteria

BOX 78-3 Home Cardiorespiratory Monitoring

Home cardiorespiratory monitoring should not be prescribed to prevent SIDS.

Monitoring may be warranted for premature infants who are at high risk of recurrent episodes of apnea, bradycardia, and hypoxemia after hospital discharge.

Monitoring may be warranted for infants who are technology dependent (tracheostomy, continuous positive airway pressure), have unstable airways, have rare medical conditions affecting the regulation of breathing, or have symptomatic chronic lung disease.

If monitor is prescribed, then monitor should be equipped with an event recorder.

Parents should be advised that home monitoring does not prevent sudden, unexpected deaths in infants.

Pediatricians should continue to promote proven practices that decrease the risk of SIDS—supine sleep position, safe sleeping environments, and elimination of exposure to tobacco smoke.

SIDS, Sudden infant death syndrome.
From American Academy of Pediatrics, Committee on Fetus and Newborn. Apnea, sudden infant death syndrome, and home monitoring. *Pediatrics.* 2003;111:914-917.

for an apnea monitor according to the insurance company may be necessary.

Sleep Position

Guidance regarding safe infant sleep and sleep position is discussed in the section on Parent Education.

Vehicle Seat Safety

Preterm infants who have achieved readiness for hospital discharge are at an increased risk of respiratory compromise (desaturation, apnea, and bradycardia caused by poor postural tone, hypoventilation, and airway obstruction) when seated in standard vehicle seats. The American Academy of Pediatrics recommends that all premature infants born at less than 37 weeks' gestation at birth be assessed for cardiorespiratory stability in their vehicle seat before discharge. Experts recommend that infants should have a vehicle seat challenge test performed several days before the infant's anticipated discharge date during which the infant is placed in the vehicle seat to be used by the family for 60 to 90 minutes of continuous monitoring. Careful attention must be given to smaller infants who require proper positioning to maintain head, neck, and trunk stability. The American Academy of Pediatrics has made specific recommendations for the positioning of preterm infants in vehicle safety seats[42] (Box 78-4). In addition, the recommendation is that infants should not be left unsupervised in vehicle seats. Tremendous variation exists among neonatal units in the practice of predischarge vehicle seat testing, and among neonatal units where vehicle seat testing is conducted, variation in the indications for testing, duration of the observation period in the vehicle seat, and criteria for *passing* the challenge test exist.

Improper positioning of preterm infants, even infants born at 35 weeks' gestation can cause respiratory compromise. Poor postural tone contributes to slouching that can cause neck flexion and airway obstruction. Consideration regarding delaying the discharge home to allow for continued growth and maturation should be given to infants who, despite proper positioning and modifying the seat with blanket rolls or inserts, exhibit desaturations or other signs of cardiorespiratory compromise during the vehicle seat test. Although the recommendation for vehicle seat testing exists, an evidence base is not currently available that confirms the clinical importance of desaturations, bradycardia, or apnea experienced by preterm infants who are classified as *failing* the challenge test or that passing a vehicle seat challenge will improve the outcome in preterm infants.[43]

An alternative transportation device for infants is the vehicle bed.[44] Vehicle beds allow the infant to travel reclining rather than positioned vertically in a vehicle seat. Vehicle beds have been suggested as being more appropriate for transportation of infants at risk for desaturation, apnea, or bradycardia when in a vehicle seat. Vehicle beds can be positioned so the infant is flat or inclined at 30 degrees to allow an infant to travel supine or prone. Vehicle beds have been recommended for infants with medical conditions requiring prone or supine position, such as premature infants, infants after repair of myelomeningocele, or infants who must lie prone to maintain an open airway (eg, those with Pierre Robin sequence).[45] A recent investigation by Salhab et al comparing vehicle seat versus vehicle bed for infant transportation found no significant difference in the incidence of apnea, bradycardia, or desaturation in very low–birth-weight infants. Each infant was tested in an infant vehicle seat and a vehicle bed. The reported incidence of one or more cardiorespiratory events was 15% and 19%, respectively. Infants with chronic lung disease were more likely to have a vehicle seat event, whereas infants with lower gestational age at birth were at greater risk for a vehicle bed event.[46]

BOX 78-4 Recommendations for Positioning of Preterm Infants in Vehicle Safety Seats

- Use infant-only, rear-facing safety seats with three- or five-point harness systems.
- The vehicle safety seat should be semi-reclined to a 45-degree angle in the rear seat of the vehicle, ideally adjacent to an adult.
- Place the infant's buttocks and back firmly against the back of the vehicle safety seat to reduce slouching.
- The distance from the crotch strap to the seat back should be $\leq$14 cm and from the lower harness strap to the seat bottom should be $\leq$25 cm.
- Shoulder straps should be in the lowest slots until the infant's shoulders are above the slots.
- Place the retainer clip over the midpoint of the chest rather than on the abdomen or near the neck.
- The vehicle safety seat should not be placed in the front passenger seat of a vehicle with a passenger-side front air bag.
- The infant should not be left unattended in a vehicle safety seat.

From American Academy of Pediatrics, Committee on Injury and Poison Prevention and Committee on Fetus and Newborn. Safe transportation of premature and low birth weight infants. *Pediatrics.* 1996;97:758-60; Pilley E, McGuire W. The car seat: a challenge too far for preterm infants? *Arch Dis Child Fetal Neonat Ed.* 2005;90:f452-f455.

IMMUNIZATIONS

Routine Immunizations

Routine immunizations are required for all infants, including preterm and sick infants. Preterm and low–birth-weight infants are at greater risk of increased morbidity from vaccine-preventable diseases than term infants.[47] Therefore gestational age and birth weight should not deter an infant from receiving immunizations on schedule, except with specific criteria for the hepatitis B vaccine. In addition, vaccine doses should not be decreased or altered for preterm or low–birth-weight infants. The anterolateral thigh is the preferred site for administering intramuscular vaccines to preterm and low–birth-weight infants.

If an infant is in the NICU at 2 months of age, then routine vaccines including diphtheria and tetanus toxoids, acellular pertussis, *Haemophilus influenzae* type B conjugate, inactivated polio vaccine, and pneumococcal conjugated vaccine (Prevnar) will have been administered according to the schedule and doses for full-term infants according to the American Academy of Pediatrics and the Centers for Disease Control and Prevention.[48] The safety of these vaccines in preterm and low–birth-weight infants is comparable to that in full-term infants, with no increase in adverse reactions noted.[49,50] Routine vaccinations should also be given at 4 and 6 months of age.

Hepatitis B Vaccine

Hepatitis B vaccine is recommended for administration at birth or before discharge home from the hospital.[48] Recommendations for administering the hepatitis B vaccine to preterm neonates depend on the maternal hepatitis B status. Infants born to hepatitis B surface antigen–positive mothers will have received monovalent hepatitis B vaccine and hepatitis B immune globulin within 12 hours after birth, regardless of birth weight or gestational age. If the infant's birth weight was less than 2000 grams, then this dose does not count toward the three-dose hepatitis series. Three additional doses are required beginning at 1 month of age. In addition, these infants should be tested for anti–hepatitis B antibodies and hepatitis B surface antigen at 9 to 15 months of age after the immunization series has been completed.[51]

Medically stable preterm infants and infants weighing less than 2000 grams demonstrate predictable hepatitis B–antibody response and should receive the first dose of monovalent hepatitis B vaccine at 30 days' chronologic age, regardless of gestational age or birth weight. If hospital discharge occurs before 30 days, then the infant should be immunized before discharge. These infants should complete the three-vaccine series, and follow-up testing is not required. Medically stable infants who receive the vaccine at birth or at 30 days may receive a hepatitis B–containing combination vaccine beginning at 6 to 8 weeks of age,[51] regardless of whether their weight is less or greater than 2000 grams.

Respiratory Syncytial Virus Prophylaxis

Respiratory syncytial virus (RSV) is an important pathogen that causes lower respiratory tract infections in infants and young children. Premature infants may develop severe, fatal lower respiratory tract infections from RSV. Palivizumab should be given to infants and children younger than 24 months who were infants born at less than 32 weeks' gestation, infants with chronic lung disease, and infants with cardiovascular complications. Infants born from 32 to 35 weeks' gestation may be considered for prophylaxis if two or more risk factors are present, including child care attendance, school-aged siblings, exposure to environmental air pollutant, congenital abnormalities of the airway, or severe neuromuscular disorders.[52] Infants with chronic lung disease, hemodynamically significant congenital heart disease, or other serious conditions that compromise respiratory or immune function should also be scheduled to receive palivizumab monthly during the RSV season. Some hospital neonatal services provide a referral to the appropriate specialty pharmacy or community-based RSV-prevention program. The pediatric care physician must be familiar with immunoprophylaxis guidelines, local resources, and specific insurer and state Medicaid eligibility requirements to ensure that infants at risk receive treatment. Seasonal variation can be found in the timing of RSV infection geographically, with additional variation in regional peak infection rates. Palivizumab use should not interfere with the standard immunization schedule.[53]

Influenza Vaccine

Preterm and other medically fragile infants with chronic medical conditions are at high risk for complications and morbidities associated with the influenza virus infection. Plans for vaccine administration to the infant and family should be included in the discharge summary. If the infant is being discharged from the hospital during influenza season, then the child's parents and household contacts should be strongly encouraged to receive the influenza vaccine, particularly if the high-risk infant is younger than 6 months and is unable to be vaccinated.

Rotavirus Vaccine

Rotavirus is the most common cause of severe gastroenteritis in infants and young children worldwide.[54] In consideration of the potential risks for and benefits of vaccinating premature infants against rotavirus, the Centers for Disease Control and Prevention Advisory Council on Immunization Practices (ACIP) has encouraged providers immunize preterm infants born at less than 37 weeks' gestation between 6 and 12 weeks of age. Limited data suggest that preterm infants are at increased risk for hospitalization from viral gastroenteritis during their first year of life. The safety and efficacy of rotavirus vaccine appears to be similar for premature and term infants, although relatively few preterm infants have been evaluated in clinical trials. A theoretical concern exists that lower levels of maternal antibody to rotaviruses in very low–birth-weight premature infants have the potential to increase the risk for adverse vaccine reactions because the vaccine is administered as a live virus. Despite this caution, the ACIP supports vaccination of prematurely born infants if they are at least 6 weeks of age, are being or have been discharged from the hospital, and are clinically stable. The ACIP considers the benefits of vaccination of preterm infants against rotavirus to outweigh the theoretical risks. No safety or efficacy data are available regarding administration of rotavirus vaccine to immunocompromised infants. Rotavirus vaccine should also be deferred for 42 days after any administration of immune globulin.[54,55]

HEARING SCREENING

Universal newborn hearing screening has become the standard of care in the United States; currently more than 90% of newborn infants are screened before hospital discharge. The overall rate of permanent hearing loss at birth is 1 to 2 per 1000 live births. The prevalence of hearing loss increases with a child's advancing age because of progressive losses caused by genetic, hereditary, and acquired conditions, as well as environmental exposures. Among healthy newborn infants the incidence of permanent childhood hearing loss is 0.9 in 1000, in comparison with a prevalence of 9 to 13 per 1000 or 5% to 10% of infants requiring neonatal intensive care. The cause of hearing loss in childhood is equally distributed among hereditary or genetic conditions and environmental hazards or acquired conditions.

Infants who are at risk from environmental and acquired causes include those born preterm, babies with persistent pulmonary hypertension (particularly if extracorporeal membrane oxygenation and inhaled nitric oxide are required), those with TORCH infections (**t**oxoplasmosis, **o**ther agents, **r**ubella, **c**ytomegalovirus, **h**erpes simplex) and bacterial meningitis, and infants with significant hyperbilirubinemia. Among infants who have experienced persistent pulmonary hypertension, 17% to 30% will develop progressive sensorineural hearing loss. As a group, high-risk neonates are 10 times more likely to experience sensorineural hearing loss. Hyperbilirubinemia, prematurity, exposure to ototoxic medications, hypoxia, and infection predispose infants to auditory neuropathy (AN) and auditory dys-synchrony (AD). Infants with AN-AD have abnormal sound transmission to the brain and will have normal otoacoustic emissions (cochlear function) but will have abnormal brainstem-evoked responses (response to sound and the auditory neural pathway). Preterm infants who are born at 23 to 28 weeks' gestation experience the highest rates of AN-AD and sensorineural hearing loss and have a higher prevalence rate for AN-AD compared with more mature infants. In addition, young-for-gestational-age and low–birth-weight preterm infants with AN-AD have increased exposure to potentially ototoxic medications, an increased incidence of bronchopulmonary dysplasia, and extended hospitalizations. Prolonged hospital courses are caused by their multiple medical complications: intraventricular hemorrhage or periventricular leukomalacia, gastroesophageal reflux, retinopathy of prematurity, cholestasis, osteopenia, and anemia.[56-58]

Newborns who require an extended period of neonatal intensive care, particularly those with additional risk factors, are at risk for delayed-onset or progressive hearing loss. In addition to a hearing screen before discharge, these newborns should receive audiologic monitoring every 6 months until 3 years of age, as recommended by the Joint Committee on Infant Hearing. The indicators are listed in Box 78-5. (See Chapter 39, Auditory Screening, for more information.) Discharge planning for NICU infants should include newborn hearing screening preferably using a two-stage screening approach, with the initial screen performed to assess the infant's auditory brainstem response. If the infant does not pass this test, then otoacoustic emission testing should be initiated. Infants may be tested as early as 30 weeks' postmenstrual age, although the optimal time for the initial hearing screen is when the infant is at least 34 weeks' postmenstrual age. Infants who are at risk must be screened because infants requiring neonatal intensive care have been found to be more likely to miss predischarge screening for hearing loss.[59,60] An important point to note is that mild (20-40 dB) and low (conductive)–to-middle frequency (‹500-2000 Hz) hearing losses will not be identified on newborn screening. Continued hearing surveillance and periodic hearing testing is necessary for infants at risk for delayed onset and progressive hearing loss. Infants who fail or miss NICU hearing screening must have follow-up testing scheduled; infants with known hereditary (genetic) or acquired conditions associated with a high risk for hearing loss should be referred for medical evaluation and comprehensive otologic evaluation.

BOX 78-5 Risk Factors or Indicators for Infants With Delayed-Onset or Progressive Hearing Loss

1. Parental or caregiver concern regarding hearing, speech, language, or developmental delay
2. Family history of permanent childhood hearing loss
3. NICU stay >5 days, assisted ventilation >10 days, prolonged exposure to ototoxic medications (gentamicin and tobramycin) or loop diuretics (furosemide)
4. Postnatal infections associated with sensorineural hearing loss, including bacterial meningitis
5. In utero infections such as cytomegalovirus, herpes, rubella, syphilis, and toxoplasmosis
6. Neonatal indicators (eg, hyperbilirubinemia at a serum level requiring exchange transfusion, conditions requiring extracorporeal membrane oxygenation)
7. Stigmata or other findings associated with a syndrome known to include a sensorineural or conductive hearing loss or eustachian tube dysfunction
8. Syndromes associated with progressive hearing loss such as neurofibromatosis, osteopetrosis, and Usher syndrome
9. Neurodegenerative disorders
10. Head trauma
11. Recurrent or persistent otitis media for at least 3 months
12. Physical findings such as a white forelock associated with a syndrome known to include a sensorineural or permanent conductive hearing loss
13. Chemotherapy

NICU, Neonatal intensive care unit.
From American Academy of Pediatrics, Joint Committee on Infant Hearing. Year 2000 position statement: principles and guidelines for early hearing detection and intervention programs. *Pediatrics.* 2000;106:798-816; American Academy of Pediatrics, Joint Committee on Infant Hearing, Year 2007 position statement: principles and guidelines for early hearing detection and intervention programs. *Pediatrics.* 2007;120(4):898-921.

NEWBORN SCREENING

Newborn blood spot testing for a variety of metabolic, endocrine, and hematologic disorders is routine through the United States, the District of Columbia, Puerto Rico, US Virgin Islands, and Guam. Premature and sick neonates will often have serial testing performed during their NICU hospitalization based on established state protocols.[61] In contrast to healthy newborns who have their newborn blood spot test obtained at 2 to 3 days of age, sick and preterm newborns have their initial newborn screening sample obtained during the first hours of life because of the need for blood product administration or early initiation of parenteral nutrition. The amino acid contained in parenteral nutrition solutions can cause elevations in various amino acids levels (eg, phenylalanine, tyrosine), leading to a false-positive test result. Blood transfusions can also result in elevation in the blood spot hemoglobin A level; this elevated level will be detected on the newborn screen in states that test for hemoglobinopathies. Therefore screening tests will need to be repeated 3 to 4 months after a transfusion.

State screening protocols require repeat blood spot screens at 1 to 2 weeks and at 1 month of age for infants requiring prolonged hospitalization. Infants transferred to another facility should have their screening test before transfer and require coordinated follow-up between the medical care providers to ensure test results are known. Sick and extremely preterm infants often exhibit transient abnormalities in thyroid function that require monitoring to ensure that persistent thyroid dysfunction is not missed.[62] Another common abnormality identified on the early newborn screening tests of premature infants are elevations in 17-hydroxyprogesterone (17-OHP) levels, suggestive of congenital adrenal hyperplasia.[63-65] However, preterm infants frequently have high blood 17-OHP levels that decline as they mature. Weight-adjusted 17-OHP values may be used to reduce the incidence of false-positive results in premature neonates. Cystic fibrosis screening is included in the newborn screening panel in many states. The test process involves detection of immunoreactive trypsinogen (IRT) activity and cystic fibrosis transmembrane conductance regulator (CFTR) mutations.[66]

Current mutation analysis encompasses the gene mutations common among white individuals but does not detect the mutations more typically occurring in black patients. IRT levels may be elevated, causing false-positive test results in many conditions, including perinatal distress and prematurity; levels may be low (false-negative test) in infants with meconium ileus. Infants with meconium ileus are at risk for cystic fibrosis and should have a follow-up sweat test, even if the newborn screen is negative. Infants with abnormal IRT levels or identified CFTR mutations require a postdischarge sweat chloride test. Any newborn with an abnormal blood spot screen should have a repeat test before hospital discharge. The need for postdischarge testing will be based on the hospital-based test results. These newborns should be monitored for any signs or symptoms of the diagnosed disorder until the repeat screening results are available. Physical or metabolic signs suggestive of the presence of a screened condition should prompt appropriate diagnostic testing for the suspected disorder immediately.

RETINOPATHY OF PREMATURITY SCREENING

Conducting a thorough ophthalmologic evaluation and ensuring close follow-up care after hospital discharge are important aspects of eye care for extremely premature infants. Infants whose birth weight was less than 1500 grams or gestational age less than or equal to 30 weeks and selected infants with a birth weight between 1500 and 2000 grams or gestational age greater than 30 weeks who experienced an unstable clinical course, including the need for cardiorespiratory support or who are believed to be at high risk require ophthalmologic evaluation for the presence of retinopathy of prematurity (ROP). If the infant is to be discharged or transferred from the NICU before the first ROP examination at 4 to 6 weeks postnatal age, then an eye examination should scheduled. If concern exists about the family's ability to comply with the appointment or the availability of ophthalmologic examination at the transfer hospital, then consideration should be given to completing the initial examination performed before the infant is discharged. Communication with the pediatric ophthalmologist and family is necessary to ensure coordination of follow-up eye care. Table 78-2 and Box 78-6 provide a summary of recommendations for continuing ophthalmologic care.

Some infants may experience adverse effects from the medications uses to dilate the infant's eyes. Side effects include sweating, tearing, eye swelling, arrhythmias, apnea and bradycardia, hypertension, and eye irritation. In addition, the examination may be uncomfortable and stressful for the infant. Consequently, medically fragile infants require close monitoring after the examination. Infants at risk for ROP are also at risk for other eye disorders: strabismus, amblyopia, and cataracts. Infants with suspected congenital infection should undergo an ophthalmologic examination before discharge. If this examination is not possible before discharge, then a follow-up appointment should be made as soon as possible after discharge.

NEUROLOGIC EVALUATION

Premature and sick infants are at risk for brain abnormalities, including intraventricular hemorrhage, periventricular leukomalacia, perinatal stroke, hemorrhagic lesions from birth trauma, or encephalopathy, among other cerebral injuries. Both preterm and term neonates are vulnerable to hemorrhagic and ischemic injury. These abnormalities may lead to poor neurodevelopmental outcome. With advancing techniques in the area of ultrasonography, computed tomography (CT), and magnetic resonance imaging (MRI), information can be obtained that may help predict the infant's neurodevelopmental outcome.

Hemorrhagic brain lesions may involve the germinal matrix and the ventricles and extend into the brain parenchyma. Routine cranial ultrasonography is frequently performed in preterm infants and babies suspected of having intracranial abnormalities. Postdischarge neurosonography for ongoing surveillance of resolving hemorrhages, residual ventriculomegaly, or evolving periventricular leukomalacia or extraaxial fluid collections may be required. The American Academy of Neurology recommends

Table 78-2 Timing of First Eye Examination Based on Gestational Age at Birth

GESTATIONAL AGE AT BIRTH (in weeks)	AGE AT INITIAL EXAMINATION (in weeks)	
	POSTMENSTRUAL	CHRONOLOGIC
22*	31	9
23*	31	8
24	31	7
25	31	6
26	31	5
27	31	4
28	32	4
29	33	4
30	34	4
31†	35	4
32†	36	4

From American Academy of Pediatrics. Policy statement. screening examination of premature infants for retinopathy of prematurity. *Pediatrics.* 2006;117:572-576.
*This guideline should be considered tentative rather than evidence-based for infants with a gestational age of 22 to 23 weeks because of the small number of survivors in these gestational-age categories.
†If necessary.

BOX 78-6 Schedule of Follow-Up Examinations for Retinopathy of Prematurity (ROP)*

- 1-week or less follow-up for stage-1 or -2 ROP in zone I, or stage-3 ROP in zone II
- 1- to 2-week follow-up in the setting of immature vascularization in zone I (no ROP), stage-2 ROP in zone II, or regressing ROP in zone I
- 2-week follow-up for stage-1 ROP in zone II or regressing ROP in zone II
- 2- to 3-week follow-up in the setting of immature vascularization in zone II and no ROP, stage-1 or -2 ROP in zone III, or regressing ROP in zone III

*Based on the examining ophthalmologist's findings.
From American Academy of Pediatrics. Screening examination of premature infants for retinopathy of prematurity. *Pediatrics.* 2006;117:572-576.

that routine cranial sonographic screening be performed between 7 to 14 days of age on all newborns less than 30 weeks' postmenstrual age. A repeat scan should be performed between 36 and 40 weeks' postmenstrual age to detect the presence of periventricular leukomalacia.[67] Screening at these times can guide clinical care and inform predictions regarding the newborn's potential long-term neurodevelopmental outcome.

The American Academy of Neurology does not currently recommend that conventional MRI of the brain be performed on preterm infants with abnormal screening cranial ultrasounds because evidence as reviewed in 2002 was insufficient to support the utility of MRI in prediction of long-term outcome. However, recent studies suggest a role for MRI at term-postmenstrual age in predicting neurodevelopmental outcome.[68]

Individual hospital policies guide the level of sedation—conscious sedation or general anesthesia—required for completion of the MRI so as to limit motion artifact caused by infant movement. In addition, hospital policies may vary if the infant is an inpatient or an outpatient. If sedation is used, then the infant should be monitored after the procedure for evidence of cardiorespiratory depression, apnea, bradycardia, or desaturations. If an MRI is to be performed before the infant's discharge, then it should be obtained a few days before the anticipated discharge if feasible.

For term newborns who experience birth trauma, neonatal encephalopathy or seizures or have evidence of a perinatal stroke or other brain injury, a noncontrast CT scan and MRI are typically performed early in the neonate's hospital care. Follow-up studies are often performed 2 to 3 weeks after birth to provide information about the evolution of the brain injury and to provide information about the infant's prognosis. Discharge planning for these newborns requires follow-up neurologic care and referral to early intervention for periodic developmental surveillance or therapeutic services based on the child's specific needs.

SPECIALTY FOLLOW-UP CARE

Many infants who are ready for discharge from the NICU have experienced medical conditions requiring consultations with pediatric specialists. For example, infants with suspected (abnormal echocardiograms) or confirmed heart disease, neurologic injury or signs of neurologic dysfunction, renal dysfunction, or chronic lung disease should have pediatric specialty follow-up appointments scheduled as feasible. Due to geographic variations, it may not be possible for parents to bring their infant for follow-up appointments with subspecialists. Often, the pediatric, primary care physician must address specialty issues while consulting with the specialists. Some tertiary-care centers offer comprehensive neonatal or condition specific follow-up programs (craniofacial center, spina bifida clinic) in which appointments provide an opportunity for the infant to be assessed by a multidisciplinary team of specialists. Though coordinated, comprehensive care is optimal, insurers and state Medicaid guidelines may not provide reimbursement for multiple visits in a single day or specific components of the child's specialty care. This circumstance can present a challenge to both the family and pediatric primary care physician.

LABORATORY STUDIES

Discharge planning of a patient from the NICU may include obtaining specific laboratory tests to provide a baseline for the infant's biochemical or hematologic status at the time of hospital discharge. Decisions about what studies are necessary should be based on the individual infant's medical issues. For example, an infant with anemia should have a recent complete blood count and reticulocyte count before discharge. If the patient will be discharged on medications that require periodic drug level monitoring, such as phenobarbital, then drug levels should be obtained before discharge to ensure appropriate medication dosing. If the infant is on medications that can cause electrolyte abnormalities, such as diuretics, then a basic metabolic profile should be obtained. The infant with residual renal or liver dysfunction or metabolic bone disease (osteopenia) should have the appropriate studies to establish the infant's biochemical status at the time of discharge. The infant with cholestasis should have a liver function profile drawn. A baby with osteopenia should have calcium, phosphorous, and alkaline phosphorus levels checked before discharge. If patients are receiving medications to treat these disorders, then the dosages may need to be adjusted before discharge. Information about the proposed timing for any follow-up testing, if required, should be included in the infant's discharge recommendations.

CIRCUMCISION

Parents of medically stable male infants may request a circumcision before hospital discharge (see Chapter 91, Circumcision). The procedure may be performed by various medical professionals, including neonatologists, pediatricians, pediatric surgeons, obstetricians, and urologists. Circumcising a very-preterm infant who may weigh less than 2000 grams at the time of discharge may present a challenge because of the infant's small size at the time of discharge. The individual person performing the circumcision should be experienced with the procedure in the preterm infant. Prematurity is not a contraindication for circumcision; however, the infant should be clinically stable before circumcision.[69] No weight criteria or requirement exists for a specific penile size for a premature infant to have a circumcision performed; however, most institutions will delay circumcision until an infant is ready for discharge. An important point to remember is that preterm infants undergoing a circumcision may exhibit cardiorespiratory compromise in response to pain and the stress of the procedure. Monitoring these infants for a brief period after the procedure may be necessary. As with any infant undergoing a circumcision, appropriate pain management should be provided.

SOCIAL SERVICES AND CASE MANAGEMENT

The majority of hospitals have mechanisms to identify infants at social and environmental risk. Many neonatal units have established policies that offer the opportunity to or require that all families meet with a social worker. Social workers and case managers play an essential role in the care of any infant admitted to the NICU. They can assess the family constellation and family dynamics, identify risk factors that have the potential to influence the infant's care and family functioning, identify resource needs, and evaluate the adequacy of future home environment. Social workers also serve a vital role as advocates and support for all family members during the infant's NICU stay and can assist in assessing the mother for perinatal depression. They may also serve as liaisons between medical caregivers and community resources, such as child welfare agencies, that service at-risk children and families or community-based home health care programs. Social workers and care managers also assist in coordinating the discharge planning process, especially ordering equipment that the infant might need at home, such as an apnea monitor or oxygen-delivery system. The social worker can facilitate the preparation of paperwork that the parents might need.

INSURANCE COVERAGE

Third Party

On admission to the NICU, hospital personnel routinely verify insurance coverage for an infant and will assist the parents in obtaining necessary coverage, depending on the child's medical needs and the specific policies governing the existing insurance policy. In preparation for discharge, important reassessments include the scope of the infant's insurance coverage, whether the policy will be changed from one parent's plan to other parent's policy, and the scope of services covered for continuing outpatient and inpatient hospital care, primary pediatric, and subspecialty care, as well as coverage for durable medical equipment. Individual states have guidelines that determine Medicaid eligibility, physically handicapped children's program eligibility and requirements regarding potential exemptions from enrollment in Medicaid managed-care programs for children with special health care needs. Insurance carrier–driven policies may alter the infant's follow-up care because subspecialty follow-up may need to be with a different medical health care provider based on physician insurance plan participation.

Medicaid

Medicaid is the single largest insurer of children and is an important health resource, especially for children with special health care needs. Medicaid functions on the state and federal level. However, eligibility requirements, as recommended by the American Academy of Pediatrics, fall under federal legislation.[70]

Social Security

Many medically complex and extremely low–birth-weight infants are eligible to receive Supplemental

Security Income in addition to Medicaid. Neonates born with birth weights less than 1200 grams or who have medical complications such as blindness, deafness, or cerebral palsy may be eligible for Supplemental Security Income. The Social Security Administration eligibility requirements are available at www.ssa.gov.

Home Health or Public Health Nurse Visit

Infants who are ready to be discharged home from the NICU should have a home nursing visit scheduled, preferably within the first 2 days of discharge. Home nursing visit allows for a medical evaluation of the NICU graduate who is at home and in the care of the infant's parents or caregivers. Home nursing is also a resource that allows parents an opportunity for follow-up immediately after discharge. In addition, some infants may require a predischarge home visit, which can provide the medical team with information of potential safety problems that the infant may encounter after discharge. For example, if electricity is not working in the home, an infant's health may then be compromised. A predischarge home visit is important to assess the adequacy of the home environment and parental readiness for the infant's homecoming and can assist parents in their preparation for the infant's discharge. Individual hospital policies guide the specific discharge planning processes and define personnel roles and care-coordination responsibilities.

PARENT EDUCATION

Ideally, parental involvement in the care of a sick infant should begin at the time of the infant's admission to the NICU. Parental participation is vital during the NICU hospitalization and can aid the transition to home at the time of discharge. Parent involvement allows the parents the opportunity to gain an understanding of their infant's medical problems and become more comfortable with caring for and nurturing their infant. Ample time should be devoted to parent and other caregiver education.

INFANT SAFETY

Cardiopulmonary Resuscitation Training

Infants being discharged home from the NICU may be at continued risk for a health crisis and other apparent life-threatening events that may require cardiopulmonary resuscitation (CPR), such as apneas, bradycardias, and choking. Teaching parents and other caregivers the basic steps in CPR is a necessary part of discharge planning. A variety of tools are available to assist in CPR training, with personal training models available to teach parents and caregivers CPR, including videos or basic course instruction. Teaching materials are available from the American Heart Association. *Infant CPR Anytime* is a self-directed learning program that allows families and caregivers to learn core skills of infant CPR and choking prevention. The kit contains an infant manikin, practice video, sanitizing wipes, and reference guide (www.aap.org/family/infantcpranytime.htm). CPR teaching should be completed before the infant's discharge.

Sleeping Position

Prone sleeping position is a risk factor that has been identified for SIDS, and importantly, can be modified. Parents of all infants should be educated about the risk factor of prone sleeping and SIDS. Not only the parents, but also all caregivers should be educated. Prone sleeping has been recognized as a major risk factor for SIDS, with odds ratios ranging from 1.7 to 12.9 in various studies.[71,72]

Discussing sleeping position with parents before discharge is extremely important because many preterm infants are maintained in a prone position during the early stages of their NICU care. Parents and caregivers must be helped to understand that while the infant is hospitalized, the infant is on a cardiorespiratory monitor and under medical supervision. This positioning is frequently used as an adjunct to improve gastrointestinal reflux and other symptoms such as apnea in some infants and to facilitate development care and flexed positioning. Consequently, parents often believe that because the infant was placed prone in the NICU, this position is optimal for the infant or that the baby *became accustomed to that position* and is uncomfortable when placed supine. Preterm and low–birth-weight infants are at an increased risk for SIDS, and data suggest that the prone sleep position is a major factor in the incidence of SIDS in these patients.[73-75] Bhat et al demonstrated that, compared with term infants, premature infants ready for discharge sleep with fewer arousals and more central apneas in the prone position. Apnea of prematurity does not increase the risk of SIDS for premature infants.[76] Premature and low–birth-weight infants should be placed supine to sleep.

Exposure to Second-Hand Smoke

Many preterm and chronically ill infants have evidence of residual lung disease at the time of hospital discharge. Infants exposed to second-hand smoke from tobacco is at risk for medical conditions such as allergies, asthma, ear infections, pneumonia, permanent lung changes, SIDS, and learning disabilities.[77] However, premature infants are especially at risk. Parents and family members should be counseled about smoking cessation long before an infant is ready for discharge. Educating the parents and providing them with resources for smoking cessation can aid them and sometimes motivate them to quit smoking. Different pharmacotherapies, nicotine replacement therapies, and behavioral-modification programs exist to help with smoking cessation.[78] In addition, the Smoke-Free Home Project is a comprehensive, national effort to teach pediatricians methods to reduce children's second-hand smoke exposure through parental smoke cessation and harm reduction.[79]

Mothers who are breastfeeding should be encouraged not to smoke and should be provided with information about smoking cessation and a referral to a smoking-cessation program. If they cannot stop smoking, then these mothers should be encouraged to reduce the number of cigarettes smoked and to switch to a low-nicotine cigarette. Mothers who continue to smoke should be instructed to breastfeed before smoking a cigarette and to delay nursing or to express milk after smoking a cigarette. Despite their tobacco use, mothers who smoke should be encouraged to continue breastfeeding because the benefits to the infant outweigh potential risks. Breastfeeding mothers who desire to quit smoking may safely use the nicotine gum or nicotine transdermal patches. Safety in lactation has not been determined with nicotine gum; however, the gum exposes the infant only to nicotine and its metabolites and not the effects of smoking. Nicotine patches are designed to deliver a precise amount of nicotine transdermally over time. The infant is exposed to the effects of nicotine in the mother's milk. However, fewer effects occur than with smoking, and compared with other forms of nicotine therapies, the patch is more predictable.[80]

Preparation for Caregiving at Home: Rooming In

One technique to support parents also affords the family the opportunity to gain confidence in caring for their infant at home is rooming in with the infant for a defined period, during which time the parents assume all caregiving responsibilities. Support from the NICU staff is immediately available for answering questions or solving problems.

PRESCRIPTIONS AND MEDICATION ADMINISTRATION

Many infants will be discharged on multiple medications. Parents should have the medications filled before the infant's discharge, and they should be able to demonstrate their ability to administer the medications at the appropriate time and in the appropriate dose. Parents should be instructed to avoid adjusting or discontinuing medications on their own. Discussion should include assessment of the parents' understanding of the reason for each medication and what adverse effects, if any, to anticipate. Many NICUs have developed medication logs and care diaries as tools to help parents and caregivers keep track of their infant's treatments and other care. This tool can be helpful for infants on multiple medications, those with technology dependence, or those in families with multiple births.

CHILD FIND AND EARLY INTERVENTION

Preterm infants and any full-term neonate who require neonatal intensive care may be at risk for developmental delays and disabilities. The Individuals with Disabilities Education Act[81] requires all states to have a "comprehensive Child Find system" to ensure that all children in need of early intervention or special education services are located, identified, and referred. State-specific eligibility requirements vary, although all programs are guided by federal regulations.[82] Some states have elected to serve children who are at risk of developmental disability, even if the actual diagnosis has not been made.

Examples of eligibility criteria for referral to the Child Find system portion of the early intervention program include the following:

- Infants born at less than 32 weeks' gestation or with birth weights less than 1500 grams
- Infants who spend 10 days or more in the NICU
- Infants with prenatal exposure to drugs of abuse
- Infants exposed prenatally to therapeutic drugs with known developmental implications (antineoplastic, anticonvulsant, and psychotropic drugs)
- Any infant at risk for a developmental delay

Infants who are also at risk for developmental delay may include infants with suspected hearing loss and infants with experienced meningitis, a birth injury, or head trauma. Many infants will automatically meet eligibility requirements. Eligibility requirements vary from state to state, however, and include infants with chromosomal abnormalities, genetic disorders, inborn errors of metabolism, disorders reflecting disorders of the nervous system (neural tube defects), congenital infections, low birth weight (criteria vary by state), extreme prematurity (criteria vary by state), severe sensory impairment, HIV and severe infectious disease, toxic exposure, cerebral palsy, grade-III and grade-IV intraventricular hemorrhage, hydrocephalus, neuromuscular disorders, disorders of sense organs, brain injury, and technology dependency (tracheostomy).

Discharge Summary

History of Present Illness:
Include pertinent maternal, pregnancy, and birth history; Apgar score; and admission assessment (infant's gestational age, weight, length, head circumference, and critical vital signs and laboratory results).

Neonatal Intensive Care Unit (NICU) Problems:
Include all of the problems the infant was diagnosed with during the admission, and indicate which problems are currently diagnoses.

NICU Course by Systems or Medical Problems:
Make sure to include a section for routine health care maintenance issues, such as immunizations, neurosonographic examinations, and newborn screening tests (newborn screen, retinopathy of prematurity, and hearing).

Assessment

Discharge Plan and Follow-Up Care:
Include appointment with primary care pediatrician, subspecialty appointments, pending laboratory or diagnostics tests, Child Find referral, and plan for discharge nutrition, medications, monitoring, and any ongoing treatments.

Figure 78-1 Sample discharge summary format.

Neonatal Intensive Care Unit Discharge Planning Checklist

Name: ______________________ Medical Record Number: ____________

Category	Item	Check	Comment
General admission	Primary care physician	☐	
	Maternal laboratory tests and blood type	☐	
	Integrated medical delivery system (IMDS)	☐	
	Medicaid or insurance for infant	☐	
	Complete physical examination	☐	
Home, placement	Discharge to rehabilitation center; send summary	☐	
	Acute coronary syndrome (ACS) clearance, if necessary	☐	
	Home care referral	☐	
	Home nursing (if necessary)	☐	
	Equipment needed for discharge (apnea monitor, pulse oximeter, oxygen)	☐	
Tests, procedures	Feeding assessment; speech referral, if necessary	☐	
	Child-Find or early interventions	☐	
	Vaccinations	☐	
	Synagis and referrals for prophylaxis	☐	
	Circumcision	☐	
	Head ultrasound	☐	
	Retinopathy of prematurity	☐	
	Hearing test: otoacoustic emissions (OAE) testing for all, and possible auditory brain-stem response (ABR), if criteria is met	☐	
	Hip ultrasound: if abnormal examination and if female and breach	☐	
	Vehicle seat challenge	☐	
Parent education	General teaching for baby care (ie, bathing, feeding)	☐	
	Medication administration	☐	
	Cardiopulmonary resuscitation	☐	
	Smoking-cessation plan, if necessary	☐	
	Feeding plans: how to mix formula, instructions for feeding	☐	
	Rooming in, if necessary	☐	
Final discharge disposition	Medical clearance	☐	
	Social work and ACS clearance	☐	
	Prescription available to parents before discharge	☐	
	Women, infants, children (WIC) program form and prescription for special formula	☐	
	Discharge physical (including weight, length, head circumference, hips, hernias, red reflex)	☐	
	Parent notification	☐	
	Primary care provider appointment	☐	
	Transfer of responsibility to provincial medical director (PMD)	☐	
	All other appointments	☐	

Figure 78-2 Neonatal intensive care unit discharge planning checklist.

DISCHARGE SUMMARY AND FOLLOW-UP CARE

Follow-up care of the discharged NICU graduate is essential to the medical care of the neonate. The primary care professional should receive a detailed summary of the infant's hospital course and continuing care needs. Optimally, the NICU staff should communicate personally with the pediatric primary care physician to discuss and evaluate the salient issues for the child and family. Consideration should be given to allocating additional time for the initial primary care visit because the primary care physician not only has to become familiar with the child's prior and current medical issues, but also has to ascertain from the parents how the first days at home have gone and what their particular concerns may be. Follow-up specialty appointments should also be scheduled before the infant's discharge. The timing of initial pediatric primary care appointment depends on individual patient medical problems. For high-risk infants the follow-up appointment should occur within a few days of NICU discharge. Parents should be given a copy of the infant's medical summary and a schedule of follow-up appointments at the time of discharge (Figures 78-1 and 78-2).

TOOLS FOR PRACTICE

Engaging Patient and Family

- *Infant CPR Anytime* (toolkit), American Heart Association (www.aap.org/bookstore).

Medical Decision Support

- *Neonatal Resuscitation Program,* American Academy of Pediatrics (www.aap.org/nrp/nrpmain.html).

RELATED WEB SITES

- California Perinatal Quality Care Collaborative (www.cpqcc.org/).
- Child Find (www.childfindidea.org/).
- National Lung Health Education Program (www.nlhep.org/).

AAP POLICY STATEMENTS

American Academy of Pediatrics, Committee on Fetus and Newborn. Hospital discharge of the high-risk neonate proposed guidelines. *Pediatrics*. 1998:102(2):411-417. (aappolicy.aappublications.org/cgi/content/full/pediatrics;102/2/411).

American Academy of Pediatrics, Committee on Fetus and Newborn. Safe transportation of premature and low birth weight infants. *Pediatrics*. 1996;97:758-760. (aappolicy.aappublications.org/cgi/content/abstract/pediatrics;97/5/758).

American Academy of Pediatrics, Committee on Injury and Poison Prevention. Transporting children with special health care needs. *Pediatrics*. 1999;104(4):988-992. (aappolicy.aappublications.org/cgi/content/full/pediatrics;104/4/988).

American Academy of Pediatrics, Committee on Practice and Ambulatory Medicine and Committee on Fetus and Newborn. The role of the primary care pediatrician in the management of high-risk newborn infants. *Pediatrics*. 1996;98(4):786-788. (aappolicy.aappublications.org/cgi/content/abstract/pediatrics;98/4/786).

Council on Children With Disabilities, Section on Developmental Behavioral Pediatrics; Bright Futures Steering Committee, and Medical Home Initiatives for Children With Special Needs Project Advisory Committee. Identifying infants and young children with developmental disorders in the medical home: an algorithm for developmental surveillance and screening. *Pediatrics*. 2006;118:405-420. (aappolicy.aappublications.org/cgi/content/full/pediatrics;118/1/405).

Saari TN, American Academy of Pediatrics, Committee on Infectious Diseases. Immunization of preterm and low birth weight infants. *Pediatrics*. 2003;112(1):193-198. (aappolicy.aappublications.org/cgi/content/full/pediatrics;112/1/193).

SUGGESTED RESOURCES

Nutrition

The Academy of Breastfeeding Medicine. Clinical Protocol #12: Transitioning the Breastfeeding/Breastmilk-fed Premature Infant from the Neonatal Intensive Care Unit to Home. Available at: www.bfmed.org/ace-files/protocol/nicugradprotocol.pdf. Accessed August 1, 2007.

The American Academy of Pediatrics. *Pediatric Nutrition Handbook*. 5th ed. Elk Grove Village, IL: American Academy of Pediatrics; 2004.

Oxygen Therapy

Kotecha S. Oxygen therapy for infants with chronic lung disease. *Arch Dis Child Fetal Neonatal Ed.* 2002;87:f11-f14.

Immunization of Premature Infants

D'Angio CT. Active immunization of premature and low birth weight infants: a review of immunogenicity, efficacy and tolerability. *Pediatr Drugs*. 2007;9:17-32.

Sen S, Cloete Y, Hassan K, et al. Adverse events following vaccination in premature infants. *Acta Paediatr.* 2001;90:916-920.

Wu S-Y, Bonaparte J, Pyati S. Palivizumab use in very premature infants in the neonatal intensive care unit. *Pediatrics*. 2004;114:e554-e556.

Hearing Screening

American Academy of Pediatrics, Task Force on Newborn and Infant Hearing. Newborn and infant hearing loss: detection and intervention. *Pediatrics*. 1999;103:527-530.

Neurologic Follow-up

Perlman JM, Rollins N. Surveillance protocol for the detection of intracranial abnormalities in premature neonates. *Arch Pediatr Adolesc Med*. 2000;154:822-826.

Volpe J. *Neurology of the Newborn*. 3rd ed. Philadelphia, PA: WB Saunders; 1995.

Woodward LJ, Anderson PJ, Austin NC, et al. Neonatal MRI to predict neurodevelopmental outcomes in preterm infants. *N Engl J Med*. 2006;355:685-694.

REFERENCES

1. American Academy of Pediatrics, Committee on Fetus and Newborn. Hospital discharge of the high-risk neonate proposed guidelines. *Pediatrics*. 1998;102(2 pt 1): 411-417.
2. American Academy of Pediatrics, Council on Children With Disabilities. Care coordination in the medical home: integrating health and related systems of care for children with special health care needs. *Pediatrics*. 2005; 116(5):1238-1244.
3. Johnson CP, Kastner TA and the American Academy of Pediatrics, Committee/Section on Children With Disabilities. Helping families raise children with special health care needs at home. *Pediatrics*. 2005;115(2):507-511.

4. Clark R, Thomas P, Peabody J. Extrauterine growth restriction remains a serious problem in prematurely born neonates. *Pediatrics.* 2003;111(5):986-990.
5. Hofman PL, Regan F, Jackson WE, et al. Premature birth and later insulin resistance. *N Engl J Med.* 2004;351:2179-2186.
6. Ong KK, Ahmed ML, Emmett PM, et al. Association between postnatal catch up growth and obesity in childhood: prospective cohort study. *BMJ.* 2000;320:967-971.
7. Griffin I. Nutritional assessment in preterm infants. In: Cooke RJ, Vandenplas Y, Wahn U, eds. *Nutrition Support for Infants and Children at Risk. Nestlé Nutrition Workshop Service Pediatric Program.* Basel, Switzerland: S. Karger AG; 2007.
8. The Academy of Breastfeeding Medicine. Clinical Protocol #12: Transitioning the Breastfeeding/Breastmilk-fed Premature Infant from the Neonatal Intensive Care Unit to Home. Available at: www.bfmed.org/ace-files/protocol/nicugradprotocol.pdf. Accessed August 1, 2007.
9. California Perinatal Quality Care Collaborative. Nutritional Support of the Very Low Birth Weight Infant: Part II Quality Improvement Toolkit. Section IV: Sustaining Nutrition and Breastfeeding Through Discharge and Beyond. Available at: www.cpqcc.org/nutritioniitoolkit2.htm. Accessed July 30, 2007.
10. California Perinatal Quality Care Collaborative. Nutritional Support of the Very Low Birth Weight Infant: Part II Quality Improvement Toolkit. Appendix S: A Guide for Breastfeeding Your Premature Baby at Home. Available at: www.cpqcc.org/nutritioniitoolkit2.htm. Accessed July 30, 2007.
11. Oregon Department of Human Services, Child Development & Rehabilitation Center, Nutrition & Health Screening—WIC Program, Oregon Pediatric Nutrition Practice Group. Nutrition Practice Care Guidelines for Preterm Infants in the Community, 2006. Available at: www.oregon.gov/dhs/ph/wic/docs/preterm.pdf. Accessed July 30, 2007.
12. Buckley KM, Charles GE. Benefits and challenges of transitioning preterm infants to at-breast feedings. *Int Breastfeed J.* 2006;1:13.
13. Smith MM, Durkin M, Hinton VJ, et al. Initiation of breastfeeding among mothers of very low birth weight infants. *Pediatrics.* 2003;111:1337-1342.
14. Sisk PM, Lovelady CA, Dillard RA, et al. Lactation counseling for mothers of very low birth weight infants: effect on maternal anxiety and infant intake of human milk. *Pediatrics.* 2006;117(1):e67-e75.
15. Ehrenkranz RA, Ackerman BA. Metocloopramide effect on faltering milk production by mothers of premature infants. *Pediatrics.* 1986;78:614.
16. Hurst NM, Valentine CJ, Renfro L, et al. Skin-to-skin holding in the neonatal intensive care unit influences maternal milk volume. *J Perinatol.* 1997;17(3):213-217.
17. Lawrence R, Lawrence R. *Breastfeeding: A Guide for the Medical Profession.* 6th ed. St Louis, MO: Mosby; 1999:1091.
18. Lawrence R, Lawrence R. *Breastfeeding: A Guide for the Medical Profession.* 6th ed. St Louis, MO: Mosby; 1999:397-402.
19. Mattison D. Safety of Herbal Supplements with Breastfeeding. 2004. Available at: www.hpakids.org/holistic-health/articles/115/1/safety-of-herbal-supplements-with-breastfeeding. Accessed August 1, 2007.
20. US Department of Agriculture, Food and Nutrition Services. Women, Infants, and Children. Available at: www.fns.usda.gov/wic. Accessed July 30, 2007.
21. Merenstein G, Gardner S, Heat balance. In: *Handbook of Neonatal Intensive Care.* 6th ed. St Louis, MO: Mosby; 2006:126.
22. Garg M, Kurner SI, Bautista DB, et al. Clinically unsuspected hypoxia during sleep and feeding in infants with bronchopulmonary dysplasia. *Pediatrics.* 1988;81:635-642.
23. Tin W, Milligan DW, Pennefather P, et al. Pulse oximetry, severe retinopathy and outcome at one year in babies less than 28 weeks gestation. *Arch Dis Child Fetal Neonatal Ed.* 2001;84(2):F106-F110.
24. Razi NM, DeLauter M, Pandit PB. Periodic breathing and desaturation in preterm infants at discharge. *J Perinatol.* 2002;22:442-444.
25. Poets CF. When do infants need additional inspired oxygen? A review of the current literature. *Pediatr Pulomonol.* 1998;26:424-428.
26. Balfour-Lynn I, Primhak R, Shaw B. Home oxygen therapy for children: who, how and when? *Thorax.* 2005;60:76-81.
27. American Academy of Pediatrics, Committee on Fetus and Newborn. Apnea, sudden infant death syndrome and home monitoring. *Pediatrics.* 2003;111:914-917.
28. American Academy of Pediatrics, Task Force on Sudden Infant Death Syndrome. The changing concept of sudden infant death syndrome: diagnostic coding shifts, controversies regarding sleeping environment, and new variables to consider in reducing risk. *Pediatrics.* 2005;116(5):1245-1255.
29. Lee AP, Yamamoto LG, Relles NL. Commercial air travel decreases oxygen saturation in children. *Pediatr Emerg Care.* 2002;18:78-80.
30. Samuels MP. The effects of flight and altitude. *Arch Dis Child.* 2004;89:448-455.
31. British Thoracic Society, Standards of Care Committee. Managing passengers with respiratory disease planning air travel: British Thoracic Society recommendations. *Thorax.* 2002;57(4):289-304.
32. Burchdahl R, Bush A, Ward S, et al. Pre-flight hypoxic challenge in infants and young children with respiratory disease. *Thorax.* 2004;59(11):1000.
33. Udomittipong K, Stick SM, Verheggen M, et al. Pre-flight testing of preterm infants with neonatal lung disease: a retrospective review. *Thorax.* 2006;61:343-347.
34. Eichenwald EC, Aina A, Stark AR. Apnea frequently persists beyond term gestation in infants delivered at 24-28 weeks. *Pediatrics.* 1997;100:354-359.
35. Baird TM. Clinical correlates, natural history, and outcome of neonatal apnoea. *Semin Neonatol.* 2004;9:205-211.
36. Subhani M, Katz S, DeCristofaro JD. Prediction of post-discharge complications by predischarge event recordings in infants with apnea of prematurity. *J Perinatol.* 2000;2:92-95.
37. Darnall R, Kattwinkel J, Nattie C, et al. Margin of safety for discharge after apnea in preterm infants. *Pediatrics.* 1997;100:795-801.
38. Eichenwald EC, Blackwell M, Llyod JS, et al. Inter-neonatal intensive care unit variation in discharge timing: influence of apnea and feeding management. *Pediatrics.* 2001;108:928-933.
39. Zupancic J, Richardson D, O'Brien B, et al. Cost-effectiveness analysis of predischarge monitoring for apnea of prematurity. *Pediatrics.* 2003;111(1):146-152.
40. Daily WJ, Klaus M, Meyer HB. Apnea in premature infants: monitoring, incidence, heart rate changes, and an effect of environmental temperature. *Pediatrics.* 1969;43:510-518.
41. Di Fiore J, Arko M, Miller M, et al. Cardiorespiratory events in preterm infants referred for apnea monitoring studies. *Pediatrics.* 2001;108(6):1304-1308.

42. American Academy of Pediatrics, Committee on Injury and Poison Prevention and Committee on Fetus and Newborn. Safe transportation of premature and low birth weight infants. *Pediatrics.* 1996;97:758-760.
43. Pilley E, McGuire W. The car seat: a challenge too far for preterm infants? *Arch Dis Child Fetal Neonat Ed.* 2005; 90:f452-f455.
44. Kinane TB, Murphy J, Bass JL et al. Comparison of respiratory physiologic features when infants are placed in car safety seats or car beds. *Pediatrics.* 2006;118: 522-527.
45. American Academy of Pediatrics, Committee on Injury and Poison Prevention. Transporting children with special health care needs. *Pediatrics.* 1999;104: 988-992.
46. Salhab WA, Khattak A, Tyson JE, et al. Car seat or car bed for very low birth weight infants at discharge. *J Pediatr.* 2007;150:224-228.
47. Long SS, Pickering LK, Prober CG, eds. *Principles and Practice of Pediatric Infectious Diseases.* New York, NY: Churchill Livingstone; 1997.
48. Centers for Disease Control and Prevention. Recommendations and Guidelines: Advisory Committee on Immunization Practices (ACIP). Available at: www.cdc.gov/vaccines/recs/acip/default.htm. Accessed August 2, 2007.
49. Khalak R, Pichichero ME, D'Angio CT. Three-year follow-up of vaccine response in extremely preterm infants. *Pediatrics.* 1998;101:597-603.
50. Pfister RE, Afschbach V, Niksic-Stuber V, et al. Safety of DTaP-based combined immunization in very low birth weight premature infants: frequent but mostly benign cardiorespiratory events. *J Pediatr.* 2004;145:58-66.
51. Saari T, American Academy of Pediatrics, Committee on Infectious Diseases. Immunization of preterm and low birth weight infants. *Pediatrics.* 2003;112:193-198.
52. American Academy of Pediatrics. Respiratory syncytial virus. In: Pickering LK, Baker CJ, McMillan J, et al, eds. *2006 Red Book: Report of the Committee on Infectious Diseases.* 27th ed. Elk Grove Village, IL: American Academy of Pediatrics; 2006:561-566.
53. American Academy of Pediatrics. Respiratory syncytial virus. In: Pickering LK, Baker CJ, McMillan J, et al, eds. *2006 Red Book: Report of the Committee on Infectious Diseases.* 27th ed. Elk Grove Village, IL: American Academy of Pediatrics; 2006:561-566.
54. Prashar UD, Alexander JP, Glass RI, Centers for Disease Control and Prevention. Prevention of rotavirus gastroenteritis among infants and children: recommendations of the Advisory Committee on Immunization Practices (ACIP). *MMWR Recomm Rep.* 2006;55(RR-12):1-13.
55. American Academy of Pediatrics, Committee on Infectious Diseases. Policy statement: prevention of rotavirus: guidelines for use of rotavirus vaccine. *Pediatrics.* 2007;119(1):171-182.
56. Rance G, Beer DE, Cone-Wesson B, et al. Clinical findings for a group of infants and young children with auditory neuropathy. *Ear Hear.* 1999;20(3):238-252.
57. Hood LJ. Auditory neuropathy: what is it and what can we do about it? *Hear J.* 1998;51:10-18.
58. Berg AL, Spitzer JB, Towers HM, et al. Newborn hearing screening in the NICU: profile of failed auditory brainstem response/passed otoacoustic emission. *Pediatrics.* 2005;116(4):933-938.
59. Spivak L, Dalzell L, Berg A, et al. New York State Universal Newborn Hearing Screening Demonstration Project: inpatient outcome measures. *Ear Hear.* 2000;21(2):92-103.
60. Prieve B, Dalzell L, Berg A, et al. The New York State Universal Newborn Hearing Screening Demonstration Project: outpatient outcome measures. *Ear Hear.* 2000; 21(2):104-117.
61. Kaye C, American Academy of Pediatrics, Committee on Genetics. Introduction to the newborn screening fact sheets. *Pediatrics.* 2006;118:1304-1312.
62. Reuss ML, Leviton A, Paneth N, et al. Thyroxine values from newborn screening of 919 infants born before 29 weeks' gestation. *Am J Public Health.* 1997;87:1693-1697.
63. King JL, Naber JM, Hopkin RJ, et al. Antenatal corticosteroids and newborn screening for congenital adrenal hyperplasia. *Arch Pediatr Adolesc Med.* 2001;155:1038-1042.
64. Linder N, Davidovitch N, Kogan A, et al. Longitudinal measurements of 17α-hydroxyprogesterone in premature infants during the first three months of life. *Arch Dis Child Fetal Neonatal Ed.* 1999;81:F175-F178.
65. Olgemöller B, Roscher AA, Liebel B, et al. Screening for congenital adrenal hyperplasia: adjustment for 17-hydroxyprogesterone cut-off values to both age and birth weight markedly improves the predictive value. *J Clin Endocrinol Metab.* 2003;88:5790-5794.
66. Comeau AM, Accurso FJ, White TB, et al. Guidelines for implementation of cystic fibrosis screening programs: cystic fibrosis foundation workshop report. *Pediatrics.* 2007;119:e495-e518.
67. American Academy of Neurology. Practice parameter: neuroimaging of the neonate. Report of the Quality Standards Subcommittee of the American Academy of Neurology and the Practice Committee of the Child Neurology Society. *Neurology.* 2002;58:1726-1738.
68. Canadian Paediatric Society. Statement FN2001-01: routine screening cranial ultrasound examinations for the prediction of long-term neurodevelopmental outcomes in preterm infants. *Paediatr Child Health.* 2001;6:39-43.
69. American Academy of Pediatrics, Task Force on Circumcision. Circumcision policy statement. *Pediatrics.* 1999;103:686-693.
70. American Academy of Pediatrics, Committee on Child Health Financing. Medicaid policy statement. *Pediatrics.* 2005;116:274-280.
71. Ponsonby AL, Dwyer T, Giboons LE, et al. Factors potentiating the risk of sudden death syndrome associated with prone position. *New Engl J Med.* 1993;329:377-382.
72. Dwyer T, Ponsonby AL, Newman NM, et al. Prospective cohort study of prone sleeping position and sudden infant death syndrome. *Lancet.* 1991;337:1244-1247.
73. Mitchell EA, Scragg RK, Stewart AW, et al. Results from the first year of the New Zealand cot death study. *NZ Med J.* 1991;104(906):71-76.
74. Irgens LM, Markestad T, Baste V, et al. Sleeping position and sudden infant death syndrome in Norway 1967-91. *Arch Dis Child.* 1995;72:478-482.
75. Taylor JA, Drieger JW, Reay DT, et al. Prone sleep position and the sudden infant death syndrome in King County Washington: a case-control study. *J Pediatr.* 1996;128:626-630.
76. American Academy of Pediatrics, Task Force on Infant Sleep Position and Sudden Death Syndrome. Changing concepts of sudden infant death syndrome: implications for infant sleeping environment and sleep position. *Pediatrics.* 2000;105:650-656.
77. Platt MJ, Pharoah POD. Child health statistical review, 1996. *Arch Dis Child.* 1996;75:527-533.
78. The National Lung Health Education Program. Available at: www.nlhep.org. Accessed August 2, 2007.
79. Kamara S, Best D. *Smoke Free Homes: Pediatric Clinicians Making Children's Homes Smoke Free, Children's Medical Currents.* Vol. 15, No. 3. Washington DC: Children's National Medical Center; 2004.
80. Lawrence R, Lawrence R. *Breastfeeding: A Guide for the Medical Profession.* 6th ed. St Louis, MO: Mosby; 1999:598-599.

81. US Department of Education, Office of Special Education Programs. Child Find. Available at: www.childfindidea.org/. Accessed August 2, 2007.
82. The National Early Childhood Technical Assistance Center, State Part C Coordinators. Available at: www.nectac.org/contact/ptccoord.asp. Accessed August 2, 2007.

Chapter 79

SUPPORT FOR FAMILIES WHOSE INFANT IS SICK OR DYING: COLLABORATIVE DECISION MAKING

Joseph A. Vitterito II, MD; George A. Little, MD

The greatest risk of dying is in the perinatal period. For expecting families, birth is usually a moment filled with surprise, joy, and some trepidation about the responsibility of caring for a new life. With the birth of a premature or sick infant, emotions become fraught with shock, sadness, and possibly anger and grief.

Premature births in the United States have risen to record levels. Since 1981, the year the government began separately reporting premature births, the rate has increased 30%. Additionally, the rates of low–birth-weight and multiple births have also increased, significantly contributing to morbidity and mortality in the newborn population (Table 79-1).[1]

Neonatal diseases range from prematurity to such entities as respiratory distress, birth asphyxia, and sepsis. Box 79-1 lists the six leading causes of infant morbidity based on common diagnoses of infants admitted for intensive care and five causes of infant mortality.

Full-term newborns account for up to 40% of neonatal intensive care unit (NICU) admissions. The remainder of advanced neonatal care is for premature infants. When a newborn requires more than general newborn care, the family will also require care beyond congratulatory support and anticipatory guidance.

ROLE OF THE PRIMARY CARE PHYSICIAN

Whether providing direct care for a sick neonate, arranging for transfer to a tertiary-care facility, or providing follow-up care, the primary care pediatrician (PCP) has important and unique responsibilities, especially providing continuity in a medical home. To best support the infant and family, the PCP should be familiar with the guidelines in Box 79-2.[2] The complete guidelines provide PCPs with specific suggestions related to initiating and coordinating acute and longitudinal care, counseling families, and, crucially, communicating with families. These combined precepts are the cornerstone for supporting families.

Trust

Trust is the fundamental premise of an effective and dynamic professional relationship with families. Trust, in turn, facilitates communication. Transparency allows for a fluid dialogue. For the family members, informed consent establishes that the infant is, in fact, their baby.

BOX 79-1 Common Causes of Infant Morbidity and Mortality

MORBIDITY*
- Birth asphyxia
- Congenital and cardiac anomalies
- Infection
- Prematurity
- Respiratory distress syndrome
- Seizures

MORTALITY†
- Congenital malformations (20%)
- Prematurity and low birth weight (17%)
- Sudden infant death syndrome (8%)
- Maternal complications (6%)
- Placenta, cord, or membrane complications (4%)

*Common diagnoses of infants admitted at Dartmouth Hitchcock Medical Center, Intensive Care Nursery.
†Leading causes of infant death from Hoyert D, Mathews TJ, Menacker, et al. Annual summary of vital statistics: 2004. *Pediatrics.* 2006;117:168-183.

Table 79-1 Percentage of Preterm, Low–Birth-Weight, and Multiple Births

CHARACTERISTIC	PERCENTAGE OF BIRTHS		
	1990	2003	2004
BIRTH WEIGHT			
Very low (<1500 g)	1.3	1.4	1.5
Low (<2500 g)	7.0	7.9	8.1
Preterm	10.6	12.3	12.5
MULTIPLE BIRTHS PER 1000 TOTAL BIRTHS			
Live births in twin deliveries	2.3	3.2	—
Live births in higher-order multiple deliveries	0.1	0.2	—

BOX 79-2 Role of Primary Care Physician (PCP) in the Management of High-Risk Newborn Infants

Guideline 1—To make timely decisions, the PCP should be knowledgeable regarding problems that may occur in the perinatal period.

Guideline 2—The PCP acts as an important communication link between the family and the personnel of the center providing critical care, whether or not they are both located in the same institution.

Guideline 3—The PCP should have the expertise to assume responsibility for the acute, although less critical, care of the infant.

Guideline 4—The PCP should understand the need for proper continuity of care and be capable of providing it.

Guideline 5—The PCP should share responsibility with the neonatologist for the development and delivery of effective services in the hospital and community for newborns.

From American Academy of Pediatrics, Committee on Practice and Ambulatory Medicine and Committee on Fetus and Newborn. The role of the primary care pediatrician in the management of high-risk newborn. *Pediatrics.* 1996;98:786-788.

Communication

In the current medical model for advanced neonatal care, as in most fields of medicine, the specialist pediatrician often consults a subspecialist (ie, a neonatologist) for guidance in medical decision making. Decision making occurs with consideration of many factors and incorporates the fields of medicine, bioethics, medical sociology, and economics. In other words, physicians draw on medical education, expertise, and experience to develop the best plan of care that suits each individual patient and family. A major part of decision making is guided by the art of medicine, which is the essence of care and decision making and which pediatricians and other physicians should consistently endeavor to refine throughout their careers. The family must be included fully and appropriately in decisions regarding their infant.

A difficulty lies with the temporal nature of information processing. In situations in which physicians may be apt to understand a disease process quickly or approach a clinical situation with volumes of clinical experience, families, with the exception of those familiar with the medical environment, are likely experiencing urgent and critical care of an infant for the first time. What a physician has learned to understand over years of training and experience, the family is struggling to comprehend instantaneously.

Communication requires sincere, forthright presentation. Parents should ideally receive most information about their baby's condition from the medical team, as opposed to secondary sources. Parents, family members, and physicians come to situations from various social and educational backgrounds. Although most families' members are not expecting to become medical experts, they deserve thorough explanations of their infant's condition and the reasoning behind decisions and care plans.[3]

Transparency

Transparency can be defined as a standard requiring "the physician to engage in the typical patient-management thought process, only to do it out loud in language understandable to the patient." Two requirements further define this standard: (1) providing full disclosure of the evidence and reasoning regarding proposed and alternative treatments and (2) encouraging and answering patient questions about proposed treatment, evidence, and reasoning.[4]

These concepts are also applicable to delivering health care in the NICU setting. Some physicians may equate transparency with letting down a person's guard. This unfortunate view implies a defensive stance as a health care provider. Parents and physicians share the common goal of doing what is best for the infant. Without knowledge, neither party can make a decision. Without shared knowledge—that is, transparency—neither can collaborate in this decision-making process. This partnership with families forms the basis and goal of family-centered care.

Informed Consent

The concept of *informed consent* in pediatrics has a unique meaning. Although informed consent is generally defined as "the exercise of the patient's moral and legal right to control over his or her bodily integrity,"[5] the infant patient is unable to comprehend information, exercise control, or make decisions. Although such a situation occurs with some adult patients, this inability is the state of any infant. Providing informed consent thus falls to the parents. Parents who are thrust into a new and overwhelming setting with a sick or premature infant for whom they can offer no immediate remedy may feel stripped of their rights to comfort and care for their infant. In this instance, parents must be assured of their role as part of the team and as primary decision makers.

FAMILY-CENTERED CARE

Transparency and communication are essential attributes of family-centered care. As neonatal, general, and inpatient pediatric practices aim to include family members in discussions and decision making, the concept of direct alliances with families has evolved from the paternalistic role of the physician and the permissive care role of the family. Parents and family members should be recognized as full partners and participants in care. The American Academy of Pediatrics states that "health care providers should engage parents as co-providers and decision-making partners and seek to ensure that every encounter builds on the family's strengths, preserves their dignity, and enhances their confidence and competence."[6] Physicians are sought for information, insight, and guidance, not for directives. In fact, all physicians involved in the care of the infant should actively seek parents' and guardians' observations and preferences for the care plan. Families should become directly involved in the general routine care of their infant, as would be done if they

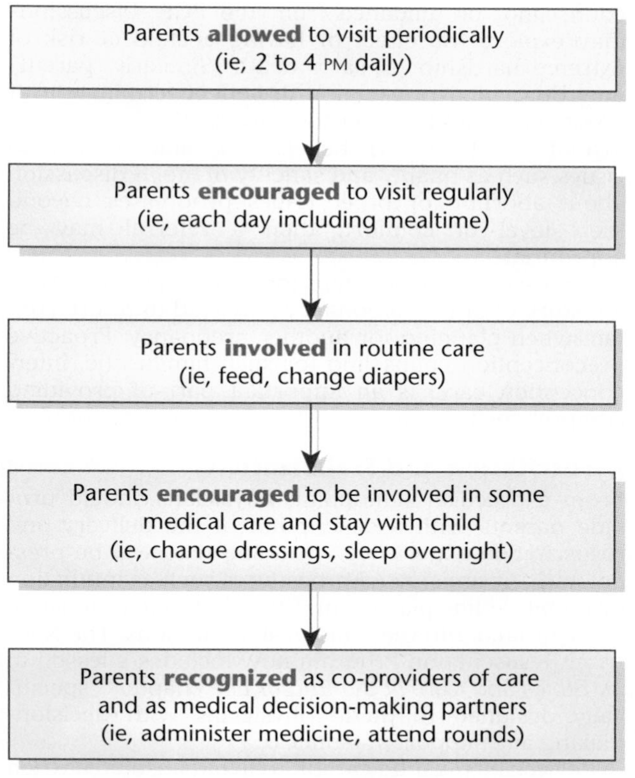

Figure 79-1 Evolution of hospital family-centered care.

BOX 79-3 Core Principles of Family-Centered Care

- Respect each child and the child's family.
- Honor racial, ethnic, cultural, and socioeconomic diversity and its effect on the family's experience and perception of care.
- Recognize and build on the strengths of each child and family, even in difficult and challenging situations.
- Support and facilitate choices for the child and family about approaches to care and support.
- Ensure flexibility in organizational policies, procedures, and provider practices so services can be tailored to the needs, beliefs, and cultural values of each child and family.
- Share honest and unbiased information with families on an ongoing basis and in ways they find useful and affirming.
- Provide and ensure formal and informal support (eg, family-to-family support) for the child and parents or guardians during pregnancy, childbirth, infancy, childhood, adolescence, and young adulthood.
- Collaborate with families at all levels of health care, in the care of the individual child, and in professional education, policy making, and program development.
- Empower each child and family to discover their own strengths, build confidence, and make choices and decisions about their health.

were at home; parents should change diapers, feed the baby, and check the infant's body temperature; parents should also record such events in the baby's bedside chart (Figure 79-1). In the neonatal realm, families may structure the day around feeding schedules or certain hospital activities, such as rounds. As they become more familiar with their infant, parents become skilled at recognizing subtle cues of illness or wellness.

The initiation of family-centered care and support optimally begins in the prenatal period. Whether the family seeks the PCP for general counsel about the newborn period or the neonatologist for information about a high-risk pregnancy, a likely premature birth, or a suspected congenital defect, involvement should initiate the development of rapport and trust. Open, evidence-based conversation with family members that uses appropriate terminology and provides ample time for questions, comments, and expression of feelings is paramount to establishing this relationship. Parents are often interested in the basic pathophysiological features of the disease process, and clear, comprehensive explanations are important.

A multidisciplinary approach to the care of an infant and family is another vital component of support in the critical care setting. The core of family-centered care is "collaboration among patients, families, physicians, nurses, and other professionals for the planning, delivery, and evaluation of health care."[7] To deal with the potential reactive stages of shock, sadness, anger, and grief, teams need skills to elicit and take care of a family's emotional and spiritual needs, as well as financial concerns, in an ongoing manner.

The core principles of family-centered care guide physicians as they assert themselves in developing compassionate collaborations with families and children. These concepts provide the backdrop in which supporting families, sharing information, and decision making can flourish (Box 79-3).[7]

NEONATAL INTENSIVE CARE UNIT ENVIRONMENT

Evidence of the importance of the environment where babies receive care has mounted.[8] Physicians and leaders need to be proactive in designing and implementing environments that enhance recovery and long-term outcomes.

The *microenvironment* around the baby is extremely important. Physical stimuli such as sound and light affect babies in ways that remain incompletely understood, and such stimuli should be managed to prevent excesses. The *macroenvironment* within which family-centered care is provided affects physicians, families, and the infants. Physical and interpersonal considerations need to be addressed. Space and privacy for comfort, communication, and deliberation are important and subject to study, implementation, and evaluation. For example, single-patient rooms that allow family members to spend 24 hours a day with their neonate in the first or second week before discharge provide family members with the opportunity to care more expertly for their infant at home.

SPECIAL SITUATIONS AND CHALLENGES

The care of a high-risk or premature infant presents PCPs with many unique situations and challenges. PCPs, acting in the patient's best interest, should be prepared to incorporate the concepts of family-centered care and initiate the development of a supportive and nurturing environment.

Consultation Before Birth

With the increasing number of extremely premature infants in NICUs, families are often facing decisions regarding the support of an infant born at the edge of viability. Although direct prenatal counseling will usually be done by obstetrical or neonatal practitioners, PCPs should possess basic knowledge of the data associated with survivability of, and morbidity associated with, extremely premature infants (Table 79-2).[9] PCPs' roles may be varied: they may initiate a consultation, offer additional support, clarify suggestions or evidence, and, in some cases, have direct involvement in resuscitation decisions and care.

Because of limitations of studies and the individuality of newborns, discussions focus not on absolutes, but rather on ranges of survival and quality of life. The American Academy of Pediatrics recommends the use of *nondirective* counseling while recognizing the role of direct suggestions in cases of extreme prematurity, congenital anomalies that result in a state incompatible with life, or situations believed to be medically futile. Physicians and members of the care team must be familiar with evidence-based and local outcome data to have a complete and accurate discussion.

For the family facing important decisions involving the possibility of poor pregnancy outcomes, the PCP should facilitate a discussion that encourages the parents to explore their perception of and ability to care for a sick or handicapped infant. If the pregnancy is early in gestation, then the parents may be considering termination and may seek further information, counseling, or guidance from the PCP. Discussions may explore the effect of having a child at risk of extreme hardship or early death. Similarly, parents may be guided to examine the effect termination of pregnancy may have on their lives. PCPs must have insight into their own beliefs and values related to issues such as quality and sanctity of life. If discussion about abortion or other issues progresses beyond their level of comfort, then a referral may be appropriate.

Professional relationships formed with families with a history of at-risk pregnancy may lead to future contact when planning for another pregnancy. Proactive preconception counseling for such families (ie, interconception care) is an important part of providing comprehensive care.

Resuscitation and Stabilization

From a practical standpoint, physicians should provide parents with a description of the delivery and resuscitation experience, including who will be present and any anticipated procedures such as intubation or umbilical line placement. Ethical principles must be incorporated into these medical discussions. The Neonatal Resuscitation Program now includes a lesson in its *Ethics and Care at the End of Life* chapter[10] specifically designed to guide physicians with decision-making and support of families.

Physicians must be careful to avoid absolutes when discussing resuscitation options, explaining the possibility of modifying decisions based on the baby's condition at birth. The care team should support parents' wishes to initiate or withhold care in cases of borderline survival or significant morbidity when the prognosis is uncertain. In cases in which the prognosis is known (eg, anencephaly or newborns born at less than 23 weeks' gestation), resuscitation is not indicated. If in the prenatal period a fetal condition is identified that necessitates palliative or comfort care, then the physician should explain options and elicit input from the family. In the event parents are not clear whether to initiate care, initial resuscitation and stabilization may provide an opportunity for further assessment, offering the family and care team more data for decision making.[10]

Table 79-2 Survival and Neurologic Disability Rates for Extremely Premature Infants

	RATE (%)			
WEEKS AT BIRTH	SURVIVAL, LITERATURE SURVEY	SURVIVAL, VERMONT OXFORD NETWORK, 2003	SEVERE NEUROLOGIC DISABILITY, LITERATURE SURVEY	MODERATE NEUROLOGIC DISABILITY, LITERATURE SURVEY
<23	~5	8	—	—
23 0/7 to 23 6/7	~15	32	~30-35	~20-30
24 0/7 to 24 6/7	~40	58	~25-30	~20-30
25 0/7 to 25 6/7	~60	76	~20-25	~20-30
26 0/7 to 26 6/7	~75	83	~15-20	~20

Death of a Baby

When resuscitation of a newborn has deliberately not been initiated or has been unsuccessful, physicians must remain supportive, caring, and professional. Whether or not they have had an opportunity before delivery to meet the family, physicians need to state clearly that the infant has died. An appropriate statement would be, "I'm sorry your daughter/son has died. I am very sorry for your loss," identifying the baby by name. If culturally acceptable and comfortable, a physical gesture (lightly touching the parent's shoulder or offering a handshake) is appropriate.

In situations in which care was withdrawn or not initiated, parents may prefer to hold the baby while the child dies. In this instance, physicians must ask parents their wishes. The emotional act of holding the baby who is in the last moments of life is an important time for many parents to bond with the infant and process the event. However, some families may decline to see or hold the infant for personal or cultural reasons. In circumstances in which family members cannot be present at the time of withdrawal of support, a health care provider may hold the infant. Nonetheless, the family should be provided with some time alone, and PCPs should offer to call support persons (eg, spiritual counselor, chaplain, bereavement specialist) as needed.

Private space for the grieving family within the hospital is important and may mean closing off the immediate area surrounding the infant's bedside. In most NICUs, suites or private rooms are available for this purpose. Finally, physicians should be present with the family in the moments surrounding the time when care is withdrawn or when an infant dies. This time is when the family will need caregivers most—if not for questions, then for emotional support.

The actual place where a child dies is of great concern to some families. Parents sometimes prefer to have a baby die in a place perceived to be closer to nature than a hospital environment—perhaps a patch of grass outside the hospital, with staff discreetly nearby. A planned death of a baby at home is an appropriate alternative. Such deaths may be anticipated to happen soon or some days or weeks ahead. Babies with conditions such as trisomy 13 or 18 might be home for weeks or months before death. Babies with shorter anticipated life spans, including those on some form of life support, might, with collaboration of medical and nursing staff, go home for a short interval. Hospital staff and physician leadership providing compassionate support and careful planning are necessary to ensure a safe transition to the home environment. This provision includes anticipating not only medical issues, but also matters such as prior notification of community services (eg, emergency response teams). Coordination between hospital and community physicians is an important general principle and is essential in these situations.

Rounds

Parent activists and opinion leaders have long expressed the belief that parents should be involved in all activities in which their child is discussed.[11] Daily rounds are the primary discussion and decision-making forum in most hospital services, including pediatrics and neonatology (Figure 79-2). They are also an opportunity for teaching. A movement toward inclusion of parents in daily rounds has recently taken place, with recognized benefits of parent involvement and satisfaction with care.

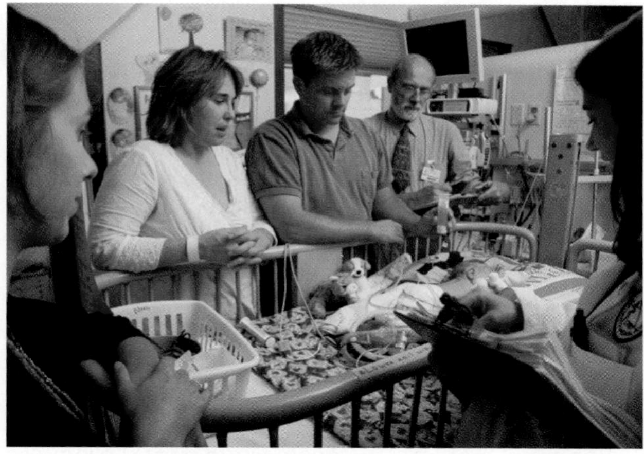

Figure 79-2 Rounds in a family-centered environment encourage participation by parents. Note the mother and father (providing expressed milk by tube feeding) joining a nurse and attending physician during presentation by a medical student.

ANTICIPATORY GUIDANCE

Adjustment to the Neonatal Intensive Care Unit Experience

As parents transition through the emotions and realities associated with the birth of a sick or premature infant, they not only learn to cope with the news, but also begin to adapt to the new challenge of life in the NICU environment. Physicians, recognizing parents' longitudinal adjustment pattern as they assimilate the role of being a parent inside the NICU, need to encourage parents to work with their lives outside the hospital. This encouragement is especially important for parents with children or other family members at home. Physicians should point out to parents that leaving the hospital as needed is acceptable; indeed, maintaining a stable and healthy family unit may be crucial. This transition is difficult for families who expected their infant, once delivered, to come home shortly thereafter.

Families with seriously ill or extremely premature infants will experience many interactions with a variety of health professionals. Their reaction has been characterized as the *model of guarded alliance*.[12] Parents progress through three stages when their infant has a prolonged hospital stay: (1) naive trust, (2) disenchantment, and (3) guarded alliance. The first stage places emphasis on the physician. It recognizes the parents' reliance, for the care of their infant, on professionals with whom they are likely unacquainted. Of utmost importance in this period is referring to the infant as a baby, using the baby's name, and encouraging family members to see the baby, despite any monitors, tubes, and wires.

Disenchantment occurs when the infant, after a period of relative stability, worsens or fails to improve rapidly. Families of stable infants (eg, those working on achieving adequate feeding and growth patterns) may also feel as though their needs are less important than select families with a more critical infant. Guarded alliance occurs as parents become more comfortable expressing needs and asking questions, mainly facilitated by the trust relationships they have formed with physicians. This alliance becomes the foundation for family-centered care. In recognizing these stages, health care providers can help normalize the family life in the unit, helping members express and prioritize needs.[13]

For many mothers, the postpartum period produces emotional, physical, and cognitive changes.[14] PCPs must recognize that this time requires intervention and support. Parental development in the NICU environment evolves over time as they become more accustomed to their baby, the NICU culture, and their role in this unique environment.

The mother's partner, be it the biological father or another person, may also experience difficulty coping with the birth of a sick or premature infant. This person may have the added burden of role confusion, identifying the person's own role with the traditionally mother-baby care dyad. Physicians can aid partners by including them as part of the care team and focusing on the family as a unit when addressing the parents.

Finally, physicians should never undermine the element of hope. This act may be inappropriately viewed as a form of denial or a coping mechanism; it may also have a deep spiritual basis. After respectfully acknowledging the parents' beliefs, the PCP can emphasize the known medical facts versus what is unknown and cannot be predicted.

Fostering Bonding in the Neonatal Intensive Care Unit

Bonding, the process of psychological intimacy and attachment that occurs between parents and infants, is recognized as an important component of the developmental changes that occur in families. Visitation policies, rounds, and care regimens, such as those incorporating kangaroo care, must promote the interaction of family members with the infant. Policies should maintain proper patient privacy, be without bias, and be sensitive to nontraditional family structures. Furthermore, incorporating family members into caregiving while preserving and building their sense of responsibility can help develop the optimal environment for the bonded family structure and help maximize outcome potentials.[6]

Siblings

Explaining the hospitalization of a sick or premature infant to a young child may prove challenging for parents. PCPs should encourage sibling visitation when appropriate and should seek opportunities to talk with children as part of routine office visits.

Sibling visitation policies vary among NICUs. Actually seeing an infant who is sick or premature may help some children understand the necessity of their parents' frequent absence. Sometimes allowing a child to simply see the hospital, describing it as the place "where mommy and daddy go every day" or "where your baby brother is living right now," may help.

As is the case with introducing a new infant into the home, children may not easily adapt to the disruption in their usual routine, or they may view the situation as a threat to time with parents. Physicians can suggest that parents keep some usual routines, such as bedtime, intact or that they specifically schedule time with the child for activities. For families with chronically hospitalized infants, providing the children at home with a calendar or schedule highlighting the times the parents will be at the hospital may be helpful.

Grandparents

The role of grandparents of a sick neonate is unique and often difficult. In the family constellation, grandmothers and grandfathers are simultaneously grandparents to the child and parents to the child's parents. The grandparents' own children are, at best, under stress and, if not physically sick themselves, are often dealing with a crisis for which they have relatively little life experience.

Grandparents need special consideration, as well as guidance and care, themselves. The natural inclination to parent may be difficult to subordinate when a grandchild is in crisis. PCPs and other members of the neonatal care team need to tend to the baby and reinforce the primacy of the parents' role. At the same time, health care providers need to provide guidance to grandparents; they can often be recruited and guided to support and assist the new parents.

Many steps consistent with family-centered care can be taken to help parents and grandparents. For example, many neonatal units permit unlimited visiting for parents and others whom the parents approve. The suggestion that grandparents might be first on the list of people to visit freely is often appreciated by all. In addition, when and if special meetings and decisions have to be faced, parents often appreciate being asked whether they would like one or more grandparents to be present.

Angry Family

Families with infants in the NICU setting experience high levels of emotional, financial, and physical stressors that may manifest as anger. Anger can be the result of distrust, unmet expectations, or fear, or it can be the result of inherent preexisting psychosocial stressors or medical or psychiatric illness. Acknowledging the presence of anger is the first step in assuaging discontent. Addressing concerns in a calm, private environment will present an opportunity for the physician to discern the underlying source. Commonly, this anger may be the result of a lapse or misunderstanding in communication. Admitting fault and ensuring better attention to the matter at hand may help regain rapport with the family.

In cases in which anger or disruptive behavior is a product of the family's psychopathological characteristics, social service support or psychiatric services, or both, should be involved to help counsel the family members and provide support while the family endures the hospitalization of the infant. Although the health care team must continue to communicate transparently and involve the family fully in the care of their infant, team members may be hesitant about sharing too much information out of concern of angering the family and perhaps precipitating an outburst. These situations are challenging tests of physician skills. Situations such as this often benefit from private discussion outside of formal rounds within the unit. The use of regularly scheduled family meetings may foster a calmer environment for discussions.

In instances of intense verbal exchanges or physical harm or threats to patients, visitors, or staff members, the first resort is the institution's security team and contact with risk-management members. Health care providers who feel insecure may be compromised in their efforts to care for patients.

CONCLUSION

When supporting a family with a sick or premature infant, the physician and other health care providers must draw on a full complement of skills and resources. These situations test a physician's strength in conveying medical knowledge in a professional, clear, concise manner while maintaining a calm, sincere, and compassionate persona. Patients, families, and health professionals benefit from family-centered care ideals. Physicians can derive a sense of fulfillment and job satisfaction from recognizing that their efforts to help and support babies and families are effective.

TOOLS FOR PRACTICE

Engaging Patient and Family

- *Newborn Intensive Care: What Every Parent Needs to Know* (book), Zaichkin J (www.aap.org/bookstore).

Medical Decision Support

- *Guidelines for Perinatal Care, 6th edition* (book), American Academy of Pediatrics and American College of Obstetricians and Gynecologists (www.aap.org/bookstore).
- *Instructor's Manual for Neonatal Resuscitation, 5th edition* (book), American Academy of Pediatrics and American Heart Association (www.aap.org/bookstore).
- *Recommendations to Improve Preconception Health and Health Care—United States: A Report of the CDC/ATSDR Preconception Care Work Group and the Select Panel on Preconception Care* (other), Centers for Disease Control and Prevention (www.cdc.gov/mmwr/preview/mmwrhtml/rr5506a1.htm).

AAP POLICY STATEMENTS

American Academy of Pediatrics, Committee on Fetus and Newborn. Levels of neonatal care. *Pediatrics*. 2004;114(5):1341-1347 (aappolicy.aappublications.org/cgi/content/full/pediatrics;114/5/1341).

American Academy of Pediatrics, Committee on Hospital Care, and Institute for Family-Centered Care. Family-centered care and the pediatrician's role. *Pediatrics*. 2003;112(3):691-696 (aappolicy.aappublications.org/cgi/content/full/pediatrics;112/3/691).

American Academy of Pediatrics, Committee on Practice and Ambulatory Medicine and Committee on Fetus and Newborn. The role of the primary care pediatrician in the management of high-risk newborn. *Pediatrics*. 1996;98:786-788 (aappolicy.aappublications.org/cgi/content/abstract/pediatrics;98/4/786).

SUGGESTED RESOURCES

American Academy of Pediatrics, Committee on Fetus and Newborn. Policy statement: levels of neonatal care. *Pediatrics*. 2004;114:1341-1347.

Fanos JH, Fahrner K, Jelveh M, et al. The Sibling Center: a pilot program for siblings of children and adolescents with a serious medical condition. *J Pediatr.* 2005;146:831-835.

Harrison H. The principles for family-centered neonatal care. *Pediatrics*. 1993;92:643-650.

Institute for Family-Centered Care. Available at: www.familycenteredcare.org/resources/pinwheel/index.htm. Accessed January 15, 2008.

Johnson K, Posner S, Biermann J, et al. Recommendations to improve preconception health and health care—United States. A report of the CDC/ATSDR Preconception Care Work Group and the Select Panel on Preconception Care. *MMWR Recomm Rep*. 2006;55:1-23.

Klerman LV, Reynolds DW. Interconception care: a new role for the pediatrician. *Pediatrics*. 1994;93:327-329.

March of Dimes. Available at: www.marchofdimes.com/. Accessed January 31, 2007.

Munch S, Levick J. "I'm special too": promoting sibling adjustment in the neonatal intensive care unit. *Health Soc Work*. 2001;26:58-64.

REFERENCES

1. Hoyert D, Mathews TJ, Menacker, et al. Annual summary of vital statistics: 2004. *Pediatrics*. 2006;117:168-183.
2. American Academy of Pediatrics, Committee on Practice and Ambulatory Medicine and Committee on Fetus and Newborn. The role of the primary care pediatrician in the management of high-risk newborn. *Pediatrics*. 1996;98:786-788.
3. Kowalski WJ, Leef KH, Mackley A, et al. Communicating with parents of premature infants: who is the informant? *J Perinatol*. 2006;26:44-48.
4. Brody H. Transparency: informed consent in primary care. *Hastings Cent Rep*. 1989;19:5-9.
5. King N. Transparency in neonatal intensive care. *Hastings Cent Rep*. 1992;22:18-25.
6. American Academy of Pediatrics and American College of Obstetricians and Gynecologists. *Guidelines for Perinatal Care*. 6th ed. Washington, DC: American College of Obstetricians and Gynecologists; 2007.
7. American Academy of Pediatrics, Committee on Hospital Care and Institute for Family-Centered Care. Policy statement: family-centered care and the pediatrician's role. *Pediatrics*. 2003;112:691-696.
8. White R, Martin G, eds. New standards for neonatal intensive care units (NICU) design. *J Perinatol*. 2006;26(suppl 3):S1-S48.
9. Kaempf J, Tomlinson M, Arduza C, et al. Medical staff guidelines for periviability pregnancy counseling and medical treatment of extremely premature infants. *Pediatrics*. 2006;117:22-29.
10. American Academy of Pediatrics and American Heart Association. Lesson 9. In: *Ethics and Care at the End of Life: Instructor's Manual for Neonatal Resuscitation Program*. 5th ed. American Academy of Pediatrics, Elk Grove Village, IL: 2006.

11. Harrison H. The principles for family-centered neonatal care. *Pediatrics.* 1993;92:643-650.
12. Thorne SE, Robinson CA. Guarded alliance: health care relationships in chronic illness. *Image J Nurs Sch.* 1989; 21:153-157.
13. McGrath J. Building relationships with families in the NICU. *J Perinat Neonatal Nurs.* 2001;15:74-83.
14. Buckwalter JG, Buckwalter DK, Bluestein DW, et al. Pregnancy and post partum: changes in cognition and mood. *Prog Brain Res.* 2001;133:303-319.

Chapter 80

PERINATAL BEREAVEMENT

Deborah E. Campbell, MD

INTRODUCTION

The birth of a sick or premature infant, a baby with life-threatening birth anomalies, or the delivery of a stillborn infant presents a significant challenge for the health professionals caring for the child's family. Few parents anticipate the birth of a sick or special needs child. However, improved diagnostic and therapeutic interventions are increasing the number of families experiencing preterm birth or prenatal diagnosis of a significant health condition in the infant. The premature birth or critical nature of the child's illness at delivery may impose separation of the infant from the infant's mother and family, impeding the bonding process. In addition, parents may need to assimilate large amounts of information quickly as they are asked to make life-and-death decisions for their newborn.

STATISTICS

Of the 4 million births that occur in the United States annually, approximately 20,000 newborns will die within the first month of life, and another 8000 will die during infancy. The 4 leading causes of death during infancy are attributed to (1) congenital malformations, (2) disorders related to short gestation, (3) sudden infant death syndrome, and (4) newborns affected by maternal complications of pregnancy. Nearly 60,000 babies are born premature or with low birth weight each year, with annual increases in the births and deaths resulting from multiple gestations, low birth weight, and prematurity.[1]

In the context of all childhood deaths, 34% occur in the neonatal period, and 28% of childhood death is due to shortened gestation, congenital anomalies that include congenital heart disease, complications of pregnancy, and respiratory disorders. Additional childbearing losses are associated with miscarriage, stillbirth, abortion, and maternal death resulting from complications of pregnancy and childbirth. Birth defects are an important contributor to years of productive life lost among children.

SUPPORT FOR THE FAMILY

Caring for the family becomes an integral component of the medical care and nurturing of the infant. Psychosocial, emotional, and spiritual support for the family are necessary elements of care as focus on the infant's quality of life and best interests frame decision making for the baby. The principles of family-centered care are interwoven in the delivery of all facets of neonatal special or intensive care. These principles form the basis for an open dialogue with families that is culturally sensitive, negotiated, and respectful of the strengths, values, and perspectives that the family brings to the discussion (Figure 80-1).

The health care professional should recognize and validate the parents' role and the range of experiences, beliefs and expectations, strengths, and needs

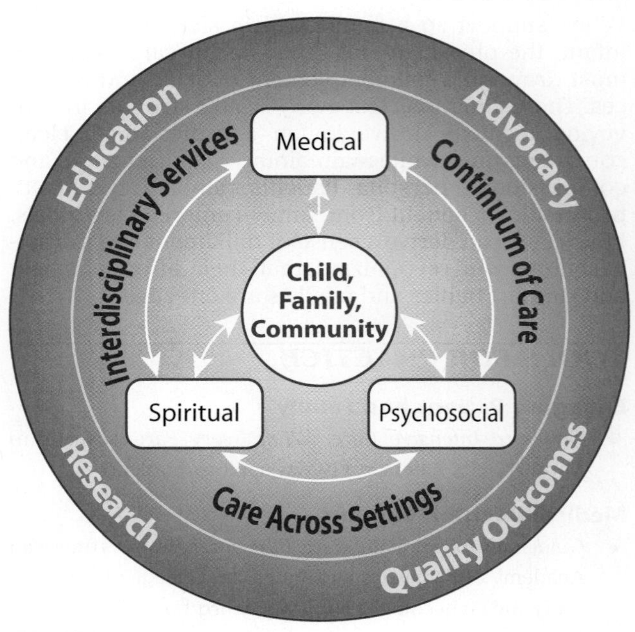

Interdisciplinary Services

Child-life specialists	Nurses
Community support	Pharmacy services
Counseling	Physicians
Durable medical supplies	Physical and occupational therapists
Expressive therapies	Speech therapy
Home health aides	Respite services

Care Across Setting	Continuum of Care
Family home	Time of diagnosis
Alternative home (eg, foster care)	Acute care
Inpatient hospice	Chronic care
Inpatient hospital	Terminal care
Long-term care nursing home	Bereavement

Figure 80-1 Scope of pediatric palliative care. *(Carter BS. Comfort care principles for the high risk newborn.* NeoReviews. *2004;5(11):e484. Data from the National Hospice & Palliative Care Organization: ChIPPS, 2001.)*

BOX 80-1 Factors That Influence a Child and Family's Adjustment to Death

Sudden, unanticipated death (birth catastrophe, undiagnosed lethal birth defect, or newborn illness)
- After a prolonged illness (extreme prematurity)
- Prenatal diagnosis of lethal or incurable condition
- Stillbirth or loss of one or more infants in a multiple gestation

Physical and emotional functioning of the surviving adults and siblings: age and cognitive understanding of death

Individual personality and temperament

Preexisting risk factors
- Mental illness
- Learning and social problems

Family structure, functioning, and relationships

Quality of prior family member relationships

Concurrent life stressors
- Finances
- Living situations
- Divorce, single parenting
- Concurrent illness in other family members

Availability of support services, resources, and interventions before, during, and after the death

expressed by the family. Family constellation and individual beliefs, values, and expectations affect a parent's ability to weather and adapt to having a premature infant or sick child. For many individuals, no greater loss exists than the death or serious disability of a child. Siblings may also exhibit a variety of feelings and responses that further influence a family's functioning and needs (Box 80-1). For many parents, their acute responses may evolve to one of chronic or recurrent sorrow and sadness, irrespective of the child's clinical condition or level of health care need. Periods of anticipated developmental transitions or high-risk periods, such as an acute illness or the need for hospitalization or surgery, may result in the need for increased family support. Recognizing that the fears and concerns exhibited by some families may seem out of proportion to the severity of the infant's medical problems is also important. The meaning of their child's condition to the parents and family should be explored, as well as their concerns and prior experiences that may be influencing their responses.

Parents confronting a perinatal or infant death often face common dilemmas: what is happening to their family; why family and friends do not understand; a sense of feeling out of balance, without boundaries or freedom; a feeling of being atypical or different for their child and family. The grief parents experience lasts a lifetime, evolves over time, and is multifaceted. Gender differences are common in terms of the distress each parent feels. Over time, individual partner needs may change. Therefore the health care professional should recognize these differences so as to facilitate long-term adjustment for parents.

Emphasis on hope, empowerment, taking action, and parent-professional partnerships are important factors in the process of adapting and healing after a high-risk birth. Parents benefit from guidance and practical tools for their day-to-day living and decision making. The health care professional should assist the family in identifying and understanding their feelings of loss and helplessness, developing their parental identity, and managing relationships (Box 80-2). The professional must also recognize the complexities of changing expectations, parental control, death, dying, multiple births, and survival with poor, unexpected, or, in the case of multiple births, varying outcomes. If their child is critically ill, then parents must learn to cope with having to make life-and-death decisions, uncertainty regarding their infant's chance for survival, or the risk for long-term disability and understanding the realities of medical decision making when viable options may not exist (Table 80-1).

PALLIATIVE CARE

When prenatal diagnosis involves identification of a life-limiting condition that will lead to an early perinatal death, hospice care should begin immediately. Perinatal hospice offers a caring, supportive program of services to families who choose not to terminate a pregnancy after a prenatal diagnosis or when the timing of the diagnosis does not allow for this option. Perinatal hospice provides information and counseling to assist families in birth planning, anticipatory grieving, and preparing for what time they may have with their infant if the child is live born. Local hospice services may be engaged to support care at home for infants with life-limiting conditions who are not expected to die immediately. Referrals may include social services, religious or spiritual services, and consultation with neonatology and maternal-fetal-medicine specialists.

Palliative care for the dying neonate includes supporting the family in finding meaning in their baby's life and death. Creating a physical environment that is family centered offers psychosocial and spiritual resources, and supports the family in decision making, advanced care planning, and the grieving process. Bereavement care begins with the infant's birth; bonding should be encouraged and families supported in their birth rituals and comfort care for their baby. Parents should be encouraged to name their infant, if this is an appropriate cultural practice for the family. The health care professional should provide the family with a private, quiet place to spend time with their dying infant and encourage them to hold, examine, and caress their infant. Families may wish to conduct cultural practices that celebrate, bid farewell, or offer protection to their infant during the dying process. Professionals may also assist families by providing resource listings that incorporate a range of media—texts, videotapes, electronic resources, and referrals to support groups—and offering information that responds to the spectrum of medical and educational information, emotional, and practical support needs of

BOX 80-2 Strategies to Support Family Coping

- Truth telling
  - Limits confusion, mistrust
  - Avoids unnecessary information
  - Avoids mixed messages
- Provide information simply and directly using correct words and language; euphemisms may cause more distress, although some cultures have specific preferences for acknowledging the deceased.
- Gain familiarity with cultural and religious beliefs and practices.
  - Families may have specific rituals and customs in response to serious illness or death.
  - Understand how to respond, tailor comfort, and what is within realm of expected behavior.
  - Understand the role of religion or spirituality in family coping.
    - Religion is a prime source of support and strength for many people when dealing with death or serious illness.
    - Religious references may cause distress for individuals for whom faith has not played an important prior role.
- Reassure children that they are not to blame.
- Understand that children make comparisons.
  - Wishing for their life before the crisis occurred
  - Comparing their life to the lives of others
- Model appropriate responses.
  - Do not hide feelings and emotions; contain strong, dramatic feelings that might frighten, confuse younger children.
  - Find ways, if feasible, to involve children in the infant's routine while in the hospital or funeral rituals.
  - Demystify events associated with illness, death, and burial.
- Encourage children to talk and ask questions.
  - What does the child think and feel?
  - Explore feelings about illness and death, and determine appropriateness of child's participation in the death process: visiting their dying sibling, the funeral, and burial and sending the child away during this time.
  - Correct misinformation and misconceptions.
- Be attuned to and respond to child's own pace for sharing feelings.
  - Provide multiple opportunities for children to express their feelings; recognize that children go through developmental stages in their understanding of death.
  - Encourage expressions of grief, collection of keepsakes, and sharing of memories.
  - Acknowledge and affirm children's expressions.
- Provide understanding, support, and extra guidance.
- Encourage families to seek support from other family members and friends and from the spiritual or faith community.

Table 80-1 Four-Quadrant Decision-Making Tool—Approach to Collaborative Decision Making

QUADRANT 1: MEDICAL FACTS	QUADRANT 2: PATIENT AND FAMILY PREFERENCES
Infant's underlying diagnoses and opportunities for recovery Goals of care—risks and benefits Response to current treatments—complications Infant's prognosis—likelihood for survival, recovery, long-term health conditions, and disability Potential additional treatment and intervention options	Parents' understanding of their child's medical problems and available treatment options Parents' desires and goals for their child and family: 1. Being involved in decisions 2. Desire for autonomy 3. Desire for privacy 4. Each specific treatment option Parents' views about illness, death, and disability
QUADRANT 3: QUALITY OF LIFE	**QUADRANT 4: CONTEXTUAL ISSUES**
Infant's current quality of life 1. Components of life that give value and meaning to the family 2. Ability to experience and control pain and suffering	Parents' cultural and spiritual beliefs/values, philosophical and psychological factors that guide their decision making 1. Parents' views about withholding or withdrawing care—spiritual and faith-based influences should also be explored

Table 80-1 Four-Quadrant Decision-Making Tool—Approach to Collaborative Decision Making—cont'd

QUADRANT 3: QUALITY OF LIFE	QUADRANT 4: CONTEXTUAL ISSUES
3. Ability to be comforted, interact, and engage with parents and other caregivers Infant's anticipated quality of life if survival is possible/probable 1. Anticipated functional outcomes 2. Anticipated ability to engage with family and caregivers—experience, comfort, pleasure 3. Anticipated life expectancy 4. Chronic pain and suffering Range of continued medical care and treatment needs and expected benefits	2. Family constellation Family and support network preferences that factor into parents' ability to make decisions Family resources and needs Needs and opinions of professional caregivers Legal issues: 1. State, local, and hospital procedural regulations that affect care options 2. Federal Child Abuse amendments that permit discontinuation of care in cases where there is irreversible coma, treatment prolongs dying, or treatment is considered inhumane

Adapted from Jonsen AR, Seigler M, Winslade WJ. *Clinical Ethics: A Practical Approach to Ethical Decisions in Clinical Medicine.* New York, NY: McGraw-Hill; 1992; Seattle Washington Pediatric Palliative Care Project, Children's Hospital and Regional Medical Center, Seattle, Washington.

families. The professional needs to be aware of specific red flags that should prompt referral of the parent for immediate medical or mental health care and assess the parent-child relationship for signs of inappropriate bonding and attachment, excessive perceived child vulnerability, and child abuse or neglect involving the infant or other children.

TOOLS FOR PRACTICE

Engaging Patients and Family

- *A Guide for Fathers: When a Baby Dies, 2004* (Web page), Nelson T (www.aplacetoremember.com/mall/prod_detail.asp?catid=1&prodid=726).
- *A Place to Remember—Uplifting support materials and resources for those who have been touched by a crisis in pregnancy or the death of a baby* (Web page), A Place to Remember (www.aplacetoremember.com/aptrfront.html).
- *At the Death of a Child: Words of Comfort and Hope* (book), Deffner DL, Concordia Publishing House (www.cph.org).
- *Coping with Holidays and Celebrations* (booklet), Ilse S, Wintergreen Press (www.wintergreenpress.com/catalog.htm).
- *Empty Arms: Coping with Miscarriage, Stillbirth and Infant Death* (book), Ilse S, Wintergreen Press (www.wintergreenpress.com/catalog.htm).
- *Empty Cradle, Broken Heart: Surviving the Death of Your Baby* (book), Davis DL, Fulcrum Publishing (www.fulcrum-books.com).
- *Giving Care, Taking Care: Support for the Helpers* (book), Ilse S, Wintergreen Press (www.wintergreenpress.com/catalog.htm).
- *Mother Care: Physical Care and Beyond After a Baby Dies* (booklet), Ilse S, Wintergreen Press (www.wintergreenpress.com/catalog.htm).
- *Peace and Remembrance: A Guide for Parents Whose Baby Dies in a Newborn Intensive Care Unit* (booklet), Shea M, Gundersen Lutheran Bereavement Services (www.bereavementprograms.com).
- *Planning a Precious Goodbye* (booklet), Ilse S, Wintergreen Press (www.wintergreenpress.com/catalog.htm).
- *Precious Lives, Painful Choices* (book), Ilse S, Wintergreen Press (www.wintergreenpress.com/catalog.htm).
- *Sibling Grief* (booklet), Ilse S, Wintergreen Press (www.wintergreenpress.com/catalog.htm).
- *Single Parent's Grief* (booklet), Ilse S, Wintergreen Press (www.wintergreenpress.com/catalog.htm).
- *What Family and Friends Can Do* (booklet), Ilse S, Wintergreen Press (www.wintergreenpress.com/catalog.htm).
- *When Hello Means Goodbye: A Guide for Parents Whose Baby Dies Before Birth, at Birth or Shortly After Birth, 1998* (booklet), Perinatal Loss (www.griefwatch.com/pl/default.htm).

AAP POLICY STATEMENTS

American Academy of Pediatrics, Committee on Psychosocial Aspects of Child and Family Health. The pediatrician and childhood bereavement. *Pediatrics.* 2000;105(2):445-447. (aappolicy.aappublications.org/cgi/content/full/pediatrics;105/2/445).

American Academy of Pediatrics, Committee on Fetus and Newborn. AAP policy statement. Noninitiation or withdrawal of intensive care for high-risk newborns. *Pediatrics.* 2007;119:401-403. (aappolicy.aappublications.org/cgi/content/full/pediatrics;119/2/401).

SUGGESTED RESOURCES

Breeze ACG, Lees CC, Kumar A, et al. Palliative care for prenatally diagnosed lethal fetal abnormality. *Arch Dis Child Fetal Neonatal Ed.* 2007;92:F56-F58.

Canadian Paediatric Society. Guidelines for health care professionals supporting families experiencing a perinatal loss. Statement FN 2001-02. *Paediatr Child Health.* 2001;6:469-476.

Carter BS. Comfort care principles for the high-risk newborn. *NeoReviews.* 2004;5(11):e484-e490. Available at: www.neoreviews.org. Accessed December 21, 2007.

Dyer KA. Identifying, understanding and working with grieving parents in the NICU. Part II: Strategies. *Neonatal Network.* 2005;24:27-48.

First Candle. Available at www.sidsalliance.org. Accessed December 18, 2007.

Hoeldtke NJ, Calhoun BC. Perinatal hospice. *Am J Obstet Gynecol.* 2001;185:525-529.

Kaempf JW, Tomlinson M, Arduza C, et al. Medical staff guidelines for periviability counseling and medical treatment of extremely premature infants. *Pediatrics.* 2006; 117:22-29. Available at: pediatrics.aappublications.org/cgi/content/full/117/1/22. Accessed December 18, 2007.

Klein SD. The challenge of communicating with parents. *Develop Behav Pediatr.* 1993;14:184-191.

Lang F, Quill T. Making decisions with families at the end of life. *Am Fam Physician.* 2004;70:719-726.

Melnyk BM, Feinstein NF. Coping in parents of children who are chronically ill: strategies for assessment and intervention. *Pediatr Nurs.* 2001;27(6):547-557.

Shah MA, Campbell D, National Perinatal Association, and University of North Carolina at Chapel Hill, Offices of Medical Education. *Transcultural Aspects of Perinatal Health Care: A Resource Guide.* Elk Grove Village, IL: American Academy of Pediatrics; 2004.

Tripp J, McGregor D. Withholding and withdrawing of life sustaining treatment in the newborn. *Arch Dis Child Fetal Neonatal Ed.* 2006; 91:F67-F71.

US Department of Health and Human Services, Health Resources and Services Administration, Maternal and Child Health Bureau, SIDS Alliance. Guidelines for Christian clergy: providing care to the family experiencing perinatal loss, neonatal death, SIDS or other infant death. 2002. Available at: www.sidsalliance.org/FC-PDF2/HHS&P/guidelines_for_christian_clergy-final2.pdf or 1-800-638-SIDS. Accessed December 18, 2007.

Vance JC, Boyle FM, Najman JM, et al. Couple distress after sudden infant or perinatal death: a 30-month follow up. *J Paediatr Child Health.* 2002;38:368-372.

Wisconsin Association for Perinatal Care [WAPC], Bereavement Loss Work Group. Position statement: childbearing loss and grief (WAPC-PS11) (Grade C; evidence level 5, expert opinion). Madison, WI: WAPC; 2002.

REFERENCE

1. Miniño A, Heron M, Smith B, et al. Deaths: final data for 2004. National vital statistics reports. Hyattsville, MD: National Center for Health Statistics; 2004. Available at: www.cdc.gov/nchs/products/pubs/pubd/hestats/infantmort/infantmort.htm. Accessed March 1, 2007.

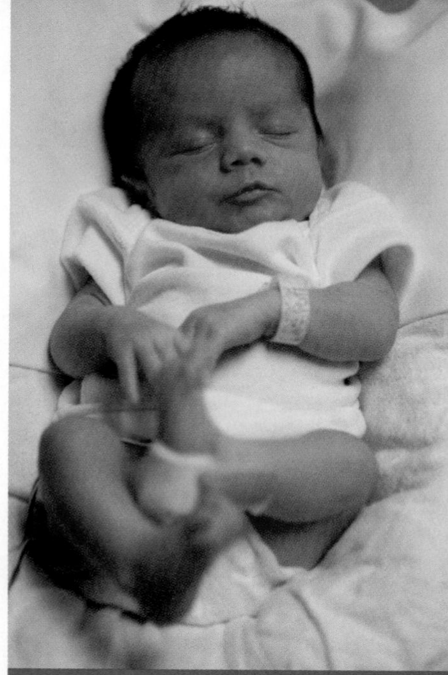

PART 5

Care of the Term and Late Preterm Infant

Section One: Assessment and Physical Examination of the Newborn

81 Medical-Legal Considerations in the Care of Newborns
82 Maternal Medical History
83 Physical Examination of the Newborn
84 Postnatal Assessment of Common Prenatal Sonographic Findings
85 Neonatal Skin
86 Common Congenital Anomalies

Section Two: Routine Care Issues

87 Prenatal Visit
88 Care of the Newborn After Delivery
89 Breastfeeding the Newborn
90 Breastfeeding: Drugs, Herbs, and Environmental Toxins
91 Circumcision
92 Care of the Late Preterm Infant

Section Three: Discharge Planning and Follow-up Care

93 Healthy Newborn Discharge
94 Follow-up Care of the Healthy Newborn
95 Health and Developmental Outcomes of Infants Requiring Neonatal Intensive Care
96 Follow-up Care of the Graduate From the Neonatal Intensive Care Unit

Section Four: Neonatal Medical Conditions

97 Abnormalities of Fetal Growth
98 Neonatal Jaundice
99 Respiratory Distress and Breathing Disorders in the Newborn
100 Evaluation of the Infant With Suspected Heart Disease
101 The Infant With Suspected Infection
102 Neonatal Hematology
103 Prenatal Drug Abuse and Neonatal Drug Withdrawal Syndrome
104 Common Metabolic Disturbances in the Newborn
105 Specific Congenital Metabolic Disorders
106 Neurologic Abnormalities

SECTION ONE

Assessment and Physical Examination of the Newborn

Chapter 81

MEDICAL-LEGAL CONSIDERATIONS IN THE CARE OF NEWBORNS

Jonathan Fanaroff, MD, JD; Robert Turbow, MD, JD

INTRODUCTION AND OVERVIEW OF MEDICAL MALPRACTICE

Approximately 4 million infants are born every year in the United States.[1] Pediatricians, family practitioners, and pediatric nurse practitioners provide the vast majority of care to these newborns. Throughout this chapter, these clinicians will be collectively referred to as pediatricians; however, the information presented here is intended for all physicians and advanced practitioners who care for infants. Although most of these newborns will be healthy, pediatricians will need to manage a variety of common but potentially harmful conditions such as hyperbilirubinemia. Furthermore, hidden among the healthy population in the newborn nursery will be infants with serious conditions, such as congenital heart disease, that have yet to occur. Delays in the initiation of resuscitation and inadequate neonatal resuscitation are the most common clinical situation leading to litigation against newborn health care providers. Missed or delayed diagnosis and management of hyperbilirubinemia, sepsis or meningitis, asphyxia, congenital hip dislocation, and congenital heart disease may also give rise to substantial medical liability. Other issues in newborn care that pose liability for pediatric primary care physicians include missed newborn (hearing) screening, improper treatment of neonatal hypoglycemia and neonatal seizures, and the timing of perinatal or neonatal injury. Factors that contribute to potential liability encompass failure to perform appropriate screening evaluations, incomplete documentation, failure to recognize high-risk conditions that may contribute to a particular neonatal condition, and inadequate or delayed follow-up care.

Unfortunately, medical malpractice liability is in the midst of a new crisis.[2] Indeed, the American Medical Association estimates that 20 states are currently in a medical liability crisis, defined as a situation in which patients lose access to care as a result of the medical liability system.[3] Although liability problems have occurred in the past, the current effect on young physicians is severe. A 2003 survey of final-year residents found that 62% of residents were significantly concerned about malpractice, up from only 15% in the 2001 survey.[4] Furthermore, many surveys have revealed physicians' increasing dissatisfaction with medical practice, in part because of liability concerns.[5]

The specialty of pediatrics ranks fourth in highest average indemnity from 1985 to 2004, behind neurology, neurosurgery, and obstetrics and gynecology. Furthermore, the Physician Insurers Association of America (PIAA) reports that the average closed pediatric malpractice claim in 2004 was at $468,000, 43% higher than the overall average for all physician specialties. The high claim amounts result because many of the common diagnostic errors in newborns, such as meningitis, lead to catastrophic and permanent injuries. Furthermore, the appearance of these permanently handicapped children in court or on video can generate enormous sympathy from juries. Finally, because neonates are at the beginning of their lives, their cost of care when permanently injured is substantial. In a study conducted by Hickson et al,[6] families whose infants experienced permanent injury or death after a perinatal event were interviewed after the end of litigation regarding their reasons for filing malpractice claims. Parents cited numerous reasons, important among these was a dissatisfaction with the physician-patient (family) communication: 13% did not believe their physician would listen to them, 32% believed that their physicians did not speak openly, and 48% expressed feeling that they were intentionally mislead. Seventy percent of participants stated that their physician did not inform them about the potential for long-term neurodevelopmental problems in their children. Families who believe that they are uninformed often assume that a complication that has occurred is a result of a mistake and that the hospital staff is afraid to acknowledge this error. Issues of blame may be compounded further by parental concerns about their own responsibility for the infant's situation; and in an attempt to avoid blaming the mother, responsibility may be ascribed to the medical caregivers.

This chapter explores relevant medical-legal issues that pediatricians encounter in the delivery room, the newborn nursery, and the office. The chapter also addresses common malpractice risks that pediatricians face in dealing with sick newborns, as well as consultation, transport, and referral issues. The final sections of the chapter examine communication issues, patient safety, and ways to minimize liability risk. The goal is to assist practicing clinicians in understanding their rights, duties, and liabilities as physicians (see also Chapter 11, Ethical and Legal Issues for the Primary Care Physician).

MEDICAL-LEGAL CONSIDERATIONS IN THE DELIVERY ROOM

Prudent pediatricians who attend deliveries will be familiar with the various clinical challenges they may face in the labor and delivery area. The care provided in the delivery room has lifelong implications. Quickly recognizing and treating potential complications can help ensure an infant's smooth transition to extrauterine life. Although a pediatrician will generally not be held to the same standard of care as that of a neonatologist, merely taking call coverage for labor and delivery mandates that the pediatrician be knowledgeable and experienced in the management of common complications of parturition. An important facet of this preparation is maintaining neonatal resuscitation certification and understanding the pitfalls associated with resuscitating a newborn.

As in other areas of medicine, appropriate preparation, intervention, and documentation are essential. The pediatrician should be well informed concerning the capabilities of the birthing facility and the training of the personnel, given that approximately 10% of newborns require resuscitation after birth. Although most newborns who will require resuscitation can be anticipated based on maternal risks, pregnancy risks, or both, 1% to 3% of low-risk pregnancies will result in an infant who requires resuscitation at birth.[7-9] If significant pregnancy complications or fetal abnormalities are noted before labor, then the newborn should be delivered at a facility that offers comprehensive care for the newborn. Pediatricians should ask themselves a series of questions. Can this facility handle this delivery? Is the appropriate equipment available and functioning? What will be the course of action if the newborn has complications that cannot be addressed at the delivering facility? If circumstances permit, the pediatrician may consult with the woman's obstetric caregiver to convey the concerns for the soon-to-be-born infant. If time permits and the safety of the mother and fetus are not compromised, then maternal transport to a facility offering a higher level of care may be possible. In cases in which this transfer is not practical the pediatrician should consider notifying the neonatologist at the affiliated regional perinatal center for assistance and preparation for transport, should the newborn require specialized or neonatal intensive care.

Pediatricians should immediately familiarize themselves with the labor and delivery room area of any hospital they will be covering. Inadequate resuscitation may result from not anticipating the need for resuscitation, lack of appropriate and functioning equipment, the presence of unskilled resuscitators, or errors in sequencing resuscitation steps. The last of these factors often includes delays in establishing an airway and initiating positive pressure ventilation, providing chest compressions, and administering the appropriate medications.[10] If the newborn is being delivered through thick meconium and the head is crowning, then this time is not the appropriate time to discover that the laryngoscope is not functioning. During a delivery room resuscitation the pediatrician is typically considered to be in charge of the newborn's care and any resuscitative measures that may be needed. If the pediatrician is not present, then the obstetrician is deemed responsible for the newborn's assessment and care. The obstetrician may delegate this responsibility to the anesthetist if one is present and if a pediatrician is not available. Much as the general surgeon may be held responsible for the negligent acts of an operating room nurse, the resuscitating pediatrician may be found to have some degree of liability for malfunctioning equipment or poorly trained staff. Because the supervising pediatrician is in a position to coordinate and direct the activities of others, this physician may have liability for persons who are assisting. Miscommunication and a perception of ineptness by close observers may further contribute to a family's decision to file a malpractice claim.

A great deal of confusion (and litigation, possibly) can be mitigated by thorough analysis, intervention, and documentation (Box 81-1). Pediatricians should document in the newborn's medical record regarding why they are attending the delivery, summarize the risks as known to them, what interventions were initiated, and the newborn's response to these interventions. Is this procedure a *repeat* caesarian section or an *emergent* caesarian section for suspected placental abruption? What is the estimated gestation? Is the mother febrile? How long have the membranes been ruptured? Is the mother on antibiotics? Does other salient maternal medical information exist that may affect the newborn or the resuscitative measures that might be necessary? What was the condition of the newborn at birth? What were the assessments, and what treatments were initiated? How did the infant respond to this intervention?

Other professionals are often in the delivery room to assist with airway management. An anesthesiologist or nurse anesthetist may be able to assist if a particular intubation is problematic. Even though the anesthesiologist's primary responsibility is the newborn's mother, fellow professionals will often be

BOX 81-1 Strategies to Minimize Delivery Room Risk

- Maintain resuscitation skills; stay current according to the Neonatal Resuscitation Program guidelines.
- Know the capabilities of the other members of the resuscitation team.
- Know the capabilities of the facility.
- Document the situation, interventions, responses, and communications.

willing to assist, as long as it does not mean jeopardizing the primary patient.

Pediatricians may have their first interaction with a family in the delivery room. The pediatrician who has had prior contact with the family can bring considerable comfort to the family. Without this prior contact the pediatrician should attempt to establish rapport with the family. Although parent (family)-professional communication under this circumstance can be quite difficult, it is nonetheless critical to helping parents understand the physician's concerns for the newborn and to engage the parents in medical decision-making plans for the newborn regarding ongoing evaluation and treatment. This factor is particularly important if the resuscitative efforts are not successful, in specific cases in which a problem was not anticipated before the newborn's delivery, and when a neonate requires transfer to another facility for care that is unavailable at the birth hospital.

MEDICAL-LEGAL CONSIDERATIONS IN THE HEALTHY NEWBORN NURSERY

One of the more challenging aspects of general pediatric practice is determining which newborns are well and which ones are sick. The differential diagnosis and initial management of a newborn can be challenging for a seasoned neonatologist who has the benefit of direct observation. Pediatricians are often at a significant disadvantage in that they may not be present in the nursery when a concern arises and they receive a call from the nursery nurse or family relaying symptoms. The most common factor that poses a liability risk for the health professional involves failure to diagnose a condition for which early diagnosis and treatment may prevent death or long-term morbidity. Among the risks are missed diagnoses of clinically significant congenital heart disease (eg, ductus-dependent cardiac lesions), detection of birth defects that result in early neonatal illness (gastrointestinal or genitourinary obstruction, congenital hydrocephalus) or require immediate intervention (congenital glaucoma, retinoblastoma, developmental dysplasia of the hip), suspected brachial plexus injuries or birth trauma and injury that may result in cerebral palsy and brain damage, congenital conditions that may be detected through newborn screening (eg, for hearing loss), and hyperbilirubinemia leading to kernicterus, signs and symptoms of hypoglycemia, infection, and seizures. Failure to follow up on prenatal information that suggests a potential health risk for the infant is an important issue as well. The use of prenatal ultrasonography, though not an American College of Obstetrics and Gynecology (ACOG) standard of care, has become a routine component of prenatal care nationwide. As a result, many infants are born with a suspected congenital problem. A high index of suspicion and appropriate follow through may prevent a tragedy.

Detailed discussion of these problems is contained in subsequent chapters in this section of the text. Appropriate counseling of the family is important, as is early postnursery follow-up care, to assess the infant's continued postnatal adaptation, evaluate for other signs or symptoms, and address parental concerns. The pediatric professional should also work with the nursery staff to ensure that home or public health nurse visits are coordinated, if covered by the family's insurance, to assist the family with the transition home and provide an objective, interim assessment of the newborn until the first follow-up office visit with the pediatrician. If this service is not available, then consideration should be given to an earlier follow-up appointment. Also essential is that the health professional assess for any barriers to compliance with recommended care and follow-up visits as required (transportation, child care, language-communication, health insurance, access to primary and specialty care). Physician documentation in the newborn's medical record of the clinical concerns, available and pending test results, the recommended plan of care, and content of discussions with the family, which includes their concerns, their understanding of their child's issues, and their expressed barriers to complying with the recommended care, will help reduce liability risks. Discharge instructions given to the parents should also be documented in the medical record.

MEDICAL-LEGAL CONSIDERATIONS IN CARING FOR SICK NEWBORNS

Before pediatricians provide care for sick newborns, they must pay close attention to their hospital's policies. Some nurseries will take care of healthy newborns only. If an infant requires supplemental oxygen beyond a defined period (perhaps greater than 4 hours), positive pressure ventilation, or ventilator assistance, then the baby must often be transferred to an affiliated hospital that can provide the scope of care required. Regionalized perinatal care varies around the country. Regional perinatal centers are typically state health department–designated tertiary-care facilities that are capable of caring for the sickest and most medically complex women and infants. Within communities, affiliation agreements will exist between the regional center and community hospitals that are able to provide varying levels of high-risk care to the pregnant women and the sick or premature infant. These relationships are often codified in individual state public health law statues. The American Academy of Pediatrics (AAP) and ACOG *Guidelines for Perinatal Care* are updated regularly and specify the requirements in facilities, personnel, expertise, and equipment for the level (scope) of care a hospital provides.

Three levels of care have been delineated: basic care (level I; routine maternity and newborn care to low risk infants and women), specialty care (level II; obstetric and newborn services to care for patients with specific high-risk conditions exclusive of the most critically ill, medically complex, and premature infants), and subspecialty care (level III; the full range of medical care to the most medically complex women and infants). In many states, subspecialty-care facilities, or level III perinatal centers, also serve as regional perinatal centers with quality assurance, education, and outreach responsibilities. However, some states have a plethora of level III facilities, with a smaller number designated as level IV regional perinatal centers in recognition of their unique role in providing the most comprehensive treatments in addition to care coordination, education, outreach, and quality-improvement activities.

In many community newborn nurseries the requirement for intravenous antibiotics will necessitate a transfer to another facility. Within larger hospitals or select institutions that are equipped to provide a broader spectrum of newborn care, transfer to another facility may not be necessary; instead the newborn may be transferred to a special-care nursery or a neonatal intensive care unit. Interhospital and regional perinatal affiliation agreements guide transfer relationships and the level of care required for particular maternal or newborn care issues. In addition to the pediatric care physician's experience and degree of comfort in caring for newborns with a variety of medical problems, hospitals have guidelines that delineate the privileges of its physicians and the scope of care that they may provide.

MEDICAL-LEGAL ISSUES RELATED TO SPECIFIC NEWBORN CONDITIONS

Pediatricians often supervise the care of a neonate who requires a higher level of care for a single organ system. Perhaps the newborn has hypoglycemia, requires antibiotics, or requires supplemental oxygen for a brief period. Although many pediatricians would choose to transfer these infants to a neonatologist, other pediatricians are quite comfortable caring for sick newborns in a specialty or level II neonatal unit. Under certain circumstances, a pediatrician may need to care for a very sick baby until the perinatal center's transport team arrives. These pediatricians may need to provide ongoing stabilization care, place umbilical lines, and supervise mechanical ventilation for brief periods. In general, most newborns who require prolonged ventilation (greater than 4 to 6 hours) or support for more than one organ system will be transferred to the care of a neonatologist.

Several common neonatal medical problems pose an increased liability risk for the pediatrician because of the potential for long-term sequelae and associated morbidities.

Hypoglycemia

Transient low serum glucose is a common issue in newborns. Pediatricians are regularly consulted about a newborn with hypoglycemia. Knowledge about the risk factors that predispose a newborn for the development of hypoglycemia and the normal physiological changes in energy metabolism and glucose utilization occurring after birth prepare the pediatric care physician to recognize, appropriately evaluate, and manage the newborn with low blood sugar. One of the challenges facing the pediatrician is the lack of a single, uniform definition of hypoglycemia and the influence of gestational and postnatal age in setting a threshold to define *clinically significant hypoglycemia*. Most nurseries have established patient-care policies that detail which infants should be screened for low blood sugar, the frequency of testing, and guidance regarding assessment, feeding, and intervention strategies. Studies reporting on the neurodevelopmental outcome of babies who develop symptomatic hypoglycemia have reported conflicting results. A recent systematic review was not able to make recommendations for clinical practice in the care of neonates experiencing hypoglycemia in the first week of life because of a paucity of quality studies and heterogeneity among the patients included in the reported studies.[11]

Among healthy, full-term newborns, transient, mild neonatal hypoglycemia has not been shown to affect later neurodevelopment.[12] The pediatrician should recognize that failure to identify, evaluate, and treat infants at risk for or exhibiting symptoms caused by hypoglycemia and failure to document the rationale for treatment or nontreatment may be a cause for later litigation if the child develops subsequent neurodevelopmental problems. For newborns experiencing clinically significant episodes of hypoglycemia, the full extent of neurologic injury may not be fully recognized for decades. Being aware of the admitting nursery's policies and documenting identified risk factors, glucose screening (and any confirmatory testing) results, and response to feeding or other interventions initiated are important. Communication with the nursery staff and the family are of paramount importance.

Perinatal Injury: Timing of Perinatal Asphyxia

Cerebral palsy (CP) is the most common injury claimed as a result of obstetric or neonatal negligence. Frequent causes cited to account for the development of CP include intrapartum or postpartum asphyxia, birth trauma, brain injury caused by intracranial hemorrhage or ischemia, peripartum infection, kernicterus, and hypoglycemia. Injury may result from chronic, subacute, or intermittent hypoxic-ischemic episodes or acute intrapartum events that may occur at various times during gestation, including the antenatal or immediate peripartum period. Substantial in-utero injury can also precede the onset of labor. A relatively common occurrence during labor is a *nonreassuring fetal monitoring strip*. A problematic monitoring strip can be associated with a variety of in-utero issues. Fetal head compression, utero-placental insufficiency, placental abruption, and other events can occur in the fetal monitoring strip. That only 12% to 23% of term infants diagnosed with CP were caused by intrapartum or peripartum events has been well described.

From a legal standpoint the statute of limitations (SOL) can last decades, which means that in many states a family can file suit against the obstetrician or pediatrician when the child is of college age. Within this context the test for SOL is generally when a reasonable plaintiff might have discovered the abnormality if they had investigated. In case of hyperimmunoglobulin E (HIE), the full extent of the injuries may not be clear for decades, which is one of the reasons that the SOL can extend so many years in these cases.

A variety of medical issues need to be considered when an infant is born with suspected HIE. Will the infant develop seizures? Was the mesenteric blood flow compromised? If so, then how long should the physician wait before the initiation of enteral feeds? Is the infant at risk for renal or other organ dysfunction? The pediatrician is well advised to consult with a neonatologist for any newborn who is born after a high-risk delivery such as this one. Many of these cases result in malpractice litigation. The pediatrician's care will likely be highly scrutinized. Did the neonate sustain additional injury after birth? Was the pediatrician's care contributory to this additional injury? Maintaining good communication with the family is particularly important in these cases. Minimally, the pediatrician should document the consultation with the family, the consultation with the neonatologist, the assessment, and the plan. Making promises to the family concerning outcome is generally not advised, given that many years may pass before the outcome is completely understood. Any assurances to the family will be based on incomplete information.

The timing of a suspected perinatal asphyxial injury sufficient to cause CP remains an issue of contention. The ACOG and AAP have published criteria to define an acute intrapartum event in a late-preterm (34 0/7 to 36 6/7 weeks' gestation) or full-term newborn that results in CP and that requires evidence of metabolic acidosis in the fetal umbilical arterial blood in conjunction with early onset moderate to severe HIE, spastic quadriplegia, or dyskinetic cerebral palsy and no underlying evidence for trauma, intrauterine drug exposure, structural brain anomaly, syndromic or genetic, infectious, or coagulation disorders.[13]

The pediatrician should be aware of the criteria that *in conjunction* suggest an intrapartum timing (within 48 hours of birth), though these criteria are not specific to asphyxial insults. These criteria include:

- Sentinel hypoxic event occurring immediately before or during labor
- Sudden and sustained fetal bradycardia or absence of fetal heart rate variability in the presence of persistent late or variable decelerations usually after an hypoxic event with a previously normal pattern
- Apgar scores of 0 to 3 beyond 5 minutes
- Onset of multisystem involvement within 72 hours of birth
- Early imaging demonstrating evidence of a nonfocal cerebral abnormality

Pediatricians should exercise care in their medical documentation and refrain from using the term *perinatal asphyxia* unless appropriate criteria exist to support using this term. Although numerous markers of intrapartum asphyxial injury have been identified, no single marker is diagnostic (Box 81-2).

BOX 81-2 Neonatal Markers of Intrapartum Asphyxial Injury

- Umbilical arterial cord or early neonatal blood gases
- Encephalopathy
- Multisystem organ dysfunction
- Seizures
- Clinical scoring systems
- Brain imaging (magnetic resonance imaging, computed tomography, neurosonography) and electroencephalographic results
- Biochemical markers (blood pH, creatine phosphokinase)
- Hematologic markers (nucleated red blood cells, platelet count)

Role of Umbilical Cord Blood Gases

Within the obstetric and risk-management communities is a growing emphasis on the role of umbilical arterial cord blood gas base deficit in timing fetal hypoxic injury. Umbilical arterial or venous blood gases or an early neonatal arterial base deficit (before administration of bicarbonate) reflect the level of acidosis at the time of delivery. Increasingly, as part of their quality-improvement and risk-management programs, hospital obstetric services are implementing protocols by which umbilical arterial cord blood gases are routinely obtained for all deliveries. Neonatal complications are associated with fetal metabolic acidosis, not as a result of respiratory acidosis. Therefore utilization of umbilical cord pH alone is not sufficient because blood pH is influenced by both respiratory and metabolic alterations. Even among newborns exhibiting severe HIE, less than 25% of cases are attributable to fetal hypoxemia.[14] At delivery the mean umbilical arterial base deficit is 4 to 5 mmol/L (if *base excess* is reported, then the respective values are 4 to 5 mmol/L).

The degree of metabolic acidosis that determines the threshold for injury is defined as greater than 2 standard deviations from the mean (10-12 mmol/L) and is accepted as greater than 12 mmol/L.[15,16] Base deficit levels exceeding 12 mmol/L occur in a less than 2% of a normal newborn population.[15,17,18] Also important to note is that the majority of newborns with a base deficit above 12 mmol/L do not demonstrate neurologic injury. Among newborns experiencing severe metabolic acidosis with base deficits above 16 mmol/L, the majority of patients either die or they are healthy if they survive.

The pediatric care physician needs to be aware of hospital protocols that require routine or risk-factor base umbilical cord blood gas analysis and have an understanding of the base deficit changes with varying fetal heart rate patterns and the normal variations in fetal base deficit attributable to mode of delivery and labor pattern in response to fetal stress and as part of the normal changes after birth.

Seizures

A pediatrician may occasionally be notified that a newborn is suspected of having had a seizure. Although this report will often place the newborn outside of the scope of general pediatric care the pediatrician may be required to provide the initial evaluation and stabilization. Although many infants will continue to breathe during a seizure, the clinician should always keep in mind the ABCs (airway, breathing, and circulation). If the newborn does not require airway management or circulatory support, then the pediatrician may give the newborn antiseizure medications. What are the complications of these drugs? Is phenobarbital the first-line drug? If the pediatrician is ordering these medications, then the potential complications, including apnea, should be considered. Incorrect dosing is a potential source of medication error; attention also needs to be paid to the medication order (loading dose or maintenance therapy), route of administration, and dosing interval. Is the seizure a result of HIE, sepsis, hypocalcemia, or a brain malformation? Is the neonate hypoglycemic? The prudent pediatrician will deal with the immediate medical needs of the newborn and promptly consult with a pediatric neurologist, a neonatologist, or both. Beyond the immediate stabilization, rarely does a general pediatrician provide continuing care for a neonate with seizures.

Medical-Legal Issues Related to Brachial Plexus Injuries

Brachial plexus injury (BPI) is relatively common in neonates, with a reported incidence of clinically significant lesions occurring at a rate of 0.5 to 2.6 per 1000 live births. Not all BPIs are the result of birth-related trauma; intrauterine malpositioning has also been implicated, especially given that BPI has been documented among healthy newborns born atraumatically by cesarean delivery. A rare nontraumatic, genetic condition—neuralgic amyotrophy—has also been described. Affected family members exhibit a similar clinical syndrome. A BPI is nonetheless an important cause of malpractice litigation against medical caregivers and therapists. The PIAA reports that nearly 60% of BPI malpractice claims result in monetary damages. Litigation may also result from a failure of the pediatric care physician to recognize medical conditions associated with BPI. These conditions include diaphragmatic paralysis, cervical spine injury, facial paralysis, shoulder subluxation and unilateral clavicular, and humeral fractures. Therefore the newborn suspected of having a BPI should have a thorough physical examination and radiographic studies to evaluate the clavicle and humerus on the involved side. Physical findings will guide the need for other studies. In general the pediatrician should carefully document normal and symmetric extremity movement and limb posture or position on the initial physical assessment and again at the time of nursery discharge.

Prognosis for recovery in BPI is typically associated with the severity of the infant's motor deficit. Infants who have moderate motor dysfunction at the time of presentation are less likely to have significant permanent weakness than infants with severe motor dysfunction. The period of recovery may continue for up to a year; however, most infants with milder injuries recover within the first few weeks. A recent meta-analysis[19] found that 20% to 30% of infants who have BPI will have residual neurologic deficits. The provision and timing of initiation of treatment are also important considerations and may also contribute to a parents' decision to initiate a claim. Initial therapy typically involves a period of immobilization to allow for resolution of edema. This therapy is followed by careful passive range-of-motion exercises to prevent contractures and muscle atrophy. Infants who are not improving by 3 to 6 months of age should be referred for further evaluation (electromyographic assessment and neurosurgery for possible nerve transplant).

Communication between the health professionals and child's parents is critical and can be an effective risk-management tool when the physician employs a proactive approach.

- The pediatrician should not assume that all BPIs are the result of birth trauma.
- Family history should be explored if the suspected BPI cannot be explained based on a difficult delivery or intrauterine malpositioning.
- Neonates with suspected BPI should be evaluated for associated conditions.
- Physical assessments should document extremity posture, position, movement, and symmetry.
- Parents should be informed about the range of recovery possible and that long-term sequelae may result from the BPI.
- Close follow-up care is important, including appropriate consultations with a pediatric neurologist and a physiatrist, as well as early intervention referrals as appropriate based on state-specific eligibility requirements.

Hyperbilirubinemia

Sixty percent of newborns develop clinical jaundice. (See Chapters 98, Neonatal Jaundice; and 197, Jaundice, for discussions on jaundice.) Consequently, most pediatricians treat newborns with elevated serum levels of indirect bilirubin. The complications of hyperbilirubinemia have been well described. Of note, kernicterus is considered a *never event* by the National Quality Forum, and cases often result in multimillion-dollar settlements. In April 2001 the Joint Commission for the Accreditation of Healthcare Organizations issued a sentinel alert about the threat posed by kernicterus, a preventable condition, to healthy newborns. In the most severe cases the newborn can sustain permanent neurologic injury or even death. Box 81-3 summarizes the factors that contribute to the risk of severe hyperbilirubinemia and kernicterus. Any of these factors can warrant more aggressive treatment of hyperbilirubinemia.

A recent publication by Beal et al[20] highlights an increasing challenge confronting health professionals who must identify and treat conditions that typically occur in higher frequencies in specific ethnic and racial groups—the increasing number of interracial infants being born. In this study conducted at the Henry Ford Health System, a major urban medical center serving a large minority population, the investigators found that racial identification in medical records did not completely overlap with maternal self-report of her infant's race. When given a single choice for their infant's race, mothers of multiracial infants overselected black race in their infants' ancestry. In general, black race places an infant in a lower-risk category for severe hyperbilirubinemia. When given the opportunity to select more than one race for their child, 41% of mothers of interracial infants described their infants as having other racial ancestry in addition to that of the mother and father. Therefore the pediatrician should consider exploring the ancestry of a newborn who exhibits clinical symptoms of a condition not common for the child's perceived race or ethnicity.

Another important cause of neonatal hyperbilirubinemia is glucose-6-phosphate dehydrogenase (G6PD)

BOX 81-3 Factors Contributing to the Risk of Severe Hyperbilirubinemia and Kernicterus

- Early discharge at less than 48 hours of age with:
  - Not recognizing that bilirubin is rising at the time of discharge
  - Inappropriate discharge of late preterm newborns
  - Failure to educate parents about the dangers of jaundice
  - Failure to ensure targeted follow up within 48 hours of nursery discharge (no appointment given)
    - Newborns with a total serum bilirubin (TSB) in the intermediate risk zone require a repeat bilirubin within 12-24 hours.
    - Newborns with a TSB in the high-risk zone should be treated.
- Failure to recognize that the severity of hyperbilirubinemia corrected for age in hours, not days of life (Bhutani curve)
- Failure to recognize risk factors
- Delay in timely or intensive intervention predischarge or at readmission
- Not recognizing the inaccuracies of visual assessment of jaundice
- Not responding appropriately to parental concerns about jaundice, poor feeding, or changes in infant behavior

The decision on whether to initiate phototherapy (or other interventions) is generally based on published algorithms and consideration of complicating factors:

- Was jaundice noticed during the first day of life?
- Does the baby have blood group incompatibility? Is the Coombs test positive?
- Does the baby have sepsis?
- Is the baby premature, between 35 and 36 weeks' gestation?
- Is the baby exclusively breastfeeding with evidence for inadequate intake?
- Is the risk for G6PD deficiency present?
- Does evidence exist of bruising or cephalohematoma?
- Is the baby's race East Asian?

G6PD, Glucose-6-phosphate dehydrogenase.

deficiency. Diverse population groups are affected by G6PD deficiency caused by many gene polymorphisms that result in decreased bilirubin conjugation. Population migration has contributed to a worldwide distribution of babies born with hyperbilirubinemia caused by G6PD deficiency. An important point to remember is that although black newborns are commonly considered as being in a lower risk group for severe hyperbilirubinemia, these babies are the largest population group affected by G6PD deficiency in North America. Documented cases of kernicterus caused by severe hyperbilirubinemia in black G6PD-deficient newborns have been reported. G6PD deficiency is an X-linked condition and is rarely considered to be a causative factor in newborn girls with hyperbilirubinemia. However, G6PD-deficient heterozygote girls have also been identified and may occur in up to 10% of heterozygote girls.

Given that hyperbilirubinemia is common, the pediatrician needs to remain current with the literature related to neonatal hyperbilirubinemia. If a particular newborn's course is complicated by serum levels that are increasing quickly, inadequate response to phototherapy, hemolysis, anemia, altered neurologic examination or mental status, or by other significant finding, then the pediatrician should strongly consider consultation with a neonatologist. The management of these cases can be complex, and the potential for liability is extremely high. If a newborn suffers a severe complication for hyperbilirubinemia, then the pediatrician's treatment will likely be scrutinized. How often were bilirubin levels checked? How quickly was therapy instituted? Was a consultation with a neonatologist obtained? The care and treatment of newborns with severe hyperbilirubinemia can lead to litigation, and the infant and the pediatrician will likely benefit from the input from a neonatologist. The key to protecting the pediatrician and ensuring optimal care for the newborn is risk assessment (performing systematic assessments on all newborns before nursery discharge for the risk of developing hyperbilirubinemia through the implementation of nursery protocols that integrate bilirubin measurement using transcutaneous bilirubin or total serum bilirubin testing and risk factor identification) and appropriate follow-up according to the time of discharge and infant risk factors.

Procedures

Pediatricians are occasionally required to perform procedures on newborn patients. General rules for procedures involve competence, training, technique, consent, and documentation. In the nonemergency setting the risk, benefits, and alternatives should be discussed with the parents, and this discussion should be documented. In the emergency setting, pediatricians should use their best judgment. Will the newborn be harmed by delaying the procedure until consent can be obtained? If a newborn requires emergency intubation in the delivery room, then obtaining consent from the parents is unnecessary. This procedure generally falls under the *emergency exception to the informed-consent doctrine*. Basically, informed consent is not necessary if the clinician's intervention is needed on an emergency basis. For example, when called to a delivery that is complicated by meconium-stained amniotic fluid the prudent pediatrician will explain to the parents that the neonate may be intubated. In many instances, time for such a discussion is not available. In this case the pediatrician is well advised to put the interest of the baby at the forefront. Proceeding without consent is acceptable if the physician can clearly demonstrate the necessity of the procedure and the emergency nature of the situation.

Procedures should be accompanied by procedure notes. Box 81-4 contains the essential elements of the procedure note. The Joint Commission for the Accreditation of Healthcare Organizations mandates a *time out* before any procedure to ensure patient safety

BOX 81-4 Essential Elements of a Procedure Note

- Name of procedure
- Indications
- Consent (if none, then explain reasons for lack of consent)
- Performance of a *time out*
- Documentation of events, including sterile technique and preparation
- Blood loss, if applicable
- Complications (if none, then document)
- Infant's tolerance
- Results of indicated follow-up studies (eg, radiograph to confirm umbilical line position)

(www.jointcommission.org). A time out is a planned period of discussion before the procedure is initiated, during which time the team verbally confirms the identification of the patient, the procedure to be undertaken, and the location. A time out can prevent a procedure from being performed on the wrong patient or the wrong side. Even if the note is added to the chart later the pediatrician should still document the indications, procedure performed, success or failure, complications, blood loss (if appropriate), and patient tolerance. If a follow-up study, such as a chest radiograph, is indicated, then the procedure note should include this information as well. Even noting that *chest x-ray is pending* documents that the clinician understands the importance of verifying the success or failure of the procedure.

Umbilical Line Complications

Some pediatricians place umbilical lines as part of their routine practice in level II neonatal intensive care units. Other pediatricians will place umbilical lines on rare occasions and only under emergency situations. In either case the attending physician needs to understand the potential complications from central venous and arterial access. The most common complications involve vasospasm, thromboembolic events, damage to the vessels being cannulated, exsanguination, and infection. Sterile technique should be used in the placement of central vascular access, and this precaution should be included in the pediatrician's procedure note. Complications, if any, should be promptly evaluated. A referral to a neonatologist is likely appropriate for any infant with a complication related to vascular access.

Transport and Referral

If a neonate requires a higher level of care, then the pediatrician will generally arrange for a transfer of service or transport to another facility. The referring pediatrician will occasionally also be the admitting physician at the receiving facility. When is the referring pediatrician no longer responsible for the decision making? Who is liable if the newborn suffers a complication after the receiving facility has been contacted? Who is liable if the newborn is harmed during transport? The answer is based, at least in part, on the role of the respective physicians. Is the referring physician making management decisions while the receiving physician is making suggestions, or has the receiving physician taken over management of the patient?

In the case of Sterling v Johns Hopkins,[21] a woman with severe preeclampsia died after transport, and the husband alleged that negligent telephone advice had been given by the receiving facility. After reviewing the facts of this case the court determined that the receiving physician was largely functioning in the role of a consultant and that the referring physician was responsible for the management decisions that were made.

MEDICAL-LEGAL CONSIDERATIONS IN OFFICE CARE OF NEWBORNS

Pediatricians spend up to 40% of their time providing preventive health care to children. During these health supervision visits, they are expected to provide an increasing number of services, from history taking and physical examination to immunizations to assessing developmental milestones to counseling, in a decreasing amount of time. Furthermore, during these visits, pediatricians need to diagnose medical problems that may not have been present or detectable in the first few days of life. For example, many ventricular septal defects are discovered only in patients older than 1 month, when pulmonary vascular resistance decreases. Failure to diagnose in a timely manner and failure to provide appropriate preventive care may give rise to liability.

Appropriate and timely follow-up of discharged newborns is essential to ensure safe and high-quality care. Several problems may not become apparent until after discharge but require intervention well before the traditional 1- to 2-week visit. Hyperbilirubinemia affects a majority of healthy term newborns, as discussed previously. Timely intervention is necessary to prevent severe and irreversible neurologic impairment. Pediatricians who wish to minimize their liability while providing the best care are advised to follow the AAP Subcommittee on Hyperbilirubinemia clinical practice guidelines published in July 2004 (see Tools for Practice).

Newborn screening programs exist in every state, and testing is performed on more than 4 million newborns each year. With the introduction of tandem mass spectrometry, the capability now exists to screen for more than 50 disorders from a single blood spot. Presently, wide variability exists among states with regard to the number and type of disorders to be screened. Pediatricians need to be aware of the specific screening tests mandated in their respective state. This awareness is particularly important for infants entering the pediatrician's practice who may have been born in a different state or outside of the United States. Comprehensive information can be found at the Web site of the National Newborn Screening and Genetics Resource Center (genes-r-us.uthscsa.edu/).

Furthermore, pediatricians must be certain that organized systems are in place so that results outside the reference range receive a timely response. Pediatricians must also be certain that newborns who missed the newborn screen before nursery discharge, who had an inadequate or untestable specimen, or who had their screens obtained before 24 hours of consuming milk (breast milk or formula) receive the appropriate follow-up testing. This approach applies to newborn hearing screening as well, given that permanent hearing loss is far more prevalent than most other conditions screened, and early intervention is key to optimizing the child's functional and educational outcomes. Certain abnormalities, such as congenital adrenal hyperplasia, are considered emergencies and require immediate attention. Finally, pediatricians must consider whether a diagnosis may affect future pregnancies for the parents or other family members; pediatricians should also refer the parents for appropriate genetic counseling when necessary.

Appropriate preventive care covers a large number of issues that vary based on age. To ensure that necessary topics are covered during a visit, as well as to ensure that appropriate documentation is maintained, pediatricians should consider using preprinted structured documentation forms. Clinicians may choose to develop these forms themselves or use the forms that are available from the AAP.

COMMUNICATION ISSUES

Communication is an integral component of providing excellent patient care. This concept is fundamental from a medical-legal standpoint, as well as an ethical perspective. The AAP and the American Board of Pediatrics recognize the importance of interpersonal and communication skills in providing quality patient care. Furthermore, a poor relationship between a patient and a physician is more likely to result in a lawsuit.[22] (Information on communicating with families is contained in Chapter 16, Disclosing a Diagnosis With Parents and Patients; and Chapter 67, Partnering With Families in Hospital and Community Settings.)

In addition to communication with the parents, clinicians must make every attempt to ensure effective communication with other members of the health care team. Effective communication and care transition is essential to safe and effective patient care (see Chapter 19, Art of Referral, Consultation, and Collaborative Management; and Chapter 64, Children With Ongoing Health Conditions).

PATIENT SAFETY

Errors in patient care are a major problem in health care. A seminal 1999 report of the Institute of Medicine, *To Err is Human: Building a Safer Health System*,[23] estimated that 98,000 deaths per year may be attributable to medical errors, and the Institute of Medicine demanded a complete shift in the health care culture. Although progress to date has been mixed, significant efforts have been made to improve patient safety. (See Chapter 6, Quality Improvement in Pediatric Primary Care.)

MINIMIZING LIABILITY RISK

Approximately one in seven physicians are sued every year.[24] The current process of litigation is expensive, time consuming, and unpleasant. Even though no guarantees exist, methods can be used to minimize the chances of being named in a malpractice suit.

Maintaining competency is an essential task, not only for risk management, but also as an ethical imperative in its own right. Medicine today is a rapidly changing field. For example, dexamethasone was frequently used 10 years ago to wean premature babies with chronic lung disease from ventilators. When long-term follow-up studies revealed poor neurologic outcomes, the use of steroids was rapidly curtailed. Failing to keep current might lead a physician to use medications or treatments even after their use has been widely abandoned. The AAP actively assists pediatricians with keeping current and has developed a Web site that provides an individualized learning plan (www.pedialink.org).

Pediatrics has become increasingly specialized, and most subspecialty and tertiary-care services are organized into a regionalized system. These systems allow all pediatricians to maintain professional ties with one another, as well as with larger medical centers. This factor becomes important when appropriate consultation, referral, and transport may be necessary to provide optimal care.

A clinician is occasionally faced with a particularly rare or challenging patient. In these situations, obtaining assistance is important. Maintaining contact with former attendees and mentors from residency can be helpful. Furthermore, academic centers with training programs will regularly discuss particularly difficult clinical cases during management conferences, morning report, grand rounds, and other meetings.

Keeping parents involved and informed is absolutely essential. Persons who feel uninformed and ignored can easily become frustrated and upset. Furthermore, they will quickly lose trust in the health care providers. Mistrust, dissatisfaction, and anger, combined with an undesirable outcome, can easily lead to a malpractice suit.

Proper documentation is an important component of risk management. One common mantra notes, "If it wasn't documented, it wasn't done." Furthermore, poor documentation reflects poorly on the clinician and can make even appropriate care appear to be shoddy and unorganized. Indeed, the PIAA found that of all the closed claims in 2004 involving a problem with the medical record, a payout occurred in 62% of them. The clinician's notes should be timed and dated, with *late entries* documented as such. All important events should be documented, along with the clinicians thought process and the rationale for the treatments.

Telephone advice can be a significant source of liability in pediatrics. Especially in the immediate newborn period, determining the clinical picture appropriately over the telephone may be especially difficult. When in doubt, the pediatrician should avoid diagnosing over the telephone. Furthermore, all telephone advice should be documented appropriately.

Finally, although United States Supreme Court cases often generate headlines, medical practice is

BOX 81-5 Strategies to Minimize Liability Risk

- Keep current through an individualized learning plan.
- Maintain professional ties with a large medical center.
- Consult with a colleague when encountering a difficult situation.
- Communicate frequently and honestly with parents.
- Document in a timely and thorough manner; include impressions and thought processes.
- Document telephone advice.
- If uncertainty exists, then do not diagnose over the telephone.
- Be aware of state laws that affect the practice.

generally regulated by each state. State government legislation and case law covers a wide variety of issues that pediatricians encounter, from the age of consent to resuscitation standards, as well as professional licensing and discipline. Furthermore, medical malpractice is controlled by the states. Therefore all practicing pediatricians need to stay up to date on the laws and regulations that affect their practice. This task can be achieved by referring to the AAP Web site, and to information disseminated by the clinician's local AAP chapter. The American Association of Family Physicians also provides its members with federal and state updates. In addition, state medical societies are a good source for current rules and regulations guiding practices. Box 81-5 summarizes strategies to minimize liability risk.

CONCLUSIONS

Clinicians should make every attempt to understand their rights, duties, and liabilities as physicians. This chapter provides an overview of medical-legal considerations in the care of newborn infants. For more detailed information, the AAP Committee on Medical Liability has published a book on *Medical Liability for Pediatricians.*

Pediatricians are appropriately concerned about the liability risks they encounter when treating newborns. Nevertheless, many steps can be taken that can minimize liability risk. Most of these steps, such as keeping current, documenting appropriately, and focusing on communication and safety, are also prerequisites for practicing good clinical medicine.

TOOLS FOR PRACTICE

Medical Decision Support

- *Bright Futures: Guidelines for Health Supervision of Infants, Children,* and *Adolescents* (book), Bright Futures (brightfutures.aap.org/web/).
- *Guidelines for Perinatal Care* (book), American Academy of Pediatrics and the American College of Obstetricians and Gynecologists (www.aap.org/bookstore).
- *Medical Liability for Pediatricians* (book), American Academy of Pediatrics (www.aap.org/bookstore).

Practice Management and Care Coordination

- *Documentation Forms* (www.aap.org/bookstore)
- *Medical Liability—AAP Member Center* (Web page), American Academy of Pediatrics (www.aap.org/moc/medicalliability/index.cfm?CFID=2065071&CFTOKEN=33319059).
- *Safer Health Care for Kids* (Web page), American Academy of Pediatrics (www.aap.org/saferhealthcare/).
- *Vaccine Administration Record* (www.aap.org/bookstore).

RELATED WEB SITES

- Joint Commission for the Accreditation of Healthcare Organizations (JCAHO) (www.jointcommission.org/).
- National Newborn Screening and Genetics Resource Center (genes-r-us.uthscsa.edu/).
- PediaLink Individualized Learning Plan, American Academy of Pediatrics (www.pedialink.org).
- Physician Insurers Association of America (PIAA) (www.piaa.us/).

AAP POLICY STATEMENTS

American Academy of Pediatrics, Steering Committee on Quality Improvement and Management. Improve the health of children: principles for the development and use of quality measures (in press).

American Academy of Pediatrics, Subcommittee on Hyperbilirubinemia. Management of hyperbilirubinemia in the newborn infant 35 or more weeks of gestation. *Pediatrics.* 2004;114(1):297-316. (aappolicy.aappublications.org/cgi/content/full/pediatrics;114/1/297).

Kaye CI, American Academy of Pediatrics, Committee on Genetics. Introduction to the newborn screening fact sheets. *Pediatrics.* 2006;118(3):1304-1312. (pediatrics.aappublications.org).

Kaye CI, American Academy of Pediatrics, Committee on Genetics. Newborn screening fact sheets. *Pediatrics.* 2006;118(3):e934-e963. (pediatrics.aappublications.org).

REFERENCES

1. DeFrances CJ, Hall MJ, Podogornik MN. *2003 National Hospital Discharge Survey. Advance Data from Vital and Health Statistics. No 359.* Hyattsville, MD: National Center for Health Statistics; 2005.
2. Mello MM, Studdert DM, Brennan TA. The new medical malpractice crisis. *N Engl Med.* 2003;348:2281-2282.
3. American Medical Association. America's Medical Liability Crisis: We All Pay for the Broken System. Available at: www.ama-assn.org/ama1/pub/upload/mm/399/mlr_fastfacts.pdf. Accessed on August 10, 2007.
4. Merritt, Hawkings & Associates. Summary Report: 2003 Survey of Final-Year Medical Residents. Available at: www.merritthawkins.com/pdf/MHA2003residentsurv.pdf. Accessed August 10, 2007.
5. Zuger A. Dissatisfaction with medical practice. *N Engl J Med.* 2004;350:69-75.
6. Hickson GB, Clayton EW, Githens PB, et al. Factors that prompted families to file malpractice claims following perinatal injuries. *JAMA.* 1992;267:1359-1363.
7. Annibale DJ, Hulsey TC, Wagner CL, et al. Comparative neonatal morbidity of abdominal and vaginal deliveries after uncomplicated pregnancies. *Arch Pediatr Adolesc Med.* 1995;149:862-867.

8. Levine EM, Ghai V, Barton JJ, et al. Pediatrician attendance at cesarean delivery: necessary or not? *Obstet Gynecol.* 1999;93:338-340.
9. Hook B, Kiwi R, Amini SB, et al. Neonatal morbidity after elective repeat cesarean section and trial of labor. *Pediatrics.* 1997;100:348-353.
10. Mitchell A, Niday P, Boulton J, et al. A prospective clinical audit of neonatal practices in Canada. *Adv Neonat Care.* 2002;2:316-326.
11. Boluyt N, van Kempen A, Offringa M. Neurodevelopment after neonatal hypoglycemia: a systematic review and design of an optimal future study. *Pediatrics.* 2006; 17:2231-2243.
12. Brand P, Molenaar N, Kaaijk C, et al. Neurodevelopmental outcome of hypoglycemia in healthy, large for gestational age, term newborns. *Arch Dis Child.* 2005;90:78-81.
13. American College of Obstetrics and Gynecology and American Academy of Pediatrics. *Monograph: Neonatal Encephalopathy and Cerebral Palsy: Defining the Pathogenesis and Pathophysiology.* Washington, DC: American College of Obstetrics and Gynecology; 2003.
14. Low JA, Galbraith RS, Muir DW, et al. The relationship between perinatal hypoxia and newborn encephalopathy. *Am J Obstet Gynecol.* 1985;152(3):256-260.
15. Helwig JT, Parer JT, Kilpatrick SJ, et al. Umbilical cord blood acid-base state: what is normal? *Am J Obstet Gynecol.* 1996;174(6):1807-1812.
16. Dellinger EH, Boehm FH, Crane MM. Electronic fetal heart rate monitoring: early neonatal outcomes associated with normal rate, fetal stress, and fetal distress. *Am J Obstet Gynecol.* 2000;182(1 Pt 1):214-220.
17. Low JA, Lindsay BG, Derrick EJ. Threshold of metabolic acidosis associated with newborn complications. *Am J Obstet Gynecol.* 1997;177(6):1391-1394.
18. Arikan GM, Scholz HS, Petru E, et al. Cord blood oxygen saturation in vigorous infants at birth: what is normal? *BJOG.* 2000;107(8):987-994.
19. Pondaag W, Malessy MJ, van Dijk JG, et al. Natural history of obstetric brachial plexus injury: a systematic review. *Dev Med Child Neurol.* 2004;46:138-144.
20. Beal A, Chou S-C, Palmer H, et al. The changing face of race: risk factors for neonatal hyperbilirubinemia. *Pediatrics.* 2006;117:1618-1625.
21. Sterling v. John Hopkins Hospital, 802 A.2d 440, 2002.
22. Vincent C, Young M, Phillips A. Why do people sue doctors? A study of patients and relatives taking legal action. *Lancet.* 1994;343:1609-1613.
23. Institute of Medicine, Committee on Quality of Health Care in America. *To Err is Human: Building a Safer Health System.* Washington DC: National Academy Press; 2000.
24. Forster HP, Schwartz J, DeRenzo E. Reducing legal risk by practicing patient-centered medicine. *Arch Intern Med.* 2002;162:1217-1219.

Chapter 82

MATERNAL MEDICAL HISTORY

Harpreet Kaur, MD; Deborah E. Campbell, MD

The maternal history is critical in identifying risk factors that can contribute to illness in the infant. The health of the mother directly affects the well being of the fetus and baby. The health professional should learn about the family constellation and the mother's physical and mental health, life stressors, support systems, and developmental adaptation to the prospect of becoming a parent. The health professional should also inquire about the family's preparations for the infant's homecoming and potential safety concerns, as well as identify resource needs and the availability of family and community supports and discuss the timing of postdischarge follow-up care for the infant.

PRECONCEPTION AND ANTENATAL HISTORY

Comprehensive care for a newborn requires a thorough review of the maternal history in preparation for examination of the newborn. Unfavorable maternal social history, poor socioeconomic status and educational history, lack of adequate prenatal care, poor nutrition and inadequate pregnancy weight gain, and exposure to nicotine, alcohol, illicit substances, domestic violence, and other environmental hazards contribute to adverse pregnancy outcomes.[1-10] The evidence of the harmful effects of maternal exposure to environmental toxins on fetal well being is increasing. Maternal race, ethnicity, and history of recent immigration are additional factors that influence pregnancy risks and outcomes. Acculturation over time moderates the benefits seen among recent immigrant women who benefit from close community support for the pregnant woman. The literature that documents the adverse health effects of chronic stress and its effect on minority, particularly black, women is also growing.[11-13] Fetal growth has also been shown to be affected by generational influences with regard to both low birth weight and cardiovascular risk.[14,15]

The practitioner examining the newborn may be alerted to suspect possible maternal drug abuse in an infant exhibiting irritability, poor feeding, vomiting, high-pitched crying, or tremors. Fetal alcohol spectrum disorders remain the largest cause of nongenetic disability worldwide and are 100% preventable. In the Western world the rate of fetal alcohol syndrome is reported as 1 in 1000 live births. In the United Kingdom, where two thirds of pregnant women admit to alcohol consumption while pregnant, 1 in 100 infants born are diagnosed with fetal alcohol syndrome. The Centers for Disease Control and Prevention 2002 Behavioral Risk Factor Surveillance System survey found that 1 in 30 pregnant women report *risk drinking* (seven or more drinks per week or five or more drinks on one occasion), with 10% of pregnant women acknowledging alcohol use during their pregnancy and 2% admitting to binge drinking. Among women of child-bearing age who are not practicing birth control, more than 50% of report using alcohol, and 12.4% report binge drinking.[16] (See Chapter 103, Prenatal Drug Abuse and Neonatal Drug Withdrawal Syndrome.)

Assisted Reproduction

The mode of conception is an additional aspect of the pregnancy history that provides the clinician with valuable information. Assisted reproduction technology (ART) has become a routine aspect of the fertility process for families worldwide, given that the rate of infertility among couples is 15%. Estimates suggest that between 1% and 5% of all neonates born are conceived through ART. Outcomes for these pregnancies vary with assistive reproductive technique, the underlying cause for the female or male infertility, and the need to use donor eggs. This information is important in determining the infant's future care and may influence the parents' adaptation to parenthood and necessitate extra care on the part of the pediatric primary care physician, should the parents choose to keep this information confidential from other family members. Singleton infants born from ART pregnancies are more likely to be preterm or low birth weight and experience similar complications related to these conditions. ART pregnancies that result in multiple births are also at risk for prematurity, low birth weight, and increased perinatal mortality and morbidity and have higher rates of congenital malformations and epigenetic alterations (imprinting defects). (See Chapter 72, Assistive Reproductive Technologies, Multiple Births, and Pregnancy Outcomes.)

Pre-existing Health Conditions

A maternal history of chronic medical conditions such as diabetes, hypertension, severe anemia, and thyroid disease can have perinatal effects on the fetus and can influence the postnatal course for the newborn. Box 82-1 provides an outline of maternal and family factors that can affect pregnancy and infant health. A woman with poorly controlled diabetes is at risk for pregnancy complications that can affect the neonate in several ways, causing fetal macrosomia that places the infant at risk for dystocia at delivery, metabolic derangements after birth, respiratory distress, hyperbilirubinemia, and, if the mother has preexisting diabetes, a variety of birth defects. Chronic hypertension and hypertensive disorders of pregnancy increase the risk of preterm delivery and fetal growth restriction. Abruptio placenta can cause neonatal anemia, perinatal distress, and permanent neurologic injury. Maternal asthma increases the risk of fetal death and spontaneous abortion. Infants born to women with Grave disease may develop neonatal thyrotoxicosis as a result of transplacental passage of maternal antibodies. Similarly, an infant born to a woman with autoimmune thrombocytopenia is at risk for intraventricular hemorrhage. An infant diagnosed with congenital heart block may be the first indication that the mother has an underlying autoimmune disorder.

The maternal medical history can also influence the counseling provided to the mother and family. A woman with a history of epilepsy, particularly if she continues to experience seizures, requires specific guidance on how to care for her infant safely, especially if she is alone with the infant. The paternal history also influences considerations regarding risks to the infant's health and need for follow-up evaluations. A paternal history of a genetic disorder or carrier status may necessitate specific infant screening. Young and advanced paternal age have been associated with the risk for infant low birth weight. Advanced paternal age has also been associated with de novo or abnormal methylation of paternally imprinted genes. Environmental exposures may affect both parents, with exposure to organic solvents, pesticides, and radiation causing the greatest concerns for fetal development.

Infants born to women on medications may experience complications from drugs that cross the placenta and accumulate in fetal tissues. A baby born to a woman with hypothyroidism who is taking propylthiouracil may exhibit transient neonatal hypothyroidism. Maternal medication use can further affect the clinical care of an infant and can aid in the diagnosis of an infant born with specific signs or stigmata. A history of antiepileptogenic medication use with carbamazepine, valproic acid, or phenytoin is associated with risk for embryopathy. Maternal depression has the potential to affect the fetus and newborn, as does the treatment of this condition in the pregnant woman.[17] The increasing use of antidepressant therapy during pregnancy, particularly selective serotonin reuptake inhibitors, for treatment of depression has not been associated with an increased risk of major congenital malformations but is linked to an increased incidence of neonatal abstinence syndrome and poor neonatal adaptation.[18-24]

PRENATAL TESTING AND DIAGNOSIS

Approximately 10% of all infants born will be found to have a birth defect. Maternal prenatal screening can therefore provide valuable information that can identify potential risk factors for the infant, as well as detect conditions that are treatable during pregnancy, with the opportunity to improve the perinatal outcome. Many pregnant women undergo sonography during their pregnancy for a variety of reasons. The information gathered from one or more sonographic studies may identify a fetal abnormality or aberrant fetal growth. In some instances, further evaluations and a diagnosis will have been known before the infant's birth. In other cases, a suspected abnormality will require evaluation after the infant's birth to confirm its presence, to identify other abnormalities, and to determine a course of care. Advances in prenatal sonography, magnetic resonance imaging, and prenatal genetic diagnosis have contributed to many more infants with suspected or confirmed anomalies at the time of their birth. Depending on the suspected anomaly or problem the infant may be cared for in the newborn nursery and undergo evaluation there rather than being separated from the mother in a neonatal unit.

For some infants, prenatal diagnosis may provide an opportunity for fetal therapy to correct an abnormality, with the goal of improving the chance for fetal survival or improving the long-term outcome for the infant after birth by preventing or reversing a process that can affect organ function. Monochorionic twins are at risk for twin-to-twin transfusion syndrome because of vascular interconnections. Fetal therapy involving laser ablation of these vessels can improve the chance for survival of the donor twin. A variety of fetal interventions for potentially life-threatening fetal malformations offer promise in improving survival rates and functional outcomes. Information obtained from the maternal testing may also provide valuable information. Discordancy in a twin gestation or abnormal umbilical vessel Doppler studies should alert the clinician to potential postnatal problems. A report of

BOX 82-1 Maternal Medical and Family History

AUTOIMMUNE DISORDERS
- Systemic lupus erythematosus
- Rheumatoid arthritis

CARDIOVASCULAR DISORDERS
- Hypertension
- Arrhythmia
- Atherosclerotic hemodialysis
- Congenital anomalies
- Rheumatic hemodialysis
- Thromboembolic disease

ENDOCRINE DISORDERS
- Thyroid
- Adrenal
- Diabetes

GASTROINTESTINAL DISEASES
- Hepatitis
- Gallbladder disease
- Inflammatory bowel disease

GYNECOLOGIC HISTORY ISSUES
- Breast or other genital tract disorders
- Breast surgery or other genital tract procedures
- Abnormal Papanicolaou smear
- Diethylstilbestrol exposure

HEMATOLOGIC-ONCOLOGIC CONDITIONS
- Anemia
- Coagulation disorders
- Thrombocytopenia (immune thrombocytopenic purpura)
- Cancer history
- Hemoglobinopathy

INFECTIOUS DISEASES
- Chlamydia
- Gonorrhea
- Herpes
- HIV
- Human papillomavirus
- Syphilis

NEUROMUSCULAR AND NEUROLOGIC CONDITIONS
- Seizure disorder
- Myotonia
- Aneurysm
- Arteriovenous malformation

PULMONARY DISORDERS
- Asthma
- Tuberculosis

RENAL CONDITIONS
- Anomalies
- Urinary tract infection
- Pyelonephritis

MENTAL HEALTH PROBLEMS
- Depression
- Eating disorder
- Domestic violence
- Psychosis
- Substance abuse

OTHER ISSUES
- Allergies
- Environmental exposures
- Medications (prescription and over the counter), complementary (herbal) products
- Prior surgeries
- History of trauma
- History of prior blood transfusion

FAMILY GENETIC HISTORY ISSUES
- Congenital anomalies
  - Neural tube defects
  - Congenital heart disease
  - Cleft lip or palate
  - Other
- Chromosomal anomalies
  - Aneuploidy—trisomy 21, 13, 18
  - Intellectual disability
    - Fragile X disease risk
    - Prader-Willi syndrome
  - Recurrent pregnancy loss
  - Other
- Maternal age older than 34 years or advanced paternal age
- Inherited disorders
  - Cystic fibrosis
  - Hemoglobinopathy
  - Hemophilia
  - Metabolic disorders
  - Neuromuscular disease
    - Muscular dystrophy
    - Huntington chorea
    - Familial dysautonomia
    - Tay-Sachs disease, Canavan disease
  - Renal disease
- Conditions linked to ethnic background or consanguinity

polyhydramnios or oligohydramnios should raise specific differential diagnoses for consideration.

FAMILY HISTORY

The family medical history provides the health professional with valuable information. Numerous hereditary conditions can affect the newborn. The clinician should obtain a detailed family history regarding illnesses or conditions that are present in family members. Congenital heart disease, pyloric stenosis, or Hirschsprung disease in a previous child increases the risk for these conditions in subsequent pregnancies. Diseases such

Table 82-1 Effect of Maternal Infections on the Newborn

INFECTION	EFFECT
Rubella	IUGR, microcephaly, rash, congenital heart disease
Tuberculin test	Asymptomatic mothers with positive purified protein derivative require a chest x-ray to rule out active tuberculosus (TB). Active TB is a contraindication to breastfeeding.
Hepatitis B surface antigen	Babies born to mothers with infection need hepatitis B vaccine immediately after birth hepatitis B immune globulin within 7 days. These infants require hepatitis B surface antigen (HBsAg) and anti–HBsAg at 9-18 month to check for infection.
Serologic test for syphilis	Increased risk of stillbirth, IUGR, hydrops, premature labor. Treatment with penicillin if (a) physical laboratory or radiographic evidence of active disease, (b) positive testing on direct fluorescent antibody staining on cord blood, (c) cerebral spinal fluid-VDRL is positive, (d) serum non–treponemal titer at least fourfold higher than the mother.
HIV	Treatment during pregnancy and delivery decreases the incidence. Newborns are screened at birth and started on prophylactic therapy.
Group B *Streptococcus*	Greatest risk for sepsis
Gonorrhea, chlamydia	Conjunctivitis

IUGR, Intrauterine growth restriction; *VDRL,* Venereal Disease Research Laboratory.

as hemophilia, sickle cell disease, Tay-Sachs disease, and cystic fibrosis are inherited. Parents should be asked if they are related because consanguinity increases the risk of autosomal-recessive disorders. The increased availability of genetic counseling and testing affords families the opportunity for a more comprehensive evaluation when a history of multiple pregnancy losses exists. As a result, genetic information is available for many more infants who have chromosome-related syndromes and balanced translocations at the time of their birth. Routine pregnancy testing includes a quad screen (see Chapter 73, Fetal Assessment) and may entail serial sonography for fetal growth, as well as a fetal evaluation for the presence of anomalies.

Review of the pregnancy history should also include the results of maternal screening during pregnancy, including maternal syphilis serology, group B *Streptococcus* colonization, and hepatitis B status, as well as possibly HIV and tuberculosis status (depending on specific state public health law requirements and maternal risk factors), blood type, and Rh and antibody (Coombs) tests. Additional test results to consider are the maternal complete blood count, blood chemistries, and studies performed in the evaluation of the mother with hypertensive disease in pregnancy, diabetes-screening studies (glucose challenge and glucose tolerance tests), and a test for thyroid disease. The clinician should inquire about a maternal history of herpes infection, treatments received, and any episodes during the current pregnancy (Table 82-1). Perinatal HIV prevention is a critical component of prenatal care required for all women, given that women are the fastest-growing group of individuals with HIV diagnoses in the United States and in many countries worldwide. Estimates indicate that 6000 to 7000 HIV-positive women give birth annually in the United States. Of particular importance is the fact that 40% of infected infants are born to women whose HIV status was not known during the pregnancy.[25] Knowledge about the woman's HIV status is also important because this status will guide breastfeeding counseling and identify infants who are in need of perinatal treatment with zidovudine to reduce the rate of HIV transmission to the infant and postnatal testing to determine whether HIV infection of the infant has occurred. Specific state public health policies augment the Centers for Disease Control and Prevention and the Institute of Medicine recommendations regarding requirements for maternal counseling and testing during pregnancy and labor and requirements for postnatal evaluation and treatment of at-risk infants.[26]

Congenital syphilis, a serious, preventable disease, continues to be an important public health and clinical care challenge.[27] Up to 40% of pregnancies in women with untreated syphilis result in fetal or perinatal death. Despite the continued increase in rates of primary and secondary syphilis among both men and women, intensive state public health surveillance programs for pregnant women have reduced the number of congenital syphilis cases. The Centers for Disease Control and Prevention recommends screening women at high risk for syphilis during the first and third trimesters of pregnancy. Screening for syphilis at delivery primarily ensures that infants born to women in whom syphilis previously was either unidentified or untreated are identified and treated. Follow-up evaluation of an at-risk infant born to a woman with positive serologic testing is necessary to ensure appropriate management.

Maternal immunization history should be reviewed. Vaccination of pregnant women is permissible with inactivated virus or bacterial vaccines or toxoids. Live-virus vaccines are generally contraindicated during pregnancy because of the theoretical risk of virus transmission to the fetus. Inactivated influenza vaccination is recommended during the winter season. Routine postpartum administration of tetanus toxoid, reduced diphtheria toxoid, and acellular pertussis (Tdap) vaccine is now recommended for women who have not previously received a dose of Tdap, even for women who are breastfeeding. Specific guidance regarding current Centers for Disease Control and Prevention Advisory Council on Immunization Practices recommendations (www.cdc.gov/vaccines/pubs/preg-guide.htm).

INTRAPARTUM COURSE

The intrapartum course can also influence the infant's care and anticipated postnatal course. A maternal history of prolonged rupture of the membranes or meconium-stained amniotic fluid provides important details that guide the newborn's initial management and alert the clinician to the level and scope of observation or assessment required. A meconium-stained neonate who exhibits intrapartum fetal distress is at increased risk for hypoglycemia, respiratory distress, pulmonary hypertension, and pulmonary air leak (pneumothorax, pneumomediastinum). Female infants born by cesarean delivery as a result of breech presentation require close surveillance for developmental dysplasia of hips.

DURATION OF PREGNANCY

Gestational age is calculated in completed weeks as the time elapsed between the first day of the last menstrual period and the day of delivery. If pregnancy was achieved using ART, then gestational age is calculated by adding 2 weeks to the conceptional age. Ultrasound in the first trimester provides a reliable estimation of the gestational age. *Full term* is defined as any neonate whose birth occurs from the beginning of the first day of the thirty-eighth week (day 260) through the end of the last day of the forty-second week (day 294) after the onset of the last menstrual period. By convention this means that an infant born from 37 0/7 to 42 0/7 weeks' gestation is classified as *term*. Prematurity is defined as less than 37 0/7 weeks' gestation. Postterm infants are at greater risk of perinatal morbidity and death.

TOOLS FOR PRACTICE

Medical Decision Support

- *Alcohol Consumption Among Women Who Are Pregnant or Who Might Become Pregnant—United States, 2002,* Centers for Disease Control and Prevention (www.cdc.gov/mmwr/preview/mmwrhtml/mm5350a4.htm).
- *Guidelines for Vaccinating Pregnant Women,* Centers for Disease Control and Prevention (www.cdc.gov/vaccines/pubs/preg-guide.htm).
- *STD Surveillance 2005,* Centers for Disease Control and Prevention (www.cdc.gov/std/stats/toc2005.htm).

AAP POLICY STATEMENTS

Mofenson LM, American Academy of Pediatrics, Committee on Pediatric AIDS. Technical Report: Perinatal human immunodeficiency virus testing and prevention of transmission. *Pediatrics.* 2000;106(6):e88. (pediatrics.aappublications.org).

American Academy of Pediatrics. Pickering LK, Baker CJ, Long SS, McMillan JA, eds. *Red Book: 2006 Report of the Committee on Infectious Diseases.* 27th ed. Elk Grove Village, IL: American Academy of Pediatrics, 2006.

Perinatal HIV Guidelines Working, G., *Public Health Service Task Force Recommendations for Use of Antiretroviral Drugs in Pregnant HIV-Infected Women for Maternal Health and Interventions to Reduce Perinatal HIV Transmission in the United States, 2007; 1-96. (aidsinfo.nih.gov/ContentFiles/PerinatalGL.pdf).*

REFERENCES

1. Luo ZC, Wilkins R, Kramer MS. Disparities in pregnancy outcomes according to marital and cohabitation status. *Obstet Gynecol.* 2004;103:300-1307.
2. Rosenberg T, Garbers S, Chavkin W, et al. Prepregnancy weight and adverse perinatal outcomes in an ethnically diverse population. *Obstet Gynecol.* 2002;102:1022-1027.
3. Rosenberg TJ, Garbers S, Lipkind H, et al. Maternal obesity and diabetes as risk factors for adverse pregnancy outcomes: differences among 4 racial/ethnic groups. *Am J Public Health.* 2005;95:1545-1551.
4. Stotland NE, Caughey AB, Lahiff M, et al. Weight gain and spontaneous preterm birth: the role of race or ethnicity and previous preterm birth. *Obstet Gynecol.* 2006;108:1448-1455.
5. Smith GCS, Shah I, Pell JP, et al. Maternal obesity in early pregnancy and risk of spontaneous and elective preterm deliveries: a retrospective cohort study. *Am J Public Health.* 2007;97:157-162.
6. Luke B, Brown MB. Elevated risks of pregnancy complications and adverse outcomes with increasing maternal age. *Hum Reprod.* 2007;22:1264-1272.
7. Wu T, Buck G, Mendola P. Maternal cigarette smoking, regular use of multivitamin/mineral supplements, and risk of fetal death. *Am J Epidemiol.* 1998;148:215-221.
8. Ulrik K, Kirsten W, Sjurur Froi, O, et al. Moderate alcohol intake during pregnancy and the risk of still birth and death in the first year. *Am J Epidemiol.* 2002;155:305-331.
9. Scannapieco RA, Bush RB. Periodontal disease as a risk factor for adverse pregnancy outcomes. A systematic review. *Ann Periodontol.* 2003;8:70-78.
10. Martin SL, Mackie L, Kupper LL, et al. Physical abuse of women before, during and after pregnancy. *JAMA.* 2001;285(12):1581-1584.
11. Hogue CJ, Bremner JD. Stress model for research into preterm delivery among black women. *Am J Obstetr Gynecol.* 2005;192:S47-S55.
12. Collins JW, David RJ, Handler A, et al. Very low birth weight in African American infants: the role of maternal exposure to interpersonal racial discrimination. *Am J Public Health.* 2004;94:2132-2138.
13. Thompson LA, Goodman DC, Chang CH, et al. Regional variation in rates of low birth weight. *Pediatrics.* 2005; 116(5):1114-1121.
14. Drake AJ, Walker BR. The intergenerational effects of fetal programming: non-genomic mechanisms for the inheritance of low birth weight and cardiovascular risk. *J Endocrinol.* 2004;180:1-16.
15. Gluckman PD, Pinal CS. Regulation of fetal growth by somatotrophic axis. *J Nutr.* 2003;133:1741S-1746S.
16. Centers for Disease Control and Prevention. Alcohol consumption among women who are pregnant or who might become pregnant—United States, 2002. *MMWR Morb Mortal Wkly Rep.* 2004;53(50):1178-1181.
17. Field T, Diego M, Dieter J, et al. Prenatal depression effects on the fetus and the newborn. *Infant Beh Dev.* 2004;27:216-229.
18. Louik C, Lin A, Werler MM, et al. First-trimester use of selective serotonin reuptake inhibitors and the risk of birth defects. *New Engl J Med.* 2007;356:2675-2685.

19. Kallen B. Neonatal characteristics after maternal use of antidepressants in late pregnancy. *Arch Pediatr Adolesc Med.* 2004;158:312-316.
20. Sanz EJ, De-las Cuevas C, Kiuru A, et al. Selective serotonin reuptake inhibitors in pregnant women and neonatal withdrawal syndrome: a database analysis. *Lancet.* 2005;365:485-487.
21. Casper RC, Fleischer BE, Lee-Ancajas JC, et al. Follow up of children of depressed mothers exposed to or not exposed to antidepressant drugs during pregnancy. *J Pediatr.* 2003;142:402-408.
22. Merlob P, Stahl B, Sulkes J. Paroxetine during breastfeeding: infant weight gain and maternal adherence to counsel. *Eur J Pediatr.* 2004;163:135-139.
23. Levinson-Castiel R, Merlob P, Linder N, et al. Neonatal abstinence syndrome after in utero exposure to selective serotonin reuptake inhibitors in term infants. *Arch Pediatr Adolesc Med.* 2006;160:173-176.
24. Ferreira E, Carceller AM, Agogué C, et al. Effects of selective serotonin reuptake inhibitors and venlafaxine during pregnancy in term and preterm neonates. *Pediatrics.* 2007;119(1):52-59.
25. Chou R, Smits AK, Hoyt Huffamn L, et al. Prenatal Screening for HIV: a review of the evidence for the US Preventive Services Task Force. *Ann Intern Med.* 2005;143:38-54.
26. Bulterys M, Jamieson DJ, O'Sullivan MJ, et al. Rapid HIV-1 testing during labor: a multicenter study. *N Engl J Med.* 2004;292(2):219-223.
27. Centers for Disease Control and Prevention. *Sexually Transmitted Disease Surveillance, 2005.* Atlanta, GA: US Department of Health and Human Services; 2006.

Chapter 83

PHYSICAL EXAMINATION OF THE NEWBORN

Harpreet Kaur, MD; Deborah E. Campbell, MD

Examining the newborn in the presence of the parents provides an opportunity to demonstrate the infant's physical and developmental characteristics and to model positive infant-caregiver interactions. This interaction with the family also affords the health professional the chance to initiate a health supervision partnership with the family.

ASSESSING THE NEWBORN IN THE DELIVERY ROOM

The first assessment is usually performed in the delivery room by a pediatrician or a nurse to identify any signs of distress or delay in the infant's initial transition and of visible malformations. Inspection of the newborn for obvious malformations is important because this inspection may guide the immediate care needs of the newborn and determine the level of nursery care required. A newborn with a cleft palate will require admission to a special or neonatal intensive care unit for evaluation and specialized feeding management. In contrast, a baby born with an isolated limb deformity may be admitted to a newborn nursery for care and evaluation. Most healthy newborns who do not exhibit transitional difficulties are able to remain with their parents in the labor-delivery-recovery suite for an extended period before admission to the newborn nursery. During the first 30 minutes after birth, infants are typically quite alert and active. This period is an opportune time to initiate skin-to-skin care and breastfeeding. The majority (85%-90%) of newborns do not exhibit any difficulty in their postnatal physiologic transition. Among the 10% to 15% of infants who do experience problems are infants who are preterm, those who are delivered by cesarean or who require instrument-assisted delivery, and newborns who exhibit signs of perinatal distress or whose mothers have pregnancy complications that affect the fetal environment and placenta function. Chapter 74, Assessment and Stabilization at Delivery, provides a comprehensive discussion about resuscitation and stabilization of the newborn who is having difficulty with the initial postnatal transition.

In the delivery room, rapid assessment of the newborn's gestational age may be performed using a rapid scoring system that assesses maturity by examining the creases in the sole of the foot, size of the breast nodule, nature of scalp hair, cartilaginous development of the earlobe, labial development in female newborns, and scrotal rugae and testicular descent in male newborns (Table 83-1). The newborn's body should be briefly inspected for obvious malformations that may necessitate admission to a special or neonatal intensive care unit.

Assessing the Gestational Age

The Ballard score provides neuromuscular and physical maturity scores to determine gestational age (Figure 83-1). Studies have shown that the Ballard score is most consistent with the prenatal ultrasound and last menstrual period in estimating the gestational age within a 2-week range and is most accurate when performed within the first 12 hours of life.[1] Newborns experiencing intrauterine stress related to a variety of maternal medical conditions (hypertension, preterm labor) or environmental exposures (nicotine, cocaine, heroin, antenatal steroids) may demonstrate accelerated neurologic maturation in comparison with the level of physical maturity.

Approach to Physical Examination of the Newborn

Clinical Observation

Initial observation of the neonate should occur with the newborn undressed and in a quiet state. The color, spontaneous movements, cry, posture, tone, and respiratory pattern should be observed. The optimal time to conduct this examination is a few hours after a feeding when the baby is in a quiet, alert state. Engaging the parents during the assessment of the infant enhances communication and parental involvement. The room should be warm and have adequate lighting available to facilitate examination of the skin for jaundice or lesions. It is important when performing the neurological examination to make sure the infant is alert and awake.

The examiner should look at the newborn's appearance. Does the baby appear normal and comfortable? What is the newborn's color? Are any skin lesions

Table 83-1 Gestational Age Assessment in the Delivery Room

PHYSICAL CHARACTERISTIC	GESTATIONAL AGE		
	≤36 WEEKS	37-38 WEEKS	≥39 WEEKS
Creases in the sole of the foot	One or two transverse creases in anterior third of the sole; posterior two thirds smooth	Multiple creases in anterior two thirds sole	Entire sole covered with creases
Ear lobe	No cartilage	Moderate cartilage	Thick cartilage, stiff ear
Scalp hair	Fine and woolly	Fine and woolly	Coarse hair; each hair single stranded
Breast nodules	2 mm	4 mm	7 mm
Testes and scrotum	Few rugae; testes partially descended	Prominent rugae; testes fully descended	Prominent rugae; testes fully descended

present? What is the newborn's tone and activity level? Is the baby alert and responsive? Are any atypical or abnormal eye movements noted? Allowing the newborn to grasp the parent's or the examiner's finger provides an opportunity to assess the strength of the newborn's grasp and reduces the tendency for reflexive startle response to exogenous stimulation. The resting posture for the healthy full-term newborn is generally symmetrically flexed. A newborn who has sustained a clavicular fracture or brachial plexus injury may appear to have an abnormal or atypical posture or limb position. Preterm newborns, babies who are ill, or neonates with conditions affecting their neurologic function may appear hypotonic.

Listening to the Cry

Physicians should train themselves to listen to and assess an infant's cry. A normal cry is strong. Hoarseness, weakness, or an unusual high- or low-pitched cry may indicate a laryngeal or neurologic abnormality. A repetitive, inconsolable cry is considered abnormal. A high-pitched cry is often related to a central nervous system problem, whereas a low, throaty cry suggests congenital hypothyroidism; a *catlike* cry is significant for cri du chat syndrome. A weak, poorly sustained cry may occur in an infant who is ill, neurologically impaired, or who is born with Down syndrome.

Body Measurements

All newborns should have measurement of weight, length, and head circumference as a part of the assessment of the appropriateness of fetal growth and as a baseline for evaluation of subsequent growth. Measurements of the length, weight, and head circumference should be plotted on standard growth charts. Measurements should be plotted on standardized, gestational age–specific growth charts. Three major sets of growth charts have been developed that are most commonly used around the world: (1) British/European (Tanner and Whitehouse), (2) the 2000 Centers for Disease Control and Prevention (CDC) Sex-Specific Growth Charts in the United States, and (3) the World Health Organization International Reference charts. Although the 2000 CDC Sex-Specific Growth Charts may be used for this initial evaluation, the physician should recognize that the data points for term gestation are a composite of data derived for infants above 1500 grams at birth and do not reflect gestation-specific data that is necessary to evaluate properly the adequacy of fetal growth and to identify infants at particular risk based on the inadequate or excessive fetal growth. This distinction is particularly important for the late preterm infant, 35 to 36 weeks' gestation, who is frequently cared for in the regular newborn nursery. No evidence has been found showing large genetic differences in birth weight among various populations and therefore does not support the use of separate, race-specific reference curves, even in situations in which race is associated with other risk factors, such as poor nutrition or low socioeconomic status. A newborn whose birth weight is below the 10th percentile or more than 2 standard deviations below the mean is considered small for gestational age. Large-for-gestational-age infants have birth weights above the 90th percentile or weights more than 2 standard deviations above the mean for their gestational age. The National Center for Health Statistics reports that the mean birth weight (+ 1 standard deviation) for singleton infants born in the United States during 2004 was 3316 grams (+ 570 grams) or 7 pounds 5 ounces. Racial and ethnic variations can be found in birthweight for infants with non-Hispanic white and Hispanic infants having higher mean birth weights than non-Hispanic black infants.[3] Mean (+ 1 standard deviation) birth weights were reported as 3375 grams (+/– 554), 3316 grams (+ 548), and 3115 grams (+ 628) for non-Hispanic white, Hispanic, and non-Hispanic black infants, respectively. Of note, since 1990 the birth weight among singleton infants has declined by 1%, with the highest declines in birth weight among non-Hispanic white infants.

Measuring the baby's head circumference requires placing a disposable measuring tape around the occipital-frontal circumference (OFC): across the forehead, just above the eyes, and over the most prominent part of the occiput. This measurement should be repeated two or three times and the results averaged to yield the OFC. A normal OFC measures 33 to 37 cm in a full-term infant. Benign familial megalencephaly, a normal variant, is the most common cause of a large head, a trait typically inherited from the father.[2] Chest

MATURATIONAL ASSESSMENT OF GESTATIONAL AGE (New Ballard Score)

NAME ____________________ SEX ____________________

HOSPITAL NO. ____________________ BIRTH WEIGHT ____________________

RACE ____________________ LENGTH ____________________

DATE/TIME OF BIRTH ____________________ HEAD CIRCUMFERENCE ____________________

DATE/TIME OF EXAM ____________________ EXAMINER ____________________

AGE WHEN EXAMINED ____________________

APGAR SCORE: 1 MINUTE ________ 5 MINUTES ________ 10 MINUTES ________

NEUROMUSCULAR MATURITY

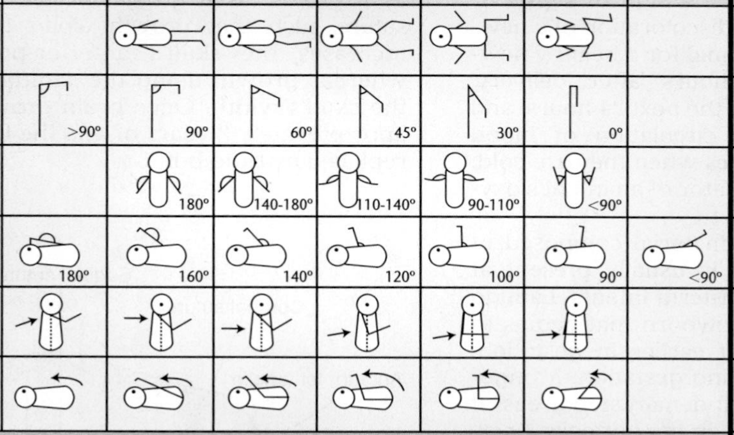

NEUROMUSCULAR MATURITY SIGN	SCORE −1	0	1	2	3	4	5	RECORD SCORE HERE
POSTURE								
SQUARE WINDOW (Wrist)	>90°	90°	60°	45°	30°	0°		
ARM RECOIL		180°	140-180°	110-140°	90-110°	<90°		
POPLITEAL ANGLE	180°	160°	140°	120°	100°	90°	<90°	
SCARF SIGN								
HEEL TO EAR								

TOTAL NEUROMUSCULAR MATURITY SCORE

PHYSICAL MATURITY

PHYSICAL MATURITY SIGN	SCORE −1	0	1	2	3	4	5	RECORD SCORE HERE
SKIN	sticky friable transparent	gelatinous red translucent	smooth pink visible veins	superficial peeling and/or rash, few veins	cracking pale areas rare veins	parchment deep cracking no vessels	leathery cracked wrinkled	
LANUGO	none	sparse	abundant	thinning	bald areas	mostly bald		
PLANTAR SURFACE	heel-toe 40-50 mm: −1 <40 mm: −2	>50 mm no crease	faint red marks	anterior transverse crease only	creases ant. 2/3	creases over entire sole		
BREAST	inperceptible	barely perceptible	flat areola no bud	stippled areola 1-2 mm bud	raised areola 3-4 mm bud	full areola 5-10 mm bud		
EYE/EAR	lids fused loosely: −1 tightly: −2	lids open pinna flat stays folded	sl. curved pinna; soft; slow recoil	well-curved pinna; soft but ready recoil	formed and firm instant recoil	thick cartilage ear stiff		
GENITALS (Male)	scrotum flat, smooth	scrotum empty faint rugae	testes in upper canal rare rugae	testes descending few rugae	testes down good rugae	testes pendulous deep rugae		
GENITALS (Female)	clitoris prominent and labia flat	prominent clitoris and small labia minora	prominent clitoris and enlarging minora	majora and minora equally prominent	majora large minora small	majora cover clitoris and minora		

TOTAL PHYSICAL MATURITY SCORE

Source: Ballard JL, Khoury JC, Wedig K, et al. New Ballard score, expanded to include extremely premature infants. *J Pediatr* 1991; 119:417-423. Reprinted by permission of Dr. Ballard and Mosby–Year Book, Inc.

SCORE

Neuromuscular ________

Physical ________

Total ________

MATURITY RATING

SCORE	WEEKS
−10	20
−5	22
0	24
5	26
10	28
15	30
20	32
25	34
30	36
35	38
40	40
45	42
50	44

GESTATIONAL AGE (weeks)

By dates ________

By ultrasound ________

By exam ________

Figure 83-1 Maturational assessment of gestational age (new Ballard score).

circumference, if measured, is usually 1 to 2 cm less than the head circumference. Length is measured by placing the baby supine on a commercially available measuring device. Care must be taken to ensure that the baby's head is touching a fixed object and the body and legs extended.

The midpoint of a newborn's body is typically considered to be at the level of the umbilicus, and the crown-pubis/pubis-heel ratio is 1.7:1. This ratio is altered in disorders such as chondrodystrophy. Normal measurements of length range between 47 and 55 cm.

Skin

Newborn skin is pink and uniform. (See Chapter 85, Neonatal Skin.) Mottling may be a sign of sepsis or shock. Acrocyanosis is a bluish discoloration of a newborn's extremities, which is normal for a healthy newborn during the first few hours after delivery, disappearing over the course of the next 24 hours, and represents relatively sluggish circulation of blood through the peripheral structures when they are cold. Acrocyanosis is not a valid indicator of an infant's oxygen status.

Vernix is white, cheesy-like material composed of cellular and other debris and is usually present at birth, though it is absent in post-term infants. Lanugo is fine body hair visible on a newborn that begins to thin after 28 weeks. Abundant earlier in gestation, lanugo diminishes with increasing gestation. Mongolian spots are bluish-green, well-demarcated areas of pigmentation visible most often on the buttocks, back, or shoulders of darker-skinned infants.

Erythema toxicum is a common neonatal rash that typically appears during the first week of life and resolves without treatment by 5 to 7 days of age. It begins as an erythematous, macular rash that develops into a small papule on an erythematous base. The papule can sometimes become vesiculopustular. Transient neonatal pustular melanosis is another common skin finding, with characteristic lesions that evolve from small vesiculopustules to hyperpigmented macules, flat dark areas that resemble freckles that may be surrounded by fine desquamating skin. Some infants will be born with hyperpigmented macules, whereas others will develop pustules after birth that rupture during the first few days, with subsequent formation of the hyperpigmented macules. These lesions fade over the course of 3 weeks to 3 months without treatment. Milia are small white, firm papules noted on the upper cheeks, nose, and chin and are caused by blockage of the sweat ducts in the skin. Nevus simplex is a pink discoloration of the skin over eyelids, glabella, and nuchal areas resulting from vascular ectasia. The skin should also be examined for evidence of jaundice, meconium staining, edema, petechiae, and hemangiomas.

Head

The newborn's head can vary in shape and symmetry, depending on the intrauterine position, presentation at delivery, degree of molding, or the need for an instrument-assisted delivery (forceps or vacuum extraction). Infants born by cesarean or breech delivery will often have a symmetric, round head, in contrast to the infant born vaginally, whose head shape is frequently elongated in the occipital area, with overriding sutures.

Sutures and Fontanels

Sutures are strong, flexible fibrous tissue connecting the six major bones of the skull. The coronal, lambdoidal, sagittal, metopic (frontal), and squamosal sutures are shown in Figure 83-2. Fontanels are the points at which the suture lines intersect. The sutures and fontanels are necessary for the infant's brain growth and development. As the brain grows, it exerts pressure on the skull bones, causing new bone deposition along the suture lines. Remolding of bone along the periosteal and dural surfaces of the sutures shapes the head as it grows. Skull growth occurs perpendicular to a suture such that growth along the coronal suture increases the skull's anterior-posterior diameter, whereas growth along the sagittal suture increases the skull's width. Once brain growth is complete at approximately 2 years of age the fibrous sutures are replaced by rigid bone.

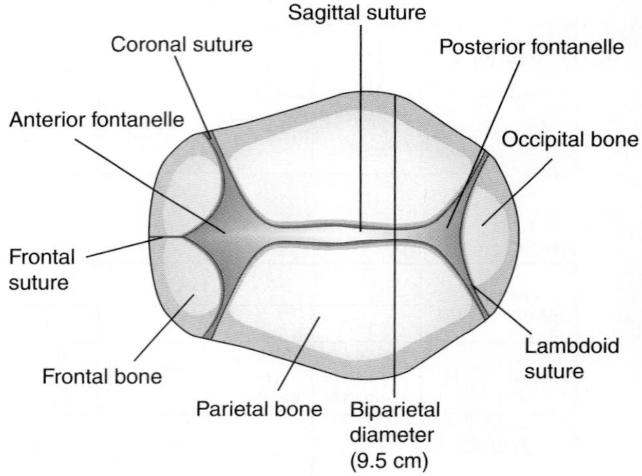

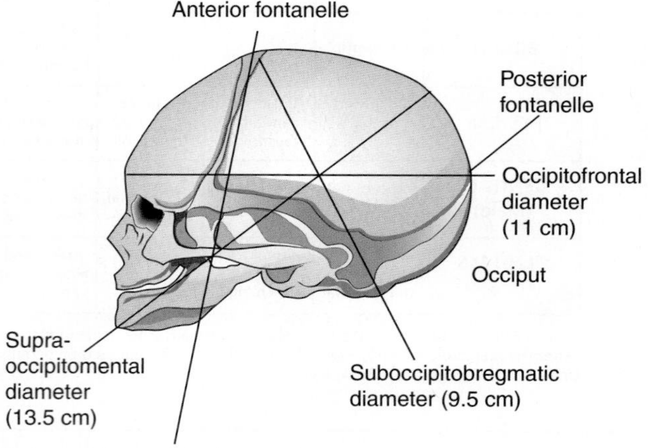

Figure 83-2 Normal skull sutures and fontanels.

During childbirth the flexibility of the fibers allows the bones to overlap their edges, without compressing and damaging the infant's brain, as the head passes through the birth canal. Sutures are easily palpable at birth when the bone edges are not widely separated. Overriding sutures palpated after delivery typically resolve with time. Premature fusion of sutures may be palpable as a prominent edge.

Fontanels, the wider spaces at the intersections of the sutures, are usually felt as *soft spots* on the head and vary in size. Large fontanels may indicate hypothyroidism, hydrocephaly, in utero malnutrition, rickets, or a genetic disorder. The posterior fontanel is located at the junction of the lambdoid and sagittal sutures. It is usually triangular, less than 0.5 cm at birth, and closes shortly after birth. The diamond-shaped anterior fontanel is located at the junction of the sagittal and coronal sutures, measures approximately 4 to 6 cm at birth, and closes around 18 months of age. A depressed anterior fontanel is a late sign of dehydration, whereas a bulging fontanel can be normal in a crying baby but may be associated with hydrocephalus, birth injury, intracranial bleeding, or infection, or it may be present as a late sign of raised intracranial pressure. A third fontanel may sometimes be present between the anterior and posterior fontanel and can be associated with congenital anomalies.

Molding is a common occurrence associated with cephalic presentation during vaginal delivery, although it may also be present in a neonate delivered by cesarean after a prolonged labor. Molding typically resolves 2 to 3 days after birth (Figure 83-3). Birth-related deformations (deformational, positional or nonsynostotic plagiocephaly) of the skull may also be present at birth. Characterized by forehead asymmetry, this deformation is caused by compressive or restrictive forces along the coronal or lambdoidal sutures in utero or during the birth or is related to subsequent positioning. Prematurity and low-birth-weight, multiple fetuses, congenital muscular torticollis, a restrictive uterine environment, congenital anomalies, neurologic disorders, and medical conditions that limit fetal head movement are risk factors for deformational plagiocephaly. Infants with positional molding will have an open suture and frontal and temporal prominence on the same side as the affected suture and frontal flattening on the opposite side. The skull has the appearance of a parallelogram.

Caput succedaneum is caused by constricting pressure on the fetal head during passage through the birth canal. It produces a diffuse subcutaneous edematous swelling of the soft tissue that may cross suture lines and usually resolves within several days. Neonatal extracranial hemorrhages occur in two forms: as a cephalohematoma or a subgaleal hemorrhage. A cephalohematoma is a subperiostal hemorrhage that is a soft, fluctuant cystlike swelling that usually occurs after a difficult or instrument-assisted delivery. Cephalohematomas occur in 1% to 2% of live births and are more common in male first pregnancies (Figure 83-4). Most resolve within a period of 6 weeks to several months. Babies who sustain a large cephalohematoma

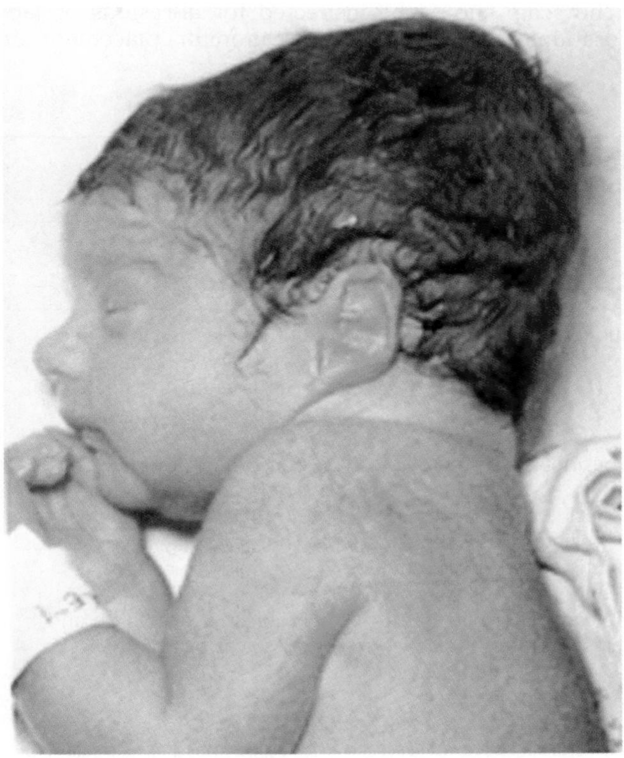

Figure 83-3 Molding.

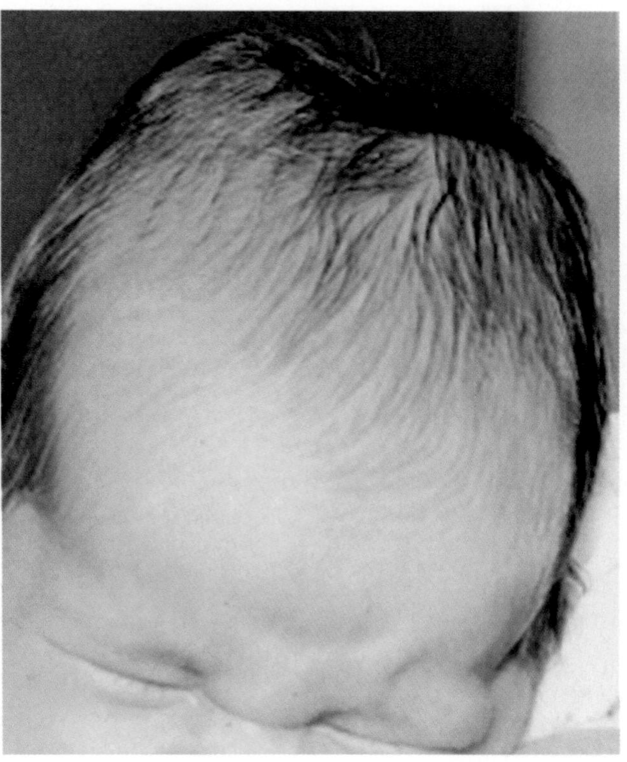

Figure 83-4 Cephalohematoma.

require monitoring of hematocrit and bilirubin levels. Cephalohematomas typically calcify at the edges during resolution, giving an impression of a depression of the skull in the center, with eggshell-like bony margins on palpation. Skull films should be obtained only if fracture is suspected.

Subgaleal hematoma is a serious, but less common, complication usually associated with vacuum-assisted delivery. It is caused by rupture of the emissary veins, which are connections between the dural sinuses and the scalp veins. Blood accumulates between the epicranial aponeurosis of the scalp and the periosteum. This potential space extends forward to the orbital margins, backward to the nuchal ridge, and laterally to the temporal fascia. This potential space can easily accommodate up to one half of the blood volume of a neonate; therefore monitoring blood pressure, hematocrit, bilirubin, and signs for hypovolemia, bleeding, and shock is necessary. Table 83-2 provides a comparison of the characteristics that differentiate caput from extracranial hemorrhages.

Craniosynostosis is the premature fusion of one or more of the cranial sutures; it can occur as part of a syndrome or as an isolated defect. Typically an infant exhibits an asymmetrical head shape and has a palpable ridge along a suture line. The premature closure or absence of one or more of the sutures prevents normal head growth and may constrain brain growth. Compensatory growth occurs along the open sutures, resulting in craniosynostosis and distortion of the head shape. Head growth is restricted in the plane that is perpendicular to the fused suture and enhanced in the plane parallel to the fused suture (Figure 83-5). Synostosis involving more than one suture is often associated with a syndrome and requires early intervention to limit the risk for increased intracranial pressure and neurologic impairment. Sagittal synostosis caused by premature closure of the metopic suture is the most frequent form of craniosynostosis, with a male predominance (3:2 male/female ratio) and occurs most commonly in white infants. Numerous syndromes and chromosomal mutations are associated with craniosynostosis. Table 83-3 describes the differences between craniosynostosis and nonsynostotic plagiocephaly.

Craniotabes is an abnormal softening or thinning primarily of the parietal bones in preterm infants and gives a sensation of a *ping-pong* ball on gentle pressure. It normally disappears in a few weeks. Persistence beyond a few weeks is considered pathological and should alert the clinician to suspect rickets, syphylis, osteogenesis imperfecta, marasmus, hypervitaminosis A, and hydrocephalus. A bruit on auscultation over the temporal arteries and anterior fontanel can be heard in cases of high-output cardiac failure or neuropathologic abnormality. Transillumination is not part of the routine examination but should be performed in a newborn with an unusually large or asymmetric head or if a widely patent suture or fontanel is present. Diagnoses associated with craniotabes include subdural effusion, subdural hematoma, hydrocephalus, hydranencephaly, porencephaly, increased intracranial pressure, and even skull fractures and nutritional deficiencies. Imaging studies such as neurosonography, computed tomography, and magnetic resonance imaging are important tools in evaluating the newborn to identify potential intracranial disease.

Scalp

The scalp should be inspected for abrasions or lacerations caused by internal monitor placement or

Table 83-2 Characteristics of Caput Succedaneum, Cephalohematoma, and Subgaleal Hematoma

FEATURE	CAPUT SUCCEDANEUM	CEPHALOHEMATOMA	SUBGALEAL HEMORRHAGE
Cause	Pressure of the fetal head on the cervix during labor. Causes decreased blood flow to the area and results in edema.	Subperiosteal hemorrhage	Suture diastasis; ruptured emissary vein caused by fragmentation parietal bone; skull fracture
Suture line	May extend suture lines	Does not cross suture line	Can extend to orbits and neck
Appearance	Localized soft-tissue edema, with poorly defined outline; pitting edema	Soft, fluctuant, localized swelling, with well-defined outline; initially firm but more fluctuant after 48 hr	Firm to fluctuant; ill-defined borders; may have crepitus or fluid waves
Timing	Usually present at birth; does not progress and resolves in 48-72 hr	Increases after birth for 24-72 hr and resolves over 2-3 wks; sometimes not evident immediately after birth	Progressive after birth and resolves over 2-3 wks
Blood loss	Minimal	Occasionally severe; coagulopathy suspected	May be massive, especially if coagulopathy is present
Complications	Rare	Intracranial bleed; jaundice	Hypovolemic shock

birth-related injury. Aplasia cutis congenita is a skin disorder in which an infant is born with a missing patch of skin. The affected area is usually covered with a thin transparent membrane, is well defined, and is not inflamed. Although aplasia cutis congenita may occur anywhere on the body, 80% of these lesions occur on the scalp. When aplasia cutis congenita occurs on the scalp, an associated skull defect may be present underneath, which may be an isolated finding or associated with other syndromes or disorders.

The clinician should examine the hair for its color, texture, distribution, and directional pattern. Reddish or blonde color of the hair in a black infant may indicate albinism. Hair color is usually uniform; random patches of white hair may be familial in origin, but a white forelock should alert the clinician to consider Waardenburg syndrome (associated pigment defect, deafness, and retardation). The frontal margin of the hairline may vary. Some infants will have extensive hair distribution involving the face, arms, and torso, which typically resolves over a few months. These infants may also have synophrys—fusion of the eyebrows in the midline—a finding that should prompt the clinician to consider if the infant has other stigmata of Cornelia de Lange syndrome. The posterior hairline has a more consistent limitation. Hair roots distributed below the neck creases, particularly at the lateral margins, can be associated with syndromes involving a short and webbed neck. Normally the direction of hair growth is consistent with a single parietal hair whorl positioned off center, 1 to 2 cm anterior to the posterior fontanel and most often to the left. If the hair whorl is in the midline, if more than one whorl is present, or if the whorl is located inferior to the posterior fontanel, then it may be associated with an underlying brain abnormality. Unusual or extremely wiry or unruly hair in a small-for-gestational-age infant with microcephaly and unusual facies suggest the presence of a genetic disorder.

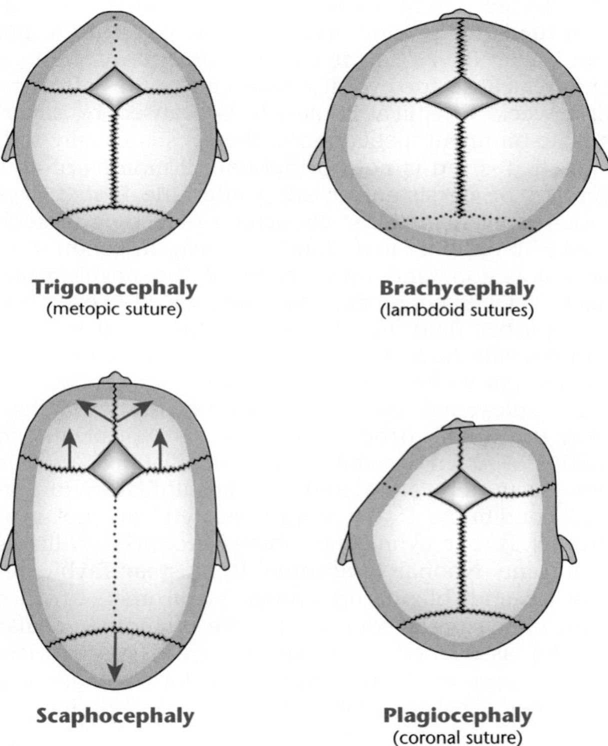

Figure 83-5 Cranial shapes associated with premature suture closure.

Face

The face should be inspected in its entirety, and the individual facial structures should be closely examined as well. The examiner should evaluate the size, shape, and position of the eyes, ears, nose, mouth, and chin. The face can be divided into thirds, with one third encompassing the forehead, one third the eyes and the nose, and one third the mouth and chin. Abnormalities of individual features in isolation are generally not significant, but a combination of atypical features increases the likelihood of an associated syndrome.

Eyes

Examination of the newborn eye can sometimes be difficult. Examining the eyes is easiest when the baby is in a quiet alert state because the eyes are often open spontaneously. The clinician can also take advantage of the vestibular reflex that is elicited by holding

Table 83-3 Features of Craniosynostosis Versus Nonsynostotic Plagiocephaly

	CRANIOSYNOSTOSIS	NONSYNOSTOTIC PLAGIOCEPHALY
Head shape	Asymmetric head because the growth is restricted perpendicular to the fused suture	Flat spot on the back or one side of the head caused by remaining in one position for too long
Cranial suture	Fusion of sutures	Normal sutures
Diagnosis	Radiographic examination or computed tomographic scan	History and physical examination
Treatment	Surgery	Positioning, helmets
Cause	Unknown	External molding caused by back sleeping, restrictive intrauterine environment, muscular torticollis, prematurity

the newborn upright, supporting the baby's head with the examiner's hand, and gently rocking the neonate back and forth. If the baby is in a quiet state, then the eyes will open. Occasionally a newborn will open the eyes when given a finger or pacifier on which to suck. Newborns typically exhibit a dysconjugate gaze, given that eye movements are frequently not coordinated until approximately 3 to 4 months of age.

The sclera is usually white, although it may appear blue in a premature newborn or yellowish in a jaundiced newborn. Neonates with osteogenesis imperfecta also have a blue sclera. Subconjuctival hemorrhages can occur normally during labor and delivery and resolve over time. These hemorrhages are the result of rupture of small blood vessels near the surface of the bulbar conjunctiva. The iris appears dark blue until 3 to 6 months of age, when eye color may change. The iris should be perfectly circular, with the pupil located centrally and visible striations radiating out from the center. The iris should be examined for evidence of a defect or coloboma. A coloboma is a hole in one of the structures of the eye, such as the lens, eyelid, iris, retina, choroids, or optic disc. The hole is present from birth and can be caused when a gap, present between two structures in the eye in the fetus, fails to close up completely before a child is born. It can be an isolated abnormality or a feature of CHARGE syndrome (coloboma, heart disease, atresia choanae, retardation of growth or development, genito-urinary tract anomalies, and ear anomalies) when it occurs in association with other anomalies. The presence of white spots may be abnormal and should prompt a formal ophthalmologic evaluation. Pupil response to a light stimulus occurs consistently after 32 weeks of gestation, but may be present from 28 weeks' gestation. The pupillary response to light and symmetry of eye movement should be checked. The cornea and lens should be clear. Opacification can occur as a consequence of congenital glaucoma, infection, cataract, or trauma. Brushfield spots, also referred to as a *speckled iris,* are small white spots that are slightly elevated on the surface of the iris arranged in a concentric ring around the pupil. These spots occur in healthy children but are far more common among children with Down syndrome.

All infants and children should have an examination of the eye's red reflex performed by a physician or trained professional before discharge from the nursery and during subsequent routine health-supervision visits. Current recommendations are that an infant's eyes should be examined for the red reflex from the newborn period through 3 months, then at 6 months, continuing on episodically through early childhood.[4] The red reflex test uses light transmitted from an ophthalmoscope through all the transparent parts of the eye, including the tear film, cornea, aqueous, and vitreous humor and the lens. An ophthalmoscope with the lens power set at zero is focused on the pupil from a distance of 18 inches away from the infant's eyes. To be considered normal the red reflex in both eyes should be symmetrical. Dark spots in the red reflex, a blunted red reflex on one side, lack of a red reflex, or the presence of a white reflex (retinal reflection) are all indications for immediate referral to an ophthalmologist for a dilated examination. Leukocoria, a white pupillary reflex visible on the ophthalmoscopic red reflex test, is the most common presenting clinical sign in retinoblastoma. Newborns in high-risk groups, including newborns with a family history of retinoblastoma, congenital cataract or glaucoma, congenital retinal dysplasia, and genetic or familial eye disease, should have a dilated eye examination, preferably by an ophthalmologist. Newborns in whom the parents or the observer describes a history suspicious for presence of leukocoria should be referred to the ophthalmologist because small retinoblastoma or other serious lesion may develop in a subtle fashion.

Congenital cataracts may result from intrauterine infection or can be inherited as a dominant trait from an affected parent. Gonococcal ophthalmia neonatorum tends to develop after first few days of life but can occur later. *Chlamydia trachomatis* infection is another cause for eye drainage and occurs after the first week. Chemical conjunctivitis caused by silver-nitrate ointment instillation in the eyes is usually self-limited. Tearing is not normal until 2 months of age. Tearing or persistent crusting after the first 2 days requires evaluation for congenital glaucoma (associated photophobia and cloudy cornea), infection, corneal abrasion, and obstruction of the nasolacrimal duct (NLD). In congenital glaucoma, elevated eye pressure pushes fluid into the cornea, causing it to swell and become hazy. Parents may be the first to notice clouding or whitening of the cornea.

An epicanthal fold, a small web of tissue overlapping the nasal corner of the eye, is typical among infants of Asian descent, may be familial in 1% of the non-Asian population, and is a clinical feature in several conditions: Down syndrome, fetal alcohol syndrome, Turner syndrome, phenylketonuria, Williams syndrome, Noonan syndrome, Rubinstein Taybi syndrome, and blepharophimosis syndrome. Upward slant of the outer edge of the eye is another ocular finding associated with trisomy 21. Hypertelorism (widely separated eyes) and hypotelorism (narrowly separated eyes) are other features to be assessed.[5]

Ears

The normal ear location is determined by drawing an imaginary horizontal line from the inner canthi of the eyes perpendicular to the vertical axis of the head. If the helix of the ears lies below this line, then the ears are low set and can be associated with other syndromes or anomalies. Hairy ears are seen in infants of diabetic mothers. Visualizing a tympanic membrane is not an essential part of a newborn examination and is often not possible because of the presence of vernix or amniotic fluid.

Abnormalities of the external ear include malformation such as microtia, malposition, preauricular pits, tags, and sinus tracts. Malformations may be familial, an isolated finding, or part of a syndrome. The degree of development of the external ear is one of the physical characteristics used in determining a neonate's maturity at birth. The clinician should examine the ears' size, shape, and position, as well as for the presence of abnormalities such as a preauricular skin tag or sinus (ear pit).

Preauricular tags and sinuses are reported to occur in 5 to 10 infants per 1000 live births. An isolated preauricular sinus is typically considered a benign malformation.[6] Although considered common minor anomalies the clinician should thoroughly examine the affected newborn and review the prenatal and family history for evidence of other malformations or a history of hearing impairment. Renal ultrasonography should be performed in any newborn with an ear anomaly accompanied by other dysmorphic features, family history of deafness, maternal history of gestational diabetes, or a defined syndrome.[7]

Although consensus exists regarding the need to evaluate the urinary tract of a newborn with a major ear malformation or a preauricular tag or sinus accompanied by other abnormalities, controversy exists regarding the need for renal sonography if the newborn's only anomaly is a preauricular tag or sinus.[8,9] Two recent publications argue against the need for renal sonography in babies with isolated minor ear anomalies, reporting that the prevalence of renal anomalies among individuals with preauricular tags and sinuses is similar to the reported incidence of renal abnormalities in the general population.[10,11] The most prudent approach in view of the current lack of a definitive conclusion is for the clinician to examine thoroughly the newborn with an isolated minor ear anomaly for evidence of other malformations or dysmorphism, the presence of which should prompt evaluation with a renal ultrasound.

Nose

Nasal flaring is a frequent finding in the neonate who is transitioning from the fetal physiological environment to independent extrauterine cardiorespiratory function and denotes the newborn's attempt to decrease airway resistance. Given that infants are obligate nose breathers, nasal patency should be verified. Gently blocking each nostril while the mouth is closed and then listening for air movement through the unobstructed nare is an important part of the physical examination. Alternatively a wisp of cotton can be placed in front of each nostril and observed for movement. If the clinician is unsure from these maneuvers that the nasal passage is patent, then a soft No. 6 French catheter may be inserted into each nare to check for patency. Babies with bilateral choanal atresia exhibit respiratory distress and cyanosis immediately after delivery; the distress is relieved with crying or if the mouth is opened.

The nasal bridge should be inspected for flattening and the presence of any midline defects. Flattened nasal bridge can be a normal variation or associated with congenital syphilis, Down syndrome, and Williams syndrome. Congenital obstruction of the nasolacrimal drainage system is common although symptomatic infants with signs of nasal obstruction or respiratory distress are rare. The two forms of lacrimal system obstruction observed are (1) NLD obstruction and (2) dacryocystocele. Reports suggest that up to 20% of newborns develop symptoms of obstruction of the nasolacrimal system. It is usually caused by persistent membranous obstruction near the lower end of the NDL; the most distal portion of the duct near its exit to the nose is most typically involved.[12,13] The obstruction may be unilateral or bilateral. Presenting signs include one or both eyes appearing moist, tearing, crusting on the eyelashes, and, over time, chronic or intermittent infections and periocular redness and irritation. Lacrimation increases during the first 2 to 3 weeks of life. Consequently, NLD obstructions may not become evident until the newborn is 3 weeks of age. Spontaneous resolution occurs in over 95% of affected infants. Differential diagnosis of the newborn with persistent tearing and mucopurulent discharge includes congenital glaucoma, an eyelash or eyelid abnormality, and conjunctivitis. Congenital dacryocystocele is a less common form of NLD obstruction that is caused by distention of the nasolacrimal sac. It is characterized by a bluish-grey cystic swelling below the medial canthus of the eye and may be confused with a vascular malformation. Acute inflammation in and around the lacrimal system develops in 20% to 60% of neonates within the first days of life.

Studies have demonstrated the efficacy of medical management with warm compresses, massage, and topical antibiotics, with 76% of dacryocystoceles resolving after 6 days of medical management.[14] Babies born with dacryocystoceles may have intranasal extension and develop respiratory distress after birth.[15] Current recommendations include early probing at 4 to 6 months of age if symptoms persist.[16]

Mouth

The mouth should open at equal angles bilaterally. Unilateral facial nerve palsy is associated with an asymmetric cry (Figure 83-6), inability to close the eye, flattening of the nasolabial fold, and drooping of the corner of the mouth on the affected side. When muscle activity of the tongue against the hard palate is limited or nonexistent during fetal life, the mandible does not develop fully, resulting in micrognathia. This anomaly occurs as part of the triad of retrognathia or micrognathia, glossoptosis, and airway obstruction in the Pierre Robin sequence. Babies with micrognathia can have respiratory distress, airway obstruction, and feeding difficulties. An important part of the mouth examination is inspection and palpation of the hard and soft palate and uvula for evidence of a cleft. A posterior cleft palate may be missed if complete

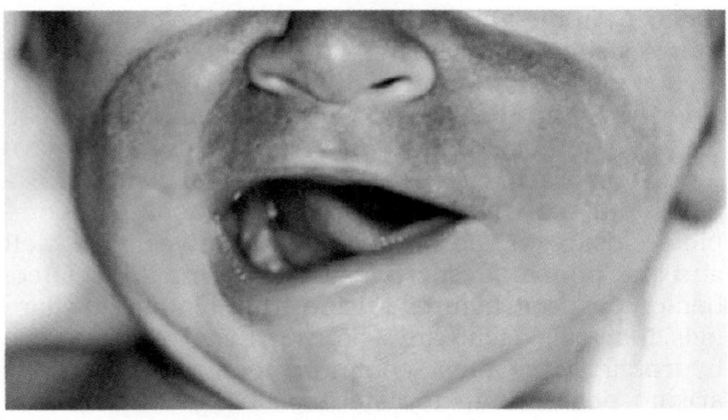

Figure 83-6 Asymmetric crying facies.

inspection of the palate is not performed. Cleft lip and palate can be hereditary or associated with syndromes. A bifid uvula may be a sign of underlying submucous cleft palate.

Natal teeth may erupt in utero or during the first month of life and, when present, require a radiographic examination to determine if it is prematurely erupted decidual teeth or supernumerary teeth. Natal teeth should be removed during the neonatal period to limit the risk of detachment and aspiration. Ankyloglossia, commonly referred to as *tongue-tie,* is caused by a short frenulum on the underside of the tongue that prevents complete protrusion of the tongue. It is an uncommon oral anomaly that can interfere with breastfeeding, speech articulation, and mechanical tasks. Macroglossia can be congenital or acquired; it can be localized when caused by a congenital hemangioma, or it can involve the entire tongue in such disorders as hypothyroidism, Beckwith-Weidemann syndrome, Pompe disease, and Down syndrome.

Mucoceles are lesions of the oral mucosa that occur as a result of leakage of salivary mucin into the surrounding soft tissues, producing a granulomatous tissue response. Mucoceles lack a true epithelial lining and are classified as pseudocysts. The most common location for a mucocele is the lower lip. Clinically, mucoceles are usually small, fluctuant, asymptomatic mucosal swellings that are benign and are believed to occur in response to salivary gland trauma. Ranulae are benign sublingual cysts that may rupture with vigorous sucking. Epstein pearls are small, white inclusion cysts present at the junction of soft and hard palate. These cysts usually resolve spontaneously with sucking. Excessive drooling from the mouth can be normal, or it may be an early sign of esophageal obstruction or isolated neuromuscular swallowing difficulties. Esophageal obstruction can be easily diagnosed by the inability to pass the feeding tube to the stomach.

Neck

A newborn should be able to turn the head to both sides of the shoulder. The rooting reflex can elicit this movement when the baby turns the head to the side when stimulated. Webbing of the neck can be associated with Turner or Noonan syndrome. The examiner should inspect the clavicles for crepitus, mass, or tenderness, which is suggestive of a fracture. Newborns with a clavicular fracture exhibit limited movement of the arm on the affected side. The sternocleidomastoid muscles should be palpated for evidence of hematoma or fibroma, and the range of rotation of head to each side should be checked. The neck should be examined for the presence of thyroid enlargement and thyroglossal or brachial cleft cysts. A brachial cleft cyst is a developmental defect that occurs as a result of incomplete closure of the brachial plate between the cleft and the pouch. Cystic hygromas are multiloculated, benign cystic structures arising from lymphatic channels that can occur anywhere in the body. A cystic hygroma is the most common neck mass, typically arising posterior to the sternocleidomastoid muscle. Thyroglossal duct cysts are caused by dilation of a remnant at the site where the primitive thyroid descended from its origin at the base of the tongue to its permanent location, low in the neck. Failure of subsequent closure and obliteration of this tract predisposes in newborn to thyroglossal cyst formation. The resulting neck mass moves during swallowing.

Cardiovascular System

Examination of the cardiovascular system includes assessment of the heart's rate, rhythm, and position; the pulse volume; adequacy of perfusion; and other signs of cardiovascular compromise. The normal heart rate is 120 to 160 beats/min in the alert newborn. Some babies, particularly those exposed to a suboptimal intrauterine environment, may have low resting heart rates when at rest and during sleep. Bradycardia in a neonate is defined as a heart rate less than 100 beats/min. Infants born to mothers with systemic lupus erythematosus will exhibit symptoms of congenital heart block and a fixed heart rate. Tachycardia occurs when the newborn heart rate exceeds 170 beats/min. A heart murmur on the first day of life is usually benign and reflects blood flow across a patent ductus arteriosus. (See Chapter 100, Evaluation of the Infant With Suspected Heart Disease.) Both femoral pulses should always be palpated and compared with the brachial pulses. Weak femoral pulses or decreased blood pressure measured in the lower extremities must be immediately evaluated for coarctation of aorta. Weak pulses may also indicate hypotension or other significant heart disease. Bounding femoral pulses may indicate hypertension or patent ductus arteriosus.

Chest and Lungs

The normal respiratory rate for a newborn is 40 to 60 breaths per minute. Newborns especially preterm babies, frequently exhibit periodic breathing, with cycles of 5- to 10-second respiratory pauses. Apnea, the cessation of respiration for more than 20 seconds, is associated with bradycardia and color change and requires rapid assessment and intervention. Newborns experiencing respiratory distress may exhibit tachypnea, nasal flaring, grunting, and intercostal retractions. Subcostal retractions occur as a result of a newborn's primary use of the diaphragm during respiration. (For a detailed discussion of respiratory disorders in the newborn, see Chapter 99, Respiratory Distress and Breathing Disorders in the Newborn.) Asymmetry of the chest may signify tension pneumothorax, diaphragmatic hernia, skeletal disorder, and intrathoracic mass. A barrel-shaped chest suggests the presence of a pneumomediastinum (particularly in the newborn with a history of meconium staining), the need for positive pressure ventilation in the delivery room, or a newborn who exhibits respiratory distress.

Malformation of the rib cage may be seen with chondrodystrophies. Pectus excavatum is a congenital depression of the sternum and is usually insignificant. Both male and female infants may have breast enlargement or may exhibit galactorrhea in the initial postnatal period. Widely spaced nipples (internipple distance is greater than 25% of the chest circumference) can be associated with congenital disorders such as Turner syndrome.

Supernumerary (or accessory) nipple, also known as polythelia, is a congenital developmental abnormality

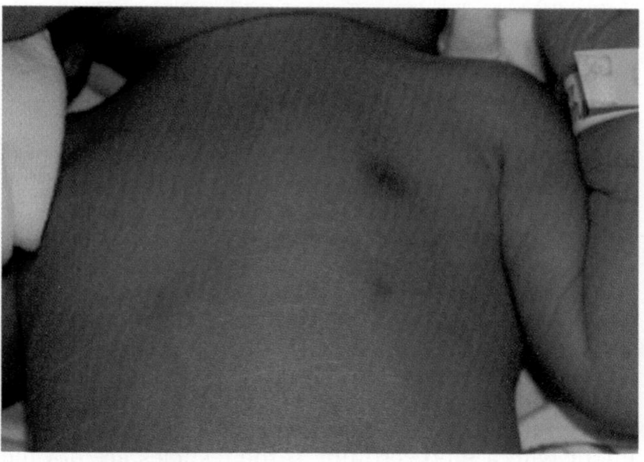

Figure 83-7 Infant with rudimentary supernumerary nipple.

that occurs most commonly over the anterior aspect of the trunk (Figure 83-7). Supernumerary nipples are found along the embryonic milk line that extends from the axilla to pubic region. Supernumerary nipples can vary in their structure, ranging from a fully developed accessory breast, areola, or nipple to a minute, rudimentary hyperpigmented structure. Incidence of supernumerary nipple is 25 per 1000 live births, with a higher prevalence for the left side and male infants.

Abdomen

The newborn abdomen is soft and slightly protuberant. Diaphragmatic hernia is a defect in the diaphragm that allows the abdominal contents to move into the chest cavity, resulting in a scaphoid abdomen. Diastasis rectus is caused by separation between the left and the right side of the rectus abdominis muscle. Diastasis recti is a common, normal condition in newborns and occurs more frequently in premature and black babies. The abdominal musculature should be examined for evidence of laxity, which can be associated with gastrointestinal and genitourinary anomalies, such as seen in infants with prune belly syndrome. The examiner should auscultate for the presence of bowel sounds. The presence of a bruit on auscultation over the liver indicates an arteriovenous malformation; if heard over the kidneys, then renal artery stenosis is suggested. The spleen is not usually palpable. The liver can be palpated 1 to 2 fingerbreadths below the right costal margin, and the lower pole of the left kidney may be felt in the pelvic gutter. Enlarged kidneys are the most frequent cause of an abdominal mass in newborns. Dilated veins are sometimes visible on the abdominal wall, indicating venous distension.

UMBILICAL CORD. The examiner needs to review the delivery history for notations regarding the umbilical cord length and abnormalities related to nuchal cord, cord wrapped around the infant's body, or other abnormalities such as knots in the cord. The average umbilical cord length is 55 to 61 cm, with 85% of cords measuring between 46 and 79 cm (18-31 inches). Six percent of umbilical cords are considered to be short (<35 cm), and 9% are long (>80 cm).[17-19] The umbilical cord length is related to the degree of fetal movements; the greater the fetal movement is, the longer the cord will be. The degree of fetal movement also correlates with the degree of twisting of the cord. Umbilical cord complications are more common when an abnormal cord length exists. Longer cords are more susceptible to knotting, entanglement, and prolapse. True knots in an umbilical cord are rare, occurring in less than 1% of live births. Knots are more common in monoamniotic twins, infants with long cords, and pregnancies complicated by polyhydramnios. Wasted umbilical cords are observed in neonates with fetal growth restriction, whereas macrosomic neonates are more likely to have bulky cords. The diameter of the umbilical cord varies in relation to the quality of Wharton jelly and is an indicator of fetal nutritional status. Abnormal marginal and velamentous cord insertion into the placenta also increases the risk for fetal growth restriction and single umbilical artery.

If the cord is broad at the base, then the newborn should be checked for the presence of a small omphalocele before the cord is cut in the delivery room. An omphalocele is a congenital malformation in which variable amounts of abdominal contents protrude into the base of the umbilical cord. The intestines are covered only by a thin layer of tissue and can be easily seen. Gastroschisis is an abdominal wall defect that occurs when the anterior abdomen does not close properly, allowing the intestines to protrude outside the fetus. Unlike the omphalocele the bowel is not covered by the membrane and is located to the right of the intact umbilicus.

An umbilical hernia is a small defect in the abdominal wall at the umbilicus. It is most often visible when a newborn cries or strains because the pressure pushes the abdominal contents or fluid through the defect, causing it to bulge. The size of the umbilical hernia is determined by palpating the opening in the abdominal muscle, not by the amount of skin protruding. Umbilical hernias are also more prevalent in black infants and typically resolve over the first years of life. Prune belly syndrome is caused by laxity of the abdominal musculature and is associated with gastrointestinal, genitourinary system, and lung hypoplasia. Edema, discharge, redness, or foul odor around the umbilical cord is a sign of omphalitis.

SINGLE UMBILICAL ARTERY. The normal umbilical cord contains two arteries and one vein. An isolated single umbilical artery (SUA) occurs in up to 2% of all live-born infants. It may be detected antenatally or identified on examination of the newborn after birth.[20,21] Prenatally, only two thirds of the SUA will be identified sonographically. An SUA is believed to result from either aplasia or atrophy of the second umbilical artery or from persistence of the normally transient early embryonic SUA. Associated structural or chromosomal anomalies are found in 27% of infants with an SUA, with renal malformations being the most common finding. SUA is seen more frequently in monoamniotic twins, and intrauterine growth restriction was observed in 15% to 18% of newborns with an SUA.

A newborn found to have an SUA should be thoroughly examined for dysmorphic features, abdominal masses, and the presence of heart disease. Postnatal screening for other malformations is warranted if additional abnormalities are present on examination or if prenatal evaluation identified other anomalies. In the absence of identified physical abnormalities on antenatal ultrasound screening the available research suggests a low yield from investigations after delivery in infants without positive examination findings, suggesting the presence of other anomalies.[22-24]

Genitalia and Anus

MALE. Usually at birth the glans is completely covered by the foreskin. The foreskin should not be retracted until the child is 3 to 10 years of age. The skin on the underside of the penis may be tethered to the scrotum, called the chordae, and may or may not be associated with hypospadias. Hypospadias is a defect of the urethra in a male infant that involves an abnormally placed urethral meatus. Instead of opening at the tip of the glans a hypospadic urethra opens anywhere along a line running from the tip along the ventral aspect of the shaft to the junction of the penis (Figure 83-8). Infants with hypospadias should not undergo circumcision as the foreskin is often used during the surgical repair. Epispadias is an opening on the dorsal surface of the penis. A malpositioned meatus may be associated with urethral or kidney abnormalities and may result in poor urinary stream.

Penile length varies from 2.5 to 3.5 cm. The penis may appear short in an obese infant with suprapubic fat. A microphallus, or micropenis, should be suspected if the stretched penile length is less than 2 standard deviations below the mean for age; measurements of less than 2.5 cm in a term newborn male meet the definition of micropenis. The examiner should observe infants with micropenis (especially if other abnormalities associated with hypopituitarism are present) for evidence of metabolic derangements. Among neonates with pituitary dysfunction an early clinical sign is hypoglycemia. If hypoglycemia occurs, then glucose, insulin, growth hormone, and cortisol levels should be immediately obtained.

The scrotum is smooth or has a rugated appearance. Confirmation of descended testes is important for the infant with a bifid scrotum. If the testicles are not felt in the scrotum, then the inguinal canal should be palpated for the testicles. Black, Asian, and Hispanic infants can have darker scrotum (Figure 83-9). Pigmentation of scrotum can be a sign of congenital adrenal hyperplasia. Discoloration of the scrotum may be present in a neonate born after breech presentation or may be caused by testicular torsion or hematoma. Testicular size, noted as a volume, is 1 to 2 mL. Transillumination should be performed if the scrotum appears distended to determine if a hydrocele is present. If the scrotum does not transilluminate, then the infant should be examined closely for a tumor or torsion.

Cryptorchidism is common in the newborn infant, given that most undescended testicles are present at

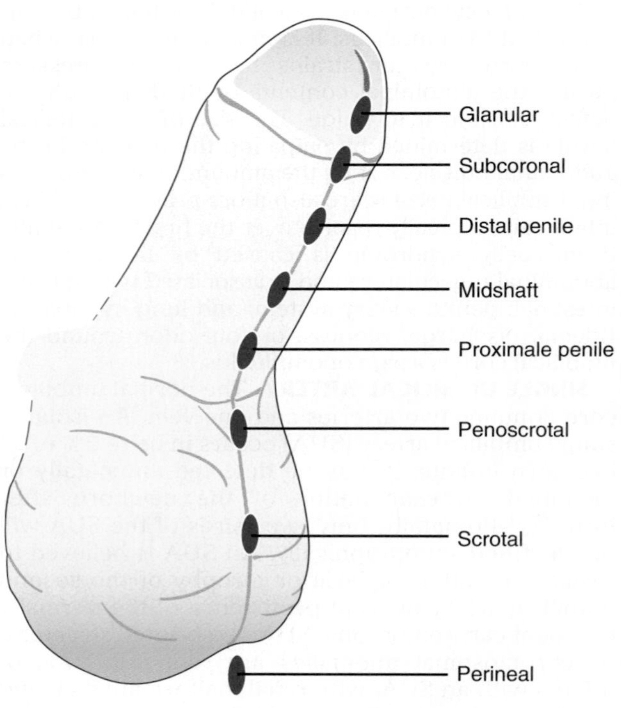

Figure 83-8 Schematic of urethral orifice in hypospadias.

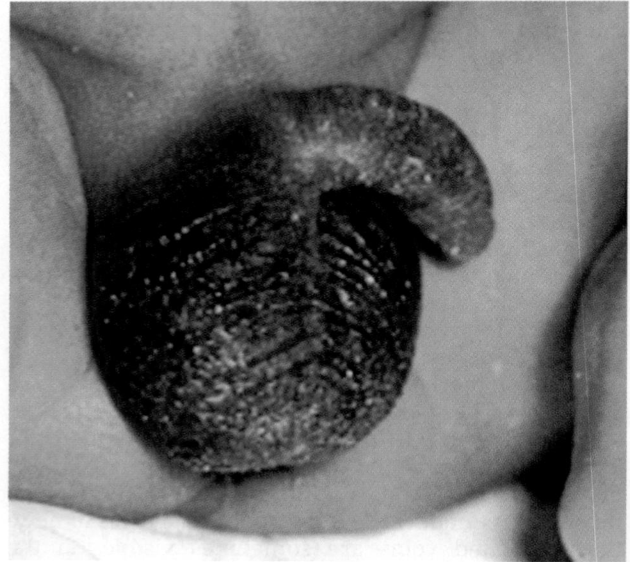

Figure 83-9 Full term male genitalia. The scrotum of the term infant with descended testes will be pendulous with well developed rugae. The scrotum of infants with deeper skin pigmentation (black, Native American and non-white Hispanic infants) will appear darker than the rest of their skin.

birth. (See Chapter 279, Hypospadias, Epispadias, and Cryptorchism.) Three to five percent of term male infants are affected. Predisposing factors include prematurity, low birth weight, twin gestation, and first-trimester exposure to estrogen. Up to 30% of premature male newborns can be affected. Undescended testicles may be true undescended testicles, ectopic testicles, or retractile testicles. A newborn who appears phenotypically male but does not have palpable testes bilaterally should be considered to be a virilized female infant with congenital adrenal hyperplasia until proved otherwise. Congenital adrenal hyperplasia may rarely produce a normal male phenotype and is a life-threatening condition.

FEMALE. The labia can be swollen or ecchymotic after a breech delivery. In a term infant the labia majora is enlarged and covers the labia minora, clitoris, urethral meatus, and external vaginal vault. Infants can have a creamy white to a slightly blood-tinged discharge 2 to 3 days after birth caused by maternal estrogen withdrawal. An enlarged bartholin gland can appear as an imperforate hymen. Vaginal mucosal skin tags are a common finding and may extend beyond the rim of the hymen. They usually disappear within the first few weeks of life. Occasionally, small vesicles with no erythema may be clustered around the genitalia, and their surface is frequently broken. Virilization of the genitalia may be difficult to identify; both labia need to be spread to ensure no labioscrotal fusion is present, and the labia majora should be palpated to be sure that no gonads are present.

Infants with ambiguous genitalia need a multidisciplinary work-up before assigning the gender. Gender assignment should be delayed if the genitalia are incompletely developed or appear indeterminate. Refer to Chapter 286, Intersex.

Anus and Rectum

The distance between the posterior fourchette and the anus divided by the distance from the coccyx to the fourchette is usually 0.44 cm (±0.05 cm) in female newborns. In male newborns the distance from the anus to the scrotum divided by the distance from the coccyx to the scrotum is 0.58 cm (±0.06 cm). Occasionally a large fistula may be mistaken for an anus. Fistulae may be located anterior or posterior to the anus and may connect to the bladder. An imperforate anus occurs in approximately 1 in 5000 newborns. The rate is slightly higher among boys than girls, and it can occur as an isolated anomaly or in association with other abnormalities of the rectum and anus.

Musculoskeletal System

SPINE. The newborn's spine should be examined with the infant in the prone position. Infants are frequently noted to have a nevus simplex *(stork bite)* at the nape of the neck that is insignificant and disappears with time. Asymmetry in the creases at the thigh or the buttock may be evident in a neonate with developmental dysplasia of the hip. The examiner should palpate the spine to check the curvature; any midline defect on the dorsal surface can be an indication of spine anomalies. A pilonadal sinus (sacral dimple) may be present at the base of the spine between the buttocks. It is typically benign; although, rarely, a true sinus tract associated with a meningomyelocele may exist. Abnormal pigmentation, overlying hemangioma, pigmented nevus, or a hair tuft over the lower spine may be associated with vertebral anomalies (Figure 83-10). Lipomas are palpable masses that move with the skin. Spinal dysraphism is usually a midline defect, whereas a sacrococcygeal teratoma tends to be located lateral to the midline. The scapulae should also be palpated to check their size, symmetry, and location. A scapula that is smaller and higher in position on one side should alert the clinician to Sprengel deformity.

EXTREMITIES. The clinician should examine the palmar creases. Simian creases (single transverse creases) occur normally in 5% to 10% of the population, although the presence of a simian crease is highly associated with a chromosomal and congenital abnormality. The upper extremities should be examined thoroughly for evidence of any brachial plexus injury; limb position, posture, symmetry, and range of motion should be assessed. Figure 83-11 provides a checklist for use in the assessment and follow-up care of an infant with a suspected brachial plexus injury.

LIMB AND DIGIT ABNORMALITIES. Syndactyly (abnormal fusion of digits) or polydactyly (supernumerary digits) and clinodactyly (radial deviation of the fifth digit) can be associated with syndromes. (See Chapter 86, Common Congenital Anomalies.) Polydactyly is usually an isolated finding in an otherwise-healthy newborn, occurring in approximately 1 in 700 live births. Postaxial polydactyly occurs more commonly than the other abnormalities, particularly among black individuals. The extra digit should be palpated for the presence of bony structures; frequently the extra digit

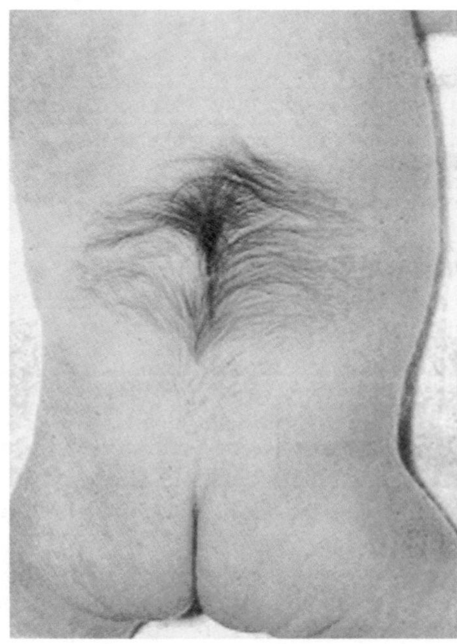

Figure 83-10 A hair tuft over the spine may be associated with vertebral anomalies.

Suspected Brachial Plexus Injury (BPI): Evaluation and Management Form

	Date ______ Admission		Date ______ Discharge		BPI Typical Clinical Findings		
					Erb's		
Physical Examination:	Left	Right	Left	Right	Palsy	Paresis	**Klumpke**
• Shoulder abduction					Absent	Decrease	Present
• Shoulder external rotation					Absent	Decrease	Present
• Elbow flexion					Absent	Decrease	Present
• Supination					Absent	Decrease	Present
• Wrist and finger extension					Present		Absent
• Biceps reflex					Absent	Decrease	Present
• Grasp reflex					Present		Absent
• Moro reflex					Abnormal		Abnormal
• Hand movement					Present		Absent
• Sensory					Varies		Varies
					"Waiter's tip position"		
Pain Management:					**Erb's + Klumpke = Total BPI**		
• Pain assessment	Present	Absent	Present	Absent	Comments:		
• Comfort care	Yes	No	Yes	No			
• Pain medication	Yes	No	Yes	No			
Diagnosis:							
• Attending name *(print)*							
• Attending signature							
Imaging:							
• Clavicles and chest x-ray							
• Upper extremity x-ray							
• Other							

Recommendations, Consultations, and Referrals

Pediatrics neurology consultation: Date ______ Time ______ Name ______
I O
NN H

Orthopedic consultation: Date ______ Time ______ Name ______
I O
NN H

Primary-care follow-up: Phone ______ Date ______ Time ______

Physical therapy and/or occupational therapy consultation: Date ______ Time ______ Name ______
Yes No

Home care referral:
Yes No

Early intervention referral:
Yes No

EIP child find (At-risk registry) referral:
Yes No

↑, Increased; U, unchanged; I, inpatient; H, HMO (referral by primary-care provider); ↓, decreased; N, normal; O, outpatient; NN, Not needed.

Developed by Carlos Vega-Rich, MD, and the Division of Neonatology, Children's Hospital at Montefiore (2003)

Figure 83-11 Suspected Brachial Plexus Injury (BPI): Evaluation and Management Form.

is attached to the hand by a thin stalk that can be easily ligated before the infant's discharge from the hospital. An x-ray examination may be necessary to evaluate for bone if the extra digit appears more fully developed. Syndactyly affects 2 to 3 per 10,000 live births and may occur sporadically or in families or in association with other abnormalities. The newborn with apparent syndactyly should be closely assessed for evidence of constriction band (amniotic band) sequence. The nails should also be examined for abnormalities.

Approximately 5 in 10,000 live-born infants will have a limb deficiency that is associated with a teratogenic

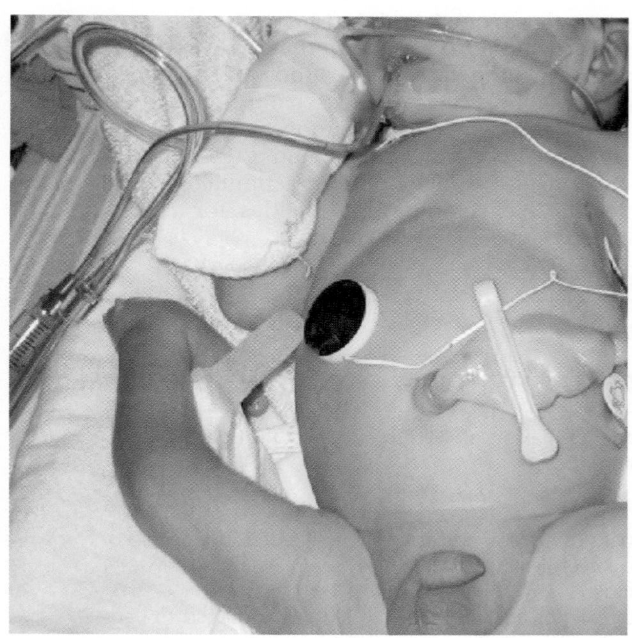

Figure 83-12 Genu recurvatum.

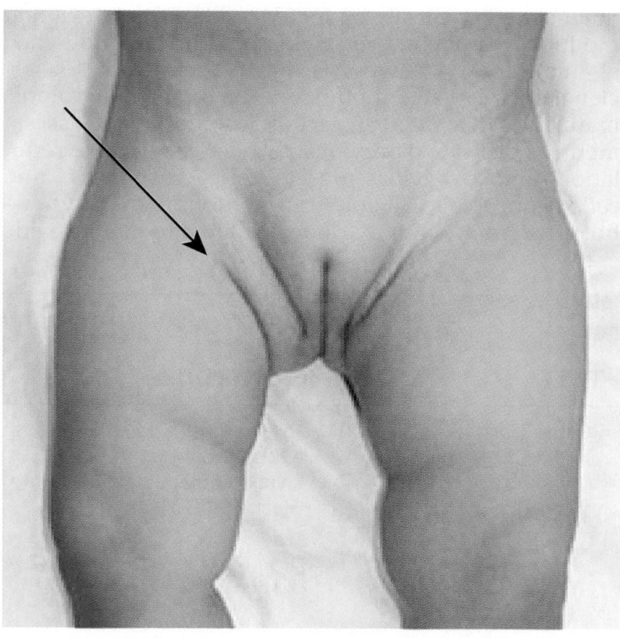

Figure 83-13 Asymmetric thigh creases in developmental dysplasia of the hip.

exposure during pregnancy, such as thalidomide and misoprostol, or caused by a prenatal diagnostic procedure (chorionic villus sampling, amniocentesis). These exposures produce a distinctive pattern of limb defects in which infants are damaged in utero by thalidomide have a symmetrical pattern of deficiency (or polydactyly) on the preaxial side of both arms and legs. Infants who are exposed early in pregnancy to misoprostol or chorionic villus sampling are at risk for developing a vascular disruption that results in asymmetrical digit loss, constriction rings, and syndactyly. Among the spectrum of radial limb deficiencies that may be seen in the newborn is an absent or hypoplastic thumb. Radial deficiencies are frequently associated with other anomalies.[25]

The presence of a dimple on the anterior leg suggests the presence of an underlying bony abnormality and warrants further evaluation. Alignment of the legs from the hips to the toes should be assessed to identify rotational misalignment. The number and appearance of the newborn's toes should be assessed for the presence of polydactyly, syndactyly, hypoplasia, overlap, and abnormal alignment. The extremities should also be observed for symmetry in limb size and muscle bulk. Genu recurvatum is a congenital anomaly of the lower limb, with hyperextension of the knees (Figure 83-12). It can be associated with congenital dislocation of hips, cerebral palsy, joint hypermobility, or clubfoot. Dislocation of the patella should be suspected if lateral displacement of the patella and limited knee motion are present.

A healthy newborn's foot is usually supinated and adducted at the forefoot, with increase in the distance between the first and the second toe. The range of motion of the ankles and subtalar joints feet should be examined. Metatarsus adductus is typically a positional deformation that occurs in varying degrees of severity and is frequently correctable with passive range-of-motion exercises. Metatarsus adductus may occur as a structural abnormality, with a fixed position that does not allow abduction of the foot beyond a neutral position. Talipes equinovarus (clubfoot) is inward with medial rotation of the foot, mild calf atrophy, and hypoplasia of the foot, tibia, and fibula. Limited dorsiflexion or a fixed equinus position of the foot occurs with congenital foot anomalies. Orthopedic evaluation and follow-up are required for a newborn with an equinovarus deformity.

All newborns should be examined for developmental dysplasia of the hip. A positive Galeazzi sign is asymmetry of the creases on the thigh and discrepancy of leg length (Figure 83-13). The Barlow test dislocates an unstable hip. With the newborn placed in a supine position and the hips in flexion, the hips are grasped and adducted with simultaneous downward pressure applied. The Ortolani test is performed to assess the relocation of a dislocated hip. In this maneuver the hip and knee are flexed while the thigh is grasped and the pelvis is stabilized by the examiner's other hand. The thigh is abducted as pressure is applied on the greater trochanter to reduce a dislocated hip. On dislocation of the femoral head against the acetabulum, a *clunk* is felt. Benign clicks are more commonly observed, caused by movement of the ligamentum teres in the acetabulum.

Neurologic Examination

The neurologic assessment includes examining the motor system, reflexes, sensory system, and cranial nerves (Table 83-4). A full-term newborn's posture in a quiet state is typically abducted, with partial flexion at the hips and knees; the arms are adducted and flexed at the elbow. Newborns have their fists loosely clenched with the thumb on the palm. Neurologic maturity is evaluated as part of gestational-age assessment, as described previously. The posture, state regulation and behavior, muscle tone, responses, and reflexes provide valuable information about the newborn's adaptation to extrauterine life and may provide clues to the newborn's intrauterine experiences. Signs on neurologic examination that warrant further evaluation include fisting or abnormal posturing of the trunk, hands, or feet; excessive tremulousness; clonus or atypical movements suggestive of seizure activity; abnormal eye movements; and a decreased or absent response to visual or auditory stimuli.[26] Refer to Chapter 106, Neurologic Abnormalities, for a more detailed discussion.

Table 83-4 Neonatal Neurologic Evaluation

TEST	TECHNIQUE	NORMAL FOR TERM	DEVIANT FOR TERM
Resting posture	Observe unswaddled infant without contact in quiet awake, quiet active, or light sleep states	Moderate flexion of 4 limbs, held off bed	Constant tight flexion
		Equal side to side and upper to lower if head is in midline	Full extension, flaccid or forced
		Extension of neck in face presentation or legs in breech	Knees abducted to bed (ie, frog leg)
			Elbows flexed with dorsum of hands on bed
			Tight, persistent fisting
			ATNR persistent 30 seconds
			Strong lateral preference
State	Deep Sleep - Light Sleep	Moves from one to the other with appropriate stimuli	Is difficult to move from one to the other
	Awake, light peripheral movements	Self calms	Stays too alert or cries without physical reason
	Awake, large movements, not crying	Modulated cry with expression	Does not come to fully awake state
	Awake, crying		Weak or monotonous cry
Motor Activity	Observe throughout physical examination	Appropriate for state of alertness	Bicycling, swatting without stimulus
		Symmetric, fairly smooth	Asymmetric, weak
		Expressive face with yawn or cry	Jittery while sucking
			Flat facial expression
Phasic (ie, passive)	Measure resistance to extension (limb recoil)	Response appropriate for gestational age	Resists too much or too little
Tone: resistance to movement	Scarf, heel to ear	Patellar reflex only one reliably present at birth	Asymmetry
Tendon reflexes	Test patellar reflex with head midline		Sustained clonus
Postural (ie, active)	Pull to sitting while grasping infant's hands	Infant pulls back with flexion at elbows, knees, and ankles	Asymmetry in pulling back
Tone: resistance to gravity		Head comes with body with minimal lag and falls forward when sitting is obtained	No resistance, Full head lag
Traction response			Pull to stand instead
			Head does not fall forward as infant goes past upright
Upright suspension	Suspend infant facing examiner with both hands in axillae	Infant supports himself then yields slowly	Infant falls through immediately
		Holds head erect, flexes hips, knees, and ankles	Legs extend, Eyes fail to open
		Eyes open	Infant fails to relax and fall through after 1 min

Table 83-4 Neonatal Neurologic Evaluation—cont'd

TEST	TECHNIQUE	NORMAL FOR TERM	DEVIANT FOR TERM
Ventral suspension	Hold infant under chest and suspend in prone position	Flexes arms, extends neck, holds back straight	Hangs limply or excessively rigidly
	Galant: Stroke adjacent to spine	Curves toward side of stimulus	Asymmetric incurving
	Landau: stroke caudocephalad along spine	Extends back, lift head and pelvis, micturates	Weak or absent response
Positive support	Hold infant to support trunk with feet touching firm, flat surface	Infant extends hips to bear his or her own weight and relaxes after 1 min	Infant fails to bear weight or extends too much or too long
Integrated Reflexes	Hold infant in supine position	Spreading: arms abduct, extend; hands open	Unequal laterality
Moro reflex	Support head & neck with hand; allow head to drop while still supporting it	Hugging: arms adduct and flex; hands close	Asymmetry; Exaggeration with disorganization in state
Tonic neck reflex	Infant in supine, neutral position; turn head to one side; repeat opposite side;	Mental extension, occipital flexion primarily of arms; does not remain in position for > 30 seconds	Exaggerated response and stays in position > 30 seconds
Withdrawal reflex	Painful stimulus to one foot	Withdrawal of stimulated foot; variable extension of opposite leg	Absence of flexion in stimulated leg

TOOLS FOR PRACTICE

Engaging Patient and Family

- *Hip Dysplasia (Developmental Dysplasia of the Hip)* (brochure), American Academy of Pediatrics (patiented.aap.org).

Medical Decision Support

- *Growth Charts,* Centers for Disease Control and Prevention (www.cdc.gov/nchs/about/major/nhanes/growthcharts/clinical_charts.htm#Clin%201) also available at AAP bookstore (www.aap.org/bookstore).
- *New Ballard Score* (Web page), Ballard JL (www.ballardscore.com/).
- *World Health Organization International Reference Charts* (growth charts), World Health Organization (www.who.int/childgrowth/en/).

AAP POLICY STATEMENT

American Academy of Pediatrics, Section on Ophthalmology. Red reflex examination in infants. *Pediatrics.* 2002;109(5):980-998. (aappolicy.aappublications.org/cgi/content/full/pediatrics;109/5/980).

SUGGESTED RESOURCE

Kozin SH. Current concepts review: upper-extremity congenital anomalies. *J Bone Joint Surg.* 2003;85(8):1564-1575. Available at: www.jbjs.org. Accessed March 18, 2007.

SUGGESTED READINGS

American Academy of Pediatrics, Susan R. Rose, and the Section on Endocrinology and Committee on Genetics, American Thyroid Association, Rosalind S. Brown, and the Public Health Committee, and Lawson Wilkins Pediatric Endocrine Society Update of Newborn Screening and Therapy for Congenital Hypothyroidism. *Pediatrics.* 2006;117:2290-2303.

American Academy of Pediatrics, Section on Ophthalmology. Red reflex examination in infants. *Pediatrics.* 2002;109:980-981.

Committee on Genetics. Maternal Phenylketonuria. *Pediatrics.* 2001;107:427-428.

American Academy of Pediatrics, Committee on Fetus and Newborn, American College of Obstetricians and Gynecologists, and Committee on Obstetric Practice. The Apgar Score. *Pediatrics.* 2006;117:1444-1447.

Committee on Quality Improvement, Subcommittee on Developmental Dysplasia of the Hip. Clinical Practice Guideline: Early Detection of Developmental Dysplasia of the Hip. *Pediatrics.* 2000;105:896-905.

Cunniff C, and Committee on Genetics. Prenatal Screening and Diagnosis for Pediatricians. *Pediatrics.* 2004;114:889-894.

Engle WA, Tomashek KM, Wallman C, and the Committee on Fetus and Newborn. "Late-Preterm" Infants: A Population at Risk. *Pediatrics.* 2007;120:1390-1401.

King SM, Committee on Pediatric AIDS, and Canadian Paediatric Society, Infectious Diseases and Immunization Committee. Evaluation and Treatment of the Human Immunodeficiency Virus-1—Exposed Infant. *Pediatrics.* 2004;114:497-505.

Lee PA, Houk CP, Faisal Ahmed S, et al, in collaboration with the participants in the International Consensus Conference on Intersex organized by the Lawson Wilkins Pediatric Endocrine Society and the European Society for Paediatric Endocrinology. Consensus Statement on Management of Intersex Disorders. *Pediatrics.* 2006;118:e488-e500.

Mofenson LM, and the Committee on Pediatric AIDS. Technical Report: Perinatal Human Immunodeficiency Virus Testing and Prevention of Transmission. *Pediatrics.* 2000;106:e88.

Noninherited Risk Factors and Congenital Cardiovascular Defects: Current Knowledge. *Pediatrics.* 2007;120:445-446.

Section on Endocrinology and Committee on Genetics Technical Report: Congenital Adrenal Hyperplasia. *Pediatrics.* 2000;106:1511-1518.

Section on Ophthalmology. Red Reflex Examination in Infants. *Pediatrics.* 2002;109:980-981.

Subcommittee on Hyperbilirubinemia. Management of Hyperbilirubinemia in the Newborn Infant 35 or More Weeks of Gestation. *Pediatrics.* 2004;114:297-316.

REFERENCES

1. Ballard JL, Khoury JC, Wedig K, et al. New Ballard score: expanded to include extremely premature infants. *J Pediatric.* 1991;119(3):417-423.
2. Day RE, Schutt WH. Normal children with large heads—benign familial megalencephaly. *Arch Disease Child.* 1979:54:512-517.
3. Martin JA, Hamilton BE, Sutton PD, et al. *Births: Final Data for 2004. National Vital Statistics Reports.* Vol 55. Hyattsville, MD: National Center for Health Statistics; 2006.
4. American Academy of Pediatrics, Section on Ophthalmology. Red reflex examination in infants. *Pediatrics.* 2002;109:980-981.
5. Hall J, Allanson J, Gripp K, et al, eds. *Handbook of Physical Measurements.* 2nd ed. New York, NY: Oxford University Press; 2007.
6. Tan T, Constantinides H, Mitchell TE. The preauricular sinus: a review of its aetiology, clinical presentation and management. *Int J Pediatr Otorhinolaryngol.* 2005;69:1469-1474.
7. Wang RY, Earl DL, Ruder RO, et al. Syndromic ear anomalies and renal ultrasounds. *Pediatrics.* 2001;108(2):e32.
8. Arora RS, Pryce R. Is ultrasonography required to rule out renal malformations in babies with isolated preauricular tags? *Arch Dis Child.* 2004;89:492-493.
9. Kugelman A, Tubi A, Bader D, et al. Pre-auricular tags and pits in the newborn: the role of renal ultrasonography. *J Pediatr.* 2002;141:388-391.
10. Deshpande SA, Watson H. Renal ultrasonography is not required in babies with isolated minor ear anomalies. *Arch Dis Child Fetal Neonatal Ed.* 2006;91:F29-F30.
11. Huang XY, Tay GS, Wansaicheong G K-L, et al. Preauricular sinus: clinical course and associations. *Arch Otolaryngol Head Neck Surg.* 2007;133:65-68.
12. Young JDH, MacEwen CJ. Fort nightly review: managing congenital lacrimal obstruction in general practice. *BMJ.* 1997;315:293-296.
13. Berkowitz RG, Grundfast KM, Fitz C. Nasal obstruction of the newborn revisited: clinical and subclinical manifestations of congenital nasolacrimal duct obstruction presenting as a nasal mass. *Otolaryngol Head Neck Surg.* 1990;103:468-471.
14. Schnall BM, Christian CJ. Conservative treatment of congenital dacryocele. *J Pediatr Opthalmol Strabismus.* 1996;33(5):219-222.
15. Hepler KM, Woodson GE, Keams DB. Respiratory distress in the neonate. Sequela of a congenital dacryocystocele. *Arch Otolaryngol Head Neck Surg.* 1995;121:1423-1425.
16. Becker B. The treatment of congenital dacryocystocele. *Am J Ophthalmol.* 2006;142(5):835-838.
17. Rayburn WF, Beyer A, Brickman DC. Umbilical cord length and intrapartum complications. *Obstetr Gynecol.* 1981;57:450-452.
18. Naeye RL. *Disorders of Placenta, Fetus and Neonate: Diagnosis and Clinical Significance.* St Louis, MO: Mosby; 1992.
19. Malpas P. Length of the umbilical cord at term. *BMJ.* 1964;1:673-674.
20. Thummala MR, Raju TN, Langenberg P. Isolated single umbilical artery anomaly and the risk for congenital malformations: a meta-analysis. *J Pediatr Surg.* 1998;33:580-585.
21. Predanic M, Perni SC, Friedman A, et al. Fetal growth assessment and neonatal birth weight in fetuses with an isolated single umbilical artery. *Obstet Gynecol.* 2005;105:1093-1097.
22. Jones TB, Sorokin Y, Bhatia R, et al. Single umbilical artery: accurate diagnosis? *Am J Obstet Gynecol.* 1993;169:538-540.
23. Gossett DR, Lantz ME, Chisholm CA. Antenatal diagnosis of single umbilical artery: is fetal echocardiography warranted? *Obstet Gynecol.* 2002;100:903-908.
24. Parilla BV, Tamura RK, MacGregor SN, et al. The clinical significance of a single umbilical artery as an isolated finding on prenatal ultrasound. *Obstet Gynecol.* 1995;85:570-572.
25. Tay S-C, Moran SL, Shin AY et al. The hypoplastic thumb. *J Am Acad Orthoped Surg.* 2006;14(6):354-366.
26. Mercuri E, Ricci D, Pane M, et al. The neurological examination of the newborn baby. *Early Human Develop.* 2005;81:947-956.

Chapter 84

POSTNATAL ASSESSMENT OF COMMON PRENATAL SONOGRAPHIC FINDINGS

Deborah E. Campbell, MD

Approximately 10% of all neonates are born with a birth defect; 3% (1 in 33) of newborns will have a serious, potentially life-threatening anomaly, and an additional 7% to 8% of neonates are born with a minor malformation. Advances in prenatal screening, diagnosis, and intervention have contributed to an increased awareness at the time of birth of newborns in need of postnatal evaluation to confirm a prenatal diagnosis. Among newborns with a confirmed prenatal diagnosis this information permits more rapid initiation of treatment and can help guide the evaluations necessary to optimize care. The patterns of malformations seen among newborns have changed over time because of prenatal diagnosis, availability of fetal interventions (including many experimental protocols), and families choosing termination of pregnancy in instances in which the fetus has multiple or complex malformations with an associated poor prognosis or a lethal chromosomal or genetic condition.[1-3]

Prenatal diagnosis, though offering the potential for earlier intervention and correction of potentially serious abnormalities, also presents a significant psychological burden on expectant women and their families that may have long-lasting effects.[4] Conversely, prenatal sonography does not identify all fetal malformations. If performed during the second trimester, prenatal sonography identifies approximately 92% of central nervous system, 80% of musculoskeletal, 60% of genitourinary, 50% of craniofacial, and 24% of cardiovascular malformations (38% if the child's underlying condition has associated congenital heart defects), with many of these findings not being of clinical significance.[5,6] Some anomalies will not yet have developed, such as microcephaly, and are identified by antenatal screening. Fetal magnetic resonance imaging and fetal karyotyping may be used to further delineate clinical findings and aid in the formulation of the initial clinical care plans for the neonate.[7] Some infants with prenatally diagnosed conditions will be healthy when evaluated postnatally. Despite explanations from obstetric caregivers and sonographers that prenatal ultrasonography will not identify all anomalies, families inherently expect that any and all problems should have been detected if the mother had one or more sonographic studies or underwent an amniocentesis. This expectation can present a challenge to the pediatric primary care physician who must assist the parents as they come to terms with their newborn's diagnosis and as they try to understand the limits of technology.

Screening ultrasonography has not been shown to be more effective in improving perinatal outcomes compared with selective use of ultrasonography based on clinical judgment. However, if fetuses with severe malformations whose pregnancies are terminated are excluded from statistical analyses, then an improvement in reported outcomes can be found. Controversy exists with regard to the benefits of prenatal diagnosis, given that decision making about the choice of delivery hospital, level of neonatal and subspecialty care, and the initial scope of care provided are influenced by the available prenatal data. The infant with a serious malformation, such as a gastroschisis or congenital diaphragmatic hernia, can benefit from delivery at a tertiary-care center, whereas knowledge that an infant has a ductus-dependent cardiac lesion can afford the pediatric primary care physician the opportunity to have prostaglandin therapy available for use during the infant's stabilization. In contrast, postnatal diagnosis of even significant birth defects, such as pulmonary atresia, may not necessarily lead to greater mortality or morbidity in comparison with infants who are identified through prenatal screening.[8] Understanding the complexities of screening is important in assisting parents as they assimilate information about their baby's condition, their awareness of the potential problem in the prenatal period, and subsequent evaluation of the infant to characterize more fully the infant's health care needs.

Surveillance programs in the United States report that orofacial clefts and Down syndrome were the most common major birth defects to occur.[9] The Metropolitan Atlanta Congenital Disorders Program is a Centers for Disease Control and Prevention (CDC)-supported initiative that tracks birth defects in that city. When all neonatal birth defects are considered, malformations involving the heart, genitourinary, and musculoskeletal systems, as well as the chromosomal anomaly, trisomy 21, are among the more common abnormalities observed. The most frequently observed cardiovascular malformations are atrial septal defects, patent ductus arteriosus, and ventricular septal defects, in increasing order of prevalence. Clubfoot or equinovarus deformity is the most common musculoskeletal defect, followed by upper limb reduction abnormalities. The CDC reports that the rate of hypospadias has increased dramatically in the last 2 decades, confirming similar findings in Europe. Rates of gastroschisis are also reported to be increasing, particularly among teen mothers. Regional variation has been reported in the incidence of these and other malformations; the causes for the changing prevalence rates are not easily determined in many instances.

POSTNATAL EVALUATION IN OTHERWISE-HEALTHY NEWBORNS

Antenatal Hydronephrosis and Pyelectasis

Antenatal hydronephrosis (ANH) has a reported incidence of 1% to 5%. A more-frequent finding on prenatal sonography is the presence of pyelectasis, mild dilation of the renal pelvis without associated dilation of the renal calyx or hydronephrosis. The reported incidence of pylectasis is 2% to 7%. Pyelectasis may be caused by vesicoureteral reflux (VUR) or a partial ureteropelvic junction obstruction. As the pregnancy progresses, pyelectasis can develop into hydronephrosis or resolve spontaneously. An association also exists between pyelectasis occurring later in gestation and Down syndrome. Wide variation can be found in the prenatal assessment and postnatal management of infants with ANH. A recent meta-analysis conducted to determine the risk of postnatal disease in infants with ANH found that the risk of any disease was 12% for mild, 45% for moderate, and 88% for severe degrees of hydronephrosis. A similar risk was noted for VUR, irrespective of the degree of hydronephrosis.[10] Among infants with ANH, 14% to 21% of affected infants will have utereropelvic junction obstruction or VUR; approximately 9% of these infants will have VUR. Posterior urethral valves are a rare, but important associated finding found in 1% of affected infants.[11]

Infants with significant hydronephrosis are more often male infants and have evidence of left kidney involvement. Additional information garnered from the prenatal evaluation that informs the diagnostic and management considerations include renal calyceal dilation, echogenicity of the kidneys, thinness of the renal parenchyma, presence of hydroureteronephrosis, bladder dilation, posterior urethral dilation, fetal gender, laterality of the involved kidney, and amniotic fluid volume. Oligohydramnios is associated with a poorer prognosis. Bladder distension or the presence of lower urinary tract obstruction suggests posterior urethral valves, particularly in a male fetus. The presence of prenatal renal dysplasia (renal cysts and hyperechoic renal parenchyma) can indicate poor kidney function. Renal cysts are highly specific for kidney dysplasia, whereas kidney hyperechogenicity is a more sensitive, but less specific, sign. Spontaneous urinary tract decompression can occur in infants with severe urethral obstruction, causing ascites or a perinephric urinoma.

The timing of the prenatal ultrasound is also important in predicting the importance of the findings. Infants with isolated ANH have varying degrees of renal pelvis or calyceal dilation, referred to as pelviectasis or pelvicaliectasis. Serial postnatal sonography has demonstrated that gradual resolution of the renal calyceal or pelvic dilation, or both, takes place. At 5 days of age, 25% of newborns with ANH showed no evidence of residual hydronephrosis. One half of the newborns with pelviectasis exhibited mild dilation. Pelviectasis resolved in 50% of the babies with dilation on the initial postnatal renal sonogram.

Newborns with ANH should be thoroughly examined for the presence of other anomalies and assessed for adequate urine output. Initiating postnatal antibiotic prophylaxis to reduce the risk of infection before performing postnatal imaging to confirm the presence of associated VUR is controversial. Current recommendations include the following:

- Newborns with bilateral severe ANH or a single kidney with any grade of hydronephrosis should undergo postnatal renal sonographic evaluation before hospital discharge.
- Newborns with any other grade of ANH should have a postnatal renal ultrasound examination performed within the first month of life (after the first 3-5 days of age).
- Newborns with persistent moderate to severe ANH should undergo a voiding cystourethrographic evaluation and functional studies as needed.
- Decisions regarding postnatal evaluation of newborns with mild persistent ANH or isolated ANH that resolves should be individualized based on the specific infant issues.
- Pyelectasis that resolves spontaneously before birth does not require postnatal evaluation.
- Newborns with persistent pyelectasis should have postnatal renal sonographic evaluation performed within the first month of life with additional evaluation (voiding cystourethrographic evaluation and functional studies) and antibiotic prophylaxis based on sonographic and clinical findings.

Antenatal Identification of Central Nervous System Variants

Ventriculomegaly and cysts of the choroids plexus and subependyma are prenatal sonographic findings with an uncertain significance that warrant postnatal evaluation and follow-up. Ventriculomegaly is the most common central nervous system abnormality identified on prenatal sonography. Seventy percent to 85% of fetuses with ventriculomegaly have associated structural or chromosomal anomalies, including neural tube defects, structural and cortical brain malformations, hemorrhage, and porencephaly.[12,13] Clinical risk is further influenced by additional factors such as maternal age and the results of maternal serum markers for aneupolidy. One third of infants with isolated ventriculomegaly have been found to subsequently exhibit developmental delay in comparison with over 84% of infants with ventriculomegaly and associated anomalies.[14,15]

Choroid plexus cysts are detected on prenatal sonography in approximately 1% of pregnancies and are associated in a small percentage of infants with aneuploidy; 40% to 50% of infants with trisomy 18 and 1.4% of babies born with Down syndrome have choroid cysts.[16] The risk for aneupolidy is unrelated to the location (laterality), size, number, complexity of the choroid plexus cysts, or whether the cysts spontaneously regress. Advanced maternal age increases the infant's risk as well. Many choroid plexus cysts regress by 28 weeks of gestation.

Subependymal cysts are believed to represent hemorrhagic-ischemic injury in a portion of the periventricular region of the brain. Infants born preterm exhibit an associated neurodevelopmental sequelae. The true incidence of cranial sonographic abnormalities in term infants is unknown; however, approximately 8% of infants have evidence of ischemic injury. The short-term neurodevelopment of these infants appears comparable with infants without cranial sonographic abnormalities at birth.[17,18]

Recommendations include the following:

- Infants with prenatal cranial sonographic abnormalities require a thorough physical examination for evidence of dysmorphism and other malformations and a postnatal neurosonographic evaluation.
- The prenatal information should be reviewed to ascertain whether the mother was evaluated prenatally for a TORCH infection (*t*oxoplasmosis, *o*ther agents, *r*ubella, *c*ytomegalovirus, *h*erpes simplex).
- Consultation with a pediatric neurologist and additional neuroimaging may be warranted based on the sonographic findings and clinical examination.
- Careful monitoring of the infant's head growth and neurodevelopment is required.

Postnatal Evaluation of Fetal Lung Masses

Fetal lung masses that cause respiratory distress are reviewed in detail in Chapter 99, Respiratory Distress and Breathing Disorders in the Newborn. Antenatally diagnosed lung lesions are most commonly congenital cystic adenomatoid malformations or bronchopulmonary sequestrations. Many echogenic fetal lung masses regress antenatally, whereas other lesions will enlarge in size. Postnatal evaluation of the asymptomatic infant with a history of an antenatal fetal lung mass should include chest computed tomographic (CT) scan. Residual lesions are often visible on CT scan despite apparent resolution on prenatal sonography.[19,20]

Recommendations include the following:

- Thorough examination of the infant for evidence of respiratory compromise
- Postnatal chest radiographs and chest CT scan
- Pediatric surgical consultation and follow-up

Postnatal Evaluation of Intraabdominal Fetal Echogenic Masses

Fetal echogenic lesions in the abdomen are common prenatal sonographic findings. Formulation of a presumptive diagnosis is based on a thorough evaluation of the lesion's characteristics, structure, and the presence of calcifications. Echogenic bowel is the most common echogenic mass in the fetal abdomen, identified in 1% of second-trimester fetuses that are evaluated. Spontaneous resolution occurs in 50% of affected infants. Echogenic bowel may be associated with fetal growth restriction. Differential diagnosis of echogenic bowel includes cystic fibrosis, chromosomal abnormalities, intra-amniotic bleeding, and congenital infection (cytomegalovirus). Bowel echogenicity seen on a third-trimester sonogram is a common variant and reflects meconium in the intestine.[21] Abdominal calcifications are often present in infants with meconium peritonitis caused by an intestinal perforation that develops in response to a vascular insult or cystic fibrosis. Infants with isolated abdominal calcifications generally have a normal outcome.

Recommendations include the following:

- Postnatal abdominal radiography with additional upper and lower gastrointestinal tract barium studies should be performed to evaluate for perforation.
- If the radiographic studies are normal and the infant passes meconium, then further evaluation is not required.

Fetal Ovarian Cysts

Fetal ovarian cysts are the most commonly identified intraabdominal cystic lesion in women; the diagnosis is typically one of exclusion. The cysts may achieve a considerable size, reaching up to 5 cm for large cysts. These cysts may be unilateral or bilateral, unilocular, or multilocular. A tendency exists for cysts less than 3 cm in size to regress near term or in the early neonatal period. Serial ultrasound of fetal ovarian cysts is indicated because approximately 35% of patients develop symptoms of torsion or rupture of the cyst, either prenatally or in the postnatal period. Torsion of cyst is suspected when changes on ultrasound findings occur that are consistent with intracystic hemorrhage. This circumstance is an indication for immediate surgical intervention.

Recommendations include the following:

- Postnatal evaluation should consist of a thorough abdominal examination for a palpable mass; abdominal sonographic evaluation is also recommended.
- Surgical consultation and follow-up are required if an ovarian cyst is identified, particularly if evidence is found of hemorrhage or torsion.

Neonatal Gastrointestinal Anomalies Causing Early Serious Illness

Gastrointestinal emergencies that may present in the newborn period in apparently healthy newborns include bowel obstruction caused by intestinal atresias, malrotation with midgut volvulus, and megacolon caused by Hirschsprung disease. Vomiting during the neonatal period should alert the clinician to a potential intestinal anomaly. Although initial symptoms may be nonspecific, the onset of bilious vomiting constitutes a medical emergency that warrants immediate assessment and intervention.[22] Prenatal sonography with evidence of dilated bowel or intraabdominal calcifications may help inform the diagnosis. A history of polyhydramnios should alert the clinician to suspect a proximal intestinal obstruction, such as duodenal or jejunoileal atresia. A thorough physical examination should be performed with emphasis on inspection and palpation of the abdomen and perineum and assessment of the infant for evidence of other anomalies.

Newborns with a malrotation and midgut volvulus exhibit bilious emesis and poor feeding and may rapidly progress to lethargy and shock. In addition to placement of a nasogastric tube and initiation of intravenous fluid resuscitation and antibiotic therapy, abdominal radiographs and an upper gastrointestinal series must be obtained immediately. Concurrent surgical consultation and arrangements for transfer to a neonatal or pediatric critical care unit are paramount.

Newborns with duodenal or jejunoileal atresias often exhibit symptoms in the immediate postnatal period with the onset of vomiting, with or without prior feeding. Duodenal atresia occurs in 1 in 5000 live births; 25% of affected infants have Down syndrome. Neonates with duodenal atresia develop bilious vomiting in the first hours after birth and may not exhibit abdominal distension. A *double bubble* is the characteristic finding on abdominal radiography. Jejunoileal atresias are caused by intrauterine vascular accidents and occur in 1 in 3000 live births. Neonates with jejunoileal atresia also are typically symptomatic within the first day of life, exhibiting vomiting and abdominal distension. Abdominal radiographs demonstrate air-fluid levels and dilated bowel.

Newborns with tracheoesophageal fistula and esophageal atresia often have a prenatal history of polyhydramnios. These babies may exhibit symptoms shortly after birth, particularly during the first attempt at feeding. Placement of a nasogastric tube before obtaining a radiograph of the chest and abdomen will show the feeding tube coiled in the upper esophageal pouch. If air is present in the stomach, then the infant has an associated tracheoesophageal fistula.

The infant with Hirschsprung disease typically exhibits failure to pass meconium in the first 24 hours of life or constipation. Infants exhibit poor feeding, vomiting, progressive abdominal distension, irritability, and bloody stools. Stabilization includes fluid resuscitation, broad-spectrum antibiotic administration, abdominal radiographs, transfer to a neonatal or critical care unit, and surgical consultation. Abdominal radiographs typically demonstrate a markedly dilated colon. A definitive diagnosis is confirmed with a rectal biopsy. Bowel obstruction may also occur as a result of meconium ileus, meconium plug syndrome, or a small left colon.

Meconium ileus occurs in 10% to 20% of infants with cystic fibrosis (CF) and may be the earliest manifestation of CF. Enemas are used to decompress the intestinal obstruction. Perforation and pseudocyst formation may complicate the infant's course. The presence of calcifications on abdominal radiography indicates an intrauterine perforation occurred.

Newborns with meconium plug syndrome are otherwise healthy neonates with plugs of meconium in the colon. Meconium plug syndrome is not associated with CF but occurs in infants with intestinal dysmotility—infants of diabetic or preeclampsia mothers, infants exposed in utero to magnesium sulfate, and infants who are preterm with sepsis or hypothyroidism. Small left colon syndrome occurs in infants of diabetic mothers. Maternal lithium use is also associated with small left colon syndrome.

RELATED WEB SITE

- Birth Defects, Centers for Disease Control and Prevention (www.cdc.gov/ncbddd/bd/default.htm).

SELECTED RESOURCES

Behnke M, Davis Eyler F, Wilson Garvan C, et al. Cranial ultrasound abnormalities identified at birth: their relationship to perinatal risk and neurobehavioral outcome. *Pediatrics*. 1999;103(4):e41.

Centers for Disease Control and Prevention. Improved national prevalence estimates for 18 selected major birth defects—United States, 1999-2001. *MMWR Morb Mortal Wkly Rep*. 2006;54(51-52):1301-1305.

Frates MC, Kumar AJ, Benson CB, et al. Fetal anomalies: comparison of MR imaging and US for diagnosis. *Radiology*. 2004;232:398-404.

Lee RS, Cendron M, Kinnamon DD, et al. Antenatal hydronephrosis as a predictor of postnatal outcome: a meta-analysis. *Pediatrics*. 2006;118(2):587-593.

McNamara A, Levine D. Intraabdominal fetal echogenic masses: a practical guide to diagnosis and management. *Radiographics*. 2005;25:633-645.

Stanton M, Davenport M. Management of congenital lung lesions. *Early Hum Dev*. 2006;82(5):289-295.

AAP POLICY STATEMENT

- Cunniff C, American Academy of Pediatrics, Committee on Genetics. Prenatal screening and diagnosis for pediatricians. *Pediatrics*. 2004;114(3):889-894. (aappolicy.aappublications.org/cgi/content/full/pediatrics;114/3/889).

REFERENCES

1. Lui S, Joseph KS, Kramer MS, et al. Relationship of prenatal diagnosis and pregnancy termination to overall infant mortality in Canada. *JAMA*. 2002; 287(12): 1561-1567.
2. Khoshnood B, De Vigan C, Vodovar V, et al. Trends in prenatal diagnosis, pregnancy termination, and perinatal mortality of newborns with congenital heart disease in France, 1983-2000: a population-based evaluation. *Pediatrics*. 2005;115(5):95-101.
3. Bell, R, Glinianaia SV, Rankin J, et al. Changing patterns of perinatal death, 1982-2000: a retrospective cohort study. *Arch Dis Child Fetal Neonatal Ed*. 2004;89: F531-F536.
4. Detraux JJ, Gillot-deVries FR, Vanden Eynde S, et al. Psychological impact of the announcement of a fetal abnormality on pregnant women and on professionals. *Ann N Y Acad Sci*. 1998;847:210-219.
5. Strauss A, Toth B, Schwab B, et al. Prenatal diagnosis of congenital heart disease and neonatal outcome—six years experience. *Eur J Med Res*. 2001;6:66-70.
6. Guariglia L, Rosati P. Transvaginal sonographic detection of embryonic-fetal abnormalities in early pregnancy. *Obstet Gynecol*. 2000;96(3):328-332.
7. Frates MC, Kumar AJ, Benson CB, et al. Fetal anomalies: comparison of MR imaging and US for diagnosis. *Radiology*. 2004;232:398-404.
8. Tzifa A, Barker C, Tibby SM, et al. Prenatal diagnosis of pulmonary atresia: impact on clinical presentation and early outcome. *Arch Dis Child Fetal Neonatal Ed*. 2007; 92:F199-F203.
9. Centers for Disease Control and Prevention. Improved national prevalence estimates for 18 selected major birth defects—United States, 1999-2001. *MMWR Morb Mortal Wkly Rep*. 2006;54(51-52):1301-1305.
10. Lee RS, Cendron M, Kinnamon DD, et al. Antenatal hydronephrosis as a predictor of postnatal outcome: a meta-analysis. *Pediatrics*. 2006;118(2):587-593.
11. Cheng AM, Phan V, Geary DF, et al. Outcome of isolated antenatal hydronephrosis. *Arch Pediatr Adolesc Med*. 2004;158:38-40.
12. Gupta JK, Bryce FC, Lilford RJ. Management of apparently isolated fetal ventriculomegaly. *Obstet Gynecol Surv*. 1994;49:716-721.
13. Vergani P, Locatelli A, Strobelt N, et al. Clinical outcome of mild fetal ventriculomegaly. *Am J Obstet Gynecol*. 1998;178:218-222.
14. Behnke M, Davis Eyler F, Wilson Garvan C, et al. Cranial ultrasound abnormalities identified at birth: their relationship to perinatal risk and neurobehavioral outcome. *Pediatrics*. 1999;103(4):e41.
15. Lee CS, Hong SH, Wang KC, et al. Fetal ventriculomegaly: prognosis in cases in which prenatal neurosurgical consultation was sought. *J Neurosurg (Suppl Pediatrics)*. 2006;105:265-270.
16. Lopez JA, Reich D. Choroid plexus cysts. *J Am Board Fam Med*. 2006;19:422-425.
17. Mercuri E, Dubowitz L, Paterson Brown S, et al. Incidence of cranial ultrasound abnormalities in apparently well neonates on a postnatal ward: correlation with antenatal and perinatal factors and neurological status. *Arch Dis Child Fetal Neonatal Ed*. 1998;79:F185-F189.
18. Haataja L, Mecuri E, Cowan F, et al. Cranial ultrasound abnormalities in full-term infants in a postnatal ward: outcome at 12 and 18 months. *Arch Dis Child Fetal Neonatal Ed*. 2000;82:F128-F133.
19. Lee HJ, Song MJ, Cho JY, et al. Echogenic fetal lung masses: comparison of prenatal sonographic and postnatal CT findings. *J Clin Ultrasound*. 2003;31(8):419-424.
20. Stanton M, Davenport M. Management of congenital lung lesions. *Early Hum Dev*. 2006;82(5):289-295.
21. McNamara A, Levine D. Intraabdominal fetal echogenic masses: a practical guide to diagnosis and management. *Radiographics*. 2005;25:633-645.
22. Kimura K, Loening-Baucke V. Bilious vomiting in the newborn: rapid diagnosis of intestinal obstruction. *Am Fam Physician*. 2000;61:2791-2798.

Chapter 85

NEONATAL SKIN

Julian J. Trevino, MD; Matthew A. Bakos, MD; Matthew P. Janik, MD

By the end of the 3rd trimester of pregnancy, the fetus's skin structure and composition are similar to those of adults. The skin contains a mature lipid bilayer, substantial subcutaneous fat, and differentiated epidermal layers. The primary functions of neonatal skin are mechanical protection, maintenance of thermoregulation, immune surveillance, and prevention of insensible loss of body fluids. Skin of premature infants is thinner and much less effective than skin of term infants in these functions.[1]

SKIN CARE OF NEWBORNS

The developmentally immature skin barrier in premature infants can result in increased transepidermal water loss, difficulties in thermoregulation, higher risk for infection, increased absorption of environmental toxins, and predisposition to injury from minor skin trauma.[2] Hand washing by caregivers is the most effective way to prevent skin colonization and nosocomial infection. Mild, alkaline to neutral pH nonantimicrobial cleanser (eg, chlorhexidine) is suggested for hand decontamination.[3]

Premature infants are at marked risk for percutaneous toxicity as compared with term infants. A conservative approach to applying topical products to the skin of preterm infants must be undertaken. Only essential products should be used, and these should be washed off once their purpose has been achieved.[2]

Sterilization of the skin before invasive procedures are performed on the neonate is assumed to eliminate pathogens from the local site and reduce the risk of subsequent bacteremia and sepsis. Chlorhexidine appears to be the safest and most effective agent for local skin sterilization.[4] Chlorhexidine has also been found to be a safe and effective agent for reducing bacterial colonization of the umbilical cord stump.[5]

Bathing of neonates should be delayed until vital signs have been stable for several hours. Excessive vernix is best left on the skin. For preterm infants, particularly those with compromised barriers, water-only nonimmersion bathing up to 3 times a week is suggested for the initial 2 to 4 weeks of life. Rubbing or scrubbing the skin should be avoided. If soap is required, then only mild, neutral-pH soaps without additives should be used in heavily soiled areas; these soaps should be promptly rinsed from the skin.[2]

Although treatment with emollient theoretically promotes the integrity and function of the stratum corneum, studies have revealed a trend toward increased risk of bacterial infection in infants prophylactically treated with emollient. Based on these studies, topical ointment should not be used routinely in preterm infants.[6]

Neonatal skin, especially that of preterm neonates, is highly susceptible to injury. Routine precautions such as care in handling, minimizing use of skin adhesives, and use of hydrogel-based cardiorespiratory monitor chest leads and masks should be routinely followed.[2]

PIGMENTARY BIRTHMARKS

Congenital Disorders of Hypopigmentation and Depigmentation

Nevus depigmentosus refers to macular hypopigmentation that is present at birth and stable throughout the lifetime (Figure 85-1). Lesions are usually unilateral and block or flag shaped.[7] Hypopigmented linear or segmental macules are seen in patients with hypomelanosis of Ito. Lesions can be present at birth, or they can develop during infancy or childhood. The spectrum of this disorder ranges from those with only cutaneous involvement (most common) to those in which cutaneous lesions are associated with ocular, musculoskeletal, or neurologic disorders.[8] This disorder is hypothesized to be the result of chromosomal mosaicism.[9]

Hypomelanotic macules are generally the 1st cutaneous clue to the diagnosis of tuberous sclerosis. These lesions are often present at birth, although in individuals with light skin types, a Wood's lamp may be needed to demonstrate their presence. The most common hypopigmented lesion is an elliptical or ash-leaf macule. Less commonly, guttate hypopigmented macules of the pretibial areas or segmental hypopigmented lesions may be present. As patients age, additional cutaneous manifestations of tuberous sclerosis (facial angiofibromas, periungual fibromas, and connective tissue nevi) often become evident.[10]

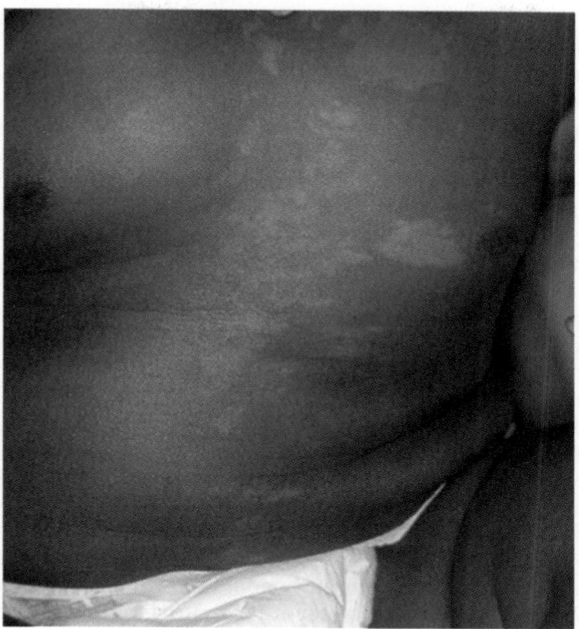

Figure 85-1 Nevus depigmentosus. (© Johnell Kolve, Dermatlas; www.dermatlas.org).

Piebaldism is an autosomal dominant disorder characterized by depigmented patches of skin on the forehead, anterior trunk, and extremities. Forehead lesions may be associated with a white forelock (poliosis).[11] In rare cases, patients with piebaldism can have associated problems, including intellectual disability. This disorder results from mutations in the *KIT* gene.[12]

Hyperpigmented Lesions

Congenital hyperpigmented lesions are the result of accumulation of melanin in melanocytes or keratinocytes, melanin incontinence, proliferation of nevus cells in the epidermis or dermis, or thickening of the stratum corneum.

Proliferation of dermal melanocytes produces brown, blue-gray, or blue-black patches. Such lesions located on the sacrogluteal area are known as *Mongolian spots.* Less commonly, they can be located on the dorsal trunk, extremities, and scalp. These lesions are the most common birthmarks in patients with highly pigmented skin, being present at birth in 85% of Asians, 96% of blacks, and 46% of Hispanics.[13] Mongolian spots typically increase in size during the 1st year and subsequently fade during childhood. *Nevus of Ota* is a blue-gray patch in the distribution of the ophthalmic or maxillary branch of the trigeminal nerve. This patch can be associated with glaucoma,[14] and rare cases of ocular melanoma have been found in these patients.[15] *Nevus of Ito* is a unilateral hyperpigmented patch over the deltoid or scapula. The nevus of Ota and nevus of Ito do not involute with time. The pathogenesis of dermal melanocytosis is thought to be caused by a defect in melanocyte migration from the neural crest to the skin.[16]

One to 3 *café au lait macules* (CALMs) are present in 10% to 28% of the general population.[17] More than 3 and particularly more than 6 CALMs nearly always indicate an underlying disorder. Neurofibromatosis type 1 is the most common associated disorder. Large, linear, or segmental CALMs are seen McCune-Albright syndrome. Additional features characteristic for McCune-Albright syndrome are polyostotic fibrous dysplasia and endocrine abnormalities, which unusually exhibit as precocious puberty.

Congenital melanocytic nevi (moles) are classified as small (<1.5 cm diameter), medium (1.5 to 19.9 cm diameter), and large (>20 cm diameter). Although small congenital nevi occur in up to 1% of infants, large congenital nevi are rare, occurring in 1 in 20,000 infants.[18] In addition to the psychosocial aspects associated with having large nevi, complications include neurocutaneous melanosis, limb hypoplasia, and cutaneous melanoma (lifetime risk of 6% to 8% in those with large congenital nevi).[19] Small- and medium-size congenital nevi should be followed with serial examinations and should be removed if they produce clinical changes that cause concern. Partial or complete excision is suggested for large congenital nevi.

Nevoid hypermelanosis is macular hyperpigmentation in a segmental or whorled pattern. This usually presents in the 1st few weeks of life and spreads until the end of the 2nd year. Nevoid hypermelanosis can be an isolated cutaneous condition or part of a genetic disease, which is the result of cutaneous mosaicism.[20]

WHEN TO REFER

- Large congenital nevi
- Small or medium congenital nevus with concerning clinical features (ie, asymmetry, border irregularity, color variegation)

VASCULAR BIRTHMARKS

Vascular birthmarks can be classified as either hemangiomas or vascular malformations.[21] *Hemangiomas* are benign proliferations of vascular endothelium characterized by a predictable growth pattern and a tendency toward spontaneous involution. *Malformations* are permanent structural lesions composed of mature vessels (arterial, venous, capillary, or lymphatic). Malformations generally do not spontaneously involute. Examples of vascular malformations include nevus simplex (salmon patch) and nevus flammeus (port wine stain).

Hemangiomas may be present at birth, but they more commonly become apparent within the first several days to weeks of life (Figure 85-2). They represent the most common tumors of infancy, occurring in 1.1% to 2.6% of newborns[22]; incidence figures at the end of 1 year are 10% to 12% of white infants.[23] Premature infants and girls are more frequently affected.[24] Many hemangiomas are heralded by precursor lesions—well-demarcated macules or papules with telangiectasia, often surrounded by an area of pallor.[25] Fully developed hemangiomas range from soft, bright-red lobulated plaques (*superficial hemangiomas,* formerly known as strawberry hemangiomas)

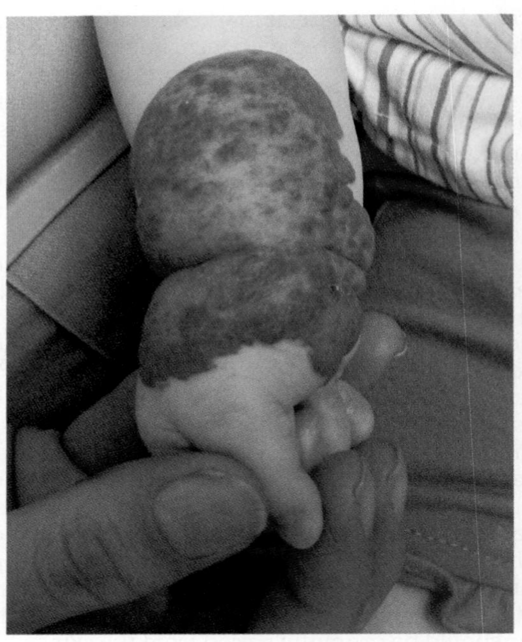

Figure 85-2 Hemangioma of infancy.

to purplish-blue, poorly defined, compressible subcutaneous nodules (*deep hemangiomas,* formerly known as cavernous hemangiomas). *Combined hemangiomas* have both superficial and deep components. A total of 15% to 30% of affected infants have more than 1 hemangioma.[26]

Most hemangiomas undergo a proliferative growth phase, followed by a period of inactivity and a final involutional phase. Superficial hemangiomas typically reach maximal size by 6 to 10 months; deep hemangiomas may continue to enlarge for several additional months. Involution generally begins during the latter part of the 1st year or the early portion of the 2nd year of life.[23] Involuting hemangiomas are characterized by loss of brilliant red color, acquisition of a grayish hue, and loss of volume. Although considerable variation exists in involution, generally, 50% of hemangiomas have completely involuted by age 5; approximately 10% involute each year thereafter such that, by age 9, approximately 90% have undergone complete involution. Approximately 10% to 20% of affected patients will have residual skin changes, most commonly telangiectasias, pallor, or redundant skin.[27]

Management for the majority of hemangiomas is watchful waiting and parental education.[28] Parents should be advised to notify the physician if any of the following occur: sudden, rapid growth; development of a hard, woody texture; prolonged bleeding from the hemangioma; or development of erosions, ulcerations, or crusts. Hemangiomas that may be associated with complications include large hemangiomas of the face or beard area, periorificial hemangiomas, and hemangiomas involving the midline spine. Additionally, infants with multiple hemangiomas may require evaluation to exclude the presence of internal hemangiomatosis (especially hepatic). Magnetic resonance imaging (MRI),

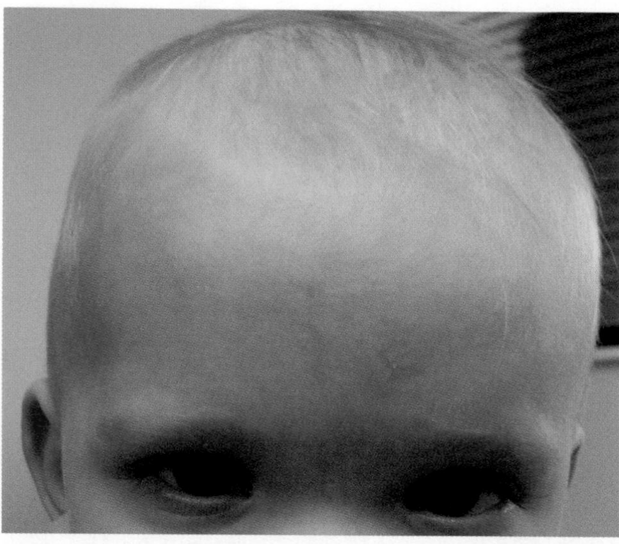

Figure 85-3 Glabellar salmon patch and nevus sebaceous.

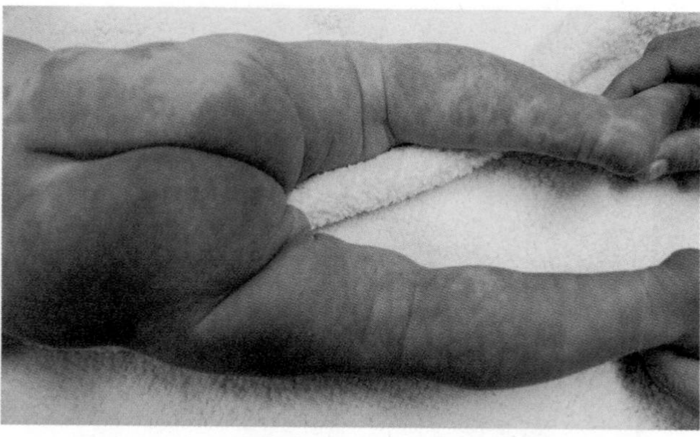

Figure 85-4 Extensive vascular malformation.

therapeutic intervention with systemic corticosteroid therapy, laser treatment, or any combination of these modalities may be necessary in severe cases.

WHEN TO REFER

- Large hemangiomas of the face or beard area
- Periorificial hemangiomas (especially perioral and periocular hemangiomas)
- Lumbosacral hemangiomas
- Ulcerated hemangiomas of the diaper area
- Multiple hemangiomas

VASCULAR MALFORMATIONS

Nevus simplex (salmon patch) is seen in approximately 40% of infants (Figure 85-3). These lesions are pink, blanch completely, have indistinct borders, and usually darken in color with crying, vigorous activity, or changes in ambient temperature. Common locations are the glabella, upper eyelids, and nape of the neck.[29] The lesion is presumed to be composed of ectatic dermal capillaries representing persistent fetal vessels. Virtually all eyelid lesions will involute; a small number of glabellar lesions will persist. Nuchal lesions generally disappear during the 1st or 2nd year, but, not uncommonly, some persist into adulthood. Persistent salmon patches will generally respond to treatment with the pulsed dye laser.

Nevus flammeus (port wine stain) is an uncommon vascular anomaly that occurs in 0.3% of newborns (Figure 85-4).[22] The initial manifestation is a red to purple-red discrete patch with irregular borders, usually unilateral in distribution. If left untreated, nevus flammeus will become purple and nodular in adulthood. It is a permanent mark and has no tendency toward involution. The most common site is the face. Nevus flammeus represents a malformation of mature capillaries of the upper dermis. Although nevus flammeus can occur as an isolated abnormality, some are associated with serious sequelae. Sturge-Weber syndrome is characterized by a nevus flammeus in the trigeminal distribution in association with cerebral calcifications, glaucoma, seizures, and mental retardation. Nevus flammeus of an extremity, venous varicosities, and hypertrophy of soft tissues and bones are seen in the Klippel-Trénaunay syndrome. The triad of findings in Klippel-Trénaunay syndrome plus the presence of an arteriovenous malformation constitutes the Parkes-Weber syndrome. Cobb syndrome is characterized by nevus flammeus in a dermatomal distribution, a vascular malformation of the corresponding segments of the spinal cord, and neurologic manifestations of cord compression. Nevus flammeus, especially facial lesions, generally improve with laser treatment. If the distribution of nevus flammeus and attendant findings suggest one of the aforementioned syndromes, then further evaluation, including MRI and consultation with a neurologist or an ophthalmologist (or both), is necessary for management.[30]

WHEN TO REFER

- Nevus flammeus in a V1 or V2 distribution
- Large nevus flammeus of an extremity or overlying the midline

HAMARTOMAS AND MISCELLANEOUS LESIONS

Hamartomas are benign growths consisting of an excess amount of tissue (eg, smooth muscle, sebaceous glands) normally found in that location. They are not cancerous or hyperproliferative.

Epidermal nevus is a benign epidermal hamartoma that usually exhibits at birth or in early childhood (Figure 85-5). It is usually an isolated, small, hyperpigmented, slightly verrucous lesion, but it can be linear or extensive. Rarely, epidermal nevi may be associated with skeletal, neurologic, cardiovascular, and ocular abnormalities (epidermal nevus syndrome). A biopsy is often performed to exclude the possibility of epidermolytic hyperkeratosis, which is a more severe skin

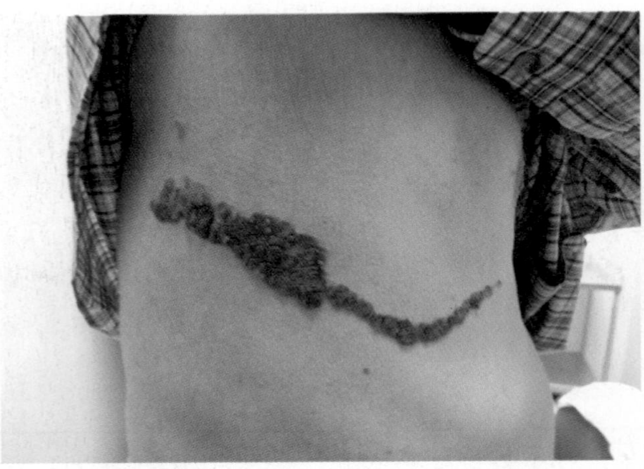

Figure 85-5 Epidermal nevus.

condition that may be passed to offspring of affected patients. In rare instances, malignant proliferation has been reported. Treatment is not necessary, but options for symptomatic or cosmetically disfiguring lesions include destructive measures such as excision, cryotherapy, laser ablation, or electrosurgery.[31]

Nevus sebaceous is a benign sebaceous hamartoma that displays at birth or early childhood. It starts as a flesh-colored to yellow smooth plaque found mostly on the face and scalp. Associated alopecia is a frequent feature of scalp lesions. During and after puberty, the nevus enlarges and becomes more verrucous, corresponding to maturation of sebaceous glands. Benign and malignant neoplasms (including basal cell carcinomas) may develop within these lesions. Prophylactic removal is no longer suggested because the rate of malignant transformation is much lower than previously reported. Close clinical observation is suggested, and any changes that cause concern should prompt biopsy.[32]

Smooth-muscle hamartoma is a congenital skin-colored to hyperpigmented plaque that is present mostly on the trunk and proximal extremities (Figure 85-6). Hypertrichosis is a frequent finding. This lesion is benign; removal is indicated if it is symptomatic or for cosmetic reasons.[33]

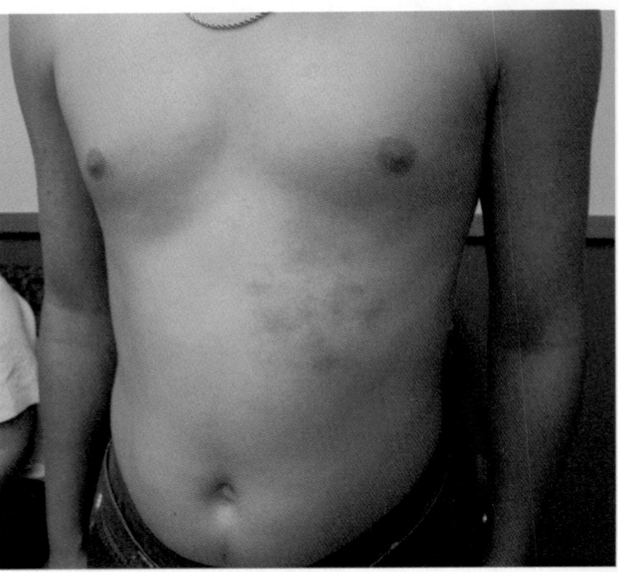

Figure 85-6 Smooth-muscle hamartoma.

DEVELOPMENTAL ANOMALIES

Developmental anomalies result from faulty morphogenesis at some point during embryonic development. These anomalies can affect any organ system, including the skin. Cutaneous defects may be an isolated, incidental finding or associated with other, possibly severe or life-threatening, abnormalities. They are also potential indicators of underlying defects or a manifesting feature of a syndrome.

Branchial cleft cysts present on the preauricular area, mandible, or lateral neck anterior to the sternocleidomastoid muscle during early childhood or adolescence. These cysts result from incomplete resolution of the 2nd and 3rd branchial clefts. Fistula or sinus formation is a common complication and must be delineated with an MRI or computed tomographic scan. These cysts must be differentiated from enlarged lymph nodes and thyroglossal duct cysts (remnants of the thyroglossal duct, which are located on the midline neck and often move with swallowing).[34]

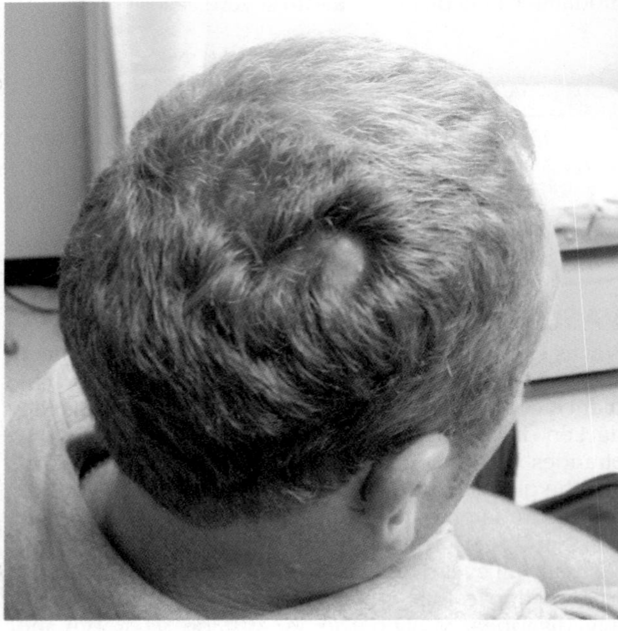

Figure 85-7 Aplasia cutis congenita.

Aplasia cutis congenita is a congenital absence of skin that occurs most commonly on the vertex of the scalp but can be found anywhere (Figure 85-7). The lesion appears as a punched-out ulceration (that heals as a scar) or scar. Within the scar, no hair or appendages are

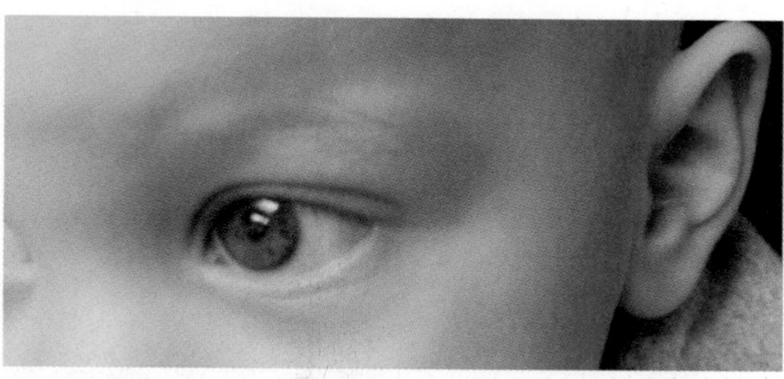

Figure 85-8 Dermoid cyst of lateral eyebrow.

present. The lesion is usually isolated, but multiple areas may be present. The lesion may involve deeper structures (absence of subcutaneous tissue or bony defects) or be associated with other congenital anomalies (neurologic, skeletal, gastrointestinal) or disorders (trisomy 13). Management involves routine wound care and prevention of infection. Once healed, no further care is necessary, but surgical excision is an option for improved cosmesis. For medicolegal reasons, the physician should recognize aplasia cutis congenita as an intrauterine event that is not related to birth trauma, electrode monitors, or forceps delivery.[35]

The skin and the nervous system are both derived from the ectoderm. Therefore any midline lesion along the posterior axial skeleton can potentially indicate an underlying spinal abnormality and a need for further evaluation. Some common cutaneous posterior midline lesions suggestive of an underlying spinal defect include congential nevi, vascular malformations, hemangiomas, hair tufts, lipomas, skin tags, dimples above the gluteal cleft, and subcutaneous nodules. An ultrasound (if within first few months) or MRI is necessary to assess for the presence of underlying spinal disease.[36]

Dermoid cysts result from trapped ectodermal-derived tissue along embryonic fusion planes. These cysts appear as subcutaneous nodules mostly on the nose or around the eyes, especially near lateral eyebrows (Figure 85-8). A small percentage of midline nasal dermoid cysts will have intracranial involvement. Such lesions require imaging before they are excised.[37]

Nasal gliomas represent ectopic neuroectoderm that was sequestered during bony fusion. No intracranial connection is found. Nasal gliomas exhibit as firm, red, telangiectatic dermal nodules located on the nasal root. Less frequently, they can be located intranasally, causing distortion of the nose and obstruction.[38]

Cephalocele is a generic term referring to herniation of any intracranial tissue through a skull defect resulting from faulty closure. Thus all cephaloceles have an intracranial connection. The most common cephaloceles are meningoceles (meninges only) and encephaloceles (meninges and brain). Most cephaloceles occur along the midline of the occiput or vertex. These appear as a soft, bluish, pulsatile nodule and rarely can be confused for deep hemangiomas or vascular malformations. If a cephalocele is clinically suspected, imaging must be done to define the extent of the tumor. Repair, often requiring collaboration between otolaryngology and neurosurgery, is indicated.[39]

Accessory tragi are common anomalies that result from an extra tubercle or remnant of the 1st branchial arch. These anomalies are most often present in the preauricular area, but they can be seen on the cheek and lateral neck. Accessory tragi are usually an isolated defect, but they can be associated with cleft lip or cleft palate or with several syndromes. The infant must be assessed for hearing loss and other dysmorphic features.[40]

Ear pits are a common congenital defect that result from defective embryonic fusion of the tubercles of the first 2 branchial arches. Cyst formation and infection are frequent complications. Rarely, ear pits are associated with hearing loss, renal abnormalities, and several syndromes.[41]

Supernumerary digits (postaxial polydactyly) are soft-tissue duplications that produce a papule or nodule most frequently on the ulnar aspect of the 5th digit. No bone development is present. These are usually isolated anomalies without systemic associations. Supernumerary digits of the hand are a common isolated finding in black children, occurring with a frequency approximately 10 times that of white children and are seen more frequently in boys. Transmission is presumed to be autosomal dominant. In contrast, when seen in white children, supernumerary digits are more commonly found in association with a syndrome and autosomal recessive inheritance. Treatment of supernumerary digits consists of surgical excision.[42]

Accessory nipple results from persistence of nipple or areola, or both, anywhere along the embryonic milk line (anterior axillary fold to medial upper thigh). These lesions are usually asymptomatic and may be single, multiple, unilateral, or bilateral. They are light brown and persist throughout life. Routine examination is essential because individuals with associated breast tissue have a similar risk of malignant transformation as normal breast tissue. No treatment is necessary.[43]

VESICULOPUSTULAR DISEASES OF THE NEWBORN

Erythema toxicum neonatorum is a benign disorder occurring in 20% to 60% of term newborns and 5% of preterm neonates. Characteristically, the eruption begins during the second 24 hours of life; it is rarely present at birth. However, this eruption may begin anytime from birth to 2 weeks of age and typically lasts several days to several weeks.[44] A polymorphous eruption is present, consisting of erythematous macules, papules, pustules, and wheals. Lesions are most commonly found on the face, trunk, proximal arms, and buttocks. The palms and soles are usually not involved. The cause is unknown, although it may represent acute graft-versus-host disease in the transiently immunosuppressed newborn by maternal lymphocytes transferred shortly before or during delivery.[45] The diagnosis is usually based on the clinical appearance of the rash in an otherwise healthy term newborn. In cases in which the diagnosis is in doubt, scrapings of pustules stained with Wright's stain will reveal large numbers of eosinophils. Fifteen percent of cases are accompanied by peripheral eosinophilia.[46] This disorder is self-limited and requires no treatment; parents should be reassured about the benign and noninfectious nature of this condition.

Transient neonatal pustular melanosis is a benign condition occurring in 0.2% to 4% of term babies and is more commonly seen in black newborns.[47] Boys and girls are equally affected. Lesions are present at birth; new lesions do not usually appear after birth. The eruption generally resolves in 24 to 48 hours. Pustules, vesicles, or pigmented macules with or without a surrounding collarette of scale are present. The eruption typically affects the chin, neck, upper back, buttocks, abdomen, thighs, palms, and soles. The cause is unknown. This diagnosis is usually based on the time of onset, clinical appearance, and absence of other findings. Gram stain of pustules demonstrates neutrophils, rare eosinophils, and an absence of bacteria. No treatment is necessary; however, hyperpigmented macules may last for several weeks to months before resolving.

Miliaria are a common finding in neonates and infants. In warm climates, they may be present in up to 15% of newborns.[48] Two types of miliaria commonly occur during the newborn period: (1) *miliaria rubra* (known as *prickly heat*) and (2) *miliaria crystallina,* with the former being more common. Incidence is equal among the sexes and races. Both types of miliaria can occur within the 1st weeks of life and can persist from hours to days. Vesicles, pustules, or papules occur in crops on the face, trunk, and intertriginous areas. Miliaria arise as a result of obstruction within the eccrine duct, followed by rupture of the duct and leakage of eccrine sweat into the skin. Precipitating factors include excessive warming in an incubator, fever, occlusive dressings, or dressing in inappropriately warm clothing. The diagnosis is usually based on lesion location, time of onset, and history of excessive warming. Miliaria usually resolve spontaneously. Providing cool baths and avoiding excessive warming can prevent recurrences.

Eosinophilic pustular folliculitis has been reported in neonates.[49] Recurrent crops of white to yellow pustules occur on the scalp and forehead. Lesions crust within 2 to 3 days of onset and resolve without scarring. The course can be months to years in duration. The cause is unknown. The strong association with HIV seen in adults is not observed in neonates, although associated immunodeficiency has been reported.[50] Multiple eosinophils are present on Giemsa stain of a lesion. Topical corticosteroids, erythromycin, or both have been reported to be effective treatments.[51]

Acropustulosis of infancy is a chronic, recurrent eruption of vesicles and pustules occurring on the hands and feet. The onset is usually hours after birth, but it can occur anytime during the 1st year of life. Lesions last 5 to 10 days; however, crops can appear every 2 to 4 weeks for 2 to 3 years in persistent cases. Erythematous papules rapidly progress to intensely pruritic vesicles or pustules (or both) on the hands, feet, ankles, and wrists, and occasionally on the chest, back, and abdomen. The cause is unknown. An association with scabies is suspected because both have similar clinical presentations.[52] Scabies preparations in acropustulosis will be negative. Gram stain reveals numerous neutrophils and occasional eosinophils. The disease usually spontaneously remits within 1 to 2 years. Symptomatic treatment includes topical corticosteroids and systemic antihistamines. Severe disease may be treated with dapsone, which requires pretreatment screening for glucose-6-phosphate dehydrogenase deficiency and monitoring of complete blood count and chemistry profile during treatment.[52]

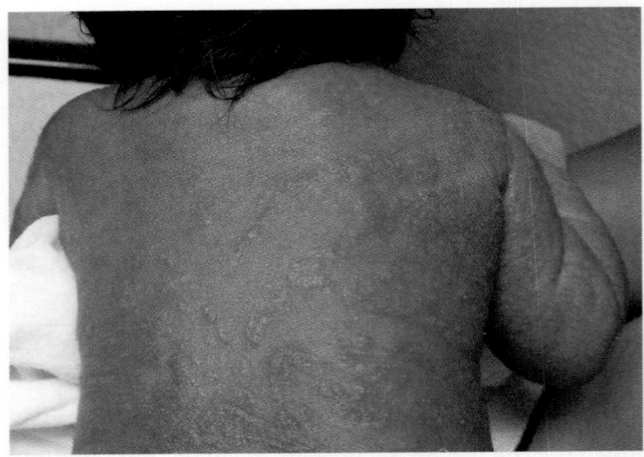

Figure 85-9 Incontinentia pigmenti—vesicular phase.

Neonatal acne occurs in 20% of healthy newborns. Onset is at approximately 2 weeks of age, and lesions generally resolve within 3 months. Small, inflamed papules occur on the nasal bridge and cheeks. Reports have implicated the fungus species *Malassezia furfur* in the pathogenesis of neonatal acneiform eruptions.[53] Given its benign and transient nature, reassuring the parents is generally adequate. If treatment is necessary, then benzoyl peroxide preparations or topical ketoconazole are effective.

Incontinentia pigmenti is an X-linked–dominant genodermatosis. More than 700 cases have been reported; 97% of those affected are girls.[54] The disease has 4 phases: (1) vesicular (Figure 85-9), (2) verrucous, (3) hyperpigmentation (Figure 85-10), and (4) hypopigmentation. In the vesicular phase, lesions are present at birth in 50% of those affected and in 90% of cases by age 2 weeks. Erythematous macules, papules, vesicles, and bullae follow the lines of Blaschko on the extremities, trunk, and scalp. The verrucous phase typically occurs between 2 to 6 weeks. Streaks of hyperkeratotic papules and pustules develop in the aforementioned areas. The 3rd phase, hyperpigmentation, usually develops by 3 to 6 months. Hyperpigmented macules and patches are present along Blaschko lines. The final phase, hypopigmentation, exhibits during the 2nd to 3rd decades of life. Previously hyperpigmented areas develop hypopigmentation with or without follicular atrophy. Additional findings include scarring alopecia, abnormal teeth (anodontia; peg or conical teeth), eye abnormalities (strabismus, cataracts, optic atrophy, retinal vascular changes), dystrophic nail changes, and seizures. These patients typically have a normal life

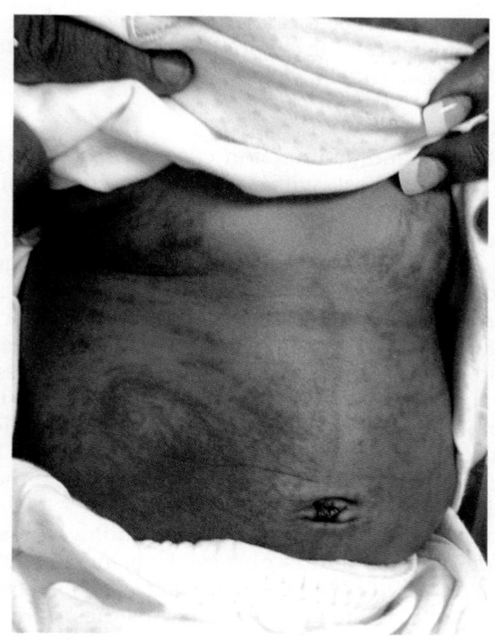

Figure 85-10 Incontinentia pigmenti—hyperpigmented phase.

span. Once diagnosis has been made, a detailed family history and complete skin examination of the mother and of the child's sisters should be performed. Patients should have periodic complete physical examinations, ophthalmologic and neurologic examinations at diagnosis, and a dental examination by 1 year.

INFECTIOUS LESIONS OF THE NEONATE

Skin infections of the neonate can be uncomplicated and benign or complex and life threatening. Most, if not all, of the cutaneous infections are part of a distinct clinical spectrum. Generally, additional clinical clues assist in making a definitive diagnosis. Following are some commonly encountered skin infections that occur either at birth or during the first few weeks of life. This list, although not all inclusive, is a starting point for an investigative workup. A complete blood count and assessment of IgM antibodies, which specifically indicate neonatal infection, are useful initial laboratory evaluations.

Sepsis is a potentially life-threatening diagnosis in the neonate. If a neonate is exhibiting signs of lethargy, irritability, fever, temperature instability, or poor feeding, then a sepsis workup is almost universally indicated. When present, cutaneous lesions of sepsis usually appear as polymorphic lesions, for example, erythematous macules, petechiae, or, less commonly, small nodules or vesicles. The workup includes cultures of blood, cerebrospinal fluid (CSF), and urine. Empiric antibiotics for the most common organisms should be initiated while awaiting culture results.

Bacterial Infections

Neonates may exhibit cutaneous infections commonly encountered in school-aged children. Impetigo is often encountered during the neonatal period. Infection presents as well-demarcated areas of erythema that progress to vesicles, which rapidly rupture or ulcerate, leaving a characteristic honey-colored crust. The most common pathogens are *Staphylococcus aureus* and *Streptococcus pyogenes*. Limited local infection may be treated with topical antibiotics such as mupirocin; more diffuse involvement is treated with mupirocin and an oral antistaphylococcal penicillin or cephalosporin.[55]

Bullous impetigo may occasionally be seen. It is caused by specific strains of toxin-producing *S aureus*. The lesion begins as an erythematous patch and progresses to bulla formation when exfoliative toxins are elaborated locally. This fluid shows gram-positive cocci in clusters. A diffuse eruption of superficial skin exfoliation is seen in staphylococcal scalded-skin syndrome. This form of staphylococcal infection is seen with the elaboration of exfoliative toxins secreted by phage-2 *S aureus* that is hematogenously disseminated. At the examination, the patient is febrile and appears ill. The patient's skin is diffusely tender and erythematous. Superficial vesicles or, more likely, bulla soon develop and quickly rupture. Application of pressure to the edge of intact skin will often result in separation of the epidermis from underlying skin layers (positive Nikolsky sign). Gram stain of this fluid will yield a sterile sample. Patients with scalded-skin syndrome can be treated with systemic antistaphylococcal antibiotics.

Syphilis

With the advent of strict perinatal surveillance, the incidence of congenital syphilis has dramatically decreased. Occasionally, mothers without prenatal care can deliver a child with congenital syphilis. In early congenital syphilis, the neonate will exhibit symptoms similar to those of a patient with secondary syphilis. A generalized papulosquamous eruption can be found, including on the palms and soles. Additional features include rhinitis, hepatosplenomegaly, lymphadenopathy, fever, pseudoparalysis, and CSF abnormalities. Evaluation of patients with congenital syphilis includes serologic studies, CSF VDRL (Venereal Disease Research Laboratory) test, and complete blood count with platelet count. The treatment of choice is intravenous penicillin G.[56]

Viral Infections

Neonatal herpes simplex virus (HSV) infection can range from a mild, self-limited disease to one with potentially devastating neurologic consequences and even death. Most neonatal HSV infections are due to HSV-2 from the primary infection of the mother who at the time of delivery has no evidence of genital herpes-like lesions. Reactivation of the virus has very low rates of transmission to the infant. Neonatal HSV infection can exhibit in several forms. First, and potentially the most deadly, is viral encephalitis. During a sepsis workup, HSV polymerase chain reaction is usually performed on CSF obtained by lumbar puncture (LP) to rule out this diagnosis. Because children generally tolerate intravenous acyclovir well, this drug should be provided after the LP while awaiting the results of viral polymerase chain reaction. Second, neonatal HSV can produce classic skin lesions of grouped vesicles on an erythematous base seen anywhere on the body that may have been exposed to HSV during delivery. Tzanck preparations will show multinucleated cells if HSV is present. Finally, and least commonly seen, is disseminated infection, the symptoms of which often overlap those described previously. The physician must think of HSV infection as a clinical spectrum. Although neonatal cutaneous HSV is possible, it is rarely seen without other organ involvement. LP should be performed in any patient suspected of having neonatal HSV because of the possibility of central nervous system involvement. Intravenous acyclovir therapy should be initiated empirically while awaiting culture results.[57]

Maternal infection with varicella zoster virus during the first 20 weeks of gestation can result in congenital varicella syndrome. Affected infants can exhibit ophthalmologic complications, neurologic defects, limb hypoplasia, and genitourinary and gastrointestinal defects. Characteristic cutaneous findings are vesicles or scarring in a dermatomal distribution. Maternal varicella with onset during the last few weeks of pregnancy or during the early postpartum period can result in neonatal varicella. Affected infants have an eruption consisting of disseminated papules, vesicles *(dewdrop on a rose petal),* and erosions. Diagnosis can be made by Tzanck preparation, viral culture, or direct immunofluorescence assay. Infants are more likely to have severe disseminated disease with systemic complications if maternal onset of varicella is within 5 days of delivery to 2 days after or if the newborn exhibits the disease between 5 to 10 days of life. Neonatal varicella is treated with intravenous acyclovir.[58]

Congenital rubella syndrome (CRS) occurs in infants of mothers exposed to rubella during the 1st portion (generally the first 16 weeks) of pregnancy. Increased risk of the CRS is associated with earlier gestational exposure. The incidence of CRS has greatly declined as a result of widespread rubella vaccination; however, occasional outbreaks continue to be reported in populations with low vaccination rates. CRS is characterized by the triad of congenital cataracts, deafness, and cardiac defects (most commonly patent ductus arteriosus). Additional features include intrauterine growth restriction, various central nervous system manifestations, jaundice, hepatosplenomegaly, thrombocytopenia, and radiolucent metaphyseal bone lesions. The characteristic cutaneous finding is a diffuse eruption of blue-red papules and nodules (so-called *blueberry muffin lesions*). These lesions generally appear at birth or appear in the first 24 hours of life. Blueberry muffin lesions are not unique to CRS and can be seen in several additional congenital infections (toxoplasmosis, cytomegalovirus, parvovirus B19), erythroblastic fetalis, and neoplastic disorders (congenital leukemia, histiocytosis). Additional nonspecific cutaneous features of CRS include nonspecific generalized maculopapular eruption, hyperpigmentation, and recurrent urticaria. The diagnosis of CRS should be suspected in infants with the appropriate constellation of findings. Confirmation is made by isolation of rubella virus from sputum, urine, CSF, or tissue, or by findings of increased titers of IgM antibodies to rubella. Treatment is supportive. A high percentage of infants with CRS will experience significant neurologic and auditory complications. Prevention is through immunization with a live rubella virus vaccine.[59]

Yeast

Congenital *Candida* infection can be present at birth, or it can manifest within the first 6 days of life. Affected neonates typically have widespread eruption of macules, papules, and pustules with relative sparing of the diaper area. Thrush is uncommon in congenital candidiasis. Pustules of the palms and soles are a helpful diagnostic sign. Changes in the fingernails, including yellow discoloration and paronychia, are occasionally present. Diagnosis is made by potassium-hydroxide test or culture. The course tends to be benign in healthy neonates, but it may be complicated by systemic involvement in preterm neonates. Treatment for skin-limited disease in otherwise healthy neonates is with topical antifungal agents.[60]

Neonatal candidiasis is most commonly caused by *Candida albicans* and is observed during the 1st and 2nd week of life. Infection should be suspected in patients with white hypertrophic plaques within the oral cavity. Another common presentation is a localized perianal eruption consisting of erythematous macules and papules that becomes confluent. This eruption is often beefy red in color and characterized by the presence of satellite lesions (papules, pustules, or vesicles). The diagnosis can be made by potassium-hydroxide test and observing the characteristic pseudohyphae. Treatment of localized disease is with topical antifungal preparations.[61]

Systemic candidiasis is typically seen in low–birth-weight infants between the 2nd and 6th weeks of life. Features include temperature instability, lethargy, hypotension, and hyperglycemia. Cutaneous involvement may or may not occur. Diagnosis is confirmed by cultures of blood, urine, and CSF. High morbidity and mortality rates are seen in patients with this condition. Treatment is with amphotericin B.[62]

TOOLS FOR PRACTICE

Medical Decision Support

- *Dermatology: Skin Essentials* (on-line course), American Academy of Pediatrics (www.pedialink.org).
- *Pediatric Dermatology: A Quick Reference Guide* (book), American Academy of Pediatrics (www.aap.org/bookstore).
- *Red Book: 2006 Report of the Committee on Infectious Diseases,* 27th edition (book), American Academy of Pediatrics (www.aap.org/bookstore).

RELATED WEB SITES

- American Academy of Dermatology (AAD) (www.aad.org).
- Society for Pediatric Dermatology (SPD) (www.pedsderm.net/index.htm).

REFERENCES

1. Schwayer T, Akland T. Neonatal skin barrier: structure, function, and disorders. *Dermatol Ther.* 2005;18:87-103.
2. Darmstadt GL, Dinulos JG. Neonatal skin care. *Pediatr Clin North Am.* 2000;47:757-782.

3. Larson E. Skin hygiene and infection prevention: more of the same or different approaches. *Clin Infect Dis.* 1999; 29:1287-1294.
4. Malathi I, Millar AR, Lemming JP, et al. Skin disinfection in preterm infants. *Arch Dis Child.* 1993;69:312-316.
5. Lacour J. Cord care: results of a survey from South France and recommendations. *Eur J Pediatr Dermatol.* 1998;8:233-234.
6. Conner JM, Soll RF, Edwards GH. Topical ointment for preventing infection in preterm infants. *Cochrane Database Syst Rev.* 2004;1:CD001150.
7. Ortonne JP, Mosher DB, Fitzpatrick TB. Vitiligo and other hypomelanoses of hair and skin. In: Ortonne JP, Moser DB, Fitzpatrick TB, eds. *Genetic and Congenital Disorders.* New York, NY: Plenum, 1983.
8. Ruiz-Maldonado R, Touissant S, Tamayo L, et al. Hypomelanosis of Ito: diagnostic criteria and report of 41 cases. *Pediatr Dermatol.* 1992;9:1-10.
9. Thomas IT, Frias JL, Cantu ES, et al. Association of pigmentary anomalies with chromosomal and genetic mosaicism and chimerism. *Am J Hum Genet.* 1989;45:193-205.
10. Harris-Stith R, Elston DM. Tuberous sclerosis. *Cutis.* 2002;69;103-109.
11. Ward KA, Moss C, Sanders DS. Human piebaldism: relationship between phenotype and site of kit gene mutation. *Br J Dermatol.* 1995;132:929-935.
12. Spritz RA. Molecular basis of human piebaldism. *J Invest Dermatol.* 1994;103:137S-140S.
13. Cordova A. The mongolian spot. *Clin Pediatr.* 1981; 20:714.
14. Teekhasaenee C, Ritch R, Rutnin U, et al. Glaucoma in oculodermal melanocytosis. *Ophthalmology.* 1990;97: 562-570.
15. Shaffer C, Walker K, Weiss GR. Malignant melanoma in a Hispanic male with nevus of Ota. *Dermatology.* 1992;1:146.
16. Smalek JE. The significance of Mongolian spots. *J Pediatr.* 1980;97:504.
17. McLean DL, Gallagher RP. "Sunburn" freckles, café-au-lait macules and other pigmented lesions of school children: the Vancouver mole study. *J Am Acad Dermatol.* 1995;32:565-570.
18. Makkar HS, Frieden IJ. Congenital melanocytic nevi: an update for the pediatrician. *Curr Opin Pediatr.* 2002;14: 397-403.
19. Gari LM, Rivers JK, Kopf AW. Melanomas arising in large congenital nevi: a prospective study. *Pediatr Dermatol.* 1988;5:151-158.
20. Simones GA. Speckled zosteriform lentiginous nevus. *J Am Acad Dermatol.* 1981;4:236.
21. Mullikin JB, Glowacki J. Hemangiomas and vascular malformations in infants and children: a classification based on endothelial characteristics. *Plast Reconstr Surg.* 1982; 69:412-422.
22. Jacobs AH, Walton RG. The incidence of birthmarks in the neonate. *Pediatrics.* 1976;67:302-305.
23. Jacobs AH. Strawberry hemangioma: natural history of the untreated lesion. *Calif Med.* 1957:83:8-10.
24. Margilth AM, Museles M. Current concepts in diagnosis and management of congenital cutaneous hemangiomas. *Pediatrics.* 1965;36:410-416.
25. Hidano A, Nakajima S. Earliest features of the strawberry mark in the newborn. *Br J Dermatol.* 1972;83: 138-144.
26. Nakayama H. Clinical and histologic studies of the classification and the natural history of the strawberry hemangioma. *J Dermatol.* 1981;8:277-291.
27. Bowers RE, Graham EA, Tomlinson KM. The natural history of the strawberry nevus. *Arch Dermatol.* 1960; 82:667-680.
28. Frieden IJ. Which hemangiomas to treat—and how? *Arch Dermatol.*1997;133:1593-1595.
29. Leung AK, Telmesani AM. Salmon patches in Caucasian children. *Pediatr Dermatol.* 1989;6:185-187.
30. Esterly NB. Cutaneous hemangiomas, vascular stains and malformations, and associated syndromes. *Curr Probl Dermatol.* 1995;7;65-108.
31. Rogers M, McCrossin I, Commens C. Epidermal nevi and the epidermal nevus syndrome: a review of 131 cases. *J Am Acad Dermatol.* 1989;20:476-488.
32. Cribier B, Scrivener Y, Grosshans E. Tumors arising in nevus sebaceous: a study of 596 cases. *J Am Acad Dermatol.* 2000;42:263.
33. Gagné EJ, Su WP. Congenital smooth muscle hamartoma of the skin. *Pediatr Dermatol.* 1993;10:142.
34. Ford GR, Balakrishnan A, Evans JN, et al. Branchial cleft and pouch anomalies. *J Laryngol Otol.* 1992;106:137-143.
35. Frieden IJ. Aplasia cutis congenita: a clinical review and proposal for classification. *J Am Acad Dermatol.* 1986; 14:646-660.
36. Drolet B. Birthmarks to worry about: cutaneous markers of dysraphism. *Dermatol Clin.* 1998;16:447-453.
37. Paller AS, Pensler J, Tomita T. Nasal midline masses in infants and children. Dermoids, encephaloceles, and nasal gliomas. *Arch Dermatol.* 1991;127;362-366.
38. Karma P, Rasanen O, Karja J. Nasal gliomas: a review and report of two cases. *Laryngoscope.* 1977;87:1169-1179.
39. Kennard CD, Rasmussen JE. Congenital midline nasal masses: diagnosis and management. *J Dermatol Surg Oncol.* 1990;16:1025.
40. Kugelman A, Tubi A, Bader D, et al. Pre-auricular tags and pits in the newborn: the role of renal ultrasonography. *J Pediatr.* 2002;141:388-391.
41. Drolet BA, Baselga E, Gosain AK, et al. Preauricular skin defects: a consequence of a persistent ectodermal groove. *Arch Dermatol.* 1997;133:1551-1554.
42. Freiden IJ, Chang MW, Lee I. Suture ligation of supernumerary digits and "tags": an outmoded practice? *Arch Pediatr Adolescent Med.* 1995;149:1284.
43. Gross NA. Supernumerary breast tissue: historical perspectives and clinical features. *South Med J.* 2000;93: 29-32.
44. Berg, FJ, Solomon LM. Erythema neonatorum toxicum. *Arch Dis Child.* 1987;62:327-328.
45. Bassukas ID. Is erythema toxicum neonatorum a mild self-limited acute cutaneous graft-versus-host reaction from maternal-to-fetal lymphocyte transfer? *Med Hypoth.* 1992;38:334.
46. Luders D. Histologic observations in erythema toxicum neonatorum. *Pediatrics.* 1960;26:219-224.
47. Ramamurthy RS, Reveri M, Esterly NB, et al. Transient neonatal pustular melanosis. *J Pediatr.* 1976;88:831-835.
48. Nanda A, Kaur S, Bhakoo ON, et al. Survey of cutaneous lesions in Indian newborns. *Pediatr Dermatol.* 1989;6; 39-42.
49. Lucky AW, Esterly NB, Heskel N, et al. Eosinophilic pustular folliculitis in infancy. *Pediatr Dermatol.* 1984;1: 202-206.
50. Rybojad M, Guibai F, Vignon-Pennamen MD, et al. Eosinophilic pustulosis in an infant accompanied by immune deficit. *Ann Dermatol Venerol.* 1999;126:29-31.
51. Duarte AM, Kramer J, Yusk JW, et al. Eosinophilic pustular folliculitis in infancy and childhood. *Am J Dis Child.* 1993;147:197-200.
52. Khan G, Rywlin AM. Acropustulosis of infancy. *Arch Dermatol.* 1979;115:831-833.
53. Rapelanoro R, Mortureux P, Couproe B, et al. Neonatal Malassezia furfur pustulosis. *Arch Dermatol.* 1996;132: 190-193.
54. Dufken A, Vollmer B, Kendziorra H, et al. Hydrops fetalis in three male fetuses of a female with incontinentia pigmenti. *Prenat Diagn.* 2001;21:1019-1021.

55. Darmstadt GL. Impetigo: an overview. *Pediatr Dermatol.* 1994;11:293-303.
56. Ikeda MK Jensen H. Evaluation and treatment of congenital syphilis. *J Pediatr.* 1990;117:843-852.
57. Jacobs RF. Neonatal herpes simplex infections. *Semin Perinatol.* 1998;22:64-71.
58. Enright AM, Prober OG. Neonatal herpes infection: diagnosis, treatment and prevention. *Semin Neonatol.* 2202; 7:283-291.
59. Murph JR. Rubella and syphilis: continuing cases of congenital infection in the 1990s. *Semin Pediatr Neurol.* 1994; 1:26-35.
60. Darmstadt GL. Dinulos JG, Miller Z. Congenital cutaneous candidiasis: clinical presentation, pathogenesis, and management guidelines. *Pediatrics.* 2000;105:438-444.
61. Chapman RL. Candida infections in the neonate. *Curr Opin Pediatr.* 2003;15:97-102.
62. Rao S, Ali U. Systemic fungal infections in neonates. *J Postgrad Med.* 2005;51:S27-S29.

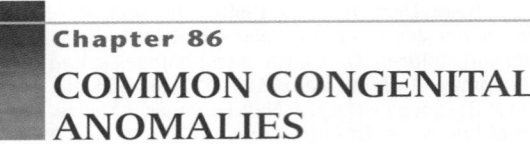

Chapter 86
COMMON CONGENITAL ANOMALIES

Orna Rosen, MD; Robert W. Marion, MD

The diagnosis of an anatomic abnormality in an infant at or around the time of delivery can be devastating for a family. From the time that a concern is raised the parents, who have been anticipating the birth of a normal, healthy newborn, must contend with a series of uncertainties. They must comprehend the meaning of their child's diagnosis, and adjust to the reality that their infant or their prospects for parenthood may be different from what they expected. Individual families handle this crisis in differing ways. The infant's primary care physician may need to assume different roles to assist and support the family.

Congenital anomalies, defined as abnormalities in form or function, occur in 2% to 4% of all infants born in the United States and are the leading cause of neonatal mortality and long-term chronic illness.[1,2]

Once a diagnosis has been made, identifying a cause for the malformation is essential for three reasons: (1) to guide the work-up in an attempt to identify associated hidden anomalies, (2) to provide anticipatory guidance for the family to aid in the decision-making process, and (3) to permit appropriate genetic counseling regarding the risk of a similar anomaly occurring in future pregnancies. In nearly 50% of cases, no clear cause can be found for the anomaly. In the other half the anomaly is caused by: (1) genetic causes, consisting of both single gene mutations and chromosomal anomalies (Table 86-1), accounting for approximately 15% of cases; (2) environmental factors (teratogens), such as drugs and infectious agents, accounting for approximately 8%; (3) multifactorially inherited conditions, anomalies caused by an interplay between genetic and environmental factors, accounting for approximately 25% of anomalies.

DEFINITIONS

Birth anomalies can be classified as malformations, deformations, or disruptions. *Malformations,* localized

Table 86-1 Common Genetic Disorders

DISORDER	MANIFESTATION	FREQUENCY PER 10,000 BIRTHS
CHROMOSOMAL		
Trisomy 21	Congenital heart disease, Brushfield spots, short hands, clinodactyly, simian crease, hypotonia, dysmorphic facies	16
Trisomy 18	Congenital heart disease, small for gestational age (SGA), clenched fist, rocker-bottom foot, dysmorphic facies	3
Trisomy 13	Congenital heart disease, small for gestational age, polydactyly, holoprosencephaly, dysmorphic facies	2
XO (Turner syndrome)	Congenital peripheral edema, webbed neck, short stature, primary amenorrhea	3
XXY (Klinefelter syndrome)	Behavior problems, small testes, infertility, clinodactyly	5
AUTOSOMAL RECESSIVE		
Sickle cell disease	Anemia, infection	20 (black)
Beta-thalassemia	Anemia	20 (Mediterranean)
Cystic fibrosis	Failure to thrive, malabsorption, cough, recurrent pneumonia	5 (white)
AUTOSOMAL DOMINANT		
Familial hypercholesterolemia	Family history of early coronary artery disease	20
Neurofibromatosis	Café-au-lait spots	3
X-LINKED RECESSIVE		
Fragile X	Mental retardation, large testes, dysmorphic facies	5
Duchenne muscular dystrophy	Muscle weakness, pseudohypertrophy of calf	1

errors in the morphogenesis of an organ that results in abnormal form or function, the damage that has occurred to the primordial tissue during the first trimester of pregnancy.[3] Malformations can be further classified as *minor* or *major*. Minor malformations, which occur in 1 of 10 newborns, are not associated with severe malfunction. They usually represent a cosmetic concern but not a functional one. In contrast, major malformations are far less common, and cause severe functional consequences.

An *association* occurs when two or more malformations occur together more often than would be expected by chance. Associations are not typically caused by a specific defect. VACTERL is an example of an association in which vertebral, anal, cardiac, renal, and limb anomalies combine with tracheoesophageal fistula.[1,3]

A congenital structural abnormality or variation that occurs as a result of external physical forces will lead to a *deformation*. Oligohydramnios, uterine fibroids, and a multifetal pregnancy may each contribute to uterine compression that can result in clubfoot. A *disruption* is a congenital abnormality that occurs because of a destructive event or process that leads to incomplete or abnormal fetal development. Disruption of blood flow to a portion of the brain may result in porencephaly, whereas rupture of the amniotic sac produces tissue strands that entangle limbs, digits, or other fetal parts, leading to amputation of the affected fetal part and amniotic band syndrome. Malformations can occur alone or with other malformations (see Chapter 178, Facial Dysmorphism). They can be a part of a *malformation sequence*, such as the Pierre Robin malformation sequence, occur as part of a multiple malformation syndrome, in which all the anomalies can be traced to a single identifiable cause (eg, an extra copy of chromosome 18 in trisomy 18, a mutation in a single copy of the *FBN1* in Marfan syndrome, exposure to alcohol in fetal alcohol syndrome).

APPROACH TO THE NEONATE WITH CONGENITAL ANOMALIES

Identifying a congenital malformation in a newborn should begin a well-defined process of evaluation and information gathering. The physician should review the pregnancy and family history with the neonate's parents, perform a thorough physical examination, and order appropriate tests that will provide the information necessary to arrive at the decisions vital to the child's future.

Appropriate care, including resuscitation, should be initiated in the delivery room after the birth of a baby with congenital anomalies. The decision to withdraw treatment should be deferred until a full diagnostic evaluation has been completed and a diagnosis has been made, unless resuscitative efforts prove unsuccessful. Under certain circumstances an advanced care plan may be developed based on a confirmed prenatal diagnosis of a condition not compatible with survival and a family's decision made in consultation with their obstetric and pediatric care physician for their newborn to receive only comfort care.[4,5] The parents must be involved from the beginning and they must have a major role in the decision-making process.

Care of the Newborn With a Condition Not Compatible With Life

When a newborn is found to have an anomaly or syndrome that, in the judgment of the physicians, is incompatible with life, some parents may have a difficult time accepting these facts and may resist the medical staff's counsel to withdraw life support or to consent to a *do not resuscitate* order. Parents may have difficulty agreeing to these types of recommendations for many reasons: some parents will be in denial about the child's condition, a normal part of the acceptance and grieving processes; others may object to withdrawal of care because of religious beliefs or personal values; still others may believe that, if given enough time, a miracle might occur or a new treatment might be developed that will save the infant's life. In such cases, to prevent the relationship between staff and family from becoming contentious, the medical staff must be as supportive of the family as possible. The care-giving team should maintain patience, empathy, and respect for the parents, their values, and preferences.

In all instances, particularly when disagreement exists between the medical team's management plan and the parents' wishes, lines of communication must be kept open. Daily meetings among the parents, their representatives (including members of the clergy), and the medical staff should be arranged; during these meetings, information about the child's condition should be discussed in detail and care options presented. The neonatal intensive care unit's social worker or hospital liaison psychologist should attend these meetings as a mediator or ombudsman. Parents may feel more comfortable discussing their feelings with a social worker or nurse than with the physician.

Under some circumstances, if no consensus can be reached, then the family may have to engage the hospital's bioethics consultation team for mediation purposes or to provide an outside assessment of the information regarding the newborn's prognosis and appropriate treatment options, including the termination of therapy. Given adequate time, however, when the situation is handled with empathy, caring, and respect, the majority of disagreements between parents and health care providers can be resolved without the intervention of a bioethics consultation committee or the involvement of the courts. In many instances, time, information, and support are the important elements that allow parents to come to terms with their child's diagnosis, with the lack of corrective or palliative treatments, and to weigh the option of continuing care without the benefit of improvement versus discontinuing treatment care except for comfort care and allowing their infant to die. If the child's death is not imminent, then the parents may choose to take their newborn home to die or consider transfer to a chronic-care hospital capable of providing hospice care. Engaging a family in a community- or hospital-based perinatal hospice program is another option. Although perinatal hospice is relatively new in the field of hospice care, the increasing frequency of prenatal diagnosis has created a need for this support for the family of the dying infant. (See Chapter 79, Support for Families Whose Infant Is Sick or Dying: Collaborative Decision Making; and Chapter 80, Perinatal Bereavement.)

Role of the Medical Geneticist and Genetic Counseling

The genetic counseling team plays an important role in the diagnosis and management of a newborn with congenital anomalies. By assisting in establishing the diagnosis and providing counseling to the family, the geneticist and genetic counselor provide an important component of care. During the process of genetic counseling the genetic counseling team supports the family, helping the parents and other family members cope with the issues that confront them. The team serves as advocates for the patient, helping the parents process medical information and treatment options and assisting as needed with decision making.[6,7] The genetic counseling team becomes an ongoing source of assistance to the child and family by providing information in written and oral forms, making referrals to family support groups, and offering assistance with care coordination, financial aid and social service needs.

DIAGNOSIS

To reach a conclusive diagnosis in a newborn with congenital anomalies, three major aspects should be pursued: (1) the medical history, (2) the physical examination, and (3) the appropriate laboratory tests.

Medical History

A comprehensive history is an essential part of the evaluation of the baby with congenital malformations. Three elements that should be included in the history are (1) the pregnancy history and prenatal course, (2) the family history, and (3) the delivery process.

Questions about the pregnancy should assess several areas (Box 86-1). First, how was the infant conceived? Evidence is growing that conditions caused by defects in gene imprinting, such as Beckwith-Wiedemann syndrome, occur more often in newborns conceived via in vitro fertilization.[8-11]

Information about the nature of fetal movements can provide clues to the functioning of the newborn's central nervous system. Decreased fetal movements or delayed quickening suggests a neuromuscular disease, whereas a mother's report that her fetus had recurrent hiccups during the second or third trimester suggests possible intrauterine seizure activity. Oligohydramnios is suggestive of anomalies of the urinary tract, such as renal agenesis and obstructive uropathy, whereas polyhydramnios may point to an obstruction in the gastrointestinal tract, such as duodenal atresia or a disorder of the central nervous system that prevents normal fetal swallowing. The possibility of fetal exposure to a teratogenic substance should also be reviewed. Intrauterine exposure to alcohol raises concern about fetal alcohol syndrome, whereas exposure to drugs such as sodium valproate, carbimazole, vitamin A analogues, warfarin, and fluconazole is associated with specific malformation syndromes.[8] Similarly, maternal infection with toxoplasmosis, rubella, cytomegalovirus, or varicella is responsible for well-defined patterns of malformations. Finally, chronic illnesses in the mother, such as poorly controlled diabetes mellitus and untreated phenylketonuria can cause multisystem abnormalities in the fetus.[1,2]

Results of prenatal testing can be helpful in determining the cause of a newborn's malformations. Prenatal karyotypes should be confirmed with a postnatal blood test from the baby. Antenatal alpha-fetoprotein levels that are too high or too low can direct the care provider toward a specific diagnosis. An alpha-fetoprotein level that is high raises a concern about a neural tube defect or gastrointestinal obstruction. If too low, then suspicion of a trisomy is raised. Ultrasound

BOX 86-1 Areas to Cover in Taking a History

ISSUES ABOUT THE PREGNANCY

1. Conception: Natural or assisted? If assisted, then what method was used to achieve this pregnancy? Were fertility issues raised related to maternal factors, paternal factors, or both?
2. Fetal movements: When did quickening occur? Were movements similar to, greater than, or less than those felt during previous pregnancies?
3. Amniotic fluid: Amount (polyhydramnios vs oligohydramnios)—color, fluid leakage
4. Exposure: To teratogenic agents or maternal illnesses (diabetes, infection), maternal drugs or chemical use (street and prescription drugs), and environmental exposure (work or community exposures, radiation, hyperthermia)
5. Prenatal testing: Biochemical screening (*quad screen*—alpha-fetoprotein, human chorionic gonadotropin, estriol, and inhibin-A), ultrasonography, amniocentesis, chorionic villus sampling
6. Other: Parity, maternal weight gain, evidence of maternal uterine pathology (bicornuate uterus, fibroids, etc), bleeding
7. Fetal growth: Appropriateness of growth, discrepancy in growth parameters—symmetric or asymmetric growth restriction, macrosomia or appropriate growth for gestational age

ISSUES ABOUT THE FAMILY

1. Complete pedigree
2. Presence of similar or dissimilar anomalies in first- and second-degree relatives
3. History of pregnancy losses: Spontaneous abortions, stillbirths, and neonatal demise in first- and second-degree relatives
4. Consanguinity in the parents

ISSUES ABOUT THE DELIVERY

1. Length of gestation
2. Type of delivery: If by cesarean section, then what was the indication?
3. Fetal presentation: Vertex, breech, or transverse lie?
4. Presence of placental or umbilical cord abnormality

Source: Marion RW, Fleischman AR. The Assessment and management of neonate with congenital anomalies. In: Evans M, ed. *Reproductive Risks and Prenatal Diagnosis*. Norwalk, CT: Appleton and Lange; 1991. Reprinted by permission of The McGraw-Hill Companies, Inc.

scans revealing shortening of long bones suggest a possible skeletal dysplasia. The presence of polyhydramnios and an ultrasound scan that shows a *double bubble* in the bowel suggest the diagnosis of duodenal atresia.

In gathering information about the family history, a pedigree consisting of at least three generations should be constructed (see Box 86-1 for questions to ask in taking the history). Detailed information about any malformations in family members should be obtained; any health problems, instances of mental retardation, or known conditions should be noted. A history of stillborn infants and spontaneous abortions suggests the presence of a balanced translocation in one of the parents, and should cause the clinician to suspect that the newborn may have an unbalanced chromosome rearrangement. Siblings with similar features may suggest that the disorder is genetic or a consequence of a teratogen. The physician should consider an inherited autosomal-recessive condition if parental consanguinity exists. Ethnic background, as well as country and city of origin, may suggest a specific genetic disorder that is more common in the specific population or gene pool. Medical records of parents, siblings, or other family members should be reviewed to corroborate any significant positive findings elicited through the history.[1,2,7,8,12]

Finally, information about the perinatal period should be obtained. How long did the gestation last? Did the mother consume any medications, vitamins, or herbal or over-the-counter products before and during her pregnancy? Did the mother smoke, drink, or use any illicit drugs. Was the mother exposed to any environmental toxins (chemicals, vapors or fumes, heavy metals or mercury, radiation)? Did the mother have any illnesses or chronic medical conditions? Did the mother have fever? Did any prenatal tests indicate a possible problem? How was the infant delivered? If delivery was via caesarean section, then what was the reason? What complications occurred during the delivery? What were the Apgar scores? Was resuscitation of the newborn needed? Was the placenta normal? Birth weight is particularly important, given that infants with chromosome anomalies, such as trisomy 18, and teratogenic syndromes, such as fetal alcohol syndrome, are typically small for gestational age, whereas babies with multifactorial disorders, such as cleft palate or meningomyelocele, or single gene mutations, such as Marfan syndrome, usually have normal birth weight, and infants born to diabetic mothers, as well as those with rare overgrowth syndromes, such as Beckwith-Wiedemann syndrome, are typically large for gestational age.[13]

Physical Examination

A detailed, systematic physical examination should be performed. The newborn's weight, height, and head circumference should be recorded and plotted on an appropriate growth curve. Measurements that are not part of the standard newborn physical examination should be included in the evaluation of the neonate with congenital anomalies. These measurements include interpupillary distance and interpalpebral distance, length of philtrum, and ear size and position.[7] Each part of the limbs should be measured.[14,15] In the newborn period the upper body/lower body ratio is approximately 1.7:1. If this ratio is too high, then the extremities are short; if the ratio is too small, then either the limbs are long or the trunk is too short. During the physical examination, when the upper extremities are in extension and adducted against the body, the tip of the fingers should reach approximately mid thigh. If the fingertips only reach the hip joint, then the limbs are too short. Comparison of limb length and the ratio of upper body to lower body segment body with standard measurements for a newborn may lead to a diagnosis of skeletal dysplasia.[14]

Features that are important in diagnosing the newborn with major congenital malformations are reviewed in the following sections.

Skull

Evaluation of the skull in the immediate newborn period may be difficult because the journey through the birth canal may produce a molded or misshapened skull. In most cases the skull will revert to its more normal shape within 48 hours.

Craniosynostosis is the premature closure of one or more sutures of the skull. The newborn with craniosynostosis will have an unusual skull shape that does not resolve during the first few days of life. The shape of the skull depends on the suture or sutures that have fused: scaphocephaly or dolicocephaly, a long, *boat-shaped* head, results from closure of the sagittal suture; brachycephaly, a short, broad skull, results from coronal suture closure; plagiocephaly, a rhomboid-shaped skull, results from premature closure of either a single lambdoidal or coronal suture (see Chapter 311, Plagiocephaly); Kleeblattschädel or cloverleaf skull occurs when multiple sutures fuse early during gestation. Craniosynostosis can be an isolated finding in an otherwise-normal infant, can arise because of an underlying metabolic or endocrinologic disorder, such as hyperthyroidism, or can be part of a multiple malformation syndrome, such as Crouzon, Apert, or Pfeiffer syndromes.[1,13,15]

An unusual skull shape is not always associated with premature closure of sutures. Brachycephaly is a feature of Down syndrome; scaphocephaly or dolicocephaly can be seen in neonatal Marfan syndrome.[13] Other malformations of the skull or scalp can provide important clues to the diagnosis. For instance, newborns with trisomy 13 frequently have aplasia cutis congenita, a punched-out–appearing scalp defect usually seen in the occipital region. The presence of such a lesion in a child with polydactyly and other malformations is virtually pathognomonic for this lethal chromosomal disorder.

Face

A detailed discussion of facial dysmorphism is found in Chapter 178, Facial Dysmorphism. The approach to evaluating infants with minor (common) facial malformations is reviewed in this chapter.

The eyes should be measured to obtain the palpebral fissure size (measured from inner to the outer canthus) and interpupillary and inner canthal distances and to determine if the infant has hypotelorism or hypertelorism that is associated with many syndromes.[16,17] Syndromes with hypotelorism as a feature include trisomy 13 and 21, holoprosencephaly, Meckel-Gruber syndrome, and Williams syndrome, among others.[13] Corneal opacity is a clue that suggests the presence of a mucopolysaccharidosis, whereas downward slanting of eyes is present in the infant with Treacher Collins syndrome. Upper slanting eyes, epicantal folds, a flat nasal bridge, and short nose with anteverted nares that occur in combination are indicative of midfacial hypoplasia and are seen in infants with Down syndrome and fetal alcohol syndrome.

The ears should be thoroughly examined. The length and shape of each ear should be measured and assessed for low set ears, preauricular skin tags or pits. Ear anomalies are commonly associated with genetic syndromes. Preauricular tags and pits are common findings on the newborn examination. Ear pits and tags can be inherited in an autosomal-dominant pattern. The physician should therefore check other family members for ear pits and tags, as well as to screen the newborn for hearing loss. Defects in middle ear and inner ear can accompany external ear abnormalities. The neck should be examined for branchial pits. If present, then it may be part of the branchio-oto-renal syndrome, and a renal ultrasound should be performed. Renal sonography should be considered when at least three minor anomalies exist that include preauricular pits or tags.[18] The diagnostic yield of renal sonography is very low for babies who have isolated pits or tags.[19]

The mouth, including philtrum length, should be measured.[20] A large mouth (macrostomia) or small mouth (microstomia) may be seen in various genetic syndromes. Some newborns will exhibit an asymmetric cry caused by the absence of the depressor anguli oris muscle. The cause of this defect is considered to be multifactorial. Research has shown that babies with asymmetric cry have a higher incidence of congenital heart disease; the most common defects include ventriculoseptal defect, atrial septal defect, patent ductus arteriosus, and tetralogy of Fallot. An asymmetric cry is associated with anomalies in other systems, including the central nervous system, gastrointestinal, urinary, and skeletal system as well. Association with velocardiofacial syndrome (22q11 deletion syndrome) has been reported. Some children have developmental disabilities and failure to thrive. Babies who are born with asymmetric cry should be checked thoroughly for cardiac and other anomalies.

Cleft lip, with or without a cleft palate, occurs approximately 1 in 750 live births among white infants and is more common in male infants than female infants. The incidence is highest among Asian infants and lowest in black infants. Cleft lip is usually located laterally at the philtrum ridges. A cleft located in the midline should alert the clinician to suspect holoprosencephaly and to assess for other midline central nervous system defects. Cleft lip and palate can occur sporadically as part of a malformation syndrome or as the consequence of maternal drug exposure or a genetic trait. Isolated cleft palate occurs less frequently at a rate of 1 in 2500 live births. Cleft defects are associated with other malformations in 25% to 50% of affected infants. An isolated cleft lip does not typically cause functional problems. The primary concern is cosmetic, and this defect may cause a great deal of anxiety for the family. Parents need support and reassurance about the frequent success with cosmetic repair. Feeding problems in the neonatal period often present a significant challenge. Infants who have a cleft palate frequently cannot generate adequately the negative pressure during sucking to feed efficiently using a standard infant nipple. Many techniques may be tried; however, use of a soft nipple with larger holes and squeezable bottle is often sufficient to solve the problem. Infants with cleft palates can successfully breastfeed with proper support, education, and assistance from a lactation consultant.[21] The mandible is usually retruded in the neonatal period. If the mandible is underdeveloped but the infant has a normal-size tongue, then space to contain the tongue properly is insufficient, leading to pressure on the palate. This process may produce a U-shaped cleft, similar to that seen in infants with Pierre Robin sequence. Prominent lips suggest Williams syndrome, whereas a thin upper lip is seen in fetal alcohol and Cornelia de Lange syndromes.

Cleft lip repairs are typically performed when the infant is 2 to 3 months of age, after the baby has gained weight and adjusted to extrauterine life. Correction of cleft palate occurs between 9 and 12 months of age.

Chest

The chest circumference and the internipple distance should be measured and plotted on an appropriate growth curve.[15] The nipples may be widely spaced in Turner and Noonan syndromes.[13] A constricted chest with a smaller-than-normal chest circumference often occurs in skeletal dysplasias involving the spine, such as Jeune asphyxiating thoracic dystrophy and Ellis van Creveld syndrome; these disorders are often associated with lung hypoplasia, a feature that may impair the infant's ability to survive. Under normal circumstances the head circumference is larger than the chest circumference by 1 to 4 cm; if these proportions are different, then a cause should be sought. Shortening of the sternum is a common feature in trisomy 18, whereas short trunk is seen in skeletal dysplasias such as osteogenesis imperfecta.[13]

Spine

Open neural tube defects are common congenital anomalies, although their frequency has decreased significantly since the advent of folic acid supplementation of the grains and grain products. Since 1998 the availability of periconceptual folic acid has decreased the occurrence of open neural tube defects by approximately 70%.[22] Open neural tube defects include meningomyelocele (the presence of both neural elements and cerebrospinal fluid in a sac protruding from the midline of the back), meningocele (the presence of just cerebrospinal fluid with no neural elements), anencephaly, and encephalocele (essentially, meningomyelocele of the skull). Spina bifida occulta, a condition in which the vertebral arches are not complete and the spinal cord is intact, is a common minor malformation that is of little clinical consequence. Not etiologically related to open neural tube defects, spina bifida occulta may, in rare cases, be associated with tethering of the spinal cord. Similarly, skin lesions or minor abnormalities such as tufts of hair in the lumbosacral region can be an occult marker of underlying cord disease, such as lipomas, or tethers.

When the primary care physician examines a neonate and observes one or more of the skin manifestations mentioned previously, the question arises as to whether an ultrasound of the spine is required to rule out a spinal anomaly. Kriss and Desai[23] described a 3.5% incidence of simple sacral dimples (less than 5 mm, midline position and not farther than 2.5 cm from anus and no other skin lesions) among 1449 term infants; none of these infants had spinal abnormalities. They did observe that the infants with other lower back skin lesions (hemangiomas, tail-like skin appendages, raised skin lesions, hairy patches, and cutis aplasia) and a more complex sacral dimple (larger than 5 mm and farther than 2.5 cm from the anus) are high risk for spinal dysraphism, more so if the baby has more than one finding.[23] (See Chapter 324, Spina Bifida.)

Trunk and Limbs

The limbs are involved in many congenital malformations syndromes. In the initial examination the newborn should be examined for symmetry, mobility, and length. Are the head and the trunk appropriate in size for the body? If not, then are the limbs too short (suggesting a skeletal dysplasia such as achondroplasia), or is the trunk too short for the limbs (suggesting a skeletal dysplasia of the spine, such as Jeune syndrome or spondyloepipheseal dysplasia congenita)?

Asymmetry of the limbs can be caused either by atrophy, often the result of either an intrauterine vascular disturbance such as Poland syndrome, or by hypertrophy, as can be seen in Beckwith Wiedemann syndrome or hemihypertrophy, each of which may be associated with Wilms tumor and other malignancies.[12,13,15]

Decreased mobility of joints and congenital contractures, often termed arthrogryposis multiplex congenita, results from conditions that interfere with normal fetal movements. Congenital contractures can result from a primary neuromuscular disorder or occur secondary to fetal crowding in the uterus (caused by oligohydramnios, bicornuate uterus, other uterine malformations, or multiple fetuses). Talipes equinovarus, more commonly known as clubfoot, is a deformity that includes hind foot plantar flexion with adduction and supination of the forefoot. It is a common anomaly, occurring in 1 to 2 per 1000 live births, that is often the consequence of restriction of intrauterine motion of the foot during the second and third trimesters of pregnancy. The cause for this anomaly is most likely the result of a combination of environmental and genetic factors. Although it is most often an isolated finding, talipes is a common feature of a number of multiple malformation syndromes, including trisomy 13 and 18.[13] Tredwell reported association of talipes equinovarus with early amniocentesis.[24] Routine care of a child with talipes equinovarus should include early consultation with a pediatric orthopedist. Early surgical procedures have not been successful, with reports of high rates of deformity recurrence.[25,26] Isolated puffiness of the hands and the feet particularly on the dorsal side suggests lymphedema, and the clinician should suspect Turner syndrome or Noonan syndrome.

Polydactyly, the presence of extra fingers or toes, is a common finding and one that is often inherited in an autosomal-dominant fashion. Polydactyly is usually an isolated finding in an otherwise-healthy newborn, occurring in approximately 1 in 700 live births.[27] However, the finding of extra digits can also be a part of a more complex multiple malformation syndrome. Classification of polydactyly is based on the position of the extra digit on the hand or foot. The extra digit can be on the radial (preaxial) side of the hand or, more commonly, on the ulnar aspect (postaxial); the digit can be represented by boneless soft tissue attached by a rudimentary pedicle (postminimus) or can be a normally functioning digit. Postaxial polydactyly occurs more frequently than preaxial polydactyly, particularly among black individuals. Preaxial polydactyly is less frequently observed. When it is present, a possible syndromic association should be sought, particularly if a triphalangeal thumb is present. Holt-Oram syndrome, short ribs–polydactyly syndromes, Carpenter syndrome, trisomy 21, VACTERL association, and Fanconi anemia are conditions that may be associated with preaxial polydactyly. Rarely, central polydactyly affecting the three central digits may occur. Central polydactyly, the least frequent type of polydactyly, is often associated with another malformation or a syndrome.

Syndactyly, an abnormal connection between adjacent digits, can involve only soft tissues (simple) or include bones (complex). It may be either complete, along the entire length of the finger, or incomplete, with sparing of the distal part of the fingers. Any number of digits can be linked. Syndactyly is relatively common; it affects 2 to 3 of 10,000 live births. The anomaly can be sporadic, familial, or associated with other abnormalities. Familial syndactyly usually affects the second and third digits and is not associated with other abnormalities; transmission is autosomal dominant, with variable expressivity and incomplete penetrance. Associated or complicated syndactyly can be syndromic or secondary to a constriction band (amniotic band) sequence. Syndromes described in association with complicated syndactyly include acrocephalosyndactylies and the Poland sequence.

Digits can be foreshortened (called brachydactyly), which can be isolated or part of a large number of syndromes, or elongated (usually referred to as arachnodactyly), a feature of Marfan syndrome. The position of digits can be abnormal. Clinodactyly, referring to an incurving of one or more digits (most often the fifth finger), is a common finding in healthy individuals but is associated with Down syndrome and Russell-Silver syndrome.[13] Camptodactyly, a contracture of the proximal interphalangeal joint most commonly affecting the third and fourth digits, is caused by shortening of the tendons, can be an isolated finding and is often inherited as an autosomal-dominant trait or part of a more complex condition such as Beals contractural arachnodactyly syndrome or trisomy 18.[13,28]

Genitalia

Immediately after birth the first question asked by parents is whether their infant is a boy or girl. When the answer to this question is not clear, the parents will be understandably anxious and confused. Because of the delicate nature of this problem and the need to communicate with the family in a timely and accurate manner, the management of the infant with ambiguous genitalia is considered a true medical emergency. The evaluation and management of the infant with ambiguous genitalia requires a coordinated approach to care that includes a neonatologist, an endocrinologist, a pediatric urologist, a geneticist, a social worker, and mental health professionals. Throughout the evaluation and treatment process, open and frequent communication with the infant's family is essential. In the past, if a baby had a micropenis or severe hypospadias, then the recommendation was for gender reassignment with genital surgery started as soon as possible. Today, controversy exists regarding gender reassignment. The current approach avoids any irreversible surgeries to the genitalia until the child's own gender identity is clear.[29-33] (See Chapter 286, Intersex.)

Hypospadias is a common malformation of the male genitalia occurring in 1 in every 200 male infants. (For a complete discussion see Chapter 83, Physical Examination of the Newborn, and Chapter 279, Hypospadias, Epispadias, and Cryptorchism.)

Testicular location is an important clue to whether hypospadias is an isolated defect or part of a more complex condition. Hypospadias is more likely to be an isolated defect in the individual in whom the testes are both descended. Isolated hypospadias, as with clefting of the lip and palate, is a multifactorial trait that shows clustering in families. As such, in these individuals, finding a positive family history is not unusual. The finding of cryptorchidism in an individual with hypospadias should trigger a more extensive work-up than would be performed on the child with isolated hypospadias. Such individuals may actually be virilized girls, caused by such underlying conditions as congenital adrenal hyperplasia resulting from 21-hydroxylase deficiency, partial androgen insensitivity, abnormalities of the sex chromosomes, or other endocrinologic or genetic syndrome. The physician should inquire about the use of progestin and other hormonal treatment in the first trimester; the child should be evaluated for the presence of ovaries and uterus, and renal and other somatic anomalies; and tested immediately to rule out congenital adrenal hyperplasia. Finally, a karyotype and endocrinologic testing are necessary if intersex is suspected.

Clitoromegaly, enlargement of the clitoris, is not a common finding. In premature babies the labia majora are not yet fully developed, and the normal-size clitoris seems unusually prominent. As described by Oberfield,[35] the paired diameter of the corpora cavernosa should be measured. When enlargement is due to trauma (edema caused by the birth process), then the diameter will be less than 6 mm. When the enlargement is due to excess of androgens, then the diameter of the paired corpora cavernosa is more than 6 mm. The infant must be evaluated for congenital adrenal hyperplasia, given that replacement therapy is lifesaving.

DIAGNOSTIC PROCEDURES

Chromosome Analysis

Polymorphisms, the most common cause of changes in DNA base pairs, do not cause disease. When an alteration in a gene leads to an alteration in function with clinical symptoms and signs, this alteration is called a *mutation*. Most genetic diseases are caused by single base pair deletions, duplications, or substitutions. Some diseases are caused by a large deletion of an entire gene that can be detected by fluorescent in situ hybridization and other molecular cytogenetic methods. DNA analysis permits the identification of a growing number of conditions caused by single gene mutations.[35,36] Updated information can be found at GeneTests (www.genetests.org), a Web site that provides information about the availability of testing for specific genetic conditions. Chromosome analysis should be performed in any newborn with two or more major anomalies, with many minor anomalies, features of a known chromosome abnormality such as Down syndrome, or with ambiguous genitalia. Chromosome analysis is performed on any cells that have the ability to actively divide in culture. As such, although the test is usually performed on lymphocytes from peripheral blood, bone marrow cells or fibroblasts from skin biopsy can also be used. When lymphocytes are used, results should be available after 3 to 4 days; karyotype from fibroblasts take much longer, on the order of 4 weeks or more. Chromosome analysis can be performed on bone marrow; the results will be ready in 1 day. This method is usually reserved for cases in which critical decisions regarding management need to be made.

If Down syndrome or another condition caused by aneuploidy is suspected, then routine chromosome analysis should be ordered. If the child's features do not fit one of these well-described conditions, then ordering high-resolution chromosome testing is more appropriate, which will provide more detailed analysis of the chromosomes.

Fluorescent in Situ Hybridization

Fluorescent in situ hybridization (FISH) is a useful technique in babies born with congenital malformations that suggest one of a group of conditions known to cause small chromosome deletions or duplications.[7,37] FISH should be ordered in infants in whom the following conditions are being considered: Prader-Willi and Angelman syndromes (deletion 15q11.2), velocardiofacial or DiGeorge syndrome (deletion 22q11.2), Williams syndrome (deletion 7q11.23), cri du chat (deletion 5p), and lissencephaly and Miller-Dieker syndrome (deletion 17p13.3).

Metabolic Tests

Metabolic tests are additional tools to confirm a diagnosis in a baby with congenital anomalies or a suspected syndrome. Increasing numbers of conditions exist in which a connection between the clinical diagnosis and the biochemical abnormality has been established. For instance, hypocalcemia is seen in velocardiofacial (DiGeorge) syndrome, whereas hypercalcemia is not uncommon in Williams syndrome; hypoglycemia, caused by hyperinsulinism, is seen in Beckwith-Wiedemann syndrome, whereas low cholesterol and increased level of 7-dehydrocholesterol is a confirmatory test for Smith-Lemli-Opitz syndrome.[8]

Imaging

Imaging studies are indicated when a baby has more than one major anomaly or several minor abnormalities. The finding of internal abnormalities will help in establishing a diagnosis and optimizing treatment of the newborn. Ultrasound of the head and abdomen may detect major anatomic defects. The kidneys should be checked as well. A magnetic resonance imaging study for the brain is the preferred diagnostic tool rather than cranial sonography; however, if a newborn is unstable, then sonography may be the appropriate first screening tool. A skeletal survey is indicated when shortening of limbs or significant short stature at birth is present. Review of a chest radiograph for the presence of the thymus is helpful if 22q11 deletion is suspected; in many syndromes the number of ribs is abnormal. In suspected craniosynostosis a skull film is helpful, whereas patellar or epiphyseal stippling can be seen in Zellweger syndrome. Periosteal cloaking of long bones is present in I-cell disease even if the baby is preterm. An echocardiogram should be obtained on any neonate with a heart murmur who has other malformations. Ophthalmologic evaluation is helpful also. Corneal opacity is seen in mucopolysaccharidosis and trisomy 18, colobomata of the iris in CHARGE syndrome (coloboma, heart disease, atresia choanae, retardation of growth or development, genitourinary tract anomalies, and ear anomalies), trisomy 13, cataracts in Sotos syndrome, and Stickler syndrome, as well as other syndromes.[13]

Other Diagnostic Tools

The diagnosis of a malformation syndrome is sometimes apparent on the basis of the infant's clinical features. A diagnosis will sometimes be determined after additional testing. To address the difficulty in determining a diagnosis, dysmorphologists have developed scoring systems for various genetic syndromes. Scoring systems have been developed for trisomy 18, as well as Down, Williams, Cornelia de Lange, and Noonan syndromes. The limitation of a scoring system is the subjective judgment of the examiner. Another helpful tool is *Smith's Recognizable Patterns of Human Malformation,*[13] which describes lists of anomalies that appear in different syndromes. Computer systems such as POSSUM (Pictures of Standard Syndromes and Undiagnosed Malformations), LDDB (London Dysmorphology Database), and SYNDROC (Syndrome Congenital Malformation Database) have been developed; these programs can be helpful in identifying malformation syndromes.

Special Concerns

Genetic testing should not occur before pretest counseling of the family. Counseling should include discussion that genetic tests results may disclose information about the extended family, including issues relates to reveal family secrets about paternity or adoption. Both family members who are carriers of the disease and family members who are healthy may experience a range of feelings, including anger and guilt. Genetic tests results can affect family members' ability to obtain health insurance, find employment, or adopt children. Many states are in the process of enacting laws to protect the privacy of genetic information. Special consideration should be given to genetic testing in children who are not capable of giving informed consent; for this reason, several national organizations, including the American Academy of Pediatrics, published recommendations[38] under which children should be allowed to have genetic testing: "(1) When there are immediate medical benefits, such as institution of measures that can prevent the disease, delay its onset, or prevent secondary disabilities; and (2) when there is benefit to another family member and no harm to the minor."[13,38] When parents request genetic testing and no benefits exist to the child, or if the genetic testing will be used solely for future reproductive decision, then in most circumstances the test should be deferred. Genetic testing brings complex social, ethical, and emotional issues, particularly in adolescents. Before ordering any genetic tests the physician must understand the above complexities, consult with the appropriate specialists, and prepare the family for the possible consequences of the genetic testing results.

TOOLS FOR PRACTICE

Medical Decision Support

- *Evaluation of Newborn with Single or Multiple Congenital Anomalies* (guideline), American College of Medical Genetics (www.health.state.ny.us/nysdoh/dpprd/index.htm).

SUGGESTED READINGS

Cassidy SB, Allanson JE, eds. *Management of Genetic Syndromes.* 2nd ed. New York, NY: John Wiley & Sons; 2005.

Gonzalez JA. Beginners guide to genetics: congenital malformations; students *BMJ.* 2004;12:437-480.

Hall J, Allanson J, Gripp K, et al, eds. *Handbook of Physical Measurements.* 2nd ed. New York, NY: Oxford University Press; 2007.

Hansen M, Bower C, Milne E, et al. Assisted reproductive technologies and the risk of birth defects—a systematic review. *Human Reproduct.* 2005;20(2):328-338.

Jones KL, Smith DW. *Smith's Recognizable Patterns of Human Malformation.* 6th ed. Philadelphia, PA: WB Saunders; 2006.

Lipson MH. Common neonatal syndromes. *Semin Fetal Neonatal Med.* 2005;10(3):221-231.

New York State Department of Health. Evaluation of Newborn With Single or Multiple Congenital Anomalies. Available at: www.health.state.ny.us/professionals/protocols_and_guidelines/index.htm. Accessed August 8, 2007.

Suri M. Craniofacial syndromes. *Semin Fetal Neonatal Med.* 2005;10:243-257.

AAP POLICY STATEMENT

American Academy of Pediatrics, Committee on Genetics. Molecular genetic testing in pediatric practice: a subject review. *Pediatrics.* 2000;106:1494-1497. (aappolicy.aappublications.org/cgi/content/full/pediatrics;106/6/1494).

REFERENCES

1. Marion RW, Fleischman AR. The assessment and management of neonate with congenital anomalies. In: Evans M, ed. *Reproductive Risks and Prenatal Diagnosis*. Norwalk, CT: Appleton and Lange; 1991.
2. New York State Department of Health. Evaluation of Newborn With Single or Multiple Congenital Anomalies. Available at: www.health.state.ny.us/professionals/protocols_and_guidelines/index.htm. Accessed August 8, 2007.
3. Gonzalez JA. Beginners guide to genetics: congenital malformations; students *BMJ*. 2004;12:437-480.
4. McDonald H, American Academy of Pediatrics, Committee on Fetus and Newborn. Perinatal Care at the threshold of viability. *Pediatrics*. 2002;110:1024-1027.
5. Bell EF, American Academy of Pediatrics, Committee on Fetus and Newborn. Non-initiation or withdrawal of intensive care for high-risk newborns. *Pediatrics*. 2007; 119:401-403.
6. Lipson MH. Common neonatal syndromes. *Semin Fetal Neonatal Med*. 2005;10(3):221-231.
7. Cassidy SB, Allanson JE, eds. *Management of Genetic Syndromes*. 2nd ed. New York, NY: John Wiley & Sons; 2005.
8. Suri M. Craniofacial syndromes. *Semin Fetal Neonatal Med*. 2005;10:243-257.
9. Dhort M, De Sutter P, Russinc G, et al. Perinatal outcome of pregnancies after assisted reproduction: a case control study. *Am J Obstet Gynecol*. 1999;181:688-695.
10. Shioto K, Yamada S. Assisted reproductive technologies and birth defects. *Congen Anom (Kyoto)*. 2005;45(2): 39-43.
11. Hansen M, Bower C, Milne E, et al. Assisted reproductive technologies and the risk of birth defects—a systematic review. *Human Reproduct*. 2005;20(2):328-338.
12. Hudgins L, Cassidy SB. Congenital anomalies. In: *Fanaroff and Martin's, Neonatal Perinatal Medicine*. 8th ed. Philadelphia, PA: Mosby Elsevier; 2006.
13. Jones KL, Smith DW. *Smith's Recognizable Patterns of Human Malformation*. 6th ed. Philadelphia, PA: WB Saunders; 2006.
14. Hall J, Allanson J, Gripp K, et al, eds. *Handbook of Physical Measurements*. 2nd ed. New York, NY: Oxford University Press; 2007.
15. Merlob P, Sivan Y, Reisner S. Anthropometric measurements of the newborn infant (27 to 41 gestational weeks). *Birth Defects Orig Artic Ser*. 1984;20(7):1-52.
16. Feingold M, Bossert WH. Normal values for selected physical parameters: an aid to syndrome delineation. *Birth Defects Orig Artic Ser*. 1974;10(13):1-16.
17. Sivan Y, Merlob P, Reisner SH. Eye measurement in preterm and term newborn Infants. *J Craniofac Genet Dev Biol*. 1982;2:239-242.
18. Adam M, Hudgins L. The importance of minor anomalies in the evaluation of the newborn. *NeoReviews*. 2003;4(4):e99-e104.
19. Kugelman A, Tubi A, Bader D, et al. Preauricular tags and pits in the newborn: the role of renal ultrasonography. *J Pediatr*. 2002;141:388-391.
20. Sivan Y, Merlob P, Reisner SH. Philtrum land intercommissural distance in newborn infants. *J Med Genet*. 1983;20(2):130-131.
21. La Leche League International. Available at: www.lalecheleague.org/. Accessed August 8, 2007.
22. Institute of Medicine. Dietary Reference Intakes for Thiamin, Riboflavin, Niacin, Vitamin B6, Folate, Vitamin B12, Pantothenic Acid, Biotin, and Choline (1998). Available at: www.iom.edu/. Accessed August 8, 2007.
23. Kriss VM, Dessai NS. Occult spinal dysraphism in neonates: assessment of high-risk cutaneous stigmata on sonography. *Am J Roentgenol*. 1998;171:1687-1692.
24. Tredwell SJ, Wilson D, Wilmink MA. Review of the effect of early amniocentesis on foot deformity in the neonate. *J Pediatr Ortho*. 2001;21:636-641.
25. Grottkau BE, Goldberg MJ. Common neonatal orthopedics ailments. In: Taeusch HW,Ballard RA,Gleason CA, eds. *Avery's Diseases of the Newborn*. 8th ed. Philadelphia, PA: Elsevier Saunders; 2005.
26. Wallach DM, Davidson RS. Lower limb disorders. In: Dormans JP, ed. *Pediatric Orthopaedics and Sports Medicine*. St Louis, MO: Mosby; 2004.
27. Talamillo A, Bastida MF, Fernandez-Teran M, et al. The developing limb and the control of the number of digits. *Clin Genet*. 2005;67:143-153.
28. Chang B, Lee BS. Upper extremity disorders. In: Dormans JP, ed. *Pediatric Orthopaedics and Sports Medicine*. St Louis, MO: Mosby; 2004.
29. Diamond M. Pediatric management of ambiguous and traumatized genitalia. *J Urol*. 1999;162:1021-1028.
30. Reiner W. Gender identity and sex assignment: a reappraisal for the 21st century. *Adv Med Biol*. 2002; 511:175-187.
31. White PC. The endocrinologist's approach to the intersex patient. *Adv Exp Med Biol*. 2002;511:107-118.
32. Lee PA, Houk CP, Ahmed SF, et al. Consensus statement on management of intersex disorders. International Consensus Conference on Intersex. *Pediatrics*. 2006; 118(2):e488-e500.
33. MacLaughlin DT, Donahoe PK. Sex determination and differentiation. *N Engl J Med*. 2004;350(4):367-378.
34. Oberfield SE, Mondok A, Shahrivar F, et al. Clitoral size in full term infants. *Am J. Perinat*. 1989;6:453.
35. Malcolm S. Molecular methodology. In: Rimoin DL, Connor JM,Pyeritz RE, eds. *Emery and Rimoin's Principles and Practice of Medical Genetics*. 3rd ed. New York, NY: Churchill Livingstone; 1997.
36. Beaudet AL, Scriver CR, Sly WS, et al. Genetics, biochemistry and molecular basis of variant human phenotypes. In: Scriver CR,Beaudet AL,Sly WS et al, eds. *The Metabolic and Molecular basis of inherited Disease*. 7th ed. New York, NY: McGraw-Hill; 1995.
37. American Academy of Pediatrics. Molecular genetic testing in pediatrics practice: a subject review. *Pediatrics*. 2000;106(6):1494-1497.
38. American Academy of Pediatrics, Committee on Bioethics. Policy statement: ethical issues with genetic testing in pediatrics. *Pediatrics*. 2001;107(6):1451-1455.

Section Two

Routine Care Issues

Chapter 87
PRENATAL VISIT

Deborah E. Campbell, MD

A prenatal pediatric visit during the third trimester of pregnancy is recommended for all expectant families as an important first step in establishing a child's medical home. The pediatric prenatal visit is often scheduled between 32 to 36 weeks' gestation. It provides an opportunity to gather basic information, provide information and advice, identify high-risk situations, and promote parenting skills.[1] A prenatal visit may be particularly valuable for first-time parents, families in which a long interval exists between births, families new to a practice, and families with high-risk pregnancies, including pregnancy complications, multiple gestation, anticipated neonatal health problems, or a prior adverse pregnancy outcome. In a randomized controlled trial of prenatal pediatric visits among a group of low-income urban families, the prenatal visit was shown to affect important health outcomes, including the breastfeeding decision, satisfaction with the initial physician-parent relationship, and reduced emergency department use.[2] The prenatal visit affords the prospective parents an opportunity to learn about the pediatric primary care physician's office practice, approach to child health care, and the newborn's initial medical care during the early weeks after the delivery. Alternatively, parents may not have the opportunity to engage with the health professional in a full prenatal office visit, but they may initiate contact with their child's prospective physician via a telephone contact or a brief office visit or through a group prenatal visit.

Group prenatal visits are an effective and efficient way to introduce prospective families to a practice and permit primary care physicians to meet with prospective parents in a relaxed setting that fosters a free flow of information and discussion. If a group prenatal pediatric visit is the venue offered, then the physician should offer individual parents an opportunity for a private conversation so they can share personal information and for individualized information gathering. Many new parents do not meet their child's primary care physician before the baby's birth. No national data exist on the number of expectant families who complete a prenatal visit. A recent study conducted by the Institute for Vaccine Safety reported that 78% of the pediatric physicians surveyed offered a prenatal pediatric visit. Among the parents surveyed, 39% of first-time mothers completed a prenatal pediatric visit.[3] Previous studies have reported that 70% to 90% of pediatricians and family physicians offer prenatal

BOX 87-1 Visit Goals and Topics to Discuss at the Prenatal Visit

1. Establish parent-physician relationship
   a. Parent perspectives on what qualities they are hoping to find in their child's health professional and their expectations of the practice and primary care physician
   b. Specific parent concerns or questions
   c. Health professional reflects on own perspectives about pediatric primary care and expectations about the parents' role in their child's care
2. Obtaining family and prenatal history
   a. Parents' age and occupation, health insurance coverage for parents and proposed coverage for the infant
   b. Specifics of family relationships, cultural beliefs, parenting beliefs and experiences
   c. Perceived impact of impending birth on the family and family functioning—family's preparation for the infant (adequacy of resources)
   d. Family social habits and potential environmental hazards, including tobacco, alcohol, and drug use
   e. Family medical and pregnancy history—known hereditary or genetic conditions
3. Provide information and support
   a. Identifying high-risk situations
      i. Prenatal evaluations, prenatal diagnoses, maternal medical conditions that may affect the timing and mode of delivery or the newborn
      ii. Multiple gestation
      iii. Previous adverse pregnancy outcome
      iv. Mental health, drug use, and domestic violence issues
   b. Delivery plans
      i. Parent concerns: *birth plan*

Continued

BOX 87-1 Visit Goals and Topics to Discuss at the Prenatal Visit—cont'd

ii. Hospital where delivery will occur: whether the practice provides the baby's care or if other clinicians will be responsible
   (1) Rooming in
   (2) What will happen if the infant requires specialized or neonatal intensive care

iii. Home birth

c. Initial newborn care after the birth
   i. Normal newborn transition
   ii. Initial assessment
   iii. Preventive care, including neonatal jaundice, immunizations, newborn screening

d. Infant feeding choices, benefits of breastfeeding

e. Circumcision decision

f. The anticipated timing of the baby's discharge from the nursery or birthing center; factors that determine when the baby can go home

4. Building parenting skills
5. Safety and anticipatory guidance including car seats, smoking, safe sleep practices, sibling responses
6. Schedule of visits: hospital care after the delivery, during the first week of life (first postdischarge follow-up visit) and subsequent well-child care visits
7. How and when the parents should contact the child's pediatric care physician and specific practice routines

Prenatal Pediatric Visit Checklist

Date ________ Name of physician ________

Name of mother ________ Name of father or partner ________

Contact information ________ Expected date of delivery ________ Home birth? Yes ☐ No ☐

History	Pertinent Details	Follow-Up and/or Action Needed
Family constellation		
Family history		
Pregnancy history		
Current pregnancy concerns including method of conception, pregnancy, and medical medical complications, fetal growth, prenatal diagnosis		
Prenatal screenng and test results		
Environmental concerns including toxic habits and exposures		
Family resources and identified needs		

Page 1 of 2

Figure 87-1

Prenatal Pediatric Visit Checklist—continued

Topics Discussed With Parent(s)	Yes	No	Follow-Up and/or Action Needed
Specific parent questions and concerns			
Process for informing the hospital about the parent's choice for the baby's pediatric care physician. Procedure for notification of the practice or physician after the infant's birth			
Initial newborn care after the delivery, including the L & D and newborn nursery routines, rooming-in, and in-hospital newborn screenings			
Feeding choice; benefits breastfeeding			
Common newborn concerns: gestational age at delivery (full-term, late preterm, preterm), transition after birth, feeding, elimination, jaundice, low blood sugar (if risks are present), presence of birth defects			
Circumcision decision			
Family functioning: adjustment to newborn, sibling reactions			
Office follow-up after nursery discharge, how and when to contact the physician, practice routines and hours of operation, insurance coverage for the infant			
Other issues			

Page 2 of 2

Figure 87-1—Cont'd

pediatric visits, with wide variation (22% to 65%) in the reported rates of mothers completing a prenatal pediatric visit. Among urban poor women, rates as low as 5% have been noted for prenatal pediatric visits.[4-6]

The National Center for Health Statistics Vital Statistics reports that 96.5% of pregnant women in the United States have entered prenatal care by the second trimester. Two thirds of pregnant women attend a child-birth class.[7] Late entry into prenatal care after the first trimester increases the risk that a child will not receive all the recommended immunizations and routine well-child care.[8]

The prenatal pediatric visit has five goals: (1) to ascertain pertinent aspects of the prenatal history, (2) to review the family history and identify disease risks for future health problems and genetic or chromosomal disorders that may affect the infant, (3) to identify psychosocial factors that may affect family functioning and the family's adjustment to the newborn, (4) to introduce anticipatory guidance about early infant care and infant safety practices, and (5) to provide a foundation on which to build a family-health professional partnership. Box 87-1 lists goals and topics for discussion. Breastfeeding promotion is another key component of this visit, particularly for expectant mothers who have not yet decided on a feeding method or are unsure about the benefits of breastfeeding or their ability to successfully breastfeed their infant. Breastfeeding education provided in the prenatal setting is a proven strategy that increases the initiation of breastfeeding.[2,9,10]

From a fiscal standpoint, debate exists within the medical community regarding whether a fee should be charged for the prenatal pediatric visit. Some advocates argue that the prenatal visit is an important marketing tool to building a physician's practice; opponents counter that the professional's time and expertise are valuable and that a charge should be levied for the visit. Individual professionals and practices will need to make their own decision regarding benefits derived from this visit and whether payment for this service is appropriate. Many insurance carriers do include a prenatal pediatric visit as a covered benefit for first-time parents, for high-risk pregnancies, and if the family requests a conference.[11]

TOOLS FOR PRACTICE

Engaging Patient and Family

- *Caring for Your Baby and Young Child: Birth to Age 5* (book), American Academy of Pediatrics (www.aap.org/bookstore).
- *Heading Home with Your Newborn: From Birth to Reality* (book), Jana L, Shu J (www.aap.org/bookstore).
- *New Mother's Guide to Breastfeeding* (book), American Academy of Pediatrics (www.aap.org/bookstore).
- *You and Your Pediatrician* (brochure), American Academy of Pediatrics (patiented.aap.org).

Medical Decision Support

- *Breastfeeding Handbook for Physicians* (book), American Academy of Pediatrics (www.aap.org/bookstore).

Practice Management and Care Coordination

- Prenatal Pediatric Visit Checklist, American Academy of Pediatrics. (practice.aap.org/content.aspx?aid=2001).

AAP POLICY STATEMENTS

American Academy of Pediatrics Committee on Fetus and Newborn. Hospital Stay for Healthy Term Newborns. *Pediatrics.* 2004;113(5):1434-1436. (aappolicy.aappublications.org/cgi/content/full/pediatrics;113/5/1434).

American Academy of Pediatrics Committee on Psychosocial Aspects of Child and Family Health. The Prenatal Visit. *Pediatrics.* 2001;107(6):1456-1458. (aappolicy.aappublications.org/cgi/content/full/pediatrics;107/6/1456).

SUGGESTED RESOURCES

American Academy of Pediatrics, Meek JY, Tippins S. *New Mother's Guide to Breastfeeding.* New York, NY: Bantam Books; 2005.

American Academy of Pediatrics. *Heading Home with Your Newborn: From Birth to Reality.* 2nd ed. Elk Grove Village, IL: American Academy of Pediatrics; 2005.

American Academy of Pediatrics. Hospital stay for healthy term infants. *Pediatrics.* 2004;113(5):1434-1436.

American Academy of Pediatrics, Schanler RJ, Dooley S eds. *Breastfeeding Handbook for Physicians.* Elk Grove Village, IL: American Academy of Pediatrics; 2005.

American Academy of Pediatrics, Shelov SP, Hannemann, RE, eds. *Caring for Your Baby and Young Child: Birth to Age 5.* 4th ed. New York, NY: Bantam; 2004.

Serwint J. The prenatal pediatric visit. *Pediatr Rev.* 2003;24:31-32. Available at: pedsinreview.aappublications.org/cgi/content/full/24/1/31. Accessed June 29, 2007.

REFERENCES

1. American Academy of Pediatrics, Committee on Psychosocial Aspects of Child and Family Health. Policy Statement: the prenatal visit. *Pediatrics.* 2001;107(6):1456-1458.
2. Serwint JR, Wilson MEH, Vogelhut JW, et al. A randomized, controlled trial of prenatal pediatric visits for inner-city families. *Pediatrics.* 1996;98:1069-1075.
3. Navar AM, Halsey N, Carter TC, et al. Missed opportunities for immunization education during the prenatal period: the pediatric prenatal visit, routine obstetric care, and hospital-based education classes. Presented at the 40th Centers for Disease Control National Immunization Conference, Atlanta, GA, March 6, 2006.
4. Sprunger LW, Preece EW. Characteristics of prenatal interviews provided by pediatricians. *Clin Pediatr.* 1981;20:778-782.
5. Sprunger LW, Preece EW. Characteristics of prenatal interviews provided by family physicians. *J Fam Pract.* 1981;13:1007-1012.
6. Berger LR, Rose E. The prenatal pediatric visit revisited. *Clin Pediatr.* 1983;22(4):287-289.
7. Lu MC, Prentice J, Yu SM, et al. Childbirth education classes: sociodemographic disparities in attendance and the association of attendance with breastfeeding initiation. *Matern Child Health J.* 2003;7(2):87-93.
8. Freed GL, Clark SJ, Pathman DE, et al. Influences on the receipt of well-child visits in the first two years of life. *Pediatrics.* 1999;103(4 pt 2):864-869.
9. Guise JM, Palda V, Westhoff C, et al. The effectiveness of primary care-based interventions to promote breastfeeding: systematic evidence review and meta-analysis for the US Preventive Services Task Force. *Ann Fam Med.* 2003;109:70-78.
10. Mattar CN, Chong Y-S, Chan Y-S, et al. Simple antenatal preparation to improve breastfeeding practice: a randomized controlled trial. *Obstet Gynecol.* 2007;109:73-80.
11. Blue Cross Blue Shield Association. *Empire's Clinical Practice Guidelines for Pediatric Health.* November 2006. Available at: www.empireblue.com/wps/portal/ehpprovider?content_path=provider/noapplication/f2/s2/t0/pw_ad067448.htm&label=Clinical%20Practice%20Guidelines. Accessed July 25, 2007.

Chapter 88

CARE OF THE NEWBORN AFTER DELIVERY

Diane Bloomfield, MD; Elaine A. Dinolfo, MD, MS; Faye Kokotos, MD

Parental concerns after the birth of their infant frequently focus on the health and *normality* of their newborn. These concerns may be heightened by a suspected fetal abnormality diagnosed prenatally, a prior adverse pregnancy outcome, or an unfavorable maternal medical condition. The mother's own health and her experiences during the labor and delivery process also affect her response to her newborn and receptivity to information about the baby. Answering questions and addressing parental concerns will reassure parents and lessen anxiety. Knowing that the health professional will be available to them, both in the nursery and after the family leaves the hospital, enhances parental satisfaction.

NEWBORNS WITH SPECIAL HEALTH CARE NEEDS

Parents of babies who are born preterm or low birth weight or who are found to have a congenital malformation or other condition that requires specialized medical care experience additional stress and anxiety. The families of otherwise healthy term and late preterm babies who develop an illness in the immediate newborn period (transient tachypnea of the newborn, hypoglycemia, infection, hyperbilirubinemia) may exhibit emotional and psychological distress equal to or exceeding that expected from parents of the most seriously ill neonates. Caring for the parents is therefore as important as caring for the newborn, especially if parents are young or have personal health problems, an inadequate personal support network, or apparent limited coping skills.

Helping parents express an understanding of their child's health needs and the effect the illness has on their family is ideal. Addressing any stated (or implied) assertions of guilt by or toward the mother as being responsible for the baby's health issues is particularly important. Searching for a reason why the newborn became sick after birth is common for mothers and families. In some cultures, illness is viewed as punishment for some wrong committed by the mother or another family member.[1] Some parents need to be given permission to ask questions, express fears, and discuss concerns regarding their hopes and dreams for their child and family and whether these hopes and dreams can remain the same or must change. Depending on the circumstances surrounding the birth and the health concerns for the mother and baby, families can be expected to express a wide range of feelings and emotions, including grief, anger, and fear. Typically these concerns must be addressed before the parents and family can engage in significant discussions about the baby and the proposed evaluation and treatment options.

INITIAL CARE OF THE NEWBORN

Care of the Healthy Newborn After Delivery

In addition to the initial assessment and any resuscitation or stabilization performed in the delivery room, the early components of newborn care are oriented toward preventing common conditions that can cause early, serious harm to the neonate. Anticipatory care includes preventing hypothermia, recognizing neonates at risk for hypoglycemia or infection, and administering topical eye care and parenteral vitamin K. Discussion of the initial assessment and care of the sick newborn are provided in Chapters 74, Assessment and Stabilization at Delivery; and Chapter 75, Identifying the Newborn Who Requires Specialized Care.

Babies who transition normally can be transported to the nursery after a period of bonding with their parents that includes the opportunity to breastfeed in the delivery room. They may also remain with the mother for the entire length of the hospital stay in centers where all care is provided in the mother's multipurpose labor-delivery-recovery-postpartum room. Irrespective of hospital maternity and newborn unit structure, mothers should be encouraged to room-in their newborns to foster frequent breastfeeding and support early caregiving activities, including adaptation to parenthood by the new parents.[2]

Breastfeeding

Initial postnatal care of the neonate should include the opportunity for breastfeeding soon after delivery.[3-5] Early initiation of breastfeeding, breastfeeding on demand, and rooming in have been shown in meta-analyses to have a positive effect on mother-infant bonding and breastfeeding in primiparous women, reducing the occurrence of maternal complications, formula use, and early breastfeeding discontinuation.[6-8] If feasible, breastfeeding should be initiated within the 1 to 2 hours after delivery, optimally within the first hour.

A recent caution has been raised regarding the need for observation of the primiparous woman who is breastfeeding for the first time immediately after delivery. Reports from Israel and France describe several infants who experienced cardiopulmonary compromise while breastfeeding, positioned prone on the mothers' abdomen.[9,10] Supporting and sustaining early breastfeeding efforts includes education regarding the newborn's early feeding skills, positioning, latch-on and suckling, and the frequency of demand feeding in the early postnatal period. Mother-baby pairs should be evaluated during the hospital stay to assess the mother's knowledge about breastfeeding and the adequacy of the breastfeeding process and to identify information and resources needed to support breastfeeding after hospital discharge. A particular challenge is encountered when women express the intent to both breast and bottle (formula) feed and desire to implement this practice while in the hospital.

Mothers receiving epidural anesthesia for postoperative pain control do not experience negative effects on breastfeeding if bupivacaine is used or if they are receiving oral ibuprofen. Buprenorphine use has been shown to affect early breastfeeding.[11-13] (See Chapter 89, Breastfeeding the Newborn, for more information on initiating breastfeeding.)

Eye Care

Prevention of ophthalmia neonatorum by providing topical prophylaxis after birth is an effective prevention strategy.[14] Ophthalmia neonatorum is inflammation of the conjunctivae in the first month of life.[15] Ophthalmia neonatorum is classified in one of 4 forms: (1) chemical conjunctivitis, (2) bacterial conjunctivitis, (3) chlamydial conjunctivitis, and (4) viral conjunctivitis. The most severe cases of ophthalmic neonatorum are due to *Neisseria gonorrhea* and *Chlamydia trachomatis* infections. Thirty percent to 40% of newborns perinatally exposed to gonococcus or *Chlamydia* will develop infection.[16] Other bacteria also cause conjunctivitis in neonates, including *Haemophilus influenza,*

Staphylococcus aureus, Streptococcus pneumoniae, Enterococcus, and other gram-negative organisms. Contamination with these organisms may occur through horizontal transmission routes postnatally and through contact with nursery and hospital staff, parents, and other caregivers. Gonococcal conjunctivitis will typically develop within 48 hours of birth, in contrast to chlamydial conjunctivitis and herpetic conjunctivitis that more commonly occur at 4 to 7 days and 1 to 2 weeks of age, respectively.

Credé, in 1881, recognized that application of silver nitrate to newborn conjunctivae greatly reduced the incidence of gonococcal ophthalmia neonatorum. The epidemiology of ophthalmia neonatorum has changed over the last century, reflecting the increase in *C trachomatis* infection worldwide. However, the routine installation of antibiotic eye drops combined with improved prenatal care and preventive treatment resulted in a significant decrease in neonatal conjunctivitis from 10% to 0.3%.[17]

With appropriate prenatal care that includes cervical cultures, the need for routine eye prophylaxis in light of the risk for chemical conjunctivitis as a complication of prophylaxis may be questioned. Bell et al in a randomized, double-blind study of low-risk infants (those whose mothers were screened for cervical infection with gonococcus and *Chlamydia*) demonstrated that 1% silver nitrate or 0.5% erythromycin ophthalmic ointment decreased the incidence of conjunctivitis (infectious or noninfectious) compared with no prophylaxis.[18] Of the 630 infants randomized to 3 groups, 17% developed conjunctivitis, with 63% of cases in the first 2 weeks. The rates of conjunctivitis were 15% in the no-treatment group, 9% with erythromycin, and 8% with silver nitrate. The authors concluded that silver nitrate had no harmful effects and may provide some benefit, although the effect on organisms of low virulence was not robust. Most states require routine eye prophylaxis of all newborns, but the data suggest that elective treatment based on maternal prenatal surveillance for infection may be a reasonable alternative. The American Academy of Pediatrics (AAP) currently recommends universal prophylaxis of all newborns with 1% sliver nitrate, 0.5% erythromycin, or 1% tetracycline.[19] A 2.5%-povidone-iodine ophthalmic solution is also effective in preventing ophthalmia neonatorum. Chemical conjunctivitis can develop during the first 24 hours of life in response to topical eye prophylaxis with silver nitrate, but the incidence has declined to approximately 1% since the concentration of the silver nitrate solution was reduced to 1%.[20]

Vitamin-K Prophylaxis

Unexpected bleeding in a healthy newborn may be caused by vitamin-K deficiency. Prophylactic administration of vitamin K reduces the incidence of bleeding.[21,22] Parenteral administration of vitamin K has been the standard of care since the 1961 AAP recommendation. Concern about the possible relationship of parenteral vitamin K and childhood cancer led to debate regarding parenteral administration, but more recent research failed to support these earlier claims. The AAP Committee on Fetus and Newborn recommends that all newborns receive vitamin-K prophylaxis via the parenteral route.[23]

Vitamin K is an essential component in the synthesis of 4 coagulant proteins—factors II, VII, IX, and X—and neither vitamin K nor the factors cross the placenta efficiently. At birth the fetal levels of these clotting factors and levels of protein C and protein S are approximately 50% of adult levels. This circumstance, combined with a sterile gut and low levels of vitamin K in human milk, increases the risk for hemorrhage in the newborn.[24,25]

Hemorrhagic disease of the newborn, also referred to as vitamin-K deficiency bleeding (VKDB) occurs in 3 forms: (1) early (first 24 hours), (2) classic (days 2-7 of life), and (3) late (after 1 week of age). Bleeding in the first hours of life is frequently associated with maternal use of drugs such as anticoagulants, barbiturates, carbamazepine, phenytoin, and some cephalosporins, as well as tuberculostatic agents such as rifampicin and isoniazid.[26] Risks to the neonate at this time are intracranial hemorrhage and gastrointestinal bleeding.

During the first week newborns with the classic form of VKDB may develop prolonged bleeding during and after circumcision, cord separation, or phlebotomy. The incidence of classic VKDB is approximately 0.25% to 1.7%, whereas late VKDB, occurring from week 2 through 12, has an incidence of 4.4 to 7.2 per 100,000 live births. Late-onset VKDB occurs primarily among exclusively breastfed infants who have not received adequate Vitamin K and in infants who have underlying diseases such as biliary atresia, cholestatic jaundice, or malabsorption syndromes. Late onset can cause cerebral hemorrhage with devastating sequelae.

Inception of vitamin-K prophylaxis worldwide has greatly reduced the incidence of classic VKDB. Controversy regarding the route of administration has led to development of alternate regimens. The disadvantages of intramuscular vitamin K include local trauma, increased cost, and concern about increased levels of the vitamin potentiating the risk of childhood cancer.[27] Oral preparations are less costly but may be difficult to properly administer. When a single dose of oral vitamin K is used the incidence of classic VKDB is nil, with a concomitant reduction in late VKDB from 4.4 to 7.2 per 100,000 live births to an incidence of 1.4 to 6.4 per 100,000.[23] However, parenteral vitamin-K prophylaxis prevents both classic and late VKDB, except for those newborns with rare severe malabsorption syndromes.

In 1990, 2 studies reported from Bristol, England, suggested an association between parenteral vitamin-K administration and childhood cancer.[28,29] Golding et al proposed as much as a 2-fold increase in childhood cancer.[28] Subsequent research performed by others has failed to confirm the association.[30] The Vitamin K Ad Hoc Task Force of the AAP reviewed the Golding study, as well as other contrary research, and concluded that a link between vitamin-K administration and childhood cancer has not been established. Current recommendations remain unchanged—all newborns receive intramuscular vitamin K at a dose of 0.5 to 1.0 mg. Continued research into the efficacy, safety, and bioavailability of oral preparations and optimal dosing regimens to prevent late VKDB remains an important need.

PHYSICAL EXAMINATION: HOW MANY EXAMINATIONS ARE NEEDED?

The purpose of the newborn examination is to assess the transition from fetal life to the extrauterine environment, to provide reassurance to parents that their newborn is healthy, and to detect potentially serious conditions in healthy-appearing neonates before discharge from the hospital. However, not all conditions that affect the newborn will be detected in the immediate postnatal period. Routine neonatal examination fails to detect the presence of heart disease in 50% of babies born with a congenital heart defect.[31,32] In addition, only one third of infants with congenital cataracts are diagnosed during the course of their newborn nursery stay.[33] This low rate of diagnosis has led some clinicians to question the number of assessments that need to be performed before the newborn's nursery discharge and the role of screening tests to assist in early diagnosis of potentially serious health conditions. An evidence review conducted in 1999 found few studies evaluating the efficacy of one versus 2 neonatal examinations in detecting congenital anomalies in low-risk, healthy newborns before hospital discharge.[34] One controlled trial did determine that more abnormalities were identified before hospital discharge if 2 examinations were conducted; however, in the group of newborns studied, no difference was noted in specific clinical outcomes evaluated.[35]

Current practice in most US hospitals providing newborn care is for the neonate to undergo at least 2 examinations before nursery discharge. However, the healthy term newborn delivered and discharged home within 24 hours may undergo only a single examination. Neonates whose delivery is attended by a clinician will typically have a brief assessment performed in the delivery room and a more comprehensive examination after admission to the newborn nursery. The majority of births, however, are not attended by a pediatric physician. Therefore most newborns will be examined by a medical professional within the first 24 hours, with a second examination occurring in preparation for the hospital discharge. Whenever possible the clinician should perform these assessments in the mother's room to facilitate history taking, to provide an opportunity to evaluate parent-infant interactions, and to promote parent involvement. It also affords the clinician the opportunity to demonstrate the newborn's abilities, answer parent questions, discuss any variations or abnormalities detected on examination, and provide anticipatory guidance and breastfeeding support.

Discussion about newborn care issues and continuity of care has been shown to enhance maternal satisfaction with early newborn care.[36] Hospitals with rooming-in policies that support complete care delivery in the mother's room facilitate this process. Studies have shown that one half of the missed abnormalities were congenital dislocation of the hip. Irrespective of whether the infant is examined once or twice before nursery discharge, a follow-up assessment at 3 to 5 days of age is paramount to ensure that conditions exhibited later during the first week of life are detected so that appropriate interventions can be initiated.

Glucose Screening

No evidence has been found to justify routine measurement of glucose in appropriately grown, healthy, term neonates. (See Chapter 104, Common Metabolic Disturbances in the Newborn.) A normal blood glucose level in a neonate during the first days of life may vary from 27 to 108 mg/dL (1.5-6 mmol/L), and approximately 10% of healthy newborns will have a blood glucose level less than 47 mg/dL (2.5 mmol/L) during the first 72 hours of life. Mean blood glucose levels for breastfed infants are slightly lower at 65 mg/dL (3.6 mmol/L) than formula-fed infants at 72 mg/dL (4 mmol/L). Glucose screening should be performed within 30 to 60 minutes of age for newborns at risk for hypoglycemia. Specific risk factors include neonates who experienced perinatal stress (perinatal depression, cold stress, delayed or prolonged transition, sepsis), newborns of diabetic mothers, newborns who are small (<10%) or large (>90%) for gestational age, or dysmature newborns with evidence of loss of subcutaneous fat, late preterm newborns, newborns whose mothers received medications that may cause in hypoglycemia in the neonate (propranolol, labetolol, oral hypoglycemic drugs, insulin, terbutaline, ritodrine), and newborns exhibiting signs suggestive of hypoglycemia (jitteriness, tremors, seizures, cyanosis, respiratory distress, apnea, poor feeding, lethargy, temperature instability, or hypothermia).

Some nurseries may perform an initial glucose screen on all newborns. Although no absolute blood glucose level exists at which intervention is mandated in a symptomatic newborn or an newborn at risk, a blood glucose level less than 47 mg/dL at 4 to 6 hours of age is accepted by consensus as being appropriate for intervention.[37] Cornblath has recommended using a threshold of 36 mg/dL (2.0 mmol/L) for intervention, with the goal of raising the blood glucose level to above 47 mg/dL (2.6 mmol/L). The frequency and duration of glucose monitoring for newborns at risk for hypoglycemia typically extends for a period of 12 to 36 hours based on the specific risk factor and the infant's response to feeding. Individual hospital protocols delineate these processes and criteria for transfer of infants to a special or neonatal intensive care unit for intravenous therapy.[38,39]

Screening for Congenital Heart Defects

Screening during both the prenatal and the postnatal period to diagnose a variety of conditions with potential short- or long-term consequences for the newborn is increasing in frequency as technology advances and parent advocacy grows. Early identification of potentially life-threatening cardiac defects before the infant develops symptoms is the rationale for considering screening for congenital heart defects. Current guidance supports the examination of a newborn's cardiovascular system at birth, recognizing that a screening physical examination will not identify all newborns with congenital heart defects, and the predictive value of a heart murmur during the first days of life is reported as 54%.[31] Some hospitals have integrated predischarge pulse oximetry into the routine care provided to all healthy newborns.

Pulse oximetry has been recommended as a screening test for the early detection of congenital heart defects based on the assumption that life-threatening heart diseases in newborns are not detected by physical examination and that many cyanotic heart defects do not have an audible murmur during the early neonatal period. An oxygen saturation level below 95% is considered abnormal, but it is important to note that poor peripheral perfusion, skin temperature, skin pigmentation, and movement may affect device readings. Several studies have evaluated the efficacy of performing pulse oximetry to identify infants at potential risk for serious heart disease.[40-43] Although pulse oximetry may have potential utility, notably, few asymptomatic infants with critical lesions are identified by pulse oximetry alone in the absence of suspected clinical disease. Furthermore, among infants referred for echocardiography, comparable detection rates of cardiac abnormalities have been reported. In a recent publication, Patton and Hey report on improved detection of suspected congenital heart disease when experienced clinicians perform the screening examinations.[44] Of the infants identified with suspected heart disease, 94% had a structural cardiac lesion (97% specificity), but only 11.4% of theses infants had a potentially life-threatening cardiac lesion. Therefore routine screening of asymptomatic newborns with pulse oximetry is not recommended. Cost-effectiveness data and larger-scale studies are required.

Newborn Blood Spot Screening

Newborn blood screening (NBS) is performed on 4 million infants each year in the United States, representing the largest application of genetic testing in medicine.[45] NBS is an essential preventive public-health program to identify disorders that may affect long-term health. Early detection and treatment of a variety of metabolic, genetic, and infectious diseases may lead to a significant reduction in death, disease, and associated disabilities.[46]

NBS began with the pioneering work of Dr Robert Guthrie, who developed a screening test for phenylketonuria by using a drop of blood placed on filter paper. In the succeeding 40 years the technology and scope of screening has lead to the ability to test metabolic, infections, and genetic conditions. In 1990, tandem mass spectrometry (MS-MS) was introduced as a more accurate and expansive mode of testing. MS-MS allows for the detection of more than 30 analyte errors. MS-MS combined with radioimmunoassay, fluoroimmunoassay, enzyme-linked immunosorbent assay, and DNA analysis has greatly expanded NBS potential. Each state public health system has a program to screen, identify, inform, and treat its newborn population. The programs require the involvement of primary care pediatricians, as well as subspecialist. The primary care physician must be aware of the tests performed, the protocols to repeat testing, and the referral base for infants with positive tests. Great interstate variability exists in the communication systems established between the newborn family, the primary care physician, and the NBS program. Interstate variation also exists in parental education, NBS consent, and diseases screened and tracking of results. Information is available at state public health Internet sites, the Health Resources and Services Administration, and the National Newborn Screening and Genetics Resource Center.[46,47]

However, universal standards exist regarding collection and storage of specimens. Only persons who are properly trained should collect specimens. Blood should be drawn from the newborn via heel stick using the medial or lateral aspect of the lower foot with saturation of the filter paper spots. Capillary tube or venipuncture is also adequate, but central lines or umbilical lines should be avoided to prevent false results. The filter paper must be handled carefully because alcohol, iodine, skin oil, petroleum jelly, urine, or feces may contaminate the specimen. Specimens should be collected before nursery discharge and before 72 hours.

NBS samples obtained before 24 hours of life can create false-positive results, although the use of MS-MS may eliminate this problem. If a specimen is collected before 24 hours, then a second specimen should be obtained by 7 days. If a neonate is to receive a blood transfusion, then the NBS sample must be drawn before blood is given and repeated 2 months later. Premature and low–birth-weight newborns may have false-positive results on several of the routine NBS tests, such as those for thyroid function, congenital adrenal hyperplasia, tyrosinemia, and galactosemia. Experts recommend that preterm, low–birth-weight, and very sick neonates be retested later, at 2 weeks of age or before discharge from a neonatal intensive care unit. Filter-paper specimens should dry for at least 3 hours in room air before placement in transport envelopes. The samples should be kept from heat and humidity, given that these environmental conditions may denature enzymes to create false results. All specimens are sent to regional, centralized laboratories where strict standards and controls must be maintained. The hospital of origin and, ideally, the medical home of the infant must be identified so that reevaluation and intervention for a positive test may happen rapidly and efficiently.

The AAP Task Force on Newborn Screening has made a series of recommendations summarized in the 2000 report *Serving the Family From Birth to the Medical Home*.[48] The Task Force emphasized that NBS is not merely a testing program but rather a tracking, diagnostic, therapeutic, and evaluation program. As technology continues to develop, the ability to recognize more potential diseases will be available through both government-sponsored programs and private industry. However, the ability to treat or alter disease may lag behind. The Task Force's key recommendations include (1) developing adequate public health infrastructure to support advanced testing, tracking, informing and treating disease, (2) advancing the involvement of health professionals, families, and the public in development and oversight of NBS, and (3) charging public health agencies with ensuring adequate infrastructure, financing, and policies for adequate surveillance and research related to newborn screening.

Prevention of Perinatal HIV Transmission

Perinatal HIV transmission remains the primary source of pediatric HIV/AIDS in the United States. The risk of infection for a neonate born to an HIV-positive mother has been reduced from 25% to less than 2% by the use of currently recommended prenatal antiretroviral therapy and obstetric interventions for women who are aware of HIV infection early in pregnancy. The Institute of Medicine and the Centers for Disease Control and Prevention recommend that all pregnant women receive counseling regarding HIV infection and perinatal HIV transmission and its prevention and that HIV testing be performed on entry into prenatal care and again in the third trimester. For women who have not been tested prenatally, rapid HIV testing in the labor and delivery unit can reduce the risk for mother-to-child transmission. HIV prophylaxis, even when begun during labor and delivery, has been shown to reduce mother-to-child HIV transmission by as much as 50%. Two states, New York and Connecticut, perform HIV screening on the newborn blood spot sample.[49-51]

Infants at Risk for Sepsis

The approach to the infant at risk for infection is discussed in detail in Chapter 101, The Infant With Suspected Infection.

Screening for Developmental Dysplasia of the Hip

Developmental dysplasia of the hip (DDH), if untreated, can lead to the development of osteoarthritis, chronic pain, and activity limitations. Although screening for DDH has been considered a standard of care for over 4 decades, conflicting recommendations remain regarding the evidence that support the efficacy of screening for DDH and the appropriate screening strategy and treatment options to improve functional outcomes. DDH represents a spectrum of anatomic abnormalities that involve improper alignment or abnormal growth of the femoral head and acetabulum. Reported rates of DDH vary between 1.5 and 20 per 1000 live births, with 1% to 10% of affected infants having an identifiable risk factor. A recent review of the available evidence by the United States Preventive Services Task Force assessed the efficacy of early detection methods and intervention outcomes.[52-54]

Breech presentation, family history of DDH, and female gender have been found in fair-quality, case-controlled and observational studies to be most consistently associated with DDH. Among affected infants, only 10% to 27% of patients diagnosed with DDH have been reported to have a risk factor other than female gender. Notably, 60% to 80% of hips assessed as abnormal on the initial newborn examinations are normal on follow-up examinations between 2 to 8 weeks later.[55] Even among neonates with evidence of mild dysplasia on ultrasonography of the hip, clinical resolution occurs between 6 weeks and 6 months of age. Studies have evaluated the efficacy of universal ultrasound screening of newborns for DDH and have found that the evidence to support this recommendation is insufficient.[56] Neither the AAP nor the Canadian Paediatric Society (CPS) recommends routine ultrasonography.

A recent retrospective, observational study reinforces the value of a positive Ortolani sign in a neonate as signifying that the femoral head is not properly within the acetabulum, warranting further evaluation.[57] Current recommendations from the AAP and the CPS are for serial clinical examination of an infant's hips at all periodic health examinations until 12 months of age and a closely monitored period of observation for newborn infants with clinically detected DDH. Positive Ortolani and Barlow tests are indicators for close surveillance by the pediatric physician, with repeat evaluation by 3 weeks of age to document either resolution or persistence of clinical findings. In those infants with spontaneous resolution, imaging, either ultrasonography at 6 weeks of age or x-ray at 4 months of age, should be performed. If the positive findings persist at the 3 weeks' visit, then the newborn should be referred to an orthopedist for management. Age appropriate imaging is also recommended by the AAP for female newborns born breech or positive family history of DDH. In contrast the CPS does not recommend imaging for high-risk infants. Due to the biologic nature of DDH, not all dislocatable hips will be detected at birth. If during periodic visits suspicions are raised by the examination or due to parental concern, confirmation by referral to an orthopedist or by imaging is recommended by the AAP.

Hearing Screening

Over 90% of newborn infants have their hearing screened before nursery discharge. A detailed discussion about infant hearing screening is available in Chapter 39, Auditory Screening.

Umbilical Cord Care

The umbilicus is rapidly colonized after birth. Up to 90% of newborns whose umbilicus is not treated with umbilical antiseptics showing evidence of colonization with *S aureus* at the time of nursery discharge. Although infants with heavy bacterial colonization are at higher risk for developing infection, the overall risk of serious infection is less than 1%. Wide variation exists in hospital practices regarding the use of antiseptics in infant cord care. The most commonly used antiseptics are chlorhexidine, triple dye, hexachlorophene, and 70% alcohol. Dry cord care is associated with higher rates of colonization with *S aureus*, whereas chlorhexidine use has been shown to decrease colonization by 33%. Cord separation typically begins by 4 to 6 days of age, with complete separation by 2 weeks of age. Separation takes longer in preterm infants than in term infants. Delayed separation beyond 3 weeks of age should alert the clinician to a possible immunologic defect or anatomic abnormality, such as a patent urachus. Cord separation has also been shown to increase with the use of chlorhexidine, alcohol, and repeated applications of triple dye.[58-60]

Antiseptic agents on the umbilical cord prevent bacterial colonization and possibly infection. However, recent changes in maternity care practice have resulted in reduced bacterial cross-contamination of infants and have made infections a rare event to the extent that many hospitals have adopted dry cord care. A recent Cochrane review concluded that evidence is insufficient to know whether antiseptics have any additional advantage over keeping the cord clean and dry.[61]

Hepatitis B Virus Vaccine

The acute and chronic consequences of hepatitis B virus (HBV) infection are major health problems. Acute HBV infection can cause liver failure, leading to death, whereas chronic HBV infection can cause long-term liver damage such as cirrhosis and hepatocellular carcinoma.[62] Approximately 12.5 million persons have been infected with HBV during their lifetime, an estimated 1.25 million Americans have chronic, lifelong HBV, and 4000 to 5000 deaths occur each year in the United States from HBV-related chronic liver disease, such as cirrhosis and liver cancer.[62]

The risk of chronic infection increases with decreasing age; people who are infected in early childhood experience a disproportionately large burden of disease attributable to HBV infection.[63] As many as 90% of newborns exposed to HBV from their mothers at birth become carriers, 30% to 50% children between 1 to 5 years of age become carriers, and by adulthood the risk of becoming a carrier is 6% to 10%. Immunization with HBV vaccine is the most effective measure of preventing HBV infection and its consequences. Universal vaccination can control vertical and horizontal transmission of HBV and the sequelae of chronic HBV infection. In populations in which the infection is highly endemic, routine childhood immunization has led to decreases in the prevalence of chronic infection, as well as declines in childhood mortality from hepatocellular carcinoma. In countries with low prevalence rates the benefits of universal neonatal vaccination will not be apparent until 2 to 3 decades later because infection in theses countries occur among adolescents and young adults through percutaneous or sexual routes. The Advisory Committee on Immunization Practices expanded its HBV immunization recommendations in 1991 to include all newborns primarily to stop HBV transmission among children and eventually to prevent HBV infections in adolescents and adults. The currently available HBV vaccines are safe and have an efficacy of above 90%.[64] The vaccines are produced by recombinant DNA technology and have been licensed in the United States in single-antigen formulations and as components of combination vaccines. Long-term studies of adults and children indicate that immune memory remains intact for 15 years or more and protects against clinical acute infections and chronic HBV infection, even though anti–hepatitis B surface antigen (HBsAg) concentrations may become low or undetectable over time. Current recommendations are to administer the first dose of the HBV vaccine to every infant at birth and no later than hospital discharge.[65] This policy eliminates the possibility of missed immunoprophylaxis in newborns of mothers who are HBsAg positive secondary to testing errors, ensures that newborns of mothers whose HBsAg status is unknown at delivery receive appropriate immunoprophylaxis, and reduces the risk of early childhood infection. This policy also protects infants who are discharged home to households with occult HBsAg-positive carriers and has been shown to significantly increase infant immunization completion rates.

Hepatitis B–Negative Mother

Experts recommend that obstetricians and family physicians routinely screen all pregnant women for HBsAg during each pregnancy regardless of the presence or absence of risk factors and regardless of history of vaccination. If the mother is HBsAg negative, then a single-antigen HBV vaccine (0.5 mL intramuscularly) should be given soon after birth and before discharge from the nursery. If the infant weighs less than 2 kg, then the first HBV vaccine dose is given at 30 days of chronologic age if medically stable or at hospital discharge before 30 days of chronologic age.[64] After the birth dose the HBV series should be completed with either single-antigen HBV vaccine (Engerix or Recombivax) or a combination vaccine (Comvax or Pediarix).[64] The second dose should be administered at age 1 to 2 months of age and the final dose at age 24 weeks or more of age. Administering 4 doses of HBV vaccine is permissible when combination vaccines are given after the birth dose.

Hepatitis B–Positive Mother

If the mother is HBsAg positive, then the baby should receive hepatitis B immune globulin (HBIg; 0.5 mL intramuscularly) and HBV vaccine (0.5 mL intramuscularly) at separate sites within 12 hours of birth. The HBV vaccination schedule should be completed on time, at 1 to 2 months, and 6 months for single-antigen vaccine; at 2, 4, and 12 to 15 months for Comvax; or 2, 4, and 6 months for Pediarix. Postvaccination testing for HBsAg and anti-HBsAg should be performed at 9 to 18 months of age to ensure immunity. If the newborn weighs less than 2 kg, then HBIg and HBV vaccine should be given within 12 hours of birth. However, this administration is not counted as the first dose; the full HBV vaccine series should be initiated at 1 to 2 months of age.

Unknown Maternal Hepatitis B Status

If the mother's HBsAg status is unknown, then HBV vaccine (0.5 mL intramuscularly) should be given within 12 hours of birth. The mother should have blood drawn as soon as possible to determine her HBsAg status. If the mother is HBsAg positive, then the infant should receive HBIg as soon as possible (no later than 1 week). The HBV vaccination series should be completed on time, and postvaccination testing should be done at 9 to 18 months of age. If the newborn weighs less than 2 kg, then HBIg and HBV vaccine should be given within 12 hours of birth. This dose is not counted as the first dose, and the full HBV vaccine series is started at 1 to 2 months of age.

Transmission of perinatal HBV infection can be prevented in approximately 95% of newborns born to HBsAg-positive mothers by early active and passive immunoprophylaxis in the newborn by vaccine and HBIg. HBV vaccine alone, initiated at or shortly after birth, is also highly effective for preventing perinatal HBV infections. HBV vaccine is extremely cost effective not only in preventing HBV infection, but also in preventing the sequelae of chronic HBV infection. Therefore the first dose of HBV vaccine should be administered to every newborn at birth and no later than hospital discharge. This approach offers the best opportunity to prevent unrecognized perinatal transmission and to prevent transmission within families caused by unrecognized chronic HBV infection in the household. It places immunization as an early and visible priority for parents and offers added insurance that an overall immunization series will be completed on time.

TOOLS FOR PRACTICE

Medical Decision Support

- *Breastfeeding Handbook For Physicians* (book), American Academy of Pediatrics (www.aap.org/bookstore).
- *Red Book: 2006 Report of the Committee on Infectious Diseases*, 27th edition (book), American Academy of Pediatrics (www.aap.org/bookstore).
- *Transcultural Aspects of Perinatal Care, A Resource Guide* (book), National Perinatal Association edited by Mary Ann Shah, CNM, MS, FACNM (www.aap.org/bookstore).

AAP POLICY STATEMENTS

American Academy of Pediatrics, Committee on Fetus and Newborn. Controversies concerning vitamin K and the newborn. *Pediatrics*. 2003;112(1):191-192. (aappolicy.aappublications.org/cgi/content/full/pediatrics;112/1/191).

American Academy of Pediatrics, Rose SR, Section on Endocrinology and Committee on Genetics; American Thyroid Association, Brown RS, Public Health Committee; Lawson Wilkins Pediatric Endocrine Society. Update of newborn screening and therapy for congenital hypothyroidism. *Pediatrics*. 2006;117(6):2290-2303. (aappolicy.aappublications.org/cgi/content/full/pediatrics;117/6/2290).

American Academy of Pediatrics, Section on Breastfeeding. Breastfeeding and the use of human milk. *Pediatrics*. 2005;115(2):496-506. (aappolicy.aappublications.org/cgi/content/full/pediatrics;115/2/496).

Kaye CI, American Academy of Pediatrics, Committee on Genetics. Introduction to the newborn screening fact sheets. *Pediatrics*. 2006;118(3):1304-1312. (aappolicy.aappublications.org/cgi/content/full/pediatrics;118/3/1304).

Kaye CI, American Academy of Pediatrics, Committee on Genetics. Newborn screening fact sheets. *Pediatrics*. 2006;118(3):e934-e963. (aappolicy.aappublications.org/cgi/content/full/pediatrics;118/3/e934).

Mofenson LM, American Academy of Pediatrics, Committee on Pediatric AIDS. Perinatal human immunodeficiency virus testing and prevention of transmission. *Pediatrics*. 2000;106(6):88. (aappolicy.aappublications.org/cgi/content/abstract/pediatrics;95/2/303).

REFERENCES

1. Shah MA, ed. National Perinatal Association. *Transcultural Aspects of Perinatal Health Care: A Resource Guide*. Elk Grove Village, IL: American Academy of Pediatrics; 2004.
2. Kennell JH, Klaus MH. Bonding: recent observations that alter perinatal care. *Pediatr Rev*. 1998;19(1):4-12.
3. Academy of Breastfeeding. Medicine Protocols #5: Peripartum Breastfeeding Management for the Healthy Mother and Infant at Term. Available at: www.bfmed.org/?menuID=139&firstlevelmenuID=139. Accessed August 10, 2007.
4. Academy of Breastfeeding. Medicine Protocols #2: Guidelines for Hospital Discharge of the Breastfeeding Term Infant and Mother: The "Going Home Protocol." Available at: www.bfmed.org/?menuID=139&firstlevelmenuID=139. Accessed August 10, 2007.
5. Academy of Breastfeeding. Medicine Protocols #3: Hospital Guidelines for Use of Supplementary Feedings in the Healthy Term Breastfed Newborn. Available at: www.bfmed.org/?menuID=139&firstlevelmenuID=139. Accessed August 10, 2007.
6. Perez-Escamilla R, Pollitt E, Lonnerdal B, et al. Infant feeding policies in maternity wards and their effect on breastfeeding success: and analytic overview. *Am J Public Health*. 1994;84:89-97.
7. Renfrew MJ, Lang S, Maryin L, et al. Feeding schedules in hospitals for newborn infants. In: *The Cochrane Library*. Issue 3. Oxford, UK: Update Software; 2000.
8. Renfrew MJ, Lang S, Woolridge MW. Early versus delayed initiation of breastfeeding. In: *The Cochrane Library*. Issue 1. Oxford, UK: Update Software; 2001.
9. Toker-Maimon O, Joseph LJ, Bromiker R, et al. Neonatal cardiopulmonary arrest in the delivery room [letter to the editor]. *Pediatrics*. 2006;118:847-848.
10. Gatti H, Castel C, Andrini P, et al. Cardiopulmonary arrest in full term newborn infants: six case reports [in French]. *Arch Pediatr*. 2004;11:432-435.
11. Walker M. Do labor medications affect breastfeeding? *J Human Lactation*. 1997;13:131-137.
12. Hirose M, Hosokawa T, Tanaka Y. Extradural buprenorphine suppresses breastfeeding after cesarean section. *Br J Anaesth*. 1997;79:120-121.
13. Hirose M, Hara Y, Hosokawa T, et al. The effect of postoperative analgesia with continuous epidural bupivacaine after cesarean section on the amount of breastfeeding and infant weight gain. *Anesth Analg*. 1996;82:1166-1169.
14. Centers for Disease Control and Prevention. *STDs in Women and Infants. Sexually Transmitted Disease Surveillance*. Atlanta, GA; Centers for Disease Control and Prevention; 1999.
15. O'Hara M. Ophthalmia neonatorum. *Pediatr Clin North Am*. 1993;40(4):715-725.
16. Schacter, J. Why we need a program for the control of Chlamydia trachomatis. *New Eng J Med*. 1989;320:802-804.
17. Toledo AR, Chandler JW. Conjunctivitis in the newborn. *Infect Dis Clin North Am*. 1992;6(4):807-813.
18. Bell TA, Grayston JT, Krohn MA, et al. Randomized trial of silver nitrate, erythromycin and no eye prophylaxis for the prevention of conjunctivitis among newborns not at risk for gonococcal ophthalmitis. Eye Prophylaxis Study Group. *Pediatrics*. 1993;92(6):755-760.
19. American Academy of Pediatrics. Prevention of neonatal ophthalmia. In: Pickering LK, Baker CJ, Long SS, et al, eds. *2006 Red Book: Report of the Committee on Infectious Diseases*. 27th ed. Elk Grove Village, IL: American Academy of Pediatrics; 2006.
20. Issenberg SJ, Apt L. Wood M. A controlled trial of povidone-iodine as prophylaxis against ophthalmia neonatorum. *New Eng J Med*. 1995;332(9):562-566.
21. Vietti TJ, Murphy T, James J, et al. Observation on the prophylactic use of vitamin K in the newborn. *J Pediatr*. 1960;56:343-346.
22. Sutherland JM, Glueck H. Hemorrhagic disease of the newborn. *Am J Dis Child*. 1967:113:524-533.
23. American Academy of Pediatrics, Committee on Fetus and Newborn. Policy statement: controversies concerning vitamin K and the newborn. *Pediatrics*. 2003;112(1) 191-192; reaffirmed May 2006.
24. Shearer MJ, Rahim S, Barkhan P, et al. Plasma vitamin K1 in mothers and their newborns. *Lancet*. 1982;1: 460-463.
25. Shearer MJ. Vitamin K and vitamin K-dependent proteins. *Br J Hematol*. 1990;75:156-162.
26. Zipursky A. Prevention of vitamin K deficiency bleeding in newborns. *Br J Hematol*. 1999;104:430-437.

27. Golding J, Greenwood R. Intramuscular vitamin K and childhood cancer: two British studies. In: Sutor AH, Hathaway WE, eds. *Vitamin K in Infancy*, New York, NY, Schauttaeur; 1995.
28. Golding J, Paterson M, Kinlen LJ. Factors associated with childhood cancer in a national cohort study. *Br J Cancer.* 1990;62:304-308.
29. Golding J, Greenwood R, Birmingham K, et al. Childhood cancer, intramuscular vitamin K and pethidine given during labour. *Br J Med.* 1992;305:341-346.
30. Ross JA, Davies SM. Vitamin K prophylaxis and childhood cancer. *Med Pediatr Oncol.* 2000;34:434-437.
31. Wren C, Richmond S, Donaldson L. Presentation of congenital heart disease in infancy: implications for routine examination. *Arch Dis Child Fetal Neonatal Ed.* 1999;80: F49-F53.
32. Meberg A, Otterstad JE, Froland G, et al. Early clinical screening of neonates for congenital heart defects: the cases we miss. *Cardiol Young.* 1999;9:169-174.
33. Rahi JS, Dezateux C. National cross sectional study of detection of congenital and infantile cataract in the United Kingdom: role of childhood screening and surveillance. The British Congenital Cataract Interest Group. *BMJ.* 1999;318:362-365.
34. Centre for Clinical Effectiveness. The Benefit of One Compared to Two Routine Neonatal Checks for the Detection of Congenital Hips, Cleft Palates, Cardiac and Eye Abnormalities in Well Neonates. Southern Health Care Network/Monash Institute of Public Health and Health Services Research, Clayton, 1999. Available at: www.mihsr.monash.org/cce/. Accessed August 16, 2007.
35. Glazener MA, Ramsay CR, Campbell MK, et al. Neonatal examination and screening trial (NEST): a randomized, controlled, switchback trial of alternative policies for low risk infants. *BMJ.* 1999;318:627-632.
36. Wolke D, Dave S, Hayes J, et al. Routine examination of the newborn and maternal satisfaction: a randomized controlled trail. *Arch Dis Child Fetal Neonatal Ed.* 2002; 86:F155-F160.
37. Canadian Paediatric Society. Position statement: screening guidelines for newborns at risk for low blood glucose. *Paedistr Child Health.* 2004;9(10):723-729.
38. Cornblath M, Hawdon JM, Williams AF, et al. Controversies regarding definition of neonatal hypoglycemia: suggested operational thresholds. *Pediatrics.* 2000;105: 1141-1145.
39. Donn SM, Fisher CW, eds. *Risk Management Techniques in Perinatal and Neonatal Practice*. Armonk, NY, Futura Publishers; 1996.
40. Hoke TR, Donohue PK, Bawa PK, et al. Oxygen saturation as a screening test for critical congenital heart disease: a preliminary study. *Pediatr Cardiol.* 2002;23: 403-409.
41. Richmond S, Reay G, Abu Harb M. Routine pulse oximetry in the asymptomatic newborn. *Arch Dis Child Fetal Neonatal Ed.* 2002;87:F83-F88.
42. Reich JD, Miller S, Brogdon B, et al. The use of pulse oximetry to detect congenital heart disease. *J Pediatr.* 2003;142:268-272.
43. Koppel RI, Druschel CM, Carter T, et al. Effectiveness of pulse oximetry screening for congenital heart disease in asymptomatic newborns. *Pediatrics.* 2003;111(3):451-455.
44. Patton C, Hey E. How effectively can clinical examination pick up heart disease at birth? *Arch Dis Child Fetal Neonatal Ed.* 2006;91:F263-F267.
45. Botkin J. Research for newborn screening: developing a national framework. *Pediatrics.* 2005;116(4):862-871.
46. National Newborn Screening and Genetics Resource Center. Newborn Screening Overview. Available at: genes-r-us.uthscsa.edu/.
47. US Department of Health and Human Services, Health Resources and Services Administration. Maternal and Child Health Bureau. Newborn Screening: Toward a Uniform Panel and System. Available at: www.mchb.hrsa.gov/screening. Accessed August 16, 2007.
48. American Academy of Pediatrics. Executive summary: Newborn Screening Task Force report: serving the family from birth to the medical home. *Pediatrics.* 2000; 106(2):386-388.
49. Chou R, Smits AK, Hoyt Huffman L, et al. Prenatal screening for HIV: a review of the evidence for the U.S. Preventive Services Task Force. *Ann Intern Med.* 2005; 143:38-54.
50. Centers for Disease Control and Prevention. *HIV/AIDS Surveillance Report 2004.* Vol 16. Atlanta, GA: US Department of Health and Human Services, Centers for Disease Control and Prevention; 2005.
51. Lampe M, Branson B, Paul S, et al. Rapid HIV-1 Antibody Test During Labor and Delivery for Women of Unknown Status: A Practical Guide and Model Protocol, 2004. Available at: www.cdc.gov/hiv/topics/testing/resources/guidelines/rt-labor&delivery.htm. Accessed August 16, 2007.
52. US Preventive Services Task Force. Screening for developmental dysplasia of the hip: recommendation statement. *Pediatrics.* 2006;117(3):898-902.
53. Shipman SA, Helfand M, Moyer VA, et al. Screening for developmental dysplasia of the hip: a systematic literature review for the U.S. Preventive Services Task Force. *Pediatrics.* 2006;117:e557-e576.
54. Agency for Healthcare Research and Quality. Screening for Developmental Dysplasia of the Hip. Evidence Synthesis No. 42. Available at: www.ahrq.gov/downloads/pub/prevent/pdfser/hipdyssyn.pdf. Accessed August 16, 2007.
55. Barlow T. Early diagnosis and treatment of congenital dislocation of the hip. *J Bone Joint Surg.* 1962;44:292-301.
56. Woolacott NF, Puhan MA, Steurer, et al. Ultrasonography in screening for developmental dysplasia of the hip in newborns: systematic review. *BMJ.* 2005;330:1413.
57. Lipton GE, Guille JT, Altiok H, et al. A reappraisal of the Ortolani examination in children with developmental dysplasia of the hip. *J Pediatr Orthop.* 2007;27:27-31.
58. Meberg A, Schoyen R. Bacterial colonization and neonatal infections. Effects of skin and umbilical disinfection in the nursery. *Acta Paediatr Scan.* 1985;74:366-371.
59. Jansen PA, Selwood BL, Donson SR, et al. To dye or not to dye: a randomized clinical trial of triple dye/alcohol regimen versus dry cord care. *Pediatrics.* 2003;111(1):15-20.
60. Pezzati M, Biagioli EC, Martelli E, et al. Umbilical cord care: the effect of eight different cord-care regimens on cord separation time and other outcomes. *Biol Neonate.* 2002;81:38-44; *NeoReviews.* 2004;5(4):e155-e163.
61. Zupan J, Garner P, Omari AAA. Topical umbilical cord care at birth. *Cochrane System Rev.* Issue 3. Oxford, UK: Update Software; 2004.
62. Centers for Disease Control and Prevention. Hepatitis B virus: a comprehensive strategy for eliminating transmission in the United States through universal childhood vaccination. Recommendations of the Immunization Practices Advisory Committee (ACIP). *MMWR Morbid Mortal Wkly Rep.* 1991;40:1-25.
63. Armstrong GL, Mast EE, Wojczynski M, et al. Childhood hepatitis B virus infections in the United States before hepatitis B immunization. *Pediatrics.* 2001;108: 1123-1128.
64. American Academy of Pediatrics. Hepatitis B. In: Pickering LK, ed. *Red Book: 2003 Report of the Committee on Infectious Diseases.* 26th ed. Elk Grove Village, IL: American Academy of Pediatrics; 2003.

65. Centers for Disease Control and Prevention. A comprehensive immunization strategy to eliminate transmission of hepatitis B virus infection in the United States. Recommendations of the Advisory Committee on Immunization Practices (ACIP). *MMWR Morbid Mortal Wkly Rep.* 2005;54:1-23.

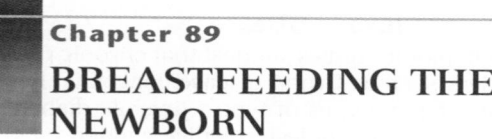

Chapter 89

BREASTFEEDING THE NEWBORN

Richard J. Schanler, MD

INTRODUCTION

Breastfeeding may be considered a natural function that every mother is able to do without preparation or support. Unfortunately, such is not the case for many women in our modern culture. Successful breastfeeding requires education, support, and an environment that values and understands breastfeeding.[1]

BREASTFEEDING RATES IN THE UNITED STATES

In 1999, by mandate of Congress, the Centers for Disease Control and Prevention began surveillance of breastfeeding rates through the National Immunization Survey.[2]

In 2004 and 2003, 70% of all US women initiated breastfeeding, which is close to the Healthy People 2010 objective of 75%.[2] Although this period had the highest rates in recent years, only 39% and 41%, respectively, were *exclusively* breastfeeding at 3 months.[3] In both years, 36% of infants 6 months of age were receiving any human milk, well below the Healthy People 2010 goal of 50%, and only 14% were exclusively breastfeeding.[3] Considerable disparity occurs among racial and ethnic groups. Although in 2004 and 2003, African-American breastfeeding rates approximated 54% at initiation and 23% at 6 months, this group had the most rapid gains in breastfeeding rates in recent years (30% increase from 1996 to 2004). Breastfeeding rates for Latino or Hispanic mothers are greater than those of the total US population (approximately 79%). Although well below the national rates, significant increases in breastfeeding rates have also been reported for mothers 20 years or younger (any breastfeeding 48% initiation, 14% at 6 months); primiparous women; participants in the Special Supplemental Nutrition Program for Women, Infants, and Children (WIC) (any breastfeeding 64% initiation and 29% at 6 months); and mothers of low-birth-weight infants.

Breastfeeding rates at 1 year of age have only recently been measured.[4] Whereas the Healthy People 2010 goal for 1 year is 25%, the total US rates in 2004 and 2003 were 17.8% and 17.2%, and the African-American rate was 9.8%. In all populations, married, older, and highly educated women not working outside the home were more likely to initiate and sustain breastfeeding for longer durations.

Considerable need to overcome obstacles and continue breastfeeding-promotion efforts still exists to reach and to maintain the modest goals set by the US Department of Health and Human Services in its Healthy People 2010 program. This effort is of particular importance for infant and maternal health because the populations at highest risk are the ones with the lowest breastfeeding rates and stand to gain the greatest health and developmental benefits from breastfeeding. The WIC program has made significant strides in increasing successful breastfeeding. Returning to employment or schooling outside the home by the mother is a major negative influence on both initiation and continuation of breastfeeding. Efforts have been made to develop breastfeeding-support programs in many work locations, often with great success.

BENEFITS OF BREASTFEEDING FOR THE INFANT

Protective Effects

Breastfeeding provides significant benefits to both infant and mother (Box 89-1). Breastfed infants experience the same infections but generally exhibit milder symptoms than formula-fed infants. Apparently, not only is the illness rate lower in breastfed infants, but the duration and severity of illness seem to be shortened as well.[5,6] These effects are observed in both developing and industrialized countries. In addition, breastfeeding limits infants' exposure to environmental

BOX 89-1 Benefits of Breastfeeding

FOR THE INFANT

- Prevents or reduces severity of gastrointestinal illness, respiratory illness, and otitis media
- Reduces incidence of necrotizing enterocolitis
- Reduces frequency of urinary tract infections
- Reduces deaths from infant botulism
- Reduces risk of developing sepsis (including in premature infants) and meningitis
- Reduces infant mortality and may reduce sudden infant death syndrome
- Increases general immune responses
- May decrease risk of Crohn's disease, leukemia, lymphoma, diabetes mellitus, hypercholesterolemia, asthma, and some allergic conditions
- Increases long-term cognitive and motor abilities
- Provides analgesia
- Increases visual acuity
- Reduces obesity in adolescents and young adults

FOR THE MOTHER

- Prevents postpartum hemorrhage
- Facilitates postpartum weight loss
- Reduces stress hormone levels
- Provides contraceptive effect if used exclusively for 4-6 months
- Decreases risk of breast cancer

pathogens (microorganisms, chemicals) that may be introduced through contaminated foods, fluids, or feeding devices.

Gastrointestinal infection is prevented and the severity is attenuated in breastfed infants, with specific effects against enteric pathogens such as rotavirus, *Giardia, Shigella, Campylobacter,* and enterotoxigenic *Escherichia coli.*[7,8] Breastfeeding may not prevent colonization of *Vibrio cholerae,* but it will protect against disease.

Respiratory illnesses, including wheezing and lower respiratory tract disease, are reduced in frequency and in duration in breastfed infants.[9,10] Breastfeeding prevents a major portion of disease from *Haemophilus influenzae* type b and *Streptococcus pneumoniae*. Fewer upper respiratory tract symptoms through 7 months' corrected age, well beyond their weaning period, have been reported in human milk–fed premature infants.[11]

Large prospective studies of children with otitis media show a protective effect of breastfeeding.[12-14] Infants exclusively breastfed for at least 4 months may experience as few as one half the number of episodes of otitis media as formula-fed infants and one half as many episodes of recurrent otitis media. These associations remained significant after controlling for a large number of confounders, including socioeconomic status, sibling factors, and maternal smoking. In many of these studies, not only is the incidence of disease diminished with breastfeeding, but also the duration of individual episodes is reduced.

Human milk protects the premature infant from necrotizing enterocolitis.[15,16] Several of the factors in human milk, such as secretory immunoglobulin A, acetylhydrolase, epidermal growth factor, and cytokines, have been identified as potential factors associated with prevention of necrotizing enterocolitis.

Urinary tract infections are more frequent among formula-fed infants than among breastfed infants.[17] Reduced adhesion by pathogens to uroepithelial cells, as mediated by oligosaccharides, secretory immunoglobulin A, or lactoferrin, has been hypothesized as a protective mechanism. Formula-fed infants are more likely to experience severe illness and sudden death from infant botulism, whereas those who were hospitalized and survived the disease were more likely to be breastfed.[18] Possible reasons as to why breastfed infants with botulism have fared better than formula-fed infants include differences in intestinal microflora between breastfed and formula-fed infants and earlier detection of illness by breastfeeding mothers because of perceived changes in infant suck. The intestinal tract pH level of breastfed infants is lower than in formula-fed infants. Proliferation of *Clostridium botulinum* declines as pH level declines.

Before the availability of *H influenzae* type b (Hib) vaccine, the risk of developing sepsis and meningitis caused by Hib was reduced among breastfed infants (particularly among those breastfed for at least 6 to 9 months) as compared with formula-fed infants. One of these studies indicated that protection lasted beyond the period of breastfeeding.[19]

A lower incidence of late-onset sepsis and a reduction in the number of positive blood cultures also has been associated with feeding human milk to premature infants.[20-22] Rates of infant mortality in the United States are also lower for breastfed infants compared with formula-fed infants.[23,24] Breastfed infants also have a significantly higher response to bacille Calmette-Guérin (BCG) vaccination and HiB conjugate vaccine and higher serum antibody titers to polio, tetanus, and diphtheria toxoid immunizations.

Prevention of Chronic Disease

Some epidemiologic studies suggest that chronic pediatric disorders such as Crohn disease, leukemia, lymphoma, specific genotypes of type 1 juvenile diabetes mellitus, obesity, hypercholesterolemia, sudden infant death syndrome, asthma, and certain allergic conditions occur less frequently among children who were breastfed as infants.[6] Immunomodulation is a benefit of breastfeeding and a common mechanism to several of these disorders.

Allergy

Data regarding the protection against allergy afforded by breastfeeding are conflicting, possibly because in some studies maternal diet did not exclude the potentially offending antigens, particularly cow milk proteins. Breastfeeding, however, appears to be protective against some food allergies. Atopic dermatitis may be lessened in infants whose mothers follow a restricted diet. A lower incidence of atopic conditions is reported in breastfed infants with a family history of atopy.[25] A lower incidence of asthma has been reported in breastfed children.[26]

Diabetes

Breastfeeding offers several potential mechanisms for protection against type 1 diabetes, including protection against infections, effects on maturation of the gut-associated lymphoid tissue, and modulation of immune response to insulin.[27] Alternatively, short duration (<3 months) of exclusive breastfeeding and early exposure (<4 months) to cow milk or complementary foods also have been implicated in increased risk of diabetes. Elevated concentrations of specific immunoglobulin G antibodies to bovine serum albumin that cross-react with β-cell–specific surface protein have been identified in children with insulin-dependent diabetes mellitus. Currently available data are inconclusive regarding the precise relationship between breastfeeding and development of β-cell autoantibodies, and research in this area remains active. Breastfeeding also is associated with a reduction in type-2 diabetes.[28,29]

Obesity and Being Overweight

Data are emerging to suggest that adolescent obesity is inversely related to the duration of breastfeeding in infancy.[30-32] Postulated mechanisms for this association relate to how food intake is regulated and to metabolic effects of human milk. The incidence of hypercholesterolemia in adolescence is less if the patient has a history of breastfeeding.[33]

Other Benefits

Maternal-infant bonding is enhanced during breastfeeding. In addition, improved long-term cognitive and motor abilities in full-term infants have been directly correlated with duration of breastfeeding.[34] Improved long-term cognitive development in premature infants has also been correlated with being fed human milk. A meta-analysis of studies in which a multitude of confounding factors (including maternal education and intelligence) were considered concluded that breastfeeding conferred a small, but significant benefit to cognitive function well beyond the period of actual breastfeeding. Some studies indicate a dose-response relationship, the longer the duration of breastfeeding being associated with a higher cognitive score. The positive effects of breastfeeding on subsequent school performance have been reported into adolescence. Breastfeeding also provides analgesia to infants during painful procedures. Human milk itself has been considered in pain-reduction regimens.

Visual acuity, particularly in premature infants, seems to be enhanced by breastfeeding compared with formula feeding. Long-chain polyunsaturated fatty acids have been implicated as factors associated with better visual acuity in breastfed infants. The visual acuity of the breastfed infant is the model for studies of long-chain polyunsaturated fatty acid supplementation.

BENEFITS OF BREASTFEEDING FOR THE MOTHER

A tendency exists to assume that only infants and children benefit from breastfeeding. (See Chapter 26, Feeding of Infants and Children.) However, positive effects of breastfeeding for the mother can be found.[6]

Breastfeeding in the first hour after delivery increases uterine contractility similar to that experienced after the administration of oxytocin. Increased uterine activity reduces maternal blood loss, supporting the World Health Organization (WHO) recommendation to decrease postpartum hemorrhage by nipple stimulation or breastfeeding (or both) in areas where oxytocics are not readily available. Breastfeeding also causes the uterus to more rapidly shrink to prepregnancy size.

Postpartum weight loss may be facilitated in breastfeeding women. Several studies indicate that the greatest effect on weight loss occurs when the duration of breastfeeding exceeds 6 months. Psychological advantages to breastfeeding are obvious, given that bonding is fostered and quiet time is enforced on the nursing mother. Human data show lactating women have decreased levels of adrenocorticotropic hormone and corticosterone in lactating women. The blunted response of stress hormones may be an adaptive mechanism for the stress of labor and delivery. Exclusive breastfeeding delays the resumption of normal ovarian cycles and the return of fertility in most mothers. As such, the contraceptive effects of breastfeeding contribute globally to increased child spacing. Amenorrhea is most likely to occur in women who are exclusively breastfeeding, particularly in the first 6 months postpartum, which allows for repletion of maternal iron stores and correction of anemia. World epidemiologic data indicate that prolonged breastfeeding into the second year, but not exclusively beyond 6 months, prolongs the interpregnancy interval to 1 year, resulting in the birth of the next infant 20 to 24 months after the previous infant. This longer interval may be a factor in reducing infant mortality.

Breastfeeding has been shown to decrease the risk of breast cancer.[35,36] The relative risk of premenopausal breast cancer was significantly reduced in women who, when younger than 20 years, breastfed their infants for at least 6 months. A reduced risk of breast cancer was also observed in women older than 20 years who breastfed for 3 to 6 months when compared with women who did not breastfeed. The anovulation associated with lactation also may protect against ovarian cancer, which has been shown to increase with greater frequency of ovulation.[6] Losses in bone density (approximately 5%) are seen during lactation, with remineralization occurring during weaning. Pharmacologic intervention and increased calcium supplementation beyond the normal intake does not prevent the bone mineral loss. Calcium needs during this time may be compensated for by decreased urinary excretion. Epidemiologic studies suggest that breastfeeding does not increase the risk of postmenopausal osteoporosis. In fact, one study showed that the incidence of hip fracture was decreased with longer duration of lactation. Researchers have suggested that the repeated cycles of demineralization-remineralization may strengthen bone.

SITUATIONS IN WHICH BREASTFEEDING MAY FAIL OR BE CONTRAINDICATED

Most women are able to establish and sustain breastfeeding for an extended period if they are motivated and if they have support from their families, employers, communities, and the medical system. Women with certain medical and psychosocial conditions, however, may not succeed at breastfeeding, and, in rare situations, an infant should not be breastfed (Boxes 89-2 and 89-3).

Breast Size

Breast size is not an indicator of breastfeeding success. Small breast size is not a predictor of lactation failure because the majority of the breast mass is fat tissue, not glandular tissue. Thus even small breasts may have enough glandular tissue to produce sufficient milk. Small breast size, however, may limit the volume of milk that can be stored and may necessitate more frequent feeding to provide the infant with sufficient milk intake. Breast maldevelopment, such as breast hypoplasia or tubular shaped breasts, although uncommon, has been associated with a high frequency of lactation failure.

Breast Surgery

Breast surgery, whether for reduction or augmentation mammoplasty, removal of a mass, or as a result of trauma, may be a cause for breastfeeding difficulties. Women who have had reduction mammoplasty with repositioning of the areolae and nipples are more likely to have difficulty producing adequate milk because of interruption of the ducts and subsequent blockage of the flow of milk into the nipple ducts.

BOX 89-2 Maternal Risk Factors for Lactation Problems

HISTORY AND SOCIAL FACTORS

- Early intention to both breastfeed and bottle feed
- History of previous breastfeeding problems or breastfed infant with slow weight gain
- History of hormone-related infertility; oral contraceptive use
- Significant medical problems (untreated hypothyroidism, diabetes, cystic fibrosis, HIV infection, active pulmonary tuberculosis)
- Maternal age (adolescent mother)
- Psychosocial problems, especially depression
- Perinatal complications (hemorrhage, hypertension, infection)

ANATOMIC AND PHYSIOLOGIC FACTORS

- Lack of noticeable breast enlargement during pregnancy
- Flat or inverted nipples
- Variation in breast appearance (marked asymmetry, hypoplastic, tubular)
- Previous breast surgery that severed milk ducts or nipple afferent nerves
- Previous breast surgery to correct abnormal appearance or developmental variants
- Previous breast abscess
- Extremely or persistently sore nipples
- Failure of lactogenesis stage 2 (milk did not noticeably *come in*)

ENVIRONMENTAL FACTORS

- Mother-baby separation or mother needing to pump

Adapted from Neifert MR. Clinical aspects of lactation. Promoting breastfeeding success. *Clin Perinatol.* 1999;26(2):281-306, v-vi. Copyright © Elsevier 1999. Used by permission.

Primary Insufficient Milk Syndrome

Breast enlargement during pregnancy is an important factor in predicting lactation success. Failure of breasts to enlarge during pregnancy often presages lactation failure. Approximately 5% of women will not produce adequate milk, the *primary insufficient milk syndrome*. Generally, breastfeeding should be encouraged and attempted if the mother so desires. The possibility of difficulty in establishing lactation should be discussed with the mother. Additional assistance, monitoring of infant milk intake or weight gain, and encouragement should be provided to ensure sustained, successful milk production.

Human Immunodeficiency Virus and Human T-Cell Lymphotropic Virus

Women in the United States who are infected with HIV and women with human T-cell lymphotropic virus type 1 should not breastfeed because of the risk of transmission to the nursing infant. In developing countries where infectious diseases and malnutrition are the predominant causes of infant mortality, the health risks of not breastfeeding must be balanced with the risk of HIV acquisition.

BOX 89-3 Infant Risk Factors for Lactation Problems

MEDICAL, ANATOMIC, AND PHYSIOLOGIC FACTORS

- Low birth weight or premature (<37 weeks)
- Multiple births
- Difficulty latching on to one or both breasts
- Ineffective or unsustained suckling
- Oral anatomic abnormalities (cleft lip or palate, micrognathia, macroglossia)
- Medical problems (jaundice, hypoglycemia, respiratory distress, infection)
- Neurologic problems (genetic syndromes, hypotonia, hypertonia)
- Persistently sleepy infant
- Excessive infant weight loss

ENVIRONMENTAL FACTORS

- Formula supplementation
- Effective breastfeeding not established by the time of hospital discharge
- Early discharge from hospital
- Early pacifier use

Adapted from Neifert MR. Clinical aspects of lactation. Promoting breastfeeding success. *Clin Perinatol.* 1999;26(2):281-306, v-vi. Copyright © Elsevier 1999. Used by permission.

Tuberculosis

Women with active pulmonary tuberculosis should not breastfeed until they have received appropriate antibiotic treatment for approximately 2 weeks and are no longer contagious, as determined by their physician or public health official. Whether the tubercle bacillus actually passes into the milk is unclear. The concern is that transmission of disease is by close contact with the mother.

Varicella-Zoster Virus

Neonates should be given varicella-zoster immune globulin if their mothers develop varicella 5 days before delivery to 2 days after delivery. Varicella vaccine may be given to susceptible breastfeeding mothers if the risk of exposure to natural varicella is high. Whether varicella virus is excreted in milk is unknown. Some clinicians recommend breastfeeding only after the exposed infant receives immune globulin. The infant should not have direct contact with lesions that have not crusted over.

Herpes Simplex Virus

Women with herpetic breast lesions should not breastfeed from that side and should cover the lesions to prevent infant contact. Women with genital herpes, however, can breastfeed. Proper hand-washing procedures should be stressed.

Cytomegalovirus (CMV) may be found in the milk of seropositive mothers. In healthy term infants, symptomatic CMV disease from transmission through human milk is uncommon. Some concern exists that premature infants may be at greater risk of symptomatic disease characterized by sepsis-like syndromes. Clinicians should consider the benefits of human milk versus the risk of CMV transmission in premature infants whose mothers are known to be CMV positive or seroconvert during lactation.

Hepatitis B

Infants born to women who are hepatitis B surface antigen positive receive hepatitis B immune globulin and hepatitis B vaccine, eliminating concerns of transmission through breastfeeding. However, even before these measures, breastfeeding was not contraindicated; thus no need exists to delay initiation of breastfeeding until after the infant in immunized.

Hepatitis C

Hepatitis C virus and hepatitis C antibody have been detected in human milk. Infant acquisition of the virus through breastfeeding has not been reported. Maternal hepatitis C infection is not a contraindication to breastfeeding.

Substance Abuse

Women ingesting drugs of abuse (amphetamine, cocaine, heroin, marijuana, phencyclidine) need counseling and should not breastfeed until they are free of the abused drugs that may harm the infant.

Alcohol

Changes in infant feeding patterns have been reported in infants soon after mothers have ingested large amounts of alcohol quickly. Mothers should be advised to limit alcohol consumption during lactation. Alcohol is one of the few substances ingested by the mother that achieves high concentrations in human milk.

Cigarette Smoking

Metabolites of cigarette smoke have been found in infants who live in an environment in which tobacco is smoked. Mothers should be discouraged from smoking during lactation. If they persist in smoking, breastfeeding should be encouraged for the protective effects in the infant, especially with respect to protection from respiratory illnesses.

Medications

Most medications are compatible with breastfeeding, or, if not compatible, a substitute medication may exist and should be sought.[37] Mothers receiving diagnostic or therapeutic radioactive isotopes or have had accidental exposure to radioactive materials should not breastfeed for as long as radioactivity in milk is present.

Cancer Therapy

Women with breast cancer should not delay treatment so they can breastfeed. Depending on the therapy, women receiving antimetabolite chemotherapy may be able to breastfeed by pumping and discarding their milk until the chemical has been cleared after each treatment. Radiation therapy is generally compatible with breastfeeding. Radiation treatment of the breast, however, may significantly damage sensitive breast tissue and be detrimental to future lactation performance of the affected breast.

Inborn Errors of Metabolism

Infants with classic galactosemia (galactose-1-phosphate uridyl transferase deficiency) cannot ingest lactose-containing milk. Therefore, because lactose is the principal carbohydrate in human and bovine milk, infants with classic galactosemia should not breastfeed or receive formula containing lactose.

Infants with other inborn errors of metabolism may ingest some human milk, but this recommendation would depend on the desired protein intake and other factors. Phenylketonuria has been managed with a combination of partial breastfeeding and phenylalanine-free formula. Human milk contains relatively low levels of phenylalanine compared with formula.

SUPPORTING BREASTFEEDING: PRENATAL VISIT

The successful management of lactation begins during pregnancy. The prenatal office visit is an ideal time to inquire about choice of infant feeding and to provide information so families can make an informed choice about the benefits of breastfeeding. Although some studies have shown that infant feeding decisions are made before the third trimester, choices may have been influenced by certain misconceptions or fears held by the expectant mother or father, such as fear of inadequate milk supply because of small breast size, possible loss of sexual breast activity during lactation, cosmetic breast changes as a result of lactation, being a failure at breastfeeding, beliefs that breast milk is not rich enough, and difficulties in learning how to breastfeed, as well as disapproval by the spouse, poor public acceptance, and possible loss of freedom or spontaneity. Because decisions are generally made early and few women have pediatric office visits prenatally, the early obstetric visit must take advantage of the opportunity to discuss and promote breastfeeding. As such, during the initial breast examination at an early obstetric visit the mother should be commended on her choice of breastfeeding and a comment added that her breasts will pose no problem.

PERIPARTUM HOSPITAL ISSUES: GETTING STARTED

The early days of lactation are critical to establishing a good milk supply and an effective let-down reflex. Ten steps to ensure breastfeeding success in the hospital are outlined in Box 89-4. Hospital staff should evaluate breastfeeding formally at least once daily per nursing shift and document their findings in the medical record. Families should have access to knowledgeable information on breastfeeding. They should be encouraged to keep in touch with physicians if questions arise. In the case of early hospital discharge, signs of hydration and the adequacy of feeding should be monitored. All breastfed infants should be seen by a knowledgeable health care professional at 3 to 5 days of age to prevent potential problems of dehydration and severe jaundice. Each hospital should establish

BOX 89-4 Ten Steps to Successful Breastfeeding

Step 1: Have a written breastfeeding policy that is routinely communicated to all health care staff.

Step 2: Train all health care staff in skills necessary to implement this policy.

Step 3: Inform all pregnant women about the benefits and management of breastfeeding.

Step 4: Help mothers initiate breastfeeding within 1 hour of birth.

Step 5: Show mothers how to breastfeed and how to maintain lactation even if they are separated from their infants.

Step 6: Give newborns no food or drink other than human milk, unless medically indicated.

Step 7: Practice rooming-in—allow mothers and infants to remain together—24 hours a day.

Step 8: Encourage breastfeeding on demand.

Step 9: Give no artificial teats or pacifiers to breastfeeding infants.

Step 10: Foster the establishment of breastfeeding support groups and refer mothers to them on discharge from the hospital or clinic.

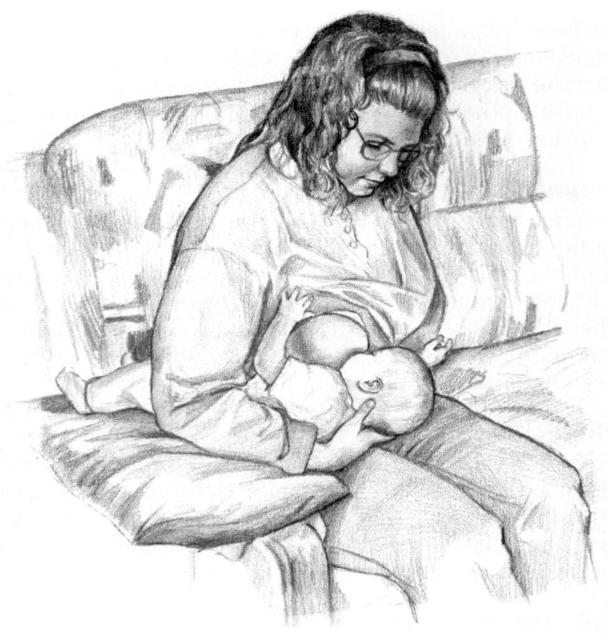

Figure 89-1 The clutch or football hold is an easy position to maintain and is particularly helpful after a cesarean delivery because it keeps the infant's weight off the incision.

breastfeeding support groups or work with organized community support groups so that families have a resource after leaving the hospital.

Initiating Breastfeeding

Early initiation of breastfeeding within the first hour after birth should be practiced unless the medical condition of the mother or infant indicates otherwise. Early nursing in the delivery room is associated with a marked increase in the percentage of mothers who continue breastfeeding at 2 to 4 months postpartum compared with initiation of nursing 2 hours after birth. Successful lactation management includes encouraging nursing in the delivery room and avoiding mother-infant separation in the first hours.

Although many infants placed on the mother's chest or abdomen during their usually alert and active first hour after delivery will spontaneously find the nipple-areola and latch on to it, others may require assistance. Although infant identification bands may be essential immediately after delivery, eye prophylaxis, vitamin K, glucose monitoring, weighing, and other procedures can be performed after the first latch-on or breastfeed has been achieved.

Positioning at the Breast

The nursing mother can use many different positions. However, regardless of position, she should be comfortable. Pillows and footstools may provide assistance. The baby should be positioned so that the head, shoulders, and hips are in alignment and the infant faces the mother's body. The *football* or *clutch* and *side-lying* positions (Figures 89-1 and 89-2) may provide an advantage for mothers who have undergone cesarean delivery by avoiding contact with the surgical incision. The football or clutch position is often used for low–birth-weight or premature infants or infants having trouble latching on because it allows for good control of the infant's head and good visibility of the infant's mouth on the breast. No matter which position is used, the mother must not push on the back of the infant's head because doing so may cause the infant to arch away from the breast.

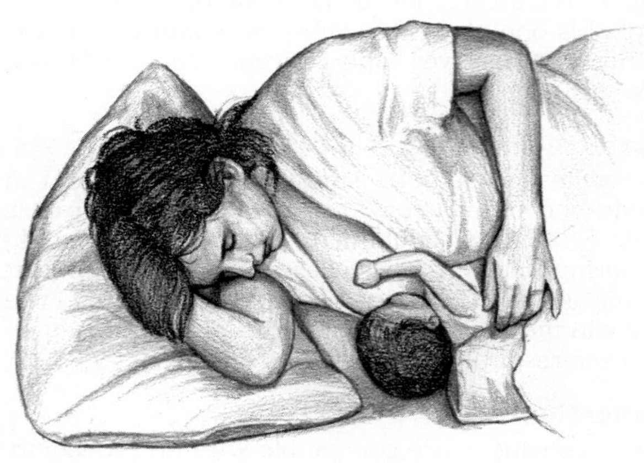

Figure 89-2 Side-lying position.

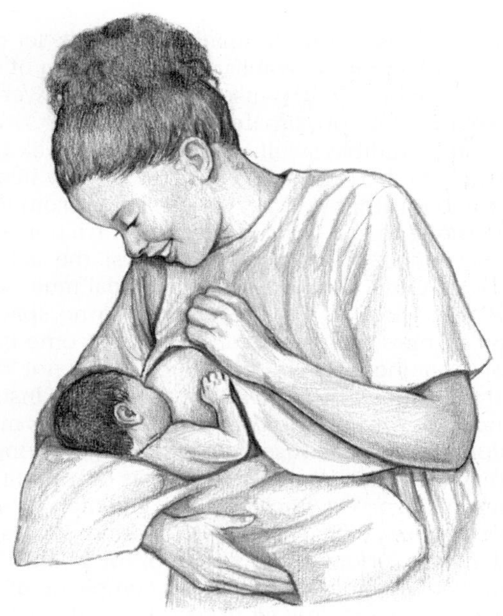

Figure 89-3 Cradle hold.

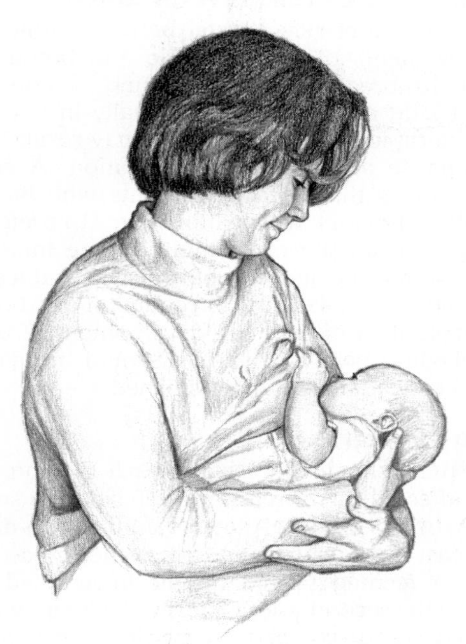

Figure 89-4 Cross-cradle or transitional hold.

In the *cradle hold* (Figure 89-3) the mother's same-sided arm supports the infant at the breast on which the infant is nursing. The infant's head is cradled near the mother's elbow while the arm supports the infant along the back, facing the mother, chest to chest. The *cross-cradle* or *transitional hold* (Figure 89-4) uses the opposite arm to support the infant with the back of the head (below the occiput) and neck held in the mother's hand. This position leaves the hand closest to the breast to support and position the breast as needed. In the *football* or *clutch hold* the infant is positioned at the mother's side. The infant's feet and body are tucked under her arm, and the infant's head is held in her hand facing the breast. If the infant pushes against the back of the chair with the feet, then the mother should angle the infant's legs and feet up the back of the chair. For the *side-lying position* the mother lies on her side facing the infant who is also in a side-lying position. The infant faces the mother with the mouth at the level of the nipple.

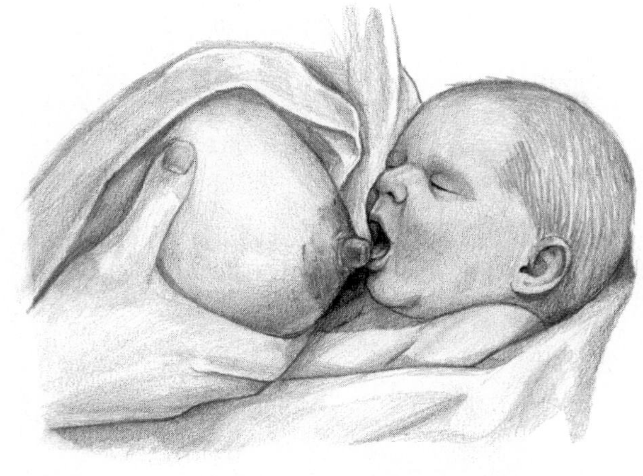

Figure 89-5 The C-hold.

Latch-On

To ensure proper latch-on, the infant should be held so that the mouth is opposite the mother's nipple and the neck is slightly extended, with the head, shoulders, and hips in alignment. While the infant is learning to nurse, proper latch-on is facilitated if the breast is supported in a clutch hold with 4 fingers underneath and the thumb on top (Figures 89-5, 89-6, 89-7). Another way to present the nipple and areola is the scissors or V-hold, but only if the mother's fingers can open wide enough to keep the areola exposed to ensure adequate latch-on. The mother's fingers should be parallel to the infant's jaws and placed well behind the areola.

The *rooting reflex* is elicited when the mother strokes the middle of the infant's lower lip with her nipple. The mother should wait patiently until the infant opens the mouth wide; the mother then quickly pulls the baby to her breast, aiming the nipple slightly upward toward the hard palate to facilitate the lower jaw taking in an adequate amount of the breast.

The infant should grasp the entire nipple and as much of the areola as comfortably possible (approximately 1 to 2 inches from the base of the nipple) and draw it into the mouth. If the infant is well positioned, then the nose and chin will touch the breast, and the lips will be flanged outward around the breast tissue. The infant's tongue should be cupped beneath the nipple-areola complex and may be visible if the infant's

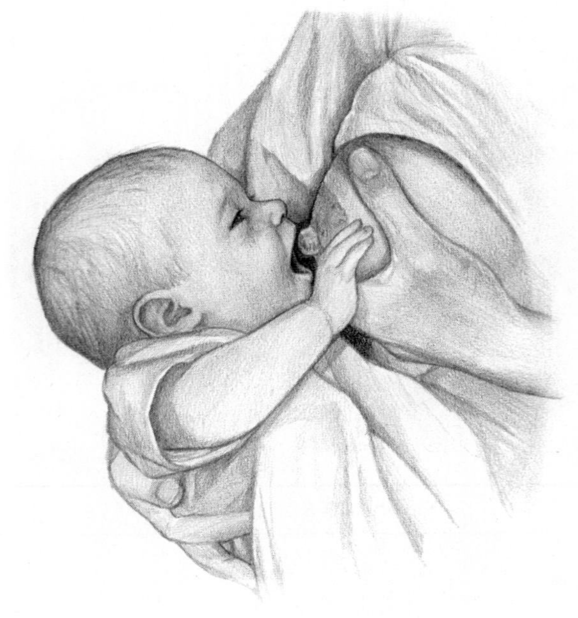

Figure 89-6 Ensure the infant's mouth is wide open.

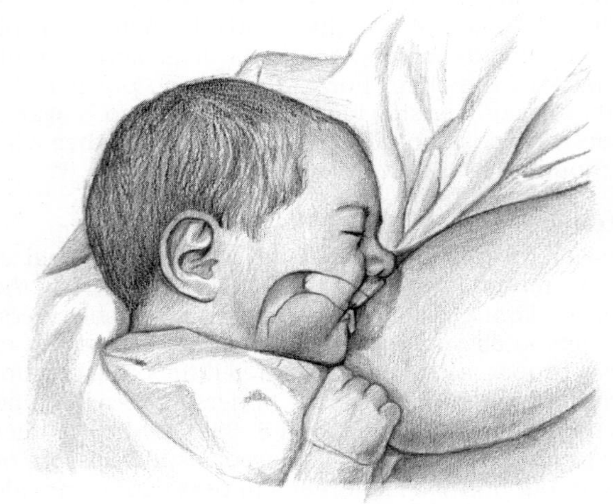

Figure 89-7 This baby is properly latched on, with lips covering the areola and the nipple well inside the mouth.

lower lip is pulled down slightly. The infant's tongue compresses the lactiferous sinuses beneath the areola against the hard palate. The new father or other family members can be helpful in looking for these signs of good positioning and latch-on. When the infant is latched correctly, the mother will feel a gentle undulating motion but no pain with each suck.

Evaluation of a Breastfeed

Once the infant is latched to the breast, suckling begins with rapid bursts and intermittent pauses. This action will assist with stimulating the milk let-down reflex. As milk flow is established, the rhythm of suckling, swallowing, and pauses becomes slower and more rhythmic, approximately one suckle or swallow per second. Audible swallowing indicates milk transfer to the infant. The milk is extracted, not by negative pressure, but rather by a peristaltic action from the tip of the tongue to the base. No stroking, friction, or in-and-out motion of the tongue occurs; the action is more of an undulating action. The buccal mucosa and tongue mold around the breast, leaving no space. At the end of nursing, the infant will often come off the breast spontaneously. If this action does not occur, then the mother can release the suction by inserting her finger gently into the corner of the infant's mouth. The nipple should be observed; it should be elongated but otherwise have no creases or areas of trauma.

Signs of incorrect latch include indentation of the infant's cheeks during suckling, clicking noises, lips curled inward, frequent movement of the infant's head, lack of swallowing, and maternal complaint of pain. Swallowing may be difficult to hear when the newborn is taking small sips of colostrum, but as milk volume increases, swallowing should be heard easily. Later signs of incorrect latch-on include trauma to the nipples, pain, poor infant weight gain, and low milk supply.

Feeding at the Breast Versus Bottle

A distinct difference exists between tongue and jaw movements of breastfeeding and bottle-feeding infants. In breastfeeding, breathing is coordinated with sucking and swallowing, usually in a 1:1:1 pattern. The rapid flow from a bottle may result in respiratory pause and shortened expiration. A common assumption is that breastfed infants who have difficulty obtaining milk will be more likely to prefer bottle feeding if given the opportunity. Some infants may simply prefer the more rapid, gravity-induced flow from a bottle. Because the introduction of a bottle has the potential to disrupt the development of effective breastfeeding behavior, its use should be minimized until breastfeeding is well established.

Feeding Patterns

Each breast should be used at each feeding. Falling asleep after the first breast and refusing the second is normal for a newborn. Allowing an infant to drain the first breast before switching to the other breast is preferable. A feeding should not be interrupted just to switch to the second side. Typically, the infant will spontaneously release the first breast after sufficient draining. Timing each side is not necessary or desirable. Limiting the time at the breast has no effect on nipple soreness, but correct latch and positioning are crucial.

Hunger Cues

Many new parents expect their baby to cry when hungry and need to be informed that crying is a late sign of hunger and can result in an infant who is difficult to calm and latch to the breast. Anticipatory guidance and rooming in 24 hours a day allows the parents to notice early infant hunger cues such as increased alertness, flexion of the extremities, mouth and tongue movements, cooing sounds, rooting, bringing the fist toward the mouth, or sucking on fingers or the hand. Rooming in provides significant benefit in promoting successful lactation. Signs of satiety also need to be taught, such as nonnutritive sucking with longer pauses between sucking bursts, the infant self-releases from the breast, disappearance of hunger cues, relaxed posture, and sleep.

Feeding Frequency

Beginning in the first 24 hours after birth, the newborn infant should breastfeed 8 to 12 times or more every 24 hours, usually for 10 to 15 minutes per breast. Frequent breastfeeding in the first few days minimizes postnatal weight loss, decreases bilirubin levels, and helps establish a good milk supply. Although every 1.5 to 3 hours is the average, a great deal of variation exists from infant to infant and during a 24-hour period. Human milk empties from the stomach faster than formula. Without anticipatory guidance, new mothers often compare their infants to bottle-fed infants and misinterpret the normal frequency of breastfeeding to mean that they have insufficient milk. As infants get older, they nurse more efficiently, and the frequency and duration of feedings decrease. (Box 89-5 highlights a feeding routine for the first week of life.)

Supplements

No reason exists to supply water, glucose water, or formula to the exclusively breastfed infant who is otherwise healthy. Supplements are likely to interfere in the process of successful initiation of breastfeeding. If the appetite or the sucking response is partially satiated by water or formula, then the infant will take less from the breast, causing diminished milk production, which may lead to lactation failure. Water and glucose water supplements may exacerbate hyperbilirubinemia because they prevent adequate milk (calorie) intake and gastrocolic stimulation. Unconjugated (indirect) bilirubin is not water soluble, must be eliminated in the feces, and is not excreted in the urine.

Separation

To support mothers in their desire to breastfeed, they should be taught how to express milk by hand or pump. If the infant is admitted to the neonatal intensive care unit, the need for this teaching will be immediate. However, it should, in any case, take place before discharge and be reinforced in early visits along with other breastfeeding skills. When mothers and infants need to be separated, expression of human milk is important not only for infant feeding, but also to initiate and maintain the woman's milk supply during the separation.

Pacifiers

The most common reason women stop breastfeeding in the hospital setting is because of perceived inadequacy of their milk supply. Offering anticipatory guidance about normal milk production and normal weight loss for the newborn in the first few days can reassure the mother. The time a newborn spends sucking on a pacifier is time not spent suckling on mother's breast, and the lack of stimulation can delay the arrival of the full milk supply, misleading the mother to think she is not making enough milk. The use of pacifiers in the early breastfeeding period has been shown to be associated with shorter breastfeeding duration and should be avoided until after breastfeeding is well established. Furthermore, the use of a pacifier may be a sign of preexisting breastfeeding difficulties or impaired milk production.

BOX 89-5 Feeding Routine for Breastfed Neonates: First Week

First hour	Infant placed skin-to-skin in delivery room
2-4 hr	Infant, mother sleep
4-24 hr	Breastfeeding every 1.5 to 3 hours (8-12 times in 24 hours)
Day 2	Breastfeeding every 1.5 to 3 hours (8-12 times in 24 hours)
Day 3	Breastfeeding every 1.5 to 3 hours (8-12 times in 24 hours)
Day 4	Breastfeeding every 1.5 to 3 hours (8-12 times in 24 hours)
Day 5	Should hear baby swallow milk; start one longer interval (up to 5 hours)
Day 6+	Continue frequent breastfeeding with one longer interval; baby appears satisfied

Adapted from Neifert MR. Clinical aspects of lactation. Promoting breastfeeding success. *Clin Perinatol.* 1999;26(2):281-306, v-vi. Copyright © Elsevier 1999. Used by permission.

ASSESSING THE BREASTFEEDING INFANT

History

The birth history, gestational age assessment, and birth weight should be reviewed. Risk factors that might herald lactation problems should be queried, such as low birth weight, prematurity (<37 weeks), multiple gestation, persistently sleepy infant, medical problems (jaundice, hypoglycemia, respiratory distress, infection, neurologic problems, genetic syndromes), difficulty latching on or ineffective or unsustained suckling, oral anatomic abnormalities (cleft lip or palate, micrognathia, macroglossia), and excessive infant weight loss. A history of formula supplementation, effective breastfeeding not established by hospital discharge, early discharge from hospital, and early pacifier use also might raise concerns about potential breastfeeding issues.

Weight Changes

The most accurate appraisal of the adequacy of breastfeeding is the serial measurement of the infant's naked weight. Nearly all infants lose weight for the first 2 to 4 days after birth. Infants who are feeding well should not continue to lose weight after the completion of lactogenesis stage 2, the time of active milk production, when the milk comes in and the mother feels somewhat engorged. When lactogenesis and milk transfer are proceeding normally, a weight loss greater than 7% of birth weight may be excessive, and, if present, milk

BOX 89-6 Elimination Patterns in Breastfed Neonates: First Week

First 24 hours	One wet diaper in 24 hr	One meconium stool in 24 hr
Day 2	2 to 3 wet diapers in 24 hr	One meconium stool in 24 hr
Day 3	4 to 6 wet diapers in 24 hr	Stool color changes
Day 4	Urine light yellow 4 to 6 times in 24 hr	Transition stools
Day 5	Urine colorless, 6 to 8 times in 24 hr	3 to 4 yellow stools
Day 6+	Urine colorless, 6 to 8 times in 24 hr	4 or more stools; once established, stool frequency may diminish

Adapted from Neifert MR. Clinical aspects of lactation. Promoting breastfeeding success. *Clin Perinatol.* 1999;26(2):281-306, v-vi. Copyright © Elsevier 1999. Used by permission.

production and transfer must be assessed. Once adequate milk supply is achieved, an infant who did not lose excessive weight and who is nursing effectively should obtain enough milk to begin gaining weight by day 4 or 5 at a rate of approximately 15 to 30 g/day (0.5 to 1 oz/day). At this rate, most breastfed infants will exceed their birth weight by 10 to 14 days and gain 150 to 210 g/week (5-7 oz/week) for the first 2 months. A breastfed infant who weighs less than birth weight at 2 weeks requires evaluation and intervention.

Elimination

Elimination patterns, such as stooling and voiding, after the first few days are good indicators of the adequacy of milk intake (Box 89-6). A journal kept by the mother recording feeding and elimination by the infant in the first few weeks can be helpful. Urine output should be colorless, dilute urine, 6 or more times per day by 5 to 7 days.

Stool output and character are also particularly useful indicators of adequate milk intake. The normal green-black meconium stool should change to transitional green, then to soft, seedy, yellow stool by day 4 or 5 after birth. By 5 to 7 days of age, well-nourished breastfed infants usually pass a medium-sized yellow stool at least 3 to 4 times a day. Some infants stool after most feedings. Anticipatory guidance is helpful because stools of the normal human milk–fed newborn may be loose and may be confused with diarrhea if parents are accustomed to seeing the firm, brown stools typical of formula-fed infants. After the first month the volume of each stool increases and the frequency decreases. Insufficient milk intake in an infant older than 5 days of age may be signaled by the presence of meconium stools, green-brown transitional stools, infrequent (<3 per day) stools, or scant stools.

Physical Examination

Physical examination of the infant should include a general examination, vital signs, growth percentiles and percent weight change from birth, and a more detailed oral-motor examination (mandible size, frenulum, rooting, sucking). Presence of congenital anomalies and overall tone should be noted.

Breastfeeding Observation

The physician should observe a feeding and evaluate infant positioning at the breast, the ability of infant to latch, quality of latch, milk let-down, presence of audible swallowing, the anatomic and physiological characteristics of the nipple, maternal responses, and whether the caregiver needs to provide assistance with feeding. The hospital staff should observe and document these breastfeeding observations in the medical record at least twice daily.

MATERNAL BREASTFEEDING ISSUES

Nipple Pain

Sore nipples is the most common complaint of breastfeeding mothers in the immediate postpartum period. Nipple pain should not be considered normal. Nipple pain beyond mere discomfort or continuing beyond the beginning of a nursing episode or after let-down should be investigated immediately. If ignored, nipple pain can then lead to other problems, such as engorgement, mastitis, or early cessation of breastfeeding. Early, mild nipple discomfort is common among breastfeeding women. Severe nipple pain, the presence of cracks and skin lesions, pain that continues throughout a feeding, or pain that is not improving at the end of the first week should not be considered a normal part of breastfeeding.

Improper breastfeeding technique, specifically, poor position and improper latch, is the most common cause of nipple pain in the immediate postpartum period. Limited milk transfer occurs when the infant is attached incorrectly, resulting in poor infant weight gain and impaired milk production. Other potential causes of nipple pain include sources of trauma that produce cracking, such as breast care rituals (overzealous breast cleansing), failing to release suction before removing the infant from the breast, climate variables, and unique skin sensitivity. Limiting the time at the breast, or gradually increasing nursing time, is inappropriate and will not prevent nipple pain. Treatment for nipple pain depends on the underlying cause. Skilled help with position and latch-on are primary interventions. Specific infections and dermatoses require directed therapy. Pain relief medications may be needed. If severe trauma exists, then either manually or mechanically expressing milk may be necessary until the tissue has healed well enough to resume breastfeeding. Nipple healing might be hastened if a small amount of milk is applied to the area after a feeding.

Sore nipples caused by fungal infections, such as *Candida,* are not uncommon. A usual source is thrush in the infant. Breast infections caused by *Candida* may produce nipple pain, itching, or burning sensation or shooting breast pains that radiate back toward the chest wall and persist or worsen after feeding is complete and the breast is drained. The nipple and areola may appear erythematous, shiny, or have white patches. However, in some cases, no external signs may be seen. Predisposing factors for *Candida* infections of the breast include diabetes, steroid use, immune deficiency, antibiotic use, nipple trauma, and the use of plastic-lined breast pads, which keep nipples moist. *Candida* breast infection can be treated.

Engorgement

Physiological breast fullness occurs because of vascular congestion during lactogenesis stage 2. Pathological engorgement is the firm, diffuse, and painful overfilling and edema of breasts usually caused by infrequent or ineffective milk removal. The woman may notice a low-grade fever. Therefore the best treatment of engorgement is prevention by frequent breastfeeding. If left untreated, engorgement may then lead to difficulties in latch and to mastitis. Engorgement should not be confused with a plugged milk duct, which can result in a localized lump in one area of the breast. Engorgement may also occur later in the course of breastfeeding related to a missed feeding or an abrupt change in feeding frequency. In severe cases, the nipples can become flattened to the point the baby cannot grasp them. The swelling and tenderness of engorged breasts are bilateral, generalized, and not unilateral or localized as in an infection, and the condition is rarely associated with high fever or systemic symptoms. Engorgement may be the result of infrequent or ineffective nursing from such causes as sore nipples, a sleepy baby, or mother-baby separation. The treatment is frequent and effective milk removal. Mothers should have ready access to an efficient pump or be trained in manual expression if separated from their infants. The breast examination will rule out related problems such as plugged ducts or mastitis.

Plugged Ducts (Milk Stasis)

A plugged duct is a localized blockage of milk, frequently characterized a painful knot in the breast. This lump may decrease in size with nursing. The condition may be caused by an abrupt change in the feeding schedule, inadequate draining of the breast, failure to vary nursing positions, or wearing tight and constricting clothing (such as a poorly fitting under-wire bra). Some anatomic variations may lead to plugged ducts, especially when the condition recurs in the same breast segment. Rarely, what is considered a plugged duct may be a tumor, benign or malignant, that is blocking the duct. Plugged ducts are easily differentiated from engorgement and mastitis and are not associated with fever or other signs of systemic illness. The treatment for plugged ducts is to apply moist heat before feeding and massage the affected area before and during the nursing.

Mastitis

Mastitis is defined typically as a unilateral bacterial infection of the breast. Mastitis most commonly produces a single area of localized warmth, tenderness, edema, and erythema in *one* breast more than 10 days after delivery. Mastitis may cause a sudden onset of breast pain, myalgia, and fever or with influenza-like symptoms such as fatigue, nausea, vomiting, and headache. The infection commonly enters through a break in the skin, usually a cracked nipple. However, milk stasis and congestion resulting from engorgement, or obstruction of milk ducts from plugged ducts, can also lead to mastitis. Most of the causative organisms are penicillin-resistant *Staphylococcus aureus*. The treatment of mastitis includes antibiotics for a 10- to 14-day course and continuation of breastfeeding with frequent feeding (or pumping) to allow the drainage of the affected breast. Manual expression or a breast pump may be needed to remove the milk from the breast caused by more severe pain prohibiting breastfeeding. Additional therapy includes the encouragement of fluid intake, best rest, and pain control.

NEONATAL ISSUES AND BREASTFEEDING

Hypoglycemia

Hypoglycemia is one of physicians' most commonly cited concerns regarding breastfed infants. The risk of hypoglycemia may be reduced by immediate and sustained mother-infant skin-to-skin contact and early initiation of breastfeeding. Blood glucose concentrations reach a nadir 1 to 2 hours after birth. An adaptive response to low blood glucose concentrations in breastfed infants is an elevated concentration of ketone bodies and other substrates that act as alternate fuels for the infant until breastfeeding is established. Routine monitoring of blood glucose in asymptomatic, not-at-risk, term neonates is unnecessary. In general, healthy term breastfed neonates do not develop symptomatic hypoglycemia. If they develop symptomatic hypoglycemia, then an underlying illness must be excluded. Infants of diabetic mothers, infants who are small for gestational age, and premature infants are among the common groups of infants at risk for hypoglycemia. At-risk infants and those with an abnormal blood glucose concentrations should be monitored every 2 to 4 hours, before a feeding, until several normal prefeeding blood glucose concentrations are obtained. Serial monitoring does not preclude routine breastfeeding.

The intervention for hypoglycemia in an asymptomatic breastfed infant involves breastfeeding and rechecking the blood glucose before the next feeding. If breastfeeding alone cannot correct and maintain an appropriate blood glucose concentration, then expressed human milk or formula should be offered. Symptomatic hypoglycemia requires treatment with intravenous glucose.

Inadequate Milk Intake

Newspaper headlines have identified isolated tragedies of breastfeeding caused by catastrophic cases of dehydration, hypernatremia, and malnutrition. Most important, the mother and the health care professional can be taught simple methods to monitor the hydration status and milk intake of the breastfed infant.

In the first few weeks after birth, an infant is adequately nourished if at least 8 to 12 feedings are

BOX 89-7 Milk Supply: First Week

First 24 hr	Some milk may be expressed
Day 2	Milk should come in (lactogenesis stage 2)
Day 3	Milk should come in (lactogenesis stage 2)
Day 4	Milk should come in (lactogenesis stage 2)
Day 5	Milk should be present; breasts may be firm or leaking
Day 6+	Breasts should feel softer after nursing

Adapted from Neifert MR. Clinical aspects of lactation. Promoting breastfeeding success. *Clin Perinatol.* 1999;26(2):281-306, v-vi. Copyright © Elsevier 1999. Used by permission.

received every 24 hours, beginning in the delivery room, and the infant sleeps contentedly between feedings. The adequacy of milk intake can be assessed daily by counting the number of wet diapers, the number and quantity of stools, and weight gain (preventing a body weight loss >7%). In the first 24 hours after birth the infant should have at least one wet diaper and one stool. On day 3, breastfed infants usually have 3 to 4 wet diapers and one to 2 stools that are no longer have the appearance of meconium, but rather are beginning to appear yellow. Later in the first week after birth, 6 pale yellow diapers per day and a yellow stool should be produced with each feeding. Later in the month the stool frequency may diminish to 3 per day. A written record can be maintained by families or health care professionals to assess the adequacy of milk intake, but it should not take the place of the physical examination of the infant if any concerns exist. Copious milk production (milk *coming in* or lactogenesis stage 2) may not peak until day 4. Therefore usual hospital discharge at 48 hours poses a concern for monitoring the breastfed infant (Box 89-7), and a knowledgeable health care professional should see the infant between 3 and 5 days of age. This first visit should be used to assess the adequacy of hydration, milk intake, and body weight, the presence of jaundice, and the state of the mother (anxiety, concerns). Breastfeeding should also be observed during this first visit. (Box 89-8 provides a checklist for the first postpartum visit.) Telephone contact should be encouraged if further questions arise. Families should be made aware of the availability of community, office, and hospital lactation resources.

Insufficient Milk Syndrome

Insufficient milk syndrome is an imprecise term because it refers to failure of mother's milk production, either primary or secondary, or failure of the infant to extract milk. Because most infants leave the hospital around 48 hours after birth, insufficient milk intake and dehydration are problems that may be seen in follow-up. However, problems that arise from insufficient intake can be prevented with appropriate interventions.

The infant with an insufficient milk intake will have delayed stool output, decreased urinary output, hyperbilirubinemia, weight loss greater than 7% of birth weight, and may be inconsolably hungry or lethargic.

BOX 89-8 The First Postpartum Office Visit: 3 to 5 Days of Age (48 to 72 Hours After Discharge)

BREASTFEEDING ASSESSMENT

- How many feedings in last 24 hours?
- How many wet diapers in last 24 hours?
- How many stools in last 24 hours?
- Does newborn need to be awakened to feed?
- Does newborn easily latch on to breast and nurse eagerly?
- Is newborn receiving any supplements?
- How is mother doing, and how is she feeling about breastfeeding?
- Are mother's breasts comfortable?
- Has mother previously breastfed?
- Is mother taking any medication?
- How is mother's nutrition?
- How do family members feel about breastfeeding?

EXAMINING NEWBORN AND MOTHER

- Calculate newborn's weight gain or loss since birth.
- Observe breastfeeding.
- Examine mother's breasts or refer for examination, if needed.
- Consider using test weight to estimate volume of human milk consumed by newborn if concern exists regarding adequacy of intake.
- Perform routine newborn examination with attention to oral-motor examination.
- Assess state of hydration.
- Observe for jaundice.

ANTICIPATORY GUIDANCE

- Encourage breastfeeding on demand.
- Review normal breastfeeding patterns.
- Discourage use of pacifiers, and discuss potential risks.
- Avoid long nighttime intervals without feeding.
- Review normal elimination patterns.
- Evaluate the need for a vitamin D supplement.
- Reinforce the importance of the care of the mother.

BREASTFEEDING INTERVENTIONS

- Attempt to determine and treat the cause of inadequate milk supply before supplementing.
- Consider referral to lactation specialist if problems are ongoing.
- Develop a support group or refer to an existing breastfeeding support group.

CLOSING THE VISIT

- Congratulate parents on decision to breastfeed their newborn.
- Review some of the benefits of breastfeeding.
- Remind mother to eat when hungry and drink when thirsty.
- Arrange for appropriate follow-up visit until weight gain is adequate and breastfeeding is going well.

Causes of insufficient milk intake may be related to either failure of the mother to produce milk or failure of the infant to extract milk. Although primary lactation failure is rare (and often heralded by a lack of breast growth during pregnancy), delayed lactogenesis stage 2 may occur with retained placental fragments, primary pituitary insufficiency, diabetes, or with certain maternal medications. Mothers who have had breast surgery are also at risk of insufficient milk production or inability to transfer the milk, especially if nipple nerves and ducts have been severed. Insufficient milk supply is more commonly caused by inappropriate early feeding routines, including infrequent feeding and the use of supplements. Occasionally, an infant with oral-motor abnormalities or neurologic problems may not be able to extract milk effectively, leading to a gradual decrease in milk supply. Premature infants, especially borderline premature infants (35 to 37 weeks), are at particular risk for insufficient milk intake. Any factor that limits milk removal may result in diminished milk synthesis because local factors in the breast govern milk production. A protein, *feedback inhibitor of lactation,* is secreted into the alveolar lumen. If not removed, then this protein interacts with the alveolar cell to alter its sensitivity to prolactin and subsequently decrease milk synthesis.

A review of the perinatal history will often identify maternal or infant factors to be addressed. A mother whose breasts did not enlarge during pregnancy or do not become full by 5 days postpartum may have structural or hormonal problems that result in inadequate milk supply. Direct observation of a breastfeeding may reveal improper latch-on, positioning, or inadequate infant effort. Manual or mechanical milk expression techniques may be needed to ascertain total milk volume before feeding or residual milk volume in the breast after a feeding. Residual milk volume that is high (>30 cc) may be a reason for concern. This assessment may contribute to the mother's feeling of inadequacy; therefore less-invasive procedures such as observing a feeding or performing a physical examination should be primary tools for evaluation.

The major goal in management is to increase milk production and milk transfer. The primary management depends on the cause but usually involves increasing the frequency and effectiveness of breastfeeding. Mothers may also need to mechanically express milk after each breastfeeding to increase stimulation and breast drainage. Insufficient milk is the primary reason for supplementation of the breastfed infant. Mechanically expressing milk is necessary if milk production does not increase with increased frequency of breastfeeding, if milk supply is markedly inadequate, or if signs of dehydration or malnutrition already are present. Fluids preferred for supplementation are expressed mother's own milk, pasteurized donor human milk (if available), or infant formula. Glucose water is not a preferred fluid. Glucose water provides significantly fewer calories, no alternate substrates, and does not stimulate intestinal motility as does milk. Depending on the circumstances, if dehydration or malnutrition are present, then the infant should be given enough supplemental milk to produce improved weight gain. Breastfeeding should continue with the addition of the supplemental milk. At the same time, mother should continue milk expression techniques to increase milk production. As milk production increases, the need for supplemental fluids will diminish.

Jaundice

The association between breastfeeding and jaundice is observed in 2 distinct entities: (1) *breastfeeding jaundice* and (2) *breast milk jaundice.*

Breastfeeding Jaundice

Severe jaundice is the most frequent reason for readmission of term and late preterm infants. Many of these infants are breastfed. Poor breastfeeding management is often a contributing factor. Severe jaundice may be part of the clinical picture of the dehydrated, malnourished breastfed infant in the first week after birth. The US Kernicterus Registry indicates that most infants with kernicterus were late preterm breastfed infants.

In their first week, infants with breastfeeding jaundice have rising total serum unconjugated bilirubin levels and poor human milk intake. A history usually exists of decreased maternal milk production or poor milk intake by the infant. Dehydration, weight loss, failure to gain weight, or hypernatremia also may be observed. Infants born at 35 to 37 weeks' gestation have been noted to be at particularly high risk for developing kernicterus, especially if breastfeeding. Clinicians cannot assume that these infants feed as do term infants. In the hospital, these infants seem to feed adequately because milk production has not maximized. Once home, as milk production increases, these premature infants may not be capable of ingesting larger volumes. Thus they often have more breastfeeding problems and have less well-developed hepatic mechanisms for disposal of bilirubin. Close observation is indicated, and slightly lower levels of bilirubin may indicate need for intervention.

Breastfed infants with an insufficient milk intake early in their first week may have an increase in serum unconjugated bilirubin caused by an exaggerated enterohepatic circulation of bilirubin. Lack of milk leads to intestinal milk stasis and intestinal action of glucuronidase enzymes to cleave conjugated bilirubin to unconjugated bilirubin, which is reabsorbed easily. This entity is also known as *breast-non-feeding jaundice* because it is similar to *starvation jaundice* in adults. The evaluation of these infants is similar to that for insufficient milk syndrome. Total serum bilirubin and conjugated bilirubin should be monitored serially. Other causes of jaundice (hemolytic, infection, metabolic) should be considered to ensure optimal overall management. The management of these infants consists of establishing good breastfeeding practices that ensure adequate milk production. Adequate intake of calories by the infant will prevent development of *breastfeeding jaundice* (see the previous section on Management of Insufficient Milk Syndrome). Close monitoring of serum bilirubin is necessary to determine when to initiate phototherapy or perform an exchange transfusion. Breastfed infant should follow the same criteria for intervention as formula-fed infants. The American Academy of Pediatrics recommendations have been published. Breastfed infants may usually continue to receive human milk if phototherapy is initiated. A plot of serum bilirubin on a bilirubin nomogram before discharge is helpful to predict future risk. The follow-up of all breastfed infants on the third to fifth day after birth to assess general health and breastfeeding competency, as well as for the presence of jaundice, is important to prevent the most serious consequences of breastfeeding jaundice. Early detection of jaundice will permit correction of any breastfeeding problems and initiation of diagnostic procedures.

Breast Milk Jaundice

In many breastfed infants, serum unconjugated bilirubin concentrations will remain elevated, and a few infants may have elevated concentrations for as long as 6 to 12 weeks. In formula-fed infants, serum bilirubin declines, reaching values of less than 1.5 mg/dL by the day 11 or 12 after birth. In contrast, by week 3, 65% of normal, thriving breastfed infants have serum bilirubin concentrations above 1.5 mg/dL, and 30% will be clinically jaundiced. Authorities have suggested that the elevation in serum bilirubin may be protective against oxidative injury because it has been shown to be an effective antioxidant *in vitro*. Given that this elevation is a normal response to breastfeeding, other than jaundice, the infants appear healthy and are thriving. The infants are growing normally and exhibit no abnormal clinical signs suggesting hemolysis, infection, or metabolic disease. Mature human milk contains an unidentified factor that enhances the intestinal absorption of bilirubin resulting in jaundice. As the production of the factor diminishes over time and the liver matures, the serum bilirubin concentration eventually returns to normal.

The clinician should ensure that no other causes of prolonged unconjugated hyperbilirubinemia (galactosemia, hypothyroidism, urinary tract infection, pyloric stenosis, low-grade hemolysis) are present. These causes may be identified on newborn screening or from the hospital records and physical examination. The total serum unconjugated bilirubin should be measured if the clinical examination indicates an elevated level. The clinician should check unconjugated and *conjugated* bilirubin if jaundice persists for more than 3 weeks.

Breastfeeding should be continued, and parents should be reassured. Persistent rise in serum bilirubin may necessitate a diagnostic challenge by interrupting breastfeeding for 24 to 48 hours. After interruption of breastfeeding, the serum bilirubin will decline markedly and not rise to prior levels with resumption of breastfeeding. If breastfeeding is interrupted, then the mother should be encouraged and helped to maintain her milk supply. The mother may be reluctant to resume breastfeeding because of the association between breastfeeding and jaundice. A positive attitude on the part of the health care providers and assurance that this circumstance will not occur later may prevent termination of breastfeeding.

Growth Patterns of Breastfed Infants

The conclusions drawn from plotting the growth of a breastfed infant on some growth charts may be erroneous if the growth chart does not adequately reflect the normal growth of the breastfeeding infant. Newer growth curves for exclusively breastfed infants, developed by the WHO, are available.

Growth faltering is a concern when the weight for age (or weight for length) is less than 2 standard deviations below the mean or a weight for age that crosses more than 2 percentile channels downward on the growth chart. Assessments of milk supply and intake, appropriateness of complementary foods, potential for micronutrient deficiencies (eg, iron, zinc, vitamin D), and the feeding environment are all part of the nutritional assessment of the infant with slow weight gain or faltering linear growth. The principles in assessing insufficient milk syndrome should also be considered for these infants. The WHO growth curve will assist in evaluating an infant whose growth is questionable.

COMPLEMENTARY FEEDING (DURATION OF EXCLUSIVE BREASTFEEDING)

The timing of introducing complementary foods into the diet of the breastfed infants is difficult to define with precision, and indeed a single optimal age for all infants may not exist. The recommendations by the WHO and other organizations for exclusive breastfeeding for approximately 6 months are intended for populations and do not dictate the management for individual infants. The American Academy of Pediatrics has supported exclusive breastfeeding for approximately 6 months, while recognizing that many infants are developmentally ready to accept complementary foods before this time, and few data exist to demonstrate any additional benefits to exclusive breastfeeding for 6 months compared with 4 months, especially in developed countries. Decisions about introducing complementary foods for individual infants need to be based on several considerations, including birth weight, postnatal growth rates, and developmental readiness. Infants who were born prematurely or small for gestational age may need micronutrients, especially iron and zinc, provided by complementary foods earlier. Delay of introducing complementary foods beyond 6 months is not recommended because of increasing risk of micronutrient deficiencies.

SUMMARY

Primary care physicians should recommend human milk for all infants in whom breastfeeding is not specifically contraindicated and should provide parents with complete, current information on the benefits and techniques of breastfeeding to ensure that their feeding decision is a fully informed one. Peripartum policies and practices that optimize breastfeeding implementation and maintenance should be encouraged. Healthy infants should be placed and remain in direct skin-to-skin contact with their mothers immediately after delivery until the first feeding is accomplished. All breastfeeding newborn infants should be examined by a pediatrician or other knowledgeable and experienced health care professional at 3 to 5 days of age.

TOOLS FOR PRACTICE

Community Advocacy

- *Supporting Breastfeeding Mothers as They Return to Work* (fact sheet), Marianne Neifert, MD, FAAP, American Academy of Pediatrics (www.aap.org/breastfeeding/BFArticle.pdf).

Engaging Patient and Family

- *Breastfeeding Your Baby: Answers to Common Questions* (brochure), American Academy of Pediatrics (patiented.aap.org).
- *Breast Pumping Video Demonstrations* (Web page), Ameda (www.ameda.com/breastpumping/videos).
- *I'm breastfeeding my baby. How can I tell if she's getting enough milk?* (fact sheet), American Academy of Pediatrics (www.aap.org/healthtopics/breastfeeding.cfm).
- *New Mother's Guide to Breastfeeding* (book), American Academy of Pediatrics (www.aap.org/bst).
- *Should I breastfeed my baby?* (fact sheet), American Academy of Pediatrics (www.aap.org/healthtopics/breastfeeding.cfm).

Medical Decision Support

- *Breastfeeding Handbook for Physicians* (book), American Academy of Pediatrics (www.aap.org/bookstore).
- *Ten Steps to Support Parents Choice to Breastfeed Their Baby* (booklet), American Academy of Pediatrics (www.aap.org/breastfeeding/tenSteps.pdf).

RELATED WEB SITES

- Academy of Breastfeeding Medicine (www.bfmed.org).
- Breastfeeding, Centers for Disease Control and Prevention (www.cdc.gov/breastfeeding/).
- Breastfeeding—Best For Baby, Best For Mom, US Department of Health and Human Services (www.womenshealth.gov/breastfeeding/index.cfm?page=home).
- Section on Breastfeeding, American Academy of Pediatrics (www.aap.org/breastfeeding/New%20SOBr.cfm).

AAP POLICY STATEMENTS

American Academy of Pediatrics, Section on Breastfeeding. Breastfeeding and the use of human milk. *Pediatrics.* 2005;115(2):496-506. (aappolicy.aappublications.org/cgi/content/full/pediatrics;115/2/496).

American Academy of Pediatrics, Committee on Drugs. The transfer of drugs and other chemicals into human milk. *Pediatrics.* 2001;108(3):776-789. (aappolicy.aappublications.org/cgi/content/full/pediatrics;108/3/776).

American Academy of Pediatrics, Subcommittee on Hyperbilirubinemia. Management of hyperbilirubinemia in the newborn infant 35 or more weeks of gestation. *Pediatrics.* 2004;114(1):297-316. (aappolicy.aappublications.org/cgi/content/full/pediatrics;114/1/297).

Read JS, American Academy of Pediatrics, Committee on Pediatric AIDS. Human milk, breastfeeding, and transmission of human immunodeficiency virus type 1 in the United States. *Pediatrics.* 2003;112(5):1196-1205. (pediatrics.aappublications.org/cgi/content/full/pediatrics;112/5/1196).

Gartner LM, Greer FR, American Academy of Pediatrics, Section on Breastfeeding and Committee on Nutrition. Prevention of rickets and vitamin D deficiency: new guidelines for vitamin D intake. *Pediatrics.* 2003;111(4):908-910. (aappolicy.aappublications.org/cgi/content/full/pediatrics;111/4/908).

REFERENCES

1. American Academy of Pediatrics, American College of Obstetrics and Gynecology. *Breastfeeding Handbook for Physicians.* Elk Grove Village, IL: American Academy of Pediatrics; 2006.
2. Center for Disease Control and Prevention. Breastfeeding Practices—Results from the National Immunization Survey. Available at: www.cdc.gov/breastfeeding/data/nis_data/data_2004.htm. Accessed August 1, 2007.
3. US Department of Health and Human Services, Office on Women's Health. *Breastfeeding: HHS Blueprint for Action on Breastfeeding.* Washington, DC: US Department of Health and Human Services; 2000.
4. Centers for Disease Control and Prevention. Breastfeeding Practices—Results from the 2005 National Immunization Survey: Any and Exclusive Breastfeeding Rates by Age. Available at: www.cdc.gov/breastfeeding/data/nis_data/2004/age.htm. Accessed August 1, 2007.
5. American Academy of Pediatrics, Section on Breastfeeding. Breastfeeding and the use of human milk. *Pediatrics.* 2005;115:496-506.
6. Ips S, Chung M, Raman G, et al. *Breastfeeding and Maternal and Infant Health Outcomes in Developed Countries.* Rockville, MD: Agency for Healthcare Research and Quality; 2007.
7. Howie PW, Forsyth JS, Ogston SA, et al. Protective effect of breastfeeding against infection. *Br Med J.* 1990;300:11-16.
8. Scariati PD, Grummer-Strawn LM, Fein SB. A longitudinal analysis of infant morbidity and the extent of breastfeeding in the United States. *Pediatrics.* 1997;99:e5.
9. Chantry CJ, Howard CR, Auinger P. Full breastfeeding duration and associated decrease in respiratory tract infection in US children. *Pediatrics.* 2006;117:425-432.
10. Friedman NJ, Zeiger RS. The role of breast-feeding in the development of allergies and asthma. *J Allergy Clin Immunol.* 2005;115:1238-1248.
11. Blaymore-Bier J, Oliver T, Ferguson A, et al. Human milk reduces outpatient upper respiratory symptoms in premature infants during their first year of life. *J Perinatol.* 2002;22:354-359.
12. Dewey KG, Heinig MJ, Nommsen-Rivers LA. Differences in morbidity between breast-fed and formula-fed infants. *J Pediatr.* 1995;126:696-702.
13. Aniansson G, Alm B, Andersson B. A prospective cohort study on breastfeeding and otitis media in Swedish infants. *Pediatr Infect Dis J.* 1994;12:183-188.
14. Duncan B, Ey J, Holberg CJ, et al. Exclusive breastfeeding for at least 4 months protects against otitis media. *Pediatrics.* 1993;91:867-872.
15. Lucas A, Cole TJ. Breast milk and neonatal necrotizing enterocolitis. *Lancet.* 1990;336:1519-1523.
16. Schanler RJ, Lau C, Hurst NM, et al. Randomized trial of donor human milk or preterm formula as supplements to mothers' own milk for extremely premature infants. *Pediatr Res.* 2002;51:319A.
17. Pisacane A, Garziano L, Mazzarella G. Breastfeeding and diarrhea morbidity. *J Pediatr.* 1992;120:87-89.
18. Arnon SS. Infant botulism: anticipating the second decade. *J Infec Dis.* 1986;154:201-206.

19. Hahn-Zoric M, Silfverdal S, Bodin L, et al. Long term enhancement of the IgG2 antibody response to Haemophilus influenzae type b by breast-feeding. *Pediatr Infect Dis J.* 2002;21:816-821.
20. Furman L, Taylor G, Minich N, et al. The effect of maternal milk on neonatal morbidity of very low-birthweight infants. *Arch Pediatr Adolesc Med.* 2003;157:66-71.
21. Schanler RJ, Shulman RJ, Lau C. Feeding strategies for premature infants: beneficial outcomes of feeding fortified human milk vs preterm formula. *Pediatrics.* 1999;103:1150-1157.
22. Ronnestad A, Abrahamsen TG, Medbo S, et al. Late-onset septicemia in a Norwegian national cohort of extremely premature infants receiving very early full human milk feeding. *Pediatrics.* 2005;115:e269-e276.
23. Chen A, Rogan WJ. Breastfeeding and the risk of postneonatal death in the United States. *Pediatrics.* 2004;113:e435-e439.
24. Bahl R, Frost C, Kirkwood BR, et al. Infant feeding patterns and risks of death and hospitalization in the first half of infancy: multicentre cohort study. *Bull World Health Organ.* 2005;83:418-426.
25. Gdalevich M, Mimouni D, David M. Breast-feeding and the onset of atopic dermatitis in childhood: a systematic review and meta-analysis of prospective studies. *J Am Acad Dermatol.* 2001;45:520-527.
26. Gdalevich M, Mimouni D, Mimouni M. Breast-feeding and the risk of bronchial asthma in childhood: asystematic review with meta-analysis of prospective studies. *J Pediatr.* 2001;139:261-266.
27. Gerstein HC. Cow's milk exposure and type I diabetes mellitus. *Diabetes Care.* 1994;17:13-19.
28. Owen CG, Martin RM, Whincup PH. Does breastfeeding influence risk of type 2 diabetes in later life? A quantitative analysis of published evidence. *Am J Clin Nutr.* 2006;84:1043-1054.
29. Taylor JS, Kacmar JE, Nothnagle M. A systematic review of the literature associating breastfeeding with type 2 diabetes and gestational diabetes. *J Am Coll Nutr.* 2005;24:320-326.
30. Harder T, Bergmann R, Kallischnigg G, et al. Duration of breastfeeding and risk of overweight: a meta-analysis. *Am J Epidemiol.* 2005;162:397-403.
31. Owen CG, Martin RM, Whincup PH, et al. Effect of infant feeding on the risk of obesity across the life course: a quantitative review of published evidence. *Pediatrics.* 2005;115:1367-1377.
32. Arenz S, Ruckerl R, Koletzko B, et al. Breast-feeding and childhood obesity—systematic review. *Int J Obesity.* 2004;28:1247-1256.
33. Owen CG, Whincup PH, Odoki K, et al. Infant feeding and blood cholesterol: a study in adolescents and a systematic review. *Pediatrics.* 2002;110:597-608.
34. Anderson JW, Johnstone BM, Remley DT. Breastfeeding and cognitive development: a meta-analysis. *Am J Clin Nutr.* 1999;70:525-535.
35. Bernier MO, PluBureau G, Bossard N. Breastfeeding and risk of breast cancer: a metaanalysis of published studies. *Hum Reprod Update.* 2000;6:374-386.
36. Collaborative Group on Hormonal Factors in Breast Cancer. Breast cancer and breastfeeding: collaborative reanalysis of individual data from 47 epidemiological studies in 30 countries, including 50,302 women with breast cancer and 96,973 women without the disease. *Lancet.* 2002;360:187-195.
37. American Academy of Pediatrics, Committee on Drugs. The transfer of drugs and other chemicals into human milk. *Pediatrics.* 2001;108:776-789.

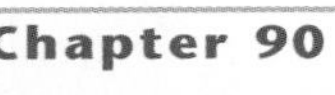

Chapter 90

BREASTFEEDING: DRUGS, HERBS, AND ENVIRONMENTAL TOXINS

Ruth Lawrence, MD

Although the notion that all medications taken by a lactating woman appear in her milk has often been stated, this is not correct. Knowledge of the pharmacologic mechanism of a given drug in general and its potential for crossing the mammary membranes in particular provides a more accurate assessment. Several reliable resources are available for obtaining specific information about a specific drug.[1-5] The American Academy of Pediatrics Committee on Drugs provides a report on drugs in human milk, which has been updated intermittently since 1985. In addition, research is being conducted on milk levels for several drugs. When specific information is not available, an estimation of the probability that the drug can reach the milk can be made by reviewing the molecular size, solubility, pH, protein binding, peak plasma time, half-life, and activity of metabolites. The drug information provided in the packaging insert and the *Physicians Desk Reference* are not good sources of information about safety of medications ingested during lactation. Several rating systems for drugs in human milk have been developed and are listed in Box 90-1.

Some generalizations can be made about drugs based on their properties. Items are passed into the milk via five general pathways: (1) by exocytosis, (2) via the fat globule, (3) as ions across the apical membrane, (4) by pinocytosis-exocytosis of immunoglobulins, and (5) via the paracellular pathway. Large molecules such as insulin or heparin do not pass. Drugs with an alkaline base are attracted across the membrane because human milk is slightly acidic (pH 7.0), whereas acidic drugs are not attracted across the membrane and are thus not actively transported. Some chemicals, such as iodine, are actively pumped across the membrane; therefore levels in milk are higher than levels in plasma. Drugs that are highly protein bound do not readily pass. When assessing the risk of a particular drug, factors that affect the infant must also be taken into account. Can the infant absorb the drug in food—that is, is it bioavailable orally? Can the infant metabolize and excrete the drug? The answer depends on the infant's gestational age, chronologic age, feeding pattern, and exclusivity of breastfeeding. An accurate assessment of any drug during lactation cannot be made with knowing the age of the infant. If a question exists about the safety of a drug, then the answer for the mother lies in its risk-benefit ratio. What is the risk of the drug versus the benefit of the child being breastfed?

The total amount of drug available to the infant through the milk also depends on the excretion curve of the drug and the infant's feeding schedule. Drugs are not stored in the breast. Milk always exists in the

BOX 90-1 Safety Ratings for Drugs During Breastfeeding

AMERICAN ACADEMY OF PEDIATRICS

- Drugs that are contraindicated during breastfeeding
- Drugs of abuse that are contraindicated during breastfeeding
- Radioactive compounds that require temporary cessation of breastfeeding
- Drugs that have unknown effects on nursing infants but may be of concern
- Drugs that have been associated with significant effects on some nursing infants and should be provided to nursing mothers with caution
- Maternal medication usually compatible with breastfeeding
- Food and environmental agents that have an effect on breastfeeding

HALE SCORING SYSTEM

- L1, safest
- L2, safer
- L3, moderately safe
- L4, possibly hazardous
- L5, contraindicated

WEINER CODE OF BREASTFEEDING SAFETY

- S, safe
- NS, not safe
- U, unknown

From Lawrence RA, Lawrence RM. *Breastfeeding: A Guide for the Medical Profession.* 6th ed. Philadelphia, PA: Elsevier; 2005. Copyright © Elsevier, 2005. Used by permission.

lactating breast in some amount because completely emptying the breast is impossible. The amount of drug in the milk depends on the amount in the maternal plasma during a feeding; therefore feedings can be scheduled to avoid peak plasma times. In the case of rapidly clearing substances such as alcohol, the feeding can be briefly postponed until the alcohol has cleared the maternal plasma. Experts usually suggest that a mother take her medication right after a feeding. In the case of medications taken once a day that have a long-delayed or prolonged peak plasma time, such as selective serotonin reuptake inhibitors, the medication should be taken when the infant is anticipated to sleep the longest (ie, the longest time between feedings). Drugs taken daily reach a steady state, but avoiding feeding during peak plasma times can decrease the infant's exposure.

When a drug is found in the milk and is of concern, but the drug is only being taken temporarily, the mother can be instructed to pump and discard the milk until the drug clears. The total time to clearance is calculated as five times the half-life of the drug.

PRESCRIBED DRUGS

Antibiotics are one of the most common medications mothers are prescribed. They all pass in some degree into milk. In general, if the antibiotic would be administered directly to a premature infant or a neonate, then it is safe for the mother to take during breastfeeding. A question arises when sulfa drugs are provided because they compete for albumin-binding sites. Until bound and unbound bilirubin can be measured clinically, sulfa drugs should not be administered during lactation in a jaundiced infant younger than 1 month because the amount of free bilirubin available to cross into the brain would be unmeasurable. Infants with glucose-6-phosphate disease should not be exposed to sulfa drugs at any time. Erythromycin appears in higher amounts in the milk than in the plasma; if provided intravenously to the mother, then the levels in milk are 10 times higher. After 1 month of age, administering erythromycin directly to the infant is usually safe. Another concern with erythromycin is the risk of cross-reaction with other drugs, such as carbimazole, cyclosporin, digoxin, triazolam, theophylline, and anticoagulants.

Aminoglycosides are poorly absorbed orally; therefore they are provided parentally. The infant does not absorb aminoglycosides from the milk because they are not orally bioavailable. Although the long-term presence of aminoglycosides in the milk can sterilize the neonatal gut, most breastfed infants will be quickly recolonized with *Lactobacillus*.

Although metronidazole (Flagyl) has been controversial, it is now provided directly to neonates. Metronidazole is not well absorbed in creams and gels used for local therapy; accordingly these substances are not an issue during lactation.

Although the American Academy of Pediatrics policy describing the effects of certain drugs in human breast milk includes well-known compounds such as methotrexate,[2] some of the newer anticancer drugs have considerably shorter half-lives. This characteristic translates to shorter clearance times; therefore women who need to start their cancer therapy can continue to breastfeed and pump and discard their milk until the drug clears her plasma. Primary care physicians should research the drug and its schedule of treatments so that clearance time can be calculated.

HERBAL MEDICINE

Herbal medicine is the use of plants or plant parts in their natural state without chemical additives or processing. The term *natural* does not necessarily mean safe; many plants have toxic parts, including such common foods as the potato or tomato. The US Food and Drug Administration (FDA) does not control herbs. The FDA has, however, warned against some herbs such as ephedra and comfrey. For an herb to be sold in the United States, it must have the following warning on the label: "This product is not intended to diagnose, treat, or prevent any disease." Many herbs are known by hearsay and historic use but not by scientific study. Herbals, especially teas, have historically been used in perinatal care, but few placebo-controlled studies of their efficacy or safety have been conducted. Because no two roots or leaves or seeds contain the same amount of ingredient, dosing is variable, even with the same amount of plant by weight. Plants also contain many chemicals in addition to the

Table 90-1 Possible Ingredients and Effects of Mother's Milk Tea

PLANT	CONSTITUENTS	EFFECTS	TOXICITY
Fennel seed	Volatile oil, anisic acid	Weak diuretic stimulant	Central nervous system disturbances
Coriander seed	Volatile oil, coriandrol	Increases flow of saliva and gastric juice	—
Chamomile flower	Volatile oil, bitter glycoside	Sudorific, antispasmodic, used to lighten hair	Vomiting, vertigo
Lemongrass	Lemon flavor	—	—
Borage leaf	Volatile oil, tannin, mineral acids	Diuretic, sudorific, euphoric	Possible
Blessed thistle leaf	Volatile oil, bitter principle	Aperitif, galactogogue, diaphoretic	Strongly emetic
Star anise	Volatile oil, anethole, resin, tannin	Stimulant, mild expectorant	—
Comfrey leaf *(Symphytum officinale)*	Protein, vitamin B_{12}, tannin, allantoin, choline, pyrrolizidine alkaloids	Used as mucilage to knit bones, weak sedative, demulcent, astringent	Venoocclusive disease, hepatotoxic
Fenugreek seed (Greek hayseed, coffee substitute, natural dye)	Mucilage, trigonelline, physterols, celery flavor	Digestive tonic, galactogogue, uterine stimulant, reduces blood sugar	Hypoglycemia, can induce labor
Coffee plant	Volatile oil, caffeine, tannin	Stimulant, diuretic, coloring	Insomnia, restlessness
Blue cohosh	Saponin, glucoside that affects muscles	Oxytocic, potent, acts on voluntary and involuntary muscles	Irritant, causes pain in fingers and toes

From Lawrence RA, Lawrence RM. *Breastfeeding: A Guide for the Medical Profession.* 6th ed. Philadelphia, PA: Elsevier; 2005.

one identified as significant. St John's wort, which is taken for mild depression, contains 25 identifiable chemicals in addition to hypericin, which was once believed to be the active ingredient.

When herbal teas are used the method of preparation alters the potency. The amount of caffeine and theobromine in common household tea has been shown to vary depending on whether the tea is made with a tea bag, loose tea, or powder. Steeping increases the concentration. A popular tea is promoted as mother's milk tea, but it may contain some potent herbals. Table 90-1 lists some possible constituents in mother's milk tea.

Galactagogues are widely used when the mother's milk supply falters. Fenugreek *(Trigonella foenum graecum)* was used by the ancient Egyptians. Fenugreek is a member of the Leguminoseae family, which includes peanuts and chickpeas, and it thus carries the same risk of allergy, including exacerbation of asthma in the mother and colic-like symptoms in the infant. Fenugreek is used as artificial maple syrup, and the mother will note that her secretions (milk, tears, and urine) and her baby will smell of maple syrup. The active ingredient appears to work for some women but not others. Fenugreek is generally regarded as safe by the FDA. Fenugreek's other effects include lowering blood sugar and cholesterol levels. It is sometimes taken for months without apparent ill effect.

Fennel seed *(Foeniculum vulgare)* is a common flavoring or spice that has some estrogenic properties. Although it is promoted as a galactogue, this designation is counterintuitive because estrogen suppresses lactation. The seeds are usually steeped for tea, but oil of fennel is highly toxic and should not be used.

Milk thistle *(Silybum marianum)* also has a reputation as a galactogogue, although with no scientific evidence. It is consumed as a tea two to three times a day. Other herbs used as galactagogues include anise, cumin, raspberry leaf, caraway, dill, and coriander. These herbs are usually taken as a steeped tea in combination with several herbs.

Herbs that suppress lactation include sage, peppermint, parsley, and even the same raspberry leaf used to stimulate supply. They are traditionally used when the child is being weaned and for the mother with an abundant milk supply that chokes her infant in the first few weeks.

For relief of engorgement, cabbage leaves have long been used. In controlled studies compared with ice packs, cabbage leaves have been found to be equally effective and considerably more comfortable. The whole leaves of a white cabbage are placed around the engorged breast until they wilt; new leaves can be applied if necessary. A poultice made of grated raw potato is also known to be effective when spread on the engorged breast. It must be rinsed off before feeding.

Some herbs have a pleasant flavor, lack known toxic properties, and provide a source of fluids for the lactating woman. These herbs include chicory (a caffeine-free coffee substitute), orange spice, and rose hips, the latter two of which contain vitamin C. Any food or drink should be consumed in moderation.

Obtaining accurate clinical information about herbals is difficult because so few blinded, randomized, controlled studies that use herbal preparations have been conducted. Dozens of books extol the benefits of herbals based on experience and historical use; the

Table 90-2 Herbal Medicine and Other Dietary Supplement–Related Sites on the Internet

ORGANIZATION	INTERNET ADDRESS	SITE INFORMATION
Center for Food Safety and Applied Nutrition, Food and Drug Administration	vm.cfsan.fda.gov/~dms/supplmnt.html	Clinicians should use this site to report adverse events associated with herbal medicines and other dietary supplements. Sections also contain safety, industry, and regulatory information.
National Center for Complementary and Alternative Medicine, National Institutes of Health	nccam.nih.gov/	This site contains fact sheets about alternative therapies, consensus reports, and databases.
Agricultural Research Service, United States Department of Agriculture	www.ars-grin.gov/duke/	The site contains an extensive phytochemical database with search capabilities.
Quackwatch	www.quackwatch.com/	Although this site addresses all aspects of health care, a considerable amount of information covering complementary and herbal therapies is provided.
National Council Against Health Fraud	www.ncahf.org/	This site focuses on health fraud with a position paper on over-the-counter herbal remedies.
HerbMed	www.herbmed.org/	This site contains information on over 120 herbal medications, with evidence for activity, warnings, preparations, mixtures, and mechanisms of action. Short summaries of important research publications with links to Medline are provided.
ConsumerLab	www.consumerlab.com/	This site is maintained by a corporation that conducts independent laboratory investigations of dietary supplements and other health products.

From Lawrence RA, Lawrence RM. *Breastfeeding: A Guide for the Medical Profession.* 6th ed. Philadelphia, PA: Elsevier; 2005.

best ones provide not only the anticipated benefits, but also the possible side effects. Table 90-2 lists Web sites that may be consulted for information about herbal medicine.

Part of a complete history for any patient, but especially those during lactation, is to inquire about the patient's use of herbal teas, capsules, or salves. The apparent medical problem can sometimes be solved by discontinuing such self-medication.

ENVIRONMENTAL TOXINS

Human milk contaminated with environmental toxins has come to public attention because of extensive press reports on the levels of certain environmental toxins in the milk of women in specific regions. These data were collected as part of a program set-up to monitor environmental toxins geographically for public health reasons. Human milk was targeted not because it was seriously contaminated, but because it is easily collected, it is continually replenished, and it is easy to analyze compared with other body fluids. However, this project had a negative effect on the public's view of the safety of human milk.

From a practical point of view, the environmental toxins of concern are persistent organochlorine compounds and the elements mercury, lead, cadmium, and silicon.

Organochlorine Compounds

The organochlorine compounds are pesticides. Within this group are the classic pesticides dichlorodiphenyltrichloroethane (DDT), hexachlorobenzene, dieldrin, hexachlorocyclohexane, and synthetic oils made from polychlorinated biphenyls, as well as polychlorinated dioxins and furans. Most of these pesticides have been discontinued; DDT has not been produced in this country since 1970. Carbamates, organophosphates, and pyrethroids are used instead. Although these substances are more toxic, they do not persist or accumulate in nature.

The safety levels for organochlorine compounds in mother's milk have been determined as an acceptable intake for the mother and child. The World Health Organization (WHO) has defined *acceptable levels* in terms of international 2,3,7,8-tetrachlorodibenzo-p-dioxin (TCDD) equivalents (TEq), or 1 to 4 pg per 1 TEq/kg/day. The Environmental Protection Agency allows 0.1 pg per 1 TEq/kg/day. The average contamination of human milk with persistent organochlorines apparently does not have negative effects and is exceeded by exposure in utero.

Elements

Mercury contamination from dental amalgam does not lead to high levels in human milk. Consumption of fish that is highly contaminated with mercury should be avoided during lactation. Canned tuna should be limited to once a week. Light tuna has less mercury than white albacore.

Lead exposure during lactation has been well studied. Levels of lead in human milk are not measurable until the maternal plasma levels exceed 40 mcg/L. Thus breastfeeding does not endanger the infant until the mother's levels are high.

Cadmium concentrations of 6 to 12 mcg/L were measured in mother's milk in Germany, but levels vary from country to country. Smoking and second-hand smoke affect cadmium levels. The WHO considers an acceptable intake value of cadmium for adults to be 1 mcg/kg. Toxic effects are unlikely, and no toxic effects have been described through mother's milk.

Silicon is ubiquitous. Silicon from breast implants has not been proven to cause real disease. Silicon is found in many common medicines, such as antacids. Exposure can be from many sources other than implants.

RELATED WEB SITES

- Agricultural Research Service, United States Department of Agriculture (www.ars-grin.gov/duke/).
- Dietary Supplements, Center for Food Safety and Applied Nutrition, US Food and Drug Administration (vm.cfsan.fda.gov/~dms/supplmnt.html/).
- Consumer Lab (www.consumerlab.com/).
- HerbMedicine (www.herbmed.org/).
- National Center for Complementary and Alternative Medicine, National Institutes of Health (nccam.nih.gov/).
- National Council Against Health Fraud (www.ncahf.org/).
- Quackwatch (www.quackwatch.com/).

AAP POLICY STATEMENTS

American Academy of Pediatrics, Committee on Drugs. The transfer of drugs and other chemicals into human milk. *Pediatrics*. 2001;108(3):776-789. (aappolicy.aappublications.org/cgi/content/full/pediatrics;108/3/776).

American Academy of Pediatrics, Section on Breastfeeding. Breastfeeding and the use of human milk. *Pediatrics*. 2005;115(2):496-506. (aappolicy.aappublications.org/cgi/content/full/pediatrics;115/2/496).

SUGGESTED RESOURCES

Berlin CM, Kacew S, Lawrence R, et al. Criteria for chemical selection for programs on human milk surveillance and research for environmental chemicals. *J Toxicol Environ Health A*. 2002;65;1839.

Berlin CM, LaKind JS, Sonawane BR, et al. Conclusions, research needs, and recommendations of the expert panel: technical workshop on human milk surveillance and research for environmental chemicals in the United States. *J Toxicol Environ Health A*. 2002;65;1929.

Briggs GG, Freeman RK, Yaffe SJ. *Drugs in Pregnancy and Lactation*. 7th ed. Philadelphia, PA: Lippincott Williams & Wilkins; 2005.

Humphrey S. *The Nursing Mother's Herbal*. Minneapolis, MN: Fairview Press; 2003.

LaKind JS, Berlin CM. Technical workshop on human milk surveillance and research on environmental chemicals in the United States: an overview. *J Toxicol Environ Health A*. 2002;65;1829.

Lawrence RA, Lawrence RM. *Breastfeeding: A Guide for the Medical Profession*. 6th ed. Philadelphia, PA: Elsevier; 2005.

Physician's Desk Reference for Herbal Medicines. 2nd ed. Montvale, NJ: Medical Economics; 2000.

Tyler VE. *The New Honest Herbal*. Philadelphia, PA: Stickly; 1999.

Weiner CP, Buhimschi C. *Drugs for Pregnancy and Lactating Women*. New York, NY: Churchill-Livingston; 2004.

REFERENCES

1. Gartner LM, Morton J, Lawrence RA, et al, and the American Academy of Pediatrics, Section on Breastfeeding. Breastfeeding and the use of human milk. *Pediatrics*. 2005; 115;496-506.
2. American Academy of Pediatrics, Committee on Drugs. Transfer of drugs and other chemicals into human milk. *Pediatrics*. 2001;108;776-789.
3. Hale TW. *Medications and Mother's Milk*. 12th ed. Amarillo, TX: Hale Publishing; 2006.
4. Lawrence RA, Lawrence RM. *Breastfeeding: A Guide for the Medical Profession*. 6th ed. Philadelphia, PA: Elsevier; 2005.
5. National Institutes of Health, National Library of Medicine. Drugs and Lactation Database (LactMed). Available at: www.nlm.nih.gov/pubs/factsheets/lactmedfs.html. Accessed August 9, 2007.

Chapter 91

CIRCUMCISION

Jack T. Swanson, MD

Circumcision is the oldest planned surgical procedure (dating back 6000 years in Egypt) and the most common operation performed in males in the United States (over 1 million annually).[1,2] Neonatal circumcision is also one of the most controversial procedures, with some advocates strongly believing that the medical evidence indicates that all male infants should undergo the procedure as a preventive health measure, whereas others passionately believing that the foreskin has its own benefits, and circumcision should be considered only when an individual has reached an age to make his own informed decision.

RATES OF CIRCUMCISION

The incidence of neonatal circumcision in the United States is estimated by hospital discharge statistics to be 61% to 65%, although rates are significantly higher in many areas of the country (greater than 80%).[3,4] Rates vary among racial and ethnic groups, with whites and blacks higher than Hispanics, and are higher among newborns born in the Northwest or Midwest, in rural locations, and in families of higher socioeconomic status.[1,4] Significant differences also exist in other countries of the world, with a lower incidence in Canada and Australia and much lower (less than 5%) in most of Europe, Asia, and South and Central America.[1,2] Cultural and religious reasons can also be found for circumcision (>95% incidence in Jewish and Islamic faiths).[1]

RECOMMENDATIONS

The American Academy of Pediatrics (AAP) has issued recommendations regarding neonatal circumcision since 1971, with the most recent policy statement written in 1999 and reaffirmed in 2005.[5,6] In 1989, reports noted the existence of potential medical benefits (especially prevention of urinary tract infections [UTIs] in the first year and penile cancer), as well as risks.[7] In 1999, an evidence-based review concluded that although potential medical benefits exist, the data are not sufficient to recommend routine neonatal circumcision for all male infants. That parents should be informed regarding the benefits and risks and should make an informed decision is acknowledged, and taking into account cultural, religious, and ethnic traditions, in addition to medical factors, is legitimate when making this choice.[5] Medical societies in other countries (Australia and Canada) have issued recommendations that do not recommend routine circumcision of male newborns.[1,5]

PROCEDURES

Circumcision in the newborn period should only be performed when the infant is stable and healthy and has urinated. Three devices are commonly used for the procedure: (1) the Gomco clamp, (2) the Mogan clamp, and (3) the PlastiBell (see Appendix B, Special Procedures for details). Contradictions to circumcision include hypospadius and other anomalies of the penis (which may require the foreskin for reconstruction), prematurity, neonatal illness, and bleeding dyscrasias or a family history of bleeding disorders. Should circumcision be performed after the newborn period (the first few weeks of life), then general anesthesia is often required, and a more extensive surgical procedure is necessary. Indications include recurrent balanitis, severe phimosis, and paraphimosis.

Complications

Complication rates for newborn circumcision are estimated to be between 0.2% and 0.6%, and these complications are usually minor.[2,5] Bleeding and infection are the most frequent. Uncommonly, postcircumcision phimosis, urethral fistula, unsatisfactory cosmesis, concealed glans, meatitis, urinary retention, skin bridges, and glans injury may occur. Rare reports include sepsis, meningitis, necrotizing fasciitis, and penile necrosis. Circumcision beyond the newborn period also has the additional risk of general anesthesia.

Pain Relief

Considerable evidence exists that infants undergoing circumcision without analgesia experience pain and stress. This evidence has been demonstrated by observing changes in physiological responses, including heart rate, blood pressure, oxygen saturation, and cortisol levels.[1,5] The AAP recommends that procedural analgesia be provided when neonatal circumcision is performed.[5] Several methods of analgesia can be used. The most effective analgesics are the dorsal penile nerve block and the subcutaneous ring block, both using injected 1% lidocaine that may be buffered with sodium bicarbonate. Bruising or hematomas are the most frequent complications, although allergic reactions, intravascular injections, and compromise to the blood supply are rare problems. Eutectic mixture of local anesthetics (EMLA cream, 2.5% lidocaine, and 2.5% prilocaine) also attenuates pain but requires application 45 to 60 minutes before the procedure and is not as effective as the nerve or ring blocks.[8] Prilocaine may produce methemaglobinemia, although the risk is very low. Sucrose (24%) given orally during the procedure (via syringe or pacifier) may offer additional benefit as well as acetaminophen in the postoperative period, although these measures are not adequate by themselves.[9-11] Firm but gentle positioning and restraining by a nurse or assistant or the use of a padded chair is less stressful than use of a rigid board.[9]

CIRCUMCISION DEBATE

Proponents of neonatal circumcision state that the benefits include reducing the risk for UTI in the first year, penile cancer, HIV and sexually transmitted infections (STIs), and phimosis, paraphimosis, and balanophosthitis.[12,13] Additionally, improved penile hygiene is suggested. Opponents point to anecdotal reports regarding decreased penile sensation and sexual satisfaction in circumcised men and their partners, although no scientific studies have been conducted that can conclusively substantiate that any significant difference exists.[1]

Circumcision and Urinary Tract Infection

Multiple studies have examined the association between UTI and circumcision status, and all studies have shown an increased risk of UTI in uncircumcised boys and men, especially in infants younger than 1 year. Results vary because of differences in methods used, samples of infants studied, methods of urine collected, and confounding variables (eg, breastfeeding, prematurity). The numbers estimate that 7 to 14 per 1000 uncircumcised infants will develop a UTI in the first year, compared with 1 to 2 per 1000 circumcised infants.[5] Although the relative risk is increased 4- to 10-fold, the absolute risk is low (at most 1%). Additionally, after the first year of life the frequency of UTI in boys and men is much lower. A possible biological explanation exists for this increased incidence, that being an increased colonization of uropathogenic organisms in the urethra and on the periurethral glans during the first 6 months of life in uncircumcised boys and men.[14]

Circumcision and Penile Cancer

Circumcision has been shown to decrease the risk for penile cancer in adulthood, with at least a 3-fold risk in uncircumcised men, although this cancer is rare in the United States (approximately 1 case per 100,000 men).[5] Phimosis increases the risk and occurs only in uncircumcised men.

Hygiene Issues

Phimosis, paraphimosis, balanitis, and inflammation of the foreskin are penile problems that are seen in uncircumcised boys and men and increase with age. Circumcised infants have a higher rate of meatitis than uncircumcised infants. Appropriate penile hygiene can decrease the incidence of phimosis and foreskin irritation. Although circumcision is often promoted as a means of improving penile hygiene, satisfactory cleanliness can be obtained in uncircumcised infants, children, and adults. The AAP has produced a fact sheet, *Care of the Uncircumcised Penis,* which discusses proper care of the foreskin.[15]

Circumcision and Sexually Transmitted Infections

Association between circumcision status and the acquisition of HIV has been increasingly noted by multiple studies, especially in heterosexual populations in Africa.[16-18] The effect is greater in high-risk groups than the general population and locations where HIV is predominately heterosexually transmitted and may be difficult to generalize to the US population. Theories for the association include viral attachment to lymphoid cells in the mucosal surface of the foreskin, an increased susceptibility to trauma of the foreskin during sexual activity, and a greater association of HIV with ulcerative sexually transmitted disease lesions.[19] Studies have also demonstrated a reduction in other STIs, especially sexually transmitted genital ulcer disease, although the issue is complex and opinions are conflicting.[5,20,21] Additionally, cancer of the cervix (human papilloma virus) and HIV transmission to women has been noted to decrease in populations in which circumcision rates are high.[22,23] Continued evaluation of these and future studies will be important for further recommendations regarding circumcision both in the United States and in other areas of the world. An important point to stress is that circumcision alone should not be a reason to lessen the practice of safe sex measures.

CONCLUSION

Because parents need to make an important decision for their male infant, including providing informed consent, a complete discussion of the potential medical benefits and the risks for circumcision needs to be provided. This discussion should ideally take place in the prenatal visit or classes and in a completely unbiased manner. Written materials can be provided, including the AAP brochure *Circumcision: Information For Parents*.[24] The importance of analgesia for the procedure should be stressed, and parents are encouraged to request this for their boys if they choose a circumcision. Additionally, the AAP strongly opposes the practice of female circumcision at any age.[24]

TOOLS FOR PRACTICE

Engaging Patient and Family

- *Care of the Uncircumcised Penis* (fact sheet), American Academy of Pediatrics (www.aap.org/bookstore).
- *Circumcision: Information for Parents* (brochure), American Academy of Pediatrics (patiented.aap.org).

Medical Decision Support

- *Trends in Circumcisions Among Newborns* (fact sheet), Centers for Disease Control and Prevention (www.cdc.gov/nchs/products/pubs/pubd/hestats/circumcisions/circumcisions.htm).

AAP POLICY STATEMENT

American Academy of Pediatrics Task Force on Circumcision. Circumcision policy statement. *Pediatrics*. 1999; 103(3):686-693 (aappolicy.aappublications.org/cgi/content/full/pediatrics;103/3/686).

REFERENCES

1. Lerman SE, Liao JC. Neonatal circumcision. *Pediatr Clin North Am*. 2001;48:1539-1557.
2. Niku DN, Stock JA, Kaplan GW. Neonatal circumcision. *Urol Clin North Am*. 1995;22:57-65.
3. Centers for Disease Control and Prevention. Trends in Circumcision Among Newborns. 2006; Available at: www.cdc.gov/nchs/products/pubs/pubd/hestats/circumcisions/circumcisions.htm. Accessed July 6, 2007.
4. Nelson CP, Dunn R, Wan J, et al. The increasing incidence of newborn circumcision: data from the nationwide inpatient sample. *J Urol*. 2005;173:978-981.
5. American Academy of Pediatrics, Task Force on Circumcision. Circumcision policy statement. *Pediatrics*. 1999; 103:686-693.
6. American Academy of Pediatrics. AAP publications retired and reaffirmed. *Pediatrics*. 2005;116:796.
7. American Academy of Pediatrics. Report of the Task Force on Circumcision. *Pediatrics*. 1989:84:388-391.
8. Butler-O'Hara M, LeMoine C, Guillet R. Analgesia for neonatal circumcision: a randomized controlled trial of EMLA cream versus dorsal penile nerve block. *Pediatrics*. 1998;101:e5.
9. Stang HJ, Snellman LW, Condon LM, et al. Beyond dorsal penile nerve block: a more humane circumcision. *Pediatrics*. 1997;100(2):e3.
10. Blass EM, Hoffmeyer LB. Sucrose as an analgesic for newborn infants. *Pediatrics*. 1991;87:215-218.
11. Howard CR, Howard FM, Weitzman ML. Acetaminophen analgesia in neonatal circumcision: the effect on pain. *Pediatrics*. 1994;93:614-646.
12. Schoen EJ, Wiswell TE, Moses S. New policy on circumcision—cause for concern. *Pediatrics*. 2000;105:620-623.
13. Schoen EJ. Ignoring evidence of circumcision benefits. *Pediatrics*. 2006;118:385-387.
14. Wiswell TE, Miller GM, Gelston HM, et al. Effect of circumcision status on periurethral bacterial flora during the first year of life. *J Pediatr*. 1988;113;442-446.
15. American Academy of Pediatrics. *Care of the Uncircumcised Penis*. Elk Grove Village, IL: American Academy of Pediatrics; 2000.
16. Halperin, DT, Bailey, RC. Male circumcision and HIV infection: 10 years and counting. *Lancet*. 1999;1813-1815.
17. Weiss HA, Quigley MA, Hayes RJ. Male circumcision and risk of HIV infection in sub-Saharan Africa: a systematic review and meta-analysis. *AIDS*. 2000;14:2361-2370.
18. Auvert B, Taljaard D, Lagarde E, et al. Randomized, controlled intervention trial of male circumcision for reduction of HIV infection risk, The ANRS 1265 Trial. *PLoS Med*. 2005;2:1112-1122.
19. Patterson BK, Landay A, Siegel JN, et al. Susceptibility to human immunodeficiency virus-1 infection of human foreskin and cervical tissue grown in explant culture. *Am J Pathol*. 2002;161:867-873.
20. Fergusson DM, Boden JM, Horwood J. Circumcision status and risk of sexually transmitted infection in young adult males: an analysis of a longitudinal birth cohort. *Pediatrics*. 2006;118:1971-1977.
21. Weiss HA, Thomas SL, Munabi SK, et al. Male circumcision and risk of syphilis, chancroid, and genital herpes: as systematic review and meta-analysis. *Sex Transm Infect*. 2006;82:101-110.
22. Castellsague X, Bosch FX, Munoz N, et al. Male circumcision, penile human papillomavirus infection, and cervical cancer in female parents. *N Engl J Med*. 2002;346:1105-1112.
23. Quinn TC, Wawer MJ, Sewankambe N, et al. Viral load and heterosexual transmission of human immunodeficiency virus type 1. *N Engl J Med*. 2000;342:921-928.

24. American Academy of Pediatrics. *Circumcision: Information for Parents*. Elk Grove Village, IL: American Academy of Pediatrics; 1999.

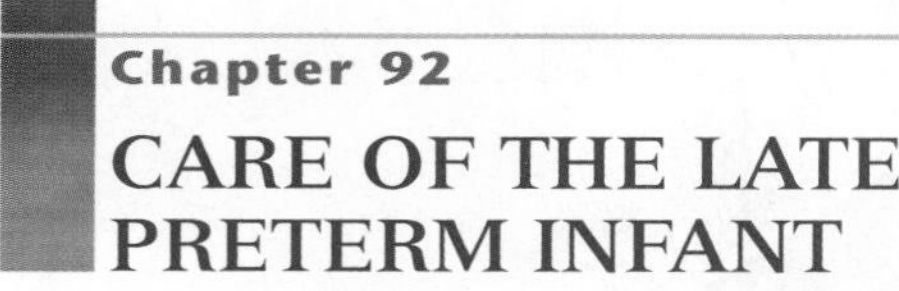

Chapter 92

CARE OF THE LATE PRETERM INFANT

Viral A. Dave, MD, DCH; Deborah E. Campbell, MD

INTRODUCTION

Prematurity continues to be an issue of major concern as the rate of preterm birth continues to rise. The significance of this change in birth demographics is the higher risk of morbidity and mortality among infants born early. In the United States alone, preterm birth accounts for over 500,000 infants born prematurely each year. Recent birth data from the National Center for Health Statistics Vital Statistics Report indicate that induction and cesarean delivery rates have increased, leading to a decline in the mean gestational age at delivery of 39 weeks (Figure 92-1). Postterm birth has also declined. Since 1990 the rate of preterm birth less than 37 weeks' gestation has risen dramatically from 10.6% to 12.7% in 2004. This increase in preterm birth has occurred among all racial and ethnic groups.[1] Shorter-than-normal gestation is the result, in part, of an increase in multiple births.[2] However, the increase in prematurity has occurred among singleton gestations as The National Vital Statistics Surveillance System continues to record an increasing rate of preterm birth for 2005 and 2006 among singleton and total pregnancies.

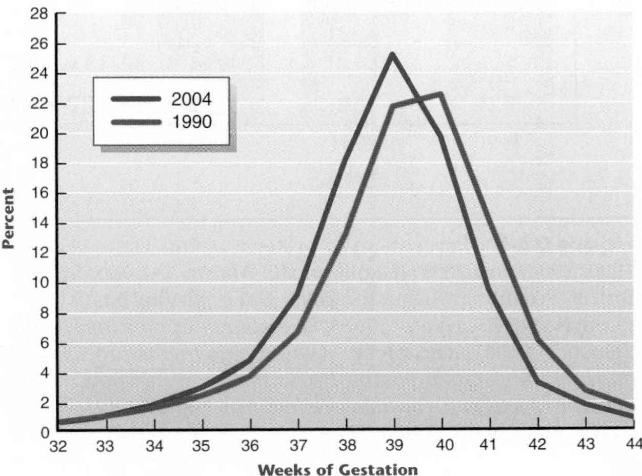

Figure 92-1 Percentage distribution births by gestational age (32-44 weeks): United States, 1990 and 2004. *(Martin JA, Hamilton BE, Sutton PD, et al.* Births: Final Data From 2004. National Vital Statistics Reports. *Vol. 55, no. 1. Hyattsville, MD: National Center for Health Statistics; 2006. Available at: www.cdc.gov/nchs/products/pubs/pubd/hestats/prelimbirths05.htm.)*

DEFINITIONS

Prematurity encompasses a broad range of infants born between 23 and 36 weeks' gestation. Within this large group of neonates, preterm babies can be grouped in categories based on their degree of immaturity. Previous convention described infants born before 28 weeks' gestation as extremely premature, whereas infants born before 32 weeks were classified as very preterm and infants born between 35 and 37 weeks were labeled near term. Recognition of the increased vulnerability associated with birth between 34 and 36 weeks' gestation and the variability in the terminology used to describe infants at different gestational and postnatal ages led to the publication of the American Academy of Pediatrics (AAP) Committee on Fetus and Newborn "Policy Statement: Age Terminology During the Perinatal Period,"[3] which defines the terms commonly used to describe the length of gestation and the age of the infant (chronologic, postmenstrual, and corrected age) (Figure 92-2). The National Institute for Child Health and Human Development during a 2005 Workshop on Optimizing Care and Long-term Outcome of Near-Term Pregnancy and Near-Term Newborn Infants (Bethesda, MD, July 18-19, 2005) refined the definition of late preterm birth to mean delivery from 34 0/7 to 36 6/7 weeks' gestation (239 to 259 days).[4]

MORBIDITY AND MORTALITY

Births between 34 and 36 weeks' gestation have increased more markedly than preterm births less than 34 weeks' gestation and now account for 71% of all premature births (Figure 92-3). In contrast, little change has occurred in the number of births between 32 and 33 weeks' gestation. Thirty-seven percent of preterm infants are born at 36 weeks' gestation. The distribution of preterm births among the remainder of babies born prematurely is 21% at 35 weeks' and 13%

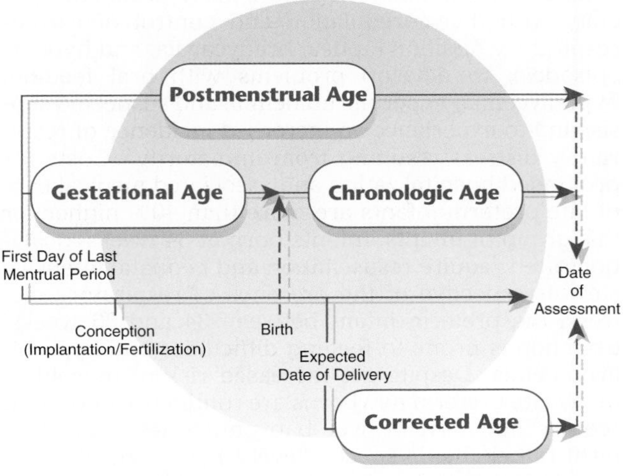

Figure 92-2 Age terminology during perinatal period.

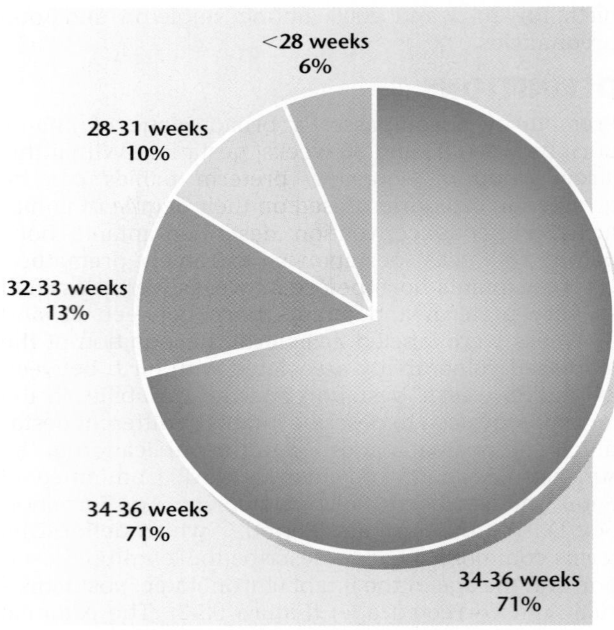

Figure 92-3 Percentage distribution preterm births, United States, 2004.

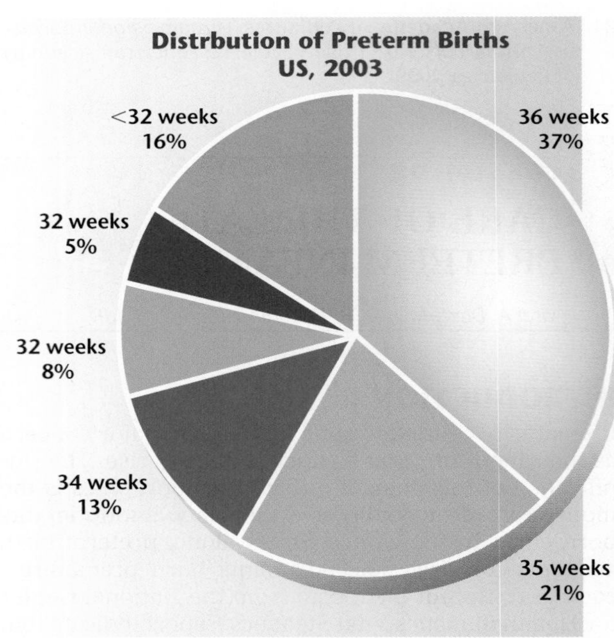

Figure 92-4 Distribution of preterm births by gestational age, United States, 2003.

at 34 weeks' gestation (Figures 92-4 and 92-5). As a group, late preterm infants experience greater mortality and morbidity than their full-term counterparts.[5] Deaths resulting from congenital malformations, immaturity, asphyxia, infection, and sudden infant death are 4 to 26 times higher among this group of babies than those born between 38 and 41 weeks' gestation. Late preterm infants represent 33% of total neonatal intensive care unit (NICU) admissions.[4] With increasing gestational maturity, the percentage of preterm infants requiring intensive care decreases. Estimates suggest that 50% of infants born at 34 weeks' gestation require NICU admission, in contrast to 15% of infants born at 35 weeks and 8% of babies at 36 weeks.[6,7]

Late preterm infants are more likely to exhibit difficulty with thermoregulation and control of cardiorespiratory function (apnea, bradycardia, and hypoxic episodes); to develop problems with oral feeding, hypoglycemia, hyperbilirubinemia, and suspected sepsis; and to experience an increased incidence of respiratory distress resulting from immaturity.[6] Costs for prolonged hospitalization and associated medical care of late preterm infants are more than 40% higher for this group of infants. Infants born at 34 weeks' gestation often require resuscitation and neonatal intensive care. Irrespective of the presence of respiratory distress, the preterm infant between 34 and 36 weeks' gestation is prone to feeding difficulties and hyperbilirubinemia. Despite the increased risk of morbidity, many late preterm newborns are routinely cared for in regular newborn or well-baby nurseries after their birth rather than a special (level II) or neonatal intensive (level III) care unit and are frequently discharged home at 2 to 3 days of age. The higher birth weights of these infants, often within the normal birth weight

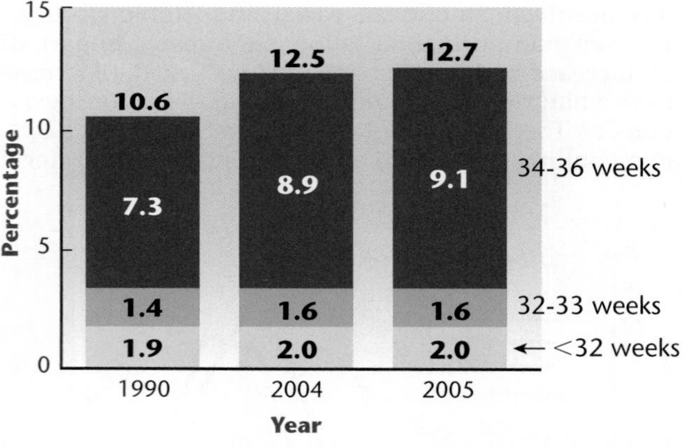

Figure 92-5 Percentage of preterm births: United States, 1990, 2004, and 2005. *(Hamilton BE, Martin JA, Ventura SJ.* Births: Preliminary Data for 2005. National Vital Statistics Reports. *Vol 55. Hyattsville, MD: National Center for Health Statistics; 2006. Available at: www.cdc.gov/nchs/products/pubs/pubd/hestats/prelimbirths05.htm; www.cdc.gov/nchs/products/pubs/hestats/prelimbirths05.htm#ref01. Accessed May 15, 2007.)*

range, over 2500 g, result in many late preterm infants being treated the same as their developmentally more mature full-term counterparts. The assumption that late preterm infants have similar risks as term infants is common. Transitional issues such as transient tachypnea of the newborn, cold stress, and hypoglycemia can be easily missed during the early hours after birth if particular attention is not paid these aspects of the transition.

The AAP-American College of Obstetrics and Gynecology[8] and the AAP Committee of Fetus and Newborn[9] specify that infants younger than 35 weeks' gestation should be cared for in a speciality nursery or NICU (level II or III neonatal unit). However, the variation in the actual scope of care within neonatal units presents a challenge to identifying best practices related to the optimal level of newborn care for the late preterm infant. Individual hospital policies and, in institutions in which regionalized perinatal health systems are in place, neonatal transfer policies currently guide when care for subsets of babies within this group occurs. The criteria determining whether an apparently healthy preterm may be cared for in a regular newborn nursery are based on the gestational age, birth weight, need for resuscitation, and transitional care.

The late preterm infant is also at increased risk for ongoing health and developmental problems. Approximately 7%-9% of newborns 34 to 36 weeks' gestation require rehospitalization within 14 days of nursery discharge.[7] The most common cause for readmission is hyperbilirubinemia. An important point to note is that late preterm newborns, particularly those between 35 to 36 weeks' gestation, are at risk for kernicterus as a complication of unrecognized and untreated hyperbilirubinemia. Less frequent, but still important, reasons for rehospitalization include dehydration and feeding difficulties, suspected sepsis, and prolonged or severe illness.[10,11] Infants born between 35 and 36 weeks' gestation account for 58% of preterm births and are reported to be four times more likely to be readmitted than a term baby, particularly if the newborn's age at discharge was less than 72 hours.[7,12]

HEALTH ISSUES INFLUENCING NURSERY CARE OF THE LATE PRETERM NEWBORN

Cold Stress and Hypothermia

Preterm newborns have an impaired ability to prevent heat loss and to increase their body heat production in response to low environmental temperatures. The risk of cold stress is greatest during the immediate transitional period after delivery and is caused by the preterm newborn's immature skin, the high ratio of surface area to birth weight, and the environmental conditions in the delivery room (large temperature gradients between the newborn's body temperature and the ambient temperature of delivery room, air flow through the room, and contact with cold surfaces that lead to significant evaporative, radiant, convective, and conductive heat losses). Wide variations in delivery room temperatures have been reported to have a significant effect on a newborn's temperature.[13,14] Approximately 50% of newborns experience some degree of cold stress after birth.

Oxidation of fatty acids is the predominant method of nonshivering heat production in newborns regardless of gestational age or birth weight. Brown fat, the major store of fatty acids in neonates, is located around the mediastinal structures, kidneys, scapulae, axillae, and nape of the neck. Cold exposure activates the sympathetic nervous system, releasing norepinephrine. Norepinephrine, in turn, stimulates the hydrolysis or breakdown of brown fat, with resultant heat production. Late preterm newborns have less brown fat in comparison with term infants. Consequently, they are more prone to develop cold stress and hypothermia. Normal core body temperature for a neonate is 36.5° to 37.4° C (97.7° to 99.3° F). Clinical manifestations of cold stress are nonspecific and may be misinterpreted as signs of sepsis. Common findings include tachypnea, peripheral vasoconstriction, pallor, mottling caused by vasomotor instability, and metabolic acidosis. Therefore maintaining thermoneutrality, keeping the newborn warm and dry while minimizing heat loss, and energy expenditure are important components of the preterm newborn's initial care.

Strategies to minimize heat loss include the following:

- Maintain the delivery room and all other patient care rooms at a temperature of 24° ±2° C (75° ±3° F) or 22° to 26° C (72°-78° F), with a humidity of 30% in the winter and 50% in the summer.[15,16]
- Rapidly dry the newborn after delivery.
- Cover the newborn's head with a hat to reduce heat loss.
- Initiate skin-to-skin contact with the mother to facilitate temperature regulation of the newborn.
- Place the newborn in an isolette when not skin-to-skin with the mother if the newborn is exhibiting difficulty maintaining the body temperature.

Respiratory Disorders and Respiratory Distress

Acute respiratory distress is the most common condition experienced by the late preterm newborn.[10,17-19] Neonates born between 34 and 36 weeks' gestation who exhibit respiratory distress after delivery are at increased risk for associated morbidities. These infants frequently require stabilization and treatments such as supplemental oxygen and assisted ventilation.[20] Late preterm newborns exhibit higher rates of low Apgar scores, transient tachypnea of the newborn (TTN), respiratory distress syndrome (RDS), persistent pulmonary hypertension, and respiratory failure. TTN and RDS are both common in the late preterm newborn and are related to delayed clearance of lung fluid, surfactant deficiency, or both. By one estimate, nearly one third of late preterm newborns will exhibit respiratory difficulties.[6] Late preterm male infants more often exhibit respiratory distress than late preterm girls. Neonates who are born by cesarean delivery before labor begins are at increased risk for respiratory distress. Labor initiates hormonal changes necessary for normal pulmonary transition and function. Hemodynamic instability caused by hypothermia or hypoglycemia may worsen the newborn's underlying respiratory distress.

Smooth respiratory transition is important to prevent respiratory distress. In utero, alveoli are filled with fluid that must clear during the initial transitional period for effective ventilation to be established. In addition, pulmonary blood flow to the lungs must increase to ensure effective pulmonary perfusion and adequate matching of perfusion and ventilation. A significant part of this process includes fluid clearance via transepithelial sodium absorption and through the mechanical *squeeze* and Starling forces that occur during the process of labor and vaginal delivery. Liquid is also driven through the pulmonary epithelium into the vasculature. Maturation and recruitment of epithelial sodium channels occur during the last few weeks of pregnancy in response to endogenous steroid and cathecholamine surges that are triggered by the onset of labor. Neonatal transition becomes difficult when the infant is born by cesarean delivery without spontaneous labor. Impaired function or inactivity of the sodium channel contributes to TTN and RDS. Although administering antenatal corticosteroids results in a significant reduction in mortality and morbidity caused by RDS in premature infants younger than 34 weeks' gestation, meta-analyses have not shown as dramatic benefit for infants older than 34 weeks' gestation, given that nearly 100 women presenting in preterm labor at this gestation would require treatment to prevent one case of RDS.[21] As a consequence, antenatal corticosteroids are not routinely used in the care of the woman in preterm labor or the woman who has a medical complication at 35 to 36 weeks' gestation that may necessitate early delivery.

Strategies to minimize the risk for respiratory morbidity include the following:

- Personnel skilled in the assessment, resuscitation, and stabilization of the preterm newborn should be present in the delivery room.
- Initial evaluation should include assessment of respiratory stability with consideration of early initiation of continuous positive airway pressure if respiratory distress is present; continuing respiratory care needs will be determined by the cause of the newborn's respiratory distress.
- Attention should be paid to maintaining thermoneutrality and glucose homeostasis to avoid additional morbidity that may prolong the newborn's physiological transition and respiratory signs.

The decision as to the site of care (regular newborn nursery versus a NICU) for the well-appearing late preterm newborn will depend on specific hospital policy and the newborn's gestational assessment. Many hospitals have policies that require the 34 weeks' gestational age newborn to be admitted to a transitional care nursery or a NICU; once the newborn completes the transitional period, shows no signs of respiratory or temperature instability, and demonstrates the ability to satisfactorily feed, the newborn may be transferred to a regular nursery to complete the required care.

Hypoglycemia

Prematurity, hypothermia, hypoxia, maternal diabetes, maternal glucose infusion in labor, and intrauterine growth restriction are each factors that contribute to the incidence of hypoglycemia. Hypoglycemia occurs more frequently in late preterm newborns than in term newborns as a result of decreased hepatic glycogen stores and delayed hepatic glucose 6-phosphatase dehydrogenase activity in response to hypoglycemia.[22-24]

The preterm newborn also has decreased availability of amino acids for gluconeogenesis and inadequate lipid stores for release of fatty acids and fat stores to maintain glucose balance. Feeding is less efficient in some late preterm infants than in term newborns because of easy fatigability and immature feeding skills. Limited enteral intake further complicates the newborn's initial transition, predisposing the late preterm newborn to hypoglycemia. Hypoglycemia has been reported to occur four to five times more frequently in newborns born at 35 to 36 weeks' gestation in comparison with infants born at term.[6] An important element of care in prevention of hypoglycemia in the late preterm newborn is appropriate risk assessment with glucose screening of babies at risk. (See Chapter 104, Common Metabolic Disturbances in the Newborn.) The late preterm newborn should be able to maintain the blood glucose level above 2.6 mmoL/L (47 mg/dL).

Strategies to minimize the risk for hypoglycemia include the following:

- Initiate early feedings to maintain glucose balance.
- Monitor glucose. Blood glucose levels should be monitored on nursery admission and every 1 to 3 hours thereafter based on the specific risk factors for a period of at least 3 to 6 hours after birth.
- Optimize enteral intake. Newborns with oral feeding difficulty should be gavage (tube) fed until effective oral feeding is achieved.
- Breastfeeding:
  - Allow feeding on demand with close attention to the newborn's state regulation and ability to express hunger cues.
  - Provide lactation consultation within 24 hours of birth.
  - The mother should initiate milk expression within 4 to 6 hours after delivery if the newborn is not able to nurse effectively.
- Provide supplemental feedings by bottle or gavage if the oral enteral intake is inadequate and the newborn exhibits excessive weight loss of greater than 10% or more than 3% per day.
- Consider increasing caloric density by feeding 22- to 24-cal/oz or fortifying expressed breast milk for newborns with excessive weight loss or persistently poor weight gain.

Risk of Infection

Late preterm infants are susceptible to infection, either congenital or acquired, because of immaturity of their immune system. (See Chapter 101, The Infant With Suspected Infection.) As a group, late preterm infants are nearly four times more likely to be evaluated for suspected sepsis than the full-term neonate and are more likely to be treated with a 7-day course of antibiotics.[6] This is related to the frequent presence of preterm birth risk factors that suggest infection. In addition, clinical signs suggestive of early systemic infection are common during the transitional period. These signs include respiratory distress, temperature instability, low tone, poor feeding, and, in some cases, evidence of hemodynamic instability.

Strategies to minimize morbidity related to infection risks include the following:

- Carefully review the maternal medical history and intrapartum course, including the administration of intrapartum antibiotics, to identify specific risk factors for infection and any treatments used to moderate infectious risks.

- Carefully monitor and thoroughly assess the infant for signs of infection, and initiate therapy as appropriate. Some hospitals use algorithms or practice guidelines based on the Centers for Disease Control and Prevention (CDC) Group B Streptococcal Disease Revised Guidelines.[25]
- Encourage early and exclusive breastfeeding, either by direct breastfeeding or the provision of expressed breast milk.

Feeding Tolerance

Maturation of the gastrointestinal tract is important not only for digestion and absorption, but for endocrine and exocrine function as well. Increases in the intestinal length and surface area including villus and microvillus growth occur during the last trimester. The majority of late preterm newborns are able to tolerate human milk and formula without difficulty despite these developmental differences. Although the late preterm newborn has low gastric acid secretion and limited pancreatic enzyme activity, preterm newborns are able to digest whole protein formulas.[26,27] Decreased bile acid secretion and enterohepatic circulation suggest that the late preterm infant might have difficulty digesting fats. However, a meta-analysis of studies comparing medium-chain triglyceride to long-chain triglyceride as the fat fed to preterm infants did not show a difference in weight gain.[28] Late preterm infants are able to digest carbohydrate despite lower lactase activity. Premature infants frequently have intestinal motor function immaturity that contributes to feeding intolerance. Intestinal dysmotility is typically present up to 34 weeks' gestation but may persist in some late preterm infants. Suck and swallow coordination is often poor before 34 weeks' gestation. Some infants may require a longer-than-normal interval between feedings because of a delay in motility and gastric emptying.

Human milk provides substantial benefits to premature infants' health. Human milk intake is associated with reduced infectious and inflammatory disease, enhanced neurodevelopmental outcome, and maintains healthy postnatal growth patterns. An important point to consider is the adequacy of the infant's intake and growth on the chosen feeding. Many late preterm infants have poor state regulation and are not able to demonstrate clear feeding cues properly. In addition, the strength and efficiency of the suck patterns and suck-swallow-breathing coordination may further impede successful oral feeding and contribute to excessive weight loss or poor weight gain. Little research has been conducted on specific feeding regimens for the late preterm infant. Most feeding recommendations are geared toward the low–birth-weight infant. Low birth weight, defined as a birth weight below 2500 g (5.5 lb), can be subgrouped into babies with a birth weight between 1501 and 2000 g (3.3 and 4.4 lb) or infants with a birth weight between 2001 and 2500 g (4.4 and 5 lb). Primary care physicians must assess the adequacy of caloric and nutrient intake and offer parents guidance. Decisions to be considered include:

1. Whether the breastfeeding infant requires supplementation as a result of excessive weight loss or inadequate weight gain
2. When appropriate, which formula should be used: a full term formula or an enriched post discharge preterm formula
3. If the late preterm infant is also small-for-gestational age (<5%), whether birth weight or gestational age should determine what feeding to use
4. Whether any red flags exist that increase concern about adequacy of the infant's intake:
    a. Feeding duration greater than 30 minutes or fewer than six feedings per day after the first 24 hours of life
    b. Fussiness, distress, or difficulty breathing during feeding; difficulty waking the infant for feeding; difficulty completing a feeding
    c. Lethargy or decreased arousal during feeding
    d. Feed refusal, arches during feeding, gags, coughs, chokes frequently while feeding

Strategies to consider when determining the feeding regimen include the following:

- Human milk should be the first choice for infants between 34 and 36 weeks' gestation.
    - Infant should be breastfed 8 to 12 times per day.
    - Supplementation with a transitional formula may be considered for the infant with a birth weight between 1500 and 2000 g until the infant is able to sustain weight gain and breastfeed fully without difficulty.
- Use of human milk fortifier is typically limited to:
    - Infants younger than 34 weeks' gestation
    - Infants with a birth weight less than 1500 g to 1800 g
    - Infants who required greater than 2 weeks of parenteral nutritional support
    - Infants with specific nutritional risks caused by chronic medical conditions or complications of prematurity
- Provide early postnursery discharge follow-up care within 48 to 72 hours to assess feeding adequacy, hydration, and weight.
- Formula-fed infants with birth weight between 1500 and 2000 g should receive an enriched post discharge formula until 6 to 9 months corrected age. Calcium and phosphorus levels should be monitored.
- Growth parameters should be plotted on a Fenton growth curve[29] (revised Babson-Benda growth curve; Figure 92-6) or a 2000 CDC growth chart. (See Chapter 14, Pediatric Physical Examination.)
- Enriched formula feeding should be discontinued if:
    - Infant is not able to tolerate it.
    - Infant demonstrates excessive weight gain greater than 40 g/day or is above the 50th percentile on the CDC growth chart.
    - Calcium and phosphorus levels exceed normal ranges for age.
- Infants with birth weight greater than 2000 g should be breastfeeding on demand or if formula feeding receive a standard (term) 20 cal/oz iron fortified formula. If supplementation is required because of inadequate weight gain or excessive weight loss, then a standard formula may be considered.

Soy formulas are not recommended for preterm infants born at less than 1800 g.[30]

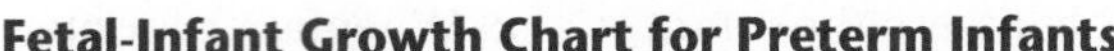

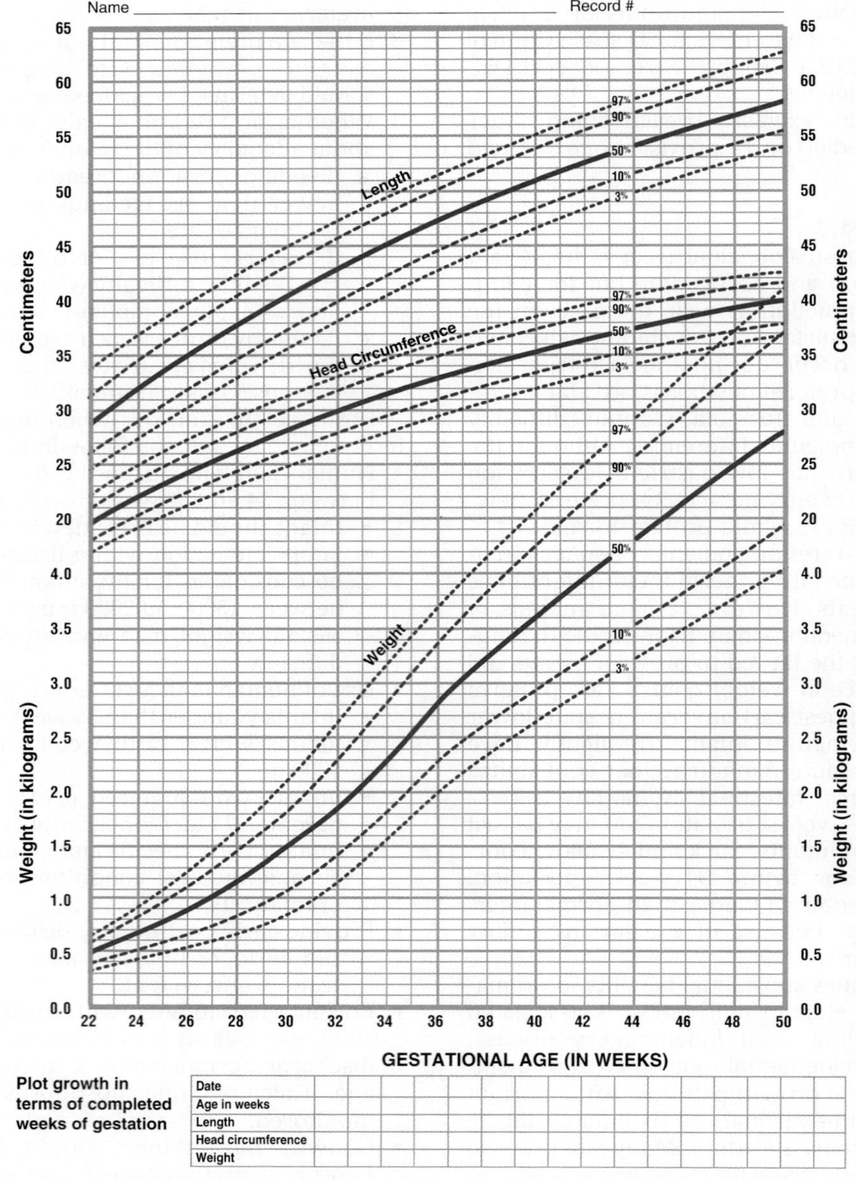

Figure 92-6 Babson-Benda growth curve.

Hyperbilirubinemia

Prematurity is the main risk factor for hyperbilirubinemia and is associated with an increased risk of kernicterus.[31,32] Jaundice in the late preterm infant often has a more severe and protracted course than in term infants. Bilirubin levels typically peak between 5 and 7 days in the premature infant and decline slowly thereafter. Kernicterus is a preventable brain injury; failure to diagnose and treat properly the late preterm infant with significant hyperbilirubinemia may place the clinician at medical-legal risk. Table 92-1 summarizes recommended interventions for various bilirubin levels in late preterm infants. In late preterm infants the progression to kernicterus can be insidious. Late preterm newborns discharged home within 72 hours of birth should have a follow-up appointment within 2 to 3 days of their discharge (within the first week of life). (See Chapter 98, Neonatal Jaundice.)

Brain Maturation and Neurodevelopment

The majority of the brain growth occurs during the last half of gestation, with 35% of the brain's weight accrued in the last 6 weeks of gestation.[33] Although neuronal proliferation and migration are considered complete by 24 weeks, the brain's gyri and sulci are

Table 92-1 Total Serum Bilirubin Levels at Which Interventions Are Recommended for Late Preterm Infants

RISK FOR BIND (AAP GUIDELINES*)	TSB THRESHOLD AT AGE 48 HR (MG/DL)		TSB THRESHOLD AT AGE ≥96 HR (MG/DL)	
	PHOTOTHERAPY	EXCHANGE	PHOTOTHERAPY	EXCHANGE
High (presence of any BIND risk factors and 35-0/7 to 37-6/7 wk)	11	18	15	19
Moderate (35-0/7 to 37-6/7 wk with no BIND risk)	13	20	18	22.5
Low (term infant with no BIND risk)	15	22	21	25

AAP, American Academy of Pediatrics; *BIND,* bilirubin-induced neurologic dysfunction; *TSB,* total serum bilirubin.
BIND risk factors: isoimmune hemolytic anemia; glucose-6-phosphate dehydrogenase deficiency: significant lethargy, sepsis, acidosis, asphyxia, temperature instability, and serum albumin level <3.0 g/dL.
*American Academy of Pediatrics. Subcommittee on Hyperbilirubinemia. Clinical practice guidelines. Management of hyperbilirubinemia in the newborn infant 35 or more weeks of gestation. *Pediatrics.* 2004;114(1):297-316.

not fully developed in the late preterm infant. In addition, a 4-fold (50%) increase in cortical brain volume occurs during the third trimester.[34] Synaptogenesis, dendritic branching, and maturation of oligodendrocytes also continue through the last weeks of gestation. These processes are extremely sensitive and susceptible to hypoxic-ischemic and free radical injury, particularly the oligodendrocytes. Cerebral palsy (CP) is the most common early neurodevelopmental impairment in infancy. Among children with CP, approximately one third will have been born between 32 and 36 weeks' gestation.[35] CP develops in response to two types of white matter injury involving (1) focal necrosis in the periventricular region (periventricular leukomalacia) and (2) diffuse injury to the surrounding central white matter, basal ganglia, and thalamus.[36] (See Chapter 245, Cerebral Palsy.)

Brainstem function and autonomic and respiratory control are also immature, contributing to periodic breathing, apnea, desaturations, and bradycardia in the preterm infant. As previously described, inefficient feeding skills in conjunction with poor coordination of suck-swallow-breathing and episodic gastroesophageal reflux precipitate these physiological responses. The incidence of sudden infant death syndrome in preterm infants between 33 and 36 weeks' gestation is 1.37/1000 live births compared with 0.69/1000 term infants.[5] For infants between 34 and 37 weeks' gestation the relative risk of experiencing an episode of prolonged apnea or bradycardia requiring intervention (apparent life-threatening event) is three times greater than the term infant. The Collaborative Home Infant Monitoring Evaluation (CHIME) study found that 30% of the study infants who experienced an apparent life-threatening event were less than 38 weeks' gestation at birth. The younger the preterm infant was, the earlier symptoms were exhibited.[37] (See also Chapter 237, Apparent Life-Threatening Events.)

Consequently, some hospital practices and primary care physicians may consider polysomnographic evaluation of the late preterm infant before nursery discharge or recommend home monitoring. However, no data are available that support the routine use of predischarge testing or home monitoring for this group of infants. Considerations regarding these care recommendations should be based on the infant's clinical and family history. Parents of late preterm infants should be counseled that their babies should be placed supine for sleep and that all other recommendations regarding safe sleep practices are applicable to their preterm infant. If the mother plans to practice bed sharing with her infant, then instructions should be provided on how to do so safely.

Long-Term Outcomes

Gestational age-specific long-term outcome data about the late preterm infant are limited. Studies have primarily reported on outcomes of infants with varying degrees of low birth weight. Care must be taken when interpreting this information because included among infants in these studies are small-for-gestational-age infants, some of whom may have been term. Population-based studies have revealed that the risk of developmental delay or disability is 40% higher for infants weighing between 1500 and 2499 g at birth in comparison with normal–birth-weight babies.[38] Educational outcomes for children born premature are similarly affected. Although the greatest effect is among the most immature infants weighing less than 1000 g at birth, heavier low–birth-weight children experience increased adverse educational outcomes in the areas of academic problems, learning disabilities, physical and sensory impairments, and mental disabilities.[39] Investigators have reported school performance outcomes for children born after 32 weeks' gestation. Reading and spelling difficulties are more frequent among children born at 33 to 36 weeks' gestation than normal–birth-weight infants.[40] Huddy et al reported on school performance at age 7 years for a population-based cohort of children born between 32 and 35 weeks' gestation. Up to one third of these children exhibited school difficulties. Nearly 25% required additional school resources. Areas of identified poor performance included writing, fine motor skills, reading, mathematics, and physical education.[41] The risk of developing attention-deficit/hyperactivity disorder is nearly two and one-half times greater than for normal–birth-weight children.[42] Behavioral difficulties are twice as common in low–birth-weight children and have been shown to be related to maternal psychological distress at term (40 weeks) postmenstrual age and a history of tobacco exposure. Whether the effects of smoking are primary or a proxy for other environmental factors or stressors that influence parental well being and their ability to support their child's maturation is unclear.[43] Therefore the clinician should monitor the child's behavioral and educational progress because the late preterm infant is not typically considered automatically eligible for early intervention services and may not even be viewed as *at-risk* under early intervention guidelines from the Child Find initiative.

Additional Routine Care Issues

Hepatitis B Vaccination

According to the CDC Advisory Committee on Immunization Practices recommendations, late preterm infants born to hepatitis B surface antigen–positive mothers should receive hepatitis B (HBV) vaccine and hepatitis B immune globulin (HBIg) within 12 hours of birth. In neonates whose birth weight is less than 2000 g, the initial vaccine dose confers lower immunogenicity than infants born at term. Therefore infants younger than 34 weeks' gestation or weighing less than 2000 g should receive a total of four doses of HBV vaccine (birth and 1-2, 3-4, and 6 months). In case of unknown maternal status at delivery, infants weighing less than 2000 g should receive both HBV vaccine and HBIg. Neonates born to hepatitis B surface antigen–negative mothers should receive the first dose of vaccine in the hospital.

Car Seat Safety

According to Federal Motor Vehicle Safety policy the maximal weight acceptable for use of an infant car seat safety is 50 lb; however, no minimal weight is specified. Preterm infants have been shown to have episodes of oxygen desaturation when placed in a standard upright infant car seat. Infants transported in car beds are less likely to exhibit desaturations. Many hospitals routinely measure the adequacy of the infant's oxygenation while in the car seat before hospital discharge to assist parents with proper positioning of the baby and to reduce the risk for cardiorespiratory compromise. Rolled towels or blankets may be placed on both sides of infant for head and neck support. Infants who exhibit apnea, bradycardia, and desaturations while upright are advised to travel in a supine position in a car bed. Babies discharged with home monitoring should also be monitored during travel. For the infant discharged on oxygen, proper storage of the oxygen tank and apnea monitor during travel includes placing the equipment below the infant seat or on the vehicle floor for safety purposes.

Newborn Screening and the Timing of Postnursery Follow-Up Care

All newborn screening procedures should be conducted. Newborn hearing screening using either automated auditory brainstem response or otoacoustic emission testing devices is feasible and should be completed before the late preterm infant is discharged from the newborn nursery. Follow-up care should include a home nurse visit or an office visit with the primary care physician within 48 to 72 hours of the newborn's discharge from the hospital. If the newborn is younger than 5 days at the time of nursery discharge, is breastfeeding, or has any risk factors for potential difficulties, then follow-up should occur within 48 hours of hospital discharge.

TOOLS FOR PRACTICE

Engaging Patient and Family

- *Care Safety Seats: A Guide for Families, 2007* (brochure), American Academy of Pediatrics (www.aap.org/family/carseatguide.htm).
- *Car Safety Seats and Transportation Safety* (Web page), American Academy of Pediatrics (www.aap.org/healthtopics/carseatsafety.cfm).
- *Safe Transportation of Children with Special Needs* (brochure), American Academy of Pediatrics (www.aap.org/bookstore).

Medical Decision Support

- *Births: Final Data for 2005* (report), National Center for Health Statistics (www.cdc.gov/nchs/data/nvsr/nvsr56/nvsr56_06.pdf).
- *Guidelines for Perinatal Care, 6th edition* (book), American Academy of Pediatrics and American College of Gynecologists and Obstetricians (www.aap.org/bookstore).

AAP POLICY STATEMENTS

American Academy of Pediatrics, Committee on Fetus and Newborn. Age terminology during the perinatal period. *Pediatrics.* 2004;114(5):1362-1364. (aappolicy.aappublications.org/cgi/content/full/pediatrics;114/5/1362).

Engle WA, Tomashek KM, Wallman C, Committee on Fetus and Newborn. "Late-preterm" infants: a population at risk. *Pediatrics.* 2007;120(6):1390-1401. (pediatrics.aappublications.org/cgi/content/full/120/6/1390).

REFERENCES

1. Martin JA, Hamilton BE, Sutton PD, et al. *Births: Final Data From 2004. National Vital Statistics Reports.* Vol. 55, no. 1. Hyattsville, MD: National Center for Health Statistics; 2006. Available at: www.cdc.gov/nchs/nvrs/nvsr55/nvsr55_01.pdf. Accessed May 18, 2007.
2. Luke B, Brown MB. The changing risk of infant mortality by gestation, plurality and race: 1989-1991 versus 1999-2001. *Pediatrics.* 2006;118(6):2488-2497.
3. American Academy of Pediatrics, Committee on Fetus and Newborn. Policy statement: age terminology during the perinatal period. *Pediatrics.* 2004;114:1362-1364.
4. Engle W. A recommendation for the definition of "late preterm" (near term) and the birth weight-gestational age classification system. *Semin Perinatol.* 2006;30:2-7.
5. Kramer MS, Demissie K, Yang H, et al. The contribution of mild and moderate preterm birth to infant mortality. Fetal and Infant Health Study Group of the Canadian Perinatal System. *JAMA.* 2000;284:843-849.
6. Wang ML, Dorer DJ, Fleming MP, et al. Clinical outcomes of near-term infants. *Pediatrics.* 2004;114:372-376.

7. Escobar GJ, Clark RH, Greene JD. Short-term outcomes of infants born at 35 and 36 weeks gestation: we need to ask more questions. *Semin Perinatol.* 2006;30:28-33.
8. American Academy of Pediatrics. Guidelines for Perinatal Care, 6th edition. Elk Grove Village, IL: American Academy of *Pediatrics*;2007.
9. American Academy of Pediatrics, Committee of Fetus and Newborn. Levels of neonatal care. *Pediatrics.* 2004;114:1341-1347.
10. Escobar GJ, Greene JD, Hulac P, et al. Rehospitalisation after birth hospitalisation: patterns among infants of all gestations. *Arch Dis Child.* 2005;90:125-131.
11. Escobar GJ, McCormick MC, Zupancic JAF, et al. Unstudied infants: outcomes of moderately premature infants in the intensive care unit. *Arch Dis Child Fetal Neonatal Ed.* 2006;91:F238-F244.
12. Paul IM, Lehman BE, Hollenbeak CS, et al. Preventable newborn readmissions since passage of the newborns' and mothers' health protection act. *Pediatrics.* 2006; 118:2349-2358.
13. Knobel RB, Wimmer JE, Holbert D. Heat loss prevention for preterm infants in the delivery room. *J Perinatol.* 2005; 25:304-308.
14. Watkinson M. Temperature control of premature infants in the delivery room. *Clin Perinaol.* 2006;33(1):43-53.
15. World Health Organization. Thermal Protection of the Newborn: A Practical Guide. 1997. Available at: www.who.org. Accessed May 18, 2007.
16. American Society of Heating, Refrigeration and Air-Conditioning Engineers, Inc, 2003. ASHRAE Handbook: Heating, Ventilating and Air-Conditioning Applications, Atlanta. Available at: www.ashrae.org. Accessed May 18, 2007.
17. Clark RH. The epidemiology of respiratory failure in neonates born at an estimated gestational age of 34 weeks or more. *J Perinatol.* 2005;25:251-257.
18. Halliday HL. Elective delivery at "term": implications for the newborn. *Arch Paediatr.* 1999;88:1180-1181.
19. National Institutes of Health. State-of-the-Science Conference Statement: Cesarean Delivery on Demand. Bethesda, MD, March 27-29, 2006.
20. As-Sanie S, Mercer B, Moore J. The association between respiratory distress and nonpulmonary morbidity at 34-36 weeks' gestation. *Am J Obstet Gynecol.* 2003;189: 1053-1057.
21. Crowley P. Prophylactic corticosteroids for preterm birth. *Cochrane Database Syst Rev.* 2002;(4):CD000065.
22. Burchell A, Gibb L, Waddell ID, et al. The ontogeny of human hepatic microsomal glucose-6-phosphatase proteins. *Clin Chem.* 1990;36:1633-1637.
23. Hume R, Burchell A. Abnormal expression of glucose-6-phosphatase in preterm infants. *Arch Dis Child.* 1993; 68: 202-204.
24. Burchell A, Allan BB, Hume R. Glucose-6-phosphatase proteins of the endoplasmic reticulum. *Mol Membr Biol.* 1994;11:217-227.
25. Centers for Disease Control and Prevention. Prevention of perinatal group b streptococcal disease: revised guidelines from CDC. *MMWR Morb Mortal Wkly Rep.* 2002; 51:1-22.
26. Hyman PE, Clarke DD, Everett SL, et al. Gastric acid secretory function in preterm infants. *J Pediatr.* 1985; 106:467-471.
27. Antonowicz I, Lebenthal E. Developmental pattern of small intestinal enterokinase and disaccharidase activities in the human fetus. *Gastroenterology.* 1977;72:1299-1303.
28. Hamosh M. Digestion in the newborn. *Clin Perinatol.* 1996;23:191-209.
29. Fenton TR. A new growth chart for preterm infants: Babson and Benda's chart updated with recent data and a new format. *BMC Pediatrics.* 2003;3:13. Available at: www.biomedcentral.com/1471-2431/3/13. Accessed May 18, 2007.
30. American Academy of Pediatrics, Committee on Nutrition. Soy protein-based formulas: recommendations for use in infant feeding. *Pediatrics.* 1998;101(1):148-153.
31. Newman TB, Xiong B, Gonzales VM, et al. Prediction and prevention of extreme neonatal hyperbilirubinemia in a mature health maintenance organization. *Arch Pediatr Adolesc Med.* 2000;154:1140-1147.
32. Ip S, Chung M, Kulig J, et al, and the American Academy of Pediatrics, Subcommittee on Hyperbilirubinemia. An evidence-based review of important issues concerning neonatal hyperbilirubinemia. *Pediatrics.* 2004;114:e130-e153.
33. Guihard-Costa AM, Larroche JC. Differential growth between the fetal brain and its infratentorial part. *Early Hum Dev.* 1990;23:27-40.
34. Huppi PS, Warfield S, Kikinis R, et al. Quantitative magnetic resonance imaging of brain development in premature and mature newborns. *Ann Neurol.* 1998;43:224-235.
35. Blair E, Watson L. Epidemiology of cerebral palsy. *Semin Fetal Neonatal Med.* 2006;11:117-125.
36. Folkerth RD. Neuropathologic substrate of cerebral palsy. *J Child Neurol.* 2005;20:940-949.
37. Ramanathan R, Corwin MJ, Hunt CE, et al. Cardiorespiratory events recorded on home monitors: comparison of healthy infants with those at increased risk for SIDS. *JAMA.* 2001;285(17):2199-2207.
38. Thompson JR, Carter RL, Edwards AR, et al. A population-based study of the effects of birth weight on early developmental delay or disability. *Am J Perinatol.* 2003; 20(6):321-332.
39. Resnick MB, Gueorguieva RV, Carter RL, et al. The impact of low birth weight, perinatal conditions and socio-demographic factors on educational outcome in kindergarten. *Pediatrics.* 1999;104(6):e74. Available at: www.pediatrics.org/cgi/content/full/104/6/e74. Accessed May 18, 2007.
40. Kirkegaard I, Obel C, Hedgegaard M, et al. Gestational age and birth weight in relation to school performance of 10-year-old children: a follow-up study of children born after 32 completed weeks. *Pediatrics.* 2006; 118(4): 1600-1606.
41. Huddy CL, Johnson A, Hope PL. Educational and behavioural problems in babies of 32035 weeks gestation. *Arch Dis Child Fetal Neonatal Ed.* 2001;85:F23-F28.
42. Elgen I, Sommerfelt, Markestad T. Population-based, controlled study of behavioural problems and psychiatric disorders in low birth weight children at 11 years of age. *Arch Dis Child Fetal Neonatal Ed.* 2000;87:F128-F132.
43. Gray RF, Indurkhya A, McCormick MC. Prevalence, stability, and predictors of clinically significant behavior problems in low birth weight children at 3, 5 and 8 years of age. *Pediatrics.* 2004;114(3):736-743.

SECTION THREE

Discharge Planning and Follow-up Care

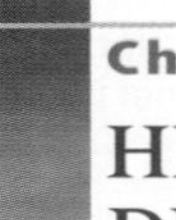

Chapter 93

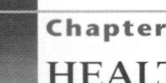

HEALTHY NEWBORN DISCHARGE

Christina Kan Sullivan, MD; Sonia Dela Cruz-Rivera, MD

NEWBORN DISCHARGE

The timing of optimal hospital discharge of the newborn and mother has been a subject of debate for the last several years. Historically, in the United States, newborn length of stay (LOS) has varied considerably in the last 50 years because of changing perinatal hospitalization practices.[1] Before 1920, hospital births were uncommon; but by 1945, 80% of births occurred in the hospital, with an average LOS after vaginal delivery ranging from 3 to 5 days.[2] The trend toward shorter LOS was first driven by a consumer-initiated movement between the 1960s and 1980s as an alternative to home delivery.[3] By the 1990s, financial constraints imposed by 3rd-party payers led to even shorter stays because insurers would not pay for hospitalizations extending beyond 24 hours for an uncomplicated vaginal delivery.[4] The average LOS in 1992 was 2.1 days.

The pressure to discharge infants early based on arbitrary financial considerations has been a source of frustration for physicians and families. In addition, many medical issues related to the transition from an intrauterine to an extrauterine environment require a longer period of observation. For instance, serum bilirubin concentration peaks at 3 to 5 days, and lactation is rarely established in fewer than 3 days. In a 1996 survey of pediatricians, 43% of respondents indicated that they had experienced adverse outcomes related to the shortened LOS.[5] The passage of the Newborns' and Mothers' Health Protection Act of 1996 prohibited payers from restricting benefits for hospital stays to fewer than 48 hours after birth for a vaginal delivery or to fewer than 96 hours for a cesarean delivery.

The American Academy of Pediatrics (AAP) first addressed the management of newborns in the hospital when the Committee on Fetus and Newborn published the 1st edition of *Standards and Recommendations for Hospital Care of Newborn Infants* in 1948. In 1977, the Committee recommended a 72 to 96 hour LOS.[6] The 1995 AAP policy statement[7] detailing the minimum discharge criteria for healthy, term newborns was issued in response to the shortened hospital stay (<48 hours) with the revised policy statement in 2004 further emphasizing the concept that the

> "...length of stay should be based on the unique characteristics of each mother-infant dyad, including the health of the mother, the health and stability of the infant, the ability and confidence of the mother to care for her infant, the adequacy of support systems at home, and access to appropriate follow-up care."[3]

The timing of the newborn's discharge is therefore best determined by the physician in consultation with the infant's family. (For further details on this subject, see Timing section.) A healthy term newborn may be ready for nursery discharge once the child exhibits stable vital signs for at least 12 hours, has a normal physical examination, voids, passes stool, demonstrates appropriate feeding skills, completes all screening tests, and has appropriate follow-up care in place. An important point to recognize is that discharge within 24 to 48 hours after birth, before completion of the normal physiological transition, may make detection of some congenital malformations difficult. Therefore the need is increased for a thorough physical examination and a careful review of the history and the nursery course. Parents should be counseled about signs of illness that warrant immediate medical attention and the importance of routine follow-up care within the first week of life.

Assessing Readiness

Whether the newborn is the firstborn or the 5th child born, all new parents experience some combination of excitement coupled with exhaustion with the new arrival. Lack of experience and the onset of medical complications impose additional stress on the family. Health professionals must be adept at identifying and addressing these issues so that, on hospital discharge, parents feel confident, knowledgeable, and well prepared to care for their newborn.

By the time of discharge, a clinician has likely examined the newborn 2 to 3 times or more. The recommended number of assessments before newborn nursery discharge is based more on accepted clinical practice rather than on data from randomized clinical trials. From an evidence-based perspective, no well-designed randomized trials have been conducted that have evaluated the efficacy of one versus two routine neonatal examinations.[8] Most important, however, is the serial assessment of the infant that permits the earliest detection of anomalies and deviations from normal and affords the clinician the opportunity for direct communication with the family to provide information, counseling, and reassurance.

Medical Factors

In addition to reviewing and verifying the maternal, family, and obstetric histories; documenting gestational age, anthropomorphic data, and the appropriateness of growth for the infant's gestational age; and monitoring vital signs and daily weights, the following systems particularly should be noted on physical examination:

- Head shape and signs of trauma (caput, cephalohematoma)
- Dysmorphic features
- Eyes (red reflex)
- Palate morphology, presence of natal teeth, and shortened frenulum
- Clavicles (crepitus suggestive of fracture)
- Cardiac system (murmurs)
- Femoral pulses
- Abdominal area (masses, distension)
- Hip (signs of dislocation or dislocatability)
- Spine (deformities)
- Foot deformities (metatarsus adductus, clubfoot)
- Genitalia and rectum
- Skin (jaundice, rash, mottling, cyanosis, birthmarks)
- General muscle tone and symmetrical reflexes
- Well-coordinated suck and swallow reflex
- Ability to fix gaze and follow a human face

Good evidence exists to support screening examination of the skin, eyes (red reflex), ears (hearing), and hips of the newborn infant. Although early detection of congenital heart defects can improve outcomes, physical examination alone will miss approximately 50% of infants with cardiac defects. Assessment of an infant's oxygen saturation through screening pulse oximetry is a promising adjunct to physical examination, but it needs further study to determine the optimal timing for this screening test.[9] All newborns should receive a hepatitis B vaccine (and hepatitis B immune globulin within 12 hours of birth if the mother is positive for hepatitis B surface antigen) and have a hearing screen and newborn screen before discharge. Good evidence exists to support the fact that universal newborn hearing screening using physiological measures (otoacoustic emission or auditory brain stem response testing) leads to earlier identification and treatment of infants with permanent hearing loss.[10,11]

Assessment of feeding adequacy irrespective of whether the infant is breastfeeding or bottle feeding is an important determinant of the newborn's readiness for discharge. Coordination of suck and swallow reflex and the frequency and duration of feeding episodes are influenced by the infant's gestation, postnatal age and physiological transition after birth, neurobehavioral state, and level of alertness. Adequacy of feeding also influences the infant's hydration status and degree of weight loss, important contributors to early or excessive hyperbilirubinemia.

Before discharge, parents should be educated about jaundice—what it is, how to assess its presence, and how to contact their physician if it is noted at home. Discharge counseling affords the clinician the opportunity to reinforce the importance of the 1st week follow-up visit, whether it is a home visit by a nurse who is under a physician's supervision or an office visit, in ensuring a safe transition for the newborn: assessing the infant's continued transition; identifying feeding, excess weight loss, or jaundice problems; and reevaluating any unusual or atypical findings. Any abnormalities requiring further testing should be discussed in detail with the family, and appropriate follow-up should be arranged. Examining the newborn at least once in the parents' presence allows the health professional to point out significant physical findings, comment on normal variations, and gives parents the chance to have their questions answered efficiently and effectively.[12] This practice also gives the physician the additional opportunity to observe parent-infant, and parent-parent interactions.

Family and Environmental Factors

Observing parents' responsiveness to their new infant and their interactions with each other can be powerful indicators of the family's comfort level with caring for their new infant. Anticipating concerns and providing thoughtful, clear answers will reassure parents and decrease any anxiety they may feel about taking their infant home.

Careful attention to the following maternal and environmental factors can further influence the physician's decision about discharge readiness and may include but is not limited to[1,3]: degree of social support (eg, single parenthood, relationship with infant's father), level of maternal fatigue and stress, young age of the mother (especially younger than 18 years), knowledge of routine infant care and breastfeeding, presence of substance abuse, the need to care for other children, and adequacy of financial resources. Although most physicians consider these factors,[1] women pediatricians are two to three times more likely than men to rate these maternal and peripartum factors as highly important determinants of discharge readiness.[1] Although significant findings in these domains may not necessarily delay hospital discharge, visiting nurse services, homes visits, or earlier follow-up plans should be instituted as appropriate.

COUNSELING THE FAMILY

Part of the newborn discharge process is counseling parents about how to care for their newborn infant and providing anticipatory guidance. No right way exists to perform newborn discharge counseling. Approaches depend on the biases and experiences of the physician.[13] Counseling can be tailored to the personality and practice patterns of the physician and the personality of the parents.[12] The style notwithstanding, certain issues (summarized in Box 93-1) need to be kept in mind.

Feeding

Physicians have the responsibility to encourage breastfeeding and should always reinforce the importance of making the decision to breastfeed.[14] Human milk is the best nutritional choice; it is economical and convenient. The most important advantage is its

BOX 93-1 Suggested Topics for Discussion: Newborn Discharge Counseling

- Feeding
  - Breastfeeding
  - Bottle feeding
- Elimination
  - Urination
  - Bowel movement
- Sleep
- Body care
  - Umbilical cord care
  - Skin care
  - Bathing
  - Nail care
- Body care—cont'd
  - Dressing
  - Genitalia care
- Safety
  - Vehicle safety
  - Environmental toxins:
    - Cigarette smoke
    - Lead
    - Carbon monoxide
    - Pesticides
- Signs of illness
- Psychosocial issues

immunologic benefits. However, supporting the mother in whatever decision she makes with regard to feeding method is also the responsibility of physicians. (See Chapter 89, Breastfeeding the Newborn.)

Breastfeeding

Physicians should work with the nursing staff to provide information to mothers to ensure successful breastfeeding. Such information should include[14]:

- Proper positioning and latch on
- What the let down reflex is
- What colostrum is and its adequacy for the early feedings
- The process and timing of the transition from colostrum to mature milk
- Ways to explore any culturally based misconceptions about giving the newborn colostrum, especially if the mother is hesitant to give the newborn colostrum (common among women from Southeast Asia, parts of Africa, and South America)
- Strategies to promote successful initiation of breastfeeding when the mother plans to breast and formula feed
- How nursing frequency affects milk supply
- How to tell if the infant is nursing properly
- How to break suction and the meaning of nipple pain or discomfort
- Basic nipple care
- How to manage engorgement
- How to express milk manually or using a breast pump
- How to store expressed milk
- Signs and symptoms of mastitis
- Breastfeeding support groups (La Leche League, lactation consultants, Special Supplemental Nutrition Program for Women, Infants, and Children)

Bottle Feeding

Commonly used infant formulas generally fall into three main categories: (1) cow's milk based, (2) soy based, and (3) elemental. Formulas are readily available in powder, concentrate, and ready-to-feed preparations, and no known advantage exists of 1 brand or form over another. If the parents are planning on formula feeding their infant, then they should determine if they have particular concerns about one category of formula or another. Vegan parents will refuse cow milk–based formulas, whereas a family with a previous child who exhibited intolerance to a particular type of formula may request another specific formula. This preference is particularly important among immigrant families who may have used animal milk (eg, goat's milk) or formulas not typical for North America. The clinicians should emphasize the importance of using iron-fortified infant formulas and the proper dilution of the powder or concentrate preparations. Parents need to be informed that sterilizing water, bottles, and artificial nipples is not necessary if the water supply is safe and if refrigeration is available. Infant formula need not be warmer than room temperature. The use of the microwave oven to warm the formula should be discouraged because it causes uneven heating. The physician should caution parents against bottle propping so as to prevent choking and aspiration.

Table 93-1 Newborn Stool Patterns

TYPE	CHARACTERISTICS	TIME FRAME
Meconium	Thick and tarry Dark green	Birth-2 days
Normal	Loose Green-brown to yellow-brown Seedy	2-5 days
Breastfed	Mushy and golden Often after each feeding Odor similar to sour milk	After 5 days

Elimination

Parents should know what normal urination and bowel patterns are for newborns. Parents need to be reassured that at least four to five wet diapers per day are normal. Bowel patterns are variable during this period and can depend on the type of feeding. Breastfed infants tend to have more frequent bowel movements than bottle-fed infants. They can initially have as much as one stool after every feeding because breast milk is more easily digestible than formula. Bottle-fed infants may have as few as one to two bowel movements per day. Stool frequency can change over the first few weeks and, by 1 month of age, can range from over 10 times per day to occurring once every 4 to 7 days. Stool appearance also can change over time. It can transition from normal meconium stools to having a seedy yellow appearance over several days (Table 93-1).

Constipation is a big concern for most parents, and the clinician should define what true constipation is. Parents need to be reassured that straining is normal and represents the effort needed to pass stools while lying down. The infant is considered constipated if the stools are becoming hard. Regardless of the amount of straining or the interval between bowel movements, as long as the stools are soft, the infant is not constipated. Parents should be encouraged to discuss their infant's stooling pattern and stool characteristics during the follow-up visit if they continue to have concerns.

Laxatives are not recommended. The clinician should emphasize that honey should not be given to infants younger than 1 year because of the risk of developing botulism.

Sleep

Newborns vary in their pattern of sleep and wakefulness. Newborns generally need 16 to 20 hours of sleep in a 24-hour period and can sleep for 2 to 4 hours at a time.[15] During the 1st few weeks of life, having day-night reversal with longer periods of wakefulness during the night is common. Not until approximately 3 to 4 months of age do most infants begin to sleep through the night.

Safe sleep should be emphasized to reduce the risk of sudden infant death syndrome (SIDS). The recommendations of the AAP Task Force on Sudden Infant Death Syndrome include the following[16]:

1. Infants should be placed for sleep in a supine position for every sleep period.
2. Use a firm sleep surface, and avoid using redundant soft bedding and soft objects in the infant's sleep environment.
3. Infants should sleep in the same room as the parents in a crib, bassinet, or cradle that conforms to the safety standards of the Consumer Product Safety Commission and the American Society for Testing and Materials.
4. Infants should be in a separate sleep space that is in close proximity to the mother or primary care giver.
5. Consider offering a pacifier at nap time and bedtime (level of evidence III-2). However, use of pacifiers should be delayed until 1 month of age in breastfeeding infants and until breastfeeding can be well established. The pacifier should not be reinserted once the infant falls asleep.
6. Breastfeeding in combination with other health practices (ie, not smoking during pregnancy, placing the infant on the back to sleep, avoiding maternal drug use, preventing second-hand smoke exposure) is recommended to ensure optimal health status for infants.

The issue of co-sleeping is controversial. Forms of co-sleeping vary and include bed sharing. The sleep surface can range from sharing a mat, futon, or the floor to sleeping on a soft mattress, quilt, waterbed, sofa, or couch. These varying surfaces may not pose an equal risk to the infant. Bed sharing is increasing in frequency throughout the United States. Studies have reported that over one third of new mothers bed shared frequently, with another 40% bed sharing with their infant sometimes.[17] Bed sharing was equally as common among mothers who smoke as those who do not in this study. Another case-controlled study found an association between bed sharing and SIDS when the infant was sleeping between two parents.[18] This association was highest for infants younger than 11 weeks. This study has been criticized for having assessed bed sharing alone as a risk factor (rather than the environment within which the bed sharing occurred) and not assessing the presence of parental alcohol use at the time of bed sharing and breastfeeding in the analysis.

Sensitivity to cultural differences is necessary when obtaining sleep histories. Additionally, the assumption should not be made that families are practicing only one sleep arrangement over the course of the day and night. Health care professionals should consider this factor when obtaining a history on infant sleep practices and encourage parents to express their views on infant sleep and recommended sleep practices.

The Academy of Breastfeeding Medicine (www.bfmed.org), an international physician breastfeeding advocacy organization, has published guidelines on co-sleeping and breastfeeding that state the following:

1. Current evidence is insufficient to support routine recommendations against co-sleeping. Parents should be educated about risks and benefits of co-sleeping and unsafe co-sleeping practices and should be allowed to make their own informed decision. Bed sharing is a complex practice.
2. Parental counseling about infant sleep environments should include the following information (some potentially unsafe practices related to bed sharing and co-sleeping have been identified either in the peer reviewed literature or as a consensus of expert opinion):
   a. Environmental smoke exposure and maternal smoking
   b. Sharing sofas, couches, or daybeds with infants
   c. Sharing waterbeds or using soft bedding materials
   d. Sharing beds with adjacent spaces that might trap an infant
   e. Placing the infant in the adult bed in the prone or side position
   f. Using alcohol or mind-altering drugs by one or more adult who are bed sharing
3. Families should also be given all the information that is known about safe sleep environments for their infants, including the following:
   a. Place infants in the supine position for sleep.
   b. Use a firm, flat surface, and avoid waterbeds, couches, sofas, pillows, soft materials, or loose bedding.
   c. Use only a thin blanket to cover the infant.
   d. Ensure that the head will not be covered. In a cold room, the infant can be kept in an infant sleeper to maintain warmth.
   e. Avoid the use of quilts, duvets, comforters, pillows, and stuffed animals in the infant's sleep environment.
   f. Never put an infant down to sleep on a pillow or adjacent to a pillow.
   g. Never leave an infant alone on an adult bed.
   h. Families should be informed that adult beds have potential risks and are not designed to meet federal safety standards for infants.
   i. Ensure that no spaces exist between the mattress and headboard, walls, and other surfaces that may entrap the infant and lead to suffocation.
   j. Placing a firm mattress directly on the floor away from walls may be a safe alternative.

4. Another alternative to sharing an adult bed or sharing a mattress is using an infant bed that attaches to the side of the adult bed and provides proximity and access to the infant but has a separate sleep surface. No current, peer-reviewed studies of such devices have been conducted, and the Consumer Product Safety Commission has not yet established safety standards for these attachable co-sleepers.

Body Care

Umbilical Cord Care

Evidence-based care of the umbilical cord in the postnatal period includes effective hand hygiene and keeping the cord dry and exposed to air or loosely covered with clean clothes, with the diaper folded below the umbilicus.[19] If the umbilical cord stump becomes soiled with urine or feces, then cleansing the area with water is adequate.[20] Studies conducted in developed countries have shown that topical antisepsis of the cord stump reduces cord colonization. However, a systematic review of randomized trials that assessed the efficacy of applying topical antimicrobial agents in the prevention of infection has not shown this practice to be superior to simply keeping the cord clean. Chlorhexidine (Hibiclens) or hexachlorophene (pHisoHex), tincture of iodine or povidone-iodine (Betadine), silver sulfadiazine, and triple dye have the most efficacy in reducing umbilical cord colonization. If topical antimicrobial agents are used, then care must be exercised because toxicity has been reported with excess or inappropriate use.

Although some hospitals and practitioners continue to recommend use of application of alcohol to the umbilical cord, alcohol use has been shown to delay umbilical cord drying, is less effective in reducing bacterial colonization, and delays cord separation. Therefore alcohol application is not recommended for routine umbilical cord care.

The umbilical cord stump usually separates between 9 and 15 days of age (up to 3 weeks may be normal).[21] Minimal discharge is to be expected thereafter. However, if significant amounts of discharge persist, it should be brought to the physician's attention. Until the cord falls off, the area should be kept dry as much as is possible to promote separation and healing. For this reason, giving infants only sponge baths is best until the cord is well healed.

Skin Care

Skin lubrication is usually not necessary; however, if it is needed, then it should be limited to the use of hypoallergenic lotions. Oil-based preparations, such as petroleum-based lubricants or barriers containing zinc oxide, are more effective than water-based preparations.[22] Talcum powder should not be used because of the danger of aspiration. The diaper area is best cleansed with warm water with each diaper change, although the use of commercially available *infant wipes* offers many conveniences. Although these wipes may contain chemicals, alcohol, and fragrances that can cause skin irritation, most of these products, particularly those designated as *hypoallergenic* or *sensitive,* are found to be as mild as using a wet washcloth and may be used even in the newborn period.[22] Wipes free of fragrance, alcohol, and other chemicals, except for lotion, have been shown to be gentler than water alone.[23] Most diaper rashes will improve with applications of zinc oxide or an antifungal preparation if the rash is not improving and has the appearance of a candidal infection. Persistent diaper rash will necessitate a consultation with a health professional. Evidence-based clinical practice guidelines on the care of neonatal skin have been published by the Association of Women's Health, Obstetric and Neonatal Nurses.[20]

Bathing

The purpose of bathing during the neonatal period is to remove debris. Daily bathing with soap is not recommended during this time. Daily bathing may contribute to excessive drying of the skin and can exacerbate skin conditions such as atopic dermatitis. Young infants can be washed with plain water. However, if use of a cleanser or soap is preferred, then it should be mild with a neutral pH. Hair can be shampooed a few times weekly using a mild shampoo or body wash.

Nail Care

Scissors should not be used. Nails should be filed using an emery board.

Dressing

Healthy, full-term infants do not need to be dressed more warmly than an older child or adult. Parents can use themselves as a guide to determine the amount of clothing to put on the infant. A good rule of thumb is to dress the infant in one more layer of clothing than an adult would be wearing in the same environment.[24] Specific guidance will need to incorporate the ambient temperature of the home where the child resides, as well as reflect the regional environmental temperatures. Questions often arise as to how warmly to dress the larger preterm (34 to 36 6/7; weeks' gestation). In general, the same principles apply in deciding how much clothing to use. The need for extra clothing or use of double blankets for these infants will primarily depend on the infant's ability to maintain temperature in the ambient environment. The infant's temperature regulation will be determined, in part, by adiposity, degree of physiological maturity, and ongoing metabolic demands. Because of high heat losses through the scalp, parents should be encouraged to cover the infant's head when going outside. Care must be exercised when swaddling a young infant. Although this method is effective for soothing a fussy infant and maintaining body temperature, an overbundled infant is at risk for hyperthermia and potentially at increased risk for SIDS if overheated during sleep.

Taking the Newborn Outdoors

As soon after discharge as the mother is ready to go outside, the newborn can go out as well. Many parents are hesitant to take their newborn outside because of fear of exposure to airborne and other communicable illnesses. A common belief among many families is that an infant cannot go outside the home until the 1st or 2nd set of immunizations has been received. Cultural prohibitions against outings before a certain age may also exist. Korean parents typically keep an infant indoors until the 100th day, the time when the infant's survival is believed to be more assured. Appropriate protection against excess sun exposure should also be discussed.

Genitalia Care—Boys

The uncircumcised penis should be cleansed simply with water with or without a mild soap or with a diaper wipe. Retracting the penile foreskin is unnecessary because adhesions will spontaneously lyse over the 1st several years of life. The newly circumcised penis can also be cleansed with warm water and gentle soap with every diaper change. An antibacterial ointment or other lubricant such as vitamin A & D ointment can be applied to the area to prevent the skin from sticking to the diaper as it heals, and can reduce the small chance of infection.[14]

Genitalia Care—Girls

Recommendations suggest washing the area between the labia gently with warm water only. Diaper wipes may be used if they do not cause skin irritation, and parents should be instructed to always wipe girls from the vagina toward the anus (front to back). Parents should be informed that a white caseous discharge or even a bloody discharge from the vagina might occur in the 1st few days. This discharge is the result of maternal hormones that are absorbed by the fetus before delivery.

Safety Issues and Injury Prevention

Vehicle Safety

Vehicle seat safety should begin with the first ride home from the hospital. The physician should emphasize to parents that a vehicle seat must be used at all times. The AAP Committee on Injury and Poison Prevention recommends that infants should face the rear of the vehicle until they are at least 1 year of age and weigh at least 20 pounds to decrease the risk of cervical spine injury in the event of a crash.[25] To provide optimal protection, the use of a convertible vehicle seat should be encouraged. Convertible vehicle safety seats can accommodate infants rear facing at higher weights.[25] For the AAP Car Safety Seats and Transportation Safety brochure and information, see Tools for Practice section.

Environmental Toxins

Several hazards exist in the home environment. Newborns have a unique vulnerability to certain environmental toxins, and their rapidly developing organ systems are particularly susceptible to the harmful effects of toxins. Toxic exposures of newborns differ from other age groups because of their own unique physical environment, food and water consumption pattern, and behavioral developmental stage.[26] Parents should be informed about common environmental toxins that can significantly affect the health of their infant.

Tobacco Smoke

Tobacco smoke is a common toxic substance that is harmful to everyone, including young infants. Parents should be educated about the harmful effects of inhaled second-hand smoke, which include increased incidence of respiratory infections, otitis media, and SIDS. The physician should stress that smoking not be allowed in the immediate environment of the infant, such as in the house or vehicle.

Carbon Monoxide and Other Sources of Indoor Air Pollution

Infants can be vulnerable to the effects of inhaled carbon monoxide. Intoxication from inhaled carbon monoxide can cause tissue hypoxia, which can affect multiple organ systems, with the central nervous and cardiovascular systems being the *prime targets*.[27] Installing smoke and carbon monoxide detectors in the home can prevent unintentional carbon monoxide inhalation (Box 93-2). The increased popularity of scented candles and incense pose another potential hazard to young children. Burning candles with lead-core wicks have been associated with lead levels above established Environmental Protection Agency standards. Even candles with nonlead wicks pose a hazard because they often release potentially harmful organic chemicals, such as formaldehyde, acetaldehyde, and acrolein. Soot from scented candles and particulate emissions from burning incense have been linked to respiratory symptoms and irritant dermatitis in vulnerable individuals.[28]

Lead

The most common route and source of exposure to lead is ingestion of lead-containing particles. These particles can be found in tap water, which is a common source of water used to reconstitute milk formula. Newborns who are given reconstituted milk are therefore particularly at risk for lead intoxication. To minimize lead exposure from drinking water, recommendations suggest flushing the water faucet in the morning for 2 minutes before using it to prepare the formula and using only cold tap water for drinking and preparing milk formula.[29]

Pesticides

More than 900 chemicals are registered in the United States as pesticides.[30] These substances include

BOX 93-2 Sources of Carbon Monoxide Exposure

- Motor-vehicle exhaust
- Unvented kerosene and propane gas space heaters
- Leaking chimneys and furnaces
- Back draft from furnaces
- Woodstoves and fireplaces
- Charcoal grills
- Gas appliances: stoves, dryers, water heaters
- Gasoline-powered generators
- Gasoline-powered equipment: lawn mowers, leaf blowers, floor polishers, snow blowers, pressure washers
- Tobacco smoke

Adapted from American Academy of Pediatrics, Committee on Environmental Health. Carbon monoxide. In: Etzel RA, ed. *Pediatric Environmental Health*, 2nd ed. Elk Grove Village, IL: American Academy of Pediatrics;2003.

insecticides, fungicides, rodenticides, fumigants, and insect repellants. The developing organ systems of young infants are especially susceptible to the harmful effects of these toxic chemicals. Routes of exposure for newborns are inhalation and skin absorption by contact. Infants of parents with occupational exposures to pesticides such as those who work on farms, as pesticide applicators, or landscapers are at increased risk of exposure to pesticides. Prevention includes washing work clothes separately from the infant's laundry, changing out of work clothing, and washing with soap and water before coming into close contact with infants and children (Box 93-3).

Signs of Illness

Parents should know when and how to contact the physician or the pediatric office in case of an emergency. Parents should be advised to contact the physician for the following reasons:

- Fever (rectal temperature ≥100.4° F [≥38° C])
- Persistent coughing or breathing difficulty
- Cyanosis (Few parents understand what the terms *cyanosis, blue,* or *dusky* skin color actually mean. Explanations should also include the differences between peripheral [acrocyanosis], circumoral, and central [body core] cyanosis. The physician should therefore explain these potential concerns and assess the parents understanding.)
- Sudden change in level of alertness, activity such as persistent irritability, or lethargy
- Feeding difficulties
- Persistent or projectile vomiting
- Diarrhea
- Jaundice
- Seizures
- Decreased urine output
- Umbilical cord problems
- Unusual skin rash or skin mottling

BOX 93-3 Safe Pesticide Practices

- Wash work clothes separately from other laundry.
- Wash work clothes with detergent and hot water before wearing them again.
- Wash hands and arms after putting clothing into washing machine.
- Change clothing and wash with soap and water before picking up or playing with your children.
- Store pesticides in an area safe from children.
- Cover children's skin if they are with you at work.
- Keep the children and their toys and playthings indoors when there is nearby aerial spraying or spraying that may drift near the house.
- Children and teenagers should avoid work that involves mixing or spraying pesticides.

Adapted from American Academy of Pediatrics, Committee on Environmental Health. Pesticides. In: Etzel RA, ed. *Pediatric Environmental Health* 2nd ed. Elk Grove Village, IL: American Academy of Pediatrics;2003.

Psychosocial Issues

The 1st few weeks at home with a newborn can be stressful to all family members but particularly new parents. The need for an adequate support system at home cannot be overemphasized. Sources of extra help might be family members, close relatives and friends, or hired help. Close support persons can assist with infant care and household chores. For families who do not have the advantage of having an adequate support system, community agencies are often available to assist them. Information on public and private groups that can provide services to these families is usually available through the social service department.

Devoting a large amount of time to discharge counseling is often difficult because of time constraints and shorter hospital stays. However, allowing sufficient time for parents to ask questions and for these questions to be addressed is important. Whether it is the initial or subsequent meeting between the physician and the parents, the physician must be able to ascertain the kind of professional relationship the family desires, as well as the anticipatory needs relative to care of their newborn and integration as a family unit.

Of paramount importance is the personal interaction between the physician and the parents before the discharge of the infant from the hospital. Providing reading materials to parents is relatively easy, but handouts can never replace the personal interaction, which can lay the groundwork for a lasting professional relationship between the physician and the parents.

FOLLOW-UP NEWBORN CARE

Timing

Follow-up of newborns within the 1st week—typically within 2 to 3 days of nursery discharge for newborns going home from the hospital within 48 hours of birth, newborns who are breastfeeding, or newborns with health concerns that place them at risk for early medical problems—is crucial to assessing the adequacy of hydration and feeding patterns and to assessing bilirubin levels and excessive weight loss. Studies have shown that newborns who receive early follow-up visits were less likely to be rehospitalized within the first 10 days of life for jaundice or dehydration.[31] The recommended timing for optimal newborn follow-up care is well established and is consistent across several organizations. According to the AAP, all healthy, singleton newborns between 38 and 42 weeks' gestation whose birthweight is appropriate for gestational age and who are discharged in fewer than 48 hours must have a follow-up appointment within 48 hours of discharge.[3] In 2001 the Joint Commission for the Accreditation of Health Care Organizations issued a Sentinel Event Alert, recommending that all newborns be followed-up within 24 to 48 hours by a physician or pediatric nurse.[32] The Bright Futures recommendation goes a step further by advising that, for mothers who are discharged within 24 to 48 hours of childbirth, a health professional should call the mother the 1st day after discharge to schedule an office visit within 3 days.[12] For infants who are discharged more than 48 hours after childbirth, the 1st office visit may occur within 2 to 4 days of discharge. In some communities, hospitals routinely offer families the option of bringing the infant back to the hospital for a postdischarge visit. These guidelines apply equally to formula-fed and breastfed infants. The AAP Section on Breastfeeding states: "All breastfeeding newborn infants should be seen by a pediatrician or other knowledgeable and experienced health care professionals at 3 to 5 days of age...and again at 2 to 3 weeks of age."[33]

Purpose

Although the main purpose of the visit is to detect problems such as jaundice, feeding difficulties, and excessive weight loss or poor weight gain, this visit also provides another opportunity for parents to have their infant examined, to be reassured about minor physical variations, and to have their questions answered.

The 2004 policy statement from the AAP states that the purpose of the follow-up visit is to[3]:

- Weigh the infant; assess the infant's general health, hydration, and degree of jaundice; identify any new problems; review feeding pattern and technique, including observation of breastfeeding for adequacy of position, latch-on, and swallowing; and obtain historical evidence of adequate urination and defecation patterns for the infant
- Assess the quality of mother-infant interaction and details of infant behavior
- Reinforce maternal or family education in infant care, particularly regarding infant feeding
- Review the results of laboratory tests performed before discharge
- Perform screening tests in accordance with state regulations and other tests that are clinically indicated, such as serum bilirubin
- Verify the plan for health care maintenance, including a method for obtaining emergency services, preventive care and immunizations, periodic evaluations and physical examinations, and necessary screenings

Families need reassurance that they are responding adequately to their infant's cues. Even a simple discussion of the normal variations in a newborn's schedule with regard to timing of feedings, sleep, and stool consistency and frequency can allay concerns and empower parents to be better observers, which can ultimately decrease stress and allow greater enjoyment of parenthood.

Barriers

On hospital discharge, physicians should ensure at a minimum that the following barriers to adequate follow-up care are addressed[3]:

- Lack of transportation to medical care services
- Lack of easy access to telephone communication
- Non–English-speaking parents

Inadequate communication from the hospital to the community-based provider about a newborn's birth, medical history, and relevant laboratory data may be the result of a lack of a clear mechanism for communication, as well as the fact that some families have not identified a postdischarge provider at the time of discharge. Gaps in parental knowledge have been attributable to a decreased opportunity for parental education with shorter LOS and lack of clinician awareness for early follow-up.

Despite the published recommendations for follow-up of newborns, many do not have a posthospital follow-up visit within the recommended time frame and do not receive appropriate management of hyperbilirubinemia.[34] Only approximately 50% of healthy term newborns who need phototherapy based on the AAP practice parameter actually receive it.[34,35] This circumstance is due, in part, to unfamiliarity with the guidelines and a well-established trend in which even guidelines based on an evidence-based approach do not translate readily into changes in standards of care and improved practice.[36] The AAP recognizes that "knowledge is essential but not sufficient to produce behavior change" and is actively working on a broad initiative, Ensuring Safe and Healthy Beginnings, which was initiated to close the gap between theory and practice in the management of issues that are critical to promoting a seamless transition from hospital discharge to home during the critical 1st week of life.[37]

TOOLS FOR PRACTICE

Engaging Patients and Family

- *Baby & Child Health—The Essential Guide From Birth to 11 Years* (book), American Academy of Pediatrics (www.aap.org/bookstore).
- *Breastfeeding Your Baby: Answers to Common Questions* (booklet), American Academy of Pediatrics (patiented.aap.org).
- *Car Safety Seats: A Guide for Families 2007* (fact sheet), American Academy of Pediatrics (patiented.aap.org).
- *Caring for Your Baby and Young Child: Birth to Age 5*, 4th edition (book), American Academy of Pediatrics (www.aap.org/bookstore).
- *Circumcision: Information for Parents* (brochure), American Academy of Pediatrics (patiented.aap.org).
- *Heading Home with Your Newborn* (book), American Academy of Pediatrics (www.aap.org/bookstore).
- *Jaundice and Your Newborn* (book), American Academy of Pediatrics (www.aap.org/bookstore).
- *One Minute Car Safety Seat Check Up* (fact sheet), American Academy of Pediatrics (patiented.aap.org).
- *Prevent Shaken Baby Syndrome* (brochure), American Academy of Pediatrics (patiented.aap.org).
- *SIDS: Important Information for Parents* (fact sheet), American Academy of Pediatrics (www.aap.org/bookstore).
- *The Wonder Years* (book), American Academy of Pediatrics (www.aap.org/bookstore).
- *Your Baby's First Year* (book), American Academy of Pediatrics (www.aap.org/bookstore).

Medical Decision Support

- *TIPP Safety Slips: REVISED! Four Steps to Prepare Your Family for Disasters* (fact sheet), American Academy of Pediatrics (www.aap.org/bookstore).

AAP POLICY STATEMENTS

American Academy of Pediatrics, Committee on Environmental Health. Environmental tobacco smoke: a hazard to children. *Pediatrics*. 1997;99(4):639-642. (aappolicy.aappublications.org/cgi/content/full/pediatrics;99/4/639).

American Academy of Pediatrics, Committee on Environmental Health. Lead exposure in children: prevention, detection, and management. *Pediatrics*. 2005;116(4):1036-1046. (aappolicy.aappublications.org/cgi/content/full/pediatrics;116/4/1036).

American Academy of Pediatrics, Committee on Fetus and Newborn. Hospital Stay for Healthy Term Newborns. *Pediatrics*. 2004;113(5):1434-1436. (aappolicy.aappublications.org/cgi/content/full/pediatrics;113/5/1434).

American Academy of Pediatrics, Committee on Injury and Poison Prevention. Safe transportation of newborns at hospital discharge. *Pediatrics*. 1999;104(4):986-987. (aappolicy.aappublications.org/cgi/content/full/pediatrics;104/4/986).

American Academy of Pediatrics, Committee on Nutrition. Iron fortification of infant formulas. *Pediatrics*. 1999;104(1):119-123. (aappolicy.aappublications.org/cgi/content/full/pediatrics;104/1/119).

American Academy of Pediatrics, Section on Breastfeeding. Breastfeeding and the use of human milk. *Pediatrics*. 2005;115(2):496-506. (aappolicy.aappublications.org/cgi/content/full/pediatrics;115/2/496).

American Academy of Pediatrics, Subcommittee on Hyperbilirubinemia. Management of hyperbilirubinemia in the newborn infant 35 or more weeks of gestation. *Pediatrics*. 2004;114(1):297-316. (aappolicy.aappublications.org/cgi/content/full/pediatrics;114/1/297).

American Academy of Pediatrics, Task Force on Circumcision. Circumcision policy statement. *Pediatrics*. 1999;103(3):686-693. (aappolicy.aappublications.org/cgi/content/full/pediatrics;103/3/686).

American Academy of Pediatrics, Task Force on Sudden Infant Death Syndrome. The changing concept of sudden infant death syndrome: diagnostic coding shifts, controversies regarding the sleeping environment, and new variables to consider in reducing risk. *Pediatrics*. 2005;116(5):1245-1255. (aappolicy.aappublications.org/cgi/content/full/pediatrics;116/5/1245).

REFERENCES

1. Britton JR, Baker A, Spino C, Bernstein HH. Postpartum discharge preferences of pediatricians: results from a national survey. *Pediatrics*. 2002;110:53-60.
2. Thilo EH, Townsend SF, Merenstein GB. The history of policy and practice related to the perinatal hospital stay. *Clin Perinatol*. 1998;25:257-270.
3. American Academy of Pediatrics, Committee on Fetus and Newborn. Hospital stay for healthy term newborns. *Pediatrics*. 2004;113:1434-1436.
4. Bradley W. Newborns' and Mothers' Health Protection Act of 1996. Pubic Law No. 104-204.
5. Danielson B, Castles AG, Damberg CL, et al. Newborn discharge timing and readmissions: California, 1992-1995. *Pediatrics*. 2000;106:31-39.
6. American Academy of Pediatrics, Committee on Fetus and Newborn. *Standards and Recommendations for Hospital Care of Newborn Infants*. 6th ed. Evanston, IL: American Academy of Pediatrics; 1977.
7. American Academy of Pediatrics, Committee on Fetus and Newborn. Hospital stay for healthy term newborns. *Pediatrics*. 1995;96:788-789.
8. Johnston R, Fennessy P, Anderson J. *The Benefit of One Compared to Two Routine Neonatal Examinations Before Discharge for the Detection of Congenital Hips, Cleft Palates, Cardiac, and Eye Abnormalities in Healthy Term Neonates*. Evidence Centre Report. Victoria, Australia: Centre for Clinical Effectiveness, Monash University; 1999.
9. Knowles R, Griebsch I, Dezateux C, et al. Newborn screening for congenital heart defects: a systematic review and cost-effectiveness analysis. *Health Technol Assess*. 2005;9(44):1-168.
10. US Preventive Services Task Force. Newborn hearing screening: recommendations and rationale. *Am Fam Physician*. 2001;64(12):1995-1999.
11. Thompson DC, McPhillips H, Davis RL, et al. Universal newborn hearing screening: summary of the evidence. *JAMA*. 2001;286(16);2000-2010.
12. Hagan JF Jr, Shaw JS, Duncan PM, eds. *Bright Futures: Guidelines for Health Supervision of Infants, Children, and Adolescents*, 3rd ed. Elk Grove Village, IL: American Academy of Pediatrics; 2008.
13. Charney E. Counseling of parents around the birth of a baby. *Pediatr Rev*. 1982;4:167-174.
14. Goldenring JM, Goldenring H. What to tell new parents before they leave the hospital. *Contempo Pediatr*. 1993; Resident Supplement:14-25.
15. Glaze DG. Childhood insomnia: why Chris can't sleep. *Pediatr Clin North Am*. 2004;51:34-50.
16. American Academy of Pediatrics, Task Force on Sudden Infant Death Syndrome. The changing concept of sudden infant death syndrome: diagnostic coding shifts, controversies regarding the sleeping environment, and new variables to consider in reducing risk. *Pediatrics*. 2005;116:1245-1255.
17. Lahr MB, Rosenberg DK, Lapidus JA. Bedsharing and maternal smoking in a population-based survey of new mothers. *Pediatrics*. 2005;116:e530-e542.
18. Tappin D, Ecob R, Brooke H. Bedsharing, roomsharing, and sudden infant death syndrome in Scotland: a case-control study. *Pediatrics*. 2005;147:32-37.
19. World Health Organization. Care of the umbilical cord: a review of the evidence, 1998; Zupan J, Garner P, Omari AAA. Topical umbilical cord care at birth. *Cochrane Database Syst Rev*. 2004;3:CD001057.
20. Association of Women's Health, Obstetric and Neonatal Nurses (AWHONN). Neonatal skin care: evidence based clinical practice guideline. Washington, DC: AWHONN; 2001.
21. Anderson JM, Philip AGS. Management of the umbilical cord: care regimen, colonization, infection, and separation. *NeoReviews*. 2004;5:e155-e162.
22. Jana LA, Shu J, *Baby Bath Basics. Heading Home with Your Newborn from Birth to Reality*. Elk Grove Village, IL: American Academy of Pediatrics; 2005.
23. Odio M, Streicher-Scott J, Hansen RC. Disposable baby wipes: efficacy and skin mildness. *Dermatol Nurs*. 2001;13:107-112, 117-118, 121.
24. American Academy of Pediatrics. Basic Infant Care. In: Shelov S, ed. *Caring for Your Baby and Young Child*. New York, NY: American Academy of Pediatrics; 1991.
25. American Academy of Pediatrics, Committee on Injury and Poison Prevention. Selecting and using the most appropriate car safety seats for growing children: guidelines for counseling parents. *Pediatrics*. 2002;109:550-553.
26. American Academy of Pediatrics, Committee on Environmental Health. Developmental toxicity: special considerations based on age and developmental stage. In: Etzel RA, ed. *Pediatric Environmental Health*, 2nd ed. Elk Grove Village, IL: American Academy of Pediatrics; 2003.

27. American Academy of Pediatrics, Committee on Environmental Health. Carbon monoxide. In: Etzel RA, ed. *Pediatric Environmental Health*. 2nd ed. Elk Grove Village, IL: American Academy of Pediatrics; 2003.
28. Knight L, Levin A, Mendenhall C. *Candles and Incense as Potential Sources of Indoor Air Pollution: Market Analysis and Literature Review*. EPA/600/SR-01/001. Springfield, VA: National Technical Information Service; 2001.
29. American Academy of Pediatrics, Committee on Environmental Health. Lead. In: Etzel RA, ed. *Pediatric Environmental Health*. 2nd ed. Elk Grove Village, IL: American Academy of Pediatrics; 2003.
30. American Academy of Pediatrics, Committee on Environmental Health. Pesticides. In: Etzel RA, ed. *Pediatric Environmental Health*. 2nd ed. Elk Grove Village, IL: American Academy of Pediatrics; 2003.
31. Meara E, Kotogal UR, Atherton HD, et al. Impact of early newborn discharge legislation and early follow-up visits on infant outcomes in a state Medicaid population. *Pediatrics*. 2004;113:1619-1627.
32. Salem-Schatz S, Peterson LE, Palmer RH, et al. Barriers to first-week follow-up of newborns: findings from parent and clinician focus groups. *Jnt Comm J Qual Safe*. 2004;30:593-601.
33. American Academy of Pediatrics, Section on Breastfeeding. Breastfeeding and the use of human milk. *Pediatrics*. 2005;115:496-506.
34. Atkinson LR, Escobar GJ, Takayama JL, et al. Phototherapy use in jaundiced newborns in a large managed care organization: do clinicians adhere to the guidelines? *Pediatrics*. 2003;111(5):e555-e561. Available at www.pediatrics.org/cgi/content/full/111/5/e555.
35. American Academy of Pediatrics, Subcommittee on Hyperbilirubinemia. Management of hyperbilirubinemia in the newborn infant 35 or more weeks of gestation. *Pediatrics*. 2004;114:297-316.
36. Christakis DA, Rivara FP. Pediatrician's awareness of and attitudes about four clinical practice guidelines. *Pediatrics*. 1998;101:825-830.
37. Lannon C, Stark A. Closing the gap between guidelines and practice: ensuring safe and healthy beginnings. *Pediatrics*. 2004;114:494-496.

Chapter 94

FOLLOW-UP CARE OF THE HEALTHY NEWBORN

Deborah E. Campbell, MD

The timing of initial follow-up care of newborns after nursery discharge is based on several factors: the newborn's gestational age and postnatal age at hospital discharge, whether the newborn is breastfeeding or formula feeding, the quality and efficiency of the newborn's feeding abilities, and the presence of risk factors that predispose to complications or an increased risk for early hospital readmission.[1] In a report by Jackson et al, 8% of indigent urban neonates monitored developed signs of illness in the early postnatal period. Of these, 31% developed symptoms after 24 hours of age, emphasizing the importance for early postdischarge follow-up care.[2] Among insured newborns with access to an integrated system of health care, follow-up care within 72 hours of nursery discharge has been found to be protective against the risk for early rehospitalization.[3] The Pregnancy Risk Assessment Monitoring System (PRAMS) collects data about newborn discharge and the timing and adequacy of postdischarge follow-up care from 27 states participating in this Centers of Disease Control and Prevention program. In 2002 the percentage of newborns discharged from the hospital within 48 hours of birth ranged from 50% to 70%.[4] Significant variation was noted among states in the receipt of follow-up within the first week, ranging from 58% to 90%. PRAMS also found that during the period between 2000 and 2002, several states improved in the proportion of infants receiving follow-up within the first week of life. Five states (Arkansas, Florida, Illinois, North Carolina, and Utah) made significant strides in improving compliance with first week follow-up care for newborns during this period of monitoring. Also notable is that only two states, New York and Rhode Island, exceeded the 90% threshold for infants having received *sufficient well-baby care* during the first 9 months of life.

Early follow-up is important in terms of reassessing the newborn for signs of illness related to congenital malformations that are not evident at birth or during the immediate newborn period. Parental adaptation to their new role and an assessment of the mother's and the newborn's readiness to leave the hospital are additional aspects to consider in determining how soon follow-up should occur. Maternal depression and the potential for peripartum abuse of the mother are additional potential risk factors that support the need for early follow-up.[5] Research regarding perceptions about mother and baby readiness for discharge from the hospital emphasizes the importance of mutual decision making about the optimal time for discharge and follow-up care.[6] Recommendations concerning the optimal timing for the initial postdischarge pediatric visit are consensus based, formulated from reported cohort and population study outcomes for newborns who have been discharged within 48 hours of birth.[7-15]

The initial follow-up visit may be provided in the newborn's home, a hospital-affiliated newborn follow-up clinic, or in the primary pediatric care physician's office. The guiding principle for this phase of care is that it should be a physician-directed source of continuing medical care for the mother and baby.[16] An important factor in the decision about where and how the initial care should occur is identification of barriers to the parents' ability to comply with early postnatal follow-up. Issues of access to care remain significant despite the 1996 Newborns' and Mothers' Health Protection Act and the Health Insurance Portability and Accountability Act of 1996, which stipulate that access of the mother and her newborn to appropriate follow-up health care must be ensured and that insurers cannot deny newborns coverage to avoid complying with these federal mandates. Numerous studies document the impact of federal regulations and the newborn's insurance status on health care utilization and the timeliness of postdischarge newborn follow-up. Common factors identified across studies are the level of maternal education, families living in poverty or residing in poor communities with limited access to care, other children at home, and immigrant or non-English–speaking status.[17-27]

Barriers to timely follow-up of newborns during the first week of life have been explored through focus groups with families and clinicians.[28] Clinicians and parents identify issues of communication and information, processes of care, and parent knowledge and education as critical factors. Parents' value and can assimilate information about early warning signs in regard to their newborn. Pediatric primary care physicians play an important role in setting office practices regarding the timing of newborn follow-up care. Despite a long-established recommendation regarding the need for early follow-up after a short newborn nursery hospitalization, many clinicians still counsel parents that follow-up within 1 to 2 weeks after nursery discharge is acceptable.[29,30] Other barriers are limited office hours or inadequate hospital and community resources to provide timely home health or pubic health nursing visits, particularly on weekends and holidays. This barrier can prevent a family's compliance with a recommended 24- to 48-hour follow-up visit or home visit. Assistance with scheduling the initial follow-up appointment, particularly among Medicaid recipients, has been shown to be an effective strategy to parental compliance with infant follow-up.[31,32]

Goals of 48- to 72-hour follow-up care include the following:

- Assess the newborn's general health, hydration, and degree of jaundice and identify any new problems.
- Review the newborn's feeding pattern and technique, including observation of breastfeeding for appropriate positioning, latch-on, coordinated sucking and swallowing, and any maternal concerns regarding clinical problems that can disrupt effective breastfeeding (newborn state regulation; cracked or sore nipples; mastitis; engorgement, flat, or inverted nipples, prior breast surgery).
- Review the pregnancy and family history, pertinent prenatal diagnostic test results, and the newborn's hospital course to ensure identification of risk factors requiring further assessment and follow-up care. (This review is particularly important if the infant is new to the physician's practice.)
- Assess the infant's voiding and stooling patterns.
- Assess maternal-infant interaction and details of newborn behavior (state regulation and adaptation), maternal and family adaptation to the infant, family functioning, and signs of maternal depression or family distress.
- Reinforce education about newborn care, feeding practices, and safety, including safe sleep practices.
- Perform necessary screening tests in accordance with state regulations and other tests as clinically indicated. Repeat blood spot testing if the newborn was initially tested before at least 24 hours of milk feedings. The optimal time for screening for congenital hypothyroidism is between 48 and 96 hours of life. Specimens collected in the first 24 to 48 hours of life may lead to false-positive thyroid-stimulating hormone elevations when using any screening test approach.
- Review with the mother or family the baby's ongoing preventive health care needs, including immunizations, completion of the newborn hearing screen, and scheduling of other evaluations as needed based on prenatal testing or postnatal assessment.
- Review with the mother or family how to access care in an emergency and for routine or nonurgent issues.
- Review with the mother or family the adequacy of family resources, including the newborn's health care coverage.
- Solicit and discuss any parent-identified concerns or issues related to the newborn or family.

Neonatal weight loss is often an issue of concern for families and clinicians, particularly because dehydration and failure to thrive are significant risks for the newborn who is experiencing feeding difficulties or whose mother has lactation failure. Controversy exists about routine monitoring of a newborn's weight, given that some clinicians have expressed concern that unnecessary interventions, interruption of exclusive breastfeeding, and parental anxiety may occur in response to early weight loss.[33,34] McKie et al noted that implementation of regular neonatal weight monitoring among a cohort of infants in Scotland did not reduce breastfeeding among the cohort of women and infants studied.[35] Another recent cohort observational study of 961 term newborns born in Scotland found that, by 5 days of age, 34% had regained their birth weight; 17 % were more than 5% below birth weight, with 3% of these infants more than 10% below birth weight. The mean weight loss for this group of babies was 50 g (1.67 oz). At 12 days of age, over 80% had regained birth weight, with the majority gaining an average of nearly 200 g. The degree of weight loss was correlated with newborn birth weight; term neonates with lower weights exhibited minimal weight loss.[36] Comparison of early neonatal weight-loss patterns between breastfeeding and formula-feeding term newborns demonstrated a median weight loss of 6.6% among breastfeeding babies versus 3.5% for formula-feeding neonates. Typically, breastfeeding babies lose more weight and take longer to regain their birth weight compared with formula-feeding babies; upper limits of weight loss were 12% of birth weight for breastfeeding babies versus 8% for formula-feeding babies. The median time of maximal weight loss and time to regain birth weight was also longer for the breastfeeding infant.[37]

A complete physical examination should be performed. Key aspects of the examination include the following:

- Eyes for opacities including cataracts (red reflex)
- Heart for congenital heart disease (cyanosis, murmur, tachypnea, femoral pulses)
- Hips for dysplasia (Barlow and Ortolani tests)
- Skin for evidence of jaundice, drying of the umbilical cord, lesions suggestive of infection, and pallor
- Nervous and musculoskeletal systems for state regulation, activity and response to stimulation, tone and reflexes, asymmetry limb posture, position, and movement
- Assessment of the newborn's hydration status, particularly for newborns at risk for feeding difficulties (prematurity, poor feeding or poor cuing in regard to hunger, signs of illness or anomalies not previously identified)

Subsequent follow-up primary care appointments are typically based on specific newborn and parent needs. Routine primary care follow-up after the first week postdischarge newborn visit for the healthy term newborn without health issues requiring interim care is scheduled for 6 to 8 weeks of age. Components of the assessment at that health visit include a thorough physical examination, with special attention focused on evaluation of the eyes for opacities, including cataracts (red reflex), heart for congenital heart disease (cyanosis, murmur, tachypnea, femoral pulses), and hips for dysplasia (Barlow and Ortolani tests). Results of newborn screening test and any other interim screening or diagnostic studies performed should be reviewed to ensure that further evaluation or treatment is not required.

TOOLS FOR PRACTICE

Medical Decision Support

- *Guidelines for Perinatal Care, 6th edition* (book), American Academy of Pediatrics and American College of Obstetricians and Gynecologists (www.aap.org/bst).
- *PRAMS 2002 Surveillance Report,* Centers for Disease Control and Prevention (www.cdc.gov/PRAMS/2002PRAMSSurvReport/PDF/2k2PRAMS.pdf).
- Cox JL, Holden JM, Sagovsky R. Detection of postnatal depression: Development of the 10-item Edinburgh Postnatal Depression Scale. *Br J Psychiatry.* 1987:150: 782-786. (www.aap.org/practicingsafety/Toolkit_Resources/Module2/EPDS.pdf).

AAP POLICY STATEMENTS

American Academy of Pediatrics, Committee on Fetus and Newborn, Subcommittee on Hyperbilirubinemia. Policy statement: clinical practice guidelines: management of hyperbilirubinemia in the newborn infant 35 weeks or more of gestation. *Pediatrics.* 2004;114(1):297-316. (aappolicy.aappublications.org/cgi/content/full/pediatrics;114/1/297).

American Academy of Pediatrics, Committee on Fetus and Newborn. Hospital stay for healthy term newborns. *Pediatrics.* 2004;113(5):1434-1436. (aappolicy.aappublications.org/cgi/content/full/pediatrics;113/5/1434).

American Academy of Pediatrics, Rose SR, and the Section on Endocrinology and Committee on Genetics; American Thyroid Association, Brown RS, and the Public Health Committee; Lawson Wilkins Pediatric Endocrine Society. Update of newborn screening and therapy for congenital hypothyroidism. *Pediatrics.* 2006;117(6):2290-2303. (aappolicy.aappublications.org/cgi/content/full/pediatrics;117/6/2290).

REFERENCES

1. Lannon C, Stark AR. Closing the gap between guidelines and practice: ensuring safe and healthy beginnings. *Pediatrics.* 2004;114:494-496.
2. Jackson GL, Kennedy KA, Sendelbach DM, et al. Problem identification in apparently well neonates: implications for early discharge. *Clin Pediatr.* 2000;39:581-590.
3. Escobar GJ, Greene JD, Hulac P, et al. Rehospitalization after birth hospitalization: patterns among infants of all gestation. *Arch Dis Child.* 2005;90:125-131.
4. Williams L, Morrow B, Shulman H, et al. *PRAMS 2002 Surveillance Report.* Atlanta, GA: Centers for Disease Control and Prevention, National Center for Chronic Disease Prevention and Health Promotion, Division of Reproductive Health; 2006.
5. Martin SL, Mackie L, Kupper LI, et al. Physical abuse of women before, during and after pregnancy. *JAMA.* 2001; 285(12):1581-1584.
6. Bernstein HH, Spino C, Finch S, et al. Decision-making for postpartum discharge of 4300 mothers and their healthy infants: The Life Around Newborn Discharge Study. *Pediatrics.* 2007;120(2):e391-e400.
7. Maisels MJ, Kring E. Length of stay, jaundice, and hospital readmission. *Pediatrics.* 1998;101(6):995-998.
8. Paul IM, Lehman EB, Hollenbeak CS, et al. Preventable newborn readmissions since passage of the Newborns' and Mothers' Health Protection Act. *Pediatrics.* 2006; 118(6):2349-2358.
9. Paul IM, Phillips TA, Widome MD, et al. Cost-effectiveness of postnatal home nursing visits for prevention of hospital care for jaundice and dehydration. *Pediatrics.* 2004;114(4): 1015-1022.
10. Wang ML, Dorer DJ, Fleming MP, et al. Clinical outcomes of near-term infants. *Pediatrics.* 2004;114(2): 372-376.
11. Madden JM, Soumerai SB, Lieu TA, et al. Length-of-stay policies and ascertainment of postdischarge problems in newborns. *Pediatrics.* 2004;113(1):42-49.
12. Britton JR, Britton HL, Gronwaldt V. Early perinatal hospital discharge and parenting during infancy. *Pediatrics.* 1999;104(5):1070-1076.
13. Malkin JD, Garber S, Broder MS, et al. Infant mortality and early postpartum discharge. *Obstet Gynecol.* 2000; 96:183-188.
14. General Accounting Office. *Maternity Care: Appropriate Follow-up Services Critical With Short Hospital Stays.* Washington, DC: General Accounting Office; 1996.
15. Danielsen B, Castles AG, Damberg CL, et al. Newborn discharge timing and readmissions: California, 1992-1995. *Pediatrics.* 2000;106:31-39.
16. American Academy of Pediatrics, American College of Obstetrics and Gynecology. *Guidelines for Perinatal Care.* 5th ed. Elk Grove Village, IL: American Academy of Pediatrics; 2002.
17. Flores G, Abreu M, Olivar MA, et al. Access barriers to health care for Latino children. *Arch Pediatr Adolesc Med.* 1998;152:1119-1125.
18. Lieu TA, Braveman PA, Escobar GJ, et al. A randomized comparison of home and clinic follow-up visits after early postpartum hospital discharge. *Pediatrics.* 2000;15: 1058-1065.
19. Escobar GJ, Braveman PA, Ackerson L, et al. A randomized comparison of home visits and hospital-based group follow-up visits after early postpartum discharge. *Pediatrics.* 2001;108:719-727.
20. Galbraith AA, Egerter SA, Marchi KS, et al. Newborn early discharge revisited: are California newborns receiving recommended postnatal services? *Pediatrics.* 2003;11:364-371.
21. Meara E, Kotagal UR, Atherton HD, et al. Impact of early newborn discharge legislation and early follow-up visits on infant outcomes in a state Medicaid population. *Pediatrics.* 2004;113(6):1619-1627.
22. Madlon-Kay DJ, DeFor TA, Egerter S. Newborn length of stay, health care utilization, and the effect of minnesota legislation. *Arch Pediatr Adolesc Med.* 2003; 157(6): 579-583.
23. Madden JM, Soumerai SB, Lieu TA, et al. Effects on breastfeeding of changes in maternity length-of-stay policy in a large health maintenance organization. *Pediatrics.* 2003;111(3):519-524.

24. Madden JM, Soumerai SB, Lieu TA, et al. Effects of a law against early postpartum discharge on newborn follow-up, adverse events, and HMO expenditures. *N Engl J Med*. 2002;347(25):2031-2038.
25. Kotagal UR, Atherton HD, Eshett R, et al. Safety of early discharge for Medicaid newborns. *JAMA*. 1999;282(12): 1150-1156.
26. Datar A, Sood N. Impact of postpartum hospital-stay legislation on newborn length of stay, readmission, and mortality in California. *Pediatrics*. 2006;118(1):63-72.
27. Madlon-Kay DJ, Asche SE. Factors that influence the receipt of well baby care in the first 2 weeks of life. *J Am Board Fam Med*. 2006;19:258-264.
28. Salem-Schatz S, Peterson LE, Palmer RH, et al. Barriers to first week follow-up care of newborns: findings from parent and clinician focus groups. *Joint Comm J Qual Safe*. 2004;30(11):593-601.
29. Maisels MJ, Kring E. Early discharge from the newborn nursery—effect on scheduling of follow-up visits by pediatricians. *Pediatrics*. 1997;100:72-74.
30. Madlon-Kay DJ. Evaluation and management of newborn jaundice by Midwest family physicians. *J Fam Pract*. 1998;47:461-464.
31. Feinberg AN, Hicks WB. Patient compliance with the first newborn visit appointment. *J Perinatol*. 2003; 23:37-40.
32. Feinberg AN, McAllister DG, Majumdar S. Does making newborn follow-up appointments from the hospital improve compliance? *J Perinatol*. 2004;24:645-649.
33. Oddie S, Richmond S, Coulthard M. Hypernatremic dehydration and breastfeeding: a population study. *Arch Dis Child*. 2001;85:318-320.
34. National Institute for Health and Clinical Excellence. *Clinical Guidelines and Evidence for Review for Postnatal Care: Routine Postnatal Care of Recently Delivered Women and Their Babies*. London, UK: National Collaborating Centre for Primary Care and the Royal College of General Practitioners; 2006.
35. McKie A, Young D, Macdonald PD. Does monitoring newborn weight discourage breastfeeding? *Arch Dis Child*. 2006;91:44-46.
36. Wright CM, Parkinson KN. Postnatal weight loss in term infants: what is "normal" and do growth charts allow for it? *Arch Dis Child Fetal Neonatal Ed*. 2004; 89:F254-F257.
37. Macdonald PD, Ross SRM, Grant L, et al. Neonatal weight loss in breast and formula fed infants. *Arch Dis Child Fetal Neonatal Ed*. 2003;88:F472-F47.

Chapter 95

HEALTH AND DEVELOPMENTAL OUTCOMES OF INFANTS REQUIRING NEONATAL INTENSIVE CARE

Deborah E. Campbell, MD; Sonia O. Imaizumi, MD; Judy C. Bernbaum, MD

Approximately 10% to 15% of newborns require specialized neonatal care after their birth. The preterm and low–birth-weight (LBW) rates in the United States continued to increase in 2005 and were reported as 12.5% and 8.2%, respectively.[1] Very preterm (<32 weeks' gestation) and moderately preterm infants (34-36 weeks' gestation) now account for 11.3% of all births nationally. Among infants born LBW, defined at less than 5.5 lb, the rates of very low–birth-weight (VLBW) infants (<1500 g, or less than 3.3 lb) and moderately LBW (1501-2499 g) infants have also increased contributing to higher neonatal and infant mortality rates. Currently, 99.6% of all newborns survive until the newborn is discharged from the hospital.

Innovations in prenatal diagnosis, fetal interventions, and neonatal intensive and surgical care have contributed to the survival of extremely premature babies and infants with malformations for which therapy was previously limited. Improved survival rates have led to increased numbers of infants and children with chronic health conditions and increased use of chronic and acute care resources. The need for neonatal intensive care after birth has long-term health-related quality-of-life implications.[2] This need is particularly true for children born preterm.[3] Rehospitalization rates for infants who have required neonatal intensive care are higher than for healthy term infants. Illness severity is typically less among late preterm infants (greater than 34 weeks' gestation) and babies who required fewer than 4 days of neonatal intensive care. As discussed in Chapter 92, Care of the Late Preterm Infant, babies born between 33 and 37 weeks' gestation are most likely to require rehospitalization for problems related to jaundice, feeding difficulties, dehydration, and suspected sepsis. Among infants younger than 32 weeks' gestation, the most common readmission diagnoses are sepsis, respiratory disease, gastroesophageal reflux or apparent life-threatening events, and hernia repair.[4,5] Normal–birth-weight (NBW) infants who require neonatal intensive care, babies with congenital anomalies, and neonates with a low 5 minute Apgar score have higher post–neonatal intensive care unit (NICU) health care utilization—physician visits, assistive technology use, and rehospitalization; over 30% of infants with malformations require rehospitalization during the first 6 months of life.[6]

The primary causes of postneonatal deaths for infants between 28 and 364 days of age have remained stable over the last decade, although the number of infants dying during the postnatal period from a specific cause has changed in frequency. During 1985 and 1986, the most common causes for postneonatal death were sudden infant death, congenital conditions, prematurity-related conditions, and nonintentional injuries. The Centers for Disease Control and Prevention reported that the five leading causes of infant mortality during 2004 were (1) congenital malformations (20%), (2) disorders relating to short gestation and LBW, (3) sudden infant death syndrome (8%), (4) maternal complications of pregnancy (6%), and (5) unintentional injuries (4%). Comparison of 2003 and 2004 data reveal that the order of the leading causes of death changed slightly when unintentional injuries moved from the sixth to the fifth leading cause. Variations also exist in the frequencies of these causes of death related to race and Hispanic origin.[1,7,8]

HEALTH-RELATED OUTCOMES DURING INFANCY AND CHILDHOOD

Health-related outcomes and health-related quality of life (HRQL) are important considerations when evaluating the consequences of neonatal illness and the cost effectiveness of care. Infancy and early childhood measures of quality of life and health status among newborns requiring neonatal intensive care reveal that preschool aged children who required NICU care had poorer health status and HRQL than newborns who did not require NICU care.[9] Among preterm children born at less than 32 weeks' gestation, parents report significantly lower HRQL, with problems affecting the lungs and stomach, eating disorders and problems with motor functioning, communication, and anxiety.[10] The range and severity of the developmental and health conditions experienced by these infants is influenced by the number of developmental domains affected. Among infants tracked prospectively who were born less than 30 weeks' gestation, 17% had a single disability, whereas 44% exhibited multiple disabilities. LBW, chronic lung disease, and evidence of disability at 2 years were associated with multiple impairments.[11] Health outcomes and HRQL of preschool children born between 29 and 32 weeks' gestation have been shown to be quite similar to children born at less than 28 weeks' gestation, despite the fact that the children younger than 28 weeks' gestation typically are sicker than the later-arriving group of infants. In addition, children born 28 to 32 weeks' gestation differ in both their health and development in comparison to children born at term.[12] Among children with intellectual disability, the prevalence of birth defects is reported to be approximately 30% in population-based data, the percentage of intellectual disability varying with the specific organ system involved.[13] A comprehensive review of outcomes for all infants requiring neonatal, special, or intensive care is beyond the scope of this chapter. However, outcomes for the broad categories of infants who require the greatest resource utilization while hospitalized are reviewed.

Respiratory Disease and Lung Function

Chronic lung disease (CLD) of infancy encompasses a heterogeneous group of pulmonary disorders that originate in the perinatal period and produce airway and parenchymal inflammation, leading to chronic airway obstruction, increased work of breathing, and airway hyperreactivity. Bronchopulmonary dysplasia (BPD) is one such condition that develops in response to the interplay of inciting factors: lung immaturity and surfactant deficiency in combination with barotrauma and stretch injury to the lung and oxygen toxicity from the therapies applied to treat the underlying disease. Extreme prematurity, the presence of intrauterine inflammation (antenatal chorioamnionitis), and changes in alveolar development caused by early extrauterine lung growth further alter lung growth and development. More mature preterm and full-term infants requiring ventilator support are also potentially at risk for developing BPD and subsequently CLD of infancy. Conditions that can cause CLD of infancy include pneumonia or sepsis, meconium aspiration pneumonia, pulmonary hypoplasia, persistent pulmonary hypertension of the newborn, apnea and various congenital malformations involving the cardiorespiratory system (tracheoesophageal fistula, congenital diaphragmatic hernia, and congenital heart disease), and congenital neuromuscular disorders.[14] (For further information, see Chapter 99, Respiratory Distress and Breathing Disorders in the Newborn.)

Child Vulnerability

The experience of giving birth to an infant who has a prenatal diagnosis or requires neonatal intensive care is traumatic for families. A prolonged hospitalization, the diagnosis of an infant with a chronic health condition, the medically fragile survivor of a complicated neonatal hospital course, and, in some instances, even a non–life-threatening, self-limited condition such as hyperbilirubinemia or transient tachypnea of the newborn can predispose the child to *vulnerable child syndrome*. Parental reactions to their child's illness or perceived vulnerability can have long-term psychological consequences, with deleterious effects for the child and family. Among the parental responses observed can be excessive concerns about the child's health and development leading to hypervigilance, medical visits for minor symptoms, separation problems, difficulty with limit setting, sleep disorders, and underestimation of the child's abilities and potential. Parental stress can also lead to family dysfunction, increase the risk for child maltreatment (either the child who is ill or a sibling), and affect the parents' own health and well being.[15]

OVERVIEW OF THE SHORT- AND LONG-TERM OUTCOMES FOR SELECTED GROUPS OF HIGH-RISK INFANTS

Prematurity

Outcomes data for preterm infants have focused principally on the very low–birth-weight (VLBW) or extremely preterm infant. The emphasis on babies born early or with a LBW is growing because of the increased understanding of the short- and long-term morbidities experienced by these children, as well as the effect on their cognitive and developmental performance. Male preterm children are reported to have more behavioral problems and higher disability rates than female preterm children.

Very Low–Birth-Weight, Extremely Preterm Infants

The National Institute of Child Health and Human Development (NICHD) Center for Research for Mothers and Children Neonatal Research Network has been prospectively collecting data regarding VLBW preterm infants and children since 1993. Survival rates for infants born during the 1990s between 23 and 32 weeks' gestation have increased. Tables 95-1 to 95-3 summarize the early outcomes data for this group of infants.[16] Rates of low mental developmental assessment scores and neurodevelopmental impairment at 18 to 22 months of age declined in infants born in the late 1990s, and the improved outcome correlated with antenatal steroid administration to promote fetal lung maturity. Among infants born weighing less than

Table 95-1 Neurodevelopmental Outcomes of Extremely Low–Birth-Weight Infants (1993-1998)

OUTCOME	22-26 WEEKS	27-32 WEEKS	*P* VALUE
Survival	61%	86%	.0001
Moderate or severe cerebral palsy	10%	6%	.0001
Mental developmental index <70	37%	23%	.0001
Psychomotor developmental index <70	26%	17%	.0001
Blind	1%	0.4%	.01
Hearing loss	1.8%	1.8%	NS
Neurodevelopmental impairment	45%	28%	.0001

NS, not significant
From: Vohr BR, Wright LL, Poole K, et al. Neurodevelopmental outcomes of extremely low birth weight infants <32 weeks' gestation between 1995-1998. *Pediatrics.* 2005;116(3):635-643.

Table 95-2 Outcomes at 18-22 Months' Corrected Age By Weight Quartile

OUTCOME (%)	QUARTILE 1	QUARTILE 4	*P* VALUE
Cerebral palsy	21	6	<.01
Abnormal neurodevelopment	30	14	<.01
MDI <70	39	21	<.01
PDI <70	35	14	<.001
Head circumference <10%	31	22	.09
Rehospitalized	63	45	.01

MDI, Mental developmental index; *PDI,* psychomotor developmental index.
Quartile 1, <25%; *quartile 4,* >75%.
From: Ehrenkrantz RA, Dusick AM, Vohr BR, et al. Growth in the neonatal intensive care unit influences neurodevelopmental and growth outcomes of extremely low birth weight infants. *Pediatrics.* 2006;117:1253-1261.

1500 g (3.3 lb), reports of survival and morbidity rates through the first 4 months of life have changed little since the mid-1990s.[17] The survival rate for infants born from 1997 to 2002 with birth weights between 501 g (1.1 lb) and 1500 g (3.3 lb) is 85%. Birth weight–specific survival for babies born during this period weighing 501 to 750 grams (1.10-1.65 lb) is 55%. The survival rate improved to 88% for infants weighing 751 to 1000 g. For infants with birth weights in the weight groups 1001 to 1250 g (2.2-2.75 lb) and 1251 to 1500 g, survival is similar at 94% and 96%, respectively. Among infants born between 1993 and 1998, extremely preterm infants with gestational ages between 27 and 32 weeks showed a significant decline in the percentage of children with a mental developmental index (MDI) less than 70 over time. In contrast, rates of cerebral palsy (CP) for all infants between 22 and 32 weeks remained stable, as did the percentage of infants with MDI less than 70 who were born 22 to 26 weeks' gestation.[16]

Factors Influencing Outcomes in Extremely Low–Birth-Weight Infants

Improvements in antenatal and postnatal care have contributed to a reduction in some sequelae. Survival without neonatal major morbidity (BPD, intraventricular hemorrhage [IVH], and necrotizing enterocolitis) has remained unchanged at 70%. A nearly 20% increase has been reported in the survival rate of VLBW infants born of a multiple gestation. Postnatal growth failure, common among immature and sick infants, has also decreased. Among the least-mature infants weighing 501 g to 750 g, morbidity rates have increased since the mid 1990s. Only 20% of these infants are reported to be morbidity free. Babies born weighing 751 to 1000 g fare somewhat better, with 33% exhibiting major neonatal morbidity; 55% of these infants are free of neonatal morbidities by 4 months of age. Similar differences are seen when the infants are grouped by gestational age (see Table 95-1). Neonatal nutrition and postnatal growth are additional factors that influence outcomes at 18 to 22 months of age, as summarized in Table 95-2.[18] Adequacy of postnatal growth also influences school-aged outcomes; infants with postnatal growth problems exhibit poorer cognitive scores and academic achievement. Preterm infants who are small for gestational age at birth but who demonstrate adequate postnatal growth do not exhibit deficits similar to those seen among appropriately grown preterm infants with poor postnatal

Table 95-3 Factors Associated With Neurodevelopmental Morbidity in Infants With Normal Head Ultrasounds

FACTOR	CEREBRAL PALSY, OR	MENTAL DEVELOPMENTAL INDEX LESS THAN 70, OR
Male	1.8	2.0
Multiple birth	1.6	1.8
Low birth weight	1.3	1.2
Pneumothorax	2.3	—
Prolonged ventilation	1.2	—
Maternal race (black/Hispanic & other)	—	1.6/1.5
Maternal education	—	1.4
Public assistance	—	1.7

OR, odds ratio

Adapted from Laptook AR, O'Shea M, Shankaran S, Bhaskar B, and the NICHD Neonatal Network. Adverse neurodevelopmental outcomes among extremely low birth weight infants with a normal head ultrasound: prevalence and antecedents. *Pediatrics.* 2005;115(3):673-680.

growth.[19] Providing human milk as part of the extremely low–birth-weight (ELBW) infant's nutritional regimen appears to have a protective effect on MDI measurements at 18 months corrected age. Every 10 mL of human milk fed was correlated with a 0.5-point increase in the MDI score.[20] Evidence indicates that all areas of brain growth, including the whole brain, cerebral and subcortical gray matter, and cerebral white matter, are affected.[21] Regions of the brain that are most vulnerable are the sensorimotor cortex, premotor cortex, and mid–temporal cortex. Cerebral volume at 8 years of age is related to the child's gestational age, irrespective of evidence of chorioamnionitis at birth or the presence of ventriculomegaly or periventricular leukomalacia.[22] High rates exists of learning and attention difficulties, as well as minor motor impairments occur in children born very preterm. Experts have speculated that perinatal brain injury or postnatal nutritional deficiencies predispose these children to abnormal brain development, causing reduced caudate and hippocampal volumes. Reduced caudate volume is associated with low IQ. Memory deficits seen among children with smaller hippocampal volume.[23]

When evaluating the outcomes for VLBW children, the three morbidities that appear to have the most significant effect on later outcomes are (1) BPD, (2) severe IVH (grade 3 to 4) or periventricular leukomalacia (PVL), and (3) severe retinopathy of prematurity (ROP).[24] The more severe the degree of CLD is, the greater the likelihood of CP or neurodevelopmental impairment. Infants who continue to require oxygen at 36 weeks' postmenstrual age have a 17% to 27% risk of CP and a 45% to 62% incidence of neurodevelopmental impairment. The need for prolonged ventilation greater than 90 days nearly triples the risk for CP from 28% to 80%. Each of the three risk factors (BPD, severe IVH or PVL, and severe ROP) independently correlates with a poor outcome; the presence of two or more of these risk factors significantly increases the likelihood of an adverse outcome that included CP, cognitive delay, severe hearing impairment, and bilateral blindness.[25,26]

Among ELBW infants, poor long-term outcome was present in 18% of children without BPD, brain injury, or severe ROP. In contrast, 88% of children with all three morbidities experienced a poor outcome. Important caveats to these findings are that not every infant who sustains a grade 3 or 4 IVH will develop CP, and, conversely, a normal neurosonogram (showing no evidence of IVH or PVL) does not always predict a good outcome. Among babies in the NICHD cohort who had normal head ultrasound examinations, 9.4% were diagnosed with CP, 25% had cognitive delay, and nearly 30% exhibited motor delays. Factors associated with neurodevelopmental impairment (CP or MDI under 70) in babies with normal neurosonography are male gender, multiple birth, lower birth weight, pneumothorax, prolonged mechanical ventilation, maternal race and education, and poverty. (Table 95-3 summarizes the degree of risk associated with each of these factors.) Late-onset sepsis has also been shown to negatively affect the outcome for ELBW neonates, increasing the risk for CP, low MDI, low psychomotor developmental index, and vision impairment.[27]

Regional and national differences have been reported in mortality and morbidity rates. European outcomes reported for infants born less than 1000 g are notable for lower survival rates and increased rates of morbidity in comparison with outcomes for infants born in the United States.[28-30] An important consideration when reviewing data from various countries is understanding the approach to perinatal and neonatal care delivery (including at what gestation and birth-weight resuscitation is offered) the scope of care available, the decision processes regarding termination of care, and whether the infants for whom outcomes are reported are population based or reflect only those infants admitted to the NICU.

Neurodevelopmental and School-Aged Outcomes

Understanding the scope and evolution of neurodevelopmental outcomes requires surveillance through childhood into adulthood. Longitudinal outcomes that reflect the effect of current approaches to perinatal care take decades to elucidate. The earliest neurodevelopmental outcomes are typically reported between 18 months and 22 months of age, with school age outcomes, particularly at age 8 years, being the most predictive of future performance. Functional outcomes have recently been reported for several cohorts of preterm young adults who have been followed longitudinally in the United States, Canada, Europe, and Australia since their birth. Sequential follow-up is necessary, given that neurodevelopmental function has been shown to improve with time for many preterm, VLBW children. Evidence of neurodevelopmental recovery with improvement in functional outcomes and verbal and IQ testing with advancing age is increasing.[31,32] Ment et al reported on full-scale, verbal and performance IQ test scores for VLBW children with and without IVH between 3 and 8 years of age. Between 4.5 and 6 years of age, improvements in mean IQ scores were evident in both groups of VLBW children. By 8 years of age, the mean full-scale IQ score was reported to be 96 for VLBW children without a history of IVH and 94 for VLBW children with a prior IVH. Verbal IQ is higher than performance IQ for both groups of children. Forty-five percent of the children monitored demonstrated at least a 10-point gain; 12.5% had a 5- to 9-point increase in their scores.[33]

Behavioral and emotional outcomes have been reported by investigators in the United States, Canada, Europe, Australia, and New Zealand. The range of problems encountered include hyperactivity, conduct problems, emotional symptoms with both internalizing and externalizing behaviors, peer difficulties, attention problems, delinquent behavior, and social problems. Generally, a 1.5- to 3-fold increase is found in these problems in comparison with healthy children born at term gestation.[34-38]

Developmental coordination disorders are also more common in preterm, LBW children. Developmental coordination difficulties correlated with poorer cognitive function and academic performance, behavior problems, and were more prevalent among EBLW and very preterm male children. Adaptive behavioral and externalizing problems are more often demonstrated. Of interest, preterm male children more frequently exhibit externalizing behaviors, whereas preterm girls demonstrate more internalizing behaviors.[39]

Neuropsychological deficits are reported to be both global and specific in nature, with greater involvement in a range of educational areas involving attention, language, sensorimotor and visuospatial abilities, and verbal memory.[40-45]

An increased incidence of nonverbal learning disabilities, borderline cognitive function, and fine-motor problems have been reported; verbal cognitive skills typically exceed nonverbal abilities. Aspects of functioning that are affected include visual-motor integration, visual perception, mathematics and spatial skills, and fine-motor speed. Beyond nonverbal learning difficulties, problems with verbal abstracting (inferences), reading comprehension, written output, and social skills are exhibited. Reading decoding has not been shown to be affected. These deficits are associated with problems in executive functioning—organization, planning, problem solving, and abstraction. Estimates of visual-perceptual and visual-motor integration problems range from 11% to 20%, Fine-motor difficulties are reported to occur in up to 70% of ELBW children. Although vocabulary and receptive language are within normal limits for LBW children, preterm children have more difficulty with more complex verbal processes such as understanding syntax, abstract verbal skills, verb production, and the length of phrases or sentences produced. Critical to academic and social success, these language difficulties are also significantly influenced by the child's environment and language experiences.

As a group, 50% to 70% of VLBW and ELBW children respectively require educational assistance in school. By middle childhood, ELBW children are three to five times more likely to have difficulties with reading, spelling, mathematics, or writing. Grade retention is reported for 23% to 39% of LBW children: up to one third exhibit school problems with particular difficulty in mathematics and reading. Fifteen percent to 28% continue to require special education. Over 50% of preterm children without any neurosensory impairment enrolled in a mainstream educational setting may require additional educational support.[46] Common factors that influence outcomes include parent involvement, parent perspectives about and approaches to the child's limitations, maternal education and socioeconomic status, and access to services.[47-49]

Longitudinal follow-up of ELBW children into late childhood and early adolescence (ages 10-14 years) continues to confirm residual effects of extreme prematurity. There is an increased trend toward depressive symptoms in the children that is more prevalent among preterm children who have poorer family functioning, social risk factors, and the coexistence of a chronic medical condition. By 10 to 12 years of age, the majority (85%) of extremely preterm children will be functioning in mainstream academic environments without significant adjustment problems.[50] VLBW children with BPD experience more significant cognitive and academic impairments than VLBW children without CLD. Decreased functioning is present in the areas of cognition (intelligence), reading, mathematics, and gross-motor skills, with greater utilization of special educational services.[51]

Chronic Conditions, Functional Limitations, and Special Health Care Needs

ELBW infants are affected by more chronic health conditions that contribute to functional limitations and increase service and technology utilization. Hack et al reported that the health conditions most prevalent at 8 years of age are asthma, mild hearing impairment, visual disability, and CP. Blindness and hearing loss requiring hearing aids also occurred but with a lower frequency.[52] These conditions correlated with school performance and academic deficiencies, including low IQ, limited academic skills, poor motor skills. and poor adaptive functioning. Farooqi et al confirmed these findings in their report on health and functional outcomes for a group of Swedish extremely immature preterm children tracked until 10 to 12 years of age.[53]

Among preterm infants with CLD, over 50% exhibit airway reactivity. Postdischarge mortality can occur as these infants are at risk for sudden death. Lung function improves between 8 and 14 years of age, at which time rates of asthma are similar to NBW children, and lung function is within the normal range. Pulmonary function testing reveals lower airflow, but no difference in lung volumes or air trapping, irrespective of whether the ELBW child had BPD.

An increased prevalence of tooth enamel defects affect both the primary and permanent teeth of preterm infants.[54] Eruption of the first tooth in preterm girls has been reported to occur later than in preterm boys. However, by the age of 2 years, no significant delays in tooth maturation are observed between preterm and full-term children. Maturation of permanent teeth was also not noted to be delayed in the preterm children. The presence of palatal grooves and a high arched palate caused by prolonged intubation and orogastric tube placement can also affect oral health, feeding, and normal speech development.

Vision Function and Retinopathy of Prematurity

Strabismus, myopia, and poor visual acuity are more common in preterm children. More than one third of ELBW children require prescription glasses compared with 10% of full-term children. Difficulties with visual-motor integration in middle childhood are strongly related to the presence of visual impairment. Mild ROP has not been shown to be correlated with decreased visual acuity at age 7 years. Stephenson et al reported on visual and cognitive outcomes in late childhood and early adolescence for a cohort of LBW children whose birth weights were less than 1701 g.[56] Among children aged 10 to 13 years with a history of ROP, 50% had an adverse ophthalmologic outcome, with reduction in visual acuity and myopia, and strabismus predominating. Additional visual abnormalities involved color vision and visual-field defects. Children between the ages of 10 and 13 years with a history of mild ROP (stages 1 and 2) did not experience adverse visual outcomes. When outcomes for children with and without treated severe ROP (threshold ROP) are evaluated, there is a 10-fold increase in the rate of functional limitations involving four or more of the following areas: vision, hearing, speech, ambulation, dexterity, emotion, cognition, and pain. Children with severe ROP showed a significant difference in the severity of functional limitations when sighted children are compared with blind or low vision VLBW children: 6.4% versus 46.5%, respectively.[57] A recent study explored the question of whether the visual problems experienced by preterm infants are the result of common associated morbidities, ROP, IVH or PVL, or the consequence of premature exposure to extrauterine visual stimulation. At 5 to 7 months corrected age, preterm infants without evidence of ROP or neurologic abnormalities exhibit visual function that is not significantly different from healthy infants born full term.[58]

Growth

Preterm children are at risk for incomplete catch-up growth, largely because of postnatal growth deficiency that develops in the weeks to months after their early birth. Achieving growth, weight gain, and nutrient accretion that parallel intrauterine accretion postnatally is not typical for many LBW infants. Four growth patterns are seen among preterm and sick infants: (1) infant is appropriate for gestational age (AGA) at birth and continues to grow along a gestation specific intrauterine growth curve; (2) the infant is AGA, but postnatal growth falls below the curve; (3) the infant is small for gestational age (SGA) at birth, but demonstrates catch-up growth; and (4) the infant is born SGA and remains below the curve. Postnatal growth failure is common among preterm and LBW children born at less than 32 weeks' gestation and less than 1500 g birth weight.[59] The incidence of extrauterine growth restriction is common, reported at 28%, 34%, and 16% for weight, length, and head circumference.[60] For each growth parameter, the incidence of extrauterine growth restriction increased with decreasing gestational age and birth weight and was influenced by the infant's illness severity. Poor physical growth is associated with suboptimal nutrition, poor feeding skills, prolonged hospitalization, chronic respiratory disease, and late-onset sepsis or infection. At 1 year of age, a significant percentage of these infants continue to demonstrate subnormal growth (<10%) for weight, length, and head circumference. The rate of neonatal hospital weight gain and head growth also influences growth and neurodevelopmental outcomes at 18 to 22 months of age.[61] Poor postnatal growth, particularly head growth, has been correlated with residual suboptimal growth and neurodevelopmental impairment at 7 years of age.[62]

Larger, more stable infants typically demonstrate catch-up growth during the first 1 to 2 years of life. VLBW and ELBW children may not exhibit catch-up growth in the first 3 years and, as a group, tend to remain permanently lighter and shorter than children born at full term. Doyle et al reported that weight measurements among VLBW children were 1 standard deviation below the mean for age at 2, 5, and 8 years of age, with catch-up achieved by 14 years of age.[63] At 8 to 12 years of age, preterm children also have lower fat mass and body mass index than full-term children.[64] Similar results have been reported by Farooqi et al on children born extremely preterm at 23 to 25 weeks' gestation.[65] At 11 years of age, these ELBW children were significantly smaller on all growth parameters than their full-term counterparts, despite evidence of catch-up growth beginning by 3 months' postnatal age. Of additional importance was the finding that, among this group of children, catch-up head growth did not occur after 6 months of age.

Pain Sensitivity

Long-term consequences occur as a result of repetitive painful and noxious stimuli during the neonatal period.[66,67] Preterm children have lower-than-normal response thresholds to tactile stimulation and appear hypersensitive to pain. At 4 to 5 years of age, significantly increased somatization occurs. Repetitive pain leads to altered pain system with decreased pain thresholds. At 8 to 10 years of age, ELBW children have similar perceptions of pain intensity, although they rated medical pain more intensely than psychological pain and ascribed higher intensity ratings to recreational pain. More preterm children report fatigue (13%) and anxiety (8%) than term infants. Preterm adolescent girls exhibit greater pain sensitivity than preterm adolescent boys.[68]

Outcomes for Moderate- to Late-Preterm Infants

Gestational age–specific long-term outcome data about late preterm and heavier LBW (1500 to 2499 grams) infants are limited. Among infants with birth weights between 1500 to 2000 g (3.3 to 4.4 lb), there is reported to be an increased risk of both behavioral and psychiatric problems.[69] Population-based studies have revealed that the risk of developmental delay or disability is 40% higher for infants weighing between 1500 and 2499 g at birth in comparison with NBW babies.[70] Educational outcomes for children born between 32 and 35 weeks' gestation are similarly affected. Although the greatest effect is among the most immature infants weighing less than 1000 g at birth, heavier LBW children experience increased adverse educational outcomes in the areas of academic problems, learning disabilities, physical and sensory impairments, and mental handicaps.[71]

School performance has been studied in children born after 32 weeks' gestation. Reading and spelling difficulties are more frequent among children born at 33 to 36 weeks' gestation than NBW infants.[72] Huddy et al reported on school performance at age 7 years for a population-based cohort of children born between 32 and 35 weeks' gestation. Up to one third of these children exhibited school difficulties; nearly 25% required additional school resources. Areas of poor performance included writing and fine-motor skills, reading, mathematics, and physical education.[73] Rates of attention-deficit/hyperactivity disorder are nearly 2.5-fold greater than for NBW children.[68] Behavioral difficulties are twice as common in LBW children and have been related to maternal psychological distress at 40 weeks' postmenstrual age and a history of tobacco smoke exposure. Whether the effects of smoking are primary or a proxy for other environmental factors or stressors that influence parental well being and their ability to support their child's maturation is unclear.[48] Among preterm children born SGA, adolescents who were under the 3% at birth were more likely than NBW term children to experience learning and attention difficulties. SGA children between the 3% and 10% for gestational age did not experience similar difficulties. Symmetry or proportionality of growth was not related to these differences.[74]

Outcomes in Adolescence and Adulthood

Longitudinal outcomes data are being reported throughout the United States, Canada, and Europe for groups of preterm children who are now adolescents and young adults.

Adolescence and Young Adulthood

Assessing outcomes during adolescence has yielded interesting data about parental and adolescent perceptions regarding the preterm teenager's health, well being, and functional abilities. In recent years, numerous publications have reported on the adolescent and young adult outcomes for preterm and LBW children born during the late 1970s and early 1980s. Most of the reports detail outcomes for very preterm infants less than 32 weeks' gestation and VLBW infants. In the last decade, particular attention has been paid to the consequences of extreme prematurity and ELBW weight. Although concerns have been raised regarding the applicability of these outcomes to preterm and LBW children born today, comparison of outcomes for children born in the late 1990s and early 2000s are similar to that reported for the older cohorts of preterm or LBW individuals. Continued reporting of the longitudinal consequence of early birth will further enhance the ability to counsel families and to develop appropriate surveillance programs for children born preterm. Overall, the transition to young adulthood is fairly comparable to young adults who were born with NBW and full term. Three areas of difference are (1) persistence of neurodevelopmental disability, (2) lower educational achievement, and (3) suboptimal growth despite catch-up growth. Table 95-4 and Box 95-1 summarize the data on young adult outcomes.

Table 95-4 Transition to Adulthood

OUTCOME	EXTREMELY LOW–BIRTH-WEIGHT GROUP (%)	COMPARISON NORMAL–BIRTH-WEIGHT GROUP (%)
Completed university education	5	14
Pursuing post–secondary education	32	33
Completed less than high school	15	11
Permanent employment	48	57
Unemployed*	26	15
Married or cohabiting	23	25
Living with parents	11	14
Visual problems†	64	37
Neurosensory impairment†	27	2

*Statistically significant, $p = .02$.
†Statistically significant, $p < .0001$.
From: Saigal S, Stoskopf B, Streiner D, et al. Transition of extremely low birth weight infants from adolescence to adulthood: comparison with normal birth weight controls. *JAMA*. 2006;295(6):667-675.

Longitudinal follow-up of growth among a group of VLBW infants at 2, 5, 8, and 14 years has been reported for a cohort of Australian youth born between 1977 and 1982. Pubertal development in these individuals was similar to that seen for full-term controls. These VLBW teenagers were significantly shorter, lighter, with smaller occipitofrontal head circumference (OFC) measurements than their NBW counterparts. Children with birth weights less than 1000 g had lower weight scores during childhood but not at 14 years in comparison with children born weighing 1000 to 1499 g. Among this latter group, lower height scores were present only at 2 years of age. However, significantly lower head circumference measurements were noted on the serial assessments.[75] Hellgren et al reported on a group of preterm Swedish youth at 15 yrs of age. Significant differences were found in visual acuity, stereo acuity, astigmatism, and full-scale (85 vs 97) and performance (87 vs 99) IQ.[76]

BOX 95-1 Adult Outcomes for Preterm and LBV Infants

INTELLIGENCE AND ACADEMIC ACHIEVEMENT

Mean IQ: 81-98

IQ < 85: 19-49%

Completed high school or obtained a general education degree: 56-85%

Post–high school: 37-38%

WORK STATUS

Full-time employment: 48%

Unemployed, not in school: 14-26%

HEALTH STATUS

Chronic illness or disability: 47%

General health
- Similar to term adults
- Increased frequency of reactive airway disease or asthma

Growth
- Weight: below normal in infancy followed by catch-up growth
- Height: shorter relative to peers and mid-parental expected height
- Body mass index: normal as teen and young adult
- Head circumference: remains below normal

Neurosensory
- Impairment (cerebral palsy, blindness, deafness): 12-28%
- Vision problems: 37%
- Retinal detachment: 4-7%

SOCIAL BEHAVIOR

Significantly less risk-taking behaviors
- Drug and alcohol use
- Sexual activity

Similar rates of conviction and incarceration

Similar rates of independent living, marriage, cohabitation, and parenting

Preterm adolescents who had evidence of brain injury performed more poorly on all achievement tests than term adolescents. Nearly 50% of teens with brain injury had associated visual dysfunction and 33% had learning disabilities. Visual dysfunction is related to white matter injury common in preterm infants causing subnormal visual acuity complicated by perceptual and cognitive visual problems. Rogers et al found significant differences in motor performance in unimpaired ELBW preterm adolescents at 17 years of age, with decreased aerobic capacity, strength, endurance, flexibility, and activity level. The teens reported a more inactive lifestyle with less previous or current sports participation, poorer coordination, and more difficulty maintaining rhythm and cadence.[77]

Parents report a high incidence of mental health problems in VLBW teens. They describe more social and attention problems and less social and school competence in boys than term adolescents. Parents also reported more internalizing (withdrawn, somatic complaints, anxious or depressed) behaviors and social and attention problems and less school competence in girls than term adolescents. Teenage VLBW boys report that they are more active and have less psychological distress and fewer problems with attention than teens that were born full term. Teenage VLBW girls also describe externalizing behaviors, being less social with fewer thought and attention problems, and higher activity levels. Discrepancies exist between parent-reported problems and competencies and teen self-reports. Notably, teens who were SGA or girls self-reported more total problems and internalizing behaviors than NBW teens and boys. These results have been seen across several studies in the United States, Canada, and Europe.[78-80] At 15 and 16 years of age, preterm teens do not rate their health status and HRQL differently than comparison group teens born at term, with the exception of reporting a higher level of cognitive difficulty (40.7% vs 25%). Teens who were born preterm exhibited wider variation in their functional abilities.[81] Saigal and colleagues found teens described similar self-worth as the full-term teens on most domains of self-esteem, although some gender effects regarding athletic competence and physical appearance were noted. Boys rated themselves more highly than girls.[82] Among another cohort of Canadian ELBW adolescents born between 1981 and 1986 lower-than-normal cognitive scores and academic skills were reported. ELBW teens reported lower-than-normal scholastic, athletic, job competence, and romantic competence. These teenagers viewed themselves as more likely to need help getting a job.

Evaluation at 12 to 16 years of age among a longitudinal cohort born in Ontario found that of the ELBW teenagers had neurosensory impairments, 28% versus 2% of term teenagers. These ELBW adolescents exhibited a higher incidence of visual problems (57% vs 21%), seizures (7% vs 1%), developmental delay (26% vs 1%), learning disabilities (34% vs 10%), and hyperactivity (9% vs 2%), as well as more use of specialists and community resources, than adolescents born at term.[83,84] Teenagers who were born weighing less than 750 g were the most disadvantaged, with 58% requiring special educational assistance or grade retention (or both), in comparison with 13% of the full-term controls, a 9-fold increase in risk for the ELBW group. A difference of 13 to 18 points was found on psychometric testing. Developmental measures at 8 years of age have been shown to predict delayed academic performance in numerous studies.[85]

The majority of very preterm and VLBW adolescents are educated in mainstream classroom settings, although a percentage of these students continue to require additional educational supports, and approximately 5% to 10% have severe motor or neurosensory impairments.[86] Parents of these extremely preterm teens attending mainstream classes report an increased incidence of problems with physical health and family functioning, and the students' teachers rated these teens as slower than normal. Only 29% of the extremely preterm adolescents attending mainstream classes were without health issues compared with 49% of their term classmates; 100% of the extreme preterm teenagers in special education classes had health problems. Asthma, vision, learning disabilities, and behavioral problems are the most frequently reported. The psychological effect on parents of these teens' health issues was greatest for those whose children were in special education. Extreme prematurity affected both family functioning and family life. Teen self-assessment of their own health did not differ from controls. In addition, no apparent difference was found in the onset of puberty in girls or boys. Similar rates of medication use (increased health service use was reported only among the special education preterm teens) and tobacco use, but decreased alcohol and recreational drug use by mainstream and special education preterm students, were reported. When future plans were queried, a lower-than-normal proportion of the extremely preterm teens were planning to continue in school or attend vocational training, with additional planning for low-skilled types of employment.

The Role of Early Intervention

Few data are available about the specific benefits of early intervention for very preterm and VLBW children. The Infant Health and Development Program is the only randomized clinical trial to evaluate the longitudinal effects of an intensive 36-month early-intervention program for LBW infants and their parents. The study population was composed of 985 LBW preterm infants (<2500 g, <37 weeks' gestational age) born between 1984 and 1985 in one of eight centers across the United States. Infants were stratified into a *light low–birth-weight* (LLBW) group at or below 2000 g and a *heavy low–birth-weight* (HLBW) group weighing 2001 to 2500 g. Infants in these groups were randomized to receive routine follow-up care or to participate in an intensive home and center-based group intervention that lasted 3 years. Major assessment points were at 3, 5, and 8 years of age. At age 36 months corrected age, children in the intervention group had higher scores than children in the follow-up–only group on tests of receptive language, cognitive development, and visual-motor and spatial skills.[87,88] The effects were the strongest for families with the greatest risk (ie, children whose parents had a high school education or less and who were of ethnic minority status).[89] The intervention was found to be effective for the HLBW infants but not for the LLBW infants.[90] McCarton et al found no overall significant differences between the intervention and follow-up groups.[91] However, a sub-sample of the HLBW children who participated in the intervention group had higher scores on several cognitive tests (receptive vocabulary, mathematics, overall IQ) than the sub-sample of HLBW children in the follow-up group. The difference between the two groups at later ages was less than that seen at age 3; thus the effects of the intervention program appeared to decline over time. Among the LLBW children in the intervention group, all of the earlier positive effects had disappeared by age 8. Reassessment of these individuals at age 18 years revealed a continued 4-point achievement advantage for the HLBW group that remained stable over time. Intervention participants also exhibited fewer risky behaviors. Similar to the results seen at age 8 years, loss of intervention benefits was demonstrated in the LLBW group. The high school drop-out rate was lower than that reported for other groups of potentially high-risk students.[92]

Young Adulthood

Examination of young adult outcomes reveals findings similar adolescent age–reported outcomes. In general, the findings related to growth, academic and employment achievement, personal satisfaction, and HRQL are comparable to the results seen during adolescence. In one report, assessing 20 year olds born with VLBW, fewer than expected graduated from high school (74% vs 83%). Furthermore, VLBW men are significantly less likely than expected to be enrolled in post–secondary education (30% vs 53%). Testing reveals lower-than-normal mean IQ scores (87 vs 92), lower-than-normal academic achievement scores, higher-than-normal rates of neurosensory impairments (10% vs 1%), and subnormal height (10% vs 5%). Less-than-expected alcohol and drug use was noted, with lower-than-expected rates of pregnancy in both the young adults with and without neurosensory impairment. When growth is evaluated, VLBW young women in this group were reported to catch up by 20 years of age, whereas VLBW young men remained significantly shorter and lighter than NBW young women. Predictors of growth attainment at 20 years included maternal education and height, race, birth weight *z* score, length of NICU stay, and chronic illness at 20 years of age.[93,94] In contrast, another study reports that among VLBW adults (20 years) weight and height were not different from the general population and were consistent with parental height. Among this group of young adults, the mean body mass index was 24.0, and findings revealed that the VLBW adults were relatively heavy for their height.[95]

Similar findings have been reported in Canada and Sweden. Assessment at 22 to 25 years of the Ontario preterm young adults revealed 27% had residual neurosensory impairments yet had similar rates of graduation (82% vs 87%) and no significant differences in educational attainment (32% vs 33% post–secondary education), employment (48% vs 57%), independent living, marriage or cohabitation, or living with parents than the NBW controls.[96] Lindstrom found that among age 23- to 29-year-old preterm adults, 13.2% of individuals born between 24 and 28 weeks' gestation and 5.6% of individuals born 29 to 32 weeks' gestation received economic aid because of handicap or chronic illness.[97] Adults who were born between 33 and 37 weeks' gestation, also exhibit significant risks for disability, accounting for 74% of the total disability associated with preterm birth in this population-based study. Preterm adults were also less likely than expected to complete post-secondary education and had a lower-than-average net income. These findings were further supported by a report from Lefebvre et al, who demonstrated that the majority of preterm adults had a mean adult IQ that was in the normal range but more than 1 standard deviation below that of NBW controls. Again, school failure, IQ less than 85, and use of special educational assistance was more prevalent than normal among the preterm group.[98]

Measurement of quality of life and social activities in preterm young adults continue to demonstrate less alcohol and illicit substance use than full term controls, although the frequency of smoking and sexual activity was similar between groups. In the United Kingdom cohort on which Cooke reported, preterm young adults had more children, were shorter, less satisfied with their appearance, more likely to use regular prescription medication and have less higher education than their term counterparts. Employment rates were similar to the adults born at term.[99] Hack et al, reporting on the Cleveland cohort of VLBW adults, determined that VLBW men exhibited fewer delinquent behaviors but showed no differences in internalizing, externalizing, or total behavior problems than NBW men. Parents continued to report significantly more-than-expected thought problems for their sons. VLBW women were more withdrawn and exhibited more internalizing behaviors (anxious or depressed) and fewer delinquent behaviors than NBW men; their parents reported significantly more-than-expected anxiety and depressive symptoms and attention problems. No differences in self-report of attention-deficit/hyperactivity disorder was noted.[100] Allin et al assessed personality among adults who had been born before 33 weeks' gestation and found different personality characteristics in the very preterm group, with lower-than-expected scores on extraversion and higher-than-normal levels of neuroticism among female participants. These results are similar to those reported by Hack: decreased risk taking and antisocial behaviors, primarily among female participants, who reported less-than-expected recreational drug use and sexual activity. Saigal confirms these findings noting that among the Ontario cohort, 27% of the ELBW adults tracked had residual neurosensory impairments (13-fold higher than NBW adults) and were more likely to have multiple impairments.[101] No overall or gender difference was noted in current health status for physical or mental health and emotional state scores between the ELBW and NBW adults. However, VLBW adults did report increased rates of seizures (8% vs 2%; odds ratio 3.8), asthma in men (18% vs 3%; odds ratio 6.3), recurrent bronchitis (6% vs 1%; odds ratio 8.5), and a higher-than-expected prevalence of chronic health conditions and functional limitations in the previous 6 months. Areas of functional impairment were broad, encompassing vision, hearing, dexterity, clumsiness, and learning disabilities. Higher-than-normal rates for use of medications for depression, prescription glasses, and home care services were noted. VLBW adults also demonstrated weaker handgrip strength, lower scores physical self-efficacy, perceived physical ability, and physical self-confidence than NBW adults. An important yet unexpected finding was a 4% incidence of late retinal detachment, with an additional 6.6% of study participants found to have retinal tears. The 15-year outcome Cryotherapy for Retinopathy of Prematurity Cooperative Group trial for threshold ROP found late retinal detachment in 4.5% treated eyes and 7.7% untreated eyes.[102]

Increasing attention is being paid to the fetal and early neonatal determinants of adult disease and potential additional risks to adult health caused by preterm or LBW birth. Hovi et al studied a group of Finnish 18 to 27 year olds who were born preterm and VLBW, two thirds of whom were AGA. Higher indexes of insulin resistance and glucose intolerance (higher fasting insulin, 2-hour insulin, and 2-hour glucose concentrations) and higher blood pressure were found in comparison with NBW adults who were born at full term.[103] No differences were found between preterm adults who were born small or AGA. VLBW men and women were shorter and had lower body mass index than controls. In contrast to Doyle et al, who reported on an Australian cohort, the Finnish VLBW men had less-than-expected lean and fat mass, and a lower-than-normal lean mass adjusted for height was found in both VLBW men and women.[104] Recent studies have also documented the continuous and independent role of LBW on adult lung function, with the lowest respiratory function among LBW adults who smoke, have a sedentary lifestyle, or are obese.[105]

Infants With Significant Congenital Heart Disease

The number of adults with congenital heart disease (CHD) is now equal to the number of children with CHD. Although the most common forms of CHD affecting adults are congenital valve defects, atrial and ventricular septal defects, and patent foramen ovale, children today are surviving increasingly complex cardiac conditions requiring staged surgical repair or orthotopic transplantation. Approximately 85% of infants with serious heart disease survive to adulthood. Many children with CHD will require a repeat operation in adolescence or adulthood, given that 50% of homografts require replacement after 15 years. Associated with improvements in survival is an increased awareness of residual neurodevelopmental abnormalities affecting survivors.[106] Sequelae are related to several factors, including (1) underlying genetic conditions, (2) an increased incidence of central nervous system abnormalities of perinatal origin caused by abnormal prenatal and postnatal hemodynamics that alter blood flow to the developing brain, and (3) specific effects of cardiopulmonary by-pass and deep hypothermic circulatory arrest during corrective or palliative surgery. Preoperative hypoxemia causes damage to the areas of the brain associated with executive functions.[107] Seizures or coma (or both) have been reported in 19% of infants (non–hypoplastic left heart syndrome, for whom the rate is higher than normal) surviving cardiac surgery.[108] Infants born with cardiac disease associated with aneuploidy and microdeletions typically exhibit neurodevelopmental deficits, with impaired cognition and visual spatial, memory, language, and attention problems. Emerging data about polymorphisms identified in some infants with CHD and an increased susceptibility to cerebral reperfusion brain injury are expanding the understanding of the heterogeneity in risk for adverse neurodevelopmental sequelae. Researchers have reported that 24% to 36% of infants born with CHD are microcephalic at birth. Preoperative evaluations have determined that over one half of neonates with serious CHD have neurologic and neurobehavioral abnormalities before their initial surgery in the newborn period. The range of abnormalities include jitteriness, seizures, abnormal or asymmetric muscle tone, poor state regulation, and various structural brain anomalies caused by brain dysgenesis.[109,110]

Developmental delay is common after cardiac surgery when infants are evaluated at 1 year of age; infants undergoing palliative procedures are more significantly delayed than their developmentally normal peers.[111] Worse neurodevelopmental outcome at 1 year of age can be predicted based on the presence of an identified genetic syndrome, LBW, and apolipoprotein E genotype. Mean MDI score is approximately 1 standard deviation below the mean for comparable infants without serious CHD (90.6 [±14.9]) and the average psychomotor developmental index score is 81.6 (±17.2). Scores for infants with an associated genetic syndrome are lower.[112] At 5 years of age, 28% of neonatal cardiac surgery survivors had neurologic abnormalities; 5% were severely affected, and 15% of the children were microcephalic. Children with hypoplastic left heart syndrome and previously documented chromosomal anomalies, brain malformations, or perinatal asphyxia were excluded from the study analysis. Nearly 50% of the studied children exhibited motor delays and 39% were developmentally delayed; 4.5% had impaired mobility, 20% moderate to severe cognitive delay, and 22% moderate to severe adaptive (self-help) delay. Children undergoing palliative surgery rather than corrective surgery have an increased risk for motor dysfunction.[113]

Parents of children with CHD report poorer school performance, more school problems and grade retention, and more social, behavioral, and attention difficulties than children without CHD. Child self-reports were similar to children without CHD, with the exception that children with CHD reported increased depressive symptoms.[114] A recent meta-analysis about the psychological and cognitive functioning of children and adolescents with CHD reported an increased risk of total, internalizing behaviors and, to a lesser degree, externalizing problem behaviors, as well as poorer cognitive performance, that remained stable over time and age groups. Perceptual organizational and visual spatial abilities were impaired.[115] Children who undergo corrective surgery often do not meet guidelines for physical activity and are typically more sedentary than children without CHD.[116]

Neurodevelopment of Infants With Severe Respiratory Failure

Extracorporeal membrane oxygenation (ECMO) is used to treat infants with reversible pulmonary disease that is refractory to standard therapy. This intervention has contributed to the survival of infants with respiratory failure and severe hypoxemia who likely would have died without intervention. Infants who experience severe respiratory failure and are treated with either conventional management strategies (conventional ventilation) or ECMO exhibit a broad range of respiratory outcomes and residual lung disease. Although ECMO, if successful, will lead to the survival of some infants who would have otherwise died, it does not prevent pulmonary sequelae from severe respiratory failure. Respiratory rates and lung tidal volumes are similar for infants treated with either strategy, although infants treated with conventional ventilation have evidence of increased impaired small airway function at 1 year of age.[117] Residual lung disease persists in late childhood.[118]

Initial reports noted that neurodevelopmental disability and developmental delay were common in infants who recovered from severe respiratory failure. Infants who survived their disease with the aid of ECMO had poorer neurodevelopment than infants treated with conventional respiratory therapies. Both mental and developmental performance indices were affected with motor scores lower than cognitive scores. Infants with sepsis exhibited higher-than-expected rates of significant impairment.[119] More recent outcomes data suggest that 75% of infants treated with ECMO survive to 1 year of age, and most will have normal neurodevelopmental assessment between 11 and 19 months of age.[120] Infants who recover from severe respiratory failure and persistent pulmonary hypertension of the newborn are at risk for delayed-onset sensorineural hearing loss and require serial evaluation of their hearing during the first 3 years of life.[121]

Neurologically Impaired Infants—Post–Hypoxic-Ischemic Encephalopathy

Perinatal hypoxia-ischemia affects approximately 2 to 4 per 1000 full-term infants; the incidence is lower than expected in resource-rich countries and higher than expected in resource-poor countries. The overall incidence of neonatal encephalopathy attributable to intrapartum hypoxia (in the absence of other identified preconceptional or antepartum abnormalities) is estimated to be 1.6 per 10,000 births. Approximately 70% of neonatal encephalopathy is caused by events that occur before the onset of labor.[122] CP remains the primary outcome of concern for infants who experience neonatal encephalopathy at birth. The worldwide prevalence rate of CP ranges between 2 and 2.5 per 1000 live births. Epidemiologic studies have determined that only approximately 10% of cases of CP are attributable to intrapartum fetal compromise. (See Chapter 245, Cerebral Palsy.)

Clinical criteria required for the diagnosis of perinatal asphyxia include evidence of cardiorespiratory and neurologic depression in conjunction with acute hypoxic compromise and acidemia (base deficit >12 mmol/L). Infants who experience hypoxic-ischemic encephalopathy all have evidence of multiorgan dysfunction involving at least one organ in addition to the brain. Renal, cardiovascular, pulmonary, or hepatic dysfunction is present in the majority of infants irrespective of outcome.[123] Despite improved methods of intrapartum monitoring and advances in neonatal care and treatment, neonatal encephalopathy and neonatal hypoxic-ischemic injury can cause significant morbidity and mortality and may lead to long-term neurologic consequences in full-term and late preterm infants. Three predictors have been identified that have high statistical correlation with outcomes: (1) administration of chest compressions for more than 1 minute, (2) onset of breathing after 30 minutes, and (3) base deficit value greater than 16 in any blood gas analysis. Severe adverse outcome rates are 46% in the absence of any of these predictors, 64% with one predictor, 76% for two, and 93% for infants with all three predictors.[124] Maternal infection has also been shown to be an important cause of neonatal brain injury; clinical chorioamnionitis is associated with CP in both preterm and full-term infants, and maternal intrapartum hyperpyrexia is associated with neonatal seizures.[125]

Neurologic sequelae of hypoxic-ischemic encephalopathy include delayed motor development, intellectual disability, learning disabilities, seizure disorders, and CP. Full-term infants who experience severe neonatal encephalopathy are at risk for neurologic sequelae. Signs of severe neonatal encephalopathy (stupor, flaccidity, seizures, brainstem and autonomic dysfunction, and abnormal electroencephalographic findings) or persistence of moderate encephalopathy (depressed responses to stimulation, hypotonia, and decreased movements with or without seizures) for more than 7 days or failure of the electroencephalographic findings to revert to normal is associated with neurodevelopmental impairment or death. Full-term newborns who develop long-term neurologic sequelae from intrapartum asphyxia may not have low Apgar scores but will demonstrate neurologic dysfunction within 48 hours.[126] Periodic neurodevelopmental surveillance is therefore an important component for the routine care for these children, with a comprehensive neurologic examination at 12 months of age and psychometric assessment between 18 and 24 months of age. Among new therapies under investigation is the use of mild hypothermia for neuroprotection. Early reports suggest a possible benefit for infants with moderate neonatal encephalopathy and higher birth weight.[127,128] Further studies and longitudinal follow-up are necessary before the full treatment efficacy and potential associated adverse effects are known.

Infants who survive severe encephalopathy are more likely to experience a poor outcome at age 2 years in comparison with infants who recover from moderate encephalopathy (62% vs 25%). Overall, nearly 40% of infants who experience neonatal encephalopathy exhibit significant developmental delay at age 2 years compared with healthy children.[129] Suboptimal head growth occurs in approximately 50% of infants surviving hypoxic-ischemic encephalopathy and is associated with white matter injury and basal ganglia and thalamic lesions. Seizures during and after the neonatal period, microcephaly at 3 months of age, and renal abnormalities are associated with an abnormal neurologic outcome at 5 years of age.[130] School performance varies with the severity of neonatal encephalopathy.[131] Severe hearing impairment is an important long-term consequence, necessitating sequential surveillance through age 3 years. Children who have 5-minute Apgar scores of 3 or less at birth and signs of neonatal encephalopathy are at increased risk of developing minor motor impairments and seizures. They demonstrate a greater-than-expected need for educational assistance during their early school years and show decreased performance in reading, mathematics, and fine-motor skills. Behavioral and emotional problems are also more prevalent.[132] Marlow et al reported on school-aged outcomes for children who survived neonatal encephalopathy and noted that 42% and 6% of children who experienced severe and moderate neonatal encephalopathy had a disability, respectively.[133] Twenty-three percent of all survivors had major disability and CP; 12% exhibited severe cognitive impairment. Among survivors without motor impairment, children who experienced severe encephalopathy had the lowest cognitive scores, on average 11 points lower than their peers. Children who recovered from moderate encephalopathy had similar performance IQ in comparison with their peers. Impairment in memory, attention, and executive function were common, as was the need for educational assistance.[134] As with preterm infants who are susceptible to periventricular injury and damage to the basal ganglia and hippocampus, full-term infants who experience an early hypoxic-ischemic insult are vulnerable to hippocampal injury.[135]

REFERENCES

1. Strobino DM, Guyer B, Hamilton BE, et al. Annual summary of vital statistics: 2005. *Pediatrics.* 2007;119: 345-360.
2. Theunissen NCM, Veen S, Fekkes M, et al. Quality of life in preschool children born preterm. *Dev Med Child Neurol.* 2001;43:460-465.
3. Slonim AD, Patel KM, Ruttimann UE, et al. The impact of prematurity: a prospective of pediatric intensive care units. *Crit Care Med.* 2000;28(3):848-853.
4. Escobar GJ, Joffe S, Gardner MN, et al. Rehospitalization in the first two weeks after discharge from the neonatal intensive care unit. *Pediatrics.* 1999;104(1):e2.
5. Stein REK, Siegel MJ, Bauman LJ. Are children of moderately low birth weight at increased risk for poor health? A new look at an old question. *Pediatrics.* 2006; 118(1):217-223.
6. Gray JE, McCormick MC, Richardson DK, et al. Normal birth weight intensive care outcomes: outcome assessment. *Pediatrics.* 1996;97(6):832-838.
7. Kempe A, Wise PH, Wampler NS, et al. Risk status at discharge and cause of death for postneonatal infant deaths: a total population study. *Pediatrics.* 1997;99(3): 338-344.
8. Miniño AM, Heron MP, Murphy SL, et al. *Deaths: Final Data for 2004. National Vital Statistics Reports.* Vol 55, no. 19. Hyattsville, MD: National Center for Health Statistics; 2007.
9. Klassen AF, Lee SK, Raina P, et al. Health status and health-related quality of life in a population-based sample of neonatal intensive care unit graduates. *Pediatrics.* 2004;113(3):594-600.

10. Theunissen NCM, Veen S, Fekkes M, et al. Quality of life in preschool children born preterm. *Dev Med Child Neurol.* 2001;43:460-465.
11. van Baar AL, van Wassenaer AG, Briët JM, et al. Very preterm birth is associated with disabilities in multiple domains. *J Pediatr Psychol.* 2005;30(3):247-255.
12. Schiariti V, Hoube JS, Lisonkova S, et al. Care-giver reported health outcomes of preschool children born at 28 to 32 weeks' gestation. *J Dev Behav Pediatr.* 2007; 28:9-15.
13. Petterson B, Bourke J, Leonard H, et al. Co-occurrence of birth defects and intellectual disability. *Paediatr Perinatal Epidemiol.* 2007;21:65-75.
14. American Thoracic Society. Statement on the care of the child with chronic lung disease of infancy and childhood. *Am J Respir Crit Care Med.* 2003;168:356-396.
15. Shandor Miles M, Holditch-Davis D, Schwartz TA, et al. Depressive symptoms in mothers of prematurely born infants. *J Dev Behav Pediatr.* 2007;28:36-44.
16. Vohr BR, Wright LL, Poole K, et al. Neurodevelopmental outcomes of extremely low birth weight infants <32 weeks' gestation between 1995-1998. *Pediatrics.* 2005; 116(3):635-643.
17. Fanaroff AA, Stoll BJ, Wright LL, et al. Trends in neonatal morbidity and mortality for very low birthweight infants. *Am J Obstet Gynecol.* 2007;196:147.e1-147.e8.
18. Ehrenkrantz RA, Dusick AM, Vohr BR, et al. Growth in the neonatal intensive care unit influences neurodevelopmental and growth outcomes of extremely low birth weight infants. *Pediatrics.* 2006;117:1253-1261.
19. Casey PH, Whiteside-Mansell L, Barrett K, et al. Impact of prenatal and/or postnatal growth problems in low birth weight preterm infants on school-age outcomes: an 8 year longitudinal evaluation. *Pediatrics.* 2006;118(3): 1078-1086.
20. Vohr BJ, Poindexter BB, Dusick AM, et al. Beneficial effects of breast milk in the neonatal intensive care unit on the developmental outcome of extremely low birth weight infants at 18 months of age. *Pediatrics.* 2006; 118(1):e115-e123.
21. Kesler SR, Ment LR, Vohr B, et al. Volumetric analysis of regional cerebral development in preterm children. *Pediatr Neurol.* 2004;31:318-325.
22. Peterson BS, Vohr B, Staib LH, et al. Regional brain volume abnormalities and long-term cognitive outcome in preterm infants. *JAMA.* 2000;284:1939-1947.
23. Abernethy LJ, Cooke RWI, Foulder-Hughes L. Caudate and hippocampal volumes, intelligence, and motor impairment in 7 year-old children who were born preterm. *Pediatr Res.* 2004;55:884-893.
24. Ehrenkranz RA, Walsh MC, Vohr BR, et al. Validation of the National Institutes of Health consensus definition of bronchopulmonary dysplasia. *Pediatrics.* 2005;116(6): 1353-1360.
25. Schmidt B, Asztalos EV, Roberts RS, et al. Impact of bronchopulmonary dysplasia, brain injury and severe retinopathy on the outcome of extremely low birth weight infants at 18 months. *JAMA.* 2003;289(9):1124-1129.
26. Kercsmar C, Baley J, Singer LT, et al. Cognitive and academic consequences of bronchopulmonary dysplasia and very low birth weight: 8-year-old outcomes. *Pediatrics.* 2003;112:e359-e366.
27. Stoll BJ, Hansen NI, Adams-Chapman I, et al. Neurodevelopmental and growth impairment among extremely low-birth-weight infants with neonatal infection. *JAMA.* 2004;292:2357-2365.
28. Tommiska V, Heinonen K, Lehtonen L, et al. No improvement in outcome of nationwide extremely low birth weight infant populations between 1996-1997 and 1999-2000. *Pediatrics.* 2007;119(1):29-36.
29. Fily A, Pierrat V, Delporte V, et al. Factors associated with neurodevelopmental outcome at 2 years after very preterm birth: the population-based Nord-Pas-de-Calais EPIPAGE cohort. *Pediatrics.* 2006;117(2):357-366.
30. Ancel P-Y. Handicap neuro-sensoriel grave de l'infant grand prématuré. *J Gynecol Obstet Biol Reprod.* 2004; 33:461-474.
31. Marlow N, Wolke D, Bracewell MA, et al. Neurologic and developmental disability at 6 years of age after extremely preterm birth. *N Engl J Med.* 2005;352(1): 9-19.
32. Wilson-Costello D, Friedman H, Minich N, et al. Improved neurodevelopmental outcomes for extremely low birth weight infants in 2000-2002. *Pediatrics.* 2007;119(1):37-45.
33. Ment LR, Vohr B, Allan W, et al. Change in cognitive function over time in very low birth weight infants. *JAMA.* 2003;289(6):705-711.
34. Saigal S, den Ouden L, Wolke D, et al. School-age outcomes in children who were extremely low birth weight from four international population-based cohorts. *Pediatrics.* 2003;112(4):943-950.
35. Mikkola K, Riatri N, Tommiska V, et al. Neurodevelopmental outcome at 5 years of age of a national cohort of extremely low birth weight infants who were born in 1996-1997. *Pediatrics.* 2005;116(6):1391-1400.
36. Delobel-Ayoub M, Kaminiski M, Marret S, et al. Behavioral outcomes at 3 years of age in very preterm infants: the EPIPAGE study. *Pediatrics.* 2006;117(6): 1996-2005.
37. Marlow N, Wolke D, Bracewell MA, et al. Neurologic and developmental disability at 6 years of age after extremely preterm birth. *N Engl J Med.* 2005; 352(1): 9-19.
38. Reijneveld SA, de Kleine MJK, van Baar AL, et al. Behavioural and emotional problems in very preterm and very low birthweight infants at age 5 years. *Arch Dis Child Fetal Neonatal Ed.* 2006;91:F423-F428.
39. Davis NM, Ford GW, Anderson PJ, et al. Developmental coordination disorder at 8 years of age in a regional cohort of extremely-low-birth-weight or very preterm infants. *Dev Med Child Neurol.* 2007;49:325-330.
40. Hoff Esbjørn B, Møholm Hansen B, Greisen G, et al. Intellectual development in a Danish cohort of prematurely born preschool children: specific or general difficulties? *J Dev Behav Pediatr.* 2006;27:477-484.
41. Taylor HG, Klein N, Drotar D, et al. Consequences and risks of <1000-g birth weight for neuropsychological skills, achievement and adaptive functioning. *Dev Behav Pediatr.* 2006;27(6):459-469.
42. Taylor HG, Burant C, Holding PA, et al. Sources of variability in sequelae of very low birth weight. *Child Neuropsychol.* 2002;8:164-178.
43. Rose SA, Feldman JF, Jankowski JJ. Recall memory in the first three years of life: a longitudinal study of preterm and term children. *Dev Med Child Neurol.* 2005; 47:653-659.
44. Aylward GE. Neurodevelopmental outcomes of infants born prematurely. *J Dev Behav Pediatr.* 2005;26:427-440.
45. Bhutta AT, Cleves MA, Casey PH, et al. Cognitive and behavioral outcomes of school-age children who were born preterm: a meta-analysis. *JAMA.* 2002;288(6): 728-737.
46. Wocaldo C, Rieger I. Educational and therapeutic resource dependency at early school-age in children who were born very preterm. *Early Hum Devel.* 2006; 82(1):29-37.
47. Smith KE, Landry SH, Swank PR. The role of early maternal responsiveness in supporting school-age cognitive development for children who vary in birth status. *Pediatrics.* 2006;117(5):1608-1617.
48. Gray RA, Indurkhya A, McCormick MC. Prevalence, stability and predictors of clinically significant behavior problems in low birth weight children at 3, 5 and 8 years of age. *Pediatrics.* 2004;114(3):736-743.

49. McCormick MC, Workman-Daniels K, Brooks-Gunn J. The behavioral and emotional well-being of school-age children with different birthweights. *Pediatrics.* 1996; 97(1):18-25.
50. Farooqi A, Hägglöf B, Sedin G, et al. Mental health and social consequences of 10 to 12-year-old children born at 23 to 25 weeks of gestation in the 1990's: a Swedish national prospective follow-up study. *Pediatrics.* 2007;120(1):118-133.
51. Short EJ, Klein NK, Lewis BA, et al. Cognitive and academic consequences of bronchopulmonary dysplasia and very low birth weight: 8-year-old outcomes. *Pediatrics.* 2003;112(3):e359-e366.
52. Hack M, Taylor HG, Drotar D, et al. Chronic conditions, functional limitations, and special health care needs of school-aged children born with extremely low birth weight in the 1990s. *JAMA.* 2005;294(3):318-325.
53. Farooqi A, Hägglöf B, Sedin G, et al. Chronic conditions, functional limitations and special health care needs in 10- to 12-year-old children born at 23 to 25 weeks' gestation in the 1990s: a Swedish national perspective follow up study. *Pediatrics.* 2006;118(5): e1466-e1477.
54. Aine L, Backström MC, Mäki R, et al. Enamel defects in primary and permanent teeth of children born prematurely. *J Oral Pathol Med.* 2000;29(8):403-409.
55. Backstrom MC, Aine L, Maki R, et al. Maturation of primary and permanent teeth in preterm infants. *Arch Dis Child Fetal Neonatal Ed.* 2000;83:F104-F108.
56. Stephenson T, Wright S, O'Connor A, et al. Children born weighing less than 1701 g: visual and cognitive outcomes at 11-14 years. *Arch Dis Child Fetal Neonatal Ed.* 2007;92:F265-F270.
57. Cryotherapy for Retinopathy of Prematurity Cooperative Group Cooperative Group. Health-related quality of life at age 10 years in very low birth weight children with and without threshold retinopathy of prematurity. *Arch Ophthalmol.* 2004;122:1659-1666.
58. Mirabella G, Kjaer PK, Norcia AM, et al. Visual development in very low birth weight infants. *Pediatr Res.* 2006; 60(4):435-439.
59. Cooke RJ, Ainsworth SB, Fenton AC. Postnatal growth retardation: a universal problem in preterm infants. *Arch Dis Child Fetal Neonatal Ed.* 2004;89:F428-F430.
60. Clark RH, Thomas P, Peabody J. Extrauterine growth restriction remains a serious problem in prematurely born neonates. *Pediatrics.* 2003;111(5):986-990.
61. Ehrenkranz RA, Dusick AM, Vohr BR. Growth in the neonatal intensive care unit influences neurodevelopmental and growth outcomes of extremely low birth weight infants. *Pediatrics.* 2006;117(4):1253-1261.
62. Cooke RWI, Foulder-Hughes L. Growth impairment in the very preterm and cognitive and motor performance at 7 years. *Arch Dis Child.* 2003;88:482-487.
63. Doyle LW, Faber B, Callahan C, et al. Extremely low birth weight and body size in early adulthood. *Arch Dis Child.* 2004;89:347-350.
64. Fewtrell MS, Lucas A, Cole TJ, et al. Prematurity and reduced body fatness at 8-12 y of age. *Am J Clin Nutr.* 2004;80:436-440.
65. Farooqi A, Hägglöf B, Sedin G, et al. Growth in 10- to 12-year-old children born at 23 to 25 weeks' gestation in the 1990s: a Swedish national prospective follow up study. *Pediatrics.* 2006;118(5):e1452-e1465.
66. Whitfield MF, Grunau, RVE. Behaviour, pain perception and the extremely low birthweight survivor. *Clin Perinatol.* 2000;27:363-379.
67. Grunau RE, Oberlander TF, Whitfield MF, et al. Pain reactivity in formerly extremely low birth weight infants at corrected age 8 months compared with term born controls. *Infant Behav Devel.* 2001;24:41-55.
68. Buskila D, Neumann L, Zmora E, et al. Pain sensitivity in prematurely born adolescents. *Arch Pediatr Adolesc Med.* 2003;157:1079-1082.
69. Elgen I, Sommerfelt K, Markestad T. Population-based, controlled study of behavioural problems and psychiatric disorders in low birth weight children at 11 years of age. *Arch Dis Child Fetal Neonatal Ed.* 2002;87:F128-F132.
70. Thompson JR, Carter RL, Edwards AR, et al. A population-based study of the effects of birth weight on early developmental delay or disability. *Am J Perinatol.* 2003; 20(6): 321-332.
71. Resnick MB, Gueorguieva RV, Carter RL, et al. The impact of low birth weight, perinatal conditions and sociodemographic factors on educational outcome in kindergarten. *Pediatrics.* 1999;104(6):e74.
72. Kirkegaard I, Obel C, Hedgegaard M, et al. Gestational age and birth weight in relation to school performance of 10-year-old children: a follow-up study of children born after 32 completed weeks. *Pediatrics.* 2006;118(4): 1600-1606.
73. Huddy CL, Johnson A, Hope PL. Educational and behavioural problems in babies of 32 to 35 weeks' gestation. *Arch Dis Child Fetal Neonatal Ed.* 2001; 85:F23-F28.
74. O'Keefe MJ, O'Callagahn M, Williams GM, et al. Learning, cognition and attentional problems in adolescents born small for gestational age. *Pediatrics.* 2003;112(2): 301-307.
75. Ford GW, Doyle LW, Davis NM, et al. Very low birth weight and growth into adolescence. *Arch Pediatr Adolesc Med.* 2000;154:778-784.
76. Hellgren K, Hellstrom A, Jaconson L, et al. Visual and cerebral sequelae of very low birth weight in adolescents. *Arch Dis Child Fetal Neonatal Ed.* 2007;92: F259-F264.
77. Rogers M, Fay TB, Whitfield MF, et al. Aerobic capacity, strength, flexibility and activity level in unimpaired extremely low birth weight (<800 g) survivors at 17 years of age compared with term-born control subjects. *Pediatrics.* 2005;116(1):e58-e65.
78. Bredrup Dahl L, Kaaresen PI, Tunby J, et al. Emotional, behavioral, social and academic outcomes in adolescents born very low birth weight. *Pediatrics.* 2006;118(2): e449-e459.
79. Saigal S, Pinelli J, Hoult L, et al. Psychopathology and social competencies of adolescents who were extremely preterm. *Pediatrics.* 2003;111:969-975.
80. Hack M, Youngstrom EA, Cartar L, et al. Behavioral outcomes and evidence of psychopathology among very low birth weight infants at 20 years. *Pediatrics.* 2004;114: 932-940.
81. Gray R, Petrou S, Hockley C, et al. Self-reported health status and health-related quality of life of teenagers who were born before 29 weeks' gestational age. *Pediatrics.* 2006;120(1):e86-e93.
82. Saigal S, Lambert M, Russ C, et al. Self-esteem of adolescents who were born prematurely. *Pediatrics.* 2002; 109(2):429-433.
83. Saigal S, Stoskopf BL, Streiner DL, et al. Physical growth and current health status of infants who were of extremely low birth weight and controls at adolescence. *Pediatrics.* 2001;108(2):407-415.
84. Allin M, Rooney M, Griffiths T, et al. Neurological abnormalities in young adults born preterm. *J Neurol Neurosurg Psychiatry.* 2006;77:495-499.
85. Saigal S, Hoult LA, Streiner DL, et al. School difficulties in a regional cohort of children who were extremely low birth weight. *Pediatrics.* 2000;105(2): 325-331.

86. Johnson A, Bowler U, Yudkin P, et al. Health and school performance of teenagers born before 29 weeks gestation. *Arch Dis Child.* 2003;88:F190-198.
87. Brooks-Gunn J, Liaw F, Klebanov PK. Effects of early intervention on cognitive function of low birth weight preterm infants. *J Pediatr.* 1992;120:350-359.
88. McCormick MC, McCarton C, Tonascia J, et al. Early educational intervention for very low birth weight infants: results from the Infant Health and Development Program. *J Pediatr.* 1993;123:527-533.
89. Brooks-Gunn J, Gross RT, Kraemer HC, et al. Enhancing the cognitive outcomes of low birth weight, premature infants: for whom is the intervention most effective? *Pediatrics.* 1992;89:1209-1215.
90. Baumeister AA, Bacharach VR. A critical analysis of the Infant Health and Development Program. *Intelligence.* 1996;23:79-104.
91. McCarton CM, Brooks-Gunn J, Wallace IF, et al. Results at age 8 years of early intervention for low-birth-weight premature infants. *JAMA.* 1997;277:126-132.
92. McCormick MC, Brooks-Gunn J, Buka SL, et al. Early intervention in low birth weight premature infants: results at 18 years of age for the Infant Health and Development Program. *Pediatrics.* 2006;117(3):771-780.
93. Hack M, Flannery DJ, Schluchter M, et al. Outcomes in young adulthood for very low birth weight infants. *N Engl J Med.* 2002;346(3):149-157.
94. Hack M, Schluchter M, Cartar L, et al. Growth of very low birth weight infants to age 20 years. *Pediatrics.* 2003;112(1):e30-e38.
95. Doyle LW, Faber B, Callahan C, et al. Extremely low birth weight and body size in early adulthood. *Arch Dis Child.* 2004;89:347-350.
96. Saigal S, Stoskopf B, Streiner D, et al. Transition of extremely low birth weight infants from adolescence to adulthood: comparison with normal birth weight controls. *JAMA.* 2006;295(6):667-675.
97. Lindstrom K, Winbladh B, Haglund B, et al. Preterm infants as young adults: a Swedish national cohort study. *Pediatrics.* 2007;120(1):70-77.
98. Lefebvre F, Mazurier E, Tessier. Cognitive and educational outcomes in early adulthood for infants weighing 1000 grams or less. *Acta Paediatrica.* 2005;94:733-740.
99. Cooke RWI. Health, lifestyle and quality of life for young adults born very preterm. *Arch Dis Child.* 2004; 89:201-206.
100. Hack M, Youngstrom EA, Cartar L, et al. Behavioral outcomes and evidence of psychopathology among very low birth weight infants at 20 years. *Pediatrics.* 2004;114:932-940.
101. Saigal S, Stoskopf B, Boyle M, et al. Comparison of current health, functional limitations and health care use of young adults who were born with extremely low birth weight and normal birth weight. *Pediatrics.* 2007;119(3):e562-e573.
102. Cryotherapy for Retinopathy of Prematurity Cooperative Group. 15-year outcomes following threshold retinopathy of prematurity. Final results from the multicentered trial of cryotherapy for retinopathy of prematurity. *Arch Ophthalmol.* 2005;123:311-318.
103. Hovi P, Andersson S, Eriksson JG, et al. Glucose regulation in young adults with very low birth weight. *N Engl J Med.* 2007;356:2053-2063.
104. Doyle LW, Faber B, Callahan C, et al. Extremely low birth weight and body size in early adulthood. *Arch Dis Child.* 2004;89:347-350.
105. Canoy D, Pekkanen J, Elliott P, et al. Early growth and adult respiratory function in men and women followed from the fetal period to adulthood. *Thorax.* 2007;62:396-402.
106. Hövels-Gürich HH, Konrad K, Skorzenski D, et al. Long-term neurodevelopmental outcome and exercise capacity after corrective surgery for tetralogy of Fallot or ventricular septal defect in infancy. *Ann Thorac Surg.* 2006;81:958-967.
107. Hövels-Gürich HH, Konrad K, Skorzenski D, et al. Attentional dysfunction in children after corrective cardiac surgery in infancy. *Ann Thorac Surg.* 2007;83:1425-1430.
108. Clancy RR, McGaurn SA, Wernovsky G, et al. Risk of seizures in survivors of newborn heart surgery using deep hypothermic circulatory arrest. *Pediatrics.* 2003;111(3):592-601.
109. Limperopoulos C, Majnemer A, Shevell MI, et al. Neurologic status of newborns with congenital heart defects before open heart surgery. *Pediatrics.* 1999;103(2):402-408.
110. Newburger JW, Bellinger DC. Brain injury in congenital heart disease. *Circulation.* 2006;113:183-185.
111. Dittich H, Bührer C, Grimmer I, et al. Neurodevelopment at 1 year of age in infants with congenital heart disease. *Heart.* 2003;89:436-441.
112. Gaynor JW, Wernovsky G, Jarvik, GP, et al. Patient characteristics are important determinants of neurodevelopmental outcome at one year of age after neonatal and infant cardiac surgery. *J Thorac Cardiovasc Surg.* 2007;133:1344-1353.
113. Majnemer A, Limperopoulos C, Shevell M, et al. Long-term neuromotor outcome at school entry of infants with congenital heart defects requiring open heart surgery. *J Pediatr.* 2006;148:72-77.
114. Miatton M, De Wolf D, Francois K, et al. Behavior and self-perception in children with surgically corrected congenital heart disease. *J Dev Behav Pediatr.* 2007;28: 294-301.
115. Karsdorp PA, Everaed W, Kindt M, et al. Psychological and cognitive functioning in children and adolescents with congenital heart disease: a meta-analysis. *J Pediatr Psychol.* 2007;32(5):527-541.
116. Massin MM, Hövels-Gürich HH, Gerard P, et al. Physical activity patterns of children after neonatal arterial switch operation. *Ann Thorac Surg.* 2006;81:665-670.
117. Beardsmore, C, Dundas I, Poole K, et al. Respiratory function in survivors of the United Kingdom Extracorporeal Membrane Oxygenation Trial. *Am J Respir Crit Care Med.* 2000;161:1129-1135.
118. Hamutcu R, Nield TA, Garg M, et al. Long-term sequelae in children who were treated with extracorporeal membrane oxygenation for neonatal respiratory failure. *Pediatrics.* 2004;114(5):1292-1296.
119. Robertson CMT, Finer NN, Sauve RS, et al. Neurodevelopmental outcome after neonatal extracorporeal membrane oxygenation. *Can Med Assoc J.* 1995;152(12):1981-1988.
120. Khambekar K, Nichani S, Luyt DK, et al. Developmental outcome in newborn infants treated for acute respiratory failure with extracorporeal membrane oxygenation: present experience. *Arch Dis Child Fetal Neonatal Ed.* 2006:91:F21-F25.
121. Hutchin ME, Gilmer C, Yarbrough WG. Delayed onset sensorineural hearing loss in a 3-year old survivor of persistent pulmonary hypertension of the newborn. *Arch Otolaryngol Head Neck Surg.* 2000;126:1014-1017.
122. American College of Obstetrics and Gynecology, American Academy of Pediatrics. *Neonatal Encephalopathy and Cerebral Palsy: Defining the Pathogenesis and Pathophysiology.* Washington, DC: American College of Obstetrics and Gynecology; 2003.

123. Shah P, Riphagen S, Beyene J, et al. Multiorgan dysfunction in infants with post-asphyxial hypoxic-ischemic encephalopathy. *Arch Dis Child Fetal Neonatal Ed.* 2004;89:F152-155.
124. Shah P, Beyene J, To T, et al. Post-asphyxial hypoxic-ischemic encephalopathy in neonates: outcome prediction rule within 4 hours of birth. *Arch Pediatr Adolesc Med.* 2006;160:729-736.
125. Greenwood C, Yudkin P, Sellers S, et al. Why is there a modifying effect of gestational age on risk factors for cerebral palsy? *Arch Dis Child Fetal Neonatal Ed.* 2005;90:F141-F146.
126. Ment LR, Bada HS, Barnes P, et al. Practice parameter: neuroimaging of the neonate: report of the Quality Standards Subcommittee of the American Academy of Neurology and the Practice Committee of the Child Neurology Society. *Neurology.* 2002;58(12):1726-1738.
127. Edwards AD, Azzopardi DV. Therapeutic hypothermia following perinatal asphyxia. *Arch Dis Child Fetal Neonatal Ed.* 2006;91:F127-F131.
128. Wyatt JS, Gluckman PD, Liu PY, et al. Determinants of outcomes after head cooling for neonatal encephalopathy. *Pediatrics.* 2007;119(5): 912-921.
129. Dixon G, Badawi N, Kurinczuk JJ, et al. Early developmental outcomes after neonatal encephalopathy. *Pediatrics.* 2002;109(1):26-33.
130. Shankaran S, Woldt E, Koepke T, et al. Acute neonatal morbidity and long-term central nervous system sequelae of perinatal asphyxia in term neonates. *Early Hum Dev.* 1991;25(2):135-148.
131. Robertson C, Finer NN, Grace PE. School performance of survivors of neonatal encephalopathy associated with birth asphyxia at term. *J Pediatr.* 1989;114(5):753-760.
132. Moster D, Lie RT, Markestad T. Joint association of Apgar scores and early neonatal symptoms with minor disabilities at school age. *Arch Dis Child Fetal Neonatal Ed.* 2002;86:F16-F21.
133. Marlow N, Rosen AS, Rands CE, et al. Neuropsychological and educational problems at school age associated with neonatal encephalopathy. *Arch Dis Child Fetal Neonatal Ed.* 2005;90:F380-F387.
134. van Handel M, Swaab H, de Vries LS, et al. Long-term cognitive and behavioral consequences on neonatal encephalopathy following perinatal asphyxia: a review. *Eur J Pediatr.* 2007;166:645-654.
135. Gadian DG, Aicardi J, Watkins KE, et al. Developmental amnesia associated with early hypoxic-ischaemic injury. *Brain.* 2000;123:499-507.

Chapter 96

FOLLOW-UP CARE OF THE GRADUATE FROM THE NEONATAL INTENSIVE CARE UNIT

Judy C. Bernbaum, MD; Deborah E. Campbell, MD; Sonia O. Imaizumi, MD

The scope of pediatric primary care for children who require neonatal intensive care will vary based on the neonate's condition and any sequelae that develop. The majority of infants requiring specialized newborn care will need routine pediatric primary care, with particular attention paid to periodic developmental surveillance for infants with risk factors for developmental delays. Among the most immature and sickest neonates, a comprehensive and coordinated approach to care is necessary that integrates routine health care, medical and surgical subspecialty care, periodic developmental surveillance to identify early intervention needs, and assessment of resources and psychosocial and emotional support needs of the family.

IDENTIFYING INFANTS REQUIRING CLOSE FOLLOW-UP

Well-defined risk groups of term and preterm infants can be found who require specialized follow-up care. Infants in these risk categories may be identified based on a biological risk, the need for particular interventions because of significant fetal or neonatal disease, and social or environmental factors that predispose the infant to an adverse outcome. The National Institute for Child Health and Human Development, National Institute for Neurological Disorders and Stroke, and the Centers for Disease Control and Prevention[1] have identified a subset of infants who require close neurodevelopmental surveillance and follow-up. This group of babies includes extremely low–birth-weight infants (≤1000 g or ≤28 weeks' gestation) and full-term infants with neonatal encephalopathy and severe hyperbilirubinemia requiring exchange transfusion. Experts further recommend that infants who have required neonatal intensive care receive periodic preventive assessments within the primary care setting.

Although many tertiary care neonatal centers will offer neonatal follow-up care for high-risk neonatal intensive care unit (NICU) graduates, funding for such surveillance programs is limited, and many families may live far from existing programs. The American Academy of Pediatrics and the National Institute of Child Health and Human Development (NICHD) have published recommendations regarding the role of the pediatric primary care physician in the follow-up care of the high-risk infant and the components of health and developmental surveillance that should be provided for high-risk, premature infants.[1-3]

Establishing a medical home for the NICU graduate encompasses the same principles applied to creating a medical home for any child with special health care needs. Parents have become acclimated to a high technology, fast-paced hospital environment and have come to rely on one set of health caregivers. When their infant is discharged from the hospital, parents must transition to a new health care provider for their child and a health care system that is complex and, at times, fragmented. Some parents will have felt supported during their infant's hospital experience and believe they were true partners in the child's care. Other families will have felt disenfranchised, will have believed that they are not actively included in their child's decision making, or will be unhappy with their child's outcome, continuing health and developmental care needs, or uncertain future. Irrespective of their NICU experience, all parents have concerns about how their child will fare at home, their role as parents, and what the future will bring. Parents of technology-dependent infants must adapt to the challenges of negotiating a vast array of home health services, medical suppliers, and early intervention services that add further stressors on family time, family functioning, parenting, and the family's economic resources.

PREPARING FOR DISCHARGE

In preparation for hospital discharge, some parents have the opportunity to meet or speak with the pediatric primary care physician. The primary care physician may have the opportunity to visit the child in the NICU or may, in some community settings, have assumed responsibility for the infant's care when the baby is transferred to a special care or level II NICU for continuing or convalescent care. In other communities, limited and fragmented care presents a challenge for both the hospital team planning for the infant's discharge and the family that must coordinate and schedule appointments and figure out transportation arrangements and how to juggle their other responsibilities to comply with their baby's health care requirements.

Comprehensive care programs, either community based or hospital based, have been shown to be effective in reducing life-threatening illness in high risk infants.[4,5] However, compliance with recommended follow-up medical care is more likely to be problematic for families of the sickest infants, particularly when multiple medical appointments are necessary. McPherson and colleagues found that children who required 3 or more medical appointments after their discharge from a pediatric intensive care unit were more likely to miss appointments.[6] Of note was the finding that, after hospital discharge, the children were more likely to complete a primary care visit than follow up with a specialist. Infants who have been transferred from tertiary care units to level I or II nurseries for continuing care are more likely to be readmitted to the hospital and fail to comply with recommended follow-up care.[7] In addition to a detailed written summary of the infant's hospital course that includes recommendations for the early follow-up subspecialty care needs of the infant, direct communication with the NICU staff can facilitate transfer of care and ensure that the pediatric primary care physician has a complete understanding of the infant's history and discharge plan. Identifying barriers that will interfere with the family's ability to comply with the child's recommended care is also important. This information will help assist the health professional in planning the visit length, given that allotting more than one new patient time slot may be necessary to properly assess the infant, address parental concerns about the transition home, adjust medications, plan follow-up appointments, and plan for and review equipment if the infant is technology dependent.

An important concern for parents bringing the medically fragile infant into a medical office, whether a private practice or clinic, is the potential exposure of the infant to individuals who are sick and the infant's risk from a possible exposure. Minimizing the time spent in the reception and waiting areas and having the office staff attuned to the unique, but common, concerns of parents of children with special health care needs can increase parental confidence and satisfaction with the primary care experience. Families also need to know the practice's policies as to how to contact their child's physician during off hours and for emergencies, as well as which hospital emergency room or urgent care facility to use. Transportation requirements need to be explored and arrangements made for ambulance or other transportation services as necessary to ensure that the child is able to keep appointments.

The degree of care coordination required by the pediatric primary care physician will vary by community, proximity to specialty care, and availability of high-risk follow-up programs for at-risk infants. Some infants will be enrolled in comprehensive follow-up programs that provide some elements of primary care, whereas other babies may be scheduled for periodic neurodevelopmental surveillance or may need to rely on their pediatric caregiver for these aspects of their care.

MANAGEMENT ISSUES DURING PEDIATRIC CARE

The specific health care needs for an individual infant or child will be based on the complications or sequelae from their original illness or health condition. The child's and the family's needs will change over time as the child transitions through different health and developmental stages; thus eliciting the family's assessment of their needs for information, resources, and support is important. Parents may be at a different transition point than the professionals involved in the child's care and may express needs that are different than what the professional perceives as necessary or important. During middle childhood through adolescence and young adulthood, parental concerns are focused primarily on the child's academic achievement and school performance, behavior, and social skills. For some families, the child's health issues will also continue to be problematic. These issues are discussed in detail in Chapter 95, Health and Developmental Outcomes of Infants Requiring Neonatal Intensive Care.

Components of care for high-risk infants from infancy through adolescence are summarized in Table 96-1. The timing for specialized or more in-depth assessments has been recommended as follows: 3 to 4 and 6 to 8 months corrected age, 12 to 14 months corrected age, 18 to 24 months corrected age, 3 to 5 years of age, and at-school age (8 to 10 years). Components of assessment during these visits should include growth and nutrition, neurologic assessment, gross-motor development, language and communication, functional behavior, and health status and health-related quality of life. Experts suggest that cognitive assessments, either comprehensive or limited using screening or abbreviated intelligence tests, be performed when the child is 12 and 24 months corrected age, 3 to 4 years of age, and at 6 and 8 years of age. Results of standardized screening or comprehensive development testing provide important information that will guide referral for diagnostic or intervention services as needed.

Table 96-1 Components of Health and Developmental Surveillance for the Preterm and High-Risk Infant

TIME FRAME	IMPORTANT HEALTH AND NEURODEVELOPMENT SURVEILLANCE
INFANCY (CORRECTED AGE)	
0-1 mo	Follow-up results of neonatal metabolic screen if repeat testing was required at hospital discharge
	Review specialty follow-up appointments:
	Refer to pediatric audiologist for initial screening if hospital screening was not documented or to follow up evaluation based on the initial screening or identified risk factors
	Refer to ophthalmology as indicated for follow-up of retinopathy of prematurity
	Assess growth and nutrition—record on standard growth charts plotting parameters using corrected age
	Infants with chronic health conditions will need condition specific assessments
	Review technologies use, adequacy of equipment function, parent comfort with use, home care support, and continuing need for the technology
	Evaluate family functioning, family stress, and parent-infant interaction
3-4 mos	Examine for strabismus; refer to pediatric ophthalmologist if present
	Examine for hip dysplasia; refer to pediatric orthopedist if hip laxity present
	Assess growth and nutrition—record on standard growth charts plotting parameters using corrected age
	Evaluate family functioning, family stress, and parent-infant interaction
4-6 mos	Refer for standardized movement, muscle tone, and movement quality assessment
	Assess growth and nutrition—record on standard growth charts plotting parameters using corrected age
	Evaluate family functioning, family stress, and parent-infant interaction
	Refer for developmental testing as indicated
8-12 mos	Refer for standardized movement assessment, assessment of muscle tone and movement quality
	Screen language, fine-motor adaptive and personal-social skills
	Refer for ophthalmologic follow-up vision surveillance
	Assess growth and nutrition—record on standard growth charts plotting parameters using corrected age
	Evaluate family functioning, family stress, and parent-infant interaction
EARLY CHILDHOOD (CORRECTED AGE)	
15-18 mos	Refer for standardized movement assessment
	Screen other areas of development and social interaction
18-36 mos	Refer for standardized assessment of speech and language skills
	Screen other areas of development and social interaction
36-48 mos	Refer for standardized assessment of cognition and social-adaptive skills
	Screen for school readiness
	Refer to ophthalmologist experienced with children for follow-up vision surveillance
MIDDLE CHILDHOOD	
6-12 yrs	Review academic achievement and school performance, attention skills, behavior, peer relationships, self-esteem, and coping skills
	Review intercurrent or continuing health care issues
	Assess for hypertension and risk for insulin resistance and metabolic syndrome
	Refer for psychometric testing as indicated
	Refer for ophthalmologic follow-up at 9-12 years of age, particularly children with a history of retinopathy of prematurity, irrespective of the need for prior laser or cryotherapy
ADOLESCENCE	
13-21 yrs	Review academic achievement and school performance, attention skills, behavior, peer relationships, self-esteem, and coping skills
	Review intercurrent or continuing health care issues
	Assess for hypertension and risk for insulin resistance and metabolic syndrome
	Refer for psychometric testing as indicated

Adapted from: Washington State Department of Health, Children with Special Health Care Needs Program. Low Birth Weight Neonatal Intensive Care Unit Graduate: Critical Elements of Care. Washington State Consensus Project. Revised 2002. Available at: www.medicalhome.org.

Transition Home Through the First Year of Life

During the initial transitional period from the hospital through the first 3 months at home, parents' primary concerns are typically focused on feeding, weight gain, elimination, sleep, and adaptation to the home environment (crying, state regulation, and social interaction). In addition, parents are worried about the child's risk for infection and other illnesses, having sufficient medical supplies if the infant is technology dependent, and managing multiple medical appointments and early intervention assessments. Common medical problems experienced by the highest-risk infants are listed in Box 96-1 on page 870. Parents often

BOX 96-1 Continuing Medical Problems

Anemia
Apnea of prematurity
Bone mineralization: osteopenia, rickets, fractures
Cholestasis
Feeding difficulties
Gallstones
Growth: incomplete catch-up growth, slow weight gain, poor or excessive head growth
Hypertension
Hypothyroidism
Malabsorption, short bowel syndrome, enterostomy losses
Nephrolithiasis
Ophthalmologic issues
  Vision loss and impairment
  Reduced visual acuity, color vision, contrast sensitivity
  Field defects, eye motility disorders
Oral health: enamel hypoplasia, delayed tooth eruption, high arch palate
Pain perception: hypo- and hypersensitivity to painful stimuli
Postanesthesia complications: apnea
Respiratory: chronic lung disease, airway complications (subglottic stenosis, laryngotracheomalacia), respiratory infections, respiratory syncytial virus, cor pulmonale, sudden death
Scars, deformations, hernias
Seizures
Sudden infant death syndrome
Use of chronic technologies: home ventilation, gastrostomy tube, tracheostomy, parenteral nutrition

report an increasing sense of isolation as family and friends return to their own routines and the parents no longer have day-to-day contact with and support from the NICU staff. Communication and partnership building with the child's pediatric primary care physician, as well as communication issues between parents and subspecialists, the pediatric care physician and specialists, the parents and their family and friends, can also present an important challenge.

Establishing routines can be challenging for families because many preterm infants exhibit sleep problems during the early weeks at home. These problems can be related to immature sleep-awake cycles (day-night cycles), disruptions in sleep patterns caused by the need to administer medications, and heightened parental concerns about the infant's vulnerability. The last of these issues can lead to the parent overresponding to the infant's nighttime behaviors, leading to further sleep disruption. Residual neurologic immaturity and emerging muscle tone abnormalities can contribute to difficulty in caring for and calming the infant. Providing the family with strategies to help calm the infant and to support the baby's state regulation will ease the family's adaptation. Swaddling the infant, keeping the infant's arms and legs close to the body, avoiding sudden movements, and gradually introducing stimuli will support the infant's ability to adapt. Demonstrating the infant's abilities can also provide the parents with valuable insights into their infant's capabilities and developmental needs.

The first follow-up pediatric visit after NICU discharge should occur within 1 week of going home. During the first years of life, infants who required neonatal intensive care have higher, though varying, rates of rehospitalization. Among the most immature infants, 58% of very preterm infants are hospitalized one or more times, with nearly 50% having 2 or more hospitalizations in this period. The most frequent causes for hospitalization include respiratory illness, apparent life-threatening events, surgery (hernia repair, laser therapy for progressive retinopathy, enterostomy closure, ventriculoperitoneal shunt revision), and failure to gain weight.

From 3 months adjusted age through 1 year of age, parent concerns continue to focus on the infant's feeding, weight gain, and catch-up growth, as well as the infant's general health. As infants mature, they exhibit improvements in state regulation and their ability to handle stimulation and social interaction. Among very preterm or chronically ill young infants, persistent difficulties with state regulation, social interactions, or continuing problems tolerating handling and stimulation may exist. Transient tone abnormalities are common during infancy among preterm infants who exhibit high, low, or mixed tone. They may also exhibit postural or movement difficulties that contribute to feeding problems, positional plagiocephaly, and delays in milestone accrual.

Emerging milestones, particularly motor skills, may be a concern as delays in development become more apparent to the parents, their families, or members of the community. Parents of infants who have experienced a neurologic injury (intraventricular hemorrhage, periventricular leukomalacia or hydrocephalus in preterm infants, neonatal encephalopathy, seizures, or microcephaly) will have ongoing concerns about the risk of cerebral palsy and other neurologic sequelae and the need for early intervention. Some families will experience continued erosion of their informal social network, further increasing their sense of isolation. Even parents who have strong family supports and well-established informal support networks will experience isolation and a lack of understanding if their support network does not include other individuals who have had similar experiences and who can empathize with their concerns and fears.

Toddler and Early Childhood Years

Parental concerns from age 1 to 3 typically focus on motor milestones, communication and language skills, and sensory issues. Generally, infants with motor problems continue to improve and make steady progress. Catch-up growth continues during this time. Infants not previously eligible for early intervention services may require referral for evaluation of speech-language or communication problems or persistent delays in other developmental domains that now meet specific state eligibility requirements for early intervention services. During the preschool years, social immaturity, attention difficulties, and hyperactivity occur in 10% to 20% of preterm and other high-risk children. Emerging learning difficulties will be evident in some children with sensory problems, and social immaturity will be a continuing concern for others. Parents should be advised to observe for learning difficulties and seek early remedial assistance from preschool, nursery, or specialized child-care programs.

Growth and Nutrition Management

Growth patterns of an infant who is born low birth weight, who is preterm, or who is ill at birth provide valuable information about the infant's health. Chronic illness, feeding difficulties, malabsorption, gastroesophageal reflux, increased metabolic and nutritional requirements with inadequate nutritional intake, and social-emotional problems can contribute to aberrant growth. Feeding difficulties may be related to poor oromotor skills, respiratory symptoms, fatigue, or reflux esophagitis. Abnormalities of growth associated with intrauterine growth restriction, genetic or chromosomal disorders, congenital infection, or other syndromes can be responsible for reduced growth potential that prevents expected catch-up growth. Growth measurements should be plotted on standard growth charts correcting for the degree of prematurity until the child is 24 to 30 months corrected age. For very low–birth-weight preterm infants born weighing under 1500 grams, the Centers for Disease Control and Prevention National Center for Health Statistics recommends using either a standard growth chart or growth curves developed for low–birth-weight infants. Irrespective of the growth chart chosen, the measurements should be plotted using the corrected rather than chronologic age. Caloric requirements for adequate growth vary.

Postdischarge Formula or Human Milk Feeding

Healthy preterm infants require 110 to 130 kcal/kg/day, whereas infants with chronic illness may need up to 150 kcal/kg/day to sustain adequate weight and growth. At the time of hospital discharge, most infants are gaining 14 to 16 g/kg/day, comparable to intrauterine growth rates. However, infants who have been born very preterm or who experience serious illness often have residual caloric and nutritional deficits at the time of discharge; the majority of these infants leave the hospital with a weight below the expected mean for their gestational and postnatal age. Preterm infants also experience greater morbidities during their first year of life, including more hospitalizations and intercurrent illnesses that can further affect their feeding and growth.

Tremendous variation often exists in an infant's milk or formula intake. Some infants will be feeding well, ingesting more than 200 mL/kg/day, whereas others are barely achieving intakes of 130 to 150 mL/kg/day. The caloric density of a feeding has been shown to influence an infant's intake because infants on lower calorie (less calorie dense) feedings will feed up to 20% more than an infant feeding on a higher calorie formula.[8,9] Preterm infants continue to need higher-than-normal protein intake to replace protein deficits that accumulate after birth. Optimal postnatal nutrient intakes for preterm infants have not been fully determined. As a consequence, recommendations regarding target intakes for calcium and phosphorus vary. Recommended mineral intakes range from 100 to 160 mg/kg/day to 150 to 175 mg/kg/day of calcium and from 60 to 90 mg/kg/day to 90 to 105 mg/kg/day of phosphorus. Similarly, the optimal intake for vitamin D has not been clearly determined. Current recommendations range from 200 to 1600 IU/day. Because of concerns about the potential for vitamin D toxicity, most clinicians recommend a maximal intake of 800 to 1000 IU/day to prevent and treat osteopenia. Importantly, if the infant is discharged receiving vitamin D doses in this range, treatment should not be maintained for a prolonged period.[10]

The heterogeneity in the nutritional status among preterm infants and the differences in growth rates related to gestation, illness severity, and gender at the time of discharge present a challenge to determining an optimal feeding regimen. Special nutrient-enriched formulas are available for postdischarge use in North America and Europe that contain additional protein, minerals, and vitamins and provide 22 cal/oz (73 kcal/dL) and 1.8 g protein/dL. However, study results on the effectiveness of these nutrient-enriched formulas in optimizing growth and development have been mixed.

In a small randomized study of preterm infants less than 35 weeks' gestation who were fed either a nutrient-enriched infant formula or a term formula after hospital discharge, Lucas and colleagues[11] found that the infants fed the enriched formula grew better and had better bone mineralization at 6 to 9 months corrected age. Similarly, Cooke and colleagues[9,12,13] demonstrated increased protein intake and greater weight, length, and head circumference and lean and fat mass in preterm infants fed nutrient-enriched formula until 6 months corrected age. Comparison infants who received the nutrient-enriched formula only until they reached term gestation or who were fed a term formula did not demonstrate these results. Between term corrected age and 6 months corrected, both boys and girls exhibited greater growth when fed a nutrient-enriched formula. Carver and colleagues[8] further refined the understanding of the benefits of feeding a nutrient-enriched formula, demonstrating better growth (weight, length, and head circumference) among infants under 1250 grams at birth (2.75 lb). In a larger randomized trial conducted by Lucas and associates,[11] preterm infants fed a nutrient-enriched formula were heavier and longer at 9 and 18 months corrected age. The effects were greater for preterm boys. No difference in neurodevelopmental outcomes was noted. These benefits are not exhibited if the nutrient-enriched formula is discontinued before the preterm infant reached at least 6 months corrected age. Infants who received enriched formulas until term or 2 months corrected age did not demonstrate any benefit.[9,11-14] In a separate study by Koo and Hockman,[15] very low–birth-weight, very preterm infants were fed a standard term formula or an enriched preterm formula. Among the infants enrolled in this study, a growth advantage at 1 year of age was noted for infants who were fed the standard term formula.

The duration of feeding is an important consideration because use of nutrient-enriched, postdischarge formulas until the preterm infant is 6 to 12 months corrected age promotes better growth.[8,9,11,12,15] The effect of diet appears the greatest in boys. A 2005 Cochrane review by Henderson and colleagues[16] that compared the growth and development of preterm infants fed an enriched preterm formula with infants fed a standard term formula found insufficient evidence to demonstrate any advantage in growth or body composition among infants fed the preterm formula. Concerns regarding the conclusions drawn by the investigators relate to the significant heterogeneity among the studies included, study sample sizes, the variation in duration of preterm infant feeding with the nutrient-enriched formula (from term to 12 months corrected age), and differences in outcome measures.

Postdischarge enriched formulas should therefore be used for feeding of preterm infants, particularly those weighing less than 1250 grams at birth and preterm babies who exhibit suboptimal catch-up postnatal growth.[17-19] Enriched formula should be continued until the infant is 9 to 12 months corrected age. Preterm infants, such as those with significant chronic lung disease, higher metabolic needs, or poor postdischarge growth (slowing growth velocity or growth failure), may require continued specialized formula use beyond 12 months corrected age.

Experts recommend that, if a standard formula is used any time during the first 12 months after discharge, supplemental vitamins and additional iron should be provided. Vitamin supplementation is recommended with a liquid multivitamin until the infant's intake reaches 600 mL/day (20 oz/day or 75 mL every 3 hours). If a postdischarge enriched formula is fed, supplemental vitamins may not be necessary for infants whose intake is more than 200 mL/kg/day (more than 500 mL/day formula). Information about the composition, usage guidelines, and preparation of available postdischarge formulas and nutritional supplements is found in Chapter 77, Continuing Care of the Infant After Transfer From Neonatal Intensive Care. For children older than 1 year who continue to exhibit inadequate growth and weight of less than 5%, nutritional supplementation can be continued using one of several specialized, complete formulas that provide 30 kcal/oz.

Supporting Breastfeeding

Supplementation of infants who successfully transition to exclusive breastfeeding and demonstrate adequate weight gain and growth is not usually necessary. (See Chapter 89, Breastfeeding the Newborn.) Studies comparing preterm infants fed unfortified human milk or standard term formula after hospital discharge demonstrated lower bone mineral content, lower serum phosphorus, and higher serum alkaline phosphatase among human milk–fed infants.[18] These differences persisted through 12 months of age, but by age 2, human milk–fed infants had caught up to their preterm formula-fed peers. Exclusively breastfeeding preterm infants should receive vitamin and iron supplementation. Adequacy of growth should be closely monitored, with consideration given to supplementation with an iron-fortified standard term or enriched postdischarge preterm formula if an infant is exhibiting a slowing growth velocity or developing signs of nutritional deficiency. A suggested strategy to support continued breastfeeding is as follows:

- Supplement exclusive breastfeeding every 2 to 3 hours during the daytime with formula feeding every 2 to 3 hours in the evening and during the night.
- Enriched preterm formula can be mixed with expressed milk to increase the caloric density and nutrient composition.
- The enriched preterm formula can be prepared in the standard dilution to provide 22 kcal/oz or concentrated to provide 27 to 30 kcal/oz.
- The enriched preterm formula is then mixed in a 1:2 ratio (1/3 enriched formula + 2/3 human milk).

Supplementation should be continued for at least 6 months or longer if the infant's growth and nutritional assessment have not normalized within that period.[18] Periodic measurement of serum phosphorus and alkaline phosphatase is also important, given that phosphorus levels under 4.5 mg/dL and an elevated alkaline phosphatase above 1000 IU/mL may warrant further evaluation and supplementation.[19]

Tube Feedings

Infants with chronic health conditions or neurologic impairment may not be able to tolerate a portion or any of their enteral feedings by mouth. In addition, infants with specific nutrient or fluid requirements may require supplementation by tube feeding to ensure an appropriate intake. If tube feedings are necessary, the caregiver should ensure that the infant has opportunities for nonnutritive sucking either by sucking on a pacifier or through partial oral feeding. Some infants may require only episodic supplemental tube feedings until their oromotor skills mature. These babies may be able to have their feedings supplemented using a nasogastric (NG) tube if the parents are comfortable inserting an NG tube. Infants who are anticipated to require a longer period without full oral feeding (more than 2 to 3 months) should have a gastrostomy tube placed. Long-term tube feeding may be required for infants with neurologic or cardiorespiratory compromise, dysfunctional feeding, or other chronic health conditions.

Infants who have gastrostomy tubes can experience problems caused by leakage or irritation and local infection at the gastrostomy insertion (stoma) site. Leakage may develop because of enlargement of the stoma site. The amount of water in the gastrostomy balloon should be checked periodically (every 2 weeks); the balloon of an infant gastrostomy should typically contain 3 to 5 mL of water; an older child's balloon should be inflated with 5 to 10 mL of water. During feeding, the infant should be positioned upright or right side down. Irritation and purulent drainage at the stoma site are common problems. Bleeding and irritation may arise as granulation tissue forms in response to tube movement. Cauterizing any granulation tissue that develops around the stoma may also reduce leakage. Localized fungal infections occur frequently and respond to topical antifungal therapy.

Local care includes (1) gentle cleansing with a mild soap and water 2 to 3 times per day, (2) ensuring that the gastrostomy balloon is properly inflated and snug against the gastric wall, (3) cauterization of granulation tissue, and (4) topical, systemic, or both forms of treatment of local infection. Tube migration may occur with slippage of the gastrostomy tube tip into the pylorus or duodenum. Measuring the tube and ensuring the external disk is secure against the abdominal wall reduce this risk. Accidental removal is more likely to occur in small infants and during the early weeks after initial gastrostomy tube placement, before complete healing has taken place. Parents can be instructed on how to replace a balloon gastrostomy that is mature (>4 weeks). If the family is uncomfortable replacing the tube themselves, they may be instructed to bring the child to the emergency room or the health professional's office. Mature gastrostomy tubes that become dislodged should be replaced within 24 hours.

Infant With Biliary Dysfunction: Cholestasis and Gallstones

Parenteral nutrition (PN) associated cholestasis develops in 40% to 60% of infants who require prolonged intravenous nutritional support.[20] Conjugated bilirubin levels typically rise above 2.0 to 2.5 mg/dL (34-43 mcmol/L), and associated abnormalities in liver transaminases and other biochemical markers may exist. Jaundice and scleral icterus can develop after 2 to 4 weeks of parental nutritional therapy. Low birth weight and prematurity-related gastrointestinal complications, prolonged delay in initiating enteral feedings, short bowel syndrome, episodes of sepsis, and continuous as opposed to cycled parenteral nutrition are factors that contribute to the development of cholestasis. Bile stasis and prolonged fasting also contribute to the development of gallstones in infants requiring prolonged PN. Medications affecting gallbladder function and bile salt malabsorption can also be contributing factors. A frequent finding on sonographic imaging of the liver and gallbladder is *biliary sludge*. Infants with cholelithiasis may be asymptomatic or can exhibit fever and signs of sepsis if cholecystitis develops. A sudden rise in bilirubin or increased jaundice may occur, as well as the onset of acholic stools. Liver function, including serum conjugated bilirubin and liver enzymes, generally return to normal levels within 1 to 4 months of discontinuing PN. Bilirubin levels may normalize within 1 week to 2 months.[16]

Evaluation of the infant with cholestasis should include assessment of liver function and testing to identify any underlying condition that may be responsible for or contributing to the liver dysfunction.[21] In addition to screening the infant for bacterial and viral infections, testing for cystic fibrosis, alpha$_1$-antitrypsin deficiency, hypothyroidism, and inborn errors of metabolism, including galactosemia, should be performed. Imaging of the liver and gallbladder should also be performed to assess the infant for anatomic abnormalities and gallstones; identification of the biliary tree is crucial to ensure that the infant does not have biliary atresia.

Treatment strategies vary based on the type of nutritional support the infant is receiving. One effective approach involves cycling the PN rather than providing it on a continuous basis, with the goal of weaning the infant to full enteral feeding as quickly as feasible. Enteral feeding, even in small quantities, stimulates bile acid flow and reduces the risk of cholestasis developing. Feeding human milk or a medium-chain triglyceride–containing formula, in addition to providing supplemental fat soluble vitamins, is preferred for infants with cholestasis. Infants on PN should have the trace elements, copper, and manganese removed from the parenteral nutrition solution. Selenium and zinc should be provided in the PN solution to prevent deficiencies of these important trace elements. Infants who have a conjugated bilirubin level above 3 mg/dL (50 mcmol/L) can benefit from treatment with ursodeoxycholic acid (ursodiol), 20 to 30 mg/kg/day in 2 divided doses. Ursodiol is beneficial in the treatment of cholestasis caused by biliary atresia, improves hepatic metabolism of essential fatty acids in cystic fibrosis, PN-associated cholestasis, and gallstone dissolution. Although early studies suggested that synthetic cholecystokinin-octapeptide was beneficial in lowering serum conjugated bilirubin concentrations, it has not been shown in more recent investigations to improve bile flow or bile acid secretion or prevent gallstone formation.[22,23] Synthetic cholecystokinin-octapeptide is not approved for the prevention or treatment of cholestasis.

Strategies to Support Tube Feeding and Transition to Oral Feeding[24]

Infants who are only tolerating partial oral feeding can be fed by mouth during the day and tube fed at night using either bolus or continuous feeds. If the presence of the NG tube causes increased gagging, consider removing the tube during the daytime to encourage oral feeding. If the infant does not appear hungry for oral feedings, consider adjusting the feeding volume or feeding interval to allow hunger cues to develop, ensuring that the infant's total daily intake is sufficient to meet nutrient, energy, and fluid needs.

If continuous feeds are given overnight, stop feeding at least 2 hours before the infant awakens in the morning to allow time for hunger cues to develop by the first morning feeding. Decrease the amounts given at night gradually to support increased appetite during the daytime.

When the oral intake is near the total required, discontinue tube feedings on a trial basis and monitor for weight changes. Temporary plateau in weight or loss of up to 5% may be acceptable for 1 to 2 weeks if the infant remains hydrated, well nourished, and otherwise healthy. If the child has a gastrostomy tube, it can be removed after an adequate period of monitoring on full oral feedings (at least 1 month).

Infants With Short Bowel Syndrome or Intestinal Failure

Increased survival among neonates developing intra-abdominal emergencies has resulted in a higher prevalence of infants with short bowel syndrome requiring long-term nutritional support. Short bowel syndrome results from surgical resection, congenital defect, or disease-associated malabsorption with loss of fluid, electrolytes, protein, and micronutrients. The range of clinical problems necessitating extensive bowel resection includes necrotizing enterocolitis, bowel atresias, midgut volvulus caused by a malrotation, and congenital intestinal aganglionosis. The loss of a significant portion of the intestines' absorptive capability can contribute to intestinal dysfunction or intestinal failure. Loss of absorptive function in existing intestinal tissue can cause intestinal failure and can develop following intestinal obstruction, dysmotility, intestinal resection, congenital defect, or disease-induced malabsorption. Infants with gastroschisis and markedly thickened bowel at delivery are at risk for developing intestinal failure. Infants who lose their ileocecal valve during surgery are at additional risk because the ileocecal valve slows intestinal transit time and prevents reflux of intestinal contents and bacteria from the colon into the small intestine. Associated complications include malabsorption of vitamin B_{12}, bile salt deconjugation, reduction in bile salt absorption, and impaired intestinal function.

Management of short bowel syndrome and intestinal failure includes minimizing fluid, electrolyte, and nutrient losses, with the goal of promoting growth and optimal nutrition and maximizing the process of bowel adaptation.[25] Long-term PN support via a secure central catheter is usually required for these infants. Intestinal failure–associated liver disease occurs in 40% to 60% of infants with short bowel syndrome. Milder liver dysfunction in the form of PN-induced cholestasis is also common in infants, with preterm infants at higher risk than term babies. Infants on long-term PN support require care from a multidisciplinary team that includes pediatric surgeons, pediatric gastroenterologists, nutritionists, clinical nurse specialists, and home care nurses to assist the parents in caring for their child. When enteral feedings are initiated, continuous feedings via a gastrostomy tube are frequently the preferred method for feeding. In cases in which the infant has a mucous fistula, refeeding of the effluent from the proximal enterostomy into a distal mucous fistula has been shown to improve weight gain. Additional important aspects of the infant's nutrition and intestinal rehabilitation are attention to nonnutritive suck, oral-motor therapy, and early oral feedings, if feasible.

Feeding Problems

Feeding difficulties are most common during the neonatal period, but can remain a problem for preterm infants, as well as babies who are recovering from severe cardiorespiratory or chronic lung disease, infants with neurologic impairments, or those with craniofacial or gastrointestinal malformations that may interfere with normal feeding. Additional factors that can contribute to feeding difficulties include tracheostomy, gastroesophageal reflux, and repetitive noxious oral stimuli caused by oral suctioning, repeated intubations, orogastric tube placement, and air flow from nasal cannulae or nasal continuous positive airway pressure. (The process of transitioning to oral feeding is discussed in Chapter 77, Continuing Care of the Infant After Transfer From Neonatal Intensive Care.) Delayed feeding skills may develop in infants who exhibit immature sucking and swallowing patterns, babies who experience frequent or prolonged illness or who fail to transition to age-appropriate feeding methods, infants with gastroesophageal reflux, or infants who are fed inappropriately. Oral reflexes that facilitate normal feeding and protect the airway from aspiration may be hypo- or hyperactive. Tongue thrusting and a hyperactive gag reflex can further interfere with effective feeding. Infants who develop oral hypersensitivity (tactile defensiveness) may be unable to tolerate any oral stimulation and refuse placement of a nipple or spoon in their mouth. Dysfunctional feeding skills may develop in infants with physical, structural, or neurologic deficits, as well as infants with severe reflux. Babies who do not receive appropriate oral stimulation during enteral or parenteral feeding are also at risk. Feeding dysfunction may also develop after Nissen fundoplication or surgical repair of a tracheoesophageal fistula. The primary care physician must recognize and intervene when a persistent plateau in weight gain or poor growth occurs.

Referral for a feeding evaluation and feeding therapy should be considered if the parents or caregivers are reporting that feeding is stressful or difficult and any of the following is persistent:

- Feedings that consistently take longer than 45 minutes
- Feeding more frequently than every 2.5 to 3 hours resulting from infant fatigue, food refusal or avoidance behaviors, or difficulty achieving an adequate feeding volume
- Parent needing to enlarge or cut a nipple hole for the infant to suck human milk or nonthickened formula successfully from the nipple
- Parents reporting that the only way the infant will complete a bottle is during sleep
- Parents having difficulty interpreting or responding appropriately to the infant's cues
- Disrupted sleep associated with crying or a parental perception of the infant being in pain
- The infant exhibiting significant discomfort during or for 30 minutes after feeding, including:
  - Arching, grimacing, grunting, leg stiffening
  - Multiple swallows, coughing, emesis
  - Significant loss of fluid during feeding, poor lip seal, wide jaw excursion
  - Heavy breathing or nasal flaring
  - The need for frequent rest periods or pacing during the feeding

Among infants who are unable to orally feed because of oromotor coordination difficulties or aspiration risk, the goal of feeding therapy is to attempt to normalize oral sensorimotor development and to develop protective reflexes and oral motor skill. Infants with significant feeding issues who are otherwise typically developing remain at risk for later communication disorders involving expressive language. Box 96-2 outlines a series of anthropometric, clinical, feeding, and dietary *red flags* that should alert the clinician to the need for evaluation of the infant's feeding ability and appropriateness of the nutritional intake. Sample questions to assist the provider in assessing the infant's feeding proficiency are provided in Box 96-3.

Management of Regurgitation

Regurgitation is common among infants and must be distinguished from the potentially more serious

BOX 96-2 Anthropometric, Clinical, Feeding, and Dietary Red Flags for High-Risk Infants

ANTHROPOMETRIC

Weight for age or weight for length <5% on the standard CDC growth chart for corrected age, or <50% on the IHDP growth charts for low birth weight, premature infants

Weight for age or weight for length >95%

Slowing growth velocity, weight loss or significant decline in percentiles, especially if decline in weight percentile precedes decline in length

Poor weight gain for age, adjusted for prematurity up to 24 mos of age

- Term (40 wk PMA) to 3 mos: <20 g/day (<5 oz/wk)
- 3 to 6 mos: <15 g/day (<3.5 oz/wk)
- 6 to 9 mos: <10 g/day (<2 oz/wk)
- 9 to 12 mos: <7 d/day (<1.5 oz/wk)
- 1 to 2 yrs: <1 kg (2 lb)/6 mos
- 2 to 5 yrs: <0.7 kg (1.5 lb)/6 mos

Disproportionate head growth

- Term to 3 mos: <0.5 cm/wk
- 3 to 6 mos: <0.25 cm/wk
- Any time during infancy: >1.25 cm/wk

CLINICAL

Vomiting

Diarrhea

Constipation

Chronic health conditions

Chronic medication use that can affect nutritional status

FEEDING

Use of technology to support nutrition

- Gastrostomy tube, nasogastric or jejunal tube feeding
- Supplemental feeding systems or lactation aids
- Home parenteral nutrition

Parents have difficulty interpreting or responding appropriately to feeding cues

Prolonged feeding duration, insufficient intake or difficulty with feeding or food progression

INFANTS

More than 30 mins to complete a feeding

Fussy or distressed during feeding

Respiratory distress during feeding

Difficult to wake for feeding

Feeding fatigue

Frequently gags, coughs, or chokes during feeding

Refuses feeding or arches backward during feeding

Limited intake

- Fewer than 5 feedings/day or less than 24 oz/day
- Older than 6 mos corrected age not yet starting spoon feeding (persistent tongue thrusting, oral sensitivity)

TODDLERS

Over 45 mins to complete a meal

Inappropriate intake

- Fewer than 4 feedings/day or less than 16 oz milk/day with no other sources of dietary dairy products
- Older than 1 yr drinking more than 32 oz cow's milk/day
- Older than 1 yr not taking finger foods

Limited dietary intake—exclusion of one or more food groups

Mealtimes are frustrating for parent or child or both

Inappropriate formula preparation or use

- Low iron formula
- Using enriched preterm formulas for nonrecommended purposes
- Adding inappropriate supplements to infant formula or breast milk
- Adding insufficient or excess water during infant formula preparation (overfeeding: more than 40 oz/day)

Adapted from: Groh-Wargo S, Thompson M, Cox JH, eds. *Nutritional care for high-risk newborns.* 3rd ed. Chicago, IL: Precept Press; 2000. Used by permission.

gastroesophageal reflux disease. Strategies for the management of infants with significant gastroesophageal reflux have been published by the North American Society for Pediatric Gastroenterology, Hepatology, and Nutrition[26] and are summarized in Chapter 77. (See also Chapter 264, Gastroesophageal Reflux Disease.) Techniques to manage the common effects of regurgitation are based on symptom reduction or symptom control. Infants who are vomiting as a result of overfeeding benefit from smaller, more frequent feedings. If the infant is not gaining adequate weight, increasing the caloric density of the infant's formula can promote weight gain without the need to increase the feeding volume. Reduction of air swallowing before or after feeding can be controlled by starting the feeding before the infant cries for a prolonged period. Use of an angled bottle or positioning the bottle so that the nipple is filled will reduce the amount of air swallowed. Proper positioning of the baby and cheek support is recommended to ensure that the infant grasps the nipple correctly and is able to maintain good lip closure on the nipple. Avoiding excessive stimulation during and after feeding is another effective strategy to limit vomiting. Prone positioning is no longer recommended unless the infant is continuously monitored. Use of hyperosmolar formulas (≥27 kcal/oz) or fat supplements should be avoided because these forms of caloric supplementation can delay gastric emptying.

Constipation

Constipation is common in premature infants. Factors that contribute to difficulty with stooling include decreased abdominal muscle strength and intestinal motility, decreased free water intake from nutrient-dense feedings, an increased incidence of mechanical

BOX 96-3 Sample Feeding Questions

Is feeding your baby unusually stressful?
How much time does it take to feed your baby?
Is there any dribbling of milk down your baby's chin while he/she is feeding?
What type of nipple are you using?
Have you made any changes or modifications to the nipple or the baby's feeding routine since the baby has come home?
Does the baby seem uncomfortable during or after the feeding? Does he/she cry or arch frequently? What about vomiting or spitting up?
Does the baby suck a pacifier? If so, can he/she keep it in his/her mouth by himself/herself while sucking? (If not, this suggests low oromotor tone or oral tactile sensitivity or both.)

gastrointestinal dysfunction after episodes of necrotizing enterocolitis or other gastrointestinal complications, and an increased incidence of muscle tone abnormalities associated with preterm birth or significant illness. A thorough examination is also important to evaluate the infant for the presence of anterior anal displacement, an anatomic cause of constipation. Dietary manipulation to provide more fiber (cereal, strained prunes, apricots, spinach) can be tried for infants older than 4 months corrected age who are tolerating complementary feedings. Milk of magnesia and osmotic laxatives such as a malt soup extract, polyethylene glycol, and lactulose can be considered in the treatment of uncomplicated constipation in older infants. Mineral oil should be avoided in young children younger than 2 years or if the child has lung disease or swallowing problems because of the risk of aspiration. Excessive stooling may lead to malabsorption of fat-soluble vitamins. Consultation with a pediatric gastroenterologist should be considered for infants with persistent symptoms.

Introduction of Solid Foods

Introduction of solid foods into the diet of the high-risk infant will depend on several factors; in particular the infant's readiness and ability to accept complementary foods by mouth. In general, introduction of solid foods can begin at 4 to 6 months corrected age, provided that the infant exhibits appropriate postural control of the head, neck, and trunk; decreased tongue thrusting; and an interest in feeding. Although some preterm infants with sucking difficulty may prefer feeding solids by spoon, others may exhibit difficulty tolerating the thickened texture of solid food or may demonstrate aversive responses to the forms of oral tactile stimulation associated with spoon feeding. Studies have shown that infants who are started on complementary feeding before 4 months of age tend to be heavier and longer and have larger head circumferences than infants who start complementary feeding after 4 months of age.[9,12,13]

Catch-Up Growth

The majority of catch-up growth occurs during the first 2 to 3 years of life, with a significant growth spurt between 36 and 40 weeks' postmenstrual age. As discussed in Chapter 95, Health and Developmental Outcomes of Infants Requiring Neonatal Intensive Care, very low–birth-weight children often remain lighter, shorter, and with smaller head size through early to middle childhood.[27-31]

Head growth is usually more rapid than weight gain and is frequently the first parameter to catch up. Rapid head growth must be distinguished from pathologic head growth caused by late-onset hydrocephalus and may require neuroimaging to ensure that progressive ventriculomegaly is not developing. Some infants exhibit head growth that crosses head circumference percentiles, but this growth should rarely exceed the 97th percentile. The head circumference should be measured at each visit during infancy. Cranial imaging is required if the rate of head growth is more than 1.25 cm/week or if any signs or symptoms are noted of increased intracranial pressure or changing neurologic status. Suboptimal brain growth, with a head circumference declining more than 2 standard deviations below the mean, considerably increases the infant's risk for developmental delays. Growth velocities for weight and length vary significantly, and an increase in weight may precede an increase in length. Growth velocity may fluctuate as the infant increases activity levels, experiences an intercurrent illness, or has feeding difficulty, worsening reflux symptoms, or has changes in diet and caloric intake. Low weight-for-length or a decline in all growth parameters suggests inadequate nutritional intake. Obesity may also develop in infants who are preterm or who experienced poor weight gain while in the hospital. Parents become hypervigilant about feeding and food intake or may be unable to read their infant's cues, interpreting crying, and fussiness as signs of hunger. Such issues can lead to overfeeding the infant.

Small-for-Gestational-Age Infants

Growth potential for infants born small for gestational age (SGA) depends on the underlying cause of the fetal growth abnormality and is most likely to be limited for specific infants who are less than the 3rd percentile for gestational age at birth. Seventy to 80% of SGA children will exhibit catch-up growth during the first years of life.[32] Investigations are ongoing about the potential benefits of hormonal therapy for the 10% of SGA children who do not exhibit catch-up growth.[33,34] In a recent consensus statement,[35] the International Societies of Pediatric Endocrinology and the Growth Hormone Research Society recommend that SGA children who do not demonstrate catch-up growth should be referred for early monitoring and evaluation for possible endocrine and metabolic disturbances and neurodevelopmental assessment for potential delays warranting early intervention. Consideration of early therapy with growth hormone should be given to children between 2 and 4 years of age whose height remains more than 2.5 standard deviations below the mean for age.

Chronic Lung Disease

Chronic lung disease (CLD), which includes bronchopulmonary dysplasia (BPD), is a significant health condition affecting many graduates of neonatal and pediatric critical care. Discussion about the pathogenesis, pathophysiologic features, and early management strategies can be found in Chapter 77, Continuing Care of the Infant After Transfer From Neonatal Intensive Care; Chapter 99, Respiratory Distress and Breathing Disorders in the Newborn; and Chapter 78, Discharge Planning for the High-Risk Newborn Requiring Intensive Care. Many infants remain symptomatic after discharge home from the hospital and may episodically exhibit the following signs: tachypnea and tachycardia, paradoxical respirations (*see-saw* pattern), retractions, cough, wheezing, pallor or cyanosis, irritability or lethargy, poor feeding, and poor weight gain or weight loss. Additional conditions that can further exacerbate CLD symptoms include gastroesophageal reflux, upper airway obstruction caused by tracheomalacia, bronchomalacia or subglottic stenosis, acute infection, high altitude for infants residing above sea level, and poor compliance with home oxygen or diuretic therapy. Optimal management for the infant with CLD involves a combination of strategies that involve optimizing the infant's nutrition, respiratory treatment (oxygen, medications), avoidance of infection and exposure to secondhand smoke, and parental education to support and optimize the child's care. Figure 96-1 provides a sample algorithm for weaning home oxygen therapy. Box 96-4 describes strategies to optimize the care of children with CLD.

If the infant is discharged home on diuretics, then the question arises as to when these medications can be weaned or when the infant can be permitted to outgrow the discharge medication dose. The diuretics can be weaned if the infant is well, exhibits adequate weight gain, has no evidence of respiratory distress, and has an improved lung examination. The lung fields should be clear to auscultation, with a heart rate and respiratory rate that is sustained in the normal range for the infant's age. The infant should not have any evidence of hepatomegaly (heart failure), should be weaning from supplemental oxygen, and should have no signs of fluid retention.

Infants who have difficulty weaning from supplemental oxygen should be evaluated for adequacy of their caloric intake because their energy and nutrient needs may have increased. Medication doses should be reviewed and doses adjusted for weight gain. Consideration should also be given to adding therapies in the event of increasing symptoms. Consultation with a pediatric pulmonary specialist can assist the pediatric care physician in optimizing the infant's respiratory care. The infant's history should be reexamined to determine if new or worsening reflux symptoms or signs of aspiration are present. The infant's oxygen saturation should be checked in all activity states and the oxygen concentration adjusted to maintain the oxygen saturation at or above 95%. The infant should be screened for significant anemia that may be contributing to the infant's symptoms. Additional testing can include obtaining a chest radiograph, an electrocardiogram, and possibly an echocardiogram to evaluate for worsening pulmonary disease (atelectasis or infiltrates) or cardiovascular sequelae (right-ventricular heart failure) associated with progressive CLD.

Gradually increase time spent at lower oxygen setting over a 7-day period.
If infant meets all weaning criteria:
1. Maintains SpO_2 ≥95% during sleep, while awake, and during feeding (obtain periodic SpO_2 readings if continuous monitoring is not available).
2. Good weight gain
3. No increase in respiratory symptoms

→ Weaning criteria are not satisfied: Poor weight gain, acute illness, hypoxemia, increased respiratory rate, increased heart rate.
→ Reinstitute oxygen.
→ SpO_2 is <95%.
→ Increase oxygen to maintain SpO_2 at ≥95%.

→ Weaning criteria are satisfied.
→ Continue to wean in 2- to 4-week intervals. Alternate daytime and nighttime weaning.
→ SpO_2 is ≥95% and clinically stable.
→ Once stable, continue to wean oxygen incrementally. ½ L/min→¼ L/min→⅛ L/min→1⁄16 L/min→room air (21% O_2)

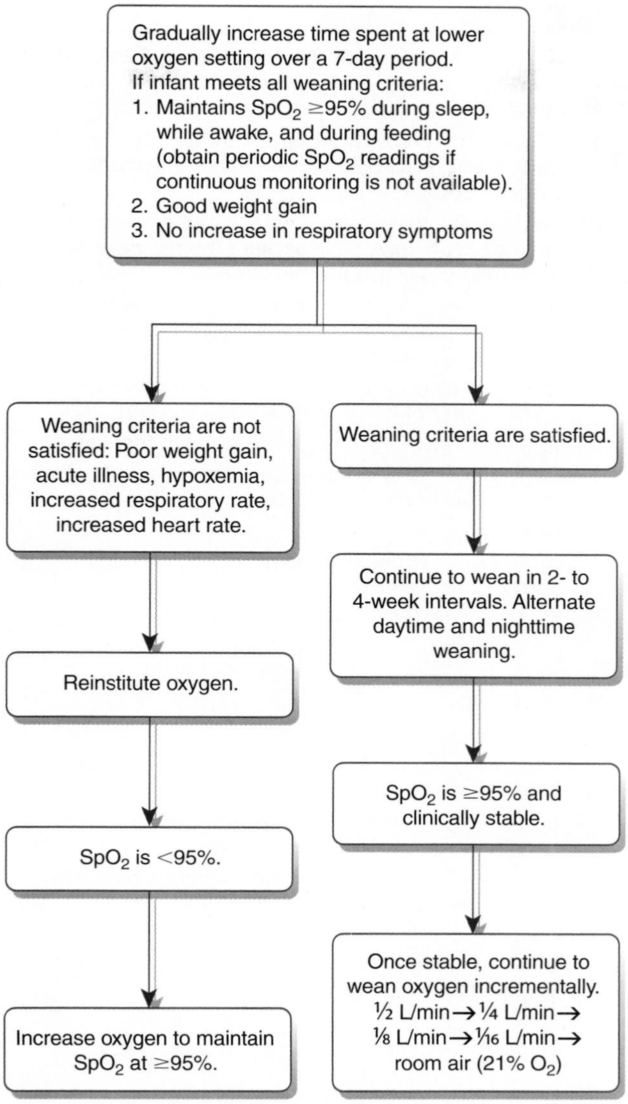

Figure 96-1 Sample protocol for oxygen weaning. *(Groothius J. Chronic lung disease. In Bernbaum J, ed.* Preterm infants in primary care: a guide to office management. *Columbus, OH: Ross Pediatrics Division of Abbott Laboratories; 2000. Used by permission.)*

Infants Discharged on Home Monitoring

Home cardiorespiratory monitoring may be required for infants with persistent apnea or apparent life-threatening events, infants discharged home on supplemental oxygen or methylxanthines, and babies with chronic conditions or malformations that impair cardiorespiratory function. If home monitoring is prescribed, an event recorder monitor capable of data storage (memory) should be used. The parents of infants discharged on home monitoring should have follow-up

BOX 96-4 Strategies to Optimize Care of Infants With Chronic Lung Disease

RESPIRATORY

An oxygen saturation over 94%-95% for infants with bronchopulmonary dysplasia who are more than 35 weeks' gestational age.

During sleep, the oxygen saturation on pulse oximetry should be kept above 93% because this has been shown to improve sleep architecture.[a]

Infants who have evidence of pulmonary hypertension should have serial echocardiography every 2 to 3 months to evaluate for development of cor pulmonale.[b]

Infants should be closely monitored for illness and acute, or subtle, signs of hypoxemia or bronchospasm.

- May need to increase or reinstitute oxygen therapy
- May need to initiate or increase the frequency of bronchodilators or corticosteroids

Medications

- Hydrochlorothiazide: 20 to 40 mg/kg/day divided every 12 hrs
- Spironolactone: 2 to 4 mg/kg/day divided every 12 hrs
- Furosemide: 2 to 4 mg/kg/dose every 12 to 24 hrs
- Potassium chloride: 1 to 4 mEq/kg/day divided every 6 to 12 hrs

Bronchodilators

- Albuterol (Proventil, Ventolin): 0.5 cc by nebulizer or 1 to 2 puffs inhaler every 6 to 12 hrs
- Ipratropium (Atrovent): 0.5 cc by nebulizer or 1 to 2 puffs inhaler every 12 hrs
- Levalbuterol (Xopenex): 0.62 mg respule by nebulizer or 1 to 2 puffs inhaler

Antiinflammatory drugs

- Cromolyn (Intal): Inhaler or nebulizer (2 to 4 weeks required for adequate trial)
- Inhaled steroids
  - Budesonide (Pulmicort): 0.25 to 0.5 mg respule every 12 to 24 hrs
  - Fluticasone (Flovent): 0.125 mg (1 puff) every 12 hrs
  - Betamethasone valerate
- Oral prednisone for serious exacerbations

Prevention of infection and reactive airway disease

- Respiratory syncytial virus and influenza virus prophylaxis
- Avoid secondhand smoke and vapor exposures: tobacco smoke, paint, kerosene, strong perfumes, aerosol sprays, incense, fireplace smoke or soot
- Limit exposure to crowds and large child-care settings

Oxygen Therapy

Can be weaned to a lower oxygen concentration (lower flow rate) when the infant exhibits (see Figure 96-1)

- No symptoms of respiratory distress
- Sustained, adequate weight gain
- No recent, intercurrent illnesses and improving overall health status
- The ability to maintain the oxygen saturation at or above 95% after 30 to 40 minutes on the proposed lower oxygen setting without any increase in respiratory symptoms
  - No compensatory tachypnea, tachycardia, pallor, cyanosis, or respiratory distress
  - No change in activity level, endurance, or increase in irritability

FEEDING AND NUTRITION

Provide adequate calories to promote a weight gain of 20-30 g/day

- Increased calorie requirements resulting from increased work of breathing and greater calorie consumption
  - 120 to 150 kcal/kg/day
  - Use nutrient dense feeding, providing 22 to 26 kcal/oz (may consider increasing to a maximum of 30 kcal/oz with caution and close monitoring of fluid and electrolyte status)
- Infants with moderate to severe chronic lung disease may require fluid restriction; attention is needed to provide appropriate calories without giving an excessive solute load that can cause additional complications
- Consider tube feeding to supplement oral feeding if inadequate weight gain occurs with oral feedings alone
- Closely monitor the infant for signs of feeding difficulties and initiate early referral for feeding therapy if feeding problems are present

Infants with signs of gastroesophageal reflux disease should be treated aggressively

[a]Fitzgerald D, Van Asperen P, Leslie G, et al. Higher SaO_2 in chronic neonatal lung disease: does it improve sleep? *Ped Pulmonol.* 1998;26:235-240.
[b]Abman SH. Monitoring cardiovascular function in infants with chronic lung disease of prematurity. *Arch Dis Child Fetal Neonatal Ed.* 2002;87:F15-F18.

contact with staff from the home monitoring program within 1 week. Subsequent follow-up contacts are often within 2 to 4 weeks and may entail a visit at the apnea center. Depending on the reason for home monitoring, many clinicians will discontinue monitoring after a symptom-free period of 4 to 6 weeks; some clinicians will obtain a monitor download or refer the infant for a diagnostic sleep study to assess the infant for any evidence of central or obstructive events that warrant continued therapy or monitoring or both. If the infant has an abnormal study 4 to 6 weeks after discharge, monitoring can be continued for an additional 4 to 6 weeks followed by repeat testing for persistent abnormalities. If a preterm infant is discharged on a methylxanthine, the medication may be discontinued when the infant reaches term gestation, provided that the baby is not having any symptoms or monitor alarms. A monitor recording or polysomnographic study should be obtained 7 to 14 days after discontinuing medication. If the study is normal, then monitoring can be stopped. If the study is abnormal, monitoring should be continued. The decision whether to reinstitute methylxanthine treatment is typically based on the severity of monitoring abnormalities.

Outpatient Screening

Follow-up care for high-risk infants should include periodic screenings beyond the routine components of care that are based on the infant's chronic conditions and risk factors.

Hearing Screening

Continued surveillance and periodic hearing testing are necessary for infants at risk for delayed-onset or progressive hearing loss.[36] Infants who fail or miss NICU hearing screening must have follow-up testing scheduled. Infants with known hereditary (genetic) or acquired conditions associated with a high risk for hearing loss should be referred for medical evaluation and comprehensive otologic evaluation. Factors to consider when determining the frequency of periodic hearing testing beyond parental concern, a family history of permanent hearing loss, or a syndrome with associated hearing loss include the need for intensive care for more than 5 days or assisted ventilation longer than 10 days and prolonged exposure to ototoxic medications (gentamicin and tobramycin) or loop diuretics (furosemide). Infants who have recovered from postnatal infections associated with sensorineural hearing loss, including bacterial meningitis and in utero infections such as cytomegalovirus, herpes, rubella, syphilis, and toxoplasmosis, also require serial hearing testing. Babies treated for severe hyperbilirubinemia (exchange transfusion) or who experience respiratory failure necessitating extracorporeal membrane oxygenation are also at high risk for progressive hearing loss and should have follow-up hearing tests every 6 months until 3 years of age.

Ophthalmologic Examinations

Follow-up of preterm infants with retinopathy of prematurity (ROP) should adhere to the screening and surveillance guidelines issued by the American Association of Pediatric Ophthalmology and Strabismus and the American Academy of Ophthalmology in collaboration with the American Academy of Pediatrics. The frequency of surveillance is based on the examining ophthalmologist's findings.[37] The Canadian Association of Pediatric Ophthalmologists and the United Kingdom have similar guidelines regarding the timing of initial screening and subsequent surveillance. The risk for vision loss from ROP is low once the preterm infant has reached 45 weeks' postmenstrual age without developing prethreshold or more severe ROP, if the infant's retina is vascularized into zone III without evidence of retinopathy in zone II, or if the retina is fully vascularized. At this point, serial ROP screening can be discontinued. However, periodic surveillance of visual acuity and other ocular morbidity should continue.[38] Preterm infants should be examined by a pediatric ophthalmologist at 6 and 12 months corrected age, before school entry, and again at 9 to 12 years of age. Robaei and colleagues recently reported on visual morbidity affecting moderately preterm and low–birth-weight children who were born between 32 to 36 weeks' gestation, weighing between 1500 and 2499 grams. Both groups of children were found to be at higher risk for development of amblyopia, strabismus, and uncorrected visual acuity in the lowest quartile of visual function. Low–birth-weight children were also more likely to exhibit anisometropia.[39]

Neurodevelopment and Behavior

Neurologic immaturity, sensory defensiveness, and transient muscle tone abnormalities can cause concern for families caring for preterm babies and infants recovering from serious illness. Strategies to support these infants' ability to tolerate stimulation and handling include (1) using calming techniques, (2) using containment positioning during bathing, and (3) cautioning parents against infant swing use because this causes sudden changes in movement patterns. Calming techniques consist of swaddling and containment (ie, holding the infant with arms and legs flexed close to the body). The infant should be swaddled or positioned using containment before moving the infant. Sudden movements should be avoided. Family members must be made aware of the early developmental needs of the infant recovering from a very preterm or traumatic birth. Recognizing and responding to the infant's neurodevelopmental cues can help the infant's adaptation to the environment and support the infant's increasing tolerance of handling and other forms of sensory stimulation. Parents benefit from guidance about their infant's ability to signal their needs through movement, facial expressions, and breathing patterns and how to interpret and respond to these behavioral cues. During the early weeks and months after hospital discharge, preterm infants may be more irritable and less responsive to their environment and social interactions. They typically need more help in calming and learning to self-soothe. The primary goal of caregiving is to match the caregiver's responses to the infant's needs without being intrusive or overwhelming the infant. Consistent caregiver responses to the infant's cues help the infant learn to anticipate and expect a response.

As the infant matures and recovers, parental concerns about infant vulnerability can affect their parenting skills and contribute to child behavior problems over time if the parents have difficulty with limit setting and discipline. Parents will benefit from support and guidance about strategies to support appropriate infant development. Many families will consult baby books and various multimedia resources and search the Internet for information and guidance about their infant's particular health issues and routine aspects in infant care. Parents should be reminded to adjust for their infant's prematurity when reading information about anticipated growth and development. Families will also benefit from assistance with sorting through the myriad materials in press, in the media, and on the Internet in terms of factual information.

Family Adjustment

The stress of a preterm or sick newborn birth can have serious effects for parents and siblings, cause significant economic hardship, and lead to family disruption and dysfunction. Parents often feel isolated and experience a wide range of emotional feelings ranging from euphoria to despair. Discord may develop between the 2 parents or between the parents and other family members or members of the infant's medical team. Each parent and family member has unique coping abilities, values, beliefs and preferences. Grandparents, extended family members, and friends can be a source of emotional support and respite for the parents. The converse may also occur when parental perspectives and wishes differ from the values and beliefs of other family members or friends. Siblings may be or feel neglected and may exhibit behavioral changes caused by disruption in the family routine and associated parent distraction and distress. Child vulnerability (vulnerable child syndrome) is discussed in Chapter 95, Health and Developmental Outcomes of Infants Requiring Neonatal Intensive Care. All the typical concerns of parents of healthy infants are exaggerated when the child is born premature, with a birth defect, or has experienced significant neonatal illness. Parents should be encouraged to normalize their care routines for their preterm or recovering infant as much as possible. Having opportunities to connect with other families of similar children is helpful for families who have a premature or sick infant because they can gain insight and support from their shared experiences. Guidance on assisting families who are confronting an unfavorable diagnosis or chronic illness for their infant is found in Chapter 67, Partnering With Families in Hospital and Community Settings; and Chapter 69, Palliative, End-of-Life, and Bereavement Care.

TOOLS FOR PRACTICE

Engaging Patient and Family

- *Respiratory Syncytial Virus (RSV)* (brochure) American Academy of Pediatrics (patiented.aap.org).

Medical Decision Support

- *Discharge Summary Form*, Transition Care of the Preterm Infant, Judy Bernbaum, MD (practice.aap.org/content.aspx?aid=2001).
- *Extremely Low Birth Weight NICU Graduate Supplement to the Critical Elements of Care for the Low Birth Weight Neonatal Intensive Care Graduate (CEC-LBW)*, Washington State Medical Home (medicalhome.org/4Download/cec/elbw.pdf).
- *Guidelines for Perinatal Care*, 6th edition (book), American Academy of Pediatrics and American College of Obstetricians and Gynecologists (www.aap.org/bookstore).
- *History Form for Premature Infants*, Transition Care of the Preterm Infant, Judy Bernbaum, MD (practice.aap.org/content.aspx?aid=2001).
- *Infant Health and Development Program (IHDP) Growth Chart for Very Low Birth Weight Premature Boys ≤1500 Grams, ≤37 Weeks' Gestation at Birth* (other), Ross Pediatrics (www.rosspediatrics.com).
- *Infant Health and Development Program (IHSP) Growth Chart for Very Low Birth Weight Premature Girls ≤1500 Grams, ≤37 Weeks' Gestation at Birth* (other), Ross Pediatrics (www.rosspediatrics.com).
- *Pediatric Nutrition Handbook*, 5th edition (book), American Academy of Pediatrics (www.aap.org/bookstore).
- *Visit Form for the Premature Infant*, Transition Care of the Preterm Infant, Judy Bernbaum, MD (practice.aap.org/content.aspx?aid=2001).

RELATED WEB SITES

- American Family Physician (www.familydoctor.org).
- Canada's Parenting Community: Canadian Parents (www.candianparents.com)/Cleft Palate Foundation (www.cleftline.org).
- ComeUnity (www.comeunity.com).
- Cystic Fibrosis Foundation (www.cff.org).
- Keep Kids Healthy (www.keepkidshealthy.com/newborn/premature_babies.html).
- Nemours Foundation: Kids Health (www.kidshealth.org).
- Lissencephaly Network (www.lissencephaly.org).
- March of Dimes (www.marchofdimes.com).
- Mothers of Supertwins (www.mostonline.org).
- National Down Syndrome Society (www.ndss.org).
- National Organization of Mothers of Twins Clubs, Inc. (www.nomotc.org).
- National Institute for Child Health and Human Development (www.nichd.nih.gov/publications/pubslist.cfm).
- Newborn Screening (www.newbornscreening.com).
- New Visions (www.new-vis.com/p-map.htm).
- Meriter: Parenting Guide for Families of Premature Infants (www.meriter.com/living/preemie/index.htm).
- Meriter: Parenting Guide for Families of Sick Newborn Infants (www.meriter.com/living/sicknewborn/index.htm).
- Parenting of Multiples (multiples.about.com/).
- Prematurity.org (www.prematurity.org).
- SIDS Network (www.sids-network.org).
- Trisomy 18, 13 and Related Disorders (www.trisomy.org).
- Twins Magazine (www.twinsmagazine.com).

AAP POLICY STATEMENTS

American Academy of Pediatrics, Section on Ophthalmology, American Academy of Ophthalmology, American Association for Pediatric Ophthalmology and Strabismus. Screening examination of premature infants for retinopathy of prematurity. *Pediatrics*. 2006;117(2)572-576. (aappolicy.aappublications.org/cgi/content/full/pediatrics;117/4/1468).

American Academy of Pediatrics, Joint Committee on Infant Hearing. Principles and guidelines for early hearing detection and intervention programs—year 2007 position statement. *Pediatrics*. 2007;120(4):898-921. (pediatrics.aappublications.org/cgi/content/full/pediatrics;120/4/898).

North American Society for Pediatric Gastroenterology, Hepatology, and Nutrition. Guidelines for evaluation and treatment of gastroesophageal reflux in infants and children. *J Pediatr Gastroenterol*. 2001;32(2):1-31. AAP Endorsed.

North American Society for Pediatric Gastroenterology, Hepatology, and Nutrition. Guideline for the evaluation of cholestatic jaundice in infants: recommendations of the North American Society for Pediatric Gastroenterology, Hepatology, and Nutrition. *J Pediatr Gastroenterol Nutr*. 2004;39(2):115-128. AAP Endorsed.

SUGGESTED RESOURCES

Kim P, Eng TR, Deering MJ, et al. Published criteria for evaluating health related web sites: review. *BMJ*. 1999;318:647-649.

Martins EN, Morse LS. Evaluation of Internet websites about retinopathy of prematurity patient education. *Br J Ophthalmol.* 2005;89:565-568.

Suchy FJ. Neonatal cholestasis. *Pediatr Rev.* 2004;25:388-396.

Wessel JJ. Short bowel syndrome. In Groh-Wargo S, Thompson M, Cox J, eds. *Nutritional care for high risk newborns,* 3rd ed. Chicago, IL: Precept Press; 2000.

REFERENCES

1. Wang CJ, McGlynn EA, Brook RH, et al. Quality-of-care indicators for the neurodevelopmental follow-up of very low birth weight children: results of an expert panel process. *Pediatrics.* 2006;117:2080-2092.
2. American Academy of Pediatrics. Follow-up care of high risk infants. *Pediatrics.* 2004;114:1377-1397.
3. American Academy of Pediatrics, Committee on Fetus and Newborn. Hospital discharge high-risk neonate—proposed guidelines. *Pediatrics.* 1998;102:411-417.
4. Broyles RS, Tyson JE, Heyne ET, et al. Comprehensive follow-up care and life-threatening illnesses among high-risk infants: a randomized controlled trial. *JAMA.* 2000;284(16):2070-2076.
5. O'Shea TM, Nageswaran S, Hiatt DC, et al. Follow-up care for infants with chronic lung disease: a randomized comparison of community- and center-based models. *Pediatrics.* 2007;119(4):e947.
6. McPherson ML, Lairson DR, O'Brian Smith E, et al. Noncompliance with medical follow-up after pediatric intensive care. *Pediatrics.* 2002;109(6):e94.
7. Lainwala S, Perritt R, Poole K, et al. Neurodevelopmental and growth outcomes of extremely low birth weight infants who are transferred from neonatal intensive care units to level I or II nurseries. *Pediatrics.* 2007;119(5): e1079.
8. Carver JD, Wu PYK, Hall TR, et al. Growth of preterm infants fed nutrient-enriched or term formula after hospital discharge. *Pediatrics.* 2001;107:683-689.
9. Cooke RJ, McCormick K, Griffin IJ, et al. Feeding preterm infants after hospital discharge: effect of diet on body composition. *Pediatric Res.* 1999;46:461-464.
10. Atkinson S, Tsang RC. Calcium and phosphorus. In: Tsang RC, Uay R, Koletzko B, Zlotkin SH, eds. *Nutrition of the preterm infant: scientific basis and practice.* 2nd ed. Cincinnati, OH: Digital Publishing; 2005.
11. Lucas A, Fewtrell MS, Morley R, et al. Randomized trial of nutrient-enriched formula versus standard formula for postdischarge preterm infants. *Pediatrics.* 2001;108:703-711.
12. Cooke RJ, Griffin IJ, McCormick K, et al. Feeding preterm infants after hospital discharge: effect of dietary manipulation on nutrient intake and growth. *Pediatr Res.* 1998;43:355-360.
13. Cooke RJ, Embleton ND, Griffin IJ, et al. Feeding preterm infants after hospital discharge: growth and development at 18 months of age. *Pediatr Res.* 2001;49: 719-722.
14. DeCurtis M, Pieltain C, Rigo J. Body composition in preterm infants fed standard term or enriched formula after hospital discharge. *Eur J Nutr.* 2002;41:177-182.
15. Koo WWK, Hockman EM. Postdischarge feeding for preterm infants: effects of standard compared with enriched milk formula on growth bone mass, and body composition. *Am J Clin Nutr.* 2006;84:1357-1364.
16. Henderson G, Fahey T, McGuire W. Calorie and protein enriched formula versus standard term formula for improving growth and development in preterm or low birth weight infants following hospital discharge (review). *Cochrane Database Syst Rev.* 2005;4(22): CD004696.
17. Bhatia J. Post-discharge nutrition of preterm infants. *J Perinatol.* 2005;25:S15-S16.
18. Schanler RJ. Post-discharge nutrition for the preterm infant. *Acta Paediatr.* 2005;94(suppl 449):68-73.
19. Greer FR. Post-discharge nutrition: what does the evidence support? *Semin Perinatol.* 2007;31:89-95.
20. Btaiche IF, Khalidi N. Parenteral nutrition-associated liver complications in children. *Pharmacotherapy.* 2002;22(2):188-211.
21. Moyer V, Freese DK, Whitington PF, et al. Guideline for the evaluation of cholestatic jaundice in infants: recommendations of the North American Society for Pediatric Gastroenterology, Hepatology and Nutrition. *J Pediatr Gastroenterol Nutr.* 2004;39(2):115-128.
22. Curran TJ, Uzoaru I, Das JB, et al. The effect of cholecystokinin-octapeptide on the hepatobiliary dysfunction caused by total parenteral nutrition. *J Pediatr Surg.* 1995;30:242-247.
23. Tsai S, Strouse PJ, Drongowski RA, et al. Failure of cholecystokinin-octapeptide to prevent TPN-associated gallstone disease. *J Pediatr Surg.* 2005;40(1):263-267.
24. Cox JH. Growth, nutrition and feeding. In Bernbaum J, ed. *Preterm infants in primary care: a guide to office management.* Columbus, OH: Ross Products Division, Abbott Laboratories; 2000.
25. Wessel JJ, Kocoshis SA. Nutritional management of infants with short bowel syndrome. *Semin Perinatol.* 2007;31:104-111.
26. North American Society for Pediatric Gastroenterology, Hepatology, and Nutrition (NASPGHN). Pediatric GE reflux clinical practice guidelines. *J Pediatr Gastroenterol Nutr.* 2001;32(suppl 2):S1-S31.
27. Ehrenkranz RA, Dusick AM, Vohr BR. Growth in the neonatal intensive care unit influences neurodevelopmental and growth outcomes of extremely low birth weight infants. *Pediatrics.* 2006;117(4):1253-1261.
28. Cooke RWI, Foulder-Hughes L. Growth impairment in the very preterm and cognitive and motor performance at 7 years. *Arch Dis Child.* 2003;88:482-487.
29. Doyle LW, Faber B, Callahan C, et al. Extremely low birth weight and body size in early adulthood. *Arch Dis Child.* 2004;89:347-350.
30. Fewtrell MS, Lucas A, Cole TJ, et al. Prematurity and reduced body fatness at 8-12 y of age. *Am J Clin Nutr.* 2004;80:436-440.
31. Farooqi A, Hägglöf B, Sedin G, et al. Growth in 10- to 12-year-old children born at 23 to 25 weeks' gestation in the 1990's: a Swedish national prospective follow up study. *Pediatrics.* 2006;118(5):e1452-e1465.
32. Karlberg J, Albertsson-Wikland K. Growth in full-term small-for-gestational-age infants: from birth to adult height. *Pediatr Res.* 1995;38:733-739.
33. Lee PA, Chernausek SD, Hokken-Koelega ACS, et al. International SGA Advisory Board Consensus Development Conference statement: management of short children born small for gestational age, April 24-October 1, 2001. *Pediatrics.* 2003;111:1253-1261.
34. Argente J, Garcia R, Ibáñez L, et al. Improvement in growth after two years of growth hormone therapy in very young children born small for gestational age and without spontaneous catch-up growth: results of a multicenter, controlled, randomized, open clinical trial. *J Clin Endocrinol Metab.* 2007;92:3095-3101.
35. Clayton PE, Cianfarani S, Czernichow P, et al. Consensus statement: management of the child born small for gestational age through adulthood: a consensus statement of the International Societies of Pediatric Endocrinology and the Growth Hormone Research Society. *J Clin Endocrinol Metab.* 2007;92:804-810.

36. American Academy of Pediatrics. Year 2007 position statement: principles and guidelines for early hearing detection and intervention programs. *Pediatrics.* 2007; 120(4):898-921.
37. American Academy of Pediatrics, Section on Ophthalmology, American Academy of Ophthalmology, American Association for Pediatric Ophthalmology and Strabismus. Policy statement: screening examination of premature infants for retinopathy of prematurity. *Pediatrics.* 2006;117:572-576.
38. Reynolds JD, Dobson V, Quinn GE, et al. Evidence-based screening criteria for retinopathy of prematurity: natural history data from the CYRO-ROP and LIGHT-ROP Studies. *Arch Ophthalmol.* 2002;120:1470-1476.
39. Robaei D, Kifley A, Gole GA, et al. The impact of modest prematurity on visual function at 6 years. *Arch Ophthalmol.* 2006;124:871-877.

Section Four

Neonatal Medical Conditions

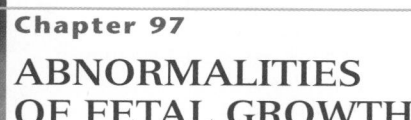

Chapter 97
ABNORMALITIES OF FETAL GROWTH

Suhas M. Nafday, MD, MRCP(Ire), DCH

Fetal growth is determined by fetal genotype and, to a large extent, by the uterine environment. The in utero environment is predominantly influenced by maternal genetics, the size of the mother, the capacity of the placenta to provide nutrients to the fetus, and, to a modest degree, paternal genetics. Although several genes have been described as maternally or paternally imprinted, two growth disorders, Beckwith-Wiedemann syndrome (macrosomia) and Russell-Silver syndrome (fetal malnutrition), represent well-characterized phenotypes that arise as a consequence of disrupted imprinting. Two protein products of genes, such as insulin-like growth factors I and II, play a specific role in the growth of trophoblastic cells, which form the placenta.[1] In a genetically abnormal fetus, genes affecting growth may result in adverse effects. Various factors affecting fetal growth are listed in Table 97-1.

INTRAUTERINE GROWTH RESTRICTION

At present, many clinicians do not distinguish between the terms *small for gestational age* (SGA) and *intrauterine growth restriction* (IUGR). However, these two clinical entities are not the same. SGA newborns traditionally have been defined as those whose birth weights are more than 2 standard deviations below the mean or less than the 10th percentile of population-based weight data obtained from newborns at the same gestational age. Conversely, a newborn with IUGR has not reached the genetic growth potential as a result of an insult that occurred in utero. An IUGR fetus may or may not be SGA, but it always implies a pathological process. IUGR is commonly defined as birth weight under the 10th percentile on intrauterine growth curves. Some perinatologists have defined IUGR as birth weight less than 2 standard deviations below the mean, which roughly corresponds to less than the 3rd percentile on intrauterine growth curves.[2] Low birth weight is defined by the

Table 97-1 Factors Affecting Fetal Growth

FACTOR	COMMENT
Fetal genetic potential	Specific genes must be expressed for fetal and placental growth.
Maternal size and uterine size	Fetal growth constraint from the maternal environment is a physiological process that includes the maternal-specific capacity of uterine size, placental implantation surface area of the uterus, and uterine circulation, which together support the growth of the placenta and its function.[a]
Patterns of gestational age	Length of gestation is proportional to fetal weight but is more strongly correlated to neural growth.
Fetal nutrient uptake and metabolism; regulation of fetal growth	Decreased rates of fetal growth represent an adaptation to inadequate nutrient supply (intrauterine growth restriction).
Maternal nutrition	Only severe starvation limits fetal growth; growth may be limited by 10-20%.
Placenta	True placental hormones, particularly placental lactogen, play an important role in fetal growth. Placental insufficiency leads to fetal growth restriction. Placental size and fetal size are directly related.[b]
Glucose, amino acids, and fat transport across placenta	Intrauterine growth restricted infants have lower glucose levels. Amino acids and energy supply are important for fetal growth. Fat accumulation occurs predominantly in the third trimester.
Maternal and fetal endocrine regulation	Maternal growth hormone and human placental lactogen increase during pregnancy, which induces insulin resistance and increased facilitated glucose transport to fetus. In infants of diabetic mothers, increased supply of glucose stimulates fetal insulin and promotes fetal adiposity (macrosomia).

[a]Regnault TRH, Limesand SW, Hay WW Jr. Factors influencing fetal growth. *NeoReviews.* 2001;6:119-128.
[b]Molteni RA, Stys SJ, Battaglia FC. Relationship of fetal and placental weight in human beings: fetal/placental weight ratio at various gestational ages and birth weight. *J Reprod Med.* 1978;21:327-334.

Table 97-2 Clinical, Genetic and Environmental Factors Associated With Intrauterine Growth Restriction

FETAL	MATERNAL	PLACENTAL
Chromosomal abnormality	Substance abuse	Partial placental separation
Aneuploidy	Smoking	Uteroplacental insufficiency:
Multifactorial congenital malformations	Alcohol	Unexplained elevated alpha feto-protein, preeclampsia
Cardiovascular abnormalities	Drugs: amphetamines, corticosteroids, heroin, hydantoin, propranolol, warfarin	Placental infarction
Renal agenesis	Chronic disease	Placenta previa
Multiple fetus pregnancy	Cyanotic heart disease, cystic fibrosis, asthma, renal disease, sickle cell disease, lupus, inflammatory bowel disease, advanced diabetes, hyperthyroidism	Multiple gestation, twin to twin transfusion
Infection	Constitutionally small mother	Small placenta
Cytomegalovirus	Lack of second-trimester weight gain	Chronic vascular disease
Toxoplasmosis	High-altitude pregnancy (hypoxia)	
Herpes simplex	Malnutrition	
Rubella		
Malaria		
Aberrant genomic imprinting		
Uniparental disomy		
Epimutations		

Modified from Peebles DM. Fetal consequences of chronic substrate deprivation. *Semin Fetal Neonatal Med.* 2004;9:379-386. Copyright Elsevier, 2004. Used by permission.

World Health Organization as a birth weight below 2500 g but does not correct for gestational age. Other weight-based definitions include *very low birth weight* (<1500 g), *extremely low birth weight* (<1000 g), and, more recently, *micropreemie* (<750 g).

However, some infants are constitutionally small. These infants have no increased obstetrical or neonatal risks. Availability of continuous fetal growth curves, developed from information gathered by ultrasound, has helped in diagnosing IUGR earlier. Race and ethnicity also play an important role. The growth curves should ideally be tailored for the patient population and geographic region.

Another concept relates to *symmetric* (proportionately small) versus *asymmetric* (relative head-sparing) growth restriction. Symmetrical IUGR is likely to result from an early fetal insult as a result of chemical exposure (eg, nicotine from cigarette smoking), viral infection, or inherent developmental abnormalities resulting from aneuploidy, whereas asymmetric IUGR is likely to be the result of utero-placental insufficiency, with preferential shunting of fetal blood to the brain. IUGR is associated with a significantly higher stillbirth rate and infant mortality rate in preterm, term, and postterm infants.

Another subset of newborns with IUGR who are born before term is at a significant risk for hypoglycemia. The risk factors that predispose preterm IUGR infants to hypoglycemia are reduced glycogen and fat stores, increased consumption of glucose, hyperinsulinism, immaturity of hepatic enzymes, reduced expression of glucose-6-phosphatase, reduced ketogenesis and failure of counterregulation. These infants require regular monitoring of blood glucose levels even after full feeds have been established.

Causes of Fetal Malnutrition and Intrauterine Growth Restriction

Fetal growth is a complex, dynamic process controlled by a wide range of factors of maternal, placental, and fetal origin. In early fetal life, the major determinant of growth is the fetal genome; however, later in pregnancy, environmental, nutritional, and hormonal influences become increasingly important. The known clinical, genetic, and environmental factors associated with IUGR are listed in Table 97-2.

Timing of Delivery

Close collaboration between obstetricians and neonatologists is essential for proper care of the growth-restricted fetus. A joint decision on the appropriate timing of delivery is made based on the risk of fetal compromise compared with that of neonatal morbidity. The management of a fetus with growth restriction must include a balance of the risks of intrauterine chronic hypoxia with those of preterm delivery.

Indications for delivery in the presence of IUGR include a gestational age of more than 37 weeks, presence of fetal distress, cessation of fetal growth over a 2- to 4-week period, oligohydramnios, and absent or reversed end-diastolic flow on Doppler velocimetry. Fetal Doppler studies give the most accurate noninvasive assessment of placental function. Although fetal lung maturity may be enhanced by treatment with prenatal corticosteroids, significant problems associated with very early delivery should deter the decision to induce early delivery unless fetal umbilical artery Doppler studies are abnormal. The guidelines for administration of prenatal corticosteroids in IUGR pregnancies are the same as with other instances of preterm labor.

Neonatal Management

Newborns with IUGR who have symptoms that result from respiratory distress, hypoglycemia, or polycythemia or who require resuscitation should be admitted to the neonatal intensive care unit. Asymptomatic newborns with IUGR of less than 35 weeks' gestation or who weigh less than 1800 g at birth should also be admitted to the neonatal intensive care unit for management.

Management in the Delivery Room

Competent staff trained in neonatal assessment and resuscitation should be present at the time of delivery. Care should be taken to prevent hypothermia. Covering the infant with plastic wrap soon after delivery maintains core body temperature well. In the event of a stillborn fetus, karyotyping, serologic testing for congenital infection, and detailed autopsy should be performed. The placenta should be examined for the presence of infarcts and gross abnormalities and sent for histopathological evaluation.

Perinatal hypoxia occurs with increased frequency among SGA infants, particularly those who have severe IUGR, which may cause fetal death or perinatal asphyxia. The rate of cesarean delivery is increased and the need for resuscitation is frequent.

Examination of Neonate

On physical examination, the skin is often dry, rough, desquamated, wrinkled, and at times covered in meconium. The skin may look plethoric, or the newborn may look pale in the presence of peripheral vasoconstriction. The neonate may appear more mature as a result of a reduced amount of vernix caseosa. Fingernails may be long. The newborn is often alert looking and jittery, even without hypoglycemia or hypocalcemia. Cranial sutures may appear wide, with large fontanelles. The umbilical cord is usually thin and can be stained yellow or green if meconium is passed in utero. Newborns can be hyperexcitable and exhibit aberrations in muscle tone. The Moro reflex may be exaggerated, with more extension and abduction. However, newborns with severe IUGR may be floppy because they become easily exhausted when they are handled. Severe symmetric IUGR neonates should be checked for chromosomal abnormalities and evidence of any intrauterine infection (skin rash, hepatosplenomegaly, and ocular abnormalities such as cloudy cornea, cataract, or chorioretinitis).

Gestational assessment may be affected by the presence of many creases on the sole of the foot, small breast nodules, less-well-formed ear cartilage, and less fat on female genitalia. The IUGR process does not greatly affect neurologic score. The weight, length, and head circumference should be recorded. In addition, the ponderal index should be calculated. In cases of asymmetric growth restriction, birth weight and occasionally length are less than the 10th percentile, but head circumference is preserved. The neonate will have a low ponderal index. Growth rates of adipose tissue and skeletal muscle are less than normal, although bone and probably brain growth are not.[4] In cases of symmetric growth restriction, a proportionate decrease weight, length, and head circumference is present; the ponderal index will be normal. Combined IUGR shares features of both asymmetric and symmetric IUGR. Skeletal shortening and some reduction in soft-tissue mass are seen. Causes include severe maternal disease from the first trimester of pregnancy, skeletal dysplasia, and metabolic bone disease. In dysmorphic IUGR, infants have disproportionately sized head, trunk, and limbs as a result of congenital abnormalities.

Evaluation of Neonate

Initial evaluation and stabilization should include preventing stress from the cold and observing the neonate for complications. If congenital infection is suspected, or if dysmorphic features are present, then appropriate evaluation should be undertaken, including laboratory testing for TORCH infections (toxoplasmosis, other agents, rubella, cytomegalovirus, herpes simplex) and genetic assessment. Temperature should be monitored every 30 minutes until stable for 2 hours, then at least every 4 hours. The infant should be kept warm with bundling, and a hat should cover the head to prevent hypothermia.

Blood glucose should be monitored within the first 1 to 2 hours of life by capillary glucose measurement, even if the child is asymptomatic. Early feedings, including breastfeeding, should be encouraged to prevent hypoglycemia in newborns who are vigorous at birth. In the presence of asymptomatic borderline hypoglycemia (25-40 mg/dL or 1.39-2.22 mmol/L), formula may be provided until adequate mother's milk is available. Newborns who are being exclusively breastfed may require intravenous glucose supplementation.

Hemoglobin level or hematocrit level should be measured at 4 to 6 hours of life by free-flowing venipuncture to exclude polycythemia. A hematocrit value of more than 65% indicates polycythemia.

PATHOPHYSIOLOGICAL FEATURES AND MANAGEMENT OF PROBLEMS ASSOCIATED WITH GROWTH-AFFECTED NEONATES

SGA and IUGR infants may experience various problems after birth that require different degrees of support based on their metabolism. Table 97-3 defines various problems and describes their management.

Nutritional Management and Follow-Up

Because SGA and IUGR infants have low muscle mass and fat content, feeding them aggressively seems logical so they can catch up in growth. Clinically, this strategy seems to work. However, animal studies of fetal IUGR caused by maternal protein restriction have demonstrated a shortened lifespan, particularly in male infants, when a catch-up strategy of markedly increased protein intake was administered after birth. Long-term clinical trials are needed to resolve this issue.

Outcomes of Growth-Restricted Infants

Growth-restricted infants have a higher incidence of sudden infant death syndrome. Compared with appropriate for gestational age infants who are the same ages, the perinatal mortality rate for SGA infants with relatively severe IUGR is 5 to 20 times higher, hospital stays are longer, and neurologic disorders and other morbidities requiring follow-up and hospitalization are more frequent among IUGR infants, occurring 5 to 10 times more often. SGA infants also are more likely to be hospitalized for serious respiratory infections.

Table 97-3 Problems Associated With Growth Affected Neonates[a]

PROBLEM	PATHOPHYSIOLOGICAL FEATURES	PREVENTION BY
Intrauterine death	Chronic hypoxia Placental insufficiency Malformation Infection Infarction or abruption	Perform careful prenatal monitoring, including biophysical profile. Perform Doppler velocimetry. Consider early delivery for worsening fetal distress.
Asphyxia	Acute and chronic hypoxia Placental insufficiency Acidosis Glycogen depletion Cord blood lactate often increased despite normal cord pH	Provide adequate neonatal resuscitation.
Meconium aspiration syndrome and persistent pulmonary hypertension of newborn	Hypoxia	See Chapter 99, Respiratory Distress and Breathing Disorders in the Newborn.
Hypothermia	Cold stress Hypoxia Hypoglycemia Decreased fat stores Decreased subcutaneous insulation Increased surface area Catecholamine depletion	Prevent heat loss. Provide thermo-neutral environment. Provide adequate nutritional support.
Hypoglycemia	Reduced fat stores Increased brain-body mass ratio (with increased consumption of glucose) Hyperinsulinism Immaturity of hepatic enzymes Reduced expression of glucose-6-phosphatase Reduced ketogenesis Failure of counterregulation[b]	Provide frequent glucose monitoring. Provide early enteral feeding. Administer intravenous glucose (4-8 mg/kg/min) soon after birth. Adjust infusion rate based on glucose measurement.[c]
Respiratory distress syndrome	Prematurity Maternal diabetes Multiple births Cesarean section Perinatal asphyxia Cold stress	Provide surfactant, respiratory support (mechanical ventilation, nasal continuous positive pressure ventilation).
Pulmonary hemorrhage	Hypothermia Polycythemia Hypoxia Disseminated intravascular coagulation	Prevent cold stress and hypoxia. Administer endotracheal epinephrine, fresh frozen plasma, administration of factor 7 (in severe, life-threatening conditions). Provide higher positive end expiratory airway pressure if patient is on mechanical ventilation.
Polycythemia and hyperviscosity	Chronic hypoxia Maternal-fetal transfusion Increased erythropoiesis	Provide hydration, glucose, and oxygen. Provide partial exchange transfusion.
Other hematologic or coagulation abnormalities	Thrombocytopenia Neutropenia Prolonged thrombin and partial thromboplastin times Increased fibrin degradation products Low iron stores	Check liver function tests for abnormalities. Check coagulation profile.
Necrotizing enterocolitis	Decreased splanchnic blood supply and hypoxia	Provide cautious enteral feeding.
Ischemia-induced necrosis leading to focal perforation	Decreased splanchnic blood supply and hypoxia	Provide cautious enteral feeding.

Table 97-3 Problems Associated With Growth Affected Neonates[a]—cont'd

PROBLEM	PATHOPHYSIOLOGICAL FEATURES	PREVENTION BY
Acute renal tubular necrosis and renal failure	Hypoxia or ischemia	Provide cardiovascular support.
Immunodeficiency	Malnutrition Congenital infection Decreased lymphocyte number and function Lower immunoglobulin levels during infancy Attenuated antibody response to oral polio vaccine	Provide early, optimal nutrition. Provide specific antibiotic and immune therapy.
Congenital, anatomical, and genetic abnormalities	Growth restriction (a feature of various syndromes)	Provide genetic consultation. Provide appropriate TORCH and genetic management.
Decreased bone mineral density	Possible substrate deficiency or altered vitamin D metabolism Low calcium stores (chronic decreased placental blood flow, insufficient nutrient supply)	Provide appropriate postnatal oral calcium and vitamin D intake.

TORCH, Toxoplasmosis, other agents, rubella, cytomegalovirus, herpes simplex.
[a]Modified from Anderson MS, Hay WW Jr. Intrauterine growth restriction and the small-for-gestational-age infant. In: Avery GB, Fletcher MS, MacDonald MG, eds. *Neonatalogy*. 6th ed. Philadelphia, PA: Lippincott Williams & Wilkins; 2006. Reprinted by permission.
[b]Hussain K, Aynsley-Green A. The effect of prematurity and intrauterine growth restriction on glucose metabolism in the newborn. *NeoReviews.* 2004;5: e365-e368.
[c]Severe hypoglycemia (<20 mg%) may require bolus of 10% dextrose 2 mL/kg followed by 10% glucose infusion at 4-8 mg/kg/min. Asphyxiated and intrauterine growth restricted infants with low ponderal index are at the highest risk of hypoglycemia; see Chapter 104, Common Metabolic Disturbances in the Newborn.

Growth and development depends on the degree of insult in utero and on the cause of growth restriction. Infants who are small as a result of family disposition will likely experience normal growth. Infants who are symmetrically growth restricted are not likely to catch up, but asymmetric IUGR infants have a reasonable chance of normal growth and development.

Infants with a small head circumference along with growth restriction have associated poor neurologic and psychological outcome, especially if the catch-up growth in head circumference has not occurred by 8 months of life. Formerly SGA infants did not exhibit delay in bone development, puberty, or sexual maturation at adolescence, although they were shorter and lighter and had smaller heads.[4]

The prognosis for preterm SGA infants is relatively poor, especially preterm infants whose brain growth failure occurred before 26 weeks' gestation. In general, subnormal intellectual outcomes are more common among preterm SGA infants than term SGA infants.[4]

IUGR infants with major chromosomal disorders have an extremely high incidence of handicap. Infants with congenital rubella or cytomegalovirus infection with microcephaly have poor outcomes, with a disability rate of more than 50%. Socioeconomic class significantly influences the school performance of children with IUGR; children from higher socioeconomic classes score better than those from low socioeconomic classes on achievement tests.

Interest in the short-term and long-term consequences of fetal growth restriction on cardiovascular, neurologic, and lung function is increasing. Catch-up growth is potentially beneficial in the short term, but it may be detrimental to long-term fitness and survival. Adults who experienced severe growth restriction in utero have an increased incidence of hypertension, insulin resistance, type 2 diabetes, and obesity. Additionally, evidence suggests that untoward metabolic events in utero that produce fetal growth restriction also may produce lifelong alterations in growth and development and contribute to the later development of metabolic syndrome with a propensity toward development of cardiovascular disease, type 2 diabetes, and stroke.[4]

Key Points

- Close collaboration between obstetricians and health professionals caring for neonates is essential for proper care of the neonate with IUGR, especially with the timing of delivery.
- Prenatal corticosteroid therapy remains effective and safe in preterm labor in the presence of IUGR.
- The cause of small size at birth carries great prognostic value.
- Close monitoring of temperature, glucose, and hematocrit is important for management. Blood glucose should be closely monitored even after full feeds have been established.
- Early feeding of these newborns should be encouraged to prevent hypoglycemia. In the event of asymptomatic hypoglycemia, formula feeding may be started until the mother's milk flow has been established.
- IUGR is associated with a significantly higher stillbirth and mortality rate in preterm, term, and postterm infants. The incidence of sudden infant death syndrome is higher.

LARGE-FOR-GESTATIONAL-AGE INFANTS AND INFANTS OF DIABETIC MOTHERS

Large for Gestational Age

At the other end of the spectrum of fetal growth abnormalities are newborns who are large-for-gestational-age (LGA) infants. LGA infants may have associated metabolic abnormalities (hypoglycemia, hypocalcemia), traumatic birth injuries, polycythemia, hyperviscosity, and hyperbilirubinemia, as well as the possibility of various congenital anomalies. Newborns are considered to be LGA if they weigh more than the 90th percentile for their gestational age or if they weigh more than 4000 g (8 lb 13 oz). *Macrosomia* is a clinical term describing excessive weight for gestational age; it results from increased adiposity caused by adipocyte hyperplasia and hypertrophy. Infants whose birth weight exceeds the 97th percentile (>4500 g, 9 lb 4 oz) are at greater risk for neonatal morbidity, with babies weighing more than 5000 g (11 lb) at highest risk for death.[5] A subpopulation of LGA infants born to mothers with diabetes mellitus (before or during pregnancy) has various abnormalities. These infants are labeled under a syndrome known as *infant of diabetic mother* (IDM). Some of the IDMs born to mothers with long-standing diabetes mellitus and vascular disease may be SGA.

LGA infants can result from being born to obese mothers (constitutional), from gestations longer than 42 weeks (postmaturity), or as the result of overstimulation of growth in utero. Additional risk factors include maternal weight gain during pregnancy, multiparity, a male fetus, and ethnicity. Infants of mothers with pregestational diabetes mellitus or gestational diabetes are exposed to high blood sugar during fetal development, or they may develop high circulating insulin levels and may therefore grow excessively. Women with gestational diabetes with glucose tolerance during late pregnancy (a positive glucose challenge test with a negative glucose tolerance test) may remain undiagnosed and may deliver a macrosomic infant with greater perinatal complications. Infants with Beckwith-Wiedemann syndrome and other genetic disorders that result in early excessive fetal growth, as well as infants with erythroblastosis fetalis, may exhibit as LGA with or without hyperinsulinism.

Infants of Diabetic Mothers

Although many IDMs have an uneventful perinatal course, other such infants have an increased risk of complications. Better management of diabetes mellitus during pregnancy has led to a marked improvement in perinatal morbidity and mortality; however, opportunities for improvement in various outcomes remain. Perinatal mortality varies directly with severity of maternal diabetes, as judged by two commonly used maternal classification schema: (1) White's revised classification of diabetes in pregnancy, based on duration of diabetes and presence of vascular complications (Table 97-4), and (2) Pedersen's Prognostically Bad Signs in Pregnancy classification, which includes complications of current pregnancy, that is, the presence of chemical pyelonephritis, precoma or

Table 97-4 White's Classification During Pregnancy

CLASSIFICATION	DESCRIPTION
Gestational diabetes	Abnormal glucose tolerance test, but euglycemia maintained by diet alone; if diet alone insufficient, insulin required
Class A	Diet alone, any duration or age at onset
Class B	Age at onset, >20 yr; duration, <10 yr
Class C	Age at onset, 10-19 yr; duration, 10-19 yr
Class D	Age at onset, <10 yr; duration, >20 yr; background retinopathy or hypertension (not preeclampsia)
Class R	Proliferative retinopathy or vitreous hemorrhage
Class F	Nephropathy, with <500 mg/dL proteinuria
Class RF	Criteria for both classes R and F coexist
Class H	Arteriosclerotic heart disease clinically evident
Class T	Prior renal transplantation

Reprinted from Cowett RM. The infant of diabetic mother. *NeoReviews.* 2002;3:e173-e189.

severe acidosis, toxemia, and so-called neglecters (pregnant diabetic women who are noncompliant with recommended care). Preeclampsia frequently complicates diabetic pregnancy and results in higher incidence of preterm delivery with consequent increased morbidity and mortality.[6]

Pathophysiological Features

Although no single pathogenetic mechanism has been clearly identified to explain the diverse problems seen in IDMs, many of the effects can be attributed to maternal metabolic control. Pedersen's maternal hyperglycemia–fetal hyperinsulinism hypothesis recognized that maternal hyperglycemia resulted in fetal hyperglycemia, which stimulates the fetal pancreas, resulting in islet-cell hypertrophy and beta-cell hyperplasia with increased insulin availability. After delivery, the neonate develops neonatal hypoglycemia as a result of the absence of continuous glucose supply across the placenta. The presence of increased C peptide and reactive immunoinsulin concentrations with hypoglycemia suggests that the control of maternal hyperglycemia in the third trimester may decrease the incidence of neonatal hypoglycemia. Other factors that may cause hypoglycemia in IDMs include decreased catecholamine and glucagon secretions, as well as diminished hepatic glucose production and decreased oxygenation of fatty acids (Box 97-1).

The pathogenesis of the increase in congenital anomalies among IDMs has remained obscure, although several causes have been proposed, including hyperglycemia (either before or after conception),

BOX 97-1 Components for Hyperinsulinism in Infants of Diabetic Mothers

Islet-cell hyperplasia and beta-cell hypertrophy
Obesity and macrosomia
Hypoglycemia with low–free-fatty-acid concentration
Rapid glucose disappearance rate
  Higher plasma insulin-like activity after glucose administration
  Umbilical vein reactive immunoinsulin increase
Increased C peptide and proinsulin concentrations

Reprinted from Cowett RM. The infant of diabetic mother. *NeoReviews*. 2002;3:e173-e189.

hypoglycemia, fetal hyperinsulinemia, uteroplacental vascular disease, and genetic predisposition. Several studies have correlated poor metabolic control of maternal diabetes in early pregnancy with an increased risk for major congenital malformations in IDMs.

Delivery

Route of delivery is determined by estimated fetal weight on ultrasound, by maternal and fetal condition, and by obstetrical history. Personnel trained in the Neonatal Resuscitation Program should be available during delivery.

The maternal blood glucose concentration is tightly controlled during labor and delivery. Blood glucose levels higher than 120 to 140 mg/dL (6.66-7.77 mmol/L) are managed with infusion of short-acting insulin.

Continuous fetal monitoring is essential during labor. Cesarean delivery is performed for obstetric reasons. Patients with advanced microvascular disease are at increased risk of delivery by cesarean.

Infants should be evaluated for presence of any birth injury, congenital malformations, evidence of macrosomia, hypoglycemia, and respiratory distress.[7]

Evaluation

IDMs with asphyxia, congenital malformations, history of maternal insulin administration, and hypoglycemia should be monitored carefully. They should be evaluated for hypoglycemia, hypocalcemia, polycythemia, and hyperbilirubinemia. Supportive care should be provided while a continuous evaluation is undertaken.

Blood glucose should be checked at 1, 2, 3, 6, and 12 hours by reagent test strip; a clinical laboratory should immediately check glucose readings less than 47 mg/dL (2.6 mmol/L). Extended monitoring beyond 12 hours of life requires consideration of transfer to a neonatal special or intensive care setting. Hematocrit levels should be checked at 4 to 6 and 24 hours. Calcium levels should be checked at 24 hours. Bilirubin levels should be checked if the baby appears jaundiced.

Physical Examination

Physical examination should focus on detection of traumatic birth injuries, including a thorough neurologic examination to detect any nerve palsies. Most facial nerve palsies will resolve without intervention, but suspected brachial plexus injuries need thorough evaluation and neurologic follow-up. Cardiac examination should focus on detecting any cardiac murmur, abnormal pulses, and cyanosis. Persistence of symptoms warrants evaluation of the newborn's electrocardiogram, chest radiograph, four-limb blood pressures, oxygen saturation, echocardiogram, and consultation with a pediatric cardiologist. Abdominal examination should be performed for detection of any masses and for evaluation for any abdominal injuries. An enlarged liver may result from glycogen deposits. Renal masses may be present, especially in the presence of a single umbilical artery.

Frequently Observed Specific Problems

Rates of adverse neonatal outcomes are three to nine times greater in infants of diabetic mothers compared with those of nondiabetic mothers. Improvement has not been significant in rates of perinatal mortality, congenital anomaly, or LGA birth in infants of diabetic mothers in 1996 to 2002 compared with 1988 to 1995.[3] Neonatal complications found in IDMs and LGA infants are listed in Table 97-5.

Hypoglycemia

The highest incidence of hypoglycemia occurs between 4 and 6 hours of age but may extend up to 48 hours after birth. Early feeding should be encouraged in IDMs and LGA newborns who are vigorous at birth to prevent development of hypoglycemia. In the presence of asymptomatic borderline hypoglycemia (25-47 mg/dL [1.39-2.6 mmol/L]), formula feeding may be initiated. If mother wishes to exclusively breastfeed and the blood sugar remains below 47 mg/dL (2.6 mmol/L) at 30 minutes after breastfeeding, then intravenous glucose supplementation should be given until mother's milk flow has been established (see Chapter 89, Breastfeeding the Newborn).

Hypocalcemia

Suppression of neonatal parathyroid function in IDMs may lead to hypocalcemia. Excessive jitteriness, alteration in muscle tone, and seizures should warrant investigations for hypoglycemia or hypocalcemia; if these symptoms are present, then ionized calcium levels should be checked. Symptomatic hypocalcemia should be treated with calcium gluconate. If symptoms are mild, then enteral supplementation may be provided. If the hypocalcemia is severe or protracted, the presence of hypomagnesemia should then be ruled out.

Macrosomia

Hyperinsulinemia in utero affects diverse organ systems, including the placenta. Insulin acts as the primary anabolic hormone of fetal growth and development, resulting in visceromegaly, especially of the heart and liver, and macrosomia. Fetal macrosomia is reflected by increased body fat, muscle mass, and organomegaly but not by increased brain or kidney size. Evaluation of nonfasting glucose rather than the fasting glucose in the third trimester

Table 97-5 Presence of Complications in Large-for-Gestational-Age Infants and Infants of Diabetic Mothers

COMPLICATION	LARGE FOR GESTATIONAL AGE	INFANTS OF DIABETIC MOTHERS
Birth trauma (shoulder dystocia, abdominal organ injury, brachial plexus injury, clavicular fracture, cephalohematoma, diaphragmatic paralysis, facial nerve palsy, ocular hemorrhage, external genitalia hemorrhage, subdural hemorrhage)	X	X
Asphyxia	X	X
Hypoglycemia	X	X
Hyperbilirubinemia	X	X
Macrosomia	X	X
Polycythemia and hyperviscosity		X
Respiratory distress syndrome, transient tachypnea of newborn, meconium aspiration, air-leak syndromes, diaphragmatic paralysis		X
Congenital anomalies (caudal regression, small left colon syndrome, hypertrophic obstructive cardiomyopathy, septal hypertrophy, double-outlet right ventricle, truncus arteriosus, anencephaly, spina bifida, hydrocephalus)		X
Neurologic instability (short and long term)		X
Hypocalcemia, hypomagnesemia		X
Organomegaly		X
Renal vein thrombosis, transient hematuria		X

Modified from Cowett RM. The infant of diabetic mother. *NeoReviews*. 2002;3:e173-e189; Cowett RM. Neonatal care of the infant of diabetic mother. *NeoReviews*. 2002;3:e190-e196.

of pregnancy is an important measure in preventing macrosomia.[8]

Traumatic Birth Injuries

As a result of their large size, LGA newborns experience complications of birth trauma, which includes shoulder dystocia, and they are also at greater risk for perinatal depression. LGA neonates are more likely to be delivered by cesarean. Injury to the brachial plexus, sometimes associated with phrenic nerve injury, may occur as a result of macrosomia and shoulder dystocia. Injury to abdominal organs may lead to hepatic and adrenal hemorrhage. Injury to external genitalia has occasionally been seen.

Asphyxia

Although the specific cause of asphyxia is unclear, it may be caused by difficulty in the intrapartum period resulting from relative macrosomia. Umbilical arterial cord blood pH and base deficit and cord lactate levels can provide early biochemical assessment of the fetus's physiological status. Asphyxia may have diverse consequences. It may acutely affect respiratory, renal, central nervous system, and gastrointestinal functioning. Restriction of fluids may be indicated until the degree of injury to the central nervous system and kidneys has been ascertained.

Polycythemia (venous hematocrit >65% [>0.65 fraction of red blood cells]) may be associated with acrocyanosis, hypoglycemia, irritability, or poor feeding. A higher-than-normal incidence of neonatal necrotizing enterocolitis is seen in IDMs with polycythemia and concurrent hypoglycemia; therefore, they should be fed cautiously. Increased erythropoietin production has been suggested to be a cause of polycythemia.

Jaundice

Hyperbilirubinemia is observed more frequently in IDMs than in healthy neonates. Management of neonatal hyperbilirubinemia in IDMs and LGA newborns is done as per the guidelines for managing jaundice in other term newborns (see Chapter 98, Neonatal Jaundice).

Respiratory Distress

IDMs born only slightly preterm (36 to 37 weeks' gestation) may have respiratory distress syndrome as a result of delayed maturation of surfactant, especially in mothers with class A, B, and C diabetes. Hyperinsulinism may adversely affect the lung maturation process in IDMs by antagonizing the action of cortisol. Newborns may also exhibit respiratory distress resulting from transient tachypnea of newborn, meconium aspiration, air-leak syndromes, or diaphragmatic paralysis.

Poor Feeding

Poor feeding is a major problem in IDMs; it occurs in almost one third of infants and is often present in the absence of other problems. Poor feeding may occasionally be related to prematurity, respiratory distress, or other problems and is a major cause of prolonged hospital stay and parent-infant separation.

Congenital Anomalies

IDMs are at three times the risk for malformations compared with infants of mothers without diabetes.

Poor metabolic control in the first trimester is correlated with major anomalies in IDMs. The recognized complications in IDMs include sacral agenesis, femoral hypoplasia, heart defects, and cleft palate. Others include preaxial radial defects, microtia, cleft lip, microphthalmos, holoprosencephaly, microcephaly, anencephaly, spina bifida, hemi vertebrae, urinary tract anomalies, and hallucal polydactyly.

Congenital Heart Disease and Cardiomyopathy

The strongest associations with maternal type 1 diabetes have been noted for double-outlet right ventricle and truncus arteriosus. No such associations have been noted with gestational diabetes. IDMs are at increased risk for congestive or hypertrophic cardiomyopathy. Hypertrophic cardiomyopathy in the neonate results from a fetal hyperinsulinemic state. Most of the infants are asymptomatic, and the diagnosis is made by echocardiography. In a small fraction of neonates, outflow tract obstruction may cause left-ventricular failure. Propranolol appears to be the therapeutic drug of choice. Resolution of symptoms occurs within 2 to 4 weeks, and resolution of the hypertrophy occurs within 2 to 12 months, with no permanent effect on the myocardium.

Renal-Vein Thrombosis

The pathogenesis of renal-vein thrombosis remains obscure, although most speculation has centered on the possible role of polycythemia. Sludging of red blood cells, combined with a further reduction in cardiac output as a result of diabetic cardiomyopathy, may be a contributing factor.

Small Left Colon

Hypoplastic left colon should be ruled out in case of feeding intolerance and inability to pass meconium. The cause of this abnormality is not clear. The condition usually resolves spontaneously with conservative medical management within the neonatal period. Vitamin E may protect against diabetic embryopathy through its well-known antioxidant effects. Further research is needed to determine the clinical applicability of these findings.

Perinatal Survival

Despite the problems associated with pregnancy, a mother with diabetes has a 95% chance of having a healthy baby if she participates in a pregnancy management and surveillance program at an appropriate perinatal center.

Follow-Up

The follow-up care should be based on the specific complications noted during the neonatal period. Pediatric cardiology follow-up should be performed for any evidence of cardiomyopathy or congenital heart disease. Newborns with repeated episodes of hypoglycemia or with any neurologic signs or symptoms should have close neurodevelopmental follow-up. Physical therapy and referral to early intervention may be required for newborns with nerve palsies. Urologic consultation may be required for those with renal abnormalities.

Long-Term Outcome

Neurodevelopment

The long-term neurodevelopment outlook is within the normal range for infants without congenital abnormalities and with good maternal metabolic control. Adverse outcomes are likely with prolonged and severe hypoglycemia. However, recommendations for clinical practice cannot be based on valid scientific evidence in this field.[9]

Psychological evaluations show that IDMs are more vulnerable to intellectual impairment, especially if the neonate was born SGA or if the pregnancy was complicated by acetonuria.[10] Children who have a history of growth delay in early diabetic pregnancy should be screened at 4 to 5 years of age by the Denver Developmental Screening Test for possible developmental impairment.

Obesity

Some evidence suggests that IDMs who are LGA at birth are more likely to be obese during late childhood. No specific guidelines are available for nutritional counseling.

Insulin-Dependent Diabetes Mellitus

The risk of developing insulin-dependent diabetes mellitus (IDDM) by 20 years of age in infants born to mothers with diabetes is 2.1% $\pm$ 0.5%. The risk of diabetes in offspring of mothers with diabetes is increased in young mothers and is independent of the risk factors for perinatal mortality.[11] The incidence of IDDM is found to be slightly increased in infants born to fathers with IDDM. The mechanism by which alterations in maternal glucose metabolism alters fetal beta cell function is unknown.

Cerebral Palsy, Epilepsy, and Intellectual Disability

The incidence of cerebral palsy and epilepsy is three to five times higher in IDMs compared with infants of mothers without diabetes, but the rate of intellectual disability does not differ.[12]

Key Points

- IDMs with asphyxia, congenital malformations, history of maternal insulin administration, and hypoglycemia should be monitored carefully.
- Transiently low blood glucose levels are common in the neonatal period and may be considered a normal feature of adaptation to extrauterine life. No evidence has been found that this condition causes brain injury in the absence of concurrent clinical manifestations.
- Persistent and severe hypoglycemia may be associated with underlying diseases that themselves predispose newborns to brain injury.
- Careful documentation of the clinical and biochemical state, response to treatment, and the pattern of any cerebral injury in neonates with hypoglycemia should be undertaken.

- Poor metabolic control in the first trimester is correlated with major anomalies in IDMs.
- Some evidence exists of increased incidence of obesity and subsequent IDDM in IDMs.

SUGGESTED RESOURCES

Bamberg C, Kalache KD. Prenatal diagnosis of fetal growth restriction. *Semin Fetal Neonatal Med.* 2004;9:387-394.

Boluyt N, Kempen AV, Offringa M. Neurodevelopment after neonatal hypoglycemia: a systematic review and design of an optimal future study. *Pediatrics.* 2006;117:2231-2236.

Cowett RM. Neonatal care of the infant of diabetic mother. *NeoReviews.* 2002;3:e190-e196.

Deshpande S, Platt MW. The investigation and management of neonatal hypoglycaemia. *Semin Fetal Neonatal Med.* 2005;10:351-361.

Hay WW Jr, Thureen PJ, Anderson MS. Intrauterine growth restriction. *NeoReviews.* 2001;2:e129-e137.

Illanes S, Soothill P. Management of fetal growth restriction. *Semin Fetal Neonatal Med.* 2004;9:395-401.

Thureen PJ, Anderson MS, Hay WW Jr. Small for gestational age. *NeoReviews.* 2001;2:e139-e148.

Williams AF. Neonatal hypoglycaemia: clinical and legal aspects. *Semin Fetal Neonatal Med.* 2005;10:363-368.

Yu VYH, Upadhyay A. Neonatal management of the growth-restricted infant. *Semin Fetal Neonatal Med.* 2004;9:403-409.

REFERENCES

1. Regnault TRH, Limesand SW, Hay WW Jr. Factors influencing fetal growth. *NeoReviews.* 2001;6:119-128.
2. Yu VYH, Upadhyay A. Neonatal management of the growth-restricted infant. *Semin Fetal Neonatal Med.* 2004;9:403-409.
3. Yang J, Cummings EA, O'Connell C, et al. Fetal and neonatal outcomes of diabetic pregnancies. *Obstet Gynecol.* 2006;108:644-650.
4. Thureen PJ, Anderson MS, Hay WW Jr. Small for gestational age. *NeoReviews.* 2001;2:e139-e148.
5. Boulet SL, Alexander GR, Salihu HM, et al. Macrosomic births in the United States: determinants, outcomes, and proposed grades of risk. *Am J Obstet Gynecol.* 2003; 188(5):1372-1378.
6. Greene MF, Hare JW, Krache M, et al. Prematurity among insulin requiring diabetic gravid women. *Am J Obstet Gynecol.* 1989;161:106-111.
7. Cowett RM. Neonatal care of the infant of diabetic mother. *NeoReviews.* 2002;3:e190-e196.
8. Jovanovic-Peterson CM, Peterson GF, Reed R, et al. Maternal postprandial glucose levels and infant birth weight: the Diabetes in Early Pregnancy Study. *Am J Obstet Gynecol.* 1991;164:103-111.
9. Boluyt N, Kempen AV, Offringa M. Neurodevelopment after neonatal hypoglycemia: a systematic review and design of an optimal future study. *Pediatrics.* 2006;117: 2231-2236.
10. Stehbens JA, Baker GL, Kitchell M. Outcome at ages 1, 3, and 5 years of children born to diabetic women. *Am J Obstet Gynecol.* 1977;127:408-413.
11. Warram JH, Krolewski AS, Kahn CR. Determinants of IDM and perinatal mortality in children of diabetic mothers. *Diabetes.* 1988;37:1328-1334.
12. Yssing M. Long term prognosis of children born to mothers diabetic when pregnant. In: Carmerini-Davalos RA, Cole HS, eds. *Early Diabetes in Early Life.* New York, NY: Academic Press; 1975.

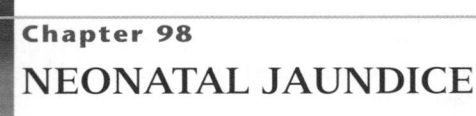

Chapter 98

NEONATAL JAUNDICE

Luc P. Brion, MD

DEFINITION

The term jaundice, derived from the French *jaune* or yellow, is defined as yellow pigmentation of sclera, skin, and urine caused by hyperbilirubinemia. Hyperbilirubinemia in the term or late preterm infant greater than 35 weeks' gestation is classified as either physiological or pathological based on age-specific statistical analysis of serum bilirubin measurements.[1]

FREQUENCY

Jaundice occurs in approximately 60% of the 4 million neonates born yearly in the United States.[2] The largest data set on neonatal bilirubin levels in term or near-term infants was obtained by Bhutani and collaborators in 2840 well newborns (Figure 98-1).[3] This nomogram is reflective of the natural history of neonatal hyperbilirubinemia during the first 48 to 72 hours of life. Thereafter the low–risk-zone threshold is less accurate because of the sampling bias that resulted in spuriously elevated levels in the lower zones (more than the high-risk zone 95th percentile in the study).[3,4] The approximate frequency of high bilirubin levels compiled from several studies[3,5-9] is shown in Table 98-1. In a population study in Denmark, hyperbilirubinemia with a serum concentration justifying an exchange transfusion occurred in 25 per 100,000 (1:4000) term or late preterm infants.[10]

DIFFERENTIAL DIAGNOSIS

Yellow skin color can develop in children with carotenemia. In contrast with jaundice, carotenemia does not affect the color of the sclera and has not been reported in neonates.

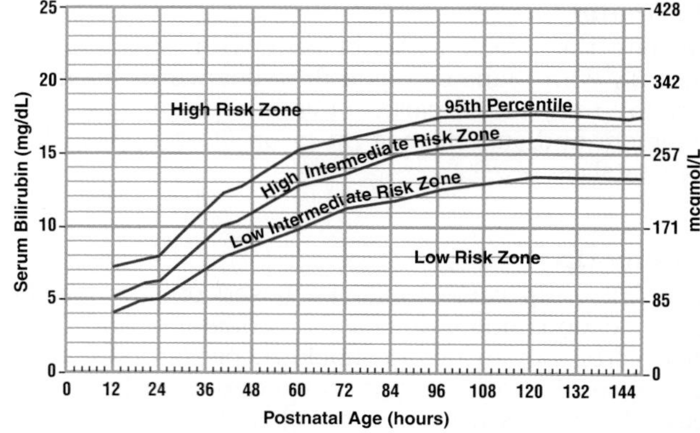

Figure 98-1 Nomogram for designation of risk in term and late preterm infants.

EVALUATION

Clinical practice guidelines for managing hyperbilirubinemia in the newborn 35 weeks or more of gestation were published by the American Academy of Pediatrics (AAP) in 2004.[2] The key elements and the diagnostic and therapeutic algorithm are shown in Box 98-1 and Figure 98-2, respectively.

Relevant History

Major risk factors for developing severe hyperbilirubinemia are listed in Box 98-2. The best documented prediction of severe hyperbilirubinemia is a total serum bilirubin or transcutaneous bilirubin level that falls within the high-risk zone of the Bhutani curve.[3] A serum or transcutaneous bilirubin level is measured and plotted on the Bhutani curve. This process allows for determination of the *degree of risk* of the infant to develop significant hyperbilirubinemia. In combination with identified risk factors for neonatal jaundice, the degree of risk can guide the clinician's treatment planning. Relevant history should also include questions about the potential use by the mother or administration to the neonate of herbs (see later discussion and Chapter 90, Breastfeeding: Drugs, Herbs, and Environmental Toxins), as well as drugs and medications (eg, sulfonamides, many cephalosporins, benzyl alcohol, paraben, methylparaben) that affect bilirubin binding. Box 98-3 lists agents that displace bilirubin from albumin. Family history may reveal one or more hereditary disorders of bilirubin production (eg, increased hemolysis), bilirubin metabolism (mutations of the promoter or of the gene coding uridine diphosphate glucuronosyl transferase, causing, respectively, Gilbert and Crigler-Najjar syndromes) or bilirubin excretion (Dubin-Johnson syndrome). The risk of neonatal jaundice is higher when the neonate has Gilbert syndrome and another factor of jaundice, for example, hemolysis or breastfeeding.[11] The risk for severe hyperbilirubinemia is increased in infants of East Asian descent and decreased in black infants.[2] Correct identification of race and ethnicity by asking the mother about the maternal and paternal ancestry is important in assessing the risk of an infant.[12]

The increased risk of severe hyperbilirubinemia in Asian neonates (with 2 parents of Asian origin)[13] may result from hemolysis, frequently caused by glucose-6-phosphate dehydrogenase (G6PD) deficiency,[14] and from abnormal bilirubin metabolism (eg, mutations affecting abundance or function of uridine diphosphate glucuronosyl transferase, thereby limiting glucuroconjugation).[15] In addition, increased risk for bilirubin toxicity in Asian neonates may result from displacement of bilirubin from albumin caused by exposure to herbals given to the neonate (eg, Chuen-Lin,

BOX 98-1 Key Elements in Managing Hyperbilirubinemia

1. Promote and support successful breastfeeding.
2. Establish nursery protocols for the identification and evaluation of hyperbilirubinemia.
3. Measure the total serum bilirubin or transcutaneous bilirubin level on newborns jaundiced in the first 24 hours.
4. Recognize that visual estimation of the degree of jaundice can lead to errors, particularly in darkly pigmented infants.
5. Interpret all bilirubin levels according to the newborn's age in hours.
6. Recognize that newborns at less than 38 weeks' gestation, particularly those who are breastfed, are at high risk of developing hyperbilirubinemia and require close surveillance and monitoring.
7. Perform a systematic assessment on all newborns before discharge for the risk of severe hyperbilirubinemia.
8. Provide parents with written and verbal information about newborn jaundice.
9. Provide appropriate follow-up based on the time of discharge and the risk assessment.
10. Treat newborns, when indicated, with phototherapy or exchange transfusion.

Table 98-1 Proposed Definitions for Severity of Hyperbilirubinemia and Its Estimated Occurrence

TSB LEVEL (MG/DL)	PERCENTILE AFTER 72 HOURS OF AGE	PROPOSED DEFINITIONS	ESTIMATED OCCURRENCE
≥17.0 (291 mcmol/L)	>95th	Significant	~1:10
≥20.0 (342 mcmol/L)	>99th	Severe	~1:70
≥25.0 (427 mcmol/L)	>99.9th	Extreme	~1:700
≥30.0 (513 mcmol/L)	>99.99th	Hazardous	~1:10,000

TSB, Total serum bilirubin.
To convert bilirubin concentration from mg/dL into mcmol/L, multiply by 17.1
Percentiles are approximate. Occurrence is estimated in screened and treated infants based on data reported in Bhutani et al, Stevenson et al, Martinez et al, and Khurana, et al. Precise data cannot be compiled because of differences in methodologies, patient selection, and thresholds for intervention.
Reproduced from Bhutani et al. *J Perinatol.* 2004;24(10):650-662. Used by permission of Nature Publishing Group.

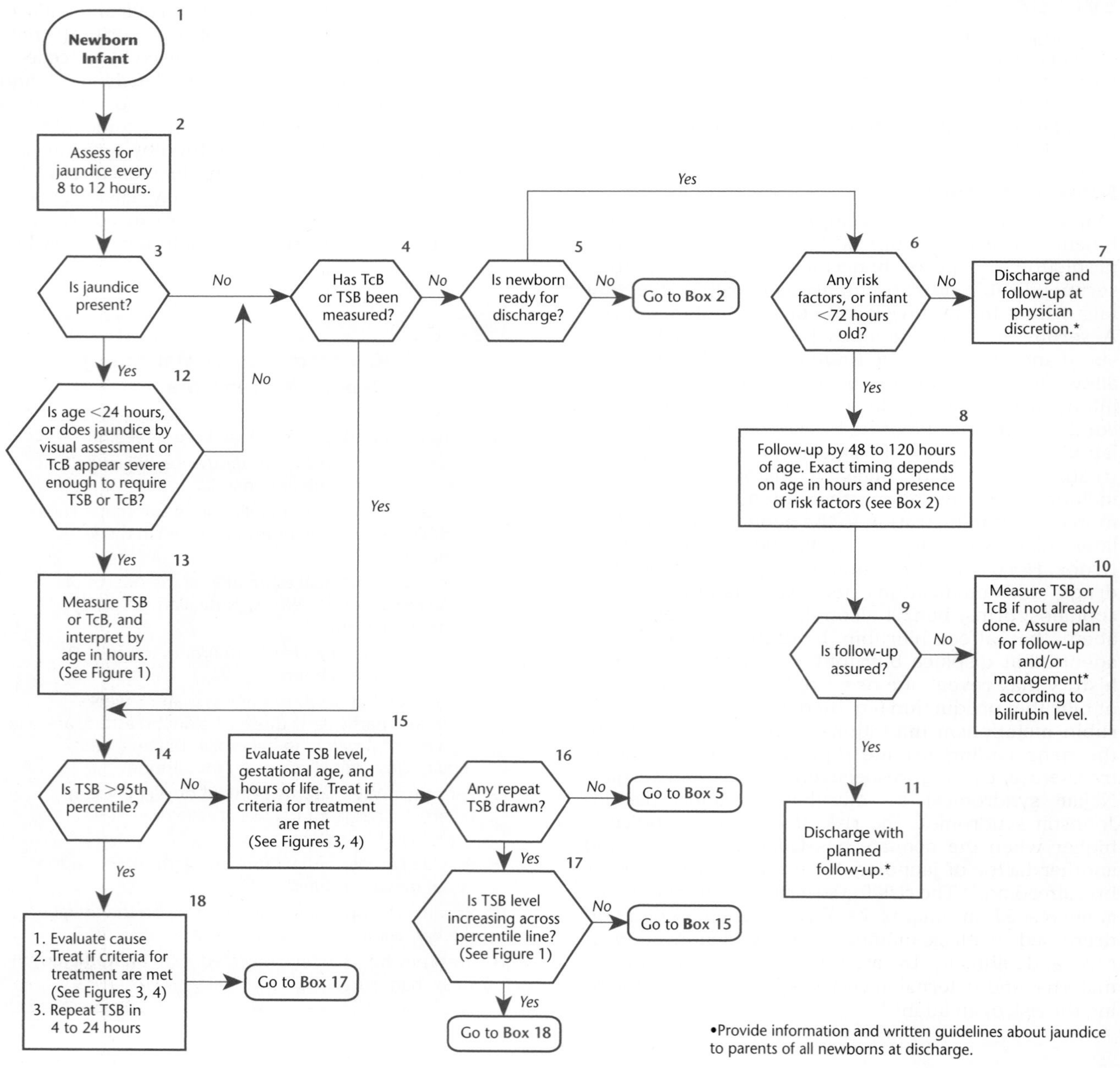

Figure 98-2 Diagnostic and therapeutic algorithm for jaundice in the newborn nursery. *TcB,* Transcutaneous bilirubin level; *TSB,* total serum bilrubin level. *(American Academy of Pediatrics, Subcommittee on Hyperbilirubinemia. Clinical practice guideline: management of hyperbilirubinemia in the newborn infant 35 or more weeks of gestation.* Pediatrics. *2004;114[1]:297-316.)*

[Coptis chinensus/japonicum], a popular herb given to 28% to 51% of Chinese neonates)[16] or taken by pregnant or breastfeeding mothers (eg, berberine, the major ingredient of the Chinese herb huanglian *[Coptis chinensis]*).[17]

Sporadic genetic mutations affecting the gene encoding G6PD on the X-chromosome occur in all ethnic and racial groups; more than 400 gene mutations have been identified. In the United States black male infants are most often affected. Although black neonates have a low risk of severe hyperbilirubinemia, a subgroup of G6PD-deficient black neonates (12.8%) has a 3-fold increase in risk for hemolysis and jaundice compared with controls.[18]

Physical Examination

Jaundice may be diagnosed at a bilirubin level of 5 mg/dL. Interobserver agreement about the presence of jaundice in neonates is only moderate (pairwise kappa, 0.48),[19] except for infants with bilirubin levels greater

BOX 98-2 Risk Factors for Development of Severe Hyperbilirubinemia in Newborns of 35 or More Weeks' Gestation (in Approximate Order of Importance)

MAJOR RISK FACTORS

Predischarge total serum bilirubin or transcutaneous bilirubin level in the high-risk zone (best documented method)

Jaundice observed in the first 24 hours

Blood group incompatibility with positive direct antiglobulin test, other known hemolytic disease (eg, glucose-6-phosphate dehydrogenase deficiency), elevated end tidal carbon monoxide

Gestational age 35-36 weeks or <38 weeks

Previous sibling required phototherapy

Cephalohematoma or significant bruising

Poor feeding

Exclusive breastfeeding, particularly if nursing is not going well and weight loss is excessive

East Asian race (race as defined by mother's description)

MINOR RISK FACTORS

Predischarge total serum bilirubin or transcutaneous bilirubin level in the high intermediate-risk zone

Gestational age 37-38 weeks

Jaundice observed before discharge

Previous sibling with jaundice

Macrosomic infant of a diabetic mother

Maternal age ≥25 years

Male gender

DECREASED RISK (THESE FACTORS ARE ASSOCIATED WITH DECREASED RISK OF SIGNIFICANT JAUNDICE, LISTED IN ORDER OF DECREASING IMPORTANCE.)

Total serum bilirubin or transcutaneous bilirubin level in the low-risk zone

Gestational age ≥41 wk

Exclusive bottle feeding

Black race (race as defined by mother's description)

Discharge from hospital after 72 hours

BOX 98-3 Common Chemicals That Displace Bilirubin From Albumin

Chuen-Lin *(Coptis chinensus/japonicum)*

Berberine *(Coptis chinensis)*

Some cephalosporins (eg, ceftriaxone, cefonicid, cefotetan, moxalactam)

Benzyl alcohol

Chloral hydrate

Ethacrynic acid

Ibuprofen

Long-chain fatty acids

Pancuronium

Salicylates

Sulfonamides—sulfisoxazole, sulfamethoxazole

Maternal intrapartum medication administration – oxytocin, diazepam, promethazine

than 12 mg/dL, which is the threshold at which all infants are correctly identified as jaundiced by all examiners. Other important parts of the physical examination include vital signs, size for gestational age, either pallor or plethora, petechiae, bruising, subcutaneous edema, blueberry muffin lesions, vasoconstriction, scalp swelling, cataract, goiter, abdominal mass, hepatosplenomegaly, activity, tone, and neurologic examination. Patients with extreme hyperbilirubinemia are at risk for bilirubin encephalopathy.[2] Acute bilirubin encephalopathy is characterized by an early phase of lethargy, hypotonia, and poor suck; an intermediate phase of stupor, irritability, fever, high-pitched cry, hypertonia alternating with hypotonia; and an advanced phase, with opisthotonos, shrill cry, lack of feeding, apnea, fever, deep stupor to coma, sometimes seizures, and death. The intermediate phase may be reversible with exchange transfusion, whereas the advanced phase is irreversible. Kernicterus (yellow discoloration of the basal ganglia and brainstem nuclei caused by bilirubin deposition), or chronic, irreversible sequela of bilirubin toxicity,[2] is characterized by athetoid cerebral palsy, auditory dysfunction, dental enamel dysplasia, paralysis of upward gaze, and, less often, intellectual and other disabilities.

Laboratory Testing

AAP recommendations for evaluating jaundiced infants are listed in Table 98-2. The World Health Organization recommends neonatal screening for G6PD in populations with a prevalence of 3% to 5% or more in boys.[20] Some neonatal screening programs also include testing for hemoglobinopathy.

The measurement of total serum bilirubin level is the most important measurement. The clinician should be aware that bilirubin measurements on automatic analyzers used in most clinical laboratories can be erroneous if the specimen is hemolyzed or turbid.[21]

If phototherapy is indicated, or if the bilirubin level crosses percentiles on the Bhutani nomogram and is unexplained by the history and physical examination, then a serum level of direct or conjugated bilirubin should be obtained.[2] Conjugated hyperbilirubinemia is defined by a serum conjugated bilirubin concentration greater than 1.0 mg/dL (17.1 mcmol/L) if the total bilirubin is less than 5.0 mg/dL (85.5 mcmol/L) or more than 20% of the total bilirubin if the total bilirubin is greater than 5.0 mg/dL (85.5 mcmol/L).[2] Neonatal cholestasis is defined as prolonged conjugated hyperbilirubinemia that occurs in the newborn period.[22] It is caused by diminished bile flow or excretion (or both) of conjugated bilirubin from the hepatocyte into the duodenum. The incidence of neonatal cholestasis is

Table 98-2 Laboratory Evaluations for the Jaundiced Newborn of 35 or More Weeks' Gestation

INDICATIONS	ASSESSMENTS
Jaundice in first 24 hr	Measure TcB, TSB, or both
Jaundice appears excessive for age	Measure TcB, TSB, or both
Infant receiving phototherapy or TSB rising rapidly (ie, crossing percentiles and unexplained by history and physical examination)	Blood type and Coombs test, if not obtained with cord blood Complete blood count and smear Measure direct or conjugated bilirubin Option: perform reticulocyte count, G6PD, and ETCOc, if available Repeat TSB in 4-24 hr depending on age and TSB level
TSB concentration approaching exchange levels or not responding to phototherapy	Perform reticulocyte count, G6PD, albumin, ETCOc, if available
Elevated direct (or conjugated) bilirubin level	Perform urinalysis and urine culture. Evaluate for sepsis if indicated by history and physical examination
Jaundice present at or beyond age 3 wk, or newborn is sick	Total and direct (or conjugated) bilirubin level; if direct bilirubin elevated, evaluate for causes of cholestasis Check results of newborn thyroid and galactosemia screen, and evaluate newborn for signs or symptoms of hypothyroidism

ETCOc, End-tidal carbon monoxide concentration; *G6PD,* glucose-6-phosphate dehydrogenase; *TcB,* transcutaneous bilirubin level; *TSB,* total serum bilirubin level.

approximately 1 per 2500 live births.[23,24] Jaundice is further discussed in Chapter 197.

The new methods of transcutaneous bilirubin assessment, valid in many populations regardless of skin color, have led to a decrease in the number of blood samples required both before and after discharge in term or late preterm infants.[25,26] Importantly, transcutaneous bilirubin assessment and clinical examination of jaundice are unreliable after phototherapy.

Additional tests indicated in newborns with early or severe hyperbilirubinemia (see Table 98-2) include blood type and Coombs test, complete blood count and smear, reticulocyte count, end-tidal carbon monoxide concentration (if available), and G6PD. Testing for G6PD deficiency is warranted when the newborn is of African, Asian, Mediterranean, or Middle-Eastern descent. Among babies with G6PD deficiency (male infants with the defective gene and homozygous female infants) the rate of hyperbilirubinemia is twice that for unaffected newborns. G6PD deficiency should be considered in neonates who develop jaundice during the first day of life, have a family history of a sibling with unexplained hyperbilirubinemia, have a bilirubin level greater than the 95th percentile on the Bhutani nomogram, and in Asian male infants.[2,14] If hemolysis is unexplained, then other causes should be considered, including infection and congenital disorders.[27] Measuring serum albumin is indicated if the bilirubin approaches exchange transfusion level. Prolonged jaundice should raise the suspicion of hypothyroidism, galactosemia, and cholestatic jaundice.

MANAGEMENT

The AAP[2] and the Joint Commission[28,29] recommend a universal systematic approach to reduce the risk of severe hyperbilirubinemia and kernicterus. The key elements of the AAP recommendations are summarized in Box 98-1.

Postnatal age–, gestational age–, and risk factor–specific criteria for phototherapy are shown in Figure 98-3. Low-intensity phototherapy can be provided at home to newborns for whom phototherapy is optional, whereas high-intensity phototherapy requires hospital care. Phototherapy reduces the risk that bilirubin levels will reach a level at which exchange transfusion is recommended. Approximately 5 to 10 newborns with serum bilirubin ranging 15 to 20 mg/dL (257-342 mcmol/L) will receive phototherapy to prevent bilirubin in one newborn from reaching 20 mg/dL (a number at which exchange transfusion may be recommended). The efficacy of phototherapy is best with special blue or with blue-green lights and increases with increasing spectrum irradiance, spectrum power (irradiance by unit of surface), and total serum bilirubin. The efficacy is reduced in patients with hemolysis and in infants with cholestasis. Side effects of phototherapy include parental anxiety related to the need for protective eye patches, development of bronze baby syndrome in newborns with cholestasis, and, rarely, purpura and bullous eruptions. Phototherapy is contraindicated in infants with congenital erythropoietic porphyria, in whom it causes severe blistering. Given that the recently developed phototherapy devices do not significantly increase insensible water loss, routine increase in fluid administration is not necessary for patients who undergo phototherapy. However, newborns with clinical or laboratory evidence for dehydration should receive additional fluid.[30]

Postnatal age–, gestational age–, and risk factor–specific criteria for exchange transfusion are shown in Figure 98-4. The ratio of bilirubin to albumin can be

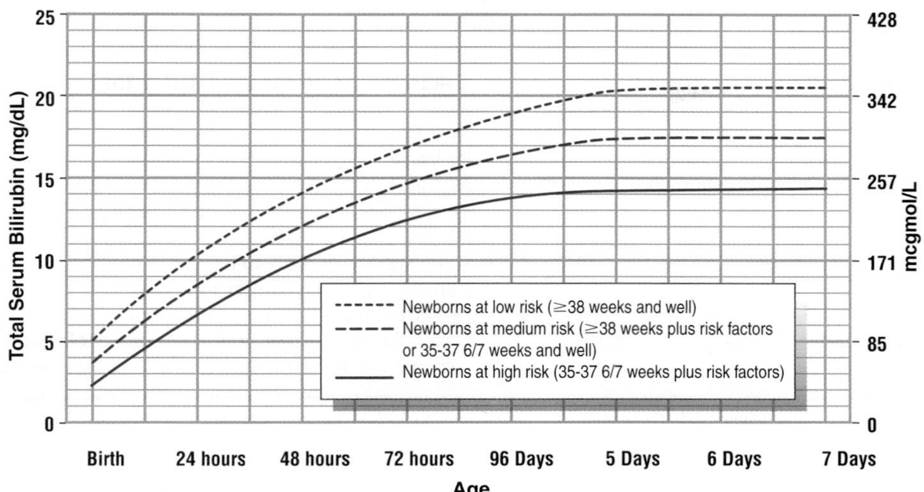

- Use total bilirubin. Do not subtract direct reacting or conjugated bilirubin.
- Risk factors: Isoimmune hemolytic disease, G6PD deficiency, asphyxia, significant lethargy, temperature instability, sepsis, acidosis, or albumin <3.0 g/dL (if measured).
- For well infants 35-37 6/7 weeks can adjust TSB levels for intervention around the medium risk line. It is an option to intervene at lower TSB levels for infants closer to 35 weeks and at higher TSB levels for those closer to 37 6/7 weeks.
- It is an option to provide conventional phototherapy in the hospital or at home at TSB levels 2-3 mg/dL (30-50 mmol/L) below those shown, but home phototherapy should not be used in any infant with risk factors.

Note: These guidelines are based on limited evidence, and the levels shown are approximations. The guidelines refer to the use of intensive phototherapy, which should be used when the TSB exceeds the line indicated for each category. Infants are designated as at high risk because of the potential negative effects of the conditions listed on albumin binding of bilirubin, the blood-brain barrier, and the susceptibility of the brain cells to damage by bilirubin.

Intensive phototherapy implies irradiance in the blue-green spectrum (wavelengths of approximately 430-490 nm) of at least 30 mcgW/cm^2 per nm (measured at the infant's skin directly below the center of the phototherapy unit) and delivered to as much of the infant's surface area as possible. Note that irradiance measured below the center of the light source is significant greater than that measured at the periphery. Measurements should be made with a radiometer specified by the manufacturer of the phototherapy system.

If total serum bilirubin levels approach or exceed the exchange transfusion line, the sides of the bassinet, incubator, or warmer should be lined with aluminum foil or white material, which will increase the surface area of the newborn exposed and will increase the efficacy of phototherapy. If the total serum bilirubin does not decrease or if it continues to rise in a newborn who is receiving intensive phototherapy, then these results strongly suggest the presence of hemolysis. Newborns who receive phototherapy and have an elevated direct-reacting or conjugated bilirubin level (cholestatic jaundice) may develop the bronze-baby syndrome.

Figure 98-3 Guidelines for phototherapy in hospitalized newborns of 35 or more weeks' gestation. *TcB,* Transcutaneous bilirubin level; *TSB,* total serum bilirubin level; *G6PD,* glucose-6-phosphate dehydrogenase. *(American Academy of Pediatrics, Subcommittee on Hyperbilirubinemia. Clinical practice guideline: management of hyperbilirubinemia in the newborn infant 35 or more weeks of gestation.* Pediatrics. *2004;114[1]:297-316.)*

used together with the total bilirubin level as an additional factor in determining the need for exchange transfusion. Double-volume exchange transfusion has a low but significant risk of complications and should be performed only by trained personnel in a neonatal intensive care unit with full monitoring and resuscitation capabilities.[2]

Intravenous gamma globulin administration is effective in reducing the need for exchange transfusion in infants with isoimmune hemolysis caused by Rh or ABO incompatibility.[31,32] It is indicated for neonates with isoimmune hemolysis if the serum bilirubin level is rising despite intensive phototherapy or if the bilirubin level is within 2 to 3 mg/dL of the level of bilirubin at which the determination is made that an exchange transfusion becomes necessary to prevent the risk of developing kernicterus.[2]

Jaundice is a frequent reason for readmission of neonates during the first 2 weeks after newborn nursery discharge. Criteria to refer and to admit are listed at the end of the chapter, and guidance for the timing of follow-up care is listed in Table 98-3. The rate of readmission for healthy infants for the treatment of jaundice in California in 1991 to 1998 ranged between 10% and 15% for full-term infants and 24% to 32% for late preterm infants.[6] The clinical pathway for management of the newborn readmitted for phototherapy or exchange transfusion is shown in Box 98-4.

The AAP recommends not delaying discharge from the hospital to observe the newborn for rebound bilirubin level.[2] Instead, a follow-up bilirubin measurement within 24 hours after discharge is recommended if phototherapy is used for hemolytic disease or initiated early and discontinued before 3 to 4 days of age. A recent study suggested a significant association with a higher rebound bilirubin level among newborns with a positive direct Coombs test, newborns with a gestational age younger than 37 weeks, and in instances in which phototherapy is initiated before 72 hours of life.[33]

PREVENTION

Because breastfeeding is the second independent risk factor for the development of hyperbilirubinemia, optimizing breastfeeding is an essential component in the prevention and management of neonatal hyperbilirubinemia.[34,35] One major aspect of prevention is early initiation and frequent breastfeeding, at least 8 to 12 times per day for the first several days. Two types of hyperbilirubinemia may be observed in breastfed

Table 98-3 Follow-Up of Newborn With Hyperbilirubinemia

NEWBORN DISCHARGED	TIMING OF FOLLOW-UP VISIT
Before age 24 hr	By 72 hr
Between 24 and 47.9 hr	By 96 hr
Between 49 and 72 hr	By 120 hr
Before 48 hr*	Two follow-up visits may be required: The first at 24-72 hr The second at 72-120 hr
Few or no risk factors*	Can be seen after longer intervals
Elevated risk factors	Earlier or more frequent follow-up
Elevated risk factors AND appropriate follow-up cannot be ensured	Delay discharge either until appropriate follow-up can be ensured or the period of greatest risk has passed (72-96 hr)

*Clinical judgment should be used in determining follow-up.

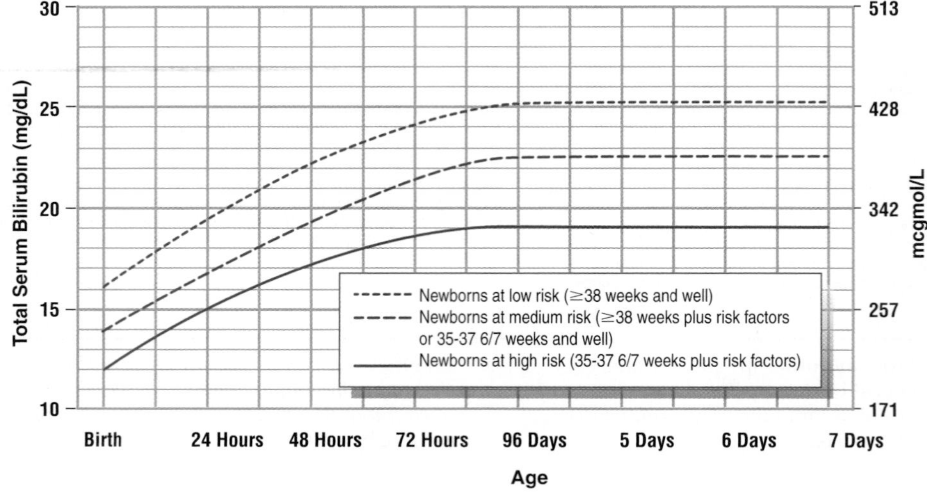

- The dashed lines for the first 24 hours indicate uncertainty as a result of a wide range of clinical circumstances and a range of responses to phototherapy.
- Immediate exchange transfusion is recommended if newborn shows signs of acute bilirubin encephalopathy (hypertonia, arching, retrocollis, opisthotonos, fever, high-pitched cry) or if TSB is ≥5 mg/dL (85 mcgmol/L) above these lines.
- Risk factors: Isoimmune hemolytic disease, G6PD deficiency, asphyxia, significant lethargy, temperature instability, sepsis, acidosis.
- Measure serum albumin, and calculate B/A ratio.
- Use total bilirubin. Do not subtract direct reacting or conjugated bilirubin.
- If newborn is well and 35-37 6/7 weeks (median risk) can individualize TSB levels for exchange based on actual gestational age.

Note: These suggested levels represent a consensus of most of the committee but are based on limited evidence, and the levels shown are approximations. During birth hospitalization, exchange transfusion is recommended if the TSB rises to these levels despite intensive phototherapy. For readmitted infants, if the TSB level is above the exchange level, then repeat TSB measurement every 2 to 3 hours, and consider exchange if the TSB remains above the levels indicated after intensive phototherapy for 6 hours.

If the TSG is at or approaching the exchange level, then send blood for immediate type and crossmatch. Blood for exchange transfusion is modified whole blood (red cells and plasma) crossmatched against the mother and compatible with the infant.

Intensive phototherapy implies irradiance in the blue-green spectrum (wavelengths of approximately 430-490 nm) of at least 30 mcgW/cm^2 per nm (measured at the infant's skin directly below the center of the phototherapy unit) and delivered to as much of the infant's surface area as possible. Note that irradiance measured below the center of the light source is significant greater than that measured at the periphery. Measurements should be made with a radiometer specified by the manufacturer of the phototherapy system.

If total serum bilirubin levels approach or exceed the exchange transfusion line, the sides of the bassinet, incubator, or warmer should be lined with aluminum foil or white material, which will increase the surface area of the newborn exposed and will increase the efficacy of phototherapy. If the total serum bilirubin does not decrease or if it continues to rise in a newborn who is receiving intensive phototherapy, then these results strongly suggest the presence of hemolysis. Newborns who receive phototherapy and have an elevated direct-reacting or conjugated bilirubin level (cholestatic jaundice) may develop the bronze-baby syndrome.

The following B/A ratios can be used together with but not in lieu of the TSB level as an additional factor in determining the need for exchange transfusion:

Risk Category	B/A Ratio at Which ExchangeTransfusion Should be Considered: TSB mg/dL/Alb, g/dL	TSB mcgmol/L/Alb, mcgmol/L
Newborns ≥38 1/7 wks	8.0	0.94
Newborns 35 0/7-36 6/7 weeks and well or ≥38 0/7 wks if higher risk or isoimmune hemolytic disease of G6PD deficiency	7.2	0.84
Newborns 35 0/7 wks if higher risk or isoimmune hemolytic disease or G6PD deficiency	6.8	0.80

Figure 98-4 Guidelines for exchange transfusion in infants 35 or more weeks' gestation. *B/A,* Bilirubin/albumin; *TcB,* transcutaneous bilirubin level; *TSB,* total serum bilirubin level; *G6PD,* glucose-6-phosphate dehydrogenase. *(American Academy of Pediatrics, Subcommittee on Hyperbilirubinemia. Clinical practice guideline: management of hyperbilirubinemia in the newborn infant 35 or more weeks of gestation.* Pediatrics. *2004;114[1]:297-316.)*

BOX 98-4 Example of a Clinical Pathway for Management of the Newborn Readmitted for Phototherapy or Exchange Transfusion

TREATMENT

Use intensive phototherapy or exchange transfusion (or both) as indicated in Figure 98-3 and Figure 98-4

LABORATORY TESTS

TSB and direct bilirubin levels

Blood type (ABO, Rh)

Direct antibody test (Coombs test)

Serum albumin

Complete blood cell count with differential and smear for red cell morphology

Reticulocyte count

End-tidal carbon monoxide (if available)

G6PD if suggested by ethnic or geographic origin or if poor response to phototherapy

Urine for reducing substances

If history or presentation (or both) suggest sepsis, perform blood culture, urine culture, and cerebrospinal fluid for protein, glucose, cell count, and culture

INTERVENTIONS

If TSB ≥25 mg/dL (428 mcmol/L) or ≥20 mg/dL (342 mcmol/L) in a sick newborn or newborn <38 weeks' gestation, obtain a type and crossmatch, and request blood in case an exchange transfusion is necessary

In newborns with isoimmune hemolytic disease and TSB level rising in spite of intensive phototherapy or within 2 to 3 mg/dL (34-51 mcmol/L) of exchange level, administer intravenous immunoglobulin 0.5 to 1 g/kg over 2 hours and repeat in 12 hours if necessary

If newborn's weight loss from birth is >12% or clinical or biochemical evidence of dehydration exists, then recommend formula or expressed breast milk. If oral intake is in question, then give intravenous fluids.

FOR NEWBORNS RECEIVING INTENSIVE PHOTOTHERAPY

Breastfeed or bottle feed (formula or expressed milk) every 2 to 3 hours

If TSB ≥25 mg/dL (428 mcmol/L), repeat TSB within 2 to 3 hours

If TSB 20 to 25 mg/dL (342-428 mcmol/L), repeat within 3 to 4 hours

If TSB <20 mg/dL (342 mcmol/L), then repeat in 4 to 6 hours. If TSB continues to fall, then repeat in 8 to 12 hours

If TSB is not decreasing or is moving closer to level for exchange transfusion or the TSB/albumin ratio exceeds levels shown in Figure 98-4, then consider exchange transfusion (see Figure 98-4 for exchange transfusion recommendations)

When TSB is <13 to 14 mg dL (239 mcmol/L), discontinue phototherapy

Depending on the cause of the hyperbilirubinemia, measuring TSB 24 hours after discharge to check for rebound is an option

G6PD, Glucose-6-phosphate dehydrogenase; *TSB,* total serum bilirubin level.

infants: (1) breastfeeding jaundice (also called *breast-non-feeding jaundice*) and (2) breast-milk jaundice.[36,37] (See Chapter 89, Breastfeeding the Newborn.) Breastfed infants who develop jaundice should be continued on frequent breastfeeding. Supplementation with expressed milk or formula is indicated only if the intake seems inadequate despite intervention, if weight loss is excessive, if the newborn appears dehydrated, or for breast-milk jaundice when levels reach greater than 20 to 25 mg/dL in an otherwise healthy infant and when a diagnostic interruption of breastfeeding may be helpful.[2,34-37]

The US Food and Drug Administration (FDA) has approved no medication for preventing hyperbilirubinemia. A small randomized trial has shown that hyperbilirubinemia in breastfed infants can be reduced by inhibiting β-glucuronidase, thereby reducing the enterohepatic cycle of bilirubin.[38] Glycerin suppositories during the first 48 hours do not significantly affect the level of bilirubin at 38 hours of life.[39] Several studies have shown that in patients with hemolytic anemia the early postnatal administration of a single dose of tin mesoporphyrin, an inhibitor of heme oxygenase, is highly effective in reducing the risk of hyperbilirubinemia.[40] However, this inhibitor is nonspecific, thereby potentially inhibiting heme oxygenase in the brain. Long-term follow-up data are required before this drug receives FDA approval for this indication.[40]

LONG-TERM OUTCOME, NEURODEVELOPMENTAL FOLLOW-UP, AND MEDICO-LEGAL RISKS

The clear guidelines of the AAP[2] and the Joint Commission[28,29] for prevention, intervention, and follow-up for hyperbilirubinemia in the term or late preterm neonate based on risk factors and total serum bilirubin levels help the clinician minimize the medico-legal risk of kernicterus.

Any term or late preterm neonate without Rh isoimmune hemolytic disease who develops acute or chronic bilirubin encephalopathy should be entered into the pilot Kernicterus Registry.[41,42] Peak or admission serum bilirubin concentrations in these patients ranged from 20.7 to 59.9 mg/dL. In this registry 8% of those who died with kernicterus or developed residual neurologic sequelae had a total serum bilirubin 20.7 mg/dL to 25.0 mg/dL, and 50% had a value less than 30.1 mg/dL.[42] Thus using a threshold of 25 mg/dL for intervention in nonhemolytic jaundice would be expected to prevent 92% of these cases of kernicterus.[42] Experimental and clinical data strongly suggest that measurement of free bilirubin may improve risk assessment for long-term neurotoxicity.[42] In a neonate exposed to an agent that unbinds bilirubin, using (measured or estimated) unbound bilirubin levels rather than total serum bilirubin levels to assess the need for phototherapy or exchange transfusion appears prudent.[42,43] Metabolic acidosis increases free bilirubin levels in the blood.

In patients readmitted with serum bilirubin concentration greater than 25 mg/dL (26.4-36.9 mg/dL) most with acute signs of encephalopathy, magnetic resonance imaging may show increased T1 signal at the level of the basal ganglia or brainstem nuclei.[40] In one series, neurologic signs normalized in 4 of 5 infants and magnetic resonance imaging results normalized in 2 of 3 infants by 2 years of age.[44]

Healthy neonates with nonhemolytic hyperbilirubinemia and moderately elevated serum bilirubin levels (13.6-26.0 mg/dL) may exhibit minor neurologic dysfunction when examined during the first year of life.[45] In one series, a strong dose-response relationship between the degree of hyperbilirubinemia and the severity of minor neurologic dysfunction was present at 12 months of age.

In contrast, in a series of 132 neonates with peak serum bilirubin levels of at least 25 mg/dL (most up to 29.9 mg/dL) and treated with phototherapy or exchange transfusion, neurodevelopment was normal beyond 2 years of age when examined at a median age of 5.8 years.[46]

Severe anomalies of the brainstem-evoked response are observed in patients with serum bilirubin greater than 20 mg/dL. Patients with hyperbilirubinemia at a serum level requiring exchange transfusion should be tested for sensorineural hearing loss by brainstem auditory-evoked response,[47] regardless of the results of hearing screening using otoacoustic emission, and should have audiologic monitoring every 6 months until the age of 3 years.[47] Long-term neurodevelopmental follow-up appears justified in patients suspected of or confirmed with bilirubin encephalopathy and those with total serum bilirubin greater than 25 mg/dL.

WHEN TO REFER

- Preparation for possible exchange transfusion: total serum bilirubin above the level recommended for exchange transfusion or total serum bilirubin above 25 mg/dL (428 mcmol/L) at any time or signs of bilirubin encephalopathy
- Need for intravenous immunoglobulin therapy: isoimmune hemolytic disease with a total serum bilirubin level rising in spite of intensive phototherapy or within 2 to 3 mg/dL (34-51 mcmol/L) of exchange transfusion level
- Sick newborn who needs to be evaluated and treated for possible sepsis
- Cholestatic jaundice, defined as a direct or conjugated bilirubin level above 1 mg/dL, if total bilirubin is below 5 mg/dL, or above 20% of total serum bilirubin if the latter is above 5 mg/dL
- Prenatal diagnosis of isoimmune hemolysis
- Newborn with poor response to high-intensity phototherapy

WHEN TO ADMIT

- Emergency admission: total serum bilirubin above the level recommended for exchange transfusion or total serum bilirubin greater than 25 mg/dL (428 mcmol/L) at any time
- Need for intravenous immunoglobulin therapy: isoimmune hemolytic disease with a total serum bilirubin level rising in spite of intensive phototherapy or within 2 to 3 mg/dL (34-51 mcmol/L) of exchange transfusion level
- Routine admission or home phototherapy: total serum bilirubin above the level recommended for phototherapy (usually total serum bilirubin >18 mg/dL)
- Sick infant who needs to be evaluated for and treated for dehydration or possible sepsis

TOOLS FOR PRACTICE

Engaging Patient and Family

- *Jaundice and Your Newborn* (brochure), American Academy of Pediatrics (www.aap.org/bookstore).
- *Questions and Answers: Jaundice and Your Newborn* (fact sheet), American Academy of Pediatrics (www.aap.org/family/jaundicefaq.htm).

Medical Decision Support

- *Algorithm for the management of jaundice in the newborn nursery* (algorithm), American Academy of Pediatrics. (aappolicy.aappublications.org/cgi/content/full/pediatrics;114/1/297).
- *BiliTool* (interactive tool), BiliTool, Inc. (www.bilitool.org/).
- *Guidelines for phototherapy in hospitalized infants of 35 or more weeks' gestation* (figure), American Academy of Pediatrics. (aappolicy.aappublications.org/cgi/content/full/pediatrics;114/1/297).
- *Kernicterus threatens healthy newborns—Sentinel Event Alert* (fact sheet), Joint Commission for the Accreditation of Healthcare Organizations (www.jointcommission.org/SentinelEvents/SentinelEventAlert/sea_18.htm).
- *Laboratory Evaluation of the Jaundiced Infant of 35 or More Weeks' Gestation* (table), American Academy of Pediatrics. (aappolicy.aappublications.org/cgi/content/full/pediatrics;114/1/297).
- *Nomogram for designation of risk in 2840 well newborns at 36 or more weeks' gestational age with birth weight of 2000 g or more or 35 or more weeks' gestational age and birth weight of 2500 g or more based on the hour-specific serum bilirubin values* (figure), American Academy of Pediatrics. (aappolicy.aappublications.org/cgi/content/full/pediatrics;114/1/297).

- *Revised guidance to help prevent kernicterus* (fact sheet), The Joint Commission (www.jointcommission.org/sentinelevents/).

AAP POLICY STATEMENT

American Academy of Pediatrics, Subcommittee on Hyperbilirubinemia. Management of hyperbilirubinemia in the newborn infant 35 or more weeks of gestation. *Pediatrics*. 2004;114(1):297-316. (aappolicy.aappublications.org/cgi/content/full/pediatrics;114/1/297).

SUGGESTED RESOURCES

American Academy of Pediatrics, Section on Breastfeeding. Policy statement: breastfeeding and the use of human milk. *Pediatrics*. 2005;115:496-506. Available at: aappolicy.aappublications.org/cgi/reprint/pediatrics;115/2/496.pdf. Accessed July 12, 2007.

Beal AC, Chou SC, Palmer RH, et al. The changing face of race: risk factors for neonatal hyperbilirubinemia. *Pediatrics*. 2006;117(5):1618-1625.

Bhutani VK, Johnson L, Sivieri EM. Predictive ability of a predischarge hour-specific serum bilirubin for subsequent significant hyperbilirubinemia in healthy term and near-term newborns. *Pediatrics*. 1999;103(1):6-14.

Kaplan M, Kaplan E, Hammerman C, et al. Post-phototherapy neonatal bilirubin rebound: a potential cause of significant hyperbilirubinaemia. *Arch Dis Child*. 2006;91:31-34.

Moyer V, Freese DK, Whitington PF, et al. Guideline for the evaluation of cholestatic jaundice in infants: recommendations of the North American Society for Pediatric Gastroenterology, Hepatology and Nutrition. *J Pediatr Gastroenterol Nutr*. 2004;39:115-128.

Thayyil S, Marriott L. Can transcutaneous bilirubinometry reduce the need for serum bilirubin estimations in term and near term infants? *Arch Dis Chil*. 2005;90:1311-1312.

The Joint Commission. Sentinel Event Alert. Revised guidance to help prevent kernicterus. Issue 31, April 31, 2004. Available at: www.jointcommission.org/sentinelevents. Accessed February 14, 2008.

REFERENCES

1. American Academy of Pediatrics, Subcommittee on Hyperbilirubinemia. Clinical practice guideline: management of hyperbilirubinemia in the newborn infant 35 or more weeks of gestation. *Pediatrics*. 2004;114:297-316.
2. American Academy of Pediatrics, Provisional Committee for Quality Improvement and Subcommittee on Hyperbilirubinemia. Practice parameter: management of hyperbilirubinemia in the healthy term newborn. *Pediatrics*. 1994;94(4):558-565.
3. Bhutani VK, Johnson LH, Sivieri EM. Predictive ability of a predischarge hour-specific serum bilirubin for subsequent significant hyperbilirubinemia in healthy term and near-term newborns. *Pediatrics*. 1999;103(1):6-14.
4. Maisels MJ, Newman TB. Predicting hyperbilirubinemia in newborns: the importance of timing. *Pediatrics*. 1999;103(2);493-494.
5. Bhutani VK, Johnson LH, Keren R. Diagnosis and management of hyperbilirubinemia in the term neonate: for a safer first week. *Pediatr Clin North Am*. 2004;51(4):843-861.
6. Bhutani VK, Johnson LH, Maisels MJ, et al. Kernicterus: epidemiological strategies for its prevention through systems based approaches. *J Perinatol*. 2004;24(10):650-662.
7. Stevenson DK, Fanaroff AA, Maisels MJ, et al. Prediction of hyperbilirubinemia in near-term and term infants. *Pediatrics*. 2001;108(1):31-39.
8. Martinez JC, Garcia HO, Otheguy LE, et al. Control of severe hyperbilirubinemia in full term newborns with the inhibitor of bilirubin production Sn-mesoporphyrin. *Pediatrics*. 1999;103(1):1-5.
9. Khurana E, Bhutani VK, Dworanczyk R, et al. Readmission rates of healthy newborns for severe hyperbilirubinemia and intensive phototherapy in USA. Abstract. *Pediatr Res*. 2003;54:1756A.
10. Ebbesen F, Andersson C, Verder H, et al. Extreme hyperbilirubinaemia in term and near-term infants in Denmark. *Acta Paediatr*. 2005;94(1):59-64.
11. Maruo Y, Nishizawa K, Sato H, et al. Prolonged unconjugated hyperbilirubinemia associated with breast milk and mutations of the bilirubin uridine diphosphate-glucuronosyltransferase gene. *Pediatrics*. 2000;06(5):E59.
12. Beal AC, Chou SC, Palmer RH, et al. The changing face of race: risk factors for neonatal hyperbilirubinemia. *Pediatrics*. 2006;117(5):1618-1625.
13. Setia S, Villaveces A, Dhillon P, et al. Neonatal jaundice in Asian, white, and mixed-race infants. *Arch Pediatr Adolesc Med*. 2002;156:276-279.
14. Frank JE. Diagnosis and management of G6PD deficiency. *Am Fam Physician*. Oct 2005;72(7):1277-1282.
15. Yamamoto A, Nishio H, Waku S, et al. Gly71Arg mutation of the bilirubin UDP-glucuronosyltransferase 1A1 gene is associated with neonatal hyperbilirubinemia in the Japanese population. *Kobe J Med Sci*. 2002;48(3):73-77.
16. Yeung CY, Lee FT, Wong HN. Effect of a popular Chinese herb on neonatal bilirubin protein binding. *Biol Neonate*. 1990;58(2):98-103.
17. Kaplan M, Herschel M, Hammerman C, et al. Hyperbilirubinemia among African American, glucose-6-phosphate dehydrogenase-deficient neonates. *Pediatrics*. 2004;114(2):e213-e219.
18. Chan E. Displacement of bilirubin from albumin by berberine. *Biol Neonate*. 1993;63(4):201-208.
19. Madlon-Kay DJ. Recognition of the presence and severity of newborn jaundice by parents, nurses, physicians, and icterometer. *Pediatrics*. 1997;100(3):e3. Available at: www.pediatrics.org/cgi/content/full/100/3/e3. Accessed July 12, 2007.
20. WHO Working Group. Glucose-6-phosphate dehydrogenase deficiency. *Bull World Health Organ*. 1989;67:601-611.
21. Grafmeyer D, Bondon M, Manchon M, et al. The influence of bilirubin, haemolysis and turbidity on 20 analytical tests performed on automatic analysers. Results of an interlaboratory study. *Eur J Clin Chem Clin Biochem*. 1995;33(1):31-52.
22. Hwang S, Shulman, R. Approach to neonatal cholestasis. *Semin Liver Disease*. 2002;18:281-286.
23. Fischler B, Papadogiannakis N, Nemeth A. Aetiological factors in neonatal cholestasis. *Acta Paediatr*. 2001;90:88-92.
24. Moyer V, Freese DK, Whitington PF, et al. Guideline for the evaluation of cholestatic jaundice in infants: recommendations of the North American Society for Pediatric Gastroenterology, Hepatology and Nutrition. *J Pediatr Gastroenterol Nutr*. 2004;39:115-128.
25. Thayyil S, Marriott L. Can transcutaneous bilirubinometry reduce the need for serum bilirubin estimations in term and near term infants? *Arch Dis Chil*. 2005;90:1311-1312.

26. Engle WD, Jackson L, Stehel EK, et al. Evaluation of a transcutaneous jaundice meter following hospital discharge in term and near-term neonates. *J Perinatol.* 2005;25:486-490.
27. Laosombat V, Dissaneevate S, Wongchanchailert M, et al. Neonatal anemia associated with Southeast Asian ovalocytosis. *Int J Hematol.* 2005;82(3):201-205.
28. Joint Commission for the Accreditation of Health Care Organizations. Sentinel Event Alert. Kernicterus threatens healthy newborns. Issue 18, April 1, 2001. Available at: www.jointcommission.org/sentinelevents/sentineleventalert/sea_18.htm. Accessed July 12, 2007.
29. The Joint Commission. Sentinel Event Alert. Revised guidance to help prevent kernicterus. Issue 31, April 31, 2004. Available at: www.jointcommission.org/sentinelevents. Accessed February 14, 2008.
30. Mehta S, Kumar P, Narang A. A randomized controlled trial of fluid supplementation in term neonates with severe hyperbilirubinemia. *J Pediatr.* 2005;147(6):781-785.
31. Gottstein R, Cooke R. Systematic review of intravenous immunoglobulin in haemolytic disease of the newborn. *Arch Dis Child Fetal Neonatal Ed.* 2003;88(5):F6-F10.
32. Alcock GS, Liley H. Immunoglobulin infusion for isoimmune haemolytic jaundice in neonates. *Cochrane Database Syst Rev.* 2002;3:CD003313.
33. Kaplan M, Kaplan E, Hammerman C, et al. Post-phototherapy neonatal bilirubin rebound: a potential cause of significant hyperbilirubinaemia. *Arch Dis Child.* 2006;91:31-34.
34. American Academy of Pediatrics, Section on Breastfeeding. Policy statement: breastfeeding and the use of human milk. *Pediatrics.* 2005;115:496-506. Available at: aappolicy.aappublications.org/cgi/reprint/pediatrics;115/2/496.pdf. Accessed July 12, 2007.
35. The Academy of Breastfeeding. ABM Clinical Protocol No. 3—Hospital Guidelines for the Use of Supplementary Feedings in the Healthy Term Breastfed Neonate. Available at: www.bfmed.org. Accessed July 12, 2007.
36. The Academy of Breastfeeding. ABM Clinical Protocol No. 10—Breastfeeding the Near-Term Infant (35-37 Weeks Gestation). Available at www.bfmed.org Accessed July 12, 2007.
37. Gourley GR. Breastfeeding, diet, and neonatal hyperbilirubinemia. *NeoReviews.* 2000;1:e25-e31.
38. Gourley GR, Li Z, Kreamer BL, et al. A controlled, randomized, double-blind trial of prophylaxis against jaundice among breastfed newborns. *Pediatrics.* 2005;116(2):385-391.
39. Bader D, Yanir Y, Kugelman A, et al. Induction of early meconium evacuation: is it effective in reducing the level of neonatal hyperbilirubinemia? *Am J Perinatol.* 2005;22(6):329-333.
40. Dennery PA. Metalloporphyrins for the treatment of neonatal jaundice. *Curr Opin Pediatr.* 2005;17(2):167-169.
41. Wennberg RP, Ahlfors CE, Bhutani VK, et al. Toward understanding kernicterus: a challenge to improve the management of jaundiced newborns. *Pediatrics.* 2006;117(2):474-485.
42. Ahlfors CE. Unbound bilirubin associated with kernicterus: a historical approach. *J Pediatr.* 2000;137(4):540-544.
43. Johnson LH, Bhutani VK, Brown AK. System-based approach to management of neonatal jaundice and prevention of kernicterus. *J Pediatr.* 2002;140(4):396-403.
44. Harris MC, Bernbaum JC, Polin JR, et al. Developmental follow-up of breastfed term and near-term infants with marked hyperbilirubinemia. *Pediatrics.* 2001;107(5):1075-1080.
45. Soorani-Lunsing I, Woltil HA, Hadders-Algra M. Are moderate degrees of hyperbilirubinemia in healthy term neonates really safe for the brain? *Pediatr Res.* 2001;50(6):701-705.
46. Newman TB, Liljestrand P, Jeremy RJ, et al. Outcomes among newborns with total serum bilirubin levels of 25 mg per deciliter or more. *N Engl J Med.* 2006;354(18):1889-1900.
47. National Center for Hearing Assessment and Management, Joint Committee on Infant Hearing. Year 2000 Position Statement: Principles and Guidelines for Early Hearing Detection and Intervention Programs. Available at: www.jcih.org/jcih2000.pdf. Accessed July 12, 2007.

Chapter 99

RESPIRATORY DISTRESS AND BREATHING DISORDERS IN THE NEWBORN

Suhas M. Nafday, MD, MRCP(Ire), DCH; Christina M. Long, DO

INTRODUCTION

The transition from intrauterine life requires major changes to the respiratory and circulatory systems of the neonate to maintain adequate respiratory gas exchange without the benefits of the placental circulation.[1] In most instances, this complex series of events goes quite smoothly. However, some babies develop respiratory distress, necessitating evaluation and possible neonatal intensive care. The incidence of respiratory distress in the newborn period ranges from 2.9% to 7.6%, and 4.3% of newborns may require supplemental oxygen therapy.[2]

Development of the respiratory system continues after birth and into childhood. Alveolar remodeling continues after delivery until a child is 6 to 7 years of age, with continued alveolar growth into adolescence. Physical, hormonal, and local factors influence fetal lung growth. Successful initiation of respiration requires sufficient pulmonary gas exchange surface in the lung in conjunction with an adequately developed pulmonary vasculature that supports transport of oxygen and carbon dioxide through the lungs. The lungs must be compliant and able to respond to the metabolic needs of the infant with minimal respiratory effort. Therefore the airways, chest wall, respiratory muscles, and neural mechanisms that control respiration must be structurally mature to allow for optimal respiratory function. Three groups of skeletal muscles—the diaphragm, intercostals and accessory muscles, and abdominal muscles—are involved in ventilation. The diaphragm is the primary muscle used during quiet breathing. Respiratory muscle fatigue occurs when work of breathing increases, when muscle strength is reduced, or when breathing is inefficient. Respiratory fatigue will lead to progressive hypercapnia and apnea. During the first 2 months after a full-term birth, significant increases occur in lung size, surface area, and lung volume. Changes in control of breathing and maturation of neural control mechanisms coincide with this rapid phase of lung growth.

Significant changes occur during the first 6 hours after birth as part of the process of cardiorespiratory adaptation. Oxygenation increases dramatically to 80 to 95 mm Hg at 6 hours of life. The arterial pressure of carbon dioxide ($Paco_2$) decreases from 45 to 65 mm Hg to 30 to 40 mm Hg. Concurrently, pulmonary blood flow increases, the foramen ovale is closed, and ductal closure begins. Throughout this period, intrapulmonary shunts persist as the lungs become air filled and the newborn's functional residual capacity is established. The initial respiratory pattern is irregular, but respiratory cycles become increasingly rhythmic with modulation of chemoreceptors and stretch receptors.

Normal physical findings in a newborn include a respiratory rate of 40 to 60 breaths per minute. During rapid eye movement (REM) sleep, infants often exhibit irregular respirations with pauses of 5 seconds or less. In contrast, during non-REM or quiet sleep, a newborn's respiratory rate is 5 to10 breaths per minute slower than in the awake or active (REM) sleep states. Respiratory distress can be defined as tachypnea with respiratory rate greater than 60 breaths per minute, nasal flaring, chest retractions (intercostal, subcostal, and substernal), and expiratory grunting. Respiratory distress may be present with or without cyanosis. Peripheral or acrocyanosis is common in the neonatal period. Central cyanosis, signifying greater than 5 gm/dL of desaturated hemoglobin, is often visible by looking at the newborn's tongue, lips, and, depending on the skin pigmentation, trunk. Decreased oxygen saturation, apnea, or both may also be present. Irregular *(see-saw)* or slow respiratory rates of less than 30 breaths per minute, particularly if associated with gasping, are a worrisome sign.

The cause of respiratory distress can be either pulmonary or nonpulmonary in origin. Nonpulmonary causes of respiratory distress include cardiac or central nervous system (CNS) abnormalities, sepsis, infection, and hematologic, metabolic, or miscellaneous conditions. Respiratory depression as the result of maternal medications or illicit substance use may also be a contributing factor. The gestational age of the newborn at birth is another factor that influences the risk for respiratory distress after birth. Newborns between 34 and 37 weeks' gestation in comparison with full-term infants experience increased respiratory difficulties. These newborns exhibit higher rates of low Apgar scores, transient tachypnea of the newborn (TTN), respiratory distress syndrome (RDS), persistent pulmonary hypertension, and respiratory failure.[3-6] Delivery by elective cesarean is also associated with higher rates of these respiratory morbidities, necessitating neonatal intensive care, oxygen therapy, and cardiorespiratory support (eg, continuous positive airway pressure [CPAP], mechanical ventilation, extracorporeal membrane oxygenation [ECMO]) because of prematurity and surfactant deficiency.

APPROACH TO THE PATIENT WITH RESPIRATORY DISTRESS

Respiratory distress can be difficult to determine immediately after birth. Many newborns may initially be cyanotic or tachypneic. These symptoms usually resolve spontaneously in the first 10 to 15 minutes after birth. A thorough history and physical examination are important to distinguish cardiac and noncardiac causes of cyanosis and respiratory distress. The pre- and perinatal histories, including maternal medication and/or substance use, are important in the evaluation for respiratory distress. Labor course and evidence of fetal distress provide important information regarding risk factors for a prolonged or difficult transition after birth. Complications occurring during delivery related to meconium passage, perinatal depression, or birth injury may also lead to transitional difficulties and respiratory distress. Many conditions that produce respiratory distress occur in preterm infants, whereas others may occur in full-term infants. In addition, many congenital anomalies may be suspected prenatally because of the presence of maternal complications that develop. Tracheoesophageal fistula, which may cause respiratory distress, is often associated with polyhydramnios, whereas an underlying condition that causes oligohydramnios may lead to pulmonary hypoplasia. Box 99-1 lists various maternal and obstetrical conditions associated with neonatal causes of respiratory distress.

After a complete history, the newborn should be examined thoroughly. Urgent evaluation and treatment are needed for the infant who is ill appearing; apneic; choking; exhibits poor, labored, or gasping respirations; or has marked retractions or stridor, poor perfusion, or cyanosis. Bradycardia and hypotension also signify serious illness. The newborn's general appearance may provide useful clues to the cause of the child's symptoms. The clinician should observe the neonate's

BOX 99-1 Maternal and Obstetrical Conditions Associated With Neonatal Causes of Respiratory Distress

MATERNAL CONDITIONS

Drug abuse: drug withdrawal

Diabetes mellitus: RDS, hypoglycemia, polycythemia, cardiomyopathy

Infections: pneumonia, sepsis

OBSTETRIC CONDITIONS

Use of general anesthesia: central depression

Hydrops fetalis: pleural effusion

Preterm delivery: RDS

PROM, maternal fever, chorioamnionitis: pneumonia, sepsis

Meconium-stained amniotic fluid: meconium aspiration syndrome

Antepartum hemorrhage: anemia, hypovolemia

PROM, Premature rupture of membranes; *RDS*, respiratory distress syndrome.

color, activity, and level of alertness, cry, posture, and perfusion and assess for dysmorphism. Upper airways obstruction should be suspected in the infant who develops inspiratory stridor. A barrel-shaped chest suggests an air leak, whereas a scaphoid abdomen should lead the clinician to consider that the newborn may have a diaphragmatic hernia. Grunting respirations and retractions signify poor lung compliance and often indicate the presence of parenchymal lung disease.

If cyanosis is present, the newborn should be examined while quiet and in a neutral thermal environment to ascertain whether the cyanosis is central or peripheral (acrocyanosis). Acrocyanosis, blue color of the hands and feet when the rest of the body is pink, is frequently seen in newborns. Acrocyanosis is usually normal, likely to be seen with exposure to cold, and in the presence of polycythemia, but it may also be a presenting sign of serious conditions such as sepsis, hypoglycemia, or hypoplastic left heart syndrome. When the baby's temperature has stabilized, it can be determined if the cyanosis is central or it is acrocyanosis. Central cyanosis of the trunk, mucosal membranes, and tongue can occur at any time after birth and is a manifestation of an underlying problem. Different conditions may affect the appearance of cyanosis, including anemia and hyperbilirubinemia. Causes of cyanosis are listed in Table 99-1. The oxygen saturation level by pulse oximetry is important to check because clinical signs of hypoxemia or cyanosis may be difficult to detect. Pulse oximetry is routinely used for this purpose. Oxygen saturations measured by pulse oximetry typically reflect an arterial pressure of oxygen ($Pa{O_2}$) between 60 and 90 mm Hg. The saturation is less than 90% when the $Pa{O_2}$ is below 40 mm Hg. In the rare condition methemoglobinemia, the infant appears cyanotic but has a high oxygen saturation level.

Accurate monitoring of respiratory rate is important. Infants attempt to minimize their work of breathing by adjusting their respiratory rate. In full-term neonates, respiratory rates average around 45 bpm when awake and 35 bpm during sleep, with wide rates of respiration variation. The respiratory rate tends to be higher in preterm infants. The clinician should look for signs of respiratory distress such as nasal flaring, intercostals or subcostal retractions, and grunting. Grunting, the result of partial closure of the glottis during expiration, may be intermittent or continuous. Suprasternal retractions may be another indication of upper airway obstruction.

Further examination of the neonate can reveal whether any obvious malformations are present, such as a barrel-shaped chest with meconium aspiration syndrome or pneumomediastinum and a small, narrow chest in cases of asphyxiating thoracic dystrophy, or a scaphoid abdomen if a congenital diaphragmatic hernia is present. The patient may have inspiratory stridor, which can be associated with vocal cord paralysis or laryngotracheomalacia.[2] Capillary refill time greater than 2 seconds may indicate poor perfusion, which may contribute to the respiratory distress. The chest must be auscultated to listen to heart and breath sounds. Heart sounds may be loud or diminished, or a heart murmur may be present. Cardiac murmur may be absent in a neonate with serious cardiac disease. Breath sounds may be unequal bilaterally, with rales, rhonchi, or wheezing. Breath sounds may be diminished or distant in situations that involve pneumothorax, atelectasis, or pleural effusion. Transillumination of the chest may be a useful tool to rule out pneumothorax. Abdominal distention may be present in cases of ascites or bowel obstructions or those caused by hepatosplenomegaly, which may contribute to respiratory distress.

Neurologic status is also important. Hypotonia is often a sign of sepsis, asphyxia, or depression as a result of maternal narcotics. Phrenic nerve injury that occurs during a difficult delivery or as a consequence of thoracic surgery may lead to paralysis of the diaphragm. The differential diagnosis of respiratory distress is listed in Box 99-2.

Table 99-1 Causes of Cyanosis in the Neonate

	ACROCYANOSIS	CENTRAL CYANOSIS	DIFFERENTIAL CYANOSIS	REVERSE DIFFERENTIAL CYANOSIS
APPEARANCE	Blue color of the hands and feet when the rest of the body is pink	Blue color of the trunk, mucosal membranes and tongue	The upper part of the body remains pink, and the lower part is cyanotic.	The upper part remains cyanotic, whereas the lower part remains pink.
POSSIBLE CAUSES	Usually normal Exposure to cold Polycythemia Serious conditions such as sepsis, hypoglycemia, or hypoplastic left heart syndrome	Serious pulmonary parenchymal, as well as nonparenchymal abnormality Persistent pulmonary hypertension of newborn Cyanotic congenital heart disease	Right-to-left shunt through the patent ductus arteriosus (PDA)	Transposition of great arteries with pulmonary hypertension and shunt through the PDA Total anomalous pulmonary venous return above the diaphragm with shunt through the PDA

BOX 99-2 Differential Diagnosis of Respiratory Distress in the Newborn

LUNG PARENCHYMAL TYPE 1 AIRWAY DISORDERS

Congenital anomalies: tracheoesophageal fistula, congenital diaphragmatic hernia, pulmonary sequestration, congenital cystic adenomatoid malformations, pulmonary hypoplasia, choanal atresia or stenosis, laryngeal web, subglottic stenosis, congenital lobar emphysema, chylothorax, external compression of upper airway (vascular ring, tumors, and cysts), laryngotracheomalacia

Acquired disorders: transient tachypnea of the newborn, respiratory distress syndrome, meconium aspiration syndrome, pneumonia, pulmonary edema, pulmonary hemorrhage, pneumatocele, pulmonary lymphangiectasia, air leak syndromes (pneumothorax, pneumomediastinum), pleural effusion including hydrops fetalis, trauma (postextubation laryngeal edema, atelectasis, and subglottic stenosis)

CARDIAC DISORDERS

Cyanotic heart lesions: transposition of the great arteries, total anomalous pulmonary venous return, truncus arteriosus, tricuspid atresia, pulmonary atresia, Ebstein anomaly

Acyanotic heart lesions: left-to-right shunts (patent ductus arteriosus, ventricular septal defect and, rarely, atrial septal defect), atrioventricular canal defect, coarctation of aorta, aortic stenosis

MECHANICAL ANOMALIES

Rib cage anomalies (Jeune syndrome), abdominal distention

CENTRAL NERVOUS SYSTEM

Cerebral edema, asphyxia, infection, vocal cord paralysis, diaphragmatic paralysis, intracranial hemorrhage

MISCELLANEOUS

Metabolic acidosis, sepsis, polycythemia, anemia, hypoglycemia, hypermagnesemia

EVALUATION OF A PATIENT WITH RESPIRATORY DISTRESS

Pulse Oximetry and Blood Gas Studies

Evaluation of a newborn with respiratory distress includes pulse oximetry and blood gas analysis. A pulse oximeter measures the oxygen saturation by comparing the amount of red light absorbed by deoxygenated hemoglobin with the amount of infrared light absorbed by oxygenated hemoglobin. If cyanosis is present, pre- (right hand) and postductal oxygen saturations (probe placed on a lower extremity) should be measured. Pre- and postductal saturation differences may indicate infracardiac shunting as a cause of respiratory distress and cyanosis. Interpreting blood gas values based on normal values for newborns is important. The reader is referred to Table 99-2 for normal blood gas values at different ages. If serial blood gas monitoring is required, then the newborn should be transferred to a special care or neonatal intensive care unit (NICU). While interpreting the blood gas results, attention must be paid to errors caused by air bubbles (high Pao_2 and low $Paco_2$), excessive heparin (metabolic acidosis), dilution of samples by intravenous fluids in samples obtained from intravascular lines, and blood gases obtained by arterial puncture (decreased $Paco_2$ with crying).

If signs of respiratory distress are present, then a hyperoxia test can aid in differentiating between cardiac and noncardiac diseases. The test consists of obtaining a baseline right radial (preductal) arterial blood gas measurement with the baby breathing room air and repeating the measurement while the baby is receiving 100% oxygen. A Pao_2 measurement greater than 300 mm Hg on 100% oxygen is normal, more than 150 mm Hg suggests pulmonary disease, and 50 to 150 mm Hg suggests cardiac disease (or severe pulmonary hypertension). Significant metabolic acidosis requires evaluation for evidence of tissue hypoxia, cold stress, an inborn error of metabolism, sepsis, acute renal failure, or loss of pH buffering ions as a result of diarrhea, parenteral nutrition, or renal insufficiency.

Table 99-2 Range of Blood Gas Values for Healthy Children

	PRETERM INFANTS (AT 15 HR)	TERM INFANTS (AT 5 HR)	PRETERM AND TERM INFANTS (AT 5 DAYS)	CHILDREN, ADOLESCENTS, ADULTS
pH	7.33	7.34	7.38	7.40
Range	7.29-7.37	7.31-7.37	7.34-7.42	7.35-7.45
$Paco_2$ (mm Hg)	47	35	36	40
Range	39-56	32-39	32-41	35-45
Pao_2 (mm Hg)	60	74	76	95
Range	52-67	62-86	62-92	85-100
HCO_3 (mEq/L)	23	19	21	24
Range	22-23	18-21	19-23	22-26
BE	−4	−5	−3	0
Range	−5 to −2.2	−6 to −2	−5.8 to −1.2	−2 to 2

$Paco_2$, arterial pressure of carbon dioxide; *Pao_2,* arterial pressure of oxygen; *HCO_3,* bicarbonate; *BE,* base excess.

Other Laboratory Tests

In addition to evaluating the newborn's blood gas, laboratory studies such as complete blood count and blood culture, calcium and magnesium levels, urine drug screen, and metabolic screening of urine and blood may be useful in finding a cause for respiratory distress.

Imaging

Any neonate with respiratory distress should also have a chest radiograph performed. The spectrum of diseases that affect the neonate's chest has significant overlap in their radiographic and clinical appearances; therefore interpreting the radiologic images with the clinical picture is important. Appropriate shielding is necessary to limit radiation-associated risks. A systematic approach to the evaluation of a chest radiograph should include review of the radiograph to confirm the patient's name and medical record number, laterality side markers, film exposure (quality), rotation, inspiratory effort, and the presence of motion and other artifact.[7] The typical radiograph view obtained is the anterior-posterior (AP) view. The utility of obtaining a lateral view chest radiograph has been questioned in the past.[8] Addition of a lateral chest radiograph does not increase the diagnostic efficacy of routine chest films in symptomatic infants. No recent studies investigating the value of the lateral chest radiograph have been conducted. However, each case should be evaluated individually, given that valuable information may be obtained for some infants.

The clinician must check the position of any tubes, catheters, and lines. The chest wall (thoracic cavity), bones (clavicles, ribs, scapulae, and vertebrae), airway, and diaphragms should also be assessed. The cardiac and thymic silhouettes often appear to be one, although careful inspection will reveal the borders of each. In a newborn the thymus is often large, but involution may occur rapidly when an infant is ill. The lung fields should be evaluated for the lung volume and position. The lungs may be hyperinflated, underinflated, opaque, or lucent. Each of these descriptors may suggest an underlying condition that aids in formulating a differential diagnosis. The clinician may suspect lung hyperinflation and possibly the presence of a pneumomediastinum in a newborn who exhibits a barrel-shaped chest in the hours after birth, particularly if positive pressure ventilation was required in the delivery room. In sick, as well as vigorous, neonates, obtaining a completely symmetric radiograph may be difficult. Radiologic findings may change over the first 24 to 48 hours after birth. Consequently, obtaining additional radiographs may be necessary to evaluate for disease progression or improvement.

Evaluating lung density includes evaluating the lungs for evidence of consolidation or collapse. In instances of lung collapse, tracheal and cardiac deviation to the side of the collapse may be seen. Lucency of the lungs is often the result of air trapping, although it may also signify the presence of air leak into the mediastinum (*sail sign* outlining the right lobe of the thymus), pleural or pericardial spaces, or hemithorax. In cases of massive air leak syndrome, lucencies (dissection of pleural air) may be seen in the neck and peritoneal spaces as well. The heart size, shape, and position and pulmonary circulation should also be assessed. The cardiac silhouette (cardiothoracic ratio) may occupy as much as 65% of the hemithorax during the first days of life. The cardiac apex, aortic notch, and gastric bubble are important orientation features that assist in determining the underlying cause for the newborn's respiratory difficulty. Evaluating the pulmonary circulation is important if congenital heart disease or persistent pulmonary hypertension is suspected. Lucent or dark lung fields suggest diminished pulmonary blood flow caused by anatomic or vascular abnormalities.

The position of the diaphragm is helpful in ascertaining lung volume, as well as identifying newborns with diaphragmatic hernias. In the latter instance the diaphragm will be elevated, and the abdominal contents are visible in the hemithorax. Pulmonary hypoplasia that results from limited thoracic space for lung growth will lead to significant respiratory compromise and distress after birth. Babies with a diaphragmatic hernia often have a characteristic scaphoid abdomen at delivery. A newborn who sustains damage to the phrenic nerve as a result of birth or surgical injury will exhibit respiratory symptoms and elevation of the diaphragm on the affected side. A nasogastric or orogastric tube should be placed before obtaining a chest radiograph. The presence of a tracheoesophageal fistula is confirmed by seeing a coiled tube in an upper esophageal pouch. Prenatal diagnosis of congenital lung masses may have included fetal sonography and fetal magnetic resonance imaging (MRI). However, most cases of congenital lung masses will be identified after birth as the newborn exhibits respiratory distress. Sonography, computed tomography (CT), or MRI of the chest is used to help characterize congenital lung lesions and aid in diagnosis.[9] These studies also assist in defining the extent of the lesion and identifying associated anomalies.

Cardiac Tests

If cardiac disease is suspected, then the clinician should obtain an electrocardiogram, 4-limb blood pressures, and pre- and postductal oxygen saturation levels. Echocardiogram is the definitive investigation for diagnosing a congenital heart disease, if available (see Chapter 100, Evaluation of the Infant With Suspected Heart Disease).

COMMON CAUSES OF EARLY RESPIRATORY DISTRESS IN THE NEWBORN

Transient Tachypnea of the Newborn

TTN is a common, relatively benign, self-limiting disease diagnosed shortly after birth (Figure 99-1). TTN is more common in newborns delivered by cesarean without labor. Other risk factors include male sex, perinatal asphyxia, history of umbilical cord prolapse, and maternal complications such as asthma, diabetes, and anesthesia or analgesia during labor.[10] Although TTN occurs in preterm infants, it is most common in

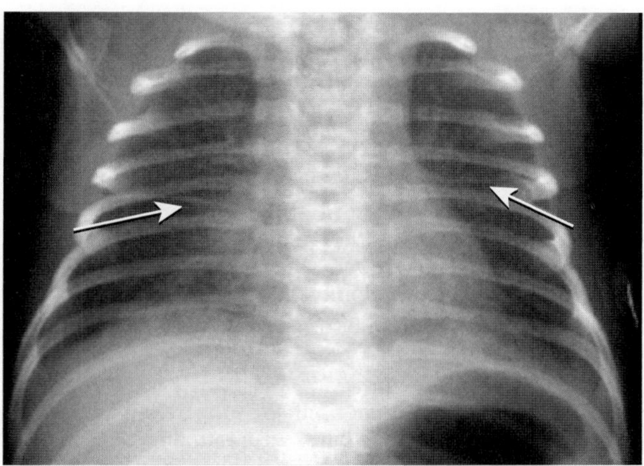

Figure 99-1 Chest radiograph of neonate with transient tachypnea of the newborn.

infants delivered between 37 and 42 weeks' gestation. The incidence in the United States is 11 per 1000 infants. Complications may occur, such as air leaks, with or without the provision of positive pressure ventilation. Neonates with mild TTN symptoms who transition quickly may be monitored closely in the regular nursery. Newborns who continue to exhibit respiratory distress after a period of transition should be admitted to the NICU for further evaluation, monitoring, and treatment. The pathophysiological mechanism of TTN involves delayed clearance of fetal lung fluid by the lymphatics and pulmonary circulation with resultant transient pulmonary edema. In addition, a delay occurs in the transition involved in the physiological shift in the lung from chlorine and water secretion in utero to sodium absorption. This process is typically mediated by the epinephrine surge associated with the onset of labor. Preterm birth is associated with further impairment in the sodium-pump activity, high pulmonary pressure, smaller lung surfaces (fewer alveoli) for fluid absorption, and lower plasma protein levels that contribute to capillary leakage. The clinical findings associated with TTN and treatment strategies are detailed in Box 99-3.

BOX 99-3 Findings and Treatment of Transient Tachypnea of the Newborn

CLINICAL PRESENTATION

Tachypnea; appears shortly after birth and resolves in 1 to 5 days

Nasal flaring, grunting, and retractions; crackles or rales heard on auscultation

Hypoxemia

Chest radiograph hyperinflation, prominent perihilar vascular markings, and fluid may be present in the fissures. Small pleural effusions may also be present (see Figure 99-1)

TREATMENT

Most infants with transient tachypnea of the newborn do not require treatment.

Supplemental oxygen: nasal canula, continuous positive airway pressure providing 5-7 cm water may be useful when fractional inspired oxygen requirements exceed 0.4-0.5 (40-50% oxygen). Mechanical ventilation is almost never required.

Antibiotics may be considered until sepsis has been excluded.

Provide intravenous hydration and nutrition.

Avoid fluid overload.

Diuretics offer little or no benefit.

Respiratory Distress Syndrome

Respiratory Distress Syndrome (RDS) is primarily a disease of preterm infants, although it may affect term infants, especially infants of diabetic mothers. RDS complicates approximately 1% of pregnancies. Approximately 50% of infants born between 26 and 28 weeks' gestation develop RDS, whereas less than 20% to 30% of premature infants at 30 to 32 weeks' gestation have the disorder. The introduction of prenatal steroids for acceleration of lung maturity and the development of exogenous surfactant have improved outcomes in patients with RDS.

Among late preterm infants born between 34 and 37 weeks' gestation the risk for respiratory distress after birth is higher than for the full-term infant. TTN and RDS are both more common in the late preterm infant related to lack of clearance of lung fluid or a degree of surfactant deficiency. Neonates who are delivered by cesarean before labor are at greater risk for respiratory distress related to the absence of the hormonal changes initiated by the onset of labor that are necessary for normal pulmonary transition and function. Hemodynamic instability caused by hypothermia or hypoglycemia may worsen preexisting respiratory difficulties. Additional risk factors for respiratory distress in the late preterm infant include maternal diabetes, multiple gestation, asphyxia, and a family history of a sibling who developed RDS. Boys are more likely to develop RDS than girls, and the disease is more prevalent among white infants.

The pathophysiological mechanism of RDS involves noncompliant, stiff lungs that are structurally immature and contain insufficient surfactant. This status leads to the development of atelectasis (alveolar collapse) at the end of expiration. Ventilation-perfusion mismatch occurs because of the relatively well-perfused, but poorly ventilated, areas of the lungs that cause hypoxemia and hypercarbia. Hypoxemia promotes pulmonary vasoconstriction that can trigger persistent pulmonary hypertension. In premature infants, respiratory muscle fatigue and a compliant chest wall further impair alveolar ventilation (Figure 99-2).

Surfactant protein (SP) deficiency results from a congenital abnormality in the SPs. SP deficiency occurs in a small group of term infants with severe respiratory distress that leads to intractable respiratory failure and death. SP deficiency type B is the most

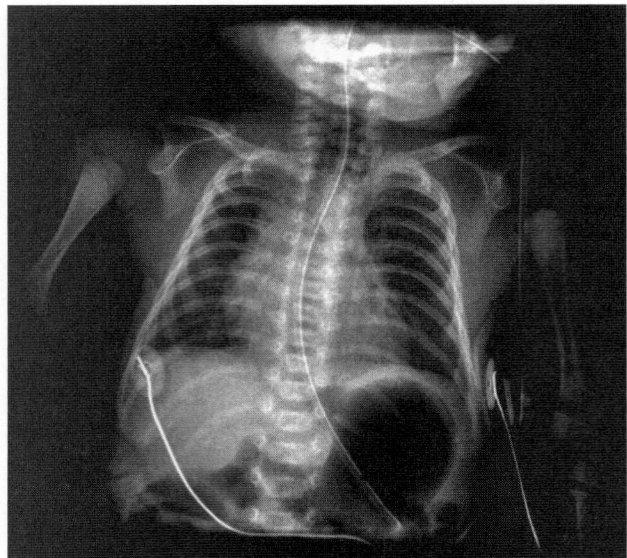

Figure 99-2 34-weeks' gestation twin born to a 28-year-old primiparous woman with preeclampsia. Baby had progressive respiratory distress requiring nasal continuous positive airway pressure and oxygen.

common form of SP deficiency and occurs as an autosomal-recessive trait. Other SPs, though present, are defective. Survival of patients with respiratory distress is inversely proportional to the gestational age at birth. Long-term morbidities are associated with RDS, including bronchopulmonary dysplasia, increased risk of pulmonary infections such as respiratory syncytial virus, and an increased incidence of retinopathy of prematurity. Treatment and prevention strategies are summarized in Box 99-4.

BOX 99-4 Treatment and Prevention Strategies for Respiratory Distress Syndrome

TREATMENT

Multidisciplinary approach: applying basic principles of neonatal care, such as thermoregulation, cardiovascular and nutritional support, treatment of early neonatal infection, and prevention of nosocomial infections

Provision of respiratory support: nasal CPAP or mechanical ventilation

Surfactant replacement therapy: meta-analysis of various trials in which natural or synthetic surfactant was used, either as a prophylactic or rescue treatment, clearly shows that surfactant improves oxygenation, decreases air leaks and reduces infant mortality due to RDS by 40%.[a]

Early administration of surfactant followed by nasal CPAP : trial stage

PREVENTION OF RDS

Prevention of prematurity, prevention of asphyxia, avoiding drug depression during preterm labor, avoidance of maternal fluid overload

Prenatal administration of a single course of corticosteroids to women in preterm labor between 24 and 34 weeks' gestation reduces the mortality and incidence of RDS.[bc]

CPAP, Continuous positive airway pressure; *RDS*, respiratory distress syndrome.

[a]Rodriguez RJ, Martin RJ. Exogenous surfactant therapy in newborns. *Respir Care Clin N Am.* 1999;5(4):595-616.

[b]American Academy of Pediatrics, Committee on Fetus and Newborn. Surfactant replacement therapy for respiratory distress syndrome. *Pediatrics.* 1999;103:684-685.

[c]Merrill J, Ballard R. Clinical use of antenatal corticosteroids: benefits and risks. *NeoReviews.* 2000;1(5):e91-e105.

Meconium Aspiration Syndrome

Meconium aspiration syndrome (MAS) is a respiratory disorder that occurs when a newborn is born through meconium-stained amniotic fluid and whose symptoms cannot otherwise be explained. MAS occurs most frequently in infants who are term, postterm, or small for gestational age. Between 10% and 26% of all deliveries will be complicated by meconium staining of the amniotic fluid. Among live births, estimates indicate that 13% of these deliveries are complicated by meconium; 4% to 5% of meconium-stained newborns develop MAS.[13,14] The incidence of MAS decreased during the last decade in response to advances in obstetric practice (reduction in deliveries weeks). Between 4% and 9% of babies who are born through meconium-stained amniotic fluid will have other causes for their respiratory distress (TTN, delayed transition, infection, persistent pulmonary hypertension, air leak, hypovolemia, pulmonary edema, or aspiration of blood). Up to one third of meconium-stained infants will exhibit perinatal depression at birth.

Meconium is composed of water and debris from the intestinal tract and skin, lanugo, bile pigments, lipids from vernix, amniotic fluid and intestinal secretions, glycoproteins, and mucopolysaccharides. Aspiration of meconium occurs during fetal gasping or with the initial breaths after delivery. Although sterile, when meconium is aspirated into the lung, it triggers an inflammatory response through stimulation of cytokine and vasoactive substance production. Respiratory failure and hypoxia develop as a result of poor lung compliance, increased airway resistance, and smaller tidal volumes. Marked ventilation-perfusion abnormality secondary to airways plugged by meconium also occurs. This condition promotes persistent pulmonary hypertension with right-to-left shunting through the ductus arteriosus or the foramen ovale. Aspirated meconium may cause airway obstruction with air trapping, chemical irritation, pneumonia, and inactivate endogenous surfactant.

The diagnosis of MAS is confirmed by radiography (Figure 99-3). Streaky, linear, or patchy infiltrates (densities) are present on the initial chest film, and the lungs may appear hyperinflated. Radiologic changes resolve over a 7 to 10 day period, though the chest radiograph may take weeks to normalize in rare instances. A 10% to 30% risk exists for air leak among newborns with MAS. These newborns may often be in the regular nursery and become acutely tachypneic or

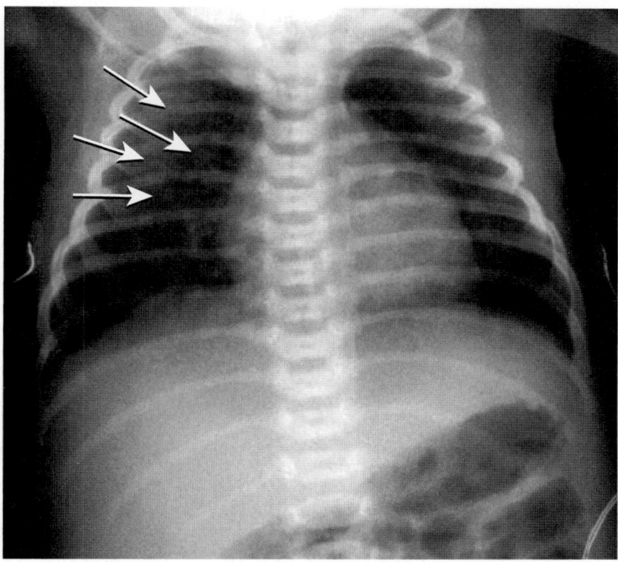

Figure 99-3 Term newborn with meconium aspiration syndrome. Arrows highlight meconium infiltrates in the lung.

cyanotic. Air leak typically occurs within 72 to 96 hours of birth. Box 99-5 summarizes treatment and prevention strategies.

Despite the increased risk of perinatal mortality, most newborns delivered through meconium-stained amniotic fluid are healthy. Perinatal depression at birth and meconium aspiration appears to be the finding most associated with death in infants with MAS. Residual lung disease during the first 6 months of life is common among infants recovering from MAS because these infants are more likely to experience episodes of wheezing and cough and require bronchodilator therapy.[15] Pulmonary function testing in later childhood shows that many children continue to have evidence of mild airway obstruction and hyperinflation and are more prone to exercise-induced bronchospasm, though they do not have increased oxygen consumption or hypercarbia. Neurologic outcomes are normal for the majority of children who had MAS as newborns. Neurodevelopmental sequelae are more commonly related to the underlying cause for the MAS (eg, infection, asphyxia).

Pneumonia

Pneumonia may be acquired in utero, during delivery, or postnatally. It is classified as early or late. Causes of neonatal pneumonia depend on whether the infection is acquired before, during, or after birth. An extensive range exists of bacterial, parasitic, and viral organisms that are responsible for infection along the pregnancy continuum and are summarized in Box 99-6. Prenatally, the fetus may be exposed to many different pathogens if a maternal infection is present. In addition, a variety of risk factors can be found related to preexisting maternal infection, premature or prolonged membrane rupture, and signs of fetal

BOX 99-5 Management Strategies in the Treatment of Meconium Aspiration Syndrome

Many newborns with meconium aspiration syndrome (MAS) at birth will transition and have no evidence of respiratory distress. Management for most newborns with MAS is supportive. For newborns with signs of respiratory distress after a meconium delivery, admission to the neonatal intensive care unit is necessary.

RESPIRATORY SUPPORT

Oxygen therapy via oxygen hood: maintain oxygen saturation >95% (Pao_2 55-90 mm Hg)

Assisted ventilation

CPAP providing 5-7 cm water may be useful when fractional inspired oxygen requirements exceed 0.4-0.5 (40-50% oxygen)

Close monitoring is important because air trapping may result in hyperinflation and air leak (pneumomediastinum, pneumothorax)

Mechanical ventilation may be needed if the Pao_2 cannot be maintained >55 mm Hg with a fractional inspired oxygen >0.6 or if severe hypercarbia develops, $Paco_2$ exceeds 55-60 mm Hg

High frequency ventilation may be used if the newborn is not responding to conventional ventilation

Exogenous surfactant and surfactant lavage

Sedation

Inhaled nitric oxide to improve oxygenation, especially in patients with persistent pulmonary hypertension of the newborn

Extra corporeal membrane oxygenation

Antibiotics

Maintain fluid and electrolyte balance

Monitor with serial chest radiographs

PREVENTION: ROLE OF SUCTIONING

Intrapartum suctioning:[a]

2006 American Heart Association Neonatal Resuscitation Guidelines[b] no longer recommend routine intrapartum suctioning of meconium stained infants.

Tracheal suctioning:

1/3 of infants born through meconium stained amniotic fluid will have meconium in their trachea after delivery even with intrapartum suctioning.

Suctioning is not recommended for the vigorous meconium-stained newborn it does not improve outcomes and may cause complications.

Tracheal suctioning should be performed before positive-pressure ventilation in meconium-stained infants who are apneic or exhibit respiratory distress, even if previously vigorous.[c]

CPAP, Continuous positive airway pressure; *Pao_2, arterial pressure of oxygen, $Paco_2$, partial pressure of carbon dioxide.*

[a]*Vain FE, Prudent LM, Wiswell T, et al. Oropharyngeal and nasopharyngeal suctioning of meconium stained neonates before delivery of their shoulders; multi-centered, randomized trial. Lancet.* 2004;364:597-602.

[b]Kattwinkel J, Ed. Textbook of Neonatal Resuscitation. Elk Grove Village, IL: American Academy of Pediatrics and American Heart Association; 2006.

[c]Dargaville PA, Copnell B, for the Australian and New Zealand Neonatal Network. The epidemiology of meconium aspiration syndrome: incidence, risk factors, therapies and outcomes. *Pediatrics.* 2006;117:1712-1772.

BOX 99-6 Pathogens Causing Pneumonia in Neonates

PRENATAL
Adenovirus
Rubella
Herpes
Mumps
Cytomegalovirus
Toxoplasma gondii
Mycobacterium tuberculosis
Listeria monocytogenes
Varicella
HIV

INTRAPARTUM
Group B *Streptococcus*
Escherichia coli
Klebsiella species
Syphilis
Neisseria gonorrhoeae
Chlamydia trachomatis—typically does not occur until after 2 weeks of age

POSTNATAL
Various gram-negative and gram-positive bacteria
Viruses (respiratory syncytial virus, adenovirus, influenza virus, and others)

BOX 99-7 Prenatal Risk Factors for Congenital Pneumonia

Unexplained preterm labor
Rupture of membranes before the onset of labor
Membrane rupture more than 18 hours before delivery
Maternal fever (>38° C [100.4° F])
Uterine tenderness
Foul-smelling amniotic fluid
Infection of the maternal genitourinary tract
Recurrent maternal urinary tract infection
Gestational history of illness consistent with an organism known to have transplacental pathogenic potential
Nonreassuring fetal well being test results
Fetal tachycardia
Meconium in the amniotic fluid
Infant with previous neonatal infection

compromise that, singly or in combination, increases the opportunity for a fetus to develop congenital pneumonia (Box 99-7).

Clinical manifestations of pneumonia are similar to other respiratory disorders in the newborn. Signs of respiratory distress may be seen. Fever or other systemic signs may be present. Systemic findings often mirror manifestations seen with sepsis or other severe infections. A variety of chest radiograph findings may be present in a newborn with pneumonia, such as air bronchograms, diffuse parenchymal infiltrates, lobar consolidation, or pleural effusions. Radiographic findings in group B streptococcal pneumonia may be similar to the reticular granular pattern seen in RDS.

Treatment includes respiratory support, including oxygen and ventilation if necessary. Broad-spectrum antibiotics must be started expeditiously. If an infecting organism is identified, then antibiotic therapy can be adjusted to the specific organism. Failure to consider the diagnosis in the absence of maternal risk factors for infection and failure to initiate neonatal antibiotics in a timely manner may be a medical-legal pitfall.

Blood counts and blood culture should be obtained. Routine culture of spinal fluid is controversial. Endotracheal culture soon after intubation may be useful. Quantitative measurements of C-reactive protein and other acute-phase reactants have limited positive predictive value. Decisions about antimicrobial treatment should not be based on inflammatory markers alone. Neonates should receive adequate nutritional support and hydration.

Apnea in Newborns

Apnea occurs in all infants and is considered normal if it occurs infrequently, is brief, and is not associated with any underlying conditions or other signs. Healthy infants have occasional apnea episodes of 10 to 12 seconds during the 1st year of life. Periodic breathing is also common during the first 6 months of life but occurs for less than 1% of the infant's sleep time. Prolonged apnea may occur as a nonspecific sign of illness in both full-term and premature infants.[16] Box 99-8 lists common conditions associated with apnea in neonates. (See also Chapter 330, Sudden Infant Death Syndrome.)

Evaluation of the neonate who exhibits apnea is warranted if apnea develops within 24 hours of birth; if the infant is born after 36 weeks of gestation or requires vigorous resuscitation; if the episode is preceded by or associated with marked cyanosis, pallor, or change in muscle tone; or if the episodes become more frequent and increase in severity. The specific diagnostic tests are chosen based on the newborn's gestational and postmenstrual age, presenting symptoms and physical examination, underlying medical problems, and the extent of resuscitation or intervention required to stabilize the newborn. Typical testing of a symptomatic neonate with unexplained apnea, bradycardia, or cyanosis includes a complete blood count, glucose and electrolyte determinations, sepsis evaluation (blood, urine, and cerebral spinal fluid cultures), and continuous multichannel recording with esophageal pH monitoring. A thorough review of the maternal history for evidence of medication use that can induce fetal CNS and respiratory depression (over-the-counter products [including herbal agents], illicit drugs, or prescribed medications and labor pain relief) is necessary. Consideration should also be given to sending a sample of the newborn's urine for toxicologic testing for drugs of abuse based on the newborn's signs and clinical history. (See Chapter 103, Prenatal Drug Abuse and Neonatal Withdrawal Syndrome.) If seizures or other CNS abnormalities are suspected, then the newborn should undergo a CT scan of the head and an electroencephalographic evaluation. If a dysrhythmia is suspected, then the newborn will require chest radiographic, electrocardiographic, and Holter monitoring studies. The newborn with a choking episode will benefit from evaluation of the newborn's airway, feeding skills, and for the presence of symptomatic gastroesophageal

BOX 99-8 Common Conditions Associated With Apnea in Neonates

ACUTE CONDITIONS
Airway obstruction
Neck flexion
Laryngospasm
Structural abnormality—glossoptosis, laryngomalacia, tracheomalacia
Central nervous system disorders
Intracranial hemorrhage
Seizures
Hypoxic-ischemic injury
Congenital malformations of the brain—Arnold-Chiari malformation
Drugs administered to the mother or to the baby
- Narcotics or central nervous system depressants
- Prostaglandin E_1-used to maintain patency of the ductus arteriosus in infants with suspected duct-dependent congenital heart disease

Infection
- Sepsis, meningitis, necrotizing enterocolitis
- Respiratory syncytial virus infection, pertussis, infantile botulism
- Impaired oxygenation, hypoxemia, severe anemia, and shock or marked systemic to pulmonary circulatory shunt (eg, patent ductus arteriosus)

Metabolic disorders
- Hypoglycemia
- Hypercalcemia
- Hyponatremia, hypernatremia
- Hyperammonemia—inborn errors of metabolism
- Postoperative status following general anesthesia
- Thermal instability (ie, rapid increase or decrease of temperature)

CHRONIC CONDITIONS
Chronic lung disease
Congenital central hypoventilation syndrome (formerly known as Ondine curse)
Gastroesophageal reflux disease
Marked anemia

Adapted from Spitzer A. Apnea syndromes. In: Donn SM, Sinha SK, eds. *Manual of Neonatal Respiratory Care*. 2nd ed. St Louis, MO: Mosby; 2006. Copyright Elsevier, 2006. Used by permission.

reflux disease. Subspecialist consultations may include cardiology, neurology, pulmonary, or other specialists as needed based on the newborn's clinical condition. The initial nursery management of the neonate with apnea will include specific therapies needed to reestablish adequate oxygenation and ventilation, as well as cardiac and hemodynamic stability. Treatment may range from simple tactile stimulation and supplemental oxygen to intubation and assisted ventilation. Pharmacologic therapy will be based on the assessment of the condition causing the apnea and may include methylxanthines, antiepileptic drugs, or medications for correcting metabolic abnormalities. Specific management strategies are beyond the scope of this chapter.[17] Commonly used terminology is defined in Box 99-9. See Chapter 330, Sudden Infant Death Syndrome, for treatment guidance including indications for methylxanthines therapy and home monitoring.

BOX 99-9 Apnea Terminology

Pathological apnea is apnea exceeding 20 seconds' duration or apnea of shorter than 20 seconds if it is accompanied by bradycardia, pallor, cyanosis, hypotonia, or oxygen desaturation. Apnea is classified as central, obstructive, or mixed.

- *Central apnea* is the cessation of both airflow and respiratory effort.
- *Obstructive apnea* is the cessation of airflow in the presence of continued respiratory effort.
- *Mixed apnea* contains elements of both central and obstructive apnea, either within the same apneic pause or at different times during a period of respiratory recording. It may start as an obstructive apnea but is followed by central apnea.

Periodic breathing is a respiratory pattern characterized by 3 or more consecutive respiratory pauses that are greater than 3 but less than 20 seconds in duration separated by less than 20 seconds of breathing between each pause. Periodic breathing is centrally mediated as a result of immaturity of the central nervous system respiratory control center.

Apnea of prematurity (AOP) usually begins after the 1st day of life and resolves when the infant reaches 37 weeks' postmenstrual age. AOP may occasionally persist to 44 to 48 weeks' postmenstrual age.

Apnea of infancy (AOI) occurs in infants who are more than 37 weeks' gestation. No specific cause is identified in infants with AOI.

Apparent life-threatening event refers to an event that is characterized by some combination of apnea, color change (pallor, cyanosis), choking, or gagging and marked change in muscle tone (limp or hypotonic or arching or hypertonic).

OTHER CAUSES OF RESPIRATORY DISTRESS IN NEWBORNS

Pulmonary Air Leak Syndrome: Pneumomediastinum and Pneumothorax

Pulmonary air leak is caused by alveolar rupture with leakage of air into extra-avleolar spaces within the lung. Air leaks occur more commonly during the newborn period than at other times in life. Forms of air leak include pneumothorax, pneumomediastinum, pulmonary interstitial emphysema, pneumopericardium, and, less frequently, pneumoperitoneum and subcutaneous emphysema.

Pneumothorax is one form of air leak syndrome that may occur in neonates either iatrogenically or spontaneously. Pneumothoraces may remain undetected in asymptomatic neonates or may cause respiratory distress. Several factors may cause a pneumothorax,

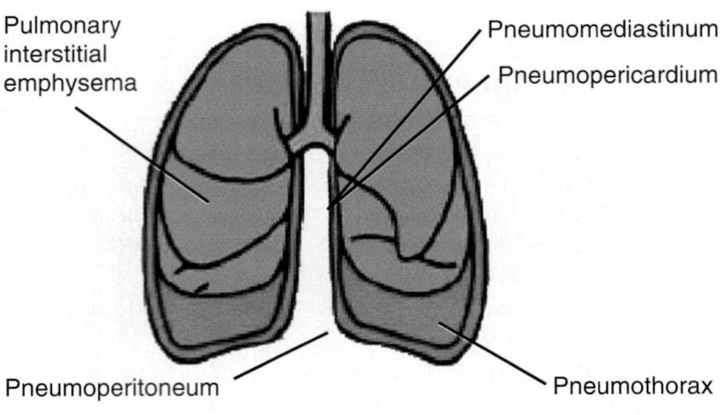

Figure 99-4 Air leak syndrome. *(Aly H. Respiratory disorders in the newborn: identification and diagnosis.* Pediatr Rev. *2004;256:201-208.)*

including overly vigorous stimulation and resuscitation at birth, RDS, MAS, pneumonia, pulmonary hypoplasia, and assisted ventilation (CPAP and positive-pressure ventilation). Generalized air trapping or uneven ventilation leads to overdistension of the lung and predisposes the infant to alveolar rupture with dissection of air along the perivascular/peribronchial tissue towards the hilum, producing a pneumomedistinum or into the pleura, thereby causing a pneumothorax. Figure 99-4 depicts the forms of air leak.

The incidence of spontaneous pneumothorax varies from 0.3% to 1.3% based on clinical symptoms or on radiographic findings. A spontaneous pneumothorax may result from rupture of alveoli secondary to high inspiratory pressures needed to expand uninflated lungs. The incidence of air leak is higher among all gestational age groups of premature infants as a result of their increased risk for lung disease and need for resuscitation and assisted ventilation.[18]

A newborn who develops a pneumothorax may exhibit signs such as tachypnea, grunting, pallor, or cyanosis. Physical examination may reveal chest asymmetry with enlargement on the affected side, decreased breath sounds on the side with the pneumothorax, and a shift of the maximal cardiac impulse away from the affected side. A newborn who develops a tension pneumothorax may deteriorate rapidly, exhibiting bradycardia, hypotension, and hypoxemia caused by decreased venous return to the heart, thereby causing a drop in cardiac output. If a pneumothorax is suspected, then transillumination of the chest is a useful technique for immediate diagnosis. Neonates diagnosed with an air leak, whether a pneumothorax or pneumomediastinum, should be admitted to the NICU for further monitoring and treatment. Although most newborns with a pneumomediastinum will not be symptomatic, newborns with larger collections of mediastinal air will exhibit tachypnea and cyanosis. The heart sounds may sound distant on auscultation. A chest radiograph will confirm the presence of a pneumothorax and other forms of air leak (Figures 99-5 and 99-6). If the infant is stable, without signs of respiratory distress or a continuous air leak, and the pneumothorax isolated and small, then the infant can be monitored closely without specific intervention. Administration of 100% oxygen to an infant with an air leak accelerates the resolution of pneumothorax. Oxygen should be administered for 8 to 12 hours and the chest radiograph repeated after oxygen therapy. The majority of infants can be managed conservatively. Thoracentesis is necessary when the infant has a tension pneumothorax or requires ventilation. A thoracostomy, or chest tube, is placed into the anterior pleural space and connected to an underwater seal with continuous-suction pressure of 10 cm to 15 cm water. The chest tube remains in place until the air leak has resolved.

Disorders of Lung Development

Congenital errors in lymphatic development are a group of rare conditions that result in primary pulmonary lymphatic disorders and are often misdiagnosed.[19] The constellation of conditions includes lymphangiomas, lymphangiectasis, lymphangiomatosis, and lymphatic dysplasia syndrome. Pulmonary lymphangiectasis is caused by pathological dilation of the lymphatics and has primary and secondary forms. The primary or congenital form occurs in neonates, is typically fatal, and is presumed to result from failure of the pulmonary interstitial tissue to regress. This form results in dilation of the lymphatic capillaries in the developing lung. Secondary lymphangiectasis in neonates is a complication that may occur after surgery, infection, or trauma. Infants with total anomalous pulmonary venous return or hypoplastic left heart syndrome may develop dilated lymphatics as a result of increased lymphatic circulation.

Lymphatic Dysplasia Syndrome

Lymphatic dysplasia syndrome is a heterogeneous group of disorders that includes idiopathic or primary lymphedema and congenital chylothorax. The neonatal form of primary lymphedema is termed *lymphedema congenita*. Abnormal lymphatic development is associated with genetic disorders and variable inheritance patterns. Most chylous effusions in neonates are congenital.

Treatment is determined by the underlying condition. Congenital lymphangiomas do not resolve spontaneously and require resection or sclerosis. Congenital chylothorax and lymphangiectasis are treated with a combination of a high-protein, low-fat diet that provides medium-chain triglycerides as the fat source. Portagen is the usual infant formula used for infant nutrition. Supplemental vitamins are also needed. Large pleural effusions need drainage and may require chest tube placement, if persistent.

Congenital Diaphragmatic Hernia

Congenital diaphragmatic hernia (CDH) is a developmental abnormality of the diaphragm that allows abdominal organs to herniate into the chest. CDH occurs in 1 in 2000 to 4000 live births and has a male predominance among affected infants. Newborns typically show signs of respiratory distress in the delivery room or during the first hours of life. The degree of respiratory distress will vary with the severity of the defect and degree of pulmonary compromise as a

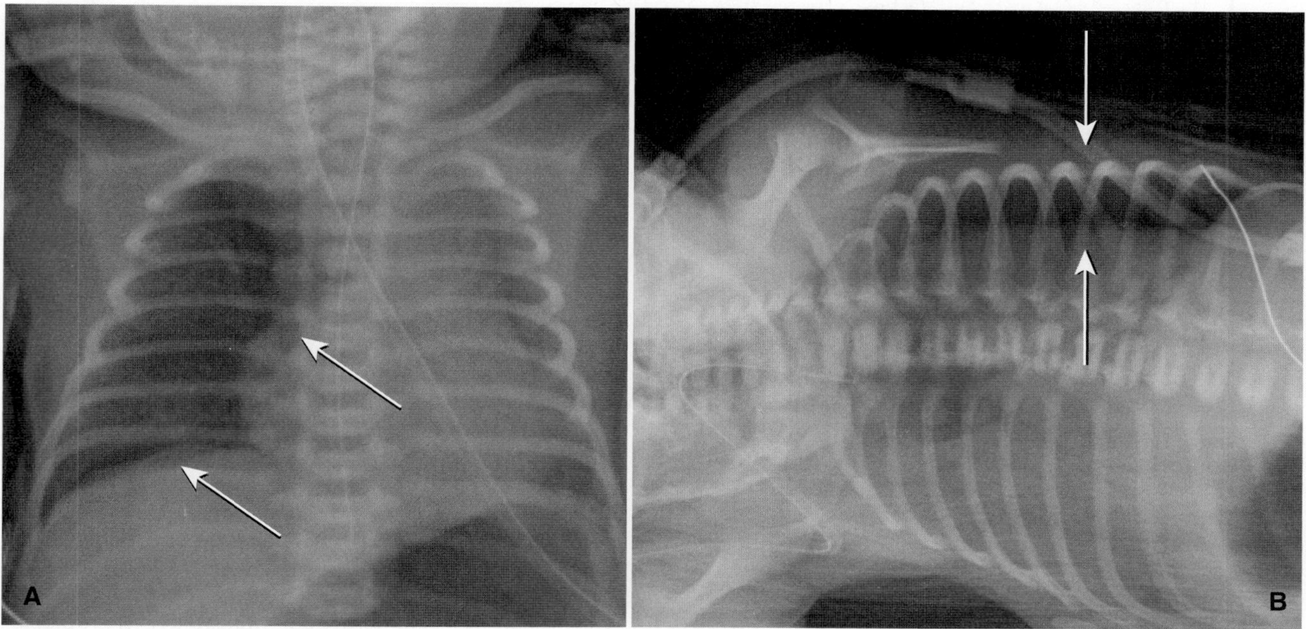

Figure 99-5 Anterior-posterior and lateral chest radiograph: full-term newborn with respiratory distress caused by right-sided pneumothorax. Note the flattening of the diaphragm and shift of the cardiothymic silhouette into the left hemithorax.

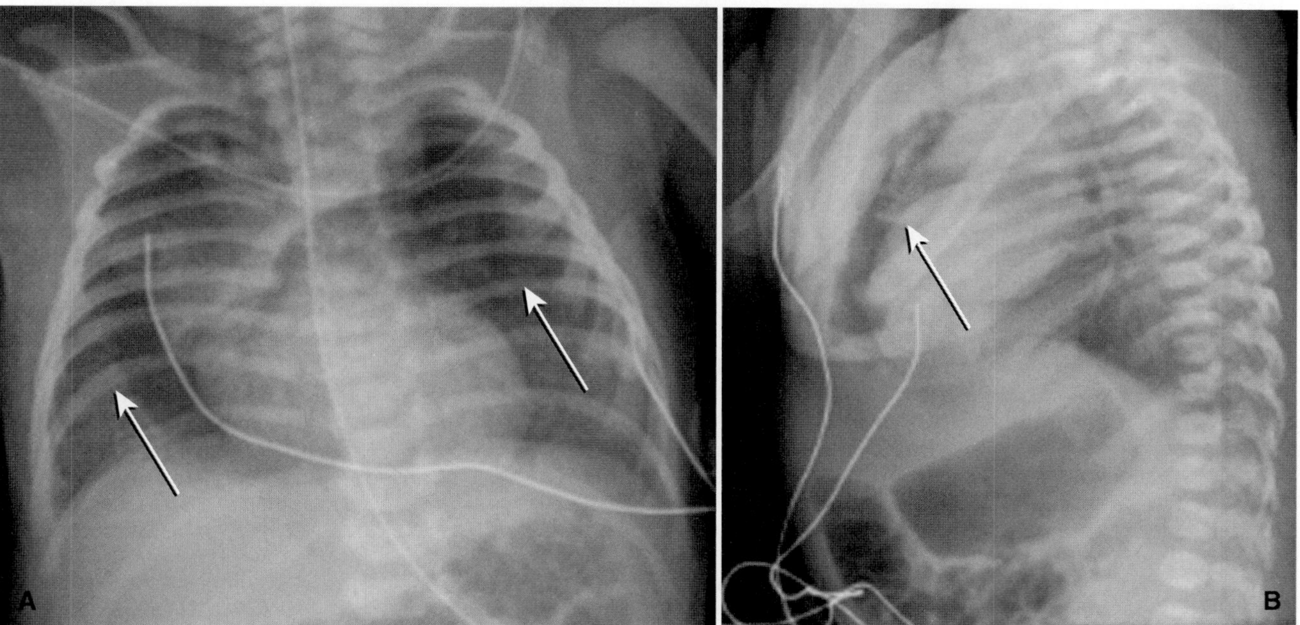

Figure 99-6 Full-term infant with large pneumomediastinum: characteristic *halo* around the heart with lifting of the right lobe of the thymus on the anterior-posterior view and lucency in the mediastinal space on the lateral film.

result of lung hypoplasia. The defect responsible for development of CDH is failure of the posterior growth of the diaphragm at the left Bochdalek foramen. This defect occurs at approximately 8 weeks' gestation during embryogenesis. The extent of abdominal organ herniation into the chest will influence the severity of lung hypoplasia and severity of infant symptoms. Lung hypoplasia is most severe on the side with the hernia, but it may also involve the contralateral side. Although the majority of CDH involves the left-sided diaphragm, right-sided lesions occur in approximately 11% of affected infants. Right-sided lesions tend to be less severe, given that the liver prevents the other abdominal organs from migrating into the chest. Bilateral diaphragm involvement occurs infrequently (2% of patients with CDH). Pulmonary hypoplasia predisposes infants born with CDH to the development of persistent pulmonary hypertension and respiratory failure.

Physical examination is notable for a barrel-shaped chest with a scaphoid abdomen. Breath sounds are absent on the affected side, and the heartbeat is displaced to the right as a result of mediastinal shift to the right. Fifty percent of infants with CDH will have associated anomalies, including chromosomal abnormalities, congenital heart disease, and neural tube defects. Many infants with CDH are diagnosed prenatally. (See Chapter 70, Prenatal Diagnosis; and Chapter 71, Fetal Interventions.) Among infants who have not been diagnosed through prenatal ultrasonography, the diagnosis is confirmed by chest radiograph. Characteristic findings include herniation of the abdominal contents (intestine, liver, and spleen) into the chest. The heart and mediastinum will be displaced, and the involved lung will appear small.

Initial treatment involves stabilization of respiration with support for hemodynamic and cardiac function as needed. Neonates with a prenatal diagnosis of CDH should be immediately intubated. Low-volume ventilation strategies using higher ventilation rates are used to minimize lung injury. The Pao_2 should be maintained above 55 mm Hg (oxygen saturation >90%) and mean arterial blood pressure should be above 50 mm Hg to reduce right-to-left shunting that will promote pulmonary hypertension. A nasogastric tube should also be placed expeditiously to reduce intestinal distension, given that this situation will further compromise respiratory function. Maintaining adequate oxygenation, blood pressure, and acid-base status are critical steps in the early care of infants with CDH. Adjunctive therapies used in conjunction with surgical repair include high frequency ventilation, inhaled nitric oxide, and ECMO. Before initiating ECMO, infants require a full evaluation that includes echocardiography, neural and renal sonography, and an electroencephalogram. Eligibility criteria for ECMO therapy require an infant to be older than 34 weeks' gestation with a weight above 2000 grams. Infants cannot have more than a grade I intraventricular hemorrhage or any congenital or chromosomal anomalies. Survival rates among neonates deemed surgical candidates are 60% to 80%.

Other developmental lung anomaly lesions should also be considered when a CDH is suspected prenatally. These congenital lung masses, often identified as echogenic structures on prenatal sonography, are congenital cystic adenomatoid malformation (CCAM), congenital lobar emphysema (CLE), pulmonary sequestrations, and bronchogenic cysts.

Congenital Cystic Adenomatoid Malformation

Congenital Cystic Adenomatoid Malformation (CCAM) is a rare anomaly that is estimated to occur at a rate of 1 in 25,000 to 35,000 pregnancies involving abnormal lung branching. The resulting hamartomas are composed of cystic and adenomatous overgrowth of the terminal bronchioles. CCAMs typically connect to the tracheobronchial tree and may be found in any lobe of either lung. The connecting bronchi are typically abnormal. Four types of CCAM have been identified, and these are classified depending on the affected area of the tracheobronchial tree and the stage of lung development when the abnormality occurs. The occurrence of CCAM is sporadic, has no racial preference, and affects male and female infants equally. Hydrops may occur in up to 40% of infants with a CCAM. Serial prenatal sonography has shown that nearly 60% of CCAMs will regress over the period of gestation.[21,22]

Approximately two thirds of neonates with a CCAM will exhibit at birth with tachypnea, grunting, retractions, cyanosis, and increased respiratory effort. The severity of the symptoms correlates with the lesion's size. The prognosis depends on the type of CCAM. Most CCAMs that occur in the neonatal period are type 1. Type 2 lesions also occur in the neonatal period but are associated with other congenital anomalies in 60% of affected infants. Type 3 CCAM is the most severe, with resultant fetal hydrops, pulmonary hypoplasia, and high mortality rate. Treatment involves resection of the CCAM postnatally.

Congenital Lobar Emphysema

Congenital Lobar Emphysema (CLE) is typically diagnosed after birth and is characterized by air trapping with progressive hyperinflation of lobar segments of the lungs that leads to airway obstruction.[23] CLE is a rare malformation that appears to have a male predominance. The reported prevalence rate is 1 in 20,000 to 30,000 births. The majority of infants with CLE will be symptomatic by 6 months of age. Up to one third of affected infants will exhibit symptoms at birth, with 50% symptomatic by 1 month of age. Respiratory distress may be mild or rapidly progressive.

Physical examination is notable for tachypnea, increased work of breathing, and wheezing. Breath sounds over the involved lobe of the lung are diminished with hyperresonance on chest percussion. If mediastinal shift is present, then the cardiac impulse may be displaced. Some infants will have associated congenital anomalies affecting the heart, kidneys, gastrointestinal tract, musculoskeletal system, and the skin. Difficulty with weight gain caused by poor feeding and recurrent pneumonias may comprise the presenting symptoms in the infant with a milder form of CLE. Diagnostic imaging includes chest radiography and CT or MRI. On chest radiograph the affected lobe may appear either consolidated or hyperinflated depending on the degree of lobar expansion. Additional findings include mediastinal shift with compression and atelectasis of the contralateral lung. CT scanning may be helpful in identifying the diagnosis in infants with persistent respiratory distress and is also useful in the postnatal assessment of the neonate with a prenatal sonographic finding of a pulmonary lesion. Included in the differential diagnosis of infants with CLE are pneumothorax, isolated pulmonary interstitial emphysema, CCAM, CDH, pulmonary sequestration, and bronchogenic cysts. Treatment in symptomatic infants is resection of the affected lobe.[24-26]

Bronchopulmonary Sequestrations

Bronchopulmonary sequestrations are lobar sequestrations of abnormal, nonfunctioning lung tissue found in the lower respiratory tract. Extremely rare, sequestrations do not connect to the tracheobronchial tree and derive their blood flow from the systemic circulation, usually through a blood vessel originating from the aorta. Sequestrations are composed on normal lung tissue that contains both airway and alveolar elements. Sequestrations are of 2 types. Intralobar sequestrations are localized within a normal lobe of the lung but without separate pleura. They are typically located in a lower lobe and are slightly more common on the left side. Intralobar sequestrations are more common than the extralobar form of sequestration. Extralobar sequestrations are composed of lung tissue encased in its own pleura that is located outside the normal lung lobe. Lesions are more likely to be found on the left side, often located between the lower lobe and diaphragm. Male infants appear more often affected than female infants, and 2 out of 3 of infants will have associated anomalies (CDH, pericardial defects, and anomalous pulmonary venous return). A gene has been identified that is necessary for normal airway development and branching.

Respiratory symptoms at birth are variable and related to the lesion's location, size, and type. Lesions may be identified on prenatal sonography. The majority of lesions regress over the course of gestation. If vascular compression develops because of a large lesion, then hydrops may develop. Extralobar sequestrations tend to present earlier than intralobar lesions. Chest radiographs show a sequestration as a dense mass in the thoracic cavity or lung parenchyma. Sonography will also demonstrate an echogenic homogeneous mass. CT scan and MRI characterize associated abnormalities and identify the aberrant arterial and venous blood supply to the sequestered lobe. Treatment involves immediate surgical resection in symptomatic infants.

Overall, developmental disorders of lung development, particularly cystic lung masses, have a favorable prognosis among infants who do not have severe respiratory distress or hydrops.[27,28] The generalized use of prenatal sonography has lead to earlier and more frequent diagnosis of suspected fetal anomalies. Questions arise as to the need for postnatal evaluation of pulmonary lesions that appear to be regressing on serial fetal sonography. In addition, investigators have reported continued postnatal regression of congenital lung lesions.[29] The current consensus is that prenatal ultrasonography is limited in its ability to assess fully echogenic lesions and that apparent involution of these lesions on prenatal sonography and postnatal chest radiography may miss residual lung lesions. Therefore, in the postnatal period, early evaluation is warranted.[24,30,31]

Tracheoesophageal Fistula and Esophageal Atresia

Esophageal atresia and tracheoesophageal fistula may occur as separate lesions but more often occur together. The classification is based on anatomy, as well as certain features that are therapeutically important. Important features are the presence or absence of a fistula and the location of the fistula. The most common type (85%) consists of an upper esophageal segment that ends in a blind pouch and the lower esophageal segment is connected to the trachea by a fistulous tract. The anomaly should be suspected in the presence of maternal polyhydramnios, excessive oral secretions, and choking, coughing, and cyanosis after the 1st feeding. Associated malformations such as cardiovascular abnormalities, imperforate anus, intestinal malrotation, and duodenal anomalies may occur. An association among vertebral anomalies, anal atresia, tracheoesophageal fistula, and radial limb dysplasia is also known as Vater syndrome. The diagnosis is confirmed by radiopaque catheter and observing coiling in the esophageal pouch on radiographic examination. The surgical correction is undertaken when the infant is stable. Follow-up complications include dysfunction of the esophageal motility, gastroesophageal reflux, chronic cough, wheezing, and recurrent pneumonia.

REFERENCES

1. Dunn MS, Reilly MC. Approaches to the initial respiratory management of preterm neonates. *Pediatr Resp Rev.* 2003;4:2-8.
2. Sasidharan P. An approach to diagnosis and management of cyanosis and tachypnea in term infants. *Pediatr Clin North Am.* 2004;51:999-1021.
3. Escobar GJ, Greene JD, Hulac P, et al. Rehospitalization after birth hospitalization: patterns among infants of all gestations. *Arch Dis Child.* 2005;90:125-131.
4. Clark RH. The epidemiology of respiratory failure in neonates born at an estimated gestational age of 34 weeks or more. *J Perinatol.* 2005;25:251-257.
5. Halliday HI. Elective delivery at "term": implications for the newborn. *Arch Paediatr.* 1999;88:1180-1181.
6. National Institutes of Health. State-of-the-Science Conference statement: Cesarean Delivery on Demand, Bethesda, MD, March 27-29, 2006.
7. Morris SJ. Radiology of the chest in neonates. *Curr Paediatr.* 2003;13:460-468.
8. Franken EA, Yu PI, Smith WL, et al. Initial chest radiography in the neonatal intensive care unit: value of the lateral view. *Am J Radiol.* 1979;133:4345.
9. Ankerman T, Oppermann HC, Engler S, et al. Congenital masses of the lung, cystic adenomatoid malformation versus congenital lobar emphysema. *J Ultrasound Ed.* 2004;23:1379-1384.
10. Bland RD. Lung fluid balance during development. *NeoReviews.* 2005;6(6):e255-e265.
11. Rodriquez RR. Management of respiratory distress syndrome: an update. *Respiratory Care.* 2003;48:279-286.
12. Merrill J, Ballard R. Clinical use of antenatal corticosteroids: benefits and risks. *NeoReviews.* 2000;1(5):e91-e105.
13. Cleary GM, Wiswell TE. Meconium-stained amniotic fluid and meconium aspiration syndrome: an update. *Pediatr Clin North Am.* 1998;45:511-529.
14. Kattwinkel J, ed. *Textbook of Neonatal Resuscitation.* Elk Grove Village, IL: American Academy of Pediatrics and American Heart Association; 2006.
15. Swaminathan S, Quinn J, Satbile MW, et al. Long-term pulmonary sequelae of meconium aspiration syndrome. *J Pediatr.* 1989;114:356-361.
16. Kelly DH, Stellwagen LM, Kaitz E, et al. Apnea and periodic breathing in normal full-term infants during the first twelve months. *Pediatr Pulmonol.* 1985;1:215-219.

17. American Academy of Pediatrics, Committee on Fetus and Newborn. Apnea, sudden infant death syndrome, and home monitoring. *Pediatrics*. 2003;111:914-917.
18. Escobar GJ, McCormick MC, Zupancic JAF, et al. Unstudied infants: outcomes of moderately premature infants in the neonatal intensive care unit. *Arch Dis Child Fetal Neonatal Ed*. 2006;91:F238-F244.
19. Faul JL, Berry GI, Colby TV, et al. Thoracic lymphangiomas, lymphangiectasis, lymphangiomatosis and lymphatic dysplasia syndrome. *Am J Respir Crit Care Med*. 2000;161:1037-1046.
20. Yost CC, Soli RF. Early versus delayed selective surfactant treatment for neonatal respiratory distress syndrome (Cochrane Review). In: *The Cochrane Library*. Issue 1. Oxford, UK: Update Software; 2002.
21. Laberge JM, Flageole H, Pugash D, et al. Outcome of the prenatally diagnosed congenital cystic adenomatoid malformation: a Canadian experience. *Fetal Diagn Ther*. 2001;16:178-186.
22. Duncombe GJ, Dickinson JE, Kikiros CS. Prenatal diagnosis and management of congenital cystic adenomatoid malformation of the lung. *Am J Obstet Gynecol*. 2002; 187:950-954.
23. Ozcelik U, Gocmen A, Kiper N, et al. Congenital lobar emphysema: evaluation and long-term follow-up of thirty cases at a single center. *Pediatr Pulmonol*. 2003; 35:384.
24. Stanton M, Davenport M. Management of congenital lung lesion. *Early Human Dev*. 2006;82:289.
25. Olutoye OO, Coleman BG, Hubbard AM, et al. Prenatal diagnosis and management of congenital lobar emphysema. *J Pediatr Surg*. 2000;35:792.
26. Truitt AK, Carr SR, Cassese J, et al. Perinatal management of congenital cystic lung lesions in the age of minimally invasive surgery. *J Pediatr Surg*. 2006:41:893.
27. Illanes S, Hunter A, Evans M, et al. Prenatal diagnosis of echogenic lung: evolution and outcome. *Ultrasound Obstet Gynecol*. 2005;26(2):145-149.
28. Davenport M, Warne SA, Cacciaguerra S, et al. Current outcome of antenatally diagnosed cystic lung disease. *J Pediatr Surg*. 2004;39(4):549-556.
29. Butterworth SA, Balir GK. Postnatal spontaneous resolution of cystic adenomatoid malformations. *J Pediatr Surg*. 2005;40(5):832-834.
30. Lee HJH, Song MJ, Cho JY, et al. Echogenic fetal lung masses: comparison of prenatal sonographic and postnatal CT findings. *J Clin Ultrasound*. 2003;31(8):419-424.
31. Blau H, Barak A, Karmazyn B, et al. Postnatal management of resolving fetal lung lesions. *Pediatrics*. 2002;109:105-108.

Chapter 100

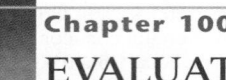

EVALUATION OF THE INFANT WITH SUSPECTED HEART DISEASE

Nicole J. Sutton, MD; Christine A. Walsh, MD

In the newborn, certain physical findings should lead to the suspicion of heart disease. The most common findings are a heart murmur, an arrhythmia, congestive heart failure, and cyanosis, and their evaluation can be performed in the primary care setting.

PREVALENCE OF CONGENITAL HEART DISEASE

The prevalence of congenital heart disease in infants in the United States is approximately 5 to 8 per 1000 live births. Of these patients, approximately 2.5 to 3 per 1000 live births will have critical heart disease that requires an intervention in the first year of life.[1] Virtually all pediatricians will see patients with congenital heart disease in their practice. The gender distribution is equal for congenital heart disease as a whole, but the male-to-female ratio varies widely among defects, with aortic stenosis; for example, more common in boys than in girls.[2,3]

Several population-based studies have been conducted in the United States to examine the prevalence of congenital heart disease. The Baltimore Washington Infant Study (BWIS)[4] is thought to be one of the most complete. The prevalence of congenital heart disease and associated risk factors were examined. The BWIS showed a significantly increased risk of congenital heart disease in children born to diabetic mothers (tetralogy of Fallot, truncus arteriosus), mothers with phenylketonuria, and mothers who abused alcohol (muscular ventricular septal defects). Overall, no racial differences were noted, but a subset analysis showed an increased proportion of white infants with Ebstein anomaly, aortic stenosis, coarctation of the aorta, transposition of the great vessels, and pulmonary atresia.[5] No difference associated with the presence or lack of early prenatal care was found, most likely because the heart is completely formed by 12 weeks of pregnancy, before most women know they are pregnant and have started prenatal care. The study also showed no effect of maternal or paternal age on the prevalence of congenital heart disease. The BWIS found a significant risk of heart disease in infants with a family history of congenital heart disease, especially if the affected relative was the mother or a full sibling. A strong correlation was found between heart disease and other congenital anomalies, with 28% of all cases having a chromosomal abnormality, a heritable syndrome, or another major organ system defect. Down syndrome was the most common association, representing 9% of all infants with congenital heart disease.

MURMURS

Murmurs are the product of turbulent blood flow. Approximately 60% of newborns will have a murmur auscultated in the newborn period. If babies were auscultated continuously from birth, nearly 100% of them would have the murmur of a closing patent ductus arteriosus (PDA). The vast majority of the murmurs of the neonatal period are benign in nature. An important point to remember is that a newborn may have a severe heart defect, for example, transposition of the great vessels, without having a murmur.

Benign Murmurs

The most common benign murmur is a peripheral pulmonary stenosis (PPS) murmur. This murmur is caused by turbulence in the branch pulmonary arteries after closure of the ductus arteriosus. It is generally a grade 1/6 to 2/6 short, early to mid systolic ejection murmur heard best over the axillae or the back. This murmur can be present bilaterally or unilaterally, and can be heard at birth or soon after. It should resolve by 6 months of age; if it does not, the infant should be referred to a cardiologist to ensure that the patient does not have pathological pulmonary artery branch stenosis, which may be associated with Williams syndrome or rubella syndrome.

The Still murmur can appear in neonates, although it is not as common in the newborn as it is in the older child. This early systolic ejection murmur is located at the left lower sternal border or near the apex and is distinguished by its low-pitched, vibratory, or humming quality. It sounds the same in the newborn and older child. If the pediatrician is comfortable with diagnosing a Still murmur, then these patients do not require a cardiologic evaluation. The murmur is not associated with any underlying pathological condition and typically disappears by puberty.

A very common cause of a murmur in the newborn period is a PDA. The PDA murmur of a newborn is different from the *machinery-type* murmur that is described in older children because the pulmonary vascular resistance is still high in the newborn period. The murmur becomes louder and longer as the ductus closes and the pulmonary vascular resistance falls. It generally starts as a short, low- to medium-pitched systolic crescendo murmur at the left upper sternal border that radiates to the left infraclavicular area. If the ductus arteriosus remains patent, the murmur will eventually become the medium- to high-pitched continuous *machinery-type* murmur of the older child. The normal PDA murmur should resolve in the first few days to weeks of life. If it persists past the first few months of life, the PDA is unlikely to close on its own, and the infant should be referred to a cardiologist.

Pathological Murmurs

The murmurs of congenital heart disease can be divided into 3 categories: (1) stenosis, (2) regurgitation, and (3) left-to-right shunt (Table 100-1).

The intensity of a murmur is not a good marker of the severity of the cardiac disease that is producing it. For example, the small amount of flow through a very small and restrictive ventricular septal defect (VSD) is very turbulent and produces a much louder murmur than the much greater but less turbulent flow through a very large VSD, which is likely to cause congestive heart failure. This feature is in sharp contrast to the murmurs of outflow tract obstruction, which become increasingly louder with increasing degrees of stenosis and turbulence. However, with a critical stenotic lesion, a complete loss of the murmur can occur because so little flow exists through the stenotic area

Table 100-1 Pathological Murmurs

LESION	PHYSICAL FINDINGS	ECG	CHEST X-RAY
STENOSIS			
Aortic stenosis	Grade 2/6-5/6 SEM at RUSB ± Systolic ejection click ± Thrill at suprasternal notch Radiates to carotids	LVH	Dilated aorta Normal PVMs
Pulmonic stenosis	Grade 2/6-5/6 SEM at LUSB ± Ejection click ± Thrill at LUSB Radiates to back	RVH, ± RAD	Dilated MPA Normal PVMs
REGURGITATION			
Mitral regurgitation	Grade 2/6-3/6 early systolic murmur, can be holosystolic at apex May be associated with midsystolic click if MVP Radiates to mid precordium	LAE, LVH	LAE, LVE
Tricuspid regurgitation	Grade 2/6-3/6 early systolic murmur, can be holosystolic at LLSB	RAE, IRBBB	Normal PVMs Possible RAE when severe
LEFT-TO-RIGHT SHUNT			
Atrial septal defect	Grade 2/6-3/6 SEM at LUSB; may not be present in infant ± Widely split, fixed second heart sound	RAD, IRBBB, RVH	Normal or cardiomegaly and increased PVMs
Ventricular septal defect	Grade 2/6-5/6 holosystolic murmur at LLSB; murmur may not be holosystolic with small VSD ± Thrill ± Loud P2	Normal or LVH, BVH	Normal or cardiomegaly and increased PVMs

BVH, Biventricular hypertrophy; *ECG,* electrocardiogram; *IRBBB,* incomplete right bundle branch block; *LAE,* left atrial enlargement; *LLSB,* left lower sternal border; *LUSB,* left upper sternal border; *LVE,* left ventricular enlargement; *LVH,* left ventricular hypertrophy; *MDR,* mid diastolic rumble; *MPA,* main pulmonary artery; *MVP,* mitral valve prolapse; *PVMs,* pulmonary vascular markings; *RAD,* right axis deviation; *RAE,* right atrial enlargement; *RUSB,* right upper sternal border; *RVH,* right ventricular hypertrophy; *SEM,* systolic ejection murmur. *VSD,* ventricular septal defect.

that the turbulence generating the murmur is very low. Newborns in severe congestive heart failure may not have a murmur until cardiac output is improved with anticongestive therapy. The loudness of the murmur must be placed in the larger context of the physical examination and presentation of the infant.

The murmur of transient tricuspid regurgitation can be heard in the newborn period. The regurgitation causing this murmur is generally not caused by a structural problem of the tricuspid valve itself, but instead by poor right ventricular function from severe pulmonary hypertension, persistent fetal circulation, neonatal asphyxia or fetal distress. It is a 1/6 to 3/6 medium-pitched regurgitant murmur best auscultated at the right lower sternal border. It is occasionally holosystolic and can be very prominent in the setting of severe pulmonary hypertension. This murmur is most frequently heard in the neonatal intensive care unit (NICU) and is generally not a murmur that is observed at an outpatient visit.

Physical Examination

In a healthy newborn, peripheral cyanosis (acrocyanosis) is common. In the normal neonatal cardiac examination, the point of maximal intensity may be at the left lower sternal border because of the hyperactivity of the right ventricle. The second heart sound may be single, and an ejection click indicative of pulmonary hypertension may be heard. Peripheral pulses are generally easy to palpate in the newborn and are accentuated in premature infants because of the lack of subcutaneous tissue.

When a murmur is heard, the examiner should analyze it in terms of intensity (grade 1/6 to 6/6), timing (systolic vs diastolic), location (of maximal intensity), transmission (eg, to the back), and quality (blowing, vibratory, harsh, or other qualities). These characteristics will suggest a differential diagnosis. For example, the Still murmur is a grade 2/6 to 3/6 vibratory, systolic ejection murmur heard best between the left lower sternal border and the apex without radiation. Abnormal physical findings that are vital to note are cyanosis, tachycardia, tachypnea, hepatomegaly, poor perfusion, and poor or discrepant pulses. These findings are discussed in more detail in the section on congestive heart failure.

Evaluation

If a murmur or other suggestion of heart disease is present, blood pressures must be obtained in the arms and a leg to rule out a coarctation of the aorta. In a healthy child the lower extremity blood pressures are approximately 10 mm Hg higher than the right arm pressure. In an infant, the right upper extremity and lower extremities may have a similar systolic blood pressure. The left subclavian artery can be involved in a coarctation; so the right arm blood pressure must be obtained. It is also important to obtain a left arm blood pressure because of the association of coarctation of the aorta with an aberrant right subclavian artery coming off the descending aorta below the coarctation, which would result in equal pressures in the right arm and the leg despite a coarctation. All of the blood pressures must be taken with the baby in the same state, for example, sleeping; otherwise, differences in the blood pressures may not be valid. In addition, the heart rate should be approximately the same throughout the process.

An electrocardiographic (ECG) evaluation should be performed on all patients with a heart murmur or other suggestion of heart disease. The ECG findings must be interpreted with regard to the axis of the P wave and QRS complex, right and left atrial and ventricular enlargement, ST-T changes, conduction abnormalities, rate, and rhythm. It must be read with knowledge of normal values for age because of the many changes that occur in the first weeks of life. The normal ECG of a newborn will show sinus rates of up to 180 beats/min. The axis can be as far rightward as plus-180 degrees. RV dominance is normal, even to the point of an occasional neonate having Q waves in V1. The examiner should make sure that any infant with a murmur or signs of congestive heart failure is in sinus rhythm (positive P waves in leads I, II, and AVF). A superior axis (0 to −150 degrees) is consistent with an endocardial cushion defect. A positive T wave in V1 after 3 days of age and a qR pattern in V1 are indicative of right ventricular hypertrophy. Specific voltage criteria exist for right and left ventricular hypertrophy at various ages. Right atrial enlargement is suggested by a P wave that is 3 mm tall or greater in any lead. In a newborn, left atrial enlargement is suggested by a P wave that is greater than 0.07 sec wide, often associated with notched P waves in the limb leads and biphasic P waves in V1. An incomplete right bundle branch block can be seen with an atrial septal defect, Ebstein anomaly, or a coarctation of the aorta in the newborn. A delta wave and short PR interval are hallmarks of Wolff-Parkinson-White (WPW) syndrome (Figure 100-1).

Oxygen saturations should be obtained in a preductal (right arm) and a postductal (foot) area to detect right-to-left shunting through the patent ductus arteriosus. This test is especially important in the immediate neonatal period. In addition, if the oxygen saturations are abnormal, a hyperoxia test should be performed. This test is described later in the discussion of cyanosis. A healthy 1-day-old infant may have an arterial pressure of oxygen (Pa_{O_2}) as low as 60 mm Hg.

Finally, a chest radiograph is frequently taken in the neonatal period when the patient is still in the hospital. A chest radiograph is less frequently performed when a murmur is detected in an office setting than it is in the hospital setting. Useful information can be gleaned from the chest radiograph, including the size, shape, and location of the heart; the status of the pulmonary vascular markings; and on which side the aortic arch is located. However, the size of the cardiac silhouette on chest radiograph is a poor predictor of the actual heart size.[6]

ARRHYTHMIAS

The easiest method of differentiating rhythm disturbances is to listen with a stethoscope. Is the rhythm too fast, too slow, or irregular but close to the normal rate?

Bradyarrhythmias

A slow heart rate is defined as being less than the 5th percentile for the age of the patient. A persistent heart

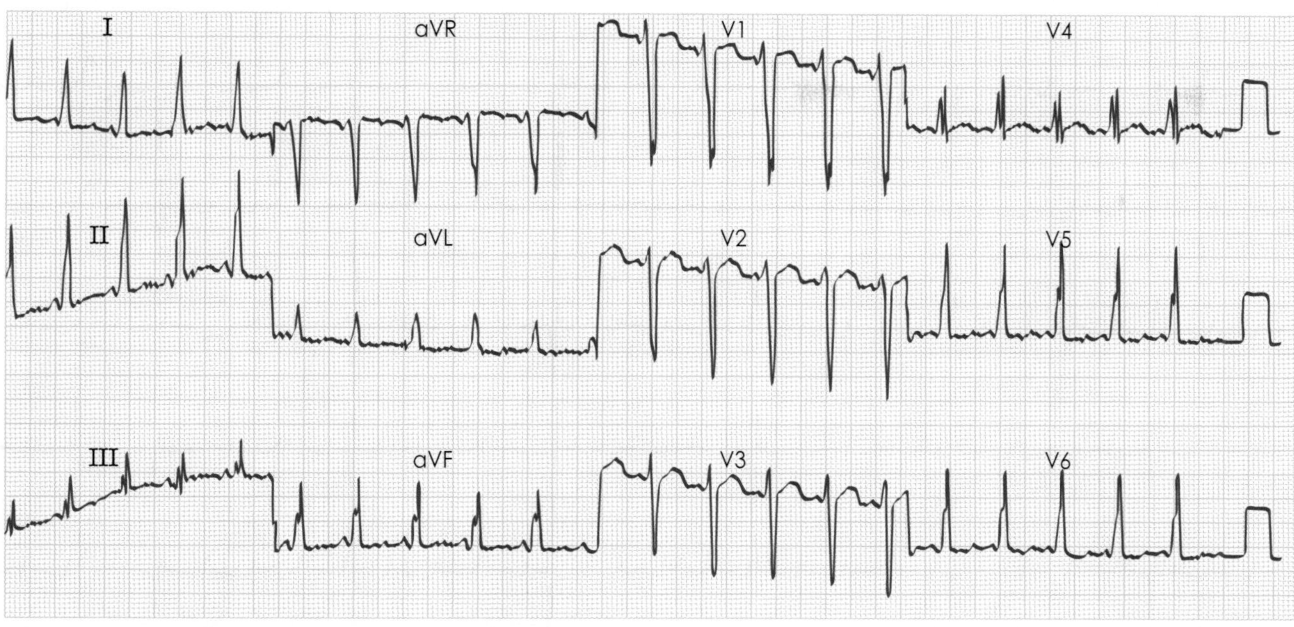

Figure 100-1 ECG showing a short PR interval and delta waves during normal sinus rhythm (Wolff-Parkinson-White syndrome) in a newborn.

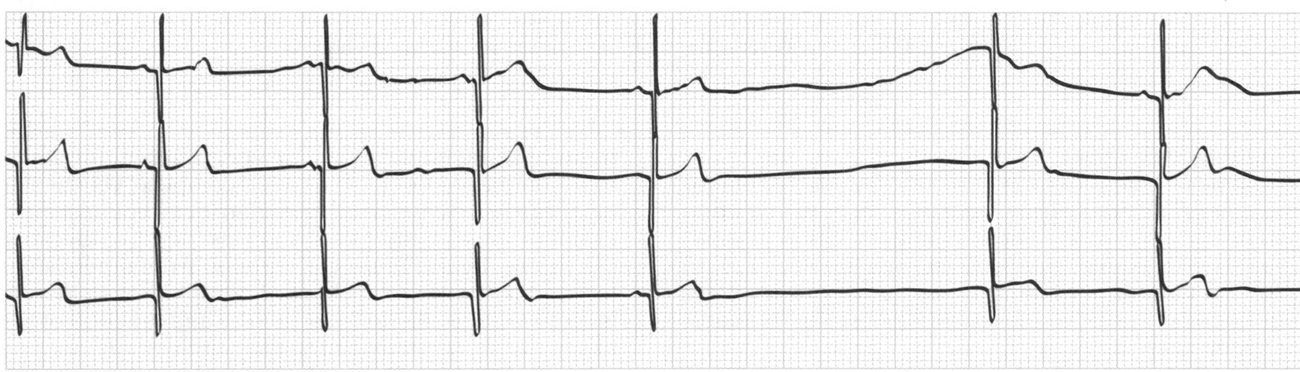

Figure 100-2 ECG showing sinus bradycardia with a 1.8-sec pause followed by a junctional escape beat in a premature newborn.

rate less than 80 beats/min is considered bradycardia in a newborn (Figure 100-2). Sinus bradycardia is seen more frequently in preterm than in term infants. Causes include maternal medication, neonatal asphyxia, increased intracranial pressure, sepsis, hypothyroidism, hypothermia, and hyperkalemia. The underlying cause of sinus bradycardia must be discovered and treated.

After sinus bradycardia, the most common cause of a slow heart rate in a neonate is congenital complete heart block (Figure 100-3), which is usually first noted during routine prenatal care. Congenital complete heart block is generally associated with maternal systemic lupus erythematosus, more specifically with anti-Ro and anti-La antibodies that attack the conduction tissue of the fetal heart. No correlation has been found between this pathological abnormality and structural heart disease. The low heart rate is generally well tolerated, and the fetus does not usually develop hydrops. When the babies are born, they appear clinically well, with a low resting heart rate, often in the 60- to 70-beats/min range. They usually do not require a pacemaker in the newborn period, but they need to be evaluated by a cardiologist when they are born. A pacemaker is indicated if the QRS is wide or if the heart rate is less than 50 to 55 beats/min in an infant with a normal heart, or less than 70 beats/min in an infant with congenital heart disease.[7] An echocardiographic examination should be performed after birth to evaluate structure and function, even if fetal echocardiograms were performed.

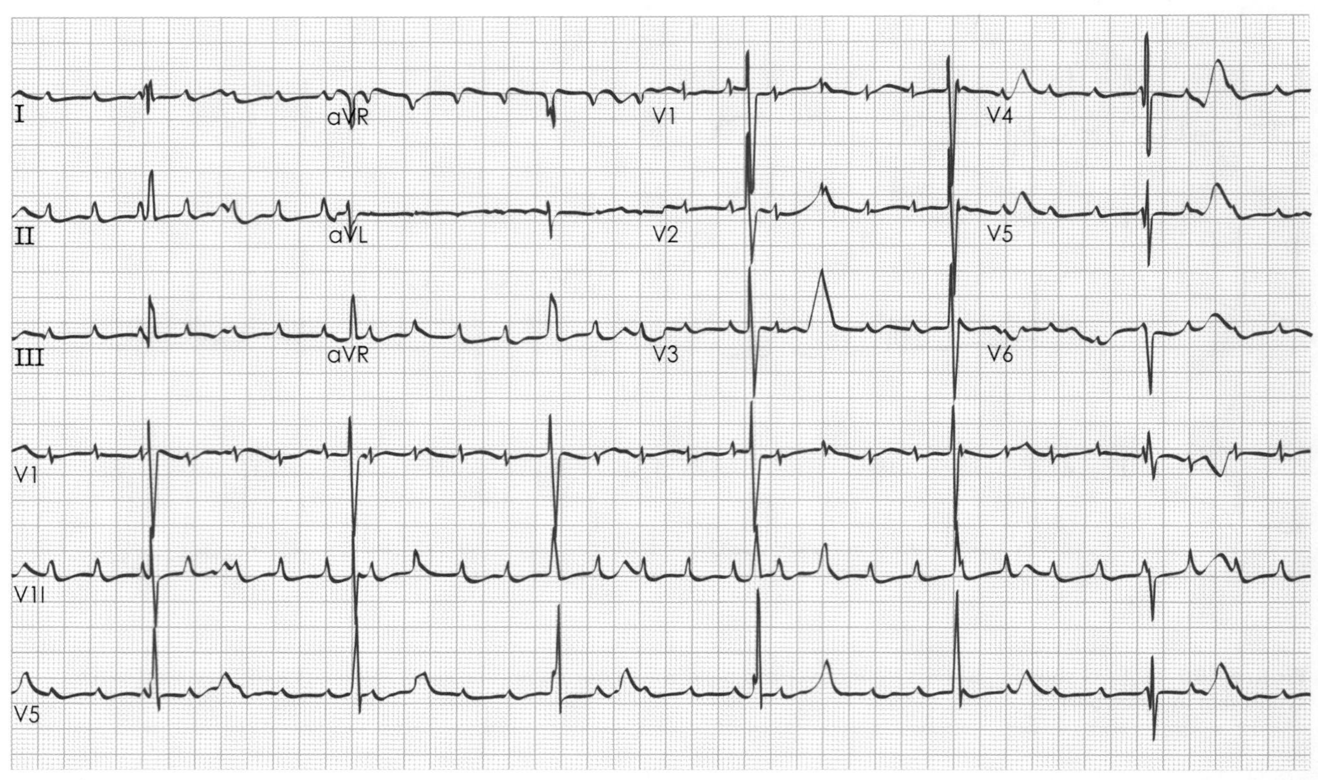

Figure 100-3 ECG reflecting complete heart block in a newborn.

Tachyarrhythmias

A fast heart rate is greater than the 95th percentile for the age of the child. Transient sinus tachycardia up to 190 beats/min is often seen in healthy newborns. However, the maximal rate should not exceed 220 to 230 beats/min in an infant. Rates above this level are not sinus because the sinus node is generally incapable of faster rates.

The most common childhood tachyarrhythmia (after sinus tachycardia) is supraventricular tachycardia (SVT), usually with a heart rate greater than 220 beats/min (Figure 100-4). The baseline ECG can be normal, or it can have a short PR interval and delta waves indicative of WPW syndrome that is present in 50% of newborns with SVT (see Figure 100-1). In addition to SVT, babies can also have atrial tachyarrhythmias such as ectopic atrial tachycardia, atrial flutter (Figure 100-5), and much less commonly atrial fibrillation. Other less common neonatal tachyarrhythmias are junctional ectopic tachycardia and ventricular tachycardia.

The normal QRS duration in a neonate is 70 ms or less, which is important when deciding whether a narrow- or wide-complex tachycardia is present. A QRS duration of 90 ms, which is normal for an adult, is wide for a baby and can indicate ventricular tachycardia (Figure 100-6). Ventricular tachycardia is often misdiagnosed as SVT in the newborn because of this feature. The rate of ventricular tachycardia can be as high as the SVT rate in neonates; therefore the rate will not differentiate between the two tachyarrhythmias. The treatment and implications are very different for a narrow-complex SVT and a wide-complex ventricular tachycardia. In either case, a pediatric cardiologist must evaluate these patients as soon as possible because congestive heart failure can develop from a persistent tachyarrhythmia. An echocardiographic examination is required to evaluate the structure and function of the heart. Acute treatment of a tachyarrhythmia may be medical or electrical cardioversion, followed by an antiarrhythmic agent to prevent recurrence. Radiofrequency ablation is not usually performed in newborns because the arrhythmia may spontaneously resolve, because of technical difficulties related to the size of the patient, and because of the possibility that radiofrequency lesions may expand with time in this age group.

Irregular Rhythms

The most common cause of an irregular rhythm in the child or adolescent is sinus arrhythmia. Sinus arrhythmia is a normal finding in which a variation exists in the heart rate with respiration. A 12-lead ECG with a rhythm strip will show positive P waves of the same morphology in leads I, II, and AVF, each followed by a QRS complex. In newborns, however, an irregular heartbeat is more often caused by premature atrial or ventricular beats, which are usually single and uniform. The overall heart rate is normal. These patients usually have structurally normal hearts. No intervention is needed, and the premature beats usually resolve with time.

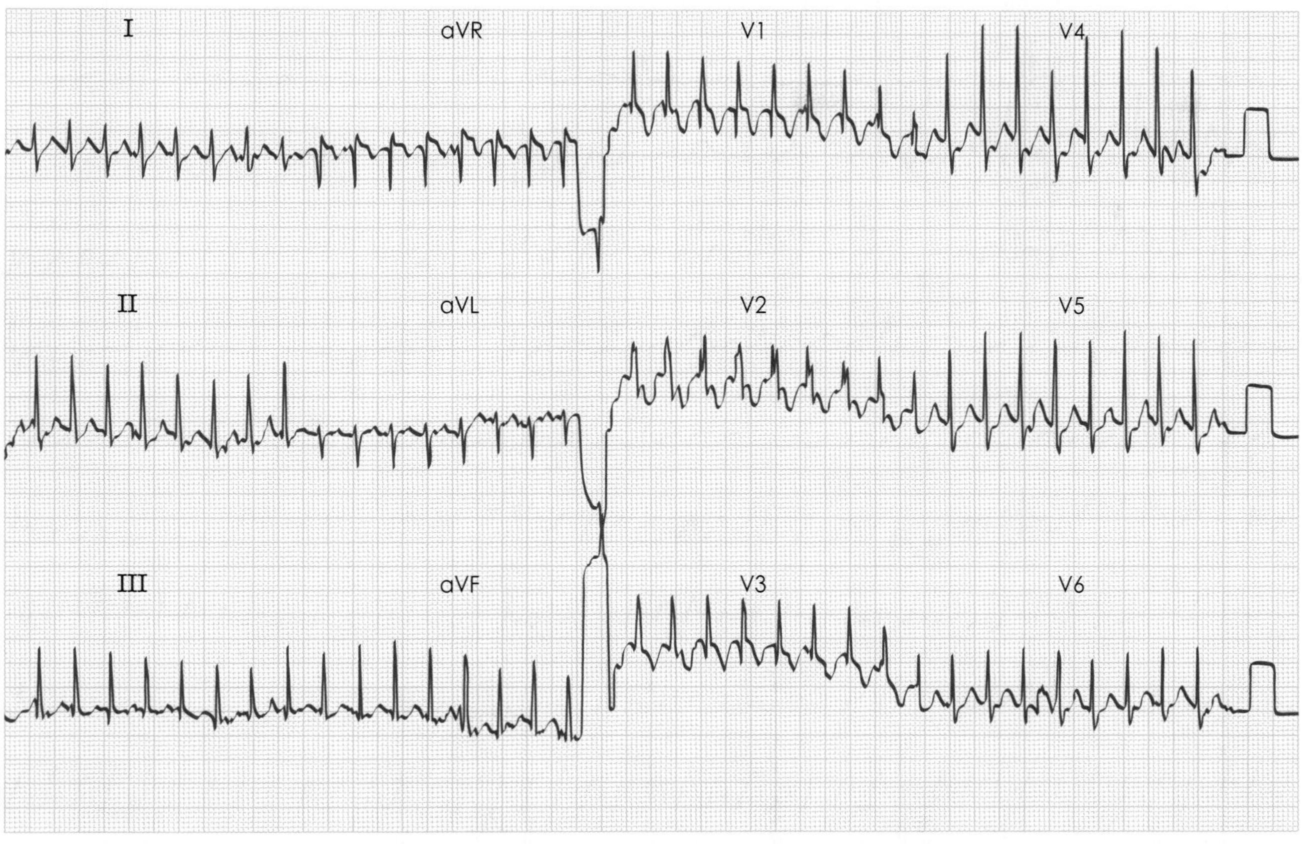

Figure 100-4 Supraventricular tachycardia in a newborn.

Atrial premature contractions (APCs) may be conducted normally resulting in a normal narrow QRS (Figure 100-7), or they may be conducted aberrantly resulting in a wide QRS (Figure 100-8). Both normally conducted and aberrantly conducted APCs have a preceding P wave, which is different from the sinus P wave. Nonconducted (blocked) APCs have an abnormal early P wave but no QRS, and if they are frequent, they may result in a low heart rate (Figure 100-9).

Premature ventricular contractions (PVCs) are early beats that are wide and not preceded by a P wave (Figure 100-10). After a PVC, a full compensatory pause usually occurs before the next sinus beat, meaning that the length of two cycles, including the premature beat, is equal to that of two normal cycles. PVCs are considered significant if they are frequent, multiform, occur as couplets or runs, or are associated with a long QT interval.

Evaluation

When an arrhythmia is appreciated, a standard 12-lead ECG evaluation should be performed with a rhythm strip that is 30 seconds to 1 minute long, preferably with 12 simultaneous leads. The rhythm strip is essential to diagnosis and can be obtained with all ECG machines or ordered specifically from any ECG laboratory. The rest of the physical examination in the baby with an arrhythmia is generally normal, but an association can be found with acquired heart disease or congenital heart disease. A common and important association is Ebstein anomaly of the tricuspid valve and SVT. These patients have an accessory pathway that can sometimes be manifested on the ECG as a short PR interval and delta wave of WPW syndrome (see Figure 100-1). Other associations are infection (eg, myocarditis), neurologic disease (eg, asphyxia), and metabolic disorders (eg, electrolyte abnormalities). Infants with heart disease often decompensate with an arrhythmia. Any sign of congestive heart failure in a baby with an abnormal rhythm requires an immediate evaluation by a pediatric cardiologist.

CONGESTIVE HEART FAILURE

Congestive heart failure (CHF) is the inability of the heart to do the work required. This inability can be caused by abnormal muscle function with a normal workload or by an increased workload with normal muscle function. (Box 100-1 lists the causes of CHF.)

The history is critical in making the diagnosis of CHF. Babies with CHF have poor feeding; they are very hungry and start to eat ravenously but tire quickly and get very short of breath. They need to rest frequently while feeding and may want to eat again

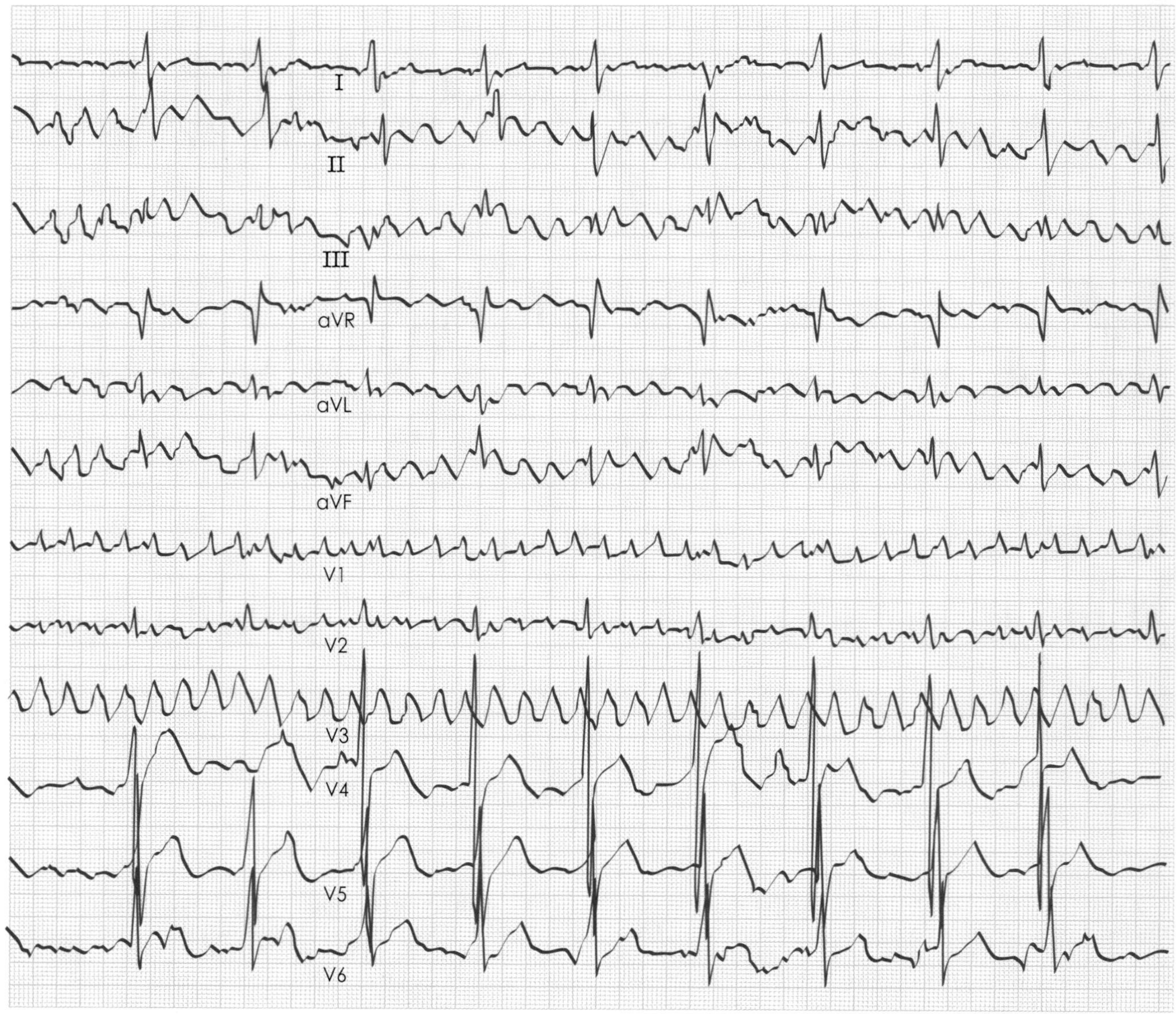

Figure 100-5 ECG showing atrial flutter in a 4-month-old boy.

shortly afterward because they cannot ingest enough at any one sitting. A detailed feeding history should be elicited, including frequency of feedings and how many minutes each feeding lasts. Babies with CHF may also have sweating with feeds, which is a sign of how hard they are working when they feed. They need more calories than normal babies but are consuming fewer. A history of poor weight gain will be found, with head circumference and length being spared to some degree.

Signs of CHF include underweight and tachypnea. Infants may exhibit retractions, nasal flaring, and grunting. A cardiac examination may show tachycardia, a gallop, or a hyperactive or hypoactive impulse. Any rhythm disturbance must be investigated to determine if the arrhythmia is the cause or result of CHF. Murmurs may or may not be appreciated in a baby with CHF. Some conditions causing CHF are not associated with heart murmurs. Even murmurs caused by structural heart disease may not be heard if the baby has low cardiac output; these murmurs become evident when anticongestive therapy is effective. Crackles in the lungs from pulmonary edema and hepatomegaly are presenting signs of CHF. Signs of poor perfusion include mottling, slow capillary refill, cool extremities, and poor pulses. Good upper extremity pulses and poor femoral pulses indicate a coarctation of the aorta; however, this difference may not be evident if low cardiac output is present. The examiner should feel the right brachial pulse and femoral pulse simultaneously to detect a delay, suggesting a coarctation.

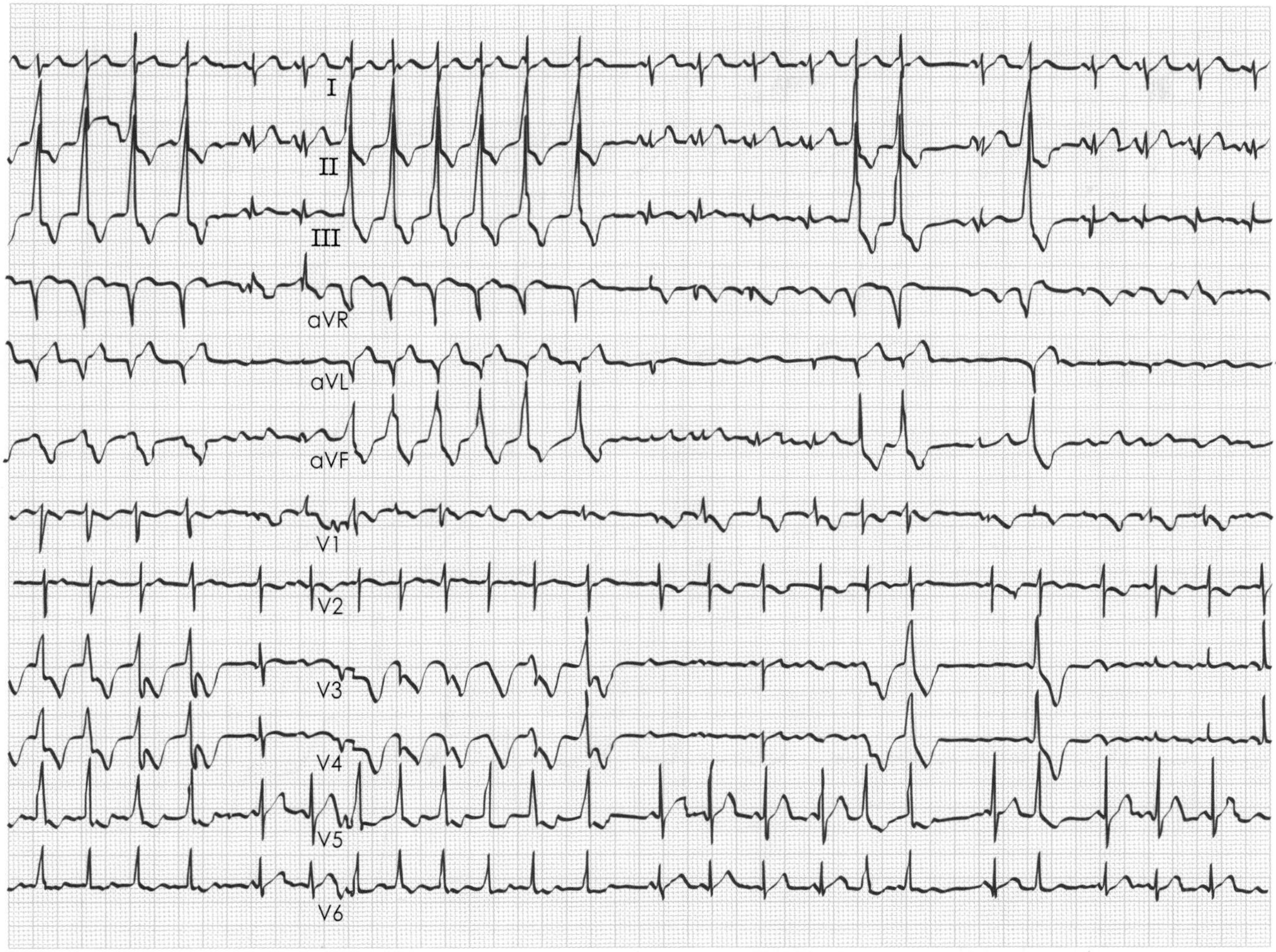

Figure 100-6 ECG reflecting nonsustained monomorphic ventricular tachycardia in a newborn.

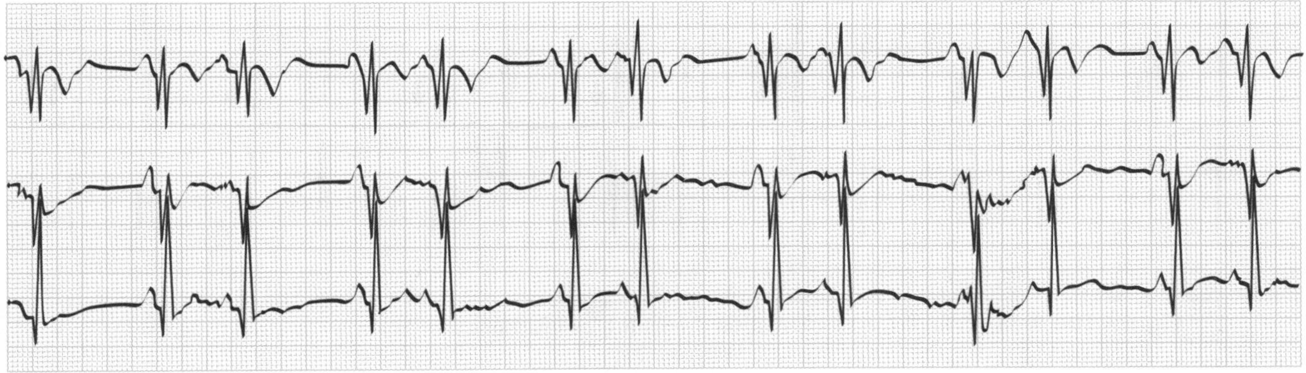

Figure 100-7 ECG showing atrial premature contractions with normal conduction as atrial bigeminy in a newborn.

A pediatric cardiologist must evaluate a baby with CHF as soon as possible. Echocardiography, ECG, and chest radiography must be performed. Some infants may need to be stabilized and transported emergently to a tertiary-care NICU or emergency room, especially if shock is present. (See Chapter 76, Care of the Sick or Premature Infant Before Transport.)

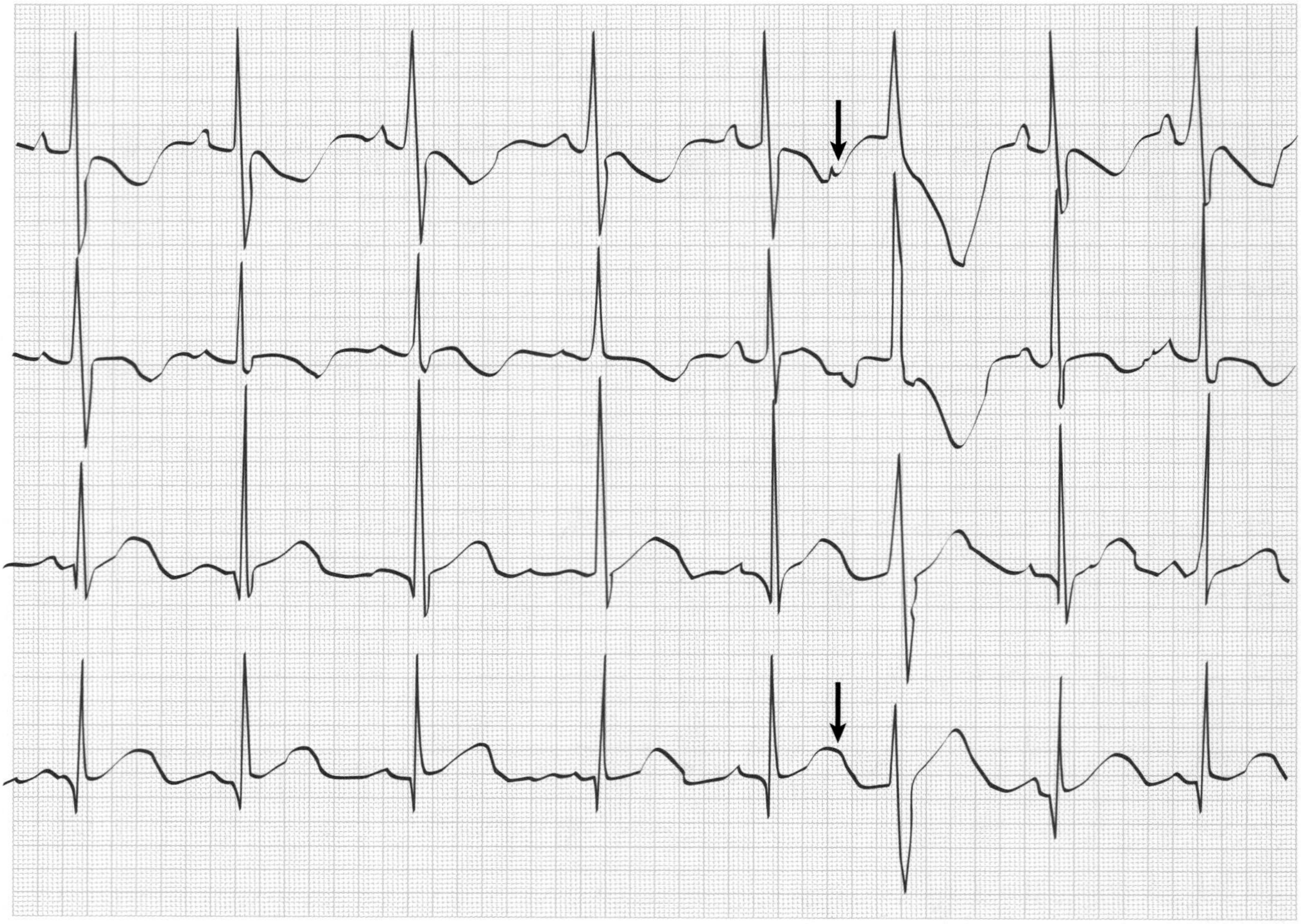

Figure 100-8 ECG showing atrial premature contractions with aberrant conduction in a newborn.

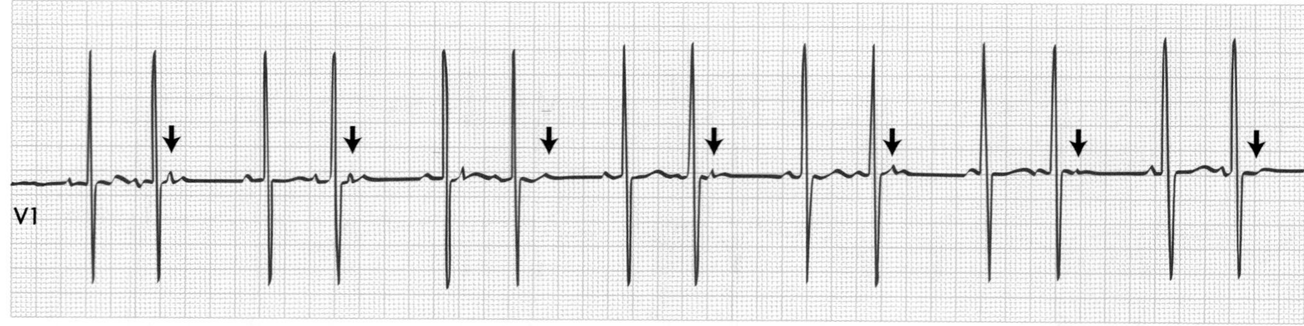

Figure 100-9 ECG showing blocked atrial premature contractions *(down arrow)* as atrial trigeminy.

Abnormal Muscle Function

Abnormal muscle function in newborns may be caused by a primary cardiomyopathy (eg, myocarditis, endocardial fibroelastosis), or it can be secondary in nature. Some causes of secondary cardiomyopathy are arrhythmias (eg, tachyarrhythmias, complete heart block), metabolic disorders (eg, adrenal insufficiency, hypocalcemia, hypoglycemia, Pompe disease), sepsis, and anemia. A gallop and the murmur of mitral or tricuspid regurgitation may be heard in these patients.

Increased Workload

The other category of patients who develop CHF have normal muscle function but have increased workload. The increased workload can be divided into pressure overload and volume overload.

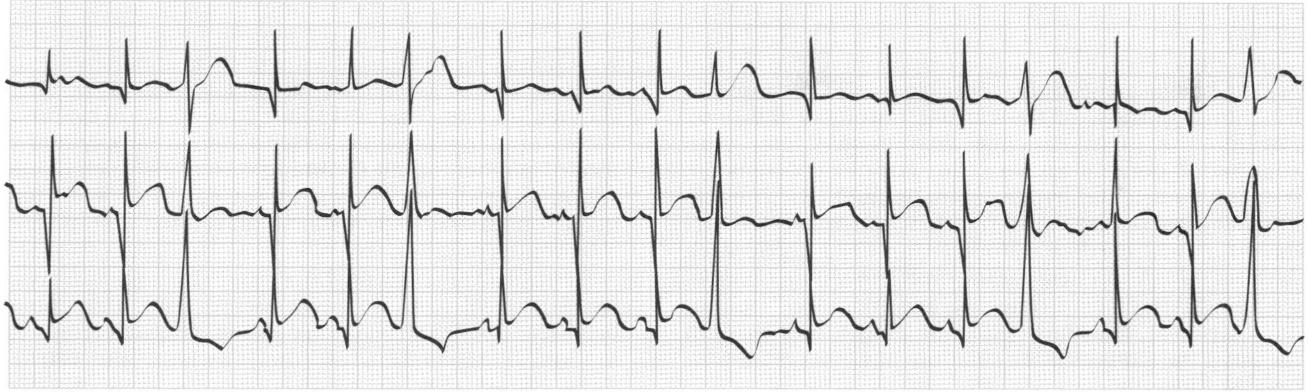

Figure 100-10 ECG reflecting single uniform premature ventricular contractions as ventricular quadrigeminy in a newborn.

BOX 100-1 Causes of Congestive Heart Failure

- Noncardiac causes
  - Birth asphyxia with myocardial ischemia
  - Sepsis
  - Anemia
  - Hypoglycemia
  - Hypocalcemia
  - Adrenal insufficiency
  - Maternal diabetes mellitus
  - Barth syndrome
  - Cerebral arteriovenous malformation
- Primary myocardial disease
  - Hypertrophic cardiomyopathy
  - Myocarditis
  - Endocardial fibroelastosis
- Arrhythmias
  - Supraventricular tachycardia
  - Ectopic atrial tachycardia
  - Atrial flutter or fibrillation
  - Junctional ectopic tachycardia
  - Ventricular tachycardia
  - Complete heart block
- Structural heart disease
  - Anomalous left coronary from the pulmonary artery
  - Pressure overload lesions:
    - Coarctation of the aorta
    - Aortic stenosis
    - Hypoplastic left heart syndrome
  - Volume overload lesions: left-to-right shunt
    - Ventricular septal defect
    - Atrial septal defect
    - Patent ductus arteriosus
    - Complete atrioventricular canal

Pressure Overload

Common causes of increased pressure work are aortic stenosis, pulmonary stenosis, and coarctation of the aorta. Hypoplastic left heart syndrome will often exhibit as a severe version of coarctation of the aorta.

Coarctation of the aorta is a stenosis of the upper thoracic aorta, usually just opposite the insertion of the ductus arteriosus (juxtaductal). Depending on the severity of the stenosis, the impact on cardiac output can vary from very minimal to severe. The degree of stenosis is hard to predict clinically or by echocardiographic evaluation before the PDA has completely closed, given that the ductal tissue can be involved in the site of the coarctation. The stenosis leads to increased pressure in the proximal aorta, causing increased systolic pressure and wall stress in the left ventricle, resulting in left ventricular hypertrophy. However, when the stenosis is severe and increases suddenly, such as occurs when the PDA closes in a patient with a critical coarctation, the left ventricular wall stress rises very sharply over a short period. The left ventricle does not have time to compensate with hypertrophy and can fail in hours or days, resulting in low cardiac output and shock. Prostaglandin is used to keep the ductus open until surgery is performed.

On cardiac examination, a suprasternal notch thrill may be present. The first and second heart sounds are generally normal. Occasionally a systolic ejection click from a bicuspid aortic valve is heard. Some newborns have a 2/6 to 3/6 systolic ejection murmur at the left upper sternal border radiating to the back from the coarctation itself, but this finding is uncommon. The most prominent finding is the discrepancy between the upper and lower extremity pulses and blood pressures. In these babies, the PDA shunts right to left and represents the only source of blood flow to the lower extremities. The saturations in the feet may therefore be lower than those in the right arm while the PDA is open. When the PDA closes, the right-to-left shunt resolves, and the saturations in the feet will be same as that in the right arm, but the perfusion will be much worse.

The ECG in the newborn is often normal without evidence of left ventricular hypertrophy. The ECG can show right ventricular hypertrophy in the neonatal period because the right ventricle is still responsible for pumping most of the cardiac output to the body through the PDA. Patients who present later with coarctation generally have a murmur or hypertension, with left ventricular hypertrophy on the ECG. They do not have as severe a coarctation and therefore still have forward cardiac output around the aortic arch without a PDA. A chest radiograph shows the nonspecific findings of cardiomegaly and increased pulmonary vascular markings. Rib notching is not present because the collateral circulation has not yet developed sufficiently.

Babies with critical aortic stenosis and hypoplastic left heart syndrome can also present in shock. In these patients the pulses are quite thready, but the brachial and femoral pulses will be equally poor, and blood pressures will be the same in upper and lower extremities. However, some babies in shock from a coarctation will have such poor pulses that detecting a difference between upper and lower extremities is difficult. Infants with coarctation often have a normal ECG or right ventricular hypertrophy, whereas neonates with aortic stenosis will have left ventricular hypertrophy, and those with hypoplastic left heart syndrome will have decreased or absent left ventricular forces with right ventricular hypertrophy.

Volume Overload

The volume overload lesions are atrial septal defect, VSD, PDA, and common atrioventricular canal. VSD is discussed here because it is the most common volume overload lesion to cause CHF in infants.

VSDs are the most common form of congenital heart disease, if bicuspid aortic valve is excluded. The amount of shunting across a VSD is determined by the size of the defect and the relative resistances of the systemic and pulmonary circulations but not the location of the VSD in the septum. CHF can occur with a moderate to large VSD.

On cardiac examination of an infant with a VSD a systolic thrill may be palpable at the left lower sternal border. A hyperactive precordium and loud P2 are present with a large shunt. A grade 2/6 to 5/6 pansystolic or early systolic murmur is audible at the left lower sternal border. An apical diastolic rumble of relative mitral stenosis may be present with a moderate to large shunt. (For a complete discussion of VSD, see Chapter 251, Congenital and Acquired Heart Disease.)

CYANOSIS

Cyanosis is a bluish discoloration of the skin and mucous membranes and is either peripheral (acrocyanosis) or central. Peripheral cyanosis can occur with hypovolemia or shock, but it is a common finding in healthy infants who are vasoconstricted from the cold or fever. Circumoral cyanosis refers to bluish skin around the mouth and, if isolated in a cold baby, is of no concern. Central cyanosis requires desaturation of 5 g/100 mL of hemoglobin and is usually not detectable until the arterial oxygen saturation is 85% or lower in an infant with a normal hemoglobin. Cyanosis can be seen at a higher level of oxygen saturation in patients with polycythemia and at a lower level in patients with anemia. Cyanosis can be difficult to detect in dark-skinned infants. The best place to assess for cyanosis is the tongue, which has a rich vascular supply and is free of pigmentation. Clubbing describes thick, wide, spoon-shaped fingertips and toes with convex nail beds; it usually does not start to develop until the child is 6 months or older.

Central cyanosis can be caused by upper airway (eg, laryngeal web) or lower airway (eg, pneumonia) disease. Upper airway disease is characterized by marked hypercarbia, inspiratory stridor, and retractions. Hypercarbia develops later in lower airway disease, and findings include tachypnea, expiratory wheezing, grunting, crackles, and retractions. Apnea or shallow irregular respirations and hypercarbia are seen in the cyanotic infant with central nervous system disease (eg, birth asphyxia). Babies with methemoglobinemia are only tachypneic; their arterial blood gas shows a normal Pa_{O_2} and low oxygen saturation. In newborns with persistence of the fetal circulation, right-to-left shunting occurs through the patent foramen ovale and PDA because of persistent pulmonary hypertension, which may be idiopathic or a result of conditions such as meconium aspiration, hypoglycemia, and perinatal asphyxia.

Infants with cyanosis from congenital heart disease can be divided into those with acyanotic congenital heart disease with CHF (eg, large VSD) producing abnormal diffusion and V/Q mismatch in the lungs (similar to lower airway disease), and those with true cyanotic congenital heart disease with a right-to-left shunt.

Patients with a true right-to-left shunt can be differentiated with a hyperoxia test. As close to 100% oxygen as possible is administered for 10 minutes. When a right-to-left intracardiac shunt is significant, the Pa_{O_2} does not usually increase to greater than 100 mm Hg, and the rise is not usually more than 10 to 30 mm Hg. However, in defects with markedly increased pulmonary blood flow, such as total anomalous pulmonary venous return, the Pa_{O_2} can rise as high as 150 mm Hg.

When possible, simultaneous blood gases should be obtained from the right upper extremity and umbilical artery or lower extremity to determine the presence of a right-to-left ductal shunt. A 10- to 15-mm Hg difference between the right radial artery and umbilical artery is considered significant.

Cyanotic congenital heart defects can be divided into those with decreased pulmonary blood flow and those with increased pulmonary blood flow (Table 100-2). Defects with decreased pulmonary blood flow have in common right-sided obstruction (eg, tricuspid atresia, pulmonary atresia, pulmonary stenosis) to pulmonary flow with a right-to-left shunt through a normal patent foramen ovale (PFO) or abnormal intracardiac communication (VSD). Tetralogy of Fallot will be discussed as an example. Defects with increased pulmonary blood flow have intracardiac mixing of saturated and desaturated blood but no obstruction to pulmonary blood flow. Transposition of the great arteries will be discussed as an example.

Table 100-2 Cyanotic Congenital Heart Disease

DISEASE	ECG	CHEST X-RAY	
		HEART SIZE	PVMS
Tetralogy of Fallot	RVH, RAD	Boot-shaped heart	Decreased
Tricuspid atresia	Superior axis, decreased RV forces, LVH	Normal to slightly increased heart size	Decreased
Pulmonary atresia	Normal axis, decreased RV forces; LVH	Normal to slightly increased heart size	Decreased
Critical pulmonic stenosis	RAD, RVH	Normal to slightly increased heart size	Decreased
Ebstein anomaly	RAE, RBBB, delta wave of WPW syndrome	Extremely enlarged heart size (mainly from RA dilation)	Decreased
Truncus arteriosus	BVH	Cardiomegaly	Increased
TGA	RAD, RVH	Egg-shaped heart with narrow superior mediastinum	Increased
TAPVR	RAD, RVH with RSR′	Cardiomegaly	Increased

BVH, Biventricular hypertrophy; *ECG,* electrocardiogram; *LVH,* left ventricular hypertrophy; *PVMs,* pulmonary vascular markings; *RA,* right atrial; *RAD,* right axis deviation; *RAE,* right atrial enlargement; *RBBB,* right bundle branch block; *RV,* right ventricular; *RVH,* right ventricular hypertrophy; *TAPVR,* total anomalous pulmonary venous return; *TGA,* transposition of the great arteries; *WPW,* Wolff-Parkinson-White.

Tetralogy of Fallot

Tetralogy of Fallot (TOF) is the most common cyanotic congenital heart defect, representing 5% to 7% of all congenital heart disease. Most patients with TOF will exhibit symptoms in the immediate newborn period with cyanosis and a murmur. The degree of cyanosis is determined by the severity of the pulmonic stenosis. Some infants will not be cyanotic at birth but will develop increasing obstruction and cyanosis over the first year of life. Other infants have such severe cyanosis that they are dependent on the PDA for blood flow to the lungs and become severely ill when the PDA closes.

On physical examination, a systolic thrill at the left upper and mid sternal borders and an increased RV impulse are usually present. The second heart sound is single, and a systolic ejection click may be heard. Typically a long, loud crescendo-decrescendo systolic murmur of right ventricular outflow tract obstruction is audible at the left upper and mid sternal borders. The infant may be tachypneic but not particularly dyspneic, and the pulses are usually good.

The ECG will show isolated right ventricular hypertrophy with a rightward axis. A chest radiograph classically shows a boot-shaped heart with decreased pulmonary vascular markings. Approximately 25% of patents with TOF have a right aortic arch.

(For a full discussion of TOF, see Chapter 251, Congenital and Acquired Heart Disease.)

Transposition of the Great Arteries

Transposition of the great arteries (TGA) represents approximately 3% to 5% of all congenital heart defects. A strong male predominance exists in this disorder, but it is not usually associated with other congenital anomalies or chromosomal abnormalities. Newborns with TGA have severe cyanosis. The rest of the physical examination is often normal except for tachypnea. The baby may be large because TGA is found more commonly in infants of a diabetic mother. The typical patient is a *big, blue, baby boy.* Murmurs are not prominent in the absence of a VSD and pulmonary stenosis.

Initially, the chest radiograph may be completely normal. With time the chest radiograph will show overcirculation of the pulmonary vasculature. The classic description of the heart on chest radiograph evaluation is an *egg on a string.* The ECG may be normal or show right ventricular hypertrophy.

The most classic, but infrequently seen, finding in TGA is reversed differential cyanosis, that is, greater cyanosis of the upper half of the body than the lower half of the body. This finding is due to shunting of blood with a higher saturation from the pulmonary artery to the descending aorta through the PDA. Usually the Pao_2 is under 35 mm Hg in room air and 35 to 40 mm Hg on 100% oxygen. (For a full discussion of TGA, see Chapter 251, Congenital and Acquired Heart Disease.)

TOOLS FOR PRACTICE

Medical Decision Support

- *ACC/AHA/ESC Practice Guidelines* (guideline), American College of Cardiology, American Heart Association Task Force, and European Society of Cardiology Committee for Practice Guidelines (circ.ahajournals.org/cgi/reprint/114/10/e385).

REFERENCES

1. Hoffman JI, Kaplan S. The incidence of congenital heart disease. *J Am Coll Cardiol.* 2002;39(12):1890-1900.
2. Campbell M. Incidence of cardiac malformations at birth and later, and neonatal mortality. *Br Heart J.* 1973;35:189-200.
3. Mitchell SC, Korones SB, Berendes HW. Congenital heart disease in 56,109 births. *Circulation.* 1971;43:323-332.

4. Ferencz C, Rubin JD, McCarter RJ, et al. Congenital heart disease: prevalence at live birth. The Baltimore-Washington Infant Study. *Am J Epidemiol.* 1985;121:31-36.
5. Correa-Villansenor A, McCarter R, Downing J, et al. *Epidemiology of Congenital Heart Disease: The Baltimore-Washington Infant Study 1981-1989.* Mount Kisco, NY: Futura; 1993.
6. Satou, GM, Lacro RV, Chung T, et al. Heart size on chest x-ray as a predictor of cardiac enlargement by echocardiography in children. *Pediatr Cardiol.* 2001;22(3):218-222.
7. Gregoratos G, Klein AJ, Moss RJ, et al. ACC/AHA/ESC 2006 guidelines for management of patients with ventricular arrhythmias and the prevention of sudden cardiac death: a report of the American College of Cardiology, American Heart Association Task Force and the European Society of Cardiology Committee for Practice Guidelines (Writing Committee to Develop Guidelines for Management of Patients With Ventricular Arrhythmias and the Prevention of Sudden Cardiac Death). *J Am Coll Cardiol.* 2006:48(5):247-346.

Chapter 101

THE INFANT WITH SUSPECTED INFECTION

Tsoline Kojaoghlanian, MD

Neonatal infections can be broadly categorized into congenital, indicating their presence at birth and likely acquisition in utero, and perinatal, indicating acquisition late in pregnancy or during the delivery. Outcomes for the neonate after infection can vary widely based on the organism involved, the time during gestation when infection occurs, and whether the mother has any protective antibodies that can provide the fetus with passive protection, reducing the disease severity for the infant.

Transplacental spread of maternal infection is the common route by which the fetus acquires infection. Placental infection is often associated with systemic illness in the neonate; thus molecular, microbiological, and pathological examination of the placenta is important in the critically ill newborn. In the perinatal period, acquired early-onset infection (before 72 hours) is almost always caused by organisms acquired in the maternal birth canal. After this period, most infections are acquired through close contact with members of the baby's environment and through human milk.[1] The manifestations of infection vary with the infecting organism. The mechanism of damage and response by the host, as well as the stage of the pregnancy determine the effects on the neonate. Some pathogens can have deleterious effects throughout gestation. Fetal organogenesis is complete by 12 weeks' gestation; thus damage incurred during this period will likely result in anomalies. The mother does not transfer T cell–specific immunity, crucial in the control of many viruses, to the fetus. Maternal IgG antibodies, conversely, are transferred to the fetus and reach one half the normal serum concentration by 30 weeks' gestation and more normal values at term. Furthermore the transferred antibodies must be of a certain concentration to be protective. In some bacterial infections the mother may not have enough circulating antibodies, and this factor is complicated by the fact that, for reasons that are poorly understood, newborns cannot mount an antibody response to polysaccharide antigens, such as those found on bacterial capsules (eg, those of group B *Streptococcus* [GBS]). Newborns who experience a sufficient period of antigenic stimulation (usually 7 to 14 days) will exhibit a measurable IgM response to some viruses and parasites, which can be used diagnostically. In addition, antigen-specific T-cell responses are significantly reduced or delayed in neonates, and this also translates to delays in B-cell and antibody responses.[2]

In the neonate, the factor associated most significantly with sepsis caused by any microorganism is low birth weight. Very low–birth-weight (VLBW) and premature infants are especially susceptible to infections. Other factors include prolonged rupture of membranes, traumatic delivery, maternal infection, chorioamnionitis, and fetal hypoxia.[3] The incidence of bacterial meningitis is greater in the neonatal period than in any other period in life.[4] The use of modern neonatal intensive care techniques that include endotracheal intubation or nasal cannula or prong use, parenteral nutrition, chronic blood vessel cannulation (umbilical, percutaneous intravenous, and other central vessel catheterization), disruption of skin integrity, delay in feeding, formula rather than human milk feedings, administration of broad-spectrum antibiotics and other medications that alter the infant's intestinal and skin flora, predispose these unique immunodeficient infants to a multitude of acquired infections. Deficiencies in mucosal barrier function and in both the innate and adaptive arms of the immune response, including serum complement components, defensins, and abnormalities in cytokine production, plus deficiencies of chemotaxis, phagocytosis, and microbial killing, contribute to the vulnerability of preterm neonates to systemic infections, including bloodstream invasion. Worldwide, the major burden of preterm birth is in the developing world, where infectious diseases such as malaria, Human Immunodeficiency Virus (HIV), tuberculosis, and intestinal parasites cause much of the mortality and morbidity.[5] Women and their infants also disproportionately bear the long-term consequences of sexually transmitted infections, including syphilis, herpesviruses, and *Chlamydia*.

Neonatal infections are caused by a variety of microorganisms. By convention, *congenital* infections have been assimilated into the acronym TORCH: toxoplasmosis, other agents (including syphilis and HIV), rubella, cytomegalovirus, and herpes simplex virus (HSV). However, unlike most TORCH infections, which are acquired transplacentally, 90% of HSV and 80% of HIV infections occur perinatally at the time of delivery. Many viruses that are transmitted from mother to child must find a way to persist in the infected mother for her to pass it on to her offspring. In addition, for several human herpesviruses, close contact is required for transmission. Infections associated with the cytomegalovirus (CMV), a herpesvirus, are the most prevalent neonatal infections.

Table 101-1 Estimated Relative Incidence of Some Neonatal Infections (per 100,000 Live Births) in the United States

INFECTIOUS AGENT	OVERALL INCIDENCE PER 100,000 LIVE BIRTHS	SYMPTOMATIC AT BIRTH
Cytomegalovirus	1000	100
Toxoplasma gondii	10-40	2-8
Rubella virus	<1	<1
Varicella virus	<1	<1
Treponema pallidum (syphilis)	13	4
Human Immunodeficiency Virus (HIV)	5	<1
Herpes simplex virus	10-40	10-40
Group B *Streptococcus*	30-50	30-50

Toxoplasma, CMV, rubella, and syphilis are the pathogens primarily acquired in utero that result in congenital infection. The most common fetal ultrasound findings to be associated with congenital infections are echogenic bowel, ascites, pleural effusions, cardiomegaly, and oligohydramnios; IUGR and ventriculomegaly coexist with other features. The yield of screening infants born with IUGR or ventriculomegaly for TORCH is low, even among infants screened for TORCH because of the presence of thrombocytopenia, neutropenia, direct hyperbilirubinemia, or dysmorphic features.[6] Maternal hypertensive disorders of pregnancy, smoking, and drug or alcohol use are more likely culprits for IUGR. In all circumstances, postnatal screening for congenital infections must be cost beneficial and cost effective to be implemented.[7] Table 101-1 summarizes the estimated relative incidence of some neonatal infections.

CONGENITAL INFECTIONS

Cytomegalovirus

Cytomegalovirus (CMV) is the leading infectious cause of damage to the developing fetus in the United States and other developed countries.[8] In the United States, 40,000 newborns (1% of births) are infected annually, 8000 of whom will have CMV-related damage. One third of sensorineural hearing loss (SNHL) cases are attributed to CMV.[9] CMV infects mainly epithelial cells but also endothelial and hematopoietic cells, from which it disseminates. As is true of herpesviruses, after primary infection, CMV establishes latency and can replicate actively at epithelial sites throughout the lifetime of the host. This factor is important because intrauterine infection after primary maternal infection is 40% to 50%, compared with 0.5% to 2% after reactivation.

The existence of multiple strains of the virus is responsible for a small number of congenital infections acquired by reinfection with a new strain during pregnancy.[10] Improved hygiene and formula feeding in the developed world have delayed acquisition of CMV to the childbearing years, at which point seropositivity is 50% to 70%. The risk of acquiring infection is higher in adolescents, in those from low socioeconomic groups, and in women who have another child in the household.[11] The infection rate is 2.5% during pregnancy, 5.5% between pregnancies.

CMV infects placental cytotrophoblasts and is transferred to the fetus through placental infection. Perinatal CMV infection occurs because CMV may be carried in the cervix during the late stages of pregnancy and in human milk. CMV is detected in 15% to 30% of lactating women. Among CMV seropositive women, 32% to 96% will excrete CMV into their milk, and the peak period of excretion is 3 to 4 weeks after delivery.[13] For congenital infection, the highest risk of transmission is during the third trimester of pregnancy (75%); however, although most of these neonates will be born asymptomatic, 25% of newborns who acquired infection during the first trimester will have central nervous system (CNS) involvement. Overall, 90% of CMV infections will be asymptomatic, but 10% to 15% of these asymptomatic infants will develop SNHL and, less commonly, other CNS sequelae. Of the 10% of newborns who have symptoms at birth, 20% will die; 70% will have hearing loss with varying degrees of developmental delay, motor or cognitive impairment, and seizures; and only 10% will survive without sequelae. Hence, overall, 20% of infected infants will have some degree of hearing or CNS disability.[14]

Most of the manifestations of congenital disease are the result of inflammation of organs caused by virus invasion. Symptomatic disease may entail premature delivery, IUGR, microcephaly, periventricular calcifications, polymicrogyria, jaundice, petechiae, hepatosplenomegaly, thrombocytopenia, hyperbilirubinemia, and mild hepatitis. CMV has a predilection to the rapidly multiplying cells of the germinal matrix. If overt CNS findings are present at birth, then 95% will have major neurodevelopmental sequelae. Microcephaly is the most specific predictor of intellectual disability and motor disability, followed by abnormal computed tomographic scan findings.[12] The developing CNS remains vulnerable to damage from persistent virus replication after birth. SNHL is characteristically progressive and thus may be missed in the newborn screening. Progressive hearing loss occurs during the first year of life.

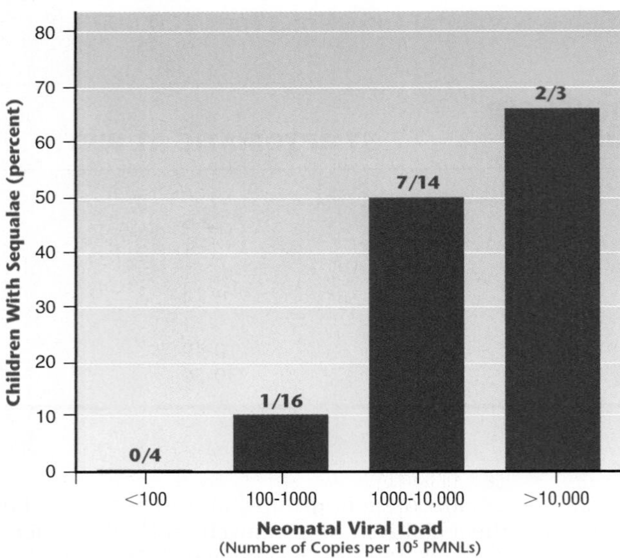

Figure 101-1 Association between neonatal blood virus load determined by quantitative polymerase chain reaction and the development of sequelae at 12 months of age (test for trend, $p = .002$). The proportion of children who developed sequelae is indicated atop of each bar. *PMNL.* Polymorphonuclear leukocytes. *(Lanari M, Lazzarotto T, Venturi V, et al. Neonatal cytomegalovirus blood load and risk of sequelae in symptomatic and asymptomatic congenitally infected newborns.* Pediatrics. *2006;117:e76-e83.)*

Perinatal disease occurs at around 2 to 8 weeks of age.

To diagnose congenital infection, urine obtained within 10 days of birth is the best sample from which to isolate the virus because of high titers, and the virus can remain stable at 4°C for up to 7 days. Saliva can also be cultured. Cultures obtained after 10 days do not differentiate congenital from perinatal disease; viral DNA detection by polymerase chain reaction (PCR) of earlier blood samples may help diagnose some cases retrospectively.[15] PCR also has great promise in providing more insight into prognosis; for example, children with asymptomatic congenital CMV who have SNHL have more CMV in urine and blood, measured by PCR, than children with asymptomatic CMV with normal hearing (Figure 101-1).[16-18]

Cord blood IgM is suggestive of intrauterine infection, but in 15%, results can be falsely negative. For prenatal diagnosis, isolated IgM titers in pregnant women are not sufficient for the diagnosis of acute infection because IgM may remain positive for 1 to 6 months after primary infection and may also be positive after reactivation. Hence viral DNA in amniotic fluid or IgM of fetal blood, together with suggestive ultrasound findings such as echogenic bowel and CNS abnormalities with IUGR, are most suggestive.

No guidelines exist for the treatment of CMV during pregnancy; the possibility of using antepartum CMV hyperimmune globulin[19] requires further assessment. Treatment of congenital infection remains limited and suboptimal.[20,21] Therapy with intravenous ganciclovir results in only modest improvement in hearing outcomes,[22] and its use is associated with adverse effects, including neutropenia, complications of prolonged central venous catheterization, and the potential for sterility (in animal models). The Institute of Medicine has classified a CMV vaccine at the highest priority to prevent congenital infections, neurologic damage, and deafness and to avoid major economic costs.[23] Assessing the risk-benefit ratio of universal screening of all infants is still difficult. Increasing awareness of CMV's public health importance will foster the development of vaccines and will drive the industry and regulatory agencies. In the meantime, education of women and health care providers about modes of transmission is key for prevention. Avoid as much as possible kissing toddlers on their mouths, sharing utensils, and lapses in effective hand-washing practices, especially after changing diapers and handling toys.[8]

Toxoplasma gondii

Although congenital toxoplasmosis is not a nationally reportable disease, it is a potentially preventable one through education, screening of mother or newborn, and treatment of the pregnant woman. The implementation of the various interventions have been debated mainly because of differences in seroprevalence rates in different geographic areas and in the true burden of disease.[24,25] The estimated seroprevalence rate in women of childbearing age in the United States is 15%. Congenital toxoplasmosis is estimated at 10 to 40 per 100,000 live births, resulting in a large economic burden caused by mental and visual disabilities. *T gondii* exposure is attributed to either consuming contaminated pork meat (the microorganism is destroyed by heating) or ingesting oocysts passed in the feces of cats in warm, moist climates, in equal percentages. A risk of transmission exists with primary infection across the placenta in utero but not if infection is acquired before conception. In women coinfected with HIV, a possibility of reactivation and transmission of infection exists. The transmission rate is higher late in gestation (50% in late gestation vs 10% early in gestation), but anomalies are most severe if infection is acquired at 10 to 24 weeks' gestation. Treatment during pregnancy has been shown to reduce the rate of transmission by 50%.

Congenital infection may exhibit as disease (toxoplasmosis) in the neonate within the first few months of life or as subclinical infection or relapse of undiagnosed infection later in life (eg, ocular toxoplasmosis). More than 75% of affected infants are asymptomatic at birth, but if untreated, up to 85% will develop visual and learning disabilities later in life. Symptomatic newborns may have one or more of the following, which overlap with symptoms of other congenital infections: chorioretinitis, hydrocephalus, intracranial calcifications, cytopenias, jaundice, and maculopapular rash. Markedly increased cerebrospinal fluid (CSF) protein concentration that results from autolysis of necrotic brain tissue is a hallmark of congenital toxoplasmosis. Adverse outcomes include intellectual disability, blindness, and epilepsy.

Serology from cord blood samples is the mainstay of diagnosis, and commercial kits detecting IgM are used for diagnosing infection in the neonate. These kits have specificities of 80%, and the test results should be interpreted with caution and confirmed. In addition, infections acquired late in the third trimester of pregnancy may be missed because antibodies have not yet been formed. IgA tests and combining serologic testing with the Western blot test increase the sensitivity of diagnosis in the neonate. Prenatal diagnosis is made based on ultrasound findings and amniocentesis between 17 to 21 weeks' gestation for detection of the organism by PCR in the presence of IgM, increased IgG, or both. Affected children who receive treatment have favorable outcomes. Treatment of infants without substantial neurologic disease at birth with pyrimethamine and sulfadiazine for 1 year results in normal cognitive, neurologic, and auditory outcomes, whereas treatment of infants who have moderate or severe neurologic disease at birth leads to normal neurologic and/or cognitive outcomes for most of the patients, and normal auditory function in all.[26]

Systematic serologic screening of either the newborn or the mother should be considered, given that improved outcomes result when infants receive proper therapy.[27] In countries such as France, where seroprevalence rates are higher than those in the United States, prenatal screening has proven cost effective. Some states, such as Massachusetts and New Hampshire, perform, and Minnesota is considering performing, newborn screening and reporting of toxoplasmosis. Until consensus is reached, raising awareness and education of health care providers and their patients (eg, using hot water to wash utensils after handling raw or undercooked meat, using gloves during gardening) are imperative to decrease the burden of disease.[28]

Rubella Virus

Although universal screening and vaccination programs have made congenital rubella syndrome (CRS) a rare occurrence in developed countries, susceptibility rates in women of childbearing age in Southern Asia, Africa, and some parts of Latin America are 20%.[29] The national objective of elimination of rubella and CRS by 2010 from the United States has been attained. Zero to 6 cases are reported per year, most born to foreign-born mothers.[30] Classically, rubella affects the heart, eyes, and ears because virus replication leads to tissue necrosis and damage to endothelium, but thrombotic thrombocytopenic purpura, osteitis (areas of translucency in metaphysis of long bones), and meningoencephalitis may occur in 25% of affected infants.[31] Manifestations can be delayed in the form of purpuric rash, persistent diarrhea, pneumonia, and diabetes. Thus, similar to congenital CMV, CRS is not a static disease, given the spectrum of time of onset of symptoms. Infants with rubella secrete virus in high titers in their urine for up to 2 years.

Syphilis *(Treponema pallidum)*

The seroprevalence rate of syphilis in the United States is 4.5%, but access to adequate prenatal care results in the relatively low number of 13 cases of congenital syphilis per 100,000 live births, with a case fatality rate (stillbirths and deaths) of 6.4%. Seroprevalence rates remain disproportionately higher in large urban areas and the rural southern states and in the African American population (8-fold). Much of Europe has low seroprevalence rates, except for rural Eastern Europe and a recent upsurge in the United Kingdom. Worldwide, congenital syphilis remains a major problem that affects 500,000 to 1 million pregnancies yearly. Seroprevalence rates in some African countries, where resources for screening and treatment are most needed, are 15%, and the disease lacks the high priority status in the global awareness on neonatal health and infectious diseases.[32]

The various manifestations of congenital syphilis depend on the stage and adequacy of treatment of maternal syphilis and the gestation and immunologic response of the fetus. Transmission can occur any time during pregnancy, and intense inflammatory responses and prostaglandins induced by disseminated fetal infection may be responsible for fetal death, preterm delivery, and severe growth retardation. Congenital syphilis is more likely to occur with maternal primary and secondary syphilis (60% to 100%), if the disease is of unknown duration or untreated, if maternal plasma nontreponemal titer (Venereal Disease Research Laboratory [VDRL] or rapid plasma reagin [RPR] test) is more than 1:16 after therapy or at delivery, and if fewer than 4 weeks have elapsed between therapy and delivery. A potentially higher rate of treatment failure exists in HIV-positive pregnant women.

Signs of congenital syphilis are nonspecific and include prematurity and low birth weight (10% to 40%); hepatomegaly, with or without splenomegaly (33% to 100%); a blistering, scaly, copper-colored skin rash (40%); periostitis and osteochondritis (75% to 100% vs 20% in asymptomatic infants); pseudoparalysis (12%); respiratory distress (35%); CNS involvement with high CSF protein and pleocytosis (25% vs 10% in asymptomatic infants); Coombs-negative hemolytic anemia with hydrops; and thrombocytopenia and fever (10% to 45%).[33] Although more than one half of affected infants are asymptomatic at birth, lumbar puncture and long bone radiographs are often justified because 60% of these infants may be infected and develop disease later in life.

Prenatal screening is cost beneficial and cost effective. Ideally, all women should be screened with nontreponemal titers during the first trimester, then early in the third trimester and again at delivery for high-risk women (HIV-infected women, women who abuse drugs, women who reside in high-prevalence areas). Thus testing of women of unknown serostatus at delivery is necessary to identify potentially infected infants. Using the same nontreponemal serologic tests for the mother-infant pair is imperative. Evaluation for congenital syphilis is warranted if the infant's titer (non-cord blood) is 4-fold higher than the mother's or if the mother's titer has increased 4-fold; nevertheless, any increase in the infant's titer should be considered for evaluation.[33,34] The presence of the treponemal antibody IgM by fluorescent treponemal antibody absorption test (FTA-ABS) in the infant indicates active infection, but this test has a high false-positive rate and will remain positive for prolonged periods after treatment.[34] Follow-up with serologic assays should be carried out for at least 6 months. In the presence of mucocutaneous skin lesions or nasal discharge, gloves should be worn until 24 hours after initiation of therapy. A vaccine is not yet available.

Parvovirus B19

Although not part of the TORCH acronym, parvovirus B19 virus is transmitted in utero and has been identified as a cause of adverse fetal and neonatal outcomes. The virus is cytotoxic to erythroid progenitor cells inhibiting erythropoiesis. Seroprevalence rates vary from 50% to as much as 70% in day care educators. Susceptible pregnant women transmit the virus (transmission rate 30%), and although most newborns are asymptomatic and healthy, some evidence suggests that a high rate of intrauterine viral infection occurs throughout gestation and the virus persists until birth and beyond.[35] Adverse outcomes such as fetal anemia, neurologic anomalies, and nonimmune hydrops fetalis, as well as fetal death (overall risk 5%), are more likely if infection is acquired in the first half of pregnancy. The virus is not transmitted through breastfeeding. Prenatal diagnosis is made by maternal IgM antibodies and viral DNA in fetal blood.

PERINATAL INFECTIONS

Human Immunodeficiency Virus

Maximal reduction of perinatal HIV infection is one of the four primary goals of the Centers for Disease Control and Prevention (CDC) Advancing HIV Prevention Initiative, which was announced in 2003. The CDC recommends that all states require public health reporting of all cases of perinatal HIV exposure in infants. Transmission of HIV can occur in utero (<20%), but it is mostly transmitted perinatally or by breastfeeding. In countries where the interventions implemented in the developed world are not in place, the rates of mother-to-child transmission are 25% to 40%. A marked decline in the number of perinatal HIV infections in the United States has occurred in response to routine HIV screening for pregnant women since 1999, to rapid testing for undocumented cases during labor and delivery since 2002, to a second test during the third trimester for high-risk women and in areas of high prevalence, and to the use of antiretroviral drugs for treatment and prophylaxis of mother and child, avoidance of breastfeeding, and elective cesarean delivery when indicated.[36] Consequently, the rate of transmission now is approximately 2%, adding to approximately 200 to 300 cases yearly, mostly because of missed prevention opportunities.[37] These infants account for more than 90% of the AIDS cases reported in children younger than 13 years, one third of them being younger than 1 year.

The American Academy of Pediatrics recommends routine education and HIV testing, with consent, of all pregnant women in the United States.[34,38] Current guidelines recommend using highly active antiretroviral therapy, preferably a regimen that includes zidovudine, for women whose plasma HIV RNA levels are greater than 1000 copies/mL. If the mother's status is unknown, then the infant's primary care physician (PCP) should recommend immediate HIV testing for the newborn by a rapid HIV antibody test. In some states, rapid testing is required by law. The PCP plays a key role in preventing mother-to-child transmission of HIV by identifying HIV-exposed infants, prescribing antiretroviral prophylaxis for these infants to decrease the risk of acquiring HIV infection, and promoting avoidance of HIV transmission through human milk.[39] Continued efforts should focus on collecting data to identify the missed opportunities and to modify practices accordingly, sustaining the commitment to reinforce recognized factors such as increased accessibility to prenatal care, enhancing counseling, and lowering barriers such as social stigma and informed consent. The preferred test for diagnosis of HIV infection in infants is HIV nucleic acid detection by PCR assay of DNA extracted from peripheral blood mononuclear cells, not umbilical cord blood. Approximately 93% of infected newborns have detectable HIV DNA by 2 weeks of age. A second PCR should be performed at 1 to 2 months of age, but a sample taken from a newborn as early as 14 days of age may facilitate decisions about initiating antiretroviral therapy.[34]

Hepatitis B Virus

Five percent of the US population and 350 million people worldwide are infected with hepatitis B virus (HBV), and 1 million people die each year of HBV-associated disease. HBV is highly endemic in China and Southeast Asia, among other places. Because only one serotype of HBV has been found, an excellent protective vaccine has been developed, and implementing routine immunization programs has decreased HBV prevalence. Most states require that all mothers be tested for serologic evidence of HBV infection. Transmission occurs through the blood of the infected mother mixing with that of her child during childbirth. Because of its lipoprotein envelope, HBV resists enzymes in the blood. The blood of carriers frequently contains approximately 100 million infectious particles per milliliter, making it one of the most infectious of all viruses: 1 mcL of blood is sufficient for spread. Thus, without intervention, 70% to 90% of infants will be infected at birth if the mother tests positive for both the hepatitis B surface antigen and the hepatitis B e antigen; the transmission rate drops if the mother tests negative for the hepatitis B e antigen.

Ninety percent of infected newborns become chronic carriers because of their immature immune system. Carriers who acquire the virus at birth comprise the largest cohort to spread the virus to others.[40] The vaccine administered within 12 hours of birth to exposed newborns, together with hepatitis B immune globulin, provides sufficient protection against any further theoretical risk.[41] This combination reduces the vertical transmission rate by almost 90% and results in less than 5% of infants becoming HBV carriers (Table 101-2).

Hepatitis C Virus

Although the exact mechanisms of pathogenesis and transmission of hepatitis C virus (HCV) are the subjects of ongoing research, 2% of the US population and 170 million people worldwide are infected with HCV. Similar to HBV, HCV is highly infectious. Maternal-fetal transmission of HCV likely occurs

Table 101-2 Hepatitis B Immunoprophylaxis Scheme by Infant Birth Weight[1]

MATERNAL STATUS	INFANT ≥2000 g	INFANT <2000 g
HBsAg positive	Hepatitis B vaccine + HBIg (within 12 hr of birth)	Hepatitis B vaccine + HBIg (within 12 hr of birth)
	Continue vaccine series beginning at 1-2 mo of age according to recommended schedule for infants born to HBsAg-positive mothers	Continue vaccine series beginning at 1-2 mo of age according to recommended schedule for infants born to HBsAg-positive mothers
		Immunize with four vaccine doses; do not count birth dose as part of vaccine series
	Check anti-HBsAg and HBsAg after completion of vaccine series[2]	Check anti-HBsAg and HBsAg after completion of vaccine series[2]
	HBsAg-negative infants with anti-HBsAg levels ≥10 mIU/mL are protected and need no further medical management	HBsAg-negative infants with anti-HBsAg levels ≥10 mIU/mL are protected and need no further medical management
	HBsAg-negative infants with anti-HBsAg levels <10 mIU/mL should be reimmunized with three doses at 2-mo intervals and retested	HBsAg-negative infants with anti-HBsAg levels <10 mIU/mL should be reimmunized with three doses at 2-mo intervals and retested
	Infants who are HBsAg positive should receive appropriate follow-up, including medical evaluation for chronic liver disease	Infants who are HBsAg positive should receive appropriate follow-up, including medical evaluation for chronic liver disease
HBsAg status unknown	Test mother for HBsAg immediately after admission for delivery	Test mother for HBsAg immediately after admission for delivery
	Hepatitis B vaccine (by 12 hr)	Hepatitis B vaccine (by 12 hr)
	Administer HBIG (within 7 days) if mother tests HBsAg positive	Administer HBIg if mother tests HBsAg positive or if mother's HBsAg result is not available within 12 hr of birth
	Continue vaccine series beginning at 1-2 mo of age according to recommended schedule based on mother's HBsAg result	Continue vaccine series beginning at 1-2 mo of age according to recommended schedule based on mother's HBsAg result
		Immunize with four vaccine doses; do not count birth dose as part of vaccine series
HBsAg negative	Hepatitis B vaccine at birth[3]	Hepatitis B vaccine dose 1-30 days of chronologic age if medically stable, or at hospital discharge if before 30 days of chronologic age
	Continue vaccine series beginning at 1-2 mo of age	Continue vaccine series beginning at 1-2 mo of age
	Follow-up anti-HBs and HBsAg testing not needed	Follow-up anti-HBs and HBsAg testing not needed

anti-HBsAg, Antibody to hepatitis B surface antigen; *HBIg,* hepatitis B immune globulin; *HBsAg,* hepatitis B surface antigen.
[1]Extremes of gestational age and birth weight are no longer a consideration for timing of hepatitis B vaccine doses.
[2]Test at 9 to 18 months of age, generally at the next well-child visit after completion of the primary series. Use testing method that allows determination of a protective concentration of anti-HBsAg (≥10 mIU/mL).
[3]The first dose may be delayed until after hospital discharge for an infant who weighs ≥2000 g and whose mother is HBsAg negative, but only if a physician's order to withhold the birth dose and a copy of the mother's original HBsAg-negative laboratory report are documented in the infant's medical record.
Source: Pickering LK, Baker CJ, Long SS, et al, eds. *Red Book: 2006 Report of the Committee on Infectious Diseases.* 27th ed. Elk Grove Village, IL: American Academy of Pediatrics; 2006, Table 3-18, p 347.

either in utero or intrapartum, and 7% to 10% of newborns of affected mothers will be infected at birth. The risk of vertical transmission is greatly increased if the mother is coinfected with HIV unless she is receiving highly active antiretroviral therapy, which eliminates the difference in risk. No current recommendations have been issued to screen mothers for HCV, given the absence of an intervention to prevent vertical transmission. Testing HIV-positive mothers in addition to those with a history of or current intravenous drug use, known HCV exposure, and history of blood transfusions before 1992 for presence of anti-HCV antibody is recommended. HCV-infected mothers can breastfeed their infants; HCV transmission rates in milk of HCV antibody-positive mothers, but HCV-RNA negative mothers are reported to be near zero. HCV antibodies in colostrum and mature human milk appear protective for infants born to HCV antibody positive, but HIV negative mothers. However, as these antibody levels wane, the risk for HCV transmission in breast milk has been documented to increase. Because of the 50% chance of viral reactivation (conversion to HCV-RNA positive status) in HCV antibody–positive women, additional HCV-RNA testing is recommended during breastfeeding.

Infected infants are asymptomatic. They may have transient viremia and maternal anti-HCV during the first year of life. PCR for HCV antibodies and HCV should be performed periodically in the infant during the first 12 to 18 months of life.[42,43] Standardizing timing for HCV-RNA testing in infants and establishing a consensus on the diagnosis of HCV in vertical transmission are being evaluated.[40] Unlike HBV, HCV has many serotypes, known as quasispecies, because of its high mutation rate; hence creating a universally effective vaccine has been difficult.

Herpes Simplex Virus Types 1 (Mucosal) and 2 (Genital)

Neonates have the highest frequency of visceral and CNS infection of any HSV-infected population of patients. The morbidity and mortality (the untreated case–fatality ratio is 60%) associated with this virus cannot be overemphasized. Early detection and treatment are required to reduce neurologic sequelae in surviving infants. A third of the world is infected with HSV.[44] Sixty percent of women of childbearing age are seropositive for HSV-1, and 25% of the US population is seropositive for HSV-2. Seroconversion rate during pregnancy is 1% to 2%. The estimated number of neonatal herpes is 10 to 40 cases per 100,000 live births, with up to one third of cases caused by HSV-1 infection.

Virus reproduction initiates rapidly in epithelial cells, and thus growth in cell culture in the laboratory generally takes 48 to 96 hours. Subsequently, the virus establishes latency in the surrounding sensory nerve cells. From time to time, reactivation occurs and leads to infection of the surrounding epithelial cells. Perinatal transmission occurs via contact between the virus produced in the epithelial cells and genital secretions (or saliva) of the mother and the baby's abraded skin, which is denuded of keratin, thus exposing epithelial cells during (or after) birth. Approximately 85% of transmission occurs during delivery and less than 10% postnatally. The transmission rate is 30% to 50% after primary HSV-1 or HSV-2 infection and 3% during reactivation; both may be subclinical in the mother.[45] Virus shedding can be continuous and subclinical such that more than 70% of infants with neonatal HSV are born to mothers with no symptoms or signs of HSV lesions at delivery.

In the immune-immature host, the virus can reproduce in very high numbers and spread systemically from the eye, skin, and mouth to the CNS, adrenals, liver, and lungs. Liver involvement is marked by fever in the newborn. Disease is most commonly evident by approximately 12 days of life (range, 3 to 21 days of life). If acquired postnatally, then it can occur as late as 28 days. HSV infection occurs in one of three forms: (1) skin, eye, and mouth disease with vesicles, which occurs at approximately 7 to 10 days; (2) CNS disease, which occurs at approximately 17 days with irritability, lethargy, poor feeding, apnea, and seizures; and (3) disseminated disease, which occurs at 9 to 12 days of life. With disseminated disease, the brain is probably infected via blood, whereas in CNS disease, infection is probably the result of neuronal spread.[45]

If untreated, 70% of skin, eye, and mouth disease progresses to CNS or disseminated disease. Disseminated disease mimics disseminated enteroviral disease in the summer months. The sequelae of CNS disease are less severe with HSV-1 than with HSV-2, but disseminated disease with either virus carries the same prognosis. Maternal IgG is somewhat protective; consequently, infants whose mothers acquired infection near delivery and preterm babies are more vulnerable. Prematurity generally predicts mortality. Thus infants born at less than 28 weeks with active maternal lesions at time of delivery may benefit from a few days of acyclovir treatment while awaiting the results of viral cultures. Cesarean delivery in a woman with active lesions significantly reduces, but does not eliminate, the risk of infection.

Skin, conjunctivae, oropharynx, rectum, and urine can be cultured for herpes. HSV PCR of CSF has significantly increased the detection of CNS disease, but a high index of suspicion should be present in all ill infants in the absence of skin lesions. Viral DNA can be detected in CSF for up to 2 weeks, although with decreasing sensitivity with time.

Despite therapy, many infants with CNS disease will have various degrees of disabilities; therefore the clinician must make an early diagnosis and promptly intervene, given the potential of timely therapy. CSF PCR is suggested for all babies with CNS disease at the end of therapy because failure to clear viral DNA warrants continuation of therapy. Yet unknown is what role suppressive oral acyclovir therapy plays as prophylaxis against recurrent skin, eye, and mouth disease that may be associated with CNS involvement in 10% of instances. However, preliminary data suggest no substantial benefits in most cases, and risks, mainly neutropenia, may outweigh the benefits. Screening of pregnant women has not been established to be cost effective. A much-needed push exists for a mandatory national surveillance system to understand better the epidemiologic factors and incidence of neonatal herpes, to identify risk determinants, and to evaluate the potential for preventions by public health interventions.[46,47]

Enteroviruses

Enteroviral infections of the neonate are common.[48] In most cases, infection is acquired from the mother perinatally in the summer months and less frequently from the hospital via caretakers in close contact with the infant. Coxsackievirus group B serotypes 2 to 5 and echovirus type 11 can cause fulminant, sometimes fatal, disease in the neonate, especially if it occurs early (between 3 and 7 days of age). Early symptoms are poor feeding and respiratory distress; generalized disease exhibits as sepsis, with myocarditis and meningoencephalitis or fulminant hepatitis. More than one half of patients may die despite adequate supportive therapy. Although neonates respond by mounting an antibody reaction, macrophage function, which is necessary to limit initial enteroviral replication, is not sufficiently mature in the neonate. Premature infants are more susceptible than term infants because of the absence of passively acquired maternal antibody. Diagnosis can be made rapidly by culturing oropharyngeal secretions, feces, or urine and detection of viral DNA by PCR.

Chlamydia and *Ureaplasma* species

Chlamydia trachomatis is the most common cause of sexually transmitted infection, resulting in 100,000 annually exposed neonates in the United States. The infant of an untreated mother has a 35% chance of developing mucopurulent conjunctivitis, which is preventable by erythromycin or tetracycline ointment within an hour of delivery, and a 15% chance of developing pneumonia in the first few months of life.[49] *Ureaplasma* species can be acquired by the fetus at any time during pregnancy or at birth by passage through an infected birth canal. Several studies have shown that *Ureaplasma* species can cause congenital and neonatal pneumonias, especially in preterm infants; however, controversy remains on whether *Ureaplasma* infection of the respiratory tract contributes to the development of bronchopulmonary dysplasia.[50] The fastidious nature and susceptibility of these organisms to drying mandate careful attention in specimen collection. Isolation from normally sterile sites in an ill infant with otherwise unexplainable causes is highly suggestive of disease. In vivo antibiotic therapy may be efficacious.

Tuberculosis

One third of the world's population is estimated to be infected with *Mycobacterium tuberculosis*. The mother-to-child transmission rate in resource-limited settings is 15%.[51] Given the increasing number of immigrants to the United States from countries where tuberculosis (TB) is endemic, a high index of suspicion for congenital and perinatal TB must be maintained for ill neonates born to women at risk for TB.[52] The incidence of TB disease among foreign-born health care providers in New York State, for example, is 18 per 100,000. Prompt treatment of disease in the mother greatly diminishes the risk of disease in the infant. Congenital TB is rare and is acquired in utero by hematogenous spread. The more frequent perinatal disease occurs at birth by aspiration of infected amniotic fluid or, more commonly, by airborne transmission from the mother or any adult in close contact with the newborn, including health care providers.[53] Such transmission of *M tuberculosis* emphasizes the importance of effective latent TB infection testing and prophylaxis programs in health care settings.[54]

Symptoms of congenital TB are nonspecific and include hepatosplenomegaly, respiratory distress with abnormal chest x-ray, fever, and lymphadenopathy, which appear at approximately 2 to 3 weeks of life. Perinatal infection exhibits similarly and, if untreated, often results in local progression and dissemination (miliary TB), including meningitis. Because treatment of the infant with multiple drugs[55] greatly improves outcome, making the correct diagnosis is imperative. Diagnosis is established by demonstrating acid-fast bacilli or isolating *M tuberculosis* from body fluids. More advanced techniques remain to be tested in this age group.[56] The tuberculin skin test (TST) is initially negative and may take 1 to 3 months to become positive. A positive TST result in infants is a sentinel indicator for recent transmission. If the mother (or household member) has received antituberculosis therapy for less than 2 weeks before delivery, then the exposed newborn should be treated with isoniazid for 3 months after TB is excluded. A TST is performed at that time, and therapy is discontinued if negative. Similar recommendations ought to be implemented in exposed infants in the nursery or neonatal intensive care unit (NICU).[57,58]

Infants suspected of having congenital TB need to be isolated and appropriate infection control precautions undertaken. Because HIV infection represents the greatest risk factor for acquisition of TB, both mother and child should be tested for HIV. Separation of the infant from the mother (or household member) is necessary only if the mother has multidrug-resistant TB[59] (or, inevitably in the future, extensively drug-resistant TB[60]) or if noncompliance is expected.

Varicella-Zoster Virus

The only herpesvirus that can also be transmitted without person-to-person contact is varicella-zoster virus (VZV). With current vaccination programs in the United States, susceptibility rates of pregnant women are low, and congenital infection with VZV (nervous system stigmata, malformed extremities), which affects 5% of exposed infants, is extremely rare. Perinatal VZV infection is associated with a high death rate if maternal disease develops within 5 days before or 2 days after delivery. Progressive pneumonitis is characteristic of perinatal disease. Postexposure prophylaxis is available and effective.

NEONATAL SEPSIS

The majority of common bacterial pathogens that cause neonatal sepsis are acquired perinatally.

Group B *Streptococcus*

Group B *Streptococcus* (GBS) was the leading cause of neonatal infections in the 1970s and 1980s, with case-fatality rates of 20% to 50%. The implementation of preventive intrapartum antibiotic prophylaxis since the 1990s has substantially reduced early-onset disease incidence by 70% to 30 to 50 cases per 100,000 live births, with case-fatality rates of 7%, except in preterm (<37 weeks' gestation) infants, in whom the rate approaches 25%.

GBS colonizes the genitourinary or gastrointestinal tract (or both), and carriage rates are higher in African American women (20% to 30%).[61] Since 2002, jointly endorsed guidelines from the CDC, American Academy of Pediatrics, and American College of Obstetrics and Gynecology recommend universal rectogenital culture–based screening at 35 to 37 weeks' gestation.[62] Pregnant carriers identified before or during pregnancy should receive intravenous penicillin or ampicillin (oral antibiotics are ineffective); in addition, if GBS status is unknown, then intrapartum antibiotics should be administered in the presence of one or more of the following: preterm labor less than 37 weeks, temperature more than 38°C during labor (maternal chorioamnionitis), rupture of membranes more than 18 hours before delivery, previous newborn with GBS disease, or GBS bacteruria during pregnancy.

GBS can be transmitted in utero, at delivery, or postnatally and results in early-onset (before the first week of life with 90% within 24 hours of life) or late-onset disease (between 1 week to 3 months of life). The incidence ratio of early-onset to late-onset disease in the era of intrapartum antibiotic prophylaxis has dropped from 3:1 to 1:1. In the neonate, early disease can cause bacteremia, sepsis, pneumonia, and meningitis (<10% of cases). Meningitis (35% of cases), occult bacteremia, and focal infections such as osteomyelitis or arthritis are more common in late-onset disease.

Ampicillin and gentamicin are provided empirically for the treatment of GBS disease and substituted with penicillin once the organism is isolated. Duration of treatment for septicemia is 10 days, for meningitis 14 days. Ampicillin and gentamicin are also recommended empirically while awaiting culture results for all infants whose mothers have intrapartum chorioamnionitis. Real-time PCR analysis of samples taken from the ear, nose, or rectum, when standardized, may hasten the speed of diagnosis and avoid unnecessary treatment.[63]

So far, maternal GBS prophylaxis has not resulted in a greater likelihood of non-GBS infections, such as invasive *Escherichia coli* infections, in newborns[64,65] except in VLBW infants.[66] In contrast, ampicillin resistance has emerged among gram-negative pathogens, and thorough evaluation and systematic monitoring for trends in various pathogen prevalence rates and resistance patterns in these infants are critical.

Escherichia coli

Escherichia coli (E coli), a member of the gram-negative Enterobacteriaceae family, which are prevalent in the maternal gastrointestinal and birth tracts, used to be the second-leading cause of neonatal bacteremia, sepsis, and meningitis. In the era of intrapartum antibiotic prophylaxis for GBS, the incidence of *E coli* infections in overall neonatal sepsis has equaled that of GBS. The incidence of *E coli* sepsis, the majority of which are ampicillin resistant, has increased in VLBW and premature infants. Many *E coli* strains isolated from neonates express capsular proteins and toxins that facilitate traversing the blood-brain barrier and attaching to brain endothelial cells. Meningitis is more likely when the level of bacteremia is high. The organism can be isolated from sterile sites, and treatment should be adjusted according to the sensitivities. Other strains cause epidemic diarrhea in newborn nurseries with listlessness, poor feeding, and watery, mucousy stools developing over 3 to 6 days. Endotoxemia, overgrowth of gram-negative bacilli in the absence of lysozyme (normally present in human milk), and many other factors have been implicated in the pathogenesis of necrotizing enterocolitis. No strategies for preventing gram-negative infections have been identified yet, and because of the diversity of neonatal pathogens, single-pathogen vaccines will have limited impact.[66]

Listeria monocytogenes

Listeria monocytogenes is a gram-positive rod that is acquired through food and can colonize the vagina and rectum of pregnant women. A nationally notifiable disease, it has characteristics similar to GBS disease; early-onset sepsis is most likely acquired in utero, and late-onset (2 weeks of age) meningitis is acquired at parturition and, less commonly, in the hospital environment. Treatment is with ampicillin and gentamicin.

Special Considerations for Infants Requiring Prolonged Hospitalization

Infants in NICUs are at increased risk of developing diseases from several other organisms. Coagulase-negative staphylococci have been the most common cause of hospital-acquired infections in the NICU since the 1980s. *Staphylococcus aureus*, a skin colonizer, is implicated in various clinical entities and outbreaks. Enterococci are isolated in 10% to 15% of neonatal cases of sepsis in the NICU. The emergence of antibiotic resistance will dictate the challenges of therapy in these newborns.[67,68] Multifaceted interventions that help ensure adherence with evidence-based infection-control practices and the judicious use of antibiotics are essential in controlling these potentially invasive pathogens.

Candida Species

Invasive *Candida* infections (incidence 1% to 15%) have been observed in recent years as a result of the larger numbers of surviving premature, VLBW babies with prolonged central vascular catheter use and prolonged use of broad-spectrum antibiotics. Death (ranging from 11% to 44% in the literature) or neurodevelopmental impairment (with and without documented meningitis) occur in young, VLBW infants who develop candidiasis.[69] Other complications include indolent arthritis, osteomyelitis, and endocarditis. *Candida albicans* is the most common and most virulent colonizing species, but it can be treated with fluconazole and is less likely to display resistance during drug exposure. *Candida galbrata* and *Candida parapsilosis* act more as opportunists, but they are capable of developing resistance to azoles under pressure of drug exposure.[70] Some NICUs have adopted prophylaxis with fluconazole to reduce colonization and subsequent invasive fungal infections.[71] Universal prophylaxis with fluconazole may lead to emergence of resistant organisms and increases in the prevalence of non-albicans species. No conclusive data exist on changes in late morbidity and mortality rates with this regimen. Targeted short-course fluconazole to VLBW infants who are to receive broad-spectrum antibiotics for more than 3 days has been shown to be cost effective and may alleviate some of the previously mentioned concerns.[72] In addition, newer antifungal agents will need to be carefully evaluated in this age group.[73]

Respiratory Syncytial Virus

Guidelines for prophylaxis against respiratory syncytial virus (RSV), the causative agent of bronchiolitis, with the monoclonal antibody palivizumab (Synagis) beginning before the onset of RSV season were last revised in 2003.[74] Breakthrough infections occur in 2% to 3% of cases, especially in particularly vulnerable preterm (<35 weeks' gestation) and VLBW infants who remain hospitalized in the NICU during RSV season, which can be partially explained by suboptimal protective serum antibody concentrations, especially after the first dose.[75] The evidence on the role of RSV immune globulin in treating severe RSV infections is limited.[76,77]

EMERGING INFECTIOUS DISEASES

Community-Acquired Methicillin-Resistant *Staphylococcus aureus*

Three molecular types account for most isolates of community-acquired methicillin-resistant *S aureus* (MRSA) in the United States, and they are genetically distinct from hospital-acquired MRSA. PCPs should be aware that community-acquired MRSA can cause skin infections among otherwise healthy newborns in nurseries and bacteremias in NICUs, and cultures and resistance testing are important to guide treatment options.[78,79] Symptoms may occur 1 to 18 days after discharge from the nursery, and some infants may need hospitalization and antibiotic treatment.[80] Maternal history is noncontributory. Prospective studies will clarify the risk factors for acquisition and transmission among neonates; in the interim, standard infection-control procedures, including consistent hand hygiene, application of dry dressings to draining lesions, and treatment of health care providers with skin lesions, should be implemented. Culture surveys for health care providers are not routinely performed, and the necessity for the universal use of gowns and gloves is debatable.

West Nile Virus

Since the initial detection of West Nile virus (WNV) in 1999 in New York, an ongoing epidemic, numbering more than 16,000 cases, has occurred in the United States because the population was immunologically naive. The first report of possible congenital infection in 2002 described a newborn with cystic destruction of the cerebrum and chorioretinal scarring. Since then, one case each of meningitis, encephalitis, and rash has been reported in infants whose mothers acquired WNV peripartum,[81] with no significant differences in growth parameters, Apgar scores, and hearing tests.[82] Cord blood anti-WNV IgM tests were negative, and the sensitivity and specificity of anti-WNV IgM in umbilical cord or amniotic fluid are not well established. Hence no conclusive laboratory evidence of congenital WNV infection exists, and more data must be gathered.

Interim guidelines for WNV were published by the CDC in 2004 and recommend reporting infections during pregnancy to local or state health departments, evaluating the fetus by ultrasound no sooner than 2 to 4 weeks after diagnosis, and providing a thorough clinical evaluation of the newborn.[83]

TOOLS FOR PRACTICE

Medical Decision Support

- *A Comprehensive Immunization Strategy to Eliminate Transmission of Hepatitis B Virus Infection in the United States* (report), Centers for Disease Control and Prevention (www.cdc.gov/mmwr/preview/mmwrhtml/rr5416a1.htm).
- *Controlling Tuberculosis in the United States: Recommendations from the American Thoracic Society, CDC, and the Infectious Diseases Society of America* (report), Centers for Disease Control and Prevention (www.cdc.gov/mmwr/preview/mmwrhtml/rr5412a1.htm).
- *Interim Guidelines for the Evaluation of Infants Born to Mothers with West Nile Virus During Pregnancy*, Centers for Disease Control and Prevention (www.cdc.gov/mmwr/preview/mmwrhtml/mm5307a4.htm).
- *Recommendations for Prevention and Control of Hepatitis C Virus (HCV) Infection and HCV-Related Chronic Disease*, Centers for Disease Control and Prevention (www.cdc.gov/mmwr/preview/mmwrhtml/00055154.htm).
- Red Book, 2006 Report of the Committee on Infectious Diseases, American Academy of Pediatrics (www.aap.org/bookstore).
- *Revised Recommendations for HIV Testing of Adults, Adolescents, and Pregnant Women in Health-Care Settings*, Centers for Disease Control and Prevention (www.cdc.gov/mmwr/preview/mmwrhtml/rr5514a1.htm).

AAP POLICY STATEMENT

King SM, American Academy of Pediatrics, Committee on Pediatric AIDS and Canadian Paediatric Society and Infectious Diseases Immunization Committee. Evaluation and treatment of the human immunodeficiency virus-1-exposed infant. *Pediatrics*. 2004;114(2):497-505. (aappolicy.aappublications.org/cgi/content/full/pediatrics;114/2/497).

SUGGESTED READINGS

Branson BM, Handsfield HH, Lampe MA, et al. Revised recommendations for HIV testing of adults, adolescents, and pregnant women in health-care settings. *MMWR Recomm Rep*. 2006;55:1-17.

Khetsuriani N, Lamonte A, Oberste MS, et al. Neonatal enterovirus infections reported to the national enterovirus surveillance system in the United States, 1983-2003. *Pediatr Infect Dis J*. 2006;25:889-893.

Lawrence RM, Lawrence RA. Breast milk and infection. *Clin Perinatol*. 2004;31:501-528.

Lopez A, Dietz VJ, Wilson M, et al. Preventing congenital toxoplasmosis. *MMWR Recomm Rep*. 2000;49:59-68.

McLeod R, Boyer K, Karrison T, et al. Outcome of treatment for congenital toxoplasmosis, 1981-2004: the National Collaborative Chicago-Based, Congenital Toxoplasmosis Study. *Clin Infect Dis*. 2006;42:1383-1394.

Ross DS, Dollard SC, Victor M, et al. The epidemiology and prevention of congenital cytomegalovirus infection and disease: activities of the Centers for Disease Control and Prevention Workgroup. *J Womens Health (Larchmt)*. 2006;15:224-229.

Saloojee H, Velaphi S, Goga Y, et al. The prevention and management of congenital syphilis: an overview and recommendations. *Bull World Health Organ.* 2004;82:424-430.
Schrag S, Schuchat A. Prevention of neonatal sepsis. *Clin Perinatol.* 2005;32:601-615.

REFERENCES

1. Lawrence RM, Lawrence RA. Breast milk and infection. *Clin Perinatol.* 2004;31:501-528.
2. Lewis DB, Wilson CB. Developmental immunology and role of host defenses in fetal and neonatal susceptibility to infection. In: Remington S, Klein J, Baker C, et al, eds. *Infectious Diseases of the Fetus and Newborn Infant.* 6th ed. Philadelphia, PA: Elsevier Saunders; 2006.
3. Schrag S, Schuchat A. Prevention of neonatal sepsis. *Clin Perinatol.* 2005;32:601-615.
4. Garges HP, Moody MA, Cotten CM, et al. Neonatal meningitis: what is the correlation among cerebrospinal fluid cultures, blood cultures, and cerebrospinal fluid parameters? *Pediatrics.* 2006;117:1094-1100.
5. Steer P. The epidemiology of preterm labor—a global perspective. *J Perinat Med.* 2005;33:273-276.
6. Abdel-Fattah SA, Bhat A, Illanes S, et al. TORCH test for fetal medicine indications: only CMV is necessary in the United Kingdom. *Prenat Diagn.* 2005;25:1028-1031.
7. Schrag SJ, Arnold KE, Mohle-Boetani JC, et al. Prenatal screening for infectious diseases and opportunities for prevention. *Obstet Gynecol.* 2003;102:753-760.
8. Ross DS, Dollard SC, Victor M, et al. The epidemiology and prevention of congenital cytomegalovirus infection and disease: activities of the Centers for Disease Control and Prevention Workgroup. *J Womens Health (Larchmt).* 2006;15:224-229.
9. Pass RF. Congenital cytomegalovirus infection and hearing loss. *Herpes.* 2005;12:50-55.
10. Ross SA, Fowler KB, Ashrith G, et al. Hearing loss in children with congenital cytomegalovirus infection born to mothers with preexisting immunity. *J Pediatr.* 2006;148:332-336.
11. Gerday E, Grose C. Demographic differences in congenital cytomegalovirus infection in the United States. *J Pediatr.* 2004;145:435-436.
12. Modlin JF, Grant PE, Makar RS, et al. Case records of the Massachusetts General Hospital. Weekly clinicopathological exercises. Case 25-2003. A newborn boy with petechiae and thrombocytopenia. *N Engl J Med.* 2003;349:691-700.
13. Maschmann J, Hamprecht K, Dietz K, et al. Cytomegalovirus infection of extremely low-birth weight infants via breast milk. *Clin Infect Dis.* 2001;33:1998-2003.
14. Vollmer B, Seibold-Weiger K, Schmitz-Salue C, et al. Postnatally acquired cytomegalovirus infection via breast milk: effects on hearing and development in preterm infants. *Pediatr Infect Dis J.* 2004;23:322-327.
15. Scanga L, Chaing S, Powell C, et al. Diagnosis of human congenital cytomegalovirus infection by amplification of viral DNA from dried blood spots on perinatal cards. *J Mol Diagn.* 2006;8:240-245.
16. Boppana SB, Fowler KB, Pass RF, et al. Congenital cytomegalovirus infection: association between virus burden in infancy and hearing loss. *J Pediatr.* 2005;146:817-823.
17. Lanari M, Lazzarotto T, Venturi V, et al. Neonatal cytomegalovirus blood load and risk of sequelae in symptomatic and asymptomatic congenitally infected newborns. *Pediatrics.* 2006;117:e76-e83.
18. Bradford RD, Cloud G, Lakeman AD, et al. Detection of cytomegalovirus (CMV) DNA by polymerase chain reaction is associated with hearing loss in newborns with symptomatic congenital CMV infection involving the central nervous system. *J Infect Dis.* 2005;191:227-233.
19. Nigro G, Adler SP, La Torre R, et al. Passive immunization during pregnancy for congenital cytomegalovirus infection. *N Engl J Med.* 2005;353:1350-1362.
20. Schleiss MR. Antiviral therapy of congenital cytomegalovirus infection. *Semin Pediatr Infect Dis.* 2005;16:50-59.
21. Tanaka-Kitajima N, Sugaya N, Futatani T, et al. Ganciclovir therapy for congenital cytomegalovirus infection in six infants. *Pediatr Infect Dis J.* 2005;24:782-785.
22. Kimberlin DW, Lin CY, Sanchez PJ, et al. Effect of ganciclovir therapy on hearing in symptomatic congenital cytomegalovirus disease involving the central nervous system: a randomized, controlled trial. *J Pediatr.* 2003;143:16-25.
23. Arvin AM, Fast P, Myers M, et al. Vaccine development to prevent cytomegalovirus disease: report from the National Vaccine Advisory Committee. *Clin Infect Dis.* 2004;39:233-239.
24. Kim K. Time to screen for congenital toxoplasmosis? *Clin Infect Dis.* 2006;42:1395-1397.
25. Gilbert R, Tan HK, Cliffe S, et al. Symptomatic toxoplasma infection due to congenital and postnatally acquired infection. *Arch Dis Child.* 2006;91:495-498.
26. McLeod R, Boyer K, Karrison T, et al. Outcome of treatment for congenital toxoplasmosis, 1981-2004: the National Collaborative Chicago-Based, Congenital Toxoplasmosis Study. *Clin Infect Dis.* 2006;42:1383-1394.
27. Boyer KM, Holfels E, Roizen N, et al. Risk factors for Toxoplasma gondii infection in mothers of infants with congenital toxoplasmosis: implications for prenatal management and screening. *Am J Obstet Gynecol.* 2005;192:564-571.
28. Lopez A, Dietz VJ, Wilson M, et al. Preventing congenital toxoplasmosis. *MMWR Recomm Rep.* 2000;49:59-68.
29. Best JM, Castillo-Solorzano C, Spika JS, et al. Reducing the global burden of congenital rubella syndrome: report of the World Health Organization Steering Committee on Research Related to Measles and Rubella Vaccines and Vaccination, June 2004. *J Infect Dis.* 2005;192:1890-1897.
30. Meissner HC, Reef SE, Cochi S. Elimination of rubella from the United States: a milestone on the road to global elimination. *Pediatrics.* 2006;117:933-935.
31. Banatvala JE, Brown DW. Rubella. *Lancet.* 2004;363:1127-1137.
32. Saloojee H, Velaphi S, Goga Y, et al. The prevention and management of congenital syphilis: an overview and recommendations. *Bull World Health Organ.* 2004;82:424-430.
33. Woods CR. Syphilis in children: congenital and acquired. *Semin Pediatr Infect Dis.* 2005;16:245-257.
34. American Academy of Pediatrics, Committee on Infectious Diseases, Pickering LK, Baker CJ, Long SS, et al, eds. *Red Book: 2006 Report of the Committee on Infectious Diseases.* 27th ed. Elk Grove Village, IL: American Academy of Pediatrics; 2006.
35. Koch WC, Harger JH, Barnstein B, et al. Serologic and virologic evidence for frequent intrauterine transmission of human parvovirus B19 with a primary maternal infection during pregnancy. *Pediatr Infect Dis J.* 1998;17:489-494.
36. Centers for Disease Control and Prevention. Achievements in public health. Reduction in perinatal transmission of HIV infection—United States, 1985-2005. *MMWR Morb Mortal Wkly Rep.* 2006;55:592-597.
37. Shetty AK. Perinatally acquired HIV-1 infection: prevention and evaluation of HIV-exposed infants. *Semin Pediatr Infect Dis.* 2005;16:282-295.
38. Branson BM, Handsfield HH, Lampe MA, et al. Revised recommendations for HIV testing of adults, adolescents, and pregnant women in health-care settings. *MMWR Recomm Rep.* 2006;55:1-17.

39. King SM. Evaluation and treatment of the human immunodeficiency virus-1–exposed infant. *Pediatrics.* 2004; 114:497-505.
40. Slowik MK, Jhaveri R. Hepatitis B and C viruses in infants and young children. *Semin Pediatr Infect Dis.* 2005;16:296-305.
41. Mast EE, Margolis HS, Fiore AE, et al. A comprehensive immunization strategy to eliminate transmission of hepatitis B virus infection in the United States: recommendations of the Advisory Committee on Immunization Practices (ACIP) part 1: immunization of infants, children, and adolescents. *MMWR Recomm Rep.* 2005; 54:1-31.
42. Polywka S, Schroter M, Feucht HH, et al. Low risk of vertical transmission of hepatitis C by breastmilk. *Clin Infect Dis.* 1999; 29:1327-1329.
43. Centers for Disease Control and Prevention. Recommendations for prevention and control of hepatitis C virus (HCV) infection and HCV-related chronic disease. *MMWR Morb Mortal Wkly Rep.* 1998;47(RR19):1-39.
44. Kimberlin DW. Neonatal HSV infections: the global picture. *Herpes.* 2004;11:31-32.
45. Kimberlin D. Herpes simplex virus, meningitis and encephalitis in neonates. *Herpes.* 2004;11(suppl 2): 65A-76A.
46. Donoval BA, Passaro DJ, Klausner JD. The public health imperative for a neonatal herpes simplex virus infection surveillance system. *Sex Transm Dis.* 2006; 33:170-174.
47. Handsfield HH, Waldo AB, Brown ZA, et al. Neonatal herpes should be a reportable disease. *Sex Transm Dis.* 2005;32:521-525.
48. Khetsuriani N, Lamonte A, Oberste MS, et al. Neonatal enterovirus infections reported to the national enterovirus surveillance system in the United States, 1983-2003. *Pediatr Infect Dis J.* 2006;25:889-893.
49. Darville T. Chlamydia trachomatis infections in neonates and young children. *Semin Pediatr Infect Dis.* 2005; 16:235-244.
50. Schelonka RL, Katz B, Waites KB, et al. Critical appraisal of the role of Ureaplasma in the development of bronchopulmonary dysplasia with metaanalytic techniques. *Pediatr Infect Dis J.* 2005;24:1033-1039.
51. Pillay T, Khan M, Moodley J, et al. Perinatal tuberculosis and HIV-1: considerations for resource-limited settings. *Lancet Infect Dis.* 2004;4:155-165.
52. Taylor Z, Nolan CM, Blumberg HM. Controlling tuberculosis in the United States. Recommendations from the American Thoracic Society, CDC, and the Infectious Diseases Society of America. *MMWR Recomm Rep.* 2005;54:1-81.
53. Ormerod P. Tuberculosis in pregnancy and the puerperium. *Thorax.* 2001;56:494-499.
54. Centers for Disease Control and Prevention. Mycobacterium tuberculosis transmission in a newborn nursery and maternity ward—New York City, 2003. *MMWR Morb Mortal Wkly Rep.* 2005;54:1280-1283.
55. Smith KC, Seaworth BJ. Drug-resistant tuberculosis: controversies and challenges in pediatrics. *Expert Rev Anti Infect Ther.* 2005;3:995-1010.
56. Starke JR. Interferon-gamma release assays for diagnosis of tuberculosis infection in children. *Pediatr Infect Dis J.* 2006;25:941-942.
57. Laartz BW, Narvarte HJ, Holt D, et al. Congenital tuberculosis and management of exposures in a neonatal intensive care unit. *Infect Control Hosp Epidemiol.* 2002; 23:573-579.
58. Crockett M, King SM, Kitai I, et al. Nosocomial transmission of congenital tuberculosis in a neonatal intensive care unit. *Clin Infect Dis.* 2004;39:1719-1723.
59. Granich RM, Oh P, Lewis B, et al. Multidrug resistance among persons with tuberculosis in California, 1994-2003. *JAMA.* 2005;293:2732-2739.
60. Centers for Disease Control and Prevention. Emergence of Mycobacterium tuberculosis with extensive resistance to second-line drugs—worldwide, 2000-2004. *MMWR Morb Mortal Wkly Rep.* 2006;55:301-305.
61. Centers for Disease Control and Prevention. Diminishing racial disparities in early-onset neonatal group B streptococcal disease—United States, 2000-2003. *MMWR Morb Mortal Wkly Rep.* 2004;53:502-505.
62. Schrag S, Gorwitz R, Fultz-Butts K, et al. Prevention of perinatal group B streptococcal disease. Revised guidelines from CDC. *MMWR Recomm Rep.* 2002;51:1-22.
63. Natarajan G, Johnson YR, Zhang F, et al. Real-time polymerase chain reaction for the rapid detection of group B streptococcal colonization in neonates. *Pediatrics.* 2006;118:14-22.
64. Schrag SJ, Hadler JL, Arnold KE, et al. Risk factors for invasive, early-onset Escherichia coli infections in the era of widespread intrapartum antibiotic use. *Pediatrics.* 2006;118:570-576.
65. Edwards RK, Duff P. Intrapartum antibiotic prophylaxis: making an evidence-based selection. *Pediatrics.* 2006;117:255-256.
66. Schrag SJ, Stoll BJ. Early-onset neonatal sepsis in the era of widespread intrapartum chemoprophylaxis. *Pediatr Infect Dis J.* 2006;25:939-940.
67. Hoehn R, Groll AH, Schaefer V, et al. Linezolid treatment of glycopeptide-resistant Enterococcus faecium in very low birth weight premature neonates. *Int J Antimicrob Agents.* 2006;27:256-258.
68. Deville JG, Adler S, Azimi PH, et al. Linezolid versus vancomycin in the treatment of known or suspected resistant gram-positive infections in neonates. *Pediatr Infect Dis J.* 2003;22:S158-S163.
69. Benjamin DK Jr, Stoll BJ, Fanaroff AA, et al. Neonatal candidiasis among extremely low birth weight infants: risk factors, mortality rates, and neurodevelopmental outcomes at 18 to 22 months. *Pediatrics.* 2006;117:84-92.
70. Long SS, Stevenson DK. Reducing Candida infections during neonatal intensive care: management choices, infection control, and fluconazole prophylaxis. *J Pediatr.* 2005;147:135-141.
71. McGuire W, Clerihew L, Austin N. Prophylactic intravenous antifungal agents to prevent mortality and morbidity in very low birth weight infants. *Cochrane Database Syst Rev.* 2004;CD003850.
72. Uko S, Soghier LM, Vega M, et al. Targeted short-term fluconazole prophylaxis among very low birth weight and extremely low birth weight infants. *Pediatrics.* 2006;117:1243-1252.
73. Muldrew KM, Maples HD, Stowe CD, et al. Intravenous voriconazole therapy in a preterm infant. *Pharmacotherapy.* 2005;25:893-898.
74. Meissner HC, Long SS. Revised indications for the use of palivizumab and respiratory syncytial virus immune globulin intravenous for the prevention of respiratory syncytial virus infections. *Pediatrics.* 2003;112:1447-1452.
75. Wu SY, Bonaparte J, Pyati S. Palivizumab use in very premature infants in the neonatal intensive care unit. *Pediatrics.* 2004;114:e554-e556.
76. Fuller H, Del Mar C. Immunoglobulin treatment for respiratory syncytial virus infection. *Cochrane Database Syst Rev.* 2006;CD004883.
77. American Academy of Pediatrics. Diagnosis and management of bronchiolitis *Pediatrics.* 2006;118:1774-1793.
78. Bratu S, Eramo A, Kopec R, et al. Community-associated methicillin-resistant Staphylococcus aureus in hospital nursery and maternity units. *Emerg Infect Dis.* 2005;11:808-813.

79. Healy CM, Hulten KG, Palazzi DL, et al. Emergence of new strains of methicillin-resistant Staphylococcus aureus in a neonatal intensive care unit. *Clin Infect Dis.* 2004; 39:1460-1466.
80. Centers for Disease Control and Prevention. Community-associated methicillin-resistant Staphylococcus aureus infection among healthy newborns—Chicago and Los Angeles County, 2004. *MMWR Morb Mortal Wkly Rep.* 2006;55:329-332.
81. Paisley JE, Hinckley AF, O'Leary DR, et al. West Nile virus infection among pregnant women in a northern Colorado community, 2003 to 2004. *Pediatrics.* 2006; 117:814-820.
82. O'Leary DR, Kuhn S, Kniss KL, et al. Birth outcomes following West Nile virus infection of pregnant women in the United States: 2003-2004. *Pediatrics.* 2006;117:e537-e545.
83. Centers for Disease Control and Prevention. Interim guidelines for the evaluation of infants born to mothers infected with West Nile virus during pregnancy. *MMWR Morb Mortal Wkly Rep.* 2004;53:154-157.

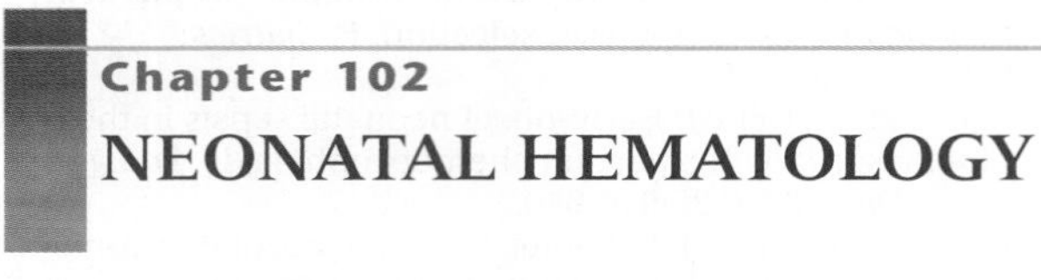

Chapter 102

NEONATAL HEMATOLOGY

M. Catherine Driscoll, MD

Evaluating hematologic disorders in newborns is fundamentally different from evaluating hematologic disorders in older children because the developmental aspects of erythropoiesis and hemostasis are not complete at birth but rather continue throughout much of the first months of life.

ANEMIA IN THE NEONATE

The fetal and neonatal erythrocyte differs from the adult erythrocyte with regard to life span, membrane structure, hemoglobin (Hb), and metabolic content. The life span of the erythrocyte in a healthy term infant is 60 to 80 days and in a preterm infant is 30 to 50 days.[1] This time span is significantly shorter than the 120 days of an adult red blood cell. At birth, the erythrocyte reflects the hypoxic environment of fetal life in which oxygen delivery is one third that of an adult. This relative hypoxia leads to increased erythropoietin and active erythropoiesis evident by increased reticulocytes and nucleated red cells during the first few days of life. At birth, when lungs become the oxygen source, Hb saturation increases to 95%, erythropoietin levels fall, and erythropoiesis significantly decreases.

Hematologic values for the term and preterm newborn reflect the active nature of erythropoiesis in late fetal development during which Hb concentration rises slowly from approximately 14.5 g/dL at 28 weeks gestation to 15.0 g/dL at 34 weeks to 16.8 g/dL at 40 weeks. The reticulocyte count is elevated for the first 3 days of life and drops to less than 1% by day 7 in the term newborn, whereas in the preterm newborn, the reticulocyte count is higher in cord blood and may remain elevated until day 7 of life.

The physiologic anemia of the term newborn is not a pathologic state but an adjustment to the state of excess capability of oxygen delivery relative to tissue needs at birth. The combination of a shortened neonatal red cell survival, decrease in erythropoiesis, and a growth-related increase in blood volume leads to a progressive decrease in Hb concentration during the first 2 months of life. This physiologic nadir may occur from week 6 to 12 of life, when the Hb concentration is between 9.5 and 11.0 g/dL. Erythropoietin will then increase as sensors in the kidney and liver detect tissue hypoxia, and an increase in reticulocytes heralds an increase in Hb concentration, which rises to a mean of 12.5 g/dL.

Anemia in premature neonates, however, is not physiologic and is multifactorial in nature. Up to 50% of premature infants younger than 32 weeks' gestation will develop symptoms associated with anemia of prematurity. Symptoms may include respiratory difficulties (apnea, periodic breathing, tachypnea), poor feeding and weight gain difficulties, tachycardia, flow murmurs, and pallor. The erythropoietin response to anemia is suboptimal in the preterm infant in whom the liver is the source of erythropoietin and hepatic oxygen sensors may be less sensitive.[2] The preterm infant's shortened red cell survival, expanding blood volume with rapid growth, and iatrogenic blood loss from frequent testing aggravates the effects of erythropoietin deficiency.

Infants weighing less than 1.2 kg will reach their Hb nadir at 4 to 8 weeks with a Hb concentration of 6.5 to 9.0 g/dL. Infants from 1.2 to 2.5 kg will reach a nadir between 5 and 10 weeks with a Hb concentration of 8.0 to 9.0 g/dL. Iron supplementation is recommended for all preterm infants, in the range of 4 to 6 mg/kg/day of elemental iron. Ensuring adequate nutritional intake of vitamin E, B_{12}, and folate is also important. Anemia of prematurity typically resolves by 3 to 6 months of age. The recently published Premature Infant in Need of Transfusion (PINT) randomized clinical trial demonstrated that transfusion to maintain a high hematocrit does not reduce mortality, morbidity, or improve long-term outcome for infants with anemia of prematurity.[3]

Approach to Anemia

Three broad classifications of anemia exist in the newborn, including blood loss, hemolysis, and decreased production. The medical history and physical examination may frequently reveal the cause of the anemia. The maternal history (ABO/Rh, infections, autoimmune disease), obstetrical history (gestation, delivery difficulties), and family history (anemia, jaundice, cholelithiasis, splenomegaly, transfusion history) may identify a cause. The age at presentation is important because a significant anemia detected within the first 24 hours of life is usually caused by blood loss or alloimmune hemolysis. Anemia detected after 24 hours of age points to hemolysis or internal hemorrhage. Anemia detected several weeks after birth may be physiologic or is compatible with Hb disorders or rare hypoplastic erythrocyte disorders. The physical examination of an infant with hemolysis may demonstrate icterus, hepatosplenomegaly, and stigmata of congenital infections. Infants with acute blood loss will exhibit hypovolemic shock, whereas those with chronic blood loss will have pallor without clinical distress.

The initial laboratory evaluation of anemia should include a complete blood count, reticulocyte count, evaluation of the peripheral smear, and a direct antiglobulin test (DAT). The diagnosis of anemia should be based on reference ranges for the newborn and must take into account gestational and postnatal age. During the neonatal period, variation in normal hematologic values is higher than at any other time of life.

Anemia Caused by Blood Loss

Hemorrhage may occur at any time during prenatal, perinatal, or postnatal life. Fetal hemorrhage is more commonly associated with fetal to maternal hemorrhage (FMH), which may occur in up to 8% of all pregnancies. The effects of FMH depend on the volume of hemorrhage and whether it is acute or chronic. Approximately 50 mL of fetal blood must be lost to produce significant anemia. Infants with chronic blood loss will exhibit pallor and anemia that can be mild normochromic, normocytic (Hb 9-12 g/dL), or hypochromic and microcytic (Hb 5-7 g/dL). Most forms are clinically stable and can be treated conservatively with iron supplementation for 3 months. Symptomatic infants (tachycardia, tachypnea, poor feeding) should be transfused with packed red blood cells (RBCs). Acute blood loss, however, may result in hypovolemic shock. These infants may have a normal Hb concentration at birth, but anemia will be present hours later as the plasma volume reexpands. FMH may be diagnosed by the presence of fetal RBCs in the maternal circulation. This task can be accomplished by either the Kleihauer-Betke test, which involves examination of a stained maternal blood smear following differential acid elution of Hb A but not fetal Hb, or by flow cytometry techniques. These studies, however, may have negative results if ABO incompatibility exists between mother and infant in which incompatible fetal RBCs may be rapidly removed. Twin-to-twin transfusion (TTS) may occur in monozygous twins and result in significant anemia for one twin and polycythemia for the other. TTS has a high rate of fetal mortality (approximately 63%). Hemorrhage occurs because of vascular anastomoses in monochorionic placentas, which allow transfer of blood from one twin to the other.[4] TTS should be thought to occur when more than 5-g/dL difference exists in Hb concentration between monochorionic twins.

Perinatal hemorrhage is associated with obstetrical complications such as placenta previa, abruptio placenta, ruptured umbilical cord, and emergency cesarean section. Placenta previa occurs more commonly in women with a history of previous cesarean birth and increased parity. The incidence is approximately 1 in 3000 deliveries, and the mortality is high in cases undetected before delivery (33% to 100%). Placental abruption occurs when the placenta separates from the uterus. The incidence is 3 to 6:1000 live births and increases with lower gestational age. Mortality is high with death in 15% to 20% of cases with significant abruption (involvement of more than 50% of the placental surface). Cord rupture can occur from traction on a shortened or abnormal umbilical cord. Cord aneurysms, varices, and cysts can lead to a weakened cord.

Postnatal blood loss is commonly caused by fetal transfusion into the placenta at birth and by birth trauma. Fetoplacental hemorrhage occurs when the infant is held above the placenta at birth. Birth trauma can result in internal hemorrhage. Cephalohematoma and subgaleal hematomas can occur with vacuum or forceps assisted births. This diagnosis should be considered when a fluid collection occurs in dependent areas of the infant's head with signs of hypovolemia. Occult hemorrhages usually occur after 24 hours of life. Breech deliveries and infants with macrosomia may develop splenic, renal, or adrenal hemorrhage into the retroperitoneal space as a consequence of a difficult delivery.

Hemolytic Anemia

Red cell hemolysis is a common cause of anemia in the newborn and has multiple causes. The neonatal red cell has intrinsic properties that lead to shortened survival. The normal neonatal erythrocyte has a less deformable membrane in the microcirculation and is more likely to be sequestered and removed by the reticuloendothelial system. Infants with mild hemolysis may have a blunted erythropoietic response and may not respond with reticulocytosis because of the excess oxygen-carrying capacity of blood. Thus hyperbilirubinemia may be the only symptom in mild anemia. Severe hemolytic anemia will also be accompanied by an elevated reticulocyte count. Hemolytic anemias can be classified based on immune-mediated disorders, acquired disorders, and hereditary disorders of the erythrocyte.

Alloimmune Hemolysis

Alloimmune hemolytic anemia, caused by maternal fetal blood group incompatibility (Rh[D] and ABO) is the most common cause of neonatal hemolytic anemia worldwide. The spectrum of alloimmune hemolysis can range from mild anemia and hyperbilirubinemia to severe anemia with hydrops fetalis. Antigens in the ABO, Rh, Kell, MN, Duffy, and Vel systems are expressed on the fetal red cell during the 1st trimester. The advent of immunoprophylaxis to prevent Rh(D) sensitization in 1968 dramatically decreased the incidence of alloimmune hemolysis.[5] Nevertheless, Rh incompatibility is still a main cause of serious alloimmunization, although ABO incompatibility is far more prevalent. Cases of alloimmunization are detected by a positive DAT, which detects the presence of antibody on fetal red cells or in the plasma (indirect antiglobulin test). Eliminating alloimmunization as a cause of hemolytic anemia is important before testing for other etiologies.

RH HEMOLYTIC DISEASE. Rh(D) hemolytic disease occurs in an Rh-negative mother and Rh-positive fetus when fetal red cells leak into the maternal circulation and sensitize the mother to the D antigen on the fetal red cell. The mother produces anti-D immunoglobulin G (IgG) antibody, which crosses into the fetal circulation, causing fetal red cell destruction. First pregnancies usually result in maternal sensitization without significant fetal hemolysis. However, subsequent pregnancies are more severely affected. A first pregnancy with significant neonatal Rh hemolytic disease usually indicates that the mother was previously exposed to Rh-positive red cells, through therapeutic abortion, ectopic pregnancy, or blood transfusion. Approximately 50% of Rh-sensitized pregnancies result in a newborn who requires transfusion postnatally; 9% of sensitized fetuses require intrauterine transfusion, and fetal death occurs in 1.5% of affected pregnancies. Concomitant ABO incompatibility decreases the risk of developing Rh alloimmune hemolysis. Rh-negative women who are not sensitized should receive Rh immune globulin at 28 weeks' gestation and then an additional dose at the birth of an Rh-positive infant.

ABO INCOMPATIBILITY. Alloimmune hemolysis associated with ABO incompatibility occurs in group O mothers and infants with blood group A or B. ABO incompatibility occurs in 12% of pregnancies, but fewer than 1% are associated with significant hemolysis.[6] First pregnancies can be affected, given that naturally occurring maternal anti-A IgG and anti-B IgG cross the placenta. The mild hemolysis of ABO incompatibility is, in part, related to the presence of A and B antigens on other tissues besides RBCs. Therefore other tissues aside from erythrocytes absorb the anti-A IgG and anti-B IgG that cross the placenta. The result of a DAT may be negative because of fewer type-specific antigens on the surface of the fetal red cell compared with adult red cells. The indirect antiglobulin test, however, is usually positive. The peripheral blood smear will show spherocytes, which are the result of reduced RBC surface area caused by the removal of antibody and membrane complexes by the reticuloendothelial macrophages. Although hemolysis in ABO incompatibility is mild, infants with evidence of hemolysis need to be monitored in the first few days of life for hyperbilirubinemia and for anemia during their first 2 to 3 weeks of life.

MINOR BLOOD GROUP INCOMPATIBILITY. The prevalence of other blood group incompatibilities is increasing because of the successful prevention of Rh immune disease. Common incompatibilities occur with Rh (c and E), Kell, Duffy, and Kidd antigens. Kell incompatibilities can result in significant hemolysis and currently account for 22% of alloimmunization cases, surpassing anti-D, which occurs in 18.4% of cases.[7]

Acquired Hemolysis (Nonimmune)

INFECTION. Congenital infections (cytomegalovirus, toxoplasmosis, rubella, syphilis) may cause hemolysis, impaired erythropoiesis, and thrombocytopenia. Hepatosplenomegaly is usually present, and an active reticuloendothelial system may account for red cell sequestration. Bacterial infections (group B streptococcus, *Escherichia coli*) may also cause hemolysis, disseminated intravascular coagulation (DIC), and hemorrhage. Malaria should also be anticipated in endemic areas and in individuals traveling from these areas.

MICROANGIOPATHIC HEMOLYSIS. Hemolysis may occur when red cells interact with fibrin deposition in the microcirculation. The red cells are sheared and form fragments (schistocytes), which lose their deformability and hemolyze. The most common cause of microangiopathic hemolysis is DIC, which is most commonly associated with infection. Other causes of microangiopathic anemia include cavernous hemangiomas, arteriovenous malformations, renal artery stenosis or thrombosis, severe valvular stenosis, and coarctation of the aorta.

Hereditary Hemolytic Anemia

Hereditary disorders of erythrocytes may cause hemolysis during the neonatal period. These disorders include membrane defects, enzyme deficiencies, and hemoglobinopathies.

MEMBRANE DEFECTS. Hereditary spherocytosis is an autosomal disease caused by mutations in genes for the membrane cytoskeleton proteins (spectrin, ankyrin, band 3).[8] These proteins are important in vertical interactions that tie the membrane cytoskeleton to the lipid bilayer. Spherocytes present on a peripheral blood smear are characteristic of the disease. Spherocytes develop when loss of membrane surface area occurs caused by microvesiculation of the lipid bilayer. The spherocyte loses flexibility and is entrapped in the microcirculation of the reticuloendothelial system. Clinical variation is significant. Some patients are transfusion dependent, whereas others have reticulocytosis without anemia. Neonatal hemolysis or hyperbilirubinemia occurs in approximately one half of patients.[9] A family history will be present in approximately 75% of patients, reflecting autosomal-dominant inheritance. Another 25% of patients with spherocytosis have no family history, and the disease may be the result of recessive inheritance or a new mutation. Given that spherocytes are prominent in ABO incompatibility as well, hereditary spherocytosis must be distinguished from ABO incompatibility.

Hereditary elliptocytosis is an autosomal-dominant disorder of the membrane proteins spectrin or protein 4.1.[10] The disease is clinically heterogeneous, and patients who are heterozygous have elliptical-shaped erythrocytes on peripheral smear but are not anemic. A transient hemolysis and poikilocytosis may occur in the newborn period in the heterozygous infant. However, patients who are homozygous or compound heterozygotes may have chronic hemolysis and splenomegaly. Hereditary pyropoikilocytosis is the severest variant and exhibits in the neonatal period with hemolysis that persists. The smear morphologic assay reveals spherocytes, poikilocytes, fragmented RBCs, and an extreme microcytosis. The inheritance may be recessive with both parents asymptomatic, or it may be that one parent has hereditary elliptocytosis and the other is a silent carrier.

ENZYME DISORDERS. Red cell enzymopathies, with the exception of glucose-6-phosphate dehydrogenase (G6PD) deficiency, are rare. They can occur in the neonatal period with hemolytic anemia and hyperbilirubinemia. G6PD is an X-linked disorder affecting millions throughout the world, primarily in areas endemic for malaria.[11] Hemolysis is, for the most part, episodic and occurs after exposure to infections or potent oxidants. G6PD is an enzyme of the hexose monophosphate shunt that is required to generate the antioxidant glutathione. The absence of glutathione leads to oxidant damage to the erythrocyte with denaturation of globin, which, in turn, damages the red cell membrane and results in red cell hemolysis. G6PD deficiency's clinical heterogeneity is dependent on race and gender. The G6PD A is a variant that occurs in Africans and results in decreased enzyme stability. It is usually mild with a transient hemolysis primarily seen with infection. The Mediterranean and Asian variant, however, results in more severe hemolysis that may be fatal, especially on exposure to fava beans. The diagnosis is suggested by a nonimmune hemolytic anemia in association with infection or administration of oxidant drugs. In the African variant, the enzyme is present in young reticulocytes such that testing after a hemolytic episode, with the presence of elevated reticulocytes, may reveal a normal G6PD activity. Neonatal jaundice is a common presentation, and in parts of the Mediterranean and Southeast Asia, G6PD deficiency is the most common cause of kernicterus. Male infants with unexplained early jaundice and no evidence for ABO or Rh incompatibility should be screened for G6PD deficiency.

HEMOGLOBINOPATHIES. Hemoglobins are developmentally regulated throughout gestation and do not complete the switch to adult Hb A until the 1st year of life. Hemoglobin consists of 2 α-like and 2 β-like globin chains. The α-like chains consist of zeta globin chains in embryonic life with a transition to adult α chains by the end of the 1st trimester. Beta-like chains consist of the embryonic ε globin, which switches to the fetal γ globin in the 1st trimester. The switch from fetal γ chains to adult β chains starts in the 1st trimester and is completed during the 1st year of life. Thus α and γ globin chains are vital to fetal Hb ($\alpha_2\gamma_2$) production, which is the major Hb throughout fetal life. Mutations in the genes encoding α and γ globins are the cause of Hb disorders that occur in the neonatal period. (See Chapter 270, Hemoglobinopathies and Sickle Cell Disease.)

Thalassemia. Alpha thalassemia is a major cause of neonatal hemolytic anemia, hyperbilirubinemia, and hydrops fetalis in Southeast Asia. It is common in areas of the world where malaria is endemic. The molecular basis of α thalassemia is deletion of 1 or more of the 4 α globin genes. Nondeletional forms of α thalassemia are known but are less common. Deletion mutants are classified as (1) silent carrier, in which 1 of the 4 genes is deleted or nonfunctional and there are no clinical or hematologic sequelae; (2) α thalassemia trait, in which deletion or nonfunction (in *cis* or *trans*) of 2 α genes results in microcytosis without anemia; (3) Hb H disease (deletion or nonfunction of 3 of the 4 genes), which results in a chronic hemolytic anemia with microcytosis; and (4) homozygous α thalassemia (deletion of all 4 α genes), which results in fetal hydrops with severe anemia, hepatosplenomegaly, and usually fetal demise. Alpha thalassemia should be thought to exist in any infant with elevation of Hb Bart's (γ_4). Infants with the silent carrier or trait status are not symptomatic. Infants with Hb H disease, however, may have neonatal hemolytic anemia and hyperbilirubinemia when exposed to oxidant drugs or infections.[12] Both Hb H and homozygous α thalassemia occur almost exclusively in infants of Asian descent who have cis gene deletions. Testing the parents of a child with Asian ancestry who has α thalassemia trait or Hb H disease is important because future pregnancies might be at risk for a fetus with homozygous α thalassemia.

Beta thalassemia is common in Southeast Asia, Africa, the Mediterranean, and India. Beta thalassemia is caused by point mutations or deletions of the adult β globin gene, which, in the homozygous state, results in transfusion dependency. Beta thalassemia may be classified as β^0 with no production of β globin or β^+, which results in decreased synthesis of normal β globin protein.[13] Neonates with homozygous β thalassemia are not symptomatic at birth because fetal Hb ($\alpha_2\gamma_2$) predominates during fetal and neonatal life. However, by 3 months of age, the switch from fetal to adult β globin chain production is approximately 80% complete, and symptoms of anemia and hepatosplenomegaly will appear.

Hemoglobin E. Hb E, common in Southeast Asia, is a structurally abnormal Hb caused by an amino acid substitution of lysine for glutamine at position 26 of the β globin protein. The Hb E mutation also results in abnormal RNA splicing, which results in decreased synthesis as well, and is considered a thalassemic phenotype. Patients homozygous for Hb E have microcytosis but little or no anemia. Patients who are compound heterozygotes for Hb E and β^0 thalassemia, however, are transfusion dependent.

Sickle Cell Disease. The sickle hemoglobinapathies are β globin chain disorders that, similar to β thalassemia, are asymptomatic at birth. The sickle Hb variants are diagnosed in newborn screening programs by Hb electrophoresis as Hb SS (FS), Hb SC (FSC), Hb Sβ^0 thalassemia (FS), and Hb Sβ^+ thalassemia (FSA). Alternatively some screening programs use DNA diagnosis. Infants with a sickle hemoglobinopathy are protected during the first months of life by the presence of fetal Hb; therefore few symptoms occur before 6 months of age. (See Chapter 270, Hemoglobinopathies and Sickle Cell Disease, for complete discussion.)

Hypoplastic Anemia

Hypoproliferative anemias caused by decreased erythrocyte production may occur in thalassemia syndromes with decreased production of globin chains, blood loss resulting in iron deficiency, congenital infections (parvovirus, rubella, cytomegalovirus), and rare bone marrow failure syndromes. Diamond-Blackfan anemia (DBA) is a rare congenital hypoplastic anemia characterized by the absence of erythroid precursor cells in the bone marrow.[14] The incidence is 2 to 7 per 1 million live births; 10% to 20% are familial and genes on chromosomes *19q1.32* and *8p23.2* have been implicated. Congenital malformations including growth retardation, skeletal anomalies, and renal anomalies are present in approximately 30% of individuals. Approximately 25% of patients will be diagnosed in the neonatal period, where DBA is suggested by a normochromic, macrocytic anemia with a reticulocytopenia. Treatment of DBA includes corticosteroids, which usually produce a remission, but chronic transfusion therapy has also been used. DBA should be distinguished from hypoproliferative anemia caused by maternally acquired parvovirus infection.

HEMOSTATIC DISORDERS IN THE NEONATE

The diagnosis and management of hemostatic disorders in the newborn is challenging because the system is dynamic and coagulant protein and inhibitor concentrations are age dependent. The hemostatic system in the newborn is thromboprotective, with an overall decrease in thrombin generation. Although the concentrations of hemostatic proteins are related to gestational age, maturation is rapid, and by 6 months of age, adult values are attained in both term and preterm infants.[15] The coagulant proteins that are vitamin K dependent (FII, FVII, FIX, FX) are approximately 50% of adult levels at birth. The inhibitors of coagulation (antithrombin, heparin cofactor II, protein C, and protein S) are also 50% of adult values at birth. The normal values for prothrombin time (PT) and activated partial thromboplastin time (aPTT) are prolonged in newborns. Platelet counts and life span in the newborn are similar to adult values.

Approach to the Newborn With Bleeding

Infants with clinically significant bleeding should be evaluated for a hemostatic disorder. Although acquired disorders predominate, hereditary deficiencies of coagulation proteins and inhibitors often present in early infancy. (See Chapter 271, Hemophilia and Other Hereditary Bleeding Disorders.)

Evaluation of the infant with a bleeding complication should include a medical history that queries familial bleeding problems, maternal illnesses (immune thrombocytopenia, infections), outcomes of previous pregnancies, obstetrical problems at delivery, and documentation that vitamin K was given. The physical examination is important in determining if bleeding is local or diffuse and if the infant has a healthy or sick appearance. Infants with hereditary deficiencies usually display ecchymosis or localized bleeding but appear healthy. However, ill infants with DIC will have diffuse bleeding and petechial hemorrhage. Infants with isolated thrombocytopenia are usually healthy appearing with petechiae or ecchymoses.

The initial laboratory evaluation should include a PT, aPTT, thrombin time, fibrinogen, and platelet count. These screening assays will direct selection of other studies, such as specific factor assays. The management of an infant with a hemostatic disorder depends on the defect identified. Replacement therapies may include specific factor concentrates, fresh frozen plasma, cryoprecipitate, and platelet transfusions.

Inherited Hemorrhagic Disorders

Hemophilia

Deficiencies of coagulation factors VIII and IX are called hemophilia A and hemophilia B, respectively. They are X-linked disorders and a family history can be obtained in two thirds of cases, but approximately one third represent new mutations. The clinical presentation is that of neonatal bleeding in 40% to 70% of cases. The most common sites of bleeding are intracranial hemorrhage (ICH), cephalohematoma, umbilical stump bleeding, and circumcision.[16] The aPTT is prolonged for age, and the specific FVIII or FIX factor assay will confirm the diagnosis. The treatment is recombinant factor specific concentrates. (See Chapter 271, Hemophilia and Other Hereditary Bleeding Disorders.)

Other Hereditary Deficiencies

The most common hereditary coagulation disorder is von Willebrand disease, which occurs in up to 1% of the population.[17] However, symptoms of this disorder do not usually appear in the newborn period because of elevation of the von Willebrand factor proteins at birth. Other, less common severe factor deficiencies (FV, FVII, FX, FXI, fibrinogen and FXIII) may produce bleeding at birth.

Acquired Hemorrhagic Disorders

Vitamin K Deficiency

Infants are at greater risk of bleeding from vitamin K deficiency because of the physiologic decrease in vitamin K-dependent factors (factors II, VII, IX, X) at birth. The 3 clinical presentations of vitamin K deficiency are early, classic, and late.[18]

The early form of vitamin K deficiency occurs in the first 24 hours of life and is linked to maternal medications that interfere with vitamin K stores or function, such as anticonvulsants and antibiotics (including those for tuberculosis). The classic form presents on days 2 to 7 of life in healthy breastfed term infants. This form occurs, in the absence of prophylactic vitamin K, in 0.25% to 1.7% of term infants. The late form manifests between 2 and 8 weeks of life and is primarily caused by disorders that result in malabsorption of vitamin K, such as biliary atresia and other hepatobiliary diseases. Infants thought to have vitamin K deficiency should receive parenteral vitamin K and fresh frozen plasma for significant bleeding.

Disseminated Intravascular Coagulation

Disseminated Intravascular Coagulation (DIC) is a secondary process related to disease states in the neonate such as asphyxia, shock, infection, necrotizing enterocolitis, and respiratory distress syndrome. DIC results from activation of coagulation factors, generation of excess thrombin, and decreased generation of the antithrombotic proteins antithrombin, protein C, and protein S. The consumption of platelets and other coagulation factors leads to diffuse bleeding. DIC occurs in sick infants, and common bleeding manifestations include oozing from mucosal membranes and puncture sites, hematuria, bruising, and ICH. Laboratory findings may include prolonged PT and aPTT, decreased fibrinogen, increased fibrin degradation products, and decreased platelets. The treatment of DIC involves treating the underlying causes, such as infection, and replacing depleted coagulation and antithrombotic factors with fresh frozen plasma, cryoprecipitate, and platelets.

Liver Disease

The coagulopathies of liver disease in neonates are caused by failure of synthetic function of the liver in combination with a physiologic immaturity of the coagulation system. The common causes of liver disease in the newborn include viral hepatitis, hypoxia, total parenteral nutrition, biliary atresia, and inherited metabolic defects. Coagulopathies related to liver disease must be distinguished from DIC.

THROMBOEMBOLIC DISEASE IN THE NEONATE

A significant increase has occurred in thromboembolic (TE) disorders in newborns because of improvement in tertiary care and the use of catheters, extracorporeal membrane oxygenation circuits, and cardiopulmonary bypass, all of which provide thrombogenic surfaces. Approximately 50% of TEs in children occur during the neonatal period; the use of catheters is the major risk factor in 90% of TEs.[19]

Genetic Risk Factors

Hereditary risk factors for TE rarely contribute to neonatal thrombosis unless a significant acquired risk factor is also present.[20] Testing for prothrombotic genetic risks should be reserved until an infant is at least 3 months of age because of the physiologic decrease in these factors (proteins C and S) at birth. Exceptions, however, would include infants with purpura fulminans, which is often a symptom of the rare homozygous or compound heterozygous state for proteins C and S or antithrombin deficiencies.[21] Besides these antithrombotic proteins, other genetic risks include factor V Leiden, which results in resistance of activated protein C proteolysis of FVa. Factor V Leiden is the most common inherited risk factor and occurs in 5% of whites. Prothrombin gene mutation 20210 is another genetic risk factor and is associated with increase in prothrombin levels.

Acquired Risks

The use of catheters, central venous lines, and umbilical lines is the most common risk factor for TE in newborns.[22] Clinical signs of TE in central venous lines include loss of patency, limb swelling and discoloration, pulmonary embolism, chylothorax, and superior vena cava syndrome. Umbilical venous and arterial catheters induce clots in 1.7% to 30% of patients; however, most are asymptomatic. Arterial clots can result in ischemia and organ dysfunction and have resulted in limb length discrepancy. The diagnosis of TE can be made by compression Doppler ultrasound, venography, and computed tomographic scan. Therapy in newborns is not guided by clinical trials data but may include short-term anticoagulation, conventionally 3 to 6 months of anticoagulation, or close monitoring.[21]

Renal Vein Thrombosis

Renal vein thrombosis (RVT) is the 2nd most common TE in neonates and accounts for 10% of neonatal venous TE, with approximately one half occurring in preterm infants. RVT usually causes hematuria, flank mass, and thrombocytopenia, and they are bilateral in approximately 20% of cases. The risk factors for RVT include asphyxia, congenital heart disease, polycythemia, dehydration, and sepsis. In a small series, the prevalence of thrombophilia was higher in neonates with RVT.[23] The long-term morbidity includes hypertension and decreased renal function. Use of anticoagulants should be considered for unilateral RVT extending into the inferior vena cava and patients with bilateral RVT.

Neonatal Stroke

Approximately 25% of arterial ischemic stroke during childhood occurs in the neonatal period, commonly in term infants. Seizures are the most common clinical presentation; approximately 50% of newborns with a seizure have an arterial infarct as reflected on magnetic resonance imaging. Acquired risk factors for arterial stroke include asphyxia, sepsis, congenital heart disease, dehydration, meningitis, and delivery complications. Outcomes reveal no sequelae in 30% to 50% of patients, and the remaining develop hemiplegia, seizures, cerebral palsy, and visual impairment.[24]

Sinovenous thrombosis (SVT) is less frequent than arterial stroke but commonly occurs in the newborn period. The major sites for SVT are the superior sagittal and transverse sinuses. The clinical presentation includes seizures, lethargy, and jitteriness. Physical examination may reveal a tense fontanel and dilated scalp veins. Acquired risk factors for SVT include asphyxia, dehydration, and sepsis. The diagnosis is made by magnetic resonance venography and Doppler ultrasound via the anterior fontanel. Seventy percent of patients are neurologically normal at 2 years of age.[25]

PLATELET DISORDERS

Thrombocytopenia

The platelet count in newborns is similar to levels in healthy adults. A platelet count fewer than 150×10^9/L is classified as thrombocytopenia. The prevalence of thrombocytopenia in the healthy newborn is 0.7% to 4%, whereas in the sick newborn it is 20% to 40%.[26] Causes of thrombocytopenia include diseases associated with decreased production, increased destruction, and a combination of both.

Decreased Production

Congenital thrombocytopenia is rare and can be seen with bone marrow diseases (amegakaryocytic thrombocytopenia, thrombocytopenia absent radii syndrome, congenital leukemia, metastatic neuroblastoma, osteopetrosis), immune disorders (Wiskott-Aldrich syndrome), neutrophil defects (Chédiak-Higashi syndrome), and giant platelet syndromes (Alport, Bernard-Soulier syndromes).

Increased Destruction

The most common mechanism leading to thrombocytopenia is increased destruction. DIC frequently occurs with bacterial infections. A localized consumption of platelets is seen with asphyxia, renal vein thrombosis, necrotizing enterocolitis, maternal eclampsia, and Kasabach-Merritt syndrome. Immune-mediated mechanisms include both alloimmune and autoimmune and should be considered in otherwise healthy infants with an isolated severe thrombocytopenia (platelets $<50 \times 10^9$/L).

Combination

Intrauterine infections (eg, toxoplasmosis, other agents, rubella, cytomegalovirus, herpes simplex; HIV; parvovirus B19) may have neonatal thrombocytopenia, in addition to other stigmata. The mechanisms are multifactorial and include bone marrow suppression and consumption in the reticuloendothelial tissues.

Approach to Neonatal Thrombocytopenia

The evaluation of a newborn with thrombocytopenia should include a review of the maternal history for infections, medications, immune disorders, previous affected pregnancies, or a family history of thrombocytopenia. Whether the newborn is sick or healthy is important, given that thrombocytopenia in most healthy newborns is caused by immune disorders. Thrombocytopenia within the first 72 hours of life is usually related to maternal or perinatal events, whereas the presentation after day 3 usually implies bacterial sepsis. The laboratory investigation should include a complete blood count with examination of the peripheral smear, a coagulation screen, and a platelet count on the mother.

Neonatal alloimmune thrombocytopenia (NAIT) occurs when the mother is sensitized to paternal antigens on the fetal platelet and produces an IgG that crosses the placenta and destroys fetal platelets. The incidence of NAIT is 0.18% of pregnancies. The 1st pregnancy can be affected because fetal platelets leak into the maternal circulation.[26] The most frequent alloantigen in the white population is human platelet antigen (HPA)-1A (PlA1), which is the cause of 80% of NAIT. However, the actual risk of developing NAIT is also related to maternal human leukocyte antigen (HLA) type, because the risk is 140-fold higher with HLA-D3 alloantigen.[27] The clinical presentation is that of severe thrombocytopenia at birth, with intracranial hemorrhage occurring in 15% to 20% of patients. Therapy consists of transfusion of maternal platelets or intravenous γ globulin. The diagnosis can be confirmed by platelet antigen typing of the parents and maternal antibody testing.

Autoimmune thrombocytopenia in the neonate occurs with maternal autoimmune disorders such as immune thrombocytopenic purpura and is milder than alloimmune disorders. Approximately 15% to 45% of infants with maternal immune thrombocytopenic purpura will have thrombocytopenia. Therapies include intravenous immunoglobulin, steroids, and platelet transfusions.

REFERENCES

1. Pearson HA. Life span of the fetal red blood cell. *J Pediatr.* 1967;70:166-171.
2. Dallman PR. Anemia of prematurity: the prospects for avoiding blood transfusions with recombinant erythropoietin. *Adv Pediatr.* 1993;40:385-403.
3. Kirpalani H, Whyte RK, Andersen C, et al. The Premature Infants in Need of Transfusion (PINT) study: a randomized, controlled trial of a restrictive (low) versus liberal (high) transfusion threshold for extremely low birth weight infants. *J Pediatr.* 2006;149(3):301-307.
4. Van Gemert MJ, Umur A, Tijssen JG, et al. Twin-twin transfusion syndrome. *Curr Opin Obstet Gynecol.* 2001; 13:193-206.
5. Freda VJ, Gorman JG, Pollack W, et al. Prevention of Rh hemolytic disease: 10 years clinical experience with Rh immune globulin. *N Engl J Med.* 1975;292:1014-1016.
6. Kaplan E, Herz F, Scheye E. ABO hemolytic disease of the newborn, without hyperbilirubinemia. *Am J Hematol.* 1976;1:279-282.
7. Geifman-Holtxman O, Wojtowycz M, Kosmos E, et al. Female alloimmunization with antibodies known to cause hemolytic disease. *Obstet Gynecol.* 1997;89:272-275.
8. Bolton-Maggs PH, Stevens RF, Dodd NJ, et al, and the General Haematology Task Force of the British Committee for Standards in Haematology. Guidelines for the diagnosis and management of hereditary spherocytosis. *Brit J Haemat.*2004;126:455-474.
9. Delhommeau F, Cynobar T, Schischmanoff PO, et al. Natural history of hereditary spherocytosis during the first year of life. *Blood.* 2000;95:393-397.
10. Gallagher PG. Update on the clinical spectrum and genetics of red blood cell membrane disorders. *Curr Hematol Rep.* 2004;3:85-91.
11. Mehta A, Mason PJ, Vulliamy TJ. Glucose-6-phosphate dehydrogenase deficiency. *Baillieres Best Pract Res Clin Haematol.* 2000;13:21-38.
12. Chen FE, Ooi C, Ha SY, et al. Genetic and clinical features of hemoglobin H disease in Chinese patients. *N Engl J Med.* 2000;343:544-550.
13. Olivieri NF. The beta-thalassemias. *N Engl J Med.* 1999;341:99-109.
14. Alter BP. The inherited bone marrow failure syndromes. In: Nathan DG, Orkin SH, eds. *Nathan and Oski's Hematology of Infancy and Childhood.* 6th ed. Philadelphia, PA: WB Saunders; 2003.
15. Andrew M, Paes B, Milner R, et al. Development of the human coagulation systems in the full-term infant. *Blood.* 1987;70:165-172.
16. Kulkarni R, Lusher J. Perinatal management of newborns with hemophilia. *Br J Haematol.* 2001;112:264-274.
17. Gill CJ. Diagnosis and treatment of Von Willebrand disease. *Hemato Oncol Clin North Am.* 2004;18:1277-1299.
18. Sutor AH, von Kries R, Cornelissen E, et al. ISTH Pediatric/Perinatal Subcommittee. International Society on Thrombosis and Haemostasis. Vitamin K deficiency bleeding in infancy. *Thromb Haemost.* 1999;81:456-461.
19. Schmidt B, Andrew M. Neonatal thrombosis: report of a prospective Canadian and international registry. *Pediatrics.* 1995;96:939-943.
20. Revel-Vilk S, Chan A, Massicotte P. Prothrombotic conditions in an unselected cohort of children with venous thromboembolic disease. *J Thromb Haemost.* 2003;1: 915-921.
21. Salonvaara M, Juismanen KM, Mononen T, et al. Diagnosis and treatment of a newborn with homozygous protein C deficiency. *Acta Paediatr.* 2004;93(1):137-139.
22. Greenway A, Massicotte MP, Monagle P. Neonatal thrombosis and its treatment. *Blood Reviews.* 2004;18:75-84.
23. Marks S, Massicotte MP, Steele B, et al. Neonatal renal venous thrombosis: clinical outcomes and prevalence of prothrombotic disorders. *J Pediatr.* 2005;146:811-816.
24. deVeber GA, MacGregor D, Curtis R, et al. Neurologic outcome in survivors of childhood arterial ischemic stroke and sinovenous thrombosis. *J Child Neurol.* 2000;15:316-324.

25. deVeber GA, Andrew M, and the Canadian Pediatric Stroke Study Group. Cerebral sinovenous thrombosis in children. *N Engl J Med*. 2001;345:417-423.
26. Burrows RF, Kelton K. Incidentally detected thrombocytopenia in healthy mothers and their infants. *N Engl J Med*. 1988;329:1463-1466.
27. Williamson LM, Hackett F, Rennie J, et al. The natural history of fetomaternal alloimmunization to the platelet-specific antigen HPA-1a as determined by antenatal screening. *Blood*. 1998;92:2280-2287.

Chapter 103

PRENATAL DRUG ABUSE AND NEONATAL DRUG WITHDRAWAL SYNDROME

Enrique M. Ostrea, Jr, MD; Neil Joseph B. Alviedo, MD; Felix P. Banadera, MD; Lilia C. De Jesus, MD

INTRODUCTION

Few barriers exist to the passage of most drugs across the placenta or to their biotransformation in the placenta.[1,2] Thus the fetus is exposed to the drugs that a pregnant woman uses. Fetal drug exposure can lead to a significant number of complications, including a high incidence of stillbirths, meconium-stained amniotic fluid, premature rupture of the membranes, maternal hemorrhage (abruptio placenta or placenta previa) and fetal distress.[3,4] In the newborn, mortality and morbidity are high, as well as an increased incidence of asphyxia, prematurity, low birth weight, infections (including sexually transmitted infections), pneumonia, congenital malformations, cerebral infarction, drug withdrawal, and acquired immunodeficiency disease.[5-7] Long-term sequelae in infants also have been reported, which include some delays in physical growth and mental development, sudden infant death syndrome, and learning disabilities.[8-10] This chapter explores one specific complication of the infant who is antenatally exposed to drugs—the neonatal drug withdrawal syndrome.

INCIDENCE

In 2004 the National Survey on Drug Use and Health estimated that approximately 19.1 million Americans, aged 12 years or older, were current illicit drug users, a figure that represents 7.9% of that age population. Among pregnant women aged 15 to 44 years, 4.6% self-reported the use of illicit drugs.[11] Significant maternal underreporting is evident; in one study population, 11% of women reported the use of illicit drugs, but meconium drug analysis revealed actual illicit drug use prevalence to be 44%.[12]

PATHOPHYSIOLOGICAL FEATURES

Two major theories about the cause of withdrawal have been presented. The theory of disuse hypersensitivity asserts that a drug may depress certain neural systems and render their targets hypersensitive to their usual stimuli, with an increase in binding sites for the drugs. When the depressant drug is removed, the drug withdrawal syndrome occurs, caused by rebound hypersensitivity of the affected targets. Morphine, for instance, has been shown to inhibit activation of nonadrenergic cells in the brain stem. Thus chronic morphine exposure results in an increase in the number of brain stem adrenergic binding sites. When morphine is withdrawn, the drug withdrawal syndrome occurs as a consequence of adrenergic hypersensitivity.[13,14] The theory of alternate pathways states that a drug may depress a primary neural pathway, and, as a result, alternate pathways, normally of minor activity, become prominent in an attempt to compensate. When the drug is removed, both the primary and alternate pathways are operative in an additive fashion and cause the withdrawal syndrome.[15]

As tolerance or addiction to drugs develops in the pregnant woman, passive dependence on the drug also develops in her fetus. Withdrawal of the infant from drugs may occur in utero or soon after birth. (Box 103-1 lists the drugs that cause withdrawal.) In utero withdrawal produces an increase in fetal movement or activity, increase in catecholamine levels in the amniotic fluid,[16] or signs of fetal distress (eg, meconium staining of the amniotic fluid, abnormal umbilical velocity waveform).[17] Undergoing rapid or self-detoxification is not safe for the pregnant addict because it will lead to withdrawal in her fetus and its concomitant complications.

DRUGS ASSOCIATED WITH THE NEONATAL DRUG WITHDRAWAL SYNDROME

Narcotics

Narcotics, or opiates, refer to a family of natural or synthetic drugs that have morphine-like pharmacologic actions. Extended use of narcotics, even in therapeutic doses, can result in psychological and physical dependence on the drug by the mother and infant.

The use of methadone in pregnant women for treating opiate addiction is associated with a drug withdrawal syndrome in their infants at birth, and its severity is related to the maternal dose,[18] cord blood level of methadone,[19] and concomitant use of heroin[18] or benzodiazepines.[20] The birth weight of infants among mothers on methadone is larger compared with those on heroin.[21] Buprenorphine has been used as a substitute treatment for maternal heroin addiction and can also induce a neonatal drug withdrawal syndrome that is less prolonged in comparison with methadone.[22-24] The neurodevelopmental outcome of buprenorphine-exposed children is normal in the majority of cases, although some infants exhibited transient motor abnormalities that resolved completely in 85% of those studied.[23,24]

The use of opiates and sedatives in the treatment of infants has been increasing, especially in the intensive care unit, because of increasing awareness of the adverse effects of pain in neonates. The drugs commonly used include fentanyl, morphine sulfate, and midazolam. Withdrawal consisting of shorter sleeping time and increased muscle tone has been observed in

BOX 103-1 Drugs That Can Cause Withdrawal in the Neonate

NARCOTICS OR OPIATES
Morphine
Codeine
Heroin
Methadone
Propoxyphene (Darvon)
Pentazocine (Talwin)
Meperidine (Demerol)
Oxycodone (Percodan, Tylox, Vicodin, Percocet)
Hydromorphone (Dilaudid)
Fentanyl (Sublimaze), Actiq, Duragesic, Wildnil, Alfenta, Sufenta
Buprenorphine (Buprenex)
Nalbuphine (Nubain)
Butorphanol (Stadol)
OxyContin
Tramadol

NONNARCOTIC HYPNOSEDATIVES
Barbiturates
Nonbarbiturate sedatives and tranquilizers
- Bromides[a]
- Chloral hydrate
- Benzodiazepines (diazepam, chlordiazepoxide, clorazepate, flurazepam, halazepam, prazepam, clonazepam, lorazepam, quazepam, estazolam, alprazolam, oxazepam, temazepam, midazolam, triazolam)
- Ethchlorvynol (Placidyl)
- Glutethimide (Doriden)

Alcohol (ethanol)

STIMULANTS
Cocaine
Amphetamines and congeners
Nicotine
Phnecyclidine (PCP)
Marijuana
SSRIs—venlafaxine, sertraline, paroxetine

INHALANT (VOLATILE SUBSTANCE) DRUGS
Paint solvents
Lacquers
Glues

OTHERS
Baclofen
Valproate

SSRIs, Selective serotonin reuptake inhibitors.
[a]Opitz JM, Grosse FR, Heneberg B. Congenital effects of bromism. Lancet. 1972;1:91-92.

these infants when the drugs are abruptly discontinued.[25,26] In one report, severe midazolam and opioid withdrawal resulted in transient myocardial ischemia, which resolved once fentanyl and midazolam were reinstituted.[27]

Nonnarcotic Hypnosedatives

Addiction in adults to nonnarcotic hypnosedatives requires prolonged and continuous use of large and partially incapacitating doses of the drugs, usually over months or years, particularly if the drugs are taken orally. On the other hand, passive addiction in the neonate to a nonnarcotic hypnosedative can occur, even at therapeutic doses taken by the mother during pregnancy. For instance, maternal use of phenobarbital for epilepsy may not cause addiction in the mother to the drug, but can induce passive addiction in her fetus. Unlike narcotic addiction, neonatal addiction to nonnarcotic hypnosedatives is often induced by physicians who treat the mother without realizing the drugs are addicting to her fetus.[28]

BARBITURATES. Although barbiturates have been used in clinical medicine for more than 50 years, their addiction potential was only recognized at a much later time. The frequent association of barbiturate use with alcohol may mask the addicting potential of barbiturates.[29] The ability of barbiturates to abolish withdrawal from alcohol may partly explain this phenomenon.

Barbiturates are classified based on their duration of action as ultrashort, intermediate, and long acting.[30] The intermediate-acting barbiturates are those abused most frequently—for example, secobarbital (Seconal), pentobarbital (Nembutal), amobarbital (Amytal), and butabarbital (Butisol). The abuse of the long-acting barbiturates (eg, phenobarbital) is not as common as the abuse of the shorter-acting forms. However, phenobarbital is involved most frequently with nonnarcotic abstinence in the newborn because it is frequently used for insomnia, for the relief of anxiety, as an anticonvulsant, or for sedation in toxemia of pregnancy.

Passive acquisition by the fetus of physical dependence on barbiturates can occur after prolonged intrauterine exposure to the drug.[29,31] Barbiturates readily cross the placenta and establish high levels in both maternal and cord blood. Relatively high levels of barbiturates have been found in the fetal brain, liver, and adrenals.[32] The manifestations of barbiturate withdrawal in the neonate are similar, regardless of which barbiturate the mother used. However, the time of onset of withdrawal may differ. Withdrawal from intermediate-acting barbiturates occurs within a day after birth[33] but approximately 3 to 7 days after birth in the case of the long-acting barbiturates.[29]

Barbiturates are metabolized principally by the liver, although a significant portion may be excreted unchanged by the kidney. In adults, for instance, up to 30% of the total dose of phenobarbital ingested is excreted in the urine in unchanged form.[34] The half-life in newborns of prenatally administered phenobarbital is almost twice that in the adult and varies inversely with the extent of the prenatal exposure to phenobarbital.[35] The prolonged half-life of phenobarbital in the neonate is due to a lower glomerular filtration rate and to a decreased capacity of the neonatal liver to metabolize drugs.

Withdrawal from barbiturates can occur in newborns even at therapeutic, nonaddicting maternal doses.[36] Withdrawal from phenobarbital has been reported in an infant born to a mother with epilepsy who was receiving phenobarbital at a dose of 60 mg per day.[29] An awareness of the possibility of late-onset withdrawal, especially after exposure to long-acting barbiturates, should alert the pediatric care physician to monitor these newborns closely during the first 2 weeks of life.

BENZODIAZEPINES. Benzodiazepines are commonly used in adults for treating generalized anxiety disorder, panic disorder, seizures, perioperative sedation, and skeletal muscle relaxation. They are frequently prescribed to women of reproductive age and to pregnant women for reducing anxiety and managing toxemia of pregnancy.[37] Benzodiazepines are classified based on their duration of action: long acting—diazepam, chlordiazepoxide, clorazepate, flurazepam, halazepam, and prazepam; intermediate acting—clonazepam, lorazepam, quazepam, and estazolam; and short acting—alprazolam, oxazepam, temazepam, midazolam, triazolam. The most commonly used benzodiazepines in the United States are diazepam, chlordiazepoxide, clonazepam, lorazepam, and alprazolam.[37] During pregnancy, benzodiazepines cross the placenta with relative ease, resulting in significant drug levels in the serum and tissues of the fetus.[2,38] Many possible effects to the fetus can occur whenever anxiolytic medications are prescribed to pregnant women. Possible effects include abortion, malformation, and intrauterine growth retardation. Benzodiazepines that are administered at or near term may cause fetal dependence and eventual neonatal drug withdrawal syndrome.[37]

Major neonatal withdrawal syndromes are observed among infants exposed to maternal parenteral diazepam for long periods or to doses exceeding 30 to 40 mg a day, especially if given intravenously or intramuscularly during pregnancy and labor. In case reports of neonatal withdrawal from diazepam,[39] withdrawal consisted of tremors, irritability, hypertonicity vigorous sucking, vomiting, and diarrhea. In these reports, phenobarbital was effective in controlling the withdrawal in the infant, although the drug had to be administered for a prolonged period. The withdrawal from diazepam can last up to several months, and the syndrome is best minimized by gradually tapering diazepam before delivery. Late 3rd-trimester use and exposure to diazepam during labor have been associated with the floppy infant syndrome. The manifestations of this syndrome are hypothermia, lethargy, apnea, cyanosis, and reluctance to suck. All of these infants appeared to recover without long-lasting sequelae.[40]

CHLORDIAZEPOXIDE. Chlordiazepoxide is a long-acting benzodiazepine frequently used in managing anxiety disorders, withdrawal symptoms from alcoholism, and preoperative anxiety. It has very low toxicity and is safe for preanesthetic use during labor. No reports have surfaced of adverse effects with the occasional use of chlordiazepoxide in the 2nd and 3rd trimester. However, case reports of neonatal drug withdrawal syndrome among infants who were either chronically exposed to chlordiazepoxide in utero or exposed to small amounts during intrapartum are well documented.[37] In a set of twins born to a mother who used chlordiazepoxide at a dose of 20 mg/24 hr during the 2nd and 3rd trimesters of her pregnancy, withdrawal occurred on the 21st day of life and consisted of severe irritability and coarse tremors.[41]

LORAZEPAM. Lorazepam, which has been suggested for pregnancy-induced hypertension, has also been used frequently during labor because of its prolonged amnestic action. Lorazepam and its metabolite do not cross the placenta as easily as other benzodiazepines. However, its elimination from the newborn is slow, and up to 8 days may be required in term babies and an even longer time in premature infants. Full-term newborns whose mothers had received oral lorazepam were noted to have no complication apart from a slight delay in establishing feeding. In contrast, intravenous use of lorazepam for severe hypertension was associated with neonatal withdrawal and significantly low Apgar scores, hypothermia, poor suck, and depressed respiration that required ventilation.[37]

ALCOHOL. Ethanol is an anxiolytic analgesic that has a depressant effect on the central nervous system (CNS).[42] It is rapidly absorbed by diffusion in the mucosa of the stomach (20%) and intestines (80%). The pregnancy does not affect the absorption rate, but blood alcohol levels may be higher in pregnancy. Alcohol is usually cleared from the bloodstream within 1 hour in adults and 2 hours in newborns. Approximately 95% is metabolized by the liver, and 5% is eliminated by the kidneys and lungs. Ethanol is metabolized to acetaldehyde and then to acetate. Acetaldehyde is more toxic than ethanol itself.

Infants can undergo withdrawal from alcohol, but this phenomenon is not often recognized because the withdrawal may be mistaken for withdrawal from narcotics or other drugs. The withdrawal from ethanol occurs early (within birth to 12 hours of life) because of its short half-life and may produce abdominal distention, opisthotonus, convulsions, tremors, hypertonia, apnea, and cyanosis. The infants are irritable, sleep restlessly, and engage in exaggerated mouthing behavior.[43,44]

Stimulants

Addiction by adults to a large number of CNS stimulants occur. These substances include cocaine, amphetamines and its congeners, indolealkylamines (eg, d-lysergic acid diethylamide, psilocyn), phenylethylamines (mescaline, peyote), cannabinoids, inhalants (solvents, aerosols), and phencyclidines. Neonatal withdrawal to some of these drugs has been described and is similar to narcotic and nonnarcotic withdrawal, although the abnormalities described in the infants also likely reflect the drug effects rather than manifestations of withdrawal.[45]

COCAINE. Data from controlled studies fail to show devastating early effects of prenatal cocaine exposure.[46] After controlling for confounders, at 40 weeks' gestation, cocaine exposure was estimated to be associated with growth deceleration and a decrease of 151 g, 0.71 cm, and 0.43 cm in birth weight, length, and head circumference, respectively.[46-48] Neurobehavioral abnormalities such as tremulousness, irritability, hypertonicity, high-pitched cry, abnormal sleep pattern, and, sometimes, seizures have been observed in infants who have been exposed prenatally to cocaine[49-52] and are similar to the manifestations of withdrawal from opiates. Separating the overlapping effects of cocaine and opiate withdrawal is difficult because abusing both drugs is not uncommon for the addicted woman. In general, the CNS manifestations in the cocaine-exposed infants are significantly milder than those observed in narcotic withdrawal. Abnormalities in cardiorespiratory patterns (increased episodes of apnea, periodic breathing),[53] electroencephalographic readings (bursts of sharp waves and spikes),[54] and neonatal behavior as assessed by the Brazelton neonatal behavioral assessment score (impairment of orientation, motor and state regulation)[49-52] also have been described. These abnormalities may be manifestations of the drug's stimulant effect rather than withdrawal.

MARIJUANA. Marijuana is the illicit drug most widely used among women of childbearing age in the United States.[11] Tetrahydrocannabinol (THC) is highly bound to the lipoprotein fraction in the blood. THC crosses the placenta within minutes of administration. The concentrations of THC in maternal and fetal sera are essentially identical.[55]

Most studies do not show a significant effect of prenatal marijuana use on fetal growth or weight.[56] An equivocal relationship exists between prenatal marijuana use and neurobehavioral outcome of the offspring. Prenatal marijuana exposure has been associated with increased fine tremors in the infant, accompanied by exaggerated and prolonged startles, both spontaneous and in response to mild stimuli, poorer visual but not auditory stimuli habituation,[57] decreased ability to regulate state, and disrupted sleep patterns.[58] Elevated serum norepinephrine levels have been observed among these infants.[59] Other reports have found no altered neurobehavioral patterns in marijuana-exposed offspring.[60,61]

NICOTINE. Nicotine is considered the compound primarily responsible for the stimulant effects of smoking. It is absorbed readily from the lungs, almost with the same efficiency as intravenous administration, and is distributed rapidly throughout the body. Nicotine is metabolized principally in the liver to its 2 principal metabolites, cotinine and trans-3′-hydroxycotinine. These metabolites have been measured in meconium with the highest concentrations found in infants whose mothers were heavy smokers (>2 packs per day). Of interest, equivalent amounts of cotinine were found in meconium of infants whose mothers were passive smokers as compared with mothers who smoked 1 pack per day, which indicates the significant exposure from passive smoking.[62]

Tobacco is used widely by women of childbearing age. The Centers for Disease Control and Prevention reported that 12.3% of mothers who gave birth during 1999 smoked.[63]

Several studies have investigated the effect of cigarette smoking during pregnancy on newborn behavior and on later child development.[64-66] Offsprings of mothers who smoked during pregnancy have been observed to perform less well compared with newborns of nonsmoking mothers on the Brazelton score in such items such as habituating to sound or orienting to a voice. Other studies indicate poorer performance with head turning and sucking; lower visual alertness; more crying, tremors, and startles; and increased lability of skin color.

In a study of 27 nicotine-exposed and 29 unexposed full-term newborns, the tobacco-exposed were more excitable and hypertonic, required more handling, and showed more stress or abstinence signs, specifically in the CNS, gastrointestinal, and visual areas. Dose-response relationships showed higher maternal salivary cotinine values related to more stress or abstinence signs among the tobacco-exposed newborns. The findings suggest neurotoxic effects of prenatal tobacco exposure on newborn neurobehavior and the dose-response relationships might indicate neonatal withdrawal from nicotine.[67] A prospective, two-group parallel study on 17 consecutive newborns of heavy-smoking mothers and 16 newborns of nonsmoking, unexposed mothers (controls) showed that neurologic scores were significantly lower in newborns of smokers than in control infants at days 1, 2, and 5 but withdrawal scores were higher. Significant correlations were observed between markers of nicotine exposure and neurologic and withdrawal scores.[68]

PHENCYCLIDINE. Phencyclidine (PCP) was first introduced as a dissociative anesthetic, but its clinical use was discontinued after reports of adverse effects that included agitation, confusion, delirium, and persistent hallucinations. PCP remains a popular drug of abuse because of its hallucinogenic and sedative effects. PCP also has strong, centrally mediated effects in animals and humans and influences many different neuronal systems. It inhibits the uptake and increases the release of monoamines in the brain, interacts with cholinergic and serotonergic systems, and antagonizes the neuronal stimulation caused by the excitatory amino acid N-methyl aspartate.

The prevalence of PCP abuse during pregnancy has not been firmly established because most reports are from urban areas and cannot be generalized nationally. In 1983 a study reported that 12% of a random sample of 200 newborns had measurable quantities of PCP in their cord blood.[69]

Early case reports of PCP-exposed newborns showed abnormal neurobehavioral findings in the infants. These effects included irritability, tremors, hypertonicity, poor attention, bizarre eye movements, staring spells, hypertonic ankle reflexes, and depressed grasp and rooting reflexes.[70-72] One of the most characteristic features in infants is a sudden and rapid change in level of consciousness, with lethargy alternating with irritability. The behavior of these newborns has been attributed to PCP intoxication rather than to withdrawal.[45]

AMPHETAMINES. The amphetamines are a group of chemically related sympathomimetic amines that have both CNS stimulant and peripheral actions. The abuse potential is very strong because of their psychic effects, which include a decreased sense of fatigue, wakefulness, alertness, mood elevation, self-confidence, and, in many instances, euphoria and elation.

Methamphetamine is the methylated derivative of amphetamine and is prepared through the reduction of ephedrine or pseudoephedrine. The ease of its synthesis, its availability and affordability, and the prolonged *high* it produces have made it an increasingly popular drug of abuse. Ice, the smokable form of methamphetamine, is claimed to produce an intense euphoria.

The newborn of an amphetamine addict exhibited diaphoresis and episodes of agitation alternating with lassitude, miosis, and vomiting.[45] Infants exposed to both cocaine and methamphetamine are described as having abnormal sleep patterns, tremors, poor feeding, hypertonia, sneezing, a high-pitched cry, frantic fist sucking, tachypnea, loose stools, fever, yawning, hyperreflexia, and excoriation.[73] In a study of 134 mother-infant pairs whose mothers used methamphetamine during pregnancy and compared with 160 unexposed newborns, exposure to methamphetamine throughout gestation was associated with decreased growth relative to newborns exposed only for the first 2 trimesters.[74] The incidence of withdrawal in newborns in the methamphetamine group was 49%, but only 4% required pharmacologic treatment for their withdrawal.

Bupropion, which is also called amfebutamone, is an amphetamine marketed to assist with smoking withdrawal and has been shown to be associated with a higher-than-expected frequency of neonatal cardiac malformations in infants born to women who have used the drug during pregnancy.[75]

ANTIDEPRESSANTS. Since the introduction of selective serotonin reuptake inhibitors (SSRIs) in 1988, they have become the drug of choice in the treatment of depression and other mood and behavioral disorders.[76] The use of SSRIs during pregnancy has also become more common.[77] Drug withdrawal syndrome associated with antidepressants, both the classic tricyclic antidepressants and the newer SSRIs, is well documented in adults. Newborns whose mothers are on tricyclic antidepressants or lithium may exhibit manifestations such as irritability, tachycardia, respiratory distress, sweating, and convulsions.[37,78,79] Case reports have surfaced of neonatal drug withdrawal syndrome associated with use of SSRIs by pregnant women.[76] Withdrawal, or discontinuation syndrome, has been described in newborns after 3rd-trimester fluoxetine, paroxetine, sertraline, and venlafaxine exposure.[80-82] These effects include acrocyanosis, tachypnea, temperature instability, irritability, and elevated drug levels among newborns exposed to fluoxetine prenatally, as well as respiratory distress, hypoglycemia, and jaundice among newborns with prenatal paroxetine exposure.[80,82]

A total of 93 cases (from 11 different countries) of SSRI use associated with either neonatal convulsions or drug withdrawal syndrome were identified. Signs included convulsions, irritability, abnormal crying, and tremors.[76] The drug withdrawal syndrome associated with SSRI use might be attributed to the cholinergic receptor or redefined in terms of dependence on the serotonin system. Nearly two thirds of reported cases of suspected SSRI-induced neonatal withdrawal are associated with paroxetine. Paroxetine is a more potent inhibitor of norepinephrine reuptake than setraline or citalopram. Paroxetine also has a distinctive effect on muscarinic receptors compared with fluoxetine and other SSRIs. These aspects of paroxetine's mechanism are more suggestive of a cholinergic withdrawal syndrome that is also described in adults.[76] Thus paroxetine should not be used in pregnancy or, if used, should be given at the lowest effective dose.[76] In another report, among a cohort of 64 infants with late-gestation fluoxetine exposure, the frequency of poor neonatal adaptation (eg, presence of jitteriness, tachypnea, hypoglycemia, hypothermia, poor tone, a weak or absent cry) was increased. These signs were observed within the 1st hours of life and had typically resolved by 48 hours of life.[82]

INHALANT (VOLATILE SUBSTANCE) ABUSE. Inhalants produce alcohol-like effects described as a *high*. It results in slurred speech, clumsy movements, dizziness, and euphoria; lightheadedness and hallucinations or delusions can also occur. Inhalants are often the 1st drugs that young children use. Between 15% and 20% of high school students report using inhalants at least once.[83]

Neonatal withdrawal from volatile substances has been described.[84] The principal products abused are paint solvents, lacquer, and glue. Nail polish remover, lighter fluid, deodorant and hair sprays, whipped cream canisters, and cleaning fluids are all widely used inhalant sources. Toluene and other hydrocarbons may be present. A characteristic chemical odor in the neonate or mother is noted that can persist for several days because the lungs are a major route for excretion, and the highly lipophilic substances are excreted slowly. The typical manifestations in the infant include excessive and high-pitched crying, sleeplessness, tremors, hypertonia, and poor feeding. Metabolic acidosis also has been described[84,85]; it occurs within the first 24 hours of life, and 2 different patterns are observed. The common form is transient and resolves spontaneously or after a single dose of sodium bicarbonate. The other type is more persistent, lasts for 1 to 2 weeks, and requires treatment with repeated doses of sodium bicarbonate or Shohl solution. The cause of the metabolic acidosis is not known, although it may be secondary to the acid load of toluene metabolite or from renal tubular acidosis.

Other Drugs

Neonatal withdrawal, consisting of seizures, has been reported in infants born to mothers who have received an antispasmodic, baclofen, during pregnancy.[86,87] Neonatal hypoglycemia and withdrawal manifestations have also been reported with maternal use of valproate for epilepsy.[88]

ONSET AND DURATION OF NEONATAL DRUG WITHDRAWAL

The onset of withdrawal is common within the first 72 hours after birth, usually within the first 24 to 48 hours. In a few instances, the onset may appear soon after birth if the drug has a short half-life or if the mother already has begun to experience withdrawal while in labor. Reports of withdrawal occurring after the 1st or 2nd week have been observed with drugs that have a longer half-life (eg, phenobarbital).[29] Among narcotics, delayed manifestations of withdrawal, sometimes as late as 6 weeks, have been observed with methadone.[89]

The onset and severity of the withdrawal is affected by several factors, among which are the amount of maternal drug use,[22] the timing of the last dose before delivery, the use of anesthesia or analgesia in the mother during labor, the maturity and nutrition of the infant, and the metabolism and excretion of the drugs and their metabolites.[21,89,90]

Neonatal withdrawal from narcotics usually peaks by the 3rd day of postnatal life and subsides between the 5th to 7th day. Manifestations include irritability, tremors, hypertonicity, sneezing, hiccups, and regurgitation but are generally milder than those of the initial withdrawal. The duration of withdrawal is related to its severity[22]; it is more prolonged in those who had severe withdrawal. Newborns treated for withdrawal also show a prolonged withdrawal period. Thus drug treatment may ameliorate the manifestations of withdrawal, but it does not shorten its duration. The mother must be made aware that her newborns's withdrawal may persist for weeks after discharge from the nursery. The unwary mother may also misinterpret her infant's irritability as hunger and then overfeed, which can lead to diarrhea and vomiting. The mother should also be instructed on how to reduce the infant's discomfort by swaddling and cuddling. She should be reassured that signs of withdrawal will subside eventually without the use of medications. In most instances, the mother who is well informed can successfully cope with the situation. If drugs are used to treat the withdrawal, then relapse may occur if treatment is discontinued abruptly. Although withdrawal manifestations diminish in intensity within the 1st week after birth, they do not disappear completely. The tremors and irritability may persist for as long as 8 to 16 weeks.[91] Withdrawal from barbiturates, diazepam, chlordiazepoxide, and even methadone may occur weeks later.[29,39,41,89]

BOX 103-2 Manifestations of Neonatal Abstinence Syndrome

CENTRAL NERVOUS SYSTEM SIGNS
Hyperactivity
Hyperirritability—excess crying, high pitch outcry
Increased muscle tone
Exaggerated reflexes
Tremors
Sneezing, hiccups, yawning
Short, nonquiet sleep
Fever

RESPIRATORY SIGNS
Tachypnea
Excess secretions

GASTROINTESTINAL SIGNS
Disorganized, poor sucking
Vomiting
Drooling
Sensitive gag
Hyperphagia
Diarrhea
Abdominal cramps

VASOMOTOR SIGNS
Stuffy nose
Flushing
Sweating
Sudden, circumoral pallor

CUTANEOUS SIGNS
Excoriated buttocks
Facial scratches
Pressure point abrasions

NEONATAL NARCOTIC WITHDRAWAL

The prototype of drug withdrawal in the neonate is withdrawal from narcotics. The manifestations are multisystemic and involve the central nervous system, respiratory, gastrointestinal, vasomotor, and cutaneous systems[91] (Box 103-2).

Central Nervous System

Neurologic signs predominate and appear early. Findings are those of CNS excitability, such as hyperactivity, irritability, tremors, and hypertonicity. Occasionally, fever may accompany these increased neuromuscular activities.

Hyperactivity exhibits as almost incessant movements of the extremities. When the newborn is supine and unrestrained, movements assume a jerky, purposeless, en masse nature apparently perpetuated by unchecked proprioceptive stimuli. When placed in the prone position, the infant's motor behavior becomes more organized. Crawling movements are observed, which may lead to displacement from the crib, abrasions or friction injuries to the knees and legs, and other motions such as chin lifting, head movement from side to side, chest elevation, and hand-to-mouth activity. The last of these movements usually quiets the infant, indicating the usefulness of pacifiers.

Hyperirritability produces an almost incessant shrill, high-pitch crying. The infant's tone is exaggerated, sometimes assuming an opisthotonic position, making the infant hard to hold. Tremors and myoclonic jerks are frequent and sustained sometimes. To distinguish from seizures, tremors can be abolished by restraint of the tremulous extremity. The reflexes of the infant such as the Moro reflex, traction response, weight bearing, placing, stepping, crawling, and Landau reflex are exaggerated. The infant's response to stimuli such as sound and light is disproportionately increased.

Electroencephalographic tracings on the addicted neonate may be abnormal and show high frequency dyssynchronous activity, suggesting CNS irritability. The prevalence of seizures is estimated to be between 5% and 21% in infants exhibiting narcotic withdrawal.

In premature newborns, neural hyperexcitability is more episodic than it is in term newborns. The neonates appear restless and overactive for short periods and then lapse into periods of lethargy and inactivity. Sustained tremors are not usually seen in premature newborns until they reach the gestational age when tone is present in the upper and lower extremities. Sweating, which is seen in the full-term newborn, is also not observed in preterm newborns.[92]

The typical patterns of active and quiet sleep periods in the newborn experiencing withdrawal are disturbed with a significant decrease in sleep from 3 to 4 hours to less than 1 hour. Heroin- and methadone-addicted infants also have fewer periods of quiet sleep.[93] Initially, these observations were thought to be related to withdrawal. However, because these abnormal sleep patterns persist beyond the period of withdrawal, they might be the result of the addiction process itself rather than to the general distress secondary to withdrawal and may be secondary to the direct effects of chronic opiate exposure on the opiate receptors in the brain involved in the regulation of sleep.[94]

Cardiorespiratory Signs

Abnormalities in ventilation have been described in infants withdrawing from narcotics, including longer and increased frequency of apneic episodes and periodic breathing. During withdrawal, these infants may also exhibit tachypnea with concomitant respiratory alkalosis.[95] Morphine has been shown, in animals, to have a dual action on fetal breathing—apnea followed by tachypnea. The postulate suggests that the dual action of morphine is secondary to the effects of the drug concentration and to the effects of the drug on two different sites involved in the control of respiration. After a bolus of morphine, its initial high concentration causes respiratory depression and apnea. As the drug is metabolized, the lower concentration is associated with stimulation of respiration, hence the tachypnea. Morphine is found to be inhibitory to the respiratory neurons in the medulla and to the neurons located more rostrally that act to inhibit respiration.

Abnormal heart rate tracings associated with elevated serum creatine phosphokinase were noted to be significantly different in infants of drug-dependent mothers compared with nonexposed infants.[96] In addition, these changes were more intense among infants who had moderate to severe withdrawal. The elevated serum creatine phosphokinase is postulated as being secondary to the excess muscular activity of infants undergoing withdrawal.

Other physiological alterations include elevated systolic blood pressure, an increase in plasma renin activity, and elevated catecholamine levels.[97] In one report, these conditions persisted for 21 days after delivery, which suggests increased beta-adrenergic activity.[98]

Gastrointestinal Signs

The suckling of the newborn who is withdrawing from narcotics is disorganized and poorly coordinated with swallowing.[22] Both suckling rate and nutrient consumption are low.[99] Frequently, milk drools around the corners of the infant's mouth. The infant appears incessantly hungry, which, when unfulfilled, leads to mounting agitation, persistent crying, hyperactivity, and exhaustion. The poor nutrient intake and increased caloric expenditure from hyperactivity may be responsible for the significant weight loss seen in these infants. Vomiting and diarrhea are also often observed, which can lead to dehydration, electrolyte imbalance, and excoriations around the buttocks.

Vasomotor Signs

Significant vasomotor instability in a newborn experiencing withdrawal produces a stuffy nose, flushing, mottling, sweating, and episodes of sudden, circumoral pallor.

Cutaneous Signs

Newborns experiencing withdrawal may be hyperactive, which may lead to facial scratches and abrasions on pressure points. Excoriations of the buttocks can occur if diarrhea is present.

NEONATAL WITHDRAWAL FROM NONNARCOTIC DRUGS

Withdrawal from nonnarcotic drugs is similar to narcotic withdrawal except that convulsions are observed more frequently in the former. Newborns of mothers who have abused stimulants during pregnancy (eg, cocaine, amphetamines) may also exhibit tremors, irritability, a high-pitched cry, and abnormal sleep patterns during the neonatal period. These signs are probably manifestations of drug effects rather than withdrawal.

DIAGNOSIS

The diagnosis of drug withdrawal is based on withdrawal signs and the verification of fetal drug exposure. However, identifying drug exposure in a newborn is not easy because of significant underreporting of maternal drug use and because of fear of the consequences stemming from such an admission. Even with maternal cooperation, information regarding the type and extent of drug usage is often inaccurate.[12] Similarly, many of the drugs to which the fetus is exposed in utero do not produce immediate or recognizable effects.[89] High-risk characteristics in the mother, which should lead to the suspicion of drug abuse, include no or little prenatal care, ethanol use, teenage pregnancy, history or presence of sexually transmitted infections or hepatitis B, and abruptio placenta. Several laboratory tests are commonly used to detect drug exposure in the infant. These tests include toxicologic analysis of the newborn's urine, hair, and meconium for drugs. Urine screening can have a high false-negative rate because only newborns who have had recent exposure will be positive. Meconium drug testing is more likely to identify babies of drug-abusing mothers than newborn urine testing.[100,101]

Newborns of drug-dependent mothers should be routinely tested for sexually transmitted infections, hepatitis B, and HIV infection.

DIFFERENTIAL DIAGNOSIS

Withdrawal from the narcotic and nonnarcotic drugs need to be distinguished from other entities such as hypoglycemia, hypocalcemia, hypomagnesemia, sepsis, meningitis, subarachnoid hemorrhage, infectious diarrhea, and intestinal obstruction. Blood chemistry, cerebrospinal fluid and radiographic studies, and cultures should be performed as indicated by the clinical circumstances.

Maternal use of phenothiazines (eg, chlorpromazine) may induce extrapyramidal dysfunctions in the newborn, such as tremors, facial grimacing, increased muscle tone, cog-wheel rigidity, increased reflexes, and torticollis, all of which can resemble the drug withdrawal syndrome.[102,103] History taking and identifying the drug's metabolites in the newborn's serum or urine are necessary to establish the diagnosis.

ASSESSMENT OF THE SEVERITY OF NEONATAL DRUG WITHDRAWAL

The manifestations of withdrawal can range in severity from none or mild to severe. Studies have shown that neither the newborn's gender, race, or Apgar score nor the mother's age, parity, or duration of heroin intake correlate with the severity of the newborn's withdrawal.[103] Similarly, control of the environment to reduce the amount of light or noise in the nursery does not improve the severity of withdrawal.[104] Given that adults who are undergoing withdrawal experience abdominal cramps, palpitation, nausea, and other discomforts, speculation asserts that the same discomforts are also experienced by a newborn, which may abolish any potential benefits from stimuli (light or noise) reduction in the nursery. The severity of withdrawal from methadone correlates significantly with the methadone dose of the mother.[104] Neonatal withdrawal tends to be more intense if the mother was on 20 mg or more of methadone per day before delivery.

The frequency of diarrhea and vomiting should be noted and the infant's weight checked at least every 8 hours. The temperature, heart rate, and respiratory rate should be taken every 4 hours. Laboratory examinations to detect serum electrolyte or pH imbalance should be performed, as indicated.

The severity of the withdrawal can be assessed clinically by several scoring systems.[91,105,106] The scoring system designed by Finnegan is an extensive evaluation system that is particularly useful for research purposes for evaluating the severity of withdrawal, as well as the response to treatment.[105] Another system[91] evaluates the newborn's need for drug treatment and focuses on manifestations of withdrawal that are life threatening, for example, irritability, tremors (convulsion), weight loss, vomiting, diarrhea and tachypnea (Table 103-1). Measurement of infant movement using a motion detector has been used to objectively measure the severity of withdrawal.[107]

The effect of polydrug abuse on the severity of withdrawal is controversial.[108] Abstinence scores of newborns whose mothers were on methadone and cocaine were similar to the scores of those newborns whose mothers were on a high methadone dose. Similarly, multiple opiates did not alter the severity of withdrawal. However, higher abstinence scores have been reported in newborns exposed to both cocaine and heroin compared to heroin or cocaine alone. In two reports, no difference was observed in the severity of withdrawal in newborns born to mothers who have used both cocaine and methadone or either drug singly,[54,109] whereas, in one report, higher abstinence scores were noted in newborns exposed to both drugs compared with one.[110]

SUPPORTIVE TREATMENT OF DRUG WITHDRAWAL

The care of drug withdrawal in the neonate is primarily supportive. This care includes swaddling the newborn, placing the newborn in a prone position, and cuddling often. Swaddling, particularly with the newborn's extremities flexed and hands placed before the mouth, enhances hand-to-mouth facility, which is soothing. A similar soothing action can be achieved with a pacifier. Other measures include frequent small feedings of hypercaloric (24 cal/oz) formula to supply the additional caloric requirements and observation of sleeping habits, temperature stability, weight loss, diarrhea, and change in clinical status that might suggest another disease process. Daily caloric intake should provide the 150 to 250 cal/kg required for proper growth in neonates exhibiting withdrawal.[108]

Pharmacologic Treatment of Drug Withdrawal

Only 25% of infants who exhibit withdrawal will need drug treatment.[22] The rest can be managed conservatively with success. The decision to use pharmacologic

Table 103-1 Assessment of the Clinical Severity of Neonatal Drug Withdrawal Syndrome

	MILD	MODERATE	SEVERE
Vomiting	Spitting up	Extensive vomiting for 3 successive feedings	Vomiting associated with imbalance of serum electrolytes
Diarrhea	Watery stools <4 times/day	Watery stools 5-6 times per day for 3 days; no electrolyte imbalance	Diarrhea associated with imbalance of serum electrolytes
Weight loss	<10% of birth weight	10%-15% of birth weight	>15%
Irritability	Minimal	Marked but relieved by cuddling or feeding	Unrelieved by cuddling or feeding
Tremors or twitching	Mild tremors when stimulated	Marked tremors or twitching when stimulated	Convulsions
Tachypnea	60-80/minute	80-100/minute	>100/minute and associated with respiratory alkalosis

From Ostrea EM. Infants of drug-dependent mothers. In: Berg FD, Ingelfinger JR, Wald ER, eds. *Current Pediatric Therapy*. Vol 14. Philadelphia PA: WB Saunders; 1993. Reprinted with permission.

Treat with pharmacologic agents (see Table 103-2) if infant has:

1. Moderate vomiting, diarrhea, or weight loss
2. Any severe sign of withdrawal (eg, convulsion or severe vomiting, diarrhea, weight loss, irritability, tachypnea)

agents to treat withdrawal is based on the assessment of the severity of withdrawal. In the system of clinical assessment shown in Table 103-1, drugs are used to treat withdrawal if a moderate degree of vomiting, diarrhea, or weight loss or any severe sign of withdrawal (convulsion, severe vomiting, diarrhea, weight loss, or irritability) is present. The use of pharmacologic agents, as compared with supportive care only, appears to reduce the time to regain birth weight and reduces the duration of supportive care but increases the duration of hospital stay.[111] The duration of treatment is also related to the severity of withdrawal, although the length of stay of newborns in the nursery is not significantly different whether treatment is with methadone or morphine.[112]

The drugs that are used to treat drug withdrawal in the newborn are listed in Table 103-2. As a rule, drug selection should match the class of agent from which the infant is withdrawing. Thus, for narcotic withdrawal, narcotics are the drugs of choice, whereas for nonnarcotic withdrawal, nonnarcotic hypnosedatives (eg, phenobarbital) are preferred. Combinations of opiate and nonopiate drugs have also been used.[113] Improved neurobehavioral scores were noted in infants treated for narcotic withdrawal with opiate and phenobarbital.[113] Although the neurologic manifestations of narcotic withdrawal may be controlled successfully by a nonnarcotic agent, the alleviation of other, non-CNS manifestations of withdrawal (eg, diarrhea) are treated more effectively with narcotics.

Paregoric, laudanum (tincture of opium), and methadone are the narcotics most commonly used to treat neonatal opiate withdrawal. However, the use of paregoric has declined because of the potential toxic effects of some of its ingredients.[108] Besides camphor, a potent CNS stimulant, paregoric contains isoquinolone derivatives (noscapine and papaverine), which are antispasmodics; it also contains a high concentration of ethanol (44% to 46%), a CNS depressant, and anise oil, which may cause habituation. Laudanum is the preferred drug for neonatal narcotic withdrawal. (Caution: Laudanum, USP, is available only as a 10% solution that contains 1.0% morphine.) Laudanum must be first diluted 25-fold to a concentration of 0.4% to reduce its morphine content to equal an amount found in paregoric. At this dilution, the recommended initial dose of 0.4% laudanum is 0.1 mL/kg (0.04 mg/kg) or 2 drops/kg with feedings every 4 hours. The dose may be increased by 2 drops/kg every 4 hours as needed to control withdrawal. After the newborn has stabilized for 3 to 5 days, the dose may be slowly decreased without altering the frequency of administration. An abrupt decrease in dose level or a discontinuance of the drug should be avoided for risk of relapse. Lower peak doses of tincture of opiate and shorter dosing intervals have been associated with shorter hospital stays for newborns with neonatal drug withdrawal syndrome secondary to maternal methadone treatment.[114]

If methadone is used, then initial doses of 0.05 to 0.1 mg/kg may be given every 6 hours, with increases of 0.05 mg/kg until withdrawal signs are controlled. Thereafter, methadone may be given every 12 to 24 hours and discontinued after weaning to a daily dose of 0.05 mg/kg per day.[115]

Nonnarcotic hypnosedatives are used to treat neonatal withdrawal from nonnarcotic drugs (see Table 103-2). The drugs that are commonly used include phenobarbital and chlorpromazine. Barbiturates can be used to treat withdrawal from nonbarbiturates (including alcohol) or vice versa. Although chlorpromazine is not a nonnarcotic hypnosedative, its ability to treat withdrawal may be the result of its ability to suppress rapid eye movement sleep, which is exaggerated during withdrawal.[116,117] However, the prolonged excretion time and many side effects of chlorpromazine, including cerebellar dysfunction, decreased seizure threshold, and hematologic problems, have limited the use of chlorpromazine in the treatment of withdrawal in the neonate.[108] Diazepam has not commonly been used because of reported side effects such as bradycardia and respiratory depression.

During the treatment of withdrawal, attention should also be focused on the nutrition and fluid and electrolyte balance of the newborn, particularly if vomiting, diarrhea, hyperpyrexia, and hyperhidrosis are present. Appropriate intravenous fluids may be required to correct deficits or prevent the occurrence of imbalances.

The aim of treatment with drugs is to render the newborn comfortable but not obtunded. Thus the drug should be titrated, starting with the smallest

Table 103-2 Common Drugs for the Treatment of the Neonatal Drug Withdrawal Syndrome

DRUGS	DOSAGE
NARCOTICS	
Paregoric	0.1 mL/kg every 4 hours, orally, and may be increased by 0.1 mL/kg every 4 hours until withdrawal manifestations are controlled
Laudanum (0.4 mg/mL morphine)	0.1 mL/kg (0.04 mg/kg) every 4 hours and may be increased by 0.1 mL/kg (0.04 mg/kg) every 4 hours to control withdrawal manifestations
Methadone	0.05-0.1 mg/kg every 6 hours, orally. Increase dose by 0.05 mg/kg until withdrawal signs are controlled
NONNARCOTICS	
Phenobarbital	3-6 mg/kg/day in divided doses, every 6 hours, orally

recommended dose and increased accordingly until the desired effect is achieved. Once the newborn has become asymptomatic for 3 to 5 days, the drug can be slowly tapered in dose until discontinued. The total detoxification period can last for 2 to 3 weeks. After discontinuance of the drug, the newborn should be observed for 1 or 2 days for possible recurrence of the withdrawal (rebound phenomenon). Once the newborn is discharged from the nursery, the mother should be informed that some jitteriness and irritability may persist for as long as 8 to 16 weeks.

Neonatal drug withdrawal syndrome can occur as well in newborns who receive narcotics for analgesia or sedation (iatrogenic neonatal drug withdrawal syndrome). The guidelines for effective weaning of newborns from opioids are not well established. A suggested strategy is that all patients in neonatal intensive care who have received opioids for more than 3 to 5 days be systematically weaned from the opioid while being regularly evaluated for signs of withdrawal.[118]

Complications

The complications in neonatal drug withdrawal are related to the severity of the withdrawal. Biochemical aberrations in the serum electrolytes and pH and dehydration may occur after vomiting and diarrhea. Weight loss may be profound as a result not only of excess fluid losses, but also of poor oral intake. Aspiration pneumonia may occur because of vomiting and incoordinate sucking and swallowing.[99,119] Respiratory alkalosis can occur because of tachypnea. Convulsions may be present and are observed more frequently in withdrawal from nonnarcotic drugs. The use of naloxone in the delivery room is contraindicated in newborns whose mothers are known to be opioid dependent. Administration of naloxone may result in neonatal seizures because of abrupt drug withdrawal.[120] However, in the absence of a specific history of opioid abuse, naloxone treatment remains a reasonable option in the delivery room management of a depressed newborn whose mother has received a narcotic drug during labor. However, the physician should be prepared to treat withdrawal in the delivery room.

Other Supportive Measures

The addicted woman has serious impediments to a successful mothering role. Similarly, the neurobehavioral abnormalities and withdrawal in her baby can prevent gratifying feedback, which is important in bonding. Thus the mother and child should have early and repeated contacts. Social services and the appropriate child welfare authorities should be engaged so as to ensure that the necessary family supports and community resources are in place to support the dyad if the baby is to be discharged to the mother's care. The determination as to the baby's disposition is predicated on local community child welfare policies. Consideration is often given to whether the mother is in recovery, what drugs she is using, if she is enrolled in drug treatment, if she has resources, and whether the extent of her family or informed support network is sufficient. Staff personnel should also discuss with the mother her infant's condition and assure her that with control of withdrawal manifestations, the infant will begin to feed better and respond more positively to her.

If plans have been made to place the infant in a foster care home, then the infant will, in the interim, need human contact and should receive stimulation through regular holding and cuddling by staff professionals.

BREASTFEEDING

Most drugs that the mother takes will cross into her milk. The concentration of illicit drugs in human milk will depend on the amount and time of drug intake by the mother.[2] The danger of transmission of HIV through human milk also exists; thus, in the United States, breastfeeding is not recommended in a mother who is HIV positive.[7,121]

For the infant whose mother has continued to use illicit substances throughout pregnancy, breastfeeding is likely to be unsafe. For the woman who is in treatment for substance abuse and is abstinent at the time of delivery, postpartum breastfeeding support and close monitoring of the mother for relapse and of the newborn for adequate weight gain, as well as frank discussions concerning the risks posed by exposure to illicit substances through milk, are essential.[122]

Methadone treatment in the mother is compatible with breastfeeding; no adverse effects have been reported in nursing infants when the mother is on a methadone dose of 20 mg per day or less.[123,124] The suggestion has been made that the mother should take the dose of methadone after the evening feeding and that she supplement breastfeeding with a bottle at the next feeding.[123]

DECISIONS REGARDING THE INFANT'S CAREGIVER

The ability of the drug-addicted woman to provide adequate care for her newborn has often been questioned. Frequently, these women are denied their rights and responsibility to care for their infants based on an unstable home and lifestyle and emotional and psychological weakness. Current evidence suggests that this practice may be counterproductive. A study that determined the outcome of such infants based on the type of caregiver[125] showed that the outcome (growth, development, and frequency of medical illnesses and child abuse) of infants cared for by their own mother with the help of a caregiver (either a husband or relative) was better than in foster care. Thus, with appropriate guidance and supervision and the presence of a supportive person, the addicted mother is capable of providing adequate care for her infant, particularly if she is highly motivated. Coordinated outpatient care also has been used to shorten the stay of the newborn in the nursery.[126] Although a high incidence of signs suggestive of child abuse (cigarette burns or hematoma) has been observed in infants born to drug-dependent mothers, these have occurred in situations in which the infant was cared for exclusively by the mother, and very few occurred in infants whose mothers had help available.[127]

Thus a support person must be available at home to help the mother in the care of her infant and to prevent child abuse or neglect.

SOCIAL AND PROTECTIVE SERVICE REFERRAL AND FOLLOW-UP

All newborns of drug-dependent mothers should have a social service referral to assess the adequacy of parenting and care of the infant at home. The discharge of the infant to the mother's care, with the help of a support person, is the primary objective, unless serious conditions dictate otherwise. The discharge of the infant to a person other than the mother (foster parent) or an agency should be attempted only when the infant will be neglected, poorly cared for, or abused. Most mothers hesitate to admit to the use of drugs during pregnancy because of fear that their infants will be taken away from them.[128] They should be assured otherwise; in fact, they should be encouraged to be responsible for the primary care of their infants. The social worker and physician should also advise the mother regarding the availability of medical and social services in the community, including substance abuse counseling and family planning.

As part of child protection laws operative in many states, newborns of drug-dependent mothers are considered to be potentially abused, and pediatric care physicians are required by law to report the mother to a child protection agency after the birth of the baby. The agency usually requires a positive drug screen in the newborn before any legal action can be taken against the mother. Maternal admission to the use of illicit drugs during pregnancy is not sufficient to generate a child protection agency referral because the mother can subsequently deny her admission of illicit drug use. Referral to a child protection agency is helpful when the intent is to ensure the adequacy of care of the infant at home. If a prenatal determination is made that the baby will be placed in foster care and the mother is informed of this determination, then she may refrain from continuing her prenatal care with her health care providers, choosing to deliver at another facility where she and her history are not known. This circumstance puts the mother (and baby) at higher risk for pregnancy-related complications and a greater risk of death or morbidity.

The infant of the drug-dependent mother is at risk for many long-term problems, including child abuse; delays in physical, mental, and motor development; and learning disabilities.[9,10] The infant is also at risk for ongoing exposure to illicit drugs in the household as a result of accidental ingestion or passive exposure, particularly to crack cocaine. Follow-up of these infants should be planned not only to assess their medical well being, but also to ascertain the occurrence of such complications and to initiate appropriate interventions.

TOOLS FOR PRACTICE

Engaging Patients and Family

- *Alcohol Use and Pregnancy* (fact sheet), Centers for Disease Control and Prevention (www.cdc.gov/ncbddd/factsheets/fas_alcoholuse.pdf).
- *Fetal Alcohol Spectrum Disorders* (fact sheet), Centers for Disease Control and Prevention (www.cdc.gov/ncbddd/factsheets/fas.pdf).

Medical Decision Support

- *Fetal Alcohol Spectrum Disorders* (Web page), Centers for Disease Control and Prevention (www.cdc.gov/ncbddd/fas/).
- *Research Reports Index* (Web page), US Department of Health and Human Services, National Institutes of Health, National Institute on Drug Abuse (www.nida.nih.gov/researchreports/).

REFERENCES

1. Ostrea EM Jr, Porter T, Balun J, et al. The effect of chronic maternal drug addiction on placental drug (xenobiotic) metabolism. *Dev Pharmacol Ther.* 1989;12:42-48.
2. Ostrea EM Jr, Mantaring JB III, Silvestre MA. Drugs that affect the fetus and newborn infant via the placenta or breast milk. *Pediatr Clin North Am.* 2004;51:539-579.
3. MacGregor SN, Keith LG, Chasnoff IJ, et al. Cocaine use during pregnancy: adverse perinatal outcome. *Am J Obstet Gynecol.* 1987;157:686-690.
4. Neerhof MG, MacGregor SN, Retzky SS, et al. Cocaine abuse during pregnancy: peripartum prevalence and perinatal outcome. *Am J Obstet Gynecol.* 1989;161:633-638.
5. Chasnoff IJ, Bussey ME, Savich R, et al. Perinatal cerebral infarction and maternal cocaine use. *J Pediatr.* 1986;108:456-459.
6. Chasnoff IJ, Hatcher R, Burns WJ. Polydrug and methadone addicted newborns: a continuum of impairment. *Pediatrics.* 1982;70:210-213.
7. Oleske J, Minnefor A, Cooper R Jr, et al. Immune deficiency syndrome in children. *JAMA.* 1983;249:2345-2459.
8. Chavez CJ, Ostrea EM Jr, Stryker JC, et al. Sudden infant death syndrome among infants of drug-dependent mothers. *J Pediatr.* 1979;95:407-409.
9. Wilson GS. Clinical studies of infants and children exposed prenatally to heroin *Ann NY Acad Sci.* 1989;562:183-194.
10. Wilson GS, McCreary R, Kean J, et al. The development of preschool children of heroin-addicted mothers: a controlled study. *Pediatrics.* 1979;63:135-141.
11. Substance Abuse and Mental Health Services Administration. *Results from the 2004 National Survey on Drug Use and Health: National Findings.* Office of Applied Studies, NSDUH Series H-28, DHHS Publication No. SMA 05-4062. Rockville, MD; US Department of Health and Human Services; 2005.
12. Ostrea EM Jr, Brady M, Gause S, et al. Drug screening of newborn infants by meconium analysis: a large-scale prospective epidemiologic study. *Pediatrics.* 1992;89:107-113.
13. Aghajanian GK. Tolerance to locus coeruleus neurons to morphine and suppression of withdrawal response by clonidine. *Nature.* 1978;276:186-188.
14. Wuster M, Schultz R, Herz A. Opioid tolerance and dependence: reevaluating the unitary hypothesis. *Trends Pharmacol Sci.* 1985;6:64.
15. Volpe JJ. Teratogenic effects of drugs and passive addiction. *Neurology of the Newborn.* 3rd ed. Philadelphia, PA: WB Saunders; 1995.
16. Zuspan FP, Gumpel JA, Mejia-Zelaya A, et al. Fetal stress from methadone withdrawal. *Am J Obstet Gynecol.* 1975;122:43-46.
17. Wong WM, Lao TT. Abnormal umbilical artery flow velocity waveform—a sign of fetal narcotic withdrawal? *Aust N Z J Obstet Gynaecol.* 1997;37:358.

18. Dashe JS, Sheffield JS, Olscher DA, et al. Relationship between maternal methadone dosage and neonatal withdrawal. *Obstet Gynecol*. 2002;100:1244-1249.
19. Kuschel CA, Austerberry L, Cornwell M, et al. Can methadone concentrations predict the severity of withdrawal in infants at risk of neonatal abstinence syndrome? *Arch Dis Child Fetal Neonatal Ed*. 2004; 89:390-393.
20. Sutton LR, Hinderliter SA. Diazepam abuse in pregnant women on methadone maintenance: implications for the neonate. *Clin Pediatr*. 1990;29:108-111.
21. Ostrea EM Jr, Chavez CJ, Strauss ME. A study of factors that influence the severity of neonatal narcotic withdrawal. *J Pediatr*. 1976;88:642-645.
22. Meyer FP, Rimasch H, Blaha B, et al. Tramadol withdrawal in a neonate. *Eur J Clin Pharmacol*. 1997;53: 159-160.
23. Auriacombe M, Fatseas M, Dubernet J, et al. French field experience with buprenorphine. *Amer J Addict*. 2004;13(1):S17-S28.
24. Kayemba-Kay's S, Laclyde JP. Buprenorphine withdrawal syndrome in newborns: a report of 13 cases. *Addiction*. 2003;98:1599-1604.
25. Dominguez KD, Lomako DM, Katz RW, et al. Opioid withdrawal in critically ill neonates. *Ann Pharmacother*. 2003;37:473-477.
26. Franck LS, Vilardi J, Durand D, et al. Opioid withdrawal in neonates after continuous infusion of morphine or fentanyl during ECMO. *Amer J Crit Care*. 1998;7:364-369.
27. Biswas AK, Feldman BL, Davis DH, et al. Myocardial ischemia as a result of severe benzodiazepine and opioid withdrawal. *Clin Toxicol*. 2005;43:207-209.
28. Ostrea EM Jr. Neonatal withdrawal from intrauterine exposure to butalbital. *Am J Obstet Gynecol*. 1982;143: 597-598.
29. Desmond MM, Schwanecke RP, Wilson GS, et al. Maternal barbiturate utilization and neonatal withdrawal symptomatology. *J Pediatr*. 1972;80:190-197.
30. Harvey SC. Hypnotics and sedatives: barbiturates. In: Gilman A, Rall TW, Goodman LS, et al, eds. *Goodman and Gilman's The Pharmacological Basis of Therapeutics*. 8th ed. New York, NY: Pergamon Press; 1990.
31. Isbell H. Addiction to barbiturates and the barbiturate abstinence syndrome. *Ann Intern Med*. 1950;33:108-121.
32. Ploman L, Persson BH. On the transfer of barbiturates to the human fetus and their accumulation in some of its vital organs. *J Obstet Gynecol Br Empire*. 1957;64: 706-711.
33. Ostrea EM Jr. Neonatal withdrawal from intrauterine exposure to butalbital. *Am J Obstet Gynecol*. 1982;143: 597-598.
34. Sharpless SK. The barbiturates. In: Goodman LS, Gilman A, eds. *The Pharmacological Basis of Therapeutics*. London, UK: MacMillan; 1970.
35. Jalling B, Boreus LO, Kallberg N, et al. Disappearance from the newborn of circulating prenatally administered phenobarbital. *Eur J Clin Pharmacol*. 1973;6: 234-238.
36. Coupey SM. Barbiturate. *Peds Rev*. 1997;18:260-264.
37. Iqbal MM, Sobhan T, Ryals T. Effects of commonly used benzodiazepines on the fetus, the neonate, and the nursing infant. *Psych Services*. 2002;53:39-49.
38. Erkkola R, Kangas L, Pekkarinen A. The transfer of diazepam across the placenta during labour. *Acta Obstet Gynecol Scand*. 1973;52:167-170.
39. Rementeria JL, Bhatt K. Withdrawal symptoms in neonates from intrauterine exposure to diazepam. *J Pediatr*. 1977;90:123-126.
40. Gillberg C. "Floppy infant syndrome" and maternal diazepam. *Lancet*. 1977;2:244.
41. Athinarayanan P, Pierog SH, Nigam SK, et al. Chlordiazepoxide withdrawal in the neonate. *Am J Obstet Gynecol*. 1976;124:212-213.
42. Pietrantoni M, Knuppel RA. Alcohol in pregnancy. *Clin Perinatol*. 1991;18:93-111.
43. Coles CD, Smith IE, Fernhoff PM, et al. Neonatal ethanol withdrawal: characteristics in clinically normal, nondysmorphic neonates. *J Pediatr*. 1984;105:445-451.
44. Robe LB, Gromisch DS, Iosub S. Symptoms of neonatal ethanol withdrawal. *Curr Alcohol*. 1981;8:485-493.
45. Rahbar F, Fomufod A, White D, et al. Impact of intrauterine exposure to phencyclidine (PCP) and cocaine on neonates. *J Natl Med Assoc*. 1993;85:349-352.
46. Eyler FD, Behnke M, Garvan CW, et al. Newborn evaluations of toxicity and withdrawal related to prenatal cocaine exposure. *Neurotoxicol Teratol*. 2001;23: 399-411.
47. Bada HS, Das A, Bauer CR, et al. Gestational cocaine exposure and intrauterine growth: maternal lifestyle study. *J Obstet Gynecol*. 2002;100:916-924.
48. Smeriglio VL, Finnegan LP, Maza PL. Gestational cocaine exposure and intrauterine growth: maternal lifestyle study. *J Obstet Gynecol*. 2002;100:916-924.
49. Eisen LN, Field TM, Bandstra ES, et al. Perinatal cocaine effects on neonatal stress behavior and performance on the Brazelton scale. *Pediatrics*. 1991;88:477-480.
50. Gingras JL, Feibel JB, Dalley LB, et al. Maternal polydrug use including cocaine and postnatal infant sleep architecture: preliminary observations and implications for respiratory control and behavior. *Early Hum Dev*. 1995;43:197-204.
51. Mayes LC, Granger RH, Frank DA, et al. Neurobehavioral profiles of neonates exposed to cocaine prenatally. *Pediatrics*. 1993;91:778-783.
52. Scafidi FA, Field TM, Wheeden A, et al. Cocaine-exposed preterm neonates show behavioral and hormonal differences. *Pediatrics*. 1996;97:851-855.
53. Silvestri JM, Long JM, Weese-Mayer DE, et al. Effect of prenatal cocaine on respiration, heart rate, and sudden infant death syndrome. *Pediatr Pulmonol*. 1991;11: 328-334.
54. Doberczak TM, Kandall SR, Friedmann P. Relationship between maternal methadone dosage, maternal-neonatal methadone levels, and neonatal withdrawal. *Obstet Gynecol*. 1993;81:936-940.
55. Ostrea EM, Subramanian MG, Abel EL. Placental transfer of cannabinoids in humans: comparison between meconium, maternal and cord blood sera. In: Chesner G, Consroe P, Musty R, eds. *Marijuana: An International Research Report: Proceedings of the Melbourne Symposium on Cannabis. Series 7*. Canberra, Australia: Australian Government Publishing Service; 1987.
56. Zuckerman B, Frank DA, Hingson R, et al. Effects of maternal marijuana and cocaine use on fetal growth. *N Engl J Med*. 1989;320:762-768.
57. Fried PA. Marijuana use during pregnancy: consequences for the offspring. *Sem Perinatol*. 1991;15:280-287.
58. Scher MS, Richardson GA, Coble PA, et al. The effects of prenatal alcohol and marijuana exposure: disturbances in neonatal sleep cycling and arousal. *Pediatr Res*. 1988;24:101-105.
59. Mirochnick M, Meyer J, Frank DA, et al. Elevated plasma norepinephrine after in utero exposure to cocaine and marijuana. *Pediatrics*. 1997;99:555-559.
60. Hayes JS, Dreher MC, Nugent JK. Newborn outcomes with maternal marihuana use in Jamaican women. *Pediatr Nurs*. 1988;14:107-110.
61. Richardson GA, Day NL, Taylor P. The effect of prenatal alcohol, marijuana and tobacco exposure on neonatal behavior. *Infant Behav Dev*. 1989;12:199.

62. Ostrea EM Jr, Knapp DK, Romero A, et al. Meconium analysis to assess fetal exposure to access fetal exposure to active and passive maternal smoking. *J Pediatr.* 1994; 124:471-476.
63. Matthews TJ. Smoking during pregnancy in the 1990s. *Natl Vital Stat Rep.* 2001;49:1-14.
64. Butler NR, Goldstein H. Smoking in pregnancy and subsequent child development. *Br Med J.* 1973;4: 573-575.
65. Dunn HG, McBurney AK, Ingram S, et al. Maternal cigarette smoking during pregnancy and the child's subsequent development: II. Neurological and intellectual maturation to the age of 6.5 years. *Can J Publ Health.* 1977;68:43-50.
66. Saxton DW. The behavior of infants whose mothers smoke in pregnancy. *Early Hum Dev.* 1978;2:363-369.
67. Law KL, Stroud LR, LaGasse LL, et al. Smoking during pregnancy and newborn neurobehavior. *Pediatrics.* 2003;111:1318-1323.
68. Godding V, Bonnier C, Fiasse L, et al. Does in utero exposure to heavy maternal smoking induce nicotine withdrawal symptoms in neonates? *Pediatr Res.* 2004; 55:645-651.
69. Kaufman KR, Petrucha RA, Pitts FN Jr, et al. Phencyclidine in umbilical cord blood: preliminary data. *Am J Psychiatr.* 1983;140:450-452.
70. Chasnoff IJ, Burns WJ, Hatcher RP. Phencyclidine: effects on the fetus and neonate. *Dev Pharmacol Ther.* 1983;6:404-408.
71. Golden NL, Kuhnert BR, Sokol RJ, et al. Neonatal manifestations of maternal phencyclidine exposure. *J Perinat Med.* 1987;15:185-191.
72. Strauss AA, Modanlou D, Bosu SK. Neonatal manifestations of maternal phencyclidine (PCP) abuse. *Pediatrics.* 1981;68:550-552.
73. Ramer CM. The case history of an infant born to an amphetamine-addicted mother. *Clin Pediatr.* 1974; 13:596-597.
74. Smith L, Yonekura ML, Wallace T, et al. Effects of prenatal methamphetamine exposure on fetal growth and drug withdrawal symptoms in infants born at term. *J Dev Behav Pediatr.* 2003;24:17-23.
75. Bupropion (amfebutamone): caution during pregnancy. *Prescrire Int.* 2005;14:225.
76. Sanz EJ, De-las-Cuevas C, Kiuru A, et al. Selective serotonin reuptake inhibitors in pregnant women and neonatal withdrawal syndrome: a database analysis. *Lancet.* 2005;365:482-487.
77. Stiskal JA, Kulin N, Koren G, et al. Neonatal paroxetine withdrawal syndrome. *Arch Dis Child Fetal Neonatal Ed.* 2001;84:134.
78. Stothers J. Lithium toxicity in the newborn. *Br Med J.* 1973;3:233-234.
79. Webster PAC. Withdrawal symptoms in neonates associated with maternal antidepressant therapy. *Lancet.* 1973;2:318-319.
80. Costei AM, Kozer E, Ho T, et al. Perinatal outcome following third trimester exposure to paroxetine. *Arch Pediatr Adolesc Med.* 2003;157:601.
81. de Moor RA, Mourad L, ter Haar J, et al. Withdrawal symptoms in a neonate following exposure to venlafaxine during pregnancy. *Ned Tijdschr Geneeskd.* 2003;147: 1370-1372.
82. Oberlander TF, Misri S, Fitzgerald CE, et al. Pharmacologic factors associated with transient neonatal symptoms following prenatal psychotropic medication exposure. *J Clin Psychiatry.* 2004;65:230-237.
83. National Institute on Drug Abuse. Monitoring the Future 1999. Available at: www.nida.nih.gov/NIDA_noks. Accessed December 23, 2006.
84. Tenenbein M, Casiro O, Seshia M, et al. Neonatal withdrawal from maternal volatile substance abuse. *Arch Dis Child.* 1996;74:F204-F207.
85. Wilkins-Haug L, Gabow PA. Toluene abuse during pregnancy: obstetric complications and perinatal outcomes. *Obstet Gynecol.* 1991;77:504-509.
86. Moran LR, Almeida PG, Worden S, et al. Intrauterine baclofen exposure: a multidisciplinary approach. *Pediatrics.* 2004;114:e267-e269.
87. Ratnayaka BD, Dhaliwal H, Watkin S. Drug points: neonatal convulsions after withdrawal of baclofen. *BMJ.* 2001;323:85.
88. Ebbesen F, Joergensen A, Hoseth E, et al. Neonatal hypoglycaemia and withdrawal symptoms after exposure in utero to valproate. *Arch Dis Child Fetal Neonatal Ed.* 2000;83:F124-F129.
89. Kandall SR, Gartner LM. Late presentation of drug withdrawal symptoms in newborns. *Am J Dis Child.* 1974;127:58-61.
90. Doberczak TM, Kandall SR, Wilets I. Neonatal opiate abstinence syndrome in term and preterm infants. *J Pediatr.* 1991;118:933-937.
91. Ostrea EM. Infants of drug dependent mothers. In: Berg FD, Ingelfinger JR, Wald ER, eds. *Current Pediatric Therapy.* Philadelphia, PA: WB Saunders; 1992.
92. Doberczak TM, Shanzer S, Senie RT, et al. Neonatal neurologic and electroencephalographic effects of intrauterine cocaine exposure. *J Pediatr.* 1988;133:354-358.
93. Reddy A, Harper R, Stern G. Observations on heroin and methadone withdrawal in the newborn. *Pediatrics.* 1971;48:353-358.
94. Pinto F, Torrioli MG, Casella G, et al. Sleep in babies born to chronically heroin-addicted mothers: a follow-up study. *Drug Alcohol Depend.* 1988;21:43-47.
95. Glass L, Rajegowda BK, et al. Effect of heroin withdrawal on respiratory rate and acid-base status of the newborn. *N Engl J Med.* 1972;286:746-748.
96. Ostrea EM Jr, Kresbach P, Knapp DK, et al. Abnormal heart rate tracings and serum creatine phosphokinase in addicted neonates. *Neurotoxicol Teratol.* 1987;9: 305-309.
97. Ward SL, Schuetz S, Wachsman L. Elevated plasma norepinephrine levels in infants of substance-abusing mothers. *Amer J Dis Child.* 1991;145:44-48.
98. Dube SK, Jhaveri RC, Rosenfeld W, et al. Urinary catecholamines, plasma renin activity and blood pressure in newborns: effects of narcotic withdrawal. *Dev Pharm Ther.* 1981;3:83-87.
99. Kron RE, Litt M, Eng D, et al. Neonatal narcotic abstinence: effects of pharmacotherapeutic agents and maternal drug usage on nutritive sucking behavior. *J Pediatr.* 1976;88:637-641.
100. Ostrea EM, Brady MJ, Parks PM, et al. Drug screening of meconium in infants of drug-dependent mothers: an alternative to urine testing. *J Pediatr.* 1989;115:474-477.
101. Ryan RM, Wagner CL, Schultz JM, et al. Meconium analysis for improved identification of infants exposed to cocaine in utero. *J Pediatr.* 1994;125:435-440.
102. Hill RM, Desmond MM, Kay JL. Extrapyramidal dysfunction in an infant of a schizophrenic mother. *J Pediatr.* 1966;69:589-595.
103. Levy W, Wisniewski K. Chlorpromazine causing extrapyramidal dysfunction in newborn infant of psychotic mother. *NY State J Med.* 1974;74:684-685.
104. Ostrea EM, Chavez CJ. Perinatal problems (excluding neonatal withdrawal) in maternal drug addiction: a study of 830 cases. *J Pediatr.* 1979;94:292-295.
105. Finnegan LP. Neonatal abstinence. In: Nelson NM, ed: *Current Therapy in Neonatal-Perinatal Medicine.* Philadelphia, PA: BC Decker; 1990.

106. Lipsitz PJ. A proposed narcotic withdrawal score for use with newborn infants. *Clin Pediatr.* 1975;14:592-594.
107. O'Brien C, Hunt R, Jeffery HE. Measurement of movement is an objective method to assist in assessment of opiate withdrawal in newborns. *Arch Dis Child Fetal Neonatal Ed.* 2004;89:F305-F309.
108. American Academy of Pediatrics, Committee on Drugs. Neonatal drug withdrawal. *Pediatrics.* 1998;101:1079-1088.
109. Rosen TS, Johnson HL. Children of methadone-maintained mothers: follow-up to 18 months of age. *J Pediatr.* 1982;101:192-196.
110. Fulroth R, Phillips B, Durand D. Perinatal outcome of infants exposed to cocaine and/or heroin in utero. *Am J Dis Child.* 1989;143:905-910.
111. Osborn DA, Jeffery HE, Cole M. Opiate treatment for opiate withdrawal in newborn infants. *Cochrane Database Syst Rev.* 2005;3:CD002059.
112. Lainwala S, Brown ER, Weinschenk NP, et al. A retrospective study of length of hospital stay in infants treated for neonatal abstinence syndrome with methadone versus oral morphine preparations. *Adv Neonatal Care.* 2005;5:265-272.
113. Coyle MG, Ferguson A, Lagasse L, et al. Neurobehavioral effects of treatment for opiate withdrawal. *Arch Dis Child Fetal Neonatal Ed.* 2005;90:F73-F74.
114. Jones HC. Shorter dosing interval of opiate solution shortens hospital stay for methadone babies. *Fam Med.* 1999;31:327-330.
115. Anand KJ, Arnold JH. Opioid tolerance and dependence in infants and children. *Crit Care Med.* 1994;22:334-342.
116. Dinges DF, Davis MM, Glass P. Fetal exposure to narcotics: neonatal sleep as a measure of nervous system disturbance. *Science.* 1980;209:619-621.
117. Shimohira M, Iwakawa Y, Kohyama J. Rapid-eye-movement sleep in jittery infants. *Early Hum Dev.* 2002;66:25-31.
118. Franck L, Vilardi J. Assessment and management of opioid withdrawal in ill neonates. *Neonatal Netw.* 1995;14:39-48.
119. Gewolb IH, Fishman D, Qureshi MA, et al. Coordination of suck-swallow-respiration in infants born to mothers with drug-abuse problems. *Dev Med Child Neurol.* 2004;46:700-705.
120. Bloom RS, Cropley C. *Textbook of Neonatal Resuscitation.* Elk Grove Village, IL: American Heart Association, American Academy of Pediatrics; 1990.
121. American Academy of Pediatrics, Section on Breastfeeding. Breastfeeding and the Use of Human Milk. *Pediatrics.* 2005;115(2):496-506. Available at: aappolicy.aappublications.org/cgi/reprint/pediatrics;115/2/496.pdf. Accessed March 7, 2007.
122. Howard C, Lawrence R. Breastfeeding and drug exposure. *Obstet Gynecol Clin North Am.* 1998;25:195-217.
123. Briggs GG, Freeman RK, Yaffe SJ. *Methadone. Drugs in Pregnancy and Lactation.* Baltimore, MD: Williams and Wilkins; 1994.
124. American Academy of Pediatrics, Committee on Drugs. The transfer of drugs and other chemicals into human milk. *Pediatrics.* 1994;93:137-150.
125. Chavez CJ, Ostrea EM. Outcome of infants of drug-dependent mothers based on the type of caregiver. *Pediatr Res.* 1977;11:375A.
126. Oei J, Feller JM, Lui K. Coordinated outpatient care of the narcotic-dependent infant. *J Paediatr Child Health.* 2001;37:266-270.
127. Ostrea EM, Chavez CJ, Stryker JS. *The Care of the Drug Dependent Woman and Her Infant.* Lansing, MI: Michigan Department of Public Health; 1978.
128. Michigan. Court of Appeals. In re Baby X. *Wests North West Rep.* 1980;293:736.

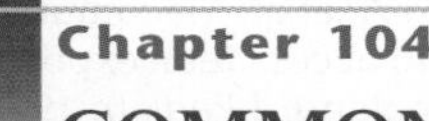

Chapter 104

COMMON METABOLIC DISTURBANCES IN THE NEWBORN

Zuzanna Kubicka, MD; George A. Little, MD

At birth, placental function, including transport of glucose, calcium, phosphorus, and magnesium, is suddenly interrupted. Usually this process occurs uneventfully; however, the primary care physician must be aware of the physiological mechanism of transition and possible problems that may occur critically.

GLUCOSE METABOLISM IN THE FETUS AND METABOLIC ADAPTATION AT BIRTH

Carbohydrate is transported to the fetus as *glucose* by transplacental facilitative diffusion across a concentration gradient. Glucose transport capacity increases with gestational age, with a portion used for placental metabolism. When placental function and fetal growth are normal, fetal glucose production is limited.

Glucose-sensing and insulin-secreting pathways are present in the human fetus as early as 14 to 18 weeks' gestation, but secretion of insulin in response to glucose is attenuated. During fetal development, pancreatic β-cells mature, with biphasic insulin release developing after birth. When the fetus is subjected to reduced glucose supply, hypoglycemia and hypoinsulinemia may develop despite fetal glucose production.

Healthy, term neonates transition to extrauterine environment without need for metabolic monitoring. Hepatic glycogen content increases with gestational age, and most deposition occurs toward the end of gestation.

Neonatal glucose requirements of approximately 5 to 8 mg/kg/min, mostly for cerebral use, must be met endogenously when the placental glucose supply ceases. Immediately after birth a three- to five-fold surge in glucagon and catecholamines takes place, which initiates glycogenolysis, gluconeogenesis, lipolysis, and ketogenesis. Endogenous growth hormone and cortisol facilitate the onset of gluconeogenesis within several hours, and insulin secretion and serum concentrations fall. Enzymatic systems for glycogen breakdown and gluconeogenesis must be in place, along with a supply of substrate in the form of fat and amino acids. Human milk has an important role in the induction of ketogenesis, which spares glucose for brain consumption and facilitates gluconeogenesis.[1-3]

Preterm and some intrauterine growth–restricted neonates have transitional metabolic processes that are not fully developed, and less glycogen stores are available for glucose mobilization after birth. Glucose regulation problems also occur with a wide range of antepartum, intrapartum, and postnatal problems such as maternal diabetes, hypoxic stress, and sepsis.

NEONATAL HYPOGLYCEMIA

The definition, significance, and management of hypoglycemia persist as controversial issues in contemporary neonatal pediatrics.

Definition

The definitive diagnosis of neonatal hypoglycemia must satisfy the Whipple triad: (1) the presence of clinical manifestations (2) coincident with reliable low plasma glucose concentrations and (3) resolution of manifestations once normoglycemia has been reestablished.[2] This definition does not include so-called *asymptomatic* hypoglycemia without clinical manifestations, even with very low plasma glucose concentrations. Controversy remains as to whether transient asymptomatic hypoglycemia causes sequelae.

Attempts have been made to identify a threshold blood glucose concentration below which a substantial likelihood of functional impairment exists. The evidence for a glucose level that causes irreversible neuronal injury remains poorly defined. Data from animal studies support the theory that sustained hypoglycemia is associated with neuronal necrosis. No prospective study in human infants has been conducted to determine such a threshold.[3-6]

Numerous textbooks and papers use the arbitrary plasma glucose level of 40 to 45 mg/dL or blood glucose value less than 35 mg/dL as a defining threshold for intervention with the range as wide as 27 to 47 mg/dL.[2,3,7-16]

An important point to remember is that a healthy term newborn exhibits an immediate postnatal fall in blood glucose concentration during the first 2 to 4 hours from values close to maternal levels to approximately 45 mg/dL (2.5 mmol/L).[1,3]

Frequency

Overall incidence has been estimated to be 1 to 5 per 1000 live births.[3] The classic Lubchenco and Bard studies of neonatal hypoglycemia illustrate that intrauterine birth-weight/gestational age status may serve as an indicator[17] (Figure 104-1).

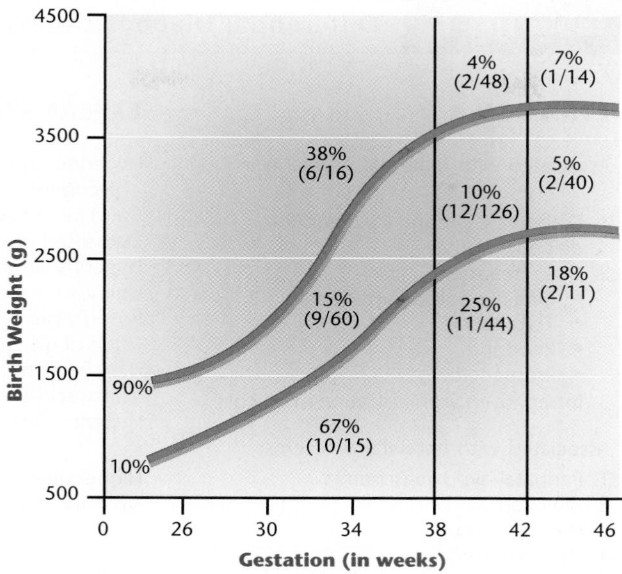

Figure 104-1 Incidence of hypoglycemia by birth weight, gestational age, and intrauterine growth. *(Lubchenco LO, Bard H. Incidence of hypoglycemia in newborn infants classified by birth weight and gestational age.* Pediatrics. *1971;47:831-838.)*

Differential Diagnosis

Table 104-1 presents the most common causes of neonatal hypoglycemia. The information provided can be used to identify at-risk infants for whom routine monitoring of blood glucose is recommended.

Transient hypoglycemia usually resolves within 2 to 3 days. A requirement of more than 8 to 10 mg/kg/min suggests hyperinsulinism and is seen most commonly in the infant of a diabetic mother. Persistence for more than 7 days or recurrence usually warrants subspecialty endocrine or metabolic evaluation.[7,16,18]

Evaluation

Physical Examination

The typical clinical manifestations of hypoglycemia are summarized in Box 104-1. Birth-weight/gestation age indicators previously discussed (see Figure 104-1), including their morphologic expressions (large for gestational age, small for gestational age, intrauterine growth restriction), must be considered.[17]

BOX 104-1 Clinical Signs Associated With Hypoglycemia*

- Changes in behavior—irritability, lethargy
- Changes in neurologic status—hypotonia, limpness, tremor, jitteriness, seizures
- Cardiovascular signs—tachycardia, bradycardia
- Abnormal respiratory patterns—apnea, cyanotic spells, tachypnea, respiratory distress
- Feeding poorly, especially after feeding well
- Hypothermia

*Clinical signs should be alleviated with concomitant correction of plasma glucose levels.
Adapted from Cornblath M, Hawdon JM, Williams AF, et al. Controversies regarding definition of neonatal hypoglycemia: suggested operational thresholds. *Pediatrics.* 2000;105:1141-1145.

An important point to realize is that the quiet or inactive newborn who is not exhibiting any of the listed symptoms may, in fact, be hypoglycemic. On the other hand these signs may occur with common neonatal disorders, including sepsis, intracranial hemorrhage, or hypocalcemia. Infants exhibiting one or more of these signs should have blood glucose screened.

Laboratory Evaluation

Glucose reagent strips screen for low blood glucose concentration and provide a valuable estimate. Diagnosis depends on plasma glucose values. Whole-blood glucose levels are 10% to 15% lower than plasma glucose levels. Blood samples should be processed quickly because of possible glycolysis. False elevation can result from line sampling without preflushing.

Table 104-1 Differential Diagnosis of Neonatal Hypoglycemia

ETIOLOGY	EXPLANATION	DURATION OF HYPOGLYCEMIA
Associated with maternal problems:		Transient (<7 days' duration)
1. Diabetes in pregnancy, infant of diabetic mother	Hyperinsulinism and resulting inhibition of glycogenolysis, lipolysis, glyconeogenesis, and increased peripheral glucose utilization Decreased glucose supply	
2. Drug treatment:		
• Oral hypoglycemic agents	Hyperinsulinism	
• Terbutaline	Unknown mechanism	
• Ritodrine		
• Propranolol	Possibly prevention of sympathetic stimulation of glycogenolysis, prevention of recovery from insulin induced, decreases in free fatty acid and glycerol	
3. Intrapartum administration of glucose	Hyperinsulinism	
Associated with neonatal problems:		
1. Perinatal hypoxia-ischemia	Higher glucose utilization or decreased production	Transient (<7 days' duration)
2. Infection		
3. Hypothermia		
4. Hyperviscosity		
5. Erythroblastosis fetalis, hydrops	Hyperinsulinism, possibly increased number of pancreatic β-cells	
6. Iatrogenic:		
• Malpositioned umbilical artery catheter	Infusion of high glucose concentration into celiac, superior mesenteric artery; hyperinsulinism	
• Abrupt cessation of high glucose infusion	Hyperinsulinism	
• Exchange transfusion	Blood containing high glucose concentration, hyperinsulinism	
Intrauterine growth restriction, prematurity, inadequate caloric intake	Limited glycogen stores Altered insulin secretion Altered hormonal response to hypoglycemia	Transient (<7 days' duration)
Genetic disorders—Beckwith-Weidemann syndrome, genetic forms of hyperinsulinism, insulin secreting tumors	Hyperinsulinism	Prolonged
Endocrine disorders: hypopituitarism, adrenal insufficiency, hypothalamic deficiency	Higher glucose utilization or decreased production	Prolonged
Inborn errors of metabolism	Higher glucose utilization or decreased production	Prolonged

Adapted from Cornblath M, Hawdon JM, Williams AF, et al. Controversies regarding definition of neonatal hypoglycemia: suggested operational thresholds. *Pediatrics.* 2000;105:1141-1145; McGowan JE. Neonatal hypoglycemia. *NeoReviews.* 1999;(July):e6-e15; Wilker RE. Hypoglycemia and hyperglycemia; Huttner KM. Hypocalcemia, hypercalcemia, and hypermagnesemia. In: Cloherty JP, Eichenwald EC, Stark AR, eds. *Manual of Neonatal Care.* 5th ed. Lippincott Williams and Wilkins, 2004; Cornblath M, Schwartz R. Hypoglycemia in the neonate. *J Pediatr Endocrinol.* 1993;6:113-129.

Blood glucose concentrations reflect enteral feeds, reaching a peak by approximately an hour afterwards and a nadir just before the next feeding. Given that the purpose of blood glucose monitoring is to identify the lowest blood glucose level, prefeed measurement is recommended.*

Management

Pragmatic operational thresholds (blood glucose concentrations at which clinical interventions should be considered) for various clinical scenarios have been recently proposed.[2]

Term Newborn

Feeding is the main preventive strategy for healthy, term newborns without risk factors or clinical signs suggesting problems. Breastfed newborns demonstrate lower blood glucose and higher ketone body concentrations than those who are formula fed.[16,20]

Newborns With Abnormal Clinical Signs

Symptomatic newborns should have a glucose reagent strip screen while awaiting laboratory determination. If the plasma value is less than 45 mg/dL (2.5 mmol/L), then clinical intervention to increase the blood glucose concentration is indicated[2] (Figure 104-2).

Enteral feeds may be continued or introduced when clinically appropriate, and parenteral treatment is not a reason to delay them. Gradual rather than rapid reductions in the rate of glucose infusion help maintain stability and avoid labile glucose concentrations.

Infants With Risk Factors for Compromised Metabolic Adaptation

Routine determination of plasma glucose concentration should be performed for newborns at risk.

*References: 2, 3, 8, 9, 16, 19.

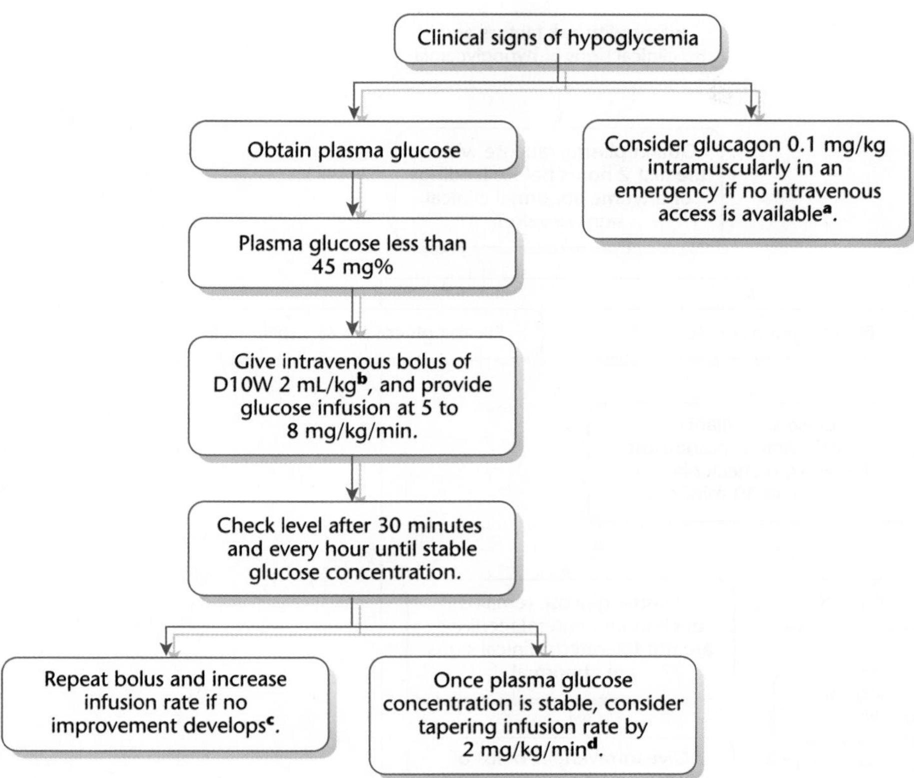
Clinical signs of hypoglycemia
Obtain plasma glucose
Consider glucagon 0.1 mg/kg intramuscularly in an emergency if no intravenous access is available[a].
Plasma glucose less than 45 mg%
Give intravenous bolus of D10W 2 mL/kg[b], and provide glucose infusion at 5 to 8 mg/kg/min.
Check level after 30 minutes and every hour until stable glucose concentration.
Repeat bolus and increase infusion rate if no improvement develops[c].
Once plasma glucose concentration is stable, consider tapering infusion rate by 2 mg/kg/min[d].

[a]Glucagon will produce a rapid rise in blood glucose only in infants with adequate glycogen stores.
[b]Boluses of hypertonic (25%, 50%) glucose solution are not recommended because they can cause a release of additional insulin and worsening hypoglycemia.
[c]Some infants (eg, with hyperinsulinism or intrauterine growth restriction) may require glucose infusion up to 12 to 15 mg/kg/min. If the need for glucose concentration is >12%, central access is necessary.
[d]At least 2 plasma glucose levels more than 50 mg% on two consecutive evaluations suggest stabilization of the plasma levels. Weaning is usually recommended after 12 to 24 hours of normoglycemia, based on preprandial plasma glucose levels.

Figure 104-2 Management of infants with clinical signs of hypoglycemia. *(Adapted from Cornblath M, Hawdon JM, Williams AF, et al. Controversies regarding definition of neonatal hypoglycemia: suggested operational thresholds.* Pediatrics. *2000; 105:1141-1145; McGowan JE. Neonatal hypoglycemia.* NeoReviews. *1999;[July]:e6-e15; Wilker RE. Hypoglycemia and hyperglycemia; Huttner KM. Hypocalcemia, hypercalcemia, and hypermagnesemia. In: Cloherty JP, Eichenwald E.C., Stark AR, eds.* Manual of Neonatal Care. *5th ed. Lippincott Williams and Wilkins, 2004; Deshpande S, Ward Platt M. The investigation and management of neonatal hypoglycemia.* Semin Fetal Neonatal Med. *2005;10:351-361.)*

Glucose monitoring should be initiated within 2 hours after birth, before feeding, and at any time abnormal signs exist. If the plasma glucose concentration remains less than 36 mg/dL (2.0 mmol/L) despite feeding, then intravenous treatments should be initiated. This approach is the initial step if the plasma glucose concentration is less than 25 mg/dL (Figure 104-3).

Asymptomatic at-risk newborns who are able to tolerate enteral feeds in the first hour after birth should receive interval feedings every 2 to 3 hours or sooner as a first-preventive strategy. If hypoglycemia develops, then increasing milk volume can be attempted, as well as strategies depicted for symptomatic newborns (see Figure 104-3).

Maintaining therapeutic levels in excess of 60 mg/dL (3.3 mmol/L) may be indicated for symptomatic newborns with documented hyperinsulinemic hypoglycemia; however, it should not be the therapeutic goal for the most newborns with transient or brief episodes of low plasma glucose concentrations.

Newborns of diabetic mothers usually express their highest incidence of hypoglycemia between 4 and 6 hours after birth but may extend initial expression to 48 hours. Early enteral feedings with human milk, if available, and regular prefeed monitoring of blood glucose concentration until stable are recommended for such infants. Excessive intravenous glucose infusions should be avoided to minimize pancreatic stimulation.[3,16]

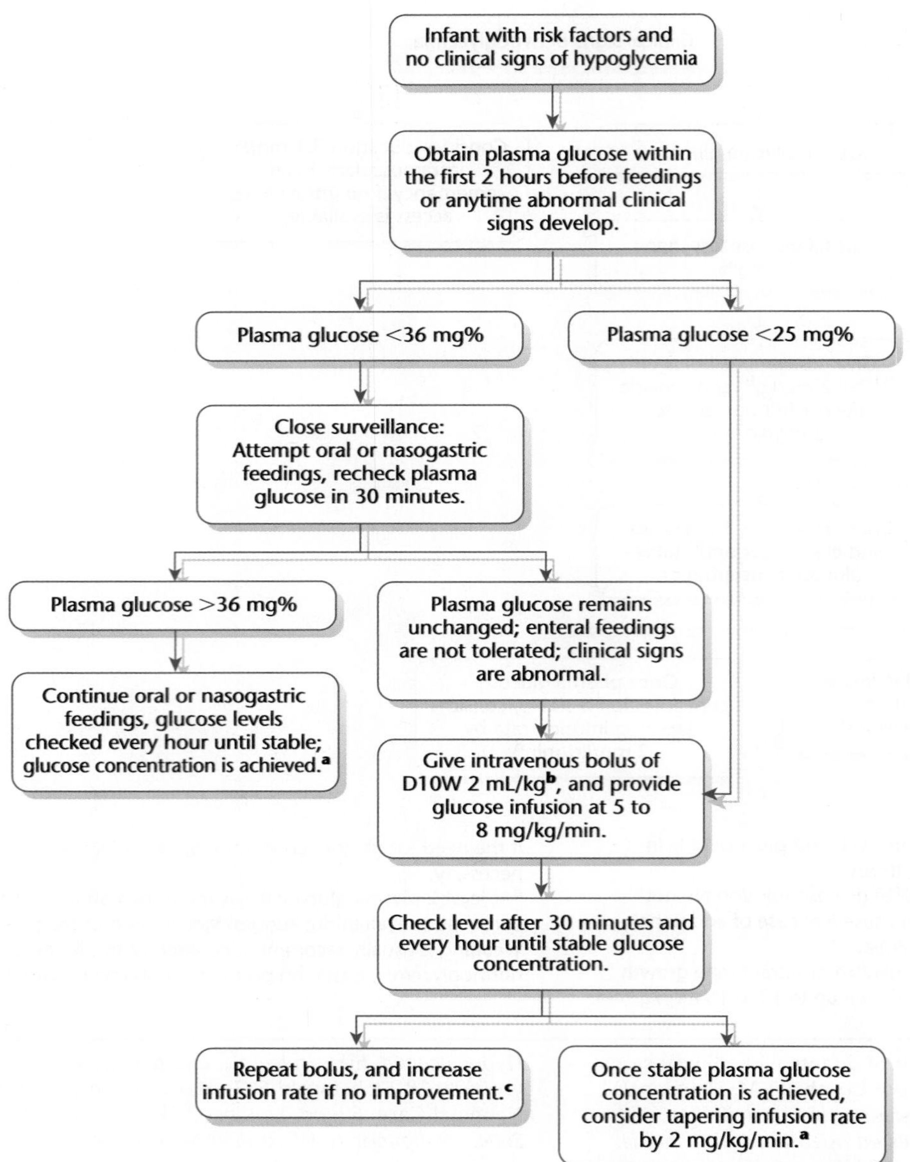

[a]At least 2 plasma glucose levels more than 50 mg% on two consecutive evaluations suggest stabilization of the plasma levels. Weaning is usually recommended after 12 to 24 hours of normoglycemia, based on preprandial plasma glucose levels.
[b]Boluses of hypertonic (25%, 50%) glucose solution are not recommended because they can cause a release of additional insulin and worsening hypoglycemia.
[c]Some infants (eg, with hyperinsulinism or intrauterine growth restriction) may require glucose infusion up to 12 to 15 mg/kg/min. If needed for glucose concentration of >12%, central access is necessary.

Figure 104-3 Management of infants with risk factors for hypoglycemia—no clinical signs. *(Adapted from Cornblath M, Hawdon JM, Williams AF, et al. Controversies regarding definition of neonatal hypoglycemia: suggested operational thresholds.* Pediatrics. *2000;105:1141-1145; McGowan JE. Neonatal hypoglycemia.* NeoReviews. *1999; [July]:e6-e15; Wilker RE. Hypoglycemia and hyperglycemia; Huttner KM. Hypocalcemia, hypercalcemia, and hypermagnesemia. In: Cloherty JP, Eichenwald EC, Stark AR, eds.* Manual of Neonatal Care. *5th ed. Lippincott Williams and Wilkins, 2004; Deshpande S, Ward Platt M. The investigation and management of neonatal hypoglycemia.* Semin Fetal Neonatal Med. *2005;10:351-361.)*

Preterm Infants

The same strategies and thresholds mentioned previously apply to preterm newborns. Intravenous glucose infusion is often necessary owing to risk factors for development of hypoglycemia, including poor glycogen stores and limited oral feeding ability. Most well-nourished but preterm infants require at least 6 to 8 mg/kg/min of glucose initially.[2]

HYPERGLYCEMIA

Definition

A whole-blood glucose level greater than 125 mg/dL or a plasma glucose level of greater than 145 mg/dL is considered to be outside normal limits by most authors.[8-10]

Differential Diagnosis

Common causes of hyperglycemia are presented in Table 104-2.

Although more common than hypoglycemia, a large portion of hyperglycemia occurs in low–birth-weight infants receiving parental glucose. Infusion rates higher than 6.6 mg/kg/min in infants less than 1100 g and more than 6 mg/kg/min in healthy, full-term newborn may cause iatrogenic hyperglycemia.[8-10]

Evaluation

Physical Examination

Clinical dehydration caused by osmotic diuresis is a serious complication of hyperglycemia; each 18-mg/dL rise in the blood glucose concentration increases serum osmolality by 1 mOsm/L and hyperosmolality of more than 300 mOsm/L. Researchers have hypothesized that hyperglycemia by increasing osmolality causes the water to move from intracellular to extracellular compartment. This *contraction* of intracellular volume may be associated risk of intracranial hemorrhage particularly in the very low–birth-weight infant.[8-10]

Laboratory Evaluation

In addition to blood determination for hypoglycemia, urine monitoring for glucosuria caused by exceeding of renal tubular reabsorption capability of glucose may be helpful.

Management

Prevention strategies and treatment of hyperglycemia are summarized in Box 104-2.

CALCIUM AND PHOSPHORUS METABOLISM IN THE FETUS AND METABOLIC ADAPTATION AT BIRTH

Active calcium and phosphorus transport to the fetus is necessary for fetal growth and increases through gestation to a peak in the third trimester. Premature newborns are therefore at risk for deficiency, which can worsen after birth as a result of renal losses and deficient intestinal absorption.

Neonatal serum calcium homeostasis is maintained by exogenous intake or absorption from bones, or by both process. In the first day, serum calcium decreases (low intake) and ionized calcium reaches the lowest level of 1.10 to 1.36 mmol/L (4.4 to 5.4 mg/dL) at approximately 24 hours of age, rising slowly thereafter.

Fetal phosphorus concentration is higher than maternal concentration. Postnatal absorption takes place primarily in the jejunum, with low excretion in the newborn. In the first day of life, neonatal serum concentration increases before increased absorption, probably related to breakdown of tissue glycogen. This increased phosphorus concentration also probably contributes to decreased calcium concentration.

Calcium is the most abundant mineral in the human body, with 99% contained in the bones. Eighty-five percent to 90% of phosphorus is found in the skeleton. Calcium-phosphorus serum concentration is tightly

Table 104-2 Differential Diagnosis of Neonatal Hyperglycemia

CAUSE	MECHANISM
Prematurity, very low birth weight (<1000 g)	Variable insulin response to persistent endogenous glucose production; high catecholamine and other stress hormone levels
Sepsis	Decreased insulin release or decreased glucose utilization; elevation of stress hormones
Hypoxia	Increased glucose production or absent increased utilization
Surgical procedures	Increased release of stress hormones; administration of intravenous glucose
Drugs: steroids, caffeine, theophylline, phenytoin	Increased glycogenolysis or gluconeogenesis Increased insulin resistance Increased insulin resistance and decreased insulin release
Hyperosmolar formula (inappropriate formula dilution)	Increased glucose load
Rare endocrine disorders: transient neonatal diabetes mellitus, diabetes related to pancreatic lesions	Decreased insulin release

Reprinted with permission from Wilker RE. Hypoglycemia and hyperglycemia; Huttner KM. Hypocalcemia, hypercalcemia, and hypermagnesemia. In: Cloherty JP, Eichenwald EC, Stark AR, eds. *Manual of Neonatal Care.* 5th ed. Lippincott Williams & Wilkins; 2004.

BOX 104-2 Prevention and Management of Neonatal Hyperglycemia

PREVENTION

Avoid sudden changes in glucose concentration.

Avoid glucose infusion rates >6 mg/kg/min in premature and full-term infants

Use initially 5%-glucose infusion concentration for the infants <1000 g.

Avoid using hypotonic fluids (<5% dextrose).

Start parenteral nutrition as soon as possible; some amino acids promote insulin secretion.

Continue enteral feedings if not contraindicated as this promotes insulin secretion.

MANAGEMENT

Decrease the glucose infusion to 4-6 mg/kg/min or by 2 mg/kg/min every 4-6 hr.

If glucose level persistent above 250 mg/dL despite all the measures to decrease the glucose intake, then consider insulin therapy.

Continuous intravenous insulin infusion of 0.01-0.1 units/kg/hr (with close monitoring of plasma glucose levels, potassium levels)

Subcutaneous insulin 0.1-0.2 units/kg every 6 hr; used most commonly in neonatal diabetes (with close monitoring of plasma glucose levels, potassium levels)

Adapted from Wilker RE. Hypoglycemia and hyperglycemia; Huttner KM. Hypocalcemia, hypercalcemia, and hypermagnesemia. In: Cloherty JP, Eichenwald EC, Stark AR, eds. *Manual of Neonatal Care*. 5th ed. Lippincott Williams and Wilkins; 2004; Pildes RS. Hypoglycemia and hyperglycemia in tiny infants. *Clin Perinatol*. 1986;3:351-375.

regulated by parathyroid hormone (PTH), vitamin D metabolites, and calcitonin.

NEONATAL HYPOCALCEMIA

Definition and Diagnosis

Calcium circulates in blood in three fractions: (1) protein bound (40% to 45%); (2) complexed with anions such as lactate, citrate, and bicarbonate (5% to 10%); and (3) ionized (50%). The last of these fractions is the only physiologically active fraction. With low serum protein the total calcium may be decreased, whereas the ionized fraction remains within normal limits. With normal total calcium the ionized fraction may be decreased by alkalosis, administration of bicarbonate, or chelating agents present in blood products.

Hypocalcemia in the term newborn is best defined as serum ionized calcium concentration of less than 1.1 mmol/L (4.4 mg/dL). (See later discussion under Laboratory Evaluation).

Differential Diagnosis

Common causes of neonatal hypocalcemia are summarized in Table 104-3.

Evaluation

Physical Examination

Physiologically the clinical signs of hypocalcemia are related to increased cell membrane excitability because low serum calcium levels increase cellular permeability to sodium ions. Signs of neonatal hypocalcemia are often nonspecific and may include jitteriness, hyperreflexia, increased tone, and generalized or focal seizures, as well as apnea and rarely laryngospasm. Occasionally the newborn may exhibit classic tetany and positive Chvostek and Trousseau signs. Electrocardiographic readings may be significant for prolonged QTc interval. These signs may also be present with other disorders, including hypoglycemia.

Laboratory Evaluation

The traditional definition of total serum calcium less than 2 mmol/L (8 mg/dL) is of limited value and should be used only if ionized calcium values are not available. Reference values for preterm infants are ionized calcium less than 1.07 mmol/L (4.28 mg/dL) or the total calcium less than 1.75 mmol/L (7 mg/dL).[21]

Measuring magnesium levels in the setting of hypocalcemia is important because correction of low serum calcium might not be possible without correcting hypomagnesemia. Low serum calcium may also be associated with seizures, although it is not the cause.

Management

Management is complicated by several factors. Most cases of neonatal hypocalcemia are asymptomatic and self-resolving by day 3 of life. Similar signs may coexist with other neonatal conditions. Asymptomatic hypocalcemia in a well newborn usually resolves spontaneously without specific treatment. With the serum calcium level below 6.5 mg/dL (usually the asymptomatic very low–birth-weight newborn), some authors recommend continuous calcium infusion with the dose of 5 mL/kg/day of 10% calcium gluconate.[8,9,21]

The treatment of symptomatic hypocalcemia consists of administering calcium salts (Table 104-4, Figure 104-4). Symptoms that are unresponsive to calcium therapy may be the result of hypomagnesemia. (See later discussion of management of hypomagnesemia.)

Bradycardia may be a serious systemic complication of intravenous calcium administration. Possible local complications include umbilical arterial spasm with rapid administration, extravasations into soft tissues, and hepatic necrosis if umbilical venous catheter lodged in the branch of the portal catheter.

The management of late-onset hypocalcemia usually consists of treating the underlying disorder.

NEONATAL HYPERCALCEMIA

Definition

Serum ionized calcium concentration greater than 1.35 mmol/L (5.4 mg/dL) with or without a total serum calcium level greater than 2.75 mmol/L (11 mg/dL) is considered outside the normal range.[21]

Differential Diagnosis

Neonatal hypercalcemia is usually iatrogenic. Excessive administration of calcium or vitamin D3 should be excluded before extensive investigation is perused for other etiology such as maternal hypoparathyroidism, neonatal hyperparathyroidism, hypophosphatemia, or drug-induced hypercalcemia (thiazides).

Table 104-3 Differential Diagnosis of Neonatal Hypocalcemia

EARLY HYPOCALCEMIA (WITHIN THE FIRST 4 DAYS AFTER BIRTH)	MECHANISM
Prematurity, intrauterine growth restriction	Low stores in more premature infants, low intake, increased phosphorus load, increased calcitonin levels, transient hypoparathyroidism, end-organ resistance to vitamin D
Maternal diabetes	Maternal hypomagnesemia during pregnancy, hypoparathyroidism, hyperphosphatemia, abnormal vitamin D metabolism
Perinatal asphyxia	Decreased intake, increased phosphorus load, increased calcitonin concentration
Maternal anticonvulsants (phenobarbital and diphenylhydantoin)	Increase hepatic catabolism of vitamin D
LATE HYPOCALCEMIA (>4 DAYS AFTER BIRTH)	**MECHANISM**
Cow milk-based formulas (particularly undiluted cow milk or evaporated milk)	Hyperphosphatemia
Hypomagnesemia	Impaired parathyroid hormone (PTH) secretion and peripheral PTH action
Hypoparathyroidism:	
• Transient congenital	Hypocalcemia and hyperphosphatemia, low PTH, with PTH improving spontaneously
• Secondary	Maternal hyperparathyroidism with maternal or fetal hypercalcemia and subsequent neonatal hypoparathyroidism
• Congenital primary—parathyroid agenesis or part of DiGeorge sequence, PTH gene mutation	Decreased PTH
Other causes:	
• Vitamin D deficiency (renal disease, hepatobiliary disease, malabsorption, maternal vitamin D deficiency)	Decreased calcium absorption
• Alkalosis	Decreased ionized calcium, decreased calcium reabsorption from bones
• Citrated blood transfusion	Chelates ionized calcium
• Lipid infusions	Enhances calcium-albumin binding
• Phototherapy	Possibly caused by increased melatonin causes increased bone calcium uptake
• Furosemide, xanthenes	Promote calciuresis

Adapted from Rigo J, De Curtis M. Disorders of calcium, phosphorus and magnesium metabolism. In: Fanaroff AA, Martin RJ, eds. *Neonatal-Perinatal Medicine.* 8th ed. St Louis, MO: Mosby; 2005. Copyright © 2004, Elsevier, with permission.

Table 104-4 Forms of Calcium Salts

FORM OF CALCIUM SALT	ELEMENTAL CALCIUM (mg/mL)
10% calcium gluconate	9.4
10% calcium chloride	27.2
Calcium glubionate syrup	23.6

Calcium gluconate administration is preferred over calcium chloride (may cause metabolic acidosis).
Adapted from Rigo J, De Curtis M. Disorders of calcium, phosphorus and magnesium metabolism. In: Fanaroff AA, Martin RJ, eds. *Neonatal-Perinatal Medicine.* 8th ed. St Louis, MO: Mosby; 2005. Copyright © 2004, Elsevier, with permission.

Evaluation

Newborns with hypercalcemia may be asymptomatic or have nonspecific signs, including poor feeding, constipation, polyuria, dehydration, decreased muscle tone, lethargy, and bradycardia. Long-term neonatal hypercalcemia may result in nephrocalcinosis.

Management

The therapy of severe, symptomatic hypercalcemia in the acute phase should include intravenous fluid (normal saline) and furosemide administration to promote urinary calcium excretion, as well as removal of excessive calcium and vitamin D from the diet.

MAGNESIUM METABOLISM IN THE FETUS AND METABOLIC ADAPTATION AT BIRTH

Most of maternal-fetal magnesium transfer occurs in the third trimester and involves active transport against a concentration gradient. Magnesium is found mostly in the skeleton and intracellular fluid, with only

1% present in the extracellular fluid, making assessment of stores difficult.

Magnesium is absorbed mainly in the small intestine; regulation of serum concentration is performed primarily by kidneys under PTH supervision. Increase in the serum magnesium will decrease PTH secretion and renal reabsorption, whereas decrease in magnesium concentration will lead to increased PTH release and decrease urinary excretion. Chronic magnesium deficiency, however, will reduce PTH secretion.

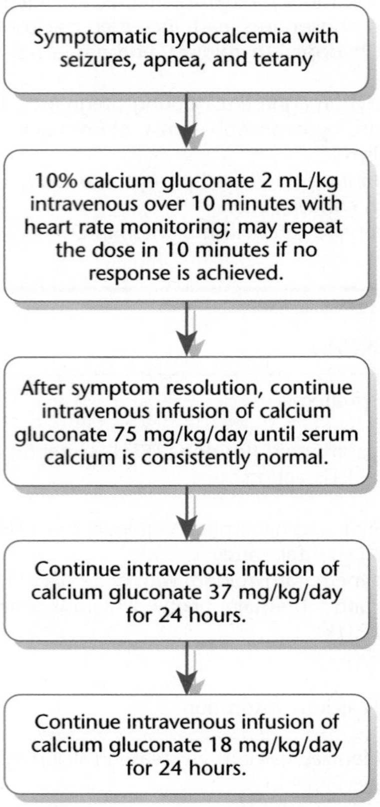

Symptomatic hypocalcemia with seizures, apnea, and tetany

↓

10% calcium gluconate 2 mL/kg intravenous over 10 minutes with heart rate monitoring; may repeat the dose in 10 minutes if no response is achieved.

↓

After symptom resolution, continue intravenous infusion of calcium gluconate 75 mg/kg/day until serum calcium is consistently normal.

↓

Continue intravenous infusion of calcium gluconate 37 mg/kg/day for 24 hours.

↓

Continue intravenous infusion of calcium gluconate 18 mg/kg/day for 24 hours.

Figure 104-4 Management of symptomatic hypocalcemia. *(Adapted from Rigo J, De Curtis M. Disorders of calcium, phosphorus and magnesium metabolism. In: Fanaroff AA, Martin RJ.* Neonatal-Perinatal Medicine. *8th ed. St Louis, MO: Mosby; 2005. Copyright © 2004, Elsevier, with permission.)*

HYPOMAGNESEMIA

Definition

The normal serum magnesium value for the newborn is 0.66 to 1.15 mmol/L (1.6 to 2.8 mg/dL). Clinical symptoms usually do not develop until serum magnesium level falls to less than 0.49 mmol/L (1.2 mg/dL). Measurement of active, ionized magnesium is usually not available; only total magnesium levels are routinely measured.[21]

Etiology

Table 104-5 summarizes the most common causes of neonatal hypomagnesemia.

Evaluation

Hypomagnesemia in the neonatal period is usually transient and asymptomatic. However, in severe cases, hypomagnesemia can cause irritability, tremor, hyperexcitability, and intractable hypocalcemic seizures that are unresponsive to calcium and anticonvulsant therapy. Electrocardiographic data may show a prolonged QT interval.

Hypocalcemia can be explained by magnesium depletion and resulting hypoparathyroidism.

Management

Management of hypomagnesemia consists of magnesium salt administration. The usual neonatal dose is 50% magnesium sulfate 0.05 to 0.1 mL/kg (2.5 to 5 mg/kg of elemental magnesium) administered intramuscularly or by slow intravenous infusion over 15 to 20 minutes. The dose may be repeated every 12 hours and eventually adjusted to oral preparations.

Table 104-5 Differential Diagnosis of Neonatal Hypomagnesemia

CAUSE	MECHANISM
Maternal diabetes	Maternal urinary losses of magnesium leading to neonatal magnesium depletion; blunted response to parathyroid hormone
Intrauterine growth restriction	Poor maternal supply or placental transfer
Hypoparathyroidism	Increased urinary losses
Malabsorption syndromes	Poor supply
Renal tubular defects: congenital or acquired (hypoxic-ischemic syndrome, nephrotoxicity) or genetic defects of renal magnesium handling	Increased urinary losses
Defects of intestinal magnesium transport	Decreased absorption
Citrated blood transfusion	Complexing of citrate with ionized magnesium

Adapted from Rigo J, De Curtis M. Disorders of calcium, phosphorus and magnesium metabolism. In: Fanaroff AA, Martin RJ, eds. *Neonatal-Perinatal Medicine.* 8th ed. St Louis, MO: Mosby; 2005. Copyright © 2004, Elsevier, with permission.

HYPERMAGNESEMIA

Definition

Hypermagnesemia is defined as a serum magnesium level more than 1.15 mmol/L (2.8 mg/dL). Hypermagnesemia does not cause hypocalcemia in the neonatal period despite PTH suppression, possibly as a result of magnesium facilitating the bony release of calcium.

Etiology

Hypermagnesemia in the neonatal period is always an iatrogenic event commonly related to maternal magnesium sulfate administration, for seizure prevention in preeclampsia, or for tocolysis. Neonatal levels do not reach problematic values and return to normal within a few days as a result of urine excretion. Less common sources of excessive magnesium are magnesium-containing antacids or excessive magnesium in parenteral nutrition.

Evaluation

The most common clinical manifestation of hypermagnesemia is hypotonia and depression at birth secondary to maternal administration of magnesium sulfate during obstetric management. Neurologic and respiratory depression may be evident on observation and examination.

Management

Usual management consists of supportive treatment, including optimal hydration. Respiratory support many be required in extreme cases. With unusually severe central nervous system depression, exchange blood transfusion may be indicated to lower the serum magnesium level.

TOOLS FOR PRACTICE

Engaging Patient and Family

- *Newborn Screening Tests—these tests could save your babies life* (brochure), Health Resources and Services Administration, US Department of Health and Human Services (test.medicalhomeinfo.org/screening/ScreenMaterials/Newborn screening tests.pdf).
- *Newborn Screening Disorders—What Parents Want to Know about Newborn Screening Disorders* (brochure), Health Resources and Services Administration, US Department of Health and Human Services (test.medicalhomeinfo.org/screening/ScreenMaterials/Newbornscreeningdisorders.pdf).

Medical Decision Support

- *Newborn Screening ACT sheets and Confirmatory Algorithms*, American College of Medical Genetics (www.acmg.net/resources/policies/ACT/condition-analyte-links.htm).
- *Newborn Screening and Related Conditions* (Web page), Centers for Disease Control and Prevention (www.cdc.gov/ncbddd/bd/genetics_screen.htm).
- *The S.T.A.B.L.E. Program: Student Manual, 5th edition* (book), Kristine A. Karlsen, MSN, RNC, NNP (www.aap.org/bookstore).
- *The S.T.A.B.L.E. Program: Learner Course Slides on CD-ROM, 5th edition*, Kristine A. Karlsen, MSN, RNC, NNP (www.aap.org/bookstore).
- *The S.T.A.B.L.E. Program: Physical Exam and Gestational Age Assessment Slide Program, CD-ROM*, Kristine A. Karlsen, MSN, RNC, NNP (www.aap.org/bookstore).
- *The S.T.A.B.L.E. Program: Quick Reference Bedside Card Set, 3rd edition*, Kristine A. Karlsen, MSN, RNC, NNP (www.aap.org/bookstore).
- *The S.T.A.B.L.E. Program: Blood Gas Interpretation Chart, 2nd edition*, Kristine A. Karlsen, MSN, RNC, NNP (www.aap.org/bookstore).

REFERENCES

1. Khalid H, Aynsley-Green A. The effect of prematurity and intrauterine growth restriction on glucose metabolism in the newborn. *NeoReviews*. 2004;5(9):e365.
2. Cornblath M, Hawdon JM, Williams AF, et al. Controversies regarding definition of neonatal hypoglycemia: suggested operational thresholds. *Pediatrics*. 2000;105(5): 1141-1145.
3. McGowan JE. Neonatal hypoglycemia. *Pediatr Rev.* 1999;20:6-15.
4. McGowan JE, Zanelli SA, Haynes-Laing AG, et al. Modification of glutamate binding sites in newborn brain during hypoglycemia. *Brain Res*. 2002;927(1):80-86.
5. Ballesteros JR, Mishra OP, McGowan JE. Alternations in cerebral mitochondria during acute hypoglycemia. *Biol Neonate*. 2003;84(2):159-163.
6. Rozance PJ, Hay WW. Hypoglycemia in newborn infants: features associated with adverse outcomes. *Biol Neonate*. 2006;90(2):74-86.
7. Sperling MA, Menon RK. Differential diagnosis and management of neonatal hypoglycemia. *Pediatr Clin North Am*. 2004;51(3):703-723.
8. Wilker RE. Hypoglycemia and hyperglycemia. In: Cloherty JP, Eichenwald EC, Stark AR, eds. *Manual of Neonatal Care*. 5th ed. Philadelphia, PA: Lippincott Williams and Wilkins; 2004.
9. Huttner KM. Hypocalcemia, hypercalcemia, and hypermagnesemia. In: Cloherty JP, Eichenwald EC, Stark AR, eds. *Manual of Neonatal Care*. 5th ed. Philadelphia, PA: Lippincott Williams and Wilkins; 2004.
10. Pildes RS, Pyati SP. Hypoglycemia and hyperglycemia in tiny infants. *Clin Perinatol*. 1986;13(2):351-375.
11. Cornblath M, Schwartz R, Aynsley-Green A, et al. Hypoglycemia in infancy: the need for a rational definition. *Pediatrics*. 1990;85(15):834-837.
12. Koh TH, Eyre JA, Aynsely-Green A. Neonatal hypoglycemia—the controversy regarding definition. *Arch Dis Child*. 1988;63(11):1386-1388.
13. Koh TH, Vong SK. Definition of neonatal hypoglycaemia: is there a change? *J Paediatr Child Health*. 1996;32(4): 302-305.
14. Schwartz RP. Neonatal hypoglycemia: how low is too low? *J Pediatr*. 1997;131(2):171-173.
15. Alkalay AL, Sarnat HB, Flores-Sarnat L, et al. Population meta-analysis of low plasma glucose thresholds in full-term normal newborns. *Am J Perinatol*. 2006;23(2): 115-120.
16. Deshpande S, Ward Platt M. The investigation and management of neonatal hypoglycemia. *Semin Fetal and Neonatal Med*. 2005;10(4):351-361.
17. Lubchenco LO, Bard H. Incidence of hypoglycemia in newborn infants classified by birth weight and gestational age. *Pediatrics*. 1971;47(5):831-838.

18. Cornblath M, Schwartz R. Hypoglycemia in the neonate. *J Pediatr Endocrinol*. 1993;6(2):113-129.
19. Leonard JV, Morris A. Diagnosis and early management of inborn errors of metabolism presenting around the time of birth. *Acta Paediatrica*. 2006;95(1):6-14.
20. Hawdon JM, Ward Platt MP, Aynsely-Green A. Patterns of metabolic adaptation for preterm and term infants in the first neonatal week. *Arch Dis Child*. 1992;67(4): 357-365.
21. Rigo J, De Curtis M. Disorders of calcium, phosphorus and magnesium metabolism. In: Fanaroff AA, Martin RJ, eds. *Neonatal-Perinatal Medicine*. 8th ed. St Louis, MO: Mosby; 2005.

Chapter 105
SPECIFIC CONGENITAL METABOLIC DISORDERS

Angel Rios, MD; Darius J. Adams, MD

When evaluating a neonate the challenge that confronts the physician is to determine whether a medical problem is a transient phenomenon that can be easily treated or whether the problem will evolve into a life-threatening condition. Neonates often exhibit nonspecific signs and symptoms that may be indicative of an array of disorders, including sepsis, delayed transition, congenital cardiac disease, endocrine disturbances, and inborn errors of metabolism.

Newborns with metabolic disease are typically healthy and asymptomatic at birth. In utero the fetus is protected by the placenta, which is responsible for removing metabolites and transferring substrates to meet fetal energy needs. Once the fetal nutrient supply is withdrawn with clamping of the umbilical cord at delivery the newborn must activate physiological mechanisms to support metabolism, remove all toxic metabolites, and maintain an endogenous energy supply. Clinical suspicion should be aroused in an infant who initially appears well and then progressively deteriorates despite appropriate therapy of the presenting clinical signs. The onset of symptoms caused by an inborn error of metabolism may range from a few hours after birth to several weeks of age, depending on the underlying disorder.

EVALUATING THE NEWBORN

Initial Approach

A complete family history is a crucial and integral part of the initial evaluation. Key items to include in the history are listed in Box 105-1. The initial assessment must also include a thorough physical examination and review of the pregnancy history. Maternal prenatal history can be useful in diagnosing inborn errors of metabolism. A newborn with a fatty acid oxidation disorder can predispose the mother to developing acute fatty liver of pregnancy and HELLP syndrome (preeclampsia with hemolysis, elevated liver enzymes, and low platelet count).

BOX 105-1 Key Items in Family History

- Prior unexplained death in sibling or siblings
- Age of death
  - Presenting symptoms
  - Seizures
  - Encephalopathy
- Hypoglycemia
- Onset of symptoms
- Sex of siblings
- Pregnancy
- HELLP syndrome—disorders of fatty acid oxidation
- Acute fatty liver of pregnancy—disorders of fatty acid oxidation
- Ethnic group with increased frequency of disorders
- Ashkenazi Jews
- African—sickle cell disease
- Mediterranean—glucose-6-phosphate dehydrogenase
- French Canadian—maple syrup urine disease
- Old Order Mennonite population of Lancaster County, PA—maple syrup urine disease
- Parental consanguinity
- Unusual family illness
- Hyperinsulinism-hyperammonemia syndrome
- Female carriers of ornithine transcarbamylase deficiency can become acutely ill during periods of stress, despite the X-linked pattern of inheritance for this disorder.

HELLP, Hemolysis, elevated liver function tests, and low platelets.

Physical Examination

A thorough physical examination can provide helpful clues in identifying the correct diagnosis. Table 105-1 lists some of the common physical findings associated with specific metabolic and endocrine disorders. Some of the disorders listed do not cause acute illness in the newborn period, but the described physical findings are present from birth, such as the coarse facies in an newborn with galactosialidosis. The presence of atypical physical findings should alert the clinician to potential problems.

HYPOGLYCEMIA IN NEWBORNS

Hypoglycemia is one of the more common signs in newborns. Hypoglycemia may be caused by many conditions that increase the infant's metabolic rate or may result from inadequate endogenous glycogen stores in infants born prematurely or small for gestational age. Box 105-2 lists signs and symptoms that may be present in the newborn who is hypoglycemic. The clinician should consider inborn errors of metabolism and endocrine abnormalities in the differential diagnosis of a newborn whose symptoms persist despite appropriate therapy. Prompt diagnosis and initiation of appropriate therapy is essential to prevent death and permanent neurological damage.

In the initial hours after delivery the typical newborn does not have fully active gluconeogenic function

Table 105-1 Physical Findings Associated With Metabolic and Endocrine Disorders in the Newborn Period

FINDING	PROBLEM	DISORDER
Odor	Maple Syrup	Maple syrup urine disease
	Sweaty feet	Isovaleric academia
		Glutaric acid type II
	Musty	Phenylketonuria
	Cat urine	Multiple carboxylase deficiency
	Cabbage	Tyrosinemia
General appearance	Mid-line defects	Smith-Lemli-Opitz syndrome
Dysmorphism	Coarse facies	Galactosialidosis
		Sialidosis
		Mucopolysaccharidosis type VII
		G_{M1} gangliosidosis
Head	Macrocephaly	Glutaric academia type I
		Canavan disease
	Microcephaly	Cobalamin disease type C
	Alopecia	Multiple carboxylase deficiency
Eye	Cataracts	Galactosemia, Zellweger syndrome
	Dislocated lens	Homocystinuria
		Electron transport–chain disorders
Heart	Cardiomyopathy	Disorders of fatty acid oxidation
		Glycogen storage disease type III
		Glycogen storage disease type IV (occasional)
		Electron transport–chain disorders
Visceromegaly	Hepatomegaly	Glycogen storage disease, Wilson disease
		Galactosemia, α_1-antitrypsin
		Disorders of fatty acid oxidation
	Hepatosplenomegaly	Lysosomal storage disorders
Neurologic	Hypotonia	Electron transport chain disorders
	Seizures	Medium-chain acyl-coenzyme A dehydrogenase deficiency
	Lethargy	Maple syrup urine disease, nonketotic hyperglycinemia
	Coma	Urea cycle defects
Genitourinary	Microphallus	Smith-Lemli-Opitz syndrome

BOX 105-2 Signs and Symptoms of Hypoglycemia

Cyanotic spells	Tremors
Apnea	Poor feeding
Respiratory distress	Hypotonia
Temperature instability	Tachypnea
Seizures	Tachycardia
Lethargy	Bradycardia
Irritability	Vomiting
Coma	

and is consequently unable to use alanine, lactate, and glycerol efficiently for endogenous hepatic glucose production. Delay in the expression of phosphoenolpyruvate carboxykinase (PEPCK), the rate-limiting step in the gluconeogenesis pathway, increases the susceptibility of the neonate to developing hypoglycemia. By 24 hours of life, PEPCK achieves adult values.[1]

Therefore, early and serial preprandial glucose monitoring in conjunction with the initiation of early feedings are important in the care of a newborn with risk factors for hypoglycemia. Other causes of hypoglycemia must be considered in neonates with persistent hypoglycemia beyond 24 hours of life, including severe refractory hypoglycemia and hypoglycemia not responding to enteral feeds, as well as newborns with persistent clinical signs as detailed in Box 105-2. Box 105-3 provides a list of factors that may contribute to neonatal hypoglycemia. Congenital hyperinsulinism occurs in the first few days of life, but cases occurring later in infancy and childhood have been reported. The hypoglycemia that occurs with congenital hyperinsulinism is severe and persistent, requiring large glucose infusion rates to maintain euglycemia. Glucose infusion rates greater than 15 mg/kg/min are usually necessary (the healthy newborn requires 5-8 mg/kg/min of glucose to remain euglycemic). This circumstance is in stark contrast to the hyperinsulinism exhibited by infants of diabetic mothers and infants who are growth restricted or who experience perinatal asphyxia. The hyperinsulinism present in these conditions is transient. Transient hyperinsulinism can also occur without any predisposing factors.

BOX 105-3 Etiologic Factors Contributing to Neonatal Hypoglycemia

PRENATAL CAUSES
Maternal diabetes
Maternal drug administration
Beta-sympathomimetics
Intrapartum intravenous dextrose bolus
Oral hypoglycemics
Propylthiouracil
Pregnancy-induced hypertension

EXCESS UTILIZATION
Hyperinsulinism
IDM
LGA
SGA
Erythroblastosis
Increase energy expenditure
RDS
Sepsis
Seizures
Drug withdrawals
Hypothermia
Increased work of breathing
Inborn errors of metabolism
Hypoxemia
Ischemia
Shock
Hemorrhage
Postexchange transfusion
Hyperviscosity, polycythemia

INADEQUATE PRODUCTION OR SUBSTRATE DELIVERY
Inadequate delivery of calories
Delayed enteral or parenteral nutrition
Transient developmental immaturity of critical metabolic pathways, reducing endogenous production of glucose or other substrates
Endocrine disorders:
  Hypothyroidism
  Hypothalamic
  Pituitary
Abrupt cessation of hypertonic parenteral glucose
Discordant twins
Cerebral hemorrhage
Perinatal asphyxia
SGA
Glucose transporter deficiency
Suppressed gluconeogenesis, glycogenolysis, lipolysis, proteolysis and ketogenesis secondary elevated insulin levels (hyperinsulinism).

IATROGENIC CAUSES
Malposition of umbilical catheter
Cold stress

IDM, Infant of diabetic mother; *LGA*, large for gestational age; *RDS*, respiratory distress syndrome; *SGA*, small for gestational age.
Table modified from Cornblath M, Ichord R. Hypoglycemia in the neonate. *Semin Perinatol.* 2000;24(2):136-149. Copyright Elsevier, 2000. Used by permission.

APPROACH TO THE INFANT WITH PERSISTENT HYPOGLYCEMIA

Ascertaining the cause of persistent hypoglycemia requires an understanding of the adaptive processes involved in the response to hypoglycemia and application of a systematic approach in identifying any underlying metabolic problems.

Clinicians often initially suspect sepsis in the infant who is ill appearing and hypoglycemic; metabolic disorders may not be considered until the infant exhibits continued deterioration despite standard therapeutic measures or when laboratory results fail to support or confirm a diagnosis of infection. Furthermore, metabolic disorders may cause other systemic manifestations. An infant affected by galactosemia may have *Escherichia coli* sepsis, whereas an infant with glycogen storage disease type Ib (glucose-6-phosphatase translocase deficiency) or organic aciduria may exhibit neutropenia, thus mimicking sepsis in the newborn in face of a metabolic disorder. A metabolic or endocrine disorder should be suspected when altered consciousness or seizures occur with profound hypoglycemia requiring greater than 10 mg/kg/min of glucose or if hypoglycemia is not responding to standard therapy.

Hypoglycemia can occur at distinct times depending on the disorder and may also occur preprandially, postprandially, or during a period of fasting. The timing of the hypoglycemic episode can be a helpful clue to its underlying cause. Five processes are responsible for maintaining normal blood glucose levels during periods of fasting in the healthy newborn infant:

1. Glycogenolysis
2. Gluconeogenesis
3. Adipose tissue lipolysis
4. Fatty acid oxidation (to synthesize glucose and ketone bodies)
5. Endocrine system capable of integrating and modulating these first four processes during periods of fasting

Sufficient endogenous gluconeogenic substrates (amino acids, glycerol, and lactate) are required for these metabolic reactions. Glycogenolysis, gluconeogenesis, adipose tissue lipolysis, and fatty acid oxidation are temporally related.[2] Figure 105-1 illustrates the relationships of these processes when prolonged starvation occurs during the newborn period. Once the endogenous supply of glucose is exhausted, glycogenolysis (process 2) takes over, usually after 4 hours. Gluconeogenesis (process 3) is activated, achieving peak activity after 12 hours of starvation. Fatty acid oxidation (process 4) begins to peak after 14 hours. Figure 105-2 reveals the relationship of the various processes after 24 hours.

Process 1: Gastrointestinal Absorption of Glucose

Glucose becomes available from gastrointestinal nutrient absorption immediately after feeding. Breastfeeding infants have a greater capacity to generate ketone bodies compared with formula-feeding neonates, suggesting that human milk augments ketogenesis in human neonates through as yet undescribed pathways.[3] Insulin and glucose levels are elevated, and glucagon is depressed as intestinal absorption of glucose takes place. Hypoglycemia occurring during this phase suggests hyperinsulinism. Excessive insulin secretion

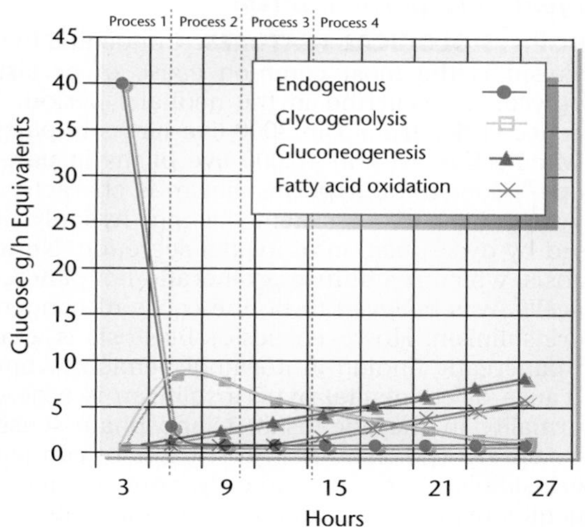

Figure 105-1 Glycogenolysis, gluconeogenesis, lipolysis, and fatty acid oxidation are temporarily related. *(Adapted from Devlin TM, ed.* Textbook of Biochemistry With Clinical Correlations. *6th ed. New York, NY; John Wiley & Sons; 2005. Reprinted by permission.)*

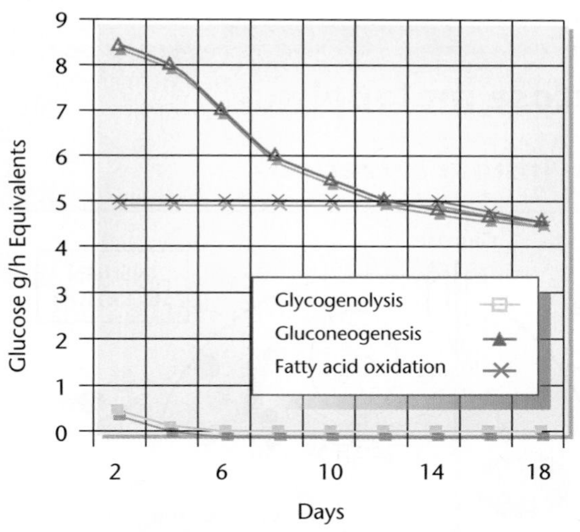

Figure 105-2 The relationship of glycogenolysis, gluconeogenesis, and fatty acid oxidation after 24 hours and beyond. *(Adapted from Devlin TM, ed.* Textbook of Biochemistry With Clinical Correlations. *6th ed. New York, NY; John Wiley & Sons; 2005. Reprinted by permission.)*

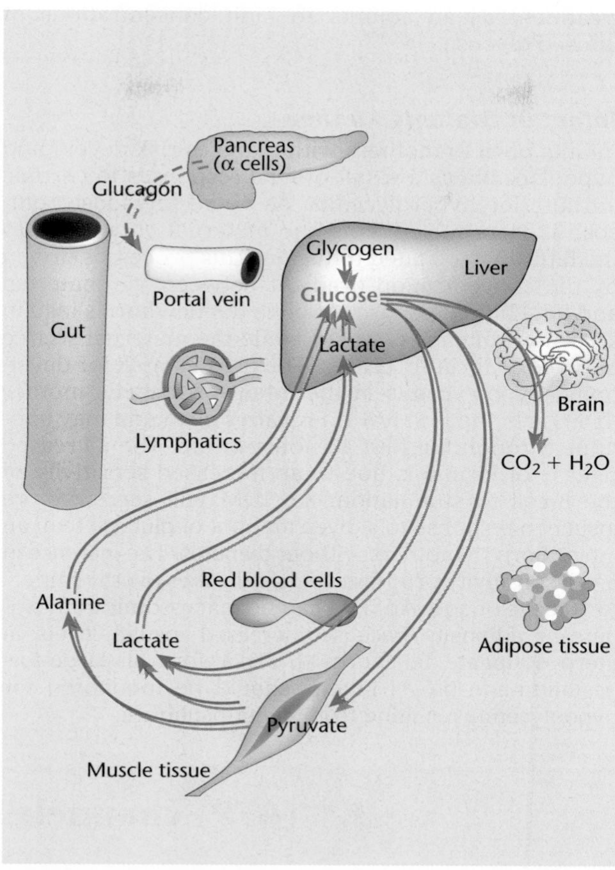

Figure 105-3 Metabolic interrelationships of major tissues in early fasting state. *(Adapted from Devlin TM, ed.* Textbook of Biochemistry With Clinical Correlations. *6th ed. New York, NY; John Wiley & Sons; 2005. Reprinted by permission.)*

BOX 105-4 Causes of Neonatal Hyperinsulinism

- Infant of diabetic mother
- Intrauterine growth restriction
- Perinatal asphyxia
- Congenital hyperinsulinism
- Beckwith-Wiedemann syndrome
- Hypopituitarism
- Rh isoimmunization

in response to an enteral feeding induces a hypoglycemic response. Consequently, hypoglycemia that is caused by hyperinsulinism is typically responsive to administration of glucagon and octreotide.

Figure 105-3 depicts how hepatic glycogenolysis preserves blood glucose homeostasis during process 1 (early fasting), during a time in which gastrointestinal absorption of glucose is predominant.

Causes of neonatal hyperinsulinism are listed in Box 105-4. Although the underlying cause of hyperinsulinism varies, the basic problem is increased glucose utilization resulting from excessive insulin secretion or, in the case of Beckwith-Wiedemann syndrome, excess tissue production of insulin-like growth factor-II. Some disorders have a genetic basis (Beckwith-Wiedemann syndrome, congenital hyperinsulinism), whereas others can be associated with adverse intrauterine events (intrauterine growth restriction, perinatal asphyxia). Infants of diabetic mothers, intrauterine growth restricted infants, and infants who experience perinatal asphyxia typically receive parenteral glucose infusions during the initial stabilization period. Congenital hyperinsulinism, Beckwith-Wiedemann syndrome, and hypopituitarism require more extensive treatment as an adjunct to high concentrations of infused glucose.

Infant of Diabetic Mother

Infants born to mothers with diabetes risk developing hypoglycemia as a result of fetal responses to chronic intrauterine hyperglycemia. As noted previously, glucose is transported from the maternal circulation to the fetus by facilitated diffusion. This process is driven by the concentration gradient between the maternal and fetal blood glucose. At birth the newborn's insulin secretion remains elevated while the maternal source of glucose abruptly ceases. The greatest risk for developing hypoglycemia in the infant of diabetic mother (IDM) is in the first few hours after birth and may continue through the first 48 hours of life. The increased release of insulin is due to an increased sensitivity of the β-cell to stimulation. An IDM will secrete more insulin in response to a given amount of glucose than an infant born to mothers without diabetes. The increase in β-cell sensitivity progressively diminishes over the first 7 to 10 days of age. An IDM can be macrosomic with significant adiposity because increased insulin levels in utero stimulate fetal growth. Therefore all large-for-gestation-age (LGA) infants should be monitored for hypoglycemia resulting from hyperinsulinism.

Congenital Hyperinsulinism

PATHOPHYSIOLOGICAL FEATURES. Congenital hyperinsulinism is the most common cause of persistent hypoglycemia occurring in the neonatal period. The incidence varies from 1 in 3000 live births in parts of the Middle East to 1 in 40,000 live births in parts of Europe.[4] Congenital hyperinsulinism is characterized by recurrent and persistent fasting hypoglycemia caused by dysregulation of insulin secretion. Nesidioblastosis, which is a diffuse proliferation of pancreatic islet cells, was believed to be the cause of congenital hyperinsulinism. However, nesidioblastosis is a common pancreatic finding in normoglycemic newborns. The cause of congenital hyperinsulinism is a genetic abnormality in the adenosine triphosphate–sensitive potassium (K^+_{ATP}) channels. Most cases of congenital hyperinsulinism occur sporadically. Some infants with congenital hyperinsulinism inherit it as an autosomal-recessive trait. In addition, autosomal-dominant transmission has been reported in some families. Several mutations have been described affecting two proteins designated as *SUR1* and *KIR6.2* (Figure 105-4). Figure 105-4 demonstrates the actions of the SUR1 and KIR6.2 in the pancreatic (β-cell secretion). The K^+_{ATP} channels are octameric complexes comprising two types of subunits—four regulatory SUR1 (sulphonylurea receptors) surrounding four KIR6.2 (pore-forming

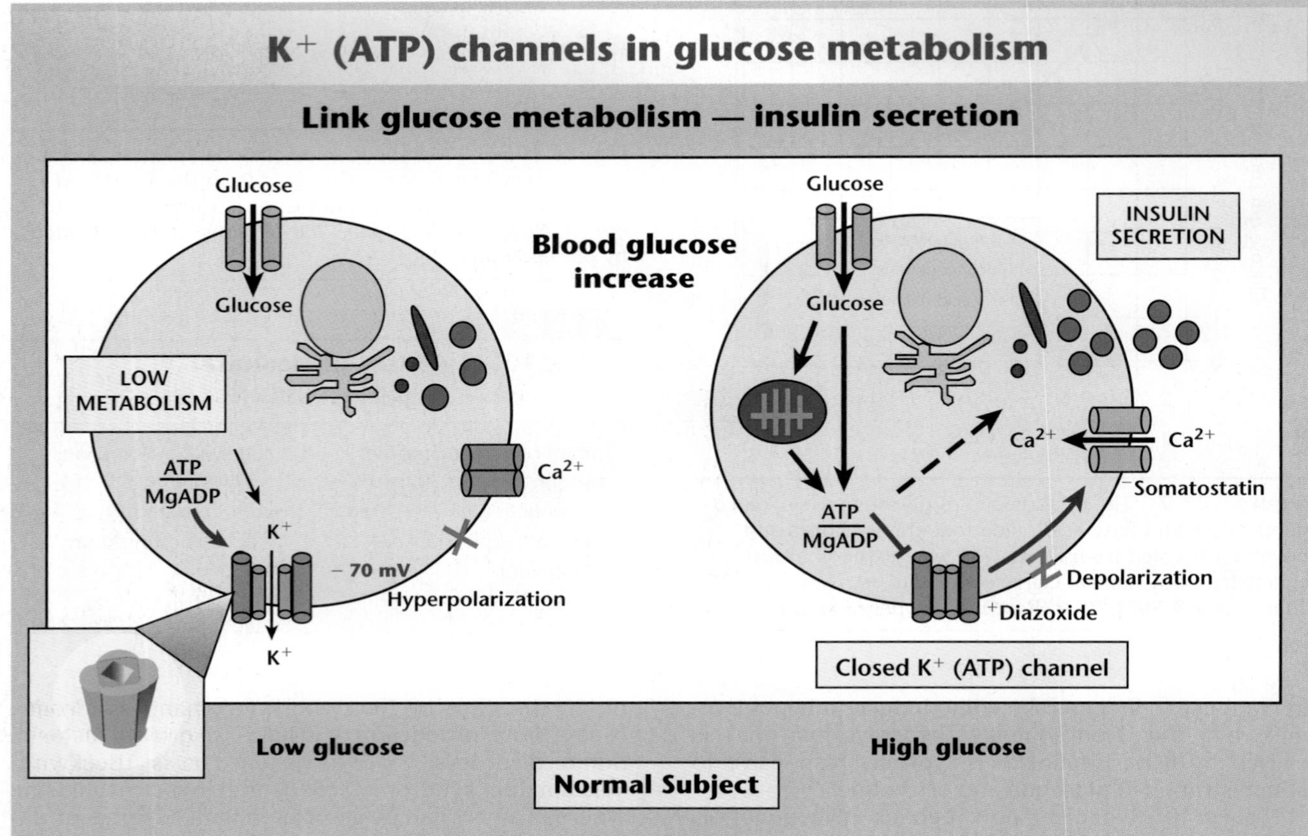

Figure 105-4 K^+_{ATP} Channels in Glucose Metabolism. *(Flechtner I, Vaxillaire M, Cavé H, et al. Neonatal hyperglycemia and abnormal development of the pancreas.* Best Pract Res Clin Endocrinol Metab. *2008;22(1):17-40. Copyright Elsevier, 2008. Reprinted by permission.)*

inwardly rectifying potassium channels) see diagram 105-6. The genes for *SUR1* and *KIR6.2* are located on chromosome 11 p. When there is a normal increase in blood glucose that results in an increase in intracellular ATP, the increase in intracellular ATP inhibits the potassium efflux through the K^+_{ATP} channels. The closure of the potassium channels depolarizes the plasma membrane, which activates calcium channels increasing the intracellular calcium resulting in the release of insulin via exocytosis. Each K^+_{ATP} channel contains at least two of these proteins. These mutations impair the function of the K^+_{ATP} channels and are inherited in an autosomal-recessive manner.

Hyperinsulinism-hyperammonemia syndrome is an autosomal-dominant condition that causes hypoglycemia. A serum ammonia level should be added to the diagnostic evaluation to determine this possibility. Hyperinsulinism-hyperammonemia syndrome is caused by mutations in the glutamate dehydrogenase gene.

LABORATORY EVALUATION. Laboratory findings include hyperinsulinemia in the presence of symptomatic hypoglycemia. Table 105-2 lists the blood and urine samples required when evaluating for hypoglycemia. The unrestricted insulin release inhibits counterregulatory mechanisms. This inhibition will affect ketone body synthesis and lipolysis, resulting in a decrease in blood ketones and fatty acids. Gluconeogenesis is also inhibited. Newborns with congenital hyperinsulinism are at risk for brain damage resulting from hypoglycemia and lack of alternate fuels for brain metabolism. Serum cortisol response is blunted, and glucocorticoid administration does not correct the hypoglycemia. A definitive diagnosis of hyperinsulinism is made based on insulin and cortisol levels obtained during the acute hypoglycemic episode, but definitive diagnoses may be difficult in mild cases. The clinician needs a high index of suspicion, otherwise the diagnosis can easily be missed.

TREATMENT STRATEGIES. Adequate carbohydrate intake can be provided with intravenous glucose or with enteral feeds, as described, and is critical to prevent brain injury. Correction of hypoglycemia may require glucose infusion rates greater than 15 mg/kg/min. A central line is required when administering glucose at concentrations greater than 12.5% dextrose because higher concentrations of intravenous glucose are particularly caustic to blood vessels. Table 105-3 provides a list of medications that may be used in the treatment of hypoglycemia. Surgery involving partial pancreatectomy or resection of localized adenomas is reserved for infants who fail to respond to medical management. Percutaneous transhepatic pancreatic venous blood sampling may be used to identify these *hot spots*.

Diazoxide and Chlorothiazide. The use of diazoxide and chlorothiazide together are the drugs of choice. Diazoxide is a ligand of the K^+_{ATP} channel, which binds to SUR1 and, in the presence of intracellular nucleotides, opens the channels. Chlorothiazide also acts on the K^+_{ATP} channels but is also used to overcome the fluid retention caused by diazoxide.

Glucagon. Glucagon may be used in the acute management of hypoglycemia. Its onset of action is 10 to 15 minutes, and its effect is transient. Glucagon should only be used as an acute therapy in infants with adequate glycogen stores. Glucagon is not appropriate for use in small-for-gestational-age and low–birth-weight infants. Subcutaneous or intravenous administration of glucagon in a dose of 0.5 to 1.0 mg will stimulate mobilization of endogenous glycogen stores and result in an increase in blood glucose greater than 30 mg/dL.

Octreotide. Octreotide is an analogue of somatostatin that can be used in the acute and chronic treatment

Table 105-2 Blood and Urine Samples Required During Hypoglycemia

BLOOD SPECIMEN	REQUIRED SAMPLE	NORMAL VALUES
Insulin	Serum	3-20 mcU/mL
Growth Hormone	Heparinized serum/plasma	5-53 ng/mL
Cortisol	Heparinized serum/plasma	1-24 mcg/dL
Glucose	Serum	40-60 mg/dL
ELECTROLYTES AND LIVER FUNCTION TEST RESULTS		
Blood gas	Heparinized whole blood	7.26-7.45 pH
Ketones	Whole blood	0.1-1.5 mmol/L
Lactate	Whole blood	1.1-2.3 mmol/L
Ammonia	Whole blood	21-95 mmol/L
Free fatty acids	Whole blood	0.5-1.6 mmol/L
Uric acid	Serum	1.7-5.8 mg/dL
Acylcarnitine profile	Blood spots on Guthrie card	Laboratory dependent
Pyruvate	Whole blood	0.3-0.7 mg/dL
Alanine (plasma amino acids)	Serum	Age dependent
URINE SPECIMEN		
Ketones	—	Negative
Organic acids	—	Laboratory dependent
Reducing substances	—	Negative

Table 105-3 Additional Medical Management for Hypoglycemia Requiring a Glucose Infusion (>15-20 mg/kg/min)

MEDICATION	MECHANISM OF ACTION	ROUTE OF ADMINISTRATION	DOSE	SIDE EFFECTS
Glucagon	Increased glycogenolysis and gluconeogenesis	SC, IV, IM Use only in the acute management.	.025-0.3 mg/kg/dose repeat 20 min as needed (max dose 1 mg)	Nausea, vomiting Do not use in SGA or low–birth-weight infants.
Diazoxide	K^+_{ATP} channel agonist decreasing insulin secretion	IV, PO	2-5 mg/kg IV push 2-105 mg/kg every 8-12 hr	Hyponatremia and fluid retention, hypertrichosis, hypotension
Chlorothiazide	Unknown	PO IV not recommended in infants and children.	<6 mo: 20-35 mg/kg PO divided twice daily (max. 375 mg) 6 mo-2 yr: 10-20 mg/kg divided twice daily (max. 375 mg) 2-12 yr: 1 g divided twice daily >12 yr: 30-60 mg/kg divided two to three times daily (max. 2 g)	Hypotension, alopecia, photosensitivity, hyperuricemia
Octreotide	Inhibits insulin and GH	SC, IV	Start 2-10 mcg/kg/day every 6-8 hours. Increase up to 40 mcg/kg/day every 4-8 hours	Tachyphylaxis, diarrhea, constipation
Hydrocortisone	Decreased peripheral glucose utilization	IV, IM	5 mg/kg every 12 hours	Immunosuppression, growth delay, gastric irritation

GH, Growth hormone; *IM*, intramuscular; *IV*, intravenous; *SGA*, small for gestational age; *PO*, oral; *SC*, subcutaneous.

of hypoglycemia. As a somatostatin analogue, octreotide has an inhibitory effect on various hormones, including growth hormone (GH), thyroid-stimulating hormone (TSH), and adrenocorticotropic hormone (ACTH). Octreotide is also used in the treatment of congenital hyperinsulinism. Octreotide's mechanisms of action include alteration in β-cell intracellular translocation of calcium and inhibition of insulin-containing granule exocytosis. Octreotide can decrease gallbladder contractility and bile secretion leading to hepatic dysfunction, steatorrhea, cholestasis, and cholelithiasis. Octreotide can also decrease splanchnic blood flow potentially increasing the risk of necrotizing enterocolitis. The following algorithm presents the clinical approach to a newborn with symptomatic hypoglycemia.

Beckwith-Wiedemann Syndrome

Beckwith-Wiedemann syndrome occurs in approximately 1 in 14,000 newborns. Most cases are sporadic, and a familial autosomal-dominant form with a variable phenotype has been described. The critical chromosomal region responsible for Beckwith-Wiedemann syndrome is located at 11p15.5. Beckwith-Wiedemann syndrome occurs when paternal uniparental disomy is present (an imprinting defect in which the maternal allele is not expressed), microdeletions involving the critical region, contiguous gene duplications in the 11p15 region, or with *CDKN1C* mutations. Characteristic findings include macrosomia (defined as a birthweight >4000 g), an abdominal wall defect, and macroglossia. Other features include hemihypertrophy, indentations on the posterior rim of the ear's helix, and linear creases of the earlobe. Treatment of the hypoglycemia is as described previously, and the hypoglycemia tends to resolve over time. Long-term management includes monitoring alpha-fetoprotein levels and abdominal sonography to monitor for tumor development, that is Wilms tumors. Figure 105-6 depicts the metabolic pathways involved in maintaining euglycemia.

In the following sections, specific metabolic pathways and their involvement in maintaining euglycemia are examined.

Process 2: Glycogenolysis—Postabsorptive and Early Catabolism

Glycogenolysis occurs when glycogen stored in the liver is broken down after completion of intestinal carbohydrate absorption and occurs approximately 3 to 4 hours postprandially. Liver glycogen stores are 50 to 75 g/kg of liver. During glycogenolysis, glucose-6-phosphate (G-6-P) is produced, which releases glucose by the action of glucose-6-phosphatase. Insulin levels return to basal levels, and increasing glucagon and

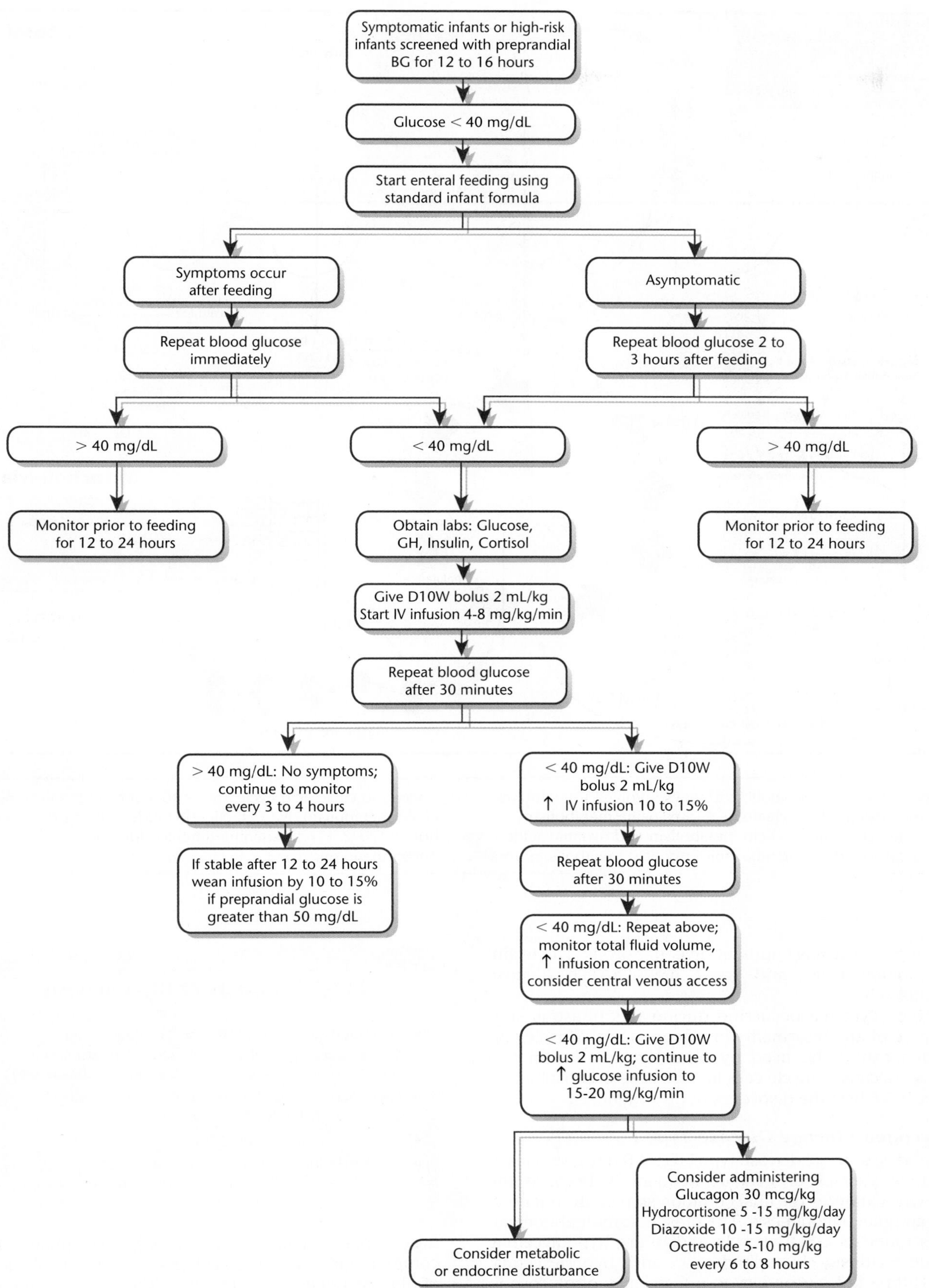

Figure 105-5 Algorithm for identifying persistent hypoglycemia in neonates. D10W IV, Dextrose 10% in water.

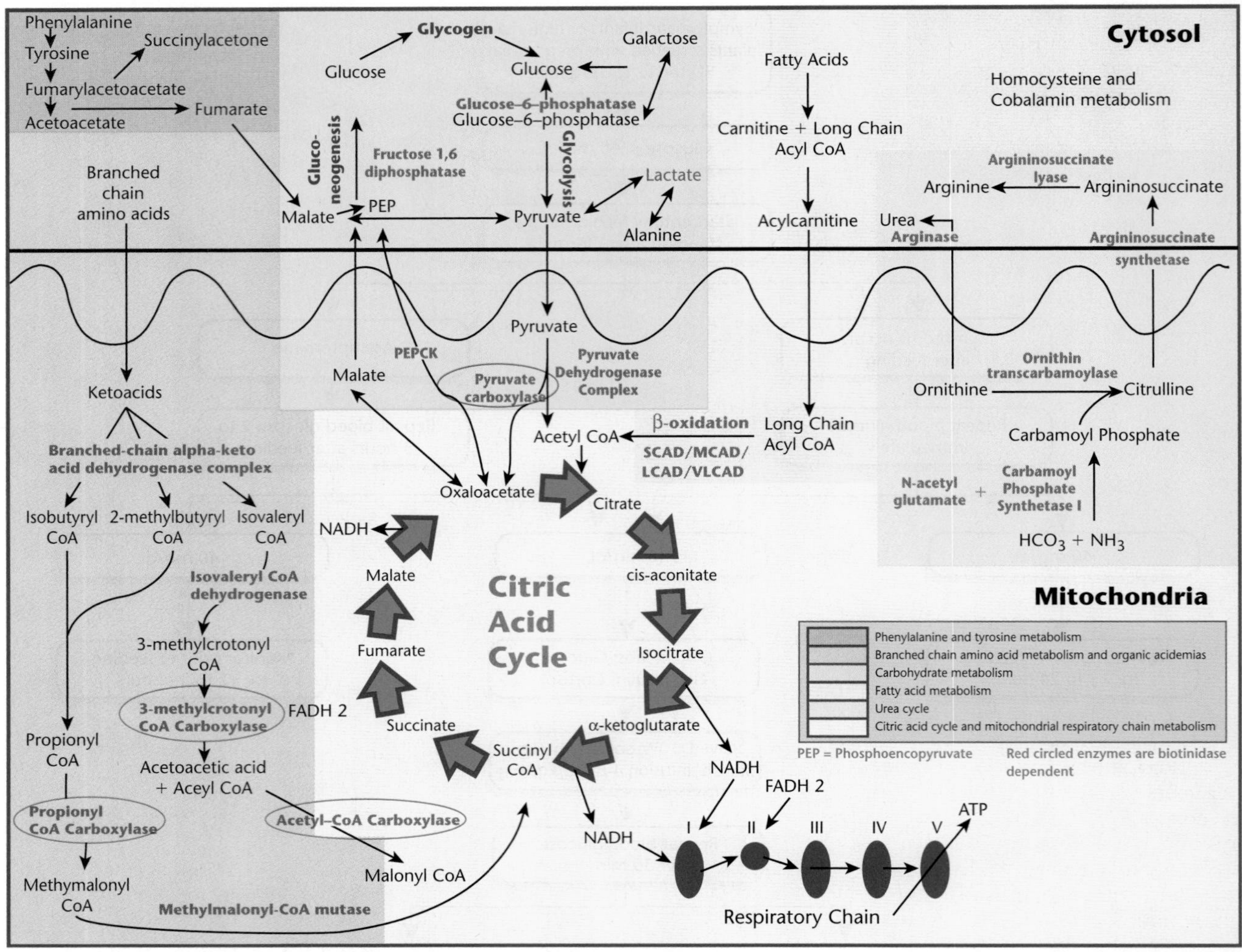

Figure 105-6 Metabolic pathways involved in maintaining euglycemia: Phenylalanine and tyrosine metabolism; branched chain amino acid metabolism and organic acidemias; carbohydrate metabolism; fatty acid metabolism; urea cycle; and citric acid cycle and mitochondrial respiratory chain metabolism. *NADH,* Nicotinamide adenine dinucleotide; *FADH2,* Flavin adenine dinucleotide; *PEP,* phosphoenolpyruvate.

epinephrine levels augment glycogenolysis. The brain, red blood cells, and renal medulla use glucose exclusively.

Hypoglycemia occurring during this phase is suggestive of an abnormality in glycogenosis. Muscle glycogen cannot be used by other tissues during this phase because muscle cells lack glucose-6-phosphatase. Box 105-5 lists the disorders of glycogenosis.

BOX 105-5 Disorders of Glycogenosis

- Glycogen storage disease type Ia (glucose-6-phosphatase deficiency, Von Gierke disease) and type Ib (glucose-6-phosphate translocase deficiency)
- Glycogen storage disease type III (debranching-enzyme deficiency)
- Glycogen synthase deficiency
- Mitochondrial respiratory-chain disorders

Glycogen Storage Disease Type I

Glycogen storage disease type I (GSD I) has been classified as a disorder of gluconeogenesis because the enzyme catalyzes the final common step in glycogenolysis and gluconeogenesis. The most common abnormalities found in GSD types Ia and Ib are hypoglycemia, lactic acidosis, hyperlipidemia, and hyperuricemia. GSD type Ia is secondary to a deficiency of glucose-6-phosphatase, whereas GSD Ib involves a defective microsomal transport of glucose-6-phosphate. The common end result of GSD types Ia and Ib is blockage of glucose release from the liver. The gene for glucose-6-phosphatase is located on chromosome 17q21. The gene for the glucose-6-phosphate transporter gene is located on chromosome 11q23. Inheritance is autosomal recessive for both forms of GSD. These enzymatic defects result in an excessive accumulation of both glycogen and fat in the liver. These two types of GSD are not clinically discernable; the major difference is that GSD Ib has an increased risk of infection and immunologic abnormalities. GSD Ib is associated with a decreased number of neutrophils and defective neutrophil and monocyte function, which increases the risk for infections. This circumstance is another example of a metabolic disease with an increased susceptibility to bacterial infection, thereby potentially masking the metabolic disorder. Definitive diagnosis is achieved by performing a liver biopsy along with enzyme analysis or by DNA analysis. As encountered in all disorders of glycogenosis, hypoglycemia becomes evident when exogenous glucose sources are depleted. Glucose-6-phosphatase has the combined effect of blocking glucose release from both the glycogenolytic and gluconeogenic pathways.

The goal of treatment is to prevent hypoglycemia-induced brain damage. Therapy consists of frequent feedings initially by continuous nasogastric feedings and then by feeding uncooked cornstarch, particularly overnight. Uncooked cornstarch has the advantage of having a more protracted release of glucose than is available from cooked cornstarch; however cornstarch use is limited to children older that 1 year. The dose of uncooked starch is 1.6 g/kg every 4 hours in patients between 1 and 2 years of age. Children unresponsive to cornstarch can be given continuous nasogastric infusion of glucose to prevent hypoglycemia. Fructose and galactose are restricted from the diet. Both galactose and fructose must be converted to glucose-6-phosphate or to fructose-6-phosphate, respectively, before forming glucose. Because glucose-6-phosphatase is deficient, glucose-6-phosphate enters glycolysis, which results in a dramatic increase in lactate levels. Allopurinol is given to control the uric acid levels and prevent uric acid crystal accumulation. For patients with GSD type Ib, granulocyte colony–stimulating factor is used to prevent neutropenia and to decrease the severity of bacterial infections. Long-term outcomes in patients with GSD types Ia and Ib can be good if diagnosis occurs early and prompt treatment is started.

Glycogen Storage Disease Type III (Debranching-Enzyme Deficiency)

GSD type III results from a deficiency of the debranching enzyme, amylo-1,6-glucosidase. The inheritance pattern is autosomal recessive. The gene for this debranching enzyme is located on chromosome 1p21. Debrancher enzyme deficiency results in an inability to degrade stored glycogen, thereby impairing the release of glucose from glycogen. Glucose production from gluconeogenesis remains unaffected. Some of the clinical features of GSD III are similar to those of GSD I. Hepatomegaly, present at birth, improves gradually during the course of childhood. Although this disorder usually occurs in infancy, severe hypoglycemia can occur at birth and steadily improves with advancing age; thus GSD III differs dramatically from GSD I in this respect. Myopathy is the major chronic morbidity associated with GSD type III. Approximately 15% of patients with GSD type III have liver involvement without any associated muscle disturbance. In comparison with GSD type I, concentrations of lactate and uric acid are normal. Unlike GSD type I, no dietary restriction of fructose and glucose is required in these patients.

Differences Between GSD Type I and GSD Type III

After a glucose challenge, lactate levels are normal in GSD type III. Alanine levels are lower in GSD III compared with GSD I, given that individuals with GSD III have increased gluconeogenesis and lower lactate levels. More robust response to a glucagon challenge can be seen in patients with GSD III compared those with GSD I after a short fast; however, this more robust response will decrease as the length of fast increases.

Definitive diagnosis is made by confirming deficiency of amylo-1,6-glucosidase in leukocytes or from a liver, muscle, or skin biopsy. Prenatal diagnosis has been accomplished by amniocyte or chorionic villus sampling using enzyme activity analysis or immunoblot analysis. In comparison with GSD I, treatment of GSD III is easier to implement.

Glycogen Synthase Deficiency

Glycogen synthase deficiency is a rare disorder that results in decreased synthesis of glycogen leading to decreased glycogen stores. Glycogen synthase deficiency is not a GSD because no accumulation of glycogen occurs. Glycogen synthase deficiency leads to ketotic hypoglycemia. Blood levels of lactate and alanine are low and no hyperlipidemia is present. Unlike GSD I and III, glycogen synthase deficiency can be observed clinically with a liver that is normal or slightly enlarged because of the decreased glycogen synthesis. Glucagon response after fasting hypoglycemia is usually reduced or absent, although it may be present in some affected infants. A minimal or absent response to glucagon suggests the diagnosis. Individuals with this condition also exhibit hyperglycemia and hyperlactatemia after feeding because of an inability to store excess glucose. Glycogen synthase is expressed only by the liver. The diagnosis is confirmed by liver enzymatic studies on a liver biopsy specimen.

Mitochondrial Respiratory-Chain Disorders

Respiratory-chain proteins are encoded by a large number of genes, resulting in several patterns of genetic inheritance that can cause mitochondrial disorders. Disorders of the respiratory chain can occur through spontaneous, autosomal-recessive, autosomal-dominant, X-linked, and maternally inherited mutations. Although these diseases can occur at virtually any age the neonatal presentation can include hypoglycemia, apnea, seizures, lethargy, muscle atrophy, hypotonia, sideroblastic anemia, lactic acidosis, coma, hepatomegaly with liver failure, and hypertrophic cardiomyopathies. Lactic acidosis is a common finding. Diagnosis is made by obtaining a muscle biopsy with mitochondrial enzyme analysis.

BOX 105-6 Disorders of Gluconeogenesis

Fructose-1,6-diphosphatase deficiency
Phosphoenolpyruvate-carboxykinase deficiency
Pyruvate carboxylase deficiency

Process 3: Gluconeogenesis During Early or Intermediate Starvation

Once hepatic glycogen stores are depleted, gluconeogenesis becomes the primary source for energy. Gluconeogenesis progressively replaces glycogen as the major source of glucose. Therefore hypoglycemia during this phase suggests impaired gluconeogenesis. Gluconeogenesis typically begins after 12 to 16 hours of fasting once glycogen stores are depleted in the term infant. This process may occur more rapidly in preterm and stressed newborn infants. Gluconeogenesis uses amino acids, lactate, and glycerol to manufacture glucose. The most characteristic feature in newborns with defects of gluconeogenesis is hepatomegaly without evidence of liver insufficiency. Important substrates for gluconeogenesis are lactate, alanine, and oxaloacetate. A hallmark of the disorders of gluconeogenesis is elevation of alanine, pyruvate, and lactate levels. Both alanine and lactate are in equilibrium with pyruvate. Abnormalities in gluconeogenesis cause an increase in downstream metabolites such as pyruvate that causes elevations in lactate and alanine. During gluconeogenesis, the brain is not yet using ketone bodies significantly. Fatty acids used for lipolysis and glycerol production become essential when prolonged fasting occurs. Box 105-6 lists the disorders of gluconeogenesis.

Fructose-1,6-Diphosphatase Deficiency

Fructose-1,6-diphosphatase deficiency is a disorder of gluconeogenesis rather than a defect in fructose metabolism. Fructose-1,6-diphosphatase deficiency is inherited in an autosomal-recessive manner. Newborns usually exhibit severe hypoglycemia and lactic acidosis during the first few days of life. These episodes are triggered by decreased oral intake. Clinical symptoms include apnea, tachycardia, hyperventilation, lethargy, and seizures. Fructose-1,6-diphosphatase deficiency has a direct effect on the formation of glucose involving gluconeogenic precursors. Hypoglycemia occurs because of the inability to make fructose-1-phosphate from fructose-1 -6-diphosphate. Fructose-1-phosphate is an important precursor to glucose formation. The enzyme deficiency results in a downstream increase in pyruvate, resulting in severe lactic acidosis. Laboratory analysis reveals increased levels of lactate, alanine, glycerol, and ketones. Definitive diagnosis is made by measuring fructose-1,6-diphosphatase activity in liver tissue. Because of the heterogeneity in expression of this disorder, deficient leukocyte activity is diagnostic; however, normal leukocyte activity does not rule out fructose-1,6-diphosphate deficiency because a form of the disorder occurs with normal leukocyte activity and isolated liver enzyme deficiency.

Treatment of acute, severe episodes involves controlling hypoglycemia and acidosis through continuous intravenous glucose infusion and administration of sodium bicarbonate. Once the hypoglycemia and acidosis are corrected, maintenance therapy is directed at preventing prolonged periods of fasting. This task can be accomplished through continuous nasogastric feedings or intake of uncooked cornstarch after 1 year of age. Dietary restriction includes elimination of fructose, sucrose, glycerol, and sorbitol, which may precipitate an acute life-threatening event. Follow-up should include monitoring growth and development. With advancing age, issues with fasting will improve, which is believed to occur because of an increased capacity for the liver to store glycogen, lowering the need for gluconeogenesis.

Phosphoenolpyruvate-Carboxykinase Deficiency

PEPCK is an important target in the regulation of gluconeogenesis. PEPCK deficiency is a rare disorder that results from a defect localized to chromosome 20q13.31. PEPCK is active in mitochondria and the cytosol. The time of clinical presentation ranges from the neonatal period to early infancy. Affected infants exhibit hypoglycemia. Other clinical features include nonspecific symptoms such as lethargy, hypotonia, and failure to thrive. Systemic manifestations include hepatomegaly with hepatocellular damage, fatty liver, renal tubular acidosis, and fatty kidneys. PEPCK is involved in the conversion of oxaloacetate into phosphoenolpyruvate. Deficiency in PEPCK blocks the conversion of pyruvate, lactate, alanine, and the citric acid–cycle intermediates to glucose. Measuring PEPCK activity from freshly obtained liver biopsy samples is necessary to make the diagnosis. Because two isoforms of PEPCK can occur, one found in the mitochondria and the other in the cytosol, liver biopsy samples require fractionating to make the diagnosis. Initial treatment involves correction of hypoglycemia with intravenous glucose and sodium bicarbonate. Once stable, avoidance of fasting and use of nasogastric feeds or uncooked cornstarch after 1 year of age at bedtime is the mainstay of therapy. Unfortunately, the long-term prognosis is poor, with patients succumbing to hypoglycemia and neurologic injury.

Pyruvate Carboxylase Deficiency (4)

Pyruvate carboxylase (PC) deficiency is an autosomal-recessive disorder. The PC gene is located on chromosome 11 and has three distinct clinical presentations: (1) a severe neonatal form, (2) a milder form occurring later with psychomotor retardation, and (3) a benign form occurring with recurrent episodes of lactic acidosis and mild neurologic deficits. In the neonatal form, infants exhibit seizures, hypotonia, spasticity, renal tubular acidosis, and hepatic dysfunction. PC is responsible for the conversion of pyruvate and carbon dioxide to oxaloacetate. PC is essential in supplying oxaloacetate to the citric acid cycle and thus in providing the necessary substrate for other metabolic pathways such as gluconeogenesis, lipogenesis, and glycerogenesis. Laboratory analysis reveals a lactic acidosis, hypoglycemia, increased ammonia, lysine, citrulline, and alanine levels. Hyperammonemia distinguishes PC deficiency from the other disorders of gluconeogenesis and should therefore be considered in any newborn infant with severe neurologic abnormalities. Diagnosis is made by measuring PC enzymatic activity in liver or skin tissue. Treatment revolves around addressing the lactic acidosis and hypoglycemia (see previous discussion). The hyperammonemia can be treated by providing an alternate source of 4-carbon intermediates (aspartate or citrate) as it replenishes oxaloacetate. The prognosis for infants presenting in the neonatal period is especially poor, given that they rarely survive beyond 3 months of life.

Process 4: Fatty Acid Oxidation and Ketogenesis

Pathophysiological Features

Fatty acid oxidation (FAO) disorders include medium-chain acyl-coenzyme A (CoA) dehydrogenase deficiency (MCADD), which is the most common of these metabolic disorders. Through the β-oxidation pathway, fatty acids provide energy-yielding substrates during periods of fasting and stress. This process is typically initiated after fasting for more than 12 hours. Normal metabolism of endogenous fats begins with lipolysis; this process, in turn, releases free fatty acids, resulting in an increase in plasma concentration. Free fatty acids are then bound to albumin and transported to other tissues. Short- and medium-chain fatty acids cross the mitochondrial membrane without esterification, unlike long-chain fatty acids. After conversion of long-chain fatty acids to their CoA esters, they react with L-carnitine to form acylcarnitine esters. The fatty acylcarnitine complex is then transported across the mitochondrial membrane. Once transported inside the mitochondria, the fatty acid–acyl-CoA complex will undergo β-oxidation, which is an important source of energy for the body during times of prolonged fasting and metabolic stress. β-Oxidation involves successive shortening by two carbon atoms ultimately releasing the end product acetyl-CoA.

In the muscle, acetyl-CoA enters the citric cycle (ATP production). While in the liver, acetyl-CoA is used to synthesize the ketone bodies 3-hydroxybutyrate and acetoacetate. These ketones can then be used as a secondary fuel source for most tissues, particularly the brain. Inborn errors involving intramitochondrial FAO diminish the supply of nicotinamide adenine dinucleotide (NADH) and flavin adenine dinucleotide (FAD) available for mitochondrial oxidative phosphorylation, decreasing the formation of ATP. Therefore disorders related to FAO may lead to multiorgan failure secondary to acute ATP deficiency. Clinical features of FAO disorders include hypotonia, cardiomyopathy, coma, and hepatomegaly (fatty liver). The clinical presentation may be confusing and misleading; for example, hyperammonemia may suggest Reye syndrome, and unexpected death may be taken as sudden infant death syndrome. Many patients have a family history of sudden death in siblings during infancy. The classic presentation is hypoketotic hypoglycemia, indicating impairment in FAO. Patients can exhibit vomiting and lethargy, which occurs after fasting. Intercurrent illness can induce prolonged fasting, potentially unmasking a primary underlying disorder of FAO. Diagnosis can be delayed considerably, given that some patients reach adulthood before experiencing a prolonged fasting episode that induces symptoms. Some affected individuals remain asymptomatic for life. This great variability in the clinical presentation can prevent prompt diagnosis in some patients. Pregnancies complicated by either acute liver failure of pregnancy or HELLP syndrome have been associated with fetuses affected with disorders of FAO. The clinician must be aware of these prenatal clues and consider all newborns delivered in mothers with acute liver failure of pregnancy or HELLP syndrome to be at risk for disorders of FAO. Box 105-7 lists the disorders of fatty acid oxidation.

BOX 105-7 Disorders of Fatty Acid Oxidation

- Medium-chain acyl-coenzyme A (CoA) dehydrogenase deficiency
- Long-chain acyl-CoA dehydrogenase deficiency
- Very long-chain acyl-CoA dehydrogenase deficiency
- Short-chain acyl-CoA dehydrogenase deficiency

Medium-Chain Acyl-CoA Dehydrogenase Deficiency

MCADD is the most common disorder in the FAO pathway. The estimated frequency is 1 in 5000 to 10,000 live-born infants. MCADD testing is currently included on newborn metabolic screening panels in many states. It is an autosomal-recessive disorder, with the *A985G* mutations occurring with the highest frequency. The worldwide prevalence is shown in Table 105-4. MCADD produces hypoketotic hypoglycemia after a fasting period of 8 to 12 hours in neonates or potentially earlier if an acute intercurrent illness is present. The most common time for presentation of MCADD is after 3 months of age when the infants typically stop night feedings. Older children may need to be fasting for 18 to 24 hours before symptoms become evident.

The first step in treatment is focused on avoiding prolonged fasts. As noted previously, avoiding prolonged fasts is not usually an issue for newborns because they generally feed every 2 to 3 hours. As individuals with this condition get older, they generally tolerate longer fasting intervals. In neonates and infants, going longer than 6 hours without a feeding should be avoided. At 1 year of age, raw cornstarch may be instituted to supply a slow release source of glucose for up to 8 hours. This approach cannot be used in children younger than 1 year because of enzyme immaturity and inability to handle the osmotic load.

Plasma L-carnitine levels should be checked as soon as the diagnosis is suspected. Some individuals may have low plasma L-carnitine levels that require supplementation with oral carnitine. Low L-carnitine levels cause a progressive cardiomyopathy. Another function of L-carnitine is to remove short-chain and medium-chain fatty acids from the mitochondria so as to maintain CoA levels. These fatty acids accumulate

Table 105-4 Worldwide Frequency of the *A985G* Mutation

LOCATION	FREQUENCY OF CARRIERS
Japan	Very low
Italy	1:333
Czech Republic	1:240
Turkey	1:216
Finland	1:191
Hungary	1:168
Spain	1:141
France	1:140
Normandy	1:118
Germany	1:116
United States	1:107
Denmark	1:101
Poland	1:98
Bulgaria	1:91
North Carolina (United States)	1:84
Belgium	1:77
Australia	1:71
United Kingdom	1:68-1:40
Holland	1:55

From Ozand PT. Hypoglycemia in association with various organic and amino acid disorders. *Semin Perinatol.* 2000;24(2):172-193.

as a result of normal and abnormal FAO. This mechanism prevents the build-up in the mitochondria of short-chain and medium-chain fatty acids that may interfere with the energy production essential to the normal function of the cell. In individuals who have normal plasma L-carnitine levels, experts have recommended that L-carnitine not be given because it may result in increased stress on the FAO pathway by its function in assisting the transport of long-chain fatty acids into the mitochondria for oxidation. Box 105-8 lists other FAO defects and characteristic findings.

BOX 105-8 Rare Fatty Acid Oxidation Defects

The prevalence of these defects are unknown, although LCADD is likely the most common. The inheritance of these conditions is autosomal recessive.

Short-chain acyl-coenzyme A (CoA) dehydrogenase deficiency (SCADD), long-chain acyl-CoA dehydrogenase deficiency (LCADD), trifunctional enzyme deficiency, long-chain hydroxyacyl-acyl-CoA dehydrogenase deficiency (LCHADD), very long-chain acyl CoA dehydrogenase deficiency (VLCADD)

CLINICAL FINDINGS

Seizures
Hypotonia
Cardiomyopathy
Sudden infant death syndrome

LABORATORY FINDINGS

Hypoketotic hypoglycemia
Abnormal liver function tests

SPECIALTY BIOCHEMICAL TESTING

Organic acids have a typical profile
Acylcarnitine profile
Plasma amino acids are normal
Enzyme testing is available but difficult

ACUTE TREATMENT

Intravenous glucose
Formula containing medium-chain triglycerides (medium-chain triglyceride oil)—Pregestimil
Supportive care for cardiomyopathy

Process 5: Disorders of Hormonal Regulation—Deficiency of Counterregulatory Hormones

When a newborn experiences hypoglycemia, a cascade of hormonal responses is activated to counter and restore blood glucose levels to normal. The first physiological response suppresses insulin secretion. This event is followed by an increase in counterregulatory hormones if hypoglycemia persists. The counterregulatory hormones are listed in Table 105-5.

These counterregulatory hormones stimulate glycogenolysis, gluconeogenesis, adipose tissue lipolysis, and hepatic ketogenesis. Some overlap in counterregulatory hormone effects occurs; thus if one system fails, partial compensation occurs by another hormone. Deficiencies in GH, glucagon, cortisol, and insulin-like growth factors may contribute to hypoglycemia. Box 105-9 describes disorders of hormonal regulation.

Pituitary Deficiency

Congenital pituitary deficiency is the second-most common cause of persistent neonatal hypoglycemia, after congenital hyperinsulinism. Physical examination may range from a normal examination to identifying abnormalities involving midline defects such as single central incisor, optic nerve hypoplasia, and cleft lip or palate. Another physical finding is the presence of a microphallus and undescended testis in male newborns secondary to gonadotropin deficiency. Therefore the association of hypoglycemia and microphallus should alert the clinician to the possibility of panhypopituitarism. Female newborns with gonadotropin deficiency have normal external genitalia because the development of the female external genitalia does not require the presence gonadotropin-releasing hormone, luteinizing hormone, follicle-stimulating hormone, or ovarian hormones. The unopposed insulin secretion found with congenital pituitary deficiency can result in clinical findings similar to hyperinsulinism.

Adrenal Deficiency

Adrenal insufficiency is rare cause of hypoglycemia in the newborn infant and occurs in cases of congenital adrenal hypoplasia or aplasia and adrenal hemorrhage. The resulting cortisol deficiency can be life threatening, making early recognition imperative.

Table 105-5 Hormonal Regulation of Fasting Metabolic Systems

	HEPATIC GLYCOGEN-OLYSIS	HEPATIC GLUCONEO-GENESIS	MUSCLE PROTEOLYSIS	ADIPOSE TISSUE LIPOLYSIS	HEPATIC KETOGENESIS
Insulin	Inhibits	Inhibits	Inhibits	Inhibits	Inhibits
Glucagon	Stimulates	—	—	—	Stimulates
Cortisol	—	Stimulates	Stimulates	—	—
Growth hormone	—	—	—	Stimulates	—
Epinephrine	Stimulates	Stimulates	—	Stimulates	Stimulates

Adapted from Polin RA, Fox WW, Abman S. *Fetal and Neonatal Physiology*. 3rd ed. Philadelphia, PA: WB Saunders; 2003. Reprinted by permission.

BOX 105-9 Disorders of Hormonal Regulation

Panhypopituitarism (adrenocorticotropic hormone deficiency)
Growth hormone deficiency
Adrenal deficiency (cortisol deficiency)

Non-Hypoglycemic Neonatal Onset Metabolic Disease

A variety of metabolic conditions exist that do not have hypoglycemia as a presenting symptom but will produce acidosis or hyperammonemia. Many of these conditions occur initially with feeding intolerance or irritability (or both) that can progress to increasing lethargy, seizures, and coma. If untreated, then the classic forms of these conditions cause severe neurologic devastation or death. Many of these metabolic conditions are now included on newborn screening programs in several states. However, screening results can take up to 7 days to return, and, in many of these conditions, onset of symptoms may begin at 3 days of life. Keeping these conditions in mind will allow the clinician to intervene and minimize the impact on an affected neonate.

An important term to clarify in regard to treatment for some of these conditions is *natural protein*, a protein obtained from complete sources, that is, standard baby formulas or table foods.

L-CARNITINE DEFICIENCY. Some individuals have low plasma L-carnitine levels that require supplementation with oral L-carnitine. Low L-carnitine levels cause a progressive cardiomyopathy. L-carnitine removes short-chain and medium-chain fatty acids from the mitochondria to maintain CoA levels. These fatty acids accumulate as a result of normal and abnormal FAO. This mechanism prevents the build-up in the mitochondria of short-chain and medium-chain fatty acids that may interfere with energy production essential to the normal function of the cell. In certain organic acidemias, L-carnitine will also bind the offending organic acid for removal, that is, propionic acid. As noted previously, in well individuals who have FAO disorders and normal plasma L-carnitine levels, experts have recommended that L-carnitine not be given because it may result in increased stress on the FAO pathway by its function in assisting the transport of long-chain fatty acids into the mitochondria for oxidation.

Peritoneal dialysis has been found to be a safe, effective, and easy way to remove excess offending metabolites in neonates and infants. Some debate has occurred over hemodialysis in neonates because of reports of poor outcomes; however, it has also been used successfully and with more efficient metabolite removal. Much can depend on the experience of persons who implement the hemodialysis in the neonatal setting.

Ammonul (sodium phenylacetate–sodium benzoate) is an intravenous plasma ammonia–binding solution that will lower ammonia levels.

GALACTOSEMIA. Galactosemia has a prevalence of 1 in 40,000 to 60,000 live births. Individuals with the classical form of galactosemia have a complete inability to metabolize galactose. Galactosemia is an autosomal-recessive condition. The primary defect in the classical form of galactosemia is deficiency of galactose-1-phosphate uridyltransferase. Deficiency in this enzyme results in an accumulation of galactose-1-phosphate and galactose. In the newborn period, galactosemia can be lethal within 2 weeks. Many states test for galactosemia as part of the newborn metabolic screening program. However, clinical signs generally emerge before the newborn screening results are available. Clinical features include jaundice, increased reducing substances in the urine, abnormalities in prothrombin time and partial thromboplastin time, and liver dysfunction. The primary cause of death at 1 to 2 weeks of age is *E coli* infection resulting from an affected infant's increased susceptibility to infection.

An important fact when considering a diagnosis of galactosemia is that urine-reducing substances will be markedly positive (four or more urine-reducing substances) in the context of a normal screening using a glucose meter, which is specific for glucose. This circumstance should alert the clinician to the fact that the infant is excreting a sugar other than glucose into the urine. Care must be taken in performing invasive procedures in a neonate such as a lumbar puncture because the associated hepatic dysfunction may cause a severe coagulopathy and bleeding. Despite the importance of evaluating the infant for possible meningitis, affected infants are at significant risk of intraspinal bleeding that may cause paralysis.

The risk of lethal *E coli* infection is high several days after birth because of increasing accumulation of abnormal metabolites. Once the galactose metabolites are lowered the risk of *E coli* infection is similar to the general neonatal population. In the past, authorities believed that tight control of galactose intake would prevent long-term sequelae. However, now apparent is that older patients with galactosemia are at high risk for specific medical issues despite minimizing galactose intake. Long-term medical complications include speech delays, premature ovarian failure in women, and, in some individuals, onset of tremor and ataxia. These complications have been associated with the *Q188R* mutation, which results in complete absence of the galactose-1-phosphate uridyltransferase enzyme.

The primary goal in management of neonates suspected of having or diagnosed with galactosemia is to minimize galactose intake. Because breast milk and standard cow milk–based infant formulas contain lactose, these feedings must be stopped. Lactose is a disaccharide that consists of glucose and galactose. Metabolism of lactose releases the galactose, resulting in elevations in galactose metabolites. Soymilk-based infant formulas do not have galactose and provide a safe alternative infant feeding. If a neonate has clinical manifestations of galactosemia, then a sepsis evaluation should be performed even after they are placed on a soymilk formula. Blood and urine cultures should be obtained, but a spinal tap should be avoided, given the risks noted previously, until results of coagulation studies confirm normal coagulation.

Long-term dietary management requires intensive nutritional counseling to avoid galactose-containing foods. The goal of the diet is to incorporate soy-based products and to avoid galactose-containing products. Individuals with galactosemia must remain on this diet for life.

FRUCTOSEMIA. Fructosemia does not occur in the neonatal period but surfaces when sucrose, fructose, or fruits are introduced in the infant's diet.

BIOTINIDASE DEFICIENCY. Biotinidase deficiency is an autosomal-recessive condition with a prevalence of approximately 1 in 60,000. Biotinidase is an enzyme involved in the generation and maintenance of biotin. Figure 105-7 reveals how biotinidase is generated. Biotin is a cofactor needed by four carboxylases—pyruvate carboxylase, 3-methylcrotonyl-CoA carboxylase, propionyl-CoA carboxylase, and acetyl-CoA carboxylase—for functional activity as shown by the red-circled enzymes in Figure 105-6. Infants with biotinidase deficiency may become symptomatic within several days to several months after birth. The deficiency can occur acutely with seizures, vomiting, diarrhea, feeding difficulties, tachypnea from acidosis, and apnea. Laboratory findings may include hyperammonemia, ketoacidosis, and elevations of characteristic organic acids. If biotinidase deficiency is not detected early and treatment initiated, then late manifestations of biotinidase deficiency may cause hypotonia, ataxia, hearing loss, optic atrophy, alopecia, abnormalities in cellular immunity, basal ganglia calcifications, intellectual disability, skin rash, and seborrheic dermatitis.

Treatment involves large doses of biotin; 20 mg/day is usually sufficient for life. Biotin supplementation

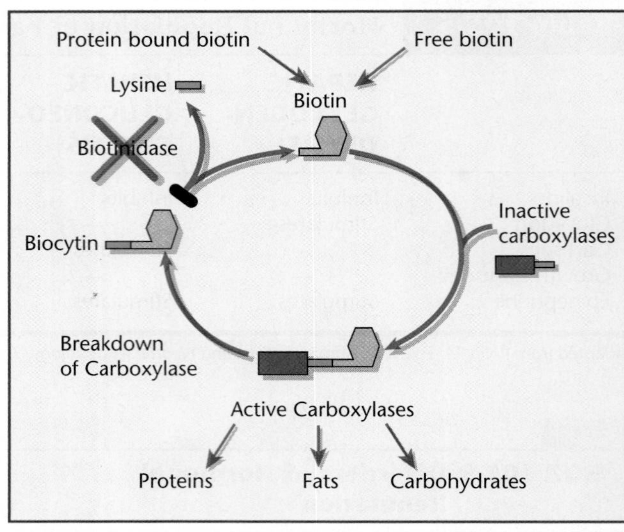

Figure 105-7 The biotin cycle has not yet been localized to a specific cellular compartment; therefore this cycle is not displayed on the master biochemical pathway figure.

prevents all of the disease manifestations. In some cases, with neonatal onset, seizures may begin during the first few days of life, necessitating antiepileptogenic medication in addition to supplemental biotin. Usually, as the biotin takes effect, the seizure medication can be discontinued.

ORGANIC ACIDEMIAS. The organic acidemias are a set of conditions that tend to occur in a similar way and have similar treatments. Organic acids form from the breakdown of branched-chain amino acids, methionine, and threonine in most cases. In individuals with enzyme deficiencies, accumulation of intermediate metabolites can cause severe illness and death. Affected infants tend to exhibit severe acidosis within several days of life. The clinician should identify the involved organic acids because treatment includes use of specialized, amino acid–modified (free) infant formulas once the infant is stabilized after acute therapies.

Methylmalonic acidemia has a prevalence of 1 in 40,000 to 50,000 live births. It is an autosomal-recessive condition that results from methylmalonyl-CoA mutase deficiency, or it may also result from a defect in cobalamin (vitamin B12) metabolism.

Propionic acidemia has a prevalence of 1 in 50,000 to 100,000 live births. It is an autosomal-recessive condition resulting from the deficiency of propionyl-CoA carboxylase, a biotin-dependent enzyme.

Isovaleric acidemia has an unknown prevalence. It is an autosomal-recessive condition that results from isovaleryl-CoA dehydrogenase deficiency. This enzyme is involved in leucine metabolism; however, leucine is not elevated in these individuals because of an irreversible step before isovaleryl-CoA dehydrogenase.

Infants with methylmalonic acidemia and propionic acidemia usually exhibit poor feeding, irritability, respiratory difficulty with tachypnea and labored breathing, severe and repetitive vomiting, cerebral edema, and progression to coma and death over a period of days to weeks. Infants affected by isovaleric acidemia can exhibit the previously listed findings along with a very strong *sweaty sock* odor. This sign may not be noticed if the neonate has been catheterized or if the urine is dilute.

Evaluation. Laboratory findings of infants with organic acidemias include metabolic acidosis on a blood gas sampling, leukopenia, thrombocytopenia, and ketosis. Hyperammonemia can be present in methylmalonic acidemia and propionic acidemia. Hyperammonemia is thought to be the result of secondary inhibition of the urea cycle by the abnormal metabolites generated. As a consequence, affected individuals may have normal blood urea nitrogen levels despite evidence of dehydration caused by a decreased ability to generate urea.

Diagnosis of an organic acidemia requires analysis of urine organic acid patterns. Characteristic excretion patterns are identifiable for various organic acidemias. Plasma amino acid analysis is significant for a marked elevation of glycine and is the reason for the categorization of methylmalonic acidemia and propionic acidemia as ketotic hyperglycinemias. In isovaleric acidemia, glycine is not elevated, which may be the result of the conjugation of isovaleryl metabolites to form isovalerylglycine. Elevations of valine, methionine, isoleucine, and threonine can be seen in methylmalonic acidemia and propionic acidemia.

Treatment. Treatment for methylmalonic acidemia and propionic acidemia involve therapy to lower the level of the elevated plasma organic acid. Beneficial therapies in the acute management of these conditions include (1) dialysis to lower potentially elevated ammonia and the offending plasma organic acid and (2) L-carnitine in a dosage of 200 to 300 mg/kg/day to bind plasma organic acids and replenish L-carnitine. Natural protein intake should also be limited to 1.0 to 1.2 g/kg/day in the acute decompensation. Additionally, though not routinely available, treatments such as *metabolic* parenteral solutions that do not contain valine, methionine, isoleucine, and threonine and administration of intravenous sodium phenylacetate–sodium benzoate (Ammonul®) to correct hyperammonemia may be helpful.

Treatment of isovaleric acidemia is as described for methylmalonic acidemia and propionic acidemia, with the following exceptions: Oral glycine is given at a dose of 500 mg/kg/day to bind isovaleryl metabolites and parenteral solutions should not contain leucine.

Long-term treatment involves use of specialty commercial formulas to prevent build-up of the offending organic acid. Natural protein is typically maintained at 1.0 to 1.5 g/kg/day, with the remainder of protein and calories provided by the specialty formula.

UREA-CYCLE DEFECTS. Urea-cycle defects are a category of conditions that involve primary dysfunction of the urea cycle. Several enzyme deficiencies cause these conditions, and most are autosomal recessive. One notable exception is ornithine transcarbamylase (OTC) deficiency, an inherited X-linked trait that is the most common urea-cycle disorder. This inheritance pattern results in a more severe presentation in male patients, with female patients typically minimally affected, if at all. The prevalence of OTC deficiency is approximately 1 in 80,000 live births. Box 105-10 lists the diagnostic criteria for OTC deficiency.

BOX 105-10 Ornithine Transcarbamylase Deficiency Diagnosis

- Low plasma citrulline
- High plasma glutamine
- Ornithine transcarbamylase urine organic acids
- High urinary orotic acid
- Specific hepatic enzyme studies
- DNA analysis

The clinical presentation of urea-cycle disorders is similar to the presentation of other metabolic conditions. However, acidosis is usually not a presenting component of these conditions. Lactic acidosis may become prominent once the patient becomes critically ill. Presenting signs frequently include anorexia, irritability, lethargy, vomiting, somnolence, asterixis (rare), obtundation, coma, cerebral edema, and combativeness and disorientation (in older individuals). Death may occur if treatment is not rapid or effective. Laboratory findings of importance are hyperammonemia (usually >150 mcmol/L; can be as high as 2000-4500 mcmol/L), low blood urea nitrogen, and respiratory alkalosis. Metabolic acidosis is *not* present unless the patient is in critical condition. Characteristic amino acid profiles confirm the specific urea-cycle defect.

Acute treatment of urea-cycle disorders involves dialysis to remove the ammonia, provision of calories by administration of 20% lipid solutions, infusions of intravenous sodium phenylacetate–sodium benzoate (Ammonul), and specially formulated formula once oral intake is possible. An infant with OTC deficiency requires infusions of arginine in doses of 200 mg/kg/day and intravenous glucose.

In certain cases, when no response or sluggish response to pharmacologic therapy occurs, the health care professional must consider hemodialysis.

Long-term urea-cycle defects are treated by providing formulas that contain essential amino acids along with natural protein at approximately 1.0 to 1.5 g/kg/day. Typically, affected infants require treatment with oral ammonia-binding agents such as sodium benzoate or Buphenyl to maintain plasma ammonia at an acceptable level. This treatment allows for maintenance of ammonia levels close to the normal range, in most cases, while the individual is well. However, affected patients remain susceptible to transient elevations of ammonia during illness even while on ammonia-binding agents. During episodes of illness, all protein should be stopped for 24 hours and a formula consisting of carbohydrates and fats administered. Protein is gradually reintroduced into the diet once the ammonia level declines. An important point to note is that protein must be given after 24 hours to prevent endogenous protein catabolism and further worsening of the hyperammonemia. If levels are dramatically elevated, then the acute management protocol described previously should be initiated. Depending on the severity of the condition, liver transplant should be considered, especially if the individual does not respond to medical management or requires frequent hospitalizations.

TYROSINEMIA TYPE 1. Tyrosine is usually metabolized to acetoacetate; however, in classical tyrosinemia type 1, fumarylacetoacetate hydrolase deficiency will result in excess succinylacetone. Succinylacetone is toxic and leads to the clinical findings in tyrosinemia type 1. Tyrosinemia type 1 has a prevalence of 1 in 1800 in certain regions of Quebec and is estimated to be approximately 1 in 100,000 elsewhere. Type 1 tyrosinemia is an acute-onset disorder that initially produces diffuse liver dysfunction, which progresses to liver failure and death without intervention. The primary defect is in the fumarylacetoacetase gene. This gene encodes the enzyme fumarylacetoacetate hydrolase. This enzyme deficiency results in accumulation of metabolites that require metabolism via alternative pathways. An important metabolite that is formed is succinylacetone, which likely contributes to the progressive hepatic dysfunction and eventual hepatic failure in affected individuals.

Acute management of tyrosinemia type 1 has been revolutionized recently with the development of Orfadin (2-[2-nitro-4-trifluoromethylbenzoyl] cyclohexane-1,3-dioneand). This medication inhibits enzyme function proximal to fumarylacetoacetate hydrolase, biochemically transforming tyrosinemia type 1 into tyrosinemia type 2. (The enzyme defect in tyrosinemia type 2 is a deficiency of hepatic cytosol tyrosine aminotransferease activity.) It also prevents the build-up of succinylacetone and the corresponding hepatotoxicity. Tyrosinemia type 2 is a milder form of tyrosinemia that results in cataract formation and skin findings without the hepatic involvement. However, even with administration of Orfadin, plasma tyrosine levels will require continued monitoring and control through dietary intervention to prevent the ocular and skin findings that are associated with tyrosinemia type 2.

Several commercial formulas are available that do not contain tyrosine. These formulas can be used to control plasma tyrosine levels. Typically, natural protein is kept at 1.0 to 1.5 g/kg/day, with the remainder of protein and calorie requirements provided by the tyrosine deficient formulas.

PHENYLKETONURIA. Phenylketonuria (PKU) does not exhibit acutely in the neonatal period; however, given that PKU is one of the most common inborn errors of metabolism, with a prevalence of 1 in 10,000 to 15,000 live births, a brief mention is provided here. The primary defect is in phenylalanine hydroxylase activity, and it results in elevations in phenylalanine. Chronic phenylalanine elevations cause brain injury that may progress to severe intellectual disability if the condition is not treated

Newborn screening for PKU does not differentiate between the classical form of PKU and rare forms that result from biopterin deficiency. The active form of biopterin, tetrahydrobiopterin, is a cofactor for phenylalanine hydroxylase. Up to 2% of affected individuals with hyperphenylalaninemia have a biopterin abnormality that disrupts neurotransmitter metabolism, in addition to phenylalanine metabolism.

PKU was one of the first conditions that was screened for on newborn screening and was the model condition for dietary management of an inborn error of metabolism. Numerous commercial formulas and low-protein products are available to aid in maintaining plasma phenylalanine concentrations at an appropriate level.

Individuals with biopterin abnormalities do not typically respond to dietary manipulations alone, given that the cofactor deficiency also adversely affects neurotransmitter production. Biopterin deficiency is treated by replacing the precursors to the affected neurotransmitters, folinic acid in some cases, and providing the active form of the cofactor, tetrahydrobiopterin. For some affected patients, treatment with tetrahydrobiopterin may make additional therapy unnecessary. A growing body of evidence indicated that up to 10% of individuals with phenylalanine hydroxylase deficiency may be responsive to tetrahydrobiopterin.

MAPLE SYRUP URINE DISEASE. Maple syrup urine disease (MSUD) has an approximate prevalence of 1 in 120,000 live births. MSUD is an autosomal-recessive condition; its primary defect is in the metabolism of the branched-chain amino acids, including isoleucine, leucine, and valine. The enzyme involved is branched-chain alpha-keto dehydrogenase complex. Acute clinical signs begin several days after birth when branched-chain amino acids accumulate as infants increase their feeding intake. Presenting signs include poor feeding, irritability, and stereotypical seizures characterized by bicycling motions of the arms and legs. In addition, the infant and the infant's urine have an odor of maple syrup. Lethargic infants rapidly progress to coma and death.

Therapy involves extracting the branched-chain amino acids from plasma, thereby reducing total body concentration of these amino acids. Dialysis is necessary to reduce the elevated amino acid levels rapidly in an affected neonate. Peritoneal dialysis has been shown to be safe and effective in lowering these amino acids; however, in severe cases, hemodialysis may be necessary. Once the leucine level is reduced to approximately 10 mg/dL, dialysis can be discontinued. Thereafter the treatment goal is to maximize caloric intake to prevent catabolic breakdown of endogenous proteins resulting in continued elevations of the branched-chain amino acids. Initially, 20% lipid solutions in a dose of 2 g/kg/day in conjunction with 12.5% to 20% dextrose are administered to prevent catabolism. Parenteral nutrition solutions without branched-chain amino acids are used to control branched-chain amino acid levels while enteral nutrition is implemented.

A thiamine (vitamin B1)-responsive form of MSUD has been identified. Thiamine supplementation corrects the enzyme deficiency, resulting in the ability to tolerate normal protein in normal amounts. Usually, 10 mg/day of thiamine will correct the hyperbranched–chain aminoaciduria without the need for dietary intervention.

In cases in which thiamine does not have any effect, several commercial formulas are available that do not contain the branched-chain amino acids, which can be used as a protein source. Additional calories can be provided by other specialty formulas that only contain fats and carbohydrates. As the branched-chain amino acids decline into the physiological range, small amounts of natural protein are required in the form of a standard formula to prevent branched-chain amino acid deficiencies. Natural protein can be started at 1.0 to 1.25 g/kg/day and then adjusted to keep the branched-chain amino acid levels within normal range. The remainder of protein requirements, 2.5 to 3.0 g/kg/day, can be achieved with the specialty formula that lacks the branched-chain amino acids.

Long-term management of MSUD involves a low-protein diet, continued use of specialty formulas, and intensive monitoring of plasma isoleucine, valine, and leucine levels.

HOMOCYSTINURIA. Homocystinuria has a prevalence of approximately 1 in 200,000. It is an autosomal-recessive condition. Most newborn screening programs test for plasma methionine concentrations to evaluate for the presence of the condition, given that methionine is elevated in individuals with homocystinuria. However, methionine can be elevated in a variety of conditions that cause liver disease, or it may occasionally be transiently elevated in the newborn. Cystathionine β-synthase is a critical enzyme in the metabolism of homocysteine. Deficiency of cystathionine β-synthase is the most common cause of homocystinuria. Cobalamin plays a critical role in the formation of cofactors for the metabolism of methylmalonic acid and homocysteine.

The acute findings in homocystinuria include thromboembolism and seizures. Homocysteine is an endothelial irritant that that cause lesions resulting in intravascular clot formation. High concentrations of plasma homocysteine can lower seizure thresholds and may be noted as a presenting symptom. Untreated or inadequately treated patients develop intellectual disability and developmental delay, psychiatric disorders, ectopia lentis, scoliosis, and osteoporosis. Fifty percent of affected individuals die before the age of 25 years.

Approximately 50% of individuals are responsive to vitamin B6. Vitamin B6 is a cofactor for cystathionine β-synthase. Individuals who respond to vitamin B6 do very well and do not required further treatment. Nonresponders to vitamin B6 therapy must be maintained on a restricted methionine and cystine diet for life. Natural protein intake at 1.0 to 1.5 g/kg/day via a low-protein diet and formula are necessary. Betaine, a trimethylglycine, is formed through the oxidation of choline and has shown promising results in the management of individuals with homocystinuria. It converts homocysteine to methionine and permits reduction of the dietary restrictions. Experts recommend that methionine levels be kept below 1000 mcmol/L to prevent cerebral edema. Studies have not yet been conducted on neonates or infants to evaluate for safety of this therapy.

COBALAMIN DISEASE. Seven subtypes of cobalamin (Cbl) disorders, designated Cbl A through G, have been identified. This group of cobalamin disorders can cause elevations in methylmalonic acid only (Cbl A and B), a combination of methylmalonic acid and homocysteine elevations (Cbl C, D, and F), or homocysteine elevations only (Cbl E and G). These disorders result from abnormal Cbl (vitamin B12) metabolism or transport.

Administration of hydroxycobalamin, the active form of Cbl, corrects the biochemical abnormalities and usually allows for a complete recovery. Hydroxycobalamin is administered subcutaneously.

PYRUVATE-DEHYDROGENASE COMPLEX DEFICIENCY. The pyruvate-dehydrogenase complex plays a critical role in metabolizing the product of glycolysis, pyruvate, to acetyl-CoA. Pyruvate-dehydrogenase complex deficiency is a mitochondrial disorder that can exhibit acutely in the neonatal period with a severe lactic acidosis. X-linked and autosomal-recessive forms have been identified. This condition is not currently screened for on state newborn metabolic testing; however, prompt intervention can minimize the effects of accumulating toxic metabolites.

Minimizing carbohydrate and glucose intake lowers the levels of lactic acid. Formulas that are high in protein and fat are commercially available. Five-percent dextrose is tolerated well; however, higher glucose concentrations can cause increased lactate levels. As long as the lactate is controlled, these infants have a good chance of surviving the neonatal period.

TOOLS FOR PRACTICE

Engaging Patient and Family

- *Newborn Screening Tests—these tests could save your babies life* (brochure), Health Resources and Services Administration, US Department of Health and Human Services (test.medicalhomeinfo.org/screening/ScreenMaterials/Newborn screening tests.pdf).
- *Newborn Screening Disorders—What Parents Want to Know about Newborn Screening Disorders* (brochure), Health Resources and Services Administration, US Department of Health and Human Services (test.medicalhomeinfo.org/screening/ScreenMaterials/Newbornscreeningdisorders.pdf).

Medical Decision Support

- *A Primer on Newborn Metabolic Screening* (Web page), Region 4 Genetics Collaborative (medhomes.region4genetics.org/primer.asp).
- *Newborn Screening ACT sheets and Confirmatory Algorithms* (algorithm), American College of Medical Genetics (www.acmg.net/resources/policies/ACT/condition-analyte-links.htm).
- *Newborn Screening and Related Conditions* (Web page), Centers for Disease Control and Prevention (www.cdc.gov/ncbddd/bd/genetics_screen.htm).

RELATED WEB SITES

- National Center of Medical Home Initiatives for Children with Special Needs, American Academy of Pediatrics: Newborn Screening (www.medicalhomeinfo.org/index.html)

- Online Mendelian Inheritance in Man, Johns Hopkins University (www.ncbi.nlm.nih.gov/sites/entrez?db=OMIM)
- Genetic Alliance (www.geneticalliance.org/)
- American College of Medical Genetics (www.acmg.net)
- Gene Test (www.genetests.org/)

SELECTED RESOURCES

Albers S, Marsden D, Quackenbush E, et al. Detection of neonatal carnitine palmitoyltransferase II deficiency by expanded newborn screening with tandem mass spectrometry. *Pediatrics*. 2001;107:e103-e104.

Burton BK. Inborn errors of metabolism in infancy: a guide to diagnosis. *Pediatrics*. 1998;102(6):e69.

Boles RG, Buck EA, Blitzer MG, et al. Retrospective biochemical screening of fatty acid oxidation disorders in postmortem livers of 418 cases of sudden death in the first year of life. *J Pediatr.* 1998;132:924-933.

Centers for Disease Control and Prevention. Mental retardation following diagnosis of a metabolic disorder in children aged 3-10 years: metropolitan Atlanta, Georgia, 1991-1994. *MMWR Morb Mortal Wkly Rep*. 1999;48: 353-356.

Chance DH, DiPerna JC, Mitchell BL, et al. Electrospray tandem mass spectrometry for analysis of acylcarnitines in dried postmortem blood specimens collected at autopsy from infants with unexplained cause of death. *Clin Chem*. 2001;47:1166-1182.

Crumrine PK. Degenerative disorders of the central nervous system. *Pediatr Rev.* 2001;22:370-379.

Davis TC, Humiston SG, Arnold CL, et al. Recommendations for effective newborn screening communication: results of focus groups with parents, providers, and experts. *Pediatrics*. 2006;117(5):S326-S340. Available at: pediatrics.aappublications.org/cgi/content/abstract/117/5/S1/S326. Accessed April 24, 2008.

Dionisi-Vici C, Deodato F, Roschinger W, et al. 'Classical' organic acidurias, propionic aciduria, methylmalonic aciduria and isovaleric aciduria: long-term outcome and effects of expanded newborn screening using tandem mass spectrometry. *J Inherit Metab Dis*. 2006;29:383-389.

Enns GM, Packman S. Diagnosing inborn errors of metabolism in the newborn: clinical features. *NeoReviews*. 2001;2: e183-e191.

Enns GM, Packman S. Diagnosing inborn errors of metabolism in the newborn: laboratory investigations. *NeoReviews*. 2001;2:e192-e200.

Gurian EA, Kinnamon DD, Henry JJ, et al. Expanded newborn screening for biochemical disorders: the effect of a false-positive result. *Pediatrics*. 2006;117:1915-1921.

Pass KA, Lane PA, Fernhoff PM, et al. US newborn screening system guidelines II: follow-up of children, diagnosis, management, and evaluation. Statement of the Council of Regional Networks for Genetic Services (CORN). *J Pediatr.* 2000;137(suppl 4):S1-S46.

Pinar H. Postmortem findings in term neonates. *Semin Perinatol*. 2004;9:289-302.

Ridel KR, Leslie ND, Gilbert DL. An updated review of the long-term neurological effects of galactosemia. *Pediatr Neurol*. 2005;33:153-161.

Tarini BA, Christakis DA, Welch HG. State newborn screening in the tandem mass spectrometry era: more tests, more false-positive results. *Pediatrics*. 2006;118:448-456.

Therrell BL, Johnson A, Williams D. Status of newborn screening programs in the United States. *Pediatrics*. 2006;117(5):S212-S252.

Waddell L, Wiley V, Carpenter K, et al. Medium-chain acyl-CoA dehydrogenase deficiency: genotype-biochemical phenotype correlations. *Mol Genet Metab*. 2006;87:32-39.

REFERENCES

1. Kalhan SC, Bier DM, Savin SM, et al. Estimation of glucose turnover and 13C recycling in the human newborn by simultaneous [1-13 C]glucose and [6,6-1H2]glucose tracer. *J Clin Endocrinol Metab*. 1980;50;456.
2. de Lonlay P, Giurgea I, Touati G, et al: Neonatal hypoglycaemia: aetiologies. *Semin Neonatol*. 2004;(9):49-58.
3. de Rooy L, Hawdon J. Nutritional factors that affect the postnatal metabolic adaptation of full-term and large-for-gestational-age infants. *Pediatrics*. 2002;109(3):E42.
4. Bruining, PD. Recent advances in hyperinsulinism and the pathogenesis of diabetes mellitus. *Curr Opin Pediatr.* 1990;2:758-765.

Chapter 106

NEUROLOGIC ABNORMALITIES

Aleksandra Djukic, MD, PhD

> *If the infant is pushed slightly and bent forward a few minutes after birth, he will make his first steps. Nevertheless, the newborn is capricious and does not always walk to order. Well disposed at one moment, he is no longer so the next. The examiner is discouraged and gives up; then he tries a last time—the baby starts walking immediately, perfectly regularly and over a long distance.*
>
> —André-Thomas and Autgaerden (1966)

Neurologic examination of the neonate is a complex task; findings depend on age, behavioral stage, and position. Neuronal mechanisms of a newborn are inconsistent, with responses occurring one moment but not the next. In spite of the objective difficulties, when the approach to the neurologically impaired neonate is well thought out and accommodates the individual baby, relevant and reliable information can be obtained (Box 106-1). A thorough knowledge and understanding of the normal development of the infant and young child is fundamental to anyone concerned with the care of children.[1]

A neonate's neurologic organization differs greatly from that of the older child. Initial assessment of the neonate should be based on the following fundamental principals: (1) developmental stage of the infant, (2) assessment adjusted to the expected level of maturity, and (3) differential diagnosis focused on treatable conditions for which a delayed response caused by awaiting consultation with a specialist might alter the prognosis.

The main stages of brain development are illustrated in Figure 106-1. During and after the third trimester of pregnancy, at the time when the fetus becomes viable, all neurons have already migrated to their final destinations. The main developmental events during this period are the following: First, glial cells proliferate in the periventricular germinal zone, which is immature and therefore exquisitely vulnerable. Second, synaptogenesis allows neurons to *talk to each other*. Insufficiency of synaptic connections is partially the basis of

BOX 106-1 Neurologic Examination of the Neonate

Observation period
- Observation of unprovoked, spontaneous activity
- Qualitative assessment
- Passive role of the examiner

Examination period
- Response to provoked external stimuli
- Quantitative approach
- Active role of examiner

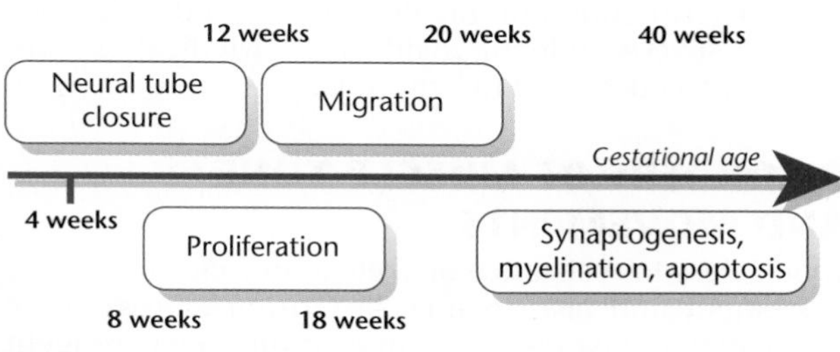

Figure 106-1 Main stages of brain development.

difficulties in the assessment. The relation between stimulus and response is often not consistent. Third, myelination develops, which will, when the child is older, enable faster and more reliable communication, not only between neurons, but also between the child and another person. Fourth, apoptosis, or the programmed elimination, of neurons which are normally produced in excess.

EVALUATION

The goal of evaluation is not only to identify pathological findings, but also to assess the degree of neurologic maturity. This task can be accomplished by careful observation of the quality of spontaneous, endogenously generated movements of the neonate.[2] A rapidly accumulating body of evidence has proved that the spontaneous motility of preterm and term infants, which is in continuity with fetal movements, is of great clinical significance. Spontaneous motility is an important functional indicator of brain dysfunction at a very early age, and it tells us more about the young nervous system than reflex testing.[3] Observation is the most important part of any examination.

The examiner plays an active role in eliciting and quantifying both behavioral and motor responses. Items included in the protocol of the assessment of the preterm and full-term newborn are listed in Box 106-2.[4] The ideal time for the examination is 2 to 3 hours after feeding, when the infant is in a period of quiet wakefulness. Except for lip, glabella, anal, and cremasteric reflexes, which can be elicited regardless of behavioral state, all other reflexes correlate with the level of alertness.[5]

BOX 106-2 Assessment of the Preterm and Full-Term Newborn

HABITUATION
- Light
- Sound

MOVEMENTS AND TONE
- Posture
- Arm and leg recoil and traction
- Popliteal angle
- Head control
- Head lag
- Ventral suspension
- Head raising in prone position
- Arm release in prone position
- Spontaneous body movements
- Tremors and startles
- Abnormal body movements

REFLEXES
- Deep tendon reflexes
- Palmar grasp
- Rooting
- Sucking
- Walking
- Moro reflex

NEUROBEHAVIORAL
- Eye appearance
- Auditory and visual orientation
- Alertness
- Defensive reactions
- Irritability
- Consolability

Developmentally, palmar grasp (weak) and Moro reflex (not full) first appear at 28 weeks' gestation. Deep-tendon reflexes are already present at this time. Asymmetrical tonic neck reflex, stepping reflex, and stronger sucking can be recorded from 34 weeks. The healthy term baby has a strong grasp (the infant can be lifted off the bed), full Moro reflex, and placing reflex. The limbs are semiflexed, and the lower limbs are in slight adduction at the hips. When the child is prone the head may be lifted off the surface and turned to the side. Visual fixation and tracking, which is still not smooth, are present.

SEIZURES

Seizures are clinical manifestations of temporary alterations in brain function that occur as a result of excessive synchronous neuronal electrical discharge. In the newborn, seizures represent an emergency for two main reasons: (1) they indicate significant dysfunction or damage to the immature brain, and (2) they can further interfere with the process of normal neurologic maturation.

The most important single determinant of prognosis in neonates with seizures is the second cause. Immediate and thorough investigation for potentially treatable causes and early institution of cause-specific therapy may mitigate the development of long-term sequelae.[6] The initial differential diagnosis is guided by two main questions: (1) Is the concerning event epileptic or nonepileptic? (2) If epileptic, then was it provoked? A detailed history and a basic laboratory work-up are often sufficient diagnostic tools with direct therapeutic implications.

Clinical suspicion that the event is a seizure should be based on the occurrence of paroxysmal, stereotypical, repetitive, and abnormal events. The signs of seizures in the neonate, when compared with those of older children and adults, may be very different; this difference is the result of the immature state of the central nervous system (CNS) before the final cortical architecture, synaptic networks, and myelination have been attained.

Newborns rarely have well-organized, generalized tonic-clonic seizures; instead, their seizures are characterized by multifocality, asynchrony, disorganized pattern of propagation, and subtle oral-buccal, bicycling, stepping, pedaling, or ocular movements. However, none of the clinical characteristics is specific; based on the characteristics of movements only, events associated with gastroesophageal reflux or those during sleep are often clinically indistinguishable from seizures. Information about the setting in which they occur, reactivity to external stimuli, associated features, and electroencephalographic (EEG) characteristics is more specific.

Jitteriness is a nonepileptic movement with rhythmical tremor as a dominant movement that can be stopped by restraint, is not accompanied by autonomic changes or ocular signs, and is especially sensitive to stimulus. Benign neonatal sleep myoclonus occurs only during sleep. The phenomenon disappears spontaneously, and the child's development is normal. Tonic fits associated with gastroesophageal reflux are linked to feeding. Hyperekplexia (familial startle syndrome) is a nonepileptic disorder characterized by abnormal response to unexpected stimuli associated with sustained tonic spasms or exaggerated startle with additional generalized hypertonia.

The main causes of epileptic seizures include hypoxia-ischemia, intracerebral hemorrhage, brain infarction, metabolic disorders (ie, hypoglycemia, hypomagnesemia, hypocalcemia), infection, inborn error of metabolism, congenital malformation, genetic predisposition, neonatal abstinence syndrome from in utero drug exposure, and pyridoxine dependency. An important point to keep in mind is that several factors that may contribute to the onset of seizures in a single infant. Because most neonatal seizures occur in a provoked setting, when the provocative factor is corrected, they are usually short lived.

Benign familial and nonfamilial neonatal seizures are neonatal epileptic syndromes defined by a favorable outcome.[7] The classical phenotype of benign familial seizures is a neonate born after an uneventful pregnancy and delivery with onset of tonic-clonic seizures during the first 2 weeks of life, intact neurologic function in between seizures, and a family history of seizures (autosomal-dominant inheritance). In the absence of family history and an identifiable cause, when seizures in an otherwise-healthy neonate appear between 3 and 7 days of age *(fifth-day fits),* diagnosis of benign neonatal nonfamilial convulsions can be proposed. The interictal EEG pattern is either normal or moderately altered.[8] Both syndromes can only be diagnosed after excluding provocative factors.

Early infantile epileptic encephalopathy and early myoclonic encephalopathy are severe neonatal epilepsies characterized by onset during the first days or weeks of life, severe seizures that do not respond to medication, a burst-suppression EEG pattern, and a poor prognosis.

In addition to the laboratory tests that should be performed urgently (determination of blood glucose sodium, potassium, calcium, phosphorus, and magnesium levels; lumbar puncture), the work-up includes EEG and imaging studies (preferably magnetic resonance imaging). The need for further, more extensive work-up is determined by the results of the initial tests.

Clinical observations and the precise characterization of neonatal seizures form the basis for their rational evaluation and therapy. Treatment strategy and duration should be based on the cause and severity of seizures. Treatment based on the specific cause of seizures should always be considered first. The initial antiepileptic medications are phenobarbital, followed by phenytoin and diazepam. Duration of treatment depends on the etiology; it is short term for a short-term condition (acute injuries) and long term for the severe epileptic syndromes. Medications are usually provided for 2 to 3 months.

DISORDERS OF MUSCLE TONE AND MOVEMENTS

Tone refers to resistance of skeletal muscles to passive movement and also to muscle tension at rest. Tone deficiency, or *hypotonia,* is one of the most frequent neurologic signs in the neonate. It can be caused by a dysfunction at any level of the nervous system, from the muscles to the cortex of the brain, and it can result from drugs administered to the mother (benzodiazepines) or from genetic or metabolic disorders (Box 106-3). Initial assessment that focuses on the presence or absence of reflexes, weakness, associated systemic signs, and dysmorphic features is helpful. Based on the combination of answers to these simple questions, planning of further work-up and treatment can be approached.

Infant botulism and some neonatal myasthenic syndromes are treatable but potentially life-threatening disorders of the neuromuscular junction. Therefore the clinician needs to recognize the symptoms of these conditions early.

BOX 106-3 Main Causes of Neonatal Hypotonia

- Muscle diseases (myopathies, dystrophies)
- Neuromuscular junction diseases (myasthenia gravis, botulism)
- Lower motor neuron or peripheral nerve diseases (spinal muscular atrophy)
- Central nervous system disorders (acute injuries or congenital)
- Metabolic disorders (amino acid, organic acid, lactic acid, glycogen storage disorder)
- Chromosomal disorders (Down syndrome, Prader-Willi syndrome)
- Endocrine disorders (hypothyroidism)

Myasthenic infants are hypotonic and weak, although their deep-tendon reflexes are present. Transient neonatal myasthenia occurs in 10% to 15% of infants born to myasthenic mothers as a result of transplacental transfer of circulating anti–acetylcholine receptor antibodies from the mother to the fetus. The severity of the mother's disease has no relationship to the severity of the neonate's disease. Symptoms typically appear within the first day of life with hypotonia, feeding difficulties, trouble breathing, feeble cry, facial weakness, and oculomotor problems. Diagnosis is confirmed by clinical response to anticholinesterase medications and, if needed, by electromyelography. The condition is self-limiting; it completely resolves within a few weeks and does not recur. Treatment is with anticholinesterase inhibitors and supportive.[9]

Congenital myasthenic syndromes represent a heterogeneous group of nonautoimmune diseases caused by genetic defects that affect neuromuscular transmission. Infants are born to nonmyasthenic mothers. Response to anticholinesterase inhibitors is variable. A classification system of congenital myasthenic syndromes based on molecular genetics is being drawn up.[10,11]

Botulism occurs when ingested spores of *Clostridium botulinum* colonize and grow in the infant's large intestine and produce botulinum neurotoxin. It causes constipation, weakness (notably of gag, cry, suck, and swallow), ptosis, autonomic (pupillary) abnormalities, loss of muscle tone, and difficulty breathing. Symptoms typically appear between 18 and 36 hours after the infant is infected by the bacteria and between 3 weeks and 6 months of life. A human-derived botulism antitoxin, intravenous botulism immunoglobulin, is a safe and effective treatment that has been licensed by the US Food and Drug Administration as BabyBIG.[12] Treatment should be provided as soon as possible because its efficacy may decrease over time as motor-nerve intoxication proceeds.

Spinal muscular atrophy is one of the most common neuromuscular disorders in childhood; it is progressive and lethal. Pathologically, spinal muscular atrophy is characterized by degeneration of anterior horn cells of the cord and of the bulbar motor nuclei. The affected infants are hypotonic, weak, and areflexic. They have problems feeding as a result of weakness of their intercostal muscles, and they have trouble breathing. Cognition and facial expression are normal. Infants rarely survive beyond the first 2 years of life. A genetic blood test confirms diagnosis and should be performed early to guide the family appropriately.

In primary disorders of the muscle (congenital myopathy, congenital dystrophy, myotonic dystrophy), neonates are weak and areflexic. Myotonic dystrophy is an autosomal-dominant condition; examination of the mother can confirm the clinical suspicion. These diseases are chronic, and the care in the neonatal period is supportive. Genetic testing is available for myotonic dystrophy. Muscle biopsy is diagnostic for congenital myopathies and dystrophies. In severely hypotonic infants with paraplegia and urinary retention, spinal cord injury should be ruled out by imaging.

Genetic or metabolic conditions in a hypotonic infant are considered based on dysmorphic features, systemic signs, presence of deep-tendon reflexes, and often absence of weakness. Neonatal hypotonia or floppiness at birth in an infant with weak cry and decreased activity are highly suggestive of Prader-Willi syndrome (PWS). This disorder occurs in 1 in 10,000 to 15,000 live births and should be considered in any neonate who exhibits generalized hypotonia. Infants with PWS frequently have a history of breech or other abnormal presentation, decreased or atypical fetal movement patterns, excessive sleepiness, poor sucking reflexes, and feeding difficulties in the newborn period. PWS is caused by abnormally imprinted genes on chromosome 15 inherited from the father. Profound hypotonia may lead to severe respiratory compromise. Other common features include a weak cry and genital hypoplasia (cryptorchidism, small penis, scrotal hypoplasia, small labia minora and clitoral hypoplasia). Molecular genetic testing is required to confirm the diagnosis.[13]

Some hypotonic infants have CNS disorders, and in these cases, hypotonia is accompanied by other signs of CNS involvement, such as lethargy or seizures. Decrease in muscle tone is an immediate response to severe CNS injury. Increased tone is a delayed consequence. Therefore hypertonia, which is a common neurologic problem in children, is far less common in neonates. Acute CNS injury of any cause (vascular, metabolic, infectious) can cause a depression of nervous functions during the initial phase. Motor responsiveness improves and an increase in tone develops over the course of weeks.

Hypertonia refers to increased resistance to passive movement and is caused by a lesion between the cerebral cortex and the anterior horn cells at the level of the spinal cord. The syndrome of upper motor-neuron dysfunction consists of increased muscle tone, weakness, and hyperreflexia. Topographic distribution of the weakness and hypertonia vary. They typically develop in the form of diplegia in the preterm neonate and in the form of either hemi- or quadriplegia in the term neonate. Catastrophic events are treated in neonatal intensive care units. The primary care physician must formulate rehabilitative strategies to reduce morbidity and to facilitate optimal development.

Hypoxia-reperfusion in both preterm and term infants is one of the main causes of upper motor-neuron syndrome.[14] Interestingly, the same pathophysiological event that causes similar long-term consequences also causes different types and patterns of cellular injury at different ages. Selective neuronal necrosis that is most prominent in the watershed areas is the pathological substrate in the term neonate. Lesions in a periventricular distribution in the white matter are the pathological equivalent in the preterm baby.

Cerebrovascular accidents (ischemic or hemorrhagic) lead to focal brain lesions and therefore focal, lateralized signs of upper motor dysfunction (hemiparesis). Contrary to the acute and catastrophic presentation of stroke in older children and adults, many neonates follow a different clinical scenario. They have normal neonatal neurologic history and remain asymptomatic during the first few months of life. Development of early hand preference during the first year of life or seizures (or both) is usually the first sign of their impairment. Of particular importance, the primary care physician should initiate a thorough neurologic evaluation of these infants immediately and promptly. Most neonatal strokes are arterial in origin but can also result from sinovenous thrombosis, coagulation abnormalities, certain genetic mutations, perinatal complications or cardiac anomalies. Neonates with stroke usually have more than one risk factor. The overall risk of recurrence is low.

Germinal matrix intraventricular hemorrhage is the most common variety of brain injury in premature infants. Its occurrence is inversely related to gestational age and birth weight. Primary injury and destruction of the glial precursors have a direct influence on the subsequent stages of brain maturation. Accelerated cell death of these reversibly injured neurons occurs through a variety of secondary injury mechanisms (excitotoxicity, oxidative stress, inflammation) and is a potential therapeutic target.

Feeding difficulties occur in a variety of clinical settings. Encephalopathies of different causes, disorders of the peripheral nerve, neuromuscular junction or muscles, congenital malformations (Möbius syndrome, Chiari malformation), focal posterior fossa tumors, and laryngeal paralysis can all cause feeding problems. Congenital isolated pharyngeal dysfunction is a self-limiting disorder that is diagnosed by exclusion; it can be severe and may persist for months.

Decreased arm movement and asymmetric Moro reflex are commonly caused by *brachial plexus injury*. Brachial plexus injury occurs typically in large babies, frequently with shoulder dystocia or breech delivery. Erb palsy (cervical roots 5 and 6) is the most common form and exhibits with the arm being adducted, prone, and internally rotated as a result of weakness of the shoulder abduction, elbow flexion, and supination. Grasp is usually present. Klumpke paralysis (C7 and C8, T1) results in the weakness of the hand muscles, absent grasp, and sometimes Horner syndrome. Total Brachial plexus palsy involves both upper and lower roots.

The site and type of brachial plexus injury determine the prognosis. Most patients have the least severe form of nerve injury neurapraxia and recover spontaneously with a 90% to 100% return of function within 3 to 4 months. Treatment includes occupational or physical therapy and is directed toward prevention of contractures. Avulsion, the most severe form of the injury, is rare. Surgical exploration should be considered in infants who do not experience sufficient recovery within 3 months.[15]

INJURIES OF THE HEAD AND SKULL

Caput succedaneum, cephalohematoma, and linear fractures are rarely associated with intracranial disease and are self-limiting. *Ping-pong fracture* is a form of depressed skull fracture associated with the inward buckling of the bone, often without a fracture line. It is rarely associated with intracranial injuries and can often be corrected by nonsurgical techniques (eg, vacuum extractor, breast pump).

Potentially dangerous and treatable conditions are growing skull fracture and subgaleal hemorrhage. Growing skull fractures result from tearing of the dura and trapping of arachnoid and brain tissue in the fracture. The pulsatile force of the brain during its maximal growth causes the fracture in the thin skull to enlarge. These fractures commonly produce a progressive, often pulsatile, scalp mass that appears some time after head trauma during infancy. Imaging is diagnostic. Surgery is required to repair the dural tear.

Subgaleal hemorrhage is a rare but potentially lethal condition found in newborns.[16] It is caused by accumulation of the blood between the epicranial aponeurosis of the scalp and the periosteum. Because this space may hold a significant volume, subgaleal hemorrhage can lead to severe hypovolemia, which may result in death. The swelling, which appears as a fluctuant, boggy mass that develops over the scalp, develops gradually 12 to 72 hours after delivery. Subgaleal hemorrhage is most often associated with vacuum extraction and forceps delivery. Treatment consists of prompt and aggressive prevention of hypovolemic shock, and treatment of any associated coagulopathy.

SUGGESTED RESOURCES

Illingworth RS. *The Development of Infant and Young Child.* Edinburgh, Scotland: Churchill Livingstone; 1960.

Einspieler C, Prechtl H, Bos A, et al. Prectl's method on the qualitative assessment of the general movements in preterm, term and young infants. In: *Clinics in Developmental Medicine.* London, UK: Mac Keith Press; 2004.

Hantai D, Richard P, Koenig J, et al. Congenital myasthenic syndromes. *Curr Opin Neurol.* 2004;17:539-551.

REFERENCES

1. Illingworth RS. *The Development of Infant and Young Child.* Edinburgh, Scotland: Churchill Livingstone; 1960.
2. Einspieler C, Prechtl H, Bos A, et al. Prectl's method on the qualitative assessment of the general movements in preterm, term and young infants. In: *Clinics in Developmental Medicine.* London, UK: Mac Keith Press; 2004.
3. Precthl H. The neurological examination of the full term newborn infant. In: *Clinics in Developmental Medicine.* Baltimore, MD: Lippincott Williams and Wilkins; 1977.
4. Dubowitz L, Dubowitz V. The neurological assessment of the preterm and full term newborn infant. In: *Clinics in Developmental Medicine.* Baltimore, MD: Lippincott Williams and Wilkins; 1981.
5. Prechtl H. State of the art of a new functional assessment of the young nervous system. An early predictor of cerebral palsy. *Early Hum Dev.* 1997;50:1-11.
6. Mirzahi EM, Wantabe K. Symptomatic neonatal seizures. In: Roger J, Bureau M, Dravet C, et al, Eds. *Epilepsy Syndromes in Infancy, Childhood and Adolescence.* London, UK: John Libbey & Co Ltd; 2002.
7. Poulin P, Anderson VE. Benign familial and non-familial neonatal seizures. In: Roger J, Bureau M, Dravet C, Genton P, et al, eds. *Epilepsy Syndromes in Infancy, Childhood and Adolescence.* London, UK: John Libbey & Co Ltd; 2002.
8. Poulin P. Benign neonatal convulsions. In: Wasterlain CG, Vest P, eds. *Neonatal Seizures.* New York, NY: Raven Press; 1990.
9. Dubowitz V. Myasthenia. In: *Muscle Disorders in Childhood.* 2nd ed. Philadelphia, PA: WB Saunders; 2000.
10. Hantai D, Richard P, Koenig J, et al. Congenital myasthenic syndromes. *Curr Opin Neurol.* 2004;17:539-551.
11. Harper CM. Congenital myasthenic syndromes. *Semin Neurol.* 2004;24:111-123.

12. Arnon SS, Schechter R, Maslanka SE, et al. Human botulism immune globulin for the treatment of infant botulism. *N Engl J Med.* 2006;354:462-471.
13. Cassidy SB, Schwartz S. Prader-Willi syndrome. GeneReviews 2006. Available at: www.genetests.org/.
14. Inder TE, Volpe J. Mechanisms of perinatal brain injury. *Semin Neonatol.* 2000;5:3-16.
15. Volpe J. *Neurology of the Newborn.* 4th ed. Philadelphia, PA: WB Saunders; 2001.
16. Chadwick LM, Pemberton PJ, Kurinczuk JJ. Neonatal subgaleal haematoma: associated risk factors, complications and outcome. *J Paediatr Child Health.* 1996;32: 228-232.

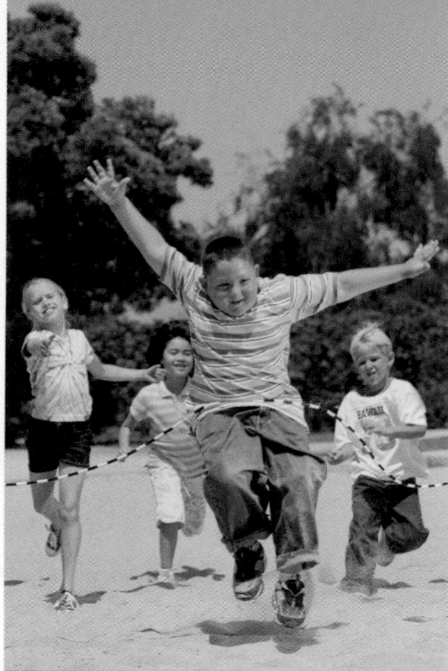

PART 6

Psychosocial Issues in Child Health Care

Section One: Psychological and Social Development of Children

107 Theories and Concepts of Development
108 Mental Health of the Young: An Overview
109 Early Education and Child Care Programs
110 Family-centered Care in Pediatric Practice
111 Principles of Effective Discipline

Section Two: Factors Influencing the Psychosocial Health of Children

112 Changing American Families
113 Adoption
114 Child Custody
115 Children of Divorce
116 Children in Foster and Kinship Care
117 Domestic Violence and the Family
118 Gay- and Lesbian-parented Families
119 Homelessness and the Family
120 Child Physical Abuse and Neglect
121 Children in Self-care
122 Sexual Abuse of Children
123 Children, Adolescents, and the Media

Section Three: School Health

124 Overview of School Health and School Health Program Goals
125 School Health Education
126 Nursing Roles in School Health
127 School Readiness
128 School Absenteeism and School Refusal
129 School Learning Problems and Developmental Differences

Section Four: Emotional and Behavioral Problems

130 A Developmental Approach to the Prevention of Common Behavioral Problems
131 Consultation and Referral for Emotional and Behavioral Problems
132 Options for the Delivery of Mental Health Services
133 Medication Management for Emotional and Behavioral Problems
134 Family Interactions: Children Who Have Unexplained Physical Symptoms
135 Anorexia and Bulimia Nervosa

Continued

Section Four: Emotional and Behavioral Problems—cont'd

136 Autism
137 Attention-deficit/Hyperactivity Disorder
138 Conduct Disorders
139 Conversion Reactions and Hysteria
140 Children With Gender-variant Behaviors and Transgender Youth
141 Substance Use Disorders: Evaluation and Management
142 Encopresis
143 Mood Disorders
144 Münchausen Syndrome by Proxy
145 Phobias and Anxiety
146 Posttraumatic Stress Disorder
147 Stuttering
148 Sleep Disturbances
149 Suicide and Suicide Attempts in Adolescents
150 Temper Tantrums and Breath-holding Spells

Psychological and Social Development of Children

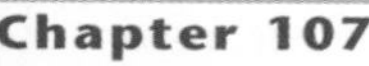

Chapter 107

THEORIES AND CONCEPTS OF DEVELOPMENT

Tasha C. Geiger, PhD; Olle Jane Z. Sahler, MD

"Developmentalists are not only interested in defining the determinants of human growth but also in changing the limits of human potential."[1]

No unified developmental theory, by itself, completely explains how individuals grow, change, and learn as they get older. A collective examination of several theories, however, enables the medical community to understand and interpret behaviors common to a particular developmental stage. With this framework, interpreting a child's behavior to parents in a developmental context and devising strategies that can help children and their families cope effectively with common stressful situations becomes possible.

The ever-developing personality style and cognitive functioning of the child require continual reevaluation and renegotiation of any treatment regimen, regardless of whether a child's problem is physical or the result of a combination of physical and emotional elements. However, this very fluidity and malleability often make it possible to intervene successfully with a child when it would be impossible with an adult. Helping the child rejoin a more adaptive developmental pathway before maladaptive behaviors become fixed is one of the rewards of working with children. Primary prevention is a realistic goal. Conversely, the child's relatively unformed and fragile sense of self is particularly vulnerable to outside influences that might have little or no effect on the adult. Thus the practitioner has an obligation to evaluate not only the child, but also the child's social network to identify and help eliminate impediments to the child's realization of his or her fullest potential. In this context, the practitioner, as developmentalist, can become a knowledgeable and effective advocate for someone who is too young, inexperienced, and politically naive to speak as an independent individual.

The generally accepted view now is that the nature versus nurture debate is moot. Asking whether a behavioral phenomenon is due to heredity *or* environment misses the point. Instead, current research supports an integrated perspective that appreciates the complex interplay among biological factors and environmental conditions (family, peers, and social group) in shaping the individual throughout development. The emphasis on genetic material as the driving force in development has been supplanted by a more comprehensive developmental systems view in which genes are only one part of the developing organism.[2] Although genes were thought to be the predominant underlying factor in species-typical development (eg, that humans generally have 2 legs, 2 arms, a visual system that operates in a particular way, a brain ready to receive important perceptual information), the role of typical experience has been identified as equally influential in terms of its effect on genetic material, brain development, and behavioral outcomes.[2-4]

Current theories of development rely on theory and research in a variety of disciplines, including genetics, embryology, and biology.[5,6] These theories incorporate a systems or organismic perspective in which development is characterized by mutual influence between different levels of the organism (eg, genes, cells, systems, organism, behavior, environment) that result in a higher level of organization. New structures, functions, systems, and behaviors occur as a result of 2 or more elements of the organism interacting over time and becoming more highly organized. Interactions occur within levels, such as cells interacting with other cells or organisms interacting with other organisms, as well as between levels, such as genes interacting with cytoplasm and the organism interacting with the environment.[2]

Before examining the interaction of biological and environmental influences in development, an important point to consider is the nature of this interaction. In developmental models, the term *transaction, mutual influence,*[7,8] or *coaction*[2] is generally used in place of *interaction*. An interaction occurs when variable A influences variable B or vice versa. In contrast, transaction refers to the idea that when variable A influences variable B, variable B is now altered in some important way. This new *altered* variable B now interacts with variable A. For example, if genes impart an influence on the surrounding cytoplasm, then this *newly changed* cytoplasm will now influence the genetic material, eliciting or hindering the development of proteins.

BEHAVIORAL GENETICS PERSPECTIVE

In recent years, the field of behavioral genetics has begun to address the issue of *how* (rather than if) heritable predispositions interact with environmental factors to influence the developmental trajectory. Key constructs include gene-environment correlation, gene-environment interaction, and shared and nonshared environment (Box 107-1 and Box 107-2).

For example, the development of intelligence, or general cognitive ability, is considered as a strong determinant of developmental outcome. What determines intelligence? Correlations among pairs of individuals show that similarity of IQ scores depend on the closeness of the genetic relationship.[9] However informative, a study of the correlation between IQ scores of genetically related individuals does not disentangle genetic and environmental contributions. For example, parents in a family study are *genetic-plus-environment* parents in that they share both heredity (through genetic transmission) and environment (living situation, experiences, resources) with their offspring.

Adoption studies offer one method of distinguishing genetic from environmental sources of family resemblance as a result of passive gene-environment correlations. Adoption results in *genetic* (birth) parents and *environmental* (adoptive) parents. Resemblance between birth parents and their adopted-away offspring directly assesses the genetic contribution to parent-offspring resemblance. Resemblance between adoptive parents and children provides an estimate of the environmental contribution to parent-offspring resemblance. In these studies, *genetic* siblings are full siblings adopted apart early in life into different homes; *environmental* siblings are genetically unrelated children adopted early in life into the same adoptive home.

Figure 107-1 summarizes adoption results for general cognitive ability. *Genetic* parents and offspring and *genetic* siblings significantly resemble each other,

BOX 107-1 Interplay of Heredity and Environment

Given the complexity of the developmental process, genetic and environmental contributions are likely interrelated. Two principal ways exist of understanding how genetic and environmental factors operate together: (1) genotype-environment correlation and (2) interaction.

GENOTYPE-ENVIRONMENT CORRELATION

Three types of genotype-environment correlation are commonly described: (1) passive, (2) evocative, and (3) active.[a,b,c]

Passive genotype–environment correlation results simply from each parent sharing 50% of either parent's genes with the children and parents providing the environment in which their children live. Therefore any correlation between the child's genotype and the environment may occur because the environment provided by the parents is also correlated with the parents' genotypes. Passive genotype–environment correlation is likely to be most important in infancy and early childhood, when the parent is the primary source of environmental influences. When the child's genotype evokes a response from the environment, *evocative* genotype-environment correlation is said to have occurred. For example, a child who has a difficult temperament is likely to elicit responses from others that signal anger or frustration.

Active genotype–environment correlation occurs when individuals actively seek out environments that are correlated with their genotype. Using the same example of difficult temperament, a child who is difficult and aggressive may be more likely to select peers who are also aggressive, increasing the likelihood not only of fitting in, but also of increasing the child's problem behaviors.

GENOTYPE-ENVIRONMENT INTERACTION

In a gene-environment interaction, a genetic factor expresses itself more readily in some environments than it does in others. For example, a study of couples at genetic risk for alcohol abuse indicated that only couples with marital dysfunction actually succumbed to the genetic predisposition.

[a]Schore AN. Affect Regulation and the Origin of the Self: The Neurobiology of Emotional Development. Hillsdale, NJ: Erlbaum Associates;1994.
[b]Rothbart J, Ahadi SA. Temperament and the development of personality. J Abnorm Pyschol 1994;103:55-66.
[c]Suomi SJ. Genetic and maternal contributions to individual differences in rhesus monkey biobehavioral development. In: Krasnegor NA, Blass EM, Hofer MA, eds. Perinatal Development: A Psychobiological Perspective. San Diego, CA: Academic Press;1987.

BOX 107-2 Shared and Nonshared Environment

SHARED ENVIRONMENT

Refers to all environmental factors that contribute to similarity among family members on some measured attribute.

NONSHARED ENVIRONMENT

Refers to all environmental factors that contribute to dissimilarity among family members on some measured attribute.

ESTIMATING SHARED AND NONSHARED ENVIRONMENT

A direct test of *shared family environment* is resemblance among adoptive relatives. Why do genetically unrelated adoptive *siblings* correlate approximately 0.25 for general cognitive ability in childhood? The answer must be *shared family environment* because adoptive siblings are unrelated genetically. Identical twins provide a direct test of *nonshared environment*. Because they are identical genetically, differences within pairs of identical twins can only be the result of nonshared environment. Genetic designs incorporating siblings varying in genetic relatedness also permit indirect estimates of nonshared environment. First, heritability is estimated by comparing correlations of pairs of identical twins, fraternal twins, full siblings, half siblings, and adoptive or step siblings. Shared family environment is estimated as family resemblance *not* explained by genetics. Nonshared environment is the rest of the variance, which also includes measurement error.

even though they are adopted apart and do not share family environment. Genetics accounts for approximately one half of the resemblance in cognitive ability for *genetic-plus-environmental* parents and siblings. The other half of familial resemblance appears to be explained by family environment, assessed by the resemblance between adoptive parents and adopted children and between adoptive siblings. Approximately one half of the environmental influence appears to be accounted for by shared environmental factors.

The effects of *shared environment* on cognitive ability decrease during childhood to negligible levels by adolescence; the heritability of general cognitive ability increases during the life span.[9] This circumstance is a prime example of the relative nature of the index of heritability. That is, the relative contributions of genetic factors and environmental factors change throughout the life span, meaning that genetic effects are *not* set in stone from the moment of conception.

Genetics studies, such as those on intelligence described previously, continue to point to the importance of the environment as directly contributing to a variety of developmental outcomes. Environmental factors also play an important indirect role through correlation and interaction with genetic factors in shaping development (see Box 107-1). For children and adolescents, most immediate environmental influences come from the family, school, and peer systems.

Family

Traditional approaches to studying the role of a child's environment in the child's development assumed that children in the same family share similar environmental influences, such as opportunities for learning and child-rearing attitudes. Behavioral genetics research, however,

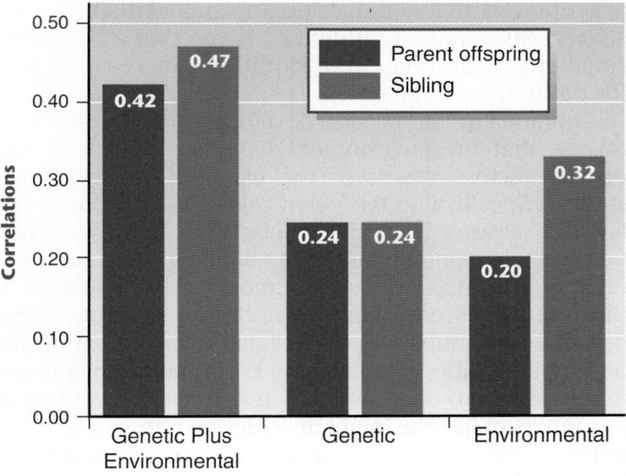

Figure 107-1 Adoption data indicate that family resemblance for cognitive ability is due both to genetic resemblance and to environmental resemblance. *Genetic* relatives refer to genetically related relatives adopted apart. *Environmental* relatives refer to genetically unrelated individuals adopted together. *(Loehlin JC. Partitioning environmental and genetic contributions to behavioral development.* Am Psychol. *1989;44:1285-1292. Reprinted by permission of the American Psychological Association.)*

consistently shows that family resemblance for various attributes is almost entirely the result of shared heredity rather than shared family environment.

Behavioral genetics research also reveals that siblings are surprisingly different from one another, despite their genetic relatedness[10] and their upbringing in the *same* family environment.[11] One factor that may contribute to sibling dissimilarity is the *difference* in the set of experiences (nonshared environment) siblings undergo, both within and outside the family. For example, within families, siblings differ in how they perceive parental affection, parenting practices, and sibling relationships; outside the family, siblings experience different relationships with teachers and peers. Thus family environment may not contribute in major ways to the *resemblance* of family members with respect to psychological or behavioral attributes, but such factors are likely to determine developmental outcome by contributing to *differences* among family members through *nonshared* influences.

Reiss et al[12] have recently reported the results of a study assessing 720 adolescents, their closest-in-age sibling, and their caregivers at 2 points in time: early and late adolescence. The adolescent outcomes studied were competency (cognitive and social competence, self-worth) and psychological compromise (depression and antisocial behavior).

Parents reported that they treat their children similarly, particularly when monitoring behavior. Parents also reported that the siblings treat each other similarly. In the siblings' eyes, parents treat them each differently, and they treat each other differently. Raters of family process tended to agree more with the children, suggesting that siblings, despite living in the same family, experience different parent-child and sibling relationship environments.[12] Furthermore, the data show strong associations between the quality of these *nonshared* aspects of various relationship environments and such domains of adolescent adjustment as antisocial behavior, depressive symptoms, sociability, autonomy, and self-worth. Negativity and conflict within the mother-child, father-child, and sibling relationship were associated with poor adjustment; in contrast, warm nurturing relationships were associated with positive adjustment. However, the most notable effect of *shared* environment was on sociability. In this instance, the most important environmental factors appeared to be school and peers.[12]

Genetic factors have been found to account for more than 50% of the variance among measures of adolescent adjustment. Previous psychosocial studies have found comparably sized influences of family process (ie, environmental effects) on adolescent adjustment. How can these potentially contradictory findings be reconciled?

Behavioral genetics studies have pointed to a genetic influence on apparently environmental factors such that genes are associated with the types of environments to which individuals are exposed.[13,14] The process by which this phenomenon occurs is through genotype-environment correlations and interactions, described in Box 107-2. In the case of the Reiss et al[12] study, the possibility exists that genetically influenced characteristics in the adolescent evoke parental responses (an example of an evocative gene-environment correlation) that, in turn, contribute to psychosocial outcomes for the adolescent. As a result, genetic influences play a role in factors typically considered *environmental.*

Shared and nonshared environments are not limited to family environments. Experiences outside the family, such as in school and with peers, also can be shared or not shared by siblings.[15]

School

The 2 basic functions of school are education and socialization. The most crucial social goals of early schooling are the facilitation of individuation from the family, control of gross-motor activity to achieve decorum in the classroom, mastery of the skills necessary to read and write, and reinforcement of qualities that promote the educational process, such as cooperation, completion of tasks, and respect for others.

In elementary school, the results of school achievement tests are influenced strongly (approximately 60%) by the shared environment and influenced modestly (approximately 30%) by genetic factors. However, later in the school years, the contribution from genetic influence increases in importance, and that from shared environment decreases. This same phenomenon is seen for cognitive ability in general.[16]

Peer Group

Peers model behavior, help determine value systems, and provide the security of group identity. Most children have developed a characteristic way of relating to peers, independently seeking friendships and engaging in social activities by approximately age 3 years. Early friendships are based on proximity (the child next door). Later, the classroom is the major source of friends. Finally, friendships become defined by mutual interests.

Friendship becomes more enduring as children grow older.[17] Friendships perceived as intimate are most likely to endure, and good friends tend to be of similar age, gender, and peer status. During adolescence, the peer group may be more influential than the family in determining social activities and values. In some instances, adolescents deliberately choose a peer group that has values antithetical to those of their parents. This process of strong group identification coupled with conflict with parents helps them individuate from the family, a major goal of late adolescence.

RECALLING A BROAD DEVELOPMENTAL PERSPECTIVE

The transaction of genetic and environmental influences in developmental outcomes is quite complex. Investigations such as the Reiss study,[12] new quantitative molecular genetics methods,[14] and complicated research designs involving genetic and psychosocial influences outlined by Bronfenbrenner and Ceci[18] will likely serve as models for genetically informed psychosocial research. Such research will provide new insights into the interplay of genetic and environmental influences on the developmental trajectory of children and have important clinical implications for pediatricians who provide anticipatory guidance.

A systems perspective is a reminder that a singular focus on proximal systems (eg, family, peers, school) may not provide a complete picture of environmental influences on development. Rather, these immediate contexts mutually influence each other and, as described by Bronfenbrenner and colleagues, are also influenced by broader, more distal environmental systems such as social class, cultural norms and beliefs, parental employment systems, neighborhoods, school boards, and community resources.[19,20]

Therefore the thorough practitioner must interpret behavioral genetics findings cautiously. Some researchers have mistakenly taken some behavioral genetics findings to indicate that parents and other family influences have little effect on children's personality, intelligence, or psychopathological characteristics.[21-23] However, current research, which takes genetic influences into account, points to the importance of general family factors and parenting strategies in children's development.[24] Furthermore, Rutter[13,14] points out the methodologic and conceptual flaws leading to such a misinterpretation of behavioral genetics studies. For example, common family influences that appear to be *shared* among family members (eg, family conflict, socioeconomic status) may actually have different effects on different family members, resulting in *nonshared* effects. Similarly, commonly studied *nonshared* effects, (eg, peer or school influences) may, in fact, result in shared effects if they impart similar influences on siblings, which may particularly be the case for twins. Additionally, shared effects play an important role in the stability of individual differences over time (not generally examined in behavioral genetics studies), whereas nonshared influences tend to show significant effects only at any one time of measurement (often examined in behavior genetics studies). Finally, Rutter cautions practitioners to avoid overlooking small effect sizes of shared environment influences, given that a relatively small effect can relate to a significant increase in risk for pathological outcomes.

Additionally, a broad developmental perspective reveals that the environment has also influenced the *genetic* factors assessed, for example, in the Reiss study.[12] Specifically, the genetically influenced characteristics assessed in the adolescents represent the *outcome* of an ongoing interplay of genetic and environmental influences from the moment of conception through adolescence (and beyond). For example, early prenatal care influences the cellular environment of the developing embryo, influencing brain development and the expression of genetic material. During the first 18 months of life, the infant develops an attachment relationship with significant caregivers, and the quality of this social-emotional bond likely influences central nervous system development,[25] as well as early emotion and behavior regulation skills—the foundation of social and psychological adjustment.[26] Therefore, as early developmentalists have aptly pointed out, "The heredity and environment of an organism can be completely separated only in analytic thinking, for in actual nature such separation would lead to instant death of the organism, even though the philosopher making the analysis might himself survive."[24,27]

APPLYING A DEVELOPMENTAL PERSPECTIVE TO GENETIC AND ENVIRONMENTAL INTERPLAY: TEMPERAMENT AND ATTACHMENT

Despite the contention that heredity and the environment are inseparable, many studies appear to be designed to present evidence falling on one side or the other of this dichotomy—reflecting perhaps the complexity of the processes by which these influences shape development. For example, consider temperament, defined as "constitutionally based individual differences in reactivity and self-regulation"[28] that likely have clear neurologic underpinnings.[29] Certainly, research supporting the heritability of temperament and even personality can be found.[30,31] Furthermore, studies show that early temperament variables are associated with later behavior problems.[32] However, several studies also provide support for the strong role of environmental influences, such as those indicating that parenting styles and the parent-child relationship are related to a variety of child outcomes.[33,34]

In this regard, Chess and Thomas[32] suggested early on that the *match* between a child's temperamental style with the demands and expectations of the child's environment influences functional outcome, with mismatches being associated with increased risk of behavioral and emotional disorders. For example, quiet, easygoing parents may have an energetic, excitable child whom they want to be similar to themselves because that is their expectation for appropriate child behavior. This situation is even more likely to arise if the child has a quiet sibling whose disposition is similar to that of the parents.

As another example of the transaction between individual child characteristics and the caregiving environment, researchers found that infants with a difficult temperament often have mothers who exhibit more negative behaviors concerning visual contact, stimulation, physical contact, soothing, and responsiveness.[35] This situation is perhaps an example of an evocative gene environment correlation. That is, these genetic predispositions (temperamental characteristics) are not the only factors that determine the child's ultimate personality. Thus understanding that, with intervention, the mothers can become more effective and responsive and their infants can become more sociable and able to soothe themselves, engage in more exploratory behavior, cry less, and exhibit more secure attachments with their caregivers is very reassuring to the practitioner.[35] This secure attachment relationship places even the child with a *difficult* temperament on a developmental pathway toward future competent outcomes.[26]

This consideration of the role of attachment (the social-emotional bond between an infant and a primary caregiver) in child development offers an ideal example of the developmental systems model. Attachment relationships are characterized in terms of the nature and quality of the mutual relationship that is created. A secure attachment develops from a pattern of consistent, sensitive caregiver responses to a variety of infant cues.[7] Research in this area consistently reveals that the pattern of mutual influence between the child and the parent (rather than the child's *genetically predisposed* temperament or the parent's *genetically predisposed* personality) plays the major role in determining, for example, the child's self-concept, internalizing and externalizing problems, and moral development.[7]

PSYCHOLOGICAL DEVELOPMENT: KEY POINTS

A behavioral genetics approach highlights that:

1. Both parents play important roles in determining developmental outcomes.
2. Given the possibility of separating genetic and environmental influences, similarities in siblings may be primarily due to heredity, whereas differences may be primarily due to nonshared environment effects.
3. Siblings' experiences with their parents appear to be different (nonshared environment), even if parents believe they treat all their children the same way.
4. Sibling dyads appear to experience each other differently (nonshared environment), whereas parents think siblings behave reciprocally with one another.

A general developmental perspective emphasizes that:

1. Each child is the product of complex interrelationships between genetic and environmental influences. Neither biological nor environmental factors are considered to be the primary influence on developmental outcomes.
2. Although the origins of some personality traits, types of psychopathology, and degree of educational attainment may lie in the genes, onset, change, and continuity of these outcomes may be the result of a "proximal risk mechanism [that] is environmentally mediated, and hence may be amendable to interventions through treatment."[14]
3. Family, school, and peers play key roles in determining developmental outcomes, as do more distal contextual factors such as social support, parental marital status, socioeconomic status, media, community resources, and neighborhoods.
4. The quality of the relationships between parent and child and between siblings influences adjustment. Thus the pediatrician should guide parents who feel a *mismatch* with their child to interventions that will optimize parent-child interaction.

The general advice would be to identify, appreciate, and encourage each child's individual strengths; address weaknesses and challenging behavior with warmth and nurturance; minimize negativity and conflict; and support siblings in being kind to one another.

THEORIES OF DEVELOPMENT

The basis for even extremely atypical or pathological behavior becomes understandable with a good understanding of typical or normative development. Because no single theory explains all aspects of psychological development, examining behavior from a variety of perspectives has become customary (see Figure 107-2 for a summary).

Several overriding concepts provide a framework for understanding developmental processes.[2,5,6] (1) Development refers to the idea that cognitive, biological, social, and emotional systems mutually influence each other and become more complexly

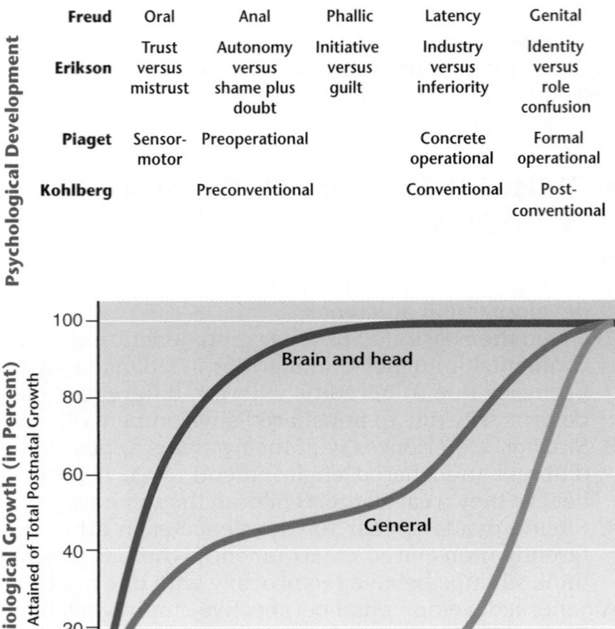

Figure 107-2 Psychological and physiological growth and development. *([Top] Sahler OJ, McAnarney ER.* The Child from Three to Eighteen. *St Louis, MO: Mosby; 1981. [Bottom, modified] Tanner JM.* Growth at Adolescence, With a General Consideration of the Effects of Hereditary and Environmental Factors Upon Growth and Maturation From Birth to Maturity. *Oxford, UK: Blackwell Scientific Publications; 1962. Reprinted by permission of Olle Jane Z. Sahler and Blackwell Publishing.)*

interdependent and organized into meaningful systems (eg, the attachment system, personality) over time. (2) The study of normative development is essential to the understanding of deviant development. (3) Certain tasks or requirements are normative for a particular age group.[5,6] During infancy, for example, an important task is the formation of an attachment relationship with the caregiver,[36] whereas during middle childhood, critical accomplishments include successful negotiation of peer relationships, academic endeavors, and appropriate conduct.[37] Some children are able to perform these tasks at a younger chronologic age (ie, they are early developers); others are unable to perform these tasks until they reach an older chronologic age (ie, they are late developers). (4) Finally, development is conceptualized as proceeding along a path, and the pattern of adaptation is examined over time.[36,38,39] Specifically, children are thought to manage current situations and challenges with the cognitive, social, biological, and emotional resources, skills, and knowledge gained through earlier negotiations with critical developmental tasks. For example, an individual who was not successful at maintaining adequate relationships with peers during childhood may lack a solid foundation for the development of later positive, fulfilling romantic relationships. The pathway model aptly depicts how failure at these important developmental tasks, though not necessarily signifying a pathological abnormality, does serve as an indicator that an individual may be on a deviant pathway, with increased risk for further maladaptive behavior. The longer an individual remains on this deviant pathway, the more difficult is the task of returning to a normal, typical developmental progression.[50] Developmental outcomes, however, are "probabilistic" (eg, Gottlieb, 1991)[2] in that movement from a deviant pathway is always possible, but the probability of this change occurring is constrained by the individual's current circumstances and previous history of adaptation.[36]

Examples of Specific Developmental Theories

The theory of psychosexual development is derived from Freud's retrospective analysis of childhood behaviors, particularly the early parent-child relationship, that he thought contributed to the neuroses for which his adult patients were seeking treatment. Based on the content of his patients' memories, Freud theorized that personality formation results from intrapsychic struggles experienced by an individual during maturation. This particular approach and the theoretical framework derived from it are limited in that (1) objective observations of current behavior are lacking, and (2) heavy emphasis is placed on explanations for the development of undesirable adult behaviors rather than on behavior in general. Despite these shortcomings, Freud and his work have had a formidable influence on generations of developmental psychologists.[40] The family triad of mother-father-child and, in particular, the early mother-child dyad were central to Freud's interpretations of later adult behaviors. Although pediatric psychology currently focuses largely on the individual in relation to a broader social unit than the family and on coping mechanisms rather than on defense mechanisms, Freud's discussions of conscious and unconscious motivations provide a unique framework for understanding observable behavior.

The total personality as conceived by Freud consists of 3 motivating forces: (1) the id, (2) the ego, and (3) the superego. The *id* is the foundation of the personality; its aim is to avoid pain and find satisfaction or pleasure. The *ego* is the intermediary system between the id and reality; it provides an accurate perception of what exists in the environment. On some occasions, fulfillment of pleasure as desired by the id may be suspended by the ego in acknowledgment of reality. The *superego* is the moral function of the personality; it is concerned with strivings for perfection rather than for pleasure or for responses that reflect reality.

Clinically, this conceptualization has relevance to psychosomatic illness, which is considered in this theoretical framework to be an example of pain or dysfunction resulting from the superego's displeasure with the individual.

Although behavior can be motivated by the drive to fulfill a variety of needs (eg, food, sleep), the major motivational system according to the psychosexual theory of development is *libido,* which is based in the instinctual (sexual) drive to preserve the species. Satisfaction of the sexual instinct is derived from stimulation or manipulation of both genital and nongenital body regions that have been called *erogenous zones.* Three primary erogenous zones, each with its associated vital need and presented in the chronologic order in which each gains prominence, are (1) the mouth and eating, (2) the anus and elimination, and (3) the genitalia and reproduction.

Activities involving the erogenous zones that individuals participate in to reduce tension (derive pleasure) may bring the child into conflict with the parents. The resulting frustrations and anxieties associated with these conflicts lead to the development of several adaptive maneuvers or defense mechanisms, such as regression or denial. Resolution of the conflict associated with a given stage allows the individual to progress to the next developmental stage. Thus Freud's conceptualization of development includes the principle that important tasks must be accomplished at each stage, and unsuccessful resolution of these tasks can lead to later emotional and behavioral difficulties. Freud conceptualized 5 psychosexual stages: (1) oral, (2) anal, (3) phallic, (4) latency, and (5) genital (adolescence or early adulthood).

Erikson and Psychosocial Development

Whereas Freud focused on internal drives as the force behind development, especially as the individual is shaped by the parent-child relationship, Erikson focused on the development of the individual within the wider context of the individual's historical-cultural-social milieu.[41] Thus Erikson's model begins to incorporate different levels of the environment, similar to Bronfenbrenner's bioecologic systems model addressed previously. For Erikson, unconscious motivation (id) exists, but the process of socialization (learning how to be an accepted and productive member of society) is key to development and determines outcome.

Erikson studied individuals and their families within the spheres of their everyday lives and at a particular moment in their cultural history. Also unlike Freudian theory, Erikson's theory focuses on an individual's potential for mastery by successfully resolving developmental crises, rather than on the potential for dysfunction from persistent psychological conflict.

Erikson conceptualized 8 ages, or stages, in human life extending, unlike Freud's theory, into late adulthood. The first 6 Eriksonian stages are a reformulation of their corresponding Freudian stages: (1) basic trust versus basic mistrust (oral), (2) autonomy versus shame and doubt (anal), (3) initiative versus guilt (phallic), (4) industry versus inferiority (latency), and the combination of (5) identity versus role confusion and (6) intimacy versus isolation (genital). The last 2 Eriksonian stages—generativity versus stagnation and ego integrity versus despair—deal with the specific developmental transitions of middle and old age. Similar to Freud, Erikson highlights central tasks that must be mastered at each stage of development.

Cognitive-Intellectual Theory: Piaget and Cognitive Development

Whereas psychodynamic theories are concerned primarily with internal, instinctual drives as a force for change, cognitive-intellectual theory is centered on the organism's active self-strivings in the process of acquiring and using knowledge.

According to Piagetian theory, cognitive development is the result of neurophysiological maturation, environmental stimulation, experience, and continual internal cognitive reorganization. Two major principles form the framework for Piaget's theory: (1) All species tend to organize or order their activities hierarchically, and (2) all species tend to incorporate new information or experiences into current cognitive structures through assimilation (incorporating new information into already existing ideas about the world) and accommodation (changing ideas about the world in response to new knowledge). For example, when infants are handed a set of small blocks for the first time, they are likely to bite or shake them. That is, they assume the new objects are similar to familiar objects (eg, nipples, rattles). This situation is an illustration of assimilation. Once children discover that blocks can be used to build a tower, they change their behavior and stack the blocks each time they are presented. This situation is an illustration of accommodation.

Piaget was concerned with describing the reasoning and conceptual ability of children of varying ages to understand how cognitive skills change over time. In seeking to identify universal developmental sequences in cognition, Piaget's theory is premised on a stepwise, ordered sequence of learning in response to experience. He defined 4 discrete stages from birth to adulthood: (1) sensorimotor, (2) preoperational, (3) concrete operational, and (4) formal operational.

Understanding the typical sequence of cognitive skills development as described by Piaget allows a person to assist individuals with learning difficulties. For example, children with autism often lack perspective-taking skills; early educational intervention can be effective in improving the outcomes of these children. An interventionist, however, should know which skills are characteristic of normally developing young children so as to identify the target child's strengths and weaknesses. This information helps determine the content and timing of the intervention. For example, attempting to teach a preschool child with autism metacognitive skills such as advanced perspective taking skills when these skills do not develop in normal children until years later would not be fruitful. Furthermore, understanding the sequence in which children acquire important conceptual skills allows the interventionist to plan academic instruction properly by ensuring that important prerequisite skills are attained before expecting the child to demonstrate competence in a more advanced area.

Finally, pediatricians with a clear knowledge of important cognitive, motor, physical, emotional, and social milestones (eg, developmental sequences and stages) would be able to determine readily when a patient's development is, indeed, atypical and in need of further evaluation or intervention.

Learning Theory

Learning theory is an outgrowth of behaviorism, or stimulus-response psychology. Following are some basic principles of learning theory:

1. Behavior (defined as observable actions of an organism) is learned; however, genetic factors and innate, involuntary reflexive behaviors influence this learning.
2. All types, patterns, and combinations of behavior can be learned as long as they are not incompatible physically.
3. Behavior can be conditioned or shaped.
4. Behavior is learned through reinforcement, which may be internal or external and positive or negative.
5. Learning results from many independent processes, including observation and imitation.

Behavior can be conditioned in 2 ways. In the process of *classical conditioning,* discovered by the Russian physiologist Pavlov, a reflex response associated in nature with one stimulus can be modified in such a way that it can be evoked by another stimulus. In Pavlov's original experiment, reflexive salivation in a dog at the sight of food could be induced eventually by the sound of a ringing bell, which, over a period, was *paired* with eating. In the process of *instrumental conditioning,* a nonreflexive behavior is learned because it is reinforced. For example, a rat in a cage might, by chance, depress a lever. If a pellet of food is released each time this action occurs, then the rat will *learn* to depress the lever and will do so with increasing frequency, especially when hungry.

Several features of conditioned behavior are important clinically. Conditioned behavior can be *extinguished,* or unlearned, if it is not reinforced; it can be *inhibited,* or counteracted, if it is followed by punishment or is not rewarded; it can be *partially reinforced* by inconsistent or random reinforcement; it can be *generalized* so that similar stimuli will elicit the same response; and it can be made *discriminatory* so that, by selective reinforcement, only one specific stimulus elicits the response.

According to this theoretical framework, an individual can be motivated to perform a certain behavior because of the positive effect (reinforcement) derived from it. Furthermore, an individual can be motivated *not* to perform a certain behavior because of the negative effect (punishment or lack of reinforcement) derived from it or because some other behavior gives more benefit. Finally, *shaping* is the process of molding a given behavior to be more similar to a desired behavior. This task is accomplished by positively reinforcing successive approximations of the desired behavior.

Social learning theory is a specialized area of behaviorism that stresses the dyadic nature of human behavior. Thus the child is in constant interaction with the environment and other individuals in this specific environment. The child's response to an environmental stimulus acts as a stimulus itself, which evokes a response from the environment or persons in this environment, and so on.[42]

Learning can also occur indirectly through observation and imitation of others who are having the actual experience. In *observational learning,* the individual watches others and modifies behavior in accord with the reinforcements others receive. *Imitative learning* occurs when the child imitates a desired model (eg, parent) and is positively reinforced with rewards that are either internal (being proud of oneself) or external (being praised by others).

If individuals learn by observational imitation, then modeling (demonstrating) is an especially important way to elicit a particular behavior. Models can be used to demonstrate everything from simple one-step behaviors to entire lifestyles (role models). Children and youth observe the behaviors of others and, based on how much they wish to identify with these others, will imitate their actions. Therefore certain behaviors often persist within families over generations, despite parental admonitions to the contrary.

RELATIONSHIP BETWEEN PHYSIOLOGICAL AND PSYCHOLOGICAL DEVELOPMENT

This section examines the child at different chronologic ages. From a broad developmental framework, psychological development and physiological maturation occur simultaneously and are interdependent. Several important principles of physical development that bear directly on psychological development can be summarized as follows:

1. Development is a continuous process that begins at conception.
2. Given that development is *canalized,* the sequence of physical development generally follows a predictable pattern. That is, individuals have a self-organizing or self-righting capacity such that biological (and psychological) development can proceed along a typical course, despite significant disruptive forces or conditions. Both biological (eg, genes) and environmental (eg, species-typical experiences) factors are responsible for this canalization.[2,3] However, the rate of acquisition of new structures, functions, and systems varies considerably, and different systems mature at different times.
3. Development of both involuntary (autonomic) and voluntary (motor) activity is related to maturation of the nervous system, and the developing nervous system is influenced by environmental factors such as maternal stress during fetal development[43] and the early caregiving environment,[25] as well as broad, species-typical experiences.[4]
4. Certain primitive reflexes (eg, stepping, grasping) must be *lost* before the corresponding voluntary (eg, walking, holding) movement is acquired.
5. Development occurs cephalocaudally.

Pregnancy

The bonds of parent-child attachment that eventually form are initiated during pregnancy. *Precursors of attachment* are physical and psychosocial changes that occur in couples anticipating the birth of their child. These changes have been researched best in pregnant women, but studies of men suggest that expectant fathers also experience emotional changes and share many of the same feelings as expectant mothers. Examples of such behaviors in pregnant women and expectant fathers[44] include changes in social patterns because of fatigue, alterations in economic planning (eg, less disposable income), and the accumulation of various material goods, such as a crib and baby clothes. Many expectant parents report a heightened sense of responsibility to keep the mother (and therefore the fetus) well and fit (eg, abstaining from tobacco, drugs, or alcohol) and to protect the father (eg, reducing risky behavior).

During pregnancy, a woman experiences physical and emotional changes within herself and the growth of the fetus. The physician can guide the expectant mother in 2 adaptive tasks: (1) acceptance of the pregnancy and (2) perception of the fetus as an individual.

Most women report strong emotional swings from positive to negative anticipation; they frequently feel ambivalent about the pregnancy. Perceiving the fetus as an individual usually commences with the first sensation of fetal movement, or *quickening*. If the original reaction to the pregnancy was predominantly negative (unplanned, unwanted), many women report heightened acceptance and noticeable changes in attitude when fetal movement is first felt. After quickening, women usually begin to have fantasies about the physical and personality characteristics they hope or fear the child will have.[45] As the time of delivery approaches, having a healthy baby is of increasing concern. Thus, should a child be born with a congenital defect, life threatening or not, the parents actually suffer the loss of their *expected* child, and some time may pass before they can reorganize their expectations and fully accept their child.

Birthing Process

Data relating to the birthing process suggest that mothers who are relaxed during labor and who have a supportive person assisting them are likely to have a shorter labor and to be more alert and interactive with their infant on first sight.[46] Being unconscious during birth does not appear to cause rejection of the infant, although systematic studies are lacking. What is known, however, is that the more difficult the labor is, the less likely the mother is to breastfeed.

Certain delivery procedures and administration of anesthetics can affect both the mother and the child at birth. For example, an infant who is physiologically depressed because of a narcotic given to the mother during delivery is more likely to respond poorly on initial contact or during feedings and be less stimulating to the mother.

Research on the behavior of fathers toward the newborn has shown that engrossment, absorption, and preoccupation with the infant occur in men as well as in women. A sense of increased self-esteem has also been reported among new fathers.[44,47]

Immediate Postpartum Period

The interval immediately after birth has been called the *maternal sensitive period*[45] and is characterized by reciprocal mother-infant interaction. The mother supplies touch, eye-to-eye (*en face*) contact, high-pitched voice, heat, and odor; the infant supplies eye-to-eye contact, odor, and entertainment and, if breastfeeding, stimulates maternal production of prolactin and oxytocin.

The mother's behaviors match certain infant needs. For example, the female voice is naturally high pitched, and the mother consciously makes it more so. This action fits the infant's sensitivity and attraction to speech in the high-frequency range. The infant's reflexive behaviors (suckling, clinging) are care eliciting; that is, they serve to bring the caregiver closer to the child and help maintain physical and emotional contact between them by mutual reinforcement. In turn, parental reinforcement behaviors (feeding, fondling) in response to the child's care-eliciting behaviors lead to further suckling and clinging. In this way, the infant's innate behaviors and the responses they generate in the caregiver initiate the attachment process.[48]

Indeed, bonding, an early manifestation of attachment, is usually discussed with reference to these mother-child interactions in the newborn period.[45] The recognition of potential impediments to bonding (use of anesthesia, separation of mother and infant) has led to major changes in obstetrical and newborn care.

Infancy

The period of infancy extends from birth to 24 months of age. The first year is marked by tremendous physical growth and the development of rudimentary skills, culminating in the ability to walk several steps unassisted and to speak 3 to 6 intelligible words. The second year is characterized by skill refinement. Some children can pedal a tricycle and speak in relatively complete, although syntactically poor, sentences. Infants also learn that other individuals inhabit their world and that these individuals come, go, and return. Finally, infants learn that they have a will and can manipulate their environment purposefully.

Emotional, social, and cognitive maturation are intricately interwoven with somatic growth. Of the many changes taking place, the principal psychological task mastered during infancy is attachment, a social-emotional bond between infant and caregiver resulting from a pattern of mutual interaction. Initially, the caregiver is responsible for regulating the emotional arousal of the infant by learning to interpret and manage the infant's physiological needs. As the infant's cognitive and physical capacities increase, emotion regulation becomes more dyadic. The infant begins to seek contact with the caregiver or display wariness at separation. Furthermore, separation anxiety—an emotional and behavioral response indicative that attachment has developed[7]—occurs after the child is cognitively able to recognize and discriminate among individuals. Therefore the display of this organized emotional attachment *system* is clearly dependent on physical maturity (to initiate proximity-seeking behaviors while exploring the environment), as well as increasing cognitive skills (to discriminate between self and others and to differentiate between caregivers).[7]

Through this dyadic regulation, in which the infant, with parental assistance, is successful at returning to a settled state after distress, the infant learns that expressing intense emotion need not be a disorganizing experience. The infant also learns to have confidence in the caregiver and to expect that personal actions will have an effect on the environment. Thus the foundation for emotion regulation, behavior regulation (eg, coping with emotional arousal), and the development of self-concept are beginning to become established.[7]

Psychosexual Development: Oral and Anal Stages

In Freudian or psychosexual terms, the child younger than 12 months is considered to be in the *oral stage* of development, so called because the mouth is the primary source of tension and pleasure. Satisfaction of hunger, as well as many comforting measures (eg, finger-sucking and mouthing), center on stimulation of the mouth.

The mouth has at least 5 primary modes of functioning that, in analytical theory, are prototypes for certain later personality types: (1) taking in (acquisitiveness), (2) holding on (tenacity), (3) biting (destructiveness), (4) spitting out (rejection), and (5) closing (negativism). The theory proposes that the extent to which any of these traits becomes part of the mature personality depends on the amount of anxiety or frustration the individual experienced with a particular function. For example, abrupt weaning may lead to a strong tendency to hold onto things; or children who are oral-aggressive and bite with their teeth may become adults who are oral-aggressive and *bite* with sarcasm.

During the second year of life, the infant moves into the *anal stage* of psychosexual development. The hypothesis asserts that as a consequence of experiencing a pleasant reduction in tension from elimination, the infant may use this action to reduce tension arising in other parts of the body. Thus expulsive elimination is considered the prototype for emotional outbursts, temper tantrums, rages, and other primitive discharge reactions. Usually, during the second to fourth year of life, involuntary expulsive reflexes are brought under voluntary control through a set of experiences known as toilet training. Toilet-training methods and caregiver attitudes about defecation, cleanliness, control, and responsibility are thought to leave indelible imprints on the child's development. For example, if the training method is strict and punitive, the child may react by soiling intentionally. When older, the child may react to authority figures by being messy, disorderly, or irresponsible.

Psychosocial Development: Basic Trust Versus Basic Mistrust and Autonomy Versus Shame and Guilt

The 1st psychosocial task, occurring early during the 1st year, is developing a sense of basic trust and overcoming a sense of mistrust. According to Erikson, to accomplish this task, the young infant needs to experience a mutually satisfying relationship based on familiarity, regularity, and predictability. The development of trust initially requires a feeling of physical comfort, which then promotes emotional comfort. If this feeling of comfort is achieved, then the infant becomes trusting (ie, anticipates receiving support and assistance) even in new environments and future relationships.

Basic trust is mutual and, according to Erikson, "implies not only that one has learned to rely on the sameness and continuity of the outer providers, but also that one may trust oneself and the capacity of one's own organs to cope with urges and that one is able to consider oneself trustworthy enough so that the providers will not need to be on guard lest they be nipped."[41]

The 2nd Eriksonian stage of psychosocial development, autonomy versus shame and doubt, is analogous to the anal stage of Freudian psychology. Erikson notes that muscular maturation during this time is important. With increasing control over both self and the environment, the child begins to experiment with manipulation and control. The manner in which successes and failures are met by caregivers helps determine how freely children express themselves. "From a sense of self-control without loss of self-esteem comes a lasting sense of good will and pride; from a sense of loss of self-control and of foreign over-control comes a lasting propensity for doubt and shame."[41]

Cognitive Development: Sensorimotor Period

According to Piagetian theory, the child from birth to approximately age 2 years is in the *sensorimotor stage,* characterized by sensory exploration, purposeful movement, manipulation of the environment, and imitation. Instrumental language (use of words to indicate needs or identify objects) develops toward the end of this phase. The sensorimotor period can be divided into 6 stages:

Stage 1: Modification of reflex activity through experience (eg, rooting evolves into active searching for the nipple)

Stage 2: Anticipation (eg, make sucking movements at the sight of the bottle)

Stage 3: Imitation (eg, clapping hands when someone else within sight claps)

Stage 4: Purposeful action (eg, removing an obstacle to a goal)

Stage 5: Production of novel behaviors (eg, trying new methods to remove an obstacle to a goal)

Stage 6 (transition phase): Thinking about problems, imitating an absent model from memory, and using words to designate ongoing events, immediate desires, or objects in view. In addition, the child has a well-developed sense of object permanence. That is, the child will look for a vanished object even if it has been displaced. Thus the child appears to understand that things exist independently of the self.

How does the individual move from one stage to the next? From a systems perspective, cognitive, biological, emotional, and social systems interact over time, becoming more complexly interdependent. These transactions bring about new forms, functions, and systems. In this case, a new system (ie, *stage*) is the result of the organism's active strivings for self-organization. In fact, Piaget thought "cognitive development during childhood was a process of extending and reorganizing the internalized action system constructed during infancy [early reflex activity which, in interaction with the environment, evolves into purposeful action] into systems of mental representation and abstract thought."[49]

Social Learning Development: Rudimentary Behavior Phase

The social learning theorists describe infancy as the period during which basic needs are met and initial learning takes place within the intimate environment of the home. Positive reinforcement in the form of attention (feeding, comforting) is the predominant mode used by the family to shape the infant's behavior. Reflexive activities (grasping in response to a parental finger in the infant's palm) are rewarded (parent plays with the infant's hand, talks, and coos, thereby giving attention). In time, true grasp is learned and is followed by lifting the arms as a signal to be played with or to be held. In this way, a naturally occurring primitive reflex evolves into a purposeful activity.

A further step takes place during later infancy when the child begins to modify behavior in response to signals that are not directly or immediately physically rewarding (eg, a smile rather than actually being held). Sensitivity to nonphysical cues is the foundation for the social component of human learning. In Freudian and Eriksonian terms, such responsiveness to the environment and acknowledgment that individuals are only part of it are indicators of ego development.

In summary, the developmental task of infancy involves the formation of an attachment relationship that paves the way for future adaptation. Achieving this milestone involves interactions among emotional, cognitive, and physical systems, which become increasingly integrated and organized over time, resulting in the host of behaviors associated with the attachment relationship. Understanding how this important developmental task unfolds is critical for the pediatrician. Individual differences in attachment quality have been predictive of later social and behavior competence, independence, and psychopathological characteristics.[50] A secure attachment is one in which the caregiver has demonstrated that this person is consistently available for the infant, even in times of stress. An insecure attachment may develop with a history of inconsistent, unresponsive, intrusive, or rejecting care. The infant who has not experienced a pattern of intense arousal coupled with attentive care and soothing may not learn that emotion can be experienced and then quelled. As a result, a smooth transition from parent-guided regulation in infancy to self-regulation during childhood may not occur, laying the groundwork for an inability to cope with intense arousal and emotions experienced later in life.[7] Variations of normal behavior, such as an infant who exhibits a *difficult* temperament, might interact with negative parenting styles to produce an insecure attachment.[51] Furthermore, a mother who is, for example, experiencing depression may not be able to provide consistent, responsive care to her infant and will need assistance in modulating her interactions with her new infant. In fact, current research supports the effectiveness of infant-parent psychotherapy for depressed parents in improving attachment quality.[52,53] In contrast, an infant with a physical or developmental disability may not signal wants, needs, or physiological states as clearly as other infants. The parent will require some guidance in learning to identify, interpret, and respond to the infant's more subtle cues and bids for attention.

Toddlerhood and Preschool Age (2 to 5 Years)

During the toddler stage, the growth rate slows, personality develops further, and important strides are made in cognitive ability. Bowel and bladder control usually evolve during the 3rd year, although the range extends from 15 months to 4 years and sometimes beyond. What the child can do physically influences the child's own perception of self, which, in turn, influences social development and independence. During infancy, the regulation of emotional arousal fell to the caregiver; it later becomes a dyadic process between infant and caregiver. During toddlerhood, the child makes the 1st strivings toward self-regulation of emotion and behavior.[7] The positive-feedback loop of testing leading to success, leading to confidence, leading to further testing is particularly significant during this stage of rapid development.

Psychosexual Development: Phallic Stage

According to Freud, the preschool-aged child derives pleasure from self-stimulation of the genitalia. The basic innocence of masturbation in both boys and girls at this age deserves repeated emphasis, especially to parents who may be highly concerned or disturbed by it. Another hallmark of the phallic stage is intense attachment to the parent of the opposite sex and hostility toward the same-sex parent. This situation has been called the *Oedipal complex* for boys and the *Electra conflict* for girls. Such behavior can be consternating to the family if the parents do not appreciate the universality of such alliances. Conflict resolution begins when the child recognizes the futility of the child's own desires and, instead of wishing to take the place of the same-sex parent, moves in the direction of trying to become more like the parent. This process has been called *identification*. This stage has resolved completely when incorporation of parental qualities (internalization of parental controls) is sufficient for what Freud has called *superego formation*, or the development of conscience. The child develops a rudimentary sense of right and wrong based on instruction and modeling by the parents.

Psychosocial Development: Initiative Versus Guilt

In Eriksonian terms, children of this age are in the initiative versus guilt stage and are moving into a larger social environment in which they are able to initiate new activities. Occasionally, the sense of personal autonomy they developed previously is challenged or frustrated by the autonomous activity of others. The ensuing conflict may lead to a sense of guilt for having gone too far in striving for initiative. This sense of guilt is overcome by learning self-modulation through the development of a conscience that reflects parental and societal values. Thus children begin to learn to put personal and social needs into perspective and to modify the one to be in concert with the other.

Cognitive Development: Preoperational Period

Extending from 2 to 7 years of age, the preoperational period, as defined by Piaget, is distinguished by the appearance of representational language and rudimentary reasoning. Problem solving during this period is intuitive rather than logical, and children cannot explain their reasoning strategies. The thought processes of the preoperational child are limited by centration (inability to consider several aspects or dimensions of a situation simultaneously), syncretism (the tendency to group several apparently unrelated things or events into a confused whole), juxtaposition (failure to perceive the real connection among several things or events), irreversibility (inability to understand successive changes or transformations), egocentrism (perception of the world only from the child's own point of view and the belief that the child is the origin of all actions in the world), and magical thinking (equation of thought and fantasy with action, feeling that a wish can cause some external event).

The thought content of the preoperational child is influenced by animism (the belief that inanimate objects are alive as people are alive), artificialism (all things are made for a purpose), and participation (some continuing connection or interaction exists between human actions and natural processes).

Social Learning Development: Secondary Motivational Systems and Family-centered Learning

As the child encounters other levels of the social system outside of the immediate family, more individuals become available to model and reinforce behavior. Discipline that is either too prescriptive or too indulgent can produce a child who has little internal sense of responsibility for personal actions.

Negative attention-seeking behaviors are common at this age. They arise most often when the child is frustrated by persistent lack of attention, such as might occur if an infant is born into the family, diverting parental time and attention away from the preschooler. Frustration at not receiving positive reinforcement for good behavior may lead to bad behavior that demands attention, even though it is negative.

Thus, during this developmental period, an important developmental task is self-regulation through internalization of parental rules and guidance. The pediatrician can assist the family in appropriate parenting styles and strategies best suited to achieving this important milestone. For example, Kochanska[54] found that children's moral development is the process of an interplay between temperamental factors and attachment. The development of a conscience, in which parental rules are internalized and exhibited as compliance, occurs when parental disciplinary style matches children's temperamental styles. Specifically, gentle discipline is associated with compliance in fearful children, whereas the quality of the attachment relationship is predictive of conscience development for temperamentally fearless children. Disciplinary styles are important at this stage of conscience development. For example, although some parents might spank their toddler to teach right from wrong, research has demonstrated that this strategy is not associated with an internalization of parental rules, but rather has been associated with increased aggressive behaviors in the child.[55]

Middle Childhood (6 to 12 Years)

The 1st major task during middle childhood is to enter school and achieve independence from home. The main developmental accomplishments include competence in the social arena (eg, the development and maintenance of friendships), in academic achievement, and in appropriate behavior or conduct.[37]

Physically, no qualitative change in the external genitalia exists, which retain their infantile appearance. Lack of observable physical change and low levels of sexually oriented drive do not mean that children are uninterested in sex, especially sex differences. Curiosity is common among 5- to 7-year-old children of both sexes. Because children have been taught to keep themselves clothed in the presence of others, *playing doctor* becomes a way of satisfying natural curiosity. Girls and boys often *kiss and run;* snapping the bra strap of a more developed girl is common. Intense *crushes,* especially those focused on an unattainable idol, occur regularly. Parents sometimes need reassurance that these practices represent normal behavior at this age. The 6-year-old child has the ability to perform most rudimentary gross- and fine-motor tasks. Therefore middle childhood is the time when skills are refined. Progress is tested less by the acquisition of new skills than by the rapidity and accuracy with which old skills are performed. Indeed, increased motor skills play a critical part in the development of the emerging personality. For the agile or athletic child, playing games and being a member of a team bring pleasure and friendship. For the child with less athletic skill, little positive reinforcement is gleaned from these activities, and the individual may need to be directed to other areas of strength. However, the group's emphasis, especially among boys, is on athletic prowess.

In more recent time, social roles have become less categorized and restrictive for both boys and girls. In addition, a new value system for social roles has emerged that encourages both athleticism in girls (eg, Title IX legislation that mandates equal support for male and female sports) and relational interests in boys.

The child who cannot excel in sports or schoolwork is a prime candidate for developing acting-out behavior. For this child, similar to the toddler who is displaced by a new baby in the family, attention (usually reprimand) comes primarily from negative attention-seeking behaviors. A boy, for example, may become famous among his friends, who marvel at his ability to get into trouble and his bravado about inviting punishment.

Psychosexual Development: Latency

Freud has described the latency stage as the period during which previously active libidinal and aggressive drives of the Oedipal stage become latent, and a truce is established between the id and the ego. At the beginning of latency, the superego (conscience) becomes more firmly internalized. The outlook of the latency-age child is black and white; notions about good and bad are clear and absolute and follow the guidelines set by the family.

Psychosocial Development: Industry Versus Inferiority

Erikson[55] has called the latency period the *age of industry versus inferiority*. The child has experienced a sense of finality in realizing that no workable future exists within the womb of the family and thus becomes ready to acquire skills and tasks that go far beyond mere physiological regulation and acquiring fine- and gross-motor skills as an end in itself. A sense of industry, or bringing a productive situation to completion, typically through the use of tools, is an aim that gradually supersedes the whims and wishes of play.

According to Erikson, the potential danger to the child at this stage lies in acquiring a sense of inadequacy or inferiority. If the child does not believe that his or her tools or skills are adequate, becoming a successful member of the group may be impossible, resulting in withdrawal back into the family and social isolation. In fact, being accepted and well liked by peers is associated with future social competence and relatively few behavioral problems,[56,57] whereas numerous studies[58,59] have demonstrated that rejection by the peer group is consistently associated with later maladjustment such as poor academic achievement, loneliness and depressive symptoms in childhood, and poor mental health and criminality in adulthood.

Cognitive Development: Concrete Operational Stage

Piaget characterized cognitive processes in the latency-aged child as concrete operational. The child is able to take an external point of view, use logic, and be objective. Thinking becomes dynamic, decentralized, and reversible; *conserving* or recognizing that certain changes (eg, physical rearrangement) do not necessarily alter other properties (eg, quantity) of a substance also becomes possible. Conservation is the result of the child's ability to focus on several aspects of a problem or situation at one time and relate them.

A child in the early concrete operational period can solve a problem only if the elements of the problem are physically present and they must often be actually manipulated. By the late concrete operational period, the child can solve problems of space and time; can conserve substance, quantity, weight, and volume; and can classify objects into hierarchical systems. Physical manipulation remains helpful but is not essential to problem solving.

In line with the organizational perspective of development, this increase in cognitive ability is closely interwoven with the development of a sense of inferiority as described by Erikson. With increasing cognitive skills, children are able to compare their behavior to that of others and to their own time, and these comparisons can influence how children feel about themselves. This new cognitive capacity of children to think abstractly and to compare themselves to their peers is closely linked with the development of self-concept.[60]

Cicchetti and Cohen[5] offer an example of the integration of emotional and cognitive processes in the development of depressive symptoms in children. Between 7 and 8 years of age, children undergo a qualitative change in cognitive abilities, moving away from thinking in absolute terms to more abstract and relative comparisons. Thus children become able to understand that their personality traits are relatively stable. Additionally, rather than associating negative feelings with absolute events that can change from situation to situation, an increasing focus on comparing self to others can influence self-evaluation by the formation of global attributions rather than event-related attributions. Thus children become capable of making global, stable, and personal attributions concerning negative events in the environment, cognitions that are associated with depressive symptoms.

Social Learning Development: Secondary Motivational Systems and Extra-Family Learning

Beginning with the child's entrance into school, the values and customs of people outside the family become increasingly important. A history of supportive caregiving, as well as early successes with peer relationships and school achievement, will pave the way for the child to act independently and in compliance with expectations made by nonfamily members of the larger social group. Admiration and approval reinforce socially acceptable behaviors. If desirable behaviors are not reinforced consistently, or if the only attention the child receives is through socially unacceptable behaviors, then undesirable behaviors will be learned at this stage just as they were at earlier ages within the home.

Thus, through understanding social, academic, and conduct or behavioral competence, pediatricians can obtain a general sense of whether their patients are on a pathway toward adaptive adult functioning or whether they are exhibiting difficulties that place them at risk for future maladjustment and warrant intervention.

Adolescence and Young Adulthood

Whereas peer relations, school success, and appropriate conduct are still important factors for the adolescent, romantic relationship and work competence also become important tasks, especially during late adolescence and young adulthood.[55] The term *adolescence* is derived from the Latin *adolescere* (to grow up) and refers to the psychological, biological, and sociologic aspects of development that occur during the second decade of life. *Puberty* refers to the condition of becoming sexually mature and capable of sexual reproduction. During early adolescence, most of the individual's physical and emotional energy is centered on physical change and its consequences. During middle adolescence, the focus is on separation from parents, and during late adolescence, the focus is on preparation for an adult identity.

Important gender-specific differences exist in both the timing of growth and final adult size. The female growth spurt occurs approximately 2 years earlier than the male growth spurt; but the final adult height of women is less than that of men because of their shorter growth period. Muscle growth appears to be influenced primarily by androgenic stimulation. Thus the mature man has greater muscle mass and strength than the mature woman.

Increase in body size and maturation of neuronal pathways contribute to the child's and the adolescent's increasing ability to perform complex motor tasks. Large muscles develop before small muscles. Therefore younger children are more skillful in activities involving gross-motor movements than they are in activities requiring fine-motor coordination. In early adolescence, differential bone and muscle growth can result in transient increases in awkwardness, particularly in gross-motor functioning. During middle and late adolescence, the growth rate slows, leading to greater stability in body proportions; motor awkwardness gradually decreases.

Throughout infancy and childhood, circulating levels of pituitary follicle-stimulating hormone and luteinizing hormone are low. For reasons that are not completely clear but that may be related to critical body weight, the hypothalamus becomes less sensitive to negative feedback from circulating gonadotropin. As a result, luteinizing hormone–releasing factor is produced, and gonadotropin secretion is enhanced, rising progressively toward adult levels. This event marks the onset of puberty.

Pubertal change can be divided into 3 stages. During the first stage—prepubescence (prepuberty)—the gonadotropin and sex steroid levels remain low; however, secondary sexual characteristics begin to appear. In girls, the earliest sign of sexual maturation is widening of the pelvic girdle. This phenomenon is followed by breast and pubic hair development and the onset of the height spurt. In boys, testicular growth precedes penile growth, development of pubic hair, and the onset of the height spurt. During the second stage—pubescence (puberty)—the reproductive organs (primary sexual characteristics) become functional, and the secondary sexual characteristics become more evident. The last stage—postpubescence (postpuberty)—includes a 1- to 2-year period of relative reproductive infertility. Skeletal growth is completed during this time.

This physical development is closely intertwined with psychological development. Caspi and Moffitt[61] clearly illustrate this point with their investigation of menses in adolescents. The researchers found that in girls who demonstrated early behavior problems, early menarche was associated with an increase in behavior problems. In contrast, no significant increase in behavior problems during adolescence was noted for girls with early-onset menarche who did not have a history of behavior problems.

Psychosexual Development: Genital Stage

According to Freudian theory, sexual impulses reemerge during adolescence, marking the onset of the genital stage. Whereas pleasure seeking through oral, anal, and genital stimulation was the aim of the infantile form of sexuality, during puberty, another sexual aim arises: reproduction.

During early adolescence, a partial recrudescence of the Oedipal conflict, or a regression to the psychosexual stage characteristic of the preschool child, is thought to be present. This partial recrudescence may occur because the adolescent feels safer expressing new and confusing sexual feelings within the familiar environment of the family. However, the adolescent recognizes that emotional closeness to the parent of the other gender is both unrealistic and unacceptable and that real competition with the parent of the same gender is hopeless.

Eventually, the adolescent seeks independence from both parents. In some cases, a period of significant alienation from the family may be necessary to gain sufficient distance for independence to be attained. During the resolution of the parent-child conflict of the genital stage, the boy completes his (adult) identification with his father by choosing a female partner. Similarly, the girl completes her (adult) identification with her mother by seeking a male partner. Thus full sexual maturity, in Freudian terms, is attained when feelings directed toward the parent of the other gender are transferred successfully to a love object that is not taboo.

In addition to whatever sexual overtones may be associated with movement into the genital stage, the process of renewed competition with the parent of the same gender also provokes questioning of the behavior, values, and judgments of the parent. To explain this phenomenon, an important point to recall is that resolution of the Oedipal phase in early childhood brought with it acceptance of the parental value system and a desire to be similar to the parent. The value system that was accepted, however, was rudimentary because the child was not cognitively capable of fully understanding such concepts as intent and competing priorities.

As becomes evident in the study of cognitive growth during adolescence, the ability to understand hypothetical situations and to argue both for and against a given point of view renders the teenager's previous value system inadequate to deal with larger moral and philosophic issues. However, rather than turn to the parent for explanation and clarification, the adolescent assumes that the parents' value system is exactly as the teenager conceived of it as a young child (eg, parents of adolescents often comment, "My teenager thinks I don't know anything"). Thus the adolescent turns to peers or adults outside the family, looking for a new, expanded set of values. In this process, the adolescent is likely to reject the parents' values. Interestingly, however, the value system the individual eventually develops is more similar than dissimilar to that of the parents. This notion is perhaps best illustrated by Mark Twain's comment: "When I was 14, I thought my father was the stupidest man alive. When I was 21, I was amazed by how much he had learned in 7 years."

The genital stage lasts from adolescence to senility. However, the personality constructs and defense mechanisms developed during the pregenital stages continue as part of the individual's permanent character structure and are displayed throughout life.

Psychosocial Development: Identity Versus Role Confusion and Intimacy Versus Isolation

The major focus of this phase of development in Eriksonian terms is the task of choosing an identity (ie, selecting a role to play within the adult community). The process of identity formation begins in early adolescence, although the developmental pathways framework is a reminder that it has its roots in the emerging sense of self-efficacy learned from the early caregiving relationship, as well as the emerging self-concept established from success or failure in earlier developmental tasks (eg, peer relations, academic achievement). The individual becomes determined to be exactly the same as the other members of the person's peer group, which is often a continuation of a latency-age *chum* group. Frequently cruel in its exclusion of others through relationally aggressive tactics,[62] the *in* group, or clique, attempts to establish its identity as a separate social unit. The rigid structure of the group provides security for individual members to identify and fulfill particular roles without feeling confused. This focus on peer group membership is particularly relevant to the pediatrician who might encounter increased reluctance on the part of young adolescents to undergo medical procedures that might make them appear *different* from peers. Chronic conditions involving extended absences from school and peer recreational activities may also place the adolescent at increased risk for depressive symptoms.

In much the same way parents did, the peer group now defines acceptable and unacceptable behavior. However, to facilitate separation from family, the rules and values of the group the adolescent chooses are often different from, if not antithetical to, those of the family. In this way, teenagers seek to demonstrate that they are their own persons, doing their *own thing*. Part of developing identity is (1) recognizing personal strengths and weaknesses, (2) aspiring to goals that are realistic and attainable, and (3) working toward these goals. The potential danger is never achieving clarity of role; closely allied to never achieving role clarity is having too many roles (identity diffusion) or choosing a role without exploring options (identity foreclosure).

Some adolescents choose a negative identity (ie, an identity counter to that suggested by society) because they see conformity as the route to being a nonentity. The positive role of the individual who has a negative identity can be social change. In such situations, even though overcoming the inertia of the status quo may require great energy and commitment, such deviance can have such a major effect on social mores that the individual perceives the effort as worthwhile. For example, many of the characteristics of the *hippie* of the late 1960s might be found in conventional youth by the mid 1970s. The danger of assuming a counterculture identity, however, is permanent ostracism: never achieving sufficient reintegration to effect desired change or to derive a satisfying sense of self from society.

During late adolescence and young adulthood, the individual moves into the stage of intimacy versus isolation. Once personal identity becomes established, the young adult is eager to fuse the identity with that of another: to develop intimacy or the capacity to commit oneself to a partnership despite personal sacrifice and compromise. Although often thought of in sexual terms, intimacy includes close friendships, inspiring teacher-student relationships, and other affiliations in which personal vulnerability and true glimpses of the self are permitted. The antithesis of intimacy, in Eriksonian terms, is the state of *distantiation*, or isolation from or the destruction of those who appear to be a danger to oneself or to the individual's intimate relations (ie, prejudices against people who are unfamiliar or foreign and thus threatening). The danger of this adolescent or young adult phase is selection of an inappropriate partner for reasons of expediency rather than for fulfillment of mutual purposes.

Cognitive Development: Formal Operational Period

Beginning in early adolescence and extending throughout adulthood, the period of formal operations is distinguished by the ability to use abstract thought. Characteristics of formal operational thought include flexibility, complex reasoning, and hypothesis formation. Not all adolescents or all adults apply formal operational thinking in all circumstances. Rather, use of formal operations is often restricted to cognitive functioning in areas of particular personal interest or professional concern and is applied most productively at times of low stress and anxiety.

The development of formal operational or abstract thought allows the adolescent to understand certain moral, political, and philosophic ideas for the 1st time. With the emergence of the ability to deal with concepts such as liberty and justice, adolescents become preoccupied with social, religious, and political issues. Because they can conceive of the ideal, be it society, religion, or family, adolescents become aware of the contradictions, falsehoods, and shortcomings embedded in their previously accepted beliefs.

Adolescents can think about thinking; they understand the thought processes of others and wonder how individuals see them and what these individuals really think about them. A belief that others may dwell on or constantly evaluate their appearance and behaviors results in the egocentrism or self-centeredness particularly characteristic of the early and middle adolescent. Self-consciousness is a direct reflection of this self-centeredness. In early adolescence, a decrease in self-esteem may be noted.[63] As formal operational thinking becomes better established, the individual begins to distinguish between personal preoccupation and the thoughts of others. This cognitive capacity may play a role in the slow increase in self-esteem, which characterizes the later adolescent years.[63] Furthermore, once this distinction can be made, the adolescent is able to enter into an intimate emotional relationship with others.

Stress, such as illness, can profoundly impair the individual's ability to use higher-order cognitive skills. Thus cognitive regression frequently accompanies the general physical and emotional regression seen in a hospitalized child. Such phenomena as magical thinking ("my wish equals action") or egocentrism ("my action caused some external unrelated event") are common. The ability to think futuristically about the potential consequences of current actions also can be impaired. Conversely, long-term illness can result in increased learning and adult-like understanding of related issues. Because this circumstance can occur in children of all ages, children who have long-term, fatal malignancies, for example, commonly have an understanding of body function or a conception of death that is surprisingly mature. This finding is in keeping with Piaget's premise that cognitive functioning is highly dependent on experience.

Social Learning Development: Secondary Motivational Systems and Extrafamilial Learning

As the individual matures, the nature and scope of interactions with others broaden. Reinforcement of rudimentary behaviors becomes less critical as socially acceptable behaviors become habitual. Rewards and punishments are based more on internal than external controls. Thus the adolescent is able to enter into relationships based on the mutuality of needs of 2 or more independent people.

"IT'S JUST A STAGE"

Although, theoretically, children and adolescents achieve biopsychosocial maturity in a predictable fashion, in reality, human variability and the complex interplay between biological and environmental influences make predictions about a given individual difficult, frustrating, and challenging. The organizational framework of development outlines development as probabilistic, rather than determined. "Individuals are neither unaffected by earlier experiences nor immutably controlled by them. Change in developmental course is always possible as a result of new experiences and reorganizations and the individual's active self-organizing strivings for adaptation."[3] When the pediatrician can offer reassurance about the temporary nature of a particular undesirable or anxiety-provoking stage of development, children and their families are often better able to cope, knowing that minor changes in parenting expectations or interpersonal relationships will result in better adjustment to the current stage and smoother transition to the next stage.

Although the spectrum of variability is broad, not all deviations from average expected development are normal. Exposure to significant risk factors and unsuccessful resolution of challenges at development stages place the child at risk for future maladaptation, but these factors do not in themselves signify a pathological abnormality.[36] The greatest challenge to the practitioner is to distinguish between adequate, although not necessarily perfect, development and true dysfunction. Passing a situation off as merely *a stage* is justified only when the true limits of acceptable behavior for that stage are clearly understood, the reasons for the behavior can be explained in such a way that the parents or child can understand what they are experiencing and why, and appropriate guidance to help them master the stage is provided.

AAP POLICY STATEMENTS

American Academy of Pediatrics, Committee on Bioethics. Sterilization of minors with developmental disabilities. *Pediatrics.* 1999;104:337-340. (aappolicy.aappublications.org/cgi/content/abstract/pediatrics;104/2/337).

American Academy of Pediatrics, Committee on Children With Disabilities. Developmental surveillance and screening of infants and young children. *Pediatrics.* 2001;108:192-195. (aappolicy.aappublications.org/cgi/content/abstract/pediatrics;108/1/192).

American Academy of Pediatrics, Committee on Children With Disabilities. Technical report: the pediatrician's role in the diagnosis and management of autistic spectrum disorder in children. *Pediatrics.* 2001;107:e85. (aappolicy.aappublications.org/cgi/content/abstract/pediatrics;107/5/e85).

American Academy of Pediatrics, Committee on Children With Disabilities. The pediatrician's role in the diagnosis and management of autistic spectrum disorder in children. *Pediatrics.* 2001;107:1221-1226. (aappolicy.aappublications.org/cgi/content/abstract/pediatrics;107/5/1221).

American Academy of Pediatrics, Committee on Early Childhood, Adoption and Dependent Care. Developmental issues for young children in foster care. *Pediatrics.* 2000;106:1145-1150. (aappolicy.aappublications.org/cgi/content/abstract/pediatrics;106/5/1145).

American Academy of Pediatrics, Committee on Quality Improvement, Subcommittee on Attention-Deficit/Hyperactivity Disorder. Clinical practice guideline: diagnosis and evaluation of the child with attention-deficit/hyperactivity disorder. *Pediatrics.* 2000;105:1158-1170. (aappolicy.aappublications.org/cgi/content/abstract/pediatrics;105/5/1158).

American Academy of Pediatrics, William L. Coleman, Craig Garfield, and Committee on Psychosocial Aspects of Child and Family Health. Fathers and pediatricians: enhancing men's roles in the care and development of their children. *Pediatrics.* 2004;113:1406-1411. (aappolicy.aappublications.org/cgi/content/abstract/pediatrics;113/5/1406).

REFERENCES

1. Sameroff A. Ecological perspectives on longitudinal follow-up studies. In: Friedman SL, Haywood HC, eds. *Developmental Follow-Up: Concepts, Domains, and Methods.* San Diego, CA: Academic Press; 1994.
2. Gottlieb G. Experiential canalization of behavioral development: *Theory Dev Psychol.* 1991;27:4-13.
3. Cicchetti D, Tucker D. Development and self-regulatory structures of the mind. *Dev Psychopathol.* 1994;6:533-549.
4. Greenough WT, Black JE, Wallace CS. Experience and brain development. *Child Dev.* 1987;58:539-559.
5. Cicchetti D, Cohen DJ. Perspectives on developmental psychopathology. In: Cicchetti D, Cohen DJ, eds. *Developmental Psychopathology. Vol. 1: Theory and Methods.* Oxford, UK: John Wiley & Sons; 1995.
6. Sroufe LA, Rutter M. The domain of developmental psychopathology. *Child Dev.* 1984;55:17-29.
7. Sroufe LA. *Emotional Development: The Organization of Emotional Life in the Early Years.* New York, NY: Cambridge University Press; 1996.
8. Sameroff A, Chandler MJ. Reproductive risk and the continuum of caretaking causality. In: Horowitz FD, Hetherington EM, Scarr-Salapatek S, et al, eds. *Review of Child Development Research.* Chicago, IL: Chicago University Press; 1975.
9. Plomin R, DeFries JC, Loehlin JC. Genotype-environment interaction and correlation in the analysis of human behavior. *Psychol Bull.* 1977;84:309-322.
10. Hetherington EM, Reiss D, Plomin R. *Separate Social Worlds of Siblings: The Impact of Nonshared Environment on Development.* Hillsdale, NJ: Lawrence Erlbaum Associates; 1994.
11. Scarr S, Grajek S. Similarities and differences among siblings. In: Lamb ME, Sutton-Smith B, eds. *Sibling Relationships: Their Nature and Significance Across the Life Span.* Hillsdale, NJ: Lawrence Erlbaum; 1982.
12. Reiss D, Neiderhiser JM, Hetherington EM, et al. *The Relationship Code: Deciphering Genetic and Social Influences on Adolescent Development.* Cambridge, MA: Harvard University Press; 2000.
13. Rutter ML. Nature-nurture integration: the example of antisocial behavior. *Am Psychol.* 1997;52:390-398.
14. Rutter M, Silberg J, O'Connor T, et al. Genetics and child psychiatry: I. Advances in quantitative and molecular genetics. *J Child Psychol Psychiatry.* 1999;40:3-18.

15. Miller BD, Wood BL. Psychophysiologic reactivity in asthmatic children: a cholinergically mediated confluence of pathways. *J Am Acad Child Adolesc Psychiatry.* 1994;33:1236-1245.
16. Plomin R, DeFries JC, McClearn GE, et al. *Behavioral Genetics.* New York, NY: WH Freeman; 1997.
17. Berndt TJ, Hawkins JA, Hoyle SG. Changes in friendship during a school year: effects on children's and adolescents' impressions of friendship and sharing with friends. *Child Dev.* 1986;57:1284-1297.
18. Bronfenbrenner U, Ceci SJ. Nature-nurture reconceptualized in developmental perspective: a bioecological model. *Psychol Rev.* 1994;101:568-586.
19. Bronfenbrenner U. The bioecological model from a life course perspective: reflections of a participant observer. In: Moen P, Elder GH, Jr., Luscher K, eds. *Examining Lives in Context: Perspective on the Ecology of Human Development.* Washington, DC: American Psychological Association; 1995.
20. Bronfenbrenner U. *The Ecology of Human Development: Experiments by Nature and Design.* Cambridge, MA.: Harvard University Press; 1979.
21. Harris JR. *The Nurture Assumption: Why Children Turn Out the Way They Do.* New York, NY: Free Press; 1998.
22. Rowe DC. *The Limits of Family Influence: Genes, Experience, and Behavior.* New York, NY: Guilford Press; 1994.
23. Scarr S. Developmental theories for the 1990s: development and individual differences. *Child Dev.* 1992;63:1-19.
24. Collins WA, Maccoby EE, Steinberg L, et al. Contemporary research on parenting. The case for nature and nurture. *Am Psychol.* 2000;55:218-232.
25. Schore AN. *Affect Regulation and the Origin of the Self: The Neurobiology of Emotional Development.* Hillsdale, NJ: Erlbaum Associates; 1994.
26. Sroufe LA, Egeland B, Carlson EA, et al. *The Development of the Person: The Minnesota Study of Risk and Adaptation From Birth to Adulthood.* New York, NY: Guilford Press; 2005.
27. Gesell A. *An Atlas of Infant Behavior: A Systematic Delineation of the Forms and Early Growth of Human Behavior Patterns.* New Haven, CT: Yale University Press; 1934.
28. Rothbart MK, Ahadi SA. Temperament and the development of personality. *J Abnorm Psychol.* 1994; 103:55-66.
29. Rutter M. Temperament, personality, and personality disorder. *Br J Psychiatry.* 1987;150:443-458.
30. Gottesman II. Heritability of personality: a demonstration. *Psychol Monogr.* 1963;77:1-21.
31. Loehlin JC, Rowe DC. Genes, environment, and personality. In: Caprara G, Van Heck GL, eds. *Modern Personality Psychology: Critical Reviews and New Directions.* New York, NY: Harvester Wheatsheaf; 1992.
32. Chess S, Thomas A. *Origins and Evolution of Behavior Disorders: From Infancy to Early Adult Life.* Cambridge, MA: Harvard University Press; 1984.
33. Maccoby EE. The role of parents in the socialization of children: an historical overview. *Dev Psychol.* 1992;28: 1006-1017.
34. Parke RD, Buriel R. Socialization in the family: ethnic and ecological perspectives. In: Damon W, Eisenberg N, eds. *Handbook of Child Psychology.* Hoboken, NJ: John Wiley & Sons; 1998.
35. van den Boom DC. The influence of temperament and mothering on attachment and exploration: an experimental manipulation of sensitive responsiveness among lower-class mothers with irritable infants. *Child Dev.* 1994;65:1457-1477.
36. Sroufe LA. Psychopathology as an outcome of development. *Dev Psychopathol.* 1997;9:251-268.
37. Masten AS, Coatsworth JD. The development of competence in favorable and unfavorable environments: Lessons from research on successful children. *Am Psychol.* 1998;53:205-220.
38. Bowlby J. *Separation.* New York, NY: Basic Books; 1973.
39. Waddington CH. The strategy of the genes: a discussion of some aspect of theoretical biology. London, UK: Allen & Unwin; 1957.
40. Hay DF, Nash A, Pedersen J. Interaction between Six-month-old peers. *Child Dev.* 1983;54:557-562.
41. Erikson EH. *Childhood and Society.* New York, NY: WWW Norton; 1963.
42. Sears RR. A theoretical framework for personality and social behavior. *Am Psychol.* 1951;6:476-482.
43. Schneider ML, Moore CF. *Effect of Prenatal Stress on Development: A Nonhuman Primate Model on Effects of Early Adversity on Neurobehavioral Development.* Mahwah, NJ: Erlbaum; 2000.
44. Parke RD. Perspectives on father-infant interaction. In: Osofsky JD, ed. *Handbook of Infant Development.* New York, NY: John Wiley & Sons; 1979.
45. Klaus MH, Kennell JH. *Parent-Infant Bonding.* St. Louis: Mosby; 1982.
46. Sosa R, Kennell J, Klaus M, et al. The effect of a supportive companion on perinatal problems, length of labor, and mother-infant interaction. *N Eng J Med.* 1980;303: 597-600.
47. Greenberg M, Morris N. Engrossment: the newborn's impact upon the father. *Am J Orthopsychiatry.* 1974;44: 520-531.
48. Korner AF. The effect of the infant's state, level of arousal, sex, and ontogenetic stage on the caregiver. In: Lewis M, Rosenblum LA, eds. *The Effect of the Infant on Its Caregiver.* Oxford, UK: Wiley-Interscience; 1974.
49. Bidell TR, Fischer KW. Beyond the stage debate: action, structure, and variability in Piagetian theory and research. In: Sternberg RJ, Berg CA, eds. *Intellectual Development.* New York, NY: Cambridge University Press; 1992.
50. Carlson EA, Sampson MC, Sroufe LA. Implications of attachment theory and research for developmental-behavioral pediatrics. *J Dev Behav Pediatrics.* 2003;24: 364-379.
51. Mangelsdorf SC, Gunnar M, Kestenbaum R, et al. Infant proneness-to-distress temperament, maternal personality, and mother-infant attachment: associations and goodness of fit. *Child Dev.* 1990;61:820-831.
52. Cicchetti D, Toth SL, Rogosch FA. The efficacy of toddler-parent psychotherapy to increase attachment security in offspring of depressed mothers. *Attach Human Dev.* 1999;1:34-66.
53. Toth SL, Rogosch FA, Manly JT, et al. The efficacy of toddler-parent psychotherapy to reorganize attachment in the young offspring of mothers with major depressive disorder: A randomized preventive trial. *J Consult Clin Psychol.* 2006;74(6):1006-1016.
54. Kochanska G. Children's temperament, mother's discipline, and security of attachment: multiple pathways to emerging internalization. *Child Dev.* 1995;66:597-615.
55. Roisman GI, Masten AS, Coatsworth JD, et al. Salient and emerging developmental tasks in the transition to adulthood. *Child Dev.* 2004;75:123-133.
56. Hymel S, Rubin KH, Rowden L, et al. Children's peer relationships: longitudinal prediction of internalizing and externalizing problems from middle to late childhood. *Child Dev.* 1990;61:2004-2021.
57. Morison P, Masten AS. Peer reputation in middle childhood as a predictor of adaptation in adolescence: a seven-year follow-up. *Child Dev.* 1991;62:991-1007.

58. Coie JD, Dodge KA, Kupersmidt JB. Peer group behavior and social status. In: Asher SR, Coie JD, eds. *Peer Rejection in Childhood: Cambridge Studies in Social and Emotional Development*. New York, NY: Cambridge University Press; 1990.
59. Parker JG, Asher SR. Peer relations and later personal adjustment: are low-accepted children at risk? *Psychol Bull*. 1987;102:357-389.
60. Harter S. The development of self-representations. In: Damon W, Eisenberg N, eds. *Handbook of Child Psychology. Vol 3. Social, Emotional, and Personality Development*. Hoboken, NJ: John Wiley & Sons; 1998.
61. Caspi A, Moffitt TE. Individual differences are accentuated during periods of social change: the sample case of girls at puberty. *J Person Social Psychol*. 1991;61:157-168.
62. Crick NR, Werner NE, Casas JF, et al. Childhood aggression and gender: a new look at an old problem. In: Bernstein D, ed. *Gender and Motivation*. Lincoln, NE: University of Nebraska Press; 1999.
63. Marsh HW. Age and sex effects in multiple dimensions of self-concept: preadolescence to early adulthood. *J Educ Psychol*. 1989;81:417-430.

Chapter 108

MENTAL HEALTH OF THE YOUNG: AN OVERVIEW

William R. Beardslee, MD; Julius B. Richmond, MD

Advances in knowledge of child development, gained through the in-depth study of healthy infants and children, as well as through observations of deviations or delays in development, have provided the primary care physician (PCP) with the conceptual framework and the empirical knowledge needed to deal effectively with the mental health needs of children and families.

Underlying this work is the core construct of developmental plasticity, which emphasizes the flexibility of the developing child in adapting to biological and environmental challenges such as low birth weight, injury, or medical illness.[1] Growing awareness of the extent to which the environment influences gene expression through different mechanisms further emphasizes the plasticity of development.[2] Another contributing factor is increasing understanding of the importance of the ecologic context in which the child is raised and how attention to various levels in the ecologic context, such as developing programs and policies to support families, can have a positive influence on development.[3] The very architecture of a developing child's brain is profoundly shaped by environmental influences, and these influences, in turn, are amenable to intervention.[4,5]

DIAGNOSIS AND TREATMENT

The last 3 decades have witnessed a dramatic increase in knowledge about the diagnosis and treatment of childhood mental disorders. One key factor was the development of reliable, standardized interview instruments scored according to criteria-based diagnostic systems (*Diagnostic and Statistical Manual*, 4th edition, of the American Psychiatric Association), and the description of the epidemiologic mechanisms and course and outcome of a large number of childhood mental disorders. Further refinements in the diagnostic system are underway. Even more important has been the recognition that treatments for child mental disorders need to be evidence based. Well-conducted empirical trials have demonstrated the effectiveness of treatments for many of the major mental disorders of childhood, including attention-deficit disorder, depression, anxiety disorder, and even psychosis. Of interest is the fact that treatments drawn from different conceptual domains (eg, pharmacology, cognitive behavioral therapy) appear to work equally well for some disorders such as childhood depression.[6] Perhaps most exciting, empirical evidence now exists to support a variety of preventive interventions with children at high risk because of parental mental illness, social demographic factors such as poverty, or the manifestation of early symptoms.[7,8] These approaches have some characteristics in common; they take account of the ecologic framework surrounding the child, and they are designed to enhance and strengthen internal and external resources rather than focus on deficits or disease.

In addition, interest is growing in ascertaining how best to translate these research findings into broad-scale programs that reach all children—in public health terms, the transition of efficacy studies to effectiveness studies and then to large-scale programs.[9] A more sophisticated understanding of the prevalence and nature of neurodevelopmental and neuropsychiatric difficulties has also substantially expanded the information available to the PCP. Expanding research in neuroscience, including molecular biology and molecular genetics, has already strengthened understanding of the cause and treatment of childhood psychiatric disorders, and more insights will be gained in the years to come.[10] For example, in Tourette syndrome and childhood depression, evidence of interference with neurotransmitter function leading to the behavioral manifestations of the disorder has been established, and this finding has helped researchers to develop drug therapies. Finally, PCPs have come to appreciate the importance of health care systems, both in terms of what can go wrong and in terms of identifying systems that are most likely to maximize the use of resources.[11]

Advances in the development of preventive and therapeutic agents over the last 40 years have brought about major reductions in infant mortality and childhood morbidity and mortality. No longer is the PCP's time consumed by providing care to children with rickets or scurvy or with acute infectious diseases such as measles, pertussis, diphtheria, and poliomyelitis. Rather, more time and energy is available to focus on the prevention of disease and on the early detection and care of children who have chronic disorders, including developmental disabilities. Given the rapid increase of knowledge, much can be done for these youngsters.

APPROACHES TO SERVICES FOR CHILDREN

The last decade has been characterized by an increasing awareness by organized consumers of the desirability of high-quality child health and child care services.

Pressure from communities for improved child health services has increased, a concern reflected in the development of programs such as *Head Start;* early periodic screening, diagnosis, and treatment for Medicaid-eligible children; and community mental health centers. The new approaches to more comprehensive services for children with disabilities also reflect intensified community sophistication, such as the Education for All Handicapped Children Act (Public Law 94-142), which emphasizes the need to mainstream such children. This Act has mandated adequate services for younger children with disabilities.

Attention to cost effectiveness and the need for broadening the base of medical and psychiatric coverage to include all Americans has also led to a reexamination of the service delivery system. An initial report emphasized the need for a wide array of services for children,[12] as has current interest in expanding *Head Start* to include children 0 to 3 years of age. In general, the need to prepare children for entrance to kindergarten has received attention; serious consideration exists for a prekindergarten year to be mandatory. In addition, awareness of the need for partnerships with parents and communities for the success of such initiatives has increased. This interest in child health in the early years will undoubtedly result in an effort to reorganize services and generate local initiatives to reflect local needs and priorities. The emphasis will increasingly be on health enhancement and disease prevention. Thus competence in the assessment and guidance of growth and development needs to be among PCPs' clinical skills. Increasing recognition has occurred that the places where mental health issues are recognized and treated are not the mental health specialists' offices but rather schools and PCPs' offices.[11]

MODELS OF MENTAL HEALTH OF CHILDREN

The PCP is and will continue to be the primary resource for parents raising their children. Consideration of mental health for both parents and children is of crucial importance in the PCPs role, as is encouraging positive health habits, encouraging effective parenting, and recognizing mental health difficulties when they occur. The PCP must have a firm grasp of child development and the early detection of developmental deviations. Piaget's work[13] provides the most useful framework within the cognitive sphere because of its emphasis on the child's actions as necessary for the acquisition of knowledge and on the predictable sequence of stages through which a child passes in developing intelligence.

Skinner's work[14] in the area of behavioral modification and its applications has proved valuable both in helping children learn and in suggesting ways to manage difficult or troublesome symptoms. Several workers in the area of early infant and child behavior[15] have helped focus attention on the importance of temperament as an early influence. Expansion of developmental frameworks to include moral development[16] and interpersonal development[17] have contributed further to the understanding of normal development. In addition, large-scale epidemiologic studies have provided valuable data about prevalence and incidence of physical and mental disorders.[8,11] (See also Chapter 107, Theories and Concepts of Development.)

The work of Erikson[18] probably provides the best integrative framework through which practicing PCPs can understand the different factors shaping the mental health of the child and then best meet the needs of their patients. Erikson stresses the importance of three domains—biological, intrapsychic, and cultural—in shaping the child's mental health. He sees the child as going through a series of stages in development and formulates the essential task or critical area to be mastered for each stage. Thus, as one example, the dilemma for the very young infant is basic trust versus mistrust; firm patterns for the solution of this dilemma must be successfully established for the infant to develop in a healthy way. As another example, the dilemma for the adolescent is identity versus role diffusion. Youths in this stage must come to understand their own physical endowments, experiences, and opportunities in a way that allows them to function in the world and have a sense of certainty about themselves. Specifically, youths must deal with 3 areas: (1) relationships with others, both sexual and nonsexual; (2) independence from family; and (3) choice of work or career. Familiarity with each stage—with its task and with its successful resolution—provides PCPs with a useful conceptual framework. More generally, a useful approach for PCPs in working with families is to conceptualize the developmental challenges and the resources available in the child, the family, and the community at a particular developmental stage. Then, PCPs will be able to recognize that a developmental stage has either been successfully accomplished or requires from a PCP either a preventive or remedial intervention.

Common to a series of investigations of youngsters at risk because of poverty or parental mental illness or other stressors is the finding that no matter how great the risk, many children do well and function effectively.[19,20] To understand this, a variety of domains needs to be considered. These areas include genetic effects, individual differences (particularly the role of temperament), inner psychological processes, and the vital role of the family, cultural influences, and influences outside of the home, especially schools. Characteristics of resilient youngsters across studies are the involvement in close, confiding human relationships and the capacity to take action outside of the home—for example, participating in school and extracurricular activities, religious and community organizations, and work or other age-appropriate developmental venues. Of particular relevance to a pediatric practice are studies that demonstrate the way that resilient individuals understand themselves and what they have accomplished—their capacity for self-reflection and the ability to use that self-reflection to form planning for the future. This crucial self-understanding involves appraisal of the stresses to be confronted, realistic assessment of the capacity to act, and actions congruent with the assessment. Self-understanding has characterized people in such diverse circumstances as survivors of cancer, civil rights workers, and children of parents with affective disorders.[21] Corresponding to an awareness of understanding at the individual level is an awareness of the importance of parenting contributing to the development of resilience. The recognition and characterization of resilient behavior in pediatric practice in high-risk families is important; the PCP must assess a child or family's strengths and capacities to adapt to adversity.[20] In many instance, the ability to mount an effective intervention depends on the recognition of strengths at the individual family and community levels and the mobilization of resources to enhance these strengths.[4,7]

PCPs have been paying increased attention to the prevention of mental disorders and psychological difficulties in addition to the treatment of the disorders once they occur. This effort requires an understanding of the developmental pathways of psychopathological conditions and healthy development and the positioning of interventions at the times of greatest likelihood of success—for example, enhancing the bond between caregiver and child early in life or assisting in an adolescent's developmental transition. An important characteristic of preventive interventions is that they may be delivered in schools or neighborhoods, as well as in physicians' offices. Equally important for PCPs is the recognition that parents may experience adversities such as bereavement, depression, or divorce and that PCPs can provide opportunities for strengthening parenting and enhancing family coping and for preventing future difficulties. One promising approach is to focus on the parent's capacity to be a good parent despite adversities such as depression and related conditions, to help build children's resilience, and to have the family understand depression together.[22]

CULTURAL COMPETENCE

Along with the rapid growth of knowledge that has led to the construction of the notion of developmental plasticity is the growing awareness of the need for cultural competence; different strategies need to be taken for members of different cultures.[23] This statement is even more true given the increase in the number of immigrants from very different cultures and the fact that demographic trends suggest that soon, the majority of children in this country will be nonwhite. Attention to cultural issues is particularly important relative to mental health. The family is the unit that perpetuates the culture in a way by carrying the chromosomes of the culture that form the cornerstone of emotional development.

In terms of a metaphor, cultural influences resemble a mainstream with many tributaries. Each tributary varies from time to time in depth, rate of flow, and course; the mainstream is modified by its tributaries but also influences them. In the United States, many variations exist in cultural patterns relating to childbearing attitudes and practices. These factors are determined, in part, by geographic, religious, educational, social, and economic backgrounds. For example, in some communities, a great premium is placed on the first-born child. Religious backgrounds definitely tend to influence the size of families. Higher educational backgrounds of parents have been correlated with later childbearing and smaller family size.

The relative rapidity of social movement tends to confuse young parents in terms of their basic group identification. Additionally, increasing educational opportunities usually generate upward social mobility for many young parents. The PCP should know how much parents identify with their old and new social groupings and their cultures. Identification with either (usually some of both) involves some reintegration on the part of the parents, who may require professional assistance. Awareness of the need to tailor interventions to a particular culture is growing, and the strategies required to do so also have expanded.[10,12]

Knowing the cultural and psychological background of a child's family is important for understanding the mental health needs of that child. The emotional climate in which a child is reared reflects the personality development of the parents. Therefore the PCP must know the developmental background of each parent and the immediate environmental factors that are important in the child's life. Because different families identify different roles for their children, the PCP should know how the child fits into the family. Just as the physiological structure and function of an infant have determinants that predate birth, the practices and attitudes that determine how the child will be cared for have comparable antecedents. PCPs may develop an understanding of these factors as they become apparent during the prenatal period or after birth, as they come to know the family as a unit.

Secular changes in family structure of the American family have occurred over the last 40 years. In 1970, 12% of children lived in single-parent homes. Now, 26% do so, with a higher percentage of black and Latino children than white children in single-parent homes. Over one half the children in the United States will spend a portion of childhood with a single parent. When poverty is added to the equation, the situation becomes dire. Eight percent of children in homes with two parents live in poverty, whereas 32% of children in single-parent homes do.[24] Over the last decade, increased emphasis has been placed on sending parents who receive public assistance to work, which means that their children must be cared for, at least part of the time, by someone other than their parents. This task requires high-quality child care or care by extended families; yet, given patterns of mobility and immigration, many parents are raising children without such supports. For all these reasons, parents, grandparents, and other caregivers rely more and more on PCPs for guidance about child rearing.

FLEXIBILITY IN GUIDANCE TO PARENTS

PCPs should learn to adjust their attitudes toward childbearing and child rearing to the cultural backgrounds and attitudes of parents who seek advice. Then, understanding that no right attitude or practice exists becomes easier. A certain practice may be effective for one family, yet its objectives will fail with another. Thus PCPs can help by being objective rather than judgmental in viewing the family. This task requires the capacity to observe, listen, and understand. PCPs can develop an objective attitude by remembering that the culture, not the physician, within certain limits, defines mental health. For example, children brought up in one Native-American culture might not be considered capable of performing the developmental tasks required of children in another tribe living in a different climate with significantly different cultural demands.[6] Many similar cross-cultural comparisons can be made. Although PCPs generally deal with more subtle contrasts, these differences, nevertheless, are real and are important for each family. In a country of people who have such varied origins and so much educational, social, economic, and geographical movement, any single stable tradition of child-rearing practices will not likely emerge in the next several decades. Therefore the objective in each instance is to help each family attain its goals in child rearing uniquely and effectively.

INTEGRATIVE ROLE FOR THE PRIMARY CARE PHYSICIAN

PCPs can combine medical findings with observations of children within their families and perceptions of larger cultural influences to evaluate and meet the mental health needs of children. The evaluation of psychological health is a vital part of the comprehensive assessment of children. Such evaluations provide the basis for helping parents become more effective in rearing their children through helping them to articulate and realize their own goals for them. Because of the increasing numbers of health professionals and disciplines that work with children, the role of PCPs has become even more integrative. As one example, the treatment of attention-deficit/hyperactivity disorder is often undertaken by a PCP, whereas childhood or adolescent depression is less frequently so; but in either case, an integrative treatment approach is needed that involves school, family, direct treatment for the child, and careful follow-up. PCPs bring together the different disciplines and different kinds of knowledge—biological, psychological, and social—in a comprehensive understanding of the treatment for the child.

PRIMARY CARE PHYSICIAN AND PSYCHOLOGICAL DEVELOPMENT

When PCPs approach the management of illness as one aspect of the total care of the child and are interested in the interpersonal relations between the PCP and family, each child can provide an intriguing study. PCPs also have the opportunity to help foster the psychological development of the child. In this regard, and in dealing with the child and parents, PCPs' attitudes toward, interest in, and curiosity about human behavior and relations are important—probably more so than formal knowledge in this area. In addition, findings on resilience have direct application to pediatric practice in that PCPs can often help parents recognize resilience in children at risk or help others who deal with such children.[20] The receptivity and alertness of PCPs in recognizing psychologically charged situations will extend, condition, or limit their effectiveness in the provision of care to many children.

PRIMARY CARE PHYSICIAN AND COMPREHENSIVE CARE

Assuming the primary responsibility for all physical and medical care of the child provides PCPs with the responsibility and opportunity to learn about and care for the psychological and mental health needs of children. PCPs who wish to provide total care should be interested in children in both intellectual and emotional terms. Such PCPs are in a unique position to encourage wholesome attitudes of child rearing during each contact with the family. Concomitantly, they can detect unwholesome attitudes and disturbances early in a child's life and endeavor to provide a more favorable setting for the child through interviews and counseling with the parents. In situations of severe distress, PCPs may decide that more extensive psychological treatment through psychotherapy or other means is needed and refer the child to psychiatric consultation. However, fundamentally, the PCP remains the key professional who comprehensively evaluates the overall health of the child, including the child's mental health, while serving as the central person in the parents' eyes for counseling and guidance and integrates the different observations and information about the child's development.

TOOLS FOR PRACTICE

Engaging Patients and Family

- *Your Child's Mental Health: When To Seek Help and Where To Get Help* (brochure), American Academy of Pediatrics (patiented.aap.org).

Medical Decision Support

- *Mental Health—AAP Mental Health Initiative* (Web page), American Academy of Pediatrics (www.aap.org/commpeds/dochs/mentalhealth/).
- *Mental Health Work Group* (Web page), Centers for Disease Control and Prevention (www.cdc.gov/mentalhealth/).
- *Surgeon General's Report on Mental Health,* US Department of Health and Human Services (www.surgeongeneral.gov/library/mentalhealth/chapter1/sec1.html).

AAP POLICY STATEMENTS

American Academy of Pediatrics, Committee on School Health. School-based mental health services. *Pediatrics.* 2004;113(6):1839-1845. (pediatrics.aappublications.org/cgi/content/full/113/6/1839).

American Academy of Pediatrics. Insurance coverage of mental health and substance abuse services for children and adolescents: a consensus statement. *Pediatrics.* 2000; 106(4):860-862. (aappolicy.aappublications.org/cgi/content/full/pediatrics;106/4/860).

SUGGESTED READINGS

Beardslee WR. Prevention and the clinical encounter. *Am J Orthopsychiatry.* 1998;68:521-533.

Beardslee WR. *When a Parent is Depressed: How to Protect Your Children from the Effects of Depression in the Family.* Originally published in hardcover under the title *Out of the Darkened Room: When a Parent is Depressed: Protecting the Children and Strengthening the Family.* New York, NY: Little, Brown and Company; 2002.

Richmond JB. An idea whose time has arrived. *Pediatr Clin North Am.* 1975;22:517-523.
Richmond JB. Child development: a basic science for pediatrics. *Pediatrics.* 1967;39:649-658.

REFERENCES

1. National Institute of Mental Health. *Advancing Research on Developmental Plasticity: Integrating the Behavioral Science and Neuroscience Of Mental Health.* Washington, DC: National Institute of Mental Health; 1998.
2. Eisenberg L. The social construction of the human brain. *Am J Psychiatry.* 1995;152:1563.
3. Bronfenbrenner U. *The Ecology of Human Development.* Cambridge, MA: Harvard University Press; 1979.
4. National Research Council and Institute of Medicine, Committee on Integrating the Science of Early Childhood Development; Board on Children, Youth, and Families, Commission on Behavioral and Social Sciences and Education. *From Neurons to Neighborhoods: The Science of Early Childhood Development.* In: Shonkoff JP, Phillips DA, eds. Washington, DC: National Academy Press; 2000.
5. National Scientific Council on the Developing Child. *Young Children Develop in an Environment of Relationships.* Working Paper 1.Waltham, MA: Heller School for Social Policy and Management at Brandeis University; 2005.
6. Evans D, Beardslee W, Biederman J, et al. Treatment of depression and bipolar disorder. In: Evans DL, Foa EB, Gur RE, et al, eds. *Treating and Preventing Adolescent Mental Health Disorders: What We Know and What We Don't Know.* New York, NY: Oxford University Press; 2005. Available at: amhi-treatingpreventing.com/anbrg/public/index.html. Accessed February 4, 2008.
7. Maton KI, Schellenbach CJ, Leadbeater BJ, et al, eds. *Investing in Children, Youth, Families, and Communities: Strengths-Based Research and Policy.* Washington, DC: American Psychological Association; 2004.
8. Mrazek PJ, Haggerty RJ, eds. *Reducing Risks for Mental Disorders: Frontiers for Preventive Intervention Research.* Report of the Committee on Prevention of Mental Disorders, Division of Biobehavioral Sciences and Mental Disorders, Institute of Medicine. Washington, DC: National Academy Press; 1994.
9. Schorr LB. *Common Purpose: Strengthening Families and Neighborhoods to Rebuild America.* New York, NY: Anchor Books, Doubleday; 1997.
10. Rutter M. The interplay of nature, nurture, and developmental influences. *Arch Gen Psychiatry.* 2002;59:996-1000.
11. US Public Health Service. *Report of the Surgeon General's Conference on Children's Mental Health: A National Action Agenda.* Washington, DC: US Department of Health and Human Services; 2000.
12. Carnegie Task Force. *Starting Points: Meeting the Needs of Our Youngest Children.* New York, NY: Carnegie Corporation of New York; 1994.
13. Piaget J. *The Origins of Intelligence in Children.* New York, NY: WW Norton; 1963.
14. Skinner BF. *Science and Human Behavior.* New York, NY: Macmillan; 1953.
15. Thomas A, Chess S, Birch H. *Temperament and Behavior Disorders in Children.* New York, NY: New York University Press; 1968.
16. Kohlberg L. Stage and sequence: the cognitive-developmental approach to socialization. In: Goslin D, eds. *Handbook of Socialization Theory and Research.* Chicago, IL: Rand McNally; 1969.
17. Selman RL, Watts CL, Schultz LH. *Fostering Friendship.* New York, NY: Aldine de Gruyter; 1997.
18. Erikson EH. *Childhood and Society,* 2nd ed. New York, NY: WW Norton; 1963.
19. Luthar SS, Cicchetti D, Becker B. The construct of resilience: a critical evaluation and guidelines for future work. *Child Dev.* 2000;71:543-562.
20. Richmond JB, Beardslee WR. Resiliency: research and practical implications for pediatricians. *J Dev Behav Pediatr.* 1988;9:157-163.
21. Beardslee WR. The role of self-understanding in resilient individuals: the development of a perspective. *Am J Orthopsychiatry.* 1989;59:266.
22. Beardslee WR, Gladstone TRG, Wright EJ, et al. A family-based approach to the prevention of depressive symptoms in children at risk: evidence of parental and child change. *Pediatrics.* 2003;112:e119-e131.
23. Rogler LH. The meaning of culturally sensitive research in mental health. *Am J Psychiatry.* 1989;146:296-303.
24. McLanahan S, Donahue E, Haskins R. Introducing the issue. *The Future of Children: Marriage and Child Wellbeing.* 2005;15(2):3-9.

Chapter 109

EARLY EDUCATION AND CHILD CARE PROGRAMS

Susan S. Aronson, MD

"High-quality early education and child care for young children improves their health and promotes their development and learning. Early education includes all of a child's experiences at home, in child care and in other preschool settings. Pediatricians have a role in promoting access to quality early education and child care beginning at birth for all children."[1]

In addition to early education programs for infants, toddlers, and preschool-aged children, many children in kindergarten through the sixth grade participate in educational and recreational child care programs that take place outside school hours. These before- and after-school programs should develop the child's skills and awareness of community while providing responsible adult supervision. Pediatricians have responsibilities for ensuring the well being of children wherever they are in care. These responsibilities include guiding families and providers of services to families and coordinating health care with other services that children receive.

ARRANGEMENTS FAMILIES CHOOSE FOR THEIR CHILDREN

In the United States the numbers and proportions of children participating in early education and child care arrangements changed little between 1995 and 2001. Approximately 12 million, or 61%, of children 0 to 6 years of age not yet in kindergarten are in some nonparental arrangement for part of the day, some days each week (Table 109-1).[2] Approximately one half of school-aged children in kindergarten through the eighth

Table 109-1 Young Children in Early Education and Child Care in 2001

TYPE	0-2 YEARS OF AGE	3-6 YEARS OF AGE
Parent only	48.0%	26.3%
Total nonparental*	52.0%	73.7%
Home-based relative	23.3%	22.7%
Home-based nonrelative	18.0%	14.0%
Center based	16.5%	56.3%

*Some children participate in more than one type of nonparental care arrangement; therefore the sum of all nonparental arrangements exceeds the total percentage in nonparental care.
From US Department of Education, National Center for Education Statistics, National Household Educations Surveys Program (NHES), Table POP8. A Child Care: Percentage of Children Ages 0-6, Not Yet in Kindergarten By Type of Care Arrangement and Child and Family Characteristics, 1995 and 2001. Available at: www.childstats.gov/americaschildren06/tables/pop8a.asp. Accessed August 14, 2007.

grade are in nonparental care outside regular school hours. In higher grades, they are more likely to be engaged in organized before- and after-school activities, most often sports.[3] An individual child may use more than one arrangement. Families may use different arrangements for siblings.

Home-based nonparental early education and child care includes care in the child's own home or in someone else's home. Services provided outside the child's own home include small-family child care homes (six or fewer children in the caregiver's home) and large-family child care homes (7 to 12 children in a caregiver's home that has more than one caregiver). Services may be provided by friends, neighbors, relatives, or employees. People who provide services in home settings call themselves caregivers, nannies, babysitters, and housekeepers. The term *teacher* is more often associated with center-based services. Center-based early education includes child care centers, nursery schools, preschools, Head Start programs, and other types of nonresidential programs. The names given to programs do not define the type of service provided or the professional competence of the staff working there.

The national organizations of early-childhood professionals describe their service as child care or early care and education. The terms *early education* and *child care* are more accurate, since all types of care involve some quality of education for the children. In addition, these terms embrace the fast-growing programs for school-aged children during nonschool hours.

American attitudes toward the navigation of work and family life are ambivalent. Parents of both genders are expected to contribute to family income and to pursue careers. Societal support in the United States for parental leave and quality early education services lags far behind most other developed countries. Whether they work outside the home or only at home, the majority of parents lack desired support for arranging education and child care services for their children.

REGULATION, ACCREDITATION, AND QUALITY OF CARE

Pediatricians should know about the core information provided in the national consensus standards for best practice on the Web site of The National Resource Center for Health and Safety in Child Care as a resource for parents and child care facilities. Information on structure, organization, and best practices for early child care is especially important for health professionals who may be the only advisors to early childhood–care professionals regarding health-related matters. Health professionals who serve as consultants for early education and child care programs can accomplish much good if they understand the constraints of the operators and engage in collaborative, constructive problem solving.

PSYCHOSOCIAL OUTCOMES

Psychosocial Outcomes for the Child

Long-term child development is not affected adversely when mothers of infants and older children work. In fact, for single mothers and low-income families, early parental employment may affect child development positively by increasing family income.[4] Promotion of exclusive early maternal care in the face of changing cultural norms feeds maternal guilt and fosters public ambivalence about necessary family support services. The majority of children thrive in a variety of reasonably nurturing child care arrangements. What children want and need is time with their parents when their parents are focused on them, which can occur when doing ordinary activities of living.[5]

Both the quality of the child care arrangement and what the family believes about the appropriateness of their child's care are strong determinants of the effect of the arrangements on the child. During infancy, most families use more than one type of care, and most children are in some type of nonparental care by 4 months of age. Children from the lowest- and highest-income families receive care of better quality than those in the middle. Family characteristics such as family income and the mother's education are much stronger predictors of children's outcomes than the amount of time they spent in a group-care setting. Low-income mothers who use full-time, higher-quality programs are more likely to be involved positively with their infants than are low-income mothers who care for their infants only at home or who use lower-quality full-time care. The behavior of children who spend more hours in group care is more of a problem at 2 years of age, but by age 3 years these children have fewer behavior problems and are more cooperative than those who spend less time in such programs.[6]

For typically developing children and those with special needs related to behavioral, social, developmental, or physical problems, early education and child care programs can function as extended family. Families with young parents, or parents who have few relatives nearby, those with children of divorce, children who are in foster care, children who are being adopted, children who are especially active, or children who have developmental delays benefit from quality group-care arrangements. These arrangements help when they are stable and involve competent, experienced adults.

Psychosocial Outcomes for the Family

Good early education and child care programs support families. Early education professionals serve as extended families for young parents by addressing everyday issues with their cumulative experience and training. In many early education and child care programs, teachers and directors refer families to community resources. They also help identify and refer children who have special needs to health professionals. When well informed by the child's health professionals, teachers or caregivers are strong partners in ensuring appropriate care for such children. By modeling and sharing strategies for healthy development of children, competent caregivers foster parent education and confidence. Because they work with children and families daily, early childhood educators can spot atypical behaviors that parents and physicians overlook.

RISKS AND OPPORTUNITIES FOR HEALTH PROMOTION

Infection, Allergy, and Asthma

Close contact in child care facilitates the spread of many respiratory, gastrointestinal, systemic, and skin infections, but the types of infections are the same as those that children and adults experience in the community.[7,8] Spread of infection in early education and child care is facilitated by children's immature immune systems and by behaviors that contaminate the environment and promote self-inoculation. Illness associated with participation in group-care settings is costly to families and staff and serves as a conduit of infection to family members and the community.

As shown in Figure 109-1 through Figure 109-3 the risk of upper respiratory infection and ear infections is higher for infants in group care compared with those cared for exclusively at home. This risk decreases as children grow older and spend more time in group care.[9-11] Attendance in center-based programs during preschool years seems to protect children against common upper respiratory infections through the elementary school years, presumably because of immunity acquired from early exposure to infectious disease agents. For gastrointestinal illness the incidence among children overall is lower than for respiratory disease, and the difference between group participants and children cared for only by their parents is less than for respiratory disease. Gastrointestinal disease is somewhat elevated for infants in center-based arrangements and for preschool-aged children who receive care in the homes of relatives.

Infectious diseases are common in all young children; every episode of childhood infection is not attributable to group-care participation. By the time children are 3 years of age, little difference can be found in the incidence of infectious diseases for children in group

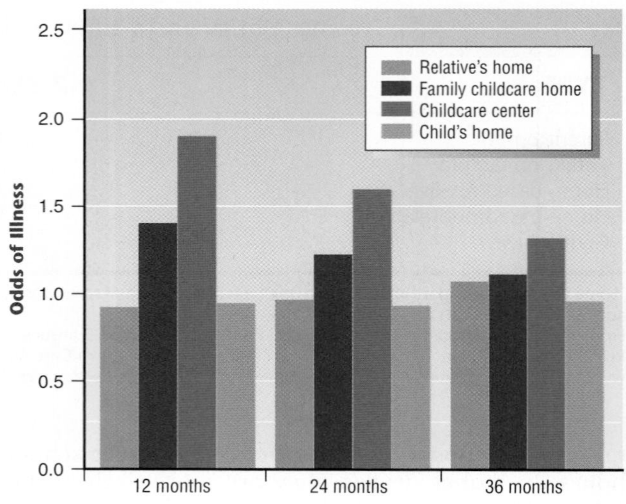

Figure 109-1 Upper respiratory infection by type of care. *(National Institute of Child Health and Human Development, Early Child Care Research Network. Child care and common communicable illnesses: results from the National Institute of Child Health and Human Development Study of Early Child Care.* Arch Pediatr Adolesc Med. *2001;155[4]: 481-488.)*

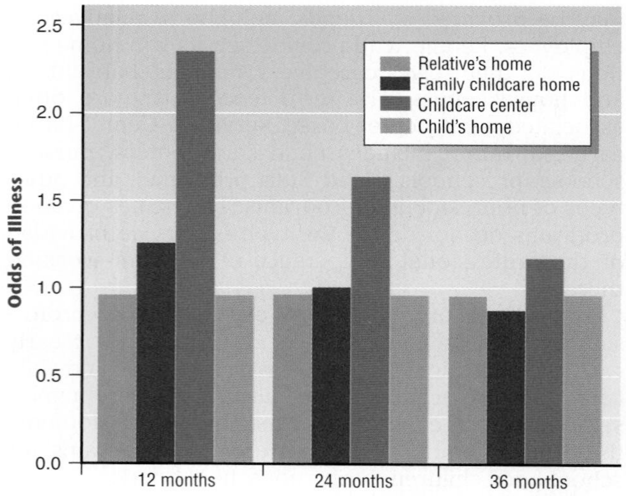

Figure 109-2 Ear infection by type of care. *(National Institute of Child Health and Human Development, Early Child Care Research Network. Child care and common communicable illnesses: results from the National Institute of Child Health and Human Development Study of Early Child Care.* Arch Pediatr Adolesc Med. *2001;155[4]:481-488.)*

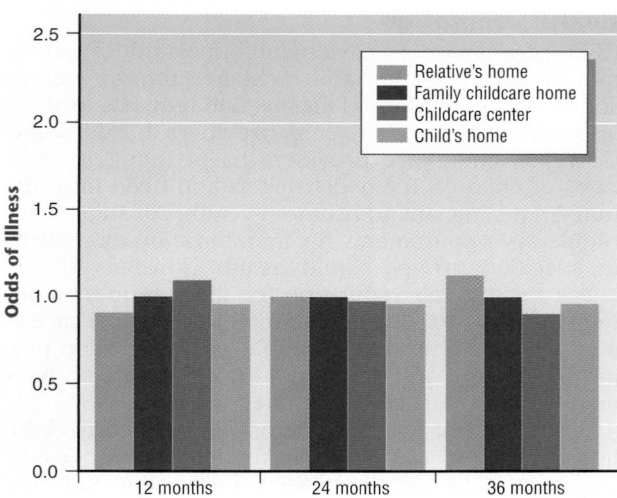

Figure 109-3 Gastrointestinal illness by type of care. *(National Institute of Child Health and Human Development, Early Child Care Research Network. Child care and common communicable illnesses: results from the National Institute of Child Health and Human Development Study of Early Child Care.* Arch Pediatr Adolesc Med. *2001;155[4]:481-488.)*

care compared with those cared for only at home. Among 3-year-old children who entered care as infants, fewer common respiratory infections occurred than for their peers who were never in group care.[12-15] In addition, the incidence of chronic illness does not seem to be increased by child care participation from infancy. Neither allergic rhinitis nor asthma is increased by group-care participation.[16] Other factors play an unexplained role in infectious disease in child care settings as well. For example, children who use pacifiers in child care have an increased risk of acquiring otitis media compared with those who suck their thumb.[17]

Although group care makes work-force participation by both parents possible, frequent illness of children in child care is a burden for children, parents, employers, and the community. Many diseases that are transmitted in group care can infect others in the community, including caregivers, parents, and family members. The most important infections transmitted to adult contacts of children in group care are hepatitis A, cytomegalovirus, and parvovirus B19.[18]

Keeping immunizations up to date, caring for children in age cohorts in which the children who make up the group at the beginning of care comprise the group for 1 or more years, and practicing good personal and environmental hygiene can reduce the risk of infectious disease in group care. Universal use of recommended vaccines can control the spread of diseases in child care. Hepatitis A vaccine has controlled outbreaks in group-care settings in states where the disease is endemic. The American Academy of Pediatrics (AAP) recommends that all children receive hepatitis A vaccine between 1 and 2 years of age.[19] The AAP and the Advisory Committee on Immunization Practices of the Centers for Disease Control and Prevention (CDC) recommend that all children between the ages of 6 months and 59 months, as well as their caregivers, receive influenza vaccine to control disease in young children and to limit dissemination of the virus to others in the community.[20,21]

Improving hand washing and environmental hygiene substantially reduces the incidence of both respiratory and gastrointestinal infections in an age-specific manner. Colds, in children younger than 24 months, were reduced by 17% when compliance with hand washing was high. Good hand hygiene reduced diarrhea episodes by two thirds in children older than 24 months.[22,23] Clinicians can advise child care providers about how to reduce the risk of spread of infectious disease. For example, clinicians can observe and advise about how educators should perform and monitor hand and surface sanitation, about the importance of using hand lotion to prevent drying and cracking of frequently washed hands, about the necessary contact time and volume of product if hand sanitizers are used, and about diapering routines to limit contamination that spreads infectious material around the facility. When properly plumbed sinks are not available where they are needed, clinicians can suggest that the facility purchase portable sinks that are commercially available.

Exclusion from Child Care

Child care workers need advice about prevention, treatment, and exclusion of ill children and adults. An infected child does not need to be excluded unless the child cannot participate in activities, requires care that exceeds caregiver resources, or the child's illness puts the other children at increased risk with continued exposure. For many infections, substantial shedding of disease agents occurs before symptoms occur; therefore removal of the symptomatic child for the sake of others is usually fruitless. On the other hand, when children have infectious diarrhea, the contamination of the environment during diaper changing and from fecal accidents is overwhelming. For the purpose of making decisions about exclusion from child care, infectious diarrhea is defined as more frequent and watery or less-formed stools not associated with changes of diet. Using this definition the national health and safety performance standards for child care require exclusion of children with diarrhea that is not contained by an ability to use the toilet.[24] To help clinicians and early educators make, implement, and communicate decisions about appropriate exclusion policies, the AAP publishes detailed guidelines and reproducible fact sheets on management of infectious diseases in child care and schools.[25]

Families need to have plans for the inevitability of their child's illness. Some communities have developed programs to care for ill children whose parents must work. Ill children benefit from familiar environments and well-established relationships for comfort and care. Arrangements that involve care by strangers in strange environments may add to the stress of illness. If strange environments are used, then special care arrangements for ill children and should be designed to meet the ill child's physical and emotional needs.

Injury

Children in center-based programs have fewer injuries during their hours at the center than do children who receive care only at home. However, children in these centers suffer more injuries during the hours they are at home than do children who are cared for only at home. This finding suggests that time spent at home may involve less supervision by tired parents or more risk-taking behavior by children making the transition from one environment to another. Children in family child care homes have a higher incidence of injury while in that setting than do either children in centers or those cared for only in their own homes. The reason for this increased risk of injury in family child care homes is unclear. Table 109-2 summarizes the incidence of injury by type of setting.

The most common and most severe injuries in early education and child care settings are falls from climbing equipment mounted over surfaces that do not absorb impact. Grass, carpeting, packed earth or sand, cement, asphalt, and ordinary gym mats do not absorb impact forces from climbers. Both indoor and outdoor climbing equipment should be installed over cushioning materials, such as 9 to 12 inches of bark mulch or a manufactured pad rated for a fall from the highest point of the equipment. Play equipment should be designed for the size and developmental abilities of the users. Too often, toddlers and preschoolers use play equipment designed for older children. Commonly, early education programs install large pieces of play equipment in relatively small areas, creating a situation in which too many children compete and interact in one place. Providing adequate supervision requires an adult stationed within arms length of the equipment and a reasonable number of children using the equipment at any one time. Children will engage in risky behavior during active play. Although some risk taking fosters child development, the equipment and supervision should keep risk taking from leading to serious injury. The US Consumer Product Safety Commission[26] (CPSC) and the CDC-founded National Program for Playground Safety at the University of Northern Iowa[27] have information for educators and health professionals, as well as links to technical resources to design and maintain safe playgrounds.

Table 109-2 Injury Rates per 100,000 Hours by Type of Setting

TYPE OF SETTING	NUMBER OF INJURIES PER 100,000 HOURS IN CARE
Center	2.18
Care only in child's own home	2.31
Care in own home (for child who also is enrolled in a center)	3.40
Family child care home	3.95

From Gunn W, Pinsky PF, Sacks JJ, et al. Injuries and poisonings in out-of-home child care and home care. *Am J Dis Child* 1991;145(7):779-781. Reprinted by permission of the American Medical Association.

Health Promotion

Child care providers have many opportunities to promote medical, dental, and mental health, as well as sound nutrition. Many clinicians find requests to share information with child care providers burdensome. However, child care providers have useful observations of children for pediatricians and need information from clinicians to promote health. All states have regulatory requirements for immunization of children in specified groups. Child health clinicians should check their state's regulation for these requirements. Requirements for documentation of preventive care as a condition of enrollment enable early education programs to serve as a safety net for children who have not sought or received recommended services.

Interdisciplinary collaboration between early childhood educators and health professionals improves the quality of care for all children. Early education and child care providers need specific instructions from pediatric practitioners to provide appropriate care for children who have special health care needs. Generally, pediatric clinicians should give direct written or verbal instructions to early childhood educators. Many parents do not recall or are unable to explain clearly to teachers/caregivers what health professionals have asked to be done for their children. Educators and health professionals need to develop efficient and effective ways to communicate with each other. Both parties need parent consent to share information about a child, and both have unpredictable, intense workday demands that make extra paperwork or telephone calls burdensome. Nevertheless, without such communication, children suffer.

Children with chronic health conditions add to the already-heavy burdens on early education and child care providers. In many instances, even small modifications of daily routines require significant effort. Nonetheless, accommodation of such children is desirable and, under the Americans with Disabilities Act, is required by federal law. Necessary equipment and supplies are the easiest to arrange. Staff who may need to administer medication or deal with emergencies usually require in-person training from a health professional, written instructions, and periodic check points to adjust the arrangements. The frequency of chronic illnesses among children in group care settings mirrors that in the child population. These conditions include allergies, asthma, developmental and behavioral problems, sensory difficulties, diabetes, and other less common conditions. Care coordination for a child with special needs should include everyone who plays a role in the child's life.

ROLES FOR CHILD HEALTH PROFESSIONALS

Child health professionals can support quality early education and child care by:

- Asking and advising families about nonparental-education and care arrangements
- Providing telephone advice and written instructions to caregivers of their patients who have special health care needs

- Offering on-site consultation to administrators and staff of early education and child care programs about decisions related to health and safety policies
- Advocating social policies that support quality early education and child care and increased access for all young children and families who need such programs
- Advocating business policies and practices to help families care for their children, such as family medical leave, flex time, and sick leave to care for an ill child

Helping Parents Make Difficult Choices

Young parents are often too stressed to consider the issues of quality and weigh them rationally against affordability and convenience. Even for middle- and upper-income families, nonparental arrangements are often made with convenience and cost as priorities. In many families, wage earners compare the cost with the mother's income, not with the pooled earnings of both parents as for other family responsibilities. The portion of family income spent on nonparental arrangements can be substantial and still grossly insufficient to purchase good services. When available options are equally convenient and costly, many parents make decisions based on the attractiveness of the facade; and few make more than walk-through observations of the staff and the parts of the program their children will experience.

By asking parents of young children about their plans and the early education and child care services they are using, health professionals can provide much-needed help to families. Topics to cover include:

- Going back to work after childbirth
- Continuing breastfeeding while working
- Parent feelings about and options for nonparental care
- How to choose among available options
- Deciding when an ill child should stay home and when a child can return after an illness
- Addressing behavior problems that occur in group settings
- Handling any special health care needs such as medication administration or other treatment required while the child is in nonparental care

In a survey of practicing pediatricians completed by the AAP in 2004, 93% of respondents reported that they asked whether children younger than 4 years of age regularly spend time in a child care setting. However, only three of the previously listed topics were reportedly initiated by more than one half of respondents. These three topics were (1) going back to work after childbirth, (2) continuing breastfeeding, and (3) deciding when a child can return after an illness.[28] Surveys of parents consistently reveal that they wish their pediatricians would bring up all these topics. Many parents do not believe their pediatricians have time or want to discuss these issues; therefore they do not ask about them during the busy well-child visits. With limited office time available, their perceptions are accurate. However, over the course of a series of visits, discussing these issues that affect the experience of nearly all children is both possible and desirable.

Bright Futures guidelines provide pediatricians two relevant handouts for parents. One resource outlines four steps parents should take when selecting child care: (1) interviewing caregivers, (2) checking references, (3) making a decision, and (4) staying involved. The other handout is a checklist for safety prepared by the CPSC. It lists hazards that a CPSC study identified in two thirds of a national sample of licensed child care facilities visited in 1998.[29]

Families should check for reliable references to confirm that teachers and other caregivers are mature and experienced in working with young children. In home-based settings with only one caregiver, special arrangements are necessary. Reliable and familiar back-up arrangements should exist when the caregiver must take time off or when an emergency occurs that requires that the caregiver care for a child who is sick or injured and also care for any other children present. In addition, plans should address possible facility emergencies that might require evacuation or shelter in place. Isolation of home-based caregivers makes monitoring of quality difficult. Occasional unannounced early pick-up of children and communication with other parents whose children are enrolled is necessary to make sure that services are provided appropriately.

Many parents will appreciate receiving information on the 13 key indicators of quality child care that research shows are predictive of overall performance of early education and child care programs. Some parents may want to read more about the research on these indicators.[30] The 13 indicators are:

- Child abuse reporting and clearances
- Up-to-date immunization status documented in early education and child care records
- Child-to-staff ratio and group size
- Director qualifications
- Teacher qualifications
- Staff training
- Supervision or discipline
- Fire drills
- Administration of medication
- Emergency contacts or plan
- Outdoor playground safety
- Inaccessibility of toxic substances
- Hand washing and diapering

From the first contact with the family, including prenatal visits, each well-child visit should include information about who is or will be involved in the child's care, both when the child is well and when the child is ill. For families who want to provide parent-only care, pediatricians can suggest options such as part-time work for both parents and jobs that permit flex-time and working at home. For parents who plan to involve others in educating and caring for their children, pediatricians should ask parents about the experience, training, and compatibility of the style of the teacher/caregiver with that of the family, as well as the child-to-staff ratio, the group size, and what observations the parents have made where their child will receive care. When asked to complete a health form for a patient's enrollment or continued participation in an early education and child care program, the child-health professional can revisit these issues to see whether further help is needed. At subsequent well-child visits, parents should be asked how the child is responding to the current arrangement for child care.

Many communities have resource and referral (R&R) agencies. These agencies help inform parents about what to anticipate in an early education and child care facility and match available services with family needs. Some R&R agencies keep track of vacancies, size of waiting lists, local sources of subsidy, requirements for providers to operate legally, and many other policy issues; some also provide training for providers of early education and child care. To determine who inspects, how often, and what they check in community child care facilities, pediatricians can call the local licensing agency. An efficient way to locate a state or local R&R and licensing agency is to call the help line of the National Association for Child Care Resource and Referral: Child Care Aware (800-424-2246).

Child Health Professional as a Parent

Parents who are health professionals have a special responsibility as community role models. They should seek competent arrangements and help improve the services they find. Those who employ in-home caregivers should pay fair wages and benefits after ensuring that in-home caregivers are supervised with frequent and unannounced visits, that cultural differences in care do not pose problems, and that literacy and language limitations are not barriers to good exchange of information between the caregiver and the family. In out-of-home care, parents who are pediatric health professionals can contribute materially to improving the program as advisors and as instructors for the children, staff, and other families.

Child Health Professional as an Advisor and Consultant for Programs

Child health professionals routinely provide advice over the telephone to families and, with parental consent, to other caregivers. In addition, pediatric clinicians can enhance compliance by providing written instructions and, when appropriate, by giving in-person training on how to carry out prescribed measures for patients who have special health care needs. Health professionals can work as paid or volunteer program consultants, advising early education and child care providers about health problems that have implications for the group. Many nurses and physicians have taken this role as a part of their commitment to the community. Training for these activities is available in every state from the graduates of the National Training Institute for Child Care Health Consultants at the School of Public Health of the University of North Carolina at Chapel Hill. In addition, a small library of excellent resources to support the health consultation role is available.[24,25,31-33]

To date, legal action against health professionals for malpractice in the role of child care health consultant has not been a problem. Nevertheless, as with any professional role, insurance against liability and legal costs for defense in the event of a suit is desirable. Liability varies with the type of work done, the relationships involved, and state law. Legal advice about the liability for this role clarified the level of risk and how to minimize exposure.[34] Individual medical liability carriers may be reluctant to modify their standard policy language to accommodate the role of the child care health consultant. However, an academic institution or large health care provider may be willing to provide a letter that affirms that service as a consultant to early education and child care in the community is within the scope of covered professional activity.

Before becoming a regular health advisor for a specific program, the health professional should visit the facility during the most active time of day, usually between early morning and mid afternoon. A visit helps the child health professional to see health and safety in context and to offer advice relevant to the program. Learning about any other health professionals who are involved with the program facilitates collaboration and avoids unnecessary conflict. Typical questions educators ask physicians are:

- When should a physician's note be required for return to care?
- How should a child who will not stop biting be managed?
- What can be done to reduce the burden for administering medicine during the day?
- How can outbreaks of lice be controlled?
- Why do physicians not keep children up to date with their immunizations?
- How can child care programs obtain information they need from physicians to provide good care for children who are the physician's patients?

Most educators are grateful for thoughtful responses to such questions and often recommend helpful pediatric practitioners to families. If asked about care for an individual child who is not a patient, then the consultant should suggest contact with that child's medical home. As a consultant, a pediatric health professional can help plan and provide training for program staff. The children's nap time or evening may be the only time when such training activities can be scheduled.

Paying for Early Education and Child Care

Care for one child on a full-day, 5-day-a-week basis costs families an amount equal to tuition and room and board at a public university.[35] Although the public routinely subsidizes college education, the cost of early education is borne primarily by parents. All but the wealthiest families spend between 9% and 23% of their income on child care, with the heaviest burden falling on those below the poverty level.[36] The supply of quality early education and child care is greatest in affluent areas where parents can afford to pay and in urban areas where government subsidies increase supply for those living in poverty. Despite recent increases in federal, state, and employer funding, financial help to pay for these services is available only to 29% of employed families with children younger than 13 years.[37] Tax credits favor families with higher incomes. Pressed to fund child care as part of welfare-to-work policies, some states offer incentives for parents to choose low-cost, low-quality arrangements.

Child Health Professional as an Advocate for Quality of Early Education and Child Care

The quality of early education programs can be improved by:

- Systematic planning to set appropriate requirements
- Good surveillance systems to measure performance
- Use of surveillance data to design interventions (technical assistance, training, linkages, and resource development)
- Use of surveillance data to determine whether interventions improve performance
- Allocation of societal resources to support quality early education and child care as support of families that benefits the entire community

Child health professionals have credibility when they speak about the importance of quality early education and child care. As respected champions of children, child health professionals can generate demand for better services by communicating about the issues in discussions with families, in three-way partnerships with families and educators, in meetings with peers and policy makers, in legislative hearings, and in contacts with the media. Without affordable and accessible early education and child care programs of good quality, many children will not come to school eager to learn. Many will lack supervision and healthful experiences. Good early education and child care can decrease socially disruptive behaviors and build children's self-esteem and competence. As effective advocates, health professionals can foster community actions that support parents and improve their early education and child care options. Of all the roles health care professionals can play, improving the quality of early education and child care is one that will make a significant difference in the lives of large numbers of children and families.

TOOLS FOR PRACTICE

Community Advocacy

- *Caring for Our Children—National Health and Safety Performance Standards: Guidelines for Out-of-Home Child Care Programs* (book), American Academy of Pediatrics (www.aap.org/bookstore).
- *Health in Child Care Manual, 4th edition* (book), American Academy of Pediatrics (www.aap.org/bookstore).
- *Managing Infectious Diseases in Child Care and Schools* (book), American Academy of Pediatrics (www.aap.org/bookstore).
- *The Pediatrician's Role in Promoting Health and Safety in Child Care* (book), American Academy of Pediatrics (www.aap.org/bookstore).

Engaging Patient and Family

- *A Parent's Guide to Choosing Safe and Healthy Child Care* (brochure), National Resource Center for Health and Safety in Child Care and Early Education (nrc.uchsc.edu/RESOURCES/ParentsGuide.pdf).
- *Child Care Safety Check List* (booklet), U.S. Consumer Product Safety Commission (www.cpsc.gov/CPSCPUB/PUBS/childcare.pdf).
- *Choosing Child Care: What's Best for Your Family* (brochure), American Academy of Pediatrics (patiented.aap.org).
- *Early Childhood Family Tip Sheet* (fact sheets), Bright Futures (www.brightfutures.org/TipSheets/pdf/ec_color.pdf).
- *Healthy Kids, Healthy Care* (Web page), National Resource Center for Health and Safety in Child Care and Early Education (www.healthykids.us/).
- *Infancy Family Tip Sheet* (fact sheets), Bright Futures (www.brightfutures.org/TipSheets/pdf/in_color.pdf).

RELATED WEB SITES

- Healthy Child Care America (www.healthychildcare.org/index.cfm).
- Healthy Child Care Consultant Network Support Center (hcccnsc.edc.org/).
- National Accreditation Commission for Early Care and Education Programs (www.naccp.org/displaycommon.cfm?an=5).
- National AfterSchool Association (www.naaweb.org/).
- National Association for the Education of Young Children (www.naeyc.org/).
- National Association of Family Child Care (www.nafcc.org/include/default.asp).
- National Child Care Association (www.nccanet.org/).
- National Early Childhood Program Accreditation (www.necpa.net/).
- National Program for Playground Safety (www.playgroundsafety.org/).
- National Resource Center for Health and Safety in Child Care and Early Education (nrc.uchsc.edu/).
- National Training Institute for Child Care Health Consultants (www2.sph.unc.edu/courses/childcare/).

AAP POLICY STATEMENT

American Academy of Pediatrics, Committee on Early Childhood, Adoption, and Dependent Care. Quality early education and child care from birth to kindergarten. *Pediatrics*. 2005;115(1):187-191. (aappolicy.aappublications.org/cgi/content/full/pediatrics;115/1/187).

REFERENCES

1. American Academy of Pediatrics, Committee on Early Childhood, Adoption, and Dependent Care. Quality early education and child care from birth to kindergarten. *Pediatrics*. 2005;115(1):187-191.
2. US Department of Education, National Center for Education Statistics, National Household Educations Surveys Program (NHES). FAM3.A Child Care: Percentage of Children Ages 0-6, Not Yet in Kindergarten By Type of Care Arrangement and Child and Family Characteristics, 1995, 2001 and 2005. Available at: www.childstats.gov/americaschildren/tables/fam3a.asp. Accessed August 14, 2007.
3. US Department of Education, National Center for Education Statistics, National Household Educations Surveys Program (NHES). FAM3.C Child Care: Percentage of Children in Kindergarten Through 8th-Grade By Weekday Care and Before- and After-School Activities By Grade Level, Poverty Status, Race, and Hispanic Origin, 2005. Available at: www.childstats.gov/americaschildren/tables/fam3c.asp. Accessed August 14, 2007.

4. Harvey E. Short-term and long-term effects of early parental employment on children of the National Longitudinal Survey of Youth. *Dev Psychol*. 1999;35(2):445-459.
5. Galinsky E. *Ask the Children: What America's Children Really Think About Working Parents*. New York, NY: William Morrow and Company; 1999.
6. Peth-Pierce R. The NICHD Study of Early Child Care. NIH Pub No 98-4318. Bethesda, MD: National Institute of Child Health and Human Development, US Department of Health and Human Services; 1998.
7. Osterholm M, Reves RR, Murph JR, et al. Infectious diseases and child day care. *Pediatr Infect Dis J*. 1992;11 (8 suppl):S31-S41.
8. Pickering L, Osterholm M. Infectious diseases in children and adults associated with out-of-home child care. In: Long S, Prober C, Pickering L, eds. *Principles and Practices of Pediatric Infectious Diseases*. New York, NY: Churchill Livingstone; 1997.
9. Hurwitz ES, Gunn WJ, Pinsky PF, et al. Risk of respiratory illness associated with day-care attendance: a nationwide study. *Pediatrics*. 1991;87(1):62-69.
10. National Institute of Child Health and Human Development, Early Child Care Research Network. Child care and common communicable illnesses: results from the National Institute of Child Health and Human Development Study of Early Child Care. *Arch Pediatr Adolesc Med*. 2001;155(4):481-488.
11. Ball TH, Holberg CJ, Aldous MB, et al. Influence of attendance at day care on the common cold from birth through 13 years of age. *Arch Pediatr Adolesc Med*. 2002; 156(2):121-126.
12. Cordell RL, MacDonald JK, Solomon SL, et al. Illnesses and absence due to illness among children attending child care facilities in Seattle-King County, Washington. *Pediatrics*. 1997;100(5):850-855.
13. Cordell RL, Waterman SH, Chang A, et al. Provider-reported illness and absence due to illness among children attending child-care homes and centers in San Diego, Calif. *Arch Pediatr Adolesc Med*. 1999;153(3): 275-280.
14. National Institute of Child Health and Human Development, Early Child Care Research Network. Child care and common communicable illnesses: results from the National Institute of Child Health and Human Development Study of Early Child Care. *Arch Pediatr Adolesc Med*. 2001;155(4):481-488.
15. Bradley RH, National Institute of Child Health and Human Development (NICHD), Early Child Care Research Network. Child care and common communicable illnesses in children aged 37 to 54 months. *Arch Pediatr Adolesc Med*. 2003;157(2):196-200.
16. Nafstad P, Brunekreef B, Skrondal A, et al. Early respiratory infections, asthma, and allergy: 10-year follow-up of the Oslo Birth Cohort. *Pediatrics*. 2005:116(2):e255-e262.
17. Niemelä M, Uhari M, Möttönen M. A pacifier increases the risk of recurrent acute otitis media in children in day care centers. *Pediatrics*. 1995;96(5 pt 1):884-888.
18. Reves RR, Pickering LK. Impact of child day care on infectious diseases in adults. *Infect Dis Clin North Am*. 1992;69(1):239-250.
19. American Academy of Pediatrics. Hepatitis A. In: Pickering LK, Baker CJ, Long SS, et al, eds. *Red Book: 2006 Report of the Committee on Infectious Diseases*. 27th ed. Elk Grove Village, IL; American Academy of Pediatrics; 2006.
20. American Academy of Pediatrics. Influenza. In: Pickering LK, Baker CJ, Long SS, et al, eds. *2006 Red Book: Report of the Committee on Infectious Diseases*. 27th ed. Elk Grove Village, IL: American Academy of Pediatrics; 2006.
21. Centers for Disease Control and Prevention. Prevention and control of influenza: recommendations of the Advisory Committee on Immunization Practices. (ACIP), 2007. *MMWR* 2007;56(NO.RRO6):1-54.
22. Roberts L, Smith W, Jorm L, et al. Effect of infection control measures on the frequency of upper respiratory infection in child care: a randomized, controlled trial. *Pediatrics*. 2000;105(4 pt 1):738-742.
23. Roberts L, Jorm L, Patel M, et al. Effect of infection control measures on the frequency of diarrheal episodes in child care: a randomized, controlled trial. *Pediatrics*. 2000;105(4 pt 1):743-746.
24. American Academy of Pediatrics, American Public Health Association, National Resource Center for Health and Safety in Child Care. *Caring for Our Children: National Health and Safety Performance Standards: Guidelines for Out-of-home Child Care Programs*. 2nd ed. Elk Grove Village, IL: American Academy of Pediatrics; 2002;124.
25. Aronson SS, Shope TR, eds. *Managing Infectious Diseases in Child Care and Schools: A Quick Reference Guide*. Elk Grove Village, IL: American Academy of Pediatrics; 2005.
26. US Consumer Product Safety Commission. Available at: www.cpsc.gov. Accessed August 15, 2007.
27. National Program for Playground Safety. Available at: www.uni.edu/playground. Accessed August 15, 2007.
28. American Academy of Pediatrics, Division of Health Services Research. AAP survey: pediatricians often address child care issues. *AAP News*. 2005;26(10):15.
29. American Academy of Pediatrics. Bright Futures: Health Professionals, Tools and Resources, Guidelines for Health Supervision of Infants, Children and Adolescents. Appendix M. pages 322-324 Available at: www.brightfutures.org/bf2/pdf/pdf/Appendices.pdf. Accessed August 17, 2007.
30. Fiene R. 13 Indicators of Quality Child Care: Research Update. US Department of Health and Human Services. Available at: aspe.hhs.gov/hsp/ccquality-ind02. Accessed August 16, 2007.
31. Murph JR. *Health in Child Care: A Manual for Health Professionals*. 4th ed. Elk Grove Village, IL: American Academy of Pediatrics; 2004.
32. Aronson SS. *Model Child Care Health Policies*. 4th ed. ECEL—Healthy Childcare Pennsylvania. Available at: www.ecels-healthychildcarepa.org/content/MHP4thEd%20Total.pdf. Accessed August 16, 2007.
33. American Academy of Pediatrics, Pennsylvania Chapter. *Health and Safety Consultation in Child Care* [DVD]. Elk Grove Village, IL: American Academy of Pediatrics; 2005.
34. Pietro J. *Legal Issues in Child Care Health Consultation*. PowerPoint Presentation delivered in Orlando, Fl, 2005. Available at: www.healthychildcare.org/TrainingConference.cfm#health. Accessed February 20, 2008.
35. Schulman K. Issue Brief: The High Cost of Quality Child Care Puts Quality Out of Reach for Many Families. Children's Defense Fund. Available at: www.childrensdefense.org/earlychildhood/childcare/basics.aspx. Accessed August 16, 2007.
36. Giannarelli L, Barsimantov J. Child Care Expenses of America's Families. Urban Institute. Available at: www.urban.org/url.cfm?ID=310028. Accessed August 16, 2007.
37. Giannarelli L, Adelman S, Schmidt SR. Getting Help with Child Care Expenses. Urban Institute. Available at: www.urban.org/url.cfm?ID=310615. Accessed August 16, 2007.

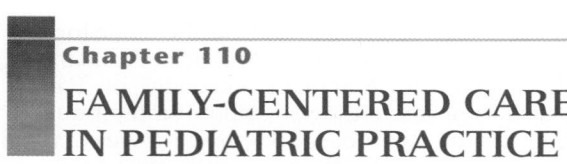

Chapter 110

FAMILY-CENTERED CARE IN PEDIATRIC PRACTICE

W. Carl Cooley, MD

CHANGING VIEW OF FAMILIES

Primary care physicians have been taught to detect deviations from normal and to recognize the occurrence of pathologic conditions. Medical training concentrates on identifying abnormalities in biological or behavioral systems, identifying causes, and providing the interventions that are necessary to correct or ameliorate altered function. In addition to appropriate emphasis on the prevention and treatment of disease, pediatric practice should extend beyond pathologic abnormalities to embrace and promote the strengths of individual children and families. Advocating for healthy lifestyles, supporting behaviors that protect children from exploitation or abuse, teaching self-care for children who have chronic conditions, and facilitating the development of self-confidence and self-esteem are important pediatric endeavors.

Most children live in the context of families. Family ecology can be portrayed as a homeostatic system in which the interrelationships among the elements (parents, siblings, extended family) exert complex, often predictable, effects on each other. This theory of family systems views families as biological systems, the equilibrium of which is disturbed by the stresses that are introduced when 1 family member is ill, disabled, stressed, or behaviorally disruptive. Although helpful in emphasizing the need to attend to the status of all family members, family systems theory and related therapeutic interventions extend to the family the same focus on pathologic conditions that has been overemphasized in our approach to individual patients.

Just as primary care physicians identify and nourish sources of strength and resilience in the individual children for whom they care, they must regard families in the same light. Most families use healthy strategies to cope with stress; characteristics of resilient families can be proactively identified (Box 110-1) and even taught to other families; and families often identify different stressors than those predicted by clinicians or researchers.[1,2]

Physicians can help families by inquiring about the family's major stressors, coping strategies the family has used, obstacles to coping or stress reduction, and sources of the family's social support (extended family, friends, place of worship). Physicians must also explore stress and coping from a cultural perspective and make an effort to extend themselves beyond their own cultural and linguistic boundaries. Difficulty with past crises or the absence of social supports is predictive of lower resilience and the potential breakdown of successful coping when multiple stressors accumulate.

DEFINITION OF FAMILY

The family is defined in many ways and takes many forms. The definition of family that we choose not only determines what we mean by family-centered care, but also incorporates the values with which we provide pediatric care. The New Mexico Coalition for Children, Youth, and Families developed the following definition of family:

> "We all come from families. Families are big, small, extended, nuclear, multi-generational, with one parent, two parents, and grandparents. We live under one roof or many. A family can be as temporary as a few weeks or as permanent as forever. We become part of a family by birth, adoption, marriage, or from a desire for mutual support. As family members, we nurture, protect, and influence each other. Families are dynamic and are cultures unto themselves, with different values and unique ways of realizing dreams. Together our families become the source of our rich cultural heritage and spiritual diversity. Each family has strengths that flow from the individual members and from the family as a unit. Our families create neighborhoods, communities, states, and nations."*

Each family enters the relationship with a pediatrician having its own personal and cultural history (see Chapter 112, Changing American Families), perceptions about health and health care, and expectations. Pediatricians must address families in a way that acknowledges and respects their uniqueness without subordinating their responsibility for the well being of their children.

FAMILY-CENTERED CARE

In the late 1970s and early 1980s, the *child life movement* began fostering new ways of caring for children in hospitals. These new methods involved making the hospital experience less threatening by incorporating age-appropriate activities into the hospital environment. Parents were invited to room in with sick children and to be involved in a child's hospital care.

BOX 110-1 Nine Aspects of Resilient Family Process

1. Balancing illness or other stressors with other family needs
2. Maintaining clear family boundaries
3. Developing communication competence
4. Attributing positive meanings to difficult situations
5. Maintaining family flexibility
6. Maintaining a commitment to the family as a unit
7. Engaging in active coping efforts
8. Maintaining social integration
9. Developing collaborative relationships with professionals

Modified from Patterson JM. Family resilience to the challenge of a child's disability. *Pediatr Ann.* 1991;20:491-499.

*From New Mexico Coalition for Children, Youth, and Families and New Mexico Young Children's Continuum, 1990.

BOX 110-2 Key Elements of Family-centered Care

- Recognizing that the family is the constant in a child's life while the service systems and personnel within those systems fluctuate
- Facilitating family and professional collaboration at all levels of health care
- Honoring the racial, ethnic, cultural, and socioeconomic diversity of families
- Recognizing family strengths and individuality and respecting different methods of coping with stressors
- Sharing with parents complete and unbiased information on a continuing basis and in a supportive manner
- Encouraging and facilitating family-to-family support and networking
- Understanding and incorporating the developmental needs of infants, children, and adolescents and their families into health care systems
- Implementing comprehensive policies and programs that provide emotional and financial support to meet the needs of families
- Designing accessible health care systems that are flexible, culturally competent, and responsive to family-identified needs

From Johnson BH, Jeppson ES, Redburn L. *Caring for Children and Families: Guidelines for Hospitals*. Bethesda, MD: Association for the Care of Children's Health; 1992.

These methods led to the formulation of the Elements of Family-Centered Care program by the Association for the Care of Children's Health in 1987 (Box 110-2).[2] In the same year, the Surgeon General of the United States published his report on children who have special health care needs, which mandated a commitment to family-centered care.[3] Since then, family-centered practice has become the standard of care among many health, mental health, early intervention, and education professionals. The elements outlined in Box 110-2 provide benchmarks against which pediatricians should measure their own behaviors, the organization of their offices, and the operation of the hospitals in which they practice.

Family-centered care is an outgrowth of the convergence of consumerism, policy developments, and research. It has led to a formulation of a new relationship between pediatric health care professionals and families, the essence of which is partnership. When families are active participants in their children's care, their sense of competence in providing care increases. The process of building a caring partnership between families and professionals is seen by some people as being as important as the outcomes of care.[4] Pediatricians can empower families by involving them as partners rather than as passive recipients of care.[5]

PEDIATRIC MEDICAL HOME

Translating the Elements of Family-Centered Care into daily primary care practice involves thoughtful planning and conscious effort.[2] This concept is an essential part of providing a primary care medical home for all children and youth.[6] Medical home is the name for primary care adopted by both the American Academy of Pediatrics and the American Academy of Family Physicians to promote the provision of a high-quality headquarters or home base for care in a welcoming, familiar, and accessible environment[7,8] (www.medicalhomeimprovement.org). Every pediatric practice should have a mission statement that is displayed cl early in the waiting area. Each practice should design and implement a method of quality improvement and consumer feedback. This effort may take the form of consumer satisfaction surveys on a periodic basis or comment forms enclosed with bills or other mailings to patients. Some practices may choose to organize a family advisory council that meets periodically to formulate suggestions for physicians and office staff about the office environment or the process of care in the office. Because 15% to 20% of the children in any pediatric practice are affected by chronic conditions, efforts should be made to hear the concerns of specific families who experience the added health care needs of such children.[9]

Families who are new to a primary care practice should be offered an initial visit during which family information is gathered and roles and expectations are made explicit. In this process, parents can define their needs for pediatric care, and the physician can explain his or her interpretation of the primary care physician's role. This meeting offers an opportunity to reconcile differences between a family's expectations and a physician's capacities and practice style. When a child is found to have a chronic illness or disability, an explicit redefinition of roles may be necessary to avoid confusion, for example, about the division of responsibility between specialists and primary care providers, about procedures for communication with schools and other agencies, and about the provision of care coordination or case management services. The medical home provides proactive care coordination that includes written care plans, planned chronic condition management visits, explicit co-management with specialists, and transition planning for adolescents about adult care needs.

Physicians in primary care need to be aware of resources for families in their communities and states. Current information about eligibility and intake procedures is available from state agencies that are responsible for special services such as clinics for children who have special health care needs, early intervention services, special education, family support services for children who have disabilities, and Medicaid programs and other entitlements. Physicians should be aware of parent support organizations in their state or region and of the availability of parent-to-parent services that link parents of children who have special needs to one another. Most states are now required to have an accessible resource guide for family services under each state's plan for early intervention services.

PEDIATRICIAN AS RELIABLE ALLY FOR FAMILIES

Families that cope successfully with challenges, such as the prolonged hospitalization of a prematurely born infant or the occurrence of a disability in a child, usually have many strengths in common. Most important among those strengths is access to social support.[7] Families without social supports not only become socially and emotionally isolated, but also fail to access tangible aid such as financial assistance and respite care and informational supports that enhance their self-confidence and mastery over their circumstances. The social supports that families require begin with the informal, natural supports of extended family, friends, and community and extend, when necessary, to include the formal supports of professionals and social service agencies.[10] History taking in the medical home should include asking parents to identify on whom they rely in critical situations, including family and friends, as well as organizations such as churches and civic groups. The primary care medical home should develop and maintain resource directories and program eligibility information. Some families may require assistance in connecting with community-based supports.

Families who have strong social support systems usually identify individuals among their formal and informal networks on whom they depend as resources. Although families naturally identify persons who are reliable allies within their support systems, pediatricians who aspire to this sort of relationship with families will not only provide more effective care, but also nourish themselves in the process.

TOOLS FOR PRACTICE

Community Coordination and Advocacy

- *Creating Patient and Family Advisory Councils* (booklet), Institute for Family Centered Care (www.familycentered care.org/advance/creatingadvisroycouncil.pdf).
- Advisory Council Workplan—Getting Started (form), Institute for Family Centered Care (www.familycenteredcare.org/advance/IFCC_Advisoryworkplan.pdf).
- Family Consultant Feedback (form), Institute for Family Centered Care (www.cshcn.org/).
- *FAQs—Serving on Advisory Boards and Councils* (fact sheet), Family Voices (www.familyvoices.org/toolbox/FAC/VT-cshnFAQ.doc).

Practice Management and Care Coordination

- Institute for Family Centered Care Resources and Publications (Web site), Institute for Family Centered Care (www.familycenteredcare.org/resources/index.html).

AAP POLICY STATEMENT

American Academy of Pediatrics, Committee on Hospital Care. Family-centered care and the pediatrician's role. *Pediatrics*. 2003;112(3):691-696. (aappolicy.aappublications.org/cgi/content/abstract/pediatrics;112/3/691).

SUGGESTED RESOURCES

Brewer EJ Jr, McPherson M, Magrab PR, et al. Family-centered, community-based, coordinated care for children with special health care needs. *Pediatrics*. 1989;83:1055-1060.

Fadiman A. *The Spirit Catches You and You Fall Down*, New York, NY: Noonday Press; 1997.

Liptak GS, Revell GM. Community physician's role in the case management of children with chronic illness. *Pediatrics*. 1989;84:465-471.

Sia CCJ. Medical home and child advocacy in the 1990s. *Pediatrics*. 1992;90:419.

REFERENCES

1. Dunst C, Trivette C, Deal A. *Enabling and Empowering Families: Principles and Guidelines for Practice*. Cambridge, MA: Brookline Books; 1988.
2. Johnson BH, Jeppson ES, Redburn L. *Caring for Children and Families: Guidelines for Hospitals*. Washington, DC: Association for the Care of Children's Health; 1992.
3. US Department of Health and Human Services. *Surgeon General's Report on Children with Special Health Care Needs*. USDHHS Publication #HRS/D/MC87-2. Rockville, MD: DHHS; 1987.
4. Cooley WC, McAllister J. Putting family-centered care into practice—a response to the adaptive practice model. *J Dev BehavPediatr*. 1999;20:120-122.
5. Cooley WC. Graduate medical education in pediatrics: preparing reliable allies for parents of children with special health care needs. In: Darling R, Peter M, eds. *Families, Physicians, and Children with Special Health Care Needs: Collaborative Medical Education Models*. Southport, CT: Greenwood Press; 1994:109-120.
6. Cooley WC. Redefining primary pediatric care for children with special health care needs: the primary care medical home. *Curr Opin Pediatr*. 2004;16:689-692.
7. Future of Family Medicine Project Leadership Committee. The future of family medicine: a collaborative project of the family medicine community. *Ann FamMed*. 2004 2004;2(suppl 1):S3-S32.
8. Medical Home Initiatives for Children With Special Needs Project Advisory Committee, American Academy of Pediatrics. The medical home. *Pediatrics*. 2002;110 (1 Pt 1):184-186.
9. Strickland B, McPherson M, Weissman G, et al. Access to the medical home: results of the National Survey of Children with Special Health Care Needs. *Pediatrics*. May 2004;113(5);1485-1498.
10. Cooley WC. The ecology of support for caregiving families. *J Behav Dev Pediatr*. 1994;15:117-119.

Chapter 111

PRINCIPLES OF EFFECTIVE DISCIPLINE

Ellen C. Perrin, MD

The word *discipline* has its root in the Latin word *disciplinare*, which means *to teach*. Discipline refers to the structure that parents create to teach their children how they are expected to behave. The term *discipline* is often used in a much more limited fashion to refer only to punishment. Punishment, however, is only a small part of the total parenting environment that helps children feel safe, capable, and lovable and helps parents feel effective.

Primary care physicians (PCPs) are in an important position to help parents create a constructive pattern of discipline, fostering optimal interaction and teaching. The PCP may be the only, or at least the most accessible, professional who knows children and their families during the preschool period. Even later in children's development, PCPs remain important anchors for parents as they negotiate the ever-changing challenges of parenting. Thus PCPs have the opportunity (and thereby the responsibility) to help parents in their efforts to provide the best possible context for growth.[1]

The longitudinal health supervision role that PCPs assume facilitates their continuing involvement in discussions of discipline, including initial guidance about effective parenting, as well as advice about specific behavioral difficulties. PCPs can empower parents, help them monitor their children's behavior and development, and provide anticipatory guidance and advice about methods to structure the family environment to avoid many common difficulties based on children's predictable developmental tasks.[2-6] PCPs also have the opportunity to recognize and advise parents about observed or described problems with children's behavior early in their course, thus preventing more serious behavioral or emotional dysfunction.

PCPs are critical participants in the management of more serious behavioral or emotional dysfunction as well. Some clinicians may be able to provide some counseling themselves, and all PCPs can help families by referring them to respected colleagues in the mental health professions (see Chapter 131, Consultation and Referral for Emotional and Behavioral Problems). Effective involvement of their PCP before and after referral makes families' work with a mental health professional more likely to be successful. Some pediatric practices have found teamwork with a mental health or child development colleague (collaborative care) to be an efficient way to deliver integrated and comprehensive pediatric care.

TIMING OF DISCUSSIONS ABOUT DISCIPLINE

Because effective discipline is so central to parenting, its discussion should be a part of every health supervision visit.[1,3,5,7] The earliest discussions about discipline can occur within the 1st few months of life. Parents' attempts to organize the family's schedule around the infant's eating and sleeping routines are among their earliest efforts at defining and agreeing on a set of rules or limits (Table 111-1). Another opportunity to help parents discuss and agree on appropriate rules occurs as children become mobile and parents begin to create and maintain safety guidelines. The responsibility to keep their child safe is universally accepted by parents, encouraging a discussion of optimal limits that must be set and a structure by which these limits can be taught and enforced. The PCP can point out to parents that in determining methods of keeping their child from falling down stairs, poking objects into electrical outlets, or spilling hot liquids, they have defined their expectations and some of their earliest rules. Developing teamwork between the parents is important at this early stage. Each parent should be explicit and clear about expectations, and parents should come to agreement about at least the basic principles and some of the details regarding the forms of discipline on which they intend to rely.

Table 111-1 Basic Rules for Effective Discipline

RULE	COMMENTS
Reward acceptable behavior.	Rewards can be tangible or symbolic. Rewards should be immediate. Hugs and praise are powerful rewards.
Use natural and logical consequences as allies.	*Natural consequences* are what would happen if you did nothing. *Logical consequences* are those you impose as a reasonable outcome of the specific behavior.
Punish unacceptable behavior.	Take away something the child values, or impose something the child dislikes. Punishment should be immediate. Frequent small punishments are more effective than occasional big ones. Spanking is effective only for the moment and has undesirable side effects.

Table 111-2 Suggested Contexts for Discussions About Discipline at Various Ages

AGE	CONTEXTS TO FRAME DISCUSSIONS ABOUT DISCIPLINE
1-4 months	Sleeping and eating schedules or routines
6-9 months	Rules to ensure safety of the environment
12-18 months	Emerging autonomy and independence
2 years	Toileting; perhaps new sibling
3 years	Entering preschool
4 years	Doing household chores
5 years	Entering a more formal school setting
6-12 years	Increasing peer activities and orientation
Adolescence	Observing curfews, guidelines for alcohol use, driving, and sexual behavior

When parents recognize that they must discuss and agree on rules to create a safe structure, they begin to recognize their own power in communicating their expectations for their child's behavior. This empowerment is one step along the arduous trail by which parents create a safe, nurturing environment and help their children learn appropriate standards of adult behavior. Table 111-2 provides some guidelines regarding other developmental periods when discussion about discipline can be woven usefully into the context of health supervision visits. Useful trigger questions can

BOX 111-1 Underlying Principles of Discipline

Parents want to do the best they can for their children.
Parents learn to parent from their experience as children.
Families are complex systems in continuous transition.
Behavior is learned primarily from its consequences.
Something keeps the problematic behavior in place.
Punishment only teaches children what is not acceptable.

become routine parts of child health supervision visits. Examples of such questions are "Are you happy with your discipline strategies?" "Do you have any questions about your child's behavior?" and "What are some situations when you and your partner don't quite agree about how to handle your child's behavior?"

BASIC PRINCIPLES AND TECHNIQUES

Parents generally want to do what is best for their children. They may be limited by inadequate knowledge of appropriate strategies and techniques, by depression or anxiety, by overwhelming challenges of their own past or present life, or by anger or a psychopathological condition. Box 111-1 outlines several basic principles underlying effective discipline.

Each child exists in the context of a complex family that is an interactive system. The behavior of any member of a family affects, in complicated ways, the behavior of all members; each time one family member moves, complicated ripples and counter ripples affect the movements of everyone else. Also important to remember is that parents work primarily on intuition and based on their experiences as children. Although parenting is among the most difficult and important jobs adults have, it is the one for which the least training and support is provided. PCPs can be important in providing support for parents, direction to parents' observations, and guidance if they need help.

BASIC PARENTING TECHNIQUES

Several specific strategies can help children feel loved and capable. The 1st strategy is *alone time* with the child (Box 111-2). This technique consists of allocating a short period (10 minutes for a 2 or 3 year old; 15 to 30 minutes as children get older; up to an hour for teens) that each parent commits to spending with each child on a predictable schedule. Each parent can plan for this time once a week or more; the important thing is the commitment to do it as scheduled. During this time, the parent and child interact one on one, and no interruptions are tolerated. The parent and child engage in an activity that is pleasurable for both of them; the activity should be chosen by the child from a list of 3 or 4 choices that the parent provides. This predictable, promised time is not contingent on the child's behavior or on the parent's mood; it occurs

BOX 111-2 Guidelines for Alone Time

Predictable, scheduled
One on one, with no interruptions
Three activity choices provided by parent; final choice by child
Interactive activity the child enjoys
Noncontingent on child's behavior or parent's mood
Time marked with a clock or timer

at its scheduled time under all circumstances. The time allotted to this activity should be monitored by an alarm clock or a kitchen timer so that the parent and child can together regret that they must stop when the time is up (rather than the parent taking the role of spoiler). Alone time should occur a minimum of once a week for each child with each parent—more often as manageable in the family's schedule. As simple and straightforward as this technique sounds, incorporating alone time into their daily and weekly life schedules is deceptively difficult for families. Parents can often benefit from making a similar arrangement between themselves.

As a 2nd strategy, parents would also do well to learn to take active notice of their child's admirable behaviors. Parents should attend to and praise their children liberally when they are playing appropriately, relating well with another adult or child, trying to be helpful, or attempting to do what the parent asks. The most effective comments are short, direct verbal messages, preferably referring directly to the parent's feelings rather than the child's behavior. An evaluative statement such as, "You did a good job," admits the possibility that the child will do a bad job the next time. In contrast, statements such as, "I really like how you cleaned up that pile of blocks," or "It makes me feel proud when I see how well you play with Johnny," refer only to the speaker's response to the behavior and do not predict potential criticism. Nonverbal messages are powerful as well, such as a hug, a smile, or a pat on the back.

A 3rd strategy involves giving children appropriate choices. In encouraging children to make and take part in appropriate decisions, parents teach them that they are capable of being responsible for their own behavior. The opportunity to make effective choices empowers children and enhances their growth. Choices must be appropriate to the child's developmental abilities, and parents must be careful to offer choices only when actual options exist from which to choose that are all acceptable to the parents. Questions such as, "Do you want orange juice or apple juice?" or "Do you want to wear your sweater or your jacket?" might be appropriate for a preschool child, whereas "Do you want to go to bed?" would not. For an older child, choices might involve choosing clothes to buy or to wear or how to organize bedtime rituals.

Many behaviors are learned, shaped primarily by their consequences. Behavior that is reinforced is likely to be repeated; behavior that results in an unpleasant consequence is much less likely to be repeated. One challenge for busy parents is to remember to notice their child when the child is quiet, content, and playing constructively. Ignoring desirable behavior is easier than ignoring disruptive behavior.

Removing reinforcement of a particular behavior (ie, ignoring it) also decreases its frequency. However, consistently ignoring unacceptable or annoying behavior is extremely difficult, and even occasional reinforcement prevents the disappearance of an undesirable behavior. The PCP should notice if an action that a parent intends as punishment may be having some reinforcing characteristics to the child. A common example of this paradox is yelling at or even spanking a child; although these are not pleasant consequences, they do reflect intense emotional involvement on the part of the parent toward the child, which may be valuable to some children.

INCREASING DESIRABLE BEHAVIOR

Attending and Praising

Parents are the most important people in children's lives; pleasing them is an important goal for most children. Furthermore, children, like the rest of us, appreciate being attended to and considered valuable company. Thus parents' attention, recognition, and praise are important reinforcers of their children's behavior. Behaviors that are rewarded or reinforced are likely to continue and even to increase in frequency.

Parents may reinforce their children's behavior directly or indirectly. Examples of direct reinforcement of behavior are a parent's praise for appropriate play or accomplishment of a task, a planned or spontaneous gift, or a joint activity contingent on the child's completion of a particular assignment. Indirect rewards for a child's good behavior may include a smile on the mother's face as she watches her child create a high tower and take pleasure in knocking it down, or the child overhearing the child's father speaking on the telephone with pride about school accomplishments.

Rewarding Behavior That Is Good

While creating a systematic solution for difficult behavior problems, parents must also attend carefully to boosting the behaviors they would prefer. Teaching children only what behavior is not acceptable without simultaneously teaching them preferred behaviors is not effective.

Parents should specify 2 or 3 particular behaviors that they appreciate and want to see the child demonstrate more often. These behaviors should be described in writing in concrete, observable terms such as "Set the table within 10 minutes after being asked" or "Read a book to your younger sister." These expectations should not be simply the absence of an undesirable behavior, such as, "Don't whine." These behaviors should be written down and posted in a visible place (eg, bulletin board, refrigerator door). For very young children, a sketch or a picture cut from a magazine will serve as useful reminders.

The child should understand that performing these activities will result in a prearranged reward. Rewards may be tangible, such as a coin or a cookie, or symbolic, such as a star or a sticker on a chart. Symbolic rewards can be accumulated toward a larger tangible prize—for example, 10 stars earns a trip to the ice cream parlor with Dad or a chance to choose a rented video. Activities that include interaction with a parent are preferable to tangible possessions.

Table 111-3 Examples of Systematic Behavior Change Plans

BEHAVIORS THAT ARE PREFERRED AND ENCOURAGED	CONSEQUENCES
Set table	Star (sticker)*
Read to sister	Star (sticker)*
Be ready for school by 7:30 AM	Watch television from 7:30 to 8:00 AM
BEHAVIORS THAT ARE UNACCEPTABLE	**CONSEQUENCES**
Hurting people	Time out
Clothes left on the floor	No clean clothes available for school
Whining	Ignore; time out
Throwing food	Dinner is over

*Ten stars (stickers) earns choice of rented video, desired toy, or breakfast out with Dad.

The particular behaviors to be encouraged, and the specific rewards offered, will differ according to the child's age, the particular issues on which the family chooses to focus, and the kinds of positive consequences the family prefers. An example is provided in Table 111-3. Parents must not promise rewards that will be difficult for them to deliver quickly. Multiple small rewards will be more effective than a large but unattainable promise. Table 111-3 outlines a summary of the use of behavioral consequences to shape children's behavior.

DECREASING UNDESIRABLE BEHAVIOR

All human beings learn faster and more effectively when they are rewarded for good behavior than when they are punished for bad behavior. Nevertheless, because all children at some time behave inappropriately, their parents must find a way to indicate that this behavior is not acceptable and to decrease its frequency. Several mechanisms can be used to decrease the likelihood of undesirable behavior. First, parents must check to be sure that they are not inadvertently rewarding behavior they find unacceptable. For example, a child who receives a cookie to head off a temper tantrum or one whose parents feed the child each time the child awakens during the night is receiving an unintentional reward for behavior the parents would rather see disappear. Similarly, some attempts by parents to punish their children's unacceptable behavior may in some way reinforce it. Even negative attention from parents is better than none at all—yelling is at least intense interaction.

Undesirable behavior will diminish if reinforcement for it is withdrawn (ie, it is ignored) or if it results in an unpleasant consequence, whether these consequences occur naturally or are imposed by adults in the environment. Common sense and common advice suggest that parents ignore the behaviors they do not like. Given enough time, behaviors that are not reinforced will indeed fade. This approach has 2 problems. First, ignoring disruptive behavior works only if the behavior is ignored 100% of the time, which is virtually impossible to do. Second, behaviors that are intrinsically rewarding, such as taking cookies from the cookie jar or staying out late at night, will not diminish simply as a result of the parent's ignoring them. Thus active punishment techniques are generally necessary some of the time to interrupt children's unacceptable behavior.

A common error is to provide to the child directives that simply define what behavior is not acceptable without providing a true goal of replacing it with acceptable behavior. For example, "Don't hit" or "No whining" are only partial goals; parents will be more successful if they provide reinforcement for asking for help to resolve a conflict instead of hitting and for asking pleasantly for a treat instead of whining. Another common error is to provide only vague directives, for example, "Be a good boy" or "Be polite." These instructions are too undefined for a child to know what is necessary to meet the requirements.

Active Punishment Strategies

Natural and Logical Consequences

The most powerful punishments are outcomes that occur naturally as a result of the child's behavior: *natural consequences*. For example, dawdling in the morning results in being late for school; if a child does not eat at mealtime, then the child may be hungry at bedtime; if the goldfish are not fed, then they will die. Parents need only refrain from interfering with the natural consequences that follow from the child's behavior. If no negative consequences would follow naturally, then parents can create some that follow logically: *logical consequences*. Scribbling on the wall might result in no crayons for a week or in the assignment of washing the walls; if toys are not put away by a prescribed time, then they are removed for several days; riding a bike without a helmet results in locking up the bike for a week.

Imposed Consequences

Some unacceptable behaviors require parents to create a more contrived intervention. For example, hitting or biting does not result in any acceptable, immediately occurring, logical, or natural negative consequence; thus a punishment needs to be imposed. Active punishment can take 2 forms: (1) privileges or pleasurable activities can be denied the child; or (2) a painful, uncomfortable, or undesirable circumstance or activity can be imposed on the child. Examples include decreasing the amount of time the child may watch television or use the family computer, decreasing the number of books a parent will read at bedtime, or forbidding the child to participate in a family activity. Commonly used methods of imposing undesirable consequences include spanking, requiring certain chores to be done, or requiring separation, such as a time out, from family activities.

Corporal Punishment

Despite its prevalence among parents and PCPs,[6,8] as well as considerable controversy,[9,10] spanking and other forms of physical punishment are not generally suggested.[1,3,4,11] Although spanking may at first appear effective as a result of children's surprise, pain, and fear, it is seldom effective in the long run and is used at great cost.[12-15]

Children learn more effectively by watching their parents' behavior than by listening passively to their words. Parents who spank model a type of behavior that they generally do not allow for the child. How can young children understand that hitting them is acceptable for their parents while they themselves are punished for hitting other children? Furthermore, spanking reduces the opportunities available for using more effective disciplinary strategies.[1,16,17]

Physical punishment undermines parents' attempts to maintain effective, cooperative, and nurturing relationships with their children. Children who are spanked learn aggressive and violent forms of conflict resolution based on power and strength. When adults are hit, they feel violated, shamed, hurt, and angry; children, too, will experience these feelings when being hit. That this action and these feelings come from the adults they trust and love most makes them even more destructive. Evidence suggests that adolescents and adults who were physically punished as children are more likely to accept and engage in violent behavior as adults.[13,14]

If parents are hesitant to punish unacceptable behaviors, then they tend to use threats and warnings to put off implementing the punishment, thus allowing the behaviors to escalate. This ambivalence often results in intense emotions that may themselves be reinforcing to the child or may lead to excessively harsh punishment. Physical punishment is difficult to modulate. If it is carried out when the parent is angry, then physical punishment carries with it the risk of excessive force and unintentional abuse. For all these reasons, spanking as a form of discipline is likely to be both ineffective and frustrating, and it may be associated with untoward long-term outcomes.

Time Out

Time out is an effective punishment strategy if used systematically and in accordance with clear guidelines. For maximal effectiveness, the guidelines for time out should first be established by parents and then described to the child at a calm time. The fact should be made clear to the child that both parents (and other consistent adult caregivers) have agreed on this plan and will respond in similar fashion to unacceptable behaviors (Box 111-3).

Two or 3 particular behaviors should be targeted initially for time out. Describing them in writing in concrete and simple terms at a central location (bulletin board, refrigerator door) is helpful. For very young children, a sketch or a picture cut out of a magazine will help remind them of the behaviors on the list. Parents and children should understand that time out will follow these specified behaviors each time they occur, without further warnings. Subsequently, time out must be enforced the 1st time and each time these behaviors occur.

A particular place should be designated for time out. This location should be in the area where the family tends to congregate (kitchen, family room) but out of sight of televisions or other stimulating activities. A particular chair, an area marked by masking tape on the floor, or a designated step of the staircase are common locations for time out. Children's bedrooms are not a good place for time out because they are too removed from the family action, they usually include toys and books, and they should remain enticing places of refuge. Once a time-out system has been perfected at home, the same procedures can be adapted to restaurants, grocery stores, and other locations. Multiple short periods of time imposed for time out are more effective than longer periods. A useful rule of thumb is 1 minute per year of the child's age. Time out should be imposed immediately when the offending behavior is noticed, not threatened for later.

Time out should begin with a short restatement by the parent of the rule that has been violated, such as, "Remember, hurting people is not OK." Then the designated time is monitored with a timer. A timer is critical because, for a parent to take responsibility for releasing the child from time out after the specified time is up, at least some amount of involvement with the child is maintained during this time, rendering the time out less effective. This period must be, as much as possible, time *out*—that is, absolutely no interaction should occur. If a sibling teases or talks to the child during the time out, then this child should be placed in time out as well. Parents must completely ignore attempts at interaction such as whining or questions such as, "Is my time up yet?" If the child leaves the designated time out place or is disruptive, then the timer should be reset for the predetermined amount of time. Parents must remain calm and controlled when supervising time out. They should reveal neither anger nor sympathy, but rather treat the time out as the inevitable consequence of the child's infraction of a predetermined family rule. When the timer rings, the child should be welcomed back into the family's positive interactions, without further comment or reprimand.

In rare instances, time out may be instituted for an unexpected episode of disruptive behavior, that is, an episode that was not anticipated in the predetermined list of unacceptable behaviors. In this case, giving the child one warning before imposing the time out is advisable, if the situation allows.

SUMMARY

An important point to remember is that punishment is never enough. At best, punishment teaches children only what behavior is not acceptable, but it cannot teach them what behavior is desirable. Thus punishment should constitute only a small part of an overall disciplinary strategy. Effective discipline results from parents' creation of an environment in which children feel safe by virtue of predictable rules and

BOX 111-3 Guidelines for Time Out

- State 2 or 3 behaviors that merit time out, using concrete descriptions.
- Time-out period takes place immediately after the behavior occurs (no exceptions, no warnings).
- Time-out period takes place each time the behavior occurs.
- Plans and place are prearranged in absence of problematic behavior.
- Length of time out is 1 minute per year of age, marked with a timer.
- Welcome the child back to *time in* without lecturing.

BOX 111-4 Preventive Strategies

- Empowerment of parents
- Discipline involving rules and consequences
- Praise and attention
- Regular experience of positive interactions
- Effective choices
- Predictable consequences (positive and negative)

BOX 111-5 Common Pitfalls Leading to Ineffective Discipline

- Inadvertent rewarding of undesirable behavior
- Failure to notice and reward desirable behavior
- Reluctance to impose time out until behavior escalates (eg, warnings, threats)
- Insufficient *time in,* positive interactions
- Inconsistent rules from day to day, situation to situation
- Too many punishable behaviors

BOX 111-6 Common Errors in Implementing Time Out

- Time out area is located in child's room.
- Duration is too long.
- Parent monitors time instead of timer
- More than one warning or threat is used.
- Child is asked to decide if time out is indicated.
- Conditions are negotiated with child.
- Parent is angry or frustrated.
- Time out is delayed for later.
- Punished behavior is too vague.
- Child is lectured or shamed.
- Time out is used unpredictably.

consequences, lovable as a result of adequate attention and praise, and capable of making decisions and taking responsibility for their own behavior. These basic preventive strategies are outlined in Box 111-4.

Common problems summarized in Box 111-5 include inadvertently rewarding undesirable behavior, failing to notice and reward desirable behavior, a family environment that is so busy or stressed that the child does not experience sufficient positive interaction with the parents *(time in),* and inconsistency in the consequences that follow *good* or *bad* behaviors. Common errors in implementing time out are featured in Box 111-6.

PCPs can provide a model for parents, teaching them the importance of empowerment in the context of a respectful and emotionally safe and nurturing environment. They also can teach parents some of the skills that will help their children know that they are lovable, capable, and responsible. In addition, PCPs can help parents construct an effective disciplinary structure by suggesting helpful reading materials and other media, such as audiotapes or videos. Some parents will benefit from discussion groups with other parents.

TOOLS FOR PRACTICE

Engaging Patient and Family

- *Discipline and Your Child* (brochure), American Academy of Pediatrics (patiented.aap.org).

AAP POLICY STATEMENT

American Academy of Pediatrics, Committee on Psychosocial Aspects of Child and Family Health. Guidance for effective discipline. *Pediatrics.* 1998;101(4):723-728. (aappolicy.aappublications.org/cgi/content/full/pediatrics;101/4/723).

SUGGESTED RESOURCES

Brazelton T. *Touchpoints.* Reading, MA: Addison-Wesley; 1992.

Clark L. *The Time-Out Solution.* Chicago, IL: Contemporary Books; 1989.

Dreikurs R. *Children: The Challenge.* New York, NY: Penguin Books; 1964.

Dreikurs R, Grey LA. *Parent's Guide to Child Discipline.* New York, NY: Hawthorn Books; 1970.

Faber A, Mazlish E. *How To Talk So Kids Will Listen and Listen So Kids Will Talk.* New York, NY: Avon Books; 1980.

Faculty of the Department of Child Development, Tufts University. *Proactive Parenting: Guiding Your Child From 2 to 6.* New York: NY: Berkley Publishing Group, 2004.

Lieberman AF. *The Emotional Life of the Toddler.* New York: NY: The Free Press, 1995.

Webster-Stratton C. *The Incredible Years.* Seattle, WA: Incredible Years Publishing; 2006.

REFERENCES

1. American Academy of Pediatrics, Committee on Psychosocial Aspects of Child and Family Health. Guidance for effective discipline. *Pediatrics.* 1998;101:723-728.
2. Christophersen ER. Discipline. *Pediatr Clin North Am.* 1992;39:395-411.
3. Howard BJ. Advising parents on discipline: what works. *Pediatrics.* 1996;98:809-815.
4. Howard BJ. Discipline in early childhood. *Pediatr Clin North Am.* 1991;38:1351-1369.
5. Olson LM, Inkelas M, Halfon N, et al. Overview of the content of health supervision for young children: reports from parents and pediatricians. *Pediatrics.* 2004;113 (6 suppl):1907-1916.
6. Regalado M, Sareen H, Inkelas M, et al. Parents' discipline of young children: results from the National Survey of Early Childhood Health. *Pediatrics.* 2004;113(6 suppl): 1952-1958.
7. Smith EE, Van Tassel E. Problems of discipline in early childhood. *Pediatr Clin North Am.* 1982;29:167-176.
8. McCormick KF. Attitudes of primary care physicians toward corporal punishment. *JAMA.* 1992;267:3161-3165.
9. Larzelere RE. A review of the outcomes of parental use of nonabusive or customary physical punishment. *Pediatrics.* 1996;98:824-828.
10. Larzelere RE. Moderate spanking: model or deterrent of children's aggression in the family. *J Fam Violence.* 1986;1:27-36.
11. Schmitt BD. Discipline: rules and consequences. *Contemp Pediatr.* June 1991:65-69.
12. McCord J. Unintended consequences of punishment. *Pediatrics.* 1996;98:832-834.
13. Straus MA. Discipline and deviance: physical punishment of children and violence and other crime in adulthood. *Soc Probl.* 1991;38:133-154.
14. Straus MA. Spanking and the making of a violent society. *Pediatrics.* 1996;98:837-842.
15. Friedman SB, Schonberg SK, editors: The short- and long-term consequences of corporal punishment. *Pediatrics.* 1996;98:803.
16. Socolar RR, Savage E, Keyes-Elstein L, et al. Factors that affect parental disciplinary practices of children ages 12 to 19 months. *South Med J.* 2005;98:1181-1191.
17. Wissow LS, Roter D. Toward effective discussion of discipline and corporal punishment during primary care visits: findings from studies of doctor-patient interaction. *Pediatrics.* 1994;94:587-593.

SECTION TWO

Factors Influencing the Psychosocial Health of Children

Chapter 112

CHANGING AMERICAN FAMILIES

Shirley A. Smoyak, RN, PhD

The family contexts in which infants, children, and adolescents are raised set the patterns for their response to illness and their expectations of caregivers. Families' beliefs about health and illness—what is preventable, what is treatable, what is natural, what is good, and what is to be avoided—are communicated to each new generation, both directly and subtly.

Because most people have experienced childhood and adolescence in a family setting, and because most people, as adults, create families of their own, the temptation is great to view their experiences as normal and to use them as a standard for understanding others. This ethnocentric tendency leads to assumptions that the familiar must be the correct or a better way and that other styles or patterns, at best, are strange and, at worst, are wrong or deviant.

Family is an elusive concept; its shape, character, and functions have been interpreted differently by historians, sociologists, psychologists, and anthropologists. Tremendous changes in American family life have occurred in the last half century. The US population is now over 300 million; new immigrants have contributed to this expansion, and their different cultures have to be understood by their caregivers. Old norms and expectations about families no longer serve clinicians well.

Privacy about matters of family life has produced what sociologists call *pluralistic ignorance*. Each person knows what goes on in their own bedrooms and how to handle a sassy 2 year old at bedtime or an adolescent who comes home drunk or smelling of pot, but they really do not know how the neighbors respond. This chapter provides an overview of changing patterns of family structure and the associated changes in functions. It attempts to explode some cherished myths about the *American family* and to provide clinicians who treat sick, injured, or well children with a more realistic understanding of families. In this chapter, a family will be viewed as a married couple or other group of adult kinfolk who cooperate economically and psychosocially in bringing up children and who share a common dwelling.

FAMILY ORIGINS

The origin of the family structure is unknown.[1] Although varying significantly in structure and function, some kind of family exists in all known human societies. The notion of *family* implies several universals: (1) that sexual relations between close relatives are forbidden; (2) that men and women cooperate through a division of labor based on gender; and (3) that marriage is a durable, although not necessarily lifelong, arrangement. The second point is disputed today as increasing numbers of gay and lesbian partners raise children.

Another universal concept, that men in general have higher status and authority than the women in their families, has generated much controversy between feminist scholars and other historians. The exact nature of family structure and gender relationships is shrouded in many layers of conjecture and scientific guesswork. Since the beginning of recorded history, no fixed pattern across cultures has been found.[2] Culture, not biology, determines the rules of organization within families. In most primitive, nomadic, communal societies, family descent was traced through the mothers, possibly because maternity could be verified, whereas paternity was often a mystery. Roughly 5000 years ago, when the development of agriculture drastically changed how people lived and organized themselves, patrilineal groups emerged. As the concept of private property developed, the transfer of such property from father to son influenced both economic and social patterns.

Historians of the family have taught that much of what people take as familiar and commonplace is a relatively recent invention.[3] Childhood as a concept did not exist before the Middle Ages. In medieval days, as soon as a child was able to live without the constant attention of the mother, the person was accorded adult status. No institution has been changed so remarkably by modernization as has the family. Until the late 18th century, families were primarily economic units. Marriages were arranged to preserve property, and children were a cheap source of labor or a hedge against poverty in old age.

Historically, all the work necessary for safety and survival was done within family units. Within the boundaries of the family, functions performed were educating the young; ensuring safety from invaders; praying to God or a superior being; providing nurturance, clothing, and shelter; and caring for the sick, infirm, young, or disabled. Every family textbook includes a discussion of the *erosion of family functions,* and predicting the eventual demise of the family as it is understood has been popular from time to time because all the reasons for its existence have been reassigned to institutions outside the family, such as schools, hospitals, welfare boards, and churches.

Several experiments have been conducted in alternative forms of living in human groups, but none has survived. Although no general societal law exists that people must live in families, most of them do. Historical perspectives help in understanding social contexts and institutions. More importantly, such understanding eliminates or dampens the tendency toward emotionality over issues of intimacy, closeness, and human relationships. Perceptions of American family life are full of myths, such as the belief that a three-generation household was once the norm. Such beliefs generate a false nostalgia—a longing for what never was.

For the first time in history, families may have 4 or 5 generations alive. Children today may have not only living grandparents, but also great-grandparents and perhaps great-great-grandparents. This increased longevity poses problems for families that they have never faced before. On a simple level, the question is raised of what the *layers* of grandparents should be called by their grandchildren. On a more complex level, great economic and psychosocial concern faces middle-aged persons who see their retirement years not as golden but as burdened by financial and social support of several elder generations.

Tracing accurate patterns and structures for families is difficult for 2 major reasons. First, upper-class or high-status families were overrepresented in the earlier literature on family structure. Second, until recently, writers tended to describe families as they *should* be, rather than as they really were. This tendency led to "the classical extended family of Western nostalgia."[4]

Families have turned over many of their previous functions, as noted previously, to institutions, organizations, and professionals outside the family, but they have maintained the functions of childbearing, primary socialization of children, and psychosocial validation or *refueling* for all their members. This last function—the provision of psychosocial verification, worth, and meaning—is probably the most important. Standards for its performance have increased tremendously in recent years, with the popular press reporting all types of help available to meet increased expectations, from individual psychotherapy and counseling to retreats and renewals, self-help books and groups, and high-priced encounters with marriage and family specialists. At the turn of the last century, the only interpersonal, behavioral requirement between husbands and wives was that they be civil to each other. The new requirement is that they love one another and continue to express this love unfailingly, even into their elder years. An associated new requirement is for increased intimacy through sexuality. Because people who marry for economic purposes have few reasons to terminate marriage, the current high rate of divorce is an indication that marriage as an economic arrangement is definitely a thing of the past.

MODERN MARRIAGE

One important marriage trend in recent decades is that "Americans have become less likely to marry, and the most recent data show that the marriage rate in the United States continues to decline."[5] Although reasons for the decline in marriages is not clear, it may be associated with delaying first marriages until older years, greater numbers cohabiting before marriage, and fewer divorced people remarrying.

College-educated women are now marrying at a higher rate than their peers, which was not the case even in the late 20th century. In addition, their divorce rate, always lower than that of non–college educated women, continues to decline. Out-of-wedlock births have always been low in this population and continue to be. People who delay marriage until past age 30 are the only group more likely to have children after marriage rather than before. The marriages of college-educated men and women are reported to be more educationally and economically matched or egalitarian, and they have similar attitudes about gender roles.

In many ways, this population matches the traditional American dream—happy, stable, two-parent families. However, these couples are not replacing themselves. In 2004, 24% of college-educated women aged 40 to 44 were childless, compared with only 15% of women without a high school degree. Pediatric practices will therefore see fewer of these *American dream* children than in the past. However, those who are more challenged economically, socially, and medically have higher fertility rates. Minority populations, especially immigrants, are in this latter group.

The divorce rate among Americans today is nearly double that in 1960, but it has declined since hitting the highest point in history in the 1980s. For the average couple marrying for the first time in recent years, the lifetime probability of divorce or separation remains between 40% and 50%. Information about new immigrants is minimal.

The background characteristics of people beginning a marriage have major implications for their risk of divorce. For instance, the probability of divorce is lower for people with incomes over $50,000 (compared with those under $25,000), who marry over age 25, have a baby 7 months or more after marriage, have a religious affiliation, have an intact family of origin, and have some college education.

Another important finding is that the number of unmarried couples living together has increased dramatically over the last 40 years and is continuing to increase.[4] Most younger Americans now spend some time living together outside of marriage; unmarried cohabitation commonly precedes marriage. Between 1960 and 2005, unmarried couples living together increased more than 10-fold.

THE AMERICAN FAMILY

The old notions of family life span no longer match reality; many families today change their structures repeatedly by marriage, divorce, and remarriage, interspersed by varying lengths of time alone or as single parents. For instance, in the first half of this century, the sequence described was courtship, marriage, childbearing and -rearing, empty nest, retirement, and death of one or both spouses. Today, many departures from this sequence take place. Among alternative family forms are unmarried couples living together (with or without children); homosexual couples (with or without children); deliberately childless couples, married or not; single-parent families with either a father or a mother as the parent; middle-aged couples whose divorced adult children return home with their young children; middle-aged couples living in very crowded situations because of the former pattern, and in addition, with their elderly parent or parents living with them; various types of blended families created by divorced or widowed parents remarrying; and group families, in which several unrelated families share a large space. A new structure is grandparents (largely grandmothers) rearing their grandchildren because the parents are victims of AIDS, are incarcerated, or are addicted to drugs or alcohol. Within each of these various structures, the rules of organization for carrying out the chores of daily living differ widely.

One trend in American families is that families are smaller than they were just 2 decades ago. In 2004 the American total fertility rate was 2.049, below the 1990 level and slightly above 2 children per woman.[6] This rate is below the replacement level of 2.1 but is still higher than other modern, industrialized societies. The total fertility rate in Germany, Spain, Italy, Greece, and Japan is 1.3.[7] In the middle of the 19th century, estimates suggested that 75% of households included children younger than 18 years of age. A century later, this level had dropped to slightly less than one half of all households. In 2000, 33% of households included children.

CHANGING FAMILY STRUCTURES AND FUNCTIONS

The US Census Bureau distinguishes between a *household* and a *family*. Households consist of units occupied by persons. A household may consist of one person living alone or several people sharing the dwelling. A family is 2 or more persons related by birth, marriage, or adoption who reside together. Relatives who may be integrally involved with the family but who do not share the dwelling are not counted. Although 70% of US households contain a family unit, family composition is quite diverse. Families include married couples with and without children, single-parent families headed by a woman or a man, siblings living together, and many other arrangements. Only one third of all families have children; but their structures, the number of generations, and the number of people in each generation varies considerably. Federal and state laws today are being rewritten to incorporate changes to ensure equal rights for gay and lesbian couples. These changes will include definitions of insurance rights, access to information, and decision making about life-and-death issues, as well as changes in definitions of what parenthood means. The issue of legal marriage for same-sex couples, however, remains controversial. At the end of 2006, only a single state, Connecticut, will issue a marriage license to a same-sex couple. New York, New Mexico, and Rhode Island have no explicit provision, and New Jersey became the seventh state to allow domestic partnership or civil union. (See Chapter 118, Gay- and Lesbian-parented Families.)

In past generations, primary care physicians were surprised if anyone other than the child's mother brought the child in for visits to the office or was the caretaker during crises. Today, primary care physicians encounter grandmothers, grandfathers, fathers, and even babysitters in increasing numbers. Primary care physicians accustomed to dealing with mothers face the challenge of adjusting their psychosocial style as they encounter men as caretakers.

Mothers who work outside the home are creating pressures for social change both inside and outside the family. The willingness of men to adjust their priorities and to shift energies from work to family is critical for producing the expected *home as haven*. Their unwillingness to change in the direction of more family involvement often produces stress, even chaos, for their wives and children. The effects of fathers' changing roles and functions as breadwinners and homemakers have been analyzed.[8] In 1991, 58% of mothers who had children younger than 6 years were employed full time. In 1960 the figure was 20%.[2] In 1994, two thirds of preschool children and three fourths of school-aged children had mothers who worked outside the home. Husbands and fathers continue to contribute less effort than what their spouses desire.[8]

DEMOGRAPHICS OF DIVERSITY

In this century, schools and health care practitioners face the challenge of delivering care to children of many cultures and faiths. By 2010, whites will account for less than 9% of the world's population, compared with 17% in 1997. Thus whites will have become the world's smallest ethnic minority. These worldwide changes will be felt in the United States as immigration patterns continue to shift. The European influence is already history; only 15% of current immigrants are European. South and Central America and Asia are the most widely represented areas in immigration statistics. People of color are the new immigrants and continue to have population growth. By 2030, most school-aged children in the United States will be *minority*, as will most Americans by 2050.[9]

The white population in the United States, as in the rest of the world, is concentrated in the northern half and is rich, well educated, and declining in number. The southern half is ethnically diverse, younger, poorer, and less well educated. Nonetheless, more than 90% of the population growth is in the South.[9]

Although general-trend data can be included in a chapter such as this, becoming better acquainted with the diversity data for the population in their specific geographic area would be well worth the time and energy for primary care physicians in practice; Web sites are particularly useful in this regard. The US Census Bureau 2000 facts are readily available at a federal Web site,[10] including information on age, gender, economic, household, and race and ethnicity data for the entire country, as well as for individual states, counties, and cities. Analysis of the data shows that for the nation, the Hispanic and Latino groups show population growth rates double than that for blacks (12.3%), who used to be the largest minority; and between 2000 and 2005 the Asian Indian population in the United States grew more than 35%. The University of Michigan Library Documents Center[11] is another excellent source for statistical resources on the Internet.

DISTINGUISHING NORMAL FROM ABNORMAL FAMILIES

Clinical theory about dysfunctional families has not kept pace with the dramatic changes that have occurred in family structures and associated functions and ways of living. Most clinical theory explicitly or implicitly upholds the ideal model of the family as intact, with father as primary wage earner and instrumental leader and mother as primary parent, homemaker, and socioemotional caretaker. However, as noted earlier, fewer American families fit this pattern today. Nonetheless, deviation from this standard is regarded in much of the literature as unquestionably pathogenic. Current textbooks used in the clinical training of health professionals virtually ignore alternative arrangements as possibly being normative. Even when divorce or separation are acknowledged as occurring in one half the marriages, the usual sequence of dissolution of ties, emotional upset, management of stress, and adaptations to community demands are not given appropriate consideration.

Clinicians thus lack knowledge about what is and is not normal in family life. When assessing normalcy, 2 types of errors are frequently made. The first error is to mistakenly identify as pathological a family pattern that is normal; the second error is to assume normality because of failure to recognize a dysfunctional pattern.[12] An example of the first error is the reaction of a clinician, reared in a family in which adults did not demonstrate affection openly and children were supposed to follow the directions of adults, who encounters a family that is noisy, affectionate, and open in expressions of joy and anguish. This clinician, seeing the solicitous concern of a mother for her child, might view this behavior as enmeshment or symbiosis instead of normal caring. Of course, clinicians do not always assume that what they experienced at home was normal. Some clinicians instead see their own upbringing as departing from normal and then apply this view to the families they see. When they encounter a family such as their own, these clinicians view it suspiciously and diagnose the behavior as pathological. An example of this view might be acceptance of the myth that healthy families are free of conflict. Such a view would preclude the clinician from exploring further an assertion by a couple that they have not disagreed in 20 years of marriage. What is common also may be accepted as normal; for instance, noncustodial fathers are so frequently cut off from their children after a divorce that clinicians may fall into the trap of seeing this as normal and thus fail to explore ways that the father and his children might spend time together.

Primary care physicians who feel uncomfortable about exploring the psychosocial aspects of their patients' families miss opportunities to suggest repairs and to help families rethink destructive relationships. Recent research demonstrates a positive association between continued supportive contact with the noncustodial parent and long-term adjustment of children. Such contact also affects the custodial mothers positively. Even when previous contact had negative consequences, continuing paternal detachment produces poorer functioning and more symptomatic behavior, especially in boys. Fathers who had negative relationships with their children before divorce have been able, in many cases, to develop improved relationships after divorce. A clinical imperative in cases of nonparticipating parents is to assess and build the coparenting alliance in postdivorce families.[12]

Clinicians need to be aware that families that exhibit similar problems may not have the same causes; no one-to-one correspondence exists between symptom and system.[12] In the past, rigid application of theories, unsubstantiated by adequate research, created additional strains for families who already were burdened by caring for a sick child. For instance, 50 years ago, removing children who had asthma from their families as a therapeutic strategy was not uncommon; this process was called *parentectomy*. The reasoning behind this action was that overinvolved, enmeshed emotionality between parent (mostly mothers) and child precipitated asthma attacks. This pattern of blaming the parent now has a trend in the opposite direction: that of blaming the child. Although families clearly have a great deal to do with influencing, even creating, the behavior of a child, particularly those who act out or cause trouble in communities and classrooms, the child is the one who is labeled disruptive or who is diagnosed with a conduct disorder.

No single pattern exists that clearly demarcates a normal from a nonnormal family. Families cannot be typed by the diagnosis of a family member or the behavior displayed by any of its members. Keeping in mind that families are tremendously complex and that a wide array of variables operate at any moment prevents jumping to faulty conclusions. A better stance is to form a tentative hypothesis and then engage the family in mutually exploring the problem and possible solutions.

When parents or caregivers refuse treatment for a child, even when sound medical evidence of its necessity can be found, they are often viewed as holding nonnormal beliefs. Nonetheless, these beliefs are often grounded in religious values or cultural norms. Religious and cultural values influence the health care treatment of children.[13]

GENOGRAMS

Increasingly, residents in family medicine programs are being taught to use family genograms as a part of the history-taking process and assessment. This technique provides valuable data for primary care physicians. A three-generation genogram can be completed within 20 minutes and is well worth the time and effort. The genogram can be focused on physical or psychosocial targets, and it can provide clues to both physical symptoms and dysfunctional behavior.[14] Genograms and a carefully executed history taking greatly improve the diagnostic process. When histories are not taken thoroughly, important facts about relatives and earlier illnesses are overlooked.[15]

When families are engaged in providing the information to construct the genogram, they often become so involved and interested in the process that they provide important information that they had not offered previously. Children can also be counted on to offer information that had not previously been shared, either about their own symptoms, feelings, or beliefs or those of other family members. The drawing is easily understood and correctible as data are drawn in. Children sometimes participate by drawing their own creations or by augmenting the master genogram. Copies of the main genogram can be given to each family member for further input and ideas.

One part of the diagnostic process is the use of Internet sources, described previously, to gather an accurate picture of the demographic profiles for patients seen in any pediatric practice. Genograms provide a way to map the cultural patterns, changes, and rules of organization within family systems. Staying focused only on biological data will not yield an accurate picture of any problems.

CHANGING SOCIALIZATION NORMS

Generations ago, parents simply bore and raised children, with almost no input from strangers and generally little, depending on ethnicity, from extended family members. Today, specialists can be found for every dimension of these functions, from specialists who help women stay healthy during pregnancy to specialists who advise parents how to respond to an adolescent's bad manners. Americans are generally the largest consumers of advice on children and health in the world. Depending on parents' social class and culture, they choose different authorities to consult. The appropriate resource for parents' questions is determined much by their social group, their level of education, and their general sense of assuredness about parenting. Most people, parents or not, tend to hear and believe what they *want* to hear and believe. Most parents measure the advice not against a standard of good research but rather against a more pragmatic one of whether the advice giver is trustworthy or has a track record of sensible advice.

A half century ago, no profession identified as one of its functions how to teach parents to be parents. Parents were supposed to know how to be good parents, either intuitively or because they learned it from growing up in large, extended families. Today, advice, counseling, and teaching about parenting are considered part of the work of primary care physicians, pediatric nurse practitioners, child study specialists, health educators, child psychologists, and behavior modifiers. Courses on effective parenting can be found in high school, college, and graduate school curricula, as well as on public television and on the Internet. Failure at socialization might be treated by an educational course or by a stay at a psychiatric hospital; some parents still see the military as a solution for offspring who fail to adopt parental values and norms. When a younger child behaves badly in the classroom or resists going to school entirely, the tendency now is to treat this behavior as a system of some kind of difficulty and to use a range of strategies to involve the parents in some type of parenting program. Programs for parents whose teenagers abuse drugs or alcohol are even available, as well as comparable programs for sibling support.

Two revolutions currently face families. One revolution is under way inside families, in which changes in sex roles resulting in increased participation in the work force, are challenging traditional marital rules. The second revolution is going on outside the family, in which unmarried people can now experience the privacy, dignity, and authority (and sometimes the loneliness) of living in their own home. A choice is now available, and some adults are choosing not to live within a family.

The first revolution is creating significant pressure to change the normative order between husbands and wives, with fathers being much more involved in homemaking and childrearing and mothers being more involved with careers and economic contributions to their families. Changes in how family roles and rules are carried out, which are now drastically departing from the traditional norms, produce new family rules of organization. Furthermore, the diversity of styles and traditions encountered with the changing demographic patterns demand taking new approaches and new strategies for problem solving. Even if the parents are from the same cultural background, their children will be encountering diversity in classroom settings and inviting children reared by different norms into their homes.

The second revolution, in which adults choose not to marry and choose instead to live independently away from families, produces the alternative of *no family at all*. Although the outcomes are different, both revolutions have the same origin—social priorities that value the workplace over the home. Men, although acknowledging the importance of families and the necessity of performing family-related tasks to provide a comfortable environment, do not see themselves as the primary workers in this arena. Women increasingly spend more of their time and energy on issues in the workplace rather than on family matters. These new directions are leading to a generation of children who know less and less about what is required to run a family, whether this includes inside tasks such as cleaning the house and preparing food or outside chores such as mowing the lawn or removing snow. The allocation of their energies mirrors that of their parents; they spend more time on schoolwork, afterschool activities, friends, and recreation than on domestic responsibilities.[8]

FAMILY TIES

A sense of personal efficacy and self-esteem is an outcome of changed family system values and practices. Until the late 18th century, families were primarily economic units. Marriages were arranged to preserve property, and children were regarded as cheap labor. Beating and whipping were commonplace, even among royalty, as approved tools to teach or extract conformity and obedience. During the Enlightenment, the standards and goals of childrearing began to change. Philosophers argued, eloquently and at length, that if children were to survive in a disorderly and unpredictable world, they could not rely passively on traditional authority. They needed reasoned judgment. To develop such judgment children needed affection and guidance rather than harsh, unreasoned discipline and brute force. Gradually, as these ideas took hold, childhood came to be recognized as a special stage of life.[3] Affection and nurturing replaced obligation and duty as the cohesive elements among family members.

Childhood mortality fell as a direct consequence of families having fewer children. Starting with the upper classes, families came to see that children had needs of their own and did not exist to serve the family. This revolutionary idea resulted in curtailing the numbers of births. Children were seen as individuals in their own right, to be paid attention to and nurtured rather than always to do for others. As lower classes also had fewer children, mortality fell among them as well. Family size is an excellent predictor of childhood survival, even today. Children in small families are strengthened by the extra nurturance and resources available to them. Several studies of infants in institutions during World War II and after demonstrated that infants who receive only physical care do not survive.

The new field of psychoneuroimmunology is pursuing the connections between emotional and physical health. Whatever the mechanism that produces greater physical health during periods of emotional well being needs to be understood. Affection and security may be considered as natural vaccines. Children who receive consistent love and attention—who grow up in situations in which self-reliance and optimism are nurtured and expected—are better equipped to survive.

LIFE WITHOUT CHILDREN

People are in the midst of a profound change in American life: "Demographically, socially and culturally, the nation is shifting from a society of child-rearing families to a society of child-free adults."[5] In 1960, one half of all households had children; today, one third of households have children, the lowest in the nation's history. The trend is expected to continue, with the 21st century perhaps becoming "the century of the child-free."[5]

Primary care physicians hear daily from parents about how difficult parenting is. Because most primary care physicians are not sociologists, they may not be paying sufficient attention to this trend of increasing complaints; nor are they necessarily aware that these complaints are validated in an enormous new literature on how burdensome childrearing can be. Childrearing, until recent decades, was what everyone expected as a large part of a person's life course.

For most of the country's history, Americans expected to devote a major portion of their adult lives to parental roles. Increased longevity and delaying having children have resulted in significant changes in the proportion of life spent in active parenting. Today, childrearing occupies a smaller share of adult lives. The end of active parenting used to occur closer to the end of life. At the beginning of the 20th century, only 41% of adults reached 65 years. Today, this figure has doubled.

In survey after survey, American parents report less happiness and more emotional and financial stress than nonparents. Troubling, too, are reports "that married couples now see children as an obstacle to their marital happiness."[5] Nonetheless, these gloomy reports do not mean that youth are rejecting parenthood entirely. Most Americans are, or will become, parents. Most women still want to have at least one child and maybe 2 children. Sixty-eight percent of today's Generation X women say that having a child is an experience every woman should have; in 1979, only 45% of baby boomer women held this view.[16]

FUTURE CONSIDERATIONS

The future of the family cannot be predicted without placing it squarely in its social context. The trends toward equality of the sexes within families and the larger society certainly have increased self-esteem for women but may cause new stresses for both men and women. Careful watching of morbidity and mortality trends will provide clues to the effect of this important social movement. Divorce rates have leveled, and marriage is again gaining in popularity. The number of dual-career or dual-job marriages and unions is growing each year. Although such arrangements improve the family's economic assets, child care becomes complex and costly, especially in the preschool years. Considering recent trend analyses and surveys, the following future directions for American families seem likely:

- Increasing value will continue to be placed on human potential, tenderness and warmth, and psychosocial needs being met, rather than on material pursuits. Human well being will be a primary goal for families, rather than economic well being.
- The trend toward decreasing numbers of children per family will continue and will result in greater attention being paid to parent-child relationships and an increased use of professionals as parenting advisers.
- Neighborhoods will reemerge along with increased numbers of community support systems.
- Extended families will gain the attention of researchers, as will grandparent-grandchild relationships.
- The new American ideal—strength without domination—will gain impetus and will influence the socialization patterns of families.

The challenge for primary care physicians will be to keep abreast of changes in family patterns and dynamics and to use this knowledge to provide humanistically oriented and enlightened patient care and advice regarding parenting.

TOOLS FOR PRACTICE

Engaging Patient and Family

- *Family Health* (Web page), American Academy of Pediatrics (www.aap.org/healthtopics/famhlth.cfm).

AAP POLICY STATEMENT

American Academy of Pediatrics, Committee on Early Childhood, Adoption, and Dependent Care. The pediatrician's role in family support programs. *Pediatrics*. 2001; 107(1): 195-197. (aappolicy.aappublications.org/cgi/content/full/pediatrics;107/1/195).

REFERENCES

1. Gough K. The origin of the family. In: Skolnick A, Skolnick J, eds. *Family in Transition: Rethinking Marriage, Sexuality, Child Rearing and Family Organization.* Boston, MA: Little, Brown; 1986.
2. Hareven T. American families in transition: historical perspectives on change. In: Walsh F, ed. *Normal Family Processes.* New York, NY: Guilford Press; 1982.
3. Aries P. *Centuries of Childhood.* New York, NY: Random House; 1962.
4. Goode WJ. *World Revolution and Family Patterns.* New York, NY: The Free Press; 1963.
5. Popenoe D, Whitehead BD. The National Marriage Project. The State of Our Unions, 2006. Available at: www.marriage.rutgers.edu/. Accessed June 19, 2007.
6. US Bureau of the Census. Births: preliminary data for 2004. *Natl Vital Stat Rep.* 2005;54:2.
7. Population Reference Bureau. *World Population Data Sheet.* Washington, DC: Population Reference Bureau; 2004.
8. Chapman V. *Working Hard or Hardly Working? An Examination of Children's Household Contributions in the 1990s* [dissertation]. Princeton, NJ: Princeton University; 1994.
9. Hodgkinson H. *Bringing Tomorrow Into Focus: Demographic Insights Into the Future,* Washington, DC: Center for Demographic Policy, Institute for Educational Leadership; 1996.
10. US Bureau of the Census. Your Gateway to Census 2000. Available at: www.census.gov/main/www/cen2000.html. Accessed June 19, 2007.
11. University of Michigan Library Documents Section. Statistical Resources on the Web. Demographics and Housing. Available at: www.lib.umich.edu/govdocs/stdemog.html. Accessed June 19, 2007.
12. Walsh F. The clinical utility of normal family research. *Psychotherapy.* 1987;24(3 suppl):496-503.
13. Linnard-Palmer L. *When Parents Say No.* Indianapolis, IN: Sigma Theta Tau International; 2006.
14. Smoyak S. Systems theory as a model to understand families. In: Burgess A. *Psychiatric Nursing: Promoting Mental Health.* Stamford, CT: Appleton and Lange; 1997.
15. Day-Salvatore D. The Genome Project: Family Systems Perspective. Lecture given at: Family Health Science, Robert Wood Johnson Medical School; Piscataway, NJ, October 20, 1999.
16. Longman P. *The Empty Cradle: How Falling Birthrates Threaten World Prosperity and What To Do About It.* New York, NY: Basic Books; 2004.

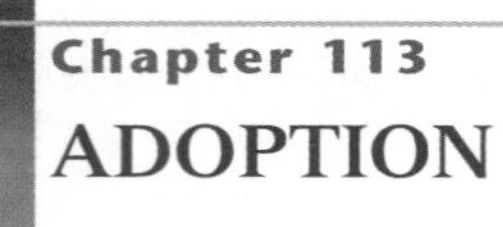

Chapter 113

ADOPTION

Sarah H. Springer, MD

WHO ARE THE CHILDREN?

The majority of children adopted in the United States today are not adopted as newborns. With easy availability of family planning and general acceptance of single motherhood, fewer newborns are placed for adoption than in generations past. Instead the majority of children join their families after being in the domestic child welfare system or out of foster or institutional care overseas. Many children with medical or developmental disabilities who were in previous times considered unadoptable are now being successfully placed with adoptive families. Today, adopted children come with histories of life before their adoptions, and this history has a tremendous effect on their needs and outcomes, both in the short term and over time.

Some children adopted from the domestic foster care system come to their adoptive families as infants, placed first as foster children then later adopted by their foster parents. These children have the benefits of nurturing care from infancy but may still experience the long-term sequelae of prenatal adversity, particularly substance exposure. More commonly, children adopted from foster care are older and have experienced significant abuse and neglect before adoption. Their long-term physical, mental, developmental, and behavioral health risks and needs are determined by the specifics of these insults but are frequently complex. (See Chapter 116, Children in Foster and Kinship Care.)

The countries from which children are adopted internationally continually change, influenced by social and political circumstances in the United States and in the sending countries. Child care circumstances vary tremendously among countries. Some children are cared for in high-quality, family-setting foster care, whereas others are cared for in institutional settings that can vary from small group homes with reasonable resources to large, extremely resource-poor orphanages. Some children enter care as newborns because of poverty, social adversity, or political circumstances; others enter as older children after experiencing the same sorts of abuse and neglect that place children into the foster care system in the United States. Most children are at least older infants or toddlers before they are eligible for international adoptive placement. Knowing how and why a child came into care is important, as is knowing the type of care a child experienced, because the history before adoption often sheds light on the physical, mental, and developmental health issues a child might be expected to face immediately and over the long term.

Children come to the United States from many countries through adoption. Although some countries have sent substantial numbers of children for many years, the list of sending countries is continually changing as a result of political and social circumstances in both in the United States and abroad. The US State Department's listing of orphan visas issued provides a concise listing of the numbers of children adopted from the top 20 sending countries each year.[1] The circumstances of individual children available in each country are varied, but general considerations are listed in Table 113-1 for the current top 10 sending countries.

Other common adoptions today include kinship placements and second-parent or coparent adoptions. Current child welfare practice emphasizes finding permanency for children more quickly than in the past and keeping children within their communities and cultures of origin whenever possible. Estimates indicate that approximately 200,000 children, or approximately one third of those in foster care, are placed in foster care with extended family members.[2] If they are not able to return to the custody of their birthparents,

Table 113-1 Top Ten Sending Countries

COUNTRY	PREDOMINANT AGE AND GENDER	REASONS IN CARE[a]	TYPE OF CARE	AVAILABILITY AND RELIABILITY OF RECORDS[b]	COMMON HEALTH CONCERNS[c]
China	Girls—infants to teens and older boys with special health care needs	One-child policy or social need for male children	Mostly institutional; some foster care	Minimal—better for children with physical disabilities	Lead intoxication, dental enamel insufficiency
Russia	Boys and girls—toddlers and older	—	Institutional	Variable quantity, minimal reliability	Prenatal alcohol exposure
Guatemala	Boys and girls—infants and older		Infants usually in foster care or small group homes, older children—institutional	Variable quantity, usually fairly reliable	—
South Korea	Boys and girls—infants and older	Lack of social acceptance of single parenthood	Foster care	Usually detailed records, very reliable	—
Ukraine	Boys and girls—toddlers and older	—	Institutional	Minimal	Prenatal alcohol exposure
Kazakhstan	Boys and girls—toddlers and older	—	Institutional	Minimal	Prenatal alcohol exposure
Ethiopia	Boys and girls—infants and older	HIV orphans	Institutional	Variable quantity Laboratories from the ICL Laboratory, Addis Ababa usually reliable	Prenatal HIV exposure, profound malnutrition
India	Boys and girls—infants and older	—	Institutional	Often detailed records, usually fairly reliable	—
Columbia	Boys and girls—infants and older	—	Small group homes or institutional	Variable	—
Philippines	Boys and girls—toddlers and older	—	Institutional—occasionally foster care	Variable	—

[a]The reasons children are eligible for adoption in all countries can include severe poverty, social adversity (maternal drug or alcohol addiction, incarceration, homelessness, mental health disabilities), and child abuse and neglect, with government termination of parental rights. The *Reasons in Care* column lists factors common to the country.
[b]Availability of reliable records does not mean that recommended new-arrival testing can be eliminated, but rather that preadoptive parents can feel reasonably confident that the information they have will accurately reflect the history of the child they are bringing home.
[c]The common health concerns column is not an all-inclusive list, but rather a note of conditions that are even more common for children from that country than for all international adoptees.

then many of these children are adopted by their extended family members or cared for in permanent legal guardianship relationships. This approach allows children to maintain family connections but can pose unique challenges to the adopting parents who must negotiate complicated relationships among the children, the birthparents, and other extended family members. Second-parent adoptions refer to the adoption of a child who already has one legal parent by the spouse or partner of that parent. Coparent adoption is the adoption of a child by 2 unmarried adults, often gay or lesbian partners.

ROLES OF THE PEDIATRICIAN IN PREADOPTION CARE

Unless the physician has a special interest in adoption medicine, a family adopting their first child might not meet the physician until the parent or parents receive information about a specific child or even until the child is home with the parents. Most pediatricians, though, will have families already in their practice who decide to adopt and can play an important role in helping the entire process to be a success. Pediatricians should be familiar with common adoption concerns[3,4] and can contact members of the American Academy of Pediatrics Section on Adoption and Foster Care for help.

Parents who are wondering what type of adoption to pursue can consider the potential needs of the children. By looking at the intersection of 3 variables, families and their physicians can anticipate at least some of the needs a child might be expected to have and some of the adoption process issues.

First, families need to consider the age of a child; children beyond infancy bring with them psychological, physical, and social consequences from previous circumstances. Professional mental health services may be needed to allow a child to reach full potential, in addition to developmental and educational supports. The second variable is whether a child is of the same or another race as the adopting parent or parents. The third variable is whether the child is in the same or a different country or culture. Although transracial adoption is not associated with poor outcomes, helping a child develop a strong sense of racial and cultural identity is important to the child's self-esteem and psychological well being and can be challenging, especially in communities with little racial or cultural diversity.[5]

Parents may also request help in deciding on an agency or facilitator to conduct the adoption. In general, parents should be encouraged to use agencies that are licensed (and therefore subject to minimal ethical and practice standards) with a mission to promote the welfare of children. Agencies with the mission of finding the right family for each child often cost more and require more of adopting parents but will also provide appropriate education for families and long-term support. Agencies with the mission of conducting an adoption rapidly may appear appealing at first glance but often do not share the complexities or risks of the children with adopting parents and are rarely there for long-term support.

Pediatricians may also be asked to review the information a family receives about a particular child whom they are considering adopting. Reviewing this information with a family is not to screen out children, but rather to help the prospective family understand the information given to them, know what additional information they need to gather, and then make a well-informed decision as to their ability to be the best parents for the child, given the predictable needs or risks. This service is often best performed by physicians familiar with all the types of adoptions, the information available for children coming from different countries, and the common risks seen in different groups of available children. Many agencies provide families with lists of physicians specializing in adoption medicine, and these can also be found through the American Academy of Pediatrics Section on Adoption and Foster Care Web site.[6] The University of Minnesota International Adoption Clinic also maintains a list of adoption medical professionals around the country (www.med.umn.edu/peds/iac/otherprofessionals.html).

Finally, pediatricians need to know the travel health issues involved for families traveling internationally to adopt. Parents should be counseled early on regarding recommended vaccinations, food and water precautions, preparing a travel first-aid kit, and emergency contact procedures (see the Centers for Disease Control and Prevention Traveler's Health Web site at wwwn.cdc.gov/travel/default.aspx) for themselves, their new child, and any other family members who are also traveling. Families traveling to very remote locations or very impoverished countries may need to bring antibiotics or other medications for themselves and their new child, given that medical care may be difficult or impossible to obtain. (Educating the family that antibiotics are being prescribed without seeing the child only for this unusual circumstance can help prevent inappropriate expectations later.) Physicians should provide a means for families to contact them in an emergency and written directions as to when and under what circumstances they might consider using the medications they are carrying.[7]

NEW-ARRIVAL ISSUES

Social and Emotional Issues

The arrival of a newly adopted child into a family brings similar joys and stresses as does the birth of a child. In addition, however, all of the circumstances that led to the adoption must be managed by adopting parents, birthparents, siblings and extended family, and the child. Adopting parents who have experienced infertility or the loss of previous children may have unresolved grief, which can complicate the feelings of joy from the arrival of this child. In addition, long waits for parenthood can create unrealistic expectations, which are often in stark contrast to the reality of parenting any child, let alone one who has lived through adversity and whose whole world has just changed. Postadoption depression is as real an entity as postpartum depression is, and pediatricians should be prepared to identify and refer affected parents.[8,9]

For children adopted outside of the immediate newborn period the transition into the new adoptive family is often bewildering, frightening, and full of loss. Ideally, children should be given as much preparation as possible, with older children even participating in the decision to join a particular family. In reality, however, many children are simply taken one day from everything that is familiar and handed to strangers. Children who have been in foster care or who have developed strong attachments to orphanage caregivers will usually grieve the loss of these significant people, and older children may worry about their well being or wonder if the caregivers are searching for them. Even children who have not been treated well by previous caregivers still have connections to them and may still grieve their loss. Adoptive parents and pediatricians need to understand this process, comfort the grieving child, and help the child develop a strong sense of connection and security with the new parents. Allowing the child to talk about the previous caregivers, to look at pictures of them, and even to telephone or write to them can help the child process this grief. Parents may need encouragement to allow children to share their grief, given that not talking about it may seem easier. Allowing children to share these strong feelings can help build strong bonds of new attachment.[8,10,11]

All children have to adjust to the arrival of a new sibling, but an adopted sibling brings challenges that a newborn does not. Most often the new child is not a helpless newborn but rather a mobile, demanding competitor for not only parental time and attention, but also for toys, food, and space. Extra love, understanding, and attention are in order, which can be hard to attain when the demands of the newly transitioning adoptee are high.

Extended family members also have a significant effect on the new-arrival period. Some may be eager to shower love and attention on the bewildered, overwhelmed, grieving child, whereas others may not accept the child as a true member of the family. Sharing information about adoption and the child's expected transition needs with extended family members before the adoption can help create a nurturing acceptance into a warm extended family without overwhelming the child.

Adopting parents should plan for plenty of quiet, uninterrupted time with their newly adopted child, regardless of the age of the child at arrival. Helping the child develop a strong attachment to the parents is of utmost importance because this groundwork is the foundation of healthy parent-child relationships and, ultimately, of all human relationships. Parents should think of their child as a newborn emotionally in an older child's body. Parents should be the ones to meet physical needs and to provide comfort so that the child learns to use them as a secure base in the world. Some parents are granted parenting leave by employers, whereas others must fight for it, given that many employers finance parenting leave through medical disability coverage, which does not apply when a woman has not given birth. Pediatricians should work with parents to convince employers that time at home with their newly adopted child is vital to the child's long-term physical and emotional health, and parents should be encouraged to use as much leave time as possible.

Medical Issues

The most important considerations in planning a child's postadoption medical evaluation are the risks inherent to the child's previous circumstances. Whether the child was adopted domestically as a newborn, from the foster care system, or internationally, the social and medical risk factors of the child's birthparents and prior circumstances should guide medical and developmental assessments.

Parents adopting newborns domestically may receive extensive records on the child, birthparents, and extended biological family, or they may receive nothing at all. Pediatricians should assess not only the available extended family medical history, but also the birthparent social history, paying special attention to risk factors for adverse outcomes for the fetus and child, including issues such as alcohol use during pregnancy, high-risk sexual behavior, and domestic violence. Records of birthmother prenatal testing for infectious diseases may or may not be available or reliable. Unknown or missing information, including unknown birthfather information, should be presumed to be high risk. Decisions regarding testing for HIV, hepatitis B and C, syphilis, and other perinatally transmissible diseases should be made on an individual basis after considering the available information.

Children adopted from the foster care system have, by definition, experienced significant abuse or neglect and are at high risk for long-term mental health and developmental sequelae. They are also, however, at very high risk for infectious exposures and malnutrition, dental problems, and physical health needs resulting from previous trauma. (See Chapter 116, Children in Foster and Kinship Care.) Medical evaluation of these risks should be guided by available records, with unknown or missing information being assumed to be high risk.

Children adopted from overseas have most often been cared for in institutional settings, where infectious diseases, including many which may not be obvious on physical examination, are easily spread. In addition, significant infectious and environmental health risks often exist in sending countries that physicians in the United States are unaccustomed to seeing. Nutrition is rarely adequate for children in institutional care, making macro- and micronutrient deficiencies common. Because a specific, detailed, reliable history is rarely available for a given child, the medical evaluation must be based on known significant risks, rather than individual history.

All newly arrived international adoptees should have a detailed, thorough evaluation soon after arrival home, including assessment of overall health, nutritional status, developmental delays, psychosocial adjustments, hearing and vision, and laboratory studies to assess for infectious diseases, nutritional deficiencies, and toxin exposures. Medical records from the child's country of origin should be reviewed but can rarely be taken as guaranteed truth, given that record keeping, transfer, and translation systems are notoriously unreliable and cannot be verified (see Table 113-1).

As outlined in the *Red Book*,[12] laboratory studies for all children should include at least hepatitis B (surface antibody, surface antigen, and core antibody), HIV, syphilis, stool for parasites, and tuberculosis testing. Most children (especially those adopted from Eastern Europe or Asia and children whose birthparents were intravenous drug abusers) should also be tested for hepatitis C. Prior bacille Calmette-Guérin vaccination is *not* a contraindication to purified protein derivative testing, and *all* internationally adopted children fall into at least the moderate-risk category when interpreting purified protein derivative test results.[12,13] All of these infections can be completely asymptomatic but have significant individual, family, and public health implications if left undetected and untreated.[14]

Deciding what to do about a child's immunizations can be challenging.[15,16] If no written records are available, then a new series should be initiated according to the consensus catch-up schedule,[17] given that even strongly positive antibody titers cannot, at one point in time, guarantee a steady-state level of immune protection. Although considerable controversy and ongoing research exists on this question, written records generally cannot be taken at face value because whether the child received the injection cannot be verified, nor can the storage or handling of the vaccines be verified, and orphanages around the world frequently receive old, outdated vaccine supplies. Records should be reviewed carefully, with attention to the timing of doses and the appearance of the records. For example, is it an original, with tattered edges and different inks, or a pristine, brand new copy? Are there doses given before the child was born? Are the vaccines stated available in the sending country? When records appear legitimate and show vaccine timing that meets the guidelines provided by the American Academy of Pediatrics and the Advisory Committee on Immunization Practices, titers can be checked,[12,15,16] and, if positive, these doses can then be counted for the child, with any remaining doses or missing vaccines following the *Red Book* catch-up schedule.

Nutritional deficiencies also are common, with the diet of most children before their international adoption being inadequate in overall calories, protein, and micronutrients. Most children are at least mildly malnourished at the time of adoption, as demonstrated by the rapid catch-up growth of even those who are on the growth curve at the time of adoption. Some children are profoundly malnourished and small for age. Most often this circumstance is the result of combined malnutrition and profound social and emotional neglect, but hypothyroidism must be ruled out, as must true growth hormone insufficiency, if rapid catch-up growth does not occur. Laboratory evaluation should include a complete blood cell count to assess for iron deficiency and calcium, phosphorus, and alkaline phosphatase assessments for rickets. Thyroid function tests should be obtained for children with significant growth or developmental delays. Lead intoxication is also common, especially in children adopted from China, and all children should have serum lead levels checked. (Box 113-1 highlights components of the medical evaluation of newly internationally adopted children.)

All newly adopted children, regardless of the type of adoption, should have a thorough assessment of development, including hearing and vision. For newborns this assessment will be the same as for any other routine well-child care, with special attention to any known long-term risk factors. Children adopted after the newborn period should have a careful assessment of all domains of development soon after placement. Most children make rapid developmental progress once they are in a nurturing family environment. Children whose delays are profound or persist beyond the first 2 to 3 months should be referred to formal developmental support services. (See Chapter 43, Identification of Developmental Delays and the Early Intervention System.)

Many children have significant medical needs on their arrival to their new families, some of which are known before the adoption and some of which will be revealed by the new-arrival evaluation. Further diagnostic work-up and treatment of these medical needs should be planned carefully, balancing medical urgency with the child and family's need for quiet nesting time in the early days of the adoption. Simple treatments, such as antibiotics or iron supplements, can begin right away. Potentially transmissible infections, such as intestinal parasites, hepatitis, and tuberculosis, should also be treated quickly. Urgent, time-sensitive or potentially life-threatening medical conditions must be treated immediately (eg, congestive heart failure, dehydration, extremely high lead levels, untreated syphilis, dense cataracts). Treatment of nonurgent medical concerns, however, can and should be deferred until the family has had some time together and the child has begun to learn to use the parents for comfort and support. Common problems in this category include repair of cleft lip and palate, orthopedic conditions, congenital heart defects, dental work, and strabismus surgery. Truly elective procedures, such as circumcision or repair of minor anomalies, should always be deferred until the child has developed a secure bond with the new family.[10]

BOX 113-1 Medical Evaluation of New Internationally Adopted Children

On arrival, *all* children should have:

- Thorough physical examination
- Purified protein derivative test (may need to alter timing if child received bacille Calmette-Guérin vaccination within the previous several months or received repeated, recent purified protein derivative tests)
- Hepatitis B surface antigen, surface antibody, and core antibody testing
- HIV-I and -II enzyme-linked immunosorbent assay (ELISA) (consider DNA polymerase chain reaction in infants)
- Assessment for syphilis—nontreponemal testing (rapid plasma reagin or Venereal Disease Research Laboratory test) for all adoptees. Treponemal testing (microhemagglutinin-treponema pallidum or fluorescent treponemal antibody absorbed) if history of exposure or positive nontreponemal test results
- Assessment of stool for ova and parasites
- Complete blood cell count
- Lead level testing
- Assessment for rickets: calcium, phosphorus, and alkaline phosphatase
- Detailed review of immunization status, with testing as needed to confirm immunity
- Detailed developmental assessment
- Assessment of hearing and vision

On arrival, risks should be assessed and the following checked appropriately:

- Hepatitis C ELISA for all children from Eastern Europe or Asia or those with history of risk factors
- Thyroid function test for children with significant growth or developmental delays
- Stool bacterial infection assessment for children with diarrhea or other gastrointestinal symptoms

Six months after arrival, *all* children should have:

- Purified protein derivative test
- Hepatitis B surface antigen, surface antibody, and core antibody testing
- HIV-I and -II ELISA
- Hepatitis C ELISA (for previously identified risk groups)

First Year Home

The first months home represent a transition time for the adopted child and the rest of the family, during which the groundwork is laid for the long-term success of the adoption.[8,10] Regardless of the age the child should be seen at least several times over the first year home to monitor catch-up in growth and development, child and family mental health needs, and the attachment of the child to the new family. In addition, all children should have age-appropriate hearing and vision screens, given that children adopted from foster care or orphanages have high rates of auditory and visual impairments.[18] These visits can be timed to accommodate catch-up on immunizations and follow-up of identified medical needs.

Perhaps most important, careful attention should be paid to attachment-related behaviors in newly adopted children. Children who have always had loving, nurturing care understand how to use an adult as a secure base in the world and will transfer this designation to a new parent quickly, usually within several weeks. Children who have never experienced one-on-one, emotionally attuned caregiving, however, have often learned to cope with life's hardships on their own, without relying on an adult. These children need to be overtly taught to use their new parents as their base in the world because secure attachments are the foundation of healthy long-term relationships. Parents may be impressed with the child's self-sufficiency, but they should be encouraged to intervene frequently, teaching the child to see the parent as the active provider of food, comfort, and entertainment. Pediatricians should closely monitor newly adopted children for signs of developing strong attachments. If after several months the child does not preferentially use the parent or parents as a source of safety, security, and joy, then the pediatrician should refer the family to a therapist experienced in attachment disturbances (see www.attach.org).[8,10,11]

The majority of children adopted out of foster care or internationally have significant developmental delays at the time of placement.[19-24] These delays usually resolve rapidly once the child is in the care of loving, nurturing parents; therefore delays that persist beyond the first 2 to 3 months should be carefully evaluated. Young children learn new languages very quickly; thus language delays that persist should not be presumed to be the result of learning a new language, but rather should be carefully investigated, with early initiation of speech and language therapy. Younger children qualify in most states for early intervention services, and older children can be evaluated and treated through local school districts or privately. For internationally adopted school-aged children, having academic assessments performed in the native language can be advantageous within the first 1 to 2 months home, before fluency in that language is lost, given that full fluency in the new language may take several years.[25,26]

Most newly adopted children struggle in some way with the routines of daily living, including eating, sleeping, bathing, and toileting, among other routines. Even a child placed as a newborn may have these issues if exposures were encountered prenatally from which the child experiences withdrawal symptoms. (See Chapter 103, Prenatal Drug Abuse and Neonatal Drug Withdrawal Syndrome.) Children who have not had enough food (particularly those cared for in institutional settings where, in addition to inadequate volumes, food is never available to satisfy individual hunger) often eat *huge* volumes of food and may hoard food, alarming parents and physicians alike. This circumstance should be recognized as an adaptive survival behavior from the prior life circumstances and should be not restricted or punished. When children are allowed unlimited access to healthy, age-appropriate food, most will learn within several months that enough is now available, that they can have it whenever they need it, and will slow down to more typical levels of intake. If, on the other hand, the child's intake is restricted, then the previously learned strategy of taking all that is available whenever it is available will continue, often developing into more secretive food-hoarding behaviors and other long-term eating disorders.[8,10,27]

Sleep problems are obviously a common concern for all children but are almost universal among newly adopted children. Many of these children have never slept alone, in a dark room, or with any notion of safety at night, and internationally adopted children may have traveled through many time zones to arrive at their new home. Sleep deprivation quickly takes its toll on parents and children alike, complicating all of the other new-arrival transitions. Until a child has developed strong attachments to the parent or parents, though, this time is inappropriate for sleep strategies that encourage parents to leave a child alone. Until the child has thoroughly internalized the notion that the parent or parents will always be available when the child needs them, parents should be encouraged to be as physically and emotionally present at nighttime as the child needs to feel safe and secure. This task can be accomplished, however, in the child's room and bed, using the desired long-term sleep routines so that parents can wean themselves out of the child's bedtime routine as the child develops a sense of safety and security. By balancing these short- and long-term goals from the beginning, most children can be helped to sleep peacefully all night in their own beds within several months.[8,10,27]

Sensory-seeking or avoiding behaviors, as well as autistic-like repetitive behaviors, are common among children who have experienced severe deprivation before adoption. As with overeating mentioned earlier, these are adaptive behaviors in a setting with little or no stimulation and usually resolve quickly when more stimulation and human interaction is made available. Many children revert to these behaviors when tired, stressed, or bored, and parents can learn to read these behaviors as cues to these feelings. Reverting to self-stimulating behaviors to cope with fatigue or stress may continue for years after adoption, with no other pathological behavioral concerns. On the other hand, children who do not respond to nurturing parenting, but instead continue to self-stimulate regularly rather than interact with the world, should have a full developmental and behavioral evaluation.[8,10,28,29]

Another common dilemma, particularly for internationally adopted children, is an uncertain date of birth. Many children come into care after being born at home, with no official record of the birth or, more commonly, after being abandoned. Assigned birthdates may or may not be accurate, particularly for older children, given that the growth and developmental delays that result from malnutrition and neglect make children appear to be younger than they really are. As previously mentioned, most children are significantly delayed in their growth and development on arrival, and these delays, combined with knowledge of an assigned birthday, often tempt new parents and pediatricians to consider changing the child's date of birth. Because these delays usually quickly resolve, however, the notion to consider legally changing the child's birth date in the first or second year after arrival is rarely advisable. Bone age testing is not helpful early on, given that both malnutrition and neglect cause delays in bone age as they do in the rest of the child's development and thus should not be used as justification for changing a birth date. When concerns about age discrepancy persist a year or more after adoption, parents and pediatricians should carefully consider what would be gained and lost for the child if the date were to be changed. This situation is more common for children adopted after the infant and toddler ages, and, as such, children should be included in the decision making about this important piece of their identity.[10,30]

Long-Term Issues

In addition to any health issues identified before or immediately after adoption, long-term health issues common to adopted children should be considered. Recognizing these risk factors in a child's history can help pediatricians maintain appropriate surveillance above and beyond the usual well-child care routine and provide referrals and support proactively.

Most importantly, the long-term effects of early adversity cannot be forgotten. Early malnutrition, abuse, neglect, or trauma can cause significant long-term cognitive, developmental, behavioral, and mental health struggles, even after years in a warm, nurturing adoptive family. Developmental disabilities, mental health problems, and substance abuse are not uncommon factors in birthparents' unplanned pregnancies in the first place, leaving adopted children as a group with a higher frequency of genetic predispositions to these diagnoses than the general population.[25,31] Prenatal substance exposure, especially to alcohol, also carries significant long-term risks.[32-34] Teasing out which of these factors is responsible for a given child's struggles is often difficult or impossible; but for most adopted children, a safe assumption is that any of these predisposing issues might be a causative factor.

Many children experience significant struggles as they enter school age. Difficulties with attention and impulse control often lead to the diagnosis of attention-deficit/hyperactivity disorder, although they frequently are far more complex. Children should have a thorough psychoeducational or neuropsychological evaluation to tease out complex visual, auditory, language and sensory processing differences, difficulties with executive functioning, and specific learning disabilities before being assumed to have simple, uncomplicated attention-deficit/hyperactivity disorder.[26,35,36] In addition, many children who spent their early lives in institutional care, lacking much direct human contact, have difficulties reading nonverbal social cues. As a result, they often have great difficulties with peer relationships and can benefit from direct teaching on social skills and reading body language.

Children who experience serious malnutrition, followed by significant catch-up growth, have a significantly higher risk of precocious puberty compared with the general population. In addition to a young age of onset, these children typically proceed through the stages of puberty at a very rapid rate, making early recognition and treatment imperative.[37]

Children who have experienced malnutrition also frequently have very weak dental enamel, which is often compounded by circumstances that lack even marginal dental hygiene. Many children experience severe dental decay despite good dental hygiene in the adoptive home. Early recognition and treatment of these conditions is obviously paramount.

Many adoptees have little or no knowledge of the biological family medical history, and those who do often have only the information that was available at the time of their birth. This missing history can be a source of social and emotional distress to adolescents and their families, but for children of any age, it can also be a significant impediment to providing appropriate health care, particularly in the case of serious illness. Some states now provide registries of birthparent and adoptee information, with access granted by mutual consent. (See Tools for Practice for resources for adoption information.) Laws vary from state to state regarding who may have access to this information and under what circumstances. Some adoption agencies also maintain and update health records of birthparents whose children they have placed, and some will help families locate birthparents (see later discussion). Children who were adopted from overseas generally have little or no information about birth family medical history, and records may or may not be maintained, thus precluding further investigation. Children who were abandoned have no way to know any family medical history. Lack of birth family medical history should be considered when determining risk factors for routine screening, for example, for hypercholesterolemia.

BILLING AND PAYMENT INFORMATION FOR ADOPTION PHYSICIAN SERVICES

Preadoption consultation services are not billable to third-party payers because the child in question is not yet part of the policy. Pediatricians with a special interest in adoption medicine who perform these services frequently have fee-for-service fee scales that reflect the time spent, the complexity of information reviewed, and local prevailing payment rates. Pediatricians who perform these services only occasionally may choose to provide these services free of charge to families who are already in their practices, or they may devise a pay scale that reflects the same variables. Some families may be able to be reimbursed for these services by employer adoption subsidy plans or flexible spending accounts.

Office visits for newly adopted children require more time than standard well-child visits, involve far more complex issues, and generally need to occur more frequently. Payment for these services can be accomplished by appropriately coding for the time spent, the diagnoses involved, and the complexity of medical decision making. Evaluation and management codes (99201-99205 for new patients and 99211-99215 for returning patients) are usually more appropriate to the services rendered than are well-child visit codes (99381-99384 and 99391-99394) and are often paid at higher rates. Practices serving a large number of adopted children may need to communicate directly with third-party payers about these children, given that differences in immunizations and well-child care billing may inadvertently hurt practices in quality or pay-for-performance measures.

Diagnostic coding for these visits should also reflect the details of the child's needs. Commonly applicable diagnostic codes for newly adopted children are listed alphabetically in Box 113-2. Many mental health diagnoses must be made first by a mental health professional before a primary care physician can use them, but domestically adopted children may already carry these diagnoses. Any other medical diagnosis that fits can also be applied.

ISSUES UNIQUE TO ADOPTIVE FAMILIES

Adoptive families come in all shapes and sizes. These families may include children by birth and adoption, children and parents of different races, single parents, gay and lesbian parents, grandparents and other relatives raising children, and stepparents adopting a new spouse's children, just to name a few. Depending on the size and diversity of the community, some of these families may stick out, and parents and children will need to learn how to handle questions from strangers and acquaintances. Parents and pediatricians need to help children learn to interpret which questions are ill intended versus simply curious, what information is appropriate to share (with whom, when, and where), and what information is private. Children can and do thrive in all of these varieties of families, especially when parents are open and honest with children about these topics that are unique to adoptive families.[5,38-42]

All pediatricians should be familiar with basic issues that are common to all adopted children and should ensure that they and the entire office staff use language that reflects respect for adopted children and their birth and adoptive families. Box 113-3 provides appropriate language to use when speaking about adoption. Numerous resources are available to help parents, professionals, and children negotiate the complexities of grief, loss, and joy that come when a child is relinquished by one set of parents and claimed by another. (See Tools for Practice for these resources.)

Pediatricians should help and encourage adoptive parents to talk with their children about adoption from a very young age, given that all available research has shown that children do far better when they come to understand adoption over time, rather than as a single, *bomb-shell* discussion.[43] Adoptive parents often struggle with how to begin these discussions and how to handle children's questions, fearing that they might jeopardize the child's sense of security or belonging in the family or that they might overwhelm the child with difficult-to-comprehend details. Just as with any other complicated matter, though, children come to understand the complexities of adoption over time and in more detail as they progress developmentally. Young children simply need to learn the language and can begin to understand that, "I didn't grow inside Mommy's tummy." Preschoolers ask many questions, and adoptive parents who respond openly to their inquiries are setting the stage for more in-depth, open dialogue as time goes on. School-aged children begin to understand that they have 2 sets of parents and spend a great deal of time

BOX 113-2 Common ICD-9* Diagnoses for Newly Adopted Children

Abnormal weight gain: 783.1
Attention-deficit/hyperactivity disorder (ADHD) with hyperactivity: 314.01
ADHD without hyperactivity: 314.00
Adjustment disorder: 309.9
Anemia: 285.9
Asperger syndrome, pervasive developmental disorder: 299.8
Attachment disorder: 313.89
Autism: 299
Bronchospasm: 519.1
Constipation: 564.0
Developmental delay: 783.40, 783.41, 783.42
Diarrhea: 787.91
Eczema: 691.8
Failure to thrive, lack of expected physiologic development: 783.4
Feeding difficulty: 783.3
Fetal alcohol syndrome: 760.71
Hypotonia, hypertonia: 781.3
Impetigo: 684
Intestinal parasites: 129
Iron deficiency: 280.9
Lack of coordination: 781.3
Lead intoxication: 984.9
Low birth weight: 765.1 (must have known birth weight)
Malnutrition:

- Mild: 263.1
- Moderate: 263.0
- Severe: 262.0

Microcephaly: 742.1
Nervousness, irritability: 799.2
Otitis media: 382.00, 382.01
Plagiocephaly: 754.0
Positive purified protein derivative test: 795.5
Prematurity: 765.1 (need gestational age or birth weight)
Prenatal drug exposure: 760.72
Rash—unspecified: 782.1
Rickets: 268.0
Scabies: 133.0
Sensation disorder: 782.0
Short stature: 783.4
Sinusitis: 461.9
Sleep disturbance: 780.5
Speech delay: 315.39
Speech disorder: 784.5
Strabismus: 378.9
Thalassemia minor: 282.4

*World Health Organization. *International Classification of Diseases*. 9th ed. Geneva, Switzerland: World Health Organization; 2007.

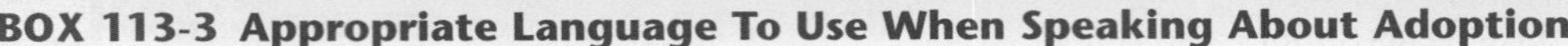

BOX 113-3 Appropriate Language To Use When Speaking About Adoption

The language used to talk about adoption can have positive or negative effects on children and their families. Physicians and office staff members who use respectful and supportive language about adoption will not only nurture the self-esteem of their patients, but also win the respect of parents and the word-of-mouth referrals of other adoptive families to the practice.

The following list discusses respectful and disrespectful ways to talk about adoption with families, with explanations of each.

- **DO:** Refer to *birth* children and *adopted* children as such when it is relevant to the discussion (eg, in discussing family medical history), and simply as *children* when it is not.
- **DO NOT:** Refer to children born to their parents as the parents' *real children, own children,* or *natural children.* Adopted children are not unreal or unnatural, and are very much their parents' *own* children.
- **DO:** Refer to the child's *birthparents* or *biological parents* when asking about them is relevant.
- **DO NOT:** Refer to the child's birthparents as a child's *real parents* or *natural parents.* Adoptive parents are very real and not at all unnatural.
- **DO:** Treat siblings who joined their families by birth or adoption equally. They are loved equally by their parents, and experience all of the usual joys and trials of *real* sibling relationships.
- **DO NOT:** Distinguish between adopted children and birth children in a family unless relevant.
- **DO:** Refer to birthparents as *making an adoption plan* for their child, or choosing to *place them for adoption.*
- **DO NOT:** Refer to children being *put up* or *given up* for adoption. Most birthparents work long and hard on their decision to place a child for adoption, and knowing that their birthparent or birthparents loved them and worked hard to reach a decision that they believed to be in the child's best interest is very important to a child's self-esteem.
- **DO:** Refer to a birthparent as *choosing to parent* the child. This term again implies to the adopted child that birthparents make their decisions based on what they believe is in the best interest of each child at the time when the decision needs to be made.
- **DO NOT:** Refer to another birthparent as choosing to *keep* a child. This term can imply to a child who was placed for adoption that he or she was not worth keeping.
- **DO:** Talk with families about how they celebrate the intercultural or interracial nature of their families. Most families today make a special effort to include a child's culture and heritage in the family's daily life and traditions, and all available research shows that children clearly benefit from this practice.
- **DO NOT:** Ignore a child's birth country, race, or genetic heritage. Especially in communities with little ethnic diversity, minority children will need family and physician support to overcome racism and develop a strong, positive racial identity.
- **DO:** Recognize that children come to understand adoption gradually as they grow, just as with all other developmental tasks. Ask if any adoption-related issues exist that may presently be difficult for the child or parent or parents, and be familiar with common issues of different developmental stages (just as with other areas of child development) so that you can be a resource for patients and their families.
- **DO NOT:** Ask "Are you going to tell the child about the adoption?" Adoptive parents are advised today to talk freely and honestly about adoption with their children from the time they are very young so that the news of the child's adoption is never shocking.
- **DO:** Be sympathetic with the long and sometimes arduous path that parents have traveled to become parents. Some parents may be suffering significant financial stresses after the expense of the adoption, some may still be grieving infertility losses, and some may be coping with extended family members who do not accept the adopted child. Recognize that even though the child may not be a newborn, the parents are new parents. Recognize that postadoption depression exists, similar to postpartum depression.
- **DO NOT:** Ask, "How much did you have to pay for the child?" Adopted children are not bought. Fees go to pay social workers, attorneys, court and government paperwork fees, travel, medical expenses, and foster or orphanage care, among others, not to *buy children.*

thinking about their birthparents. They often fear talking about this subject with their adoptive parents, worrying that these questions will hurt the feelings of or minimize their love for their adoptive parents. Parents need to offer many opportunities for children to talk and clearly tell them that this topic of conversation is acceptable. Teens begin to incorporate what they know about their birthparents and their own stories into their developing identity and may experiment with lifestyles that they know or imagine their birthparents to be living. Anticipatory guidance for adopted children should include encouraging parents to talk openly and honestly in simple, direct, developmentally appropriate language to help the children understand and deal with the specific details of their own life's story.[43]

Many adoptions, particularly domestic adoptions, include some degree of openness or ongoing contact between children and their birthparents. Although this idea is frightening at first to many prospective adoptive parents and might seem harmful to those unfamiliar with adoption, research and experience has shown that children thrive when birth and adoptive parents carefully and lovingly maintain relationships over time. Although these relationships can at times be complicated the benefit to children of being able to know exactly why their birthparents chose not to raise them and of knowing details such as who they resemble, whose musical talent or crooked toes they inherited, and how their birthparents are doing today is beyond measure.

Children who do not have ongoing contact with their birthparents often, as they become adolescents or adults, choose to search for them. Many adoption agencies and therapists offer help and support to adopted persons and their families as they proceed through this process. The emotional and legal complexities of this process vary from family to family and state to state, with some states allowing adoptees full access to records, some having mutual consent registries, and some allowing limited or no information to be obtained from sealed records. Pediatricians can help parents understand that the desire to search does not imply a rejection of the adoptive parents, but rather a need for the adopted person to fully understand him or herself. Some adoptees find and develop good relationships with their birth families, some find them but do not develop strong relationships, and others are never able to locate biological relatives. Pediatricians need to support families as they negotiate all of these possibilities. (See Tools for Practice.)

Although most adoptive placements generate positive outcomes for both children and their families, not all adoptive placements achieve permanency for children or happy long-term outcomes. Although exact numbers are unclear because of variable state reporting systems, estimates indicate that between 10% and 25% of adoptive placements are disrupted (ended before the adoption is finalized), and 1% to 10% are dissolved (legally reversed, similar to a divorce, after the adoption was final).[44] Most commonly this event happens with children who are older, with complicated, traumatic histories and complex behavioral and mental health needs, who were placed with families who were either unaware of these needs or inadequately prepared to meet them. Such occurrences are traumatic for everyone involved, most especially the child, and are best avoided by full disclosure of information before the adoption and long-term, ongoing support for the family after the adoption is finalized. Families who are considering or pursuing a disruption or dissolution of their adoption should be referred to an experienced adoption professional.[38,45] (See Tools for Practice for parent resources about disruption and dissolution.) These same stresses, combined with unrealistic expectations, can also leave children at risk for abuse or neglect in their adoptive homes, just as can occur in any other family. Pediatricians should maintain the same surveillance for these possibilities as they would for any other child and family.

CONCLUSION

Caring for adopted children and their families can be among the most rewarding experiences of a pediatrician's career. By working closely with parents to address the special needs of their adopted children, pediatricians can help ensure a bright future for children whose futures might otherwise have been bleak.

TOOLS FOR PRACTICE

Engaging Patient and Family

- *Access to Adoption Records* (brochure), Child Welfare Information Gateway (www.childwelfare.gov/systemwide/laws_policies/statutes/infoaccessap.cfm).
- *Adoption: Guidelines for Parents* (brochure), American Academy of Pediatrics (patiented.aap.org).

Medical Decision Support

- *Adoption Disruptions and Dissolutions: Numbers and Trends* (fact sheet), Child Welfare Information Gateway (www.childwelfare.gov/pubs/s_disrup.cfm).
- *Centers for Disease Control and Prevention Travelers' Health* (Web page), Centers for Disease Control and Prevention (wwwn.cdc.gov/travel/default.aspx).
- *Fostering Health: Health Care for Children and Adolescents in Foster Care, 2nd edition* (book), Task Force on Health Care for Children in Foster Care, American Academy of Pediatrics, District II, New York State (www.aap.org/bookstore).
- *Openness in Adoption: A Bulletin for Professionals* (brochure), Child Welfare Information Gateway (www.childwelfare.gov/pubs/f_openadoptbulletin.cfm).
- *Red Book: 2006 Report of the Committee of Infectious Diseases* (book), American Academy of Pediatrics (www.aap.org/bookstore).

RELATED WEB SITES

- Adopting.org (www.adopting.org).
- Adoptive Families Magazine (adoptivefamilies.com/).
- American Academy of Pediatrics, Section on Adoption and Foster Care (www.aap.org/moc/memberships/section/adoption/mission%20statement.htm).
- American Adoption Congress (americanadoptioncongress.org/).
- Association for Treatment and Training in the Attachment of Children (attach.org/).
- Child Welfare League of America (cwla.org/).
- Hague Convention on Intercountry Adoption (travel.state.gov/family/adoption/convention/convention_462.html).
- Joint Council on International Children's Services (www.jcics.org/).
- North American Council on Adoptable Children (nacac.org/).
- Perspectives Press (www.perspectivespress.com/index.php).
- Tapestry Books (tapestrybooks.com/Default.asp?c=283340).
- United States Department of Health and Human Services: Child Welfare Information Gateway (www.childwelfare.gov/adoption/).
- United States Department of State: Intercountry Adoption (travel.state.gov/family/adoption/adoption_485.html).
- University of Minnesota International Adoption Clinic (www.med.umn.edu/peds/iac/otherprofessionals.html).

AAP POLICY STATEMENT

American Academy of Pediatrics, Committee on Psychosocial Aspects of Child and Family Health. Coparent or second-parent adoption by same-sex parents. *Pediatrics.* 2002;109(2):339-340. (aappolicy.aappublications.org/cgi/content/full/pediatrics;109/2/339).

REFERENCES

1. US Department of State. Immigrant Visas Issue to Orphans Coming to the U.S. Available at: travel.state.gov/family/adoption/stats/stats_451.html. Accessed August 14, 2007.
2. US Department of Health and Human Services; Administration for Children and Families; Administration for Children, Youth, and Families, Children's Bureau. Report to the Congress on Kinship Foster Care. Available at: aspe.hhs.gov/HSP/kinr2c00/#execsum. Accessed on August 13, 2007.
3. Chambers J. Preadoption opportunities for pediatric providers. *Pediatr Clin North Am.* 2005;52(5):1247-1269.
4. Miller LC. Pre-adoption counseling and evaluation of the referral. In: Miller LC, ed. *The Handbook of International Adoption Medicine: A Guide for Pediatricians, Parents, and Providers.* New York, NY: Oxford University Press; 2004.
5. Steinberg G, Hall B. *Inside Transracial Adoption.* Indianapolis, IN: Perspectives Press; 2000.
6. American Academy of Pediatrics. Member Center. Available at: www.aap.org/moc/memberships/section/adoption/mission%20statement.htm. Accessed August 17, 2007.
7. Barnett ED, Chen LH. Prevention of travel-related infectious diseases in families of internationally adopted children. *Pediatr Clin North Am.* 2005;52(5):1271-1286.
8. Miller LC. Immediate behavioral and developmental considerations for internationally adopted children transitioning into families. *Pediatr Clin North Am.* 2005;52(5):1311-1330.
9. Miller LC. After the adoption: unspoken problems. In: Miller LC, ed. *The Handbook of International Adoption Medicine: A Guide for Pediatricians, Parents, and Providers.* New York, NY: Oxford University Press; 2004.
10. Schulte EE, Springer SH. Health care in the first year after international adoption. *Pediatr Clin North Am.* 2005;52(5):1331-1349.
11. Miller LC. Attachment. In: Miller LC, ed. *The Handbook of International Adoption Medicine: A Guide for Pediatricians, Parents, and Providers.* New York, NY: Oxford University Press; 2004.
12. American Academy of Pediatrics. Medical evaluation of internationally adopted children for infectious diseases. In: Pickering LK, Baker CJ, Long SS, et al, eds. *Red Book: 2006 Report of the Committee on Infectious Diseases.* 27th ed. Elk Grove Village, IL: American Academy of Pediatrics; 2006.
13. American Academy of Pediatrics. Tuberculosis. In: Pickering LK, Baker CJ, Long SS, et al, eds. *Red Book: 2006 Report of the Committee on Infectious Diseases.* 27th ed. Elk Grove Village, IL: American Academy of Pediatrics; 2006.
14. Curtis AB, Ridzon R, Vogel R, et al. Extensive transmission of mycobacterium tuberculosis from a child. *N Engl J Med.* 1999;341(2):1491-1495.
15. Barnett ED. Immunizations and infectious disease screening for internationally adopted children. *Pediatr Clin North Am.* 2005;52(5):1287-1309.
16. Miller LC. Immunizations and vaccine-preventable diseases. In: Miller LC, ed. *The Handbook of International Adoption Medicine: A Guide for Pediatricians, Parents, and Providers.* New York, NY: Oxford University Press; 2004.
17. The American Academy of Pediatrics. Catch-up immunization schedules for children and adolescents. In: Pickering LK, Baker CJ, Long SS, et al, eds. *Red Book: 2006 Report of the Committee on Infectious Diseases.* 27th ed. Elk Grove Village, IL: American Academy of Pediatrics; 2006.
18. Knauf L, Iverson S, Johnson D. *International Adoptees are at High Risk for Vision and Hearing Problems.* Paper presented at annual meeting of the Pediatric Academic Societies, 2004. Abstract No. 1382.
19. Johnson DE, Dole K. International adoptions: implications for early intervention. *Infants Young Child.* 1999;11(4):34-45.
20. Miller LC, Hendrie NW. Health of children adopted from China. *Pediatrics.* 2000;105(6):E76.
21. Albers LH, Johnson DE, Hostetter MK, et al. Health of children adopted from the former Soviet Union and Eastern Europe: Comparison with preadoptive medical records. *JAMA.* 1997;278(11):922-924.
22. Miller LC. Developmental delay. In: Miller LC, ed. *The Handbook of International Adoption Medicine: A Guide for Pediatricians, Parents, and Providers.* New York, NY: Oxford University Press; 2004.
23. Simms MD, Dubowitz H, Szilagyi MA, et al. Health care needs of children in the foster care system. *Pediatrics.* 2000;106(4 suppl):909-918.
24. American Academy of Pediatrics, Task Force on Health Care for Children in Foster Care. District II, New York State. Practice parameters for developmental and mental health care. In: *Fostering Health: Health Care for Children and Adolescents in Foster Care.* Elk Grove Village, IL: American Academy of Pediatrics; 2004.
25. Weitzman C, Albers L. Long-term developmental, behavioral, and attachment outcomes after international adoption. *Pediatr Clin North Am.* 2005;52(5):1395-1419.
26. Dole KN. Education and internationally adopted children: working collaboratively with schools. *Pediatr Clin North Am.* 2005;52(5):1445-1461.
27. Miller LC. Travel and transition to the adoptive family. In: Miller LC, ed. *The Handbook of International Adoption Medicine: A Guide for Pediatricians, Parents, and Providers.* New York, NY: Oxford University Press; 2004.
28. Miller LC. Dysfunction of sensory integration. In: Miller LC, ed. *The Handbook of International Adoption Medicine: A Guide for Pediatricians, Parents, and Providers.* New York, NY: Oxford university Press; 2004.
29. Costello E. Complimentary and alternative therapies: considerations for families after international adoption. *Pediatr Clin North Am.* 2005;52(5):1463-1478.
30. Miller LC. Uncertain age. In: Miller LC, ed. *The Handbook of International Adoption Medicine: A Guide for Pediatricians, Parents, and Providers.* New York, NY: Oxford University Press; 2004.
31. Nalven L. Strategies for addressing long-term issues after institutionalization. *Pediatr Clin North Am.* 2005;52(5):1421-1444, viii.
32. Davies JK, Bledsoe JM. Prenatal alcohol and drug exposures in adoption. *Pediatr Clin North Am.* 2005;52(5):1369-1393.
33. Miller LC. Fetal alcohol syndrome. In: Miller LC, ed. *The Handbook of International Adoption Medicine: A Guide for Physicians, Parents, and Providers.* New York, NY: Oxford University Press; 2004.
34. Miller LC. Prenatal drug exposure. In: Miller LC, ed. *The Handbook of International Adoption Medicine: A Guide for Physicians, Parents, and Providers.* New York, NY: Oxford University Press; 2004.
35. Miller LC. School issues. In: Miller LC, ed. *The Handbook of International Adoption Medicine: A Guide for Physicians, Parents, and Providers.* New York, NY: Oxford University Press; 2004.
36. Meese RL. *Children of Intercountry Adoption in School: A Primer for Parents and Professionals.* London, UK: Bergin and Garvey; 2002.

37. Mason P, Narad C. Long-term growth and puberty concerns in international adoptees. *Pediatr Clin North Am.* 2005;52(5):1351-1368.
38. Jenista JA. Special topics in international adoption. *Pediatr Clin North Am.* 2005;52(5):1479-1494.
39. Cox SS, Loeberthal J. Intercountry adoption: young adult issues and transition to adulthood. *Pediatr Clin North Am.* 2005;52(5):1495-1506.
40. Kang JE. International adoption: a personal perspective. *Pediatr Clin North Am.* 2005;52(5):1507-1515.
41. American Academy of Pediatrics, Committee on Psychosocial Aspects of Child and Family Health. Coparent or second-parent adoption by same-sex parents. *Pediatrics.* 2002;109(2):339-340.
42. Pawelski JG, Perrin EC, Foy JM, et al. The effects of marriage, civil union, and domestic partnership laws on the health and well-being of children. *Pediatrics.* 2006;118(1): 349-364.
43. Riley D, Meeks J. *Beneath the Mask: Understanding Adopted Teens.* Silver Spring, MD: C.A.S.E. Publications; 2005.
44. US Department of Health and Human Services; Administration for Children and Families; Administration on Children, Youth, and Families, Children's Bureau. Adoption Disruption and Dissolution: Numbers and Trends. Child Welfare Information Gateway. Available at: childwellfare.gov/pubs/s_disrupt.cfm. Accessed August 13, 2007.
45. Miller LC. After the adoption: unspoken problems. In: Miller LC, ed. *The Handbook of International Adoption Medicine: A Guide for Pediatricians, Parents, and Providers.* New York, NY: Oxford University Press; 2004.

Chapter 114
CHILD CUSTODY

Elizabeth Meller Alderman, MD

Child custody arrangements at the time of a divorce have evolved over a long period, being a judicial issue only since the early 19th century. Changes in child custody laws reflect the social mores of the times. This chapter reviews the history of child custody statutes, different custody arrangements, and the role of mediation. The pediatrician is often called to court to assess the family and child's situation in determining custody arrangements and thus should be familiar with these aspects of family law.

HISTORY

Roman law dictated that the wife and children were under the absolute control of the father. This power was also the case in feudal England, British common law, and courts in the United States until the 19th century. With the advent of developmental and psychological studies of infants and children that highlighted the importance of the mother-child bond, the concept of *parens patriae*, or judicial consideration of the best interest of the child, became the law in the United States. Both parents received equal consideration in cases of child custody.

The *tender years doctrine* subsequently evolved and was first introduced in the United States in the 1900s. This interpretation of the law gave custodial preference to the mother because of the perceived notion that mothers were the best caretakers for young children. The growing women's rights movement also advocated for maternal custody. However, this concept has fallen out of favor in the last 20 years, with laws forbidding discrimination based on gender because such statues violate fathers' rights. Thus, according to judicial standards, the pendulum has swung back. The best interests of the child are now given the greatest consideration. Current laws and court decisions try to preserve the parenting rights of both parents and provide for their ongoing commitment.

Over the last 3 decades, the total number of children younger than age 18 years involved in a divorce has tripled. Each year, more than 1 million children experience their parents' divorce.[1] Fifty percent of first marriages end in divorce. In the year 1995, less than 60% of children in the United States were living with both biological parents; most were living with their mother. Approximately 75% of black children in families in which both parents were previously married experienced divorce before age 18 years, and this is true for 38% of Americans of European descent.[2] This increased divorce rate has forced the courts, as well as pediatricians and mental health professionals, to evaluate the effect of different custody arrangements on children and adolescents. Additionally, new considerations in awarding child custody have surfaced as lifestyles and the definition of family have changed. In most cases, both parents have joint legal custody, but the primary physical residence is with the mother.[2] However, fathers are now more likely to demand a greater role in the child's life. Issues that may have impeded a parent receiving custody in the past, such as sexual orientation, parental health, psychiatric history, lifestyle, religion, and cohabitation out of wedlock, are now being scrutinized. In determining child custody, the best interests of the child are overriding. In fact, organizations such as the American Psychiatric Association have published a resource document stating that sexual orientation of the parent should not be used to determine child custody arrangements.[3] Grandparents and nonbiological parents may also wish to obtain some degree of custody or visitation privileges.

CUSTODY ARRANGEMENTS

Two dimensions of child custody are legal custody and physical custody. Legal custody refers to who will make the major decisions that will affect the life of the child, such as those involving health, dental care, emergency care, religion, and other activities. Physical custody refers to individuals with whom the child will live and spend time. Specifically, physical custody describes people with whom the child spends weekdays, weekends, holidays, and summers and who will supervise the child's daily activities.

Sole custody had been the traditional settlement in the past and still exists if 1 parent deserts a family or is judged to be unfit or if the parents cannot agree on what is best for the child. The custodial parent has legal and physical custody and thus is legally responsible for all major decisions regarding the child.

Split custody, in which each parent assumes custody of 1 or more of their children, is rarely awarded. This arrangement is usually not made because it is considered to be important to keep children together to provide consistency and mutual support.

Joint custody, which encompasses either joint legal or joint physical custody, is the most common arrangement and occurs in 80% to 90% of all custody arrangements.[4] Joint legal custody is the most popular and allows both parents equal responsibility in important decisions regarding the child's life. One parent is awarded physical custody of the child, with the other receiving liberal visiting privileges. In more than 70% of the cases, the children's primary residence is with the mother. Less than 10% result in primary custody granted to the father. Joint physical custody provides for the child to live with both parents for significant amounts of time, but not simultaneously.

The majority of states in the United States have enacted joint custody laws.[5] Some states have ordered joint custody as the preferred arrangement; others have the legal assumption of joint custody if agreed on by both parents. Advocates of joint custody, such as fathers' rights activists and family mediators, believe that children living solely with mothers have less paternal contact and that mothers are overburdened physically and financially if they are the sole caretakers.

Research examining whether joint physical custody is preferable to sole custody has shown mixed results. Joint custody provides the best continuity for the child with both the parents. Parents in joint custody arrangements have better cooperation with former spouses and greater financial resources than those who obtain sole custody.

Joint custody is an expensive option because each parent must provide full physical facilities for the child. Joint physical residence is best if parents are cooperative and have minimal conflict. This custody arrangement may be detrimental if conflict over childrearing and discipline arise, and children get caught in the middle.[2] In addition, as children grow older, especially during adolescence, their primary residence may need to be reevaluated. At that point, the adolescent's wishes need to be respected. Many times adolescents wish to have a single home so that they may maintain contact with their friends. This arrangement may not preclude weekend or vacation visitation with the noncustodial parent.

Most parents demonstrate high satisfaction with joint custody. Success of such an arrangement depends on geographic proximity, valuing the other parent as the child's parent, lack of guilt, and low levels of anger.

Contrary to popular belief, only a small percentage of child custody decisions are made in the courtroom; most cases are settled by attorneys and clients or go to mediation. Cases that do go to court result from different motivations. A parent may wish to establish the incompetency of the other in a public forum such as the courtroom. Custody of the child may be a way to seek revenge on a former spouse or fulfill a parent's emotional needs after the divorce. From a financial standpoint, the parent providing child support may wish to have full custody to have greater control over the child's life, as well as decreased support payments. In addition, a continued court battle may allow former spouses to maintain a relationship although their marriage has been dissolved. Child custody may become a bargaining chip in a divorce settlement. Unfortunately, some parents use desperate measures, such as allegations of child abuse, to obtain custody of a child. If abuse does exist, the courts must be informed of it. However, if the allegation is unfounded, then it will lengthen the proceedings and might cause undue emotional harm to an already fragile family constellation.

In the last decade, the legal system has moved away from litigation and toward mediation as a method of resolving child custody disputes. In fact, many states have statutes that mandate mediation as the first step in determining child custody to facilitate communication and conflict resolution and encourage exploration of all alternatives to reach a compromise that is acceptable to both parties. The benefits of mediation are that (1) the needs of both parties are heard, (2) the spouse feels more competent because a third party (lawyer or judge) is not relied on to arrive at a decision, (3) it is less expensive, and (4) the process is shorter. Mediated settlements are usually stable because they have been obtained by consensus rather than mandated from the courts.

Mediation encourages parental cooperation and thus better outcomes for children. Usually, this increased parental satisfaction translates to better compliance with mediated agreements. Studies have shown that with successful mediation, the risk of relitigation is reduced and communication between parents is increased.[6] Benefits of mediation also include greater involvement with children and greater compliance with visitation by noncustodial parents. In terms of long-term effects, these parents also have more frequent communication during the period following the dispute.

The majority of couples who use mediation are able to reach a mutually acceptable agreement, which is usually joint custody. The key variables that predict successful conflict resolution are commitment, communication, and the experience of the mediator. A situation of great conflict, such as allegations of child abuse or domestic violence, is less likely to be resolved by mediation. In fact, mediation is not appropriate in cases of domestic violence. Mediation is also not appropriate if a spouse has a serious psychiatric illness or is intellectually disabled.

ROLE OF THE PEDIATRICIAN

The pediatrician may be asked by the attorney to evaluate the family and by the court to help determine the best custody arrangement. In fact, evaluation by a health or mental health professional is one of the most influential factors that judges consider in disputed child custody cases. Appropriate permissions from the custodial parent or parents for the mental health professional to share information must be provided to the pediatrician before disclosing any health-related information regarding the child.[7]

Several considerations should be kept in mind in determining the best custody arrangement: health, safety, and welfare of the child; maintenance of a consistent living arrangement; quality of the parent-child relationship; degree to which a parent has been a caretaker; the child's preference; the parent's physical and mental health; styles of parenting and discipline; conflict resolution; and the parent's ability to provide emotional support for the child. Practical factors include location of the child's school, the parent's work schedule and location, parental finances, and availability of social support systems.[8] The health professional should consider all aspects of a child's life by interviewing the child and the parents and observing their interactions. The physician may also need to gather information from the child's school, friends of the family, relatives, and other community organizations with which the family is involved. Medical and mental health records also might be important.

The pediatrician needs to know the exact custody arrangements. As the child's health care provider, the pediatrician must clarify who has the right to medical information regarding the child, who can give consent for medical treatment, and who must be informed about the child's medical needs. The American Academy of Pediatrics recommends that the pediatrician be given a copy of the custody agreement to keep in the child's health file.[9] Arrangements as to which parent may legally provide informed consent, who is responsible for payment for the child's health care, and with whom the pediatrician may discuss health information should be clear. If joint physical custody has been granted, then both parents must be instructed to coordinate health care regimens for the child.[10] Moreover, if the noncustodial parent has visiting rights, then this parent should also have a copy of the child's immunization record and other important health records in the case of a medical emergency.[1] If the child is visiting the noncustodial parent in another state, then it must be clarified whether the state law permits the noncustodial parent to give consent for health care.[9]

The pediatrician should reassess custody situations periodically; children's needs may change as they change physically and developmentally. The physician may need to refer some children and families for psychological support. The pediatrician can also offer developmentally appropriate advice to parents who are helping their child cope with divorce and a new living situation.

TOOLS FOR PRACTICE

Engaging Patients and Family

- *Divorce and Step-Parenting* (Q&A), American Academy of Pediatrics (www.aap.org/healthtopics/divorce.cfm).
- *Divorce and Children* (brochure), American Academy of Pediatrics (patiented.aap.org).

AAP POLICY STATEMENTS

American Academy of Pediatrics, Berger, JE, Committee on Medical Liability. Consent by proxy for nonurgent pediatric care. *Pediatrics.* 2004;112(5):1186-1195. Available at: aappolicy.aappublications.org/cgi/content/full/pediatrics;112/5/1186.

American Academy of Pediatrics, Cohen GJ, Committee on Psychosocial Aspects of Child and Family Health. Helping children and families deal with divorce and separation. *Pediatrics.* 2002;110(5):1019-1023. Available at: aappolicy.aappublications.org/cgi/content/abstract/pediatrics;110/5/1019.

American Academy of Pediatrics, Committee on Psychosocial Aspects of Child and Family Health. The child in court: a subject review. *Pediatrics.* 1999;104(5):1145-1148. Available at: aappolicy.aappublications.org/cgi/content/abstract/pediatrics;104/5/1145.

SUGGESTED RESOURCES

American Psychiatric Association Task Force on Clinical Assessment in Child Custody. *Child Custody Consultation.* Washington, DC: American Psychiatric Association; 1988.

Brems C, Carssow KL, Shook C, et al. Assessment of fairness in child custody decisions. *Child Abuse Negl.* 1995;19:345-353.

Cancian M, Meyer DR. Who gets custody? *Demography.* 1998;35:147-157.

Emery RE. *Marriage, Divorce and Children's Adjustment.* London, UK: Sage; 1988.

Emery RE. *Renegotiating Family Relationships: Divorce, Child Custody and Mediation.* New York, NY: Guilford; 1994.

Griffith DB. The best interest standard: a comparison of the state's *parens patriae* authority and judicial oversight in best interests determinations for children and incompetent patients. *Issues Law Med.* 1991;7:283.

Hlady LJ, Gunther EJ. Alleged child abuse in custody access disputes, *Child Abuse Negl.* 1990;14:591.

Kappelman MM, Black J. Children of divorce: the pediatrician's responsibility. *Pediatr Ann.* 1980;9:50.

Kunin CC, Ebbesen EB, Konecni VJ. An archival study of decision-making in child custody disputes, *J Clin Psychol.* 1992;48:564.

Wallerstein JS, Kelly JB. *Surviving the Breakup: How Children and Parents Cope with Divorce.* New York, NY: Basic Books; 1980.

REFERENCES

1. Cohen GJ, Committee on Psychosocial Aspects of Child and Family Health. Helping children and families deal with divorce and separation. *Pediatrics.* 2002;110(6):1019-1023.
2. Emery RE, Coiro MJ. Divorce: consequences for children. *Pediatr Rev.* 1995;16:306-310.
3. American Psychiatric Association. *Controversies in Child Custody: Gay and Lesbian Parenting; Transracial Adoptions; Joint versus Sole Custody; and Custody Gender Issues.* Resource Document 970008. Washington DC: American Psychiatric Association; 1997.
4. Binder RL. American Psychiatric Association resource document on controversies in child custody: gay and lesbian parenting, transracial adoptions, joint versus sole custody, and custody gender issues, *J Am Acad Psychiatry Law.* 1998;26:267-276.
5. Coller DR. Joint custody: research, theory, and policy. *Fam Process.* 1988;27:459-469.
6. Dillon PA, Emery RE. Divorce mediation and resolution of child custody disputes: long-term effects, *Am J Orthopsychiatry.* 1996;66:131-140.
7. American Academy of Pediatrics, Committee on Psychosocial Aspects of Child and Family Health. The child in court: a subject review. *Pediatrics.* 1999;104(5):1145-1148.
8. American Academy of Child and Adolescent Psychiatry. Practice parameters for child custody evaluation. *J Am Acad Child Adolesc Psychiatr.* 1997;36:57S-67S.
9. Berger JE, American Academy of Pediatrics, Committee on Medical Liability. Consent by proxy for nonurgent pediatric care. *Pediatrics.* 2003;112(5):1186-1195.
10. American Academy of Pediatrics. The pediatrician's role in helping children and families deal with separation and divorce. *Pediatrics.* 1994;97:119-121.

Chapter 115

CHILDREN OF DIVORCE

Rhonda M. Graves, MD; Lori Legano, MD; Michael L. Weitzman, MD

Approximately 1 million children experience divorce in the United States each year.[1] In the early 1960s, almost 90% of children spent their childhood and adolescence with two biological parents. Now, that number has decreased to 40%.[2] For adults, divorce is second only to the death of a spouse or a parent in terms of its intensity as a stressor and the length of time required to adjust to it.[3] Divorce often produces anger and a sense of failure for parents; conflicted loyalties, guilt, grief, and anxiety for children; and concern on the part of all about whether the children will suffer long-term harm. Most children of divorce experience it, at the least, as a potent transient stress. It should never be viewed therefore as an isolated event, but rather as a step in a series of family transitions that significantly affects both of the parents and the children.[4] Many people accommodate to their new circumstances successfully; but a substantial percentage suffer long-term negative effects. Many of the problems of these children and their families can be anticipated, prevented, or alleviated by thoughtful and timely intervention.

FAMILY CHANGES PRECIPITATED BY DIVORCE

In most cases, both parents are awarded joint legal custody, but the children's primary physical residence is with their mother in more than 80% of cases.[1] Divorce often has devastating financial consequences for these children and their mothers, and children in postdivorce families are four times as likely to live in poverty compared with children overall. A significant number of divorced mothers have few financial and personal resources to direct toward the children, and many take on new employment arrangements. This circumstance may result in new child-care arrangements for younger children, older children taking care of themselves or siblings for greater parts of the day, and curtailment of certain activities because of expense or parental time constraints.

For nonresidential parents, who are most often fathers, problems range from what to do with children on visiting days to profound concern about the emotional consequences for their children. Some nonresidential parents fear that their children will abandon them, some have unrealistic expectations about the kind of relationship they will have with their children, and some believe divorce deprives them of the right to exercise authority and discipline the children. Much public attention has deservedly focused to issues of failed child support, nonresidential fathers who do not visit, and the economic plight of single-parent households. The importance of long-term paternal involvement in a meaningful and unconflicted relationship with their children cannot be overstated.

STAGES OF DIVORCE

The period immediately before and after the separation is referred to as the acute stage; it is characterized by maximal turmoil and generally lasts up to 2 years. The family then moves into the transitional stage, which is characterized by more controlled changes. The final stage is the postdivorce stage, when major family restructuring ceases.

During the acute stage, all family members are confronted with disruptions of their expectations, relationships, and support systems. Parents may be depressed, may be preoccupied with personal concerns, and may exhibit diminished parenting abilities. During this stage, two events appear to be most stressful to most children: (1) learning about the divorce and (2) the actual departure of a parent. The 1st year after divorce is the year of maximal negative behavior by children and the poorest parenting by parents. The apparent intensity of a child's reaction to this stage, however, does not predict long-term adjustment. Initially, many parents make fewer demands on the children, communicate less effectively, are less affectionate, and have difficulty disciplining children. In a significant minority of divorces, the troubled relationship between parents continues indefinitely. In these cases, children have the greatest incidence of postdivorce maladjustment.[1,5-9]

The transitional stage is marked by new undertakings for the single-parent household and more stability than the acute stage. Children must accommodate to their parents' new relationship with each other, to new friends, and often to new romantic partners of one or both parents. During this stage, children are often concerned about the well being of, and their relationship with, the nonresidential parent. Visitation patterns tend to have become more stable, whether they are acceptable to all parties or not. The major exception to the general pattern of increased stability is the family in which the parents still are actively in conflict, either informally with each other and the children or formally through the legal system.

In the postdivorce stage, relative stability is achieved. The family may still be headed by one parent, or a stepparent may now be present. Remarriage does not convey automatic stability but requires new adjustments as a result of the reawakening of unresolved issues and to new roles in the new family.

EFFECTS OF DIVORCE ON CHILDREN

On average, small but detectable negative emotional, cognitive, social, and physical effects, both short term and long term, are found among children of divorce. Of course, these effects vary greatly and depend on many factors.

Initial Effects

Initial responses are greatly influenced by the developmental level of the child; the child's temperament[10]; the level of parental conflict; and the emotional, cognitive, and economic support available to the child. The effects of divorce on children are similar for male and female family members.[11]

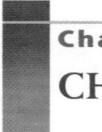

Infants and toddlers have minimal to no comprehension that divorce has occurred and may not have a direct reaction to the divorce.[12] Preschoolers, aged 2 to

5 years, initially tend to display regressive behaviors that can be highly stressful for parents, such as sleep disturbances, temper tantrums, separation anxiety, loss of bowel and bladder control, and increased need for parental attention. School-aged children, 5½ to 12 years of age, may experience sadness, grief, or intense anger at one or both parents. School performance and peer relationships may deteriorate, and phobias may emerge among both early and late school-aged children. Adolescents of divorcing parents find themselves without the expected home base from which to move away. This situation may result in insecurity, loneliness, decreased self-esteem,[13] and depression. These feelings may be overtly or covertly expressed in diminished school performance, school failure, truancy, violent and nonviolent criminal behavior, substance use, eating disorders, or sexual promiscuity. Children of any age may exhibit psychosomatic symptoms as a reaction to the stressors placed on them by the divorce. These children may play one parent against the other to gain more control.[14]

Long-Term Effects

Prior studies revealed long-lasting effects of parental divorce in a significant minority of cases.[1,5-9] Adults who experienced divorce as children tend to score lower on a variety of indicators of psychological, interpersonal, and socioeconomic well being. Although the majority of adults who experienced divorce as children appear to do well, as a group overall, they have higher rates of depression, job changes, premarital pregnancies, and divorce. The degree of marital conflict before the divorce has been shown to be a stronger predictor of adjustment than the divorce itself or the conflicts after the divorce.[15]

In the last decade, further study has been conducted about the long-term effects of divorce. A 25-year follow-up study confirmed that children of divorced parents are less likely to marry and when they do marry are more likely to divorce.[16] They are also less likely to enter and complete college.[16] The gap between children of divorced and married parents with respect to academic achievement, psychological well being, self-concept, and social relations was small in both the 1980s and 1990s, although a trend for a wider gap occurred in the 1990s.[11] The differences in outcomes between children of married and divorced parents may be influenced by ethnicity, with smaller differences seen in black families than in European-American families.[17] The long-term negative effects of divorce are mitigated by a variety of social factors: support of parents[18] and grandparents,[19] social support in adulthood,[18] educational attainment by the child[18] and mother,[20] and socioeconomic status of the family.[20]

Not all effects of divorce are negative, however. Children from divorced families demonstrate less stereotyped sexual behavior, greater maturity, and greater independence.[21]

TASKS FOR THE CHILDREN AND PARENTS OF DIVORCE

Children of divorce have several specific tasks on which they work simultaneously and with varying degrees of success.[22] These tasks are very dependent on the child's development and age. Mastery of these tasks is greatly facilitated by support and cooperation of both parents. Parents can better help children cope with divorce if they are aware of the child's developmental age and respond to them accordingly.

Understanding the Meaning of Divorce and Custody

Toddlers and preschoolers may have a difficult time understanding the meaning of divorce. Because these children view their world very concretely, they may not be able to comprehend the changes in relationships and the alterations within their household. Confusion about the actual meaning of divorce is the rule rather than the exception.[23] Parents should provide simple explanations about the meaning of divorce and custody and should never avoid the subject. Parents should maintain routines so that the child does not equate divorce with instability or loss of normalcy.

Accepting the Permanency of Divorce

The task of acceptance requires the child to accept the reality of the divorce despite tendencies to deny the dissolution of the family and fears of abandonment. These tendencies and fears may persist, leading to repeated efforts by children to persuade their parents to reconcile, even after one or more has remarried. Young school-aged children fantasize about being able to reunite their parents. Parents need to recognize that their children have these fantasies and that they will try to get them to interact with each other in any way and as often as possible. Older children and adolescents, however, who have lived in persistent high-conflict or violent marriages are more likely to be relieved about parental separation and are less likely to wish for parental reunion.[24]

Regaining a Sense of Direction

Immediately after divorce, many children experience emotional and behavioral difficulties, and many seem to lose interest in school, friends, and leisure time activities. Approximately one third of adolescents, particularly boys, in divorced and remarried families separate from the family unit, spend little time at home, and avoid interactions with family members.[4] Generally, the return to more typical activities for the child takes approximately 1 year. If this transition has not occurred within this period, then referral of the child or family for psychotherapy may be indicated. During this time, parents must maintain discipline and avoid allowing their own emotions surrounding the divorce cloud their judgment and authority. If a child is having a particularly difficult time adjusting in one home, parents may then consider a trial of living with the noncustodial parent. Children who are better adjusted before the marital breakup, those who are not enmeshed in a prolonged battle between the parents, and those who are supported in their efforts to understand their feelings are better able to accomplish this task.

Dealing With Painful Feelings

Departure of a parent through divorce is experienced by children of all ages as a major assault on their self-esteem and sense of security. Because of preschoolers' egocentric thinking, they may believe that they are responsible for the divorce, must therefore be bad, and consequently believe that they are at risk for further abandonment by the other parent. Older children, appreciating that the departing parent is exercising a choice to leave, often feel anger, as well as other negative aspects of grief. These feelings result in a complex interplay of negative emotions and their consequences. Parents should explain the situation to the child in simple, age-appropriate language and assure them that they are not the cause of the divorce. Despite parents' best efforts, however, long-term follow-up studies indicate that this important task may never be accomplished by a significant number of individuals who experienced divorce as children.[22]

Not Choosing Sides

Children, especially school-aged children, may see divorce as posing a problem of conflicting loyalties. Parents must consistently reassure children that they are equally loved by both of them and that divorce is not going to change these feelings. Parents should also refrain from buying excessive gifts to prove their affection.

Remaining a Child

Divorce leads to many changes, but one of the most obvious is the physical absence of one parent in the home. Older adolescents often feel responsible for the happiness of their parents and the well being of their younger siblings. They may make attempts to comfort and console their parents. Parents should avoid treating their children as adults. Boys should not be expected to become the man of the house, and girls should not be expected to become the cooks.[12] Children's lives will undergo enough changes without also relinquishing their childhood.

Forgiving the Parents

Forgiving the parents is often a task for older children. Adolescents often struggle with chaos in their own lives and are often angered by having to deal with their parents' lives. Forgiving their parents therefore requires their ability to appreciate the parents' need to separate as being more important than any reason to stay together, including the desires of the children. Children must then overcome grief over the loss of the intact family, as well as the anger and resentment generated by the resulting changes in their life. Parents should be flexible and understanding of the adolescent's need for space, as well as available for comfort and maintenance of discipline.

Resolving Issues of Relationship

Divorce often leaves children fearful and unable "... to reach, sustain, and support the personal vision that love, mutual understanding, and constancy are expectable components of human relationships. Perhaps the major developmental task posed by divorce is this: to achieve realistic hope regarding future relationships and the enduring ability to love and be loved."[3] "At young adulthood, when love, sexual intimacy, commitment and marriage take center stage, children of divorce are haunted by the ghosts of their parent's divorce and are frightened that the same fate awaits them."[16] This task is difficult for a significant number of adults who experienced divorce as children. As children get older, parents should discuss the reasons for the divorce so that the young person learns to view the divorce "not as inevitable but as a result of avoidable human error."[25]

CUSTODY

Chapter 114, Child Custody, contains a detailed discussion of the range of custody arrangements and the pediatrician's role in determining what sorts of arrangements are in the child's best interest. If the noncustodial or nonresidential parent has not abandoned the family and wants to remain involved with the children, then the custodial or residential parent must not attempt to sabotage this relationship.

REMARRIAGE AND STEPFAMILIES

Within 4 years, 50% of divorced adults remarry, and one third of American children will eventually become members of a stepfamily. Over 80% of these stepfamilies are composed of a biological mother and a stepfather.[4] In many cases, it restores a secure, two-parent environment, and it may provide children with a model of a loving, caring adult relationship. Despite the wicked stepmother figure portrayed in fairy tales, most stepchildren like their stepparents and report that they get along with them well. Most studies have shown that stepchildren do not appear to differ from other children in personality characteristics or in cognitive or intellectual accomplishments.[26]

Remarriage does, however, have the potential of creating new tensions and stresses for both the parent and the child. When one parent remarries, the other may fear that the children will abandon the other for the new stepparent. Lutz's interviews of adolescents living in stepfamilies between 12 and 18 years of age revealed that the areas causing the most difficulty are those of divided loyalty and discipline. Many children may feel conflicted about loving their stepparent and may even see it as a source of betrayal of their biological parent. In addition, many children may continue to wish for parental reunion. Regarding discipline, stepparents are often unsure of their roles and may feel awkward in these situations. Discussing these issues with the custodial biological parent and conforming to their approaches is important for stepparents.[27]

Adults can help children adapt better to remarriage. Children adjust better to remarriage with decreased conflict among family members and a supportive residential parent and stepparent. The stepparent should not exert authority immediately but instead be supportive of the residential parent. Social support from peers, grandparents,[19] and school personnel may positively influence the child's adjustment.[28]

Two other factors may play significant roles in the adjustment of children within stepfamilies. First, the child's age is an important aspect to consider in the evaluation. Although a toddler may not fully understand the implications of a stepparent, the school-aged child has been found to be the most vulnerable to the stresses associated with the remarriage. Second, timing is equally important to the overall adjustment.

If the remarriage occurs abruptly or before the child is ready to accept a new parent in the child's life, the stress may be magnified. Unfortunately, the divorce rate of second marriages is still higher than in 1st marriages.[12]

PREVENTIVE INTERVENTIONS FOR DIVORCING FAMILIES

Different interventions have recently been attempted to help alleviate the deleterious effects of divorce on families. Court-connected divorce education programs have been developed to inform parents how children respond to divorce and to help parents respond to the child's needs. Evaluations of these programs are sparse.[11] Mediation of divorce and custody issues promote higher levels of agreement among parents before the court hearing than the adversarial process.[17] Therapy for the mother and child can reduce symptoms of mental disorders; reduce marijuana, alcohol, and other drug use; and reduce sexual promiscuity.[29]

PEDIATRICIAN'S ROLE

The pediatrician can help the family anticipate, prevent, or address problems that frequently accompany divorce by providing anticipatory guidance, counseling for problems as they arise, and assessing and referring children and family members for more extensive or detailed psychosocial intervention when needed. Parents and courts also may ask that pediatricians offer expert witness testimony when custody is questioned.[30]

The 1st year after divorce is often the worst; parents often feel depressed and angry. If the parents are not otherwise receiving counseling, then the pediatrician may offer to meet with one or preferably with both of them to facilitate cooperation regarding child-related issues, such as helping the parents formulate an approach to informing the children about the divorce. Pediatricians need to be the advocate for the child, they should avoid taking sides between parents, and they should be aware that one parent may manipulate the other by using the pediatrician.[14]

Parents should be encouraged to avoid placing the child in the difficult position of which parent to believe or side with when the two most significant adults in their lives have widely differing views. They should also be informed that behind many of their questions, children are asking "Do you still love me, and can I trust you?" Parents should explain the divorce process to children in a developmentally appropriate manner. Also suggested is that parents be *concrete* about the children's future: Where they will live, who will care for them, where the nonresidential parent will live, and how often he or she will visit. Parents should be encouraged to maintain children's routines, including going to school and taking on responsibilities in and outside the home. Parents should maintain consistent discipline strategies.

Both before and after the divorce, children need reassurance that they are not unique as offspring of divorced parents. They may find comfort in discovering that many other children have divorced parents, live in stepfamilies, have the feelings they are having, and that nothing is wrong with feeling this way. They should also be encouraged to ask questions and express feelings, and they should be brought to realize that expending a great amount of energy hoping their parents will be reunited is useless. Visitation with the nonresidential parent may be court mediated. Pediatricians need to be aware of the visitation agreement that is permitted; the pediatrician can then offer guidance about how to make visits more comfortable for the child. Suggestions that can be given to make this visitation easier is to let the child bring a friend along so that the child will not be bored, to set up the child's room as it was in the original home, and to spend time with the child and to avoid expecting the child to fit into the noncustodial parent's new world.

If a child does not wish to visit, then parents should be informed that the child should not be made to feel guilty, and the offer to visit soon should be extended. The nonresidential parent should be counseled to avoid forcing visitation if the child refuses. Persistent refusals to visit the nonresidential parent may suggest that the child is enmeshed in parental difficulties, siding with the residential parent, or that the residential parent may be using the child to hurt the nonresidential parent.

Pediatricians should work with both parents; if abuse by a parent is thought to exist, however, then the appropriate action should be taken. Pediatricians should be knowledgeable about confidentiality laws; sharing medical information with any party during a divorce proceeding requires written permission by both parents or a court order.[31] Pediatricians should maintain an accurate record of the custody arrangements.

Visits for well-child care and for acute illnesses can be used routinely to screen children's adjustment and to assess the need for further counseling by the primary care physician or for referral for individual or family therapy.

TOOLS FOR PRACTICE

Engaging Patients and Family

- *Divorce and Children* (brochure), American Academy of Pediatrics (patiented.aap.org).
- *Marital Problems and Divorce* (fact sheet), American Academy of Pediatrics (www.dbpeds.org/articles/detail.cfm?TextID=280).
- *Divorce and Step-Parenting* (Q&A), American Academy of Pediatrics (www.aap.org/healthopics/divorce.cfm).

AAP POLICY STATEMENTS

American Academy of Pediatrics, Committee on Psychosocial Aspects of Child and Family Health. Helping children and families deal with divorce and separation. *Pediatrics.* 2002;1019-1023. Available at: aappolicy.aappublications.org/cgi/content/full/pediatrics;110/5/1019.

American Academy of Pediatrics, Committee on Psychosocial Aspects of Child and Family Health. The child in court: a subject review. *Pediatrics.* 1999;104(5 pt 1):1145-1184. Available at: aappolicy.aappublications.org/cgi/content/full/pediatrics;104/5/1145.

American Academy of Pediatrics, Committee on Psychosocial Aspects of Child and Family Health. The pediatrician's role in helping children and families deal with separation and divorce. *Pediatrics*. 2005;115(4):1092-1094. Available at: aappolicy.aappublications.org/cgi/content/abstract/pediatrics;94/1/119. Accessed July 7, 2006.

SUGGESTED RESOURCES

Books for children

Brown LK, Brown M. *Dinosaur's Divorce—A Guide for Changing Families*. Boston, MA: Little Brown and Company; 1986.

Girard LW. *At Daddy's on Saturdays*. Morton Grove, IL: Albert Whitman and Company; 1987.

Hazen BS. *Two Homes to Live in—A Child's Eye View of Divorce*. New York, NY: Human Sciences Press, Inc; 1983.

Lansky V. *It's Not Your Fault Koko Bear*. Minnetonka, MN: Publishers Group West; 1998.

Prestine JS. *Mom and Dad Break Up*. Torrance, CA: Fearon Teacher Aids; 1996.

Thomas P. *My Family's Changing*. Hauppauge, NY: Barron's Educational Series, Inc; 1999.

Additional resource recommendation for parents and children

American Academy of Pediatrics, Cohen GJ, and the Committee on Psychosocial Aspects of Child and Family Health. Helping children and families deal with divorce and separation. *Pediatrics*. 2002;110(5):1019-1023.

Useful Web sites

Active Parenting Publishers. Resources for parents and children on Divorce, Loss and Grief [a source for books on divorce for parents]. Available at: www.activeparenting.com/PCloss.htm.

Compassion Books [a source for children's books about divorce]. Available at: www.compassionbooks.com.

Divorcenet. 10 Holiday Tips for Divorced Parents [a source of useful advice about how to handle holidays]. Available at: www.divorcenet.com/states/nationwide/10_holiday_tips_for_divorced_parents/view.

Other recommended reading

Emery R. *Renegotiating Family Relationships: Divorce, Child Custody, and Mediation*. New York, NY: Guilford Press; 1994.

REFERENCES

1. Shiono P, Quinn L. Epidemiology of divorce. *The Future of Children: Children and Divorce*. 1994;4:15-28.
2. Hetherington EM, Stanley-Hagan M. The adjustment of children with divorced parents: a risk and resiliency perspective. *J Child Psychol Psychiatr*. 1999;40:129-140.
3. Wallerstein JS. Children in divorce: stress and developmental tasks. In: Garmezy N, Rutter M, eds. *Stress, Coping and Development in Children*. New York, NY: McGraw-Hill; 1983.
4. Hetherington EM. Divorce and the adjustment of children. *Pediatr in Rev*. 2005;26:163-169.
5. Amato P. Life-span adjustment of children to their parents' divorce. *The Future of Children: Children and Divorce*. 1994; 4:143-164.
6. Amato P, Keith B. Parental divorce and the well-being of children: a meta-analysis. *Psychol Bull*. 1991;110:26-46.
7. Chase-Lansdale P, Cherlin A, Kiernan K. The long-term effects of parental divorce on the mental health of young adults: a developmental perspective. *Child Dev*. 1995;66:1614-1634.
8. Emery R, Forehand R. Parental divorce and children's well-being: a focus on resilience. In: Haggerty RJ, Sherrod LR, Garmezy N, et al, eds. *Risk and Resilience in Children*. London, UK: Cambridge University Press; 1994.
9. Fincham F. Child development and marital relations. *Child Dev*. 1998;69:543-574.
10. Lengua L, Sandler I, West S, et al. Emotionality and self regulation, threat appraisal and coping in children of divorce. *Dev Psychpathol*. 1999;11:15-37.
11. Amato P. Children of divorce in the 1990's: an update of the Amato and Keith 1991 meta-analysis. *J Fam Psychol*. 2001;15:355-370.
12. Bryner C. Children of divorce. *J Am Board Fam Pract*. 2001;14:201-210.
13. Emery R. Laumann-Billings L. Practical and emotional consequences of parental divorce. *Adolesc Med*. 1998;9:271-282.
14. American Academy of Pediatrics, Cohen GJ, and the Committee on Psychosocial Aspects of Child and Family Health. Helping children and families deal with divorce and separation. *Pediatrics*. 2002;110:1019-1023.
15. Kelly J. Children's adjustment in conflicted marriage and divorce: a decade review of research. *J Am Acad Child Adolesc Psychiatry*. 2000;39:963-973.
16. Wallerstein J, Lewis J, Blakeslee S. *The Unexpected Legacy of Divorce: Report of a 25-Year Landmark Study*. New York, NY: Hyperion Press, 2000.
17. Shaw DS, Winslow EB, Flanagan C. A prospective study of the effects of marital status and family relations on young children's adjustment among African American and European American families. *Child Dev*. 1999;70:742-755.
18. O'Connor TG, Thorpe K, Dunn J, et al, and the ALSPAC study team. Parental divorce and adjustment in adulthood: findings from a community sample. *J Child Psychol Psychiatry*. 1999;40:777-789.
19. Lussier G, Deater-Deckard K, Dunn J, et al. Support across two generations: children's closeness to grandparents following parental divorce and remarriage. *J Fam Psychol*. 2002;16:363-376.
20. DeGarmo DS, Forgatch MS, Martinez CR Jr. Parenting of divorced mothers as a link between social status and boys' academic outcomes: unpacking the effects of socioeconomic status. *Child Dev*. 1999;70:1231-1245.
21. Emery R, Coiro M. Divorce: consequences for children. *Pediatr Rev*. 1995;16:306-310.
22. Zill N, Morrison D, Coiro M. Long-term effects of parental divorce on parent-child relationships, adjustment, and achievement in young adulthood. *J Fam Psychol*. 1993;7:91-103.
23. Pruett KD, Pruett MK. "Only God decides": young children's perceptions of divorce and the legal system. *J Am Acad Child Adolesc Psychiatry*. 1999;38:1544-1550.
24. Kelly J. Marital conflict, divorce and children's adjustment. *Child and Adolesc Psychol Clin North Am*. 1998;7:259.
25. Wallerstein JS, Blakeslee S. *What About the Kids? Raising your Children Before, During and After Divorce*. New York, NY: Hyperion; 2003.
26. Dubowitz H, Newberger CM, Melnicoe LH, et al. The changing American family. *Pediatr Clin North Am*. 1988;35:1291-1311.
27. Lutz P. The step-family: an adolescent perspective. *Fam Relat*. 1983;32:367.
28. Isaacs A. Children's adjustments to their divorced parents' new relationships. *J Paediatr Child Health*. 2002;38:329-331.
29. Wolchik SA, Sandler IN, Millsap RE, et al. Six-year follow-up of a preventive interventions for children of divorce: a randomized controlled trial. *JAMA*. 2002;288:1874-1881.

30. Emery R. *Renegotiating Family Relationships: Divorce, Child Custody, and Mediation*. New York, NY: Guilford Press; 1994.
31. Committee on Psychosocial Aspects of Child and Family Health. The child in court: a subject review. *Pediatrics*. 1999;104:1145-1148.

Chapter 116

CHILDREN IN FOSTER AND KINSHIP CARE

Moira Szilagyi, MD, PhD; Sandra H. Jee, MD, MPH

In an ideal world, every child would be reared by nurturing and caring birth parents. Many children and adolescents, however, cannot reside with their birth families for reasons of health and safety, and they require care in other settings. Every year, approximately 3.3 million reports involving 6 million children are made to child protective services, resulting in 899,000 founded investigations. In 2005 this incidence resulted in 317,000 children being removed from their families for child maltreatment as a result of investigation into allegations of child abuse and neglect.[1] Adolescents frequently enter out-of-home care because of parental inability to cope with their behavioral or emotional issues, although abuse and neglect often precede removal. When children or adolescents are removed from their family of origin by child welfare services, they may be placed in either foster or kinship care. In most states, kinship care remains a less-formal arrangement, in which a child is cared for by extended family, neighbors, or friends, frequently without child welfare services oversight. Foster and kinship care are intended to be temporary respites for a family in crisis, and most of what is discussed in this chapter relates to children and adolescents in foster and kinship care.

In the United States, as of September 30, 2005, approximately 513,000 children and adolescents resided in foster care, with approximately 30% in care with extended family members.[2] Furthermore, estimates suggest that approximately four times as many children and teens live in informal, unregulated kinship care.[3,4] These children are, by and large, the children of the indigent, and 70% have a documented history of child abuse, neglect, or both. Over 80% have been exposed to high levels of violence in their homes or communities, with over 40% living in homes with active domestic violence at the time of removal.[5,6] Close to one half (48%) have a caregiver with a significant mental health impairment, and rates of parental substance and alcohol abuse are enormous, ranging up to 80% for the youngest children.[7] These children have often had multiple caregivers even before removal and have not experienced the typical, predictable, responsive parenting that fosters well being.[8] Removal from their family of origin and all that is familiar is traumatic for almost all children. Placement in foster or kinship care is intended to nurture and heal children while facilitating the rehabilitation of their families. In reality, foster care has become a system of last resort for the most vulnerable children and challenging families.

The foster care system is in crisis. The system is burdened by huge caseloads, families with multiple intractable problems, lack of funding, and complex and often conflicting bureaucratic, legal, and ethical demands. The system is also in transition since passage of the Adoption and Safe Families Act in 1997,[9] shifting the emphasis in foster care from parental rights toward the best interests of the child, with the goal of reunification now offset by the need to transition a child into an appropriate, permanent family setting in a timely manner. A secondary goal remains the rehabilitation of parents and reunification of families when goals of health and safety can be met. Approximately 58% of children in foster care are reunited with their families, whereas 18% are adopted, 18% *age out* of foster care, and the remaining are transferred to the care of other agencies.[2] Children in kinship homes achieve permanency in these placements at a higher rate than those in foster care, although an unknown percentage of kinship homes are disrupted, leading to subsequent foster care placement.[3,4] Of adolescents who are transferred to other agencies from foster care, some are intellectually disabled youth for whom the state retains guardianship in adulthood, whereas others run away or end up in the criminal justice system.

Most pediatric practitioners will encounter children and adolescents in foster or kinship care during the course of their practice; thus familiarity with the effect of child abuse and neglect, removal, and placement in foster or kinship care on children, adolescents, and their families is important.

HISTORY OF THE FOSTER CARE SYSTEM

The foster care system is a 20th-century institution rooted in England's Elizabethan Poor Laws of 1601. Foster care evolved out of the dedicated efforts of many individuals to improve the lot of destitute and abandoned children. Designed to protect children previously left to their own resources, the charity of the community, or warehoused in institutions, foster care is rooted in the belief that society has a responsibility for such children and that children fare best when they are reared in nurturing family-based settings.[10]

Government funding and regulation of the foster care system in the United States is relatively recent. As part of the Social Security Act of 1935, Aid to Dependent Children provided economic support to widowed parents left with young children. Beginning in the 1960s, amendment of Title IV-A of the Social Security Act allowed states to use federal matching funds to support children placed in foster care whose parents qualified for public assistance. With the increased public awareness of child abuse dating from the 1960s the population of children in foster care expanded rapidly over the next several decades because of increased admissions and long lengths of stay. The recognition that separating children from their families only to leave them lingering in foster care without permanency was harmful to children, coupled with burgeoning costs of the foster care system, led to several attempts at reform. In 1980 the Adoption Assistance and Child Welfare Act (PL-96-272)[11] mandated states to provide preventive services (eg, counseling, child care, parenting education, drug rehabilitation) to avert the removal of children from their birth families. Agencies were also mandated to conduct semiannual case reviews and to develop permanency plans within 18 months of placement. Adoption subsidies were funded so that a marginal family income would be less of a barrier to the adoption of children out of foster care.

After enactment of PL-96-272 the size of the foster care population transiently declined. Unfortunately, the cocaine epidemic in the inner cities led to a dramatic increase in the number of very young children in foster care in the late 1980s and early 1990s, offsetting the effects of earlier reforms. The Adoption and Safe Families Act (ASFA) of 1997[10] was meant to address several issues. The focus on parental rights and reunification placed some children at considerable risk of injury, neglect, or prolonged stays in foster care. ASFA shifted the emphasis in child welfare toward the health and safety of the child and timely permanency planning. States are now obligated to pursue termination of parental rights for any child who has been in foster care for 15 of the prior 22 months, unless a compelling reason exists, such as impending reunification, not to. Under ASFA, adoption subsidies were further enhanced, leading to a surge in adoptions in many states in the late 1990s and the early years of this century.

Other important trends in foster care include the increased emphasis on assessing extended family and *kin* as potential placement resources for a child when removal is necessary, leading to a dramatic increase (300%) in kinship care placements in the last decade.[3,4] Given that many removals are urgent, increasing numbers of children are entering foster care for very short stays while child welfare identifies and investigates kinship resources. Parental methamphetamine abuse has become an increasingly important reason for removing children, especially in rural areas.[11] Finally, the Chafee Foster Care Independence Act of 1999 allowed states the option of extending certain benefits, such as Medicaid, to youth aging out of foster care until they turned 21 years of age. Many states have taken advantage of this option to enhance their independent living programs, providing some resources to this vulnerable population of youth.

RISK FACTORS FOR PLACEMENT

Families whose children reside in foster care are, in general, impoverished and living on the fringes of society, with few social supports. Children and adolescents are removed from their family of origin when imminent risk exists to the health and safety of the child. Although child abuse and neglect account for 70% of removals, children and teens entering out-of-home care have commonly experienced a multiplicity of adversities. Child neglect, including neglect of basic nutritional needs, educational and medical neglect, and lack of supervision, is the most commonly cited reason for placement.[12] Reports of child physical abuse and sexual abuse have declined in the last decade[13] but, along with abandonment, remain reasons for placement.[1,13] Many children, however, experience multiple forms of abuse and neglect. Although child abuse and neglect occur in all sociodemographic groups, young people placed in foster care come from the most economically deprived segments of society; thus extreme poverty remains the pervasive common factor underlying foster care placement. Parental mental illness, substance abuse, active domestic violence, and criminal activity permeate the environments in which children have lived before removal. More than 80% of young children entering foster care have a parent who abuses drugs, alcohol, or both.[6] Many children come from homes and neighborhoods in which drug sales and the presence of drug paraphernalia are common. National data indicate that 48% of parents have a mental illness, and 10% are cognitively impaired.[13] Before foster care, 44% of children were living in homes with active domestic violence, and 84% experienced significant levels of violence in their homes, schools, or neighborhoods.[6] In one national dataset, child protective caseworkers identified 80% of birth parents as having significantly impaired parenting skills at the time of the child protective investigation.[13] Other social stressors in these families include single parenthood and lack of education and unemployment. Approximately one third of birth parents admit to being abused or neglected as children, and approximately the same number spent time in foster care. Removal of a child often occurs after prolonged involvement with social service agencies, including child protective services, after preventive strategies have been exhausted, and the child's health and safety are at imminent risk.

Admission to foster care is and should be difficult. Almost all children entering foster care are placed involuntarily by court order, either for reasons of child abuse and neglect (approximately 70%) or by the juvenile justice system as person in need of supervision (PINS) or juvenile delinquent placements (27%). Fewer than 1% are placed voluntarily by families who are temporarily unable to care for them.[2] Many voluntary placements are by families who have exhausted other options and opt for placement as a means of accessing residential treatment services for a child or teen with severe mental health issues. In rare instances, parents who are unable to cope may opt to place a child with catastrophic medical illness. Infants and children with multiple-handicapping chronic health conditions resulting from extreme prematurity, genetic disorders or syndromes, chronic illness, or trauma are overrepresented in foster care. The numbers of HIV-infected infants entering foster care have declined dramatically since the mid-1990s, mostly because of improved perinatal interventions and longer survival of their infected parent.

Although the genders are fairly equally represented in foster care, the preponderance of children of black and mixed racial heritage in out-of-home care is dramatic, reflecting, in part, their numbers in the poorer segments of this society. However, concern exists that the overrepresentation of minority children in foster care reflects overselection in investigation and removal.[14] Unaccompanied refugee minors, especially from Africa and Haiti, represent a very small proportion of the total foster care population.

FOSTER CARE SYSTEM

The foster care system, simple in its conception of providing needy children with nurturing families, is, in fact, a complex bureaucracy. Federal legislation determines patterns of funding and regulatory guidelines, but responsibility for the structure and implementation of foster care programs resides with state social service agencies, which may delegate daily management to county or private child welfare agencies.

Role of Caseworkers

Each child welfare agency retains the responsibility for hiring and training caseworkers and foster families. Child welfare casework is a demanding job, requiring multiple skills. Although the professional demands of casework are more commensurate with masters'-level social work skills, casework positions are entry-level jobs in most child welfare agencies, requiring no more than 2 years of college education. As advocates for the biological family, caseworkers must engage the parent around the care of their child while undertaking a *diligent effort* to rehabilitate the parent or parents, ensuring the accessibility of whatever educational or service resources are necessary (eg, housing, counseling, medical care, drug and alcohol rehabilitation) for reunification. Meanwhile, they must also coordinate educational, developmental, medical, and mental health services for children and teens in their care. When birth parents are noncompliant or unable to undertake the work necessary for reunification, caseworkers have the delicate task of supporting them through the process of developing an alternate permanency plan and enabling the child to develop secure attachments and a sense of belonging in a different family than the family of origin. Caseworkers also recruit, train, monitor, annually recertify, and investigate minor complaints about foster homes.

Caseworkers must also develop a working familiarity with the legal system in their state, particularly the family court and the juvenile justice systems. Within 72 hours the caseworker must prepare a petition for the court documenting the reasons for removal. Many children are returned within this time frame if the court finds insufficient basis for the removal. When the child or adolescent remains in foster care the caseworker must return to court at intervals to provide ongoing documentation for the continuation of placement and to detail their own efforts at rehabilitation of parents, reunification, and alternate permanency planning.

Other Child Advocates

Every child in foster care is represented in court by a law guardian (guardian ad litem), who may or may not be an attorney, depending on the state. In some states the court may also designate a court-appointed special advocate (CASA) worker to advocate on behalf of the child in particularly difficult cases. As trained volunteers who are not attorneys, CASA workers devote many hours to investigating the child's circumstances for presentation to the court. Most children in foster care, however, do not have such a designated advocate, except for the caseworker, who is more accurately regarded as the case manager for the entire family.

Termination of Parental Rights

Legally, parents retain guardianship of their children who are residing in *the care and custody* of the state or county commissioner of social services. Guardianship can only be terminated as part of a legal process, in which the commissioner then becomes the child's legal guardian until the child either reaches the age of majority or is adopted. Parents sometimes choose to surrender their children for adoption, but more often, termination of parental rights (TPR) occurs involuntarily after all efforts at reunification have failed. The TPR process can take years, during which time concurrent, but conflicting, efforts at reunification and alternative permanency planning occur. The time constraints imposed by ASFA legislation on beginning the TPR process and the increased focus on the child's health and safety were intended to shorten the time between placement and TPR (and thus adoption) for children for whom reunification is not an option.

CHILDREN IN FOSTER CARE

Entry into foster care is fraught with uncertainty, upheaval, and losses. The family, no matter how dysfunctional, is the center of the child's world. The child or adolescent is removed from all that is familiar. Removal, even though required for the child's health and safety, is an emotionally traumatizing experience for all children except the youngest infants and should be treated accordingly.[8,15,16]

Agencies may first place children in a shelter, an emergency foster home, or home of a relative, pending the availability of a traditional foster home. Most foster parents are kind and welcoming but are unfamiliar to the child. Placement with kin caregivers can be less traumatic if the child already has a meaningful relationship with them. Within the first few days the child meets a variety of strangers, from child protective service personnel and foster care caseworkers to police officers, physicians, and members of the foster home. Little privacy is afforded, and most children, grieving the loss of their home and families, are uncertain when they will see them again, are afraid to ask questions, and feel alone and isolated. Children are often wary for the first several weeks, the poorly termed *honeymoon period*, viewed by most child welfare professionals as a time of emotional withdrawal for the overwhelmed and confused child. However, as children and teens adjust to their new environments, some of them begin to act out their anger, frustration, and sadness. Children sometimes act out, thinking that if they are bad enough, then they will be returned to their parents; others believe that they will prove to the new parent that they are not worthy of their affection and care. The majority of children, however, may simply be overwhelmed by feelings they do not understand and cannot control.

Children removed from their families spend varying lengths of time in foster care. Although many children (approximately 50%) cycle through foster care in weeks to months,[2] approximately 10% to 20% remain in the system for years—as their families repeatedly fail to meet the goals set for reunification—and resist other permanency options. The largest determinant of length of stay is the biological family's level of cooperation with the individualized case plan for their child or children, although reports indicate that minorities, older children, and children with developmental disabilities are almost twice as likely to remain in care.[17] The average length of stay in the foster care system has declined from its high of just over 5 years to approximately 2.5 years, attributed in part to increased efforts at reunification, greater dependence on relatives as resources, and more intensive permanency planning.[2,17] Select children who remain in foster care for a long time are likely to have behavioral or mental health problems or have complex medical needs, reducing the likelihood of their adoption.

Longer stays in foster care are associated with a reduced likelihood of reunification and an increased number of placements. Changes in foster care placement are almost always traumatic for children,[18] given that each transition involves a loss that reinforces feelings of rejection and worthlessness. Approximately 50% of children and teens will experience more than one foster care placement, with approximately 25% having three or more placements. Reasons for disrupted placements vary; however, most frequently, a child's behavior problems are beyond the skills of a particular foster parent or deteriorate to the point at which the child needs a higher level of care. Stable foster care is associated with improved outcomes.[17,18] Less often, foster parents may retire, become ill or die, feel threatened by the birth parent, or move out of a child's location of residence. Approximately 20% of all foster homes close each year, with approximately one half of this number closed by child welfare agencies for inadequate care.

Uncertainty, powerlessness and guilt pervade the life of the child in foster care. Children in foster care often deny awareness of the reason for placement, and younger children may blame themselves for the disruption of their families. Children do not know how long they will be in care, whether their parent will arrive for visits, or when their parent will get out of jail or rehabilitation. Most children worry about the well being of their parents and siblings. Birth parents may make promises they do not or cannot keep. Children are sometimes discharged from foster care or transitioned between placements without preparation. Other children tease them about being in foster care, contributing to their already-poor self-regard and sense of alienation. Younger children and infants quickly form attachments to foster parents and may view their seldom-seen birth parent as a stranger. Differences in parenting style, as well as outright conflict between birth parents and current caregivers, creates confusion for children and teens.

ADOLESCENTS IN FOSTER CARE

Adolescents in foster care are a varied group; most enter foster care through juvenile detention or PINS or when a parent who is unable to afford appropriate mental health care places their teen in foster care. Some adolescents have grown up in foster care, and this group is likely to have experienced a variety of foster care settings over time. Some members of this group are intellectually disabled or developmentally delayed, with significant behavior issues. They may have lingered in care because a suitable adoptive home was never identified. Pregnant or parenting teens are another small group who may be living with their children in foster care or placed separately if they have significant mental health issues or constitute a risk to their offspring. A small group enters foster care as emancipated refugee minors, having immigrated to the United States from a variety of war-torn countries after surviving war, rape, injury, or the death of their families. Most emancipated refugee minor teens are now arriving from various regions of Africa and Haiti.

The majority of adolescents in foster care reside in group-home or residential treatment facilities where their activities are restricted, education is structured, and they receive mental health services and substance-abuse treatment, if needed. However, many teens also reside in foster families. In general, adolescents in foster care have had similar adverse life experiences as younger children entering foster care but have also experienced many transitions and engaged in high-risk behaviors, including substance abuse, sexual activity, school truancy, and petty criminal mischief.

Adolescents in foster care are less likely to be adopted than younger children. When they do leave foster care, they do so to return home or because they *age out* at age 18 years (several states allow teens who are in school or job training to remain in foster care until age 21 years), run away, or are moved to another agency or placement setting (residential care or group home care, jail, or inpatient mental health or drug and alcohol treatment). Foster care caseworkers are charged with preparing adolescents who are aging out of care for independent living by offering them education regarding finances, job training, and health insurance. However, resources for this approach are limited, transitional services are few, and youth aging out of care often find their way back to their family of origin if they have no sense of belonging elsewhere. Foster or kin families who remain invested in youth are their best resource.

Little is known about the outcomes of youth who have aged out, and what *is* known is discouraging. Young adults who are a decade removed from foster care are underemployed, undereducated, have difficulty with trust in intimate relationships, and blame the child welfare system for the disruption of their families. In prevalence studies, adults with a history of foster care are overrepresented among the homeless and the incarcerated.[18,19]

Adolescence is the time during which the individual is supposed to form a stable identity rooted in self-esteem, a sense of autonomy rooted in self-efficacy, and a larger sense of commitment and comfort in relatedness to peers. For young people in foster care, especially minority youth, negative self-concept, lack of self-esteem, and a lack of self-efficacy are likely outcomes because of early adverse experiences, the accrual of multiple losses over time, and a sense of helpless dependence developed from living in the uncertain world of foster care. Early abuse and neglect coupled with impaired caregiving, repeated separation and losses, unpredictability, and a lack of role models for healthy relationships result in young adults who are isolated, alienated, dependent, and prone to distrust.

VISITATION

For the child who remains in foster care, even in a stable placement, major issues need to be addressed. Although consistent visitation with the biological family is the best predictor of reunification, visits are laden with difficulty for the child. The tenor of the parent-child relationship is variable. Children who have been abused or severely neglected by their parents may not feel safe even in a supervised visitation setting. Birth parents may attempt to sabotage the relationship of the child with their current caregivers, and vice versa. Parents may visit inconsistently, which is confusing and frightening for children. When the parent does come, the visit ends with the child reliving the initial separation from their parent. When the parent fails to show, feelings of rejection and abandonment are reinforced.

Visitation usually progresses through stages, beginning with visits supervised by caseworkers in a neutral setting. Visits then transition to the parent's home, where they may be monitored before eventually becoming unsupervised. Kinship placement may allow for more frequent contact with the birth parent, but kin caregivers may also be in a particularly difficult situation regarding visitation if they harbor resentment toward the birth parent or are conflicted about visitation.

FOSTER FAMILIES

Foster families are the unsung heroes of the foster care system. Most of these families are warm, caring, dedicated individuals who open their homes to society's most fragile and needy children, taking them into their own families and nurturing them through multiple crises. Although foster parents vary in the skills they bring to caring for children, they are generally motivated by religious conviction, altruism, or personal need. They tend to be *child centered,* often having raised children of their own, and see foster care as a mission because of their love for children. Some families become foster parents as a path to adoption, although a guarantee that a child placed with them will become eligible for adoption seldom exists. Foster parents are usually married, have a middle or lower-middle income, come from tradition-rich backgrounds, are deeply religious, and have a fairly open definition of whom constitutes family. A very small percentage of foster parents are same-sex couples. In some states, laws allow same-sex couples to foster but not adopt. Approximately 5% of foster families have specialized training or skills and act as resources for severely emotionally disturbed or medically fragile children. Many states now have designated skilled homes that provide care for children with HIV infection or other complex medical problems.

Reimbursement for foster parenting varies widely. Families are paid a daily *board rate* for each child in their care. The rate, set by individual states, is determined by the child's age, health needs, and the complexity of the parenting tasks. Average monthly board rates for uncomplicated children hover around approximately $300 per month and are expected to cover food, shelter, personal needs, recreation, and most transportation and educational costs. A recent study shows that board subsidies cover about two-thirds of the cost of caring for a child and that most foster parents "chip in" their own funds.[20] Many agencies reimburse for some transportation (involving medical or mental health visits) and pay an additional stipend for clothing. The highest foster family board reimbursements are for children with extremely complex medical conditions or severe behavioral and emotional issues and may exceed $1000 per month in foster family care. Approximately 20% of children in foster care, mostly adolescents, reside in residential or group home placements, the most costly form of care, which can cost upwards of $90,000 per child annually.

Recruitment, adequate training, and retention of suitable foster families are some of the most compelling tasks facing child welfare agencies. Agencies provide potential foster parents with education in the areas of child development, child abuse and neglect, behavior problems, discipline, safety issues, and their roles in relation to the agency and birth families, but the training is minimal. Certification does not occur until the agency has conducted a home visit and a criminal background check and a review of the state's child abuse registry. Agencies lack adequate staff to scrutinize foster homes carefully, and annual recertification is less rigorous than the original certification process.

Boundaries are blurred in the foster care system in terms of authority, responsibility, and accountability. Foster families retain the bulk of the daily responsibility for children and teens but are accountable to caseworkers, the legal system, and the birth family for the child's care. Foster parents may feel excluded from planning on the child's behalf, given that birth parents retain legal custody, and child welfare agencies have authority to make decisions on behalf of the child and generate permanency plans, and courts make placement decisions. However powerless, foster families remain the individual child's strongest advocate.

Foster parents often have only limited information about children in their care. Placement in a foster home is often regarded as the only necessary therapeutic intervention a child needs, and agencies vary widely in the amount of guidance and services they provide to foster parents and children in their care. Foster families may be overwhelmed, and placements may fail when foster families feel isolated in dealing with a child's complex behavioral and emotional problems. Because of foster home shortages in many areas, particularly large urban centers, most homes maintain the maximum number of children allowed under regulations, further stressing a family's emotional resources.

Foster families, like children in foster care, experience multiple separations and losses as children enter and then leave their homes, often for a living situation that the foster parent deems unsuitable. Relationships with birth families range from adversarial to mutually supportive. Foster parents often bear the brunt of a child's anger over a failed visit or a parent's telephone call, or they may be unjustly accused of neglect or abuse by an angry birth parent. They may feel scrutinized, but simultaneously unsupported, by child welfare staff.

However, the foster family is the entity to which the system turns for adoption when reunification is no longer considered an option. Over 60% of children adopted out of foster care are adopted by their foster parents.[2] Long-term foster care placement is no longer an option under ASFA, although some foster families make a long-term commitment to one or several of the 110,000 children and teens who have been freed for adoption but for whom belonging in a *forever family* remains an elusive goal.

KINSHIP CARE

In the last decade, the numbers of children placed in kinship care increased dramatically (over 300%). Unofficial placement with kin caregivers is more common than *relative resource care,* defined as care provided by a relative who has become certified as a foster parent. Although driven by a commitment to maintaining a child within their family of origin, kinship care providers have often made this choice under some duress and with recognition that a member of their own family, who is often their adult child, has neglected or abused the child. They are often older, poorer, and have access to fewer resources than foster caregivers. Unless they have become certified foster parents, they are not subject to the same review or oversight as foster caregivers, nor do they have access to the same supports.

Placement with a relative, however, offers significant advantages to children, the most obvious of which is that it maintains their ties with their larger family of origin, their community, and their culture.[3,4] A few studies have also shown that kinship care is associated with fewer placement disruptions and, in one study, a reduced incidence of abuse or neglect, when compared with placement with a nonrelative provider. Relative caregivers with marginal income have the option of applying for foster care certification in many states, making them eligible for foster care stipends, but with all the oversight of foster care.

BIRTH FAMILIES

Removal of a child is a traumatic event for the birth parent. For some of these parents the shock of the removal is sufficient to precipitate cooperation with child welfare and family court and improved parenting behaviors, resulting in speedy reunification. Approximately one half of children in foster care are returned to their birth families within the first 6 months. For other families, even the removal of a child does not alter ingrained patterns of substance abuse, violence, and child neglect.

Parents, while battling addiction, mental illness, and poverty, often have to contend with feelings of guilt, powerlessness, inadequacy, anger, frustration, and resentment when children are removed. Even though they retain legal custody, their contact with their children is constrained, with only several hours of supervised visitation per week initially. Parents may fail to show for visitation, whether because of substance use, mental illness, guilt, the pain of separation, fear of confronting their child or children, or barriers such as transportation.

Although one of the goals of the foster care system is reunification, and although caseworkers are mandated to provide a range of services supporting this goal, some birth parents become locked in an adversarial relationship with child welfare staff, resentfully refusing all help offered. In the past, some parents effectively abandoned their children to the system, maintaining contact just sufficient to prevent termination of their rights. Many of these same parents refused to surrender their children for adoption, even when reunification was clearly not an option. ASFA legislation has made the TPR process easier in such situations. This legislation also reinforces the concept of open adoptions, believed to benefit the child by providing some ongoing limited supervised contact with the family of origin.

DEVELOPMENTAL AND EDUCATIONAL ISSUES

Multiple studies have shown that approximately 60% of young children entering foster care have developmental delays, especially in the areas of language, social, and self-help skills, although they have been shown to benefit from placement in a nurturing foster home and early intervention services.[20] Before foster care placement, children and teens have experienced high rates of absenteeism, suspension, school failure, grade retention, and multiple school transitions.[22] Children and youth in foster care are an educationally vulnerable population who continue to perform below grade level (75%), perform poorly on standardized testing, and exhibit significant behavior issues.[22] Forty-four percent of children and youth in foster care are in special education settings, one half for behavioral concerns. Stable placement in foster care has been shown to result in predictable school attendance for the first time and is often accompanied by improved academic performance for younger children.[4] A national study of 20,000 young adults who had aged out of foster care in 1998 showed that only 35% graduated from high school, and only 11% went on to college or vocational school; 37% of foster teens in another study dropped out of high school.[21] Of seniors in high school who were also in foster care, 65% said that a parent or guardian had never attended a parent-teacher conference. Teens in foster care are as likely to drop out or attain a general education degree as to graduate from high school.[21]

OUTCOMES FOR CHILDREN IN FOSTER CARE

Ultimately, almost 60% of children are reunified with their parents, and another 11% return to a relative. An overall 20% recidivism (return to foster care) rate exists in the first year after reunification; recidivism approaches 30% for infants.[2]

Approximately 18% of children in foster care are eventually adopted, usually by their foster parent or parents or by a member of their extended family.[2] Almost all adoptions out of foster care involve some subsidy, reflecting the child's physical health, mental health, and developmental needs. Many children also retain their Medicaid insurance, although this retention depends on laws in individual states. Adoption subsidy, once granted, continues until the child reaches 18 years of age.

Of the 113,000 children and teens currently residing in foster care who are free for adoption, only one half of them have an adoptive home identified. Persons who are waiting for adoptive homes are mostly adolescents, children considered difficult to adopt by virtue of their significant medical or behavioral problems, older minority children, or those who are part of large sibling groups. Studies indicate that even older adolescents in foster care continue to dream of the permanency and sense of belonging to a family that adoption means for them.

Approximately 20,000 children per year age out of foster care's independent living programs[2]; many leave the system without any permanent family resources, whereas others maintain some contact with their families of origin or their foster families. Most adolescents age out at 18 years of age, although a few states allow adolescents to remain in care until 21 years of age. A small percentage (3% of adolescents) are lost to care through elopement, and a similar number become involved with the criminal justice system or are placed in long-term residential care.

TERMINATION OF PARENTAL RIGHTS

For children whose families will never be able to resume their care, the TPR process can create significant conflict. Termination of rights severs the child's legal ties to the birth family, but not their emotional ones, and the child may be torn between conflicting loyalties to birth and adoptive families. If the parent surrenders the child, then the child may view this action as the ultimate rejection. Behavior problems often escalate around the time when children are freed for adoption, whether voluntarily or involuntarily, and when the adoption process is begun in earnest.

HEALTH CARE ISSUES AND RECOMMENDATIONS FOR CHILDREN IN FOSTER AND KINSHIP CARE

Children in foster care represent a highly vulnerable, medically complex population, suffering high rates of chronic medical illness, developmental disabilities, educational disorders, and behavioral, emotional, and mental health problems (Table 116-1). All children in foster care should be considered as *children with special health care needs.* In general, for older children and adolescents, these conditions predate placement. Prenatal drug exposure, poor maternal nutrition, and poor prenatal care lead to an increased incidence of premature and small-for-gestational-age infants. Postnatally, psychosocial deprivation, poor nutrition, and failure to attend to the child's health and developmental needs exacerbate problems. Limited use of preventive health services, fragmentation of health care, and underimmunization are typical of children entering foster care, and 70% have a history of physical abuse, neglect, sexual abuse, or any combination. Children enter foster care with a history of complex trauma and chronic stress that affects their physical, emotional, and developmental well being.[16]

Studies of the health status of the foster care population have yielded fairly bleak results. Approximately 45% have at least one chronic medical condition, with approximately one quarter of all children in care having three or more chronic problems.[22-24] The most commonly encountered diagnoses are listed in Table 116-2.[22] Respiratory problems affect approximately 18% of children in foster care, with asthma being the most commonly encountered diagnosis (15%); the high prevalence is attributed partially to a higher incidence of premature birth and attendant lung disease and partially to the concentration of the foster care population in urban settings. Approximately 10% of children in foster care have short stature, with an additional 6% to 10% of infants and toddlers meeting criteria for failure to thrive. At the other extreme, approximately 15% of children in foster care meet the criteria for obesity. Hematologic disorders, mostly attributable to anemia, are present in approximately 20% of children. Dermatologic diagnoses are commonly noted, especially atopic dermatitis. Burn scars or scars from physical abuse are encountered commonly (10% to 15% of children younger than 12 years). Visual and hearing impairment, recurrent otitis media, gastroesophageal reflux, neurologic disorders

Table 116-1 Prevalence of Health Conditions for Children in Foster Care

CONDITION	FOSTER CARE (%)
Chronic medical	35-60%
Mental health	48-80%
Developmental delay	60% children <5 yr
Educational issues	45% in special education
Dental concerns	35% significant dental needs

Table 116-2 Common Medical Diagnoses for Children in Foster Care in Oakland, California

DIAGNOSIS	PERCENTAGE OF CHILDREN IN FOSTER CARE
Growth failure	43%
Height under the 5th percentile	23%
Weight under the 5th percentile	15%
Head circumference under the 5th percentile	19%
Failure to thrive	9%
Infections, parasites	17%
Recurrent otitis media	10%
Congenital infections	8%
Hematologic, anemia	20%
Neurologic	30%
Respiratory	18%
Asthma	16%
Gastroesophageal	15%
Gastroesophageal reflux	6%
Encopresis	3%
Genitourinary	10%
Enuresis	7%
Dermatologic	23%
Congenital anomaly	8%

From Halfon N, Mendonca A, Berkowitz G. Health status of children in foster care: the experience of the Center for the Vulnerable Child. *Arch Pediatr Adolesc Med.* 1995;149:386-392. Reprinted by permission of the American Medical Association.

(varying from mild motor delay to seizures and cerebral palsy), and congenital anomalies are more prevalent than in the general pediatric population. Sexually transmitted infections and other infectious diseases are also commonly encountered. Approximately 8% of children in foster care are high-cost patients because they are technology dependent, multiply handicapped, or heavy users of ancillary services.

Once children enter foster care, their overall health does not appear to improve. The transient nature of the population dramatically increases the likelihood that they will continue to have poor access to health care, and this access will be fragmented. Health information on admission is almost universally lacking, and identifying who previously provided medical care is a cumbersome and often fruitless task. Neither caseworkers nor foster parents have the level of knowledge necessary to serve as the health care manager, yet the system relies on them to perform this complex task. Inadequate health care management underlies the pattern of inadequate, fragmented, and, occasionally, redundant care received. Medicaid limits access to health care because of inadequate financing, delays in payment, and limited numbers of medical subspecialists willing to accept it. Medicaid-managed care may increase access to medical subspecialists, but it significantly reduces mental health access for these children who often have immense mental health needs. Complex consent and confidentiality issues limit access, delay evaluations and treatment, and confound communication among professionals. Failure to support and educate foster parents about a child's medical, developmental, and mental health needs and failure to secure appropriate treatment can lead to disruptions in placement, when foster parents are overwhelmed. The pediatric practitioner has the opportunity to improve outcomes for children in foster care by working with agencies as a health care consultant around health care management issues or by providing a *medical home* for children and teens in foster care (Box 116-1).

BOX 116-1 Guidelines for Health Care for Children Entering Foster or Kinship Care

Children entering foster care should have an admission health evaluation, which includes:

1. Health screen within 72 hours of placement to assess and document:
   - Symptoms or signs of child abuse and neglect, with referral as needed
   - Growth parameters
   - Symptoms or signs of acute illness
   - Symptoms or signs of chronic illness
   - Developmental screening results and referral for evaluation
   - Behavioral and mental health screening results (focusing on suicidal or homicidal ideation or intent, history of aggressive behaviors) and referral for evaluation
   - Appropriate referral for emergent health issues or sexual abuse evaluation
   - Appropriate treatment of identified issues
   - Health education of foster or kinship caregiver
2. Health information gathering: an ongoing process that begins at admission to foster care
3. Comprehensive health evaluation within 30 days of placement to:
   - Review all available health history
   - Address health concerns
   - Assess adjustment to foster or kinship care, child care, school, and visitation
   - Address behavior concerns and daily schedule
   - Assess growth parameters
   - Review systems
   - Perform a developmental or educational evaluation, or review of evaluation, or referral for evaluation if not previously completed
   - Perform a mental health evaluation or review of evaluation or referral for evaluation if not previously completed
   - Perform a complete physical examination
   - Screen for signs and symptoms of child abuse and neglect
   - Undertake all recommended screening tests (hearing, vision, lead, complete blood count and differential, purified protein derivative, rapid plasma reagin, hepatitis B and C, and HIV)
   - Administer immunizations (consider catch-up immunizations if no history is available)
   - Provide age-appropriate anticipatory guidance, focusing on transition issues
   - Provide appropriate or indicated treatment and referrals, including dental treatment
   - Provide communication in writing of health plan to foster care agency
4. Follow-up admission assessment within 90 days of placement to:
   - Review all available health history, including results of mental health assessment, developmental and educational evaluations, and dental assessment
   - Address interval concerns
   - Document growth parameters
   - Assess adjustment to foster care, child care, school, and visitation
   - Conduct behavioral screening
   - Conduct developmental screening and review
   - Perform a focused physical examination
   - Screen for child abuse and neglect
   - Administer immunizations as indicated
   - Ensure that all referrals and recommended treatments are in process or have been completed
   - Schedule or plan next visit

OPTIMIZING HEALTH CARE FOR CHILDREN IN FOSTER CARE

Standards for health care of children in out-of-home care were published by the Child Welfare League of America and the American Academy of Pediatrics in 1988.[25] Unfortunately, many states have only broad guidelines governing the provision of health services to children in foster care, and multiple barriers exist (including inadequate funding, insufficient caseworker and foster family knowledge, limited understanding of the foster care experience by health professionals, blurred boundaries over who has responsibility of health care management for this complex population) to translating these guidelines into accessible, effective, and efficient health care (Box 116-2). Recently, District II (New York State) of the American Academy of Pediatrics published a more detailed set of standards, which more clearly defines the parameters for health care for this complex population and describes the components of health care management.[26,27]

Recommendations for optimizing health care in the medical home and promoting healing for children and adolescents in foster care (Box 116-3) include the following:

1. The pediatrician should establish a relationship with the foster care agency (Box 116-4). The caseworker is the case manager. Establishing methods of communication and information exchange will facilitate the child's care.
2. The caseworker should obtain appropriate releases of information and medical consents from the birth family and make copies available to the pediatric primary care physician. The pediatrician should become familiar with the foster care agency's

BOX 116-2 Guidelines for Periodic Preventive Health Care for Children in Foster or Kinship Care

Periodic preventive health care should occur according to the American Academy of Pediatrics schedule, with the following exceptions:

1. Children younger than 6 months should be seen monthly if they are considered high risk for developmental, growth, or illness problems (includes all premature infants or infants with risk factors for poor outcomes).
2. Children ages 12 to 24 months should have periodic preventive health visits every 3 months.
3. Children between 2 and 21 years should have periodic preventive health visits every 6 months.

Every preventive health visit with a child in foster care should include anticipatory guidance around issues specific to foster care: transition issues, visitation issues, the need for routines and reasonable expectations, the impact of prior trauma on emotional and developmental well being, and appropriate discipline, among other issues.

BOX 116-3 Special Considerations in Caring for Children and Adolescents in Foster Care

Every health encounter in foster care requires extra diligence on the part of the pediatric primary care physician, including the following:

- Children in foster care should be screened for abuse and neglect at each health care encounter, and the physician should bear in mind that inadequate weight gain is often the first sign of inadequate parenting in a foster home.
- Children entering foster care should have a full mental health and behavioral health evaluation performed by professionals in the field of mental health within 60 to 90 days of entry to foster care.
- Children entering foster care should have a full developmental or educational evaluation performed by professionals in the field within 60 to 90 days of entry to foster care.
- Children in foster care should be referred for dental care at the first health encounter or by 1 year of age.
- The physician should review *goodness of fit* in foster care placement at each preventive health or behavioral health encounter and should monitor the child more closely during transitions.
- The physician should review recent changes in child's visitation and contact with birth family, school attendance and performance, and participation in normalizing activities, among other issues.
- Every encounter should be considered an opportunity to immunize the child.
- The physician should maintain a well-documented health record for the child in foster care.
- The pediatric practitioner should offer appropriate anticipatory guidance with additional focus on school issues, normalizing activities, predictable routines, dealing with transitions, visitation, and the impact of trauma and separation on emotional and developmental well being, among other issues.
- The physician should have a system for tracking health care utilization and compliance for the child in foster care and should alert the agency when noncompliance exists.
- Referrals should be made promptly when an issue is identified.
- Children leaving foster care should have a discharge health visit, and health information should be summarized and transferred to the new health care provider and caregiver.
- Systems for information exchange should be established by the foster care agency and the physician.
- The physician should provide a summary of each health encounter to the foster care agency, with recommendations for treatment and follow-up.
- The foster care agency should provide the physician with a complete health history that is available for the child, copies of appropriate consents and releases, notification of changes in placement or caseworker assignment, and notification of referrals made by the agency shortly after the child enters foster care.

BOX 116-4 Pediatrician's Role in Caring for Children in Foster Care

This list is meant to show two possible separate, but overlapping roles for pediatricians. Of course, the pediatrician who is the medical home health care provider may choose to serve any or all of the consulting roles.

CONSULTANT ROLE[a]

1. Ensure that the foster care agency understands all American Academy of Pediatrics standards for health care.
2. Help the foster care agency ensure that each child has a medical home with access, insurance, consents, continuity, and other avenues of support.
3. Develop systems for communication and information exchange among caseworkers, mental health professionals, the court system, other health care providers, and school personnel.
4. Provide or refer to health-education resources to the foster parents, caseworkers, the court system, attorneys, and school personnel.
5. Develop systems for merging health information and planning into child welfare permanency plan.
6. Develop systems for transitioning health care when the child or teen transitions or leaves foster care.
7. Develop systems for tracking patients that include information on their health needs and health data, monitoring outcomes, and any other information.

MEDICAL HOME ROLE[b]

1. Deliver care by the American Academy of Pediatrics Foster Care Standards. Identify and attend to the child's health care needs.
2. Accept patients in foster care, and provide a medical home for them.
3. Communicate and coordinate with caseworker, foster parents, school personnel, subspecialists, and the court system regarding individual patients in foster care.
4. Educate the foster parents, caseworkers, or anyone else involved regarding the child's health care needs.
5. Advocate on behalf of patients in foster care to ensure that health care needs are met.
6. Shared health information and plan for the child with the caseworkers, foster parents, the court system, and older children in foster care.
7. Ensure that information on the patient is transmitted to the appropriate professionals when the patient transitions.
8. Monitor and track the patient's health needs and care.

[a]Health care resource: consultant for child welfare regarding children in foster care
[b]Medical home provider for children in foster care

guidelines regarding consent and confidentiality and, whenever possible, should obtain a signed consent to provide medical treatment. The foster care agency should have the authority to provide consent in the absence of the birth parent. Certain adolescent health issues, such as pregnancy, sexually transmitted infections, birth control, and substance abuse, are governed by separate confidentiality laws in most states.

3. As much health history as possible should be gathered. The caseworker will be invaluable in this respect, although this person may also be stymied by a dearth of records. The foster care agency and the physician's office should both attempt to access records from prior health care providers that include prenatal and perinatal history, developmental history, growth curves, immunization records, risk factors for HIV, and accounts of other vertically transmitted infections. For older children, additional information should also include any chronic illnesses, medications, allergies, educational problems, and mental health problems. A paucity of such information may exist because the child may not have received adequate services before foster care or may have had multiple providers.
4. Children entering foster care should have a series of health care encounters over the first two months (see Box 116-1). Multiple encounters during this transitional phase often reveals more than one isolated evaluation.[25-27] Children entering foster care are encouraged to have an initial medical screen performed within 72 hours to document growth parameters, signs and symptoms of abuse or neglect, and the presence of acute or chronic illness. Children should have a comprehensive medical evaluation within 30 days of placement, including recommended screening tests, HIV-risk assessment, and developmental and behavioral screening. A follow-up to this visit should occur within 60 to 90 days of placement to continue monitoring the adjustment to foster care and the *goodness of fit* in the placement.
5. Routine primary preventive health care should be scheduled, according to American Academy of Pediatrics guidelines, between birth and 18 months, although experts recommends that infants in foster care be seen monthly until age 6 months. Toddlers in foster care should be seen every 3 months until age 24 months. After age 2 years, children should have a comprehensive health visit at least every 6 months until they exit foster care (see Box 116-2).
6. Comprehensive preventive health care in the foster care population requires diligent effort on the part of the physician. Extended appointment slots and a tracking system are strongly suggested. Ideally the agency should inform the physician about changes in placement and casework assignment and about any referrals made by the caseworker. The health care practitioner should communicate with the caseworker around each health care encounter about the assessment and recommended plan.
7. Approximately 70% of children and adolescents entering foster care have been physically abused, sexually abused, or neglected. Physicians should be familiar with the signs and symptoms of abuse and neglect and should screen all children and teens at the time of admission to care. Children who may have been sexually abused should be referred to a center specializing in child sexual abuse to prevent the trauma of repeated interviews and examinations. The pediatrician should monitor the child for

possible abuse or neglect at every health encounter and address any concern about the adequacy of parenting in a foster home with the foster care agency. *Inadequate weight gain in a foster home is often the first sign of neglect.*

8. Children in foster care have a high prevalence of dental problems, especially dental caries and malocclusion. Changes in placement may result in a lapse in dental care; therefore continued monitoring of dentition and reminders to foster parents about the importance of routine dental care are important. Referral for dental care should begin at age 1 year.
9. Children entering foster care tend to be underimmunized, even compared with other poor children, and every health encounter should be viewed as an opportunity to immunize a child in foster care.
10. Underutilization of routine preventive health care services before foster care placement implies a deficiency of screening for lead, iron-deficiency anemia, and tuberculosis exposure. Many children in foster care reside in or have resided in older housing stock, and pica is a commonly encountered behavioral issue in this population, increasing the risk for elevated plasma lead levels. Poor nutrition before foster care places children at risk for iron-deficiency anemia; thus clinicians should obtain plasma lead levels and screen all children younger than 6 years for anemia at least annually. Adolescent girls should also have annual hemoglobin screening. Universal tuberculosis screening is recommended using the Mantoux test at admission and every 3 to 5 years thereafter while in foster care. Hemoglobin electrophoresis in at-risk children with no documentation of sickle cell screening at birth should be considered.
11. Maternal lifestyles during pregnancy, including substance abuse and promiscuity, place children in foster care at increased risk for a variety of vertically transmitted infectious diseases, including HIV, hepatitis B and C, congenital syphilis, and herpes. Every child placed in foster care should have a rapid plasma reagin and hepatitis C antibody screen. Up to 80% of young children placed into foster care are at high risk for vertically transmitted HIV infection, but fewer than 10% are screened because of the complexities of risk-assessment, obtaining informed consent, and confidentiality barriers.[28] Guidelines for HIV-risk assessment and screening for children in foster care vary from state to state. Some agencies use risk-assessment tools to determine a child's risk for HIV infection, although the accuracy of such tools depends on the birth parent's availability and veracity. In general the biological parent retains the right to consent to testing or not, unless the child has been freed for adoption or parental rights have been terminated. Agencies vary in their policies regarding consent procedures when a parent declines screening but the child meets high-risk criteria. Identification of children who are HIV positive is critical to appropriate medical management, including pneumocystis pneumonia prophylaxis, modification of the immunization schedule, and early antiretroviral therapy. Practitioners should become familiar with the HIV policies in their state and should promote appropriate risk assessment and screening for the individual child.
12. Adolescents in foster care also represent a high-risk group for HIV infection, usually because of unprotected sex with multiple partners. In general, adolescents in foster care may give consent for HIV testing, unless they are cognitively impaired. Confidentiality laws vary. However, in some states the adolescent has the right to designate who has access to HIV-related information, whereas in others, social service agencies and their representatives have access to such data on any child in their care and custody, including adolescents.
13. Approximately 60% of preschool children in foster care have a developmental disability, especially language disorders and delayed social-adaptive and fine-motor skills. Older children have increased rates of educational disorders, including learning disabilities, behavioral disorders, and limited cognitive ability to the extent that upwards of 40% qualify for special education services. Many of these children are placed in special education settings for emotional rather than for cognitive concerns, given that attentional difficulties, poor impulse control, and aggressive behaviors often preclude placement in a regular classroom. Children younger than 5 years should undergo developmental screening at admission and at each well-child care visit, with a formal developmental evaluation within 3 months of admission to foster care. The high prevalence of language disorders (50% to 60% of preschool children) implies that universal hearing and speech evaluations of toddlers and preschool children may be beneficial in identifying children who would benefit from such services. Children older than 5 years should be referred in a timely manner for an educational evaluation. The primary care physician should maintain contact with the case manager for developmental or educational services (or both) and should obtain copies of all evaluations.
14. **Mental health care is the single overwhelming health care need of most children in foster care.** Prevalence of severe disturbance ranges from 35% to 85%.[29,30] Children in foster care use both inpatient and outpatient mental health services at rates 15 to 20 times the rate that other children of similar backgrounds use but are still believed to be underserved. Conduct disorder, oppositional defiant disorder, attention-deficit/hyperactivity disorder, attachment disorder, and anxiety disorders are the most commonly cited mental health diagnoses for children in foster care (Table 116-3). Experienced professionals in foster care believe that the prevalence and severity of mental health disabilities have increased dramatically in the last decade. Preplacement issues, such as prenatal drug exposure, poor maternal nutrition, inappropriate parenting, violence exposure, and abuse and neglect during early childhood, all contribute to the poor emotional health of children in foster care.[17] Entry to foster care, instead of remediating emotional

Table 116-3 Common Mental Health Diagnoses in Children in Foster Care

PROBLEM	PERCENTAGE OF POPULATION
Conduct disorder	30-52%
Oppositional defiant disorder	17-35%
Attention-deficit disorder	18-32%
Anxiety disorders	8-20%
Depression	3-5%

Modified from Stein E, Rae-Grant N, Ackland S, et al. Psychiatric disorders of children "in care": methodology & demographic correlates. *Can J Psychiatry.* 1994;39(6):341-347. Reprinted by permission.

disorders, may exacerbate them because of the trauma of separation from families and the emotional turmoil of living as a child in an uncertain world. Physicians should screen for emotional and behavioral issues at admission and at each preventive health care visit. Every child in foster care older than 2 years should have a full mental health evaluation within 3 months of placement. Children with identified mental health or behavioral issues should be referred appropriately for mental health services. All children in foster care have to deal with ongoing separation and loss issues, as well as their feelings of anger, sadness, rejection, powerlessness, alienation, and guilt. Even children who do not initially appear to need mental health services should be rescreened at intervals to assess for changes in their emotional well being. Some of the common stressors that up-end the lives of children in foster care include inconsistent visitation, resumption of regular visits after a prolonged lapse, cessation of visitation, incarceration of a parent, illness of a foster parent, and being freed for adoption. These critical junctures are times at which resumption of lapsed counseling or increased frequency of counseling visits are beneficial.

15. Many foster families have a wealth of child-rearing experience, but the clinician should not presume that knowledge about child development, behavior, discipline, and safety are adequate. Anticipatory guidance should be a routine part of well-child care and should include issues specific to foster care, such as behavior problems related to visitation and the permanency planning process, significant sleep disorders, confused loyalties, attachment, violence, and coercion. Adolescents should be counseled not only about safe behaviors, but also about healthy activities, planning for their futures, and developing relationships with adult mentors. Support for foster families and older children in foster care around transitions and other stressors can stabilize a foster care placement for a child.
16. All medical information, unless specifically prohibited by law, should be shared with the child's caseworker and foster parent or parents in appropriate lay language. The caseworker has the responsibility for communicating the information to the birth parent in the likely event that the parent was not present at the medical visit. If possible the physician should provide a written summary of each health encounter, including the assessment, the treatment plan, and any scheduled follow-up. Caseworkers are required to have at least semi-annual *Child and Family Service Reviews,* during which health information can be incorporated into planning for the child.
17. In caring for a child in foster care the pediatric primary care physician must sometimes assume the role of advocate for appropriate health care for the child.

PSYCHOTROPIC MEDICATION

The use of psychotropic medication has become controversial in the foster care population. Studies show that children and teens in foster care are more likely to be on psychotropic medications than peers not in foster care; they are also more likely to be on multiple medications and sometimes on medications from the same class. Studies also indicate that psychotropic medications may not match the major symptom of concern or diagnosis. At least two states (Texas and New York) have developed comprehensive guidelines regarding the prescription and management of psychotropic medications in the foster care population, and the reader is directed to these or their individual states for further information. In general, psychotropic medications should be use as part of a comprehensive mental health treatment plan and are best prescribed for patients in foster care by a qualified pediatric mental health professional or a primary care physician with extensive foster care experience. A detailed health history, including mental health, behavior, development, trauma history, medication use, social and family history, and a full mental health evaluation should be obtained before beginning medication. Therapy should be initiated with a single agent in the lowest dose. Dosage increases should be gradual and closely monitored for efficacy and side effects. Single-agent therapy should be used whenever possible. Close monitoring is the essence of good care for children and teens who are prescribed psychotropic medication.[32-39]

SUMMARY

Children and adolescents removed from their families for reasons of health and safety enter foster or kinship care having experienced multiple synergistic adversities that negatively affect their health and well being. As a result, these children and adolescents have a high prevalence of medical, mental health, developmental, educational, and dental conditions. Pediatric professionals should use foster care as a window of opportunity in which the child or teen can heal. The pediatrician can provide the medical home while the child or teen is in foster care, following recommended standards of health care to identify and treat all of the child's health needs. The pediatrician will need to be proactive in engaging child welfare agencies to ensure that health planning is integrated into the child's permanency plan in a meaningful way. Pediatric professionals also have a role in educating child welfare professionals, foster parents, and birth parents and youth about health issues and in advocating and coordinating health care for this vulnerable population.

The authors gratefully acknowledge the children and families they serve for their inspiration and the staffs of Starlight Pediatrics and Child Welfare for their compassion, dedication, and caring.

TOOLS FOR PRACTICE

Community Advocacy and Coordination

- *Child Maltreatment 2005*, U.S. Department of Health and Human Services (www.acf.dhhs.gov/programs/cb/pubs/cm05/index.htm).
- *Meth and Child Welfare: Promising Solutions for Children, Their Parents and Grandparents*, Generations United (ipath.gu.org/documents/A0//Meth_Child_Welfare_Final_cover.pdf).
- *Northwest Foster Care Alumni Study Improving Family Foster Care*, Casey Family Programs (www.casey.org/Resources/Publications/NorthwestAlumniStudy.htm).
- *Traumatic Stress/Child Welfare*, Focal Point (www.rtc.pdx.edu/PDF/fpW07.pdf).

Medical Decision and Support

- *Fostering Health: Health Care for Children and Adolescents in Foster Care, 2nd edition* (book), American Academy of Pediatrics, Task Force on Health Care for Children in Foster Care, District II, New York State (www.aap.org/bookstore).
- *Standards of Excellence for Health Care Services for Children in Out of Home Care*, Child Welfare League of America (cwla.org/programs/standards/cwsstandardshealthcare.htm).

Other

- *Adoption and Foster Care Analysis and Reporting System (AFCARS) Report*, U.S. Department of Health and Human Services (www.acf.hhs.gov/programs/cb/stats_research/afcars/tar/report13.htm).

RELATED WEB SITE

- Casey Family Programs (www.casey.org/Home/).

AAP POLICY STATEMENTS

American Academy of Pediatrics, Committee on Early Childhood Adoption and Dependent Care. Developmental issues for young children in foster care. *Pediatrics*. 2000; 106(5):1145-1150. (aappolicy.aappublications.org/cgi/content/full/pediatrics;106/5/1145).

American Academy of Pediatrics, Committee on Early Childhood Adoption and Dependent Care. Health care of young children in foster care. *Pediatrics*. 2002;109(3):536-541. (aappolicy.aappublications.org/cgi/content/full/pediatrics;109/3/536).

American Academy of Pediatrics, Committee on Pediatric AIDS. Identification and care of HIV-Exposed and HIV-infected infants, children, and adolescents in foster care. *Pediatrics*. 2000;106(1):149-153. (aappolicy.aappublications.org/cgi/content/full/pediatrics;106/1/149).

REFERENCES

1. US Department of Health and Human Services, Administration for Children and Families. Child Maltreatment, 2005. Available at: www.acf.dhhs.gov/programs/cb/pubs/cm05/index.htm. Accessed August 6, 2007.
2. US Department of Health and Human Services, Administration for Children and Families. The AFCARS Report, 2005. Available at: www.acf.hhs.gov/programs/cb/stats_research/afcars/tar/report13.htm. Accessed August 6, 2007.
3. Barth RP, Green R, Guo S. *Kinship Care and Foster Care: Informing the New Debate*. Paper presented at the National Survey of Child and Adolescent Well-Being (NSCAW) Conference: "Child Protection: Using Research to Improve Policy and Practice." Washington DC; 2005.
4. Taussig H, Clyman R. *Kinship Care and Foster Care: Differential Outcomes Following Six Years in Care*. Presented at the International Congress on Child Abuse and Neglect. Denver, CO; 2002.
5. Barbell K, Freundlich M. *Foster Care Today*. Washington DC: National Center for Resource Family Support, Casey Family Programs; 2001.
6. Stein BD, Zima BT, Elliott MN, et al. Violence exposure among school-age children in foster care: relationship to distress symptoms. *J Am Acad Child Adolesc Psychiatry*. 2001;40(5):588-594.
7. Leslie LK, Landsverk J, Ezzet-Lofstrom R, et al. Children in foster care: factors influencing outpatient mental health service use. *Child Abuse Negl*. 2000;24:465-476.
8. American Academy of Pediatrics, Committee on Early Childhood, Adoption, and Dependent Care. Developmental issues for young children in foster care. *Pediatrics*. 2000;106(5):1145-1150.
9. US Department of Health and Human Services, Administration for Children and Families. Adoption and Safe Families Act of 1997. Pub Law No. 105-89 (1997).
10. Simms MD. Foster children and the foster care system. I. History and legal structure. *Curr Probl Pediatr*.1991;21:297-321.
11. Generations United. Meth and Child Welfare: promising solutions for children, their parents and grandparents—2006. Available at: ipath.gu.org/documents/a0//meth_child_welfare_final_cover.pdf. Accessed August 6, 2007.
12. Jones LM, Finkelhor D, Halter S. Child maltreatment trends in the 1990s: why does neglect differ from sexual and physical abuse? *Child Maltreat* 2006;11(2):107-120.
13. Szilagyi MA, Jee S, Nilsen W, et al. Under-utilization of specialty mental health services by young children in foster and kinship care. Presented at Pediatric Academic Society Meetings. May 2006.
14. Hill RB. Synthesis of research on disproportionality in the child welfare system: An update. Washington DC. The Casey CSSP Alliance for Racial Equity in Child Welfare, 2006. Available at: www.cssp.org/major_initiatives/racialEquity. Accessed July 18, 2008.
15. Szilagyi M. The pediatrician and the child in foster care. *Peds Rev*. 1998;19(2):39-50.
16. Walker JS, Weaver A, Gowen LK, et al. Focal point: research, policy and practice in children's mental health. *Traumatic Stress/Child Welfare*. 2007;21(1). Available at: www.rtc.pdx.edu/pgfpw07toc.php. Accessed August 6, 2007.
17. Rubin DM, O'Reilly ALR, Luan X, et al. The impact of placement stability on behavioral well-being for children in foster care. *Pediatrics*. 2007;119:336-344.

18. Reilly T. Transition from care: status and outcomes of youth who age out of foster care. *Child Welfare.* 2003;82: 727-745.
19. The Northwest Foster Care Alumni Study. Improving Family Foster Care: findings from the Northwest Foster Care Alumni Study—2005. Available at: www.casey.org. Accessed August 6, 2007.
20. Children's Rights, National Foster Parent Association, University of Maryland School of Social Work. *Hitting the MARC—establishing foster care minimum adequate rates for children.* Accessed at www.childrensrights.org.
21. Horwitz SM, Balestracci KMB, Simms MD. Foster care placement improves children's functioning. *Arch Pediatr Adolesc Med.* 2001;155:1255-1260.
22. Smithgall C, Gladden M, Yang D, et al. *Behavior Problems and Educational Disruptions Among Children in Out-Of-Home Care.* Chicago, IL: University of Chicago, Chapin Hall Center for Children; 2005.
23. Halfon N, Mendonca A, Berkowitz G. Health status of children in foster care. The experience of the Center for the vulnerable child. *Arch Pediatr Adolesc Med.* 1995; 149:386-392.
24. Simms MD, Dubowitz H, Szilagyi MA. Health care needs of children in the foster care system. *Pediatrics.* 2000;106: 909-918.
25. Leslie LK, Gordon JN, Meneken L, et al. The physical, developmental, and mental health needs of young children in child welfare by initial placement type. *Develop Behavior Pediatr.* 2005;26:177-185.
26. Child Welfare League of America. *Standards of Excellence for Health Care Services for Children in Out-of-Home Care.* Washington, DC: Child Welfare League of America; 1988.
27. American Academy of Pediatrics, Committee on Early Childhood, Adoption, and Dependent Care. Health care of children in foster care. *Pediatrics.* 1994;93:335-338.
28. American Academy of Pediatrics, Task Force on Health Care for Children in Foster Care. *I. Fostering Health: Health Care for Children and Adolescents in Foster Care.* Elk Grove Village, IL: American Academy of Pediatrics; 2005.
29. American Academy of Pediatrics, Committee on Pediatric AIDS. Identification and care of HIV-exposed and HIV-infected infants, children, and adolescents in foster care. *Pediatrics.* 2000;106:149-153.
30. Simms MD, Freundlich M, Battistelli ES, et al. Delivering health and mental health services to children in family foster care after welfare and health care reform. *Child Welfare.* 1999;78:166-183.
31. Leslie LK, Hurlburt MS, Landsverk J, et al. Outpatient mental health services for children in foster care: a national perspective. *Child Abuse Negl.* 2004;28:697-712.
32. Zito JM, Safer DJ, Sai D, et al. Psychotropic medication patterns among youth in foster care. *Pediatrics,* 2008; 121(1):e157-163.
33. American Academy of Child and Adolescent Psychiatry. AAAP Position Statement on Oversight of Psychotropic Medication Use for Children in State Custody: A Best Principles Guideline, 2003. Available at: www.aacap.org/galleries/PracticeInformation/FosterCare_BestPrinciples_FINAL.pdf
34. Coyle JT. Psychotropic drug use in very young children. *JAMA.* 2000;283(8):1025-1030.
35. Malkin M. *Psychotropic medication for children and adolescents.* Los Angeles, CA: Los Angeles County Department of Mental Health, Juvenile Court Mental Health Services. 2005.
36. Irwin M. *Understanding the use of psychiatric medication in foster care and residential treatment.* Saratoga Springs, NY: New York Public Welfare Association Summer Conference. 2004.
37. New York State Office of Children & Family Services. Informational Letter 08-OCFS-INF-02—The Use of Psychiatric Medications for Children and Youth in Placement; Authority to Consent to Medical Care Available on-line at www.ocfs.state.ny.us/main/sppd/health_services/manual.asp
38. New York State Office of Mental Health. Clinical Advisory and Issue Analysis Regarding Antidepressant Use in Children and Adolescents. 2004. Available at: www.omh.state.ny.us/omhweb/advisories/clinicaladvisory.htm
39. Texas Department of State Health Services. Psychotropic Medication Utilization Parameters for Foster Children. 2005. Available at: www.dshs.state.tx.us/mhprograms/PsychotropicMedication UtilizationParametersFoster Children.

Chapter 117

DOMESTIC VIOLENCE AND THE FAMILY

Peter G. Sherman, MD; Abraham C. Rice, MD

The environment created by domestic violence has profound short- and long-term effects on the well being of children, in addition to harmful consequences for the victim. Because the abuser is not always present at the pediatric visit, this setting may be one of the few places where an adult victim can feel safe disclosing that she or he is being battered. The immediate safety of a child or parent may depend on physician intervention. Children living in environments where domestic violence occurs are at increased risk of abuse. Pediatricians need to be adept at addressing this issue because children living in households where violence occurs are likely to need evaluation, referral, and treatment.

Domestic violence can be defined as a pattern of behaviors used by an adult to establish and maintain power and control over another adult. These behaviors, which can occur sporadically or continually, include physical violence, verbal abuse, psychological abuse, nonconsensual sexual behavior, and economic coercion.[1] Contrary to stereotypes, men are also abused by women, and violence occurs within same-sex couples. For example, in 2001, 15% of the victims of domestic violence were men.[2] The departure of the abuser from the relationship does not necessarily mean that the abuse has stopped. In fact, terminating or attempting to terminate a relationship frequently results in an increase in abuse.

The incidence of domestic violence against women has declined over the last decade, with a decrease from 1.1 million nonfatal violent crimes reported in 1993 to 588,490 in 2001.[2] In 2001, 5:1000 women and 0.9:1000 men experienced nonfatal intimate-partner violence.[2] However, these statistics are derived from police reports, and only 25% of intimate-partner assaults and 20% of intimate-partner rapes are reported.[1] Though the conclusion can be made that domestic violence has been declining, the actual number of victims is certainly higher than what is officially reported. Nearly one third of women have experienced battering at least once by an intimate partner during her lifetime, though given current trends this number should show a decrease.[3] Those at highest risk are more likely to be 16 to 24 years of age, low income, black, divorced or separated, and living in urban areas.[4] The decrease in domestic violence over the last 10 years is most likely due to more effective law enforcement, legal system intervention, and improved resources for victims.

The number of women killed by intimate partners has also declined; 1596 women were murdered by an intimate partner in 1976, which decreased to 1159 in 2004.[5] This number represents a 56% decline for black women but only a 5% decline for white women. Given that the relationship between victim and perpetrator is not identified in nearly 30% of the homicide cases in which the perpetrator is known, this number is a conservative estimate.

Domestic violence is a familiar event in the lives of many children. Forty percent of female victims of domestic violence live in households with children younger than 12 years.[2] Approximately 15.5 million children live in homes where domestic violence has recently occurred and 7 million where recent severe domestic violence has occurred.[6] These figures do not include children in single-parent households, separated couples, and homosexual couples, which would significantly increase this estimate. Violence directed toward a parent may place a child at increased risk for injury or even death.[7] Though the extent of this problem is not well documented, the Department of Justice found that in a cohort of 84 children younger than 12 years murdered by a parent, 6 were the unintended consequence of a conflict between parents.[8] The exact number of children who are injured unintentionally during incidents of domestic violence is unknown.

DOMESTIC VIOLENCE AND CHILD ABUSE

Domestic violence places a child at increased risk for abuse and is considered the single major precursor to child abuse.[9] In 35 studies reviewed by Edelson, concurrence between domestic violence and abuse was as high as 60%.[10] The risk of physical abuse of children increases with the level of violence in the household. With 1 self-reported act of domestic violence per year, child abuse occurs 5% of the time. However, in households with 50 or more episodes of domestic violence per year, nearly 100% of children are physically abused by their father, and 30% are abused by their mother.[11] The converse is also true; domestic violence occurs in 40% to 60% of households where an abused child resides, a figure far higher than the 13% overall prevalence of domestic violence.[12] Domestic violence also places children at increased risk of sexual abuse. One study found a 150% increase in the risk of child sexual abuse in households where domestic violence took place.[13]

Thus the primary care physician must screen for child abuse in cases in which domestic violence is identified and complete a thorough, unclothed head-to-toe examination to look for signs of abuse. Any suspected abuse must be reported to the appropriate local child welfare agency. In addition, the child should be referred to a pediatric child abuse center or to a pediatrician who specializes in this area.

A child may be injured or even killed when caught between a batterer and parent. All threats made against a parent or children have to be taken seriously, and a plan should be created to alleviate the threat. This plan may involve, in addition to contacting domestic violence shelters or agencies, communicating with law enforcement, child welfare agencies, and the court system. If children are in immediate danger and their mother is not willing to leave the batterer, then a report needs to be made to the local child welfare agency that a child is living in an unsafe environment. Some states go as far as defining a child's witnessing of domestic violence as maltreatment.[14] Ascertaining at what point a child's witnessing domestic violence becomes maltreatment may be difficult. This issue often places children's advocates in disagreement with domestic violence advocates who may view reporting as further victimizing the victim. The goal of reporting is to ensure children's safety, as well as to access and implement needed services. Knowledge of state reporting laws and guidelines is essential when determining whether to make a report because laws vary among states. Certainly a report is required when a child is injured during a domestic dispute or when a determination has been made that a child is at risk for future injury. If a child's basic medical, educational, emotional, or safety needs are not being met because of a domestic violence situation, then a report is warranted. Factors that may lower the threshold to report include younger children (increased risk of abuse and increased psychological trauma from witnessing violence) and children who are already displaying emotional, behavioral, or developmental problems because of previous exposure to domestic violence. If the pediatrician is uncertain as to whether the witnessing of domestic violence constitutes child abuse, then they should consult local child abuse authorities by calling the state child abuse reporting hotline or contacting a local child advocacy center. A local child advocacy center can be identified through the National Children's Alliance telephone number or Web site (listed in the resource section at the end of this chapter).

DOMESTIC VIOLENCE AND THE HEALTH CARE SYSTEM

Health care providers are uniquely positioned to identify victims of domestic violence. One half of female victims of domestic violence report a physical injury, and 40% seek medical care.[2] The American Academy of Pediatrics, the American Medical Association, and the American College of Obstetricians and Gynecologists recommend that physicians routinely screen for domestic violence.[15-17] On a cautionary note, the US Preventive Services Task Force recommendation on *Screening for Family and Intimate Partner Violence* found only limited evidence as to whether intervention reduces harm to women and did not find any studies that addressed the issue of whether intervention increased risk. As a consequence, they did not recommend for or against routine screening for intimate-partner violence.[18] Further study is needed to improve the ability to detect and safely treat victims. Resources for screening and intervention protocols are listed at the end of this chapter.

IDENTIFYING VICTIMS

Although identifying parents who are victims of domestic violence has not traditionally been considered part of the pediatric assessment, this view is changing. The American Academy of Pediatrics (AAP) recommends that domestic violence training be incorporated into residency and continuing medical education programs, that screening for domestic violence be a part of routine anticipatory guidance, and that pediatricians should be capable of intervening when necessary.[17] AAP surveys measuring pediatrician attitudes toward screening for domestic violence found that from 1998 to 2003 the percentage of pediatricians who believed screening for domestic violence should be routinely increased from 66% to 72%.[19] Pediatricians' confidence in identifying and managing domestic violence remained low; lack of education and training were identified as significant barriers to screening.[20] Pediatricians and family practitioners screen less than 10% of their patients at routine health visits for domestic violence.[21] Educational interventions positively affect pediatricians' knowledge and practice regarding screening for domestic violence.[22] Greater effort must be made to expose primary care physicians to domestic violence training.

Pediatricians are in an ideal position to identify domestic violence. Women in their childbearing years are at the highest risk for domestic violence,[23] most likely because the 1st years of parenthood are financially, physically, and emotionally stressful. This period has the most frequent visits to the pediatrician. The perpetrator may isolate a woman, thereby limiting access to family, friends, community, and social service agencies. However, mothers who are domestic violence victims are just as likely to seek routine well-child care for their children as women who are not victims.[24] Maternal victims of domestic violence do disclose in significant numbers when appropriately screened in a pediatric office setting.[25]

The Family Violence Prevention Fund's consensus recommendations in the pediatric setting are to screen for domestic violence in parents at new patient visits, at least once per year, when they disclose a new intimate relationship, and when signs and symptoms raise concerns.[26] Adolescents should be similarly screened for exposure to family violence, as well as intimate-partner violence.[26] Questions should be direct, clear, easy to understand, and nonjudgmental. They should be asked whether or not signs or symptoms are present and whether or not the provider suspects abuse has occurred. Box 117-1 and Table 117-1 highlights examples of screening questions.

Providers should look for signs or symptoms of domestic violence in a parent such as bruising, depression, anxiety, failure to keep appointments, reluctance to answer questions about discipline, and frequent office visits for complaints not substantiated by the medical evaluation.[17] Particular attention should be given to children who are in homes with factors that put the child at increased risk of exposure to violence: parental mental illness, alcohol and substance abuse, parental social isolation, and financial difficulties.

In addition to screening, establishing an environment of trust and safety by communicating concern nonjudgmentally is essential. Several visits may be required for a parent to feel safe enough to discuss the situation; thus the clinician needs to maintain an index of suspicion and a commitment to inquiry, not only at the 1st visit, but during subsequent visits as well.

Children can also be questioned in a developmentally appropriate manner, though they may be reluctant to talk about what they have seen or heard. In addition to information that can be elicited by directly interviewing the child, the pediatrician should be alert to nonverbal cues that indicate child distress. Although nonspecific, they may indicate possible exposure, such as a child who demonstrates aggressiveness to a parent or physician while being examined or interviewed, a child who is overly protective of a parent when the physician engages the parent in conversation, or a child who demonstrates an excessive fear-of-stranger anxiety when introduced to the physician.

DATING VIOLENCE

A related form of domestic violence is dating violence. Adolescents are frequent victims of dating violence that includes verbal abuse, as well as physical and sexual assault. The percentage of adolescents who report physical or sexual violence in the context of dating is startling. Whether this circumstance is a recent phenomenon or a longstanding epidemic is not clear, given that this problem has only recently been studied. The Youth Risk Behavior Survey is conducted every 2 years by the Centers for Disease Control and Prevention on a national representative sample of over 15,000 adolescents across the country ages 12 to 21 years. Its latest survey in 2005 demonstrated high rates of physical violence, with 9.3% of female adolescents and 9.0% of male adolescents reporting being "hit, slapped, or physically hurt on purpose by their boyfriend of girlfriend during the past 12 months."[27] No racial or ethnic differences were found, though teenagers living in urban and rural environments were at greater risk than those in suburban locations.[28] Other studies revealed even higher rates of violence, with 1 study showing 30% of 14- to 23-year-old female victims in an urban setting reporting an unwanted sexual experience during the previous 12 months[29] and another with 20% of female high school students reporting physical or sexual abuse by a dating partner.[30] The rates of dating violence follow a similar pattern among gay, lesbian, and bisexual youth, with 14% of gay and lesbian youths reporting physical or sexual violence by a date or partner.[31]

Though awareness of adolescent dating violence has increased over the last decade, no clear consensus has formed on how to address this issue in the clinical setting.[32] Given the prevalence of violence in the context of dating, even in the absence of consensus, asking teenagers who are dating about their exposure to violence would be prudent. Inquiries should be made in a nonjudgmental manner by letting the patient know that this is an area of concern for all patients who are dating. Suggested questions are included in Box 117-2.

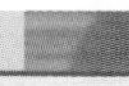

BOX 117-1 How to Assess for Domestic Violence

Ask direct questions, whether or not signs or symptoms are present and whether or not the provider suspects abuse has occurred.
Inform patient about the limits of practitioner-patient confidentiality related to intimate-partner violence before assessing.
Use language that is direct, specific, and easy to understand.
Conduct assessment in a private room.
For a parent, assessment should take place without the intimate partner or other adult family members present.
For adolescents, assessment should take place without the parent (or partner) in the room.
Inquiries can be included as part of a written health questionnaire or health history but should not replace face-to-face assessment.
Assessment should be conducted in patient's primary language.
If an interpreter is used, then this person should not be an acquaintance or relative of the family. Children should never be used as interpreters.

WHAT TO ASK

Intimate-partner violence questions can be framed within discussion of other safety issues such as vehicle safety, bicycle helmet safety, guns at home, or community violence.

FOR ADULTS WHO ACCOMPANY THEIR CHILDREN

Introductory statements or questions might include:

"I have begun to ask all of the women [parents, caregivers] in my practice about their family life as it affects their health and safety and that of their children. May I ask you a few questions?"

"Violence is an issue that unfortunately affects everyone today, and thus I have begun to ask all families in my practice about exposure to violence. May I ask you a few questions?"

Indirect questions:

"What happens when a disagreement occurs with your partner [husband, boyfriend] or other adults in your home?"

"Do you feel safe in your home and in your relationship?"

Direct questions:

"Have you ever been hurt or threatened by your partner [husband, boyfriend]?"

"Do you ever feel afraid of (or controlled or isolated by) your partner [husband, boyfriend]?"

"Has your child witnessed a violent or frightening event in your neighborhood or home?"

FOR ADOLESCENTS

Introductory statements or questions:

"Many teens your age experience threats, name calling, uninvited touching, sex or violence, so I ask all my teen patients about it. May I ask you a few questions?"

"I don't know if this is a concern for you, but many teens I see are dealing with violence or bullying issues, so I've started asking questions about violence routinely."

"When I see an injury like yours, sometimes it's because somebody got hit. How did you get this injury [bruise]?"

"Now I am going to ask you confidential questions. The answers are confidential, unless your health is in immediate danger."

"How are disagreements handled in your family?"

Indirect questions:

"Are you in a relationship or seeing anyone?" or "Do you have a boyfriend or girlfriend?"

"How are your parents getting along?"

"How often do you have yelling or screaming fights? Do any of them involve pushing or slapping?"

Direct questions:

"If someone is being hurt in her or his own relationship, this person may have seen it happen in her or his own family. Have you seen anyone get hurt in your home?"

"Teens see a lot of violence these days. Seeing parents or other adults fight can feel as bad as being hit yourself. Has this happened to you?"

"We all have disagreements sometimes with family members or friends. Have you ever been hurt or threatened by anyone?"

"Have you ever been hurt—hit, kicked, slapped, shoved, or pushed—by a friend or person you know?"

"Have you ever been forced to do something sexual that you didn't want to do?" (Assessed as part of sexual history.)

"Do you ever feel afraid of or controlled by someone you're dating or a friend?"

"Has anyone hit you at home in the last year?"

Questions based on indicators:

"I noticed that you have an injury. Injuries like that sometimes come from someone hurting you. What happened to you?"

ASKING ABOUT INTIMATE PARTNER VIOLENCE WITH A CHILD IN THE ROOM

If seeing the parent without the child is possible (eg, the child is older enough to wait alone, the child is in a supervised waiting area, the child is having laboratory work or vision or hearing screening done), questions can be asked in the manner mentioned in the previous section "What to Ask."

For children under age 3 years, asking the mother questions about safety and relationships in the presence of the child is generally not an issue.

Continued

BOX 117-1 How to Assess for Domestic Violence—cont'd

IF THE CHILD IS IN THE ROOM

Begin inquiry with an indirect question (see previous section "What to Ask")

If the parent appears uncomfortable or upset and seeing the parent alone is not possible in this visit, then ask if another time is available to speak by telephone or to follow up.

If parent appears comfortable with the questions, then proceed to ask more specific questions about intimate partner violence.

Produced by The Family Violence Prevention Fund, 383 Rhode Island Street, Suite 304, San Francisco, CA 94103-5133. Telephone: 415-252-800; TTY 1-800-595-4889. Available at: www.endabuse.org. First printing September 2002; updated August 2004. Reprinted by permission.

Table 117-1 Who and How Often to Assess for Domestic Violence

TYPE OF VISIT	WHO TO ASSESS	WHEN TO ASSESS
Newborn	Caregiver	At postpartum visit
New patient	Caregiver and adolescent	At 1st visit
Well child: child, adolescent	Caregiver	At 2, 6, and 12 months, then yearly
	Adolescent	Yearly
Prenatal	Adolescent mother	Once per trimester
Mental health	Caregiver and adolescent	At initial visit
Emergency	Caregiver and adolescent	At every visit
Other visits	Caregiver and adolescent	Whenever physical or behavioral indicators or chronic somatic complaints are present

Produced by The Family Violence Prevention Fund, 383 Rhode Island Street, Suite 304, San Francisco, CA 94103-5133. Telephone: 415-252-800; TTY 1-800-595-4889. Available at: www.endabuse.org. First printing September 2002; updated August 2004. Reprinted by permission.

Since dating violence, by definition, does not involve family members, most cases are addressed by criminal law statutes and through law enforcement intervention. Intervention is dependent on the adolescent victim's willingness to press criminal charges against the perpetrator, and whether this person is another adolescent or an adult. In high-risk situations, such as an abuser threatening to kill the victim, an adolescent may need to access the same domestic violence resources that adults use. However, this task may be a challenge because most domestic violence shelters only accept adult victims. Intervention can also be a challenge in cases in which the teenagers are reluctant to accept help and request confidentiality regarding parental involvement. It all cases, clinicians must be familiar with state laws regarding adolescent consent and confidentiality. In cases when an adolescent refuses intervention and when a clear-cut safety mandate exists to break confidentiality, the patient should have frequent follow-up. Over time, the teenager may become more open to assistance.

Discussing intervention in cases of adolescent rape is beyond the scope of this chapter. Further information in regard to this subject can be found in Chapter 356 on Rape.

ASSISTING VICTIMS AND THEIR CHILDREN

The most immediate concern of the pediatrician is the safety of the child and family. Protocols should be established to ensure a clinician's ability to respond to a parent who discloses a history of domestic violence. Community resources should be identified ahead of time so that the family can be moved quickly into a safe environment. Contacts may include the police, domestic violence shelters, social service agencies, or hotlines. An excellent 24-hour national resource for clinicians and victims is 1-800-799-SAFE. Web sites that contain useful information for the clinician are listed in the resource section at the end of this chapter. The Family Violence Prevention Fund's *Identifying and Responding to Domestic Violence: Consensus Recommendations for Children and Adolescent Health* provides a detailed protocol for use in a pediatric clinic (see resource section). In instances in which the abuser is also threatening clinic staff, the clinician may be required to ensure that office personnel are safe by working with local law enforcement personnel.

A parent may not be ready or willing to leave an abuser. In this case, once the determination has been made that any involved children are safe, the pediatrician should give the parent appropriate assistance with creating a contingency plan. This plan should include what to do in case of further episodes of battering or if the parent decides to leave the batterer. Police, domestic violence hotline, and shelter contact information should be provided to the parent. The clinician should be aware that a victim might not be safe in carrying such information because the abuser may be provoked by it.

A parent can be instructed to do concrete things regarding family safety.

- Prepare an emergency bag and place it in a safe location that contains clothing, money, identification, and other important papers. Items to include are medications, prescriptions, birth certificates, and immunization records.[33]

BOX 117-2 Questions for Detecting Dating Violence

Are you in a relationship or seeing anyone? or

Do you have a boyfriend or girlfriend?

What happens when you disagree with your boyfriend [girlfriend]?

How are your parents getting along? (In case of same-sex relationships, using the term *partner* or mirroring the language of the adult being screened is recommended. For example, if a parent refers to her same sex partner as *roommate,* then the term *roommate* should be used. If the sexual orientation is unknown, then the term *partner* is recommended.)

How often do you have yelling or screaming fights? Do any of them involve pushing or slapping?

If someone is being hurt in her or his own relationship, they may sometimes have seen it happen in their own family.

Have you seen anyone get hurt in your home?

Teens see a lot of violence these days. Seeing parents or other adults fight can feel as bad as being hit yourself. Has this happened to you?

We all have disagreements sometimes with family members or friends. Have you ever been hurt or threatened by anyone?

Have you ever been hurt—hit, kicked, slapped, shoved, pushed—by a friend or person you know?

Have you ever been forced to do something sexual that you didn't want to do?

Do you ever feel afraid of or controlled by someone you're dating or a friend?

I noticed that you have an injury. Injuries like that sometimes come from someone hurting you. What happened to you?

Produced by The Family Violence Prevention Fund, 383 Rhode Island Street, Suite 304, San Francisco, CA 94103-5133. Telephone: 415-252-800; TTY 1-800-595-4889. Available at: www.endabuse.org. First printing September 2002; updated August 2004. Reprinted by permission.

- Establish a code word that can be used by the victim to signal family or friends to call the police. Children can be instructed on how to call for help as long as they can do so safely.[34]
- Make sure schools and child care providers know who has permission to pick up children.
- Remove firearms from the home if this task can be done safely. The presence of firearms increases the risk of homicide.[35]
- If the parent is open to mental health counseling, then the parent and children should be referred to someone who is experienced working with victims of domestic violence.

The clinician may have to counsel the parent without children present so as to prevent a child from inadvertently communicating to the abuser that the victim is seeking help or to prevent emotional trauma to the child that may occur when discussing violence between parents. Clinicians should keep in mind that the highest period for risk of injury or death is when the victim attempts to leave.

A parent who is being battered may choose not to leave for many reasons. In many instances, the batterer creates an atmosphere of financial and emotional dependence or threatens to harm the victim and children or to take custody of the children. Depression and denial may also be important factors. Though this situation may be frustrating to the clinician, communicating an understanding for a parent's decision and being available to assist when the patient is ready and able to leave can be extremely effective.

TREATMENT

Children exposed to domestic violence exhibit increased rates of emotional, behavioral, developmental, and medical problems. Infants, toddlers, children, and adolescents demonstrate increased rates of anxiety, social withdrawal, depression, suicidal ideation, aggressiveness, hyperactivity, conduct problems, reduced social competence, school difficulties, truancy, bullying, clinging behaviors, speech disorders, bed wetting, disturbed sleep, failure to thrive,[36] headaches, asthma, allergies, and gastrointestinal problems.[37] Mothers who are victims of domestic violence during their pregnancy are more likely to have low–birth-weight infants.[38] Witnessing violence can be extremely traumatic[39] and can result in a child displaying characteristics of posttraumatic stress disorder (PTSD). PTSD may include symptoms such as sleep disturbance, difficulty concentrating, flashbacks, and reenactment of the trauma through play. These may interfere with school, social relationships, and emotional development. Female children who have PTSD have increased odds of a wide range of adverse health conditions.[40]

Helping a parent understand the relationship between a child's witnessing violence and the child's behavior is important because a parent may not be aware or deny the impact that this situation has. This circumstance is especially true in the case of infants and toddlers, in which the parent may think that the child is too young to be cognizant of what is occurring. This awareness may be instrumental in motivating a parent to leave the batterer.

The pathophysiological effects of witnessing domestic violence and the effects on children are complex. In all likelihood, it is a combination of the direct effects of violence on the development and emotional state of the child and the impairment of the parental victim as a caregiver to their child. Decreased attachment to children, depression, and an inability to access services are problems that can interfere with the parental victims of domestic violence meeting their children's needs. The children of mothers who are identified and referred for domestic violence advocacy have less depression, anxiety, aggressiveness, and attention problems than children of mothers without intervention.[41] Developmentalists, psychologists, psychiatrists, domestic violence advocates, social workers, child welfare workers, and law enforcement personnel are some of the people who can be involved in assisting a child and parent.

A child who lives or has lived in a household where domestic violence occurs requires a thorough medical, developmental, and psychological evaluation, regardless of whether the child has witnessed any such events. Living in a home where violence occurs may produce an increased need for services. This need can be the result of a parent not accessing care regularly because of the impact of domestic violence on the parent's mental health, as may be seen with maternal depression or a child requiring mental health evaluation and treatment. A health maintenance visit may require additional time to gather a more detailed history concerning the child's exposure to violence, to catch-up on routine health care maintenance such as immunizations, and to refer to medical and behavioral health specialists. The clinician should have a low threshold for referring for psychological evaluation and treatment, for either the parent or the child. This willingness to refer is particularly important when symptoms persist after physician intervention, in cases in which trauma was particularly violent, or when the parent unrealistically minimizes the impact that domestic violence has had on the parent's children. For the clinician to identify a family in which domestic violence is occurring, yet have the victim repeatedly decline any intervention, is a common scenario. This situation must be closely monitored to ensure that any children are not endangered or show any manifestations of exposure to violence that warrants reporting caregivers to child abuse authorities. If such is not the case, in addition to close monitoring, patience is warranted, given that victims with ongoing support may eventually choose to remove themselves and their children from the situation.

The clinician needs to be aware that an abuser can request a child's medical chart. Any information in the chart regarding the victim's communication with the child's physician about domestic violence can endanger the victim. Possible solutions to this dilemma are using code words such as *family problems* or *difficult home situation* or documenting information in the victim parent's chart or social work notes.

BREAKING THE CYCLE OF DOMESTIC VIOLENCE

Children who witness domestic violence are at increased risk as adults for being battered or battering.[42-44] By identifying children who live in households where domestic violence occurs, creating safe environments, treating and appropriately referring, and enlisting the strengths of parents and children, pediatricians are not only providing for their well being, but also putting an end to a cycle of violence that is passed from generation to generation.

TOOLS FOR PRACTICE

Community Coordination and Advocacy

- *National Children's Alliance* (hotline), National Children's Alliance (800-239-9950).
- *National Domestic Hotline* (hotline), National Domestic Violence Hotline (800-799-SAFE).
- *Children and Domestic Violence State Statutes* (database), US Department of Health and Human Services: Child Welfare Information Gateway (www.childwelfare.gov/systemwide/laws_policies/state/index.cfm).
- *Directory of Crime Victim Services* (Web page), Department of Justice (ovc.ncjrs.org/findvictimservices/).

Engaging Patient and Family

- *Family Conflicts* (fact sheet), American Academy of Pediatrics (www.aap.org/parents.html).
- *Domestic ViolenceSafety Plan: Tips for you and your family* (fact sheets), American Bar Association (www.abanet.org/domviol/safety_tips.html).
- *Expect Respect: Healthy Relationships* (brochure), American Academy of Pediatrics (www.aap.org/bookstore).
- *Preventing Child Abuse* (fact sheet), American Academy of Pediatrics (www.aap.org/healthopics/.childabuse.cfm).

Medical Decision Support

- *AAP Intimate Partner Violence Screening Questions* (questionnaire), American Academy of Pediatrics.
- *Abuse Assessment Screen (AAS),* (questionnaire), Centers for Disease Control and Prevention (www.ispub.-com/ostia/index.php?xmlFilePath=journals/ijapa/vol4n1/violence.xml).
- *American Medical Association recommended 3 screening questions* (questionnaire), American Medical Association.
- *HITS: A Short Domestic Violence Screening Tool* (questionnaire), Kevin Sherin.
- *How to Assess for Domestic Violence,* (questionnaire) Family Violence Prevention Fund.
- *Identifying and responding to domestic violence: consensus recommendations for child and adolescent health* (report), Family Violence Prevention Fund, AAP endorsed (www.endabuse.org/programs/healthcare/files/Pediatric.pdf).
- *Intimate Partner Violence* (fact sheet), Centers for Disease Control and Prevention (www.cdc.gov/ncipc/factsheets/ipvfacts.htm).
- *Questions for Detecting Dating Violence* (questionnaire), Family Violence Prevention Fund. (practice.aap.org/content.aspx?aid=2001).

RELATED WEB SITES

- Centers for Disease Control and Prevention: Violence Prevention (www.cdc.gov/ncipc/dvp/dvp.htm).
- Family Violence Prevention Fund (endabuse.org/).
- Feminist Majority Foundation: Domestic Violence Information Center (www.feminist.org/other/dv/dvhome.html).
- National Children's Alliance (www.nca-online.org/pages/page.asp?page_id=4028).
- US Department of Justice: Office for Victims of Crime (www.ojp.gov/ovc/ovcres/welcome.html).
- *Temper Tantrums: A Normal Part of Growing Up* (brochure), American Academy of Pediatrics (patiented.aap.org).
- *Connected Kids—Teaching Good Behavior: Tips on How to Discipline* (brochure), American Academy of Pediatrics (www.aap.org/bookstore).

AAP POLICY STATEMENTS

American Academy of Pediatrics, Committee on Injury and Poison Prevention. Firearms-related injuries affecting the pediatric population. *Pediatrics*. 2000;105(4):888-895. (aappolicy.aappublications.org/cgi/content/full/pediatrics;105/4/888).

Kairys SW, Johnson CF, American Academy of Pediatrics, Committee on Child Abuse and Neglect. The psychological maltreatment of children. *Pediatrics*. 2002;109(4):e68. (aappolicy.aappublications.org/cgi/content/full/pediatrics;109/4/e68).

American Academy of Pediatrics, Task Force on Violence. The role of the pediatrician in youth violence prevention in clincal practice and at the community level. *Pediatrics*. 1999;103(1):173-181. (aappolicy.aappublications.org/cgi/content/full/pediatrics;103/1/173).

SUGGESTED RESOURCES

Publications

Children's Safety Network. *Domestic Violence: a Directory of Protocols for Health Care Providers*. Newton, MA: Education Development Center; 1992.

Family Violence Prevention Fund. *Identifying and Responding to Domestic Violence: Consensus Recommendations for Child and Adolescent Health*. San Francisco, CA: Family Violence Prevention Fund; 2004. Available at: www.fvpf.org.

Organizations

National Children Alliance (1-800-239-9950; www.nca-online.org)

National Domestic Violence Hotline (1-800-799-SAFE)

Web Sites

American Bar Association, Commission on Domestic Violence (www.abanet.org/domviol/)

Child Welfare Information Gateway, US Department of Health and Human Services, Administration for Children and Families (www.childwelfare.gov/systemwide/laws_policies/statutes/domviolall.pdf)

Domestic Violence Information Center (www.feminist.org/other/dv/dvhome.html)

Family Violence Prevention Fund (www.fvpf.org)

Office for Victims of Crime (ovc.ncjrs.org/findvictimservices/)

US Department of Justice (www.ojp.gov/ovc/help/dv.htm)

REFERENCES

1. Tjaden P, Thoennes N. *Extent, Natures, and Consequences of Intimate Partner Violence*. Washington, DC: National Institute of Justice Statistics; 2000.
2. Bureau of Justice Statistics. *Intimate Partner Violence, 1993-2001*. (NCJ 197838). Washington, DC: Bureau of Justice Statistics; 2003.
3. Wilt S, Olson S. Prevalence of domestic violence in the United States. *J Am Med Womens Assoc*. 1996;51(3):77-82.
4. Bureau of Justice Statistics. *Intimate Partner Violence*. NCJ 178247. Washington, DC: Bureau of Justice Statistics; 2000.
5. US Department of Justice, Bureau of Justice Statistics. Homicide trends in the U.S., Intimate Homicide. Available at: www.ojp.usdoj.gov/bjs/homicide/intimates.htm. Accessed March 4, 2007.
6. McDonald R, Jouriles EN, Ramisetty-Mikler S, et al. Estimating the number of American children living in partner-violent families. *J Fam Psychol*. 2006;20:137-142.
7. Nelson KG. The innocent bystander: the child as the unintended victim of domestic violence involving deadly weapons. *Pediatrics*. 1984;73(2):251-252.
8. Dawson J, Langan P. *Murder in Families*. Washington, DC: Bureau of Justice Statistics; 1994.
9. US Department of Health and Human Services, Advisory Board on Child Abuse and Neglect. A Nation's Shame: Fatal Child Abuse and Neglect in the United States. Available at: ican-ncfr.org/documents/Nations-Shame.pdf. Accessed February 13, 2008.
10. Edelson JL. The overlap between child maltreatment and woman battering. *Violence Against Women*. 1999;5:134-154.
11. Ross SM. Risk of physical abuse to children of spouse abusing parents. *Child Abuse Negl*. 1996;20:589-598.
12. McKibben L, DeVos E, Newberger E. Victimization of mothers of abused children: a controlled study. *Pediatrics*. 1989;84:531-535.
13. Rumm PD, Cummings P, Krauss MR, et al. Identifying spouse abuse as a risk factor for child abuse. *Child Abuse Negl*. 2000;24:1375-1381.
14. US Department of Health and Human Services. Children and Domestic Violence: Summary of State Laws. Available at: www.childwelfare.gov. Accessed February 13, 2008.
15. American College of Obstetricians and Gynecologists. Policy Statement on Domestic Violence. Available at: www.acog.org/. Accessed February 13, 2008.
16. American Medical Association. Policy Statement on Abuse of Spouses, Children, Elderly Persons, and Others at Risk E2.02. Available at: www.ama-assn.org/ama/pub/category/8387.html. Accessed February 13, 2008.
17. American Academy of Pediatrics, Committee on Child Abuse and Neglect. The role of the pediatrician in recognizing and intervening on behalf of abused women. *Pediatrics*. 1998;101(6):1091-1092.
18. US Preventive Services Task Force. Screening for Family and Intimate Partner Violence—Recommendation Statement. Available at: www.ahrq.gov. Accessed February 13, 2008.
19. Trowbridge MF, Sege RD, Olson L, et al. Intentional injury management and prevention in pediatric practice: results from 1998 and 2003 American Academy of Pediatrics Periodic Surveys. *Pediatrics,* 2005;116(4):996-1000.
20. Gadomski AM, Wolff D, Tripp M, et al. Changes in health care providers' knowledge, attitudes, beliefs, and behaviors regarding domestic violence, following a multifaceted intervention. *Acad Med*. 2001;76(10):1045-1052.
21. Erickson MJ, Hill TD, Siegel RM. Barriers to domestic violence screening in the pediatric setting. *Pediatrics*. 2001;108(1):98-102.
22. Johnson CD, Fein JA, Campbell C, et al. Violence prevention in the primary care setting: a program for pediatric residents. *Arch Pediatr Adolesc Med*. 1999;153(5):531-535.
23. Ross SM. Risk of physical abuse to children of spouse abusing parents. *Child Abuse Negl*. 1996;20(7):58.
24. Thompson RS, Krugman R. Screening mothers for intimate partner abuse at well-baby care visits: the right thing to do. *JAMA*. 2001;285(12):1628-1630.
25. Siegel RM, Hill TD, Henderson VA, et al. Screening for domestic violence in the community pediatric setting. *Pediatrics*. 1999;104(4:1): 874-877.
26. Groves BM, Augustyn M, Lee D, et al. *Identifying and Responding to Domestic Violence: Consensus Recommendations for Child and Adolescent Health*. San Francisco, CA: Family Violence Prevention Fund; 2002.
27. Centers for Disease Control and Prevention. Youth Risk Behavior Survey. Available at: www.cdc.gov/HealthyYou/partner/funded/yrbs.htm. Accessed February 13, 2008.
28. Silverman JG, Raj A, Clements K. Dating violence and associated sexual risk and pregnancy among adolescent girls in the United States. *Pediatrics*. 2004;114:e220-e225.

29. Rickert VI, Wiesmann CM, Vaughn RD, et al. Rate and risk factors for sexual violence among an ethnically diverse sample of adolescents. *Arch Pediatr Adolesc Med.* 2004;158:1132-1139.
30. Silverman JG, Raj A, Mucci LA, et al. Dating violence against adolescent girls and associated substance use, unhealthy weight control, sexual risk behavior, pregnancy, and suicidality. *JAMA.* 2001;286:572-579.
31. Freedner N, Freed LH, Yang W, et al. Dating violence among gay, lesbian, and bisexual adolescents: results from a community survey. *J Adolesc Health Care.* 2002;31:469-474.
32. Omar H, Griffith JR. Screening for dating violence: should we screen or not? *J Pediatr Adolesc Gynecol.* 2004;17:53-55.
33. Family Violence Prevention Fund. Personal Safety Plan. Available at: endabuse.org/resources/gethelp/personal_plan.php3. Accessed February 13, 2008.
34. Knapp JF, Dowd MD. Family violence: implications for the pediatrician. *Pediatr Rev.* 1998;19:316-321.
35. Kellerman AL, Rivara FP, Somes G, et al. Gun ownership as a risk factor for homicide in the home. *N Engl J Med.* 1993;329:1084-1091.
36. McFarlane JM, Groff JY, O'Brien JA, et al. Behaviors of children who are exposed and not exposed to intimate partner violence: an analysis of 330 black, white, and Hispanic children. *Pediatrics.* 2003;112(3:1):e202-e207.
37. Graham-Bermann SA, Seng J. Violence exposure and traumatic stress symptoms as a additional predictors of health problems in high-risk children. *J Pediatr.* 2005; 146(3):349-354.
38. Murphy CC, Schei B, Myhr TL, et al. Abuse: a risk factor for low birth weight? A systematic review and meta-analysis. *CMAJ.* May 2001;164(11):1567-1572.
39. Abbott J, Johnson R, Koziol-McLain J, et al. Domestic violence against women: incidence and prevalence in an emergency department population. *JAMA.* 1995;273: 1763-1767.
40. Seng JS, Graham-Bermann SA, Clark MK, et al. Post-traumatic stress disorder and physical comorbidity among female children and adolescents: results from service-use data. *Pediatrics.* 2005;116:e767-e776.
41. McFarlane JM, Groff JY, O'Brien JA, et al. Behaviors of children following a randomized controlled treatment program for their abused mothers. *Issues Compr Pediatr Nurs.* 2005;28(4):195-211.
42. Ehrensaft MK, Cohen P, Brown J, et al. Intergenerational transmission of partner violence: a 20 year prospective study. *J Consult Clin Psychol.* 2003;71:741-753.
43. Bensley L, Van Eenwyk J, Simmons WK. Childhood family violence history and women's risk for intimate partner violence and poor health. *Am J Prev Med.* 2003;25:38-44.
44. Kwong MJ, Bartholomew K, Henderson AJZ, et al. The intergenerational transmission of relationship violence. *J Fam Psychol.* 2003;17:288-301.

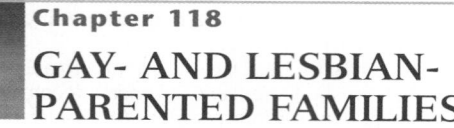

Chapter 118

GAY- AND LESBIAN-PARENTED FAMILIES

Cindy M. Schorzman, MD; Melanie A. Gold, DO

Family structures in the United States, as in much of the world, are changing. The traditional structure of a working father, a homemaker mother, with 1 or more children no longer describes the majority of families in the United States.

BOX 118-1 Glossary of Terms

Gender identity: Personal sense of one's integral maleness or femaleness

Gender role: Behaviors within a culture commonly thought to be associated with maleness or femaleness

Homophobia: Unprovoked fear, distrust, and/or hatred of lesbian, gay, and/or bisexual persons

Sex: Classification as either male or female based on external anatomy such as the penis and testes or vulva

Sexual orientation: Persistent pattern of emotional and/or physical attraction to members of the same or opposite sex. Included are homosexuality (same-sex attractions), bisexuality (attractions to members of both sexes), and heterosexuality (opposite-sex attractions)

Alternate family structures are diverse. Unmarried couples may live together with or without children. Single mothers and fathers, stepparents, and blended families may be created by design, by divorce, or by death. These family structures may include gay men and lesbian women, with or without children.

Recent estimates of children in the United States with at least one gay or lesbian parent range from 1 to 10 million.[1] According to US Census data from 2000, same-gender couples live in over 99% of US counties, and nearly one quarter of all same-gender couples are raising children.[2] These estimates are limited by barriers to obtaining accurate numbers, in part, because many gay and lesbian parents fear discrimination and do not report their sexual orientation.

Specific research on issues regarding gay and lesbian parenting has been driven by legal issues, chiefly concerning custody.[3] This research has focused on assessing the development and well-being of children raised by gay or lesbian parents. (Box 118-1 contains a glossary of terms.).

CHILD DEVELOPMENT IN THE CONTEXT OF GAY- AND LESBIAN-PARENTED FAMILIES

No consistent differences exist in the psychological profiles of children raised by gay and lesbian parents compared with children raised by heterosexual parents. During the 1990s, research became increasingly available on children conceived in the context of gay and lesbian relationships.

Children who have gay or lesbian parents do not differ from children who have heterosexual parents in terms of psychological health, social relationships, or cognitive or emotional functioning.[4-6] The best predictors of child behavior problems are higher levels of parental stress and interparental conflict.[7]

The sexual orientation of parents has not been found to affect the gender identity of their children.[4,8,9] Furthermore, adolescent sexual orientation is similar among adolescents raised by gay or lesbian parents and those raised by heterosexual parents.[3,4,10] Children raised by lesbian mothers are more likely to explore same-gender sexual relationships, particularly if their childhood family environment is characterized by an openness and acceptance of lesbian and gay relationships. These children are no more likely than the children of heterosexual mothers to identify themselves as gay or lesbian.[5]

Clinicians should be aware that the psychological experience might differ for children raised in heterosexual versus homosexual parenting environments. The greatest difference reported is bullying. Although no overall increase in stigmatization may exist, children of nonheterosexual couples are more likely than those of heterosexual couples to be teased and to be concerned about being harassed. Some children experience shame because of conflicts between loyalty to their parent and the perceived need to conceal their parents' sexual orientation for self-preservation.[11]

The conclusion that research to date demonstrates few discernible differences in parenting based on parental sexual orientation is not universally accepted. Outspoken critics of the literature have highlighted the limitations of these studies. Important limitations included small sample size (these studies may be more likely to conclude that no differences exist when some differences do indeed exist), lack of generalizability (participants were mostly lesbian, white, well-educated, and upper-middle class), lack of randomization of study populations, and lack of appropriate comparison groups.[12]

However, no studies have been published in the peer-reviewed literature that demonstrate differences in a child's development based on the sexual orientation of their parents or show any evidence that gay and lesbian parenting causes significant deleterious effects on children. Taken together, the overwhelming numbers of studies (despite their limitations) demonstrate no differences in children's development based on the sexual orientation of their parent or parents.[13]

The American Academy of Pediatrics (AAP) Committee on Psychosocial Aspects of Child and Family Health reviewed the available data on children of gay and lesbian parents and published a technical report in 2002 with a policy statement supporting co-parent or 2nd-parent adoption by same-gender parents. Their conclusion was that "a growing body of scientific literature demonstrates that children who grow up with one or two gay and/or lesbian parents fare as well in emotional, cognitive, social, and sexual functioning as do children whose parents are heterosexual," and that "children's optimal development seems to be influenced more by the nature of the relationships and interactions within the family unit than by the particular structural form it takes."[14] Despite some reservations based on the limitations of the studies, such as those noted previously, the Committee believed that the weight of the available evidence was strong enough to demonstrate "that there is no systematic difference between gay and nongay parents in emotional health, parenting skills, and attitudes toward parenting."[14]

SOCIAL RELATIONSHIPS AND DISCLOSURE

All children, especially as they reach school age, must develop a wide range of relationships outside their nuclear family. Children who have gay or lesbian parents may be assumed to be homosexual and experience stigmatization by peers when their parents' sexual orientations become known. The difference between dominant cultural values in the community and the family constellation may be distressing to children and add to their social isolation and uncomfortable relationships with peers.[15] Gay and lesbian parents frequently fear that school staff will treat their children differently if they disclose their sexual orientation. As a result, many parents help children learn *differential disclosure*—to be open about their parents' sexual orientation to some people but not to others—so that harassment and social isolation can be minimized. Parents should understand that both secrecy and disclosure represent potential burdens for their children.

Clinicians can act as supportive listeners for families with difficult interactions with their school system. Some clinicians with longstanding school relationships may choose to act as intermediaries between the family and the school to help make the educational environment more supportive. They can educate child care providers and teachers and encourage schools to include information about diverse family structures in their libraries and curricula. Clinicians can also encourage families to develop a social support network in the interest of their children. In many larger cities, an active network of gay and lesbian parents work to create an environment of peer support in which their children feel more accepted than they might in other social contexts. Parent-child discussion or playgroups, story hours, and periodic communal meals have helped some parents and children seeking mutual support.

LEGAL ISSUES

Controversy regarding securing legal parental rights for gay and lesbian parents is ongoing.

Legislation constantly shifts the parameters of parental rights and responsibilities. Currently, the spectrum ranges from co-parent adoption being recognized by statute, in states such as California, Connecticut, and Vermont, to laws such as those in the state of Florida, which prohibit single gay men and lesbian women, as well as same-gender couples, from adopting. Many states have no formal statutory policy on adoption by a gay or lesbian, and this ambiguity often leaves decisions in the hands of individual judges.[16]

Because courts have continuing legal authority to protect children until they reach majority (18 years of age), questions of custody can be reopened in any state in which the child resides, leaving the family vulnerable if they move to another state. If a court finds it to be in the child's best interest, then it can remove the child from the home when parental custody is challenged (eg, by a former spouse or grandparents), particularly when a gay or lesbian parent's sexual orientation was unknown in a previous custody decision. Furthermore, even with court precedents declaring that parents cannot be deprived of child custody based solely on parental sexual orientation, a heterosexual parent is still more likely than a gay or lesbian parent to be granted custody and visitation rights unless the heterosexual parent is unavailable or obviously unfit.

In the frequent circumstance that only one of the same-gender couple is legally recognized as a child's parent, the clinician should clarify how responsibility for the medical decisions and consent for treatment for the child will be shared and document this in the medical record. In the event of serious injury, illness, death, or voluntary separation of the legal parent, a prior written agreement giving the other parent power of attorney in making medical decisions for the child is necessary.

In general, when gay or lesbian couples first contemplate raising a child together, they should agree in writing on issues concerning child custody, support, and consent for treatment. Curry, Clifford, and Leonard give guidelines for writing agreements that specify parental rights and responsibilities.[17] Without a written agreement, nonbiological or nonadoptive parents may have difficulty proving their status as parents.

CLINICAL ISSUES IN PROVIDING PEDIATRIC CARE

The challenge for the clinician who cares for these children lies in addressing practical concerns faced by individual families. Meeting the needs of children of gay and lesbian parents means addressing the needs of the children themselves, as well as understanding the particular issues within the context of their family as a whole. Gay or lesbian parents may choose not to identify their sexual orientation to their child's clinician. They may worry that latent homophobia or bias in professional or nonprofessional staff will jeopardize the care their children receive or that the clinician will not honor their confidentiality, particularly if the parents are concerned about legal threats to their custody rights. The challenge for the clinician caring for these children often lies in creating an environment in which the family feels comfortable enough to disclose and discuss their sexual orientation and family constellation. Health care professionals have traditionally received little or no training about homosexuality.[18-20] In fact, evidence suggests that gay and lesbian adults find the health care system to be unresponsive and sometimes antagonistic to their unique needs and concerns.[18,21,22]

Little information exists about how lesbian and gay parents view pediatric care. One study found that most gay and lesbian parents perceived that their children received pediatric care that was affirming, supportive, and satisfactory. However, many specific deficiencies were noted, such as heterosexist assumptions on office forms, exclusion of the nonbiological parent from the evaluation and treatment process, and explicit insensitivity to particular family involvements.[22] In addition, parents who had not disclosed their sexual orientation to their child's clinician had concerns that such disclosure might compromise their child's care, result in negative judgments about their parenting, and infringe on their confidentiality. They described a significant number of concerns regarding health care providers such as prejudice against their children, providing disparate care, lack of communication about the child's health with the nonbiological parent, and accusing parental lifestyle as the cause of any child physical or behavioral problems.[22]

Clinicians should create a safe and inclusive environment for same-gender parents and their children.

BOX 118-2 Questions to Clarify the Family Constellation

- Is there anything about your family that would be helpful for me to know?
- Who are the adults who make up your family?
- Who are the important people in your child's life?
- Who lives at home? What is your relationship with each child caretaker?
- By what name does your child call each family member?
- Who are the other important members of your family or support system who help care for your child?
- Do you share parenting responsibilities with anyone else?
- Who helps you with parenting?
- Is there anyone else who participates in parenting?
- Do(es) the biological parent(s), if not part of the current constellation, have any involvement in child care?
- Which of your child's caretakers can give legal consent for medical care?
- Do any of your child's biological relatives have any medical conditions?

Establishing a supportive health care environment requires, first and foremost, that clinicians examine their own attitudes toward gay and lesbian parenting. Health care providers "who cannot reconcile their personal beliefs with their professional obligation to provide supportive, understanding, and respectful care to gay and lesbian families should recognize this limitation and refer these families to a clinician who can better meet their needs."[22] Once the clinician has addressed these issues personally, then health care staff attitudes should be similarly addressed with interventions such as diversity training and strict guidelines regarding confidentiality.

Clinicians should convey their support of all forms of families and avoid assuming that all parents are heterosexual. The office environment should reflect a supportive, safe environment for children of diverse families. Hospital and office policies regarding the use of gender-neutral language and the inclusion of nonbiological parents during the child's office visits should be discussed and enforced. Box 118-2 illustrates examples of questions to clarify family constellation in nonheterosexist ways. In their work, Perrin and Kulkin identified several changes in the office or hospital environment that demonstrate support for a diversity of family structures. These efforts include displaying posters, magazines, books, and pamphlets that portray a wide range of family constructs. A nondiscrimination policy, prominently displayed in the waiting area, can do much to assure both gay and lesbian parents and adolescents that the office is a safe environment for disclosure of sensitive issues (Figure 118-1). Standard office forms should be modified to include gender-neutral terms, such as parent, caregiver, and family member.[20,23] Other resources should be available in the office, such as books about gay and lesbian parenting, information regarding community and national

Office Nondiscrimination Policy

This office appreciates diversity and does not discriminate based on race, national origin, age, religion, ability, sexual orientation, or perceived gender.

Figure 118-1 Example of nondiscrimination policy for the pediatric office.

resources, and standard medical forms such as medical power of attorney designation.

As the child grows and develops, in addition to standard anticipatory guidance issues, particular concerns tend to surface at different developmental stages. In the preschool period, common concerns include how to explain the composition of their own family and the methods of reproduction.[24] Gold and colleagues suggest that early childhood "is a good time to initiate explanations to the child about his or her own origin and to introduce concepts of the variety of loving relationships."[21] Clinicians can help parents empower their children to deal with these issues by encouraging them to allow the child to control the information they disclose to friends or teachers; parents should simultaneously help their children prepare for the possible negative consequences of disclosure.[20]

Parents should be encouraged to help their children come up with their own creative ways to describe their family in positive terms.[22] A gay or lesbian couple might celebrate their essential roles as two loving supportive parents while additionally recognizing the other important adult role models and caretakers who comprise the child's extended family. For example, in the context of a lesbian couple with children, one approach to Father's Day might be to redefine it as a celebration of the child's male role models, such as writing cards to an uncle or close male family friend.

The transition to school years also poses particular challenges for children from a nontraditional family background.[22] For parents and children alike, this transition involves whether to disclose their nontraditional family status to teachers and the families of the child's friends. During the early school years, peer acceptance and teasing often become concerns. In the National Lesbian Families Study, 18% of children had experienced some form of discrimination by age 5, and 43% had experienced homophobia by age 10.[24,25] Empathic listening, role playing about how to respond to teasing, and providing information to parents and their children through support groups can assist both parents and children in coping with stigma and discrimination.[21,23]

During adolescence, issues of sexuality tend to come to the forefront regardless of family structure; teenagers in households with lesbian and gay parents are certainly no exception, and they may have their own unique challenges. Early adolescents may feel marginalized and stigmatized by being seen as part of a nontraditional family.[21] Teenagers may feel guilty, torn between their loyalty to their family and pride in their family structure, and their intense desire to form and maintain relationships and fit in with their peers. Health care providers can help adolescents and their parents by listening in a nonjudgmental fashion and by offering lists of resources and support groups.[21] Although individual situations vary, some evidence supports encouraging adolescents to disclose their nontraditional family status to their friends. Gershon and colleagues found that adolescents who disclosed their mother's lesbianism to their friends reported closer friendships and higher self-esteem than those who did not.[26]

To meet the ever-changing needs of their patients and their families, clinicians should have available a list of local and national support groups and community resources (see Tools for Practice). They might also consider taking a proactive approach in their patient's lives by not only providing a safe, nurturing office environment, but also by taking steps in the community to help counteract the generalized homophobia that children of gay and lesbian parents continually face.

PHYSICIAN ADVOCACY

Although no evidence has been found that children raised by gay or lesbian parents will develop abnormally or be maladjusted any more than other children, these children may be faced with criticism and isolation, which may affect their self-esteem. Clinicians have an opportunity to help change social attitudes and restrictive legal codes that are damaging to their patients with gay and lesbian parents. Clinicians who care for these children should be informed about community resources and may choose to be available as consultants to schools and to gay and lesbian support groups. They can learn which community and national programs are receptive and supportive of alternative family lifestyles and can provide guidance to gay and lesbian parents regarding child care and school selection. Clinicians can also provide a bibliography of books for children and parents and a list of local and national resource groups. Above all, clinicians have the opportunity and the responsibility to support and advise all families in achieving their maximal nurturing potential.

CONCLUSION

Children will flourish in various family environments as long as these settings include adequate nurturance and guidance for optimal development. Although no data have been found to suggest that children with gay or lesbian parents are different from other children with regard to their cognitive, psychosocial, and sexual development, these children and their families face social challenges that clinicians can help address. These challenges are best addressed within the context of the child's life as a whole, and the routine medical care of children and adolescents should not be overshadowed by their nontraditional family status. The diversity of the family structures of the gay and lesbian community should be recognized, and anticipatory guidance and care should be tailored to individual needs.

The authors gratefully acknowledge the expert contributions of Debra L. Bogen, MD, and Mark S. Friedman, PhD.

TOOLS FOR PRACTICE

Community Coordination and Advocacy

- *The Effects of Marriage, Civil Union and Domestic Partnership Statutes and Amendments on the Legal, Financial and Psychosocial Health and Well-Being of Children* (article), American Academy of Pediatrics (www.aap.org/securemoc/docs/pediatrics_v118_349.pdf).

Engaging Patients and Family

- *Gay, Lesbian or Bisexual Parents* (brochure), American Academy of Pediatrics (www.aap.org/bookstore).

Medical Decision Support

- *Questions to Clarify the Family Constellation* (questionnaire), American Academy of Pediatrics.

Practice Management

- *Consent by Proxy for Nonurgent Pediatric Care Form*, American Academy of Pediatrics (aappolicy.aappublications.org/cgi/content/full/pediatrics;112/5/1186).

RELATED WEB SITES

- COLAGE: Children of Lesbians and Gays Everywhere (www.colage.org).
- Family Pride Coalition (formerly Gay and Lesbian Parents Coalition International [GLPCI]) (www.familypride.org).
- Human Rights Campaign (www.hrc.org/familynet).
- Pinkbooks (www/pinkbooks.com).
- Parents of Friends of Lesbians and Gays (www.pflag.org).
- Families Like Ours (www.familieslikeours.org/modules/news/).
- Gay, Lesbian and Straight Education Network (www.glsen.org/cgi-bin/iowa/home.html).
- Rainbow Families (www.rainbowfamilies.org).

SELECTED BOOKS AND RESOURCES FOR FAMILIES

Stories of Lesbian, Gay, Bisexual, and Transgender Families

Drucker J. *Families of Value*. New York, NY: Plenum Press; 1998. A collection of stories depicting LGBT parents and their children.

Gillespie P, ed. Kaeser G, photog. *Love Makes a Family: Portraits of Lesbian, Gay, Bisexual, and Transgender Parents and Their Families*. Amherst, MA: University of Massachusetts Press; 1999. Combines interviews and photographs to document the experiences of LGBT parents and their children.

Herrera D, Seyda B, photog. *Women in Love: Portraits of Lesbian Mothers & Their Families*. Boston, MA: Bulfinch Press; 1998. A collection of photographs and stories of lesbian mothers and their families.

Rizzo C, Schneiderman J, Schweig L, et al, eds. *All The Ways Home*. Norwich, VT: New Victoria Publishers; 1995. A collection of stories written for and by lesbian and gay parents exploring what it means to be a parent in the LGBT community.

Strah D, Margolis S. *Gay Dads: A Celebration of Fatherhood*. Putnam, MA: JP Tarcher; 2003. The stories of 24 families, including family-building resources for gay men.

Coming out:

MacPike L. *There's Something I've Been Meaning to Tell You*. Tallahassee, FL: Naiad Press; 1989. True-life stories from 25 lesbians and gay parents who have come out to their children.

Legal issues:

Curry H, Clifford D, Hertz F. *A Legal Guide For Lesbian and Gay Couples*. 13th ed. Berkeley, CA: Nolo Press; 2005. An excellent resource for all lesbian and gay couples; includes information on custody, parental rights, and domestic partner benefits.

Lambda Legal Defense and Education Fund. A national organization focusing on full recognition of the civil rights of LGBT people, including legal resources such as examples of hospital visitation documentation for LGBT family members. Available at: www.lambdalegal.org/cgi-bin/iowa/index.html.

American Civil Liberties Union. A national organization with state-by-state reference information regarding legislation affecting LGBT families. Available at: www.aclu.org/lgbt/index.html.

The Evan B. Donaldson Adoption Institute. Resources regarding adoption, including specific section on gay and lesbian adoption. Available at: www.adoptioninstitute.org/index.php.

Parenting resources:

Davis L, Keyser J. *Becoming The Parent You Want To Be: A Sourcebook of Strategies for the First Five Years*. New York, NY: Broadway Books; 1997. A guide to parenting that addresses a broad range of issues including toilet training, punishment, parenting with a partner, and gender roles.

Clunis DM, Green GD. *The Lesbian Parenting Book: A Guide to Creating Families and Raising Children*. Washington, DC: Seal Press; 2003. Detailed, chapter-by-chapter information on each stage of parenthood and child development.

Martin A. *Lesbian and Gay Parenting Handbook*. New York, NY: Harper Collins; 1993. A guide to parenting, with many examples of gay and lesbian parents and their children.

Books For Children

Aldrich A, Motz M. *How My Family Came to Be: Daddy, Papa and Me*. Oakland, CA: New Family Press; 2003. For ages 4-8. Loving story of how two men and a baby came together to make a family.

de Haan L, Nijland S. *King & King*. Berkeley, CA: Tricycle Press; 2000. For ages 4-8. A prince "who has never cared much for princesses" finds true love with another prince.

Newman L. *Heather Has Two Mommies*. 10th ed. Los Angeles, CA: Alyson Publications; 2000. For ages 2-6. Originally self-published in 1989, the story of a little girl named Heather and her two lesbian mothers.

Parnell P, Richardson J. *And Tango Makes Three*. New York, NY: Simon & Schuster Children's Publishing; 2005. For ages 4-8. This tale is based on a true story about Roy and Silo, two male penguins living in New York City's Central Park Zoo who raise a penguin daughter.

AAP POLICY STATEMENT

American Academy of Pediatrics, Perrin EC, and the Committee on Psychosocial Aspects of Child and Family Health. Technical Report: Coparent or 2nd-parent adoption by same-sex parents. *Pediatrics*. 2002;109(2):341-344. (aappolicy.aappublications.org/cgi/content/full/pediatrics;109/2/341).

REFERENCES

1. Patterson CJ, Friel LV. Sexual orientation and fertility. In: Bently G, Mascie-Taylor N. *Infertility in the Modern World*. Cambridge, UK: Cambridge University Press; 2000.
2. Simmons T, O'Connell M. US Census Bureau. Married-Couple and Unmarried-Partner Households: 2000. Available at: www.census.gov/prod/2003pubs/censr-5.pdf. Accessed December 18, 2006.
3. Patterson CJ. Children of lesbian and gay parents. *Child Dev*. 1992;63:1025-1042.
4. Allen M, Burrell N. Comparing the impact of homosexual and heterosexual parents on children: meta-analysis of existing research. *J Homosex*. 1996;32:19-35.
5. Golombok S, Tasker F, Murray C. Children raised in fatherless families from infancy: family relationships and the socioemotional development of children of lesbian and single heterosexual mothers. *J Child Psychol Psychiatry*. 1997;38:783-791.
6. Flaks D, Ficher I, Masterpasqua F, et al. Lesbians choosing motherhood: a comparative study of lesbian and heterosexual parents and their children. *Dev Psychol*. 1995; 31:105-114.
7. Chan RW, Raboy B, Patterson CJ. Psychosocial adjustment among children conceived via donor insemination by lesbian and heterosexual mothers. *Child Dev*. 1998; 69(2):443-457.
8. Brewaeys A, Ponjaert I, Van Hall EV, et al. Donor insemination: child development and family functioning in lesbian mother families. *Hum Reprod*. 1997;12(6): 1349-1359.
9. Tasker F, Golombok S. Adults raised as children in lesbian families. *Am J Orthopsychiatry*. 1995;65:203-215.
10. Bailey JM, Bobrow D, Wolfe M, et al. Sexual orientation of adult sons of gay fathers. *Dev Psychol*. 1995;31: 124-129.
11. O'Connell A. Voices from the heart: the developmental impact of a mother's lesbianism on her adolescent children. *Smith Coll Stud Soc Work*. 1993;63:281-299.
12. Cameron P, Cameron K, Landess T. Errors by the American Psychiatric Association, the American Psychological Association, and the National Educational Association in representing homosexuality in amicus briefs about Amendment 2 to the U.S. Supreme Court. *Psychol Rep*. 1996;79:383-404.
13. Golombok S. Adoption by lesbian couples. *BMJ*. 2002; 324:1407-1408.
14. Perrin EC. Technical report: coparent or second-parent adoption by same-sex parents. *Pediatrics*. 2002;109: 341-344.
15. Casper V, Schultz S, Wickens E. Breaking the silences: lesbian and gay parents and the schools. *Teach Coll Rec*. 1992;94(1):109-137.
16. Human Rights Campaign. Adoption Laws: State by State. Available at: www.hrc.org/issues/parenting/adoptions/ 2375.htm. Accessed February 14, 2008.
17. Curry H, Clifford D, Leonard R. *A Legal Guide for Lesbian and Gay Couples*. 7th ed. Berkeley, CA: Nolo Press; 1993.
18. Harrison AE. Primary care of lesbian and gay patients: educating ourselves and our students. *Fam Med*. 1996; 28:10-23.
19. Kelley TF, Langsang D. Pediatric residency training and the needs of gay, lesbian, and bisexual youth. *J Gay Lesbian Med Assoc*. 1996;3(1):5-9.
20. Perrin EC. *Sexual Orientation in Child and Adolescent Health Care*. New York, NY: Plenum Publishers; 2002.
21. Gold MA, Perrin EC, Futterman D, et al. Children of gay or lesbian parents. *Pediatr Rev*. 1994;15: 354-358.
22. Perrin EC, Kulkin H. Pediatric care for children whose parents are gay or lesbian. *Pediatrics*. 1996;97:629-635.
23. Ahmann E. Working with families having parents who are gay or lesbian. *Pediatr Nurs*. 1999;25:531-535.
24. Gartrell N, Banks A, Reed N, et al. The National Lesbian Family Study: 3. Interviews with mothers of five-year-olds. *Am J Orthopsychiatry*. 2000;70:542-548.
25. Gartrell N, Deck A, Rodas C, et al. The National Lesbian Family Study: 4. Interviews with the 10-year old children. *Am J Orthopsychiatry*. 2000;75:518-524.
26. Gershon TD, Tschann JM, Jemerin JM. Stigmatization, self-esteem, and coping among the adolescent children of lesbian mothers. *J Adolesc Health*. 1999;24:437-445.

Chapter 119

HOMELESSNESS AND THE FAMILY

Peter G. Sherman, MD; Rosemarie A. Pezzullo, MD

Although homelessness brings to mind the stereotype of a man panhandling on a street corner, in fact, single women and their children comprise a significant proportion of people who are homeless. Pediatricians will likely encounter children in their practices who are experiencing or have experienced homelessness. Knowledge of a patient's past and present housing status is important to clinical care. Homelessness can affect the health, psychologic, and developmental well being of a child and can present barriers to accessing health care and adherence to treatment.

NUMBERS OF HOMELESS

Although homelessness is well substantiated as a major problem for many communities, determining exactly how many people are homeless is difficult because comprehensive studies are dated. One of the best approximations uses data extrapolated from the National Survey of Homeless Assistance Providers and Clients by the US Census. This study surveyed homeless service providers and estimates that 1% of the US population experiences homelessness each year, and 39% of homeless individuals are children.[1] This estimate translates into 3.5 million homeless individuals each year, of whom more than 1.3 million are children. However, this study markedly underestimates the number of homeless individuals because it counts only those connected to homeless programs.

Trends in homelessness can be difficult to monitor because no mechanism exists for tracking this population. The US Conference of Mayors has collected data on people who are homeless since 1990 in selected cities and provides a surrogate for monitoring trends. Encouragingly, the demand for emergency shelter has been decreasing since 2002.[2] The percentage of homeless families with children peaked in 2002 at 41% and dropped to 33% in 2005.[1] Whether this trend is a significant reversal of the decade-long trend of increasing numbers of homeless families remains to be seen.

Homeless youth, in contrast to homeless families, are individuals younger than 18 who leave their place of residence without permission of a parent or legal guardian. An important subgroup, throwaway youth, consists of persons who are asked to leave home or are not allowed back home by a parent or guardian.[3] The US Department of Justice estimated in 1999 that over 1.6 million youth were runaways or throwaways. Seventy-one percent of these youths were categorized as being in immediate danger because of factors such as substance dependency, sexual or physical abuse, living in an area of criminal activity, or young age (13 or younger).[4] According to the US Conference of Mayors, the percentage of the homeless population that consisted of runaway youth between 1990 and 2005 varied from a low of 3% to a high of 7%. In 2005, 3% of homeless individuals were youth.[2]

CAUSES OF HOMELESSNESS

A 2005 study by the Vera Institute of Justice found that families who entered the New York City shelter system experienced remarkably high rates of disruption in their lives in the 5 years before becoming homeless. Sixty-nine percent had a job loss, 43% had physical health problems, 39% had emotional health problems, and 21% were victims of domestic violence.[5]

Poverty

A clear and direct correlation exists between poverty and homelessness. The majority of homelessness in the United States is caused by the gap between income and the cost of housing. The US Department of Housing and Urban Development places families who rent, have incomes less than 50% of the median family income in their community, pay more than one half of their income for housing, and do not receive federal housing assistance in the category of worst-case housing needs. These families are at the highest risk for becoming homeless. Since this statistic was tracked in 1991, approximately 5% of households have fallen within this category.[6] Children reside in 36% of households with worst-case housing needs and 41% of these families have at least 1 full-time worker.[6]

Full-time employment is not a guarantee against homelessness. More and more individuals are employed by service industries, such as hotels and restaurants, that pay minimum wage and often provide only part-time work, with few or no benefits. This circumstance puts housing out of reach for many families. The federal office of Housing and Urban Development calculates fair market rent as "the amount that would be needed to pay the gross rent (rent plus utilities) of privately owned, decent, and safe housing of a modest (non-luxury) nature with suitable amenities."[7] The National Low-Income Housing Coalition defines housing wage as the "hourly wage necessary to pay the fair market rent for a 2-bedroom home while spending no more than 30% of income on housing costs."[8] Nationally, the housing wage in 2005 was $15.78, with a range of $8.10 to $29.54.[9] The national housing wage is more than triple the minimum federal wage.

Housing Shortage

A serious gap continues in the number of units needed to house families in this country that has been exacerbated by the federal government's decreased role in low-income housing over the last 20 years. Federal support for low-income housing fell 49% between 1980 and 2003,[9] and only 30% of persons who are eligible for low-income housing assistance receive this subsidy.[10] Since 1995, over 200,000 subsidized housing units have been lost.[11]

Domestic Violence

The clinician needs to be aware that domestic violence is an important cause of homelessness for families. Fifty percent of cities surveyed in 2005 identified domestic violence as the leading cause of homelessness.[2]

EFFECT OF HOMELESSNESS ON CHILDREN'S HEALTH

Homeless children are 2.5 times as likely to have health problems and 3 times as likely to have severe health problems as compared with housed children. In 1 study, the most common health problems identified in the homeless children were asthma (33%), problems with vision (13%), mental health problems (9%), and acute illness (8%). Lack of medical coverage was evident in 58% of homeless children compared with 15% of housed children.[12]

Health risks related to homelessness begin during the prenatal period. Statistics show an increase in morbidity and mortality caused by a lack of prenatal care, poor nutrition, stress, and exposure to violence; and increased substance abuse. One study revealed that preterm birth occurred in 20% of infants born to homeless mothers. The risk of a homeless woman giving birth to an infant weighing less than 2 kg was 6 to 7 times that of the control group.[13] Severity of homelessness predicts low birthweight and preterm births beyond its correlation with delayed prenatal care and other risk factors.[14] Among pregnant homeless adolescents, a frequent history of severe sexual abuse and early injection drug abuse correlates with poor health outcome in the newborn.[15]

Homeless Children and Rates of Illness

Homeless children are sick 4 times as often as middle-class children. They also experience higher rates of acute and chronic illness. Homeless children suffer from twice as many ear infections, 4 times as many asthma attacks, and 5 times more stomach problems.[16] They are also at increased risk for elevated lead levels.[17]

Because homeless families live in crowded conditions, the risk of acquiring upper respiratory tract infections, diarrhea, and otitis media is increased. One study revealed that homeless children had a 50% increased rate of otitis media when compared with the national average (27% versus 18%). This increase was probably the result of greater exposure to upper respiratory tract infections and second-hand smoke. Because of a lack of consistent medical care among the homeless, otitis media is often undiagnosed and untreated, leading to possible hearing loss.[18] The prevalence of asthma among a random sample of homeless children in New York City was found to be 39.8%, more than 6 times the rate for other children. Asthma in homeless children was more likely to be severe and undertreated.[19] The risk of homeless children acquiring ectoparasitic infections such as lice and scabies is also increased.[20]

Homeless Adolescents

Among homeless adolescents, the incidence and prevalence of human immunodeficiency virus infection, chlamydia, herpes, and hepatitis B and C is increased. This increase may be caused by lack of access to educational and prevention programs, lack of condom use, and increased drug use.[21] Homeless youth are at high risk of substance abuse, mental illness, and blood-borne infections.[22] Mortality among homeless youth is approximately 11 times the expected rate based on age and sex and is mainly caused by suicide and drug overdose.[23]

Homeless Children and Nutrition

Homeless children are 3 times more likely to experience iron deficiency anemia caused by poor nutrition.[24] One study reported a 52% rate of obesity, 45% rate of anemia, and a 36% rate of failure to thrive among homeless children.[25] Given the importance of adequate nutrition for development in the infant and young child and the risk factors associated with obesity in later life, these findings are disturbing. According to the National Health Care for Homeless Providers, the rates of poor dentition and dental caries are approximately 10 times greater among homeless children than among the general population.[26]

EFFECT OF HOMELESSNESS ON CHILDREN'S BEHAVIORAL HEALTH

Developmental, educational, and psychological outcomes in homeless children are equally worrisome. Compared with other children, homeless children are 4 times as likely to have developmental delays, twice as likely to have learning disabilities, and twice as likely to repeat a grade because of frequent absences and school changes.[27] The majority of both homeless mothers and their preschool children exhibit delays in at least one of the following areas: auditory comprehension, verbal expression, reading, and writing.[28]

School and Homeless Children

Buckner compared the school experiences and academic achievement of adolescents in families who experienced homelessness with permanently housed adolescents whose families received public assistance. Formerly homeless students had more school mobility, were more likely to repeat a grade, and had worse school experiences by maternal report and lower plans for post-secondary education by self-report. Homelessness was associated with declines in achievement during the period of maximal residential disruption. Days absent from school were hypothesized as the mediating link between homelessness and academic achievement.[29]

In an effort to improve the educational opportunities of homeless children, the McKinney-Vento Homeless Assistance Act of 2001 was created. It requires that children and youths experiencing homelessness are immediately enrolled in school and have educational opportunities equal to those of their nonhomeless peers. The statute requires every public school district and charter holder to designate a *homeless liaison* to ensure that homeless students are identified and that their needs are met.[30]

Homeless Children and Behavioral Health

Twenty percent of homeless preschoolers have emotional problems requiring intervention. One third of homeless school-age children have a major mental disorder that interferes with daily activity compared with 19% in the general population. Forty-seven percent have anxiety and depression compared with 18% in the general population, and 36% are aggressive compared with 17% in the general population. Less than one third who might benefit from treatment are receiving assistance.[31]

Evidence that homeless youth may suffer disproportionately from behavioral and psychological problems is persuasive. Trauma is a common experience among homeless youth, and once homeless, an increase can be found in the number of psychological diagnoses, including drug and alcohol diagnoses. Trauma resulting from exposure to violence may be a mediating factor, with 83% of homeless youth older than 12 years who are exposed to violence and 25% having witnessed violence in their family.[31]

The risk of sexual and physical victimization is increased among homeless adolescents, leading to increased risk of posttraumatic stress syndrome.[32] One half of homeless youth report being physically abused, and one third experience sexual abuse.[33] Homeless adolescents are 6 times more likely to meet criteria for conduct disorder, major depressive disorder, posttraumatic stress syndrome, alcohol abuse, or drug abuse.[34] After homelessness, involvement in criminal activity is common.[35]

Clinical Care Issues

Once a family is identified as homeless, the most important issue is ascertaining that all children are living in a safe environment. If not, then the family should be assisted with making contacts that will enable them to access a local family homeless shelter system, welfare agency, or charitable institution that can provide temporary housing.

All children need a thorough medical, developmental, and psychological history and a physical examination to identify medical conditions that result from homelessness, the factors leading to homelessness, and the lack of access to medical care. Particular attention should be paid to health care maintenance, including immunizations and lead testing, and to the diagnosis and treatment of chronic medical conditions. Clinic care that is offered to children while they are homeless should be comprehensive, meeting the criteria of a medical home. In addition to primary pediatric care, clinic care should include 24-hour telephone access, referral to subspecialty care, developmental and psychological evaluation and treatment, medication and medical devices, and case management.[17]

Asthma is overrepresented among homeless children. Children often require aggressive treatment, and parents may need comprehensive education to avoid hospitalization, excessive emergency department use, and school absenteeism for their children. A child who is not sleeping at night or keeping other family members awake because of coughing can exacerbate the stress of being homeless.

If a family is living in a shelter, then children may have frequent acute illnesses as a result of living in close quarters with other families. In treating upper respiratory infection, gastroenteritis, otitis media, and tinea, a helpful approach would be to instruct parents about infection control measures in addition to applying standard treatment regimens. Outbreaks of certain illnesses, such as varicella or hepatitis, may require contacting shelter personnel or the local department of health to initiate infection-control measures.

It is important when a parent brings in a child who has a minor acute illness to use this visit as an opportunity to perform a thorough medical assessment and initiate any needed treatment and referral. Follow-up can be problematic for homeless families, and any delay in initiating a comprehensive treatment plan may impede needed health care.

In addition to referrals that need to be made for developmental assessment or psychological problems found in children, referring parents for counseling may also be necessary. Some families are homeless because of severe parental mental health problems or substance abuse. A parent may become depressed as a result of being homeless. All of these issues need to be addressed so as to optimize the environment needed for a child's well being.

One of the most common reasons for a woman and her children becoming homeless is domestic violence. Women must be queried about this issue. (See Chapter 117, Domestic Violence and the Family.) Clinicians should be aware of local resources for victims of domestic violence so that any necessary referrals can be made. Moving a family into a domestic violence shelter may be necessary if the batterer is a threat.

Chronic medical conditions are often not treated properly because families who are homeless frequently move, which results in being cared for by multiple providers, thus preventing continuity of care. This circumstance leads to underreferral, overreferral, and undertreatment. A child may be referred multiple times to specialists for the same problem, with a diagnostic workup being restarted with each referral. Because of this delay, the specialist often never reaches the point of implementing an adequate treatment plan. A useful approach is to initiate the medical workup in the primary care setting and provide education about these issues while the patient is homeless to allow for the orderly transfer of medical care when the family enters permanent housing.

When a family is moving out of a shelter into permanent housing, they will often need assistance in locating medical care in their new community. This involves helping to identify a new medical home and transferring medical records to the new practitioner.

Long-Term Effects of Homelessness on Women and Children

Whether the experience of homelessness, in itself, has long-term effects on the health of a child is unknown. Although differences in the psychological and developmental characteristics of homeless children compared with housed-poor children have been identified, whether this difference is the result of events that occurred before or during homelessness is not clear.

Although the long-term effects of homelessness on children are not established, providing needed educational, medical, and psychological services would be prudent to limit the potential damaging effects of homelessness on a child and to prevent long-term sequelae that may increase a child's risk for becoming a homeless adult. It is important to keep in mind that many homeless families demonstrate an enormous amount of strength and resilience under adverse conditions and respond positively to the resources found in a medical home. A clinician, in addition to identifying problems, must also reinforce these qualities as they are crucial to helping a family get through the crisis of being homeless.

AAP POLICY STATEMENTS

American Academy of Pediatrics, Committee on Community Health Services. Health needs of homeless children and families. *Pediatrics*. 1996;98(4):789-791. (pediatrics.aappublications.org/cgi/content/abstract/98/4/789).

American Academy of Pediatrics, Committee on Community Health Services. Providing care for immigrant, homeless, and migrant children. *Pediatrics*. 2005;115(4):1095-1100. (aappolicy.aappublications.org/cgi/content/full/pediatrics;115/4/1065).

REFERENCES

1. The Urban Institute. A New Look at Homelessness in America. Available at: www.urban.org/publications/900366.html. Accessed January 21, 2006.
2. The United States Conference of Mayors, Sodexo, Inc. Hunger and Homelessness Survey. Available at: www.usmayors.org/uscm/hungersurvey/2005/HH2005FINAL.pdf. Accessed January 23, 2006.
3. Levin-Epstein J, Greenberg MH, eds. Leave No Youth Behind: Opportunities for Congress To Reach Disconnected Youth. Center for Law and Social Policy. July 2003. Available at: www.clasp.org/publications/Disconnected_Youth.pdf. Accessed January 25, 2006.
4. Hammer H, Finkelhor D, Sedlak A. Runaway/Thrownaway Children: National Estimates of Characteristics. US Dept of Justice. Available at: www.ncjrs.gov/html/ojjdp/nismart/04/index.html. Accessed January 27, 2006.
5. Smith N, Flores ZD, Lin J, et al. Understanding Family Homelessness in New York City. Vera Institute of Justice. February 2005. Available at: vera.org/publications/publications_5.asp?publication_id=308. Accessed January 29, 2006.
6. US Department of Housing and Urban Development. Affordable Housing Needs: A Report to Congress on the Significant Need for Housing. December 2005. Available at: www.huduser.org/Publications/pdf/AffHsgNeedsRpt2003.pdf. Accessed on February 5, 2006.
7. Department of Housing and Urban Development. Final Fair Market Rents for the Housing Choice Voucher Program and Moderate Rehabilitation Single Room Occupancy Program for Fiscal Year 2005 (Docket No. FR-4995-N-03). Available at: www.huduser.org/datasets/fmr.html. Accessed February 6, 2006.
8. National Coalition for Low Income Housing. Out of Reach 2006. Available at: www.nlihc.org. Accessed February 6, 2006.

9. Hockett D, McElwee P, Pelletiere D, et al. *The Crisis in America's Housing: Confronting Myths and Promoting Balanced Housing Policy*. Washington, DC: Center for Community Change; 2005.
10. National Law Center on Homelessness and Poverty. Poverty in America. Available at: www.nlchp.org. Accessed February 11, 2006.
11. National Housing Trust. HUD Assisted, Project Based Losses by State. Available at: www.nhtinc.org/pre payment/State_Loss_Report.pdf. Accessed February 11, 2006.
12. Berti LC, Zylbert S, Rolnitzky L. Comparison of health status of children using a school based health center for comprehensive care. *J Pediatr Health Care*. 2001;15: 244-250.
13. Little M. Adverse perinatal outcomes associated with homelessness and substance use in pregnancy. *CMAJ*. 2005;173:615-618.
14. Stein JA. Severity of homelessness and adverse birth outcomes. *Health Psychol*. 2000;19:524-534.
15. Haley N, Roy E, Leclerc P, et al. Characteristics of adolescent street youth with a history of pregnancy. *J Pediatr Adolesc Gynecol*. 2004;17:313-320.
16. National Center on Family Homelessness. *America's Homeless Children*. Available at: www.familyhomelessness.org/ pdf/fact_children.pdf. Accessed January 22, 2007.
17. Karr C. Homeless children. What every clinician should know. *Pediatr Rev* 2004;25:235-241.
18. Bonin E. *Adapting Your Practice: Treatment and Recommendations for Homeless Children with Otitis Media*. Nashville, TN: National Health Care for the Homeless Council, Inc; 2003.
19. McLean DE, Bowen S, Drezner K, et al. Asthma among homeless children. *Arch Pediatr Adolesc Med*. 2004;158: 244-249.
20. Estrada B. Ectoparasitic infestations in homeless children. *Sem Pediatr Infect Dis*. 2003;14:20-24.
21. Beech BM, Myers L, Beech DJ, et al. Human immunodeficiency syndrome and hepatitis B and C infections among homeless adolescents. *Sem Pediatr Infect Dis*. 2003;14:12-19.
22. Nyamathi AM, Christiani A, Windokun F, et al. Hepatitis C virus infection, substance use and mental illness among homeless youth: a review. *AIDS*. 2005;19:S34-S40.
23. Boivin JF, Roy E, Haley N, et al. The health of street youth: a Canadian perspective. *Can J Public Health*. 2005;96:432-437.
24. Ligon B. Infectious diseases among homeless children and adolescents: a national concern. *Sem Pediatr Infect Dis*. 2000;11:220-226.
25. Kourgialis N, Wendell J, Darby P, et al. *Improving the Nutrition Status of Homeless Children: Guidelines for Homeless Family Shelters. A report from the Children's Health Fund*. New York: Children's Health Fund; 2001.
26. Karr C. Homeless children: what every clinician should know. *Pediatr Rev*. 2004;25:235-241.
27. Buckner JC, Bassuk EL, Weinreb LF. Predictors of academic achievement among homeless and low-income housed children. *J School Psychol*. 2001;39:45-69.
28. Oneil-Pirozzi TM. Language functioning of residents in family homeless shelters. *Am J Speech Lang Pathol*. 2003;12:229-242.
29. Buckner J, Bassuk EL, Weinreb LF. Predictors of academic achievement among homeless and low-income housed children. *J School Psychol*. 2001;39:45-69.
30. National Law Center on Homelessness and Poverty. McKinney-Vento Reauthorization at a Glance. Available at: www.nlchp.org/FA_Education/mckinneyGlance.cfm. Accessed May 14, 2006.
31. Buckner J, Beardslee W, Bassuk EL. Exposure to violence and low-income children's mental health. Directed, moderated and mediated relations. *Am J Orthopsychiatry*. 2004;74:413-423.
32. Stewart AJ, Steiman M, Cauce AM, et al. Victimization and posttraumatic stress disorder among homeless adolescents. *J Am Acad Child Adolesc Psychiatry*. 2004; 43:325-331.
33. Tyler KA, Cauce AM. Perpetrators of early physical and sexual abuse among homeless and runaway adolescents. *Child Abuse Neglect*. 2002;26:1261-1274.
34. Whitbeck LB, Johnson KD, Hoyt DR, et al. Mental disorder and comorbidity among runaway and homeless adolescents. *J Adolesc Health*. 2004;35:132-140.
35. Martijn C. Pathways to youth homelessness. *Soc Sci Med*. 2006;62:1-12

Chapter 120

CHILD PHYSICAL ABUSE AND NEGLECT

Howard Dubowitz, MD, MS; Martin A. Finkel, DO

INTRODUCTION

The abuse and neglect (maltreatment) of children are pervasive problems, with short- and long-term physical and mental health and social consequences.[1,2] Primary care physicians have an important role in helping address this problem. In addition to their responsibility to identify maltreated children and help ensure their protection and health, primary care physicians can also play vital roles related to prevention, treatment, and advocacy.[3]

DEFINITIONS

Abuse is generally defined as acts of commission and neglect as acts of omission. The federal government as a guide to the states defines child abuse as "any recent act or failure to act on the part of a parent or caretaker, which results in death, serious physical or emotional harm, sexual abuse or exploitation, or an act or failure to act which presents an imminent risk of serious harm."[4] Children may be found in situations in which no imminent risk of serious harm exists but rather the potential for harm (ie, endangered). Although the term *endangerment* is not included in the definition of abuse, debate continues around its inclusion; the potential for harm allows consideration of situations in which harm is possible or may only be apparent later. When primary care physicians identify potentially harmful situations, they can prevent abuse and neglect.

Predicting potential harm is inherently difficult. Two aspects should be considered. One is the likelihood of harm; the other is the severity. In some situations, the history is helpful. For example, patients with severe asthma are known to be at substantial risk of returning to the intensive care unit if they do not adhere to the treatment plan. In contrast, the risks associated with not being fully immunized are small. The potential severity also can vary. Leaving an infant alone in a bathtub poses a potentially fatal risk, whereas the risks associated with not keeping a follow-up appointment for pneumonia are probably minor.

Physical Abuse

Physical abuse includes beating, shaking, scalding, and biting. Given that corporal punishment is widely accepted in the United States, what is the threshold for considering spanking or hitting as being abusive? One approach is to consider any injury beyond immediate redness of the skin as abuse. Any punishment that leaves a bruise or imprint beyond the initial redness should be considered excessive and abusive. If parents spank a child, then the spanking should be limited to the buttocks, should occur over clothing, and should never involve the head and neck. When parents use objects other than a hand, the potential for serious harm increases. Acts of serious violence (eg, throwing a rock at a child, slapping an infant's face) should also be seen as abusive even if no injury ensues; significant risk of harm exists.

Forty percent of primary care physicians surveyed on the use of corporal punishment believed that "it was acceptable to use corporal punishment only under limited circumstances and/or with specific conditions or rules,"[5] whereas 98% of primary care physicians believed that positive reinforcement for good behavior and the use of time outs and withholding privileges for negative behaviors were preferable to corporal punishment. In community surveys, approximately 3% of parents report using very severe violence (eg, hitting with fist, burning, using gun or knife) against their child in the prior year.[6]

Sexual Abuse

Sexual abuse has been defined as "the involvement of dependent, developmentally immature children and adolescents in sexual activities which they do not fully comprehend, to which they are unable to give consent, or that violate the social taboos of family roles."[7] Sexually abusive experiences include exposure to sexually explicit materials, oral-genital contact, genital-to-genital contact, genital fondling, and genital-to-anal contact. Any touching of private areas that occurs in a context other than necessary care is inappropriate. Any inappropriate sexual contact regardless of the degree of physical intrusiveness has the potential for significant psychological consequences. (See Chapter 122, Sexual Abuse of Children.)

Child Neglect

Child neglect refers to parental omissions in care regarding health care, education, supervision, protection from hazards in the environment, physical needs (eg, clothing, food), and emotional support resulting in actual or potential harm.[8] An alternative view to focusing on caregiver omissions in care is to instead consider the basic needs of children (ie, adequate food, clothing, shelter, health care, education, nurturance); neglect occurs when one of these needs is not adequately met, whatever the reasons. This broader perspective encompasses the role of caregivers and other factors (eg, lead in the environment, lack of access to health care, costs of medications) that may contribute to the child neglect. This perspective points to the need for broad strategies to address problems underpinning neglect. In addition, the outcomes of neglect are often not immediately apparent. For this reason, situations of actual and potential harm should be carefully considered. Child protective services (CPS) is increasingly diverting *less serious cases*, including many involving neglect, to an alternative response. Instead of investigating a report of child abuse, the family's needs are assessed, and an attempt is made to meet these needs with community resources. Most state laws exclude cases in which children's needs are unmet as a result of poverty, yet poverty remains a major factor in a parent's ability to provide adequate food and shelter. In many states, the threshold for CPS accepting a report of neglect is high, requiring actual harm to the child.

Psychological Abuse

Psychological abuse includes verbal abuse and humiliation and acts that scare or terrorize a child. Although this form of abuse may be extremely harmful to children, resulting in depression, anxiety, estrangement, poor self-esteem, or lack of empathy, CPS seldom becomes involved. Therefore primary care physicians must consider this area of children's care.

Primary care physicians routinely see children and families in situations in which they have legitimate concerns that children are at risk, but the concern fails to reach a legal or agency threshold for reporting. These children and families can benefit from counseling by primary care physicians and referrals to social support, as well as behavioral, educational, and mental health services in the community. Children experiencing abuse, neglect, or both rarely fit neatly into the aforementioned categories. Children who experience one form of maltreatment have commonly had other experiences of abuse or neglect, which also need to be assessed and addressed.

INCIDENCE

Child abuse and neglect is not rare. In 2003, 2.9 million reports were made to CPS at a rate of 39.1 per 1000 children. Sixty-eight percent of these reports were considered appropriate for investigation. Between 1990 and 2003 the overall rate dropped from 13.4 to 12.4 per 1000 children. The highest rate of maltreatment, 16.4 per 1000, was for children 0 to 3 years old. The rate for black children was almost twice that of white children (20.4 vs 11.0 per 1000). This rate is likely due, in part, to professional bias in reporting low income and minority families for maltreatment.[9] In 2003, physicians accounted for 8.2% of all child abuse reports investigated by CPS. Approximately 906,000 children were determined to have been abused or neglected, a substantiation rate of approximately 1 in 3 children reported.[10] These cases involved the following: neglect, 60.1%; physical abuse, 18.9%; sexual abuse, 9.9%; emotional abuse, 4.9%; and medical neglect, 2.7%. Rates of sexual abuse have remained relatively stable, with studies continuing to suggest that as many as 1 in 4 girls and 1 in 10 boys have been sexually abused. Reported cases reflect only the tip of the iceberg; child abuse and neglect usually occur behind closed doors and are often not detected.[11]

ETIOLOGY

Risk Factors

Child maltreatment seldom has a single cause; rather, multiple and interacting biopsychosocial risk factors usually exist.[12,13] The following discussion illustrates factors at 4 levels. At the individual level, a child's disability[14] or a parent's depression[15] predispose the child to maltreatment. At the familial level, intimate partner (or domestic) violence[16] presents risks for children. Influential community factors include stressors such as dangerous neighborhoods or the lack of recreational facilities.[17] Broad societal factors, such as poverty and its associated burdens, also contribute to maltreatment.[18] Children in all social classes, however, can be maltreated, and primary care physicians need to guard against biases concerning low-income families.[9]

Protective Factors

In contrast, resources are available that may buffer the influence of risk factors and protect children from maltreatment. Clinical experience suggests that protective factors include a parent's recognition of a problem and interest in help, a supportive grandparent, and accessible mental health care. Child maltreatment generally results from a complex interplay among risk and protective factors. For example, a single mother who has a colicky baby and who recently lost her job is at risk for maltreatment, but a loving grandmother may be protective. A good understanding of what is contributing to the maltreatment, as well as the family's strengths, is key to intervening effectively.

PREVENTION

In general, medical responses to child maltreatment have been after the fact; preventing the problem is preferable. Primary care physicians can help in several ways.[19] An ongoing relationship in primary care offers opportunities to develop trust and knowledge of a family's circumstances. Astute observation of parent-child interactions can reveal useful information. For example, does the relationship appear warm and comfortable or tense and hostile?

Parent Education

Parent education regarding medical conditions helps to ensure implementation of the treatment plan and to prevent neglect.[8] Possible barriers to treatment should be addressed. Practical strategies such as writing down the plan can help. In addition, anticipatory guidance may help with childrearing, diminishing the risk of maltreatment. Hospital-based programs that educate parents of newborns about infant crying and the risks of shaking the infant appear beneficial in preventing abusive head trauma.[20]

Screening

Risk factors for maltreatment are described later in this chapter. Screening for some of these risk factors and helping address identified problems—often via referrals—may strengthen families and reduce maltreatment. This role fits well with a broad view of health and a professional mandate to help ensure children's health and safety.[21] Regular checkups—focused on prevention—offer excellent opportunities to screen briefly for psychosocial problems. The review of systems is standard in these visits. Its traditional focus on the organ systems can be expanded to probe briefly areas such as feelings about the child, the parent's own functioning, possible depression, substance abuse, intimate partner violence, disciplinary approaches, and stressors and supports. Beginning with questions that are familiar to physicians and parents, such as inquiries about the presence of smoke detectors helps broach more sensitive areas gradually.

Considering information that can or should be obtained directly from children or youth is also important, especially given that separate interviews with teens have become the norm. Sample questions include:

"How do you get along with your parents?"

"If you're really upset about something, whom can you talk to?"

"Is anyone giving you a hard time at home?" If yes, "How so?"

"Most kids get punished sometimes. How do you get punished?"

"Are you sometimes hungry, and there's no food at home?"

Any concerns raised on such screens require at least brief assessment and initial management, which may involve a referral for further evaluation and treatment. More frequent office visits can be scheduled for support and counseling while monitoring the situation. Other key family members (eg, fathers) might be invited to participate, thereby encouraging informal support. Practices might arrange parent groups through which problems and solutions are shared. Primary care physicians also need to recognize their limitations and when other professional intervention is indicated, making knowledge of community resources essential.

Finally, the problems underpinning child maltreatment, such as poverty, parental stress, substance abuse, and limited resources related to child rearing, require policies and programs to enhance families' abilities to care for their children adequately. Primary care physicians can help advocate for such policies and programs.

EVALUATION

Primary care physicians who face questions of abuse and neglect often need to decide whether the history reasonably explains a child's injury. This decision requires understanding the clinical and biomechanical aspects of trauma and the context in which maltreatment occurs. Carefully considering alternative explanations for the injury is essential. A thorough history that includes comprehensive psychosocial information, a physical examination, and appropriate laboratory and radiologic studies are needed. The medical history may reveal evidence of noninflicted injuries suggestive of poor supervision, abuse, or inadequate adherence to medical advice (ie, medical neglect). CPS may have information on past or current involvement. Their investigation can offer helpful information on the home and family situation.

Pediatricians are accustomed to consulting with subspecialists; pediatrician experts in child maltreatment should also be viewed this way. Pediatricians should identify a local specialist in child maltreatment with whom they can consult. When the pediatrician's concern meets jurisdictional or agency criteria for suspected maltreatment, a need exists to refer to CPS. Typically, the statutory requirement is a *reason to believe* rather than a certainty.

Interdisciplinary practice provides the optimal approach to the complex problem of child maltreatment. Pediatricians focus on the medical piece of the puzzle; colleagues from mental health, CPS, law enforcement, and schools can add important perspectives and information. This interdisciplinary evaluation is optimal not only for determining whether maltreatment has occurred, but also for clarifying the needs of the child and family. For example, law enforcement officers or CPS workers who have visited the home may provide useful information on the circumstances surrounding the injury (eg, the temperature of the hot water) and insight into the functioning of a family. Ultimately, the collective insight of several professionals is generally required to substantiate abuse, and this collaboration results in shared decision making and liability in these complex cases.

In understanding what happened to a child, doing so objectively and empathically is important. Pediatricians need to control their responses to seeing a clearly abused child and to modulate their feelings. They should not be accusatory or confrontational. Being a concerned, helping professional with a mandate to protect children will best serve the child's and the family's interests. Most maltreated children are not removed from their caregivers. Maintaining a constructive relationship with the child's parents, without compromising the statutory requirement to report suspected maltreatment, is best.

Obtaining a History of an Injury

Whenever possible, primary care physicians should obtain a history from the child's caregivers and from the child separately. Children can frequently explain how their injuries occurred. Questions should be open ended, encouraging a detailed explanation. Questions that are least directive (leading) and not suggestive are always preferable.

The physical findings may be nonspecific, making the history especially important. A history that does not reasonably explain an injury is key to determining abuse. Caregivers may state that they did not witness the incident, which may be true. Primary care physicians generally believe that parents provide an accurate history. Unfortunately, when abuse occurs, deliberate or unconscious motives for not disclosing what happened may exist. Therefore primary care physicians need to assess carefully the likelihood that the history adequately explains the findings. Information collected by CPS and law enforcement professionals regarding the scene in which the injury occurred can be useful.

Physical Examination of an Injury

Just as great care is needed when obtaining a history, the physical examination must be comprehensive and meticulous, with detailed and legible documentation. Whenever possible, injuries should be photographed, providing a permanent and objective record and enabling second opinions. Primary care physicians naturally wish to make a clear diagnosis, prescribe treatment, and see their patient improve. Unfortunately, ambiguity often exists in child abuse cases.

Cutaneous Manifestations of Abuse

Bruises

Bruises are the most common manifestation of physical abuse. Primary care physicians are often faced with the dilemma of whether the bruise was caused by noninflicted (unintentional) trauma. Bruising in preambulatory children is rare (2.2%). Cruising children (18%) and walking children (52%) experience more bruises.[23] Noninflicted bruises are characteristically anterior and over bony prominences, such as shins and forehead,[23] usually resulting from falls. Well-padded areas such as the buttocks, cheeks, and thighs are less likely to bruise during most childhood activities, as are the neck, ears, and genitalia. Bruises of these areas may suggest abuse.[24] Some bruises carry the imprint of the implement used. Circumferential marks around the wrists, ankles, and neck may result from squeezing, grabbing, or ligatures.

Primary care physicians may be asked to determine the age of a bruise to identify possible perpetrators, corroborate explanations for injuries, or confirm that injuries occurred at different times. However, precisely dating bruises is difficult.[25] Many factors determine the color of a bruise, including the depth of the injury, location, force employed, vascularity of the tissues, time since the injury, skin color, and ambient lighting. Previously published tables on dating bruises therefore should be ignored.[26] If a bruise is red, then it is likely to be less than a week old. If it is yellow or green, then the injury is probably more than 24 to 48 hours old. Hence an explanation that a red bruise resulted from an injury 2 weeks earlier would be worrisome. However, these time frames indicate the wide range that limits usefulness.

Bruises are the most common manifestation of physical abuse. However, in some instances, an underlying medical explanation for bruises can be found, such as blood dyscrasias or connective tissue disorders. The history or examination usually provides clues to these conditions. Henoch-Schönlein purpura, the most common vasculitis in young children, may be confused with abuse. If an underlying bleeding disorder is suspected, then a platelet count, prothrombin time, international normalized ratio (the ratio of a patient's prothrombin time to a normal [control] sample, raised to the power of the International Sensitivity Index [ISI]), and partial thromboplastin time should be obtained. However, the pattern and location of bruises caused by abuse are usually different from those resulting from a coagulopathy. The presence of a medical disorder does not preclude possible abuse. Birthmarks and mongolian spots can be confused with bruises; however, these skin markings are not tender and do not rapidly change color or size.

Cultural practices need to be considered in the differential diagnosis. Cao Gio, commonly known as *coining*, is a Southeast Asian folkloric therapy.[22] A coin or other object is vigorously rubbed on the skin in a linear fashion, causing petechiae or purpura. Cupping is another approach that is popular in the Middle East. A heated glass is applied to the skin, often on the back. As it cools, a vacuum results, leading to perfectly circular bruises. The context here is important, and such circumstances should not be considered abusive.

Bites

Bites have a characteristic pattern of 1 or 2 opposing arches with multiple bruises. They can be inflicted by an adult, another child, an animal, or the patient. Bites by a child (younger than approximately 8 years with primary teeth) typically have a distance of less than 2.5 cm between the canines—often the most prominent bruises. Animal bites vary and usually have narrower arches than human bites and are often deep. Self-inflicted bites are on accessible areas, particularly the hands. Adult bites raise concern for abuse. Multiple bites by another child suggest inadequate supervision and neglect.

Burns

Childhood burns are often caused by abuse (Box 120-1).[27] Many other burns involve inadequate supervision or neglect. Scalding burns may be immersion or splash. Immersion burns, when a child is forcibly held in hot water, have clear delineation between the burned and the healthy skin and uniform depth and may have a sock or glove distribution. In many instances, no splash marks are evident, as might be expected if a child inadvertently encountered hot water.[28] Symmetrical burns are especially suggestive of abuse,[28] as are burns of the buttocks and perineum.[29] A splash burn may be the result of abuse.

Burns from hot objects such as curling irons, radiators, steam irons, metal grids, hot knives, and cigarettes have shapes that reflect the object. A child is likely to try to escape from a hot object; thus burns that are extensive and deep and reflect more than fleeting contact are suggestive of abuse. Other unusual causes of abusive burns include hair dryers, microwave ovens,[30] and stun guns.[31]

Neglect frequently contributes to childhood burns.[32] Children, home alone, may be burned in house fires. A parent taking drugs may cause a fire and may be unable to protect a child. Exploring children may pull hot liquids left unattended onto themselves.[33] Liquids cool as they flow downward so that the burn is most severe and broad proximally. If the child is wearing a diaper or clothing, then hot water may be soaked up into the fabric and cause burns worse than otherwise might be expected, with patterns that follow what the child is wearing. Children may stick objects into an electrical outlet, usually resulting in no external burn, unless the child touched the electrical source. Burns may occur from electric water heaters.[34] Some circumstances are difficult to foresee, and a single burn resulting from a momentary lapse in supervision should not automatically be seen as neglectful parenting.

Several conditions mimic abusive burns, such as brushing against a hot radiator, car seat burns, impetigo, hemangiomas, and folk remedies such as moxibustion.[27,35] Impetigo may resemble cigarette burns. Cigarette burns are usually 7 to 10 mm across,[36] whereas impetigo has lesions of varying size. Noninflicted cigarette burns are usually oval and superficial.

Concluding whether a burn was inflicted depends on the history, burn pattern, and the child's capabilities. A delay in seeking health care may be the result of the burn initially appearing minor, before blistering or becoming infected. This circumstance may represent reasonable behavior and should not be automatically deemed neglectful. A home investigation can be valuable (eg, testing the water temperature). Severe burns can lead to lifelong scarring and serious psychosocial sequelae.[37] Prevention is key, such as setting hot water cylinders under 125°F.[38,39]

BOX 120-1 Characteristics of Burns Suggestive of Abuse

- History does not adequately explain the burn
- Burn reflects shape of an object
- Multiple burn sites
- Deep or extensive burn
- Extremities on both sides burned
- Clear, regular edge, uniform depth, no splash marks
- Other history or examination findings suggestive of abuse
- Glove- or sock-pattern burns of distal extremities

Skeletal Trauma

Any bone can be fractured as a result of abuse; however, fractures strongly suggestive of abuse are classic metaphyseal lesions, posterior rib fractures, and fractures of the scapula, sternum, and spinous processes, especially in young children.[39] These fractures all require more force than would be expected from a minor fall or routine handling and activities of a child. Rib and sternal fractures rarely result from cardiopulmonary resuscitation, even when performed by untrained adults.[40] These fractures are likely caused by excessive compression of a young child's thorax. Commonly fractured long bones, in order of decreasing frequency, as seen in abuse are the femur, humerus, tibia, and forearm. In abused infants, rib, metaphyseal, and skull fractures are most common.

Clavicular, femoral, supracondylar humeral, and distal extremity fractures in children older than 2 years are most likely noninflicted unless they are multiple or accompanied by other stigmata of abuse. Spiral fractures of the femur in nonambulatory infants are highly suggestive of abuse. With increasing mobility and running, toddlers can fall with enough rotational force to cause a spiral, femoral fracture, reducing the specificity of this type of injury for abuse under these circumstances. Few fractures are pathognomonic of abuse, and all must be considered in light of the history.

The possible causes of fractures include conditions that increase susceptibility to fractures, such as osteopenia, osteogenesis imperfecta, metabolic and nutritional disorders (eg, scurvy, rickets), renal osteodystrophy, osteomyelitis, congenital syphilis, and neoplasia. Multiple fractures in various stages of healing are suggestive of abuse; nevertheless, underlying physical abnormalities need to be considered.[40]

A skeletal survey should be routine in children younger than 2 years who have a fracture, especially if a possibility of abuse exists. In children between 2 and 5 years of age, the usefulness of a skeletal survey depends on specific circumstances. *Babygrams* (1 or 2 radiograph examinations of the entire body) do not provide adequate visualization of the entire skeleton and should be avoided. If the survey is negative for fracture but concern for an occult injury remains, then a radionucleotide bone scan should be performed.[41] A scan will be generally positive for fracture within 24 to 48 hours after an injury and will remain positive throughout the stage of callous formation. Subsequent skeletal survey at approximately 2 weeks may significantly increase the identification of fractures that were not apparent initially. Standards for a skeletal survey and other forms of imaging have been developed by the American College of Radiology.[42]

In corroborating the history and the injury, the age of the fracture can only be crudely estimated.[40] Soft-tissue swelling generally subsides in 2 to 21 days. Periosteal new bone can be seen as early as 4 days after injury but up to 21 days later. Loss of definition of the fracture line occurs between 10 and 21 days. Soft callus on a long bone can first be observed 10 days after an injury. Hard callus is evident between 14 and 90 days. The child's age, the type of bone, and the nature of the fracture can influence the healing process. Remodeling of bone can continue until epiphyseal closure. These time frames are shorter in infancy and longer when the child has poor nutritional status or a chronic underlying disease. Subperiosteal new bone formation is a nonspecific finding and can be seen in infectious, traumatic, and metabolic disorders. In young infants, new bone formation may be a normal physiologic finding, usually bilateral, symmetric, and less than 2 mm. Fractures of flat bones such as the skull do not form callus and cannot be aged.[42]

Central Nervous System

Of all inflicted injuries, those to the central nervous system (CNS) result in the most significant morbidity and mortality.[43] Injuries resulting from direct impact, asphyxia, or shaking (shaken baby syndrome) are referred to as abusive head trauma (AHT). Direct trauma may be the result of punching, slapping, or the child's head being struck against a hard surface. Many instances of AHT appear to result from a combination of shaking and direct trauma. Subdural hematomas, retinal hemorrhages (especially when extensive and involving multiple layers), and diffuse axonal injury, although not exclusively the result of AHT, are critically important markers and should always raise the question of AHT.

Infants with their poor neck muscle tone and relatively large heads are most vulnerable to AHT. Simple linear skull fractures in the absence of other traumatic brain injuries such as subdural hematomas and retinal hemorrhages are not uncommon and can be associated with an noninflicted injury. Frequently, different explanations are offered for the child's injuries, such as a rolling off a sofa. A fall from a height of 4 feet or less by children younger than 2 years rarely results in a skull fracture.[44-46] Several studies have found that short falls rarely lead to severe neurologic problems. CNS injuries in association with cutaneous, visceral, and skeletal findings suggestive of abuse, in the absence of a readily verifiable major accidental trauma, strongly point to AHT. With multiple caregivers, obtaining the history from all parties independently would be best. An investigation of the site where the injury occurred helps clarify the possible mechanism of a child's injury.[47]

Obtaining a History of Abusive Head Trauma

In AHT, the patient's history commonly reveals an insidious onset of symptoms or that the infant appears well before suddenly having severe symptoms (eg, not breathing).[48] Lucid periods after severe head injuries are rarely seen after witnessed trauma (eg, motor vehicle crashes). Most infants lose consciousness at the time of injury; those who remain lucid are still symptomatic.[49] Severe CNS injury in the absence of a credible account of a major incident must be considered inflicted until proven otherwise. In a study of children younger than 3 years with head trauma, one third of these children were not correctly diagnosed as having AHT; 28% of them were abused again.[50] Children with AHT were found to have had earlier symptoms or signs suggestive of AHT (eg, vomiting without fever or diarrhea). Children whose abuse was missed were younger and had milder and nonspecific symptoms.

Evaluation of Patients With Abusive Head Trauma

Children may lack external signs of injury, even with serious intracranial trauma. Signs and symptoms may be nonspecific, ranging from lethargy, vomiting (without diarrhea), changing neurologic status or seizures, and coma. In all preverbal children, an index of suspicion for AHT should exist. Metabolic and toxicology screens must be considered to explain nonspecific symptoms. *Raccoon eyes* occurs in association with subgaleal hematomas after traction on the hair and scalp or after a single impact to the forehead, but neuroblastoma should be considered. Bruises from attempted strangulation may be visible on the neck.[51,52] Choking or suffocation results in asphyxia and hypoxic brain injury, often with minimal external signs.

Retinal hemorrhages are a key marker of AHT.[53] Whenever AHT is being considered, a dilated indirect ophthalmologic examination by a pediatric ophthalmologist should be performed. If available, retinal photographic documentation can be useful. Although retinal hemorrhages can be found in other conditions, hemorrhages that are bilateral and extensive, involve all layers of the retina, and extend to the periphery beyond the immediate perinatal period and in the absence of a known medical cause, are most often the result of the AHT. Severe noninflicted head trauma rarely results in retinal hemorrhages; and when this result does occur, the hemorrhages tend to be few in number and confined to the posterior retina (posterior pole).[54] The indirect trauma, most commonly caused by repeated acceleration-deceleration (eg, shaking), seems to be critical in the development of more extensive retinal or vitreous hemorrhages. One particular unique form of hemorrhage is called *traumatic retinoschisis:* The retina layers are sheared apart as a result of traction from the repeatedly accelerating-decelerating vitreous gel to which it is firmly attached. Blood accumulates between the layers. Given that the resolution rates of different types and locations of retinal hemorrhages are highly variable, retinal injury is rarely useful in helping to estimate when the injury occurred.[55] The postmortem examination may demonstrate patterns of posterior orbital hemorrhage and intraorbital optic nerve injury, helping to differentiate noninflicted head injury from AHT. The presence of ocular injury (eg, optic nerve injury, retinal hemorrhage), CNS injury, and skeletal trauma strongly suggests abusive shaking, with or without impact, as the mechanism of injury.

Many other causes of retinal hemorrhages exist, including coagulopathy, in particular leukemia, retinal diseases, carbon monoxide poisoning, and metabolic disorders such as glutaric aciduria. Birth retinal hemorrhages are very common, but superficial *(flame)* and deeper intraretinal (*dot* or *blot*) hemorrhages are well known to resolve by 1 and 6 weeks, respectively. Severe accidental life-threatening direct crush injury to the head can rarely cause an extensive hemorrhagic retinopathy. Cardiopulmonary resuscitation rarely, if ever, causes retinal hemorrhage in infants and young children, and, if so, reports suggest that very few hemorrhages would be present in the area around the optic nerve. Hemoglobinopathies, diabetes mellitus, routine play, minor accidental head trauma, and vaccinations do not appear to be causes of retinal hemorrhage. Almost all of the medical causes of retinal hemorrhage are readily diagnosed based on history, eye examination, full physical examination, and, when indicated, laboratory testing.

Direct trauma to the orbital region may result in corneal abrasions, subconjunctival hemorrhages, hyphema, globe rupture, and periorbital edema or ecchymosis.[53]

Intracranial trauma is best evaluated via initial and follow-up imaging with computed tomography (CT) as the 1st study of choice. Magnetic resonance images (MRIs) are helpful in differentiating extraaxial fluid, determining timing of injuries, assessing parenchymal injury, and identifying vascular anomalies. MRIs are best obtained 5 to 7 days after an acute injury. When AHT is suspected, a skeletal survey should be routine. CT scans of the abdomen and thorax are obtained as dictated by the clinical condition. Additional laboratory tests can assist in identifying metabolic diseases such as glutaric aciduria type 1 or conditions such as osteogenesis imperfecta. All of these entities are rare, but they should be considered depending on the clinical circumstances.

Orofacial Injuries

Injuries to the head, neck, and oral cavity may be seen in physically abused children. Soft-tissue injuries to the upper lip or the frenulum are seen in forced feeding but can also occur when a toddler trips, especially with a hard object in the child's mouth. The forceful introduction of hot or caustic liquid into a child's mouth may result in intraoral lacerations or mucosal injury.[56] Noninflicted trauma to the forehead, lower lip, chin, and nose is common in toddlers and should be differentiated from abuse. A dentist can help manage the injuries and detect subtle injuries such as fractured teeth.

Blunt trauma to the ear may produce subperichondrial hematoma and intracranial injury resulting from rotational acceleration of the head. A slap to the face or choking may leave a hand imprint. A slap to the face not only can cause injuries; it also has a strong associated psychological component. Long-term dental neglect may result in multiple dental caries, eating difficulties, chronic pain, and periodontal infection.

Abdominal Trauma

Abdominal trauma accounts for significant morbidity and mortality in abused children.[57] Young children are especially vulnerable because of their relatively large abdomens and lax abdominal musculature. Hollow organs can be ruptured by a blow or kick. Solid organs such as the pancreas, which can be compressed against the spine when the abdomen is struck, can be injured. Intraabdominal bleeding may result from trauma to an organ or from shearing of the vascular supply. Children may have cardiovascular failure or an acute abdomen often after a delay in care.[57] Bilious vomiting in a young child without fever or peritoneal irritation suggests a duodenal hematoma, often the result of abuse. Indeed, any of the abdominal organs may be injured because of abuse.[58]

The manifestations of abdominal trauma are often subtle, even with severe injuries. Bruising of the abdominal wall is unusual, and symptoms may evolve slowly. Delayed perforation may occur days after the injury, or bowel strictures or a pancreatic pseudocyst may occur weeks or months later. Primary care physicians should consider screening for occult abdominal trauma when other evidence of physical abuse exists. Physicians should screen urine and stool samples for blood and check liver[59] and pancreatic enzyme levels.[60] A screening abdominal ultrasound should also be considered,[61] although CT is preferable for detecting trauma to solid organs.[57] Children with abusive abdominal injuries may also have fractures and head injuries.[62] Possible noninflicted mechanisms should be considered, such as trauma in a bicycle handlebar injury, but caution is needed in accepting unlikely explanations.[63]

Child Neglect

Neglect is the most prevalent form of child maltreatment,[64] with potentially severe and long-lasting sequelae.[65] Primary care physicians may encounter several manifestations of possible neglect (Box 120-2). Initial questions include, "Is this neglect?" "Have the circumstances harmed the child, or jeopardized the child's health and safety?"[66] For example, adherence to the

BOX 120-2 Manifestations of Possible Neglect

- Nonadherence to treatment
- Delay or failure in obtaining health care—medical, mental, dental
- Nonorganic failure to thrive; obesity that is not being addressed
- Recurring injuries or ingestions suggesting inadequate supervision
- Drug-exposed newborns and children
- Exposure to environmental hazards, in and out of the home
- Poor hygiene, sanitation
- Inadequate attention to emotional and cognitive needs

treatment may be suboptimal without clearly impairing a child's health. Inadequacies in the care children receive naturally fall along a continuum, inviting a range of responses tailored to the individual situation. Legal considerations or public agency guidelines may discourage physicians from labeling many circumstances as neglect. Even if a report is not made to CPS, primary care physicians can still help ensure children's needs are adequately met.

In most instances, multiple and interacting contributors to neglect exist. Therefore a comprehensive biopsychosocial assessment of the possible underpinning problems—at the levels of child, parent, family, and community—is necessary.[67] Biopsychosocial refers to a view that certain phenomena such as child neglect may result from a complex interplay of biological, psychological, and social factors. The system of health care should also be examined. Do barriers to health care exist? Does a problematic relationship exist between the pediatrician and the parent or child? Poor adherence to treatment for asthma may be the result of not understanding the treatment plan; the primary care physician may not have clearly communicated the plan. The pediatrician needs to be cautious not to assume that the parents are responsible. For example, a complicated medical course does not prove poor adherence to treatment; the disease may be inherently difficult to control. In addition to probing for risk factors, strengths and resources (protective factors) should also be assessed; these factors are often crucial to intervening effectively. A parent's interest to keep a child out of the hospital, for example, may motivate adherence to treatment.

Primary care physicians may face other forms of neglect.[8] For example, a child may have inadequate clothing, or the family may be homeless—conditions that can affect children's health. Children may not be enrolled in school. A child's learning may be problematic and the school's response inadequate. A broad view of health and an interest in children's health and development require attention to such facets of their environment. Neglect is a heterogeneous phenomenon that calls for varied responses to address the specific circumstances. Some key principles are outlined later in this chapter.[68]

OUTCOMES OF CHILD MALTREATMENT

Child maltreatment often has significant short- and long-term medical, mental health, and social sequelae. Physically abused children are at risk for behavioral and functional problems, including conduct disorders, aggressive behaviors, decreased cognitive functioning, and poor academic performance.[69,70] Neglect is similarly associated with many potential problems.[65] A wide range of possible psychosocial problems exists; the limited specificity of these problems means that they are not useful in diagnosing maltreatment. However, the need for behavioral interventions for maltreated children should always be considered. Even if such children appear to be functioning well, primary care physicians and parents need to be sensitive to the possibility of later problems. Maltreatment is associated with increased risk in adulthood for several health risk behaviors and physical and mental health problems.[71] Maltreated children are at risk for becoming abusive parents.[72] Preliminary research showing lasting neurobiological effects of child abuse on the developing brain may explain some of these sequelae.[73]

Some children appear to be resilient and may not exhibit sequelae of maltreatment, perhaps owing to protective factors or interventions. The benefits of intervention have been found in even the most severely neglected children, such as those from Romanian orphanages, who were adopted—the earlier the better.[74] Children who were adopted when younger than 6 months fared better than those adopted at an older age.

LEGAL ISSUES

Whenever a primary care physician is involved in a case of possible abuse or neglect, the potential exists for legal involvement, although few cases are tried in court. Many more cases are not prosecuted because of the difficulty of proving who was responsible, or the cases are plea bargained. Neglect is rarely considered a criminal offense and is seldom prosecuted. The best way to prepare for testifying in court is to practice good medicine. For example, being able to justify an impression or diagnosis carefully is important. This justification may mean rendering a tentative or preliminary opinion (eg, *possible abuse*) and not being more definitive than justified pending further laboratory results or information. Having a sound basis for opinion protects the pediatrician from feeling intimidated by the adversarial court system.

Most primary care physicians provide their opinion in their capacity as the treating physician. This circumstance is important because much of what the child tells the primary care physician (ie, hearsay) may be admissible in criminal court proceedings as an exception to hearsay rules of evidence. A requirement for admissibility of these out-of-court statements is that patients understand that they are being examined for diagnosis and treatment. A simple explanation of this circumstance and documentation in the medical record helps ensure admissibility of a child's statements as an exception to hearsay. This initial history may be crucial to understanding a child's experience. As cases proceed, children may recant their initial statements regarding their abuse because of either direct threats or fears of consequences following disclosure.

Reporting and Documenting for Court

State laws mandate that primary care physicians report suspected child abuse or neglect to the designated public agency. Some states penalize mandated reporters who fail to do so. All reporting statutes supersede any ethical duty to protect confidentiality. As long as the report of suspected abuse or neglect is made in good faith, primary care physicians are immune from both civil and criminal liability. Whether the level of suspicion meets the threshold for reporting is sometimes a judgment call. The pediatrician does not need to be certain that maltreatment has occurred to make a report; reasonable suspicion is adequate, although *reasonable* is not defined in most regulations. If possible, an interdisciplinary child-maltreatment or child-protection team or a primary care physician with expertise in this field can provide useful guidance. Similarly, a call to CPS may help assess whether the circumstances warrant a report, as well as ascertain possible past or current family involvement with CPS.

Reporting child maltreatment is never easy. Parental inadequacy or culpability is at least implicit, and considerable anger may result. Primary care physicians should supportively inform families directly of the report; it can be explained as an effort to clarify the situation and provide help or as a professional (and legal) responsibility. Explaining what the ensuing process is likely to entail (eg, a visit from a CPS worker and sometimes a police officer) and what will not happen is useful. Parents are frequently concerned that they might lose their child. Primary care physicians can cautiously reassure parents that CPS is responsible for helping children and families and that, in most instances, children remain with their parents. Even when CPS does not accept a report or when a report is not substantiated, they may offer voluntary supportive services such as food, shelter, homemaker services, and child care.

Clear documentation is crucial to the admissibility of all evidence. Appropriate verbal or photographic documentation preserves evidence for future reference. The medical history is the verbal evidence; thus it is important in discerning how an injury likely occurred and may be as important as physical evidence. Written documentation should include both the questions and the responses, and important parts should be recorded verbatim in quotation marks. This practice enables careful evaluation of the evidence. A comprehensive and legible record may obviate the need to testify. Whenever possible, obtaining photographic documentation of injuries that are suggestive of abuse is helpful.

Testifying

Primary care physicians may be called to testify before a grand jury or law enforcement officials, which in many states is a preliminary step to indictment. It is an opportunity for the prosecution alone to present its case. A grand jury indictment implies that sufficient evidence exists to justify a trial, and it determines what charges will be filed. If the case proceeds to trial, then most primary care physicians who then testify do so to provide the medical history and examination findings. A fact witness should not be asked to render an opinion regarding the likelihood of abuse. The court may, however, determine that the primary care physician can testify as an expert, thus allowing opinion. In some cases, another expert in child maltreatment will be asked to interpret the findings for the court.

A subpoena is often the 1st notice of the need for involvement in the legal system. Different subpoenas may be generated on behalf of the state, the child, and the defendant. When a subpoena is received, the person issuing the subpoena should be asked to clarify what is being requested and to prepare for the legal proceeding. Prosecutors and the court generally try to accommodate primary care physicians' time constraints.

Any information a primary care physician has should be considered privileged and confidential and should be disclosed only when the client or legal guardian consents or a subpoena requires such disclosure. In general, state laws grant CPS access to medical records pertaining to a maltreatment report. State laws concerning confidentiality and reporting responsibility in suspected child abuse and neglect cases vary; primary care physicians need to know their state's laws; these are available on the Child Welfare Information Gateway Web site at www.childwelfare.gov (state statute search) or by contacting their local CPS agency.

In the pretrial process of discovery, both the prosecutor and the defense attorney have an opportunity to learn what evidence the other possesses. The defense attorney may contact the examining primary care physician directly to discuss the case as part of discovery. The primary care physician is not legally obligated to comply unless the request is accompanied by a subpoena. If a primary care physician is going to testify for either the prosecution or the defense, the physician obtains the permission of counsel before speaking to the opposing counsel, and counsel may wish to be present. During cross-examination, however, failure to have met with the defense attorney if requested may be used to demonstrate a lack of objectivity. An important point to remember is that the defense is responsible for representing the accused; the interests of the child are secondary. Even though the court process is clearly adversarial, providing a balanced, objective, and defensible opinion is the responsibility of the fact or expert witness. This opinion should be the same whether testifying at the request of the prosecution or defense.

TREATMENT

The specific treatment depends on the specific problems contributing to a child's maltreatment, as well as the consequences. The following discussion reflects important general principles. Primary care physicians are naturally responsible for helping address any medical problem. Approaching problems of neglect should begin with less-intrusive interventions. For example, if an infant's failure to thrive is due to an error in mixing the formula, then parent education and perhaps a visiting nurse should be the initial strategy. At the same time, ensuring a child's safety is paramount. Therefore severe failure to thrive requires hospitalization, and, if the contributing factors are particularly serious (eg, a psychotic mother), out-of-home placement may be needed. Thus, in situations in which less-intrusive efforts have not succeeded or in which the circumstances of the maltreatment are severe, a report to CPS should be made. CPS can conduct a home assessment that can provide valuable insights that help develop a fuller picture of the family situation. Primary care physicians can be a valuable liaison between the family and the public agencies, and they should make every effort to remain involved after reporting to CPS. Families are typically under great duress after a report, and the involvement of different professionals and agencies can be confusing. With more frequent office visits, primary care physicians can offer support and guidance.

In families in which maltreatment occurs, the parents may need to be nurtured before they are able to nurture their children. The parents, even if suspected as perpetrators, remain "patients" of the pediatrician and should be presumed for the purpose of delivery of care to the family until such time as when CPS or law enforcement may temporarily or permanently abrogate their parental rights. Therefore a comprehensive assessment of the child, parent or parents, and family is important to guide appropriate interventions. The use of informal supports such as family members, neighbors, and friends (eg, inviting the father to an office visit) should be encouraged. Families also may need other professional interventions (eg, drug treatment, mental health services); primary care physicians can help with referrals.

The importance of addressing concrete needs should not be overlooked. Accessing nutrition programs, obtaining health insurance, enrolling children in preschool programs, and helping with housing can make a valuable difference. The problems contributing to child maltreatment often require long-term professional support and monitoring; few quick fixes are available.

ADVOCACY AND PREVENTION

The primary care physician is well positioned to assist in understanding the factors that contributed to the child's maltreatment. When advocating for the best interest of the child and family, addressing risk factors at the individual, family, and community levels would be optimal. At the individual level, an example of advocating on behalf of a child is explaining to a parent that an active toddler is behaving normally and not intentionally challenging the parent. Learning about a parent's response to a child's difficult behavior also allows an opportunity to educate the parent regarding appropriate responses. Encouraging a mother to seek help dealing with a violent spouse, saying, "You and your life are very important," asking about substance abuse and smoking and assisting parents in seeking health care coverage for their children are all forms of advocacy.

Primary care physicians advocate on behalf of families when they try to enhance the functioning of families. Encouraging the involvement of fathers in child care, strengthening ties with extended family, and, in some instances, facilitating family therapy are examples of advocacy. Remaining involved after a report to CPS and helping ensure appropriate services are provided are other examples.

In the community, primary care physicians can be influential advocates for resources for children and families. These resources may include parenting programs, services for battered women and their children, and recreational facilities. Primary care physicians have many opportunities to share their knowledge of children's physical, developmental, and emotional needs. They can participate on local multidisciplinary child death review teams or as advisors to organizations concerned with child abuse. Engaging in such activities provides opportunities to understand better the issues concerning child maltreatment and to help build safe and nurturing environments for children.

Finally, primary care physicians can play an important role in advocating for policies and programs at the local, state, and national levels that will benefit children and families. Primary care physicians can advocate for community-wide maltreatment prevention efforts at the primary, secondary, and tertiary levels. Primary care physicians can share their knowledge on the health and welfare of children and families with CPS colleagues. This contribution can lead to system changes that are responsive to children and to families entrusted to protect children. Such efforts may include involvement with state officials along with outreach to legislators and organizations involved in child advocacy. The American Academy of Pediatrics has an advocacy office in Washington, DC, engaged in legislative advocacy on a range of important child health issues and conducts an annual training on legislative advocacy. Child maltreatment is a complex problem that has no easy solutions. Through partnerships with colleagues in child protection, mental health, education, and law enforcement, primary care physicians can make a valuable difference in the lives of many children and families.

TOOLS FOR PRACTICE

Community Advocacy and Coordination

- *Child Welfare Information Directory* (Web page), Child Welfare Information Gateway (www.childwelfare.gov/).
- *Recognition of Child Abuse for the Mandated Reporter, 3rd ed* (book), American Academy of Pediatrics (www.aap.org/bst/showdetl.cfm?&did=15&product_id=2848&catid=132).
- *State Statutes Child Welfare Information Gateway* (interactive tool), Child Welfare Information Gateway (www.childwelfare.gov/systemwide/laws_policies/search/index.cfm).

Engaging Patients and Family

- *Child Abuse* (fact sheet), American Academy of Pediatrics (www.aap.org/topics.html).

- *Child Maltreatment: Prevention Strategies* (fact sheet), Centers for Disease Control and Prevention (www.cdc.gov/ncipc/factsheets/cmprevention.htm).
- *Prevent Shaken Baby Syndrome* (brochure), American Academy of Pediatrics (patiented.aap.org).

Medical Decision Support

- *Child Maltreatment: Fact Sheet* (fact sheet), Centers for Disease Control and Prevention (www.cdc.gov/ncipc/factsheets/cmfacts.htm).
- *Practicing Safety* (Web page), American Academy of Pediatrics (www.aap.org/practicingsafety/index.htm).
- *The Shaken Baby Syndrome* (book), Haworth Maltreatment & Trauma Press (www.aap.org/bookstore).
- *Treatment of Child Abuse* (book), American Academy of Pediatrics (www.aap.org/bookstore).
- *Visual Diagnosis of Child Abuse on CD-ROM, 2nd ed* (CD-ROM), American Academy of Pediatrics (www.aap.org/bookstore).

AAP POLICY STATEMENTS

American Academy of Pediatrics, Committee on Child Abuse and Neglect, and Committee on Children With Disabilities. Assessment of maltreatment of children with disabilities. *Pediatrics*. 2001;108(2):508-512. (pediatrics.aappublications.org/cgi/content/full/108/2/508).

American Academy of Pediatrics, Committee on Child Abuse and Neglect, and the National Association of Medical Examiners. Distinguishing sudden infant death syndrome from child abuse fatalities. *Pediatrics*. 2006;118(1):421-427. (aappolicy.aappublications.org/cgi/content/full/pediatrics;118/1/421).

American Academy of Pediatrics, Committee on Child Abuse and Neglect, Committee on Nutrition. Failure to thrive as a manifestation of child neglect. *Pediatrics*. 2005;116(5):1234-1237. (aappolicy.aappublications.org/cgi/content/full/pediatrics;116/5/1234).

American Academy of Pediatrics, Committee on Child Abuse and Neglect. Oral and dental aspects of child abuse and neglect. *Pediatrics*. 2005;116(6):1565-1568. (aappolicy.aappublications.org/cgi/content/full/pediatrics;116/6/1565).

American Academy of Pediatrics, Committee on Child Abuse and Neglect. Shaken baby syndrome: rotational cranial injuries-technical report. *Pediatrics*. 2001;108(1):206-210. (aappolicy.aappublications.org/cgi/content/full/pediatrics;108/1/206).

American Academy of Pediatrics, Committee on Child Abuse and Neglect. The psychological maltreatment of children-technical report. *Pediatrics*. 2002;109(4):e68. (aappolicy.aappublications.org/cgi/content/full/pediatrics;109/4/e68).

American Academy of Pediatrics, Committee on Child Abuse and Neglect. When inflicted skin injuries constitute child abuse. *Pediatrics*. 2002;110(3):644-645. (pediatrics.aappublications.org/cgi/content/full/110/3/644).

American Academy of Pediatrics, Committee on Child Abuse and Neglect. When is lack of supervision neglect? *Pediatrics*. 2006;118(3):1296-1298. (pediatrics.aappublications.org/cgi/content/full/118/3/1296).

American Academy of Pediatrics, Committee on Hospital Care, Committee on Child Abuse and Neglect. Medical necessity for the hospitalization of the abused and neglected child. *Pediatrics*. 1998;101(4):715-716. (aappolicy.aappublications.org/cgi/content/full/pediatrics;101/4/715).

SUGGESTED RESOURCES

Dubowitz H, DePanfilis D, eds. *The Handbook for Child Protection*. Thousand Oaks, CA: Sage Publications; 2000.

Finkel MA, Giardino AP. *Medical Evaluation of Child Sexual Abuse: A Practical Guide*. Newbury Park, CA: Sage Publications; 2002.

Reece R, Nicholson C. *Inflicted Childhood Neurotrauma*. Chicago, IL: American Academy of Pediatrics; 2003.

Reece RM, Ludwig S, eds. *Child Abuse: Medical Diagnosis and Management*. 2nd ed. Philadelphia, PA: Lea & Febiger; 2001.

REFERENCES

1. Edwards VJ, Holden GW, Felitti VJ, et al. Relationship between multiple forms of childhood maltreatment and adult mental health in community respondents: results from the adverse childhood experiences study. *Am J Psychiatry*. 2003;160:1453-1460.
2. Schuck AM, Widom CS. Understanding the role of neighborhood context in the long-term criminal consequences of child maltreatment. *Am J Community Psychol*. 2005;36:207-222.
3. Dubowitz H, Guterman N. Prevention of physical abuse and child neglect. In: Giardino A, Alexander R, eds. *Child Maltreatment: A Clinical Guide and Reference*. 3rd ed. St Louis, MO: GW Medical; 2005.
4. The Child Abuse Prevention and Treatment Act. 42 U.S.C. 5101 et seq. Available at: www.acf.hhs.gov/programs/cb/laws_policies/cblaws/capta03/capta_manual.pdf. Accessed November 27, 2006.
5. American Academy of Pediatrics, Division of Child Health Research. *AAP Survey on Corporal Punishment*. AAP Periodic Survey #38. Evanston, IL: American Academy of Pediatrics; 1998.
6. Wauchope BA, Straus MA. Physical punishment and physical abuse of American children. In: Straus MA, Gelles RJ, eds. *Physical Violence in American Families: Risk Factors and Adaptations to Violence in 8145 Families*. New Brunswick, NJ: Transaction Publishers; 1990.
7. Kempe CH. Sexual abuse: another hidden pediatric problem. *Pediatrics*. 1978;62:382.
8. Dubowitz H, Giardino A, Gustavson E. Child neglect: guidance for pediatricians. *Pediatr Rev*. 2000;21(4):111-116.
9. Lane WG, Rubin DM, Monteith R, et al. Racial differences in the evaluation of pediatric fractures for physical abuse. *JAMA*. 2002;288(13):1603-1609.
10. US Department of Health and Human Services, Administration on Children, Youth and Families. *Child Maltreatment 2003*. Washington, DC: US Government Printing Office; 2005.
11. Faller KC. *Understanding Child Sexual Maltreatment*. Newbury Park, CA: Sage Publications; 1990.
12. Molina JA. Understanding the biopsychosocial model. *Int J Psychiatry Med*. 1983;13(1):29-36.
13. Wu SS, Ma CX, Carter RL, et al. Risk factors for infant maltreatment: a population-based study. *Child Abuse Negl*. 2004;28(12):1253-1264.
14. Kendall-Tackett K, Lyon T, Taliaferro G, et al. Why child maltreatment researchers should include children's disability status in their maltreatment studies. *Child Abuse Negl*. 2005;29(2):147-151.
15. Wilson SL, Kuebli JE, Hughes HM. Patterns of maternal behavior among neglectful families: implications for research and intervention. *Child Abuse Negl*. 2005;29(9):985-1001.
16. Hazen AL, Connelly CD, Kelleher KJ, et al. Female caregivers' experiences with intimate partner violence and behavior problems in children investigated as victims of maltreatment. *Pediatrics*. 2006;117(1):99-109.

17. Korbin JE. Neighborhood and community connectedness in child maltreatment research. *Child Abuse Negl.* 2003;27(2):137-140.
18. Sedlack AJ, Broadhurst DD. *Third National Incidence Study of Child Abuse and Neglect: Final Report.* Washington, DC: US Department of Health and Human Services; 1996.
19. Dubowitz H. Preventing child neglect and physical abuse: a role for pediatricians. *Pediatr Rev.* 2002;23(6): 191-196.
20. Dias MS, Smith K, DeGuehery K, et al. Preventing abusive head trauma among infants and young children: a hospital-based, parent education program. *Pediatrics.* 2005;115(4):e470-e477.
21. Hoekelman RA. Child health supervision. In: Hoekelman N, Friedman SB, Nelson NM, et al, eds. *Primary Pediatric Care.* 3rd ed. St Louis, MO: Mosby; 1997.
22. Davis RE. Cultural health care or child abuse? The Southeast Asian practice of cao gio. *J Am Acad Nurse Pract.* 2000;12(3):89-95.
23. Sugar NF, Taylor JA, Feldman KW. Bruises in infants and toddlers: those who don't cruise rarely bruise. Puget Sound Pediatric Research Network. *Arch Pediatr Adolesc Med.* 1999;153(4):399-403.
24. Naidoo S. A profile of the oro-facial injuries in child physical abuse at a children's hospital. *Child Abuse Negl.* 2000;24(4):521-534.
25. Johnson CF, Sahuers J. Injury variables in child abuse. *Child Abuse Neglect.* 1985;9:207.
26. Maguire S, Mann MK, Sibert J, et al. Can you age bruises accurately in children? A systematic review. *Arch Dis Child.* 2005;90(2):187-189.
27. Jenny C. Cutaneous manifestations of child abuse. In: Reece RM, Ludwig S, eds. *Child Abuse: Medical Diagnosis and Management.* 2nd ed. Philadelphia, PA: Lea & Febiger; 2001.
28. Renz BM, Sherman R. Abusive scald burns in infants and children: a prospective study. *Am Surg.* 1993;59(5):329-334.
29. Angel C, Shu T, French D, et al. Genital and perineal burns in children: 10 years of experience at a major burn center. *J Pediatr Surg.* 2002;37(1):99-103.
30. Surrell JA, Alexander RC, Cohle SD, et al. Effects of microwave radiation on living tissues. *J Trauma.* 1987; 27(8):935-939.
31. Frechette A, Rimsza ME. Stun gun injury: a new presentation of the battered child syndrome. *Pediatrics.* 1992; 89(5 pt 1):898-901.
32. Chester DL, Jose RM, Aldlyami E, et al. Non-accidental burns in children—are we neglecting neglect? *Burns.* 2006;32(2):222-228.
33. Drago DA. Kitchen scalds and thermal burns in children 5 years and younger. *Pediatrics.* 2005;115(1):10-16.
34. Chuang SS, Yang JY, Tsai FC. Electric water heaters: a new hazard for pediatric burns. *Burns.* 2003;29(6): 589-591.
35. Feldman KW. Pseudoabusive burns in Asian refugees. *Am J Dis Child.* 1984;138(8):768-769.
36. Forjuoh SN. Pattern of intentional burns to children in Ghana. *Child Abuse Negl.* 1995;19(7):837-841.
37. Holter JC, Friedman SB. Etiology and management of severely burned children. Psychosocial considerations. *Am J Dis Child.* 1969;118(5):680-686.
38. Erdmann TC, Feldman KW, Rivara FP, et al. Tap water burn prevention: the effect of legislation. *Pediatrics.* 1991;88(3):572-577.
39. Feldman KW, Schaller RT, Feldman JA, et al. Tap water scald burns in children. *Pediatrics.* 1978;62(1):1-7.
40. Kleinman PK. *Diagnostic Imaging of Child Abuse.* Baltimore, MD: Mosby; 1998.
41. Mandelstramm SA, Cook D, Fitzgerald M, et al. Complementary use of radiological skeletal survey and bone scintigraphy in detection of bone injuries in suspected child abuse. *Arch Dis Child.* 2003;88:387-389.
42. American College of Radiology. Practice guideline for skeletal surveys in children. *AJR.* 2002;178:119-123.
43. Bonnier C, Nassogne MC, Evard P. Outcome and prognosis of whiplash shaken infant syndrome: late consequences after a symptom-free interval. *Dev Med Child Neurol.* 1995;37:973.
44. Helfer RE, Slovis TL, Black M. Injuries resulting when small children fall out of bed. *Pediatrics.* 1997;60:533-535.
45. Nimityongskul P, Anderson LD. The likelihood of injuries when children fall out of bed. *J Pediatric Ortho.* 1987;7: 184-186.
46. Lyons TJ, Oakes RK. Falling out of bed: a relatively benign occurrence. *Pediatrics.* 1993;92:125-127.
47. Hanzlick R. On the need for more expertise in death investigation. *Arch Path Lab Med.* 1996;120:329-332.
48. Arborgast KB, Margulies SS, Christian CW. Initial neurologic presentation in young children sustaining inflicted and no intentional fatal head injuries. *Pediatrics.* 2005; 116:180-184.
49. Willman KY, Bank DE, Senac M, et al. Restricting the time of injury in fatal inflicted head injuries. *Child Abuse Negl.* 1997;21:929.
50. Jenny C, Hymel KP, Ritzen A, et al. Analysis of missed cases of abusive head trauma. *JAMA.* 1999;281:621.
51. Maxeiner H, Bockholdt B. Homicidal and suicidal ligature strangulation: a comparison of postmortem findings. *Forensic Sci Int.* 2003;137:60-66.
52. Plattner T, Bollinger S, Zollinger U. Forensic assessment of survived strangulation. *Forensic Sci Int.* 2005;153(2-3): 202-207.
53. Levin AV. Retinal hemorrhages and child abuse. In: David TJ, ed. *Recent Advances in Paediatrics.* 18th ed. London, UK: Churchill Livingstone; 2000.
54. Odom A, Christ E, Kerr N, et al. Prevalence of retinal hemorrhages in pediatric patients after in-hospital cardiopulmonary resuscitation: a prospective study. *Pediatrics.* 1997;99:e3.
55. Massicotte SJ, Folberg R, Torczynski E, et al. Vitreoretinal traction and perimacular retinal folds in eyes of deliberately traumatized children. *Ophthalmology.* 1991;98: 1124.
56. Ambrose JB. Orofacial signs of child abuse and neglect: a dental perspective. *Pediatrician.* 1989;16:188.
57. Ludwig S. Visceral manifestations of child abuse. In: Reece RM, Ludwig S, eds. *Child Abuse: Medical Diagnosis and Management.* 2nd ed. Philadelphia, PA: Lippincott, Williams and Wilkens; 2001.
58. Roche KJ, Genieser NB, Berger DK, et al. Traumatic abdominal pseudoaneurysm secondary to child abuse. *Pediatr Radiol.* 1995;25:s247-s248.
59. Hennes HM, Smith DS, Schneider K, et al. Elevated liver transaminase levels in children with blunt abdominal trauma: a predictor of liver injury. *Pediatrics.* 1990;86: 87-90.
60. Coant PN, Kornberg AE, Brody AS, et al. Markers for occult liver injury in cases of physical abuse in children. *Pediatrics.* 1992;89:274-278.
61. Partan G, Pamberger P, Blab E, et al. Common tasks and problems in paediatric trauma radiology. *Eur Radiol.* 2003;48(1):103-124.
62. Barnes PM, Norton CM, Dunstan FD, et al. Abdominal injury due to child abuse. *Lancet.* 2005;366:34-235.
63. Huntimer CM, Muret-Wagstaff S, Leland NL. Can falls on stairs result in small intestine perforations? *Pediatrics.* 2000;106(2 pt 1):301-305.

64. US Department of Health and Human Services, Administration on Children. *Youth and Families. Child Maltreatment 2004*. Washington, DC: US Government Printing Office; 2006.
65. Hildyard KL, Wolfe DA. Child neglect: developmental issues and outcomes. *Child Abuse Negl*. 2002;26(6 pt 7):679-695.
66. Dubowitz H, Black M. Child neglect. In: Reece RM, Ludwig S, eds. *Child Abuse: Medical Diagnosis and Management*. 2nd ed. Philadelphia, PA: Lea & Febiger; 2001.
67. Dubowitz H. The neglect of children's health care. In: Dubowitz H, ed. *Neglected Children: Research, Practice and Policy*. Thousand. Oaks CA: Sage Publications; 1999.
68. Dubowitz H. *Child Neglect: the Long-Term Medical Management. The Treatment of Child Abuse*. Baltimore, MD: The Johns Hopkins University Press; 2000.
69. Kolko DJ. Characteristics of child victims of physical violence: research findings and clinical implications. *J Interpers Viol*. 1992;7:244-276.
70. Perez CM, Widom CS. Childhood victimization and long-term intellectual and academic outcomes. *Child Abuse Negl*. 1994;18(8):617-633.
71. Dube SR, Felitti VJ, Dong M, et al. The impact of adverse childhood experiences on health problems: evidence from 4 birth cohorts dating back to 1900. *Prev Med*. 2003;37(3):268-277.
72. Kaufman J, Zigler E. Do abused children become abusive parents? *Am J Orthopsychiatry*. 1987;57(2):186-192.
73. van der Kolk BA. The neurobiology of childhood trauma and abuse. *Child Adolesc Psychiatr Clin North Am*. 2003;12(2):293-317, ix.
74. Rutter M, O'Connor TG. Are there biological programming effects for psychological development? Findings from a study of Romanian adoptees. *Dev Psychol*. 2004;40(1):81-94.

Chapter 121

CHILDREN IN SELF-CARE

Robert D. Needlman, MD

The widespread entry of women into the labor force during World War II raised concerns about parental supervision for children who wore their house keys around their necks to let themselves into their homes after school, so-called "latchkey children." Care for children and adolescents continues to pose a dilemma for many parents whose occupations preclude them from being available outside of school hours. Pediatricians, aware of the potential stresses and dangers associated with unsupervised care, can help parents find acceptable solutions.

The typical family is now a working family, with both parents, or the only parent, employed outside of the home. This circumstance is the case in 60% of 2-parent families with school-age children, 70% of single-mother families, and 80% of single-father families.[1] According to a recent national survey, among working families, approximately 31% of children in kindergarten through 12th grade are in self-care on a regular basis, and only 14% participate in organized after-school programs.[2] With increasing age, the rate of self-care rises and program participation falls (Figure 121-1). In rural areas, self-care is more prevalent and after-school programs are less available (Figure 121-2).

The true prevalence of unsupervised care is difficult to estimate. Parents may underreport children in self-care to avoid stigma or feared legal action[3]; they may even be reluctant to disclose self-care arrangements to their child's physician. Unsupervised care actually represents a spectrum of arrangements. For example, a parent may telephone home every hour, may be reachable by telephone at any time, reachable only in emergencies, or not reachable at all. The nearest responsible neighbor may be across the hall or a mile away. A child may be home alone, or in the care of an older sibling, or caring for a younger one. Many children spend the after-school hours at the library, which may provide a formal after-school program, informal guidance by a concerned librarian, or merely grudging toleration. Some children go to friends' homes, where a responsible adult may be present, or not. Others

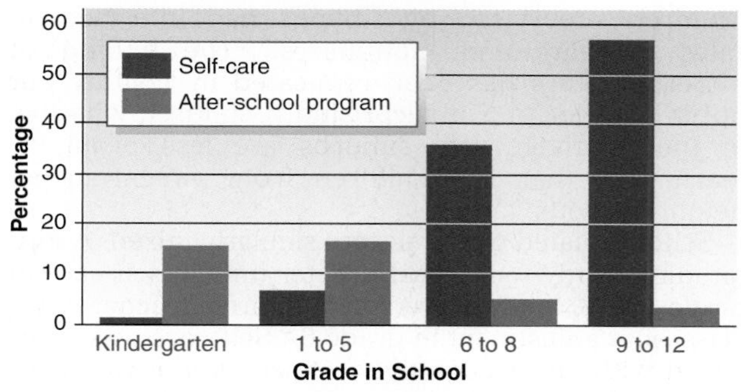

Figure 121-1 With increasing age, the percentage of children in after-school programs declines while the percentage in self-care increases.

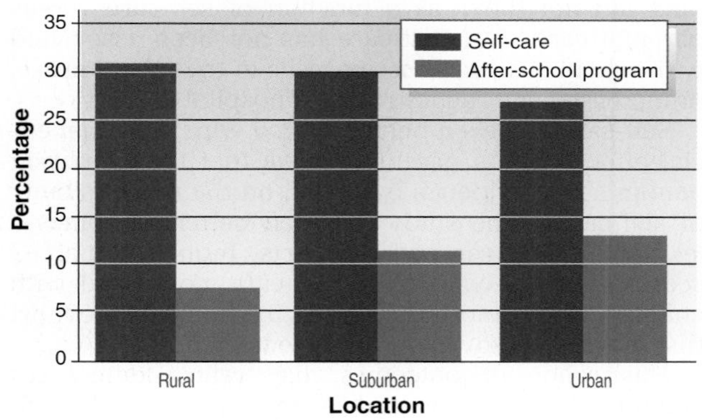

Figure 121-2 In rural areas, self-care is more prevalent and after-school programs are less available.

meet at the mall, in parks, or elsewhere in the community. It is typical for a child to experience different arrangements on different days of the week and for arrangements to change from year to year, if not more frequently.[4] This considerable variability needs to be taken into account when counseling parents and when interpreting the research literature.

EFFECTS OF SELF-CARE: SCHOOL-AGE CHILDREN

Many parents and professionals believe that self-care is harmful. James Garbarino, a well-known researcher and author, has suggested that children in self-care suffer in 4 ways: (1) they feel bad (emotional effects), (2) act badly (high-risk behaviors), (3) develop badly (academic deficits), and (4) are treated badly (risk of victimization).[3] The research literature, however, is equivocal.

Parents often worry that their children will be scared to stay alone. Indeed, a 1981 study of low-income children in 1st through 6th grades in Washington, DC, reported higher rates of fearfulness and nightmares among children who were unsupervised after school, compared with those in parental care. Children supervised by siblings had intermediate rates of fears and nightmares.[5] The finding of increased fears has been replicated in 1 study but not in another.[6,7] Not surprisingly, children who live in the relatively safe suburbs are less prone to fearfulness than are children from violent urban neighborhoods.[4,8]

School-related outcomes are similarly mixed. A longitudinal study found that greater time in self-care in grades 1, 3, and 5 predicted poorer teacher-rated classroom adjustment in grade 6.[9] Self-care was associated with lower cognitive test scores in a cohort of lower-income girls (but not boys)[10] but was *not* associated with poorer grades, either among suburban 3rd graders,[11] rural 5th and 7th graders,[12] or urban 8th graders.[6] A 1992 study found no difference in children's self-rated competence between self- and parent care, although children in the care of siblings had lower self-rated competence.[13]

In cross-sectional studies, children's self-esteem, locus of control, peer relationships, and classroom conduct did not differ as a function of self-care versus parental care.[7,12,14] Self-care has not been associated with school absence, obesity, visits to the school nurse, or increased emergency room or hospital use.[10,15]

Self-care has even been credited with some beneficial effects. Some parents believe that their children gain in self-confidence by taking on the responsibility of self-care.[4] One study reported better outcomes—less anxiety, fewer peer conflicts, higher verbal IQ scores—among children in self-care, compared with children whose mothers were in the home, in a cohort that included many lower-income teen mothers.[16]

This range of outcomes may reflect differences among the populations studied, among the various definitions of self-care, or among the selection of outcome measures. Most of the studies are cross-sectional, limiting conclusions about causality. Multiple factors go into determining whether a child might be exposed to after-care and if so, what type. The salient factors are likely to be hard to quantify, such as a parent's sense that his or her child is mature enough to handle self-care or the strength of a parent's guilt or fear about leaving his or her child unsupervised. No randomized studies are available to provide definitive answers.

EFFECTS OF SELF-CARE: TEENS

One area in which a fairly high level of agreement exists concerns the association of less adult supervision and increased substance use and other risk-taking behaviors among teens. The number of hours of self-care per week has been correlated consistently with rates of cigarette, alcohol, and marijuana use among adolescents.[17-20] Adolescents who are unsupervised at friends' homes are more at risk of succumbing to negative peer pressure than are those who stay in their own homes. Those who hang out with friends without a set location are at greatest risk.[21] Nonpermissive parenting style, family rules prohibiting substance use, and increased supervision (eg, through required telephone calls) lower, but do not eliminate, the risk associated with self-care.[17,21]

Early adolescents may be particularly vulnerable to the stresses and temptations of self-care. Compared with parent-supervised 8th graders, those in self-care for 11 or more hours per week reported 1.5 to 2 times higher levels of risk taking, anger, family conflict, peer influence, attendance at parties, and substance use. Moreover, earlier initiation of self-care was associated with increased rates of these negative behaviors. For example, 11% of 8th graders in parental care reported heavy alcohol use compared with 19.5% in self-care since junior high school and 25.5% in self-care since elementary school.[6]

AFTER-SCHOOL PROGRAMS

Alternatives to self-care include care provided by relatives or hired sitters or by structured after-school programs. Evidence suggests that high-quality after-school programs can improve children's academic and personal growth, particularly for economically disadvantaged children.[22] A growing movement advocates after-school programming for everyone, and such programs are increasingly available.[23] However, a 2003 survey by the US Conference of Mayors found that after-school programs were still only serving approximately 35% of the children who might have benefited from them.[23] Cost and the lack of transportation to the program from school often limits access. Fewer programs are offered for teens,[4] and older children are more likely to find structured programs uninteresting or crave the freedom of self-care.[23,24] High-quality after-school programs may be especially sparse in lower-income neighborhoods, where higher crime levels also tend to make self-care less acceptable.[25]

DECISIONS ABOUT AFTER-SCHOOL CARE

Parents' decisions about after-school care can be relatively straightforward, or they can be difficult and fraught with guilt and worry.[4] Self-care can be a positive experience, assuming that the child is mature

BOX 121-1 Signs of Readiness for Self-Care

Age: A sensible 8 year old should be fine for a half hour or so once in a while, but most children will not be mature enough to manage alone on a regular basis until they are 10 or 11 years of age.

Interests: The child is able to keep busy reading, drawing, making music, doing homework, and playing with toys among other things (not just watching television or playing video games).

Memory: The child remembers common-sense safety rules, such as not opening the door and not telling telephone callers that they are alone.

Common sense: The child can relate how to respond to a fire or gas leak or other emergency.

Caution: The child generally shows caution, thinking before acting. This is particularly important for young teens, who are tempted to engage in sexual and other experimentation.

Comfort: The child seems to be truly OK with the idea of being home alone.

enough, the neighborhood safe enough, and the hours short enough. Box 121-1 presents a common-sense checklist to help parents decide if self-care is right for them.[26] Many states have adopted guidelines that attempt to help draw the line between acceptable unsupervised care and neglect, although the wording of these documents is sometimes vague; actual laws on the subject exist only in few states.[27] In many communities, service agencies offer "survival training" to prepare children to cope with self-care. The efficacy of such classes has been questioned, however.[3,28]

PEDIATRICIAN'S ROLE

Pediatricians can ask about child-care arrangements at health supervision visits for children of all ages. Parents of school-age and adolescent children may have questions about care outside of school hours but may hesitate to bring up the subject. Parents need to understand that the effect of self-care varies depending on the child and the specific circumstances. Pediatricians can help parents think through the issues as they apply to their individual situation. Awareness of the increased rates of substance use and other risk taking among unsupervised adolescents may lead parents to reconsider self-care for their teenage children. To date, the efficacy of pediatric guidance about out-of-school care has not been demonstrated empirically.

Pediatricians can also help connect parents with community resources, such as high-quality after-school programs, latchkey training programs, and telephone "warm lines" that provide safe human contact and support to children alone after school. Locally, service agencies such as the YMCA and Boys and Girls Clubs are likely to be good resources, as are public libraries. Guidance and referrals can be found through the Child Care Resource and Referral Programs in most states. The National Child Care Information Center (www.nccic.org) maintains computerized links to these programs; the national toll-free number is 1-800-424-2246. Where local services are inadequate, pediatricians can play an important role in advocating for more high-quality out-of-school programs for school-age children and adolescents.

AAP POLICY STATEMENT

American Academy of Pediatrics, Committee on Early Childhood, Adoption, and Dependent Care. Quality early education and child care from birth to kindergarten. *Pediatrics*. 2005;115(1):187-191. (aappolicy.aappublications.org/cgi/content/full/pediatrics;115/1/187).

REFERENCES

1. United States Department of Labor, Bureau of Labor Statistics. Table 4. Families with Own Children: Employment Status of Parents by Age of Youngest Child and Family Type, 2003-04 Annual Averages. Available at: www.bls.gov/news.release/famee.t04.htm. Accessed April, 20, 2006.
2. Afterschool Alliance. America After 3 PM: Working Families and Afterschool: A Special Report: A Household Survey on Afterschool in America. Available at: www.afterschoolalliance.org/america_3pm.cfm. Accessed April, 20, 2006.
3. Lamorey S, Robinson BE, Rowland BH, et al. *Latchkey Kids: Unlocking Doors for Children and Their Families*. 2nd ed. Thousand Oaks, CA: Sage Publications; 1999.
4. Belle D. *The After-School Lives of Children: Alone and With Others While Parents Work*. Mahwah, NJ: Lawrence Erlbaum Associates; 1999.
5. Long T, Long L. *Latchkey Children. The Child's View of Self-Care* [ED 211 229]. Urbana, IL ERIC Clearinghouse on Elementary and Early Childhood Education; 1981.
6. Dwyer KM, Richardson JL, Danley KL, et al. Characteristics of eighth-grade students who initiate self-care in elementary and junior high school. *Pediatrics*. 1990;86(3): 448-454.
7. Posner JK, Vandell DL. Low-income children's after-school care: are there beneficial effects of after-school programs? *Child Dev*. 1994;65(2 spec no.):440-456.
8. Padilla ML, Landreth GL. Latchkey children: a review of the literature. *Child Welfare*. 1989;68(4):445-454.
9. Pettit G, Laird R. Patterns of after-school care in middle childhood: risk factors and developmental outcomes. *Merrill-Palmer Quarterly*. 1997;43:515-538.
10. Woods M. The unsupervised child of the working mother. *Dev Psychol*. 1972;6:14-25.
11. Vandell DL, Corasaniti MA. The relation between third graders' after-school care and social, academic, and emotional functioning. *Child Dev*. 1988;59(4):868-875.
12. Galambos NL, Garbarino J. Identifying the missing links in the study of latchkey children. *Child Today*. 1983;12(4): 2-4, 40-41.
13. Berman BD, Winkleby M, Chesterman E, et al. After-school child care and self-esteem in school-age children. *Pediatrics*. 1992;89(4 Pt 1):654-659.
14. Rodman H, Pratto D, Nelson R. Child care arrangements and children's functioning: a comparison of self-care and adult-care children. *Dev Psychol*. 1986;21:413-418.
15. Williams RL, Boyce WT. Health status of children in self-care. *Am J Dis Child*. 1989;143(1):112-115.
16. Vandell D, Ramanan J. Children of the national longitudinal survey of youth: choices in after-school care and child development. *Dev Psychol*. 1991;27(4):637-643.
17. Mott JA, Crowe PA, Richardson J, et al. After-school supervision and adolescent cigarette smoking: contributions of the setting and intensity of after-school self-care. *J Behav Med*. 1999;22(1):35-58.

18. Mulhall P, Stone D, Stone B. Home alone: is it a risk factor for middle school youth and drug use? *J Drug Educ.* 1996;26:39-48.
19. Richardson JL, Radziszewska B, Dent CW, et al. Relationship between after-school care of adolescents and substance use, risk taking, depressed mood, and academic achievement. *Pediatrics.* 1993;92(1):32-38.
20. Richardson JL, Dwyer K, McGuigan K, et al. Substance use among eighth-grade students who take care of themselves after school. *Pediatrics.* 1989;84(3):556-566.
21. Steinberg L. Latchkey children and susceptibility to peer pressure: an ecological analysis. *Dev Psychol.* 1986;22: 433-439.
22. Miller B. *Critical Hours: Afterschool Programs and Educational Success.* Brookline, MA: Nellie Mae Education Foundation; 2003. Available at: www.nmefdn.org/ Accessed April 22, 2006.
23. National Institute on Out-of-School Time. Making the case: a fact sheet on children and youth in out-of-school time. Wellesly, MA: National Institute on Out-of-School Time; 2006. Available at: www.niost.org. Accessed April 21, 2006.
24. Larner M, Zippiroli L, Behrman R. When school is out: analysis and recommendations. *The Future of Children: When School is Out.* 1999;9(2):10-12.
25. Halpern R. After-school programs for low-income children: promises and challenges. *The Future of Children: When School is Out.* 1999;9(2):81-95.
26. Needlman R. Latchkey Arrangements. Available at: www.drspock.com. Accessed April 25, 2006.
27. National Child Care Information Center. Children Home Alone and Babysitter Age Guidelines. Available at: nccic.acf.hhs.gov/poptopics/homealone.html. Accessed April 25, 2006.
28. Kraizer S, Witte S, Fryer GE, et al. Children in self-care: a new perspective. *Child Welfare.* 1990;69(6):571-581.

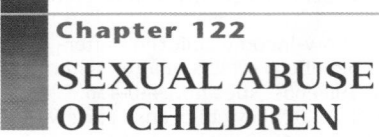

Chapter 122

SEXUAL ABUSE OF CHILDREN

John M. Leventhal, MD; Andrea Gottsegen Asnes, MD, MSW

Although sexual abuse of children has existed for centuries, only in the last 30 years have clinicians come to recognize the scope of the problem, including its epidemiologic factors, clinical characteristics, approaches to management, and consequences to children and families.

DEFINITION AND EPIDEMIOLOGIC FACTORS

Sexual abuse is defined as the involvement of children or adolescents in sexual activities that they do not fully understand, to which they cannot give informed consent, and that violate the social taboos of families or society.[1] This type of abuse includes activities such as the sexual touching of a child's genitals by an adult or adolescent, sexual intercourse between an adult and child, the exposing of children to pornography, or involvement of children in prostitution. Sexual abuse should be distinguished from sexual play or exploration by preschool or young school-age children or sexual activities between consenting adolescents.

Child protection laws that were passed in the 1960s in each state initially required the reporting of cases of suspected physical abuse or neglect but were shortly after broadened to include children suspected of being sexually abused. Since 1976, national statistics of cases reported to each state's child protection agency have been compiled. When reports of sexual abuse are examined, the most dramatic increase in reports occurred in the 1980s as a result of increased publicity and increased recognition by parents and clinicians. In the 1990s, substantiated reports of sexual abuse peaked at more than 150,000 cases per year (representing approximately 13% of almost 1.2 million substantiated cases of child maltreatment). Since then the number has decreased to a total of 84,398 substantiated reports of sexual abuse in 2004, the latest year for which complete data were compiled. These reports represent 9.7% of all substantiated reports of child maltreatment that year.[2]

In 2004, of all reports made to protective services, approximately 26% were substantiated after investigation. The failure to substantiate an allegation does not necessarily mean that the abuse did not occur, but rather that protective services did not have enough evidence to confirm the allegation.

Approximately 75% of children evaluated for suspected sexual abuse are girls. The age range is from 6 months to 18 years, with a median age of approximately 8 years.

Although such cases represent those reported to child protective services, an alternative approach to estimating the frequency of the problem has been to interview adults about their childhood experiences of sexual abuse. These studies provide information about lifetime prevalence. A review of 19 studies conducted on community samples in the United States or Canada since 1980 found that the rates of sexual abuse reported by women were 2% to 62% and by men were 3% to 16%.[3] Finkelhor has suggested that a summary statistic for women of 20% would be reasonable.[3] Multiple studies of adults conducted in other countries, including developing countries, have yielded similar prevalence rates.[4] Because only 9 of the studies in Finkelhor's review surveyed men, less certainty existed about a summary statistic for men, but a conservative estimate would be 5% to 10%.[3] The prevalence of sexual abuse reported by adults in different studies varies because of the population studied, the response rate, the number and types of questions asked, the definition of sexual abuse, the age used to define childhood, the accuracy of the adults' memories, and the willingness of the adults to report past events.[5]

Unlike cases of physical abuse or neglect, which are reported much more commonly in families who are poor and have limited education, cases of sexual abuse occur in families from all social classes and educational backgrounds. Perpetrators of sexual abuse are almost all boys and men, and nearly one third of them are adolescents. Most children who have been sexually abused know the perpetrator, who may be the father, stepfather, another male relative, family friend, or an adult in the child's community. Although female perpetrators are unusual in most clinical series, these rates may be falsely low because of underrecognition. A small number of sexually abused children do not know the perpetrator; these victims are usually older children or adolescents who are victims of forceful sexual assault or rape.

ETIOLOGY

Although clinicians are able to understand how a parent might lose control and physically abuse a child, understanding how an adult can move from close bodily contact and even sensual feelings toward sexually abusing a child is much more difficult. Two prerequisites for sexual abuse to occur include the offender's sexual arousal to children and the willingness to act on this arousal.[6] Studies have attempted to examine adults' sexual attraction to children. For example, 21% of male college students in an anonymous questionnaire indicated that they felt sexual attraction toward children.[7] Some offenders may focus their attention on children of a certain age or gender; others may find themselves aroused only by children in certain circumstances. Factors that influence the offender's willingness to act on the aroused feelings toward the child include a lack of conscience about such behaviors, a lack of empathy for the child, a belief that such sexual behaviors are acceptable and not harmful to the child, poor impulse control, and the use of drugs or alcohol that might further decrease the ability to control behavior.[6] Additional contributors to the likelihood that sexual abuse may occur include the history of the perpetrator (eg, having experienced sexual abuse during childhood), circumstances that allow the perpetrator to have increased contact with the child (eg, a mother hospitalized for a lengthy period), and the particular vulnerabilities of the child (eg, intellectual disability).

Children who are sexually abused are often selected because they seem particularly vulnerable or needy. Such children may initially enjoy and appreciate the attention that they receive from the offender, who may begin by giving the child gifts, attention, and special hugs and touches. These behaviors may progress to special secrets and eventually from nonsexual to sexual activities that lead to sexual intercourse. This process has been labeled the child sexual abuse accommodation syndrome,[8] which describes 5 stages that occur in the sexual abuse of children: (1) secrecy; (2) helplessness; (3) entrapment and accommodation; (4) delayed, unconvincing disclosures; and (5) later retraction of the alleged abuse.

CLINICAL MANIFESTATIONS

Similar to other forms of family violence, sexual abuse of children often occurs in the privacy of a home or in a setting that involves only the abused and the abuser and is seldom witnessed by another person. A child who has been sexually abused may have experienced other forms of maltreatment, including physical abuse or neglect, and certainly has been emotionally abused as well.

A clinician's concerns about the possibility of sexual abuse occur because of reports of specific statements made by the child, usually to a parent or other adult, about uncomfortable experiences such as being touched on the genitalia, reports of specific behaviors of the child such as sexualized behaviors with a sibling, symptoms such as encopresis or vaginal discharge or bleeding, or a genital or anal injury noted on physical examination.

Clear statements by the child (or occasionally accidental direct observations of the sexual abuse) are the best indicators that sexual abuse has occurred. These statements are usually told to a parent or trusted adult, such as a schoolteacher. Young children, however, may not have the necessary vocabulary to describe what has happened to them. They may use words that the perpetrator used to encourage their participation (eg, "We played the hugging game") or words that describe their experience of what happened or how it felt but are confusing to the adults (eg, "He stuck a knife in my pee-pee"). Older children may begin by offering a guarded, vague disclosure (eg, "My uncle kisses too hard"). If the adult reacts in a concerned manner with appropriate exploratory questions, then more details may follow. The older child may be embarrassed about what happened, feel partially responsible, have experienced pleasurable feelings, or be concerned about the threats that the perpetrator made (eg, "If you tell your mother, I will punch you" or "If you tell, you know they will think you are a liar"). Even after a clear disclosure, once children realize how upsetting the information is to the family, they may retract the statement. Older children also may feel responsible for holding the family together: If the child tells, then the father will go to jail, the house will be sold, and everyone will be angry at the child; on the other hand, if nothing is said, then the sexual abuse will continue, but at least the family will be saved. Some children consciously or unconsciously sacrifice themselves for their family.

Children who have been sexually abused may demonstrate a variety of symptoms and behaviors. Some may be relatively asymptomatic and be able to function reasonably well in social settings and in school. Many children exhibit nonspecific symptoms, such as sleep problems, generalized anxiety, suicidal gestures, or poor school performance, which are seen in response to other childhood stresses as well. Sexualized behaviors, such as excessive masturbation, the use of adult words associated with sexuality, or simulation of sexual intercourse with another child, animal, or doll, are more suggestive of sexual abuse. Other concerning symptoms include vaginal pain, bleeding, or discharge or rectal bleeding. Even a symptom such as a vaginal discharge, however, has a low likelihood of being caused by sexual abuse. Several studies of premenarcheal girls who have complained of vaginal discharge have shown that the occurrence of sexual abuse is infrequent (fewer than 5% to 10% of girls who have this complaint) and that the most common cause is poor hygiene.[9]

Only a small percentage of sexually abused children will have an abnormal genital or anal finding. For example, a study of 2384 children referred for possible sexual abuse to a tertiary referral center found that only 4% of the children had an abnormal examination at the time of evaluation.[10] Acute findings such as genital or anal abrasions may be more likely to be seen in the emergency department setting. The absence of physical findings, however, does not rule out sexual abuse because no injury may have occurred to the genital area, or if an injury did occur, then it may have healed without leaving any physical signs. Even in cases in which the perpetrator has been convicted of sexual abuse, having had an abnormal examination is unusual for the victim. For example, in a series of 236 child abuse cases in which the perpetrators were convicted, only 23% of the victims' genital examinations were considered suspicious or abnormal in girls and only 7% of anal examinations were considered so in boys and girls.[11] Even in adolescents who are pregnant and examined for suspected sexual abuse, physical findings indicating sexual abuse are unusual. In a case review of 36 pregnant adolescents evaluated for sexual abuse, only 2 of the 36 girls had definitive findings of penetration.[12] The authors of this study suggest 2 possible explanations for this finding: Penetration does not result in visible tissue damage, or acute injuries occur with penetration but heal completely. These studies highlight both the limited role of physical findings in the investigations of sexual abuse and the crucial role of the child's history of the abuse.

Over the last several years, research has defined normal and abnormal genital and anal anatomic features in prepubertal children and adolescents. Several studies have described the variations in the anatomic features of the hymen in female newborns and have concluded that the hymen is present in all normally developed newborns.[13] The appearance of the hymen is often thickened early in life because of the effects of maternal estrogen in utero; in preschool and school-age girls, the hymenal tissue becomes thinner until the effects of estrogen during puberty result in a thickening of the tissue and the development of redundant folds. Studies of normal prepubertal girls have described the shapes of the hymen as crescentic, annular, and fimbriated (or redundant) and have noted the frequency of normal variations, including hymenal mounds, intravaginal ridges, and adhesions of the labia minora.[14,15] These studies have provided data on the means and ranges of the vertical and horizontal diameters of the hymenal orifice in different age groups, the variations in diameter depending on how the genital examination is performed (eg, separation versus traction of the labia majora),[16] and the width of the posterior hymenal rim.

Children who have been sexually abused may have acute injuries of the genitalia, including acute lacerations, abrasions, or hematomas.[17] Most children who have been sexually abused, however, do not disclose until weeks or months after the occurrence of the abuse. In such children, findings that are considered suspicious or suggestive of past abuse include U- or V-shaped clefts (or notches) of the posterior rim (from 3 o'clock to 9 o'clock) of the hymen, which occur in the healing process after an acute laceration, and attenuation or decreased width of the hymenal tissue posteriorly (<1 mm). These findings should persist when the child is examined in the prone, knee-chest position.[17,18] A study of 192 prepubertal girls between the ages of 3 and 8 years who had a history of penetrating sexual abuse and 200 who denied prior abuse detected few differences in anatomic findings between the abused and nonabused samples. A few specific hymenal findings were evident, however, that were noted in 4 girls in the abused group and not in the comparison group. These were hymenal deep notches, perforations, or transections, and each was noted in a girl who disclosed penetration.[19] Scarring, such as of the posterior fourchette, is also indicative of previous trauma.[17,18] Although, in the past, investigators have considered an enlarged horizontal diameter of the hymen of greater than 4 mm to be suspicious of previous sexual abuse in prepubertal children, studies of normal children have indicated that this demarcation is incorrect and that the size of the opening varies with the child's age and different examination techniques,[16] as well as with the child's state of relaxation. A horizontal diameter of greater than 10 mm may concern a clinician about the possibility of sexual abuse but should not be used by itself to make a diagnosis.

Data about normal physical findings in adolescence have been limited; 1 study compared 3 groups of female adolescents: (1) those who denied sexual intercourse and used only pads for menses, (2) those who denied sexual intercourse and used tampons, and (3) those who had experienced sexual intercourse.[20] Although significant differences were found in the median horizontal diameters of the hymenal orifice in the 3 groups (1.2, 1.5, and 2.5 cm, respectively), overlap certainly existed among the groups. In addition, a striking difference among the groups was that of the sexually active teenagers: 81% had a complete cleft (or V-shaped notch) between the 2 o'clock and 10 o'clock positions on the hymenal border compared with 11% in tampon users and 5% in pad users.

A 2004 study of 85 girls between the ages of 13 and 19 years improved on these data by using a colposcope for magnification and photographic documentation of hymenal morphologic features. In this study, posterior hymenal notches and clefts were more common in girls admitting past intercourse (48%) than in girls who denied intercourse (3%). The 3% of girls who denied intercourse and had posterior hymenal clefts described a painful first experience with tampon insertion. Of note, the mean width of the posterior hymenal tissue was not significantly different between girls who admitted and those who denied past intercourse.[21]

Abnormalities of the male genitalia caused by sexual abuse are unusual. Acute abrasions, lacerations, or bruises caused by physical abuse, however, can be seen.

Acute anal findings, such as lacerations resulting from anal penetration or injury, have been noted in sexually abused children, but few systematic studies of perianal findings in chronically abused children have been conducted. Worrisome findings include thickening of the rugae, distorted anatomy secondary to scarring, and dilation greater than 2.0 cm (when the child is in the prone, knee-chest position and no stool is visible in the rectal ampulla). In a study of children with documented anal injuries followed from acute injury to healing, 29 of the 31 children healed completely, with scar formation only in the 2 cases requiring acute surgical repair.[22] A study of normal prepubertal children highlighted common normal findings that were noted when the child was examined in the prone, knee-chest position; these included skin tags in the midline, fan-shaped areas in the midline superiorly, perianal erythema, venous congestion, and anal dilation up to 2.0 cm.[23]

Children who have been sexually abused may acquire a sexually transmitted infection (STI).[17] Controversy continues about how children acquire such diseases, in part, because of the social and legal implications and because of the difficulty in believing that a young child's infection is from sexual contact. Approximately 5% of sexually abused children acquire an STI from the perpetrator of the abuse.[24] According to a 2005 clinical report published by the American Academy of Pediatrics, the presence of *Neisseria gonorrhea*, syphilis, or *Chlamydia trachomatis* is diagnostic of sexual abuse in prepubertal children in whom perinatal transmission and rare, nonsexual vertical transmission are excluded.[17] The presence of human immunodeficiency virus (HIV) infection in prepubertal children is diagnostic of sexual abuse in those in whom perinatal and transfusion related acquisition are excluded.[17]

Human papillomavirus (HPV) presents a special case in the evaluation for possible sexual abuse. Condylomata noted in 12- to 24-month-old infants were previously believed to be the result of perinatal transmission. Recent work has determined that vertical transmission is either not a common source of HPV infection or not a source of infection at all.[25,26] Recent epidemiologic data suggest that many preadolescent children acquire HPV from nonsexual horizontal transmission, either by autoinoculation if a child has common skin warts or horizontally from nonabusive contact by a person who has common warts, and that the likelihood of sexual abuse as a possible cause increases with age.[27,28] History and full medical evaluation are of particular importance in ascertaining the possibility of sexual abuse in a child with HPV.

Pubertal female victims are at risk of pregnancy from sexual abuse. Adolescents who become pregnant from sexual abuse often try to hide the pregnancy and can be extremely reluctant to name the perpetrator. If the perpetrator is a family member, then the psychological consequences for the adolescent and nonoffending family members can be particularly complex and debilitating.

ASSESSMENT AND DIAGNOSIS

A primary care physician may learn about suspected sexual abuse from concerns raised by parents, direct statements from the child, or abnormalities noted on physical examination or laboratory tests. When sexual abuse is suspected, an important decision point is whether the concerns or suspicions meet the requirement of mandatory reporting to the local child protective service agency. In most states, the requirement to report is based on the level of reasonable suspicion.

When initially evaluating possible sexual abuse, the primary care provider should take 5 important clinical steps. First, a careful decision about how much history to obtain directly from the child should be made. Many locales can provide timely, subspecialty level evaluation for suspected sexual abuse. When such care is available, only a minimal history or, in some circumstances, no direct history will be necessary because the child will be interviewed by a specially trained forensic interviewer (with representatives of the police and child protective services observing).

Second, the primary care provider should decide the extent of the physical examination to be performed and whether the collection of laboratory or forensic data is indicated. A brief external examination to rule out acute trauma can be performed with referral for emergency care only in the event that acute trauma is present. If the child has symptoms of a sexually transmitted infection, then appropriate laboratory tests should be obtained. If the primary care physician evaluates the child within 72 hours of the last occurrence of sexual abuse, then forensic evidence may need to be collected in an emergency department setting. Parents should be advised to reserve any unwashed clothing or bedding with which a suspected perpetrator may have been in contact in a paper bag for possible forensic evaluation.

Third, careful documentation in the medical record of collected information must be performed.

Fourth, the physician should meet with nonoffending parents (and the child, if old enough) to explain that a report will be made to child protective services and that an investigation will be conducted in the community.

Fifth, and finally, follow-up with the family should be arranged so that the primary care physician can offer ongoing support during the ensuing forensic evaluation.

Many communities have children's advocacy centers (CACs), multidisciplinary teams (MDTs), or both that provide a rational and coordinated approach to the evaluation of children who may have been sexually abused. CACs provide comprehensive, multidisciplinary assessments of abused children in an environment designed to be both neutral and child friendly. In addition to medical evaluations, CACs may house needed mental health services for children and their families. MDT members can include representatives from the local police, prosecutors' office, and protective services, and experts in interviewing and examining the child. MDT meetings provide an opportunity for discussion of specific cases resulting in coordinated investigative and treatment efforts for each abused child and a forum for community wide efforts in prevention and early detection of child sexual abuse. Shared goals of CACs and MDTs are minimizing secondary trauma experienced by the child and family resulting from the investigation and improving case investigations leading to more successful prosecutions.

As part of the evaluation, the subspecialty clinicians should consider alternative explanations, including an unintentional injury (or *accident*), a medical problem, or a false allegation.[29] Because evaluations for suspected sexual abuse usually include the child protection and legal systems, care should be taken to provide an unbiased assessment and one that provides documentation that can be reviewed by professionals outside the medical system.

History

The purpose of the history is to understand what may have happened to the child. This history should include the events that led to the evaluation, the child's health status and level of development, and the family's strengths and weaknesses. The parents (or guardians) should be asked what the child has said, how the child reacted when telling about the abuse, and whom the child told. Information should be obtained about (1) the child's behaviors, such as changes in behaviors or attitudes toward a specific person or situation, recurrent fears or nightmares, or sexualized behaviors; (2) specific symptoms, such as vaginal bleeding or discharge, dysuria, anal bleeding, constipation, and encopresis; and (3) where the child spends time and who cares for the child. Also to be determined is who the alleged perpetrator is, the relationship with the child, and the amount of time spent with the child. In preparation for interviewing the child, knowing about the child's developmental history is important, for example, whether a language delay is present.

The family history should include information about the parents' physical and mental health, including a history of sexual abuse during childhood; the health and developmental status of the siblings; the presence of family violence, substance abuse, or recent stresses; and the resources and supports available to the family. Understanding how family members view the allegations and how they have reacted is important. Because allegations that arise during a custody fight between parents are often difficult to sort out, the clinician should determine whether the parents are separated or divorced, the custody arrangements, the kind of visitation schedule, and any dispute about custody or visitation. Distinguishing whether the allegations of abuse occurred before the separation or divorce, during the process of separation and divorce, or after the divorce had been finalized is helpful.

A child who is old enough to be interviewed directly should be asked about what may have happened.[30,31] Pediatric primary care physicians should perform minimal interviewing so as to obtain enough information to warrant a report to child protective authorities. Trained, forensic interviewers can then obtain a full disclosure that can then be used as evidence in any legal proceedings stemming from the allegations. The recent development of forensic interview protocols, such as the National Institute of Child Health and Human Development Protocol for Investigative Interviews of Alleged Sex-Abuse Victims, allow for standardization of techniques, more elicited detail, and minimalization of trauma to the interviewed child.[32,33] This interview or series of interviews should be conducted with the child alone, if possible. The interviewer should be comfortable and skilled at interviewing young children about the possibility of sexual abuse, use simple questions, and be aware of the child's nonverbal responses and direct statements. Leading questions, such as, "Didn't he touch your pee-pee?" should be avoided, when possible. Nonleading questions are preferable, such as, "Can you tell me what happened?" or "Where did he touch you?" In many instances, however, children are reluctant to talk because of a variety of reasons, including fear and embarrassment; in such cases, questions with forced choice responses, such as, "Was it your mother or father or teacher who did that?" or "Was his pee green or pink or white?" can be helpful.

To help young children during the interview, anatomic drawings or anatomically correct dolls have been used. Considerable controversy has occurred about the sexual nature of the dolls and whether their use suggests to children that they can talk about sex, thus leading to false allegations. Research, however, indicates that few non-sexually abused children respond in sexual ways with the dolls and that the dolls can be helpful to children in describing what happened.[34] Because of the controversy involving the dolls, most interviewers prefer not to use them. Some older children who have difficulty verbalizing acts of sexual abuse may be able to draw pictures of or write out a description of what occurred.

Physical Examination

The purposes of the physical examination are to determine the presence or lack of (1) signs of physical abuse or neglect, (2) anogenital injuries that are consistent with or suggestive of sexual abuse, and (3) conditions that need medical treatment. In addition, the examination provides an opportunity for the clinician to reassure the child and family about the child's physical condition. In premenarcheal girls, the genital examination is performed best in both the supine and the prone, knee-chest positions; a speculum is seldom used. To visualize the hymen, 2 physical examination maneuvers should be used: (1) labial separation (separating and pulling posteriorly at an angle of 45 degrees) and (2) labial traction (gently pinching the labia and pulling out and toward the examiner). Evaluations conducted in specialty centers rely on the use of a colposcope during the anogenital examination to provide 5- to 30-fold magnification and documentation through photographs or videotape recordings. A study comparing examinations with and without the use of the colposcope indicated that more than 95% of physical findings can be detected without its use.[35] A handheld magnifying lens that provides 2.5- to 3-fold magnification or an otoscope (without a speculum) can provide reasonably good magnification.

Laboratory Tests

When the child is at risk of acquiring an STI from suspected sexual contact, appropriate tests should be obtained for gonorrhea, herpes simplex, trichomonas, bacterial vaginosis, chlamydia, syphilis, HIV infection, and hepatitis B and C. Historically, cultures for *N gonorrhea* and *C trachomatis* have been considered the gold standard for diagnosing infection with these organisms. Many medical settings have forgone culture in favor of newer tests, such as nucleic acid amplification tests that detect the presence of the organism's DNA or RNA. A particular advantage of these tests is that they may be run on urine samples as opposed to vaginal or urethral swabs. Data regarding the use of these tests in prepubertal children are scarce, and the prevalence of these infections in children is very low. As nucleic acid amplification tests are increasingly used, their importance both clinically and legally can be expected to increase. Currently, the Centers for

Disease Control and Prevention suggests the use of nucleic acid amplification tests for the detection of *N gonorrhea* and *C trachomatis* because of these tests' increased sensitivity over culture.[36] That many medical centers no longer offer culture for *C trachomatis* suggests that newer tests will take on increasing significance in the future. For a child who has a vaginal discharge, additional studies may be performed to test for trichomonas or bacterial vaginosis. Serologic samples may be analyzed for HIV, hepatitis B and C, and syphilis. Although universal screening is recommended for postpubertal children, the decision to screen for these infections in prepubertal children should be guided by the nature of the sexual contact and the signs and symptoms in the child, the presence of another STI, the risk status of the perpetrator, family wishes, and the discretion of the medical provider.[17]

Studies have attempted to determine which children should be tested for STIs. For example, in a review of 2731 preteens who had vaginal cultures, 84 (3.1%) had gonorrhea, and 80 of these had a vaginal discharge.[37] No data, however, are available to help determine which children should have cultures taken from all 3 sites: the genitals, throat, and anus. If the child has evidence of 1 STI, conducting a full range of tests for other STIs would then be reasonable.

The collection of forensic evidence is an important component of evaluating victims of sexual assault. When an adolescent is evaluated within 72 hours of an episode of suspected sexual abuse, appropriate forensic information, such as swabs to detect semen, should be collected[38] (see Chapter 356, Rape). The epidemiologic factors of forensic evidence findings in prepubertal victims of sexual abuse, however, suggest that the collection of this evidence has a low yield. A study of forensic evidence findings in 273 prepubertal children in whom abuse was suspected revealed that the likelihood of useful evidence collection 24 hours after an acute assault is extremely low. Swabbing a child's body for evidence is therefore indicated within the 24-hour period immediately after an acute sexual assault. The same study showed that clothing and linens from sexually abused children provided a significantly higher yield of forensic evidence after an acute sexual assault than samples taken directly from the child. These items should be rigorously pursued for analysis in the setting of an acute sexual assault.[39] In pubertal girls, a pregnancy test may be necessary.

Documentation

Documentation of the evaluation should include direct quotations, when appropriate, from the parents and the child and a clear description of the findings from the physical examination, with sketches, if necessary. In many states, the information is recorded on a specific form for suspected sexual assault. A videotape of the child's interview and videotape or photographs of the examination provide additional detailed information; these should be labeled with the date, child's name, physician's name, and the child's medical record number.

DIFFERENTIAL DIAGNOSIS

Conditions that need to be considered in the differential diagnosis depend on the child's symptoms and physical findings.[40] Some of the physical findings that can be seen in sexually abused children also are nonspecific findings, such as erythema of the vulva or introitus. Bruises to the genital or anal area should raise concern about physical abuse, but if bruising is more widespread, then medical conditions, such as bleeding disorders, need to be considered. Straddle injuries, which can affect the genitalia, are usually witnessed, thus the history is clear. These types of injuries are usually unilateral or anterior and produce obvious bruising and swelling of the external genitalia; affecting the hymen is unusual for such injuries because of the protection provided by the labia and bones of the pelvis.

An important dermatologic condition that may exhibit genital soreness and subependymal hemorrhages is lichen sclerosus.[40] This condition usually affects the vulva and perianal region and produces an hourglass appearance, with areas of subependymal hemorrhage, decreased pigmentation, and tissue friability. Urethral prolapse can produce vaginal bleeding and dysuria, and the abnormalities noted on physical examination might be considered the result of trauma from sexual abuse. Another condition that may be mistaken for sexual abuse is a streptococcal infection that can cause marked redness of the perianal region and a vaginal discharge. For children who have a foul-smelling vaginal discharge, a foreign body should be considered in the differential diagnosis.

A critical challenge for the examiner is to identify abnormalities that are due to trauma from sexual abuse versus normal variations. Studies have shown that physicians do not always agree on their descriptions or interpretations of genital findings. For example, Paradise and colleagues used 7 simulated cases to compare the assessments of 206 US physicians who considered themselves skilled at examining sexually abused children with the assessments of a panel of experts.[41] Not surprisingly, the most experienced physicians were more likely than the less experienced physicians to agree with the ratings of the expert panel. In a related study, the history provided in a simulated case was noted to have an influence on physicians' interpretations of findings: when the history did not suggest sexual abuse, the physicians (especially those who had little experience) were more likely to consider the examination normal. The opposite effect was found as well: when the history suggested sexual abuse, physicians were more likely to consider the same examination as abnormal.[42]

The possibility of a false allegation also should be considered in the differential diagnosis.[29] Although false allegations seem to occur infrequently, controversy exists about the accuracy of young children's memory, under what circumstances they can be asked leading questions that result in false reports of what happened, and how relevant these studies are to children's reports of sexual abuse.[43] False allegations should be carefully considered if the child has a serious mental health problem or if the child's statements lack detail about the event, have important inconsistencies, or appear rote in nature. If the child is part of a bitter dispute between the parents (eg, a custody fight), a false allegation, though rare, must also be carefully considered.[44,45]

MANAGEMENT AND TREATMENT

Management of children who are suspected of having been sexually abused includes action in 3 domains: (1) providing appropriate medical care, (2) reporting the case to protective services, and (3) ensuring mental health services for the child and family.

Guidelines for the treatment of STIs are highlighted in Chapter 356, Rape. In addition, counseling may be necessary about the implications of certain infections, such as HPV or HIV. Occasionally, surgical repairs of genital or anal injuries are necessary, and adolescents may need counseling about terminating a pregnancy that was due to sexual abuse. A major purpose of the physical examination is to provide reassurance to children and families that their bodies are physically intact. When abnormalities are noted on the physical examination, reassurance often can be provided by indicating that these likely will heal and be of little functional importance to children.

Clinicians who suspect sexual abuse are mandated to report their findings to the state's child protection agency. Because sexual assault is a criminal offense, the local police also participate in the investigation. Issues that need to be considered include the following: to what extent the children should be interviewed further, by whom, and in what setting; where the children should go to ensure their safety; and whether other children in the home need an evaluation.

The period after the child's disclosure can be emotionally upsetting to everyone involved and especially confusing to the child. Repeated interviews of the child (by well-meaning professionals, such as police or a protective service worker) may upset the child, who may be confused about why so many people are asking questions, embarrassed about talking about private parts, and worried about the family's reactions. Family members may blame themselves for allowing the abuse to happen and be furious at the suspected perpetrator. If the abuser is a relative, then the family may be divided, with the child's side believing the child and the abuser's side believing that the abuse could not happen and that the child is lying. If the abuser is in the immediate family, then the psychological issues are even more complicated. A mother will have to decide between siding with and supporting her child or believing that her child lied and supporting her husband. If her husband did sexually abuse their child, then the mother may question her ability to protect her child, her own sexuality, and her ability to choose a partner; at the same time, she may be concerned about how the family will be supported with the father in jail.

The clinician can be helpful by maintaining contact with the family, advocating for a reasonable approach by protective services (eg, having the alleged abuser leave the home rather than place the child in foster care), and helping the family to recognize and discuss the various emotional issues that surface.

When a child discloses sexual abuse, a chain of events is set in motion that has immediate and often distressing consequences for the child. What was once a secret for the disclosing child becomes a very public and emotionally charged event. Not only do children feel guilty for causing this upheaval, but they must also endure potentially terrifying interactions with child protective services and law enforcement. Parents are often overwhelmed by their own reactions to a child's disclosure; intense anger, fear, blame, and helplessness can be very strong and can cause acute distress and significant disturbances in functioning.

A majority of sexually abused children and their parents need short- or long-term counseling to help come to terms with what happened to the child. Recent work has shown that a cognitive behavioral treatment model that focuses specifically on the sexual abuse of the child and involves both the child and nonoffending parents has achieved measurable improvement in children's functioning in the wake of sexual abuse.[46] Furthermore, the presence or absence of parental support is directly correlated with children's functioning, even as much as a year after disclosure.[47] This finding highlights the importance of involving nonoffending parents, especially those in obvious distress, in counseling.

Because sexual abuse of a child is a criminal offense, the child and family are often involved in the criminal justice system. Despite this involvement, however, most cases do not actually result in a trial in criminal court for a variety of reasons, including lack of clear evidence that abuse has occurred, the young age of the victim, a confession of the perpetrator, or the willingness of the perpetrator to plea bargain for a lighter sentence. In approximately 3% to 5% of cases, a criminal trial is held in which the child actually testifies. Additionally, sexual abuse cases sometimes are tried (1) in family court when allegations of sexual abuse occur as a part of a divorce or custody proceeding or (2) in juvenile court when protective services are concerned about the child's safety in the home.

PSYCHOSOCIAL CONSEQUENCES

Sexual abuse can have a long-lasting and devastating impact on the development of children, adolescents, and adults.[48,49] Domains of functioning that can be affected include the survivor's emotional state (eg, depression, anxiety, suicide), sense of self (eg, feeling worthless or powerless, viewing one's self as a victim), and relationships with others (eg, setting poor boundaries, being promiscuous, using inappropriate sexual behaviors, mistrusting others). Important targets for long-term treatment include self-blame for allowing the abuse to happen, the child's sexuality and sexual awareness, poor self-esteem and feelings of powerlessness, and mistrust of adults. For example, school-age and adolescent boys may be very concerned about their own masculinity and whether, because they were abused by an older boy or a man, they are gay. At the same time, because of changes in the family (eg, the child no longer visits the grandfather), the child has to come to terms with the losses created by the disclosure and the upset and anger in the family.

Teenage girls and young women appear to be at an increased risk of other mental health problems, such as eating disorders, multiple personality disorders, and posttraumatic stress disorders. They are also more likely to become pregnant at a young age.

Men who were sexually abused as children are at increased risk of having mental health or substance abuse problems. They are also more apt to perpetrate sexually coercive acts, including victimizing children sexually.[50]

PREVENTION

Attempts to prevent sexual abuse have been directed toward developing programs to teach children, usually at school, about good and bad touches and what to do if bad touches occur. Children as young as 4 to 6 years are able to learn these concepts and retain them, at least over a short period. In general, evaluations have focused on the children's increased knowledge resulting from participation in a teaching program but have not been able to provide conclusive evidence that such programs actually have resulted in the prevention or earlier recognition of sexual abuse.

TOOLS FOR PRACTICE

Engaging Patients and Family

- *Child Sexual Abuse: What It Is and How To Prevent It* (brochure), American Academy of Pediatrics (patiented.aap.org).

Medical Decision Support

- *Treatment of Child Abuse* (book), Johns Hopkins University Press, American Academy of Pediatrics (www.aap.org/bookstore).
- Visual Diagnosis of Child Abuse on CD-ROM-2nd Edition (CD-ROM), American Academy of Pediatrics (www.aap.org/bookstore).

Community Coordination and Advocacy

- *Recognition of Child Abuse for the Mandated Reporter,* third edition (book), GW Medical Publishing, Inc. (www.aap.org/bookstore).

AAP POLICY STATEMENTS

Kairys SW, Johnson CF, American Academy of Pediatrics, Committee on Child Abuse and Neglect. The psychological maltreatment of children—technical report. *Pediatrics.* 2002;109(4):e68. (aappolicy.aappublications.org/cgi/content/full/pediatrics;109/4/e68).

Kellogg N, American Academy of Pediatrics, Committee on Child Abuse and Neglect. The evaluation of sexual abuse in children. *Pediatrics.* 2005;116(2):506-512. (aappolicy.aappublications.org/cgi/content/full/pediatrics;116/2/506).

REFERENCES

1. Kempe CH. Sexual abuse, another hidden pediatric problem: the 1977 C. Anderson Aldrich lecture. *Pediatrics.* 1978;62:382-389.
2. US Department of Health and Human Services, Administration on Children, Youth and Families. *Child Maltreatment 2004.* Washington, DC: US Government Printing Office; 2006.
3. Finkelhor D. Current information on the scope and nature of child sexual abuse. *The Future of Children: Sexual abuse of children.* 1994;4:31-53. Available at: www.futureofchlidren.org. Accessed October 15, 2007.
4. Vogeltanz ND, Wilsnack SC, Harris TR, et al. Prevalence and risk factors for childhood sexual abuse in women: national survey findings. *Child Abuse Negl.* 1999;23:579-591.
5. Leventhal JM. Epidemiology of sexual abuse of children: old problems, new directions. *Child Abuse Negl.* 1999;22:481-491.
6. Faller KC. *Understanding Child Sexual Maltreatment.* Newbury Park, CA: Sage Publications; 1993
7. Briere J, Runtz M. University males' sexual interest in children: predicting potential indices of pedophilia in a nonforensic sample. *Child Abuse Negl.* 1989;13:65-75.
8. Summit RC. The child sexual abuse accommodation syndrome. *Child Abuse Negl.* 1993;7:177-193.
9. Paradise JE, Campos JM, Friedman HM, et al. Vulvovaginitis in premenarcheal girls: clinical features and diagnostic evaluation. *Pediatrics.* 1982;70:193-198.
10. Heger A, Ticson L, Velasquez O, et al. Children referred for possible sexual abuse: medical findings in 2384 children. *Child Abuse Negl.* 2002;26:645-659.
11. Adams JA, Harper K, Knudson S, et al. Examination findings in legally confirmed child sexual abuse: it's normal to be normal. *Pediatrics.* 1994;94:310-317.
12. Kellogg ND, Menard SW, Santos A. Genital anatomy in pregnant adolescents; "normal" does not mean "nothing happened." *Pediatrics.* 2004;113:e67-e69.
13. Berenson A, Heger A, Andrews S. Appearance of the hymen in newborns. *Pediatrics.* 1991;87:458-465.
14. Berenson AB, Heger AH, Hayes JM, et al. Appearance of the hymen in prepubertal girls. *Pediatrics.* 1992;89:387-394.
15. McCann J, Wells R, Simon M. Genital findings in prepubertal girls selected for nonabuse: a descriptive study. *Pediatrics.* 1990;86:428-439.
16. McCann J, Voris J, Simon M, et al. Comparison of genital examination techniques in prepubertal girls. *Pediatrics.* 1990;85:182-187.
17. Kellogg N, American Academy of Pediatrics, Committee on Child Abuse and Neglect. The evaluation of sexual abuse in children. *Pediatrics.* 2005;116:506-512.
18. Adams JA. Approach to the interpretation of medical and laboratory findings in suspected child sexual abuse: a 2005 revision. *APSAC Advisor.* 2005;17(3):7-13.
19. Berenson AB, Chacko MR, Weimann CM, et al. A case-control study of anatomic changes resulting from sexual abuse. *Am J Obstet Gynecol.* 2000;182:820-834.
20. Emans SJ, Wood ER, Allred EN, et al. Hymenal findings in adolescent women: impact of tampon use and consensual sexual activity. *J Pediatr.* 1994;125:153-160.
21. Adams JA, Botash A, Kellogg N. Differences in hymenal morphology between adolescent girls with and without a history of consensual sexual intercourse. *Arch Pediatr Adolesc Med.* 2004;158:280-285.
22. Heppenstall-Heger A, McConnell G, Ticson L, et al. Healing patterns in anogenital injuries: a longitudinal study of injuries associated with sexual abuse, accidental injuries, or genital surgery in the preadolescent child. *Pediatrics.* 2003;112:829-837.
23. McCann J, Voris J, Simon M, et al. Perianal findings in prepubertal children selected for nonabuse: a descriptive study. *Child Abuse Negl.* 1989;13:179-193
24. American Academy of Pediatrics. Sexually transmitted infections in adolescents and children. In: Pickering LK, ed. *Red Book: 2006 Report of the Committee on Infectious Diseases.* 27th ed. Elk Grove Village, IL: American Academy of Pediatrics; 2006:172.
25. Smith EM, Ritchie JM, Yankowitz J et al. Human papillomavirus prevalence and types in newborns and parents: concordance and modes of transmission. *Sex Transm Dis.* 2004;31:57-62.
26. Watts DH, Koutsky LA, Holmes KK, et al. Low risk of perinatal transmission of human papillomavirus: results from a prospective cohort study. *Am J Obstet Gynecol.* 1998;178:365-373.

27. Sinclair KA, Woods CR, Kirse DJ, et al. Anogenital and respiratory tract human papillomavirus infections among children: age, gender, and potential transmission through sexual abuse. *Pediatrics*. 2005;116: 815-825.
28. Sinal SH, Woods CR. Human papillomavirus infections of the genital and respiratory tracts in young children. *Semin Pediatr Infect Dis*. 2005;16:306-316.
29. Bernet W. False statements and the differential diagnosis of abuse allegations. *J Am Acad Child Adolesc Psychiatry*. 1993;32:903-910.
30. Bourg W, Broderick R, Flagor R, et al. *A Child Interviewer's Guidebook*. Thousand Oaks, CA: Sage Publications; 1999.
31. Leventhal JM, Bentovim A, Elton A, et al. What to ask when sexual abuse is suspected. *Arch Dis Child*. 1987;62: 1188-1193.
32. Orbach Y, Hershkowitz I, Lamb ME, et al. Assessing the value of structured protocols for forensic interviews of alleged child abuse victims. *Child Abuse Negl*. 2000;24: 733-752.
33. Lamb ME, Sternberg KJ, Esplin PW. Conducting investigative interviews of alleged sexual abuse victims. *Child Abuse Negl*. 1998;22:813-823.
34. Everson MD, Boat BW. Putting the anatomical doll controversy in perspective: an examination of the major uses and criticisms of the dolls in child sexual abuse evaluations. *Child Abuse Negl*. 1994;18:113-129.
35. Muram D. Child sexual abuse: genital tract findings in prepubertal girls: comparison of colposcopic and unaided examination. *Am J Obstet Gynecol*. 1989;160: 333-335.
36. Centers for Disease Control and Prevention. Sexually transmitted diseases treatment guidelines 2006. *MMWR Recomm Rep*. 2006;55 (RR-11):1-94.
37. Ingram DL, Everett VD, Flick LAR, et al. Vaginal gonococcal cultures in sexual abuse evaluations: evaluation of selective criteria for preteenaged girls. *Pediatrics*. 1997; 99:E8.
38. Bechtel K, Podrazik M. Evaluation of the adolescent rape victim. *Pediatr Clin North Am*. 1999;46:809-823.
39. Christian CW, Lavelle JM, DeJong AR, et al. Forensic evidence findings in prepubertal victims of sexual assault. *Pediatrics*. 2000;106:100-104.
40. Bays J. Conditions mistaken for child sexual abuse. In: Reece RM, ed. *Child Abuse: Medical Diagnosis and Management*. Philadelphia, PA: Lippincott Williams & Wilkins; 2001;287-306.
41. Paradise JE, Finkel MA, Beiser AS, et al. Assessments of girls' genital findings and the likelihood of sexual abuse: agreement among physicians self-rated as skilled. *Arch Pediatr Adolesc Med*. 1997;151:883-891.
42. Paradise JE, Winter MR, Finkel MA, et al. Influence of the history on physicians' interpretations of girls' genital findings. *Pediatrics*. 1999;103:980-986.
43. Ceci SJ, Bruck M. *Jeopardy in the Courtroom: A Scientific Analysis of Children's Testimony*. Washington, DC: American Psychological Association; 1995.
44. Trocme N, Bala N. False allegations of abuse and neglect when parents separate. *Child Abuse Negl*. 2005;29:1333-1345.
45. Faller KC. False allegations of child maltreatment: a contested issue. *Child Abuse Negl*. 2005;29:1327-1331.
46. Cohen JA, Mannarino AP. Predictors of treatment outcome in sexually abused children. *Child Abuse Negl*. 2000;24:983-994.
47. Cohen JA, Mannarino AP. A treatment study for sexually abused preschool children: outcome during a one-year follow-up. *J Am Acad Child Adolesc Psychiatry*. 1997;36:1228-1235.
48. Briere J. *Child abuse trauma: theory and treatment of the lasting effects*. Newbury Park, CA: Sage Publications; 1992.
49. Kendall-Tacket TA, Williams LM, Finkelhor D. Impact of sexual abuse on children: a review and synthesis of recent empirical studies. *Psychol Bull*. 1993;113:164-180.
50. Holmes WC, Slap GB. Sexual abuse of boys: definition, prevalence, correlates, sequelae, and management. *JAMA*. 1998;280:1855-1862.

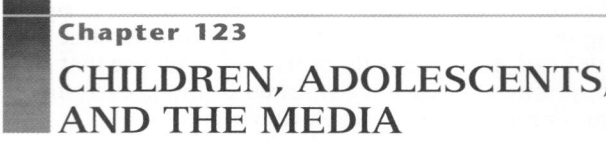

Chapter 123

CHILDREN, ADOLESCENTS, AND THE MEDIA

Victor C. Strasburger, MD

The media play a role in virtually *every* concern that a pediatrician or parent has about children and adolescents. Sex, drugs, violence, suicide, obesity, eating disorders, school problems—the media substantially contribute to each of these problems.[1,2] By asking 2 questions during a well-child visit, pediatricians can take the first step in protecting young people against harmful media influence: "How much time do you spend with different media such as TV or the Internet in an average day?" and "Do you have a TV set or Internet connection in your bedroom?"[3]

TYPES OF MEDIA

By the time today's children and teens reach age 70, they will have spent 7 to 10 *years* of their lives watching television and a variety of other media.[1] Although television remains the predominant medium for children and teens of all ages, a bewildering array of media are available for young people to use and abuse—television, movies, radio, video games, the Internet, cell phones, text messaging, iPods, and more. A 2005 sample of more than 2000 third through twelfth graders nationwide found that young people spend an average of nearly 6.5 hours a day with a variety of different media (Figure 123-1).[4] Despite the American Academy of Pediatrics' recommendation that children under the age of 2 years should not watch television, a separate study of 6 month to 6 year olds found that young children average 2 hours of screen time per day, which is as much as they spend playing and 3 times as much as they spend reading or listening to someone reading to them.[5] One of the most significant findings is that two thirds of American children and teens have a television set in their own bedroom, one half have a VCR or DVD player, one half have a video game console, and nearly one third have a computer (Figure 123-2).[4]

CONTENT ANALYSES

Content analyses are studies of exactly what children and teens view in different media. Although the studies do not address the issue of causality, they do give an accurate snapshot of the content being viewed. All these studies contain worrisome data about the amount

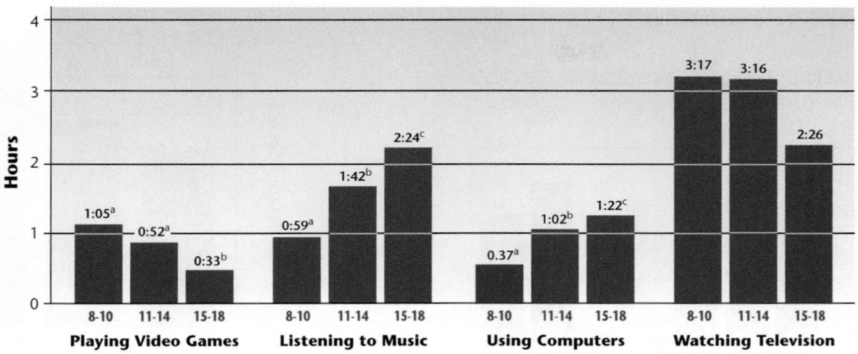

Figure 123-1 Young people spend an average of 5 to 6 hours per day using different media; television use predominates at any age. *(Roberts DF, Henriksen L, Christenson PG.* Substance Use in Popular Movies and Music. *Washington, DC: Office of National Drug Policy Control Policy; 2000.)*

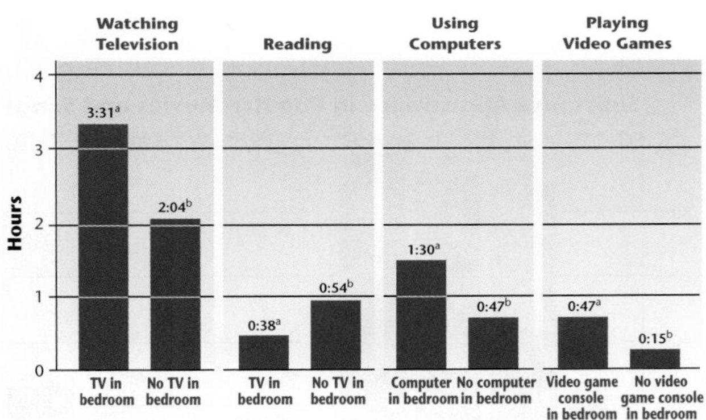

Figure 123-2 When media move into the children's bedrooms, their media use increases significantly. *(Roberts DF, Henriksen L, Christenson PG:* Substance Use in Popular Movies and Music. *Washington, DC: Office of National Drug Policy Control Policy; 2000.)*

of sex, drugs, and violence to which young people are exposed.

Violence

The average American child sees an estimated 10,000 acts of violence per year on television alone.[6] Of the 10,000 acts, 500 or more are considered very high risk: (1) the perpetrator is an attractive role model; (2) the violence is portrayed as being realistic, justified, or unpunished; or (3) the consequences of the violence are not shown[6] (see also Chapter 31, Violence Prevention, and Chapter 117, Domestic Violence and the Family).

Sex

The average American child sees more than 14,000 sexual references and innuendoes a year on television, of which fewer than 170 deal with abstinence, birth control, or the risk of pregnancy or sexually transmitted infection.[7] According to the most comprehensive analysis of American television ever performed, more than 75% of all prime time shows contain sexual content, 1 of every 10 shows includes a portrayal of sexual intercourse or implied intercourse, and only 14% of shows with sexual content mention any of the risks or responsibilities that go with having sex (Figure 123-3).[8] Almost counterintuitively, teen shows seem to contain more sex (Figure 123-4) and less mention of risks than adult shows.[8] In addition, movies, music videos, and advertising have all become increasingly suggestive.[9] Two thirds of teenagers have *accidentally* stumbled across pornography online.[10] At the same time, the media far outrank parents or schools as a source of information about birth control.[11]

Drugs

Alcohol, tobacco, or illicit drugs are present in 70% of prime time television programming, 95% of top-grossing movies, and 50% of music videos.[12,13] Despite the federal government's pronouncements, the 2 legal drugs—alcohol and tobacco—pose the greatest threat to youth, not illicit drugs; alcohol and tobacco are far more prevalent in mainstream media than illicit drugs (Figure 123-5). Cigarette smoking, in particular, seems to be making a big comeback in Hollywood movies: The prevalence of smoking among lead characters is 4 times the prevalence of people in real life.[14] Even G-rated animated children's movies contain high levels of tobacco and alcohol use.[15]

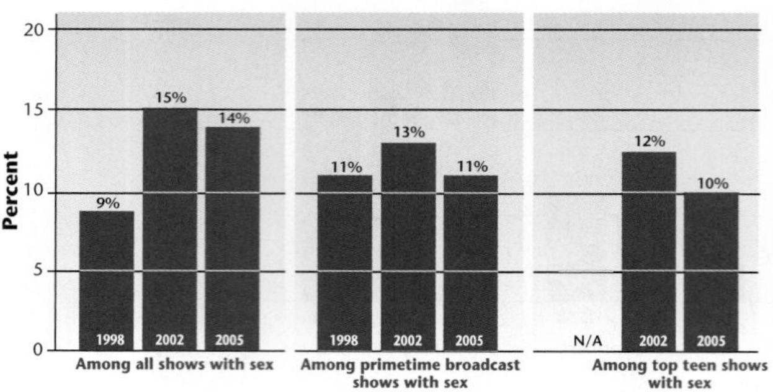

Figure 123-3 Fewer than 14% of prime time shows with sexual content include mentions of the risks or responsibilities of having sex. *(From "Sex on TV 4," a Kaiser Family Foundation Report. The Henry J. Kaiser Family Foundation, November 2005. This information was reprinted with permission from the Henry J. Kaiser Family Foundation. The Kaiser Family Foundation, based in Menlo Park California, is a nonprofit, private operating foundation focusing on the major health care issues facing the nation and is not associated with Kaiser Permanente or Kaiser Industries.)*

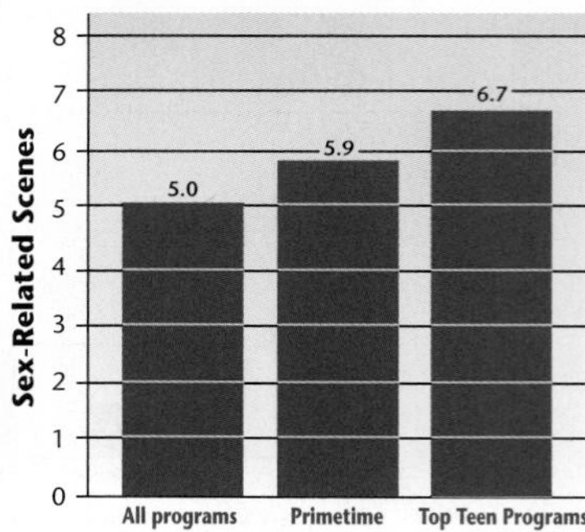

Figure 123-4 Teen television shows have more sexual content than adult television shows. *(From "Sex on TV 4," a Kaiser Family Foundation Report. The Henry J. Kaiser Family Foundation, November 2005. This information was reprinted with permission from the Henry J. Kaiser Family Foundation. The Kaiser Family Foundation, based in Menlo Park California, is a nonprofit, private operating foundation focusing on the major health care issues facing the nation and is not associated with Kaiser Permanente or Kaiser Industries.)*

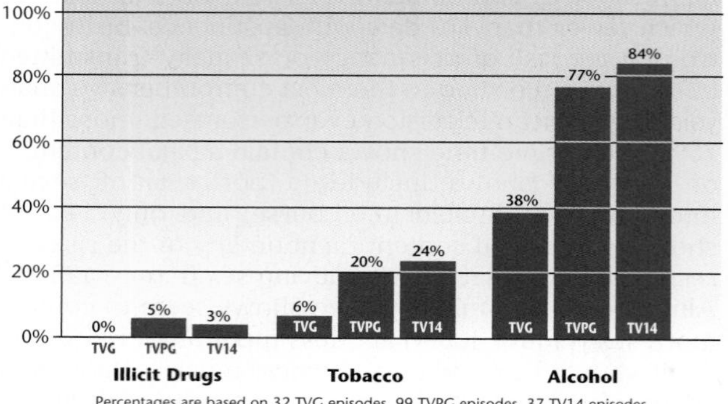

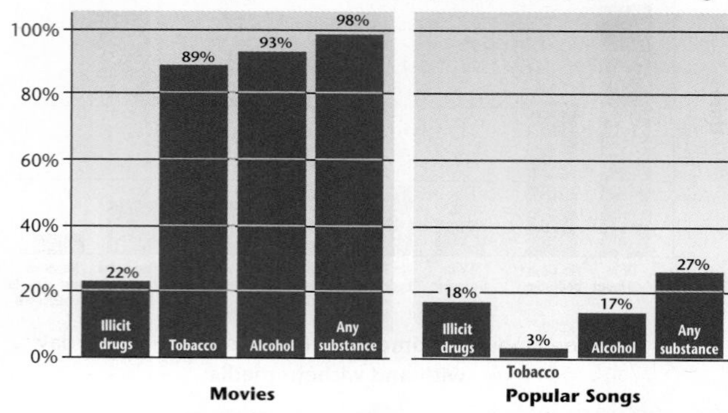

Figure 123-5 Although marijuana and cocaine are targets of federal antidrug advertisements, the 2 most significant drugs for teenagers are tobacco and alcohol; they are the 2 drugs most often portrayed in mainstream media. *(Christenson PG, Henriksen L, Roberts DF.* Substance Use in Popular Prime-Time Television. *Washington, DC: Office of National Drug Control Policy; 2000, and Roberts DF, Henriksen L, Christenson PG.* Substance Use in Popular Movies and Music. *Washington, DC: Office of National Drug Policy Control Policy; 2000.)*

HOW MEDIA AFFECT CHILDREN AND ADOLESCENTS

By sheer numbers, the media are a powerful influence on young people. Six hours a day spent with media are 6 hours *not* spent reading, exercising, or playing with friends. This phenomenon is known as the *displacement effect.* Most young people spend more time watching screen media than in any other activity except sleeping.[16] Television alone accounts for 15,000 hours by the time teens graduate from high school, compared with only 12,000 hours spent in formal classroom instruction.

Many theories have been offered about how media affect youth. According to the *social modeling theory,* the media expose young people to a variety of different role models who demonstrate potential behaviors to young and sometimes impressionable viewers.[17] Role modeling may be a crucial factor in whether preteens or teens begin smoking cigarettes, drinking alcohol, or having sex. In this sense, the media function as a kind of *super-peer*, making unhealthy behavior appear as normative behavior ("everyone's doing it").[16,18] According to the *cultivation hypothesis*, people who view a lot of television and other media tend to think that they depict real behavior in the real world or that the real world should conform to media rules.[19] Clearly, the media represent a powerful teacher of children and adolescents. The question is this: What is the media teaching them? One group of researchers worries about the media's ability to influence young people's attitudes and perceptions about the world and the media's "stalagmite effects—cognitive deposits built up almost imperceptibly from the drip-drip-drip of television's electronic limewater."[20]

MEDIA VIOLENCE

The controversy about whether media violence influences aggressive behavior should be over.[21] More than 1000 studies and 2500 reviews document the effect of media violence on children's and adolescents' behavior.[22] By contrast, fewer than 30 studies have found no relationship.[22] Given the difficulty of undertaking social science research and of pinpointing influences on human behavior, these numbers seem rather remarkable.[23]

High levels of television viewing are related causally to aggressive behavior in *some* children and teens and the acceptance of aggressive attitudes in nearly everyone (desensitization).[1,21-24] Exposure to media violence at young ages has been found to be a highly significant risk factor for adolescent or young adult aggressive behavior and criminal violence.[25,26] Children appear to learn their attitudes about violence at a very young age, and these attitudes apparently persist throughout their lives.[25] American media are uniquely problematic in 2 important ways[1]: Screen media are rife with portrayals of *justified* violence (the *good guy* beats up or kills the *bad guy*),[2] and guns are glorified in the media. Portraying interpersonal violence as being justified is the strongest positive reinforcer known. Guns contribute heavily to the second and third leading causes of death among teenagers (homicide and suicide); glorifying their use in the media seems unwise. On television alone, 25% of all violent episodes involve gun play.[6] First-person shooter video games are used by the military and by law enforcement agencies to teach new recruits how to shoot. In one of the school shootings during the 1990s, a teenager walked into his school in Paducah, Kentucky, and opened fire on a prayer group. In spite of never having fired a gun in his life, Michael Carneal hit 8 different teens with 8 shots, all in the head and upper torso, resulting in 3 deaths and 1 case of paralysis. He had learned to fire a gun from playing first-person shooter video games.[27] Overall, the research suggests that media violence may contribute to between 5% and 15% of all violence in the United States.[23] The connection between media violence and real-life aggression is nearly as strong as the connection between smoking and lung cancer (Figure 123-6).[1]

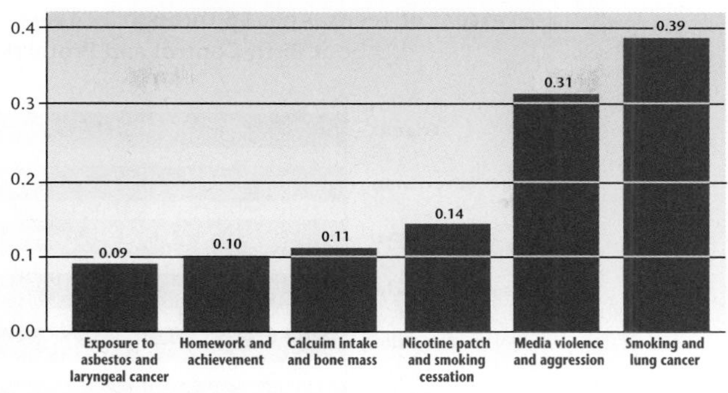

Figure 123-6 The connection between media violence and real-life aggression is nearly as strong as the link between smoking and lung cancer and is stronger than many other known associations. *(Strasburger VC, Wilson BJ. Children, Adolescents, and the Media. Thousand Oaks, CA:Sage Publications;2002. Reprinted by permission of Sage Publications.)*

SEX AND THE MEDIA

American media have become the leading sex educator of teenagers today in the United States.[9] With parents traditionally reluctant to discuss sexual matters in detail with their teens, and with abstinence-only sex education beginning to dominate the landscape, the media have picked up the slack. Teenagers who want more information about sex, sexuality, and contraception increasingly look to the media for information. A 2004 national survey of teenagers ages 15 to 17 years found that the media are a leading source of information about birth control, for example (Figure 123-7).[11] Unfortunately, what is available to them is sexually suggestive material without a lot of factual information or portrayals of sexual responsibility.[9]

Unlike the thousands of studies about media violence, only a handful of studies have been conducted on the media and sex and sexuality. The 2 most important studies are also the most recent. A 2004 RAND study of nearly 1800 teens ages 12 to 17 years found that teens who are exposed to sexual media were more likely to begin having intercourse or engaging in other sexual activities at a young age. Exposure to media that contain sexual images or dialogue doubled their risk.[28] A unique 2006 study of more than 1000 North Carolina 12 to 14 year olds found that exposure to sexual content in a wide variety of media (television, movies, music, magazines) accelerates white adolescents' sexual activity and doubles their risk of early intercourse.[29]

Given the suggestiveness of American media, one might think that advertising birth control products would not be a problem. After all, the majority of American adults (even Catholics) *favor* the advertising of birth control products on television.[30,31] Nevertheless, drug companies advertising Viagra, Levitra, and Cialis spent $343 million in 2004 to advertise their products—probably 10 times the amount spent on television advertisements for birth control products.

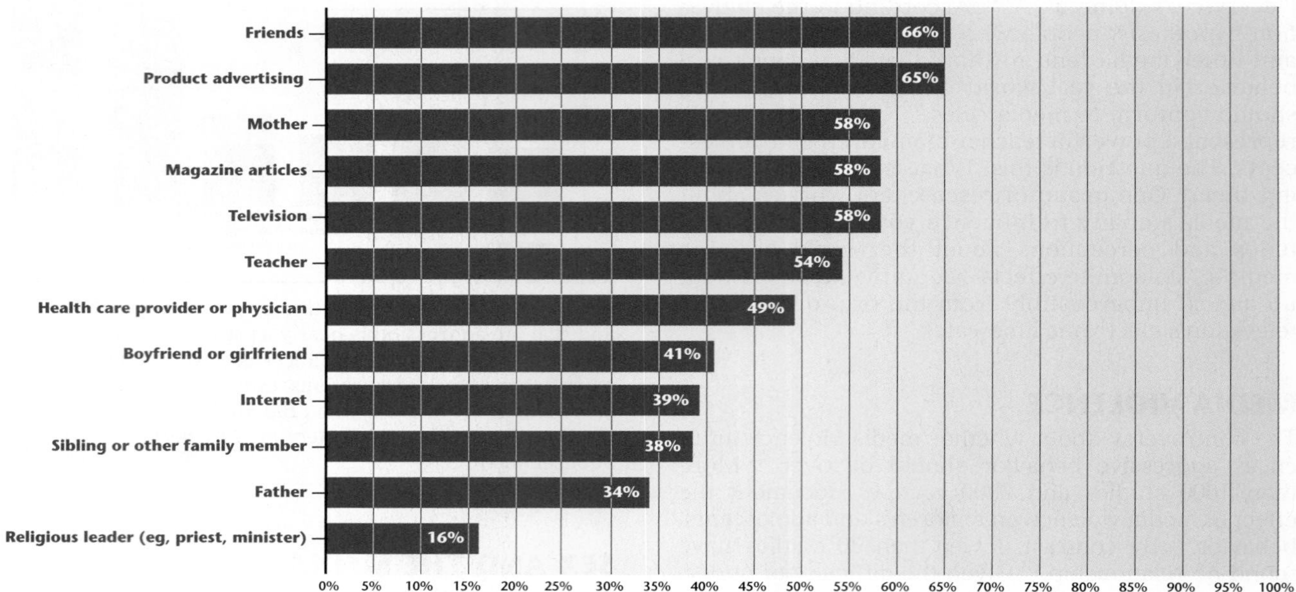

Figure 123-7 The media represent a leading source of information about birth control for teens. *(From "SexSmarts Survey – Birth Control and Protection," The Henry J. Kaiser Family Foundation and Seventeen Magazine, July 2004. This information was reprinted with permission from the Henry J. Kaiser Family Foundation. The Kaiser Family Foundation, based in Menlo Park California, is a nonprofit, private operating foundation focusing on the major health care issues facing the nation and is not associated with Kaiser Permanente or Kaiser Industries.)*

Three of the 6 major television networks refuse to air ads for oral contraceptives, and a different 3 refuse to air ads for condoms.[9]

OBESITY AND EATING DISORDERS

The media play a crucial role in the development of young girls' body self-image. For example, a large study of nearly 7000 9 to 14 year olds found that girls who want to mimic the appearance of television or movie stars were twice as likely to be concerned about their weight, to be constant dieters, or to engage in purging behavior.[32] A study of nearly 3000 Spanish 12 to 21 year olds over a 19-month period found that respondents who read girls' magazines had a doubled risk of developing an eating disorder[33]; and the Pacific isle of Fiji had virtually no problems with eating disorders until American television shows were introduced. Two years later, 75% of the teen girls surveyed reported feeling "too big or fat."[34]

At the opposite end of the spectrum, an important connection appears to exist between television viewing and obesity, although the exact nature of it remains to be elucidated. Nearly one half of the approximately 40,000 advertisements per year that children and teens see on television are for food, especially sugared cereals and high-caloric snacks.[35] Five national, cross-sectional studies have found a significant association between television viewing and obesity.[16] Children with a television set in their own bedroom have a 30% increased risk of being overweight.[36] Furthermore, a simple 6-month curriculum that reduced media use resulted in significant decreases in 3rd and 4th graders' body mass index.[37] What is unknown is whether the connection exists because of food advertising, snacking while watching television, displacement of exercise, or the fact that children burn less calories while watching television than they do while sleeping or reading a book.[16]

DRUGS AND THE MEDIA

American society wants children and teens to *just say no* to drugs, yet it allows more than $20 billion of cigarette, alcohol, and prescription drug advertising to air that is designed to get kids to *just say yes*. Frequently, alcohol and tobacco advertisers use sex to sell their products (Figure 123-8).

US tobacco manufacturers spend more than $11 billion a year on advertising and promotion. Tobacco advertising may, in fact, exceed the influence of family members and peers on a teenager's decision to smoke.[38] Approximately one third of all adolescent smoking can be attributed to tobacco advertising and promotions.[39,40] In addition, cigarette smoking seems to be making a comeback on prime time television and in the movies. In the last 15 years, 85% of the 250 top-grossing movies have depicted smoking.[41] A child or teen who sees a lot of R-rated movies has double the risk of beginning smoking[42]; and a child or teen who views more than 4 hours of television per day is 5 times more likely to

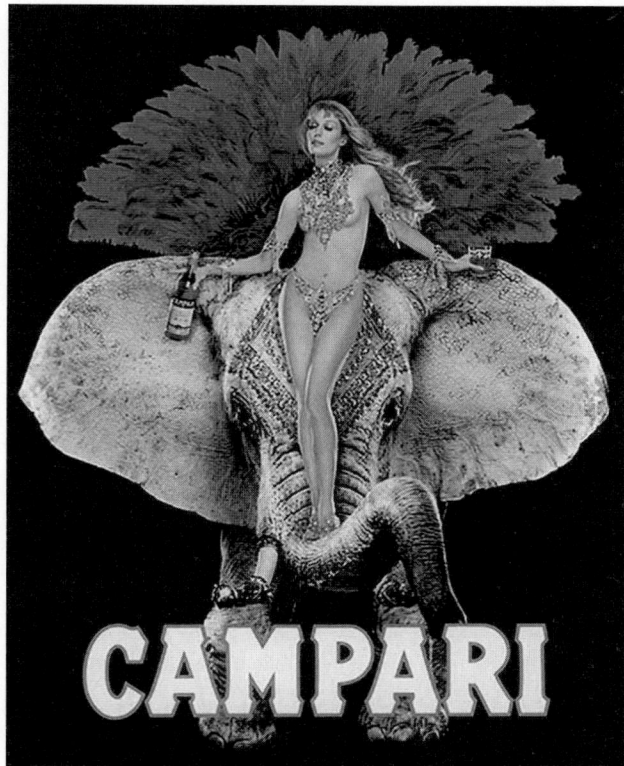

Figure 123-8 Alcohol manufacturers routinely use sexual images to sell their products.

begin smoking than one who watches less than 2 hours per day.[43]

Beer and wine manufacturers spend nearly $6 billion a year on advertising.[44] The average American teen sees 2000 beer and wine commercials per year, with most of them concentrated during sports programming.[45] On prime time television, 71% of programs depict alcohol use.[12] Music videos are filled with alcohol use; more than one half of all videos on networks such as MTV, VH-1, and BET depict alcohol use.[46,47] As with cigarette advertising and program content, research suggests that adolescents who are exposed to alcohol advertising and depictions are more likely to become drinkers.[16,48]

Relatively new to the media scene is advertising for prescription drugs. Currently, $4 billion is spent on it, and this figure is likely to continue increasing.[49] Prescription drug advertising gives young people the message that a drug is available to cure all ills, heal all pain, and that a drug is available for every occasion (including sexual intercourse, "when the time is right").

ROLE OF THE PEDIATRICIAN

Although they sometimes may feel inundated with the amount of counseling that they need to do, pediatricians must realize that the media have a significant role in nearly every health issue about which they are concerned. Consequently, a minute or 2 of counseling about media and its effects may pay rich dividends.

Counseling Parents

Asking 2 short questions may give an important glimpse into a child or teenager's risk:

1. How much media such as television and video games does he or she consume in an average day?
2. Does he or she have a television set or Internet connection in the bedroom?

The current American Academy of Pediatrics (AAP) recommendation is that parents be counseled to limit their child's total entertainment media time to no more than 2 hours per day, that children under the age of 2 should not view television, and that television sets should not be present in children's bedrooms.[50] Nonetheless, a recent survey of 365 pediatricians found that only one half recommended limitations on total screen time, and nearly one half were not interested in learning about media effects on young people through continuing medical education programs.[51]

Media Education

A hundred years ago, to be literate meant that you were able to read and write. In 2006, to be *literate* means that you can decipher and decode a bewildering array of media and media messages.[52] Media education programs can teach young people how to use media properly, how to understand media, and can help them avoid harmful media influences. In particular, media education programs have been successful in reducing violence, obesity, and drug use.[37,53,54] The United States is one of the few Western nations lacking a comprehensive, school-based media education program for children.

Advocacy

Since it formed its Task Force on Children and Television in 1983, the AAP has been a leader in trying to create a healthful media environment for children and adolescents.[55] Pediatricians can become involved at the local, state, or national level. Specific public health proposals that practitioners might support include:

- Mandating media education for all school children from kindergarten through the 12th grade
- Mandating a media education component for all sex education and drug education programs
- Greater dialogue between public health organizations and the creative community in Hollywood, including topics such as cigarette smoking on television and in the movies, use of profanity in movies, media violence, and sexual suggestiveness
- Greater restrictions on cigarette and alcohol advertising, including the creation of more aggressive counter-advertisements
- Support for the television industry to air contraceptive ads during prime time programming
- Creation of voluntary standards for the advertising industry regarding the use and depiction of anorectic or severely underweight models
- Greater pressure on Congress to restrict fast-food advertising on television
- Creation of a universal ratings system. Currently, each medium has its own idiosyncratic ratings system, which is confusing to parents. A universal system would provide actual content information to

parents, not just age-based categories (eg, PG-13, TV-Y7).

- More funding for a variety of much-needed media research

Fifty years ago, no one was able to have anticipated that limitations would be placed on tobacco advertising; that workplaces, restaurants, and airplanes would be smoke free; that a multimillion-dollar settlement against the tobacco industry would occur; or that public opinion would be solidly mobilized against the unhealthy practice of cigarette smoking. Nonetheless, public health activism has created all of these circumstances. Media are different from tobacco in that media can, at times, be a powerful positive tool. Nevertheless, the negative effects are widespread and have been well documented. Despite the power of the new multinational media conglomerates and the reluctance of the entertainment industry, pediatricians *can* make a difference in the future.

TOOLS FOR PRACTICE

Engaging Patient and Family

- *Pulling the Plug on TV Violence—Connected Kids* (brochure), American Academy of Pediatrics (www.aap.org/connectedkids/samples/tvviolence.htm).
- *Media Guidelines for Parents* (fact sheet), American Academy of Pediatrics (www.aap.org/connectedkids/samples/tvviolence.htm).
- *SafetyNet* (Web page), American Academy of Pediatrics (safetynet.aap.org).
- *Internet/Media Use* (Web page), American Academy of Pediatrics (www.aap.org/healthtopics/mediause.cfm).
- *Television and the Family* (brochure), American Academy of Pediatrics (patiented.aap.org).
- *Internet and Family* (brochure), American Academy of Pediatrics (patiented.aap.org).
- *The Ratings Game, Choosing Your Child's Entertainment* (brochure), American Academy of Pediatrics (patiented.aap.org).

Medical Decision Support

- Media History Questionnaire, American Academy of Pediatrics (www.aap.org/bookstore).

SELECTED READINGS

Broughton, Daniel D. Keeping kids safe in cyberspace: Pediatricians should talk to patients, parents about Internet dangers. *AAP News* 2005 26: 11-12.

Gonzalez, Rosario. Pediatricians should not ignore impact of music on youths. *AAP News* 2005 26: 41.

Milteer, Regina M. My house, my rules: Parents should control kids' media exposure. *AAP News* 2005 26: 38.

Shifrin, Donald L. Bombarded by media: As TV, computers and videos become ubiquitous in children's lives, pediatricians are urged to help change media habits. *AAP News* 2005 26: 21.

AAP POLICY STATEMENTS

American Academy of Pediatrics, Committee on Public Education. Media education. *Pediatrics*. 1999;104:341-343. (aappolicy.aappublications.org/cgi/content/full/pediatrics;104/2/341).

American Academy of Pediatrics, Committee on Public Education. Sexuality, contraception, and the media. *Pediatrics*. 2001;107:191-194. (aappolicy.aappublications.org/cgi/content/full/pediatrics;107/1/191).

American Academy of Pediatrics, Committee on Public Education. Media violence. *Pediatrics*. 2001;108(5):1222-1226. (aappolicy.aappublications.org/cgi/content/full/pediatrics;108/5/1222).

REFERENCES

1. Strasburger VC, Wilson BJ, Jordan A. *Children, Adolescents, and the Media*. Thousand Oaks, CA: Sage Publications; 2002.
2. Strasburger VC. Risky Business: What primary care practitioners need to know about the influence of the media on adolescents. *Prim Care*. 2006;33:317-348.
3. Strasburger VC. Adolescents & the media: why don't paediatricians and parents "get it"? *Med J Aus*. 2005;183:425-426.
4. Rideout V, Roberts DF, Foehr UG. *Generation M: media in the lives of 8-18 year-olds*. Menlo Park, CA: Kaiser Family Foundation; 2005.
5. Rideout VJ, Vandewater EA, Wartella EA. *Zero to Six: Electronic Media in the Lives of Infants, Toddlers, and Preschoolers*. Menlo Park, CA: Kaiser Family Foundation; 2003.
6. Federman J, ed. *National Television Violence Study*. Vol 3. Thousand Oaks, CA: Sage Publications; 1998.
7. Harris L, and Associates. *Sexual Material on American Network Television during the 1987-1988 Season*. New York, NY: Planned Parenthood Federation of America; 1988.
8. Kunkel D, Eyal K, Finnerty K, et al. *Sex on TV 4*. Menlo Park, CA: Kaiser Family Foundation; 2005.
9. Strasburger VC. Adolescents, sex, and the media: ooooo, baby, baby—a Q&A. *Adolesc Med Clin*. 2005;16:269-288.
10. Rideout V. *Generation Rx.com: how young people use the Internet for health information*. Menlo Park, CA: Kaiser Family Foundation; 2001.
11. Kaiser Family Foundation/Seventeen Magazine. *Sex Smarts: Birth Control and Protection*. Menlo Park, CA: Kaiser Family Foundation; 2004.
12. Christenson PG, Henriksen L, Roberts DF. *Substance Use in Popular Prime-Time Television*. Washington, DC, Office of National Drug Control Policy, 2000.
13. Roberts DF, Henriksen L, Christenson PG. *Substance Use in Popular Movies and Music*. Washington, DC: Office of National Drug Control Policy; 2000.
14. Stockwell TF, Glantz SA. Tobacco use is increasing in popular films. *Tob Control*. 1997;6:282-284.
15. Goldstein AO, Sobel RA, Newman GR. Tobacco and alcohol use in G-rated children's animated films. *JAMA*. 1999;281:1131-1136.
16. Strasburger VC. Children, adolescents, and the media. *Curr Probl Pediatr Adolesc Health Care*. 2004;34:54-113.
17. Bandura A. Social cognitive theory of mass communication. In: Bryant J, Zillman D, eds. *Media Effects: Advances in Theory and Research*, Hillsdale, NJ: Lawrence Erlbaum; 1994:61-90.
18. Brown JD, Halpern CT, L'Engle KL. Mass media as a sexual super peer for early maturing girls. *J Adolesc Health*. 2005;36:420-427.
19. Gerbner G, Gross L, Morgan M, et al. Growing up with television: the cultivation perspective. In: Bryant J, Zillmann D, eds. *Media Effects: Advances in Theory and Research*. Hillsdale, NJ: Lawrence Erlbaum; 1994:17-41.
20. Bryant J, Rockwell SC. Effects of massive exposure to sexually-oriented prime time television programming on adolescents' moral judgment. In: Zillmann D, Bryant J, Huston A, eds. *Media, Children, and the Family: Social Scientific, Psychodynamic, and Clinical Perspectives*. Hillsdale, NJ: Lawrence Erlbaum, 1994:183-195.

21. Bushman BJ, Anderson CA. Media violence and the American public. Scientific facts versus media misinformation. *Am Psychol*. 2001;56:477-489.
22. Wartella E, Olivarez A, Jennings N. Children and television violence in the United States. In: Carlsson U, von Feilitzen C, eds. *Children and Media Violence*. Goteborg, Sweden: UNESCO International Clearinghouse on Children and Violence on the Screen; 1998:55-62.
23. Comstock GA, Strasburger VC. Media violence. *Adolesc Med*. 1993;4:495-509.
24. Hogan MJ. Adolescents and media violence: six crucial issues for practitioners. *Adolesc Med Clin*. 2005;16:249-268.
25. Huesmann LR, Moise-Titus J, Podolski CL, et al. Longitudinal relations between children's exposure to TV violence and their aggressive and violent behavior in young adulthood 1977-1992. *Dev Psychol*. 2003;39:201-221.
26. Johnson JG, Cohen P, Smailes EM, et al. Television viewing and aggressive behavior during adolescence and adulthood. *Science*. 2002;295:2468-2471.
27. Strasburger VC, Grossman D. How many more Columbines? What can pediatricians do about school and media violence? *Pediatr Ann*. 2001;30:87-94.
28. Collins RL, Elliott MN, Berry SH, et al. Watching sex on television predicts adolescent initiation of sexual behavior. *Pediatrics*. 2004;114:e280-e289.
29. Brown JD, L'Engle KL, Pardun CJ, et al. Exposure to sexual content in music, movies, television and magazines predicts Black and White adolescents' sexual behavior. *Pediatr*, 2006;117:1018-1027.
30. Harris L, and Associates. *Attitudes about Television, Sex and Contraceptive Advertising*. New York, NY: Planned Parenthood Federation of America; 1987.
31. Kaiser Family Foundation. *Condom Ads on Television: Unwrapping the Controversy*. Menlo Park, CA: Kaiser Family Foundation; 2001.
32. Field AE, Cheung L, Wolf AM, et al. Exposure to the mass media and weight concerns among girls. *Pediatrics*. 1999;103:E36-E40.
33. Martinez-Gonzalez MA, Gual P, Lahortiga F, et al. Parental factors, mass media influences, and the onset of eating disorders in a prospective population-based cohort. *Pediatrics*. 2003;111:315-320.
34. Becker AE, Burwell RA, Gilman SE, et al. Eating behaviours and attitudes following prolonged exposure to television among ethnic Fijian adolescent girls. *Br J Psychiatry*. 2002;180:509-514.
35. American Academy of Pediatrics, Committee on Communications. Strasburger VC. Children, adolescents, and advertising. *Pediatrics*. 2006;118(6):2563-2569.
36. Dennison BA, Erb TA, Jenkins PL. Television viewing and television in bedroom associated with overweight risk among low-income preschool children. *Pediatrics*. 2002;109:1028-1035.
37. Robinson TN. Reducing children's television viewing to prevent obesity: a randomized controlled trial. *JAMA*. 1999;282:1561-1567.
38. Evans N, Farkas A, Gilpin E, et al. Influence of tobacco marketing and exposure to smokers on adolescent susceptibility to smoking. *J Natl Cancer Inst*. 1995;87:1538-1545.
39. Pierce JP, Choi WS, Gilpin EA, et al. Industry promotion of cigarettes and adolescent smoking. *JAMA*. 1998;279: 511-515.
40. Biener L, Siegel M. Tobacco marketing and adolescent smoking: more support for a causal inference. *Am J Public Health*. 2000;90:407-411.
41. Sargent J, Tickle JJ, Beach ML, et al. Brand appearances in contemporary cinema films and contribution to global marketing of cigarettes. *Lancet*. 2001;357:29-32.
42. Sargent J, Beach ML, Dalton MA, et al. Effect of seeing tobacco use in films on trying smoking among adolescents: cross sectional study. *BMJ*. 2001;323:1394-1397.
43. Sargent JD. Smoking in movies: impact on adolescent smoking. *Adolesc Med Clin*. 2005;16:345-370.
44. Gidwani PP, Sobol A, DeJong W, et al. Television viewing and initiation of smoking among youth. *Pediatrics*. 2002; 110:505-508.
45. Center on Alcohol Marketing and Youth. *Alcohol Advertising and Youth*. Washington, DC: CAMY; 2003.
46. Robinson TN, Chen HL, Killen JD. Television and music video exposure and the risk of adolescent alcohol use. *Pediatrics*. 1998;102:E54.
47. Roberts DF, Christenson PG, Henriksen L, et al. *Substance Use in Popular Music Videos*. Washington, DC, Office of National Drug Control Policy; 2002.
48. Grube JW, Waiters E. Alcohol in the media: content and effects on drinking beliefs and behaviors among youth. *Adolesc Med Clin*. 2005;16:327-343.
49. Rubin A. *Prescription Drugs and the Cost of Advertising Them*. November 6, 2004. Available at: www.therubins.com. Accessed July 28, 2005.
50. American Academy of Pediatrics, Children, adolescents, and television. *Pediatrics*. 2001;107:423-426.
51. Gentile DA, Oberg C, Sherwood NE, et al. Well-child visits in the video age: pediatricians and the American Academy of Pediatrics' guidelines for children's media use. *Pediatrics*. 2004;114:1235-1241.
52. Rich M, Bar-On M. Child health in the information age: media education of pediatricians. *Pediatrics*. 2001;107: 156-162.
53. Huesmann LR, Eron LD, Klein R, et al. Mitigating the imitation of aggressive behaviors by changing children's attitudes about media violence. *J Pers Soc Psychol*. 1983; 44:899-910.
54. Austin EW, Johnson KK. Effects of general and alcohol-specific media literacy training on children's decision making about alcohol. *J Health Commun*. 1997;2:17-42.
55. American Academy of Pediatrics, Task Force on Children and Television. Children, adolescents and television. *News and Comment*. 1984;35:8.
56. American Academy of Pediatrics, Committee on Public Education. Media violence. *Pediatrics*. 2001;108:1222-1226. Available at: aappolicy.aappublications.org/cgi/content/abstract/pediatrics;108/5/1222. Accessed April 20, 2006.

School Health

Chapter 124

OVERVIEW OF SCHOOL HEALTH AND SCHOOL HEALTH PROGRAM GOALS

Howard L. Taras, MD; Philip R. Nader, MD

"Health Care is not equivalent to Health. Education is not the same as learning. Health and learning must be defined by more than the current performance of the institutions that claim to serve these ends."

I. ILLICH, *DESCHOOLING SOCIETY*, NEW YORK, 1972, HARPER AND ROW

Almost 98% of school-aged children attend public, charter, or private schools.[1] With this penetration, not surprisingly, schools have an enormous influence, both positive and negative, on the health and well being of the nation's children. The nature and quality of school health programs are germane to primary care physicians' success with disease management, as well as illness and injury prevention. Moreover, pediatric primary care physicians have the ability to influence the nature and quality of school health programs. Familiarity with how schools work and how to work with schools and knowledge of advocacy techniques that help improve school health programs for all students in a community are some of the tools primary care physicians require to influence the health of their own school-aged patients and that of all youth in a community.

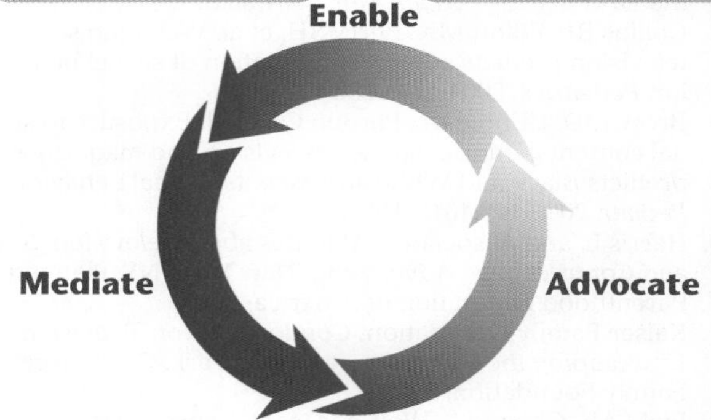

Figure 124-1 Three components interact dynamically to create a health-promoting school.

SCHOOL HEALTH PROGRAM GOALS

Various ways exist of describing the goals of a school health program. The *health-promoting school,* a term used by the World Health Organization's Healthy Schools initiative, describes the goals for school health in many countries around the world. This initiative stresses starting with school culture and ethos, moving to policy organization and procedures, and then addressing curriculum, teaching, and community involvement. The components in a health-promoting school are illustrated in Figure 124-1.

One of the most widely used models for school health goals in the United States is the *coordinated school health program,* a model originating in, and endorsed by, the Division of Adolescent and School Health at the Centers for Disease Control and Prevention.[2] The model recognizes 8 major components to any coordinated school health program (Figure 124-2). The term *coordinated* replaces the term *comprehensive* and refers to the need for better linkages between available services and education and training. For example, teaching students about proper nutrition in the classroom is counterproductive if they are offered few healthy choices in the cafeteria. Equally nonsensical is to encourage school counselors and other staff members to help students with emotional issues reach appropriate mental health services if staff members themselves do not believe they are supported by school personnel policies for their own mental health needs. Coordination among all 8 components of a school health program strengthens each one of them.

The 8 components of a coordinated school health program are each described in this chapter in terms of (a) what is recommended for schools and (b) how a primary care physician can relate to each component. Further details of each component are available in

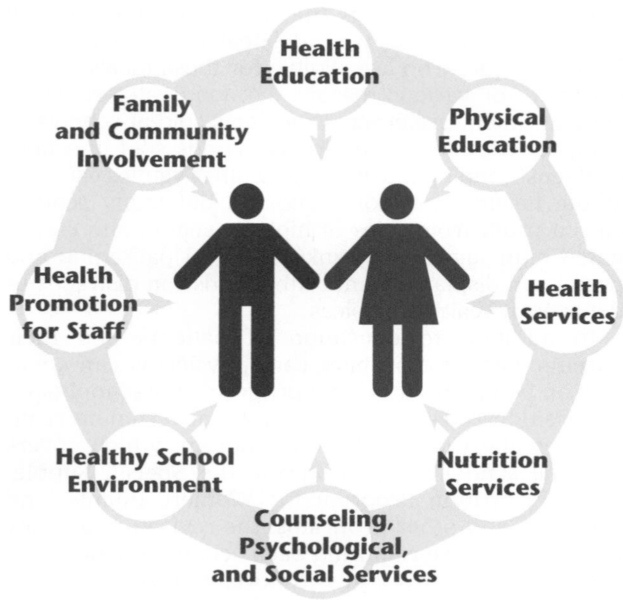

Figure 124-2 Coordinated school health programs: an eight-component model.

2 publications of the American Academy of Pediatrics: *Health, Mental Health and Safety Guidelines for Schools* and the 6th edition of *School Health Policy and Practice*.[3,4]

Health and Safety Education

Under ideal circumstances, health education would be part of any school districts' core academic curriculum and have the same budgetary and scheduling prioritization as literacy, mathematics, and other traditional basics. Not surprisingly, such a situation is highly atypical. Among physicians and other primary care physicians for school-aged children who recognize this predicament are some who try to correct the situation by volunteering to teach a health class (eg, a nutrition class, a class on prevention of drug abuse). Although this effort is well intended, often enjoyed by students and lecturers, and possibly successful at increasing short-term knowledge of healthful practices, such interventions by themselves are unlikely to change student health behaviors.[5] Schools must be encouraged to adopt student health and safety curricula that have evidence of effectively changing student behavior. To be effective, a curriculum should be planned and sequential (ie, each class builds on previously taught skills and knowledge of a previous class, and each year builds on the previous year), be interactive, have skills-based instruction, optimally involve the family, and be consistent with established health education standards. Ideally, health education is integrated with other content areas. School or curricular health education is addressed more fully in Chapter 125, School Health Education.

Physical Education and Activity

Physical education should be provided daily, with no substitutions allowed for participation in other courses or activities, and should meet national standards for physical education.[6] Ample resources should be available for the entire class in physical education so that skill building and aerobic fitness are optimized. Physical educators should be appropriately trained. Recess, active play during and after school, sports, and other activities should be provided as well. Safety gear should be provided when appropriate, and safety should be one of the educational goals for this program.

Most primary care physicians interact with physical education programs through their role in preparticipation physical examinations for sports and by providing medical cause for exemption and resumption of physical activity in school. As such, health care providers need to recognize that schools must make physical education available to all children, including those with special needs (eg, severe asthma, physical, emotional disabilities, developmental delays), either through modifications of a regular physical education class or through an adaptive physical education program. Written excuses from medical offices that exempt children from physical education should be reserved for severe and temporary conditions (such as children on chemotherapy). Rather, health care providers should work with the school to find an appropriate physical education curriculum for patients with chronic health conditions.

Health and Mental Health Services

Each school district must provide students with basic first-aid services, mandated health screens (eg, vision screening, hearing screening), immunization monitoring, and medical services that are necessary to accommodate safely a student with special medical needs in a school setting (eg, gastric tube feeding, observation and suctioning for a student with a tracheostomy, administration of medications during the school day).[7] In addition to expected instances of emergencies or trauma requiring immediate medical attention (eg, crisis episodes of asthma or seizures), the school health service must be prepared to deal with life-and-death situations of medically fragile children who may be located on school campuses, as well as the unfortunate eruption of violence, shootings and suicide, and community disasters. Most schools have ready access to emergency 911 systems, but trained personnel, standing policies and procedures, and key decision makers need to be identified before such crises arise. Beyond these basic services, schools and students often benefit from a much broader range of health and mental health services. Although forces within the educational system reflect an emphasis on traditional academics, school administrators are volunteering or are feeling obliged to provide additional services and involve community health partners to meet student educational and support needs. At least 2 major gaps exist in today's health care system: (1) inadequate access to health care and (2) lack of preventive services for youth. School health is rapidly being recognized as a linchpin for the system to ensure a way to deal with these deficiencies. The recent proliferation of school-linked services is a direct outgrowth of these educational, health, and welfare reform movements. These services develop most frequently in urban settings and target disadvantaged populations. Typically, private-public partnerships seed these new services and coordinate a wide range of human services for all children and their families. A chronology of school health in relation to health care issues and public health is shown in Figure 124-3.

The most important health service a school can provide is identifying student health problems and making appropriate referrals. The completeness and effectiveness of problem identification and solutions depend, to a large degree, on the numbers and quality of school health personnel. The more trained and sophisticated the personnel are, the more they can achieve. Differentiated staffing with appropriate use of aides, nurses, nurse practitioners, and physician-consultant back-up is likely to be the most cost-effective way of responding to the identified needs of a population.[8] An analysis of frequent visits to the school health room, of underachieving students, or of students with frequent problem behaviors can identify students who may need medical or mental health attention.

For school health programs to be effective, linkages must be formed between the school and the source of primary health care for the child. All pediatric care physicians might benefit from the ability to link their primary care services to schools for treatment of minor conditions, follow-up and screening, medication administration, immunization delivery systems, the monitoring of school absenteeism, and achievement for selected patients. Major difficulties arise when no regular source of care or insurance coverage exists or when multiple school systems overlap a pediatric practice. Primary care physicians would be wise to examine ways to use school-based personnel to provide cost-effective services at school sites when it is deemed desirable for a given community. Although a school-based clinic might become a medical home for a family without other options in a community, developing additional resources so that each family has an ongoing medical home that would be available independent of school hours and locations is preferable. All school-based services should be linked to 24-hour 7-days-per-week back-up resources that extend beyond the school day and the school year. Systems of managed care need to examine the potential benefits of linking health services and education to families through schools.[9]

Nutrition and Food Services

Schools should provide foods that (1) are prepared using specifications that guarantee its safety, (2) are composed of competitively priced selections that are low in fat and simple sugars, and (3) are served in an appetizing way that appeal to its ethnic student populations. Foods should never be used as a reward or punishment in school. This tactic does occur frequently, with staff providing a pizza party for a classroom that completed an assignment, for example. The National School Meal Program, sponsored by the United States Department of Agriculture, provides free or reduced-cost lunches to low-income students and is available in a majority of public schools.[10] In some schools, breakfasts and snacks are also provided under the program. The standards for foods that fall under the national lunch program are well delineated. Unfortunately, many students who are eligible for these meals do not eat them for various reasons (eg, long cafeteria lines, stigmatization, preferences for items sold at schools to compete with subsidized foods). Foods sold in school canteens, vending machines, and other venues can constitute healthy nutritional choices, but many schools earn a profit from sales of high-fat snacks and carbonated high-sugar soft drinks. Colorful packaging and prominent displays of unhealthy foods can distract students from healthier choices.

In addition to education of patients and their parents, pediatric primary care physicians can advocate on behalf of nutritional programs for school-aged children. In 2004, when the federal government reauthorized the Child Nutrition Program, which covers national school lunch program, the Special Supplemental Nutrition Program for Women, Infants, and Children, and other programs, the revised public law included a clause requiring each school or school district with these programs to develop a *local wellness policy* that addresses childhood obesity. Schools must comply with this law if they participate in these federal school lunch or breakfast programs. They must set goals (and take action to meet goals) for nutrition education, physical activity, and other school-based activities that promote student wellness. Schools must involve a broad group of community members to set and oversee these goals, often in the form of a school health council (also referred to as a school wellness council). Pediatric primary care physicians can make excellent reference sources for these councils, as well as enthusiastic advocates. Policies of the American Academy of Pediatrics, for example, on soft drinks in schools,[11] can provide helpful guidance to pediatric primary care physicians. See end of chapter for a listing of American Academy of Pediatrics policy statements regarding school health.

Physical Environment and Transportation

An overzealous focus on basic academic skills that coincides with limitations or reductions in school budgets can lead to a compromising effect on the physical infrastructure that supports a safe and pleasing school environment. Heating, ventilation, and air conditioning systems can easily fall into disrepair when funds are not set aside for adequate maintenance personnel or supplies. Health ramifications occur, but they are not always obvious to students or their parents. Accumulation of mold and dust, attraction of vermin (cockroaches, rodents), and decay of organic materials can be causes of unhealthy buildings that first affect persons with specific allergies but eventually cause health problems for a broad population of students and staff. Pediatric primary care physicians should be aware of the general condition of schools in their area and should look for patterns of avoidable illness or symptoms.

Other health-related matters related to the physical environment are specific safety precautions that schools must take in designated play areas (eg, for recess) and in classes for science, physical education,

1850 1880 1910 1920 1930 1940 1950 1960 1970 1980 1990

Civil War — World War I — Great Depression — World War II — Great Society

Key Health System Issues

Key Health Problems: Professionalism — Infrastructure Building — Improving Access — Cost Control — Market Forces — Reinventing Government

Infectious Diseases — Chronic Diseases — Modern Challenges

Key Health Strategies:

Quarantine — Sanitary Reform — Maternal and Child Health Programs — Antibiotics — Screen and Treat — Managed Care

Water Systems — Pasteurization — Personal Hygiene — Hospital as Center of Care — Categorical Health Programs — Healthy Communities

Education Compulsory (Rhode Island) (1840)
Founding of American Medical Association (AMA) (1847)
Shattuck Report (1850)
Smallpox outbreak, New York City (1860)
Metropolitan Board of Health, New York City (1866)
Massachusetts Board of Health (1869)
Smallpox vaccination required for school attendance (1870)
Founding of American Public Health Association (APHA)
Koch Discovery-Age of Bacteriology (1876)
Hygienic Lab (forerunner of National Institutes of Health) (1887)
NYC nurses reduce absenteeism by 50% in several weeks (1902)
Pure Food and Drug Act (1906)
Flesner Report on Medical Education (Carnegie Foundation) (1910)
Joint NEA-AMA Committee on Health Problems (1911)
The Open Air Classrooms (1915)
Welch-Rose Report on Schools of Public Health (Rockefeller Foundation) (1915)
Cardinal Principles of Education (1918)
Maternity and Infancy Act (Sheppard-Towner) (1921)
All states with laws regarding school health, safety, nutrition, health screenings (1921)
Blue Cross Insurance (1929)
School Health Study American Child Health Association (1930)
Social Security Act (Title V and Title VI) (1935)
Astoria Plan (NYC) (1936)
Garfield/Kaiser Prepaid Group Practice (forerunner Kaiser Permanente)
Center for Control of Malaria in War Areas (forerunner of Centers for Disease Control) (1940s)
Kark Community-Oriented Primary Care Clinic—South Africa (1940s)
Hospital Survey and Construction Act (Hill-Burton) (1946)
Separation of primary health services from schools. AMA-NEA, scattered services to indigent populations (1920s-1950s)
Salk Polio Vaccine (1952)
Recognition of social morbidities (1960s)
SHES-School Health Education Study—10 conceptual areas (1960)
Surgeon General's Report on Smoking (1964)
Community Health Centers Program (1964)
Medicare and Medicaid Act (1965)
Health Professions Educational Assistance (1965)
Robert Wood Johnson Foundation Demonstration School Health (1970-1980)
US Health and Nutrition Projects (1970-1980)
Health Maintenance Organization (HMO) Act (1973)
LaLonde Report on Health of Canadians (1974)
Healthy People: Surgeon General's Report on Health Promotion and Disease Prevention (1979)
Medicare Payment Reform (1983, 1989)
Community-Oriented Primary Care (1984)
Health of the Public Program (1985)
DASH-CDC (1988)
The Future of Public Health (Institute of Medicine) (1988)
Healthy People 2000 (1988)
US Preventive Services Task Force: Guide to Clinical Preventive Services (1989)
Healthy Schools, Healthy Communities (1990)
HEDIS-Health Plan Employer Data and Information Set (1993)
Failure of Federal Health Reform (1993-1994)
National Education Goals (1994)
National Congress of the Medicine/Public Health Initiative (1996)
Institute of Medicine Report: Schools and Health (1997)
GWU Comprehensive School Health Initiative (1998)

Figure 124-3 Medicine and public health timeline (1840-1998) and school health timeline.

and shop. Traffic-safety around schools (sidewalks, crosswalks, traffic lights, and monitored intersections), availability of racks to lock bicycles, and places at school to store helmets and other safety gear might appear on the surface to be important primarily for student safety. However, these factors are equally important to encourage children to be more physically active because they remove barriers to students' walking and riding to and from school.

Social Environment

Schools must have violence-prevention strategies, suicide-prevention strategies, actions against bullying, and policies on student discipline. Clear, written and well-known rules can contribute to a social environment that makes staff and students feel safe. The teaching staff must learn to recognize signs of student distress and know how to direct these children to staff resources within the school (eg, a school counselor, psychologist, nurse, or site administrator trained for this purpose), who, in turn, must feel comfortable with initial assessment and working with children's primary care physicians. Teachers should be as knowledgeable as possible about principles of child development. Teaching strategies need to be matched to the developmental and cognitive capabilities of children. School systems that espouse noncoercive discipline and high academic expectations have the best educational outcomes.

The potential for spillover of neighborhood violence onto school campuses always exists. Students who carry a weapon, possess an illicit drug, or threaten violence typically fall under a school's *zero-tolerance rule* and are promptly suspended or expelled. Unfortunately, schools rarely insist on a referral to the primary care physician of the suspended or expelled student whenever a suspension or expulsion based on such aberrant behavior occurs.[1,12] Many of these students have unrecognized health, mental health, and family-dynamic problems that not only underlie their school behavior, but are also amenable to therapeutic interventions. Schools' policies must be geared toward correcting problems, not solely toward punishing students.

Drug screening for students who want to enroll in extracurricular activities (eg, chess club, football team) became legal with a US Supreme Court decision in 2002.[13] Although well intended, school districts and pediatric care physicians must consider the ramifications of such screening. Will screening discourage students to join extracurricular activities if they experiment with illicit substances? Can this effort lead to fewer healthy connections to school and exacerbate, rather than ameliorate, substance abuse? Has any research found screening to be a deterrent? Has screening changed the social atmosphere of a school and, if so, for the better or worse? Are false positives possible, and, if so, what will the effect of a false-positive result be on the student and family until it is demonstrated to be false? As with any proposed screening program performed or suggested to be performed in the school setting (vision screening, cholesterol screening), the benefits of early identification must be established, clear benefits-costs analysis of the screen must be established, and, most important, potential harm must be known and gauged against potential benefits.

Health Promotion for Staff

Employees' mental health and physical health are integrated with achieving student health. School employees who exercise often and eat well are probably more likely to encourage others to do so enthusiastically, including their students. Employees who have taken advantage of wellness programs offered through their school district employment's insurance or a workplace program (eg, smoking cessation, stress management) may be more likely to recognize the value of such programs for students.

Family and Community Involvement

Success in achieving school health goals depends largely on how well these goals are communicated with and endorsed by parents, health care providers, and health and social agencies in the school's communities.

Pediatric primary and secondary care physicians need to take an active role in developing and implementing school policies. Busy health care professionals can do so by annually asking school-aged patients (and then documenting in the patient's record) the name of the child's school. This approach allows for interaction, should the necessity arise. Eliciting patient histories from parents and patients, as well as from school personnel, is essential, particularly when a behavioral problem or a learning problem exists. Obtaining a history is important because children may act differently at home and at school (itself, an important piece of diagnostic information), parents may have a different perspective than other adults in the child's life, and schools often need to become part of a management plan, if the medical management is to be optimal. Pediatric primary care physicians and specialists often need to interact with schools on behalf of children with special health care or special learning needs. The pediatrician may be effective as an advocate not only for a particular patient, but also for better school policies and practices that affect all students in the community.

EVALUATION

Because school health programs are linked closely to systems of health care delivery in a community, evaluation is an integral part of program planning and assessment. A community needs assessment can determine the challenges and resources present in a particular community. The needs assessment should involve all key child health, education, and social services leaders in the community and be broadly based across both private and public sectors. A needs assessment can guide the development and nature of school-linked or school-based health services and guide which agencies need to partner with schools. Selection of outcome indicators to be measured at periodic intervals can demonstrate to program planners and funding agencies the usefulness of the programs established. For example, monitoring problem identification and outcomes can be useful by providing rationale and justification for services, as well as assessing needs for additional services. Other examples are illustrated in Table 124-1.

Table 124-1 Potential Outcome Measures for Sample School Health Goals

GOAL	EXAMPLE OF AN OUTCOME MEASURE
Access to primary care	Number (%) of students who have an identifiable medical care home (ongoing source of primary health care)
	Decrease in use of emergency departments for nonemergent care
Critical medical situations	Number (%) of staff who have active CPR certification
	Presence of standing emergency medical orders
	No preventable deaths
	Reduction in school accidents
Mandated screening and immunization	Number (%) of vision referrals made, confirmed to need correction, and fitted (using corrective lenses)
	Number (%) of false-positive screening results (referred but found not to have needed referral)
	Number (%) referred and not reaching a source of care
	Number (%) of students who are up to date on required immunizations
Identification or solution of problems	Number (%) of problems identified that are corrected or being treated
	Absenteeism rates; dropout rates
	Number (%) at risk of academic failure (retention)
Obesity prevention	More healthful school lunches (decreased fat and salt)
	More aerobic or active physical education classes
	Existence of parental programs in health
	Existence of one or more comprehensive sexual education course
School environment	Smoke-free school
	No incidents of violence in school
	Soap, water, paper towels, and toilet paper available
Evaluation	Existence of a plan for evaluation and publication of an annual report

CPR, Cardiopulmonary resuscitation.

KNOWLEDGE REQUIRED FOR PATIENT ADVOCACY AND CONSULTATION TO SCHOOLS

Many large school districts have district physicians. These professionals are typically pediatricians, family physicians, or adolescent medicine specialists. In some states, such as Maine, school districts are mandated to have such consultants. Time for physicians to acquire experience and skills is necessary to attain a consistent high quality of service delivery. In the best of these arrangements, physicians provide numerous services that become indispensable and efficient for schools.

School physicians' roles include communicating on behalf of the school or school district to students' own physicians when the school administrators need information and interaction to accommodate complex health and safety problems. School physicians should help administrators design ongoing communication systems between the school health office and primary care physicians, assist administrators with the development and interpretation of school health-related policies (eg, exclusion policies for illness, nutrition policies), be on call for school nurses who have questions, and design and update protocols for medical procedures delivered in school (eg, gastric-tube feeding, administration of rectal diazepam).

Pediatric primary care physicians may also serve as directors of comprehensive school-based or school-linked health programs. In these roles, pediatric care physicians should (1) have experience in planning, managing, and evaluating systems of care; (2) be knowledgeable about funding and programmatic requirements in both health and education; and (3) be able to establish quality-assurance programs. These skills will build on a solid clinical expertise in child and youth health issues, as well as firsthand knowledge and expertise with schools and educational systems. Guidelines for physicians as school consultants have been suggested (Table 124-2). Boxes 124-1 to 124-3 illustrate examples of activities and suggested guidelines and approaches to be used by primary or secondary care physicians interested in working with local schools.

Any role of the physician in school requires knowledge of the educational system and laws that protect students' rights in the health system. In the United States, the Individuals with Disabilities Education Act (IDEA) addresses children with special educational needs. In many instances, associated health needs exist with special education. For example, a child with cerebral palsy often has severe developmental delay. A girl with a chronic illness (cancer, for example) may not be able to learn to the extent of her full ability if she is expected to learn within the schedule of regular classroom instruction. These situations are examples of how health problems often coexist with the need for special education considerations. The school must address both the educational and health needs in the child's written individualized education program. Laws require schools to place students in the least-restrictive environment. In some cases, this requirement means bringing in one-to-one nurse coverage in the classroom for a student (for example, when the child is tracheostomy dependent and requires frequent suctioning and continuous observation). In other circumstances, a child's specialized health needs

Table 124-2 Examples of a Physician's Role in Schools

CLINICAL ISSUE OR PROBLEM	EXAMPLES OF PHYSICIAN'S ACTIVITIES AS CHILD'S PRIMARY HEALTH CARE PRACTITIONER	EXAMPLES OF PHYSICIAN'S ACTIVITIES AS CONSULTANT TO SCHOOL OR SCHOOL SYSTEM
Learning disability	1. Requests teacher's perception of child's learning and behavior, as well as results of individualized testing 2. Shares results of medical evaluation of child with the school 3. Works cooperatively with school personnel and parents to develop educational and behavioral management plan for child (may include school visit) 4. Sets up mechanism for follow-up on behavioral and educational progress of child	1. Serves on district committee to accomplish biannual review of disabled children's progress 2. Assists in setting up mechanism for providing follow-up behavioral and academic information to physicians who have placed students on psychoactive medication 3. Provides in-service session for classroom teachers on new concepts in attention deficit disorder 4. Advises school board on need for movement training for children who have learning disabilities
Asthma (school-age)	1. Requests school information on absenteeism, communicates with school nurse; obtains evidence of nonparticipation in physical education activities 2. Sets up mechanism for regular administration of bronchodilator at school 3. Sets up follow-up mechanism for continued monitoring of school attendance, medication-taking compliance, and participation in appropriate physical activities	1. Reviews absenteeism data to identify groups of students who have excessive absences that might be amenable to some intervention 2. Assists curriculum director and nurse in developing educational program for children who have asthma and their parents 3. Helps publicize program and communicates directly with students; solicits primary care physicians' input and support for the educational program by reinforcing concepts in their patient visits

Adapted from Nader P. A pediatrician's primer for school health activities. *Pediatr Rev.* 1982:4:82-92.

require training of non–health staff members that are already in the school or classroom. Physicians should describe the child's health need (for example, "my patient needs someone trained to recognize a seizure and be able to record the incident and administer rectal diazepam if it is prolonged longer than 5 minutes") and refrain from prescribing how the school should meet this need (eg, avoiding comments such as, "my patient needs a full-time 5-day a week nurse" or "my patient needs a one-on-one aid"). School administrators need to be able to choose from an assortment of safe solutions. Working with the school in a cooperative manner is the best way to meet the student's needs without compromising the student's safety and without unnecessarily compromising the school's budget.

Section 504 of the Rehabilitation Act of 1973 is another law relevant for primary care physicians. To receive special services under Section 504, a student does not need to have any special learning needs. Schools must provide any service within reason if the service is required to accommodate a student's disabling condition safely. When more than one possible way exists to accommodate a student to provide access to the student's education, administrators are permitted to make the choice. Unlike IDEA laws addressing special education, disabling conditions under Section 504 can be purely medical or physical, with no problem that affects learning. However, the condition must be severe enough to *substantially limit a major life activity.* A concrete example of an accommodation that a school must make to address a student's special need would be to build a ramp if a ramp is necessary to accommodate a student with muscular dystrophy confined in a wheelchair. However, Section 504 also applies to less concrete forms of access to a student's education. An example would be a young male student who has diabetes and requires someone trained to assist him to test and interpret the significance of serum glucose levels during the school day. Without this service, the student could not be educated safely. A 504 Plan is an individualized plan that describes what the school will do for a specific student to provide access to the student's education. The 504 Plan describes the actions a school will take to support the student in overcoming any limitation in a student's major activities. In this example, the district may relocate this child to a nearby school that has a 5-day-a-week nurse. Alternatively, the district may choose to keep the child in the home school and teach lay-staff members to recognize hypoglycemia and respond to it (ie, test blood sugar, administer oral sucrose, even inject glucagon). The district can arrange for a licensed nurse to come to the school each day at lunch hour to administer insulin.

Pediatric health care physicians are advised to refrain from prescribing special services for their patients

BOX 124-1 Guidelines for the Physician as Child's Health Care Provider

1. Always obtain permission from the parents to communicate with the school, and keep them informed of their child's progress.
2. Approach all school personnel as coprofessionals who have skills and interests that complement your expertise and that can provide you with information you do not have. Recognize their interest in helping the children in their charge.
3. When contacting a school for the first time, contact the principal initially.
4. When calling a teacher, find out the best time for the teacher to talk.
5. Encourage direct school-parent and parent-school communication.
6. Be willing to attend a school meeting, if necessary, to share information and develop treatment plans.
7. Listen carefully to ascertain the school personnel's main concerns and questions, and attempt to respond to them.

BOX 124-2 Guidelines for the Physician as School Health Consultant

1. Distinguish between roles of a primary health care practitioner and those of a school consultant.
2. Become aware of laws and regulations affecting schools, including those related to school finance, education for handicapped children, bilingual education, and other educational mandates.
3. Become knowledgeable about the formal and informal decision-making processes in schools regarding *regular* and *special* education of children (including health education).
4. Be a liaison to the rest of the medical community.
5. Establish a contract with the school that defines mutually agreed-on expectations and objectives.
6. Provide a regular report on your consultation to the school district.
7. Attempt to establish relationships with all levels and departments of the school system to permit access from the board and superintendent level to that of the classroom teacher.
8. Become aware of group process dynamics and decision making in groups.

BOX 124-3 A Checklist

STATE POLICIES AND PROGRAMS

- Have you apprised yourself of state policies and programs related to comprehensive school health programs?
- Have you checked to see whether health outcome objectives exist, and, if so, how they are assessed?

LOCAL POLICIES AND PROGRAMS

- Have you apprised yourself of district policies and programs related to comprehensive school health programs?
- Have you determined what health curriculum, textbooks, and materials are actually being used in the schools?
- Have you ascertained the following parameters?
  - Policies and programs that need strengthening
  - Serious gaps or deficits
  - Opportunities for health professionals to contribute meaningfully

INFLUENCING LOCAL POLICIES AND PROGRAMS

- Do you know how the local education system works? Who makes decisions? Who has authority? Who actually does the work?
- Do you know who supports (and who is concerned with) various aspects of comprehensive school health programs and their reasons for doing so?
- Have you contacted appropriate officials about your ideas and obtained their support for working with schools?
- Have you refined your ideas in consultation with key parties—teachers, administrators, school health professionals, public health professionals, school board members, and parents?
- Have you provided for periodic progress reports and changed direction or emphasis based on their results?

From National Association of State Boards of Education. *How Schools Work and How to Work With Schools.* Alexandria, VA: The Association; 1989.

after having communicated with only the student and the student's parents. Too often parents encourage physicians to write notes to schools, often scribbled on prescription pads, that demand that a school provide a student with "door-to-door transportation" or "air conditioned classroom for heat intolerance" when these services are convenient but not medically necessary or essential. Interaction with a school representative, that is, a school nurse, if a nurse is on site, or a school principal can help the physician find a perfectly appropriate intervention without unnecessarily taxing the school budget and jeopardizing other worthwhile school programs. For more information on these laws, the Internet (especially the US Department of Education Web site) provides continuously updated resources. For information on IDEA, the reader is referred to www.ed.gov/offices/osers/policy/idea/index.html. For Section 504, the reader is referred to www.ed.gov/about/offices/list/ocr/504faq.html.

Pediatric clinicians must be current with new approaches and use school-linked human services programs to reach families in need. They should understand the basic principles of community organization and the need for increased public policy support for school-linked preventive care. Second, pediatric clinicians need to be aware of the seven major goals of a comprehensive school health program. Third, primary care physicians need to be aware of the multitude of health care and non–health care personnel who play key roles. Unless pediatric clinicians are aware of the child development principles from preschool through adolescence, they cannot help implement comprehensive school health programs effectively.

Because medications, including psychoactive drugs, are sometimes needed to keep children in school and on task, the clinician must master ways to ensure medication compliance. Standardized procedures for medication administration in schools are available.[14]

CONCLUSION

School health programs must reach their potential in ensuring a safe, healthy, and nurturing environment. They are a logical access point for required health and mental health referrals, as well as a good system to provide preventive health care and education. Pediatric care physicians need to become integral parts of these systems; only in this way will the school health programs achieve these goals.

TOOLS FOR PRACTICE

Community Advocacy and Coordination

- *Adolescent & School Health Tools* (Web page), Centers for Disease Control and Prevention (www.cdc.gov/HealthyYouth/SchoolHealth/tools.htm).
- *State School and Health Contacts* (Web page), American Academy of Pediatrics (www.schoolhealth.org/section_contacts.cfm).
- *School Health: Training for the Pediatrician* (tool kit), American Academy of Pediatrics and American Medical Association (www.schoolhealth.org/trnthtrn/trainmn.html).
- *The National School Lunch Program (NSLP)* (Web page), US Department of Agriculture (www.fns.usda.gov/cnd/lunch/).
- *What is a Coordinated School Program* (fact sheet), Centers for Disease Control and Prevention (www.cdc.gov/HealthyYouth/CSHP/#model).

Medical Decision Support

- *School Health: Policy & Practice, 6th edition* (book), American Academy of Pediatrics (www.aap.org/bookstore).

Practice Management and Care Coordination

- *Authorization of Health Information to and from School Districts (HIPPA form)* (form), University of California, San Diego (www.schoolhealth.org/content/HIPAAform.pdf).
- *Example Job Description for School Physician/Medical Consultant* (fact sheet), Department of Public Health School Health (www.schoolhealth.org/content/physiciantemplate.doc).
- *Frequently Asked Questions About Section 504 and the Education of Children with Disabilities* (fact sheet), US Department of Education (www.ed.gov/about/offices/list/ocr/504faq.html).
- *Individuals with Disabilities Education Act (IDEA)* (Web page), US Department of Education (idea.ed.gov/).

RELATED WEB SITES

- American Academy of Pediatrics: School Health Resources (www.schoolhealth.org/index.cfm).
- American Association of School Administrators (www.aasa.org/).
- American School Health Association (www.ashaweb.org/).
- Centers for Disease Control and Prevention: Healthy Schools Healthy You (www.cdc.gov/HealthyYouth/index.htm).
- National Association for Sport and Physical Education (www.aahperd.org/naspe/).
- National Association of School Nurses (www.nasn.org/).
- National Center on Physical Activity and Disability: Disabilities and Condition (www.ncpad.org/disability/).
- National School Board Association (www.nsba.org/site/index.asp).

AAP POLICY STATEMENTS

American Academy of Pediatrics, Committee on Children With Disabilities. The pediatrician's role in development and implementation of an individual education plan (IEP) and/or an individual family service plan (IFSP). *Pediatrics*. 1999;104(1):124-127. (aappolicy.aappublications.org/cgi/content/full/pediatrics;104/1/124).

American Academy of Pediatrics, Committee on Injury, Violence, and Poison Prevention and Council on School Health. School transportation safety. *Pediatrics*. 2007;120(1):213-220. (aappolicy.aappublications.org/cgi/content/full/pediatrics;120/1/213).

American Academy of Pediatrics, Committee on School Health. Guidelines for emergency medical care in school. *Pediatrics*. 2001;107(2):435-436. (aappolicy.aappublications.org/cgi/content/full/pediatrics;107/2/435).

American Academy of Pediatrics, Committee on School Health. Guidelines for the administration of medication in school. *Pediatrics*. 2003;112(3):697-699. (aappolicy.aappublications.org/cgi/content/full/pediatrics;112/3/697).

American Academy of Pediatrics, Committee on School Health. Out-of-school suspension and expulsion. *Pediatrics*. 2003;112(5):1206-1209. (aappolicy.aappublications.org/cgi/content/full/pediatrics;112/5/1206).

American Academy of Pediatrics, Committee on School Health. School-based mental health services. *Pediatrics*. 2004;113(6):1839-1845. (aappolicy.aappublications.org/cgi/content/full/pediatrics;113/6/1839).

American Academy of Pediatrics, Committee on School Health. School health centers and other integrated school health services. *Pediatrics*. 2001;107(1):198-201. (aappolicy.aappublications.org/cgi/content/full/pediatrics;107/1/198).

American Academy of Pediatrics, Committee on School Health. Soft drinks in schools. *Pediatrics*. 2004;113(1):152-154. (aappolicy.aappublications.org/cgi/content/full/pediatrics;113/1/152).

American Academy of Pediatrics, Committee on School Health. The role of the school nurse in providing school health services. *Pediatrics*. 2001;108(5):1231-1232. (aappolicy.aappublications.org/cgi/content/full/pediatrics;108/5/1231).

American Academy of Pediatrics, Council on Sports Medicine and Fitness and Council on School Health. Active healthy living: prevention of childhood obesity through increased physical activity. *Pediatrics*. 2006;117(5):1834-1842. (aappolicy.aappublications.org/cgi/content/full/pediatrics;117/5/1834).

National Association of School Nurses and American Academy of Pediatrics. *Health, Mental Health and Safety Guidelines for Schools*. Silver Spring, MD: National Association of School Nurses; 2005.

REFERENCES

1. US Department of Education, Institute of Education Sciences, National Center for Health Statistics. 1.1 Million Homeschooled Students in the United States in 2003. Washington DC: US Department of Education; 2003. Available at: http://nces.ed.gov/nhes/homeschool. Accessed June 6, 2007.
2. Allensworth DD, Kolbe LJ. The comprehensive school health program: exploring an expanded concept. *J Sch Health*. 1987;57(10):409-412.
3. Taras H, Duncan P, Luckenbill D, et al. *Health, Mental Health and Safety Guidelines for Schools*. Elk Grove Village, IL: American Academy of Pediatrics; 2004.
4. American Academy of Pediatrics, Committee on School Health. *School Health: Policy and Practice*. 6th ed. Elk Grove Village, IL: American Academy of Pediatrics; 2004.
5. American Cancer Society, Joint Committee on National Health Education Standards. *National Health Education Standards: Achieving Health Literacy*. New York, NY: American Cancer Society; 1995.
6. National Association for Sports and Physical Education. *Moving into the Future: National Standards of Physical Education*. 2nd ed. Reston, VA: The Association; 2004.
7. American Academy of Pediatrics, Committee on School Health. Guidelines for emergency medical care in school. *Pediatrics*. 2001;107:435-436.
8. Marx E, Wooley SF, Northrup D. *Health is Academic: A Guide to Coordinated School Health Programs*. New York, NY: Teachers College Press; 1998.
9. American Academy of Pediatrics, Committee on School Health. School health centers and other integrated school health services. *Pediatrics*. 2001;107:198-201.
10. US Department of Agriculture, Food and Nutrition Services. School Meal Programs. Available at: www.fns.usda.gov/cnd/. Accessed June 13, 2007.
11. American Academy of Pediatrics, Committee on School Health. Soft drinks in school. *Pediatrics*. 2004;113:152-154.
12. American Academy of Pediatrics, Committee on School Health. Out-of-school suspension and expulsion. *Pediatrics*. 2003;112(5):1206-1209.
13. Pottawatomie County School District v. Earls. Citation: 536 U.S. 822 (2002).
14. American Academy of Pediatrics, Committee on School Health. Guidelines for the administration of medication in school. *Pediatrics*. 2003;112:697-699.

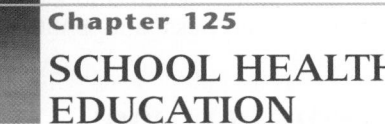

Chapter 125

SCHOOL HEALTH EDUCATION

Guy S. Parcel, PhD; Sharon S. Cummings, MPH

Schools have become a logical place for children to learn about health and to develop the skills needed to make effective health-related decisions. Success in school health education must involve a cooperative effort between educational and health care personnel. For example, the pediatrician's knowledge of child health and development is much greater than that of most educational personnel in the schools. Therefore the child health care professional has an essential role in school health-education programs. On the other hand, most educational personnel have more refined and effective skills in teaching and greater opportunities to reach children than do pediatricians. They also have more time to devote to health education itself.

Including health education as part of the instructional program in schools is by no means a new concept. Through the involvement of a school nurse or school physician, health-education activities have become part of school health services. For example, while screening for vision and hearing, the school nurse can discuss with the children, either individually or in groups, the purpose of the screening and the importance of health care in terms of sight and hearing. The school nurse might also go into the classroom and instruct the students in particular health habits, such as dental health (brushing and flossing teeth) or hand washing. Health instruction that is incorporated into the curriculum of the regular classroom teacher or the special health-education teacher is referred to as *curricular health education*. Health education is either integrated into the classroom curriculum or established as a separate curriculum in the total instructional program of the school.

TRENDS IN SCHOOL HEALTH EDUCATION

Early approaches to curriculum development in health education focused primarily on specific types of health problems, particularly those associated with risky or illicit behavior. In the 1950s, drinking alcoholic beverages was recognized as a serious health and social problem. School personnel were called on to provide instruction, pointing out the dangers and health hazards associated with alcohol consumption. The assumption was that if students knew about these dangers and were told about the health hazards, they would avoid alcohol abuse. Some states went so far as to enact laws requiring public schools to instruct students in the prevention of alcohol abuse.

Even when information is presented effectively, it does not necessarily lead to a change in behavior. Many drug-education programs were developed that effectively taught the pharmacologic aspects, legal penalties, and physical risks of drug abuse; however, evaluations of these programs revealed that they had a limited effect on alcohol abuse and other drug use.[1] Similar results from nutrition and tobacco-education programs in the late 1960s, 1970s, and early 1980s further demonstrated the weaknesses of health-education programs based primarily on a cognitive approach.[2,3]

This failure reinforced what many educators had been suggesting for years—that health behavior is related not only to knowledge, but also to factors such as expectations and values associated with health behavior. That health-related problems might not be resolved effectively on a *crisis* basis also became apparent; if health problems were to be prevented through education, then a means of addressing these problems had to be developed long before they reached a state of crisis. Teaching methods that focus on the learners' attitudes and feelings fall into the realm of *affective education*. Teaching in this area is related more to personal development than to learning facts and concepts. Affective education programs hypothesize that children who feel good about themselves, who can develop effective relationships with others, and who clearly understand what is important to them are less likely to have problems with drug abuse or other high-risk behaviors. For the teacher, this approach involves helping students build self-esteem, to learn interpersonal skills, and to develop effective decision-making and problem-solving techniques.

As an outgrowth of the increased interest in affective education, in the 1970s, many school health-education programs were expanded or redirected to focus more on attitudes, feelings, and values. Some programs tended to deemphasize the importance of information, whereas others emphasized an integration of cognitive and affective learning. However, a review of affective approaches to preventing substance abuse concluded that, in general, they made no significant difference on student substance use.[4]

In the 1980s, school-based interventions were grounded in social learning, which typically involved training students to resist social pressure to engage in unhealthy behavior (eg, smoking cigarettes), as well as creating a social environment that encouraged the development of healthy behavior (healthful diet and physical activity).[5,6] Social learning methods were expanded to the health-education curriculum, which led to development of the *social influences approach*. This approach recognized the importance of preparing students to resist the pressures of an environment that encouraged risk-taking behavior. Teaching strategies in this approach include augmenting students' knowledge about the short-term consequences of risky behavior, training in resisting peer pressure, *inoculation* against mass media messages, establishing normative expectations for healthful behavior, using peer leaders as role models, and having students make a personal commitment to avoid risk-taking behavior or to engage in healthy behavior. These methods have been applied successfully to smoking prevention[7] and drug abuse prevention.[8] Evaluations of the social influences approach find a significant effect in reducing risk-taking behavior.

Another approach in school health education from the 1980s is the use of skill-development methods to prevent risky behavior. The *skills approach* assumes that a set of social and behavioral skills is essential for making effective decisions about health behavior. Furthermore, if students are able to develop these skills, know the consequences of risky behavior, and have opportunities to practice these skills, then they will be more likely to avoid risk-taking behavior and develop healthier patterns. The skills usually addressed in these types of programs involve decision making, problem solving, communication, and stress management or relaxation. The skills approach has been shown especially effective when applied to smoking; it has also proved effective in other areas of health behavior, such as prevention of substance abuse.[9]

Youth empowerment is a recent model of school health education. The underlying principle of this model is that students must be responsible for identifying and defining the problem to be addressed and determining what action should be taken. Because many of the issues addressed by school health education have roots in community and social problems, the health-education process should enable students to recognize these roots and determine appropriate social or community actions to effect positive changes.

Besides the health-education curriculum, the concept of school-based health promotion and disease prevention has expanded to include other components of the school that influence or facilitate healthy behavior.[10] Such programs have been developed to coordinate classroom health instruction with changes in school food services and physical education, thus improving the diet and amount of physical activity of elementary schoolchildren.[11] Efforts have also been made to involve parents and to focus on the family as a critical component in influencing changes in health behavior through school-based programs.[12-14] Linking school-based programs with community programs and agencies has shown potential for improving the effectiveness of existing programs concerned with promoting healthy behavior and preventing health problems.[8,15,16]

The latest multiple-component approach for school health education is based on the *comprehensive school health education* (CSHE) *model*. CSHE programs involve health education; physical education; health services; nutrition services; health promotion for staff; counseling, psychological, and social services; a healthy school environment; and parent and community members' involvement. CSHE programs involve a set of strategies, activities, and services that provide a sequence of events at each grade level to address each designated content area (eg, intentional and unintentional injuries, alcohol and other drug use, tobacco use, dietary behaviors, physical activity, sexual behaviors). (See Chapter 124, Overview of School Health and School Health Program Goals.) In 1997 the Institute of Medicine examined the status of school health-education programs and made recommendations regarding 4 topics of school health: (1) education, (2) services, (3) infrastructure, and (4) research and evaluation.[17] Although many components of the CSHE program exist in schools across the country, the Institute of Medicine reported that many programs lack the involvement of critical community stakeholders (eg, parents, students, educators, health and social service personnel, insurers, business and political leaders).

PEDIATRICIAN'S ROLE IN SCHOOL HEALTH EDUCATION

Community pediatrics involves expanding the focus from one child to focusing on all children in the community.[18] Pediatricians can benefit many children in a community setting by working together with educators on school health education.

The goal of school health education is to help students develop skills and confidence that will enable them to make good choices about their health behavior and about appropriate use of health care resources.

If this goal is to be achieved through a school health program, then a cooperative effort by health care and educational personnel will be required. In structured classroom activities and in noncurricular health education activities, the physician can contribute to school health education in 5 distinct ways: (1) by helping to determine which health risk behaviors are prevalent in the community; (2) by helping the school or district choose health-education curricula; (3) by conducting health-education activities for children, parents, teachers, and school nurses; (4) by helping evaluate health-education activities; and (5) by reinforcing health-education messages taught in school during pediatric office visits.

Physicians are usually aware of the health issues related to specific age groups, as well as health risk behaviors in their community. Specific topics that may be important to address include physical fitness and activity in schools,[19] healthful eating habits,[20] and safer sex education.[21]

Pediatricians should consider participating in the implementation of curricula. Physicians, particularly pediatricians, can help teachers understand child development and help them identify children's developmental needs. Teachers are required to master a broad spectrum of information related to health behavior, and staying current in all these areas is difficult for them. The pediatrician can be especially helpful by alerting teachers to recent information about specific areas of health and by suggesting resources for additional information. A gap usually exists between data generated by the health sciences and the information available for use in instructional programs. The physician can help narrow this gap.

Physicians may be called on to serve as guest lecturers in classrooms. When a teacher is faced with complicated or sensitive material, such as information on HIV or AIDS, contraception and family planning, substance abuse, or specific diseases, the physician may be asked to talk to students. The easiest way for physicians to handle such a request is to visit the classroom. However, this approach has some obvious drawbacks. The physician may not be prepared to present the material at a level appropriate for the students, and the physician's time will be limited. A better approach is for the physician to work with the teacher to identify the information students need and together plan an ongoing program that the teacher can then present. In this way, a larger number of students can benefit from the physician's contribution over a longer period.

Pediatricians can advocate for program evaluation and assist schools in evaluating health-education activities. Evaluations are based on how well the program was implemented and whether the goals and objectives were met.

The time, effort, and resources devoted to the school health-education curriculum depend on the priority a school district places on health education. When the discussion involves health, physicians enjoy considerable influence and prestige in a community. Spending time with school board members and administrators can encourage a high priority for the school health education curriculum.

APPROACH TO DEVELOPING SCHOOL HEALTH-EDUCATION PROGRAMS

Forming Planning Committees

Two planning committees should be formed. The first committee should comprise top school administrators and school staff members who are likely to have responsibility for the health program. Planning committees' charge should be to establish the process for program planning and make final programmatic decisions. Regardless of the level of community enthusiasm and support for health education, school administrators and staff members should always be included at the highest levels of the decision-making process to approve and support program development officially. A second group, the program planning group, should consist of administrators, teachers, students, parents, and experts or consultants from the community and should establish strong communication links with the first group.

Assessing Needs and Resources

The program planning group will need information to determine the scope and direction of the proposed program. Useful information can be obtained from a review of the literature and of programs from other school districts. However, information about the local situation is essential to direct the program toward meeting local needs. Standardized survey questionnaires can be used to measure students' current health knowledge, attitudes, and behaviors. This information can be useful in setting priorities for the program and is often already available through the local health department or school district.

Information should also be obtained about the resources available for a health-education program. Individuals who have training and experience in health education, effective educational techniques, the development of interpersonal skills, and methods of social learning are invaluable resources. Identifying potential sources of funding (local, state, federal, and philanthropic) and available instructional materials and consultants is important.

Developing Program Goals and Objectives

Goals, the outcomes expected from the program, should be realistic and achievable. The goals should preferably be stated in such a way that the extent of their achievement can be measured. For example, (1) at the end of 5 years, the number of youths younger than age 19 arrested for driving under the influence of alcohol or drugs will be reduced by 30%; or (2) at the end of 3 years, the number of youths who begin smoking in the eighth grade will be reduced by 50%. Goals that include statements about *when, how much, of what,* and *by whom* add specificity that provides more direction and focus for the education program.

The next step is to state specific objectives for each goal by student grade level. Objectives are accomplished by students and are therefore usually stated in behavioral terms. They address what the student is expected to do as a result of this instruction. For example, the student will be able to (1) demonstrate how to use techniques to resist peer pressure, (2) apply steps in decision making to resolve a conflict about food selection in a social situation, and (3) use relaxation techniques to cope with feelings of stress.

Conducting Program Activities

Activities are the experiences that provide the knowledge, skills, practice, reinforcement, and confidence for performing the behaviors stated in the objectives. Activities are linked to objectives and should not be developed until after the specific goals and objectives for the health education program have been identified. Attention should be given to activities outside the classroom that will support and reinforce classroom learning. Activities for parents, teachers, and other school staff members are valuable in providing the social support and environment for reinforcing the learning of new behaviors.

Conducting a pilot program in one school or a few schools should be considered to test ideas and techniques and to make changes before a district wide program is implemented. A pilot program that has worked effectively and is accepted is relatively easy to implement in other schools in the district. The pilot program should be evaluated in such a way that components requiring modification can be identified.

Preparing Teachers

In-service training for teachers is essential for implementing a new curriculum. Such training should include attitudinal support for the curriculum and specific teaching skills. Attention should be given to involving other school personnel who might not teach the curriculum but whose support for it is important. For example, the school principal, nurse, counselor, or social worker should be involved in planning the implementation of the program.

IMPLEMENTING CHANGE

Change in school systems tends to occur slowly, often because of the lack of a systematic approach. One model for implementing change in schools has 4 phases: (1) organizational commitment, (2) change in policies and practices, (3) alteration of roles and actions of the staff, and (4) implementation of learning.[5] This model is intended to provide a systematic approach to change that includes school components that support and facilitate behaviors addressed by health-education programs in the classroom.

In the first phase, commitment from key decision-makers in the school system should be obtained to proceed with the planning of a new or modified health-promotion program. A top-down approach involves school board members, superintendents, and program directors deciding to commit to the proposed program. The proposal for the new program can come from an agency outside the district, such as a health department or voluntary health agency, or from inside groups, such as curriculum planning committees or task force groups appointed to address specified problems. Commitment is usually obtained through a series of meetings with key decision makers. These meetings typically involve a written or verbal presentation on the importance of and need for the proposed program. Physicians can provide information to help establish a high priority for proposed health-promotion programs.

Commitment also needs to be obtained from a bottom-up, or grassroots, approach in which the individuals who implement the program (teachers and staff members) are involved in making decisions about planning new or modified programs. This method often results in a strong personal and professional commitment for health-promotion programs.

SETTING EXPECTATIONS FOR SCHOOL HEALTH EDUCATION

The health professional may expect that, to be effective, health education must influence behavior to reduce the risk of disease or to improve health status. The educator, however, might argue that the role of the school is to increase knowledge and develop critical-thinking skills and not necessarily to change student behavior, which may be greatly influenced by factors outside the classroom. Both perspectives might be considered correct, and each will influence how programs are designed and evaluated.

School health-education programs can help students learn about their health. Evaluations of school health-education programs have demonstrated their effectiveness in influencing a variety of outcomes, including knowledge, attitudes, health practices, behavior, and physiological factors.[8,16,22,23] The program's effect on learning, and eventually on behavior, depends on the quality of the planning and the input of sufficient resources, including teacher training and adequate classroom instructional time.[22] Behavioral change, however, is complex, and simplistic approaches that do not effectively use what has been learned both in research and in the field are unlikely to succeed.

Expecting school-based educational programs alone to influence behaviors that are not supported by the child's larger social environment is unreasonable. See Chapter 124 for an overview of school health program goals of which health education is a part. Health education should relate to other parts of the school curriculum and programs. Students need numerous opportunities to experience personal development, and the social environment of the school should be structured to support students in their practice of decision-making and related skills.

TOOLS FOR PRACTICE

Community Advocacy and Coordination

- *Coordinated School Health Program* (fact sheet), Centers for Disease Control and Prevention (www.cdc.gov/healthyyouth/CSHP/).

Medical Decision Support

- *School Health: Policy & Practice, 6th edition* (book), American Academy of Pediatrics (www.aap.org/bookstore).

RELATED WEB SITES

- American Alliance for Health, Physical Education, Recreation & Dance (aahperd.org/index.cfm).
- Centers for Disease Control and Prevention: Healthy You Healthy Schools (www.cdc.gov/healthyyouth).

AAP POLICY STATEMENTS

American Academy of Pediatrics and National Association of School Nurses. *Health, Mental Health and Safety Guidelines for Schools*. Elk Grove Village, IL: American Academy of Pediatrics; 2005. AAP endorsed.

American Academy of Pediatrics, Committee on Community Health Services. The pediatrician's role in community practice. *Pediatrics*. 2005;115(4):1092-1094. (aappolicy.aappublications.org/cgi/content/full/pediatrics;115/4/1092).

American Academy of Pediatrics, Committee on Psychosocial Aspects of Child and Family Health and Committee on Adolescence. Sexuality education for children and adolescents. *Pediatrics*. 2001;108(2):498-502. (aappolicy.aappublications.org/cgi/content/full/pediatrics;108/2/498).

American Academy of Pediatrics, Council on Sports Medicine and Fitness and Council on School Health. Active healthy living: prevention of childhood obesity through increased physical activity. *Pediatrics*. 2006;117(5):1834-1842. (aappolicy.aappublications.org/cgi/content/full/pediatrics;117/2/1834).

REFERENCES

1. Bangert-Drowns RL. The effects of school-based substance abuse education: a meta-analysis. *J Drug Educ*. 1988;18:243-264.
2. Contento IR, Manning AD, Shannon B. Research perspectives on school-based nutrition education. *J Nutr Educ*. 1992;24:247-260.
3. Perry CL, Kelder SH. Models for effective prevention. *J Adolesc Health*. 1992;13:355-363.
4. Hansen WB. School-based substance abuse prevention: a review of the state of the art in curriculum, 1980-1990. *Health Educ Res*. 1992;7:403-430.
5. Parcel GS, Simons-Morton BG, Kolbe LJ. Health promotion: integrating organizational change and student learning strategies. *Health Educ Q*. 1988; 15:435-450.
6. Perry CL, Parcel GS, Stone E, et al. The Child and Adolescent Trial for Cardiovascular Health (CATCH): overview of the intervention program and evaluation methods. *Cardiovasc Risk Factors*. 1992;2: 36-44.
7. Perry CL, Luepker RV, Murray DM, et al. Parent involvement with children's health promotion: a one-year follow-up of the Minnesota home team. *Health Educ Q*. 1989;16:171-180.
8. Pentz MA, Dwyer JH, MacKinnon DP, et al. A multicommunity trial for primary prevention of adolescent drug abuse. *JAMA*. 1989;261:3259-3266.
9. Botvin GJ. Prevention of adolescent substance abuse through the development of personal and social competence. In: Glynn T, ed. *Preventing Adolescent Drug Abuse: Intervention Strategies*. NIDA Research Monograph Series, No. 47. Washington, DC: US Government Printing Office; 1983.
10. Kolbe LJ. Increasing the impact of school health promotion programs: emerging research perspectives. *Health Educ Q*. 1986;17:47-52.
11. Parcel GS, Simons-Morton B, O'Hara NM, et al. School promotion of healthful diet and physical activity: impact on learning outcomes and self-reported behavior. *Health Educ Q*. 1989;16:181-199.
12. Kelder SH. The Students for Peace Project: a comprehensive violence-prevention program for middle school students. *Am J Prev Med*. 1996;12:22-30.
13. Nader PR, Sallis JF, Patterson TL, et al. A family approach to cardiovascular risk reduction: results from the San Diego Family Health Project, *Health Educ Q*. 1989;16:229-244.
14. Nader PR, Sellers DE, Johnson CC, et al. The effect of adult participation in a school-based family intervention to improve children's diet and physical activity: the Child and Adolescent Trial for Cardiovascular Health. *Prev Med*. 1996;25:455-464.
15. Pentz MA. Community organization and school liaisons: how to get programs started. *J Sch Health*. 1986;56:382-388.
16. US Department of Health and Human Services. *Preventing Tobacco Use among Young People: A Report of the Surgeon General*, Atlanta, GA: Centers for Disease Control and Prevention; 1994.
17. Institute of Medicine. *Schools & Health: Our Nation's Investment*. Washington, DC: National Academies Press; 1997.
18. American Academy of Pediatrics, Committee on Community Health Services. The pediatrician's role in community pediatrics. *Pediatrics*. 2005;115:1092-1094.
19. American Academy of Pediatrics, Committee on Sports Medicine and Fitness and Committee on School Health. Physical fitness and activity in schools. *Pediatrics*. 2000;105:1156-1157.
20. American Academy of Pediatrics, Committee on School Health. Soft drinks in schools. *Pediatrics*. 2004;113:152-154.
21. American Academy of Pediatrics, Committee on Psychosocial Aspects of Child and Family Health and Committee on Adolescence. Sexuality education for children and adolescents. *Pediatrics*. 2001;108:498-502.
22. Connell DB, Turner RR, Mason EF. Summary of findings of the school health education evaluation: health promotion effectiveness, implementation, and costs. *J Sch Health*. 1985;55:316-321.
23. Parcel GS, Taylor WC, Brink SG, et al. Translating theory into practice: intervention strategies for the diffusion of a health promotion innovation. *Fam Community Health*. 1989;12:1-13.

Chapter 126

NURSING ROLES IN SCHOOL HEALTH

Bernadette Mazurek Melnyk, PhD, RN, CPNP/NPP;
Karen Teeple Reuter, MS, BSN, RN, CAzSN

R. W. Blum states, "We need to understand that health and education are closely intertwined and that school failure needs to be viewed as a health as well as an education crisis."[1] When children are not mentally and physically healthy, their academic performance and attendance at school are adversely affected.[2] The impact of children's health on school outcomes was first recognized more than a hundred years ago, when school absenteeism in Boston schools was related to the incidence of communicable diseases in children. As a result of the high absenteeism rates, Lillian Wald, a public health nurse, challenged New York officials and the New York Board of Education to allow her to place a public health nurse in selected schools as a pilot project.[3] The outcome of this intervention was a startling decrease in the number of students sent home from school over a 1-year period.[4] Subsequently, school nursing became a specialty.

Today, the role of the school nurse has expanded and is more complex. The continually evolving school nurse role is both driven and guided by advances in health care, federal mandates, and societal changes. For example, health care advances have resulted in viable premature newborns, some of whom go on to become medically fragile students in schools. Federal education mandates accompany these and other children who have unique learning and health care needs.[5,6]

The notion that healthy children learn better is now recognized. If this premise is accepted, then it follows that physical, mental, emotional, and social health problems compromise a child's ability to learn and to be academically successful.[7,8]

Schools are a reflection of changes in society. Recent trends in American society and family life can place children at risk for academic failure. A growing number of children live in poverty, have limited access to health care, are affected by mental health disorders, or are limited by long-term disabilities, each influencing and being influenced by schools.[9,10] Traditional 2-parent families are no longer the norm for many children. Single-parent families, blended families, and gay and lesbian families, as well as traditional 2-parent biological families, are faced with a variety of challenges that often express themselves in the school setting.[11] Conversely, educational failure may contribute to adverse health conditions (eg, stress correlates with the development of health problems).[12]

School nursing is a critical component in assessing, coordinating, planning, providing, and evaluating school health service programs. School nurses develop team relationships within the school and with community health care providers so that student health needs are met and replication of services is prevented. School nurses serve as the liaison among the school, home, and the medical community regarding concerns that may affect a child's ability to learn.[8]

DEFINITION AND PREPARATION FOR SCHOOL NURSING

According to the National Association of School Nurses,

> "School nursing is a specialized practice of professional nursing that advances the well-being, academic success, and life-long achievement of students. To that end, school nurses facilitate positive student responses to normal development; promote health and safety; intervene with actual and potential health problems and actively collaborate with others to build student and family capacity for adaptation, self-management, self-advocacy, and learning."[8]

Until recent years, school districts sought health care employees for their students primarily to care for emergencies and acute illness. Emergency medical technicians, health aides or assistants, and licensed practical nurses provided health care to students in some schools. With increased accountability for students' academic success, the introduction of school-based health care clinics, and an increase in chronic health conditions among school-aged children, an increasing number of schools provide their school health services through a professional registered nurse. Although approximately 58,000 school nurses practice in the United States, many schools do not have full-time nurses, even though the Centers for Disease Control and Prevention has recommended that a nurse in every school would facilitate better asthma management in children.[3]

Educational preparation of the school nurse varies from a 2-year associate of arts degree registered nurse to a master's-prepared pediatric, family, or school nurse practitioner. The generalist school nurse must hold a current license to practice as a registered nurse. The nurse practitioner must hold current licensure as an advanced practice nurse in the state in which the nurse practices. Because of the complexity of issues addressed by school nurses, the National Association of School Nurses recommends that the minimal educational preparation level for a school nurse be a baccalaureate degree (bachelor of science in nursing [BSN]) and school nurse certification.[13] The independent nature of the school practice and the advanced skill and critical thinking required for demanding and unstable situations command this minimal level of educational preparation.[1,13] For nurses in management, supervisory, or consultant positions, a master's degree is essential.[14]

A school nurse needs expertise in pediatric, community health, and mental health nursing with strong health-promotion, assessment, referral, communication, leadership, organization, and time-management skills. Knowledge of health education laws that affect children is essential, as are teaching strategies for the delivery of health education to students and staff.[8]

SCHOOL HEALTH PROGRAMMING

Harrington states, "The school nurse is challenged to collaborate in the development, implementation, coordination, and evaluation of a school health services program that promotes optimal health and students who are healthy and able to learn, and thereby facilitates the learning process and student success."[8] The model for coordinated school health programs provides a structure and process to support health-related knowledge, skills, values, and practice. A coordinated school health program consists of 8 components:

1. School health services
2. Health education
3. Health-promotion programs for faculty and staff
4. Counseling, psychological, and social services
5. School nutrition services
6. Physical education programs
7. Health school environment
8. Family and community involvement[8]

This model has been promoted by the Centers for Disease Control and Prevention, Division of Adolescent and School Health.

The 8 components of a coordinated school health program provide a framework for school nurse practice. Additionally, models from community and public health nursing, epidemiology, and the social sciences are incorporated in the provision of quality school health services and programming. The framework for the practice of the professional school nurse is provided through the National Association of School Nurses' "Scope and Standards of Practice," which describe standards of practice or the steps in the nursing process: assessment, diagnosis, outcome identification, planning, implementation, and evaluation and through the standards of professional performance, which describe a competent level of behavior in the professional role composed of quality of care, performance appraisal, education collegiality, ethics, collaboration, research, resource use, communication, program management, and health education.[15]

Students are more broadly defined today than the traditional public K-12 school. Today, school nurses work in variety of settings, including preschools, juvenile detention centers, college campuses, boarding schools, drug rehabilitation facilities, schools for the deaf, alternative education schools, schools for emotionally disturbed students, and international programs for children of members of the armed forces.[5]

The focus of this discussion will be the school nurse's role in the traditional school setting. The function of the school nurse is to promote academic success and provide optimal nursing care to the entire school community, including the staff. Student health status includes the well student and those with urgent health needs, chronic health problems, psychosocial or mental health problems, medically fragile conditions, and technology-dependent students with multiple health problems.[5] In school settings where the professional nurse cares for the health needs of students, primary, secondary, and tertiary levels of prevention are implemented.[16,17]

Primary prevention, the promotion of health and prevention of disease is routinely provided to students either individually, when a student visits the health office (eg, teaching about the relationship of adequate sleep to academic performance, providing information about how to cope with stress),[18,19] or in support groups (eg, weight loss, grief and loss, teen issues). In addition, school nurses often provide classroom presentations on such topics as human growth and development, HIV/AIDS, nutrition, stress management, coping strategies, cognitive behavioral skills building, and bullying and harassment prevention.

Secondary prevention is provided through screening programs that assess hearing, vision, scoliosis, blood pressure, dental needs, and height and weight. In addition, as a result of the increase in mental health problems that affect 1 in 4 children and adolescents,[20] school nurses must be knowledgeable of how best to screen for mental health problems such as anxiety and depression.[2] They must also be aware of excellent resources, such as the National Association of Pediatric Nurse Practitioners' (NAPNAP) KySS (Keep Your Children/Yourself Safe and Secure) Program, a national mental health–promotion campaign that assists health care providers to screen for and intervene early for children and adolescents with mental health problems.[2]

Each state determines which screenings are mandated. School districts also establish health-screening policies, which further determine the grade level that additional screening programs will be performed with their students. When health problems are identified, the school nurse makes a referral to the parent or guardian for follow-up. Preferably, telephone contact should be made at the same time that a referral letter is sent in the mail. The telephone contact provides the nurse with the opportunity to discuss the findings, to interpret them, and to determine whether the family needs financial assistance or social services to enable them to follow through with the referral for their child. The form letter states what the outcome of the screening test was and usually provides a space for the physician's response and diagnosis. If the parent or guardian has signed a release of information, then the nurse will be able to make contact with the examining physician to discuss any suggested academic accommodations at school. The school nurse would then communicate and coordinate any academic accommodations with the student's teachers.

The school nurse works closely with families, school staff, physicians, and health care agencies to provide tertiary prevention for students with chronic physical and mental health conditions. Specifically, the school nurse must be knowledgeable of the assessment, early intervention, and prevention for the changing morbidities of childhood, particularly chronic health conditions, including obesity, and mental health problems.

Chronically ill children and children with complex medical needs are guaranteed a free and appropriate education in schools through the Individuals with Disabilities Education Improvement Act (2004),[7] the Americans with Disabilities Act (1990), and the Section 504 of the Vocational Rehabilitation Act (1973).[12,21] These laws provide educational opportunities, protection, and support for students in both special and regular education programs who have special needs related to their disability.[22] Applicable students must complete an evaluation process by the school team to determine whether they qualify for the services under the Individuals with Disabilities Education Improvement Act or Section 504. The school nurse is an integral participant of the school team, which includes the teachers, school psychologist, parents or guardians, school counselor, and, depending on the disability, speech therapist, occupational therapist, physical therapist, or teachers of hearing- or vision-impaired students. Pending the outcome of the qualification process, an *individual education plan,* also known as a *504 Accommodation Plan,* may be written. The medical or nursing services are coordinated by the school nurse, and depending on the disability, an *individual health care plan* or an *emergency care plan* (or both) is completed with input from the physician and parent. A physician's order may be required for some aspects of the required medical care provided by the school nurse. To provide maximal safety for the student and to provide an increased level of comfort for the parent or guardian and the classroom teacher, the school nurse will educate the classroom teacher regarding any signs or symptoms that should be anticipated relative to the student's presenting health condition.

Sociodemographics, student illness acuity (eg, chronically ill, medically fragile), and size of the student population all determine the school nurse's focus and programming emphasis. The National Association of School Nurses recommends a nurse-to-student ratio of 1:750 in general school populations, 1:225 in mainstreamed special education populations, 1:125 in severely chronically ill or developmentally disabled populations, and a ratio based on individual needs in medically fragile populations.[15] However, school districts determine the school nurse-to-student ratio.

MODELS OF SCHOOL NURSE SERVICES

Many models have been developed for the provision of health services in schools, with varying levels of educational preparation. Some districts have BSN and master's degree-prepared nurses for each school, and a health assistant who may travel between schools. Some school districts are staffed with health assistants in their schools with one 1 supervising professional registered nurse. Other school districts have a mix of licensed practical nurses and health assistants with a supervising registered nurse. The determinants of the health services model include school district budgetary constraints, school district priorities, and availability of registered professional nurses in a given community.

Some school districts have incorporated telemedicine into their health services model. School nurses have been on the forefront of telemedicine. This process allows students to receive an evaluation from a health care professional without the student leaving school. Fundamental to its effectiveness is the presence of a licensed professional on the sending and receiving ends of the transmission to ensure accurate input and a directed intervention. However, school districts can be found that use this service model with health assistants providing the telemetry input to the physician. Although school-based health care centers can provide a similar service, the challenge of keeping them funded led to this technology-driven approach.[23]

Some states provide school health services through their state and county health departments. In this model, the public health nurse provides primarily consulting services. A health assistant or other nonmedical school employee provides the daily care given to students.

The role of the nurse practitioner in school-based health care clinics has developed in response to the health care crisis and the development of managed health care.[24,25] The reform of health care was driven by the goals of quality, access, and cost containment. Schools were recognized as an effective conduit for delivering health services to school-aged children and youth.[26] Similarly, schools were aware that many children have unrecognized health and psychological disorders because they lack access to health care.[24] A significant decrease in emergency department visits as a result of availability of a school-based health care center has been documented.[27] According to a 2002 survey, 1498 school-based health care centers have been established across the country.[28-30] Working with a pediatric primary care physician colleague, the nurse practitioner may assume an effective primary care role that involves providing comprehensive well-child care, assessing and managing minor illnesses, and performing initial assessments of more serious acute and chronic conditions.

School districts have recognized that through the provision of specific health services to qualified students, they can be reimbursed by Medicaid. Medicaid reimburses schools for services provided under 1 of 3 different models. The 1st model provides the following categories of nursing services and procedures[31]: case finding, nursing care procedures, care coordination, patient-student counseling or instruction, and emergency care.

The 2nd model provides for an increase in service provision. In this model, a nurse practitioner provides comprehensive primary and preventive care. According to the NAPNAP's scope and standards of practice, the pediatric nurse practitioner is an advanced practice registered nurse who provides health care to children from birth through 21 years of age and has a minimum of a master's degree.[32] The nurse practitioner provides comprehensive health care to children through assessment, diagnosis, management, and evaluation of care, with emphases on health promotion and disease prevention.[32]

In the 3rd model, school-based health care centers—made up of an interdisciplinary team of physicians, nurses, counselors, laboratory and medical assistants, and other health professionals—provide comprehensive services in a clinical setting licensed at the school site.

When a primary care clinic is present, activities of the school health program are often altered based on the type of primary care services provided. The scope of the school nurse's role is related to the organizational structure under which health services are provided. The school nurse may be fully integrated into the functioning of the clinic or remain separate from the clinic and serve as a liaison with the school health program.

No matter which model a school health system provides, the role of the school involves collaboration on interdisciplinary teams. An awareness of some of the variations in the school nurse's role can help the physician establish a collaborative relationship with the nurse and become familiar with the school program.

PHYSICIAN AND SCHOOL NURSE COLLABORATION

Although communication between the physician and school personnel may occur in many contexts, the school nurse is the person who most often initiates interaction with the primary care physician. School and health care agencies have different priorities and backgrounds. The school nurse can help the physician bridge the gap; at the same time, the nurse may gain valuable consultation and support for health-related activities in the school. Mutual respect, open communication, and some understanding of each other's views can enhance cooperation between the physician and the school nurse. Collaboration in pursuit of common goals ultimately improves the health of schoolchildren. A collaborative school nurse–physician relationship is critical in the provision of continuity and quality of care for children who have unstable chronic illnesses and for the care of medically fragile children.

QUALITY SCHOOL HEALTH SERVICES

The provision of quality school health services requires a team approach among the school nurse, parent, physician, community agencies, teacher, administration, and other school personnel who affect children's potential for optimal health and learning. Judith Vessey states,

> "In today's educational arena, community leaders, legislators, and parents are concerned about student academic performance, school safety, and fiscal responsibility. These concerns have led to calls for improved educational accountability. For school nurses to be seen as a requisite, integral part of the education system, they must show that school nursing makes a difference in students' academic performance."[33]

Evidence-based practice provides a framework to facilitate a practice model that promotes quality care for students, facilitates school nurses ability to contain costs, and demonstrates the clinical efficacy of school nursing practice.[34,35] Evidence-based practice is a problem-solving approach to the delivery of care that integrates the best evidence from well-designed studies in combination with a clinician's expertise and patient preferences.[36] The results of evidence-based studies help the school nurse or nurse practitioner provide the highest quality of care to students. For example, school nurses have an opportunity to apply evidence-based practice to management of asthma control in their students and thereby improve school attendance.[12] The "Health and Education Leadership Project: A School Initiative for Children and Adolescents With Chronic Health Conditions" is another example of evidence-based practice in school nursing, and the use of this research is both an individual and organizational responsibility.[37] With the support of their administration, school nurses can greatly enhance their students and families' health and developmental outcomes through the application of evidence-based practice.

TOOLS FOR PRACTICE

Medical Decision Support

- *Health, Mental Health, and Safety Guidelines for Schools,* American Academy of Pediatrics and National Association of School Nurses (www.nationalguidelines.org/).
- *Healthy Schools Healthy Youth* (Web page), Centers for Disease Control and Prevention (www.cdc.gov/HealthyYouth/index.htm).
- *Managing Infectious Diseases in Child Care and Schools* (book), American Academy of Pediatrics (www.aap.org/b).
- *School Health: Policy & Practice, 6th edition* (book), American Academy of Pediatrics (www.aap.org/bookstore).

RELATED WEB SITES

- American School Health Association (www.ashaweb.org/index.html).
- National Association of Pediatric Nurse Practitioners (NAPNAP) (www.napnap.org/index_home.cfm).
- National Association of School Nurses (www.nasn.org/).
- US Department of Education: Individuals with Disabilities Education Act 2004 (www.ed.gov/policy/speced/guid/idea/idea2004.html).

AAP POLICY STATEMENTS

Taras H, Duncan P, Luckenbill D, et al, eds. *Health, Mental Health, and Safety Guidelines for Schools.* Elk Grove Village, IL: American Academy of Pediatrics; 2004. AAP endorsed.

American Academy of Pediatrics, Committee on School Health. School health assessments. *Pediatrics.* 2000;105(4):875-877. (aappolicy.aappublications.org/cgi/content/full/pediatrics;105/4/875).

American Academy of Pediatrics, Committee on School Health. The role of the school nurse in providing school health services. *Pediatrics.* 2001;108(5):1231-1232. (aappolicy.aappbulications.org/cgi/content/full/pediatrics;108/5/1231).

REFERENCES

1. Blum RW, Beuhring T, Rinehart PM. *Protecting Teens: Beyond Race, Income, and Family Structure.* Minneapolis, MN: University of Minnesota; 2000. Available at: http://allaboutkids.umn.edu/kdwbvfc/beyondrace.pdf. Accessed April 11, 2007.
2. DeSocio J, Hootman J. Children's mental health and school success. *J Sch Nurs.* 2004;20:189-196.
3. Kennedy MS. School nursing. A successful experiment: celebrating 100 years of service. *Am J Nurs.* 2003;103:102-103.
4. Wrightslaw. IDEA 2004 Statute and Regulations. Available at: www.wrightslaw.com/idea/law.htm. Accessed April 1, 2007.
5. US Department of Health and Human Services, Substance Abuse and Mental Health Services Administration. Child and Adolescent Mental Health. Available at: www.mentalhealth.samhsa.gov/publications/allpubs/CA-0004/default.asp. Accessed April 2, 2007.
6. Wolfe LC. Roles of the school nurse. In: Selekman J, ed. *School Nursing: A Comprehensive Textbook.* Philadelphia, PA: FA Davis; 2006.
7. American Academy of Pediatrics. *School Health Policy and Practice.* 6th ed. Elk Grove Village, IL: American Academy of Pediatrics; 2004.
8. Harrington JF. Overview of school health services. Castle Rock, CO: National Association of School Nurses Inc; 2002.
9. At Health Inc. Mental health information. 2000. Available at: www.athealth.com/Consumer/newsletter/FPN_4_5.html. Accessed April 11, 2007.
10. Centers for Disease Control and Prevention, National Advisory Committee on Children and Terrorism. Schools and terrorism. *J School Health.* 2004;74:39-51.
11. Conlin M, Hempel J. Unmarried America. *Business Week.* 2003;(3854):106-116.
12. Zaiger DS. *School Nursing Practice: An Orientation Manual.* 2nd ed. Castle Rock, CO: National Association of School Nurses Inc; 2001.
13. National Association of School Nurses. *Coordinated School Health Program.* Position statement. Scarborough, ME: National Association of School Nurses; 2001.
14. Constante C. Requirements for school nurse practice and certification. In: Selekman J, ed. *School Nursing: A Comprehensive Textbook.* Philadelphia, PA: FA Davis; 2006.
15. National Association of School Nurses. *Scope and Standards of Professional School Nursing Practice.* Washington, DC: National Association of School Nurses; 2003.
16. Wold SJ. *School Nursing: A Framework for Practice.* St Paul, MN: Sunrise River Press; 1981.
17. Cooper P. The Whole Child in a Coordinated School Health: There Is Life After Tests, and Before. Keynote speech presented at the Arizona Public Health Association Conference, 2006, Phoenix, AZ.
18. Kelman BB. The sleep needs of adolescents. *J Sch Nurs.* 1999;15:14-19.
19. Taras H, Potts-Datema W. Sleep and student performance at school. *J Sch Health.* 2005;75:248-254.
20. Melnyk BM, Moldenhauer Z. *The KySS Guide to Child and Adolescent Mental Health Screening, Early Intervention, and Health Promotion.* Cherry Hill, NJ: National Association of Pediatric Nurse Practitioners; 2006.

21. Council for Exceptional Children. CEC's Update on IDEA Reauthorization. August 2005. Available at: www.cec.sped.org/content/navigationmenu/policyadvocacy/ideare sources/ideareauthtimeline.pdf. Accessed April 11, 2007.
22. Zimmerman B. Student health and education plans. In: Selekman J, ed. *School Nursing: A Comprehensive Textbook.* Philadelphia, PA: FA Davis; 2006.
23. Marcontel-Shattuck M, Gregory EK. Dealing with controversy in the practice of school nursing. In: Selekman J, ed. *School Nursing: A Comprehensive Textbook.* Philadelphia, PA: FA Davis; 2006.
24. Texas Department of State Health Services. School-Based Health Centers. Available at: www.dshs.state.tx.us/schoolhealth/healctr.shtm. Accessed April 11, 2007.
25. Zaiger DS. Historical perspectives of school nursing. In: Selekman J, ed. *School Nursing: A Comprehensive Textbook.* Philadelphia, PA: FA Davis; 2006.
26. Federal Interagency Forum on Child and Family Statistics. America's Children: Key National Indicators of Well-Being, 2006. Available at: www.childstats.gov/index.asp Accessed April 11, 2007.
27. Young TL, D'Andelo SL, Davis J. Impact of a school-based health center on emergency department use by elementary school students. *J Sch Health.* 2001;71:196-200.
28. Centers for Disease Control and Prevention. Children and teens told by doctors that they were overweight—United States, 1999-2002. *MMWR Morb Mortal Wkly Rep.* 2005;54:848-849. Available at: www.cdc.gov/mmwr/PDF/wk/mm5434.pdf. Accessed February 27:2007.
29. Salmon ME. School nursing in the era of health care reform: what is the outlook? *J Sch Health.* 1994;12:23.
30. Yates S. The practice of nursing: integration with new models of health service delivery. *J Sch Nurs.* 1994;13:4.
31. Gaffrey EA, Bergren MD. School health services and managed care: a unique partnership for child health. *J Sch Nurs.* 1998;14:5-22.
32. National Association of Pediatric Nurse Practitioners. *Scope and Standards of Practice: Pediatric Nurse Practitioner (PNP).* Cherry Hill, NJ: National Association of Pediatric Nurse Practitioners; 2004.
33. Vessey J. The school nurse's role related to research. In: Selekman J, ed. *School Nursing: A Comprehensive Textbook.* Philadelphia, PA: FA Davis; 2006.
34. Denehy J. Developing a program of research in school nursing. *J Sch Nurs.* 2003;19:125-126.
35. Hootman J. The importance of research to school nurses and school nursing practice. *J Sch Nurs.* 2002;18:18-24.
36. Melnyk BM. Fineout-Overholt E. *Evidence-Based Practice in Nursing and Healthcare.* Philadelphia, PA: Lippincott, Williams & Wilkins; 2005.
37. Thies KM, McAllister JW. The health and education leadership project: a school initiative for children and adolescents with chronic health conditions. *J. Sch Health.* 2001;71:167-172.

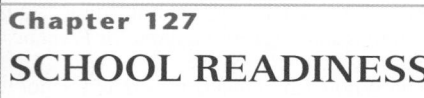

Chapter 127
SCHOOL READINESS

Karen Ratliff-Schaub, MD

Kindergarten is typically viewed as the beginning of school, given that almost all children in the United States attend kindergarten.[1] School readiness, how prepared a child is to learn at school, is an important but complex issue. No standard definition of readiness exists. Parents and teachers do not always agree on what makes a child ready for school. States have varying educational requirements; standards and expectations may be different from one school district to another. More than one million Web sites pertain to kindergarten readiness. Some of these resources are state and school Web sites, outlining entrance criteria and providing readiness questionnaires. Although many sites offer products for sale designed to prepare a child for kindergarten, few of them attempt to define readiness.

DEFINITION

In general, school readiness means a child has the prerequisites to succeed in school. These prerequisites include a large number of gross-motor, fine-motor, and cognitive skills, as well as knowledge and social attributes, listed in Box 127-1. The US Department of Education's Early Childhood Longitudinal Study, Kindergarten Class of 1998-1999 (ECLS-K) collected data on 19,000 children entering kindergarten in 1998. ECLS-K found that most children can recognize numbers and letters, count more than 10 objects, identify simple shapes, and demonstrate basic print familiarity. The majority of children can interact appropriately with peers and are fairly well behaved, although a substantial minority were reported by parents and teachers to be overly active and have difficulty paying attention. Boys were more likely than girls to be judged as having behavior problems and difficulty paying attention.[1]

Parents and teachers often disagree about which factors are most important. Parents tend to emphasize academic and cognitive skills, whereas teachers, particularly experienced ones, are more concerned with emotional factors.[2]

Teachers also tend to view children who are shy or withdrawn as less ready than other children.

BOX 127-1 Readiness Skills

- Knows colors
- Counts to 10
- Retells story
- Plays cooperatively with peers
- Identifies some letters
- Listens quietly to a story
- Goes to bathroom independently
- Demonstrates curiosity and persistence
- Talks in sentences
- Follows directions
- Completes an activity
- Separates easily from parents

From Nader P. Five years: entering school. In: Dixon SD, Stein MT, eds. *Encounters with Children: Pediatric Behavior and Development.* 3rd ed. Philadelphia, PA: Mosby; 2000; Schor EL, American Academy of Pediatrics. *Caring for Your School-Age Child: Ages 5 to 12.* Rev ed. New York, NY: Bantam Books; 1999; Kaplan-Sanoff M. School readiness. In: Parker S, Zuckerman B, Augustyn M, eds. *Developmental and Behavioral Pediatrics.* 2nd ed. Philadelpia, PA: Lippincott Williams & Wilkens; 2005.

Well-developed social skills and adaptability are other characteristics of readiness according to teachers.[3] Both parents and teachers agree that children should enter school healthy and socially competent. Parents, however, tend to put more emphasis on certain skills such as being able to communicate in English. Some research has suggested different levels of expectations regarding readiness from parents, depending on their own level of education, but other studies have not found any difference.[4]

Teachers do not necessarily agree about which qualities are important. In general, kindergarten teachers from the ECLS-K placed a strong emphasis on the social aspects of learning (ie, ability to tell thoughts and wants, turn taking, following directions, displaying nondisruptive behavior). However, younger teachers in the study were more likely to value academic skills, whereas teachers from southern states had higher social and academic expectations of their students.[2]

Parents tend to agree with teachers that children should be healthy, socially competent, and compliant with teacher demands. They actually place a higher value on compliance than teachers do. Parents believe that the child should be able to communicate in English and have certain basic skills and knowledge. These findings were true regardless of level of education or ethnicity.[4] McBryde concluded that parents and teachers were less concerned with developmental status and more focused on chronologic age, adaptability, persistence, and social skills.[3] Interestingly, little evidence has been found that teachers or parents put much stock or emphasis on the types of qualities measured by kindergarten screening tests.

Some professionals view readiness as an intrinsic, child-centered factor; a child is ready when certain skills are displayed. If not ready, then the child simply needs more time to mature. Eighty-eight percent of teachers hold this view, although 94% also believed that experiences might help these skills develop.[5] A corollary of this view is that readiness skills can be measured by some sort of assessment.

The National Education Goals Panel (NEGP)[6] identified 3 components of school readiness:

1. The child's readiness
2. The school's readiness
3. Family and community supports

This concept is an emerging viewpoint that sees readiness as more of an interaction between the school and the child, with additional influences from the community, culture, and society. An increasing number of educators are emphasizing that not only should children be ready for school, but also schools should be prepared to meet the learning needs of the children they serve.[7] As the Policy Report of the National Institute for Early Education Research (NIEER) states, "The exact definition of readiness depends on who is doing the defining."[8]

AGE ELIGIBILITY

Part of the definition of readiness in most states includes age eligibility. Forty-four states and the District of Columbia have a date by which children must turn 5 years to be eligible for kindergarten. These cutoff dates range from July 1st to January 1st, with the most popular date falling in September. Overall, three quarters of states require children turn 5 years by October 16th.[8] To complicate matters further, some states allow individual school districts to select a cutoff date earlier than the one required by the state.

Some states have raised the official age for school entry, citing evidence that older students possess more skills and do better on standardized testing.[9] This practice does not, however, address age-related variability. Making the state age requirement for kindergarten entry higher simply increases the average age. The age span remains the same.[10] Increasing the age of kindergarten entry also encourages schools to make the kindergarten curriculum more demanding, particularly in states where the primary motive was to improve standardized test scores. This practice also has the potential to cost families more money because of extra time in child care or private preschool. Raising the age for kindergarten eligibility may also delay access to quality education for some children, potentially those with the greatest need.[9]

Many schools perform some sort of kindergarten readiness screening. Several issues are involved in screening. Screening often involves the use of standardized tests, most of which were designed for other purposes, usually as developmental screening tests. The validity of using these tests for kindergarten screening has been questioned. Performance on these tests predicts little about outcomes in first and second grade.[11]

The American Academy of Pediatrics (AAP) recommends against using readiness tests to deny entrance to kindergarten or to determine special-education placement. Children who appear to have special needs should have a full multifactored assessment with standardized tools designed for this purpose.[12]

FACTORS AFFECTING SCHOOL SUCCESS

Medical Factors

Most children enter school in excellent health, something parents and teachers agree is important. Box 127-2 lists some of the more common health issues related to school readiness and learning. Chronic medical conditions can affect school readiness in several ways. Some conditions such as recurrent otitis media can cause hearing impairment. Other conditions may result in increased medical care, resulting in less time for other more typical and stimulating activities. Children with chronic conditions may

BOX 127-2 Health Risk Factors

Prematurity	Lead toxicity
Attention-deficit/hyperactivity disorder	Iron-deficiency anemia
Otitis media	Dental caries
Sensory impairment	Asthma
	Allergies

experience pain or fatigue, which interfere with learning. Medications used to treat some conditions can also interfere with learning. For example, children with seizures may require treatment with certain medicines that cause cognitive dulling. Chronic conditions also change the parent-child dynamic, which might result in parents having lower expectations and placing fewer demands on children who have chronic conditions. Parents may also become overprotective and prevent the child from participating in activities that foster skills and character development important for learning.[13]

The degree of effect a given condition may have is not always clear. For example, much debate exists about the presence and size of any effect of otitis media with effusion (with or without hearing loss) on language skills. Because language is a large component of learning skills, anything that affects language development is likely to decrease learning and readiness to learn. A meta-analysis has shown some effect, but the clinical relevance was deemed *uncertain*.[14] A prospective study of otitis media with effusion and the relationship to school readiness found that children with more frequent otitis media with effusion did have lower scores on some measures of school readiness, but the associations were moderate. Home environment variables were more strongly related to school readiness scores.[15]

Prematurity is clearly a risk factor for developmental and learning difficulties, but the effects are modified to some extent by the home environment.

Genetics is also important. Genetic differences are important determinants of differences in academic achievement. The exact role and degree of importance is not known but is estimated to be in the range of 30% to 40%.[16] Genes seem to exert their effect on readiness via their effect on cognitive ability.

Environmental Factors

Overall, environment has been shown to play a large role in multiple aspects of school readiness. Language development is a key example. Children from language rich homes have 2 times the vocabulary by age 4 compared with children in less-stimulating environments.[17] Vocabulary has the potential to directly affect school readiness and learning.

High-quality educational preschool programs promote development and readiness. The AAP Committee on Early Childhood, Adoption, and Dependent Care has concluded that high-quality early education and child care for young children promotes development and learning,[18] especially for children from high-risk environments. Children whose family income is at or below the poverty level are eligible for Head Start, a federally funded preschool program designed to improve school readiness, as well as meet several of other needs. Head Start services are designed to promote physical, emotional, and cognitive development, all deemed necessary for true school readiness.

One study comparing children attending Head Start with those on the waiting list found that children in the program made significantly greater progress in receptive vocabulary and phonemic awareness. Parents of children attending Head Start were also more likely to have addressed dental, immunization, and other health needs for their children.[19] In general, studies show that Head Start narrows the gap for disadvantaged children, especially in vocabulary, writing skills, and social skills.[20]

Early intervention improves outcomes for young children with developmental delays. At-risk families benefit from home visits from paraprofessionals and nurses in the first 2 years of life. Research shows that parents who received these home visits were more supportive of their child's learning. The children had more advanced language and superior executive functioning during the preschool years. They also had higher intellectual functioning and receptive vocabulary scores and fewer behavior problems at 6 years of age. These findings suggest long-term benefits to academic performance.[21,22]

Societal Influences

The media exert strong influence on the learning capacity of young children. Children 2 to 7 years of age are exposed to media an average of 4 hours per day. On the one hand, preschoolers who are exposed to violent television shows were more aggressive and displayed less imaginative play. The flip side was that watching educational programming such as Sesame Street and Mr. Rogers Neighborhood was associated with better letter and number recognition, larger vocabulary, and more prosocial behavior than those who did not view such programs.[23] Other aspects of learning including attention may be adversely affected by television. Christakis et al found a correlation between amount of television viewing at 1 and 3 years of age and attention problems at age 7.[24] The AAP recommends that children younger than 2 years avoid watching television and that parents limit viewing for older children to less than 2 hours per day.[25]

Additional sources of media exposure are available for children. Computers are increasingly common in preschool classrooms, and many preschoolers have access to a computer. Computer programs and related activities can help 3 to 4 year olds acquire verbal skills, increase manual dexterity, and improve long-term memory.[26]

CONSEQUENCES OF BEING UNPREPARED FOR SCHOOL ENTRY

Being prepared for school is important. Educational achievement or attainment can have long-lasting and far-reaching effects on various aspects of life, including health. Poor school performance is linked to behaviors such as smoking, unprotected sex, and drug and alcohol use.[27] Educational level is also a significant contributor to many adult causes of morbidity and disability. Increasing educational level is one way to decrease risk of disability and increase life span.

Children who wind up old for grade, either because of retention or starting school late, are at risk for a significant number of poor outcomes. Children who are old for their grade level have an increased rate of behavioral difficulties as adolescents.[28] Children who are held back once are 20% to 30% more likely than age-appropriate children to drop out of school before graduation, and if held back 2 or more times the risk increases to close to 100%.[29] Retention is also damaging to a child's self-esteem.[30] Retention does not appear to help children's learning. Children who are retained typically get the same instruction again and do not receive services that might correct the learning difficulty they are experiencing. Children who are retained typically seem to do better in school for only part of the following year, after which time their academic achievement appears to revert to the same level as before the retention.[30] In fact, children who are retained learn less than if they had been promoted.[30,31] Similarly, children who are held out of school despite being age eligible do not do any better than children who start school on time. Although the youngest children in the class do score slightly lower on vocabulary and reading in the first few grades, these differences disappear by the fourth grade.[28] Thus neither retention nor delayed school entry seem to be practices that benefit children and may actually put them at risk for unintended negative consequences.

For the child who does poorly on the screening or has a birthday near the cutoff date, some schools offer placement in a kindergarten readiness class (also sometimes called *developmental kindergarten*). The structure of these classes varies, but many offer smaller class size and slower-paced instruction. Most, however, do not count as kindergarten; therefore children in these placements are essentially delaying entry to kindergarten for another year. Research about these classes has not found any benefits in terms of social and emotional development. Children in these classes are still more likely to be placed in special education or drop out of school. These findings suggest that developmental placement is similar to delayed entry and may be an inadequate response to the initial signs of a learning disability.[32]

PHYSICIAN'S ROLE IN PREPARING CHILDREN FOR SCHOOL

Given that school readiness is important, yet complex, what can a busy physician do to promote it? Some suggestions for such anticipatory guidance are listed in Box 127-3.[33] Helping children stay (or get) healthy is a direct way that pediatricians can positively affect school readiness. Prevention and treatment of lead poisoning, iron-deficiency anemia, sensory impairments, and optimal management of any chronic conditions are key roles that pediatricians can play. Anticipatory guidance regarding reading, language stimulation, and media control should start early.

The AAP urges pediatricians to promote access to quality child-care and preschool programs.[18] A survey of pediatricians found that most of them discuss such issues with families. Pediatricians were also interested in learning more about office-based methods to assist families in accessing Head Start programs.[34] Additional evidence suggests that families are more likely to enroll their children in Head Start if the pediatrician's office plays an active role.[35]

Reach Out and Read is a useful tool to illustrate the importance of early preliteracy activities. Research shows that Read Out and Read promotes literacy skills that are highly linked to school readiness and results in improved language development.[36] Asking about literacy activities (ie, reading aloud, trips to the library) and about media exposure sends parents the message that these issues are important and can affect health outcomes.

Another way physicians can influence school success is by identifying children with suspected developmental delays and referring them for early intervention. Early intervention has been shown to improve cognitive and behavioral outcomes, especially for children from high-risk environments.[37] Success, of course, depends on physicians to recognize delays, something that can be accomplished by developmental screening. Clinical judgment alone detects only one half of children with delays, contributing to the fact that up to 70% of children with a disability are not recognized until they begin school.[38] Besides allowing for possible remediation, early recognition of delays allows schools to be better prepared, helping ensure that children with special needs receive the most appropriate educational services.

Pediatricians can also serve as advocates, pressing school systems, as well as local, state, and federal governments, for changes that help ensure that all children enter school ready to learn in schools that are prepared to teach them. Some of the issues will be local, whereas others more universal. Retention, entry requirements, developmentally appropriate curriculums, and safer schools are just some of the issues that may require advocacy in the pediatrician's local community or beyond. Obviously, more widespread issues such as quality child care and preschool, prevention of preterm

BOX 127-3 ***Bright Futures* Recommendations: Preparing Children for School**

1. Screen vision and hearing.
2. Screen for lead and anemia (if indicated).
3. With child:
   a. Discuss preschool or child-care experiences.
   b. Ask about child's feelings about school.
   c. Talk about how child will get to or from school.
4. With parents:
   a. Inquire about parents' thoughts toward school.
   b. Ask if the school needs to know anything in particular.
   c. Ask about before- and after-school care.
   d. Find out what the parents have done to prepare child for school.
   e. Discuss safety skills for walking to school or riding bus.
5. Anticipatory guidance to promote successful school entry:
   a. Suggest that parents and child meet with teacher.
   b. Encourage discussions between child and parents about new opportunities and activities at school.
   c. Recommend a tour of the school.
   d. Encourage parental involvement at school.

births, and early media exposure might also benefit from professional advocacy efforts and attention.

One of the most promising approaches to increasing school success is by increasing access to high-quality, center-based, early childhood programs, especially for poor 3 to 4 year olds.[6] Some states are considering or already have universal preschool. Because not all eligible families participate in already available programs, pediatricians can help promote preschool involvement by asking if children are in preschool and exploring reasons children are not enrolled. Additionally, pediatricians can guide families in choosing high quality programs, given that quality certainly seems to matter.

CONCLUSION

No simple answer exists to the question, "Is my child ready for kindergarten?" Parents should be encouraged to also ask, "Is the school ready to teach my child?" Children should start kindergarten when they are eligible to do so and be schooled with their age-level peers. Children who appear to have special needs should have a full assessment with standardized tools designed for this purpose. Pediatricians can help ensure best-learning outcomes for children by detecting and treating chronic conditions, conducting developmental screening, and referring the child for early intervention and providing ongoing anticipatory guidance to help parents build early literacy, learning, behavior, and attention skills that will prepare children to enter school ready for the challenges of learning.

RELATED WEB SITES

- American Academy of Pediatrics: Bright Futures (Web page), Bright Futures (brightfutures.aap.org/web/).
- American Academy of Pediatrics: Developmental Pediatrics Online (www.dbpeds.org/).
- Reach Out and Read (ROR) (www.reachoutandread.org/).
- US Department of Education: No Child Left Behind (www.ed.gov/nclb/landing.jhtml).
- US Department of Health and Human Services: Head Start Information and Publication Center (www.headstartinfo.org).

AAP POLICY STATEMENTS

American Academy of Pediatrics, Committee on Early Childhood, Adoption, and Dependent Care. Quality early education and child care from birth to kindergarten. *Pediatrics*. 2005;115:187-191. Available at: aappolicy.aappublications.org/cgi/content/full/pediatrics;115/1/187.

American Academy of Pediatrics, Committee on School Health and Committee on Early Childhood, Adoption, and Dependent Care. The inappropriate use of school "readiness" tests. *Pediatrics*.1995;95:437-438. Available at: aappolicy.aappublications.org/cgi/reprint/pediatrics;95/3/437.pdf.

REFERENCES

1. Zill N, West J, National Center for Education Statistics, Educational Resources Information Center. *Entering Kindergarten*. Washington, DC: US Department of Education, Office of Educational Research and Improvement, National Center for Education Statistics, Educational Resources Information Center; 2001.
2. Lin H, Lawrence FR, Gorrell J. Kindergarten teachers' views of children's readiness for school. *Early Child Res Q*. 2003;18:225-237.
3. McBryde C, Ziviani J, Cuskelly M. School readiness and factors that influence decision making. *Occup Ther Int*. 2004;11:193-208.
4. Piotrkowski CS, Botsko M, Matthews E. Parents' and teachers' beliefs about children's school readiness in a high-need community. *Early Child Res Q*. 2000;15:537-558.
5. Heaviside S, Farris E, Carpenter JM, US Office of Educational Research and Improvement, National Center for Education Statistics. *Public School Kindergarten Teachers' Views on Children's Readiness for School: Contractor Report*. Washington, DC: US Department of Education, Office of Educational Research and Improvement; 1993.
6. Halle T, Zaslow M, Zaff J, et al. Background for Community-Level Work on School Readiness: A Review of Definitions, Assessments, and Investment Strategies. Available at: www.childtrends.org. Accessed February 25, 2006.
7. Meisels S. Assessing readiness. In: Pianta RC, Cox MJ, eds. *The Transition to Kindergarten*. Baltimore, MD: National Center for Early Development & Learning, Paul H. Brookes; 1999.
8. Ackerman DJ, Barnett WS. Prepared for Kindergarten: What Does "Readiness" Mean? Available at: nieer.org/resources/policyreports/report5.pdf. Accessed July 20, 2007.
9. Datar A, Rand Graduate School. *The Impact of Changes in Kindergarten Entrance Age Policies on Children's Academic Achievement and the Child Care Needs of Families*. Vol RGSD-177. Santa Monica, CA: Rand; 2003.
10. Lewit E, Baker LS. Child Indicators: School readiness. *The Future of Children: Critical Issues For Children and Youths*. 1995;5:128-139.
11. Meisels SJ. Should we test 4-year-olds? *Pediatrics*. 2004;113:1401-1402.
12. American Academy of Pediatrics, Committee on School Health and Committee on Early Childhood, Adoption, and Dependent Care. The inappropriate use of school "readiness" tests. *Pediatrics*. 1995;95:437-438.
13. Currie J. Health disparities and gaps in school readiness. *The Future of Children: School Readiness: Closing Racial and Ethnic Gaps*. 2005;15:117-138.
14. Roberts JE, Rosenfeld RM, Zeisel SA. Otitis media and speech and language: a meta-analysis of prospective studies. *Pediatrics*. 2004;113:e238-e248.
15. Roberts JE, Burchinal MR, Jackson SC, et al. Otitis media in childhood in relation to preschool language and school readiness skills among black children. *Pediatrics*. 2000;106:725-735.
16. Dickens WT. Genetic differences and school readiness. *The Future of Children: School Readiness: Closing Racial and Ethnic Gaps*. 2005;15:55-69.
17. Hart B, Risley T. *Meaningful Differences in the Everyday Experiences of Young American Children*. Baltimore, MD: Paul H. Brooks; 1995.
18. American Academy of Pediatrics, Committee on Early Childhood, Adoption, and Dependent Care. Quality early education and child care from birth to kindergarten. *Pediatrics*. 2005;115:187-191.
19. Abbott-Shim M, Lambert R, McCarty F. A comparison of school readiness outcomes for children randomly assigned to a head start program and the program's wait list. *Journal of Education for Students Placed At Risk*. 2003;8:191-214.
20. Zigler E, Styfco SJ. Head start's national reporting system: A work in progress. *Pediatrics*. 2004;114:858-859.
21. Olds DL, Kitzman H, Cole R, et al. Effects of nurse home-visiting on maternal life course and child development: Age 6 follow-up results of a randomized trial. *Pediatrics*. 2004;114:1550-1559.

22. Olds DL, Robinson J, Pettitt L, et al. Effects of home visits by paraprofessionals and by nurses: age 4 follow-up results of a randomized trial. *Pediatrics*. 2004;114:1560-1568.
23. Zimmerman FJ, Christakis DA. Children's television viewing and cognitive outcomes. *Arch Pediatr Adolesc Med*. 2005;159:619-625.
24. Christakis DA, Zimmerman FJ, DiGiuseppe DL, et al. Early television exposure and subsequent attentional problems in children. *Pediatrics*. 2004;113:708-713.
25. American Academy of Pediatrics, Committee on Public Education. Media education. *Pediatrics*. 1999;104:341-343.
26. Li X, Atkins MS. Early childhood computer experience and cognitive and motor development. *Pediatrics*. 2004; 113:1715-1722.
27. Byrd RS. School failure: Assessment, intervention, and prevention in primary pediatric care. *Pediatr Rev*. 2005; 26:233-243.
28. Byrd RS, Weitzman M, Auinger P. Increased behavior problems associated with delayed school entry and delayed school progress. *Pediatrics*. 1997;100:654-661.
29. Shepard LA, Smith ML. Synthesis of research on grade retention. *Educ Leadersh*. 1990;47(8):84-88.
30. Pagani L, Tremblay RE, Vitaro F, et al. Effects of grade retention on academic performance and behavioral development. *Dev Psychopathol*. 2001;13:297-315.
31. Hong G, Raudenbush SW. Effects of kindergarten retention policy on children's cognitive growth in reading and mathematics. *Educ Eval Pol Analys*. 2005;27:205-224.
32. Matthews LL, May DC, Kundert DK. Adjustment outcomes of developmental placement: A longitudinal study. *Psychol Sch*. 1999;36:495-504.
33. National Center for Education in Maternal and Child Health. *Bright Futures: Guidelines for Health Supervision of Infants, Children, and Adolescents*. 2nd ed rev. Arlington, VA: National Center for Education in Maternal and Child Health; 2002.
34. Silverstein M, Grossman DC, Koepsell TD, et al. Pediatricians' reported practices regarding early education and head start referral. *Pediatrics*. 2003;111:1351-1357.
35. Silverstein M, Mack C, Reavis N, et al. Effect of a clinic-based referral system to head start: a randomized controlled trial. *JAMA*. 2004;292:968-971.
36. Needleman R, Silverstein M. Pediatric interventions to support reading aloud: how good is the evidence? *J Dev Behav Pediatr*. 2004;25:352-363.
37. Gray R, McCormick MC. Early childhood intervention programs in the US: recent advances and future recommendations. *J Prim Prev*. 2005;26:259-275.
38. Glascoe FP. Early detection of developmental and behavioral problems. *Pediatr Rev*. 2000;21:272-279; quiz 280.

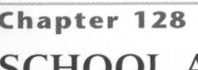

Chapter 128

SCHOOL ABSENTEEISM AND SCHOOL REFUSAL

Ronald V. Marino, DO, MPH

A major developmental task of childhood is the child separating from the child's family and accepting the functional demands of society. One of the most obvious indicators that this process may not be occurring normally is lack of attendance at school. Assessing the child's school attendance and functioning in the context of biopsychosocial health supervision is the responsibility of child health professionals.

Nonattendance may be due to a variety of underlying reasons. *Absenteeism* is generally considered to be parentally sanctioned nonattendance, most commonly attributed to medical illness. *Truancy* is nonattendance without parental consent, in which the time allegedly spent at school is often spent engaging in antisocial behaviors or rebelling against authority. *School refusal* is characterized by inappropriate fear about leaving home, inappropriate fear of school, or both.

ABSENTEEISM

Excessive absenteeism is important to health care professionals because it is an excellent marker for both physical and mental health problems (Box 128-1). It also is negatively correlated with social adjustment and academic performance. In fact, excessive absenteeism and failure to read at the appropriate level in the 3rd grade are the 2 strongest predictors of subsequent dropping out of school. National surveys indicate that healthy children average 4 or 5 absences a school year, whereas children who have a chronic disease typically are absent at least twice as often.[1,2] Educators believe that missing more than 10 days in a 90-day semester results in difficulty staying at grade level.[3]

Acute physical health problems are given as the reason for nonattendance 75% of the time. However, the variability in absenteeism among children who have the same medical condition suggests that individual and family responses to the physical condition are more important than the actual condition in determining attendance.[3] The decision not to attend school reflects subtle and complex relationships among the physical, social, and psychological states of the student, family, and community. Individual rates of absenteeism tend to be stable for a given child and also for a given school district.

The health conditions most commonly associated with nonattendance include upper respiratory tract infections, headaches, abdominal distress, menstrual cramps, and sleep disorders.[3,4] Parental characteristics associated with excessive absenteeism include

BOX 128-1 Chronic School Absence: Differential Diagnosis

- School refusal
- Overresponse to minor illnesses
- Chronic physical disease with poor adaptation
- Learning disability with poor adaptation
- Truancy
- Substance abuse
- Psychosis
- Teenage pregnancy
- Family dysfunction

Modified from: Nader P, ed. *School Health: Policy and Practice*. Elk Grove Village, IL: American Academy of Pediatrics; 1993.

lower socioeconomic class, cigarette smoking, chronic parental illness (including mental illness), lower educational expectations, and vulnerable child syndrome.[5-7] A plethora of nonmedical conditions, including transportation difficulties, illness of other family members, religious holidays, family vacations, inclement weather, and professional appointments, are also reasons children miss school. Chronically ill children typically miss more school than their healthy peers. This tendency may result from a wide variety of causes, including acute exacerbations of the underlying condition, health care visits, side effects of medications, and parental misconceptions about the child's ability to attend school. Healthy adjustment by the child and family to the chronic condition minimizes the potential impact of the increase in school days missed. A significant increase in absenteeism over baseline is always a warning sign. Exploring the reasons why a particular child seeks to avoid school is the clinician's responsibility. Sudden changes in school attendance may be the first concrete symptom of family dysfunction, mental illness, physical deterioration of the student or a family member, alcohol or drug abuse, or school refusal.

SCHOOL REFUSAL

Difficulties attending school despite caretakers' support for it have been a problem for children, families, schools, and clinicians for most of the 20th century. Initial views of school refusal focused on truancy and its link to delinquency. In 1932, Broadwin[8] focused attention to the frequent role of anxiety in attendance difficulties, and in 1939, Patridge[9] labeled this clinical condition *psycho-neurotic truancy*. Johnson et al[10] introduced the term *school phobia* in 1941, stressing that the child's anxiety about separating from mother was displaced to fear of attending school. This view was strengthened further in the 1950s when Estes et al[11] concluded that school phobia was a variant of separation anxiety.

This view and nomenclature persisted until the late 1970s, when the term *school refusal* was introduced. The term has descriptive merits that recognize the heterogeneity of the underlying disorders. These disorders include, but are not limited to, major depression, simple and social phobia, or separation anxiety disorder. Criteria for making this diagnosis include (1) severe difficulty in attending school or refusal to attend school, (2) severe emotional upset when attempting to go to school, (3) absence of significant antisocial disorders, and (4) staying at home with the parent's knowledge.

A variety of physical symptoms frequently accompany the child's request to not attend school. Symptoms can be quite impressive to parents and may emulate organic medical problems.

PREVALENCE

The prevalence of school refusal has been estimated to be between 0.4% and 18%.[12,13] Two peaks can be found in the incidence of school refusal. The first peak is associated with entering primary school (4 to 6 years), and the second is at the age of 11 to 12 years, a time of change from elementary to intermediate school, as well as the onset of early adolescence. The American Academy of Pediatrics estimates that 5% of elementary school children and 2% of junior high students have this disorder.[12]

CHILD-RELATED FACTORS

Children who have school refusal usually have at least average intelligence and academic achievement. Cultural norms encourage girls to admit fear and discourage boys from doing the same. The actual incidence of school refusal is nearly identical between the sexes.[13,14] Younger children report more fear of being scolded or of performing before a group, whereas older children seem to be more intimidated by tests and the possibility of failure. Vague somatic symptoms, which is typically offered as a rationale for nonattendance, may belie the underlying anxiety that is frequently present. Symptoms may amplify in response to parental pressure to attend and/or excel in school. Overdependency or concern about the well being of a parent is also a common underlying dynamic. Depression has often been noted, as have panic disorder and agoraphobia. Some reports of suicide among school refusers have also been noted. Thus any reference to this possibility must be addressed seriously.

FAMILY FACTORS

The family context is always a major factor in understanding the symptoms. Marital conflict or constricted communication patterns are frequently found in families who have school refusers. The child's presence at home as a result of physical illness may provide a cohesive force to an otherwise unstable marital relationship.

Three common patterns of communication in families in which school refusal occurs have been described[15]: (1) Both parents are overly concerned and solicitous of the child's medical problem; (2) 1 parent, usually the mother, is overprotective and concerned, whereas the other overtly disagrees; and (3) 1 parent, typically the mother, is overinvolved in caring for the child's every need, whereas the other parent is emotionally absent.[14] Understanding and clarifying the family dynamics are important in developing an effective treatment plan.

SCHOOL ENVIRONMENT FACTORS

The role of the school environment in school refusal has received little attention. Institutional factors such as changing classrooms or lack of privacy in the school bathroom have been associated with fear of school. Humiliation caused by an insensitive teacher may also be a precipitating stressor in the onset of clinical symptoms. Temperamental mismatch among teacher, student, and parents may serve a maintaining role.

Violence in secondary schools provides children a seemingly appropriate reason for refusing to attend school. Twenty-six percent of junior and senior high school students have been assaulted on school grounds, 20% of students admitted bringing a knife or gun to school, and 10% admitted not going to school because of fear of violence.[16] Media attention to school violence may provide a rationale that might further accelerate a child's anxiety and school refusal. Clearly, school-associated stressors are emerging as a concern in understanding and treating school refusal.

ASSOCIATED STRESSORS

While exploring child, parent, family, and school environment factors, the clinician must also search for a precipitating event or stress that may have tipped the balance in causing a child to refuse to attend school. Illness or injury of a family member or of the child may be the initial reason for nonattendance. Similarly, the death of a relative or close friend may precipitate the refusal. Moving to a new home, community, or school also may contribute to refusal. The longer a child has been out of school, the more potentially difficult and stressful returning becomes.

CLINICAL MANAGEMENT

In 1958, Eisenberg[17] stated, "[I]t is essential that the paralyzing force of the school phobia on the child's whole life be recognized. The symptom itself serves to isolate him from normal experience and makes further psychological growth almost impossible. If we do no more than check this central symptom, we have nonetheless done a great deal." The foundations of any clinical treatment plan are rapport, trust, and respect. The initial interview should serve not only as a means of gathering data, but also as the start of a therapeutic alliance. Clinicians should use a sensitive, holistic approach to data gathering because the history-taking technique provides the first opportunity for creating a therapeutic alliance. Factors related to the child, parents, family, and school environment must be investigated when exploring school maladaptation. An open mind that recognizes the unique and complex interactions of temperament, stressful life events, family systems function, learning style, parental medical conditions or psychopathological disorder, and school system variables will be helpful in solving this problem. The child must understand that involving a physician in treatment reflects the seriousness of the symptoms and marks a turning point in changing the avoidant behavior.

Organic disease should be ruled out through a thorough history and physical examination, coupled with judicious laboratory evaluation. Time spent in conducting a thorough medical examination communicates the physician's sincere acceptance of the child's symptoms as being real. Parents are better able to confront the lack of organic disease when a clinician who is completely familiar with the child's history and physical examination discusses the subject with them. A biopsychosocial approach from the outset also aids family acceptance of psychiatric concerns. The laboratory should be used in a symptom-specific, noninvasive, cost-effective manner consistent with ruling out possible organic disease. Additionally, addressing the potential contributions of parental psychopathological disorders or specific environmental problems will be helpful in formulating a treatment plan.

The parents, physician, and school personnel must all agree that returning to school as quickly as possible is the immediate goal of treatment. Allowing the child to stay home while awaiting laboratory data results or using home tutors only delays the inevitable and makes the return to school more difficult. A specific plan must be developed to respond to clinical symptoms. Objective criteria such as an increase in temperature for school absence should be consistently used in modifying performance expectations, both at home and in school. Parents in doubt should seek the guidance of the child's physician regarding the significance of acute symptoms before keeping the child home. In addition, the patient must understand that the significant attachment figures in the patient's life will adhere to the therapeutic program consistently and persistently. In most cases of school refusal, especially in the elementary years, the aforementioned program, carried out by the primary care physician, is curative. Other treatment modalities, typically used by a mental health professional, include desensitization, psychotherapy, hypnotherapy, cognitive restructuring, and behavior modification. Psychopharmacologic agents have been used as aids in the management of school refusal. However, lack of double-blinded, placebo-controlled studies limits the use of psychopharmacologic agents in the management of school refusal. Current concerns relating selective serotonin reuptake inhibitors to risk of suicide in children and adolescents reduced the number of primary care physicians prescribing these medications. Children who are recalcitrant to behavioral interventions may require referral to a mental health specialist. Suggested criteria for mental health referral are listed in Box 128-2.

BOX 128-2 Criteria for Mental Health Referral

- Unresponsive to management
- Out of school for 2 months
- Onset in adolescence
- Psychosis
- Depression
- Panic reactions
- Parental inability to cooperate with treatment plan

PROGNOSIS

Experience suggests that most children who refuse to attend school quickly overcome the difficulty with appropriate clinical management. Intermittent relapses associated with stress or new separation experiences, such as camp or sleepovers, occur in approximately 5% of children. Children who require psychiatric management do not fare as well.[16] Most published series in the psychiatric literature reveal significant cohorts of patients requiring ongoing therapy and having persistent difficulties in emancipating themselves from their family.[17,18] Phobias, depression, and anxiety are more common in adults who have a history of childhood school refusal.[19] Table 128-1 lists long-term sequelae in children with school refusal.[20]

PREVENTION

Anticipatory guidance is an excellent means of primary prevention, which allows the primary care physician to advise parents on developmentally appropriate separation guidelines. For example, by the time an infant is 6 months of age, the parents should be able to spend some evenings out alone. By 1 year of age, peer contact should be encouraged. Toddlers should

Table 128-1 Long-Term Sequelae in Children With School Refusal

OUTCOME	PREVALENCE
Interrupted compulsory school	18%
Did not complete high school	45%
Adult psychiatric outpatient care	43%
Adult psychiatric inpatient care	6%
Criminal offense	6%
Still living with parents after 20-year follow-up	14%
Married at 20-year follow-up	41%
PERCENTAGE OF CHILDREN AT 20-YEAR FOLLOW-UP	
None	59%
One or more	41%

From Fremont WD. School refusal in children and adolescents. *Am Fam Physician.* 2003;68(8):1555-1568. Data from Bernstein GA, et al. *J Am Acad Child Adolesc Psychiatry.* 2001;40:206-213; Flakierska-Praquin N, et al. *Compr Psychiatry.* 1997;38:17-22. Reprinted by permission.

experience babysitters while awake. By age 3 years, the child should experience being away from home without a parent, such as in a playgroup or at a neighbor's home. Age 4 years is a good time to consider preschool for the child. Such guidance can be shared in the context of routine health supervision. Parents should also be discouraged from keeping children home because of minor illness, and physicians must avoid unnecessary medical restrictions.

Preventing vulnerable child syndrome is also important when caring for ill children. This disorder arises when parents believe that their child's life has been threatened significantly, and it results in separation difficulties, overprotection, bodily concerns, and underachievement in school.[7] Parents need to be informed about the true significance and prognosis of any medical difficulty the child has experienced. Practitioners have a responsibility to avoid creating iatrogenic misconceptions about a child's health. They can accomplish this task by using everyday language as much as possible, rather than medical jargon, and by demystifying anxiety associated with insignificant findings, such as a functional murmur. Parents need to be reassured that children who have recovered fully from an acute illness are at no increased risk for future illness. By inquiring about children's school attendance and promoting healthy parenting styles, primary care physicians can help prevent school refusal.

TRUANCY AND DROPPING OUT

Truancy is a good predictor of dropping out at a later date. Many schools in inner cities report daily absence rates above 20%, with most of this thought to be the result of truancy; an equal or greater percentage of these children never finish high school. Truancy is a serious social problem that has potentially lifelong consequences. Unemployment or underemployment, criminal behavior, marital problems, and chronic social maladjustment are often seen in children with truancy or children who drop out. These same long-term outcomes have been identified in groups of children who have learning disabilities. One risk factor for truancy is learning disability and its associated school failure.

Truancy also has been noted among children who have a history of having been sexually abused. Other risk factors are low socioeconomic status, conduct disorder, gang membership, substance abuse, cigarette smoking, and family discord. Early recognition of children at risk should prompt immediate intervention to promote optimal adjustment. Mobilization of resources in the school, community, and family is critical to help prevent progression from truancy to dropping out. Creative programs to foster school attendance and success have been conducted with variable results. An emerging new truancy variant is the child who goes to school or its immediate environment but does not attend class. This child is participating in the social aspects of the school community but is shunning the academics. Medical clinicians can assume an advocacy role in guiding and supporting therapeutic interventions in the educational and social welfare arenas.

CONCLUSION

Absenteeism is a simple symptom that has multiple causes. Because success in school is often the foundation for continuing success in life, health care professionals must devote thoughtful attention to understanding and treating absentees. Using a biopsychosocial model and mobilizing multidisciplinary resources are the keys to clinical success.

TOOLS FOR PRACTICE

Medical Decision Support

- *School Health* (Web page), American Academy of Pediatrics (www.schoolhealth.org/).
- *Healthy Schools Healthy Youth* (Web page), Centers for Disease Control and Prevention (www.cdc.gov/HealthyYouth/index.htm).
- *Managing Infectious Diseases in Child Care and Schools* (book), American Academy of Pediatrics (www.aap.org/bookstore).
- *School Health: Policy & Practice, 6th edition* (book), American Academy of Pediatrics (www.aap.org/bookstore).

RELATED WEB SITE

- American School Health Association (ASHA) (www.ashaweb.org/index.html).

AAP POLICY STATEMENTS

American Academy of Pediatrics, Committee on School Health. Home, hospital, and other non-school–based instruction for children and adolescents who are medically unable to attend school. *Pediatrics.* 2000;106:1154-1155. (aappolicy.aappublications.org/cgi/content/full/pediatrics;106/5/1154).

American Academy of Pediatrics, Committee on School Health. Out-of-school suspension and expulsion. *Pediatrics.* 2003;112:1206-1208. (aappolicy.aappublications.org/cgi/content/full/pediatrics;112/5/1206).

Taras H, Duncan, P, Luckenbill D, et al, eds. *Health, Mental Health, and Safety Guidelines for Schools.* Elk Grove Village, IL: American Academy of Pediatrics; 2004. AAP endorsed.

REFERENCES

1. Fowler MG, Johnson MP, Atkinson SS. School achievement and absence in children with chronic health conditions. *J Pediatr.* 1987;106:683-687.
2. Klerman LV. School absence—a health perspective. *Pediatr Clin North Am.* 1988;35:1253-1269.
3. Weitzman M, Klerman Lu, Albert JJ, et al. Factors associated with excessive school absence. *Pediatrician.* 1986; 13:74.
4. Bernstein GA, Massie ED, Thuras PD, et al. Somatic symptoms in anxious depressed school refusers. *J Am Acad Child Adolesc Psychiatry.* 1997;36:661-667.
5. Charlton A, Blair U. Absence from school related to children's and parental smoking habits. *BMJ* 1989; 298:90-92.
6. Cassino C, Auerbach M, Kammeran S, et al. Effect of asthma on performance of parenting tasks and children's school attendance. *J Asthma.* 1997;34:499-507.
7. Green M Solnit AJ. Reactions to the threatened loss of a child: a vulnerable child syndrome. *Pediatrics.* 1964; 34:58.
8. Broadwin IT. A contribution to the study of truancy. *Am J Orthopsychiatry.* 1932;2:253-259.
9. Patridge JM. Truancy. *J Mental Sci.* 1939;85:45-81.
10. Johnson AM, Falstein EI, Szurek SA, et al. School phobia. *Am J Orthopsychiatry.* 1941;11:702-711.
11. Estes HR, Haylett CH, Johnson M. Separation anxiety. *Am J Orthopsychiatry.* 1956;10:682-695.
12. Aldaz EG, Vivas E, Gelfand DM, et al. Estimating the prevalence of school refusal and school related fears. *J Nerve Mental Dis.* 1984;172:722-729.
13. Nader PR, ed. *School Health: Policy and Practice.* Elk Grove Village, IL: American Academy of Pediatrics; 1993.
14. Hersov L. School refusal. *BMJ.* 1972;3:102-104.
15. Nader PR, Bullock D, Caldwell B. School phobia. *Pediatr Clin North Am.* 1975;22:605-617.
16. New York State Education Department, Division of Criminal Justice Services. Study: 1 in 5 Students Were Armed. *Newsday.* February 14, 1994, p. 19.
17. Eisenberg L. School phobia: a study on the communication of anxiety. *Am J Psychiatry.* 1958;114:712.
18. Flaierska-Paquin N, Lindstrom M, Gillberg C. School phobia with separation anxiety disorder: a comparative 20- to 29-year follow-up study of 35 school refusers. *Compar Psychiatry.* 1997;38:17-22.
19. Bernstein GA, Hektner JM, Borchadt CM, et al. Treatment of school refusal: one-year follow-up. *J Am Acad Child Adolesc Psychiatry.* 2001;40:206-213.
20. Fremont WD. School refusal in children and adolescents. *Am Fam Physician.* 2003;68:1555-1568.

Chapter 129

SCHOOL LEARNING PROBLEMS AND DEVELOPMENTAL DIFFERENCES

Paul H. Dworkin, MD

School learning problems are complex issues that defy traditional methods of pediatric assessment and management. Learning problems are not the exclusive responsibility of the primary care physician (PCP) but rather are a multidisciplinary concern. Furthermore, PCPs neither diagnose definitively nor treat learning disabilities independently. Nonetheless, PCPs assume critical roles when their patients develop learning problems. Such roles include clarifying the reasons for poor school performance and facilitating appropriate intervention. The importance of such pediatric involvement has become evident; parents and educators regard such problems as learning disabilities to be within the PCP's area of responsibility and demand their attention to the needs of children who perform poorly in school. Unfortunately, many PCPs view themselves as inadequately prepared to deal with school learning problems.

REASONS FOR LEARNING PROBLEMS

Causes of school failure may be classified into *intrinsic* and *extrinsic* causes.[1] Intrinsic causes comprise the inherent characteristics of the failing child, such as specific learning disabilities, intellectual disability, and sensory impairment. Extrinsic causes are adverse external influences, such as family dysfunction, social stressors within the home, and ineffective schooling.

Actually, however, learning problems are typically the consequence of a complex interaction of variables related to the child, the family, and the school (Figure 129-1). For example, even a subtle learning disability can be devastating for a child reared in poverty who attends a school of inferior quality. Furthermore, learning problems often coexist with clusters of adverse influences. For example, a child with a learning disability may be at a particular disadvantage if this child has a *slow to warm up* temperament that precludes active classroom participation or if the child is confronted with the trauma of parental divorce. Thus the PCP's assessment of school learning problems must include the child's capabilities and weaknesses within the context of social and environmental circumstances.

Specific Learning Disabilities

Of the many causes of school learning problems, specific learning disabilities are the most prevalent and perplexing. Learning disabilities are regarded as a heterogeneous group of disorders demonstrated by significant difficulties in the acquisition and use of listening, speaking, reading, writing, reasoning, or mathematical abilities. These disorders are presumed to be the result of central nervous system dysfunction and not directly the result of other disabling conditions or environmental influences.[2] The hallmark of learning disabilities is a discrepancy between a student's potential for academic achievement, as suggested by cognitive abilities, and actual performance, as documented by achievement tests. The prevalence of learning disabilities is estimated to be 3% to 5% of students.

No single cause of learning disabilities has been identified. Family, genetic, cognitive, and neuroanatomic factors are all implicated in learning disabilities.[3] Learning disabilities are both familial and heritable, as evidenced by studies documenting that 23% to 65% of children whose parents have reading disability also have the disorder, a 40% rate of reading disability among siblings of affected children, and a higher

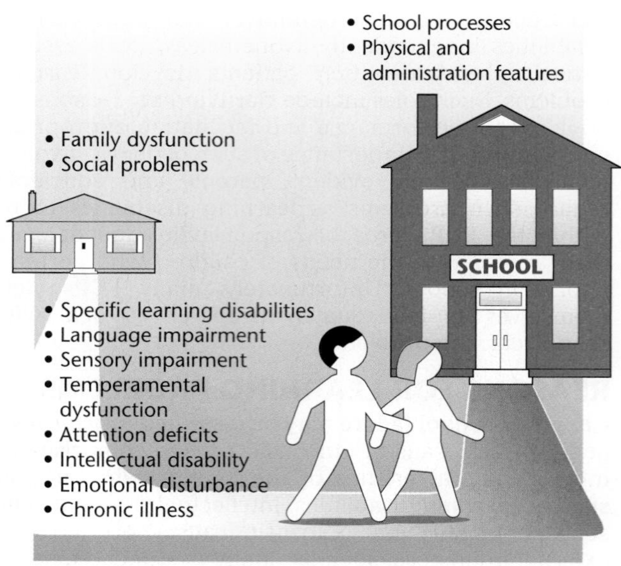

Figure 129-1 Learning problems typically stem from a complex interaction of variables related to the child, family, and school. (*Dworkin PH. School failure.* Pediatr Rev. *1989; 10:301-312.)*

concordance rate among monozygotic twins. Evidence exists for single locus, polygenic, and multifactorial modes of transmission, with linkage studies implicating chromosomes 6 and 15. Postmortem studies, functional magnetic resonance imaging, and electrophysiological studies have suggested such neuroanatomic factors as changes in temporo-parieto-occipital brain regions among children with reading disability, the involvement of both hemispheres (especially the left parietotemporal areas) among children with mathematics disorder, and disruption of white matter association fibers among children with nonverbal learning disabilities. Learning disabilities may not be discrete disorders but rather represent the extreme lower end of a continuum of learning abilities.[4]

Research has emphasized the critical importance of language development in learning. Many children with learning disabilities have experienced delayed or disordered language acquisition, supporting the belief that learning disabilities may be the expression of a more general linguistic disability. The phonologic deficit hypothesis for reading disability proposes a deficiency within the phonologic module engaged in processing the sounds of speech, characterized by difficulty reading single words in isolation. More recently, the importance of weaknesses in higher-order cognitive functions (ie, thinking and reasoning processes, memory) attributed to the prefrontal region of the brain have been implicated in nonverbal learning disabilities. Deficits in so-called metacognitive skills, such as being able to access acquired knowledge when needed and knowing how to apply learned skills, may be the reason that children with learning disabilities are unable to focus attention on the salient features of tasks or effectively devise problem-solving strategies.[5] Such children have been described as passive learners because of their difficulty with strategy selection and problem solving.

Children with learning disabilities typically display deficits in various areas of developmental functioning. When developmentally assessed, these children are more likely than their learning-normal peers to be confused by sequences and time relationships (temporal-sequential deficits), to confuse left from right (directional disorientation), to fail to appreciate spatial relationships and visual detail (visuoperceptual difficulties), and to have difficulty integrating auditory and visual stimuli, such as the sounds of words and the visual configurations of letters (deficits in intersensory integration). These children also are more likely to be clumsy and awkward (motor abnormalities) and neurologically immature (ie, to exhibit neuromaturational delay or so-called soft neurologic signs). In addition, behavioral or emotional problems, such as diminished self-esteem, are more common among such students. Up to 50% of children with learning disabilities may have comorbid emotional disorders.

Except for language and cognitive deficits, the extent to which these clinical correlates contribute to, result from, or merely coexist with learning disabilities is uncertain. For example, extensive research failed to substantiate a causal relationship between faulty visuoperceptual skills and academic deficits. The presence of such correlates should not form the basis of a diagnosis of learning disability. Rather, findings such as temporal-sequential deficits and directional disorientation should serve as warning signs that increase the clinician's suspicion about the possibility of learning disabilities and prompt a referral for psychoeducational evaluation to document the potential-performance disparity required for diagnosis.

Children with learning disabilities most commonly have problems with the language arts (reading, spelling, and written expression). They may also have difficulties with arithmetic and handwriting skills, although isolated problems with arithmetic are less common. A child's pattern of academic performance may change over time. For example, some children with learning disabilities may cope satisfactorily during the first 3 years of school, only to experience increasing problems with academic achievement and organization of assignments by the third or fourth grade, as classroom expectations increase and demands for the rapid retrieval of information and work productivity escalate.[6] Learning disabilities are not outgrown and require a lifespan approach.

Other Reasons for Learning Problems

Whether attention-deficit disorders represent a specific clinical syndrome (attention-deficit/hyperactivity disorder) or result from complex interactions between child-related and environmental factors is controversial. Regardless, for a group of children, difficulties such as inattention, distractibility, lack of persistence, and impulsivity impair school functioning. These attention deficits are often associated with other causes of learning problems, such as specific learning disabilities.

Mild intellectual disability is not usually identified until the child is confronted with the cognitive demands of school. The academic performance of such children is characterized by slow learning and acquisition of skills to at most the fifth- or sixth-grade level. Intellectual disability and learning disabilities may coexist, and both contribute to a child's learning problems.

Sensory impairment may contribute to school learning problems. Of the five senses, hearing and vision are the most crucial for academic learning. Of these two, hearing loss results in the more profound educational disability, primarily because of impaired language acquisition and communication skills. The learning problems of children with hearing impairments are characterized by difficulties in reading, mathematical reasoning, and problem solving. Deaf students also may struggle with classroom maladjustment, behavioral problems, and social immaturity. Children who have visual disturbances usually fare better than their peers with hearing impairments in the classroom. In general, such children tend to perform rather well; thus their academic achievement has not received much scrutiny.

Although 30% to 80% of emotionally disturbed students have problems with academic achievement and classroom behavior, emotional illness (eg, depression, conduct disorders) is the primary cause of learning problems for only a small percentage of children facing school failure. Emotional factors may be far more important in the exacerbation of academic difficulties caused by other problems. For example, the inevitable feelings of diminished self-esteem and frustration that accompany school failure because of learning disabilities may serve to further impair classroom functioning.

One fourth to one third of children who have a chronic illness have problems achieving academically. Chronic illness may contribute to school learning problems as a consequence of limited alertness or stamina, chronic pain, side effects of medication, absenteeism, altered or inappropriate expectations of teachers or parents, maladjustment, or inappropriate placement in special classes. Low intelligence and learning disabilities may be problems for children who have certain neurologic disorders.

A child's behavioral style, or temperament, may contribute to school learning problems. The temperamentally difficult child may quickly become frustrated and angry when confronted with material that is not easily mastered; or the initial reluctance of the *slow to warm up* child to participate and the child's tendency to withdraw may be misinterpreted as anxiety or a limited capability for learning. Although children with easy temperaments usually fare well in the classroom, problems may arise when expectations for behavior markedly differ between home and school.

Social and environmental factors can also contribute to school learning problems. These factors include parental divorce or separation, child abuse or neglect, illness or death of immediate family members, parental emotional illness, early parenthood, substance abuse, and poverty. Ineffective schooling itself may contribute to learning problems. Some studies have revealed that school processes (eg, academic emphasis, use of rewards and praise, teachers' actions during lessons) are more important than physical or administrative features.[7] Factors such as school climate and social environment may be particularly important for children from disadvantaged homes who attend schools that have limited resources.

For children of ethnocultural minorities, additional factors may influence school performance. Cultural factors include differences in concepts necessary to learn such subjects as math and science, teaching and learning styles, assumptions about interpersonal relations, and language. The influence of bilingual education is controversial. Select studies report that acquisition of English as a second language may interfere with school achievement, but other studies indicate that acquisition of a second language facilitates school achievement and cognitive development in the bilingual child.[8] A review from the National Research Council found effects favorable to bilingual education when such confounding factors as socioeconomic status are taken into account.[9]

EVALUATION OF LEARNING PROBLEMS

The goal of evaluation of school learning problems depends on the specific circumstances of a child's referral. When school-based assessment has already raised the possibility of a child being learning disabled, evaluation assumes a fairly small role in excluding medical problems that may contribute to poor school functioning. Alternatively, evaluation is far more challenging when a child is experiencing unsuspected or unexplained learning problems. The goals of such evaluation are diagnosing medical conditions that may contribute to school problems (eg, sensory impairment, a seizure disorder) and identifying clinical correlates (medical, neurophysiological, and psychological) of other causes of learning problems, such as specific learning disabilities.

The PCP should follow certain guidelines when evaluating children for school learning problems. For example, the many factors that can contribute to school failure must be considered. Communication with school personnel is invaluable in obtaining information about classroom functioning, past assessments, and school resources. The child must be evaluated within the context of the learning environment; for example, the expectations of a 5 year old entering an academically oriented kindergarten class are quite different from those of a child entering a more developmentally and socially oriented program.

History

Important historical information should be sought from parents, teachers, and the child (Table 129-1); questionnaires such as the ANSER System (www.epsbooks.com/) may facilitate the gathering of necessary information. Certain aspects of school functioning should be examined in detail, including the child's academic achievement, classroom behavior, school attendance, past psychoeducational testing, and special school services provided. Findings that suggest the possibility of specific learning disabilities are listed in Box 129-1.

Other aspects of the traditional medical history should also be examined in detail. The perinatal history of children with learning disabilities is characterized

Table 129-1 Role of the History in Evaluating School Learning Problems

ASPECT	FINDINGS SUGGESTING SPECIFIC LEARNING DISABILITIES
Academic achievement	Discrete delays in select subjects (eg, language); adequate early performance with difficulties emerging later (eg, mathematics, writing)
Classroom behavior	Longstanding, pervasive problems with inattention, impulsivity, overactivity; disorganization and poor strategy formation; depression, moodiness
Attendance	Excessive absenteeism; school avoidance
Past psychoeducational testing	Discrepancy between cognitive abilities and academic achievement
Special required school services	Response to *diagnostic teaching*
Perinatal history	*Clusters* of adverse events; maternal alcohol or drug intake
Medical history	Recurrent or persistent otitis media; iron-deficiency anemia; lead poisoning; seizures; frequent accidents; chronic use of medication
Development	Delayed or disordered language acquisition and communication skills; subtle delays in select milestones; uneven pattern of skills and interests
Behavioral history	Longstanding problems with attention span, impulsivity, overactivity; sadness; acting out; poor self-esteem
Family history	Learning problems, school failure among first-degree relatives
Social history	Child abuse or neglect; other stressors

BOX 129-1 Findings That Suggest the Possibility of Specific Learning Disabilities

- Discrete delays in select subjects, such as the language arts, or an adequate early performance with later emergence of difficulties
- Behavioral problems such as longstanding, pervasive problems with inattention, impulsivity, overactivity; acting out; disorganization and poor strategy formation; or depression, sadness, and moodiness resulting from frustration and diminished self-esteem
- School avoidance because of frustration
- Discrepancy between cognitive abilities and academic achievement on past psychoeducational testing
- Poor response to special teaching techniques, which suggests special learning requirements

by a somewhat increased incidence of clusters of adverse events, such as anoxic encephalopathy, prematurity, and bronchopulmonary dysplasia, as well as maternal alcohol and drug intake (eg, substance abuse, anticonvulsants). The medical history may indicate the presence of recurrent or persistent otitis media, iron-deficiency anemia, lead poisoning, seizures, frequent injuries as a result of overactivity, or chronic use of medication (eg, phenobarbital, theophylline, antihistamines). The developmental history of children with learning disabilities may suggest delayed or disordered language acquisition and communication skills; subtle delays in select milestones, such as speaking, sitting, or walking; or an uneven pattern of skills and interests, with discrete areas of strength and weakness. The behavioral history may reveal longstanding problems with attention span, impulsivity, and overactivity; sadness; acting out; or poor self-esteem. The family history may corroborate the increased incidence of learning problems and school failure among first-degree relatives of children with learning disabilities. The social history may reveal such stressors as child abuse or neglect, which are known to be associated with specific learning disabilities.

Physical Examination

The physical examination plays a small but important role in evaluating children who have learning problems (Table 129-2). The physician's general observation of the youngster may note sadness, anxiety, a short attention span, impulsivity, or overactivity. Tics may indicate Tourette syndrome, which is sometimes associated with learning disabilities. Physical features may be observed that suggest syndromes associated with learning disabilities, such as fragile X syndrome, fetal alcohol effects, or Turner syndrome. Alternatively, an increased incidence of so-called minor congenital anomalies (epicanthal folds, hypertelorism, low-set ears, high-arched palate, clinodactyly, and syndactyly of the toes) has been observed among some children who have specific learning disabilities and attention deficits, although the significance of such findings is uncertain.

Certain specific aspects of the physical examination deserve special emphasis. Examination of the skin should include a search for multiple café-au-lait spots (neurofibromatosis), as well as ash-leaf spots and adenoma sebaceum (tuberous sclerosis); these conditions are associated with learning problems. Examination of the tympanic membranes may reveal signs suggesting recurrent or chronic otitis media. Among older boys, examination of the genitalia may reveal delayed sexual maturation, which has been correlated with learning

Table 129-2 Role of the Physical Examination in Evaluating School Learning Problems

ASPECT	FINDINGS SUGGESTING SPECIFIC LEARNING DISABILITIES
General observations	Sadness, anxiety, short attention span, impulsivity, overactivity; tics
Phenotypical features	Stigmata of genetic syndromes (eg, sex chromosome abnormalities, fetal alcohol syndrome); minor congenital anomalies
Skin	Multiple cafe-au-lait spots; ash-leaf spots; adenoma sebaceum
Tympanic membranes	Signs of recurrent or chronic otitis media
Genitalia	Delayed sexual maturation in boys
Growth measurements	Short stature; microcephaly and macrocephaly
Sensory screening	Poor hearing or vision

problems. Growth measurements may indicate problems such as short stature, microcephaly, and macrocephaly, which have also been associated with learning disabilities. Sensory screening should exclude hearing impairment or vision defects.

Examination of Mental Status

Simple projective testing may identify emotional issues as either the cause or, more likely, the consequence of school learning problems. Techniques such as asking the child for three wishes, asking the child to draw a picture of the child's family, or playing the Winnicott Squiggle Game[10] may reveal the child's sadness, diminished self-esteem, or concerns regarding family functioning.

Neurodevelopmental Assessment

Surveying the child's functioning in different areas of development may help identify factors that contribute to learning problems. As noted previously, children who have specific learning disabilities are more likely to have deficits in language functioning and cognitive abilities. Furthermore, the developmental profile of children with learning disabilities is characterized by an uneven pattern, with discrete areas of relative strength and weakness.

Instruments

A few tools have been developed for assessing the development of school-aged children. The Pediatric Early Elementary Examination (PEEX 2) is for children ages 6 to 9 years, and the Pediatric Examination of Educational Readiness at Middle Childhood (PEERAMID 2) is for children ages 9 to 15 (www.epsbooks.com/). These tools survey the following areas of development: fine motor skills, graphomotor function, language function, gross motor skills, memory, visual processing, and selective attention and activity.

Laboratory Studies

Laboratory tests should be used only to assess children who are at specific risk for conditions known to be associated with learning disabilities. Examples include anemia screening for children at risk because of nutritional or socioeconomic factors, lead screening for those at risk because of their home environment or a history of pica, thyroid function studies if signs or symptoms of thyroid disease are noted or if the possibility is suggested by family history, and chromosome analysis (and molecular genetic testing for fragile X syndrome in all children with intellectual disability) if the child has phenotypical features or several congenital anomalies that are associated with intellectual disability. Older children and adolescents who have shown a precipitous decline in school performance or erratic, unpredictable behavior should be tested for drug use.

Neuroanatomic and neurophysiological studies should be performed only for specific indications. For example, an electroencephalogram should be reserved for children suspected of having a seizure disorder; computed tomography or magnetic resonance imaging is indicated for suspected central nervous system malformations, microcephaly, or macrocephaly.

Further Investigations and Referrals

Referral for psychoeducational evaluation is indicated when the assessment suggests the possibility of learning disabilities as a cause of learning problems. For example, learning disabilities may be suspected if (1) the child's history reveals difficulties with discrete subjects such as reading and spelling; (2) developmental testing indicates an uneven profile, with areas of strength and weakness; and (3) a child demonstrates poor self-esteem and poor self-image. The goals of psychoeducational evaluation are to examine the child's academic strengths and weaknesses, to determine cognitive ability, to assess perceptual strengths and weaknesses, to examine communicative ability, and to assess social and emotional adaptation. Ideally, such evaluations are performed by the child's school system, although specific circumstances may dictate a private referral. School personnel participating in such evaluations may include psychologists, special educators and learning disability specialists, speech-language pathologists, and social workers. Tests typically administered include those for intelligence; general learning abilities; academic achievement in reading, mathematics, and writing; perceptual and motor function; and speech and language skills. Diagnostic teaching also may be an effective test.

Assessment of the child may indicate the need for referral to other professionals. For example, concern about language functioning may result in direct referral to a speech-language pathologist, and emotional disturbance or family dysfunction may suggest the need for referral to a mental health professional, such as a psychologist, social worker, or psychiatrist. Concern about sensory impairment may suggest referral to an ophthalmologist, otolaryngologist, or audiologist.

INTERVENTION

A variety of actions may follow assessment of the child who has school learning problems. Although educational programming is the mainstay of treatment for specific learning disabilities, the PCPs participation may involve a variety of traditional and nontraditional roles.

Examples of traditional roles include specific medical intervention for underlying conditions, such as treatment of a seizure disorder that may contribute to learning problems, as well as pharmacologic management of attention deficits. Counseling is another traditional role, which may include clarifying a child's strengths and weaknesses; alleviating undue concern, guilt, and anxiety; explaining the legal rights of children and families under state and federal regulations (eg, the Individuals with Disabilities Education Act); offering guidance on such alternative treatment strategies as diet, megavitamins, and optometric training; and, depending on the PCP's expertise, giving advice about such specific behavioral management strategies as positive reinforcement and time out. Arranging for further investigations and referrals is yet another traditional role, and it may involve coordinating indicated laboratory studies and referring the child for psychoeducational testing and other evaluations.

With their access to young children and families and their responsibility for monitoring children's growth and development during the preschool years, PCPs are well positioned to contribute to early detection of potential school dysfunction.[11] Developmental surveillance may be the most effective process enabling the PCP to predict school readiness. Surveillance has four components. (1) Eliciting and attending to parents' concerns acknowledges the importance of their opinions and descriptions of their child's development. Clinicians may use parent-completed questionnaires to efficiently solicit this information. (2) Observing the child's development may be done longitudinally by using an informal collection of age-appropriate tasks and by periodically administering a developmental screening test. (3) Obtaining the opinion of preschool teachers is important because such opinions are the single best predictor of kindergarten success. (4) Interpreting findings, including social and environmental circumstances, must be accomplished within the context of the child's overall well being.

A less traditional but nonetheless important role is serving as an ombudsman to help students and families use community services and resources effectively. Specific measures may include facilitating communication with school systems, introducing families to helpful parent and peer support groups, and initiating referrals to mental health and social service agencies. PCPs may also assist families by referring them to educational and advocacy organizations such as the International Dyslexia Society (www.interdys.org/), the Learning Disabilities Association of America (www.ldaamerica.org/), the National Center for Learning Disabilities (www.ncld.org/), and the National Institute of Neurological Disorders and Stroke (www.ninds.nih.gov/). Although PCPs are unlikely to have the expertise to suggest educational strategies for learning disabilities, participation as a member of a multidisciplinary planning team is both helpful and feasible. Such participation is often reassuring to the parents and children, who regard the PCP as an effective child advocate.

TOOLS FOR PRACTICE

Engaging Patient and Family

- *How do I know if my child has a learning disability?* (fact sheet), American Academy of Pediatrics (www.aap.org/publiced/BR_LearningDisabilities.htm).
- *Learning Disabilities: What Parents Need to Know* (brochure), American Academy of Pediatrics (patiented.aap.org).

Medical Decision Support

- *Attention Deficit Disorders Behavior Rating Scales (ADDBRS),* Ned Owens and Betty White (buros.unl.edu/buros/jsp/reviews.jsp?item=06000218).
- *Brown Attention-Deficit Disorder Scales,* Thomas Brown (harcourtassessment.com/haiweb/cultures/en-us/productdetail.htm?pid=015-8029-240).
- *Child Behavior Checklist (CBC) and Revised Child Behavior Profile* (assessment), Quay-Peterson (www.iprc.unc.edu/longscan/pages/measures/Ages5to11/Child Behavior Checklist 4-18.pdf).
- *Connors Parent and Teacher Rating Scales,* C. Keith Conners (cps.nova.edu/~cpphelp/CRSR.html).
- *Infant Temperament Questionnaire* (questionnaire), Behavioral-Developmental Initiatives (www.temperament.com/).
- *Pediatric Early Elementary Examination (PEEX 2)* (assessment), Melvin D. Levine, MD, FAAP (www.epsbooks.com/dynamic/catalog/series.asp?seriesonly=1795M).
- *Pediatric Examination of Educational Readiness at Middle Childhood (PEERAMID 2)* (assessment), Melvin D. Levine, MD, FAAP. (www.epsbooks.com/dynamic/catalog/series.asp?seriesonly=1795M).

RELATED WEB SITES

- International Dyslexia Society (www.interdys.org/).
- Learning Disabilities Association of America (www.ldaamerica.org/).
- National Center for Learning Disabilities (www.ncld.org/).
- National Institute of Neurological Disorders and Stroke (www.ninds.nih.gov/).

AAP POLICY STATEMENT

American Academy of Pediatrics, Committee on Children With Disabilities; American Academy of Ophthalmology; American Association for Pediatric Ophthalmology and Strabismus. Learning disabilities, dyslexia, and vision: a subject review. *Pediatrics.* 1998;102(5)1217-1219. (aappolicy.aappublications.org/cgi/content/full/pediatrics;102/5/1217).

SUGGESTED RESOURCES

Dworkin PH. *Learning and Behavior Problems of Schoolchildren.* Philadelphia, PA: WB Saunders; 1985.

Dworkin PH. School failure. *Pediatr Rev.* 1989;10:301-312.

Levine MD. *Educational Care.* Cambridge, MA: Educators Publishing Service Inc; 1994.

Lindsay RL. School failure/disorders of learning. In: Bergman AB, ed. *Common Problems in Pediatrics.* New York, NY: McGraw-Hill; 2001.

Shaywitz S. Dyslexia. *N Engl J Med.* 1998;338:307-312.

Wender ED, ed. *School Dysfunction in Children and Youth: The Role of the Primary Care Provider for Children Who Struggle in School.* Report of the Twenty-Fourth Ross Roundtable on Critical Approaches to Common Pediatric Problems. Columbus, OH: Ross Products Division, Abbott Laboratories; 1993.

REFERENCES

1. Bax M. Looking at learning disorders [editorial]. *Dev Med Child Neurol.* 1982;24:731-732.
2. Hammill DD. On defining learning disabilities: an emerging consensus. *J Learning Disabil.* 1990;21:74-84.
3. Pennington BF. Toward an integrated understanding of dyslexia: genetic, neurological, and cognitive mechanisms. *Dev Psychopathol.* 1999;11:629-654.
4. Shaywitz SE. Evidence that dyslexia may represent the lower tail of a normal distribution of reading ability. *N Engl J Med.* 1992;326:145-150.
5. Denckla MB. Biological correlates of learning and attention: what is relevant to learning disability and attention-deficit hyperactivity disorder? *J Dev Behav Pediatr.* 1996; 17:114-119.
6. Levine MD, Oberklaid F, Meltzer L. Developmental output failure: a study of low productivity in school-aged children. *Pediatrics.* 1981;67:18-25.
7. Rutter M, et al. *Fifteen Thousand Hours: Secondary Schools and Their Effects on Children.* Cambridge, MA: Harvard University Press; 1979.
8. Baca L, Amato C. Bilingual special education: training issues. *Except Child.* 1989;56:168-173.
9. National Research Council. *Improving Schooling for Language-Minority Children: A Research Agenda.* Washington, DC: National Academy Press; 1997.
10. Berger LR. The Winnicott Squiggle Game: a vehicle for communication with the school-aged child. *Pediatrics.* 1980;66:921-924.
11. Dworkin PH. Ready to learn: a mandate for pediatrics. *J Dev Behav Pediatr.* 1993;14:192-196.

Emotional and Behavioral Problems

Chapter 130

A DEVELOPMENTAL APPROACH TO THE PREVENTION OF COMMON BEHAVIORAL PROBLEMS

Joshua Sparrow, MD; T. Berry Brazelton, MD

Pediatric primary care physicians are uniquely positioned to prevent common behavioral problems through the relationships they make with young children and their families in the course of well-child care visits and to identify and refer—effectively and early—problems that cannot be prevented.[1-5] Such opportunities can spare the child and family unnecessary suffering, and they can conserve scarce health care resources, including primary pediatric provider time and tertiary mental health services.[6-9] These considerations are particularly important in locations where access to mental health services is limited. The savings that result extend beyond health care to education, social services, and the criminal justice system.

REGRESSION AND PROGRESSION IN PRIMATE DEVELOPMENT AND ITS NEUROBIOLOGIC UNDERPINNINGS: IMPLICATIONS FOR PEDIATRIC ANTICIPATORY GUIDANCE AND PREVENTION

Although predictably unfurled by neurobiological forces, development—once considered linear and continuous—is now widely understood to be a precarious process in which vulnerable periods of regression are necessary for new and more advanced motor, cognitive, and social-emotional skills to displace earlier ones.[3,10-16] Developmental events characterized by regression and disorganization in the child and, as a result, in the family, followed by a predictable new acquisition of skill or ability are referred to here and in our other work[17,18] as touchpoints. As our knowledge about these touchpoints grows, it likely will lead to new interventions to aid children, parents, and families.

Neurobiologic processes (for example, neurohormonal regulatory mechanisms affecting infant, mother and father, synaptogenesis, myelinization, and pruning, among others)[19-23] are critical to understanding mechanisms of developmental change; yet these processes are insufficient to account for widely divergent outcomes unless embedded in a broader view of the child's interactions with the environment. The developing brain allows the young infant to process critical environmental input and to send mediating signals to the environment; the brain must adapt, structurally and functionally, to this interaction, a process best accounted for by a *systems theory* approach.[6,10,24-33] The infant brain shapes and is shaped by the environment in which it evolves. As a result, primary care physicians can make a major contribution to a child's development—including optimal brain development—when they position themselves to enhance these interactions.[6,7,34-38] This approach demands that physicians redefine their roles to enter into the family system and become part of the child-parent team.

Nonlinear, discontinuous development marked by predictable episodes of regression that precede leaps to new mastery have been observed both in human infants and nonhuman primates in their first years of life.[39,40] Across these species, development is a costly affair in which the prerequisite periods of regression expose the infant to increased vulnerability: to developmental deviation, to parent-infant conflict that may result in abuse,[41] and to heightened immunologic fragility that increases the likelihood of illness.[42-45] Consequently, an understanding of the mechanisms of developmental change, and of the predictable cycles of regression and developmental leaps, or touchpoints, permits primary care physicians to offer anticipatory guidance that targets these periods of vulnerability and to screen for the earliest signs of developmental derailment parsimoniously.

For 1 to 4 weeks before early major developmental achievements, according to some authors,[11,12] regressive periods may cause more frequent and prolonged crying, clinging, and bids for physical contact in both human and nonhuman primate infants. Although chimpanzee mothers immediately remove their infants from the social group at the first signs of these regressions to avoid male castigation, human mothers more often first interpret the behavioral change as a possible sign of illness.[40,41,43] This finding should come as no surprise to seasoned pediatric practitioners who have already noted a predictable developmental pattern to the anxious calls of parents who wonder if their child may be ill when they note such changes in behavior. "He just isn't acting the way he usually does," is one common expression of this parental observation. These periods of crying are often attributed to teething, even when evidence to support this explanation is nonexistent.[42,46] Instead, however, they are routinely associated with the approach of new developmental challenges, for example, the onset of the perceptual and cognitive capacities for stranger anxiety, pulling to stand, or the first step.

After parents have reassured themselves that their child is not sick, they often shift from acceptance of the regressive behavior to a range of other attitudes, which we have clinically observed to vary from one temperamental fit to another, and from culture to culture, including annoyance and decreased indulgence of infant demands for physical contact and attention. These stances can effectively discourage regressive behaviors while reinforcing new skills.[47] Nonetheless, this shift in the parent—from initial acquiescence to efforts to propel the child's development—leads to conflict between parent and child. Although conflict may be necessary to the child's progress, and a wide range of parental response to regression may be adaptive in fostering the child's development, difficulties in negotiating these conflicts may sometimes lead to developmental deviation, or abuse.

The developmental processes of attachment, self-regulation, feeding, sleep, and toilet training are among the opportunities for primary pediatric prevention of common behavioral problems and child abuse. Regressions accompanying developmental advances in each of these areas occur at predictable times in the first years of life. We present here one touchpoint in each of these areas (although several occur in each) as examples of heightened vulnerability to developmental deviation and abuse, along with practical preventive strategies that can be used in primary pediatric care settings.

ANTICIPATORY GUIDANCE AT BIRTH OR AT THE 4-MONTH WELL-CHILD CARE VISIT: PREDICTABLE LOSS OF INTEREST IN FEEDING ACCOMPANYING IMPROVED VISUAL ACCOMMODATION AT 4 TO 5 MONTHS

Inevitably, the birth of a new baby disorganizes any family; all members must reconfigure their previous roles and arrive at a new level of organization to adjust to a new member, one with particularly pressing new demands. Fortunately, newborns are endowed with attachment behaviors that shape neurohormonally mediated parental responses, helping adults learn to become parents.[48] However, the newborn period, with its disorganization and opportunities for rapid new growth, is a vulnerable one, a period when primary care physicians can be more influential than at any other time.

Impaired attachments have long been recognized as risk factors in child abuse and child psychiatric disorders; yet much can be done to support healthy attachments and to identify early threats to this critical developmental process.[49-52] Primary care physicians can readily assess the attachment behaviors of the newborn and parental responses during the earliest routine well-child care visits.[53-55] The Neonatal Behavioral Assessment Scale[56] and the abbreviated version, the Neonatal Behavioral Observation, include an inventory of predictable newborn behaviors that elicit nurturing responses in parents.[57,58] A few of these are:

- The alert state visual gaze and visual communication between newborn and parent
- Reflexive reaching toward parent's voice and face
- Turning the head toward parent's voice, and arching toward parent's face
- Molding into parent's body when cuddled
- Responses to parent's soothing
- Crying
- Smiling
- Suckling

Attachment depends not only on parental responses to these and other behaviors, but also on each newborn's individual ability to mobilize effective attachment behaviors in parents.[59] This ability varies from one newborn to another and may be affected by a wide range of circumstances, for example, prematurity, illness, or in utero exposures. In addition, the *goodness of fit*[60] of infant attachment behaviors and parental sensibilities is a factor in this critical process.

Physicians also will be able to observe protective parental reactions to noxious aspects of the routine examination of the newborn as further possible evidence of the progress of attachment. They can also reinforce this process by sympathetically commenting on parents' distress, for example, when their baby cries when being undressed or with heel sticks. Parental reactions may be influenced by many factors, for example, parity and culture, but they may also reveal potential interferences with attachment such as postpartum depression[61] or overwhelming life events. When parents do respond to their infant's distress cues with efforts to soothe, physicians will have an opportunity to assess and, if needed, respectfully offer to supplement parental repertoires for comforting. In addition, an infant who is particularly difficult to soothe should be noted because parents will need extra support and encouragement to avoid taking such challenges personally.

Physicians should consider an early referral to developmental specialists for families in which a young infant shows an impaired ability to exhibit attachment behaviors, is irritable and challenging to console, or when parents fail to respond to these behaviors or to demonstrate protective reactions when their infant shows signs of distress. Early interventions to support attachment in such circumstances may prevent child abuse, behavioral problems, and later psychopathologic abnormalities in the child.[62-65] A pediatric provider's sincere praise for parents' expertise and dedication can help enforce parents' self-perceptions of competence and thereby help protect the attachment process. This quick and simple intervention can be readily offered to all parents during this vulnerable period.

UNEXPLAINED END-OF-THE-DAY CRYING AND SELF-REGULATION FROM 3 TO 12 WEEKS

Unexplained end-of-the day fussiness and crying is a predictable phenomenon, initiated in the majority of infants at approximately 3 weeks of age, peaking at approximately 8 weeks, and subsiding by 12 to 16 weeks of age, usually lasting for 1 to 3 hours at the end of the day.[46,66] Prolonged crying that does not follow this pattern and time course or is accompanied by other symptoms should, of course, prompt further medical investigation. Fussing and crying are challenging for any parent but can become intolerable when parents interpret this behavior as a rejection of their efforts to comfort or as the baby's reproach for their failure as parents. First-time parents and those who are isolated, multiply stressed, or struggling with postpartum depression may be particularly vulnerable to such interpretations of colic. The incidence of sudden infant death syndrome (SIDS) peaks in the month or 2 after the typical climax of colic. Some small subgroup of presumed SIDS deaths may be attributable to intentional suffocation by overwhelmed parents.

The 2- to 3-week well-child care visit is an ideal opportunity for anticipatory guidance for colic. Although checklists of anticipated developmental steps abound, predictably exhausted parents are unlikely to absorb such information at this point. During this visit, a simple and more effective strategy than simply telling or offering a brochure is to note when the baby cries and to observe the parents' reaction to it, valuing their sensitivity to the baby's distress and their intense dedication to offering comfort. This approach may be novel for many physicians who have had to listen to and indeed make so many babies cry! Nonetheless, when pediatricians demonstrate their own sensitivity to a baby's distress and to parents' commitment to mitigate it, they have positioned themselves and readied parents to face unexplained end-of-the-day fussing as a team.

Pediatricians who understand that some parents may interpret the predictable developmental phenomenon of unexplained end-of-the-day crying in ways that may make it harder for them to bear can anticipate this new challenge and what it may mean to parents during the brief 2- to 3-week visit: "I noticed how you leaned in to comfort your baby as soon as she began to cry. She's so responsive to your soothing! In another week or 2, you may want to watch and see whether she, like many babies, starts to fuss and cry at the end of the day." Pause to allow parents to express their concerns or doubts ("Not my baby!") or to assert their mastery and their baby's precocity ("She already does!"). A pediatrician can then let parents know that this period is a predictable but trying time for parents, and the hardest part may be that none of the skillful soothing strategies parents have learned seem to work. In fact, at the end of the day, infants may be overstimulated by attempts to soothe them; they will often calm briefly while being jiggled or rocked, but as soon as a parent stops, they will cry out even more lustily than before. Ask the parent, "What is that going to be like for you?" Listen, and then ask, "Will you call me and let me know?" (Any experienced pediatrician knows they will call anyway during the colicky period, but now they will be more likely to listen if the pediatrician concludes that, in fact, no gastrointestinal disturbance exists or that there is no need to switch to a soy-based formula, for example.)

After these brief maneuvers, parents will be ready for the recommendation that they may be able to decrease the length of fussing during this period if they can limit their efforts to soothe: After checking for other possible causes for crying (hunger, fatigue, or wet diaper), too much jostling and handling may overstimulate the infant and prolong the end-of-the-day fussing.[46,67] (Infant massage, swaddling, or carrying the baby close in a serape-like snuggler may soothe with less stimulation and help parents feel certain that they are doing all they can.)

At the very least, anticipatory strategies such as these will save the pediatrician time, but they can also prevent noncompliance, unnecessary treatment, physician shopping, and possibly abuse. At the end of the 2- to-3-week visit, you can reassure parents that this colicky period may be an important step in the development of self-regulatory functions and that the reward will be the 2 or 3 month old who is more available, responsive, and seems to have become more of a real person than before.

ANTICIPATORY GUIDANCE AT THE 4-MONTH WELL-CHILD CARE VISIT: PREDICTABLE LOSS OF INTEREST IN FEEDING ACCOMPANYING IMPROVED VISUAL ACCOMMODATION AT 4 TO 5 MONTHS

The succession of steps through which the infant, toddler, and young child acquire the range of motor and other skills that are necessary for autonomous feeding includes several readily identifiable vulnerable periods before which anticipatory guidance can prevent predictable behavioral problems. Some of these skills pertain not specifically to eating, but rather to balancing other interests and impulses to prevent them from interfering with eating. For example, at approximately 4 months of age, a period of regression can be expected when previously acquired feeding habits seem to be shoved aside by new, though predictable, behaviors: At the breast or on the bottle, the 4 to 5 month old abruptly seems to lose interest in feeding and is suddenly distracted by a wider range of visual stimuli now perceptible to the infant.[68]

Experienced pediatricians expect telephone calls from mothers of 4 or 5 month olds who misinterpret this behavioral change as a sign that their milk is no longer sufficient and ask whether it is time to wean or to introduce solids. In the absence of acute medical illness interfering with appetite and intake, the neurobiologic process accounting for this behavioral change is the child's expanding visual accommodation that now results in the ability to focus on objects that are farther away than the breast or the nurturer's face. In this instance, new neurobiological capabilities disrupt previously established adaptations, leading to a period of instability during which the infant must learn to handle new levels of environmental stimulation and to balance these with other ongoing and changing demands. This new challenge can be predicted for parents at the 4-month well-child care visit. (Similarly, at the 12-month well-child care visit, pediatricians can predict that the burgeoning drive to use new motor skills and walk are likely to set off other parenting challenges—temporary sleep disturbances, tantrums at any interference with mobility, or another bout of flagging interest in feeding.) When they have been advised to expect this new turn of events as a marker of a new developmental accomplishment, parents will be less likely to interpret temporary feeding resistance as a failure on their part or as a sign to wean or introduce solids prematurely.

At the 4-month visit, pediatricians can suggest nursing or bottle feeding the infant in a quiet, darkened room when distractibility at feeding commences, and they can offer reassurance that this phenomenon is transient and a positive sign that the child is developing appropriately. In a few days or weeks, when parents find that their infant does display the predicted behavior, their confidence in the provider is likely to deepen. If their baby, however, does not become more difficult to feed, then they are less likely to question the physician's expertise than to share the pride they feel in their exceptional baby who has traversed this new challenge so unperturbedly and spared them the predicted inconvenience. A few parents might wonder whether such a child is still developmentally on track but can be easily reassured if they have noticed or can be prompted to observe the baby's new, more widely roaming gaze as the infant follows objects in motion across a room.

The period between 4 and 5 months is a vulnerable time that can lead to premature introduction of solids and discontinuation of breastfeeding, or even forced feedings. With the *normalization* of this predictable touchpoint through anticipatory guidance, pediatricians may be able to avert such consequences or, at the very least, to open a dialogue that will increase the likelihood that parents will disclose such concerns and seek help.

ANTICIPATORY GUIDANCE FOR THE 6-MONTH WELL-CHILD CARE VISIT: PREDICTABLE SLEEP DISTURBANCES FROM 9 TO 12 MONTHS AS THE HARBINGER OF THE FIRST STEP

Experienced primary care physicians expect anxious calls from parents about their 9 and 10 month olds who seem driven and tense, will not settle for bed at night, and wake up several times during the night despite having slept all the way through during the preceding months. After establishing that the child is healthy and is already pulling to stand, some physicians have learned to suggest that in the majority of cases the new sleep disturbance is temporary and represents the sign of a child who will take the first step in a matter of weeks.[69,70] Parents, eager for this much-awaited event, relax, or even rejoice and often recast the baby's disrupted sleep and their own as an acceptable though annoying nuisance.

Here, again, a regression to earlier behavior (waking during the night) or temporary loss of a recently acquired skill (self-settling for sleep and managing sleep cycles) disorganizes the child and indeed the entire family—the price for the next developmental step to come. The anxiety of parents as they struggle to understand this sudden, unexplained change renders them more vulnerable while making the physician's support even more deeply valued. How much more reassured parents may be to learn that infants this age spend proportionally more of their sleeping hours in light sleep than at other times in these early years! No wonder they wake more often. Some scientists currently hypothesize that this sleep-phase shift is necessary so that the brain can lay down the memory traces for each of the motor movements that will soon come together as the child's first step.[69,71]

If this predictable sleep disturbance occurs a few weeks or more before consultation with the pediatrician, then preventive opportunities for anticipatory guidance may be missed. Parents may begin to take a child who had been sleeping alone in his or her bed—not necessarily a problem for families who choose to co-sleep with a child this age. However, choosing to co-sleep will likely lead to difficulties in reestablishing independent sleep at a later time. In addition, parents, who are once again sleep-deprived, exhausted, and frustrated by their child's reversion to old behavior, may react more harshly than they would have otherwise wanted to, or more desperately, and perhaps abusively when other risk factors are present. However, if parents are forewarned at the 6-month well-child care visit of this trying harbinger of new steps ahead, then they are far more likely to take the child's disrupted sleep and their own sleep deprivation in stride. The physician will have helped them shape their own behavior, even infusing it with pride, as they have been given a new, more constructive way of understanding the child's behavior—a laudable goal for anticipatory guidance. Parents are then more likely to be open to, and retain a few suggestions about how to respond to their driven, motor-focused infant.

ANTICIPATORY GUIDANCE AT 12 MONTHS: WAITING FOR TOILET TRANING READINESS FROM 24 TO 36 MONTHS

Toilet training is another developmental acquisition that is often accompanied by predictable parent-child conflict and with it another peak in the risk for developmental derailment and child abuse. Opportunities for prevention begin with anticipatory guidance at the 12-month visit when pediatric primary care providers can provocatively ask, "So, have you started to think about toilet training yet?" Most parents will say, "Toilet training? She's too young for that. She's just a baby." "Good," practitioners can reply. "Will you remember that you said that when you get the potty chair in the mail in a few months?" "What potty chair?" a parent will ask, again surprised. At this point, a brief discussion can ensue about the pressures for premature toilet training from family and friends and parents' own beliefs about when to toilet train.

Parents may cite a particular chronologic age for toilet training, and this age may vary among parents of different cultures, but parents can be encouraged to consider the signs of readiness (eg, interest in putting things away in their proper place, ability to sit still) that appear with some variability beginning at the end of the second year.[72] They can also be warned against the risks of responding too soon and too eagerly to the earliest signs—pointing to the diaper, grunting, or going off to a corner while defecating—that often appear at 18 months and before the child is truly ready. Parents can be asked about the approach to toilet training they believe to be best suited to their child's temperament and to consider the risks of a non–child-centered approach versus the rewards to the child of setting up this process as the child's achievement rather than that of the parents.[72,73]

At the 1-year visit, the groundwork will have been laid to protect parent and child from external pressure and premature toilet training. These matters can then be productively elaborated on in later visits. Unless parents have undertaken *elimination communication* (a kind of physiologic conditioning that is dependent on extensive close physical contact, careful cue reading, and consistent responses) in the first year, toilet training can be effectively begun only when a child is cognitively and emotionally ready. This function, similar to feeding, is one that parents cannot control. Excessive parental pressure arising from unrealistic developmental expectations is likely to set off struggles and developmental derailment, which can take the form of withholding stools and encopresis, for example.

The peak in child abuse associated with toilet training is often associated with such misguided expectations and an ensuing belief that the child is wetting, soiling, or smearing in retaliation. In some instances, this action may indeed be the child's way of attempting to exert control, or to assert him or herself in response to pressure that interferes with the establishment of autonomy. This attempt, of course, only heightens the frustrated parent's sense of being at the child's mercy and the exasperation that may spill over into abuse. As in all other instances, once abuse has occurred or is seriously suspected, referrals to mental health and child protection specialists become necessary. Anticipatory guidance, however, can prepare parents for the child's need for control in this area and for their own understandable feelings of frustration—magnified by the expense and inconvenience of diapering into the third year. These concerns can be reduced with a preventive readjustment of expectations. When early anticipatory guidance includes normalizing predictions about parental reactions to the child's refusal to cooperate and insistence on control of his or her own bodily functions, parents are also more likely to confide in pediatric providers later as parents experience potentially destructive though understandable antagonism toward the child. This early shared understanding will set up further opportunities to intervene before such feelings intensified.

ROLE OF THE THERAPEUTIC RELATIONSHIP IN ANTICIPATORY GUIDANCE AND PREVENTION: TOUCHPOINTS AS DEVELOPMENTAL OPPORTUNITIES FOR RELATIONSHIP BUILDING

The influence of pediatric practice on critical child-family interactions in the contexts of crying, feeding, sleeping, and toilet training may be underestimated by providers who limit their approach to teaching, giving advice, or providing information. Extensive research on adult learning and behavioral change[38,74-78] calls into question widespread yet unexamined assumptions about the effects of simply telling parents what to do. Physicians' offer of information is often insufficient unless parents are open to accept it. In addition, consensus on the benefits of intentional relationship building is emerging from the expanding literature on the therapeutic effects of the physician-patient relationship.

In the context of a physician-patient relationship in which both parties are active participants and in which patients feel respected, listened to, and cared for, patients are far more likely to:

- Share important information critical to medical-decision making.
- Reveal concerns about treatment that may lead to noncompliance if unstated and unaddressed.
- Undergo positive behavioral change.[35,79-87]

The healing effects of the physician-patient relationship are magnified for parents of chronically ill children who must spend more time in provider offices and for isolated parents, without other supports, who are at increased risk of neglecting and abusing their children.[88]

Intentional strategies for relationship building and the resulting increase in trust and communication are especially salient to preventing pediatric behavioral problems. Parents have many reasons for not sharing information that is relevant to prevention and health promotion:

- Parents' feelings about their children's progress and their own parental competence are central to their fundamental sense of self-worth and to their effectiveness in parenting. These feelings are often fragile and defensively protected, especially when a child is not thriving or when a child is in the midst of the regressive period of a developmental touchpoint.
- Parents' childrearing practices are often unconscious or unexamined.
- Parents' views on parenting are deeply personal, strongly held, and emotionally charged, given that they are for the most part derived from their own childhood, from their own experience of being parented (or lack thereof).

Parents are more likely to reveal their concerns and struggles in the context of an intentionally elaborated physician-patient relationship.

Parents' profound investment in their child's health and well being, independent of whatever challenges and limitations they may face, offers a unique opportunity for pediatric care providers to establish and deepen relationships by valuing their passion and commitment and by sharing developmentally based observations of their children's behavior, including predictable, temporary regressions. Such carefully initiated and managed relationships are a potent diagnostic and therapeutic tool that can:

- Encourage parents to provide more complete and accurate information pertinent to diagnosis, treatment planning, and adherence.
- Prepare parents to be more open to anticipatory guidance.
- Ready parents to reflect on their attitudes and consider the possibility of change.
- Decrease parental isolation, a risk factor for child abuse and other pathologic conditions, for example, parental depression. (Parental depression may in some cases increase the risk of prematurity, child abuse, and interfere with optimal child development.)

An accurate assessment of parent-child conflict, one that can be readily shared with parents (and with the old-enough child), requires that parents confide in a nonjudgmental and trusting climate and that difficult-to-acknowledge child behaviors can be safely opened up for shared observation. Every opportunity to strengthen the provider-family relationship in the course of routine care will make these challenging dialogues more effective.

Understanding parental development is as essential as knowledge of child development for pediatric practitioners. When both areas have been mastered, primary pediatric care physicians will recognize the meanings of a child's struggles and progress to parents. They can then elicit parents' beliefs, rather than imposing their own, to build therapeutic relationships that help parents optimize their responses to the demands of their child's development. As parents are invited to share their own interpretations of their child's challenging behaviors—for example, food refusal, tantrums, or bedtime battles—they have a chance to rework them, to consider what they bring from their own childhood that may interfere with their sensitivity to the child, or hamper effective responses, and then to consider the child's perspective. In this process of sharing the meaning of the child's behavior with the pediatrician in a short visit (or in longer ones, when necessary, that may be separately billable as counseling), parents will feel less alone and freer to redefine the behavior in ways that make them feel more hopeful and effective, less personally targeted by the behavior, and less prone to power struggles that can lead to more serious and more chronic behavioral problems.

The tendency for medical providers to underestimate the preventive and therapeutic power of their relationships with their patients has been reinforced by shortened visits and related financial pressures. Nonetheless, effective physician-patient relationships can likely reduce some costs, for example, by improving appropriate health care resource utilization and treatment adherence, decreasing litigation rates, and preventing physician demoralization and burnout (in physicians who no longer reap their own rewards from the therapeutic relationship and who must pay the price for poorly managed ones). Even with the limited time to devote to each family, choices need to be made about how to use it. We can squander the precious time we have by offering advice to deaf ears, or we can prepare parents to take it to heart. We can ignore parents' heightened vulnerability and openness to our support during their children's touchpoints, or we can present anticipatory guidance at precisely the moments when they are most ready to hear it. We can intimidate parents with our expertise, rather than welcoming theirs. We can tell them what we think first, or we can start by inviting their observations about their children. We can describe and value the behaviors that we know matter deeply to parents to show rather than tell them that we too are committed to their children's well being. We can focus on intentionally building relationships that parents can take with them beyond the confines of our offices and conjure up in moments of doubt and loneliness. We can focus on their "failings" and their children's "deficits," or we can help them see their own strengths through our eyes when they are unable to see them through their own.

TOOLS FOR PRACTICE

Engaging Patients and Family

- *Parenting Skills: Nurturing and Guiding* (fact sheet), American Academy of Pediatrics (www.aap.org/topics.html).
- *Children's Mental Health, When To Seek Help* (fact sheet), American Academy of Pediatrics (www.aap.org/topics.html).
- *Your Child's Mental Health: When to Seek Help and Where to Get Help.* (brochure), American Academy of Pediatrics (patiented.aap.org).

REFERENCES

1. Schor EL. Rethinking well-child care. *Pediatrics*. 2004; 114(1):210-216.
2. Brazelton TB. How to help parents of young children: the touchpoints model. *J Perinatol Suppl*. 1999;19:6-8.
3. Brazelton TB. How to help parents of young children: the touchpoints model. *Clin Child Psychol Psychiatry*. 1998; 3:481-483.
4. Brazelton TB, O'Brien M, Brandt KA. Combining relationships and development: Applying touchpoints to individual and community practices. *Infants Young Child*. 1997;10:74-84.
5. Brazelton TB. Working with families: opportunities for early intervention. *Pediatr Clin North Am*. 1995;42(1):1-9.
6. Shonkoff J, Phillips D. *From Neurons to Neighborhoods: The Science of Early Childhood Development 2000*. Washington, DC: National Academies Press; 2000.
7. Beckwith L, Sigman MD. Preventive interventions in infancy. *Infant Psychiatry*. 1995;4(3):683-700.
8. Beeghly M, Brazelton TB, Flannery KA, et al. Specificity of preventative pediatric intervention effects in early infancy. *J Dev Behav Pediatry*. 1995;16:158-166.
9. Brazelton TB. Touchpoints: opportunities for preventing problems in the parent-child relationship. *Acta Pediatrica Supplement*. 1994;394:35-40.

10. Brazelton TB, Sparrow JD. *Touchpoints of Anticipatory Guidance in the First Three Years: A Preventive Approach to Pediatric Primary Practice. Developmental and Behavioral Pediatrics*. 2nd ed. Parker S, Zuckerman B, Augustyn M, eds. Philadelphia, PA: Lippincott Williams and Wilkins; 2005.
11. Sadurni M, Rostan C. Reflections on regression periods in the development of Catalan infants. In: Heimann M, ed. *Regression Periods in Human Infancy*. London, UK: Lawrence Erlbaum Associates; 2003:7-22.
12. Lindahl LB, Heimann M, Ullstadius E. Occurrence of regressive periods in the normal development of Swedish infants. In: Heimann M, ed. *Regression Periods in Human Infancy*. London, UK: Lawrence Erlbaum Associates; 2003:411-458.
13. Trevarthen C, Aitken K. Regulation of brain development and age-related changes in infants' motives: the developmental function of regressive periods. In: Heimann M, ed. *Regression Periods in Human Infancy*. London, UK: Lawrence Erlbaum Associates; 2003:107-184.
14. Bateson, PPG, Hinde RA. Developmental changes in sensitivity to experience. In: Bornstein MH, ed. *Sensitive Periods in Development: Interdisciplinary Perspectives*. Hillsdale, NJ: Lawrence Erlbaum; 1987:19-34.
15. Fischer KW, Pipp SL, Bullock D. Detecting developmental discontinuities. Methods and measurement. In: Emde RN, Harmon RJ, eds. *Continuities and Discontinuities in Development*. New York, NY: Plenum Press; 1984:94-121.
16. Bever TG, ed. *Regressions in Mental Development: Basic Phenomena and Theories*, Hillsdale, NJ: Lawrence Erlbaum; 1982.
17. Brazelton TB, revised with Sparrow JD. *Touchpoints 0-3: Your Child's Emotional and Behavioral Development*. Vol. I. Cambridge, MA: Da Capo; 2006.
18. Brazelton TB, Sparrow JD. *Touchpoints Three to Six: Your Child's Emotional and Behavioral Development*. Vol. II, Cambridge, MA: Perseus Books; 2001.
19. Thompson PM, Giedd JN, Woods RP, et al. Growth patterns in the developing brain detected by using continuum mechanical tensor maps. *Nature*. 2000;40:190-193.
20. Nelson CA, Bloom FE. Child development and neuroscience. *Child Dev*. 1997;68(5):970-987.
21. Giedd J, Snell JW, Lange N, et al. Quantitative magnetic resonance imaging of human brain development: ages 4-18. *Cerebral Cortex*. July/Aug 1996;6:551-560.
22. Shatz CJ. The developing brain. *Sci Am*, Sep 1992;267(3): 60-67.
23. Purves D, Lichtman JW. Elimination of synapses in the developing nervous system. *Science*. 1980;210:153-157.
24. Bronfenbrenner U, ed. *Making Human Beings Human: Bioecological Perspectives on Human Development*. Thousand Oaks, CA: Sage Publications; 2005.
25. Senge P. *Presence: Exploring Profound Change in People, Organizations, and Society*. New York, NY: Doubleday; 2005.
26. Fogel A, Maria CDP, Lyra, JV. *Dynamics and Indeterminism in Developmental and Social Processes*. Mahwah, NJ: Lawrence Erlbaum Associates; 1997.
27. Moen P, Elder GHJr, Lüscher K. *Examining Lives in Context: Perspectives on the Ecology of Human Development*. Washington, DC: American Psychological Association; 1995.
28. Thelen E., Smith L. *A Dynamic Systems Approach to the Development of Cognition and Action*. Cambridge, MA: MIT Press; 1994.
29. Senge PM. *The Fifth Discipline: The Art and Practice of the Learning Organization*. New York, NY: Doubleday; 1994.
30. Fogel A. *Developing Through Relationships: Origins of Communication, Self, and Culture*. New York, NY: Harvester Wheatsheaf; 1993.
31. Gunnar MR, Thelen E. *Systems and Development*. Hillsdale, NJ: Lawrence Erlbaum; 1989.
32. Bronfenbrenner U. *The Ecology of Human Development: Experiments by Nature and Design*. Cambridge, MA: Harvard University Press; 1979.
33. Peterfreund E. *Information, Systems, and Psychoanalysis: An Evolutionary Biological Approach to Psychoanalytic Theory*. New York, NY: International University Press; 1971.
34. Ong LM, de Haes JC, Hoos AM, et al. Doctor-patient communication: a review of the literature. *Soc Sci Med*. 1995;40(7):903-918.
35. Kurtz SM. Doctor-patient communication: principles and practices. *Can J Neurol Sci*. 2002;29(Suppl 2):S23-S29.
36. Skelton JR, Kai J, Loudon RF. Cross-cultural communication in medicine: questions for educators. *Med Educ*. 2001;35(3);257-261.
37. van Dulmen AM, Holl RA. Effects of continuing paediatric education in interpersonal communication skills. *Eur J Pediatr*. 2000;159(7);489-495.
38. Brazelton TB. Reaching out to new parents. *Child Today* 1978;27.
39. Horwich RH. Regressive periods in primate behavioral development with reference to other mammals. *Primates*. 1974;15:141-149.
40. Van de Rijt-Plooij HC, Plooij F. Growing independence, conflict, and learning in mother-infant relations in free-ranging chimpanzees. *Behaviour*. 1987;101:1-86.
41. Van de Rijt-Plooij HC, Plooij F. Distinct periods of mother-infant conflict in normal development: sources of progress and germs of pathology. *J Child Psychol Psychiatr*. 1993;34(2):229-243.
42. Plooij FX, Van de Rijt-Ploiiij, Van d Stelt JM, et al. Illness peaks during infancy and regression periods. In: Heimann M, ed. *Regression Periods in Human Infancy*. London, UK: Lawrence Erlbaum; 2003:81-96.
43. Van de Rijt-Plooij HC, Plooij F. Mother-infant relations, conflict, stress, and illness among free-ranging chimpanzees. *Dev Med Child Neurol*. 1988;30, 306-315.
44. Laudenslager M, Reite M, AHrbeck RJ. Immune status during mother-infant separation. *Psychosom Med*. 1982; 44:303.
45. Michaut RJ, Dechambre RP, Doumerc S, et al. Influence of early maternal deprivation on adult humoral immune response in mice. *Physiol Behav*. 1981;26:189-191.
46. Brazelton TB. Crying in infancy. *Pediatrics*. 1962;29:579-588.
47. Plooij FX. Périodes de transition et de vulnérabilité: conflits et progressions. In: Busnuel MC, ed. *Le Langage des Bébés: Savons-Nous L'entendre?* Paris, France: Éditions Jacques Grancher; 1993.
48. Brazelton TB. The remarkable talents of the newborn, *Birth Fam J*. 1978;5:187-191.
49. Lyons P, Doueck HJ, Wodarski JS. Risk Assessment for child protective services: a review of the empirical literature on instrument performance. *Social Work Res*. 1996; 20(3):143-155.
50. Lyons-Ruth K, Alpern L, Repacholi B. Disorganized infant attachment classification and maternal psychosocial problems as predictors of hostile-aggressive behavior in the preschool classroom. *Child Dev*. 1993;64: 572-585.
51. Main M, Solomon C. Discovery of a new insecure-disorganized, disoriented attachment pattern. In: Brazelton BT, Yogman MW, eds. *Affective Development in Infancy*. Norwood, NJ: Ablex; 1986.
52. Ainsworth MDS, Blehar MC, Water E, et al. *Patterns of Attachment: A Psychological Study of the Strange Situation*, Hillsdale, NJ: Lawrence Erlbaum; 1978.
53. Brazelton TB. Demonstrating infant's behavior. *Children Today 10*. 1981;4:5.

54. Brazelton TB. Behavioral competence of the neonate. *Sem Perinatol*. 1979;3:35-44.
55. Brazelton TB, Als H. Clinical uses of the Brazelton neonatal scale. *Birth Fam J*. 1975;2:12.
56. Brazelton TB, Nugent JK. *The Neonatal Behavioral Assessment Scale*. 3rd ed. Mac Keith PressCambridge, MA 1995.
57. Parker S, Brazelton TB. Newborn behavioral assessment: research, prediction and clinical uses. *Child Today*. 1981;10:4-5.
58. Brazelton TB, Scholl MS, Robey JS. Visual responses in the newborn. *Pediatrics*. 1966;37:284-290.
59. Kochanska G. Mother-child relationships, child fearfulness, and emerging attachment: a short-term longitudinal study. *Dev Psychol*. 1998;34(3):480-490.
60. Chess S, Thomas A. *Temperament: Theory and Practice*. New York, NY: Brunner Mazel; 1996.
61. Lyons-Ruth K, Zoll D, Connell D, et al. The depressed mother and her one year old infant: environment, interaction, attachment, and infant development. *New Direct Child Dev*. 1986;34:61-82.
62. Ogawa JR, Sroufe LA, Weinfeld NS, et al. Development and the fragmented self: longitudinal study of dissociative symptomatology in a nonclinical sample. *Dev Psychopathol*. 1997;6:77-98.
63. Warren S, Huston L, Egeland B, et al. Child and adolescent anxiety disorders and early attachment. *J Am Acad Child Adolesc Psychiatry*. 1997;36(5):637-644.
64. Zuravin S, McMillen C, DePanfilis D, et al. The intergenerational cycle of child maltreatment: Continuity vs. discontinuity. *J Interper Viol*. 1996;11(3):315-334.
65. Carlson EA, Jacobvitz D, Sroufe LA. A developmental investigation of inattentiveness and hyperactivity. *Child Dev*. 1995;66(1):37-54.
66. Brazelton TB. Crying and colic. *Infant Ment Health J* 1991;11:349-356.
67. Brazelton TB, Sparrow JD. *Calming Your Fussy Baby the Brazelton Way*. Cambridge, MA: Perseus Books; 2003.
68. Brazelton TB, Sparrow JD. *Feeding Your Child the Brazelton Way*. Cambridge, MA: Perseus Books; 2004.
69. Brazelton TB, Sparrow JD. *Sleep the Brazelton Way*. Cambridge, MA: Perseus Books; 2003.
70. Kawasaki C, Nugent JK, Miyashita H, et al. The cultural organization of infants' sleep, *Child Environ* 1994;11: 135-141.
71. Matthew Walker (in personal communication), and in Cromie W. Matthew Walker: sleep researcher. *Harvard Gazette*. October 17. 2002.
72. Brazelton TB, Sparrow JD. *Toilet Training Your Child the Brazelton Way*. Cambridge, MA: Perseus Books; 2004.
73. Brazelton TB. A child oriented approach to toilet training. *Pediatrics*. 1962;29:121.
74. Weiner SJ, Barnet B, Cheng TL, et al. Processes for effective communication in primary care. *Ann Intern Med*. 2005;142(8);709-714.
75. Coulehan J. Viewpoint: today's professionalism: engaging the mind but not the heart. *Acad Med*. 2005;80(10); 892-898.
76. Clark PA. Medical practices' sensitivity to patients' needs: opportunities and practices for improvement. *J Ambul Care Manage*. 2003;26(2);110-123.
77. Charon R. Narrative medicine: a model for empathy, reflection, profession, and trust. *JAMA*. 2001;286(15); 1897-1902.
78. O'Keefe M, Sawyer M, Roberton D. Medical student interviewing skills and mother-reported satisfaction and recall. *Med Educ*. 2001;35(7):637-644.
79. Teutsch C. Patient-doctor communication. *Med Clin North Am*. 2003;87(5);1115-1145.
80. Skelton JR, Kai J, Loudon RF. Cross-cultural communication in medicine: questions for educators. *Med Educ*. 2001;35(3);257-261.
81. Roter D. The enduring and evolving nature of the patient-physician relationship. *Patient Educ Counsel*. 2000;39(1);5-15.
82. Lingard L, Haber RJ. Teaching and learning communication in medicine: a rhetorical approach. *Acad Med*. 1999;74(5):507-510.
83. Lutfey KE, Wishner WJ. Beyond "compliance" is "adherence". Improving the prospect of diabetes care. *Diabetes Care*. 1999;22(4):635-639.
84. Stewart M, Brown JB, Boon H, et al. Evidence on patient-doctor communication. *Cancer Prevent Control*. 1999;3(1):25-30.
85. DiMatteo MR. Enhancing patient adherence to medical recommendations 1994; *JAMA* 271(1):79, 83.
86. Novack DH, Suchman AL, Clark W, et al. Calibrating the physician: physician personal awareness and effective patient care. *JAMA*. 1997;278(6):502-509.
87. Plack MM. The reflective practitioner: reaching for excellence in practice. *Pediatrics*. 2005;116(6):1546-1552.
88. Guterman N. *Stopping Child Maltreatment Before it Starts*. Thousand Oaks, CA: Sage Publication; 2000.

Chapter 131

CONSULTATION AND REFERRAL FOR EMOTIONAL AND BEHAVIORAL PROBLEMS

Jason E. Jones, MD; Richard M. Sarles, MD

INDICATORS FOR CONSULTATION OR REFERRAL

Certain types of behavior are such clear indicators of psychosocial disorders that a single occurrence should signal the pediatrician to consider referral. For example, some children with schizophrenia typically display such bizarre behavior or preoccupations and such grossly impaired emotional relationships that they are readily identifiable. In fact, a major shortcoming of even relatively successful therapy is the inability to make the psychotic child socially inconspicuous. Similarly, identifying certain acting-out behaviors as clear signals for referral is also easy. These behaviors include those that are dangerous to the child or others, vandalism, fire setting, and cruelty to animals. Unfortunately, most problems requiring referral cannot be readily identified by the occurrence of a single behavior or event. Rather, identifying the child or adolescent for referral to behavioral specialists most often requires differentiating matters of degree and severity. Probably the most difficult determination is whether certain behaviors, such as mood swings in adolescence, represent merely the normal developmental process or are manifestations of a more serious problem. This very dilemma prompted the development of the *Diagnostic and Statistical Manual for Primary Care* (DSM-PC)[1] sponsored by the American Academy of

Pediatrics. A task force of primary care clinicians and behavioral specialists was convened to describe and distinguish normal developmental variation versus behavior problems versus psychiatric disorders. DSM-PC provides helpful guidelines for separating children along this continuum depending on the presentation of various symptoms and youth functioning. However, other factors such as the family and youth beliefs and attitudes, availability and capabilities of the specialty system, and comfort level of the primary care clinician must also be considered. Although the DSM-PC provides specific guidelines in particular symptom areas, the following reviews a general framework around youth symptoms and functioning that should raise consideration for referral, barriers that often interfere with referral decisions, and general approaches to the referral process.

Signals for Concern

In general, the difference between normal and problematic behavior is not the actual behavior but rather the quantity (frequency of occurrences), distribution (different manifestations), and duration (generally, at least 4 weeks). Two additional factors also determine when behavior warrants attention: (1) if it is maladaptive, impairing social or cognitive functioning; or (2) when the concomitant level of distress is inappropriate (either elevated distress or a total lack of distress when some would be anticipated). For example, any sudden change in behavior, such as a significant drop in grades or withdrawal from peers or family may be related to a change in environment (eg, moving to a new school or neighborhood) and may be transient, with the child's behavior returning to normal in 1 or 2 weeks. If the change persists for more than a month, however, then the child probably needs special assistance to cope with the new environment or other stressor.

Similarly, all 5 factors (quantity, distribution, duration, maladaptiveness, and level of distress) are relevant in discriminating between a very energetic child and one who is hyperactive. In other instances, the problem behavior may be more circumscribed but still of concern because of its frequency, duration, or maladaptiveness (eg, drug abuse, sexual promiscuity, stealing, poor academic performance). Children often have conduct problems at home but not at school or at school but not at home.[2] The degree of maladaption of the behavior, however, may signal a need for intervention, even though the behavior occurs in only one setting.

The problems that health professionals most likely miss are the quiet ones that do not make life difficult for parents or teachers, such as poor peer relationships, emotional and social withdrawal, apathy, dysphoria, and poor self-esteem. Children at risk of depressive and anxiety disorders are more likely to be missed than other children requiring specialty care.

Determining the Need

A biopsychosocial model provides the framework for discriminating between problems that do and those that do not warrant referral. For example, in the case of a closed head injury, the pediatrician would assess for 4 parameters: (1) severity of the injury, (2) biological risk factors that might predispose the patient to a coexisting psychological disorder (eg, whether a significant family history of or genetic predisposition exists for depression), (3) psychological risk factors that may affect the treatment course and outcome (eg, whether this patient has previously documented cognitive deficits or behavior problems), and (4) social stressors that may prevent the patient from achieving an optimal recovery (eg, whether a lack of financial resources or family support systems plays a role). Using this framework will ensure that factors possibly inhibiting treatment will not be missed.

When deciding whether to refer patients, the pediatrician must consider not only the current maladaptiveness of the problem, but also the potential benefit of early intervention, which may prevent severe problems or significantly improve the quality of life for a child or family. Some disorders are more amenable to early intervention than others or may have treatments more available in the community.

BARRIERS TO REFERRAL

Many barriers to behavioral consultation or referral exist in primary care. The most commonly mentioned barrier is family or patient reluctance to accept mental health diagnoses or services. However, other factors exist as well. For example, the primary care practitioner may feel pressured to comply with the current medical trend to treat all the patient's needs in the primary care setting. However, any individual physician may not have the time, expertise, or interest to do so. Generally, parents acknowledge a physician's honesty in delineating the physician's own area of expertise and concomitant limitations and appreciate the concern and interest exhibited by the physician in suggesting appropriate consultation or referral.

Another barrier to behavioral referrals is confusion about the origin of particular symptoms or impairments. In such cases, joint assessments or concurrent evaluations are often helpful. Conversion disorder[3] illustrates the advisability of simultaneously exploring organic and psychosocial factors (see Chapter 139, Conversion Reactions and Hysteria). First, when a patient is admitted to the hospital for diagnostic evaluation, behavioral consultation should be requested at the outset of the hospitalization. Completing medical work-ups before consulting with behavioral specialists may lead to delays in diagnosis, prolonged hospitalization, and poor family interactions.

Primary care physicians may also avoid referring a child who has a behavioral problem because they are reluctant to label a child or adolescent as having such a problem. Such worries about labeling may stem from concerns about a child's future insurability or about a family's acceptance. In addition, a behavioral diagnosis may reduce payment rates for pediatricians and prevent accurate reporting of conditions.

Pediatricians frequently have complaints about accessing mental health services promptly and effectively.[4] Most of these concerns are legitimate, reflecting the often incompatible structures of pediatric and mental health services, as well as some attitudinal differences regarding what constitutes an emergency.

These obstacles can be partially reduced, however, if pediatricians (1) become more familiar with behavioral services and how to access them[4] and (2) clearly communicate their expectations regarding referral questions, reports, and ongoing feedback. Good mutual communication of expectations and needs appears to be the key. For example, evaluation of suicidal risk is often missing in psychiatric reports, whereas the family's attitude and involvement of other agencies (important data for mental health specialists) are often missing in referrals from primary care practitioners.[4]

Pediatricians may also hesitate to refer patients if the former are concerned about the effectiveness of behavioral intervention; that is, how much good it will do. Studies of the effectiveness of behavioral health services in community settings are not encouraging. However, an increasing number of evidence-based practices are available. A related concern, which is also appropriate, is the effort involved for physicians, parents, and children in going to a different place and person for consultation then possibly having to adapt to yet another professional. Financial considerations may present another difficulty. In general, the question is whether a referral involves much more effort and expense than it is worth.

Although no therapeutic approach or therapist can be totally effective, a skilled therapist is generally at least helpful, often successful, and unlikely to be harmful. Many behavioral specialists now routinely generate a treatment contract with their patients by which both parties agree to an initial series of sessions (usually between 4 and 6), after which they jointly assess whether progress has been made. If the parents or patient believe that the initial experience has been productive, then they may continue with the intervention plan; if not, then a change should occur in either the plan or the therapist. This practice ensures that patients will not continue in a long and expensive course of treatment that the therapist or the family deems as unnecessary or unproductive. However, the length and intensity of appropriate intervention vary tremendously with the particular patient and problem. Even a highly effective and responsible therapist will have a range of cases, some requiring 4 sessions or fewer and others 100 sessions or more. The key is to select and use a behavioral specialist to provide optimal care while maintaining contact with the primary care physician.

GENERAL CONSIDERATIONS

The physician ideally selects a consultant who can both assess and treat the patient. This approach reduces the chances that the child must first relate to a consultant and then adjust to another professional for treatment. In some cases, selection will not be possible, nor would it always represent optimal use of specialized skills. Knowledge of available behavioral resources, however, enables the physician to refer appropriately.

Another consideration is how best to structure interaction with behavioral specialists. One possibility is to include behavioral specialists within general pediatric practices. Increasingly, pediatricians have invited mental health professionals to base their practices in adjacent offices. Even better, such professionals have become members of group practices. This approach has obvious advantages for providing many behavioral services to patients naturally and efficiently. This approach also allows the behavioral specialist the opportunity to provide a variety of other services. The specialist may offer suggestions to office staff concerning aspects of patient treatment (eg, behavioral techniques or interventions for reducing anxiety during painful procedures). One or 2 brief sessions with this specialist before an inpatient hospitalization for treatments or procedures, such as chemotherapy, magnetic resonance imaging, and computed tomography scans, to familiarize the patient and family with these events would also be an excellent use of the specialist's consultation skills. Another example would be short-term group sessions for those with common problems such as young mothers or diabetic teenagers. Although one particular professional cannot possess the entire range of skills required, this person can enhance the effective use of other resources in the community.

Preparing the Parents

Preparing parents for behavioral consultation begins during the first discussion of the differential diagnosis, when both physical and emotional factors are included as potential causes of the symptoms. Even when the primary care physician has correctly introduced the possibility of emotional issues early in the diagnostic work-up, parents may resist exploring emotional factors. Such resistance is most likely when the symptoms appear to have an organic origin or when no overt behavioral disruption has occurred.

In some instances, parents may be encouraging some maladaptive behavior by children and not be aware that they are doing so; instead, they often blame the school or their child's peers. In other instances, parents may deny any problems with their child, partly to avoid revealing their own interpersonal or marital difficulties or a problem such as alcoholism. In other situations, parents may be relieved to understand that clinicians are also concerned with some behaviors. Nevertheless, the physician should present an honest appraisal of the situation (with appropriate recommendations for behavioral consultation) without trying to please or appease the parents by avoiding a discussion of the physician's true assessment of the clinical situation.

If parents are reluctant to consider a behavioral consultation, addressing their concern for their child's health and welfare may help. In explaining the need for such consultation, the pediatrician should suggest that this service is an important one for complete, comprehensive care of their child. The pediatrician should emphasize that behavioral consultation suggests that emotional factors may totally or partly account for their child's difficulty.

When the complaint is somatic, a useful example most parents can understand is the feeling of *butterflies in the stomach* or sweating before an examination, when speaking in public, during a marriage ceremony, or at other times of stress. A tension headache is another common symptom that can be used to demonstrate that a person can experience physical distress or pain without actual structural or physical disease being present.

The pediatrician can reduce the stigma of many emotional or behavioral problems by conceptualizing them as an absence of skills rather than deep-seated pathological condition. Furthermore, treatment that improves a child's coping skills or social skills can have lifelong benefits, going well beyond resolution of the current problem. Finally, the good news is that behavioral problems are generally treatable; from this perspective, they are better problems to have than many organic disorders that are less responsive to intervention.

If the parents agree to the consultation, then the pediatrician should give them the consultant's name and the reasons for this selection, the consultant's credentials, and how closely the consultant works with the primary care physician. Contacting the consultant initially and discussing the reasons for consultation are the pediatrician's responsibility.

The parents should be informed that the consultant will probably want to see both parents together to collect important data about the child's development and to obtain a detailed family history. The number of visits generally required for a consultation and its approximate cost should be discussed with the parents. After the consultation, the primary care physician should meet with the parents to discuss the consultant's findings and recommendations. Including the consultant and the child in this meeting is often useful as well. If treatment is recommended, then similar details should be provided regarding the nature of therapeutic activity and probable length of treatment (see Chapter 132, Options for the Delivery of Mental Health Services).

If the parents are reluctant to follow a consultant's recommendation for intervention, then the primary care physician should be careful to avoid supporting the parents' hesitation. Such a stance engenders lack of faith in the consultant the physician has recommended. If, however, both parents and pediatrician drastically disagree with the findings and recommendations of the consultant, then a second opinion is indicated.

Preparing the Child

The child should be told that the child's parents and the physician are concerned about aspects of the child's behavior, such as an inability to get along with friends, anger, nightmares, or difficulty coping with a physical illness. In the case of a psychosomatic symptom, the child needs to be told that pain or illness is often caused by emotional feelings or worries. Children should be informed that they will be seeing a professional who is an expert in helping with these kinds of problems; the fact that the consultant helps children by playing with them and by talking with them about their thoughts and feelings should be emphasized.

With an older child or adolescent, the pediatrician should prepare the patient for consultation even while obtaining a physical and psychosocial history. As the physician concentrates on social and emotional aspects, some teenagers may become indignant and confront the physician about the personal nature of the questions.

The physician should avoid retreating or becoming defensive but should emphasize the need for such probing personal questions to understand the symptoms or illness troubling the patient. As with parents, relating everyday examples can help the older child or adolescent understand the connection between emotions and physical well being. Teenagers, because they are struggling with the developmental tasks of adolescence, may be concerned about confidentiality. In addition, given the normal mood swings during this period, wondering about their own mental health is common for teenagers. Suggesting behavioral consultation can trigger a protest that may reflect their own worst fear—that they really are different or crazy. In most cases the pediatrician can reassure teenage patients that they indeed are not.

However, the physician must convey concern if a significant psychopathological condition is suspected. Not to do so is frightening to the patient or parent, who may recognize that reassurance is premature and inappropriate. If severe problems are present, then the pediatrician should explain that the teenager's behavior signals a departure from normal and indicates some excessive stress, which may be interfering with optimal well being. Also extremely useful is to identify some specific potential benefit of intervention that is likely to be meaningful to the patient (eg, better relationships with peers), as well as the alleviation of a problem (eg, reducing conflict with parents or feelings of anxiety).

The physician should be firm but not argumentative about the need for referral. While acknowledging the adolescent's anger or dismay, the physician needs to assert professional responsibility to render the best medical opinion, even if it is not to the patient's liking. It seems paradoxical that a sturdy posture in this regard is often reassuring, but it does convey the idea that someone is listening and hearing the patient's troubles and is concerned about the patient's behavior.

In most instances, the child or adolescent should be informed of the approximate number of visits usually required and the type of interaction to expect. If the patient inquires about the cost of the consultation and evidences concern, then the physician can assure the patient that only the parents can make this decision. In most situations, the physician can emphasize that the patient's parents are concerned enough and care enough to be willing to spend whatever it may take to obtain proper help.

In cases of overt psychosis, in which reality testing is seriously impaired, psychological preparation of the patient may be ineffective. However, the physician cannot assume that the patient is totally oblivious to the surroundings. In fact, the pediatrician can provide a stabilizing, reliable, and predictable influence for the patient. The physician can introduce the consultant as an expert in helping patients whose thoughts are confused or jumbled. Offering to be present during the first consultative session as a source of security for the patient may even be helpful for the primary care physician.

Selecting a Consultant

Choosing the appropriate professional or agency probably is the most important service that the primary care physician can provide to a patient who has psychosocial or learning problems. Although the common practice of suggesting a list of specialists protects the physician from any accusation of favoritism, it is actually not helpful to parents. A specific referral is preferable because it relieves the family of wondering whether they made the best choice.

A common issue is whether the best course of action is to use a pediatrician interested and expert in behavioral disorders, a child psychiatrist, a clinical psychologist, a psychiatric nurse, or a social worker.[4] Although a thorough discussion of this issue is beyond the scope of this chapter, a brief review of relevant training and credentials may be helpful.

Pediatricians who are well versed in managing behavioral disorders generally have had training in behavioral or developmental pediatrics (or both) after their pediatric residency. Their specialized training typically consists of a 1- to 3-year fellowship in behavioral pediatrics or child development, or both, including academic and clinical experience. Such fellowships vary greatly in their emphasis, some focusing almost exclusively on infants and young children, others covering a broad range of ages and problems. The behavioral pediatrician's area of expertise, theoretical orientation, and interests obviously reflect the specific training received.

Most physicians formally engaged in psychotherapy have been trained in psychiatry. The internship year can be the first year of a 4-year residency in psychiatry, or it can consist of a year in internal medicine, pediatrics, or neurology. Three additional years of psychiatric residency are required for board eligibility in psychiatry. Two years of child and adolescent psychiatric training (1 year of which can constitute the fourth year of psychiatric residency) are needed for board eligibility in child and adolescent psychiatry. Certification in child and adolescent psychiatry is allowed only after an individual has been certified in general psychiatry.

Psychologists vary greatly in their educational background and may have a master's or doctoral degree. Persons who are qualified to provide clinical service, both diagnostic assessment and therapy, have received a degree in clinical psychology (as opposed to developmental, experimental, physiological, or social psychology) or have completed a formal, accredited respecialization program in clinical psychology. Such training includes, in addition to a dissertation, 3 or 4 years of graduate coursework, with accompanying practicum experience, and a year of clinical internship. Graduate programs in clinical psychology and clinical internships are reviewed and accredited by the American Psychological Association.[5] In addition, the referring physician may wish to determine whether the consultant is listed in the *National Register of Health Service Providers,* which is published biannually.[6] Finally, all states now have licensing procedures for psychologists, and the physician should not use an individual who is unlicensed. In addition, licensure is often generic and does not distinguish areas of training in psychology (eg, clinical, developmental, experimental, industrial).

A clinical specialist in child and adolescent psychiatry and mental health nursing (psychiatric nurse) is required to have earned a 4-year bachelor's degree in nursing, to have obtained registered nursing licensure, and to have been involved in direct clinical nursing practice. Completion of a master's degree in psychiatric nursing is then necessary; this program consists of academic and clinical work focused on children, adolescents, and families. On providing evidence of post-master's degree, clinical experience, and access to supervision, these clinicians must pass a national examination, which results in certification by the American Nurses Association. These clinicians must be recertified every 5 years.

Social workers may have a bachelor's degree (BSW), a master's degree (MSW), or a doctoral degree (DSW or PhD). Social workers are accredited nationally by the Academy of Certified Social Workers (ACSW), a component of the National Association of Social Workers (NASW), the primary professional association. The ACSW accreditation requirements include (1) a master's degree from a school of social work accredited by the Council of Social Work Education; (2) 2 years of supervised, post-master's degree social work practice; and (3) successful completion of a written examination. All states now have licensing procedures for social workers, most with requirements similar to those of the ACSW. The ACSW and most state licenses are generic, however, and do not distinguish among practitioners in clinical social work, administration, and community organization. The NASW maintains a national register of clinical social workers who have demonstrated clinical training and experience.

Accreditation and organizational affiliations indicate only minimal standards of professional competence. Even in their original training, behavioral specialists vary substantially with regard to orientation and areas of expertise (see Chapter 132, Options for the Delivery of Mental Health Services). For example, many child psychiatry programs have a largely organic focus and emphasize psychopharmacology, whereas others provide more training in psychotherapy. Similarly, some psychologists have more expertise in assessment, whereas others have focused on intervention; some are much better trained in behavioral or cognitive-behavioral intervention than others. Mental health specialists diverge even more after their training because their knowledge and skills are influenced by their professional activities and the continuing education experiences they select.

The lines between disciplines can become blurred, with individuals developing expertise in other areas.[4] Such blurring is exacerbated by individual differences in dedication and talent.[4] Each mental health discipline has individuals who are inadequate and those who are superb. This unevenness of skill simply highlights the importance of the referring physician's systematic evaluation of consultative resources.

Knowing what behavioral resources are available in a particular community and arranging ongoing contact with appropriate individuals requires deliberate effort. Pediatricians should meet with an experienced and respected mental health professional to discuss appropriate referral resources within the community. Acquiring appropriate sophistication about available referral sources is undoubtedly time consuming, but it will ensure more meaningful referrals and, ultimately, save time.

The role of the primary care physician does not end once the referral has been made. The physician should contact the family to determine that an appointment has been made. With the appropriate permission, the physician should provide a summary of the pertinent information to the professional or agency and, in turn, expect periodic reports. It is helpful if the primary care physician clearly states at the time of referral the physician's expectations for feedback and how often this feedback is to occur. Ongoing communication allows the pediatrician to maintain an integral role in providing total care to patients. Over time, the approach also allows evaluation of the quality of service available from a particular professional or agency.

TOOLS FOR PRACTICE

Engaging Patient and Family

- *Facts for Families* (Web page), American Academy of Child & Adolescent Psychiatry (AACAP) (www.aacap.org/cs/root/facts_for_families/facts_for_families).

Practice Management and Care Coordination

- *State Mental Health Resources* (Web page), American Academy of Pediatrics (www.aap.org/commpeds/dochs/mentalhealth/chapterMap.cfm).

RELATED WEB SITES

- American Nursing Association (www.nursingworld.org/).
- American Psychological Association (www.apa.org/).
- National Association of Social Workers (www.socialworkers.org/).

AAP POLICY STATEMENTS

American Academy of Pediatrics, Committee on Quality Improvement and Subcommittee on Attention-Deficit/Hyperactivity Disorder. Diagnosis and evaluation of the child with attention-deficit/hyperactivity disorder. *Pediatrics*. 2000;105(5):1158-1170. (pediatrics.aappublications.org/cgi/content/full/105/5/1158).

American Academy of Pediatrics. Insurance coverage of mental health and substance abuse services for children and adolescents: a consensus statement. *Pediatrics*. 2000;106(4):860-862. (aappolicy.aappublications.org/cgi/content/full/pediatrics;106/4/860).

REFERENCES

1. Wolraich ML, Felice ME, Drotar D, eds. *The Classification of Child and Adolescent Mental Diagnoses in Primary Care: Diagnostic and Statistical Manual for Primary Care (DSM-PC) Child and Adolescent Version*. Elk Grove Village, IL: American Academy of Pediatrics; 1996.
2. Ammerman RT, Hersen RT. *Handbook of Child Behavior Therapy in the Psychiatric Setting*. New York, NY: Wiley; 2001.
3. American Psychiatric Association. *Diagnostic and Statistical Manual of Mental Disorders (DSM-IV-TR)*. 4th ed, text revision. Washington, DC: the Association; 2000.
4. Phillips S, Clawson L, Osinski A. Pediatricians' pet peeves about mental health referrals. In Friedman SB, DeMaso D, eds. *Adolescent Psychiatric and Behavioral Disorders, Adolescent Medicine: State of the Art Reviews*. Vol 9. Philadelphia, PA: Hanley and Belfus; 1998.
5. American Psychological Association. *General Guidelines for Providers of Psychological Services*. Washington, DC: The Association; 1987.
6. Council for the National Register of Health Service Providers in Psychology. *National Register of Health Service Providers in Psychology*. Washington, DC: The Council; 2006.

Chapter 132

OPTIONS FOR THE DELIVERY OF MENTAL HEALTH SERVICES

David J. Kolko, PhD

WHY ASSESS AND TREAT BEHAVIOR PROBLEMS IN PEDIATRIC PRIMARY CARE?

The pediatric primary care physician (PCP) is an increasingly important provider of mental health services for several reasons. Although the prevalence of emotional and behavioral problems in children is quite high, access to specialty mental health services is limited by a lack of specialists, insufficient insurance coverage, and inefficient networks. PCPs believe they have a responsibility to recognize common pediatric mental disorders[1] especially behavioral problems such as attention-deficit/hyperactivity disorder (ADHD).[2]

Providing mental health services to children in the primary care setting has challenges, including the existence of few standard psychiatric diagnostic criteria or tools,[3] limited time for clinicians, concerns about psychotropic medications by patients and clinicians, limited ability to follow-up, and limited referral options.[1,2]

Although challenging to incorporate initially, the use of structured screening programs and newer models of primary care or specialty care integration can overcome some of the aforementioned barriers and enhance the likelihood that children in need will receive services.[4] The next section reviews screening tools, and the following section discusses models of care integration.

SCREENING AND ASSESSMENT TOOLS

Overview of Tools

Despite their primary use in research applications, the measures described here may lend themselves to efficient or focused clinical assessment of an array of mental health concerns and disorders, along with related contextual contributors to such patient problems (Table 132-1 provides a summary of

Table 132-1 Representative Assessment Measures and Their Key Characteristics

PRIMARY SYMPTOMS	SOURCE	METHOD
Master screening or demographic form	CL	I
Pediatric Symptom Checklist (PSC-17)	P	SR
K-SADS Diagnostic/Needs Assessment-Brief	C, P	I
Child Health and Illness Profile—Adolescent and Child Editions (CHIP)	C	SR
Vanderbilt ADHD Diagnostic Parent Rating Scale	P, T	SR
Strengths and Difficulties Questionnaire (SDQ)	P, T	SR
Mood and Feelings Questionnaire (MFQ)	C	SR
SCARED	C	SR
FUNCTIONAL STATUS, IMPAIRMENT AND SKILL, COMPETENCY		
Clinical Global Impressions Scale (C-GAS)	CL, P, C	SR
Brief Impairment Scale (BIS)	P	I
Pediatric Quality of Life Inventory (PEDS-QL)	C	SR
ENVIRONMENTAL CONTEXT		
Patient Health Questionnaire (PHQ)	P	SR
Caregiver Strain Questionnaire (CGSQ)	P	SR
Alabama Parenting Questionnaire (APQ)	P	I, SR
Family Adaptability and Cohesion Scale	P, C	SR, or I
CLIENT CONSUMER SATISFACTION, PRACTICE CHARACTERISTICS		
Client Satisfaction Questionnaire-8 (posttreatment only)	C, P	SR
Barriers to Treatment Participation Scale (posttreatment only)	P	I
Therapist Evaluation Inventory-Revised (posttreatment only)	CL	O
SERVICE USE, INVOLVEMENT		
Individualized Goal Achievement Ratings	C, P	I
SKIP-2 Family Feedback Form	P	I
Service provider log, process of treatment	CL	O
OFFICE PRACTICE OR SYSTEM		
Physician Belief Scale	PCP	R
Mental Health Services in Primary Care Survey	PCP	SR
Chart review of pediatric services or visits	R	A

ADHD, Attention-deficit/hyperactivity disorder; *A,* archival records; *C,* child; *CL,* clinician; *I,* interview; *K-SADS,* Schedule for Affective Disorders and Schizophrenia for School-Age Children; *O,* observation; *P,* parent; *PCP,* primary care physician; *R,* researcher; *SCARED,* Scale for Anxiety and Related Emotional Disorders; *SKIP,* Services for Kids in Primary-Care study; *SR,* self-report; *T,* teacher.

characteristics of selected tools.) Assessment may permit more accurate triage and selection of appropriate treatments and referral, and may facilitate an evaluation of treatment response or outcomes. For example, office staff may use certain forms during intake in the office. Children and their caregivers may use various data collection methods (eg, tablet PC [notebook- or slate-shaped mobile computer], interview, take-home packet). The PCP may be able to request the completion of these forms at discharge to document important changes in targeted outcomes.

Representative Assessment Tools—Child Symptoms, Functioning, and Adjustment

Pediatric Symptom Checklist

The Pediatric Symptom Checklist (PSC-17)[5,6] is one of the more practical screening instruments because of its brevity and good psychometric properties such as strong internal reliability and face validity. It includes a small set of items that screen for externalizing, attentional, and internalizing problems using continuous scores and clinical cutoffs.[7] The PSC-17 compares with the Child Behavior Checklist (CBCL) in predicting child functional impairment.[8]

Vanderbilt ADHD Diagnostic Parent Rating Scale

The Vanderbilt ADHD Diagnostic Parent Rating Scale (VADPRS) evaluates ADHD (all 18 *Diagnostic and Statistical Manual of Mental Disorders,* fourth edition [DSM-IV] items), oppositional defiant disorder (ODD) (8 of 9 items), and conduct disorder (CD) (12 of 15 items) symptoms and includes 7 items that screen for anxiety and depression.[9] Parent ratings on 4-point scales are used to derive overall severity scores and diagnoses based on symptom counts. An 8-item performance scale evaluates impairment in key domains (eg, academics, peers, siblings, parents, activities). The measure has acceptable reliability and sensitivity to change, and a parallel teacher version of this scale (the Vanderbilt ADHD Diagnostic Teacher Rating Scale [VADTRS]) is available.

Child Health and Illness Profile—Child Edition

The 45-item Child Health and Illness Profile—Adolescent and Child Editions (CHIP-CE) is a brief assessment of 5 factors (physical or health satisfaction, physical and emotional discomfort, behavioral risks, achievement threats, and resilience).[10] The measure has good psychometric properties, but it awaits an evaluation of its sensitivity to treatment outcome. An adolescent version that contains additional items in various life domains has also been developed.

Mood and Feelings Questionnaire

The Mood and Feelings Questionnaire (MFQ)[11] is a 32-item self- and parent-report inventory of depressive symptoms in children and adolescents. It has sound psychometric properties and good sensitivity to symptomatic change over time. Although the MFQ was developed for epidemiologic studies, its brevity may make this screening tool useful in evaluating response to treatment.

Scale for Anxiety and Related Emotional Disorders

The Scale for Anxiety and Related Emotional Disorders (SCARED)[12] is used to assess self-reported severity of anxiety in children and adolescents. It includes 37 items rated on 3-point scales to assess the severity and presence of DSM-IV anxiety disorders. The scale has excellent psychometric properties and normative data for comparison purposes. The authors have also reported an abbreviated SCARED subscale with 5 items that can be used for general screening purposes.

Pediatric Quality of Life Measurement Model

The Pediatric Quality of Life Inventory (PEDS-QL) assesses specific health-related quality of life items from the child's perspective.[13] The measure includes 23 items in 4 dimensions (eg, physical, emotional) and has very good reliability and treatment validity for school-aged children.

Representative Assessment Tools: Environmental Context and Services

Patient Health Questionnaire

The primary caretaker completes the Patient Health Questionnaire (PHQ)[14] to screen for and evaluate the severity of a primary adult psychiatric disorder (eg, depression, substance abuse).

Caregiver Strain Questionnaire

The Caregiver Strain Questionnaire (CGSQ) evaluates changes in perceived caregiver burden resulting from having a child with a developmental or behavior disorder,[15] which is an important moderator of treatment outcome.

Alabama Parenting Questionnaire

The Alabama Parenting Questionnaire (APQ)[16] evaluates positive (eg, involvement, positive parenting) and negative (poor monitoring, corporal punishment) parenting practices related to antisocial behavior. This scale has very good psychometrics and will help evaluate any changes in primary parenting practices.

MENTAL HEALTH INTERVENTION

Efficient Referral Procedures and Materials

Indications for referral to specialty services include diagnostic uncertainty, failure to respond to treatment, presence of severe affective symptoms, and the need for continued psychotherapy.[17] By some estimates, only one third of patients follow through with recommendations to receive mental health treatment.[17] The referral process may be facilitated by providing an information packet (physician referral letter, physical examination form, immunization record) sent directly to the specialist or agency. A clinic-based automated referral system such as this was found to increase subsequent attendance in local Head Start programs.[18]

Social Support and Information

To address the burden associated with caring for and managing children with chronic health and/or mental health needs, some studies have examined the benefits of support services for this population. Mothers of children with ongoing or chronic health conditions (eg, asthma, anemia, epilepsy) were assigned to either a 12-month community-based social support intervention (the Parent-to-Parent network) or usual care.[19] The support intervention included 6 face-to-face or telephone meetings with lay interventionists whose children had similar health problems; access to information, services, and advisors; and a realistic discussion of common issues related to parenting and linkages to community services. Parental distress showed a greater change in the experimental condition but only for mothers with the highest levels of stress. The authors not only suggested that a longer series of meetings may have been helpful, but also indicated the importance of maintaining an individualized approach to meet the needs of the mothers in this study.

Internet-Based Parenting Materials or Discussion

Despite their considerable potential, few applications of interventions for mental health problems have been reported with pediatric primary care patients. In terms of the few studies reporting child mental health problems, one recent study examined a telephone-based parent-directed intervention for 7- to 15-year-old children who met the clinical cutoff on at least one of the scales of the PSC-17 or its total score.[20] The intervention consisted of a discussion of key parenting principles and review of a workbook delivered via the internet. Compared with controls, children in the intervention showed significant reductions in externalizing problems (eg, aggression, delinquent behavior, attentional problems) and were more likely to receive a mental health referral but did not differ in primary care clinic visits or medication use. Improvements in parenting (reduced corporal punishment and depression) were also found in the experimental group. This study focused on the delivery of parenting information via telephone visits, which served as a highly efficient mechanism for service delivery, and it resulted in improvement in a broad array of behavioral and emotional measures. Whether outcomes would be improved by directly involving the child's pediatrician in services or by including any specific child and parent interventions to address the child's behavior problems and related diagnostic comorbidities is unclear.

On-Site Services and Collaborative Care Management

Guidance for treating chronic mental disorders in adult primary care emphasizes the importance of several collaborative methods designed to augment service delivery and clinical response that can be organized within the pediatric setting: (1) a prepared practice (trained PCPs and available materials or tools); (2) a care manager (someone to coordinate and administer intervention plans); (3) a mental health interface to provide consultation and invoke relevant evidence-based practices[21,22]; (4) the use of stepped care procedures to address differences in severity and individual needs; (5) patient choice in selecting care management options; (6) an accessible delivery system; (7) the use of methods to address comorbidity; (8) ongoing patient follow-up; and (9) increased capacity building among PCPs.[23,24] Such methods have shown enhanced outcome for several chronic conditions, such as depression,[25-28] anxiety,[24,29] and bipolar disorder.[30-32]

These methods are applicable to managing pediatric mental health disorders and merit further empirical application with younger populations.[33] In fact, a few applications of related procedures with children and youth have been conducted to address ADHD and its correlates.[34,35] Lozano et al[36] found that peer leader education plus a nurse care manager improved asthma care and functional status in children, relative to peer leader education alone or existing care.[36] In addition, Asarnow et al[37] found that a care management approach (Youth Partners in Care [Y-PIC]) to treating adolescent depression (expert leader teams, care manager, cognitive-behavioral therapy, medication options) in 5 primary care offices was more effective than treatment as usual in reducing depressive symptoms or disorders, enhancing adjustment, and increasing satisfaction. No differences were found in the mental health practices (therapy, medication) of the PCPs, which remained at a low level. The work by Campo et al[33] describes an integrated approach to treating mental health services in pediatric primary care using a trained care manager, consistent with other recent descriptions of the role of quality improvement guidelines for the management of ADHD[34] and recommendations for the use of pathways in pediatric primary care.[38]

Promoting Service Input and Engagement Via Participatory Management

Pediatricians interested in incorporating mental health screening and collaborative care might use participatory management (PM) theory to help them customize, standardize, and pilot test interventions in primary care.[39,40] This approach incorporates translational research principles used to facilitate primary care delivery and implementation. PM consists of 3 processes that ensure that front-line staff and stakeholder input are incorporated into the development of the treatment model to address their own priorities and any barriers to quality improvement. The phased approach—customization, evaluation and refinement, and implementation—is accomplished through the use of periodic in-services at key times to obtain and exchange information (eg, just before initiation, immediately after the start of training, several months later). PM can be used to socialize pediatric colleagues in the use of novel clinical models and methods, and to obtain feedback regarding necessary adaptations of new material.

Enhanced Care Using Expanded Evidence-Based Clinical Content

Several common conditions affecting children and adolescents have new evidence about effective treatment in primary care and other community settings. One advance relates to the enhanced treatment of ADHD[41-43] that is based on a set of empirically supported practices superior to typical community care.[43] These recommendations address preparing the family for medication, arranging for a visit to review medication options, initiating a medication trial using medications with which the PCP feels most comfortable, and formally monitoring treatment responses and side effects via information from patients, parents, and teachers with standard forms (eg, target behaviors, school performance, side effects, adherence). Adequate parental preparation may facilitate acceptance and understanding of the role of medication for this condition or its more careful monitoring by the PCP, especially given high rates of poor medication adherence or follow-up.[7,35] In addition, the PCP must have preparation for the use of effective pharmacotherapy (eg, use or dosing, side effects, monitoring, alternatives), given that many PCPs report a lack of training in the management of psychosocial problems.[2,44] PCP implementation of mental health services may be enhanced via in-service training, ongoing consultation, and collaborative programming using the PM procedure.[45]

Developments in the brief treatment of children's anxiety have also been adapted for use in the primary care setting.[46] Derived from a review of the empirical literature,[47] this primary care content extends work in the area of anxiety.[48] Thus, for mild anxiety or fears, methods involve self-monitoring of anxiety or fear levels using an abbreviated scale (0 to 10), discussion of the basis for the child's anxiety or fears (cognitive restructuring), relaxation training, and suggestions to children using parent-mediated assistance to expose themselves to anxiety-eliciting situations (including direct parental reinforcement of *brave behavior*). In cases of more emergent symptoms, plans for more immediate care via referral can be made with the PCP. Such procedures may serve as a useful adjunct designed to address children's behavior problems. In a more formal and extensive treatment for adolescent depression, the incremental benefit of a cognitive-behavioral treatment (CBT) program was evaluated beyond the effects of a treatment as usual control condition consisting of selective serotonin reuptake inhibitor medication delivered outside of an experimental protocol.[49] Modest improvements occurred for the CBT and medication condition on a few outcomes (eg, depressive symptoms, outpatient visits). This study shows the feasibility of combining these methods in the context of the primary care setting.

Attention to Parental Distress or Partner Conflict

Although not directly within the purview of pediatric primary care, efforts to address parental functioning and the partner relationship are important because their influence on parenting skills can clearly affect the impact of any effort to modify their children's behavior problems. For example, one recent article provides a compelling overview of the prevalence, characteristics, consequences, and treatment of postpartum depression and concludes that many women with this condition are not receiving mental health services.[50] Recent work by Weissman et al[51] indicates that effective medication treatment of maternal depression in primary care can improve children's disorders and symptoms. This finding suggests that more active treatment of depressed mothers may enhance the functioning of both the mothers and their children. Accordingly, screening for parental dysfunction or impairment (eg, depression, anxiety, substance abuse) and developing plans to either manage parental distress or facilitate outside referral may be necessary in some cases. As noted earlier, several brief screening measures to identify psychological distress and other materials may be used (eg, list of adult referral sources, handout describing the impact of parental dysfunction on child behavior and treatment response) to prompt a discussion of parental preferences for addressing their own clinical problems. Possibly, greater focus on parental functioning or skills may enhance a parent's overall consistency and appropriateness with parenting practices at home and, ultimately, reduce the severity of a child's symptoms. Of course, any successful effort to address children's mental health must also address issues of initial treatment engagement and attention to self-management, as well as general behavior management and routines to facilitate their maintenance after treatment ends.

Incorporation of Technological Innovation and Advances

Applications of any treatment or collaborative care model may be enhanced using various technological developments designed to increase access to and the efficiency of all aspects of the service delivery process (eg, screening, assessment, monitoring, education, treatment, referral) in primary care. To promote their effectiveness, generalizability, and sustainability, the use of brief and automated efficient screening procedures that yield an immediate summary for the PCP before a visit is encouraged, perhaps using tablet PCs or internet-based data collection methods. Psychoeducational materials have been found to be both feasible and effective when posted on a Web-based platform or when made available via telephone sessions. A mental health service delivery system that includes efficient options for identifying patient needs or receiving subsequent care (eg, telephone, internet, on-site visits) might also enhance participation by larger segments of the practice who can *have it their way*.[52]

KEY PROCEDURES AND PROCESSES IN A COLLABORATIVE CARE APPROACH TO TREATMENT

Table 132-2 outlines some proposed components for implementation of a collaborative care model for the management of behavior problems in the pediatric primary care setting based on an integration of much of the work with adults and children that was described earlier in this chapter. This information may facilitate efforts to plan for, incorporate and operate, evaluate, and revise collaborative approaches designed to enhance the provision of on-site mental health services. Many of these elements have been included in a treatment effectiveness study being conducted by the author (see National Institute of Mental Health grant MH063772).

Identification and Assessment (Diagnostic Review or Triage)

To identify patient needs, an abbreviated diagnostic evaluation or related screening forms (or both) may be used. A case manager (CM) and the PCP might briefly review the case, selected targets, clinical concerns, and a proposed intervention plan (see Table 132-2). The CM might prepare an evaluation summary (eg, diagnostic status, exacerbating conditions, treatment status, service plan, treatment tasks or roles) that will be entered into the medical record and provided to the caregiver.

Patient Self-Management Promotion (Psychoeducation)

Psychoeducational materials should be provided to inform parents, children, and PCPs about relevant clinical and psychiatric conditions or issues, as needed. Sample materials can be found in several expert sources (see end of chapter Tools for Practice) and include such topics as DSM-IV disorders (ADHD, ODD, MDD), treatment methods (CBT, medication), and brief suggestions for dealing with common pediatric behavioral and emotional problems. This material should be organized for efficient administration in each office practice to facilitate routine distribution to address the family's unique needs (via handouts, Web site, or tablet PC). General information can also be furnished efficiently through any program or office Web site. One example of such a resource is provided through a local network of university researcher-practitioners and community pediatric practices called Child and Adolescent Research Network (CARE-NET; see *www.care-netpgh.org*). This Web site offers information on psychiatric disorders and clinical services, among other treatment and research resources, available to families and PCPs.

Treatment Facilitation

Once treatment targets are identified, the PCP must select relevant treatment procedures. Because no simple risk-stratification algorithm exists, certain guides may help identify key priorities[53]: (1) medication management and monitoring guidelines should be integrated for ADHD and other disorders[54]; (2) parental engagement should be promoted, parenting skills

Table 132-2 Key Components of a Proposed Collaborative Care Model for the Management of Behavior Problems in the Pediatric Primary Care Setting

GOAL	FUNCTION	AGENT	TASK OR ACTIVITY
Identify or assess	Announcements, screens Assess, diagnose	All CM	Case finding using established behavior problems scale (eg, PSC-17; 6 items) and brief diagnostic interview (K-SADS PL)
Enhance patient self-management	Educate or destigmatize (psychoeducation)	CM, PCP	Education about diagnosis, behavior problems, and treatment options (eg, handouts, DVDs, Web site, etc.)
	Motivate or activate	CM, PCP	Brief motivational interview or target behavior selection (IGAR)
Facilitate treatment	Track behavioral outcomes (via tablet PC, medical record, etc.)	CM	Regular contacts to track effectiveness and identify need for treatment changes or clinical emergencies (IGAR, VADPRS)
	Case supervision, quality monitoring	CM	Regular reviews patient outcomes with supervisor and PCP (weekly case review; calls; tablet PC notes or records)
	Deliver or support services or treatment with revised primary (phase I) protocol materials	CM, PCP	Deliver protocol material (brief, focused on behavior management) via telephone or on site. Focus on adherence, any side effects, gains, and need for any changes in plans or methods.
	Medication management by PCP (consider stimulants first)	PCP	Prescribe medication for comorbid ADHD with input from CM using medication protocol and consultation with tablet PC.
	Facilitate, coordinate case using revised treatment algorithm	CM	Coordinate with PCP or specialty mental health provided to address priorities in order (ADHD → ODD → parental functioning → serious problems); monitor and maintain registry.
Establish primary care linkage	Communicate with patient	CM, PCP	Educate about diagnosis; arrange PCP visit; re: ADHD. Monitor status (calls) and link patient to PCP.
	Communicate, consult with PCP; re: patient's behavioral or clinical status and treatment outcomes	CM, PCP	Provide information to PCP via meeting, telephone, fax, letter; review patients not improving within 4-8 wk; make recommendations to change plan; refer back to PCP.
	Communicate with PC	CM, PC	Review records of services provided; other monitoring materials.
Mental health specialty linkage (therapy, consultations, etc.)	Communicate with patient	CM, PCP	Review referral to metal health specialist; re: alternative treatment. Encourage or facilitate follow-up visits.
	Communicate with mental health specialist; re: behavioral status and treatment outcomes	CM, MHS, PCP, CP	Review patients with minimal progress after 4-8 wk; discuss possible referral and CM involvement with CP. Refer, provide information (telephone, fax) and support treatment.
	Communicate with PC	CM, PC	Review monitoring forms.

ADHD, Attention-deficit/hyperactivity disorder; *CM,* case manager; *CP,* community provider; *IGAR,* Individualized Goal Achievement Rating; *K-SADS,* Schedule for Affective Disorders and Schizophrenia for School-Age Children; *MHS,* Mental Health Specialist; *ODD,* oppositional defiant disorder; *PC,* psychiatric consultant; *PCP,* primary care physician; *PSC-17,* Pediatric Symptom Checklist; *VADPRS,* Vanderbilt ADHD Diagnostic Parent Rating Scale.

Sources: Hegel MT, Imming J, Cyr-Provost M, et al. Role of behavioral health professionals in a collaborative stepped care treatment model for depression in primary care: Project IMPACT. *Fam Sys Health.* 2002;20(1):265-277; Oishi SM, Shoai R, Katon W, et al. Improving mood: promoting access to collaborative treatment: impacting late life depression: integrating a depression intervention into primary care. *Psychiatr Q.* 2003;74(1):75-89; Saur CD, Harpole LH, Steffens DC, et al. Treating depression in primary care: an innovative role for mental health nurses. *J Am Psychiatr Nurs Assoc.* 2002;8(5):159-167; Unutzer J, Katon W, Williams JW Jr, et al. Improving primary care for depression in late life: the design of a multicenter randomized trial. *Med Care.* 2001;39(8):785-799.

taught, and home contingency management routines developed; (3) the PCP should help older children learn self-control and social skills; (4) brief relaxation should be offered and fear-eliciting thoughts countered with mildly anxious children; and (5) the PCP should screen and refer for significant parental or partner dysfunction (eg, promoting positive relationships, reducing coercion via problem solving, communication).

The PCP or a CM can deliver focused intervention and case management services based on family preferences (on site, telephone) and in collaboration with the operations of each practice to enhance feasibility and sustainability. In general, common treatment methods seek to develop consequences for various child behaviors, to teach skills to the child and parent, and to establish positive parent-child interactions using treatment guidelines. When applicable, a CM should recommend involvement in community-based activities or provide crisis management.

Linkages—Consultation With the Primary Care Physician

The CM may consult with the PCP at several junctures. PCPs should be informed of the findings of the diagnostic evaluation to familiarize CMs with the clinical targets of the case and treatment options and discuss collaborative arrangements for initiating intervention in the practice. PCPs also want to be kept informed as to the status of the patients they refer for mental health services and to discuss arrangements for possible co-location with a mental health care provider.[17] The CM will provide the PCP with updated information about key targets or conditions (eg, ADHD ratings from teachers) to facilitate intervention and provide feedback regarding the initial effects of psychosocial or medication treatment. Finally, the CM should discuss potential aftercare and follow-up plans with the PCP so as to promote continuity of care.

Linkages—Consultation With Specialty Services

The PCP should develop clear criteria for making a facilitated referral into specialty care and to develop a relationship to key community providers.[55] Such criteria may vary by level of clinical severity or condition and may reflect cases needing alternative treatments not adequately addressed in the office. Criteria should also be designated for existing cases that may need a referral to a community resource provider as a result of showing a poor clinical response to treatment after a reasonable period (eg, symptoms got worse, child's functionality has deteriorated, parents or family system are unable to ensure safety or efficacy). Routine follow-up telephone calls can be supplemented by updated disposition plans to provide written documentation of all aftercare services and recommendations.

FUTURE DIRECTIONS

This chapter describes some of the potential benefits and challenges associated with both the standardization of assessment procedures and implementation of practice-based interventions in primary care that can address children's psychosocial symptoms or disorders, functional or health status, and treatment compliance. A development that has been encouraged involves the use of collaborative care treatments that include elements of the chronic care model of disease or disorder management. Indeed, collaborative care models provide a helpful organizing framework for expanding the initial intervention model by delivering more coordinated mental health services to treat developmental and behavioral disorders in primary care and by placing greater responsibility on the practice for the implementation of these services. Several programmatic and practice developments were recommended to enhance the integration, use, impact, and maintenance of this intervention in the pediatric setting, notably, advances in conceptual models, clinical materials or content, and technological innovations or developments that we have successfully applied in the pilot work.

Additional collaborative care intervention studies are needed in primary care with children and adolescents to learn the specific care elements that are needed to improve the quality of treatment for specific psychiatric conditions and the degree of infrastructure needed to support a collaborative care approach. Finally, understanding how these interventions can be sustained and financed in the long run is also important.

SUMMARY

Many psychiatric problems in youth are clinically and socially significant concerns embedded in vulnerable families that require innovative models of service delivery. Primary care provides a child- and family-friendly setting in which efficacious interventions can be employed to reduce children's symptoms, enhance adjustment, and promote child and family well being. Moreover, coordinated on-site services may also convey beneficial preventive effects (eg, fewer office or emergency room visits, reductions in delinquency and school failure, placement, system involvement). Such outcomes may help promote the ultimate goal of implementing integrated collaborative care for common child mental health disorders.

The author expresses his appreciation to the clinical and research staff of the Services for Kids in Primary-Care study (SKIP), to Elizabeth Austin Holden and Carrie Fascetti, Megan Griuas, H. Eric Hinrichson, Heather Bragg, to the physicians and staff of Children's Community Pediatrics, and to Drs. David Brent, John Campo, Kelly Kelleher, Amy Kilbourne, Harold Pincus, Evelyn Reis, Dana Rofey, Bruce Rollman, Abby Schlesinger, Stephen Wisniewski, and David Wolfson. Preparation of this chapter was supported, in part, by National Institute of Mental Health grants MH63772, MH57727, and MH66371.

TOOLS FOR PRACTICE

Engaging Patient and Family

- *Facts for Families* (fact sheet), American Academy of Child and Adolescent Psychiatry (AACAP) (aacap.org/cs/root/facts_for_families/facts_for_families).

Medical Decision Support

- *Alabama Parenting Questionnaire* (questionnaire), Frick P (fs.uno.edu/pfrick/APQ.html).
- *Child Behavior Checklist* (checklist), Thomas Achenbach, Ph.D. (www.aseba.org/products/forms.html).
- *Child Health and Illness Profile (CHIP)* (questionnaire), Johns Hopkins Bloomberg School of Public Health (www.chip.jhu.edu/).
- *Client Satisfaction Questionnaire* (questionnaire), Attkisson, C (web.mac.com/cliffattkisson/iWeb/TamalpaisMatrix/CSQ%20Scales.html).
- *Clinical Global Impressions Scale* (form), (www.neurotransmitter.net/CGI.pdf).
- *Family Adaptability & Cohesion Scale* (questionnaire), Olsen D et al (www.facesiv.com/studies/fip.html#inventories).
- *Mood and Feelings Questionnaire* (questionnaire), Adrian Angold and Elizabeth J. Costello (devepi.mc.duke.edu/mfq.html).
- *NICHQ Vanderbilt Assessment Scale—Parent Informant* (questionnaire), American Academy of Pediatrics (www.aap.org/bookstore).
- *NICHQ Vanderbilt Assessment Scale—Teacher Informant* (questionnaire), American Academy of Pediatrics (www.aap.org/bookstore).
- *Patient Health Questionnaire (PHQ)* (questionnaire), Spitzer R, Williams J, Kroenke K (www.pdhealth.mil/guidelines/downloads/appendix2.pdf).
- *Pediatric Quality of Life (PEDS-QL)* (other), James Varni, Ph.D. (www.pedsql.org/).
- *Pediatric Symptom Checklist* (checklist), Michael Jellenik, MD, and J. Michael Murphy, EdD (www.mgh.harvard.edu/allpsych/PediatricSymptomChecklist/psc_home.htm).
- *Scale for Anxiety and Related Emotional Disorders (SCARED)* (questionnaire), Birmaher B et al (www.wpic.pitt.edu/research/city/Family/Anxiety/OnlineAnxietyScreen_files/PDF%20Files/Scared%20Child-final.pdf).
- *Strength and Difficulties Questionnaire* (questionnaire), Goodman (incredibleyears.com/Resources/pathfinders-teacher-questionnaire-strength-difficulties.pdf).

RELATED WEB SITES

- American Academy of Pediatrics: AAP Children's Health Topic: Mental Health (www.aap.org/healthtopics/behavior.cfm).
- National Initiative for Children's Healthcare Quality (NICHQ): Chronic Conditions: ADHD (www.nichq.org/NICHQ/topics/chronicconditions/ADHD).

AAP POLICY STATEMENT

American Academy of Pediatrics, Committee on Quality Improvement and Subcommittee on Attention-Deficit/Hyperactivity Disorder. Clinical practice guideline: diagnosis and evaluation of the child with attention-deficit/hyperactivity disorder. *Pediatrics*. 2000;105(5):1158-1170. (aappolicy.aappublications.org/cgi/content/full/pediatrics;105/5/1158).

REFERENCES

1. Kelleher K, Scholle SH, Feldman HM, et al. A fork in the road: decision time for behavioral pediatrics. *J Dev Behav Pediatr.* 1999;20(3):181-186.
2. Rushton JL, Forcier M, Schectman RM. Epidemiology of depressive symptoms in the National Longitudinal Study of Adolescent Health. *J Am Acad Child Adolesc Psychiatry.* 2002;41(2):199-205.
3. Gardner W, Kelleher K, Pajer K, et al. Primary care clinicians' use of standardized psychiatric diagnoses. *Child Care Health Dev.* 2004;30(5):401-412.
4. Ringeisen H, Oliver KA, Menvielle E. Recognition and treatment of mental disorders in children: considerations for pediatric health systems. *Paediatr Drugs.* 2002;4(11):697-703.
5. Jellinek M, Murphy M, Little M, et al. Use of the pediatric symptom checklist to screen for psychosocial problems in pediatric primary care. *Arch Pediatr Adolesc Med.* 1999;153:254-260.
6. Jellinek M, Murphy JM. The recognition of psychosocial disorders in pediatric office practice: the current status of the Pediatric Symptom Checklist. *J Dev Behav Pediatr.* 1990;11(5):273-278.
7. Gardner W, Murphy M, Childs G, et al. The PSC-17: a brief pediatric symptom checklist with psychosocial problem subscales. A report from PROS and ASPN. *Ambulatory Child Health.* 1999;5:225-236.
8. Gardner WP, Lucas A, Kolko DJ, et al. Comparison of the PSC-17 and alternative mental health screens in an at-risk primary care sample. *J Am Acad Child Adolesc Psychiatry.* 2007;46(5):611-618.
9. Wolraich ML, Lambert W, Doffing MA, et al. Psychometric properties of the Vanderbilt ADHD diagnostic parent rating scale in a referred population. *J Pediatr Psychol.* 2003;28(8):559-567.
10. Rebok G, Riley A, Forrest C, et al. Elementary school-aged children's reports of their health: a cognitive interviewing study. *Qual Life Res.* 2001;10:59-70.
11. Angold A, Costello E. The Child and Adolescent Psychiatric Assessment (CAPA). *J Am Acad Child Adolesc Psychiatry.* 2000;39(1):39-48.
12. Muris P, Merckelbach H, Moulaert V, et al. Associations of symptoms of anxiety disorders and self-reported behavior problems in normal children. *Psychological Reports.* 2000;86(1):157-162.
13. Varni JW, Katz ER, Seid M, et al. The Pediatric Cancer Quality of Life Inventory (PCQL). I. Instrument development, descriptive statistics, and cross-informant variance. *J Behav Med.* 1998;21(2):179-204.
14. Lowe B, Grafe K, Zipfel S, et al. Diagnosing ICD-10 depressive episodes: superior criterion validity of the Patient Health Questionnaire. *Psychother Psychosom.* 2004;73(6):386-390.
15. Brannan AM, Heflinger CA. The Caregiver Strain Questionnaire: measuring the impact on the family living with a child with serious emotional disturbance. *J Emotional Behav Disord.* 1997;5(4): 212-222.
16. Shelton KK, Frick PJ, Wooten J. Assessment of parenting practices in families of elementary school-age children. *J Clin Child Psychol.* 1996;25:317-329.
17. Williams J, Palmes G, Klinepeter K, et al. Referral by pediatricians of children with behavioral health disorders. *Clin Pediatr.* 2005;44(4):343-349.
18. Silverstein M, Mack C, Reavis N, et al. Effect of a clinic-based referral system to head start: a randomized control trial. *JAMA.* 2004;292(8):968-971.
19. Silver EJ, Ireys HT, Bauman LJ, et al. Psychological outcomes of a support intervention in mothers of children with ongoing health conditions: the parent-to-parent network. *J Comm Psychol.* 1997;25(3):249-264.

20. Borowsky IW, Mozayeny SM, Stuenkel KN, et al. Effects of a primary care-based intervention on violent behavior and injury in children. *Pediatrics.* 2004;114:392-399.
21. Oxman TE, Dietrich AJ, Schulberg HC. The depression care manager and mental health specialist as collaborators within primary care. *Am J Geriatr Psychiatry.* 2003; 11(5):507-516.
22. Oxman TE, Dietrich AJ, Williams J, et al. A three-component model for reengineering systems for the treatment of depression in primary care. *Psychosomatics.* 2002;43(6):441-450.
23. Rollman BL, Belnap BH, Reynolds CF, et al. A contemporary protocol to assist primary care physicians in the treatment of panic and generalized anxiety disorders. *Gen Hosp Psychiatry.* 2003;25:74-82.
24. Rollman BL, Weinreb L, Korsen N, et al. Implementation of guideline-based care for depression in primary care. *Admin Policy Ment Health and Mental Health Serv Res.* 2006;33(1):47-57.
25. Dietrich AJ, Oxman TE, Williams J, et al. Going to scale: re-engineering systems for primary care treatment of depression. *Ann Fam Med.* 2004;2:301-304.
26. Hunkeler EM, Meresman JF, Hargreaves WA, et al. Efficacy of nurse telehealth care and peer support in augmenting treatment of depression in primary care. *Arch Fam Med.* 2000;9:700-708.
27. Katzelnick DJ, Simon GE, Pearson SD, et al. Randomized trial of a depression management program in high utilizers of medical care. *Arch Fam Med.* 2000;9:345-351.
28. Simon G, Von Korff M, Rutter C, et al. Randomized trial of monitoring, feedback, and management of care by telephone to improve treatment of depression in primary care. *BMJ.* 2000;320:550-554.
29. Roy-Byrne P, Katon W, Cowley DS, et al. A randomized effectiveness trial of collaborative care for patients with panic disorder in primary care. *Arch Gen Psychiatry.* 2001;58:869-876.
30. Bruce ML, Ten Have TR, Reynolds CF, et al. Reducing suicidal ideation and depressive symptoms in depressed older primary care patients. *JAMA.* 2004;291(9):1081-1091.
31. Simon G, Ludman E, Unutzer J, et al. Randomized trial of a population-based care program for people with bipolar disorder. *Psychologic Med.* 2005;35:13-24.
32. Unutzer J, Katon W, Callahan C, et al. Collaborative care management of late-life depression in the primary care setting: a randomized controlled trial. *JAMA.* 2002; 288(22):2836-2845.
33. Campo JV, Shafer S, Strohm J, et al. Pediatric behavioral health in primary care: a collaborative approach. *J Am Psychiatr Nurse Assoc.* 2005;11(5):276-282.
34. Leslie L, Weckerly J, Plemmons D, et al. Implementing the American Academy of Pediatrics attention-deficit/hyperactivity disorder diagnostic guidelines in primary care settings. *Pediatrics.* 2004;114(1):129-140.
35. Rushton JL, Fant KE, Clark SJ. Use of pediatric guidelines in the primary care of children with attention-deficit/hyperactivity disorder. *Pediatrics.* 2004;114(1): 23-28.
36. Lozano P, Finkelstein JA, Carey VJ, et al. A multisite randomized trial of the effects of physician education and organizational change in chronic-asthma care: health outcomes of the Pediatric Asthma Care Patient Outcomes Research Team II study. *Arch Pediatr Adolesc Med.* 2004;158:875-883.
37. Asarnow JR, Jaycox LH, Duan N, et al. Effectiveness of a quality improvement intervention for adolescent depression in primary care clinics. *JAMA.* 2005;293(3):311-319.
38. Sayal K. Pathways to care for children with mental health problems. *J Child Psychol Psychiatry.* 2005;47:649-659
39. Valentine NM. A national model for participative management and policy development. *Nurs Admin Q.* 1996; 21:24-34.
40. Leana C, Florkowski G. Employee involvement programs: implementing psychological theory and management practice. *Res Pers Hum Resour Manage.* 1992;10: 233-270.
41. American Academy of Child and Adolescent Psychiatry. Practice parameter for the use of stimulant medications in the treatment of children, adolescents, and adults. *J Am Acad Child Adolesc Psychiatry.* 2002;41(2 suppl): 26S-49S.
42. American Academy of Pediatrics. Clinical practice guidelines: treatment of the school-aged child with attention-deficit/hyperactivity disorder. *Pediatrics.* 2001;108: 1033-1044.
43. Jensen PS, Hinshaw SP, Swanson JM, et al. Findings from the NIMH Multimodal Treatment Study of ADHD (MTA): implications and applications for primary care providers. *J Dev Behav Pediatr.* 2001;22:60-73.
44. Leaf P, Owens P, Leventhal J, et al. Pediatricians' training and identification and management of psychosocial problems. *Clin Pediatr.* 2004;43:355-365.
45. Kilbourne AM, Schulberg HC, Post JA, et al. Translating evidence-based depression management services to community-based primary care pediatrics. *Milbank Q.* 2004;82(4):631-659.
46. Weersing VR. Brief CBT for Pediatric Internalizing Disorders. Presented at the Child Depression Consortium Meeting, sponsored by the Division of Pediatric Translational Research and Treatment Development, National Institutes of Health, and the Department of Psychiatry, University of Pittsburgh, Pittsburgh, PA, 2005.
47. Compton SN, March JS, Brent D, et al. Cognitive-behavioral psychotherapy for anxiety and depressive disorders in children and adolescents: an evidence-based medicine review. *J Am Acad Child Adolesc Psychiatry.* 2004;48(8): 930-959.
48. Campo JV, Perel J, Lucas A, et al. Citalopram treatment of pediatric recurrent abdominal pain and comorbid internalizing disorders: an exploratory study. *J Am Acad Child Adolesc Psychiatry.* 2004;43:1234-1242.
49. Clarke G, Debar L, Lynch F, et al. A randomized effectiveness trial of brief cognitive-behavioral therapy for depressed adolescents receiving antidepressant medication. *J Am Acad Child Adolesc Psychiatry.* 2005;44(9): 888-898.
50. Logsdon MC, Wisner K, Billings DM, et al. Raising awareness of primary care providers about postpartum depression. *Issues Ment Health Nurs.* 2006;27(1):59-73.
51. Weissman MM, Pilowsky DJ, Wickramaratne PJ, et al. Remissions in maternal depression and child psychopathology: a STAR*D-Child Report. *JAMA.* 2006;295(12): 1389-1398.
52. Kelleher K. Prevention and intervention in primary care. In: Remschmidt H, Belfer M, Goodyear I, eds. *Facilitating Pathways: Care, Treatment and Prevention in Child and Adolescent Mental Health.* Heidelberg, Germany: Springer-Verlag; 2004.
53. Arnold LE, Hoagwood K, Jensen PS, et al. Toward clinically relevant clinical trials. *Psychopharmacol Bull.* 1997; 33:135-142.
54. Dulcan MK, Lizarralde C, eds. *Helping Parents, Youth, and Teachers Understand Medications for Behavioral and Emotional Problems: A Resource Book of Medication Information Handouts.* 2nd ed. Vol. 2. Washington, DC: American Psychiatric Publishing; 2003.
55. Hacker K, Weidner D, McBride J. Integrating pediatrics and mental health: the reality is in the relationships. *Arch Pediatr Adolesc Med.* 2004;158(8):833-834.

Chapter 133

MEDICATION MANAGEMENT FOR EMOTIONAL AND BEHAVIORAL PROBLEMS

Matthew B. Perkins, MD, MBA; Peter S. Jensen, MD

Prescribing medications for emotional and behavior problems in children and adolescents has moved into the purview of the primary care physician (PCP). The advent of new medications that have less risk and simpler management profiles as compared with the older generation of medications accelerated the PCP's prescribing of psychiatric medication to children and adolescents.[1]

Recent warnings[2,3] from the US Food and Drug Administration (FDA) regarding the use of antidepressant and stimulant medications may make PCPs reluctant to engage in medication management for emotional and behavioral problems in children. Another deterrent is the lack of training for PCPs in the use of these medications.

Although psychotherapies are excellent treatment modalities, they are sometimes insufficient to bring an affected child to a normal range of functioning when impairment exists, and they are not effective for all children.[4] Furthermore, psychotherapeutic regimens can be difficult to sustain over a long period. In the treatment of emotional and behavioral problems, PCPs should have several treatment options on which to draw, including medications when appropriate. This chapter discusses the role of the PCP and optimal medication management strategies for children and adolescents with emotional and behavioral problems. The chapter also discusses obstacles to medication use and suggests techniques for overcoming these obstacles.

OBSTACLES TO EFFECTIVE MEDICATION USE

A variety of barriers can act as obstacles to effective medication use in primary care settings (Box 133-1).

Lack of Time

PCPs' time with each patient is both valuable and limited. One complicated and time-consuming case can disrupt the office schedule, resulting in frustrated patients and clinicians. Clinicians may think the time involved to manage medications effectively for emotional or behavioral issues comes at too great a cost to the rest of their practice.

Lack of Training

PCPs have often had little or no formal training in child and adolescent psychiatry and the use of psychiatric medications. Those who have received training find keeping up on new drugs, recent FDA warnings, and concerns about the use of psychoactive medications in children and adolescents challenging. Furthermore, the options for further medical education are often limited.

BOX 133-1 Obstacles to Effective Medication Use

- PCP's lack of time
- PCP's lack of training
- Lack of adequate insurance payment to PCP
- Limited parental knowledge about disorders and medication treatment strategies
- Negative parental beliefs about medication treatment strategies
- Limited family resources
- Teacher's knowledge and beliefs and school policies and resources
- Therapist's lack of training or beliefs

PCP, Primary care physician.

Payment

The current system is not designed to pay PCPs adequately for the time they spend working on complex and challenging cases. Although PCPs are often willing to help and extend themselves for their patients, the less well-defined and poorly paid billing options for clinicians may act as powerful disincentives to PCPs' willingness to provide these services.

Limited Parental Knowledge

At the time of an emotional or behavioral disorder diagnosis, parents may not know much about the disorder, the treatment, or how to access needed services. Years may pass before parents learn to navigate the mental health system effectively so as to get the care and services that their child needs.

Negative Parental Beliefs

Either from the media or from personal experience, parents may have negative beliefs about medication use to treat emotional and behavioral problems. A growing literature documents both the stigma among parents associated with psychiatric medications and the increasing use of these medications by physicians treating children and adolescents. The PCP must take the time to identify these beliefs and parental concerns. If they go unaddressed, these concerns will interfere with effective medication management.

Family Financial Resources

The cost of medications for emotional and behavioral problems can be high. Parents may be reluctant or embarrassed to admit that they cannot pay for the medication. In such situations, parents may take the prescription and simply never have it filled. Parents may also have to make difficult choices between paying for a medication and purchasing items of necessity. Parents may be unaware of programs offered by pharmaceutical companies to aid families in need with prescription expenses or may not ask the PCP to consider a less-expensive option. The family's insurance company will often refuse to cover the medication that may be most effective for a particular child. Additionally, the insurance company may request preauthorization for nonformulary medications or require that the medication be prescribed by a mental health specialist. Insurance payment constraints may also limit the amount of time that the PCP has available to spend with a family.

Teacher's Knowledge and Beliefs and School Policies and Resources

A teacher's knowledge and beliefs about psychiatric medications, and a teacher's training in classroom management may be obstacles to effective medication use. Although rating scales that teachers complete are an important component of diagnosis and effective medication management, teachers may be reluctant to complete them. Additionally, some states prohibit teachers and schools from explicitly recommending medications. Although physicians may make medication suggestions, these laws may have chilling effects on teacher-parent and teacher-physician communications by discouraging teachers from being candid with parents about the problems they see in the classroom. Communication with the school provides important diagnostic and therapeutic information.

Therapist's Lack of Knowledge and Beliefs About Medication

The PCP prescriber will often work with the patient's mental health care provider whose medication knowledge and beliefs might be a potential barrier to compliance and response. For example, a psychotherapist may have a particular bias in favor of psychotherapy over medication. This bias may be important, given data from several recent major studies[5-7] in attention-deficit/hyperactivity disorder (ADHD) and depression that therapy alone may not be nearly as effective as medication, either alone or in combination with therapy.

OVERCOMING OBSTACLES

In the medical home, the PCP should be the point person for treatment planning and implementation. This task requires determining what resources are available in the community for school and home behavioral interventions, identifying the family's performance goals, and determining the family's preference and experience with interventions. The PCP must anticipate these obstacles and work to overcome them.

Lack of Time

PCPs need to be proactive and creative about scheduling time to address the pharmaceutical management of emotional or behavioral problems. One way clinicians are able to maintain their schedule is to arrange particularly difficult cases before planned breaks, before lunch, or as the last appointment of the day. If these cases last longer than expected, then the rest of the schedule may still be maintained. If PCPs find that most of their time is spent in collecting data, then they might train staff to retrieve relevant information through the use of questionnaires that capture the key diagnostic and follow-up issues. The systematic gathering of information may not only improve the information that clinicians obtain, it may also result in more thorough evaluations. Furthermore, as PCPs become more adept at addressing these cases, many find they become more efficient. In many instances, a nurse or receptionist can play helpful roles in gathering initial data or in providing the needed additional information and support to families.

Lack of Training

PCPs may need to look to colleagues from child psychiatry and developmental and behavioral pediatrics to develop a network of consultation and referral for psychiatric medications. These relationships may prove to be beneficial to all parties because PCPs may learn more about the management of emotional or behavioral problems, and establish partnerships to address mental health care appropriately in a variety of settings. Furthermore, innovative collaborations and trainings are being developed to assist PCPs in managing mental health issues. In Massachusetts and Minnesota, innovative collaborations have been established, with ongoing training and back-up support for PCPs being provided by mental health specialists. Even when such solutions are not available locally, innovative PCPs may often find that they can approach mental health specialist colleagues and ask them to provide back-up for specific cases. In other situations, approaching this problem strategically may make sense, such as working to encourage a local pediatric organization to form special relationships with appropriate local mental health care providers and organizations.

Payment

Payment is another area that requires creative and ethical energy. One option is to learn from PCPs who have been successful in achieving appropriate payment rates. Another option is appropriate referral of complex and challenging cases that require the services of specific mental health care providers. PCPs need to know when more services and support are needed than the PCP can provide. PCPs might also encourage their patients and families to write their insurance companies or employers' insurance purchasing agent to address payment issues. Ultimately, these problems will need to be addressed at state and national levels, and strategic partnerships between family advocacy organizations and national pediatric societies will be needed. Such efforts are already underway in the area of ADHD.

Limited Parental Knowledge

After identifying a child's mental health disorder, the PCP should provide written information about the diagnosis, treatment goals, and interventions, as well as resources where the family can obtain more information. PCPs should educate the parents about the disorder and address any misconceptions or stigmas about the disorder or treatment. Many Web sites are available that offer such information. The PCP should also encourage the parents to be active partners in obtaining information. Parents have the responsibility of becoming their child's case manager, just as a parent must be an active partner in caring for children with other chronic diseases such as diabetes, cystic fibrosis, or asthma.

When providing information to parents, the clinician should state that medication alone may not solve the child's problem. Helping parents see themselves as part of the solution is critical in helping parents to see their role as active partners in life-long care. As partners in care, parents will learn about the disorder and how to access available help and services, including psychotherapy. Establishing regular communication with parents and school personnel to monitor the child's progress is necessary. Determining target behaviors of concern to the family and the child with input from teachers and others helps provide measures of the effectiveness of the treatment. PCPs must be comfortable in telling parents, "I can't do this without you. The medication may be helpful, but treatment will not be nearly as effective unless you learn all you can about this disorder and learn how you can best help your child. No one knows your child as well as you do. As your child's doctor, I can help a lot; but I need you to become the expert on how this disorder affects your child." Just as asthma medications may not be effective if the parent does not take steps to eliminate allergens from food and from the house, the parent with a child with a mental health disorder must become equally savvy in learning what triggers or mitigates a child's emotional and behavioral symptoms.

The range of potential therapeutic options needs to be explained to the parent. The benefits and drawbacks of medication and other treatments must be explained to both the parents and the patient. The family must arrive at a choice, and the PCP must help everyone in the family do so. In severe cases, or when prior treatment has failed, combined treatment options should be encouraged in consultation with specialists. In addition, the prescriber should work to involve the child in the process at a developmentally appropriate level and help the child to believe that children have an active role in their recovery. The clinician should help the child understand that the medications are not to control behavior but to help the child have increased self-control, which will allow the child to be successful in achieving goals.

Families will often have concerns about medication. These concerns must be anticipated and actively elicited. At the start, telling the parents "I don't put your child on medication; that will be your decision" may be helpful. Understanding a family's specific needs and values will encourage the expression of concerns and questions. Successfully involving the family takes knowledge, effort, and time. Additionally, the clinician should encourage participation in parental support groups, such as Children and Adults With Attention Deficit/Hyperactivity Disorder (CHADD) and the National Alliance on Mental Illness. One strategy might be to tell parents, "I need you to attend a CHADD meeting before our next visit, read the following book, and to go online to a certain Web site and download such-and-such fact sheet"; or write out a prescription to parents that says, "Instructions: Attend one CHADD meeting every month."

Negative Parental Beliefs

Psychotherapy combined with pharmacologic intervention is often associated with better outcomes than either treatment alone. Educating families about the benefits of interventions and helping them understand how these combined approaches can result in better outcomes are important tasks for PCPs. Combined interventions typically produce additive effects in many domains, thus bringing children closer to normal functioning. For example, in the case of ADHD, maximal improvement may be reached in school with less-complex and less-restrictive behavioral interventions (eg, special class placement can often be avoided) and with a lower dose of medication.

Family Resources

The first step for the PCP is to ask the family whether financial issues may get in the way of providing a medication. The PCP must have a good understanding of the costs of the medications if the family is purchasing the medication out of pocket. Additionally, the PCP should consider using resources within the office to help parents request or apply for medication from pharmaceutical companies that offer programs to assist families. Furthermore, the PCP should be prepared to consider alternative medications or forms when prescribing. For example, the generic drug fluoxetine is available for treating depression and anxiety disorder, and it is cheaper than comparable brand-name medications.

Insurance coverage is another area in which the PCP must be proactive and get involved. If a medication that is proven to be effective and safe is not authorized by the insurance company, then the PCP or the PCP's office might directly engage the insurer and provide a clinical justification for the use of the medication. Although this process can be time consuming, it also helps build an alliance with the family. The family will recognize that the PCP is working for the best clinical outcome for the patient. Sample letters that PCPs may use are available.[8]

Limited Teacher's Knowledge

Teachers may not have enough information about mental illness among youth. Issues such as school resources, lack of knowledge about mental illness, and difficulties with physician-parent-teacher communication should be considered at local pediatric society meetings. Possible solutions may include more in-services in the form of community service by PCPs, alone or in combination with child and adolescent psychiatrists. Another option that some PCPs use is a personalized form letter sent to teachers, informing them about a child's condition (ADHD, for example) and asking for their help and cooperation in the child's treatment plan.

Therapist's Lack of Knowledge and Beliefs About Medication

When referral to mental health care providers is appropriate, then the clinician should negotiate roles and responsibilities between the PCP and the mental health care provider. Continuing to monitor the patient is often necessary in the primary care setting after referral to the mental health specialist and to maintain contact with the mental health care provider.

OPTIMAL MEDICATION MANAGEMENT STRATEGIES

A PCP can use several strategies to ensure that medication treatment is effective and safe for the child (Box 133-2). Following are general guidelines that constitute optimal medication management strategies.

Conduct an Initial Evaluation to Diagnose the Child Properly

The first step in managing the medication of a child or adolescent is to conduct an initial evaluation to determine the appropriate diagnosis. Although clinical experience and judgment has no substitute, the use of standardized measures such as the Vanderbilt ADHD Diagnostic Rating Scale or the Pediatric Symptom Checklist provides a systematic way to evaluate symptoms. Additionally, standardized measures allow for a common language for consultation and discussion among colleagues, and it serves as a baseline that permits progress to be tracked. Even highly trained clinicians produce unreliable assessments without the use of a systematic, structured format.[9]

Ensure an Adequate Trial of an Appropriate Medication

Every child with a well-diagnosed psychiatric disorder deserves an adequate trial of appropriate medications. Stimulants work in up to 96% of children with ADHD.[10] Other agents (selective serotonin reuptake inhibitors, atypical antipsychotics) are effective for specific conditions (Box 133-3). All medications must be titrated to effect, which requires close follow-up. The frequency and immediacy of the follow-up depends on the potential side effects, the coadministration of other medications, and the clinical condition of the child. For antidepressant medication, the FDA suggests weekly monitoring for 4 weeks after initiating therapy. Such an approach is optimal, but if circumstances do not allow for a child to be seen this frequently, then follow-up with a care manager or telephone follow-up should be considered. In other words, the method and the frequency of the monitoring should be individualized to the needs of the patient and the family. Once the medication is stabilized and the child is doing well, follow-up visits every 1 to 3 months are generally consistent with high-quality care. The FDA has developed a medication guide for physicians and parents (available at www.parentsmedguide.org) that describe the risks and benefits, as well as important signs, that would warrant more immediate follow-up.

BOX 133-2 Optimal Medication Management Strategies

- Conduct an initial evaluation, establish diagnoses in accordance with *Diagnostic and Statistical Manual of Mental Disorders*, fourth edition, and identify target symptoms.
- Ensure an adequate trial of an appropriate medication before changing or adding medications.
- Start low, go slow, but do not stop short.
- Avoid polypharmacy.
- Systematically monitor side effects.
- Systematically monitor symptoms and progress.
- Consider a washout period.
- If no effect, then reconsider diagnosis.
- Involve the family and patient.
- Give clear guidance about expectations to parents to improve adherence.

Start Low, Go Slow, but Do Not Stop Short

Although the *try it and see* approach is unavoidable, the clinician needs to ensure that an adequate dose has been provided before changing medications or adding another. A *start low, go slow* policy is often the best approach. Starting low can minimize potential side effects of medications and can provide time for other psychosocial interventions to have an effect. Going slow allows the PCP and parents an appropriate period at a particular dose to determine whether it provided any benefit. The goal should be to achieve the desired effect at the lowest possible dose. Although this rule must be respected, PCPs should also remember that available data suggest that most physicians typically start low but often *stop short*.[6,7] This undesirable outcome can be minimized by using rating scales and by working to achieve full remission of symptoms. In the case of ADHD, most children can be helped to achieve symptomatic remission with adequate doses of medication, but available evidence suggests that most doses are inadequate.[6,7]

Avoid Polypharmacy

Polypharmacy should be avoided as much as possible. Although instances occur when multiple psychotropic drugs must be administered, alternatives should be considered whenever possible. For example, if a child is having trouble sleeping as a side effect of a medication, then its dose or time should be adjusted first, rather than switching to another medication to combat the side effect. Better yet, environmental or behavioral interventions should be considered that might minimize the side effect or target symptom.

Systematically Monitor Side Effects and Symptoms

To assess a drug's benefits and drawbacks, the PCP must systemically measure both the response and the possible side effects to the treatment. A variety of feasible no-cost, reliable methods are available that can be used to monitor the side effects of the drug, as well as the child's response, carefully. Thus the use of scales, diaries, and checklists not only provide a baseline measure of a particular condition, they also allow for the condition to be monitored over time. Additionally, the use of these tools has been shown to increase physician-patient alliance and reassure the patient and family about the quality of care being received.

Consider a Washout Period

If multiple drugs are having little effect, a washout—a total withdrawal of all medications so as to start over—should be considered. Some medications may cause side effects that mimic psychiatric symptoms. In

BOX 133-3 Fast Facts for Psychoactive Medications for Primary Care Physicians

ADHD

- Several classes of medication have evidence of efficacy for the treatment of ADHD. Eleven medications have scientific support: methylphenidate, pemoline, mixed salts of amphetamine, desipramine, imipramine, nortriptyline, imipramine, bupropion, atomoxetine, clonidine, and guanfacine.
- For the stimulants (methylphenidate, pemoline, dextroamphetamine, amphetamine or mixed salts of amphetamine), common side effects include nervousness, insomnia, abdominal pain, nausea, anorexia, motor tics, headache, palpitations, dizziness, blurred vision, tachycardia, weight loss, fever, depression, transient drowsiness, dyskinesia, angina, rash, urticaria, and blood pressure changes. Serious side effects include growth suppression (long term), seizures, dependency, abuse, arrhythmia, leukopenia (rare), thrombocytopenic purpura (rare), toxic psychosis (rare), Tourette syndrome (rare), exfoliative dermatitis (rare), erythema multiforme (rare), neuroleptic malignant syndrome (rare), cerebral arteritis (rare), and hepatotoxicity (rare).
- The noradrenergic modulators (atomoxetine, clonidine, guanfacine) are often used when stimulants present a problem or are ineffective. Common side effects include dizziness, light-headedness, drowsiness, dry mouth, constipation, reduced appetite, and weight loss. Uncommon side effects include nausea. Rare side effects include liver damage and allergic reactions (eg, swelling, hives).
- Antidepressants (desipramine, imipramine, nortriptyline, bupropion) are used less often than other medication for ADHD but might be needed when other agents fail. Common side effects include nausea, somnolence, headache, diarrhea, dry mouth, ejaculatory dysfunction, dyspepsia (stomachache), decreased libido, constipation, anorexia, sweating, and tremor. Serious side effects include suicidality, depression, serotonin syndrome, withdrawal syndrome, mania, hyponatremia, hypoglycemia (rare), anaphylactoid reaction (rare), and extrapyramidal symptoms (rare).

ANXIETY DISORDERS

- For anxiety disorders, including obsessive-compulsive disorder, studies show four SSRIs (fluoxetine, sertraline, fluvoxamine, and paroxetine) that can significantly reduce anxiety symptoms and are generally well tolerated in children and adolescents. Common side effects include nausea, somnolence, headache, diarrhea, dry mouth, ejaculatory dysfunction, dyspepsia, decreased libido, constipation, anorexia, sweating, and tremor. Serious side effects include suicidality, depression, serotonin syndrome, withdrawal syndrome, mania, hyponatremia, hypoglycemia (rare), anaphylactoid reaction (rare), and extrapyramidal symptoms (rare).

DEPRESSIVE DISORDERS

- Fluoxetine is approved for treatment of depression. Some evidence exists for the use of sertraline and citalopram for mood disorders. The common side effects of these medications are listed above.

CONDUCT DISORDERS OR AGGRESSION

- Six medications may improve symptoms of conduct disorder including methylphenidate, risperidone, mood stabilizers such as lithium (but not carbamazepine), $\alpha 2$-agonists, and possibly β-blockers. These medications do not alter the underlying course of illness.
- Atypical antipsychotics (risperidone, clozapine, olanzapine, quetiapine, ziprasidone, and aripiprazole) can reduce aggression associated with a variety of psychiatric disorders, including those among children with below-average IQ. Risperidone has been particularly effective in producing sustainable improvements in conduct problems and aggression. Common side effects of atypical antipsychotics include insomnia, agitation, extrapyramidal symptoms, headache, anxiety, rhinitis, constipation, nausea and vomiting, dyspepsia (stomachache), dizziness, tachycardia, somnolence, increased dream activity, dry mouth, diarrhea, weight gain, visual disturbances, sexual dysfunction, hyperprolactinemia, and menstrual irregularities. Serious side effects include hypotension, severe syncope (rare), extrapyramidal symptoms, severe tardive dyskinesia, neuroleptic malignant syndrome, hyperglycemia, severe diabetes mellitus, seizures (rare), priapism (rare), stroke, and transient ischemic attack.

CHILDHOOD SCHIZOPHRENIA

- Since 1999, only one randomized, controlled trial has been published testing the efficacy of three atypical antipsychotics (olanzapine, haloperidol, and risperidone) on childhood schizophrenia. Although the study reported overall reduction in negative psychotic symptoms, no change was reported for positive symptoms. Side effects of atypical antipsychotics are reported above.

AUTISM

- Four medications may be helpful in treating symptoms of autism (risperidone, clomipramine, haloperidol, and methylphenidate). Side effects for atypical antipsychotics, antidepressants, and stimulants are reported above.

TOURETTE SYNDROME AND TICS

- For Tourette syndrome and tics, five medications may improve tic frequency or severity: risperidone, clonidine, ziprasidone, pimozide, and pergolide. Side effects for atypical antipsychotics and noradrenergic modulators have been reported above.

BIPOLAR DISORDER

- Two mood stabilizers (lithium and valproic acid) and combination treatment with quetiapine-divalproex or lithium-divalproex have been studied for the treatment of bipolar disorder. Side effects for atypical antipsychotics and mood stabilizers are reported above.

ADHD, Attention-deficit/hyperactivity disorder; *SSRI,* selective serotonin reuptake inhibitor.
From New York State Office of Mental Health, The Research Foundation for Mental Hygiene, Inc., and the Center for Advancement of Children's Mental Health.
For copies of *10 Tips: Navigating Child and Adolescent Inpatient and Residential Services in New York State,* contact New York State Office of Mental Health.

many instances, medications have been added to treat side effects of medications, and carefully monitoring of benefit and side effects at each stage has been neglected. In these situations, consider starting at a point from which the effect of each medication can be measured. Because side effects are possible, the PCP should decide whether the potential benefit of the added medication is greater than the potential risk. If the additive benefit is unclear, then starting from scratch may be a better way to not only understand the effects of the medication, but to clarify the diagnosis and target symptoms.

Reconsider Diagnosis and Condition If No Effect Is Seen

Overreliance on previous labels and diagnoses should be avoided. If a child does not respond to a medication, then the diagnosis and coexisting conditions should be reexamined, along with the treatment and the child's adherence to it. Because many conditions are comorbid and diagnostic categories do not always reflect complex reality, understanding the child and the child's diagnosis can be challenging and frustrating. PCPs should consider arranging regular discussions or follow-up assessments with a physician who is expert in the use of these medications in children with complex emotional or behavioral problems.

Involve the Family and Patient

When considering the range of proven therapeutic options, the entire family must be involved in decision making, including the patient. This process is completed by providing informed decision making in regard to the medication by explaining both the benefits and drawbacks for the use of the medication and other treatments. Involving the family also allows the PCP to gauge the attitudes and abilities of the family. Addressing misconceptions parents may have toward the use of treatments and offering assistance to family members as they arrive at a decision about which treatment option is best for them may be necessary. Parents should be provided with clear directions about the use of the medication, about what medication can be expected to accomplish, and about what the dangers of taking the medication are.

Another important principle is to help parents identify the symptoms that are being targeted and what the goal of the medication will be. By using input from teachers and others, the PCP may determine target behaviors of concern to both the parents and the child. Education and encouragement about how to increase self-management effectively and how to track target symptoms are necessary. Helping families to be aware of side effects that may be encountered is the first step in the identification of such side effects.

SUMMARY

The close relationships with children and families combined with the shortage of mental health care providers for children and adolescents has left the PCP to play a lead role in addressing emotional and behavioral problems. By obtaining extra training and providing extra support when needed, involving the family, conducting a systematic diagnostic evaluation, providing adequate trials of appropriate medications, and providing objective and thoughtful monitoring, the PCP can successfully manage many emotional and behavioral disorders. PCPs should develop relationships with experts in medication management for consultation and referral when necessary.

TOOLS FOR PRACTICE

Engaging Patient and Family

- *Treatment of Children with Mental Disorders* (booklet), National Institute of Mental Health, National Institutes of Health (www.nimh.nih.gov/publicat/childqa.cfm).
- *What Kind of Mental Health Professionals are Trained to Help Children?* (fact sheet), American Academy of Pediatrics (www.aap.org/publiced/BR_MentalHealth.htm).

Medical Decision Support

- *Antidepressant Use in Children, Adolescents, and Adults* (Web page), US Food and Drug Administration (www.fda.gov/cder/drug/antidepressants/default.htm).
- *FDA Asks Attention-Deficit Hyperactivity Disorder Drug Manufacturers to Develop Patient Medication Guides* (Web page), US Food and Drug Administration (www.fda.gov/cder/drug/infopage/ADHD/default.htm).
- *Pediatric Prescribing Update: Psychoactive Medications* (on-line course), American Academy of Pediatrics (www.pedialink.org/cme/).

RELATED WEB SITES

- American Academy of Child and Adolescent Psychiatry (www.aacap.org/).
- Center for the Advancement of Children's Mental Health at Columbia University (www.kidsmentalhealth.org/).
- Children and Adults with Attention Deficit/Hyperactivity Disorder (CHADD) (www.chadd.org/).
- National Alliance on Mental Illness (NAMI) (www.nami.org).
- National Institute of Mental Health, National Institutes of Health (www.nimh.nih.gov/).
- Parents MedGuide (www.ParentsMedGuide.org).
- US Food and Drug Administration: Drug Information (www.fda.gov/cder/drug/default.htm).

REFERENCES

1. Martin A, Leslie D. Trends in psychotropic medication costs for children and adolescents, 1997-2000. *Arch Pediatr Adolesc Med.* 2003;157(10):997-1004.
2. US Food and Drug Administration. Public Health Advisory: Suicidality in Children and Adolescents Being Treated With Antidepressant Medications. October 15, 2004. Available at: www.fda.gov/cder/drug/antidepressants/ssripha200410.htm. Accessed June 25, 2007.
3. Rosack J. Panel urges FDA to clarify ADHD label warnings. *Psychiatr News.* 2006;41(5):1-74.
4. Weisz JR, Jensen PS. Efficacy and effectiveness of child and adolescent psychotherapy and pharmacotherapy. *Ment Health Serv Res.* 1999;(3)1:125-157.
5. Treatment for Adolescents With Depression Study Team. Treatment for Adolescents With Depression Study (TADS): rationale, design, and methods. *JAMA.* 2004; 292(7):807-820.

6. The MTA Cooperative Group. A 14-month randomized clinical trial of treatment strategies for attention-deficit/ hyperactivity disorder. Multimodal Treatment Study of Children with ADHD. *Arch Gen Psychiatry.* 1999; 56(12): 1073-1086.
7. The MTA Cooperative Group. Moderators and mediators of treatment response for children with attention-deficit/ hyperactivity disorder. *Arch Gen Psychiatry.* 1999; 56(12): 1088-1096.
8. Jensen PS. *Making the System Work for Your Child With ADHD.* New York, NY: Guilford Press; 2004.
9. Piacentini J, Shaffer D, Fisher P, et al. The Diagnostic Interview Schedule for Children—Revised Version (DISC-R): III. Concurrent criterion validity. *J Am Acad Child Adolesc Psychiatry.* 1993;32(3):658-665.
10. Elia J, Borcherding BG, Rappoport JL, et al. Methylphenidate and dextroamphetamine treatments of hyperactivity: are there true nonresponders? *Psychiatry Res.* 1991;36(2): 141-155.

Chapter 134

FAMILY INTERACTIONS: CHILDREN WHO HAVE UNEXPLAINED PHYSICAL SYMPTOMS

A. John Sargent III, MD

Children with unexplained physical symptoms after a complete history and thorough physical examination often cause frustration for the primary care physician, the parents, and the child. These children have symptoms that are labeled somatoform, functional, or psychosomatic symptoms, leading to increased use of health care services and increased risk for psychiatric illness. The antecedents and causes of such symptoms are often not identifiable. Illnesses and symptoms are physical, psychological, and social events. The family, as the child's primary social context, is affected significantly by a child's physical condition; in turn, the family affects both the child's physical status and psychological well being.[1] This chapter discusses the importance of family evaluation and intervention for some children with unexplained physical symptoms, especially when these symptoms are persistent.

The parents, in collaboration with health care providers, are responsible for managing appropriate treatment and promoting the child's psychosocial adaptation.[1] Because of the importance of the family, the investigation and treatment of unexplained physical symptoms should include examining interactions between the family and the child. Evaluating family interactions is especially important in situations in which the unexplained symptoms are chronic and unremitting, in which the parents have sought opinions and treatment from several physicians, and in which the symptoms interfere with developmentally appropriate and important behaviors such as attending school, pursuing out-of-school activities, or engaging in normative peer relationships.

CHARACTERISTICS OF SOME FAMILIES WITH CHILDREN WHO HAVE PSYCHOSOMATIC DISORDERS

Liebman, Minuchin, and Baker[2] and Minuchin et al[3,4] investigated the influence of a child's family in treating the symptoms of chronic illness and functional physical symptoms. Their work involved children who had recurrent diabetic ketoacidosis and intractable asthma and adolescents who had anorexia nervosa. They studied the patterns of interaction of these families and identified five specific characteristics of family interaction that typified their daily responses and manner of reacting to the child's physical symptoms: (1) enmeshment, (2) overprotection, (3) rigidity, (4) lack of resolving family conflict, and (5) involvement of the symptomatic child in unresolved parental conflict.

Enmeshment refers to an extremely high degree of involvement and responsiveness among family members. Members are exquisitely sensitive to one another, and minor upsets of one individual may lead to rapid attempts of another to restore calm. Relationships can be overly close to the point that individuation and autonomy are sacrificed. Family members report that they feel for one another and that they know what other family members are thinking. In situations in which parents and infants are concerned, enmeshment is an appropriate and necessary quality. However, as a child grows and develops, more distance in family relationships and independence for the child are required. Pathological enmeshment always entails excessive parental involvement for the child's developmental stage. Enmeshment between parents and child also interferes with the child's development of problem-solving skills because the parents act rapidly to relieve the child's distress rather than require the child to respond to stressful situations. Family members also accommodate viewpoints of others excessively, even when they disagree. Therefore family cohesion is based on submerged and denied family conflict rather than on negotiation, compromise, and agreement.

A child who has a chronic illness, such as diabetes, may become angry about the need for medical treatment and dietary discretion. Parents in adaptive families learn to allow the child to become upset while continuing to require necessary adherence to the treatment regimen. In the pathologically enmeshed family, the parents become upset when the child attempts to deny the disease and the need to comply with its treatment regimens. Furthermore, parents attempt to rationalize their nonadherence to the restrictions of the illness and its treatment.[5] The parents may also carry out illness-management tasks that the child can perform. Finally, one or both parents may become so involved with the ill child that they recognize the symptoms before the child does. In summary, these family responses seriously inhibit the child's acceptance of the illness and autonomy in learning to manage and control the child's own body.

The *overprotectiveness* seen in these families refers to an overly high degree of concern of all family members for one another. Although the ill child is the most obviously vulnerable member of the family, all members are perceived as vulnerable and in need of protection. Evidence of distress in any one family member induces protective responses from the rest of the family. The father may be perceived as explosive and in need of calming, the mother as depressed and in need of paternalistic support, and the ill child as sick and weak and in need of care and attention. Immature behavior on the child's part is allowed, and any difficulties that the child might experience at school or with peers lead to pity and excuses from the parents. The parents may try to shield the child from unpleasant events, such as medical procedures, even to the child's physical detriment.

The *rigidity* of these families is demonstrated not only in their attempts to deny family problems and to repeat the same ineffective solutions over and over, but also in their desire to maintain fixed relationships among one another, even when development or stress requires change. Each family member states steadfastly that the behavior of other members or of the person's own cannot be altered, regardless of the need for change. A mother will report that she cannot bring her husband to the physician's office or hospital no matter how ill the child is. A father will insist that he cannot assist his wife in following through with illness treatment for their child (eg, giving insulin injections by himself). The child will state that the child cannot help the parents understand the child's feelings about his chronic illness. These protestations of incompetence persist, increasing the overall family stress and leading to a deterioration in the child's condition and further ineffective family responses; a circular pattern results. These families appear to be in a tenuous balance, with any change seen as highly threatening.

Disagreement and conflict exist in all families. Psychosomatic disorders in a child may arise in families in which rigid patterns of extreme closeness and protectiveness exist. In these families, these rigid patterns are prominent and persist even though conflict and disagreements are not resolved. In many instances the existence of conflict is denied. Family members contradict themselves to maintain a facade of agreement, and immediate consensus develops concerning even small issues of disagreement. If a consensus cannot be achieved immediately, then distractions occur that dissipate the conflict, or the disagreeing family members avoid one another until the situation calms. An air of chronic tension exists in the family, which is reinforced by avoidance, denial, or outright capitulation by one member. These unresolved disagreements may involve any aspect of family life; however, the physician should note in particular that the parents do not resolve differences of opinion about the ill child and management of the child's disease.[5]

Finally, when conflict occurs between the parents, the ill child becomes involved in the disagreement, distracting attention to the child and thus reducing the disagreement significantly. The balance of harmony and consensus is then restored. The child is often asked to mediate between the parents; at times the child sides with one parent against the other; at other times the parents unite (leaving their disagreement) either to protect and nurture the sick child or to attack the child and blame the child for all family troubles. Chronic marital strife is reinforced as more and more disagreements remain unresolved. Nonetheless, often because of the child's illness or symptoms, neither parent leaves the family. The ill child remains highly vigilant to future family disagreements and experiences, increasing stress as family tension persists. Precisely at the point of parental disagreement and personal stress does the child become symptomatic, requiring medical care and sometimes hospitalization. The cycle then begins again.

Thus the child's participation in parental conflict reduces physical and psychological distress in the parents but induces symptoms in the labile child. The family's patterns of interaction induce symptoms in the child, while the child's symptoms assist the family in maintaining stability. Minuchin et al[3,4] found that these family characteristics occurred in families who had children who had unexplained (functional) physical symptoms, regardless of the child's primary diagnosis. Although all families engage in enmeshed, protective, and conflict-avoiding interactions, some families engage in these patterns inordinately, even when such patterns are unproductive. This circumstance does not mean that the family causes the insulin deficiency of diabetes or the reactive airway diathesis of asthma. The physiological differences in these children are specific vulnerabilities that are affected by the family and other factors to become repeatedly symptomatic. Thus functional or unexplained symptoms become a circular process, reinforced by the child's vulnerability and the family's characteristic patterns of interaction.

Criticisms of this model have pointed out the lack of consistent data supporting the existence of all of these features in families of children who have unexplained physical symptoms.[6,7] Minuchin's description of the family also has been interpreted as blaming parents for the child's physical difficulties and psychosocial problems. These authors have emphasized that the family does not cause the child's symptoms and that unexplained symptoms in a child often cause significant stress for a family and worsen any interactional difficulties a family might have. Furthermore, many of these family relationship characteristics are noted in families that have children with other emotional and behavioral difficulties. Possibly, these relationship characteristics are prominent in families with poor marital cooperation and a child who has a challenging physical, emotional, or behavioral problem.[8,9] This fact further underscores the importance of being aware that the child's problem is not caused by problematic family interaction. It does highlight, though, that for treatment to be effective, appropriate family involvement is essential.[8]

Wood[10-12] has suggested that families who have children with unexplained physical symptoms have two features in common: (1) biobehavioral reactivity among members, which renders them exquisitely sensitive, physically and emotionally, to one another and (2) poor collaboration among parental figures, leading to marked difficulty dealing with the uncertainty, stress, and confusion associated with persistent unexplained physical symptoms. Lock and colleagues[13,14] have developed a treatment manual using family therapy for anorexia nervosa in adolescents based on the principles of encouraging parental collaboration and parents encouraging adolescent weight gain and enhanced maturity. They also tested this treatment in a randomized controlled trial[13] and demonstrated its effectiveness, further reinforcing the use of family assessment and family-based treatment for children and adolescents with unexplained physical symptoms and psychosomatic disorders.

IMPLICATIONS FOR THE PEDIATRICIAN

Diagnosis

Assessment of the family, including both parents, is essential in evaluating situations in which a child's illness becomes repeatedly symptomatic at home and yet is controlled easily in the hospital.[15,16] The pediatrician should note how family members behave with one another and should question each member directly about the member's own impressions of the causes of the child's frequent symptoms. The pediatrician can suggest to family members that they discuss the problem together and can observe their nonverbal responses when other members are talking. The pediatrician will need to pay attention to the process of family interaction, as well as to the content of their statements.

These families are typically well informed about their child's medical condition, and they understand and carry out treatment. However, they often appear helpless and defeated, relating to the physician in a dependent and demanding fashion. Parental overprotectiveness is common, and the enmeshment within the family is demonstrated as parent and child constantly maintain eye contact, speak for each other, and sit very close together. Therefore the physician will often find difficulty in developing an independent relationship with the child. The father may also be devalued and thus may appear disinterested and unsympathetic. The parents may present differing views of the situation, and when asked to reconcile these different perceptions, they are unable to do so. The child is often immature or pseudomature and frequently clings to one parent. The child usually has limited peer relationships and is the primary focus of parental attention because of the symptoms. The child's lack of insight and general sense of helplessness are often striking. Finally, both family and symptomatic child readily deny psychological difficulties, and all maintain a strongly somatic orientation.

Pediatric Interventions

The pediatrician's primary goal in these situations is to gain the family's trust and collaboration in the evaluation and with treatment. The physician should not challenge the reality of the child's physical symptoms and should ensure that the appropriate medical evaluation is completed. Results of medical evaluations should be presented clearly and directly and with compassion and support. Through honesty and empathy the pediatrician can enlist the family's trust, accept family difficulties, and create, with family and child involvement, a plan for further assessment and treatment that will foster the child's development.

When caring for a physically symptomatic child, the pediatrician, noting significant parental involvement and protectiveness, can help the parents require more independence from their child. If the physician determines that the parents disagree about how to accomplish this task and thus are rendered ineffective, then the need for parents to act cooperatively can be emphasized. The pediatrician can also ensure that the child is participating in school and in activities with peers. Regular follow-up will be necessary to determine if the parents can cooperate and encourage more maturity from their child and if this maturity leads to improvements in the child's physical condition.[8] If the child improves, then the pediatrician will need to watch for signs of marital distress in the parents. The clinician can then discuss with the parents the need to resolve their differences either independently or through psychotherapy. Three principles should guide the efforts:

1. Pediatricians should attend first to the physical and psychological difficulties of the ill child before attempting to address stress in the marriage directly.
2. In working with the family, pediatricians should develop and maintain an attitude that places responsibility on them to ensure their child's physical and psychosocial adjustment.
3. Pediatricians should pursue regular follow-up care with the family to ensure that progress is maintained.

Referral for family psychotherapy is indicated in situations in which the ill child demonstrates serious emotional and behavioral immaturity or in which the child's illness is so labile that hospitalization is repeatedly necessary, which leads to school absence, further social isolation, and worsening parental concern.[9,15] Referral is also indicated when the parents are unable to decrease overinvolvement and overprotectiveness with the physician's assistance or to develop and carry out cooperative methods of dealing with the ill child. Before referral, the pediatrician must identify the child's physical condition accurately and outline appropriate medical treatment. All physicians involved in the child's care must agree on the diagnosis, treatment, and recommendation for family therapy. The therapist should be familiar and comfortable with family-oriented treatment of serious physical and emotional disorders in children[9] and should work collaboratively with the physician. The therapist can best be introduced to the family as a professional who will help them manage their child's illness or symptoms effectively and assist them in reducing the stressful effects of the child's symptoms on both child and family. The physician can further state that psychotherapy is a highly important part of treatment and that without psychotherapy the physician will continue to be ineffective in reducing the symptoms. The family should not perceive the referral for psychotherapy as implying blame for their problems. Rather, it can be described as an opportunity for the family and physician to improve the child's condition. Treatment may be aided by assisting the family in understanding the role and effect of physical illness, medical problems, and medical care within their family throughout its history.[17] Awareness of other family concerns about illness, disability, and death may free the family to attend to this child and the child's problems more effectively. In addition, attending to the specific developmental, emotional, and physical concerns and needs of the child in question leads to more appropriate treatment and more respectful engagement of the family in the treatment.[18]

Pediatrician-Therapist Collaboration

The pediatrician assists the course of psychotherapy by answering the medical questions of the family directly and by informing the family of the improvements that should be achieved through their work with the therapist. Both professionals will need to support each other's efforts and encourage the family to resolve differences straightforwardly with each of them. The physician should avoid answering psychological questions that the family raises and should inform the parents that these issues will need to be addressed with the therapist. This support enables the parents to work directly with the therapist and resolve any disagreements they may have straightforwardly. It also prevents the parents from pitting the therapist against the physician during treatment. The therapist, in turn, refers any medical questions the parents raise to the physician. During the initial phases of family treatment, the child's medical condition may worsen, and short-term emergencies may develop at stressful points during the psychotherapy. Both the therapist and the physician need to be available to the family at these times. By maintaining a mutually supportive relationship and open communication, the pediatrician and the family therapist can assist each other through difficult phases of treatment. Working together, pediatrician, therapist, and parents can improve the child's physical and psychological condition dramatically.

RELATED WEB SITES

- American Academy of Child & Adolescent Psychiatry (AACAP) (www.aacap.org).
- American Psychosomatic Society (www.psychosomatic.org/).

REFERENCES

1. Sargent J. The sick child: family complications. *J Behav Develop Pediatr.* 1983;4:50-56.
2. Liebman R, Minuchin S, Baker L. The use of structural family therapy in the treatment of intractable asthma. *Am J Psychiatry.* 1974;131:535-540.
3. Minuchin S, Baker L, Rosman BL, et al. A conceptual model of psychosomatic illness in childhood. Family organization and family therapy. *Arch Gen Psychiatry.* 1975;32:1031-1038.
4. Minuchin S, Rosman BL, Baker L. *Psychosomatic Families: Anorexia Nervosa in Context.* Cambridge, MA: Harvard University Press; 1978.
5. Baker L, Minuchin S, Milman L, et al. Psychosomatic aspects of juvenile diabetes mellitus: a progress report. *Mod Probl Paediatr.* 1975;12:332-343.
6. Coyne JC, Anderson BJ. The "psychosomatic family" reconsidered. I. Diabetes in context. *J Marital Fam Ther.* 1988;14:113-123.
7. Coyne JC, Anderson BJ. The "psychosomatic family" reconsidered. II. Recalling a defective model and looking ahead. *J Marital Fam Ther.* 1989;15:139-148.
8. Nichols MP, Schwartz RC. *Family Therapy: Concepts and Methods.* 4th ed. Boston, MA: Allyn and Bacon; 1998.
9. Sargent J. Physician-family therapist collaboration: children with medical problems. *Fam Syst Med.* 1985;3:454-465.
10. Wood BL. A developmental biopsychosocial approach to the treatment of chronic illness in children and adolescents. In: Mikesell RH, Lusterman DD, McDaniel SH, eds. *Integrating Family Therapy: Handbook of Family Psychology and Systems Theory.* Washington, DC: American Psychological Association; 1995.
11. Wood BL. Beyond the "psychosomatic family": a biobehavioral family model of pediatric illness. *Fam Process.* 1993;32:261-278.
12. Wood B. Proximity and hierarchy: orthogonal dimensions of family interconnectedness. *Fam Process.* 1985;24:487-507.
13. Lock J, Agras WS, Bryson S, et al. A comparison of short- and long-term family therapy for adolescent anorexia nervosa. *J Am Acad Child Adolesc Psychiatry.* 2005;44:632-639.
14. Lock J, Le Grange D. Family-based treatment of eating disorders. *Int J Eat Disord.* 2005;37(suppl):s64-s67.
15. Sargent J. The family and childhood psychosomatic disorders. *Gen Hosp Psychiatry.* 1983;5:41-48.
16. Sargent J, Liebman R. Childhood chronic illness: issues for psychotherapists. *Community Ment Health J.* 1985;21:294-311.
17. McDaniel SH, Hepworth J, Doherty WJ. Medical family therapy with somatizing patients: the co-creation of therapeutic stories. *Fam Process.* 1995;34:349-361.
18. Friedrich WU. A customized approach to the treatment of anorexia and bulimia. In: Mikesell RH, Lusterman DD, McDaniel SH, eds. *Integrating Family Therapy: Handbook of Family Psychology and Systems Theory.* Washington, DC: American Psychological Association; 1995.

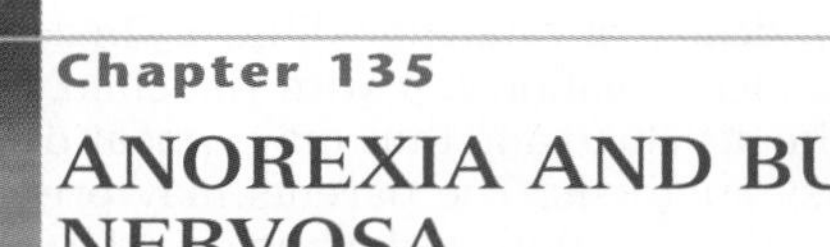

Chapter 135

ANOREXIA AND BULIMIA NERVOSA

Marcie B. Schneider, MD; Martin M. Fisher, MD

INTRODUCTION

The eating disorders, a group of conditions that affect primarily adolescents and young adults, increased significantly in prevalence during the last 3 decades. Marked by a combination of medical and psychological factors in their etiology and outcome, they include predominantly the well-known entities of anorexia and bulimia nervosa. Anorexia nervosa is viewed most simply as the purposeful loss of weight beyond a healthy state, whereas bulimia nervosa is marked by recurrent episodes of binge eating along with purging behaviors. The diagnosis and prevalence of these disorders are much debated, and many questions remain about their etiology and outcome. Nevertheless, the growing incidence and prevalence of eating disorders in adolescents and adults requires that the primary care physician has some knowledge of the principles involved in the evaluation and treatment of both anorexia and bulimia nervosa essential for the primary care physician.

BOX 135-1 Criteria for the Diagnosis of Eating Disorders

ANOREXIA NERVOSA

- Refusal to maintain body weight at or above a minimally normal weight for age and height (eg, weight loss, leading to maintenance of body weight less than 85% of that expected, or failure to make expected weight gain during period of growth, leading to body weight less than 85% of that expected)
- Intense fear of gaining weight or becoming fat, even though underweight
- Disturbance in the way in which body weight or shape is experienced, undue influence of body weight or shape on self-evaluation, or denial of seriousness of the current low body weight
- In postmenarchal girls, amenorrhea, that is, the absence of at least 3 consecutive menstrual cycles (a woman is considered to have amenorrhea if her periods occur only following hormone [eg, estrogen] administration)
- Restricting type: during the current episode of anorexia nervosa, person has not regularly engaged in binge-eating or purging behavior (ie, self-induced vomiting or the misuse of laxatives, diuretics, or enemas)
- Binge-eating or purging type: during the current episode of anorexia nervosa, person has regularly engaged in binge-eating or purging behavior (ie, self-induced vomiting or the misuse of laxatives, diuretics, or enemas)

BULIMIA NERVOSA

- Recurrent episodes of binge eating; episode of binge eating characterized by both of the following:
  Eating, in a discrete period (eg, within any 2-hour period), an amount of food that is definitely larger than most people would eat during a similar period and under similar circumstances
  A sense of lack of control over eating during the episode (eg, a feeling that the person cannot stop eating or control what or how much the person is eating)
- Recurrent inappropriate compensatory behavior so as to prevent weight gain, such as self-induced vomiting; misuse of laxatives, diuretics, enemas, or other medications; fasting; or excessive exercise
- The binge eating and inappropriate compensatory behaviors both occur, on average, at least twice a week for 3 months
- Self-evaluation is unduly influenced by body shape and weight
- The disturbance does not occur exclusively during episodes of anorexia nervosa
- Purging type: during the current episode of bulimia nervosa, person has regularly engaged in self-induced vomiting or the misuse of laxatives, diuretics, or enemas
- Nonpurging type: during the current episode of bulimia nervosa, person has used other inappropriate compensatory behaviors, such as fasting or excessive exercise, but has not regularly engaged in self-induced vomiting or the misuse of laxatives, diuretics, or enemas

EATING DISORDERS NOT OTHERWISE SPECIFIED*

- All criteria for anorexia nervosa, except has regular menses
- All criteria for anorexia nervosa, except weight still in normal range
- All criteria for bulimia nervosa, except binges less than twice a week or less than 3 times a month; patient with normal body weight who regularly engages in inappropriate compensatory behavior after eating small amounts of food (ie, self-induced vomiting after eating 2 cookies)
- A patient who repeatedly chews and spits out large amounts of food without swallowing
- Binge eating disorder: recurrent binges but does not engage in the inappropriate compensatory behaviors or bulimia nervosa

*In patients who do not meet criteria for anorexia nervosa or bulimia nervosa, per DSM-IV.
Reprinted with permission from the Diagnostic and Statistical Manual of Mental Disorders Editions, (Copyright 2000). American Psychiatric Association.

ETIOLOGY

Several factors most likely converge in the development of an eating disorder. The adolescent girl who is culturally primed, biologically at risk, and psychologically vulnerable may begin dieting or vomiting in response to a particular precipitant (often an insult by family or friends, exposure to another individual who has an eating disorder, or a stressful situation). The positive psychological feedback that initially accompanies a perceived improved appearance and the biochemical changes that occur in response to decreased nutrition may serve to perpetuate the behavior.

DEFINITIONS

The current criteria for both anorexia nervosa and bulimia nervosa are listed by the American Psychiatric Association in the *Diagnostic and Statistical Manual of Mental Disorders DSM-IV,* 4th edition (DSM-IV),[1] as shown in Box 135-1. In addition, large numbers of adolescents, and even children, display abnormal attitudes toward weight and food, with many showing evidence of subclinical eating disorders.[2] Included in this category are adolescents who lose enough weight to cause irregular periods but not enough to meet DSM-IV criteria for anorexia nervosa and those who use vomiting to control their weight[2] but do not binge and therefore do not meet specific criteria for bulimia nervosa. These adolescents often have medical and psychological difficulties similar to those described in patients whose eating disorders are more overt and generally require similar treatment.[3] These patients are categorized as having *eating disorders not otherwise specified* and represent as many as one half of the patients treated for eating disorders in pediatric and adolescent medicine settings.[3,4]

CLINICAL MANIFESTATIONS

Incidence

Anorexia Nervosa

Conservatively, anorexia nervosa occurs in 0.5% to 1% of girls and young women and 0.2% of boys and young men.[5,6] A bimodal peak of onset occurs during the adolescent years at 14.5 and 18 years.[7] Increasingly, the onset of anorexia nervosa has been seen in both prepubertal children and adults.[8] Mortality is higher than in any other psychiatric illness, up to 5% per decade after the onset of the eating disorder.[9]

Bulimia Nervosa

Up to 15% of adolescents report binge eating, purging, or both.[10,11] However, only 2% of female adolescents and 0.3% of male adolescents actually meet full diagnostic criteria for bulimia nervosa.[6,12,13] The peak prevalence of lifetime bulimia nervosa is reported to be 2% to 4% among white Western girls and women aged 17 to 25 years,[13,14] with a modal age of onset of 18 to 19 years.[15,16] Bulimia nervosa occurs in patients under the age of 14 years, but this situation is very rare.[17]

Risk Factors

Anorexia Nervosa

The serotonergic system likely plays a role in the development of anorexia nervosa, with areas on chromosomes 1 and 10 that may relate to susceptibility.[18] Low self-esteem, perfectionism, and obsessiveness are associated with anorexia nervosa.[19] Additionally, a family history of eating disorders, family dieting, and a focus on weight in the family are all linked to the onset of anorexia nervosa.[20] Interestingly, very preterm small-for-gestational-age infants have a higher risk of developing anorexia nervosa.[21] Psychiatric illnesses can coexist with anorexia nervosa, including depression, anxiety, and obsessive-compulsive disorder.[22]

Bulimia Nervosa

Dieting has been documented as a risk factor for the development of bulimia nervosa.[16] Bulimia nervosa is associated with early menarche, early sexual experiences, and increasing age in girls and with very early or late puberty and early sexual experiences in boys.[23] Personal and parental obesity are each risk factors for bulimia nervosa.[24] Urbanization,[25] not socioeconomic status,[26] has been found to be a risk factor for bulimia nervosa, which occurs at a rate 5 times higher in large cities than in rural areas. Because bulimia nervosa occurs in all ethnic and racial groups, being a member of an ethnic subculture does not apparently protect against the sociocultural factors that promote body dissatisfaction among teenage girls.[27,28] Childhood sexual abuse has been reported to be a significant risk factor for bulimia nervosa, especially when psychiatric comorbidity is present.[29] Premorbid negative self-evaluation, parental alcoholism, low parental contact, and high parental expectations have each been associated with a higher risk of development of the disorder.[30] In addition, bulimia nervosa is associated with impulsivity, stressful life events, high levels of family conflict, inadequate expression of emotions, lack of parental warmth and care, inappropriate parental control, and a family history of affective disorders or eating disorders.[30]

A family history of eating disorders increases the risk for having an eating disorder by 7 to 12 fold.[31] A greater prevalence of eating disorders in monozygotic versus dizygotic twins is present, and 54% to 83% of the variance in bulimia nervosa can be accounted for by genetic factors.[31] Molecular genetic research on several genes (the *5 HT 2A* receptor gene, the *UCP2/UCP-3* gene, and the estrogen receptor-beta gene) provides a new and exciting area of study aimed at gaining an understanding of the genetics of anorexia and bulimia nervosa.[18,31]

DIFFERENTIAL DIAGNOSIS

The differential diagnosis of the eating disorders includes possible medical causes of weight loss or vomiting and other psychiatric causes of poor appetite. Included in the differential diagnosis are malignancies and central nervous system tumors; gastrointestinal problems, including malabsorption, celiac disease, and inflammatory bowel disease; endocrinologic problems such as diabetes mellitus, hyperthyroidism, and hypopituitarism; chronic illnesses and chronic infections; and the superior mesenteric artery syndrome. The history, physical examination, and baseline laboratory tests should help rule out most of these diagnoses; further testing may be necessary if the weight loss or vomiting cannot be explained adequately. A magnetic resonance image (MRI) of the brain, gastrointestinal series, or other tests may be considered in some cases for patients who claim to be eating well or not vomiting on purpose. In some instances, a patient may show obvious pleasure in the weight loss or vomiting brought on by another disorder; however, this circumstance must not be confused with a positive diagnosis of anorexia or bulimia nervosa.

Psychiatric causes of weight loss can include depression, obsessive-compulsive disorder, and psychosis (especially schizophrenia). The patient who refuses to eat because of a desire to lose weight must be differentiated from the patient who cannot eat because of depression or the patient who will not eat because of delusional fears (eg, that the food is poisoned). Although patients may have concomitant depression or psychosis with anorexia or bulimia nervosa, separate criteria must be used to establish each entity. A full psychosocial history must be obtained as part of the initial evaluation to establish both the diagnosis and the psychosocial severity of the disorder. The patient's functioning in the family, in school, and among peers must be evaluated, and possible psychiatric symptoms such as sleep disorders, hallucinations, delusions, or obsessions should be elicited. Almost all patients with eating disorders exhibit psychosocial changes with the onset of the illness. These changes generally include fighting with the family, withdrawing from friends, and performing less optimally in school, although some patients paradoxically report improved school performance as they withdraw from friends and family. If additional psychiatric symptoms are found, the possibility of an additional diagnosis should be pursued.

EVALUATION

Evaluation of the specific diagnostic criteria for eating disorders listed in Box 135-1 serves to both elucidate the diagnosis and determine the severity of the illness. Distortion of body image, a hallmark in the diagnosis of anorexia nervosa, may be evaluated by exploring the patient's views of initial, current, and desired weight. Establishing the patient's eating and exercise patterns and use of vomiting or medications designed to promote weight loss (including diet pills, laxatives, diuretics, or ipecac) provides hints to both the diagnosis and the possibility of medical complications. Care must be taken to avoid being misled by the patient who is not completely forthright; the results of the physical examination and laboratory tests often suggest the true extent of the patient's disorder.

Anorexia Nervosa

History

Initial evaluation of the patient with weight loss includes a determination of the diagnosis and its severity, an evaluation of other possible causes of weight loss and the effects of malnutrition, an analysis of the psychological context of the illness, and a decision about treatment. Relevant history includes patients' recollection of height, maximum weight, minimum weight, current weight, and desired weight. Additionally, evaluation for a distortion in body image, a history of binging or purging, and overexercising is necessary. On the review of systems, symptoms of malnutrition, including alopecia, cold hands and feet, dry skin, constipation, fatigue and amenorrhea, may be present (Box 135-2). For girls, a full menstrual history should be obtained, including age at menarche, last normal menstrual period, usual length of menses, heaviness of flow, presence of dysmenorrhea, and regularity of menses.

Physical Examination

The first steps in the physical examination of the patient who is thought to have anorexia nervosa include calculation of the percentage below ideal body weight (IBW) and determination of vital signs. The percentage below IBW, which may be calculated by comparing the patient's current weight with the average weight expected for height, age, and sex (as determined by standard pediatric growth charts), serves both as one of the diagnostic criteria and as a gross estimate of the degree of malnutrition. In general, body weight more than 25% below IBW represents severe malnutrition, 20% below IBW represents moderate malnutrition, and weight not yet 20% below IBW represents mild malnutrition. For example, a 16-year-old girl who is 5 feet 4 inches tall would be expected to have a body weight of 120 pounds, plus or minus 10%; she would be 20% below IBW at 96 pounds and 25% below IBW at 90 pounds. Body mass index is being used increasingly to describe nutritional status. In addition, pediatric growth charts[32] (www.cdc.gov/growthcharts) are needed for premenarchal girls and growing boys to determine previous heights and weights to establish appropriate weight goals for achievement of expected adult height.

BOX 135-2 Medical Complications of Anorexia Nervosa and Bulimia Nervosa

ANOREXIA NERVOSA

Acrocyanosis
Dry skin
Lanugo
Ecchymosis
Fatigue
Muscle wasting
Decreased subcutaneous fat
Decreased deep-tendon reflexes
Constipation
Delayed gastric emptying
Delayed gastric motility
Orthostatic hypotension
Bradycardia
Mitral valve prolapse
Pericardial effusion
Electrocardiographic abnormalities
Decreased left-ventricular mass and contractility
Psychomotor retardation
Growth delay
Pubertal delay
Amenorrhea
Osteopenia, osteoporosis

BULIMIA NERVOSA

Hypertension or hypotension
Electrolyte abnormalities
Dehydration
Erosion of dental enamel
Calluses on the dorsum of the hand
Parotid enlargement
Acute pancreatitis
Acute gastric dilatation or rupture
Mallory-Weiss tears
Gastric and esophageal irritation
Gastric and esophageal bleeding
Gastric esophageal reflux disease
Barrett esophagus
Aspiration pneumonia
Diarrhea, constipation, steatorrhea
Emetine cardiomyopathy
Menstrual irregularity
Polycystic ovarian syndrome
Osteopenia, osteoporosis

Vital signs provide further evidence of the degree of malnutrition because chronic malnutrition is accompanied by declines in blood pressure, pulse, and electrocardiographic (ECG) voltage.[33] Other cardiovascular changes can include sinus bradycardia, prolonged QTc, orthostatic hypotension, increased vagal tone, poor myocardial contractility, mitral valve prolapse, pericardial effusion, and decreased left-ventricular mass.[34] To document orthostatic changes accurately, the patient's blood pressure and pulse should be checked in the sitting position, followed by standing for 2 minutes. An increase of 20 beats per minute in pulse, a decrease of 20 mm Hg in systolic blood pressure, or a decrease of 10 mm Hg in diastolic blood pressure is considered significant.[35] Other physical findings associated with malnutrition include scaphoid abdomen, muscle wasting, acrocyanosis, decreased subcutaneous fat, lanugo hair similar to that seen in newborns, ecchymoses, diminished reflexes, and dry skin.

Laboratory Evaluation

Laboratory tests further elucidate the severity of the illness. Most patients who have anorexia nervosa have normal laboratory results initially, although all organ systems are probably affected by the malnutrition. The laboratory abnormalities found on routine testing are related generally to the individual's particular nutritional pattern. Thus the patient who is chronically malnourished usually has leukopenia, occasionally thrombocytopenia, and in rare cases severe anemia (being protected for some time from iron-deficiency anemia by the concomitant amenorrhea). The patient who restricts fluid intake may show evidence of dehydration (including an elevated sodium or blood urea nitrogen), whereas the patient who drinks excessive fluids to satisfy hunger or the physician's scale may show signs of hyponatremia and dilute urine. Conversely, the patient who vomits or uses laxatives may show evidence of hypokalemia, which is often severe in persons who use both methods of weight control. Nutrient values, including levels of zinc, calcium, magnesium, copper, vitamin B12, and folate, may all be altered in the malnourished patient, but are usually normal.

Hormonal testing may produce evidence of dysfunction in endocrine systems.[36] Development of a relative hypothyroidism caused by a combination of euthyroid sick syndrome and decreased production on a hypothalamic basis is believed to be an adaptive response to inadequate nutrition. Hypothyroidism is generally evident by low-normal levels of triiodothyronine, thyroxine, thyroid-stimulating hormone, or any combination. Amenorrhea, a hallmark of the disorder, generally develops when the patient's weight reaches approximately 15% below IBW but may be seen earlier; it is accompanied by low levels of luteinizing hormone (LH) and follicle-stimulating hormone (FSH). Hypercortisolemia with loss of diurnal variation and low levels of insulin-like growth factor 1 (IGF-1) are seen in patients with anorexia nervosa, although these tests need not be performed in most patients.[37]

In general, the initial laboratory work-up of patients with anorexia nervosa includes a complete blood cell count, evaluation of serum electrolytes, liver and thyroid function tests, and levels of LH, FSH, estradiol, and prolactin in patients who have amenorrhea. Obtaining a urinalysis for specific gravity and ketonuria is often helpful. An ECG is performed for persons with bradycardia. This battery of tests is generally sufficient to provide a barometer of current status, a baseline to monitor further changes, and screening for other possible causes of weight loss. Data have demonstrated that patients who have eating disorders, especially those whose amenorrhea is prolonged because of malnutrition, show evidence of osteopenia on bone density studies.[38] Initial studies have shown that this effect may not be preventable, even with calcium supplementation or hormonal replacement, or completely reversible, even after patients regain their normal weights.[39] A 3-fold increase in the long-term risk of fracture development has been seen in patients with a history of anorexia nervosa.[40] Studies are under way to determine the possible causes of osteopenia, including hypoestrogenemia, hypercortisolemia, and decreased IGF-1. Bone density values in patients with anorexia nervosa are correlated with body mass index, age at onset, and duration of illness.[41] Bone densitometry, using dual-energy x-ray absorptiometry, has become a common test in the evaluation of patients who have eating disorders and amenorrhea of at least 6 to 12 months' duration.[42]

Evidence of abnormalities may be found on computed tomography and MRI scans of the brain, but these tests are generally reserved for evaluating other possible causes when the diagnosis is in question. MRI changes in the brain, including gray matter deficits and elevated cerebrospinal fluid volumes, may not be reversible.[43] Additionally, delayed gastric emptying and decreased gastrointestinal motility can be seen in anorexia nervosa. Gastric emptying studies can be done to evaluate these abnormalities if necessary.

Bulimia Nervosa

History

Initial evaluation of a patient with bulimia nervosa includes determining the diagnosis and its severity and evaluating other causes of the symptoms. Relevant history includes frequency of binging; frequency of purging behaviors, including laxative, diuretic, diet pill or ipecac use; and frequency of vomiting or exercising. History of maximum, minimum, and usual weight are also obtained. Similar to patients with anorexia nervosa, symptoms of malnutrition, including cold hands and feet, hair loss, and irregular menses, may be present. Symptoms related to purging that include heartburn, hematemesis, constipation, and diarrhea should be explored.

Physical Examination

Patients with bulimia nervosa may be underweight, overweight, or normal weight. Specific abnormalities on the physical examination are rarely found; therefore more subtle changes in vital signs, the complete physical examination, and laboratory tests should be sought (see Box 135-2). Vital signs will vary depending on the substances used to control weight. For example, persons using diet pills may have tachycardia, hypertension, or both, whereas those using substances that cause dehydration, such as stimulant laxatives or diuretics, may have tachycardia, hypotension, or both. Vomiting can cause hypovolemia and, in turn, tachycardia and hypotension. For persons who exercise excessively, resting heart rates may show significant bradycardia. Thus the initial physical examination generally begins with measurements of weight, height, blood pressure, and pulse. If dehydration needs to be ruled out, then measuring blood pressure for orthostatic changes as previously described is needed. Hands should be examined for Russell sign (ie, irritation on the dorsum of the joints of the fingers used to induce vomiting); teeth should be examined for erosion of enamel as a result of vomiting; parotid enlargement from vomiting may also be seen.

Laboratory Evaluation

Blood tests include a complete blood cell count with differential, electrolytes, lipid studies, liver function tests, and serum chemistries. Amylase levels and urinary pH may be elevated in some patients who have bulimia. The urinalysis may reveal an elevated specific gravity in dehydration, ketones in starvation, increased pH in the presence of vomiting, or any combination. A hormonal work-up is performed if menstrual periods are problematic; these tests include thyroid function tests, as well as assessments of LH, FSH, estradiol, and prolactin (if amenorrheic). If potassium levels are abnormal, or if a history of ipecac use exists, then an ECG should be performed. If patients are oligomenorrheic or amenorrheic, then a bone density assessment looking for osteopenia should be pursued.

TREATMENT

The patient who has an eating disorder may seek medical care in a variety of ways. Some of these patients visit their pediatrician or family physician because of concern about weight loss, vomiting, or abnormal eating attitudes noticed by family, friends, or school authorities; others visit a gynecologist because of the menstrual irregularities that characteristically accompany the disorder. Many patients are seen first by a psychiatrist, psychologist, or social worker; others may be seen for the 1st time in an emergency department because of dehydration or other medical complications. Some patients may be seen within weeks of the disorder's onset; others avoid medical care for months or even years. Being brought in for their initial evaluation against their will is common for many patients, although some may seek help willingly. Many patients who have mild to moderate eating disorders, both anorexia and bulimia nervosa, avoid medical care altogether by hiding or denying their illness.[5]

Team Approach

The combination of medical and psychological treatment required in the treatment of eating disorders makes the task of being proficient in all aspects of care difficult for any single professional.[44] No single individual can be responsible totally for any patient's care beyond the initial evaluation or for the most straightforward of cases.[44,45] Rather, a team approach is most often used. The team may consist of a primary care physician; a psychiatrist, psychologist or social worker; and a nutritionist, with the exact combination determined by local expertise, availability, and preference. Generally, each team member manages specific aspects of care, and team meetings and discussions are held frequently to prevent miscommunication that can sabotage the treatment.

Multimodal Therapy

The treatment team may use several modalities, including medical management, nutritional rehabilitation, behavior therapy, individual psychotherapy, family and group therapy, and psychopharmacology. The fact that a *multimodal therapy* that includes aspects of each of these approaches holds the best promise for successful treatment is generally acknowledged.[46,47] The degree to which each of these approaches is incorporated into the treatment varies, both with the preferences of the treatment team and the requirements of the individual patient. Each of these approaches may be used for inpatients, day-program patients, and outpatients.

Medical and Nutritional Rehabilitation

The malnutrition that accompanies anorexia nervosa is directly responsible for most, if not all, of the physical abnormalities noted in the disorder, as well as for some of the mental deterioration. Accordingly, medical and nutritional rehabilitation is crucial in the treatment of the patient who has anorexia nervosa. Restoration of body weight, generally to within 10% of IBW, with restoration of menses, should be among the main goals of treatment. For many patients whose malnutrition is mild to moderate (15% to 25% below IBW), this task may be accomplished on an outpatient basis; patients who have moderate to severe malnutrition (more than 25% below IBW) can rarely accomplish the required weight gain without hospitalization. Medical treatment includes management of electrolyte abnormalities, cardiovascular issues, endocrine disorders, and other organ system dysfunction. These aspects of care are managed simultaneously with and are abetted by nutritional rehabilitation, which is generally achieved through oral feedings. Whether in the inpatient or outpatient setting, a daily intake of 3 substantial meals and 3 to 4 snacks is usually sufficient to bring about required weight gain and improvement of medical parameters. On inpatient units, meals are generally provided as part of a strict regimen, and snacks generally consist of high-calorie supplements, available as liquids or puddings in various brands and flavors. Care is taken to avoid overfeeding patients whose malnutrition is severe because a too-rapid weight gain has been associated with severe metabolic abnormalities in some patients, that is, the refeeding syndrome.[48] Slow refeeding and phosphorus supplementation are required in patients with severe malnutrition to prevent this syndrome, which may result in cardiac failure, hemolysis, coma, and death.

Dietary Plan

In the outpatient setting, an appropriate meal pattern may be developed based on the patient's and the family's prior eating habits or on a specific dietary plan offered by the physician or a nutritionist. The dietary plan should be specific so that ambiguities that can lead to family fighting are avoided; it should provide approximately 2000 to 3000 calories a day. Some of these calories may be supplied in the form of high-calorie supplements. The plan should be well balanced and include foods from each of the major food groups. Outpatient gains should be 1 to 2 pounds per week,[49] whereas inpatient gains may be 2 to 4 pounds per week.[50] Compliance with the dietary regimen may be evaluated by having the patient keep a diet diary; however, many patients do not always keep these records accurately and honestly.

A similar dietary plan, without the high-calorie supplements, may be offered to healthy-weight patients who have bulimia because these patients generally require nutritional adjustment rather than nutritional rehabilitation. Caloric requirements for persons with bulimia will depend on the need for weight gain, loss, or maintenance. Because caloric restriction may often spark binge-eating episodes, the implementation of a nonrestrictive well-balanced diet is warranted. If hospitalization is necessary for uncontrolled binge or purge cycles, abnormal electrolytes, or unstable vital signs, then supervision after meals, locked bathrooms, and restricted access to food are often necessary.

Menses Restoration

Menses restoration generally requires an estradiol level above 30 mg/dL.[51] Although estrogen replacement may be able to increase bone density in select situations or help maintain bone density in others,[52,53] estrogen replacement has not been shown to reverse or prevent bone loss in adolescents with anorexia nervosa.[54] Researchers are exploring other treatments, such as recombinant human IGFs, dehydroepiandrosterone, bisphosphonates, and testosterone,[55,56] in an effort to find ways to protect the bones of patients with eating disorders.

Behavioral Therapy

Merely offering a nutritious diet to a patient who has either anorexia or bulimia nervosa is unlikely to result in a drastic change in the patient's status. For this reason, behavioral therapy is normally a necessary component of treatment. The goal of behavioral therapy in the treatment of eating disorders is to offer a set of external positive and negative reinforcements to replace specific internal sensors that usually control appetite and weight gain but that are currently missing. Behavioral therapy is not intended to be definitive but rather to accomplish specific goals in the areas of weight and diet stabilization, thus allowing the psychological modalities of treatment to proceed in a more *medically healthy* patient.

Inpatient Settings

Various behavioral approaches may be used. The strict behavioral plans used on some psychiatric units involve removal of all *privileges,* including use of the telephone, television, and regular clothing, if a particular weight goal is not achieved each day. A somewhat less strict plan used on some adolescent medicine units includes the use of several phases of treatment, with patients moving from 1 phase to another based on achievement of progressively higher weight goals. Each phase incorporates additional privileges into the patient's daily activities (eg, mobility on the unit, exercise, meals, snacks, passes) in such a way that improved weight and eating patterns lead to additional privileges and responsibilities. For patients unable to respond to the positive reinforcements provided by such a phased system, an all-liquid diet, provided by mouth or, more rarely, nasogastric tube, may be substituted. Use of such methods ultimately achieves the necessary weight goals in almost all patients. However, behavioral therapy alone cannot be considered adequate treatment, and controlled studies have been unable to distinguish among the effects of the various behavioral approaches.

Outpatient Settings

Applying behavioral principles may be somewhat more difficult when treating eating disorders in the outpatient setting. For many patients who have anorexia nervosa, the usual approaches to behavioral therapy in outpatient settings (eg, use of monetary or similar rewards) may not be strong enough to overcome the fear of eating. Fear of hospitalization itself may be the sole motivation. Similarly, classic approaches may not be effective for the patient who has bulimia because the symptom of vomiting cannot be measured readily. More sophisticated cognitive-behavioral approaches have therefore been developed so that patients who have bulimia may understand and participate in their own behavioral therapy.[57] These approaches make use of diaries and changes in daily patterns to effect change.

Individual, Family, and Group Therapy

Individual Therapy

Individual psychotherapy remains an essential part of the treatment for most patients who have an eating disorder. Although therapeutic styles differ based on the treatment team and the individual therapist, exploration of underlying psychological features and determination of possible mechanisms for change are appropriate for most patients who have either anorexia or bulimia nervosa. Although several common themes have been noted in many of these patients—including poor self-esteem, family conflicts, difficulties with friends, and fear of sexuality—great individual variety exists in the way these themes are expressed and exhibited. For many patients, the eating disorder apparently serves as a defense against other difficult aspects of life; an important secondary gain also may be involved. Psychological change is generally acknowledged to be a necessary precursor to significant improvement in the disordered thinking and behavior exhibited by most patients who have an eating disorder.

Family Therapy

Family therapy is a particularly important component of treatment, especially for younger patients, because of the major role that family conflicts and problems play in symptom continuation.[58] Family sessions, arranged in varying combinations to include parents and siblings, generally focus on the disordered communication patterns that often accompany the eating disorder. Resolving specific conflicts arising from the presence of the eating disorder itself also becomes an important area for discussion. The course of the eating disorder is much more difficult for adolescent patients whose families are unable or unwilling to make necessary changes in their customary patterns of communication and parenting. An approach to outpatient treatment (developed at the Maudsley Hospital in London, England) in which families provide and supervise all meals, similar to what would be done by the staff in a hospital setting, has increasingly been used for younger patients with anorexia nervosa with positive results.[59]

Group Therapy

Many patients who have eating disorders participate in group therapy during their treatment. For some patients whose anorexia nervosa is mild and for college-aged patients who have bulimia, group therapy may be the only approach used. Groups may be organized in many different ways, some focusing on a psychotherapeutic approach, others concentrating more specifically on behavioral changes. Initial fears that patients who have eating disorders will *learn bad habits* from one another in the group have been outweighed by the apparent benefit most patients derive from group therapy. This circumstance is especially true for patients who have had social difficulties during their adolescence.

Types of Therapy

Psychotherapy has been associated with improved weight gain and improved psychosocial functioning in patients with anorexia nervosa. However, no specific type of therapy has been shown to be better than another.[60,61] For patients with bulimia nervosa, cognitive behavior therapy has been documented to be more effective than psychotherapy in decreasing binge eating and vomiting behaviors initially,[62] but interpersonal psychotherapy has efficacy similar to cognitive behavior therapy in long-term studies.[63,64] Cognitive behavior therapy (CBT) was formulated by Fairburn in 1981.[65] CBT for eating disorders is aimed at decreasing nutritional restriction, normalizing eating, developing skills for coping with situations that trigger binge eating or purging (or both), and changing perceptions and overconcern with body weight and shape. Neither CBT nor interpersonal therapy has been studied in adolescents with bulimia.

Psychopharmacologic Therapy

The use of medication to treat eating disorders has a long history of decidedly mixed results. Numerous medications have been tried, from thyroid hormone and insulin in the 1940s and 1950s to phenytoin (Dilantin) and hydroxyzine (Atarax) in the 1960s and 1970s, as attempts were made to improve appetite, increase weight gain, and reverse physiological abnormalities. More recently, pharmacologic treatment of the eating disorders has concentrated on psychoactive medications, especially the selective serotonin reuptake inhibitor (SSRI) antidepressants. Two specific lines of reasoning have guided the use of these medications. In patients who are diagnosed as having an eating disorder along with, or as part of, another psychiatric diagnosis, medication for the associated diagnosis is offered with the expectation that the eating disorder will improve as other psychiatric symptoms are relieved. Alternately, more recent evidence has demonstrated that use of these medications diminish the urge to binge and purge in patients who have bulimia nervosa and help treat obsessive-compulsive symptoms in patients with either anorexia or bulimia nervosa.[66] Only physicians who are familiar with the use of psychopharmacologic agents should prescribe these medications as part of the treatment, given the recent concerns about the potential for SSRI medications to increase the risk of suicide in a minority of children and adolescents treated for depression.

The SSRI medications have not been shown to be effective in promoting weight gain in anorexia nervosa or treating symptoms of depression or obsessive-compulsive disorder when body weight is low; some questions remain about whether they may be effective in preventing relapse in patients initially treated successfully for anorexia nervosa.[67] Atypical antipsychotic agents at low doses can improve weight gain and treat symptoms of depression and obsessional thoughts in patients with severe eating disorders, including both anorexia and bulimia nervosa.[68-70]

Various types of antidepressant medications have been studied for the treatment of bulimia nervosa, including tricyclics, monoamine oxidase inhibitors. and SSRIs. All of these agents seem to be roughly equivalent in decreasing bulimic behaviors at the end of short-term treatment; with any of these medications, approximately 30% of patients are abstinent and 70% have decreased bulimic behaviors.[70] Fluoxetine has been the most intensively studied medication; a dose of 60 mg per day has been found to yield the best treatment outcome for decreasing bulimic symptoms, relieving symptoms of depression and anxiety, and decreasing concerns with shape, weight, and desire to restrict food intake. Other drugs, including anticonvulsants, serotonergic agents, and lithium, have also been studied, with modest (anticonvulsants) or no significant (serotonergic agents or lithium) changes in symptoms.[70] CBT, followed by the introduction of medication if necessary, has been suggested as a logical treatment approach in the treatment of bulimia.[71,72]

OUTCOME AND PROGNOSIS

Eating disorders must be viewed as a chronic illness, similar to other medical or psychiatric chronic illnesses. A wide range of outcomes can be expected.[73] Adolescents who have severe anorexia nervosa have a protracted disease course, yet recovery estimates 10 to 15 years later vary from 76%[74] to 24%.[75] Although many different approaches are used to evaluate outcome, at least an estimated 50% of patients do well in the long term, 30% show varying degrees of improvement, and 20% do poorly despite adequate treatment. Patients who are younger, as well as those whose forms of the disease are milder, appear to have a better prognosis than these general numbers indicate.[76] Follow-up of patients with bulimia nervosa has also shown that approximately 50% recover, 30% experience relapse, and 20% continue to meet the full criteria for bulimia nervosa 5 years after diagnosis.[76,77]

Numerous personal, family, and treatment factors may predict the outcome of an eating disorder; none of these may be predictive for an individual patient. For instance, a poorer outcome in anorexia nervosa has been associated with factors such as older age, vomiting, and premorbid personality problems, yet any particular patient who has this constellation of findings may do well with treatment. Furthermore, no specific treatment has been shown by controlled studies to be more effective than others, in general or for any particular type of patient.

PREVENTION

Although a focus on both primary and secondary prevention has increased of late, the best strategies for the prevention of eating disorders remain unclear.[78] To date, several programs geared toward both teenage boys and girls, primarily in school settings, have been implemented. These programs generally provide factual information and are aimed at maintaining a healthy body image, healthy eating, and promoting self-esteem without relation to weight, and they appear to succeed in terms of increasing awareness and knowledge about eating disorders.[79] However, whether these programs prevent or actually promote eating-disordered behavior is debatable.[80,81] The concept of preventing eating disorders through more generic programs focused on building self-esteem is currently being explored. In keeping with this effort, the concept of a comprehensive school-based approach has been advocated.[82] This approach would include classroom interventions, staff training throughout the school, informal discussions between staff and students, integration of material about eating issues into the curriculum, more intensive work with persons at high risk, changes within the school with respect to cafeteria food and physical education, and referrals and outreach, both within the school and to the community. Early case detection remains the most effective preventive measure currently available. For most patients, the earlier an eating disorder is treated, the easier the treatment will be and the less entrenched the disease becomes. Therefore families, friends, school personnel, and health professionals must be vigilant for the signs and symptoms of an eating disorder so that early treatment be initiated.

WHEN TO REFER

- Refer to a dietician if the primary care physician or staff does not have the expertise, or time, to set a nutritional plan with the patient.
- Refer to a psychotherapist if the patient is open to therapy.
- Refer to a psychotherapist if the patient is unable to attain goals set by the physician, even if the patient is resistant.
- Refer for psychopharmacologic evaluation if both the physician and the therapist believe that the patient might benefit from medication (if the patient is binging and open to medication or if obsessive-compulsive symptoms are interfering with treatment).
- Refer to adolescent medicine if the physician is not comfortable with treating the patient or does not have the time to do so or if the patient does not adhere to the physician's treatment plan.

WHEN TO ADMIT

Any 1 or more of the following:

- Severe malnutrition (weight <75% IBW)
- Dehydration
- Electrolyte disturbances
- Cardiac disturbances
- Physiological instability (bradycardia, hypotension, hypothermia, orthostatic changes)
- Arrested growth and development
- Failure of outpatient treatment
- Acute food refusal
- Uncontrollable bingeing and purging
- Acute medical complication of malnutrition (eg, syncope, seizures, cardiac failure, pancreatitis)
- Acute psychiatric emergencies (eg, suicidal ideation, acute psychosis)
- Comorbid diagnosis that interferes with the treatment of the eating disorder (eg, severe depression, obsessive-compulsive disorder, severe family dysfunction)

TOOLS FOR PRACTICE

Engaging Patient and Family

- *Eating Disorders: What You Should Know* (brochure), American Academy of Pediatrics (patiented.aap.org).

Medical Decision Support

- *Pediatric Nutrition Handbook* (book), American Academy of Pediatrics (www.aap.org/bookstore).

RELATED WEB SITES

- Academy for Eating Disorders (www.aedweb.org/index.cfm).
- National Association of Anorexia Nervosa and Associated Disorders (ANAD) (www.anad.org/).

AAP POLICY STATEMENT

American Academy of Pediatrics, Committee on Adolescence. Identifying and treating eating disorders. *Pediatrics.* 2003;111(1):204-211. (aappolicy.aappublications.org/cgi/content/full/pediatrics;111/1/204).

REFERENCES

1. American Psychiatric Association. *Diagnostic and Statistical Manual of Mental Disorders DSM-IV.* 4th ed. Washington, DC: APA Press; 1994.
2. Fisher M, Schneider M, Pegler C, et al. Eating attitudes, health-risk behaviors, self-esteem and anxiety among adolescent females in a suburban high school. *J Adolesc Health.* 1991;12:37.
3. Bunnell OW, Shenker IR, Nussbaum MP, et al. Subclinical versus formal eating disorders: differentiating psychological features. *Int J Eat Disord.* 1990;9:357.
4. Fisher M, Burns J, Symons H, et al. Treatment of eating disorders in a division of adolescent medicine. *Int J Adolesc Med Health.* 2002;14:283-295.
5. Lucas AR, Beard CM, O'Fallon WM, et al. Fifty-year trends in the incidence of anorexia nervosa in Rochester, Minnesota: a population-based study. *Am J Psychiatry.* 1991;148:917.
6. Carlat OJ, Camargo CA Jr, Herzog DB. Eating disorders in males: a report on 135 patients. *Am J Psychiatry.* 1997; 154:1127-1132.
7. Halmi K, Casper R, Eckert E, et al. Unique features associated with age of onset of anorexia nervosa. *Psychiatry Res.* 1979;1:209-215.
8. Beck O, Casper R, Andersen A. Truly late onset of eating disorders: a study of 11 cases averaging 60 years of age at presentation. *Int J Eat Disord.* 1996;20:389-395.

9. Sullivan P. Mortality in anorexia nervosa. *Am J Psychiatry.* 1995;152:1073-1074.
10. French SA, Leffert N, Story M, et al. Adolescent binge/purge and weight loss behaviors: associations with developmental assets. *J Adolesc Health.* 2001;28:211-221.
11. Stice E, Killen JD, Hayward C, et al. Age of onset for binge eating and purging during late adolescence: a 4-year survival analysis. *J Abnorm Psychol.* 1998;107(4):671-674
12. Kaltiala-Heino R, Rimpela M, Rissanen A, et al. Early puberty and early sexual activity are associated with bulimic-type eating pathology in middle adolescence. *J Adolesc Health.* 2001;28:346-352.
13. Flament M, Ledoux S, Jeamet P, et al. A population study of bulimia nervosa and subclinical eating disorders in adolescence. In: Steinhausen HC, ed. *Eating Disorders in Adolescence: Anorexia and Bulimia Nervosa*. New York, NY: De Gruyter; 1995.
14. McCallum K. Eating disorders. *Curr Opin Psychiatry.* 1993;6:167-173.
15. Fairburn CG, Cooper PJ. Clinical features of bulimia nervosa. *Br J Psychiatry.* 1984;44:238-246.
16. Fairburn CG, Beglin SJ. Studies of the epidemiology of bulimia nervosa. *Am J Psychiatry.* 1990;147:401-408
17. Stein S, Chalhoub N, Hodes M. Very early-onset bulimia nervosa: report of two cases. *Int J Eat Disord.* 1998;24: 323-327.
18. Klump KL, Gobrogge KL. A review and primer of molecular genetic studies of anorexia nervosa. *Int J Eat Disord.* 2005;37S:343-348.
19. Fairburn CG, Cooper Z, Doll HA, et al. Risk factors for anorexia nervosa. *Arch Gen Psychiatry.* 1999;56: 468-476.
20. Lilenfeld LR, Kaye WH, Greeno CH, et al. A controlled family study of anorexia nervosa and bulimia nervosa. *Arch Gen Psychiatry.* 1998;55:603-610.
21. Cnattingius S, Hultman CM, Dahl M, et al. Very preterm birth, birth trauma and the risk of anorexia nervosa among girls. *Arch Gen Psychiatry.* 1999;56:634-638.
22. Yager J, Andersen AE. Anorexia nervosa. *N Eng J Med.* 2005;353:1481-1488.
23. Kaltiala-Heino R, Rissanen A, Rimpela M, et al. Bulimia and bulimic behavior in middle adolescence: more common than thought? *Acta Psychiatr Scand.* 1999;100: 33-39.
24. Fairburn CG, Welch SL, Doll HA, et al. Risk factors for bulimia nervosa; a community-based case-control study. *Arch Gen Psychiatry.* 1997;54:509-517.
25. Hoek HW, Bartelds AIM, Bosveld JJF, et al. Impact of urbanization on detection rates of eating disorders. *Am J Psychiatry.* 1995;152:1272-1278.
26. Hoberman HM, Opland E, Garfinkel BD. *Psychiatric Characteristics of Adolescents With Eating Disordered Behavior.* Paper presented at the annual meeting of the American Academy of Child and Adolescent Psychiatry, Chicago, IL, 1990.
27. French SA, Story M, Neumark-Sztainer D, et al. Ethnic differences in psychosocial and health behavior correlates of dieting, purging, and binge eating in a population-based sample of adolescent females. *Int J Eat Disord.* 1997; 22:315-322.
28. Steinhausen HC, Boyadjieva S, Grigoroiu-Serbanescu M, et al. A transcultural outcome study of adolescent eating disorders. *Acta Psychiatr Scand.* 2000;101:60-66.
29. Wonderlich SA, Brewerton TO, Jocic Z, et al. Relationship of childhood sexual abuse and eating disorders. *J Am Acad Child Adolesc Psychiatry.* 1997;36:1107-1115.
30. Schmidt U, Tiller J, Treasure J. Psychosocial factors in the origins of bulimia nervosa. *Int Rev Psychiatry.* 1993; 5:51-60.
31. Klump KL, Kaye WH, Strober M. The evolving genetic foundations of eating disorders. *Psychiatr Clin North Am.* 2001;24(2):215-225.
32. Ogden CL, Kuczmarski RJ, Flegal KM, et al. Centers for disease control and prevention 2000 growth charts for the United States: improvements to the 1977 National Center for Health Statistics version. *Pediatrics.* 2002;109:45.
33. Fisher M. Medical complications of anorexia and bulimia nervosa. *Adolesc Med.* 1992;3:487.
34. Katzman OK. Medical complications in adolescents with anorexia nervosa: a review of the literature. *Int J Eat Disord.* 2005;37S:S52-S59.
35. Engstrom JW, Aminoff MJ. Evaluation and treatment of orthostatic hypotension. *Am Family Physician.* 1997;56(5): 1378-1386.
36. Newman MW, Halmi KA. The endocrinology of anorexia nervosa and bulimia nervosa. *Neurol Clin.* 1988;6:195.
37. Misra M, Aggarwal A, Miller KK, et al. Effects of anorexia nervosa on clinical, hematologic, biochemical, and bone density parameters in community-dwelling adolescent girls. *Pediatrics.* 2004;114:1574-1583.
38. Wong JCH, Lewindon P, Mortimer R, et al. Bone mineral density in adolescent females with recently diagnosed anorexia nervosa. *Int J Eat Disord.* 2001;29:11-16.
39. Bachrach LK, et al. Recovery from osteopenia in adolescent girls with anorexia nervosa. *J Clin Endocrinol Metab.* 1991;72:602.
40. Lucas AR, Melton LJ 3rd, Crowson CS, et al. Long term fracture risk among women with anorexia nervosa: a population-based cohort study. *Mayo Clin Proc.* 1999; 74:912.
41. Castro J, Lazaro L, Pons F, et al. Predictors of bone mineral density reduction in adolescents with anorexia nervosa. *J Acad Child Adolesc Psychiatry.* 2000;39: 1365-1370.
42. Grinspoon S, Thomas E, Pitts S, et al. Prevalence and predictive factors for regional osteopenia in women with anorexia nervosa. *Ann Intern Med.* 2000;133:790-794.
43. Katzman OK, Zipursky RB, Lambe EK, et al. A longitudinal magnetic resonance imaging study of brain changes in adolescents with anorexia nervosa. *Arch Pediatr Adolesc Med.* 1997;51:793.
44. American Academy of Pediatrics, Committee on Adolescence. Identifying and treating eating disorders. *Pediatrics.* 2003;111:204-211.
45. Becker AE, Grinspoon SK, Klibanski A, et al. Eating disorders. *N Engl J Med.* 1999;340:1092-1098.
46. Powers PS. Initial assessment and early treatment options for anorexia nervosa and bulimia nervosa. *Psychiatry Clin North Am.* 1996;19:639-655.
47. Yager J, Andersen A. Anorexia nervosa. *N Engl J Med.* 2005;353:1481-1488.
48. Fisher M, Simpser E, Schneider MB. Hypophosphatemia secondary to oral refeeding in anorexia nervosa. *Int J Eat Disord.* 2000;28(2):181-187.
49. American Psychiatric Association. Practice guidelines for the treatment of patients with eating disorders (revision). *Am J Psychiatry.* 2000;157(suppl):1-39.
50. Howard WT, Evans KK, Quintero-Howard CV, et al. Predictors of success or failure of treatment for inpatients with anorexia nervosa. *Am J Psychiatry.* 1999;156:1697-1702.
51. Golden N, Jacobson MS, Schebendach J, et al. Resumption of menses in anorexia nervosa. *Arch Pediatr Adolesc Med.* 1997;151:16-21.
52. Hergenroder AC, Smith EO, Shypailo R, et al. Bone mineral changes in young women with hypothalamic amenorrhea treated with oral contraceptives, medroxyprogesterone, or placebo over 12 months. *Am J Obstet Gynecol.* 1997; 176:1017-1025.
53. Klibanski A, Biller BMK, Schoenfeld DA, et al. The effects of estrogen administration on trabecular bone loss in young women with anorexia nervosa. *J Clin Endocrinol Metab.* 1995;80:898-904.

54. Golden N, Lanzkowsky L, Schebendach J, et al. The effect of estrogen-progestin treatment on bone mineral density in anorexia nervosa. *J Pediatr Adolesc Gynecol.* 2002;15: 1325-1343.
55. Gordon CM, Grace E, Emans, SJ, et al. Use of DHEA to prevent osteoporosis in patients with anorexia nervosa. *J Adolesc Health.* 1998;22:176.
56. Miller KK, Grieco KA, Klibanski A. Testosterone administration in women with anorexia nervosa. *Clin Endocrinol Metab.* 2005;90:1428-1433.
57. Fairburn CG, Jones R, Peveler RC, et al. Psychotherapy and bulimia nervosa: longer-term effects of interpersonal psychotherapy, behavior therapy, and cognitive behavior therapy. *Arch Gen Psychiatry.* 1993;50:41.
58. Eisler I, Dare C, Russel GFM, et al. Family and individual therapy in anorexia nervosa: a 5-year follow-up. *Arch Gen Psychiatry.* 1997;54:1025-1030.
59. Lock J, Le Grange D, Agras S, et al. *Treatment Manual for Anorexia Nervosa: A Family-Based Approach.* New York, NY: Guilford; 2001.
60. Hay P, Bacaltchuk J, Claudina A, et al. Individual psychotherapy in the outpatient treatments of adults with anorexia nervosa. *Cochrane Database Syst Rev.* 2003;4: CD003909.
61. Dare C, Eisler I, Russell G, et al. Psychological therapies for adults with anorexia nervosa: randomized controlled trial of out-patient treatments. *Br J Psychiatry.* 2001;178: 216-221.
62. Wilson GT. Cognitive behavior therapy for eating disorders: progress and problems. *Behav Res Ther.* 1999; 37(supp):S79-S95.
63. Fairburn CG, Norman PA, Welch SL. A prospective study of outcome in bulimia nervosa and the long-term effects of three psychological treatments. *Arch Gen Psychiatry.* 1995;52:304-312.
64. Agras WS, Walsh T, Fairburn CG, et al. A multicenter comparison of cognitive-behavioral therapy and interpersonal psychotherapy for bulimia nervosa. *Arch Gen Psychiatry.* 2000;57(5):459-466.
65. Fairburn CG. A cognitive behavioural approach to the management of bulimia. *Psychol Med.* 1981;11:707-711.
66. Attia E, Schroeder L. Pharmacologic treatment of anorexia nervosa: where do we go from here? *Int J Eat Disord.* 2005;27(suppl):60-63.
67. Walsh BT, Kaplan AS, Attia E, et al. Fluoxetine after weight restoration in anorexia nervosa: a randomized controlled trial. *JAMA.* 2006;295:2605-2612.
68. Barbarich NC, McConaha CW, Gaskill J, et al. An open trial of olanzapine in anorexia nervosa. *J Clin Psychiatry.* 2004;65:1480-1482.
69. La Via MC, Gray N, Kaye WH. Case reports of olanzapine treatment of anorexia nervosa. *Int J Eat Disord.* 2000; 27(3):363.
70. Powers PS, Santana CA, Bannon YS. Olanzapine in the treatment of anorexia nervosa: an open label trial. *Int J Eat Disord.* 2002;32:146-154.
71. Agras WS. Pharmacotherapy of bulimia nervosa and binge eating disorder: longer term outcomes. *Psychopharmacol Bull.* 1997;33(3):433-436.
72. Walsh BT, Agras WS, Devlin MJ, et al. Fluoxetine for bulimia nervosa following poor response to psychotherapy. *Am J Psychiatry.* 2000;157(8):1332-1334.
73. Fisher M. The course and outcome of eating disorders in adults and in adolescents: a review. *Adolesc Med.* 2003; 14:149-158.
74. Strober M, Freeman R, Morrell W. The long-term course of severe anorexia nervosa in adolescents: survival analysis of recovery, relapse and outcome predictors over 10-15 years in a prospective study. *Int J Eat Disord.* 1997; 22:339.
75. Eckert ED, Halmi KA, Marchi P, et al. Ten year follow-up of anorexia nervosa: clinical course and outcome. *Psychol Med.* 1995;25:143-156.
76. Steinhausen HC. Outcome of anorexia nervosa in the younger patient. *J Child Psychol Psychiatry.* 1997;38:271.
77. Keel PK, Mitchell JE. Outcome in bulimia nervosa. *Am J Psychiatry.* 1997;154:313.
78. Rosen DS, Neumark-Sztainer D. Review of options for primary prevention of eating disturbances among adolescents. *J Adolesc Health.* 1998;23:354.
79. Story M, Neumark-Sztainer D. Promoting healthy eating and physical activity in adolescents. *Adolesc Med.* 1999; 10:109.
80. Mann T, Nolenhoeksema S, Huang K, et al. Are two interventions worse than none? Joint primary and secondary prevention of eating disorders in college females. *Health Psychol.* 1997;16:215.
81. Neumark-Sztainer D, Butler R, Palti H. Eating disturbances among adolescent girls: evaluation of a school-based primary prevention program. *J Nutr Educ.* 1995;27:24.
82. Neumark-Sztainer D. School-based programs for the prevention of eating disturbances. *J Sch Health.* 1996; 66:64.

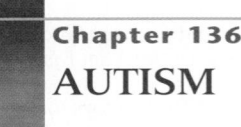

Chapter 136
AUTISM

Eric M. Butter, PhD; James A. Mulick, PhD

Autism is a neurobiologic developmental disorder characterized by significant developmental delays in language and communication skills, abnormalities in language when it does develop, significant impairments in reciprocal social behavior, a restricted and narrow repertoire of interests and behaviors, ritualized and repetitive behavior patterns, and stereotyped, destructive, and disruptive behavior problems. The diagnosis is made based on the child's behavior, in part historically and in part by concurrent observation or behavior reporting.[1] Children with autism often function within the mentally retarded range of general intellectual ability and have limited adaptive behavior. Autism is most often a pervasive and lifelong disability that is difficult to treat.

More common in boys than in girls, autism is not a rare childhood disorder. Historically, autism was thought to occur at a rate of 2 to 5 in every 10,000 children[2]; however, recent reports indicate that the incidence of autism may be far greater, at 10 to 20 per 10,000 children.[3] Despite controversy over recent reports of increasing rates of autism, it is unclear whether the reported increase in autism cases is related to a truly greater incidence or to other factors, such as greater awareness, broader diagnostic criteria, improved diagnostic methods, and even increased parent demand for the diagnosis so the child can meet treatment and educational service eligibility criteria.[4]

The most debilitating aspect of autism is comorbid mental retardation (MR). Although some experts have argued that intellectual disabilities are not as common among children diagnosed with autism as has been previously thought, MR is reported to occur in approximately 70% of all cases of autism.[3] MR remains the most difficult aspect of autism to ameliorate, and the presence of MR with autism has the poorest prognosis. Children with both autism and MR fail to benefit from conventional social and educational experiences—the same experiences that allow other children opportunities for cognitive growth and learning. Other comorbid conditions include seizures, gastrointestinal problems, and sleep difficulties. Children with autism also often have associated behavioral problems, including pica, self-injury, and aggression.[1]

No known, single cause of autism has been found, and most researchers have accepted that autism likely has multiple causes.[5] Evidence is growing for a genetic link to autism that affects neurologic development as early as the prenatal period, and the search for autism susceptibility genes is ongoing.[6] Neurologically, brain imaging and head circumference studies have suggested an increase in brain growth coinciding with the development of autistic symptoms.[7] Outside of a specific biological cause, several medical and genetic conditions have been associated with autism, including fragile X syndrome, Cornelia de Lange syndrome, and tuberous sclerosis.[8]

DIFFERENTIAL DIAGNOSIS

Three diagnoses encompass the cluster of symptoms most often associated with autism: (1) *autistic disorder,* (2) *Asperger disorder,* and (3) *pervasive developmental disorder not otherwise specified* (PDD-NOS). Autistic disorder describes a child who meets full diagnostic criteria in terms of language, social interaction, and repetitive, restricted behaviors. Asperger disorder is diagnosed when typical language development is present in the context of impaired social interactions and repetitive, restricted behaviors. The diagnosis of PDD-NOS is reserved for cases in which the central features of language delay, impaired reciprocal social interaction, or restricted, repetitive behaviors are present but not in the degree that would warrant a more specific diagnosis. These diagnostic categories are conventionally referred to as *autism spectrum disorders* (ASDs). This term is not a clinical diagnosis; rather, it is descriptive and refers to the wide range of impairments and different abilities present among children with autism, Asperger disorder, and PDD-NOS.

Additionally, the fourth edition of the American Psychiatric Association's *Diagnostic and Statistical Manual of Mental Disorders* places childhood disintegrative disorder and Rett syndrome within the category of pervasive developmental disorders.[2] *Childhood disintegrative disorder* may be distinguished from ASDs in that it is marked by a period of developmental regression after at least 2 years of normal development. *Rett syndrome* may be distinguished from ASDs in most cases by a deceleration of head growth before 48 months, loss of purposeful hand movements before 30 months, development of stereotyped hand movements (hand wringing), and severe to profound language and cognitive delays. Rett syndrome is associated with mutations of the *MECP2* gene on the X chromosome. It is predominately expressed in girls, but a few cases in boys have been identified.[9]

Finally, autism and PDD-NOS should be distinguished from a *developmental language disorder.* Language disorders are characterized by significant delays in receptive or expressive language skills (or both), but social interaction skills are not qualitatively impaired. Children with language disorders do not usually demonstrate repetitive, restricted behavior patterns.

EVALUATION

Diagnosing autism is not a straightforward process. No single biological marker or laboratory test or procedure exists to identify children with autism. Although the diagnosis of autism is primarily a behavioral one based on a comprehensive history, direct observation, and standardized assessment, several medical procedures should be followed to rule out specific known causes of expressed behaviors. Guidelines for medical screening and diagnosis have been widely recognized by scientific and professional societies.[1]

History

A comprehensive medical, developmental, and psychosocial history is the most important aspect of an evaluation for autism. An evaluator should document birth and neonatal history, developmental milestones, and any developmental regression. History that indicates excessive irritability, self-injury, feeding or sleeping problems, or any combination would imply a diagnosis of autism, as would extreme hyperactivity, pica, or seizures. Family history of autism, MR, learning difficulties, language delays, mental health problems, and social difficulties should also be explored.

Physical Examination

General physical examinations for children with suspected autism should consider several suggestive factors. Among children with autism, head circumference is sometimes larger than in typically developing children.[10] Motor stereotypies of a nonfunctional character (eg, hand flapping) are the most common motor impairments in autism, although hypotonia and limb apraxia have been reported. The latter impairments are more common among children with isolated MR and other developmental disabilities than among children with autism.

Tuberous sclerosis, a neurocutaneous disorder affecting the brain and other organs, can account for 0.4% to 3% of children diagnosed with autism.[1] Although 2 gene loci have been identified, the most common initial signs are ash leaf–shaped depigmented macules observed with exposure to ultraviolet light. Any child being assessed for autism should be exposed to ultraviolet light to exclude tuberous sclerosis. If the assessment is positive, then the child should be referred to a geneticist.

Laboratory Evaluation

No single test for autism exists. Lead screening is indicated for most children with developmental disabilities because pica is a common comorbidity and is associated with lead toxicity. Commonly, DNA analysis and high-resolution chromosomal (karyotype) testing is completed to rule out fragile X syndrome; children diagnosed with fragile X syndrome often meet the criteria for autism. Metabolic and expanded genetic testing should be performed when additional physiological signs (eg, unusual and dysmorphic features, seizures, abnormal growth) are observed. Electrophysiological testing is only necessary in cases of suspected comorbid seizure disorder, severe sleep problems, or developmental regression.[1]

Imaging Studies

No imaging evaluation procedures are needed in a routine evaluation for autism. When other neurologic findings co-occur with suspected autism, such as seizure, asymmetric motor functioning, cranial nerve dysfunction, or severe headache, principles of standard clinical assessment apply.

MANAGEMENT

The physician's role in managing ASDs involves screening and referring for specialist evaluation, managing unique medical comorbidities, identifying the need and perhaps managing psychopharmacologic interventions, and advocating for effective psychosocial interventions.

Screening and Referral

Children must be diagnosed as early as possible and referred to appropriate, effective intervention services because of advances in the psychological and educational treatment of children with autism over the last 20 years. Primary care physicians are most likely to be the initial public health care providers to see a child with autism. Primary care assessment for high-risk cases at 18 to 24 months is the most important step health care providers can make toward identifying children with autism.

Several measures are available for evaluating and diagnosing autism, and a sampling of these are listed in Table 136-1. Primary care physicians are most likely to make use of pen-and-paper parent report measures such as the Modified Checklist for Autism in Toddlers (M-CHAT).[11] This measure and several others presented in Table 136-1 are brief questionnaires that help determine whether children should be referred for further evaluation. A much longer and more comprehensive questionnaire, the Pervasive Developmental Disorders Behavior Inventory (PDDBI),[12] provides more information and may be sensitive to changes in symptom presentation over time and as related to intervention and treatment. The PDDBI has a computer scoring program available to help with interpretation of the results and scoring. The Autism Diagnostic Interview Revised (ADI-R)[13] and the Autism Diagnostic Observation Schedule (ADOS)[14] are 2 measures widely used among specialists and in research settings, but the time and training involved with these instruments make them impractical for primary pediatric care settings.

Psychopharmacology

Children with autism often have behavioral problems that can be partially managed with medication. Risperidone, an atypical antipsychotic medication, has been reported to be safe and effective for use among children with autism to treat irritability, as well as aggression, self-injury, and tantrums.[15] To date, risperidone is the only medication approved by the US Food and Drug Administration for autism.[16] Selective serotonin reuptake inhibitors (eg, fluoxetine, sertraline) and medicines designed to improve attention and limit distractibility (eg, stimulants, atomoxetine) have been used with varying degrees of success.[17]

Advocating for Treatment

Effective psychosocial interventions for autism have been developed, and early intervention is critical.[18] Primary care physicians are often placed in the role of advocate for a child's placement within highly intensive, behaviorally oriented intervention programs that are based on several decades of research. Up to nearly one half of children with autism who receive at least 2 years of one-on-one behavioral instruction for 40 hours a week have been reported to achieve age-level functioning, including normal intelligence, average adaptive behavior, and regular educational placement.[19] These findings have been partially replicated by other research groups, suggesting that early and intensive behavioral intervention can lead to improved outcomes for children with autism.[20-23] This psychosocial intervention is known by many names, including *applied behavior analysis* (ABA), *discrete trial training* (DTT), *intensive behavioral intervention* (IBI), or *early intensive behavioral intervention* (EIBI). EIBI is probably the most descriptive of terms; this intervention occurs early (between the ages of 2 and 7 years), is intensive (30 to 40 hours per week), and is based on the principles of applied behavior analysis.[24]

In an EIBI program, teaching methods and curricula are specially designed. This type of program consists of multiple teachers, sometimes called aides or therapists, working in 2- or 3-hour sessions, one on one with a child for up to 40 hours a week. Each session includes structured, teacher-directed activities and free play. EIBI sessions are initially implemented within the child's home, but as treatment progresses, sessions are conducted in community and school settings. The child is taught new skills in a systematic, step-by-step fashion that is designed to not be too difficult. Instruction is quickly paced, which helps keep the child engaged and interested. Teaching methods are derived from ABA and involve reinforcing children with favorite foods, preferred activities, and praise for successfully completing developmental tasks. The teachers help the children perform tasks that are too hard for them with a system of prompts that are gradually faded to promote an independent response. The curriculum used in EIBI programs is individually designed, hierarchically sequenced, and paced at each child's learning rate. The curriculum includes learning the prerequisites to language (eg, imitation, matching), expanding language and communication, play skills, self-help skills, and social skills, as well as early school-related concepts. Parents are also trained in the behavioral teaching methods and work to generalize the child's learning from the EIBI teaching sessions into everyday situations at home. The most successful children in EIBI programs are those who eventually discover how to learn from

Table 136-1 Advantages and Disadvantages of Measures for Diagnosing Autism Spectrum Disorders

MEASURE	AGE AT DIAGNOSIS	METHOD	MAJOR ADVANTAGES	MAJOR DISADVANTAGES
Asperger Syndrome Disorder Scale[a]	5-18 yr	Parent or teacher questionnaire	Brief administration (5 min)	Dichotomous response scale Inadequate reliability
Autism Diagnostic Interview: Revised (ADI-R)[b]	18 mo to adult	Semistructured parent interview	Comprehensive and historical	Requires specialized training Long administration (> hour)
Autism Diagnostic Observation Schedule (ADOS)[c]	18 mo to adult	Standardized observation of child-adult interactions	Behavioral observations coded by examiner Brief administration (30 min)	Requires specialized training High rate of false-positive results
Childhood Autism Rating Scale (CARS)[d]	3 yr to adult	Parent or teacher report or observation	Brief administration (20 min)	Inadequate reliability
Gilliam Asperger's Disorder Scale (GADS)[e]	3-22 yr	Parent or teacher questionnaire	Brief administration (5 min)	Inadequate reliability
Gilliam Autism Rating Scale (GARS)[d]	3-22 yr	Parent or teacher questionnaire	Brief administration (5 min)	Inadequate reliability
Modified Checklist for Autism in Toddlers (M-CHAT)[f]	18 mo	Parent or teacher questionnaire	Brief administration (5 min) Widely adopted in research and clinical settings for surveillance	Dichotomous response scale Lacks specificity as a diagnostic measure
Pervasive Developmental Disorders Behavior Inventory (PDDBI)[g]	18 mo to 12.5 yr, 5 mo	Parent or teacher questionnaire	Comprehensive May be sensitive to treatment effects	Long administration (30-45 min)
Social Communication Questionnaire (SCQ)[h]	4 yr to adult	Parent or teacher questionnaire	Based on the ADI-R	Not useful for early childhood assessment Lacks adequate specificity
Social Responsiveness Scale (SRS)[i]	4-18 yr	Parent or teacher questionnaire	Brief administration (20 min) Emphasizes social disability	Not useful for early childhood assessment

[a]Myles BS, Bock SJ, Simpson RL. *Asperger Syndrome Diagnostic Scale.* Austin, TX: Pro-Ed; 2001.
[b]Lord C, Rutter M, Le Couteur A. Autism Diagnostic Interview—Revised: a revised version of a diagnostic interview for caregivers of individuals with possible pervasive developmental disorders. *J Autism Dev Dis.* 1994;24:659-685.
[c]Lord C, Rutter M, Goode S, et al. Autism Diagnostic Observation Schedule: a standardized observation of communicative and social behavior. *J Autism Dev Dis.* 1989;19:185-212.
[d]Schopler E, Reichler RJ, Rochen Renner B. *Childhood Autism Rating Scale.* Los Angeles, CA: Western Psychological Services; 1986.
[e]Gilliam JE. *Gilliam Asperger's Disorder Scale.* Austin, TX: Pro-Ed; 2001.
[f]Robins DL, Fein D, Barton ML, et al. The Modified Checklist for Autism in Toddlers: an initial study investigating the early detection of autism and pervasive developmental disorders. *J Autism Dev Dis.* 2001;31:131-144.
[g]Cohen IL, Sudhalter V. *Pervasive Developmental Disorders Behavior Inventory: Professional Manual.* Lutz, FL: Psychological Assessment Resources; 2005.
[h]Rutter M, Bailey A, Lord C. *Social Communication Questionnaire.* Los Angeles, CA: Western Psychological Services; 2003.
[i]Constantino JN, Gruber CP. *Social Responsiveness Scale.* Los Angeles, CA: Western Psychological Services; 2000.

natural environments and typical educational experiences.[24] EIBI has been recognized as an effective treatment by the US Surgeon General in a report issued in 1999.[25]

PROGNOSIS

The future is not as dark for children diagnosed with autism as it was 20 or 30 years ago. Home childrearing and the availability of community special educational services for all developmentally disabled children since the early 1980s has decreased behavioral morbidities associated with institutionalization and restricted access to learning experiences. Parents and professionals have learned how to advocate effectively for these children,[26] and these efforts have resulted in much wider adoption of empirically validated interventions in schools and health service settings. Intense study of these disorders has become a federal research priority, and several private research advocacy groups have formed to support research and information dissemination efforts. Advances in epigenetics will likely shed light on the various causes of the ASDs, thus permitting some prevention options.

WHEN TO REFER

Children between 18 and 24 months of age should be referred to a developmental specialist if any one of the following exists:

- A lack of simple pretend play
- A lack of pointing out objects of interest
- An inability to direct a child's attention
- Little interest in other children
- An inability to follow simple instructions
- Little or no expressive language, including single words by 18 months and phrases by 24 months

WHEN TO ADMIT

- Severe malnutrition related to restricted food interests
- Evaluation for gastrointestinal problems
- Evaluation for seizure disorder
- Evaluation for sleep disorder
- Life-threatening self-injurious behavior or aggression
- Psychopharmacologic toxicity

TOOLS FOR PRACTICE

Community Advocacy and Coordination

- *Life Journey Through Autism: An Educator's Guide* (booklet), Organization for Autism Research (www.researchautism.org/resources/OAR_EducatorsGuide.pdf).
- *Life Journey Through Autism: An Educator's Guide to Asperger Syndrome* (booklet), Organization for Autism Research (www.researchautism.org/resources/OAR_Guide_Asperger.pdf).

Engaging Patient and Family

- *Autism Spectrum Disorders Fact Sheets* (fact sheet), Centers for Disease Control and Prevention (www.cdc.gov/ncbddd/autism/ActEarly/autism.html).
- *Is Your One Year Old Communicating with You?* (brochure), American Academy of Pediatrics (patiented.aap.org).
- *Life Journey Through Autism: A Parent's Guide to Research* (booklet), Organization for Autism Research (www.researchautism.org/resources/parents%20guide.pdf).
- *Understanding Autism Spectrum Disorders (ASD)* (brochure), American Academy of Pediatrics (patiented.aap.org).

Medical Decision Support

- *Asperger Syndrome Diagnostic Scale* (scale), Myles BS, Bock SJ, Simpson RL (proedinc.com/customer/productView.aspx?ID=1842).
- *Autism Diagnostic Interview: Revised (ADI-R)* (interview), Lord C, Rutter M, Le Couteur A (portal.wpspublish.com/portal/page?_pageid=53,70436&_dad=portal&_schema=PORTAL).
- *Autism Diagnostic Observation Schedule (ADOS)* (package), Lord C, Rutter M, DiLavore P, Risi S (portal.wpspublish.com/portal/page?_pageid=53,70384&_dad=portal&_schema=PORTAL).
- *Autism—Members Only Channel* (Web page), American Academy of Pediatrics (www.aap.org/moc/mmrautismres.cfm).
- *Caring for Children with Autism Spectrum Disorders: A Resource Toolkit for Clinicians* (tool kit), American Academy of Pediatrics (www.aap.org/bookstore).
- *Childhood Autism Rating Scale: CARS* (scale), Schopler E, Reichler R, Renner B (portal.wpspublish.com/portal/page?_pageid=53,69417&_dad=portal&_schema=PORTAL).
- *Gilliam Asperger's Disorder Scale*, Gilliam JE (proedinc.com/customer/productView.aspx?ID=822).
- *Gilliam Autism Rating Scale*, Gilliam JE (proedinc.com/customer/productView.aspx?ID=3754).
- *Pervasive Developmental Disorders Behavior Inventory (PDDBI)*, Cohen I, Sudhalter V (www3.parinc.com/products/product.aspx?Productid=PDDBI).
- *Screening for Autism in Young Children: The Modified Checklist for Autism in Toddlers (M-CHAT)*, Dumont-Mathieu T, Fein D, Kleinman J (www.dbpeds.org/articles/detail.cfm?TextID=377).
- *Social Communication Questionnaire: SCQ* (other), Rutter M, Bailey A, Lord C (portal.wpspublish.com/portal/page?_pageid=53,70432&_dad=portal&_schema=PORTAL).
- *Social Responsiveness Scale: SRS*, Constantino JN (portal.wpspublish.com/portal/page?_pageid=53,70492&_dad=portal&_schema=PORTAL).
- *The Modified Checklist for Autism in Toddlers (M-CHAT)* (checklist), Robins DL, Fein D, Barton ML, Green JA (www.dbpeds.org/media/mchat.pdf).

RELATED WEB SITES

- American Academy of Pediatrics—Children's Health Topics: Autism (www.aap.org/healthtopics/autism.cfm).
- American Academy of Pediatrics: Autism Spectrum Disorders (www.medicalhomeinfo.org/health/autism.html).
- Autism Speaks (www.autismspeaks.org/).
- Cambridge Center for Behavioral Studies (www.behavior.org/autism/).
- Centers for Disease Control and Prevention: Autism Information Center (www.cdc.gov/ncbddd/autism/index.htm).
- Organization for Autism Research (www.researchautism.org/index.asp).

AAP POLICY STATEMENTS

- Johnson CP, Myers SM, American Academy of Pediatrics, Council on Children With Disabilities. Identification and evaluation of children with autism spectrum disorders. *Pediatrics*. 2007;120(5):1183-1215.
- Myers SM, Johnson CP, American Academy of Pediatrics, Council on Children With Disabilities. Management of children with autism spectrum disorders. *Pediatrics*. 2007;120(5):1162-1182.

SUGGESTED RESOURCES

Autism Speaks, Inc. Available at: www.autismspeaks.org/. This organization and their Web site are dedicated to increasing public awareness about autism, providing advocacy, and supporting autism research. The Web site provides text and video segments to educate about autism.

Cambridge Center for Behavioral Studies. Autism and ABA, Introduction to the CCBS Autism Section. Available at: www.behavior.org/autism/. This organization along with their Web site provides resources and articles describing science-based information on effective autism treatment.

Jacobson J, Mulick JA, Foxx RM. *Fads, Controversies, and Politically Correct Treatment in Developmental Disabilities*. Hillsdale, NJ: Lawrence Erlbaum Associates; 2004.

Maurice C, Green G, Luce S. *Behavioral Intervention for Young Children With Autism*. Austin, TX: Pro-Ed; 1996.

Organization for Autism Research. Available at: www.researchautism.org/. This organization along with their Web site is dedicated to promoting science in autism treatment. Several parent- or teacher-oriented publications on autism and Asperger disorder are available that can be downloaded free of charge. including the "Life Journey Through Autism" series.

Volkmar FR, Wiesner LA. *Healthcare for Children on the Autism Spectrum: A Guide to Medical, Nutritional, and Behavioral Issues*. Bethesda, MD: Woodbine House; 2004.

REFERENCES

1. Filipek PA, Accardo PJ, Baranek GT, et al. The screening and diagnosis of autistic spectrum disorders. *J Autism Dev Disord*. 1999;29:439-484.
2. American Psychiatric Association. *Diagnostic and Statistical Manual of Mental Disorders*. 4th ed, text revision. Washington, DC: American Psychiatric Association; 2000.
3. Fombonne E. Epidemiological surveys of autism and other pervasive developmental disorders: an update. *J Autism Dev Disord*. 2003;33:365-382.
4. Jacobson JW. Early intensive behavioral intervention: emergence of a consumer-driven service model. *Behavior Analyst*. 2000;23:149-171.
5. Happe F, Ronald A, Plomin R. Time to give up on a single explanation for autism. *Nat Neurosci*. 2006;9:1218-1220.
6. Rutter M. Genetic influences in autism. In: Volkmar F, Klin A, Paul R, eds. *Handbook of Autism and Pervasive Developmental Disorders*. 3rd ed. New York, NY: J Wiley; 2005.
7. Minshew NJ, Sweeney JA, Bauman ML, et al. Neurologic aspects of autism. In: Volkmar F, Klin A, Paul R, eds. *Handbook of Autism and Pervasive Developmental Disorders*. 3rd ed. New York, NY: J Wiley; 2005.
8. Towbin KE. Pervasive developmental disorder not otherwise specified. In: Volkmar F, Klin A, Paul R, eds. *Handbook of Autism and Pervasive Developmental Disorders*. 3rd ed. New York, NY: J Wiley; 2005.
9. Van Acker R, Loncola JA, Van Acker EY. Rett syndrome: a pervasive developmental disorder. In: Volkmar F, Klin A, Paul R, eds. *Handbook of Autism and Pervasive Developmental Disorders*. 3rd ed. New York, NY: J Wiley; 2005.
10. Redclay E, Corschene E. When is the brain enlarged in autism? A meta-analysis of all brain size reports. *Biol Psychiatry*. 2005;58:1-9.
11. Robins DL, Fein D, Barton ML, et al. The Modified Checklist for Autism in Toddlers: an initial study investigating the early detection of autism and pervasive developmental disorders. *J Autism Dev Dis*. 2001;31:131-144.
12. Cohen IL, Sudhalter V. *Pervasive Developmental Disorders Behavior Inventory: Professional Manual*. Lutz, FL: Psychological Assessment Resources; 2005.
13. Lord C, Rutter M, Le Couteur A. Autism Diagnostic Interview—Revised: a revised version of a diagnostic interview for caregivers of individuals with possible pervasive developmental disorders. *J Autism Dev Dis*. 1994;24:659-685.
14. Lord C, Rutter M, Goode S, et al. Autism Diagnostic Observation Schedule: a standardized observation of communicative and social behavior. *J Autism Dev Dis*. 1989;19:185-212.
15. Research Units on Pediatric Psychopharmacology (RUPP) Autism Network. Risperidone in children with autism and serious behavioral problems. *N Engl J Med*. 2002;347:314-321.
16. Johnson & Johnson, Inc. News release: FDA Approves RISPERDAL (risperidone) for Treatment of Irritability Associated with Autistic Disorder. Available at: www.jnj.com/news/jnj_news/20061006_135241.htm. Accessed June 19, 2007.
17. Scahill L, Martin A. Psychopharmacology. In: Volkmar F, Klin A, Paul R, eds. *Handbook of Autism and Pervasive Developmental Disorders*. 3rd ed. New York, NY: J Wiley; 2005.
18. National Research Council. *Educating Children with Autism*. Washington DC: National Academy Press; 2001.
19. Lovaas OI. The UCLA Young Autism Model of service delivery. In: Maurice M, Green G, Luce S, eds. *Behavioral Intervention for Young Children With Autism*. Austin, TX: Pro-Ed; 1996.
20. Howard JS, Sparkman CR, Cohen HG, et al. A comparison of behavior analytic and eclectic treatments for young children with autism. *Res Dev Dis*. 2005;26:359-383.
21. Sallows GO, Graupner TD. Intensive behavioral treatment for children with autism: four-year outcome and predictors. *Am J Ment Retard*. 2005;110:417-437.
22. Cohen H, Amerine-Dickens M, Smith T. Early intensive behavioral treatment: replication of the UCLA model in a community setting. *J Dev Behav Pediatr*. 2006;27:S145-S155.
23. Butter EM, Mulick JA, Metz B. Eight case reports of learning recovery in children with pervasive developmental disorders after early intervention. *Behav Intervent*. 2006;21:227-243.
24. Butter EM, Wynn J, Mulick JM. Behavioral intervention for autism. *Pediatr Ann*. 2003;32:677-684.
25. US Department of Health and Human Services. *Mental Health: A Report of the Surgeon General*. Rockville, MD: US Department of Health and Human Services; 1999.
26. Mulick JA, Butter EM. Educational advocacy for children with autism. *Behav Intervent*. 2002;17:57-74.

Chapter 137

ATTENTION-DEFICIT/ HYPERACTIVITY DISORDER

Laurel K. Leslie, MD, MPH; James P. Guevara, MD, MPH

CASE REPORT

Bethany, a 12-year-old black girl, arrives for her first visit at your office with her aunt, Cassandra. Cassandra is Bethany's legal guardian and is concerned that Bethany is failing school. Cassandra, who has raised Bethany from birth, tells you that Bethany was born 2 months early to a mother who abused drugs and alcohol during pregnancy. Although Bethany was a colicky infant who was difficult to feed, she had no major problems after birth and has been healthy except for a few early ear infections. She has since developed into a very social child with endless energy and is currently active with cheerleading. Bethany's talkativeness appeared in first grade and has been noted by every teacher since then. At age 6, she was unable to read simple words but subsequently made adequate progress on reading through elementary school. Although Bethany has never received evaluations or services through school, Cassandra has been helping significantly by structuring Bethany's approach to her schoolwork and by paying for private tutoring. Lately, Bethany has been very low about her academic performance, is having trouble falling asleep, and is difficult to arouse in the morning. Her appetite has been poor, although she insists that she is just not hungry. She denies any suicidal thoughts. Her grades had been average until last year when she began middle school and started failing. On physical examination, Bethany is at the 75th percentile for height, weight, and head circumference. Her vital signs, vision screening, and hearing screening are normal. She has no dysmorphic features, and her physical examination is normal. Bethany is articulate and answers your questions willingly.

DEFINITION OF TERMS

Bethany illustrates one of the frequently occurring presentations to pediatric primary care offices—the child or adolescent with school problems of unclear cause. Attention-deficit/hyperactivity disorder (ADHD), one of the most common neurodevelopmental disorders in children and adolescents, is frequently diagnosed in children with academic underachievement or behavioral problems.[1]

According to the *Diagnostic and Statistical Manual of Mental Disorders,* fourth edition, text revision DSM-IV-TR, the hallmarks of this disorder are hyperactivity, impulsivity, and inattention that are beyond normal developmental expectations for a child's age.[2] The criteria, as depicted in Box 137-1, require that a child meet a minimum of six of nine inattention criteria or six of nine hyperactivity or impulsivity criteria for at least 6 months' duration. Furthermore, the criteria stipulate that symptoms must be present before age 7 years, result in clinically significant impairment in two or more settings (eg, home and school), and not be better explained by another mental health disorder. The definition of clinically significant impairment is not provided but presumably entails academic underachievement or social disruption. The current diagnostic criteria do not account for differences in presentation by age, gender, or race or ethnicity. Therefore clinicians will need to exercise judgment in their use of the criteria.

PREVALENCE

A review of community-based epidemiologic studies has estimated the prevalence of ADHD at 6.8% of school-aged children.[3] Boys are diagnosed at rates 3 times that of girls (9.2% vs 3.0%). The rates of diagnosed ADHD increase with age up to 9 years of age and level off or decline depending on whether youth are taking medications. Differences exist in diagnosed prevalence by race or ethnicity; white children are diagnosed at a greater rate (8.6% vs 7.7% and 3.7%) than black or Hispanic children, respectively.[4]

CLINICAL MANIFESTATIONS

The core symptoms associated with ADHD interfere with attainment of many of the normal developmental milestones of childhood and adolescence, such as academic, fine-motor, and social and adaptive skills. Youth identified with ADHD and monitored into adolescence demonstrated an increased risk for poor academic attainment, impaired familial and peer functioning, lower self-esteem, substance abuse, delinquency, and driving-related accidents.[5-7] Some evidence suggests that treatment may ameliorate some of this risk, particularly for substance abuse.[8] Although many youth with ADHD continue to experience symptoms into adulthood,[6] an age-dependent decline appears to exist in apparent symptoms as children grow older.[9] Hyperactivity and impulsivity tend to remit at a greater rate than inattention.

DIAGNOSIS

Although the diagnosis of ADHD can be made reliably in children using a standardized approach, concerns regarding the validity of the diagnosis of ADHD often arise.[10,11] At present, no biological marker or gold standard diagnostic test exists that can reliably identify persons with and without ADHD. Furthermore, whether the symptoms of ADHD represent a unique disorder or merely one end of the continuum of age-appropriate behavior is unclear.[12] Data that support the validity of ADHD as a unique disorder come from multiple sources. First, cohort studies have consistently shown similar long-term outcomes for youth identified with ADHD (predictive validity).[6] Second, twin studies have demonstrated higher concordance rates of ADHD among monozygotic twins than among dizygotic twins or related siblings, suggesting a genetic predisposition.[13] Third, genetic studies have shown higher rates of gene alterations involving dopamine neurotransmission in subjects with ADHD,[14] and, finally, brain imaging and physiological studies have shown a greater proportion of abnormalities among persons with ADHD than similar controls without ADHD, which suggest a neurodevelopmental process leading to ADHD.[3]

Diagnosing ADHD is complicated by the fact that presentations of ADHD in clinical practice can vary substantially. The core symptoms of ADHD result in three distinct subtypes of ADHD recognized in the DSM-IV-TR (see Box 137-1): (1) a predominantly inattentive subtype (ADHD-IA), (2) a hyperactive/impulsive subtype (ADHD-HI), and (3) a subtype that includes a combination of both inattentive and hyperactive/impulsive features (ADHD-CT). Youth with ADHD-IA often have school underachievement and may go unrecognized by parents and teachers. Contrastingly, youth with ADHD-HI or ADHD-CT commonly demonstrate school underachievement and disruptive classroom behavior and poor relationships with both peers and family members. In addition, many conditions can

BOX 137-1 DSM-IV-TR Criteria for Attention-deficit/Hyperactivity Disorder

A. Either 1 or 2
   1. Six (or more) of the following symptoms of inattention have persisted for at least 6 months to a degree that is maladaptive and inconsistent with developmental level:
      Inattention
      a. Often fails to give close attention to details or makes careless mistakes in school work, work, or other activities
      b. Often has difficulty sustaining attention in tasks or play activities
      c. Often does not seem to listen when spoken to directly
      d. Often does not follow through on instructions and fails to finish schoolwork, chores, or duties in the workplace (not caused by oppositional behavior or failure to understand instructions)
      e. Often has difficulty organizing tasks and activities
      f. Often avoids, dislikes, or is reluctant to engage in tasks that require sustained mental effort (eg, schoolwork, homework)
      g. Often loses things necessary for tasks or activities (eg, toys, school assignments, pencils, books, tools)
      h. Is often easily distracted by extraneous stimuli
      i. Is often forgetful in daily activities
   2. Six (or more) of the following symptoms of hyperactivity or impulsivity have persisted for at least 6 months to a degree that is maladaptive and inconsistent with developmental level:
      Hyperactivity
      a. Often fidgets with hands or feet or squirms in seat
      b. Often leaves seat in classroom or in other situations in which remaining seated is expected
      c. Often runs about or climbs excessively in situations in which doing so is inappropriate (in adolescents or adults, may be limited to subjective feelings of restlessness); often has difficulty playing or engaging in leisure activities quietly
      d. Is often *on the go* or often acts as if *driven by a motor*
      e. Often talks excessively
      Impulsivity
      f. Often blurts out answers before the questions have been completed
      g. Often has difficulty awaiting turn
      h. Often interrupts or intrudes on others (eg, butts into conversations or games)

B. Some hyperactive-impulsive or inattentive symptoms that caused impairments were present before 7 years of age.

C. Some impairment from the symptoms is present in 2 or more settings (eg, at school [or work] or at home).

D. Clear evidence exists of clinically significant impairment in social, academic, or occupational functioning.

E. The symptoms do not occur exclusively during the course of a pervasive developmental disorder, schizophrenia, or other psychotic disorder and are not better accounted for by another mental disorder (eg, mood disorder, anxiety disorder, dissociative disorder, a personality disorder).

   Code based on type:
   314.00 Attention-Deficit/Hyperactivity Disorder, Predominantly Inattentive Type: if criterion A1 is met but criterion A2 is not met for the past 6 months
   314.01 Attention-Deficit/Hyperactivity Disorder, Predominantly Hyperactive-Impulsive Type: if criterion A2 is met but criterion A1 is not met for the past 6 months
   314.01 Attention-Deficit/Hyperactivity Disorder, Combined Type: if both criterion A1 and A2 are met for the past 6 months
   314.9 Attention-Deficit/Hyperactivity Disorder, Not Otherwise Specified

coexist with ADHD, further adding to variation in presentation.

Despite these complexities, the American Academy of Pediatrics (AAP) has encouraged increasing responsibility for the care of youth with ADHD in primary care settings and has recently published evidence-based diagnostic and treatment guidelines for pediatric clinicians.[10,15] This decision reflects the high prevalence rates of ADHD in the community, families' perception of the approachability of primary care physicians, an insufficient supply of child mental health care professionals, and the fact that more than 50% of youth with ADHD currently receive their care in primary care settings.[16,17] To support clinicians in caring for youth with ADHD, the AAP has developed an on-line, interactive training program on ADHD and has partnered with the National Initiative for Children's Healthcare Quality (NICHQ) and the North Carolina Center for Children's Healthcare Improvement to develop an ADHD toolkit. In addition, Bright Futures in Practice: Mental Health, has published a variety of tools for the early identification of childhood behavioral problems.[18] This chapter reviews ADHD diagnosis and treatment within the context of the AAP and Bright Futures initiatives and offers practical resources for the primary care clinician caring for youth with this disorder.

DIFFERENTIAL DIAGNOSIS

Because no definitive biological or imaging markers exist for ADHD, a diagnosis of ADHD requires determining if a child meets DSM-IV-TR diagnostic criteria for ADHD (see Box 137-1) and ascertaining if any other disorders or factors exist that may better explain a child's symptoms and impairment. Many medical, psychosocial, psychiatric, or neurologic conditions may exhibit symptoms similar to ADHD (Box 137-2). These conditions may be the primary cause of the child's behavioral and attention difficulties or may increase a child's level of impairment if comorbid with ADHD. The primary care clinician is responsible for determining if these conditions are present and, if so, whether they are the primary cause of the child's dysfunction or whether they coexist with ADHD. Determining the cause of a child's difficulties and any conditions that may coexist is a complicated process, but the evaluation can be streamlined through a complete history and thorough physical examination, as reviewed here.

Although other professionals may assist in identifying mental health or educational disorders, establishing whether any medical conditions are present is paramount for primary care clinicians. For instance, poor visual acuity or hearing loss can contribute to academic difficulties.[19] Obstructive sleep apnea caused by enlarged tonsils or adenoids or both can be associated with daytime somnolence, hyperactivity, and academic problems.[20] Medication side effects may also explain unusual drowsiness and lack of attention in the classroom. Dermatologic findings such as café au lait spots may suggest neurofibromatosis or other neurologic disorders associated with learning and behavioral difficulties. A history of 20 to 50 episodes a day of repeated staring pauses lasting several seconds in both the home and the school setting may lead a clinician to consider absence seizures.

BOX 137-2 Conditions That May Mimic or Co-Occur With Attention-deficit/Hyperactivity Disorder*

Developmental differences or normal variants
- *Normal variation; giftedness;* sociocultural differences in expectations or parenting or both

Medical disorders:
- *Medication side effects; substances of abuse; hearing impairment; visual impairment; obstructive sleep apnea;* toxins (eg, chronic lead exposure or acute lead intoxication; chronic iron-deficiency anemia); thyroid disorders; chronic disease complications

Neurologic or developmental disorders
- *Learning disabilities; pervasive developmental disorders; tic disorders (Tourette syndrome); communication disorders; processing disorders; intellectual disability; neurodevelopmental syndromes (eg, fetal alcohol syndrome, fragile X syndrome);* cerebral palsy; seizure disorders (petit mal or developmental delays); sequelae of central nervous system trauma or infection; neurodegenerative disorders; motor coordination disorders

Psychosocial or environmental problems
- *Stress in family situation (marriage, separation or divorce, birth of sibling, death); stress in environment (new home, new school); family dysfunction; parenting dysfunction; neglect, abuse, or both; parental psychopathology; parental substance abuse; inappropriate educational program*

Emotional or behavioral disorders
- *Oppositional defiant disorder; conduct disorder; depressive disorders; anxiety disorders;* bipolar disorder; obsessive-compulsive disorder; posttraumatic stress disorder; adjustment reaction; schizophrenia

*Conditions that in general occur more commonly are *italicized*. Notably, the prevalence of any of these conditions will vary depending on the characteristics of the setting in which a youth is being evaluated.

COEXISTING CONDITIONS

Coexisting conditions found commonly in youth with ADHD include oppositional defiant disorder, conduct disorder (see Chapter 138), mood disorders (see Chapter 143), anxiety and depressive disorders (see Chapter 145), and learning disabilities. A recent review of these disorders found high rates of comorbidity with ADHD across multiple studies. Oppositional defiant disorder was the most common, with an average prevalence rate of 35.2% (range, 27.2% to 43.8%). Conduct disorder 25.7% (range, 12.8% to 41.3%), anxiety disorders 25.8% (range, 17.6% to 35.3%), and depressive disorders 18.2% (range, 11.1% to 26.6%) were also common.[3] Rates of coexisting learning disabilities are also high, ranging from 12% to 50%.[4] For many of these disorders, a complete history will provide important clues for further evaluation. For example, a history of speech delay in early childhood, family history of learning disabilities, problems with decoding words in the early elementary school years, or disparate skill acquisition across math, reading, and spelling suggests a learning disability. Psychosocial and environmental factors are common and essential to consider (see Box 137-2).

EVALUATION

The AAP recommends that children ages 6 to 12 years who exhibit inattention, hyperactivity, impulsivity, academic underachievement, or behavior problems should undergo an evaluation for ADHD.[10] The evidence supporting this recommendation is strong and was derived from clinical studies showing a high prevalence of ADHD among school-aged children exhibiting developmental and behavioral concerns.[21] In the opening case report, Bethany's talkativeness and high energy level may represent hyperactivity, impulsivity, or both. This situation combined with her history of academic difficulties, particularly on entry to middle school when attention to detail and organizational skills are increasingly necessary, should prompt an evaluation for ADHD and related conditions.

History

A comprehensive history with particular attention to the presenting complaint, development, school history, family history, and social history is essential to the evaluation and can help identify other problem areas or provide clues to other diagnoses. For a sample comprehensive pediatric intake form, see Tools for Practice at the end of the chapter. The physical examination, though usually normal, can help identify other problems that may contribute to or represent the cause of a child's behavior problems. In addition, the physical examination may allow the opportunity to assess a child's mental status and interaction with caregivers.

Laboratory and Imaging Studies

Laboratory or imaging tests are not indicated in the routine assessment of ADHD but may be appropriate if the review of symptoms or physical examination suggests an alternative diagnosis.[10] For example, plumbism and thyroid dysfunction are often thought to be associated with behavioral problems. However, a systematic review of blood lead levels and thyroid hormone levels are infrequently abnormal in youth with ADHD, and little evidence exists that these tests adequately discriminate between youth with ADHD and those without ADHD.[3] Youth with ADHD often have abnormalities noted on brain imaging or electroencephalography. The abnormalities are not consistent, do not usually represent clinically significant findings, and, again, do not adequately discriminate youth with and without ADHD.[3] Continuous performance tests are often touted as scientific measures of vigilance and distractibility that can help confirm a diagnosis of ADHD. However, systematic reviews of these tests find that their sensitivity and specificity (<70%) are inadequate to distinguish reliably between children with and those without ADHD.[22]

Diagnostic Criteria and Diagnostic Tools

The AAP guidelines recommend that a child must meet DSM-IV-TR criteria to receive a diagnosis of ADHD.[10] The AAP supports use of these criteria to ensure a valid diagnosis is made in primary care and to decrease variation in the diagnostic process among clinicians. ADHD-specific behavior rating scales probe for the presence of ADHD diagnostic criteria and other behavioral problems and can be used to ensure uniformity in how diagnostic criteria are met (Table 137-1). In addition, ADHD rating scales provide cut-point scores that when exceeded increase the likelihood that ADHD is present.[3] Several excellent ADHD rating scales for parent and teacher respondents are commercially available to clinicians (see Tools for Practice), such as the Vanderbilt Rating Scales, the ADHD Rating Scale, the Conners' Rating Scales, and the SNAP Rating Scales.[23-26] The Vanderbilt Rating Scales are also available in the public domain at no cost. Other more general behavioral rating scales, such as the Child Behavior Checklist[27,28] and the Behavior Assessment System for Children,[29] do not include ADHD diagnostic criteria and lack adequate sensitivity and specificity (approximately 86%) for the diagnosis of ADHD and related disorders. However, they may be used to triage children for specific

Table 137-1 Sensitivity and Specificity of Rating Scales for the Diagnosis of Attention-deficit/Hyperactivity Disorder*

RATING SCALE	AGE (YEARS)	GENDER	EFFECT SIZE	95% CI
Conners Parent Rating Scale- 1997 Revised Version: Long Form, ADHD Index Scale (CPRS-R:L-ADHD Index)	6-17	MF	3.1	2.5, 3.7
Conners Teacher Rating Scale- 1997 Revised Version: Long Form, ADHD Index Scale (CTRS-R:L-ADHD Index)	6-17	MF	3.3	2.8, 3.8
Conners Parent Rating Scale- 1997 Revised Version: Long Form, DSM-IV Symptoms Scale (CPRS-R:L-DSM-IV Symptoms)	6-17	MF	3.4	2.8, 4.0
Conners Teacher Rating Scale- 1997 Revised Version: Long Form, DSM-IV Symptoms Scale (CTRS-R:L-DSM-IV Symptoms)	6-17	MF	3.7	3.2, 4.2
ACTeRS- Parent Version ADD-H: Comprehensive Teacher Rating Scale, Hyperactivity Subscale	6-14	MF	1.5	1.3, 1.7
ACTeRS- Parent Version ADD-H: Comprehensive Teacher Rating Scale, Attention Subscale	6-14	MF	2.0	1.8, 2.2
SNAP-III (Hyperactivity Subscale)	7-12	MF	5.1	3.9, 6.3
SNAP-III (Inattention Subscale)	7-12	MF	4.2	3.2, 5.2
SNAP-III (Impulsivity Subscale)	7-12	MF	5.5	4.3, 6.7
School Situations Questionnaire- Original Version, Number of Problem Settings Scale (SSQ-O-I)	6-11	F	1.3	0.5, 2.2
School Situations Questionnaire- Original Version, Mean Severity Scale (SSQ-O-II)	6-11	F	2.0	2.2, 3.5
Vanderbilt AD/HD Diagnostic Parent Rating Scale (VADPRS)	6-12	MF	N/A	N/A
Vanderbilt AD/HD Diagnostic Teacher Rating Scale (VADTRS)	6-12	MF	N/A	N/A

*Green M, Wong M, Atkins D, Taylor J, Feinleib M. *Diagnosis of Attention-Deficit/Hyperactivity Disorder. Technical Review No. 3.* Rockville, MD: Agency for Health Care Policy and Research; 1999. AHCPR Publication No. 99-0050.
M, male; *F*, female.

diagnostic interviews[30] or to give a more global impression of a child's functioning. The use of these tools does not indicate that a youth has a particular disorder; only a trained clinician should make a diagnosis after a thorough assessment. Any symptoms suggestive of possible harm to self or others warrant immediate evaluation by a skilled clinician.

An algorithm that may be helpful in assessing ADHD is shown in Figure 137-1. Patients with behavior problems or academic difficulties are scheduled for

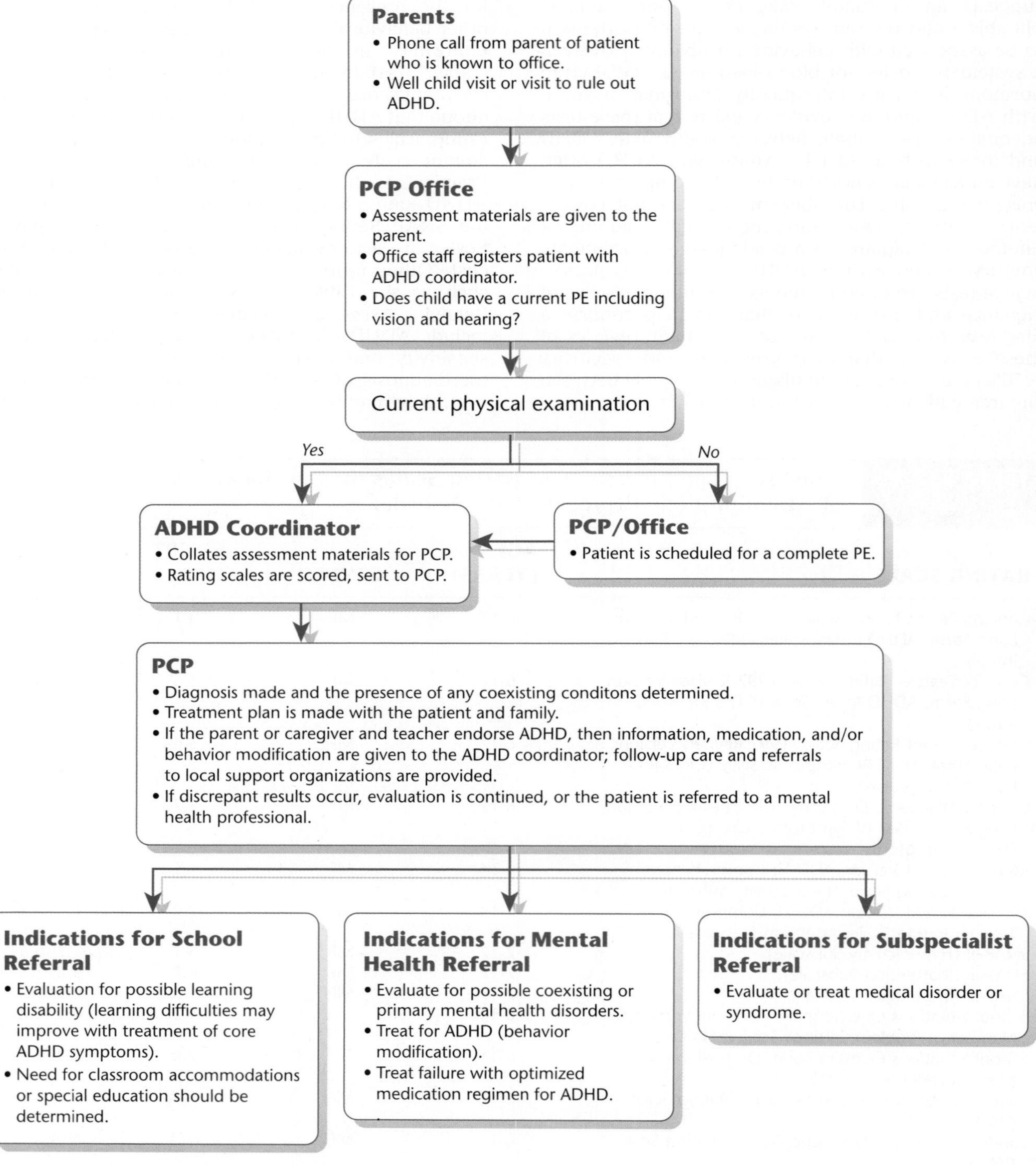

Figure 137-1 Sample attention-deficit/hyperactivity disorder flowchart for the primary care office. *PCP,* Primary care provider; *ADHD,* attention-deficit/hyperactivity disorder; *PE,* physical examination.

a complete physical examination, including hearing and vision assessments, and are given assessment materials. The assessment materials may contain a pediatric intake history form, a request for school records, behavior rating scales, or educational materials. Once the assessment materials have been completed, rating scales scored, and a current physical examination documented, patients may be scheduled for an evaluation. The number of visits needed to complete the evaluation depends on the complexity of complaints and the amount of time available at each visit. The time reported to complete the overall evaluation, review background records, provide patient and family education, and establish a treatment plan may take from 90 to 240 minutes.[31] Offices have found multiple solutions for obtaining assessment materials and completing an evaluation, including the use of written assessment or computerized packets, longer appointments scheduled at designated times (eg, evenings, Saturday mornings, one particular clinic session every other week), partnerships with local schools, or the use of affiliated health care personnel, including social workers or mental health professionals. The ADHD toolkit includes the Vanderbilt Rating Scales, both parent and teacher initial assessment and follow-up forms, and a sample cover letter to assist physicians in creating an office-based system for efficiently evaluating a child for ADHD.

Given that children spend a substantial amount of time in the classroom, the AAP guidelines stipulate that clinicians should obtain data from schools on children's level of functioning and academic achievement.[10] Data that may be helpful in formulating a diagnostic impression of children include information on the DSM-IV-TR diagnostic criteria for ADHD and results of multidisciplinary evaluations, individual educational plans (IEPs), achievement tests, grades, and written or verbal teacher narratives. Many of the ADHD rating scales discussed previously employ teacher versions that can be used to facilitate endorsement of diagnostic criteria or to assess for other conditions by school or after-school personnel (see Table 137-1). For children who are home schooled or who spend a fair amount of time in after-school programs, clinicians may want to obtain information from adults overseeing these programs, such as coaches, religious educators, after-school caregivers, and tutors.

Evaluating Children Who Fail to Meet Attention-deficit/Hyperactivity Disorder Criteria

Some children may not meet diagnostic criteria for ADHD because they have fewer than the required number of DSM-IV-TR criteria or because of conflicting reports among parents and school staff. The *Diagnostic and Statistical Manual for Primary Care, Child and Adolescent Version* (DSM-PC), can assist clinicians in identifying subclinical conditions or normal variations in behavior and in considering environmental stressors that may influence behaviors (Table 137-2).[32] The manual provides descriptions of problematic behaviors from normal variations and problem behaviors to the level of the disorder. These descriptions are accompanied by *The International Classification of Diseases, Ninth Revision, Clinical Modification* codes to assist the clinician in billing; however, the acceptability

Table 137-2 Attentional-Hyperactivity Variations That Do Not Meet DSM-IV-TR Criteria[*]

DEVELOPMENTAL VARIATION	COMMON DEVELOPMENTAL PRESENTATIONS
V65.49 Inattention Variation A young child will have a short attention span that will increase as the child matures. The inattention should be appropriate for the child's level of development and not cause any impairment.	*Early childhood:* The preschooler has difficulty attending, except briefly, to a storybook or a quiet task such as coloring or drawing. *Middle childhood:* The child may not persist very long with a task the child does not want to do, such as read an assigned book, homework, or a task that requires concentration such as cleaning something. *Adolescence:* The adolescent is easily distracted from a task that the child does not desire to perform.
V65.49 Hyperactive/Impulsive Variation Young children in infancy and in the preschool years are normally very active and impulsive and may need constant supervision to avoid injury. Their constant activity may be stressful to adults who do not have the energy or patience to tolerate the behavior. During school years and in adolescence, activity may be high in play situations and impulsive behaviors may normally occur, especially in peer pressure situations. High levels of hyperactive/impulsive behavior do not indicate a problem or disorder if the behavior does not impair function.	*Early childhood:* The child runs in circles, does not stop to rest, may bang into objects or people, and asks questions constantly. *Middle childhood:* The child plays active games for long periods. The child may occasionally do things impulsively, particularly when excited. *Adolescence:* The adolescent engages in active social activities (eg, dancing) for long periods, may engage in risky behaviors with peers.

[*]American Academy of Pediatrics. *The Classification of Child and Adolescent Mental Diseases in Primary Care.* Washington, DC: American Academy of Pediatrics; 1996.

of such diagnostic codes by insurance carriers is not clear. An additional resource containing *Current Procedural Terminology* billing codes for mental health services in the primary care setting is provided at the Bright Futures in Practice: Mental Health Tool Kit Web site.

Evaluating Co-Occurring Conditions

Many children with ADHD have co-occurring behavioral or developmental conditions that may impair functioning and the AAP guidelines recommend that all youth undergoing an evaluation for ADHD be assessed for these conditions. In addition to taking a complete history, several excellent tools are available that can aid the primary care clinician in assessing for these conditions. Several of the ADHD ratings scales (ie, Vanderbilt Rating Scales, the Conners' Rating Scales-Revised, and the SNAP-IV rating scales) include items that query for symptoms of depression or anxiety, oppositional-defiant, and conduct disorders.[23,25,26] Rating scales also exist that specifically target the assessment of particular conditions including depression, anxiety, and disruptive behaviors. Some examples include the Center for Epidemiological Studies Depression Scale for Children (CES-DC),[33] the Multidimensional Anxiety Scale for Children,[34] and the Eyberg Child Behavior Inventory.[35] A detailed table of screening tools and rating scales specific to a variety of childhood mental health symptoms are available on line that is a superb reference for clinicians. Questionnaires are also available that review DSM-IV-TR criteria for most common childhood mental health disorders in one instrument, such as the Child Symptom Inventory (CSI)[36] and the DISC Predictive Scales.[37] Global behavioral rating scales such as the Pediatric Symptom Checklist, Child Behavior Checklist (CBCL), and the Behavior Assessment System for Children (BASC) can provide an overall perspective on a youth's functioning although they do not identify specific co-occurring conditions.

The algorithm (see Figure 137-1) directs the clinician to refer to another professional (ie, mental health or school-based) if a comorbid condition is suspected and if the clinician is not equipped to evaluate sufficiently for these types of disorders in the office setting. Compiling a mental health resource list in the office can assist families in identifying local mental health care providers on their insurance plans who can evaluate the youth for possible comorbid mental health disorders. Bright Futures provides a template for mental health referrals that can be used to structure referral information. For school referrals, parents should be directed to draft a letter requesting a multidisciplinary evaluation, including psychoeducational testing, if the history suggests a possible learning disability such as a reading disorder (dyslexia), mathematics disorder (dyscalculia), a disorder of written expression, or a communication disorder. An example of such a letter is included in the AAP ADHD toolkit. Handouts regarding school problems are also available from Bright Futures, including one on common signs of learning disorders. Public schools are required to respond to family requests for evaluations within a specified period, determined by local school district policies; even children attending private schools or who are home schooled are eligible to receive an evaluation through their local school district. Families may also be referred to independent psychologists for psychoeducational evaluations through their insurance plans, but clinicians should inquire whether their local school district accepts outside evaluations before making any referrals. In any event, the algorithm recommends that treatment for ADHD not be delayed while awaiting the results of referrals, given that symptoms of many of these conditions may improve with treatment of the ADHD core symptoms.

MANAGEMENT

The AAP treatment guidelines[15] recommend that families, school personnel, and clinicians first recognize that ADHD is a chronic condition that will require ongoing, collaborative care. The Chronic Care Model, developed by Wagner and colleagues[38] and then modified for children by NICHQ, highlights the importance of patient and family education in the management of any chronic condition. Youth and family education is particularly important in treating ADHD for several reasons. First, ADHD affects youth across multiple domains of functioning, and understanding the implications of this disorder across these domains is important for youth and families. Second, parents are important partners in treatment because they ultimately implement any treatment programs in the home setting. Third, youth with ADHD are often cared for by a spectrum of health and school professionals; parents, especially with latency-age children, function as essential case managers in any ADHD management plan. As youth age, it becomes increasingly important that they take on the role of case manager, with the ultimate outcome that they are ready to assume management of their ADHD in adulthood. Handouts, book or Web site reference lists or evening or weekend informational sessions in the office for youth and families with ADHD are some educational mechanisms that have been used successfully by primary care clinicians (see Tools for Practice at the end of the chapter). Additional strategies include educational and support groups such as Children and Adults with ADD (CHADD) or the Learning Disabilities Association (LDA) that provide important information to youth and families regarding ADHD and its comorbid disorders, access to mental health and school-based services, and day-to-day lifestyle strategies to address the impact of ADHD on the youth and family.

The AAP recommends that clinicians, parents, and the child, in collaboration with school personnel, should identify specific target outcomes in youth functioning that they hope to effect through a treatment management plan. Treatment strategies of choice delineated in the guidelines include evidence-based medication strategies or psychosocial interventions (or both) and are discussed in more detail later in this chapter. The guidelines also comment that youth functioning should be systematically monitored over time to evaluate whether target outcomes are achieved or adverse side effects to treatment develop. If a youth is not meeting targeted outcomes, then clinicians, parents, and school personnel should collaboratively determine the validity of the diagnosis, adherence to all components of the treatment plan, and the possibility of any previously unidentified coexisting conditions. The ADHD toolkit includes sample management plans and follow-up parent and teacher assessment forms to assist clinicians in monitoring treatment.

Although the AAP guidelines specifically discuss medications and psychosocial interventions, three broad treatment modalities have been recommended in the literature, most often combined in what is commonly referred to as *multimodal treatment*. These modalities include (1) medications, (2) psychosocial interventions directed at the child in the home and school settings, and (3) classroom assistance. These treatment types are reviewed in the subsections later in this chapter. Data are drawn from four sources: (1) the Agency for Healthcare Research and Quality's 1999 evidence report and technology assessment on the treatment of ADHD,[39] (2) Jensen and Cooper's 2002 volume reviewing the state of the evidence regarding diagnosis and treatment of ADHD,[40] (3) publications from the Children's Medication Algorithm Project,[41,42] and (4) results from the recent Multimodal Treatment Study of Children with Attention Deficit Hyperactivity Disorder (MTA).[43-48] In general, solid evidence exists for the use of stimulant medication, behavioral-modification strategies, and their combination in the treatment of ADHD. Other treatments such as other psychotropic medications and school-based services have been studied although not as extensively, and the evidence supporting their use is present but less robust.

Medication

Psychostimulants (methylphenidate, dextroamphetamine, and the mixed salts of amphetamine) with careful medication management are the most commonly prescribed medications for ADHD (Table 137-3). Although the mechanism of attentional enhancement is unknown, the psychostimulants are believed to have putative effects on central catecholamine pathways.[49] In short-term studies, psychostimulants have been found to address the core symptoms of ADHD and improve sustained attention, organization, and motor inhibitor control.[50] They also decrease disruptive behaviors (eg, fidgetiness, impulsive interrupting, aggression, relational interactions, oppositionality) in the classroom, on the playground, in social settings, and at home.[51-53] With respect to cognitive functioning, these medications increase the accuracy of performance and improve short-term memory, reaction time, and seatwork computation; however, the effect size is smaller than that seen for behavioral challenges (see review by Spencer et al, 1996).[54] An initial trial of stimulants with careful medication management has been shown to be effective for approximately 70% of children diagnosed with ADHD.[55,56] This percentage increases to over 90% if an alternative stimulant is tried after failure of an initial stimulant.[57]

The most rigorous long-term trial of stimulant medications is the National Institute of Mental Health–funded MTA Study. This study was designed to compare the effects of four 14-month treatments for school-aged children with ADHD-CT: (1) stimulants and medication management alone, (2) behavioral interventions, (3) combination therapy (stimulants plus behavioral interventions), or (4) assessment and referral to community care. The stimulant medication and management arm included careful titration of methylphenidate to the maximal dose that improved functioning with the fewest side effects, a three-times-daily schedule, manualized algorithm for dose adjustment and trial of alternative medications, and monthly pharmacotherapist-performed clinical assessments with parent and teacher. Results demonstrated that carefully managed stimulant medication, either alone or in combination with behavioral interventions, was effective in reducing the core symptoms of ADHD, reducing oppositional-aggressive and anxiety symptoms, and in improving social skills.[43-48]

The effects of the stimulants are compensatory and not curative. The effect lasts only as long as the youth takes the medication. Unfortunately, very few long-term studies of the efficacy of the stimulant medications have been conducted; specific studies that are available are limited by their retrospective study design, lack of adherence measures, limited use of titration, and poor identification of comorbid conditions. A meta-analysis by Swanson and colleagues[58] concluded that the effect of stimulant medications over time on academic achievement was significantly less than the effect on behavior and cognition. In addition, many children with ADHD continue to show symptoms as they enter adult life, including troublesome interpersonal relationships with family members and peers, career underachievement, and poor self-esteem.[1,59] However, these earlier studies have not adjusted for the onset of treatment and the intensity of intervention offered. More recent retrospective studies demonstrate that treatment may be protective against poor outcomes. For example, children treated for ADHD with stimulant medication may be less likely to experiment with substances during adolescence compared with their untreated peers with ADHD.[60]

The decision regarding the use of psychostimulants requires careful consideration of the associated benefits and risks. Common side effects of the psychostimulants include headaches, stomachaches, insomnia, and anorexia. Growth delay of approximately 1 cm in height lost per year has been documented in the MTA Study.[61] Recent data suggest that the medications do not appear to consistently exacerbate tics.[62] Less commonly reported adverse events include irritability, emotional lability or constriction, and compulsive picking of the nose or skin. These medications are also classified as schedule II medications with possible high abuse potential, although the research does not suggest a preferential use of stimulants in individuals with ADHD and substance use disorders.[63,64]

Other safety concerns were the focus of a US Food and Drug Administration (FDA) review in 2006 and included cardiovascular and psychiatric complications related to the stimulant medications.[65] Cardiovascular concerns included elevations in heart rate and blood pressure, as well as rare cardiovascular events such as stroke, myocardial infarction and sudden death, particularly in youth with preexisting cardiac disease. The panel concluded that youth should be monitored for

Table 137-3 Stimulant Medications, Dosing, and Duration of Effects

ACTIVE INGREDIENT	DRUG NAME	DOSING	DURATION OF BEHAVIORAL EFFECTS
Mixed salts of amphetamine (dextroamphetamine/ levoamphetamine)	ADDERALL Tablets (*scored*): 5, 7.5, 10, 12.5, 15, 20, 30 mg	Start with 5 mg 1-2 times per day and increase by 5 mg each week until good control achieved. Maximal recommended dose: 40 mg	4-6 hr
	ADDERALL RX Extended-Release Capsule (*sprinkable*): 5, 10, 15, 20, 25, 30 mg extended-release capsules	Start at 5 mg in the morning and increase by 5 mg each week until good control is achieved. Maximal recommended dose: 30 mg	10-12 hr
Dextroamphetamine	DEXEDRINE Tablet: 5 mg DEXTROSTAT Tablet (*scored*): 5, 10 mg	Tablet: Start with 5 mg 1-2 times per day and increase by 5 mg each week until good control achieved. Maximal recommended dose: 40 mg	4-6 hr
	DEXEDRINE SPANSULES Sustained-Release Capsule (*cannot be chewed*): 5, 10, 15 mg	Capsule: start with 5 mg one time per day and increase by 5 mg each week until good control is achieved.	6-10 hr
Methylphenidate	RITALIN METHYLIN Tablets (*scored*): 5, 10, 20 mg METHYLIN Chewable Tablets: 5, 10, 20 mg METHYLIN Oral Solution: 5, 10 mg/ 5 mL	Start with 5 mg 1-2 times per day and increase by 5 mg each week until good control is achieved. May need third reduced dose in the evening. Maximal recommended dose: 60 mg	
	FOCALIN Tablets (*scored*): 2.5, 5, 10 mg	Start with 2.5 mg 1-2 times per day and increase by 2.5 mg each week until good control is achieved. May need third reduced dose in the evening. Maximal recommended dose: 30 mg	4-5 hr
	RITALIN-LA Capsule (*can be sprinkled*): 10, 20, 30, 40 mg RITALIN-SR Tablet: 20 mg SR METADATE ER Tablet: 10, 20 mg extended release METHYLIN ER Tablet: 10 mg extended release METADATE CD Capsule (*can be sprinkled*): 10, 20, 30 mg extended release	Start with 10-20 mg in the morning and increase each week until good control is achieved. Alternatively, titrate using short-acting methylphenidate and then switch over to a longer-acting form. May need second dose or regular methylphenidate dose in the evening. Maximal recommended dose: 60 mg	6-10 hr
	FOCALIN XR Capsule (*can be sprinkled*): 5, 10, 20 mg	Start with 5 mg in the morning and increase by 5 mg each week until good control is achieved. Maximal recommended dose: 30 mg	8-10 hr
	CONCERTA Capsule (*noncrushable*): 18, 27, 36, 54 mg	Start at 18 mg in the morning and increase by 18 each week until good control is achieved. Maximal recommended dose: 72 mg	8-12 hr
	DAYTRANA Patch 1.1, 1.8, 2.2, 3 mg/hr	Worn daily for 9 hours. Patch is to be replaced once a day in the morning. Skin sensitization as compared with contact rash may occur rarely, causing FDA advisory board to recommend oral methylphenidate use before the patch.	Approximately 12 hr
Lysdexamfetamine	VYVANSE Capsule (*sprinkle in water and drink immediately*): 30, 50, 70 mg	Start at 30 mg in the morning and increase by 20 mg each week until good control is achieved. Maximal recommended dose: 70 mg	Approximately 12 hr

FDA, US Food and Drug Administration.

the emergence of hypertension. In addition, children starting on medication should have a complete history taken (including a family history of heart disease or arrhythmias, as well as symptoms of shortness of breath, chest pain, dizziness, or palpitations on exertion) and a physical examination. Psychiatric concerns raised included new onset or acute exacerbation of aggressive symptoms and rare hallucinogenic symptoms, particularly visual hallucinations related to bugs. Although all of these complications are rare, as with any medication, careful monitoring and vigilance regarding safety is essential.

If parents, in concert with the clinician, decide to try a psychostimulant, all must realize that medication choice, dose, and time interval must be carefully titrated to meet the needs of the individual child. In fact, several trials may be necessary before the most effective medication type and dose with the fewest side effects are identified. Carefully monitored titration that includes documentation of changes in ADHD symptoms and target outcomes and the development of any side effects is essential. Once a child is stable on a medication, the AAP treatment guidelines recommend an office visit every 3 to 6 months to reassess academic performance, behavior, and side effects. More intensive visits may be necessary around predictable periods of change such as entry into middle or high school or the onset of puberty. Trials off medication are important to conduct but should be scheduled so as to not overlap with the beginning of school terms, examinations, or family stressors. Families, youth, and clinicians should consider carefully the use of medication in the afternoons and evenings, on weekends, and during the summer, taking into account the severity of a youth's dysfunction, the effect on family and peers, cultural expectations, and the presence of any decrease in weight or height velocity. Sample follow-up forms are included in the ADHD toolkit. Management of possible side effects is delineated in Table 137-4.

Although not mentioned in the AAP guidelines, preschoolers and children with pervasive developmental disorders or intellectual disability may also benefit from the psychostimulants if they have symptoms of hyperactivity or impulsivity. However, their response is less predictable, and they often experience more adverse events such as tics, anxiety, and social withdrawal. At this point, most clinicians stress behavioral management in the treatment of these children.

Other medications have been used as second-line treatment of ADHD, including a selective norepinephrine reuptake inhibitor (atomoxetine), the tricyclic antidepressants (desipramine, nortyptiline), the atypical antidepressants (bupropion), and the alpha-agonists (clonidine and guanfacine) (Table 137-5). These medications are currently considered second-line treatment because of fewer rigorous research trials, more adverse side effects, or less efficacy in comparison with the stimulants.[66] The Texas Medication Algorithm Project, a large state-wide implementation program on ADHD in public mental health, has published algorithms for the possible use of these medications in the management of ADHD.[41,42] In brief, the alpha-agonists, clonidine and guanfacine, have moderate effects on the hyperactivity and impulsivity associated with ADHD, aggression, and on tics.[62,67] Given their effect on the cardiovascular system, care must be taken to avoid stopping these medications abruptly, which might result in rebound hypertension. In addition, sedation, particularly with clonidine, can be a significant problem. Bupropion has few studies relating to its use in ADHD[68] but has been suggested as an option in youth with comorbid depression. Atomoxetine was approved for the treatment of ADHD in 2003; common side effects include stomachache, nausea, appetite suppression, and weight loss. With increasing use in the community over the last several years, warnings have surfaced regarding aggression, suicidality, reversible hepatotoxicity, and cardiac effects.[69,70] The tricyclics have some effect on ADHD, but their low toxic-to-therapeutic ratio has limited their widespread use.[71] Modafinil is currently approved for treatment of narcolepsy, and recent studies suggest its possible use in ADHD, although the FDA denied its application for approval for treatment of ADHD in 2006.[72] No long-term studies on these medications in the management of ADHD have been completed. As with all medications, clinicians should continue to monitor new scientific information about efficacy and adverse events.

Psychosocial Interventions

Several studies show that psychosocial interventions, predominantly using behavioral-management principles, decrease ADHD symptoms and impairment.[73] Behavioral interventions usually consist of parent training programs, youth-focused intensive summer camp programs, and behavioral consultation in the classroom and, in general, have focused less on improving the core symptoms of ADHD (inattention, impulsivity, and hyperactivity) and instead have sought to improve parenting practices, school functioning, and peer relationships. Common to many of these approaches is the use of behavioral techniques such as positive reinforcement, time-out, response costs, or token economies (Table 137-6). Individual psychotherapy, play therapy, and cognitive therapy have not been shown to reduce core ADHD symptoms; these nonbehavioral therapies may benefit some children with ADHD who have associated mental health conditions responsive to these therapies.

The MTA Study examined the efficacy of behavioral interventions compared with stimulant medication alone or in combination with behavioral therapy. Components of the behavioral interventions in the MTA Study included 27 group and 8 individual parent training sessions, youth participation in an 8-week intensive therapeutic all-day summer camp program, and teacher consultation plus 12 weeks of a half-time behaviorally trained paraprofessional aide in the classroom.[43] The results of this trial have been interpreted in conflicting manners, with some suggesting that the MTA Study demonstrates the superiority of medication either alone or in combination as showing the best outcomes[74] and others highlighting the potential importance of psychosocial interventions among persons receiving the behavioral intervention.[75] Medication in combination with behavioral approaches was found to be particularly effective for children with

Table 137-4 Common Side Effects of Stimulant Medications and Recommended Clinical Management

SIDE EFFECTS	RECOMMENDED CLINICAL MANAGEMENT
General	For mild side effects, allow seven to 10 days for tolerance to develop. Evaluate time-action, and determine if timing of administration can be adjusted to minimize side effect. Determine whether side effects are related to other disorders or current environmental stressors and adjust accordingly. If these strategies fail, consider an alternative stimulant.
Weight Loss/Anorexia	Administer medication at or after a meal. Try calorie enhancement strategies, such as high protein instant breakfasts, protein bars, etc. Get eating started with any highly preferred food before giving regular foods. Allow grazing in the evening when appetite suppression wanes. Change stimulant medications. Consider drug holidays.
Dizziness	Monitor blood pressure and pulse. Encourage adequate hydration. If associated only with peak drug effect, then try longer-acting preparation.
Insomnia/nightmares	Establish bedtime routine. Omit or reduce last dose or change to standard, short-acting version if using longer-acting preparation. Administer medication earlier in the day. Try a different stimulant. Give "Sleep Problems" handout (sample available at http://www.dbpeds.org). Consider additional medication as a last resort.
Dysphoric Mood, Emotional Constriction	If peak effect, reduce dose, or switch to longer-acting preparation. Evaluate when it occurs. If rebound, see below. Try a different stimulant. Consider co-morbid anxiety or depression disorders requiring alternative or adjunctive treatment. Consider additional medication as a last resort.
Rebound	Try to decrease precipitous dTry to decrease precipitous drop in blood levels by using a "stepped down" dosage at the end of the day through increasing morning long-acting dose or adding a smaller dose of short-acting medication towards the end of the day. Switch to longer-acting preparation. Combine longer-acting and short-acting preparations. Overlap stimulant dosing.
Tics	Conduct drug trial at different doses, including no medication, to be sure tics are drug related. For mild tics that abate after 7 to 10 days, reconsider risk vs. benefit, and negotiate a new informed consent with the parent/guardian. Conduct drug trial to see if tics abate with another stimulant. Consider nonstimulant treatment, such as clonidine, alone or in combination with a stimulant, or refer to mental health specialist or neurologist skilled in the management of tics.
Psychosis	Check that correct dose is being administered. Discontinue stimulant treatment. Assess for presence of co-existing bipolar or thought disorder. Consider alternative treatments, or referral to mental health specialist.

Adapted from Conners CK, Jett JL. *Attention Deficit Hyperactivity Disorder (In Adults and Children): The Latest Assessment and Treatment Strategies.* Kansas City, MO: Compact Clinicals; 1991; Block SL. Attention-deficit disorder: a paradigm for psychotropic medication intervention in pediatrics. *Pediatr Clin North Am.* 1998;45(5):1053-1083; and Wilens TE. *Straight Talk About Psychiatric Medications for Kids.* New York, NY: Guilford Press; 1999.

ADHD and with associated anxiety disorder, ADHD anxiety with associated oppositionality, or children in single parent households or from low-income families.[44-47] Combined treatment was also superior to medication alone for outcomes such as parent-child relations and consumer satisfaction.[44-48,76]

Several advantages of behavioral interventions that deserve mention include (1) use in combination with medication may allow for a reduced dose of medication;[77] (2) the therapeutic benefits of stimulant medication usually occur during the day, whereas behavioral interventions may be used in the late afternoon or evening in place of an additional dose of medication; (3) disruptive disorders that commonly co-occur with ADHD have been shown to respond to behavioral modification;[46] (4) psychosocial treatment may help to enhance parents' positive perception of their children and of their own parenting abilities; and

Table 137-5 Additional Medications for Treatment of Attention-deficit/Hyperactivity Disorder (in Alphabetical Order by Drug Class)

DRUG	FORM	DOSING	COMMON SIDE EFFECTS	DURATION OF BEHAVIORAL EFFECTS	BENEFITS	PRECAUTIONS
ALPHA-AGONISTS						
CATAPRES Clonidine HCl	Tablets: 0.1, 0.2, 0.3 mg Patches TTS-1 TTS-2 TTS-3 Cream by special order	Start with one quarter to one half of 0.1-mg tablet; 0.025-0.3 mg/day for up to four doses	Sleepiness, irritability, hypotension, dizziness, dry mouth, constipation, localized skin reactions with patch	Tablet: 3-6 hr Patch: 1-5 days	Helpful for patients with ADHD who have significant comorbid tics; may be helpful for patients with ADHD and aggression or insomnia.	Sudden discontinuation might result in rebound hypertension; to avoid daytime tiredness, starting dose should be given at bedtime and increased slowly.
TENEX Guanfacine	Tablet: 1, 2 mg	Start with one-half tablet given twice daily. Can give up to 2 mg 2 times per day	Irritability, tiredness, confusion at higher doses, agitation	Approx 12 hr	May be helpful for patients with ADHD who exhibit aggression. Causes less sedation and irritability than clonidine.	Sudden discontinuation might result in rebound hypertension; to avoid daytime tiredness, starting dose given at bedtime and increased slowly.
ATYPICAL ANTIDEPRESSANTS						
WELLBUTRIN Bupropion	Tablets: 75, 100 mg Sustained-release tablets: 100, 150, 200 mg Extended (XL): 150, 300 mg	Start with 75 mg given twice per day; sustained-release can be given in 1-2 doses. Maximum, 450 mg/day.	Irritability, decreased appetite, insomnia, worsening tics, seizures, rash	8-24 hr, depending on formulation	Helpful as second line treatment for ADHD or for patients with ADHD and comorbid anxiety or depression.	Contraindicated in patients with a history of seizures or eating disorders. May increase risk of suicidality.
SELECTIVE NOREPINEPHRINE REUPTAKE INHIBITORS						
STRATTERA Atomoxetine	Capsules: 10, 18, 25, 40, 60, 80, 100 mg	Start with a dose of 0.5 mg/kg and increase gradually to 0.5 mg/kg or 100 mg, whichever is less.	Nausea, vomiting, fatigue, decreased appetite, dizziness, tiredness, aggression, constipation, dry mouth, insomnia, decreased libido, and mood swings	18-24 hr	Helpful as second line treatment for ADHD or for patients with ADHD and comorbid anxiety	May increase risk of suicidality. Should not be used within 2 weeks of a monamine oxidase inhibitor or in a patient with narrow-angle glaucoma.
TRICYCLIC ANTIDEPRESSANTS						
NORPRAMIN Desipramine HCl	Tablets: 10, 25, 50, 75, 100, 125 mg	Start with 10-25 mg/day; up to 5 mg/kg/day; 25 to 150 mg daily	Dry mouth, decreased appetite, headache, stomachache, dizziness, constipation, and mild tachycardia	12-24 hr	Helpful for patients with ADHD and comorbid depression or anxiety disorders.	May take 2-4 weeks for clinical response; discontinue gradually.
PAMELOR Nortriptyline	Capsules: 10, 25, 50 mg Elixir	Start with 10-25 mg/day; 25 to 150 mg daily	Dry mouth, decreased appetite, headache, stomachache, dizziness, constipation, mild tachycardia	12-24 hr	Helpful for patients with ADHD and comorbid depression or anxiety disorders.	May take 2-4 weeks for clinical response; discontinue gradually.
OTHER						

ADHD, Attention-deficit/hyperactivity disorder.

Table 137-6 Effective Behavioral Techniques for Children With Attention-deficit/Hyperactivity Disorder

TECHNIQUE	DESCRIPTION	EXAMPLE
Positive reinforcement	Providing rewards or privileges contingent on the child's performance	Child completes an assignment and is permitted to play on the computer.
Time-out	Removing access to positive reinforcement contingent on performance of unwanted or problem behavior	Child hits sibling impulsively and is required to sit for 5 minutes in the corner of the room.
Response cost	Withdrawing rewards or privileges contingent on the performance of unwanted or problem behavior	Child loses free time privileges for not completing homework.
Token economy	Combining positive reinforcement and response cost. The child earns rewards and privileges contingent on performing desired behaviors and loses rewards and privileges based on undesirable behavior.	Child earns stars for completing assignments and loses stars for getting out of seat. The child cashes in the sum of stars at the end of the week for a prize.

From American Academy of Pediatrics. Clinical practice guideline: treatment of the school-aged child with attention-deficit/hyperactivity disorder. *Pediatrics* 2001;108:1033-1044.

(5) the results for medication last only as long as a youth continues to take the medication, whereas behavioral interventions may extend over time. In addition, not all children and families accept the use of long-term medication treatment for ADHD or respond to stimulants.[54] Finally, medications may be more expensive than behavioral interventions in the long run.

Disadvantages regarding the use of behavioral interventions primarily reflect challenges related to accessing these services. The psychosocial interventions with demonstrated effectiveness in the literature are usually quite intensive, including the behavioral intervention in the MTA Study, 9-week summer day camp for children with ADHD,[78] and intensive social skills training sessions for parents and children.[79] These types of intensive interventions are often difficult to access for the majority of youth because of a lack of identified mental health care providers trained in these programs, lack of insurance payment, and limited services available through schools.

Clinicians caring for youth with ADHD can access these types of services through several mechanisms. First, mental health professionals are increasingly being trained in behavioral modification techniques; knowing which providers in the community offer these types of services is essential. Clinicians may also choose to provide parenting programs in their office setting or through their health plan. Several practices that participated in a year-long quality improvement program on ADHD care sponsored by the NICHQ, AAP, and Carolina Center for Children's Healthcare Improvement chose to implement behavioral-intervention programs for parents in their office setting using available protocols.[10,15,80] Behavioral intervention programs for the school setting have also been published and are available on line (see Tools for Practice at the end of the chapter).

School-Based Services

School-based services are a critical part of a comprehensive management plan for multiple reasons. First, the behaviors observed in ADHD are contextually driven and often display themselves more in concentration-demanding situations such as school. Communication with school personnel is essential for making the diagnosis of ADHD and for optimal titration of medication, if prescribed.[10,11] Second, a solid evidence base exists for the effectiveness of highly structured behavioral-management strategies implemented by school staff in addressing many of the behavioral and organizational challenges experienced by youth with ADHD.[73,81] These interventions can range from daily report cards to point or token systems with primary outcomes consisting of following classroom rules, complying with teacher requests, improving peer interactions, and increasing classwork productivity. The effects tend to be greater for more intensive programs in special class settings, though gains are also seen in regular classrooms.[81] Third, comorbid learning disabilities are not uncommon, and clinicians, families, and school personnel should closely monitor each child to ensure that the problems associated with ADHD are not masking coexisting learning disabilities that would require formal testing for learning problems, identification of areas of disability, and specific learning interventions under an IEP, as stipulated under the Individuals with Disabilities Education Act (IDEA) (Public Law 94-142, amended in 1997 under Public Law 105-17).[82] Learning disabilities coexistent with ADHD usually fall into the category of language-based disorders of learning or impaired mathematics performance.

Even if a youth does not meet criteria for a specific learning disability, challenges with academic work are quite common in youth with ADHD. They may demonstrate motor challenges, including dysgraphia, with resultant poor handwriting, and problems related to poor visual-motor abilities (eg, copying materials off of a board or textbook onto paper). Other challenges include inconsistent performance, delayed acquisition of core reading and math skills, low productivity, delay in rapid retrieval of facts, difficulty with higher-level problem solving involving multiple steps, impaired reading comprehension, and poor meta-cognitive abilities (eg, organization, time management, breaking tasks down into smaller components). These problems can often be inappropriately attributed to laziness or lack of motivation. Education of the youth, parents, and school personnel regarding the inadvertent labeling of behaviors related to these difficulties as oppositionality rather than as cognitive challenges associated with ADHD is critical. Interventions such as direct remediation of learning problems, bypass strategies, and meta-cognitive skills training are all-important academic tools in planning curricula for children with ADHD.[83] Intervention practices not specific to ADHD have been developed and are reviewed in Kavale and Forness' recent monograph entitled *Efficacy of Special Education and Related Services*.[84]

Youth can access school-based services through their local public school system through several mechanisms. Individual teachers will often modify the curriculum or classroom environment to address a child's needs. Many schools have an interdisciplinary council (eg, student study team, multidisciplinary assessment team) that informally reviews a child's academic performance and behavior and suggests possible remediation. Through Section 504 of the Rehabilitation Act,[85] school systems are mandated to provide accommodations in the mainstream classroom. Under IDEA,[85] school systems also provide a continuum of special education services, ranging from accommodations in the mainstream classroom to a special day class in a public or private, nonpublic placement. Youth with ADHD often qualify for special education services because of a coexisting specific learning disability, language disorder, or severe emotional disturbance. In 1991, the US Department of Education also stated that individuals with ADHD might be considered disabled under the "Other Health Impaired" categorization under IDEA,[86] potentially increasing access to school-based special education services for youth with ADHD.

Because academic underachievement is so commonly seen in ADHD, clinicians need some comfort level with the types of interventions available through the public school system. Accommodations requested through a 504 plan or IEP should address youth's individual areas of need. For example, youth with ADHD often need preferential seating close to teacher and daily or weekly progress reports for both behavior and academic performance sent to the home to allow for close monitoring of school success. Youth may also need reduction of the amount of written work, modified homework assignments, or extra time to complete assignments or tests. Organizational difficulties may require supervision of the writing of homework assignments in a planner, an extra set of books at home, and assistance breaking large projects into small steps. Youth problems with handwriting may need access to a computer for written work, copies of teacher lectures, or electronically recorded textbooks. If behavior interferes with the individual child's academic performance or the ability of other children in the classroom to learn, then a behavioral intervention plan is necessary that delineates what behaviors a youth displays, factors that escalate or dampen the behavior, and appropriate behavioral interventions. If a child does have a coexisting learning or language disorder, then specific interventions for these disorders should also be included in any plan. Consideration should be given to the appropriate educational placement of a child (eg, mainstream classroom with or without assistance from a resource specialist, special day class, private nonpublic placement). Sample letters requesting a 504 plan or IEP, as well as additional information on these programs, are available in the ADHD toolkit and the Bright Futures Web site.

Concerns are often raised by clinicians, parents, and teachers that these types of accommodations may lead to youth who feel entitled to extra assistance and who will not be able to function adequately in college or the workplace setting. For these reasons, accommodations must be provided within the context of teaching a youth to understand the child's own strengths and weaknesses and develop compensatory strategies for addressing their areas of challenge.

Alternative Treatments for Attention-deficit/Hyperactivity Disorder

Alternative approaches to treatment for ADHD abound and have included dietary recommendations, ocular training, and hypnotic and biofeedback regimens. Some treatments have been demonstrated to be efficacious (oligoantigenic diet in children who have ADHD and food sensitivities), disproven (sugar in the diet), or are potentially unsafe (megavitamin doses), but the majority lacks any real evidence for or against their use at this time. A full discussion of these modalities is beyond the scope of this chapter, but an excellent review is available.[87]

CASE REPORT: RESOLUTION

Bethany's talkativeness, endless energy, and poor school performance may represent ADHD. You are concerned that her mood and somatic complaints may represent depression, and her early reading difficulties may represent a learning disability. You decide to have her guardian and teacher or teachers complete the Vanderbilt Assessment Scales, given that they are available in the public domain, facilitate documentation of diagnostic criteria, and can be used to explore the possibility of a comorbid depressive disorder. You compose a brief letter to her teachers using the sample form in the ADHD toolkit as a guide to request their assistance in completing the scales and sending any additional school information such as grades, achievement test results, or narrative summaries to you. You also instruct Bethany's guardian to draft a letter to her school to request a multidisciplinary assessment for learning disabilities. You elect not to pursue any laboratory or imaging tests, given that Bethany's history and physical examination are not suggestive of another diagnosis that would be assessed by such tests.

On a follow-up visit, you review the results of the Vanderbilt Assessment Scales and school information obtained from her teacher with Bethany and her guardian. You note that in both her parent and teacher scales she meets 6 of 9 criteria for the predominately hyperactive/impulsive subtype. You also note that she screens positive on 3 of 7 anxiety or depression symptoms. Narrative information from her homeroom teacher corroborates the rating scales and affirms her guardian's concerns that her grades have been slipping. The letter also informs you that the school has scheduled Bethany for psychoeducational testing in the near future. You inform Bethany and her guardian that she meets criteria for ADHD and discuss cause and possible treatment options. You provide educational materials on ADHD for them that you have compiled from the AAP and other selected sites. You relate your concerns that Bethany might be suffering from a depressive disorder. In collaboration with the family, you structure a treatment plan and goals for Bethany using the sample management plan in the ADHD toolkit. The treatment plan includes a prescription for a psychostimulant, a referral to a child psychologist to assess for depression, and a community referral to a local health center that sponsors parent behavioral training courses. With Bethany and her guardian's permission, you draft a letter to the school to inform them of Bethany's diagnosis and to encourage their ongoing collaboration with you in Bethany's care. You also distribute Vanderbilt Assessment Follow-Up Scales to her guardian and teachers to document any changes in her symptoms that will assist you in titrating her medication dosage optimally.

At her next visit, you review Bethany's progress in meeting her goals. You note substantial improvement in her total symptom scores and in her average performance scores on the Vanderbilt Scales. Bethany relates that she initially had stomach pain and headaches with the medication, as you had anticipated with them, but that these symptoms have resolved. You also check and find that her pulse and blood pressure are within normal limits. Bethany states that she is feeling better about her academic work. Her aunt states that Bethany has been less talkative at home and more organized and focused with her homework since she implemented a behavioral-management plan. Next, you review the results of the psychology referral with the family, which confirms a diagnosis of ADHD but does not support a diagnosis of depression or anxiety. Her anxious and depressive symptoms have also decreased as her ability to succeed at school and on homework have improved with medication. Several weeks later, you receive the results of the psychoeducational testing from the school. You note that Bethany meets criteria for a reading disability and that an IEP has been established to assist Bethany in improving her reading abilities and to provide classroom accommodations (eg, seating in front, reduction in distractions, a daily homework report card). You are pleased with Bethany's progress to date, and you make plans with the family to continue to monitor her closely in the future.

Over time, your goal is to help Bethany and her aunt identify Bethany's strengths, as well as areas of challenge related to her ADHD. In concert with any mental health professionals and school personnel involved in her care, everyone will partner to help Bethany develop strategies to address her areas of challenge and to best manage her ADHD symptoms so that she can be a productive, healthy adult.

CONCLUSION

ADHD is a common, chronic disorder of childhood and adolescence affecting multiple domains of functioning and often continuing into adulthood. Diagnosis and treatment are complicated by the lack of a biological marker, high rates of comorbid conditions, and the need to coordinate care across multiple settings. Youth with ADHD, however, can successfully function in the home and school settings. Families, school personnel, and clinicians often observe that children whose symptoms are recognized, assessed, and managed at an early age will show improved self-esteem and success in the classroom, both of which are essential for normal psychosocial and educational development. Although as many as 70% of children and adolescents continue to be symptomatic in adulthood, outcomes are improved with familial stability and support, an ongoing therapeutic relationship with a health care professional, and a higher IQ. The primary care clinician's role is to help youth, in partnership with their families and teachers, achieve this goal.

General guidelines for referral are provided in Figure 137-1. These guidelines should be modified depending on the constellation of ADHD symptoms and coexisting conditions with which a particular child exhibits and the skill-set and comfort level of the primary care clinician in managing the treatment of ADHD and any coexisting conditions. If assistance is needed in evaluating a child, then referral to a mental health professional, school professional, or medical specialist might be indicated. Referral to a mental health professional is indicated for pharmacological management of treatment-resistant ADHD, more intensive behavioral-modification training for the home setting than can be provided in the primary care office, or psychosocial or pharmacological interventions for a coexisting mental health disorder. Mental health professionals may also play an important role if significant familial stress related to a child's ADHD or psychopathology exists in the family, including domestic violence, substance abuse, and other conditions. Schools are essential partners in the diagnosis and management of ADHD, whether a child has a coexisting learning disability or not. Children with severe emotional impairment secondary to any mental health disorder, including ADHD, are also eligible for development of an intensive behavioral management plan under the IEP mechanism through their local school district. Referral to a medical subspecialist is indicated if the history or physical suggest evaluation for an additional medical disorder is indicated.

WHEN TO REFER

- Evaluation (if discrepant results or complicated clinical picture exists and the primary care physician is uncomfortable continuing evaluation)
- Psychological testing
- Intensive parent training in behavior modification

- Significant social and family issues
- Coexisting conditions that are unresponsive to treatment for ADHD (oppositionality, depression, and anxiety may improve with treatment of ADHD core symptoms)
- Pharmacologic management of treatment resistant ADHD or severe side effects

WHEN TO ADMIT

The core symptoms of ADHD should not necessitate admission to a medical or psychiatric hospital. Indications for admission result from:

- Symptoms related to any of the mental health conditions that may co-occur with ADHD
- Adverse event secondary to medication for the treatment of ADHD
- A medical condition resulting from the core symptoms of inattention, hyperactivity, or impulsivity associated with ADHD (eg, accidental injury)

SUGGESTED RESOURCES

American Academy of Pediatrics. Clinical practice guideline: diagnosis and evaluation of the child with attention-deficit/hyperactivity disorder. *Pediatrics.* 2000;105:1158-1170.

American Academy of Pediatrics. Clinical practice guideline: treatment of the school-aged child with attention-deficit/hyperactivity disorder. *Pediatrics.* 2001;108:1033-1044.

Jellinek M, Patel BP, Froehle MC, eds. *Bright Futures in Practice: Mental Health—Volume I. Practice Guide.* Arlington, VA: National Center for Education in Maternal and Child Health; 2002.

Jellinek M, Patel BP, Froehle MC, eds. *Bright Futures in Practice: Mental Health—Volume II. Tool Kit.* Arlington, VA: National Center for Education in Maternal and Child Health; 2002.

Jensen PS, Cooper JR, eds. *Attention Deficit Hyperactivity Disorder: State of the Science, Best Practices.* Kingston, NJ: Civic Research Institute; 2002.

TOOLS FOR PRACTICE

Community Advocacy and Coordination

- *Teaching Children with ADHD: Instructional Strategies and Practices* (booklet), US Department of Education (www.ed.gov/teachers/needs/speced/adhd/adhd-resource-pt2.doc).

Engaging Patient and Family

- *ADHD: A Complete and Authoritative Guide* (book), American Academy of Pediatrics (www.aap.org/bookstore).
- *ADHD and Your Health Insurance Plan* (brochure), American Academy of Pediatrics (patiented.aap.org).
- *Living and Thriving with ADHD: A Guide for Families Video,* American Academy of Pediatrics (www.aap.org/bookstore).
- *How to Establish a School-Home Daily Report Card* (report), American Academy of Pediatrics (www.aap.org/bookstore).
- *Parent Page: ADHD and Your School Age Child* (fact sheet), American Academy of Pediatrics (pediatrics.aappublications.org/cgi/data/108/4/1033/DC1/1).
- *Sleep Tips* (brochure), Henry Shapiro, MD (dbpeds.org/articles/detail.cfm?TextID=34).
- *Understanding the Child with ADHD: Information for Parents on ADHD* (brochure), American Academy of Pediatrics (patiented.aap.org).
- *Understanding the Child with ADHD: Information for Parents on ADHD (Spanish)* (brochure), American Academy of Pediatrics (patiented.aap.org).
- *What About Medicines for ADHD? Questions From Teens Who Have ADHD* (brochure), American Academy of Pediatrics (patiented.aap.org).
- *What Is ADHD, Anyway? Questions From Teens* (brochure), American Academy of Pediatrics (patiented.aap.org).

Medical Decision Support

- *ADHD Management Plan—Sample 1,* American Academy of Pediatrics (www.aap.org/bookstore).
- *ADHD Management Plan—Sample 2,* American Academy of Pediatrics (www.aap.org/bookstore).
- *ADHD Rating Scale-IV: Checklists, Norms, and Clinical Interpretation* (checklist), DuPaul GJ, Power TJ, Anastopoulos AD, Reid R (www.guilford.com/cgi-bin/cartscript.cgi?page=pr/dupaul2.htm&dir=pp/adhdr&cart_id=496674.7708).
- *Bright Futures: Guidelines for Health Supervision of Infants, Children, and Adolescents* (book), Bright Futures (brightfutures.aap.org/web).
- *Caring for Children with ADHD: A Resource Toolkit for Clinicians (English only)* (tool kit), American Academy of Pediatrics (www.aap.org/bookstore).
- *Caring for Children with ADHD: A Resource Toolkit for Clinicians (English and Spanish)* (tool kit), American Academy of Pediatrics (www.aap.org/bookstore).
- *Clinician ADHD Economy Pack (English and Spanish Tools)* (tool kit), American Academy of Pediatrics (www.aap.org/bookstore).
- *Conner's Rating Scales—Revised,* Conners CK (https://www.mhs.com/ecom/(igbqcj55zn3nutq4gqkkgs55)/product.aspx?RptGrpID=CRS).
- *Cover Letter to Teachers* (letter), American Academy of Pediatrics (www.aap.org/bookstore).
- *Diagnosis of Attention-Deficit/Hyperactivity Disorder* (Web page), Agency for Health Care Policy and Research (www.ahrq.gov/clinic/epcsums/adhdsutr.htm).
- *Managing Your Patients with ADHD* (interactive tool), American Academy of Pediatrics (www.eqipp.org).
- *NICHQ ADHD Primary Care Initial Evaluation Form,* American Academy of Pediatrics (www.aap.org/bookstore).
- *NICHQ Vanderbilt Assessment Follow-up—Parent Informant* (questionnaire), NICHQ (www.aap.org/bookstore).
- *NICHQ Vanderbilt Assessment Follow-up—Teacher Informant* (questionnaire), NICHQ (www.aap.org/bookstore).

- *NICHQ Vanderbilt Assessment Scale—Parent Informant* (scale), American Academy of Pediatrics (www.aap.org/bst).
- *NICHQ Vanderbilt Assessment Scale—Teacher Informant,* American Academy of Pediatrics (www.aap.org/bookstore).
- *Scoring Instructions for the SNAP-IV Rating Scale* (fact sheet), Swanson JM (www.adhd.net/snap-iv-instructions.pdf).
- *The Classification of Child and Adolescent Mental Diagnoses in Primary Care* (book), American Academy of Pediatrics (www.aap.org/bst).
- *The SNAP-IV Teacher and Parent Rating Scale* (scale), Swanson JM (www.adhd.net/snap-iv-form.pdf).
- *Vanderbilt Teacher Behavior Evaluation Scale* (VTBES), Vanderbilt Child Development Center (www.vanderbiltchildrens.com/uploads/documents/ccdr_behavior_scale.pdf?PHPSESSID=647c127d6c143df09f80bb31ff02392e).

Practice Management and Care Coordination

- *ADHD Complete Practice Management Package,* American Academy of Pediatrics (www.aap.org/bookstore).

RELATED WEB SITE

- American Academy of Pediatrics: Children's Health Topics: ADHD (www.aap.org/healthtopics/adhd.cfm).

AAP POLICY STATEMENTS

American Academy of Pediatrics, Committee on Quality Improvement and Subcommittee on Attention-Deficit/Hyperactivity Disorder. Clinical practice guideline: diagnosis and evaluation of the child with attention-deficit/hyperactivity disorder. *Pediatrics.* 2000;105(5):1158-1170. (aappolicy.aappublications.org/cgi/content/full/pediatrics;105/5/1158).

American Academy of Pediatrics, Committee on Quality Improvement and Subcommittee on Attention-Deficit/Hyperactivity Disorder. Clinical practice guideline: Treatment of the School-Aged Child With Attention-Deficit/Hyperactivity Disorder. *Pediatrics.* 2001;108(4):1033-1044.

Schechter MS, American Academy of Pediatrics, Section on Pediatric Pulmonology, Subcommittee on Obstructive Sleep Apnea Syndrome. Diagnosis and management of childhood obstructive sleep apnea syndrome. *Pediatrics.* 2002;109(4):e69. (aappolicy.aappublications.org/cgi/content/full/pediatrics;109/4/e69).

REFERENCES

1. Goldman LS, Genel M, Bezman RJ, et al. Diagnosis and treatment of attention-deficit/hyperactivity disorder in children and adolescents. Council on Scientific Affairs, American Medical Association. *JAMA.* 1998;279:1100-1107.
2. American Psychiatric Association. *Diagnostic and Statistical Manual of Mental Disorders (DSM-IV).* 4th ed, text revision. Washington, DC: American Psychiatric Association; 2000.
3. Green M, Wong M, Atkins D, et al. *Diagnosis of Attention-Deficit/Hyperactivity Disorder. Technical Review No. 3.* Rockville, MD: Agency for Health Care Policy and Research; 1999. AHCPR Publication No. 99-0050.
4. Centers for Disease Control and Prevention. Mental health in the United States. Prevalence of diagnosis and medication treatment for attention-deficit/hyperactivity disorder—United States, 2003. *MMWR Morb Mortal Wkly Rep.* 2005;54:842-847.
5. Robin AL. *ADHD in Adolescents: Diagnosis and Treatment.* New York, NY: Guilford Press; 1998.
6. Mannuzza S, Klein RG. Long-term prognosis in attention-deficit/hyperactivity disorder. *Child Adolesc Psychiatr Clin North Am.* 2000;9:711-726.
7. Hechtman L, Weiss G, Perlman T. Young adult outcome of hyperactive children who received long-term stimulant treatment. *J Am Acad Child Psychiatry.* 1984;23:261-269.
8. Wilens TE, Faraone SV, Biederman J, et al. Does stimulant therapy of attention-deficit/hyperactivity disorder beget later substance abuse? A meta-analytic review of the literature. *Pediatrics.* 2003;111:179-185.
9. Biederman J, Mick E, Faraone SV. Age-dependent decline of symptoms of attention deficit hyperactivity disorder: impact of remission definition and symptom type. *Am J Psychiatry.* 2000;157:816-818.
10. American Academy of Pediatrics. Clinical practice guideline: diagnosis and evaluation of the child with attention-deficit/hyperactivity disorder. *Pediatrics.* 2000;105:1158-1170.
11. American Academy of Child and Adolescent Psychiatry. Practice parameters for the assessment and treatment of children, adolescents, and adults with attention-deficit/hyperactivity disorder. *J Am Acad Child Adolesc Psychiatry.* 1997;30:85-121.
12. Carey WB. Problems in diagnosing attention and activity. *Pediatrics.* 1999;103:664-667.
13. Faraone SV, Biederman J. Neurobiology of attention-deficit hyperactivity disorder. *Biol Psychiatry.* 1998;44:951-958.
14. Biederman J, Faraone SV, Keenan K, et al. Family-genetic and psychosocial risk factors in DSM-III attention deficit disorder. *J Am Acad Child Adolesc Psychiatry.* 1990;29:526-533.
15. American Academy of Pediatrics. Clinical practice guideline: treatment of the school-aged child with attention-deficit/hyperactivity disorder. *Pediatrics.* 2001;108:1033-1044.
16. Wolraich ML. *Current Assessment and Treatment Practices.* Paper presented at the NIH Consensus Conference on Diagnosis and Treatment of ADHD, Washington, DC, November 1998.
17. Hoagwood K, Kelleher KJ, Feil M, et al. Treatment services for children with ADHD: a national perspective. *J Am Acad Child Adolesc Psychiatry.* 2000;39:198-206.
18. Jellinek M, Patel BP, Froehle MC. *Bright Futures in Practice: Mental Health—Volume 1, Practice Guide.* Arlington, VA: National Center for Education in Maternal and Child Health and Georgetown University; 2002.
19. Reiff MI, Banez GA, Culbert TP. Children who have attentional disorders: diagnosis and evaluation. *Pediatr Rev.* 1993;14:455-465.
20. Schechter MS. Technical report: diagnosis and management of childhood obstructive sleep apnea syndrome. *Pediatrics.* 2002;109:e69.
21. Mulhern S, Dworkin PH, Bernstein B. Do parental concerns predict a diagnosis of attention-deficit hyperactivity disorder? *J Dev Behav Pediatr.* 1994;15:348-352.
22. Losier BJ, McGrath PJ, Klein RM. Error patterns on the continuous performance test in non-medicated and medicated samples of children with and without ADHD: a meta-analytic review. *J Child Psychol Psychiatry.* 1996;37:971-987.
23. Wolraich M. *Vanderbilt Teacher Behavior Evaluation Scale (VTBES).* Nashville, TN: Vanderbilt Child Development Center; 1998.

24. DuPaul GJ, Power TJ, Anastopoulos AD, et al. *ADHD Rating Scale–IV: Checklists, Norms, and Clinical Interpretation*. New York, NY: Guilford Press; 1998.
25. Conners CK. *CRS-R, Conners' Rating Scales-Revised: Instruments for Use With Children and Adolescents*. Toronto, Canada, North Tonawanda, NY: Multi-Health Systems; 1997.
26. Swanson JM. *The SNAP-IV Teacher and Parent Rating Scale*. Irvine, CA: University of California; 1991.
27. Achenbach TM. *Manual for the Child Behavior Checklist/2-3 and 1991 Profile*. Burlington, VT: University of Vermont, Department of Psychiatry; 1991.
28. Achenbach TM. *Manual for the Teacher's Report Form and 1991 Profile*. Burlington, VT: University of Vermont, Department of Psychiatry; 1991.
29. Reynolds C, Kamphaus R. *Behavioral Assessment System for Children Manual*. Circle Pines, MN: American Guidance Service; 1992.
30. Rishel CW, Greeno C, Marcus SC, et al. Use of the Child Behavior Checklist as a diagnostic screening tool in community mental health. *Res Soc Work Pract*. 2005;15: 195-203.
31. Gephart HR. A managed care approach to ADHD. *Contemp Pediatr*. 1997;14(5):123-139.
32. American Academy of Pediatrics. *The Classification of Child and Adolescent Mental Diseases in Primary Care*. Washington, DC: American Academy of Pediatrics; 1996.
33. Faulstich ME, Carey MP, Ruggiero L, et al. Assessment of depression in childhood and adolescence: an evaluation of the Center for Epidemiological Studies Depression Scale for Children (CES-DC). *Am J Psychiatry*. 1986;143(8):1024-1026.
34. March JS, Parker JD, Sullivan K, et al. The Multidimensional Anxiety Scale for Children (MASC): factor structure, reliability, and validity. *J Am Acad Child Adolesc Psychiatry*. 1997;36:554-565.
35. Eyberg SM, Pincus D. *Eyberg Child Behavior Inventory and Sutter-Eyberg Student Behavior Inventory-Revised*. Odessa, FL: Psychological Assessment Resources; 1999.
36. Sprafkin J, Gadow KD, Salisbury H, et al. Further evidence of reliability and validity of the Child Symptom Inventory-4: parent checklist in clinically referred boys. *J Clin Child Adolesc Psychol*. 2002;31:513-524.
37. Lucas CP, Zhang H, Fisher PW, et al. The DISC Predictive Scales (DPS): efficiently screening for diagnoses. *J Am Acad Child Adolesc Psychiatry*. 2001;40:443-449.
38. Wagner EH, Glasgow RE, Davis C, et al. Quality improvement in chronic illness care: a collaborative approach. *Jt Comm J Qual Improv*. 2001;27:63-80.
39. Jadad A, Boyle M, Cunningham C, et al. *Treatment of Attention-Deficit/Hyperactivity Disorder. Evidence Report/Technology Assessment No. 11*. Rockville, MD: Agency for Healthcare Research and Quality; 1999. AHRQ Publication No. 00-E005.
40. Jensen P, Cooper J. *Attention Deficit Hyperactivity Disorder: State of Science, Best Practices*. Kingston, NJ: Civic Research Institute; 2002.
41. Pliszka SR, Greenhill LL, Crimson ML, et al. The Texas Children's Medication Algorithm Project: report of the Texas Consensus Conference Panel on medication treatment of childhood attention-deficit/hyperactivity disorder. Part I. *J Am Acad Child Adolesc Psychiatry*. 2000; 39(7):908-919.
42. Pliszka SR, Greenhill LL, Crimson ML, et al. The Texas Children's Medication Algorithm Project: report of the Texas Consensus Conference Panel on medication treatment of childhood attention-deficit/hyperactivity disorder. Part II: tactics. *J Am Acad Child Adolesc Psychiatry*. 2000;39(7):920-927.
43. Arnold LE, Abikoff HB, Cantwell DP, et al. National Institute of Mental Health Collaborative Multimodal Treatment Study of Children with ADHD (the MTA). Design challenges and choices. *Arch Gen Psychiatry*. 1997;54(9): 865-870.
44. Jensen PS, Hinshaw SP, Kraemer HC, et al. ADHD comorbidity findings from the MTA study: comparing comorbid subgroups. *J Am Acad Child Adolesc Psychiatry*. 2001;40:147-158.
45. Jensen PS, Hinshaw SP, Swanson JM, et al. Findings from the NIMH multimodal treatment study of ADHD (MTA): implications and applications for primary care providers. *J Dev Behav Pediatr*. 2001;22:60-73.
46. Swanson JM, Kraemer HC, Hinshaw SP, et al. Clinical relevance of the primary findings of the MTA: success rates based on severity of ADHD and ODD symptoms at the end of treatment. *J Am Acad Child Adolesc Psychiatry*. 2001;40:168-179.
47. MTA Cooperative Group. Moderators and mediators of treatment response for children with attention-deficit/hyperactivity disorder: The Multimodal Treatment Study of Children with Attention-Deficit/Hyperactivity Disorder. *Arch Gen Psychiatry*. 1999;56:1088-1096.
48. MTA Cooperative Group. A 14-month randomized clinical trial of treatment strategies for attention-deficit/hyperactivity disorder. *Arch Gen Psychiatry*. 1999;56: 1073-1086.
49. Pliszka SR, McCracken JT, Maas JW. Catecholamines in attention-deficit hyperactivity disorder: current perspectives. *J Am Acad Child Adolesc Psychiatry*. 1996;35: 264-272.
50. Solanto MV. Neuropsychopharmacological mechanisms of stimulant drug action in attention-deficit hyperactivity disorder: a review and integration. *Behav Brain Res*. 1998;94:127-152.
51. Gadow KD, Nolan EE, Sverd J, et al. Methylphenidate in aggressive-hyperactive boys. I. Effects on peer aggression in public school settings. *J Am Acad Child Adolesc Psychiatry*. 1990;29:710-718.
52. Hinshaw SP, Heller T, McHale JP. Covert antisocial behavior in boys with attention-deficit hyperactivity disorder: external validation and effects of methylphenidate. *J Consult Clin Psychol*. 1992;60:274-281.
53. Klein RG, Abikoff H, Klass E, et al. Clinical efficacy of methylphenidate in conduct disorder with and without attention deficit hyperactivity disorder. *Arch Gen Psychiatry*. 1997;54:1073-1080.
54. Spencer T, Biederman J, Wilens T, et al. Pharmacotherapy of attention-deficit hyperactivity disorder across the life cycle. *J Am Acad Child Adolesc Psychiatry*. 1996;35(4): 409-432.
55. Swanson JM, Sergeant JA, Taylor E, et al. Attention-deficit hyperactivity disorder and hyperkinetic disorder. *Lancet*. 1998;351:429-433.
56. Wolraich ML, Lindgren S, Stromquist A, et al. Stimulant medication use by primary care physicians in the treatment of attention deficit hyperactivity disorder. *Pediatrics*. 1990;86(1):95-101.
57. Jensen PS, Payne JD. *Behavioral and Medication Treatments for Attention Deficit Hyperactivity Disorder: Comparisons and Combinations*. Paper presented at the NIH Consensus Conference on Diagnosis and Treatment of ADHD, Washington, DC, November 1998.
58. Swanson JM, McBurnett K, Wigal T, et al. Effect of stimulant medication on children with attention deficit disorder: a "review of reviews". *Except Child*. 1993;60(2):154-163.
59. Frankel F, Cantwell DP, Myatt R, et al. Do stimulants improve self-esteem in children with ADHD and peer problems? *J Child Adolesc Psychopharmacol*. 1999;9: 185-194.

60. Biederman J, Wilens T, Mick E, et al. Pharmacotherapy of attention-deficit/hyperactivity disorder reduces risk for substance use disorder. *Pediatrics.* 1999;104(2):e20.
61. MTA Cooperative Group. National Institute of Mental Health Multimodal Treatment Study of ADHD follow-up: changes in effectiveness and growth after the end of treatment. *Pediatrics.* 2004;113(4):762-769.
62. Tourette's Syndrome Study Group. Treatment of ADHD in children with tics: a randomized controlled trial. *Neurology.* 2002;58(4):527-536.
63. Carroll KM, Rounsaville BJ. History and significance of childhood attention deficit disorder in treatment-seeking cocaine abusers. *Compr Psychiatry.* 1993;34:75-82.
64. Wilens TE, Biederman J, Spencer TJ, et al. Comorbidity of attention-deficit hyperactivity and psychoactive substance use disorders. *Hosp Community Psychiatry.* 1994;45:421-423.
65. Abikoff H. *Matching Patients to Treatments.* Paper presented at the NIH Consensus Conference on Diagnosis and Treatment of ADHD, Washington, DC, November 1998.
66. Hoagwood K. *A National Perspective on Treatments and Services for Children with Attention Deficit Hyperactivity Disorder.* Paper presented at the NIH Consensus Conference on Diagnosis and Treatment of ADHD, Washington, DC, November 1998.
67. Connor DF, Fletcher KE, Swanson JM. A meta-analysis of clonidine for symptoms of attention-deficit hyperactivity disorder. *J Am Acad Child Adolesc Psychiatry.* 1999;38:1551-1559.
68. Conners CK, Casat CD, Gualtieri CT, et al. Bupropion hydrochloride in attention deficit disorder with hyperactivity. *J Am Acad Child Adolesc Psychiatry.* 1996;35:1314-1321.
69. Spencer T, Heiligenstein JH, Biederman J, et al. Results from 2 proof-of-concept, placebo-controlled studies of atomoxetine in children with attention-deficit/hyperactivity disorder. *J Clin Psychiatry.* 2002;63:1140-1147.
70. US Food and Drug Administration. Patient Information Sheet: Atomoxetine (marketed as Strattera). Available at: www.fda.gov/cder/drug/InfoSheets/patient/atomoxetinept.htm. Accessed March 9, 2006.
71. Spencer TJ, Biederman J, Wilens T. Pharmacotherapy of ADHD with antidepressants. In: Barkley R, ed. *Attention-Deficit Hyperactivity Disorder: A Handbook for Diagnosis and Treatment.* 2nd ed. New York, NY: Guilford Press; 1998.
72. Biederman J, Swanson JM, Wigal SB, et al. Efficacy and safety of modafinil film-coated tablets in children and adolescents with attention-deficit/hyperactivity disorder: results of a randomized, double-blind, placebo-controlled, flexible-dose study. *Pediatrics.* 2005;116:e777-e784.
73. Pelham WE, Wheeler T, Chronis A. Empirically supported psychosocial treatments for attention-deficit hyperactivity disorder. *J Clin Child Psychol.* 1998;27:190-205.
74. Jensen PS. Fact versus fancy concerning the multimodal treatment study for attention-deficit hyperactivity disorder. *Can J Psychiatry.* 1999;44:975-980.
75. Pelham WE. The NIMH multimodal treatment study for attention-deficit hyperactivity disorder: just say yes to drugs alone? *Can J Psychiatry.* 1999;44:981-990.
76. MTA Cooperative Group. A 14-month randomized clinical trial of treatment strategies for attention-deficit/hyperactivity disorder. *Arch Gen Psychiatry.* 1999;56(12):1073-1086.
77. Pelham WE, Burrows-Maclean L, Gnagy EM, et al. Transdermal methylphenidate, behavioral, and combined treatment for children with ADHD. *Exp Clin Psychopharmacol.* 2005;13:111-126.
78. Pelham WE, Hoza B. Intensive treatment: a summer treatment program for children with ADHD. In: Hibbs ED, Jensen PS, eds. *Psychosocial Treatments for Child and Adolescent Disorders.* Washington, DC: American Psychological Association; 1996.
79. Frankel F, Myatt R, Cantwell DP, et al. Parent-assisted transfer of children's social skills training: effects on children with and without attention-deficit hyperactivity disorder. *J Am Acad Child Adolesc Psychiatry.* 1997;36(8):1056-1064.
80. Center for Children and Families at the University of Buffalo. CTADD: Comprehensive Treatment for Attention Deficit Disorder. Available at: summertreatmentprogram.com. Accessed February 11, 2008.
81. DuPaul G, Eckert T. The effects of school-based interventions for attention deficit hyperactivity disorder: a meta-analysis. *School Psychol Rev.* 1997;26(1):5-27.
82. US Department of Education. IDEA '97: The Individuals with Disabilities Education Act Amendments of 1997. Available at: www.ed.gov/offices/osers/idea/. Accessed February 11, 2008.
83. Smith C, Strick L. *Learning Disabilities: A to Z.* New York, NY: Free Press; 1997.
84. Kavale K, Forness S. Efficacy of special education and related services. In: Siperstein G, ed. *Monographs of the American Association on Mental Retardation.* Washington, DC: American Association on Mental Retardation; 1999.
85. US Department of Justice. A Guide to Disability Rights Laws. Available at: www.usdoj.gov/crt/ada/cguide.htm. Accessed February 11, 2008.
86. US Department of Education. Children with ADD/ADHD—Topic Brief. Available at: www.ed.gov/print/policy/speced/leg/idea/brief6.html. February 11, 2008.
87. Arnold L. Treatment alternatives for attention deficit hyperactivity disorder. Jensen P, Cooper J, eds. *Attention Deficit Hyperactivity Disorder: State of Science, Best Practices.* Kingston, NJ: Civic Research Institute; 2002.

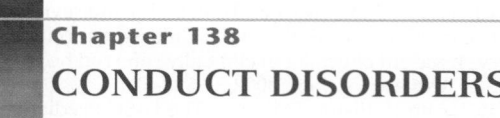

Chapter 138

CONDUCT DISORDERS

Michael S. Jellinek, MD

OPPOSITIONAL AND CONDUCT DISORDERS

One of the most common behavioral issues facing pediatricians is a child's oppositional, violent, or potentially delinquent behavior[1-3] (Box 138-1). Parents who are confronted with such situations are upset at feeling that they have failed, are powerless, and feel disrespected; all parents worry that their child may be destined for school dropout, delinquency, or criminal behavior.

A useful point to remember is that some forms of aggressiveness are part of a developmental trajectory to autonomy and independence; they are often socially sanctioned, as in football and other competitive circumstances, including academics, job hunting, and even making plans for the high school prom. Such aggression is socially accepted and achievement oriented. On the other hand, oppositional behavior for

BOX 138-1 Examples of Parental Behavioral Concerns

Jimmy runs out of the house while I am telling him not to.

Sally will not stay in her room for a time out.

My husband and I cannot get Billy to sit down and start his homework.

Jason lied to me about where he was.

Peter used my credit card to buy a violent videogame on the Internet.

Tom drove the car, despite having only a learner's permit, to see his girlfriend, even though he was grounded.

Mike may be using and even selling marijuana to his friends.

Jared is getting into fist fights at school.

many children is a sign of or a solution to a hidden problem. Disrupting a class may be the solution to an underlying fear of appearing stupid, a sign that they need treatment for attention deficit hyperactivity disorder (ADHD), or a reaction to tension or even violence in the home. Violating rules to see a girlfriend may be simply oppositional, a reasonable attempt to assert autonomy in the face of overly restrictive parents, or sensible in the context of a private adolescent crisis. The pediatrician is faced with a difficult challenge. How does the pediatrician differentiate common behaviors from the serious disorders that portend long-term risk? How does the pediatrician help a parent differentiate the prognosis and needs of a 7 year old lying about a bad grade from one who steals the change off the bedroom dresser or from one who coldly and aggressively beats up a classmate? What are the diagnostic criteria for oppositional and conduct disorders? How are they relevant to primary care practice? How does the pediatrician evaluate these behaviors and assess the severity? What are the critical clinical steps to take to help the child and family?

Diagnostic Criteria

Oppositional and conduct disorders are bushel-basket terms for a wide range of behaviors. Commonly used—and misused—terms for children and adolescents with these behaviors are violent, conduct disordered, oppositional, delinquent, sociopathic, psychopathic, and antisocial.[4] The formal psychiatric criteria are listed in Boxes 138-2 and 138-3.[5] Using these criteria, approximately 5% of children will be diagnosed as having oppositional or conduct disorder. In addition, diagnoses that are commonly co-morbid or co-occurring diagnoses will be made, such as learning disabilities, ADHD, depression, substance use, and anxiety. Oppositional and conduct disorders in combination with the impulsivity of ADHD or the use of alcohol increase the risk of accidental injury, especially in adolescence; adding depression increases the risk of suicidal behavior; and learning disabilities increases the risk of school dropout and running away. Therefore understanding and tracking these behaviors is a critical aspect of primary care pediatrics. Fortunately, most children who demonstrate oppositional behavior do not progress to conduct disorder as adolescents, and most adolescents with conduct disorder do not become criminals.

Prevalence

The prevalence of conduct disorder is approximately 5% (3:1 or 4:1 ratio of boys to girls).[6] The criteria used, severity, overlap of co-morbid disorders such as ADHD, poor agreement among informants, and length of follow-up confound studies aiming to provide a precise estimate. The prevalence of oppositional disorder is higher, but declines substantially, between early childhood and school age compared with other age groups. Even aggressive behavior seems to decline after early childhood but is more stable and worrisome when still evident in school age and adolescence. By late adolescence, another substantial decline in conduct disorder occurs but, again, a distinct subsample becomes criminal. The specific profile of causes and symptoms that are prognostic for a persistent course from early childhood to adulthood is not well defined. However, oppositional and conduct disordered symptoms at any age cause dysfunction in the child and family and are potentially dangerous to others.

Etiology

Genetics seem to play a role in conduct disorder, but defining this role specifically is difficult because the behaviors are broad. The genetics of alcohol and substance use, depression, and impulsivity are better defined by and relate to aspects of conduct disorder. Other neuronal substrates to these behaviors such as autonomic underarousal may also have genetic roots. Learning disabilities, whether genetic or related to complications of pregnancy, may contribute. Conduct disorder results from genetic vulnerability that is subjected to psychosocial stressors: insecure early attachment between young child and caretaker; harsh discipline, abuse, or neglect; family dysfunction and conflict; mental illness in parents; paternal criminality; and low income. Clearly the broader social environment can have a major impact; peer group influences such as gangs compete with more adaptive opportunities to feel connected to meaningful relationship or activities (eg, sports teams, religious institutions).[7]

Paralleling these risk factors are protective factors that likely improve the prognosis for oppositional conduct disorders; adaptable temperament, higher IQ, competence in at least one area (academic, social, athletic, or activities), warm relationship with a parent or adult, opportunities to connect to the community (clubs, town teams, religious programs, community centers), and financial resources to facilitate opportunities are all protective factors.

Primary Care Assessment

Pediatricians will commonly hear about oppositional children from parents who are frustrated and angry.[8] Given the range of behaviors that can broadly raise the concern of oppositional or conduct disorder, a thorough history assessment of each behavior and its circumstances, including the child's functioning at home, at school, with peers, and in activities, is critical.

BOX 138-2 Diagnostic Criteria for Conduct Disorder

A. A repetitive and persistent pattern of behavior in which the basic rights of others or major age-appropriate societal norms or rules are violated, as exhibited by the presence of 3 (or more) of the following criteria in the last 12 months, with at least one criterion present in the last 6 months:

Aggression to people and animals

1. Often bullies, threatens, or intimates others
2. Often initiates physical fights
3. Has used a weapon that can cause serious physical harm to others (eg, a bat, brick, broken bottle, knife, gun)
4. Has been physically cruel to people
5. Has been physically cruel to animals
6. Has stolen while confronting a victim (eg, mugging, purse snatching, extortion, armed robbery)
7. Has forced someone into sexual activity

Destruction of property

8. Has deliberately engaged in fire setting with the intention of causing serious damage
9. Has deliberately destroyed others' property (other than fire setting)

Deceitfulness or theft

10. Has broken into someone else's house, building, or car
11. Often lies to obtain goods or favors or to avoid obligations (ie, *cons* others)
12. Has stolen items of nontrivial value without confronting a victim (eg, shoplifting, but without breaking and entering; forgery)

Serious violations of rules

13. Often stays out at night despite parental prohibitions, beginning before age 13 years
14. Has run away from home overnight at least twice while living in parental or parental surrogate home (or once without returning for a lengthy period)
15. Is often truant from school, beginning before age 13 years

B. The disturbance in behavior causes clinically significant impairment in social, academic, or occupational functioning

Specify severity:

- Mild: few if any conduct problems in excess of those required to make the diagnosis and conduct problems cause only minor harm to others
- Moderate: number of conduct problems and effect on others intermediate between *mild* and *severe*
- Severe: many conduct problems in excess of those required to make the diagnostic or conduct disorder problems cause considerable harm to others

For many children, the oppositional or defiant behavior is not the core problem but is the solution that emerges to the child feeling overwhelmed, frustrated, or angry. Although parents will have worries of delinquency or even criminality, the focus of primary care efforts will be a review of risk factors, assessing severity, counseling on childrearing, and co-management with mental health, school, and legal professionals. Generally, when assessing parental concerns, reactive behavior such as arguing or losing one's temper after feeling unfairly punished or exhausted by a long school day is less serious than proactive anger. A younger child occasionally blaming others or even lying as a means of coping with what the child believes is an unsolvable situation is not as serious as a more consistent pattern of annoying or blaming others. Reacting to bullying with violence or destroying property as part of a group prank is very different from proactively initiating fights, using weapons, or acting cruel. Therefore the pediatrician should consider a hierarchy of severity: reactive, nonviolent, proactive nonviolent, reactive violent, and proactive violent.[9] Of course, the younger the age, the more violent, and the less the child experiences a sense of responsibility (remorse) or guilt (having failed the trust of a loved one), the more serious the pattern and prognosis. Behaviors exhibited as part of a group are, in general, not as serious as acts performed alone. Adolescents who demonstrate a sense of feeling connected to a school, team, peers, or family likely have a better prognosis than those who are isolated, unfeeling, or alone.

Pediatricians should examine the following areas to help explain the evolution or change in the child's behavior: (1) childrearing practices (inconsistent discipline, harsh discipline, domestic violence, child abuse and neglect), (2) acute family stressors (maternal depression, marital conflict, frequent family moves, birth of a sibling, financial stresses), and (3) characteristics of the child (rigid temperament, poor fit between child's temperament and parenting styles, academic difficulties, struggles concerning autonomy, and co-morbid conditions such as ADHD, depression, or substance use). Even the simplest symptoms require some thoughtful assessment. Is refusing to go to

BOX 138-3 Diagnostic Criteria for Oppositional Defiant Disorder

A. A pattern of negativistic, hostile, and defiant behavior lasting at least 6 months, during which four (or more) of the following are present:
   1. Often loses temper
   2. Often argues with adults
   3. Often actively defies or refuses to comply with adults' requests or rules
   4. Often deliberately annoys people
   5. Often blames others for his or her mistakes or misbehavior
   6. Is often touchy or easily annoyed by others
   7. Is often angry and resentful
   8. Is often spiteful or vindictive

   Note: A criterion is considered as being met only if the behavior occurs more frequently than typically observed in individuals of comparable age and developmental level.

B. The disturbance in behavior causes clinically significant impairment in social, academic, or occupational functioning

school an issue of anxiety, emerging learning disabilities, fear of a bully, a consequence of rejection by peers, or a reaction to parental conflict? Mild-to-moderate, short-term defiant behaviors may well yield to the pediatrician's assessment and recommendations. Persistent, escalating, violent, and remorseless behavior requires a comprehensive mental health evaluation, psychosocial and behavioral treatments, and appropriate use of medication to treat associated conditions such as depression, ADHD, or anxiety.

Conduct disorder is a more serious concern than oppositional behavior, although maintaining an appropriate sense of optimism is important because most adolescents with quite disturbing behaviors emerge as productive adults. However, the risks for self-injury, injury to others, academic discipline, and intervention by legal authorities are real, with serious consequences. We do not know which interventions will alter the course of children and adolescents who demonstrate disturbing and dangerous conduct, and we do not know which patient will go on to lifelong difficulties. Therefore behaviors that meet the criteria of conduct disorder require comprehensive pediatric attention and action.

Behaviors can be conceptualized as related to property (vandalism, theft, fire setting), interpersonal aggression (bullying, cruelty, fighting, assault), and high personal risk (truancy, substance use, running away from home). Aggressive and dangerous behaviors are likely more worrisome than truancy or marijuana use. These behaviors are more worrisome if they are severe, repeated, done alone, and done without remorse; however, even the more serious conduct disorders do not necessarily lead to criminality, addiction, or lifelong disorders. Therefore the pediatrician must prioritize assessment, referral, and comprehensive follow-up to optimize the prognosis. In addition to the family and behavior interventions, increasingly, one of the newer antipsychotic drugs such as Risperdol[10] is prescribed off label to address violent conduct disordered behavior. Use of this potent and complex medication should not be initiated without a comprehensive treatment plan and collaboration with a child and adolescent psychiatrist.

Pediatricians should assess the severity, frequency, and context of the behavior.[11] What family (eg, abuse, marital discord), personal (depression, academic failure), and social (peer influence, limited opportunities) factors may be underlying the behavior? What is the parental reaction, and do any legal ramifications exist? Given the complexity of the behavior and likely contributing circumstances, no easy questionnaires or tools have been developed that substitute for interviews of the child and family.

In the context of an office visit, the following is an outline of issues and actions that may be helpful in the initial management if conduct disordered behavior is a serious concern:

- Patient safety: Does the child experience abuse or violence from peers or gang members? Does the child exhibit self-destructive behaviors, including use of substances? Does the child exhibit suicidal risk caused by depression, severe embarrassment, or shame, intensified by a sense of being trapped with no escape and no solution? Does the child have access to guns or life-threatening medications?
- Family safety: Does the home have guns, patterns of domestic violence, or patient-initiated violence to parents or peers? Does the child's home life have escalating, physical confrontations between the child and the parent as part of the emerging behavior? The clinician should consider structured family agreements or having the child stay with a relative or friend.
- Support structure: The clinician should provide access to mental health consultation for patient, parent, or family work and should determine the need for other urgently needed services, such as legal representation, liaison with school guidance or probation officer, or state department of social services.
- Limit setting and negotiation: The clinician should suggest limit setting that decreases stress, such as limiting contact to provocative peers, limiting access to substances (or substance abuse treatment), and tracking of where the patient is when not in school.
- Building on strengths: The clinician should reinforce any positive supports, such as area of competence, relationship with a caring adult (coach, teacher, parent, sibling, grandparent), and behaviors that will elicit parental praise.
- Establishing rules: The clinician should encourage consistency and unanimity of parental discipline and overall response to conduct disordered behaviors. (Support by a behavioral psychologist is often critical.)[12]
- School interventions: The clinician should help the child reduce academic stress with the help of the school psychologist or guidance counselor, through a teacher conference, by eliminating a stressful class, or by implementing an education plan. The clinician should consider if school-based peer pressures such

as bullying, threats, humiliation, or clique or gang group behavior are contributing factors. If others are involved, then the clinician should support contacting relevant parents.

- Legal interventions: The clinician should facilitate parents contacting a lawyer or public defender to deal with potential legal issues, arrests, or pressure from local law enforcement. Lawyers may also appropriately engage police who are assigned as youth officers, work with probation departments, or negotiate with the court and local agencies to ensure the availability of services in the context of legal proceedings.
- Department of social services: A comprehensive plan often needs to be mobilized to provide safety. The clinician should consider a referral to the local department of social services to coordinate legal, mental health, and school resources.

The initial goals of management are to increase safety and to decrease the level of tension, discord, and stress. Long-term goals are, of course, to eliminate the conduct disordered behavior, help the patient make amends, relieve underlying stressors or comorbid conditions, restore trust, and build on the child's adaptive strengths in school, activities, with friends, and in the family.

Prevention

Pediatricians can encourage prevention of conduct disorders by encouraging efforts focused on high-risk populations.[13] Early identification of at-risk infants can be accomplished through postpartum home visits or screening young children in child care settings for young mothers who are vulnerable to depression, domestic violence, conflictual relationships, or using harsh disciplinary techniques; identifying and providing services for school-aged children who demonstrate aggression, bullying, learning disabilities, and ADHD; and identifying high-risk adolescents who might be failing in school, depressed, using substances, or fighting. Broad-based prevention efforts include comprehensive services for abused and neglected children; community efforts directed against substance use or development of gangs; adequate opportunities for connecting children and adolescents to their community through sports, activities, and religious affiliation; and access to mental health services when needed. Sadly, financial pressures on community services and schools have caused a decrease in preventive services in many communities, and pressures to control health care spending have further lowered the priority of mental health services for children and their families. The cost to a community of an adolescent with conduct disorder who elicits mental health, social service, school-based, and legal attention is $70,000 over a 7-year period.[14] Despite this high cost, prevention, early intervention, and mental health services in most communities are poorly funded, with the result being that primary care pediatricians shoulder more of the burden for mental health problems such as oppositional and conduct disorders.

CONCLUSION

Patients with oppositional and conduct disordered behaviors are part of every primary care practice. Most of these behaviors are mild to moderate and respond to guidance and short-term stress-reduction or behavioral treatment. Some behaviors increase the risk of danger through violence, legal consequences, or high-risk behavior, leading to serious accidents. Pediatricians can often offer hope, a sense of calm, preliminary assessment, and a plan of action that helps worried parents and reduces the risks and dysfunctions of their patients.

TOOLS FOR PRACTICE

Engaging Patients and Family

- *Attention, Consistency, and Violence Prevention* (fact sheet), American Academy of Pediatrics (www.aap.org/topics.html)
- *Aggressive Behavior* (fact sheet), American Academy of Pediatrics (www.aap.org/topics.html)
- *Building Healthy Family Communication* (fact sheet), American Academy of Pediatrics (www.aap.org/topics.html)
- *Connected Kids—Bullying is Not Okay* (brochure), American Academy of Pediatrics (www.aap.org/bookstore)
- *Children's Mental Health—When to Seek Help* (fact sheet), American Academy of Pediatrics (www.aap.org/topics.html)
- *Communication With Your Adolescent* (fact sheet), American Academy of Pediatrics (www.aap.org/topics.html)
- *Dealing With Family Conflicts* (fact sheet), American Academy of Pediatrics (www.aap.org/topics.html)
- *Development and Behavior* (fact sheet), American Academy of Pediatrics (www.aap.org/topics.html)
- *Discipline and Young Children* (fact sheet), American Academy of Pediatrics (www.aap.org/topics.html)
- *Discipline and Your Child* (brochure), American Academy of Pediatrics (patiented.aap.org)
- *Discipline Methods* (fact sheet), American Academy of Pediatrics (www.aap.org/topics.html)
- *Expect Respect: Healthy Relationships* (brochure), American Academy of Pediatrics (patiented.aap.org)
- *Family Disruptions—Arguments and Conflicts* (fact sheet), American Academy of Pediatrics (www.aap.org/topics.html)
- *Connected Kids—How Do Infants Learn?* (brochure), American Academy of Pediatrics (www.aap.org/bookstore)
- *How Parenting Styles Influence Temperament* (fact sheet), American Academy of Pediatrics (www.aap.org/topics.html)
- *How Temperamental Traits Can Be Expressed—Living with a "Difficult" Child* (fact sheet), American Academy of Pediatrics (www.aap.org/topics.html)
- *Keys to Effective Discipline* (fact sheet), American Academy of Pediatrics (www.aap.org/topics.html)
- *Connected Kids—Parenting Your Infant* (brochure), American Academy of Pediatrics (www.aap.org/bookstore)
- *Connected Kids—Playing is How Toddlers Learn* (brochure), American Academy of Pediatrics (www.aap.org/bookstore)
- *Connected Kids—Pulling the Plug on TV Violence* (brochure), American Academy of Pediatrics (www.aap.org/bookstore)

- *Connected Kids—Teaching Good Behavior: Tips on How to Discipline* (brochure), American Academy of Pediatrics (www.aap.org/bookstore)
- *Teaching the Basics of Violence Prevention* (fact sheet), American Academy of Pediatrics (www.aap.org/topics.html)
- *VIPP and Connected Kids CD-ROM* (CD-ROM), American Academy of Pediatrics (www.aap.org/ConnectedKids/)
- *Types of Mental-Health Professionals* (fact sheet), American Academy of Pediatrics (www.aap.org/topics.html)
- *Understanding Disobedience* (fact sheet), American Academy of Pediatrics (www.aap.org/topics.html)
- *Connected Kids—Young Children Learn a Lot When They Play* (brochure), American Academy of Pediatrics (www.aap.org/bookstore)
- *Connected Kids—Your Child is On the Move: Reduce the Risk of Gun Violence* (brochure), American Academy of Pediatrics (www.aap.org/bookstore)
- *Youth Violence: Overview* (Web page), Centers for Disease Control and Prevention (www.cdc.gov/ncipc/factsheets/yvoverview.htm)
- *Connected Kids—Welcome to the World of Parenting* (brochure), American Academy of Pediatrics (www.aap.org/bookstore)

Medical Decision Support

- *Bright Futures in Practice: Mental Health* (Web page), Bright Futures (www.brightfutures.aap.org/mentalhealth/)
- *Connected Kids—Clinical Guide* (booklet), American Academy of Pediatrics (www.aap.org/ConnectedKids/ClinicalGuide.pdf).
- *Connected Kids—Full Training Module* (PowerPoint), American Academy of Pediatrics (www.aap.org/ConnectedKids/CKtrain.ppt).
- *Connected Kids—Introduction and Tips for Use* (PowerPoint), American Academy of Pediatrics (www.aap.org/ConnectedKids/CKtrain-intro.ppt).
- *Connected Kids—Infancy and Early Childhood Training* (PowerPoint), American of Pediatrics (www.aap.org/ConnectedKids/CKtrain-green.ppt).
- *Connected Kids—Middle Childhood Training* (PowerPoint), American Academy of Pediatrics (www.aap.org/ConnectedKids/CKtrain-blue.ppt).
- *Connected Kids—Adolescent Training* (PowerPoint), American Academy of Pediatrics (www.aap.org/ConnectedKids/CKtrain-red.ppt).
- *Connected Kids* (Web page), American Academy of Pediatrics (www.aap.org/ConnectedKids/).
- *Violence Intervention and Prevention Program Database* (Web-based database), American Academy of Pediatrics (www.aap.org/vipp/).
- *Youth Violence* (fact sheet), Centers for Disease Control and Prevention (www.cdc.gov/ncipc/factsheets/yvfacts.htm).

Community Coordination and Advocacy

- *ASK (Asking Saves Kids) Campaign* (Web page), American Academy of Pediatrics (www.paxusa.org/ask/index.html).
- *Stop Bullying Now!* (Web page), US Department of Health and Human Services (www.stopbullyingnow.hrsa.gov/index.asp?area=main).

AAP POLICY STATEMENTS

American Academy of Pediatrics. Firearm-related injuries affecting the pediatric population. *Pediatrics.* 2000; 105(4):888-895. (aappolicy.aappublications.org/cgi/content/abstract/pediatrics;89/4/788).

American Academy of Pediatrics. The role of the pediatrician in youth violence prevention in clinical practice and at the community level. *Pediatrics.* Jan 1999;103(1):173-181. (aap policy.aappublications.org/cgi/content/full/pediatrics;103/1/173).

REFERENCES

1. Jellinek M, Patel BP, Froehle MC, eds. *Bright Futures in Practice: Mental Health—Volume 1, Practice Guide.* Arlington, VA: National Center for Education in Maternal and Child Health; 2001.
2. Jellinek M, Patel BP, Froehle MC, eds. *Bright Futures in Practice: Mental Health—Volume 2, Tool Kit.* Arlington, VA: National Center for Education in Maternal and Child Health; 2001.
3. Connor DF. *Aggression and Antisocial Behavior in Children and Adolescents.* New York, NY: The Guilford Press; 2002.
4. Steiner H, Remsing L. Practice Parameter for the Assessment and Treatment of Children and Adolescents With Oppositional Defiant Disorder. *J Am Acad Child Adolesc Psychiatry.* 2007;46(1):126-141.
5. American Psychiatric Association. *Diagnostic and Statistical Manual of Mental Disorders,* Text Revision. Washington, DC: American Psychiatric Association; 2000.
6. Earls F, Mezzacappa E. Conduct and oppositional disorders. In: Rutter M, Taylor E, eds. *Child and Adolescent Psychiatry.* 4th ed. Oxford, England: Blackwell Publishing Company; 2002:419-436.
7. Burke JD, Loeber R, Birmaher B. Oppositional defiant disorder and conduct disorder: a review of the past 10 years, part 11. *J Am Acad Child Adolesc Psychiatry.* 2002;42:1275-1293.
8. McMahon Rick P. Evidence-based assessment of conduct problems in children and adolescents. *J Clin Child Adolesc Psychol.* 2005;34:477-505.
9. Connor DF. *Aggression and Antisocial Behavior in Children and Adolescents.* New York, NY: The Guilford Press; 2002.
10. Reyes M, Buitelaar J, Toren P, Augustyns I, Eerdekens M. A randomized, double-blind, placebo-controlled study of Risperidone maintenance treatment in children and adolescents with disruptive behavior disorders. *Am J Psychiatry.* 2006;163:402-410.
11. Jellinek M, Patel BP, Froehle MC, eds. *Bright Futures in Practice: Mental Health—Volume 2, Tool Kit.* Arlington, VA: National Center for Education in Maternal and Child Health; 2001.
12. Greene RW. *The Explosive Child: A New Approach for Understanding and Parenting Easily Frustrated Chronically Inflexible Children.* New York, NY: Harper-Collins; 2001.
13. Connor DF, Carlson GA, Chang KD, et al. Juvenile maladaptive aggression: a review of the prevention, treatment, and service configuration and a proposed research agenda. *J Clin Psychol.* 2006;67(5):808-820.
14. Foster EM, Jones DE. The high costs of aggression: public expenditures resulting from conduct disorder. *Am J Public Health.* 2005; 95:1767-1772.

Chapter 139

CONVERSION REACTIONS AND HYSTERIA

Gregory E. Prazar, MD

DEFINITION, INCIDENCE, AND ETIOLOGY

The amalgamation of emotions and physical symptoms in patients challenges the primary care physician to formulate priorities in history taking, diagnosis, and management. Some somatic complaints, such as headaches, nausea, and vomiting, can result directly from emotional upsets. Indeed, anxiety is often associated with palpitations, sweating, and tremulousness; depression is often exhibited by symptoms of fatigue and weakness. Other somatic complaints reflect organic disorders, such as neuromuscular headaches, which may be associated with emotional turmoil. Still other physical problems are attributed to conversion symptoms. The terms *conversion symptom, conversion reaction,* and *conversion disorder* are often used interchangeably. Somatic or functional complaints differ from conversion symptoms in that patients with somatic or functional complaints are aware of emotional distress associated with the symptom. Patients with conversion symptoms are not cognizant of any associated emotional distress.

Conversion reactions are a way of communicating the uncomfortable, or as Engel writes,

> ...a psychic mechanism whereby an idea, fantasy, or wish is expressed in bodily rather than in verbal terms and is experienced by the patient as a physical symptom rather than as a mental symptom.[1]

The idea or wish is psychologically threatening to individuals or is unacceptable for them to express directly. A conversion symptom serves as a form of decompression whereby unpleasant affects associated with acknowledgment of the wish are dissipated through the use of a somatic symptom. Because the wish is completely unconscious, patients in no way relate any psychological stigmata to the somatic complaint. As Hollender succinctly states, "The conversion symptom is a code that conceals the message from the sender as well as from the receiver."[2]

To understand why a wish or thought is represented by a bodily symptom, exploring patterns of everyday behavior and infant development is necessary. Body activity (ie, gestures) is used to express ideas during verbal interaction. Common conversational phrases frequently allude, metaphorically, to the intermixing of emotion and body functioning. "I'm fed up" and "He is a pain in the neck" are 2 such examples. Developmentally, infants express feelings and communicate through visible behavior long before spoken language becomes their dominant mode of communication. Furthermore, infants explore and learn about their environment, including the people in it, by using their bodies as investigative tools (eg, placing new objects in the mouth) and as a means of making contact. Any bodily process that can be perceived by the individual can serve as the focus for conversion symptoms. Similarly, somatic symptoms of relatives or close friends also can serve as the source of a patients' complaints. The patients' interpretation of the other person's symptom provides a model for the somatic complaint. When the symptom is adapted from one observed in the other person, that person frequently evokes strong feelings in the patient. Because the patient expresses guilt about feelings or impulses toward that person, the patient may take the other person's symptoms as a form of self-punishment while at the same time psychologically expressing the forbidden idea or wish.

All body systems may be invoked in a conversion reaction. The sensory system frequently is involved (eg, paresthesia, anesthesia, diffuse pain), although typically these symptoms are not distributed in the correct pattern of innervation of the implicated cutaneous nerves. Motor system involvement can be represented by paralysis, tremors, or weakness of an extremity. Hyperventilation and dizziness are other common conversion symptoms, as are nausea and vomiting and visual problems.

A common conversion symptom seen in children and young adolescents is abdominal pain. After an extensive investigation of 100 children who had abdominal pain, Apley[3] found an organic cause in only 8 cases. Another study by Oster[4] revealed abdominal pain in 14% of the children studied. The incidence was highest in individuals 9 years of age and lowest in those 16 to 17 years of age. Recurrent abdominal pain and its causes remain controversial (see Chapter 159, Abdominal Pain). However, an important point to remember is that many patients who have recurrent abdominal pain may have emotional concerns of which they are unaware. Many of these patients may be suffering from conversion symptoms.

Although the incidence of certain individual somatic complaints has been studied, the specific overall incidence of conversion symptoms in children and adolescents is not known. Available data suggest an incidence of 5% to 13%.[5] Lack of more definitive data reflects the difficulty in ascertaining whether a somatic complaint indeed represents a conversion symptom. Conversion symptoms may appear to be more common among adolescents than among younger children because the former more often have alarming somatic complaints, such as chest pains and fainting spells, whereas younger children frequently suffer from more indolent complaints, such as sporadic abdominal pains. Conversion symptoms are 2 to 3 times more common in girls than in boys and may appear as early as 7 or 8 years of age.[1] No correlation appears to exist between the occurrence of conversion symptoms and socioeconomic status; less sophisticated patients, however, tend to have rare or very unusual and physiologically unexplained symptoms. Therefore the more classic conversion symptoms (eg, paralysis, blindness) are less likely to be seen by practitioners in Western societies. These practitioners are more likely to diagnose conversion symptoms in patients presenting with chronic abdominal pain or chronic headaches.

Conversion symptoms can appear as a group phenomenon. Such a situation is often referred to as *epidemic hysteria*. Adolescent girls swooning and fainting at rock concerts is an easily appreciated example. In this situation, the unacceptable wish relates to sexualized thoughts involving rock stars. Other examples of epidemic hysteria are explained less easily. Episodes of epidemic hysteria appear to have several characteristics in common: (1) audiovisual cues (eg, seeing ambulances arrive to care for accident victims) seem to be important as precipitators, (2) adolescent girls are involved more often than adolescent boys, (3) the reaction is more likely if it is initiated by a group member identified either as a leader (of a large subgroup) or as an outsider, and (4) episodes are likely to involve larger numbers of adolescents if the youngsters are allowed to confer among themselves without adults present. Entire school populations may be involved in mass conversion reactions.[6,7]

Although conversion symptoms have no organic basis by themselves, their perpetuation may result in biochemical or physiological body changes, known as conversion complications. These events can include changes such as muscle atrophy caused by longstanding paralysis and respiratory alkalosis secondary to acute hyperventilation.

INTERVIEW TECHNIQUES

Because symptoms caused by conversion and somatic processes can be easily confused, the practitioner evaluating any patient who has a somatic complaint should always consider the possibility of a conversion symptom. Attention to personal history (family functioning, school performance, and peer relationships) and to physical functioning demonstrates to the patient and family that the physician appreciates without prejudice the importance of all elements that may be contributing to ill health. Showing respect for the importance of emotional-physical interaction is thereby suggested so that this concept will not be foreign if it is later presented to the family in a diagnostic framework. Such an approach also contributes to the physician's understanding, as Engel[1] states, "of those personal, family, and social circumstances that are most relevant to the understanding of the illness and the care of the patient, whether or not the ultimate diagnosis is conversion."

Nondirective interviewing proves more rewarding than direct questioning. For example, asking the patient to describe the pain ("Tell me how it feels.") almost always provides insight into the emotions that the patient associates with the symptom. Suggesting how the symptom feels to the patient ("Is it dull or sharp pain?") limits possible responses. If the patient spontaneously offers information about recent events, then the interviewer should obtain further data related to such changes in the patient's life. However, care should be taken to avoid suggesting a cause-and-effect relationship between the patient's feelings and the symptoms. Because patients who have conversion symptoms have no conscious knowledge of such an association, the suggestion of such a relationship may alienate them and prevent establishing a trusting relationship.

DIAGNOSTIC CRITERIA FOR CONVERSION SYMPTOMS

The conversion symptom has a specific, but unconscious, symbolic meaning to the patient. In other words, the conversion symptom is often related to an unconscious wish, and the physical impairment serves to prevent acting out the wish. For example, the adolescent boy who has hand paralysis may have anxieties about masturbating. The physician treating children and adolescents may not always be aware of the symbolic meaning of the symptom. Indeed, the concept that conversion symptoms have a symbolic meaning to the patient was formulated only after a series of these patients had undergone extensive psychotherapy. Although being cognizant of the presence of the symbolic meaning may be intellectually rewarding for the physician, ignorance of the specific symbolism does not prevent adequate treatment of the patient (Box 139-1).

Adolescents who have conversion symptoms frequently display characteristic patterns of behavior, sometimes designated as traits of the *hysterical personality*. Such characteristics include egocentricity; labile emotional states (quick shifts from sadness to elation and from anger to passivity); dramatic, attention-seeking behavior; and sexual provocativeness (displayed in gestures and in dress). Patients who have such characteristics are also usually demanding, display an air of pseudomaturity, and are dependent in personal interactions. Their personal relationships, however, are rarely intimate or satisfying. Although many aspects of the hysterical personality are seen in adolescent patients who have conversion symptoms, such characteristics are also demonstrable in adolescents who do not have such symptoms. Therefore hysterical behavior traits in adolescents are not synonymous with conversion symptoms and, in isolation, are not indicative of a psychopathologic condition.

The manner in which patients who have a conversion symptom describe their problem is often distinctive. The account frequently is dramatic. A pain may be described as "thousands of burning needles thrust into my leg" or as "a giant spike being driven into my chest." Because these patients are suggestible, any symptom description alluded to by the physician may be adopted readily and thereafter reported, which again emphasizes the importance of a nondirective approach in the interview.

BOX 139-1 Case Report

Jane, a 12 year old, suddenly developed an inability to walk. Physical examination, including a neurologic evaluation, revealed no abnormalities. Interviews by a psychiatrist and a pediatrician working as a team revealed no apparent symbolic causative factor. The pediatrician formulated a system to reward Jane's progress in walking and implemented this approach; the psychiatrist was similarly supportive with the patient. Over a period of 3 weeks, the patient regained her ability to walk.

Conversion symptoms are adopted unconsciously in an attempt to reduce unpleasant affects, especially anxiety, depression, and guilt. Therefore, although patients may describe incapacitating pain, they often affect an air of unconcern. Psychiatrists refer to this as *la belle indifference*. The extent to which the conversion symptom diminishes the unpleasant affect and symbolically communicates the forbidden wish for the patient is referred to as the primary gain. Patients who have conversion reactions are often stubborn in their belief that the symptom is caused by organic problems, which reflects denial of the underlying emotional problem. Conversely, insistence (especially by an adolescent) that a symptom is psychological in origin may indicate denial of a physical problem. Therefore differentiating between conversion symptoms and physical disease in adolescent patients cannot depend solely on the patient's emotional response.

Conversion symptoms not only affect a primary gain for patients, but they also help them cope with the environment. In this respect, the conversion symptom achieves a secondary gain for patients. For example, patients who have a conversion symptom defending against homosexual thoughts may be excused from attending school, where anxiety may have been intensified (eg, in the locker room). Limitations imposed by the symptom may contradict patients' verbalized wishes to participate in activities but, nevertheless, remove them from potentially threatening social interactions. Interference with daily activities also provides a secondary gain for patients in that attention and more frequent expressions of love are elicited from concerned parents and friends. This situation may be resistant to change, not only because the symptom is reinforced continually, but also because the symptom meets the parents' psychological needs. In effect, the symptom may provide the parents with a reason for inappropriately attending to or infantilizing their children. Consequently, patients and their entire families may fall into a vicious circle of dependence on the symptom.

Demonstration of a secondary gain does not ensure a diagnosis of conversion. To an extent, all illness is involved with some secondary gain. Bedridden patients must accept increased attention to cope with their physical confinement. Therefore a degree of secondary gain is necessary for adequate adaptation to a physical disability. However, in the case of a conversion symptom, secondary gain not only intensifies symptoms, but may also be associated with further occurrence of somatic complaints. Because perpetuation of secondary gain depends on concern from others, a conversion symptom is exhibited more readily in the presence of individuals meaningful to the patient.

Children and adolescents who develop conversion symptoms are often overprotected and become extremely dependent on their parents. Daily familial communication may have been invested heavily in somatic complaints, children recognizing how often activities may have been canceled because of a father's headaches or a mother's cramps. Therefore a patient's symptoms may conform to the unspoken interactional rules of the family. Family members indirectly reinforce patient problems, although the family may assume an air of indifference with respect to the patient's symptoms (Box 139-2).

BOX 139-2 Case Report

James was a 13 year old who had severe abdominal pain and was referred to a pediatrician by his family practitioner. Physical examination revealed little objective evidence of abdominal pain in the physician's office. However, his return home quickly resulted in intensified pain. Abdominal pain appeared to be well controlled during a subsequent 4-day hospitalization (all organic tests were unremarkable). His return home again produced an immediate exacerbation of the abdominal discomfort. Furthermore, John, James' identical twin, began exhibiting signs of abdominal pain. The boys' mother admitted feeling trapped by the demands of her children and volunteered that in the past she had been treated for chronic abdominal pain. The appearance of abdominal pain in both twins reassured her that the pain was "probably a virus." She chose not to pursue further counseling for the boys.

BOX 139-3 Case Report

Chip, a 13 year old, was brought by his mother to his pediatrician because of chronic abdominal pain, which appeared to be precipitated by his competing in horse-riding events. His history revealed the death of a grandparent 4 months previously, but his mother related that her son's pain preceded the onset of the fatal illness. Other family stresses were denied. The teenager did not appear for follow-up care but returned 6 months later, primarily because his mother wanted to discuss her son's reaction to her upcoming divorce. At this visit, the mother volunteered that marital stress had been ongoing for several years.

Precipitation of a conversion symptom may be related to specific stressful events. A change of school, final examinations, new social experiences, and parental conflict are examples of events that may induce a conversion symptom. Unresolved grief reactions may represent a source of stress that can precipitate a conversion symptom. Examples of grief reactions include loss of a parent through death, divorce, or moving. Furthermore, adolescent and adult patients experience pseudoseizures more often in families in which *an unspeakable dilemma* was present[8] Specifically, the dilemma was often associated with a fear of physical or sexual assault. Even though other family members were aware of the specific dilemma, they often underestimated how severely the family member who experienced the pseudoseizures was affected by the dilemma. Because the patient's association between conflict and the conversion reaction is unconscious, a history is helpful only if the interviewer elicits details about daily activities. The stressful event precipitating a conversion symptom often becomes apparent only after many visits (Box 139-3).

BOX 139-4 Case Report

During a routine physical examination, Jeff, a 14 year old, mentioned that he experienced "migraine headaches," which appeared to be focused "behind my left eye" and occurred approximately once a month. Jeff's mother attached more importance to the symptoms than did Jeff. Initially, exploration of the family history proved unremarkable. Persistent questioning about stress led the mother to mention almost parenthetically that she had recently been diagnosed as having multiple sclerosis. She felt that the case was mild and therefore had not told Jeff and her other children directly about the diagnosis, although she sensed that the children knew. Her initial symptom that precipitated the diagnosis of multiple sclerosis was temporary loss of vision in her left eye.

BOX 139-5 Case Report

Terry, a 15-year-old girl, recently had been treated for otitis media, which was characterized by pain and some dizziness. After the ear appeared adequately healed, her dizziness persisted. By encouraging Terry to discuss her daily schedule, the fact that she was under significant academic pressure became apparent, having recently transferred to an extremely competitive private school. In addition, extracurricular pressures were heavy, including her fervent commitment to gymnastics and her hope to achieve professional status. On further questioning, Terry related that she had had dizzy spells in past years just before competitions.

Symptom selection is based on the unconscious remembrance of the patient's own body function or understanding of symptoms in others. The patient's conversion symptom may appear quite dissimilar to that displayed by the other (often a parent or a close relative) because the patient's perception of disease governs the display of symptoms. Parents and relatives often misinform children and adolescents about diseases, fearing that the truth would be too frightening. However, such misinformation may actually potentiate the adolescent's fantasies and result in the development of a symptom quite different from the one actually experienced by the individual serving as the model (Box 139-4).

The choice of a symptom may also be based on a physical illness the patient had suffered previously. Thus patients who have a history of seizures may, after many years of adequate anticonvulsant control, have atypical and physiologically unexplainable seizures. Unfortunately, these patients often receive only a physiological workup for seizures. Despite the atypical history, the physician assumes that the diagnosis rests *where the money is, or was,* in the past (Box 139-5).

Because the somatic complaint expressed by the patient is based on a model symptom, a physical disease often is mimicked. Close scrutiny of the symptom's history and description often reveals anatomic and physiological discrepancies. The child or adolescent who has a stocking anesthesia—an anesthesia confined to a specific area of an extremity without any relationship to cutaneous nerve innervation—demonstrates an example of such symptom inaccuracy. It is based on the concept of the patient's own body rather than on anatomic principles.

BOX 139-6 Criteria for Diagnosis of Conversion Symptoms

The symptom has symbolic meaning to the patient.

The patient frequently exhibits characteristic interpersonal behaviors.

Conversion symptoms are more common in girls than boys.

Reporting symptoms has a characteristic style.

The symptom helps patients cope with their environment *(secondary gain)*. Health issues and symptoms frequently are used in family communication.

Symptoms occur at times of stress.

The symptom has a model.

History and physical findings often are inconsistent with anatomic and physiological concepts.

From Prazar G. Conversion reactions in adolescents. *Pediatr Rev.* 1987;8:279-286.

A thorough history may not only elicit symptom inconsistencies in the present illness, but may also reveal a record of inexplicable or recurrent bouts of illness associated with life events. A history of chronic abdominal pain that occurs only on school days, a history of somatic complaints associated with stressful social events, or documentation of abdominal surgery with equivocal findings should raise suspicion that the patient's current problem represents conversion. A list of the diagnostic criteria for conversion symptoms appears in Box 139-6. No one criterion can be confirmatory, and each patient who has a conversion symptom may not display every criterion listed. However, a conversion symptom cannot be diagnosed solely based on negative physical and laboratory findings; it is not a diagnosis of exclusion.

DIFFERENTIAL DIAGNOSIS

Other psychosomatic disorders at times may be confused with conversion symptoms. Patients exhibiting hypochondriasis, a common entity, especially in adolescents, view their symptoms with extreme concern. None of the apparent indifference seen in patients who have conversion symptoms exists. Patients who have conversion symptoms frequently seem relieved when an organic cause is considered; patients who have hypochondriasis become more concerned if an organic diagnosis is suggested because they suspect and fear a serious or fatal disease. However, neither type of patient is reassured more than transiently by being informed that the patient has no disease.

Malingering is an uncommon problem in adolescents, except in institutionalized adolescents or those who are in restrictive situations (eg, military service). Malingering may even be regarded as an appropriate means of avoiding threatening or unpleasant circumstances. Attempts to feign illness often are naive, especially in younger patients. As Engel states, malingerers exhibit "an intense need to be nurtured or suffer."[1] Many of these individuals appear to be accident prone and may submit to painful procedures readily and without objection. Malingering adolescents are aloof and hostile to the physician; thus discovery of their deception often is delayed. In contrast, patients who have conversion symptoms are often appropriately fearful of procedures and may appear charming and garrulous with the physician. Malingerers and patients who have conversion symptoms are similar in that their parents may have an unconscious psychological need to have their children be ill and therefore may reinforce their children's symptoms.

Somatic delusions are symptoms of psychosis and usually are not confused with conversion symptoms. Other signs of severe mental illness are usually present, such as an inability to relate to peers, visual or auditory hallucinations, and stereotypical behaviors. Furthermore, the symptoms described sometimes are intermittent and are often extremely bizarre. For example, patients who have somatic delusions may express the conviction that their heart is shriveling or that something is wrong with the blood that is running from the head to the leg.

Psychophysiological symptoms may occur when conversion symptoms have failed to dissipate anxiety. Thus continuing anxiety activates biological systems (especially the autonomic nervous system), resulting in physiological changes such as tachycardia, hyperperistalsis, and vasoconstriction. A patient's cognizance of these changes is exhibited by palpitations, diarrhea, and sweating. In this situation, the symptom itself has no organic symbolic meaning and results from a reaction to actual body changes. Therefore psychophysiological symptoms can occur when conversion symptoms have failed. Similarly, conversion symptoms can replace psychophysiological symptoms.

CARE OF THE PATIENT WHO HAS CONVERSION SYMPTOMS

Adolescents who have conversion symptoms are seen most often initially, and eventually treated, by pediatricians or other primary care physicians. Families see this course of action as appropriate because the obvious aspect of the problem is physical. They typically will accept a diagnosis of conversion only from a medical professional they consider an expert in physical disease. Nevertheless, when physicians undertake a case of suspected conversion, their interviewing acumen and sensitivity to the patient's feelings are paramount. The initial interaction between the physician and the patient is crucial to the degree of success achieved in dealing with a conversion symptom. In essence, treatment of the patient begins before a definitive diagnosis is made. Some considerations involved in the initial evaluation of patients suspected of having conversion symptoms appear in Box 139-7.

The physician should advise the patient and family that the cause of any disorder involves both physical

BOX 139-7 Important Considerations in the Initial Evaluation of Patients Suspected of Having Conversion Symptoms

From the outset, the parents and patient should be told that everyone's body has a certain physical way of responding to emotional stress. The parents and patient should be encouraged to suggest diagnostic tests that they may want performed and to suggest possible diagnoses for consideration by the physician.

The parents and patient should understand that the symptom may persist but that the goal is to help maintain normal daily functioning in school and with peers. The parents and patient should understand that referral to a psychiatrically trained professional may be necessary if progress is not made in coping with the symptom.

Modified from Prazar G. Conversion reactions in adolescents. *Pediatr Rev.* 1987;8:279-286.

and emotional factors. As Schmitt[9] states, the family should be told that "everyone's body has a certain physical way of responding to emotional stress." Similarly, every individual has an emotional response to physical stress. Simple examples should be given (eg, most people have learned that headaches often are intensified when they are upset). If the physician communicates an appreciation of the role of emotions in physical disease, then the family may volunteer information more readily about psychosocial functioning. Furthermore, an eventual diagnosis involving emotional aspects may be more acceptable because the family has been prepared for the possibility. Focusing only on a strictly physical diagnosis intimates to the parents that psychological involvement is unlikely, unimportant, and improbable. Turning to psychological issues after all physical tests prove unremarkable implies to parents that this approach was chosen as a last resort because the physician was unable to ascertain an organic cause. A concurrent physical-psychological diagnostic approach not only prepares the physician to consider the problem with some psychotherapeutic intent, but may also save the family time and money because multiple laboratory tests can often be avoided.

After the evaluation has been completed, the physician must develop a treatment plan. Before embarking on this venture, the physician must be satisfied with the completeness of the medical evaluation. Common sense should dictate when the physician believes that further organic tests will be futile. The patient and family can often sense a physician's uncertainty, especially if the family is averse to accepting a psychological diagnosis. Therefore a prudent step would be to ask the family what additional tests they might expect to have performed and what other diagnoses they may have considered. Involvement of the patient and family in this diagnostic process frequently dissipates anxiety and allows eventual psychological counseling.

Although patients who have conversion symptoms are suggestible, reassurance that the symptom will go away rarely is effective and also does not contribute to a psychological investigation of the symptom. On the contrary, suggesting that the symptom will persist allows time to work out a therapeutic relationship with the patient and sometimes has a paradoxical effect. Because the symptom is unlikely to disappear after 2 or 3 visits, the patient will retrospectively view the physician's suggestion as sound. Trust in the physician will be reinforced, and the patient may be more comfortable communicating information about feelings. Anxiolytic medications may reduce attendant anxiety transiently in some cases of conversion symptoms; however, using medication as the sole therapy rarely results in lasting improvement. Because medication does not relieve the underlying conflict responsible for the symptom, another symptom eventually may appear. Furthermore, a risk that the medication's side effects may become the model for new conversion symptoms—or that new symptoms may be confused with side effects—does exist.

At the conclusion of the evaluation, the number of anticipated follow-up sessions should be discussed with the family. The number of sessions should be flexible so that it can be renegotiated if needed. Follow-up sessions with the teenager can usually be limited to 15 to 20 minutes every 2 to 4 weeks. More frequent visits may be necessary if symptoms interfere with school attendance, peer relationships, or family functioning. During follow-up sessions, the teenager should be encouraged to talk about daily life (eg, school, friends, family, dating). If the teenager volunteers information about recurrence of the somatic complaint, then the physician should inquire about events that were transpiring concurrently when the symptom occurred and how the teenager felt about these events. In this way, the physician can help the adolescent become reacquainted with how daily events and feelings are related. Suggesting that the adolescent keep a symptom diary may be helpful. The patient records when the symptom occurred and what was happening at the time the symptom began. Such a record may illustrate to the patient the association of the symptom with feelings or emotionally charged life events.

When physicians feel comfortable acting as both therapist for the teenager and provider of acute medical care, occasions may arise when the teenager has a new physical symptom or complaint that requires attention. If the physician suspects a physical illness that is unrelated to the conversion symptom, whatever evaluation that is indicated must be performed, including a full or partial physical examination. However, an overzealous search for disease should be avoided. Treatment goals need to be realistic. Conversion symptoms seldom disappear completely. However, adolescents often acquire increased coping skills so that their daily functioning is unimpaired, and dependence on secondary gain is minimized.

For physicians with sufficient expertise, follow-up visits with parents should take place every 4 to 6 weeks. Such meetings should serve to elicit persistent or new concerns that parents may have about their teenager's progress and should attempt to assess the parents' reaction to their teenager's continuing complaints. The practitioner should emphasize the validity of the teenager's concerns so that misconceptions about the symptom being faked are dispelled. Furthermore, positive reinforcement needs to be offered so that parents believe they are doing what is best for their child. Selected follow-up sessions with the parents should include the teenager. Not only do such family meetings demonstrate to the patient that confidentiality of individual sessions is not being violated, but they also offer the physician an opportunity to observe parent-adolescent interaction. These observations may provide an important index to the effectiveness of ongoing therapy.

REFERRAL

Referral to mental health professionals is indicated if symptoms continue to interfere with the patient's daily activities or functioning or when the physician or school personnel believe that the teenager's symptoms have not diminished. School officials can provide valuable information about the effect of the conversion symptom on school functioning and peer interaction. Referral is indicated if the family believes that inadequate progress has been made after an agreed-on duration of therapy.

Referral also is indicated if the patient's symptom creates uncomfortable feelings in the pediatrician. Situations involving seductive adolescent behavior in association with a conversion symptom may create feelings in the pediatrician that can prevent effective intervention. Assuming that a pediatrician can treat all psychological and medical problems adequately is unrealistic. Cognizance of one's own limitations is an important professional attribute. Another situation requiring referral involves the patient or family member who is a social acquaintance or a relative of the pediatrician. Dealing with the emotional problems of friends' or relatives' children is inappropriate. Obtaining personal details of family or sexual functioning is often indicated in the evaluation and may jeopardize the social relationship. Conversely, failure or hesitancy to obtain appropriate data may jeopardize subsequent resolution of the problem.

In all cases when referral is suggested, parental and patient compliance with the referral is improved if the possibility has been mentioned as a contingency early in the evaluation. The pediatrician should always help families understand that seeing a psychiatrically trained professional does not connote *craziness*. Rather, the pediatrician may suggest that a mental health professional might help because a physician or professional trained in mental health can help teenagers understand feelings about prolonged or unusual symptoms better than can most pediatricians. The physician should recommend a specific counselor rather than offering a list of suggested therapists. Before the name of the therapist is given to the family, the physician should verify that the counselor feels comfortable with the referral and has time available to see the patient.

After the referral is made, continued pediatrician contact with the family concerning the conversion symptom promotes adherence with the therapy. Indications for referring patients who have conversion symptoms are listed in Box 139-8.[10]

BOX 139-8 Indications for Referral of Patients Who Have Conversion Symptoms

The symptom continues to interfere with daily functioning (school attendance, participation in extracurricular activities, involvement with peers). Parents and patient believe that no progress is being made in dealing with the symptom.

The physician feels uncomfortable with the patient's symptom or behavior (eg, patients exhibiting seductive behavior).

The patient's family includes a social friend or relative of the physician.

From Prazar G. Conversion reactions in adolescents. *Pediatr Rev.* 1987;8:279-286.

The prognosis for patients who have conversion reactions is unknown. In a report of 74 children who had psychogenic pain, many patients were judged to be improved after several years regardless of whether professional intervention took place. In a 7-year followup of patients hospitalized with conversion, 23 of 41 patients no longer suffered from their presenting physical symptom, were free of underlying stress, and had experienced no symptom substitution or new associated complaint.[11] Patients who have conversion symptoms, indeed, may have an encouraging future. On the other hand, in some patients, adolescent conversion symptoms mark the beginning of a lifelong course of conversion illness.

SUMMARY

Conversion reactions represent an emotionally charged issue not only literally for the adolescent, but also figuratively for the physician because patients displaying such symptoms often elicit a wide range of emotions from their physician. The physician's emotional response results from the frustration in dealing with such difficult patients. Patients who have a somatic complaint have feelings about their symptoms. An evaluation of any somatic complaint should involve inquiry into aspects of the patient's family, school attendance and performance, and peer relationships. A better understanding of the patient's baseline emotional functioning can be achieved in this way. The physician must advise both parents and patient that having feelings about somatic complaints is acceptable. Both family and patient may be much more accepting of primary emotional involvement if permission for expressing feelings is given early in the physician-patient relationship. The diagnosis of a conversion reaction should never be one of exclusion and should follow specific diagnostic criteria.

Care of the adolescent patient who has a conversion reaction involves establishing a renegotiable number of regular visits, encouraging the patient to discuss daily activities and interrelated feelings, meeting with parents regularly to provide them with emotional support and counseling, and knowing that palliation rather than a cure may be the end goal. When the physician feels uncomfortable treating a patient who has a conversion reaction, or when ongoing follow-up care appears to have made no progress in reducing the symptom, the patient should be referred to a mental health professional. However, referral should not end the pediatrician's contact with the patient because ongoing physician interest may improve patient adherence with the referral source and may increase the physician's ability to resume responsibility later for the patient's care. The patient who has a conversion symptom usually will not outgrow it in the short term. Such patients severely tax the primary care physician's diagnostic and therapeutic acumen. However, the physician who respects the involvement of emotions with somatic complaints can help patients who have conversion symptoms cope with their disorders.

TOOLS FOR PRACTICE

Engaging Patients and Family

- *A Parent's Guide to Building Resilience in Children and Teens* (book), American Academy of Pediatrics (www.aap.org/bookstore).
- *Stressed Read This* (brochure), American Academy of Pediatrics (patiented.aap.org).
- *Helping Your Child Cope with Life* (brochure), American Academy of Pediatrics (patiented.aap.org).

AAP POLICY STATEMENT

American Academy of Pediatrics. Insurance coverage of mental health and substance abuse services for children and adolescents: a consensus statement. *Pediatrics.* 2000;106(4):860-862. (aappolicy.aappublications.org/cgi/content/full/pediatrics;106/4/860).

REFERENCES

Engel GL. Conversion symptoms. In: MacBryde CM, Blacklow RS, eds. *Signs and Symptoms: Applied Pathologic Physiology and Clinical Interpretation.* 6th ed. Philadelphia, PA: JB Lippincott; 1983.

Hollender MH. Conversion hysteria: a post-Freudian reinterpretation of nineteenth century psychosocial data. *Arch Gen Psychiatr.* 1972;26:311-314.

Apley J. *The Child with Abdominal Pains.* 2nd ed. Oxford, UK: Blackwell Scientific; 1975.

Oster J. Recurrent abdominal pain, headache, and limb pains in children and adolescents. *Pediatrics.* 1972;50:429-436.

Friedman SB. Conversion symptoms in adolescents. *Pediatr Clin North Am.* 1973;20:873-882.

Levine RJ. Epidemic faintness and syncope in a school marching band. *JAMA.* 1977;238:2373-2376.

Moffett MEK. Epidemic hysteria in a Montreal train station. *Pediatrics.* 1982;70:308-310.

Griffith JL, Polles A, Griffith ME. Pseudoseizures, families and unspeakable dilemmas. *Psychosomatics.* 1998;39:144-153.

Schmitt BD. School phobia—the great imitator: a pediatrician's viewpoint. *Pediatrics.* 1971;48:433-438.

Prazar G. Conversion reactions in adolescents. *Pediatr Rev.* 1987;8:279-286.

Maisami M, Freeman JM. Conversion reactions in children as body language: a combined child psychiatry/neurology team approach to the management of functional neurologic disorders in children. *Pediatrics.* 1987;80:46-52.

Chapter 140

CHILDREN WITH GENDER-VARIANT BEHAVIORS AND TRANSGENDER YOUTH

Robert J. Bidwell, MD

Throughout history and across many cultures, children and adolescents have, through their gender expression and gender identity, transcended cultural expectations about the meaning of being a girl or a boy.[1-4] In some times and places, as these children and youths grew into adulthood, they became respected and even revered members of their societies. In others, including the current culture in this country, they have been ridiculed or reviled and seen as legitimate targets of discrimination and persecution. Issues related to gender-variant behaviors and gender identity are highly controversial. Although the American Academy of Pediatrics has issued clinical guidelines on working with gay, lesbian, and bisexual (GLB) adolescents,[5] it has no policy statements or clinical guidelines related to addressing issues of gender-variant behaviors or gender identity in pediatric practice.

Gender is a complex concept that is still not well understood. Researchers and theorists have attempted to study and explain various aspects of gender to understand better this important part of being human. Gender role represents a set of behaviors, attitudes, and interests that a society or culture believes are typically female or male. A child's gender role is usually established by the age of 3 to 5 years. When a child displays behaviors, attitudes, or interests outside the cultural norm for the child's biologic (genetic and anatomic) sex, it is referred to as *gender-variant behavior* (or gender-nonconforming behavior). For example, boys with gender-variant behavior may prefer playing house to playing football, enjoy dressing up in their mothers' clothes or trying on their makeup, prefer long hair, and be more stereotypically feminine in their mannerisms and speech. Girls with gender-variant behavior may avoid wearing girls' clothes, enjoy more physically aggressive play with boys, prefer short hair, and have the stereotypic mannerisms of a tomboy.

In contrast, gender identity refers to a person's deepest inner sense of being female or male (or even something other than female or male) and is often established by age 2 to 3 years. For most individuals, gender identity is congruent with biological sex, although for some, it is not. Although their bodies tell them and the world around them that they are female or male, their inner identity is either of the opposite gender or a sense of gender separate from female or male. These individuals are referred to as transsexual or transgender.

Gender identity is distinct from sexual orientation, which refers to an individual's affectional, romantic, or sexual attraction to others of the same sex (homosexual), opposite sex (heterosexual), or both sexes (bisexual), as discussed in Chapter 157, Gay, Lesbian, and Bisexual Youth.

DEFINITIONS

Transgender has become an umbrella term encompassing everyone who does not conform to cultural norms of being female or male. This group includes transsexual persons, whose gender identity does not match their biological gender and who seek to physically change their bodies to make them more consistent with their inner sense of gender. Also included in this group are cross-dressers (transvestites), drag kings and queens, and persons who perceive themselves to be of both genders. It can also include individuals who are simply gender nonconforming in terms of their attitudes, interests, and behaviors.

Transgender may also be used in a narrower sense, synonymous with transsexual. It is primarily in this sense that transgender is used in this chapter. Transgender individuals often refer to themselves as trans, TG, or T. Many transgender people, but not all, experience significant gender dysphoria, a persistent discomfort with the gender assigned to them at birth and the societal gender role expectations that accompany it. These dysphoric feelings often begin in early childhood and increase with the appearance of unwanted physical changes at puberty. Many transgender individuals gradually let go of the need to conform to societal expectations attached to their biological gender and increasingly present themselves to the world in a manner consistent with their gender identity. This process is known as *transition*. The terms male-to-female (MTF) and female-to-male (FTM) transgender are used to describe the direction of transition from biological gender to actual gender identity. The transition process may include hormone treatment and sex-reassignment surgery.

The prevalence of gender-variant behaviors among children and adolescents is uncertain. Occasional or single gender-variant behaviors among elementary school children are common.[6] During the development of the well-known Child Behavior Checklist,[7] mothers of 4- to 5-year-old children described 6% of boys and 11.8% of girls as sometimes or frequently behaving in a manner more typical of the opposite sex. Furthermore, 1.3% of the boys and 5.0% of the girls sometimes or frequently wished to be the opposite sex. The prevalence of transgenderism is also uncertain. Although few people seek hormonal and surgical sex reassignment,[8] the true prevalence of transgenderism remains unknown because some transgender individuals do have access to or do not want sex-reassignment treatments.

One of the most debated issues related to gender expression and gender identity during childhood and adolescence is whether gender nonconformity, gender-variant behaviors, and even transgenderism are causes for concern.[9-13] Do they represent a pathological abnormality, or are they simply part of the continuum of normal human development? Similar debates occurred around homosexuality until it was officially removed from the American Psychiatric Association's list of mental disorders in 1973. Although controversial, transsexualism is represented in the fourth edition of the *Diagnostic and Statistical Manual of Mental Disorders* (DSM-IV) under the diagnostic category of *gender identity disorder* (GID).[14] To make a diagnosis of GID in childhood or adolescence, 4 criteria must be met: (1) evidence of a strong and persistent cross-gender identification (eg, the desire to be or the insistence that one is of the other sex); (2) persistent discomfort with an individual's assigned sex or a sense of inappropriateness of the gender role assigned to that sex; (3) no concurrent physical intersex condition (eg, androgen insensitivity syndrome, congenital adrenal hyperplasia); and (4) evidence of clinically significant distress or impairment in social, occupational, or other important areas of functioning.

The DSM-IV also describes separate specific clinical features for boys and girls, as well as for children and adolescents or adults. Based on these criteria, a child or adolescent with gender-variant behaviors who identifies with the gender assigned at birth would not be diagnosed with GID. Furthermore, the diagnosis of GID requires discomfort and distress or impairment. Much of the controversy arising from the creation of GID as a DSM-IV diagnostic category is the observation that any gender-variant child or adolescent raised in a society that enforces a binary view of gender will predictably experience discomfort related to gender expression and identity. Given the overt discrimination and violence against transgender individuals in US society, distress or impairment in social and other areas of functioning should be expected. Evidence suggests that transgender individuals growing up in more accepting societies experience less discomfort and distress related to their gender identity and gender role than those in the United States.

Several developmental trajectories have been described for children with GID. Most boys diagnosed with GID eventually self-identify as homosexual or bisexual as adolescents or adults and no longer report gender dysphoria. A smaller percentage of children with gender-variant behaviors later self-identifies as heterosexual and also reports no gender dysphoria. Approximately 15% continue to experience discomfort with their biologic sex and self-identify as transgender. Research data for girls diagnosed with GID is less certain. Most girls eventually self-identify as heterosexual or bisexual. A smaller percentage report being homosexual, and only a small percentage continue to have gender dysphoria.

ETIOLOGY

Several theories have been proposed suggesting possible causes for the development of gender-variant behavior and transgender identity. Because many children diagnosed with GID later identify themselves as homosexual and are no longer gender dysphoric as adolescents or adults, research on GID in childhood overlaps with research on the origins of sexual orientation.[12,15] No clear biological marker for GID has yet been found, although animal studies suggest that prenatal hormones may influence a fetus's developing brain and lead to sexually dimorphic behaviors. Studies of girls who were exposed to large levels of androgens prenatally—for example, those with congenital adrenal hyperplasia—found that they had gender roles more masculine than those of control peers. Studies of girls with congenital adrenal hyperplasia have indicated a possible higher incidence of bisexuality and homosexuality than expected. One possible explanation is that children with GID, whose anatomic sex is consistent with genetic sex, may be exposed to subtle increases or decreases in prenatal androgens at critical points in fetal psychosexual development that later result in gender-variant behaviors and transgender identity. Some studies, mostly related to boys, have found an association between GID and handedness, sibling sex ratio, birth order, and birth weight, which may also provide indirect evidence of prenatal events predisposing a child to gender variance.[12]

Psychosocial theories have also attempted to explain variations in gender expression and gender identity.[12,15] These theories often focus on familial, and particularly parental, psychopathology, and aberrant parenting practices that may interact with biological factors and predispose a child to GID. Such theories are controversial because similar psychosocial theories were offered in the past, then abandoned, as explanations for homosexuality. This fact is especially relevant because most boys and many girls diagnosed with GID later identify themselves as homosexual or bisexual. Psychosocial theories have also been criticized because they appear to identify presumed negative factors, such as parental failure to discourage a son's feminine behaviors, that might be modified through family therapy to prevent undesirable gender-variant behaviors in a child. In addition to a growing belief that gender-variant children should be permitted to express their gender-variant behaviors and identities freely and without shame,[13,16-19] a belief exists among some investigators that GID diagnosis has been used as an indirect means of treating children to prevent the development of a later homosexual orientation.[11,20] Finally, controversy exists because much research *pathologizes* gender-variant behavior and transgenderism, yet has not invited the participation of the transgender community into a discussion of what research questions are important to ask and how results of those studies are to be interpreted and used. By trying to answer the question, "What went wrong?" the focus on individuals and their families may be misdirected. Instead, the most revealing and helpful inquiry might be that which is focused on observing gender-variant children and families within the context of a disapproving and often violently retributive society.

In most ways, children with gender-variant behaviors and transgender youths are exactly the same as their peers. They have the same needs for protection, nurturance, and love and the same hopes and dreams for the future. They grow up in the same families and communities and attend the same schools and places of worship. Similar to other children, they face the fundamental task of achieving a sense of identity that integrates all aspects of who they are, including their gender identity. This integration of identity, accompanied by a growing sense of comfort with that identity, is essential for the optimal health and well being of each child and adolescent.

However, the experience of growing up as a child with gender-variant behaviors or a transgender youth is different in several important ways.[9,21,22] First, unlike their peers, these young people face an often lonely and sometimes frightening journey of self-discovery, attempting to understand two of the most fundamental aspects of who they are as human beings: (1) their gender identity and (2) their sexual orientation. Most children with significant gender-variant behaviors eventually identify themselves as gay, lesbian, or bisexual; their experience and the special challenges they face are discussed in Chapter 157, Gay, Lesbian, and Bisexual Youth. Some of these children will recognize, often at a young age, that their inner sense of being female or male differs from the gender that was assigned to them at birth. Some children and adolescents accommodate themselves to this growing awareness. Most, however, experience significant confusion and distress, wondering what their feelings mean and uncertain of who they are (male? female? gay? lesbian? homosexual? bisexual? none of the above?). Growing up in a society that believes that a person is either male or female and that gender expression and identity must strictly reflect biological sex undoubtedly intensifies their sense that something inside them has gone terribly wrong. Many of these individuals become filled with an overwhelming mix of shame, anger, self-hatred, and despair.

ADVERSE EFFECTS

Transgender youths often experience a profound isolation that intensifies their feelings of confusion and distress. They and everyone in their lives, including parents, teachers, counselors, clergy, and health care providers, know little or nothing about gender identity or what it means to be transgender. In many instances, gender identity is confused with sexual orientation, a much different concept. Many primary care physicians (PCPs) and counselors were trained at a time when gender-variant behaviors and transgender identity were seen as aberrant or pathological, and they conduct their practices accordingly. Few transgender youths have adult role models or mentors for support or validation, and few know another transgender youth. When transgender youths have no access to accurate information, supportive counselors, or health care providers, and when they have no opportunity for healthy interactions with transgender peers and adults, the negative messages that surround them in their daily lives go unchallenged.

The most harmful reality in the lives of these children and youths is that they grow up in a society that deeply disapproves of who they are and how they present themselves to the world. Social stigma, and the violence and discrimination it engenders, permeates their daily lives. It makes completing the expected developmental tasks of childhood and adolescence related to identity and self-esteem enormously difficult. Many of these children and youths are viewed by their families with shame and disgust. They are often forced to change their behaviors and renounce their declared inner sense of being female or male. Many of them are taken to therapists for the express purpose of changing their gender expression or gender identity. Many transgender adolescents and adults recall being ridiculed, ostracized, or beaten for being true to who they were. As a result, many gender-variant children and transgender youths run away or are thrown out of their homes; many end up in the child welfare or juvenile justice systems.[23,24] The harassment and abuse against gender-variant and transgender young people often continue in these settings, perpetrated by other youths and by staff members.

Schools are an especially dangerous place for gender-variant children and transgender youths.[25-28] Many of these individuals experience daily verbal, physical, and sexual harassment on the playground and in the classroom. In many instances, this harassment is not addressed by teachers, counselors, or other school staff, or it is dealt with by blaming the victim. Sometimes, disapproving teachers and other school staff members engage in harassing behaviors themselves. Most schools have no specific policies prohibiting harassment or bullying based on gender identity or expression, even though these, along with sexual orientation, are among the most common targets of harassment on school campuses. Many of these children and youth are equally unsafe in their own neighborhoods. When society as a whole disapproves of who a child is, simply stated, no place of refuge exists.

Societal stigma is also reflected in daily discrimination. They are told with which toys they can and cannot play, and what interests they may or may not pursue. They are told by what names they will be called and by what pronouns they will be referred, in spite of their protests that these names and pronouns do not reflect who they really are. Their genitalia rather than their inner identity as female or male are referenced in assigning them to bathrooms, lockers, physical education classes, athletic teams, and other school activities in which gender is still seen as relevant. School dress codes often limit transgender students' ability to wear clothes that are consistent with their gender identity. Many gay, lesbian, bisexual, and transgender (GLBT) students across the United States have sought to start *gay-straight alliances*—school-sanctioned support groups for GLBT students and their friends—and although some administrations permit them, many others do not.

As transgender youths age, they begin to experience broader societal forms of discrimination. Their driver's licenses and other forms of identification, as well as their school, employment, and health records, usually reflect their biological sex rather than their gender identity. Because fear, embarrassment, and potential humiliation accompany the presentation of these documents to others, many transgender adolescents may avoid applying for school or a job or accessing health care. Transgender individuals have been denied access to educational opportunities, community programs, social services, and health care because of their gender identity. Because only a few states have enacted laws that prohibit discrimination based on gender identity and expression in the areas of housing, employment, public accommodations, and health care, transgender individuals, particularly adolescents, have little recourse when faced with discrimination. They have few advocates outside their own community. Even the GLB community, which has made great strides in securing its civil rights over the last decades, has often failed to provide supportive services and advocacy for the transgender community, including its youth.

Children with GID have more mental health problems,[12] particularly depression, separation anxiety, and a variety of behavior problems when compared with those without GID. Although rates of psychopathological conditions are higher among referred children with GID, they are no higher than in other referred but non-GID children. Although the distress experienced by younger children with GID may not be primarily the result of social stigma, many of the mental health problems that transgender adolescents encounter likely result from the stigmatization, peer rejection, and discrimination they face. Behavior problems among children diagnosed with GID can be predicted by poor peer relationships, which supports the notion that much of the distress that these young people experience is the result of environmental factors.[29] *Psychopathological condition* may be an inaccurate term when applied indiscriminately to gender-variant and transgender youths; depression, anxiety, and behavior problems are expected, and perhaps even adaptive, responses to growing up in an unaccepting and hostile society.

Many transgender youths face significant risks to their health and well being from violence.[9,30] Because of the pervasive violence they face at school, many transgender students are constantly fearful for their safety, find it impossible to concentrate on their studies, and eventually drop out of school. Because of rejection or violence within their families, many of these individuals are thrown out or run away from homes and end up living on the streets. Once on the streets, youths often survive by exchanging sex for money, drugs, or shelter.[24] Some of them may find validation of their gender identity in these and other sexual encounters. Because life on the streets often involves sexual activity with multiple and often older and anonymous sexual partners that is often unprotected by condoms, these youths are at high risk for sexually transmitted infections (STIs) and infection with HIV.[31] Street life also brings with it the threat of physical and sexual assault. Some youths deal drugs to survive, and many are engaged in multisubstance use, in part, to numb their emotional pain. In larger towns, a community of transgender adults may take in runaway transgender youths and provide them with shelter, food, protection, basic survival skills, and validation. Unfortunately, this new *family* is often a conduit into commercial sex work, substance use, and underground acquisition of transition hormones (estrogen and testosterone) and injectable silicone. Given these experiences, not surprisingly, many transgender adolescents and adults have attempted suicide.[32]

The risks described previously are not inherent in being a gender-variant child or transgender youth. They are the common experience of any young person who is stigmatized, fearful, and alone. The genuine distress experienced by some children diagnosed with GID and some transgender youths over the perceived dissonance between their biological sex and gender identity should not be dismissed or minimized. Nevertheless, evidence from other cultures and the experience of many counselors and clinicians suggest that when provided loving, supportive validation, these young people thrive and can expect to grow into happy, healthy, and productive adults. Perhaps the most important role that PCPs can play in the lives of gender-variant children and transgender youths is to ensure that they grow up in safe and nurturing environments.

EVALUATION

The American Academy of Pediatrics and the American Academy of Child and Adolescent Psychiatry have issued no policy or position statements related to the provision of care and counseling to children with gender-variant behaviors and transgender youths. The American Academy of Family Practice has issued policies reaffirming its opposition to *all discrimination in any form* based on actual or perceived sexual orientation or gender identity and encouraging physicians to ask open questions about sexuality to initiate a dialogue on issues facing GLBT adolescents in a sensitive and accepting atmosphere.[33,34] In addition, several resources are available to PCPs on providing culturally sensitive and relevant care to gender-variant children and transgender adolescents and adults.[35,36]

PCPs should not presume the sexual orientation or gender identity of any patient. Children with gender-variant behaviors, many who will later identify as GLB, have often learned or have been pressured to change their behaviors, particularly in public settings such as health clinics. Many transgender youths will also hide their true gender identity. Even when asked in a sensitive and nonjudgmental manner about their inner feelings of being female or male, they will often deny these feelings because they are fearful of PCP disapproval, uncertain about confidentiality, or still confused about the meaning of their emerging feelings. Perhaps one of the greatest barriers to appropriate health care for transgender youths is providers' assumption that they have no children or youths in their practices who are dealing with issues of gender identity. Another mistaken assumption is that significant gender-variant behavior in childhood accurately predicts sexual orientation. Although most children with gender-variant behaviors will later identify as GLB, at least 25% will not. Although many PCPs understand that some gender-variant individuals are heterosexual, many do not consider the possibility that a child may be transgender. Many transgender youths are thought by their PCPs, and sometimes by themselves, to be GLB. However, the distinctions between sexual orientation and gender identity are important for the provision of care because of the different issues they face. In addition, gender identity does not predict sexual orientation. Transgender youths may be gay, lesbian, heterosexual, or bisexual. For example, an MTF-transgender adolescent who falls in love with a boy is considered heterosexual.

The goal of PCPs is not to identify every child with gender-variant behaviors or transgender identity; instead, it is to create a safe and accepting clinical setting where children, adolescents, and their families know they can discuss any topic of concern, including gender identity and expression, without discomfort or disapproval. Some patients and parents do not know that PCPs may have expertise in discussing issues of sexual and gender development. Specific messages can be provided through clinic posters and brochures informing patients that these issues are appropriate topics of discussion. The most important signal that these topics are a natural part of pediatric practice is in the PCP's own history taking and anticipatory guidance, in which issues of child and adolescent sexuality and gender should be routinely discussed.

After patients have identified themselves as transgender, the PCP should create an accepting and supportive clinical environment by using pronouns consistent with their patients' gender identity and asking by what name they would like to be called by clinic staff. Although medical records must retain the patient's legal name, the notice "Also Known As [preferred name]" can be added to the front of the chart, and all clinic staff members should use this name in personal encounters with the patient. Patients should use either a unisex restroom or a restroom consistent with their gender identity while in the clinic. As with all adolescents, transgender patients should be seen alone and their confidentiality respected. A patient's gender identity should not be revealed to parents without the patient's permission. Patients should also be asked how they would like their gender identity recorded in the chart, if at all, because medical records containing confidential information are sometimes accessible to parents.

PCPs should reflect on their own feelings about gender-variant behaviors and gender identity issues. As products of their own society, many health care providers may initially approach these issues with discomfort or disapproval. However, discomfort with or disapproval of gender-variant children or transgender youths will diminish the ability to care for these patients. Most transgender patients have had profoundly negative experiences with the health care system.[36,37] These patients are labeled as *disordered* and are often treated as such. Transgender patients report how staff in clinical settings often display fear or open disapproval of them or joke about them, even within hearing of the patient. At times, these patients have been refused medical care. PCPs who receive little training about transgender health issues often do not understand the transgender adolescent's unique life experiences and needs. Most PCPs are unfamiliar with community resources that might help their transgender patients. Health insurance companies almost universally refuse to pay for transition treatments, including hormone therapy, surgery, and the laboratory studies needed to monitor treatment.

PCPs are in a position of power relative to their transgender patients. As gatekeepers, PCPs decide who does or does not receive transition treatments.[38] Many, often through ignorance or disapproval, have barred transgender patients from passing through that gate, preventing them from receiving appropriate and necessary transition treatment and care. PCPs must understand the history of tension between the transgender and medical communities. PCPs can improve this strained relationship by listening carefully and respectfully to their patients' life stories and expressions of need and by providing care that addresses these needs in a compassionate and comprehensive manner.

History

Gender and sexuality are important parts of a child's life. At each well-child visit, beginning in early childhood, the PCP should ask parents how they think their child is developing compared with other children. Parents and child should be asked how the child is getting along with siblings and peers. Does their child appear happy? Is the child teased or harassed by other children, and over what issues? All parents should be asked if they have any concerns over their child's sexual development or gender expression. Many parents who have such concerns are hesitant to bring them up on their own but are often relieved when the PCP does so. If a child with gender-variant behavior is happy and safe from teasing and parents have no concerns about these behaviors, no reason exists for the PCP to question further. Gender-variant behavior is not a problem in this situation.

If parents express concerns about their child's gender expression or gender identity, then the PCP should ask what they have noticed or heard from the child and what their concerns or fears might be. Parents' concerns are often related to their own embarrassment because of their child's behavior; they may also fear for their child's safety in a nonaccepting world. Many of them fear that their child's behavior or verbal expressions of wanting to be the opposite gender signal an eventual lesbian or gay sexual orientation or transgender identity. PCPs may gently question gender-variant children if they feel safe from teasing at home and school and about their feelings of being more like a girl or a boy inside. However, care must be taken to avoid conveying the message that anything is wrong with the child because of the child's gender variance. In addition to the well-child visit, any visit suggesting an unhappy child or a child in distress should lead the PCP to consider discussing issues of gender-variant behaviors and gender identity with parents and child.

Transgender adolescents may come to the PCP's office either because of parental concerns or through school or child welfare agency referral. Transgender youths may also seek care themselves, often to discuss issues of safety and acceptance at home or school, concerns about STIs, or to request hormone treatment. However, many transgender patients see their PCPs not through referrals or acute care visits but rather in the context of routine well-teen evaluations. Many transgender patients hide any evidence of their inner gender identity; others are presumed, perhaps even by themselves, to be lesbian or gay. PCPs should initiate discussion of sexuality with all adolescents at each well-teen visit. Although many PCPs routinely discuss sexual activity and safer sex practices, fewer discuss sexual orientation, and almost none of them address gender identity. However, as noted earlier, most transgender adolescents face significant confusion and distress related to their gender identity and major risks from growing up in a nonaccepting world. PCPs must be willing to open the door to discussion of gender so as to reduce the turmoil and dangers that these youths face.

The PCP can begin to approach the issue of gender identity in the broader context of obtaining a HEADSSS (home, education, activities, drugs, sexuality, suicide, and safety) interview.[39] This approach will provide a sense of how things are going in various aspects of an adolescent's life, recognizing that many transgender youths face serious issues in each of these areas. To address gender identity within a broader sexual history, the PCP might say, "Sexuality and sexual feelings can be confusing things sometimes. During puberty, bodies change in lots of different ways. Sexual feelings are changing as well. Some of my patients are not sure if they are attracted to guys or girls or maybe both; and some of my patients even wonder if they're more like a girl or a boy inside. All of this is completely normal but can be really confusing. So I'm wondering what it's been like for you." After asking about attractions (sexual orientation), the PCP can simply ask, "And how about inside? Does it seem to feel more like a girl or a boy or maybe somewhere in between?" For the patient who is not dealing with gender identity issues, these questions may seem odd. This aspect can be addressed by a simple statement such as, "These are questions I ask all my patients, and for some, they're really important." For transgender youths, the questions may be life saving. Even if they decide not to acknowledge their gender identity concerns at the current visit, they have learned that someone is available with whom they can talk when the time is right.

If adolescents acknowledge their transgender identity, the PCP should thank them for their trust in sharing this important and personal part of who they are. Patients should be reassured that the discussion of gender identity will remain confidential unless given permission to share it with others or unless a risk of danger to someone exists. The history may then focus on the adolescents' path to recognizing their transgender identity. When were they first aware of feeling more like a girl or a boy? What was this experience like? How comfortable are they with their transgender identity now? What do they know about gender identity and what it means to be transgender? What are their hopes and dreams for the future? Do they see their futures as enhanced or limited by being transgender? The history may then focus on the adolescent in the context of the world around them. Have they told others (family, peers, teachers, or counselors) about their inner feelings of gender? Have these people responded in a supportive or negative way? Have they been scolded, teased, harassed, or ridiculed because of their gender identity? With whom do they spend time, and what kinds of things do they do together? Have they met other transgender adolescents or adults? Have they been in relationships, and have these relationships been healthy ones? Have they been sexually active, and do they use safer-sex practices? Have they ever been pregnant, impregnated anyone, or had an STI? How many different sexual partners have they had, and what have been their genders? Have they ever been touched sexually or forced to have sex without their permission?

Understanding that transgender youths often are subjected to rejection and harassment at home and school, the PCP should ask if they have run away from home or dropped out of school. Have they needed to sell their bodies, deal drugs, or engage in other illegal activities to survive on the streets? Have they been involved with the child welfare or juvenile justice systems, and how have they been treated within them? As with other youths in distress, have they ever used drugs or contemplated suicide? How do they believe their physical health has been, and do they have any health needs they believe are not being addressed? Finally, have they begun the transition process from male to female or female to male? Have they chosen a new name, and would they like the PCP to call them by that name? Have they begun to cross-dress? Have they begun hormone therapy, and, if so, where have they obtained their hormones? Have they injected silicone? Have they thought about sex-reassignment surgery or other transition-related procedures in the future?

Not all of these questions need to be addressed at the first visit. Follow-up visits should be made to address these issues on an ongoing basis. The PCP should be aware that the history, beyond providing specific information about the experience and needs of a transgender adolescent, is an opportunity for the PCP to interact with the patient in a comfortable, respectful, and caring manner that validates who the adolescent is as a human being. Most transgender adolescents have never experienced such acceptance before, and it is one of the most fundamentally important things a PCP can do.

Physical Examination

The physical examination of children with gender-variant behaviors or who express the desire to be other than their anatomic gender is the same as that for other children. A complete examination, including the genitals, should be a routine part of every well-child visit. On occasion, the PCP may observe a child wearing clothes or exhibiting behaviors or interests that are more typical of the opposite gender. These behaviors or interests may or may not relate to the child's gender identity as female or male.

Similarly, the physical examination of transgender adolescents does not differ significantly from that of other adolescents. It should be guided by a comprehensive and accurate health history, including sexual and other risk behaviors. The PCP should remember that transgender youths may be heterosexually, homosexually, or bisexually active or not sexually active at all. Many transgender youths hide all public expressions of their gender identity. Some may have already begun the transition process and come to clinic displaying dress, hairstyles, makeup, and mannerisms usually associated with the opposite gender but consistent with their gender identity. Occasionally, transgender patients may wear non–gender-defining street clothes but underwear appropriate for their gender identity. If patients have already begun transition hormone treatment, then they may show evidence of breast development (MTF), appearance of facial hair (FTM), and other expected changes of estrogen and testosterone treatment.

PCPs should understand and respect the significant discomfort that many transgender youths have related to their pubertal changes, which feel alien to their gender identity. Some MTF-transgender adolescents may tuck their genitals, placing them between their legs so they are less visible. Some FTM-transgender youths may wear chest binders or baggy tops to make their breasts less visible. In preparing for the examination, the PCP should discuss the rationale for suggesting the parts of the examination that might be particularly uncomfortable for a transgender adolescent, especially the breast and genital examinations. PCPs should explain that their intention is to make the examination as comfortable as possible for the patient and to elicit the patient's guidance in how best to accomplish this task. The patient should be informed that they have a right to refuse any part of the examination. The PCP should ask transgender patients what words they would like used in referring to various body parts—for example, *genitals* instead of *penis* or *vagina*. An FTM-transgender patient may prefer the term *chest* rather than *breast*. MTF-transgender patients should be treated the same as other female patients, and FTM-transgender patients like other male patients in conducting the examination. Conducting all comprehensive physical examinations of MTF- and FTM-transgender patients with the patient in a gown and draped appropriately to minimize exposure is best. At the same time, acknowledging that the patient's anatomic gender may suggest gender-specific evaluation such as breast, testicular, or pelvic examinations is appropriate. For example, suggesting a pelvic examination for any FTM adolescent with unexplained vaginal discharge or bleeding would be appropriate. Most transgender patients will agree to the suggested examination if the medical rationale is presented in a factual and respectful manner, inviting the patient's questions and input on how to make the examination as comfortable as possible.

Laboratory Evaluation

The child with gender-variant behaviors who has an unremarkable history and normal physical examination requires no special laboratory evaluation. Laboratory evaluation of transgender adolescents should be based on an accurate and comprehensive history, including sexual and other risk behaviors, and physical examination, not on gender identity. The evaluation and treatment of STIs and of adolescents engaged in homosexual and bisexual activity is discussed in Chapter 322, Sexually Transmitted Infections; and Chapter 157, Gay, Lesbian, and Bisexual Youth. Several clinical guidelines provide information on the appropriate laboratory evaluation and monitoring of those patients who elect to begin hormonal transition therapy.[40,41]

MANAGEMENT

The goal of care in working with gender-variant children and transgender youths is to promote optimal physical, emotional, and social development and well being. The challenge faced by PCPs is to achieve this goal within a context of nonacceptance and stigmatization by many people in society. In this sense, gender-variant children and transgender youths have life experiences and needs that are similar to those of GLB youths; management approaches addressing these are discussed in Chapter 157, Gay, Lesbian, and Bisexual Youth.

Physical Well Being

Gender-variant children and transgender youths face the same health issues as do other young people. The health care they receive should be based on a comprehensive history, physical examination, and evaluative studies, not on their gender expression or identity. Nevertheless, the PCP should recognize that these children and youths often grow up in hostile environments that may have a negative impact on their physical well being.

Developmental, Social, and Emotional Well Being

The PCP's role as educator and counselor is as important as that of medical provider in caring for gender-variant children, transgender youths, and their families. Each child and adolescent will be affected by issues of gender expression and identity in the child's or the adolescent's own individual way, and the PCP should listen carefully to understand best each patient's unique experience and needs. In general, the counseling of gender-variant and transgender youths will address 6 areas: (1) self-acceptance and validation of gender expression and identity, (2) safety, (3) connectedness to supportive others, (4) self-disclosure or *coming out*, (5) healthy relationships and sexual decision making, and (6) optimism for the future. Addressing each of these areas is essential in ensuring their healthy development.

Self-Acceptance and Validation

The PCP can play an important role in countering the effects of disapproval and the pathologizing of gender-variant expression and identity. For the gender-variant child, the PCP should state that although being different in this society can be painful, the child's gender-variant behavior is healthy for that child. For transgender youths, the PCP should acknowledge the controversy around the use of GID as a diagnostic category. Although the medical profession at present includes transsexualism within this categorization, the PCP should inform the patient that many professionals, including some physicians, disagree that being transsexual or transgender is a disorder. PCPs who can honestly state that they view being transgender as part of the tapestry of normal human sexuality should share this belief with their patient. This reassurance of healthiness is perhaps the most powerful statement that a PCP can make to a transgender youth.

Most gender-variant children and transgender youths know little about the concepts of gender expression and gender identity. Gender-variant children can be reassured that many ways exist of being a boy or a girl and that their way is one of these many ways. They can also be told that some children feel more like a girl inside and some more like a boy, or perhaps somewhere in between, and that however they feel is all right. Transgender youths should be provided information on sexual orientation, gender identity, and what it means to be transgender. Some of these adolescents may go through a period of uncertainty, not knowing whether they are gay, lesbian, bisexual, straight, transgender, or a combination of these. The PCP should inform the adolescent that such confusion is normal and that over time they will have a clearer understanding of who they are. The PCP may also provide brochures to adolescents facing issues of gender identity.[42]

Ethnic and other minority youths who are transgender may have an especially difficult time. The PCP should discuss these issues with their patients openly and connect them to appropriate supportive resources within their various communities.

Safety

Because gender-variant children and transgender youths endure physical and sexual assault, harassment, discrimination, and social rejection, PCPs should ask gender-variant children and transgender youths about their safety at home, school, or church, within the peer group, and within the broader community. If harassment or other harmful treatment is acknowledged, then the PCP should work with the youth to identify and implement appropriate strategies to end the violence. Many of these children and youths feel shame and are afraid to advocate for their own safety. They may believe that they deserve the harm inflicted on them, or they may simply accept that this is the way the world is. The PCP should tell children and adolescents that they do not deserve such treatment and that they should expect and demand safety and respect from everyone in their lives and in all settings. Because gender-variant children and transgender youths have so few advocates, the PCP should offer to join with them in approaching every venue in which they experience violence, including the home and school, to work out a plan to end violence immediately and completely. If necessary, the PCP should call on the state child protective services or advocacy organizations such as the American Civil Liberties Union to join in the effort to keep these young people safe.

Isolation

Because gender-variant children and transgender youths experience profound isolation and loneliness, physical and emotional health may be compromised. PCPs should address the issue of isolation by giving accurate information about gender expression and gender identity. They should provide supportive and reassuring counseling, or they should refer the child or adolescent to colleagues who have the time, comfort, and expertise to provide accepting and supportive care and counseling to these young people. PCPs should connect these children and youths to local community resources such as support groups and other youth programs. Children, youths, and families who do not have access to local programs should be informed about national organizations and Web sites created specifically for gender-variant children, transgender youths, and their families. PCPs can also point out positive gender-variant and transgender role models in the community or nationally. In certain circumstances, for transgender PCPs to present themselves as role models to transgender youths and their families may also be appropriate.

Self-Disclosure and Coming Out

Transgender adolescents often reach a point in their development at which they feel a strong urge to disclose their gender identity to others. Unlike most GLB adolescents, transgender youths often have a history of gender-variant expression as children. Therefore others may have already assumed or sensed that they may be transgender or perhaps, more often and usually mistakenly, gay or lesbian. Some transgender youths, however, successfully conceal their gender identity, either by adapting their gender expression to fit societal expectations consistent with their biologic sex or by labeling themselves or allowing others to perceive them as gay or lesbian. The process of disclosure to family and friends is often emotional and traumatic. Transgender youths who disclose their gender identity (come out) risk condemnation and rejection by family and peers. Therefore coming out should be considered carefully, weighing the risks and benefits. It is sometimes suggested that if an adolescent expects a negative response from parents, then the adolescent should wait to disclose until legally and financially independent. However, many adolescents believe that continuing to live a lie is intolerable and harmful to their self-esteem, and they come out earlier. A PCP should never reveal an adolescent's gender identity to parents without permission unless risk of harm exists. A PCP can play an important role in the process of disclosure by helping adolescents decide whether they are ready to come out to family or friends and helping them choose an appropriate time, place, and approach for disclosure.

Relationships and Sexual Decision Making

Most transgender youths have difficulty in meeting other transgender adolescents to establish friendships and share mutual support. PCPs should help connect transgender youths to local GLBT teen support groups and GLBT-supportive programs in the community, if they exist. This task can be accomplished ethically without parental notification. PCPs can suggest national telephone hotlines or Web sites where transgender youths can receive accurate information and supportive counseling and can communicate with other transgender youths. If these options are not available, then the PCP can serve as a supportive and reassuring lifeline until the adolescent is old enough to become independent and possibly move away to attend school or work in a community more accepting of transgender people.

The fact that most transgender adolescents are heterosexual—that is, they are attracted to people whose gender is opposite from their own gender identity—poses a particularly difficult problem for transgender youths hoping to find girlfriends or boyfriends. Whereas GLB youths can establish dating relationships within the GLB community, most transgender individuals are attracted to those within the heterosexual community. Given the prevailing societal antipathy toward transgender individuals, many transgender youths are afraid to reveal their gender identity to those in whom they might be interested in establishing a relationship. Therefore some transgender youths find that their only options for exploring emotional and physical intimacy are through anonymous sexual encounters on the streets, in parks, or through Internet hook-ups. These encounters are often accompanied by feelings of shame and degradation, which are harmful to an adolescent's sense of identity and self-worth. Many transgender youths wish they had the opportunity to engage in the same courting rituals as other adolescents in safer and more affirming circumstances.

Transgender youths who are in relationships face many of the same questions as their nontransgender peers. "Am I in love?" "What do I want from a relationship?" "Do I really want to be in this relationship?" "How do I know if this is a good relationship?" "How do I get out of this relationship?" In addition, transgender youths face the exceedingly difficult questions of how and when to tell their potential boyfriend or girlfriend about their gender identity. A transgender-supportive PCP or counselor can help adolescents reflect on and find answers to these questions.

As with other adolescents, many transgender youths know little about sexuality and how to make healthy sexual choices. Abstinence is always the appropriate option for adolescents who do not feel ready for a sexual relationship. Transgender adolescents should understand that when they are ready for a sexual relationship, they can expect to lead healthy and fulfilling sexual lives. All adolescents who have decided they are ready for a sexual relationship should be advised to limit their number of sexual partners and avoid mixing sex and alcohol or drugs so as to reduce their risk for infection, trauma, and sexual assault. Safer sex practices related to oral, vaginal, and anal sex should be reviewed in detail. Transgender youths should also be aware that *no* always means *no* in negotiating sex, and any forced or coerced sexual experience represents sexual assault.

Optimism for the Future

PCPs should not only focus on the risks that transgender youths face, but also identify specific strengths that have allowed them to survive and sometimes thrive in the face of an often hostile environment. They should also challenge the belief of many transgender adolescents that their futures will be significantly limited by their gender identity. Although some communities are more accepting of transgender people than others, many transgender adults lead happy, healthy, and productive lives. Although growing up transgender is often challenging, the future should be seen as hopeful and exciting.

TRANSITION CARE

Transition represents the emotional, psychological, social, physical, and legal processes transgender persons experience to assume a body and role consistent with their gender identity. The transition process often begins in childhood and continues through adolescence into adulthood. Hormone therapy and surgery are usually the final steps in this process. PCPs play an important role in facilitating the patient's transition from female to male or male to female, either by referring patients or by providing transition medical care and counseling themselves. Pediatric PCPs generally refer transgender patients for transition-related care and counseling but should retain their central role as PCP and medical home. Many larger communities have adolescent medicine, family practice, and internal medicine physicians, as well as mental health care providers, who provide transition medical care and supportive counseling to transgender patients. These providers can be located through local GLBT community centers or national organizations such as the Gay and Lesbian Medical Association.

Guidelines exist to help PCPs and other health care providers facilitate the transition process.[40,43] After a diagnosis of GID, the therapeutic approach progresses through 3 stages: (1) a real-life experience consistent with gender identity, (2) hormones of the desired gender, and (3) surgery to change genitalia and other sexual characteristics. Before initiating hormone treatment during adolescence, these standards require a minimal age of 16 (preferably with parental consent if under 18) and the involvement of a mental health professional with both patient and family for at least 6 months. When these requirements have been met, the patient's therapist will write a letter to the physician authorizing the initiation of hormone treatment. Once hormone therapy has begun, the patient continues to meet with both the physician and the therapist regularly to monitor the patient's successful adaptation to the physical and psychosocial changes. These guidelines are perceived by some as reflecting an underlying assumption that transgenderism is a mental disorder and imposing gatekeepers to decide who may and who may not receive treatment. In addition, strict eligibility requirements might force some patients to access hormones and other treatments on the streets, without medical monitoring. Individual providers may need to modify the guidelines on a patient-to-patient basis.

Transition is not the same for everyone. Some individuals are satisfied to live their lives consistent with their gender identity in a social sense but have no urge to initiate hormone therapy or undergo surgery. Others seek hormone treatment but think that surgical alteration of their bodies is unnecessary. Still others may choose partial surgical gender reassignment; for example, many FTM transgender individuals choose mastectomy but not genital reconstruction. In addition, the transition process is not necessarily a linear one. Some individuals move back and forth between feelings of being more feminine or masculine and may present themselves differently to the world at different times in terms of gender role and expression. This fluidity of identity should be expected and supported by the PCP.

Hormone Therapy

Several treatment protocols have been used to facilitate transition.[40,41] Although transgender identity is often established in childhood, hormone therapy is usually withheld until at least 16 years of age, when puberty is complete, because younger adolescents may not be mature enough to have a clear understanding of their gender identity and may not be in the best position to make an important decision about whether to change their bodies. At the same time, puberty-associated changes are distressing to many transgender youths, and earlier transition may lead to better physical and psychological outcomes and reduced gender dysphoria.[44]

Because the physical changes of puberty are so distressing to transgender youths, several medical centers have developed protocols to suppress progression of puberty in younger adolescent who are likely to be transgender.[45] This approach allows adolescents time to understand better their gender identity and to decide later whether they wish to proceed with hormone therapy or surgery. Suppression treatment consists of a gonadotropin-releasing hormone analogue (GnRHa), which suppresses endogenous gonadal stimulation, resulting in a delay in progression of secondary sexual characteristics. Eligible patients are usually at least 12 years of age and have achieved a sexual maturity rating of 2 or 3. If an adolescent later decides not to pursue hormone therapy or surgical sex reassignment, then suppression can be discontinued and puberty allowed to progress consistent with biological sex. If, however, at age 16 the adolescent wishes to begin hormone treatment, then estrogen or testosterone can be added to GnRHa to initiate pubertal changes consistent with gender identity.

Male-to-Female Hormone Treatment

Estrogen is the mainstay of MTF-transgender hormone therapy. It may be provided in oral, injectable, or transdermal forms. Expected changes include breast development, softening of skin, increase in subcutaneous fat and its redistribution to the thighs and buttocks, diminished body hair, fewer erections, testicular atrophy, and possible infertility. Patients may also experience decreased libido, weight gain, and emotional changes. Some of these changes may be permanent, continuing even after discontinuation of treatment, particularly if treatment is lengthy. Estrogen treatment is generally safe in adolescents.[46] Although PCPs should be aware of the precautions generally noted for estrogen therapy,[41] medical contraindications to estrogen treatment in adolescents are rare. Occasionally, antiandrogens, such as spironolactone, are added to the regimen to suppress the action of endogenous testosterone, augment breast development, and soften facial and body hair.

Female-to-Male Hormone Treatment

The FTM transition is facilitated through use of testosterone administered through injection, patch, or topical gel. Testosterone treatment is generally safe in adolescents. Expected changes include increased facial and body hair, clitoral enlargement, cessation of menses, possible infertility, increased acne, male-pattern baldness, deepening of voice, and redistribution of fat and increased muscle mass leading to a more masculine body shape. Patients may also notice increased libido, mood changes, increased weight, more prominent veins, coarser skin, and mild breast atrophy.

Other Treatments

Some transgender individuals will seek other treatments to facilitate the physical and psychosocial transition to their appropriate gender. Usually these treatments will occur after the adolescent years, partly because these procedures are expensive and seldom covered by insurance. MTF-transgender individuals may seek reconstructive surgery, including orchiectomy, vaginoplasty, breast augmentation, tracheal shaving, and facial reconstruction. Electrolysis or other hair-removal procedures may be sought. FTM-transgender individuals may seek chest reconstruction surgery, hysterectomy, oophorectomy, and genital reconstruction. Both MTF and FTM individuals may seek voice therapy and professional guidance in how to present themselves to the world as male or female through body language, gait, and mannerisms. Although these surgical, cosmetic, and other procedures often take place after adolescence, discussing these options or making appropriate referrals should be part of the PCP's anticipatory guidance of transgender youths.

PARENTS

Parents who come to recognize their child's gender-variant behavior may experience a variety of emotions: confusion, concern, fear, guilt, anger, and disgust. Many parents fear for their child's safety. Many of them fear that their child may eventually self-identify as lesbian or gay. In many instances these concerns and fears are not raised on visits to the PCP or are referred to only indirectly ("My son is a sensitive child," or "My daughter is definitely a tomboy"). The PCP should be sensitive to any cues of parental worry about gender variance and ask parents simply, "Do you have any concerns about your child's behaviors?" or more directly, "Have you had any concerns that your son's [daughter's] behaviors or interests are more feminine [masculine] than other children's his [her] age?" Most concerned parents, although perhaps embarrassed, are relieved to have such a discussion. The PCP's primary role in working with parents is to help them understand and accept their gender-variant child for who the child is and to ensure their child's safety.

Parents should be referred to Web sites, list serves, books, and brochures geared to parents of gender-variant children.[47] In addition to defining the meaning of gender variance, PCPs should discuss what is known about the possible causes of gender-variant behaviors, including genetic and environmental influences. They should explain that many, but not all, boys with gender-variant behaviors will grow up to recognize their homosexual orientation as adolescents or adults. Most, but not all, girls with gender-variant behaviors identify themselves as heterosexual or bisexual as they grow older. A small percentage of gender-variant children will continue to have a cross-gender identification into adolescence and adulthood and will identify themselves as transgender. They may eventually seek hormone therapy or surgery to make their biological gender more consistent with their inner gender identity. Parents should be informed that although gender-variant behavior may diminish as a result of social pressure when a child enters school at age 5 or 6 years, or as a result of parental pressure to conform, a child's core traits usually remain unchanged. Efforts to change a child's behavior to conform to stereotypic notions of appropriate behaviors for girls or boys should be avoided.

Box 140-1 lists ways parents can support their child, and Box 140-2 lists pitfalls parents should try to avoid.

BOX 140-1 Children's National Medical Center Outreach Program Guidelines for Parents of Gender-variant and Transgender Youth

Love their child for who the child is. Love, acceptance, understanding, and support are especially important when peers and society are often intolerant of difference.

Question traditional assumptions about gender roles and sexual orientation. Do not allow societal expectations to come between them and their child.

Create a safe space for their child, allowing the child always to be who the child is, especially in the child's own home.

Seek out socially accepted activities (sports, arts, hobbies) that respect their child's interests while helping the child fit in socially.

Validate their child and the child's interests, supporting the idea that more than one way exists to be a girl or boy. Speak openly and calmly about gender variance with their child. Talk about these subjects in positive terms, and listen as their child expresses feelings of being different.

Seek out supportive resources (books, videos, Web sites, support groups) for parents, families, and children.

Talk about gender variance with other significant people in their child's life, including siblings, extended family members, baby sitters, and family friends.

Prepare their child to deal with bullying. Let the child know that the child does not deserve to be hurt. Be aware of behaviors that suggest that bullying may be occurring, such as school refusal, crying excessively, or complaining of aches and pains.

Be their child's advocate. Expect and insist on acceptance, respect, and safety wherever their child is. Parents may need to educate school staff and others about the special experience and needs of gender-variant children.

Recognizing that a child has gender-variant behaviors and may one day self-identify as lesbian, gay, or bisexual is difficult for most parents. Learning that a person's daughter or son is transgender is usually extremely challenging. With the protection, acceptance, and love of parents, and with the reassurance and support of PCPs, transgender adolescents should look forward to happy, healthy, and fulfilling adult lives.

ADVOCACY

Because of their expertise and position of respect, PCPs are in an advantageous position to advocate on behalf of children with gender-variant behaviors, transgender youths, and their families. PCPs should encourage parents, siblings, and extended family to accept and love these young people unconditionally. The PCP should also be willing to meet with school personnel, child and youth welfare program staff, church groups, and others to share information about gender variance and transgenderism. For PCPs seeking to advocate for societal change, encouraging the development and implementation of policies, procedures, and programs that recognize and respect the individuality of these children and youth and address their special needs for nurturance and safety is important. The PCP may also provide testimony at official meetings and hearings on proposals to add gender identity and expression to laws and school policies prohibiting discrimination and harassment. The PCP may also advocate for the inclusion of meaningful medical school, residency training, and continuing education curricula on the life experience and health needs of children with gender-variant behaviors and transgender individuals and how to meet these needs in a respectful and effective manner. Finally, the PCP should encourage professional organizations to develop policy statements and clinical guidelines to support them in their work with these young people and their families.

BOX 140-2 Children's National Medical Center Pitfalls to Avoid as Parents of Gender-variant and Transgender Youth

Avoid finding fault. No blame exists. Their child's gender variance came from within, not from them as parents. Blame will get in the way of enjoying their child.

Do not pressure their child to change, because this will cause much pain and harm.

Do not blame the victim.

Do not accept bullying as *just the way things are.* No one has the right to torment or criticize others because they are different.

WHEN TO REFER

- When an adolescent has acute or recurrent suicidal ideation
- When an adolescent is engaged in multiple high-risk behaviors
- When the PCP believes that time, expertise, or comfort is insufficient to provide care and counseling to gender-variant children and transgender youths
- Referral should be made only to health care providers and counselors who have experience in working with gender-variant children and transgender youths and who accept gender variance as normal. Referrals for therapy to change a child's or adolescent's gender expression or gender identity are unethical and potentially harmful.

TOOLS FOR PRACTICE

Community Advocacy and Coordination

- *TransYouth Family Advocates* (Web page), TransYouth Family Advocates (imatyfa.org).

Engaging Patient and Family

- *If You Are Concerned About Your Child's Gender Behaviors: A Parent Guide* (booklet), Children's National Medical Center: Outreach Program for Children with Gender-Variant Behaviors and Their Families (www.dcchildrens.com/dcchildrens/about/subclinical/subneuroscience/subgender/guide.aspx).
- *I Think I Might Be Transgender, Now What Do I Do?* (booklet), Youth Resource (www.advocatesforyouth.org/youth/health/pamphlets/transgender.pdf).

Medical Decision Support

- *Guidelines for the Care of Lesbian, Gay, Bisexual, and Transgender Patients* (guideline), Gay and Lesbian Medical Association (ce54.citysoft.com/_data/n_0001/resources/live/GLMA guidelines 2006 FINAL.pdf).

RELATED WEB SITES

- Centers for Disease Control and Prevention: Transgender Persons (www.cdc.gov/lgbthealth/transgender.htm).
- Gay and Lesbian Medical Association (www.glma.org).
- Gay, Lesbian, and Straight Educational Network (GLSEN). Available at: www.glsen.org/. Accessed July 5, 2007.
- Parents, Families, and Friends of Lesbians and Gays (PFLAG) Transgender Network. Available at: www.pflag.org/tnet.tnet.0.html/. Accessed July 5, 2007.
- PFLAG Transgender Network (www.pflag.org/PFLAG_s_Transgender_Network.tnet.0.html).
- TransYouth Family Advocates. Available at: www.imatyfa.org/. Accessed July 5, 2007.
- World Professional Association for Transgender Health (www.wpath.org).
- World Professional Association for Transgender Health (WPATH). Available at: www.wpath.org/. Accessed July 5, 2007.
- Youth Resource (www.youthresource.com/).

AAP POLICY STATEMENT

Frankowski BL, American Academy of Pediatrics, Committee on Adolescence. Sexual orientation and adolescents. *Pediatrics*. 2004;113(6):1827-1921. (aappolicy.aappublications.org/cgi/content/full/pediatrics;113/6/1921).

SUGGESTED RESOURCES

Children's National Medical Center Outreach Program for Children With Gender-Variant Behaviors and Their Families. *If You Are Concerned About Your Child's Gender Behaviors: A Guide for Parents*. Washington, DC: Children's National Medical Center; 2003. Available at: www.childrensnational.org/DepartmentsandPrograms. Accessed February 29, 2008.

REFERENCES

1. Peletz MG. Transgenderism and gender pluralism in Southeast Asia since early modern times. *Curr Anthropol*. 2006;47:309-340.
2. Lang S. Lesbians, men-women, and two-spirits: homosexuality and gender in Native American cultures. In: Blackwood E, Wieringa S, eds. *Female Desires: Same-Sex Relations and Transgender Practices Across Cultures*. New York, NY: Columbia University Press; 1999.
3. Nanda S. Hijras: an alternative sex and gender role in India. In: Herdt G, ed. *Third Sex, Third Gender*. New York, NY: Zone Books; 1993.
4. Matzner A. *'O Au No Kea: Voices from Hawai'i's Mahu and Transgender Communities*. Philadelphia, PA: Xlibris; 2001.
5. Frankowski BL, American Academy of Pediatrics, Committee on Adolescence. Sexual orientation and adolescents. *Pediatrics*. 2004;113:1827-1832.
6. Sandberg DE, Meyer-Bahlburg HFL, Ehrhardt AA, et al. The prevalence of gender-atypical behavior in elementary school children. *J Am Acad Child Adolesc Psychiatry*. 1993;32:306-314.
7. Achenbach TM, Edelbrock C. *Manual for the Child Behavior Checklist and Revised Child Behavior Profile*. Burlington, VT: University of Vermont Department of Psychiatry; 1983.
8. Bakker A, van Kesteren PJM, Gooren LJG, et al. The prevalence of transsexualism in the Netherlands. *Acta Psychiatr Scand*. 1993;87:237-238.
9. Mallon GP, DeCrescenzo T. Transgender children and youth: a child welfare practice perspective. *Child Welfare*. 2006;85:215-241.
10. Richardson J. Response: finding the disorder in gender identity disorder. *Harvard Rev Psychiatry*. 1999;7:43-50.
11. Zucker KJ, Spitzer RL. Was the gender identity disorder of childhood diagnosis introduced into DSM-III as backdoor maneuver to replace homosexuality? A historical note. *J Sex Marital Ther*. 2005;31:31-42.
12. Zucker KJ. Gender identity development and issues. *Child Adolesc Psychiatr Clin North Am*. 2004;13:551-568.
13. Pleak R. Ethical issues in diagnosing and treating gender-dysphoric children and adolescents. In: Rottnek M, ed. *Sissies and Tomboys: Gender Nonconformity and Homosexual Childhood*. New York, NY: New York University Press; 1999.
14. American Psychiatric Association. *Diagnostic and Statistical Manual of Mental Disorders (DSM-IV)*. 4th ed. Washington, DC: American Psychiatric Association; 2000.
15. Zucker KJ. Gender identity disorders. In: Lewis M, ed. *Child and Adolescent Psychiatry: A Comprehensive Textbook*. Philadelphia, PA: Lippincott Williams & Wilkins; 2002.
16. Menvielle EJ. Gender identity disorder [letter to the editor]. *J Am Acad Child Adolesc Psychiatry*. 1998;37:243-245.
17. Menvielle EJ, Tuerk C. A support group for parents of gender-nonconforming boys. *J Am Acad Child Adolesc Psychiatry*. 2002;41:1010-1013.
18. Rosenberg M. Children with gender identity issues and their parents in individual and group treatment. *J Am Acad Child Adolesc Psychiatry*. 2002;41:619-621.
19. Children's National Medical Center. *If You Are Concerned About Your Child's Gender Behaviors: A Guide for Parents*. Washington, DC: Children's National Medical Center. 2003.
20. Bem SL. *The Lenses of Gender: Transforming the Debate on Sexual Inequality*. New Haven, CT: Yale University Press; 1993.
21. DeCrescenzo T, Mallon GP. *Serving Transgender Youth: The Role of Child Welfare Systems*. Arlington, VA: Child Welfare League of America; 2002.
22. Woronoff R, Estrada R, Sommer S. *Out of the Margins: A Report on Regional Listening Forums Highlighting the Experience of Lesbian, Gay, Bisexual, Transgender, and Questioning Youth in Care*. Washington, DC: Child Welfare League of America Inc, and New York, NY: Lambda Legal Defense and Education Fund Inc; 2006.
23. Wilber S, Ryan C, Marksamer J. *CWLA Best Practices Guidelines for Serving LGBT Youth in Out-of-Home Care*. Washington, DC: CWLA Press; 2006.

24. National Gay and Lesbian Task Force Policy Institute, National Coalition for the Homeless. *Lesbian, Gay, Bisexual, and Transgender Youth: An Epidemic of Homelessness*. 2007. Available at: www.thetaskforce.org/downloads/homelessyouth.pdf/. Accessed June 20, 2007.
25. Kosciw JG. *The 2003 National School Climate Survey: The School-related Experiences of Our Nation's Lesbian, Gay, Bisexual, and Transgender Youth*. New York, NY: Gay, Lesbian, and Straight Education Network; 2003.
26. California Safe Schools Coalition, 4-H Center for Youth Development, University of California, Davis. *Safe Place to Learn: Consequences of Harassment Based on Actual or Perceived Sexual Orientation and Gender Non-Conformity and Steps for Making Schools Safer*. 2004. Available at: www.casafeschools.org/20040112.html. Accessed June 16, 2007.
27. Ryan C, Rivers I. Lesbian, gay, bisexual and transgender youth: victimization and its correlates in the USA and UK. *Cult Health Sex*. 2003;5:103-119.
28. Sausa LA. Translating research into practice: trans youth recommendations for improving school systems. *J Gay Lesbian Issues Educ*. 2005;3:15-28.
29. Cohen-Kettenis PT, Owen A, Kaijser VG, et al. Demographic characteristics, social competence, and behavior problems in children with gender identity disorder: a cross-national, cross-clinic comparative analysis. *J Abnormal Child Psychol*. 2003;31:41-53.
30. Garofalo R, Deleon J, Osmer E, et al. Overlooked, misunderstood and at-risk: exploring the lives and HIV risk of ethnic minority male-to-female transgender youth. *J Adolesc Health*. 2006;38:230-236.
31. Nemoto T, Operano D, Keatley J, et al. HIV risk behaviors among male-to-female transgender persons of color in San Francisco. *Am J Public Health*. 2004;94:1193-1199.
32. Clements-Nolle K, Marx R, Katz M. Attempted suicide among transgender persons: the influence of gender-based discrimination and victimization. *J Homosex*. 2006;51:53-69.
33. American Academy of Family Practice. Discrimination: Family Practice Residency Guidelines. Available at: www.aafp.org/online/en/home/policy/policies/d/discrimination2.html. Accessed May 28, 2007.
34. American Academy of Family Practice. Adolescent Health Care. Available at: www.aafp.org/online/en/home/policy/policies/a/adol3.html. Accessed May 28, 2007.
35. Gay and Lesbian Medical Association. Guidelines for the Care of Lesbian, Gay, Bisexual, and Transgender Patients. 2006. Available at: ce54.citysoft.com. Accessed May 28, 2007.
36. Kaiser Permanente National Diversity Council, Kaiser Permanente National Diversity Department. *A Provider's Handbook on Culturally Competent Care: Lesbian, Gay, Bisexual, and Transgendered Population*. 2nd ed. Oakland, CA: Kaiser Permanente; 2004.
37. Dean L, Meyer IH, Robinson K, et al. Lesbian, gay, bisexual, and transgender health: findings and concerns. *J Gay Lesbian Med Assoc*. 2000;4:101-151.
38. Lev AI. *Transgender Emergence: Guidelines for Working With Gender-Variant People and Their Families*. Binghamton, NY: Haworth Clinical Practice Press; 2004.
39. Goldenring JM, Rosen DS. Getting into adolescents' heads: an essential update. *Contemp Pediatr*. 2004;21:64-90.
40. de Vries ALC, Cohen-Kettenis PT, Delemarre-Van de Waal H, et al. *Caring for Transgender Adolescents in BC: Suggested Guidelines*. Vancouver, BC: Transcend Transgender Support & Education Society and Vancouver Coastal Health's Transgender Health Program; 2006.
41. Tom Waddell Health Care Center. Tom Waddell Health Center Protocols for Hormonal Reassignment of Gender, 2006. Available at: www.sfdph.org/dph/default.asp. Accessed June 21, 2007.
42. Advocates for Youth. *I Think I Might Be Transgender, Now What Do I Do?* Washington, DC: Advocates for Youth; 2004. Available at: www.advocatesforyouth.org/. Accessed June 20, 2007.
43. Harry Benjamin International Gender Dysphoria Association. Standards of Care for Gender Identity Disorders, 2001. Available at: www.wpath.org/. Accessed June 20, 2007.
44. Smith YLS, van Goozen SHM, Kuiper AJ, et al. Sex reassignment: outcomes and predictors of treatment for adolescents and adult transsexuals. *Psychological Med*. 2005;35:89-99.
45. Delamarre-van de Waal HA, Cohen-Kettenis PT. Clinical management of gender identity disorder in adolescents: a protocol on psychological and paediatric endocrinology aspects. *Eur J Endocrinol*. 2006;155:S131-S137.
46. van Kesteren PJM, Asscheman H, Megens JAJ, et al. Mortality and morbidity in transsexual subjects treated with cross-sex hormones. *Clin Endocrinol*. 1997;47:337-342.
47. Parents, Families, and Friends of Lesbians and Gays Transgender Special Outreach Network. *Our Trans Children*. 3rd ed. Washington, DC: Parents, Families, and Friends of Lesbians and Gays; 2001.

Chapter 141

SUBSTANCE USE DISORDERS: EVALUATION AND MANAGEMENT

Susan M. Coupey, MD; Sara Buchdahl Levine, MD, MPH

Pediatricians caring for adolescents are often faced with issues of substance use and abuse. Identifying substance use, assessing its effect on the patient's overall health, and planning appropriate interventions when indicated are important tasks for the primary care physician (PCP).[1] The PCP is well served by an understanding of substance-use patterns and prevalence, skills for screening and evaluation, and the ability to recognize both acute intoxication and abstinence syndromes.

Substance use and abuse continue to threaten the well being of adolescents and young adults. Sporadic substance use contributes to accidents and unintentional trauma and plays a significant role in the major causes of adolescent mortality: motor-vehicle injuries, homicide, and suicide. Substance use is also related to behavioral choices that carry significant risk, such as unprotected or unwanted sexual activity. Frequent or long-term use is associated with impairments of health and daily functioning. Screening for substance use should be a routine component of adolescent health care, and anticipatory guidance should be provided to both patients and families, with the goal of minimizing substance-related morbidity and mortality.

PREVALENCE OF SUBSTANCE ABUSE

The use of alcohol, tobacco, and other drugs by adolescents in the United States has been monitored for decades, and surveys such as the University of Michigan's *Monitoring the Future* and the Centers for Disease Control and Prevention's *Youth Risk Behavior Surveillance* allow identification of trends over time. Patterns of substance use evolve and change in response to fluctuating popularity and perceived harm. The mid-1990s showed a peak in adolescent use of most illicit drugs, including marijuana, cocaine, amphetamines, inhalants, and hallucinogens. Since that time a gradual decline has occurred in the use of marijuana and other illicit drugs; however, a sharp increase in the use of ecstasy and other *designer* or *club* drugs was noted in 2000.[2]

Alcohol, cigarettes, and marijuana are the drugs most commonly used by adolescents. The 2007 *Monitoring the Future* survey found that nearly three quarters of high school seniors had used alcohol, 46% had smoked cigarettes, and 42% had used marijuana. Though use was less common among younger students, 40% of 8th graders had used alcohol, 22% had smoked cigarettes, and 14% had used marijuana (Figure 141-1). The prevalence of current drug use among high school students is also impressive. Among 12th graders, 44% reported alcohol use, 22% reported cigarette use, and 19% reported marijuana use in the previous 30 days.[2]

High school students also report a significant amount of other illicit drug use. In 2007, 26% of 12th graders and 11% of 8th graders reported any use of illicit drugs other than marijuana. The most commonly used substances were inhalants (particularly by younger students), hallucinogens, cocaine, amphetamines, narcotics, sedatives, and tranquilizers.[2]

Though all of the substances used and abused by adolescents may be associated with episodic illnesses and emergencies, teenagers using these agents most often are encountered when they seek routine health maintenance or care for an illness unrelated to drugs. Only through routine questioning is such drug use discovered (see Chapter 50, Substance Use Disorders: Early Identification and Referral). Even in the setting of a drug-related illness or acute intoxication, adolescents rarely seek care because of a particular drug habit or the impairment of a specific body organ, but rather they exhibit symptoms mandating medical attention. In this respect, adolescents are similar to all other patients; determining the etiological factors and the pathological conditions of their illnesses requires a comprehensive analysis of all possibilities. If drug abuse, of either one or several agents, is not considered along with other possible etiological factors to explain the symptoms, then the physician may miss an opportunity for meaningful therapeutic intervention.

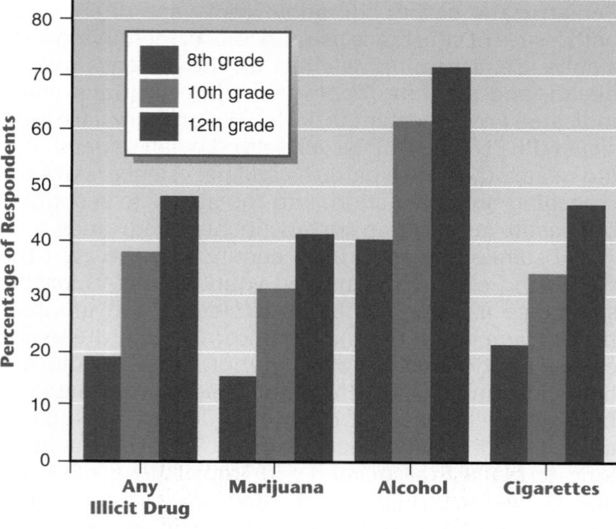

Figure 141-1 Prevalence of lifetime substance use among US students reported by grade level. *(Johnston LD, O'Malley PM, Bachman JG, et al.* Monitoring the Future: National results on adolescent drug use: Overview of key findings, 2007. *(NIH Publication No. 08-6418). Bethesda, MD: National Institute on Drug Abuse; 2008.*

MEDICAL HISTORY AND ANTICIPATORY GUIDANCE

During each health-supervision visit with an adolescent or preadolescent patient, pediatricians should assess drug involvement. Such inquiries should be a natural adjunct to the assessment of other psychosocial indicators, including family and peer relationships, academic progress, recreational activities, and sexual behavior, captured by a complete psychosocial history represented by the acronym *HEADSSS* (**h**ome, **e**ducation, **a**ctivities, **d**rugs, **s**afety, **s**exuality, **s**uicide or depression). An accurate substance use history can be obtained only in an atmosphere of confidentiality and privacy, with parents excluded from the interview. Information should be obtained about not only the specific type of drug used, but also the frequency of use, the setting in which use occurs, and the degree of social, educational, and vocational disruption attributable to the drug use behavior.

Simple screening tools are available to help the pediatrician assess a patient's substance use. The *CRAFFT* screening tool (Box 141-1) has been validated

BOX 141-1 CRAFFT Screening Tool

C—Have you ever ridden in a *car* driven by someone (including yourself) who was high or had been using alcohol or other drugs?

R—Do you ever use alcohol or drugs to *relax*, feel better about yourself, or fit in?

A—Do you ever use alcohol or drugs while you are by yourself *(alone)*?

F—Do you ever *forget* things you did while using alcohol or drugs?

F—Do your *family* or *friends* ever tell you that you should cut down on your drinking or drug use?

T—Have you ever gotten into *trouble* while you were using alcohol or drugs?

From Knight JR, Shrier LA, Bravender TD, et al. A new brief screen for adolescent substance abuse. Arch Pediatr Adolesc Med 1999;153(6):591-596. Reprinted by permission of the American Medical Association.

for adolescents and consists of 6 items aimed at identifying specific adolescents with problematic substance use. Positive answers to 2 or more items suggest that intervention is necessary.[3] (See Chapter 50 for more information on screening for substance abuse.)

All teenagers, including those who do not drink or use drugs at all, need to be counseled about the relationship between intoxicants and injuries, the leading cause of death among adolescents. The majority of these fatal injuries are vehicle related, and substance use is implicated in many, if not most, of these injuries. Adolescents should also be counseled regarding the connections among substance use, intoxication, and unprotected or unwanted sexual activity.

COUNSELING ABOUT COMMONLY USED SUBSTANCES

Alcohol

The prevalence of drinking among youth has been declining for several years, though measures of self-reported *drunkenness* have not changed as much. Data from 2007 demonstrate that of the nearly three quarters of high school seniors who had ever used alcohol, 55% had been drunk, and 22% had been drunk in the previous 30 days. The numbers are lower for 8th graders; but even among these young students, 18% report having ever been drunk, and 5.5% report being drunk in the previous 30 days.[2] Episodic heavy drinking, or binge drinking, is a particular problem for many high school and college students. Twenty-six percent of 12th graders and 10% of 8th graders reported consuming 5 or more drinks in a row on at least 1 occasion in the prior 2 weeks.[2] Teenage binge drinkers are at especially high risk for injuries and for significant developmental, educational, and emotional difficulties.

Marijuana

Prevalence of marijuana use increased dramatically during the 1990s, reaching a peak in 1996. Since 2002, use among high school students has been declining, though the declines have not necessarily reached statistical significance each year. In 2007, 42% of 12th graders, 31% of 10th graders, and 14% of 8th graders reported ever having used marijuana. Current use (the prior 30 days) was reported by 19%, 14%, and 6% of 12th, 10th, and 6th graders, respectively.[2] Though marijuana's role as a gateway drug has been debated, studies have shown that youth who use marijuana are more likely than their nonusing peers to use other illicit substances.[4] Therefore even casual use of marijuana should be noted by the pediatrician and, at a minimum, monitored over time.

Although the intoxicating effects of alcohol and the importance of its role in causing motor-vehicle injuries are well known, the effects of marijuana *(Cannabis)*, the active ingredient of which is tetrahydrocannabinol, are understood less widely. The drug is a euphoriant and most often produces feelings of relaxation and enhanced well being, with behavioral effects mediated by specific cannabinoid receptors in the brain and interaction with other neurochemical systems. Similar to other drugs that have addictive potential, such as heroin and nicotine, tetrahydrocannabinol has been shown in experiments with rats to result in a release of dopamine in the brain's *reward* pathway in the nucleus accumbens, and long-term administration alters the limbic system in the brain similarly to other drugs of abuse.[5]

In addition to euphoria, the marijuana *high* causes a loss of critical judgment, distortions in time perception, impairment of tracking (the ability to follow a moving object accurately), and poor performance on *divided-attention* tasks, such as driving. The infrequent correlation between marijuana intoxication and mishaps may be because users show no specific signs of drug abuse and authorities lack a quick, convenient method to detect marijuana. Other behavioral effects include impaired short-term memory, interference with learning, and difficulty with oral communication, all of which can affect school performance adversely. Occasionally, a physician will encounter a patient who has an acute adverse reaction to marijuana characterized by a toxic psychosis with depression or panic. Both the symptoms and the treatment of these reactions are similar to those for hallucinogen abuse. Prolonged (and possibly permanent) personality changes have been reported in long-term marijuana users. This amotivational syndrome is marked by lethargy and a lack of goal-directed activity.[6,7]

Physiological effects do occur with marijuana use but are generally less worrisome than the behavioral effects of the drug. Respiratory effects with more prolonged exposure include bronchodilation with acute inhalation and subsequent chronic intermittent bronchoconstriction. Thus adolescents who have asthma may experience either relief or exacerbation of symptoms. Allergic reactions to marijuana do occur and may cause asthmatic attacks. Furthermore, chronic marijuana use has been found to cause exercise-induced dyspnea and chronic cough that may be mistaken for new-onset asthma in an adolescent.[8,9] Cardiovascular effects include both tachycardia and a transient low-grade elevation of systolic and diastolic blood pressure. Neither of these cardiac consequences is clinically significant. Marijuana has been reported to have numerous effects on the endocrine system in boys and men who have histories of prolonged and frequent use, including depression of testosterone levels in the blood, diminished sperm counts, impaired sexual function, and gynecomastia. The associated clinical problems of impotence and infertility should respond to abstinence from marijuana.

Other Drugs of Abuse and Designer Drugs

Increasing attention is being paid to less commonly used substances that are playing a larger role in adolescent substance use. Among these substances are anabolic steroids and other *performance-enhancing* drugs, *club drugs* such as ecstasy and Rohypnol®, and misuse of prescription drugs such as oxycodone.

Steroids and other performance-enhancing drugs are receiving increased attention in both professional athletics and college and high school competition. Adolescents are faced with an understandable drive for success that may be exacerbated by normal developmental feelings of invulnerability. The use of substances, both pharmacologic and *nutritional* that help a person control weight (either increase or decrease), improve stamina, or mask the effects or detection of other substances used to improve performance in athletics, carries many risks for the adolescent patient. The American Academy of Pediatrics (AAP) policy statement regarding the use of such substances stresses the role of the pediatrician in educating patients and parents about the risks of such substance use and recommends a system that provides positive reinforcement of healthy decisions rather than a simply punitive detection practice.[10]

Club drugs such as ecstasy, Rohypnol (also known as the *date-rape drug*), gamma-hydroxybutyrate, and ketamine (also known as *special K*) have also entered the adolescent drug scene. These drugs share the common desired effects of disinhibition, altered states of consciousness, and, often, increased energy or euphoria.[7,11] Many of these drugs were introduced as part of *rave* culture, being used by young people attending all-night, traditionally alcohol-free, dance parties.[11] However, when combined with other substance use, particularly alcohol, use of these drugs may be fatal. Although national data for use of several of these specific drugs are lacking, lifetime ecstasy use was reported by 6.5% of 12th graders and 2.3% of 8th graders in 2007.[2]

Signs of 3,4-methylenedioxymethamphetamine (MDMA, or *ecstasy*) toxicity include sympathetic overactivity, disturbed behavior, and increased temperature. Serious complications such as delirium, seizures, and coma are more common when MDMA is used in combination with other substances, especially other stimulants. Rhabdomyolysis and acute renal failure have been reported with MDMA use by adolescents who use the drug in the setting of prolonged physical activity such as raves. Gamma-hydroxybutyrate, ketamine, and Rohypnol are all associated with disinhibition and varying levels of relaxation. Adverse effects include nausea, respiratory depression, delirium or delusions, and, potentially, coma. All of these effects are potentiated by alcohol, benzodiazepines, and other drugs.

Misuse and abuse of prescription drugs by adolescents has also been receiving increasing attention both in the lay media and in the medical community. According to data from the 2007 *Monitoring the Future* study, in the previous year, 10% of 12th graders had used Vicodin, and 5% had used OxyContin without a prescription.[2] Abuse of prescription drugs poses significant health risks for adolescents and can lead to high levels of addiction and dysfunction.

PHYSICAL EXAMINATION

The medical complications of chronic substance use, although sometimes severe, usually do not appear until after adolescence. Acute intoxication is typically encountered by the emergency department physician rather than the primary care pediatrician. Findings particular to various drugs are summarized in Box 141-2. Some physical findings may be more subtle manifestations of chronic drug use, such as gynecomastia in heavy marijuana users. Young women abusing opiates may develop secondary amenorrhea secondary to anovulation.

BOX 141-2 Physical Findings Potentially Indicating Substance Use and Abuse

GENERAL APPEARANCE

Altered mood
Poor dress or hygiene
Inappropriate or strange behavior

VITAL SIGNS

Weight loss
Hypertension (cocaine, amphetamine)
Hypotension (heroin)
Hyperthermia (cocaine, amphetamine, ecstasy)
Hypothermia (heroin)
Tachycardia (marijuana, cocaine, amphetamine)

EAR, NOSE, THROAT

Conjunctival injection (marijuana, inhalants)
Dilated pupils (cocaine, amphetamine)
Constricted pupils (heroin, morphine, other opiates)
Sluggish pupillary response (barbiturates)
Nasal irritation

CARDIAC

Arrhythmias (heroin, cocaine, amphetamine)

CHEST

Gynecomastia (marijuana, anabolic steroids)

ABDOMEN

Hepatomegaly

GENITOURINARY

Testicular atrophy (anabolic steroids)
Clitoromegaly (anabolic steroids)

SKIN

Acne (anabolic steroids)
Abscesses (intravenous use, or *skin popping*)
Hirsutism (anabolic steroids)
Tattoos
Needle track marks
Jaundice

NEUROLOGIC

Altered sensorium
Poor coordination
Ataxia (alcohol, barbiturates)
Nystagmus (barbiturates)
Hyporeflexia or hyperreflexia (marijuana, cocaine, amphetamine)

From Duffy A, Millin R. Case study: withdrawal syndrome in adolescent chronic cannabis users. *J Am Acad Child Adolesc Psychiatry.* 1996;35:1618-1621. Reprinted by permission of Lippincott Williams & Wilkins.

Less-specific physical complaints frequently accompany substance use. Frequent alcohol users may complain of abdominal pain and can even develop gastritis, ulcers, and pancreatitis. Constipation is common among chronic opiate users. Users of inhalational drugs may complain of chronic cough, nasal irritation, and rhinorrhea. Jaundice may accompany hepatitis secondary to the use of inhalants (acute toxic hepatitis), anabolic steroids (cholestatic hepatitis), or ecstasy (fulminant hepatic failure).

LABORATORY TESTING

Laboratory tests for blood or urine drug levels in the context of substance use and abuse should be used only as an adjunct to the history and physical examination. Obviously, toxicologic screens may be indicated in the acute setting of an adolescent with altered mental status. However, the use of screening tests in asymptomatic patients has less utility and has many associated ethical and legal concerns. The AAP 1996 statement on testing for drugs of abuse in children and adolescents addresses many of the issues surrounding consent and notification. Generally, the older competent adolescent should be tested only with the patient's explicit consent and after a discussion of the reasons for testing and the possible outcomes.[12]

If laboratory testing for drugs of abuse is pursued, then the pediatrician should be familiar with various screening panels and diagnostic tests used to confirm positive screens. Pediatricians should also be familiar with the sensitivity and specificity of the various tests so as to interpret potential false-positive or false-negative results. False positives are generally the result of cross-reactivity with other substances, including foods or over-the-counter medications, and false negatives may be the result of pharmacokinetics and length of time since last use or deliberate alterations of the testing substrate (substitution or dilution of urine, for example). At any rate, testing can only provide information about a given moment in time and does not necessarily contribute to the evaluation of chronic use or dysfunction.[13]

ABSTINENCE SYNDROMES

Although acute intoxication is generally obvious, and even chronic signs of substance use and abuse can be easily recognized by the clinician who maintains a high degree of suspicion, abstinence syndromes and withdrawal may produce more subtle signs and symptoms, often mimicking a viral illness. Withdrawal from significant abuse habits can be uncomfortable and even dangerous. Adolescents may voluntarily stop using drugs, or withdrawal may be precipitated by circumstances outside of the teenager's control by life events such as moving, changing schools, or even hospitalization. In either case, efforts should be made to minimize the associated withdrawal symptoms and provide reinforcement of abstinence.

In many instances, adolescents do not reach levels of alcohol use that would precipitate acute withdrawal or abstinence syndromes. Regular heavy drinking can, however, lead to physical dependence, resulting in withdrawal syndromes of varying severity, most commonly associated with nausea, vomiting, insomnia, autonomic hyperactivity, and a mild confusional state. If found to be in acute alcohol withdrawal, then teenagers may require hospitalization and management with benzodiazepines.

Nicotine withdrawal is not uncommon among daily cigarette smokers and may be seen in the context of acute hospitalization. Nicotine withdrawal is characterized by irritability, restlessness, increased appetite, anxiety, impatience, digestive problems and nausea, palpitations, headaches, and tobacco cravings. Replacement therapy can mitigate many of these symptoms and may be useful during hospitalizations of adolescents with significant tobacco use habits.

Often exhibiting more subtly and frequently overlooked are the clinical symptoms produced by *Cannabis* withdrawal. Marijuana produces pharmacologic tolerance after several days of regular use and addiction after long-term daily use. A clinical withdrawal syndrome begins within 24 to 48 hours of discontinuing the drug. Withdrawal symptoms peak in intensity by the 4th day and gradually resolve by 10 to 14 days. The *Cannabis* abstinence syndrome is characterized by an influenza-like illness. Adolescents who are heavy *Cannabis* users report withdrawal symptoms including malaise, irritability, agitation, insomnia, drug craving, shakiness, diaphoresis, night sweats, and gastrointestinal disturbance. The most persistent symptoms appear to be insomnia and irritable mood and, to a lesser extent, drug cravings.[6]

Withdrawal syndromes from other drugs such as opiates, barbiturates, and stimulants can occur with varying levels of medical urgency. If a known user is hospitalized or for another reason voluntarily or involuntarily ceases to use the given substance, then the clinician must maintain a vigilant watch for signs and symptoms of abstinence syndromes and may decide to treat the patient preemptively to prevent the full-blown syndrome from developing.

MANAGEMENT OF THE ADOLESCENT WITH SUSPECTED SUBSTANCE ABUSE

The challenge continually posed to pediatricians is to recognize when a patient's substance use becomes significant enough to warrant referral to a treatment program or facility rather than being monitored in the primary care setting. An understanding of the definitions of *substance abuse* and *substance dependence* can be helpful in guiding treatment decisions.[13] The AAP statement regarding the management and referral of substance-abusing patients provides specific guidance as to when a patient requires intensive drug treatment, either as an outpatient or as an inpatient.[14] An important point to recognize is that resistance and denial are often key elements of substance use disorders and may be exhibited by both patients and parents. Although avoiding an adversarial relationship with the family can be difficult, appropriate medical treatment and referrals must be recommended.

SUMMARY

Whether the adolescent voluntarily comes for treatment for a drug abuse problem, is compelled to seek medical attention because of a drug- or alcohol-related illness, or is discovered to be using drugs or alcohol during a routine evaluation, the primary care physician is in a position to provide education, guidance, and treatment. State and federal guidelines allow for confidentiality in drug abuse treatment of minors, and the physician who uses a nonjudgmental, empathetic approach to these teenagers may be able to establish trust and thereby gather sufficient information to make a knowledgeable decision as to the need for further intervention. Such information must include not only the history of past and present drug or alcohol abuse, but also the nature of peer and family relationships, the extent of involvement with law enforcement authorities, the degree of educational or vocational disruption, and the adolescent's own interpretation of the need for therapy.

The extent of substance abuse and related disruption is often minimal such that no further action beyond the counsel of the physician is required. Such counsel should address the potential somatic effects of the teenager's current drug practices, the potential for escalation of drug-taking behavior, and the risk of injuries and death from even occasional intoxication. At the other extreme are adolescents who have severe mental health disorders and who are in obvious need of psychiatric care.

Perceived limitations of time for adequate psychosocial evaluation, discomfort addressing sensitive issues, or lack of familiarity with available therapeutic resources often prevent practitioners from thoroughly and appropriately addressing substance use and abuse with adolescents. Occasionally, referrals may need to be made to other professionals or agencies that have expertise and interest in the field of adolescent drug and alcohol abuse. In this regard, substance abuse does not differ from other behavioral problems for which specific therapeutic interventions are beyond the primary care physician's professional scope. However, assessing adolescent substance use, determining the level of danger or dysfunction associated with an individual patient's use, and counseling and referring appropriately is well within the scope of primary care pediatricians' skill and responsibility. More often than not, sensitivity to these issues, attention to adolescents' risk behaviors in general, and periodic follow-up in the primary care setting are adequate to help keep adolescents safe and healthy.

TOOLS FOR PRACTICE

Engaging Patient and Family

- *Alcohol: Your Child and Drugs* (brochure), American Academy of Pediatrics (patiented.aap.org).
- *Inhalant Abuse: Your Child and Drugs* (brochure), American Academy of Pediatrics (patiented.aap.org).
- *National Institute on Drug Abuse Information for Parents and Teachers* (Web page), National Institute on Drug Abuse (www.drugabuse.gov/parent-teacher.html).
- *The Risks of Tobacco Use: A Message to Parents and Teens* (brochure), American Academy of Pediatrics (patiented.aap.org).
- *Steroids: Play Safe, Play Fair* (brochure), American Academy of Pediatrics (patiented.aap.org).
- *Substance Abuse: A Guide for Health Professionals* (book), American Academy of Pediatrics (www.aap.org/bookstore).
- *Substance Abuse Prevention: What Every Parent Needs To Know* (brochure), American Academy of Pediatrics (patiented.aap.org).
- *Testing Your Teen for Illicit Drugs: Information for Parents* (brochure), American Academy of Pediatrics (patiented.aap.org).
- *Tobacco: Straight Talk for Teens* (brochure), American Academy of Pediatrics (patiented.aap.org).

Medical Decision Support

- *CRAFFT: A Brief Screening Test for Adolescent Substance Abuse* (questionnaire), John Knight and Boston Children's Hospital (www.ceasar-boston.org/clinicians/crafft.php).
- *Monitoring the Future National Results in Adolescent Drug Use: Overview of key findings, 2006* (book), National Institute on Drug Abuse (www.monitoringthefuture.org/pubs/monographs/overview2006.pdf).
- *National Institute on Drug Abuse Information for Medical and Health Professionals* (Web page), National Institute on Drug Abuse (www.drugabuse.gov/medstaff.html).
- *Youth Risk Behavior Surveillance, United States—2005*, Centers for Disease Control and Prevention (www.cdc.gov/mmwr/PDF/SS/SS5505.pdf).

AAP POLICY STATEMENTS

American Academy of Pediatrics, Committee on Sports Medicine and Fitness. Use of performing-enhancing substances. *Pediatrics.* 2005;115(4):1103-1106. (aappolicy.aappublications.org/cgi/content/full/pediatrics;115/4/1103).

American Academy of Pediatrics, Committee on Substance Abuse. Indications for management and referral of patients involved in substance abuse. *Pediatrics.* 2000; 106(1):143-148. (aappolicy.aappublications.org/cgi/content/full/pediatrics;106/1/143).

American Academy of Pediatrics, Committee on Substance Abuse. Testing for drugs of abuse in children and adolescents. *Pediatrics.* 1996;98(2):305-307. (aappolicy.aappublications.org/cgi/content/abstract/pediatrics;98/2/305).

Kulig JW, American Academy of Pediatrics, Committee on Substance Abuse. Tobacco, alcohol, and other drugs: the role of the pediatrician in prevention, identification, and management of substance abuse. *Pediatrics.* 2005; 115(3):816-821. (aappolicy.aappublications.org/cgi/content/full/pediatrics;115/3/816).

REFERENCES

1. American Academy of Pediatrics, Kulig JW, Committee on Substance Use. Tobacco, alcohol, and other drugs: the role of the pediatrician in prevention, identification, and management of substance abuse. *Pediatrics.* 2005;115: 816-821.
2. Johnston LD, O'Malley PM, Bachman JG, et al. *Monitoring the Future—Illicit Drug Use by American Teens Continues Gradual Decline in 2007.* University of Michigan News Service: Ann Arbor, MI; 2007. Available at: www.monitoringthefuture.org; accessed March 21, 2008.
3. Knight JR, Shrier LA, Bravender TD, et al. A new brief screen for adolescent substance abuse. *Arch Pediatr Adolesc Med.* 1999;153:591-596.
4. Morral AR, McCaffrey DF, Paddock SM. Reassessing the marijuana gateway effect. *Addiction.* 2002;97:1493-1504.
5. Tanda G, Pontieri FE, Di Chiara G. Cannabinoid and heroin activation of mesolimbic dopamine transmission by a common μ1-opioid receptor mechanism. *Science.* 1997; 276:2048-2050.

6. Duffy A, Millin R. Case study: withdrawal syndrome in adolescent chronic Cannabis users. *J Am Acad Child Adolesc Psychiatry.* 1996;35:1618-1621.
7. Coupey SM. Specific drugs. In: Schydlower M, ed. *Substance Abuse: A Guide for Health Professionals,* 2nd ed. Elk Grove Village, IL: American Academy of Pediatrics; 2000.
8. Tashkin DRP. Airway effects of marijuana, cocaine, and other inhaled illicit agents. *Curr Opin Pulmon Med.* 2001;7:43-61.
9. Taylor DR, Poulton R, Moffitt TE, et al. The respiratory effects of Cannabis dependence in young adults. *Addiction.* 2000;95:1669-1677.
10. American Academy of Pediatrics, Committee on Sports Medicine and Fitness. Use of performing-enhancing substances. *Pediatrics.* 2005;115:1103-1106.
11. Rome ES. It's a rave new world: rave culture and illicit drug use in the young. *Cleveland Clin J Med.* 2001;68: 541-550.
12. American Academy of Pediatrics, Committee on Substance Abuse. Testing for drugs of abuse in children and adolescents. *Pediatrics.* 1996;98:305-307.
13. Kaul P, Coupey SM. Clinical evaluation of substance abuse. *Pediatr Rev.* 2002;23:85-93.
14. American Academy of Pediatrics, Committee on Substance Abuse. Indications for management and referral of patients involved in substance abuse. *Pediatrics.* 2000;106:143-148.

Chapter 142 ENCOPRESIS

Barton D. Schmitt, MD

DEFINITION

Encopresis (soiling) is the voluntary or involuntary passage of feces into the clothing. Most children who have encopresis leak fecal material involuntarily from an impaction (retentive encopresis). Some children simply pass normal movements into their underwear rather than use the toilet (nonretentive encopresis). Retentive and nonretentive encopresis should be separated because the treatment for each type is radically different. The minor fecal staining that occurs when children do not wipe themselves adequately after using the toilet should not be mistaken for encopresis.

PATHOPHYSIOLOGICAL FEATURES OF IMPACTION

To understand retentive encopresis, the pathophysiologic features of an impaction, which occurs when constipation has gone unrelieved for approximately a week, must also be understood. By then, the rectum is so distended with stool that the sacrospinal defecation reflex is no longer energized, and the mass is so wide that voluntary effort alone cannot force it through the anal canal. Hence an impaction is almost irreversible by natural events. The pressure of the impaction dilates the internal anal sphincter and makes it incompetent. Small amounts of the impaction are extruded intermittently through the external sphincter as a result of gravity, exercise, and relaxation.

INCIDENCE

Encopresis affects approximately 2% of kindergarten and 1st-grade students. The *Diagnostic and Statistical Manual of Mental Disorders,* 4th edition, inclusion criteria for encopresis require the child to be 4 years of age or older, although any child older than 3 years who is not toilet trained may be considered encopretic. Without professional advice for this age range, many parents mistreat encopresis with coercion or punishment, and the condition worsens.[1] Most children who have encopresis are brought in for examination by 5 years of age when their symptom interferes with school entry.[2] Affected boys outnumber affected girls by a ratio of 3:1.

DIFFERENTIAL DIAGNOSES

Retentive encopresis has an organic basis in fewer than 5% of encopretic children. Organic causes of constipation and retentive soiling often are noted on physical examination (Table 142-1). Most children hold back stool in an attempt to avoid the pain associated with passage or because they are enmeshed in a control issue with a parent.

Approximately 10% to 20% of children who are encopretic are not constipated. Frequently, preschoolers who are of this type are resisting bowel training deliberately. Most school-aged children who have this type are postponing bowel movements (BMs) *(waiting too long)* because they do not want to leave some enjoyable activity (eg, video games) or they do not want to use public toilets (eg, school bathrooms).

All encopretic children (of either type) eventually develop secondary emotional problems; encopresis takes a great toll in shame. The unpredictable nature of the symptom in retentive children causes constant fear of exposure. Many of these children are *scapegoated* at home, teased by peers, and ostracized at school.

EVALUATION

History

A thorough history usually distinguishes between retentive and nonretentive encopresis (Table 142-2). The clinician asks about size and consistency of stools and soiling intervals. In the retentive form, leakage occurs many times a day or even continuously. Commonly, the primary care physician elicits a history of periodic pain or crying with BMs, blood on the toilet tissue, passage of a huge BM that clogs the toilet, or posturing that suggests deliberate holding back. By contrast, the child who has nonretentive soiling passes a BM of normal size and consistency into the underwear once or twice a day; all symptoms of constipation are denied.

Other helpful parts of the history are diet and use of the toilet. The intake of milk products, fruit juice, and fiber should be recorded, as should information about sitting on the toilet: how many times per day and if sitting is spontaneous or prompted by parents or teachers. If the stool pattern is unknown, then sending the parent home with an encopresis diary to complete for the child can be most illuminating.

Table 142-1 Organic Causes of Constipation and Retentive Soiling

ENTITY	DIAGNOSTIC CLUE
Constipating medication	History positive
Constipating diet	History positive
Chronic anal fissure	Examination positive
Perianal cellulitis	Examination positive
Hypothyroidism	Linear growth delayed
Anal or rectal stenosis	Finger cannot enter rectum
Pelvic mass	Mass found on rectal examination (usually posteriorly)
Hirschsprung disease	Rectal ampulla repeatedly empty; rectum is tight

Table 142-2 Differentiation of Retentive Soiling From Nonretentive Soiling

	RETENTIVE SOILING	NONRETENTIVE SOILING
HISTORY		
Symptoms of constipation	Yes	No
Interval	Many times per day	Once per day
Size	Small	Normal
Consistency	Loose	Normal
Previous need for laxatives, suppositories, or enemas	Yes	No
EXAMINATION		
Abdominal mass	Yes	No
Abdominal distention	Often	No
Anal canal	Sometimes full	Empty
Rectum	Packed	Normal

Physical Examination

The physical examination provides definitive information. In retentive soiling, an abdominal mass is usually palpable. Although the mass sometimes extends throughout the entire colon, it more commonly involves only the rectosigmoid area. The mass is midline, suprapubic, irregular, and moveable. The mass can be missed if the rectus abdominis muscles are not relaxed. The backup of gas and stool can cause a protuberant abdomen.

A rectal examination must be performed on every patient; it can be done with minimal pain and distress in most children. Overlooking this procedure can lead to an erroneous diagnosis. Inspection of the anal opening often reveals protruding fecal material in children who are deliberate stool holders. The rectum in all impacted children is dilated and packed with wall-to-wall stool (often 6-10 cm across). The consistency of the impaction more commonly is similar to wet clay, rather than hard. By contrast, the child who has nonretentive soiling has a normal abdominal examination, and the rectal vault contains either a stool of normal caliber or nothing if the child has evacuated recently.

Laboratory Studies

Children who are encopretic generally need no routine laboratory confirmation of this diagnosis. Because an impaction can cause partial bladder emptying and urine retention, a urinalysis for nitrite and pyuria may be helpful to screen for urinary tract infection, especially if any associated enuresis exists. Any abnormal perianal erythema should be cultured for group A *Streptococcus*. Occasionally, thyroid function tests are warranted.

Radiographic Findings

If the examiner cannot determine if the patient is impacted (eg, abdominal fullness but empty rectum), a plain film postvoiding, supine abdominal radiograph can be helpful. Other indications include sexually abused children who might be emotionally traumatized by a rectal examination and those who refuse a rectal examination. A child who is impacted will demonstrate on radiograph a rectum grossly dilated with granular stool and increased stool in the transverse and descending colon, which normally is empty.[2] A healthy child has granular stool in the ascending colon that is formed of normal diameter in the rectosigmoid area. A barium enema or rectosigmoid manometric study is indicated only if Hirschsprung disease is strongly suspected. Children who have retentive soiling and experience repeated treatment failures may occasionally warrant a barium enema to reassure the family (and physician) that some rare diagnosis has not been overlooked.

MANAGEMENT OF RETENTIVE ENCOPRESIS

In recent years, the treatment of constipation has become more uniform.[3-6] The need for chronic medications to allow the lower bowel adequate time to

BOX 142-1 Treatment of Retentive Encopresis

- Hyperphosphate enemas (one daily for 2 or 3 days) to remove impaction
- Mineral oil, polyethylene glycol, or lactulose for 3 months to keep the stools soft
- Senna laxatives if stool softeners are ineffective
- Sitting on the toilet for 10 minutes after meals
- Nonconstipating high-fiber diet

return to normal diameter and function has gained acceptance. Most children older than 5 years want to stay clean. However, they may not understand how to do so. Physicians should tell these children that they need to have a BM every day. They need to keep their rectum empty. Physicians should help them understand that holding back BMs is the main cause of leaking or messing their pants. (Box 142-1 outlines the treatment of encopresis.)

INITIAL DISIMPACTION

Unless the impaction is removed, the child will be unable to maintain any bowel control. The traditional way to remove an impaction is to give a daily sodium phosphate enema for 2 or 3 days. Warn the parents that phosphate enemas given in excessive doses can cause tetany, dehydration, or even death.[7] For children who refuse enemas, administering high-dose mineral oil or polyethylene glycol (Miralax) orally can also dislodge the impaction if the treatment is continued for approximately 4 days.[8,9] A combination of these 2 approaches, starting with mineral oil or polyethylene glycol orally and followed by enemas on day 3, may be useful. Occasionally, enemas have to be administered in the office or clinic.

HOSPITALIZATION

Hospitalization rarely is needed for children with constipation. For severe impactions involving the entire colon, however, the child may need to be hospitalized for polyethylene glycol-electrolyte solution by nasogastric tube for 8 to 24 hours.[10]

Stool Softeners

As soon as the impaction is eliminated, the long-term treatment of constipation should be administered orally. Mineral oil, polyethylene glycol, or lactulose is prescribed (Table 142-3). The goal is the passage of 1 or 2 normal-sized BMs per day. Stool softeners must be continued for 3 months because bowel diameter and tone require this amount of time to return to normal. If the child refuses to take straight mineral oil, then parents should consider a better-tasting (though more expensive) emulsified derivative of mineral oil.

Laxatives

Stool softeners are the 1st line of therapy for constipation. If stool softeners (eg, polyethylene glycol) are not effective, then laxatives (bowel stimulants) to help the child keep the rectum empty should be recommended. Laxatives are usually needed for children who deliberately hold back BMs or for those who have acquired megarectum and megacolon (for dose levels, see Table 142-3).[11,12]

Undermedicating is the main cause of treatment failure and recurrences.[12,13] If the child is not having a normal-sized BM daily, then the dose should be increased. Some children temporarily require doses that exceed the standard dose recommended by textbooks and the package insert. Many parents worry unnecessarily about laxative dependency. They should be reassured that children can be tapered off laxatives successfully, even after 6 months of taking them.[14] All affected children need stool softeners or laxatives for at least 3 months, and many for 6 months or longer. Many parents are in a hurry to stop the medications; they should be told on the 1st visit that to achieve a cure, medications need to be continued until the child has gone at least 1 month without any soiling. The medications then can be tapered gradually over 1 to 2 months.

Toilet Habits

The child must sit on the toilet for at least 10 minutes once a day with a timer. The gastrocolic reflex, which takes effect 20 to 30 minutes after a meal (especially breakfast), should be used to advantage. Any treatment that neglects this opportunistic timing will fail.

Children who have been impacted for many months have no urge to defecate. The defecation urge may not return until the rectum is kept empty for 1 to 2 weeks. Other important tips to impart to children are to flex the hips to open the rectum, to use a footstool for leverage, and to apply some pressure to the abdomen while pushing down. If they have no BM for 24 hours, then these children need to sit on the toilet more often and longer each time. Soiling (leakage) also requires sitting on the toilet, as well as cleanup.

Some preschoolers and toddlers adamantly refuse to sit on the toilet, holding back their stools when they are forced to do so. The overriding goal is to produce a BM daily. Passing it into the diaper is better than holding it in. In cases such as these, pediatricians and parents need to lower their expectations. The child can be told that the "poop wants to come out every day and it needs your help." Going in the diaper is fine. Rather than putting the child back in diapers or pull-ups fulltime, the child should be given access to them when the need to release a stool exists. This approach prevents the child from regressing with bladder control.

Nonconstipating High-Fiber Diet

All constipated children need more fiber in their diet, as is found in foods such as popcorn, grains, fruits, and vegetables. However, diet therapy alone will cure only specific children who have mild constipation. The only foods that have been shown to be constipating are milk products. Identifying the 10% or so of children who have impactions and who are drinking great amounts of milk (>32 oz per day) is critical. Milk intake can be limited to 16 oz per day in children older than 1 year. Fluid requirements for these children can be met with fruit juices, especially those that have a high sorbitol content

Table 142-3 Medications for Constipation

MEDICATION	DOSAGE	COMMENTS
STOOL SOFTENERS		
Mineral oil	1-2 mL/kg/dose twice daily Adolescents: 60 mL/dose (max 8 oz/day)	Do not use in children who have gastroesophageal reflux or vomiting or who are not yet walking. Emulsified types (Petrogalar, plain Agoral, Kondremul) taste better.
Lactulose	0.5-1.0 mL/kg/dose twice daily Adolescents: 15 mL twice daily (max 3 oz/day)	This is a prescription item.
Polyethylene glycol (Miralax)	0.5 g/kg/day Adolescents: 17 g/day	This is a prescription item.
Milk of Magnesia	1-2 mL/kg/dose Adolescents: 30-60 mL	1 Milk of Magnesia tablet = 2.5 mL liquid.
STIMULANT LAXATIVE		
Senokot (senna)	<5 yr: 1-2 tsp syrup/day >5 yr: 2-3 tsp syrup Adolescents: 1 tbsp/day (max 2.5 tbsp or 8 tablets)	1 tablet = 3 mL granules = 5 mL syrup.
Fletcher's Castoria	<5 yr: 1-2 tsp/day >5 yr: 2-3 tsp Adolescents: 2 tbsp max	—
Ex-Lax (senna)	>5 years: 1 square/day Adolescents: 2 squares	Chewable squares
Dulcolax, 5-mg tablet	>5 yr: 5 mg/day >12 yr: 10 mg (2 tablets) Adolescents: 4 tablets max	Liquid form not available.
RECTAL SUPPOSITORIES		
Glycerin suppository	1 or 2 suppositories	
Dulcolax suppository 10 mg	>2 yr: 1 suppository	
ENEMA FOR DISIMPACTION		
Mineral oil enema	1-2 oz/20 lb of weight/day Adolescents: 4 oz	Squeeze-bottle size: 4.5 oz
Sodium phosphate enema (Fleet)	1 oz/20 lb of weight/day Adolescents: 4 oz (max 8 oz)	Squeeze-bottle size: 2.25 oz children, 4.5 oz adult
ORAL DISIMPACTION		
Mineral oil	1 oz/yr of age/day Max dose: 8 oz/day	—
Polyethylene glycol (Miralax)	0.5 gm/kg/dose 3 times daily Max 25 g or 1½ cap 3 times daily	—

such as pear, peach, or prune juice. Sorbitol can increase the frequency of stools.

Follow-Up Visits

All children who have impactions need follow-up approximately 1 week into treatment; over 30% still will be impacted.[12] The abdominal examination should be repeated even if patients tells you that they are having normal BMs and no soiling. Children who have an impaction actually can keep themselves clean temporarily by making a superhuman effort at control and sitting on the toilet several times a day. If the history and abdominal examination leaves uncertainty, then the rectal examination should be repeated.

If a child still is impacted at the follow-up examination, then a more detailed explanation of the disimpaction process is necessary. Some children need enemas in the office at this point.

Back-Up Plan for Recurrence of Constipation or Encopresis

Back-up plans are critical for preventing all-too-frequent relapses. If the child goes for longer than 48 hours without a normal-size BM, then the parents should be instructed to increase the dose of stool softener or laxative.[10,12] This approach is critical to prevent impactions from recurring.

If soiling occurs more than twice over a few days, then the child is at risk for recurring impaction. At this point, the parents should intervene vigorously by giving a double dose of laxative, a suppository, or an enema. Merely mentioning an enema sometimes results in the child sitting on the toilet and producing a BM. For older children who are cooperative about sitting on the toilet, sitting there for 10 minutes out of every hour will usually relieve an early impaction. Again, the family should be made to realize that soiling

BOX 142-2 Treatment of Nonretentive Encopresis

Medications are not needed.
Stop all reminders, lectures, or punishments.
Give incentives for bowel movements into the toilet.
For soiling, insist on immediate cleanup.
Refer treatment failures.

always means that the rectum is full and the impaction is returning.

Failure of these primary care interventions is likely due to rectal hyposensitivity and inability to relax the external anal sphincter.[15] Both of these pathophysiological conditions probably are gradually acquired, the former caused by prolonged stretching of the rectum and the latter resulting from voluntary attempts to prevent stool leakage or pain. Both of these conditions usually recede once stool impaction is permanently resolved with more aggressive interventions.

MANAGEMENT OF NONRETENTIVE ENCOPRESIS

For children who simply postpone BMs, a simple admonition "to find a toilet whenever you feel rectal pressure" or "don't make your body wait" usually removes the symptom. Most children with nonretentive encopresis, however, are resistant to toilet training, and they need more intensive intervention (Box 142-2).[16]

Medications

Stool softeners, laxatives, and enemas are clearly not needed for cases of nonretentive encopresis.

Reminders and Lectures

The parents should be reassured that nothing more can be taught to their child. To eliminate the control issue, the parents should be told to stop all reminders about using the toilet and to let the child decide when the need exists to go to the bathroom. Children should neither be reminded to go to the bathroom nor be asked if they need to go. Reminders, inquiries, and lectures are a form of pressure, and pressure does not work. The parents should not threaten punishment. Many young children try to hold back all BMs to avoid punishment, such as being spanked or grounded for soiling. They are under the mistaken impression that not passing any BMs is the best way to avoid punishment. The parents should be told about the importance of not punishing their child for soiling. The child should be reassured that soiling will no longer incur punishment.

Incentives

Incentives for passing BMs into the toilet should be given and the parents reassured that this approach is how they can turn the tide. If the child passes a BM into the toilet, then the parents should give immediate positive feedback such as praise, a hug, and a sticker.

BOX 142-3 When to Refer Encopresis to a Mental Health Professional

Unresponsive to pediatric management
Refuses to sit on the toilet and is older than 5 years
Refuses to take medications
Has nonretentive encopresis and is older than 8 years
Has nonretentive encopresis and deliberately passes bowel movements on family possessions or at school (overt anger)
Is depressed
Parent-child relationship is severely disturbed

To achieve a breakthrough with some children who have never had a BM into a potty chair or toilet, the parent should offer major incentives such as going out to their favorite fast-food restaurant, watching their favorite video, or giving them treats.[1] A star chart also helps many children stay focused on the goal of releasing stool into the potty chair or toilet. Incentives are also helpful in younger children who deliberately hold back BMs and refuse to sit on the potty.

Changing Soiled Underwear

Soiling should not be ignored. The parents' only remaining assignment is to help the child change clothes when they become soiled. As soon as the parents notice that the child has messy pants, they should clean the child up immediately. Changing should be made a neutral, timely interaction.

PROGNOSIS

Pediatric management can cure 99% of children who have mainly pain-related impaction. The physician will be successful with approximately 70% of children who have psychogenic impaction and will need to work with a mental health professional for the others. Levine studied 127 encopretic children for more than 1 year.[17] At that time, 51% were cured and 27% had marked improvement.

Nonretentive encopresis is much easier to treat than retentive encopresis. These children have good results if the problem is recent and poor results if the problem is longstanding (>5 years). In mildly resistive children, primary care management can achieve a 90% to 95% cure rate. Children who have severe resistance need early referral. Box 142-3 lists the reasons for referral of encopretic children to a mental health professional.

SUMMARY

The primary care pediatrician plays a critical role in evaluating children with encopresis. Most people who are not physicians cannot distinguish between the retentive and nonretentive types. The physician can also treat many of these children successfully by using combined therapy (stool softeners, laxatives, diet, altered toilet habits, and positive reinforcement). If a child who has retentive soiling is referred to a mental health professional, then the pediatrician should remain involved in titrating medications with the child's symptoms.

TOOLS FOR PRACTICE

Engaging Patients and Family

- *Constipation and Your Child* (brochure), American Academy of Pediatrics (patiented.aap.org).
- *Guide to Toilet Training* (book), American Academy of Pediatrics (www.aap.org/bookstore).

Medical Decision Support

- *Soiling Diary* (form), Barton D Schmitt MD (www.med.umich.edu/1libr/pa/pa_soildiar_art.htm).

AAP POLICY STATEMENTS

American Academy of Pediatrics, Kellogg N, Committee on Child Abuse and Neglect. The evaluation of sexual abuse in children. *Pediatrics*. 2005;116(2):506-512. (aappolicy.aappublications.org/cgi/content/full/pediatrics;116/2/506).

American Academy of Pediatrics, Subcommittee on Chronic Abdominal Pain. Technical report: Chronic abdominal pain in children tech report. *Pediatrics*. 2005;115(3):e370-e381. (aappolicy.aappublications.org/cgi/content/full/pediatrics;115/3/e370).

American Academy of Pediatrics, Subcommittee on Chronic Abdominal Pain. Clinical report: Chronic abdominal pain in children clinical report. *Pediatrics*. 2005;115(3):812-815. (aappolicy.aappublications.org/cgi/content/full/pediatrics;115/3/812).

REFERENCES

1. Schmitt BD. Toilet training problems: underachievers, refusers, and stool holders. *Contemp Pediatr.* 2004;21(4):71-82.
2. Nolan T, Oberklaid F. New concepts in the management of encopresis. *Pediatr Rev.* 1993;14:447.
3. Barr RG, Levine MD, Wilkinson RH, et al. Chronic and occult stool retention: a clinical tool for its evaluation in school-aged children. *Clin Pediatr.* 1979;18:674.
4. Liptak GS, Baker SS, Colletti RB, et al. Constipation. In: Moyer V, Davis RL, Elliott E, et al, eds. *Evidence Based Pediatrics and Child Health*. London, UK: BMJ Publishing Group; 2000.
5. North American Society for Pediatric Gastroenterology and Nutrition. Constipation in infants and children: evaluation and treatment. *J Pediatr Gastroenterol Nutr.* 1999;29:612-626.
6. Nurko S, Baker SS, Colletti RB, et al. Managing constipation: evidence put to practice. *Contemp Pediatr.* 2001;18(12):56-65.
7. Craig JC, Hodson EM, Martin HC. Phosphate enema poisoning in children. *Med J Aust.* 1994;160:347-351.
8. Gleghorn EE, Heyman MB, Rudolph CD. No-enema therapy for idiopathic constipation and encopresis. *Clin Pediatr.* 1991;130:669.
9. Youssef NN, Peters JM, Henderson W, et al. Dose response of PEG 3350 for the treatment of childhood fecal impaction. *J Pediatr.* 2002;141:410-414.
10. Abi-Hanna A, Lake AM. Constipation and encopresis in childhood. *Pediatr Rev.* 1998;19:23.
11. Nolan T, Debelle G, Oberklaid F, et al. Randomised trial of laxatives in treatment of childhood encopresis. *Lancet.* 1991;338:523.
12. Schmitt BD, Mauro RD. 20 common errors in treating encopresis. *Contemp Pediatr.* 1992;9:47.
13. Borowitz SM, Cox DJ, Kovatchev B, et al. Treatment of childhood constipation by primary care physicians: efficacy and predictors of outcome. *Pediatrics.* 2005;115:873-877.
14. McClung HJ, Boyne LJ, Linsheid T, et al. Is combination therapy for encopresis nutritionally safe? *Pediatrics.* 1993;91:591.
15. Loening-Baucke V. Modulation of abnormal defecation dynamics by biofeedback treatment in chronically constipated children with encopresis. *J Pediatr.* 1990;116:214.
16. Brazzelli M, Griffiths P. Behavioral and cognitive interventions with or without other treatments for defecation disorders in children. *Cochrane Database Syst Rev.* 2001;(4):CD002240.
17. Levine MD, Bakow H. Children with encopresis: a study of treatment outcome. *Pediatrics.* 1976;58:845.

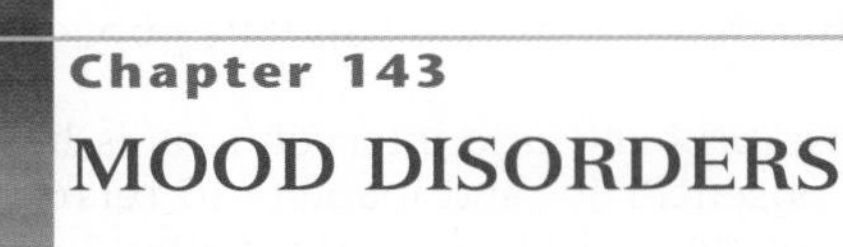

Chapter 143
MOOD DISORDERS

David A. Brent, MD

Mood disorders are important contributors to the morbidity and mortality of children and adolescents. As the focus of pediatric practice shifts to accommodate a greater emphasis on psychosocial issues, the pediatrician should recognize and share in the management of these relatively common and serious problems of childhood and adolescence.[1,2]

CLASSIFICATION

Mood disorders are classified on the basis of 3 factors: (1) severity, (2) course, and (3) presence or absence of mania. In terms of depressive symptoms, the diagnosis of major depressive disorder requires at least 2 weeks of depressed mood more than one half of the time and 4 additional depressive symptoms[3] (Box 143-1). A more chronic, intermittent disorder such as dysthymic disorder may have periods of depression interspersed with normal mood (Box 143-2). Adjustment disorder is a still milder and self-limited disturbance of mood that follows a serious life stressor (Box 143-3). A history of manic symptoms in a person who has major depression or dysthymia confers a diagnosis of bipolar affective or cyclothymic disorder respectively (Boxes 143-4 and 143-5).

EPIDEMIOLOGIC DESCRIPTION

Mood disorders are relatively rare in prepubertal children, with estimates of point prevalences ranging from 1.8% to 2.9%.[4] The incidence of mood disorder is estimated to be 3 to 4 times more common in adolescence (approximately 3% to 8% for depression, 1% to 2% for bipolar disorder, and 5% to 7% for bipolar spectrum.[5] Whereas the gender ratio for affectively ill prepubertal children approaches unity, depression among adolescents is approximately 2 to 3 times more common among girls than boys. Earlier onset of puberty may be associated with an increased risk of depression, especially in girls.[6] Retrospective studies in adults show the rates of bipolar disorder are twice as high in adolescents than in prepubertal children.[7]

RISK FACTORS

The most potent risk factor for developing a depressive disorder in childhood is having at least 1 parent

BOX 143-1 Criteria for the Diagnosis of a Major Depressive Episode

A. Five (or more) of the following symptoms have been present during the same 2-week period and represent a change from previous functioning; at least 1 of the symptoms is either (1) depressed mood or (2) loss of interest or pleasure. Note: Do not include symptoms that are clearly due to a general medical condition or mood-incongruent delusions or hallucinations:
   1. Depressed mood most of the day, nearly every day, as indicated by either subjective report (eg, feels sad or empty) or observation made by others (eg, appears tearful). Note: In children and adolescents, can be irritable mood.
   2. Markedly diminished interest or pleasure in all, or almost all, activities most of the day, nearly every day (as indicated by either subjective account or observation made by others).
   3. Significant weight loss when not dieting or weight gain (eg, a change of more than 5% of body weight in a month) or decrease or increase in appetite nearly every day. Note: In children, consider failure to make expected weight gains.
   4. Insomnia or hypersomnia nearly every day.
   5. Psychomotor agitation or retardation nearly every day (observable by others, not merely subjective feelings of restlessness or being slowed down).
   6. Fatigue or loss of energy nearly every day.
   7. Feelings of worthlessness or excessive or inappropriate guilt, which may be delusional nearly every day and not merely self-reproach or guilt about being sick.
   8. Diminished ability to think or concentrate, or indecisiveness, nearly every day (either by subjective account or as observed by others).
   9. Recurrent thoughts of death (not just fear of dying), recurrent suicidal ideation without a specific plan, or a suicide attempt or a specific plan for committing suicide.

B. The symptoms do not meet criteria for a mixed episode (see p. 365).

C. The symptoms cause clinically significant distress or impairment in social, occupational, or other important areas of functioning.

D. The symptoms are not due to the direct physiologic effects of a substance (eg, a drug of abuse, a medication) or a general medical condition (eg, hypothyroidism).

E. The symptoms are not better accounted for by bereavement (ie, after the loss of a loved one), the symptoms persist for longer than 2 months, or are characterized by significant functional impairment and a morbid preoccupation with worthlessness, suicidal ideation, psychotic symptoms, or psychomotor retardation.

who has a history of depression. Anxiety disorders also predispose the individual to developing depression. The risk of depression is greater and the age of onset of depression is younger with a greater familial loading for depression, an earlier age of onset of depression in parents, and a family history of either bipolarity or recurrent unipolar disorder. Physical or sexual abuse and exposure to family and community violence are also associated with depressive symptoms. Certain medications may lead to depression, namely, antihypertensive agents, steroids, and phenobarbital. The incidence of depression may be increased in patients who have some chronic illnesses, such as epilepsy, inflammatory bowel disease, and juvenile-onset diabetes. Childhood depression is associated with abnormalities in serotonergic and noradrenergic neurotransmission, as demonstrated by altered response to neuroendocrine challenges. Neuroimaging studies show structural and functional alterations in the prefrontal cortex and the limbic system.[8,9] Adoption, twin, and linkage studies support a genetic cause, and genetic epidemiologic studies suggest that depression results from an interaction between genetic vulnerability and accumulated stressful life events.[10-12]

CLINICAL PICTURE

The clinical picture of depressive disorders in children and adolescents is similar to that described in adults. Children and adolescence may describe *depressed mood* as sadness, irritability, or boredom. The pediatrician's index of suspicion for depression should be high when a patient exhibits substantial alteration of mood along with evidence of a decline in function. Pediatricians should consider referring patients who have chronic, complex, or severe disorder, exhibited by comorbidity, suicidality, psychosis, and bipolar-type depression. Depressed children and depressed adolescents exhibit similarly, although depressed adolescents are more likely to have made a suicide attempt and to be using illicit drugs. However, suicidal thoughts are a very frequent symptom in both pre- and postpubertal depression. Patients who have either dysthymia or major depression frequently have other comorbid psychiatric disorders (anxiety disorders, attention deficit disorder, conduct disorder, and substance abuse). Prepubertal depression segregates into 2 subpopulations. The first subgroup is characterized by comorbid behavioral disorders, history of parental criminality, parental substance abuse, family adversity, and increased risk in adulthood of antisocial disorder and substance abuse without an increased risk of mood disorder. The second, smaller subsample has familial mood disorder and an increased risk for recurrent depression and for the development of bipolar disorder. The depressive picture for patients who have bipolar illness often includes psychotic features, along with hypersomnia, hyperphagia, and anergia.

Mood in the manic or hypomanic phase may be characterized by expansive mood, euphoria, and grandiosity or by anger and irritability. Symptoms of mania and hypomania (a milder form of mania without severe functional impairment) may occur separately from

BOX 143-2 Criteria for the Diagnosis of Dysthymic Disorder

A. Depressed mood for most of the day, for more days than not, as indicated either by subjective account or observation by others, for at least 2 years. Note: In children and adolescents, mood can be irritable and duration must be at least 1 year.
B. Presence while depressed of 2 (or more) of the following:
   1. Poor appetite or overeating
   2. Insomnia or hypersomnia
   3. Low energy or fatigue
   4. Low self-esteem
   5. Poor concentration or difficulty making decisions
   6. Feelings of hopelessness
C. During the 2-year period (1 year for children or adolescents) of the disturbance, the person has never been without the symptoms in Criteria A and B for more than 2 months at a time.
D. No major depressive episode (see Box 143-1) has been present during the first 2 years of the disturbance (1 year for children and adolescents); that is, the disturbance is not better accounted for by chronic major depressive disorder, or major depressive disorder, in partial remission. Note: A previous major depressive episode may exist provided a full remission occurred (no significant signs or symptoms for 2 months) before development of the dysthymic disorder. In addition, after the initial 2 years (1 year in children or adolescents) of dysthymic disorder, episodes of major depressive disorder may be superimposed, in which case both diagnoses may be given when the criteria are met for a major depressive episode.
E. The patient has never had a manic episode, a mixed episode, or a hypomanic episode (see Box 143-5), and criteria have never been met for cyclothymic disorder.
F. The disturbance does not occur exclusively during the course of a chronic psychotic disorder, such as schizophrenia or delusional disorder.
G. The symptoms are not due to the direct physiological effects of a substance (eg, a drug of abuse, a medication) or a general medical condition (eg, hypothyroidism).
H. The symptoms cause clinically significant distress or impairment in social, occupational, or other important areas of functioning.

depressive episodes or may co-occur with them. The simultaneous occurrence of manic and depressive symptoms is known as a *mixed state*. Early-onset bipolar disorder is characterized by frequent presentation with mixed states, mood lability, rapid cycling, and greater frequency of episodes than is seen in adult patients who are bipolar. Mixed states pose a high risk for suicide attempt and completed suicide. Delusions associated with either grandiosity or paranoia often accompany severe mania, particularly if prolonged sleep deprivation has occurred.

BOX 143-3 Criteria for the Diagnosis of Adjustment Disorder with Depressed Mood

A. The development of emotional or behavioral symptoms in response to an identifiable stressor(s) occurring within 3 months of the onset of the stressor(s).
B. These symptoms or behaviors are clinically significant as evidenced by either of the following:
   1. Marked distress that is in excess of what would be expected from exposure to the stressor
   2. Significant impairment in social or occupational (academic) functioning
C. The stress-related disturbance does not meet the criteria for another specific axis I disorder and is not merely an exacerbation of a preexisting axis I or axis II disorder.
D. The symptoms do not represent bereavement.
E. Once the stressor (or its consequences) has terminated, the symptoms do not persist for more than an additional 6 months.

DIFFERENTIAL DIAGNOSIS

Within depressive disorders, the main differential diagnosis is among the triad of dysthymia, depression, and adjustment disorder with depressed mood. Dysthymia is more chronic and intermittent depression than major depression, although the 2 disorders can coexist (major depression developing *on top* of dysthymia, so-called *double depression*). Adjustment disorder with depressed mood has less severe mood disturbance and fewer symptoms and is self-limited in course compared with dysthymia or major depression. However, if a life stressor precedes a syndrome of depression, then the presence of the stressor does *not* invalidate the diagnosis of major depressive disorder. The symptoms of bereavement may be hard to distinguish from depressive symptoms. Depression in a bereaved patient is diagnosed if bereavement is associated with functional impairment, suicidal ideation, psychotic features, feelings of worthlessness, and prolonged course. A previous psychiatric disorder and a family history of depression predispose to the development of depression following bereavement.

Various other psychiatric disorders also may have associated mood disturbances. Patients who have learning disabilities or attention deficit disorder may have poor self-esteem and feel demoralized but should not be diagnosed as being depressed unless they meet the criteria for the syndrome. Poor concentration is characteristic of both attention deficit hyperactivity disorder and depression, but the former usually has an earlier onset and is not associated with anhedonia or social withdrawal. Children who have separation anxiety disorder are often dysphoric when separated from their parents, but, in the absence of premorbid depression, the dysphoria will be relieved by reunion with the parent. Patients who are anorectic, particularly if malnourished, may

BOX 143-4 Criteria for the Diagnosis of Bipolar Disorder

Past or current history of a manic episode, characterized by:

A. A distinct period of abnormally and persistently elevated, expansive, or irritable mood, lasting at least 1 week (or any duration if hospitalization is necessary).
B. During the period of mood disturbance, 3 (or more) of the following symptoms have persisted (4 if the mood is only irritable) and have been present to a significant degree:
   1. Inflated self-esteem or grandiosity
   2. Decreased need for sleep (eg, feels rested after only 3 hours of sleep)
   3. More talkative than usual or pressure to keep talking
   4. Flight of ideas or subjective experience that thoughts are racing
   5. Distractibility (ie, attention to easily drawn to unimportant or irrelevant external stimuli)
   6. Increase in goal-directed activity (either socially, at work or school, or sexually) or psychomotor agitation
   7. Excessive involvement in pleasurable activities that have a high potential for painful consequences (eg, engaging in unrestrained buying sprees, sexual indiscretions, or foolish business investments)
C. The symptoms do not meet criteria for a mixed episode.
D. The mood disturbance is sufficiently severe to cause marked impairment in occupational functioning or in usual social activities or relationships with others or to necessitate hospitalization to prevent harm to self or others, or psychotic features are present.
E. The symptoms are not due to the direct physiological effects of a substance (eg, a drug of abuse, a medication) or a general medical condition (eg, hyperthyroidism). Note: Manic-like episodes that are clearly caused by somatic antidepressant treatment (eg, medication, electroconvulsive therapy, light therapy) should not count toward a diagnosis of bipolar I disorder.

BOX 143-5 Criteria for the Diagnosis of Cyclothymic Disorder

A. For at least 2 years, the presence of numerous periods with hypomanic symptoms (see p. 368) and numerous periods with depressive symptoms that do not meet criteria for a major depressive episode. Note: In children and adolescents, the duration must be at least 1 year.
B. During this 2-year period (1 year in children and adolescents), the person has not been without the symptoms in Criterion A for more than 2 months at a time.
C. No major depressive episode, manic episode, or mixed episode has been present during the first 2 years of the disturbance. Note: After the initial 2 years (1 year in children and adolescents) of cyclothymic disorder, manic, or mixed episodes may be superimposed (in which case both bipolar I disorder and cyclothymic disorder may be diagnosed) or major depressive episodes (in which case both bipolar II disorder and cyclothymic disorder may be diagnosed).
D. The symptoms in Criterion A are not better accounted for by schizoaffective disorder and are not superimposed on schizophrenia, schizophreniform disorder, delusional disorder, or psychotic disorder not otherwise specified.
E. The symptoms are not due to the direct physiological effects of a substance (eg, a drug of abuse, a medication) or a general medical condition (eg, hyperthyroidism).
F. The symptoms cause clinically significant distress or impairment in social, occupational, or other important areas of functioning.

show a markedly depressed affect. However, depression should not be diagnosed until nutritional status has been normalized. Patients who abuse drugs and alcohol often show disturbances of mood. At times, the mood disorder may antedate and even predispose the individual to substance abuse, but the mood disorder is often secondary to substance abuse and subsides within a month of detoxification.[13]

Distinguishing depression from chronic medical illness can be difficult, given that the incidence of depression may be higher in certain illnesses and that chronic illness may affect sleep, appetite, and energy similarly to depression. Feelings of guilt, worthlessness, hopelessness, and suicidal thoughts are unlikely to be attributable to the illness itself and, if present, strongly suggest the presence of a depressive disorder.

Mania can be mimicked by stimulant abuse (eg, cocaine, amphetamine). The irritability of mania also can be seen in depression; thus distinguishing depression from mania rests on whether the preponderance of associated symptoms is more consistent with mania or with depression. Euphoria, increased energy, and increase in sexuality are 3 symptoms that are much more common in bipolar than in unipolar (ie, only experiencing depression and not mania) depressed patients. Irritability, anger, and poor judgment also may be prominent features of conduct disorder, but the lack of changes in energy, sleep, sexuality, and thought patterns in conduct disorder will generally exclude mania as a diagnosis. Similarly, the features of attention deficit disorder may suggest mania, but patients with mania are more likely to have mood swings and alterations in sleep and appetite and to show hypersexuality and inappropriate joking and punning. A severe clinical deterioration of a patient with an attention deficit disorder after a trial of stimulants, particularly with some of the manic clinical features mentioned earlier or with a positive family history of mania, also suggests bipolar disorder. Sexually abused children may show sexually provocative behavior and depressed mood, but euphoria or increased energy in the absence of bipolar disorder is rarely seen. The differential diagnosis notwithstanding, mood and behavioral disorders frequently co-occur.

CLINICAL COURSE

Naturalistic studies indicate that depressive disorders in children and adolescents run a chronic and recurrent course. Untreated major depressive disorder lasts an average of 7.2 months and dysthymic disorder an average of 45.9 months. Patients who have both major depressive disorder and nonaffective morbidity (eg, additional diagnoses of conduct disorder, attention deficit disorder) may show a more prolonged course, as do depressed youth whose parents also are depressed. On the average, 40% of depressed children experience a recurrence within 2 years, and nearly 75% have a recurrence within 5 years.[14] Earlier age of onset and co-occurrence of a preexisting dysthymic disorder increase the risk for major depressive recurrences. As depressed adolescents make a transition into adulthood, they show a greater risk of academic, occupational, and interpersonal impairment, tobacco and substance abuse, and obesity than their nondepressed peers. Residual social impairment may be related to unresolved depression, but many of the other adverse outcomes are due to risk factors that are shared between depression and these other conditions (eg, abuse, family discord, parental substance abuse). Moreover, depression confers a substantially increased risk for completed and attempted suicide, in both male and female adolescents.[11] Whereas girls are more likely to attempt suicide, boys are more likely to complete suicide.[15]

IDENTIFICATION OF DEPRESSED PATIENTS IN PEDIATRIC SETTINGS

Any disturbance in mood that is associated with functional impairment (ie, impairment in fulfilling developmentally appropriate roles in school, home, or community) should be considered a psychiatric disorder until proved otherwise. Parents and children alike frequently have a tendency to mislabel *bona fide* depressive disorders as *the ups and downs* of childhood or adolescence. Mood disorder should be a strong consideration for any child who presents with unexplained somatic complaints, drop in school performance, apathy and loss of interest, social withdrawal, increased irritability or tearfulness, sleep and appetite changes, or suicidal ideation or behavior. Moreover, depressive illnesses frequently accompany tobacco, alcohol, and drug abuse, as well as promiscuous sexual and risk-taking behavior. Depressive disorders may follow bereavement, particularly if the patient has a personal or family history of depression. Depression also may follow other severe stressors, such as physical or sexual assault. The pediatrician should be aware of a family history of depression because such a history will increase the risk of depressive disorder at least 3-fold. A family history of bipolar disorder greatly increases the risk that other biological family members will develop this disorder.

Both the child and the parent will usually contribute important information to be used by the pediatrician in diagnosing depression. The child is likely to be the most accurate reporter of symptoms that refer to an internal state such as depressed mood, anhedonia, guilt, worthlessness, and suicidal thoughts.[16,17] The parent, by contrast, may be able to note such externally validated symptoms as irritability, decline in school performance, listlessness, withdrawal from social and other pleasurable activities, and weight loss. An important issue in identifying mood disorder in children is to recognize that the depressed mood in children may be described as grouchy, mad, or bored rather than sad. A brief self-report, the *Mood and Feelings Questionnaire* can be useful in identifying which children have depression and need more specialized treatment.[18]

MANAGEMENT

Children and adolescents who have mood disorders are best managed by a collaboration among pediatrician, mental health specialist, and child psychiatrist. Generally, psychiatric intervention has 3 components: (1) psychoeducation, (2) psychotherapy, and (3) pharmacotherapy. Most patients with mood disorder can be managed as outpatients. Inpatient admission should be reserved for people who are psychotic, acutely suicidal, acutely manic or in a mixed state, abusing substances, or unresponsive to outpatient intervention.

FAMILY PSYCHOEDUCATION

Family psychoeducation approaches depression as a chronic illness, with its aim to instruct family members about the nature and course of the illness. Such an approach is likely to improve adherence with treatment and may reduce the rate of relapse. Psychoeducation also is aimed at reducing the tensions of living with a person with mood-disorder by altering familial expectations. This alteration involves parents' accepting the illness and making appropriate expectations of the patient and of themselves. Finally, psychoeducation should enable the child and family to identify early signs of recurrence of the disorder and to seek treatment before the recurrent mood disorder becomes severe and chronic. Identification and treatment of parental depression is critical because evidence suggests that parental depression may prolong the child's depressive episodes and interfere with recovery.

PSYCHOTHERAPY

Individual, brief (3 months) cognitive behavior treatment (CBT) has been shown to be more efficacious than credible alternative treatments (family, supportive, or relaxation therapies) for the relief of adolescent depression.[19] Group CBT has also been shown to be helpful both for treating depression and for preventing depression in at-risk youth.[20] In 1 notable exception, the Treatment of Adolescent Depression Study,[21] found CBT to be no better than placebo and markedly inferior to fluoxetine in relieving adolescent depression. The combination of CBT and medication results in the highest remission rate and a trend toward lower rates of suicidal adverse events, but in more severe depression, the combination may not be better than fluoxetine alone.[22] Another type of psychotherapy, interpersonal psychotherapy, has also been shown to be efficacious in treating adolescent depression but has not yet been compared with antidepressant medication.[23]

PHARMACOTHERAPY

Selective serotonin reuptake inhibitors (SSRIs) have been shown to be more effective than placebo for child and adolescent depression, with the strongest and most consistent data supporting the use of fluoxetine, the only 1 of the SSRIs that has US Food and Drug Administration (FDA) approval for the treatment of pediatric depression.[24] Other drugs for which some data exist to support efficacy are sertraline and citalopram.[25,26] A standard approach for the treatment of depression is to prescribe the equivalent 10 mg of fluoxetine for 1 week, then increase to 20 mg for 3 more weeks, and, if the patient does not show an adequate clinical response to increase, the dose is increased to 40 mg. Pharmacokinetic studies in children and adolescents who are taking SSRIs indicate shorter drug half-lives than in adults, meaning that the doses should be at least as high in pediatric patients.[27,28]

The FDA has determined that SSRIs are associated with an increased risk of suicidality (ie, suicidal ideation and behaviors) compared with placebo and recommends close monitoring for clinical response and adverse events during the early phase of treatment (weekly for the first month, every other week for the next 2 months, and monthly thereafter).[29] This adverse effect emerges early in treatment and is most often characterized by new-onset or worsening suicidal ideation, a suicidal threat, or much more rarely, a suicide attempt. In the FDA's review of clinical trials involving over 4300 pediatric patients, no suicides occurred. The rate of emergent or worsening suicidality in the antidepressant group was on average 4% versus 2% in the placebo group. Although many more patients will benefit from SSRIs than will experience suicidality, SSRIs should be prescribed only when patients and families understand the risks and benefits and the physician can monitor progress and side effects on a regular basis. Between 2% and 5% of patients treated with SSRI develop manic symptoms (expansive mood, racing thoughts, increased energy, decreased need for sleep, increased risk taking).[21] The risk is higher in younger patients and in persons with a positive family history for bipolar disorder.[30,31] An older type of antidepressant, tricyclic antidepressants, should *not* be prescribed as a first-line treatment because they are not efficacious for treating pediatric depression and are potentially fatal in overdose.

Depressed patients with a positive family history for bipolar disorder should be treated initially with psychotherapy; if they require an antidepressant, then these patients should be monitored closely for emergent manic symptoms. Other side effects include drowsiness, extrapyramidal symptoms, galactorrhea, and, more rarely, tardive dyskinesia.

For adolescents who fail to respond to a first SSRI, standard practice is to try another SSRI at an adequate dose for 6 to 8 weeks. Establishing adherence and ruling out possible medical problems, such as hypothyroidism that might contribute to lack of response, are important. If the patient shows a partial response, then one may consider augmentation with lithium, which has been shown to be effective in adults. With a complete lack of response, clinical guidelines[32,33] recommend a switch to another type of agent, such as bupropion. The addition of psychotherapy may also enhance treatment response. However, none of these strategies have yet been empirically validated in younger populations, although some have been proven efficacious in adults.[34]

CONTINUATION TREATMENT

After termination of either CBT or pharmacotherapy, the risk of relapse is high; therefore continued treatment is recommended at a lower frequency of contact for 6 months after recovery is achieved. For CBT, this approach consists of monthly visits or *booster sessions;* for pharmacotherapy, this involves continued treatment at the same dose of medication for at least 6 months *after* recovery. This phase is critical in treating early-onset depression because simply getting depressed patients well is not enough; *keeping* them well is also crucial.

BIPOLAR DISORDER

Treatment of bipolar disorder consists of the use of mood stabilizers for prophylaxis and for acute treatment of manic or depressive episodes.[35] One of the most challenging aspects of the management of the disease is encouragement of continued treatment after normalization of mood. Therefore psychoeducation for the patient and family are key.

For the patient who is bipolar and who exhibits acute mania, empirical evidence supports the use of lithium, anticonvulsant mood stabilizers (divalproex or carbamazepine), or atypical neuroleptics (risperidone and quetiapine). When patients exhibit psychotic mania, then lithium, divalproex, or carbamazepine in combination with an atypical neuroleptic agent is recommended. If a patient achieves partial response to monotherapy, then adding a second agent from the previously noted group is recommended. Treatment of the depression in a patient who bipolar is always a balancing act between relief of the depression and prophylaxis against mania. Mood stabilizers and atypical neuroleptics have some antidepressant properties, although depressed patients with bipolar disorder often require the addition of an antidepressant, but this should always be prescribed *after* adequate coverage with a mood stabilizing agent. Although only open trials have been conducted, family interventions to improve communication, problem solving, and coping with having a bipolar family member may improve outcome as well.

All of the mood-stabilizing agents have significant medical complications that require close medical management. Lithium causes weight gain, acne, hypothyroidism, and, rarely, renal damage. Therapeutic lithium levels are between 0.6 and 1.0 mEq/L and should be monitored to assess compliance and prevent toxicity. Patients should be monitored every 4 to 6 months for hypothyroidism and annually to monitor renal function with a blood urea nitrogen test, creatinine test, urinalysis, and a creatinine clearance test. Divalproex causes weight gain, can affect hepatic and hemopoietic function, and has been associated with polycystic ovarian disease. Therefore use of this agent requires periodic assessment of liver function and blood and platelet counts. Carbamazepine is less frequently used because of its greater sedative effects and risk of hemopoietic side effects. The main concern of the atypical neuroleptics is weight gain; before prescribing these medications, weight and body mass index should be documented, along with a fasting blood sugar and lipid profile, and weight and body mass index should be monitored closely.

Lamotrigine is an anticonvulsant that has been demonstrated to be helpful for treating and preventing adult bipolar depression[36] but has not yet been carefully studied in children. It has a very benign side effect profile except for rare but very serious complication, Stevens-Johnson syndrome. For this reason, practitioners titrate this medication very slowly and monitor carefully for rashes.

TOOLS FOR PRACTICE

Engaging Patients and Family

- *Teen Suicide, Mood Disorder, and Depression* (brochure), American Academy of Pediatrics (patiented.aap.org)
- *Your Child's Mental Health: When to Seek Help and Where To Get Help* (brochure), American Academy of Pediatrics (patiented.aap.org)
- *Some Things You Should Know About Preventing Teen Suicide* (fact sheet), American Academy of Pediatrics (www.aap.org/healthopics/depression.cfm)
- *What Are the Warning Signs of Suicide?* (fact sheet), American Academy of Pediatrics (www.aap.org/healthopics/depression.cfm)
- *Behaviorial/Mental Health* (Web page), American Academy of Pediatrics (www.aap.org/healthopics/behavior.cfm)
- *Help Stop Teenage Suicide—Connected Kids* (brochure), American Academy of Pediatrics (www.aap.org/bookstore)
- *Suicide and Guns* (brochure), American Academy of Pediatrics (www.aap.org/bookstore)

Medical Decision Support

- Mood and Feelings Questionnaire (questionnaire), Duke University (devepi.mc.duke.edu/MFQ.html).
- Table of Screening Tools and Ratings Scales (table), Massachusetts General Hospital (www.massgeneral.org/schoolpsychiatry/screeningtools_table.asp).
- Detail Information from Table on Depressive Disorders (table), Massachusetts General Hospital (www.massgeneral.org/schoolpsychiatry/screening_depression.asp).
- *Bright Futures in Practice: Mental Health* (book), National Center for Education in Maternal and Child Health at Georgetown University, AAP endorsed (www.brightfutures.org/mentalhealth/).

AAP POLICY STATEMENT

American Academy of Pediatrics, Committee on Adolescence. Suicide and suicide attempts in adolescents. *Pediatrics*. 2000;105(4):871-874. (aappolicy.aappublications.org/cgi/content/abstract/pediatrics;105/4/871).

SUGGESTED RESOURCES

Birmaher B, Axelson D, Strober M, et al. Clinical course of children and adolescents with bipolar spectrum disorders. *Arch Gen Psychiatry*. 2006;63:175-183.

Birmaher B, Brent DA, Benson RS. Summary of the practice parameters for the assessment and treatment of children and adolescents with depressive disorders. *J Am Acad Child Adolesc Psychiatry*. 1998;37:1234-1238.

Birmaher B, Ryan ND, Williamson DE, et al. Childhood and adolescent depression: a review of the past 10 years. Part I. *J Am Acad Child Adolesc Psychiatry*. 1996;35:1427-1439.

Birmaher B, Ryan ND, Williamson DE, et al. Childhood and adolescent depression: a review of the past 10 years. Part II. *J Am Acad Child Adolesc Psychiatry*. 1996;35:1575-1583.

Botteron KN, Raichle ME, Drevets WC, et al. Volumetric reduction left subgenual prefrontal cortex in early onset depression. *Biol Psychiatry*. 2002;51:342-344.

Brent DA, Holder D, Kolko D, et al. A clinical psychotherapy trial for adolescent depression comparing cognitive, family, and supportive treatments. *Arch Gen Psychiatry*. 1997;54:877-885.

Drevets WC. Functional anatomical abnormalities in limbic and prefrontal cortical structures in major depression. *Prog Brain Res*. 2000;126:413-431.

Kowatch R, Fristad M, Birmaher B, et al. Treatment guidelines for children and adolescents with bipolar disorder. *J Am Acad Child Adolesc Psychiatry*. 2005;44:213-235.

Lewinsohn PM, Rohde P, Seeley JR. Major depressive disorder in older adolescents: prevalence, risk factors, and clinical implications. *Clin Psychol Rev*. 1998;18:765-794.

March JS, Silva S, Petrycki S, et al. Fluoxetine cognitive-behavioral therapy, and their combination for adolescents with depression. Treatment for Adolescent Depression Study (TADS) randomized controlled trial. *JAMA*. 2004;292:807-820.

Mufson L, Weissman MM, Moreau D, et al. Efficacy of interpersonal psychotherapy for depressed adolescents. *Arch Gen Psychiatry*. 1999;56:573-579.

Riggs P, Baker S, Mikulich SK, et al. Depression in substance-dependent delinquents. *J Am Acad Child Adolesc Psychiatry*. 1995;34:764-771.

Thomas KM, Drevets WC, Dahl RE, et al. Amygdala response to fearful faces in anxious and depressed children. *Arch Gen Psychiatry*. 2001;58:1057-1063.

Weersing VS, Brent DA: Cognitive-behavioral therapy for adolescent depression comparative efficacy, mediation, moderation, and effectiveness. In: Kazdin AE, Weisz JR, eds. *Evidence-Based Psychotherapies for Children and Adolescents*. New York, NY: The Guilford Press; 2003:135-147.

REFERENCES

1. Ryan ND, Williamson DE, Iyengar S, Orvaschel H, Reich T, Dahl RE, Puig-Antich J. A secular increase in child and adolescent onset affective disorder. *J Am Acad Child Adolesc Psychiatry*. 1992;31(4):600-605.
2. Kovacs M, Gatsonis C. Secular trends in age at onset of major depressive disorder in a clinical sample of children. *J Psychiat Res*. 1994;28:319-329.
3. American Psychiatric Association. *Diagnostic and Statistical Manual of Mental Disorders (DSM-IV-TR)*. 4th ed. Washington, DC: The Association; 2000.
4. Angold A, Costello EJ. The Epidemiology of Depression in Children and Adolescents. In: Goodyer IM, ed. *The Depressed Child and Adolescent*. 2nd ed. Cambridge University Press; 2001:143-178.
5. Lewinsohn PM, Klein DN, Seeley JR. Bipolar disorders in a community sample of adolescents: Prevalence, phenomenology, comorbidity and course. *J Am Acad Child Adolesc Psychiatry*. 1995;34:454-463.

6. Angold A, Costello EJ, Erkanli A, Worthman CM. Pubertal changes in hormone levels and depression in girls. *Psychol Med.* 1999;29:1043-1053.
7. Pavuluri MN, Birmaher B, Naylor MW. Pediatric bipolar disorder: A review of the past 10 years. *J Am Acad Child Adoles Psychiatry.* 2005;44:846-871.
8. Todd RD, Botteron KN. Etiology and genetics of early-onset mood disorders. *Child Adolesc Psychiatr Clin North Am.* 2002;11:499-518.
9. Thomas KM, Drevets WC, Dahl RE, Ryan ND, Birmaher B, Eccard CH, Axelson D, Whalen PJ, Casey BJ. Amydgala response to fearful faces in anxious and depressed children. *Archives of General Psychiatry.* 2001;58:1057-1063.
10. Caspi A, Sugden K, Moffitt TE, Taylor A, Craig IW, Harrington H, McClay J, Mill J, Martin J, Braithwaite A, Poulton R. Influence of life stress on depression: Moderation by a polymorphism in the 5-HT gene. *Science.* 2003;301: 386-389.
11. Thapar A, McGuffin P. A twin study of depressive symptoms in childhood. *Br J Psychiatry.* 1994;165:259-265.
12. Eaves L, Silberg J, Erkanli A. Resolving multiple epigenetic pathways to adolescent depression. *J Child Psychol Psychiatry.* 2003;44:1006-1014.
13. Riggs P, Baker S, Mikulich SK, et al. Depression in substance-dependent delinquents. *J Am Acad Child Adolesc Psychiatry.* 1995;34:764-771.
14. Kovacs M. Presentation and course of major depressive disorder furing childhood and later years of the life span. *J Am Acad Child Adolesc Psychiatry.* 1996;35(6): 705-715.
15. Bridge JA, Goldstein TR, Brent DA. Adolescent suicide and suicidal behavior. *J Child Psychol Psychiatry.* 2006; 47:372-394.
16. Walker M, Moreau D, Weissman MM. Parents' awareness of children's suicide attempts. *Am J Psychiatry.* 1990; 147(10):1364-1366.
17. Kendall PC, Cantwell DP, Kazdin AE. Depression in children and adolescents: Assessment issues and recommendations. *Cog Ther Res.* 1989;13:109-146.
18. Thapar A, McGuffin P. Validity of the shortened Mood and Feelings Questionnaire in a community sample of children and adolescents: A preliminary research note. *Psychiatry Res.* 1998;81:259-268.
19. Compton SN, March JS, Brent D, Albano AM, Weersing VR, Curry J. Cognitive behavioral psychotherapy for anxiety and depressive disorders in children and adolescents: An evidence based medicine review. *J Am Acad Child Adolesc Psychiatry.* 2004;43:930-959.
20. Lewinsohn PM, Rohde P, Seeley JR. Major depressive disorder in older adolescents: Prevalence, risk factors, and clinical implications. *Clinical Psychology Review.* 1998;18:765-794.
21. March JS, Silva S, Petrycki S, Curry J, Wells K, Fairbank J, Burns B, Domino M, McNulty S. Fluoxetine, cognitive-behavioral therapy, and their combination for adolescents with depression. Treatment for Adolescent Depression Study (TADS) randomized controlled trial. *J Am Med Assoc.* 2004;292:807-820.
22. Curry J, Rohde P, Simons S, Silva S, Vitiello B, Kratochvil C, Reinecke M, et al. Predictors and moderators of acute outcome in the treatment for adolescents with depression study (TADS). *J Am Acad Child Adolesc Psychiatry.* 2006 (in press).
23. Mufson L, Weissman MM, Moreau D, Garfinkel R. Efficacy of interpersonal psychotherapy for depressed adolescents. *Archives of General Psychiatry.* 1999;56:573-579.
24. Cheung A, Emslie G, Mayes T. Review of the efficacy and safety of antidepressants in youth depression. *J Child Psychol Psychiatry.* 2005;46:735-754.
25. Wagner KD, Ambrosini P, Rynn M, Wohlberg C, Yang R, Greenbaum MS, Childress A, Donnelly C, Deas D. Efficacy of sertraline in the treatment of children and adolescents with major depressive disorder: two randomized controlled trials. *J Am Med Assoc.* 2003;290:1033-1041.
26. Wagner KD, Robb AS, Findling RL, Jin J, Gutierrez MM, Heydorn WE. A randomized, placebo-controlled trial of citalopram for the treatment of major depression in children and adolescents. *Am J Psychiatry.* 2004;161:1079-1083.
27. Axelson D, Perel J, Birmaher B, Rudolph G, Nuss S, Brent D. Sertraline pharmacokinetics and dynamics in adolescents. *J Am Acad Child Adolesc Psychiatry.* 2002;41:1037-1044.
28. Findling RL, Preskorn SH, Marcus RN, Magnus RD, D'Amico F, Marathe P, Reed MD. Nefazodone pharmacokinetics in depressed children and adolescents. *J Am Acad Child Adolesc Psychiatry.* 2000;39:1008-1016.
29. Hammad TA, Laughren T, Racoosin J. Suicidality in pediatric patients treated with antidepressant drugs. *Archives of General Psychiatry.* 2006;63:332-339.
30. Geller B, Craney JL, Bolhofner K, DelBello MP, Williams M, Zimmerman B. One year recovery and relapse rates of children with a prepubertal and early adolescent bipolar disorder phenotype. *Am J Psychiatry.* 2001;158:303-305.
31. Martin A, Young C, Leckman JF, Mukonoweshuro C, Rosenheck R, Leslie D. Age effects of antidepressant-induced manic conversion. *Arch Pediatrics Adolesc Medicine.* 2004;158:773-780.
32. Birmaher B, Brent DA, Benson RS. Summary of the practice parameters for the assessment and treatment of children and adolescents with depressive disorders. *J Am Acad Child Adolesc Psychiatry.* 1998;37:1234-1238.
33. Hughes CW, Emslie GJ, Crismon L, Wagner KD, Birmaher B, Geller B, et al. The Texas Consensus Conference Panel on Medication Treatment of Childhood Major Depressive Disorder. The Texas children's medication algorithm project: Report of the Texas consensus conference panel on medication treatment of childhood major depressive disorder. *J Am Acad Child Adolesc Psychiatry.* 1999;38:1442-1454.
34. Thase M. Therapeutic alternatives for difficult-to-treat depression: What is the state of the evidence? *Psychiatr Ann.* 2003;33:813-821.
35. Kowatch R, Fristad MA, Birmaher B, Wagner KD, Findling R, Hellander M. Treatment guidelines for children and adolescents with bipolar disorder. *J Am Acad Child Adolesc Psychiatry.* 2005;44:213-235.
36. Calabrese JR, Bowden CL, Sachs GS, Ascher JA, Monaghan E, Rudd GD. A double-blind placebo-controlled study of lamotrigine monotherapy in outpatients with bipolar I depression. *J Clin Psychiatry.* 1999;60:79-88.

Chapter 144

MÜNCHAUSEN SYNDROME BY PROXY

Donna Andrea Rosenberg, MD

Münchausen syndrome by proxy (MSBP) is a somewhat bizarre form of abuse involving the persistent fabrication of illness in a child by an adult. It was first described in 1977 by Meadow,[1] an English pediatrician, and the name is derived from Münchausen syndrome, the condition of self-inflicted illness in adults. Compared with other forms of child abuse, MSBP has proven to be a form of child maltreatment that is fraught with rather different diagnostic and legal problems. The perpetrator of MSBP, usually the child's mother, often evades the early detection of her noxious ministrations because the symptoms and signs she reports seem plausible and because she appears attentive and concerned. The perpetrator's history often sounds cogent to the physician, bespeaking a serious illness. Although physicians are educated to evaluate critically the reliability of a historian, pediatricians do not expect that a history is an elaborate lie. Once the diagnosis has been considered, definitive inclusion or exclusion may be technically problematic. In consequence, ensuring civil court–ordered protection of a victim and any siblings may also prove difficult and is uneven from location to location. Evaluation of the family, information which helps shape therapy and which is useful only when the perpetrator is forthcoming, is often stymied by the mother's refusal to participate or her indignant denial of her malfeasance, however compelling the evidence may be.[2] Awareness of MSBP also varies significantly among mental health professionals,[3] and the mother may be very persuasive, even to experienced evaluators.[4] Criminal court proceedings undertaken against the perpetrator are still relatively rare,[5] even in homicidal MSBP. Medical professionals continue to struggle with this form of child abuse, which now goes by various names, including pediatric condition falsification[6] or fabricated or induced illness.[7]

DEFINITIONS

In MSBP, illness in a child is persistently and secretly simulated (lied about or faked), produced, or both by a parent or someone who is *in loco parentis* and the child is repeatedly brought for medical assessment and care. This circumstance often results in multiple medical procedures, both diagnostic and therapeutic. The definition specifically excludes physical abuse only, sexual abuse only, and nonorganic failure to thrive that is solely the result of nutritional or emotional deprivation.

In the context of this syndrome, the term *simulated* means that the mother tells lies about the child's symptoms. For example, the mother may repeatedly report that her child has episodes of stiffening, shaking, or decreased level of consciousness, when, in fact, these episodes never occurred; or she may tell the pediatrician that the child has hematuria and bring in a urine sample that she has contaminated with her own menstrual blood. The term *produced* means that the mother secretly interferes with the child's body (eg, by surreptitious suffocation, by administering unprescribed and unnecessary medicines or substances) to produce symptoms or signs in the child, the fact or the extent of which are not proffered on history.

DEMOGRAPHICS

Hundreds of cases of MSBP have been reported worldwide, although most cases of MSBP likely go unreported in the literature. Most of the literature concerning this form of maltreatment originates in the United Kingdom and the United States. Cases of MSBP have also been reported from Canada; Australia; New Zealand; Western, Central, and Eastern Europe; Scandinavia; the Middle East; South America; the Indian subcontinent; Central America; Africa; Sri Lanka; Japan; and Singapore.[8] Clearly, MSBP is not a culture-specific disorder, nor is it confined to either a socialized or privatized medical system. In addition, apparently, the perpetration of MSBP is not as uncommon as originally thought, although actual incidence is unknown. One study in the United Kingdom estimated the combined annual incidence of MSBP, nonaccidental poisoning, and nonaccidental suffocation as at least 2.8 per 100,000 in children younger than 1 year.[9] Extrapolation of this data to the United States suggests somewhere between 200 new cases of serious MSBP per year[10] to at least 600 new cases per year of suffocation or intentional poisoning.[6] A New Zealand study reported an incidence rate of 2 per 100,000 in children younger than 16 years.[11]

In the overwhelming majority of cases of MSBP, the perpetrator is the biological mother,[12] although fathers,[13,14] adoptive mothers,[15] other relatives,[16,17] babysitters,[18] and nurses[19] are occasionally implicated.

Boys and girls are victims almost equally, and no special trend is noted as to birth order.[20] Curiously, however, although several children in a family may be victimized sequentially, for more than one child to be victimized within any given period is unusual,[21] except during relatively brief transition periods. Typically, if the original victim survives, then the child's medical troubles melt away when another child comes along and develops unusual and inexplicable troubles.

Most victims of MSBP are infants and toddlers.[9,12,20] Presumably, the younger children are more commonly affected than older children because they are preverbal or semiverbal and relatively helpless physically; they are therefore easier to manipulate and assault. Although victimization of the children commonly begins in infancy or toddlerhood, a delay in making the correct diagnosis usually occurs. In 2 series, the average time from onset of symptoms and signs to diagnosis was 15 to 22 months,[12,20] but the time span might be as long as 20 years[20] or never.[22] A rare report describes cessation of MSBP not because of medical diagnosis, but rather because the school-aged victim threatened to disclose the mother's longstanding, painful, and disfiguring abuse.[23] Older child victims of MSBP, whose abuse may have begun years earlier, may adopt the false symptoms and signs as their own.[24] These children are less likely than young children to have illness produced and are more likely to have falsified reports of symptoms and medical history.[25] Some evidence suggests that these children may go on to develop Münchausen syndrome themselves[26] or some type of personality disorder.[27,28]

In one series, 25% of MSBP cases involved simulation only, 25% involved production only, and 50% involved both simulation and production of illness.[20] Another larger series showed that 57% of illness was produced.[12] In 50% to 95% of cases, depending on the meta-analytic series, the perpetrator continued victimizing the child in the hospital,[12,20] often in the most egregious ways,[29] and even in closely monitored settings, such as the pediatric intensive care unit.[30] Short-term morbidity for the children, by definition, is

100%, much of it related to the diagnostic and therapeutic procedures ordered by the physician. Long-term morbidity, defined as pain, illness, or both that causes permanent disfigurement or impairment, is harder to assess statistically than short-term morbidity. Approximately 8% of the surviving victims of MSBP have some kind of long-term morbidity as a result of complications of the attack or, rarely, complications from medical procedures.[12,20,31] This figure is probably an underestimate, however, and does not include long-term psychological morbidity, which may be considerable.[32]

Although assessing the mortality rate from MSBP is currently impossible for methodologic reasons, an important point to state is that some children die because of an ultimate fatal attack. Perhaps the perpetrator accidentally goes too far, having meant to make the child ill but not to kill the child. Perhaps the attack is a final act of unbridled hostility toward the child. Whatever the intent, children are at some risk of death. Series death rates vary from 6% to 33%.[12,20,31] In the largest series to date, apnea was the most common repeated symptom that preceded death.[12] Almost all victims were infants and toddlers, and the causes of death notably featured suffocation and poisoning. Other causes of death have been described,[20] and still others, as yet undescribed, are possible. Children as old as 8 years have been killed in the context of MSBP.[12] Furthermore, siblings of victims of MSBP tend to die in alarming numbers, often with the misdiagnosis of sudden infant death syndrome (SIDS), and every reason exists to believe that they died in a homicidal manner.[12,31,33-36] Child fatality review teams are now common throughout the country and, with the availability to these teams of multidisciplinary records and expertise, they are occasionally discovering cases of MSBP that had been previously but incorrectly designated as accidental, natural, or undetermined manner of death.

A few cases of adult victims of adult perpetrators of MSBP have been reported.[37-40] The methods of assault included repeated injection of gasoline or turpentine under the skin, injection of insulin, and poisoning with benzodiazepines.

CLINICAL AND LABORATORY FINDINGS

Although symptoms and signs and laboratory findings in MSBP cover an enormous spectrum, the most common serious presentation seems to be apnea. Seizures, feeding problems, bleeding, central nervous system depression, diarrhea, vomiting, fever (with or without sepsis or other localized infection), rash, allergy, and behavioral problems are also reported quite commonly.[12,20] At no time, however, should any list be considered inclusive because the understanding of the breadth of presentations of this syndrome is continually expanding. Table 144-1 lists some of the presentations of MSBP.

Nissen fundoplications are unnecessarily performed with distressing frequency in victims of MSBP, as are operations for the installation of a central venous catheter. Both procedures result in direct-line access to the child and therefore the possibility of further intraluminal assaults on the child with feces, saliva, contaminated water, drugs, salt, air, and many other substances.[41] Some child victims of MSBP are developmentally delayed as a result of the damage done by the inflicted illness or as a result of chronic hospitalization, enforced invalidism, or lack of stimulation. Malnutrition may be the result of the chronically inflicted illness; surreptitious withholding of food; prolonged emetic, laxative, or other drug assault; or other causes. MSBP may also exhibit in the context of a bona fide chronic disease, when the caretaking parent has intentionally and surreptitiously withheld treatment to significantly exacerbate the child's illness.[42,43]

The perpetration of MSBP may terminate with the homicide of the child. Probably the most common cause of death in homicidal MSBP is suffocation, but death occurs from many causes, among which are poisoning with various drugs, inflicted bacterial or fungal sepsis, hypoglycemia, and salt or potassium poisoning. Too frequently, suffocation and other homicidal deaths are signed out incorrectly as to cause and manner. The significantly positive clinical history is either undiscovered or ignored; a scene investigation is delayed or inadequate; or the autopsy, if performed, has not included all necessary dissections or tests.

A significantly positive clinical history of a deceased child would feature one or more items listed in Box 144-1. If any of these factors figure in the clinical history, then MSBP should be included in the differential diagnosis, along with possible genetic, metabolic, other natural, toxicologic, or environmental causes of death. These factors are not diagnostic criteria for MSBP; they are historical flags that should spur further investigation and, in particular, an exhaustive autopsy.

The usefulness of the autopsy as an investigative tool for determining cause and manner of death is obviously enhanced when it is performed in the most thorough manner. Specifically, evidence of poisoning should be diligently sought, with the necessary toxicologic studies performed from vitreous, blood, urine, gastric contents, tissues, and other sources. A *routine toxicology study* may be inadequate, and different laboratories include different tests in their routine toxicology study.[44] Specific requests may be necessary to have certain tests done. For example, though ipecac is no longer recommended as a household staple, intentional ipecac poisoning still occurs. A useful fact to know is that alkaloids persist in urine for weeks, whereas they are detectable in blood for only a few hours.[45] Consulting with the laboratory director as to the best method to detect suspected agents or drugs is often useful. Identifying a substance may be more specifically delineated with gas chromatography or mass spectrophotometry. The laboratory should be asked to preserve the samples securely, with proper chain of evidence documented, because they may be needed later for repeated studies or other studies not originally considered. If both serum sodium and urine sodium are elevated and the child is not dehydrated, then salt poisoning should be suspected. The premortem blood sodium or the postmortem vitreous sodium is useful. Postmortem vitreous urea nitrogen is a reliable study and may be useful as a reflection of hydration status. This finding is interpreted in the context of other renal function studies, in the same way as is

Table 144-1 Some Clinical Presentations of Münchausen Syndrome by Proxy*

SYSTEM	SYMPTOM AND SIGN OR LABORATORY FINDING
Head, eyes, ears, nose, throat, mouth	Bleeding from ears, nose, throat
	Conjunctivitis
	External otitis
	Hearing or speech impairment
	Nasal excoriation
	Nystagmus
	Otorrhea
	Parotitis or orbital cellulitis
	Tooth loss
Respiratory	Apnea or acute life-threatening event
	Asthma
	Bleeding from upper respiratory tract
	Choking or dyspnea
	Cyanosis (and other color changes, including pallor)
	Cystic fibrosis
	Hemoptysis
	Respiratory arrest
	Respiratory infection
	Sleep apnea
Cardiovascular	Bradycardia
	Cardiomyopathy
	Cardiopulmonary arrest
	Hypertension
	Rhythm abnormalities (including bradycardia, tachycardia, ventricular tachycardia, and others)
	Shock
Gastrointestinal	Abdominal pain
	Anorexia
	Bleeding from nasogastric tube or ileostomy
	Celiac disease
	Chronic intestinal pseudoobstruction
	Crohn disease
	Diarrhea
	Esophageal burns
	Esophageal perforation
	Feculent vomiting
	Feeding problems
	Gastrointestinal ulceration
	Hematemesis
	Hematochezia or melena
	Hemorrhagic colitis
	Malabsorption syndromes
	Polyphagia
	Pseudomelanosis coli
	Retrograde intussusception
	Vomiting (cyclic or otherwise)
Genitourinary	Bacteriuria
	Hematuria
	Menorrhagia
	Nocturia
	Polydipsia
	Polyuria or impaired urinary concentrating ability
	Proteinuria
	Pyuria
	Renal failure
	Urination from umbilical micropenis
	Urethral stones
	Urine gravel
Neurologic, musculoskeletal, developmental, psychiatric	Arthralgia
	Arthritis
	Ataxia
	Behavioral or personality disorders (including anxiety, autistic-spectrum disorders, panic reactions, rage, disorientation, and others)

Table 144-1 Some Clinical Presentations of Münchausen Syndrome by Proxy*—cont'd

SYSTEM	SYMPTOM AND SIGN OR LABORATORY FINDING
	Cerebral palsy
	Developmental delay (failure to attain or loss of milestones, or both)
	Headache
	Hyperactivity
	Irritability
	Learning or attention-deficit disability
	Lethargy
	Morning stiffness
	Psychotic symptoms
	Sleep disturbances: prolonged sleep, other sleep problems
	Seizures
	Syncope
	Tourette syndrome
	Unconsciousness
	Weakness
Skin	Abscesses
	Burns
	Eczema
	Excoriation
	Rash
Infectious, immune, allergic	Allergies (to food, drugs, or other substances)
	Bacteremia (unimicrobial or polymicrobial)
	Fevers
	Immunodeficiency
	Osteomyelitis
	Septic arthritis
	Sinopulmonary disease
	Soft-tissue or skin infection
	Urinary tract infection
Abnormalities of growth	Failure to gain weight or weight loss
Hematologic	Anemia
	Bleeding diathesis
	Bleeding from specific sites (see system)
	Easy bruising
	Leukopenia
Metabolic, endocrine, fluid and electrolyte	Acidosis
	Alkalosis
	Biochemical chaos
	Creatine kinase and aldolase increase
	Cystinosis
	Dehydration
	Diabetes
	Glycosuria
	Hyperglycemia
	Hyperkalemia
	Hypernatremia
	Hypochloremia
	Hypoglycemia
	Hypokalemia
	Hyponatremia
	Mitochondrial encephalopathy lactic acidosis and stroke-like (MELAS) syndrome
Other	Abuse (sexual, physical, or other)
	Diaphoresis
	Fatigue
	Foreign-body ingestions
	Hypothermia
	Pain
	Peripheral edema
	Poisonings
	Premature birth

*Including items reportedly observed by mother or actually observed by medical staff.

BOX 144-1 Review of Clinical History in a Dead Child: Circumstances Suggestive of Münchausen Syndrome by Proxy

A history of repeated medical visits for unusual, poorly defined, unpredictable, or unresponsive illness, especially apnea and seizures, which had never been confirmed to be witnessed at their starting moment by anyone other than the mother; *and* a full medical evaluation of the child that revealed no organic abnormality that might *fully* account for the child's reported illness, *or* a partial medical evaluation of the child that excluded major causes for the child's reported illness, *or* any medical evaluation that led to a conclusion about the child's diagnosis but the accuracy of which, on review, is seriously questioned; *OR*

Ill sibling of decedent, especially if the person were ill or is ill with chronic, poorly defined medical problems; *OR*

Dead sibling of decedent or dead unrelated child in the same home as decedent, especially if any of the following is found: (a) Other child's death was signed out as sudden infant death syndrome; (b) death followed a poorly defined or chronic illness; (c) cause of death was allegedly an illness that overwhelmingly is nonfatal in childhood; (d) cause of death was related to poisoning or intoxication; (e) cause of death was the result of an unusual accident; (f) death followed a presumed illness that was either unsubstantiated or excluded at autopsy; *or* (g) explanation for the death was inadequate; *OR*

Mother with chronic, poorly defined medical problems

blood urea nitrogen. As with all children suspected of having been maltreated, a skeletal survey should be performed to look for fractures. Classic physical abuse injuries have been reported in victims of MSBP.[12] Microbiological studies may be central to determining whether the child was the victim of inflicted microbial assault. When postmortem microbiologic studies of blood samples are positive, care must be taken to discriminate between those that reflect infection in the child and those that are the result of postmortem blood contamination with bowel, skin, or other organisms. The condition and contents of any lines into the child (central venous catheter, gastrostomy, endotracheal tube, shunt, or pacemaker, among others) should be examined closely, and preserving them would be prudent. As in a clinical situation, careful attention should be paid to chain of evidence for laboratory specimens and biomedical appliances.

Homicidal suffocation deaths[36,46] deserve further comment because they are still too commonly misdiagnosed as SIDS. The notion is reemphasized here that if any significant history precedes death, then SIDS, by definition, is excluded. The current definition of SIDS is the unexpected death of an infant younger than 1 year that remains unexplained after a complete review of the clinical history, death scene investigation, and autopsy. What this definition really means is that, after a thorough evaluation, although certain causes and manners have been definitively excluded, the cause and manner of death remain undetermined. Despite this explanation, and for reasons having more to do with a combination of good intentions or politicking (or both) than with scientific durability, using the term SIDS as a cause of death on a death certificate is still common practice, with manner of death as natural. The physician must always be concerned when sudden death occurs in a child who had repeated apnea or acute life-threatening events before death, especially episodes that featured attacks beginning only in the mother's presence and, when the mother called someone to see the infant, the child was hypoxic (ie, cyanotic, gray, gasping, and limp).[36,47] The physical findings of suffocation more commonly seen in adult victims (head and neck petechiae or bruising [or both], defensive marks) are almost always absent in young children.[48] Intraalveolar hemosiderin found at autopsy may be a marker of past smothering,[49] but this situation is not definitive.[50]

PERPETRATORS

What are the characteristics of the perpetrator of MSBP, and why does she do this? First, an important point to make is that no psychological test can include or exclude perpetration of MSBP. Second, no classic profile exists for a perpetrator, meaning that possessing certain characteristics does not entirely implicate a suspect, and lacking certain characteristics does not entirely exclude a suspect.

The perpetrator of MSBP is usually the mother. She sometimes has had nursing, medical, or paramedical training, perhaps never completed. She may be married, single, or divorced; but if she is married, then the relationship with her husband, although perhaps seemingly satisfactory, is often shallow, with the husband at arm's length from the child's illnesses. In some instances, the husband vehemently endorses his wife's history of the child, even when it is proven definitively to have been untrue. Although she was originally described as generally affable with medical and nursing staff, broader experience shows that she may have a hostile, difficult, and demanding personality. Some mothers, in their roles as champions of their ill children, have had good success at enlisting the admiration of their communities; making useful, powerful, or lucrative contacts; or obtaining benefits consequent on the child's illness, including wish-fulfillment trips.[51] Features of Münchausen syndrome[20,52] and a history of problems related to her reproductive system (including spontaneous abortions during motor vehicle crashes), unsubstantiated by her medical records, are not uncommon in these mothers, but they may lack a documented psychiatric history, or it may be unavailable. (Finding out if psychiatric records exist, much less what they contain, is often difficult.)

Mothers have been variably diagnosed psychiatrically as normal, depressed, borderline personality disorder, hysterical personality disorder, narcissistic personality disorder, or various other personality disorders.[12,53] MSBP in the context of postpartum depression has also been reported.[54] This circumstance does not mean that the mother has some kind of disease that renders her incapable of discerning right from wrong, that she compulsively performs acts outside her consciousness, or that she is either the unwilling or the unwitting captive of an irresistible impulse. Only rarely is the mother deemed to be psychotic or delusional.[12,20] Some reports cite a history of significant childhood maltreatment in these mothers,[55] including physical and sexual abuse,[32] with the generational legacy of abuse in some way *medicalized,* from the mother's exposure to the medical field, either as a patient or a close party to a sick person. One fascinating single case study proposed that the perpetration of MSBP is related to transgenerational transmission of an attachment disorder; the perpetrator, having been insecurely attached as a child then demonstrating abnormalities of caregiving and care eliciting when she, herself, became a mother.[56] When the behavior of mothers who suffocated their infants was recorded on covert video surveillance, 3 groups emerged: (1) normal, (2) hostile, and (3) paucity of interaction.[57] These interpretations are psychodynamic. Other authors emphasize observable maternal behavior, with the perpetrator first needing to *discharge dysphoric affects* (anger, anxiety, and others), next, having a breakdown in internal inhibitions, and, finally, neutralizing external inhibition, all resulting in the *habit strength* of the assaultive behavior.[58] The primary motivation, according to another, is the "use of a sick child as a vehicle to maintain and regulate a relationship with physicians and other medical personnel and later with other people seen as powerful,"[51] with motivation going beyond needing to be in the limelight; it is, rather, "a dare, a challenge, engaged in compulsively about who is going to be able to outsmart whom."[51] The personality styles, backgrounds, and motivations to perpetrate MSBP (when inferable) are quite diverse, though, "(T)he difficulty that besets the endeavor to understand Münchausen by Proxy is how to judge the veracity of a person who repeatedly dissimulates."[51]

The mother may become suicidal when her duplicity is uncovered or when she becomes aware of professional suspicions. Psychiatric interventions should be offered and available. Why MSBP is overwhelmingly a female-perpetrated form of child abuse is not clear, although female patterns of learned behavior and expression of hostility have been proposed. It certainly stands in contrast to almost every other form of child abuse and neglect (except sexual abuse), in which male and female perpetrators figure in approximately equal numbers.

No evidence whatsoever suggests that the perpetrator of MSBP is unaware of her actions. On the contrary, the planning and organization involved, the minute attention to secrecy, the fact that the assaults are committed without witnesses, and the carefully woven fabric of lies presented to the physician all suggest great awareness. The perpetration of MSBP is volitional; it is also violent. The fact that the violence is encased in duplicity only hides, but does not diminish, its aggression.

Most mothers do not have a criminal history, but a mother occasionally does. They may break into their own homes to stage thefts or set fires, sometimes collecting insurance settlements. They may also be dangerous to others in their midst, with the homicide of relatives or children in their charge, for example, having occasionally been proven or highly suspected. Fabricating factitious illness in pets has also been reported.[59,60]

Perpetrators may also be dangerous to medical professionals. They have been known to undertake criminal behavior such as stalking, breaking and entering, theft, fraud, destruction of property, and death threats. It is no longer uncommon for the perpetrator of MSBP to make false allegations of malpractice by the physician to professional or licensing bodies, or to sue the physician, hospital, or both on one or several of a number of pretexts: defamation of character, malicious reporting, malpractice, wrongful detention of the child, or wrongful death.

DIAGNOSTIC STRATEGIES

Failure to diagnose MSBP means that a fundamentally healthy child and the child's siblings might be irreversibly damaged or killed. Conversely, the failure to exclude MSBP may mean that necessary treatment is withheld from an ill child, a family is not offered prognostic information or genetic counseling, or the child is separated from the family. The single largest impediment to making a diagnosis of MSBP is the failure to include it in the differential diagnosis. Once the diagnosis is entertained and a diagnostic strategy designed, the diagnosis is usually included or excluded relatively quickly.

Once MSBP is considered, the difficulties in pursuing the diagnosis generally revolve around the dilemma of not wishing to expose the child to any more potential risk and yet needing reasonably definitive proof. This clinical judgment call is best made with the assistance of the director of medical services, the head nurse, the primary care nurse, the hospital child-protection team, and, if necessary, the hospital lawyer. At this point, social services and their representative lawyer should be notified of a possible child abuse case. The diagnostic strategy (or strategies) must maximize diagnostic capability while minimizing risk to the child and must obviously take into account access to, and condition of, the child.

When MSBP is suspected, confirmation or elimination of the diagnosis may be undertaken through one of several strategies: the search for evidence of illness fabrication, the search for evidence of an explanation other than MSBP, the separation of the child from the suspected perpetrator, and records review.

The 1st diagnostic strategy, the search for evidence of illness fabrication, includes tests such as toxicology studies if poisoning is suspected, blood group typing, subtyping, or DNA typing if contamination with exogenous blood is suspected, or hidden video monitoring if surreptitious suffocation is suspected. The medical literature contains some fascinating accounts in which evidence of commission has been thus captured: Ipecac poisoning is uncovered by finding a postmortem blood sample that is positive for the alkaloids in ipecac[61] or by toxicologic studies in a living child[62]; factitious bleeding is exposed by minor blood group typing of erythrocytes in urine,[63] injecting radiolabeled erythrocytes as comparisons to the child's *bleeding sites,*[64] DNA typing of the bloody towel presented by the parent compared with that of the child's buccal cells,[65] and comparing the hemoglobin F concentration of an infant's blood to that of the blood stains on the child's bedclothes[66]; factitious diabetes mellitus is confirmed by using ascorbic acid as a marker for the child's own urine[67]; factitious hyperinsulinemic hypoglycemia is discovered by finding simultaneous low C-peptide and high insulin levels in a 1st critical blood sample of a hypoglycemic child[68,69]; and factitious intractable apnea is uncovered by covertly videotaping mothers suffocating their children.[29,70-72]

To a great extent, the physician must choose, or even design, the test, depending on the fabrication that is suspected. The search for evidence of illness fabrication must be carefully planned and executed. Depending on the situation, this search involves setting up the proper chain of evidence, preserving laboratory specimens, continuous monitoring and recording of video units with plans to intervene immediately and decisively if assault is seen, and establishing precise coordination with law enforcement, social services, or both. The advantage of this diagnostic strategy is that, if positive evidence is uncovered and is reliable, it is more likely to be accepted as definitive, medically and legally. The disadvantage is that the child is potentially exposed to at least one more assault. If the test is negative, then distinguishing among absence of assault, failure to capture the assault, or a false-negative test is often impossible.

One diagnostic strategy in the search for evidence of illness fabrication is covert video monitoring. This strategy is highly useful, if somewhat controversial. A video camera with its lens, for example, in what seems to be a sprinkler head or smoke alarm, may be installed and linked to a monitoring and recording unit in a nearby room. Administrators in tertiary care hospitals should seriously consider the diagnostic benefits of such a system, especially when undertaking remodeling. Obviously, this type of system must be in place before the child's admission. If the hospital room has a private bathroom, then closing it off to avoid the possibility of an assault to the child outside the range of the video camera would be prudent.

Useful clinical data may be accrued with videotaping.[29,70-73] One investigator who videotaped mothers smothering their children noted that smothering has been labeled *gentle* battering. The author of this chapter rejects this notion. The video and physiologic recordings showed that both children struggled violently until they lost consciousness. Considerable force was used to obstruct their airways, and this force was needed for at least 70 seconds before electroencephalographic changes, probably associated with loss of consciousness, occurred. Interestingly, in both cases, a soft garment was used to smother the children, and no marks were seen on the lips or around the nose.

The authors further delineated features of the multichannel recordings, "a combination of which may in the future prove to be pathognomonic of this type (smothering) of apnea. . . ."[29] The features included the sudden onset of large body movements during a relatively regular breathing pattern (from struggling induced by airway obstruction); a series of large breaths at approximately 1 minute after the onset of the episode, with a characteristically prolonged expiratory phase, at a relatively slow rate (a response to severe arterial hypoxia); a severe degree of sinus tachycardia; and, last, at approximately 1 minute after the onset of the episode, large slow waves and a subsequent isoelectric baseline on the electroencephalogram typical of hypoxia.[29]

If videotaping is planned, then the multidisciplinary team may want to consult with the hospital attorney. Continuous observation of the video-tape by real-time monitoring is essential, and notifying hospital security and the local police department would be wise because their participation may be needed.

The subject of diagnostic, covert video monitoring in the hospital has engendered some animated debate, with authors addressing the legal, ethical, and logistic aspects of videotaping.[72,74-82] Some authors are concerned with the rights of privacy of parents in the hospital or suggest that a warrant for covert video monitoring be obtained beforehand.[78] Other authors point out that the parental rights to privacy are abrogated when that parent is the agent of the child's possible destruction. In this pediatrician's opinion, the videotape may be considered the equivalent of other tests undertaken in the usual diagnostic process that do not individually require consent; the general medical consent form signed on behalf of the child at the time of admission to the hospital covers most procedures. Furthermore, child abuse statutes in every state permit the taking of pictures without parental consent if child abuse is suspected. In 1 covert video monitoring study of 41 patients, the authors note that

> "specific permission to monitor was included in the admission form for consent to treat given to families on admission to the hospital. Contained within this form is the statement, 'Closed circuit monitoring of patient care may be used for educational or clinical purposes.' In addition, a sign at the entrance to the hospital informs visitors that this facility is monitored and recorded by hidden cameras."[72]

The authors also note that in 4 of 41 cases, MSBP was definitely excluded, a very useful diagnostic milestone that informs further investigation.

The 2nd diagnostic strategy, the search for an explanation other than MSBP, has often been extensive by the time that MSBP is suspected, but it has not necessarily been exhaustive. Certain situations can be found in which an exhaustive search for an explanation other than MSBP is the best diagnostic strategy: when no opportunity or the diagnostic test exists that might capture evidence of commission or when the search for evidence of illness fabrication would expose the child to grave risk. The contending diagnoses on the differential should be those that are subject to definitive inclusion or exclusion. For example, if a child is repeatedly presented to the hospital with apnea that begins only in the presence of the mother, then the disorders that might be causing the child's apnea (however unlikely, for example, a cerebral space–occupying lesion or gastroesophageal reflux) can be sought and can therefore be definitively included or excluded. Positive test results must be carefully scrutinized to ensure that they are positive neither as a result of maternal contamination or intervention nor as a result of being *overcalled;* that is, the range of normal for the test is not reliably delineated, or minimally positive findings are said to account for the massive number of symptoms. Certain gastrointestinal tests seem to be especially vulnerable to this problem, in particular gastrointestinal motility studies[83] and esophageal pH probe studies. Normal gastrointestinal motility excludes the diagnosis of chronic intestinal pseudo-obstruction.[84,85] The advantage of this diagnostic strategy is that the gathering of diagnostic evidence does not involve exposing the child to the possibility of another assault. The disadvantage is that it can be time consuming and expensive, and risks exist to the patient of various diagnostic procedures or prolonged hospitalization.

The 3rd diagnostic strategy, the separation of the child from the parent, may be a very useful diagnostic strategy. In certain circumstances, this action carries the most diagnostic weight and is the least malignant. Having a baseline against which to compare the child's subsequent course during separation is important, whether the separation occurs in the hospital or in a foster home. The baseline is the well-documented history of the child's symptoms and signs as provided by the mother. Therefore the only major change that is made in the child's care during the separation should be the presence of the caretaker. In some instances, the fabrication of illness causes irreversible medical problems or that the fabrication of illness is piled onto an already-existing illness. Only reversible conditions of the child can be expected to improve and these only to the degree and at a rate that is consonant with the condition itself. The advantage of this diagnostic strategy is that it can be definitive without exposing the child to further risk. The disadvantage is that, if MSBP is not present, then an ill child has been separated unnecessarily and perhaps harmfully from the mother, and correct diagnosis has been delayed. One way to minimize the possible disadvantages is to have supervised visits with the mother. The supervision must be constant and scrupulous, with no foods, medications, or candy permitted. The 4th diagnostic strategy is records review. This diagnostic strategy involves the reformulation of a differential diagnosis—one that is comprehensive without being promiscuous. This strategy follows from the observation that the pivotal facts, although present in the medical record, are frequently obscured by the sheer volume of information. In other words, the crucial data are there, but they are buried.

Furthermore, the importance of a comprehensive survey of the child's medical presentation has been repeatedly overshadowed by the immediacy of the crises. Curiously, the more chronic and intractable the child's problem is, the less the likelihood is that the problem is given a fresh, comprehensive look. Finally, a sort of colonial system of medical care sometimes evolves, with fragments of the child's condition being parceled off to subspecialists, whose purview extends only to the edge of their organ systems of interest. They accept without question the *fact* of abnormalities in another system. Overview is neglected. The totality of the presentation is lost. Records review may be the preferred diagnostic strategy because it is low risk and often definitive. Records review may be the only diagnostic strategy available when, for example, the child is alive but is unavailable for some reason, when the symptoms and signs of fabrication are long gone, or when the child is dead.

For most pediatric patients, a thorough records review is straightforward; the examiner reads and remembers. Records are relatively brief and come from a small number of medical facilities. That a substantially different approach to records review is in order when MSBP is suspected is a consequence of 3 typical features: (1) the record is mammoth, (2) the legal implications are broad, and (3) the stakes are high. Records often run to thousands of pages, sometimes from dozens of medical facilities. The physician may be called to testify in civil or criminal proceedings, or both, where the medical facts—perhaps hundreds of thousands of them—may be minutely tracked and challenged, as may the process by which the diagnosis was distilled from the facts. A computerized system for data entry, storage, organization, and retrieval is often indispensable, and any one of several commercially available database-management systems can be adapted for this purpose. Records pages should be numbered immediately so that data can be noted with their corresponding page numbers and later found again.

Because the medical and nursing records are often complicated, using someone (or several people) experienced in both inpatient and outpatient pediatrics to review the records would be best. Advantages and disadvantages exist to working with original medical records. The advantages are that poor quality or missed duplication of records is not an issue and that vital information on oversized pages is accessible. The disadvantages are considerable: Pages cannot be numbered, and accessibility, space, and the simultaneous availability of the record and the necessary computer equipment are generally problematic.

In reality, reviewing original records is usually impossible because of geographic or logistic problems. In these usual circumstances, care must be taken to ensure, as far as possible, that photocopied records, or records scanned onto a CD-ROM, are complete. In the process of the records review, compiling a cumulative dated list of factors such as prescribed medications, operations, consultations, hospitalizations, diagnoses explored, diagnostic tests performed and their results, interventions attempted, and school days missed is often helpful.

The diagnostic strategies used to detect MSBP in its most common presentations are outlined in Table 144-2. These diagnostic strategies will not fit every type of suspected event, and the physician must tailor the diagnostic strategy to the type of perpetration suspected. This effort may involve contacting colleagues in related fields so as to gather information or to seek help. Commonly, various diagnostic strategies must be combined. An excellent example of evaluating seizures by Barber and Davis[86] appears in Box 144-2, and the comprehensive approach can be adapted to many presentations.

DIFFERENTIAL DIAGNOSIS

Most children who are persistently presented to the physician for medical care are not victims of MSBP.[87]

Table 144-2 Symptoms, Methods of Fabricating Illness and Corresponding Diagnostic Strategies in Münchausen Syndrome by Proxy

PRESENTATION	METHOD OF SIMULATION OR PRODUCTION OR BOTH	METHOD OF DIAGNOSIS
Apnea	Manual suffocation	Video monitoring
		Implantable ECG recorder
		Diagnosis by exclusion
		Patient with pinch marks on nose
		Witnessed
	Poisoning	Toxicology (gastric or blood)
	Tricyclic antidepressants	Toxicology of IV fluid
	Hydrocarbon	
Seizures	Lying	Diagnosis by exclusion
	Poisoning	Toxicology or assay of blood, urine, IV fluid, milk
	Phenothiazines	Serum and urine sodium concentrations
	Hydrocarbons	
	Salt	
	Sulfonylurea	
	Tricyclic antidepressants	
	Suffocation or carotid sinus pressure	Witnessed
		Forensic photographs of pressure points
Diarrhea	Phenolphthalein or other laxative poisoning	Stool or diaper positive
	Salt poisoning	Assay of formula or gastric contents
Vomiting	Emetic poisoning	Assay for drug
	Injection of air into gastrostomy tube	Video monitoring
	Lying	Hospital observation
CNS depression	Drugs	Assays of blood, gastric contents, urine, IV fluid, hair; analysis of insulin type; video monitoring
	Diphenoxylate and atropine (Lomotil)	
	Insulin	
	Chloral hydrate	
	Clonidine	
	Barbiturates or narcotics	
	Benzodiazepines	
	Aspirin	
	Diphenhydramine	
	Tricyclic antidepressants	
	Acetaminophen	
	Hydrocarbons	
	Chlordiazepoxide	
	Phenytoin	
	Phenobarbital	
	Carbamazepine	
	Suffocation	See Apnea and Seizures
Bleeding	Rodenticide (warfarin) poisoning	Toxicology
	Phenolphthalein poisoning	Diapers positive
	Exogenous blood applied	Blood group antigen profiling; DNA typing
		^{51}Cr labeling of erythrocytes
	Exsanguination of child	Single-blind study
		Witnessed
	Addition of substances (paint, cocoa, dyes)	Testing; washing
Rash	Drug poisoning	Assay
	Scratching	Diagnosis of exclusion
	Caustics applied/painting skin	Assay or wash off
Fever	Contamination with infected material	Witnessed
	Materials	Improper taping of line discovered
	Saliva	Type of organism growing from infected sites
	Feces	
	Dirt	Trial separation
	Contaminated water	Epidemiologic assay (relative-risk assessment)
	Coffee grounds	Diagnosis by exclusion
	Vaginal secretions	
	Target tissues	

Table 144-2 Symptoms, Methods of Fabricating Illness and Corresponding Diagnostic Strategies in Münchausen Syndrome by Proxy—cont'd

PRESENTATION	METHOD OF SIMULATION OR PRODUCTION OR BOTH	METHOD OF DIAGNOSIS
	Blood Skin Bones Bladder	
	Falsifying temperature	Careful charting, rechecking (especially urine for core body temperature)
	Falsifying chart	Careful charting, rechecking Duplication (ghost record) of temperature chart in nursing station

Adapted with permission from Elsevier from Rosenberg DA. Web of deceit: a literature review of Münchausen syndrome by proxy. *Child Abuse Negl.* 1987;11:547-563. *ECG,* Electrocardiographic; *IV,* intravenous; *CNS,* central nervous system.

BOX 144-2 Practical Guidance: How to Avoid Making a False Diagnosis of Epilepsy

- The starting point is obtaining a meticulous history supplemented by carefully chosen diagnostic tests.
- Consider first the differential diagnosis of paroxysmal events (gastroesophageal reflux, gratification phenomena, breath-holding attacks, cardiac arrhythmia, syncope, metabolic disturbances, reflex anoxic seizures, and pseudoseizures).
- Look for clinical epilepsy syndromes with typical supporting electroencephalogram (EEG) findings.
- Ask the caregiver to video *episodes.* Most families have the means to perform this task, and some hospitals may be able to loan equipment.
- Do not start treatment until sure. At a minimum, seek independent corroboration of a parent's history or supportive EEG findings. Starting anticonvulsant medication immediately is rarely necessary, and having EEG information beforehand is good practice.
- Be especially wary of making the diagnosis if the EEG is normal. Seek confirmation from purported witnesses early on in the course of investigations, preferably an independent 3rd party.
- Beware of the caregiver who uses the threat of harm coming to the child so as to influence clinical decision making.
- Consider hospital admission if the reported episodes are frequent. Cessation of episodes during periods of observation is suspicious.
- Actively seek to verify details given by the caregiver regarding seizures or other aspects of history.
- Question discrepancies; children with severe, polymorphic epilepsy do not generally have normal neurodevelopment.
- Take and analyze blood and urine from any child being presented for the 1st time with a seizure; they may have been poisoned. Ensure that the urine is screened for relevant substances, not just drugs of abuse. Store serum so that future quantitative analysis is possible.
- In the sick child, glucose and electrolytes will usually be checked. An electrocardiogram should also be routine; it may provide a clue to poisoning with tricyclic antidepressants.
- If poisoning is suspected, then collect other body fluids (eg, vomitus, fluid from gastric lavage).
- Look for subtle signs of smothering (eg, petechial bruising to the face, nasal bleeding).
- Arrange appropriate supportive investigations, including prolactin levels, raised glucose level, and white blood count (after prolonged generalized seizures), prolonged EEG or video-EEG records, pH studies, or tilt-table tests.

Adapted with permission from Elsevier from Barber M, Davis P. Fits, faints, or fatal fantasy? Fabricated seizures and child abuse. *Arch Dis Child.* 2002;86:230-233.

Waring discusses the 2 questions that the physician must consider with any child: "What is the matter with the patient?" and "Why is this child being brought for care at this moment?" The answer to the 1st question is taught in medical schools and during residency training, whereas the ability to answer *both* questions, in Yudkin's words, is "the beginning of real medicine."[87,88]

Most children have a primary organic illness that accounts for the totality of their presentation, but other possibilities exist that may account for the persistence. Box 144-3 gives the differential diagnosis of persistent presentation.

Genuine illness and MSBP may coexist. The discovery of a real illness in a child who is persistently presented does not exclude MSBP. The question then becomes, "Does this illness reasonably explain the severity, extent, and type of the child's symptoms and signs?" Occasionally, the distinction between MSBP and pathological physician shopping, or magnification

BOX 144-3 Differential Diagnosis of Persistent Presentation

Organic illness
Anxious parent
Developmentally delayed parent
Vulnerable child syndrome
Psychogenic illness
Münchausen syndrome by proxy
Münchausen syndrome

BOX 144-4 Münchausen Syndrome by Proxy: Criteria for a Definitive Diagnosis by Inclusion

1. Child has been repeatedly presented for medical care.

AND

2. Test or event is positive for tampering with child or with child's medical situation.

AND

3. Positivity of test or event is not credibly the result of test error or misinterpretation or of miscommunication or specimen mishandling.

AND

4. No explanation for the positive test or event other than illness falsification is medically possible.

AND

5. No findings credibly exclude illness falsification.

Reprinted with permission from Elsevier from Rosenberg DA. Münchausen syndrome by proxy: medical diagnostic criteria. *Child Abuse Negl.* 2003;27:421-430.

of a child's real but minimal illness for the parent's own psychological or fiscal gain, may not be clear. For specific cases that seem to fall at the edges of the definition of MSBP, a point worth remembering is that the name applied to the child's circumstances is not so material as a careful assessment of the threatened harm to the child.

DIAGNOSTIC CRITERIA

When MSBP is suspected, the strength of the known facts may extend from weak to definitive. Thus different degrees of diagnostic conviction may be found, not only from case to case, but also within a case, depending on the stage of the assessment. Here are diagnostic criteria for a definitive diagnosis and a possible diagnosis of MSBP. Because the gathering of evidence in a case may ultimately diminish the likelihood or altogether exclude MSBP, diagnostic criteria for the uncertain diagnosis and the definitely excluded diagnosis are also given below.[89]

Diagnostic criteria serve to discriminate efficiently between one particular diagnosis and all others. Collectively, the diagnostic criteria for a disorder are the smallest set of findings that must be present to make a diagnosis.

Each diagnostic criterion must be present to make a diagnosis. Each criterion must be pivotal, meaning that its presence is required for, and its absence excludes, the diagnosis. Each finding must be credibly observable. Other competent observers, using the same method, would observe the finding the same way. Thus the observation would be replicable. To summarize, each criterion is necessary, and the criteria collectively are sufficient, for diagnosis.

Definitive Diagnosis

The definitive diagnosis of MSBP can be made in 1 of 2 ways: (1) by inclusion or (2) by exclusion.

A diagnosis by inclusion is one supported by incontrovertible evidence of commission. For example, if a mother smothers the child that she had previously and repeatedly presented for apnea, and if her act were captured with covert videotaping in hospital, then the definitive diagnosis of MSBP would be one by inclusion. Box 144-4 lists the criteria for the definitive diagnosis by inclusion of MSBP.

A diagnosis by exclusion is one in which all other possible explanations for the child's condition have been considered and excluded. A diagnosis by exclusion is the only diagnosis left standing after an exhaustive investigation. For example, if a child is presented with recurrent apnea that begins exclusively in one person's presence and results in observable clinical compromise, if the child is conclusively shown to not otherwise exhibit apnea, and if all possible medical conditions that might account for the apnea are properly investigated and definitively excluded, then the definitive diagnosis of MSBP would be one by exclusion. Box 144-5 lists the criteria for the definitive diagnosis by exclusion of MSBP.

Possible Diagnosis

A possible diagnosis of MSBP is one among several likely diagnoses. Box 144-6 lists the criteria for the possible diagnosis of MSBP. Medical professionals are legally mandated to report child abuse to the local authority when they have a reasonable suspicion of it. *Reasonable suspicion* is not a term of art in medicine, but rather roughly translates into the set of diagnostic criteria here noted as a possible diagnosis.

Inconclusive Determination: Cannot Know

Rather than increasing the weight of medical evidence in support of a diagnosis of MSBP, accumulating data may instead diminish its likelihood. Medical criteria for inconclusive findings—that is, for MSBP being indeterminate—are therefore articulated here. *Cannot know* means that, although the collection of data is complete, the data are insufficient to determine the diagnosis. The investigator can confidently neither establish nor eliminate MSBP as the diagnosis. *Cannot know* differs from possible diagnosis because implicit in a *cannot know* determination is the assertion that all relevant and available strategies for diagnosis have been exhausted. This position is in contrast to a possible diagnosis, in which an expectation of further diagnostic strategy can be found. Box 144-7 lists the criteria for an inconclusive *(cannot know)* determination.

BOX 144-5 Münchausen Syndrome by Proxy: Criteria for a Definitive Diagnosis by Exclusion

1. Child has been repeatedly presented for medical care.

AND

2. All diagnoses other than illness falsification have been credibly eliminated so that:
   a. If the child is alive, then the competing diagnoses are those that took into account the child's major medical findings, and that account for the entirety of the child's presentation. (A major medical finding is one that is objectively observed, sufficiently specific as to help formulate the range of diagnoses, and verifiable in the record.)

   OR

   b. If the child is alive, then separation of the child from the alleged perpetrator results in resolution of the child's reversible medical problems, in accordance with their degree and speed of reversibility. No variable other than the separation can logically and fully account for the child's improvement.

   OR

   c. If the child is dead, then autopsy examination does not reveal a cause of death that is credibly of accidental, natural, or suicidal manner.

AND

3. No findings credibly exclude illness falsification.

Reprinted with permission from Elsevier from Rosenberg DA. Münchausen syndrome by proxy: medical diagnostic criteria. *Child Abuse Negl.* 2003;27:421-430.

BOX 144-6 Münchausen Syndrome by Proxy: Criteria for Possible Diagnosis

1. Child has been repeatedly presented for medical care.

AND

2. Test or event is presumptively positive for tampering with child or with child's medical situation. No other explanation is readily apparent. No findings seem to exclude illness falsification.

   OR

   Child has a condition that cannot be fully explained medically, despite a respectable initial evaluation, at least. Cogent hypothesis suggests a faked medical condition. No findings seem to exclude illness falsification.

Reprinted with permission from Elsevier from Rosenberg DA. Münchausen syndrome by proxy: medical diagnostic criteria. *Child Abuse Negl.* 2003;27:421-430.

Definitely Not

Definitely not MSBP means that the diagnosis can be absolutely eliminated because a wholly credible alternative explanation is at hand. To allow degrees of certainty within this diagnostic option, the physician might want to use some kind of qualifier, for example, *probably not* MSBP. *Probably not* MSBP is about the same as saying that, in all likelihood, an alternative explanation is at hand. The fact that diagnostic criteria for the exclusion of MSBP are included means that, as with other pediatric disorders, inevitably, more suspected cases than actual cases exist. Recognizing this situation means also recognizing the need for the swiftest and most decisive diagnostic test but one in which the risk to the child does not seem to be excessive. Extreme care must be taken not to overdiagnose MSBP or to be married to the diagnosis in the absence of sufficient evidence. Cases of misdiagnosed MSBP[90] are a real tragedy for the family and child. Box 144-8 lists the criteria for excluding the diagnosis of MSBP.

BOX 144-7 Münchausen Syndrome by Proxy: Criteria for Inconclusive Determination

1. Child has been repeatedly presented for medical care.

AND

2. The relevant and available information has been reviewed, the child has been appropriately evaluated, or both.

AND

3. Physician is left with a differential diagnosis, rather than a single diagnosis.

AND

4. Conclusively affirming one diagnosis is not possible.

AND

5. Excluding all but one diagnosis conclusively on the differential is not possible.

AND

6. Conclusively excluding all but one diagnosis on the differential diagnosis is not possible.

Reprinted with permission from Elsevier from Rosenberg DA. Münchausen syndrome by proxy: medical diagnostic criteria. *Child Abuse Negl.* 2003;27:421-430.

BOX 144-8 Münchausen Syndrome by Proxy: Criteria for Excluding the Diagnosis

1. Child has been repeatedly presented for medical care.

AND

2. What had seemed to be possible falsification of illness has been wholly and credibly accounted for in some other way.

Reprinted with permission from Elsevier from Rosenberg DA. Münchausen syndrome by proxy: medical diagnostic criteria. *Child Abuse Negl.* 2003;27:421-430.

INTERVENTION

A list of treatment directives for all cases in which MSBP is suspected is not possible. The reader, however, may find the following considerations useful:

1. **Optimally, the child can be protected and the definitive data to either include or exclude the diagnosis can be simultaneously collected.**

Professionals find themselves poised between weighing the eventual usefulness of these data against the possibility of a mishap occurring to the child during the data-collection process. When further diagnostic procedures place the child in a situation of untenable risk, the protection of the child is always the paramount consideration. Because child protection is a civil matter, the legal burden of proof is preponderance of the evidence. Thus absolute diagnostic proof is not necessary, and, in its absence, epidemiologic evidence pertaining to the case may be sufficiently compelling.

2. **A multidisciplinary team should be involved early in the investigation.**

The county department of social services should be contacted before any discussion with the family so that the medical concerns are understood and the county is involved in the plan development, including the possibility of being prepared with a restraining order. Contacts, meeting, and planning must sometimes be done on an emergency basis so that the child is not exposed to potential harm.

Some individuals who are not customarily members of a hospital child-protection team might be included. The social worker from the county to which the case has been reported is a pivotal person. Much will depend on the social worker's communication with the medical staff and understanding of the case. Given the volume and complexity of the data and the generally high rate of staff turnover among county social workers, these individuals should work in pairs. Any way to circumvent the widespread and inefficient practice of having an *intake worker* start the case and then an *ongoing worker* continue it should be pursued. The supervisor of the social workers and the county attorney should be similarly included in the multidisciplinary team from the start.

Two psychiatrists or 2 psychologists (or 2 from both disciplines) should be engaged to participate. Optimally, one party is assigned to the family and the other to the medical and nursing staff. The family needs extend not only to evaluation, but also to support. After confrontation of the family with the suspected diagnosis, the mother, who is generally the alleged perpetrator, is at increased risk for suicide.[20,91] The child also needs to be developmentally and, if of sufficient age, psychologically evaluated. Interactional assessments by an experienced developmental psychologist may be fruitful.

Police and other law-enforcement personnel should also be involved early, especially if videotaping in the hospital is anticipated. Should an episode of intentional infliction of harm come to light during the videotaping, then the police generally prefer to have prior knowledge of the case and may want to be prepared with an arrest warrant. A decision must be made between the hospital and law enforcement as to which entity will undertake video monitoring.

The primary care nurse and the head nurse should be included in the multidisciplinary child-protection team. The primary care nurse is often the person who has spent the most time with the child and the family over an extended period and multiple hospitalizations. This person often has valuable information about a case that may not be known to the others on the team, and this individual certainly must be included in any plans that involve diagnostic procedures for MSBP. The primary care nurse often becomes responsible for important items such as documentation and chain of evidence of specimens.

Finally, having a good clinical epidemiologist participating with the multidisciplinary team from the beginning is often advisable because data of commission (eg, a videotape showing the mother suffocating the infant, a definitive blood test showing exogenous insulin in the child's body) are often unobtainable. The diagnostic alternative to these data is the calculation of the relative risk to the child of being in the maternal care. For example, if the child has an unspecified illness characterized by vomiting, failure to thrive, and multiple hospitalizations, then an epidemiologist can review the child's records and calculate the relative risk to the child of losing weight at home compared with that of losing weight in the hospital. In the absence of data of commission, relative-risk data may be the most compelling evidence to present to the court. Data that can be interpreted to the court in lay language by the epidemiologist or by the attending clinician is helpful.

The multidisciplinary child-protection team is under no obligation to include the mother's attorney (if she has engaged one) or any other professionals who may divulge either the diagnostic strategies planned or the content of the proceedings to the family. Care must be taken in this regard.

Because medical records in cases of suspected MSBP are often voluminous, efficient review must be organized prospectively. Otherwise, the result of the records review is a mass of detail from which no trends can be elicited and therefore no conclusions drawn. Therefore, in beginning the review of the records, certain patterns are shortly recognized, and these preliminary observations can then be formalized into questions the investigator asks. In a child with a chief complaint of intractable vomiting, did the child have any documented episodes of vomiting while in the presence of a physician or nurse? In a child with repeated episodes of apnea, how many episodes, if any, actually began in the presence of someone other than the mother? In a child with recurrent fevers in the hospital, who actually took and charted the temperatures when the child was febrile?

3. **All medical records of all siblings must be reviewed, including autopsy reports and death certificates.**

The process often requires some vigor to obtain these records, but they are vital. Neither police summaries nor social work records are sufficient.

4. **Review of the parents' medical, educational, and work history, as far as possible, from documents should take place, especially if the parent claims various illnesses or medical education.**

5. **Several methods may be used, singly or in combination, to gain access to records.**

In some instances, having signed parental consent to obtain the records is possible.

Otherwise, the attorneys on the multidisciplinary team may advise canvassing the area with subpoenas or requesting court-ordered discovery of records.

6. **Presentation of the review of records to the multidisciplinary team should include, as briefly as possible, a chronologic review followed by a review of discrepancies, if any.**

How does the mother's history compare with the observed clinical findings in the child? How do the laboratory test results compare with the given histories (eg, are drug levels continually subtherapeutic or toxic with a history of absolute compliance)? Listing all of the possible questions is impossible, but the data will lead the reviewer to which questions are important. In reviewing a case of suspected MSBP, considering and exploring all possible organic explanations is essential.

7. **When presenting a case of MSBP to the civil or juvenile court, some strategies of presentation may assist in coming to a conclusion.**

Despite the many hours spent in reviewing records and making an extensive chronologic compilation of the child's medical history, presentation of the information to the court in long, narrative form often only confuses, rather than elucidates, the material. A short summary is often better. Questions may then be asked to clarify or expand on particular events.

Graphs and charts, clearly readable and with a single issue to illuminate, often better illustrate a complex issue than a long, verbal narrative. For example, a growth chart may show that the child consistently gains weight in the hospital but loses weight at home. A histogram may show the number of apnea episodes that originated in the presence of the mother compared with the number that originated in the presence of the nursing staff or grandmother.

Cases typically involve conflicting medical opinions, and the parents usually have medical experts testify in their behalf. These experts may be the person's colleagues. A clear grasp of the medical and epidemiologic evidence and a professional, nonadversarial attitude is always best.

The perpetrator only rarely admits to MSBP; however, curiously, she will more often agree to voluntary services as long as the court is not involved and a dependency petition is not filed. No success with this approach has been reported. Experience has shown that court-ordered intervention is necessary if any hope of successful protection of the child can be found.

8. **Recommending out-of-home placement for the child is prudent.**[20,32]

This measure ensures protection of the child and a diagnostic period of separation to see how the child's health fares. If a mother has hitherto only simulated but not produced illness this is no guarantee that she will not do something more harmful to the child in the future. *Simulators* may become *producers* of illness. Confrontation of the parent with the news of the suspected diagnosis does not, in and of itself, ensure safety for the child.[20,32,92]

The reader is cautioned in particular about the dangers of placing the child with a family member or friend. This situation is always difficult because, for the child, the easiest transition may be to an aunt or grandmother, but the perpetrator may have access to the child, despite the relative's or the friend's promises to the contrary. This decision places the child at potential dire risk.

9. **If the child is to remain in the hospital for a time, then a medically experienced person must supervise all visits with all family members to ensure that no one is tampering with the child's medical care.**

In some instances, the best course of action is to ask the court for a short (ie, 10-day to 2-week) period of hospitalization with only supervised parental visits as a diagnostic trial to determine if the child's symptoms floridly persist. If they do not, then concern about MSBP is heightened. If they do, then the court should be asked to vacate the order and turn attention to a fresh look for an organic diagnosis. This approach is useful only if the child's symptoms and signs, if induced, would reasonably be expected to abate rather quickly in the absence of ongoing assault.

10. **Recommending out-of-home placement of siblings is prudent because they may become the next victims if they remain in the home.**

All siblings must at least have court-ordered medical evaluations and review of records.

11. **Once the child is in foster care, the health status of the child must be monitored and documented closely by the same physicians.**

Although having the original physician or set of physicians involved in the child's ongoing care is often optimal, this arrangement is sometimes not practical for reasons of geographic circumstances or temperament.

12. **Deciding when to send the child home is difficult.** If the diagnosis is indeed MSBP, then the same guidelines that apply to other forms of child abuse and neglect should be applied in consideration of when to send the child home; that is, the perpetrator must acknowledge that she committed these acts, she must have some insight into the reasons for it, and she must provide reasonable assurance that not only insight, but also sufficient change has occurred to ensure the safety of the child. Very little information is available on family reunification after psychiatric intervention. In one study, family reunification was thought to be feasible in certain cases, but the authors cautioned that long-term follow-up is necessary to monitor the safety of the child and assess whether the perpetrator's mental health has deteriorated.[92] The mother's therapist will discuss with the court and the child-protection team specific issues that concern the safety of the child. If the mother and the psychiatrist insist that all the information is privileged, then the court has no way to determine that the children will be safe at home, and other permanent arrangements must be made for them.

13. **Even if the children are removed permanently and parental rights are terminated, subsequent children born to the mother are at high risk of being victims of MSBP.**

In some instances, no formal method is available by which to keep track of the mother's pregnancies; but every effort must be made to protect future children.

LEGAL CONSIDERATIONS

In a courtroom or out, physicians are not required to translate the degree of diagnostic conviction into a legal equivalent. Terms such as *probable cause, reasonable suspicion, preponderance of the evidence, clear and convincing evidence,* and *evidence beyond a reasonable doubt* have a specific meaning in the law. If asked whether the evidence conforms to any of these burdens, or if a reasonable degree of medical certainty exists about the diagnosis (a popular question), the medical language that is meaningful to the physician should be used and distilled into lay terms that best embody the physician's meaning. Legal terminology should be avoided unless definitions have been precisely rendered and are in the court record.

The physician should be alert to attempted manipulation by lawyers. The disputatious lawyer is no more a threat, in this regard, than the pleasingly respectful lawyer. The physician should not be badgered, flattered, or lulled into a small, but medically unjustifiable, resizing of opinion or into being persuaded that the physician is a standard-bearer for a good and righteous cause. The lawyer must be reminded that the court appearance is meant only to provide as balanced, thorough, and comprehensible an interpretation of the medical data as is possible. An important point to remember is that practicing attorneys have jobs that are different from those of physicians.

A diagnosis of MSBP may have been based, at least in part, on the information that the physician reviewed in records. The physician may be asked if the professional opinion would change given different or additional information. In reality, few instances exist in which the physician can be absolutely sure that all existing records have been reviewed. If asked whether a change of diagnosis would occur, or degree of conviction about it, should new information be given, the most accurate answer is often that the possibility exists but, absent the information and the time to think it over, the likelihood of that possibility is impossible to determine.

One of the responsibilities of the judge or jury, not the physician, is to determine if the conclusion and the reasons for the conclusion contribute to a finding that the burden of proof has been met.

PHYSICIANS AND MÜNCHAUSEN SYNDROME BY PROXY

The pathogenic role of a health care system that over-investigates and prescribes unnecessarily something that, in short, promotes false illness has been rightly identified as contributing to MSBP.[93] However, this notion is perhaps too abstract. After all, what is a system other than people? Physicians see many children with persistent illness, most of which are identifiably organic, some of which follow an expected course, but some of which are peculiar or do not conform tidily to textbook descriptions. Physicians do not expect a false history. Young physicians are worried by the cautionary tales of missed diagnoses that they have absorbed throughout training; seasoned physicians are haunted by their own experiences of having missed a timely diagnosis of serious illness because this circumstance is almost universal in a long and busy primary care practice. Most physicians want to be thorough. The hierarchy in the medical world places the opinion of a subspecialist above that of the generalist. Indeed, a curious and paradoxical weakness of famous children's hospitals is the greater likelihood of attributing exotic, but wrong, organic diagnosis when the real problem is MSBP. Relief can be found at having a consultant label a hitherto inexplicable child with an organic diagnosis, even when the label is doubtful. A well-founded fear of litigation pervades the practice of medicine. What used to be known as *defensive medicine* has now become almost mainstream medicine. Little time exists for pondering.

Personal vulnerabilities of some physicians may make it difficult for them to say, "I don't know." Or, some may have a certain pride that "Only I can manage this case"[94] or become married to a obscure or pet diagnosis, even when the accumulating evidence is against it.

These realities, combined with the diversity of perpetrators of MSBP, have led to the sensible suggestion that the prevention of MSBP "might not be from understanding perpetrators better, but from better understanding of physicians and the health system."[95] How is this task accomplished? Escaping the culture of investigation and subspecialty referral is nearly impossible. Besides which, such a culture is often helpful to a patient. Therefore, because the most useful warning sign for MSBP are symptoms, signs, and tests that are incongruent, perhaps the most practical answer is that MSBP should routinely be on the differential diagnosis for *persistence with incongruence,* just as pneumonia is routinely on the differential for dyspnea. Every physician knows that most possible diagnoses on a differential will be wrong, hopes that one diagnosis will be right, and realizes that, as the old saying goes, "If you never think of it, you'll never see it." Importantly and by corollary, the physician will never exclude it. Warning signs are not diagnoses; rather, they are features that might mean one of several possibilities. However, if a child's presentation does not make sense, then the reason may be that it does not make sense.

CONCLUSION

A child who is a victim of MSBP is at high risk of harm. The fact that the perpetrator abruptly desists from the assault does not ensure that the situation is even minimally adequate for the child. The impetus to attack the child repeatedly and the ability to objectify the child in the first place and to use the child as a tool generally reflects a lack of empathy so profound as to likely hobble the overall capacity for mothering. Regrettably, cases involving MSBP may first be identified by a multidisciplinary child-fatality review board. However, although help for the child who has died is too late, other children in the family may be protected as a result. The dangerousness of perpetrators of MSBP should never be underestimated.

SUGGESTED RESOURCE

Hymel KP, American Academy of Pediatrics, Committee on Child Abuse and Neglect, National Association of Medical Examiners. Distinguishing sudden infant death syndrome from child abuse fatalities. *Pediatrics.* 2006;118(1):421-427.

REFERENCES

1. Meadow R. Munchausen syndrome by proxy: the hinterland of child abuse. *Lancet*. 1977;2:343-345.
2. Feldman MD. Denial in Munchausen syndrome by proxy: the consulting psychiatrist's dilemma. *Int J Psychiatry Med*. 1994;24:121-128.
3. Ostfeld BM, Feldman MD. Factitious disorder by proxy: awareness among mental health practitioners. *Gen Hosp Psychiatry*. 1996;18:113-116.
4. Szajnberg NM, Moilanen I, Kanerva A, et al. Munchausen-by-proxy syndrome: countertransference as a diagnostic tool. *Bull Menninger Clin*. 1996;60:229-237.
5. Freckelton I. Munchausen syndrome by proxy and criminal prosecutions for child abuse. *J Law Med*. 2005;12:261-266.
6. Ayoub CC, Schreier HA, Keller C. Munchausen by proxy: presentations in special education. *Child Maltreat*. 2002; 7:149-159.
7. Royal College of Pediatrics and Child Health. *Fabricated or Induced Illness by Carers—Report of the Working Party*. London, UK: Royal College of Pediatrics and Child Health; 2002.
8. Feldman MD, Brown RM. Munchausen by proxy in an international context. *Child Abuse Negl*. 2002;26:509-524.
9. McClure RJ, Davis PM, Meadow SR, et al. Epidemiology of Munchausen syndrome by proxy, non-accidental poisoning, and non-accidental suffocation. *Arch Dis Child*. 1996;75:57-61.
10. Schreier HA. Error in Munchausen by proxy defined. *Pediatrics*. 2004;113:1851-1852.
11. Denny SJ, Grant CC, Pinnock R. Epidemiology of Munchausen syndrome by proxy in New Zealand. *J Paediatr Child Health*. 2001;37:240-243.
12. Sheridan MS. The deceit continues: an updated literature review of Munchausen syndrome by proxy. *Child Abuse Negl*. 2003;27:431-451.
13. Makar AF, Squier PJ. Munchausen syndrome by proxy: father as perpetrator. *Pediatrics*. 1990;85:370-373.
14. Meadow R. Munchausen syndrome by proxy abuse perpetrated by men. *Arch Dis Child*. 1998;78:210-216.
15. Wright M. *A Mother's Trial*. New York, NY: Bantam Books; 1984.
16. Atoynatan TH, O'Reilly E, Loin L. Munchausen syndrome by proxy. *Child Psychiatry Hum Dev*. 1988;19:3-13.
17. Lasher LJ, Feldman MD. Celiac disease as a manifestation of Munchausen by proxy. *South Med J*. 2004;97:67-69.
18. Richardson GF. Munchausen syndrome by proxy. *Am Fam Physician*. 1987;36:119-123.
19. Carrell S. Texas nurse found guilty of killing child. *Am Med News*. 1984;1-27.
20. Rosenberg D. Web of deceit: a literature review of Munchausen syndrome by proxy. *Child Abuse Negl*. 1987; 11:547-563.
21. Alexander R, Smith W, Stevenson R. Serial Munchausen syndrome by proxy. *Pediatrics*. 1990;86:581-585.
22. Meadow R. Mothering to death. *Arch Dis Child*. 1999; 80: 359-362.
23. Bryk M, Siegel PT. My mother caused my illness: the story of a survivor of Munchausen by proxy syndrome. *Pediatrics*. 1997;100:1-7.
24. Janofsky JS. Munchausen syndrome in a mother and daughter: an unusual presentation of folie á deux. *J Nerv Ment Dis*. 1986;174:368-370.
25. Awadallah N, Vaughan A, Franco K, et al. Munchausen by proxy: a case, chart series, and literature review of older victims. *Child Abuse Negl*. 2005;29:931-941.
26. Conway SP, Pond MN. Munchausen syndrome by proxy abuse: a foundation for adult Munchausen. *Aust N Z J Psychiatry*. 1995;29:504-507.
27. Raymond CA. Munchausen's may occur in younger persons. *JAMA*. 1987;257:3332.
28. Roth D. How "mild" is mild Munchausen syndrome by proxy? *Isr J Psychiatry Rel Sci*. 1990;27:160-167.
29. Southall DP, Plunkett BM, Banks MW, et al. Covert video recordings of life-threatening child abuse: lessons for child protection. *Pediatrics*. 1997;100:735-760.
30. Kamerling LB, Black XA, Fiser RT. Munchausen syndrome by proxy in the pediatric intensive care unit: an unusual mechanism. *Pediatr Crit Care Med*. 2002;3:305-307.
31. Meadow R. Suffocation, recurrent apnea, and sudden infant death. *J Pediatr*. 1990;117:351-357.
32. McGuire TL, Feldman KW. Psychologic morbidity of children subjected to Munchausen syndrome by proxy. *Pediatrics*. 1989;83:289-292.
33. Beal SM, Blundell HK. Recurrence incidence of sudden infant death syndrome. *Arch Dis Child*. 1988;63:924-930.
34. Bools CN, Neale BA, Meadow SR. Co-morbidity associated with fabricated illness (Munchausen syndrome by proxy). *Arch Dis Child*. 1992;67:77-79.
35. Meadow R. Recurrent cot death and suffocation [letter]. *Arch Dis Child*. 1989;64:179-180.
36. Truman TL, Ayoub CC. Considering suffocatory abuse and Munchausen by proxy in the evaluation of children experiencing apparent life-threatening events and sudden infant death syndrome. *Child Maltreat*. 2002;7:138-148.
37. Ben-Chetrit E, Melmed RN. Recurrent hypoglycaemia in multiple myeloma: a case of Munchausen syndrome by proxy in an elderly patient. *J Intern Med*. 1998;244:175-178.
38. Sigal M, Altmark D, Gelkopf M. Munchausen syndrome by adult proxy revisited. *Isr J Psychiatry Rel Sci*. 1991;1:33-36.
39. Sigal MD, Altmark D, Carmel I. Munchausen syndrome by adult proxy: a perpetrator abusing two adults. *J Nerv Ment Dis*. 1986;174:696-698.
40. Chodorowski Z, Anand JS, Porzezinska B, et al. Consciousness disturbances: a case report of Munchausen by proxy syndrome in an elderly patient. *Przegl Lek*. 2003;60:307-308.
41. Feldman KW, Hickman RO. The central venous catheter as a source of medical chaos in Munchausen syndrome by proxy. *J Pediatr Surg*. 1998;33:623-627.
42. Masterson J, Dunworth R, Williams N. Extreme illness exaggeration in pediatric patients: a variant of Munchausen's by proxy? *Am J Orthopsychiatry*. 1988;58:188-195.
43. Meadow R. Neurological and developmental variants of Munchausen syndrome by proxy. *Dev Med Child Neurol*. 1991;33:270-272.
44. Osterhoudt KC. A toddler with recurrent episodes of unresponsiveness. *Pediatr Emerg Care*. 2004;20:195-197.
45. Yamashita M, Yamashita M, Azuma J. Urinary excretion of ipecac alkaloids in human volunteers. *Vet Hum Toxicol*. 2002;44:257-259.
46. Meadow R. Unnatural sudden infant death. *Arch Dis Child*. 1999;80:7-14.
47. Rosen CL, Frost JD, Glaze DG. Child abuse and recurrent infant apnea. *J Pediatr*. 1986;109:1065-1067.
48. DiMaio VJ, DiMaio D. *Forensic Pathology*. Boca Raton, FL: CRC Press; 2001.
49. Milroy CM. Munchausen syndrome by proxy and intra-alveolar haemosiderin. *Int J Legal Med*. 1999;112:309-312.
50. Forbes A, Acland P. What is the significance of haemosiderin in the lungs of deceased infants? *Med Sci Law*. 2004;44:348-352.
51. Schreier H. On the importance of motivation in Munchausen by proxy: the case of Kathy Bush. *Child Abuse Negl*. 2002;26:537-549.
52. Meadow R. Different interpretations of Munchausen syndrome by proxy. *Child Abuse Negl*. 2003;27(4): 353-355.
53. Bools C, Neale B, Meadow R. Munchausen syndrome by proxy: a study of psychopathology. *Child Abuse Negl*. 1994;18:773-788.
54. Gojer J, Berman T. Postpartum depression and factitious disorder: a new presentation. *Int J Psychiatry Med*. 2000; 30:287-293.

55. Lesnik-Oberstein M. Munchausen syndrome by proxy [letter]. *Child Abuse Negl*. 1986;10:133.
56. Adsheaad G, Bluglass K. A vicious circle: transgenerational attachment representations in a case of factitious illness by proxy. *Attach Hum Dev*. 2001;3:77-95.
57. Adshead G, Brooke D, Samuels M, et al. Maternal behaviors associated with smothering: a preliminary descriptive study. *Child Abuse Negl*. 2000;24:1175-1183.
58. Rand DC, Feldman MD. An explanatory model for Munchausen by proxy abuse. *Int J Psychiatry Med*. 2001; 31: 113-126.
59. Tucker HS, Finlay F, Guiton S. Munchausen syndrome involving pets by proxies. *Arch Dis Child*. 2002;87:263.
60. Munro HM, Thrusfield MV. 'Battered pets': Munchausen syndrome by proxy (factitious illness by proxy). *J Small Anim Pract*. 2001;42:385-389.
61. Schneider DJ, Perez A, Knilamus TE, et al. Clinical and pathological aspects of cardiomyopathy from ipecac administration in Munchausen's syndrome by proxy. *Pediatrics*. 1996;97:902-906.
62. Feldman KW, Christopher DM, Opheim KB. Munchausen syndrome-bulimia by proxy: ipecac as a toxin in child abuse. *Child Abuse Negl*. 1989;13:257-261.
63. Outwater KM, Lipnick RN, Luban NLC, et al. Factitious hematuria: diagnosis by minor blood group typing. *J Pediatr*. 1981;98:95-97.
64. Kurlandsky L, Lukoff JY, Zinkham WH, et al. Munchausen syndrome by proxy: definition of factitious bleeding in an infant by ^{51}Cr labeling of erythrocytes. *Pediatrics*. 1979;63:228-231.
65. Wenk RE. Molecular evidence of Munchausen syndrome by proxy. *Arch Pathol Lab Med*. 2003;127:e36-e37.
66. Bolz WE, Brouwer HG, Schoenmakers CH. Measurement of HbF concentration for diagnosing a case of Munchausen by proxy syndrome. *J Pediatr*. 2006;148:145-146.
67. Nading JH, Duval-Arnould B. Factitious diabetes mellitus confirmed by ascorbic acid. *Arch Dis Child*. 1984;59:166-167.
68. Edidin DV, Farrell EE, Gould VE. Factitious hyperinsulinemic hypoglycemia in infancy: diagnostic pitfalls. *Clin Pediatr*. 2000;39:117-119.
69. Giurgea I, Ulinski T, Touati G, et al. Factitious hyperinsulinism leading to pancreatectomy: severe forms of Munchausen syndrome by proxy. *Pediatrics*. 2005;116:e145-e148.
70. Rosen CL, Frost JD Jr, Bricker T, et al. Two siblings with cardiorespiratory arrest: Munchausen syndrome by proxy or child abuse? *Pediatrics*. 1983;71:715-720.
71. Southall DP, Stebben VA, Rees SV, et al. Apnoeic episodes induced by smothering: two cases identified by covert video surveillance. *Br Med J (Clin Res Ed)*. 1987;294:1637-1641.
72. Hall DE, Eubanks L, Meyyazhagan LS, et al. Evaluation of covert video surveillance in the diagnosis of Munchausen syndrome by proxy: lessons from 41 cases. *Pediatrics*. 2000;105:1305-1312.
73. Epstein MA, Markowitz RL, Gallo DM, et al. Munchausen syndrome by proxy: considerations in diagnosis and confirmation by video surveillance. *Pediatrics*. 1987; 80: 220-224.
74. Evans D. The investigation of life-threatening child abuse and Munchausen syndrome by proxy. *J Med Ethics*. 1995; 21:9-13.
75. Johnson P, Morley C. Spying on mothers. *Lancet*. 1994; 344:132-133.
76. Feldman MD. Spying on mothers [letter]. *Lancet*. 1994; 344:132.
77. Samuels MP, Southall D. Covert surveillance in Munchausen's syndrome by proxy: welfare of the child must come first [letter]. *BMJ*. 1994;308:1101-1102.
78. Connelly R. Ethical issues in the use of covert video surveillance in the diagnosis of Munchausen syndrome by proxy: the Atlanta study—an ethical challenge for medicine. *HEC Forum*. 2003;15:21-41.
79. Howe EG. Criteria for deceit. *J Clin Ethics*. 2004;15:100-110.
80. Leuthner SR. Covert video surveillance in pediatric care: the fiduciary relationship with a child. *J Clin Ethics*. 2004; 15:173-175.
81. Vaught W. Parents, lies, and videotape: covert video surveillance in pediatric care. *J Clin Ethics*. 2004;15: 161-172.
82. Flannery MT. First, do no harm: the use of covert video-surveillance to detect Munchausen syndrome by proxy—an unethical means of "preventing" child abuse. *Univ Mich J Law Reform*. 1998;32:105-194.
83. Baron HI, Beck DC, Vargas JH, et al. Overinterpretation of gastroduodenal motility studies: two cases involving Munchausen syndrome by proxy. *J Pediatr*. 1995;126: 397-400.
84. Cucchiara S, Borrelli O, Salvia G, et al. A normal gastrointestinal motility excludes chronic intestinal pseudoobstruction in children. *Dig Dis Sci*. 2000;45:258-264.
85. Hyman PE, Bursch B, Beck D, et al. Discriminating pediatric condition falsification from chronic intestinal pseudo-obstruction in toddlers. *Child Maltreat*. 2002; 7:132-137.
86. Barber MA, Davis PM. Fits, faints, or fatal fantasy? Fabricated seizures and child abuse. *Arch Dis Child*. 2002; 86: 230-233.
87. Waring WW. The persistent parent. *AJDC*. 1992;146: 753-755.
88. Yudkin S. Six children with coughs. *Lancet*. 1961;2: 561-563.
89. Rosenberg DA. Munchausen syndrome by proxy: medical diagnostic criteria. *Child Abuse Negl*. 2003;27:421-430.
90. Rand DC, Feldman MD. Misdiagnosis of Munchausen syndrome by proxy: a literature review and four new cases. *Harv Rev Psychiatry*. 1999;7:94-101.
91. Vennemann B, Perdekamp MG, Weinmann W, et al. A case of Munchausen syndrome by proxy with subsequent suicide of the mother. *Forensic Sci Int*. 2006; 158:195-199.
92. Berg B, Jones DP. Outcome of psychiatric intervention in factitious illness by proxy (Munchausen's syndrome by proxy). *Arch Dis Child*. 1999;81:465-472.
93. von Hahn L, Harper G, McDaniel SH, et al. A case of factitious disorder by proxy: the role of the health-care system, diagnostic dilemmas, and family dynamics. *Harv Rev Psychiatry*. 2001;9:124-135.
94. Jureidini JN, Shafer AT, Donald TG. "Munchausen syndrome by proxy": not only pathological parenting but also problematic doctoring? *Med J Aust*. 2003;178:130-132.
95. Eminson M, Jureidini J. Concerns about research and prevention strategies in Munchausen syndrome by proxy (MSBP) abuse. *Child Abuse Negl*. 2003;27:413-420.

Chapter 145

PHOBIAS AND ANXIETY

Pieter le Roux, D Litt et Phil; Christina M. McCann, PhD

DEFINITION OF TERMS

A phobia is an extreme and persistent fear of an object, event, or situation that, in reality, is not dangerous to the individual and would not be of concern to most people. Phobias are divided into 3 categories: (1) specific phobia, (2) social phobia, and (3) agoraphobia (often associated with panic disorder), all of which may occur in children and adolescents.[1] The following diagnoses are defined according to the *Diagnostic and Statistical Manual of Mental Disorders,* fourth edition, text revision (DSM-IV-TR).[2]

Specific Phobia

Specific phobias are defined as fears being related to a single stimulus for at least 6 months. Categories of feared stimuli commonly include animals, insects, certain situations (eg, health care or dental care procedures), and objects in the natural environment. Exposure to the feared stimulus or even thoughts of the feared stimulus result in an immediate anxiety response that can include physiological (tachycardia, sweating), cognitive (thoughts of being harmed), and emotional reactivity (crying, tantrums).

Social Phobia

Social phobia is a more complex and potentially more disabling diagnosis than specific phobia. This disorder, which often begins in late childhood or early adolescence, is characterized by an evident fear of social or performance situations for at least 6 months. The child has fears of doing or saying something that will be socially inappropriate and thus humiliating. Some typical situations that trigger these fears include reading aloud in front of the class, making a telephone call, joining in a conversation with peers, going to parties, or even ordering at a restaurant. Because of the fear of social situations, such children limit contacts and become at risk for social immaturity and stigmatization by other children.

Agoraphobia

Agoraphobia is the fear of being in places from which escape may not be possible or where help might not be available and often begins in late adolescence. It may be associated with panic disorder or fears of panic or embarrassing happenings such as the loss of bowel or bladder control. Because of these fears, individuals will often progressively limit outside activities. This disorder is usually persistent and disabling if left untreated.

PREVALENCE

In large-scale population studies of adults, phobias and other anxiety disorders are the most frequent psychiatric disorders occurring in the general population.[3] Although no comparable studies of the frequency of psychiatric disorders in childhood or adolescence have been conducted, phobias are clearly common in these age groups.[4,5] In Rutter's Isle of Wight Study, approximately 2.5% of children had disabling specific fears or phobias.[6] A more recent community study found specific phobias in 2.6% of children.[4] In a study of children and adolescents who have anxiety disorders, except for separation anxiety disorders, specific phobias and social phobias were extremely common.[7]

The most common specific phobias occurring in children and adolescents involve animals, insects, and objects in the natural environment (eg, storms, water) and are likely to begin before the age of 7 years. Other common phobias of closed spaces *(claustrophobia)* and heights *(acrophobia)* are much less frequent and tend to have their origins in adulthood.

Phobias associated with injury, blood, and health care (eg, injections, other invasive medical procedures) are also common and should not be dismissed as trivial.[8] Extreme responses such as panic, fainting, or vomiting as a reaction to injury, venipuncture, or injection (even when such events happen to another person) may interfere with a phobic person seeking health care.

PHOBIAS AND DEVELOPMENT

Some fears are common and expected at various developmental levels. For example, stranger anxiety is seen at approximately 8 months of age and usually decreases around the middle of the 2nd year. Toddlers are commonly fearful of being left alone or with babysitters, and preschool children are afraid of the dark. Because such fears are common and readily recognized as part of childhood, parents often do not consult physicians about them.

Many children have fears that technically meet the criteria for a diagnosis of specific phobia but that then disappear without specific intervention. However, the avoidance behavior associated with a phobia may interfere with usual activities and productive social relationships. Animal phobias may prevent a child from playing with neighbors or attending after-school activities because of a need to avoid the feared object. Even when a particular specific phobia disappears spontaneously, the consequences of the missed opportunities, embarrassment, or interference with social development may linger.

Social phobias commonly occur in adolescence as the importance and impact of peer interactions emerges. Teenagers turn toward peers to help with identity development, but this process can be interrupted if the adolescent has intense fears about social interactions.

ETIOLOGY

The literature offers various theoretic speculations about the cause of phobias.[9-11] Early theories postulated unconscious conflicts as the source; others suggest that phobias are learned responses in the context of a child's experience. According to classical and operant conditioning theories, once a child experiences fear and physiological arousal in association with the stimulus (classical conditioning), the phobia is maintained and strengthened by avoiding the feared stimulus (negative reinforcement). Empirical research indicates that early correlates of anxiety disorders may be present. In very young children, behavioral inhibition, the tendency to exhibit withdrawal, and autonomic arousal to challenge or novelty is correlated with the later risk for anxiety and phobic disorders.[12]

In recent years, increased emphasis has been placed on the way in which factors such as genetic influences, temperamental predispositions, parental functioning, and practices affect the development of childhood anxiety disorders.[11,13] Thus a multidimensional understanding of the cause of such childhood disturbances is crucial to best practices in diagnostic and treatment approaches.[11,13]

DIFFERENTIAL DIAGNOSIS

The following psychiatric disorders, as defined by the DSM-IV-TR,[2] have several overlapping symptoms with phobias. A thorough clinical interview with the patient and parents will help determine the appropriate diagnosis or diagnoses.

Separation Anxiety Disorder

Children suffering from separation anxiety are afraid of leaving parents or others to whom they are attached and often fear that something may happen to parents when they are not present. Fear of the dark, animals, or objects may be present; however, unlike a specific phobia, the added fear of separation from loved ones exists. School phobia or school refusal is a specific manifestation of this disorder. (See Chapter 128, School Absenteeism and School Refusal.)

Selective Mutism

Selective mutism is a child's persistent failure to speak in certain social situations, even though the child will talk in other situations. A rare condition, selective mutism usually occurs by 5 years of age and lasts for at least 1 month, with a typical life course of a few months. However, the disorder can last several years, although this pattern is uncommon. Selective mutism should not be diagnosed if a child is encountering some type of significant transition, such as the first month of a school term or recent immigration to a new country with a different dominant language, especially for shy children. This disorder should be diagnosed only in a child who has demonstrated ability to speak at the appropriate developmental level in other more familiar social situations. Social anxiety and social avoidance associated with social phobia may also be present in children with selective mutism. In this case, both diagnoses would be appropriate if the child's symptoms also meet the criteria for social phobia.

Generalized Anxiety Disorder

The essential feature of generalized anxiety disorder is excessive or unrealistic anxiety or worry for a period of 6 months or longer. The worries are considered uncontrollable by the patient and significantly interfere with daily functioning. Although phobias are often present, generalized anxiety disorder is more global and has fewer focused fears.

Obsessive-Compulsive Disorder

When ruling out the presence of obsessive-compulsive disorder, avoidance behaviors associated with obsessive-compulsive disorder are associated specifically with the content of the obsession, such as dirt and contamination, rather than a feared stimulus. Repetitive, purposeful, and intentional behavior may also develop to neutralize or prevent the occurrence of anxiety or worry, in addition to the development of anxiety and avoidance behaviors.[14] (See Chapter 138, Conduct Disorders.)

Posttraumatic Stress Disorder

Posttraumatic stress disorder develops subsequent to experiencing a traumatic stressor. In addition to avoidance behaviors that are typical for phobias, symptoms of posttraumatic stress disorder include reexperiencing the trauma (eg, flashbacks, being retraumatized by witnessing a similar event, frightening dreams, repetitive play in which the child expresses themes or aspects of the trauma), and restricted affect. Acute stress disorder may be diagnosed if disturbances related to the trauma persist for a minimum of 2 days and a maximum of 4 weeks and occur within 4 weeks of the traumatic event. (See Chapter 146, Posttraumatic Stress Disorder.)

Hypochondriasis

Distinguishing between specific phobia (blood-infection-injury type) and hypochondriasis depends on the presence or absence of disease conviction. People with hypochondriasis are preoccupied with fears of having a disease, whereas individuals who have a specific phobia fear contracting disease but do not believe it is already present. A vasovagal fainting response is also typical for a phobia of the blood-infection-injury type, whereas this event is not common for hypochondriasis.

Additional Psychiatric Factors

Avoidance behaviors or phobias themselves may be present with other anxiety disorders, depressive disorders, substance abuse, and psychotic disorders. However, the symptoms of these other disorders are typically the focus of treatment because they tend to produce more distress and impairment of daily functioning than symptoms of phobias.

EVALUATION

Relevant History

A complete history will usually help define possible diagnoses in the primary care setting. The report of fearful behavior, the symptoms of anxiety, or the development of avoidance behavior or compulsions (repetitive, purposeful, intentional behaviors in response to fears or obsessions) should prompt further assessment. Some important areas to screen include:

- Onset of symptoms, including review of recent life changes (deaths, births, moves, etc.)
- Specific history of symptoms and associated behaviors
- Circumstances in which symptoms occur
- Responses of parents, teachers, peers, and others to the symptoms
- Review of the patient's general pattern of psychosocial development

Because children, and more commonly adolescents, may recognize that their fear is irrational, they may invent another reason for their avoidance behavior. The possibility of traumatic experience with the phobic object, such as having been frightened by even a playful dog, being lost, threatened, or abused, should be explored.

Social anxiety can sometimes produce depressive symptoms that mask the anxiety symptoms. Therefore use of a brief screening instrument can help the primary care physician identify anxiety symptoms. Depending on the level of impairment, the primary care physician can decide whether to intervene, consult with, or refer to a mental health specialist. Numerous screening instruments are available to use in primary care setting (see end-of-chapter materials).

Practitioners should review available screening instruments to determine which one fits best in their practice. Consultation with a mental health care provider can also help with selecting such instruments, such as the Self-Report for Childhood Anxiety Related Emotional Disorders (SCARED), which consists of 41 items, takes an average of 5 minutes to complete, and can be used with children ages 8 and older. The Liebowitz Social Anxiety Scale—Child Adolescent Version (LSAS-CA) screens for social anxiety symptoms and consists of 24 items, takes an average of 10 to 20 minutes to complete, and can be used with children ages 7 and older. Providing the results of the initial screening and assessment to the mental health care specialist is helpful, especially if the primary care practitioner has an established relationship with the patient.

Physical

Although the history may seem to define the problem clearly, particularly if the patient can describe the object of the fear, a thorough physical examination should be completed if physical problems are likely. Hypoglycemia, hyperthyroidism, and pheochromocytoma can all produce symptoms similar to anxiety. Additionally, withdrawal from some abused substances may be associated with episodes of severe anxiety, and side effects from prescribed medications may also produce similar symptoms.

The key symptoms of phobias include avoidance of the fear-provoking object or situation and fear often associated with sweating, tachycardia, difficulty in breathing, and light-headedness or dizziness.

According to the DSM-IV-TR,[2] children may express anxiety by crying, tantrums, clinging, or freezing, and they do not typically realize that their fears are unreasonable. In extreme cases, panic may occur for adolescents. The degree to which avoidance or anticipatory anxiety occurs is often the critical factor in parents' seeking help.

Prognosis

Most phobias in children and adolescents seem to respond to treatment, at least in terms of relief of major symptoms. However, the lack of controlled studies creates difficulty in attributing remission clearly to treatment. Although follow-up studies are limited, those that exist suggest a positive long-term outcome.[5,11,13] However, adults seeking treatment for phobias and other anxiety disorders often report a childhood onset of a phobia or similar symptoms during childhood or adolescence that diminished or disappeared for some time.

The prognosis for children and adolescents who have social phobia is less clear, but experience suggests that these disorders are less likely to remit spontaneously or as a consequence of treatment. Agoraphobia also has a more guarded prognosis than social phobia, although outcome studies and long-term follow-up information are lacking.

MANAGEMENT

Treatment of phobias includes thorough assessment, initial intervention, and short-term follow-up. If the phobia persists, then further assessment and potential consultation and referral to a mental health specialist may be necessary. The primary care physician should inform the patient and parents of the diagnosis and treatment because the parents need to be partners in the treatment, and their responses are usually crucial to the outcome. For example, without intending to do so, parents can reinforce and perpetuate symptoms by allowing the child to avoid the feared stimulus.[11] Family therapy can provide additional treatment opportunities by offering education to parents about the diagnosis, strengthening the child's coping skills, improving familial support, helping the family cope with any recent life transitions, and addressing best-parenting practices.[15]

When evaluating and treating the patient, developmental issues should be considered. For example, children may exhibit *phobic* behaviors, such as a fear of the dark, that are common and likely to be self-limited. Providing a nightlight and using simple cognitive self-control strategies (eg, relaxation, visualizing a pleasant scene, teaching the child positive self-statements such as "I am brave; I can take care of myself in the dark.") may be all that is needed.[16] More likely the phobia will abate spontaneously over time.

Cognitive-Behavioral Therapy

Patients who have phobias are typically treated by a mental health specialist with systematic desensitization. This approach includes a combination of progressive exposure to the feared stimulus using a hierarchy of fears (ranked by the patient according to level of anxiety) paired with relaxation techniques. As anxiety occurs in response to the actual feared stimulus (in vivo) or imagined (in vitro) stimulus, the relaxation techniques are invoked and the stimuli or image removed. The feared stimulus will gradually become paired with a relaxed state instead of an anxious state, resulting in a decrease or absence of the fear response.[5]

Other behavioral approaches used by the mental health specialist can enhance the effectiveness of systematic exposure, including the use of behavioral contracts and modeling procedures.[14] Getting a child to participate in deliberate exposure to the feared stimulus is often difficult for parents. Contracts can increase the patient's compliance by using specific contingencies to reinforce positively the desired behavior toward the feared stimulus (eg, the child earns stickers when allowing the dog the child fears to come closer). Contracts can also ensure that treatment plans are followed consistently outside of the office by the patient and the family. Modeling includes direct observation of the desired behavior (eg, not avoiding the feared stimulus) demonstrated by the practitioner, family members, or peers, who initially show a comparable level of fear, which they are able to overcome.

Psychopharmacologic Therapy

Psychiatric consultation is typically considered when the child is in so much distress that the child's ability to function is significantly impaired, which also prevents success with cognitive-behavioral treatment. Medications are usually used in combination with behavioral interventions to achieve the best treatment outcomes. If medications are contemplated, then anxiolytics or antidepressants are the medications of choice for the vast majority of children and adolescents. (See Chapter 133, Medication Management for Emotional and Behavioral Problems.)

Other Therapy

Social phobia and agoraphobia are difficult to treat and often require psychological treatment and pharmacotherapy. Systematic desensitization can be difficult to establish because of the complexity of the anxiety-provoking stimuli and social immaturity of the patient. A range of psychotherapeutic interventions, including cognitive-behavioral individual therapy, family therapy, and group therapy with age-appropriate peers, may be used to promote socialization and improve social skills. In vivo exposure with response prevention is the most effective treatment for agoraphobia with and without panic attacks, with effectiveness ranging from 60% to 70%. Booster sessions for symptoms of panic are usually necessary when panic and anxiety are still present once treatment has been completed.[16]

Anticipatory guidance plays an important role in recognizing, diagnosing, and treating childhood fears and phobias. In many instances the child would rather avoid discussing fears, and in some cases the parents may not recognize avoidant and anxious behavior as something that should be reported to the pediatrician. Therefore routine screening for fears that might interrupt or impair normal development should be included when treating children and adolescents in primary care. Well-child visits may provide a good opportunity for such screening.

WHEN TO REFER

Psychological consultation is indicated if the initial treatment does not result in symptom relief, which may result in a need for further assessment, including referrals for cognitive-behavioral psychotherapy, psychiatric consultation, or both. Maintaining collaboration with referral sources helps coordinate treatment planning.[14]

WHEN TO ADMIT

If a comorbid condition exists that is threatening the safety of the patient or others, then psychiatric admission may be necessary to stabilize the patient.

TOOLS FOR PRACTICE

Engaging Patient and Family

- *Anxiety Disorders* (fact sheet), National Institute of Mental Health (www.nimh.nih.gov/publicat/anxiety.cfm).
- *A Parent's Guide to Building Resilience in Children and Teens* (book), American Academy of Pediatrics (www.aap.org/bookstore).
- *Fears* (Web page), Keep Kids Healthy (www.keepkidshealthy.com/parenting_tips/fears.html).
- *Fears and Phobias* (fact sheet), American Academy of Pediatrics (www.aap.org/publiced/BK5_Fears.htm).
- *Separation Anxiety* (fact sheet), American Academy of Pediatrics (www.aap.org/publiced/BK0_SeparationAnxiety.htm).
- *Soothing Your Child's Separation Anxiety* (article), American Academy of Pediatrics (www.aap.org/family/healthychildren/06fall/Separationanxiety.pdf).
- *Stress and Your Child* (fact sheet), American Academy of Pediatrics (www.aap.org/publiced/BK5_Stress.htm).
- *Stressed? Read This* (brochure), American Academy of Pediatrics (patiented.aap.org).

Medical Decision Support

- *Child Form—Screen For Child Anxiety Related Disorders* (SCARED) (questionnaire), Western Psychiatric Institute and Clinic, Boris Birmaher, MD, et al (www.wpic.pitt.edu/carenet/care-netproviders/pdfforms/scaredchild-final.pdf).
- *Liebowitz Social Anxiety Scale for Children and Adolescents (LSAS-CA)* (brochure), Liebowitz, MR (healthnet.umassmed.edu/mhealth/LiebowitzSocialAnxietyScale.pdf).
- *Parent Form—Screen For Child Anxiety Related Disorders* (SCARED) (questionnaire), Western Psychiatric Institute and Clinic, Boris Birmaher, MD, et al (www.wpic.pitt.edu/carenet/care-netproviders/pdfforms/scaredparent-final.pdf).
- *Pediatric Prescribing Update: Psychoactive Medications* (online course), American Academy of Pediatrics (www.pedialink.org).
- *Screening Tools & Rating Scales* (Web page), School Psychiatry Program and Mood and Anxiety Disorders Institute Resource Center, Massachusetts General Hospital (www.massgeneral.org/schoolpsychiatry/screeningtools_table.asp).

RELATED WEB SITES

- American Academy of Child and Adolescent Psychiatry (www.aacap.org).
- American Psychological Association (www.apa.org).
- Anxiety Disorders Association of America (www.adaa.org/anxietydisorderinfor/childrenado.cfm).
- College of Community Health Sciences, University of Alabama: Digital Library (cchs-dl.slis.ua.edu/patientinfo/psychiatry/anxiety/phobic-disorders/).
- Emedicine (www.emedicine.com/ped).
- Keep Kids Healthy (www.keepkidshealthy.com/parenting_tips/fears.html).
- School Psychiatry Program and Mood and Anxiety Disorders Institute Resource Center, Massachusetts General Hospital: Screening Tools & Rating Scales (www.mgh.harvard.edu/madiresourcecenter/schoolpsychiatry/screeningtools_table.asp).
- Virtual Children's Hospital (www.vh.org/pediatric/patient/pediatrics/cqqa/anxiety.html).

AAP POLICY STATEMENTS

American Academy of Pediatrics, Committee on School Health. School-based mental health services. *Pediatrics*. 2004;113(6):1839-1845. (aappolicy.aappublications.org/cgi/content/full/pediatrics;113/6/1839).

Hagan JF, American Academy of Pediatrics, Committee on Psychosocial Aspects of Child and Family Health, and Task Force on Terrorism. Psychosocial implications of disaster or terrorism on children: a guide for the pediatrician. *Pediatrics*. 2005;116(3):787-795. (aappolicy.aappublications.org/cgi/content/full/pediatrics;116/3/787).

SUGGESTED RESOURCES

American Psychiatric Association. *Diagnostic and statistical manual of mental disorders (DSM-IV-TR)*. 4th ed. Text revision. Washington, DC: The Association; 2000.

Berent J, Lemley A. *Beyond Shyness: How to Conquer Social Anxieties*. New York, NY: Fireside; 1993.

Garber SW, Garber MD, Spizman RF. *Monsters Under the Bed and Other Childhood Fears: Helping Your Child Overcome Anxieties, Fears, and Phobias*. New York, NY: Villard; 1993.

Morris TL, March JS, eds. *Anxiety Disorders in Children and Adolescents*. 2nd ed. New York, NY: Guilford Press; 2004.

REFERENCES

1. Chung E, Cheng T. In brief: childhood fears and phobias. *Pediatr Rev*. 2003;24(12):431-432.
2. American Psychiatric Association. *Diagnostic and Statistical Manual of Mental Disorders*. 4th ed. Washington, DC: The Association; 2000.
3. Robius L. Lifetime prevalence of specific psychiatric disorders in three sites. *Arch Gen Psychiatry*. 1984;41: 949-958.
4. Kashani JH, Orvaschel H. A community study of anxiety in children and adolescents. *Am J Psychiatry*. 1990;147(3): 313-318.
5. Ollendick T, King N, Yule W. *International Handbook of Phobic and Anxiety Disorders in Children and Adolescents*. New York, NY: Plenum Press; 1994.
6. Rutter M, Tizard J, Yule W, et al. Research report: Isle of Wight Studies, 1964-1974. *Psychol Med*. 1976;6(2): 313-332.
7. Last CG, Perrin S, Hersen M, et al. DSM-III-R anxiety disorders in children: sociodemographic and clinical characteristics. *J Am Acad Child Adolesc Psychiatry*. 1992;31(6):1070-1076.
8. Marks I. Blood-injury phobia: a review. *Am J Psychiatry*. 1988;145(10):1207-1213.
9. Merckelback H, de Jong PJ, Muris P, et al. The etiology of specific phobias: a review. *Clin Psychol Rev*. 1996; 16(4): 337-361.
10. Schowalter JE. Fears and phobias. *Pediatr Rev*. 1994; 15(10):384-388.
11. King N, Muris P, Ollendick T. Specific phobia. In: Morris T, March J, eds. *Anxiety Disorders in Children and Adolescents*. New York, NY: Guilford Press; 2004.
12. Rosenbaum JF, Biederman J, Hirshfeld DR, et al. Further evidence of an association between behavioral inhibition and anxiety disorders: results from a family study of children from a non-clinical sample. *J Psychiatr Res*. 1991; 25(1-2):49-65.
13. Ollendick T, King N, Muris P. Fears and phobias in children: phenomenology, epidemiology, and aetiology. *Child Adolesc Ment Health*. 2002;7(3):98-106.
14. Albano AM, Chorpita BF. Treatment of anxiety disorders of childhood. *Psychiatr Clin North Am*. 1995;18(4):767-784.
15. Ziegler R. Anxiety disorders in children: applying a cognitive-behavioral technique that can be integrated with pharmacotherapy or other psychosocial interventions. In: Ellison J, ed. *Integrative Treatment of Anxiety Disorders*. Washington, DC: American Psychiatric Association; 1996.
16. Craske M, Brown T, Barlow D. Behavioral treatment of panic disorder: a two-year follow-up. *Behav Ther*. 1991; 22(3):289-304.

Chapter 146

POSTTRAUMATIC STRESS DISORDER

Judith A. Cohen, MD; David J. Kolko, PhD

Posttraumatic stress disorder (PTSD) is a psychiatric disorder that some children and adolescents develop in response to being the direct victim of or witnessing traumatic events (eg, child abuse; domestic, community, or school violence; vehicular or other accidents; fires or natural disasters; terrorism or war; traumatic medical conditions). In the Great Smokey Mountain Study, 25% of children and adolescents in North Carolina had experienced at least 1 serious traumatic event by their 16th birthday.[1] Among inner-city children, this proportion is even higher, with as many as 90% of inner-city adolescents reporting significant exposure to traumatic events.[2] The prevalence of PTSD after such events has been estimated based on studies of various types of stressful events, and thus, not surprisingly, the rates vary considerably by type of event. Other characteristics that are related to prevalence are demographics, family characteristics, and research methods. Among the few nationally representative studies, early studies of adolescents and young adults reported overall lifetime PTSD rates of 9.2%,[3] with some rates reported separately for boys (2.8%) and girls (10.3%).[4] A more recent study of adolescents (ages 12 to 17 years) reported different rates than previous studies, with slightly higher rates for boys (3.7%) and lower rates for girls (6.3%).[5] The rates of PTSD vary across types of traumatic events,[6-11] such as exposure to acute physical injury (23%),[6] natural disasters (24%-39%),[7,8] and community violence (27%).[9] Many children may not meet full criteria for PTSD but may show heightened posttraumatic stress symptoms after exposure to various events, including family violence (15%)[12] and natural disasters (24%).[7,8]

PTSD is often underrecognized, particularly in young children who have difficulty reporting certain PTSD symptoms and in those who have experienced traumas associated with shame, secrecy, or stigma, such as sexual abuse or domestic violence or being the victim of bullying. Although reliance on parental reports of child's symptoms greatly improves diagnosis,[13] parents who are themselves traumatized or who are the perpetrators of the child's traumatic experience may not wish to provide accurate reports of children's trauma exposure or symptoms.

Left untreated, childhood trauma and PTSD are associated with serious and long-lasting negative outcomes, including impairments in learning, memory, and academic performance[14]; increased risk for depression, suicide attempts, and completed suicide in adolescence and adulthood[15]; increased risk for substance abuse, self-injury, and risky sexual behaviors[16,17]; and impaired physical health and immunity with increased health care use in adulthood.[17,18] Children who have significant PTSD symptoms without meeting the strict psychiatric criteria of this disorder often have comparable functional impairment to those with the full disorder.[19] However, these outcomes are not inevitable. Effective treatment is available for children with PTSD symptoms. If these children are identified and treated with optimal interventions, then PTSD symptoms generally remit relatively quickly and cost effectively and do not return. The most tested treatment leads to reduction of depressive, anxiety, shame, and behavioral difficulties in addition to remission of PTSD symptoms.[20]

Because many traumatized children do not spontaneously report their traumatic experiences or trauma symptoms, primary care physicians (PCPs) may be in the best position to identify these children and to influence developmental trajectory positively. For these reasons, PCPs should be aware of the high prevalence of child trauma exposure and be willing and able to assess children for the presence of PTSD symptoms in the primary care setting. This chapter presents basic information about assessing trauma exposure and PTSD symptoms in children and adolescents in the primary care setting, as well as referral sources for evidence-based treatments for PTSD.

COMPONENTS OF POSTTRAUMATIC STRESS DISORDER

To receive a diagnosis of PTSD, the child must have experienced a traumatic event that qualifies as a serious traumatic stressor. Although the American Psychiatric Association *Diagnostic and Statistical Manual* (DSM-IV)[21] requires specific criteria for a PTSD-level stressor—that is, that it threatens the child's or significant others' life or physical integrity—a realistic understanding of child development dictates that events that objectively are not threatening to life or physical integrity might be perceived in this way by a young, frightened child, particularly if the child fears for the safety of a primary attachment figure, even if this fear is not based in reality. Children's perceptions of threats to their primary caretakers have been found to predict significantly the children's PTSD symptoms.[13,22] Thus, for children, more leeway exists in defining PTSD-level traumas. In reaction to the traumatic exposure, the child must have experienced subjective fear, helplessness, or horror. In children, this reaction may be expressed as disorganized behavior.

The 3 core symptom clusters of PTSD are (1) reexperiencing, (2) avoidance or numbing, and (3) hyperarousal. To meet full PTSD criteria, children must have at least 1 reexperiencing symptom, 3 avoidance symptoms, and 2 hyperarousal symptoms. However, as noted previously, children who do not meet these criteria (eg, those who have at least 3 PTSD symptoms and at least 1 in each cluster) are still considered to have significant PTSD symptoms and should still be referred for mental health evaluation and treatment. Even if a child has only a few PTSD symptoms, if they are of sufficient severity to cause functional impairment, then they may warrant a referral for further evaluation.

Reexperiencing symptoms occurs when upsetting feelings are experienced after memories or reminders of the traumatic event recur. These symptoms may be idiosyncratic and hard for parents and PCPs to identify. For example, that a child who saw her father shot to death began reliving the shooting in her mind whenever a thunderstorm occurred would not be difficult to understand; the sound of thunder reminded this child of the sound of the gunshots that killed her father. However, another child's grandmother was stymied when her grandson started hitting her and screaming whenever she sang what she thought was his favorite lullaby. The story gradually emerged that the boy's mother had sung this song to him before she was hit by a car and killed. To him, the song was not a reminder of comfort and happy times with his mother, but rather a traumatic reminder of the night she died. Reexperiencing symptoms include the following:

- Recurrent and distressing memories or thoughts of the event, including repetitive play
- Recurrent distressing or frightening dreams, including nonspecific scary dreams in younger children
- Feeling as though the traumatic event is occurring again in the present (flashbacks; rare in younger children)
- Intense psychological distress when reminded of the trauma
- Physiological reactions to trauma reminders, including upset stomach, headaches, and school refusal[21]

The 2nd PTSD cluster includes avoidance and numbing symptoms. Children's trauma reminders are accompanied by strong, upsetting feelings. When trauma reminders are present in many environments, to escape the upsetting feelings, children may develop avoidance coping strategies. For example, children will try to avoid talking about the traumatic experience or will avoid thinking about it. They will avoid places, people, and situations that serve as trauma reminders. For some children, these avoidant strategies become generalized—that is, they not only avoid the place where the traumatic event happened, but also avoid all similar places. For example, a child who was beaten up on the way to school becomes avoidant of going to school at all. A child who was sexually abused in the bathroom at home is now afraid of all bathrooms and becomes enuretic because the child is unable to use the toilet without becoming overwhelmed with fear. Children who deal with fear through avoidance are reinforcing their fears rather than extinguishing them. As these avoidance strategies become increasingly ineffective, some children may become emotionally numb to escape the overwhelming fear they feel. Avoidance and numbing symptoms include the following:

- Efforts to avoid thoughts, feelings, or talking about the traumatic event
- Avoiding activities, places, people, or situations that serve as trauma reminders
- Inability to remember an important aspect of the trauma
- Loss of interest or participation in significant activities
- Detachment or estrangement from others
- Restricted affect
- In older children and teens, a sense of a foreshortened future[21]

The 3rd PTSD cluster includes hyperarousal symptoms that were not present before the traumatic event. In children who have experienced chronic trauma, such as ongoing domestic or community violence or child abuse, assessing the onset of these symptoms or distinguishing them from other syndromes such as attention-deficit/hyperactivity disorder may be difficult. Increased arousal symptoms include the following:

- Difficulty falling or staying asleep
- Irritability or temper outbursts
- Trouble concentrating
- Hypervigilance
- Increased startle response
- In young children, the development of new fears not previously present[21,23]

Finally, these symptoms must be present for at least a month, and they must cause functional impairment in social, school, family, health, or another important area of daily living.[21]

ASSESSING TRAUMA EXPOSURE

PCPs who have a favorable relationship with their patients will feel comfortable asking the child directly about possible exposure to a variety of different types of traumas at well-child care appointments. Generally, children and parents should be asked these questions in private, rather than together, because many types of traumas are believed by children or parents to be stigmatizing and shameful or things that should be kept secret within the family. Children may be less likely to disclose such information in the presence of the parent than alone with the PCP. Reporting requirements in the case of child maltreatment are discussed elsewhere in this volume, and these guidelines should be followed if the child discloses maltreatment in this context. (See Chapter 120, Child Physical Abuse and Neglect.) Some general questions designed to elicit information about a child's potential exposure to traumatic events are as follows:

- Has any significant change occurred in the child's life or functioning since the last visit?
- Since the last time the child was seen, has something really scary or upsetting happened to the child or someone in the child's family?
- Has any significant change occurred in the child's behavioral or emotional functioning?
- Has anyone reported or observed any sudden changes in the child's behavior or mood?

The PCP is also encouraged to monitor a child's potential exposure to specific traumatic events or experiences. Box 146-1 lists some key domains that should be included in an interview. Self-report instruments are also available for inquiring about trauma exposure. Commonly used exposure instruments include the Trauma Exposure Structured Interview for Children,[24] which can be administered as a self-report instrument; and the UCLA PTSD Index for DSM-IV.[25]

BOX 146-1 Key Domains That Should Be Included in an Interview

Bad accidents (vehicular, falls, fires)

Medical trauma, illness, or related procedures (eg, long hospitalization stay, painful procedures)

Natural disasters (storm, hurricane, blizzard, earthquake, flood, hit by lightning)

Physical violence (toward child or other, threatened or happened, including bullying)

Domestic violence (adults fighting, attacking, shooting, stabbing, beating each other up at home)

Sexual abuse (unwanted touches in private parts, taking pictures, Internet abuse)

Physical abuse at home (beating, punching, hitting by parent or older sibling)

Traumatic death (knew or observed someone die—ask about circumstances: was death sudden, shocking, terrifying, gory?)

Other scary, frightening events (eg, kidnapping, terrorism)

ASSESSING POSTTRAUMATIC STRESS DISORDER SYMPTOMS

When assessing children for the presence of PTSD symptoms, the symptoms should be anchored to a specific stressor. If the PCP is interviewing the child, then the child should be asked whether any of the specific experienced events was upsetting or scary to the child. If the child reports that any of these events were distressing, then the clinician should determine which one was most traumatic from the child's perspective and then assess the child for the presence of the PTSD symptoms described previously. However, interviewing children for PTSD symptoms is a challenging task, particularly when asking about avoidance. Children and parents should ideally be asked about the child's symptoms separately to obtain optimal information because inclusion of parental report has been shown to improve the rate of accurate diagnosis.[13]

Given all of these requirements, in most PCP practices, time demands will preclude PCPs from conducting personal interviews to assess PTSD symptoms. However, a child self-report PTSD screening measure can be used in office settings. The 9-item Abbreviated UCLA PTSD Index[25] (Figure 146-1) has been used in school settings after disasters such as the September 11, 2001, terrorist attacks[22] with good results. A score of 20 on the Abbreviated UCLA PTSD Index highly correlates with a diagnosis of PTSD.[25] Accordingly, children with scores of greater than or equal to 20 should be referred for evaluation. Clinical judgment should be used to determine whether children with scores between 10 and 19 should also be referred for evaluation, especially if they have clinically meaningful symptoms of PTSD, and if these are accompanied with functional impairment (ie, if the child or parent reports that the child is having difficulty getting along with people at school or at home, or if the child has trouble sleeping, eating, or concentrating), then the child should be referred for further mental health evaluation. If a child has a score that is even lower than 10 but the parent or PCP has concerns based on the child's clinical symptoms or history after exposure to a traumatic event, then the child should be referred for

Item	None	Little	Some	Much	Most
1. I get upset, afraid, or sad when something makes me think about what happened.	☐ 0	☐ 1	☐ 2	☐ 3	☐ 4
2. I have upsetting thoughts or pictures of what happened come into my mind when I do not want them to.	☐ 0	☐ 1	☐ 2	☐ 3	☐ 4
3. I feel grouchy, or I am easily angered.	☐ 0	☐ 1	☐ 2	☐ 3	☐ 4
4. I have trouble going to sleep, or I wake up often during the night.	☐ 0	☐ 1	☐ 2	☐ 3	☐ 4
5. I try not to talk about, think about, or have feelings about what happened.	☐ 0	☐ 1	☐ 2	☐ 3	☐ 4
6. I have trouble concentrating or paying attention.	☐ 0	☐ 1	☐ 2	☐ 3	☐ 4
7. I try to stay away from people, places, or things that make me remember what happened.	☐ 0	☐ 1	☐ 2	☐ 3	☐ 4
8. I have bad dreams, including dreams about what happened.	☐ 0	☐ 1	☐ 2	☐ 3	☐ 4
9. I feel alone inside and not close to other people.	☐ 0	☐ 1	☐ 2	☐ 3	☐ 4

Figure 146-1 Abbreviated UCLA Posttraumatic Stress Disorder Reaction Index for DSM-IV. (*Steinberg A, Brymer MJ, Decker KB, et al. University of California PTSD reaction index.* Curr Psychiatr Rep. *2004;6:96-100.* © Robert S. Pynoos and Alan M. Steinberg, 2001.)

further mental health evaluation because avoidant children are likely to underreport PTSD symptoms.[13]

An alternative self-report method for evaluating the severity of posttraumatic symptoms is the Trauma Symptom Checklist for Children (TSCC).[26] The TSCC was developed to evaluate children's responses to unspecified traumatic events in an array of symptom domains by using several scales, such as posttraumatic stress, anger, anxiety, depression, sexual concerns and preoccupation, and dissociation. Thus the TSCC includes several scales relevant to the assessment of posttraumatic stress symptoms and other symptoms related to PTSD. The TSCC was standardized on a large sample of racially and socioeconomically diverse children from urban and suburban settings, and it provides norms according to age and sex, as well as clinical cutoff scores. The child is asked to indicate how often each item happens by using a 4-point scale (0 = never; 1 = sometimes; 2 = lots of times; 3 = almost all the time). The posttraumatic stress subscale consists of 10 items reflecting posttraumatic stress symptoms (eg, intrusive recollections of traumatic events, sensory reexperiencing and nightmares, dissociative avoidance, fears). This particular subscale has high internal consistency and good criterion validity.

OTHER TRAUMA-RELATED MENTAL HEALTH PROBLEMS

Childhood traumatic grief (CTG) is another condition that PCPs should be prepared to recognize and refer for specialized intervention if indicated. CTG occurs in a minority of children who lose significant others to death under traumatic (frightening, unexpected) circumstances. These children get stuck on the traumatic circumstances of the death and are unable to move through the typical stages of grieving. They may seem less sad than children who are mourning in a more usual fashion because they develop PTSD symptoms of avoidance and numbing. For example, these children may not talk about the deceased, may avoid visiting the cemetery, or seem detached from parents and friends; or they may become easily angered and irritable when others want to reminisce about the deceased. Parents may become angry in response because they may interpret this behavior to mean that the child is not mourning the loss of the deceased or does not seem to care about the death. The PCP can be of help to the child and family by recognizing the signs and presentation of CTG and educating the family about this condition.

Additionally, PCPs should be aware that PTSD is not the only, or even the most common, outcome for children to experience after trauma exposure. PTSD most typically co-occurs with other difficulties such as depression, as well as anxiety and behavioral problems.[5] Consequently, the PCP may have to include other assessments or instruments to evaluate these potential comorbidities. In some cases, parents may initially identify other clinical concerns that may relate to the child's recent exposure to traumatic events. Children may develop these problems in the absence of PTSD symptoms as well, and substance abuse, self-injury, and serious behavior problems are common sequelae of traumatic experiences, particularly child physical abuse and domestic violence.

MAKING REFERRALS TO SPECIALIZED MENTAL HEALTH SERVICES

As noted previously, children with scores above 8 to 10 on the Abbreviated UCLA PTSD Index should be considered for specialized mental health evaluation. PCPs should be aware that, in addition to current PTSD symptoms, additional risk factors exist for developing PTSD and other mental health difficulties after traumatic exposure. These risk factors include female sex; more frequent or intense exposure to the traumatic event; having a preexisting anxiety disorder; lack of parental or other support; parental psychopathological abnormality, including parental PTSD related to the index trauma; and past trauma exposure.[27,28] Children who have several of these risk factors may need more prompt mental health referrals or closer PCP follow-up (or both) after exposure to traumatic life events. PCPs may be particularly well placed to follow up on such children and to monitor them for the later emergence of mental health difficulties.

Effective treatment is available for children who have significant PTSD symptoms, and with optimal interventions, most children are able to recover in as few as 12 treatment sessions.[20] (See Tools for Practice at the end of the chapter for resources.)

Most children are remarkably resilient in the face of trauma and do not go on to develop PTSD. However, many exposed children may experience subclinical PTSD, with or without symptoms that interfere with their functioning or cause impairment in other domains (eg, behavioral dysfunction or aggression, hypersexuality, social incompetence, anger or explosiveness, relationship conflicts or problems). Improvements in such clinical problems have been reported among physically abused children by using Parent-Child Interaction Therapy[29] or Abuse-Focused Cognitive-Behavioral Therapy,[30] among children exposed to domestic violence by using parent-child psychotherapy,[31] and in adolescents exposed to community violence by using the Cognitive Behavioral Intervention for Trauma in Schools project tools.[32]

In terms of specific efforts that can be made in the office, the PCP is in a unique position to promote an initial response to the child who may have been exposed to traumatic events and who exhibits the symptoms of PTSD. Opportunities to observe the child during routine physical examinations provide both observational and physical evidence that may be relevant to the identification of traumatic exposure and symptoms. These impressions may be confirmed through parental interview when questions about the child's experiences and the timing of any recent or sudden reactions to these events can be ascertained. The PCP may also be in a position to work toward preventing PTSD by noting when children appear to be at risk for traumatic exposure or experiences. Potential high-risk scenarios that may be reported by the family include sudden and frequent moves, major disruptions in caregiving environment or caregiver functioning or status, reports of increased frustration or physical force during child management or disciplinary interactions, exposure to or knowledge of age-inappropriate sexual activities, child reactions to a caregiver that have changed suddenly, exposure to drugs and alcohol, and spending a lot of time with nonbiologically related men. Certainly the PCP can offer advice regarding steps that may minimize a child's exposure to high-risk situations and encourage parents to monitor and promote child safety, both in and out of the home.

SUMMARY

PCPs are in a critical position to recognize, respond to, and refer traumatized children. The PCP may possibly be the first adult or professional to learn about a child's potential exposure to traumatic events or to obtain evidence consistent with this clinical impression. Consequently the PCP may be an initial responder in terms of understanding and addressing PTSD in young children. An understanding of the material described herein may provide the PCP with some of the basic tools designed to promote the assessment and treatment of the traumatized child.

The authors acknowledge the support of grant MH074737 (National Institutes of Mental Health) and grant SM54319 (Substance Abuse and Mental Health Services Administration) in the preparation of this chapter.

TOOLS FOR PRACTICE

Engaging Patient and Family

- *What is child traumatic stress?* (fact sheet), National Child Traumatic Stress Network (NCTSN) (www.nctsnet.org/nctsn_assets/pdfs/what_is_child_traumatic_stress.pdf).
- *What kind of mental health professionals are trained to help children?* (fact sheet), American Academy of Pediatrics (www.aap.org/publiced/BR_MentalHealth.htm).

Medical Decision Support

- *Pediatric Medical Traumatic Stress Toolkit for Health Care Providers* (tool kit), National Child Traumatic Stress Network (NCTSN) (www.nctsnet.org/nccts/nav.do?pid=typ_mt_ptlkt).
- *Responding to Children's Emotional Needs During Times of Crisis: An Important Role for Pediatricians* (fact sheet), American Academy of Pediatrics (www.aap.org/terrorism/topics/parents.pdf).

- *The UCLA PTSD Index for DSM-IV (UPID)* (interview), University of California, Los Angeles (www.ncptsd.va.gov/ncmain/ncdocs/assmnts/the_ucla_ptsd_index_for_dsmiv.html).
- *Trauma and Disaster Mental Health Resources* (Web page), Centers for Disease Control and Prevention (www.bt.cdc.gov/mentalhealth/).
- *Trauma Symptom Checklist for Children (TSCC)* (checklist), John Briere (www.swin.edu.au/victims/resources/assessment/ptsd/tscc.html).

RELATED WEB SITES

- National Child Traumatic Stress Network (NCTSN) (www.nctsnet.org).
- Substance Abuse and Mental Health Services Administration (SAMHSA) (www.SAMHSA.gov).
- National Crime Victims Research and Treatment Center Department of Psychiatry and Behavioral Sciences, Medical University of South Carolina: Trauma Focused Cognitive Behavioral Therapy (TF-CBT) (tfcbt.musc.edu/).

AAP POLICY STATEMENTS

American Academy of Pediatrics, Committee on Psychosocial Aspects of Child and Family Health. The pediatrician and childhood bereavement. *Pediatrics*. 2000;105(2):445-447. (aappolicy.aappublications.org/cgi/content/full/pediatrics;105/2/445).

Hagan JF, American Academy of Pediatrics, Committee on Psychosocial Aspects of Child and Family Health, and Task Force on Terrorism. Psychological implications of disaster or terrorism on children: a guide for the pediatrician. *Pediatrics*. 2005;116(3):787-795. (aappolicy.aappublications.org/cgi/content/full/pediatrics;116/3/787).

REFERENCES

1. Costello EJ, Erklani A, Fairbank J, et al. The prevalence of potentially traumatic events in childhood and adolescence. *J Trauma Stress*. 2002;15:99-112.
2. Singer M, Anglin T, Son L, et al. Adolescents' exposure to violence and associated symptoms of psychological trauma. *JAMA*. 1995;273:477-482.
3. Breslau N, Davis GC, Andreski P, et al. Traumatic events and posttraumatic stress disorder in an urban population of young adults. *Arch Gen Psychiatry*. 1991;48(3):216-222.
4. Kessler R, Sonnega A, Bromet E, et al. Posttraumatic stress disorder in the National Comorbidity Survey. *Arch Gen Psychiatry*. 1995;52:1048-1060.
5. Kilpatrick DG, Ruggiero KJ, Acierno R, et al. Violence and risk of PTSD, major depression, substance abuse/dependence, and comorbidity: results from the national survey of adolescents. *J Consult Clin Psychol*. 2003;71(4):692-700.
6. Aaron J, Zaglul H, Emery RE. Posttraumatic stress in children following acute physical injury. *J Pediatr Psychol*. 1999;24(4):335-343.
7. Foa EB, Johnson KM, Feeny NC, et al. The child PTSD symptom scale: a preliminary examination of its psychometric properties. *J Clin Child Psychol*. 2001;30(3):376-384.
8. La Greca AM, Silverman WK, Vernberg EM, et al. Symptoms of posttraumatic stress in children after Hurricane Andrew: a prospective study. *J Consult Clin Psychol*. 1996;64(4):712-723.
9. Fitzpatrick KM, Boldizar JP. The prevalence and consequences of exposure to violence among African-American youth. *J Am Acad Child Adolesc Psychiatry*. 1993;32(2):424-430.
10. Ackerman PT, Newton JE, McPherson WB, et al. Prevalence of post traumatic stress disorder and other psychiatric diagnoses in three groups of abused children (sexual, physical, or both). *Child Abuse Negl*. 1998;22:759-774.
11. Saigh P, Yasik A, Oberfield R, et al. An analysis of the internalizing and externalizing behaviors of traumatized urban youth with and without PTSD. *J Abnorm Psychol*. 2002;111(3):462-470.
12. McCloskey LA, Walker M. Posttraumatic stress in children exposed to family violence and single-event trauma. *J Am Acad Child Adolesc Psychiatry*. 2000;39(1):108-115.
13. Scheeringa MS, Wright MJ, Hunt JP, et al. Factors affecting the diagnosis and prediction of PTSD symptomatology in children and adolescents. *Am J Psychiatry*. 2006;163:644-651.
14. Runyon MK, Deblinger E, Behl L, et al. Post-traumatic stress disorder. In: Ammerman RT, ed. *Comprehensive Handbook of Personality and Psychopathology*. Vol 3. Hoboken, NJ: John Wiley & Sons; 2006.
15. Brent DA, Oquendo M, Birmaher B, et al. Familial pathways to early-onset suicide attempts: risk for suicidal behavior in offspring of mood-disordered suicide attempters. *Arch Gen Psychiatry*. 2002;59:801-807.
16. Nelson EC, Heath AC, Madden PAF, et al. Association between self-reported childhood sexual abuse and adverse psychosocial outcomes. *Arch Gen Psychiatry*. 2002;59:139-145.
17. Warshaw MG, Fierman E, Pratt L, et al. Quality of life and dissociation in anxiety disorder patients with histories of trauma or PTSD. *Am J Psychiatry*. 1993;150:1512-1516.
18. Walker EA, Unutzer J, Rutter C, et al. Costs of health care use by women HMO members with a history of childhood abuse and neglect. *Arch Gen Psychiatry*. 1999;56(7):609-613.
19. Carrion VG, Weems CF, Ray R, et al. Toward an empirical definition of pediatric PTSD: the phenomenology of PTSD symptoms in youth. *J Am Acad Child Adolesc Psychiatry*. 2002;41:166-173.
20. Cohen JA, Deblinger E, Mannarino AP, et al. A multisite, randomized controlled trial for children with sexual abuse-related PTSD symptoms. *J Am Acad Child Adolesc Psychiatry*. 2004;43:393-402.
21. American Psychiatric Association. *Diagnostic and Statistical Manual of Mental Disorders*. 4th ed, text revision. Washington, DC: The Association; 2000.
22. New York Board of Education. *Effect of the World Trade Center Attack on New York City Public School Students. Initial Report*. New York, NY: Applied Research and Consulting, LLC, Columbia Mailman School of Public Health, New York State Psychiatric Institute; 2002.
23. Dyregrov A, Yule W. A review of PTSD in children. *Child Adolesc Ment Health*. 2006;11(4):176-184.
24. Ford JD, Racusin R, Daviss WB, et al. Trauma exposure among children with oppositional defiant disorder and attention deficit-hyperactivity disorder. *J Consult Clin Psychol*. 1999;67:786-789.
25. Steinberg A, Brymer MJ, Decker KB, et al. University of California PTSD reaction index. *Curr Psychiatr Rep*. 2004;6:96-100.
26. Briere J. *Trauma Symptom Checklist for Children: Professional Manual*. Odessa, FL: Psychological Assessment Resources; 1996.
27. Bisson JI, Cohen JA. Disseminating early interventions following trauma. *J Trauma Stress*. 2006;19(5):583-595.

28. Pine DS, Cohen JA. Trauma in children: risk and treatment of psychiatric sequelae. *Biol Psychiatry.* 2002;51: 519-531.
29. Chaffin M, Silovsky JF, Funderburk B, et al. Parent-child interaction therapy with physically abusive parents: efficacy for reducing future abuse reports. *J Consult Clin Psychol.* 2004;72(3):500-510.
30. Kolko DJ. Individual cognitive-behavioral treatment and family therapy for physically abused children and their offending parents: a comparison of clinical outcomes. *Child Maltreat.* 1996;1(4):322-342.
31. Lieberman AF, Van Horn P, Ozer EJ. Preschooler witnesses of marital violence: predictors and mediators of child behavior problems. *Dev Psychopathol.* 2005;17(2): 385-396.
32. Stein BD, Zima BT, Elliot MN, et al. Violence exposure among school-age children in foster care: relationship to distress symptoms. *J Am Acad Child Adolesc Psychiatry.* 2001;40(5):588-594.

Chapter 147

STUTTERING

Pearl A. Payne, PhD

Because of their early and frequent contacts with preschool children, primary care physicians are often the first professionals asked to respond to parental concerns about stuttering. *Stuttering* is a speech disorder that typically emerges in the early preschool years (2-5 years of age), and onset is rarely observed after puberty.[1] Similar to many other speech and language disorders, stuttering is more prevalent in boys than in girls. First-grade children who stutter demonstrate a 3:1 male-female ratio, which increases to 5:1 by the 5th grade.[1] The male-female ratio is closer to 1:1 in the earliest ages of onset.[1]

Stuttering is marked by involuntary interruptions or breaks in the fluency of speech. The breaks, or disfluencies, include part-word repetitions (eg, "pi-pi-picture," "mo-mother"), single–syllable-word repetition (eg, "but-but," "he-he-he"), prolongations of speech sounds (eg, "winnnter, "annnnd"), and blocks or abnormal pauses (eg, "be...because"). Typically, stuttering is first observed during the preschool years as children are progressing through the stages of speech and language development. Although all children are disfluent or have some breaks in their speech, the children who stutter have more than 2 times the number of stuttered disfluencies as their nonstuttering peers. Only 4% to 5% of children demonstrate persistent or chronic stuttering at some point in their lives. The lifetime prevalence of stuttering is approximately 5% of the general population, although the point prevalence estimate is 1%. These figures also hold true for the preschool population.[2] Approximately 80% of affected individuals experience recovery from stuttering. Natural recovery occurs, and some individuals recover after receiving treatment. Most children will be disfluent only for a few months and will show no reaction to these temporary disfluencies. In children, critical clinical questions to be asked are (1) which of these children will naturally recover, and (2) which of them will require intervention services from speech-language pathologists (SLPs)?

Approximately 20% to 30% of persons who begin to stutter will have a lifelong problem.[2] In general, the longer the stuttering continues, the greater the likelihood is that the disorder will become chronic and that it will increase in complexity and severity. This complexity usually includes an individualized pattern of reactions to the disorder, including fear and avoidance of speech. This pattern of chronic and worsening stuttering is sometimes called *developmental stuttering* distinguishing it from the much rarer type, *acquired stuttering*. The latter type usually appears suddenly, long after speech and language skills have been developed; acquired stuttering disorders are associated with neurologic or psychological trauma.

Common risk factors associated with development of chronic stuttering include a family history of stuttering, the presence of other speech or language disorders, male sex, age at the time of identification of stuttering, and the child's temperament.

When developmental stuttering is treated appropriately, especially in its beginning stages, the prognosis for recovery is generally good. The types of behaviors typically seen in advanced stuttering (severe struggling and fear of talking) can usually be prevented. Even adults who have stuttered for years can learn to decrease the severity of their stuttering and improve their attitudes about speaking. The prognosis for acquired stuttering is much less certain. The small number of cases and the wide differences in type of cortical damage or psychogenic trauma make prediction of recovery much more tenuous.[3]

At one time, SLPs were hesitant to treat young children who stuttered, and health care professionals were generally of the opinion that the problem of stuttering would resolve itself without intervention. Today, SLPs commonly practice early intervention with young children, and results of effective early intervention have been reported. The Lidcombe Program[4] is a treatment approach developed in Australia and is used in the United States and other countries. It uses a highly systematic direct intervention approach, and it has an extensive research base. Efficacy of this program has been well studied. Many therapy approaches are based on play and use parental participation to facilitate the transfer of the treatment effect to the child's daily speaking.

Box 147-1 summarizes the characteristics and features of stuttering in children as the disorder develops.

ETIOLOGY

Despite ongoing research, the specific causes of developmental stuttering are still unknown. However, some evidence exists to support a genetic component in the transmission and development of stuttering.[5-8] Genomic linkage studies have identified genes on chromosomes 1, 13, 16, and 18 as loci associated with stuttering. Research is just beginning to study inheritance patterns and the specifics of what is inherited, but this line of research will eventually contribute to a better understanding of the disorder, its onset, and perhaps

BOX 147-1 Characteristics and Features of Stuttering

PRESCHOOL YEARS (2-6 YEARS)

Word, but primarily sound and syllable, repetitions, produced with some tension and effort occur.

Some reactions to stuttering occur; child may experience mild tension.

EARLY SCHOOL YEARS (6-10 YEARS)

Syllable repetitions continue; child exhibits more tension and struggles at point of stutter; blocks appear; child pushes to get *unstuck*.

Some reactions to stuttering occur; child exhibits mild tension at point of stutter; tongue protrusions, jaw tremors, grimaces, and other involuntary behaviors occur, varying from individual to individual; these behaviors may become habituated and part of the disorder.

Child is at risk for developing negative feelings of self as a speaker and a person.

EARLY TEENS AND ADOLESCENTS

Blocks (eg, getting stuck) are the most common type of stuttering or disfluencies; sound prolongations ("...mmmmouse pad") may also be part of stuttering.

Child exhibits frequent use of escape and avoidance behaviors (teen hides the stuttering).

Some fear and avoidance of specific words, speaking situations, or both occur.

Teen exhibits feelings of shame and embarrassment; may begin to have significant negative self-concept.

its prevention. In addition to its genetic component, physiological and environmental factors play a role in the origin and progression of stuttering.[2]

Considerable evidence shows that developmental stuttering is related to children's efforts to learn to talk. This effort may be characterized by physical, cognitive, emotional, or motor effort. Parents frequently report that their children have difficulty getting started or frequently repeat a word, especially at the beginning of a sentence, or the children repeat a sound at the beginning of a word. This pattern usually appears between the ages of 2 and 5 years when children are rapidly mastering speech and language skills. When low in frequency and loose in tension, these disfluencies are considered normal; but for some young children, they are the 1st signs of early stuttering. The disfluencies that mark the onset of early stuttering but that also describe normal disfluencies displayed by all children present a problem for parents and professionals in the diagnosis of stuttering.

One explanation of childhood stuttering, useful for counseling parents, explains its cause by a *demands and capacities* model.[9] This model states that stuttering develops when either internal or external demands for fluency exceed the child's capacities for fluent speech. This model allows for the variability of environmental demands (eg, parental or self-imposed pressures for speech performance) that might exceed the child's capacities (eg, motor speech skills, cognitive or language ability or development) for fluent speech.

In contrast to the lack of definitive known causes for developmental stuttering, acquired stuttering usually has a neurogenic or, more rarely, a psychogenic origin. Neurogenic stuttering usually results from brain damage. No consistent pattern in type of damage (eg, stroke, tumor, disease) or site of lesion (eg, brain hemisphere or lobe) has been found.

DIFFERENTIAL DIAGNOSIS

At its onset, stuttering is variable and often difficult to diagnose. Some days the child is highly disfluent; other days the child barely stutters at all. Additionally, many young children are hesitant to talk with unfamiliar people, particularly in a medical setting. As a result, the primary care physician may not hear a sample of the speech that concerns the caregiver. All speakers are disfluent sometimes, and young children are even more likely to have interruptions in their speech because they are mastering the intricate motor, linguistic, and cognitive skills related to speech and language development. Because stuttering frequently varies among children who stutter, obtaining information about disfluent speech by questioning the parents or caregivers may be necessary.

Normally Disfluent Speech

In normally disfluent speech, the repetitions are usually brief (typically 1 second or less) and occur infrequently (only one syllable or less in 10 syllables spoken), and no signs of struggle in speaking exist. Repetitions of a word or phrase (rather than of a sound or syllable) are considered normal and are often associated with the search for a word (eg, "Mommy, where is my, where is my—you know, my, uh, twicycle?"). Disfluencies often increase when a child is excited or tired.

Early Stuttering

Early stuttering occurs on the initial word or syllable of an utterance, and repetitions are a common behavior. However, the repetitions of the child who is beginning to stutter are produced with more tension and effort. This tension may be seen as signs of struggle and effort around the child's face or mouth, or it may be heard as brief vocal strain or cry. Despite the effort, these children usually have little or no awareness about their speech, although they may show signs of frustration and exasperation with their inability to get the word out. For the young child, stuttering is considered severe when the following conditions are found: (1) stuttering is very frequent (10% or more of the syllables spoken); (2) the repetitions are rapid and uneven; (3) sound prolongations or blockings last 1 second or longer; (4) the child appears to struggle in an attempt to say a word; and (5) fear or avoidance of speaking is evident.

EFFECTS OF STUTTERING

A child's initial reactions to stuttering are usually surprise and frustration. If the stuttering continues, then the frustration can change to a fear of *being stuck*. Some young children react to their stuttering.

Children as young as 2 or 3 may react by hiding or twisting their faces or showing other signs of struggle. Because severe stuttering occurs in only approximately 1% of the population, many young children have difficulty understanding why they are different from others. As the child who stutters enters school, a stuttering problem can make reading aloud difficult and can interfere with academic performance or learning in other ways. Many stuttering children will not ask or answer questions of a teacher even when they want information or know the answers. The psychosocial aspects of stuttering are particularly insidious. School-aged stutterers are frequent targets of teasing.[2] The embarrassment about stuttering usually increases in adolescence, and teens may begin to avoid speaking or participating in specific speaking and social situations. Even adults who formerly stuttered often report feeling embarrassed and guilty about their use of tactics to avoid or conceal a problem, such as pretending to have not heard a question or substituting one word for another when stuttering is anticipated.

REFERRAL

Referring the child whose speech is considered normally disfluent is unnecessary. Parents should be advised to reduce communication time pressure. This technique includes pausing briefly before speaking, avoiding bringing attention to the disfluencies, giving the child their full attention, and allowing the child plenty of time to say what the child wants to say.

Children who stutter mildly should be referred to an SLP if they have stuttered for 3 months or longer or if the stuttering continues after the parents have tried to follow the suggestions previously mentioned. The SLP should hold a certificate of clinical competence from the American Speech-Language-Hearing Association and a license by the state board of examiners in speech-language pathology in the required state of practice. Experience working with childhood stuttering is preferred.

If a child's speech meets the criteria for severe stuttering, then the child should be referred to a qualified SLP as soon as possible. The course of treatment may well last a year or more. The primary care physician can assist teenagers who stutter by showing an understanding for the difficulties they encounter but should urge them not to let the stuttering prevent them from engaging in activities they would otherwise attempt. In the case of this older child who stutters, a qualified SLP is essential in aiding the child and parents to identify an appropriate course of speech therapy.

In the past, parents who were worried about their child's stuttering were often advised to ignore the problem and were told that the child would eventually outgrow it. Although many young children who have incipient stuttering become fluent without treatment, children whose speech is appropriately diagnosed as stuttering usually require professional attention from an SLP to avoid the long term embarrassment and frustration of a stuttering problem that gets worse rather than better as the child grows. The primary care physician is often the 1st professional to recognize stuttering in a child. If a child can undergo therapy when the problem consists primarily of easy, effortless repetitions, then the chances for success are much better than when the stuttering has become complicated by habitual struggle, fear of speaking, and avoidance behaviors. The key to early success is early identification and intervention.

WHEN TO REFER

- No referral necessary for normally disfluent speech.
- Mild stuttering requires a referral to an SLP.
- Severe stuttering requires immediate referral to an SLP

TOOLS FOR PRACTICE

Engaging Patient and Family

- *Stuttering* (Web page), American Speech-Language-Hearing Association (ASHA) (www.asha.org/public/speech/disorders/stuttering.htm).

Medical Decision Support

- *Lidcombe Program* (guideline), The Australian Stuttering Research Centre (www3.fhs.usyd.edu.au/asrcwww/treatment/lidcombe.htm).
- *The Child Who Stutters: To the Pediatrician* (booklet), The Stuttering Foundation (www.stutteringhelp.org/Portals/english/0023tped.pdf).

RELATED WEB SITE

- The Stuttering Foundation (www.stutteringhelp.org/Default.aspx?tabid=4).

SUGGESTED RESOURCES

Australian Stuttering Research Centre. Available at: www3.fhs.usyd.edu.au/asrcwww/. Accessed January 31, 2007.

Guitar B, Conture E, Williams D, et al. *Do You Stutter? A Guide for Teens.* 4th ed. Memphis, TN: Stuttering Foundation of America; 2004.

Stuttering Foundation of America. 3100 Walnut Grove Road, Suite 603, Memphis, TN 38111-0749; 1-800-992-9392. Available at: www.stutterhelp.org/. Accessed January 31, 2007.

Guitar B, Conture E. *The Child Who Stutters: To the Pediatrician.* 4th ed. Memphis, TN: Stuttering Foundation of America; 2004.

REFERENCES

1. Bloodstein O. *A Handbook on Stuttering.* Chicago, IL: National Easter Seal Society; 1995.
2. Guitar B. *Stuttering: An Integrated Approach to Its Nature and Treatment.* Baltimore, MD: Lippincott Williams & Wilkins; 2006.
3. Helm-Estabrooks N. Stuttering associated with acquired neurological disorders. In: Curlee RF, ed. *Stuttering and Related Disorders of Fluency.* 2nd ed. New York, NY: Thieme Medical Publications; 1999.
4. Australian Stuttering Research Centre. The Lidcombe Program. Available at: www3.fhs.usyd.edu.au/asrcwww/treatment/lidcombe.htm. Accessed June 8, 2007.
5. Shugart YY, Mundorff J, Kilshwa J, et al. Results of a genome-wide linkage scan for stuttering. *Am J Med Genet.* 2004;124A:133-135.

6. Cox N. *Genetics of Stuttering: Insights and Recent Advances*. Presented at the annual national convention of the American Speech-Language-Hearing Association. Washington, DC, 2000.
7. Ambrose NG, Cox NJ, Yairi E. The genetic basis of persistent stuttering. *J Speech Lang Hear Res*. 1997;36: 701-706.
8. Felsenfeld S, Plomin R. Epidemiological and offspring analyses of developmental speech disorders using data from the Colorado Adoption Project. *J Speech Lang Hear Res*. 1997;40:778-791.
9. Starkweather CW, Gottwald SR, Halfond MM. *Stuttering Prevention: A Clinical Method*. Englewood Cliffs, NJ: Prentice-Hall; 1990.

Chapter 148
SLEEP DISTURBANCES

Mark L. Splaingard, MD

Sleep problems are common during childhood, occurring in approximately 25% of healthy children younger than 5 years and in up to 80% of children with special needs. Many of these difficulties can be managed successfully in the primary care setting; other problems require evaluation and treatment by a sleep specialist. The pediatrician is in an ideal position to anticipate, recognize, and treat most sleep problems and to refer the patient to a specialist when appropriate. Successful management of pediatric sleep problems often results in improved sleep and daytime function for all members of the household.[1]

A strong subjective component can be found to many pediatric sleep problems. Consider the typical case of the toddler with night awakenings who wants to get in the parental bed.

- The parents in family A do not consider this desire as a problem. Both parents are good sleepers and do not care if the child sleeps in their bed.
- The parents in family B believe strongly that the child does not belong in the parents' bed and that the adult bedroom is the only place the adults have to themselves.
- The mother in family C lives with her own mother and is raising two children. They live in a small apartment in which the two children share a bed.
- The parents in family D own a bed-and breakfast business and live on the premises. They do not want their child in their bed but cannot afford to have a crying child wake the guests.
- The parents in family E have been willing to let the child into their bed in the past, but another infant is due in 3 months, and the parents would like the child to make the transition to spending the night in her own bed.

These examples illustrate the variety of responses to a common sleep issue in the young child. All of these families have caring parents and normally developing toddlers. Some of the parents consider the behavior as a sleep problem, whereas others do not. The parents in family B are more likely to consult a pediatrician about the child's sleep than the parents in family A.

Other sleep problems such as obstructive sleep apnea (OSA) are more likely to be acknowledged as problems by most families, although perceptions may vary. A hearing-impaired parent may not complain of a child's snoring. A parent who is a light sleeper is more likely to take note of a child's sleep disruptions than a parent who is a sound sleeper. Parents frequently consult pediatricians about sleep issues, and the pediatrician should recognize the range of sleep problems and the variability in parental perception of these problems.[2]

DEVELOPMENT OF SLEEP

The development of physiologic sleep patterns is predictable (Table 148-1). It begins in utero; by 28 weeks gestational age, rapid eye movement (REM, or active) sleep can be discerned via fetal ultrasound. Nonrapid eye movement (NREM, or quiet) sleep appears at 32 weeks gestational age. At term, newborns have discrete sleep cycles, lasting 50 to 60 minutes, with awakenings every 2 to 6 hours. These sleep cycles are composed of alternating periods of equal amounts of quiet and active sleep. Quiet sleep is characterized by body stillness, regular respirations, and normal muscle tone. During active sleep, the infant has decreased muscle tone with frequent body movements, including eye movements, and irregular respirations. The total daily amount of sleep at birth ranges from 11 to 23 hours, with an average of 16.5 hours (Table 148-2).

By 4 months of age, mature sleep stages begin to emerge, and day-night sleep patterns are well consolidated. Infants have their longest sleep periods at night and have 3- to 4-hour periods of wake during the day. By 6 months, circadian rhythms begin to display activity similar to rhythms in adults and are well established by 1 year of age. By 3 years of age, the child reaches an adult pattern of sleep, with each discrete cycle of NREM and REM sleep lasting 70 to 100 minutes.[3]

At the beginning of the night, a child progresses rapidly through stage 1 and stage 2 sleep and enters slow-wave sleep (stages 3 and 4) for much of the first third of the night. During slow-wave sleep, the child is difficult to awaken. (Many parents will recognize this period as the time of night that they can vacuum or listen to loud music without waking the child.) Subsequent sleep cycles have decreased amount of slow-wave sleep and increased amounts of stage 2 sleep and REM sleep. Dreaming takes place during REM sleep. REM sleep episodes become longer and more intense later in the sleep period; thus children are more likely to complain of bad dreams during the last portion of the night. In addition, sleep-disordered breathing (SDB) is likely to be most prominent during REM sleep. This tendency is important to recognize, given that this time of night is when parents are least likely to be awake and watching the sleep patterns of their children.

The amount of sleep that children need varies by age, but most children in the early school years need at least 10 hours of sleep. Children who are sleep deprived are sometimes sleepy but are more often irritable, inattentive, or hyperactive. Adolescents need sleep as much as younger children do, but they are less likely to get as much sleep as they need.

Table 148-1 Sleep Developmental Milestones

GESTATIONAL AGE	SLEEP PATTERNS
10 weeks	Spontaneous fetal movements are identified.
24	Neither quiet nor active sleep can be identified between 24 and 26 weeks. Early premature (24 to 27 weeks) toddlers have atypical sleep state characteristic of active and quiet sleep.
28	Active sleep identified by 28 to 30 weeks by eye, body, and irregular respiratory movements. Chin tone does not become tonic before 36 weeks. Rhythmic cycling period of activity and quiescence is identified between 28 to 32 weeks.
30	Typical sleep states begin to emerge at 30 weeks.
32	*Tracé alternant* pattern associated with quiet sleep appears at 32 to 34 weeks. Occipital predominance of delta activity is striking at 31 to 32 weeks. At 32 weeks, EEG differences among wakefulness, active sleep, and quiet sleep develop.
34	Active sleep is 60% of total sleep time (TST).
37	Sleep organization at 37 weeks similar to term newborn.
40	Sleep onset thru REM (REM within 15 minutes of sleep onset). Three distinct sleep states in term newborn: (1) REM (active), (2) NREM (quiet), and (3) indeterminate. Newborn sleeps 16 to 17 of 24 hours. Active sleep 50% of TST in term infant. Newborn sleep cycle is 50 to 60 minutes (range 30 to 70), 58% active, and 39% quiet. Periodic breathing is noted, particularly in active sleep.
46	*Tracé* alternant present in quiet sleep in normal infants is not seen after 46 weeks.
48	Sleep spindles appear. Premature infants show spindle development approximately 4 weeks in advance of full term. Periodic breathing becomes rare after 48 weeks.
3 months	NREM sleep stages begin to appear. By 3 months, sleep-onset REM is no longer present. By 3 months, 60% of sleep is quiet sleep, and 40% is active sleep. Lack of sleep spindles after 3 months is associated with hypothyroidism.
4 months	Sleep shifts to nighttime *settling* by 12 to 16 weeks. Slow-wave sleep recognized at 3 to 4 months. Adult sleep stages at 4 to 5 months. Infant asleep 14 to 15 hours a day by 4 months. By 16 weeks, sustained wake periods are as long as 3 to 4 hours.
6 months	By 6 months, 90% of infants have more NREM sleep than REM sleep.
8 months	REM sleep occupies 30% of TST. Sleep lasts 13 to 14 hours a day by 6 to 8 months of age.

Table 148-2 Average Sleep by Age (Hours)

AGE	NIGHTTIME SLEEP	DAYTIME SLEEP
1 week	8.25	8.25
1 mo	8.5	7.0
3 mo	9.5	5.5
6 mo	10.5	3.75
9 mo	11.0	3.0
12 mo	11.25	2.5
18 mo	11.5	2.0
2 yr	11.5	1.5
3 yr	11.0	1.0
4 yr	11.5	0
5 yr	11.0	0
6 yr	10.75	0
7 yr	10.5	0
8 yr	10.25	0
9 yr	10.0	0
10 yr	9.75	0
11 yr	9.5	0
12 yr	9.25	0
13 yr	9.25	0
14 yr	9.0	0
15 yr	8.75	0
16 yr	8.5	0
17 yr	8.25	0
18 yr	8.25	0

Humans have internal clocks that operate on a cycle of approximately 24 hours. These 24-hour cycles are known as *circadian rhythms*. They are controlled by the hypothalamic suprachiasmatic nucleus. Most people have cycles that are not exactly 24 hours in length, and external time cues help reinforce the 24-hour schedule. The time cues are known as *zeitgebers* (German, *time givers*). The most powerful cue is exposure to bright light; others cues include social interaction, food, and exercise. Circadian rhythms are usually synchronized or *entrained* with light-dark cycles. Infants develop these circadian rhythms over the first few months of life. Circadian rhythm sleep disorders occur when a person's sleep is of normal duration but occurs at a time that does not allow adequate sleep in the context of the person's life. For example, an adolescent who is unable to fall asleep until 4 AM and cannot wake before noon is said to have a circadian rhythm disorder (sleep-phase delay) and is likely to have problems functioning in a usual school environment. If, however, a person with the same sleep-phase delay works at night, then the sleep-phase delay is not considered a disorder.

SLEEP EVALUATION

Children rarely complain of sleeping problems. A parent or other caregiver usually initiates the diagnostic evaluation. The most common complaints are the child's inability to fall asleep or remain asleep, daytime sleepiness, and abnormal behaviors during sleep (snoring, gasping, or yelling). In sorting out a sleep concern, history is the major initial diagnostic tool.

Table 148-3 Questions to Clarify Sleep Problems

QUESTIONS	TO CLARIFY
TO THE PARENTS	
Do you have any concerns about the child's sleeping?	Problem versus disorder
How do you think the child is sleeping compared with other children of similar age?	Traumas or stress
When and how did the child's sleep problems start?	Secondary gain
Did other changes in the child's life occur around this time?	Traumas or stress
• What have you tried to solve this problem?	
• What ideas have you had about solving this problem?	
• What have others told you about this problem?	
What is the atmosphere in the room where the child sleeps with regard to temperature, darkness, noise, presence of siblings, and type of bed?	Environmental sleep disorder
When is the last time the child eats before falling asleep?	Inadequate sleep hygiene Sleep-onset association disorder
Does the child consume any caffeine or nicotine in the evening?	Insomnia caused by substance or drug effects
What is the child doing just before bedtime?	Inadequate sleep hygiene Limit-setting disorder Bedtime resistance
What routines do you use to put the child to bed?	Inadequate sleep hygiene Limit-setting disorder Bedtime resistance
What exactly do you do at bedtime?	Sleep-association disorder
How does the child act at bedtime?	Bedtime resistance
Where and with whom does the child sleep?	Sleep-association disorder
What does your spouse or partner think about this arrangement?	Family conflict
Who else has something to say about the child's sleeping?	Family conflict
Is the child already asleep when you put him or her in the crib or bed?	Sleep-association disorder
What time is the child put in bed?	Limit-setting disorder Inadequate sleep hygiene Circadian disorders
What time is the child asleep?	Limit-setting disorder Inadequate sleep hygiene Circadian disorders
Does the child do anything unusual during sleep?	Sleep-disordered breathing
Snoring, gasping, apnea?	
Leg kicking, thrashing?	Periodic limb movements, restless leg syndrome
Bedwetting?	Nocturnal enuresis
Shaking, screaming?	Nocturnal seizures Parasomnias
What times does the child wake up?	Night feeders Sleep-association disorder
How does he appear, or what does he or she do after waking?	Parasomnias Developmental night waking Trained night feeders Seizures
What works to resettle the child?	Sleep-association disorder Trained night waking Trained night feeding Gastroesophageal reflux
How is that process for you?	Secondary gain
Does the child snore or seem to stop breathing during the night?	Sleep-related breathing disorder
What time is the child up for the day?	Circadian disorders Mood disorders
Is the schedule the same on weekends, or does the child sleep in?	Limit-setting disorder or sleep-phase delay
How does the child wake up in the morning?	Circadian disorder or sleep-phase delay
When you wake the child, does he or she seem rested and cheerful?	Circadian disorder or sleep-phase delay Inadequate sleep
What time does the child eat in the morning?	Circadian disorder or sleep-phase advance Limit-setting disorder

Table 148-3 Questions to Clarify Sleep Problems—cont'd

QUESTIONS	TO CLARIFY
If older than 3 years, does the child remember what happened during the night?	Parasomnia (not remembered) Nightmares (remembered) Panic attacks (remembered)
Does the child fall asleep during the day? If so, then when, where, and for how long?	Circadian disorders Idiopathic hypersomnia or narcolepsy
How is the child settled for naps?	Sleep-association disorder Limit-setting disorder
Does the child sleep differently at other people's houses? If so, then how?	Sleep-association disorder Limit-setting disorder
Has the child ever been given any medications for sleep?	Insomnia caused by a psychiatric or behavioral condition
What was the medication? How did it work?	
Has anyone in the family ever had sleep problems? Did either of you have sleep problems as kids?	Genetic factors (short or long sleeper)
TO THE CHILD	
What do you think about before you go to sleep?	Anxiety or mood disorder Limit-setting disorder
How do you feel when you wake up in the night?	Nightmares Disorders of arousal Anxiety or mood disorders
Do you still feel sleepy in the morning?	Inadequate sleep Circadian disorder or sleep-phase delay
How do you feel about this sleeping problem?	Anxiety Secondary gain
What do you think your parents should do about this?	Secondary gain
How are your concentration and grades at school?	Sleep-related breathing disorder Sleep-phase delay Periodic limb movements disorder Narcolepsy Idiopathic hypersomnia

EEG, Electroencephalogram; *NREM*, nonrapid eye movement; *REM*, rapid eye movement.

Questionnaires for general screening or for evaluating sleep complaints may be helpful in gathering data in busy practices. One simple, 5-item pediatric sleep screening instrument is BEARS (**B**edtime problems, **E**xcessive daytime sleepiness, **A**wakenings at night, **R**egularity and duration of sleep, and **S**noring).[4] The key areas explored on the BEARS parent questionnaire can lead to further open-ended questions by the practitioner to determine the level of parental concern (or to elicit maladaptive patterns if no concern is expressed) and to help formulate a differential diagnosis (Table 148-3). Having the parents keep a sleep chart is helpful (Figure 148-1 on pages 1298-1299). It may demonstrate a consistent pattern, which may improve with use of guidelines for sleep hygiene (Box 148-1 on page 1300). A general medical, developmental, and mental health history assessment should include any medications, herbal products, drugs, alcohol, or tobacco use. Given that many sleep disorders have a strong familial component; family history of parent sleep issues may be helpful.

Parental perceptions and differences of opinion about sleep often are critical in problem-solving efforts. Co-sleeping (one or both parents sharing a bed with one or more children) serves as a good example of this point. Co-sleeping is a common practice in many households. When it is agreeable to both parents, co-sleeping is not associated with greater-than-average behavioral or emotional problems in the child. If, however, co-sleeping is a source of discord between parents or reflects a parent's inability to manage the child's behavioral bedtime problems, then it should be addressed as a sleep problem. When co-sleeping is planned, parents should agree on the desired duration. The pediatrician may help the parents by telling them that this arrangement is easier to change before 6 months of age (if an end is intended during infancy). Purported cases of death by overlying have almost always been the result of adult intoxication, extremely deep sleep or obesity in the adult, or child abuse.

Parental mental health needs to be screened in assessing sleep difficulties because the emotional stability of parents may affect both the perception of problems in children and the ability to carry out a treatment plan. Histories from babysitters or relatives who observe the child's sleep may be diagnostic, especially when problems seen at home are not seen in these settings. The family may provide audiotapes or videotapes that may be helpful.

The history is often diagnostic, but some patients need an overnight sleep study for further assessment.

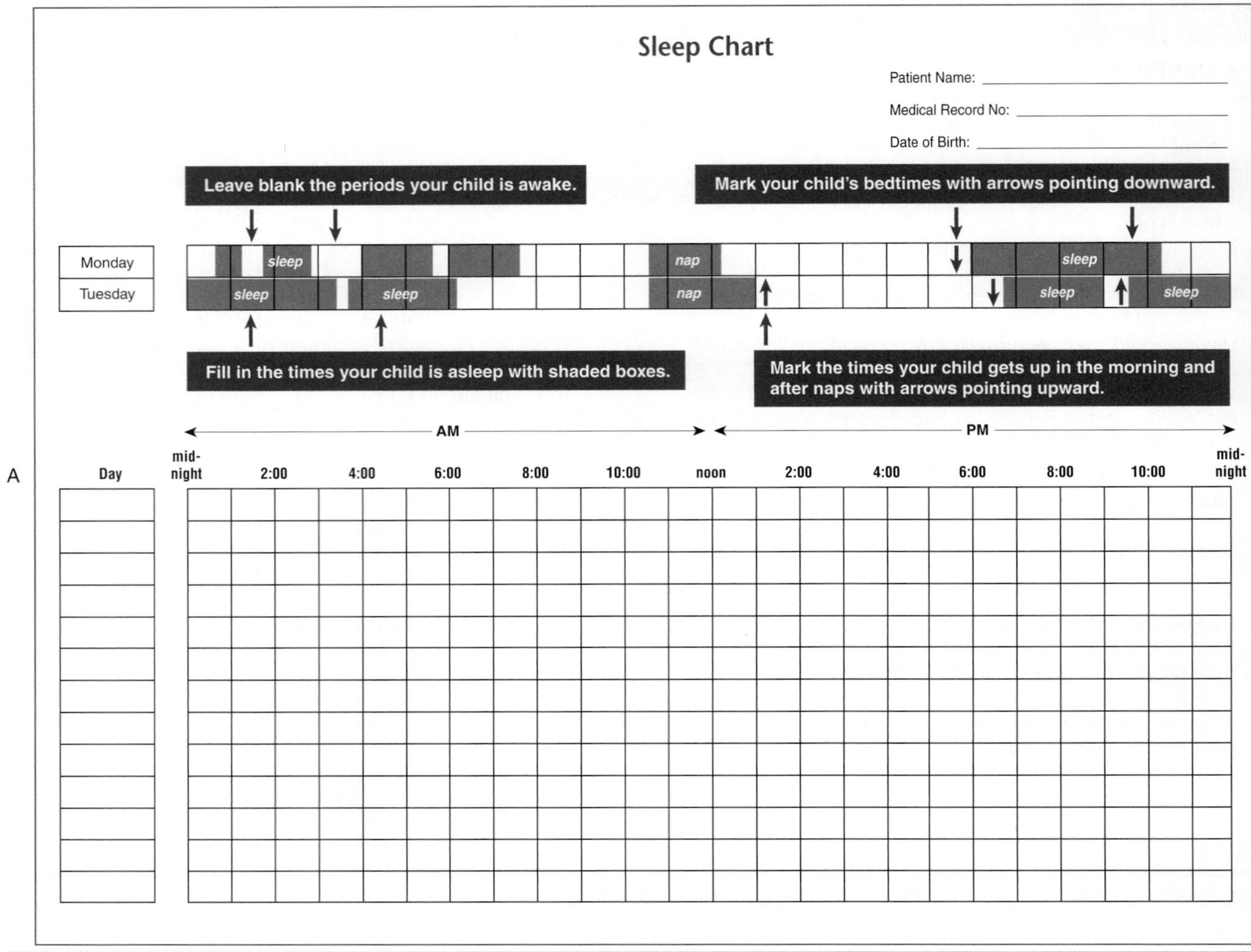

Figure 148-1 **A**, Sleep log. **B**, Sleep log showing sleep phase delay.

An overnight sleep study or polysomnogram consists of the following:

- Electroencephalogram (EEG) to identify sleep stages
- Electromyelogram of chin activity to help identify decreased tone during REM sleep
- Leg electromyelogram to measure leg movements
- Electrooculogram to identify eye movements seen in REM sleep
- Electrocardiogram to monitor cardiac rate and rhythm
- Nasal and oral thermistors to measure airflow
- Thoracic and abdominal belts to measure chest and abdominal movements during breathing (helpful in demonstrating increased or decreased respiratory effort)
- Pulse oximetry to measure oxygen saturation
- End-tidal carbon dioxide monitoring to indirectly measure hypoventilation

All of these measurements provide clinically useful information about sleep stages, sleep disruption, respiratory status during all sleep stages, leg movements, and changes in cardiac rate and rhythm during sleep. The sleep study also provides a picture of the relationship of sleep-related measurements. For instance, OSA may cause arousals, cardiac deceleration, and oxygen desaturation; these findings may be mild during NREM sleep but profound during REM sleep.

Overnight sleep studies are attended by a sleep technologist who attaches monitoring sensors and adjusts them during the night. The technologist also provides observations about the child's sleep that may be invaluable in making an accurate diagnosis.

Extended-montage video electromyelograms may be incorporated into polysomnogram to diagnose nocturnal seizures. Haplotyping, karyotyping, or fluorescent in situ hybridization studies can be helpful for diagnosing some of the genetic conditions associated with sleep disorders such as congenital central hypoventilation syndrome, Rett syndrome, Smith-Magenis syndrome, and Prader-Willi syndrome.

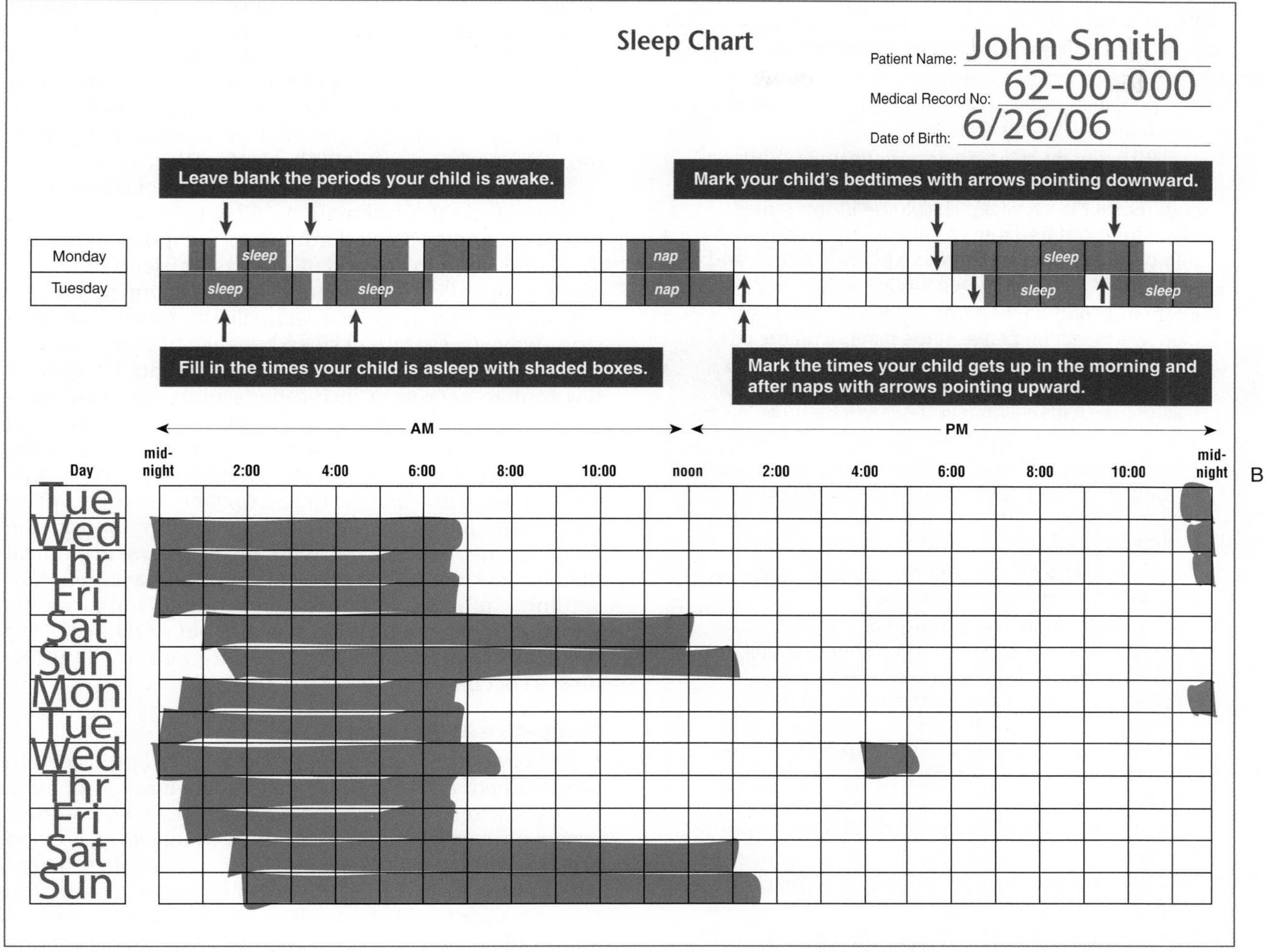

Figure 148-1—*cont'd* **A**, Sleep log. **B**, Sleep log showing sleep phase delay.

CLASSIFICATION OF SLEEP DISTURBANCES

Sleep disturbances in children can be categorized according to the *International Classification of Sleep Disorders*, second edition[5]:

- Maturational or behavioral sleep issues
- SDB
- Circadian rhythm disorders
- Parasomnias
- Sleep-related movement disorders
- Hypersomnia

MATURATIONAL OR BEHAVIORAL ISSUES

Day-Night Reversals

The earliest parent complaint about sleep is often day-night reversal, occurring around 2 weeks of age. This problem is predictable because consolidated nocturnal sleep has not yet developed. Parent concerns provide the pediatrician a valuable opportunity to assess parental coping skills and help parents understand the normal unfolding of the child's physiologic regulation. Day-night reversals can be shifted by establishing a general bedtime, keeping the lights off or low, and keeping handling and interaction to a minimum during nighttime feedings. In the morning, lights should be bright and social interaction encouraged. Lack of sleep at this age is unusual and should alert the clinician to medical problems, especially if associated with irritability.

Delayed Settling

Another common problem is a delay in the much-desired milestone of sleeping through the night. One definition of settling or sleeping through the night is 5 hours of continuous sleep after midnight for 4 consecutive weeks. Unrealistic parental expectations for sleeping through the night are common, and pediatricians need to address carefully misperceptions about how well a child should sleep. Anders observed that 44% of parents of 2 month olds reported that their child slept throughout the night when, in fact, actual recording on time-lapse videotape showed that only 15% actually slept throughout the night without awakening.[6] This issue of sleeping through the night may

BOX 148-1 Sleep Hygiene Principles

General principles of sleep hygiene apply at any age but specifics may vary by the child's age.

1. Establish a good sleep environment that is dark, quiet, and comfortable and has a steady, slightly cool temperature. Sleep should be in the same place for night and naps as much as possible. The bed or crib should be used as a place for sleep and not as play area or playpen while awake.
2. Establish a soothing bedtime routine that involves friendly interaction between the parent and the child. This routine may include a snack and then tooth brushing, use of the toilet, and then story, prayer, or talking time with children in their own bed. The parent should leave the room while the child is still awake.
3. Infants should be fed in a parent's arms and placed in the crib without a breast or a bottle in their mouth. Avoid excessive feeding close to bedtime to reduce the need to void during the night.
4. The child should be put to bed when moderately tired to reduce bedtime resistance.
5. For children whom the parents would like to have sleep in their own crib, teach the child the skill of falling asleep on his or her own by avoiding pacifiers or body contact with the parent as the child drifts to sleep (self-soothing). This method enables the child to go back to sleep on his or her own after waking during the night.
6. Avoid changing the routine because of demands or tantrums at bedtime, which can quickly develop into a pattern.
7. No television or computer should be in the child's room.
8. Try to keep a consistent schedule for bedtime, naps, and morning wake-up. This consistency will help the child maintain regular circadian rhythms. Naps should not be taken too close to bedtime.
9. Remember that television programs and movies may be frightening or stimulating. Arguments between parents or other family members may also be distressing. Try to keep the household atmosphere calm in the evening.
10. Keep track of activities that seem to lead to sleeping problems. If active play or video games lead to problems, then stop them an hour or 2 before bedtime. Caffeine and nicotine can disrupt sleep. Avoid caffeine at least 6 hours before bedtime.

have important ramifications regarding the breastfeeding infant. Despite the widely recognized and undisputed advantages of human milk for infants, the duration of lactation in the United States is still well below the recommended goal of 50% at 6 months in all ethnic groups.[7] The perceptions of normal maternal and infant sleep patterns may be an important factor in failure to sustain lactation. Although breastfed infants are typically assumed to feed more frequently and have shorter meal intervals than bottle-fed infants, widely disparate differences in sleep patterns, crying, fussiness, and colic behavior between breastfed and bottle-fed infants have been reported. The perception that breastfed infants typically *settle* at an older age than bottle-fed infants and awake more frequently at night is quoted in the popular press as an *advantage* of formula feeding. A corollary, a mother's need for an uninterrupted night's sleep, may inadvertently promote the early cessation of breastfeeding.

In fact, breastfeeding need not be associated with increased night wakening by 12 weeks of age; both breastfed and bottle-fed infants can respond to behavioral interventions aimed at increasing sleep time during the night.[8-10] Additional evidence is emerging that continuing lactation can actually increase maternal slow-wave (restorative) sleep because of increased circulating prolactin levels.[11] The circadian rhythm of tryptophan secretion in mother's milk may help promote nocturnal infant sleep.[12] Infants who appear to have a low threshold of sensitivity by temperamental disposition also tend to settle later. Premature infants tend to settle around the time expected for their gestational age, although variability is greater than in the full-term group. Infants who have delays in central nervous system (CNS) maturation often have delays in settling. Infants with frank neurologic impairments may not only be delayed in settling, but also have other medical issues that need to be addressed to allow settling to occur.

Sleep-Onset Associations

Infants and children develop habits of falling asleep in accustomed circumstances, such as in a bed, in a parent's arms, or while being fed. These sleep-onset associations may begin in the first 2 months of life and are one of several behavioral causes for insufficient sleep outlined in Table 148-4. Sleep-onset association may be viewed as a problem by the family when a child older than 6 months needs prolonged parental assistance to fall asleep at the beginning of the night and after each nocturnal arousal. This pattern is a conditioned response, and the child is unable to fall asleep unless the conditions allowing sleep onset are recreated. Parents may complain of severe disruption of their own sleep because of the need to help the infant resettle several times per night. Treatment is straightforward. The child learns to make the transition from wake to sleep without expecting a parent's participation. Parents should be advised to place the infant while still awake into bed for both night and naps starting by 48 weeks postgestational age. A helpful tactic is for the infant's bedding to have mother's scent for comfort. If a problematic sleep-onset association has already developed, then the parent may need to institute a graduated extinction program to help the infant older than 6 months to learn to fall asleep on his or her own over several weeks.[13]

Limit-Setting Disorder

Bedtime routines should take 30 minutes or less. If bedtime routines are consistently longer than this, then it may reflect parental difficulty in setting limits. Prolonged bedtime routines are often associated with multiple curtain calls for stories, hugs, water, and trips to the toilet. Toddlers and preschool children no longer sleeping in a crib may reappear after being put to

Table 148-4 Causes of Insufficient Sleep in Children

	PREVALENCE	TREATMENT
Behavioral	30%-40%	
Sleep-onset association disorder		Education, extinction strategy
Limit-setting disorder		Education, family counseling
Adjustment disorder		Education, family counseling
Chronic sleep deprivation	Common	Education in sleep hygiene
Early school starting times		Education; advocacy (petition school boards and legislature for later school start times)
Parent work schedule		Education
Social activities		Education
Idiopathic insomnia (diagnosis of exclusion; often made retrospectively)	Unknown	Good sleep hygiene; hypnotics under investigation
Circadian rhythm disorder		Education, morning light therapy
Delayed sleep phase		Advance sleep phase
Sleep entrainment		Intense sensory clues; regular or strict daily schedule; melatonin
Hypothalamic tumor		Intense sensory clues; regular or strict daily schedule; melatonin
Blindness		Intense sensory clues; regular or strict daily schedule; melatonin
Mental retardation		Intense sensory clues; regular or strict daily schedule; melatonin

bed, thus prolonging the routine. These curtain calls are unintentionally reinforced by the parental attention needed to return the child to bed, even if done with obvious displeasure.

The best management of prolonged bedtime routines is prevention through reasonable daily schedules, assurance of adequate special individual time with each parent every day, and careful limit setting. This approach reduces the child's separation anxiety, as well as parental guilt. The bedtime routine should be limited to a defined set of activities or length of time. The parent may then either notify the child that they will not respond to further requests, or say "only one more" and adhere to this declaration. Parents should be warned to avoid responding to the excuses that will likely ensue. Having the parent promise to check the child frequently can also be reassuring. Bedtime should occur when the child is tired to enhance the child's tendency to fall asleep. Naps should not occur close to bedtime.

Positive reinforcement may enhance limit setting. Children succeeding in staying in bed without calling out may be motivated by simple rewards with stickers in the morning or an extra story the following night. Parents may need coaching on limit setting or referral to a psychologist if discipline is a major problem. Parents may benefit from marital counseling if significant discord exists regarding family life.

Bedtime Fears

Preschool and early school-age children often have bedtime fears, frequently generated by stresses such as separation from parents, aggressive peers, sibling birth, or the death of a grandparent. Exposure to frightening movies or video games can also contribute. The child's fears should be acknowledged, and the child should be reassured that the parents will be able to keep the child safe. A ritual of the adult *spraying for monsters* may be helpful. Having the child help the parent buy a special flashlight to use to check out the room at night provides a sense of mastery. Older children benefit from relaxation exercises accompanied by empowerment stories. A night-light may be helpful.

BOX 148-2 Symptoms and Signs of Inadequate Amount of Sleep

1. Excessive daytime sleepiness (rare in young children)
2. Hyperactivity—impaired attention
3. Poor school performance—impaired concentration, vigilance
4. Behavior problems—bad mood, irritability
5. Obesity—link to inadequate sleep
6. Failure to thrive

Primary Insomnia

Primary insomnia can be seen in normal children but is generally transient and is a diagnosis of exclusion. It must last at least 1 month, interfere significantly with functioning or cause significant distress, and not be part of another medical, sleep, or mental disorder. The symptoms and signs of inadequate sleep are listed in Box 148-2.

Table 148-5 Causes of Sleep Fragmentation in Children

	PREVALENCE	TREATMENT
Behavioral	30-40% of persons with sleep fragmentation	
Sleep-onset association		Education
PARASOMNIAS		
Sleep terrors		Education, good sleep hygiene, medication (rarely)
Sleep talking		Education, good sleep hygiene
Somnambulism		Education, good sleep hygiene, review safety issues
Confusional arousals		Education, good sleep hygiene
SLEEP-RELATED BREATHING DISORDER		
Sleep apnea	2%	Adenotonsillectomy, nasal continuous positive airway pressure (CPAP)
Upper airway resistance syndrome	Unknown	Adenotonsillectomy, nasal CPAP
OTHER MEDICAL		
Asthma		Medical management
Cystic fibrosis		Medical management
Gastroesophageal reflux		Medical management
Nocturnal seizure		Anticonvulsants
Periodic leg movements of sleep	3.9-10% of adults; 2% children; 20% of children with attention deficit hyperactivity disorder	Iron replacement therapy; dopamine agonists; gabapentin
ENVIRONMENT		
Co-sleeping, noise, pets		Education, safety issues

Medication for primary insomnia in healthy children is controversial, but medications such as diphenylhydramine, clonidine, and melatonin have been used in pediatric insomnia. Indiscriminate medication usage can mislead physicians and families about the causes of insomnia and ignore the behavior management needed.[14]

Other Difficulties Falling Asleep

Dyssomnia is the term for insomnia that does not meet disorder criteria, occurring mainly in preschool and older children. This problem includes environmental sleep disorder caused by chaotic or noisy households. Revising the household routine to allow quiet for adequate sleep is necessary to resolve this dilemma. Periodic limb movement disorder has been reported in children, causing either leg discomfort when the child is still at night or arousing the child during sleep and causing sleep-maintenance insomnia and sleep fragmentation (Table 148-5).

Awakenings from Sleep

Waking at night occurs in more than 80% of children and, of course, in infants who still need to feed at night. Night waking is only problematic when the child cannot return to sleep on his or her own. As many as 20% of 2 year olds, 14% of 3 year olds, and 6.5% of 5 to 12 year olds have problematic night awakenings.[15] Common causes and treatment of sleep fragmentation and disrupted sleep continuity are outlined in Table 148-5.

Sleep-Onset Association Disorder

TRAINED NIGHT FEEDING. In Western industrialized societies, between 60% and 70% of either breastfed or bottle-fed infants are reported to be settling or sleeping through the night by 12 weeks of age without any specific behavioral interventions.[9,16] Nonetheless, some infants older than 6 months who wake up during the night are immediately fed to encourage their return to sleep. Their sleep cycle may be changed by the introduction of food to produce an arousal—basically, learned hunger—and they will consume a full feeding during the night. Trained night feeding should generally not be diagnosed before 6 months postterm because of the frequent need for a feeding during the night in younger or in premature infants. Infants who have learned to sleep through the night and subsequently begin waking during the night appearing genuinely hungry are probably ready for solids (if they are older than 4 to 6 months) or need increased volumes or number of feeds during the day and evening if they are formula fed. Breastfed infants may respond better to more frequent evening feedings (cluster feeding) of smaller but richer (higher lipid content) human milk.

Trained night feeding can be prevented by teaching parents ways to recognize when an infant is fussy because of hunger and when fussiness arises from other causes, such as boredom. Parents should not automatically feed a fussy infant unless the infant appears hungry. Parents who go to their infants older than 4 months at the first sound of the infant stirring should also be encouraged to allow their infants the opportunity to return to sleep without parental intervention. Expectations of the appropriate need for a late (eg, 10 PM) feeding should be clarified. Daytime feeding intervals can be adjusted gradually and any sleep associations retrained simultaneously. If night feedings are an established pattern, then the formula-fed infant can be bottle-fed 1 oz less. This tactic will usually help resolve trained night feeding in approximately 1 week.

TRAINED NIGHT WAKING. Waking at night without requiring a feeding in the infant between 4 and 8 months of age is called trained night waking. This pattern often begins when the infant is ill or has been subjected to travel or some other change in routine, but the pattern may persist because the child gets a secondary reward by the parent's attention. One parent may believe that quieting the infant quickly is necessary so as to avoid disturbing other family members or neighbors. In some instances, parents who have little time to spend with the child during the day enjoy this time with the child and reinforce the night waking by playing with the child. Trained night waking is also increasingly common in infants who have difficult temperaments.

Management of trained night waking that causes persistent family disruption requires management of the precipitant stress and, ideally, collaboration with spouse or neighbors to tolerate some crying during treatment. Bedtime routines need to be established, perhaps with bedding or infant clothing with a maternal scent, and the infant should be put into bed awake. Daytime naps should be limited to 2 hours to consolidate the longest sleep period at night. When the infant awakens during the night, he or she should be allowed 1 to 2 minutes of crying before being checked, but not fed, then checked every 2 to 5 minutes in most circumstances. The infant may be touched but not picked up, rocked, or cuddled. This approach may require the more involved parent to take a shower, turn up music, go out of the house, or otherwise distract themselves for this tactic to be successful. Brief sedation with diphenylhydramine for the infant should rarely be needed to help modify this habit if the graded extinction techniques described previously are strictly applied.

DEVELOPMENTAL NIGHT WAKING. Although most infants are sleeping through the night by 6 months of age, many begin awakening again starting around 8 to 10 months of age. This new behavior, called *developmental night waking,* corresponds to several coincident developmental processes, including increased mobility, fear reactions to strangers, and object permanence (ability to remember and seek something once it is out of sight).

The best management is advising parents at the 6-month health supervision visit to expect a recurrence of night waking. Because of differences in cultures, not all parents will see this circumstance as a problem. For parents who do, they should be advised to wait a few minutes before going in to the infant but to avoid feeding or other reinforcement. If waking is already established, then the parents should have the contributing developmental forces explained and be advised to create a bedtime routine, including a transitional object and a dim night-light. When the infant awakens, he or she should be given at least 2 minutes to self-soothe, with some fussing tolerated as part of the process. If fussing continues, then one parent can go to the child, reassure him or her briefly, without touching or feeding, and settle down within sight to sleep the rest of the night without talking to the child. The child often becomes enraged instead of fearful, which is more tolerable to the parent, who can see that the child is safe. Some parents are more comfortable than others with this plan. For children who are no longer constrained to a crib, the parent must prevent body contact with the child by giving the child the alternative that the parent will leave the room to avoid establishing a sleep association. Further interactions should be brief and minimally interactive. Eventually, the child will no longer require the parent's presence to return to sleep after nocturnal awakenings.

Sleep-Related Breathing Disorder

The pediatrician is often confronted with the problem of what to do with the child who snores. Snoring is common; obstructive sleep apnea (OSA) is less common. For a discussion of evaluating snoring in children and for details on treating OSA, please see Chapter 331, Tonsillectomy and Adenoidectomy.

Young children with sleep disordered breathing (SDB) are usually not obese, unlike typical adult patients. Some groups of children are at particularly high risk for SDB, including those with craniofacial anomalies, chromosomal syndromes, and neuromuscular disorders. Children with Down syndrome, Prader-Willi syndrome, cleft palate, achondroplasia, muscular dystrophy, cerebral palsy, and other underlying disorders should be routinely screened for sleep problems.[17] Many people assume that children with Down syndrome, for instance, have difficulty learning because of the syndrome, but treatment of SDB may result in improved daytime performance.

Most children with obstructive SDB improve after adenotonsillectomy. On occasion, tracheostomy or nasal continuous positive airway pressure (CPAP) may be needed.

The question of which children should have sleep studies is controversial. However, certain groups of children are clearly at risk for perioperative complications and should have polysomnograms as part of a preoperative evaluation. Children younger than 3 years of age, children with morbid obesity or chromosomal or craniofacial anomalies, children with underlying neuromuscular disorders, and those with other underlying medical conditions should all be considered as higher-risk surgical patients and should probably have preoperative polysomnograms.[18,19]

Circadian Rhythm Sleep Disorder

The most common circadian rhythm disorder causing insomnia is a sleep-phase delay that is seen in adolescents. Because the natural circadian cycle is approximately 24.5 hours, some individuals are vulnerable to shifting sleep cycles by approximately 30 minutes a day. This shift often results in difficulty waking in time for school in the morning. Morning battles with parents about waking for school are common. Phase-delayed adolescents often sleep very late on weekends and vacations and then find falling asleep at a reasonable bedtime even more difficult. This pattern can be altered with the use of bright light exposure in the morning and very consistent wake times 7 days per week. Changing adolescent sleep-phase delay is very difficult and requires intense commitment and active participation of the adolescent and parents.

Some children who are deprived of normal circadian stimuli develop circadian rhythm disorders. Because zeitgebers that entrain normal circadian rhythm include light (especially sunlight that may be 100,000 lux), exercise, social activities, and eating, the fact that a child with cerebral palsy who is blind, wheelchair dependent, and fed by gastrostomy tube has difficulty with a wandering sleep time throughout the month is not surprising.

Other children have circadian rhythm problems that reflect a chaotic home life. Some families do not adhere to predictable routines. They may allow the child to set his or her own schedule, resulting in seemingly bizarre sleep patterns. A circadian rhythm disorder may be differentiated from an oppositional disorder by the child's behavior pattern. A child with a circadian rhythm disorder may not resist going to bed but is unable to fall asleep. In the morning, the child is difficult to arouse and does not feel rested.

A sleep-phase advance usually occurs in infants or toddlers who fall asleep early (7 PM) but then awaken early in the morning (3 AM). Different types of circadian shift can be adjusted by simultaneously shifting naps, bedtime, waking time, and meals to a desired schedule that matches the child's total daily sleep needs.

In difficult cases, the child can wear an actigraph, a small portable device similar to a large wristwatch, for several weeks. The device senses physical motion by means of an accelerometer and stores the information. Actigraphy provides a graphic illustration of a child's sleep-wake schedule and can be a useful, noninvasive method for assessing specific sleep disorders such as insomnia, excessive daytime sleepiness, and circadian rhythm disorders (Figure 148-2).

Parasomnias (Partial Arousal Disorders)

Parasomnias are unusual behaviors or experiences that occur during sleep or the transition between sleep and wake. Parasomnias associated with partial arousal from slow-wave sleep are common in children. They include confusional arousals, sleep terrors, and sleepwalking disorder (somnambulism). All of these episodes arise during arousal from slow-wave sleep, usually occurring in the first third of the night. The child appears confused or frightened and is unresponsive to parental intervention. The child is not fully awake and does not remember the event in the morning.

Symptoms most often begin in childhood and resolve spontaneously, occasionally persisting into adulthood (0.5%). Diagnosis is based on the timing of these symptoms (generally during the first third of the night), the typical presentation, and the child's lack of recall of the events when awake the next morning (morning amnesia). A strong familial component exists, and history often reveals that one or both parents had similar behaviors as youngsters.

CONFUSIONAL AROUSALS. Young children may experience partial arousals from slow-wave sleep, during which they sit up, mumble, and may appear awake; they appear confused and nonresponsive to parental questions. The prevalence of confusional arousals was 17% between ages 3 and 13 years in one study.[20] Children may sometimes thrash about and respond combatively to parental attempts to intervene. Confusional arousals usually occur in the first third of the night, but a child may occasionally have multiple arousals, extending into the second half of the night, generally decreasing in intensity. Confusional arousals are most common when children are overtired or ill. Management includes reassurance that the episodes are generally benign, minimal intervention during episodes, and removal of potential safety hazards from the child's bedroom. Treating disorders that may fragment sleep and adequate time for sleeping are also suggested. In severe cases, a few weeks of a benzodiazepine, such as lorazepam, at bedtime may interrupt the sequence by reducing slow-wave sleep. However, rebound occurs with discontinuation of the medication often with an increasing number of events. A sleep study may be helpful to confirm the diagnosis and detect precipitating events such as OSA in severe or atypical cases.

SLEEP TERRORS. Sleep terrors are partial awakenings from slow-wave sleep characterized by physiologic arousal including pallor, sweating, pupillary dilation, piloerection, and tachycardia. The child may sit up and scream and may appear terrified. The child may thrash or run and is not responsive to attempted parental comforting. The child does not remember the event in the morning. Sleep terrors occur in 3% of children, usually starting between 18 months and 5 years. These episodes do not reflect emotional disturbance, although, as with all NREM parasomnias, occurrence is increased with illness, stress, or sleep deprivation. A family history of sleep terrors, enuresis, somnambulism, or sleep talking is often present. Sleep terrors may be precipitated by fatigue, stress, a full bladder, or loud noises. They tend to occur in bouts for several weeks and then disappear only to recur several weeks later. Parents need reassurance about the benign nature of sleep terrors and their tendency to resolve in approximately 95% of children by 8 years of age. The bladder should be emptied routinely before bedtime, and the environment should be kept dark and quiet. The bouts may occasionally be interrupted by waking the child 15 minutes before the expected episode, generally occurring approximately 1 hour into sleep each night for approximately a week. A 30- to 60-minute afternoon nap can also reduce the depth and amount of stage IV sleep and may decrease the number of episodes. Treatment with benzodiazepines can reduce the frequency of these events by altering stage 4 sleep, but episodes may recur when the child is weaned or when tolerance occurs. An investigation for nocturnal seizures with full EEG as part of a sleep study is indicated in intractable cases or those that have their onset in adolescence.

SLEEPWALKING DISORDER (SOMNAMBULISM). Approximately 15% of children sleepwalk at some time. Between 1% and 6% have 1 to 4 episodes per week, mostly between ages 4 and 12 years.[21] Sleepwalking, as with other disorders of arousal, occurs mainly during

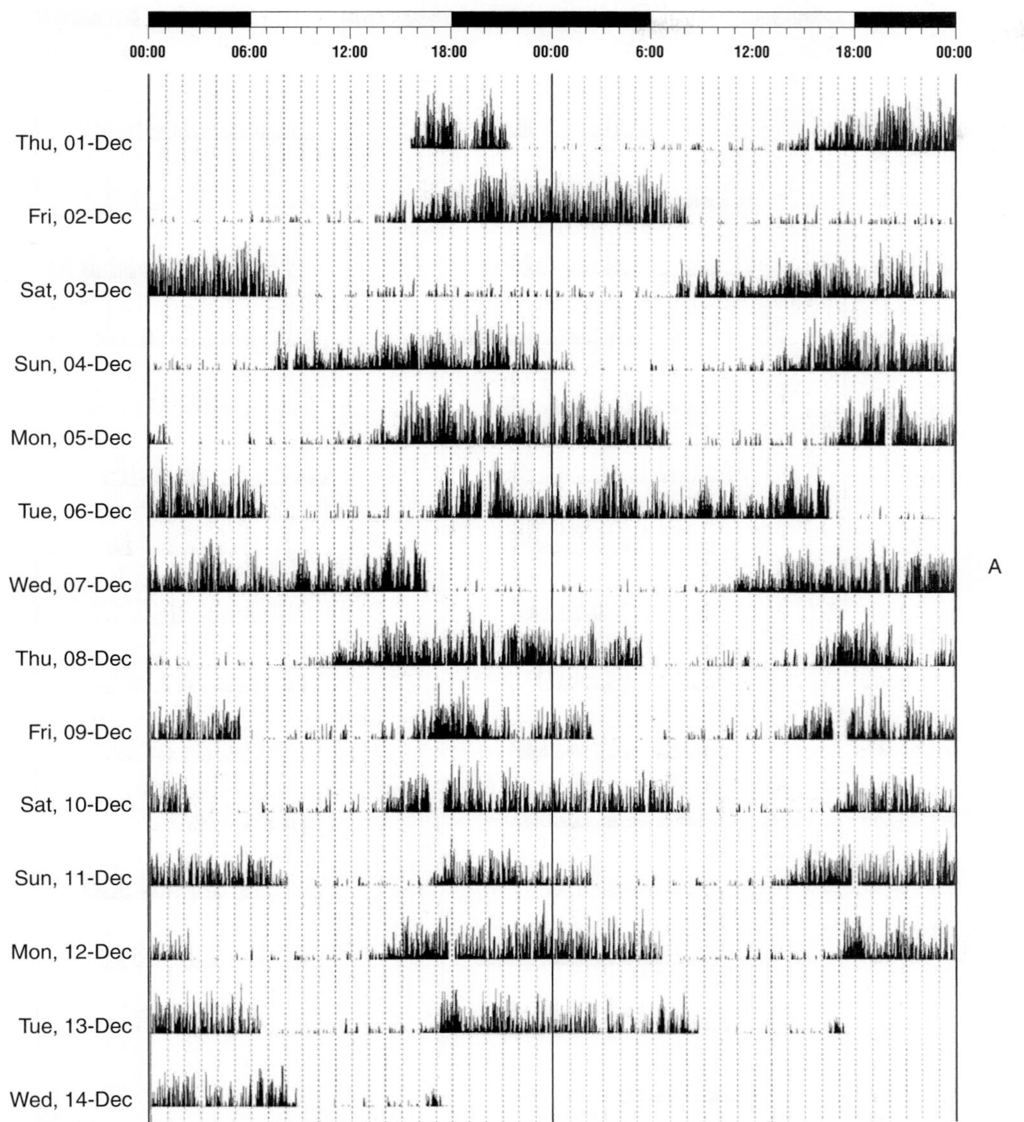

Figure 148-2 Ten-year-old child with Down syndrome and nighttime G-tube feeding after brain injury. **A**, Random sleeping pattern with the child frequently awake at night.

stage 4 sleep, generally in the initial 120 minutes of sleep. During sleepwalking, children are difficult to arouse, are uncoordinated, and tend to wander in illogical places, often urinating outside the toilet. Chronic sleepwalkers need to be carefully safeguarded so that they do not injure themselves. Door and window alarms and locks may be necessary. Amnesia of the event in the morning is common. Sleepwalking can usually be differentiated by history (regular timing, same movements) or videotapes from dissociative states or seizures; however, occasionally, extended EEG as part of a sleep study may be necessary.

Nightmare Disorder

Nightmares are an extremely common parasomnia occurring during REM sleep and are most common in the last third of the sleep period. The dream content often is recalled as frightening and reflects daytime stresses. Although children clearly dream by 14 months of age, nightmares are most common between 3 and 6 years, occurring in 10% to 50% of children. At these ages, children have the verbal skills to describe dreams. They also have vivid imaginations and fears.

Nightmares are uniformly part of posttraumatic stress disorder. Nightmares may increase after withdrawal of REM-suppressing substances such as alcohol and antidepressants.

A child who wakes from a frightening dream should be briefly comforted, keeping intervention brief to avoid secondary gain by adult attention. The same concerns listed for bedtime fears should be addressed when nightmares are frequent. Children who have

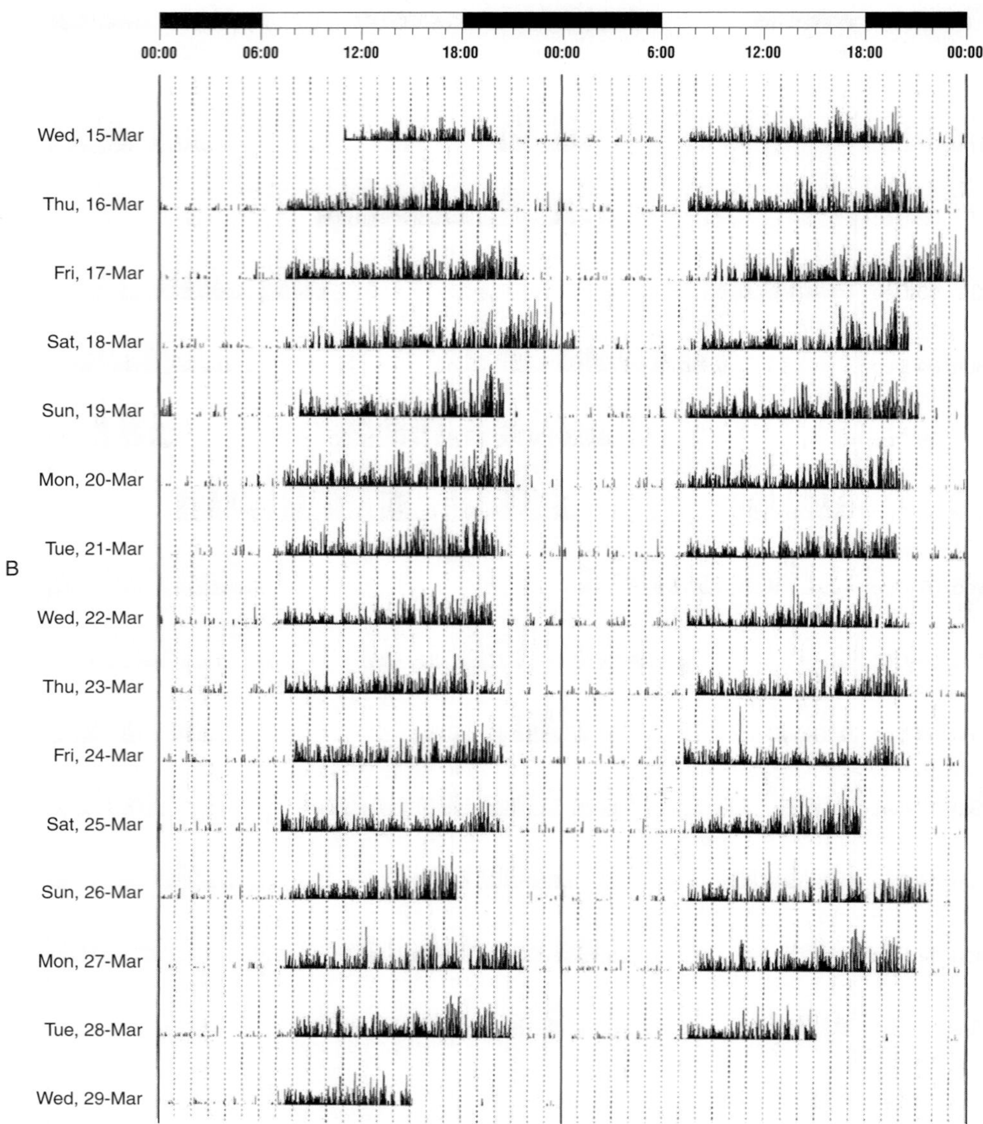

Figure 148-2—*cont'd* **B**, Stabilized sleeping pattern using nighttime melatonin, morning phototherapy, and stopping G-tube feedings at night.

chronic nightmares have been shown to improve with targeted relaxation exercises and stories in which the child masters a situation. Children can prepare to have good dreams through rehearsal and imaging at bedtime. Severe nightmares may respond to bedtime medications such as diphenylhydramine or trazodone, although counseling is mandatory if the condition is of severity to warrant medication.

Violent Behavior During Sleep

A REM behavior disorder (RBD) has been described in which normal REM atonia does not occur. Dream content can be physically acted out, sometimes in violent ways. RBD is rare in healthy children but has been seen in autistic children or in association with neurologic disorders. A clue to diagnosis is that abnormal behaviors occur during the last third of the night, unlike NREM motor parasomnias, which typically occur during slow-wave sleep during the first third of the sleep period. Diagnosis requires a sleep study and neuroimaging studies. Treatment with clonazepam has been beneficial in autistic children and is the most common treatment in adults.

Other Parasomnias

Bruxism is grinding the teeth during sleep and has been reported in over 50% of children, with a mean age of onset of 10.5 years. No longitudinal studies demonstrating the natural history of bruxism have been conducted, but dental evidence of bruxism can be identified in 10% to 20% of the general population. Bruxism can also be caused by dental malocclusion or

Table 148-6 Excessive Sleepiness in Children—Causes of Increased Sleep Drive

DIAGNOSIS	PREVALENCE	TREATMENT
Narcolepsy	0.2%	Stimulant medication, attention to sleep hygiene, treatment of coexisting sleep problems (periodic limb movement disorder, obstructive apnea)
Temporary hypersomnolence		None specifically
Acute medical illness		
Illicit drug use		
Medications		
Recurrent hypersomnolence		
Depression	Common	Antidepressants
Kleine-Levin syndrome	Rare	Lithium; carbamazepine; monitor serum levels for both drugs
Menstrual related	Rare	Oral contraceptives
Idiopathic hypersomnolence		Stimulant medication

neurologic or psychiatric conditions. Tooth guards can protect the teeth and reduce potential damage to the temporomandibular joint. If stress or anxiety is a trigger, then relaxation exercises at bedtime may be helpful.

SLEEP-RELATED MOVEMENT DISORDERS

Restless Legs Syndrome and Periodic Limb Movements of Sleep

Restless legs syndrome is a common (2% to 5% of the general population) condition seen in children and adults. It is characterized by uncomfortable sensations in the legs ("like worms crawling under my skin"). These sensations are present in the evening, are associated with the need to move, and are temporarily relieved by movement. They are sometimes confused with growing pains. They may interfere with the child's ability to fall asleep. A strong familial component exists. Periodic limb movements of sleep are repetitive, brief leg twitches, occurring more than 5 times per hour in children. They may cause arousals, fragmenting the continuity of sleep and leading to a complaint of sleep maintenance insomnia. Although the two syndromes are not identical, many patients experience both. In children, limb movements may be exacerbated by iron deficiency or the use of antidepressant medication. They are more common in children with attention deficit hyperactivity disorder (ADHD).[22] Treatment may include iron supplements, clonidine, gabapentin, or dopaminergic agents, depending on the age of the child.

Sleep-Wake Transition Disorder

Rhythmic movements while falling asleep are common in infants and toddlers. Rhythmic movement disorders include head banging and body rocking. Some rhythmic activity at bedtime occurs in 58% of 9 month olds, decreasing to 33% at 18 months, and 22% at 2 years. Head banging is typically monotonous, occurring 60 to 80 times per minute, usually for less than 15 minutes. Head banging is usually benign but may occasionally be caused by CNS injury, headache, inner ear abnormality, sensory deprivation (including visual or hearing impairment), neglect, or abuse. Children of intense temperament are especially likely to bang. Although head banging usually does not cause brain injury, it can be traumatic if the bed is unstable or if safety precautions are not taken in the environment. The condition may be reduced by kinesthetic stimulation during the evening and holding the child as part of the bedtime routine. Sleep restriction (ie, limiting the time the child lies in bed before falling asleep) and mild sedation has been shown to be helpful in difficult cases. Parents may need reassurance of the generally benign nature of these behaviors.

HYPERSOMNIA

Excessive daytime sleepiness (EDS) can be caused by insufficient sleep (see Table 148-4), fragmented sleep (see Table 148-5), or increased sleep drive (Table 148-6). Although some sleepy children appear to have difficulty remaining awake, many sleepy children may exhibit hyperactivity, restlessness, poor concentration, impulsivity, aggressiveness, or irritability. Sleepiness needs to be differentiated from weakness or fatigue. The major sleep disorders causing primary hypersomnia in children are narcolepsy and idiopathic hypersomnia.

Narcolepsy

Narcolepsy is a potentially disabling syndrome of irresistible daytime sleep attacks, abnormally fast transitions to REM sleep from awake, and disrupted nighttime sleep. It occurs in 0.04% of whites and 0.07% of blacks. Up to 34% of adults with narcolepsy report onset of symptoms before 15 years of age, but diagnosis is frequently delayed at least a decade.[23] Loss of muscle tone with emotions while awake (cataplexy), inability to move for a few seconds to minutes on awakening (sleep paralysis), and visual aura or dream states while falling asleep (hypnagogic hallucinations) along with EDS comprise the complete narcolepsy tetrad seen in 30% of persons with narcolepsy. Approximately 90% of patients with narcolepsy with cataplexy are positive for HLA DQB1*0602. Narcolepsy is seen in children but peak age of onset of symptoms is 15 to 25 years. Cataplexy—brief episodes of bilateral muscle weakness that may result in falling, head bobbing, or jaw sagging—is highly specific to narcolepsy but may not be seen in more than 50% of cases. These episodes are usually associated with laughter or strong emotion. Diagnosis of narcolepsy without documented cataplexy can be made by overnight polysomnography showing absence of other sleep diagnoses and a multiple sleep latency test (5 nap opportunities, separated by 2 hours, immediately following the overnight sleep study) showing rapid sleep onset periods (mean less than 8 minutes) with at least 2 naps containing REM sleep. Differential diagnosis includes hydrocephalus, postviral infection (mononucleosis), previous CNS trauma, or idiopathic hypersomnia. Absence of HLA DQB1*0602 does not exclude the diagnosis of narcolepsy, especially without cataplexy. Given that 20% of the general population is positive for HLA DQB1*0602, this test is not specific for possible narcolepsy patients with EDS.

Treatment of narcolepsy includes daytime stimulants such as modafinil or methylphenidate, regular adequate sleep, 2 to 3 planned 30-minute daytime naps, and timing activities at optimal hours of alertness. Education of the patient, family members, and school personnel is important. Support for handling the difficulties of this lifelong chronic condition is such that referral to a pediatric sleep disorders center is indicated. Medications including antidepressants can help eliminate cataplexy.

Idiopathic Hypersomnia

Idiopathic hypersomnia is a disorder of constant and severe EDS, despite adequate nocturnal sleep. Idiopathic hypersomnia is, by definition, a diagnosis of exclusion. A complete evaluation for other causes of hypersomnia must be undertaken, including neurologic disorders (hydrocephalus or CNS tumors), primary sleep disorders (OSA), mood disorders, chronic fatigue syndrome, and medical disorders (acute and chronic infections including mononucleosis, metabolic disorders, or muscle diseases). Although the mean sleep latency on the mean sleep latency test is short in idiopathic hypersomnia, similar to narcolepsy, the patients do not have the 2 sleep-onset REM periods that characterize the diagnosis of narcolepsy. Treatment of idiopathic hypersomnia includes attention to sleep hygiene issues, use of stimulant medications, and thorough review of safety issues such as driving or operating machinery.[24]

SLEEP DISORDERS ASSOCIATED WITH PSYCHIATRIC OR BEHAVIORAL DISORDERS

Sleep problems may occur in association with almost any mental health disorder (Table 148-7). Mood disorders are among the most common mental health disorders affecting sleep. Depression may cause sleep-onset insomnia, although this condition is less common in young children than other age groups. The early-morning waking of depressed adults is usually not seen prepubertally and rarely in adolescents. Hypersomnia

Table 148-7 Behavioral and Psychiatric Disorders Associated With Sleep Problems in Children

DIAGNOSIS	SLEEP PROBLEMS
Depression	Sleep-onset or maintenance insomnia seen in 50% Early morning awakenings Excessive daytime sleepiness (EDS) seen in 25% Sleep complaints are the most prevalent symptoms of major depression in adolescents
Bipolar disorder	Decreased need for sleep without fatigue Insomnia
Seasonal affective disorder	Prevalence 3-4% in children with EDS, fatigue in winter
Anxiety disorder	Increase night awakenings, night time fears Increase sleep-onset insomnia, bedtime problems Increased EDS
Obsessive compulsive disorder	Decrease total sleep time
Autism, pervasive developmental disorder	Sleep-onset insomnia, difficulty settling at night, prolonged and frequent nocturnal awakenings Shortened duration of sleep Irregular sleep-wake pattern Parasomnia (including rapid eye movement behavioral disorder)
Attention deficit hyperactivity disorder	Sleep-onset or maintenance insomnia Nocturnal wakening, obstructive sleep apnea, excessive periodic limb movements

Reprinted from *Pediatric Clinics of North America*, v51, Ivananko A, Crabtree VM, Gozal D, Sleep in children with psychiatric disorders, pp. 51-68, Copyright 2004, with permission from Elsevier.

is a more common complaint than insomnia in depressed adolescents.[25] The sleep problems that are intrinsic to depression are complicated by intrusive thoughts or worries that may interfere with sleep maintenance.

Children with bipolar disorder may have dramatically reduced need for sleep (less than 4 hours a day) during the manic phase. Anxiety and panic disorders may result in difficulties falling asleep because of specific or nonspecific fears, as well as difficulties returning to sleep if aroused during the night. Children who have been abused have frequent sleep problems, including nightmares, increased activity during sleep, and sleep-onset and sleep-maintenance insomnia.[26]

Personality disorders in adolescence have been associated with sleep-onset insomnia. Psychoses may include troubling intrusive thoughts, especially at night.

Insomnia or hypersomnia caused by substance abuse should be considered in sleep disorders in older children and adolescents. Alcohol can induce sleep, but it causes sleep fragmentation in the latter portion of the night. When alcohol is metabolized (1 beer, 5 oz of wine, or 1 oz of liquor per hour), sympathetic tone increases, leading to abrupt arousals and sleep maintenance insomnia. Withdrawal from chronic alcohol abuse may cause severe insomnia. Stimulants such as cocaine and amphetamines can cause severe insomnia. Some antidepressants such as fluoxetine may cause insomnia, whereas others such as tricyclics, trazodone, or mirtazapine may cause EDS. Antidepressants may eliminate REM atonia, thus precipitating RBD. Atypical antipsychotics such as aripiprazole may cause stimulation, whereas others such as olanzapine cause sedation.

DEVELOPMENTAL DISORDERS

Learning disabilities are associated with elevated rates of sleep disturbance, including night waking and troubles falling asleep. One half of these sleep difficulties persist for more than 3 years.[27] Systematic review of the literature suggests that children who have ADHD have higher daytime sleepiness, more movements during sleep, and higher apnea-hypopnea indexes compared with controls. Reported sleep problems also include troubles settling to sleep and multiple awakenings from sleep.[28] Medications used to treat ADHD may prolong sleep-onset latency. Clonidine at bedtime has been found to be effective in improving the sleep of 85% of these children when behavioral measures failed.[29]

Many children with autism have serious sleep problems with difficulties falling asleep, waking in the night, and early-morning waking. Asperger syndrome has been associated with insomnia and RBD. Children who have Tourette syndrome have increased parasomnias.

SLEEP DISORDERS ASSOCIATED WITH MEDICAL PROBLEMS

Sleep problems are seen in a variety of medical conditions (Table 148-8).

Neurologic Disorders

Any CNS impairment can result in dysregulation of the sleep cycle. As many as 85% of children who have major developmental disabilities may experience chronic sleep problems.[30] Behavioral sleep problems in these children can be improved by establishing a bedtime routine and putting the child to bed when sleep onset is likely to occur quickly. If the child has persistent difficulty falling asleep, then establishing a new pattern may be helpful by delaying the usual bedtime for 30 minutes and then removing the child from bed if sleep does not occur in 15 to 20 minutes. After removing the child from bed, the parent should keep him or her awake and play with the child for 1 hour. This procedure is repeated until the child falls asleep within 15 minutes of being put in bed. Wake-up time is kept constant. Daytime naps are not allowed for children older than 4 years.

Other factors such as timing of medications, need for repositioning during the night, pain, nighttime feedings, and caregiver anxiety can contribute to sleep problems in the neurologically impaired child. Melatonin at bedtime has been shown to be helpful in some children who have CNS problems or blindness as the cause of their sleep disturbance. Melatonin should be used cautiously in children with seizure disorders.

Kleine-Levin syndrome, a rare disorder with episodes of severe daytime sleepiness, hyperphagia, and hypersexuality lasting hours to weeks, may be seen in adolescence. Tumors of the third ventricle or posterior hypothalamus may also cause daytime sleepiness. Brainstem lesions or Chiari malformation type II, which are common in children with myelomeningoceles, can cause severe central apnea or vocal cord paralysis causing obstructive apnea.

Sleep-Related Epilepsy

Approximately 20% of seizure patients have seizures only during sleep. Seizures are most likely to occur at the time of sleep-wake transitions. Seizures occurring during the night may disrupt sleep by causing multiple awakenings. The possibility of a seizure disorder should be considered in adolescents with new-onset parasomnias. Atypical seizures may produce EDS.

Sleep-Related Headaches

Most headaches occurring during sleep occur during REM sleep. Cluster headaches are more frequent at night than in the daytime and often disrupt sleep. Headaches on awakening are unusual; the child should be evaluated carefully for the presence of increased intracranial pressure or hypercapnia caused by hypoventilation (eg, Duchenne muscular dystrophy).

Degenerative Disorders

Degenerative brain disorders result in frequent awakenings, difficulty falling asleep, early-morning waking, sleep deprivation, and daytime sleepiness.

Other Medical Disorders

Any condition causing pain at night, such as juvenile rheumatoid arthritis, can result in disrupted sleep.[31] Eczema that causes associated scratching results in frequent awakenings. Painful menstrual cramps may also disrupt sleep.

Sleep-Related Asthma

Asthma episodes are increased during sleep, presumably because the neuroendocrine regulators of respiration are sensitive to diurnal regulation. Children

Table 148-8 Medical Disorders Associated With Sleep Problems in Childhood

DIAGNOSIS	SLEEP PROBLEMS
Asthma	Circadian variation in: • Peak expiratory flow (nadir at 4 AM) • Cutaneous immediate hypersensitivity to house dust allergen • Airway inflammation Sleep-related changes: • Decrease in lung volumes and increase airway resistance • Increase airway resistance and decrease intrapulmonary blood volume • Decrease mucociliary clearance • Nocturnal gastroesophageal reflux Frequent nocturnal awakenings and decrease stage 4 sleep
Cystic fibrosis	Obstructive sleep apnea (OSA) can be common in children <7 years Nocturnal oxygen desaturation in children >7 years: • Hypoventilation, especially in rapid eye movement (REM) sleep caused by derecruitment of ventilatory muscles • Ventilation perfusion mismatch caused by decreased functional residual capacity • Occurs more frequently with forced expiratory volume <65% or resting oxygen saturation while sitting <94%
Craniofacial abnormalities (Pierre Robin syndrome, Goldenhar syndrome, Down syndrome, Treacher Collins syndrome, velocardiofacial syndrome, cleft lip and palate)	Upper airway obstruction Nocturnal hypoventilation
Gastroesophageal reflux	Increased night awakening and pain Delayed sleep onset May result in nocturnal stridor, cough, and wheezing
Down syndrome	Upper airway obstruction with OSA in 30-60% Decreased REM sleep associated with low IQ
Sickle cell disease	Episodic and continuous nocturnal hypoxemia in 40% of children caused by either OSA or primary lung disease
Obesity	OSA Obesity hypoventilation syndrome: • Hypercapnia, hypoxemia, and daytime somnolence • 95% of children with Prader-Willi syndrome have excessive daytime sleepiness
Scoliosis or congenital neuromuscular disorder (Duchenne muscular dystrophy, spinal muscular atrophy)	Nocturnal hypoventilation Nocturnal hypoxemia—excessive daytime sleepiness, morning headaches OSA Restless sleep Frequent awakenings
Traumatic brain injuries	Sleep-onset and maintenance insomnia Excessive daytime sleepiness Dreaming disturbances Nocturnal hypoventilation
Spina bifida	Obstructive, central, or mixed apnea Nocturnal hypoventilation may cause severe excessive daytime sleepiness

who have sleep-related asthma have fragmented sleep and may develop anxiety associated with breathing discomfort. This disruption may lead to bedtime resistance and insufficient nocturnal sleep, leading to problems outlined in Box 148-2. In one study of children with asthma, 34% awakened at least once a week, and 5% awaken every night from asthma symptoms. Daytime sequelae were common, with 59% reporting daytime sleepiness and 51% reporting difficulty with concentration. These complaints all improve with successful asthma management.[32]

Gastroesophageal Reflux Disease

Gastroesophageal reflux disease may produce sleep problems in a variety of ways. The reflux can be painful, resulting in night waking and crying. Reflux has also been associated with either central or obstructive apneas or apparent life-threatening event in infants and young children. The diagnosis of gastroesophageal reflux disease may not always be obvious, owing to lack of usual signs, including excessive spitting up, reswallowing motions, increased fussiness, refusal of feedings, and failure to thrive. Esophagoscopy, assessing for esophageal erosions, may be needed to determine the cause of nighttime pain. Failure to be consoled while being held can be a clue that the child is suffering pain. Holding the child upright reduces the amount of acid in the esophagus and may comfort a child with reflux. See Chapter 229, Vomiting, for further discussion of gastroesophageal reflux.

WHEN TO REFER

If the clinician is unable to relieve a sleep disturbance after working with the family over the course of 6 weeks, then assistance may be needed either from a sleep specialist or from a family therapist or psychologist. The clinician should always consider, and generally respect, a family that really does not care to change a sleeping situation that would seem to be a sleep disturbance to others. Children with chronic, physically based sleep disorders, such as narcolepsy and SDB requiring CPAP, benefit from referral to a sleep disorders center for treatment and group support.

Alternative therapies have been devised by many cultures to restore the essential health-giving function of sleep. Herbal remedies such as chamomile and other soothing teas are common. Any treatment that involves scheduled rest and mental expectation of sleep would be expected to result in improvement.

WHEN TO ADMIT

Primary sleep disturbances rarely require hospitalization, other than the overnight stay needed for a sleep study. Exceptions may include severe SDB with life-threatening oxygen desaturations, arrhythmias, or cor pulmonale. Hospitalization may be needed for some of the underlying disorders, such as CNS tumors or serious depression that may initially present symptoms of a sleep disorder.

TOOLS FOR PRACTICE

Engaging Patients and Family

- *Fostering Comfortable Sleep Patterns in Infancy* (fact sheet), Bright Futures (www.brightfutures.org/mentalhealth/pdf/families/in/sleep_patterns.pdf).
- *Guide to Your Child's Sleep* (book), American Academy of Pediatrics (www.aap.org/bookstore).
- *Sleep Apnea and Your Child* (brochure), American Academy of Pediatrics (patiented.aap.org).
- *Sleep Hygiene Principles* (fact sheet), American Academy of Pediatrics.
- *Sleep Problems in Children* (brochure), American Academy of Pediatrics (patiented.aap.org).
- *Sleep Tips* (fact sheet), American Academy of Pediatrics (www.dbpeds.org/articles/detail.cfm?TextID=34).

Medical Decision Support

- *Questions (to Parents) to Clarify Sleep Problems or Disorders* (questionnaire), American Academy of Pediatrics.
- Questions (to Child) to Clarify Sleep Problems and Disorders (questionnaire), American Academy of Pediatrics.

AAP POLICY STATEMENTS

American Academy of Pediatrics, Millman RP, Working Group on Sleepiness in Adolescents/Young Adults, and Committee on Adolescence. Excessive sleepiness in adolescents and young adults: causes, consequences, and treatment strategies. *Pediatrics*. 2005;115(6):1774-1786. (aappolicy.aappublications.org/cgi/content/full/pediatrics;115/6/1774).

American Academy of Pediatrics, Schechter MS, Section on Pediatric Pulmonology, and Subcommittee on Obstructive Sleep Apnea Syndrome. Diagnosis and management of childhood obstructive sleep apnea syndrome. *Pediatrics*. 2002;109(4):e69. (aappolicy.aappublications.org/cgi/content/full/pediatrics;109/4/e69).

American Academy of Pediatrics, Section on Pediatric Pulmonology and Subcommittee on Obstructive Sleep Apnea Syndrome. Clinical practice guideline: diagnosis and management of childhood obstructive sleep apnea syndrome. *Pediatrics*. 2002;109(4):704-712. (aappolicy.aappublications.org/cgi/content/full/pediatrics;109/4/704).

SUGGESTED RESOURCES

Sheldon SH, Ferber R, Kryger MH. *Principles and Practice of Pediatric Sleep Medicine*. Philadelphia, PA: WB Saunders; 2005.

Splaingard M, ed. Sleep medicine. *Pediatr Clin North Am*. 2004;51(theme issue):XIII-XIV.

REFERENCES

1. Minde K, Faucon A, Falkner S. Sleep problems in toddlers: effects of treatment on their daytime behavior. *J Am Acad Child Adolesc Psychiatry*. 1994;33(8):1114-1121.
2. Riter S, Wills L. Sleep wars: research and opinion. *Pediatr Clin North Am*. 2004;51(1):1-13, v.
3. Sheldon SH. *Evaluating Sleep in Infants and Children*. Philadelphia, PA: Lippincott-Raven Publishers; 1996.
4. Owens JA, Dalzell V. Use of the 'BEARS' sleep screening tool in a pediatric residents' continuity clinic: a pilot study. *Sleep Med*. 2005;6(1):63-69.
5. Sateia MJ. *The International Classification of Sleep Disorders: Diagnostic and Coding Manual*. 2nd ed. Westchester, IL: American Academy of Sleep Medicine; 2005.
6. Anders TF. Night-waking in infants during the first year of life. *Pediatrics*. 1979;63(6):860-864.
7. Gartner LM, Morton J, Lawrence RA, et al. Breastfeeding and the use of human milk. *Pediatrics*. 2005;115(2):496-506.
8. Pinilla T, Birch LL. Help me make it through the night: behavioral entrainment of breast-fed infants' sleep patterns. *Pediatrics*. 1993;91(2):436-444.
9. St James-Roberts I, Sleep J, Morris S, et al. Use of a behavioural programme in the first 3 months to prevent infant crying and sleeping problems. *J Paediatr Child Health*. 2001;37(3):289-297.
10. Nikolopoulou M, St James-Roberts I. Preventing sleeping problems in infants who are at risk of developing them. *Arch Dis Child*. 2003:88(2):108-111.
11. Blyton DM, Sullivan CE, Edwards N. Lactation is associated with an increase in slow-wave sleep in women. *J Sleep Res*. 2002;11(4):297-303.

12. Cubero J, Valero V, Sanchez J, et al. The circadian rhythm of tryptophan in breast milk affects the rhythms of 6-sulfatoxymelatonin and sleep in newborn. *Neuro Endocrinol Lett*. 2005;26(6):657-661.
13. Kuhn BR, Elliott AJ. Treatment efficacy in behavioral pediatric sleep medicine. *J Psychosom Res*. 2003;54(6): 587-597.
14. Pelayo R, Chen W, Monzon S, et al. Pediatric sleep pharmacology: you want to give my kid sleeping pills? *Pediatr Clin North Am*. 2004;51(1):117-134.
15. Blader JC, Koplewicz HS, Abikoff H, et al. Sleep problems of elementary school children. A community survey. *Arch Pediatr Adolesc Med*. 1997;151(5):473-480.
16. Parmelee AH Jr, Wenner WH, Schulz HR. Infant sleep patterns: from birth to 16 weeks of age. *J Pediatr*. 1964; 65:576-582.
17. Marcus CL. Sleep-disordered breathing in children. *Am J Respir Crit Care Med*. 2001;164(1):16-30.
18. McColley SA, April MM, Carroll JL, et al. Respiratory compromise after adenotonsillectomy in children with obstructive sleep apnea. *Arch Otolaryngol Head Neck Surg*. 1992;118(9):940-943.
19. Rosen GM, Muckle RP, Mahowald MW, et al. Postoperative respiratory compromise in children with obstructive sleep apnea syndrome: can it be anticipated? *Pediatrics*. 1994;93(5):784-788.
20. Laberge L, Tremblay RE, Vitaro F, et al. Development of parasomnias from childhood to early adolescence. *Pediatrics*. 2000;106(1 Pt 1):67-74.
21. Anders TF, Eiben LA. Pediatric sleep disorders: a review of the past 10 years. *J Am Acad Child Adolesc Psychiatry*. 1997;36(1):9-20.
22. Picchietti DL, Walters AS. Moderate to severe periodic limb movement disorder in childhood and adolescence. *Sleep*. 1999;22(3):297-300.
23. Challamel MJ, Mazzola ME, Nevsimalova S, et al. Narcolepsy in children. *Sleep*. 1994;17(8 suppl):S17-S20.
24. Sheldon SH, Ferber R, Kryger MH. *Principles and Practice of Pediatric Sleep Medicine*. Philadelphia, PA: Elsevier Saunders; 2005.
25. Dahl RE, Ryan ND, Matty MK, et al. Sleep onset abnormalities in depressed adolescents. *Biol Psychiatry*. 1996; 39(6):400-410.
26. Glod CA, Teicher MH, Hartman CR, et al. Increased nocturnal activity and impaired sleep maintenance in abused children. *J Am Acad Child Adolesc Psychiatry*. 1997;36(9): 1236-1243.
27. Wiggs L, Stores G. Severe sleep disturbance and daytime challenging behaviour in children with severe learning disabilities. *J Intellect Disabil Res*. 1996;40(pt 6):518-528.
28. Cortese S, Konofal E, Yateman N, et al. Sleep and alertness in children with attention-deficit/hyperactivity disorder: a systematic review of the literature. *Sleep*. 2006; 29(4):504-511.
29. Prince JB, Wilens TE, Biederman J, et al. Clonidine for sleep disturbances associated with attention-deficit hyperactivity disorder: a systematic chart review of 62 cases. *J Am Acad Child Adolesc Psychiatry*. 1996;35(5): 599-605.
30. Piazza CC, Fisher WW, Sherer M. Treatment of multiple sleep problems in children with developmental disabilities: faded bedtime with response cost versus bedtime scheduling. *Dev Med Child Neurol*. 1997;39(6): 414-418.
31. Zamir G, Press J, Tal A, et al. Sleep fragmentation in children with juvenile rheumatoid arthritis. *J Rheumatol*. 1998;25(6):1191-1197.
32. Stores G, Ellis AJ, Wiggs L, et al. Sleep and psychological disturbance in nocturnal asthma. *Arch Dis Child*. 1998; 78(5):413-419.

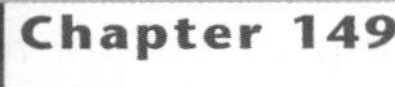

Chapter 149

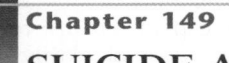

SUICIDE AND SUICIDE ATTEMPTS IN ADOLESCENTS

American Academy of Pediatrics Committee on Adolescence

Suicide is the third-leading cause of death for adolescents 15 to 19 years of age.[1] Pediatricians can help prevent adolescent suicide by knowing the symptoms of depression and other presuicidal behavior. The extent to which pediatricians provide appropriate care for suicidal adolescents depends on their knowledge, skill, comfort with the topic and on ready access to appropriate community resources. All teenagers with suicidal symptoms should know that their pleas for assistance are heard and that pediatricians are willing to serve as advocates to help resolve the crisis.

The number of adolescent deaths from suicide in the United States has increased dramatically during the last few decades. In 1997, 4186 suicides were reported among people 15 to 24 years of age, 1802 suicides among those 15 to 19 years of age, and 2384 among those 20 to 24 years of age.[1] In 1997, 13% of all deaths in the 15- through 24-year-old age group were attributable to suicide.[1] The true number of deaths from suicide actually may be higher because some of these deaths are recorded as *accidental*.[2]

From 1950 to 1990 the suicide rate for adolescents in the 15- to 19-year-old group increased by 300%.[3] Male adolescents 15 to 19 years of age had a rate 6 times greater than the rate for female adolescents.[1] The ratio of attempted suicides to completed suicides among adolescents is estimated to be 50:1 to 100:1, and the incidence of unsuccessful suicide attempts is higher among girls than among boys.[4] Suicide affects young people from all races and socioeconomic groups, although some groups seem to have higher rates than others. Native-American boys and men have the highest suicide rate, black women the lowest. A statewide survey of students in the seventh through the twelfth grades found that 28.1% of bisexual and homosexual boys and 20.5% of bisexual and homosexual girls had reported attempting suicide.[5] The National Youth Risk Behavior Survey of students in the ninth through the twelfth grades indicated that nearly one fourth (24.1%) of students had seriously considered attempting suicide during the 12 months preceding the survey, 17.7% had made a specific plan, and 8.7% had made an attempt.[6]

Firearms, used in over 67% of suicides, are the leading cause of death for male and female victims of suicide.[7] More than 90% of suicide attempts involving a firearm are fatal because little chance for rescue exists. Firearms in the home, regardless of whether they are kept unloaded or stored in a secure location, are associated with an increased risk for adolescent suicide.[8,9] Parents must be warned about the lethality of firearms in the home and be advised strongly to remove them from the premises, especially if an adolescent has had a previous attempt.[10] Ingestion of pills is the most common method among adolescents who attempt suicide.

Youth may imitate suicidal behavior seen on television.[11] Media coverage of a teenage suicide may lead to cluster suicides, additional deaths from suicides in youths within a 1- to 2-week period afterward.[11-13]

ADOLESCENTS AT INCREASED RISK

Adolescents at higher risk for suicidal behavior commonly have a history of depression, a previous suicide attempt, a family history of psychiatric disorders (especially depression and suicidal behavior), family disruption, and certain chronic or debilitating physical disorders or psychiatric illness.[14] Alcohol use and alcoholism increase the risk for suicide.[15] Alcohol use has been associated with 50% of suicides.[16] Living out of the home (in a correctional facility or group home) and a history of physical or sexual abuse are additional factors more commonly found in adolescents who exhibit suicidal behavior.[17] Psychosocial problems and stresses, such as conflicts with parents, breakup of a relationship, school difficulties or failure, legal difficulties, social isolation, and physical ailments (including hypochondriacal preoccupation), are commonly reported or observed in young people who attempt suicide. These precipitating factors are often cited by youths as reasons for attempting suicide. Gay and bisexual adolescents have been reported to exhibit high rates of depression and have been reported to have rates of suicidal ideation and attempts 3 times higher than other adolescents. Studies of twins show that monozygotic twins have significantly higher concordance for suicide than dizygotic twins.[15] Long-term high levels of community violence may contribute to emotional and conduct problems and add to the risk of suicide for exposed youth.[18] Adolescent and parent questionnaires that cover these risk factors listed previously may be useful in the office setting to assist in obtaining a complete history.[19]

APPROACHING THE ADOLESCENT

All adolescents with symptoms of depression should be asked about suicidal ideation, and an estimation of the degree of suicidal intent should be made. No data indicate that inquiry about suicide precipitates the behavior. In fact, adolescents are often relieved that someone has heard their cry for help. For most adolescents this cry for help represents an attempt to resolve a difficult conflict, escape an intolerable living situation, make someone understand their desperate feelings, or make someone feel sorry or guilty. Suicidal thoughts or comments should never be dismissed as unimportant. Pediatricians must tell adolescents that their plea for assistance has been heard and that they will be helped.

Serious depression, as one of the most important risk factors, may show in several ways. For some adolescents, symptoms may be similar to those in adults, with signs such as depressed mood almost every day, crying spells or inability to cry, discouragement, irritability, a sense of emptiness and meaninglessness, negative expectations of self and the environment, low self-esteem, isolation, a feeling of helplessness, markedly diminished interest or pleasure in most activities, significant weight loss or weight gain, insomnia or hypersomnia, fatigue or loss of energy, feelings of worthlessness, and diminished ability to think or concentrate.[20] However, a more common circumstance is for an adolescent with serious depression to exhibit psychosomatic symptoms or behavioral problems. Such a teenager may seek care for recurrent or persistent complaints such as abdominal pain, chest pain, headache, lethargy, weight loss, dizziness and syncope, or other nonspecific symptoms.[21] Behavioral problems that may be manifestations of masked depression include truancy, deterioration in academic performance, running away from home, defiance of authorities, self-destructive behavior, vandalism, alcohol and other drug abuse, sexual acting out, and delinquency.[22] Episodic despondency leading to self-destructive acts can occur in any adolescent, including high achievers. These adolescents may believe that they have failed or disappointed their parents and family and perceive suicide as their only option. Other adolescents may believe that suicide is a better option than life as they experience it.

One approach to initiate an inquiry into suicidal thoughts or concerns is to ask a general question, such as, "Have you ever felt so unhappy or depressed that you thought about killing yourself or wished you were dead?" If the response is positive, then the pediatrician should inquire about thoughts of death, thoughts of suicide, suicide plans (eg, method, time, place), securing the available means (eg, firearms, medication), previous attempts (and whether the attempts were discovered), and the response of the family. These basic questions can help pediatricians construct an assessment of suicidal risk. In addition, they should assess individual coping resources, accessible support systems, and attitudes of the adolescent and family toward intervention and follow-up.[23] Another option is to include routine screening questions about suicidal thoughts or behaviors as part of a global health-risk survey to be completed by the adolescent. Such questions may reassure adolescents that inquiries about suicide are part of care that can be addressed by primary care physicians. Regardless of the method used to solicit such information from youth, the physician and staff should be prepared with well-considered plans for assessing severity of the threat and options for immediate referral and treatment if needed.

Although confidentiality is important in adolescent health care, for adolescents at risk of suicidal behavior, confidentiality must be breached. Pediatricians need to inform the appropriate persons when they believe an adolescent is at risk of suicide. In all cases, determining the sequence of events that preceded the threat, identifying current problems and conflicts, and assessing the degree of suicidal intent must be completed.

MANAGEMENT OF THE SUICIDAL ADOLESCENT

Adolescents with a well-thought-out plan that includes method, place, time, and clear intent are at high risk. The degree of intent can be inferred from the actual and perceived lethality of the intended means. Use of firearms, for example, has a high degree of lethality and

BOX 149-1 Examples of Adolescents at Low, Moderate, and High Risk for Suicide

LOW RISK

Took 5 ibuprofen tables after argument with girlfriend

Impulsive; told mother 15 minutes after taking pills

No serious problems at home or school

Occasionally feels *down* but has no history of depression or serious emotional problems

Has several good friends

Wants help resolving problems and is no longer considering suicide after interview

MODERATE RISK

Suicidal ideation precipitated by recurrent fighting with parents and failing grades in school

Wants to *get back* at parents

Cuts both wrists while at home alone; called friend 30 minutes later

Parents separated, changed school this semester, history of attention-deficit/hyperactivity disorder

Symptoms of depression for the last 2 months, difficulty controlling temper

Binge drinking on the weekends

Answers all the questions during the interview, agrees to see a therapist if parents get counseling, will contact the interviewer if suicidal thoughts return

HIGH RISK

Thrown out of house by parents for smoking marijuana at school, girlfriend broke up with him last night, best friend killed in auto crash last month

Wants to be dead, sees no purpose in living

Took parent's gun, is going to shoot himself where "no one can find me"

Gets drunk every weekend and uses marijuana daily

Hates parents and school, has run away from home twice and has not gone to school for 6 weeks

Hospitalized in the past because he says he "lost it"

Does not want to answer many of the questions during the interview and hates *shrinks*

poor chance of rescue. An adolescent who takes pills in the presence of others, however, has a good chance of rescue (Box 149-1).[24] Even adolescents who may initially seem at low risk, joke about suicide, or seek treatment for repeated somatic complaints may be asking for help the only way they can. Their concerns should be assessed thoroughly and follow-up arranged for additional evaluation and treatment. For adolescents who seem to be at moderate or high risk for suicide or have attempted suicide, a mental health professional should be consulted immediately during the office visit. Options for immediate evaluation include hospitalization, transfer to an emergency department, or an appointment the same day with a mental health professional.

The safest course of action for an adolescent at risk of immediate suicidal behavior is hospitalization, placing the adolescent in a safe and protected environment. An inpatient stay will allow time for a complete medical and psychiatric or psychologic evaluation and initiation of therapy in a controlled setting. The choice of hospital unit depends on available facilities in the area, health and mental health insurance, and managed-care policies. Adolescent medicine units must be staffed to manage the medical and psychiatric needs of suicidal adolescents.[25] Proper medical intervention and treatment are essential for stabilization and management of patients' conditions. After the adolescent's condition has been stabilized medically a comprehensive emotional and psychosocial assessment must be initiated before discharge. Inquiry should be made into the events that preceded the attempt, the adolescent's current problems, and the presence of current or previous psychiatric illness and self-destructive behavior. In addition to an in-depth psychological evaluation of the adolescent, family members should be interviewed to obtain additional information to help explain the adolescent's suicidal thoughts or attempt. This information includes detailed questions about the adolescent's medical, emotional, social, and family history, with special attention to signs and symptoms of depression, stress, and substance abuse. With parental permission and adolescent assent, teachers and family friends also may provide useful information if confidentiality is not breached.

Intervention should be tailored to the adolescent's needs. Adolescents with a responsive intact family, good peer relations and social support, hope for the future, and a desire to resolve conflicts may require only brief crisis-oriented intervention.[26] In contrast, adolescents who have made previous attempts, exhibit a high degree of intent to commit suicide, show evidence of serious depression or other psychiatric illness, are abusing alcohol and other drugs, and have families who are unwilling to commit to counseling are at high risk and may require psychiatric hospitalization.

All adolescents who attempt suicide need a comprehensive outpatient treatment plan before discharge. Specific plans and careful monitoring are needed because compliance with outpatient therapy is often poor. Most adolescents examined in emergency rooms after suicide attempts and referred to outpatient facilities fail to keep their appointments. Such is especially the case when the appointment is made with someone other than the family pediatrician or the person who performed the initial assessment.[27] Continuity of care is therefore of paramount importance. Pediatricians can enhance continuity and compliance by maintaining contact with suicidal adolescents even after referrals are made. All firearms should be removed from the home because adolescents may still find access to locked firearms stored in the home.

Adolescents with suicidal ideation judged in the office setting not to be at high risk for suicide should be followed up closely, referred for mental health evaluation in a timely manner, or both.

Recommendations are as follows:

1. Pediatricians need to know the risk factors (eg, signs and symptoms of depression) associated with adolescent suicide and serve as a resource for parents, teachers, school personnel, clergy, and community groups that work with youth about the issue of adolescent suicide.

2. Pediatricians should ask questions about depression, suicidal thoughts, and other risk factors associated with suicide in routine history taking, through screening tools. or both throughout adolescence.
3. During routine evaluations, pediatricians need to ask whether firearms are kept in the home and discuss with parents the risks of firearms as specifically related to adolescent suicide. Specifically for adolescents at risk of suicide, parents should be advised to remove firearms and ammunition from the house.
4. Pediatricians should recognize the medical and psychiatric needs of the suicidal adolescent and work closely with families and health care professionals involved in the management and follow-up of youth who are at risk or have attempted suicide.
5. Pediatricians should become familiar with community, state, and national resources that are concerned with youth suicide, including mental health agencies, family and children's services, crisis hotlines, and crisis-intervention centers. Working relationships should be developed with colleagues in child and adolescent psychiatry, clinical psychology, and other mental health professions to manage the care of adolescents at risk for suicide optimally. Because mental and physical health services are often provided through different systems of care, extra effort is necessary to ensure good communication, continuity, and follow-up.
6. Pediatricians should advocate for benefit packages in health insurance plans to ensure that adolescents have access to preventive and therapeutic mental health services that adequately cover the treatment of clinically significant mental health disorders.*

*Modified from American Academy of Pediatrics, Committee on Adolescence. Policy statement: suicide and suicide attempts in adolescents. *Pediatrics.* 2000;105(4):871-874. Available at: aappolicy.aappublications.org/cgi/content/full/pediatrics;105/4/871.

TOOLS FOR PRACTICE

Engaging Patient and Family

- *Facts for Families: Teen Suicide* (fact sheet), American Academy of Child and Adolescent Psychiatry (www.aacap.org/cs/root/facts_for_families/teen_suicide).
- *Teen Suicide, Mood Disorder, and Depression* (brochure), American Academy of Pediatrics (patiented.aap.org).

Medical Decision Support

- *The Classification of Child and Adolescent Mental Diagnoses in Primary Care* (book), American Academy of Pediatrics (www.aap.org/bookstore).

RELATED WEB SITE

- Centers for Disease Control and Prevention Injury Topics: Suicide (www.cdc.gov/ncipc/dvp/suicide/).

AAP POLICY STATEMENTS

American Academy of Pediatrics, Committee on Injury and Poison Prevention. Firearm-related injuries affecting the pediatric population. *Pediatrics.* 2000;105(4):888-895. (aappolicy.aappublications.org/cgi/content/full/pediatrics;105/4/8880).

Shain BN, American Academy of Pediatrics, Committee on Adolescence. Suicide and suicide attempts in adolescents. *Pediatrics.* 2007;120(3):669-676. (aappolicy.aappublications.org/cgi/content/full/pediatrics;120-3/669).

REFERENCES

1. Centers for Disease Control and Prevention, National Center for Health Statistics. *Death Rates From 72 Selected Causes by 5-Year Age Groups, Race, and Sex—United States, 1979-1997.* Table 291A. Atlanta, GA: Centers for Disease Control and Prevention, National Center for Health Statistics; 1999.
2. Committee on Adolescence, Group for the Advancement of Psychiatry. *Adolescent Suicide.* Washington, DC: American Psychiatric Press; 1996.
3. Centers for Disease Control and Prevention. Programs for prevention of suicide among adolescents youth adults. *Morb Mortal Wkly Rep Surveill Summ.* 1994;43 (RR-6):1-7.
4. Husain SA. Current perspective on the role of psychological factors in adolescent suicide. *Psychiatr Ann.* 1990;20: 122-127.
5. Remafedi G, French S, Story M, et al. The relationship between suicide risk and sexual orientation: results of a population-based study. *Am J Public Health.* 1998;88: 57-60.
6. Centers for Disease Control and Prevention. Youth risk behavior surveillance—United States, 1995. *Morbid Mortal Wkly Rep Surveill Summ.* 1996;45(SS-4): 1-84.
7. Kachur SP, Potter LB, James SP, et al. *Suicide in the United States: 1980-1992: Violence Surveillance.* Summary Series 1. Atlanta, GA: National Center for Injury Prevention and Control; 1995.
8. Brent DA, Perper JA, Allman CJ, et al. The presence and accessibility of firearms in the homes of adolescent suicides. A case-control study. *JAMA.* 1991;266:2989-2995.
9. American Academy of Pediatrics, Committee on Injury and Poison Prevention. Firearm injuries affecting the pediatric population. *Pediatrics.* 1992;89:788-790.
10. American Academy of Pediatrics, Committee on Adolescence. Firearms and adolescents. *Pediatrics.* 1992;89: 784-787.
11. Bollen KA, Phillips DP. Imitative suicides: a national study of the effects of television news stories. *Am Sociol Rev.* 1982;47:802-809.
12. Gould MS, Wallenstein S, Kleinman M. Time-space clustering of teenage suicides. *Am J Epidemiol.* 1990;131: 71-78.
13. Phillips DP, Carstenson LL. Clustering of teenage suicides after television news stories about suicide. *N Engl J Med.* 1986;315:685-689.
14. Bennett DS. Depression among children with chronic medical problems: a meta-analysis. *J Pediatr Psychol.* 1994;19:149-169.
15. Roy A, Segal NL, Centerwall BS, et al. Suicide in twins. *Arch Gen Psychiatry.* 1991;48:29-32.
16. Frances RJ, Franklin J, Flavin DK. Suicide and alcoholism. *Am J Drug Alcohol Abuse.* 1987;13:327-341.
17. Hodgman CH, McAnarney ER. Adolescent depression and suicide: rising problems. *Hosp Pract (Off Ed).* 1992; 27:73-76, 81, 84-85.
18. Cooley-Quille MR, Turner SM, Beidel DC. Emotional impact of children's exposure to community violence: a preliminary study. *J Am Acad Child Adolesc Psychiatry.* 1995;34:1362-1368.
19. Remafedi G, Farrow JA, Deisher RX. Risk factors for attempted suicide in gay and bisexual youth. *Pediatrics.* 1991;87:869-875.

20. American Psychiatric Association. *Diagnostic and Statistical Manual of Mental Disorders*. 4th ed. Washington, DC: American Psychiatric Association; 1994.
21. Wolraich ML, Felice ME, Drotar D, eds. *The Classification of Child and Adolescent Mental Diagnoses in Primary Care: Diagnostic and Statistical Manual for Primary Care (DSM-PC) Child and Adolescent Version*. Elk Grove Village, IL: American Academy of Pediatrics; 1996.
22. McIntire MS, Angle CR, Wikoff RL, et al. Recurrent adolescent suicidal behavior. *Pediatrics*. 1977;60:605-608.
23. Gispert M, Wheeler K, Marsh L, et al. Suicidal adolescents: factors in evaluation. *Adolescence*. 1985;20:753-762.
24. Jellinek MS, Snyder JB. Depression and suicide in children and adolescents. *Pediatr Rev*. 1998;19:255-264.
25. Marks A. Management of the suicidal adolescent on a nonpsychiatric adolescent unit. *J Pediatr*. 1979;95:305-308.
26. Hodgman CH, Roberts FN. Adolescent suicide and the pediatrician. *J Pediatr*. 1982;101:118-123.
27. Hawton K. *Suicide and Attempted Suicide Among Children and Adolescents*. Beverly Hills, CA: Sage Publications; 1986.

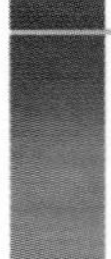

Chapter 150

TEMPER TANTRUMS AND BREATH-HOLDING SPELLS

Gregory E. Prazar, MD

TEMPER TANTRUMS

Children exhibit temper tantrums almost inevitably during the 2nd through 4th years of life. Therefore a temper tantrum is generally a *problem behavior* rather than a *behavioral problem*. Helping parents cope with temper tantrums involves providing anticipatory guidance, sharing information on developmental psychology, and offering strategies to deal with tantrums.

Temper tantrums usually become part of the child's emotional repertoire during the 2nd and 3rd years of life. Early signs of the negativism that is part of tantrums can be appreciated as early as 12 months of age. Some children continue to display occasional tantrums until the age of 5 or 6 years. Tantrums typically reappear in a slightly less intense form during adolescence, when independence once more becomes an issue for the developing child.

Several aspects of the toddler's development appear to make tantrums almost inevitable. First, because the 1 year old can walk and climb, the child begins to achieve physical mastery over the environment. This increased physical independence and an insatiable curiosity frequently place the child in dangerous situations that require parental intervention. Imposition of adult safety limits thwarts and frustrates the child, often precipitating tantrums. Second, the child's increased exploration of the environment immediately creates a conflict because the child must adapt to rules of an adult world. The child enters an environment of adult social values, in which people are expected to use the bathroom appropriately, verbalize dissatisfactions rather than *act* them out physically, sit quietly while eating, and sometimes subjugate their own wants to those of others. This process is too much for the egocentric toddler to bear, and frustration is inevitable. Third, between the ages of 1 and 4 years, the toddler begins to develop an increased awareness of how the child is separate and different from the mother. The child experiences a conflict between desires for autonomy and desires to remain close to the mother. Frustration in dealing with these intense feelings frequently results in tantrums.

Tensions are created in "establishing ego boundaries as separate from those of parents," as Brazelton[1] states, and in coping with physical limitations placed on exploring an adult world. Adults frequently deal with their own tensions and frustrations by verbalizing their feelings; the toddler, however, lacks a sophisticated ability to verbalize. A toddler's frustration with the adult world may be displayed in doing the exact opposite of what the adult requests, by saying "no, no" yet following through with the adult request (what Fraiberg[2] refers to as the "cheerful no"), by dawdling, or by displaying physical behavior outright (eg, kicking, screaming, lying on the floor, hitting, throwing, biting).

Most parents would probably agree that intellectual appreciation of the cause of tantrums does not necessarily aid in coping with a screaming and inconsolable child. Reasons for parental frustration are understandable. Well-meaning relatives and friends (who have likely forgotten their experience as young parents) may propagate myths about tantrums, which intensify parental anxiety and confusion. Myths of causation suggest that children who display tantrums are underdisciplined or parented inadequately. Myths of management suggest that tantrums can be quelled by spanking, dousing with cold water, or threats.

ANTICIPATORY GUIDANCE FOR TANTRUMS

The primary care physician should provide anticipatory guidance about temper tantrums. Such guidance may forestall events that precipitate tantrums and prevent future parental confusion in dealing with negative behaviors. The physician has many opportunities during the child's first 2 years to provide behavioral counseling.

At the 6-month well-child visit, the importance of parental time away from the infant can be emphasized. Parents who occasionally leave their infants and toddlers with responsible baby-sitters provide their children with the security that adults can leave and will come back; they also provide themselves with important mental health holidays from the rigors of parenting.

At the 9- or 12-month infant visit, environmental engineering should be discussed.[3] Home safety (eg, safety plugs in outlets, safety latches on drawers), removing valuables or breakables from the child's reach, and ensuring a safe place for the child to play (playpen or enclosed area) are examples of such engineering. Therefore this visit not only may reduce chances for childhood accidents, but also may forestall potential adult-toddler power struggles over environmental dangers.

The 15- or 18-month visit provides the physician another opportunity to offer the parent alternatives to negative interactions with the toddler. Afternoon naps (to allow for renewal of toddler and parental energy), the importance of praising cooperative toddler efforts, and the concept of limited decision making for the toddler ("Do you want to wear the green or blue shirt today?" versus "Which shirt do you want to wear today?") represent issues that may help parents minimize hostile encounters with their toddler.

The approach here should be one that encourages parents to describe how they believe tantrums should be handled rather than one that displays the physician's personal biases about child rearing. Several excellent books describing turbulent toddlerhood can be suggested to parents, including Brazelton's *Toddlers and Parents,*[1] Ilg and Ames' *Child Behavior,*[4] and Schmitt's *Your Child's Health.*[5] Furthermore, general guidelines concerning tantrums can be given. Tantrums are best ignored unless, as Fraiberg[2] states, "they encroach on rights of others or potentially endanger." If safety is the issue, then either environmental engineering should take place or the child should be restricted to the child's bedroom for 2 to 3 minutes (a kitchen timer is helpful to remind both parent and toddler of the time). If the child hits, bites, or throws in anger, then room restriction for 2 to 3 minutes should once again be suggested. Some behavioral psychologists suggest 1 minute of time out for each year of age (therefore a 5-year-old child would have a 5-minute time-out). Other behaviorists recommend that the time-out not be fixed. Because the goal is to help the child develop self-regulation, the time-out should end when the tantrum subsides.[6] The child should receive a brief hug or be praised and then be allowed to resume previous activity.

Parents may be reluctant to use bedroom restriction because they worry either that the child will associate the bedroom with unpleasant experiences or that the child will not feel adequately remorseful if placed in a room full of toys. Parents should be reassured that room restriction does not cause bedroom fears. Similarly, goals of discipline are to teach rules and to help the child understand which behaviors are acceptable. Discipline does not need to be severe to be effective.

Time-outs are an effective method of dealing with temper tantrums. Time-ins represent a method to reward acceptable behavior. Specifically, when a toddler is playing quietly, the parent should pat the child on the shoulder, give a brief hug, or otherwise offer some form of nonverbal affection. Such attention from the parent simply but effectively indicates approval of the current behavior. Some behavioral psychologists believe that time-ins are a more powerful method of encouraging acceptable behavior than time-outs.

Temper tantrums occur much more frequently in the presence of parents; they are much less common in the presence of alternative child care providers. Most experienced child care providers feel comfortable dealing with temper tantrums. If the child care provider expresses concern to a parent about a child's temper tantrums, then several questions should be considered. Does the child care provider have adequate training to deal with such a common behavior? Is this child care setting the most appropriate for the child (in terms of adult-child ratio, philosophy of discipline used by the provider, and realistic developmental expectations for the child's behavior in the child care setting)? Are the child's temper tantrums much more severe or frequent than those of the child's peers? These questions should be addressed with the child care provider. Subsequently, parents and the child care provider should formulate a plan for dealing with the tantrums that is followed consistently at home and at the child care location. If the parent and the child care provider cannot agree on such a plan, then the child's primary care physician should be consulted.

More specific guidelines for managing tantrums may be necessary in other individual situations. Parents should be encouraged by the physician to ventilate their feelings (to the physician) about tantrums and be reassured that they are doing the best job they can for their toddler.

MANAGEMENT OF PROBLEM TANTRUMS

Although tantrums represent a stage of the normal developing toddler's personality, several factors may suggest that further professional intervention is advisable. Toddlers who display persistent negativism or tantrums may suffer from too restrictive parenting, may receive too little positive reinforcement and affection, or may have parents who place unreasonable behavioral expectations on them. One study of 3 year olds defined severe temper tantrums as "episodes of shouting, banging, kicking, or screaming occurring 3 or more times a day or lasting more than 15 minutes."[7] Approximately 50% of these children had behavior problems. Furthermore, such severe tantrums were associated with specific psychosocial issues, including maternal depression, use of corporal punishment, marital stress, and low maternal education.

Children who display tantrums regularly beyond 5 or 6 years of age may be displaying signs of depression or poor self-esteem, or they may be children who live in a family in which emotional problems exist. When temper tantrums regularly occur at school, academic problems should be suspected, because peer pressure usually inhibits displays of tantrums.

Children exhibiting persistent tantrums along with other associated behaviors (eg, inability to concentrate, stereotypical behaviors, unrealistic fears, inability to display affection) may have more significant underlying problems, such as attention-deficit disorder, oppositional defiant disorder, or autism spectrum disorder. Similarly, parents who verbalize persistent frustration with tantrums or an inability to cope with age-appropriate tantrums may need more comprehensive counseling than the primary practitioner can provide.

Many parenting groups are available to help parents cope with negative behaviors. Programs such as Systematic Training for Effective Parenting (STEP) and Parent Effectiveness Training (PET) provide valuable community referral sources for families. If such services are not available, or if more sophisticated professional counseling is obviously warranted, then the family should be referred to a psychiatrically trained counselor.

Referral should be discussed as soon as the physician anticipates its necessity and should stress the involvement of both parents. The physician should maintain contact with the family about the problem after the referral has been made. Such ongoing contact may solidify the family's commitment to obtain and adhere with the counseling (see Chapter 131, Consultation and Referral for Emotional and Behavioral Problems).

BREATH-HOLDING SPELLS

Breath-holding spells cause particular anxiety for parents. Spells occur between ages 4 months and 5 years, with most occurring between 12 and 36 months of age. According to Menkes,[8] approximately 5% of all children display breath-holding spells. A positive family history of breath-holding spells occurs in approximately 25% of cases.

Such spells are precipitated by anger, frustration, fear, or minor injury (often a very minor head injury) and are categorized as cyanotic or pallid. Both types of spells are unlikely to occur more often than once a day and are not associated with an increased predisposition to epilepsy (although brief seizure-like activity can occur as a terminating event in either form of spell).

Cyanotic breath-holding spells are precipitated more often by anger or frustration than by fear or injury. The child emits a short, loud cry, takes a deep breath, and holds it. Cyanosis occurs after approximately 30 seconds. Either the episode terminates at this point or the child becomes rigid or limp and loses consciousness (loss of consciousness occurs in approximately 50% of all children who have breath-holding spells). In rare situations, mild clonic movements of the extremities follow.

Pallid breath-holding spells are similar to cyanotic spells in most respects but are more often precipitated by fear or minor injury. The initial cry is brief or silent. The spell then proceeds as with a cyanotic spell. Toddlers who suffer from pallid spells are often from families that have a history of syncope, and, in fact, these toddlers have an increased chance (approximately 15%) of syncopal attacks as adults.

Both cyanotic and pallid breath-holding spells are caused by autonomic nervous system dysregulation. Cerebral anoxia is responsible for spells that terminate with loss of consciousness. Furthermore, both forms of spells are involuntary and reflexive, despite spells often being precipitated when the child is angry or frustrated.

Children who display pallid breath-holding spells may, as adults, suffer from neurocardiogenic syncope. Neurocardiogenic syncope is a form of vasovagal response to postural changes. Adults who suffer from neurocardiogenic syncope are more likely to faint at the sight of blood or when injured than are adults who do not have this disorder.

Because both forms of breath-holding spells potentially can terminate with seizure-like movements, differentiation between spells and epilepsy is important. The occurrence of a precipitating factor (eg, minor injury, being frustrated) before the onset of the spell indicates that the episode is a breath-holding spell. Patients who have epilepsy display cyanosis during or after the seizures, not before seizure onset. Furthermore, electroencephalograms performed on patients who suffer from breath-holding spells are normal during non–breath-holding periods; patients who have epilepsy often have abnormal electroencephalograms during seizure-free periods.

MANAGEMENT OF BREATH-HOLDING SPELLS

No effective medical therapy exists for breath-holding spells, although some toddlers who experience seizure-like activity along with spells are prescribed anticonvulsant therapy. However, the decision to use medication remains controversial among pediatric neurologists.

Iron-deficiency anemia has been associated with breath-holding spells. A study involving 67 children who had breath-holding spells revealed that iron therapy reduced spells in the treatment group by 88%. These results suggest that iron may be important in the regulation of the autonomic nervous system.[9]

Coping with breath-holding spells can be extremely difficult for parents. Spells that terminate with loss of consciousness or with seizure-like movements are obviously frightening. Convincing parents that no harm will come to their child is important. Nevertheless, parents of a breath holder will frequently avoid enforcing limits for fear of precipitating the child's anger and a subsequent attack. Such parents need repeated reassurance and encouragement to continue age-appropriate limits on their child's behavior. To do otherwise will create an overindulged child who subsequently may fear loss of parental love because limits have been rescinded.

When to refer a breath-holding patient to a neurologist or a psychiatrically trained professional may not be an easy decision for the physician. If parents request further consultation, then their wish certainly should be respected, even if the physician is confident that further evaluation is unnecessary. If parents indicate agreement with the physician that spells are of no consequence yet continue to withhold appropriate limit-setting, then referral to a mental health professional should take place. The physician who is unsure of the diagnosis of breath-holding (especially in situations in which loss of consciousness or seizure-like activity occurs) should always refer the family to a pediatric neurologist. Referral must not end the physician-parent communication concerning the spells, however, because an ongoing dialogue may ensure adherence with the referral.

SUMMARY

Temper tantrums and breath-holding spells usually represent benign forms of childhood behavior evolving from the child's preverbal attempts to express feelings of frustration and anger. Unfortunately, parents frequently have difficulty appreciating the benign course of such behaviors when they daily must face a screaming, inconsolable toddler who may even lose consciousness and then display seizure-like movements. Parents can best deal with negative behaviors when they are adequately prepared by the physician before such behaviors occur and when they are offered empathic guidance and positive reinforcement during regular office visits.

TOOLS FOR PRACTICE

Engaging Patient and Family

- *Caring for Your Baby and Young Child: Birth to Age 5* (book), American Academy of Pediatrics (www.aap.org/bookstore)
- *Managing Normal Tantrums: 10 Tips for Parents* (fact sheet), North Carolina ABCD Project (dbpeds.org/media/managing-tantrums-tips.pdf).
- *Temper Tantrums: A Normal Part of Growing Up* (brochure), American Academy of Pediatrics (patiented.aap.org).

Medical Decision Support

- *Bright Futures: Guidelines for Health Supervision of Infants, Children, and Adolescents* (book), Bright Futures (brightfutures.aap.org/web/).
- *Bright Futures Toolkit* (toolkit), Bright Futures (brightfutures.aap.org/web/).

REFERENCES

1. Brazelton TB. *Toddlers and Parents*. New York, NY: Dell; 1989.
2. Fraiberg S. *The Magic Years*. New York, NY: Charles Scribner's Sons; 1996.
3. Hagan JF Jr, Shaw JS, Duncan PM, eds. *Bright Futures: Guidelines for Health Supervision of Infants, Children, and Adolescents*. 3rd ed. Elk Grove Village, IL: American Academy of Pediatrics; 2008.
4. Ilg FL, Ames LB. *Child Behavior*. New York, NY: Harper & Row; 1992.
5. Schmitt B. *Your Child's Health*. New York, NY: Bantam Books; 1991.
6. Levine MD, Carey WB, Crocker AC. *Developmental and Behavioral Pediatrics*. Philadelphia, PA: WB Saunders; 1993.
7. Needlman R, Stevenson J, Zuckerman B. Psychosocial correlates of severe temper tantrums. *J Dev Behav Pediatr.* 1991;12:77-83.
8. Menkes JH. *Textbook of Child Neurology*. 2nd ed. Philadelphia, PA: Lea & Febiger; 1995.
9. Daoud AS, Batieha A, al-Sheyyab M, et al. Effectiveness of iron therapy on breath-holding spells. *J Pediatr.* 1997;130:547-550.

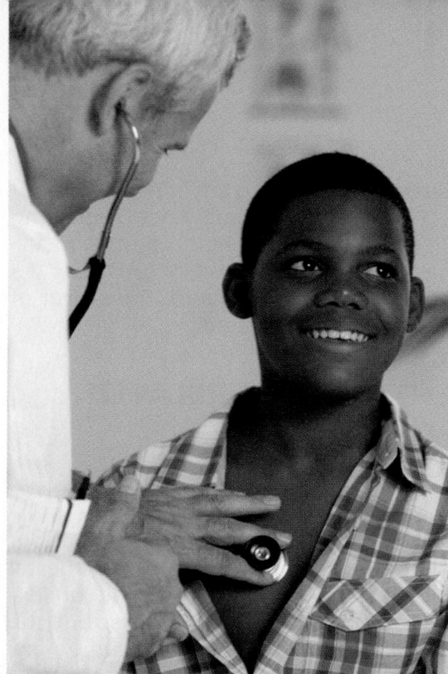

PART 7

Adolescence

151 Challenges of Health Care Delivery to Adolescents
152 Counseling Parents of Adolescents
153 Interviewing Adolescents
154 Adolescent Sexuality
155 Adolescent Pregnancy and Parenthood
156 Contraception and Abortion
157 Gay, Lesbian, and Bisexual Youth

Chapter 151

CHALLENGES OF HEALTH CARE DELIVERY TO ADOLESCENTS

Richard E. Kreipe, MD

Several challenges threaten health care delivery to contemporary adolescents. First, adolescence itself is an unsteady transitional stage between childhood and adulthood.[1] Developmentally, adolescents share characteristics of both children and adults, often vacillating from one extreme to the other, depending on circumstances. Therefore a health care system designed for younger individuals (who depend on their parents) and adults (who act entirely autonomously) does not easily accommodate adolescents. Second, the major threats to adolescent health are closely related to their behavior and environment. The causes of mortality and morbidity for adolescents in the 21st century can be traced to modifiable behaviors more than to diseases. The federal blueprint for the health of all Americans has identified 21 *critical health objectives* covering 6 domains for adolescents and young adults: (1) mortality, (2) unintentional injury, (3) violence, (4) mental health and substance abuse, (5) reproductive health, and (6) chronic diseases.[2] Even the objectives within the chronic disease category are related to behavior (smoking, being overweight, and lacking physical activity). Thus primary health care for adolescents should focus more on prevention than on diagnosing illness or prescribing treatment.

A growing body of knowledge focused on changing health-related behaviors in adolescents is emerging. However, the highly variable contexts of health care delivery, both the settings in which it occurs and as the health care providers who render the care, represent a third challenge.[3] For example, ambulatory settings include private physician's offices, hospital clinics, school-based clinics, or private agencies. In addition, adolescents may receive care in free clinics that emphasize confidential services, whereas homeless youth receive care from a mobile van. Similarly, clinicians providing these services can range from a board-certified adolescent medicine physicians to youth workers. The wide variety of settings and health care providers, with little in the way of standardization or best-practice models, represents a major challenge to delivering consistently high-quality health care to adolescents.[4] A fourth factor challenging adolescents is the *system* in which health care is delivered.[5] Issues related to health insurance, time spent in visits, and other factors need to be addressed in a realistic manner.

This chapter addresses each of these challenges and points to the opportunities in each of these areas for improving health care delivered to adolescents. The dedication to improving the health of infants and children must be carried forward for adolescents and young adults. Improving the health of adolescents and young adults often requires strong advocacy and innovative methods. However, the challenges regarding health care delivery to adolescents are not insurmountable, if the emphasis is on the word *care*. As Peabody noted more than 70 years ago, the secret of patient *care* is in *caring* for the patient.[6]

DEVELOPMENTAL ISSUES RELATED TO HEALTH CARE DELIVERY TO ADOLESCENTS

Puberty

Tanner observed that the only thing constant about adolescence is change.[7] Within the realm of pubertal changes, a well-recognized *sequence* of events of sexual maturation exists for boys and for girls, but the *timing* of the onset and the velocity of the *tempo* are highly variable from individual to individual. Thus healthy 12-year-old children can range from having no secondary sex characteristics to full sexual maturity. Girls are now experiencing the onset of breast development (thelarche) up to 2 years earlier than they were a generation ago.[8] This factor is important because earlier-developing girls are at greater risk of engaging in high-risk health behaviors than are those who develop later and because girls who develop precociously sexually may not be mature cognitively. Similarly, endogenous androgen levels (or exogenous anabolic steroids) may account for some aggressive behaviors in boys. However, the psychosocial aspects of adolescence are not necessarily synchronous with each other, or with sexual maturation.

Autonomy

The hallmarks of adolescence—the emergence of independence and autonomy—also affect health care delivery. Adolescents who have not yet reached the age of majority (18th birthday in most jurisdictions) have legal rights to seek health care without parental consent as determined by several factors, including (1) their status as an emancipated or as a mature minor, (2) the nature of the condition for which they are seeking confidential care, and (3) the laws governing their state of residence.[9] Confidential health care tends to be most commonly sought for conditions that are highly charged emotionally, such as reproductive health care. To the degree that an adolescent's right to confidential health care is honored, the adolescent's parents may feel excluded and argue that their parental rights and responsibilities are being denied. Health care providers, especially family practitioners, family nurse practitioners, and physician's assistants who provide primary care for both adolescents and adults in a family, may be caught in the middle of this conflict. Determining what is in the best interest of the adolescent is sometimes difficult in such situations. A balanced approach, honoring the rights and needs of both adolescents and parents, is most productive.[9] Nonadherence to treatment, especially for chronic illnesses such as diabetes, HIV infection, or cystic fibrosis often emerges during adolescence as a manifestation of autonomy. Adolescents may not want to be told what to do, or they may use the disease as a means of exerting control in conflict with parents.

Cognition

Nonadherence to a treatment regimen may be related to cognitive limitation imposed by an adolescent being *concrete operational* in thinking. For example, a 15 year old with pelvic inflammatory disease might be encouraged by a physician to complete a 14-day course of antibiotics to prevent infertility. After taking the medication for 2 days, she might stop treatment because she feels well. However, she might also interpret the warning about infertility after a treatment course of less than 14 days to mean that she no longer needs to use birth control. A better method to increase adherence would be to warn about the possibility of chronic pain or internal scarring if she does not complete treatment. These situations are concrete and immediate realities that may have greater effect than warning about a future, abstract concept such as infertility. The delivery of health care to adolescents should take into consideration the cognitive functioning (including the literacy level) of each patient and adapt education and interventions accordingly.

Identity

Identity development, sometimes characterized as the essence of adolescence, can present a challenge to professionals delivering health care to individuals in this age group. As the major task of adolescence, identity development generally occurs in the context of a peer group, which can have either health-promoting (eg, Students Against Drunk Driving) or health-threatening, risky behaviors. Not only can the latter predispose individuals to sexually transmitted infections, unintended pregnancy, violence, or substance abuse, but it can also make obtaining the history extremely difficult. For example, if a girl has been forbidden by her parents to see her boyfriend, then she may deny sexual activity with him, or if a boy is a member of an athletic team that uses drugs, then he may not be willing to admit to substance use. Similarly, a boy who has an emerging homosexual orientation may have numerous concerns related to health and be engaging in high-risk behaviors but be unable to bring these issues up spontaneously with a health care provider. Thus the developmental aspects of adolescence itself present significant challenges to the delivery of health care in several domains.

Not all identity developmental challenges represent barriers to the delivery of care, however. For example, adolescents focusing on their own identities are normally very self-centered or egocentric. Instead of viewing this focus as a narcissistic shortcoming of the patient, the clinician can make use of it by offering authoritative advice to help the adolescent feel better, rather than an authoritarian prescription of what *must* be done. Alternatively, adolescents often modify their physical appearance as a personal statement reflecting their identity. Multicolored hair, body piercings, tattoos, and clothes all relate to the emerging individual's sense of self (even if the person assumes an appearance that is remarkably similar to peers). For health care providers, the challenge is to continue to respect the person, regardless of how unusual the adolescent may appear, and to seek the positive qualities and assets of each adolescent.[10,11]

MORBIDITY AND MORTALITY IN ADOLESCENTS

More than 75% of the mortality among adolescents is caused by motor-vehicle accidents, homicide, or suicide, most of which are potentially preventable and generally related to behavior. The morbidity caused by violence, sexually transmitted infections (including HIV), pregnancy, substance abuse, eating disorders, and obesity are linked to modifiable behaviors. In addition, mental health concerns, such as depression, are important threats to the health of adolescents. However, effective means of preventing many of these conditions remain elusive.[12] The content of adolescent health care must focus on behavior, knowledge, and attitudes, rather than on disease because adolescents are generally healthy and notably free of disease. The conditions affecting the health of adolescents are not readily preventable, may be resistant to treatment, or may require interventions that clinicians are unable to provide. Therefore clinicians need to involve other segments of society, such as social workers, educators, and law enforcement individuals, to assist them in providing an environment that encourages healthy behaviors.

Given the nature of health problems facing contemporary adolescents, health care providers commonly feel unprepared to address either the problems or the adolescents who must contend with them.[13] A recent analysis of a national ambulatory dataset showed that counseling regarding nutrition, exercise, HIV or sexually transmitted infections, or birth control was 2 to 3 times more likely at an acute visit than at a well visit, which is designed to include such counseling.[14] Thus adolescent health care requires a high degree of flexibility and willingness to use every encounter with adolescents as an opportunity for providing anticipatory guidance. Moreover, they need to have training and experience related specifically to the care of adolescents. This training and experience is available through publications, continuing-education services, and programs by professional organizations such as the American Academy of Pediatrics (www.aap.org) and the Society for Adolescent Medicine (www.adolescenthealth.org), as well as numerous universities that provide hands-on or distance-learning opportunities in adolescent health.

In response to the need for greater efforts at prevention of morbidity and mortality among adolescents, different comprehensive preventive strategies have been developed, most notably the American Medical Association's *Guidelines for Adolescent Preventive Services* (GAPS)[15] (www.ama-assn.org/ama/pub/category/1980.html) or the American Academy of Pediatrics' and Maternal and Child Health Bureau's *Bright Futures Guidelines* (brightfutures.aap.org). These resources structure both initial and follow-up health-supervision visits by providing paper forms that patients and parents complete, as well as providing specific questions that clinicians can use in assessment and management.

CONTEXTS (SETTINGS AND PROVIDERS) OF HEALTH SERVICE DELIVERY TO ADOLESCENTS

Outpatient Settings

As health care expands to include preventive adolescent services, the settings in which health services are delivered to adolescents have appropriately expanded beyond the physician's office or the hospital bed. A wide variety of service settings and an even wider variability of service providers are available. For example, within the category of private office, the physician might be a pediatrician, internist, or family practitioner, each of whom will have different training in adolescent health, ranging from an optional elective to a 3-year fellowship in adolescent medicine. In addition, nurse practitioners and physician's assistants often provide health care to adolescents, depending on the setting (eg, college health or institution-based care) and geographic location.

School-based clinics offer many advantages to the other settings, most notably convenience, ready access, and the ability to minimize school absence.[16,17] Because schools represent a focal point of youth activity, authorities argue for full-service schools that offer education, health services, after-school activities, and family services.[12] This model has special advantages for inner-city communities that offer little in the way of quality health care or safe out-of-school activities to their residents. The challenge is to get the community involved in the program, which generally requires a dedicated leader in the school.

Because of the public nature of schools, political controversy often surrounds school-based health services, especially those related to reproductive health care.[18] For example, many health care professionals consider that the use of condoms is a central element in reducing unintended pregnancy and sexually transmitted infections for sexually active adolescents. Proponents of abstinence-only programs argue that providing condoms to sexually active adolescents encourages all adolescents to be sexually active. An option that proponents of condom use may consider is to let adolescents know where condoms are available, if distribution in school is not allowed.

Multiple service settings can be seen as a challenge or as an opportunity. For example, homeless youth constitute a high-risk, underserved group with respect to health. Because their needs cannot be met in traditional medical settings, leaders in cities such as Seattle, Los Angeles, and New York have established programs that include free clinics with late evening hours, linkages with community-based youth workers, mobile units providing information and services, and telephone hotlines, as well as job-training, high school equivalency education, and referral to adolescent-friendly specialists. Similarly, obstetric or gynecologic services are often clustered in a clinic specifically for adolescents, but with adolescent obstetric services provided at different times than adolescent gynecologic services. This model recognizes the differences between pregnant teens and adults (eg, greater need for assistance with high school education, nutrition assistance, child care, and transportation), as well as the different obstetric and gynecologic needs of teens.

Regardless of the outpatient setting, several considerations need to be given to the needs of adolescents.[19] Having a waiting area with space that is adolescent oriented, apart from space for young children is optimal, if space allows. Contemporary posters, magazines, and patient-education materials should consistently focus on adolescents in a positive light. The American Academy of Pediatrics has a large number of health brochures and pamphlets for adolescents (www.aap.org/healthtopics/stages.cfm#adol). With respect to appointments, arranging clinic schedules at times when teens will not need to miss school and when only other adolescents will be in the waiting room is optimal.

Perhaps the most important aspect of making an outpatient setting attractive to adolescents, however, is the attitude of the receptionist toward adolescents. When adolescents perceive that they are welcomed and respected, a positive tone is set for their visit. If teens feel negatively regarded, then they may approach the visit with a negative attitude or fail to keep appointments. In such circumstances, the skills and training of the health care provider are irrelevant because the staff has made the provider inaccessible to the adolescent. Unfortunately, this circumstance often is most likely to occur for patients who are most in need of care.

Researchers are developing interactive computer programs that obtain medical history and provide immediate feedback to the adolescent waiting for a scheduled appointment. The information is available to the physician during the visit. Such innovative technology can serve several purposes simultaneously: entertaining, educating, and medical record keeping.[20]

Inpatient Settings

Most hospitals, even large university-based facilities, do not have a separate adolescent inpatient unit. Despite the advantages of creating an adolescent-oriented therapeutic environment and developing professional staff with expertise in working with adolescents in an adolescent unit,[21] most institutions do not have the critical mass of specialists with experience (or interest) in adolescent health care nor an average census of adolescent patients to sustain such a unit. Thus adolescents tend to be admitted to hospital units based on their age (to pediatrics) or their admitting diagnosis (eg, to orthopedics for a fractured femur or to psychiatry for depression). This tendency can result in additional challenges in delivering appropriate inpatient services. For example, in some hospitals the age limit for pediatrics is 16 years, resulting in middle adolescents being admitted to a unit where the average patient is older than 50 years.

Hospitalizing adolescents on units based on their admitting diagnosis can present other challenges. For example, orthopedic units may be unprepared to address the psychosocial needs of a 15-year-old boy with attention-deficit/hyperactivity disorder who breaks his femur driving a car while intoxicated and without a license. He would benefit from staff understanding his need for concrete, concise, and clear explanations of any treatment planned and for consistent and reasonable limits on behavior in the hospital.

This model enhances his sense of control over the environment in which he is rendered relatively vulnerable and addresses his need to express his feelings in socially acceptable and productive ways. Otherwise the hospital unit staff may respond to typical behavior with escalating frustration or punitive restrictions.

Even when adolescents are admitted to a pediatric unit, they may not have their psychosocial needs met if they have chronic symptoms or undiagnosed conditions. If staff members do not understand the mental health needs of these adolescents, especially those with life-threatening conditions or somatic symptoms such as headache or abdominal pain, then opportunities to help the patient may be missed. For example, the rule-out approach, in which an adolescent is admitted for a battery of tests or procedures but is finally judged to have a psychosomatic condition because of a negative work-up, is rarely of benefit. The biopsychosocial model recognizes the complex interplay among biological, psychological, and social factors and includes mental health issues in both the differential diagnosis and the treatment planning for each patient.[22]

Even if a hospital does not have a geographically distinct adolescent unit, several factors can improve adolescent inpatient services. First, having a recreation room where adolescents can congregate for social interaction and leisure activity, sufficiently far away from patient rooms that noise levels will not bother other patients, is advisable. A child-life professional on staff will ensure that developmentally appropriate activities are available and that the psychosocial needs of hospitalized adolescents (eg, keeping up with schoolwork) are identified. A daily schedule, particularly for anyone in the hospital for more than 3 days, provides structure and predictability and enhances the adolescent's sense of control. Regardless of the length of stay, a unit should have clear rules for adolescents regarding visitors, timing of various activities, leaving the unit, and schoolwork, among others. Emphasis should be on what the adolescent may do, rather than a series of rules on what *not* to do.

In the absence of a geographically distinct unit, cohorting adolescents together is best, rather than distributing them throughout a pediatric inpatient service. A close working relationship with one or more physicians who have subspecialty training in adolescent medicine provides important support in staff development and consultation services. Because pediatric residency requirements include a 1-month elective in adolescent medicine, most institutions have such a specialist, albeit often as a part-time faculty member. Mental health consultation should be readily available as well. Such consultation may be patient or staff oriented; that is, the mental health services are often requested not only to address diagnosis and treatment for the adolescent, but also to address staff concerns about their response to behavior and how an adolescent's behavior affects other patients and staff on the unit. Similarly, when a simple behavior modification program needs to be established for an adolescent inpatient, the hospital staff may need assistance in developing and implementing it.

HEALTH CARE SYSTEM AND THE DELIVERY OF SERVICES TO ADOLESCENTS

The National Adolescent Health Information Center (NAHIC)[5] has proposed 5 recommendations to improve health care for adolescents: (1) ensure the delivery of high-quality services (by improving training in adolescent health, by improving workforce distribution for providing adolescent-related services, and by enhancing coordination and support for adolescent health services); (2) provide access to comprehensive health services (by ensuring appropriate services are readily available and by implementing strategies to overcome adolescents' barriers to access); (3) improve financial access to comprehensive health services (by improving existing health coverage and by expanding coverage for adolescents beyond existing parameters); (4) ensure the legal right to health care and confidentiality (by improving legal access to health services and by ensuring legal protection of confidential care); and (5) ensure that services are available, accessible, and appropriate.

In addition, the NAHIC described 5 crosscutting themes related to the adolescent health care systems. These themes include (1) the need for prioritizing the health and well being of adolescents on a national level; (2) coordination to reduce fragmentation and to maximize existing resources at the local, state, and federal levels; (3) effective use of resources, joint collaborative efforts, and additional sustainable funding to meet major gaps in adolescent health; (4) greater programmatic focus on primary prevention and early intervention that is substantiated by rigorous research; and (5) increased role of families and other meaningful adults who play a critical role in the lives of young people as they transition to adulthood.

PRACTICAL ISSUES IN PROVIDING ADOLESCENT HEALTH SERVICES

Much of the discussion about challenges to delivering health care to adolescents focuses on adolescents[4] rather than health care providers. Some specific suggestions have been made in each of the preceding sections of this chapter to enhance services. However, additional practical considerations exist that deserve consideration. These considerations include the structure and format of the adolescent visit, billing issues, referrals, and transition of patients with chronic illness. Recognizing the multiplicity of service sites and professional training previously mentioned, this section addresses these issues in the context of traditional office visit, but the principles apply widely.

Ideally, patients enter adolescence having been in the care of a physician who will provide continuity of care across the transition from childhood to adulthood. In anticipation of the inevitable emergence of puberty, clinicians often advise parents of patients around age 8 or 9 of an office policy to begin to provide the patient with some time alone with the physician around the age of 10 years. This policy can be framed in the context of preparing the adolescent to take increasing responsibility for the adolescent's own health (paralleling the increasing responsibility in other domains, such as school and work). Then, at the next visit, the parent can be reminded of the physician's desire to talk to the emerging adolescent alone, usually at the end, rather than the beginning of the visit.

Confidentiality

As adolescents progress developmentally, an increasing need for, and right to, confidential care exists. This area is best discussed at the outset of the visit; however, the subject, in most instances, needs to be addressed only once. Two points regarding confidentiality deserve emphasis. First, the principle underlying confidentiality is respect for the person, not keeping secrets from parents. Second, absolute confidentiality should never be offered. A physician might say to the patient in the presence of the parent or parents, "It is important for my adolescent patients to have time alone with me because by the time they get to be 18 years old, they can see me completely on their own. To help you prepare for that, you will have time at each visit when we can talk alone. What we talk about will be between us, unless I believe that you or others are in danger—like if you were seriously thinking about hurting yourself. I would only do what I think is in your best interest and I will not go behind your back; but most things we talk about will remain private." Parents are usually comfortable with this policy. If they are not, then a serious problem with trust in their relationship usually exists, which itself might be a focus for intervention.

Private Time With Patients

A question commonly asked by clinicians is, "How do I get the parent to leave the room?" A useful technique is to get some background history from the accompanying parent or parents, then give the patient an examination gown while saying, "Please put on this gown so that I can do your physical. Your mom and dad and I will step out to give you some privacy." Then, after shepherding the parents out of the room, the physician asks if either parent has any concerns. This approach gives the parents an opportunity to mention concerns privately. The parents can then be asked to have a seat in the waiting room while the adolescent is examined privately. Again, most parents accept this approach readily. Parents who refuse to leave the room may have serious problems trusting their adolescent or the physician. The physical examination is a fairly low-yield procedure in an asymptomatic adolescent, but the patient and parents often expect one to be performed. A history and brief physical examination can be performed simultaneously.[22]

Most clinicians allow at least 30 minutes for follow-up adolescent visits, more for an initial visit. Using structured survey forms, such as *GAPS* or *Bright Futures,* greatly facilitates data gathering, but the information contained in such formats needs to be reviewed before the patient leaves the office. The adolescent must know what is going to happen at the visit, how much time has been allotted, and that additional visits may be necessary if all concerns cannot be addressed at once.

Financial Considerations

Billing issues need to be discussed openly and early in the delivery of services to adolescents. Although many adolescents are without health care insurance, the federal State Child Health Improvement Program (SCHIP) promises to provide much needed coverage for a large portion of uninsured teenagers. One in six adolescents 15 to 18 years of age and one in three 18 to 24 year olds lack health insurance coverage, private or public.[23] Adolescents who are living in poverty or are members of racial or ethnic minority groups are even more likely to be uninsured.

Billing appropriately for services is necessary to avoid viewing the adolescent as a source of lost revenue. For persons who do have health insurance, some insurance companies or managed care organizations allow for confidential billing.[24] Alternatively, services can be provided under a broad generic code (such as 99215) when the medical decision making is of high complexity. For example, a pelvic examination might be recorded in the chart but not be noted on the bill. The fees for counseling sessions should reflect the time spent. In addition, parents may be willing to pay for bills that do not have a detailed list of services, reassured that their adolescent is acting responsibly toward health maintenance. Adolescents who prefer to pay out of pocket generally need an installment plan but are often more than willing to pay for services with their own money. Finally, patients who cannot pay for services can be referred to free clinics, if they are available locally.

Specialty Referral

The referral of an adolescent to a subspecialist is most likely to represent a challenge when the subspecialist is a mental health care provider. Adolescents tend to interpret the referral to a psychiatrist, psychologist, social worker, or counselor as an indication that they are *crazy.* To minimize resistance, the physician should let the adolescent know the reason for the referral ("I am concerned that you seem to be feeling very sad, at times hopeless, and recently thinking that life's not worth living"), to frame the referral in terms of bringing the consultant onto the treatment team ("I need the help of Dr. Smith. He's a psychiatrist who helps me help my patients who are feeling the way you are"), and to plan a follow-up so that the referral does not evoke feelings of rejection or abandonment ("I want to schedule a visit in 2 weeks, after you had a chance to talk to him. I want to make sure that things are improving. You also know you can call me if you feel like you're going to hurt yourself before you see him").

Patients with chronic conditions, previously fatal during childhood or adolescence, are now living into adulthood. As a result, an increasing awareness exists of the need for the transition from pediatric to adult health care. The transition of care needs to be anticipated and a plan made for this process. This transition of care should occur early in the patient's life. Hearing from a pediatrician the statement, "and when Jenny gets to be an older adolescent or young adult, we will need to make sure that the physician who will be assuming care for her knows about her cystic fibrosis" is interpreted by parents as positive because it reflects an expectation that she will live to adulthood. Combined training in medicine and pediatrics prepares physicians especially well for the care of such patients, given that no need exists for transfer of care as the patient grows out of the pediatric age group. Physicians with such training are especially well prepared to address the needs of adolescents with complex medical and surgical problems as they progress toward adulthood.

CONCLUSION

Although caring for adolescents can be challenging, following the principles outlines here will enable the clinician to provide sensitive, effective care for a group of patients who are often desperately in need of sound health care, thus providing a great service to these patients, as well as a sense of satisfaction for the clinician.

TOOLS FOR PRACTICE

Community Advocacy and Coordination

- *Helping Teens Stay Healthy and Safe: Health Care, Birth Control and Confidential Services* (brochure), Center for Adolescent Health and the Law (www.cahl.org/helpingteensstayhealthyandsafe.htm).
- *Improving the Health of Adolescents & Young Adults* (report), Centers for Disease Control and Prevention (nahic.ucsf.edu/index.php/companion/index/#complete).

Engaging Patient and Family

- *Caring for Your Teenager* (book), American Academy of Pediatrics (www.aap.org/bookstore).
- *Developmental Stages* (Web page), American Academy of Pediatrics (aap.org/healthtopics/stages.cfm#adol).
- *For Today's Teens: A Message From Your Pediatrician* (brochure), American Academy of Pediatrics (patiented.aap.org).
- *What is an Adolescent Health Specialist?* (fact sheet), American Academy of Pediatrics (www.aap.org/family/WhatisAdolHealthSplt_Eng.pdf).

Medical Decision Support

- *Adolescent Medicine: State of the Art Reviews* (book), American Academy of Pediatrics (www.aap.org/bookstore).
- *Caring for Adolescent Patients, 2nd edition* (book), American Academy of Pediatrics (www.aap.org/bookstore).
- *Guidelines for Adolescent Preventive Services* (guideline), American Medical Association (www.ama-assn.org/ama/pub/category/1980.html).

RELATED WEB SITE

- Society for Adolescent Medicine (www.adolescenthealth.org/).

AAP POLICY STATEMENT

Hagan JF, Shaw JS, Duncan PD, eds. *Bright Futures: Guidelines for Health Supervision of Infants, Children, and Adolescents*. Elk Grove Village, IL: American Academy of *Pediatrics*; 2007. AAP endorsed. (brightfutures.aap.org).

REFERENCES

1. Steinberg L. *Adolescence*. 8th ed. New York, NY: McGraw-Hill; 2007.
2. Centers for Disease Control and Prevention, National Center for Chronic Disease Prevention and Health Promotion, Division of Adolescent and School Health; Health Resources and Services Administration, Maternal and Child Health Bureau, Office of Adolescent Health; National Adolescent Health Information Center, University of California, San Francisco. *Improving the Health of Adolescents & Young Adults: A Guide for States and Communities*. Atlanta, GA: Centers for Disease Control and Prevention; 2004.
3. Weinstein J. School-based health centers and the primary care physician: an opportunity for collaborative care. *Prim Care*. 2006;33:305-315.
4. Morreale MC, Kapphahn CJ, Elster AB, et al. Access to health care for adolescents and young adults. Position paper of the Society for Adolescent Medicine. *J Adolescent Health*. 2004;35:342-344.
5. Brindis CD, Irwin CE, Ozer EM, et al. *Improving Adolescent Health: An Analysis and Synthesis of Health Policy Recommendations*. San Francisco, CA. University of California at San Francisco, National Adolescent Health Information Center; 1997.
6. Peabody FW. The care of the patient (1927). Reprinted. *JAMA*. 1984;252:813-818.
7. Tanner JM. Issues and advances in adolescent growth and development. *J Adol Health Care*. 1987;8:470-478.
8. Herman-Giddens ME, Slora EJ, Wasserman RC, et al. Secondary sexual characteristics and menses in young girls seen in office practice: a study from the Pediatric Research in Office Settings network. *Pediatrics*. 1997;99: 505-512.
9. Center for Adolescent Health Law, and Healthy Teen Network. Helping Teens Stay Healthy and Safe: Health Care, Birth Control and Confidential Services (2007). Available at: www.cahl.org/helpingteensstayhealthyandsafe.htm. Accessed July 17, 2007.
10. Alexander B, Schrauben S. Outside the margins: youth who are different and their special health care needs. *Prim Care*. 2006;33:285-303.
11. McManus RP. Adolescent care: reducing risk and promoting resilience. *Prim Care*. 2002;29:557-569.
12. Dryfoos JG, Barkin C. *Adolescence: Growing Up in America Today*. New York, NY: Oxford University Press; 2006.
13. Hedberg VA, Bracken AC, Stashwick CA. Long-term consequences of adolescent health behaviors: implications for adolescent health services. *Adolesc Med*. 1999; 10:137-151.
14. Rand CM, Auinger P, Klein JD, et al. Preventive counseling at adolescent ambulatory visits. *J Adolescent Health*. 2005;37:87-93.
15. American Medical Association, Department of Adolescent Health. Guidelines for Adolescent Preventive Services (GAPS) Recommendation Monograph. Available at: www.ama-assn.org/ama/pub/category/1980.html. Accessed July 17, 2007.
16. Fisher M. Adolescent health assessment and promotion in office and school settings. *Adolesc Med*. 1999:10: 71-86.
17. Johnson V, Hutcherson V. A study of the utilization patterns of an elementary school-based health clinic over a 5-year period. *J School Health*. 2006;76:373-378.
18. Santelli JS, Nystrom RJ, Brindis C, et al. Reproductive health in school-based health centers. *J Adolesc Health*. 2003;32:443-451.
19. Reif C, Warford A. Office practice of adolescent medicine. *Prim Care*. 2006;33:269-284.

20. Mackenzie RG. Adolescent medicine: a model for the millennium. *Adolesc Med.* 2000;11:13-18.
21. Fisher M. Adolescent inpatient units. *Arch Dis Child.* 1994;70:461-463.
22. Joffe A. Evaluation and management of adolescent illness. *Adolesc Med* (in press).
23. English A. *Health Insurance for Older Adolescents and Young Adults: Policy Options to Expand Coverage.* Chapel Hill, NC: Center for Adolescent Health & the Law; 2006.
24. Newacheck PW, Park MJ, Brindis CD, et al. Trends in private and public health insurance for adolescents. *JAMA.* 2004;291:1231-1237.

Chapter 152

COUNSELING PARENTS OF ADOLESCENTS

Jonathan D. Klein, MD, MPH

Adolescence is often characterized by dramatic, uneven integration of development into the daily lives of young people. Teenagers are simultaneously experiencing changing body image, mood swings, burgeoning sexuality, intense need for peer acceptance, increasing independence from family, expectations to achieve and to act maturely, and fragile egos. At the conclusion of adolescent development, the emergent young adult is expected to comprehend the nuances of complex issues, arrive at decisions, develop an ethical and moral value system, prepare for a chosen field of work, and be capable of intimacy. These tasks begin and are realized within family units (see Chapter 107, Theories and Concepts of Development). Parents view their pediatrician as a person from whom to seek advice about both physiological and behavioral issues. The pediatrician's ongoing relationship with families allows the opportunity to provide anticipatory guidance and to support parents as children enter and move through adolescence.

Autonomy and independence evolve over time, progressing from and within an environment of continuous connectedness to parents and family. This process rarely leads to adolescents achieving independence through a sudden break with their parents; rather, the process is a gradual redefinition of relationships to a state of adult interdependence.[1] The adolescent years are one phase of a developmental continuum as young people continually renegotiate their place within their families. Experimentation and risk-taking behaviors are often perceived negatively, as something to be avoided. Nonetheless, some risks, such as those faced by athletes, performers, or peer leaders, have positive development effects, leading to competence and mastery. Most adolescents need to experience the tension created by experimenting with ideas and lifestyles that contrast with those of their family. However, during this time of *trying on* diverse personalities, the adolescent also needs to know that return to the safety and refuge of the family is assured.

A parent or guardian's greatest challenge is to maintain the delicate balance between fostering the adolescent's independent behavior and supporting the adolescent's sense of trust and security in the family. The tension created by adolescents experimentation with ideas and behaviors can be a source of conflict and emotional distress experienced simultaneously by parents and adolescents. The parents may feel a loss of control provoked by the young person's independent behavior; the adolescent's discomfort may be caused by feelings of loss of childhood security as the young person struggles to cope with greater freedom and responsibility. The emotional conflict and pain is often unrecognized and unarticulated; yet these issues underlie many confrontations between parents and adolescents. Helping parents understand the developmental basis for this conflict may reduce their frustration, as does acknowledging and empathizing with the parents' emotional separation, which may be more painful for them than it is for the adolescent.

PARENTING GOALS

Pediatricians can help parents navigate their children's adolescence. Clinicians can begin by providing parents information about the physical, cognitive, and psychosocial developmental tasks of adolescence and by helping parents realize that adolescent development is a fluctuating process. Parenting styles are often described as authoritative, authoritarian, permissive or indulgent, and uninvolved.[2] *Authoritarian* parents are demanding and directive, expecting their orders to be obeyed without explanation. *Authoritative* parents are both demanding and responsive, monitoring and communicating standards for children's conduct and expecting their children to be self-regulated. *Permissive* parents are nontraditional, do not require or expect mature behavior, and generally avoid confrontation. *Uninvolved* parents are neither responsive nor demanding, and they may be neglectful. Although both authoritarian and authoritative parenting styles appear to result in good social and vocational outcomes,[3] the former style is often associated with much greater conflict and turmoil for all family members.[4] Parents should be encouraged to set clear expectations for their adolescents; however, parents should also be encouraged to assume the role of facilitator and teacher for their adolescent, with 2 major goals. The first goal is to promote communication and resolution of conflict through *mutual respect.* Parents should maintain the adolescent's trust in the family by speaking respectfully to their chid and ensuring that their child speaks respectfully to them. The second goal for parents is to be able to tolerate adolescent's expression of differing views. When parents can demonstrate this ability, the teenager's perception of parental support is heightened and the adolescent's ego is nurtured. In this way, parents become leaders in a process in which collaboration and mutuality are affirmed and the ultimate goal of interdependent adult partnership can be achieved.

PARENT-ADOLESCENT COMMUNICATION

Open communication is probably the most important skill for parents to develop and maintain with their maturing child (Box 152-1). Adolescents need a trusted

BOX 152-1 Dos and Don'ts of Parent-Adolescent Communication

Listen more, speak less.
Respond empathetically rather than intellectually.
Resist saying "I told you so!"
Clarify expectations.
Discuss consequences.
Allow adolescents to participate in decision making.

sounding board, and, as facilitators, parents should *listen* more than speak. When parents lecture, adolescent's shut down. The axiom *actions speak louder than words* makes a more useful parental motto than *do as I say, not as I do*. This latter philosophy seems hypocritical, often diminishing the adolescent's respect for the parent. Such a situation may result in angry confrontations and weakens parent-teen relationship.

Adolescents' need for parental affection and acceptance, plus their not yet fully developed sense of self, makes them vulnerable to perceived injustices, put-downs, and negative innuendoes. Parents gain immeasurably when they respond to their adolescents' feelings with empathetic rather than intellectual responses. For example, during the teen years, peer relationships are characterized by intense emotions consistent with adolescents' egocentricity. Should a break occur in a heretofore close friendship, then the wise parent demonstrates support by empathizing with their child's hurt feelings. Statements such as, "I'm sorry that you are in such pain," "I can imagine how bad you might be feeling," or "It seems that your friend has really hurt you; do you want to talk about it?" express empathy and allow for continued discussion. Sometimes in an attempt to *make it better*, parents tend to minimize the adolescent's pain, perceiving it as *only* a short-lived adolescent drama. They respond with statements such as, "You'll find other friends," or "Don't worry; you're young and have your whole life ahead of you." Rather than finding this approach helpful, the adolescent may feel misunderstood and may cut off communication, saying, "You just don't understand!"

If the parent did not approve of the friend, then the end of the relationship may be a source of relief for the parent. Telling a teenager to "forget about it" may represent the parent's wish, rather than the teen's. The ultimate negative scenario is a parent who adds, "I told you so!" Thoughtful parents refrain from statements that belittle the adolescent. In fact, adolescents feel devastated when berated by a parent, despite attempts to defend themselves against the hurt by false bravado or an "I don't care!" response. When parents empathize with their teenagers' emotional intensity and allow their youngsters to express emotions without restraint or embarrassment, adolescents are comforted and feel supported. This approach reinforces open communication with parents and minimizes the need for adolescents to act out their angry or hurt feelings.

Parents also have an obligation to clarify expectations, responsibilities, and privileges. However, these decisions are not made in a vacuum, and the parents of adolescents should allow teens to participate as a member of the contractual, decision-making team. The success of any contract between 2 or more parties requires that each person express *without dissent* what each person wants. Also important is that both sides *gain something* from the outcome. Win-lose outcomes breed discontent and nonadherence by the person who perceives no gain. These guidelines can be useful when thinking about interactions between parents and adolescents. Open communication and decision making founded on mutual respect are skills that are best learned within a family and ensure a win-win outcome.[5]

The consequences of breaking a contract should be discussed by all involved family members. Few parents have difficulty grounding their adolescent for nonadherence to an agreement, but many have difficulty acknowledging that they, themselves, have failed to abide by an agreement. As an example of this situation consider a family in which the parents conceded that they nagged their daughter about not spending enough time on school work, fearing her academic failure. The parents agreed with their physician's counsel that they respect the adolescent's privacy and give her responsibility for her school work. A contract was signed by the pediatrician (as mediator), parents, and the adolescent. The terms included the adolescent's decision about the time to set aside for study and the parents agreement to permit her to experience her decision and to avoid questioning her. If the adolescent's grades declined, then she would be grounded; if the parents continued to harangue, then they agreed to be grounded, too, for that weekend.

ASSESSING THE PARENT-ADOLESCENT RELATIONSHIP

Pediatricians can assess how families are coping with their adolescents' development by asking parents how parent-teen decision making is handled. Curfews are a good issue to discuss with parents because they are a frequent source of conflict. The conflict about curfew decisions highlights the different jurisdictions at issue. Curfew decisions include safety issues (subject to parental authority) and the issues of adolescent choice of friends and social functions (decisions within the adolescent's jurisdiction). Physicians should explore whether parents are able to have open discussions with their adolescent about the young person's plans. Do the parents routinely ask about the location of the social function and travel plans? Do they easily agree on curfews with which everyone is reasonably satisfied? In the event of a disagreement, how are compromises negotiated? (See Box 152-2.) Parents should try to avoid arbitrarily rigid limits. An example of the type of statement best avoided is, "I have decided that you are to be home no later than midnight." Such unilateral decisions usually end in angry, unresolvable confrontations. Sometimes the rigidity of the curfew time is confounded by the parents' feelings about the adolescent's choice of friends or activities.

BOX 152-2 Guidance for Parents

***P**articipate as partners with the adolescent.*
***A**cknowledge your parental authority.*
***R**espect each other's differences.*
***E**ncourage open communication.*
***N**egotiate win-win agreements.*
***T**olerate the adolescent's separateness.*

Not infrequently, parental disapproval of an adolescent's friends or activities may be the *expressed* reason for parental inflexibility about the teen's curfew. However, the *underlying* cause for concern may have more to do with the parents' fear that their adolescent might be engaged in sexual activity or substance use. The pediatrician might ask the parents whether they and their adolescent have been able to share their views about alcohol and drug use or about sexual activity and relationships and, if so, whether the discussion resulted in mutual understanding. The pediatrician can suggest to both parent and teen that such discussions take place to make sure that parents have made their values clear and to encourage communication about responsible behavior and safe decision making.

Parents may also feel anxious because they fear adverse outcomes from their adolescent's behavioral choices. In particular, parents may be afraid that such behavior will become permanent or will threaten the teen's opportunity to mature into a responsible, productive adult. Knowing that extremes of adolescent behavior are generally transient and that most adolescents mature into adults whose lifestyles, values, and mores are similar to those of their families may reassure parents.[6] However, rigid parental control may lead to greater adolescent rebellion. The adolescent's perception of parental acceptance, interest, warmth, and respect is associated positively with the adolescent's self-esteem. Nevertheless, parents should be supported in their efforts to protect adolescents from injuries and dangerous behavior that may occur during experimental ventures.

Parents are also well advised to avoid abdicating their authority abruptly. Rather, they need to be encouraged to maintain confidence in their authority to negotiate limits, particularly when true issues of safety are involved. An example is presented by a mother and her 14-year-old son at a routine visit. In response to a question about how things were going, the mother angrily reported that her son thought he no longer needed a parent. The boy silently reacted by rolling his eyes upward. Each person was given an opportunity to explain. The mother focused on her son's defiant behavior after the parents had denied his request for an extended curfew to join a friend's birthday celebration at a downtown urban center. The pediatrician encouraged the mother to explain her main objection. She cited her fear for their son's safety, given the lateness of his planned return. At this statement the boy blurted, "Why didn't you just say that!" The parents' perceived loss of control undermined their authority; as a result, their son's immaturity became the focus of the confrontation. In this instance the pediatrician facilitated a reframing of the problem to highlight the safety issues, on which both the parents and the son agreed.

MANAGEMENT OF PARENT-ADOLESCENT CONFLICT

Some families are intuitively or purposefully flexible and reasonable, and others are able to achieve this with their pediatricians' counsel. However, some families require the intervention of a mental health professional. For example, some parents resist understanding adolescent development and have difficulty acknowledging the *mutuality* of parent-adolescent interactions. Instead, they chronically respond to the adolescent's point of view with "Yes. . .but," followed by a litany of the adolescent's misdeeds. Other parents are themselves immature and needy and may thus rely inappropriately on the adolescent for their nurturance and support. The unmet needs of such adolescents may result in chronic acting-out behaviors, marked by poor school performance, loss of friends, somatic complaints, and, in some situations, in depression or suicide attempts. For serious adjustment issues and depressive symptoms, referral and support by mental health professionals is appropriate. For less-serious adjustment issues, some pediatricians may choose to meet with the parents to assess their willingness and capacity to understand the developmental and family communication issues and to manage change within the family. If parents are refractory to counseling after 1 or 2 meetings, then the pediatrician will be in a better position to make appropriate mental health referrals than he or she would have been at the initial visit (see Chapter 131, Consultation and Referral for Emotional and Behavioral Problems).

Pediatricians who counsel parents and adolescents about developing mutually satisfying working relationships can make a significant difference in these families' lives. By enhancing the parents' knowledge and increasing their coping abilities, pediatricians can help parents provide a safe harbor for their adolescent patients; they can also help promote appropriate development of responsibility and autonomy as teens mature into adults.

TOOLS FOR PRACTICE

Engaging Patient and Family

- *Caring for Your Teenager* (book), American Academy of Pediatrics (www.aap.org/bookstore).
- *Dealing With Family Conflicts* (fact sheet), American Academy of Pediatrics (www.aap.org/topics.html).
- *How can I keep the lines of communication open with my teenager?* (fact sheet), American Academy of Pediatrics (www.aap.org/topics.html).
- *Tips for Parents of Adolescents* (brochure), American Academy of Pediatrics (patiented.aap.org).

SUGGESTED RESOURCES

Bendtro L, Brokenleg M, Van Brockern S. *Reclaiming Youth At Risk: Our Hope for the Future.* Bloomington, IN: National Educational Service; 2002.

DeVore KR, Ginsburg ER. The protective effects of good parenting on adolescents. *Curr Opin Pediatr.* 2005;17(4): 460-465.

McCurdy SJ, Scherman A. Effects of family structure on the adolescent separation-individuation process. *Adolescence.* 1996;31:122, 307.

Rueter MA, Conger RD. Interaction style, problem-solving behavior, and family problem-solving effectiveness. *Child Dev.* 1995;66:l.

Smetana JG, Asquith P. Adolescents' and parents' conceptions of parental authority and personal autonomy. *Child Dev.* 1994;65:1147.

Smetana JG, ed. *New Directions for Child Development: Changing Boundaries of Parental Authority During Adolescence* (No. 108). San Francisco, CA: Jossey-Bass; 2005.

REFERENCES

1. Baumrind D. Patterns of parental authority and adolescent autonomy. In: Smetana J, ed. *New Directions for Child Development: Changes in Parental Authority During Adolescence.* San Francisco, CA: Jossey-Bass; 2005.
2. Baumrind D. The influence of parenting style on adolescent competence and substance use. *J Early Adolesc.* 1991;11(1):56-95.
3. Steinberg L, Lamborn SD, Dornbusch SM, et al. Impact of parenting practices on adolescent achievement: authoritative parenting, school involvement, and encouragement to succeed. *Child Dev.* 1992;63(5):1266-1281.
4. DeVore KR, Ginsburg ER. The protective effects of good parenting on adolescents. *Curr Opin Pediatr.* 2005;17(4): 460-465.
5. Fish LS. Hierarchical relationship development: parents and children. *J Marital Fam Ther.* 2000;26(4):501-510.
6. Gecas V, Seff MA. Families and adolescent: a review of the 1980s. *J Marriage Fam.* 1990;52(4):941-958.

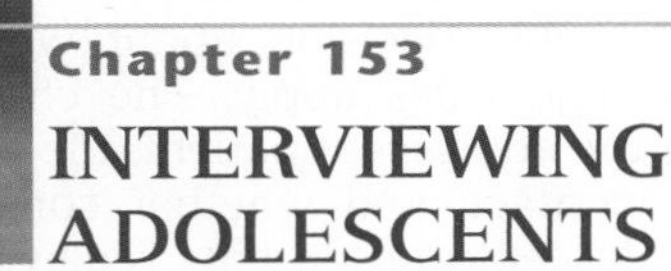

Chapter 153

INTERVIEWING ADOLESCENTS

Melanie A. Gold, DO; Aimee E. Seningen, MD

The skill of interviewing is put to the test in the practice of adolescent medicine because the relationship between the adolescent patient and the adult in a position of authority changes rapidly and is often fragile. Good interviewing requires establishing a relationship that enhances communication between the interacting parties. The information most relevant and useful to both people emerges when the relationship promotes communication and respect. Conversely, the questions most skillfully formulated do not yield useful information if the interaction between the conversing parties is tense, rushed, hostile, or judgmental.

WHOM TO INTERVIEW

During adolescence, a transition from dependence to independence should be made by the teenager and should be facilitated by the parents. In early adolescence, the parents are still largely responsible for their teen's health care, although by late adolescence, these patients are often managing their own medical needs completely. These changes occur over a relatively brief period; therefore the health care professional is faced with assessing the stage of transition toward independence each time the adolescent patient is seen. Whom to interview should be decided in the context of this transition, and the following several potential issues need to be considered.

ADOLESCENT'S DEVELOPMENTAL LEVEL

Nothing is more upsetting to adolescents than feeling that they are being treated as younger children. This perception is a particular problem in early adolescence when lack of sexual maturation on the part of teens causes insensitive adults to underestimate the youth's psychological age. Adolescent patients are often sensitive to the atmosphere of the primary care professional's office that emphasizes the interests of the young child. Therefore the health care professional should arrange the office waiting room with a section that contains reading material and decor appropriate for adolescent patients. At least one examining room should be equipped and decorated with the adolescent patient in mind. The hospital ward should also have a section furnished and decorated specifically for adolescent patients, and an interviewing room to be used exclusively for teens should be available.

The need for privacy during the interview is never more important than in the practice of adolescent medicine. If the adolescent believes that the conversations will be interrupted or overheard, then important information may not be revealed. Privacy may be particularly difficult to find on the hospital ward or in the emergency department, but every effort should be made to achieve it.

The interview room should be arranged with the health care professional, the patient, and the parents seated at the same level, at comfortable conversational distances, and without desks between the professional and the other person or persons to whom the professional is speaking. The few moments needed to rearrange the furniture to meet these requirements are well spent.

ESTABLISHING RAPPORT

Establishing rapport with an adolescent can be difficult; therefore the health care professional should take a genuine interest in the adolescent from the beginning of the interview. Establishing a partnership with the adolescent patient is important to building trust and setting the stage for developing an effective therapeutic relationship. Greeting the adolescent patient before greeting the parent or guardian is best. Asking the patient to introduce the others in the room can be helpful. The adolescent is then given the message that the primary focus is on the adolescent. Also helpful is to chat informally with the adolescent patient briefly before the interview begins, being careful to gear the conversation to the appropriate developmental level for that patient. To accomplish this task, the health care professional should know enough about normal adolescent development to judge the appropriateness of this preinterview conversation (see Chapter 107, Theories and Concepts of Development). This initial conversation with the adolescent patient can help establish rapport and possibly relieve anxiety the patient may have about the visit.

PARENTS' ROLE

Although creating an environment in which the adolescent feels comfortable is essential, the health care professional should not ignore the importance of the parents' role. In early and middle adolescence, the parents' input is critical for a thorough evaluation because adolescents may have limited insight about themselves or inadequate perspective on the timing and importance of symptoms. Adolescents may not be familiar with their own perinatal and birth history, developmental history, previous illnesses, hospitalizations, surgeries, allergies, medications, immunizations, and family history. A portion of the interview conducted with the parent present may help elicit important health history information while giving the adolescent the opportunity to learn these important aspects of the adolescent's own medical history. Interviewing the patient and parent together initially also gives insight into family dynamics and interaction.

Confidentiality issues should be addressed with both the adolescent patient and the parents early on before sensitive topics are discussed. The health care professional should also explain that the adolescent will be interviewed alone for part of the medical history and that the adolescent may have the physical examination conducted without the parents to ensure confidentiality. Confidentiality and the limits of confidentiality based on state laws or health care professional comfort should be made clear to the adolescent and the family. The health care professional should be aware of the particular state's laws regarding the adolescent's rights to confidential evaluation, and these rights must be respected. State-specific guidelines are available from the American Medical Association and the National Center for Adolescent Health and Law. For more information on confidentiality laws by state, see *State Minor Consent Laws: A Summary,* available from the Center for Adolescent Health and Law, or visit their Web site at www.adolescenthealthlaw.org/.

Although the adolescent's independence should be encouraged, and although time should always be set aside to see the health care professional alone, the appropriate role of the parents should not be ignored. Because of adolescents' possible limited perspective and their need for emotional and financial support, the health care professional would be wise in most cases to encourage younger adolescents to involve their parents in their medical decision making. When parents are involved, allowing them time to discuss their concerns without their child present may also be helpful because they may be reluctant to discuss some concerns openly, such as parental conflict or mental health issues.

HEALTH CARE PROFESSIONAL NEUTRALITY

If a significant disagreement exists between an adolescent and the adolescent's parents, then the health care professional must avoid the appearance of taking sides on these issues. This task can best be accomplished by interviewing the adolescent and parents together, concentrating on understanding and clarifying their disagreements and thus conveying an appropriately neutral attitude about the conflict. The following vignette illustrates this technique. The evaluation was initiated by the parents, who were concerned that their 15-year-old son has behavioral problems.

Mr Jones: We think his choice of friends leaves a lot to be desired.

Jim: What's the matter with my friends?

Mr Jones: Most of them have no ambition. They don't care about school and spend their time just hanging around.

Jim: It's just that we're not like you. You don't care about anything except work. At least my friends know how to have fun.

Health Care Professional: Jim, you think your father devotes too much time to work.

Jim: Yeah.

HCP: And, Mr Jones, you wish Jim were more ambitious and that he would pick friends who are ambitious too.

Mr Jones: Yes. I worry that Jim isn't going to succeed.

Jim (to his father): I'll succeed in my own way.

HCP: What are your ideas about success, Jim?

In this interaction, the health care professional has facilitated communication between the father and son by using reflections and open-ended questions without stating an opinion that would appear to commit to either person's point of view. A review of these issues before the interview helps the health care professional make a reasonable decision about whom to interview first; no rigid rules apply. The choice depends on the age of the adolescent patient, the person who initiates the contact, and whether conflict exists between the adolescent and parents regarding the problem.

INTERVIEWING TECHNIQUE

The key to good interviewing is building a trusting relationship among the health care professional, patient, and parents. This goal can be accomplished if the health care professional makes an effort to understand how the adolescent patient perceives the problem and relationships with important people in the patient's life. Most health professionals would say that they attempt to understand their patients. However, health care professionals can often become involved in their own agenda of asking questions and obtaining answers to specific medical questions and thus miss important clues about their patients' feelings and perspectives. The following vignette illustrates the insensitivity that results when medical issues are pursued vigorously and when the health care professional becomes more interested in the answers than in establishing a therapeutic relationship. The patient is a 16-year-old girl who has diabetes.

Physician: How much insulin do you take?

Sarah: Sixteen units of NPH and four units of regular each morning.

Physician: Do you test your urine?

Sarah: Yeah.

Physician: How often?

Sarah: Every morning and in the late afternoon, when my mother doesn't bug me.

Physician: Do you ever spill sugar?

Sarah: Sometimes; not too often.

Physician: How much? One plus, two plus?

Sarah: Just one plus a couple of times a week. Mom's always asking me that, but I tell her to leave me alone.

Physician: Do you ever have insulin reactions?

Sarah: Not for a long time.

Physician: How's school?

The casual observer can sense the physician's urgency to fill in the blanks of the medical history and that a rushed demanding of information is taking place illustrated by the series of closed-ended questions asked of the patient without eliciting more elaboration from the patient. In the process, this physician has failed to pick up the clues of the mother-daughter conflict. The physician completed the agenda and then turned to a question about the adolescent's life that will probably be perceived by the patient as a mechanical question because the physician did not *hear* the previous comments.

Rapport can be better established by using techniques to further open communication. These strategies include using open-ended questions, affirmations, reflections, and summaries (the mnemonic is *OARS*). Open-ended questions encourage adolescents to voice their thoughts or concerns and avoid the feeling of being interrogated by numerous closed-ended questions asked in a row. Affirmations are noncriticizing statements showing support for the patient's participation in sharing information, such as, "I really appreciate that you are able to share that information with me" and "That sounds like a really difficult time for you. I'm impressed that you have taken care of yourself so well." Reflections indicate to adolescents that their perspective is being understood. They can be a simple restatement of what the adolescent has said, or they can be made more complex by extending the meaning of the words or emotions that the adolescent has used. Summaries are often helpful to clarify the problem and pull together the discussion, and they can often help encourage the adolescent to make additional comments.

Techniques that promote the acquisition of useful information fall into two main categories: (1) listening skills and (2) facilitative responses (see interviewing techniques in Chapter 24, Communication Strategies; and Chapter 12, The Pediatric History). Component aspects of these two techniques, discussed briefly in the next two sections, are outlined in Box 153-1.

BOX 153-1 Listening Skills

Clarification of meaning
Verbal asides
Nonverbal communication
Facilitative responses
Repetition and review
Acknowledgment of feelings
Periods of silence

Listening Skills

Unless health care professionals pay attention to the meaning of words, they often think that they understand the patient's perspective when they really do not. Every time patients use words that are abstract or unclear, health care professionals should ask for clarification by using open-ended questions or reflections. Skilled interviewers continually ask themselves if they understand what has just been said. In the following vignette, the importance of this technique is illustrated. The patient is a 15-year-old boy who has problems with school.

Nurse Practitioner: Your parents seem concerned about how you are doing in school. What do you think?

Dave: Sometimes I think I'm a wreck.

NP: A wreck?

Dave: Yeah, you know, like I'm a mess.

NP: I don't know, Dave. What does that feel like?

Dave: Like I get these funny feelings, and I think I'm falling apart.

NP: Tell me about one of these funny feelings.

Dave: Well ... sometimes it's like my fingers are growing really big, or small. It's weird.

NP: You mean like parts of your body are changing size?

Dave: Yeah.

NP: What else?

Dave: Sometimes I feel like I'm walking just a little off the ground, like I am floating.

If the nurse practitioner did not pursue the meaning of Dave's words, she might have been left with the vague statement that Dave believes he is a *wreck*, which many people would assume means that he thinks he is a failure. Instead, the nurse practitioner now has evidence that Dave is experiencing somatic symptoms of anxiety or psychotic thinking, and the practitioner can pursue the source of these feelings.

Verbal asides are parenthetical statements that often reveal the patient's true feelings but that are stated as though they are unimportant. They usually reflect the adolescent's ambivalence about exposing real feelings. The patient with diabetes described earlier, who said that she tested her urine twice a day "when my mother doesn't bug me," is giving a verbal aside. Statements about her mother constitute unsolicited and important information. Health care professionals often focus only on the solicited information, and therefore they fail to hear such asides. All that is usually required to facilitate further communication is to echo the phrase back to the patient in a simple or complex reflection, such as, "It sounds like you are annoyed at your mom. What do you mean when you said she bugs you? Tell me more about that."

Nonverbal communication consists of body movements and facial expressions that reveal a person's feelings. A health care professional who is preoccupied with asking the right questions, accumulating the answers, and documenting them on the record will miss these important clues. The skilled interviewer learns to divide attention between the words that are being said and the body language of the person being interviewed. Because body language usually is outside the patient's awareness, commenting immediately on such observations may be premature, which may impart discomfort or anxiety on the patient. Part of the art of interviewing is to sense when such comments may be useful. A good rule to remember is that when body language reveals something that the person seems to be trying to hide, it should be left alone. For example, a person's clenched fists may indicate tension when the patient's words suggest calm. However, when a facial expression suggests an inner thought or feeling, then commenting is often useful by using a reflection of emotion. The patient may say something funny, for example, and then appear sad. In this instance, saying something such as, "It looks as if that thought suddenly made you feel sad" is often helpful.

Facilitative Responses

The person who is talking usually feels good when the listener can synthesize what the speaker has just said into a summary that reflects the speaker's thoughts accurately. If, for example, the patient has had difficulty finding the right words to describe symptoms and the health care professional then restates these symptoms briefly and accurately, then the patient realizes that the professional heard what the patient has been experiencing. People like to be understood, and this type of repetition and review using summaries greatly facilitates further communication.

An important component of repetition and review is the acknowledgment of feelings, as well as the recognition of facts. In many instances, patients make a series of statements that are really meant to build a case for the underlying feelings they are experiencing. If the health care professional can hear and then acknowledge these feelings with a reflection of emotion or meaning, then the relationship may be significantly enhanced. The following segment of an interview illustrates this interaction. The patient is a 13-year-old girl brought in by her parents because of acting-out behavior.

> Physician: Your parents are upset over some of the things you have done. What do you think?
>
> Jen: They really bug me. Last week, Mom wouldn't let me go to the mall with my friends. She said that we were too young to go by ourselves; but all of my friends' parents let them go. Then, a couple of nights ago, I wanted to stay at Katie's house for dinner, and Dad made me come home. He said that it's getting too dark at night. You'd think I was a baby!
>
> Physician: You don't feel that your parents trust you.
>
> Jen: I know they don't trust me. It makes me feel like doing whatever I want, since they don't trust me anyway.
>
> Physician: It makes you angry that they don't give you more freedom.

Another important facilitative response is the carefully timed use of silences, or pauses. This tactic is particularly important when the patient has difficulty with self-expression. Health care professionals are usually highly verbal people and respond to such patients by asking more and more questions. When a question has been asked and the response is not immediate, the interviewer should look closely for cues that the patient is processing the question. If the patient appears to be thinking about the answer, then the health care professional should learn to pause to allow a response. Further statements might include facilitative responses, such as, "What thoughts are you having?" or "It's hard, sometimes, to find the right words." Such replies tend to encourage the response. Similarly, the periods of silence should not be so long that the patient is made to feel uncomfortable. In psychiatric interviews, long silences are sometimes used purposefully; but this approach would be too threatening for most medical interviews, especially with younger adolescents. Instead, the suggested approach is to allow time for the person whose verbal responses are slow.

APPROACHING THE SENSITIVE ISSUES OF DRUGS, SEX, AND EMOTIONAL PROBLEMS

Vital issues in adolescent medicine include a healthy response to emerging sexuality and avoidance of addiction to drugs or alcohol. Health care professionals should address these issues from the perspective of prevention. This approach requires inquiring about these topics throughout the period of adolescent development. However, adolescents and health care professionals often feel uncomfortable with these issues. Questions about sexual activity, the use of drugs and alcohol, and the possibility of serious emotional problems often seem intrusive and embarrassing. Reassuring the adolescent again about confidentiality is important at this stage of the medical interview. In addition, a useful way to begin the discussion is to explain to the adolescent why these questions are being asked—for example, "I am asking you these questions to help me find out if there is anything that may be putting your health at risk and to tell me what kind of exam and tests I should do."

A tool for assessing the psychosocial history in adolescents is known by the acronym HEEADSSS, used to address issues of *h*ome, *e*ducation or employment, *e*ating, *a*ctivities in the peer group, *d*rugs, *s*exuality, *s*uicide or depression, and safety. The HEEADSSS assessment was developed in 1972, refined in 1988, and then updated in 2004. Examples of HEEADSSS questions are summarized in Table 153-1.

Table 153-1 The HEEADSSS Interview

TOPIC	SAMPLE QUESTIONS
Home	• Who lives with you at home? • Do you live in a house or apartment? • Do you share a room or have your own? • Do any new people live in your home? • How are your relationships with parents, siblings, other important relatives? • What are the rules like at home? □ Have you ever been homeless or in shelter care? □ Have you ever been in foster care or a residential group home?
Education	• What school do you go to? What is your grade level? • Are you in gifted, regular, or special education classes? • How do you do in school in terms of grades? • What are your best and worst subjects? • In the last year, how many days of school have you missed? Why? □ Have you ever had to repeat a year of school? Why? □ Have you ever been suspended? Why? ▲ What are your educational goals? ▲ Do you feel connected to your school? Do you feel as if you belong? ▲ Are there adults at school who you feel you could talk to about something important? Who?
Employment	• Do you work after school? • What type of work do you do? • How many hours a week do you work? • What are your future career goals? What do you want to do when you grow up in terms of a job? □ Do you have any home chores? Do you get an allowance?
Eating	• How do you feel about your weight? Do you want to weigh more or less or stay the same? • What do you think your ideal or perfect weight should be? • How many meals and snacks do you eat per day? • Tell me what you would eat in a typical day. □ Do you ever skip meals? Why? How often? □ How do you control your weight? With exercise, vomiting, diuretics, laxatives? □ How often do you have a bowel movement? Do you have any problems with your bowel movements? ▲ What would it be like if you gained (lost) 10 pounds?
Activities	• How do you like to spend your free time? What do you like to do for fun? □ What hobbies, clubs, church, or school activities do you have? • Do you play any sports? Which ones, and how many hours a week? □ How many hours of television per week do you watch? How many hours a week are you on the computer (sedentary)?
Drugs	• How many of the people with whom you hang out smoke cigarettes, drink alcohol, or use drugs? • Do you smoke or chew tobacco? • Do you drink alcohol? What kind? Beer, wine, wine coolers, hard liquor? • How often do you use tobacco, alcohol, or drugs? How much and how often? □ Have you ever blacked out or passed out? □ Have you ever done anything you regretted while drunk or high? □ When do you most often use alcohol or drugs? Socially? Alone? Time of day? Day of week? □ How do you feel about cutting back or quitting? • What other drugs have you used or tried? Marijuana, inhalants, cocaine or crack, heroin, pills, LSD, ecstasy, crystal meth, or other drugs? • Do you use anabolic steroids? ▲ Have you ever received drug treatment or counseling? ▲ How do you support your alcohol or drug use? Have you ever had any arrests? • (Ask the CRAFFT questions in Box 153-2)
Depression and suicidality	• How do you usually feel: happy, sad, or a bit of both? • What makes you feel stressed? • What do you do to relieve stress? How do you cope? • Have you ever thought about trying to hurt or kill yourself? □ Have you ever tried to hurt or kill yourself? What did you do? Whom did you tell? □ Have you ever gotten counseling or therapy? ▲ Have you ever been in a psychiatric hospital? Why? How long did you stay?

Continued

Table 153-1 The HEEADSSS Interview—cont'd

TOPIC	SAMPLE QUESTIONS
Sexuality	For female adolescents: • How old were you when you started your menstrual periods? • How often do you have a period? • How long are your periods, and how heavy is your flow? • Do you have menstrual cramps? • How often do you miss school because of cramps? For all adolescents: □ When you think of people to whom you are attracted, are they guys, girls, both, neither, or are you not sure? How comfortable are you with your feelings? □ When you think of yourself as a person, do you think of yourself as male, female, neither, or both? Are you comfortable with your feelings? • Have you ever had the kind of sex in which [add specific type of contact: penis in vagina, mouth on penis, mouth on vagina, penis in rectum, etc]? • How old were you when you first [describe sexual contact]? • How often do you have pain during sexual intercourse or other sexual activities? • Are you satisfied with how often you have sexual relations, and with what you do with your sexual partner? □ Any problems becoming aroused, getting an erection, getting lubricated (wet), or having an orgasm? □ Have you ever been pregnant or gotten someone pregnant? What concerns do you have about being able to get pregnant or get someone else pregnant? □ What have you used in the past to prevent pregnancy? What are you using now? For methods that you stopped, why did you stop them? □ How many people have you had sexual relationships with in your lifetime? What about the last 3 months? □ Have you ever had a sexually transmitted infection (STI) such as gonorrhea, *Chlamydia,* trichomonas, herpes, or warts? What concerns do you have about STIs? □ Have you ever exchanged sex for drugs, money, food, or a place to stay?
Safety	• Have you ever been forced to have sex or been touched in a sexual way against your will? By whom, and is this still going on? • In what ways does that experience affect your day-to-day life? • In what ways does that experience affect your sexual relationships now? • How often do you wear protective sports gear when you play sports? • Have you ever been a victim of violence in your home, neighborhood, or school? • Do you have access to weapons? Is there a gun in your home? □ Do you ever ride in a stolen car, in a car with a drunk driver, in a car late at night? □ Do you use sunscreen when in the sun?
Spirituality	• What do you consider to be your religion? ▲ How often do you participate in religious activities? ▲ How important are your spiritual beliefs in your day-to-day life? • How do your beliefs influence your health and attitudes about drug and alcohol use, sex, and contraception?

• = *essential questions* □ = *as time permits* ▲ = *when situation requires*

Reprinted with permission from *Contemporary Pediatrics*, Vol. 21, January 1, 2004, p. 64-90. *Contemporary Pediatrics* is a copyrighted publication of Advanstar Communications Inc.

Providing an anonymous questionnaire to the adolescent to fill out is another method to help facilitate questioning on more sensitive issues. Such questionnaires usually begin with questions that are medical, such as questions about the adolescent's perception of the patient's own weight, skin condition, and development of secondary sexual characteristics. Such questionnaires should include a review of systems with questions about the major organ systems: head, eyes, ears, nose, and throat, as well as cardiac, pulmonary, gastrointestinal, genitourinary, gynecologic, endocrine, musculoskeletal, neurologic, hematologic, dermatologic, and psychiatric issues, in addition to general complaints such as fatigue and change in appetite. Questions may then move to more sensitive areas such as sexual orientation and activity, use of alcohol and drugs, and exposure to violence and abuse. Questions should also address mental health problems such as feelings of depression, suicidal thoughts, and symptoms of anxiety. The questionnaire should also ask about school performance, including possible problems with teachers or peers. The health care professional can then use the questionnaire to address issues that are pertinent to the adolescent at the visit. For example, if the adolescent indicates sexual activity is occurring, then the physician can address issues of preventing pregnancy and sexually transmitted infections. If the patient is not sexually active, then the health care professional can emphasize making informed choices about abstinence and sexual activity in the future. However, a questionnaire should not substitute for addressing these issues in person and conducting a thorough history. The questionnaire can be a helpful tool to open up conversation; but questions unanswered or answered as no problem should be readdressed during the interview because problems may be revealed that the adolescent was uncomfortable writing down, especially related to sexuality, substance use, sexual or physical abuse, and mental illness.

When addressing the issue of sexuality with adolescents, care must be taken to avoid making assumptions regarding their sexual orientation. Such assumptions may dissuade adolescents from discussing important medical problems related to their sexual health. The use of gender-neutral terms such as *partner* can keep communication open for discussion of same gendered attractions. One way of opening a conversation about sexual orientation is to ask, "Many people have sexual experiences with members of the same sex at some point in their lives. Have you had any experiences with other men [women]?" This question can be followed up with questioning regarding whether adolescents consider themselves attracted to men, women, or both, or if they are unsure. The health care professional should recognize that people who have sex with those of the same gender may not consider themselves to be homosexual. In addition, the health care professional should be aware that a person's sexual orientation may change throughout the person's life and that adolescents can go through periods of confusion in which they may be unsure or questioning of their sexual orientation.

Another helpful approach, especially in addressing issues of drug and alcohol use, is to precede any direct questions about such use with indirect normative statements about the possible use of such substances by others. The following vignette illustrates this approach. The patient is a 15-year-old boy.

Nurse Practitioner: Sometimes kids your age try alcohol, like beer, wine, or mixed drinks, when they're at parties or hanging out together. Have you ever had anything with alcohol?

Justin: Yeah, like, a couple of times.

NP: What was it like?

Justin: Once I was with a friend who was driving and I thought he was, like, kind of crazy. I was really afraid he might get us in an accident.

NP: Was there anything you felt you could do to protect yourself?

Justin: Well, no, but I sure wish there was.

NP: How about yourself? Did you ever feel you drank too much?

Justin: Well, yeah, once I woke up the next day and I couldn't remember anything that happened.

These responses would probably not have been forthcoming had the nurse practitioner asked directly, "Do you drink alcohol or take drugs?" The indirect approach is face saving and is therefore likely to yield more truthful information. The nurse practitioner can now give more targeted advice. The importance of possible drug or alcohol abuse has also led to screening questionnaires that may be helpful in a population of adolescents at particularly high risk of abuse. Such questionnaires usually assume some alcohol or drug use and are designed to measure the severity of that use and indicate when a referral might be needed. One such method of assessing the severity of drug and alcohol use is the CRAFFT questions outlined in Box 153-2. Two or more *yes* answers suggest a high risk of a serious substance use problem or disorder.

BOX 153-2 CRAFFT Questions

Two or more *yes* answers suggest high risk of a serious substance use problem or disorder.

Have you ever ridden in a CAR driven by someone who was high or had been using drugs or alcohol?

Do you ever use alcohol or drugs to RELAX, feel better about yourself, or fit in?

Do you ever use drugs or alcohol when you are ALONE?

Do you FORGET things you did while using drugs or alcohol?

Do your FRIENDS ever tell you that you should cut down your drinking or drug use?

Have you ever gotten into TROUBLE while using drugs or alcohol?

From Knight J, Sherritt L, Shrier L, et al. Validity of the CRAFFT Substance Abuse Screening Test among adolescent clinic patients. *Arch Pediatr Adolesc Med.* 2002;156:607. Reprinted by permission of the American Medical Association.

SUMMARY

The interviewing techniques described provide some suggestions for the practitioner who provides health care for adolescents. Effective interviewing requires practice. However, the skill is well worth learning because it leads to the completion of better medical and psychosocial histories and improved patient compliance. The result is improved health care for adolescents and their families.

The authors acknowledge the substantive contributions of Esther Wender and Susan Coupey in authoring the previous versions of this chapter.

TOOLS FOR PRACTICE

Community Advocacy and Coordination

- *Helping Teens Stay Healthy and Safe: Health Care, Birth Control, and Confidential Services* (brochure), Center for Adolescent Health and the Law (www.cahl.org/helpingteensstayhealthyandsafe.htm).
- *Improving the Health of Adolescents & Young Adults* (other), Centers for Disease Control and Prevention (nahic.ucsf.edu/index.php/companion/index/#complete).
- *State Minor Consent Laws: A Summary Second Edition (2003)* (book), Center for Adolescent Health & the Law (www.adolescenthealthlaw.org/MC%20Monograph.htm).

Engaging Patient and Family

- *Caring for Your Teenager* (book), American Academy of Pediatrics (www.aap.org/bookstore).

- *Developmental Stages* (Web page), American Academy of Pediatrics (http://aap.org/healthtopics/stages.cfm#adol).
- *For Today's Teens: A Message From Your Pediatrician* (brochure), American Academy of Pediatrics (www.aap.org/bst).
- *What Is an Adolescent Health Specialist?* (fact sheet), American Academy of Pediatrics (www.aap.org/family/WhatisAdolHealthSplt_Eng.pdf).

Medical Decision Support

- *Adolescent Medicine: State of the Art Reviews* (book), American Academy of Pediatrics (www.aap.org/bst).
- *Caring for Adolescent Patients, 2nd Edition* (book), American Academy of Pediatrics (www.aap.org/bst).
- *Covering the Bases: Adolescent Sexual Health*, American Academy of Pediatrics (www.pedialink.org/cme/_coursefinder/CMEdetail.cfm?aid=32003&area=liveCME).
- *Guidelines for Adolescent Preventive Services (GAPS)* (guideline), American Medical Association (www.ama-assn.org/ama/pub/category/1980.html).
- *HEADSS Guide* (booklet) (www.bcchildrens.ca/NR/rdonlyres/6E51B8A4-8B88-4D4F-A7D9-13CB9F46E1D6/11051/headss20assessment20guide1.pdf).
- *Sample HEADSSS Questions* (Long Form) Minnesota Department of Health (www.health.state.mn.us/youthproviders/headssslong.html).
- *Motivational Interviewing* (Web page), The Mid-Atlantic Addiction Technology Transfer Center; Motivational Interviewing Resources, LLC (www.motivationalinterview.org/).
- *The CRAFFT Questions: A Brief Screening Test for Adolescent Substance Abuse* (questionnaire), Knight J and Boston Children's Hospital (www.netwellness.org/healthtopics/substanceabuse/crafft.cfm).

AAP POLICY STATEMENTS

American Academy of Pediatrics. Confidentiality in Adolescent Health Care. AAP News. 1989;5(4):9. (aappublications.org/cgi/content/abstract/5/4/9).

Hagan JF, Shaw JS, Duncan PD, eds. Bright Futures: Guidelines for Health Supervision of Infants, Children, and Adolescents. Elk Grove Village, IL: American Academy of Pediatrics; 2007. AAP endorsed. (brightfutures.aap.org).

SUGGESTED RESOURCES

Center for Adolescent Health and Law. Available at: www.adolescenthealthlaw.org/. Accessed February 22, 2007.

Coupey SM. Interviewing adolescents. *Pediatr Clin North Am.* 1997;44:1349.

Ginott HG, Ginott A, Goddard HW. *Between Parent and Child.* New York, NY: Three Rivers Press; 2003.

Goldenring JM, Cohen E. Getting into adolescent heads. *Contemp Pediatr.* 1988;5:75.

Goldenring JM, Rosen DS. Getting into adolescent heads: an essential update. *Contemp Pediatr.* 2004;21:64-90.

Knight J, Sherritt L, Shrier L, et al. Validity of the CRAFFT Substance Abuse Screening Test among adolescent clinic patients. *Arch Pediatr Adolesc Med.* 2002;156:607.

Marks A, Fisher M. Health assessment and screening during adolescence. *Pediatrics.* 1987;80(suppl):135.

Miller WR, Rollnick S. *Motivational Interviewing: Preparing People for Change.* 2nd ed. New York, NY: Guilford Press; 2002.

Motivational interviewing: resources for clinicians, researchers, and trainers. Available at: www.motivationalinterview.org/. Accessed February 22, 2007.

Rollnick S, Mason P, Butler C. *Health Behavior Change: A Guide for Practitioners.* London, UK: Churchill Livingstone; 1999.

Society of Adolescent Medicine (Web page), Society for Adolescent Medicine (http://www.adolescenthealth.org/).

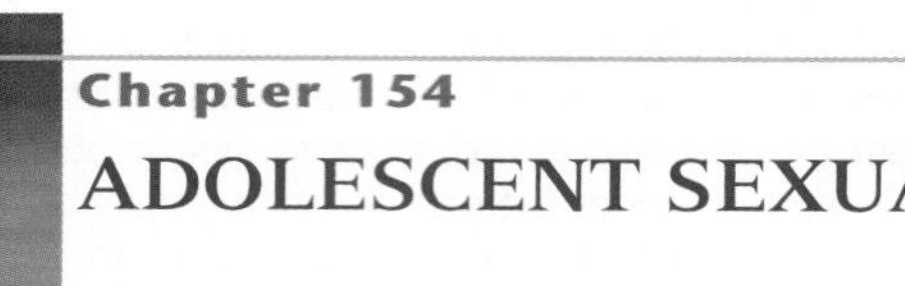

Chapter 154

ADOLESCENT SEXUALITY

Susan M. Coupey, MD; Unab I. Khan, MD

Adolescent sexuality and sexual behavior are best viewed within the context of overall adolescent development. Sexuality is a multidimensional construct and includes ethical, psychological, biological, and cultural dimensions. The overt expression of sexuality depends on the biopsychosocial environment in which the individual exists.[1] Biological changes at puberty prime the adolescent brain and body for reproduction, and individual and family psychodynamics influence sexual behavior. The larger sociocultural environment sets the norms for sexual behaviors and controls them through its institutions, including churches, schools, government, and the media. As adolescents experiment with sexual expression, they inevitably make errors of judgment. Most such errors are minor, but many have significant health consequences.

Pediatricians and other primary care physicians are in an ideal position to provide longitudinal sexual health care to children and adolescents as part of preventive care and to help adolescent patients maintain their sexual health (Box 154-1).[2] Traditionally, monitoring pubertal changes and providing anticipatory guidance to adolescents and their parents regarding timing of the growth spurt or onset of menstruation have been viewed as appropriate tasks for pediatricians. However, with initiation of sexual intercourse at younger ages, clinicians caring for teens should also be able to provide preventive care related to sexual behavior, including contraceptive counseling and prescription, screening for sexually transmitted infections (STIs), and counseling related to issues of sexual orientation and abuse. In addition, because of a high prevalence of health problems stemming from sexual behavior in the adolescent age group, clinicians must be able to diagnose and manage conditions such as pregnancy, STIs, sexual dysfunction, and sexual victimization. The physician's role is not limited to providing direct care—schools and other community organizations can often benefit from the expertise of health care providers who may help design sexuality education classes, pregnancy prevention programs, or HIV-AIDS prevention initiatives. This expanded societal role gives clinicians a broader influence on adolescent sexuality than is possible within the patient-physician-family relationship.

PUBERTAL DEVELOPMENT AND SEXUALITY

In the United States, most girls enter puberty at age 9 or 10 years, reach menarche on average at 12½, and achieve full fertility by age 15 or 16. The mean age for pubarche is approximately 1 year earlier for black girls than white girls.[3,4] Boys begin pubertal development somewhat later than girls, at age 11 or 12 years, produce sperm (spermarche) and have their first ejaculation on average at age 13 or 14, and achieve full fertility at approximately age 16.[5] Thus, by middle adolescence, most boys and girls have completed the biological developmental requirements for reproduction. Puberty is accompanied by a surge of hormones in both sexes. Androgenic hormones are primarily responsible for sexual motivation (libido) and pubic and axillary hair growth in both boys and girls and for the increase in muscle mass and skeletal growth in boys. Estrogenic hormones are important for skeletal growth in both sexes and for breast and uterine development and body fat redistribution in girls. (See Chapter 212, Puberty: Normal and Abnormal.) Sex hormones have a direct effect on the brain, and as their levels increase during puberty the adolescent's sexual interest is stimulated. Most adolescents report their first experience of sexual attraction occurred between ages 10 and 12 years, with the first sexual fantasy occurring several months to a year later.[6,7] Changes in the adolescent's outward appearance signals to others in the environment the individual's readiness for sexual intercourse (Figure 154-1). Hence girls who are early developers are at risk for early initiation of intercourse.[8]

Social factors can either facilitate or inhibit sexual expression. Researchers who propose a biopsychosocial model have identified individual attributes correlated with adolescent sexual behavior, such as testosterone levels,[9] physical maturation,[10] and temperament and personality,[11] as well as social influences such as religiosity[12] and friends' behaviors.[13] Differences by race and ethnicity are found for some, but not all, adolescent sexual behaviors. Black and Hispanic adolescents are more likely to report early initiation of sexual intercourse than are white adolescents, and boys report sexual intercourse at an earlier age than girls.[14,15] Santelli et al found an association among parental educational attainment and family

BOX 154-1 Adolescent Sexuality: Role of the Primary Care Physician

ANTICIPATORY GUIDANCE
- Pubertal development
- Postponing coitus
- Safer sex practices
- Family planning
- Sexual victimization
- Genetic counseling

PREVENTIVE CARE
- Screening for sexually transmitted infections (STIs)
- Prescribing contraceptives
- Providing psychological support (sexual orientation and abuse)

DIAGNOSING, TREATING, AND REFERRING
- STIs
- Pregnancy
- Sexual dysfunction
- Sexual victimization

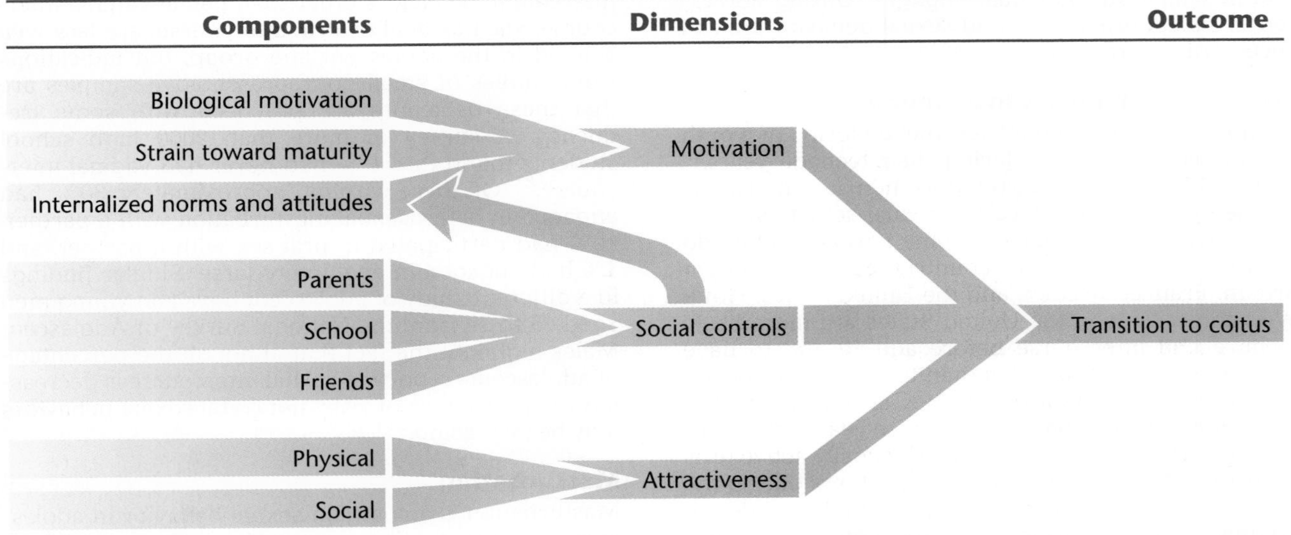

Figure 154-1 Conceptual model of transition to coitus in adolescence. *(Modified from Udry JR. Hormonal and social determinants of adolescent sexual initiation. In: Bancroft J, Reinisch JM, eds.* Adolescence and Puberty. The Kinsey Institute Series. *Vol 3, New York, NY: Oxford University Press; 1990. By permission of Oxford University Press, Inc.)*

structure and sexual debut, with higher parental education and two-parent families associated with older age at initiation of sexual intercourse.[14] Factors shown to be significantly associated with postponing initiation of coitus to later adolescence or adulthood in girls include later pubertal development (menarche at age 13 or older), careful parental supervision, good communication with the mother, and high educational aspirations.[8] Few studies have examined postponing coitus in boys, and sociocultural influences are less well understood for male coital behavior. A program developed by Howard and McCabe[16] entitled *Postponing Sexual Involvement: Educational Series for Young Teens* was used with all 8th-grade students in 24 Atlanta city schools and was evaluated in the mid-1980s. The evaluation found that the program was helpful to both boys and girls. By the end of the 9th grade, boys who had not had sexual intercourse before they participated in the program were significantly more likely to postpone sexual involvement than were similar boys who had not participated. This result indicates that boys do respond to educational intervention aimed at helping them control their sexual behavior. However, in this study, 44% of the 8th-grade boys (ages 13 and 14) had already initiated sexual intercourse before the program was given, and these sexually experienced boys did not benefit from it.

ADOLESCENT SEXUAL BEHAVIOR

Definitions

Gender identity refers to an individual's innate sense of being male or female and develops in early childhood. Gender role is influenced by societal and cultural norms and refers to the outward expression of the individual's sense of maleness or femaleness to the outside world. *Sexual orientation* refers to an individual's pattern of physical and emotional arousal toward others.[17] *Sexual behavior* refers to the actual sexual acts in which an individual engages. During adolescence, sexual orientation and sexual behavior are not necessarily congruent.

Prevalence of Sexual Intercourse

In most developed countries the majority of youth become sexually active during their teenage years.[18] At least 75% of girls and young women have had intercourse by age 20. The levels of sexual activity and the age at which adolescents become sexually active do not vary much across such countries as Canada, Great Britain, France, Sweden, and the United States. However, adolescents in the United States are more likely to have had intercourse before age 15 and to have shorter sexual relationships than teens in other developed countries.[18] As a result, they are more likely to have more than one partner in a given year and to contract an STI. In one survey, 46% of sexually active girls aged 15 to 19 years had 2 or more partners during the year.[19] US adolescents also have the highest rates of pregnancy, childbearing, and abortion when compared with peers in other developed countries.

Large changes in adolescent sexual behavior have occurred since the 1960s and continue to evolve. Several high-quality longitudinal data sets exist linking sexual behavior to demographic characteristics in adolescents in the United States. These data sets include the National Survey of Family Growth for Females, the National Survey of Adolescent Males, and the Youth Risk Behavior Survey (YRBS). Although findings vary somewhat among individual studies the trends are consistent. From 1982 to 1988 the percentage of teen girls and young women aged 15 to 19 years living in metropolitan areas nationwide and who ever had sexual intercourse increased from 47% to 53%.[20] However, from 1990 to 1997, as measured by the YRBS, the proportion of male and female high school students in the United States reporting any sexual intercourse fell from 54% to 48%, with the greatest drop seen among white adolescent boys.[21] Data from the 2005 YRBS survey of US high school students are summarized in Table 154-1.[15] The survey found that, nationwide, 47% of high school students in 2005 report having had sexual intercourse at least once. This prevalence has not changed since the 2003 survey.

Details about the patterns of sexual behaviors among adolescents who have made the transition to sexual intercourse have also been studied. Of adolescents who are sexually active the overwhelming majority practice serial monogamy; that is, they have only one sexual partner at a time. Nevertheless, boys and girls who begin having intercourse in early or middle adolescence will often accumulate three to five different sexual partners before they leave their teens. The percentage of young people who have intercourse once or twice and then stop the behavior for months or years is unknown. Some studies indicate that younger adolescents who are unlikely to be living with a sexual partner have intercourse infrequently. For example, sexually active 15-year-old boys report spending an average of nearly 8 months of the year without a sexual partner.[22]

Noncoital Sexual Behaviors

Intercourse behaviors other than penile-vaginal intercourse, such as anal or oral intercourse, are less well studied in the adolescent age group, but indications from studies of small nonrepresentative samples are that these behaviors are practiced with some frequency. A survey of more than 2000 high school students found that 47% had never had vaginal intercourse.[23] Of these virgins, approximately 30% had engaged in heterosexual masturbation with a partner, 10% had participated in oral sex with a partner, and 1% had engaged in anal intercourse. Similar findings in a different study of adolescent boys and young men aged 15 to 19 from the National Survey of Adolescent Males highlight the fact that although the percentage of adolescents reporting sexual intercourse is decreasing the prevalence of risky noncoital sexual behaviors may be increasing.[24]

Masturbation

Masturbation is a common sexual behavior in adolescents.[1] Smith et al[25] surveyed 15- to 18-year-old Australian adolescents and found 59% of boys and 43% of girls reported having masturbated. Reviewing a sample of university students, Leitenberg et al[26] found that twice as many young men reported masturbation

Table 154-1 Sexual Behaviors Among High School Students in the United States, 2005

INFORMATION SURVEYED	ALL (%)	BOYS (%)	GIRLS (%)
EVER SEXUALLY ACTIVE			
Students who have ever had sexual intercourse	47	48	46
RACE-ETHNICITY			
White	43	42	44
Black	68	75	61
Hispanic	51	58	44
GRADE			
9th grade	34	39	29
12th grade	62	61	62
Students who had first sexual intercourse before age 13 years	6	9	4
Students who have ever been physically forced to have sexual intercourse	8	4	11
CURRENTLY SEXUALLY ACTIVE			
Students who have had sexual intercourse within the previous 3 months	34	33	35
HIGH-RISK SEXUAL BEHAVIORS			
Students who have had 4 or more lifetime sexual partners	14	17	12
Currently active students who used drugs or alcohol at last intercourse	25	31	19
HEALTHY BEHAVIORS			
Currently active students who used a condom at last intercourse	63	70	56
Students who were ever tested for HIV	12	11	13

Data from Eaton DK, Kann L, Kinchen S, et al. Youth risk behavior surveillance—United States, 2005. *MMWR Surveill Summ.* 2006;55(SS05):1-108. Available at: www.cdc.gov/mmwr/preview/mmwrhtml/ss5505a1.htm. Accessed August 6, 2007.

activity than women, and men also reported engaging in the activity more frequently than women. Despite high prevalence of the behavior, masturbation is still not generally viewed as a normative sexual behavior, and it is given little attention in research, clinical settings, and in sexuality education curricula.

Homosexual Behavior

Homosexual behavior is often overlooked in studies of adolescent sexuality. Although research has shown that a portion of the population, variously estimated at between 2% and 10%, grow up to be homosexual adults, only in the last few decades have any studies of large representative populations tackled the issue of sexual orientation in adolescence. (See Chapter 157, Gay, Lesbian, and Bisexual Youth.) In the late 1980s a representative sample of nearly 35,000 high school students (grades seven through twelve) in Minnesota responded to survey questions pertaining to sexual attraction, fantasy, behavior, and affiliation.[27] Overall, 1% of students described themselves as bisexual or homosexual, and 11% were unsure of their sexual orientation. Boys were significantly more likely than girls to label themselves as *mostly* or *100%* homosexual. Uncertainty about sexual orientation gradually diminished with increasing age, from 26% of 12 year olds to 5% of 18 year olds, with corresponding increases in heterosexual and homosexual affiliation. Nearly 5% of students reported homosexual attractions, but only 1% reported such behavior. Boys were more likely than girls to report homosexual behavior (1.6% vs 0.9%), and the prevalence of homosexual behavior increased with increasing age in boys, from 0.4% at age 12 to 2.8% at age 18 years.

Much less is known about the adolescence of lesbian women. The pathways by which girls develop a same-sex sexual orientation are more diverse than those of boys. In the past, girls tended to develop a homosexual identity at an older age than boys, often not until young adulthood or later. However, this pattern may be changing as the stigma of lesbian identity is reduced. Rust[28] surveyed nearly 400 women who identified as either lesbian (76%) or bisexual (10%). She found that many women moved between the two sexual identities with frequent periods of doubt and questioning. Lesbians reported their first homosexual attraction around age 15 years, and they adopted their lesbian or bisexual affiliations by age 22 years. These findings do not support the widely held concept that homosexual behavior is common among early adolescents and gradually diminishes with age. Rather, the opposite may be true that a gradual unfolding of sexual orientation occurs during adolescence and that the behavior follows the awareness of homosexual attraction.

HEALTH CONSEQUENCES OF ADOLESCENT SEXUAL BEHAVIOR

Sexually Transmitted Infections

Adolescents account for 25% of the 12 million new cases of STIs in the United States each year.[29] Young people who begin to have sexual intercourse in early or middle adolescence are more likely to develop an STI than those who postpone intercourse until later adolescence or adulthood. This tendency is due to both anatomic and behavioral factors. Cervical ectopy, a normal feature of the anatomy of the cervix in adolescent girls, increases the risk for acquisition of STIs. Asymptomatic STIs are prevalent in both boys and girls and contribute to the spread of infections. Because of the many barriers adolescents face in obtaining routine STI screening and gynecologic care, asymptomatic infections are likely to go undetected and untreated unless or until they become symptomatic. Newer nucleotide amplification tests that can be performed on urine and do not require genital examination should help with the detection and control of asymptomatic infections. For young adolescents, love relationships may last for only a few days or weeks, and younger sexually active teens may accumulate several different sexual partners by the time they reach adulthood. Thus they are more likely to be exposed to STIs than are their peers who wait until they are older to initiate sexual intercourse.

Some STIs are associated with a high rate of permanent damage to the reproductive tract, especially for girls. For example, salpingitis caused by *Chlamydia trachomatis* is the leading cause of acquired infertility in women. In a study of more than 3000 inner-city 12- to 19-year-old black female adolescents and young adults who were sexually active, 14 year olds had the highest age-specific chlamydia prevalence rate, with more than one of every four girls (28%) infected.[30] Human papillomavirus, the most common STI in adolescents, can cause cancer of the cervix, vulva, anus, and penis, as well as genital warts; studies of adolescents report that up to one third of sexually active girls are infected with this virus, although most are completely asymptomatic. However, with the approval and anticipated widespread use of a new vaccine against several different types of human papillomavirus, many infections and their consequences will be prevented. Infection with HIV continues among adolescents, especially those in certain subgroups of the population. Factors found to be significantly associated with HIV seropositivity in adolescents include having been sexually abused, engaging in survival sex, having sex under the influence of drugs, using multiple drugs, having sex with casual partners, having had an STI, and engaging in multiple problem behaviors.[31]

Unintended Pregnancy

One of the most socially significant issues related to adolescent sexual activity is unintended pregnancy. Adolescent mothers are more likely to drop out of school, face unemployment, live in poverty, and rely on public assistance than are their peers who do not have children. The children of adolescent mothers have more health and social problems than children of adult women as well. From 1999 to 2000, both the teenaged pregnancy and the birth rates in the United States declined by 2%, and the abortion rate declined by 3%.[32] Data from the Alan Guttmacher Institute indicate that in 2000, 84 pregnancies, 48 births, and 24 abortions per 1000 women aged 15 to 19 occurred.[32] Although showing a significant decline throughout the 1990s the adolescent pregnancy rate in the United States is still very high in comparison with other developed countries.[33] Japan and most western European countries have low teenaged pregnancy rates (less than 40 per 1000), whereas Australia, Canada, and New Zealand have moderate rates (40 to 69 per 1000).[18] The primary reasons for the high teenage pregnancy rate in the United States include less overall contraceptive use and less use of the most effective contraceptives, that is, hormonal methods. Other reasons include negative societal attitudes toward teenage sex, restricted access to reproductive health services, and ambivalence toward contraceptive methods.[18] Part of the reduction in teen pregnancy rates in the United States can be explained by increased condom use. As shown in Table 154-1, nearly two thirds of currently sexually active high school students in 2005 used a condom at last intercourse, and this number represents a significant increase from the 46% using condoms in 1991.[15]

Depression and Suicide

Depression and suicide attempts are very common in the adolescent population, and sexuality issues are often linked to these mental health problems. In community samples the 6-month prevalence of depressive disorders in adolescents is 5% to 6%, with the lifetime prevalence reaching 15% to 20%.[34] Depression is the leading risk factor for youth suicide. According to the 2005 YRBS, nationwide, 17% of high school students had seriously considered suicide in the previous year, and 8% had made an attempt.[15] Forced sexual activity is a risk factor for suicide, and 8% of students surveyed in the 2005 YRBS reported being physically forced to have sex (see Table 154-1). In a school-based survey of a representative sample of nearly 8000 students in Vermont, 30% of the girls reported ever being forced or pressured to have sex, and they were twice as likely to report seriously considering suicide than were girls who had not experienced forced sex.[35] Homosexual sexual orientation is also a risk factor for suicide in adolescents. Because of the social stigma associated with homosexuality, adolescents who are questioning their sexual orientation or who know they are gay or lesbian are under considerable psychological stress. Initial parental reaction to disclosure of a teenager's homosexuality is usually negative and may lead to withdrawal of family support. Among 104 self-identified gay, lesbian, and bisexual high school students responding to a survey of more than 4000 students in Massachusetts, 35% had attempted suicide in the previous 12 months compared with 10% of heterosexual youth.[36]

Sexual Victimization

Sexual abuse should always be considered a possibility when an adolescent has very early onset of sexual activity. Both adolescent boys and girls who have been victims of forced sex, either as young children by an adult perpetrator or as adolescents, have higher-than-normal rates of health-risk behaviors and mental health problems. Prevalence rates of child and adolescent sexual abuse vary in the literature depending on the definition of abuse. A telephone survey conducted in 1995 of a national household probability sample of more than 4000 adolescents aged 12 to 17 years using a very clear and explicit definition of sexual abuse found 8% of adolescents reported being victims of sexual abuse.[37] A prior history of sexual abuse correlates significantly with young age at onset of voluntary sexual intercourse, unintended pregnancy, suicide attempts, drug and alcohol abuse, eating disorders, and violence.[37,38] Girls who have been sexually abused are twice as likely as those not abused to have had intercourse by age 15 and three times more likely to have been pregnant.[39] Thus exploring the possibility of sexual abuse is important when an adolescent has very early onset of sexual intercourse or has multiple behavioral problems.

Sexual Dysfunction

Sexual dysfunction is an area not well studied in adolescence, although the prevalence in both boys and girls is probably quite high. Clinical reports indicate that many sexually active adolescent girls do not enjoy sexual intercourse and have never reached orgasm. Reasons for engaging in the behavior have more to do with intimacy and closeness to the partner than with personal sexual gratification.[40] Occasionally a girl who is anxious and unsure about sexual activity or who has previously been abused develops vaginismus. Large numbers of adolescent boys are thought to have premature ejaculation, but they rarely complain of the problem. Erectile dysfunction does occur in adolescence, often as a result of performance anxiety and other psychogenic causes.[41] Heavy alcohol or marijuana use can be responsible for erectile dysfunction and should be explored in the medical history. Prescription medications are often implicated in erectile dysfunction in men and anorgasmia in women. Frequent offenders in this regard are antihypertensives, antipsychotics, and antidepressants. Other drugs that cause sexual dysfunction and that may be taken by adolescents are cimetidine, ranitidine, sulfasalazine, and some anticonvulsants.

ADOLESCENT SEXUALITY AND THE PATIENT-PRACTITIONER-PARENT RELATIONSHIP

Even though sexual feelings and behaviors are of great concern to adolescents and their families and adverse effects of sexual behavior are common in this age group, most patients and parents will avoid introducing the subject at the health care visit. Primary care clinicians must set the stage for frank, honest discussions of feelings and behaviors that are often embarrassing, shameful, and psychologically painful. The clinician should help parents communicate clearly to their adolescents about sexual issues because this may have the added benefit of making teenagers less likely to rely on peers for advice and less likely to conform to peer norms. Helping parents develop the skills to communicate effectively with their teenage children is the clinician's role. Studies have shown that parent-child connectedness and clear communication about sexual issues have been associated with delay of sexual initiation.[42]

All medical care providers should pay particular attention to privacy for both adolescent patients and parents. In general, the medical interview with the adolescent should take place in private. To give optimal care to adolescents, clinicians should be open, honest, interested, concerned, and supportive and should tailor their communication style to the developmental level of the adolescent.[43] Asking questions that do not make assumptions or presuppose certain behaviors is important, given that adolescents are more likely to disclose closely guarded information when interviewed in this way. For example, if the clinician assumes that everyone is heterosexual and asks girls if they have a boyfriend and boys if they have a girlfriend, adolescents who are questioning their sexual orientation or who know they are homosexual will be unlikely to offer this information. If, on the other hand, the question pertains to sexual attraction to women, men, or both men and women or includes a gender-neutral term, such as *sexual partner*, then the patient is more likely to understand that the clinician is ready to hear nontraditional information.

Assuming that just because a question has been asked and answered, the full story has been told is a mistake. Such is especially true of questions about sexual abuse. Some adolescents who have been abused are afraid to disclose painful secrets because they have not yet developed a secure, trusting relationship with the health care provider. The clinician should understand this factor, should avoid pushing too hard and too soon for disclosure, and should explore the topic in more depth at a later visit when the relationship has had a chance to develop.

Negotiating confidentiality between adolescents and parents around sexual issues is a thorny area for the patient-clinician-parent relationship. Studies show that giving assurance of confidentiality increases the number of adolescents willing to return for future visits.[44] Every medical care provider should be aware of the individual state laws that exist regarding diagnosis and management of STIs, contraception, and termination of pregnancy. When a problem is diagnosed the specifics of what will be disclosed to parents need to be negotiated in advance with the patient. Clinicians should refuse to lie to parents because this sets a bad example and is unprofessional. However, disclosing all of the details of the situation is usually unnecessary. For example, a 16-year-old girl being seen for her annual checkup reveals that she has recently become sexually active. She reports that she has had two partners in the last 8 months. She complains of a slight vaginal discharge. The clinician discovers mucopurulent cervicitis during a pelvic examination and prescribes appropriate antibiotics. What should the mother be told? Most adolescents would agree to allow the clinician to tell the mother that a pelvic examination was performed and an infection was noted that is easily treated with antibiotics. The clinician can tell the adolescent beforehand that if the mother asks directly whether the infection is sexually transmitted, she will be told that information about her daughter's sexuality is kept in confidence. However, the adolescent patient should know that the clinician will encourage a dialogue between mother and daughter about sexual behavior. The clinician must resist acting as a go-between in the mother-daughter relationship and should emphasize the necessity of direct communication between parent and child.

An integral part of taking care of adolescents is providing developmentally appropriate anticipatory guidance. An important point to remember is that the early adolescent still retains concrete thinking. Given the increased awareness of physical changes, these factors need to be addressed and explored during this stage. If the adolescent is not sexually active, then the adolescent should be encouraged to postpone coitus to a later stage. In middle adolescence an increase in risk-taking behaviors often occurs. Counseling at this stage should focus on safer sex practices and contraception, as well as postponing intercourse. Anticipatory guidance should also include a discussion of signs and symptoms of STIs and the need for regular screening. By late adolescence, patients should be encouraged and empowered to negotiate the health care system and make decisions regarding their reproductive health. Pregnant adolescents should be offered options counseling in a safe, nonjudgmental, and trusted environment.

SUMMARY

Providing health care related to adolescent sexuality is one of the more difficult tasks of the primary care clinician. It demands in-depth knowledge of pubertal and psychosexual development, familiarity with the norms of adolescent sexual behavior, knowledge of pertinent gynecologic and urologic medicine, and superior communication skills. Adolescents are in great need of this type of care and are appreciative when it is done well; the large majority wants to be sexually healthy and eventually to have children and raise healthy families themselves.

TOOLS FOR PRACTICE

Community Advocacy and Coordination

- *Condom Effectiveness—Fact Sheet for Public Health Personnel: Male Latex Condoms and Sexually Transmitted Diseases* (fact sheet), Centers for Disease Control and Prevention (www.cdc.gov/condomeffectiveness/latex.htm).
- *Facts at a Glance* (Web page), Child Trends (www.childtrends.org/_docdisp_page.cfm?LID=D6F165A5-00B3-4D76-ABACFD97F248817C).
- *Helping Teens Stay Healthy and Safe: Health Care, Birth Control, and Confidential Services* (brochure), Center for Adolescent Health and the Law (www.cahl.org/helpingteensstayhealthyandsafe.htm).
- *Improving the Health of Adolescents & Young Adults*, Centers for Disease Control and Prevention (nahic.ucsf.edu/index.php/companion/index/#complete).
- *State Minor Consent Laws: A Summary, 2nd edition* (book), Center for Adolescent Health and the Law (www.adolescenthealthlaw.org/MC%20Monograph.htm).

Engaging Patient and Family

- *1 800 NOT 2 LATE* (hotline), National Emergency Contraception Hotline.
- *Caring for Your Teenager* (book), American Academy of Pediatrics (www.aap.org/bookstore).
- *Developmental Stages* (Web page), American Academy of Pediatrics (aap.org/healthtopics/stages.cfm#adol).
- *Deciding to Wait: Guidelines for Teens* (brochure), American Academy of Pediatrics (patiented.aap.org).
- *Emergency Contraception* (fact sheet), American Academy of Pediatrics (www.aap.org/family/ecparentpage.pdf).
- *For Today's Teens: A Message From Your Pediatrician* (brochure), American Academy of Pediatrics (patiented.aap.org).
- *Making Healthy Decisions About Sex* (brochure), American Academy of Pediatrics (patiented.aap.org).
- *The Pelvic Exam* (brochure), American Academy of Pediatrics (patiented.aap.org).
- *What is an Adolescent Health Specialist?* (fact sheet), American Academy of Pediatrics (www.aap.org/family/WhatisAdolHealthSplt_Eng.pdf).

Medical Decision Support

- *Adolescent Medicine: State of the Art Reviews* (book), American Academy of Pediatrics (www.aap.org/bookstore).
- *Caring for Adolescent Patients, 2nd edition* (book), American Academy of Pediatrics (www.aap.org/bookstore).
- *Covering the Bases: Adolescent Sexual Health*, American Academy of Pediatrics (www.pedialink.org/cme/_coursefinder/CMEdetail.cfm?aid=32003&area=liveCME).
- *Guidelines for Adolescent Preventive Services (GAPS)*, American Medical Association (www.ama-assn.org/ama/pub/category/1980.html).
- *Motivational Interviewing* (Web page), The Mid-Atlantic Addiction Technology Transfer Center; Motivational Interviewing Resources, LLC (www.motivationalinterview.org/).

RELATED WEB SITES

- Boston Children's Hospital: Center for Young Women's Health (www.youngwomenshealth.org/).
- Centers for Disease Control and Prevention: Teen Pregnancy (www.cdc.gov/reproductivehealth/AdolescentReproHealth).
- Centers for Disease Control and Prevention: Unintended Pregnancy Prevention: Contraception (www.cdc.gov/reproductivehealth/UnintendedPregnancy/Contraception.htm.
- Guttmacher Institute (www.guttmacher.org/sections/pregnancy.php).
- National Center for Health Statistics (NCHS) (cdc.gov/nchs).
- Planned Parenthood: Teenwire (www.teenwire.com/).
- Society for Adolescent Medicine (www.adolescenthealth.org/).

AAP POLICY STATEMENTS

American Academy of Pediatrics, Committee on Adolescence and Committee on Early Childhood, Adoption, and Dependent Care. Care of adolescent parents and their children. *Pediatrics*. 2001;107(2):429-434. (aappolicy.aappublications.org/cgi/content/full/pediatrics;107/2/429).

American Academy of Pediatrics, Committee on Adolescence. Care of the adolescent sexual assault victim. *Pediatrics*. 2001;107(6):1476-1479. (aappolicy.aappublications.org/cgi/content/full/pediatrics;107/6/1476).

American Academy of Pediatrics, Committee on Adolescence. Condom use by adolescents. *Pediatrics*. 2001;107(6): 1463-1469. (aappolicy.aappublications.org/cgi/content/full/pediatrics;107/6/1463).

American Academy of Pediatrics, Committee on Adolescence. Contraception and adolescents. *Pediatrics*. 2007; 120(5):1135-1148. (aappolicy.aappublications.org/cgi/content/full/pediatrics;120/5/1135).

American Academy of Pediatrics, Committee on Adolescence. Counseling the adolescent about pregnancy options. *Pediatrics*. 1998;101(5):938-940. (aappolicy.aappublications.org/cgi/content/full/pediatrics;110/5/938).

American Academy of Pediatrics, Committee on Adolescence. Emergency contraception. *Pediatrics*. 2005;116(4): 1026-1035. (aappolicy.aappublications.org/cgi/content/full/pediatrics;116/4/1026).

American Academy of Pediatrics, Committee on Adolescence. The adolescent's right to confidential care when considering abortion. *Pediatrics*. 1996;97(5):746-751. (aappolicy.aappublications.org/cgi/content/abstract/pediatrics;97/5/746).

American Academy of Pediatrics, Committee on Psychosocial Aspects of Child and Family Health and Committee on Adolescence. Sexuality education for children and adolescents. *Pediatrics*. 2001;108(2):498-502. (aappolicy.aappublications.org/cgi/content/full/pediatrics;108/2/498).

American Academy of Pediatrics, Committee on Public Education. Sexuality, contraception, and the media. *Pediatrics*. 2001;107(1):191-194. (aappolicy.aappublications.org/cgi/content/full/pediatrics;107/1/191).

American Academy of Pediatrics. Confidentiality in adolescent health care. *AAP News*. 1989;5(4):9. (aapnews.aappublications.org/cgi/content/abstract/5/4/9).

Frankowski BL, American Academy of Pediatrics, Committee on Adolescence. Sexual orientation and adolescents. *Pediatrics*. 2004;113(6):1827-1921. (aappolicy.aappublications.org/cgi/content/full/pediatrics;113/6/1827).

Klein JD, American Academy of Pediatrics, Committee on Adolescence. Adolescent pregnancy: current trends and issues. *Pediatrics*. 2005;116(1):281-286. (aappolicy.aappublications.org/cgi/content/full/pediatrics;116/1/281).

Murphy NA, Elias ER, American Academy of Pediatrics, Council on Children With Disabilities. Sexuality of children and adolescents with developmental disabilities. *Pediatrics*. 2006;118(1):398-403. (aappolicy.aappublications.org/cgi/content/full/pediatrics;118/1/398).

REFERENCES

1. DeLamater J, Friedrich WN. Human sexual development. *J Sex Res*. 2002;29(1):10-14.
2. American Academy of Pediatrics, Committee on Psychosocial Aspects of Child and Family Health and Committee on Adolescence. Sexuality education for children and adolescents. *Pediatrics*. 2001;108(2):498-502.
3. Herman-Giddens ME, Slora EJ, Wasserman RC, et al. Secondary sexual characteristics and menses in young girls seen in office practice: a study from the Pediatric Research in Office Settings Network. *Pediatrics*. 1997; 99(4):505-512.
4. Chumlea WC, Schubert CM, Roche AF, et al. Age at menarche and racial comparisons in US girls. *Pediatrics*. 2003;111(1):110-113.
5. Sun SS, Schubert CM, Chumlea WC, et al. National estimates of the timing of sexual maturation and racial differences among US children. *Pediatrics*. 2002;110(5): 911-919.
6. Bancroft J, Herbenick D, Reynolds M. Masturbation as a marker of sexual development: two studies 50 years apart. In: Bancroft J, ed. *Sexual Development*. Bloomington, IN: Indiana University Press; 2003.
7. Rosario M, Meyer-Bahlburg H, Hunter J, et al. The psychosexual development of urban lesbian, gay and bisexual youths. *J Sex Res*. 1996;33(2):113-126.
8. Rosenthal SL, Von Ranson KM, Cotton S, et al. Sexual initiation: predictors and developmental trends. *Sex Transm Dis*. 2001;28(9):527-532.
9. Halpern CT, Udry JR, Campbell B, et al. Testosterone and pubertal development as predictors of sexual activity: a panel analysis of adolescent males. *Psychosom Med*. 1993;55(5):436-437.
10. Halpern CT, Udry JR, Suchindran C. Testosterone predicts initiation of coitus in adolescent females. *Psychosom Med*. 1997;59(2):161-171.
11. Udry JR, Talbert LM. Sex hormones effects on personality at puberty. *J Pers Soc Psychol*. 1988;54(2): 291-295.
12. Halpern CT, Udry JR, Campbell B, et al. Testosterone and religiosity as predictors of sexual attitudes and activity among adolescent males: a biosocial model. *J Biosoc Sci*. 1994;26(2):217-234.
13. Smith EA, Udry JR, Morris NM. Pubertal development and friends: a biosocial explanation of adolescent sexual behavior. *J Health Soc Behav*. 1985;26(3):183-192.
14. Santelli JS, Lowry R, Brener ND, et al. The association of sexual behaviors with socioeconomic status, family structure, and race/ethnicity among US adolescents. *Am J Public Health*. 2000;90(10):1582-1588.
15. Eaton DK, Kann L, Kinchen S, et al. Youth risk behavior surveillance—United States, 2005. *MMWR Surveill Summ*. 2006;55(SS05):1-108. Available at: www.cdc.gov/mmwr/preview/mmwrhtml/ss5505a1.htm. Accessed August 6, 2007.
16. Howard M, McCabe JB. Helping teenagers postpone sexual involvement. *Fam Plann Perspect*. 1990;22(1): 21-26.
17. Frankowski BL and American Academy of Pediatrics, Committee on Adolescence. Sexual orientation and adolescents. *Pediatrics*. 2004;113(6):1827-1832.
18. Guttmacher Institute. Facts in Brief. Teenagers' Sexual and Reproductive Health: Developed Countries. Available at: www.guttmacher.org/pubs/fb_teens.html. Accessed August 6, 2007.
19. Finer LB, Darroch JE, Singh S. Sexual partnership patterns as a behavioral risk factor for sexually transmitted diseases. *Fam Plann Perspect*. 1999;31(5):228-236.
20. Forrest JD, Singh S. The sexual and reproductive behavior of American women: 1982-1988. *Fam Plann Perspect*. 1990;22(5):206-214.
21. Centers for Disease Control and Prevention. Trends in sexual risk behaviors among high school students—United States, 1991-2001. *MMWR Morb Mortal Wkly Rep*. 2002;51(38):856-859.
22. Sonenstein FL, Pleck JH, Ku LC. Levels of sexual activity among adolescent males in the United States. *Fam Plann Perspect*. 1991;23(4):162-167.
23. Schuster MA, Bell RM, Kanouse DE. The sexual practices of adolescent virgins: genital sexual activities of high school students who have never had vaginal intercourse. *Am J Public Health*. 1996;86(11):1570-1576.

24. Gates GJ, Sonenstein FL. Heterosexual genital sexual activity among adolescent males: 1988 and 1995. *Fam Plann Perspect*. 2000;32(6):295-297.
25. Smith AM, Rosenthal DA, Reichler H. High schoolers masturbatory practices: their relationship to sexual intercourse and personal characteristics. *Psychol Rep*. 1996;79(2):499-509.
26. Leitenberg H, Detzer MJ, Srebnik D. Gender differences in masturbation and the relation of masturbation experience in preadolescence and/or early adolescence to sexual behavior and sexual adjustment in young adulthood. *Arch Sex Behav*. 1993;22(2):87-98.
27. Remafedi G, Resnick M, Blum R, et al. Demography of sexual orientation in adolescents. *Pediatrics*. 1992;89 (4 pt 2):714-721.
28. Rust PC. The politics of sexual identity: sexual attraction and behavior among lesbian and bisexual women. *Soc Prob*. 1992;39(4):366-386.
29. Weinstock H, Berman S, Cates W. Sexually transmitted diseases among American youth: incidence and prevalence estimates, 2000. *Perspect Sex Reprod Health*. 2004; 36(1):6-10.
30. Burstein GR, Gaydos CA, Diener-West M, et al. Incident Chlamydia trachomatis infections among inner-city adolescent females. *JAMA*. 1998;280(6):521-526.
31. Hein K, Dell R, Futterman D, et al. Comparison of HIV+ and HIV− adolescents: risk factors and psychosocial determinants. *Pediatrics*. 1995;95(1):96-104.
32. Guttmacher Institute. US Teenage Pregnancy Statistics: Overall Trends, Trends by Race and Ethnicity, and State-by-State Information. Available at: www.guttmacher.org/pubs/state_pregnancy_trends.pdf. Accessed June 25, 2006.
33. Singh S, Darroch JE. Adolescent pregnancy and childbearing: levels and trends in developed countries. *Fam Plann Perspect*. 2000;32(1):14-23.
34. Klein DN, Dougherty LR, Olino TM. Toward guidelines for evidence-based assessment of depression in children and adolescents. *J Clin Child Adolesc Psychol*. 2005;34(3): 412-432.
35. Shrier LA, Pierce JD, Emans SJ, et al. Gender differences in risk behaviors associated with forced or pressured sex. *Arch Ped Adolesc Med*. 1998;152(1):57-63.
36. Garofalo R, Wolf RC, Kessel S, et al. The association between health risk behaviors and sexual orientation among a school-based sample of adolescents. *Pediatrics*. 1998;101(5):895-902.
37. Kilpatrick DG, Acierno R, Saunders B, et al. Risk factors for adolescent substance abuse and dependence: data from a national sample. *J Consult Clin Psychol*. 2000;68(1):19-30.
38. Nagy S, Adcock AG, Nagy MC. A comparison of risky health behaviors of sexually active, sexually abused, and abstaining adolescents. *Pediatrics*. 1994;93(4):570-575.
39. Stock JL, Bell MA, Boyer DK, et al. Adolescent pregnancy and sexual risk-taking among sexually abused girls. *Fam Plann Perspect*. 1997;29(5):200-203.
40. Cohen MW. Adolescent sexual activity as expression of nonsexual needs. *Pediatr Ann*. 1995;24(6):324-329.
41. Farrow JA. An approach to the management of sexual dysfunction in the adolescent male. *J Adolesc Health Care*. 1985;6(5):397-400.
42. Sieving RE, McNeely CS, Blum RW. Maternal expectations, mother-child connectedness, and adolescent sexual debut. *Arch Pediatr Adolesc Med*. 2000;154(8):809-816.
43. Coupey SM. Interviewing adolescents. *Pediatr Clin North Am*. 1997;44(6):1349-1364.
44. Ford CA, Millstein SG, Halpern-Felsher BL, et al. Influence of physician confidentiality assurances on adolescents' willingness to disclose information and seek future health care. A randomized controlled trial. *JAMA*. 1997; 278(12):1029-1034.

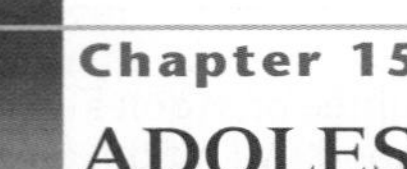

Chapter 155

ADOLESCENT PREGNANCY AND PARENTHOOD

Dianne S. Elfenbein, MD; Marianne E. Felice, MD

Teenage pregnancy and parenthood are a national concern because of the resulting societal, economic, and educational disadvantages for teen mothers and their babies. These disadvantages lead to and exacerbate emotional stressors for teen parents and their families. Although the United States has higher rates of births to teen mothers than any other industrially developed nation, births to teen mothers in the United States have decreased since the late 1950s, with the exception of a steep increase in rates from the late 1980s until 1991, after which a steady decline has continued[1-4] (Figure 155-1). Declines in birthrates have been accompanied by declines in *rates* of pregnancy, induced abortion, and fetal loss. From 1990 to 2000, declines occurred in the teen birthrates of all racial and ethnic groups, with the greatest decline for black teens (31%). Birthrates to European-American descent dropped 24%, and rates among Hispanic girls dropped approximately 15%. As of 2000, rates for Hispanic and black teens continued to be the highest of all population groups.[3] The future will tell if this trend continues over the next decade.

The decrease in the rates of adolescent pregnancies and births appears to be the result of several factors, including delayed initiation of sexual activity, increased use of contraception (eg, condoms) at first coitus, and a greater efficacy of hormonal contraceptive methods.[5,6] All hormonal methods remove the act of pregnancy

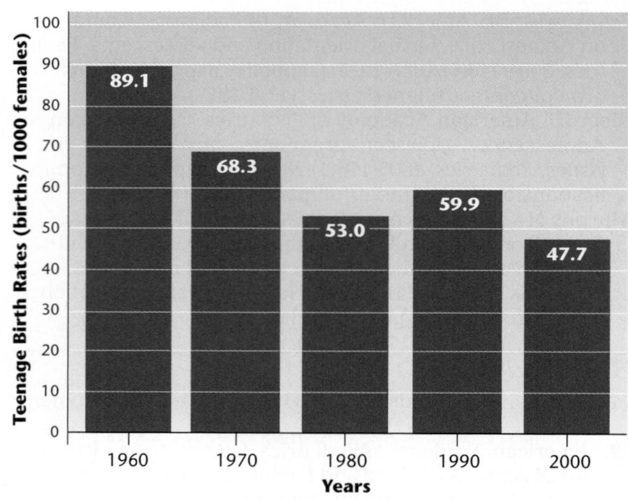

Figure 155-1 Teen birth rates (births/1000 females aged 15-19 years), 1960-2000. *(Modified from Child Trends: Facts at a Glance 2003. Available at www.childtrends.org/Files/FAAG2003.pdf; accessed July 29, 2008. Reproduced by permission of Child Trends.)*

prevention from the act of sexual intercourse and are more effective than barrier methods, spermicides, or methods based on the periodicity of the menstrual cycle. Methods such as injectable or implantable contraception and newer hormonal delivery systems such as patches and intravaginal rings do not require the need to take a pill every day, which may be difficult for young women who may not have regular life routines. Although intrauterine devices are also available, they are not generally used in young teens or women who have never borne children.

CHARACTERISTICS OF TEEN PARENTS

Teens growing up in conditions of poverty are known to be at the highest risk for early pregnancy.[7] In addition, pregnancy rates differ for young women of different racial and ethnic groups; marked changes in the rates of each group have occurred over the last 40 years. Data from 2004 indicate that Hispanic teens aged 15 to 19 years had the highest birthrates of their age group (82.6 live births per 1000), in contrast to black teens (62.7) and European-American teens (26.8).[8] Two thirds of all births in the age range 15 to 19 years were to 18- to 19-year-old women. Numerically, births to young women under age 15 represented a small proportion of overall births; however, in this age group, black mothers have consistently had the highest rate.[3] Birthrates also varied geographically, with the highest rates of teen pregnancy in Washington, DC (83.5) and Mississippi (72.5) and the lowest rate in New Hampshire (24.0) in 1999.[1] Geographic rates generally reflect the racial, ethnic, and socioeconomic status of those living in the area.

Early childbearing is associated with educational disadvantages.[7] Girls who become pregnant as teens are educationally behind their peers before the pregnancy, and girls with intellectual disability appear to be at particularly high risk of pregnancy.[9,10] In addition, the educational aspirations of girls who bear childen appear to be lower than those of their peers; such teens do not regard early pregnancy or parenting as undesirable life options.[11-13] Other associations with pregnancy in teens include increased rates of alcohol, tobacco, and drug use; early initiation of sexual activity; family history of adolescent pregnancy in the mother or in siblings; and adverse childhood experiences such as abuse, exposure to violence, substance abuse, mental illness, criminal household member, or having divorced or separated parents.[14,15]

Fathers of infants born to teen mothers have the same backgrounds and many of the same characteristics as their partners, although many of the men are older and are legally adults. In most instances, male sexual partners are approximately 3 years older than their female partners, whatever their ages. In some racial and ethnic groups, the age difference between fathers and their teen partners may be greater than average.[16,17] Each state has its own definition of statutory rape, and some pregnancies clearly fit into this official category, although most teen mothers view their sexual activity as voluntary and consensual. The younger the pregnant teen is, the greater the likelihood will be that the pregnancy is a result of either forced sex or statutory rape.[18] In general, the men who father the infants of teen women are frequently from disadvantaged socioeconomic classes, are often educationally behind their peers, are more likely to have legal difficulties, are more likely to use illegal substances, and are more likely to acquire a sexually transmitted infection than age-matched peers. If they work, these men usually have lower-paying jobs than their age-matched peers.[16,17,19-21] Many of these young men have mothers or sisters who were pregnant as adolescents. These characteristics may not apply to young men whose pregnant partners choose to terminate their pregnancies.

EVALUATION

Physical Examination

Pregnant teenagers may not seek care for the classic symptoms of pregnancy, such as a missed menstrual period, morning nausea, and breast tenderness. Instead, teens may seek care for other physical complaints, some of which are entirely unrelated to pregnancy (eg, sore throat). Primary care physicians who care for young women of childbearing age must always consider pregnancy, regardless of the symptoms the teen exhibits. The last menstrual period should be routinely determined and recorded at every office visit then noted by the clinician before seeing the patient. The validity of the stated last menstrual period should be questioned if any clinical suspicion of pregnancy exists, and a urine or serum pregnancy test should be performed.

Pregnancy should always be considered in any young woman who has secondary amenorrhea. Other symptoms that suggest pregnancy are fatigue, nausea (particularly nausea that is relieved by eating), dizziness or syncope, urinary frequency, weight gain, breast tenderness or enlargement, and abdominal tenderness or enlargement.

Pelvic and breast examinations may be performed to confirm the diagnosis. Breast fullness and tenderness may be noted. Uterine enlargement varies with the gestational age of the pregnancy (Box 155-1). In addition, the clinician may note cervical softening and cyanosis during the pelvic examination during early pregnancy. A pregnancy test should be performed in these cases.

Laboratory Evaluation

Currently available urine pregnancy tests, most of which use enzyme-linked immunosorbent assay techniques

BOX 155-1 Uterine Changes With Pregnancy

4 weeks: cervical softening and cyanosis is noted.

8 weeks: uterus is the size of an orange.

12 weeks: uterus is grapefruit sized and palpable suprapubically.

20 weeks: uterus is at the umbilicus.

and monoclonal antibodies to human chorionic gonadotropin (hCG), are sensitive and are able to detect pregnancy as early as 3 to 3.5 weeks after the last menstrual period (1 to 1.5 weeks after ovulation in a woman with 28-day cycles), although they are more accurate at 4 to 4.5 weeks because the low level of hCG seen at 1 week's gestation is at the lower level of detection and may be missed. These tests are easy to perform in an office setting. Serum hCG determination can be performed if any question exists of urine tampering, inaccurate urinary hCG, spontaneous or threatened abortion, or ectopic pregnancy.

Imaging Studies

If the dating of the pregnancy is in question, or suspicion of an abnormal pregnancy exists, then a pelvic ultrasound may be useful. Pelvic ultrasound performed transabdominally can detect a gestational sac as early as 5 to 6 weeks after the last menstrual period. If the ultrasound is performed transvaginally, then a gestational sac may be determined as early as 4 to 5 weeks' gestation.[22]

MANAGEMENT

Once a teen pregnancy has been confirmed, several complicated issues need to be addressed with the patient. To address these issues appropriately, primary care clinicians must be familiar with the pertinent laws of the state in which they are practicing, with their local school system's policies in dealing with pregnant teens and teen parents, and with local medical, financial, and social resources. Box 155-2 lists the ways a primary care physician can help the pregnant teenager.

The teen must first be privately informed of her pregnancy. Her reaction will depend on several factors—whether the pregnancy was suspected or not suspected, wanted or unwanted, planned or unplanned. Next, a determination must be made as to whether informing the patient's parents and the father of the infant will cause any difficulties, and then the patient must be helped to address the difficulties. The age of the father of the baby and the teen's relationship to the father should always be asked to determine whether the clinician should inform local authorities of abuse or statutory rape. See Chapter 356, Rape, for more information. In addition, the patient should be helped to understand the social, emotional, educational, and financial implications of the pregnancy. Addressing all of these issues may require referral of the patient to an outside counselor such as a social worker skilled in these issues or several office visits for a patient with few other resources.

All patients should be presented with the options legally available to them: abortion, adoption, or parenthood. Some pregnant teens will decide that they are not ready to parent, and they may decide to terminate the pregnancy or to make a plan for adoption. Physicians who have moral or religious objections to discussing these issues should refer their patients to other physicians who can support the possible patient choices. Patient coercion of any kind in this matter is not appropriate professional behavior. Primary care physicians should refer patients who choose termination to the appropriate local resources. Patients who choose adoption should be referred to agencies that have policies in place to safeguard the rights of the pregnant mother, her infant, the father of the baby, and the prospective parents. Teens who choose to terminate the pregnancy and those who opt for adoption may continue to need emotional support from their primary care clinician or their counselor, just as the young mother who decides to parent will.

BOX 155-2 How a Primary Care Clinician Can Help a Pregnant Teenager

Help the teenager think through her options for the pregnancy.
Facilitate an appointment for prenatal care.
Help the teen's parents cope with the pregnancy.
Facilitate the teen's return to school.

Although the social aspects of the pregnancy are addressed, and although the patient is awaiting her first obstetric visit with a clinician who is knowledgeable about and accepting of teenage pregnancy, the primary care physician must be sure that the young mother has no disorders that might constitute a risk to herself or her unborn child and that she can appropriately care for herself during her pregnancy. In addition, the risk of violence to the young mother should be determined. Baseline height, weight, and blood pressure should be obtained. Screening for HIV, syphilis, chlamydia, gonorrhea, bacterial vaginosis, and trichomonas should be carried out, and treatment should be initiated as appropriate. The adolescent should be counseled about proper nutrition and rest; she should also be encouraged to avoid exposure to tobacco, alcohol, and drugs, including both drugs of abuse and excessive over-the-counter medications. Any medications taken for chronic illnesses should be reviewed for teratogenic potential. Prenatal vitamins should be prescribed.

OUTCOMES

Pregnancy outcomes in teens include not only the physical outcomes to mother and child, but also the social, educational, emotional, and financial outcomes for everyone affected by the pregnancy. An abundance of information exists regarding the infants' and the mothers' health, but the lives of the infant's father and grandparents will also be affected.

The physical outcomes of pregnancies in teenagers are generally good. However, very young mothers are at increased risk for toxemia of pregnancy, maternal anemia, infant death, prematurity, and low–birth-weight infants.[1,7,23-25] Many of these effects appear to be ameliorated by early prenatal care and appropriate maternal weight gain.[26] Although poor outcomes are influenced by the lower socioeconomic status of the adolescent mother, age itself may be a moderating factor as well.[24] Adolescent mothers generally do well in labor and recover easily from the effects of childbirth.

Other risk factors exist for the adolescent mother. One short-term concern is violence. Pregnant teens appear to be at increased risk for becoming victims of family or intimate partner violence.[9,27,28] Another short-term concern is depression; postpartum adolescents appear to be at higher risk than their adult counterparts, although this may be ameliorated by the presence of social supports from the teen's mother and from the father of the infant.[29] Women who become pregnant during adolescence also appear to have a higher than normal long-term risk for depression and other emotional difficulties.[14,30] In addition, although most women who become pregnant as teenagers eventually complete their high school education, they continue to remain educationally behind their age-matched peers; many of their peers elect participation in post–high school training, and teen mothers are less likely to do so.[7,31] Mothers who live with the father of their infant or who do not return to school to complete their education are most likely to have a repeat pregnancy soon after the first.[9,32] The second pregnancy is more likely to end in elective termination than the first. If it does not, then the mother frequently enters into prenatal care later than she did with her first infant, and the second infant is at greater risk for low birth weight. The second infant is also at greater risk for death by homicide[33] with the mother's current boyfriend (not the infant's father) being the most common perpetrator. Marriages formed in response to pregnancy generally fail with time, leaving the young mother with children and few resources for their support. These issues clearly produce significant financial implications for the young mother, her children, and society. Clinics specializing in the care of pregnant adolescents have been shown to improve the outcomes of pregnancy, reduce premature delivery, and reduce subsequent teenage pregnancies.[34]

For the child born to a teen mother, the long- and short-term effects of the mother's lower educational status, lower financial status, developmental immaturity, emotional stress, and adverse environment are significant. Adolescent mothers generally appear to lack knowledge of normal infant behavior, misinterpreting infant behavior as indicating that their child is more capable than is the case. They also appear to offer less infant stimulation than older mothers and to use harsher methods of discipline.[9,35] The higher than normal rate of postpartum depression in teen mothers may influence maternal-child bonding and that the developmentally immature mother finds difficulty with putting sufficient energy into guiding and teaching her infant.[9] Infants of teenage mothers also appear to have an increased risk of abuse and neglect, although this appears to be related to family stress, socioeconomic circumstances, and the presence of a new boyfriend in the mother's life. Children born to teen mothers appear to have a higher than normal incidence of early behavior problems and to be less secure in their maternal-child bond than their peers.[36-39] They also have higher rates of school failure, legal difficulties, and adolescent parenthood than their age-matched peers.[9,34-39] Some of the problems teen mothers encounter with parenthood can be addressed by providing social supports such as visiting nurses on a regular basis.[40] Box 155-3 lists ways to help a teen mother.

BOX 155-3 How a Primary Care Clinician Can Help the Teen Mother and Her Infant

Teach the teen mother the meaning of her child's developmental progression.

Teach positive parenting to the teen mother.

Discuss ways to improve the infant's safety.

Watch closely for postpartum depression.

Encourage contraceptive use.

Include the infant's grandmother and the father of the baby, if possible, in discussions of modern trends in child rearing (eg, newest immunizations, feeding, discipline).

Encourage the young mother to continue her education.

Refer the family to support services as needed.

Watch for early behavioral and school problems in the child.

PREVENTION

Physicians can facilitate pregnancy prevention by routinely providing education about risks and prevention methods to all pubertal patients. However, prevention appears to require more than education and readily available contraception. Facilitating parent-child discussions about sexuality and childbearing may also be an effective strategy. Community programs, particularly those that foster positive youth development, may be an effective adjunct. Effective programs need to identify specific youth at greatest risk—school dropouts, risk takers, delinquents—and concentrate their efforts on these individuals. Much has been learned about the prevention of adolescent pregnancy in the last 40 years, and, clearly, no sole program is appropriate for all communities or for all teens and their families. However, some characteristics are common to most successful programs.[41] These characteristics include:

1. A focus on specific behavioral goals
2. A program based on theoretical approaches
3. Delivering clear messages about sexual activity and contraceptive use
4. Providing basic information about risks associated with teen sexual activity
5. Addressing social pressure to have sex
6. Providing activities to practice communication and refusal skills
7. Incorporating multiple teaching methods
8. Tailoring the program to participants' age-level, culture, and level of sexual experiences
9. Providing an appropriate length of time to cover all the activities
10. Providing appropriate training for teachers or peer leaders who are involved in the program[41]

Programs to reduce repeat births (secondary prevention) need a different emphasis than the programs for primary prevention (preventing the first birth). Successful secondary prevention programs require effective personnel who maintain close, sustained relationships with teen mothers with an emphasis on school completion and family planning.[42] Regardless of the type of program developed for secondary prevention, clinicians should always remember that the pregnant teenager is an adolescent who happens to be pregnant, not a pregnant woman who happens to be an adolescent.

TOOLS FOR PRACTICE

Community Advocacy and Coordination

- *Facts at a Glance* (Web page), Child Trends (www.childtrends.org/_docdisp_page.cfm?LID=D6F165A5-00B3-4D76-ABACFD97F248817C).

Engaging Patient and Family

- *Deciding to Wait* (brochure), American Academy of Pediatrics (patiented.aap.org).
- *Making Healthy Decisions About Sex* (brochure), American Academy of Pediatrics (patiented.aap.org).

RELATED WEB SITES

- Centers for Disease Control and Prevention: Teen Pregnancy (www.cdc.gov/reproductivehealth/AdolescentReproHealth/).
- Guttmacher Institute (www.guttmacher.org/sections/pregnancy.php).
- National Center for Health Statistics (NCHS) (cdc.gov/nchs/).

AAP POLICY STATEMENTS

American Academy of Pediatrics, Committee on Adolescence and Committee on Early Childhood, Adoption, and Dependent Care. Care of adolescent parents and their children. *Pediatrics*. 2001;107(2):429-434. (aappolicy.aappublications.org/cgi/content/full/pediatrics;107/2/429).

American Academy of Pediatrics, Committee on Adolescence. Condom use by adolescents. *Pediatrics*. 2001;107(6):1463-1469. (aappolicy.aappublications.org/cgi/content/full/pediatrics;107/6/1463).

American Academy of Pediatrics, Committee on Adolescence. Counseling the adolescent about pregnancy options. *Pediatrics*. 1998;101(5):938-940. (aappolicy.aappublications.org/cgi/content/full/pediatrics;101/5/938).

Klein JD, American Academy of Pediatrics, Committee on Adolescence. Adolescent pregnancy: current trends and issues. *Pediatrics*. 2005;116(1):281-286. (aappolicy.aappublications.org/cgi/content/full/pediatrics;116/1/281).

SUGGESTED RESOURCES

Centers for Disease Control and Prevention, National Center for Health Statistics. Available at: www.cdc.gov/nchs.

East PL, Felice ME. *Adolescent Pregnancy and Parenting: Findings From a Racially Diverse Sample*. Mahwah, NJ: Lawrence Erlbaum Associates; 1996.

English A, Kenney KE. *State Minor Consent Statutes: A Summary*. Prepared by the National Center for Youth Law for the Center for Continuing Education in Adolescent Health. Cincinnati, OH: The Center, Division of Adolescent Medicine, Children's Hospital Medical Center; 2003.

Guttmacher Institute. Available at: www.guttmacher.org.

REFERENCES

1. Ventura SJ, Mathews TJ, Hamilton BE. Births to teenagers in the United States, 1940-2000. *Natl Vital Stat Rep*. 2001;49(10):1-23.
2. Hamilton BE, Ventura SJ, Martin JA, et al. Preliminary births for 2004. Health E-stats. US Department of Health and Human Services, Centers for Disease Control and Prevention, National Center for Health Statistics. October 28, 2005. Available at: www.cdc.gov/nchs/products/pubs/pubd/hestats/prelim_births/prelim_births04.htm Accessed June 26, 2007.
3. Ventura SJ, Abma JC, Mosher WD, et al. Estimated pregnancy rates for the United States, 1990-2000: an update. *Natl Vital Stat Rep*. 2004:52(23):1-9.
4. Child Trends. Facts at a Glance 2005. Publication No. 2005-02. Available at: www.childtrends.org/files/facts_2005.pdf. Accessed June 26, 2007.
5. Santelli JS, Abma J, Ventura S, et al. Can changes in sexual behaviors among high school students explain the decline in teen pregnancy rates in the 1990s? *J Adolesc Health*. 2004;35(2):80-90.
6. Sonenstein FL. What teenagers are doing right: changes in sexual behavior over the past decade. *J Adolesc Health*. 2004;35(2):77-78.
7. American Academy of Pediatrics, Committee on Adolescence. Adolescent pregnancy—current trends and issues: 1998. *Pediatrics*. 1999;103(2):516-520. Available at aappolicy.aappublications.org/cgi/content/full/pediatrics;103/2/516. Accessed June 26, 2007.
8. Child Trends. Facts at a Glance, 2006. Publication No. 2006-03. Available at: www.childtrends.org/files/faag2006.pdf. Accessed June 25, 2007.
9. American Academy of Pediatrics, Committee on Adolescence and Committee on Early Childhood and Adoption, and Dependent Care. Care of adolescent parents and their children. *Pediatrics*. 2001;107(2):429-434.
10. Shearer DL, Mulvihill BA, Klerman LV, et al. Association of early childbearing and low cognitive ability. *Perspect Sex Reprod Health*. 2002;34(5):236-243.
11. Stevens-Simon C, Kelly L, Singer D, et al. Why pregnant adolescents say they did not use contraceptives prior to conception. *J Adolesc Health*. 1996;19(1):48-53.
12. Unger JB, Molina GB, Teran L. Perceived consequences of teenage childbearing among adolescent girls in an urban sample. *J Adolesc Health*. 2000;26(3):205-212.
13. Rosengard C, Phipps MG, Adler NE, et al. Adolescent pregnancy intentions and pregnancy outcomes: a longitudinal examination. *J Adolesc Health*. 2004;35(6):453-461.
14. Hillis SD, Anda RF, Dube SR, et al. The association between adverse childhood experiences and adolescent pregnancy, long-term psychosocial consequences, and fetal death. *Pediatrics*. 2004;113(2):320-327.
15. Elfenbein DS, Felice ME. Adolescent pregnancy. *Pediatr Clin North Am*. 2003;50(4):781-800.
16. Taylor D, Chavez G, Chabra A, et al. Risk factors for adult paternity in births to adolescents. *Obstet Gynecol*. 1997;89(2):199-205.
17. Lindberg LD, Sonenstein FL, Ku L, et al. Age differences between minors who give birth and their adult partners. *Fam Plann Perspect*. 1997;29(2):61-66.
18. Taylor DJ, Chavez GF, Adams EJ, et al. Demographic characteristics in adult paternity for first births to adolescents under 15 years of age. *J Adolesc Health*. 1999;24(4):251-258.
19. Spingarn RW, DuRant RH. Male adolescents involved in pregnancy: associated health risk and problem behaviors. *Pediatrics*. 1996;98(2 pt 1):262-268.

20. Fagot BI, Pears KC, Capaldi DM, et al. Becoming an adolescent father: precursors and parenting. *Dev Psychol.* 1998;34(6);1209-1219.
21. Guagliardo MF, Huang Z, D'Angelo LJ. Fathering pregnancies: marking health-risk behaviors in urban adolescents. *J Adolesc Health.* 1999;24(1):10-15.
22. Emans SJ, Laufer MR, Goldstein DP. *Pediatric and Adolescent Gynecology.* 5th ed. Philadelphia, PA: Lippincott Williams & Wilkins; 2005.
23. DuPlessis HM, Bell R, Richards T. Adolescent pregnancy: understanding the impact of age and race on outcomes. *J Adolesc Health.* 1997;20(3):187-197.
24. Fraser AM, Brockert JE, Ward RH. Association of young maternal age with adverse reproductive outcomes. *N Engl J Med.* 1995;332(7):1113-1117.
25. Menacker F, Martin JA, MacDorman MR, et al. Births to 10-14 year old mothers, 1990-2002: trends and health outcomes. *Natl Vital Stat Rep.* 2004;53(7):1-17.
26. Chang SC, O'Brien KO, Nathanson MS, et al. Characteristics and risk factors for adverse birth outcomes in pregnant black adolescents. *J Pediatr.* 2003;143(2): 250-257.
27. Covington DL, Justason BJ, Wright LN. Severity, manifestations, and consequences of violence among pregnant adolescents. *J Adolesc Health.* 2001;28(1):55-61.
28. Wiemann CM, Agurcia CA, Berenson AB, et al. Pregnant adolescents: experiences and behaviors associated with physical assault by an intimate partner. *Matern Child Health J.* 2000;4(2):93-101.
29. Barnet B, Joffe A, Duggan AK, et al. Depressive symptoms, stress, and social support in pregnant and postpartum adolescents. *Arch Pediatr Adolesc Med.* 1996;150(1): 64-69.
30. Kalil A, Kunz J. Teenage childbearing, marital status, and depressive symptoms in later life. *Child Dev.* 2002;73(6): 1748-1760.
31. Hofferth SL, Reid L, Mott FL. The effects of early childbearing on schooling over time. *Fam Plann Perspect.* 2001; 33(6):259-267.
32. East PL, Felice ME. *Adolescent Pregnancy and Parenting: Findings From a Racially Diverse Sample.* Mahwah, NJ: Lawrence Erlbaum Associates; 1996.
33. Overpeck MD, Brenner RA, Trumble AC, et al. Risk factors for infant homicide in the United States. *N Engl J Med.* 1998;339(17):1211-1216.
34. Klerman LV, Horwitz SM. Reducing the adverse consequences of adolescent pregnancy and parenting: the role of service programs. *Adolesc Med.* 1992;3(2):299-316.
35. Parks PL, Arndt EK. Differences between adolescent and adult mothers of infants. *J Adolesc Health Care.* 1990;11(3): 248-253.
36. Leadbeater BJ, Bishop SJ, Raver CC. Quality of mother-toddler interactions, maternal depressive symptoms, and behavior problems in preschoolers of adolescent mothers. *Dev Psychol.* 1996;32(2):280-288.
37. Hubbs-Tait L, Hughes KP, Culp AM, et al. Children of adolescent mothers: attachment representation, maternal depression, and later behavior problems. *Am J Orthopsychiatry.* 1996;66(3):416-426.
38. Spieker SJ, Larson NC, Lewis SM, et al. Developmental trajectories of disruptive behavior problems in preschool children of adolescent mothers. *Child Dev.* 1999;70(2): 443-458.
39. Andreozzi L, Flanagan P, Seifer R, et al. Attachment classifications among 18-month-old children of adolescent mothers. *Arch Pediatr Adolesc Med.* 2002;156(1): 20-26.
40. Eckenrode J, Zielinski D, Smith E, et al. Child maltreatment and the early onset of problem behaviors: can a program of nurse home visitation break the link? *Dev Psychopathol.* 2001;13(4):873-890.
41. Solomon J, Card JJ. *Making the List: Understanding, Selecting, and Replicating Effective Teen Pregnancy Prevention Programs.* Washington, DC: The National Campaign to Prevent Teen Pregnancy; 2004.
42. Klerman LV. *Another Chance.* Washington, DC: The National Campaign to Prevent Teen Pregnancy; 2004.

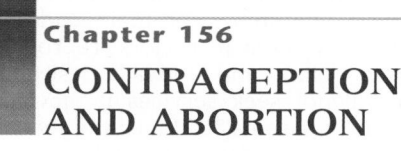

Chapter 156

CONTRACEPTION AND ABORTION

Eric A. Schaff, MD

In 2002 the number of 15- to 19-year-old female adolescents in the United States was approximately 10 million, of which approximately 750,000 became pregnant, one half resulted in births, one third had abortions, and the remaining had failed pregnancies.[1] Although the rate of unintended pregnancies in the United States continues to decline slowly, it is higher than most developed countries. An estimated one third of teens will experience a pregnancy by age 20.[2] The *Healthy People 2010 Guidelines* established by the US Department of Health and Human Services include the goal of reducing adolescent pregnancies by targeting 100% of those who are at risk to use contraception.[3]

An unintended pregnancy has significant consequences socially, physically, and financially for an unprepared teen, her family, and the community. The American Academy of Pediatrics, American College of Obstetrics and Gynecology, and the American Medical Association's *Guidelines for Adolescent Preventive Services* have guidelines[4] for teens that include the routine screening for sexual activity, support for sexual abstinence, the need for contraception, and the importance of counseling about the risks of unintended pregnancy and sexually transmitted infections (STIs). The National Campaign to Prevent Teenage Pregnancy in "No Easy Answers: Research Findings on Programs to Reduce Teen Pregnancy"[5] found that no single strategy exists to reduce teen pregnancy rates significantly. Approaches need to be targeted to both abstinent and sexually active youth.

Pediatricians are particularly attuned to preventive public health measures that decrease morbidity and decrease costs.[6] They need to play an important role in preventing unintended pregnancies and ensuring access to contraceptive methods and emergency contraception for sexually active teens. Teenagers who are sexually abstinent need encouragement and reassurance, emphasizing that being abstinent is normal, common, and prevents both pregnancy and STIs.[7] For sexually active youth, using contraception and reducing the number of sexual contacts should be encouraged.

The rights of teens to receive services without parental consent to different types of health care vary widely among states. These situations include emergency medical care, specific state-mandated health issues, the emancipated minor, and the mature minor. To be emancipated, an adolescent must generally be of a state-defined minimal age (often 16), live apart from her parents, and be economically self-sufficient. In addition, emancipation includes teens who are married, parenting, or serving in the military. State-mandated situations include contraceptive care, abortion services, and treatment for STIs.

The US Supreme Court has extended the constitutional right to privacy to include the right of minors to obtain contraception without parental consent. Although parental involvement in minors' reproductive decisions may be helpful and is ideally desirable, some adolescents will not seek services if they are required to inform their parents.[8,9] Under the federal Health Insurance Portability and Accountability Act, health care providers must follow state guidelines for confidentiality and may require the consent of the adolescent before releasing information to anyone, including her parents.[10]

Significant advances have been made in early abortion services. Detection of early pregnancy has been simplified by inexpensive home and office pregnancy tests that are positive 4 weeks after the last menstrual period. Earlier and more accurate pregnancy dating is now possible through vaginal probe sonography. Earlier and safer abortion procedures are now available with the medical abortion pill, mifepristone, and suction abortion.

This chapter provides information basic to the pediatrician's task of providing reproductive health care to teenagers.

CONTRACEPTION

Two methods are used to describe the effectiveness of contraception to prevent pregnancy: (1) typical use rate and (2) perfect use rate. Typical use rate refers to the effectiveness of a method when used by the average woman (ie, not using the method correctly or every time). Perfect use rate refers to the ability of the method to prevent pregnancy when the method is used perfectly (ie, according to manufacturer's directions and every time required).

In general, all contraceptive methods are highly effective when used correctly, and their benefits outweigh their health risks. When considering a contraceptive method, the short- and long-term medical risks and financial costs should also be compared with the risks and costs associated with not using the method, that is, an unintended pregnancy.

Hormonal Methods

Hormonal methods involve using combined synthetic estrogen and progestin or progestin-only agents. While progesterones are sufficient and necessary for contraception, estrogens help to regulate the menstrual cycle. As a group, these methods have many features in common that include their mechanism of action, effectiveness, advantages, disadvantages, and side effects. To a varying degree, these methods prevent pregnancy by 3 main mechanisms: (1) suppressing luteinizing and follicle-stimulating hormones, thereby inhibiting ovulation; (2) thickening cervical mucus, making it less penetrable by sperm; and (3) altering the endometrium, making it less receptive to implantation of a fertilized ovum.[11] Inhibiting ovulation is the primary mechanism of action of hormonal methods, but ovulation can occur occasionally. When used correctly, these methods are 99% effective in preventing pregnancy, and ovulation returns quickly when stopped (except for intramuscular progesterone that often delays ovulation beyond 3 months). When hormonal methods are started within 5 days of the onset of a normal menses, ovulation is usually suppressed, and pregnancy is prevented.

While using combined hormonal contraception, menses are usually more regular, shorter in duration, sometimes absent, and avoided altogether for convenience by delaying the hormonal-free time period. These methods are associated with less acne, less dysmenorrhea, less benign breast disease, less pelvic inflammatory disease (because of the thickened cervical mucus and the blocking of ascending infection), and less ovarian and endometrial cancer. Women who use oral contraceptive pills (OCPs) for as little as 6 to 12 months experienced a 40% reduction in the risk of ovarian cancer, and long-term OCP users (>10 years) experienced an 80% reduction.[12] No evidence has been found that OCPs increase mortality from breast cancer, even with prolonged use.[13]

The progestin-only methods (progestin-only oral contraceptives, the 3-month injectable depomedroxyprogesterone acetate, and the 3-year subdermal rod implant) are not associated with venous thromboembolic events. Therefore these methods are indicated for women with a contraindication to estrogen use or preferred because of their inherent properties.

Oral Contraceptives

OCPs are one of the most popular methods of birth control used by young women. Unfortunately, compliance continues to be a concern; over one half of teens will stop taking the pill during the first year of use.[14]

All low-dose combination pills consist of only one estrogen ethinyl estradiol, with the dose ranging from 20 to 35 mcg/day, and one of many different synthetic progestins derived from estranes, gonanes, or unclassified group. Estranes were marketed first and consist of norethindrone or compounds that convert to norethindrone. Gonanes consist of norgestrel, levonorgestrel, norgestimate, and desogestrel. The latter 2 agents are newer and have the advantage of being potent progestins but producing fewer androgenic side effects. Norgestimate and desogestrel also increase high-density lipoprotein, which is protective against atherosclerosis, and have a slightly longer half-life that makes vaginal spotting and pregnancy less likely if a woman forgets to take her daily pill. An unclassified progestin is drospirenone derived from spironolactone and may possess antimineralocorticoid with fewer premenstrual bloating symptoms and mild antiandrogenic activity. No clinical difference in effectiveness has been found in pregnancy prevention among the different OCPs.

The disadvantages of OCPs include (1) need for daily compliance, (2) theoretical decreased effectiveness caused by some antibiotics (eg, rifampin, doxycycline) and antiseizure medications (eg, phenobarbital and phenytoin), and (3) increased risk of rare venous thromboembolic disease.

The risk of venous thromboembolism for healthy teenagers not using hormonal contraception is very low, approximately 3 per 100,000 women. The risk increases to 7 to 10 per 100,000 when using combined oral contraceptives that is proportional to the amount of estrogen. Of note, the dose of synthetic estrogens have decreased significantly since the original pill formulations. The risk should be compared with the greater risk of thromboembolism in pregnancy. Some confusion exists in attempting to quantify the exact risk attributed to different birth control pills because these adverse events are rare and the studies are not randomized but observational after the products have been marketed. Newest methods may seem to have higher risks than older methods because of a known bias to prescribe the newest and lowest dose oral contraceptives to women having complications on older OCPs and women at higher risk for medical complications.[15]

PRESCRIBING ORAL CONTRACEPTIVES

Relevant History. Before prescribing OCPs, the clinician should be certain that no contraindications to their use exist, which are very few. In general, healthy teens are excellent candidates for hormonal contraceptives. A summary of the recommendations for prescribing combined hormonal contraception is noted in Table 156-1 by the World Health Organization.[16,17]

Physical Examination. Hormonal contraception can safely be provided based on complete medical history and blood pressure measurement. A physical examination that included breast and pelvic examinations were commonly accepted practices before prescribing hormonal contraception. These examinations may be feared and avoided by teens and therefore may reduce access to highly effective contraceptive methods and increase a teen's overall health risks. In general, expert medical opinion has shifted away from requiring a general examination that includes breast and pelvic examinations before initiating hormonal contraception.[18] Of note, breast cancer is rare in women younger than 30 years and occurs in less than 4 per 100,000 annually in the United States.[19] The US Preventive Services Task Force recommends breast cancer screening with mammography, with or without clinical breast examination, starting at age 40.[20]

Unrelated to hormonal contraception, routine screening at regular health visits for all sexually active teens is recommended for chlamydia and for gonorrhea if the community prevalence is high.[21] A significant advance, especially for pediatric practices that are not prepared for pelvic examinations or male penile cultures, is the screening for chlamydia and gonorrhea by urine testing.[22]

Cervical cancer screening with either Papanicolaou tests or liquid cytologic assessment should also not be directly tied to hormonal contraceptive provision. Current cervical screening guidelines recommend starting after 3 years of sexual activity or, if not sexually active, by age 21.[23]

Management. To improve compliance with contraception, pediatricians need to ensure confidentiality.[24] They must also assess their patient's understanding of the effectiveness, benefits, and risks of the chosen method; their concerns about becoming pregnant; and their motivation to use the method selected. Counseling and handouts are key to supporting teens dealing with or anticipating minor side effects, such as breakthrough vaginal bleeding, nausea, headaches, bloating, mood changes, and irritability, all of which are likely to resolve spontaneously after several menstrual cycles. Many of these side effects may be unrelated to contraception but rather the usual stresses in a teen's life. Weight gain caused by an increase in

Table 156-1 World Health Organization's Contraindications and Precautions for Prescribing Hormonal Contraception

NO CONTRAINDICATIONS	CAUTION ADVISED	CONTRAINDICATIONS
Mild headaches	Hyperlipidemia	Pregnancy
Benign breast disease	Less than 21 days postpartum	Hypertension
Obesity	Breastfeeding from 6 weeks to 6 months postpartum using medications that affect liver enzymes (eg, rifampin, griseofulvin, phenytoin, carbamazepine, barbiturates, primidone)	Certain heart and liver diseases
Pelvic inflammatory disease	Undergoing major surgery with prolonged immobilization	Diabetes mellitus when either long-standing or with end-organ involvement
Thyroid disorders	Unexplained vaginal bleeding	History of thromboembolic disease or stroke
Epilepsy		Migraine headaches with focal, neurologic symptoms
Iron deficiency anemia		Less than 6 weeks postpartum and breastfeeding
Use of antibiotics		
Dysmenorrheal		
Endometriosis		
HIV		
Viral hepatitis carrier		
Irregular menstrual bleeding		
History of ectopic pregnancy		
History of gestational diabetes		
Family history of breast cancer		
Gestational trophoblastic disease (benign or malignant)		
Benign ovarian tumors		

appetite can be countered by good eating habits. Persistent mood changes or depression will require stopping the hormonal method for further evaluation. Although effective at preventing pregnancy, these methods do not protect against STIs, and therefore the use of condoms must always be encouraged.

Considerable flexibility exists regarding which brand of OCPs to prescribe. Most commonly, a 28-day-cycle pack (21 days of active hormones and 7 days of placebo) is used. Despite claims by manufacturers, clinical differences among brands of low-dose pills are minimal regardless of whether the hormones are fixed (monophasic) or varied (triphasic) throughout the month. Clinicians can choose any one of the following strategies in prescribing oral contraceptives: (1) an inexpensive generic brand, (2) a low-estrogen preparation containing 20 mcg of ethinyl estradiol, (3) a weak progestin such as norethindrone, or (4) a new-generation progestin that has weak androgenic effects (norgestimate or drospirenone). OCPs containing desogestrel probably carry a small increased risk (1.5-2.7 times) for venous thromboembolism.[25]

To improve compliance, the physician should prescribe a sufficient number of packs to prevent running out of pills. The first few months should serve to identify any health concerns or problems the teen may identify in taking the pills. After this initial prescription, 12-month supplies should be prescribed to increase compliance.

OCPs can be started (1) on day 5 of the cycle, (2) on the Sunday after the menstrual bleeding starts (Sunday start), or (3) on the quick-start method. The quick start allows hormonal methods to be started on any day, if the clinician is reasonably certain that the teenager is not pregnant; for example, she has not had sex since her last normal menses or has been using another birth control method correctly and every time. For the quick start, if more than 5 days have elapsed since the menses started, then the teenager will need to abstain from sex or use additional contraceptive protection such as condoms for the next 7 days. These 3 options ensure that the teen is not pregnant and should suppress ovulation that first cycle except for the quick-start method.

The OCP should be taken at the same time each day. Taking OCPs before bedtime allows for the peak concentration of the hormones to occur during sleep, thereby masking some symptoms such as nausea. If one pill is forgotten (particularly during the first 7 days that are needed to suppress ovulation), then it should be taken as soon as it is remembered. If 2 pills are missed, then 2 pills should be taken each day for 2 days, and a barrier birth control method should be used for the next week. If more than 2 pills are missed, then another barrier contraceptive method should be used, and another pill pack should be started on the first Sunday after the next menses begins. (If pregnancy is likely from unprotected intercourse, then emergency contraception should be considered.) Withdrawal bleeding usually occurs 2 or 3 days after the last OCP is taken.

If mild side effects do not resolve after several cycles from one OCP, then the brand can be changed to another containing a different progestin. If menstruation does not occur, the pills should be continued and a pregnancy test obtained for reassurance and to detect the rare pregnancy.

The most recent products are OCPs that contain ethinyl estradiol and levonorgestrel that provide 84 days of active pills, followed by either placebo pills (Seasonale) or pills with small dose of estrogen (Seasonique), which reduce the number of menses from 13 to only 4 per year. A low-dose pill is also available that is taken for 365 days without stopping, having 0.09 mg of levonorgestrel and ethinyl estradiol 20 mcg (Lybrel). These products with fewer or no menses may be of benefit for teens who prefer to have fewer menses or who have menorrhagia, menstrual migraine, and endometriosis. Break-through bleeding may be encountered.

Other Hormonal Methods of Contraception

Newer hormonal methods that change the route of administration of hormones do not require daily use, have improved compliance, and have higher typical effectiveness rates. These methods include the weekly transdermal patch[26] and the monthly vaginal contraceptive ring.

The transdermal patch (Ortho Evra Patch) has the advantage of once-weekly application. This product contains norelgestromin, the active metabolite of norgestimate, and ethinyl estradiol. The patch is worn weekly for 3 consecutive weeks; the 4th week is patch free, allowing for withdrawal bleeding. The patch may be applied to the abdomen, buttocks, upper outer arm, or upper torso (excluding breasts). The patch's pregnancy failure rate is increased for women who weigh more than 200 pounds.

The vaginal ring (NuvaRing) is a combination of ethinyl estradiol (15 mcg/day) and etonogestrel (120 mcg/day). The ring consists of a flexible plastic, ethylene vinyl acetate, and is available in 1 size (2 inches in diameter and ⅛-inch thick). Because the ring is *1 size fits all,* it requires no specific placement techniques. The ring should be placed in the vagina within the first 5 days of the menstrual cycle and remain in place for 3 consecutive weeks. It is then removed and discarded. A new ring is inserted after 7 days, allowing for withdrawal bleeding. If the user and her partner prefer, the ring may be removed to allow for intercourse as long as it is replaced within 2 to 3 hours. However, if the ring is left out for more than 3 hours, then she can reinsert the ring but either abstain from sex or use a condom for the next 7 days.

PROGESTERONE-ONLY INJECTION. A highly effective and popular method is the 3-month injectable progestin, depo-medroxyprogesterone acetate (DMPA; Depo-Provera). As many as 10% to 15% of teens report using DMPA. Each 150-mg injection provides 12 weeks of effective contraceptive protection plus an additional 1-week grace period (for a total of 13 weeks). It requires vigorous shaking to suspend all the particles and is given deep intramuscularly in either the deltoid or upper outer quadrant of the gluteal muscle. The site should not be massaged because the rate of absorption and metabolism may be increased and thereby decrease effectiveness. A generic product is available that reduces the cost.

A new route of medroxyprogesterone acetate is subcutaneous administration, the same as insulin injections. This 104-mg dose can be given at home if the teen or a support person can be taught how to give the injection, thereby avoiding an office visit.

The advantages of the progesterone-only injection include (1) long-acting protection, (2) avoidance of estrogen and venous thromboembolic disease, (3) lack of interference with breastfeeding, (4) possible reduction in both the incidence of seizures and the painful hemolytic crisis of teens with sickle cell disease, (5) continued contraceptive effectiveness when using antibiotics or antiseizure medicines, and (6) a thinning of the endometrium, causing amenorrhea in up to 50% of women after the first year and an even higher percentage of women thereafter. The disadvantages of this injection include (1) the need for repeated injections every 3 months, (2) a hypoestrogen state that causes a reversible decrease in bone density though significantly less than pregnancy, and (4) delay in clearance of DMPA for as long as 12 months, resulting in reduced fertility after discontinuation.

Managing side effects is important in supporting continued use of injectable progesterone. Irregular vaginal bleeding can be managed by offering a 28-day cycle of OCPs or conjugated estrogens, such as Premarin™.

THREE-YEAR SUBDERMAL ROD IMPLANT. In 2006 a subdermal implantable hormonal contraceptive became available (Implanon™).[27] It is highly effective at providing low-dose and continuous contraception up to 3 years. It involves only the progesterone etonogestrel with ethylene vinyl acetate. (Both components are also used with the vaginal ring.) Etonogestrel is the active metabolite of desogestrel, a progestin in oral contraceptives. With training, insertion and removal are easy skills to learn.

The advantages of the implantable rod include the (1) long-acting protection, (2) avoidance of estrogen and venous thromboembolic disease, (3) the low dose of progestin allowing for continuous endogenous estrogen production thereby not affecting bone demineralization, and (4) quick reversibility. The major disadvantages of this method include the unpredictability of menstrual patterns, the costs, and the need for a minor procedure.

EMERGENCY CONTRACEPTION. Emergency contraception pills (ECPs) prevent pregnancy after unprotected intercourse[28] and may also be referred to as postcoital or morning-after pills. They consist of a high dose of the oral progestin levonorgestrel (Plan B).

ECPs are indicated when other methods fail, when no contraception is used, or when rape occurs. ECPs are available over the counter for women 18 and over. One strategy to increase access to ECPs for younger teens is to give them a prescription in anticipation of an unprotected intercourse.[29]

ECPs reduce the risk of pregnancy by 88%.[30] For example, if 100 women have unprotected intercourse in the second or third week of their cycle, 8 will become pregnant without ECPs, but one will become pregnant using progestin-only ECPs, an 88% reduction. If a current pregnancy is possible, then a pregnancy test should be performed before the ECPs are taken, though taking ECPs have not been known to harm an established pregnancy. A nationwide hotline (800-NOT-2-LATE) and Web site (opr.princeton.edu/ec/) have been established to increase public awareness of emergency contraception.

Two tablets of PlanB can be taken as soon as possible after unprotected intercourse up to 5 days.[31] Nausea and rarely vomiting can occur and may require antinausea treatment. Breast tenderness, irregular bleeding, fluid retention, and headaches occasionally occur. Hormonal contraceptives can be started on the first Sunday after the onset of the next menstrual period or the same day as the ECPs (quick-start method) with 7 days of condom use. If the next menses is delayed, then the teen should be instructed to return for a pregnancy test.

Barrier Methods

Condoms

Throughout the world, condom use has increased significantly from social marketing campaigns attempting to address the HIV epidemic.[32] Latex condoms work by containing the ejaculate. Condoms are effective in pregnancy prevention and in reducing the spread of all STIs, including HIV. Making condoms readily available increases their use.[33,34] Even if teens prefer a hormonal birth control as their primary method for preventing pregnancy, they should be encouraged to use condoms if they are at risk for STIs.

Condoms are (1) inexpensive, (2) available over the counter, (3) a means to involve the male in sharing responsibility for contraception, (4) lubricated for comfort, (5) associated with minimal side effects, and (6) simple to use.[35] The disadvantages of condoms are the diminished genital sensation noted by some individuals and the lack of 100% protection against STIs.

Lubricated latex condoms offer the best protection. Condoms should be placed on the erect penis before any sex. To prevent condom breakage, condoms should (a) not be stored in warm places (eg, a wallet) for long periods, (b) not be lubricated with oil-based lubricants such as Vaseline, and (c) not be reused. An alternative, the polyurethane condom is stronger and thinner than latex condoms, is odorless, and can be used with oil-based lubricants.

To prevent accidental spillage, teens should be instructed that the condom should be removed shortly after ejaculation while holding the rim of the condom on the base of the penis. If spillage occurs or a condom breaks, then the penis and vagina should be washed with soap and water and a spermicide, as well as ECPs, should be used.

Diaphragm, Female Condom, and Cervical Cap

The diaphragm is a thin, rubber, 6.5- to 8-cm dome that is inserted into the vagina. It covers the cervix and blocks sperm from entering. It must be used with a spermicidal contraceptive jelly, the active ingredient of which is nonoxynol-9. When used correctly and consistently, the diaphragm's effectiveness can be quite high, although the typical use failure rate ranges from 6% to 16%. It also offers some protection from STIs and has minimal side effects. A diaphragm is a reasonable choice for a motivated teen who has contraindications or wants to avoid taking contraceptive hormones. The disadvantages of the diaphragm include (1) the skill needed for placement, (2) the need to leave it in place 6 hours after intercourse, (3) the need for a second application of spermicidal jelly if intercourse is repeated after 6 hours, and (4) the slight increase in vaginitis and urinary tract infections. Disadvantages for the health care provider include keeping a set of diaphragm rings for sizing, as well as learning and maintaining the skill to fit one when the requests are likely to be few.

The female condom is readily available in pharmacies without a prescription but is not widely used. It is made from polyurethane with 2 flexible polyurethane rings. One ring is placed inside the vagina to cover the cervix, similar to a diaphragm; the 2nd open ring remains on the outside of the perineum to protect against STIs. The female condom should not be used concomitantly with latex condoms, nor should it be reused.

Spermicidals: Vaginal Foam, Vaginal Sponge, and Vaginal Suppository

Vaginal foam, sponges, and suppositories contain nonoxynol-9, which has in vitro and in vivo protective properties against some STIs. These methods are relatively simple, effective, and inexpensive and can be obtained without a prescription. The spermicidals are important complementary methods (1) when used with condoms, (2) when intercourse is infrequent and hormonal methods are not used, and (3) when used as a backup for other birth control methods.

The vaginal sponge, which is moistened with water before use, can be inserted several hours before intercourse and remains effective for 24 hours. Suppositories must be in the vagina at least 10 to 15 minutes before intercourse to allow them to dissolve.

Natural Family Planning

Natural family planning methods identify the most fertile time during the menstrual cycle in order to avoid sexual intercourse. Methods include (1) charting of menstrual cycles on the calendar, (2) recording basal body temperatures to document the rise of at least 0.4°C after ovulation, and (3) monitoring cervical mucus to detect when ovulation occurs. Advantages include (1) the lack of side effects, (2) acceptance by religious groups opposed to hormonal and barrier methods, (3) knowledge gained about reproductive physiology, and (4) its practicality when barriers exist to accessing other methods. Disadvantages for teenagers include their irregular menstrual cycles, which make predicting ovulation difficult, the high degree of motivation required for effective use, and a 20% annual typical failure (pregnancy) rate.

Intrauterine Device

Advances in the intrauterine device (IUD) (with copper wire [Paragard] or containing the progestin levonorgestrel [Mirena]) have made both the typical and perfect use approximately 99% in preventing pregnancy. The mechanism of action is not clear but involves irritation of the endometrium, making it unsuitable for implantation of a fertilized egg, copper's effects on enzymes that inhibit sperm migration, and additional atrophic endometrial changes from the progestin-containing method that also reduces menstrual bleeding. The IUD is indicated for women interested in highly effective, nonhormonal, long-term, and reversible contraception. Once in place, the IUD requires no effort for continued effectiveness and has no additional costs.

The IUD has traditionally not been offered to teens because of their increased risk for STIs. Women with IUDs and STIs have a higher incidence of pelvic inflammatory disease that can lead to infertility. Resurgence in interest in this method has occurred for a subset of teenagers at low risk for STIs. Compared with other countries, the prevalence of IUD use in the United States is low mainly because of its high initial costs.

ABORTION

Over a third of pregnant teens in the United States choose abortion. The earlier the abortion is performed, the safer it is. Unfortunately, teens are more likely than older women to delay an abortion. The reasons cited most often by teens for choosing an abortion are how having a baby will negatively affect their lives, financial concerns, and feeling that they are not mature enough to have a child.

Most young teenagers involve their parents in these decisions. Some states require parental consent or notification for a minor to obtain an abortion. In these states, a minor who does not want to involve her parents must be able to obtain a judicial or administrative bypass.

Suction Curettage

Surgical abortion is greater than 99% effective and has an excellent safety record of approximately one death per million early first-trimester procedures. Unfortunately, mortality rates remain high in developing countries where a need exists for safe, legal, and accessible abortion services.

Complications of abortion can include excessive bleeding, infection, perforation of the uterus, and adverse anesthetic events.

Medical Abortion

Mifepristone (Mifeprex, formerly known as RU 486, the *French abortion pill*), available in over 2 dozen countries, was approved in the United States in 2000. Mifepristone blocks the action of progesterone, detaches the pregnancy from the endometrium, and sensitizes the uterus to the uterotonic effects of synthetic prostaglandins. The second required medication, misoprostol, is a synthetic prostaglandin given 2 days later and causes the uterus to contract and a pregnancy to be expelled. The prescribing clinician must be able to confirm the gestational age is no greater than 7 weeks gestation, to make sure it is not an ectopic pregnancy, and to perform or refer for a surgical abortion if needed. Because of the high cost of mifepristone, evidence-based regimens in the United States have been developed that use a lower dose of mifepristone, require a higher dose of misoprostol taken either buccally or vaginally, and are effective up to 8 or 9 weeks pregnant, depending on the regimen. Approximately 5% of women will need an aspiration curettage for a continuing pregnancy or persistent or heavy bleeding.

The major advantages of a medical abortion include (1) its early use in pregnancy; (2) avoidance of a surgical procedure; and (3) perception of being more natural, less invasive, and private. Disadvantages of medical abortion include (1) the side effects from misoprostol of nausea, vomiting, and diarrhea; (2) cramping; (3) unexpected heavy or persistent bleeding requiring suction curettage in up to 4% of women; (4) continuing pregnancies requiring suction curettage in 1% of women; and (5) serious infections from clostridium species that have a mortality rate of approximately 1 per 100,000 medical abortions, similar to miscarriage.

SUMMARY

Sexually abstinent teens need support and reassurance. Sexually active teens are at high risk for an unintended pregnancy and need contraception information and services. Current contraceptive methods are highly effective and safe. Hormonal methods have important noncontraceptive benefits such as regulated menses and reduced risks of endometrial and ovarian cancer. Easy access to emergency contraception is an important back-up method to reduce unintended pregnancies and can be prescribed in advance at pediatric visits. Early abortion should be readily available with minimal obstacles because of its safety over later abortions. Mifepristone is an important alternative to suction abortion for teens fearful of a surgical abortion. Pediatricians continue to play an important role in supporting the reproductive health care needs of their teen patients.

TOOLS FOR PRACTICE

Community Advocacy and Coordination

- *Condom Effectiveness—Fact Sheet for Public Health Personnel: Male Latex Condoms and Sexually Transmitted Diseases*, Centers for Disease Control and Prevention (www.cdc.gov/condomeffectiveness/latex.htm).
- *Facts at a Glance* (Web page), Child Trends (www.childtrends.org/_docdisp_page.cfm?LID=D6F165A5-00B3-4D76-ABACFD97F248817C).

Engaging Patient and Family

- *Cervical Cancer—Basic facts on screening and the pap test* (fact sheet), Centers for Disease Control and Prevention (www.cdc.gov/cancer/cervical/pdf/cc_basic.pdf).
- *Deciding to Wait* (brochure), American Academy of Pediatrics (patiented.aap.org).
- *Emergency Contraception* (fact sheet), American Academy of Pediatrics (www.aap.or/family/ecparentpage.pdf).
- *Making Healthy Decisions About Sex* (brochure), American Academy of Pediatrics (patiented.aap.org).
- *National Emergency Contraception Hotline* (hotline) (800-NOT-2-LATE).
- *The Pelvic Exam* (brochure), American Academy of Pediatrics (patiented.aap.org).

Medical Decision Support

- *Guidelines for Adolescent Preventive Services (GAPS)*, American Medical Association, Elster A, and Kuznets N (www.ama-assn.org/ama/pub/category/1980.html).

RELATED WEB SITES

- Boston Children's Hospital: Teen Pregnancy Center for Young Women's Health (www.youngwomenshealth.org/).
- Centers for Disease Control and Prevention: Teen Pregnancy (www.cdc.gov/reproductivehealth/AdolescentReproHealth).
- Centers for Disease Control and Prevention: Unintended Pregnancy Prevention: Contraception (www.cdc.gov/reproductivehealth/UnintendedPregnancy/Contraception.htm.
- Guttmacher Institute (www.guttmacher.org/sections/pregnancy.php).
- National Center for Health Statistics (NCHS) (cdc.gov/nchs).
- Planned Parenthood: Teenwire (www.teenwire.com/).

AAP POLICY STATEMENTS

American Academy of Pediatrics, Committee on Adolescence and Committee on Early Childhood, Adoption, and Dependent Care. Care of adolescent parents and their children. *Pediatrics*. 2001;107(2):429-434. (aappolicy.aappublications.org/cgi/content/full/pediatrics;107/2/249).

American Academy of Pediatrics, Committee on Adolescence. Condom use by adolescents. *Pediatrics*. 2001; 107(6):1463-1469. (aappolicy.aappublications.org/cgi/content/full/pediatrics;107/6/1463).

American Academy of Pediatrics, Committee on Adolescence. Contraception and adolescents. *Pediatrics*. 2007; 120(5):1135-1148. (aappolicy.aappublications.org/cgi/content/full/pediatrics;120/5/1135).

American Academy of Pediatrics, Committee on Adolescence. Counseling the adolescent about pregnancy options. *Pediatrics*. 1998;101(5):938-940. (aappolicy.aappublications.org/cgi/content/full/pediatrics;101/5/938).

American Academy of Pediatrics, Committee on Adolescence. Emergency contraception. *Pediatrics*. 2005;116(4): 1026-1035.

American Academy of Pediatrics, Committee on Adolescence. The adolescent's right to confidential care when considering abortion. *Pediatrics*. 1996;97(5):746-751. (aappolicy.aappublications.org/cgi/content/abstract/pediatrics;97/5/746).

Klein JD, American Academy of Pediatrics, Committee on Adolescence. Adolescent pregnancy: current trends and issues. *Pediatrics*. 2005;116(1):281-286. (aappolicy.aappublications.org/cgi/content/full/pediatrics;116/1/281).

SUGGESTED RESOURCE

Hatcher RA. *Contraceptive Technology*. 18th ed, rev. New York, NY: Ardent Media; 2004.

REFERENCES

1. Guttmacher Institute. US Teenage Pregnancy Statistics National and State Trends by Race and Ethnicity. Available at: www.guttmacher.org/pubs/2006/09/12/ustpstats.pdf. Accessed July 19, 2007.

2. National Campaign to Prevent Teen Pregnancy. *How is the thirty-four percent calculated?* [fact sheet]. Vol 2004. Washington, DC: National Campaign to Prevent Teen Pregnancy; 2004.
3. Grunbaum J, Kann L, Kinchen S, et al. Youth risk behavior surveillance—United States, 2003. *MMWR Surveill Summ.* 2004;53:1-95.
4. American Medical Association. *Guidelines for Adolescent Preventive Services (GAPS).* Chicago, IL: American Medical Association; 1997.
5. Kirby D. *No Easy Answers: Research Findings on Programs to Reduce Teen Pregnancy (Summary).* Washington DC: The National Campaign to Prevent Teen Pregnancy, Task Force on Effective Programs and Research; 1997.
6. Trussel J, Koenig J, Stewart F, et al. Medical care cost savings from adolescent contraceptive use. *Fam Plann Perspect.* 1997;29:248-255, 295.
7. Jemmott JB, Jemmott LS, Fong GT. Abstinence and safer sex: HIV interventions for African Americans. *JAMA.* 1998;279:1529-1536.
8. American Academy of Pediatrics, Committee on Adolescence. Adolescents' right to confidential care in abortion. *Pediatrics.* 1996;96:747-751.
9. Jones RK, Boonstra H. Confidential reproductive health services for minors: the potential impact of mandated parental involvement for contraception. *Perspect Sex Reprod Health.* 2004;36(5):182-191.
10. Gudeman R. Adolescent Confidentiality and Privacy Under the Health Insurance Portability and Accountability Act. Youth Law News. July-Sept 2003. Available at: www.youthlaw.org/fileadmin/ncyl/youthlaw/publications/yln/2003/issue_3/03_yln_3_gudeman_confidentiality.pdf. Accessed July 19, 2007.
11. Hatcher RA, Guillebaud J. The pill: combined oral contraceptives. In: Hatcher RA, ed. *Contraceptive Technology.* New York, NY: Ardent Media Publishers; 1998.
12. Burkman RT, Kauntiz AM, Shulman LP, et al. Oral contraceptives and noncontraceptive benefits: summary and application of data. *Int J Fertil.* 2000;45(suppl 2):134-147.
13. Collaborative Group on Hormonal Factors in Breast Cancer. Breast cancer and hormonal contraceptives: collaborative reanalysis of individual data of 53,297 women with breast cancer and 100,239 women without breast cancer from 54 epidemiological studies. *Lancet.* 1996; 237:1713.
14. Brooks TL, Shrier LA. An update for contraception for adolescents. *Adolesc Med.* 1999;10:211-219.
15. Pymar HC, Creinin MD. The risks of oral contraceptive pills. *Seminars Reprod Med.* 2001;19:305-312.
16. World Health Organization. *Improving Access to Quality Care in Family Planning-Medical Eligibility Criteria for Contraceptive Use.* Geneva, Switzerland: World Health Organization; 1996.
17. World Health Organization. *Medical Eligibility Criteria For Initiating and Continuing Use of Contraceptive Methods.* Geneva, Switzerland: World Health Organization; 2000.
18. Schachter J, Shafer MA, Young M, et al. Routine pelvic examinations in asymptomatic young women. *N Engl J Med.* 1996;335:1847-1848.
19. Ries LAG, Kosary CL, Hankey BF, et al. *SEER Cancer Statistics Review, 1973-1994.* Bethesda, MD: National Cancer Institute; 1997.
20. US Preventive Services Task Force. Screening for Breast Cancer. Avaiable at: www.ahrq.gov/clinic/uspstf/uspschlm.htm. Accessed July 19, 2007.
21. US Preventive Services Task Force. Screening for Chlamydial Infections, 2001. Available at: www.ahrq.gov/clinic/uspstf/uspschlm.htm. Accessed July 19, 2007.
22. Cook RL, Hutchison SL, Ostergaard L, et al. Systematic review: noninvasive testing for Chlamydia trachomatis and Neisseria gonorrhoeae. *Ann Int Med.* 2005;142: 914-925.
23. US Preventive Services Task Force. *Guide to Clinical Preventive Services.* 2nd ed. Baltimore, MD: Williams & Wilkins; 1996.
24. American Academy of Pediatrics, Committee on Adolescence. Contraception and adolescents. *Pediatrics.* 1999; 104:1161-1166.
25. Mishell DR Jr. Oral contraceptives and cardiovascular events: summary and application of data. *Int J Fertil.* 2000;45(suppl 2):121-133.
26. Archer DF, Bigrigg A, Smallwood GH, et al. Assessment of compliance with a weekly contraceptive patch among North American women. *Fertil Steril.* 2002;77(suppl 2): S27-S31.
27. Darney PD. Everything You Need to Know About the Contraceptive Implant. Available at: www.jfponline.com/pages.asp?aid=4431. Accessed July 24, 2007.
28. American Academy of Pediatrics, Committee on Adolescence. Emergency contraception. *Pediatrics.* 2005;116(4): 1026-1035.
29. Glasier A, Baird D. The effects of self-administering emergency contraception, *N Engl J Med.* 1998;339:1.
30. World Health Organization, Task Force on Postovulatory Methods of Fertility Regulation. Randomised controlled trial of levonorgestrel versus the Yuzpe regimen of combined oral contraceptives for emergency contraception. *Lancet.* 1998;352:428-433.
31. von Hertzen H, Piaggio G, Ding J, et al. for the WHO Research Group on Post-Ovulatory Methods of Fertility Regulation. Low dose mifepristone and two regimens of levonorgestrel for emergency contraception. *Lancet.* 2002;360:1803-1810.
32. Family Health International. Condom Use Increases. Available at: www.fhi.org/en/rh/pubs/network/v18_3/nw183ch6.htm. Accessed July 19, 2007.
33. Schuster MS, Bell RM, Berry SH, et al. Impact of a high school condom availability program on sexual attitudes and behaviors. *Fam Plann Perspect.* 1998;30:67, 88.
34. Guttmacher S, Lieberman L, Ward D, et al. Condom availability in New York City public high schools: relationships to condom use and sexual behavior. *Am J Public Health.* 1997;87:1427.
35. Warner DL, Hatcher RA. Male condoms. In: Hatcher RA, ed. *Contraceptive Technology.* New York, NY: Ardent Media Publishers; 1998.

Chapter 157

GAY, LESBIAN, AND BISEXUAL YOUTH

Robert J. Bidwell, MD

In 2004 the American Academy of Pediatrics (AAP) issued its clinical report on sexual orientation and adolescents. This report gives guidance to clinicians on providing care to gay, lesbian, and bisexual (GLB) adolescents and "reaffirms the physician's responsibility to provide comprehensive health care and guidance in a safe and supportive environment for all adolescents, including nonheterosexual adolescents and young people struggling with issues of sexual orientation."[1] Because GLB adolescents are present in every pediatric setting, an understanding of sexual orientation and the unique experiences and needs of GLB youth is an essential part of the practice of pediatrics.

DEFINITIONS

Sexual orientation is an integral part of human sexuality; it refers to an individual's pattern of affectional, romantic, or sexual attractions to the same sex (homosexual), opposite sex (heterosexual), or both sexes (bisexual). Homosexual men are generally referred to as *gay*, homosexual women as *lesbian* (or gay), heterosexual individuals as *straight*, and bisexual individuals sometimes as *bi*. Sexual orientation is generally represented as a continuum from completely homosexual to completely heterosexual, with many individuals finding themselves somewhere in between. Gender identity is another important aspect of human sexuality, distinct from sexual orientation; it refers to a person's inner sense of being female or male. Although too simplistic a definition, *transgender* individuals are generally described as those whose genetic and anatomic sex may be female or male but whose inner identity is of the opposite gender. Although the experiences and needs of transgender youths are not discussed in this chapter, a growing number of clinical guidelines address these issues (see Chapter 140, Children with Gender-variant Behaviors and Transgender Youth).[2,3] Although the term *queer* has historically been considered pejorative, an increasing number of GLB and transgender individuals are claiming this term as a positive descriptor of their nonheterosexual identity.

PREVALENCE

The percentage of adolescents who already or one day will recognize their GLB identities is uncertain. Estimates range from approximately 3% to 10%.[1,4] Whatever the exact percentage might be, GLB adolescents are present in all pediatric practices. They exist within all ethnic, religious, and socioeconomic groups and may be more highly represented among homeless and runaway youths and youths in the juvenile justice and child welfare systems. However, GLB adolescents are often invisible, either because they do not fit GLB stereotypes, because they have not yet labeled their orientation as GLB, or because they are reluctant to reveal in health care settings their sexual orientation for fear of primary care physician (PCP) disapproval or lack of confidentiality. Many of these individuals likely remain invisible because PCPs do not routinely address sexual orientation with their adolescent patients.

DEVELOPMENT

The process of GLB identity acquisition is long, complex, and often difficult because of the generally negative societal stance toward nonheterosexual orientations. Several models of GLB identity formation have been proposed, each citing stigma as a major factor influencing development. Troiden[5] has defined a 4-stage process that begins in childhood, proceeds through the confusion and 1st sexual explorations of adolescence, and culminates in a healthy and open self-acceptance sometime in adulthood. More recently, developmental theorists have suggested that no typical developmental trajectory exists for GLB individuals.[6,7] Instead, they posit multiple possible developmental pathways that, in addition to societal stigma, are shaped by gender, ethnicity, social class, family and community environment, region of residence, life experiences, intelligence, attractiveness, sex drive, and personality factors such as self-esteem and self-confidence. The PCP should therefore not assume a predefined developmental trajectory for any given patient.

As reflected in the 2004 AAP clinical report, the pediatric profession views heterosexuality, homosexuality, and bisexuality as equally valid and healthy developmental outcomes for youth. This view is consistent with the American Psychiatric Association position that homosexuality is part of the spectrum of normal human sexuality.[8] Homosexuality and bisexuality appear to be well established by early childhood and are not a choice or a matter of *something gone wrong*. Sexual orientation is likely shaped by biological, genetic, and environmental factors, and these influences may differ for different individuals.[9,10] Biological theories appear to have received the strongest research support in recent years. Nevertheless, significant sectors of American and other societies do not accept the normalcy of homosexuality and bisexuality, seeing them as shameful, sinful, or pathological. This negative view has significant implications for the development of GLB youths.

ENVIRONMENTAL EFFECTS

GLB youths are ordinary adolescents in every regard, except that most grow up in environments that are deeply disapproving of their sexual orientation, a fundamental part of who they are. Research strongly suggests that societal stigma and the resultant victimization and discrimination under which GLB youths grow up are the primary reasons for the unique physical, emotional, and social problems they face.[1,11-18] Many GLB youths experience an adolescence of profound isolation, believing they are absolutely alone in their feelings of same-sex attraction. They have little or no access to accurate information about sexual orientation, yet they are surrounded by a multitude of negative messages about homosexuality coming from their families, schools, churches, and communities and often from people they love and respect. Most GLB youths have no access to GLB-supportive PCPs, counselors, or community programs. Many of these people grow up in families and communities where prejudice, discrimination, and violence against GLB individuals is approved or tolerated. Home and school can be especially dangerous places for GLB youths whose sexual orientation is known or presumed.

Given the stigma related to homosexuality and their own fears about their emerging same-sex attractions, many GLB youths repress their same-sex feelings or decide to keep them hidden from others. Many of them expend great energy attempting to pass as heterosexual. They often avoid any exploration of their GLB orientation, thereby delaying an essential part of their identity development. Most GLB youths are denied socially approved dating rituals through which heterosexual youths begin to explore, understand, and become comfortable with their sexuality. Many GLB youths have never had sex with another person; others have been only heterosexually active. Some GLB youths realize that the only way to begin exploring their same-sex attractions is through secretive or anonymous sexual encounters; such encounters are increasingly facilitated through the Internet. Although these situations are understandable given the lack of opportunities for sexual socialization enjoyed by heterosexual youths, they are potentially dangerous and may engender feelings of anxiety, guilt, and self-hatred. A very small minority of GLB youths are fortunate to live in communities where schools and agencies have begun to provide safe, healthy, and accepting venues, such as support groups, drop-in centers, dances, and leadership retreats, for GLB adolescents to meet one another and engage in a process of healthy peer socialization.

GLB youths of color, immigrant youths, disabled youths, rural youths, and youths belonging to conservative religious faiths may have an especially difficult time understanding and accepting their sexual orientation. In many instances, they have few GLB-supportive resources within their communities and risk rejection if they openly acknowledge or explore their GLB identity.

Some GLB youths, as with other adolescents who are alone, fearful, and stigmatized, respond in predictable ways, by dropping out of school, running away from home, engaging in risky sex, using drugs, and turning to street life and prostitution.[1,12,13,19-22] Persons struggling for survival on the streets often encounter violence and sexual exploitation, with the attendant risks of sexually transmitted infections (STIs) and pregnancy. A significant percentage of GLB youths consider suicide to be their only choice.[23-25] PCPs should realize that these risky behaviors are not a necessary part of the script for growing up GLB. Research has shown that vulnerable adolescents who grow up in stigmatizing or risky environments thrive when they are connected to safe and supportive families, friends, and communities.[25-27] One of the most important roles for PCPs in working with GLB youths is to participate in creating safe environments and supportive networks of family, peers, teachers, counselors, PCPs, and others to buffer the generally hostile society in which GLB youths grow up.

EVALUATION

The AAP clinical report on sexual orientation and adolescents and the *Bright Futures* guidelines call on PCPs to address the issue of sexual orientation with all adolescents.[1,28] These and other guidelines also describe ways in which clinicians can provide care that is respectful of GLB patients and relevant to their needs.[2,3] PCPs should not presume an adolescent's sexual orientation on the basis of stereotypes or reported sexual behaviors. One of the greatest barriers GLB youths face in receiving appropriate health care is PCPs' belief that they have no GLB adolescents in their practices. Many GLB adolescents will deny same-sex attractions or behaviors even when directly asked. This tendency may be the result of fear of physicians' disapproval or lack of confidentiality or to their own uncertainty about their sexual feelings. Fortunately, the goal of pediatric practice is not to identify all GLB adolescents. Instead, the objective is to create a safe and comfortable clinical setting in which adolescents can discuss sexual orientation issues when they are ready to do so. This task can be accomplished indirectly through posters, brochures, health questionnaires, and other clinic forms that demonstrate respect for diversity, including diversity of sexual orientation and gender identity. More direct messages come from office staff and PCPs who model respectful attitudes and make no assumptions about sexual orientation or gender identity in their interactions with patients.

Perhaps the strongest message that would allow a GLB adolescent to open up and discuss these issues is when these issues are raised routinely, in a genuinely interested and nonjudgmental manner, at all well-teen visits and any visit suggestive of an adolescent in distress. A candid discussion of sexuality and other personal issues is facilitated further by meeting with the adolescent alone, without parents or friends present, and accompanied by appropriate assurances of confidentiality. Revealing an adolescent's GLB orientation to others, including parents, without the person's consent is unethical and potentially dangerous. If issues of GLB orientation arise, then adolescents should be asked whether they are comfortable with the PCP recording these in the chart. Even with permission, these notations should be made carefully and perhaps indirectly because parents often have the ability to obtain or review their adolescent's medical record, including specific parts that should remain confidential.

PCPs must reflect on their own attitudes and comfort around issues of sexual orientation. Research has shown that many pediatric PCPs are uncomfortable in discussing sexuality, including sexual orientation, with their adolescent patients, and this discomfort limits their ability to provide appropriate care.[29-31] Studies of GLB adolescents reveal that only a small minority of them have ever been asked about or discussed sexual orientation with their health care providers.[32] Research has also demonstrated that many PCPs disapprove of homosexuality.[2,15,33-35] This disapproval makes the provision of appropriate health care and counseling to GLB youths nearly impossible. The failure of PCPs to discuss relevant health issues knowledgeably, comfortably, and nonjudgmentally has been a major barrier to accessing health care for GLB youths. Only when issues of sexual orientation are addressed openly and supportively can appropriate medical screening, treatment, education, counseling, and advocacy be provided.

History

Every annual well-teen health evaluation should include a sexual history.[36] Sexual activity, sexual orientation, and sexual decision-making skills should be routinely assessed at these visits.[37,38] Sexual orientation also should be addressed at any acute care visit suggestive of an adolescent in distress (eg, parent-teen conflict, school problems, substance use, increased heterosexual or homosexual activity, depression, self-harm, unusual displays of anger or frustration). Signs and symptoms of STIs should also prompt an inquiry into sexual practices and orientation.

In addressing sexuality with an adolescent patient, the PCP should begin by using gender-neutral language, letting the adolescent know that no assumptions are made about the patient's sexual orientation or practices. For example, the use of terms such as *partner* rather than *boyfriend* or *girlfriend* and *protection* rather than *birth control* is important until a more complete history has been obtained. The PCP can approach the issue of sexuality first by asking if an adolescent has ever been in a dating or romantic relationship with another person. If yes, have these relationships been with girls, boys, or both girls and boys? To learn whether an adolescent has been in a dating or romantic relationship, the patient also should be asked, "Have you ever had sex with another person, including just kissing or touching?" If the answer is yes, again, the PCP should ask, "Has this been with girls, boys, or both boys and girls?" An important point to remember is that the question, "Have you ever had sexual intercourse?" may be interpreted as meaning only vaginal intercourse and may not identify youths who have engaged only in petting, oral sex, or anal intercourse.

PCPs should remember that many GLB youths may only have been heterosexually active or not sexually active with others at all. Youths who have been homosexually active may be afraid to acknowledge same-sex behaviors. Therefore the PCP should search beyond dating relationships and sexual behaviors and ask all adolescents if their feelings of attraction are generally to girls, boys, or both boys and girls and their comfort around these feelings. Many GLB adolescents have not yet labeled their sexual feelings, and therefore asking patients early in the interview whether they consider themselves gay, lesbian, or bisexual is usually an ineffective and sometimes frightening screening approach for GLB adolescents. However, as part of a broader discussion over time, asking an adolescent in a supportive and nonjudgmental manner, "Have you ever wondered if you might be lesbian (gay, bisexual)?" may be appropriate at some point. Finally, use of the word *homosexual* as a label ("Are you a homosexual?") is generally believed to be stigmatizing by many GLB patients and should be avoided.

In interviewing adolescents who acknowledge same-sex behaviors or attractions, the PCP should not focus only or even primarily on their sexual practices and the degree to which they employ safer sex. Because most of the health risks faced by GLB youths are related not to their sexual behavior but to growing up in a hostile environment, the PCP should address these latter issues in depth before engaging in a detailed discussion of sexual behaviors. For example, the PCP should ask how comfortable GLB adolescents feel regarding their same-sex attractions and relationships. How do family background, religion, ethnicity, or community norms play a role in their degree of self-acceptance? The PCP should also inquire whether the patient has told others of the patient's GLB orientation and whether family members, friends, school counselors, and others have been supportive or rejecting in their response. In other words, knowing whether a GLB youth is isolated or has a network of supportive family, friends, and adults already in place is important. Another area to explore with GLB adolescents is the degree to which they believe their sexual orientation will limit or enhance their future in terms of career, relationships, or acceptance in the community. Can they envision themselves as happy, healthy, and productive GLB adults? What are their fears, if any? What are their hopes and dreams?

Because some GLB adolescents respond to stigmatization and rejection by engaging in risky behaviors, the PCP should inquire directly about the possibility of parent-teen conflict, school problems, runaway behavior and street life, substance use, eating disorders, depression, and involvement in the child welfare or juvenile justice systems. Because most GLB adolescents grow up in nonaccepting—even hostile—environments, the PCP should ask specifically about their experience of violence in the home, school, and community.

As with other sexually active adolescents, the PCP should ask sexually active GLB youths how comfortable they are with their sexual behaviors and relationships. Specifically, have these behaviors and relationships been healthy and fulfilling or unpleasant and exploitative in nature? A comprehensive health history should also include a detailed sexual history. It should be preceded by an explanation from the PCP that obtaining personal information about sexuality is helpful in providing patients quality care that meets their specific needs. At the same time, the adolescent patient should be assured that they have a right to answer only specific questions they are comfortable answering. The sexual history should include a discussion of specific sexual behaviors in which the adolescent is engaged, frequency of activity, consensual and nonconsensual encounters, safer-sex practices, number and nature of partners (age; boyfriend or girlfriend vs acquaintance or anonymous), and how contact with potential partners is made (school, church, malls, parties, the Internet). Few sexual practices exist that are unique to GLB youths; thus history taking related to this specific issue is similar for both GLB and heterosexual youths. Symptoms of STIs also should be elicited, as should any history of combining substance use and sexual activity or exchanging sex for money, drugs, or shelter.

Physical Examination

The physical examination of GLB adolescents, whether sexually active or not, does not differ from that of heterosexual adolescents. At the same time, PCPs should remember that many GLB youths are *invisible,* so that any adolescent may have a history of same-sex activity, although it may not always be acknowledged. PCPs should also remember that some gay and lesbian youths have been heterosexually active. The content of the physical examination should be determined by a comprehensive health history, including sexual and other risk behaviors, and not by sexual orientation. If indicated by history, a thorough anal examination should be performed because people of both sexes with a history of anal intercourse are at higher risk for human papilloma virus infection leading to anal dysplasia, anal warts, and subsequent anal carcinoma.

Lesbian adolescents should be offered the same gynecologic care as other young women, as guided by a complete and accurate general health and sexual history.[2,39] However, PCPs should be aware that among lesbian patients who exclusively have sex with other women, STIs are uncommon. Nevertheless, some lesbian youths are bisexually active, have bisexual female partners, or may be victims of sexual assault, which make pregnancy and STI testing advisable for some lesbian patients. Furthermore, many lesbians, including some adolescents, choose pregnancy as a route to parenthood and will require prenatal care that takes into account their specific life circumstances. Present guidelines suggest routine Papanicolaou tests (Pap smears) for all sexually active lesbian patients because women who have sex exclusively with other women are apparently at risk for many STIs, including human papilloma virus. Having sex with bisexual female partners increases their risk for other infections, including bacterial vaginosis and candidal vulvovaginitis.[2]

Laboratory Evaluation

Any decision to offer laboratory or other diagnostic testing to GLB adolescents should be based on a complete and accurate health history and physical examination and not on sexual orientation. Nevertheless, in considering laboratory and other evaluative studies, the PCP should remember that any adolescent may have a history of same-sex encounters and yet be fearful of disclosing them. For sexually active gay and bisexual male adolescents, some researchers suggest screening for hepatitis A, B, and C.[2] If screening indicates no exposure and no immunity to hepatitis A or B, then immunization should be suggested. Also based on history and symptoms, adolescents should be offered gonorrhea, chlamydia, syphilis, and HIV testing. Anal Pap smears have been suggested for any male or female patient with active anal warts or a history of anal warts and current HIV infection.[2] The evaluation and treatment of STIs are discussed in Chapter 322, Sexually Transmitted Infections.

MANAGEMENT

As stated in the 2004 AAP clinical guidelines, the goal of care in working with GLB youths is "to promote normal adolescent development, social and emotional well-being, and physical health."[1]

Physical Well Being

GLB adolescents face the same kinds of health issues as other adolescents. The health screening, immunizations, and treatment provided to GLB adolescents should not be based on sexual orientation, but rather on information obtained from an accurate history, physical examination, and evaluative studies. Nevertheless, many GLB youths face increased risks to health because of societal nonacceptance. Patients who show evidence of drug dependency, eating disorders, depression, and other mental health concerns should be referred to appropriate GLB-supportive community resources. As a GLB adolescent approaches adulthood, discussions about transition to a GLB-supportive adult health care provider should begin.

Developmental, Social, and Emotional Well Being

Although providing appropriate health care is important, for many GLB adolescents, the most important role a PCP can play is that of supportive counselor. Adolescents who acknowledge same-sex or bisexual attractions exhibit varying levels of self-acceptance and differing issues of concern. Therefore a 1st step in counseling GLB adolescents is to listen carefully to their stories because these will help shape the content of issues to be discussed during the present and subsequent visits. In general, the counseling of GLB adolescents addresses the following 6 areas: (1) self-acceptance and validation of same-sex attractions, (2) safety, (3) connectedness to supportive others, (4) self-disclosure, or *coming out,* (5) healthy relationships and sexual decision making, and (6) optimism for the future. PCPs often focus their counseling of GLB adolescents only on sexual activity, risk for STIs, and safer-sex practices. However, addressing each of the 6 areas previously listed is important in ensuring the healthy development of GLB adolescents.

Self-Acceptance and Validation

Most adolescents grow up surrounded by negative messages about GLB sexual orientation and the presumption that heterosexuality is the only acceptable orientation. These messages often come from people they love and respect and have a profoundly negative effect on the health and development of GLB youths. GLB adolescents often believe that they are sick or sinful because of their emerging sexual feelings and are filled with shame and self-hatred. The PCP should try to determine the degree of comfort each GLB youth has with emerging sexual feelings and discuss the adolescent's specific concerns or fears. While acknowledging that some cultures and communities may view a GLB orientation as unhealthy or wrong, the PCP should state clearly that the pediatric profession considers homosexuality and bisexuality to be healthy and normal. They are not a choice and do not represent *something gone wrong.* This emphatic reassurance of normalcy from the pediatric perspective is perhaps the most powerful and important statement that a PCP can make to a GLB youth. The PCP should also determine an adolescent's accuracy of knowledge about sexual orientation and correct any misconceptions. Some GLB youths are frightened by GLB stereotypes, thinking these somehow represent who they are as a person. The PCP should remind GLB adolescents that the stereotypes do not define who they are; rather, they, in their own individuality, help define what it means to be GLB. Ethnic and other minority GLB youths may have an especially difficult time as they try to manage more than one type of stigma. The PCP should recognize and discuss this difficult reality with the patient. Letting the GLB adolescent know that growing self-acceptance of a person's sexual orientation is an evolutionary process would be helpful. The uncertainty and discomfort they experience now will likely diminish or disappear as they move into adulthood.

If an adolescent denies same-sex attractions, and yet the PCP or others believe that it is an issue that may emerge later in an adolescent's life, then the PCP can simply say, "This may or may not ever be a part of your life, and I hear you telling me clearly today that it is not. I just want you to know that, as your doctor, I will always be here for you and available to discuss any issues that come up in your life as you grow older."

For adolescents who express uncertainty about their sexual orientation, the PCP can say, "It's not my place to tell you if you are gay, lesbian, bisexual, or straight; only you can decide this for yourself. What I can do is provide you information and support, and let you know that whoever you finally discover you are is all right. The most important thing is that you are happy and comfortable with who you are, no matter what your sexual orientation might be." For some adolescents to go through stages during which they believe they are gay, then straight, then bisexual, then gay again is not unusual. This uncertainty is part of the normal process of self-discovery and will eventually be resolved, although not necessarily during adolescence. The PCP should not tell adolescents who are experiencing same-sex attractions that they are "just going through a phase." For a significant percentage of adolescents, these feelings do, in fact, represent an emerging GLB identity, and false *reassurances* to the contrary can be harmful.

SAFETY

Most GLB youths grow up in environments that are potentially harmful to their physical, emotional, and developmental health. Many of these individuals endure harassment and bullying, discrimination, or social rejection; at the very least, many are surrounded by negative messages about GLB orientation. These dangers may arise at home, school, or church, and within the peer group or the broader community. PCPs should ask GLB adolescents about their safety in each of these settings. If an adolescent acknowledges harassment or other harmful treatment, then the PCP should work with the youth to identify and implement appropriate strategies to end the violence. Unfortunately, many GLB adolescents are filled with shame and are afraid to advocate for their own safety. They often believe that they deserve the harm inflicted on them, or they simply accept that *this is the way the world is*. The PCP should tell adolescents clearly that they have done nothing to deserve such treatment and that they should expect and demand safety and respect from everyone in their lives and in all settings. Because GLB youths have so few advocates, the PCP should offer to join with the adolescent in approaching every venue in which the adolescent experiences violence, including the home and school, to work out a plan to end violence immediately and completely. If necessary, the PCP should call on the state child protective services or advocacy organizations such as the American Civil Liberties Union to join in the effort to keep the adolescent safe.

ISOLATION

GLB adolescents are among the most isolated of youths. Many of them have little or no access to accurate and supportive information about sexual orientation, and most know of no accepting and supportive counselors in their schools or communities. At a time when they should begin exploring their sexuality, most GLB adolescents have no safe venues in which to meet other GLB youths. Many of them have distanced themselves emotionally or become estranged from their parents and siblings. Many GLB adolescents believe they are the only ones they know who are experiencing same-sex attractions. Few of them have visible GLB adult role models in their communities to provide reassurance that a happy and rewarding adulthood is attainable. As with any other adolescents, isolation and loneliness can lead to compromised physical and emotional health. PCPs should address the issue of isolation by giving accurate information about sexual orientation. They should provide supportive and reassuring counseling, or they should refer the adolescent to GLB-supportive colleagues who have the time, comfort, and expertise to do so. They should connect GLB youths to local community resources such as support groups and other youth programs for GLB adolescents. GLB youths who do not have access to local programs should be informed about Web sites created for GLB adolescents where they can receive accurate information and communicate with other GLB youths in a safe, monitored setting. PCPs can also point out positive GLB youth and adult role models in the community or nationally. In certain circumstances, for GLB PCPs to present themselves as role models to GLB youths and their families is also appropriate.

SELF-DISCLOSURE, OR *COMING OUT*

GLB adolescents often reach a point in their development at which they feel a strong urge to disclose their sexual orientation to others, referred to as *coming out*. The process of disclosure to family and friends is often emotional and frequently traumatic. Adolescents who come out risk condemnation and rejection by family and peers. Disclosure can also result in physical violence both at home and at school. Therefore coming out should be considered carefully, weighing the risks and benefits. If an adolescent expects a negative response from the youth's parents, then the adolescent should wait to disclose until legally and financially independent. However, many adolescents believe that continuing to *live a lie* is intolerable and harmful to their self-esteem, and therefore they come out to their parents much earlier. Under no circumstances should a PCP reveal an adolescent's orientation to parents without permission. A PCP can play an important role in the process of disclosure by helping adolescents decide whether they are ready to come out to family or friends and helping them choose an appropriate time, place, and approach for disclosure.

HEALTHY RELATIONSHIPS AND SEXUAL DECISION MAKING

Although some GLB youths manage to meet other GLB adolescents and establish friendships and dating relationships, most do not. PCPs should help connect GLB adolescents to local GLB teen support groups and GLB-supportive programs in the community if they exist. This task can be accomplished ethically without parental notification. PCPs can suggest national telephone hotlines or Web sites where GLB youths can receive accurate information and supportive counseling and communicate with other GLB youths. If these options are not available, then the PCP can serve as a supportive and reassuring lifeline until the adolescent is old enough to become independent and possibly move away to work or go to school in a community more accepting of GLB people.

GLB youths who are in relationships face many of the same questions as their heterosexual peers. "Am I in love?" "What do I want from a relationship?" "Do I really want to be in this relationship?" "How do I know if this is a good relationship?" "How do I get out of this relationship?" A GLB-supportive PCP or counselor can help adolescents reflect on and find answers to these questions.

As with other adolescents, many GLB youths know little about sexuality and how to make healthy sexual choices. Abstinence is always the appropriate option for adolescents who do not feel ready for a sexual relationship. GLB adolescents should understand that when they are ready for a sexual relationship, they can expect to lead healthy and fulfilling sexual lives. All adolescents who have decided that they are ready for a sexual relationship should be advised to limit their number of sexual partners and avoid mixing sex and alcohol or drugs so as to reduce their risk for infection, trauma, and sexual assault. Safer sex practices related to oral, vaginal, and anal sex should be reviewed in detail. GLB youths should also be aware that *no always means no* in negotiating sex, and any forced or coerced sexual experience represents sexual assault. GLB youths should also understand that no set GLB repertoire of sexual behaviors exists and that they should engage only in those sexual practices with which they are comfortable.

OPTIMISM FOR THE FUTURE

PCPs should not only focus on the risks that GLB youths face, but also identify specific strengths that have allowed them to survive and sometimes thrive in the face of an often hostile environment. They should also challenge the belief of many GLB adolescents that their futures will be significantly limited by their sexual orientation. Although some communities are clearly more accepting of GLB people than others, most GLB adults lead happy, healthy, and productive lives. GLB youths should be encouraged to pursue any career they wish. They should expect to have deep, long-lasting, and fulfilling relationships throughout their lives. They should expect to be respected and valued members of their communities. They also should understand that marriage and parenthood are enhancing the lives of thousands of GLB adults across the United States. Although growing up GLB is often challenging, the future should be seen as hopeful and exciting.

PARENTS

Parents who learn of their child's GLB orientation often experience an intense mix of emotions, including guilt, shame, fear, anger, repulsion, and profound sadness. Many of these individuals go through a deep mourning period, feeling as if they have lost the child they knew and loved. Some parents will reject or physically and emotionally abuse a GLB child. Parents are often as isolated from accurate information and supportive resources as are their children. PCPs should listen patiently and respectfully to parents' concerns and fears, acknowledging their pain and sense of loss. The PCP should emphasize the importance of their continued expressions of love for their child, especially at this time when many adolescents believe that they will lose their parents' love and support. At the same time, the PCP can acknowledge that understanding and acceptance of their child's sexual orientation is an evolutionary process and will take time. Parents should be reassured that they did nothing wrong and that the pediatric profession has come to accept homosexuality and bisexuality as normal and healthy developmental outcomes. To decrease their isolation, parents should be given the AAP brochure titled *Gay, Lesbian, and Bisexual Teens: Facts for Teens and Their Parents.*[40] They should be referred to supportive books, Web sites, and support programs for parents and families of GLB children. One of the most prominent national parent support organizations is Parents, Friends, and Families of Lesbians and Gays (PFLAG), which has many local affiliate groups across the country. Parents should be reassured that American society as a whole is becoming increasingly accepting of GLB people. By providing love, support, and protection, parents should expect their child to achieve a happy, healthy, and rewarding adulthood.

The PCP should discourage any parental search for *treatment* that is directed at changing their child's sexual orientation. Such *reparative therapy* or similar religion-based *transformational ministries* are considered by the pediatric profession to be both unethical and dangerous. Finally, PCPs who believe that they are unable to give GLB-supportive counseling to families should refer them to colleagues who have the time, comfort, and expertise to provide such support.

ADVOCACY

One of the most important roles that PCPs can play in ensuring the health and safety of GLB adolescents is that of advocate. The advocacy role is essential, even life saving, because most GLB youths grow up in extremely hostile environments and have few if any advocates in their families or communities. PCPs' expertise is respected, and their offering of visible and confidant support for GLB adolescents can promote increased community awareness, understanding, and acceptance, which are essential for the healthy development of these youths.

Advocacy can take place on many levels. On an individual patient level, PCPs can meet with families, school officials, social welfare agency staff, mental health care providers, and others to ensure that their individual patient is safe and accepted in the home, school, and community. They should also ensure that clinic and hospital policies and practices reflect respect for GLB patients. At a community level, PCPs can participate in educational forums that present the pediatric perspective that GLB orientations are normal and healthy. PCPs should be willing to go to schools and school boards, churches, child welfare agencies, juvenile detention and correctional institutions, city councils, and legislatures to advocate for policies and programs that specifically ensure the respectful treatment and address the special needs of GLB adolescents. National guidelines have been developed recently addressing these issues.[41]

In addition, PCPs can advocate for school curricula and library holdings that reflect the diversity of students and their families, including diversity of sexual orientation and gender identity. Furthermore, they should advocate for the development and implementation of robust medical school, residency training, and continuing medical education curricula that include an in-depth consideration of the development, life experiences, and health needs of GLB adolescents and adults and provide the skills to work with these populations respectfully and effectively. This effort is especially important because, for many GLB youths, a supportive PCP may be the only lifeline they have ensuring safe passage into a happy, healthy, and rewarding adulthood.

WHEN TO REFER

- When an adolescent has acute or recurrent suicidal ideation
- When an adolescent is engaged in multiple high-risk behaviors
- When the PCP believes that time, expertise, or comfort is insufficient to provide GLB-supportive care and counseling

Referral should be made only to PCPs who have experience in working with GLB adolescents and who accept same-sex attractions as normal and healthy. Referrals for *reparative therapy* or to *transformational ministries* are unethical and potentially dangerous.

TOOLS FOR PRACTICE

Engaging Patients and Family

- *Gay, Lesbian, and Bisexual Teens: Facts for Teens and Their Parents* (brochure), American Academy of Pediatrics (patiented.aap.org).
- *National Gay, Lesbian, Bisexual Youth Hotline 1-800-347-TEEN* (Hotline), National Gay, Lesbian, Bisexual Youth Hotline.
- *Parents, Families, and Friends of Lesbians and Gays (PFLAG)* (Web page), Parents, Families, and Friends of Lesbians and Gays (PFLAG).
- *Youth Resource* (Web page), Youth Resource.

Medical Decision Support

- *Gay and Lesbian Medical Association (GLMA)* (Web page), Gay and Lesbian Medical Association (GLMA).
- *Gay, Lesbian, and Straight Educational Network (GLSEN)* (Web page), Gay, Lesbian, and Straight Educational Network (GLSEN) (www.glsen.org/cgi-bin/iowa/all/home/index.html).

AAP POLICY STATEMENTS

American Academy of Pediatrics, Committee on Adolescence. Sexual orientation and adolescents. *Pediatrics.* 2004;113(6):1827-1832. (aappolicy.aappublications.org/cgi/content/full/pediatrics;113/6/1827).

American Academy of Pediatrics, Committee on Psychosocial Aspects of Child and Family Health, Committee on Adolescence. Sexuality education for children and adolescents. *Pediatrics.* 2001;108(2):498-502. (aappolicy.aappublications.org/cgi/content/full/pediatrics;108/2/498).

REFERENCES

1. Frankowski BL, American Academy of Pediatrics, Committee on Adolescence. Sexual orientation and adolescents. *Pediatrics.* 2004;113:1827-1832.
2. Kaiser Permanente National Diversity Council, Kaiser Permanente National Diversity Department. *A Provider's Handbook on Culturally Competent Care: Lesbian, Gay, Bisexual, and Transgendered Population.* 2nd ed. Oakland, CA: Kaiser Permanente; 2004.
3. Gay and Lesbian Medical Association. Guidelines for the Care of Lesbian, Gay, Bisexual, and Transgender Patients. 2006. Available at: ce54.citysoft.com/_data/n_0001/resources/live/GLMA%20guidelines%202006%20FINAL.pdf. Accessed March 4, 2007
4. Seidman SN, Rieder RO. A review of sexual behavior in the United States. *Am J Psychiatry.* 1994;151:330-341.
5. Troiden RR. Homosexual identity development. *J Adolesc Health Care.* 1988;9:105-113.
6. Diamond LM, Savin-Williams RC. The intimate relationships of sexual minority youths. In: Adams GR, Berzonsky MD, eds. *Blackwell Handbook of Adolescence.* Malden, MA: Blackwell Publishing; 2003.
7. Maguen S, Floyd FJ, Bakeman R, et al. Developmental milestones and disclosure of sexual orientation among gay, lesbian, and bisexual youths. *Appl Dev Psychol.* 2002;23:219-233.
8. American Psychiatric Association. *Diagnostic and Statistical Manual of Mental Disorders* (DSM-IV). 4th ed. Washington, DC: American Psychiatric Association; 2000.
9. Bailey JM, Pillard RC. Genetics of human sexual orientation. *Annu Rev Sex Res.* 1995;6:126-150.
10. Savin-Williams RC, Cohen KM. Homoerotic development during childhood and adolescence. *Child Adolesc Psychiatr Clin North Am.* 2004;13:529-549.
11. Bontempo DE, D'Augelli AR. Effects of at-school victimization and sexual orientation on lesbian, gay, or bisexual youths' health risk behaviors. *J Adolesc Health.* 2002;30:364-374.
12. Garofalo R, Wolf RC, Kessel S, et al. The association between health risk behaviors and sexual orientation among a school-based sample of adolescents. *Pediatrics.* 1998;101:895-902.
13. Savin-Williams RC. Verbal and physical abuse as stressors in the lives of lesbian, gay male, and bisexual youths: associations with school problems, running away, substance abuse, prostitution, and suicide. *J Counseling Clin Psychol.* 1994;62:261-269.

14. Gwadz MV, Clatts MC, Leonard NR, et al. Attachment style, childhood adversity, and behavioral risk among young men who have sex with men. *J Adolesc Health.* 2004;34:402-413.
15. Perrin EC. *Sexual Orientation in Child and Adolescent Health Care.* New York, NY: Kluwer Academic/Plenum; 2002.
16. Ryan C, Futterman D. *Lesbian and Gay Youth: Care and Counseling.* New York, NY: Columbia University Press; 1997.
17. Hershberger SL, D'Augelli AR. The impact of victimization on the mental health and suicidality of lesbian, gay, and bisexual youth. *Dev Psychol.* 1995;31:65-74.
18. Ryan C, Rivers I. Lesbian, gay, bisexual and transgender youth: victimization and its correlates in the USA and UK. *Cult Health Sex.* 2003;5:103-119.
19. Saewyc EM, Skay CL, Bearinger LH, et al. Sexual orientation, sexual behaviors, and pregnancy among American Indian adolescents. *J Adolesc Health.* 1998;23:238-247.
20. Faulkner AH, Cranston K. Correlates of same-sex sexual behavior in a random sample of Massachusetts high school students. *Am J Public Health.* 1998;88:262-266.
21. Lock J, Steiner H. Gay, lesbian, and bisexual youth risks for emotional, physical, and social problems: results from a community-based survey. *J Am Acad Child Adolesc Psychiatry.* 1999;38:297-304.
22. Noell JW, Ochs LM. Relationship of sexual orientation to substance use, suicidal ideation, suicide attempts, and other factors in a population of homeless adolescents. *J Adolesc Health.* 2001;29:31-36.
23. Remafedi G. Suicidality in a venue-based sample of young men who have sex with men. *J Adolesc Health.* 2002;31:305-310.
24. Garofalo R. Sexual orientation and risk of suicide attempts among a representative sample of youth. *Arch Pediatr Adolesc Med.* 1999;153:487-493.
25. Eisenberg ME, Resnick MD. Suicidality among gay, lesbian, and bisexual youth: the role of protective factors. *J Adolesc Health.* 2006;39:656-661.
26. Blum RW, McNeely C, Nonnemaker J. Vulnerability, risk and protection. *J Adolesc Health.* 2002;31:28-39.
27. Bell CC. Cultivating resiliency in youth. *J Adolesc Health.* 2001;29:375-381.
28. Green M, Palfrey JS, eds. *Bright Futures: Guidelines for Health Supervision of Infants, Children, and Adolescents.* 2nd ed, rev. Washington, DC: National Center for Education in Maternal and Child Health, Georgetown University; 2002. Available at: www.brightfutures.org/bf2/pdf/pdf/AD.pdf. Accessed March 4, 2007.
29. Gans Epner J, Levenberg P, Schoeny M. Primary care providers' responsiveness to health-risk behaviors reported by adolescent patients. *Arch Pediatr Adolesc Med.* 1998;152:774-780.
30. East JA, El Rayess F. Pediatricians' approach to the health care of lesbian, gay, and bisexual youth. *J Adolesc Health.* 1998;23:191-193.
31. Lena SM, Wiebe T, Ingram S, et al. Pediatricians' knowledge, perceptions, and attitudes towards providing health care for lesbian, gay, and bisexual adolescents. *Ann R Coll Phys Surg Can.* 2002;35:406-410.
32. Allen LB, Glicken AD, Beach RK, et al. Adolescent health care experience of gay, lesbian, and bisexual young adults. *J Adolesc Health.* 1998;23:212-220.
33. Peterson KJ. Preface: developing the context: the impact of homophobia and heterosexism on the health care of gay and lesbian people. *J Gay Lesbian Social Serv.* 1996; 5:xix–xxii.
34. Tellez C, Ramos M, Umland B, et al. Attitudes of physicians in New Mexico toward gay men and lesbians. *J Gay Lesbian Med Assoc.* 1999;3:83-89.
35. Schwanberg SL. Health care professionals' attitudes toward lesbian women and gay men. *J Homosexual.* 1996;31:71-83.
36. Goldenring JM, Rosen DS. Getting into adolescent heads: an essential update. *Contemp Pediatr.* 2004;21:64-90.
37. Garofalo R, Harper GW. Not all adolescents are the same: addressing the unique needs of gay and bisexual male youth. *Adolesc Med State Art Rev.* 2003;14:595-611.
38. Catallozzi M, Rudy BJ. Lesbian, gay, bisexual, transgendered, and questioning youth: the importance of a sensitive and confidential sexual history in identifying the risk and implementing treatment for sexually transmitted infections. *Adolesc Med Clin.* 2004;15:353-367.
39. Waitkevicz HJ. Lesbian health in primary care. *Women's Health Prim Care.* 2004;7:134-141.
40. American Academy of Pediatrics. *Gay, Lesbian, and Bisexual Teens: Facts for Teens and Their Parents.* Elk Grove Village, Ill: American Academy of Pediatrics; 2001.
41. Wilber S, Ryan C, Marksamer J. *CWLA Best Practice Guidelines: Serving LGBT Youth in Out-of-Home Care.* Washington, DC: Child Welfare League of America; 2006.

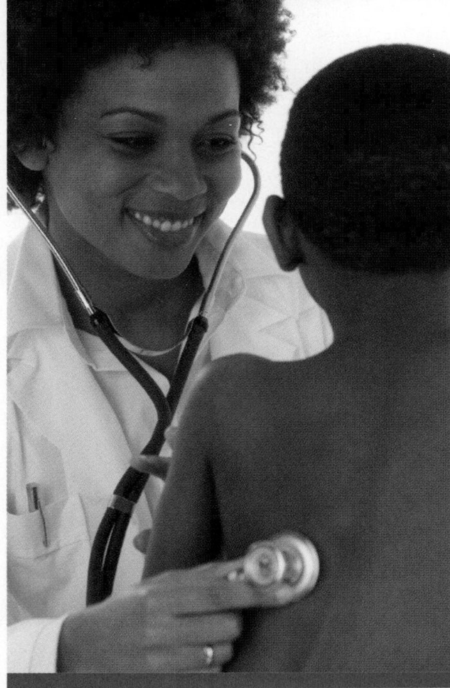

PART 8

Presenting Signs and Symptoms

158 Abdominal Distention
159 Abdominal Pain
160 Alopecia and Hair Shaft Anomalies
161 Amenorrhea
162 Anemia and Pallor
163 Back Pain
164 Cardiac Arrhythmias
165 Chest Pain
166 Constipation
167 Cough
168 Dental Stains
169 Diarrhea and Steatorrhea
170 Dizziness and Vertigo
171 Dysmenorrhea
172 Dysphagia
173 Dyspnea
174 Dysuria
175 Edema
176 Epistaxis
177 Extremity Pain
178 Facial Dysmorphism
179 Failure to Thrive
180 Fatigue and Weakness
181 Fever
182 Fever of Unknown Origin
183 Foot and Leg Problems
184 Gastrointestinal Hemorrhage
185 Headache
186 Hearing Loss
187 Heart Murmurs
188 Hematuria
189 Hemoptysis
190 Hepatomegaly
191 High Blood Pressure in Infants, Children, and Adolescents
192 Hirsutism, Hypertrichosis, and Precocious Sexual Hair Development
193 Hoarseness
194 Hyperhidrosis

Continued

195 Hypotonia
196 Irritability
197 Jaundice
198 Joint Pain
199 Limp
200 Loss of Appetite
201 Lymphadenopathy
202 Macrocephaly
203 Malocclusion
204 Microcephaly
205 Nervousness
206 Nonconvulsive Periodic Disorders
207 Odor (Unusual Urine and Body)
208 Petechiae and Purpura
209 Polyuria
210 Proteinuria
211 Pruritus
212 Puberty: Normal and Abnormal
213 Rash
214 Recurrent Infections
215 Red Eye/Pink Eye
216 Scrotal Swelling and Pain
217 Self-stimulating Behaviors
218 Short Stature
219 Splenomegaly
220 Strabismus
221 Strange Behavior
222 Stridor
223 Syncope
224 Tics
225 Torticollis
226 Vaginal Bleeding
227 Vaginal Discharge
228 Visual Development, Amblyopia, and Vision Testing
229 Vomiting
230 Weight Loss
231 Wheezing

Chapter 158

ABDOMINAL DISTENTION

Peter F. Belamarich, MD

The child with abdominal distention can be a formidable clinical challenge. The number of possible diagnoses is large, and the most likely diagnosis varies greatly with the child's age. Furthermore, not all distention is pathological. Healthy infants may have variable degrees of abdominal distention caused by aerophagia during feeding or crying or from transient constipation; healthy toddlers have a potbelly resulting from a combination of lumbar lordosis and hypotonia of the abdominal rectus muscles. The nonpathological distention often seen in infants and toddlers may exceed the mild distention seen with some intraabdominal malignancies. Thus, not surprisingly, numerous cautionary tales exist of parents being reassured by a physician that a child's mild and otherwise asymptomatic abdominal distention was normal, only later to learn that it was a tumor. Therefore a careful systematic approach should be used whenever concerns about abdominal distention are raised.

APPROACH TO THE CHILD WITH ABDOMINAL DISTENTION

History

Historical clues to the cause of distention in newborns are often absent, although they may at times be found in the pregnancy history; oligohydramnios suggests distal urinary obstruction, whereas polyhydramnios is seen with upper gastrointestinal obstruction. Although the use of routine prenatal sonography has led to the increased antenatal recognition of numerous congenital intraabdominal anomalies, particularly hydronephrosis, sonography is not as sensitive or diagnostically accurate when done prenatally as is sonography done on the newborn; a report of a normal prenatal sonogram does not rule out congenital causes of abdominal distention.

In older infants and children, the history should establish the duration and pattern of the child's distention. Whereas intermittent distention suggests intermittent gastrointestinal obstruction, progressive distention suggests an intraabdominal tumor, progressive hepatosplenomegaly, or ascites.

The primary care physician must be careful to differentiate a parent's question about whether a toddler's potbelly appearance is normal from more ominous reports of progressive or marked distention. When parents report that they have felt an abdominal mass, radiologic evaluation is indicated even if the physician does not appreciate the mass. Constitutional symptoms such as fever, weight loss, failure to thrive, anorexia, fatigue, irritability, or bone pain suggest a malignancy; however, their absence does not exclude one. Next, a systematic review of symptoms referable to the intraabdominal organs should be sought. Symptoms of gastrointestinal obstruction (vomiting, distention, pain, obstipation, delayed passage of meconium at birth) or malabsorption (diarrhea or greasy, bulky, malodorous stools) should be sought. The possibility of occult hydronephrosis should be considered, which, in the newborn, may exhibit initially as an asymptomatic flank mass. In older infants and children, recurrent fever from urinary tract infection (often misdiagnosed as viral illness or otitis media), gross hematuria after minor trauma, and voiding difficulty in boys who have posterior urethral valves are possible presentations.

A confidential history of sexual activity in all female adolescents who have abdominal distention should be obtained, as well as a history of the onset of puberty and menarche.

Given the number of possible diagnoses, a comprehensive medical and surgical history and review of systems is warranted. Medication use, including herbal and alternative therapies, should be reviewed, with particular attention paid to laxative use and to agents that can cause gastrointestinal ileus and constipation.

The family history should include questions about cystic fibrosis (meconium ileus), polycystic kidney disease, metabolic diseases, and whether any history exists of fetal demise or early neonatal deaths that might indicate an unrecognized metabolic disease, some of which produce hepatomegaly, splenomegaly, and congenital ascites.

Although rare, the presence of inherited syndromes that predispose a child to an intraabdominal malignancy should be remembered.[1] In the case of Wilms tumor, these include the WAGR syndrome (Wilms tumor, aniridia, genitourinary anomalies, and intellectual disability), Denys-Drash syndrome, and Beckwith-Wiedemann syndrome. An increased incidence of hepatoblastoma and adrenal carcinoma is also observed in children who have Beckwith-Wiedemann syndrome. Children with DNA fragility syndromes and immunodeficient states are at risk for lymphoma and leukemia.

Physical Examination

The profile of the abdomen should be inspected with the child in a supine position, noting whether the distention is generalized (maximal at the umbilicus) or localized. Box 158-1 presents commonly encountered causes for focal abdominal distention and common masses. The pattern and prominence of the abdominal veins should be noted. Prominent superficial veins on the abdomen may indicate portal hypertension or obstruction to the systemic venous return. The abdomen should be auscultated for hyperactive bowel sounds (malabsorption, acute obstruction), rushes (incomplete obstruction), and absence of sounds (paralytic ileus), as well as for bruits (vascular malformation).

Percussion can be used to differentiate diffuse versus more focal epigastric tympani and to identify shifting dullness in older children.

Gentle palpation should begin from the lower quadrants and progress upward so that the inferior edge of the liver and spleen are appreciated (massive hepatomegaly may be missed if the liver is compressible and the liver's edge is near the child's pelvis). The abdomen should be assessed for focal or generalized tenderness. Involuntary guarding noted on gentle palpation is a sensitive sign of peritoneal inflammation; assessment of rebound tenderness in young children is rife with false-positive results.

When an abdominal mass is appreciated, the examiner should note its location and whether it is painful, is mobile (intraabdominal) or nonmobile (retroperitoneal, malignant), moves with respiration (liver and spleen), is cystic or solid or malleable (fecal masses), is smooth or nodular, and whether it crosses the midline (often seen with neuroblastoma). Renal ballottement—lifting the kidney anteriorly with a finger in the costovertebral angle while palpating with the other hand—can help elicit and define features of masses in the flank. Although rectal examination is often avoided, properly done, this examination can add considerable information to the evaluation of children who have constipation, anal stenosis, Hirschsprung disease, and pelvic masses.

Infants who have ascites will have bilateral bulging flanks in the supine position. In older children who have ascites, the examiner may be able to elicit shifting dullness and a fluid wave. An acquired umbilical hernia may indicate massive ascites.

In female patients, a genital examination is necessary to exclude imperforate hymen with hydrometrocolpos or, in adolescents, hematocolpos and pregnancy. In both sexes, lower genitourinary tract malformation raises the question of upper genitourinary tract malformation.

BOX 158-1 Causes of Focal Abdominal Distention or Mass

EPIGASTRIUM
- Duodenal atresia
- Pyloric stenosis
- Malrotation
- Gastric duplication
- Bezoar

FLANK
- Wilms tumor
- Hydronephrosis
- Multicystic kidney
- Polycystic kidney
- Neuroblastoma
- Renal vein thrombosis
- Adrenal hemorrhage

RIGHT UPPER QUADRANT
- Choledochal cyst
- Hepatomegaly
- Hepatic tumors
- Acute hydrops of the gallbladder

LEFT UPPER QUADRANT
- Splenomegaly
- Splenic cyst

RIGHT LOWER QUADRANT
- Ovarian mass
- Intussusception
- Appendiceal abscess
- Crohn disease
- Fecal mass

LEFT LOWER QUADRANT
- Ovarian mass
- Fecal mass

HYPOGASTRIUM
- Hydrometrocolpos
- Hematocolpos
- Fecal mass
- Presacral teratoma
- Obstructed bladder
- Urachal cyst

DIFFERENTIAL DIAGNOSIS

The differential diagnosis can be narrowed based on whether the child has a tympanitic abdomen and/or prominent gastrointestinal symptoms, a palpable mass, ascites, or hypotonia of the abdominal wall (Table 158-1). Hepatomegaly and splenomegaly are reviewed in Chapters 190 and 219, respectively.

Tympanitic Abdomen in Newborns and Neonates

Tympanitic abdominal distention may occur in healthy infants, in infants who have systemic conditions, and in newborns who have congenital causes of intestinal obstruction.

Some healthy infants experience mild distention because of air swallowing with crying or feeding. This distention is variable, greatest after feeding or fussing, and absent at other times. Vomiting is absent, and the stooling pattern and physical examination are normal. This transient generalized distention responds to changes in feeding technique and burping and in consoling techniques for the crying infant.

In the ill newborn, many systemic conditions cause a paralytic intestinal ileus characterized by quiet, nontender abdominal distention: sepsis, birth asphyxia, hypothyroidism, and electrolyte imbalance. Newborns who have pneumonia or respiratory distress may also develop distention from aerophagia.

Table 158-1 Differential Diagnosis of Abdominal Distention Based on Physical Examination Findings

PHYSICAL SIGN	POSSIBLE CAUSES
Tympanitic abdomen	Gastrointestinal ileus Gastrointestinal obstruction Peritonitis Malabsorption Aerophagia Pneumoperitoneum
Palpable mass	Renal Adrenal, sympathetic Hepatic Gastrointestinal Mesenteric, omentum Uterine, vaginal, ovarian Splenic, lymphatic
Ascites	Urinary Idiopathic Cardiac Hepatic Biliary, gastrointestinal Chylous
Abdominal wall hypotonia	Generalized hypotonia Rickets Hypothyroidism
Peritonitis	Gastrointestinal perforation Bacterial peritonitis Chemical peritonitis

The most common cause of acquired abdominal distention in premature infants is necrotizing enterocolitis (NEC). Definitive radiographic evidence of NEC includes findings of (1) pneumatosis intestinalis and (2) gas visible in the portal venous system of the liver (Figure 158-1).

Congenital causes of proximal gastrointestinal obstruction causing distention in the newborn include intestinal atresias, annular pancreas, abnormalities of intestinal rotation, and fixation (see Chapter 266, Gastrointestinal Obstruction). The most common proximal gastrointestinal obstruction is duodenal atresia,[2] characterized by polyhydramnios in 50% of patients and the onset of bilious vomiting in the 1st hours of life in conjunction with focal epigastric distention (Figure 158-2). Upright plain-film radiographs are diagnostic of duodenal obstruction when they demonstrate the double-bubble sign. Occasionally, evacuating the stomach of bile and amniotic fluid and instilling air are necessary to appreciate duodenal obstruction. Intestinal atresias are medical emergencies in so far as urgent decompression via nasogastric suction is indicated to diminish the risk of aspiration and gastrointestinal perforation. Malrotation is seen in up to 19% of patients who have intrinsic duodenal obstruction; a barium enema should establish normal intestinal rotation in infants whose surgery is deferred.

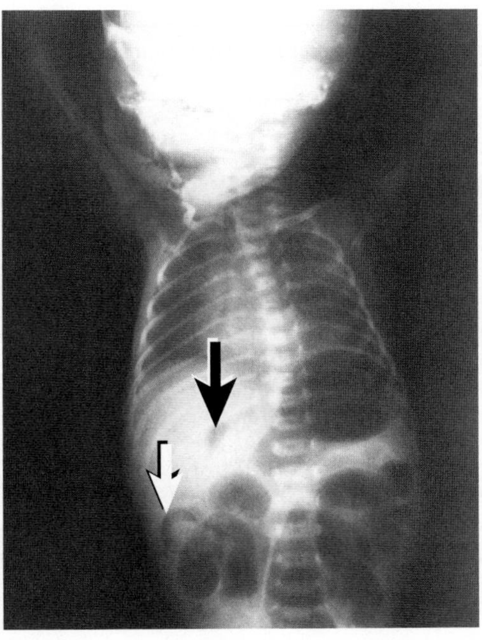

Figure 158-1 Radiograph of a premature infant with necrotizing enterocolitis showing gas in the wall of the intestine (white arrow) and portal venous gas (black arrow).

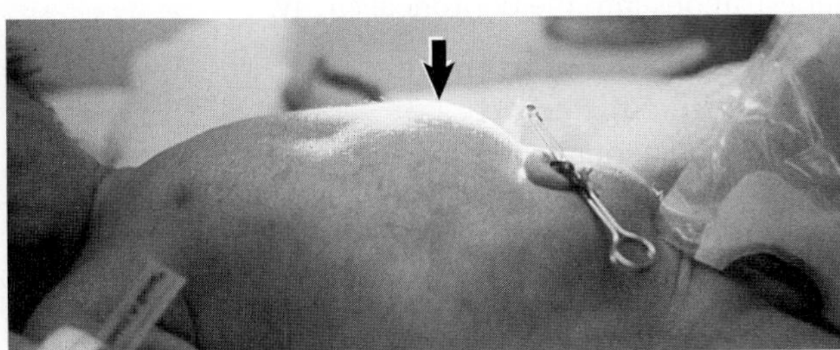

Figure 158-2 Newborn infant with duodenal atresia and upper abdominal distention.

Upper abdominal distention is a common, though not universal, finding in newborns and infants who have symptomatic intestinal malrotation,[3] the majority of whom will have bilious vomiting in the first 4 weeks of life. Approximately 25% of infants who have malrotation may have nonbilious vomiting; a high index of suspicion is warranted, given the severe morbidity of a delay in diagnosis. Plain-film radiographs may demonstrate a distended stomach or duodenal distention that has a paucity of gas distally (Figure 158-4). Most significantly, plain-film radiographs may appear normal. Therefore a stable infant thought to have malrotation should undergo an upper gastrointestinal series, which is diagnostic when the duodenal-jejunal junction is seen on the right side of the midline or when a beak or corkscrew obstruction is noted in the 2nd or 3rd part of the duodenum. Symptomatic malrotation is an operative emergency whether or not signs of intestinal ischemia (hematochezia, acidosis, shock, a blue-gray tinge to the abdomen, or peritonitis) have developed.

Congenital causes of lower intestinal obstruction include distal intestinal atresias, meconium ileus (Figure 158-5), Hirschsprung disease, small left colon syndrome, and anorectal malformations (see Chapter 266, Gastrointestinal Obstruction). Newborns who have lower intestinal obstruction typically develop generalized tympanitic distention over the course of 24 to

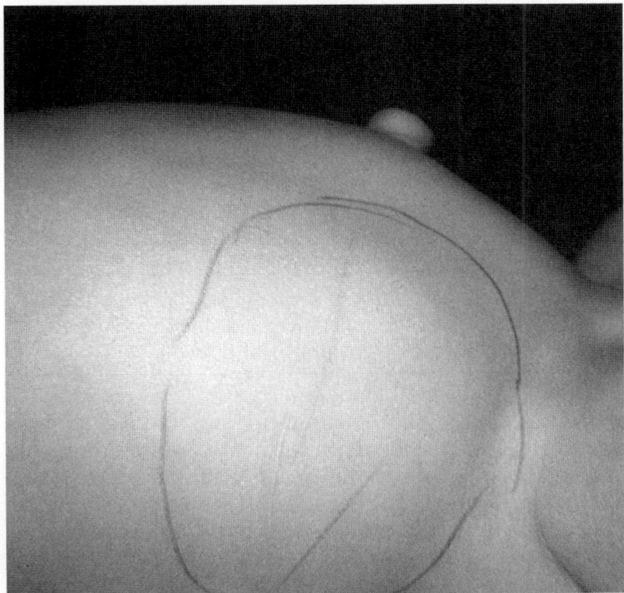

Figure 158-3 Newborn with distention secondary to torsion.

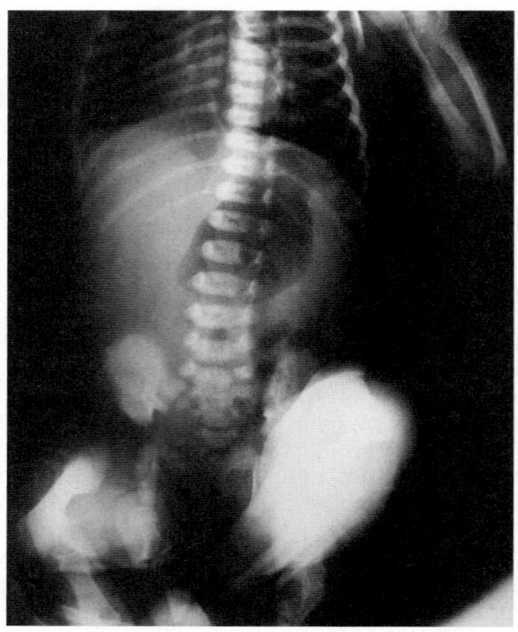

Figure 158-4 Malrotation with distended stomach and paucity of distal gas.

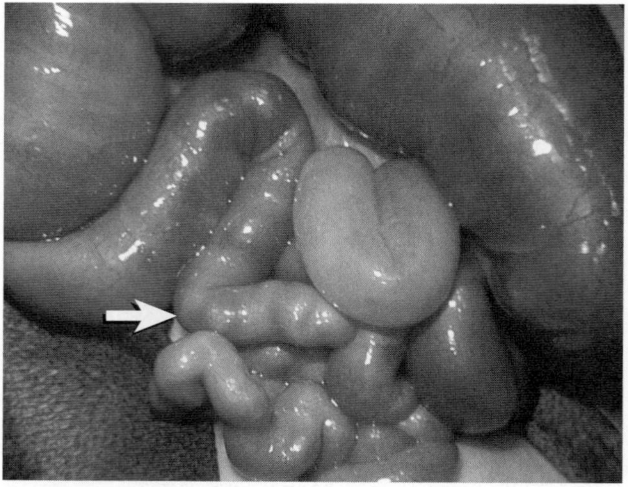

Figure 158-5 Distal ileum segment with inspissated meconium secondary to meconium ileus (arrow) surrounded by dilated proximal loops of bowel.

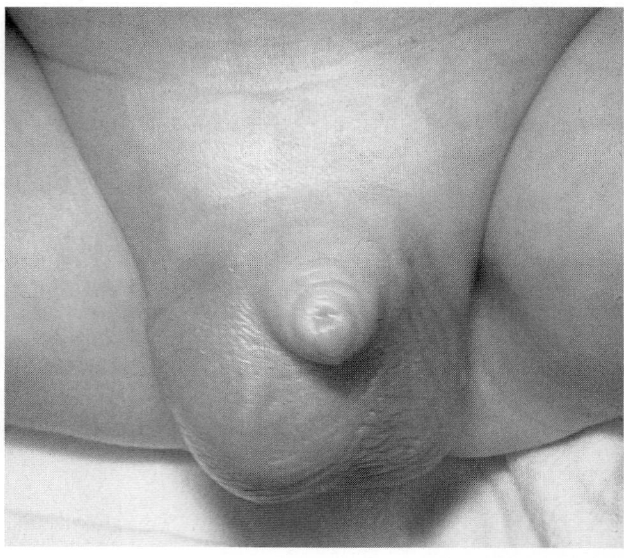

Figure 158-6 Incarcerated right inguinal hernia in a newborn.

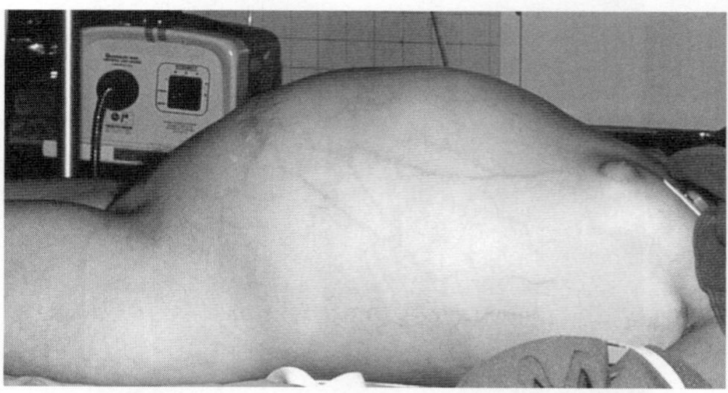

Figure 158-7 Thirteen-year-old girl with severe fecal impaction.

48 hours, with bilious vomiting and failure to pass meconium. Although an imperforate anus or an incarcerated hernia (Figure 158-6) will be apparent on physical examination, differentiation of the remaining causes of lower intestinal obstruction involves radiographic evaluation.

Marked tympanitic abdominal distention can be a manifestation of pneumoperitoneum, which is demonstrated by upright and cross-table lateral abdominal radiographs revealing free air within the peritoneum. When pneumoperitoneum is associated with peritonitis, intestinal perforation is likely, and the causes include NEC, volvulus, an intestinal obstruction causing perforation, appendicitis, and spontaneous perforations. In infants on a respirator, pneumoperitoneum may occur without peritonitis as a complication of pneumomediastinum when air tracks down through diaphragmatic fenestrations into the peritoneal cavity.

Tympanitic Abdomen Beyond the Neonatal Period

Beyond the neonatal period, the causes of a tympanitic abdomen includes constipation, mechanical obstruction, paralytic ileus, and malabsorption.

Idiopathic constipation is extremely common throughout childhood but is accompanied only infrequently by abdominal distention (Figure 158-7). The diagnosis is supported by a history of hard or large, infrequent stools beginning after the neonatal period. Frequently, periumbilical pain is present. Rectal examination should reveal a hard, large fecal mass in a generous rectal vault. The child's distention should be relieved completely by an enema or laxative therapy. Persistent distention should not be attributed to functional constipation (see Chapter 166, Constipation).

Gastrointestinal obstructions that cause a tympanitic abdomen beyond the neonatal period can be a result of late presentations of congenital problems or of acquired causes, including intraluminal obstructions such as pyloric stenosis, intussusception, bezoars, meconium ileus equivalent, intestinal polyps, ascariasis, and intrinsic tumors. Extraluminal obstructions include postoperative adhesions, appendiceal abscesses, a Meckel diverticulum, and extrinsic compression by abdominal or pelvic masses.

Children with paralytic ileus have a clinical picture similar to that seen with distal mechanical bowel obstruction; however, bowel sounds are diminished or absent, and plain-film radiographs demonstrate air throughout the gastrointestinal tract. Common precipitants include abdominal surgery, peritonitis, trauma, shock, sepsis, hypokalemia, and anesthesia, as well as numerous medications. Recurrent attacks of unexplained ileus characterize intestinal pseudoobstruction syndrome.

Finally, tympanitic distention occurs in conjunction with the fat malabsorption syndromes, cystic fibrosis, and celiac disease. These conditions are characterized by steatorrhea and variable degrees of malnutrition and growth failure with muscle wasting, creating the picture of a thin-limbed child who has a bloated abdomen.

Abdominal Masses in Newborns and Neonates

Two thirds of abdominal masses in neonates originate from the kidney or the urinary tract.[4] Renal masses are retroperitoneal, nonmobile, and appreciated either in the flank or on deep abdominal palpation. Cystic masses predominate and have a slightly compressible quality. A multicystic kidney is the single most common neonatal flank mass. It is unilateral in 70% to 80% of cases. The affected kidney lacks parenchyma, is associated with ipsilateral ureteral atresia, and is composed of macroscopically visible, variably sized, fluid-filled cysts that may be appreciable on physical examination as a soft mass with a slightly irregular contour.

The next most frequently encountered renal mass is caused by hydronephrosis (see Chapter 300, Obstructive Uropathy and Vesicoureteral Reflux). A smooth flank mass in an otherwise well newborn is usually from a ureteral-pelvic junction obstruction. Posterior urethral valves, a common cause of bilateral hydronephrosis and hydroureters in male infants, may exhibit as a low-pressure urinary stream and bilateral flank masses or a palpable bladder. Newborns who have autosomal-recessive polycystic kidney disease may have palpable bilateral firm flank masses, oliguria, hematuria, and hypertension. Ultrasonography reveals the kidneys to be enlarged. Renal vein thrombosis is a rare but important cause of a smooth flank mass and hematuria, which develop concurrently in an ill newborn after an episode of asphyxia, sepsis, or dehydration or in an infant whose mother has diabetes.

Finally, the most common renal tumor encountered in the newborn is not Wilms tumor but mesoblastic nephroma, a surgically curable tumor that may cause massive unilateral nephromegaly.

The remaining one third of neonatal abdominal masses arise outside of the urinary tract. Of these, neuroblastoma, gastrointestinal duplications, hydrometrocolpos, and ovarian cysts account for a large proportion.[4] Gastrointestinal duplications, which may be found as mobile asymptomatic abdominal masses in the newborn, arise most often from the jejunum, ileum, or cecum. Duplications may obstruct the gastrointestinal tract by direct compression or by acting as a lead point for an intussusception or for a volvulus, or they may contain heterotopic gastric mucosa that produces enough acid to cause an ulceration, resulting in lower gastrointestinal bleeding and sometimes perforation with peritonitis.

Female newborns may have a lower abdominal or pelvic mass from hydrometrocolpos, which develops as a result of an upper or lower vaginal obstruction in combination with a secretory response to a high level of maternal estrogens in utero. An imperforate hymen will be evident on the genital examination as a bulging round membrane within the introitus. Rectal examination can be diagnostic for the presence of a dilated vagina in higher obstructions. Maternal estrogens may also induce the development of a large functional or follicular ovarian cyst in newborns.

When a neonate has a palpable flank mass after a traumatic or breech delivery, the possibility of an adrenal hemorrhage should be considered, as should hepatic and splenic hematomas. Other hepatic masses and hepatomegaly are discussed in Chapters 190, Hepatomegaly, and 219, Splenomegaly. Although rare, a significant number of benign epithelial cysts may arise in the neonatal period, including choledochal cysts (right upper quadrant), splenic cysts (left upper quadrant), mesenteric cysts (mid-abdominal, mobile in the transverse plane), and urachal cysts (hypogastrium). Retroperitoneal cysts include abdominal lymphangiomas and pancreatic cysts.

Abdominal Masses in Infants and Children

The differential diagnosis of masses in infants and older children includes late presentations of congenital masses, malignancies, fecal masses, bezoars, and pancreatic pseudocysts. Of the congenital masses, gastrointestinal duplications, mesenteric cysts, and choledochal cysts may enlarge slowly and become apparent in later infancy or childhood. Similarly, an adolescent who has an imperforate hymen or vaginal septum may not become symptomatic with a pelvic mass from hematocolpos until the onset of cyclical uterine bleeding.

The abdomen is the site of origin of Wilms tumor, hepatic tumors, ovarian tumors, approximately 70% of neuroblastomas, and 30% of non-Hodgkin lymphomas (see Chapter 244, Cancers in Childhood). Neuroblastoma, Wilms tumor, and hepatoblastoma in particular have a propensity to produce asymptomatic abdominal distention that is frequently noted by the parent during bathing or dressing the child or by the physician on routine physical examination. Wilms tumor tends to occur in older infants and toddlers, with a peak incidence in 2- to 5-year-old children (Figure 158-8). Hypertension is

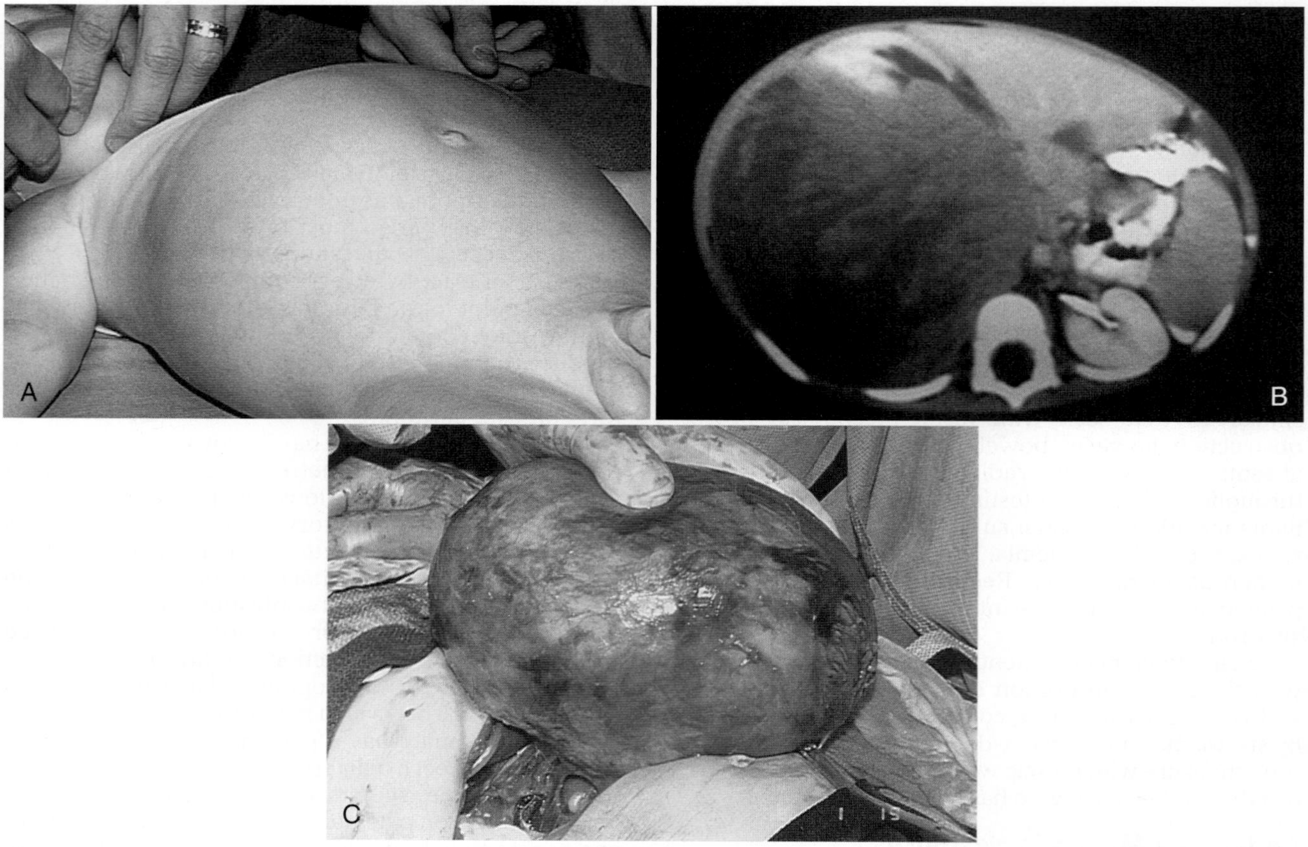

Figure 158-8 **A,** Abdominal distention because of right-sided Wilms tumor. **B,** Computed tomographic scan of tumor. **C,** Tumor exposed during surgery.

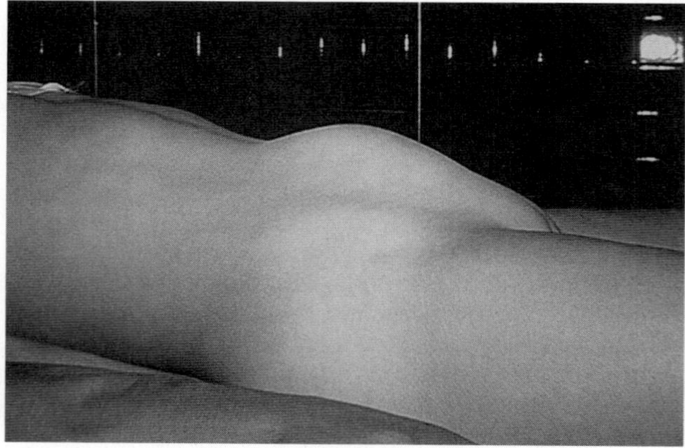

Figure 158-9 Lower abdominal distention caused by ovarian teratoma.

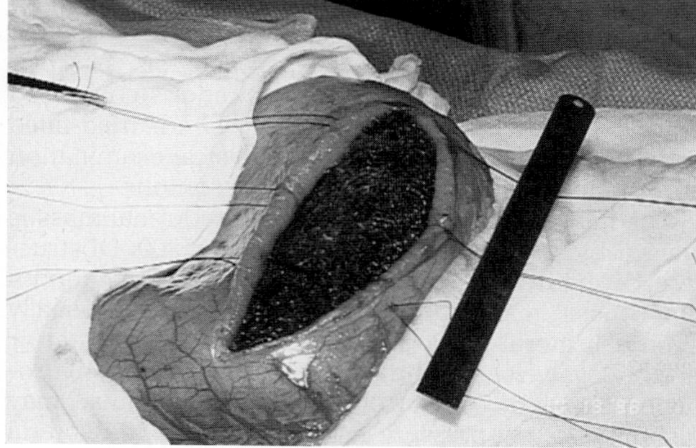

Figure 158-10 Trichobezoar in the stomach.

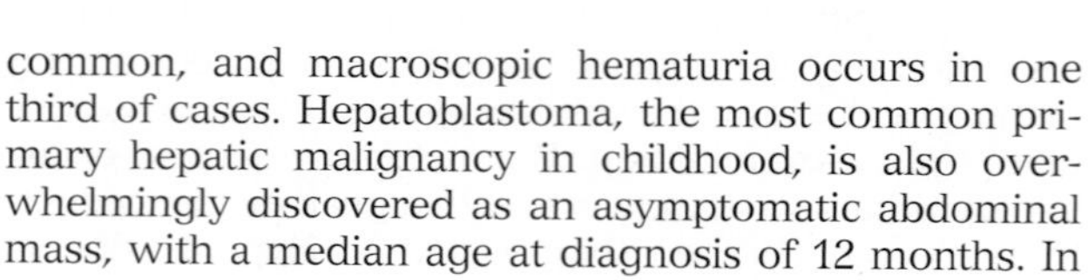

common, and macroscopic hematuria occurs in one third of cases. Hepatoblastoma, the most common primary hepatic malignancy in childhood, is also overwhelmingly discovered as an asymptomatic abdominal mass, with a median age at diagnosis of 12 months. In the 2nd decade, tumors exhibiting as an abdominal mass are predominantly ovarian (Figure 158-9) or non-Hodgkin's lymphoma (see Chapter 244, Cancers in Childhood).

Fecal masses are extremely common in childhood and adolescence and may be found in the right lower

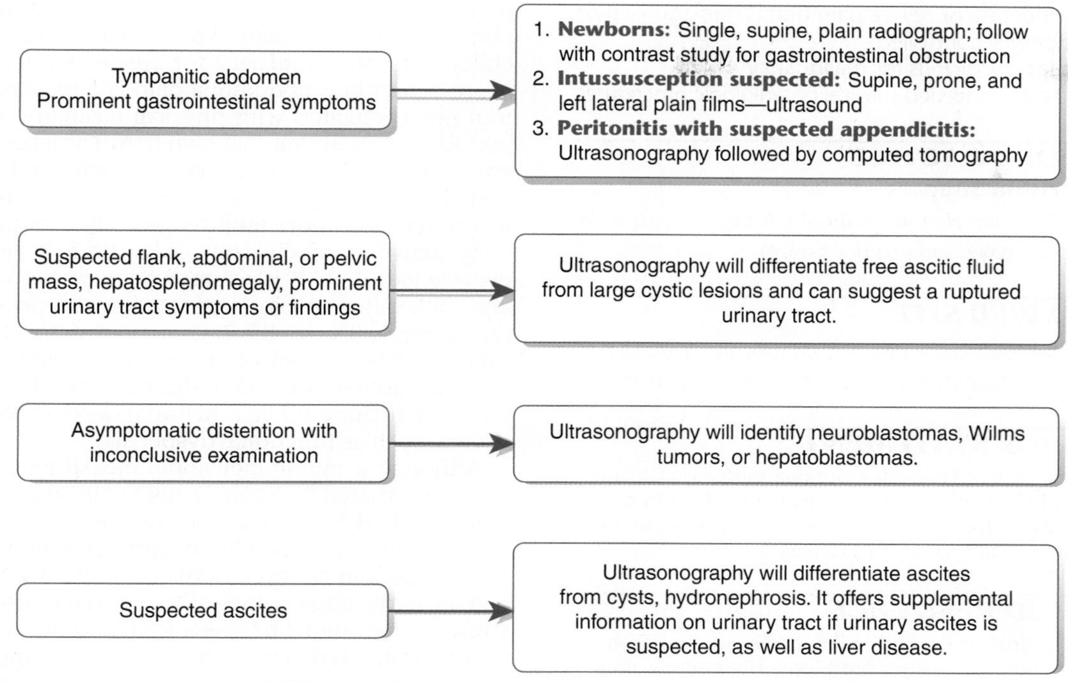

Figure 158-11 Initial radiographic approach to abdominal distention in infants and children.

quadrant (when a redundant sigmoid colon loops to the right), in the hypogastrium, or in the left lower quadrant. They are mobile, nontender, and malleable. In questionable cases, plain-film radiographs can confirm the diagnosis. Reexamination is indicated after laxative therapy to confirm that the masses are no longer present.

Bezoars, which are intragastric concretions of indigestible material, can cause a large array of gastrointestinal complications, including upper abdominal discomfort and a large mass. Most bezoars are seen in girls with psychiatric disorders, commonly resulting from the ingestion of hair (Figure 158-10).

Ascites in Newborns and Neonates

The newborn with ascites has a distended, nontympanitic abdomen with bulging and dullness in the flanks, findings that may be mimicked by a massively dilated bladder, a severely hydronephrotic kidney, or a large ovarian cyst. In the newborn, ascites results most often from a perforation within an obstructed urinary tract; in boys, posterior urethral valves are a common precipitant.[5] Ascites also occurs as a complication of congestive heart failure or of liver disease caused by congenital infections, galactosemia, or a lysosomal storage disease, and it has been reported in association with intestinal malrotation. Chylous ascites is a rare condition that occurs when lymphatic fluid leaks directly into the peritoneum because of a malformation or perforation of the intestinal lymphatics occurring in utero. The diagnosis is made by paracentesis, when the characteristic milky-appearing ascitic fluid is found to have a high level of triglycerides. Idiopathic or benign ascites is a diagnosis of exclusion and resolves without treatment.

Beyond the neonatal period, ascites occurs most commonly as a consequence of chronic liver disease with cirrhosis and portal hypertension.

Abdominal Wall Hypotonia

Abdominal distention is frequently encountered in healthy infants and may also be seen in infants with a variety of neuromuscular conditions that produce generalized hypotonia. Hypothyroidism and rickets are treatable conditions in which abdominal distention may be part of a subtle symptom complex that develops insidiously.

Radiographic Approach

Although the history and physical examination sometimes provide the diagnosis, many children who have abdominal distention require radiographic imaging. The choice of initial imaging modality is dictated both by clinical suspicion and by locally available resources and expertise. Therefore consulting with the radiologist is helpful (see Chapter 15, Pediatric Imaging).

Some general guidelines for choosing an initial radiologic study are presented in Figure 158-11.

The author wishes to thank Kenneth Kenigsberg, MD, for providing the photographs used in this chapter.

WHEN TO ADMIT

A child with abdominal distention in the presence of:

- Refractory vomiting, dehydration
- Peritonitis
- Toxic or septic appearance

- Moderate or severe pain that is undiagnosed or not well controlled
- Mass suspicious for malignancy
- Urgently needed surgical or radiologic procedures

TOOLS FOR PRACTICE

Medical Decision Support

- *Pediatric Nutrition Handbook* (book), American Academy of Pediatrics (www.aap.org/bookstore).

RELATED WEB SITE

- National Association for Pediatric Gastroenterology Hepatology and Nutrition (NASPGHAN) (www.naspghan.org/).

AAP POLICY STATEMENT

American Academy of Pediatrics, Subcommittee on Chronic Abdominal Pain. Chronic Abdominal Pain in Children. *Pediatrics.* 2005;115(3):812-815. (aappolicy.aappublications.org/cgi/content/full/pediatrics;115/3/812).

SUGGESTED RESOURCE

Constipation Guideline Committee of the North American Society for Pediatric Gastroenterology, Hepatology, and Nutrition. Evaluation and treatment of constipation in infants and children: recommendations of the North American Society for Pediatric Gastroenterology, Hepatology, and Nutrition. *J Pediatr Gastroenterol Nutr.* 2006; 43(3):e1-13.

REFERENCES

1. Worth L. Molecular and cellular biology of cancer. In: Berman RE, Kliegman RM, Jensen HB, eds: *Nelson Textbook of Pediatrics.* 17th ed. Philadelphia, PA: WB Saunders; 2004.
2. Escobar MA, Ladd AP, Grosfeld KW, et al. Duodenal atresia and stenosis: long-term follow-up over 30 years. *J Pediatr Surg.* Jun 2004;39(6):867-871.
3. Torres MA, Ziegler MM. Malrotation of the intestine. *World J Surg.* 1993;17:326-331.
4. McVicar M, Margoulett D, Chandra M. Diagnosis and imaging of the fetal and neonatal abdominal mass: an integrated approach. *Adv Pediatr.* 1991;38:135-147.
5. Griscom NT, Colodny AH, Rosenberg HK, et al. Molecular and cellular biology of cancer diagnostic aspects of neonatal ascites: report of 27 cases. *AM J Roentgenol.* 1977;128: 961-969.

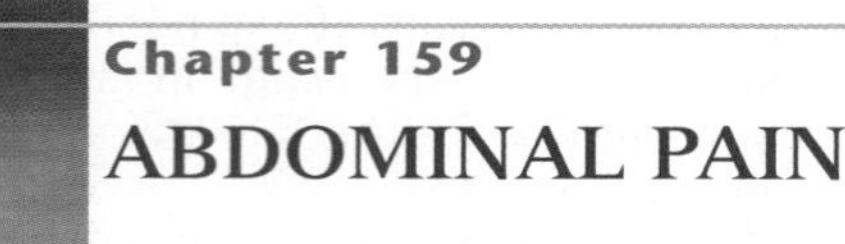

Chapter 159

ABDOMINAL PAIN

Anthony M. Loizides, MD; Barry K. Wershil, MD

Abdominal pain is one of the most common symptoms in children and adolescents and is estimated to account for approximately 5% of unscheduled office visits.[1] Acute abdominal pain may require medical or surgical intervention to prevent disability or even death. The precise number of children who experience acute abdominal pain is unknown, but each year, 4 in 1000 children undergo surgery for suspected appendicitis. More commonly, abdominal pain is a recurrent symptom not associated with physical disability or mortality.[2] Recurrent abdominal pain (RAP) as a recognizable entity in childhood was first characterized by Apley and Naish as pain that occurs at least three times over a period of 3 or more months severely enough to affect daily activities in children older than 3 years.[3] The prevalence of RAP is estimated to be between 0.3% and 19%, although in large studies the prevalence is far lower, 0.3% to 8%.[4] One reason for the broad range may be the lack of uniformity of criteria for making the diagnosis of RAP; definitions may be too broad and may include other functional gastrointestinal disorders, such as functional dyspepsia.[4]

Although a multidimensional measurement of RAP has been created,[5] no consensus exists on an exact definition of RAP. Some trends have been noted, such as a higher prevalence of RAP in girls. The highest prevalence occurs in children between 4 and 6 years of age and in early adolescence. Studies have also demonstrated associations between RAP and the child's family dynamics (eg, children living in a single-parent household are more likely to experience RAP[6]), psychological comorbidity such as anxiety,[7] and socioeconomic environment in which children living in low-income, low-educated–worker families were more likely to experience pain.[8]

Criteria have been established in adults to categorize abdominal pain: the Rome I criteria, later updated as Rome II to improve the definition of functional gastrointestinal disorders. Although this classification system can help categorize patients so appropriate treatment options can be considered, not all children can be clearly placed in these categories. Some authorities have argued against using the classification in children,[9] with one major reason being that the most common location of RAP is periumbilical pain, and this is not considered in the Rome II criteria. Twenty-seven percent of children with abdominal pain do not meet Rome II criteria.[10]

Pediatric gastroenterologists have identified and developed similar criteria for childhood functional disorders, including RAP.[11] These criteria—the Rome III Criteria for Functional Bowel Disorders Associated With Abdominal Pain or Discomfort in Children—are based on symptom classification. Four classes were identified, including (1) functional dyspepsia, (2) irritable bowel syndrome, (3) childhood functional abdominal pain (with a subgroup of children having childhood functional abdominal pain syndrome), and (4) abdominal migraine. The usefulness of the Rome III criteria has yet to be established.

Along with the difficulty in characterizing different types of functional abdominal pain, assessing the effectiveness of various treatments is also difficult. For example, a well-known fact is that significant inconsistencies exist in the methodologic approaches currently used to assess pain.[12] The influence of age and developmental maturation, individual differences (eg, temperament, coping patterns), family interactions, and community and cultural contexts may

BOX 159-1 Differential Diagnosis of Recurrent Abdominal Pain Based on Symptom Subtype Associated With Symptoms of Dyspepsia

- Associated with upper gastrointestinal inflammation
  - Gastroesophageal reflux disease
  - Peptic ulcer
  - *Helicobacter pylori* gastritis
  - Nonsteroidal antiinflammatory drug ulcer
  - Crohn disease
  - Eosinophilic gastroenteritis
  - Ménétrier disease
  - Cytomegalovirus gastritis
  - Parasitic infection *(Giardia, Blastocystis hominis)*
  - Varioliform gastritis
  - Lymphocytic gastritis or celiac disease
  - Henoch-Schönlein purpura
- Motility disorders
  - Idiopathic gastroparesis
  - Biliary dyskinesia
  - Intestinal pseudo-obstruction
- Other
  - Obstructive disorders
  - Chronic pancreatitis
  - Chronic hepatitis
  - Chronic cholecystitis
  - Ureteropelvic junction obstruction
  - Abdominal migraine
  - Psychiatric disorders
- Associated with altered bowel pattern
  - Idiopathic inflammatory bowel disorders
  - Ulcerative colitis
  - Crohn disease
  - Microscopic colitis with crypt distortion
  - Lymphocytic colitis
  - Collagenous colitis
  - Infectious disorders
  - Parasitic *(Giardia, Blastocystis hominis, Dientamoeba fragilis)*
  - Bacterial *(Clostridium difficile, Yersinia, Campylobacter, tuberculosis)*
  - Lactose intolerance
  - Complication of constipation—megacolon, encopresis, intermittent sigmoid volvulus
  - Drug-induced diarrhea, constipation
  - Gynecologic disorders
  - Neoplasia (lymphoma, carcinoma)
  - Psychiatric disorders
- Presenting as isolated paroxysmal abdominal pain
  - Obstructive disorders
  - Crohn disease
  - Malrotation with or without volvulus
  - Intussusception with lead point
  - Postsurgical adhesions
  - Small bowel lymphoma
  - Endometriosis
  - Infection (tuberculosis, *Yersinia*)
  - Vascular disorders
  - Eosinophilic gastroenteritis
  - Angioneurotic edema
  - Appendiceal colic
  - Dysmenorrhea
  - Musculoskeletal disorders
  - Uteropelvic junction obstruction
  - Abdominal migraine
  - Acute intermittent porphyria
  - Mental disorders (factitious disorder, conversion reaction, somatization disorder, school phobia)
  - Functional abdominal pain

From Boyle JT. Pediatric gastrointestinal disease. In: Walker WA, ed. *Pathophysiology, Diagnosis, Management.* 4th ed. Hamilton, Ontario, Canada: BC Decker; 2004. Reprinted by permission.

influence the expression of RAP. To address some of these issues, a multidimensional analytic approach has been developed to assess the primary outcome in clinical trials.[5]

In light of suboptimal classification and assessment tools, a symptom-based differential diagnosis with an emphasis on identifying the warning signals for organic disease is currently the most useful approach to patient care. However, primary care physicians must recognize that functional abdominal pain can lead to significant dysfunction and disability, with school absences, repeated visits to health care professionals, and secondary psychological problems if assessment and initiation of treatment are either ignored or delayed.[13] Box 159-1 lists the causes of RAP by symptom subtype.

DIFFERENTIAL DIAGNOSIS

The differential diagnosis of acute abdominal pain can be subdivided into three broad categories: (1) conditions that require immediate surgical intervention (Box 159-2), (2) conditions that may be managed medically at first but may require surgical involvement (Box 159-3), and (3) specific conditions that can be managed medically (Box 159-4).[14] The differential diagnosis, evaluation, and management of the acute surgical abdomen are discussed in Chapter 238, Appendicitis. The differential diagnosis of acute abdominal pain based on age is provided in Box 159-5.

Entities that may require a combined surgical and medical management are primarily associated with the gastrointestinal lumen and its associated organs (see Box 159-3) and can include postsurgical complications

BOX 159-2 Differential Diagnosis of Acute Surgical Abdomen

- Closed loop intestinal obstruction
- Volvulus (gastric, midgut, sigmoid)
- Incarcerated hernia (inguinal, internal, external)
- High-grade bowel obstruction
- Nonreducible intussusception
- Malrotation with Ladd bands
- Ovarian torsion
- Testicular torsion
- Acute appendicitis
- Perforated viscus with diffuse peritonitis or toxicity
- Ruptured tumor
- Ectopic pregnancy

From Boyle JT. Pediatric gastrointestinal disease. In: Walker WA, ed. *Pathophysiology, Diagnosis, Management*. 4th ed. Hamilton, Ontario, Canada: BC Decker; 2004. Reprinted by permission.

BOX 159-3 Differential Diagnosis of Acute Abdominal Pain That May Require a Combined Surgical and Medical Approach

- Partial small bowel obstruction
- Postsurgical adhesions
- Crohn disease
- Lymphoma
- Periappendiceal abscess
- Abdominal abscess
- Cholecystitis
- Gallbladder hydrops
- Pancreatitis
- Pancreatic pseudocyst
- Toxic megacolon or typhlitis

From Boyle JT. Pediatric gastrointestinal disease. In: Walker WA, ed. *Pathophysiology, Diagnosis, Management*. 4th ed. Hamilton, Ontario, Canada: BC Decker; 2004. Reprinted by permission.

BOX 159-4 Differential Diagnosis of Acute Abdominal Pain That Requires Medical Management

- Upper respiratory infection, pharyngitis
- Viral gastroenteritis (mesenteric adenitis)
- Pneumonia
- Partial bowel obstruction
- Paralytic ileus
- Fecal impaction
- Meconium ileus equivalent in cystic fibrosis
- Bacterial enterocolitis
- Acute gastritis or peptic ulcer
- Acute constipation
- Flare of functional abdominal pain
- Acute hepatitis
- Perihepatitis (Fitz-Hugh–Curtis syndrome)
- Inflammatory bowel disease (Crohn disease and ulcerative colitis)
- Henoch-Schönlein purpura
- Hemolytic uremic syndrome
- Collagen vascular disease
- Hereditary angioedema
- Pyelonephritis
- Renal calculi
- Pelvic inflammatory disease
- Sickle cell crisis
- Diabetic ketoacidosis
- Dysmenorrhea
- Mittelschmerz
- Poisoning
- Porphyria
- Intestinal gas pain

From Boyle JT. Pediatric gastrointestinal disease. In: Walker WA, ed. *Pathophysiology, Diagnosis, Management*. 4th ed. Hamilton, Ontario, Canada: BC Decker; 2004. Reprinted by permission.

such as abdominal abscess or pancreatitis. Pancreatitis deserves special mention as a possible cause of abdominal pain. Acute pancreatitis is defined as the abrupt commencement of abdominal pain associated with an increase of acinar digestive enzymes detected in the blood or urine, which resolves with total restoration of pancreatic structure and function. In contrast with adults, in whom over three quarters of cases are associated with alcoholism and biliary tract disease, the causes of acute pancreatitis in children, which are diverse and which have shifted over time,[15] are as follows: idiopathic causes (23%), trauma (22%), structural anomalies (15%), multisystem disease (14%), drugs and toxins (12%), viral infections (10%), hereditary (2%), and metabolic disorders such as hyperlipidemia and hypercalcemia (2%).[16]

Injury of the acinar cells and the premature activation of trypsinogen to trypsin in the pancreas caused by obstruction of ductal flow (in most cases) precipitates an aggressive immune response, resulting in the clinical entity of pancreatitis. Its manifestation ranges from mild abdominal pain to severe systemic involvement exemplified by metabolic derangements and shock. Abdominal pain is present in nearly everyone, and it can be sudden in onset or insidious. Although the most common location is the epigastrium, pain can be described as in either the right or the left upper quadrant. The classic radiation of the pain to the back described in the adult population is not present in most children.[17] Other accompanying symptoms are vomiting, anorexia, and nausea. Commonly, food aggravates pain and vomiting. On assessment, children may be sick, irritable, quiet or exhibit all of these signs. They usually lie still because movement intensifies the pain.

BOX 159-5 Main Causes of Acute Abdominal Pain by Age

NEONATE
- Necrotizing enterocolitis
- Spontaneous gastric perforation
- Hirschsprung disease
- Meconium ileus
- Intestinal atresia or stenosis
- Peritonitis owing to gastroschisis or ruptured omphalocele
- Traumatic perforation of viscus (difficult birth)

INFANT (<2 YEARS)
- Colic (<3 months)
- Acute gastroenteritis or viral syndrome
- Traumatic perforation of viscus (child abuse)
- Intussusception
- Incarcerated hernia
- Volvulus (malrotation)
- Sickling syndromes

SCHOOL AGE (2-13 YEARS)
- Acute gastroenteritis or viral syndrome
- Urinary tract infection
- Appendicitis
- Trauma
- Constipation
- Pneumonia
- Sickling syndromes

ADOLESCENT
- Acute gastroenteritis or viral syndrome
- Urinary tract infection
- Appendicitis
- Trauma
- Constipation
- Pelvic inflammatory disease
- Pneumonia
- Mittelschmerz

From Boyle JT. Pediatric gastrointestinal disease. In: Walker WA, ed. *Pathophysiology, Diagnosis, Management.* 4th ed. Hamilton, Ontario, Canada: BC Decker; 2004. Reprinted by permission.

Examination of the abdomen may reveal decreased bowel sounds, guarding, rebound tenderness, or any combination, and systemic signs may be present such as fever, hypotension, and tachycardia. Gray Turner and Cullen signs—discoloration of the flanks and umbilicus, respectively—are typical of hemorrhagic pancreatitis, but they are seldom present in children.

The concept of *referred pain* is especially relevant when discussing acute abdominal pain in children. A complete history may provide crucial information that suggests the abdominal pain may originate outside the abdomen. For example, a 3-year-old who has pneumonia may have inflammatory irritation of the diaphragm, resulting in acute abdominal pain as the presenting complaint. In addition, perihepatitis (Fitz-Hugh–Curtis syndrome) can produce acute abdominal pain, and the physician should be sensitive to an adolescent girl's possible reluctance to disclose spontaneously a history of sexual intercourse. The differential diagnoses of medical entities, including those that are extraabdominal or systemic, are listed in Box 159-4.

Box 159-5 lists some of the major diagnostic considerations for acute abdominal pain by children.[14] Although diagnostic considerations overlap for each age group, the child's age and physiological development can help the physician focus the differential diagnosis. For example, Hirschsprung disease should be considered more likely in an infant in the first weeks of life; Mittelschmerz should most certainly be in the differential diagnosis for an adolescent girl.

EVALUATION

History

The approach to the evaluation of abdominal pain begins with a complete history and a thorough physical examination, which should direct the use of selected laboratory studies that are based on a reasonable differential diagnosis and that will permit a clear therapeutic strategy to be created. Figure 159-1 summarizes the evaluation of the child or adolescent who has abdominal pain.[18,19] The history alone accounts for most of the data the physician uses in making a diagnosis.

A systematic history should elicit information about the location, onset, and severity of the pain; alleviating and precipitating factors; and associated symptoms. The timing of the onset and changes in the intensity, location, and quality of pain over time are essential factors in determining its cause. For children or adolescents who have recurring abdominal pain, information about the timing of the onset of the pain in relation to other events (eg, mealtime, school days), as well as the duration of each episode and the frequency of recurrence, is helpful. Additional information about family (inherited disorders, concurrent illnesses, chronic pain disorders), medical history (prior surgery, chronic medication, faltering growth), and environmental or behavioral factors (recent changes in family or school, travel, unusual food) should also be obtained.

Pain frequency, severity, location, and effects on lifestyle cannot be used to distinguish between an organic or a functional cause for chronic abdominal pain. However, children with RAP are more likely than children without RAP to have headache, joint pain, anorexia, vomiting, nausea, excessive gas, and altered bowel symptoms. However, the presence or absence of associated symptoms does not help the physician distinguish between functional and organic disorders. The presence of alarming symptoms or signs suggests a higher probability or prevalence of organic disease and may justify performing diagnostic tests and referring the child to a subspecialist. Alarm symptoms or signs include, but are not limited to, involuntary weight loss, deceleration of linear growth, gastrointestinal blood loss, significant vomiting, chronic severe diarrhea, persistent right upper or right lower quadrant pain, unexplained fever, and family history of

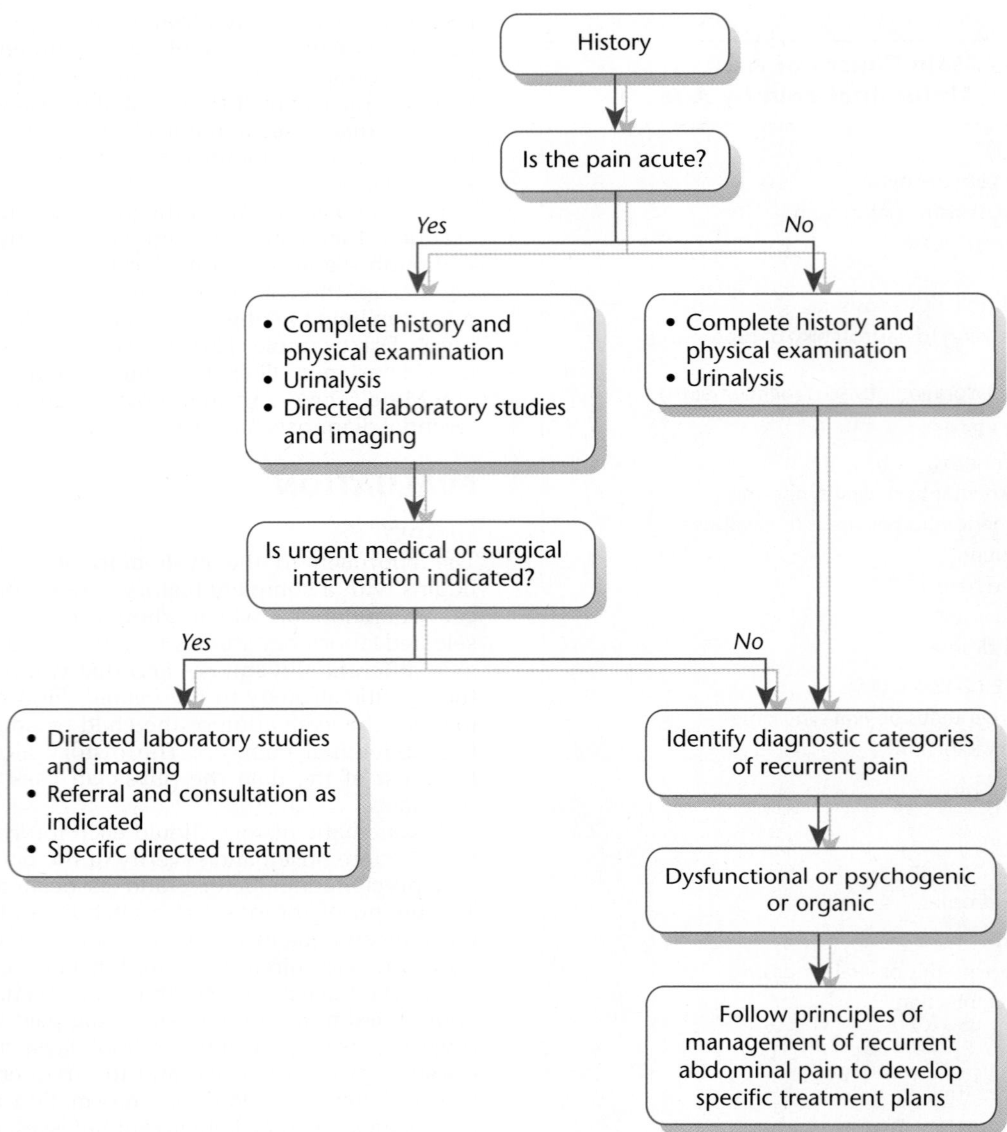

Figure 159-1 Evaluation of child or adolescent who has abdominal pain.

inflammatory bowel disease (see When to Refer).[20] No single test can diagnose functional abdominal pain. In patients with RAP a component of pain can be visceral hyperanalgesia,[21] which provides a physiological explanation of symptoms in children who have distinct functional gastrointestinal disorders.

The physician should help the family understand the importance of the history during the assessment. Both the parents and the patient should be interviewed (see Chapter 13, Interviewing Children). The patient must feel comfortable in discussing the person's own symptoms and concerns, even if these are different from those expressed by the parents. Obtaining a history from the patient without the parents present is therefore often useful; similarly, the parents may want to relate some of their concerns without the child being present. Important diagnostic information can be missed if the primary care physician does not give the child and parents the opportunity to provide separate histories.

In addition to the presence of specific symptoms and positive history, negative aspects of the history can provide important information to narrow the differential diagnosis. For example, the absence of dysuria in an older child or adolescent would make the diagnosis of urinary tract infection unlikely.

Physical Examination

Physical examination of children with recurrent or chronic abdominal pain has rarely been described. The presence of tenderness on abdominal palpation has been reported to be characteristic of children with recurrent episodes of abdominal pain without evidence of organic disease,[22] but most children's physical examination will be normal. A normal examination

BOX 159-6 Suggested Screening Laboratory Tests

ALL PATIENTS
- Complete blood count with differential
- Erythrocyte sedimentation rate
- Comprehensive metabolic panel
- Stool hemoccult

DIARRHEA
- Stool ova and parasite
- *Giardia* enzyme-linked immunosorbent assay
- *Clostridium difficile* toxin
- Celiac panel
- Lactose breath test

DYSPEPSIA
- *Helicobacter pylori* serologic test

and the absence of alarm signals point toward a functional diagnosis for abdominal pain. A complete physical examination, however, including a careful external examination of the urethral orifice and vaginal orifice and a rectal examination, should always be part of an initial assessment of abdominal pain. The history of the presenting symptoms will alert the primary care physician to consider more specific aspects of the physical examination (see Chapter 14, Pediatric Physical Examination).

Laboratory Evaluation

Laboratory and diagnostic studies performed without any medical indications are generally not helpful and may actually hinder the therapeutic suggestions made by the primary care physician. The common pitfall of overtesting occurs when the physician responds to the parents' initial request to rule everything out by performing a battery of laboratory or radiographic studies.[23] Maintaining a systematic approach to RAP will not only minimize the use of expensive, unnecessary laboratory studies, but will also decrease recurrent emergency visits and, most importantly, prevent a delay in beginning effective treatment.

Dysfunctional and psychogenic causes account for most diagnoses of RAP, with organic causes identified in only approximately 5% to 8% of cases. However, diagnostic testing is indicated when alarm signals or abnormal physical findings suggest the possibility of an organic disorder. Suggested tests are listed in Box 159-6. When the history and physical examination indicate a dysfunctional or psychogenic cause, urinalysis should suffice as the initial laboratory study.

Laboratory and other diagnostic studies such as urine, stool, or genital tract cultures; serum chemistries or erythrocyte sedimentation rate; radiographic studies (eg, barium swallow, upper or lower gastrointestinal series, gallbladder series); and abdominal or pelvic ultrasound or computed tomographic scans should be directed to evaluate specific concerns identified in the history and physical examination. For example, when pancreatitis is suspected, laboratory investigations should include amylase and lipase. Serum lipase is usually high in acute pancreatitis and remains high for longer than serum amylase. In addition, lipase has greater sensitivity and specificity than amylase. A more than three-fold level of lipase increase is considered consistent with pancreatitis, and in children, the simultaneous measurement of both amylase and lipase has a high sensitivity for the diagnosis of pancreatitis. However, the extent of the increase in either amylase or lipase does not correlate with disease severity.

When indicated, abdominal and pelvic ultrasound provide a safe, noninvasive way to assess bowel and pelvic organ structures and help clarify the need for urgent surgical intervention (eg, intussusception, ovarian torsion, kidney abscess).[24] In general, the physician should consider the least-invasive procedures first, keeping in mind the cost of special studies in terms of pain, discomfort, and time.

Common laboratory tests (complete blood cell count, erythrocyte sedimentation rate, comprehensive metabolic panel, urinalysis, stool parasite analysis) are not helpful in distinguishing between organic and functional abdominal pain. The coexistence of abdominal pain and an abnormal test result does not necessarily indicate a cause-and-effect relationship. For example, eliminating dietary lactose as the treatment for patients with demonstrable lactose malabsorption does not necessarily result in the resolution of abdominal pain. Children found to have *Helicobacter pylori* infection are not more likely to have abdominal pain than children without *H pylori*.[20]

Imaging Studies

Ultrasound of the abdomen or pelvis is not useful in the absence of alarm symptoms.[20] When atypical symptoms are present, such as jaundice, urinary symptoms, back or flank pain, vomiting, or abnormal findings at physical examination, abdominal and pelvic ultrasound is more likely than not to detect an abnormality. Endoscopy and biopsy in the absence of alarm symptoms similarly fail to discover organic disease.[20] Insufficient evidence exists to suggest that the use of esophageal pH monitoring in the absence of alarm symptoms results in finding organic disease.[20] In patients who experience recurrent vomiting, an upper gastrointestinal series should be considered to define potential anatomic abnormalities such as gastric outlet disorder or malrotation. The choice of radiologic test should be guided by the differential diagnosis generated by the history and the physical examination. To use pancreatitis again as an example, imaging is important for diagnostic purposes but may also identify the cause (eg, gallstone-induced pancreatitis). Imaging can also assess the development of potential complications, such as pseudocyst formation. The most useful and frequently used imaging studies are abdominal ultrasound and computed tomographic scans. Ultrasound has a specificity of approximately 62% to 67% for the diagnosis of pancreatitis,[25] but it is the most sensitive of the available methods to appraise the biliary tract for evidence of the cause of acute pancreatitis. Ultrasound is indicated when the patient has a history of major blunt trauma to stage severe pancreatitis (predominantly to assess for substantiation of necrosis, which is often not noted for 48 to 72 hours after onset and to learn whether noteworthy intraabdominal complications of pancreatitis are present).

TREATMENT

The treatment of abdominal pain that results from an organic process should be pursued according to accepted practice guidelines for that condition. The treatment of functional abdominal pain should be approached as a biopsychosocial phenomenon. Functional abdominal pain is still real pain. However, the response to pain can be subjective, experienced through the lens of life experience. The treatment may therefore be a combination of psychotherapy, pharmacology, or alternative medicine techniques and must always begin with educating the child and parent about the cause of the pain and the treatment plan. This approach not only improves the adherence to the treatment plan, but also has been shown to affect the outcome. Treatment response may be influenced by whether the parents perceived the pain to have an organic cause.[26] Similarly, children of parents who are open to a psychiatric consultation are more likely than not to report less pain.[26]

MANAGEMENT

A discussion of functional abdominal pain as a real entity that is a product of an alteration in the brain-gut axis makes understanding the cause of the pain easier for parents. A good analogy is that of a migraine headache: no specific test exists to confirm the diagnosis, but stress and other inciting events may trigger a headache. When explained this way, parents may be better able to understand that the current thinking of autonomic dysfunction and visceral hypersensitivity as causes of the child's recurrent functional abdominal pain does not mean that the pain is purely in the child's head or solely the effect of an undiagnosed physical ailment. Equally important is to inform the parents that the goal of therapy is not so much to arrive at a diagnosis, but rather to be able to have the child resume the lifestyle the child had before the onset of the abdominal pain, including school attendance, sleep patterns, and appetite.

Psychosocial Treatment

Several psychological therapies have been tried in various conditions associated with functional pain. These therapies have included treatments delivered to individuals or parent-child couples in one-to-one contacts with a therapist, group-based interventions, or a mixture of individual and group treatment. Psychological treatments, principally relaxation and cognitive-behavioral therapy, are effective in reducing the severity and frequency of chronic headache in children and adolescents. No evidence has been found for the effectiveness of psychological therapies in attenuating pain in conditions other than headache.[27,28]

Cognitive-behavioral therapy that combines operant elements and stress management may provide an effective treatment for RAP.[29] Cognitive-behavioral therapy results in short-term improvement, with more than one half of patients experiencing freedom from pain.[30,31] The child's coping skills and the parent's caregiving strategies predict the effectiveness of treatment.[32] Disengagement and involuntary engagement are correlated with increased anxiety, depression, and somatic symptoms. Anxiety as a comorbidity has also been an associated with RAP,[33] and therefore psychological therapy may be used as a strategy in treating RAP.

Alterative medical techniques for the treatment of functional gastrointestinal disorders, including functional abdominal pain of childhood, are becoming more common.[34] Specific mind-body techniques include various breathing techniques, guided imagery, progressive muscle relaxation, biofeedback, hypnosis, cognitive-behavioral training, and music therapy, with guided imagery, relaxation, biofeedback, and hypnosis showing the most promise in treating functional abdominal pain of childhood. Reported improvement in the pain, fewer school absences, better engagement in social activities, and fewer visits to the physician's office may result from guided imagery and progressive-relaxation techniques taught over approximately four office visits.[35] Such techniques are easy to learn and teach and are office friendly, even in children.

Medication

Several drugs have been used to treat RAP in childhood, including famotidine, pizotifen, and peppermint oil.[36] Of these, the only one that appears to be of specific use for abdominal pain is peppermint oil in the form of a pH-dependent, enteric-coated capsule. Other commonly used medications are anticholinergics, antiemetics, antidepressants, and simethicone, but they have not yet been adequately studied. Citalopram, a selective serotonin reuptake inhibitor, may be administered to treat functional abdominal pain. Children who receive this agent improve in terms of abdominal pain, anxiety, depression, and functional impairment.[33]

Dietary Interventions

Dietary manipulation has been used as a means to treat the pain in functional disorders. Common dietary changes include eating a high-fiber diet, avoiding lactose, eating an oligoantigenic diet, and eating a low-oxalate diet in abdominal migraine.[37] A high-fiber diet may be suggested, primarily in constipated children, to substitute for nutrient-poor, high-fat, high-calorie diets. Dietary manipulation is something that parents and children can understand, and suggesting this intervention can empower the family.

CONCLUSION

The causes of abdominal pain range from acute, life-threatening disease to chronic, functional conditions. Regardless of the cause, the consequences of abdominal pain can be far reaching and can affect not only the mental and psychological well being of the child, but also the social and economic dynamics of the family. The need to diagnose and treat emergent conditions quickly must be balanced with not overtesting when a functional cause appears likely. In the case of functional conditions, a caring approach that educates and reassures the patient and parents is essential for good compliance and an effective therapeutic relationship.

WHEN TO REFER

- Involuntary weight loss
- Deceleration of linear growth
- Gastrointestinal blood loss
- Significant vomiting
- Chronic severe diarrhea
- Persistent right upper or right lower quadrant pain
- Unexplained fever
- Family history of inflammatory bowel disease
- Extraintestinal symptoms
- History of psychiatric disorder
- Abnormal test results
- Anemia or low mean corpuscular volume
- Peripheral eosinophilia
- Increased erythrocyte sedimentation rate
- Increased transaminases
- Increased blood urea nitrogen or creatinine
- Hypoalbuminemia
- Low complement-4 protein
- Intestinal infection

WHEN TO ADMIT

Hospitalization is seldom indicated for patients with functional abdominal pain. Fifty percent of patients experience relief of symptoms during hospitalization. However, no data suggest that the natural history of the pain is affected. Hospitalization does not help the fundamental goals of environmental modification and will likely reinforce pain behavior. Hospitalization is required in the following circumstances:

- Surgical or medical emergency as determined by diagnostic or therapeutic intervention
- Inability to tolerate enteral nutrition
- Inability to maintain hydration and oral feeds fail in the emergency department
- Diagnosis that requires observation to evaluate the progress or natural history of the illness

TOOLS FOR PRACTICE

Medical Decision Support

- *Pediatric Nutrition Handbook, 5th edition* (book), American Academy of Pediatrics (www.aap.org/bookstore).

AAP POLICY STATEMENT

American Academy of Pediatrics, Subcommittee on Chronic Abdominal Pain, and the North American Society for Pediatric Gastroenterology, Hepatology, and Nutrition. Technical Report: Chronic Abdominal Pain in Children. *Pediatrics.* 2005;115(3):e370-e381. (aappolicy.aappublications.org/cgi/content/full/pediatrics;115/3/e370).

REFERENCES

1. Scholer SJ, Pituch K, Orr DP, et al. Clinical outcomes of children with acute abdominal pain. *Pediatrics.* 1996; 98(4 pt 1):680-685.
2. Caty MG, Azizkhan RG. Acute surgical conditions of the abdomen. *Pediatr Ann.* 1994;23:192-194, 199-201.
3. Apley JNN. Recurrent abdominal pains: a field survey of 1000 school children. *Arch Dis Child.* 1957;33:165-170.
4. Chitkara DK, Rawat DJ, Talley NJ. The epidemiology of childhood recurrent abdominal pain in Western countries: a systematic review. *Am J Gastroenterol.* 2005;100: 1868-1875.
5. Malaty HM, Abudayyeh S, O'Malley K, et al. Development of a multidimensional measure for recurrent abdominal pain in children: population-based studies in three settings. *Pediatrics.* 2005;115:e210-e215.
6. Bode G, Brenner H, Adler G, et al. Recurrent abdominal pain in children: evidence from a population-based study that social and familial factors play a major role but not Helicobacter pylori infection. *J Psychosom Res.* 2003;54: 417-421.
7. Hyams JS, Burke G, Davis PM, et al. Abdominal pain and irritable bowel syndrome in adolescents: a community-based study. *J Pediatr.* 1996;129:220-226.
8. Groholt EK, Stigum H, Nordhagen R, et al. Recurrent pain in children, socio-economic factors and accumulation in families. *Eur J Epidemiol.* 2003;18:965-975.
9. Christensen MF. Rome II classification—the final delimitation of functional abdominal pains in children? *J Pediatr Gastroenterol Nutr.* 2004;39:303-304.
10. Walker LS, Lipani TA, Greene JW, et al. Recurrent abdominal pain: symptom subtypes based on the Rome II criteria for pediatric functional gastrointestinal disorders. *J Pediatr Gastroenterol Nutr.* 2004;38:187-191.
11. Rasquin-Weber A, Hyman PE, Cucchiara S, et al. Childhood functional gastrointestinal disorders. *Gut.* 1999; 45(suppl 2):II60-II68.
12. Ball TM, Weydert JA. Methodological challenges to treatment trials for recurrent abdominal pain in children. *Arch Pediatr Adolesc Med.* 2003;157:1121-1127.
13. Stone RTBG. Recurrent abdominal pain in childhood. *Pediatrics.* 1970;45:732.
14. Boyle JT. Pediatric gastrointestinal disease. In: Walker WA, ed. *Pathophysiology, Diagnosis, Management.* 4th ed. Hamilton, Ontario, Canada: BC Decker; 2004.
15. Nydegger A, Couper RT, Oliver MR. Childhood pancreatitis. *J Gastroenterol Hepatol.* 2006;21:499-509.
16. Benifla M, Weizman Z. Acute pancreatitis in childhood: analysis of literature data. *J Clin Gastroenterol.* 2003;37: 169-172.
17. Haddock G, Coupar G, Yaungsor GG, et al. Acute pancreatitis in children: a 15-year review. *J Pediatr Surg.* 1994;29:719-722.
18. Green M. Diagnosis and treatment: psychogenic, recurrent, abdominal pain. *Pediatrics.* 1967;40:84.
19. Poole SR, Schmitt BD, Mauro RD. Recurrent pain syndromes in children: a streamlined approach. *Contemp Pediatr.* 1995;12:47-50, 52, 58.
20. Di Lorenzo C, Bridge J, Ehman M, et al. Chronic abdominal pain in children: a technical report of the American Academy of Pediatrics and the North American Society for Pediatric Gastroenterology, Hepatology and Nutrition. *J Pediatr Gastroenterol Nutr.* 2005;40:249-261.
21. Di Lorenzo C, Youssef NN, Sigurdsson L, et al. Visceral hyperalgesia in children with functional abdominal pain. *J Pediatr.* 2001;139:838-843.
22. Alfven G. The pressure pain threshold (PPT) of certain muscles in children suffering from recurrent abdominal pain of non-organic origin. An algometric study. *Acta Paediatr.* 1993;82:481-483.
23. Coleman WL, Levine MD. Recurrent abdominal pain: the cost of the aches and the aches of the cost. *Pediatr Rev.* 1986;8:143-151.
24. Bhisitkul DM, Listernick R, Shkolnik A, et al. Clinical application of ultrasonography in the diagnosis of intussusception. *J Pediatr.* 1992;121:182-186.

25. Neoptolemos JP, Hall AW, Finlay DF, et al. The urgent diagnosis of gallstones in acute pancreatitis: a prospective study of three methods. *Br J Surg.* 1984;71:230-233.
26. Crushell E, Rowland M, Doherty M, et al. Importance of parental conceptual model of illness in severe recurrent abdominal pain. *Pediatrics.* 2003;112(6 pt 1):1368-1372.
27. Eccleston C, Morley S, Williams A, et al. Psychological therapies for the management of chronic and recurrent pain in children and adolescents. *Cochrane Database Syst Rev.* 2003;(1):CD003968.
28. Huertas-Ceballos A, Macarthur C, Logan S. Psychosocial interventions for recurrent abdominal pain (RAP) in childhood (protocol for the Cochrane Review). In: *The Cochrane Library.* Issue 3, Chichester, UK: John Wiley & Sons; 2004.
29. Blanchard EB, Scharff L. Psychosocial aspects of assessment and treatment of irritable bowel syndrome in adults and recurrent abdominal pain in children. *J Consult Clin Psychol.* 2002;70:725-738.
30. Sanders MR, Rebgetz M, Morrison M, et al. Cognitive-behavioral treatment of recurrent nonspecific abdominal pain in children: an analysis of generalization, maintenance, and side effects. *J Consult Clin Psychol.* 1989;57:294-300.
31. Sanders MR, Shepherd RW, Cleghorn G, et al. The treatment of recurrent abdominal pain in children: a controlled comparison of cognitive-behavioral family intervention and standard pediatric care. *J Consult Clin Psychol.* 1994;62:306-314.
32. Thomsen AH, Compas BE, Colletti RB, et al. Parent reports of coping and stress responses in children with recurrent abdominal pain. *J Pediatr Psychol.* 2002;27:215-226.
33. Dorn LD, Campo JC, Thato S, et al. Psychological comorbidity and stress reactivity in children and adolescents with recurrent abdominal pain and anxiety disorders. *J Am Acad Child Adolesc Psychiatry.* 2003;42:66-75.
34. Gerik SM. Pain management in children: developmental considerations and mind-body therapies. *South Med J.* 2005;98:295-302.
35. Youssef NN, Rosh JR, Loughran M, et al. Treatment of functional abdominal pain in childhood with cognitive behavioral strategies. *J Pediatr Gastroenterol Nutr.* 2004;39:192-196.
36. Weydert JA, Ball TM, Davis MF. Systematic review of treatments for recurrent abdominal pain. *Pediatrics.* 2003;111:e1-e11.
37. Huertas-Ceballos A, Macarthur C, Logan S. Dietary interventions for recurrent abdominal pain (RAP) in childhood (protocol for the Cochrane Review). In: *The Cochrane Library.* Issue 3, Chichester, UK: John Wiley & Sons; 2004.

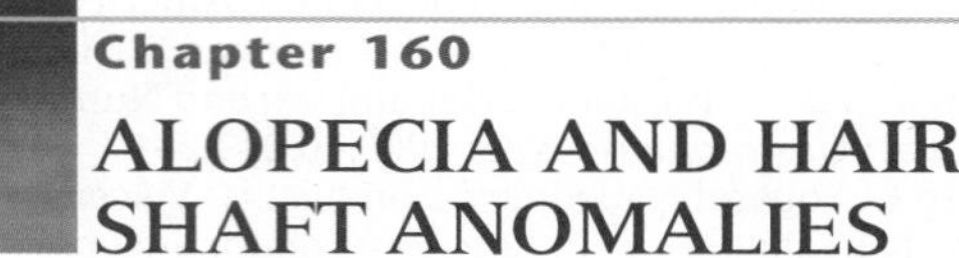

Chapter 160

ALOPECIA AND HAIR SHAFT ANOMALIES

Nancy K. Barnett, MD

Hair matters. It does not serve an essential function, inasmuch as people can live without it. Nevertheless, the symbolism over the ages, from Samson to John Lennon, and the emotional investment people have in their hair make any of its abnormalities a matter of concern. This anxiety is particularly so with alopecia; loss of hair is a disturbing event.

DEFINITIONS

A sequence of events makes up the life of a single hair, from active growth over 2 to 6 years, a busy period known as the *anagen phase,* to passivity, a resting period of approximately 3 months, known as the *telogen phase.* As many as 15% of scalp hairs may be in the telogen phase at any 1 time. These hairs are soon lost in the constant turnover of scalp hair, a continuous shedding that is hardly apparent to a casual observer. Surprisingly, approximately 50% of the hair must be shed for loss to be noticeable. Normally, up to 100 hairs are lost from the scalp daily and 200 with shampooing.[1]

Hair loss may increase to as much as 60% during a period known as a *telogen effluvium.* During such a period, the situation is similar to that of animals, which shed seasonally. In humans, this change in the normal anagen/telogen ratio may occur after a stress, such as a prolonged fever, a pregnancy, or a severe illness. It may appear in either gender and results in a diffuse, nonpatterned and nonscarring loss of hair. The diagnosis of telogen effluvium can be confirmed simply by plucking a group of hairs and examining them microscopically (see Evaluation, later in this chapter). Notably, plucking these hairs does not hurt because they are in the resting phase, with the number of resting hairs increased well beyond the usual 10% to 15%.

Excessive hair loss is a matter deserving careful attention. A precise, pointed history and physical examination are necessary. Determining if an alopecia is scarring or nonscarring is important. The pediatrician must not limit the examination simply to the site of hair loss. The whole body and all its hair-bearing parts must be observed and hairs themselves examined microscopically. Under the light microscope, the normality of the individual hair and the ratio of anagen to telogen hairs can be judged. The pediatrician may need to consult with a dermatologist.

Lanugo, the 1st hair made by hair follicles in utero, feels *silky* and covers the entire body of the fetus. It is most often shed in utero, to be replaced by hair that begins to grow on the scalp in the 3rd trimester and continues to grow after birth, which is lost a few months after birth in a normal process that results in a temporary near baldness. In many instances, parents are concerned with the thinning or with a more markedly localized area of loss, usually over the occiput, once thought to be the result of the pressure of the head as the infant lies in the crib. Finally, however, the lost early hair is gradually replaced by new hair, which has more of a *feel* to it; thicker, usually darker, and more stable, it grows longer before loss and does not shed quite so readily.

The constant ebb and flow of growth and shedding and the extreme activity of the hair follicle puts it at great risk when exposed to antimetabolites and mitotic inhibitors. When a child loses scalp hair rather suddenly, the physician should be concerned with the possibility of a toxic event. Children treated with antimetabolites for a malignancy suffer hair loss because of the damage done by the drugs during the anagen phase, resulting in an anagen effluvium. Occasionally, similar hair loss is caused by accidental poisoning, as with rat poison that contains thallium or coumarin. In most instances, over a period of several months, new hairs will replace lost hairs, unless the exposure to the toxic element is chronic.

The prognosis for the return of hair depends, in large part, on elimination of the toxic stimulus and on whether the loss is accompanied by scarring. Loss with scarring (eg, from iatrogenic scalp injury during delivery or from a burn) is permanent. Additionally, hair will not grow at the site of most nevi and hemangiomas. In children, alopecia of both known and unknown cause usually occurs without scarring: alopecia areata (spotty loss of scalp hair), alopecia totalis (loss of all scalp hair), and alopecia universalis (loss of all scalp and body hair); drug-induced, postfebrile, and postpartum alopecias; and alopecias associated with an endocrinopathy (hypothyroidism, hyperthyroidism, or hypoparathyroidism) or a nutritional deficiency (vitamins A, B, and C, or kwashiorkor).

When scarring is present, as with a kerion associated with tinea capitis, keloid formation, or discoid lupus erythematosus, little hope exists for hair recovery.

EVALUATION

Appropriate diagnosis requires microscopic differentiation of the hair and its root in both the anagen and the telogen stages. Anagen hairs have fat, healthy follicle bulbs and an attached emerging long terminal hair, whereas telogen hairs have a small bulb and an attached hair with a club shaped appearance. Deformities of the hair shaft can be seen, particularly with aminoacidopathies and in a variety of rare syndromes, including Menkes kinky hair syndrome. The clinician can differentiate microscopically monilethrix (usually an inherited, autosomal-dominant disorder in which the diameter of the hair shaft varies) from pili torti (a disorder in which the hair is twisted on its long axis).

DIFFERENTIAL DIAGNOSIS

A variety of congenital and hereditary disorders can produce hair loss, either total or less obviously with thinning (Table 160-1). True congenital alopecia is rare and may be inherited as an autosomal-recessive trait. If the loss is not due to this genetic circumstance but is

Table 160-1 Distinguishing Characteristics of Alopecias

CONDITION	PATTERN OF LOSS	PULLED HAIR CHARACTERISTICS AS EXHIBITED WITH LIGHT MICROSCOPY
NONSCARRING WITH HAIR SHAFT ABNORMALITIES		
Trichorrhexis nodosa	Fragile, short hair with grayish-white nodules	Nodes along hair shaft similar to interlocking broom or brush ends
Monilethrix	Fragile, short stubblelike growth	Variable shaft thickness gives beaded appearance with internodal breakage
Pili torti	Fragile, short, light-colored hair appears spangled as a result of light reflection	Irregularly spaced twists along the shaft appear flattened
NONSCARRING WITHOUT HAIR SHAFT ABNORMALITIES		
Alopecia areata	Sharply demarcated, round, nearly bald patches appearing suddenly	Exclamation point hairs from periphery of patches with poorly pigmented shaft and tapered attenuated bulb
Adrogenetic alopecia	Thinned scalp hair in common male baldness pattern or diffuse thinning with retained frontal hair in the female	Increased telogen:anagen ratio Biopsy shows miniaturized anagen bulbs
Trichotillomania	Irregularly shaped areas of thinned stubble of varying lengths	Normal cuticle, shaft and anagen bulb of varying lengths
Traumatic alopecia	Bizarre patterns conforming to site and method of injury (eg, head trauma, braiding)	Normal cuticle, shaft and anagen bulb of varied lengths
Telogen effluvium	Diffuse, thinning with easy epilation from all areas of scalp	More than 25% of pulled hairs are telogen club hairs with no pigment
Anagen effluvium	Significant thinning	Tapered anagen bulbs
Loose anagen syndrome	Slight diffuse or patchy thinning	Anagen hairs have misshapen pigmented bulbs with ruffled cuticle
POTENTIALLY SCARRING WITHOUT HAIR SHAFT ABNORMALITIES		
Tinea capitis and kerion	Varied ranging from round, minimally inflamed alopecic area with slight seborrheic scale to the boggy, tender often pustular, severely inflamed kerion	Potassium hydroxide preparation of broken hairs (black dot hairs) reveals clusters of chains of arthrospores around or in hair shaft and bulb
Lupus erythematous	Discoid, well-demarcated erythematous plaques with scale, plugging of follicles and becoming atrophic and/or thinning as a result of broken, fragile hair with acute flares (lupus hair)	Not applicable if scarred Short, broken (frayed) anagen hairs

congenital, then it is most often evidence of a significant hereditary disorder. Hairs may be thin or poorly anchored to the scalp or have a variety of shaft abnormalities. The pediatrician must look for signs of ectodermal dysplasia and thus consider radiographic exploration for skeletal defects (as with cartilage-hair hypoplasia, congenital ectodermal dysplasia, or orofaciodigital syndrome), as well as for evidence of inherited metabolic or endocrine disorders such as phenylketonuria, homocystinuria, and congenital hypothyroidism. Children with serious chromosomal defects (de Lange syndrome or trisomy 13 syndrome) obviously provide a surfeit of signs and symptoms beyond simple loss of hair.

Hair Shaft Anomalies

Anomalies of the hair usually result in a stubbly growth of broken hair rather than true alopecia. Ectodermal defects, brittle fingernails, or perhaps cataracts and tooth anomalies may accompany hair shaft anomalies. Actually, fragile hair with resultant breakage (trichorrhexis) and stubble can be seen in a variety of rare conditions. Trichorrhexis nodosa is a familial condition in which the hair is fragile without other associated findings. Children with argininosuccinic aciduria, a rare inborn error of metabolism, have stubbly hair and show evidence of severe intellectual disability in the 1st year of life.

The texture of hair may be helpful in finding the source of difficulty. In an infant who has hypothyroidism, the hair may be coarse, brittle, and without luster; with progeria and cartilage-hair hypoplasia syndrome, it may be fine and even silky. In all these circumstances, the hair may break off, and apparent baldness increases. Whenever the hair is abnormal, it becomes weakened, fragile, and fractured, and it may be lost or unevenly shortened, often resulting in a stubbly, ragged *alopecia*. Given that a variety of abnormalities (congenital, traumatic, or endocrine) can lead to such fragility and loss, referral to a dermatologist is appropriate so that a specific diagnosis can be pursued.

Loose Anagen Syndrome

Loose anagen syndrome is characterized by hairs that are quite easily and painlessly pulled from the scalp.[2] Generally, but not always, affected children are blond and female preschoolers between 2 and 5 years of age.[2] Their hair appears sparse. The individual hairs are not fragile. On examination, they have misshapen anagen bulbs with a cuffed cuticle and no external root sheath. Hairs are not firmly anchored because of an inner root sheath defect.

Typically, the child's hair is said to be slow growing, seldom requiring cutting. The hair over the occiput often is matted and sticky. The condition may wane with time, although adult-onset cases have been reported.[3] The hair grows thicker and longer, and its pigmentation increases. Nonetheless, even in adulthood, it may pull out easily and painlessly. A hereditary factor may be involved, but most cases are sporadic. The diagnosis can be made from the history and examination, the painless *pull test* (when hair is growing normally, it usually hurts to pull it), and light microscopy to view the recovered hairs. Management is limited to reassurance and the passage of time.

Trichorrhexis Nodosa

Trichorrhexis nodosa is a common abnormality of the hair shaft that becomes obvious under the light microscope, where the *nodes* resemble the effect observed when the ends of 2 brushes are pushed together. Most often congenital, trichorrhexis nodosa results in breakage of hair and short stubble over the scalp; it may also be a genetic predisposition in some black patients who experience hair breakage over large areas of the scalp and whose hair will not grow beyond a relatively short length. Trichorrhexis nodosa is usually accompanied by a history of hair straightening or repeated vigorous brushing and combing. Avoiding this kind of steady abuse and using a more gentle cosmetic approach can result in some gradual improvement. White and Asian individuals can experience the same difficulty, probably without congenital or familial relationship, and the breakage occurs most often at the distal end of the hair. White specks marking the *nodes* may appear after some physical and chemical injuries. Here again, a gentle approach and elimination of any noxious exposure are appropriate.

Monilethrix

Monilethrix (beaded hair syndrome) is a condition in which scalp hairs have regularly spaced differences in their circumference, suggesting a chain of beads. The cause is unknown but is probably genetic, and no treatment is known. Although some degree of recovery may occur spontaneously, particularly after puberty or during pregnancy, this period is a long time to wait, inasmuch as hair breakage becomes obvious during infancy. Variable expressivity was noted in 3 kindreds in whom monilethrix was mapped to the type II keratin gene cluster at chromosome *12q13*.[4] Occasionally, associated problems (cataracts, brittle nails, faulty teeth) are suggestive of a more widespread ectodermal defect.

Pili Torti

Pili torti simply means *twisted hair*, which indeed is the way this hair appears under the microscope. The color is *off*, and the hair is coarse and lusterless. It is as though straight and curly hair were competing for a place in the same strand. In cross-section, a straight hair appears round, and a curly hair appears oval. In pili torti, both configurations may be seen in a single strand, an abnormality that can be an important clue to Menkes kinky hair syndrome, an X-linked disease characterized by low serum copper, progressive cerebral degeneration, arterial degeneration, and the suggestion of scurvy in the bones.

Alopecia Areata

Alopecia areata, most often seen as an acute problem, results in a sudden and total loss of hair in sharply circumscribed, round areas, often several centimeters in diameter, usually on the scalp, but possibly anywhere on the body where hair is found (Figure 160-1). Hairs at the periphery of an area are plucked easily and may be particularly colorless and thin. *Exclamation point* hairs may appear throughout the patch, which is sometimes salmon colored as a manifestation of the presumed inflammation seen histologically around the

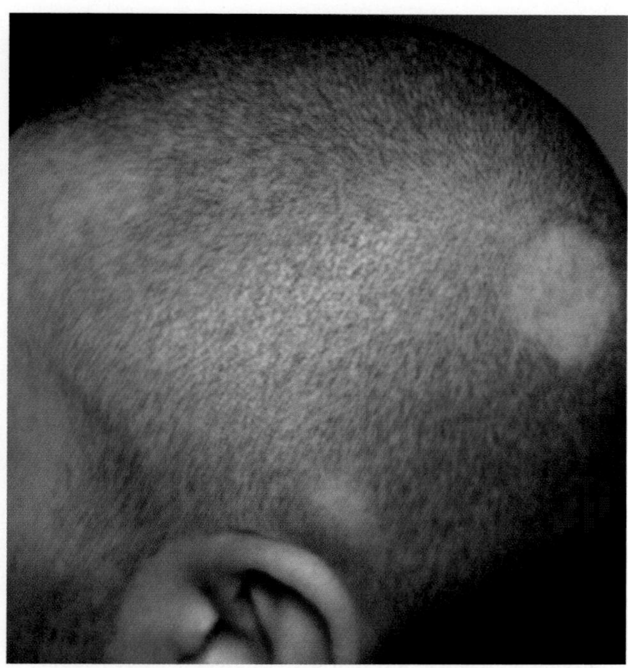

Figure 160-1 This 30-year-old man developed slow expanding hair loss on the scalp one month earlier. Although a potassium hydroxide preparation was supposedly positive, he did not improve on topical ciclopiron shampoo and oral itraconazole. At a subsequent visit a month later, several new patches were also noted and the diagnosis was switched to alopecia areata. *(Reprinted with permission from DermAtlas.org. Courtesy of Manoj Ram, MD.)*

hair follicle. The fingernails may be pitted, possibly indicating a more extensive ectodermal problem.

Just a few patches of loss may be found, or a total absence of body hair (alopecia universalis) may occur, including eyebrows and eyelashes. The more extensive the loss and the younger the child, the less likelihood there is of a full recovery. The prognosis is best when the loss is less widespread, and only 1 or 2 patches are present. Although the cause is unknown, some suggestion has been made of a T-cell mediated autoimmune process against the anagen hair follicle. Occasionally, autoimmune antibodies are identified in patients who have alopecia areata when no other clinical evidence exists of autoimmune disease. An increased incidence of alopecia areata also occurs in persons who have acute autoimmune thyroid disease and vitiligo. An association with certain class II genes in the human leukocyte antigen locus suggests a genetic predisposition to alopecia areata.

Approximately one third of patients who have alopecia areata will regrow hair spontaneously in 6 months and approximately one third in 5 years. For the remaining one third, treatments must be given to stimulate hair growth.

Cortisone creams applied topically have been used with some success. In the older more cooperative child, direct injection into the scalp or eyebrow hair follicles with corticosteroids can be effective, but the process is painful. The primary care pediatrician should seriously question the appropriateness of this procedure, carefully assessing the impact of the disease and of the treatment on the child, and should refer the patient to a dermatologist for consideration of this intervention. Large areas (more than 50% scalp hair loss) that require infiltration present obvious difficulty. Oral steroid therapy has the risk of serious complications but is occasionally used, as is 5% minoxidil solution twice daily, which can be effective for small stubborn alopecic areas.

For extensive alopecia, some irritants (dinitrochlorobenzene immunotherapy and tars such as short-contact anthralin) and psoralen with ultraviolet A light (known as PUVA therapy) have been used. These agents should be used only in children older than 12 years and only by a knowledgeable dermatologist in controlled circumstances.

An oddity of alopecia areata is that when hair does regrow, it may initially be white. Eventually, color returns, and casual observers cannot identify the formerly affected area.

The efficacy of treatment is difficult to assess because of the waxing and waning nature of alopecia areata. The National Alopecia Areata Foundation (www.naaf.org) offers education and support to families and sponsors an annual children's camp. In counseling patients and their families, primary care pediatricians should remind them that this process is nonscarring, which always has the potential for full regrowth.

Androgenetic Alopecia

Androgenetic alopecia is a genetically determined loss of hair that begins most often with a receding hairline and some thinning over the vertex. It occurs most often in men, but it can happen to women. The fullest expression is most common in the mature adult, but pediatricians are confronted with the problem in 15% of adolescents over age 14. Hairs from affected follicles do not epilate easily on pulling, but they are shorter and finer as a result of normal pubertal androgen increase in susceptible individuals. No therapy is reliably effective, although topical minoxidil twice daily and hair transplant micrografts may help some individuals.[1] Finasteride can be given after 18 years of age in male patients but is contraindicated in female patients because of the possibility of genital defects in exposed male fetuses if a pregnancy occurs.

Trichotillomania

Some children have a compulsive need to pull out their hair or even their eyebrows or eyelashes. Although not always of emotional significance, trichotillomania may provide a major clue to an underlying psychosocial problem. The hair loss often appears in large, patchy, ill-defined patterns. The family structure and the interaction with siblings and parents and with friends at home and at school should be explored in an effort to find stressors. Consulting a psychiatrist should also be considered. The primary care pediatrician can paint the attacked areas with petroleum jelly in an attempt to frustrate the habit; however, without attention to the possibility of an underlying emotional issue, this

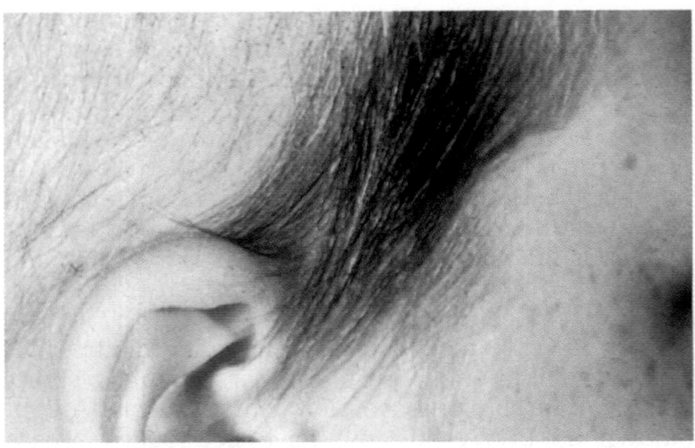

Figure 160-2 Trichotillomania in a 7-year-old boy.

approach is quite obviously temporary. Both imipramine and fluoxetine have been used successfully to control trichotillomania in certain children.[5]

The hair lost is that which is most accessible to the probing hand. In some cases, enough is pulled to simulate alopecia areata (Figure 160-2). The patient who eats hair may accumulate it in the stomach and create a trichobezoar (hairball), which may ultimately lead to acute intestinal obstruction or, most often, to the complaint of abdominal pain. A trichobezoar may be palpable as an abdominal mass and is demonstrable on a radiograph. Referral for either endoscopic or surgical removal is indicated.

Traumatic Alopecia

Hair is fragile. It should be handled gently and without physical or chemical assault. In children, hair is probably best left alone, except for simple washing and, to suit the fashion, simple cutting.

Constant teasing or straightening with heat or chemicals may seriously damage hair. Some hairstyles, particularly with barrettes, ponytails, braids, or cornrows, cause constant and prolonged traction, especially along the hairline. The hair may then fall out, accompanied by redness and inflammation, even with pustular involvement of the follicles. Generally, simply discontinuing the stress will help. In childhood, the hair will almost always return, although the regrowth can be slow. Injured hair follicles, whether from trichotillomania or simple traction, do not heal quickly, often taking 3 months or longer to return to an anagen phase.

Tinea Capitis

Whenever a child has patches of alopecia or stubbly hair growth, even in the absence of crusting, scaling, redness, or other inflammatory signs, the practitioner should consider the possibility of tinea capitis, along with seborrheic dermatitis, atopic dermatitis, or psoriasis (Figure 160-3). Certainly, seborrhea and atopy are more common in children than fungal scalp infection; but particularly when alopecia is accompanied by local adenopathy, tinea capitis should be in the differential diagnosis.[6] Obviously, if crusting, scaling, or redness is present, then the likelihood of alopecia areata is diminished because inflammation is not a symptom of that condition. In any event, the practitioner should perform a mycologic examination, looking particularly for the usual fungus, *Trichophyton tonsurans*. Clinically, the lesions tend to be more elevated than in other forms of tinea and may be characterized by black dots. In rare cases, the endothrix fungi *Microsporum canis* and *M audouinii* can invade the hair shaft and cause breakage and stubbiness. *M canis* tends to cause much more inflammation than does *M audouinii*. Endothrix fungal infections, but not *T tonsurans*, can produce a greenish fluorescence under Wood light in a darkened room.

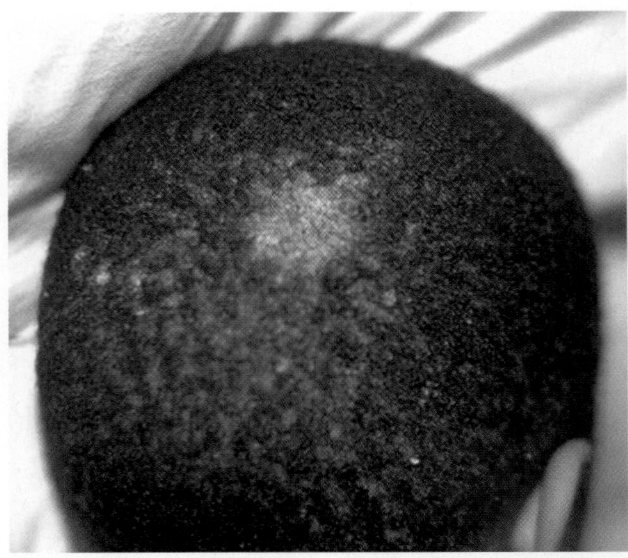

Figure 160-3 A young boy admitted for asthma therapy was incidentally noted to have a scalp lesion. The scaling and focal alopecia suggested the diagnosis of tinea capitis. The child was successfully treated with griseofulvin.

On occasion, particularly with *M canis* or after treatment with an irritant, the affected area may become secondarily infected and seriously inflamed, requiring treatment with an antibiotic. Kerion, a delayed hypersensitivity reaction to the fungus, may develop, and if it is unchecked, then the resultant scarring interferes with the regrowth of hair (Figure 160-4). Early diagnosis and treatment are therefore helpful.

Topical antifungal agents do not provide adequate treatment. Several systemic fungistatic agents are effective in treating tinea capitis, but griseofulvin remains the standard of care. The long course of oral therapy with griseofulvin, usually approximately 2 months, may present difficulties with compliance in a young child. The fungicidal drug terbinafine appears effective for tinea capitis when given for 6 weeks but is currently approved only for children 4 years and older for this use by the US Food and Drug Administration; neither itraconazole nor fluconazole are approved but may be similarly safe for short courses in children.[7] These agents provide alternatives if griseofulvin therapy fails or is not tolerated. Liquid itraconazole has been associated with diarrhea in children and with

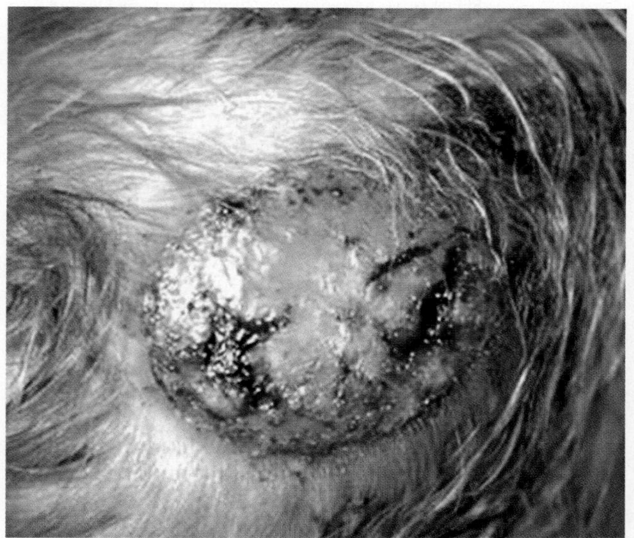

Figure 160-4 A 2½-year-old boy with a kerion caused by chronic, progressive tinea capitis.

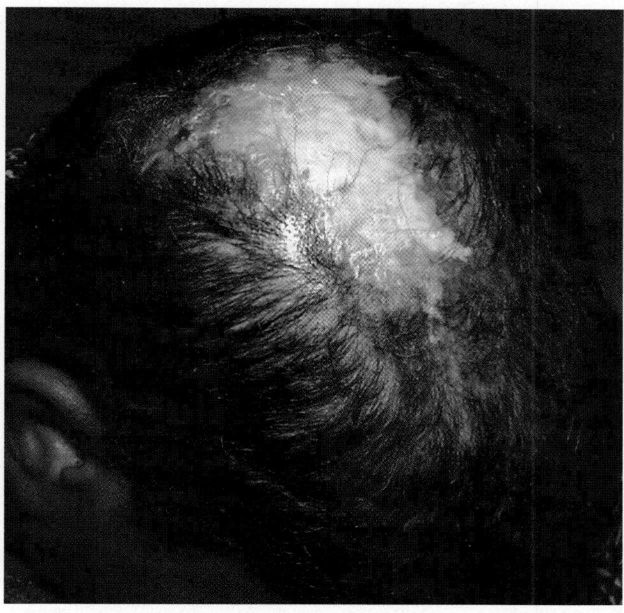

Figure 160-5 This 48-year-old woman had discoid lesions for over 10 years with lesions restricted to sun exposed sites. She had large areas of scarring alopecia. *(Reprinted with permission from DermAtlas.org. Courtesy of Kosman Sadek Zikry, MD.)*

pancreatic adenocarcinoma in laboratory animals and should be avoided.[8] Liver function should be tested if antifungal medications are used for longer than 12 weeks and at the start of therapy if any suggestion of preexisting liver disease exists. Oral prednisone tapered over 10 days may help rapidly decrease the tenderness and inflammation of a kerion and prevent a widespread id reaction. (For medication dosage information, consult the *Red Book*.)

Acrodermatitis Enteropathica

Acrodermatitis enteropathica, an autosomal-recessive disorder characterized by abnormal zinc absorption, has several important cutaneous manifestations, simulating, at times, psoriasis, epidermolysis bullosa, pyoderma, or candidiasis. Zinc deficiency can result in abdominal pain and diarrhea, as well as a wispy alopecia and dystrophic development of the fingernails, suggesting widespread ectodermal involvement. Oral zinc sulfate is the treatment of choice.

Discoid and Systemic Lupus Erythematosus

Discoid lupus erythematosus can be disfiguring to the scalp and, with scarring, can cause a permanent loss of hair (Figure 160-5). Early treatment with topical or intralesional steroids may prevent scarring. Systemic lupus erythematosus can also cause alopecia, and the scalp itself can be erythematous; however, the loss of hair is generally temporary and does not involve the scarring characteristic of discoid disease.

MANAGEMENT

Treatment for alopecia depends, of course, on the cause. Practitioners are accustomed to seeing children who are being treated with antimetabolites wearing baseball caps or bandanas to hide their full or partial baldness from anagen arrest. A noticeable loss of hair from any cause may be disturbing to both patient and parent; therefore the suggestion that the child wear a baseball cap or other concealing adornment may be appropriate. Even a hairpiece can be designed for a child. These steps serve in the interim while practitioners attempt potentially helpful treatments or wait expectantly in circumstances in which their role is diagnostic and supportive. The possibility that hair will not regrow must be considered when loss (1) follows high fever or chronic toxicity, (2) is accompanied by scarring, or (3) occurs in the areas of nevi, aplasia cutis, or persistent hemangiomas. The practitioner must talk this through with the child who is old enough and with the parents as well, exploring the emotional reaction and discomfort and, if recovery of hair is questionable, working with them to achieve an emotional balance consistent with reality and to adopt suitable coping mechanisms. In most instances, this goal is achievable, and the pediatrician should not back away from trying. The practitioner, sometimes frustrated by the lack of a practical, successful management regimen, should not forget the value of a willing, listening ear. Plastic surgery expertise should be sought for consideration of hair transplants and scalp reduction (for scarred areas) when possible.

WHEN TO REFER

- Rapid, diffuse hair loss
- Chronic, progressive, localized, or diffuse hair loss without regrowth
- Scarring alopecia

- Inability to grow hair as a result of breakage, loss, or abnormal texture of hair
- Appearance of scalp mass or plaque affecting localized hair loss

TOOLS FOR PRACTICE

Engaging Patients and Family

- *National Alopecia Areata Foundation* (Web page), The National Alopecia Areata Foundation (www.naaf.org/default2.asp).
- *Teens—Alopecia Areata Fact Sheet* (fact sheet), The National Alopecia Areata Foundation (www.naaf.org/kids/teen-facts.asp).

Medical Decision Support

- *Pediatric Dermatology: A Quick Reference Guide* (book), American Academy of Pediatrics (www.aap.org/bookstore).

SUGGESTED RESOURCES

Atton A, Tunnessen W. Alopecia in children: the most common causes. *Pediatr Rev.* 1990;12:25-30.

Price VH. Androgenetic alopecia in adolescents. *Cutis.* 2003;71:115-121.

Price VH. Office diagnosis of structural hair anomalies. *Cutis.* 1975;15:231-240.

Roberts BJ, Friedlander SF. Tinea capitis: a treatment update. *Pediatr Ann.* 2005;43(3);191-200.

REFERENCES

1. Price VH. Androgenetic alopecia in adolescents. *Cutis.* 2003;71:115-121.
2. Price VH, Gummer CL. Loose anagen syndrome. *J Am Acad Dermatol.* 1989;20:249-256.
3. Tosti A, PelusoAM, Misciali C, et al. Loose anagen hair. *Arch Dermatol.* 1997;133:1089-1093.
4. Birch-Machin AM, Healy E, Turner R, et al. Mapping of monilethrix to the type II keratin gene cluster at chromosome 12q13 in three new families, including one with variable expressivity. *Br J Dermatol.* 1997;137:339-343.
5. Sheikha SH, Wagner KD, Wagner RF. Fluoxetine treatment of trichotillomania and depression in a prepubertal child. *Cutis.* 1993;51:50-52.
6. Williams JV, Eichenfield LF, Burke BL, et al. Prevalence of scalp scaling in prepubertal children. *Pediatrics.* 2005;115:e1-e6.
7. Gupta AK, Soloman RS, Adam P. Itraconazole oral solution for the treatment of tinea capitis. *Br J Dermatol.* 1998;139:104-106.
8. Roberts BJ, Friedlander SF. Tinea capitis: a treatment update. *Pediatr Ann.* 2005;43:191-200.

Chapter 161
AMENORRHEA

Maria Trent, MD, MPH; Alain Joffe, MD, MPH

Amenorrhea is a common clinical complaint; its frequency varies based on the gynecologic age of the young woman (the number of months or years elapsed since menarche). For example, in a study of high school adolescent girls, the percentage of girls who missed 3 consecutive menstrual periods in a single year was 12.5 in the first year postmenarche and 5.4 after 7 years postmenarche.[1] Traditionally, amenorrhea has been classified as being either primary or secondary. Primary amenorrhea is defined as the failure to initiate menstruation, whereas secondary amenorrhea refers to cessation of menses in an adolescent who has previously menstruated. Although some value can be found in knowing if the absence of menses is due to a disruption or lack of initiation, this distinction is of limited clinical utility because many diseases and clinical states cause both primary and secondary amenorrhea.

The mean age of menarche among girls in the United States has decreased slightly in recent years. In 1973 the average age of menarche was 12.76 among participants in the National Health Examination Survey (NHES). Recent analyses using the combination of NHES and National Health and Nutrition Examination Surveys (NHANES) has documented that the current age of menarche in the United States is 12.54 years, with some variation by race or ethnicity.[2] Further analyses from the NHANES data demonstrated that 90% of girls will have menstruated by age 13.75 years and that fewer than 10% menstruate before 11 years of age.[3]

Amenorrhea is a symptom, not a disease, and has a variety of causes. The differential diagnoses for the patient with amenorrhea includes maturational (constitutional) factors, disorders of the central nervous system (CNS), adrenal and ovarian disease, congenital abnormalities of the reproductive tract (primary amenorrhea), thyroid disease, nutritional disorders, systemic illness, and pregnancy. Therefore a thoughtful, systematic approach to the patient who has a menstrual disorder usually identifies the cause. The major causes of amenorrhea are listed in Box 161-1.

Menstruation usually begins approximately 2 years after breast budding; however, the interval between the 2 events can be as short as 6 months or as long as 4 years. Given this broad range of individual variation in the onset of puberty and menarche, the physician first must assess pubertal status noting breast and pubic hair development. An evaluation is warranted if:

1. No signs of secondary sexual development are present by 13 years of age. In this instance, the evaluation should include an assessment for delayed puberty. (See Chapter 212, Puberty: Normal and Abnormal.)
2. Menarche has not occurred by 16 years of age even if the patient has experienced development of secondary sexual characteristics and growth has been normal.
3. Three consecutive menstrual cycles are absent, or the patient who has previously menstruated has had amenorrhea for more than 6 months.[4] (See Chapter 212, Puberty: Normal and Abnormal.)

Gynecologic age is important when evaluating an adolescent who appears to have secondary amenorrhea. After the onset of menarche, many teenagers will menstruate sporadically; regular monthly cycles often are not established until 1 to 2 years after menarche.[5] Clearly, the abrupt cessation of menstruation in a teenager who has established regular cycles is of

BOX 161-1 Major Causes of Amenorrhea in Adolescent Girls by Organ System

- Central nervous system
  - Familial-physiologic delay
  - Systemic illness
  - Developmental defects (eg, Kallmann syndrome)
  - Laurence-Moon-Bardet-Biedl syndrome
  - Prader-Willi syndrome
  - Infiltrative disease
  - Head trauma
  - Sheehan syndrome (postpartum necrosis)
  - Primary empty sella syndrome
  - Irradiation
  - Surgery
  - Depression
  - Drugs (eg, hormonal contraception, cocaine, phenothiazines)
  - Psychologic stressors
  - Eating disorders (eg, anorexia nervosa)
  - High-level athletic training with low weight for height (eg, female athlete triad)
  - Psychosocial stress
  - Central nervous system tumor (eg, prolactinoma)
- Thyroid
  - Hyperthyroidism
  - Hypothyroidism
- Adrenal
  - Addison disease
  - Cushing syndrome
  - Late-onset congenital adrenal hyperplasia (21-hydroxylase deficiency)
  - Tumor
- Ovaries
  - Gonadal dysgenesis
  - Premature ovarian failure
  - Radiation or chemotherapy
  - Ovarian removal or destruction
  - Polycystic ovary syndrome
  - Tumor
- Uterus
  - Pregnancy
  - Uterine synechiae
  - Congenital abnormalities (müllerian agenesis, androgen insensitivity)
- Vagina, cervix, hymen
  - Agenesis
  - Imperforate hymen
  - Transverse septum

greater concern than the absence of menses for 3 to 4 months in a teenager who has a gynecologic age of 6 months to 1 year. The point at which the clinician elects to pursue an evaluation depends on the anxiety of the patient and her family, the possibility of pregnancy, and the likelihood that a potentially serious disease is responsible for the amenorrhea. For a general approach to the evaluation of amenorrhea, see Figure 161-1 on page 1392.

HISTORY

The history and physical examination are critical elements in the diagnostic approach. Although the adolescent should always be interviewed alone during the visit, many adolescent girls may have difficulty with the details of their own medical and family medical histories, making maternal involvement during the visit extremely useful. Mothers are able to provide detailed medical histories for their daughter from infancy to the present and the details of their own menstrual and medical history and usually that of 1st-degree female relatives. Finally, mothers are often acutely aware of behavioral factors within the home, such as the daughter's menstrual patterns, symptoms associated with menstrual cycles, consumption of pads or tampons, dietary and exercise patterns, stressors on the family and their daughter, and the subtle development of physical features such as weight gain, acne, or hirsutism. Detailed discussions of personal lifestyle factors such as sexual activity should be conducted without the parent present. Use of the HEADDSS assessment (**h**ome situation, **e**ducational status of the patient, **a**ctivities, **d**iet, **d**rug use, **s**uicidality or depression, and **s**exuality or sexual behavior) facilitates this portion of the interview.

The hypothalamic-pituitary-ovarian axis of the adolescent is more sensitive to physical and psychologic stress than is that of the adult woman. Stress, emotional upset, fever accompanying viral illness, and changes in weight or environment (eg, going away to college) all can induce amenorrhea. Comments about weight or body image may be a clue to anorexia nervosa. The history also should include questions about drug or medication use, including any forms of hormonal contraception that the patient may be using. Most women who develop amenorrhea while using combined estrogen-progesterone contraceptive methods resume menstruation within 6 months of discontinuing their use. Pregnancy should be the primary consideration in patients who have a history of sexual intercourse. Unfortunately, denial of sexual activity does not exclude pregnancy, inasmuch as many teenagers are reluctant to admit to something they believe will be met with condemnation from adults. Sudden cessation of menstruation is more likely to indicate pregnancy or stress as a cause, whereas a gradual cessation suggests polycystic ovary disease or premature ovarian failure. A history of uterine surgery or abortion raises the possibility of uterine synechiae. Given that many women are involved in sports, questions about exercise patterns or participation in athletics (frequency, duration, intensity) are essential. The clinician must be sure to seek clues to any of the endocrine abnormalities (eg, galactorrhea), a history of past CNS insults (eg, meningitis), or symptoms of an intracranial tumor. The age at which the patient's mother and sisters first

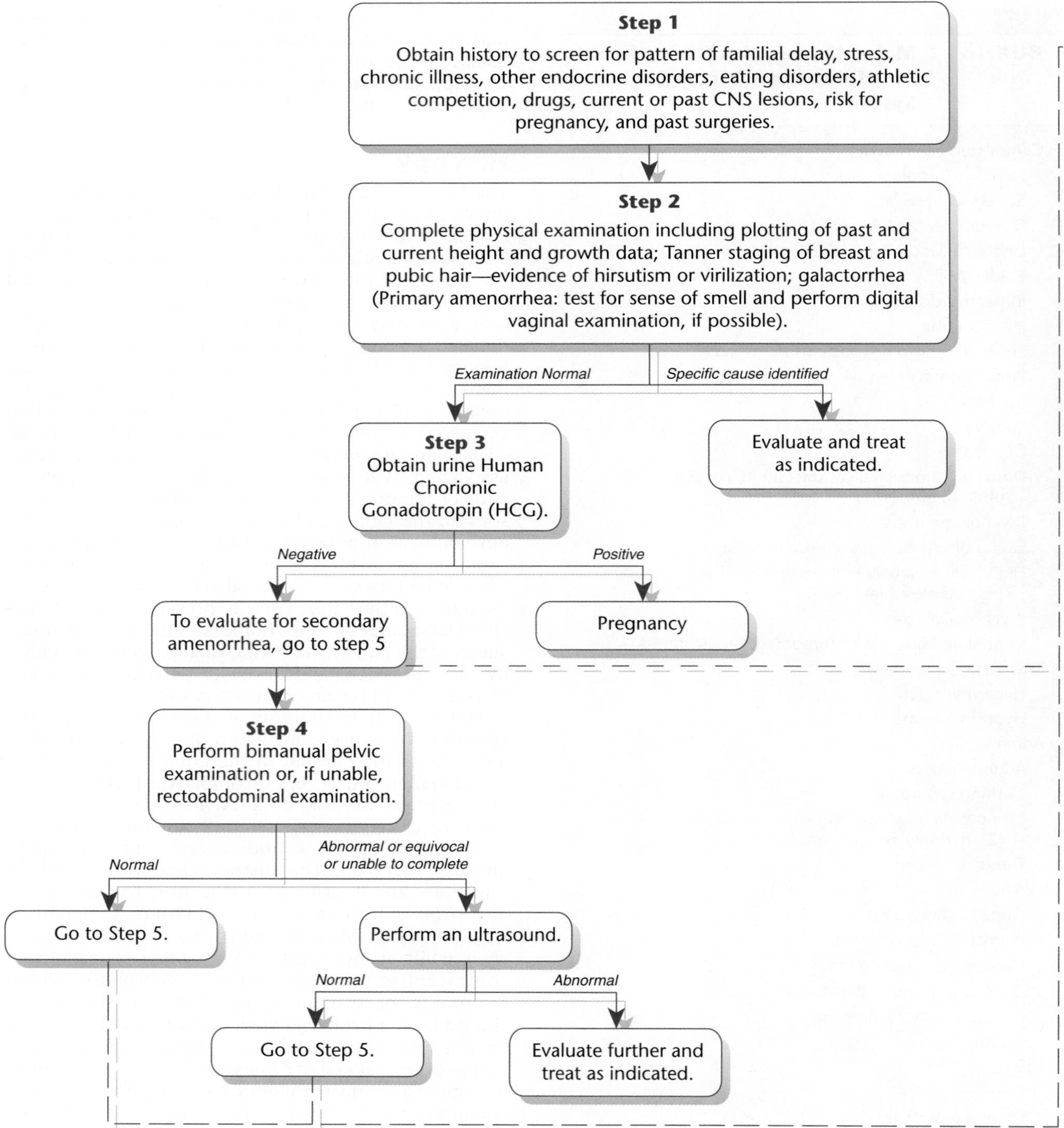

Figure 161-1 Evaluation of patients who have amenorrhea in whom secondary sex characteristics are present.

menstruated is also helpful information because such a pattern may be familial.[2] Finally, chronic diseases such as inflammatory bowel disease or renal failure may be subtle in their early presentation; hence questions aimed at uncovering these illnesses must be included in the review of systems.

PHYSICAL EXAMINATION

Plotting of previous growth data (both height and weight) is essential. A short girl who has amenorrhea should prompt a search for the other physical characteristics of Turner syndrome.[1] Diagnostic criteria for anorexia nervosa include loss of weight or failure to

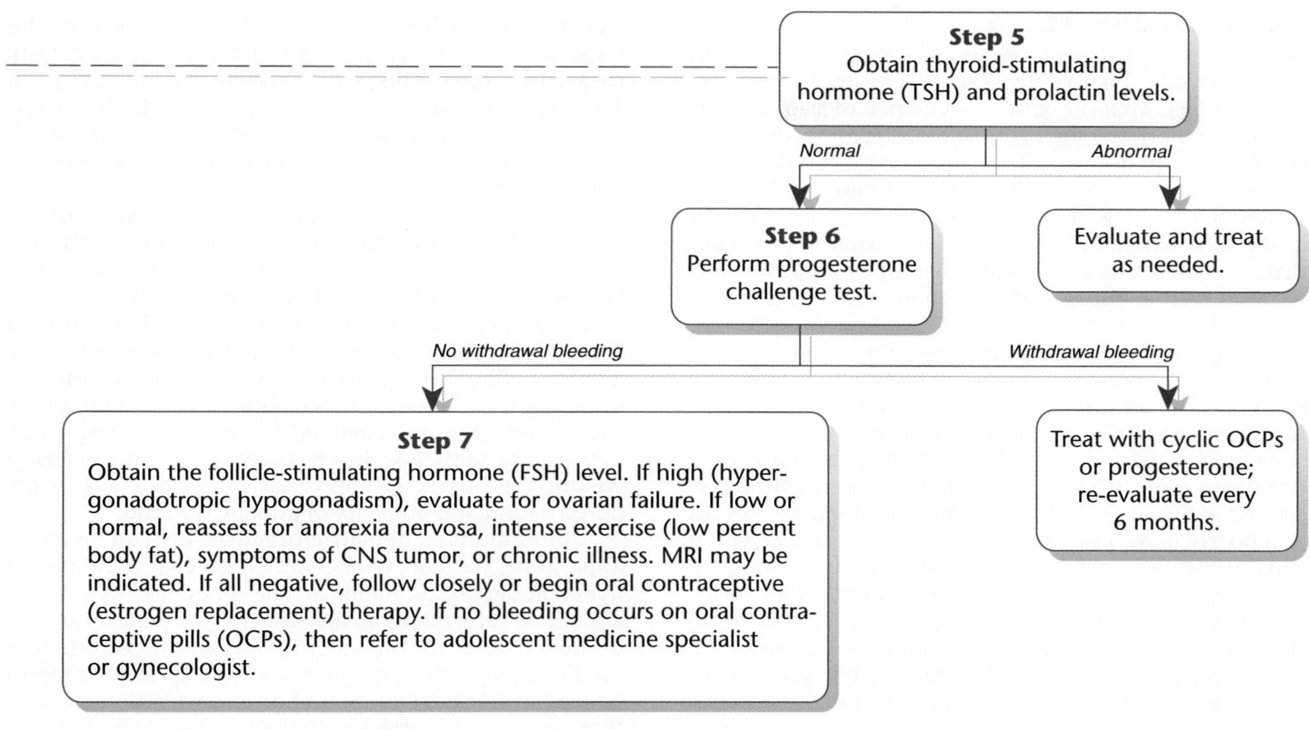

Figure 161-1 Evaluation of patients who have amenorrhea in whom secondary sex characteristics are present.

gain the weight expected with pubertal development (see Chapter 135, Anorexia and Bulimia Nervosa). A complete physical examination, which in most cases will include a pelvic examination, should be performed. Obesity or excessive thinness can result in amenorrhea. Abnormalities of the visual field, smell, or other cranial nerve function; papilledema; or disturbances of reflexes suggest a CNS tumor. Hirsutism, a receding hairline, excessive acne, moon facies, striae, an enlarged thyroid, or buffalo hump suggests an endocrine disorder. A webbed neck, short stature, or widely spaced nipples suggest Turner syndrome. Nipple discharge may indicate elevated prolactin levels, and lack of or scant pubic hair in a girl who has Tanner stage 3 to 4 breast development suggests androgen insensitivity syndrome.

A pelvic examination is essential to ensure the presence of normal internal and external female genitalia. An imperforate hymen or transverse vaginal septum prevents menstrual blood from escaping. If the hymenal opening is patent, then the examination should proceed to determine the presence of a normal vagina, cervix, and uterus. If the hymenal opening is very small, then the cervix and uterus can be palpated by means of a bimanual rectoabdominal examination. The size of the clitoris should be noted because clitoromegaly indicates the presence of excess androgens (eg, partial 21-hydroxylase deficiency). In the few cases in which a pelvic or rectoabdominal examination cannot be performed to determine the presence or absence of a uterus, an ultrasound may be necessary.

Although a pink vaginal mucosa indicates the presence of some degree of estrogenization, the patient's estrogen status can be assessed using a progesterone challenge, vaginal maturation index, or measurement of serum estradiol levels. The progesterone challenge is particularly useful because a positive result indicates an estrogen-primed uterus. The progesterone challenge is conducted by administering 10 mg of medroxyprogesterone acetate for 5 to 10 days. Any spotting or bleeding in the week afterward is considered a positive test. Some experts in the field recommend measuring follicle-stimulating hormone (FSH) levels before performing a progesterone challenge because some women who have hypergonadotropic amenorrhea will have a withdrawal bleed.[6] A vaginal maturation index is performed by collecting cells from the upper lateral sidewall of the vaginal wall using a moistened cotton-tipped applicator, rolled on a glass slide, and fixed using the same technique in Papanicolaou smear preparation (see Chapter 322, Sexually Transmitted Infections). Cytologic assessment will determine the number of parabasal, superficial, and intermediate cells present. Samples can be scored using Meisels modified scoring system to interpret results in terms of estrogen and pubertal status.[7]

LABORATORY TESTS

For the girl with primary amenorrhea who has an unremarkable history, review of systems, general physical examination, and no evidence of vaginal outlet obstruction, the next step is to determine, either by pelvic examination or ultrasound, or both, whether a uterus is present. If not, then karyotyping and serum testosterone levels should be determined to screen for müllerian agenesis or androgen insensitivity syndrome. If a uterus is present, then an evaluation comparable to that for secondary amenorrhea should be pursued.

Patients with primary or secondary amenorrhea who have a history of sexual activity should first be screened for pregnancy using a urine pregnancy test. If negative, then initial laboratory evaluation includes FSH, prolactin, and thyroid-stimulating hormone. Low or normal FSH levels are usually associated with physiologic delay, hypothalamic and pituitary causes of amenorrhea, and chronic illnesses. Elevated levels of FSH indicate ovarian failure. Follow-up testing in patients with elevated FSH levels should include karyotyping and screening for autoimmune endocrinopathies. Patients with amenorrhea and clinical evidence of androgen excess most likely have polycystic ovary syndrome (PCOS)[8] or, less commonly, late-onset congenital adrenal hyperplasia (21-hydroxylase deficiency). Additional useful laboratory tests to assess for PCOS and other disorders associated with androgen excess include serum testosterone (total and free) and dehydroepiandrosterone (DHEA) and its sulfate (DHEA-S). Measurement of the first morning 17-hydroxyprogesterone levels is also indicated for patients with elevations in DHEA-S to further assess for late onset congenital adrenal hyperplasia. If the patient has evidence of virilization (eg, clitoromegaly), or if the androgens are elevated in the tumor range, then adrenal and ovarian imaging are indicated, depending on the source of androgens. Isolated elevations of testosterone are suggestive of ovarian origin, whereas DHEA-S is suggestive of adrenal origin. (See also Chapter 192, Hirsutism, Hypertrichosis, and Precocious Sexual Hair Development.)

Imaging is indicated for other specific presentations of amenorrhea. Pelvic sonography is indicated if abnormalities are noted on bimanual examination or if bimanual examination is not possible. Magnetic resonance imaging of the pelvis is indicated for patients with possible congenital abnormalities. Dual-energy radiograph absorptiometry bone density evaluations should be obtained in girls with hypoestrogenic amenorrhea, given the association with low bone mineral density.[9] Hypoestrogenic amenorrhea is commonly seen in patients with restrictive eating disorders, athletic amenorrhea, and ovarian failure.[10-13]

MANAGEMENT

Definitive recommendations for treatment of secondary amenorrhea depend on the underlying cause. When adolescent girls initiate puberty late, but progression through puberty appears normal and the findings of a thorough history and physical examination are also normal, the patient can be reassured that she should anticipate menarche 2 to 3 years after the initiation of puberty. This probability is particularly true when family history suggests late menarche in 1st-degree female relatives. Regularly scheduled follow-up visits until menarche occurs are warranted. Any halt in development or absence of menarche by age 16 merits an evaluation.

In patients with secondary amenorrhea and normal estrogen levels, medroxyprogesterone 5 to 10 mg for 12 to 14 days can be used every 1 to 3 months to stimulate withdrawal bleeding. For sexually active patients and patients with PCOS, treatment with combined contraceptives is indicated. Patients with PCOS may also benefit from additional medications to address underlying metabolic abnormalities or clinical findings associated with androgen excess (hirsutism and acne). In patients with low levels of estrogen, normalizing weight for height is important by addressing disordered eating and intensity of athletic training.

Although many pediatric practices provide gynecologic care, patients who cannot receive a thorough gynecologic assessment in the pediatrician's office should be referred to an adolescent medicine specialist or pediatric gynecologist for evaluation. Adolescent medicine physicians may be particularly well suited to address other developmental or endocrinologic issues that may also be present. Patients who have evidence of complicated endocrine disease; evidence of a CNS, adrenal, or androgen tumor; genetic disorder; eating disorder; or structural abnormality should also be referred to the appropriate specialty team for further evaluation and management.

WHEN TO REFER

- If the amenorrhea appears secondary to a chronic illness that the pediatrician is unable to manage
- If the pediatrician feels uncomfortable performing a pelvic examination
- If long-term hormonal therapy is required
- If the patient has an eating disorder
- If evidence exists of anatomic or chromosomal abnormality
- If evidence exists of a complicated endocrine disorder
- If evidence exists of a CNS, adrenal, or ovarian tumor

REFERENCES

1. Johnson J, Whitaker AH. Adolescent smoking, weight changes, and binge purge behaviors: association with secondary amenorrhea. *Am J Public Health*. 1992;82:47-54.
2. Anderson SE, Dallal GE, Must A. Relative weight and race influence average age at menarche: results from two nationally representative surveys of US girls studied 25 years apart. *Pediatrics*. 2003;111:844-850.
3. Chumlea LC, Schubert CM, Roche AF, et al. Age at menarche and racial comparisons in US girls. *Pediatrics*. 2003; 111:110-113.
4. Speroff L, Glass RH, Kase NG. *Clinical Gynecologic Endocrinology and Infertility*. 6th ed. Baltimore, MD: Lippincott Williams and Wilkins; 1999.

5. World Health Organization, Task Force on Adolescent Reproductive Health. World Health Organization multicenter study on menstrual and ovulatory patterns in adolescent girls. *J Adolesc Health Care*. 1986;7(4): 229-235.
6. Rebar RW, Connolly HV. Clinical features of young women with hypergonadotropic amenorrhea, *Fertil Steril*. 1990;53:804.
7. Meisels A. Computed cytohormonal findings in 3,307 healthy women. *Acta Cytol*. 1965;9:328-333.
8. The Rotterdam ESHRE/ASRM-Sponsored PCOS Consensus Workshop Group. Revised 2003 consensus on diagnostic criteria and long-term health risks related to polycystic ovary syndrome (PCOS). *Hum Reprod*. 2004; 19:41-47.
9. White CM, Hergenroeder AC, Klish WJ. Bone mineral density in 15- to 21-year-old eumenorrheic and amenorreheic subjects. *Am J Dis Child*. 1992;146:31-35.
10. Golden NH, Jacobson MS, Schebendach J, et al. Resumption of menses in anorexia nervosa. *Arch Pediatr Adolesc Med*. 1997;151(1):16-21.
11. Yeager KK, Augustine R, Nattiv A, et al. The female athlete triad: disordered eating, amenorrhea, and osteoporosis. *Med Sci Sports Exerc*. 1993;25:775-777.
12. Hetland ML, Haarbo J, Christiansen C. Running induces menstrual disturbances but bone mass is unaffected, except in amenorreheic women. *Am J Med*. 1993;95: 553-558.
13. Gidwani GP. Amenorrhea in the athlete. *Adolesc Med*. 1999;10:275-290.

Chapter 162

ANEMIA AND PALLOR

E. Anders Kolb, MD; Adam S. Levy, MD

INTRODUCTION

Anemia is a laboratory finding reflecting a decrease in red blood cell (RBC) mass below an age-appropriate normative value. Anemia may be associated with pallor, but it is more likely a silent symptom and detected only on routine screening studies. Pallor and anemia are not diagnoses; rather, they are signs and symptoms of an underlying disease process requiring a thorough evaluation by the primary care physician.

DEFINITIONS AND CLINICAL MANIFESTATIONS

Pallor

Pallor, derived from the Latin *pallere*, meaning *to be pale*, is a clinical sign associated with a variety of systemic illnesses resulting in a decrease in the amount of oxygenated hemoglobin visible through the superficial and translucent layers of the skin and mucosa. Accurate assessment of pallor may be hindered by fluorescent lighting, dark skin color, jaundice, or cyanosis. Although a common finding in children with moderate to severe anemia, pallor does not necessarily indicate a low hemoglobin level. Sepsis may cause pallor resulting from a decrease in peripheral perfusion. Vasoconstriction from sepsis or exposure to cold or febrile illnesses may also result in pallor. Diseases such as heart failure, hypoproteinemia, or myxedema that lead to an accumulation of fluid in the interstitium may result in pallor.

Anemia

Anemia can be defined as a reduction in RBC number, RBC mass (hematocrit), or hemoglobin concentration.[1] For each value, the lower limit of the normal range is defined as 2 standard deviations from the mean for age and gender (Table 162-1). Normal ranges for hemoglobin and hematocrit vary with age and gender. Racial differences exist as well. Black children on average have normal hemoglobin values that are approximately 0.5 g/dL lower than white and Asian children.[2]

CLASSIFICATION AND DIFFERENTIAL DIAGNOSIS

Anemias can be systematically evaluated based on RBC size (mean corpuscular volume [MCV]). Normal MCV values vary with age, but microcytic anemias generally have an MCV less than 70 fL, normocytic anemias have an MCV of 72 to 79 fL, and macrocytic anemias have an MCV of greater than 85 fL. Subclassification of anemias as microcytic, normocytic, and macrocytic will greatly reduce the differential diagnosis and limit the number of laboratory tests needed to attain the diagnosis. Figures 162-1 and 162-2 contain guidelines for a diagnostic approach to children and newborns with anemia. Box 162-1 lists the differential diagnoses of specific pathological RBC features.

Microcytic Anemia

The differential diagnosis of a microcytic anemia is listed in Table 162-2, and the main causes are reviewed in detail here.

Iron Deficiency

Iron-deficiency anemia is the most common cause of anemia in the United States.[3] Iron deficiency may be attributed to poor iron intake, poor iron absorption, or blood loss. Full-term neonates are born with sufficient iron stores to last for the first 6 months of life. Iron deficiency is rare during this period. The incidence of iron-deficiency anemia peaks at age 12 to 24 months and then again in adolescence. The peak in childhood corresponds to the transition of children from human milk or iron-containing formulas to whole milk. Iron deficiency in adolescents is typically due to a poor dietary intake of iron, whereas adolescent girls may also have significant blood and iron loss with menstrual bleeding.

In children of all ages, occult blood loss must be considered as a source for iron loss leading to deficiency. Blood loss may be acute, chronic, or intermittent. A thorough history should be obtained to rule out melena, hematochezia, tarry stools, and bloody or coffee-ground emesis. Stool guaiac tests for occult blood should be performed at several different times

Table 162-1 Mean Values for Hemoglobin, Hematocrit, and Mean Corpuscular Volume

AGE	HEMOGLOBIN (g/dL)	HEMATOCRIT (%)	MCV (fL)
Cord blood	15.3	49	112
1 day	19.0	61	119
1 wk	17.9	56	118
1 mo	17.3	54	112
2 mo	10.7	33	100
3 mo	11.3	33	88
6 mo-2 yr	12.5	37	77
2-4 yr	12.5	38	79
5-7 yr	13	39	81
8-11 yr	13.5	40	83
12- to 14-year-old girls	13.5	41	85
12- to 14-year-old boys	14	43	84
15- to 17-year-old girls	14	41	87
15- to 17-year-old boys	15	46	86

Modified from Nathan DG, Orkin SH. *A Diagnostic Approach to the Anemic Patient in Nathan and Oski's Hematology of Infancy and Childhood.* 5th ed. Philadelphia, PA: WB Saunders; 1998. Copyright © 1998, Elsevier, with permission.

to capture any intermittent bleeding. Common causes of gastrointestinal bleeding include gastric and duodenal ulcers, Meckel diverticulum, polyps, hemorrhoids, and gastritis. Signs and symptoms of inflammatory bowel disease should also be considered in the history and physical examination. Patients with iron-deficiency anemia have symptoms similar to those in other forms of anemia. However, occasionally, pica is reported, particularly cravings for ice.

When iron deficiency is sufficient to cause anemia, other abnormalities may be seen on routine laboratory testing. In addition to being microcytic, the RBCs will be hypochromic, with target cells and elliptocyte forms visible on the peripheral blood smear. These features and a low reticulocyte count are sufficient to make the diagnosis of iron-deficiency anemia. In many instances, further testing is not necessary but may be helpful in some settings. Serum iron and ferritin levels will be low, whereas the total iron-binding capacity will be elevated. Many children will also have an elevated platelet count.

When a primary care physician is treating a child with hypochromic, microcytic anemia found on a routine screening blood cell count and a history of poor iron intake or excessive milk intake is elicited, a reasonable approach would be to give a trial of supplemental iron (6 mg/kg of iron per day divided into 2 or more doses) rather than to draw additional blood for biochemical analysis. The reticulocyte count should increase within 5 to 7 days once therapy is initiated. Assuming the dietary deficiency is corrected, supplemental iron should continue for 2 to 3 months after the hemoglobin concentration has normalized. For patients with a hypochromic microcytic anemia who do not appear to be at risk based on diet alone, and for those who do not respond to supplemental iron, additional testing is required. Iron deficiency, although common, is still abnormal, and the etiology of the deficiency should be clearly defined.

Thalassemias

The thalassemias are a heterogenous group of disorders of hemoglobin production. The alpha-thalassemias have deficient production of the alpha chain, and beta-thalassemia deficient production of the beta chain. The normal chains are made in excess of the abnormal chains, resulting in precipitation and destruction of the RBCs.

BETA-THALASSEMIA. Thalassemia minor (or thalassemia trait) is common among black patients and results from a mutation of 1 of the 2 genes on chromosome 11 encoding for the beta chain. When only 1 gene is affected, a mild decrease in beta-chain production occurs, resulting in a mild anemia. Patients with thalassemia trait frequently have a hypochromic, microcytic anemia found on a routine complete blood count, similar to patients with iron-deficiency anemia. Target cells are also common to both diseases. However, patients with thalassemia trait will usually have an increase in the number of RBCs, whereas patients with iron deficiency will commonly have a decrease in RBC number. A hemoglobin electrophoresis may also be helpful in diagnosing thalassemia trait. Both the hemoglobin F and hemoglobin A_2 levels are commonly elevated. Although treatment is not necessary, diagnosing thalassemia trait is important so that appropriate genetic counseling may be offered to patients and families.[4]

THALASSEMIA MAJOR. Thalassemia major (Cooley anemia) results from defects in both beta-globin genes and exhibits as a severe hemolytic anemia. Marked compensatory erythropoiesis resulting in expansion of the medullary space will result in a prominence of the cheeks and frontal bossing.[4] Long-term transfusion therapy is required for these patients, and immediate referral to a hematologist is necessary.

ALPHA-THALASSEMIA. Each chromosome 16 contains 2 identical genes (4 genes total) for the alpha chain. Abnormalities in these genes, most commonly seen in

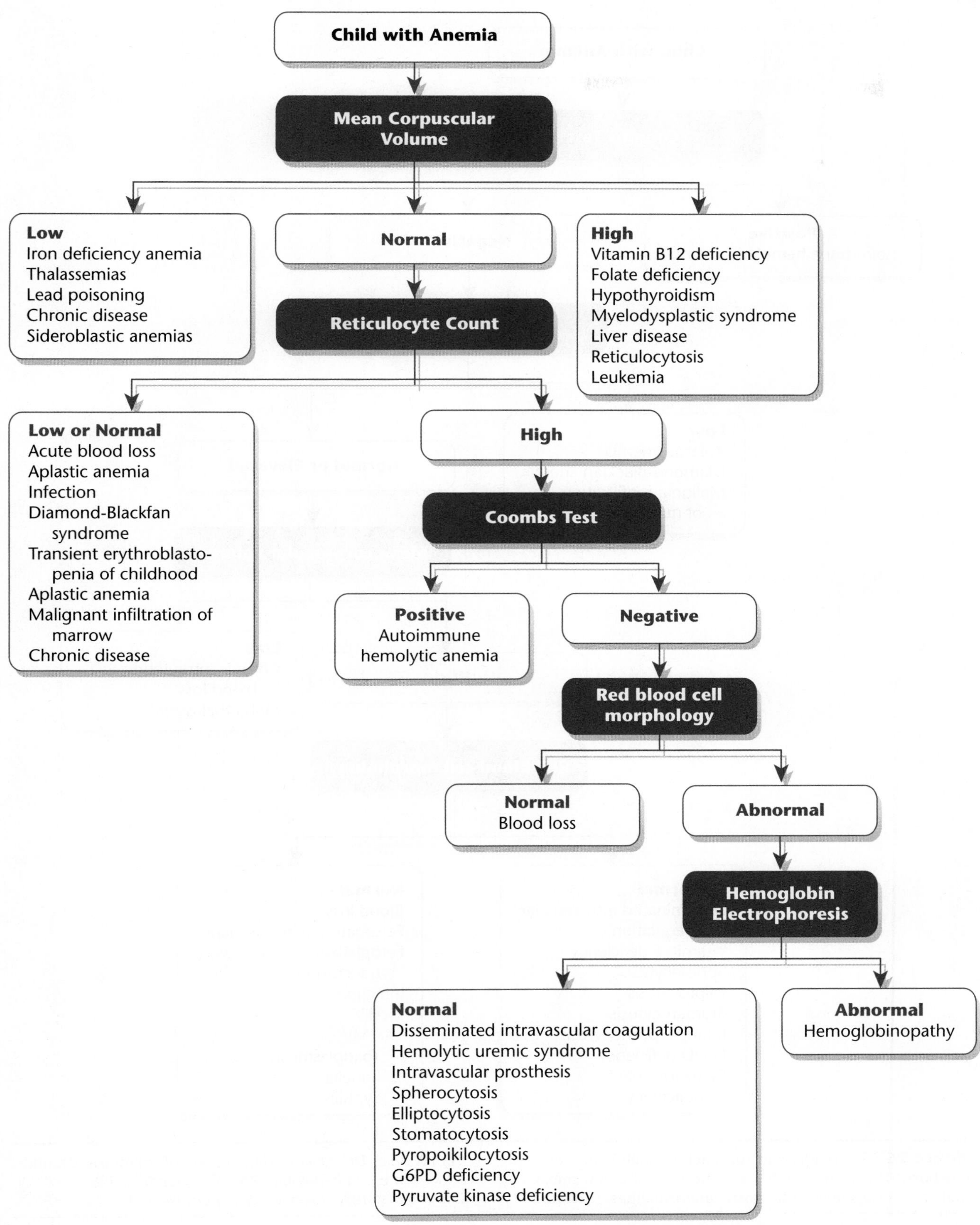

Figure 162-1 Diagnostic approach to anemia in childhood based on red blood cell mean corpuscular volume. *(Adapted from Nathan DC, Oski F:* Hematology of Infancy and Childhood. *3rd ed. Philadelphia, PA: WB Saunders; 1987. Copyright © 1987, Elsevier, with permission.)*

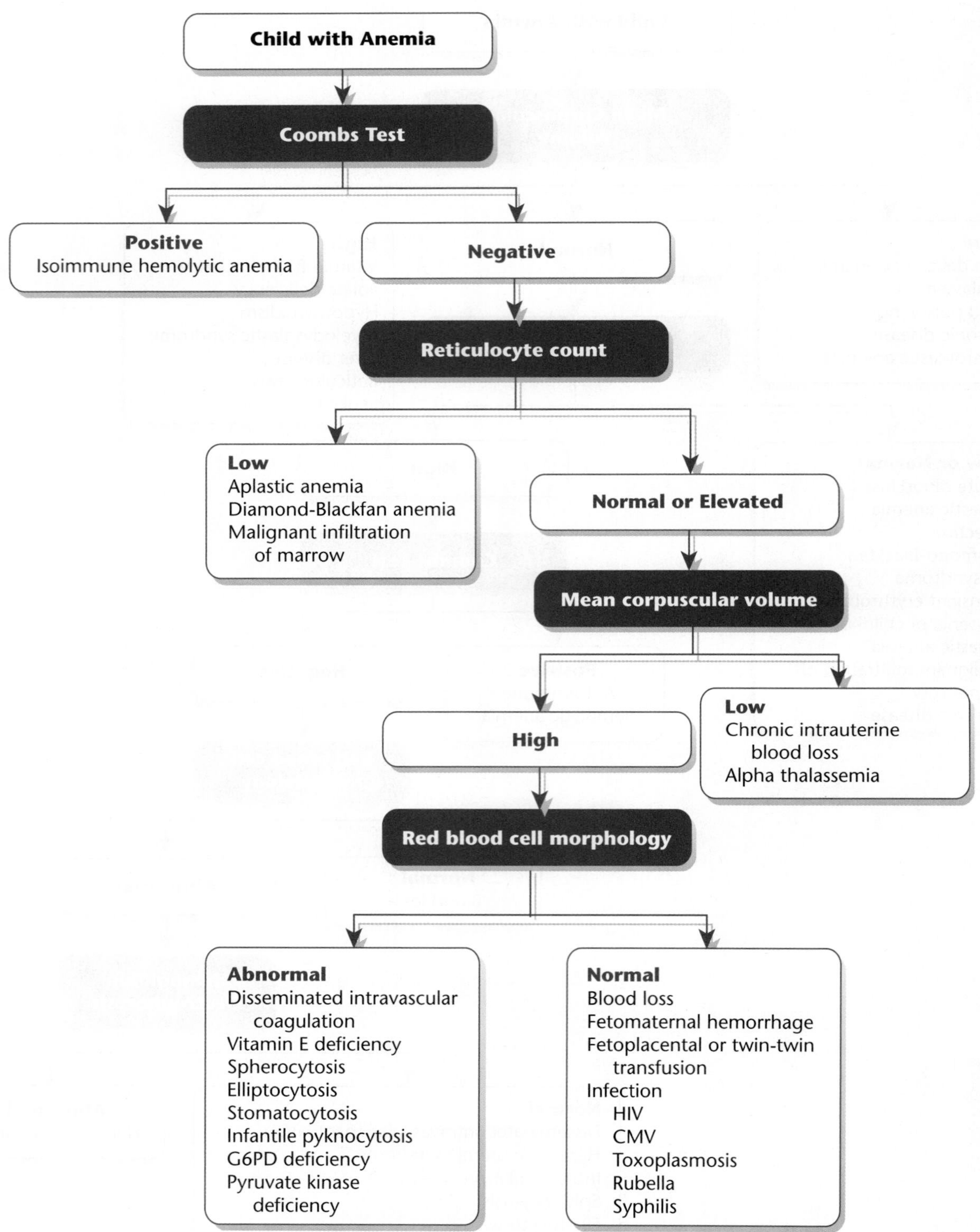

Figure 162-2 Diagnostic approach to anemia in the newborn. The asterisk indicates a peripheral blood smear that shows no specific diagnostic abnormalities. *(Adapted from Nathan DC, Oski F:* Hematology of Infancy and Childhood. *3rd ed. Philadelphia, PA: WB Saunders; 1987. Copyright © 1987, Elsevier, with permission.)*

BOX 162-1 Differential Diagnosis of Specific Pathological Red Blood Cell Features

TARGET CELLS

Surface-to-volume ratio increased
Thalassemia
Hemoglobinopathies
Hemoglobin E disease
Hyposplenism or postsplenectomy
Hepatic disease
Severe iron-deficiency anemia
Abetaproteinemia
Lecithin or cholesterol acyltransferase deficiency

SPHEROCYTES

Hyperdense cells with a decrease in surface-to-volume ratio and an increased mean corpuscular hemoglobin concentration
Hereditary spherocytosis
Hemolytic anemia (autoimmune, ABO incompatibility, water dilution)
Microangiopathic hemolytic anemia
Hemoglobin SS disease
Hypersplenism
Burns
After RBC transfusions
Pyruvate kinase deficiency

ACANTHOCYTES (SPUR CELLS)

Cells with 10-15 spicules that are typically irregular in length, spacing and width; cells usually smaller than normal RBCs
Disseminated intravascular coagulation
Microangiopathic hemolytic anemia
Hyposplenism or postsplenectomy
Hepatic disease
Hypothyroidism
Vitamin E deficiency
Abetalipoproteinemia
Malabsorption

ECHINOCYTES (BURR CELLS)

Cells with 10-30 spicules that are typically of comparable size and distributed evenly
Dehydration
Renal disease
Hepatic disease
Pyruvate kinase deficiency
Peptic ulcer disease
After RBC transfusion

PYKNOCYTES

Hyperchromic RBCs with a decreased volume and distorted shape
Similar to acanthocytes and echinocytes

BLISTER CELLS

Contain a clear area in RBCs that contains no hemoglobin
Hemoglobin SS disease
G6PD deficiency
Pulmonary emboli

BASOPHILIC STIPPLING

Retention of RNA resulting in fine blue inclusions in the cytoplasm
Iron-deficiency anemia
Lead poisoning
Hemolytic anemias
Pyrimidine 5′-nucleotidase deficiency

ELLIPTOCYTES

Elliptical-shaped cells
Hereditary elliptocytosis
Iron-deficiency anemia
Thalassemia
Hemoglobin SS disease
Sepsis
Megaloblastic anemia
Malaria
Leukoerythroblastic reaction

TEAR DROP CELLS

Microcytic and hypochromic cells that are in the shape of a teardrop
Normal finding in newborns
Thalassemia
Myeloproliferative diseases
Leukoerythroblastic reaction

SCHISTOCYTES

RBC fragments that result from trauma
Disseminated intravascular coagulation
Hemolytic anemia and microangiopathic hemolytic anemia
Kasabach-Merritt syndrome
Purpura fulminans
Hemolytic uremic syndrome
Uremia, glomerular nephritis, acute tubular necrosis
Cirrhosis of the liver
Malignant hypertension
Thrombosis
Thrombotic thrombocytopenia purpura
Amylosis
Chronic relapsing schistocytic hemolytic anemia
Burns
Connective tissue disorders

STOMATOCYTE

Area of central pallor is more slitlike than round
Present in small numbers in normal individuals
Stomatocytosis (hereditary)
Thalassemia

BOX 162-1 Differential Diagnosis of Specific Pathological Red Blood Cell Features—cont'd

NUCLEATED RBCS

Normal on a peripheral blood smear in the 1st week of life only

Normal newborns

Significant bone marrow stimulation

Congenital infections

Hyposplenism or postsplenectomy

Leukoerythroblastic reaction, particularly with severe infections and leukemias or metastatic tumors in the bone marrow

Megaloblastic anemia

Dyserythropoietic anemias

Frequently, normal blood smears will contain abnormal-appearing RBCs that are simply an artifact of trauma during the blood draw or ex vivo processing of the blood.

G6PD, Glucose-6-phosphate dehydrogenase; *RBC*, red blood cell.

Modified from Nathan DG, Orkin SH. *A Diagnostic Approach to the Anemic Patient in Nathan and Oski's Hematology of Infancy and Childhood.* 5th ed. Philadelphia, PA: WB Saunders; 1998. Copyright © 1998, Elsevier, with permission.

Table 162-2 Classification of Anemia in Childhood

MICROCYTIC	NORMOCYTIC	MACROCYTIC
Iron-deficiency anemia	Infection	Megaloblastic anemias from vitamin B_{12} or folate deficiency
Lead poisoning	Acute blood loss	Reticulocytosis
Copper deficiency	Renal disease	Postsplenectomy
Malnutrition	Connective tissue disorder	Myelodysplastic syndrome
Chronic disease	Hepatic disease	Aplastic anemia
Thalassemia	Hemolysis	Fanconi anemia
Hemoglobin E trait	Hypersplenism	Diamond-Blackfan syndrome
Sideroblastic anemia	Malignancy	Persons syndrome
Atransferrinemia	Aplastic anemia	Dyskeratosis congenita
Inborn errors of metabolism	Dyserythropoietic anemia	Paroxysmal nocturnal hemoglobinuria
	Drugs	Down syndrome
		Hypothyroidism
		Hepatic disease, jaundice
		Drugs (eg, phenytoin, methotrexate)

blacks and Asians, result in alpha-thalassemia.[5] When 1 gene is affected, the patient will be asymptomatic, with little or no abnormality on routine testing. Alpha-thalassemia trait is the result of a mutation in 2 genes. Patients with alpha-thalassemia trait are also asymptomatic. They will have laboratory findings similar to patients with beta-thalassemia trait or iron deficiency (microcytic, hypochromic anemia). However, unlike beta-thalassemia trait, the anemia is usually less severe, and the hemoglobin electrophoresis will be normal. No confirmatory test is readily available for alpha-thalassemia. The diagnosis is empiric and based on the findings of a microcytic, hypochromic mild anemia in patients of Asian or black descent with a normal electrophoresis and no evidence of iron deficiency. When 3 of the 4 genes are affected, hemoglobin H disease is the result. Patients with hemoglobin H disease may be asymptomatic but with moderate to severe anemia (hemoglobin in the range of 7 to 10 g/dL). The anemia will be microcytic and hypochromic, with RBC fragments visible on review of the peripheral blood smear. A hemoglobin electrophoresis will show 5% to 30% hemoglobin H (hemoglobin consisting of 4 beta chains). Patients with mutations in all 4 genes will not make any normal hemoglobin. Survival of the fetus is possible only with intrauterine transfusions.[4]

Lead Poisoning

Any measurable lead in the plasma is abnormal, but clinically significant lead poisoning occurs at lead levels greater than 10 mcg/dL. In most instances, lead poisoning is diagnosed on routine screening tests.[6] The anemia in lead poisoning is microcytic and hypochromic, similar to iron deficiency. However, intense basophilic stippling of the RBCs may also be observed. Lead inhibits the insertion of iron into the protoporphyrin ring, thus inactivating heme synthesis and leading to an accumulation of free erythrocyte protoporphyrin, the levels of which can be elevated in both iron deficiency and lead poisoning.

Chronic Inflammation

Chronic illness may be associated with anemia, likely the result both of decreased production and shortened RBC survival. Iron flow from the reticuloendothelial cells to the erythroblasts may also be diminished, resulting in a hypochromic, microcytic anemia. Anemia of chronic disease can be associated with malignancies, autoimmune diseases, renal failure, and chronic infections. Frequently, RBCs in chronic disease are normocytic and normochromic, but microcytic and hypochromic anemias are seen as well. The hemoglobin will typically be in the range of 7 to 10 g/dL with a normal to low reticulocyte count.

Sideroblastic Anemias

The sideroblastic anemias, caused by the retention of iron in the mitochondria of immature erythrocytes, are rare forms of anemia in childhood. Acquired sideroblastic anemia is a disease primarily of adulthood, whereas inherited forms of the disease occur in childhood.

Normocytic Anemia

Normocytic anemia is defined as a decreased circulating RBC mass with an MCV in the appropriate range for age.[7,8] As noted previously, the distinction of age-appropriate normative values is well established and important to consider lest the clinician misinterpret a child's results and pursue an unnecessary evaluation (see Table 162-1).

The differential diagnosis of normocytic anemia (see Table 162-2) is broad and can be divided into primary hematologic disorders or systemic disorders with secondary anemia. Primary hematologic causes of normocytic anemia include early iron-deficiency anemia, aplastic anemia and other bone marrow failure syndromes, and hemolytic anemias (most commonly sickle cell disease). Systemic disorders with secondary normocytic anemia include anemia of chronic disease, systemic infection, acute blood loss, renal failure, and other disorders.[9] The clinician can also classify normocytic anemia as a disorder of decreased RBC production or increased RBC destruction.[7] Whichever way is chosen to develop a diagnostic algorithm, approaching the diagnosis of anemia in a structured way that can consistently consider the broad range of diagnostic possibilities is useful.

Primary Hematologic Causes of Normocytic Anemia

For many patients, the diagnosis of anemia is made on routine screening. Iron-deficiency anemia is the most common cause of nutritional anemia in childhood discovered by routine screening. Although the classic indices for iron-deficiency anemia include a low MCV and a high red cell distribution width, early iron-deficiency anemia may appear as a normocytic anemia. A reticulocyte count will be lower than expected for a patient with anemia because RBC production will be decreased. Iron studies should corroborate the diagnosis of iron-deficiency anemia, but a trial of supplemental iron should be both diagnostic and therapeutic.

Aplastic anemia and bone marrow failure syndromes can result in normocytic anemia as a result of decreased RBC production.[10] Examples include congenital or acquired aplastic anemia, transient erythroblastopenia of childhood,[11,12] pure red cell aplasia (Diamond-Blackfan anemia), and viral infections (eg, parvovirus, Epstein-Barr virus).[13]

Bone marrow infiltration from a malignant process (either leukemia or metastatic solid tumors) can result in decreased RBC production and cause a normocytic anemia. Again, the reticulocyte count will be lower than expected for the degree of anemia. Abnormalities in the white blood cell count and platelet count may also be noted. Immature cells may be noted on review of a peripheral blood smear. Evidence of hemolysis and increased RBC turnover should be absent.

Hemolytic anemias result from RBC membrane defects (eg, hereditary spherocytosis, elliptocytosis),[4] enzyme defects (eg, glucose-6-phosphate dehydrogenase [G6PD] deficiency, pyruvate kinase deficiency),[14] hemoglobin defects (eg, sickle cell disease, thalassemias), and autoimmune hemolytic anemias. In general, the hemolytic anemias are characterized by an elevated reticulocyte count and evidence of increased RBC destruction (elevated serum bilirubin level). A patient with or family history of early cholecystectomy or intermittent jaundice may suggest a familial hemolytic anemia. Obtaining the complete blood count results of immediate family members may help confirm the diagnosis. Although routine newborn screening will identify patients with sickle cell disease born in the United States, for children born in an area without routine screening to have sickle cell disease diagnosed later in life is not uncommon.[15]

Rarely, normocytic anemia may result from a combination of a microcytic anemia (iron deficiency) and a macrocytic anemia (folate deficiency). The MCV is a mean and, as such, 2 populations of RBCs may average out to a normal MCV.

Systemic Causes of Normocytic Anemia

Acute blood loss will result in a normocytic anemia. Patients with chronic blood loss (eg, gastrointestinal bleeding) will likely become iron deficient and develop a microcytic anemia. However, in the early stage of the process, the patient will have normocytic RBCs. Testing the stool for occult blood is indicated in the evaluation.

Anemia of chronic disease is a poorly understood but well-recognized cause of normocytic anemia in children and adults. Anemia of chronic disease can be associated with a variety of illnesses, including rheumatologic conditions, systemic infections, endocrine dysfunction, liver failure, lung disease, and renal disease.[7,16,17]

Evaluation of Normocytic Anemia

In general, normocytic anemias that are nonresponsive to supplemental iron and not clearly associated with a systemic illness warrant referral to a pediatric hematologist. A reticulocyte count and review of the peripheral blood smear are indicated for every child with normocytic anemia referred to a hematologist. The smear may help identify morphologic features to aid in the diagnosis (eg, spherocytosis, sickle cells) or reveal evidence of hemolysis (schistocytes, RBC fragments).

The percentage reticulocyte count must be considered within the context of the patient's hemoglobin level and hematocrit. A high percentage reticulocyte count is expected in a child who can mount an appropriate response to anemia. An apparently normal reticulocyte percentage (1.1% to 3.5%) in a child with severe anemia is actually relatively lower than it should be to compensate for the anemia. For this reason, the reticulocyte index is a useful calculation: the reticulocyte count multiplied by the ratio represented by the patient's hematocrit divided by the normal hematocrit.[10]

A relatively low reticulocyte count suggests decreased RBC production. The primary care physician must then consider aplastic anemia, malignancy, transient erythroblastopenia of childhood, and other causes of bone marrow suppression. A bone marrow aspirate and biopsy are rarely indicated but must be considered to rule out malignancy, especially when more than 1 blood cell line is abnormal.

An elevated reticulocyte count suggests that the bone marrow is compensating for blood loss either from hemolysis or from hemorrhage. Causes of blood loss must be considered. Patients with an elevated reticulocyte count and an elevated bilirubin level likely have ongoing hemolysis. A positive Coombs test (direct antiglobulin test) suggests an autoimmune hemolytic anemia. Without evidence of an autoimmune process, hemoglobinopathies (sickle cell disease and variants and thalassemias) must be evaluated by hemoglobin electrophoresis.

Other specialized assays may define specific RBC disorders that result in hemolysis. G6PD deficiency is the most common enzyme defect. Many variants have been found, and the assay may be falsely negative in patients with a high reticulocyte count immediately after a hemolytic crisis. Families need to be educated regarding the triggers for hemolysis in G6PD deficiency, including a variety of medications, infections, and, for some variants, fava beans (favism). A positive osmotic fragility test helps confirm the diagnosis of hereditary spherocytosis and should be considered in patients with RBC morphology consistent with the diagnosis.[18]

Macrocytic Anemias

Macrocytic anemias in childhood are extremely rare and are typically due to deficiencies in folate and vitamin B_{12}.[1] Folate deficiency can be associated with inborn errors of metabolism, poor dietary intake, increased utilization in patients with hemolytic anemias, malabsorption, and drugs that inhibit folate metabolism (methotrexate). Vitamin B_{12} deficiency may be caused by inborn errors of metabolism, poor dietary intake, and malabsorption. In cases of significant deficiencies, these anemias can be quite severe, with an MCV between 100 and 140 fL. In addition to normochromic macrocytic RBCs, hypersegmented neutrophils may be visible on the peripheral blood smear. Serum folate and B_{12} levels may help confirm the diagnosis, but the underlying etiology of the vitamin deficiency must be determined.

A macrocytic anemia in a child is always concerning for an underlying disorder in bone marrow production. Myelodysplasia, early aplasia, and leukemia may all exhibit as macrocytosis with or without anemia. In the absence of a clear vitamin B_{12} or folate deficiency, a referral to a hematologist is warranted for assessment of macrocytosis to rule out myelodysplasia or malignancy.

Anemia of the Newborn

The differential diagnosis of anemia in a newborn is distinctly different from that of older children. Peripartum hemorrhage and maternal factors, such as alloantibodies, are important in deciphering neonatal anemias. Iron deficiency in the newborn period is quite rare. Anemias with similar origins may also be displayed differently in infants and children.

Table 162-1 lists the normal hematologic parameters for infants and children. Hematologic parameters in children evolve over the 1st couple of months of life. Typically, a normal hemoglobin level in a term newborn is approximately 19 g/dL. The hemoglobin concentration will fall gradually to a nadir at 10 to 11 g/dL by 8 to 12 weeks of age. This nadir, termed *physiologic anemia of the newborn,* is more pronounced in preterm infants with nadirs as low as 7 to 8 g/dL. Despite the low nadir, transfusions are necessary only if the anemia is uncompensated, although early supplementation with iron may be indicated.[1]

When considering the differential diagnosis and etiology of anemia in newborns, classifying the cause of the anemia into 1 of 3 broad classifications is helpful: (1) blood loss, (2) hemolysis, or (3) decreased production.[19,20] Blood loss may occur at any time during a pregnancy. Common causes include fetomaternal transfusion, twin-to-twin transfusion, placental abruption, placenta previa, or internal hemorrhage (eg, intraventricular hemorrhage, cephalohematoma, caput succedaneum). The Betke-Kleihauer test will detect the presence of fetal RBCs in the mother. Fetal cells can be detected in the circulation of 50% of pregnancies; however, rarely is the hemorrhage significant enough to cause anemia in the newborn. Mothers who are blood type O with infants who are not type O may have a false-negative Betke-Kleihauer test.

At least 15% of monochorionic twins will develop significant twin-to-twin transfusions, with differences in hemoglobin concentrations of 5 g/dL or more. At birth, the donor twin will typically be smaller and may have pallor, oligohydramnios, and even shock. Polycythemia, polyhydramnios, and congestive heart failure may be present at birth in the recipient twin.[21]

The clinical manifestation of infants with anemia from blood loss is dependent on the severity and rapidity of the blood loss. Infants with chronic blood loss throughout pregnancy may have pallor and microcytic, hypochromic anemia but appear otherwise well and hemodynamically stable. Infants with acute blood loss may have pallor, tachypnea, tachycardia, hypotension, and decreased tone. A normocytic, normochromic anemia with a reticulocytosis will be detectable soon after birth.[19,20]

The most common cause of hemolytic anemia in the newborn is isoimmune hemolytic anemia caused by an incompatibility in maternal and fetal RBC antigens, including Rh, ABO and minor blood groups. Mothers who are Rh negative may become immunized against the Rh antigen when pregnant with an Rh-positive fetus. During subsequent pregnancies, if the fetus is Rh positive, then maternal anti-Rh antibodies will readily cross the placenta and destroy the Rh-positive RBCs in the fetus. In utero and perinatal hemolysis may be rapid and severe, resulting in life-threatening hemolysis and hyperbilirubinemia. However, with the prenatal administration of Rh immune globulin to Rh-negative mothers, life-threatening Rh incompatibility is rare today. In cases of hemolytic anemia from ABO or minor blood group antigen incompatibility, the mechanism of immunization and hemolysis is similar in Rh incompatibility, but the hemolysis is rarely severe.[1] Hemolytic anemia in the newborn may also occur as a result of maternal drug use and neonatal infections, including bacterial sepsis, cytomegalovirus, toxoplasmosis, herpes, and rubella. Microangiopathic hemolysis may occur in infants with thrombi, disseminated intravascular coagulation, and Kasabach-Merritt syndrome (multiple cavernous hemangiomas).

Hemolysis from hemoglobinopathies rarely causes symptomatic anemia in newborns. Anemia from beta chain defects (eg, sickle cell disease, beta-thalassemias) may not appear until later in infancy when the hemoglobin concentration is more dependent on beta-chain production. Alpha-thalassemia major will exhibit as erythroblastosis fetalis in the newborn period. RBC membrane and enzyme defects may be apparent at birth but more commonly appear later in the newborn period.

RBC production deficiencies are rare in the newborn period and are typically the result of infection or drugs. Diamond-Blackfan anemia is a rare congenital pure RBC precursor aplasia. However, affected patients are typically not anemic until 3 to 12 months of age. Congenital leukemias and osteopetrosis may also result in deficient RBC production but are also typically associated with disorders in the other cell lines and are extremely rare.

EVALUATION

Anemia is frequently identified in the 1st or 2nd year of life and in adolescence on routine screening performed by primary care physicians. By using information obtained from a thorough history and physical examination, as well as results of routine laboratory studies, most causes of anemia can be accurately diagnosed in the primary care physician's office. Diseases leading to anemia and pallor in infants and children are listed in Table 162-2, Figure 162-1, and Figure 162-2.

History

Many children with anemia are asymptomatic and have their conditions diagnosed only on routine screening evaluations. Nonetheless, a thorough history may help identify patients most at risk for developing anemia, as well as help identify the cause of an existing anemia. Demographic factors such as age, gender, and ethnicity will identify risk groups for specific types of anemia. Toddlers and adolescent girls account for most cases of iron-deficiency anemia. Blacks are at greatest risk for sickle cell anemia, whereas the thalassemias occur primarily in patients of Mediterranean and Southeast Asian descent. A diet history is crucial in identifying children most likely to develop iron-deficiency anemia. Sulfa drugs can produce a hemolytic anemia in patients with G6PD deficiency. Many common acute bacterial and viral infections may result in a mild anemia from decreased RBC production or increased RBC destruction, or both. Anemias resulting from such infections are typically short-lived but are commonly the cause of abnormalities identified on routine screening. Acute or chronic blood loss (or both) should be considered in all patients with anemia. Common sites of blood loss in otherwise asymptomatic patients include the gastrointestinal tract for all patients and the genitourinary tract for female patients. Anemia may be the benign manifestation of an underlying systemic disease such as autoimmune disorders and may be associated with signs of systemic illness (fevers, weight loss, among other signs). Finally, a family history may help guide the workup for a patient with anemia. In addition to a family history of hemoglobinopathies, a history of jaundice during systemic illnesses or infections, cholecystectomy at a young age, or splenectomy may suggest a hereditary hemolytic anemia. Historical factors worthy of note in evaluating an anemic patient are listed in Table 162-3.

Physical Examination

Infants and toddlers may experience fatigue, irritability, pallor, increased periods of sleep, poor feeding, and failure to thrive. Older children and adolescents may experience fatigue, pallor, exercise intolerance, dizziness, headaches, shortness of breath, or palpitations. However, most mild to moderate anemias in childhood are asymptomatic as they develop slowly over time, and patients are usually well compensated. In fact, seeing a child for a routine physical examination only to find out later that routine laboratory studies reveal anemia is not uncommon.

Pallor is the classic physical examination finding suggestive of anemia but is rare in mild anemias and frequently only seen reliably with hemoglobin concentrations less than 8 g/dL. Pallor may be more easily identified in the nail beds, mucosa, conjunctiva, and palmar creases than in a cursory examination of the skin. Splenomegaly, scleral icterus, and jaundice in the setting of anemia are highly suggestive of a hemolytic process. In chronic hemolytic anemia such as thalassemia, frontal bossing and maxillary prominence are indicative of the marrow expansion necessary to keep pace with ongoing hemolysis. Leukemia or lymphoma may exhibit as an anemia associated with focal lymphadenopathy and hepatosplenomegaly. Regardless of the cause of the anemia, a mild to moderate decrease in RBC mass may result in a pulmonary valve flow murmur, whereas more severe anemias may be associated with signs and symptoms of congestive heart failure. Compensated anemia usually refers to anemia associated with sufficient cardiovascular compensation to preserve normal oxygen delivery to tissues. Patients in whom the anemia develops or persists over a long period may have hemoglobin concentrations less than 6 g/dL but no signs or symptoms of anemia other than pallor. Cardiac stroke volume is increased, allowing patients to maintain normal oxygen delivery

Table 162-3 Pertinent Historical Factors in the Diagnosis of Childhood Anemia

Age	Nutritional anemias are rare in infancy in term infants but are more common in infants born preterm, as well as in school-aged children and adolescents. Significant anemia diagnosed in the first 6 months of life in a term infant is most likely due a congenital anemia.
Gender	G6PD deficiency and pyruvate kinase deficiency are X-linked disorders.
Race and ethnicity	Thalassemias are more common in patients of African or Asian descent, whereas thalassemia syndromes are more common in patients of Mediterranean descent.
Nutrition	Sources of iron, folate, vitamin B_{12}, and vitamin E should be documented. A history of pica suggests iron deficiency.
Medications	Phenytoin and methotrexate can induce a megaloblastic anemia. Oxidants can induce hemolytic anemias.
Family history	Document a history of anemia, jaundice, gallstones, cholecystitis, splenomegaly, splenectomy or hemolytic crisis, which may suggest an inherited hemolytic anemia.
Infection	Infections may induce hemolysis or red blood cell hypoplasia or aplasia (parvovirus B19), whereas hepatitis may induce aplastic anemia.
Gastrointestinal	The gastrointestinal tract is a common source of blood loss. Nutritional deficiencies may result from malabsorption syndromes.

G6PD, Glucose-6-phosphate dehydrogenase.
Modified from Nathan DG, Orkin SH. *A Diagnostic Approach to the Anemic Patient in Nathan and Oski's Hematology of Infancy and Childhood.* 5th Ed. Philadelphia, PA: WB Saunders; 1998.

to tissues with normal or near-normal heart rates. Patients who lose blood more rapidly, from hemolysis or hemorrhage, may not have time for compensatory mechanisms to maintain tissue perfusion and oxygenation. Tachycardia will be an early sign followed by orthostasis, headache, dizziness, and hypotension, all of which are reasons to hospitalize a patient with anemia.

Laboratory Findings

In addition to a determination of the hemoglobin level and hematocrit, which may be done exclusively in some practice settings, RBC morphology and reticulocyte count should be assessed. Anemias may be classified by RBC size as determined by the MCV and RBC production as determined by the reticulocyte count. An elevated reticulocyte count implies bone marrow compensation for chronic blood loss or hemolysis, whereas a low reticulocyte count may suggest impaired RBC production or acute blood loss. Although not necessary in the initial diagnosis of all patients with anemia, iron studies may be performed and erythrocyte sedimentation rate, serum bilirubin, and serum lactate dehydrogenase levels may be assessed easily in most practice settings and may provide clues to the cause of the anemia. The mean corpuscular hemoglobin (MCH) and mean corpuscular hemoglobin concentration (MCHC) are generally of minimal value in the classification and diagnosis of an anemia. Changes in the MCH typically parallel changes in the MCV. The MCHC is a measure of RBC hydration status. Higher MCHC values (>35/dL) are seen in dehydrated red cells associated with spherocytosis, and low MCHC values may be seen in iron deficiency.

TREATMENT

Treatment of a compensated anemia will be dictated by the cause of the anemia. Patients with uncompensated anemia should be admitted to the hospital for observation and possible transfusion. Effective treatment of the anemia is best accomplished by treating the underlying disorder. A substantial number of patients with a microcytic anemia or a normocytic anemia will have early iron-deficiency anemia, and a course of supplemental iron is appropriate. However, for patients with anemia that is nonresponsive to nutritional supplements and not clearly related to a systemic illness, referral to a pediatric hematologist is warranted. Referral to a pediatric oncologist is also warranted for management of most macrocytic anemias that are not related to nutritional deficiencies. Specific treatment will be predicated on the underlying hematologic disorder.

WHEN TO REFER

- Hemoglobin level less than 8 g/dL or hematocrit less than 25%
- Anemia of unknown origin
- When anemia is associated with disorder in white blood cells or platelets
- If diagnosis of hemoglobinopathy or RBC membrane defect is suspected or confirmed

WHEN TO ADMIT

- Profound anemia (hemoglobin level <5 to 6 g/dL or hematocrit level <15% to 20%)
- Uncompensated anemia or anemia associated with a rapidly dropping hemoglobin level
- Anemia in an ill child

TOOLS FOR PRACTICE

Engaging Patient and Family

- *Anemia and Your Young Child* (brochure), American Academy of Pediatrics (patiented.aap.org).

- *Iron Deficiency* (fact sheet), Centers for Disease Control and Prevention (www.cdc.gov/nccdphp/dnpa/nutrition/nutrition_for_everyone/iron_deficiency/index.htm).

Medical Decision Support

- *Pediatric Nutrition Handbook* (book), American Academy of Pediatrics (www.aap.org/bookstore).

REFERENCES

1. Nathan DG, Orkin SH. *A Diagnostic Approach to the Anemic Patient in Nathan and Oski's Hematology of Infancy and Childhood*. 5th ed. Philadelphia, PA: WB Saunders; 1998.
2. d'Onfrio G, Chirillo R, Zini G, et al. Simultaneous measurement of reticulocyte and red blood cell indices in healthy subjects and patients with microcytic and macrocytic anemia. *Blood*. 1995;85:818-823.
3. Dallman PR, Yip R, Johnson C. Prevalence and causes of anemia in the United States. *Am J Clin Nutr*. 1984;49: 437-445.
4. Weatherall DJ, Clegg JB. *The Thalassemia Syndromes*. 3rd ed. Oxford, UK: Blackwell Scientific Publications; 1981.
5. Higgs DR, Vickers MA, Wilkie AO, et al. A review of the molecular genetics of the human alpha-globin gene cluster. *Blood*. 1989;73:1081-1104.
6. Piomelli S, Seaman C, Zullow D, et al. Threshold for lead damage to heme synthesis in urban children. *Proc Natl Acad Sci U S A*. 1982;79:3335-3339.
7. Brill JR, Baumgardner DJ. Normocytic anemia. *Am Fam Physician*. 2000;62(10):2255-2264.
8. Dallman PR, Siimes MA. Percentile curves for hemoglobin and red cell volume in infancy and childhood. *J Pediatr*. 1979;94(1):26-31.
9. Lanzkowsky P. Classification and diagnosis of anemia during childhood. In: *Manual of Pediatric Hematology and Oncology*. 4th ed. Burlington, MA: Elsevier Academic Press; 2005.
10. Perkins SL. Pediatric red cell disorders and pure red cell aplasia. *Am J Clin Pathol*. 2004;122:S70-S86.
11. Mupanomunda OK, Alter BP. Transient erythroblastopenia of childhood (TEC) presenting as leukoerythroblastic anemia. *J Pediatr Hematol Oncol*. 1997;19(2):165-167.
12. Gerrits GP, van Oostrom CG, de Vaan GA, et al. Transient erythroblastopenia of childhood. A review of 22 cases. *Eur J Pediatr*. 1984;142(4):266-270.
13. Irwin JJ, Kirchner JT. Anemia in children. *Am Fam Physician*. 2001;64(8):1379-1386
14. Prchal JT, Gregg XT. Red cell enzymes. *Hematology Am Soc Hematol Educ Program*. 2005;:19-23.
15. Carreiro-Lewandowski E. Newborn screening: an overview. *Clin Lab Sci*. 2002;15(4):229-238.
16. Abshire TC. The anemia of inflammation. A common cause of childhood anemia. *Pediatr Clin North Am*. 1996; 43(3):623-637.
17. Christensen RD, Hunter DD, Goodell H, et al. Evaluation of the mechanism causing anemia in infants with bronchopulmonary dysplasia. *J Pediatr*. 1992;120(4:1): 593-598.
18. Deters A, Kulozik AE. Hemolytic anemia. In: Sills RH, ed: *Practical Algorithms in Pediatric Hematology and Oncology*. Basel, Switzerland: Kargar; 2003.
19. Lubin B, Vichinsky E. Anemia in the newborn period. *Pediatr Ann*. 1979;8(7):416-434.
20. Oski FA, Naiman JL. *Hematologic Problems of the Newborn*. 3rd ed. Philadelphia, PA: WB Saunders; 1982.
21. Blickstein I. The twin-twin transfusion syndrome. *Obstet Gynecol*. 1990;76:714-722.

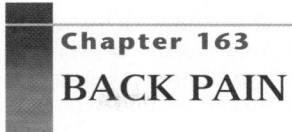

Chapter 163

BACK PAIN

Joel S. Brenner, MD, MPH; Robert A. Pendergrast Jr, MD, MPH

DEFINITION

The back encompasses the region from the upper thoracic vertebra (T1) and shoulder girdle to the sacrum and surrounding musculature. The patient who complains of pain in this region may have a specific sense of localization to a muscle group or vertebral body, for example, or the pain may be more diffuse or sensed by the patient as deep and difficult to localize. Allowing patients to define in their own words the nature, location, and duration of the pain is an important first step in arriving at a clinical diagnosis. Confirmation of the pain history should be obtained from parents, especially for young children but also for teens, who may minimize the pain out of imagined fears of diagnostic or therapeutic procedures. Any functional disability that accompanies pain, such as interference with sports or play, also lends urgency to the diagnostic evaluation, and the corroboration of other observers, such as parents, coaches, and school personnel, can assist the clinician at this point.

EPIDEMIOLOGY

Back pain is an uncommon presenting symptom in pediatric practice. Population-based data on back pain in children are limited, and estimates of prevalence vary considerably depending on sample size and method used. At the least, most studies have consistently shown that prevalence of back pain increases with age. In nonclinical populations, prevalence is less than 10% in preteens, progressing to nearly 50% of 18 to 20 year olds reporting at least one episode of low-back pain.[1] Clearly, most people who experience such pain do not seek medical care, and in preadolescent children, back pain is not only unusual, but also likely to indicate serious underlying illness when severe or persistent enough to prompt a medical visit.[2] One 6-year study in a tertiary orthopedic setting found that back pain constituted fewer than 2% of referrals in children ages 15 years or younger but that roughly 50% of these children had serious underlying diseases.[3] From early adolescence onward, back pain not only becomes more common as a presenting complaint, but also is more likely to be a benign condition related to acute injury or repetitive stress. The clinician presented with a child or adolescent complaining of back pain may use a careful history and physical examination to guide any further laboratory or radiologic evaluation but should be aware of the relatively higher risk of serious underlying disease in younger children, even without specific physical findings.

DIFFERENTIAL DIAGNOSIS

Infants

From infancy through the 3rd or 4th year of life, the patient is not capable of localizing or complaining of pain in the back. Unexplained fever or toxicity, along with refusal to walk or stand, may be the presenting signs of diskitis.[4,5] Leukemia, lymphoma, vasoocclusive crisis, vertebral osteomyelitis in a child who has sickle cell disease, or trauma (especially intentional injury) may exhibit as disease localized to the back in this age group.

Children

As children mature and become more capable of localizing symptoms, a specific history of the duration, quality, associated symptoms, and radiation of back pain becomes possible, but back pain before adolescence remains an uncommon presenting complaint. The differential diagnosis in this age group includes diskitis, an inflammatory process presumed to be a bacterial infection in the intervertebral disk space. An unusual, if not rare, condition, diskitis is most common in children younger than 10 years (mean age approximately 6 years). Vertebral osteomyelitis usually affects school-age children and teenagers, and it causes severe back pain and systemic symptoms. A family history of rheumatoid disease should prompt consideration of ankylosing spondylitis. In the presence of sickle hemoglobinopathy, a vasoocclusive crisis is a strong consideration. Acute leukemia, lymphoma, and primary vertebral tumors, such as Ewing sarcoma, aneurysmal bone cyst, benign osteoblastoma, and osteoid osteoma, must also be considered as possible diagnoses.[4] Back pain on walking may be the only sign of a tethered cord.[4] Only after a thorough diagnostic evaluation should the clinician consider the diagnosis of muscular or ligamentous strain as a cause of back pain in younger children.

Adolescents

Classifying the causes of back pain in adolescents as acute or chronic would be helpful (Table 163-1). In adolescent patients, a diagnostic consideration of acute back pain caused by muscular or ligamentous strain is reasonable. Other causes of acute back pain include lumbar disk disease, vertebral osteomyelitis, epidural abscess, and sciatica caused by piriformis syndrome. The adolescent who has chronic pain (more than 3 weeks) may still have a strain, but stronger consideration should be given at this point to rule out spondylolysis or spondylolisthesis, which are the most common identifiable causes of low-back pain in this age group.[2] The most frequent cause of spondylolysis is a stress fracture of the pars interarticularis (posterior arch) of the spine, thought to be acquired through repetitive extension loading. Athletes who participate in gymnastics, dance, cheerleading, football, and diving are at highest risk. For example, ballet dancers, as a group, have great flexibility but may be predisposed to lumbar lordosis by postural demands and relatively weak core musculature, possibly making them prone to spondylolysis and to disk disease.[6] Less commonly, spondylolysis can be an asymptomatic congenital deformity. Spondylolisthesis is the anterior movement of 1 vertebral body on top of another, usually L5 on S1, as a result of bilateral spondylolysis. Chronic low-back pain, especially in adolescent athletes or others who have cumulative trauma, may indicate lumbar disk disease. Other chronic causes of back pain in this age group include Scheuermann kyphosis, facet or vertebral dysfunction, sacroiliac dysfunction, spinal stenosis, the spondyloarthropathies (ie, ankylosing spondylitis, psoriatic arthritis, Reiter syndrome, arthritis of inflammatory bowel disease), and a tumor or malignancy. Chronic back pain can also be a disorder of the soft tissues of the back, perhaps caused by repetitive strain coupled with genetic predisposition and environmental factors, such as prolonged seated posture or forward bending of the spine, as with studying or reading while sitting at a desk for long periods or carrying an excessively heavy backpack (10% to 20% of bodyweight).[7-9]

Table 163-1 Differential Diagnosis of Back Pain

INFANTS	CHILDREN	ADOLESCENTS
Diskitis	Diskitis	Acute:
Leukemia, lymphoma	Tethered cord	Lumbar disk disease
Vasocclusive crisis	Osteomyelitis	Muscle, ligament strain
Osteomyelitis	Ankylosing spondylitis	Sciatica, piriformis syndrome
Trauma	Vasocclusive crisis	Osteomyelitis
	Leukemia, lymphoma	Epidural abscess
	Ewing sarcoma	Spinal tuberculosis
	Osteoid osteoma	Chronic:
	Spinal tuberculosis	Spondylolysis
		Spondylolisthesis
		Scheuermann kyphosis
		Facet, vertebral dysfunction
		Sacroiliac dysfunction
		Lumbar disk disease
		Spinal stenosis
		Spondyloarthropathy
		Tumor or malignancy
		Soft tissue strain
		Functional (nonorganic)

PSYCHOSOCIAL CONSIDERATIONS

Although malingering or the use of pain symptoms for secondary gain may be relatively common in adults, it should not be a strong consideration in the diagnosis of back pain in children or adolescents. However, whereas back pain is not as common a somatoform symptom among adolescents as is headache, abdominal pain, or chest pain, if a thorough diagnostic evaluation of chronic back pain in an adolescent is unrevealing and the usual management involving exercise and stretching is not beneficial, then a psychosocial or nonorganic cause should be considered. The Wadell test, a series of 5 questions, may be used to help determine if significant psychologic stress is associated with chronic low-back pain.[10] If 3 or more of the following 5 criteria are present, then the test is considered positive:

1. Inappropriate tenderness that is superficial or wide spread
2. Pain on pressing the top of the head or on passive rotation of shoulders and pelvis
3. Distraction signs such as inconsistent performance between straight leg raising in the seated and the supine position
4. Strength and sensory loss patterns that do not fit a directional distribution
5. Overreaction during the physical examination[10]

EVALUATION

Infants, Children, and Adolescents

The age of the patient is a critical factor in determining the diagnostic evaluation, with the extent and urgency of evaluation usually being greater for preadolescent patients.[11,12] Another factor is the duration of symptoms; chronic pain, even in adolescent patients, is uncommon and may indicate structural or serious underlying disease and should prompt a diagnostic evaluation possibly to include rectal examination for sphincter tone loss, radiographs of the spine (anteroposterior, lateral, and oblique views), blood count, uric acid, lactate dehydrogenase, sedimentation rate, C-reactive protein, and urinalysis and culture. Evaluation of acute or chronic back pain should always include motor, sensory, and reflex examination to help differentiate any nerve root involvement (Figure 163-1).

Infants, young children, or adolescents who have fever and back pain must be considered as having an infectious, inflammatory, or neoplastic process until proven otherwise: diskitis, vertebral osteomyelitis, ankylosing spondylitis, pyelonephritis, vasoocclusive crisis in a patient who has sickle cell anemia, acute lymphoblastic leukemia, Ewing sarcoma, or Hodgkin lymphoma.[4,11] Spinal tuberculosis (Pott disease), fortunately, is rare but should be considered when back pain is accompanied by low-grade fever.[12]

A child with diskitis is typically uncomfortable in an upright posture, may refuse to walk or may have pain when bending forward. Even in the absence of fever, a child who refuses to walk, particularly a preschooler, should be evaluated promptly for diskitis. Typically, diskitis is associated with an elevated erythrocyte sedimentation rate and a high white blood cell count; plain radiographs of the spine may show narrowing of the disk space. If a second radiologic test is needed, then magnetic resonance imaging is generally thought to be a sensitive test in evaluating for diskitis.[4,5]

Weight loss, bone pain in other locations, bruising, organomegaly, or adenopathy should prompt aggressive diagnostic evaluation for malignancies such as leukemia, lymphoma, or sarcomas. Especially in the presence of fever or other systemic signs and symptoms, acute leukemia and lymphoma are serious concerns and must be ruled out.

A child with nocturnal back pain, even if relieved by nonprescription analgesics, should be evaluated for osteoid osteoma or osteoblastoma with bone scans if plain radiographs are normal.[2,4] Primary vertebral tumors almost always will be visible on plain radiographs, but computed tomography or magnetic resonance imaging may be needed.

Fever accompanied by back pain should prompt an aggressive diagnostic evaluation and orthopedic surgery consultation because aspiration and culture to evaluate for possible vertebral osteomyelitis should be considered.[2] Dysuria, urinary urgency, or urinary frequency, especially if accompanied by fever, warrants consideration of pyelonephritis.

Idiopathic scoliosis usually does not cause back pain[12]; thus scoliosis with pain should raise concern about a malignancy in the region of the spine or a benign osteoid osteoma.

Adolescents

Muscular or ligamentous strain begins to become common during adolescence. The typical presentation is low-back pain of 3 weeks' or less duration, with or without

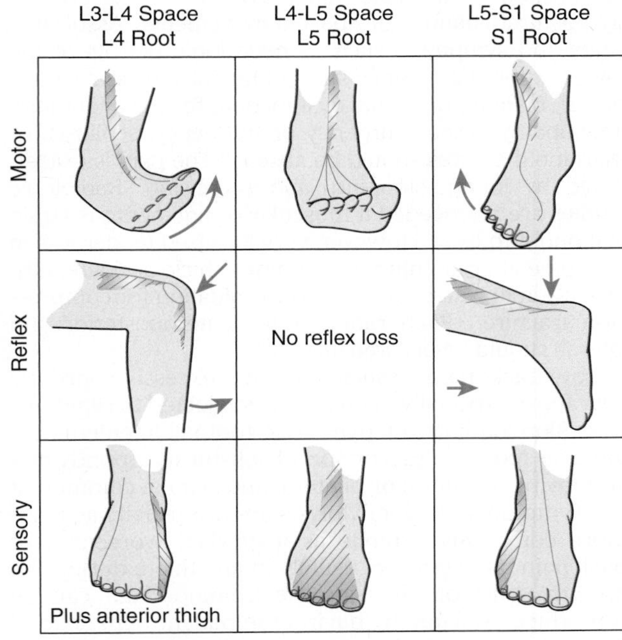

Figure 163-1 Sensory, motor, reflex grid. (*Lewis RC.* Primary Care Orthopedics. *Copyright © 1988, Elsevier, with permission.*)

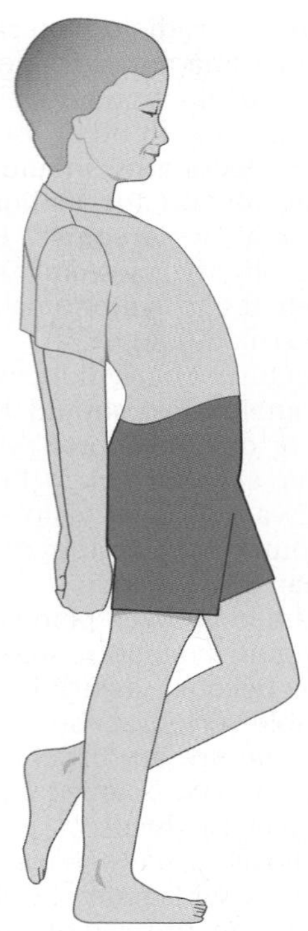

Figure 163-2 One leg hyperextension test (stork test). *(Jackson DW, Wiltse LL, Dingeman RD, et al. Stress reactions involving the pars interarticularis in young athletes.* Am J Sports Med. *1981;9(5):304-312. Reprinted by permission of Sage Publications Inc.)*

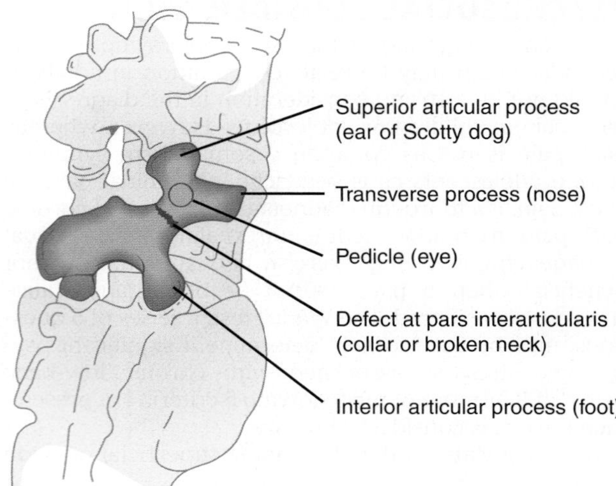

Figure 163-3 Scotty dog with a collar. *(Smith JA, Hu SS. Management of spondylolysis and spondylolisthesis in the pediatric and adolescent population.* Orthopedic Clinics of North America. *1999;30(3):487-499, ix. Copyright © 1999, Elsevier, with permission.)*

recollection of an acute injury and that is exacerbated by postural changes or specific movements. Associated signs and symptoms such as neurologic deficits of the lower extremities, limited straight leg raising, sciatic pain, bowel, bladder, or sexual dysfunction, fever, weight loss, adenopathy, urinary urgency or frequency, scoliosis, or marfanoid habitus should be absent.[3] The pain is exacerbated by lifting, stooping, and exercising. Radiologic studies are not needed if muscular or ligamentous strain is thought to exist. However, very localized tenderness in the spine after an injury (eg, motor vehicle accident, athletic trauma) warrants radiologic evaluation for compression fracture.[4] Plain radiographs (anteroposterior and lateral) should be ordered initially.

Low-back pain associated with excessive lordotic curvature, especially in an athlete subjected to repetitive extension loading (eg, gymnasts, football linemen) may indicate spondylolysis or spondylolisthesis. Spondylolysis may be unilateral or bilateral and is most common at L5. Symptoms of spondylolysis are not usually acute; it more commonly exhibits as a gradual worsening of back pain on extension, usually in an athlete during the growth spurt or after intense training. Pain can be reproduced reliably by having the patient hyperextend the back while standing on one leg (the stork test) (Figure 163-2).[2,13] The patient usually has no pain with flexion, rotation, or lateral bending of the back. Hamstring tightness is a common associated finding.[4] Plain radiographs of the lumbar spine should be ordered (anteroposterior, lateral, oblique views). The *Scotty dog with a collar* is visualized on the oblique radiographs (Figure 163-3). Normal plain radiographs alone do not rule out spondylolysis completely, and a single-photon emission computed tomography (SPECT) scan should be ordered if the diagnosis is highly suggested. A positive plain radiograph with a negative SPECT scan is indicative of a nonmetabolically active spondylolysis that may not be the cause of the patient's back pain. Back pain on extension with normal plain radiographs and SPECT scan is usually from facet or vertebral dysfunction.

Spondylolisthesis may be accompanied on physical examination not only by excess lumbar lordosis but also by the sensation of a shelf at the base of the lordotic curvature, where the lower of the 2 affected vertebrae has held its position while the upper vertebral body slipped forward. The anterior slippage is diagnosed and staged for treatment purposes on the lateral plain radiographs. In rare cases, radiographs will reveal congenital absence of a lumbosacral articular process.[14]

Accompanying neurologic symptoms, including radicular pain down the leg, numbness or tingling, bowel or bladder problems, erectile dysfunction, or loss of sphincter tone on rectal examination, may indicate lumbar disk herniation or other nerve compression and should prompt an urgent evaluation and referral.[4,11] Symptoms are typically worsened by mechanical strain, as with lifting or coughing.[4] A positive straight leg-raising test or a *slump test* (Figure 163-4) is highly suggestive of nerve root compression.[13] Using cervical flexion to accentuate the patient's symptoms during straight leg raising may add to the test's sensitivity. Any reproduction of the patient's usual symptoms during testing before 60 degrees of hip flexion, or marked asymmetry in symptoms, should be considered a positive test.[15,16] Pain after 60 degrees or limited to the posterior thigh is more likely caused by hamstring tightness.

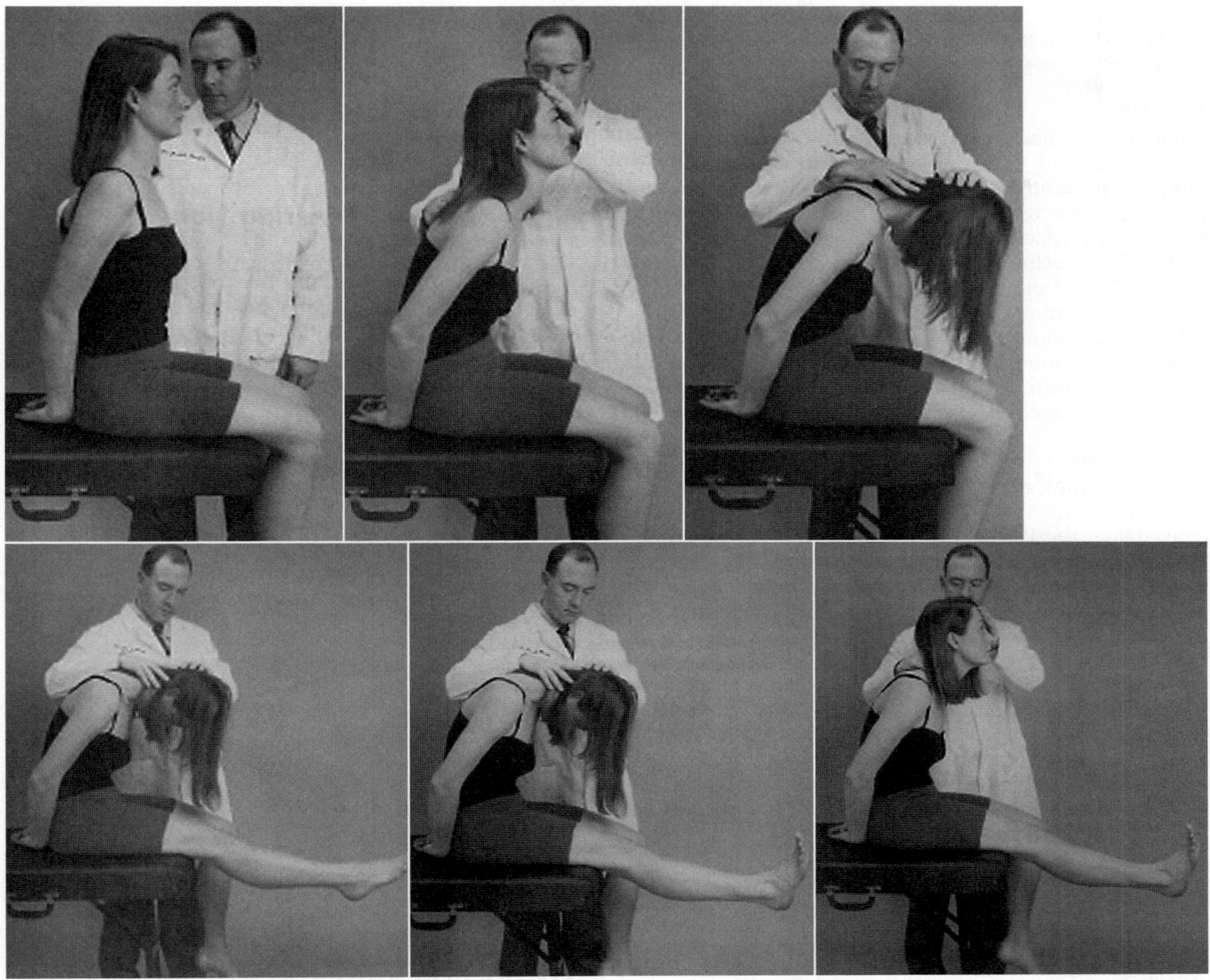

Figure 163-4 Slump test. *(Reider B.* The Orthopedic Physical Examination. *Philadelphia, PA: WB Saunders; 1999. Copyright © 1999, Elsevier, with permission.)*

Scheuermann disease, or butterflyer's back, typically exhibits in an adolescent, particularly a competitive swimmer, with thoracic back pain after exercise or late in the day, rigid thoracic kyphosis on examination, and pain worsened by forward flexion.[2,4,17] It must be differentiated from postural kyphosis, commonly seen in adolescents, which is a flexible kyphosis (disappearing on forward flexion and conscious postural straightening). The diagnosis is confirmed by anterior wedging of 5 degrees or greater in three or more contiguous vertebrae shown on lateral plain spine radiographs.[17] Oblique radiographs also should be obtained because spondylolysis is associated with Scheuermann disease.[18]

Stigmata of Marfan syndrome include joint hyperextensibility, pectus excavatum, pes planus, dislocated lenses, hernias, arachnodactyly, and scoliosis. The scoliosis may result from a dural ectasia or widening of the subarachnoid space in the lumbar area, which has been associated with low-back pain in adolescents and young adults.[19] Patients who have Marfan syndrome are also at increased risk of spondylolysis.[12]

MANAGEMENT

Pain that is acute and lasting fewer than 3 weeks, especially with a history of musculoskeletal injury, may be managed expectantly in many cases, whereas more chronic pain in a child or adolescent demands further investigation.[11,12] When back pain results from an underlying disorder, treatment of the pain itself should occur in addition to treatment of the primary condition.

Infants

Treatment for diskitis is variable, depending on its cause. Most experts recommend parenteral followed by oral antibiotic administration, if evidence of bacterial infection exists, and relative rest to promote pain control.[20,21] Staphylococcal infection is the most common cause of vertebral osteomyelitis and should be treated with antibiotics, rest, and a prompt orthopedic surgery consultation.[2]

Children

Treatment for diskitis and osteomyelitis in children is the same as that for infants. Management of patients with ankylosing spondylitis is best coordinated by a pediatric rheumatologist who will use antiinflammatory medications with physical and occupational therapy.[22] Treatment of vasocclusive crisis entails pain management, hydration, and physical therapy. Leukemia, lymphoma, and Ewing sarcoma should be managed by a pediatric oncologist. Pain from osteoid osteoma is typically relieved with nonsteroidal antiinflammatory agents, and patients should be referred to a pediatric orthopedic surgeon for possible excision or ablation.[23,24]

Adolescents

When the adolescent exhibits back pain acutely after an injury that is thought to be a muscular or ligamentous strain, the PRICEMMMS mnemonic (**p**rotection, **r**elative rest, **i**ce, **c**ompression, **e**levation, **m**edication, **m**otion, **m**odalities, **s**trength) should be used. Bed rest, which has been shown to delay recovery, should be discouraged.[25] Continuous frequency ultrasound and massage are often helpful. Pain-free activity may be resumed gradually, and low-back and hamstring flexibility, as well as the strengthening of the core musculature (abdominal area, hip, and back) with an exercise ball or Pilates exercises should be emphasized.

Evidence indicates that full sit-ups with the feet fixed and the knees bent, by using hip flexors rather than abdominal muscles, increase intervertebral disk pressure and should be discouraged. The goal of abdominal muscle strengthening is to reduce pelvic tilt and its accompanying tendency toward lordosis and low-back strain. Because decreased strength and endurance of spinal extensor muscles is associated with low-back pain, extensor exercises such as raising the torso and head off the floor or exercise ball while lying prone are recommended. These same exercises, and stretching after warming the muscles by gentle exercise or moist heat, are recommended for chronic low-back pain of muscular origin. Proper posture should also be taught, and backpack weights should not exceed 15% to 20% of the person's bodyweight.[7-9]

The treatment of spondylolysis is controversial and may best be managed by a pediatric sports medicine specialist or orthopedic surgeon. All regimens include the initial cessation of extension-loading activities while providing symptomatic relief and physical therapy that promotes abdominal strengthening and hamstring stretching (the Williams program). Thoracolumbar bracing to prevent extension has been shown to be helpful, but some experts advocate restricting extension activities without a brace.[26-28] Bracing should be used up to 6 months or until the patient is pain free with extension. Bone stimulators have been used as adjunctive therapy.[29,30]

Treatment for Scheuermann disease is usually conservative, including physical therapy with strengthening and stretching exercises, avoiding painful activities, and analgesic medication if needed.[17] Thoracolumbar bracing and surgery may be indicated if kyphosis is more than 60 degrees.[2,17] Patients should be referred to an orthopedic surgeon (pediatric or spinal) for failure of conservative management, intractable pain, or progression of the kyphotic deformity.

Referral to a mental health professional may not be necessary for functional or nonorganic back pain. If the family has a high degree of trust with the physician, then a sensitive evaluation of family and social factors may be an effective first step. In these cases, the clinician should not assume that the pain is feigned, but rather is a very real physical symptom rooted in psychologic or emotional distress. At the very least, chronic pain and its accompanying disability can, of itself, lead to psychologic distress, which should be addressed openly by the clinician.

WHEN TO REFER

- Abnormality of posture or gait
- Neurologic findings
- Persistent pain in a preteen
- Pain unrelated to activity or on awakening from sleep
- Functional disability (decreased play or sports activity)
- Diagnosis and evaluation is outside of the primary care physician's scope of expertise

WHEN TO ADMIT

- Whenever a prompt and thorough outpatient diagnostic assessment cannot be completed for a child who has back pain and associated fever or neurologic findings

TOOLS FOR PRACTICE

Engaging Patients and Family

- *Backpack Safety* (fact sheet), American Academy of Pediatrics (www.schoolhealth.org/content/backpackSafety.pdf).
- *Sports Shorts: Lower Back Pain in Athletes* (fact sheet), American Academy of Pediatrics (www.aap.org/family/SportsShorts_10.pdf).

Medical Decision Support

- *Care of the Young Athlete* (book), American Academy of Pediatrics (www.aap.org/bookstore).
- *Essentials of Musculoskeletal Care,* 3rd edition (book), American Academy of Pediatrics (www.aap.org/bookstore).
- *Sports Shorts: Lower Back Pain in Athletes* (fact sheet), American Academy of Pediatrics (www.aap.org/family/SportsShorts_10.pdf).

AAP POLICY STATEMENT

American Academy of Pediatrics, Committee on Psychosocial Aspects of Child and Family Health, Task Force on Pain in Infants, Children, and Adolescents. The assessment and management of acute pain in infants, children, and adolescents. *Pediatrics*. 2001;108:793-797. (aappolicy.aappublications.org/cgi/content/full/pediatrics;108/3/793).

REFERENCES

1. Leboeuf-Yde C, Kyvik K. At what age does low-back pain become a common problem? *Spine*. 1998;23:228-234.
2. Hollingsworth P. Back pain in children. *Bri J Rheumatol*. 1996;35:1022.
3. Turner P, Green J, Galasko C. Back pain in childhood. *Spine*. 1989;14:812-814.
4. Payne W, Ogilvie J. Back pain in children and adolescents. *Pediatr Clin North Am*. 1996;43:899-918.
5. Staheli L. Pain of musculoskeletal origin in children. *Curr Opin Rheumatol*. 1992;4:748-752.
6. Bryan N, Smith B. Back school programs: the ballet dancer. *Occup Med*. 1992;7:67-75.
7. Mackenzie W, Sampath J, Kruse R, et al. Backpacks in children. *Clin Orthop Rel Res*. 2003;409:78-84.
8. Negrini S, Carabalona R, Sibilla P. Backpack as a daily load for schoolchildren. *Lancet*. 1999;354:1974.
9. Brackley H, Stevenson J. Are children's backpack weight limits enough? A critical review of the relevant literature. *Spine*. 2004;29(19);2184-2190.
10. Wadell G, Kummel E, Venner R. Nonorganic physical signs in low back pain. *Spine*. 1980;5:117-125.
11. Dyment P. Low back pain in adolescents. *Pediatr Ann*. 1991;20:170.
12. Sponseller P. Evaluating the child with back pain. *Am Fam Phys*. 1996;54:1993.
13. Reider B. *The Orthopaedic Physical Examination*. Philadelphia, PA: WB Saunders; 1999.
14. Ikeda K, Nakayama Y, Ishii S. Congenital absence of lumbosacral articular process: report of three cases. *J Spin Dis*. 1992;5:232-236.
15. Farrell J, Drye C. Back school programs: the young patient. *Occup Med*. 1992;7:55.
16. Epstein J, Epstein N, Marc J. Lumbar intervertebral disk herniation in teenage children: recognition and management of associated anomalies. *Spine*. 1984;9:427-432.
17. Lowe T. Scheuermann's disease. *Orthop Clin North Am*. 1999;30:475-487.
18. Ogilvie J, Sherman J. Spondylolysis in Scheuermann's disease. *Spine*. 1987;12:251-253.
19. Schlesinger E. The significance of genetic contributions and markers in disorders of spinal structure. *Neurosurgery*. 1990;26:944-951.
20. Ring D, Johnston C, Wenger D. Pyogenic infectious spondylitis in children: the convergence of discitis and vertebral osteomyelitis. *J Pediatr Orthop*. 1995;15: 652-660.
21. Cushing A. Diskitis in children. *Clin Infect Dis*. 1993; 17:1-6.
22. Cassidy J, Petty R, Laxer R, et al. *Textbook of Pediatric Rheumatology*. 5th ed. Philadelphia, PA: Elsevier Saunders; 2005.
23. Lindner N, Ozaki T, Roedl R, et al. Percutaneous radiofrequency ablation in osteoid osteoma. *J Bone Joint Surg Brit Vol*. 2001;83(B3):391-396.
24. Wenger D, Rang M. *The Art and Practice of Children's Orthopaedics*. New York, NY: Raven Press; 1993.
25. Malmivaara A, Hakkinen U, Aro T, et al. The treatment of acute low back pain—bed rest, exercises, or ordinary activity? *N Engl J Med*. Feb 1995;332(6):351-355.
26. Anderson K, Sarwark J, Conway J, et al. Quantitative assessment with SPECT imaging of stress injuries of the pars interarticularis and response to bracing. *J Pediatr Orthop*. 2000;20(1);28-33.
27. Steiner M, Micheli L. Treatment of symptomatic spondylolysis and spondylolisthesis with the modified Boston brace. *Spine*. 1985;10(10):937-943.
28. Smith J, Hu S. Management of spondylolysis and spondylolisthesis in the pediatric and adolescent population. *Orthop Clin North Am*. 1999;30:487-499.
29. Zimmerman J, Simmons S. Bony healing in a patient with bilateral L5 spondylolysis. *Curr Sports Med Rep*. 2005;4:35-37.
30. Stasinopoulos D. Treatment of spondylolysis with external electrical stimulation in young athletes: a critical literature review. *Bri J Sports Med*. 2004;38(3);352-354.

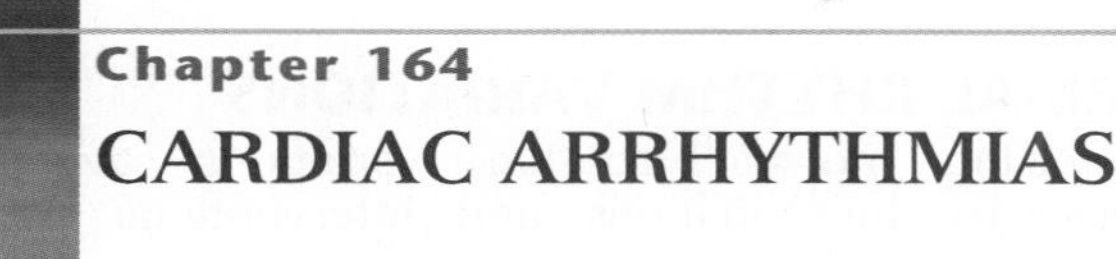

Chapter 164
CARDIAC ARRHYTHMIAS

J. Peter Harris, MD

Arrhythmias in the young are common and usually benign but may be life altering or lethal. Arrhythmias may begin at any age, from in utero up to the later teenage years, with a higher incidence in early infancy and mid-adolescence. Newer investigative modalities such as event recorders to capture infrequent episodes have enhanced our ability to detect and treat arrhythmias. Empirical therapy without detecting arrhythmia does not meet the current standard of practice. A 12-lead electrocardiogram (ECG) should always be obtained when an arrhythmia is being considered because rhythm alterations may be quite subtle and not always identified on a rhythm strip. In addition, a thorough family history is required, with particular emphasis on sudden and premature death, syncope, and recurrent arrhythmias.

Depending on the age of the patient and the rate and type of rhythm disturbance, children with arrhythmias may have nonspecific signs and symptoms such as fatigue, malaise, poor feeding, nausea, and pallor, or they may have more typical symptoms of cardiac dysfunction such as palpitations (the disquieting awareness of the person's own heartbeat), lightheadedness, syncope, visceral chest pain, and dyspnea.

Premature beats are infrequently noted by young patients. Supraventricular tachyarrhythmias in infancy may be noted incidentally on a visit for other reasons, but, more commonly, infants with supraventricular tachycardia (SVT) have signs and symptoms of congestive heart failure: tachypnea, dyspnea, truncal diaphoresis, diminished pulses, pallor, hepatomegaly, and poor feeding, in addition to tachycardia. Older children and adolescents are able to verbalize discomfort, including palpitations, chest pain, dyspnea, and nausea, from various forms of SVT. Ventricular tachyarrhythmias frequently compromise cardiac output to a greater degree than SVT and have more overt signs of congestive failure, chest pain, syncope, dyspnea, and palpitations. Infants and children with moderate or greater bradycardia from advanced 2nd-degree and complete heart block also display signs and symptoms of inadequate cardiac output, including fatigue, reduced exercise capacity, pallor, presyncope, and syncope.

APPROACH TO ARRHYTHMIAS

As a part of the systematic approach to ECG interpretation, the cardiac rhythm should be analyzed in an organized fashion. The answers to the following 4 questions will define the majority of arrhythmias:

1. Is the rhythm fast or slow?
2. Is the rhythm regular or irregular?
3. Are the QRS complexes narrow or wide?
4. What is the relationship between the P waves and the QRS complexes?

NORMAL RHYTHM VARIATIONS

Recognizing normal rhythm variations avoids unnecessary investigations and interventions and allays patient and parental anxiety. For instance, sinus arrhythmia (phasic respiratory variations of sinus rate with inspiratory slowing and expiratory acceleration) is common in childhood; so too is wandering atrial pacemaker, usually noted with slower heart rates and characterized by different P wave morphologies. These rhythm variations are related to alterations in vagal tone.

A wide range of heart rates is present in the young. Sinus tachycardia has been documented at rates of 230 to 250 beats per minute (bpm) during infancy, but a rate in excess of 200 bpm in a teenager who is not involved in maximal exertion would be abnormal. Greater consternation occurs with slow heart rates than with fast rates. Sinus bradycardia is a sinus rate below what is expected for a patient's age. A sinus rate below 100 bpm in an awake neonate would be abnormal, but during sleep, rates down to 80 bpm are commonly observed on ECG monitoring. Brief dips into the 60 to 80 bpm range are also observed in sleeping neonates during normal, vagally induced episodes of junctional rhythm that arise from either the atrioventricular node or the bundle of His and that are characterized by a narrow QRS without a preceding P wave. A highly conditioned adolescent endurance athlete may have a resting heart rate of 40 bpm or less. Table 164-1 provides guidelines for the diagnosis of sinus bradycardia on the surface ECG and during ambulatory monitoring.

Table 164-1 Bradycardia by Age and State

AGE	HEART RATE
SURFACE ELECTROCARDIOGRAM	
Neonates and infants	<100 bpm, awake
Children to 3 years	<100 bpm
Children 3 to 9 years	<60 bpm
Adolescents 9 to 16 years	<50 bpm
Adolescents >16 years	<40 bpm
AMBULATORY (HOLTER) MONITORING	
Neonates and infants	<60 bpm, sleeping, 80 bpm, awake, quiet
Children 2 to 6 years	<60 bpm
Children 7 to 11 years	<45 bpm
Adolescents >11 years	<40 bpm
Athletes	<30 bpm

PREMATURE BEATS

Premature beats are common but are usually benign arrhythmias, which may arise in the atria, the atrioventricular junction, or the ventricles. By definition, premature beats are early and thus are distinguished from escape or late beats occurring when higher pacemaker cells fail to produce an impulse at the expected interval. Two premature beats in a row constitute a couplet. If every 2nd or 3rd beat is a premature impulse, then a bigeminal or trigeminal rhythm is present.

Atrial Premature Contractions

Atrial premature contractions (APCs) are characterized by premature P waves with an axis and morphology that are different from the sinus P waves. If an APC occurs when one of the bundle branches is refractory, then the premature beat will be conducted down the other bundle branch, resulting in an aberrant APC with a QRS morphology wider and different from sinus QRS complexes (Figure 164-1). If both bundle branches are refractory, then the APC will not be conducted to the ventricles (blocked APC) but may reset the sinus node with a resultant pause greater than the previous RR interval. If every other beat is a blocked APC (blocked atrial bigeminy) in a newborn, then slowing of the heart rate sufficient to alter feeding and arousal time may be present. T waves are usually smoothly inscribed, and consistent sharp deflections in the T waves may represent P waves (Figure 164-2). APCs usually occur with normally conducted QRS complexes; but if wide beats are also noted, then the apparently prolonged QRS beats are likely to be aberrant APCs because premature atrial and ventricular contractions rarely occur together, especially in the newborn period.

The incidence of APCs in pediatric patients is 50% to 75%. Although associated with myocarditis, atrial stretch, sympathomimetic or other stimulant drugs, intracardiac catheters, and electrolyte disturbances,

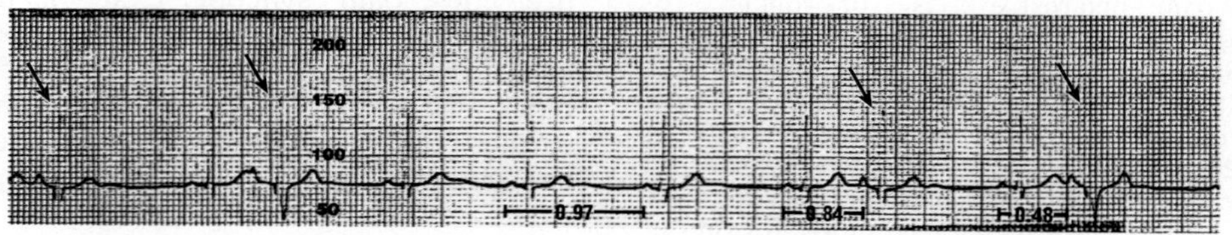

Figure 164-1 Atrial premature contractions *(arrows)* with normal and aberrated conduction.

the majority do not have an obvious incitant, and these are usually not recognized by the child or adolescent. Therapy is not necessary unless the APCs initiate SVT or result in blocked impulses in a newborn that is dependent, in part, on heart rate to maintain an adequate cardiac output. If suppressive therapy is required, then either digoxin or propranolol is suitable.

Premature Ventricular Contractions

Premature ventricular contractions (PVCs) are less common than APCs but, on Holter monitoring, may affect up to 25% of healthy infants, children, and adolescents. PVCs are characterized by a QRS morphology that is different from sinus QRS beats, occur before the next expected sinus beat, and are not preceded by a premature P wave. The QRS duration may be only slightly prolonged. Uniform PVCs have similar morphology in contrast to multiform beats. The designations *unifocal* and *multifocal* are no longer used because PVCs that have different origins may appear similar, and depending on the direction of exit from a particular location in the myocardium, PVCs arising from the same focus may have different morphologies. If a PVC occurs late, at the beginning of the next expected sinus beat, then it will produce a hybrid or fusion beat derived, in part, from the normal conduction pathways and, in part, from the PVC. Fusion beats have a morphology that is intermediate between the sinus QRS and PVC.

Although observed most often in healthy children and adolescents, PVCs occur in patients who have underlying heart disease, especially cardiomyopathic processes such as myocarditis, hypertrophic and dilated cardiomyopathies, and ventricular dysfunction in congenital cardiac malformations. Other causes include sympathomimetic and street stimulant drugs, electrolyte imbalances, and intraventricular catheters. A 12-lead ECG should always be obtained to assess the premature beat morphology and to look for chamber enlargement but also to calculate the corrected QT interval.

$$\text{QTc} = \frac{\text{QT interval (seconds)}}{\sqrt{\text{Preceding RR interval (seconds)}}}$$

PVCs are considered benign if no evidence for heart disease exists, the QTc is normal ($\leq$0.44 seconds), the family history is not adverse (no sudden premature deaths or cardiac arrests, important arrhythmias, or cardiomyopathies), and the PVCs are uniform in appearance and are either suppressed or not aggravated with exercise. On the other hand, the presence of any of these risk factors defines worrisome PVCs and prompts the need for referral and further investigation. The new appearance of PVCs in the setting of a febrile illness should raise the question of myocarditis. Because underlying heart disease may be subtle, an echocardiogram to assess cardiac structure and function is usually obtained in referred patients. Benign PVCs do not require treatment or curtailment of exercise, even if a bigeminal rhythm is present. However, if very frequent PVCs persist, then long-term yearly follow-up should be instituted to detect the unusual situation of arrhythmia-induced ventricular dilatation or dysfunction, or both.[1] If worrisome PVCs are present, then the need for therapy should be determined by a pediatric cardiologist. Ventricular couplets or pairs are assessed in the same manner, but triplets represent ventricular tachycardia and are discussed later in this chapter.

SUPRAVENTRICULAR TACHYCARDIA

Supraventricular tachycardia (SVT) is very common in the young, affecting as many as 1 out of every 250 children. More than 90% of pediatric SVT is reentrant in nature, involving 2 distinct pathways that have different conduction characteristics and unidirectional blocks in one pathway. The impulse enters the second unblocked pathway and then reenters the blocked pathway from the opposite direction. Most of the reentrant SVT encountered in infants and children is due to an accessory pathway, but the incidence of atrioventricular (AV) nodal reentry increases during adolescence with further development of the atrioventricular node. Unlike reentrant SVT, automatic ectopic SVTs cannot be initiated or terminated by a premature beat or pacing and tend to be incessant with a variable rate dependent on autonomic tone. Automatic tachycardias account for less than 10% of SVT in children.

In decreasing order of frequency, the mechanisms underlying SVT in the young include:

- Atrioventricular reentry tachycardia through an accessory pathway (preexcitation)
- AV nodal reentry tachycardia using the fast and slow pathways in the AV nodal region
- Primary atrial tachycardias such as automatic SVT, atrial flutter, and atrial fibrillation[2]

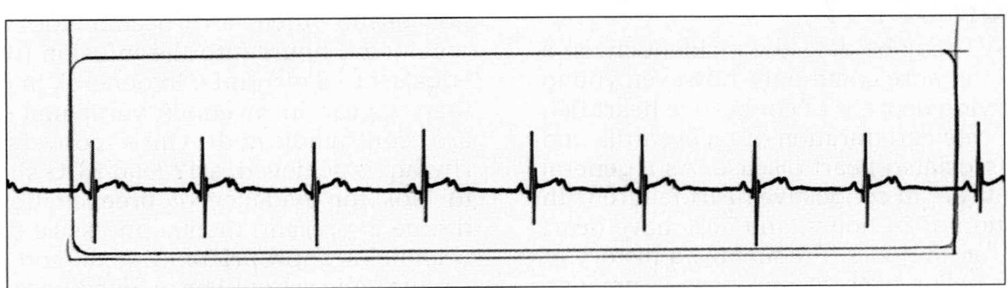

Figure 164-2 Every other beat is a blocked atrial premature contraction (blocked atrial bigeminy) represented by a consistent sharp deflection in the T waves.

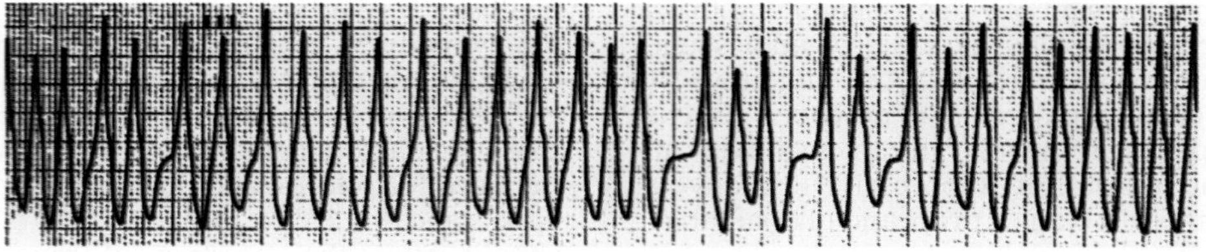

Figure 164-3 Antegrade conduction over an accessory pathway during atrial fibrillation in a 15-year-old boy with syncope. The short RR intervals represent rapid conduction over the accessory connection and a risk for ventricular fibrillation.

Approximately 50% of patients with SVT will have the onset of tachycardia during the first 4 months of life, and 60% of this group will have recurrences, especially if overt preexcitation or Wolff-Parkinson-White (WPW) syndrome is present. Although potentially still inducible at an electrophysiologic study, more than 90% will be free of clinical episodes of tachycardia by 1 year of age. However, as many as one third of children who have a history of SVT in early infancy and clinical resolution by 1 year of age may have a recurrence at a mean age of 8 years. The age range of 1 to 5 years is usually electrically quiescent. If SVT occurs for the first time in a child 5 years old or older, then the chance of recurrent episodes of tachycardia is 75% to 80%.[3] SVT is usually initiated by an APC or sinus tachycardia in early infancy, but in childhood and adolescence, PVCs and sinus pauses with junctional escape beats are additional initiators. Most children with SVT have a structurally normal heart, but if WPW syndrome is present (shortened PR interval, delta wave, and wide QRS on the ECG), an echocardiogram should be performed to look for subtle congenital cardiac defects such as Ebstein malformation of the tricuspid valve or levo-transposition of the great vessels. If surgery for a cardiac defect is contemplated and episodes of SVT have occurred, then preoperative assessment and ablation should be considered to reduce arrhythmia-related postoperative morbidity and potential mortality.

The incidence of WPW in the general population is 0.15%, but in many affected individuals, no SVT occurs. WPW syndrome (with tachycardia) may be inherited in an autosomal-dominant fashion in which situation the risk of sudden death substantially increases (Figure 164-3).

PRESENTATION OF SVT

During infancy, SVT may be detected incidentally on a routine examination; more commonly, however, young infants exhibit varying degrees of congestive heart failure related to the rate and duration of tachycardia and the presence of associated heart disease. As a general rule, 25% of infants are in congestive heart failure with tachycardia duration of 24 hours, and 50% have heart failure after SVT for 48 hours. Frequently, a history of poor feeding and pallor over several days is present, culminating in respiratory distress. Children older than 5 years are usually able to communicate their distress soon after the onset of SVT, hence the relative paucity of congestive heart failure caused by SVT in older children. The duration of SVT in children and adolescents ranges from a few seconds to several hours. Palpitations may be the only symptom in some children; others have initial lightheadedness, as well as subsequent chest discomfort, pallor, diaphoresis, and nausea. SVT-induced syncope is rare. In infancy, the rate of SVT may range from 230 to 300 bpm but is usually between 260 and 280 bpm, in contrast to older patients who typically have rates between 180 and 240 bpm. The QRS complexes are usually narrow but may be transiently wide at initiation, especially with aberrant left bundle branch morphology in early infancy as a consequence of aberrancy (Figure 164-4). However, as a general rule, wide QRS tachycardias should be considered ventricular in origin until proven otherwise. A 12-lead ECG should be obtained with careful attention paid to the T waves for sharp deflections representing retrograde conduction from the ventricles to the atria via an accessory pathway (Figure 164-5).

MANAGEMENT OF SVT

If cardiogenic shock is present with SVT, then direct current synchronized cardioversion should be performed by using ½ to 2 watt-seconds or J/kg with the largest paddles allowing effective chest contact. Adenosine can be administered via intravenous bolus, followed by a second doubled dose if the first dose is ineffective. Adenosine always should be administered with ECG monitoring to detect the rare conversion to a more malignant arrhythmia. Adenosine is effective in approximately 90% of episodes. If adenosine is ineffective, or if SVT quickly recurs, then an infusion of procainamide can be administered to infants and young children after appropriate loading, with a subsequent repeat trial of adenosine. If conversion does not ensue, then a procainamide level should be obtained 4 hours into the infusion (therapeutic range equals 4 to 8 mcg/mL). In general, in children younger than 1 year intravenous verapamil and propranolol are contraindicated. Once conversion to a sinus rhythm is achieved, a 12-lead ECG should be repeated to look for evidence of preexcitation. If WPW syndrome is present, then suppressive therapy with propranolol is appropriate. Digoxin and verapamil in this circumstance should be avoided because both medications may shorten the antegrade refractory period of the accessory pathway, allowing more rapid conduction to the ventricles, a potentially fatal scenario if atrial fibrillation develops. If preexcitation is not

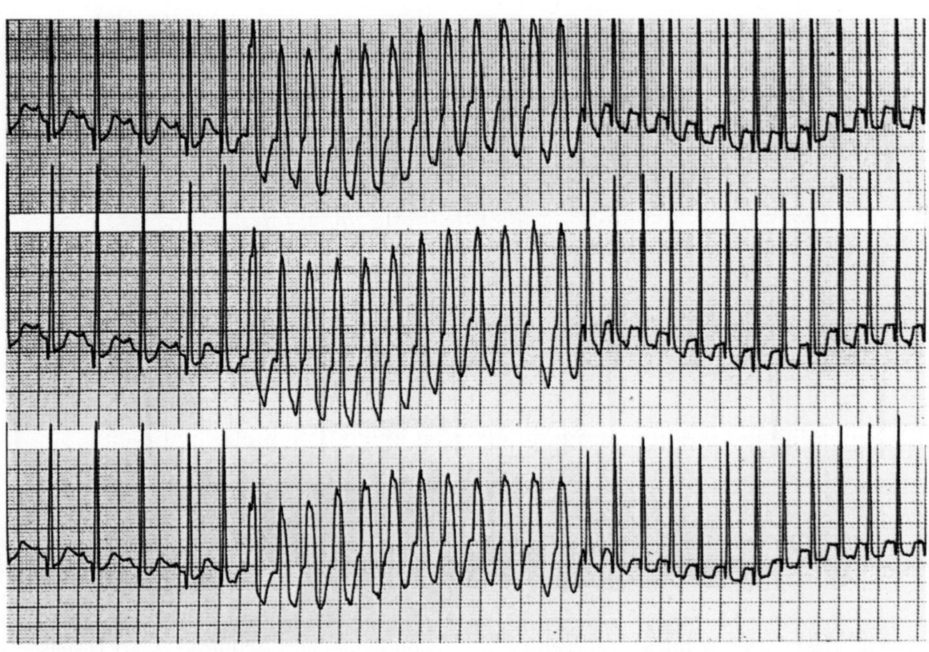

Figure 164-4 Transient aberrant conduction at the onset of SVT during an exercise test in a 14-year-old adolescent. The QRS duration then returns to normal.

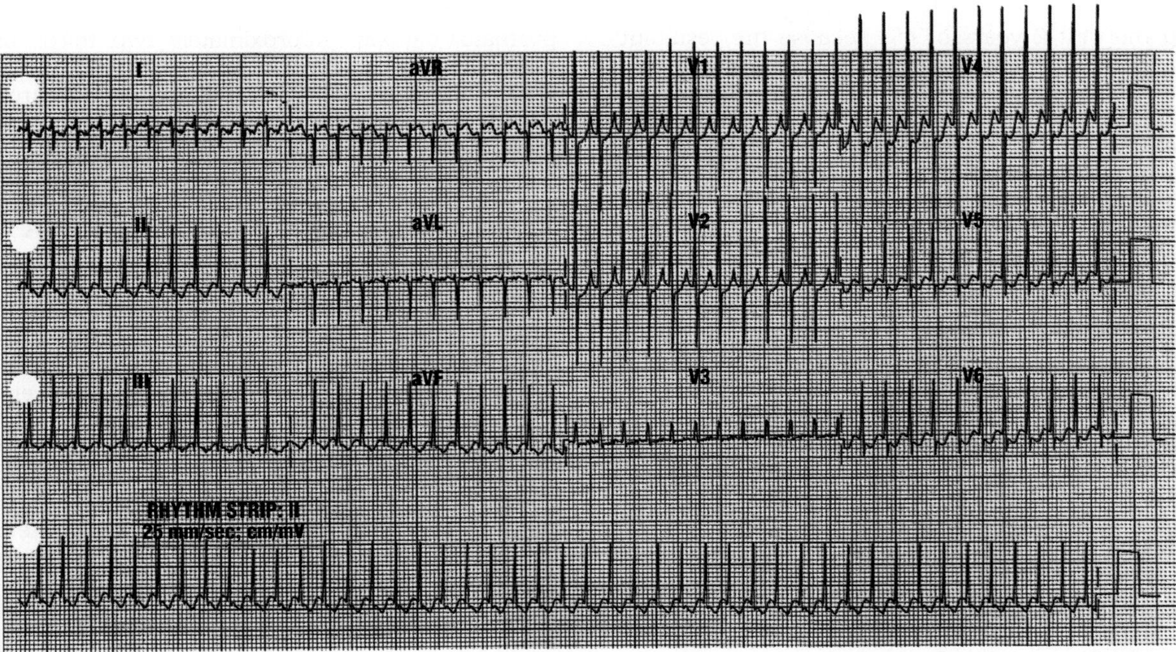

Figure 164-5 Twelve-lead ECG of SVT in a 2-week-old infant. Consistent sharp deflections in the T waves are present in lead III, indicating retrograde atrial activation via an accessory pathway. A repeat ECG after conversion to sinus rhythm did not reveal any preexcitation; therefore a concealed accessory pathway is present.

present, then either digoxin or propranolol can be used to prevent recurrences. Beta-blockers should be avoided in the presence of congestive heart failure, sick sinus syndrome, or a history of bronchospasm. If these agents are ineffective, then other medical therapies include flecainide, sotalol, or amiodarone, all of which require hospitalization for drug initiation.

Infants who have SVT are usually treated for 6 to 12 months and then observed in view of the risk of later recurrence. Ablations are not recommended

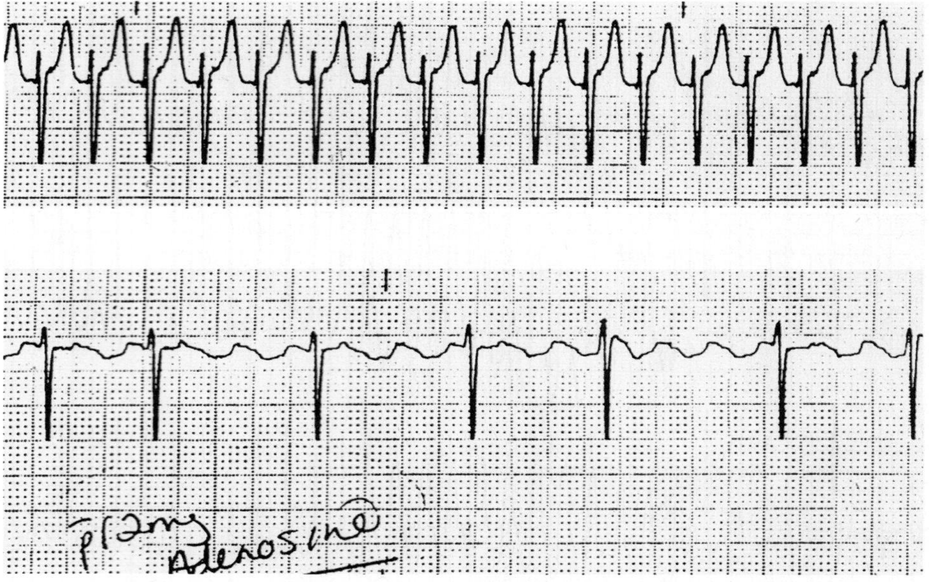

Figure 164-6 Atypical atrial flutter or intraatrial reentry tachycardia before and immediately after adenosine treatment in a 12-year-old boy after a Mustard repair of transposition of the great arteries in infancy (see Chapter 251, Congenital and Acquired Heart Disease). Adenosine produces high-grade AV block revealing but not converting the underlying atypical atrial flutter.

during the first 2 years of life because the resultant myocardial scar may grow with the patient and become a subsequent nidus for malignant, often drug-refractory arrhythmias. Depending on the frequency and ease of conversion of episodes, older children and adolescents have 3 therapeutic choices:

1. No therapy other than self-conversion via a Valsalva maneuver or headstand
2. Drug therapy, although the duration, compliance issues, and cost of this approach need to be addressed with the family
3. Radio-frequency ablation, currently at least 90% successful but with a chance of a later recurrence

Automatic ectopic tachycardias in childhood are often incessant and relatively drug resistant with the eventual possible outcome of a tachycardia-induced cardiomyopathy if conversion is not achieved. However, spontaneous resolution may occur.[4]

ATRIAL FLUTTER

Atrial flutter, a primary atrial reentrant tachycardia, is seen in a bimodal distribution in newborns and in older children, the latter usually with cardiomyopathies and after repair of complex congenital heart malformations.

In the newborn, the characteristic rapid saw-tooth pattern with inverted P waves in the inferior limb leads is found with an atrial rate typically between 350 and 500 bpm with 2:1 atrioventricular conduction and brief interruptions caused by higher degrees of AV block. If the onset is in utero, then hydrops fetalis may develop. After birth, congestive heart failure may be seen but not as dramatically as in infants who have the usual variety of SVT. Structural cardiac problems are uncommon. One third of very young patients respond to in utero or postnatal digoxin. Approximately two thirds usually require electrical cardioversion. Chronic therapy is usually unnecessary because recurrences are rare.

Although the typical form of atrial flutter may be seen in older children and adolescents, more commonly, an atypical variety called intraatrial reentrant tachycardia is found. The atypical form is characterized by a slower atrial rate and distinct P waves separated by isoelectric periods and is usually seen after repair of complex congenital cardiac lesions (Figure 164-6).[5] Management is often difficult, but if conversion to and maintenance in a sinus rhythm cannot be achieved, then morbidity is substantial and a 4- to 5-fold increase in the risk of sudden death ensues.[6] Commonly, after atrial repair of transposition of the great vessels or after a Fontan procedure* for underlying single ventricular morphology and physiology, the patient's resting heart rate is in the 50- to 70-bpm range. If such a patient is then seen with a rate of 100 to 140 bpm, then a 12-lead ECG should be obtained to look for atypical atrial flutter.

ATRIAL FIBRILLATION

Atrial fibrillation, an irregular tachycardia with variable atrioventricular conduction, is much less common than the other forms of SVT and is seen in older patients with structural heart disease and cardiomyopathies. However, the incidence of lone (no underlying cause) and paroxysmal atrial fibrillation in adolescence

*The Fontan procedure is a complex reconstruction of the heart in 3 stages such that, on completion, venous blood flows passively to the lungs, and oxygenated blood is actively pumped by a single ventricular chamber into the aorta.

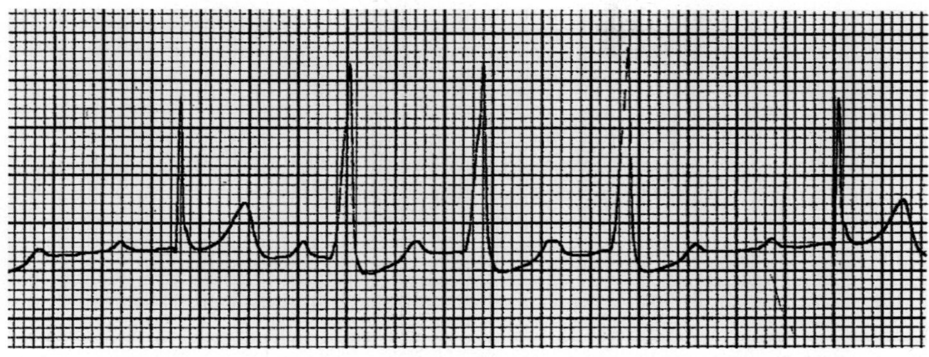

Figure 164-7 Accelerated ventricular rhythm with a ventricular rate of 110 bpm in a healthy 7-year-old girl. First-degree block is present in the sinus beats.

may be underestimated. If preexcitation (WPW syndrome) is present and the accessory pathway is capable of rapid antegrade conduction, then atrial fibrillation may conduct quickly to the ventricles, with a resultant decrease in cardiac output, syncope, and the potential for ventricular fibrillation and sudden death (see Figure 164-3).

VENTRICULAR TACHYCARDIA

Ventricular tachycardia (VT) is defined as three or more repetitive excitations arising from the ventricles with a rate more than 120 bpm or 25% faster than the sinus rate. The QRS complexes are different from the sinus QRS complexes and are typically wide, except in young infants in whom minimal QRS prolongation (0.08 to 0.09 seconds) may be seen. VT may be extremely rapid, up to 500 bpm, and slightly irregular because of intermittent sinus capture beats. The differential diagnosis includes SVT with persistent aberrancy (see Figure 164-4) and SVT with antegrade conduction across an accessory pathway (see Figure 164-3), both of which are relatively uncommon. Safety dictates that all wide QRS tachycardias be considered VT until proven otherwise. The presence of similar but isolated PVCs and fusion beats in sinus rhythm assists in establishing the diagnosis, but VT is confirmed by the presence of atrioventricular dissociation.

VT in the newborn and young infant is rare, but if it is drug resistant and incessant, then a ventricular tumor may be present. Mitochondrial fatty acid β-oxidation disorders may also cause VT in neonates.[7] Predisposing factors in older children and adolescents include myocarditis, repaired and unrepaired congenital cardiac lesions, cardiomyopathies, long QT syndrome, catecholamine- or exercise-induced VT, marked electrolyte imbalances, and use of street drugs (eg, cocaine). In general, VT is a marker for myocardial disease.

Acute management depends on the patient's clinical status, which is determined by the rate and duration of VT and the presence of structural cardiac lesions or prior myocardial dysfunction. Hemodynamic compromise dictates electrical cardioversion with 1 to 2 watt-seconds/kg. If reasonable clinical stability is present, then intravenous lidocaine, procainamide, magnesium, or amiodarone can be administered.

Chronic suppressive therapy is predicated on the risk of recurrence, the morbidity and mortality of the type of VT, and the risk-benefit ratio of treatment. Beta-blockers, sotalol, and amiodarone are commonly used antiarrhythmic agents to prevent VT recurrences. Other treatments include implantation of an automatic cardioverter-defibrillator and VT ablation. One form of VT, accelerated ventricular rhythm, is characterized by a rate of 120 bpm or less. This is less than 25% faster than the basic sinus rate and is benign, requiring observation only (Figure 164-7). Relatively benign forms include right ventricular outflow tract and idiopathic left VT. These entities occur in structurally normal hearts and have a substantial incidence of spontaneous resolution in childhood.

CONDUCTION ABNORMALITIES

First-degree AV block is a prolongation of the PR interval beyond the upper limit of normal for age, with all impulses conducted. It may be seen in patients who have congenital cardiac malformations (especially AV septal defects), electrolyte disorders, rheumatic fever, myocarditis, and congenital muscular disorders. Patients on antiarrhythmic agents frequently exhibit 1st-degree AV block, which is a benign finding that does not require therapy.

Type I 2nd-degree AV block (called Wenckebach block or Mobitz type I block) is a progressive prolongation of the PR interval until a dropped ventricular beat (nonconducted P wave) occurs. It is a normal finding in healthy children during sleep and in highly conditioned athletes at rest, circumstances that are associated with a predominance of vagal tone. In general, this entity is benign, but if syncope occurs, especially with exertion, then cardiologic referral is mandated.

On the other hand, type II 2nd-degree AV block (Mobitz type II block) is characterized by intermittent loss of AV conduction without preceding lengthening of the PR interval. In contrast to type I in which the site of block is in the AV node and little risk of progression to complete block is present, the site of block in Mobitz type II is more distally located in the bundle of His. Symptoms are more common, and progression to higher levels of AV block does occur. The presence of

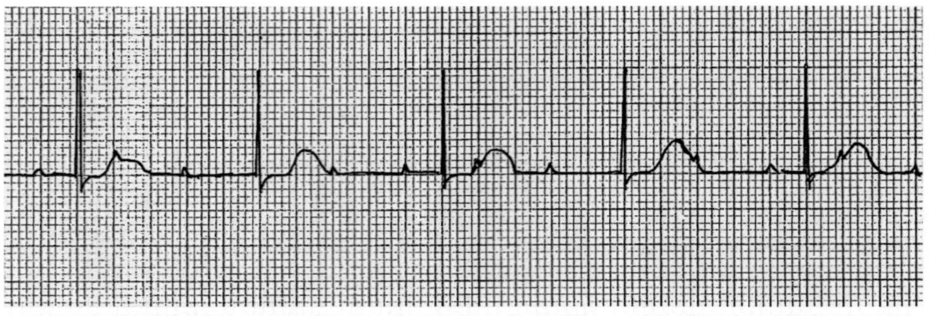

Figure 164-8 Complete congenital AV block in a newborn infant whose mother has Sjögren syndrome. The atrial rate is 150 bpm. The QRS duration is normal.

type II block implies an abnormal conduction system with a need for referral, ongoing medical surveillance, and a potential need for pacemaker implantation.

Complete AV block, in which no atrial impulses are conducted to the ventricles, may be acquired or congenital. Acquired block is usually a consequence of conduction system injury at the time of repair of congenital cardiac malformations but can also be seen in myocarditis, including Lyme disease. The need for pacemaker insertion in these situations depends on the presence of symptoms, the ventricular rate, and the stability of the ventricular escape rhythm. Approximately 50% of newborns who have complete congenital AV block (CCAVB) have underlying complex congenital heart malformations, particularly levo-transposition of the great vessels and complex AV septal defects. The other 50% of neonates with CCAVB have immune-mediated block caused by the passage in utero of immunoglobulin G SS-A/Ro and SS-B/La antibodies from the mother who has overt or occult autoimmune disease. When the fetus is exposed to these maternal antibodies, especially between 15 and 24 weeks of gestation, the result may be fibrotic replacement of AV nodal tissue (Figure 164-8). Fewer than 5% of infants born to mothers who have autoimmune disease develop CCAVB.[8] Infants without CCAVB born to anti-Ro/SS-A–positive mothers with autoimmune disease may have QT prolongation and sinus bradycardia.[9] If a mother bears 1 child who has CCAVB, then the risk in future pregnancies is 15%.[10] An immune-mediated myocarditis may also occur in fetuses exposed to maternal anti-Ro and anti-La antibodies, with possible development of a postnatal dilated cardiomyopathy (endocardial fibroelastosis).

Risk factors for fetal, neonatal, or late death with CCAVB include fetal hydrops, premature birth, the presence of complex structural heart disease, a prolonged QT interval seen in up to 25% of affected patients, congestive heart failure, ventricular ectopy, atrioventricular valve insufficiency, and a low or decreasing ventricular rate (55 bpm or less in a neonate).[11] In view of the 20% risk of mortality, early pacemaker implantation is advised if any of these risk factors or symptoms of an inadequate cardiac output are present. An infusion of isoproterenol can be administered, if necessary, to increase the heart rate while awaiting pacemaker therapy but should not delay implantation. In patients who do not require pacemaker implantation in early infancy, pacing usually becomes necessary in adolescence.

SUDDEN CARDIAC DEATH

Sudden cardiac death, a rare but devastating event in the young, strikes approximately 1:100,000 children and teenagers, with the highest incidence in mid-adolescence. In decreasing order of frequency, predisposing factors include:

1. Repaired complex congenital heart malformations
2. Cardiomyopathies
3. Myocarditis
4. Congenital coronary artery anomalies (especially origin of the left main coronary artery from the right sinus of Valsalva)
5. Primary arrhythmias such as long QT syndrome (LQTS), WPW syndrome, and catecholamine-sensitive polymorphic VT

LQTS is a familial, clinically and genetically heterogeneous ion channel cardiac disorder that prolongs repolarization and may cause syncope, seizures, and sudden death as a consequence of polymorphic VT (torsades de pointes). The Romano-Ward subcategory, which accounts for 95% of patients with LQTS, is related to a heterozygotic mutation on chromosomes 11, 7, 3, 4, or 21. The remaining 5% are characterized by homozygotic mutations on chromosome 11 leading to the Jervell and Lange-Nielsen (JLN) syndrome, which is characterized by marked prolongation of the corrected QT intervals and congenital deafness.[12] Patients with JLN syndrome have a greater degree of QTc prolongation and a substantially higher incidence of sudden death compared with patients with the much more common Romano-Ward variant.[13] Potassium-channel function is affected by mutations on chromosomes 11, 7, 4, and 21, whereas the sodium channel is perturbed as a consequence of mutations on chromosome 3.

The incidence of LQTS is estimated at 1 in 10,000 individuals, with no gender preference, but the incidence may be underestimated because of incomplete genetic ascertainment. The annual mortality after onset of symptoms in untreated young patients is 1% to 5%, with a nearly 10% risk of sudden death as the initial symptom. The cumulative probability of a cardiac event (predominantly syncope) occurring in patients who are genotyped LQT1, 2, and 3 by 15 years of age ranges between 10% for patients with LQT3 and 69% for those with LQT1.[14] The highest risk for sudden death occurs in patients with a history of syncope and a QTc more than 530 ms. Syncope, atypical seizures, or cardiac arrest usually occur during exertion or emotional stress, except for long QT3 subtype events, which predominantly occur at rest. Other than bradycardia, the physical examination is usually normal. LQTS is defined by a corrected QT interval in excess of 460 ms, with a borderline QTc defined by an interval of 440 to 460 ms. In general, the longer the QTc is, the greater the risk of polymorphic VT will be. The differential diagnosis includes electrolyte abnormalities such as hypokalemia, hypocalcemia, and hypomagnesemia. Myocardial ischemia or injury, acute central nervous system events, and cardiomyopathies may be associated with mild QTc prolongation. Cisapride, imipramine, pentamidine, and intravenous erythromycin may also prolong the QT interval. Therapy for LQTS includes avoidance of competitive sports, β-blocker therapy, avoidance of drugs capable of prolonging the QTc and sympathomimetics, and avoidance and rapid correction of electrolyte abnormalities, followed by cardiac pacing, a left stellate ganglionectomy, and implantation of cardioverter-defibrillator, if necessary. Gene-specific therapy with potassium-channel opening agents and sodium-channel blockers is on the horizon.

LQTS has been identified as a rare cause of the sudden infant death syndrome.

Beyond infancy, 25% of sudden deaths in the young occur during exercise; the vast majority of occurrences are electrical in nature, with ventricular fibrillation as the final common pathway. For any child or adolescent who collapses suddenly with no discernible cardiac output, rapid resuscitation including early defibrillation is mandated. The availability of automatic external defibrillators in some school systems has already begun to decrease the incidence of sudden cardiac death in the young. In addition, risk reduction may be achieved by asking 2 critical questions in presports clearance evaluations: (1) Has the patient ever passed out, had visceral chest pain, or experienced symptomatic palpitations during strenuous exercise? (2) Has any family member died suddenly and unexpectedly before the age of 35 years? An affirmative answer to either question should prompt a cardiologic referral before participation in competitive sports.

WHEN TO REFER

- Arrhythmias associated with presyncope, syncope, chest pain, or a sense of doom
- Underlying heart disease
- Family history of premature (before age 35 years) sudden cardiac death
- Persistent or repetitive bradycardias or tachycardias
- Premature ventricular beats that increase with exercise

WHEN TO ADMIT

- Arrhythmias associated with syncope or low cardiac output
- Symptomatic high-grade AV block
- Difficult-to-control SVT, atrial flutter
- VT
- LQTS with syncope, aborted sudden death

TOOLS FOR PRACTICE

Engaging Patients and Family

- *Sports Shorts: Sudden Cardiac Death* (fact sheet), American Academy of Pediatrics (www.aap.org/family/SportsShorts_09.pdf).

Medical Decision Support

- *Preparticipation Physical Evaluation*, 3rd edition (book), American Academy of Pediatrics (www.aap.org/bookstore).
- *Preparticipation Physical Evaluation Forms* (questionnaire), American Academy of Pediatrics (www.aap.org/bookstore).
- *Sports Shorts: Sudden Cardiac Death* (fact sheet), American Academy of Pediatrics (www.aap.org/family/SportsShorts_09.pdf).

AAP POLICY STATEMENTS

American Academy of Pediatrics, American Heart Association, and American College of Cardiology Foundation. ACC/AHA/AAP recommendations for training in pediatric cardiology. *Pediatrics*. 2005;116(6):1574-1575.

American Academy of Pediatrics, Committee on Sports Medicine and Fitness. Cardiac dysrhythmias and sports. *Pediatrics*. 1995;95(5):786-788. (aappolicy.aappublications.org/cgi/content/abstract/pediatrics;95/5/786).

American Academy of Pediatrics. Committee on Sports Medicine and Fitness. Medical conditions affecting sports participation. *Pediatrics*. 2008;121:841-848. (aappolicy.aappublications.org/cgi/content/full/pediatrics;121/4/841).

American Academy of Pediatrics. Guidelines for pediatric cardiovascular centers. *Pediatrics*. 2002;109(3):544-549. (aappolicy.aappublications.org/cgi/content/full/pediatrics;109/3/544).

Hazinski MF, Markenson D, Neish S, et al. Response to cardiac arrest and selected life-threatening medical emergencies: the medical emergency response plan for schools. a statement for healthcare providers, policymakers, school administrators, and community leaders. *Pediatrics*. Jan 2004;113(1):155-168. AAP Endorsed. (pediatrics.aappublications.org/cgi/content/full/113/1/155).

SUGGESTED RESOURCES

Deal BJ, Wolff GS, Gelband H, eds. *Current Concepts in Diagnosis and Management of Arrhythmias in Infants and Children*. Armonk, NY: Future Publishing; 1998.

Zeigler VL, Gillette PC, eds. *Practical Management of Pediatric Cardiac Arrhythmias*. Armonk, NY: Future Publishing; 2001.

REFERENCES

1. Yarlagaddi RK, Iwai S, Stein KM, et al. Reversal of cardiomyopathy in patients with repetitive monomorphic ventricular ectopy originating from the right ventricular outflow tract. *Circulation*. 2005;112:1092-1099.

2. Ko JK, Deal BJ, Strasburger JF, et al. Supraventricular tachycardia mechanisms and their age distribution in pediatric patients. *Am J Cardiol*. 1992;69:1028-1032.
3. Perry JC, Garson A Jr. Supraventricular tachycardia due to Wolff-Parkinson-White syndrome in children: early disappearance and late recurrence. *J Am Coll Cardiol*. 1990;16:1215-1220.
4. Bauersfeld U, Gow RM, Hamilton RM, et al. Treatment of atrial ectopic tachycardia in infants <6 months old. *Am Heart J*. 1995;129:1145-1148.
5. Cecchin F, Johnsrude CL, Perry JC, et al. Effect of age and surgical technique on symptomatic arrhythmias after the Fontan procedure. *Am J Cardiol*. 1995;76: 386-391.
6. Garson A Jr, Bink-Boelkens M, Hesslein PS, et al. Atrial flutter in the young: a collaborative study of 380 cases. *J Am Coll Cardiol*. 1985;6:871-878.
7. Bonnet D, Martin D, de Lonlay P, et al. Arrhythmias and conduction defects as presenting symptoms of fatty acid oxidation disorders in children. *Circulation*. 1999;100: 2248-2253.
8. Brucato A, Frassi M, Franceschini F, et al. Risk of congenital complete heart block in newborns of mothers with anti-Ro/SSA antibodies detected by counterimmunoelectrophoresis. *Arthritis Rheum*. 2001;44:1832-1835.
9. Cimaz R, Strambi-Badiale M, Brucato A, et al. QT interval prolongation in asymptomatic anti-SSA/R_0 positive infants without congenital heart block. *Arthritis Rheum*. 2000;43:1049-1053.
10. Buyon JP, Hiebert R, Copel J, et al. Autoimmune-associated congenital heart block: demographics, mortality, morbidity and recurrence rates obtained from a national neonatal registry. *Am J Cardiol*. 1998; 31:1658-1666.
11. Michaelsson M, Riesenfeld T, Jonzon A. Natural history of congenital complete atrioventricular block. *Pacing Clin Electrophysiol*. 1997;20:2098-2101.
12. Weintraub R, Gow RM, Wilkinson JL. The congenital long QT syndromes in childhood. *J Am Coll Cardiol*. 1990;16:674-680.
13. Komsuoglu B, Goldei O, Kulan K, et al. The Jervell and Lange-Nielsen syndrome. *Int J Cardiol*. 1994;47:189-192.
14. Zareba W, Moss AJ, Schwartz PJ, et al, and the International Long QT Syndrome Registry Research Group. Influence of the genotype on the clinical course of the long QT syndrome. *N Engl J Med*. 1998;339:960-965.

Chapter 165

CHEST PAIN

Scott A. Schroeder, MD

Although chest pain from cardiac disease in children is extremely rare, few symptoms result in more fear and anxiety in children and their parents. Undiagnosed cardiac disease causes chest pain in less than 5% of patients, and if children with preexisting heart disease are excluded, then cardiac abnormalities are found in less than 1% of patients. Although chest pain from cardiac disease occurs in a few children, much of the primary care physician's evaluation and teaching will be focused on convincing families that the heart is normal. If the care of a child with chest pain is managed inappropriately, then grief, anxiety, restriction of activities, and distrust by the family may result. However, a thorough history and physical examination will usually uncover the cause of the chest pain and will allow the clinician to state emphatically that chest pain in healthy children is rarely from heart disease.

DIFFERENTIAL DIAGNOSIS

Of children and adolescents with chest pain, by far the largest number has musculoskeletal chest wall trauma or other conditions identified as the source of the pain. Pulmonary diseases—pneumonia, asthma, pneumothorax, and cough itself—account for approximately a fifth of cases, and the rest are the result of hyperventilation or psychiatric causes, gastrointestinal disorders, and, finally, cardiac disease.[1-6] Approximately 15% of cases remain idiopathic. However, studies have not rigorously looked for the presence of esophageal disorders or reactive airway disease, both of which have been shown to be common in children with idiopathic chest pain.[7,8]

PATHOPHYSIOLOGICAL FEATURES OF CHEST PAIN

Because numerous organ systems are within the thorax, and because of the confusing overlap of sensory inputs from the various tissues in the chest, a systematic approach to the thorax is essential to determine the source of the child's pain. Pain from the chest wall and the supporting musculoskeletal structures is transmitted from these inflamed or irritated tissues to the central nervous system via the primary sensory afferents that terminate in the dorsal root ganglia. Spinal neurons then transmit the sensation from the inflamed chest wall tissues to the brain, where it is perceived as a sharp, localized pain. This feature is why chest wall pain (eg, from costochondritis or trauma) is sharp, localized, and easily reproduced on palpation.

Spinal neurons that receive input from the organs within the thorax also receive sensory input from the thoracic dermatomes. This overlap of sensory input leads to the phenomenon of *referred pain*, which often makes the evaluation of chest pain challenging. Diffuse, poorly localized chest pain can originate from any of the organs within the thorax. Inflammation of the structures that pass through the mediastinum results in pain over dermatomes T1 to T4, from the retroclavicular to the retrosternal regions. Pain over dermatomes T5 to T8, especially in the xiphoid area, suggests lower chest wall or diaphragmatic irritation or even intraabdominal disease. Because both the intercostal nerves and the phrenic nerve innervate the diaphragm, peripheral diaphragmatic irritation causes pain in the lower anterior chest or epigastric regions, and central diaphragmatic inflammation results in ipsilateral shoulder pain because of its innervation by the phrenic nerve. The pericardium, positioned on the central diaphragm, has pleural connections and is innervated by the phrenic, vagus, and recurrent laryngeal nerves. Therefore, when the pericardium is inflamed or infected, sharp substernal pain can occur. The pain of pericarditis may be limited to the sternal and precordial areas; however, if the left lobe of the diaphragm is irritated, then pain will be referred to the ipsilateral shoulder or neck. Pleural pain results from distension or inflammation of the pleura that can occur during the course of a pneumonia, pneumothorax, or empyema. Pain from pleural inflammation is aggravated by respiratory movements. The pain is characterized as well-localized and sharp, exaggerated by coughing or deep inspiration. The pain associated with a pneumothorax can be pleuritic in nature, or it can be referred to the ipsilateral shoulder.

The pain associated with esophageal disorders can seem indistinguishable from that associated with myocardial ischemia because the sensory afferents from the esophagus are through the cardiac and esophageal plexi, as well as the sympathetic trunk. Within the lungs, sensory input exists only from the larger airways and parietal pleura; thus the pain arising from pulmonary parenchymal disease results from inflammation of or traction on contiguous structures.

EVALUATION

History

Because pathognomonic findings are rare on physical examination in the evaluation of a child with chest pain, a detailed history will help focus the differential diagnosis, develop a logical intervention, and allow the child and family to voice their concerns. A meticulous history should address the nature of the pain, as well as the child's response to the pain. If possible, children should describe the pain in their own words, and they should be asked what they think is causing the pain. Along with a description of the location, duration, radiation, and quality of the pain, the primary care physician should elicit any associated signs and symptoms, as well as any aggravating and alleviating factors, and attempt to uncover the family history and dynamics. To many adolescents, chest pain is synonymous with heart disease; therefore this issue should be addressed; and if no cardiac cause is discovered, then the physician should unequivocally state to the adolescent and the family that the heart is normal.

Pain that occurs with exercise points toward either a cardiac or a respiratory cause. If the pain awakens the child from sleep, then the cause might be respiratory, cardiac, musculoskeletal, or gastroesophageal, but it is never psychological. When the pain is poorly localized, associated with recurrent somatic complaints or family or school stress, and when a family history of chest pain can be found, a psychogenic source of the pain is likely. Conversely, deep, poorly localized pain that radiates to the neck or shoulders is characteristic of visceral pain. Superficial sharp pain that is exacerbated by lifting or movements of the torso suggests musculoskeletal pain.

Peripheral pain that increases with inspiratory efforts originates from pleural inflammation. Questions regarding trauma to the chest wall should always be asked, and even if the trauma occurred 1 to 3 months before the pain, it should not be discounted because the pain might represent a posttraumatic pericardial effusion. Sharp pain that decreases when the child leans forward is characteristic of pericardial inflammation. Children with a family history of Marfan or Turner syndromes, as well as those with a history of Kawasaki disease or congenital heart disease, warrant referral to a pediatric cardiologist.

Even if the history is highly suggestive of the cause for the chest pain, the primary care physician should be careful and thorough because the potential exists of 2 different causes for the pain. Children with asthma can also have gastroesophageal reflux. Children with sickle cell disease who develop acute chest syndrome may have chest pain as a result of medication-induced gastritis or vasoocclusive crisis.

Laboratory Evaluation

Laboratory tests are usually not helpful in establishing a specific diagnosis; therefore a thorough history and physical examination should guide the clinician in ordering tests. In most cases, chest radiographs and electrocardiographs will only confirm what is suspected clinically. If a child has a fever, acute onset of chest pain, and an abnormal cardiac examination suggestive of pericarditis, then a chest radiograph and electrocardiogram are indicated. If a child has fever, tachypnea, chest pain, and decreased breath sounds over a segment of the lungs, then a chest radiograph is appropriate to determine whether pneumonia, a pleural effusion, or other pulmonary disease is present. If the pain occurs with exercise, then exercise testing or spirometry may help uncover underlying asthma or exercise-induced bronchospasm. One cause of idiopathic chest pain may be an esophageal disorder.[7] Signs and symptoms of children with chest pain who warrant hospitalization or specialty evaluation are listed in Box 165-1.

BOX 165-1 Signs and Symptoms That Accompany Chest Pain That Warrant Referral or Hospitalization

SIGNS

- Syncope
- Fevers, chills, weight loss, malaise, anorexia
- History of Kawasaki disease, Turner syndrome, Marfan syndrome, sickle cell disease, or cystic fibrosis
- Recent elective abortion, calf pain, oral contraceptive use
- Family history of hypertrophic obstructive cardiomyopathy or unexplained syncope
- Pica
- Foreign body aspiration
- Conversion disorder

SYMPTOMS

- Cyanosis, toxic appearance, or respiratory distress
- Murmur that increases with Valsalva maneuver
- Pleural or pericardial friction rub
- Pulsus paradoxus
- Cardiac clicks, thrills, gallop, or 3rd heart sound
- Chest pain with exercise
- Palpitation or tachycardia

SPECIFIC CAUSES OF CHEST PAIN IN CHILDREN

Musculoskeletal and Chest Wall Conditions

After a determination has been made that the child is in no distress, inspection of the thorax will determine the presence of bruising, swelling over joints, splinting, signs of trauma, or an abnormal breathing pattern. Palpation and percussion are extremely important to localize and reproduce the pain because disturbances in the chest wall are the most common diagnoses in children with chest pain. Each rib cartilage should be palpated with only 1 finger or with the child's finger because palpation with 2 or more digits may cause splinting and will not recreate the pain. Reproduction of point tenderness at the origin of the spontaneous pain is the strongest evidence favoring the diagnosis of chest wall disease. Pain from the thoracic cage that can be elicited by movements of the torso or by flexion of the arms is highly suggestive of a musculoskeletal chest wall injury. The pain of costochondritis causes tenderness over the affected costochondral or costosternal junctions and can occur at rest or with movement. Adolescents with gynecomastia or breast pain may experience chest pain that is easily discernible on inspection and palpation of the developing breast tissue. No laboratory testing is needed if any of the these conditions is identified as a cause of the chest pain. Table 165-1 lists common, uncommon, and rare causes of chest pain and their associated signs and symptoms.

Pulmonary Conditions

Children with asthma may have chest pain from excessive coughing and overuse of their intercostal muscles. Having pain alone as a manifestation of asthma is unusual for a child with asthma; usually, nocturnal cough, adventitial breath sounds, abnormal pulmonary function tests, or other signs of atopic diseases can exist. The presentation of asthma is further discussed in Chapter 239.

A variety of other diseases of the airways, pleurae, and parenchyma can cause substernal or pleuritic chest pain. Pneumonia, asthma, exercise-induced bronchospasm, pleural effusions, and air in the pleural space can cause pain, but the chest pain is never the sole sign

Table 165-1 Common, Uncommon, and Rare Causes of Chest Pain and Associated Signs and Symptoms

CAUSE OF CHEST PAIN	SIGNS AND SYMPTOMS
MUSCULOSKELETAL	
Costochondritis (common)	Localized, superficial, reproducible pain over rib cartilage
Exercise, overuse, muscle strain (common)	Reproducible pain with use of involved muscle group
Protracted coughing or vomiting (common)	Intercostal muscle tenderness
Trauma	Localized pain; pain with movement of involved areas
Stitch (common)	Sharp, crampy costal pain that occurs with running
Precordial catch (uncommon)	Transient, stabbing pain at left sternal border; relieved by forced inspiration
PULMONARY	
Asthma (common)	Associated with cough, shortness of breath, wheezing, abnormal pulmonary function tests; relief with inhaled antiinflammatory drugs or bronchodilators
Exercise-induced bronchospasm (common)	Abnormal exercise tests; improvement with bronchodilators
Pneumonia (common)	Crackles, fever, cough
Pleural effusion (uncommon)	Pleural rub, fever, decreased breath sounds
Pneumothorax (uncommon)	Sudden pain, referred shoulder pain, dyspnea
Pulmonary embolus (rare)	Contraceptive use or recent abortion, pleuritic pain
GASTROINTESTINAL	
Esophagitis (common)	Retrosternal pain; relief with antacids
Gastroesophageal reflux (common)	Retrosternal burning pain; worse after eating and when reclining; relief with antacids
CARDIAC	
Hypertrophic cardiomyopathy (rare)	Syncope, family history, systolic ejection murmur
Pericarditis (rare)	Associated fever with acute onset of pain; pain increases with movement; narrow pulse pressure, distant heart sounds; alleviated by leaning forward
Myocarditis (rare)	Precedent viral illness, anorexia, shortness of breath, 3rd heart sound or gallop, cardiomegaly
NONORGANIC	
Psychogenic (common)	Normal physical examination, trouble sleeping, family or school problems, life stresses, family history of chest pain, other somatic complaints
Hyperventilation (common)	Associated light-headedness, paresthesias, underlying anxiety

of the underlying disease process. A child with a parapneumonic effusion will classically have fever, tachypnea, tachycardia, a pleural friction rub or crackles (or both) on auscultation, and dullness to percussion in addition to the pleuritic chest pain that heightens with inspiration.

Exercise-induced chest pain or chest tightness that resolves with the cessation of the exercise or the administration of bronchodilators may be a manifestation of cardiac disease but is more commonly related to exercise-induced bronchospasm. Exercise testing, cold air challenge, or a therapeutic trial of bronchodilators can confirm the diagnosis of exercise-induced or cold air–induced bronchospasm. Treatment with bronchodilators will help these children participate in sports and allow them to lead normal, active lives.

Spontaneous pneumothorax can occur in teenagers with chronic illnesses such as cystic fibrosis, asthma, and Marfan syndrome but can also occur in healthy teenagers. A child with cystic fibrosis who experiences chest pain should be assumed to have a pneumothorax until proven otherwise. Dyspnea, shoulder pain, and tachypnea are often observed in addition to the chest pain in tall, thin adolescents who develop a spontaneous pneumothorax.

Gastrointestinal Conditions

Acid reflux to the esophagus can mimic the pain of angina and can cause both acute and chronic chest pain. Pain that originates from the esophagus or stomach is described as an uncomfortable, gnawing substernal burning sensation. The pain can last for hours, and it intensifies after meals and on reclining. Any inflammation of the esophagus, abnormalities of peristalsis, esophageal foreign body, or trauma can cause chest pain. The most common gastrointestinal cause of chest pain is esophagitis. However, because the clinical presentation of esophagitis can be nonspecific, children with idiopathic chest pain may benefit from a trial of antacids or H_2-receptor antagonists before embarking on an exhaustive evaluation.

Cardiac Conditions

The least likely but most worrisome causes of chest pain in children are cardiac disorders that cause myocardial ischemia. Cardiac disease in children rarely produces isolated chest pain and is always associated with other findings at evaluation. Sudden death from cardiac disease in children is caused by a small subgroup of disorders: abnormalities of the myocardium or coronary vessels, specific congenital heart lesions, and arrhythmia and conduction disorders.[9] Signs and symptoms that identify children with these disorders and warrant cardiology evaluation include exertional nonrespiratory dyspnea, syncope, and palpitations. A pediatric cardiologist should also see children with chest pain and a family history of sudden death.

A child with chest pain from myocarditis or pericarditis usually appears ill, with fever, dyspnea, changes in the pain associated with the respiratory cycle, and abnormal ausculatory findings. In most instances, the echoviruses, especially coxsackievirus type B, are identified as the culprit responsible for myocarditis. Pericarditis can result from either an infectious agent or an autoimmune process.

Aortic stenosis and idiopathic hypertrophic cardiomyopathy, which are the most important lesions that cause left-ventricular outflow obstruction, can cause chest pain as a result of the heart's inability to increase the cardiac output with exercise. These disorders cause syncope and chest pain with exertion. Mild aortic stenosis does not cause chest pain.

Chest pain may be, but is not usually, the primary complaint of children with arrhythmias unless they perceive the palpitations as painful. More commonly, older children complain of light-headedness or dizziness along with the palpitations. The arrhythmia can usually be detected on auscultation and confirmed by resting electrocardiogram. If the palpitations or chest pain occur infrequently or are not associated with exercise, then referral to a pediatric cardiologist is indicated for Holter monitoring.

Although mitral valve prolapse (MVP) is commonly thought to cause chest pain in adolescents, most children with MVP are asymptomatic. Chest pain has been found to be no more common in teenagers with MVP than it is in those without MVP.[10]

Findings on auscultation that point to a cardiac source of pain include clicks, rubs, and systolic murmurs. A murmur can be worrisome if it increases in intensity with the Valsalva maneuver or any other procedure that expands the degree of left-ventricular outlet obstruction. A 3rd heart sound or gallop is heard in myocarditis and congestive heart failure. Pleural friction rubs, wheezes, tachypnea, and crackles suggest a pulmonary cause. Conversely, hyperventilation associated with light-headedness, paresthesias, dizziness, and a high level of stress or anxiety suggest a hyperventilation syndrome.

Idiopathic Causes

Especially among adolescents, as many as 39% of patients complaining of chest pain will not have a readily identifiable cause.[3,4] Children with chronic chest pain, no history of respiratory or cardiac disease, and a normal physical examination are unlikely to have a serious cause for their pain. In teenagers, a careful explanation of the pathophysiological features in concrete terms is a fundamental part of their therapeutic regimen. Several studies of children with idiopathic chest pain have shown that most of them have no further pain 1 to 2 years after their initial evaluation.[11]

Psychogenic Chest Pain

A child with a long history of chest pain, other recurrent somatic problems, school or sleep problems, a family history of chest pain, or any combination of these factors may have a psychogenic cause for the pain. If a psychogenic cause is entertained, then the diagnosis should not be made by exclusion of organic disease; rather, the diagnosis should be based on positive psychiatric evidence. As with any somatic illness, if the family or the child is able to articulate a relationship between the chest pain and stress or emotional upheaval, then the diagnosis will be easier for them to comprehend and accept.[12] Emotional causes for chest pain seem to be more common in adolescents than in children younger than 12.[1] Hyperventilation can be associated with the chest wall syndrome but is more commonly seen in teenagers with underlying anxiety. The diagnosis is usually made by history alone because the child may need to hyperventilate for 20 minutes to reproduce the pain.

Almost all children with hyperventilation syndrome have associated paresthesias, carpopedal spasm, and light-headedness. For a child with an acute episode of hyperventilation, the treatment is to have the child breathe into a paper bag to relieve the hypocapnia. Resolution of the chronic problem is based on techniques to allow the children to understand the nature of their anxiety and allow them to regain control of their emotional state. The treatment of other forms of psychogenic chest pain should be focused on the family's comprehension of the cause of the pain and reassurance that no long-term sequelae exist, all while acknowledging that the pain is real. For children with severe psychiatric problems, referral to a psychiatrist may be necessary.

WHEN TO ADMIT

Rarely will a child with chest pain need to be hospitalized because, for the most part, chest pain is usually benign, self-limited, and not associated with severe intrathoracic illness. Box 165-1 provides guidance for when to refer and when to admit. However, children with the following should be hospitalized:

- Myocarditis
- Pericarditis
- Empyema
- Pneumothorax
- Significant thoracic trauma
- Acute chest syndrome
- Esophageal foreign bodies
- Coronary artery anomalies or other cardiac lesions
- Myocardial ischemia
- Chest pain and palpitations
- Cyanosis
- Distress

REFERENCES

1. Selbst SM, Ruddy RM, Clark BJ, et al. Pediatric chest pain: a prospective study. *Pediatrics.* 1988;82:319-323.
2. Rowe BH, Dulberg CS, Peterson RG, et al. Characteristics of children presenting with chest pain to a pediatric emergency department. *CMAJ.* 1990;143:388-394.
3. Pantell R, Goodman B. Adolescent chest pain: a prospective study. *Pediatrics.* 1983;71:881-887.
4. Driscoll D, Glicklich L, Gallen W. Chest pain in children: a prospective study. *Pediatrics.* 1976;57:648-651.
5. Massin MM, Bourguignont A, Coremans C, et al. Chest pain in pediatric patients presenting to an emergency department or to a cardiac clinic. *Clin Pediatr.* 2004;43:231-239.
6. Fyfe DA, Moodie DS. Chest pain in pediatric patients presenting to a cardiac clinic. *Clin Pediatr.* 1984;23(6):321-324.
7. Glassman M, Medow MS, Berezin S, et al. Spectrum of esophageal disorders in children with chest pain. *Dig Dis Sci.* 1992;37:663-666.
8. Weins L, Sabath R, Ewing L. Chest pain in otherwise healthy children and adolescents is frequently caused by exercise-induced asthma. *Pediatrics.* 1992;90:350-353.
9. Liberthson R. Sudden death from cardiac causes in children and young adults. *N Engl J Med.* 1996;334:1039-1044.
10. Savage D, Garrison R, Devereux R. MVP in the general population-epidemiological features: the Framingham study. *Am Heart J.* 1983;106:571-576.
11. Rowland T, Richards M. The natural history of idiopathic chest pain in children: a follow-up study. *Clin Pediatr (Phila).* 1986;25:612-614.
12. Green M. *Sources of Pain.* Philadelphia, PA: WB Saunders; 1983.

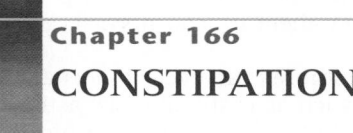

Chapter 166

CONSTIPATION

Peter F. Belamarich, MD

The term *constipation,* which denotes both a symptom and a chronic condition, refers to the infrequent elimination of large or hard stools that cause pain on defecation. In childhood, chronic constipation that is not caused by another condition is known by several different names, including dysfunctional stool retention, psychogenic constipation, and idiopathic, chronic, and functional constipation. The last group of terms, which reflects our lack of understanding of the cause and is not pejorative, is used in this chapter. Given that constipation encompasses both objective and subjective complaints that vary by age, it has defied a comprehensive standard definition. Several consensus groups have developed definitions of constipation; however, none of these definitions seems entirely satisfactory to all.[1] One expert consensus definition of constipation is presented in Box 166-1.[2]

Constipation is a common symptom among children in the industrialized world. In parental surveys, from 16% to 37% of toddlers are reported to suffer from it.[3] Most often, constipation is a self-limited symptom relieved by dietary changes or transient laxative use. Functional constipation presents a challenge to the pediatrician, as suggested by the observation that the evaluation and treatment of constipation occupies a

BOX 166-1 Definition of Constipation

Defined by any of the following:

- Passage of hard scybalous pebblelike or cylindrical cracked stools
- Straining or painful defecation
- Passage of large stool that may clog the toilet
- Stool frequency less than 3 times per week, unless breastfed

Can manifest as pain, fecal soiling, urinary tract infection, and enuresis significant percentage of all referrals to pediatric gastroenterologic services, although these children rarely require an invasive procedure.[4] To pediatricians caring for chronically constipated children, treatment failure raises the question of Hirschsprung disease. Among referral populations, more than 90% of childhood constipation is functional; ultimately, 50% to 90% of these children are cured.[5]

The approach to chronically constipated children used by gastroenterologists is well within the scope of the primary care pediatric practice and represents a therapeutic opportunity with a good cure rate. The focus of this chapter is on identifying and treating children who have functional constipation. An evidence-based guideline, endorsed by the American Academy of Pediatrics, has been published on evaluating and treating constipation.[6]

PATHOPHYSIOLOGIC MECHANISM OF FUNCTIONAL CONSTIPATION

Normal Colonic Function

The role of the colon is to reclaim water from the liquid ileal effluent. This task is accomplished, in part, by a motility pattern that includes focal circular contractions, which impede the progress of the luminal contents while solutes and water are absorbed. Subsequently, forward progress of the relatively dehydrated fecal stream is achieved by coordinated contractile waves, which propel the bolus of stool to the next colonic segment and ultimately to the rectum. The final elimination of stool is controlled by defecation, a coordinated sequence of neuromuscular events with both reflexive and conscious components. Control of defecation, continence, is a critically important social achievement in early childhood. At rest, continence is maintained by the involuntary resting tonic contraction of the smooth muscle cuff of the internal anal sphincter and by the posterior turn of the anal canal in relation to the anterior angulation of the rectal vault. This angle is modulated by the puborectalis sling muscle, which loops posteriorly around the anorectal junction and is anchored anteriorly on the pubic bone.

When stool arrives in the rectal ampulla, causing distention of the rectal walls, a reflexive relaxation of the internal anal sphincter occurs, which lowers the pressure of the anal canal and allows the stool bolus to descend to the anal canal, a phenomenon known as the *rectoanal inhibitory reflex*. Control of defecation then occurs by the voluntary (and learned) deliberate contraction of the striated muscle of the external sphincter and puborectalis sling muscles, which increase the pressure in the anal canal and make the exiting angle more acute. Conversely, a Valsalva maneuver in combination with relaxation of the external anal sphincter and the puborectalis sling permit defecation to proceed.

Factors in Functional Constipation

The cause of functional constipation is not clear. Based on current knowledge, functional constipation may likely result from several distinct initiating pathophysiologic events,[7] which include a disorder of the dynamics of defecation; problem with rectal sensation; or disorder of colonic transit, leading to impacted, overly desiccated stool in the colon.

Stool withholding, the act of voluntarily deferring defecation to avoid pain, significantly contributes to the chronicity of constipation in childhood independently of the primary cause.

Stool Withholding

In practical terms, several commonly recognized clinical scenarios can result in constipation, including painful anal fissures, perianal streptococcal cellulitis, traumatic toilet-training experiences, and transient periods of dehydration, illness, or immobility. Stool withholding likely figures prominently in the perpetuation of constipation when pain or an aversive experience is the primary insult. Withholding behavior in the toddler or child is strongly self-reinforcing. The child is avoiding painful bowel movements, which makes the stool harder and more painful to pass. Parents who focus with great concern on the withholding crisis, often believing that the child is valiantly trying to defecate rather than to withhold, also reinforce stool withholding unwittingly. Toddlers love the worried attention of their parents! The lack of privacy commonly found in some school lavatories can engender withholding by older children. Anorectal manometric studies have documented abnormalities in the dynamics of defecation in a large series of chronically constipated children, the most common being a paradoxic contraction of the external anal sphincter and the puborectalis sling in response to the rectoanal inhibitory reflex.

This commonly identified abnormality is known variously as rectoanal pelvic floor dyssynergia, abnormal defecation dynamics, and anismus.[8] Most experts consider dyssynergia a learned phenomenon. For a large proportion of chronically constipated children, painful defecation and withholding antedate the clinical presentation of constipation by 1 to 5 years.[9] In a significant subset of children who experience persistent constipation, withholding becomes entrenched and particularly difficult to unlearn. In fact, initial enthusiasm over manometrically based biofeedback training was based on its potential to help patients identify and unlearn this withholding behavior. However, controlled studies have not documented greater improvements in the outcome for patients who have undergone biofeedback training than for those given a standard treatment regimen.[8]

Sensory Abnormalities

Another common manometric abnormality found in chronically constipated children is known as megarectum. As the name implies, the rectum is dilated with a chronic impaction, a finding associated with an increase in the sensory threshold to minimal rectal distention, as well as an increase in the minimal volume required to initiate the urge to defecate. These sensory abnormalities persist for several years in some patients after successful treatment, suggesting that ongoing sensory abnormalities contribute to relapses and perhaps to the initial pathogenesis of constipation in some children.

Slow Transit

Constipation from abnormally slow transit of the fecal stream through the colon occurs predominantly in young women but can occur in children.[10] Whether slowed colonic transit is the primary problem or an acquired epiphenomenon of more distal difficulties with defecation is unclear. Slow-transit constipation in children is not easily differentiated clinically from normal-transit constipation. A unique therapeutic approach to slow-transit constipation has not emerged.

Despite experimental evidence that documents the varieties of abnormal anorectal or colonic pathophysiologic factors in children who have chronic constipation, no studies identify any of these abnormalities prospectively.

Dietary Factors

Whether dietary factors alone can cause constipation is unclear. Despite broad agreement that dietary fiber has an important role in promoting a regular bowel habit, very little literature and no prospective studies support this belief. A case control study has documented decreased fiber intake as a risk factor for childhood constipation; however, substantial overlap exists in the fiber intake between cases and controls.[11] Nonetheless, many clinicians have remarked that, in infancy, the transition from human milk or formula to whole cow's milk or periods of excess protein intake such as occur in toddlers with excessive whole cow's milk consumption are associated with constipation. The tenacious and harmful myth that iron-containing formula causes constipation has been disproved many times.

DIFFERENTIAL DIAGNOSIS

The differential diagnosis of chronic childhood constipation includes many conditions (Box 166-2). Despite the large number of possible diagnoses, at least 90% of affected children have functional constipation.

Frequently, the foremost consideration in the differential diagnosis of chronic constipation is Hirschsprung disease (see Chapter 266, Gastrointestinal Obstruction). The most common basis for this concern is treatment failure, an appropriate concern in early infancy when functional constipation is unusual and is easily treatable. However, treatment failure in the toddler and the school-age child more often reflects the complexity and duration of intervention required to treat functional constipation adequately than a missed diagnosis of Hirschsprung disease. Fortunately, several findings in the history have an extremely high negative predictive value in ruling out Hirschsprung disease. Perhaps most useful is that almost all children with functional constipation withhold stool in response to the rectoanal inhibitory reflex, whereas this reflex is absent with Hirschsprung disease. Simply stated, *doodie dancing* is a historical finding that almost always rules out Hirschsprung disease. Conversely, Hirschsprung disease should be considered in any child with refractory constipation who has had any of the following:

1. Failure to pass meconium in the first 24 hours of life
2. Onset of constipation before 3 months of age
3. Symptoms of intestinal obstruction at any time (distention, pernicious emesis)
4. Lifelong dependence on laxatives, enemas, or mechanical manipulation to initiate defecation
5. History of enterocolitis in early infancy (sometimes misdiagnosed as gastroenteritis)

See Table 166-1 for a summary of features that distinguish Hirschsprung disease from functional constipation.

Other conditions that specifically affect the neuromuscular function of the colon include the pseudo-obstruction syndromes, which are characterized by intermittent episodes of functional intestinal obstruction. Furthermore, a large percentage of children who have generalized neuromuscular disabilities (eg, cerebral

BOX 166-2 Differential Diagnosis of Constipation in Childhood

FUNCTIONAL CONSTIPATION
Disorders of intestinal neuromuscular function

ANAL AND RECTAL DISORDERS
Anal fissure
Anterior ectopic anus
Anal stenosis
Rectal duplication
Anal trauma (abuse)
Pelvic tumor (presacral teratoma, ganglioneuroma, ovarian cyst, hematocolpos)

NEUROLOGIC—NEUROMUSCULAR
Hirschsprung disease
Pseudoobstruction syndromes
Spinal cord lesions
Cerebral palsy
Neuromuscular diseases with hypotonia

METABOLIC AND ENDOCRINE
Hypothyroidism
Diabetes insipidus
Hypercalcemia
Hypokalemia

MEDICATION AND TOXIN RELATED
Antihistamines
Anticholinergics
Anticonvulsants
Opioids
Bismuth, aluminum hydroxide
Tricyclic antidepressants
Iron preparations (not iron-fortified formulas)
Plumbism
Infant botulism

MISCELLANEOUS
Celiac disease
Cystic fibrosis
Cow's milk allergy
Sclerodema
Systemic lupus erythematosus

Table 166-1 Comparison of Hirschsprung Disease to Functional Constipation

CHARACTERISTIC	HIRSCHSPRUNG DISEASE	FUNCTIONAL CONSTIPATION
Prevalence	~1 in 6000 births	1.5% of 7-year-old boys
Failure to pass meconium <24 hr	58-94%	~5%
Constipation in first 3 mo	90%	Rare
Obstruction	Common	Absent
Abdominal distention	Common	Mild or absent
Stool size	Narrow, ribbon-like	Intermittent large-caliber stools
General appearance	Chronically ill	Well
Stool-withholding behavior	Rare	Extremely common
Soiling	Unusual	Common
Stool in ampulla	Unusual	Common
Plain roentgenograms	Empty rectum	Dilated enlarged rectum
Rectal manometry	Recto-anal reflex absent	Recto-anal reflex present
Typical barium enema	Distal spasm, proximal dilatation	Diffusely dilated colon and rectum

palsy, muscular dystrophy, generalized hypotonia) have refractory constipation that is frequently multifactorial and difficult to treat.

Anorectal disorders producing constipation include anal fissures, anal stenosis, anterior ectopic anus, and extrinsic masses that partially obstruct the rectum. Fissures may induce a self-perpetuating cycle of withholding and worsening constipation that causes reinjury. Congenital anal stenosis is characterized by straining during the production of small-caliber stools; it is frequently diagnosed during infancy. The anal canal is noted to be narrow and not distensible during digital examination. Occasionally, chronic constipation is caused by a subtle anorectal malformation known as anterior ectopic anus,[12] in which the anal orifice is misplaced anteriorly so that the stool bolus must turn anteriorly at the perineum to exit. The parents may report seeing a perineal bulge when the infant attempts to defecate. Surgical reconstruction may be necessary in children who fail to improve with medical therapy. In rare cases, constipation is a manifestation of an intermittent or partial extrinsic obstruction of the rectum by a rectal duplication cyst or by a pelvic mass such as a neuroblastoma, presacral teratoma, or ovarian tumor.

Spinal cord lesions affecting the 2nd, 3rd, and 4th sacral nerves are associated with both sensory and motor deficits affecting defecation. Trauma to the sacral cord, intraspinal and extraspinal tumors, and congenital malformations that can tether the spinal cord should be thought to exist when constipation is accompanied by abnormalities in bladder function or gait or when visible abnormalities overlying or palpable deformities of the lumbosacral spine exist.

Metabolic and endocrine disorders associated with constipation include hypothyroidism, hypercalcemia, diabetes insipidus, hypokalemia, and plumbism. These conditions generally do not exhibit with chronic constipation as a sole symptom.

Both cystic fibrosis and celiac disease can cause constipation. Clinicians should be alert to these possibilities in children with poor growth in weight or height, recurrent respiratory complaints, anemia, or hypoproteinemia.

BOX 166-3 Studies in Children With Constipation

For growth failure, failure to thrive, short stature:
- Thyroid function tests
- Celiac panel
- Sweat test

For delayed passage of meconium:
- Anorectal manometry
- Rectal suction biopsy
- Unprepared barium enema
- Sweat test

For hair tufts, lipomas, hemangiomas, overlying the lumbosacral spine and for abnormalities of gait, urination, absence of anal wink or cremaster reflex:
- magnetic resonance image of the lumbosacral spinal chord

For refractory constipation:
- Thyroid function tests
- Serum calcium
- Potassium
- Lead
- Celiac panel
- Sweat test

Routine studies of children who are thought to have functional constipation are not recommended.

Many medications and toxins are reported to cause constipation (see Box 166-2).

Recently, 2 reports have linked constipation to cow's milk protein allergy.[13,14] In a study of a referral population of 65 children who had treatment-resistant chronic constipation, 44 had a positive therapeutic response to the substitution of soy milk for cow milk. Questions remain, however, about the generalizability of these findings to the primary care setting.

Box 166-3 presents a diagnostic approach for children thought to have an organic cause of their constipation.

COMMON PRESENTATIONS OF FUNCTIONAL CONSTIPATION

Infancy

Particularly in the first 6 months of life, parental notions of what constitutes constipation may be incorrect. Breastfed infants may have a mushy stool as infrequently as once a week. In the otherwise healthy infant, this situation does not deserve the label constipation and requires no intervention. In general, stool consistency rather than frequency is the critical determinant of constipation in the infant. Parents also worry about infants who strain or grunt excessively (often turning deep red) in the course of producing a soft stool of normal caliber. Manometric studies have documented the presence of a functioning rectoanal inhibitory reflex at birth, and infants exhibiting this behavior are likely attempting, unsuccessfully, to coordinate the voluntary with the involuntary components of defecation.

The truly constipated infant, who does require treatment, typically displays a pattern of straining associated with either the production of a desiccated plug of stool followed by loose stool or by the production of a consistently desiccated stool that has a pebbly consistency.

Toddlers

Although parents of toddlers are usually aware of when their child is constipated, they frequently do not recognize stool withholding. During the act of withholding, the child may hide quietly, clinging to an inanimate object, while squeezing the buttocks together. Numerous variations of stool withholding behavior exist, including crouching, dancing or walking on tiptoes, and crying out in anticipation of the pain. Not infrequently, these episodes are misinterpreted by the parents as valiant attempts to defecate, and they generate great concern. Eliciting a history of stool withholding is critical for both diagnostic and therapeutic purposes.

Childhood

Once the child has attained privacy in the bathroom, parents are not likely to be involved in the toilet routine, and constipation becomes occult. The child often goes to the bathroom with a regular or increased frequency but during defecation passes only a small, hard piece of desiccated stool. Not infrequently, the child emerges from the bathroom not terribly bothered. The parent inquires, "Did you go?" The child answers, "Yes." Thus both parties are happy. This stooling pattern, known as incomplete evacuation, is common in school-age children and is punctuated episodically by the passage of massive bowel movements. Many children do not seem terribly bothered by their constipation and are brought in by their parents for associated phenomena rather than for the constipation itself: soiling, recurrent abdominal pain, blood streaks seen on the stool, excessive flatus, or anorexia. Finally, pelvic floor dyssynergia seen in children with stool withholding can affect urinary voiding dynamics, predisposing some to enuresis or urinary tract infection.[15] Box 166-4 lists features that support the diagnosis of functional constipation.

BOX 166-4 Findings That Support the Diagnosis of Functional Constipation

Onset after infancy
Presence of stool-withholding behavior
Absence of red flags
Episodic passage of large caliber stools

EVALUATION

Functional constipation frequently can be diagnosed by history, physical examination, and therapeutic response to a comprehensive treatment regimen. The history should incorporate the frequency, consistency, and caliber of the stools that the child passes, as well as the age of the child at the onset of constipation. The newborn history should specifically establish whether the child passed meconium in the first day of life. A history of the child's toilet-training experience and whether traumatic toileting experiences occurred is critical in toddlers and preschool children. The diet history can establish whether the onset of constipation occurred concurrently with the transition to cow's milk or with periods of high protein intake (excessive cow's whole milk consumption).

Common complications of constipation should be assessed: fissures, bleeding, abdominal pain, anorexia, enuresis, and urinary tract infection. A history of distention and vomiting are explored because they are not caused by functional constipation. Eliciting a history suggesting stool withholding is critical because it strongly supports the diagnosis of functional constipation and should be addressed in the therapeutic plan. Details of prior evaluations and treatments should be explored, including over-the-counter medicines, home remedies, alternative therapies, and culturally specific therapies that can be incorporated in the treatment plan, if they pose no harm.

Specific questions should address the differential diagnosis. Symptoms of Hirschsprung disease, as well as endocrine, metabolic, and neurologic disease, should be sought. The possibility of an occult spinal process affecting the sacral nerves can be addressed by inquiring about any changes in the urinary voiding pattern (urinary stream or urinary continence) or in the child's gait. The family history covers heritable conditions in the differential diagnosis and a family history of functional constipation, which has been shown to have a heritable component.

On physical examination, the child's growth parameters, including recent growth velocity, should be normal. The child should appear well and not wasted or malnourished. The abdomen should not be distended, and the examination should establish the presence or absence of a fecal impaction in the lower quadrants or in the hypogastric area. The external examination of the perineal area is performed to establish normal placement of the anal orifice and to look for evidence

BOX 166-5 Red Flags in Childhood Constipation

Failure to thrive, weight loss, poor growth
Vomiting
Abdominal distension
Persistent anal fissures, perianal disease
Persistent blood in stool or guaiac-positive stool
Delayed passage of meconium
Weak urinary stream, diurnal enuresis

of soiling, fissures, skin tags, and a normal anal wink in response to touch.

When a rectal examination can be done with the child's cooperation, it should be part of the evaluation. In the majority of children who have functional constipation, desiccated stool is found in the rectal vault on rectal examination. For older children who have longstanding constipation and a megarectum, chronic rectal distention may efface the internal sphincter along the rectal wall, making the anal canal feel foreshortened. Children who soil from chronic constipation with a megarectum have only a sensory disorder; thus the tone of the internal sphincter should be normal. The examiner should be alert during the digital examination for the rare situation in which an extrinsic mass is compressing the rectum. A patulous anus is indicative of a neurologic lesion or of sexual abuse involving the anus. Especially in infants, an empty rectum on digital examination raises the possibility of Hirschsprung disease, particularly in conjunction with an explosive gush of stool on withdrawal or a hard impacted mass palpated in the pelvis or lower abdomen. Impactions in infancy are unusual and may indicate Hirschsprung disease. In the older child who has functional constipation, an empty rectum may be found occasionally if the child has just defecated. Nonetheless, the possibility of Hirschsprung disease should be considered carefully.

The evaluation should continue with an examination of the spine, looking for a dimple, hair tuft, or palpable vertebral deformity (signs of spina bifida occulta), and from this evaluation to a thorough neurologic examination that explicitly assesses the tone, strength, symmetry, and reflexes of the lower extremities and to an analysis of the patient's gait.

Routine laboratory tests are not indicated in evaluating for functional constipation.[6] In addition, a recent systematic review has shown that plain abdominal radiographs do not have significant diagnostic value.[16] Nonetheless, plain radiographs of the abdomen can be used selectively for confirmation that an abdominal mass appreciated on physical examination is indeed a fecal impaction and for children with a questionable diagnosis who are unable to cooperate with a rectal examination.

Children thought to have Hirschsprung disease should be discussed with a consulting surgeon and radiologist to decide on the choice of initial diagnostic testing, keeping in mind that rectal biopsy is the gold standard. Box 166-5 presents red flags in constipation.

TREATMENT

Treatment of constipation involves parental education, laxatives, diet, and behavioral modification. Consideration must be given to the age of the patient and the duration of symptoms. Whereas transient constipation of several days' duration typically can be managed with 1 to a few days of laxative use and dietary change, the majority of patients who have functional constipation are affected for weeks to months before coming to attention and require a phased approach and months of treatment. Successful treatment of functional constipation in older children may even require 1 to 2 years of laxative therapy. Ultimately, the goals of treatment are to establish a pattern of soft bowel movements at a regular frequency (at least 3 per week), to wean the child from pharmacotherapy, and to have the child and family manage the problem on their own with diet and behavioral modification.

Treatment of Infants

Before they are introduced to infant food, constipated infants can be treated by the addition to the diet of undigestible, osmotically active carbohydrates; either dark corn syrup or malt soup extract can be added to the formula in a dose of 2 to 6 teaspoons divided in several bottles per day. Once juice and infant food are introduced, apple or prune juice and fruits can be added to the diet. Infant glycerin suppositories can be used at the beginning of therapy to remove a desiccated rectal plug but should not be the mainstay of therapy because infants can become behaviorally conditioned to depend on rectal stimulation to initiate defecation. Infants should not receive mineral oil because of the risk of pneumonia from aspiration. Externally visible anal fissures should be treated with petroleum jelly. Two studies have established the efficacy of polyethylene glycol (PEG) in infants.[17,18] Infants whose constipation is refractory to these measures should be referred to a pediatric gastroenterologist.

Treatment in Toddlers and Older Children

A highly successful treatment paradigm for toddlers and children who have longstanding functional constipation was developed by Dr. Murray Davidson in the 1960s and was refined by Dr. Melvin Levine in the 1970s. This method divides the treatment of established constipation into 3 phases: (1) education and disimpaction, (2) maintenance, and (3) weaning. This method has been adopted widely by pediatric gastroenterologists and advocated in published guidelines.[6]

Education

The treatment of constipation begins with parental education. Particular focus is given to the concept that, once established, constipation frequently engenders withholding, which is self-perpetuating. Toddlers, in particular, require several months of laxative treatment that produces soft stools before they abandon this behavior. A corollary to this point is to address the widely held parental fear that long-term laxative use in childhood is not safe or engenders laxative dependence. This fear, compounded by a general reluctance to medicate children for what is widely perceived as a transient problem, almost always leads to premature

Table 166-2 Regimens for Older Toddlers and Children Who Have Chronic Constipation**

	LAXATIVE DOSAGES
DISIMPACTION	
Enema	
Hypertonic sodium phosphate*	3 mL/kg/dose, once daily via rectum for 1-6 days
Mineral oil	30-60 mL, once daily via rectum for 1-6 days
Oral	
Polyethylene glycol electrolyte free	1.5 g/kg/day, maximum 100 g for 3 days
Mineral oil	30 mL/year of age to maximum 8 oz twice daily for 3 days
Polyethylene glycol with electrolytes	10-40 mL/kg/hr, via nasogastric tube (maximum 2 L/hr) until stool effluent clear
MAINTENANCE	
Polyethylene glycol–electrolyte free powder	0.8gm-1.5gm/kg/day
Mineral oil	1-3 ml/kg/day
Milk of magnesia	1-3 ml/kg/day
Lactulose 10 g/15 mL	1-2 ml/kg/day
Senna syrup 218 mg/5 mL*	10-20 mg/kg/dose po qhs

*See maximum doses in the PDR.
**Not recommended for children younger than 2 years of age.

discontinuation of therapy. In fact, innumerable studies have established that nonstimulant laxatives such as mineral oil, milk of magnesia, PEG, and lactulose do not result in dependence. On the other hand, experts discourage the prolonged use of stimulant laxatives (Senna, Bisacodyl),[6,19] but the limited use of Senna, an anthraquinone-stimulant laxative, as an adjunct to an osmotic agent or as rescue therapy for children who have transient relapses is acceptable. Concerns that prolonged periods of mineral oil use may impair fat-soluble vitamin absorption have not been substantiated.[20]

Some time must be spent educating parents on the nearly universal behavioral phenomenon of stool withholding. As difficult as it may be, parents should be instructed to ignore these events, as they would a temper tantrum. Parents should talk directly to toddlers and engage them in the therapeutic program: "I want you to push the poo-poo out of your body; don't hold it in. That's how you will get better, and it will stop hurting!"

Disimpaction

Treatment begins with disimpaction in the toddler or child who has had months to years of symptoms or an impaction on examination. For older children, disimpaction treatment (Table 166-2) should be deferred until the weekend; in the interim, the child can be treated with mineral oil to lubricate the impacted stool. Enemas once a day for 3 to 6 days are simple and effective and, with some important caveats, are safe. Dose guidelines should be followed, and the child should be brought to medical attention in the rare event of failure to stool following an enema. Sodium phosphate enemas are contraindicated in children who weigh less than 10 kg, in those who have any cardiac or renal impairment or electrolyte disorders, and in those who may have any form of intestinal obstruction.[21] Oral PEG has been used successfully for disimpaction, and the choice of enemas versus the oral route should be made with the child and the family's input.

The goal of disimpaction is to remove all the hard-formed stools throughout the colon. A follow-up telephone call after 2 days can ascertain whether the child is still passing hard stools. Any questions about whether the disimpaction phase of treatment is complete should prompt a revisit for an abdominal, rectal examination or an abdominal radiograph. Last, children who have extremely hard or treatment-resistant impactions can be admitted for nasogastric administration of a polyethylene glycol solution. Failure to achieve a thorough disimpaction, a common therapeutic mistake, undermines successful treatment because laxatives given in maintenance doses do not penetrate or remove the impaction. For the same reason, fiber is withheld during the disimpaction phase of treatment.

Maintenance

The maintenance phase of treatment follows disimpaction and incorporates laxative use and behavioral and dietary advice. Maintenance doses of laxatives are listed in Table 166-2. Telephone follow-up within 2 to 3 days of starting therapy is essential so that the laxative can be titrated to a dose that induces a daily soft bowel movement. Choice of laxative is less important than close follow-up for dose adjustment.

If mineral oil is used, then it should not be prescribed to children younger than 2 years or to children who are at risk for pulmonary aspiration.[22] For the same reason, parents should be counseled explicitly never to force the child to take mineral oil.

Recently, PEG has gained wide use for the treatment of functional constipation. PEG, an osmotic laxative, is a polymer of ethylene glycol that is not absorbed or fermented by colonic bacteria. One appeal of PEG is that it is a fairly tasteless, water-soluble powder that can be disguised when mixed into a child's drink. Pediatric studies of PEG have established clinical tolerance, effective dose, and the absence of unanticipated or serious adverse effects in small groups of study subjects.[23,24] No difference was found between the prevalence of abnormal electrolyte or nutritional parameters in a 3-month study that compared a low dose PEG with lactulose.[25] Despite its popularity (and several claims of its superiority) the question of whether PEG is truly superior to and safer than other commonly used (and frequently less expensive laxatives) awaits more rigorous studies than are currently available. The same cautions that would be applied to the use of mineral oil should be applied to the use of PEG. A case report has documented the successful use of bronchioalveolar lavage for severe pulmonary edema as a consequence of PEG aspiration.[26]

The addition of dietary fiber is a widely advocated adjunct to the treatment of childhood constipation, and a recent randomized controlled trial has shown benefits of a fiber supplement when prescribed with a laxative.[27] Alternatively, dietary changes that increase the child's fiber intake can be made and include the introduction of whole-grain breads and of cereals and increasing the child's fruit and vegetable intake.

The maintenance phase of therapy incorporates behavioral modification as well. For toddlers, the focus is on replacing stool-withholding behavior with deliberate attempts to defecate. Toilet-training efforts are deferred until the child stops withholding. For older children, a behavioral modification program of sitting on the toilet for 5 to 10 minutes after meals to capitalize on the gastrocolic reflex is effective, with success rewarded by the use of a star-chart system: The child should be rewarded for the targeted behavior (sitting). The physician is responsible for titrating the laxative dose to achieve the desired effect (a soft bowel movement every day), which requires an active partnership with the child and parents, who need to report to the physician frequently. Referral to a child behavior specialist or psychiatrist is warranted when toileting is the focus of a power struggle or when a significant mental health problem complicates the treatment regimen.

Weaning From Maintenance Therapy

Weaning, as opposed to abrupt cessation, of laxative therapy is the next phase of treatment. Successful weaning can occur following 6 to 12 weeks of maintenance treatment in some toddlers but may not be possible for 6 to 12 months in older children. Typically, the daily laxative dose is decreased to 75%, 50%, and 25% of the initial dose over successive months, or the full dose is given every second day for 6 to 8 weeks and then every third day for another 6 to 8 weeks. Efforts to increase the child's fiber intake and to comply with the behavioral program are redoubled during weaning. The older school-age children are encouraged to practice self-monitoring of the frequency and adequacy of their bowel movements, and a rescue plan for an enema, a suppository, or a dose of stimulant laxative must be in place for a transient relapse (no stool for longer than 3 days) that may occur during weaning. The inability to wean from laxatives following 12 months of therapy is not uncommon in functional constipation but may reasonably justify referral to a pediatric gastroenterologist. Box 166-6 presents common reasons for treatment failure of functional constipation. Remaining optimistic and involved at this point is important because improvement beyond 12 months of therapy is well documented.[5,28]

BOX 166-6 Common Reasons for Treatment Failure of Functional Constipation

- Inadequate disimpaction
- Failure to escalate laxative dose to achieve 1 to 2 soft stools per day
- Failure to address widely held notion that laxatives are addictive leading to premature discontinuation
- Relying on dietary fiber alone

WHEN TO REFER

- Abnormal studies
- Findings that are inconsistent with functional constipation (growth failure, distension, vomiting, bleeding)
- Significant behavioral, emotional, and parenting problems complicating treatment
- Refractory to comprehensive treatment regimen

WHEN TO ADMIT

- Constipation associated with obstruction or enterocolitis
- Failure of disimpaction as an outpatient

TOOLS FOR PRACTICE

Engaging Patients and Family

- *Constipation and Your Child* (brochure), American Academy of Pediatrics (patiented.aap.org).

Medical Decision Support

- *Constipation in Infants and Children: Evaluation and Treatment* (guideline), North American Society for Pediatric Gastroenterology and Nutrition (aappolicy.aappublications.org/misc/Constipation_in_Infants_and_Children.dtl).

AAP POLICY STATEMENTS

American Academy of Pediatrics. Technical report: Chronic abdominal pain in children. *Pediatrics*. 2005;115(3):e370-e381. (aappolicy.aappublications.org/cgi/content/full/pediatrics;115/3/e370).

American Academy of Pediatrics. Clinical report: Chronic abdominal pain in children. *Pediatrics*. 2005;115(3):812-815. (aappolicy.aappublications.org/cgi/content/full/pediatrics;115/3/812).

REFERENCES

1. Maffei HVL, Moreira FL, Oliveira WM Jr, et al. Defining constipation in childhood and adolescence: from Rome, via Boston, to Paris and...? *J Pediatr Gastroenterol Nutr.* 2005;41:485-486.
2. Hyams J, Colletti R, Faure C, et al. Functional gastrointestinal disorders: working group report of the first World Congress of Pediatric Gastroenterology, Hepatology and Nutrition. *J Pediatr Gastroenterol Nutr.* 2002; 35(suppl 2):S110-S117.
3. Issenman RM, Hewson S, Pirhonen D, et al. Are chronic digestive complaints the result of abnormal dietary patterns? Diet and digestive complaint in children at 22 and 40 months of age. *Am J Dis Child.* 1987;141:679-682.
4. Taitz LS, Wales JK, Urwin OM, et al. Factors associated with outcome in management of defecation disorders. *Arch Dis Child.* 1986;61:472-477.
5. Loening-Baucke V. Chronic constipation in children. *Gastroenterology.* 1993;105:1557-1564.
6. Baker SS, Liptak GS, Colletti RB, et al. Constipation in infants and children: evaluation and treatment. A medical position statement of the North American Society for Pediatric Gastroenterology and Nutrition. *J Pediatr Gastroenterol Nutr.* 1999;29:612-626.
7. Croffie JM, Fitzgerald JF. Idiopathic constipation. In Walker WA, Goulet OJ, Kleinman RE, et al, eds. *Pediatric Gastrointestinal Disease* 4th ed. St Louis: Mosby; 2003.
8. Loening-Baucke V. Biofeedback training in children with functional constipation: a critical review. *Dig Dis Sci.* 1996;41:65-71.
9. Partin JC, Hamill SK, Fischel JE, et al. Painful defecation and fecal soiling in children. *Pediatrics.* 1992;103:1007-1009.
10. Benninga MA, Buller HA, Staalman CR, et al. Colonic transit time in constipated children: does pediatric slow transit constipation exist? *J Pediatr Gastroenterol Nutr.* 1996;23:241-251.
11. Morrais MB, Vitolo MR, Aguirre AC, et al. Measurement of low dietary fiber intake as a risk factor for chronic constipation. *J Pediatr Gastroenterol Nutr.* 1999;29:132-135.
12. Leape LL, Ramenofsky ML. Anterior ectopic anus: a common cause of constipation in children. *J Pediatr Surg.* 1978;13:627-630.
13. Iacono G, Cavataio F, Montalto G, et al. Intolerance of cow's milk and chronic constipation in children. *N Engl J Med.* 1998;339:1100-1104.
14. Daher S, Sol D, Nuspitz CK, et al. Cow's milk protein intolerance and chronic constipation in children. *Pediatr Allergy Immunol.* 2000;12:399-342.
15. Erickson BA, Austin C, Cooper CS, et al. Polyethylene glycol 3350 for constipation in children with dysfunctional elimination. *J Urol.* 2003;107:1518-1520.
16. Reuchlin-Vroklage LM, Bierma-Zienstra S, Benninga MA, et al. Diagnostic value of abdominal radiography in constipated children: a systematic review. *Arch Pediatr Adolesc Med.* 2005;159:671-678.
17. Michail S, Gendy E, Preud'Homme D, et al. Polyethylene glycol for constipation in children younger than eighteen months old. *J Pediatr Gastroenterol Nutr.* 2004;39: 197-199.
18. Loening-Baucke V, Krishna R, Pashankar DS. Polyethylene glycol 3350 without electrolytes for the treatment of functional constipation in infants and toddlers. *J Pediatr Gastroenterol Nutr.* 2004;39:536-539.
19. Benninga MA, Voskuijl WP, Taminiau JAJM. Childhood constipation: is there new light in the tunnel? *J Pediatr Gastroenterol Nutr.* 2004;39:448-464.
20. McClung HJ, Boyne LJ, Linsheid T, et al. Is combination therapy to treat encopresis nutritionally safe? *Pediatrics.* 1993;91:591-594.
21. Harrington L, Schuh S. Complication of Fleet enema administration and suggested guidelines for use in the pediatric emergency department. *Pediatr Emerg Care.* 1997;13:225-226.
22. Hari R, Baudla R, Davis SH, et al. Lipoid pneumonia: a silent complication of mineral oil aspiration. *Pediatrics.* 1999;103:e19.
23. Youssef NN, Peter JM, Henderson W, et al. Dose response of PEG 3350 for treatment of childhood fecal impaction. *J Pediatr.* 2002;141:410-414.
24. Bell EA, Wall GC. Pediatric constipation therapy using guidelines and PEG 3350. *Ann Pharmacother.* 2004;38: 686-693.
25. Dupont C, Leluyer B, Maamri N, et al. Double-blind randomized evaluation of clinical and biological tolerance of polyethylene glycol 4000 versus lactulose in constipated children. *J Pediatr Gastroenterol Nutr.* 2005;41:625-633.
26. Liangthanasarn P, Nemet D, Sufi R, et al. Therapy for pulmonary aspiration of a polyethylene glycol solution. *J Pediatr Gastroenterol Nutr.* 2003;37:192-194.
27. Loening-Baucke V, Miele E, Staiano A. Fiber (glucomannan) is beneficial in the treatment of childhood constipation. *Pediatrics.* 2004;113:259-264.
28. Nolan T, Debelle G, Oberklaid F, et al. Randomized trial of laxative in the treatment of childhood encopresis. *Lancet.* 1991;338:523-527.

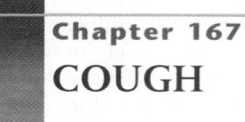

Chapter 167

COUGH

Michael G. Marcus, MD

INTRODUCTION

Cough is one of the most common complaints of children. Although generally resulting from acute viral infections and therefore self-limited, cough may be the harbinger of a more serious problem. Because cough can be exceedingly disruptive to the child and family, it can lead to significant anxiety for all involved parties. Allaying this anxiety through appropriate diagnosis and management is of prime importance to the primary care physician.

PATHOPHYSIOLOGICAL FEATURES

Cough can be described as a forceful exhalation. Its primary purpose is to facilitate the removal of inhaled irritants and secretions from the airway. The cough reflex can be triggered by stimulation of the cough receptors located at all levels of the respiratory tract, beginning at the sinus level and extending caudally throughout the respiratory tree and ending at the terminal bronchi. Impulses from these airway cough receptors travel through the cranial nerve afferent pathway to the medullary cough center. The reflexive efferent response of this activation causes the coordinated activity of glottic closure and diaphragmatic, chest wall, abdominal, and pelvic floor contraction, resulting in cough.[1]

CLASSIFICATION

The cough sequence can be divided into 3 classic phases. The 1st phase, termed the inspiratory phase, results in a deep inspiration ending in glottic closure. During the short 2nd phase, termed the compressive phase, intrathoracic pressure increases as a result of coordinated contraction of the expiratory muscles. With the expiratory 3rd phase, the glottis opens rapidly, leading to the sudden, sometimes explosive, release of the pent-up intrathoracic air (ie, cough). Coupled with this 3rd phase, secretions and irritants are expelled from the airway. Incomplete or inefficient removal of these materials will result in recurrence of the cough sequence, as will ongoing irritation or inflammation.[2]

DIFFERENTIAL DIAGNOSIS

Many classification schemes for cough have been developed over the years, and each has its benefits and limitations.[3] Ultimately, any useful classification scheme must help in planning an efficient and successful evaluation and management plan. When classifying cough, 2 basic questions need to be addressed. The 1st question is whether the cough is acute or chronic (greater than 3 weeks' duration), with chronic cough likely requiring a more extensive evaluation plan. The 2nd question is whether the cough is of upper, lower, or mixed airway origin. This is not always apparent, especially in younger children, but is critical to determine, in order to minimize unnecessary testing, treatment or both.

The character of the cough can sometimes be helpful in answering this question, with *croupy, throaty,* and *honking,* or *foghorn* coughs being more likely upper airway in origin; however, young children with asthma (clearly a disease of the lower airways) may initially exhibit a croupy cough, presumably from the physiological narrowing of the subglottic space in children younger than 4 years.

At the other extreme, although a productive cough with expectoration of sputum is classically the result of bacterial pneumonia, children with severe chronic sinusitis (a disease of the upper airway) will frequently cough and expectorate or swallow thick sputum, which may even be blood tinged at times. Therefore cough character, although helpful, should not limit the differential diagnosis. A variety of qualities attributed to cough character have been described that can be useful starting points in the evaluation of cough, including paroxysmal for pertussis, staccato for *Chlamydia* infection, barking for laryngotracheal infection, throat clearing for postnasal secretions, and honking for psychogenic cough.[4] History and pattern of illness progression are crucial for putting these cough qualities into perspective. For example, cough that occurs only during the daytime, increases when more attention is paid to it, and does not limit or change with physical activity is more likely psychogenic. In contrast, if the cough clearly increases with activity and limits the child from participating in desired physical activities, then asthma is a likely diagnosis. Night cough with nasal symptoms suggests allergy or sinusitis (or both), cough during feeding suggests swallowing dysfunction or tracheoesophageal fistula with aspiration, and cough after feeding with spitting up, retching, or arching of the back suggests gastroesophageal (GE) reflux. [5]

Age of onset is also an important feature in planning a workup. Chronic or recurrent cough that begins in early infancy, especially in children younger than 3 months, suggests congenital or anatomic origins and clearly requires a more aggressive approach toward evaluation. Cough that begins relatively suddenly in toddlers might suggest foreign-body aspiration, with a similarly active approach toward testing (ie, bronchoscopy). Cough beginning at more than 6 months of age may suggest airways hyperreactivity, and a therapeutic trial of treatment with a beta-2 agonist may be a reasonable 1st step. Cough beginning relatively suddenly in adolescents, especially at times of psychosocial stress, might indicate a psychogenic origin.[6-8]

Classifying cough provides a starting point in developing a differential diagnosis and suggests important pieces of historical information that should be gleaned from the patient. In addition, classifying cough helps focus the physical examination to the key features necessary in making a presumptive diagnosis and developing an appropriate plan of management.

EVALUATION

History

Personal and Family History

The history from a patient complaining of cough should begin with an accurate description of the cough, with a focus on the pattern and progression of symptoms. The duration of cough, the frequency of discrete cough episodes, quiet periods between cough (daily cough vs days or weeks between cough episodes), and the quality, timing, and triggers of the cough are all important pieces of information to help make an accurate diagnosis. Associated fever suggests a respiratory tract infection; cough worsening with exercise suggests reactive airways disease; and night cough suggests a postnasal drip, as with sinusitis. Past history is also important. Previous episodes, especially with seasonal variation, suggest allergy, and chronic cough with poor weight gain suggests a more severe systemic illness such as cystic fibrosis or an immune deficiency. Family history can be especially helpful with more chronic symptoms. A family history of allergies, atopy, or asthma makes these diagnoses far more likely in the child with chronic or recurrent cough, given that a history of asthma or atopy in 1st-degree relatives confers a 2- to 4-fold increase in risk of asthma in the child.[9] Similarly, a family history of early childhood death related to infection makes an immune deficiency more likely.[10]

Neonatal History

Neonatal history is similarly important because preterm infants are more likely than full-term infants to have persistent airways hyperreactivity, laryngotracheomalacia, and GE reflux. Infants with poor Apgar scores, perinatal hypoxia, or a difficult postnatal course may have central nervous system sequelae and therefore have suck or swallow dysfunction, increasing the risk of aspiration. Finally, associated congenital abnormalities (eg, diaphragmatic hernia) may result in pulmonary hypoplasia, leading to chronic respiratory dysfunction and recurrent pneumonia.

Environmental History

Environmental history is also important in determining the source of cough. Children who live in households with smokers have significantly more respiratory infections and asthma symptoms than children not exposed to secondhand smoke. Exposure to molds from household water leaks, decaying garbage, or ineffective cleaning of bathroom tile; dust mites from old mattresses, stuffed animals, or forced air heating systems; and roaches, mice, and household pets all increase the risk of allergy and asthma symptoms.[11] Exposure to other children through school, child care, babysitters, or school-aged siblings all make recurrent respiratory tract infections far more common.

Physical Examination

The physical examination plays a critical role in pinpointing the origin of the cough and identifying signs of a more serious underlying, chronic condition. A nasal speculum examination can help determine the color and quality of the nasal mucosa, coupled with the presence or absence of nasal secretions, which can help determine if the cause of the cough is upper airway disease. Inflamed nasal mucosa, coupled with thick secretions, suggests rhinitis and, when the symptoms have been prolonged, sinusitis. Associated maxillary, ethmoid or frontal sinus tenderness, and pharyngeal drip with a cobblestone appearance (lymphoid hyperplasia) further support the diagnosis of sinusitis.[12] Halitosis may also be present. In contrast, pale, boggy, swollen nasal mucosa makes allergic rhinitis far more likely. Associated atopic symptoms, such as eczema, further support this diagnosis. Other features of the pharyngeal examination can also be helpful. Chronic pharyngeal inflammation, in the absence of other signs of acute infection, suggests GE reflux. Oral mucosal ulcerations or thrush suggests an immune deficiency. When pertussis is a consideration, cough paroxysms triggered by a tongue depressor support the diagnosis. Signs of an acute infectious process, such as fever, adenopathy, pharyngitis, or rash, are important to appreciate but do not necessarily rule out a predisposing condition, especially when the pattern of illness suggests chronicity or frequent recurrence. A thorough assessment of other body systems is important in judging whether a more global workup is necessary. Growth failure, poor developmental milestone achievement, clubbing, heart murmurs, hepatosplenomegaly, and chronic lymphadenopathy are all potential clues to a more severe underlying process.

A thorough examination of the respiratory system is critical in making an accurate diagnosis. Stridor and inspiratory rhonchi or wheeze suggest upper and large central airway disease, whereas rales, expiratory rhonchi, and wheeze are indicative of lower or distal airway inflammation. Similarly, a change in the quality of air exchange can be an early finding in asthma and other diseases of airways obstruction.[13,14]

An accurate lower airway examination depends on the cooperation of the patient. Wheeze and distal airways sounds can be masked by a patient's vocalization or crying. Similarly, force of airflow insufficient to uncover milder changes may mask both inspiratory and expiratory findings in infants and children who do not take deep breaths on command. Every effort should be made to place the child at ease during the examination. Game playing, such as blowing on a feather or blowing up a balloon, can be helpful. In younger children and infants, the examiner can mimic a forced expiratory maneuver by firmly but gently compressing the anterior-posterior chest wall inward once the child has begun voluntary exhalation. This approach will frequently uncover milder degrees of wheezing previously not appreciated with passive breathing. The examiner should allow the child to begin exhalation passively before performing this maneuver to ensure that the glottis is relaxed and the procedure proceeds safely and effectively.

Laboratory Evaluation

Hematologic Tests

Acute cough rarely needs extensive laboratory assessment. A detailed history and physical examination are usually sufficient to reach an accurate presumptive diagnosis, and response to empiric therapy will confirm this assessment. In cases in which this approach does not lead to a resolution of symptoms, or when the cough is either recurrent or chronic, a few tests can be helpful. A complete blood cell count with differential may help distinguish a bacterial from a viral cause if infection is suspected. However, localized infections such as sinusitis are not always accompanied by an elevated white blood cell count with a shift to the left. The total eosinophil count on the complete blood cell count may be an important clue to atopy. Similarly, an elevated IgE level or positive nasal smear for eosinophils would further corroborate the diagnosis of allergy and suggest the possibility of asthma. Although increased polymorphonuclear leukocytes on a nasal smear may suggest rhinosinusitis, the result is difficult to quantify, and the test may be misleading. Ultimately, if sinusitis is suspected, then a computed tomographic scan of the sinuses may be necessary to confirm the diagnosis. Alternatively, empiric therapy may be initiated based on history and physical examination, and response to therapy may be monitored.[12]

Gastroesophageal Tests

When aspiration or GE reflux is a consideration, a barium swallow (modified for aspiration and standard for GE reflux) may be useful. Although barium swallow is of limited use in diagnosing GE reflux (approximately 40% false negative), looking for anatomic causes of partial obstruction, for tracheoesophageal fistulae, and for vascular rings is important in infants. Monitoring with a pH probe is the gold standard for diagnosing GE reflux; however, many experts suggest a period of empiric therapy if reflux is suggested by history and physical examination findings, with the pH probe being reserved for patients in whom primary empiric treatment fails.[15-17]

Pulmonary Function Tests

Pulmonary function testing can be a useful tool in making the distinction between upper and lower airways disease and differentiating obstructive from restrictive changes. Children must be old enough to exhale fully and inhale forcefully on command, and the test should be reproducible to ensure accuracy and reliability of results.[18]

Changes on the inspiratory loop of the flow-volume curve suggest upper airway obstruction, whereas changes in the ratio of the forced expiratory volume in the first 1 second to the forced vital capacity of the lungs (FEV_1/FVC) or the forced midexpiratory flow rate over the middle half of the FVC (FEF25%-75%) indicate airways obstruction consistent with distal disease. Reversibility of these changes (20% improvement) with a beta-2 agonist confirms the diagnosis of asthma and leads to effective therapy.[19]

Other Tests

Other tests, such as the sweat test, chest x-ray examination, tuberculin skin test, immunologic studies, and alpha-1 antitrypsin levels, can all be useful in the proper clinical setting. Bronchoscopy can also be useful to diagnose structural abnormalities of both the upper and lower airways and should be considered in patients with chronic symptoms not responsive to empiric treatment. Furthermore, it is the test of choice when a foreign body or chronic aspiration is considered a likely diagnosis. In cases in which an upper airways origin is likely, flexible bronchoscopy can make a definitive diagnosis. The bronchoscopist must always look beyond the vocal cords in this setting, given that lesions to the level of the thoracic inlet can cause symptoms suggestive of upper airways obstruction.[20,21]

TREATMENT

Once the history and physical examination have led to an initial assessment, the fact that cough is a symptom of an underlying condition should be discussed with the patient and family. Treatment of the underlying disorder (if necessary) should always be the prime focus.[22-25] Empiric therapy, based on primary assessment, can be a reasonable starting point. Judicious use of laboratory testing, as previously discussed, can be helpful in confirming the diagnosis and allaying parental anxiety. Furthermore, in some conditions, cough is an important component of the body's natural response to the primary illness, and suppressing the cough, in the absence of effective therapy of the primary disorder, may actually worsen the problem.

Treatment of the underlying disorders causing cough is discussed in other sections of this book; this chapter is limited to a review of medications used to treat cough itself. The decision to use a cough medicine as an adjunct to the treatment of the primary disease is left to the primary care physician and family. When cough is limiting or otherwise debilitating the patient, symptomatic treatment may be reasonable. Over-the-counter cough and cold medications should not be used in children younger than 2 years because serious and potentially life-threatening side effects can occur from their use.[26] Furthermore, studies have shown that these medications are generally ineffective in children younger than 6 years.[27]

Expectorants

Expectorants such as guaifenesin (formerly known as glyceryl guaiacolate) may be used to make secretions more fluid and reduce sputum thickness.[28] This therapeutic approach may be useful when drainage of secretions is important, as with sinusitis. Because expectorants work by increasing the fluid content of secretions, water is probably the most effective expectorant. Whether administering water by nasal spray, inhalation, or orally, saline solutions are safe adjuncts to primary therapy. Despite widespread use, expectorants have not been shown to decrease cough in children. Other older expectorants, such as potassium iodide and ammonium chloride, are no longer prescribed to children because of their adverse effects when used at effective doses.

Mucolytic Agents

Acetylcysteine was previously used as a mucolytic agent to help liquefy thick secretions, especially in diseases such as cystic fibrosis; however, its propensity for inducing airway reactivity and inflammation has lately made it less popular.[29,30]

Cough Suppressants

Cough suppressants, which can be divided into peripheral and centrally acting agents, can be effective in transiently decreasing cough severity and frequency. Peripheral agents include demulcents (eg, throat lozenges), which soothe the throat, and topical anesthetics, which can be sprayed or swallowed. Topical agents block the cough receptors, but their effects are short-lived because oral secretions rapidly wash them away. Centrally acting cough suppressants, including both narcotic and nonnarcotic medications, suppress the cough reflex at the brain stem level. The narcotic agent most commonly used in children is codeine and it has been shown to be effective in adults. Studies on its safety and efficacy in children are lacking. Furthermore, the metabolic clearance pathway of codeine in babies is immature and therefore data in adults should not be extrapolated to children, particularly those younger than 2 years. In older children, codeine should be used with appropriate instructions and cautions to avoid overuse and abuse. Other agents, such as hydrocodone have no demonstrated advantage and pose a greater risk of dependency. Dextromethorphan (the dextro isomer of codeine) is the most commonly used nonnarcotic antitussive, and despite evidence in adults, efficacy data in children are lacking.

Decongestants

Decongestants, such as pseudoephedrine, can be used either topically or systemically to decrease nasal mucosal swelling. Decongestants, which can also facilitate sinus drainage by decreasing sinus ostia obstruction may work well in combination with expectorants to optimize treatment of chronic sinusitis. Care should be taken in the use of these agents because they have been shown to lead to tachyarrhythmias in individuals who use them in excess. In addition, these agents have not been studied in children and should be avoided in children younger than 2 years. A review of the data in children between the ages of 2 and 6 years is presently underway by the U.S. FDA with further recommendations forthcoming.

Antihistamines

Antihistamines, which can be helpful in the treatment of cough triggered by allergy, have minimal effect when cough is the result of viral or bacterial infection and may actually be detrimental because they can increase the thickness of secretions. First-generation H_1-receptor antagonists may decrease nasal drip by exerting an anticholinergic effect. Additionally, diphenhydramine may have a modest direct effect on the medullary cough center. The clinical benefits of these findings are unclear.[31]

WHEN TO REFER

- When cough persists despite adequate therapy
- When cough recurs more than every 6 to 8 weeks
- When associated with failure to thrive
- When associated with other systemic illness

WHEN TO ADMIT

- When patient has respiratory distress
- When infant is unable to feed
- When associated with bacterial pneumonia not responsive to oral antibiotic trial

TOOLS FOR PRACTICE

Engaging Patient and Family

- *Cover Your Cough* (flyers and posters), Centers for Disease Control and Prevention (www.cdc.gov/flu/protect/covercough.htm).
- *Information for Parents Complaining of Cough: A Guide for Parents* (brochure), American College of Chest Physicians (www.chestnet.org/downloads/patients/guides/cough/adult.pdf).

Medical Decision Support

- *Managing cough as a defense mechanism and as a symptom: a consensus panel report of the American College of Chest Physicians* (report), American College of Chest Physicians (www.chestjournal.org).

AAP POLICY STATEMENT

American Academy of Pediatrics, Committee on Drugs. Use of codeine- and dextromethorphan-containing cough remedies in children. *Pediatrics.* 1997;99(6):918-920. Reaffirmed January 1, 2007. (aappolicy.aappublications.org/cgi/content/full/pediatrics;99/6/918).

SUGGESTED RESOURCES

American Academy of Pediatrics, Committee on Drugs. Use of codeine- and dextromethorphan-containing cough remedies in children. *Pediatrics.* 1997;99(6); 918-920. (aappolicy.aappublications.org/cgi/content/full/pediatrics;99/6/918).

American Academy of Pediatrics. Treating coughs and colds. Available at: (www.aap.org/new/kidscolds.htm).

Brooke AM, Lambert PC, Burton PR, et al. Recurrent cough: natural history and significance in infancy and early childhood. *Pulmonology.* 1998;26:256-261.

Chang AB, Phelan PD, Sawyer SM, et al. Airway hyperresponsiveness and cough-receptor sensitivity in children with recurrent cough. *Am J Respir Crit Care Med.* 1997; 155:1935-1939.

Chang AB, Gaffney JT, Eastburn MM, et al. Cough quality in children: a comparison of subjective vs. bronchoscopic findings. *Respir Res.* 2005;6:3.

Chang AB, Lasserson TJ, Kiljander TO, et al. Systemic review and meta-analysis of randomized controlled trials of gastro-oesophageal reflux interventions for chronic cough associated with gastro-oesophageal reflux. *BMJ.* 2005; 332:11-17.

Chawla S, Seth D, Mahajan P, et al. Gastroesophageal reflux disorder: a review for primary care providers. *Clin Pediatr.* 2006;45:7-13.

Irwin RJ, Cloutier F, Gold H, et al. Managing cough as a defense mechanism and as a symptom: a consensus panel report of the American College of Chest Physicians. *Chest.* 1998;114(2):133S-181S.

Petty JL. Testing patient's lungs: spirometry as part of the physical examination. *Clin Ther.* 1999;21:1908-1922.

Saito J, Harris WT, Gelfond J, et al. Physiologic, bronchoscopic, and bronchoalveolar lavage fluid findings in young children with recurrent wheeze and cough. *Pediatr Pulmonol.* 2006;41:709-719.

Schroeder K. Over-the-counter medications for acute cough in children and adults in ambulatory settings. *Cochrane Database Syst Rev.* 2004;4:CD001831.

Steel RW: Rhinosinusitis in children. *Curr Allergy Asthma Rep.* 2006;6:508-512.

Wright AL, Holberg CJ, Morgan WJ, et al. Recurrent cough in childhood and its relation to asthma. *Am J Respir Crit Care Med.* 1996;153:1259-1265.

REFERENCES

1. Chang AB, Phelan PD, Sawyer SM, et al. Airway hyperresponsiveness and cough-receptor sensitivity in children with recurrent cough. *Am J Respir Crit Care Med.* 1997;155:1935-1939.
2. Guilbert TW, Tuussig LM. Chronic cough. *Contemp Pediatr.* 1998;15:155.
3. Irwin RJ, Cloutier F, Gold H, et al. Managing cough as a defense mechanism and as a symptom: a consensus panel report of the American College of Chest Physicians. *Chest.* 1998;114(2):133S-181S.
4. Chang AB, Gaffney JT, Eastburn MM, et al. Cough quality in children: a comparison of subjective vs. bronchoscopic findings. *Respir Res.* 2005;6:3.
5. Callahan C. Etiology of chronic cough in population of children referred to a pediatric pulmonologist. *J Am Board Fam Pract.* 1996;9:324-327.
6. Chang AB, Powell CV. Non-specific cough in children: diagnosis and treatment. *Hosp Med.* 1998;59:680-684.
7. Doull IJ, Williams AA, Freezer NJ, et al. Descriptive study of cough, wheeze and school absence in childhood. *Thorax.* 1996;51:630-631.
8. Brooke AM, Lambert PC, Burton PR, et al. Recurrent cough: natural history and significance in infancy and early childhood. *Pulmonology.* 1998;26:256-261.
9. Burke W, Fesinmeyer M, Reed K, et al. Family history as a predictor of asthma risk. *Am J Prev Med.* 2003;24(2): 160-169.
10. Marchant JM, Masters IB, Taylor SM, et al. Evaluation and outcome of young children with chronic cough. *Chest.* 2006;129:1132-1141.

11. Wilson NW, Robinson NP, Hogan MB. Cockroach and other inhalant allergies in infantile asthma. *Ann Allergy Asthma Immunol.* 1999;83:27-30.
12. Steel RW. Rhinosinusitis in children. *Curr Allergy Asthma Rep.* 2006;6:508-512.
13. Faniran AO, Peat TK, Woolrock AJ. Persistent cough: is it asthma? *Arch Dis Child.* 1998;79:411-414.
14. Wright AL, Holberg CJ, Morgan WJ, et al. Recurrent cough in childhood and its relation to asthma. *Am J Respir Crit Care Med.* 1996;153:1259-1265.
15. Chawla S, Seth D, Mahajan P, et al. Gastroesophageal reflux disorder: a review for primary care providers. *Clin Pediatr.* 2006;45:7-13.
16. Sontag SJ. The spectrum of pulmonary symptoms due to gastroesophageal reflux. *Thorac Surg Clin.* 2005;15: 353-368.
17. Callahan CW. Primary tracheomalacia and gastroesophageal reflux in infants with cough. *Clin Pediatr.* 1998;37: 725-731.
18. Zanconato S, Meneghelli G, Braga R, et al. Office spirometry in primary care pediatrics: a pilot study. *Pediatrics.* 2005;116:e792-e797.
19. Petty JL. Testing patient's lungs: spirometry as part of the physical examination. *Clin Ther.* 1999;21:1908-1922.
20. Nicolai T. Pediatric bronchoscopy. *Pediatr Pulmonol.* 2001;31:150-164.
21. Saito J, Harris WT, Gelfond J, et al. Physiologic, bronchoscopic, and bronchoalveolar lavage fluid findings in young children with recurrent wheeze and cough. *Pediatr Pulmonol.* 2006;41:709-719.
22. Chang AB, Phelan PD, Carlin JB, et al. A randomized, placebo-controlled trial of inhaled albuterol and beclomethasone for recurrent cough. *Arch Dis Child.* 1998; 79:6-11.
23. Cochrane D. Diagnosing and treating chesty infants: a short trial of inhaled corticosteroids is probably the best approach. *BMJ.* 1998;316:1546-1547.
24. O'Brien KL, Dowell SF, Schwartz B, et al. Cough illness/ bronchitis: principles of judicious use of antimicrobial agents. *Pediatrics.* 1998;101:178-181.
25. Chang AB, Lasserson TJ, Kiljander TO, et al. Systemic review and metaanalysis of randomized controlled trials of gastro-oesophageal reflux interventions for chronic cough associated with gastro-oesophageal reflux. *BMJ.* 2005;332:11-17.
26. US Food and Drug Administration. Public Health Advisory. Nonprescription Cough and Cold Medicine Use in Children: FDA recommends that over-the-counter (OTC) cough and cold products not be used for infants and children under 2 years of age. Department of Health and Human Services. Available at: www.fda.gov/cder/ drug/advisory/cough_cold_2008.htm. Accessed March 4, 2008.
27. American Academy of Pediatrics, Committee on Drugs. Use of codeine- and dextromethorphan-containing cough remedies in children. *Pediatrics.* Jun 1997;99(6); 918-920.
28. Schroeder K. Over-the-counter medications for acute cough in children and adults in ambulatory settings. *Cochrane Database Syst Rev.* 2004;4:CD001831.
29. Duijvestijn YC. Systemic review of N-acetykysteinc in cystic fibrosis. *Acta Paediatr.* 1999; 88:38-41.
30. Duijvestijn YC, Gerritsen J, Brand PL. [Acetylcysteine in children with lung disorders prescribed by one third of family physicians: no support in the literature] (Dutch). *Ned Tijdschr Geneesk.* 1997;141:826-830.
31. Arroll B. Non-antibiotic treatments for upper-respiratory tract infections (common cold). *Respir Med.* 2005;99: 1477-1484.

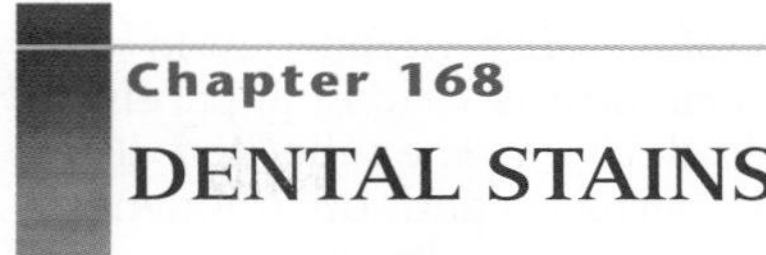

Chapter 168

DENTAL STAINS

Lindsey K. Grossman, MD

Parental concerns about changes in tooth color, often the cause of much anxiety, are frequently first brought to the pediatrician. An important point to remember is that normal tooth color varies greatly from 1 tooth to another, from 1 individual to another, and between the usual blue-white of the primary dentition and the yellowish ivory of the permanent teeth.

EXTRINSIC STAIN

Teeth are often discolored as a result of staining from external deposits on their surface layer. These extrinsic stains are usually removable by careful daily brushing and professional oral prophylaxis (scaling). Chromogenic bacteria in plaque biofilm can result in green, orange, or black stains along the gingival margin of the teeth. Although in most cases chromogenic bacteria is associated with poor oral hygiene, black stains may be associated with good hygiene and a low incidence of dental caries. Although excessive use of certain foods or beverages and smoking can stain the teeth, the discoloration will usually disappear with oral prophylaxis and avoidance of the staining substance. Children who are receiving certain liquid medications, especially iron preparations, may have teeth with a dark stain, which also resolves with professional scaling after the medication is discontinued but may be completely prevented if the medication is administered through a straw from the onset. A new dental calculus was first reported in 1995 in children who are intensive swimmers.[1] Spanish investigators demonstrated an increased prevalence of this yellow to dark-brown stain, most noticeable on the facial and lingual surfaces of the anterior teeth, in competitive school-aged and adolescent swimmers years compared with other athletes living in the same area and of similar age, with a trend toward higher risk with increasing hours in the pool.[2] Professional oral prophylaxis appeared to be protective.

INTRINSIC STAIN

When a staining substance is incorporated into the deep structures of the tooth (ie, enamel, dentin, or both), it cannot be removed by scaling and is referred to as an intrinsic stain. Neonatal conditions resulting in high serum concentrations of bilirubin pigments, such as erythroblastosis fetalis, biliary atresia, and neonatal hepatitis, can cause yellow-green or blue-green staining of primary teeth resulting from pigment deposition in the structures of these teeth. As many as 50% of children who have cyanotic congenital heart disease may have dull, pale, bluish-white teeth, the color of which resembles skim milk, believed to be caused, at least in part, by the hypoxemia associated with these conditions.

Intrinsic stains may be associated with certain rare childhood conditions. The erythrodontia of porphyria caused by deposition of red-brown porphyrin pigments into the tooth structure is readily apparent in ultraviolet light if not in daylight. The inherited disorders amyelogenesis imperfecta and dentinogenesis imperfecta are associated with hypoplastic enamel and a yellow, opalescent, blue-gray or brown-violet tooth color. Major dental work is required to restore normal appearance with any of these disorders.

Common pedodontic problems often result in a change in tooth color. Tooth trauma and associated bleeding into dentin can cause a pink color that fades, first to gray as pulp degenerates and eventually to yellow. In certain cases, the dentin resorption will result in a permanent pink hue. Active dental caries may appear chalky white or yellow but gradually convert to shiny black as the dental caries converts to the arrested state. An unusual secondary complication of local infection or trauma is Turner tooth, a brown or yellow-brown discoloration of a single tooth associated with hypoplasia of the enamel in a tooth undergoing odontogenesis at the time of the illness.

Fluoridated water is protective against dental caries.[3] However, as the fluoride content rises over 1.5 parts per million (ppm), many individuals in the area will begin to demonstrate hypoplastic enamel, with characteristic dull, opaque, white mottled patches in the permanent teeth. If the amount of fluoride consumed is extremely high (>5 ppm), then the teeth will show a blotchy brown or black-brown color that is highly disfiguring and requires extensive restoration of the dental surfaces.

In recent years the application of fluoride varnish by pediatricians during routine visits with young children has been promoted as a cost-effective measure to prevent early dental caries even in children as young as 12 months with their first primary teeth. There is no evidence that this or other professionally applied topical fluoride preparations results in enamel fluorosis. However, concern does exist that sufficient fluoride may be ingested from daily tooth brushing with fluoride toothpaste or the use of fluoride mouthwash to be a concern in children less than 6 years.[4]

As with significant intrinsic staining from enamel fluorosis, a similarly involved course of treatment is often required for the severe intrinsic staining caused by tetracycline, a dose-dependent and duration-linked problem caused by the incorporation of tetracycline itself into the mineral complex at the dentinoenamel junction during odontogenesis. If the tetracycline was ingested by the mother during pregnancy or by the child in the 1st months after birth, then the primary teeth will be affected. Permanent teeth will be stained if drug ingestion occurs between 3 months and 7 to 8 years of age. The result may be yellow, gray, or brown tooth discoloration in a linear pattern that, without restoration, may be quite disfiguring. Tetracycline should be avoided in pregnant or lactating women and in young children.

MANAGEMENT

After allaying parental anxieties, the pediatrician should consider referring any child who has extrinsic or intrinsic stains. Simple office dental procedures and preventive education can resolve all extrinsic staining problems, and esthetic improvement is possible with the majority of intrinsic discoloration problems. Table 168-1 outlines causes and treatment of dental staining.

Table 168-1 Common Colorations of Primary and Permanent Teeth

COLOR	DISTRIBUTION AND PATTERN	CAUSES	TREATMENT
Green	Several teeth; gingival third of crowns; extrinsic stain	Chromogenic bacteria in plaque biofilm, associated with poor oral hygiene	Oral prophylaxis; preventive education
Orange	Several teeth; gingival third of crowns; less common than green stain; extrinsic stain	Chromogenic bacteria in plaque biofilm, associated with poor oral hygiene	Oral prophylaxis; preventive education
Black	Several teeth; gingival third of crowns; less common than green and orange stains; extrinsic stain	Chromogenic bacteria in plaque biofilm, associated with poor oral hygiene	Oral prophylaxis; preventive education
	Several teeth; extrinsic stain	Oral medications, especially iron	Oral prophylaxis after discontinuing medication
	One or several teeth; occlusal or interproximal surfaces; hard, shiny	Arrested dental caries	Dental evaluation, observation, or restoration
Brown black	Several teeth; occlusal pits and fissures or smooth surfaces	Accumulation of tin or staining of demineralized enamel after strontium fluoride topical treatment	None or esthetic restoration
Pink	Single tooth; entire crown	Posttraumatic change	None or observation
		Within 1-2 days—bleeding into dentin; changes to gray in 1-3 wk	
		After several months—internal resorption of dentin	Minor resorption—endodontics
			Severe resorption—extraction

Table 168-1 Common Colorations of Primary and Permanent Teeth—cont'd

COLOR	DISTRIBUTION AND PATTERN	CAUSES	TREATMENT
Gray	Several teeth; linear pattern or entire crown, depending on stage of tooth development	Tetracycline incorporation in tooth and subsequent oxidation by sunlight; exhibits other colors	Esthetic improvement—endodontic therapy and bleaching, esthetic restoration, or both
	All primary and permanent teeth; entire crown	Dentinogenesis imperfecta (autosomal dominant)	Esthetic improvement and protection from wear—prosthetic coverage
	Single tooth; entire crown	Posttraumatic change	Observation
		Within 1-3 wk—hemosiderin pigment in dentin	
		After several months—pulpal necrosis	Endodontic treatment or extraction
Yellow	Several teeth; entire crown	Natural color of permanent compared with primary teeth	None necessary
	Several teeth; linear pattern or entire crown	Tetracycline; systemic infections	Esthetic restoration
	All primary and permanent teeth; entire crown	Amelogenesis imperfecta (various inheritance patterns)	Esthetic restoration and protection from occlusal wear
	Single tooth; entire crown	Posttraumatic change—pulpal obliteration by dentin	Observation or esthetic restoration
	Several teeth; gingival third of crown; extrinsic stain	Food debris and chromogenic bacteria in plaque biofilm, associated with poor oral hygiene	Oral prophylaxis; preventive education
	Several teeth; extrinsic stain; part of or entire crown	Tea, coffee, cola, tobacco	Oral prophylaxis; avoid excessive use of substance
Yellow brown	Several teeth	Premature birth; enamel disturbance—hypoplasia and hypocalcification	None
	One or several teeth; 1 or more surfaces with cavitations	Advanced active dental caries	Restoration
Brown	Several teeth; entire crown	Amelogenesis imperfecta; dentinogenesis imperfecta; premature birth; jaundice	As suggested above under gray and yellow colorations
	Individual teeth; localized area	Turner hypoplasia secondary to infection	None or esthetic restoration
		Hypocalcified or hypoplastic area—traumatized primary tooth affecting permanent crown	None or esthetic restoration
	Several teeth; linear or generalized distribution; associated hypoplasia	Fluorosis; systemic infections, especially with high fever; nutritional deficiencies	None or esthetic restoration
	Several teeth; generalized or linear	Tetracycline	Esthetic restoration
	Several teeth; 1 or more surfaces; loss of tooth structure	Advanced active dental caries	Restoration
Red brown	Several teeth; primary and permanent; generalized	Porphyria	None or esthetic restoration
Blue	Several teeth; extrinsic stain; part of or entire crown	Berries	Oral prophylaxis; avoid excessive use of substance
Blue green or yellow green	All primary teeth; entire crown	Bilirubin pigments incorporated into dentin—erythroblastosis fetalis, biliary atresia, neonatal hepatitis	None; generally fades; permanent teeth not affected if condition does not continue
White or cream	Several teeth; linear or entire crown	Fluorosis; systemic infections	None; generally fades; permanent teeth not affected if condition does not continue
	All primary and permanent teeth; entire crown	Amelogenesis imperfecta	
	Individual teeth; localized area	Turner hypoplasia	
	One or several teeth; occlusal or gingival third of smooth surface	Early active dental caries—demineralization of enamel	Preventive therapy
	Several teeth; any surface; extrinsic stain	Plaque biofilm and food debris (materia alba)—removed easily with gauze	Oral hygiene instruction

Modified from Abrams RG, Josell SD. Common oral and dental emergencies and problems. *Pediatr Clin North Am.* 1982;29(3):681-715.

TOOLS FOR PRACTICE

Community Coordination and Advocacy

- *Making Oral Health Supervision Accessible* (booklet), Bright Futures (www.brightfutures.org/oralhealth/pdf/MOHSA_87to94.pdf).

Engaging Patient and Family

- *A Guide to Children's Dental Health* (brochure), American Academy of Pediatrics (patiented.aap.org).
- *Brush Up on Healthy Teeth—a quiz for parents* (fact sheet), Centers for Disease Control and Prevention (www.cdc.gov/oralhealth/pdfs/BrushUpQuiz.pdf).
- *Brush Up on Healthy Teeth—simple steps* (fact sheet), Centers for Disease Control and Prevention (www.cdc.gov/oralhealth/pdfs/BrushUpTips.pdf).
- *Brushing Up on Oral Health: Never Too Early to Start* (article), American Academy of Pediatrics (www.aap.org/family/healthychildren/07winter/oralhealth.pdf).
- *How To Prevent Tooth Decay in Your Baby's Teeth* (fact sheet), American Academy of Pediatrics (www.aap.org/bookstore).
- *Oral Health* (Web page), American Academy of Pediatrics (www.aap.org/healthtopics/oralhealth.cfm).
- *What is a Pediatic Dentist* (fact sheet), American Academy of Pediatrics (www.aap.org/sections/peddentist/PediatricDentist_Eng.pdf).

Medical Decision Support

- *CDC Oral Health* (Web page), Centers for Disease Control and Prevention (www.cdc.gov/oralhealth).
- *Oral Health Risk Assessment Training for Pediatricians and Other Child Health Professionals* (Web page), American Academy of Pediatrics (www.aap.org/commpeds/dochs/oralhealth/screening.cfm).

AAP POLICY STATEMENT

American Academy of Pediatrics, Section on Pediatric Dentistry. Oral health risk assessment timing and establishment of the dental home. *Pediatrics.* 2003;111(5):1113-1116. (aappolicy.aappublications.org/cgi/content/full/pediatrics;111/5/1113).

RELATED WEB SITES

- American Academy of Pediatric Dentristy (www.aapd.org/).
- American Dental Association (www.ada.org/).

SUGGESTED RESOURCES

Acosta F, Carrel R, Binns WH. Dental stains and their relationship to periodontal diseases in children. *Acta Odontol Pediatr.* 1982;3(1):13-18.

Creighton PR. Common pediatric dental problems. *Pediatr Clin North Am.* 1998;45:1579.

Faunce F. Management of discolored teeth. *Dent Clin North Am.* 1983;27:657-670.

McDonald RE, Avery DR, Weddell JA. Gingivitis and periodontal disease. In: McDonald RE, Avery DR, eds. *Dentistry for the Child and Adolescent.* St Louis, MO: Mosby; 2000.

Sweeney EA. Pediatric dentistry. *Curr Probl Pediatr.* 1981;11(4):1-51.

REFERENCES

1. Rose LI, Carey CM. Intensive swimming: can it affect your patients' smiles? *JADA.* 1995;126:1402-1406.
2. Escartin JL, Arnedo A, Pinto V, et al. A study of dental staining among competitive swimmers. *Community Dent Oral Epidemiol.* 2000;28:10-17.
3. Lewis CW, Milgrom P. Fluoride. *Pediatr Rev.* 2003;24:327-336.
4. Centers for Disease Control, Morbidity and Mortality Weekly Report, 2001;50:1-42.

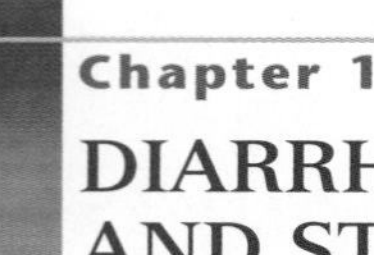

Chapter 169

DIARRHEA AND STEATORRHEA

Martin H. Ulshen, MD

Diarrhea, similar to vomiting, is a common symptom in the young child, especially during infancy. Loosely defined, diarrhea is characterized by an increase in the frequency and water content of stools. Normal daily stool volume varies with the size of the child. Adults and older children have a normal daily stool weight up to 250 g (consisting of 60% to 85% water); infants weighing fewer than 10 kg can have approximately 5 g/kg/day of stool. An intermediate range of 50 to 75 g/day is an appropriate approximation for the preschool-age child. In infancy, the frequency and quality of normal stools depend very much on diet.

During the first weeks of life, breastfed infants commonly have up to 8 loose stools per day, which, at times, may contain mucus. These stools frequently follow feedings, as a result of the *gastrocolic reflex*, and do not constitute diarrhea. Infants receiving cow milk or soy formula usually have firmer and somewhat less frequent stools. After the first few weeks of life, normal breastfed infants tend to have less frequent stools, occasionally even less than once a week, although the stools remain soft. Commonly, the stool of the nursing infant becomes firm when solids or cow milk is introduced into the diet.

Steatorrhea signifies an excess of fat in the stool and is a symptom of malabsorption. However, disorders associated with malabsorption, such as gluten-sensitive enteropathy, do not always produce steatorrhea. Stools that contain an increased quantity of fat can be greasy, bulky, and foul smelling; however, with mild steatorrhea, the stool may appear normal. The stool can be evaluated quickly for fat content by using light microscopy with Sudan staining (known as qualitative analysis for stool fat). Fat excretion can be measured more precisely by quantitative chemical analysis of a 72-hour collection of stool. A record of the diet is kept during this period, and fat intake is calculated. The percentage of the ingested fat that is absorbed is called the *coefficient of absorption:*

$$\frac{\text{Fat Intake} - \text{Fat Output}}{\text{Fat Intake}} \times 100$$

Absorption of fat by young infants varies with the type of fat that is fed and with the maturity of the infant. A healthy premature infant may absorb as little as 65% to 75% of dietary fat, but this amount improves to 90% in the term infant. Furthermore, neonates absorb vegetable fat much more efficiently than butterfat but human milk fat best of all. Children and adults typically absorb at least 95% of the fat in a normal diet.

PATHOPHYSIOLOGIC FACTORS

Advances in the understanding of the pathophysiologic mechanism of diarrhea allow a more rational approach to diagnosis and treatment. Normally, the gastrointestinal tract processes a large volume of fluid (Figure 169-1 lists adult data). An infant can rapidly become fluid depleted from diarrhea when such large gastrointestinal fluid shifts take place each day. Under normal circumstances, approximately 90% of fluid absorption takes place in the small bowel. However, the colon has a reserve capacity for fluid absorption that must be overcome before diarrhea results. In adults, the colon can reabsorb as much as 2 L of ileal fluid daily without diarrhea occurring.

Movement of water across the gastrointestinal tract mucosa is passive, following osmotic gradients created by electrolytes and other osmotically active solutes such as glucose and amino acids. Nutrients are absorbed by active transport, facilitated transport, or passive diffusion; some solutes first require digestion to simpler compounds. The flux of electrolytes across the mucosa is bidirectional. The net result of absorption and secretion of these osmotically active solutes is net water retention or loss in the stool. In this sense, diarrhea can be considered as the result of either malabsorption or net secretion of osmotically active substances.

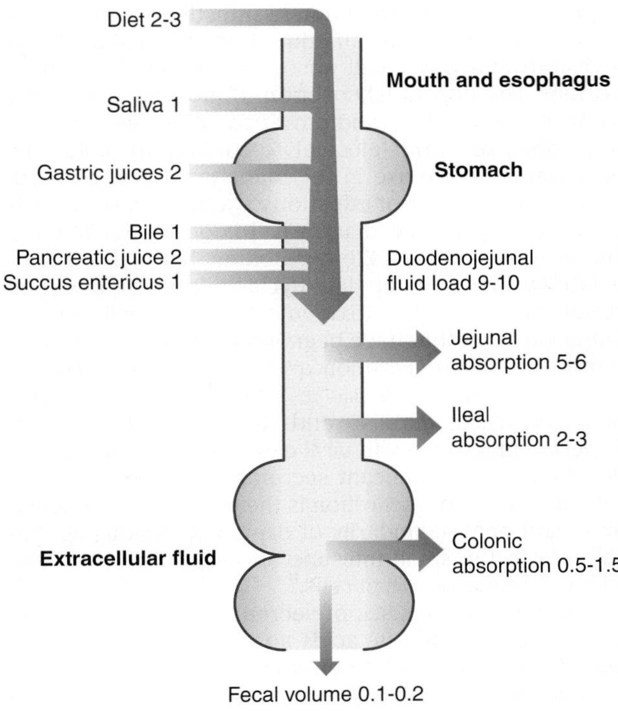

Figure 169-1 Ingestion, secretion, and absorption of water in the gastrointestinal tract of an adult. Numbers refer to liters of water.

Many nutrients, including glucose and most amino acids, are absorbed by active, carrier-mediated transport, which is coupled with sodium transport. The osmotic gradient created promotes the absorption of water. Movement of water, in turn, also carries small solutes such as sodium and chloride. This process is known as *solvent drag* and appears to be an important route for sodium absorption during normal digestion. These mechanisms of sodium movement associated with carrier-mediated nonelectrolyte transport are important to preserve normal fluid and electrolyte balance during some episodes of diarrhea (see discussion on oral rehydration).

Active absorption of chloride in exchange for bicarbonate takes place in the ileum and colon. Potassium moves passively along electrochemical gradients in the small intestine, but both active absorption and secretion of potassium occur in the colon. The permeability of the intestinal mucosa to passive fluid and electrolyte movement is high in the duodenum and proximal jejunum and decreases distally to the ileum and colon, which are poorly permeable. This feature allows the proximal intestinal contents to equilibrate rapidly with the isotonic extracellular fluid and facilitates the rapid absorption of water and small solutes by diffusion (ie, solvent drag). Conversely, the ileum and colon are poorly permeable and are able to absorb water and sodium against high electrochemical gradients.

The pathophysiologic mechanisms for diarrhea fall into four basic groups[1,2]: (1) osmotic diarrhea, (2) diarrhea resulting from secretion or altered absorption of electrolytes, (3) exudative diarrhea, and (4) diarrhea resulting from abnormal intestinal motility. Each mechanism has unique clinical characteristics and requires a different therapeutic approach. Therefore, for the physician considering an individual patient who has diarrhea, this framework provides a rational approach for both diagnosis and treatment. Frequently, more than one mechanism of diarrhea will be involved in an episode of diarrhea, but this variation will be apparent in the evaluation.

Osmotic Diarrhea

The ingestion of a poorly absorbable, osmotically active substance and its presence in the bowel lumen create an osmotic gradient that encourages movement of water into the lumen and subsequently into the stool. Electrolyte losses increase because electrolytes will follow water into the lumen through solvent drag and will tend not to be reabsorbed because of unfavorable electrochemical gradients.

Two main groups of poorly absorbed solutes exist, the ingestion of which result in osmotic diarrhea. The first group includes normal dietary components that may be malabsorbed either transiently or permanently. For example, disaccharides are usually hydrolyzed to monosaccharides before they are absorbed. If a mucosal disaccharidase (eg, lactase) is deficient, then the disaccharide (in this case lactose) will be malabsorbed and will represent an osmotic load that will produce diarrhea. Similarly, monosaccharides may, at times, be poorly absorbed. Medium-chain triglycerides are also osmotically active and may lead occasionally to diarrhea when ingested in high concentration, such as when infants who have compromised mucosal function are given an elemental formula containing medium-chain triglycerides. Malabsorption of long-chain triglycerides (LCTs) does not lead to osmotic diarrhea because LCTs are large hydrophobic molecules and therefore have little osmotic activity. Malabsorption of LCTs, however, may lead to secretory diarrhea, as described later in this chapter. In addition, any osmotically active solute may produce diarrhea in healthy persons if given in quantities great enough to surpass the intestinal capacity for absorption.

Thus some infants whose bowel function is normal will not tolerate the high osmolality of an elemental formula, especially if it is undiluted. Similarly, older children may develop functional gastrointestinal symptoms, including diarrhea, from ingesting large amounts of fructose in fruits and juices.[3] Patients who have decreased mucosal surface area may have decreased functional capacity and resultant osmotic diarrhea, a problem seen in infants after small-bowel resection. Protein malabsorption does not appear to be associated with diarrhea except in the rare instance of congenital trypsinogen or enterokinase deficiency. For example, Hartnup syndrome, with its malabsorption of primary amino acids, is not associated with diarrhea.

The second group of poorly absorbed solutes includes substances that are transported in limited amounts, even by healthy individuals. This group includes magnesium, phosphates, and sulfates. Because these ions invariably lead to diarrhea when given in large enough quantities, they are used as cathartics. The introduction of lactulose in the treatment of hepatic encephalopathy takes advantage of its being a nondigestible disaccharide that leads to acidification of colonic contents by bacterial fermentation of nonabsorbed sugar. Its side effect is diarrhea. In fact, lactulose has become a popular alternative for the treatment of constipation. Sorbitol, an artificial sweetener, causes osmotic diarrhea when ingested in large quantities.

The key characteristic of an osmotic diarrhea is its association with the ingestion of the offending solute. When a patient who has an osmotic diarrhea is given no oral or enteral feeding, the diarrhea will stop dramatically within 24 hours or less. If the agent is reintroduced, as in a lactose tolerance test, the diarrhea will reappear. The diarrhea is of a moderate volume compared with that in secretory diarrhea. The sodium and potassium ion concentrations in the stool fluid are useful in establishing a diagnosis. As ileal and colonic sodium absorption continue to function against a concentration gradient, stool sodium concentration will be lower than it is in the plasma. Normally, the electrolyte concentration in the stool is roughly twice its combined sodium and potassium concentration. When this number is much less than the total stool osmolality (usually approximately 290 mOsm/kg), osmotically active nonelectrolytes must be in the stool, and osmotic diarrhea is present.[4] An osmotic gap of more than 50 mOsm/kg indicates osmotic diarrhea. In some instances, the clinician may be able to find the osmotic component in the stool, such as a reducing substance in lactose malabsorption.

Diarrhea Secondary to Secretion or Altered Electrolyte Absorption (Secretory Diarrhea)

Under normal circumstances, opposing active and passive secretory and absorptive processes result in normal luminal electrolyte and water content. Secretory diarrhea occurs when a physiologic electrolyte secretory process is pathologically stimulated. Under such circumstances, a net increase in luminal electrolytes and, subsequently, a secondary increase in water occur. In addition, an associated decrease in absorptive processes may occur. The electrolytes that have been implicated are sodium, chloride, and perhaps bicarbonate. Diarrhea also may result from a decrease in active electrolyte absorption in the absence of any change in secretory function. Distinguishing increased electrolyte secretion from decreased absorption is clinically difficult; the results are similar.

The prototype for a secretory diarrhea is cholera. Cholera enterotoxin increases intestinal secretion of chloride and inhibits the absorption of sodium by stimulating surface epithelial adenylate cyclase, leading to an increase in cellular levels of cyclic 3′5′-adenosine monophosphate. The intestinal mucosa appears normal during cholera infection, without evidence of cell necrosis, inflammation, or local bacterial invasion; and other cell absorptive functions remain normal. The normal absorption of glucose provides a route for secondary sodium absorption; as a result, oral glucose- and electrolyte-containing solutions have gained wide use in the management of cholera. A growing number of infectious agents may be associated with secretory diarrhea. Toxigenic *Escherichia coli* produces at least 2 enterotoxins that activate adenylate cyclase or guanylate cyclase. Infantile diarrhea resulting from enterotoxigenic *E coli* is well known. Other bacteria that have been associated with stimulation of intestinal secretion are strains of *Shigella, Salmonella, Yersinia, Klebsiella, Clostridium perfringens, Staphylococcus aureus,* and *Pseudomonas* species. Experimental work with viral enteritis suggests that this diarrhea has a significant secretory component.[5] With rotavirus infection, secretion is the result of viral enterotoxin and only secondarily of damage to villous epithelial cells in the small intestine and repopulation of the villi with immature crypt cells.[6]

Noninfectious causes of secretory diarrhea exist as well. Malabsorbed bile acids and long-chain fats have been shown to stimulate a colonic secretory diarrhea.[7] Certain prostaglandins have been shown to activate adenylate cyclase and produce intestinal secretion in experimental models. Because prostaglandins are released during inflammation, researchers have hypothesized that diarrhea associated with certain inflammatory states may be caused by these hormones.

This hypothesis is a particularly appealing way to explain the small-bowel secretion that may take place with chronic inflammatory bowel disease. Prostaglandins have also been suggested as possible mediators for the activation of adenylate cyclase by *Salmonella* organisms in the absence of an enterotoxin. Secretory diarrheas may occur in association with increased levels of certain gastrointestinal hormones, most notably vasoactive intestinal polypeptide (VIP).

Isolated decrease of electrolyte absorption is much less frequent. The best-known example, although extremely rare, is congenital chloride-losing diarrhea. This autosomal-recessive abnormality results from the apparent lack of normal, active chloride absorption by the distal small intestine. Great quantities of chloride are lost in the stool and lead to diarrhea from birth onward. A metabolic alkalosis results, in contrast to other causes of diarrhea.

The stool in secretory diarrheas tends to be watery and large in volume. Unlike osmotic diarrhea, secretory diarrhea persists despite discontinuing oral intake. The stool electrolyte concentration (ie, twice the sum of the sodium and potassium concentrations) is approximately equal to the stool water osmolality because no significant osmotic nonelectrolyte component is present.[4]

Exudative Diarrhea

A break in the integrity of the mucosal surface of the intestine can result in water and electrolyte loss, driven by hydrostatic pressure in blood vessels and lymphatics. The exudate contains mucus, protein, and blood cells. Examples include infectious, allergic, or ulcerative colitis.

Motility Diarrhea

The intestine has a cyclical, orderly pattern of motility. Increased, decreased, or disordered movement can lead to diarrhea. Rapid intestinal transit often occurs in association with osmotic and secretory diarrheas. Increased intraluminal volume has been implicated in stimulating increased peristaltic action. Increased motility may cause diarrhea by allowing less time for the contact of intraluminal contents with absorptive surfaces. When bowel function is compromised, as with the short-bowel syndrome, the time of contact with the limited functioning surface may be a crucial factor. In irritable bowel syndrome, disordered motility may also play a role.[8] Slowed transit and severely disordered motility lead to intraluminal stasis. In the normal bowel, steady, progressive movement of chyme is one of the mechanisms that prevent the development of bacterial overgrowth, whereas stasis encourages overgrowth. Certain bacteria deconjugate bile acids in the upper small bowel and produce fat malabsorption. In addition, bacterial proteases may damage the small-bowel surface. Stasis may result from an anatomic obstruction, as well as from functional motor disorders. Disordered motility frequently is an associated factor in chronic inflammatory bowel disease. Stools associated with motility diarrhea, except those secondary to fatty acid malabsorption, tend to be small in volume. The response to feeding is variable, and the gastrocolic reflex may be heightened. Patients who have chronic inflammatory bowel disease may find that meals stimulate intestinal activity, resulting in postprandial abdominal cramps and bowel movements.

ACUTE DIARRHEA

Acute diarrhea is common in children, is transient and usually self-limited, and is caused most often by infection. In the United States, children in the first few years of life average 1 or 2 episodes per year.[9] The role of the physician is to rule out causes that require specific treatment, to advise parents in supportive management, and to provide follow-up for possible complications. Box 169-1 lists some of the more frequent causes of acute diarrhea categorized by the usual presentation with or without gross blood in the stool. Transmission of diarrheal organisms is commonly food borne, by water, person-to-person, and by exposure to animals at home, fairs, and petting zoos. Child care centers are likely sites for the spread of enteric pathogens. Pathogens that have been associated with epidemics include *Giardia lamblia*, rotavirus, *Norovirus*, *Shigella*, *Campylobacter*, *Cryptosporidium*, and *Clostridium difficile* organisms.[10-13]

BOX 169-1 Causes of Acute Diarrhea

USUALLY WITHOUT BLOOD IN STOOL

Viral enteritis C rotavirus, orbivirus, noroviruses (includes Norwalk virus), other caliciviruses, enteric adenovirus, astrovirus, sapoviruses

Enterotoxin C *Escherichia coli*, *Klebsiella* organisms, cholera, *Clostridium perfringens*, *Staphylococcus* organisms, *Bacillus cereus*, and *Vibrio* species

Parasitic C *Giardia*, *Cryptosporidium*, *Cyclospora*, *Dientamoeba fragilis*, and *Blastocystis hominis* organisms

Extraintestinal infection C otitis media and urinary tract infection

Antibiotic-induced and *Clostridium difficile* toxin (without pseudomembranous colitis)

COMMONLY ASSOCIATED WITH BLOOD IN STOOL

Bacterial C *Shigella*, *Salmonella*, and *Campylobacter* organisms, *Yersinia enterocolitica*, invasive *E coli*, gonococcus (venereal spread), enteroadherent *E coli*, enteroaggregative *E coli*, *Aeromonas hydrophilia*, and *Plesiomonas* shigelloides

Cytomegalovirus (especially in immunocompromised individuals)

Amebic dysentery, *Trichuris trichiura* (whipworm)

Hemolytic-uremic syndrome (enterohemorrhagic *E coli*—*E coli* O157:H7 and other Shiga toxin-producing *E coli*)

Henoch-Schönlein purpura

Pseudomembranous enterocolitis (*C difficile* toxin)

Ulcerative or granulomatous colitis (acute presentation)

Necrotizing enterocolitis (neonates)

Neonatal Diarrhea

Neonates with acute diarrhea must be considered differently from older infants and children because of both lower tolerance to the associated fluid shifts and the greater likelihood of severe infection or of a congenital anomaly. In addition, signs of necrotizing enterocolitis, including gastric retention (frequently bilious), distention, and occult or bright red blood in the stool, should raise concern. Although this disease usually occurs in premature infants, it also has been reported in full-term infants. The presence of pneumatosis intestinalis, gas in the portal vein, or free intraperitoneal gas seen on abdominal radiographs supports this diagnosis. Epidemics of diarrhea associated with rotavirus, enteropathogenic *E coli*, salmonellae, and other organisms, including *Klebsiella* organisms, have been reported in nurseries. If the onset of diarrhea is associated with initial feedings, then the clinician should consider congenital digestive defects, especially sugar intolerance. Hirschsprung disease may produce acute diarrhea and enterocolitis in the neonatal period and should be considered, especially in the infant who has not passed meconium in the first 24 hours. Bloody diarrhea that results from cow milk or soy protein intolerance may develop as early as the first few days of life. Resolution and exacerbation on removal and reintroduction of cow milk or soy formula, as well as an atopic family history, are clues to the diagnosis.

Differential Diagnosis in the Older Infant and Child

Most episodes of acute diarrhea are transient and benign. On the initial visit, the physician must evaluate the course in terms of both possible causes and the status of hydration. The diarrhea is usually the result of viral enteritis, typically occurring with low-grade fever, vomiting, and frequent watery stools. Generally, the stools are without blood or white blood cells. Enterotoxin-producing organisms (eg, toxigenic *E coli*) are associated with watery stools and are without evidence of mucosal invasion (no high fever or blood in the stool). *G lamblia* produces watery diarrhea associated with intestinal gas and crampy abdominal pain. Diarrhea in association with extraintestinal infections, most notably otitis media and pyelonephritis, has been called *parenteral diarrhea*; its mechanism is obscure. An associated viral enteritis may occur in some cases of otitis media. Certain antibiotics, especially ampicillin, have been associated with transient diarrhea. Less common but of greater danger is antibiotic-associated pseudomembranous colitis,[10] which may occur acutely or as a more chronic illness of 1 or 2 months' duration.[14] *C difficile* toxin, the cause of most cases of pseudomembranous colitis, may also be associated with chronic childhood diarrhea in the absence of colitis.[15]

The presence of blood in the stool, especially with symptoms of colonic involvement (tenesmus, urgency, and crampy lower abdominal pain), should make the clinician think of infection with *Campylobacter, Shigella*, or *Salmonella* organisms or with *C difficile* toxin-associated pseudomembranous colitis. The symptoms of dysentery may be less striking with *Salmonella*. When the *Shigella* is an enterotoxin-producing organism, watery diarrhea may actually precede the onset of dysentery.

BOX 169-2 Food-Borne Diarrhea (US incidence per 100,000 persons*)

Campylobacter	13
Salmonella	15
Shigella	5
Escherichia coli O157	0.9
Cryptosporidium	0.013
Yersinia	0.004
Vibrio	0.003
Cyclospora	0.003±

*Incidence of food-borne infection at 10 US sites under surveillance by the Foodborne Diseases Active Surveillance Network (total of 15,806 laboratory-diagnosed cases of infections from a surveillance population of 44.1 million persons). Centers for Disease Control and Prevention. Preliminary FoodNet data on the incidence of infection with pathogens transmitted commonly through food—10 sites, United States, 2004. *MMWR* 2005;54: 352-356.

Patients who have *Shigella* organisms tend to appear severely ill and may have meningismus or seizures. The stools tend to be foul smelling. Up to 40% of individuals who have Guillain-Barré syndrome have evidence of a *Campylobacter* infection occurring before the onset of neurologic symptoms.[16] *Yersinia* enterocolitis also may be associated with blood in the stool, but *Yersinia* appears to be incriminated less commonly as an etiologic agent in the United States. *E coli* can produce diarrhea by several pathogenic mechanisms; the enteroadherent, enteroinvasive, enterohemorrhagic, and enteroaggregative forms can all be associated with blood in the stool.[17] Hemolytic-uremic syndrome is the result largely of enterohemorrhagic *E coli* (especially serotype O157) and less commonly *Shigella* infections.

Amebiasis is unusual in the United States, but *Entamoeba histolytica* can produce a picture of acute colitis. Causes of bloody diarrhea that are not obviously infectious include intussusception and immune deficiencies. Chronic inflammatory bowel disease can produce an initial episode of acute dysentery, although the history may reveal previous episodes; arthralgia or growth failure may have preceded the diarrhea. A history of recent similar diarrheal illness in family members or friends suggests an infectious diarrhea.

Food-borne spread of organisms or toxins is an important cause of acute diarrheal illness[18,19] (Box 169-2). Improperly prepared poultry and eggs are the major source for both campylobacteriosis and salmonellosis, and the major source for *E coli* O157 infection is ground beef. Preventive measures include safe food-handling practices, pasteurization of in-shell eggs, and irradiation of ground meat and raw poultry. Explosive diarrhea after ingesting seafood is likely to be due to infection with *Vibrio* species.

Evaluation

At the initial evaluation (Box 169-3), the physician should establish the quantity of the diarrhea, the child's ability to maintain oral intake, and the presence

BOX 169-3 Evaluation of Acute Diarrhea

HISTORY

1. Length of illness
2. Characterization of stools: frequency, looseness (watery versus mushy), and presence of gross blood
3. Oral intake: diet, quantity of fluids and solids taken
4. Presence of vomiting
5. Associated symptoms: fever, rash, and arthralgia
6. Urine output: frequency and qualitative amount
7. Possible exposure to diarrheal illness

PHYSICAL EXAMINATION

1. Hydration status: weight (stable or loss), mucosa (moist or dry), saliva and tears (present or absent), skin turgor (normal or poor), eyeballs and fontanelle (normal or sunken), and vital signs
2. Alertness
3. Infant: vigor of suck

LABORATORY (PERFORMED AS INDICATED)

1. Stool evaluation: culture, ova and parasites, smear for white blood cells, *Clostridium difficile* toxin assay, occult blood, and reducing substances
2. Complete blood count
3. If hydration status is in question: blood urea nitrogen (BUN) and serum electrolyte levels
4. Urinalysis
5. If child is lethargic or has had a seizure, culture for sepsis: measure the BUN and serum electrolyte and glucose levels and examine and culture the cerebrospinal fluid

of associated vomiting. On physical examination, the state of hydration should be estimated. The presence of tears and saliva is usually evidence of adequate hydration. A simple guideline to hydration is that the absence of tears and the presence of a dry mouth suggest 5% dehydration; the addition of sunken eyes, sunken fontanelle, and poor skin turgor suggests 10% dehydration. Shock indicates at least 15% dehydration. In the presence of hypernatremia, the state of dehydration is typically more severe than suggested on physical examination inasmuch as extracellular fluid volume tends to be preserved at the expense of intracellular volume (see Chapter 341, Dehydration). A recorded weight is essential; it can be compared with previous weights and will also be available to reevaluate the state of hydration during the illness. Information about the frequency and quantity of urination is important. A history of good urine output is reassuring. Parents may underestimate or overestimate urine output (frequency and volume), especially when urine becomes mixed with liquid stool.

A stool culture should be obtained if blood or leukocytes are noted in the stool and the child is severely ill. Examination of the stool for leukocytes is helpful in establishing the presence of colitis. In the presence of both infectious and noninfectious colitis, white blood cells (WBCs) are usually found in high numbers, frequently in sheets. Polymorphonuclear leukocytes usually account for at least 60% to 80% of the cells; the presence of only occasional cells is considered a negative finding. The absence of WBCs in grossly bloody diarrheal stool occurs with enterohemorrhagic *E coli* infection but should also direct attention to entities such as intussusception and Meckel diverticulum when these diagnoses seem clinically appropriate. Amebic colitis also may not be associated with WBCs in the stool, although the trophozoites and numerous red blood cells may be visible on a saline wet mount preparation of the stool. Invasive bacterial diarrhea frequently is associated with a peripheral blood leukocytosis.

Treatment

The cornerstone of treatment in acute gastroenteritis is good fluid and electrolyte management (Box 169-4). Commercial oral hydration solutions provide more sodium and lower carbohydrate concentration than traditional clear liquids.[20] Human milk contains low concentrations of sodium (6 to 7 mEq/L); therefore a supplemental rehydration solution should be used when diarrhea is persistent or severe.

Electrolyte content in diarrheal stool varies widely, with the highest concentrations occurring in secretory diarrheas such as cholera. Fecal sodium levels may range from 40 to 100 mEq/L and may occasionally be as high as 150 mEq/L. In rotavirus diarrhea, fecal sodium concentration is typically 20 to 40 mEq/L.

Viruses cause at least 40% to 50% of acute diarrheal illnesses in childhood. Rotavirus is most common, followed, in descending frequency, by noroviruses, astroviruses, and enteric adenoviruses. Viral enteritis has been shown to result in a transient, patchy, mucosal lesion of the small intestine, which may be associated with temporary lactose and fat malabsorption. Decreased mucosal lactase levels may be seen. In experimental viral diarrhea in piglets, intestinal glucose-stimulated absorption of sodium, and therefore water, is impaired.[5] Rotavirus produces an enterotoxin (known as NSP4), which is of much greater importance in the production of diarrhea than virus-induced mucosal damage.[5,6] Abnormal glucose absorption has also been observed in infants who have rotavirus enteritis. Nevertheless, secretion can be converted to net absorption in most children by providing oral glucose electrolyte solution because of the patchy nature of the lesion in viral gastroenteritis.

Oral rehydration solutions have been used safely and successfully to treat acute diarrhea with dehydration.[21,22] Infants who have diarrhea are usually able to drink large volumes of salty-tasting liquids ad libitum appropriate for the stool output. Episodes of diarrhea in previously healthy, well-nourished children are often mild; nevertheless, the use of oral rehydration solutions to replace diarrheal loss is encouraged in infants. Liquids can be offered ad libitum, although smaller volumes per feeding may be tolerated better when diarrhea is associated with vomiting. Guidelines for rehydration are described in Box 169-4. The most recent World Health Organization recommendation is for a lower osmolarity (245 mOsm/L) solution for rehydration (containing 75 mEq/L sodium and 75 mmol/L glucose). The contents of commercially available rehydration solutions have evolved with advances in the understanding of optimal absorption during oral rehydration; thus the clinician

BOX 169-4 Fluid and Electrolyte Management of Acute Diarrhea

A. General rules for management of acute diarrhea
   1. Oral rehydration therapy with glucose-electrolyte solution (oral rehydration solution [ORS]) is the preferred treatment of fluid and electrolyte loss, except as noted below. These solutions generally contain 25 g/L glucose (or ≥30 g/L rice starch), 45 to 90 mEq/L sodium, 20 to 25 mEq/L potassium, and 30 mEq/L bicarbonate. The higher sodium concentration is appropriate for rehydration; the lower concentration is usually adequate for rehydration with mild diarrhea and is appropriate for maintenance.
   2. Moderate-to-large stool output should be replaced with ORS at 10 mL/kg/stool, if losses cannot be estimated. Losses from emesis should be replaced with ORS at 2 mL/kg/episode of emesis or replace estimated losses.
   3. The use of ORS is labor intensive. If a caregiver is not available to give small amounts of fluid frequently, then intravenous therapy may be necessary. If the child is not severely dehydrated, then oral rehydration may be completed at home with close follow-up. Otherwise, intravenous fluids should include replacement of deficit, ongoing losses, and maintenance fluids. Addition of intravenous potassium should wait until urine output is established.
   4. ORS therapy is effective for hypernatremic dehydration, as well as hyponatremic and isotonic dehydration.
   5. Age-appropriate feedings should be continued during acute diarrhea, except as noted below. Formula should be offered full strength. Diet may be better tolerated if fatty foods and foods high in simple sugars (eg, undiluted juices and soft drinks) are avoided.
   6. Breastfeeding should be continued when possible.
   7. Lactose-free diet is generally unnecessary. If stools worsen on reintroduction of lactose (human milk, cow milk, or lactose-containing formula), then lactose intolerance should be considered. If stools become acid and contain reducing substances, then lactose intolerance is likely.

B. No dehydration
   1. Continue age-appropriate feeding (see A.5, A.6).
   2. Use ORS only to replace excessive stool output (see A.2).

C. Mild-to-moderate dehydration (3% to 9% of body weight)
   1. Correct dehydration with 50-100 mL/kg ORS over 3-4 hours, and replace continuing losses from stool and emesis with additional ORS (see A.2). See section E for special considerations for vomiting.
   2. Reevaluate hydration and replacement of losses at least every 1-2 hours. This process may require medical supervision (emergency department, hospital outpatient unit, or physician's office).
   3. Once dehydration is corrected, begin feeding (see A.5, A.6) and continue to correct losses as above.

D. Severe dehydration (at least 10%)
   1. Resuscitate with intravenous or intraosseous normal saline or lactated Ringer's solution 20 mL/kg of body weight over 1 hour. Monitor vital signs closely. Repeat until pulse and state of consciousness return to normal. Larger volumes and shorter periods of administration may be required. Delay giving intravenous potassium until urine output is established.
   2. Determine serum electrolyte levels.
   3. Lack of response to initial resuscitation suggests an underlying problem such as septic shock, toxic shock syndrome, myocarditis, myocardiopathy, or pericarditis. Persistently poor urine output may be a sign of hemolytic-uremic syndrome.
   4. ORS may be initiated when the child's condition has stabilized and mental status is satisfactory. An intravenous line should be maintained until no longer needed. See section E for special considerations for vomiting.
   5. Feeding may be restarted when rehydration is complete (see A.1, A.2).

E. Special considerations
   1. Vomiting
      a. Vomiting occurs commonly during acute gastroenteritis.
      b. Children who are dehydrated and vomit usually tolerate ORS.
      c. Intractable, severe vomiting, unconsciousness, and ileus are contraindications to ORS treatment.
      d. ORS should be started at 5 mL every 1 to 2 minutes.
      e. Vomiting usually decreases as dehydration improves; larger amounts can be given at less frequent intervals.
      f. Nasogastric tube can be used for continuous ORS infusion for persistent vomiting or feeding refusal secondary to mouth ulcers (do not use in comatose child or one who has ileus or intestinal obstruction).
      g. Intravenous fluids should be used if ORS treatment is unsuccessful.
   2. Refusal to take ORS
      a. Children who are not dehydrated may not take ORS because of the salty taste. However, dehydrated children generally take it well.
      b. Giving ORS in small amounts at first allows the child to become accustomed to the taste.
      c. ORS can be frozen in ice-pop form.

Modified from American Academy of Pediatrics, Provisional Committee on Quality Improvement, Subcommittee on Acute Gastroenteritis. Practice parameter: the management of acute gastroenteritis in young children. *Pediatrics* 1996;97:424-435; and King CK, Glass R, Bresee JS, et al. Managing acute gastroenteritis among children: oral rehydration, maintenance, and nutritional therapy. *MMWR* 2003;52:1-16.

should consult current manufacturer specifications before choosing a product. Continuing regular feedings with supplemental oral rehydration solution is generally tolerated and thought to lead to quicker recovery.[23] Vomiting is usually not a contraindication for oral rehydration.

Oral rehydration appears to be associated with shorter hospitalization and lower medical costs. Infants who have hypernatremic dehydration have fewer problems with seizures during oral rehydration, as compared with intravenous rehydration.[21] Oral rehydration therapy, however, requires the constant presence of a caretaker, although this individual need not have previous medical experience. The use of starches, amino acids, and probiotics in oral maintenance or rehydration solution to improve sodium and water absorption has been considered. For further discussion of oral rehydration, see Chapter 59, Fluids and Electrolytes in Clinical Practice, and Chapter 341, Dehydration.

Indications for medications in the treatment of acute gastroenteritis in infants and children are limited. As already noted, the key mechanisms involved are intestinal secretion and transient malabsorption; physiologically, no apparent rationale exists for medications that slow gut motility (diphenoxylate, loperamide, and anticholinergics). In fact, pooling of fluid in the intestinal lumen after treatment may give a false impression that the diarrhea has improved. Slowing intestinal transit with drugs may allow greater mucosal contact with pathogens and thereby allow for local mucosal invasion. Bismuth subsalicylate, which may decrease the duration of diarrhea, has been shown to be a safe adjunct to oral rehydration but is not used routinely.[24] Antibiotics are useful in specific situations: *Shigella* dysentery *Yersinia* or *Campylobacter* gastroenteritis, pseudomembranous colitis, *Salmonella* infections in infants younger than 6 months, and *Salmonella* infections in older patients who have enteric fever, typhoid fever, or complications of bacteremia.[25] *Campylobacter* gastroenteritis must be identified very early for antibiotics to shorten the illness. For the individual patient, the presence of an *E coli* serotype previously labeled enteropathogenic correlates poorly with the presence of diarrhea and is not alone an indication for antibiotic treatment.[17] *Lactobacillus* or other probiotics may be useful to prevent infectious diarrhea but are probably not effective as treatment.[26,27]

Most episodes of gastroenteritis are self-limited and of short duration. Symptoms of rotavirus enteritis typically last 4 to 10 days. However, prolonged secretion of rotavirus in stool (up to 8 weeks) has been demonstrated in association with severe gastroenteritis in immunocompetent children.[28] The current approach to treatment is to restart the previous full-strength formula and solids early after the onset of diarrhea. If diarrhea recurs on the introduction of lactose-containing formula, then the child may have transient lactose intolerance. In this situation, a lactose-free formula should be offered. (The sugar in this formula can be either sucrose or a glucose polymer.) Sugar malabsorption (see malabsorption syndromes) can be identified by the determination of reducing substance in the stool. (Sucrose must be hydrolyzed first with hydrochloric acid.) Transient lactose intolerance usually lasts only a week or less but can, at times, persist for months. If the degree of dehydration is 5% or greater, then use of oral rehydration solution should be instituted, if possible, in the manner presented in Box 169-4. For severe dehydration or shock, rapid intravenous administration of 10 to 20 mL/kg of isotonic fluid or colloid is required initially and may need to be repeated early. Hyponatremia and hypernatremia must be corrected slowly to prevent complications of the central nervous system. Oral solutions are better tolerated and result in fewer central nervous system complications than intravenous solutions in infants who have hypernatremia.[21] Potassium should not be added to intravenous fluids until adequate urine output is established. Urine specific gravity may be misleading inasmuch as kidney-concentrating ability may be poor as a result of reduced renal urea or whole body potassium. Inability to acidify the urine during acute diarrhea occurs commonly in infants despite the presence of metabolic acidosis.[29] This finding is thought to be caused by sodium deficiency and the resulting inadequate delivery of sodium to the distal nephron. Complete discussion of intravenous treatment is presented in Chapter 59, Fluids and Electrolytes in Clinical Practice.

CHRONIC DIARRHEA

Although chronic diarrhea occurs in children of all ages, it is most frequent and often most challenging to diagnose in infants.[30] Both healthy and ill infants can develop diarrhea in response to a variety of stresses. The younger the infant is, the more likely he or she will be to enter the cycle of diarrhea and secondary malnutrition that leads to further diarrhea, malnutrition, and susceptibility to infection (known as protracted diarrhea of infancy). Many of the causes of chronic diarrhea may appear at any time during childhood. Certain diseases, however, occur much more commonly in infancy; others are more likely to begin in later childhood. Dividing the causes of diarrhea between infancy and older childhood is arbitrary because the groups overlap; but this method is a helpful guide in initiating the evaluation of the child who has chronic diarrhea (Box 169-5).

Infants

The physician who is confronted with an infant who is reported to have chronic diarrhea must decide first whether the stool pattern is abnormal. A nursing mother who has not been forewarned may become concerned about the appearance and frequency of her child's transitional stools. The infant's weight gain and healthy appearance, combined with an explanation about stools of breastfed infants, should dispel these concerns.

In the latter half of the first year and in the second year, the most common cause for persistent diarrhea is chronic nonspecific diarrhea (also called *toddler's diarrhea*).[3,31] Affected infants and toddlers have intermittent loose stools for no apparent reason. In many instances, the stools occur early in the day and typically not overnight. These children appear healthy and are thriving according to weight and length growth curves, unless inappropriate treatment with clear fluids

BOX 169-5 Causes of Chronic Diarrhea

COMMON CAUSES

- Chronic enteric infection: *Salmonella* organisms; *Yersinia enterocolitica; Campylobacter, Giardia, Cryptosporidium,* and *Cyclospora* organisms; *Clostridium difficile* toxin; enteroadherent *Escherichia coli*; rotavirus (in immunodeficient patients); cytomegalovirus; adenovirus; and HIV
- Food allergy
- Chronic nonspecific diarrhea (toddler's diarrhea, irritable colon of childhood)
- Disaccharide intolerance
- Chronic constipation with overflow *diarrhea*
- Cystic fibrosis
- Celiac disease (gluten-sensitive enteropathy)
- Inflammatory bowel disease: Crohn disease and ulcerative colitis
- Hirschsprung disease
- Immunodeficiency states
- Monosaccharide intolerance
- Eosinophilic (allergic) gastroenteritis
- Short-bowel syndrome
- Urinary tract infection
- Postenteritis bile acid malabsorption
- Factitious causes

LESS COMMON CAUSES

- Autoimmune enteropathy
- Hormonal: adrenal insufficiency and hyperthyroidism
- Vasoactive intestinal polypeptide-secreting tumor
- Neural crest tumor and carcinoid
- Intestinal lymphangiectasia
- Acrodermatitis enteropathica
- Intestinal stricture or blind loop
- Pancreatic insufficiency with neutropenia
- Trypsinogen or enterokinase deficiency
- Congenital chloride-losing diarrhea
- Congenital sodium-secretory diarrhea
- Abetalipoproteinemia
- Microvillus inclusion disease
- Tufting disease
- Immunodysregulation, polyendocrinopathy, enteropathy, X-linked syndrome (IPEX)
- Intestinal pseudoobstruction
- Ileal bile salt receptor defect
- Congenital disorders of glycosylation

has led to caloric deprivation. This condition represents a stool pattern rather than a pathologic state and requires minimal or no laboratory evaluation. Symptoms may begin initially after an apparent acute enteritis (postinfectious irritable bowel).

Treatment may include (1) restricting the frequency of feedings, whether liquids or solids, in an effort to decrease stimulation of the gastrocolic reflex (in the toddler, three meals and a bedtime snack with nothing by mouth in between); (2) restricting the volumes of fluids ingested when excessive; (3) avoiding excessive intake of juices; and (4) reassuring the parents of the benign nature of this entity. A high-fat diet may be helpful in some children, although probably is of less importance.[31] Cholestyramine (2 g by mouth 1 to 3 times daily) is also effective at times; however, the duration of use should be restricted because of the potential for interference with fat-soluble vitamin absorption. In any event, this condition is self-limited and typically resolves by 3.5 years of age. The only danger is that well-intentioned parents may restrict oral intake to clear liquids repeatedly in an effort to treat the child; this action may result in poor weight gain. Bile acid malabsorption is an occasional sequela of gastroenteritis that can produce persistent, watery diarrhea. This condition also will respond to cholestyramine therapy.

Protracted Diarrhea of Infancy

The syndrome of protracted diarrhea of infancy is poorly understood,[32] probably representing the final pathway for multiple causes, including gastrointestinal infections and, perhaps, food intolerances. This condition is defined somewhat arbitrarily as occurring in infants younger than 3 months and persisting for more than 2 weeks. Historically, this syndrome, previously called intractable diarrhea of infancy, has been associated with a high mortality from irreversible diarrhea and related malnutrition. However, the outcome has improved markedly with the advent of elemental diets and total parenteral nutrition. Now, intractable diarrhea is rare and related to more specific causes, such as microvillus inclusion disease.

Generally, malnutrition develops and, in concert with the protracted diarrhea, leads to alteration of gastrointestinal flora sometimes associated with bacterial overgrowth of the small intestine. Altered mucosal function of the small intestine and transient pancreatic insufficiency may occur with malnutrition and protracted diarrhea. Bile salts may be deconjugated as a result of bacterial overgrowth. In many instances, the initiating cause of protracted diarrhea is not found; it may likely be no longer present when the diarrhea has become chronic. The small-bowel biopsy specimen may show patchy villous shortening with a decreased villus/crypt ratio and marked inflammation, as well as a damaged surface epithelium. However, the results of the small-bowel biopsy also may be normal. Similarly, a rectal biopsy specimen may show evidence of inflammation, including crypt abscesses, or it may be normal. The presence or absence of these biopsy findings may not correlate with the severity of the clinical syndrome.[33] Affected infants are severely malnourished and have low serum protein and hemoglobin levels. In many instances, they have had repeated treatment with oral clear liquids and peripheral intravenous fluids, all of which provide inadequate nutrient intake.

When evaluating a young infant who has protracted diarrhea, the physician must rule out causes that require urgent treatment while correcting hydration and nutrition. Rehydration is similar to the treatment of acute diarrhea, although estimating the level of dehydration accurately is difficult in the presence of malnutrition, and initial oral therapy is less likely to be successful. Stool output should be measured. If the urine is collected in a urine bag, then diapers can be weighed before and after stools to give an accurate measure of stool output. Urine specific gravity and volume may be deceptive because of poor concentration by the kidneys in the presence of malnutrition and total body hypokalemia. The infant should be weighed at least daily.

Infection should be ruled out as a cause of diarrhea early in the evaluation. Several stools should be collected for culture, for examination for parasites, and for *C difficile* toxin assay when indicated; blood and urine cultures should also be ordered. Consideration of Hirschsprung disease with enterocolitis is important because infants who have this disorder are prone to perforation of the colon unless a decompression colostomy is performed. In such infants, eliciting a history of early obstipation and of the absence of stools in the first 24 hours of life is usually possible. In Hirschsprung disease, a flat plate radiograph of the abdomen may show a dilated colon with absence of air in the rectum. Toxic megacolon may also be seen in infectious colitis or in chronic inflammatory bowel disease in infancy. Air-fluid levels throughout the bowel are common in infants who have gastroenteritis, and this sign is not helpful in defining a cause. A barium enema under low pressure in the unprepared patient may show the narrow distal segment of rectum; however, this finding may not be present in neonates, and evaluation for ganglion cells on rectal biopsy is often necessary. The transition zone of Hirschsprung disease may be more obvious on a delayed radiograph (24 to 48 hours after the barium enema).

For a child who has chronic diarrhea and has been fed recently, the presence of reducing substance or an acid stool pH (less than 5.3) suggests carbohydrate malabsorption.[4] The stool pH is not a good measure of the effect of diarrhea on total body acid-base balance. If stool concentration of sodium and potassium minus chloride is greater than the plasma bicarbonate, then the infant is losing bicarbonate. WBCs or gross blood in the stool usually indicates colonic inflammation; occult blood in the stool suggests loss of blood across the mucosa anywhere in the gastrointestinal tract.

Nutritional rehabilitation should begin at once. The best choices are either enteral alimentation with an elemental or modular formula[34] or total parenteral nutrition (TPN), peripheral or central (see Chapter 59, Fluids and Electrolytes in Clinical Practice). In many instances, enteral nutrition is tolerated best by the continuous drip method, and recovery may be more rapid when enteral alimentation is used.[35] Nevertheless, unsuccessful attempts at enteral feeding necessitate initiation of TPN therapy in some infants. Initial treatment with TPN and a gradually increasing, continuous enteral drip is a good approach to patients who do not tolerate elemental diet alone. Elemental formulas are composed of predigested components in fixed proportions; modular formulas allow the clinician to vary the components. Stool output and weight gain may be measured to assess the infant's response.

During the treatment, further work-up, including an upper gastrointestinal series with small-bowel radiograph, barium enema, small-bowel biopsy, proctoscopy, the measurement of sweat electrolytes, and other specific tests to rule out the entities noted later in this chapter, should be conducted as indicated. If disaccharidase levels are abnormal on small-bowel biopsy, then disaccharides should be avoided.

Malabsorption Syndromes

Infants and children who have malabsorption syndromes typically have diarrhea, steatorrhea, growth failure, or a combination of these conditions. Celiac disease and cystic fibrosis (see Chapter 254, Cystic Fibrosis) are the most common chronic disorders that cause malabsorption in children in the United States. Steatorrhea is much more striking with cystic fibrosis, resulting from pancreatic insufficiency and secondary maldigestion. Infants who have cystic fibrosis who nurse or are fed soy formula, but not cow milk formula, may exhibit protein malabsorption in the first months of life.

Although cystic fibrosis is thought of primarily as a respiratory disease, some infants and children have malabsorption and little history of respiratory symptoms; these patients typically have voracious appetites. The diagnosis must be confirmed by sweat electrolyte studies or genetic testing. Other diseases much less common than cystic fibrosis may be associated with prominent steatorrhea in early infancy, including congenital pancreatic insufficiency with cyclic neutropenia (Shwachman-Diamond syndrome),[36] intestinal lymphangiectasia, and abetalipoproteinemia. Transient steatorrhea may follow an acute enteritis.[37] Measurement of stool elastase or serum trypsinogen is a useful screening test for pancreatic insufficiency.

Celiac disease (gluten-sensitive enteropathy) is now appreciated to be a much more frequent disorder than previously recognized.[38] Presentation may occur at any age, and the manifestations may be subtle. In infancy, celiac disease becomes apparent 1 to several months after the introduction of gluten-containing products (eg, wheat, rye, barley) into the diet (see Chapter 265, Gastrointestinal Allergy).[39] The classic symptoms in an infant with celiac disease are irritability, loose stools, poor appetite, and poor weight gain. Vomiting may occur as well. In older children, features such as growth retardation or iron deficiency anemia may be more striking than diarrhea.[40] In many patients, steatorrhea is not present, and results of absorptive studies such as the D-xylose tolerance test may be normal. Gluten-free dietary trials and antigliadin antibody studies may be misleading. The presence of endomysial antibody (EMA) or tissue transglutaminase (tTG) antibody in the serum is a much more reliable predictor of celiac disease.[40,41] tTG has been identified as the antigen recognized by endomysial antibody[42,43] In individuals with IgA deficiency, the absence of these serum antibodies does not rule out celiac disease. A diagnosis of celiac disease should be confirmed by small-bowel biopsy. In the past, the diagnosis was often reconfirmed by a challenge with gluten and a repeat biopsy. Currently available antibody studies make this strategy unnecessary. Measuring endomysial IgA or tTG antibody is useful in evaluating compliance with diet. *Giardia* infection can produce small-bowel malabsorption that mimics celiac disease.

Carbohydrate (monosaccharide or disaccharide) intolerance may be primary or more commonly secondary to other gastrointestinal disorders.[44] The congenital form of lactase deficiency is much less common than congenital sucrase-isomaltase deficiency,[45] which typically appears after introduction of sucrose into the diet in solids. In carbohydrate intolerance, the extent of symptoms varies directly with the quantity of the offending sugar in the diet. Similarly, the age at presentation varies with the age at which the sugar is introduced into the diet. Infants who have congenital sucrase-isomaltase deficiency may have diarrhea when fed formula containing glucose polymers.[46] The diagnosis can be established by conducting standard sugar tolerance tests, measuring hydrogen excretion in the breath, or assaying the enzymes present in tissue obtained by a small-bowel biopsy. Examination of the stool for reducing sugars is an imprecise screening test for stool carbohydrate content.[47] A stool pH less than 5.3 is suggestive of carbohydrate malabsorption, whereas a stool pH more than 5.6 is evidence against this diagnosis. Sorbitol,[48] an artificial sweetener, as well as fructose,[49] may produce diarrhea when ingested in large amounts, and both are present in fruits. Oral enzyme supplements are available for both lactase and sucrase deficiency.

The congenital deficiency of trypsinogen, the zymogen precursor of the pancreatic protease trypsin, has been reported to be a very rare cause of congenital diarrhea. The absence of trypsin in the stool suggests the diagnosis (in the absence of cystic fibrosis and congenital pancreatic insufficiency), but evaluation of the pancreatic proteases in the duodenal aspirate is necessary to confirm this impression. Congenital deficiency of enterokinase, the intestinal enzyme that activates trypsinogen to trypsin, appears in a similar fashion to that of congenital trypsinogen deficiency and is reversed with very small amounts of pancreatic replacement.

Infection

Acute bacterial or viral enteritis may be an important initiator of protracted diarrhea in infancy.[50,51] If the initial infection is no longer present at the time of evaluation for chronic diarrhea, then this association will be difficult to prove. Infections at distant sites, especially urinary tract infections, have also been implicated as a cause of chronic diarrhea in infancy. A urinalysis and urine culture should be obtained routinely in the evaluation of children who have chronic diarrhea. *Salmonella* enteritis is commonly associated with a chronic asymptomatic carrier state, especially in infancy. *Salmonella* infection, however, may also be associated with persistent diarrhea in infants. *Yersinia enterocolitica* enteritis has been associated with a chronic relapsing diarrhea although not commonly in the United States; however, the microbiology laboratory must look specifically for this organism, or it will be missed. *Campylobacter* enteritis also may have a protracted course. Persistence of rotavirus excretion has been identified in immunocompromised individuals but also rarely in immunocompetent children after severe gastroenteritis.[28] *Candida* has been described as a rare cause of persistent diarrhea in immunocompetent individuals.[52] However, the incidental finding of *Candida* is so common that the clinician must be cautious before identifying it as the cause of diarrhea. A dramatic response to treatment for *Candida* would support this diagnosis.

Parasites

The principal parasite that causes diarrhea in the United States is *G lamblia*, which may be associated with watery diarrhea and crampy abdominal pain and may occur in epidemic form. This protozoon may be difficult to detect in stools, although stool antigen testing has improved diagnosis. The best yield of organisms comes from a duodenal fluid aspirate or a small-bowel biopsy. Diarrhea from *Cryptosporidium* occurs in immunocompetent individuals.[53,54] *Cyclospora* has been introduced into the United States on contaminated fruits. *Blastocystis hominis* and *Dientamoeba fragilis* may cause persistent diarrhea. Amebic dysentery may be indistinguishable from the colitis of inflammatory bowel disease and must be considered along with bacterial colitis before a diagnosis of inflammatory bowel disease can be made.

Hirschsprung Disease

Hirschsprung disease is a congenital abnormality involving the submucosal and myenteric plexuses of the colon (rarely involving the small intestine) and accounts for approximately 25% of intestinal obstructions in newborns. Affected neonates almost invariably fail to pass meconium early and have persistent obstipation and recurrent abdominal distention. These features may be overlooked, however, and the infants may subsequently have chronic diarrhea. The diarrhea is secondary to enterocolitis, which can be a surgical emergency that demands rapid diagnosis and treatment. A barium enema in the neonate may reveal false negative findings. Anorectal manometric examination may be helpful, but an adequate rectal biopsy specimen showing absence of ganglion cells and presence of nerve fiber hypertrophy confirms the diagnosis. Acetylcholinesterase staining is useful as well. Properly performed, suction biopsy of the rectum is highly reliable.[55]

Food Allergy

Dietary protein hypersensitivity occurs in 6% to 8% of children during the first 5 years of life and most commonly is a hypersensitivity to cow milk protein. Food allergy is present in approximately 4% of the adult population. In 85% of children who have dietary protein intolerance, the symptoms resolve by 3 years of age.[56,57] This entity should be considered when an infant who has chronic diarrhea has any of the following manifestations:

- Occult or gross blood in the stool (colitis)
- Protein-losing enteropathy
- Peripheral eosinophilia
- Other extraintestinal manifestations of allergy such as eczema, hives, or asthma.[58]

Continued or recurrent manifestations when the infant is fed a soy formula diet (free of cow milk) do not rule out the diagnosis, inasmuch as 30% to 50% of children who have cow milk protein intolerance will also be intolerant to soy protein. Typically, symptoms improve when the feeding is changed to a protein hydrolysate formula, although the response to specific protein hydrolysate formulas may not be equivalent. Occasionally, an amino acid formula will be necessary.[59]

Most food allergic reactions are IgE mediated and include immediate gastrointestinal hypersensitivity, with nausea, abdominal pain, and vomiting within 1 to 2 hours and diarrhea in 2 to 6 hours. Implicated food proteins include milk, egg, peanut, soy, cereal, and fish. Eosinophilic (allergic) gastroenteropathy is considered a mixed IgE-mediated and non–IgE-mediated disorder. It is characterized by infiltration of the stomach and intestine with eosinophils and often a peripheral eosinophilia. Symptoms include vomiting, abdominal pain, growth failure, and diarrhea (often with gross blood). Eosinophilic gastroenteropathy may respond to elimination diet, but corticosteroid treatment may be necessary. Non–IgE-mediated hypersensitivity includes dietary protein enterocolitis, which occurs most commonly in the first year of life. Diet-induced proctitis causes gross blood in stool and often diarrhea in the first few days to months of life. Symptoms usually resolve within 72 hours with removal of the offending food allergen. Bloody diarrhea can develop in some infants while they are nursing; resolution when cow milk is removed from the mother's diet or when a protein hydrolysate formula is substituted for nursing suggests an allergic basis.[60]

Short-Bowel Syndrome

Short-bowel syndrome follows extensive resection of the small intestine with the presentation of chronic malabsorption and diarrhea.[61] It begins most commonly in the newborn period in association with necrotizing enterocolitis or a congenital anomaly involving small intestine (eg, gastroschisis, intestinal atresia, malrotation with secondary midgut volvulus). Recovery may be prolonged, requiring the use of TPN for the first several years of life.[62] The factors that appear to contribute to persistence of symptoms in neonates include the cause, decreased intestinal absorptive surface, altered intestinal motility, intraluminal bacterial overgrowth[63] (with secondary deconjugation of bile salts and hydroxylation of fatty acids), malabsorption of bile salts secondary to terminal ileal resection, and disaccharidase deficiency. Among neonates, infants with necrotizing enterocolitis or gastroschisis tend to have a more prolonged course than those with other causes of short bowel. In infants, symptoms of colitis commonly occur during the initiation of enteral feedings.[64] Later in life, volvulus, trauma, and Crohn disease are the most common causes of short-bowel syndrome.

Intestinal Lymphangiectasia

Intestinal lymphangiectasia is a syndrome of dilated intestinal lymphatic vessels and is associated with protein-losing enteropathy, steatorrhea, lymphocytopenia, and chronic diarrhea. As a result of the bowel protein loss, affected children may have hypogammaglobulinemia and hypoalbuminemia, usually with peripheral edema. Primary intestinal lymphangiectasia appears to be a developmental anomaly of unknown origin and is frequently associated with lymphatic abnormalities of the extremities. Secondary lymphangiectasia may result from chronic volvulus secondary to malrotation with malfixation of the bowel, constrictive pericarditis, tumor, lymphatic malformation, elevated right atrial pressure associated with the Fontan procedure for congenital heart disease, or any other factor that leads to obstruction of intestinal lymphatic flow. The diagnosis is suggested by a history of chronic diarrhea and poor growth and the presence of peripheral edema, hypoalbuminemia, hypogammaglobulinemia, and lymphocytopenia. The last 2 abnormalities may lead to a decreased immune defense and an increased risk for infections. A radiologic small-bowel follow-through study may show generalized thickening of the intestinal folds. The diagnosis is confirmed by the presence of characteristically dilated lymphatics on a small-bowel biopsy specimen. The treatment includes the dietary use of medium-chain triglycerides and avoidance of long-chain fat. Protection from and early treatment of infection also are important.

Acrodermatitis Enteropathica

The cause of acrodermatitis enteropathica, a rare familial disease that typically appears when breastfed infants are weaned, is poorly understood. The infant has chronic diarrhea, intermittent vomiting, and an intractable erythematous, raw, and crusty rash, which is most prominent in the perianal and perioral regions but may be seen on the extremities. Alopecia is characteristically present, and conjunctivitis and dystrophic changes of the nails may occur. Infants who have acrodermatitis enteropathica are usually irritable and unhappy. The disorder is associated with a zinc deficiency (perhaps secondary to malabsorption) and responds dramatically to zinc salts given orally.[65] Nutritional zinc deficiency (eg, TPN without zinc supplementation or cystic fibrosis) may produce a syndrome similar to acrodermatitis enteropathica.

Factitious Diarrhea

Factitious diarrhea is undoubtedly more common than pediatricians recognize. Screening a stool specimen for laxative abuse is reasonable when an infant has persistent diarrhea that does not seem to fit any known pattern. Surreptitious administration of laxative to an infant is a symptom of the caretaker's psychosocial dysfunction; problems in other areas often become apparent during the social history. Frequently a parent is a medically knowledgeable person (eg, nurse, laboratory technician) and often seems to prefer staying in the hospital to being at home. These parents are usually helpful to the nursing staff, often to the degree of excessive involvement in the nursing care, and are commonly described by the nurses as caring and concerned parents. The pediatrician may note that the parent seems to encourage invasive diagnostic studies and treatment even beyond the medical plan and does not show an appropriate degree of hesitancy. When a stool osmolality well below 290 mOsm/L is noted, this can only occur by surreptitious dilution of stool with water. Another form of factitious diarrhea occurs among teenage girls who take laxatives surreptitiously to lose weight.

Hormone-Related Diarrhea

Adrenal insufficiency caused by either adrenogenital syndrome or adrenal hemorrhage may be associated with significant diarrhea, as may congenital thyrotoxicosis. VIP-secreting tumors of the pancreas have been reported as a rare cause of diarrhea in adults and an even rarer cause in children.

Ganglioneuroma and ganglioneuroblastoma have been associated with chronic secretory diarrhea. The tumors are usually abdominal but have also been reported in the mediastinum. Although these tumors are catecholamine secreting, prostaglandins or VIP may be the mediator of the diarrhea. A workup of the infant who has persistent, undiagnosed, secretory diarrhea should include urinary catecholamine studies, prostaglandin and VIP levels, and computed tomographic scans of chest and abdomen. Even when the results of these studies are negative, the clinician must strongly consider further studies if severe secretory diarrhea persists. When a tumor is found and is completely excised, the diarrhea usually resolves abruptly.

Immune Disorders

Immunodeficiency should be considered in any child who has chronic diarrhea. AIDS has become a major cause of immunodeficiency in childhood, and its first manifestation may be diarrhea. Several mechanisms of diarrhea have been described in infants and children who have AIDS.[66] In addition to the organisms the clinician usually considers in individuals who have persistent diarrhea (especially *Giardia*), cytomegalovirus, *Mycobacterium avium*-intracellulare, *Cryptosporidium parvum, Isospora belli,* and *Enterocytozoon bieneusi* must also be considered. Astrovirus, calicivirus, and adenovirus have been associated with diarrhea in HIV-infected individuals and may be more important than rotavirus as agents of AIDS diarrhea.[67] HIV may be a primary pathogen in the bowel of these patients as well. Lactose intolerance occurs commonly in individuals who have AIDS, presumably occurring as a result of injury to small-bowel mucosa. Pancreatic insufficiency with steatorrhea also has been noted in these patients.

The 2 major inborn disorders of immunity associated with diarrhea in early infancy are severe combined immunodeficiency and Wiskott-Aldrich syndrome. The most common primary disorder seen in later childhood is late-onset, variable hypogammaglobulinemia. Pure T-cell abnormalities (DiGeorge syndrome and other T-cell deficiencies) are also associated with diarrhea. Patients with selective IgA deficiency have an increased risk of celiac disease. Measurement of Ig levels should be a routine part of the workup of any patient who has chronic diarrhea. If the diagnosis remains unclear, then a T-cell evaluation should be conducted. Chronic parasitic, adenovirus, or rotavirus infection can be seen with immunodeficiencies. Diarrhea in association with granulomas of the intestinal tract has been noted in chronic granulomatous disease of childhood. These children may have perianal fistulas or gastric outlet obstruction; the disorder may initially be mistaken for Crohn disease.

The clinician must consider the full range of enteric infections associated with immunosuppression in children who have received organ transplants. Diarrhea may also be the presentation of tacrolimus toxicity or of lymphoproliferative disease. In bone marrow transplant recipients, graft-versus-host disease is a common cause of diarrhea as well.

Autoimmune Enteropathy

Autoimmune enteropathy is a poorly understood disorder, with chronic diarrhea beginning in the first year of life, and is often associated with failure to thrive.[68] Intestinal biopsies demonstrate villous atrophy and increased T-cell infiltrate in the lamina propria. Serum antienterocyte antibodies are identified in at least 50% of these patients. Extraintestinal autoimmune disorders (eg, diabetes mellitus, arthritis, thrombocytopenia, hemolytic anemia) are common and help make the diagnosis. Celiac disease, food allergy, and gastrointestinal infection must be ruled out. Treatment is immunosuppressive therapy, and a response confirms the diagnosis.[69]

IPEX Syndrome

Immune dysregulation, polyendocrinopathy, enteropathy, and X-linked inheritance (thus the condition is known as the IPEX syndrome) exhibits a presentation similar to autoimmune enteropathy and similar biopsy findings.[68] This disorder is the result of a mutation in the *FOXP3* gene.

Idiopathic Intestinal Pseudoobstruction

Idiopathic intestinal pseudoobstruction constitutes a group of rare disorders characterized by widespread gastrointestinal dysmotility. When this syndrome occurs in early infancy, vomiting and diarrhea are often major components. Diarrhea may alternate with constipation. In older children, the presentation is frequently more insidious; a long history of constipation may precede the onset of diarrhea. Persons who have this syndrome usually have intermittent or constant abdominal distention. The syndrome is characterized by the radiographic findings of bowel dilation with disordered motility; urinary bladder dysfunction is also often present. These disorders, which can be sporadic or transmitted in an autosomal-dominant fashion, can result from a visceral myopathy or neuropathy or from a combination of both. Bacterial overgrowth is an important cause of diarrhea in this disorder.

Microvillus Inclusion Disease

Microvillus inclusion disease (familial enteropathy) is a rare disorder that is present from birth and causes severe intractable secretory diarrhea with malabsorption.[68,70] It is the most common cause of intractable diarrhea in the neonatal period. Affected infants have small-bowel villous atrophy in the absence of crypt hyperplasia. The villous surface epithelial cells lack a normal brush border, and on electron microscopic examination the microvilli are absent or severely abnormal. The defective enterocytes and colonocytes contain intracytoplasmic inclusions, which, in turn, contain the components of the brush border. Microvillus inclusions are not found in every enterocyte. Fecal sodium and chloride concentrations are similar to those found in serum. Several families have been identified with more than one child with this disorder.

Tufting Enteropathy

In contrast to microvillus inclusion disease, symptoms of tufting enteropathy are not present at birth. Affected infants develop chronic watery diarrhea in the first few months of life.[68] The name derives from a typical light microscopic *tufted* configuration of the small-bowel mucosal epithelium.[71]

Congenital Disorders of Electrolyte Absorption

Congenital chloride-losing diarrhea and congenital sodium-secretory diarrhea are very rare, autosomal-recessive disorders associated with maternal polyhydramnios. The small-bowel mucosa is histologically normal, and absorption of other nutrients is normal. Infants with congenital chloride-losing diarrhea have persistent diarrhea resulting from absence of the normal ileal mechanism for active absorption of chloride in exchange for bicarbonate. They have acidic stools and a chronic metabolic alkalosis instead of the metabolic acidosis usually seen in chronic diarrhea. Stool chloride concentration is high, usually exceeding the sum of concentrations of sodium and potassium. The stool chloride of children who have this disorder may be in the range of 100 to 150 mEq/L, although it may be 30 to 100 mEq/L in infants. (Adult stool chloride is normally less than 20 mEq/L.) Although no satisfactory treatment exists, support with oral fluids and potassium chloride is recommended. Congenital sodium diarrhea is also a rare cause of watery diarrhea from birth. However, these infants are acidotic, and stool chloride concentration is not excessive. The disorder is the result of defective mucosal Na^+/H^+ exchange in the small and large bowel.

Congenital Disorders of Glycosylation

Congenital disorders of glycosylation exhibit in the 1st year of life, often with multisystem dysfunction.[72,73] In addition to hepatic, neurologic, cardiac, and optic manifestations, they can be associated with chronic diarrhea or severe protein-losing enteropathy, or both. Diagnosis is suggested if levels of serum glycoproteins such as haptoglobin and transferrin are low. Screening for this diagnosis has been performed with serum transferrin isoelectric focusing.

Infant of a Drug-Addicted Mother

Diarrhea may be a prominent manifestation of neonatal drug abstinence syndrome, and this diagnosis should be entertained in newborns who have persistent diarrhea, especially when other symptoms of neonatal drug withdrawal are present (see Chapter 103, Prenatal Drug Abuse and Neonatal Drug Withdrawal Syndrome).

Older Children

A pediatrician will see fewer older children with chronic diarrhea than they will infants, but older children are more likely to have chronic diarrhea associated with significant underlying disease compared with toddler's diarrhea in young children. As in infancy, the association of poor growth, weight loss, or other systemic manifestations suggests a serious organic cause. Older children commonly tend to deny symptoms, and the true effect of the disorder may not be immediately apparent. Clues are subtle changes in personality, diminished sense of well being, or loss of appetite. Children may hesitate to talk about their stooling pattern, and the degree of deviation from the norm may become apparent only after improvement occurs following initiation of appropriate therapy.

Causes of diarrhea differ somewhat after infancy, although many of the causes seen in infancy, even congenital anomalies, may exhibit first in childhood and therefore must still be considered. Factors that determine the age at diagnosis include (1) variability of presentation of signs and symptoms, (2) parental expectations of normality, and (3) the index of suspicion of the physician who is consulted. However, certain diseases, including inflammatory bowel disease and chronic constipation with encopresis, are much more likely to be seen in childhood than in infancy. Symptoms of celiac disease may begin at any age, and the high occurrence rate of celiac disease is now recognized. Cystic fibrosis may be associated with only mild manifestations in infancy and may be overlooked until frequent, bulky, foul-smelling stools become intolerable at home. AIDS is seen in older children, as well as in infants.

Irritable Bowel Syndrome

Irritable bowel syndrome (IBS) similar to that occurring in adults may be seen in children and adolescents.[8] Stools may alternate from diarrhea to constipation. In addition, the patient may have recurrent, crampy, abdominal pain. Late-onset lactose intolerance and fructose or sorbitol ingestion are important to rule out as causes of symptoms that may mimic IBS.[48,49] Symptoms of inflammatory bowel disease or celiac disease may also be mistaken at first for IBS. Treatment includes increased fiber in the diet, anticholinergics, and amitriptyline for diarrhea-predominant IBS.

Inflammatory Bowel Disease

The manifestations and presentation of Crohn disease and ulcerative colitis are so variable that these diseases should be considered whenever the clinician sees an older child who has chronic diarrhea.[74] Systemic evidence of inflammation (fever, weight loss, and leukocytosis), abdominal pain, blood in the stool (gross or occult), perianal disease, anemia, or extraintestinal manifestations (arthralgia, arthritis, or erythema nodosum) are helpful in suggesting this diagnosis. Growth failure can occur with or precede other symptoms. An elevated sedimentation rate also is a clue; however, normal sedimentation rates may occur in as many as 50% of patients who have inflammatory bowel disease. Thrombocytosis and elevated C-reactive protein, both acute-phase reactants, have been associated with inflammatory bowel disease as well and may be present in the absence of an elevated sedimentation rate. Suggestive signs and symptoms require evaluation, including a complete blood count, platelet count, erythrocyte sedimentation rate, serum protein levels, radiographic contrast studies of the upper bowel (including good views of the terminal ileum) or a CT of the abdomen and pelvis, and colonoscopic examination with biopsy. Capsule endoscopy is useful when, despite negative radiographic and colonoscopic evaluation, a strong suggestion of small-bowel Crohn disease is present. Newer antibody screening studies may be helpful in identifying the need for further evaluation for Crohn disease or ulcerative colitis. Currently, these antibodies include (1) anti-*Saccharomyces cerevisiae* antibody, (2) an antibody directed against outer membrane porin C of *E coli* known as anti-OmpC, and (3) an anti-neutrophil cytoplasmic antibody known as pANCA. Elevations of the former 2 antibodies tend to be associated with Crohn disease, whereas elevation of the last antibody tends to suggest ulcerative colitis. Management of inflammatory bowel disease includes an array of medical, nutritional, and surgical measures.[74]

Chronic Constipation

Chronic constipation with overflow incontinence may be mistaken for diarrhea. A thorough history and physical examination, including a rectal examination, should make the diagnosis apparent. A large amount of stool may be palpable in the abdomen, but a hard mass of stool is usually found in the rectal ampulla. This presentation is treated in the usual fashion of chronic constipation (as noted in Chapter 166, Constipation).

WHEN TO REFER

- Persistent diarrhea when the workup for routine infectious causes is negative
- Steatorrhea
- Diarrhea or steatorrhea (or both), causing weight loss or failure to thrive
- Diarrhea associated with fevers, chronic anemia, or abdominal pain without an obvious explanation

WHEN TO ADMIT

- Acute or chronic diarrhea with mild-to-moderate dehydration that cannot be managed successfully with outpatient rehydration solution
- Dehydration greater than 10% of body weight
- Diarrhea with intractable vomiting
- Severe electrolyte imbalance, including hypernatremic dehydration or serum potassium level less than 3.0 mEq/L
- Laboratory evidence suggesting hemolytic-uremic syndrome
- Chronic diarrhea or steatorrhea (or both) with persistent signs of malnutrition that is unresolved with outpatient management

TOOLS FOR PRACTICE

Engaging Patients and Family

- *Chronic Diarrhea* (fact sheet), Centers for Disease Control and Prevention (www.cdc.gov/ncidod/dpd/parasites/diarrhea/factsht_chronic_diarrhea.htm).
- *Common Childhood Infections* (brochure), American Academy of Pediatrics (patiented.aap.org).
- *Cryptosporidium Infection Cryptosporidiosis* (fact sheet), Centers for Disease Control and Prevention (www.cdc.gov/ncidod/dpd/parasites/cryptosporidiosis/factsht_cryptosporidiosis.htm).
- *Diarrhea and Dehydration* (brochure), American Academy of Pediatrics (patiented.aap.org).
- *Escherichia coli O157:H7* (fact sheet), Centers for Disease Control and Prevention (www.cdc.gov/ncidod/dbmd/diseaseinfo/escherichiacoli_g.htm).
- *Escherichia coli Infection and Farm Animals* (fact sheet), Centers for Disease Control and Prevention (www.cdc.gov/healthypets/diseases/ecoli.htm).
- *Giardia—Recreational Water Safety* (fact sheet), Centers for Disease Control and Prevention (www.cdc.gov/healthyswimming/giardiafacts.htm).
- *Giardiasis* (fact sheet), Centers for Disease Control and Prevention (www.cdc.gov/ncidod/dpd/parasites/giardiasis/factsht_giardia.htm).
- *Norovirus: Q&A* (fact sheet), Centers for Disease Control and Prevention (www.cdc.gov/ncidod/dvrd/revb/gastro/norovirus-qa.htm).
- *Rotavirus* (brochure), American Academy of Pediatrics (patiented.aap.org).
- *Salmonella Infection (salmonellosis) and Animals* (fact sheet), Centers for Disease Control and Prevention (www.cdc.gov/healthypets/diseases/salmonellosis.htm).
- *Salmonella enteritidis* (fact sheet), Centers for Disease Control and Prevention (www.cdc.gov/ncidod/dbmd/diseaseinfo/salment_g.htm).
- *Salmonellosis* (fact sheet), Centers for Disease Control and Prevention (www.cdc.gov/ncidod/dbmd/diseaseinfo/salmonellosis_g.htm).
- *Shigellosis* (fact sheet), Centers for Disease Control and Prevention (www.cdc.gov/ncidod/dbmd/diseaseinfo/shigellosis_g.htm).
- *Treating Diarrhea and Dehydration* (fact sheet), American Academy of Pediatrics (www.aap.org/topics.html).
- *Viral Gastroenteritis* (fact sheet), Centers for Disease Control and Prevention (www.cdc.gov/ncidod/dvrd/revb/gastro/faq.htm).
- *When You Swim, Swim Healthy! Recreational Water Illnesses* (Web page), Centers for Disease Control and Prevention (www.cdc.gov/healthyswimming/).

Medical Decision Support

- *Cryptosporidium—Lab Assistance* (Web page), Centers for Disease Control and Prevention (www.dpd.cdc.gov/dpdx/HTML/Cryptosporidiosis.htm).
- *Diarrheagenic Escherichia coli (non-Shiga toxin-producing E coli)* (fact sheet), Centers for Disease Control and Prevention (www.cdc.gov/ncidod/dbmd/diseaseinfo/diarrecoli_t.htm).
- *Giardiasis—Lab Assistance* (Web page), Centers for Disease Control and Prevention (www.dpd.cdc.gov/dpdx/HTML/Giardiasis.htm).

- *Managing Acute Gastroenteritis Among Children* (guideline), Centers for Disease Control and Prevention (www.cdc.gov/mmwr/PDF/RR/RR5216.pdf).
- *Norovirus: Technical Fact Sheet* (fact sheet), Centers for Disease Control and Prevention (www.cdc.gov/ncidod/dvrd/revb/gastro/norovirus-factsheet.htm).
- *Practice Guidelines for Management of Infectious Diarrhea* (guideline), Infectious Diseases Society of America (www.idsociety.org).
- *Rotavirus (Rotavirus Infection)* (fact sheet), Centers for Disease Control and Prevention (www.cdc.gov/rotavirus).
- *Salmonellosis* (fact sheet), Centers for Disease Control and Prevention (www.cdc.gov/ncidod/dbmd/diseaseinfo/salmonellosis_t.htm).
- *Shigellosis—Technical Information* (fact sheet), Centers for Disease Control and Prevention (www.cdc.gov/ncidod/dbmd/diseaseinfo/shigellosis_t.htm).

AAP POLICY STATEMENTS

American Academy of Pediatrics, Committee on Nutrition. The use and misuse of fruit juice in pediatrics. *Pediatrics*. 2001;107(5):1210-1213. (aappolicy.aappublications.org/cgi/content/full/pediatrics;107/5/1210).

Centers for Disease Control and Prevention. Managing acute gastroenteritis among children: oral rehydration. *Pediatrics*. 2003;52(RR16):1-16. AAP Endorsed. (www.cdc.gov/mmwr/pdf/rr/rr5216.pdf).

SUGGESTED RESOURCES

Centers for Disease Control and Prevention. Diagnosis and management of foodborne illnesses: a primer for physicians and other healthcare professionals. *MMWR*. 2004;53:1-33.

Centers for Disease Control and Prevention. Preliminary FoodNet data on the incidence of infection with pathogens transmitted commonly through food—10 sites, United States, 2004. *MMWR*. 2005;54:352-356.

Eherer AJ, Fordtran JS. Fecal osmotic gap and pH in experimental diarrhea of various causes. *Gastroenterology*. 1992;103:545-551.

Fasano A, Berti I, Gerarduzzi T. Prevalence of celiac disease in at-risk and not-at-risk groups in the United States: a large multicenter study. *Arch Intern Med*. 2003;163(3):286-292.

Field M. Intestinal ion transport and the pathophysiology of diarrhea. *J Clin Invest*. 2003;111:931-943.

Hill ID, Dirks MH, Liptak GS. Guideline for the diagnosis and treatment of celiac disease in children: recommendations of the North American Society for Pediatric Gastroenterology, Hepatology and Nutrition. *J Pediatr Gastroenterol Nutr*. 2005;40:1-19.

Kim SC, Ferry GD. Inflammatory bowel diseases in pediatric and adolescent patients: clinical, therapeutic, and psychological considerations. *Gastroenterology*. 2004;126:1550-1560.

King CK, Glass R, Bresee JS, et al. Managing acute gastroenteritis among children. Oral rehydration, maintenance and nutritional therapy. *MMWR*. 2003;52:1-16.

Scurlock AM, Lee LA, Burks AW. Food allergy in children. *Immunol Allergy Clin North Am*. 2005;25:369-388.

Sherman PM, Mitchell DJ, Cutz E. Neonatal enteropathies: defining the causes of protracted diarrhea of infancy. *J Pediatr Gastroenterol Nutr*. 2004;38:16-26.

REFERENCES

1. Phillips SF. Diarrhea: a current view of the pathophysiology. *Gastroenterology*. 1972;63:495-518.
2. Field M. Intestinal ion transport and the pathophysiology of diarrhea. *J Clin Invest*. 2003;111:931-943.
3. Lifshitz F, Ament ME, Kleinman RE, et al. Role of juice carbohydrate malabsorption in chronic nonspecific diarrhea in children. *J Pediatr*. 1992;120:825-829.
4. Eherer AJ, Fordtran JS. Fecal osmotic gap and pH in experimental diarrhea of various causes. *Gastroenterology*. 1992;103:545-551.
5. Kerzner B, Kelly MH, Gall DG, et al. Transmissible gastroenteritis: sodium transport and the intestinal epithelium during the course of viral enteritis. *Gastroenterology*. 1977;72:457-561.
6. Morris AP, Estes MK. Microbes and microbial toxins: paradigms for microbial-mucosal interactions. VIII. Pathological consequences of rotavirus infection and its enterotoxin. *Am J Physiol Gastrointest Liver Physiol*. 2001;28:G303-G310.
7. Oelkers P, Kirby LC, Heubi JE, et al. Primary bile acid malabsorption caused by mutations in the ileal sodium-dependent bile acid transporter gene (SLC10A2). *J Clin Invest*. 1997;99:1880-1887.
8. Drossman DA, Whitehead WE, Camilleri M. Irritable bowel syndrome: a technical review for practice guideline development. *Gastroenterology*. 1997;112:2120-2137.
9. Glass RI, Lew JF, Gangarosa RE, et al. Estimates of morbidity and mortality rates for diarrheal diseases in American children. *J Pediatr*. 1991;118:S27-S33.
10. Alpert G, Bell LM, Kirkpatrick CE, et al. Outbreak of cryptosporidiosis in a day-care center. *Pediatrics*. 1986;77:152-157.
11. Bartlett AV, Reves RR, Pickering LK. Rotavirus in infant-toddler day care centers: epidemiology relevant to disease control strategies. *J Pediatr*. 1988;113:435-441.
12. Bartlett AV, Moore M, Gary GW, et al. Diarrheal illness among infants and toddlers in day care centers. I. Epidemiology and pathogens. *J Pediatr*. 1985;107:495.
13. Hutson AM, Atmar RL, Estes MK. Norovirus disease: changing epidemiology and host susceptibility factors. *Trends Microbiol*. 2004;12:279-287.
14. Schwarz RP, Ulshen MH. Pseudomembranous colitis presenting as mild, chronic diarrhea in childhood. *J Pediatr Gastroenterol Nutr*. 1983;2:570-573.
15. Sutphen JL, Grand RJ, Flores A, et al. Chronic diarrhea associated with Clostridium difficile in children. *Am J Dis Child*. 1983;137:275-278.
16. Allos BM. Association between Campylobacter infection and Guillain-Barré syndrome. *J Infect Dis*. 1997;176:S125-S128.
17. Canadian Paediatric Society, Infectious Diseases Committee. Escherichia coli gastroenteritis: making sense of the new acronyms. *Can Med Assoc J*. 1987;136:241-244.
18. Centers for Disease Control and Prevention. Diagnosis and management of foodborne illnesses: a primer for physicians and other healthcare professionals. *MMWR*. 2004;53:1-33.
19. Centers for Disease Control and Prevention. Preliminary FoodNet data on the incidence of infection with pathogens transmitted commonly through food—10 sites, United States, 2004. *MMWR*. 2005;54:352-356.
20. King CK, Glass R, Bresee JS, et al. Managing acute gastroenteritis among children. Oral rehydration, maintenance and nutritional therapy. *MMWR*. 2003;52:1-16.
21. Santosham M, Daum RS, Dillman L, et al. Oral rehydration therapy of infantile diarrhea. A controlled study of well-nourished children hospitalized in the United States and Panama. *N Engl J Med*. 1982;306:1070-1076.

22. Tamer AM, Friedman LB, Maxwell SRW, et al. Oral rehydration of infants in a large urban U.S. medical center. *J Pediatr.* 1985;107:11-19.
23. Duggan C, Nurko S. "Feeding the gut": the scientific basis for continued enteral nutrition during acute diarrhea. *J Pediatr.* 1997;131:801-808.
24. Figueroa-Quintanilla D, Salazar-Lindo E, Sack RB, et al. A controlled trial of bismuth subsalicylate in infants with acute watery diarrheal disease. *N Engl J Med.* 1993;328: 1653-1658.
25. Wolfe DC, Giannella RA. Antibiotic therapy for bacterial enterocolitis: a comprehensive review. *Am J Gastroenterol.* 1993;88:1667-1683.
26. DuPont HL. Prevention of diarrhea by the probiotic. Lactobacillus GG. *J Pediatr.* 1999;134:1-2.
27. Costa-Ribeiro H, Ribeiro TC, Mattos AP, et al. Limitations of probiotic therapy in acute, severe dehydrating diarrhea. *J Pediatr Gastroenterol Nutr.* 2003;36:112-115.
28. Richardson S, Grimwood K, Gorrell R, et al. Extended excretion of rotavirus after severe diarrhoea in young children. *Lancet.* 1998;351:1844-1848.
29. Izraeli S, Rachmel A, Fishberg Y, et al. Transient renal acidification defect during acute infantile diarrhea: the role of urinary sodium. *J Pediatr.* 1990;117:711-716.
30. Branski D, Lerner A, Lebenthal E. Chronic diarrhea and malabsorption. *Pediatr Clin North Am.* 1996;43:307-331.
31. Cohen SA, Hendricks KM, Mathis RK, et al. Chronic nonspecific diarrhea: dietary relationships. *Pediatrics.* 1979;64: 402-407.
32. Larcher VF, Sheperd R, Francis DEM, et al. Protracted diarrhea in infancy. *Arch Dis Child.* 1977;52:597.
33. Goldgar CM, Vanderhoof JA. Lack of correlation of small bowel biopsy and clinical course of patients with intractable diarrhea of infancy. *Gastroenterology.* 1986;90: 527-531.
34. Klish WJ, Potts E, Ferry GD, et al. Modular formula: an approach to management of infants with specific or complex food intolerances. *J Pediatr.* 1976;88: 948-952.
35. Orenstein SR. Enteral versus parenteral therapy for intractable diarrhea of infancy: prospective, randomized trial. *J Pediatr.* 1986;109:277-286.
36. Mack DR, Forstner GG, Wilschanski M, et al. Shwachman syndrome: exocrine pancreatic dysfunction and variable phenotypic expression. *Gastroenterology.* 1996; 111:1593-1602.
37. Jonas A, Avigad S, Diver-Haber A, et al. Disturbed fat absorption following infectious gastroenteritis in children. *J Pediatr.* 1979;95:366-372.
38. Fasano A, Berti I, Gerarduzzi T, et al. Prevalence of celiac disease in at-risk and not-at-risk groups in the United States: a large multicenter study. *Arch Intern Med.* 2003; 163:286-292.
39. Janatuinen EK, Pikkarainen PH, Kemppainen TA. A comparison of diets with and without oats in adults with celiac disease. *N Engl J Med.* 1995;333:1033-1037.
40. Green PHR, Jabri B. Coelic disease. *Lancet.* 2003;326: 383-391.
41. Hill ID, Dirks MH, Liptak GS, et al. Guideline for the diagnosis and treatment of celiac disease in children: recommendations of the North American Society for Pediatric Gastroenterology, Hepatology and Nutrition. *J Pediatr Gastroenterol Nutr.* 2005;40(1);1-19.
42. Dieterich W, Laag E, Schoepper H, et al. Autoantibodies to tissue transglutaminase as predictors of celiac disease. *Gastroenterology.* 1998;115:1317-1321.
43. Sulkanen S, Halttunen T, Laurila K, et al. Tissue transglutaminase autoantibody enzyme-linked immunosorbent assay in detecting celiac disease. *Gastroenterology.* 1998;115:1322-1328.
44. Ulshen MH: Carbohydrate absorption and malabsorption. In: Walker WA, Watkins JB, Duggan C, eds. *Nutrition in Pediatrics: Basic Science and Clinical Applications.* Hamilton, Ontario: BC Decker; 2003.
45. Treem WR. Congenital sucrase-isomaltase deficiency. *J Pediatr Gastroenterol Nutr.* 1995;21:1-14.
46. Newton T, Murphy MS, Booth IW, et al. Glucose polymer as a cause of protracted diarrhea in infants with unsuspected congenital sucrase-isomaltase deficiency. *J Pediatr.* 1996;128:753-756.
47. Ameen VZ, Powell GK, Jones LA. Quantitation of fecal carbohydrate excretion in patients with short bowel syndrome. *Gastroenterology.* 1987;92:493-500.
48. Hyams JS. Sorbitol malabsorption. An unappreciated cause of functional gastrointestinal complaints. *Gastroenterology.* 1983;84:30-33.
49. Riby JE, Fujisawa T, Kretchmer N. Fructose absorption. *Am J Clin Nutr.* 1993;58:748S-753S.
50. Mitchel DK, Van R, Morrow AL, et al. Outbreaks of astrovirus gastroenteritis in day care center. *J Pediatr.* 1993;123: 725-732.
51. Yolken RH, Lawrence F, Leister F, et al. Gastroenteritis associated with enteric type adenovirus in hospitalized infants. *J Pediatr.* 1982;101:21-26.
52. Kane JG, Chretien JH, Garagusi VF. Diarrhea caused by Candida. *Lancet.* 1976;1:335-336.
53. Phillips AD, Thomas AG, Walker-Smith JA. Cryptosporidium, chronic diarrhoea and the proximal small intestinal mucosa. *Gut.* 1992;33:1057-1061.
54. Wolfson JS, Richter JM, Waldron MA. Cryptosporidiosis in immuno-competent patients. *N Engl J Med.* 1985;312: 1278-1282.
55. Andrassy RJ, Isaacs H, Weitzman JJ. Rectal suction biopsy for the diagnosis of Hirschsprung disease. *Ann Surg.* 1981;193:419-424.
56. Bock SA. Prospective appraisal of complaints of adverse reactions to foods in children during the first 3 years of life. *Pediatrics.* 1987;79:683-688.
57. Scurlock AM, Lee LA, Burks AW. Food allergy in children. *Immunol Allergy Clin North Am.* 2005;25:369-388.
58. Odze RD, Bines J, Leichtner AM, et al. Allergic colitis in infants. *J Pediatr.* 1995;126:163-170.
59. Vanderhoof JA, Murray ND, Kaufman SS, et al. Intolerance to protein hydrolysate infant formulas: an underrecognized cause of gastrointestinal symptoms in infants. *J Pediatr.* 1997;131:741-744.
60. Lake AM, Whitington PF, Hamilton SR. Dietary protein-induced colitis in breast-fed infants. *J Pediatr.* 1982;101: 906-910.
61. Goulet OJ, Revillon Y, Jan D, et al. Neonatal short bowel syndrome. *J Pediatr.* 1991;119:18-23.
62. Goulet O, Ruemmele F, Lacaille F, et al. Irreversible intestinal failure. *J Pediatr Gastroenterol Nutr.* 2004;38: 250-269.
63. Kaufman SS, Loseke CA, Lupo JV, et al. Influence of bacterial overgrowth and intestinal inflammation on duration of parenteral nutrition in children with short bowel syndrome. *J Pediatr.* 1997;131:356.
64. Taylor SF, Sondheimer JM, Sokol RJ, et al. Noninfectious colitis associated with short gut syndrome in infants. *J Pediatr.* 1991;119:24-28.
65. Neldner KH, Hambridge KM. Zinc therapy of acrodermatitis enteropathica. *N Engl J Med.* 1975;292:879-882.
66. Winter H, Chang TI. Gastrointestinal and nutritional problems in children with immunodeficiency and AIDS. *Pediatr Clin North Am.* 1996;43:573-590.
67. Grohmann GS, Glass RI, Pereira HG, et al. Enteric viruses and diarrhea in HIV-infected patients. *N Engl J Med.* 1993;329:14-20.

68. Sherman PM, Mitchell DJ, Cutz E. Neonatal enteropathies: defining the causes of protracted diarrhea of infancy. *J Pediatr Gastroenterol Nutr.* 2004;38:16-26.
69. Bousvaros A, Leichtner AM, Book L, et al. Treatment of pediatric autoimmune enteropathy with tacrolimus (FK506). *Gastroenterology.* 1996;111:237-243.
70. Cutz E, Rhoads JM, Drumm B, et al. Microvillus inclusion disease: an inherited defect of brush-border assembly and differentiation. *N Engl J Med.* 1989;320:646-651.
71. Patey N, Scoazec JY, Cuenod-Jabri B, et al. Distribution of cell adhesion molecules in infants with intestinal epithelial dysplasia (tufting enteropathy). *Gastroenterology.* 1997;113:833-843.
72. Jaeken J. Congenital disorders of glycosylation (CDG): update and new developments. *J Inherit Metab Dis.* 2004; 27:423-426.
73. Mention K, Michaud Left, Dobbelaere D, et al. Neonatal severe intractable diarrhea as the presenting manifestation of an unclassified congenital disorder of glycosylation (CDG-x). *Arch Dis Child Fetal Neonatal Educ.* 2001; 85:F217-F219.
74. Kim SC, Ferry GD. Inflammatory bowel diseases in pediatric and adolescent patients: clinical, therapeutic, and psychological considerations. *Gastroenterology.* 2004; 126:1550-1560.

Chapter 170

DIZZINESS AND VERTIGO

Ruby F. Rivera, MD; Catherine R. Sellinger, MD

Dizziness and vertigo, although often confused and placed together, are very different symptoms that have very different clinical implications. Distinguishing these symptoms in young children may be especially difficult because much of the distinction depends on the patient's account of the history.

DIZZINESS

Definition

Dizziness, a relatively common complaint in childhood and adolescence, is "an imprecise term commonly used by patients in an attempt to describe various peculiar subjective symptoms such as faintness, giddiness, light-headedness, or unsteadiness."[1] Patients who have simple dizziness do not describe the room spinning around them, and they do not have nystagmus.

Causes of Dizziness

Dizziness is commonly seen as a symptom of presyncope in children and adolescents with fever, dehydration, orthostatic hypotension, and vasovagal syncope. It is also commonly associated with anemia, either from acute or chronic blood loss or from a congenital condition such as sickle cell disease.[2] Any heart disease or dysrhythmia that affects cardiac output can cause dizziness, as can hypertension. Hypoglycemia, which may be associated with altered mental status or seizures, can first manifest as dizziness. Hyperthyroidism, hypothyroidism, and Addison disease can also cause dizziness. In female adolescents, pregnancy should be considered in the differential diagnosis of dizziness. Ocular disorders such as refractive errors, astigmatism, amblyopia, and strabismus can cause dizziness.[3] Dizziness is often a symptom of anxiety and as part of panic attacks. Dizziness may also be caused by medications such as aminoglycosides, phenytoin, loop diuretics, and nonsteroidal antiinflammatory drugs. An algorithm to aid in narrowing the differential diagnosis of dizziness is shown in Figure 170-1.

When young children cannot describe dizziness or vertigo, observers tend to apply these terms to a child who is unsteady while standing. Disequilibrium in this age group may reflect acute cerebellar problems, such as postviral acute cerebellar ataxia and posterior fossa tumors. In adolescents, particularly girls, ataxia as part of multiple sclerosis may be described as dizziness.[4] Another common cause of disequilibrium in young children is middle-ear disease. Several studies have shown deterioration in vestibular balance and motor function in children with middle-ear effusion. If not self-limited, symptoms usually resolve after placement of tympanostomy tubes.

VERTIGO

Definition

Vertigo is "a sensation of spinning or whirling motion. Vertigo implies a definite sensation of rotation of the subject or of objects about the subject in any plane."[1] True vertigo almost always is accompanied by nystagmus, at least at the time of the episode.[5] Thus the primary care physician should ask observers about the presence of nystagmus and should ask them to watch for it in future episodes.

Causes of Vertigo

The causes of vertigo can be differentiated based on 3 elements in the history: (1) whether the vertigo is acute or chronic, (2) whether episodes are recurrent, and (3) whether it is accompanied by hearing loss. The causes of vertigo in children vary greatly from those in adults. Acute episodic vertigo is the most common type encountered by pediatricians and is usually not accompanied by hearing loss (Figure 170-2).

The most common causes of acute episodic vertigo are migraine headaches and related syndromes. Benign paroxysmal torticollis of infancy is thought to be a migraine variant that begins in infancy and generally resolves spontaneously by 2 to 3 years of age. It is characterized by episodes of recurrent head tilt, which may last for hours or days and is often associated with vomiting, agitation, pallor, and ataxia. Benign paroxysmal vertigo of childhood is also considered a migraine variant and is typically seen in children younger than 5 years. These children have the sudden onset of extreme unsteadiness and inability to stand, usually with nystagmus and sometimes with vomiting. The episodes last seconds to minutes. In many cases, the family has a history of migraine headaches, and many of these patients develop more typical migraine headaches in later life. Older children and adolescents may have episodic vertigo as a result of basilar artery migraines. Affected patients often have scintillating scotomas or visual obscuration, oral paresthesias, tinnitus, and

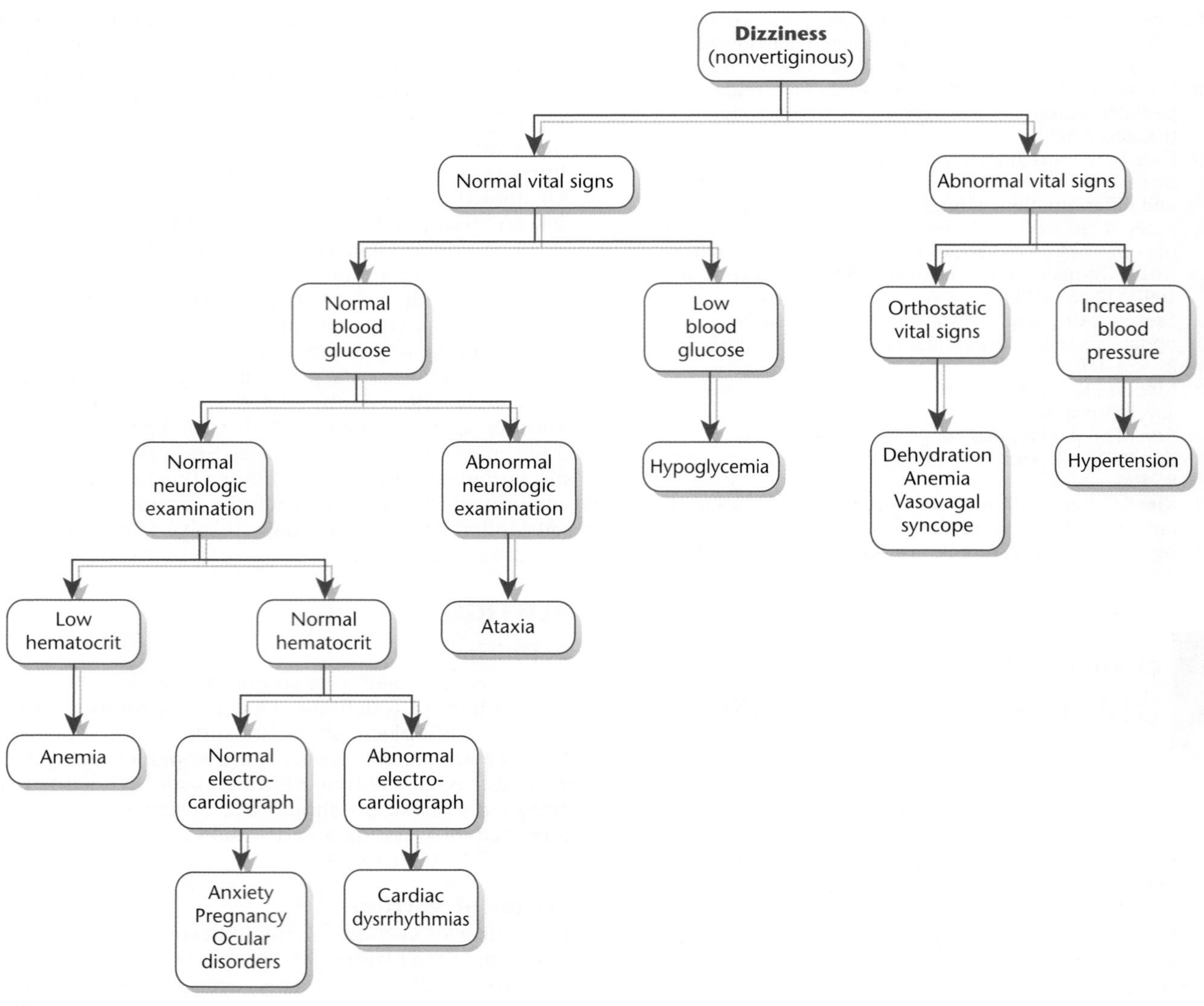

Figure 170-1 Algorithm for the differential diagnosis of dizziness.

occasionally *drop attacks* with or without loss of consciousness. These early symptoms are commonly but not always followed by a pounding headache. Other causes of acute recurrent vertigo include seizures, perilymph fistula, and benign paroxysmal positional vertigo. Seizures that are associated with vertigo are followed by an alteration or loss of consciousness. A perilymph fistula is an abnormal connection between the inner- and middle-ear spaces. Although some fistulas are congenital, most are acquired from trauma, such as direct penetrating trauma, head trauma, or barotrauma. Flying, diving, coughing, sneezing, or any type of excessive strain or exertion may tear the oval or round window, causing a sudden onset of vertigo associated with hearing loss. Benign paroxysmal positional vertigo (BPPV), although extremely common in adults, is rare in children. BPPV is believed to be caused by otoconia (debris or *ear rocks*) that have been deposited in a sensitive location in the semicircular canal. Acute episodes of severe vertigo are precipitated by a change of head position and are associated with nystagmus, nausea, and vomiting. The Epley and Semont maneuvers at tempt to relocate the otoconia into a less-sensitive location. (A helpful Web site that illustrates these maneuvers is www.tchain.com/otoneurology/disorders/bppv/bppv.html.) Vestibular neuritis exhibits similar symptoms to BPPV and, although uncommon in children, should be considered if vertigo is preceded by a viral infection. Neither BPPV nor vestibular neuritis is associated with hearing loss.

Vertigo with hearing loss in childhood is usually associated with severe otitis media leading to labyrinthitis. Affected patients are acutely uncomfortable, both from ear pain and from severe vertigo, usually with nausea, vomiting, and nystagmus. Less common causes of hearing loss together with vertigo in children include head trauma or ear trauma. Ménière disease, consisting of vertigo, fluctuating hearing loss,

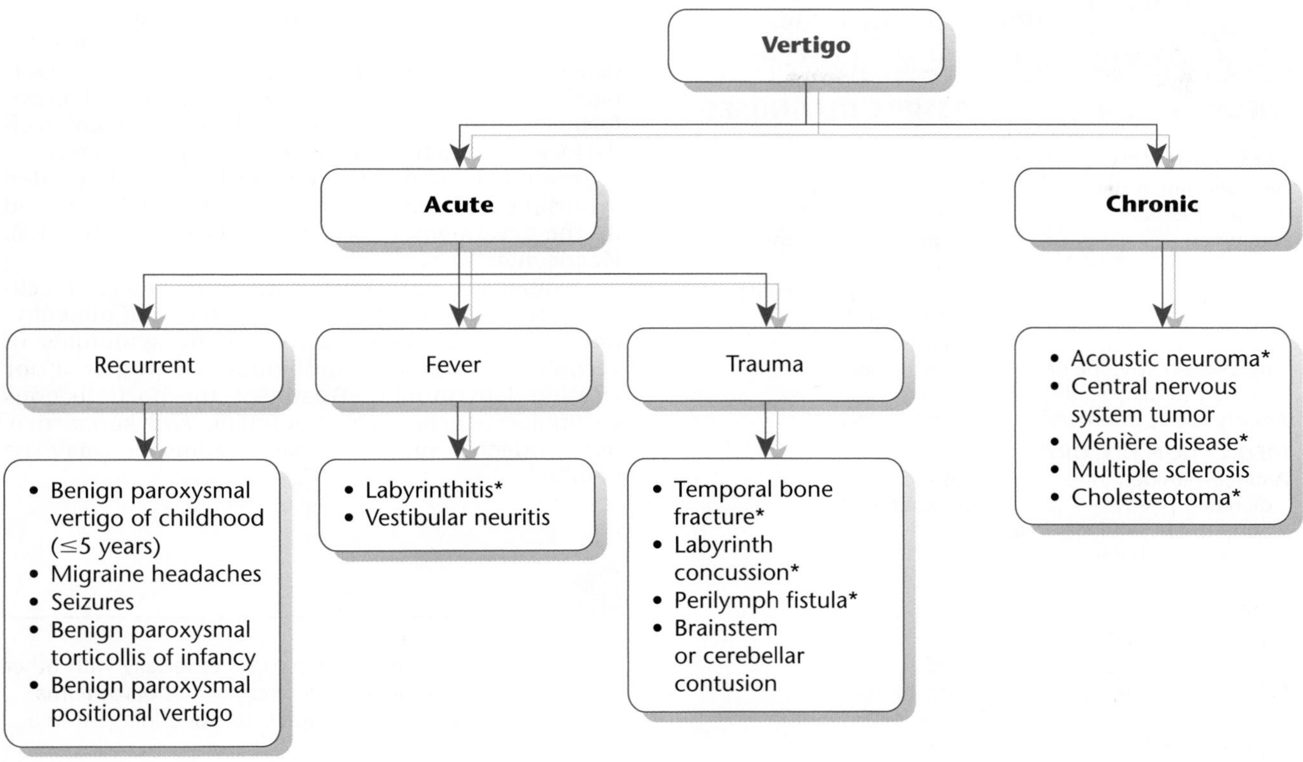

Figure 170-2 Algorithm for the differential diagnosis of vertigo. Asterisk denotes an associated hearing loss.

pressure in the ear, and tinnitus, is rare in young children, usually occurring after 11 years of age.

Chronic persistent vertigo, especially if accompanied by neurologic signs, is usually indicative of central nervous system disease, including tumors, acoustic neurinomas (seen in neurofibromatosis type II), and demyelinating and degenerative disorders.

EVALUATION OF DIZZINESS AND VERTIGO

History

Most episodes of dizziness and vertigo can be diagnosed on history and physical examination. Useful information, which may lead to a particular diagnosis, is listed in Table 170-1.

Physical Examination

On physical examination, the physician should document orthostatic vital signs, look for evidence of anemia or dehydration, and pay particular attention to the head, neck, cardiac, and neurologic findings. The Dix-Hallpike maneuver (Nylan-Barany test) can help localize the source of nystagmus or vertigo. To provoke an episode, the child is moved rapidly from a sitting to supine position with the head 45 degrees below the edge of the table and turned 45 degrees to 1 side. The ear that is facing the floor when the nystagmus is elicited is the affected side. Nystagmus that resolves when the child fixates on an object is suggestive of a peripheral or vestibular disease, as opposed to persistent nystagmus that is seen in central nervous system disorders.

Examine the ears for vesicles of herpes zoster (Ramsay-Hunt syndrome); a distorted tympanic membrane may be seen with otitis media, cholesteatoma, and perilymph fistula. Two useful maneuvers that may help in the diagnosis of perilymph fistula are applying pressure to the tragus to occlude the external auditory canal and pneumatic otoscopy; they may induce nystagmus or vertigo and transiently worsen a hearing loss.

Laboratory Testing and Imaging

With a limited role in the evaluation of dizziness and vertigo, laboratory tests such as complete blood count, metabolic panel, thyroid function tests, electrocardiogram, electroencephalogram, and magnetic resonance imaging should be guided by the history and physical examination. In adolescent girls, a pregnancy test should also be considered. A formal audiometry and an electronystagmogram may be warranted for the evaluation of vertigo.

MANAGEMENT OF DIZZINESS AND VERTIGO

For patients who have presyncopal or orthostatic dizziness, reassurance and instructions about adequate hydration, about care when arising suddenly, and

Table 170-1 Differential Diagnoses of Dizziness and Vertigo

INFORMATION	POSSIBLE DIAGNOSES
FAMILY HISTORY	
Neurofibromatosis	Acoustic neuroma
Seizure disorder	Seizure
Migraines	Benign paroxysmal torticollis of infancy Benign paroxysmal vertigo of childhood Migraine
Unexplained syncope or sudden cardiac death	Dysrhythmias
Anxiety, panic disorders	Anxiety
MEDICATION HISTORY	
Aminoglycosides, loop diuretics, phenytoin, nonsteroidal antiinflammatory drugs, chemotherapeutic agents, quinine	Ototoxicity Intoxication
MEDICAL HISTORY	
Acute or chronic blood loss	Anemia
Palpitation or chest pain	Dysrhythmias Anxiety, panic disorder
Recent life stressor	Anxiety
Last menstrual period	Pregnancy
Motion sickness	Benign paroxysmal vertigo of childhood Migraine
Recent upper respiratory infection	Vestibular neuritis
Fever	Otitis media Labyrinthitis
Ear trauma, barotrauma	Perilymph fistula
Headache	Migraine CNS disease
Head trauma	Temporal bone fracture Labyrinth or brain stem concussion Cerebellar contusion Perilymph fistula
Neurologic deficits	CNS tumor Multiple sclerosis
Hearing loss	Cholesteatoma Acoustic neuroma Temporal bone fracture Perilymph fistula Labyrinth concussion Labyrinthitis Ramsay-Hunt syndrome Ménière disease
Triggered by change in head position	Benign paroxysmal positional vertigo Perilymph fistula Vestibular neuritis Acute labyrinthitis
Loss of consciousness or altered mental status	Seizure Dysrhythmia Vasovagal syncope CNS disease Hypoglycemia

CNS, Central nervous system.

about the necessity of putting the head lower than the heart when symptoms occur generally suffice for patient management. For patients in whom dizziness is part of a panic attack or a marker of significant stress, further history should be obtained, including any suicidal ideation, and referral for counseling considered.

Treatment for migrainous vertigo and its related syndromes should be symptomatic and targeted to the treatment of migraines (see Chapter 185, Headache).

Vestibular suppressants such as diazepam, meclizine (for children older than 12 years), and dimenhydrinate may be used to relieve the symptoms of vertigo and nausea. Antibiotics are required for treating labyrinthitis. Treatment for postinfectious vestibular neuritis is symptomatic and supportive, but evidence suggests that prednisone may be helpful.[6]

WHEN TO REFER

- Acute ataxia
- A clear history of vertigo, especially with other neurologic signs or after head or barotrauma
- Suspected perilymph fistula or cholesteatoma
- Suspected seizure
- Complicated migraine

WHEN TO ADMIT

- Bacterial or suppurative labyrinthitis
- Head trauma with temporal bone fracture
- Space-occupying lesions
- Potential life-threatening cardiac dysrhythmias
- Labile hypertension

TOOLS FOR PRACTICE

Medical Decision Support

- *BPPV: Benign Paroxysmal Positional Vertigo* (Web page), Timothy C. Hain, MD (www.dizziness-and-balance.com/disorders/bppv/bppv.html).

REFERENCES

1. *Stedman's Medical Dictionary*. 27th ed. Baltimore, MD: Lippincott Williams and Wilkins; 2000.
2. Walker JS, Barnes SB. The difficult diagnosis. *Emerg Med Clin North Am.* 1998;16:846-875.
3. Anoh-Tanon MJ, Bremond-Gignac D, Wiener-Vacher SR. Vertigo is an underestimated symptom of ocular disorders: dizzy children do not always need MRI. *Pediatr Neurol.* 2000;23:49-53.
4. Casselbrant ML, Mandel EM. Balance disorders in children. *Neurol Clin.* 2005;23:807-829.
5. Tusa RJ, Saada AA, Niparko JK. Dizziness in childhood. *J Child Neurol.* 1994;9:261-274.
6. Strupp M, Zingler VC, Arbusow V, et al. Methylprednisolone, valacyclovir, or the combination for vestibular neuritis. *N Eng J Med.* 2004;351:354-361.

Chapter 171

DYSMENORRHEA

Linda Meyer Dinerman, MD; Alain Joffe, MD, MPH

Dysmenorrhea, meaning painful menstruation, is a syndrome characterized by varying degrees of crampy, lower abdominal pain, and other symptoms such as nausea, vomiting, urinary frequency, low back pain, diarrhea, fatigue, thigh pain, nervousness, dizziness, sweating, and headache. The pain typically begins just after menses and lasts for approximately 1 to 2 days, but it can also begin 1 to 2 days before the onset of menses and can last up to 4 days into menstruation.[1] Cramps may be more severe among teenagers who smoke. At least 40% to 60% of adolescent girls suffer some degree of discomfort during menstruation, with approximately 15% reporting severe symptoms and 14% reporting that they frequently miss school as a result of menstrual symptoms.[1] Most affected teenage girls have primary dysmenorrhea, that is, a syndrome not associated with pelvic or other pathologic conditions; however, causes of secondary dysmenorrhea always should be considered when the patient is evaluated.

PRIMARY DYSMENORRHEA

Increased amounts of prostaglandins E_2 and $F_{2\alpha}$ in the endometrium of women with dysmenorrhea[1] lead to smooth-muscle contractions along with other symptoms such as vomiting and diarrhea. This biological explanation correlates with the clinical observation that women who have anovulatory cycles usually do not have dysmenorrhea. Adolescent girls typically develop dysmenorrhea 1 to 2 years after menarche, correlating with the onset of ovulatory cycles.[2]

The incidence of dysmenorrhea increases with gynecologic age (as does the percentage of ovulatory cycles), with up to 31% of girls reporting dysmenorrhea in their first year of menses and 78% in their 5th year.[2] The increase in prostaglandin synthesis may be related to changes in serum progesterone levels not seen in anovulatory women. Additional confirmation comes from the dramatic response women experience with use of either prostaglandin synthetase inhibitors or oral contraceptives, which inhibit ovulation. Increased levels of prostaglandin activity are associated with increased uterine tone and high-amplitude myometrial contractions, both of which result in reduced uterine blood flow and pain.

The assessment of a teenager with dysmenorrhea should include the following:[1]

- Complete menstrual history
- Timing of cramps or pain
- Missed school or other activities
- Ability to participate in social events
- Presence of nausea, vomiting, diarrhea, dizziness, or other symptoms
- Medications used, including doses
- Factors that improve or worsen symptoms
- Family history of dysmenorrhea or endometriosis

In some cases, dysmenorrhea may be the presenting complaint when the true agenda is otherwise.[1] For example: Is the patient reluctant to attend school? Does the patient have a history of physical or sexual abuse? Does the patient have significant psychosocial problems? Is the teen secretly sexually active, and is this a way for her to obtain oral contraceptives for the purpose of contraception?

A careful history usually excludes most pathologic causes of dysmenorrhea. Physicians differ in their opinions regarding what examination is necessary to evaluate a patient with dysmenorrhea. In general, for a non–sexually active teenager who has mild to moderate menstrual cramps relieved by nonsteroidal antiinflammatory drugs (NSAIDs), only an external genital examination to rule out hymenal abnormalities is indicated. Some clinicians would also initiate oral contraceptive pills without first performing a pelvic examination for a few cycles if the dysmenorrhea is unresponsive to NSAIDs. For any sexually active teenager or, in the opinion of some experts, for one who is having significant pain that is unresponsive to NSAIDs, a thorough pelvic examination is necessary. In sexually active teenagers, evaluating for sexually transmitted infections and pregnancy should be included. If a pelvic examination is not possible, then a rectoabdominal examination will provide some useful information about the presence of masses or adnexal tenderness. A pelvic ultrasound may be useful in defining uterine and vaginal abnormalities associated with obstruction but is not helpful in the detection of pelvic or abdominal adhesions or endometriosis.[1]

Although treatment of primary dysmenorrhea is likely to include drug therapy, the physician also should take the valuable opportunity to teach the patient about her body. Many teenagers do not understand the physiologic mechanisms of menstruation fully or may have inaccurate beliefs that have been passed on from mother to daughter.

Although teenagers who have very mild discomfort benefit from almost any analgesic, prostaglandin synthetase inhibitors in the form of NSAIDs are the treatment of choice for most young women with dysmenorrhea. Doses, both in terms of amount and timing, vary from patient to patient. Establishing not only prior use of specific medications, but also doses is important, given that most patients use them in subtherapeutic amounts.[1] Some need medication only for part or all of the first day of menstruation; others require medication for up to 4 days or more.[1] Ibuprofen (200 to 800 mg every 6 to 8 hours) is highly effective for dysmenorrhea, as is naproxen sodium (550 mg immediately and then 275 mg every 6 to 8 hours). Mefenamic acid, an NSAID that blocks the effect of prostaglandin at the end-organ level and inhibits its production, can be used in a dose of 500 mg administered immediately followed by 250 mg every 6 hours. In 1 study, 57% of adolescents used medications less often than the maximal daily frequency; thus advising patients of the range of correct doses is important.[2] These medications are most effective if started at the first sign of menstrual bleeding; women who experience significant nausea with menses may benefit from starting treatment at the earliest symptom of menses, even before bleeding occurs. If the adolescent fails to respond to 1 type of NSAID (eg, ibuprofen), another (eg, naproxen sodium) should be tried because variability is noted in response to different NSAIDs.[1] Between 70% and 80% of girls will respond to one NSAID or another. The patient should be reevaluated after 2 to 3 menstrual cycles to determine effectiveness of the treatment.

Some patients (perhaps as many as 20% to 30%) will not respond to these measures. In these young women, a trial of oral contraceptive pills (OCPs) used in the same way as for contraception usually provides relief. OCPs work by suppressing ovulation and decreasing endometrial prostaglandin production. Patients should be told that 2 to 3 cycles may elapse before contraceptives exert their maximal effect. If the patient is sexually active, then oral contraceptives are continued on a routine basis; for the non–sexually active teenager, therapy can be reassessed at 6 to 12 month intervals.

Low-dose OCPs significantly decrease the symptoms of dysmenorrhea in adult women and adolescents.[3,4] After 3 cycles, adult patients using OCPs with 20 mcg of ethinyl estradiol and 150 mcg of desogestrel or adolescent patients using OCPs with 20 mcg of ethinyl estradiol and 100 mg of levonorgestrel experienced significant relief of dysmenorrhea compared with those using placebo.[3,4]

In a study of adolescent girls using the patch (Ortho Evra) for contraception, dysmenorrhea decreased in 39%, increased in 11%, and resulted in no change in 50%.[5] Depot-medroxyprogesterone acetate (Depo-provera, DMPA) is also used to prevent ovulation and menstrual flow when OCPs are not tolerated or estrogen is contraindicated.[2] An extended oral contraceptive regimen in which OCPs are taken for up to 12 consecutive weeks followed by 1 hormone-free week is another treatment approach.[6] DMPA and extended oral contraceptive regimens decrease dysmenorrhea, and they decrease the frequency of menses.[7,8]

The efficacy of other treatments is still unproven. Some experts believe that heat, pelvic exercise, general exercise, biofeedback, relaxation therapy, massage, vitamin E, or various herbal remedies are effective; other authorities remain skeptical of these alternatives. Magnesium has been shown to be beneficial in some studies.[1] To the extent that smoking exacerbates dysmenorrhea, it provides yet another reason for clinicians to urge their patients to stop smoking. The adolescent with dysmenorrhea should be encouraged to exercise, eat a well-balanced diet, decrease stress, and decrease caffeine consumption.[7]

Women who fail to respond to any of these measures should be referred to an adolescent medicine specialist or gynecologist for evaluation; they probably have secondary rather than primary dysmenorrhea.

SECONDARY DYSMENORRHEA

Causes of secondary dysmenorrhea, such as pelvic inflammatory disease (PID), endometriosis, or conditions arising in a variety of other organ systems, can usually be excluded by a careful history and physical examination. Underlying pathologic conditions should be anticipated in a young woman whose pain begins after 20 years of age, who has a history of surgery related to the genitourinary or gastrointestinal tract, or who has pain that is dull and constant rather than crampy.

Endometriosis is the presence of functional endometrial glands and stroma outside the normal anatomic location in the uterus.[9] Patients who have endometriosis will have failed therapy with NSAIDs and oral contraceptives, and their pain may be acyclic rather than cyclic. Menstrual bleeding may be irregular, gastrointestinal symptoms may be present, and a family history of endometriosis can often be elicited. Endometriosis also may be associated with dyspareunia, tenesmus, and rectal pain. Some studies of teenagers with chronic pelvic pain show 25% to 38% of those undergoing laparoscopy have endometriosis. In yet other studies, 52% to 73% of teenagers with chronic pelvic pain have evidence of endometrial implants.[7,9] PID can cause dysmenorrhea acutely, and women often develop chronic pelvic pain as a consequence of PID. Even with assurances of confidentiality, some young women may still not admit to sexual activity. Hence clinicians must maintain a high index of probability if other historical and physical examination findings suggest PID. Teenagers who have a history of genital tract surgery, including abortions, may have outflow tract obstruction. A variety of müllerian anomalies with incomplete obstruction of the outflow tract also produce dysmenorrhea.[1] Depending on the type of obstruction, a pelvic mass may be palpable. Endometrial polyps or fibroids are rare in women younger than 20 years but should be anticipated if the menstrual bleeding is heavy, prolonged, or associated with the passage of clots. Whether these entities alone cause dysmenorrhea is unclear.

A pelvic examination that reveals cervical motion tenderness, or adnexal tenderness, or masses strongly suggests PID. If the cervical os is stenotic or the cervix or uterus feels atretic or abnormally shaped, then outflow obstruction is possible (eg, a uterus with a blind horn). Among adult women, physical findings such as small fixed nodules in the rectovaginal septum or cul de sac or fixation of the uterus indicated by the sensation of pain on stretching of the uterosacral ligaments suggest endometriosis. However, most adolescents generally have normal examinations; hence endometriosis can be extremely difficult to detect on clinical grounds alone.[10] If a secondary cause of dysmenorrhea is thought to be present, then consultation with an adolescent medicine specialist or gynecologist is warranted. Ultrasound examination of the uterus will rule out uterine anomalies but cannot exclude endometriosis. Confirmation of endometriosis requires laparoscopy. Because the lesions of endometriosis in adolescents may differ from the typical lesions seen in adults, a gynecologist who is experienced in evaluating adolescents should perform this procedure. Endometriosis may be difficult to manage, and women who have this condition are at increased risk for infertility.

PID should be treated according to standard antibiotic regimens (see Chapter 322, Sexually Transmitted Infections). Follow-up is critical because young women, once infected, are at risk for further episodes of PID, as well as for chronic pelvic pain, ectopic pregnancy, and infertility.

WHEN TO REFER

The point at which a clinician chooses to refer depends on his or her experience. For dysmenorrhea, referral might be appropriate:

- If the clinician feels uncomfortable prescribing oral contraceptive pills for the treatment of primary dysmenorrhea
- If the patient fails to respond to NSAIDs and OCPs
- If the clinical presentation or course suggests that the patient has secondary rather than primary dysmenorrhea
- If the patient is sexually active and the clinician feels uncomfortable performing a pelvic examination

WHEN TO ADMIT

If the cause of the dysmenorrhea is determined to be pelvic inflammatory disease, some clinicians would recommend hospitalization of all adolescents for treatment. Others recommend hospitalization under certain but not all circumstances (see Chapter 322, Sexually Transmitted Infections).

RELATED WEB SITES

- Center for Young Women's Health (www.youngwomenshealth.org).
- Teenwire.com (www.teenwire.com).

REFERENCES

1. Emans SJ, Laufer MR, Goldstein DP. *Pediatric and Adolescent Gynecology*, 5th ed. Philadelphia, PA: Lippincott Williams & Wilkins; 2005.
2. Iglesias EA, Coupey SM. Menstrual cycle abnormalities: diagnosis and management. *Adolesc Med*. 1999;10(2): 255-273.
3. Callejo J, Diaz J, Ruiz A, et al. Effect of a low-dose oral contraceptive containing 20 mcg ethinylestradiol and 150 mcg desogestrel on dysmenorrhea. *Contraception*. 2003;68:183-188.
4. Davis AR, Westhoff C, O'Connell K, et al. Oral contraceptives for dysmenorrhea in adolescent girls. *Obstetr Gynecol*. 2005;106 (1):97-104.
5. Harel Z, Riggs S, Vaz R, et al. Adolescents: experience with the combined estrogen and progestin transdermal contraceptive method ortho evra. *J Pediatr Adolesc Gynecol*. 2005;18:85-90.
6. Sulak PJ, Carl J, Gopalakrishnan I, et al. Outcomes of extended oral contraceptive regimens with a shortened hormone-free interval to manage breakthrough bleeding. *Contraception*. 2004;70:281-287.
7. Greydanus DE, Patel DR, Pratt HD. *Essential Adolescent Medicine*. New York, NY: McGraw-Hill; 2006.
8. Westoff C. Depot-Medroxyprogesterone acetate injection (Depo-provera): a highly effective contraceptive option with proven long-term safety. *Contraception*. 2003;68(2):75-87.
9. Attaran M, Gidwani G. Adolescent endometriosis: *Obstet Gynecol Clin North Am*. 2003;30:379-390.
10. Schroeder B, Sanfilippo JS. Dysmenorrhea and pelvic pain in adolescents. *Pediatr Clin North Am*. 1999;46: 555-571.

Chapter 172

DYSPHAGIA

Mohammad F. El-Baba, MD

Feeding and swallowing disorders are common complaints in children. *Dysphagia* is defined as *difficulty swallowing,* which derives from the Greek root, *dys,* meaning *difficulty,* and *phagia,* meaning *to eat.* It is not synonymous with the term *odynophagia,* which refers to painful swallowing.

NORMAL DEVELOPMENT OF SWALLOWING

A sucking reflex, present as early as 18 weeks' gestation, is initially disorganized but becomes more organized and efficient for feeding by 34 to 36 weeks' gestation. For the term newborn the suck is mature and efficient for liquid feedings.[1,2] During early infancy the infant develops a more rapid suck rate and higher suck pressure. Tongue movements are differentiated and become more coordinated, preparing the infant for pureed food by 5 to 6 months of age.[3] After this stage, sensory experience with food increases, and oral motor skills expand to handle more textured food. The gag reflex decreases to allow swallowing of an increasing amount of food with more texture. By age 2 years, chewing and tongue movements become more proficient.

NORMAL PHASES OF SWALLOWING

Swallowing is divided into three phases: (1) oral, (2) pharyngeal, and (3) esophageal.[4] These phases allow the food and liquid to move from mouth to stomach efficiently and safely. In the oral phase the food is mixed with saliva and chewed if needed. A single bolus of food is collected between the roof of the mouth and tongue. The bolus is propelled to the posterior of the tongue and then to the pharynx. In infants and young children the suckling swallow allows the liquid to fall from mouth into the pharynx.

The pharyngeal phase is the actual reflexive swallow stimulated by the presence of food on the posterior tongue. During this phase the soft palate raises to keep the food from the nasal passage. The larynx moves up and forward, closing the glottis. The vocal cords come together, the epiglottis closes over the airway, and respirations cease. Food is propelled further by contraction of the pharyngeal muscles and relaxation of the upper esophageal sphincter.

During the esophageal phase, esophageal peristalsis moves the food down the esophagus into the stomach through the relaxed lower esophageal sphincter. The lower esophageal sphincter then returns to the closed tonic state to prevent regurgitation of gastric contents.

CAUSES OF DYSPHAGIA

Any anatomic or functional disorder in the well-coordinated act of swallowing can result in dysphagia,[5] which can be for liquids, solids, or both. In general,

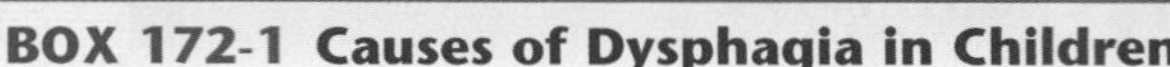

BOX 172-1 Causes of Dysphagia in Children

- Prematurity
- Congenital abnormalities
  - Congenital anomalies of the nasal and oral cavity
    - Cleft lip or palate
    - Choanal atresia or stenosis
    - Craniofacial anomalies (Crouzon syndrome, Apert syndrome, Möbius sequence, Pierre Robin syndrome, Treacher Collins syndrome)
    - Congenital nasal masses (dermoids, encephaloceles)
  - Congenital anomalies of the larynx, trachea, and esophagus
    - Laryngomalacia
    - Laryngeal clefts
    - Laryngeal stenosis and webs
    - Vocal cord paralysis
    - Tracheoesophageal fistula
    - Esophageal atresia
    - Esophageal duplication
- Vascular rings
  - Double aortic arch
  - Right aortic arch with left ligamentum from a descending aorta
  - Innominate artery tracheal compression
- Infectious causes
  - Acute pharyngitis or tonsillitis
  - Peritonsillar and retropharyngeal abscesses
  - Epiglottitis
  - Esophagitis (cytomegalovirus, herpesvirus, *Candida albicans*)
- Inflammatory
  - Esophagitis secondary to gastroesophageal reflux disease
  - Eosinophilic esophagitis
- Neurologic or neuromuscular disorders
  - Hypoxic-ischemic encephalopathy
  - Head trauma
  - Cerebral palsy
  - Congenital malformations (Arnold-Chiari malformation, absent corpus callosum)
  - Degenerative diseases of white and gray matter
  - Brainstem tumors
  - Syringomyelia
  - Infantile spinal muscular atrophy (Werdnig-Hoffmann disease)
  - Diseases of neuromuscular junction
    - Myasthenia gravis
    - Guillain-Barré syndrome
    - Botulism
- Muscular
  - Congenital myopathies
  - Mitochondrial diseases
  - Glycogen storage diseases
  - Congenital muscular dystrophy and myotonic dystrophy
- Traumatic
  - External trauma
  - Intubation injury
- Neoplastic
  - Hemangioma
  - Lymphangioma
- Miscellaneous
  - Foreign-body aspiration
  - Caustic ingestion
  - Motor dysfunction of esophagus (achalasia)
  - Epidermolysis bullosa

mechanical or obstructive factors result in dysphagia for solids. Dysphagia for liquids is more pronounced in patients with neurologic disorders. The causes of dysphagia in children are widespread and include congenital, inflammatory, infectious, systemic, neoplastic, and traumatic reasons (Box 172-1).

Infants born before term or with a birth weight below the 10th percentile for gestational age are at increased risk for developing dysphagia and feeding difficulties.[6]

Central nervous system impairment and developmental delay are common causes of dysphagia in infants and children. Children with gastroesophageal reflux disease often experience some feeding problems and food refusal.[7] Reflux can lead to nausea, vomiting, and esophagitis, all of which may cause feeding to be perceived as an aversive experience. Eosinophilic esophagitis has become a recognized entity that causes dysphagia in adults and children,[8,9] and it should be considered in the differential diagnosis of children with unexplained oral aversion, feeding difficulties, and poor weight gain.

Prolonged tube feeding in infancy or childhood can lead to long-term feeding difficulties. Several factors are implicated in such difficulties and include age at which oral feeding commences, underlying medical conditions, exposure to taste and textures during sensitive periods, aversive experiences, and different methods of delivering tube feeds.[10]

CLINICAL MANIFESTATION

Feeding disorders are commonly seen in early childhood. Minor feeding problems are reported in 25% to 35% of healthy young children, with major feeding disorders observed in 40% to 70% of infants born prematurely or children with chronic medical problems.[4,11] Affected infants or children commonly exhibit feeding difficulties, food refusal, failure to thrive, or sensation of food stuck in the throat or chest. These children may also have drooling, difficulty initiating swallowing, change in dietary habits, aversions to certain food textures, and unexplained weight loss.

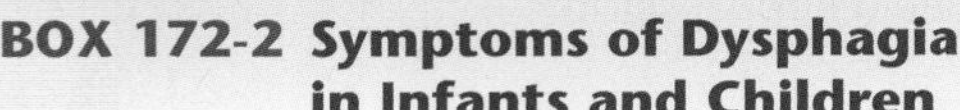

BOX 172-2 Symptoms of Dysphagia in Infants and Children

ORAL PHASE
Failure to initiate or maintain sucking
Prolonged feeding time
Drooling

ORAL HYPERSENSITIVITY
Exaggerated gag reflex
Difficulty making the transition to textured foods
Sensitivity to touch in and around mouth

ORAL HYPOSENSITIVITY
Retaining food in the mouth
Increased drooling

PHARYNGEAL PHASE
Coughing
Choking
Noisy breathing during feeding
Nasopharyngeal reflux

ESOPHAGEAL PHASE
Spitting up or vomiting
Irritability or arching during feeding
Preference for liquid food
Sensation of food stuck in the throat

Some children may experience change in voice, recurrent coughing, or noisy breathing during feeding. Oropharyngeal dysphagia should be considered in young children with recurrent aspiration or unexplained respiratory symptoms.[12] Respiratory symptoms that result from dysphagia vary and may be associated with coughing, chronic congestion, recurrent choking, acute life-threatening events, recurrent pneumonias, and chronic lung disease. The different symptoms of dysphagia in infants and children are summarized in Box 172-2.

EVALUATION

History and Physical Examination

A complete history and thorough physical examination of the child with dysphagia usually leads to the diagnosis and guides the selection of further diagnostic tests. Emphasis should be placed on birth history, neurodevelopmental history, and medical comorbidities. Detailed feeding history should include the type of current diet, texture, route of administration, meal duration, and specific food aversion or aversions. General examination should document any orofacial malformation. The combination of micrognathia and glossoptosis seen in Pierre Robin sequence may cause feeding difficulty in an infant. Cleft lip and palate, including submucous cleft, are important causes of dysphagia. Newborns with choanal stenosis may experience difficulty feeding because of the obligate nasal breathing in the first few months of life. Neurologic examination should include assessment of muscle tone and strength and evaluation of cranial nerve function.[1,13]

A clinical feeding evaluation should be performed by an experienced occupational therapist or speech pathologist. This clinical evaluation includes assessment of posture, positioning, oral structure and function, patient motivation, and interaction between the infant and feeder. A variety of foods, different positions, and adaptive utensils may be used during the examination. Specific symptoms observed during feeding can help identify the underlying disorder. Gagging, coughing, or emesis is usually present in infants with a structural or neurologic disorder. Repeated swallowing after feeding, fussiness, crying, or regurgitation are usually noted in infants with gastroesophageal reflux disease and require further investigation.

Laboratory Evaluation

A complete blood count can be useful as a screening test for infectious or inflammatory conditions. Serum protein and albumen are useful for nutritional assessment. Chromosomal karyotyping, metabolic analysis, or specific DNA tests may be required for a specific diagnosis as directed by physical and neurologic examination. Electromyography, nerve conduction studies, and muscle biopsy may be needed in infants with suspected neuromuscular disorders.

Imaging Studies

Chest radiography is indicated in patients with suspected pneumonia or chronic lung disease. Infants or children with recurrent stridor or upper airways obstruction may require magnified airway radiography. Computed tomography or magnetic resonance imaging of the brain may be especially helpful in patients with suspected central nervous system injury or structural abnormalities.

Diagnostic Studies

Upper Gastrointestinal Barium Study

Barium radiography plays a role in evaluating esophageal dysphagia. It is valuable in assessing anatomic or structural abnormalities, such as strictures, fistulas, masses, or intestinal rotational anomalies. Barium studies are usually more sensitive than endoscopy in the evaluation of patients suspected to have achalasia or vascular ring. In most cases, vascular rings appear as a persistent indentation of the esophagus.[14]

Videofluorographic Swallowing Study

The videofluorographic swallowing study (VFSS), also known as the modified barium study, is considered the gold standard for assessment of the oral and pharyngeal stages of swallowing and allows the clinician to determine the risk of aspiration.[14-16] Conducted jointly by a radiologist and a speech pathologist or occupational therapist, the VFSS provides evidence of all categories of oropharyngeal swallowing dysfunction, which include inability or excessive delay in initiation of pharyngeal swallowing, aspiration of food, nasopharyngeal regurgitation, and residue of food within the pharyngeal cavity after swallowing.

During this study the child will drink or eat foods mixed with barium while radiographic images are observed and recorded. Patients' difficulties with different food textures can be identified and compatible diets planned. The definitive finding of aspiration will permit the clinician to make suggestions to avoid the offending consistency, usually thin liquids. Furthermore, the study allows for testing of the efficacy of compensatory dietary modifications, postures, and swallowing maneuvers so that the observed dysfunction can be corrected.

Fiberoptic Endoscopic Evaluation of Swallowing

In fiberoptic endoscopic evaluation of swallowing (FEES) a fiberoptic endoscope is introduced into the nose and advanced into the laryngopharyngeal area, permitting observation of the pharyngeal phase of swallowing. A swallowing assessment is performed with liquids and a variety of textures, if developmentally appropriate. Typically, dye is added to the food to provide better visualization and to determine residual pooling of food versus saliva. The feeding parameters evaluated in this study are laryngeal penetration and aspiration.[16] FEES, combined with laryngopharyngeal sensory testing, has shown that patients with a higher laryngopharyngeal sensory threshold are more likely to experience laryngeal penetration and aspiration during a feeding assessment.[17,18] The ability to initiate airway closure with stimulation demonstrates airway protection. FEES and sensory testing may be particularly valuable for the evaluation of swallowing safety in children who refuse to ingest adequate amounts of barium to perform VFSS.

Esophagogastroduodenoscopy

Endoscopy is suggested for most patients with dysphagia of esophageal origin to establish or confirm a diagnosis, to seek evidence of esophagitis, and, when appropriate, to implement therapy.[19] It is particularly useful in evaluating patients suspected of having strictures, webs, mucosal inflammatory lesions, or specific infections. Endoscopic and histologic features are required for the diagnosis of eosinophilic esophagitis. A normal appearance of the esophagus during endoscopy does not exclude histopathological esophagitis; subtle mucosal changes such as erythema and pallor may be observed in the absence of esophagitis. During endoscopy, esophageal biopsy should be performed to detect microscopic esophagitis and to exclude causes of esophagitis other than gastroesophageal reflux.

Esophageal Manometry

Esophageal manometry, the standard test for disorders of esophageal motility, is especially useful in establishing a diagnosis of achalasia and for detecting esophageal motor abnormalities associated with autoimmune diseases.

Esophageal pH Probe Study

Esophageal pH monitoring, a valid and reliable measure of acid reflux, is useful to establish the presence of abnormal acid reflux, to determine whether a temporal association exists between acid reflux and frequently occurring symptoms, and to assess the adequacy of therapy in patients who do not respond to treatment with acid suppression.

Scintigraphy

Scintigraphy is useful in the evaluation of gastric emptying and can also demonstrate episodes of aspiration detected during a 1-hour study or on images obtained up to 24 hours after the test feeding is administered. The role of scintigraphy in diagnosing gastroesophageal reflux disease in infants and children is unclear.

MANAGEMENT

Management of children with dysphagia often involves a multidisciplinary approach, the aims of which are to identify and characterize dysphagia and identify the underlying cause whenever possible. Special emphasis should be placed on detection of treatable conditions, which include surgically or endoscopically treatable structural abnormalities, inflammatory conditions (eg, reflux esophagitis, eosinophilic esophagitis), specific infections, and underlying systemic conditions.

The goals of managing dysphagia are to reduce aspiration, improve the ability to eat and swallow, and optimize nutritional status. Feeding therapy for infants and children may include the strategies described in the following subsections.[1,20]

Normalization of Posture and Tone

Head and trunk control are crucial to the development of oral motor skills. Children with neurologic abnormalities frequently have poor head control and poor trunk stability. Occupational and physical therapy can be used to improve head control, and neck and trunk tone and posture as a basis for improved oral motor function.

Adaptation of Food and Feeding Equipment

Food and feeding equipment may be adapted by changing the attributes of food and liquids, such as bolus volume, consistency, temperature, and taste. Adjustments in feeding schedule may be beneficial for children receiving continuous tube feeds with supplemental food orally. The feeds can be changed gradually to bolus feeds to stimulate the child's appetite. The rate of feeding should be paced to allow sufficient time to swallow before giving another bite. In addition, the bottle or utensils may be changed according to the child's needs.

Oral Motor Therapy

Oral motor therapy is focused on improving the oral phase of feeding and may include stimulation with stroking, stretching, brushing, icing, tapping, and vibrating areas of the face and mouth.

Nutritional Support

Management of dysphagia must focus on meeting the child's nutritional needs for adequate growth. When a patient is unable to achieve adequate nutrition and hydration by mouth, supplemental feedings through a nasogastric tube or a percutaneous endoscopic gastrostomy may be necessary. The presence of a feeding tube is not a contraindication for therapy. Many children with feeding disorders have neurologic or anatomic abnormalities that cannot be corrected, making oral feeding difficult or unsafe.

MANAGEMENT OF ASSOCIATED DISORDERS

Associated disorders, such as gastroesophageal reflux disease, eosinophilic esophagitis, and chronic lung disease, may also need to be specifically managed. Application of synchronized neuromuscular electrical stimulation to cervical swallowing muscles (VitaStim™ therapy) has been shown to improve oral intake and help restore normal swallowing mechanism in adults,[21,22] but empirical data are lacking to support its use in children.

WHEN TO REFER

A referral to a pediatric dysphagia center, if available, provides the most complete method to establish a diagnosis and render a management plan. Members of the team vary from center to center and usually include a gastroenterologist, otolaryngologist, physical medicine and rehabilitation specialist, surgeon, occupational therapist and pediatric dietitian. Referral is warranted:

- When symptoms are persistent
- When the cause of dysphagia is unclear
- On evidence of aspiration

WHEN TO ADMIT

- Severe feeding difficulties
- Malnutrition
- Failure to thrive
- Dehydration
- Aspiration

SUGGESTED RESOURCES

Arvedson JC. Management of pediatric dysphagia. *Otolaryngol Clin North Am.* 1998;31(3):453-476.

Dusick A. Investigation and management of dysphagia. *Semin Pediatr Neurol.* 2003;10(4):255-264.

Kosko JR, Moser JD, Erhart N, et al. Differential diagnosis of dysphagia in children. *Otolaryngol Clin North Am.* 1998; 31(3):435-451.

Miller CK, Willging JP. Advances in the evaluation and management of pediatric dysphagia. *Curr Opin Otolaryngol Head Neck Surg.* 2003;11(6):442-446.

Rudolph CD, Link DT. Feeding disorders in infants and children. *Pediatr Clin North Am.* 2002;49(1):97-112, vi.

REFERENCES

1. Dusick A. Investigation and management of dysphagia. *Semin Pediatr Neurol.* 2003;10(4)255-264.
2. Bu'Lock F, Woolridge MW, Baum JD. Development of co-ordination of sucking, swallowing and breathing: ultrasound study of term and preterm infants. *Dev Med Child Neurol.* 1990;32(8):669-678.
3. McGowan JS, Marsh RR, Fowler SM, et al. Developmental patterns of normal nutritive sucking in infants. *Dev Med Child Neurol.* 1991;33(10):891-897.
4. Rudolph CD, Link DT. Feeding disorders in infants and children. *Pediatr Clin North Am.* 2002;49(1):97-112, vi.
5. Kosko JR, Moser JD, Erhart N, et al. Differential diagnosis of dysphagia in children. *Otolaryngol Clin North Am.* 1998;31(3):435-451.
6. Rommel N, De Meyer AM, Feenstra L, et al. The complexity of feeding problems in 700 infants and young children presenting to a tertiary care institution. *J Pediatr Gastroenterol Nutr.* 2003;37(1):75-84.
7. Mathisen B, Worrall L, Masel J, et al. Feeding problems in infants with gastro-oesophageal reflux disease: a controlled study. *J Paediatr Child Health.* 1999;35(2):163-169.
8. Pentiuk SP, Miller CK, Kaul A. Eosinophilic esophagitis in infants and toddlers. *Dysphagia.* 2007;2(1)2:44-48.
9. Furuta GT, Straumann A. Review article: the pathogenesis and management of eosinophilic oesophagitis. *Aliment Pharmacol Ther.* 2006;24(2):173-182.
10. Mason SJ, Harris G, Blissett J. Tube feeding in infancy: implications for the development of normal eating and drinking skills. *Dysphagia.* 2005;20(1):46-61.
11. Hawdon JM, Beauregard N, Slattery J, et al. Identification of neonates at risk of developing feeding problems in infancy. *Dev Med Child Neurol.* 2000;42(4):235-239.
12. Lefton-Greif MA, Carroll JL, Loughlin GM. Long-term follow-up of oropharyngeal dysphagia in children without apparent risk factors. *Pediatr Pulmonol.* 2006; 41(11):1040-1048.
13. Garg BP. Dysphagia in children: an overview. *Semin Pediatr Neurol.* 2003;10(4):252-254.
14. Furlow B. Barium swallow. *Radiol Technol.* 2004; 76(1): 49-58.
15. Palmer JB, Drennan JC, Baba M. Evaluation and treatment of swallowing impairments. *Am Fam Physician.* 2000;61(8):2453-2462.
16. Cook IJ, Kahrilas PJ. AGA technical review on management of oropharyngeal dysphagia. *Gastroenterology.* 1999;116(2):455-478.
17. Link DT, Willging JP, Miller CK, et al. Pediatric laryngopharyngeal sensory testing during flexible endoscopic evaluation of swallowing: feasible and correlative. *Ann Otol Rhinol Laryngol.* 2000;109(10 pt 1):899-905.
18. Willging JP, Thompson DM. Pediatric FEESST: fiberoptic endoscopic evaluation of swallowing with sensory testing. *Curr Gastroenterol Rep.* 2005;7(3):240-243.
19. Spechler SJ. AGA technical review on treatment of patients with dysphagia caused by benign disorders of the distal esophagus. *Gastroenterology.* 1999;117(1): 233-254.
20. Arvedson JC. Management of pediatric dysphagia. *Otolaryngol Clin North Am.* 1998;31(3):453-476.
21. Shaw GY, Sechtem PR, Searl J, et al. Transcutaneous neuromuscular electrical stimulation (VitalStim) curative therapy for severe dysphagia: myth or reality? *Ann Otol Rhinol Laryngol.* 2007;116(1):36-44.
22. Miller CK, Willging JP. Advances in the evaluation and management of pediatric dysphagia. *Curr Opin Otolaryngol Head Neck Surg.* 2003;11(6):442-446.

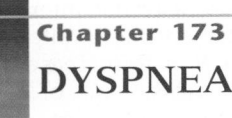

Chapter 173 DYSPNEA

Jay H. Mayefsky, MD, MPH

Dyspnea is the uncomfortable feeling of not being able to satisfy *air hunger.* Patients may complain of not being able to catch their breath or of a suffocating feeling. Dyspnea is a symptom, a subjective complaint by the patient that describes the sensation caused by an underlying disorder. As with any subjective complaint, the diagnosis of dyspnea and its cause in an infant or young child can be problematic. Therefore, to evaluate fully a child in respiratory distress, the pediatric health care professional must be familiar with the pathophysiological features, signs, and common causes of dyspnea. With the aid of the medical history, physical examination, and appropriate laboratory tests, the condition can be diagnosed and therapy initiated.

PATHOPHYSIOLOGICAL FEATURES

Dyspnea is seen most commonly with exercise because of the increased work of breathing necessary to keep up with the body's increased metabolic demands. The sensation is probably transmitted from stretch receptors in the chest wall muscles to the central nervous system (CNS). Chemoreceptors, sensing changes in arterial pH, oxygen, and carbon dioxide concentrations, as well as chest wall proprioceptors, lung stretch receptors, and mechanoreceptors in the heart, skeletal muscles, and upper airway, play a role.[1-4] The transmission is processed in the CNS, causing the individual to experience the sensation of dyspnea. With exercise, the person who has dyspnea is aware of an increased ventilatory effort. A person who has obstructive or restrictive lung disease also experiences difficulty breathing, as will someone who has a neuromuscular disease who believes that insufficient air is being received.

To satisfy their oxygen needs, children who have dyspnea must increase their minute ventilation ($\dot{V}_E$), working harder to do so. In normal breathing, respiratory muscles work only during inspiration, and the diaphragm does most of the work. The work of inspiration is the sum of the work necessary to overcome the elastic forces of the lung, the tissue viscosity of the lung and chest wall, and airway resistance.[5] When any of these factors is increased (eg, elastic force and tissue viscosity in restrictive pulmonary disease, resistance in obstructive airway disease), the work of inspiration must increase to maintain adequate $\dot{V}_E$. The accessory muscles of inspiration (the sternocleidomastoid, anterior serratus, and external intercostal muscles) are recruited to accomplish this task. Contraction of these muscles causes forceful expansion of the thorax, resulting in an unusually large negative intrathoracic pressure. This negative pressure draws in the soft tissues of the chest wall and creates one of the classic signs of dyspnea: retractions. Retractions may be seen in the suprasternal, infrasternal, intercostal, subcostal, and supraclavicular areas. An alternative way to maintain an adequate $\dot{V}_E$ is to increase the rate of breathing, hence the 2nd classic sign of dyspnea: tachypnea. Nasal flaring and grunting are other signs seen and heard during respiration.

Little energy is expended during normal expiration. Relaxation of the diaphragm, elastic recoil of the lungs and chest wall, and compression of the lungs by the intraabdominal organs force air from the lungs. In obstructive airway disease the force generated by these processes may not be great enough to effect adequate expiration. In a child who has tachypnea the elastic recoil may not be fast enough to allow adequate exhalation between breaths. In either instance the accessory muscles of expiration are used. The abdominal recti muscles contract and force the abdominal contents against the diaphragm to compress the lungs, and the internal intercostal muscles contract to pull the ribs downward and to create a positive intrathoracic pressure to force the air from the lungs. The contractions of these muscles provide the most important expiratory sign of dyspnea.

Although dyspnea is a respiratory symptom, it may be caused by primary disorders in other body systems. Cardiac, hematologic, metabolic, circulatory, and psychogenic causes must be considered in the differential diagnosis of dyspnea. The child's age is also important because various disorders occur with different frequency at different ages.

History

The history is essential. It starts with a complete description of the dyspnea. The patient or parent should be asked whether the onset was sudden (eg, inhaled foreign body, lung collapse) or evolved over several hours (eg, asthma, diabetic ketoacidosis). The patient should also be asked about the duration of the illness, the frequency of attacks of dyspnea, and whether a trigger or event is apparent that is temporally related to the onset of dyspnea. An attempt should be made to quantify the severity of the dyspnea. This task may be accomplished by asking to what degree daily activities are restricted by shortness of breath. However, given that dyspnea is a subjective sensation, its perceived severity can be affected by the patient's anxiety level, previous experiences, perceived control over the symptom, perceived consequences of the symptom, and available coping resources.[6] The chronic use of medications such as inhaled corticosteroids and β_2-agonists have also been shown to have an effect on the patient's perception of dyspnea.[7,8] Therefore, whenever possible, objective measures as discussed here should be obtained.

An inquiry should also be made as to whether the dyspnea is affected by the patient's position. With unilateral lung disease, dyspnea may get worse when the patient lies with the affected lung down. Dyspnea that worsens with the recumbency is often due to left-ventricular failure, obstructive airway disease, or muscle weakness. Dyspnea in the upright position relieved by lying down usually is due to intracardiac, vascular, or parenchymal lung shunts.

The patient should also be asked about associated symptoms such as cough, wheezing, sputum production, and pleuritic pain. In addition, a history of other known illnesses, allergies, illnesses in the family, medication, and environmental exposure must be obtained.

Clinical Evaluation

A thorough physical examination is always indicated, with special attention paid to the aforementioned systems. The most useful laboratory tests are the complete blood count and peripheral blood smear, arterial blood gas measurement, and radiographic studies of the airways and lungs. Measurement of arterial oxygen saturation by pulse oximetry is invaluable for its ability to assess oxygenation status quickly and noninvasively. Pulmonary function tests are helpful but may not be immediately available for evaluation of an acutely ill patient.

ETIOLOGY AND CLINICAL PRESENTATION

Pulmonary Disease

Pulmonary disease that causes dyspnea can be classified as obstructive, restrictive, or vascular.

Obstructive Pulmonary Disease

Obstructive disease is characterized by narrowing of airways that can be caused by intraluminal objects (mucus, foreign bodies, or tumor), intramural factors (smooth-muscle contraction, edema, or bronchomalacia), or extramural compression (tumor or lymph nodes). The narrowing increases both airway resistance and turbulent flow in the airways. If a fixed obstruction is present, then affected areas of the lungs will become atelectatic. With a ball valve–type obstruction (ie, air can get into the lungs but not out), air is trapped, and affected areas become hyperinflated. In either case, an imbalance occurs between pulmonary ventilation and perfusion, and oxygen exchange is adversely affected.[9] All of these processes force the patient to work harder to maintain adequate ventilation; hence dyspnea ensues.

During normal respiration, inspiration and expiration are of equal length. With a fixed degree of obstruction, both processes are equally prolonged. If the obstruction varies and is extrathoracic (ie, above the vocal cords), then inspiration is affected more because the negative intraairway pressure during inspiration tends to collapse the extrathoracic airway. The characteristic sign of such an obstruction is inspiratory stridor (see Chapter 222, Stridor).

If the obstruction varies and affects the intrathoracic airways, then expiration is prolonged because the positive intrathoracic pressure tends to collapse these airways during expiration. If larger airways are involved, then rhonchi are present. Airflow across an obstruction in smaller airways generates wheezing.

A paradoxical pulse and cyanosis are sensitive, but nonspecific, signs of severe obstruction. Patients who have chronic obstructive disease may be barrel chested and have signs of chronic hypoxia, such as clubbing. Children who have a systemic disease, such as cystic fibrosis, will also show the extrapulmonary manifestations of this disease. The common causes of obstructive airway disease in childhood are shown in Box 173-1. Obstruction in the nose or nasopharynx should not be overlooked, especially in infants who are obligatory nasal breathers.

Blood gas values may be normal with mild obstructive disease. As the disease progresses, hypoxemia is the 1st sign of abnormality seen. Hypocapnia, initially

BOX 173-1 Causes of Obstructive Pulmonary Disease

NEWBORNS
- Choanal atresia or stenosis
- Dermoid cyst
- Encephalocele
- Nasolacrimal duct cyst
- Hemangioma
- Vocal cord paralysis
- Pierre Robin syndrome
- Ankyloglossia (tongue tie)
- Pertussis
- Tracheal stenosis (postintubation)

INFANTS
- Foreign body
- Vascular ring
- Tracheal web
- Bronchiolitis
- Asthma
- Cystic fibrosis
- Bronchomalacia
- Pyogenic thyroid
- Accessory thyroid

CHILDREN AND ADOLESCENTS
- Foreign body (airway or esophagus)
- Asthma
- Adenopathy:
  - Lymphoma
  - Systemic lupus erythematosus
  - Tuberculosis
  - Sarcoidosis
- Croup
- Epiglottitis
- Retropharyngeal abscess
- Enlarged tonsils or adenoids
- Cystic fibrosis
- Anaphylaxis
- Laryngeal tumor
- Vocal cord tumor
- Tracheal tumors
- Mediastinal tumors
- Vocal cord polyp
- Laryngeal trauma
- Supraglottitis
- Diphtheria
- Bacterial tracheitis
- Ingestion of caustic substance
- Crack cocaine
- Trauma
- Environmental or occupational inhaled toxin exposure

Modified from Mukai S, Mukai C, Asaoka K. Ankyloglossia with deviation of the epiglottis and larynx. *Ann Otol Rhinol Laryngol* 1991;153:3-20; Reino AJ, Lawson W. Upper airway distress in crack cocaine users. *Otolaryngol Head Neck Surg* 1993;109:937-940.

seen as a reflection of increased $\dot{V}_E$, is replaced by hypercapnia as the maldistribution of ventilation and perfusion increases. The patient then tires, and respiratory failure occurs.

The chest radiograph may reveal whether the cause of the obstruction is inside or outside the airway. In many instances, hyperinflation with an increased anteroposterior chest diameter and flattened diaphragm are seen. Atelectasis may appear with a fixed obstruction. Fluoroscopic examination or inspiratory and expiratory radiographs may be useful in localizing a ball valve–type obstruction. However, an important point to remember is that many foreign bodies are radiolucent and will not be seen on radiographic examination. If a radiolucent foreign body is suspected, then laryngoscopy, bronchoscopy, or even esophagoscopy may be required.

Restrictive Pulmonary Disease

The cardinal features of restrictive pulmonary disease are a reduction in lung volume and pulmonary compliance secondary to pathological changes in the lung parenchyma or the pleura, deformities of the chest wall, or neuromuscular disease. Decreased volume necessitates an increase in respiratory rate to maintain a normal $\dot{V}_E$. The work of breathing must be increased to overcome the reduced compliance. Because breathing rapidly with small tidal volumes is more energy efficient than breathing slowly and attempt to expand the chest against great restrictive forces, children who have restrictive diseases characteristically have rapid, shallow respirations.[9] The common pediatric causes of restrictive pulmonary disease are listed in Box 173-2.

Observation of the child often reveals skeletal and neuromuscular causes. Pleural and parenchymal diseases are detected best by palpation, percussion, and auscultation of the chest. Tactile fremitus can demonstrate pulmonary consolidation or pleural effusion. Careful percussion reveals effusions, consolidation, and abnormal diaphragmatic excursion. On auscultation, rales characteristic of alveolar disease may be heard, and changes in whispered pectoriloquy and egophony can be detected.

The complete blood count may be helpful in diagnosing an infectious cause. Arterial blood gases have a characteristic pattern of hypoxemia and hypocapnia. The chest radiograph is useful in that it can demonstrate decreased lung volume, pleural thickening and effusions, increased interstitial markings, parenchymal consolidation, skeletal deformities, and abnormal movement of the diaphragm.

Vascular Pulmonary Disease

Vascular lung disease is characterized by a decrease in the size of the pulmonary vascular bed. In the neonate, this disease is often due to persistent pulmonary hypertension of the newborn.[10] Microemboli have also been reported in the lungs of infants who are in severe respiratory distress.[11] In older children, the most common cause of vascular pulmonary disease is intimal hyperplasia after persistent left-to-right shunting and resultant pulmonary hypertension. The size of the pulmonary vascular bed can also be reduced by obstruction caused by thromboembolic disease, obliteration (eg, vasculitis),[12] or destruction, as in emphysema. The reduced blood flow through the lungs results in arterial hypoxemia and hypercapnia, which, in turn, lead to the symptoms and signs of dyspnea.

In addition to the common signs of dyspnea, the child who has vascular lung disease may have signs of pulmonary edema and pleural effusion. Systemic signs of right-sided heart failure caused by pulmonary hypertension or left-sided heart failure that was the cause of the pulmonary hypertension may be present. The cardiac findings observed with pulmonary hypertension are an accentuated P_2, paradoxical splitting of 2nd and 3rd heart sound, a pulmonary ejection click, and a right-ventricular heave.

An electrocardiogram is helpful in the diagnosis of right-ventricular hypertrophy. A chest radiograph may reveal increased right-ventricular size, enlargement of the pulmonary artery silhouette, decreased pulmonary blood flow in advanced disease, or increased flow early in the course of disease, with a left-to-right shunt.

Exercise-Induced Dyspnea

As described earlier, dyspnea is a normal sensation felt during exercise, especially for children with a sedentary lifestyle and poor cardiovascular conditioning. However, if the dyspnea is severe, occurs after only minimal exertion, or is troublesome to the patient, then investigations into the cause of exercise-induced dyspnea (EID) are warranted.

Asthma is the most common cause of pathological EID. However, when other signs and symptoms of asthma are absent, or when pretreatment with beta-agonistic medications does not prevent EID, then other causes must be considered. These causes include vocal cord dysfunction, exercise-induced laryngomalacia, exercise-induced hyperventilation, restrictive airway disease caused by skeletal abnormalities such as scoliosis and pectus deformities, or cardiac arrhythmias that occur only during exercise.[13,14]

Cardiac Disease

Dyspnea occurs with cardiac disease when insufficient blood is pumped to the lungs as a result of congenital structural anomalies in the heart, pump failure (myocarditis or cardiomyopathy), restrictive pericarditis, arrhythmia, or, as already described, secondary pulmonary hypertension. Heart disease must be considered in all dyspneic newborns and older children who have a history of congenital heart disease. In the neonate, pulmonary disease can often be differentiated from cyanotic heart disease through a hyperoxia test. The nature of the cardiac defect can be delineated with the help of a thorough cardiac examination, an electrocardiogram, a chest radiograph, and an echocardiogram.

A trivial respiratory infection in a healthy child may cause severe respiratory insufficiency in a child who has cardiopulmonary disease. Indeed, the mortality of infants who have respiratory syncytial viral pneumonia and congenital heart disease has been shown to exceed significantly the mortality of children who have normal hearts.[15]

BOX 173-2 Causes of Restrictive Pulmonary Disease

NEWBORNS

Hyaline membrane disease
Hypoplastic lungs
Pulmonary agenesis
Eventration of the diaphragm
Meconium aspiration
Pneumonia (group B streptococci or gram-negative organisms)
Diaphragmatic paralysis
Osteogenesis imperfecta
Central nervous system depression:
- Hypoxia
- Congenital
- Maternal drugs

Congenital myasthenia gravis
Aspiration
Pulmonary edema:
- Septicemia
- Congenital heart disease

INFANTS

Pneumonia:
- Bacterial
- Viral
- Aspiration

Bronchopulmonary dysplasia
Wilson-Mikity syndrome
Hamman-Rich syndrome
Pulmonary edema
Infantile botulism
Congenital lobar emphysema

CHILDREN AND ADOLESCENTS

Skeletal:
- Kyphoscoliosis
- Ankylosing spondylitis
- Pectus excavatum
- Crush chest injury

Parenchymal:
- Pneumonia
- Hypersensitivity pneumonitis
- Systemic lupus erythematosus
- Scleroderma
- Fibrosis
- Toxin inhalation
- Granulomatous disease
- Drugs (eg, antineoplastic agents, narcotics)
- Carcinoma
- Fat embolus
- Pneumothorax
- Pneumomediastinum

Smoke inhalation
Pulmonary infarction
Pulmonary edema:
- Congestive heart failure
- Sepsis
- Intracranial disease
- Croup
- Epiglottitis

Neuromuscular:
- Cord transection
- Myasthenia gravis
- Muscular dystrophy
- Multiple sclerosis
- Guillain-Barré syndrome
- Pickwickian syndrome
- Toxins

Pleural effusion:
- Pneumonia
- Malignancy
- Cardiac disease
- Hepatic disease
- Renal disease
- Rheumatologic disease

Hypoproteinemia
Renal failure
Tumor
Pulmonary infarction

Modified from Rietveld S. Paradoxical breathlessness in asthma. *Behav Res Ther* 2000;38:1193-1203; Ducker TB, Simmons RL, Martin AM. Pulmonary edema as a complication of intracranial disease. *Am J Dis Child* 1969;118:638-641; Kanter RK, Watchko JF. Pulmonary edema associated with upper airway obstruction. *Am J Dis Child* 1984;138:356-358.

Hematologic Disease

If the oxygen-carrying capacity of the blood is reduced sufficiently, then tissue hypoxia ensues. The resultant drop in arterial pH signals the CNS and stimulates the onset of dyspnea. Severe anemia, whether chronic or acute, congenital or acquired, can cause dyspnea. The oxygen-carrying capacity can also be lowered when the hemoglobin's ability to bind oxygen is reduced, seen most commonly with carbon monoxide poisoning but also with cyanide poisoning and methemoglobinemia. In any of these cases the child will not be cyanotic. The blue color of cyanosis is caused by at least a 5-g/dL reduction of hemoglobin in the blood.[9] Such a concentration of reduced hemoglobin is not found in anemia uncomplicated by other diseases or in the other conditions cited. Conversely, an infant with polycythemia whose blood is hyperviscous may have dyspnea from poor perfusion. Because such an infant has an increased hemoglobin concentration and more oxygen is removed from the hemoglobin as a result of decreased flow, the child may be cyanotic (having more than 5-g/dL unsaturated hemoglobin) and not hypoxic. An extreme elevation of leukocyte or platelet counts can also cause blood hyperviscosity and dyspnea.

Children with anemia, even though they may have tissue hypoxia and be dyspneic, are usually not hypoxemic; that is, the arterial oxygen tension measured by blood gas analysis is in the normal range.

Metabolic Disease

Disorders that increase the body's rate of metabolism and therefore oxygen consumption can cause dyspnea. Examples are hyperthyroidism[16] and fever. Metabolic disorders associated with an increased production of hydrogen ion and carbon dioxide cause a dyspnea-like breathing pattern to help rid the body of the carbon dioxide. The classic example is Kussmaul breathing with diabetic ketoacidosis. Aspirin poisoning can be characterized similarly. In addition, children who have various muscle enzyme deficiencies, especially those affecting the mitochondria, may have dyspnea as a result of their increased acid production and decreased work tolerance.[17,18] In chronic renal failure the kidney's inability to remove acid from the blood adequately is the underlying cause of dyspnea. The history, physical examination, and appropriate laboratory tests should facilitate the proper diagnosis of these diseases.

If oxygen cannot reach the tissues, then the body responds with dyspnea, cardiovascular collapse, and shock.

Obesity

Dyspnea, especially with exertion, is a common complaint of obese children because their metabolic requirement for a given amount of work is increased.[19] In addition, the diaphragm of an obese child must move against increased abdominal pressure, and the chest wall is heavier; thus more energy must be expended to maintain $\dot{V}_E$.

Asthma does not appear to play an important role as a cause of dyspnea in obese individuals. Although obesity is a risk factor for self-reported asthma, bronchodilator use, and dyspnea on exertion, obese individuals have a lower risk of objective airway obstruction as compared with persons who are not obese.[20]

Treatment of dyspnea in obesity should include dietary regulation and an exercise program graded to keep pace with the child's level of exercise tolerance.

Pregnancy

Dyspnea is normal during pregnancy[21] and occurs during the 1st or 2nd trimester. Seventy-six percent of women complain of dyspnea by the 31st week of gestation. The sensation is due to a subjective awareness of the hyperventilation normally present during pregnancy.

The normal dyspnea of pregnancy can be differentiated easily from dyspnea arising from heart or lung disease. First, the woman who has dyspnea of pregnancy has no other symptoms of cardiac or pulmonary disease. Second, dyspnea of pregnancy begins early and plateaus or improves as term approaches. Dyspnea resulting from heart disease begins during the 2nd half of pregnancy and is worst during the 7th month. Finally, dyspnea of pregnancy is rarely severe, rarely occurs at rest, and does not interfere with the activities of daily life.

Intravenous Drug Use

Several causes of dyspnea must be considered with a history of intravenous drug use. Heroin can cause bronchospasm that responds to bronchodilator medications. In addition, heroin and other opioids may precipitate pulmonary edema.[22] Therapies consist of oxygen, diuretics, and naloxone.

Infections also may cause dyspnea in intravenous drug users. The most common infection is community-acquired pneumonia. However, opportunistic pulmonary infections, tuberculosis, and bacterial endocarditis with associated septic pulmonary emboli or heart failure must be considered.

Finally, talc granulomatosis, which can lead to chronic mild to moderate dyspnea, must be considered. It is caused by intravenous injection of dissolved opioid tablets, with deposition of foreign bodies in the pulmonary vasculature and granuloma formation.

Psychogenic Cause

Stress or hysteria may cause dyspnea.[23] A complete history and thorough physical examination are keys to the diagnosis. Affected patients are tachypneic and complain of air *hunger*. When dyspnea is caused by pulmonary or cardiac conditions, the shortness of breath worsens with increasing activity and improves with rest. However, when dyspnea is due to hysteria, it does not improve with rest and may worsen. The patients also often complain of chest pain and sigh more often. Contrary to previous belief, tetany is an uncommon accompaniment of hysterical dyspnea.

The findings of the physical examination are usually normal. However, stress-induced paradoxical adduction of the vocal cords during inspiration has been reported.[24] Patients who have this disorder may have either stridor or wheezing. In this instance the diagnosis of hysterical dyspnea is one of exclusion, and it can be made only after pathological lesions in the airways and lungs have been ruled out.

In most instances, the only laboratory abnormality found with hysteria-induced dyspnea is a diminished arterial carbon dioxide tension.

Treatment consists of calm reassurance and, occasionally, mild sedation. If the condition is chronic, then interventions to reduce stress and gain insight into the cause of the dyspnea such as psychotherapy and hypnosis[25] may be required. When paradoxical vocal cord motion is the cause, the patient should also be taught laryngeal relaxation techniques.

MANAGEMENT

Severe dyspnea is a medical emergency. If not treated promptly, a child who has dyspnea may then progress rapidly to respiratory failure and death. First, the adequacy of the airway must be assessed. Foreign bodies must be removed and anatomic obstructions bypassed with endotracheal intubation or, in rare cases, tracheotomy. Bronchospasm, when present, should be treated with beta-agonistic drugs.

Subsequently, the efficacy of the child's ventilation must be evaluated. Normally, breathing uses 2% to 3% of the total body energy expenditure. When the work of breathing is increased during dyspnea, this amount may rise to 30% or more. Such a degree of energy expenditure cannot be continued indefinitely, and the child tires. Even after an obstruction is removed, the child may still be unable to effect adequate ventilation.

In this instance, or in the case of neuromuscular disease, the child requires mechanical ventilation.

Once ventilation is established, the cardiovascular system's ability to deliver oxygen to the tissues must be appraised by evaluating the heart, peripheral circulation, intravascular volume status, and the blood's oxygen-carrying capacity. Therapy with vasopressors, fluids, blood transfusions, or diuretics should be initiated when indicated. Although not all children who have dyspnea require supplemental oxygen, every child should have oxygen administered until the cause of the dyspnea is known. Once the patient's condition has stabilized, the search for the underlying cause of the dyspnea should progress urgently, but calmly. At this point, a detailed history can be elicited, a full physical examination can be performed, and a chest radiograph and appropriate blood tests can be obtained. When the diagnosis is made, specific therapy can be initiated.

When dyspnea is caused by a chronic illness, no satisfactory therapy may be available to treat the underlying disease. However, simply relieving the dyspnea can improve the child's functional ability and quality of life significantly.[26] Several modalities can be used to treat the symptom of dyspnea in a chronically ill child.[27,28] Sedatives and narcotics reduce $\dot{V}_E$ and thereby diminish the intensity of the breathless feeling.[29,30] Prostaglandin inhibitors and beta-agonists may blunt the perception of dyspnea without affecting ventilation.[31] Theophylline may improve diaphragmatic contractility. Continuous supplemental oxygen with or without continuous positive airway pressure reduces ventilatory drive.[32] Children who have chronic obstructive pulmonary disease may be taught to breathe through pursed lips, reducing respiratory rate, increasing tidal volume, and diminishing the sensation of dyspnea. Hypnosis has proved useful in some patients, and others have reported a decrease in dyspnea when seated next to an open window or a blowing fan.[33]

Exercise and proper nutrition are helpful in maintaining or increasing inspiratory muscle mass and thereby in reducing the perceived magnitude of dyspnea.[26,34,35] Finally, because dyspnea is a subjective complaint, a significant psychological contribution exists to its perceived severity.[36] The child's emotional state, behavior, and personality must be monitored because psychosocial intervention may be indicated.

WHEN TO REFER

- Chronic pulmonary disease
- Congenital or acquired heart disease
- Metabolic disease
- Conditions requiring endoscopy or surgical procedures

WHEN TO ADMIT

- Respiratory failure
- Impending respiratory failure
- Hypoxia while breathing room air

SUGGESTED RESOURCES

Abu-Hasan M, Tannous B, Weinberger M. Exercise-induced dyspnea in children and adolescents. If not asthma then what? *Ann Allergy Asthma Immunol.* 2005;94:366-371.

Anbar RD. Stressors associated with dyspnea in childhood: patients' insights and a case report. *Am J Clin Hypn.* 2004; 47:93-101.

Killian KJ, Campbell EJ. Dyspnea and exercise. *Annu Rev Physiol.* 1983;45:465-479.

Manning HL, Schwartzstein RM. Pathophysiology of dyspnea. *N Engl J Med.* 1995; 333:1547-1553.

Ottanelli R, Rosi E, Romagnoli I, et al. Do inhaled corticosteroids affect perception of dyspnea during bronchoconstriction in asthma? *Chest.* 2001;120:770-777.

Rosenow EC. The spectrum of drug-induced pulmonary disease. *Ann Intern Med.* 1972;77:977-991.

Sin DD, Jones RL, Man SF. Obesity is a risk factor for dyspnea but not for airflow obstruction. *Arch Intern Med.* 2002; 62:1477-1481.

Tobin MJ. Dyspnea: pathophysiologic basis, clinical presentation, and management. *Arch Intern Med.* 1990; 150(8): 1604-1613.

Zeldis SM. Dyspnea during pregnancy: distinguishing cardiac from pulmonary causes. *Clin Chest Med.* 1992; 13(4): 567-585.

REFERENCES

1. Angelillo VA. Evaluation of dyspnea. Is it really present and, if so, why? *Postgrad Med.* 1983;73:336-339, 343-345.
2. Killian KJ, Campbell EJ. Dyspnea and exercise. *Annu Rev Physiol.* 1983;45:465-479.
3. Manning HL, Schwartzstein RM. Pathophysiology of dyspnea. *N Engl J Med.* 1995;333:1547-1553.
4. Wasserman K, Casaburi R. Dyspnea: physiological and pathophysiological mechanisms. *Annu Rev Med.* 1988; 39:503-515.
5. Guyton AC. *Textbook of Medical Physiology.* Philadelphia, PA: WB Saunders; 1981.
6. Spinhoven P, Van Peski-Oosterbaan AS, VanderDoes AJW. Association of anxiety with perception of histamine-induced bronchoconstriction in patients with asthma. *Thorax.* 1997;52:149-152.
7. Ottanelli R, Rosi E, Romagnoli I, et al. Do inhaled corticosteroids affect perception of dyspnea during bronchoconstriction in asthma? *Chest.* 2001;120: 770-777.
8. Bijl-Hofland ID, Cloosterman SG, Folgering HT, et al. Inhaled corticosteroids, combined with long-acting β_2-agonists, improve the perception of bronchoconstriction in asthma. *Am J Respir Crit Care Med.* 2001;164: 764-769.
9. Tisi GM. *Pulmonary Physiology in Clinical Medicine.* Baltimore, MD: Williams & Wilkins; 1980.
10. Fox WW, Duara S. Persistent pulmonary hypertension in the neonate: diagnosis and management. *J Pediatr.* 1983; 103:505-514.
11. Levin DL, Weinberg AG, Perkin RM. Pulmonary microthrombi in newborn infants with unresponsive persistent pulmonary hypertension. *J Pediatr.* 1983:102: 299-303.
12. Goffman TE, Bloom RL, Dvorak VC. Acute dyspnea in a young woman taking birth control pills. *JAMA.* 1984; 16(251):1465-1466.
13. Abu-Hasan M, Tannous B, Weinberger M. Exercise-induced dyspnea in children and adolescents. If not asthma then what? *Ann Allergy Asthma Immunol.* 2005; 94:366-371.

14. Seear M, Wensley D, West N. How accurate is the diagnosis of exercise induced asthma among Vancouver schoolchildren? *Arch Dis Child.* 2005;90:898-902.
15. MacDonald NE, Hall CB, Suffin SC, et al. Respiratory syncytial virus infection in infants with congenital heart disease. *N Engl J Med.* 1982;307:397-400.
16. Leigh M, Holman G, Rohn R. Dyspnea as the presenting symptom of thyroid disease. *Clin Pediatr (Phila).* 1980; 19:773-774.
17. Robinson BH, De Meirleir L, Glerum M, et al. Clinical presentation of mitochondrial respiratory chain defects in ADH-coenzyme Q reductase and cytochrome oxidase: clues to pathogenesis of Leigh disease. *J Pediatr.* 1987; 110:216-222.
18. Scholte HR, Busch HF, Luyt-Houwen IE, et al. Defects in oxidative phosphorylation: biochemical investigations in skeletal muscle and expression of the lesion in other cells. *J Inherit Metab Dis.* 1987;10(1):81-97.
19. Wasserman K, Casaburi R. Dyspnea: physiological and pathophysiological mechanisms. *Annu Rev Med.* 1988; 39:503-515.
20. Sin DD, Jones RL, Man SF. Obesity is a risk factor for dyspnea but not for airflow obstruction. *Arch Intern Med.* 2002;62:1477-1481.
21. Zeldis SM. Dyspnea during pregnancy: distinguishing cardiac from pulmonary causes. *Clin Chest Med.* 1992; 13(4):567-585.
22. Rosenow EC. The spectrum of drug-induced pulmonary disease. *Ann Intern Med.* 1972;77:977-991.
23. Tobin MJ. Dyspnea: pathophysiologic basis, clinical presentation, and management. *Arch Intern Med.* 1990;150(8): 1604-1613.
24. O'Hollaren MT. Masqueraders in clinical allergy: laryngeal dysfunction causing dyspnea. *Ann Allergy.* 1990; 65(5):351-356.
25. Anbar RD. Stressors associated with dyspnea in childhood: patients' insights and a case report. *Am J Clin Hypn* .2004;47:93-101.
26. Altose MD. Assessment and management of breathlessness. *Chest.* 1985;88(2):77S-83S.
27. Belman MJ. Factors limiting exercise performance in lung disease: ventilatory insufficiency. *Chest.* 1992; 101(5):253S-254S.
28. Sweer L, Zwillich CW. Dyspnea in the patient with chronic obstructive pulmonary disease: etiology and management. *Clin Chest Med.* 1990;11(3): 417-445.
29. Williams SG, Wright DJ, Marshall P, et al. Safety and potential benefits of low dose diamorphine during exercise in patients with chronic heart failure. *Heart.* 2003; 89:1085-1086.
30. Cohen SP, Dawson TC. Nebulized morphine as a treatment for dyspnea in a child with cystic fibrosis. *Pediatrics.* 2002;110:e38.
31. Starck RD. Dyspnoea: assessment and pharmacological manipulation. *Eur Respir J.* 1988;1:280-287.
32. Younes M. Load responses, dyspnea, and respiratory failure. *Chest.* 1990;97(3):59S-68S.
33. Schwartzstein RM, Lahive K, Pope A, et al. Cold facial stimulation reduces breathlessness induced in normal individuals. *Am Rev Respir Dis.* 1987;136: 58-61.
34. Carter R, Coast JR, Idell S. Exercise training in patients with chronic obstructive pulmonary disease. *Med Sci Sports Exerc.* 1992;24(3):281-291.
35. Olopade CO, Beck KC, Viggiano RW, et al. Exercise limitation and pulmonary rehabilitation in chronic obstructive pulmonary disease. *Mayo Clin Proc.* 1992;67(2):144-157.
36. Cherniak NS, Altose MD. Mechanisms of dyspnea. *Clin Chest Med.* 1987;8;207-214.

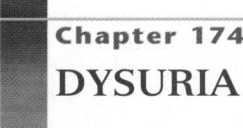

Chapter 174

DYSURIA

Katarina Supe-Markovina, MD; Frederick J. Kaskel, MD, PhD

Dysuria is pain or burning associated with urination that stems from irritation of the bladder, the urethra, or both. Although any condition that leads to inflammation, irritation, or obstruction of the urinary tract can cause dysuria, it usually stems from one of several common disorders of childhood and adolescence, such as urinary tract infections, urethritis, and chemical or traumatic irritants. Box 174-1 lists infectious and noninfectious causes of dysuria.

Young children may complain of painful urination when they are instead experiencing related symptoms, such as the pruritus seen with pinworms. In addition, victims of sexual abuse may complain of dysuria, or they may exhibit behaviors that are interpreted by caretakers as indicative of genital pain. Identifying the cause of dysuria requires a complete history, a thorough physical examination, and a planned laboratory evaluation. Failure to follow this routine usually leads to unnecessary expense, incorrect diagnosis, and improper management (Figures 174-1 and 174-2).[1,2]

EVALUATION

History

Although dysuria is occasionally the only complaint, identifying the cause of dysuria is often aided by considering the associated symptoms. Regardless of the patient's age, the associated symptoms can be placed into two major categories: (1) nonspecific symptoms and (2) specific urinary symptoms. For example, symptoms outside the genitourinary tract might include conjunctival erythema, oral lesions, joint pain or swelling, or a generalized rash, which would suggest a systemic inflammatory condition such as Stevens-Johnson, Reiter, or Behçet syndrome.[1] In addition, fever indicates a systemic infectious condition such as

BOX 174-1 Causes of Dysuria

SYSTEMIC
- Stevens-Johnson syndrome
- Behçet syndrome
- Reiter syndrome
- Varicella

INFECTIOUS
- Cystitis
- Pyelonephritis
- Vulvovaginitis
- Balanitis
- Balanoposthitis
- Pelvic inflammatory disease

NONINFECTIOUS
- Labial adhesions
- Urethral strictures
- Dysfunctional voiding
- Meatal stenosis
- Urethral prolapse
- Nephrolithiasis

pyelonephritis or pelvic inflammatory disease. Although patients with a systemic condition may have dysuria as one of their many symptoms, it is rarely the principal reason for seeking care.

Symptoms more specific to the urinary tract include hematuria, malodorous urine, frequency, urgency, incontinence, and refusal to void. The physician should ask about exposure to chemicals (detergents, perfumed soaps, bubble baths, and medications) that may irritate the mucosal lining of the urethra or bladder. Symptoms suggesting a voiding dysfunction, such as delayed toilet training, enuresis, and constipation, should be identified. Although children are usually open about giving a history of trauma, masturbation or abuse is frequently denied. Sexually transmitted infections, a common cause of dysuria in adolescents, may be suspected by obtaining a history of sexual activity. A family history of nephrolithiasis or a history of high dietary intake of salt, dairy products, or vitamins suggests hypercalciuria.

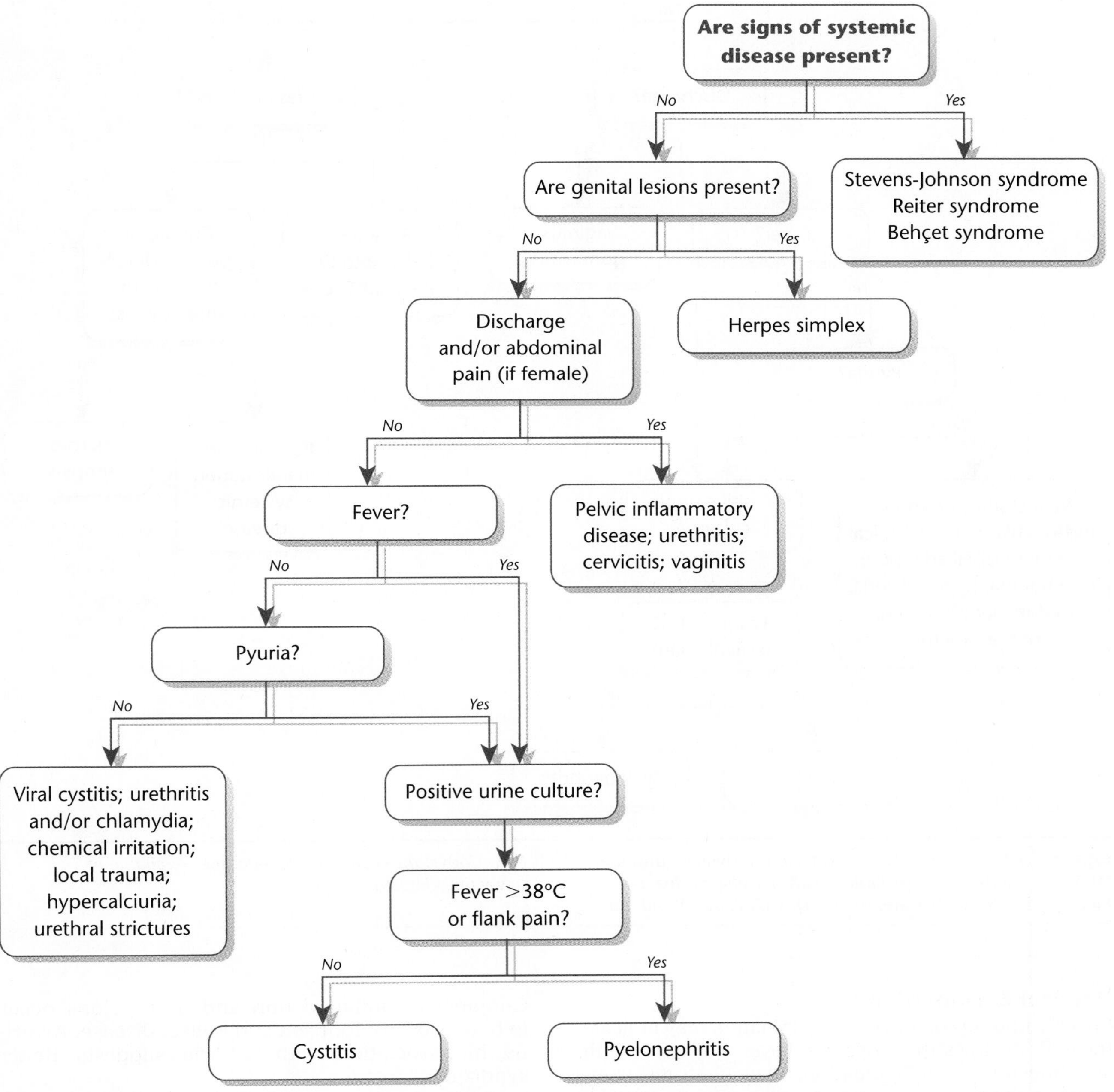

Figure 174-1 Algorithmic approach to dysuria in prepubertal males and females. *(Adapted with permission from Fleisher GR. In:* UpToDate, *Rose BD;* UpToDate, *Waltham MA. Copyright © 2006 UpToDate, Inc. Available at www.uptodate.com.)*

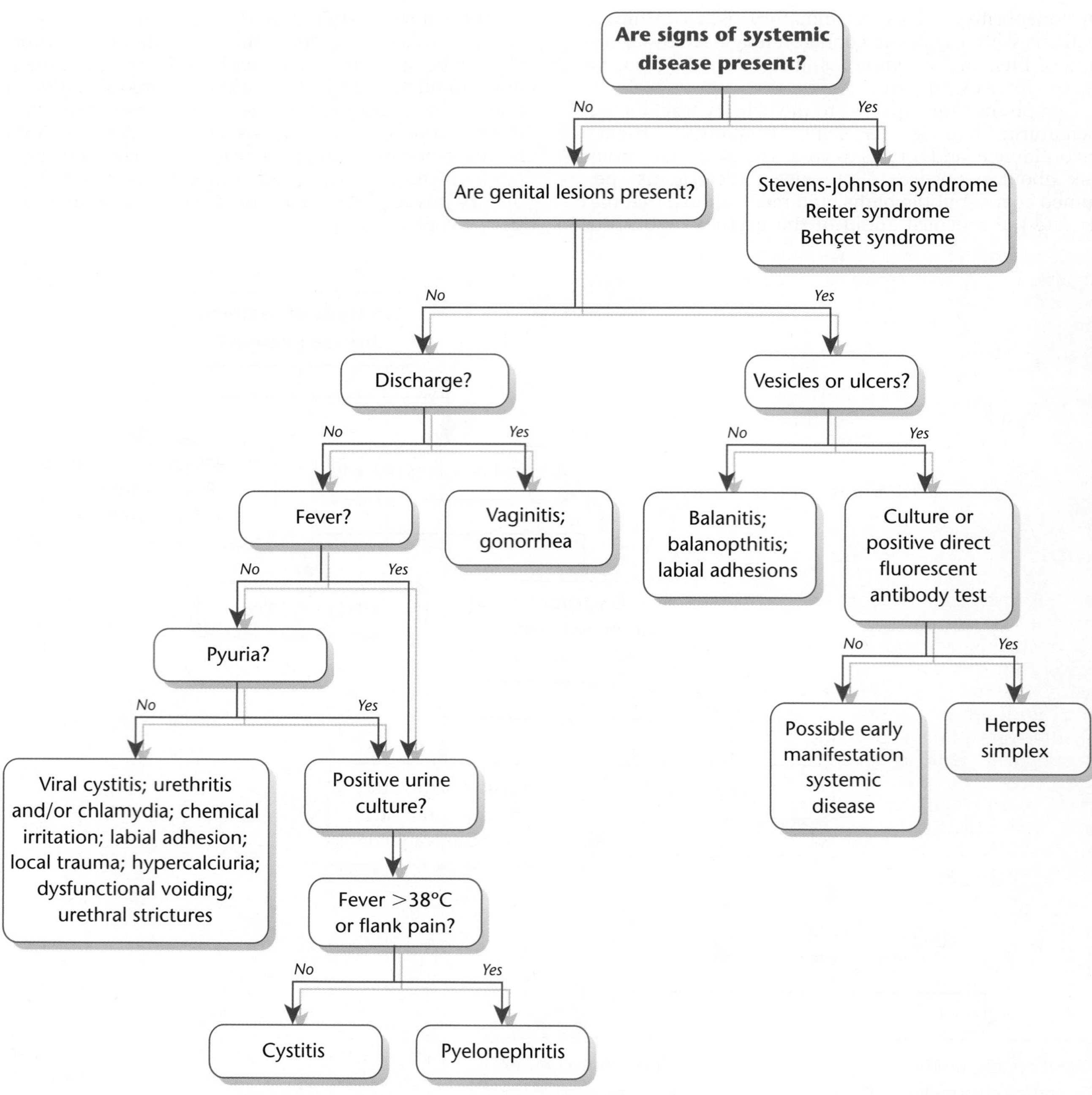

Figure 174-2 Algorithmic approach to dysuria in pubertal males and females. *(Adapted with permission from Fleisher GR. In:* UpToDate, *Rose BD;* UpToDate, *Waltham MA. Copyright © 2006 UpToDate, Inc. Available at www.uptodate.com.)*

Physical Examination

Specific findings on physical examination may indicate the underlying cause of dysuria. Fever may occur with any infection or inflammation. Pyelonephritis commonly produces fever greater than 38.5°C (101°F), whereas cystitis only occasionally produces fever.[3] Infectious, chemical, or traumatic urethritis usually does not mount a febrile response.

Generalized target lesions and vesicles may suggest Stevens-Johnson syndrome or varicella. Conjunctival inflammation and oral lesions occur in both Stevens-Johnson and Behçet disease. Arthritis in association with dysuria suggests Reiter syndrome.[1]

If a patient has symptoms of voiding dysfunction along with dysuria, then the lower back should be observed for any midline defects. Neurologic examination of the lower extremities and evaluation of the bulbocavernosal reflex indicates the neurologic integrity of the lower motor neuron reflex arcs.

In addition to a routine physical examination, special attention should be directed to the genitourinary tract. Palpation of the abdomen may elicit costovertebral angle and suprabupic tenderness, suggesting pyelonephritis and cystitis, respectively. In patients with urethral obstruction, the bladder and kidneys may be enlarged. Findings to note in the genital area include labial adhesions, vesicles, and ulcerations. In boys, the physician should note if the child is circumcised. The meatus should be examined for size and location in boys for meatal stenosis. In girls, a urethral prolapse is seen as a reddened or dark circumferential protrusion of the mucosa from the urethral orifice. Furthermore, a urethral or vaginal discharge indicating infection may be found on inspection. The character of the discharge might help reveal the specific pathogen. For instance, a cheesy discharge is found in candidal vaginitis, whereas a green discharge is usually associated with gonorrhea.

COMMON CONDITIONS

Urinary Tract Infections

Urinary tract infection (UTI) is the most common cause of dysuria.[4] In older children, pyelonephritis may be clinically differentiated from cystitis by the presence of systemic features such as fever, chills, vomiting, flank pain, and costovertebral angle tenderness. Patients with cystitis frequently complain of suprapubic pain. Cystitis may or may not cause fever, which is usually low grade if present. The clinical picture of urinary tract infections in infants and young children may be nonspecific, with fever and other symptoms present in upper and lower tract disease. All children younger than 5 years should be evaluated for congenital anatomic abnormalities (eg, vesicourethral reflux) after their first UTI.[3] For boys, a UTI at any age requires evaluation. For more information on UTIs, see Chapter 334.

Urethritis

Urethritis may result from infection, trauma, allergy, or foreign body. In adults and adolescents, urethritis usually has an infectious cause, which is always the result of sexual contact. *Neisseria gonorrhoeae* and *Chlamydia trachomatis* are the most common pathogens.[5] Infectious urethritis in the pediatric age group is uncommon, except in sexually active adolescents or children who have been sexually abused by an infected adult. Therefore a concern for sexual abuse should be raised in prepubertal children if a sexually transmitted pathogen is discovered. Children with urethritis may note dysuria, urethral discharge, or blood spots on their underwear. Vesicles or ulcers may appear in the genital area if herpes simplex is the pathogen. Patients suspected of having urethritis should have a urethral smear and urine culture included as a part of their evaluation. (See Chapter 122, Sexual Abuse of Children.)

Irritants and Trauma

Local irritants (bubble baths, detergents, perfumed soaps) may produce only mild erythema or no physical findings on examination. Trauma from sexual abuse, voluntary sexual activity, or masturbation may cause dysuria.

Vulvovaginitis

Vaginitis is erythema and inflammation of the vaginal mucosa, usually associated with vaginal discharge, which varies from scant whitish to green with a foul odor.[6] It can be the result of poor hygiene, allergy, or infection. Pathogens causing vulvovaginitis in younger girls are group A *Streptococcus* and *Shigella,* which are associated with vulvar bleeding.[7,8] Sexually transmitted pathogens are frequently isolated in postpubertal girls. *Candida albicans* is usually seen in the setting of recent antibiotic use, diabetes mellitus, or children who are in diapers. Candidal vaginitis frequently causes pruritis in addition to dysuria. Vaginal discharge should be sent for pH, wet preparation, potassium hydroxide, Gram stain, and culture to identify the pathogen so appropriate antibiotic treatment may be initiated. (See Chapter 227, Vaginal Discharge.)

Dysfunctional Voiding

Dysfunctional micturition can be categorized into neuropathic and nonneuropathic voiding disorders. Nonneuropathic voiding encompasses functional problems with the act of micturition. In general, dysfunctional voiders exhibit a dyscoordination between the bladder and the bladder outlet that results in inefficient bladder emptying. Clinical manifestions range from incontinence to UTIs. Constipation is common because of the inability to relax the pelvic floor musculature. Neuropathic voiding is associated with neurologic conditions such as spina bifida, transverse myelitis, or spinal cord trauma.[9] (See Chapter 236, Anuria and Oliguria.)

LESS COMMON CONDITIONS

Pelvic Inflammatory Disease

Although pelvic inflammatory disease may be associated with dysuria, it usually causes fever, abdominal pain, and pelvic discomfort in adolescent girls.[10,11] For more information on sexually transmitted infections in the adolescent, see Chapter 322.

Balanitis and Balanoposthitis

Inflammatory lesions involving the glans penis (balanitis) or both the glans penis and the prepuce (balanoposthitis) may occur in younger boys. They are most common in uncircumcised boys with infection from the entrapped smegma beneath the foreskin. These lesions may be the result of local trauma or poor penile hygiene.[12] Treatment involves warm soaks and an appropriate antibiotic.

Pinworms

Enterobius vermicularis, the parasite that causes pinworms, infests the perianal area. The anal pruritus that is accompanied by this infestation may be incorrectly expressed as dysuria in children. (See Chapter 310, Pinworm Infestations.)

Labial Adhesions

Labial adhesions are common in prepubertal girls. Recurrent irritation or infection of the hypoestrogenized epithelium of the labia minora causes the mucosa to adhere to the midline. Severe fusion may cause dysuria, postvoid dribbling, or UTIs. The adhesions are easily visualized in young girls on inspection.[13,14] (See Chapter 290, Labial Adhesions, for more information.)

Urethral Strictures

Urethral strictures in children are divided into two categories: (1) acquired and (2) congenital. Acquired urethral strictures result from urethral instrumentation, trauma, or inflammation. Congenital urethral strictures are rare. Children with urethral strictures have obstructive and irritative urinary symptoms such as urinary retention, dysuria, or a weak urinary stream. Diagnosis is usually made with retrograde urethrography or cystoscopy.[14]

Meatal Stenosis

Meatal stenosis is a relatively common acquired condition in circumcised boys. It is characterized by an upward, deflected, and difficult-to-aim urinary stream. It is sometimes accompanied by dysuria, urgency, frequency, and prolonged urination.[14] Consultation with a pediatric urologist for a surgical meatomy is recommended.

Urethral Prolapse

Urethral prolapse is a circular protrusion of the distal urethra through the external meatus. It is a relatively uncommon condition and almost exclusively occurs in black girls; the average age at presentation is 4 years. Vaginal bleeding is the most common presenting symptom. Diagnosis is made by verifying that a central opening is present within the prolapsed tissue and that this opening is the urethral meatus, which can be determined by observation during voiding or catherization of the central opening. If medical therapy fails (sitz baths, antibiotics, estrogen cream), then surgical intervention is warranted.[15]

Hypercalciuria (Kidney Stones)

Nephrolithiasis may produce dysuria, but it frequently causes intense flank pain that occurs suddenly and radiates toward the lower abdomen or groin, often accompanied by hematuria. Hypercalciuria, on the other hand, commonly causes dysuria. Experts have suggested that microcrystallization of calcium with urinary anions leads to injury of the uroepithelium. Therefore patients may complain of symptoms related to the urinary tract such as frequency, urgency, hematuria, and recurrent UTIs along with dysuria.[16] A positive family history of nephrolithiasis may be present.

WHEN TO REFER

- Voiding dysfunction
- Nephrolithiasis
- Girl younger than 5 years with a UTI for the first time
- Boy with a UTI (any age)
- Genitourinary tract anomalies

WHEN TO ADMIT

- Systemic inflammatory or infectious cause of dysuria
- Suspicion of sexual abuse

TOOLS FOR PRACTICE

Engaging Patient and Family

- *What is a Pediatric Urologist?* (fact sheet), American Academy of Pediatrics (www.aap.org/sections/sap/he3010.pdf).

AAP POLICY STATEMENTS

American Academy of Pediatrics, Committee on Quality Improvement and Subcommittee on Urinary Tract Infection. Practice parameter: the diagnosis, treatment, and evaluation of the initial urinary tract infection in febrile infants and young children. *Pediatrics*. 1999;103(4):843-852. (aappolicy.aappublications.org/cgi/content/full/pediatrics;103/4/843).

Downs S, American Academy of Pediatrics. Technical report: urinary tract infections in febrile infants and young children. *Pediatrics*. 1999;103(4):e54. (aappolicy.aappublications.org/cgi/content/full/pediatrics;103/4/e54).

REFERENCES

1. Fleisher GR, Ludwig S. *Synopsis of Pediatric Emergency Medicine*. 4th ed. Philadelphia, PA: Lippincott Williams & Wilkins; 2002.
2. American Academy of Pediatrics, Committee on Quality Improvement, Subcommittee on Urinary Tract Infection. Practice parameter: the diagnosis, treatment, and evaluation of the initial urinary tract infection in febrile infants and young children. *Pediatrics*. 1999;103(4):843-852. Available at: http://aappolicy.aappublications.org/cgi/content/full/pediatrics;103/4/843. Accessed June 22, 2007.
3. Hellerstein S. Urinary tract infections. Old and new concepts. *Pediatr Clin North Am*. 1995;42(6):1433-1457.
4. Eichenwald HF. Some aspects of the diagnosis and management of urinary tract infection in children and adolescents. *Pediatr Infect Dis*. 1986;5:760-765.
5. Best D, Ford CA, Miller WC. Prevalence of Chlamydia trachomatis and Neisseria gonorrhoeae infection in pediatric private practice. *Pediatrics*. 2001:108(6):E103.
6. Paradise JE, Campos JM, Friedman HM, et al. Vulvovaginitis in premenarcheal girls: clinical features and diagnostic evaluation. *Pediatrics*. 1982;70(2):193-198.
7. Straumanis JP, Bocchini JA Jr. Group A beta-hemolytic streptococcal vulvovaginitis in prepubertal girls: a case report and review of the past twenty years. *Pediatr Infect Dis J*. 1990;9(11):845-848.
8. Murphy TV, Nelson JD. Shigella vaginitis: report of 38 patients and review of the literature. *Pediatrics*. 1979; 63(4):511-516.
9. Austin PF, Ritchey ML. Dysfunctional voiding. *Pediatr Rev*. 2000;21(10):336-341.
10. Banikarim C, Chacko MR. Pelvic inflammatory disease in adolescents. *Semin Pediatr Infect Dis*. 2005;16(3):175-180.
11. Lappa S, Moscicki AB. The pediatrician and the sexually active adolescent. A primer for sexually transmitted diseases. *Pediatr Clin North Am*. 1997;44(6):1405-1445.
12. Vohra S, Badlani G. Balanitis and balanoposthitis. *Urol Clin North Am*. 1992;19(1):143-147.
13. Baldwin DD, Landa HM. Common problems in pediatric gynecology. *Urol Clin North Am*. 1995;22(1):161-176.
14. Farhat W, McLorie G. Urethral syndromes in children. *Pediatr Rev*. 2001;22(1):17-21.
15. DeSai SR, Cohen RC. Urethral prolapse in a premenarchal girl: case report and literature review. *Aust N Z J Surg*. 1997;67(9):660-662.
16. Alon US, Berenbom A. Idiopathic hypercalciuria of childhood: 4- to 11-year outcome. *Pediatr Nephrol*. 2000;14(10-11):1011-1015.

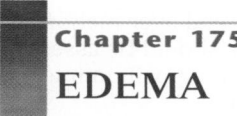

Chapter 175

EDEMA

Paul A. Levy, MD

At birth, as much as 70% of the newborn's body weight is water. This level decreases to approximately 60% of total body weight in older children, adolescents, and adults.[1] The body water is distributed into several compartments. Intracellular water represents two thirds of the total volume. The remaining one third is considered extracellular and is distributed between the vascular compartment (25%) and the interstitial spaces between the cells (75%). The distribution of water in these various body compartments is tightly controlled. Failure of this control can result in the accumulation of extra fluid in the interstitium, which is *edema*.

PATHOPHYSIOLOGICAL FEATURES

Water movement across a semipermeable membrane (osmosis) is governed by the number of particles (osmolarity) on either side of the membrane. Water moves to establish equilibrium between the two compartments. In blood vessels, such as capillaries, the osmolarity is generated, in part, by the electrolytes in plasma; however, because the concentrations of electrolytes in plasma and the interstitium are relatively equal, the osmotic force is largely determined by charged protein molecules, with albumin being the most predominant. The plasma proteins are referred to as *colloids,* and the osmotic force they generate is the *colloid osmotic pressure,* or *oncotic pressure.* Movement of fluid across a capillary wall is controlled by a combination of oncotic pressure, hydrostatic pressure, and the permeability of the capillary wall. The capillary oncotic pressure draws fluid into the capillary; the interstitial oncotic pressure draws capillary fluid out. The capillary hydrostatic pressure, which is related to blood pressure, is highest at the arteriole end of the capillary and drops off as blood moves toward the venule. The capillary hydrostatic force pushes fluid into the interstitium. Interestingly, systemic (arterial) hypertension does not result in edema because arteriolar sphincters protect the capillary bed from increased blood pressure.[2] The interstitial hydrostatic pressure is related to the pressure of the fluid in the interstitium, which depends on the lymphatic drainage, the amount of fluid present in the interstitium, and the compliance of the tissue. This force counteracts the capillary hydrostatic pressure and pushes fluid back into the capillaries. Finally, the permeability of the capillary wall contributes to the leakage of fluid into the interstitium.[2,3]

In normal circumstances, the interplay of these forces results in fluid exiting the capillaries at the arteriolar end and entering the capillaries at the venule end. Approximately 90% of fluid that leaves the capillaries is reabsorbed before reaching the venule. The lymphatic system returns the remaining 10%, along with its associated proteins, to the circulation.

CAUSES OF EDEMA

Fluid distribution between the intravascular compartment and the interstitial compartment results from the interplay of oncotic pressure, hydrostatic pressure, and capillary membrane permeability. Disruption of these forces can result in edema, but sodium concentration is usually the ultimate controller of this fluid movement[2,4-6] (Box 175-1).

Change in Capillary Membrane Permeability

An increase in capillary membrane permeability is often the result of cytokines released from inflammation. Infections and burns tend to cause localized edema. An allergic reaction may cause more generalized edema. Hereditary angioedema can cause localized edema of the gastrointestinal tract and larynx. Trauma causes local edema.

Decreased Capillary Oncotic Pressure

A decrease in the capillary oncotic pressure can be caused by decreased levels of protein, usually of albumin in the blood. Decreased synthesis of albumin occurs in cirrhosis or as a result of malnutrition or intestinal malabsorption. Protein loss by the kidneys in

BOX 175-1 Causes of Edema

RENAL
Nephrotic syndrome
Glomerulonephritis
Renal failure

CARDIOVASCULAR
Congestive heart failure
Deep-vein thrombosis
Embolic disease
Vasculitis
Constrictive pericarditis

HEMATOLOGIC (SEVERE ANEMIA)
Hemolytic disease of the newborn

ENDOCRINE OR METABOLIC
Thyroid disease
Starvation
Hereditary angioedema

GASTROINTESTINAL
Cirrhosis
Protein-losing enteritis
Cystic fibrosis
Celiac disease
Enteritis
Lymphangiectasis
Lymphatic abnormalities
Milk protein allergy
Inflammatory bowel disease

nephrotic syndrome may also contribute to edema. Albumin levels below 2 mg/dL are usually associated with generalized edema.[2] The mechanism of edema formation with decreased oncotic pressure results in extravasation of fluid into the interstitium, but it also results in poor kidney perfusion, which activates renin-aldosterone secretion and results in increased sodium reabsorption, fluid retention, and eventually increased capillary hydrostatic pressure, which compounds the formation of edema.

Increased Capillary Hydrostatic Pressure

Systemic Venous Hypertension

Systemic venous hypertension can be the result of heart failure, constrictive pericarditis, cardiomyopathy, tricuspid valvular disease, and cirrhosis. All of these conditions increase the capillary hydrostatic pressure and result in edema from increased extravasation of fluid into the interstitium. Left-ventricular heart failure results in pulmonary edema; right-ventricular heart failure results in venous congestion, hepatomegaly, and peripheral edema.

Localized Venous Hypertension

Localized edema may result from increased venous pressure with deep-vein thrombosis or from compression of the inferior vena cava or iliac vein by a tumor. The increased venous pressure raises the capillary hydrostatic pressure.

Increased Plasma Volume

Renal disease (glomerulonephritis, nephrotic syndrome, renal failure), heart failure, and liver disease (cirrhosis) all lead to increased plasma volume through a similar mechanism.[2,4-6] Increased sodium reabsorption in the kidney from activation of the renin-angiotensin-aldosterone system leads to increased water reabsorption and increased plasma volume. Sympathetic nervous stimulation can also result in increased sodium reabsorption in the kidney.

Increased Interstitial Hydrostatic Pressure

Increased interstitial hydrostatic pressure, although rare, may result from lymphatic obstruction by a tumor or large lymph nodes, from damage to the lymphatic system by radiation or surgery, or from parasitic infections such as filariasis.

EVALUATION

History

A detailed history must be obtained to discover the cause of the edema. The time course of the edema—whether its onset is recent or chronic—is particularly important. If chronic, then the parents and child may report weight gain, tight clothing, or snug-fitting shoes, findings they may have attributed to the growth of the child. The history of a recent illness, such as pharyngitis, is important for the diagnosis of glomerular nephritis. In addition to the edema, other systemic complaints may be present, such as shortness of breath, tachypnea, or cough, which may indicate the presence of heart failure and pulmonary edema. Ascites, a form of localized edema, is seen with liver failure or cirrhosis and with some congenital liver malformations. The child's nutritional status should be assessed because malnutrition may result in hypoalbuminemia, which can, in turn, result in edema.

Physical Examination

Edema may be generalized or localized. If localized, then it may be easily apparent when it affects an extremity (deep-vein thrombosis, cellulitis, burn) or when it is more occult (pulmonary edema from left-ventricular heart failure, ascites from liver disease). Physical examination should begin with close observation of the vital signs. Tachypnea may indicate pulmonary edema. Increased blood pressure may be present in glomerular nephritis and renal failure. Fever and localized edema may be present with cellulitis.

Periorbital edema is generally found with nephrotic syndrome and glomerular nephritis. Crackles or rales may indicate the presence of pulmonary edema. A gallop may indicate heart failure. Abdominal distention, shifting dullness, or a fluid wave may be present with ascites. Generalized edema may include scrotal or labial edema. Findings related to generalized edema may depend on whether the patient has been lying down (sacral edema) or standing (feet and lower legs). Chronic edema may result in bedsores. A distinction may be made between pitting and nonpitting edema. *Nonpitting edema* is often the result of lymphedema, whereas *pitting edema* is the result of increased membrane permeability, increased hydrostatic pressure, or decreased oncotic pressure.[7]

Laboratory Evaluation

Initial testing may include a urinalysis, complete blood count, electrolytes with blood urea nitrogen and creatinine, liver function tests with albumin, thyroid function tests, an electrocardiogram, and chest x-ray examination, depending on the clinical circumstances. Renal and abdominal ultrasound examination can be helpful. Testing for fecal fat is appropriate if intestinal malabsorption is suspected, and α1-antitrypsin may be helpful for diagnosing protein-losing enteropathy. With angioedema, whether hereditary or acquired, levels of C1 esterase inhibitor are low.

INTERPRETATION OF TESTS

Hematologic Abnormalities

Severe anemia can result in edema, especially in a newborn. The edema can be the result of hemolysis from ABO blood type or Rh incompatibility or from glucose-6-phosphate dehydrogenase deficiency.

Renal Disease

The presence of proteinuria with low serum albumin is highly suggestive of nephrotic syndrome. If red cell casts and hematuria (especially cola-colored urine) are present, then glomerular nephritis may be the cause of the edema. C3 levels may be needed to help distinguish between the types of glomerulonephritis. For nephrotic syndrome, levels of C3, C4, or antinuclear antibody can help exclude lupus or membranoproliferative glomerulonephritis. Bilateral hydronephrosis, usually demonstrated on a renal ultrasound, in an infant boy with edema may be the result of posterior urethral valves. Congenital renal anomalies may produce ultrasound results of small or malformed kidneys and clinical findings of renal failure. Children with undiagnosed reflux nephropathy may have severe hydronephrosis and renal failure.

Liver Disease

Hypoalbuminemia without proteinuria suggests either a synthesis defect found with chronic liver disease or a protein-losing enteropathy. Prothrombin time, which is a good marker of the liver's ability to synthesize protein, should be assessed when hypoalbuminemia is present without proteinuria. Liver function tests may also provide helpful information. Analysis of stool α1-antitrypsin will help diagnose protein-losing enteropathy.

Venous Thrombosis

If venous thrombosis is suspected, then coagulation studies should be conducted, especially if no predisposing factor, such as an indwelling catheter, is present. A Doppler ultrasound examination should be performed to assess the blood flow in the area that may be affected by the thrombosis.

Enteropathy

The presence of increased fat in fecal matter strongly suggests intestinal malabsorption. Determining which intestinal disorder (cystic fibrosis, inflammatory bowel disease, milk protein allergy, enterokinase deficiency, celiac disease, or intestinal lymphangiectasia) may be the cause of the hypoalbuminemia requires further testing and consultation with a gastroenterologist.

MANAGEMENT

Initial management involves determining whether the patient should be admitted to the hospital. Many causes of edema require admission. Patients with signs of respiratory distress that result from edema of the airway, heart failure with pulmonary edema, and tachypnea should be admitted. Renal causes, such as previously undiagnosed renal failure, acute glomerular nephritis, or nephrotic syndrome, may also require admission. Oliguria from renal failure or poor renal perfusion should result in emergent admission. Edema that results from cirrhosis may require admission if the cirrhosis had been unrecognized or if respiratory distress resulting from the ascites is present. Localized edema that results from venous thrombosis or lymphatic obstruction requires admission to assess and treat the underlying cause. Further management depends on the underlying cause of the edema.[2,7,8]

Anemia

Severe anemia may need to be treated with transfusion. A hematologist should be consulted if the cause of the anemia is not readily apparent.

Renal Disease

Most patients with renal disease benefit from a low-sodium diet. Fluid restriction may help, but it should be used cautiously on an individual-patient basis in consultation with a nephrologist. Diuretics may also be needed but should be used cautiously. If plasma volume is decreased, then fluid expansion with colloid followed by diuretics may be necessary.

Liver Disease

A low-sodium diet is generally helpful if ascites is present. Diuretics, especially spironolactone, may also be beneficial. When possible, treating the underlying cause of the ascites is critical.

Heart Disease

Treating heart failure may require inotropic medications such as digoxin or dobutamine. An angiotensin-converting enzyme inhibitor may help with afterload reduction. If congenital heart disease is causing the heart failure, then surgical repair of the underlying structural lesion is the ultimate treatment.

Venous Thrombosis

When a venous thrombosis is present, anticoagulation therapy may be indicated. Consultation with a hematologist and possibly a vascular surgeon may be necessary. In the absence of an obvious predisposing factor, investigation for an underlying coagulopathy is appropriate.

Enteropathy

Treatment depends on the cause of the enteropathy. A gastroenterologist should be consulted.

Myxedema

Generally, myxedema is found with hypothyroidism and responds to treatment with thyroid hormone replacement.

SUMMARY

Edema is the accumulation of fluid in the interstitial tissues resulting from disruption of the forces that control normal fluid movement out of and into capillaries and may be the result of many different disease states. Diagnosis of the underlying cause is generally apparent, although sometimes subtle. Intervention may initially need to be supportive; but once a patient is stable, efforts to treat the underlying cause of the edema should be pursued, often with the help of a specialist.

WHEN TO REFER

Many disorders that cause edema may require the assistance of a specialist. A referral to a specialist should be considered if evidence exists of:

- Liver disease (ie, ascites)
- Renal disease (glomerular nephritis, nephritic syndrome)
- Anemia
- Protein losing enteropathy or increased fecal fat with malabsorption with secondary hypoalbuminemia
- Heart failure

WHEN TO ADMIT

Many of the causes of edema are serious medical problems that often require admission. This approach may initially be for support. Once a diagnosis is established and the patient is stable, further treatment usually continues on an outpatient basis with the assistance of a specialist. Signs of any of the following may require admission:

- Respiratory distress
- Heart failure
- Tachypnea
- Renal failure
- Acute glomerular nephritis or nephrotic syndrome
- Oliguria from renal failure
- Edema caused by previously unrecognized cirrhosis
- Localized edema that results from venous thrombosis or lymphatic obstruction
- Anemia severe enough to require a transfusion

REFERENCES

1. Ruth JL, Wassner SJ. Body composition: salt and water. *Pediatr Rev.* 2006;27:181-187.
2. Cho S, Atwood JE. Peripheral edema. *Am J Med.* 2002; 113:580-586.
3. Starling EH. On the absorption of fluids from the connective tissue spaces. *J Physiol.* 1896;19:312-326.
4. Cárdenas A, Arroyo V. Mechanisms of water and sodium retention in cirrhosis and the pathogenesis of ascites. *Best Prac Res Clin Endocrinol Metab.* 2003;17:607-622.
5. Koomans HA. Pathophysiology of oedema in idiopathic nephrotic syndrome. *Nephrol Dial Transplant.* 2003; 18(suppl 6):vi30-vi32.
6. Schrier RW. Water and sodium retention in edematous disorders: role of vasopressin and aldosterone. *Am J Med.* 2006;119(7A):S47-S53.
7. O'Brien JG, Chennubhotla SA, Chennubhotla RV. Treatment of edema. *Am Fam Physician.* 2005;71:2111-2117.
8. Diskin CJ, Stokes TJ, Dansby LM, et al. Towards an understanding of oedema. *BMJ.* 1999; 318:1610-1613.

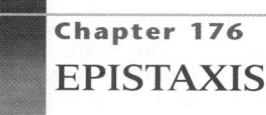

Chapter 176

EPISTAXIS

Miriam B. Schechter, MD; David M. Stevens, MD

Epistaxis, from the Greek *epistazō*, to bleed at the nose (from *epi*, on, + *stazō*, to fall in drops) is defined as acute bleeding from the nostril, nasal cavity, or nasopharynx. A nosebleed is a relatively common and usually self-limited occurrence in childhood; yet when profuse or recurrent, it can be extremely distressing to children and parents and can at times be a sign of a more serious condition.

EPIDEMIOLOGIC FACTORS

The incidence of epistaxis has a bimodal distribution with peaks in children under 10 years and in adults over 50 years. It is more common in boys and men than it is in girls and women.[1] From 5% to 14% of Americans have a nosebleed each year, and approximately 10% of them seek care from a physician.[2] Although common in children, epistaxis is rare under the age of 2 years, peaks between the ages of 3 and 8 years, and is infrequent after puberty.[3] Nosebleeds also are more common in children living in dry climates and occur more frequently in winter months.[4] Approximately 30% of children from birth to age 5, 56% of children ages 6 to 10, and 64% of children ages 11 to 15 have had at least 1 nosebleed in their lifetime.[5] In a study of the epidemiology of epistaxis in US emergency departments from 1992 to 2001, approximately 1 in 200 of all emergency department visits were for epistaxis. Peaks were found in children under age 10 and in older adults between the ages of 70 and 79. A higher proportion of emergency department visits occurred during the winter months, and 83% of cases were from atraumatic causes.[6]

DEFINITIONS AND ANATOMIC FEATURES

Nosebleeds are usually classified as anterior or posterior based on the location of the vessels that are the source of the bleed. The blood supply to the nose originates in both the internal and the external carotid arteries (Figure 176-1). The ophthalmic branch of the internal carotid gives off the anterior and posterior ethmoid arteries, which supply the superior nasal septum and the lateral nasal wall. The internal maxillary and facial arteries, which are branches of the external carotid, further divide to supply the nose. The internal maxillary artery splits into the sphenopalatine artery, the posterior nasal artery, and the greater palatine artery, and the facial artery gives off the superior labial artery. The branches of the sphenopalatine provide blood flow to the turbinates laterally and the anterior and posterior septum, the greater palatine supplies the anterior septum, and the superior labial artery supplies the anterior nose and anterior nasal septum.

The anastomoses of vessels in the anterior 2 to 3 cm of the nasal septum, just 0.5 cm from the tip of the nose, also known as Little area, make up Kiesselbach plexus, the primary source of anterior nosebleeds. The delicate vessels that comprise Kiesselbach plexus include the septal branches of the anterior ethmoid, sphenopalatine, greater palatine, and superior labial arteries. These vessels are superficial because the nasal mucosa is closely adherent to the perichondrium and periosteum. Posterior bleeds usually originate in Woodruff plexus, a convergence of the sphenopalatine, posterior nasal, and ascending pharyngeal arteries, located over the posterior middle turbinate. Specifically, the sphenopalatine is the most frequent source of posterior epistaxis.

Anterior bleeds are by far the most common type, accounting for greater than 90% of epistaxis in children.[7] The rich vasculature under the thin mucosa in the area most exposed to trauma and dry air makes Kiesselbach plexus the most vulnerable to bleeding. During anterior epistaxis, almost all the blood exits anteriorly through the nares. However, with posterior epistaxis, most of the blood flows into the nasopharynx and mouth, making the degree of bleeding difficult to assess. Anterior bleeds are therefore much easier to visualize and easier to control than posterior bleeds, which are generally much more profuse and are more likely to lead to hemodynamic instability.

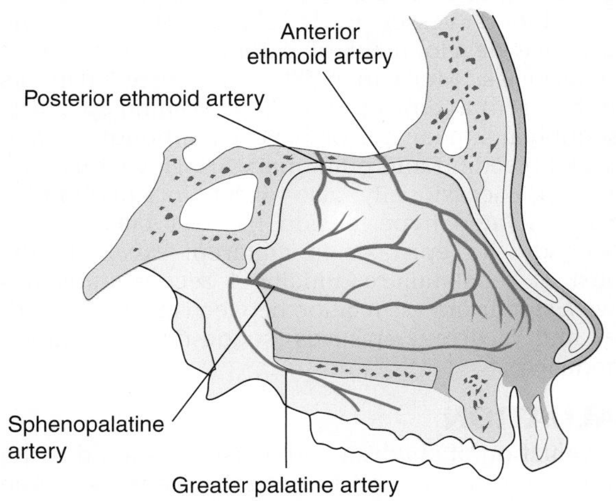

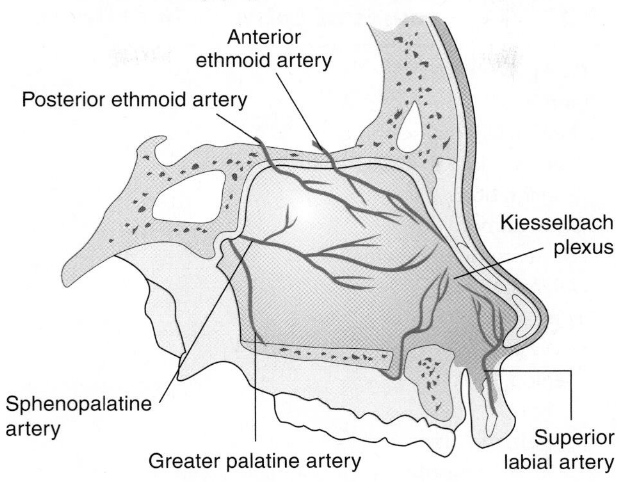

Figure 176-1 Blood supply to the nose (septum and lateral wall). *(Adapted from Massick D, Tobin E. Epistaxis. In: Cummings C Schuller DE, Thomas JR, et al, eds.* Otolaryngology/Head and Neck Surgery. *4th ed. Philadelphia, PA: Elsevier Mosby; 2005. Copyright © 2005, Elsevier, with permission.)*

DIFFERENTIAL DIAGNOSIS

The causes of epistaxis can be categorized into local and systemic causes (Box 176-1). More than 1 factor often plays a role in the bleeding.

Trauma from nose picking or nose rubbing accounts for most cases in children, particularly in association with inflammation from infection or allergy. Epistaxis resulting from blunt external trauma is generally acute and self-limiting but should prompt evaluation for fractures of the facial bones and an anterior septal hematoma. Trauma from a foreign body is an occasional cause in toddlers, often resulting in unilateral bleeding accompanied by foul-smelling or bloody discharge.

Upper respiratory infection and allergic rhinitis are commonly associated with childhood epistaxis. The resultant rhinorrhea leads to digital manipulation or forceful sneezing and nose blowing, and the vascular congestion and mucosal irritation promote easy injury to the blood vessels of the anterior septum. Positive allergy skin tests and recurrent epistaxis are associated in children.[8]

Exposure to low environmental humidity, especially in winter months, has clearly been associated with an increased frequency of nosebleeds.[4,6] A deviated nasal septum can contribute to recurrent epistaxis by causing a change in normal airflow, leading to mucosal drying and irritation.[9]

Neoplasms are uncommon causes of epistaxis in children but should be considered in certain circumstances. Polyps in children are usually associated with cystic fibrosis. Juvenile nasopharyngeal angiofibroma is a benign vascular tumor originating in the lateral nasopharynx that occurs only in male adolescents because of its hormonal sensitivity. Although unilateral progressive obstruction or discharge are clues to this diagnosis, recurrent epistaxis is the most frequent presenting complaint in these patients.[10] Rhabdomyosarcoma of the nasal cavity or nasopharynx is a rare malignant cause of severe episodic epistaxis and may be associated with signs of eustachian tube dysfunction such as unilateral middle ear effusion. Nasal hemangioma is also a rare cause of epistaxis but should be considered in infants. Nasopharyngeal carcinoma is an extremely uncommon but serious disease in children.[11] Epistaxis is the presenting complaint in approximately 50% of children,[12] although it is nearly always accompanied by a neck mass or neck pain.[13]

Systemic causes of epistaxis should be considered whenever nosebleeds are recurrent or persistent in the absence of any obvious local cause. Hematologic disorders include platelet disorders and coagulation defects and may be either congenital or acquired. Thrombocytopenia as a cause of epistaxis is almost always accompanied by petechiae or ecchymoses. The most common cause of isolated thrombocytopenia in otherwise healthy children is idiopathic thrombocytopenic purpura, which presents as acute mucosal hemorrhage, often epistaxis, in approximately 30% of patients, although the bleeding is rarely severe.[14,15] By contrast, epistaxis rarely is the first symptom of leukemia, but this diagnosis should be considered in an ill-appearing child with epistaxis, especially with fever, pallor, lymphadenopathy, or hepatosplenomegaly. Thrombocytopenia can also be an adverse reaction to a variety of medications, including anticonvulsants such as carbamazepine and chemotherapeutic agents.

Platelet dysfunction from aspirin or nonsteroidal antiinflammatory drugs can also predispose the individual to epistaxis. Bernard-Soulier syndrome, a disorder of platelet aggregation, is an occasional diagnosis in children evaluated for isolated epistaxis.[16,17] Primary coagulation defects may result in persistent and

BOX 176-1 Causes of Epistaxis in Children

LOCAL
- Trauma
  - Nose picking or rubbing
  - Blunt trauma or facial fractures
  - Foreign body
- Inflammation
  - Upper respiratory infection
  - Allergic rhinitis
- Dry air
- Neoplasms
  - Benign
    - Polyps
    - Hemangiomas
    - Juvenile nasopharyngeal angiofibroma
  - Malignant
    - Nasopharyngeal carcinoma
    - Rhabdomyosarcoma
- Nasal septal deviation
- Intranasal drugs
  - Steroids
  - Cocaine
- Systemic/Bleeding Disorders
  - Thrombocytopenia
    - Immune thrombocytopenic purpura
    - Leukemia
  - Platelet dysfunction
    - Bernard-Soulier syndrome
    - Aspirin; nonsteroidal antiinflammatory drugs
  - Coagulopathies
    - von Willebrand disease
    - Hemophilias
    - Liver disease
  - Vascular abnormalities
- Osler-Weber-Rendu disease

longstanding epistaxis; a positive family history is often present. Up to one third of children with isolated recurrent epistaxis have a diagnosable coagulopathy.[17,18] Von Willebrand disease (VWD) is the most commonly identified inherited coagulopathy. In fact, 60% of patients with VWD suffer from recurrent epistaxis; other mucosal bleeding (eg, menorrhagia or postsurgical or postdental extraction) is also a common complaint in older children and adolescents. Much less common are the hemophilias, which in mild cases may cause isolated epistaxis (factors VII, VIII, IX or XI deficiency).[17]

Acquired coagulopathies are a rare cause of epistaxis in children, unlike adults, but include various liver diseases (eg, chronic active hepatitis) with consequent depletion of clotting factors. In addition, an acquired form of VWD has been described in children receiving valproic acid.[19]

Osler-Weber-Rendu disease (hereditary hemorrhagic telangiectasia) is an autosomal-dominant disorder of blood vessel walls characterized by the progressive development of cutaneous and mucosal telangiectasias. More than 90% of affected patients have recurrent and progressively worsening epistaxis, presenting at a mean age of 12 years, although gastrointestinal bleeding and pulmonary arteriovenous malformations occasionally also occur in childhood.[20] Primary isolated hypertension has not been clearly associated with epistaxis in children, except in the context of renal failure. Finally, 1 recent study has shown a significant association between migraine headaches and recurrent epistaxis, suggesting a common pathogenesis.[21]

EVALUATION

The evaluation of children with epistaxis should begin with a careful history and physical examination. The season and associated environmental conditions should be noted. The degree of chronicity may suggest an inherited systemic cause. Unilaterality may suggest a local anatomic cause. A history of nose picking or blunt trauma should be sought. One half of children treated in an emergency room for intranasal foreign body admitted placing the object in the nose; therefore young children should be questioned.[22] A family history of bleeding symptoms or diagnosed disorder is useful in identifying children with a bleeding diathesis.[17]

Associated symptoms should be sought. Unilateral progressive obstruction suggests a mass. The presence and character of any associated rhinorrhea should be noted. Clear, watery rhinorrhea with associated sneezing suggests allergic rhinitis, and mucosal discharge with cough suggests upper respiratory infection. Unilateral foul smelling discharge in a young child may indicate a retained foreign body. A history of petechiae or easy bruising or other mucosal bleeding (eg, menorrhagia, postsurgical) may point to a bleeding disorder. Associated fever or pallor may suggest leukemia. A history of medication use, particularly aspirin or nonsteroidal antiinflammatory drugs should be sought.

The physical examination should include a blood pressure and pulse if the history suggests significant acute or chronic blood loss. A careful examination of the nose should attempt to identify the source of any active bleeding (see Management later in this chapter) and to note any discharge, obstructing mass, or foreign body. The skin should be checked for petechiae or unusual location or number of ecchymoses. The neck should be examined for the presence of a mass. If the child is ill, a full examination, including a search for lymphadenopathy and hepatosplenomegaly, should be performed.

The need for and extent of laboratory testing should be guided by the history and physical examination. Frequent and prolonged episodes may warrant ruling out anemia caused by blood loss. Persistent or recurrent epistaxis in the absence of an obvious cause may warrant testing to search for an underlying pathologic condition. A complete blood count is always indicated in the presence of petechiae or unusual ecchymoses to

Table 176-1 Epistaxis Scoring System

COMPONENT	SCORE*
FREQUENCY	
5-15/yr	0
16-25/yr	1
>25/yr	2
DURATION	
<5 min	0
5-10 min	1
>10 min	2
AMOUNT†	
<15 mL	0
15-30 mL	1
>30 mL	2
EPISTAXIS HISTORY AND AGE‡	
33%	0
33%-67%	1
>67%	2
SITE	
Unilateral	0
Bilateral	2

*Mild, 0-6; severe, 7-10.
†Estimation of average blood loss per episode, based on fractions or multiples of teaspoons, tablespoons, or cups.
‡Proportion of the child's life that nosebleeds had been recurrent (>5/yr).
(From Katsanis E, Luke K, Hsu E, et al. Prevelance and significance of mild bleeding disorders in children with recurrent espistaxis. *J Pediatr* 1988;113: 73-76. *Copyright © 1988, Elsevier, with permission.*)

rule out thrombocytopenia. In an ill child with pallor, fever, lymphadenopathy, or hepatosplenomegaly, a complete blood count will help rule out leukemia.

The frequency, duration, amount, age at onset, and site of epistaxis have been used in an epistaxis scoring system (Table 176-1) to determine which patients should be evaluated for an underlying bleeding disorder.[23,24] Prothrombin time and partial thromboplastin time are useful as initial screening tests. However, given that these results may be within the normal range in some patients with VWD, further evaluation with von Willebrand factor studies may be necessary. If this relatively common coagulopathy is being considered, then referring the patient to a hematologist may be prudent.

Rarely, imaging studies are indicated, but plain films can rule out an associated fracture of the facial bones in the setting of blunt trauma. If a mass is thought to be present, then a computed tomography scan or referral to an otolaryngologist should be considered.

MANAGEMENT

Management of nosebleeds can be divided into 3 general phases. The initial first aid measures that often are performed at home should also be the first line of treatment on presentation to the physician. Next is the acute management of persistent bleeding, which may be initiated by a pediatrician in an office or emergency room but may have to be continued by an otolaryngologist if initial measures are unsuccessful. This phase may involve medical or surgical intervention, or both (Figure 176-2). Finally, long-term preventive treatment of recurrent epistaxis is necessary, including evaluation and treatment of underlying causes. Although most episodes of epistaxis in childhood are self-limited, they create parental concern and anxiety, and pediatricians must therefore be aware of the treatment options.

Many health care physicians and patients are unaware of the proper spot for applying direct pressure to the nose to stop a nosebleed.[25,26] Given that a vast majority of bleeds originate anteriorly, in Little area, the first step is to apply pressure to the alar nasi using the first and second fingers. Pressure should be held by pinching the nostrils without interruption for 5 to 10 minutes. The child should sit up with the head bent forward slightly, to minimize blood dripping posteriorly and being swallowed,[27] which can cause nausea and hematemesis. Some providers suggest placement of ice packs to the forehead, bridge of the nose, nape of the neck, or upper lip to promote vasoconstriction, although only theory supports this practice.[28]

In the health care setting, initial treatment measures should occur simultaneously with assessment and history taking. Basic equipment should be readied (Box 176-2). Most anterior nosebleeds in children will stop after basic first-aid measures. However, if bleeding persists, then additional measures are available. As in any acute situation, an initial *ABCD* assessment should be made. Evaluation for major hemorrhage includes evaluating for tachycardia, hypotension, and orthostasis. Although uncommon in children, a child with airway compromise or hemodynamic instability (or both) requires emergency management.

A history should quickly be obtained (see discussion under "Evaluation" earlier in this chapter). The pediatric care physician should attempt to locate the source of bleeding. The bleeding has often stopped by the time medical attention is sought. The child should be asked to blow out all clots. If this is not possible, then blood in the nose can be suctioned out. To try to visualize the source of bleeding, one of the following three tools could be used: (1) a flashlight, while applying gentle upward pressure to the nasal tip, (2) an otoscope with speculum, or (3) a headlight and nasal speculum. Because the anterior septum is the most common location of epistaxis in children, this area should be inspected first. Anterior bleeds on the septum, or lateral wall, should be evident by active bleeding, clots, crusts, ulcerations or prominent blood vessels.[7] If an anterior source is not found and a posterior bleed is thought to exist, then an otolaryngologist should be consulted immediately because posterior bleeds are usually profuse and difficult to stop. Luckily, posterior bleeds are rare in children. If an anterior bleed has not ceased with application of pressure alone, then topical vasoconstrictors such as oxymetazoline, phenylephrine, or epinephrine (1:1000) can be applied with a cotton pledget to shrink the nasal mucosa to improve visualization and possibly to slow down or even stop the bleeding.[29] Pressure, again by pinching, should be applied for another 5 to 10 minutes.

The next step to attempt to stop persistent hemorrhage is chemical cauterization, with silver nitrate on

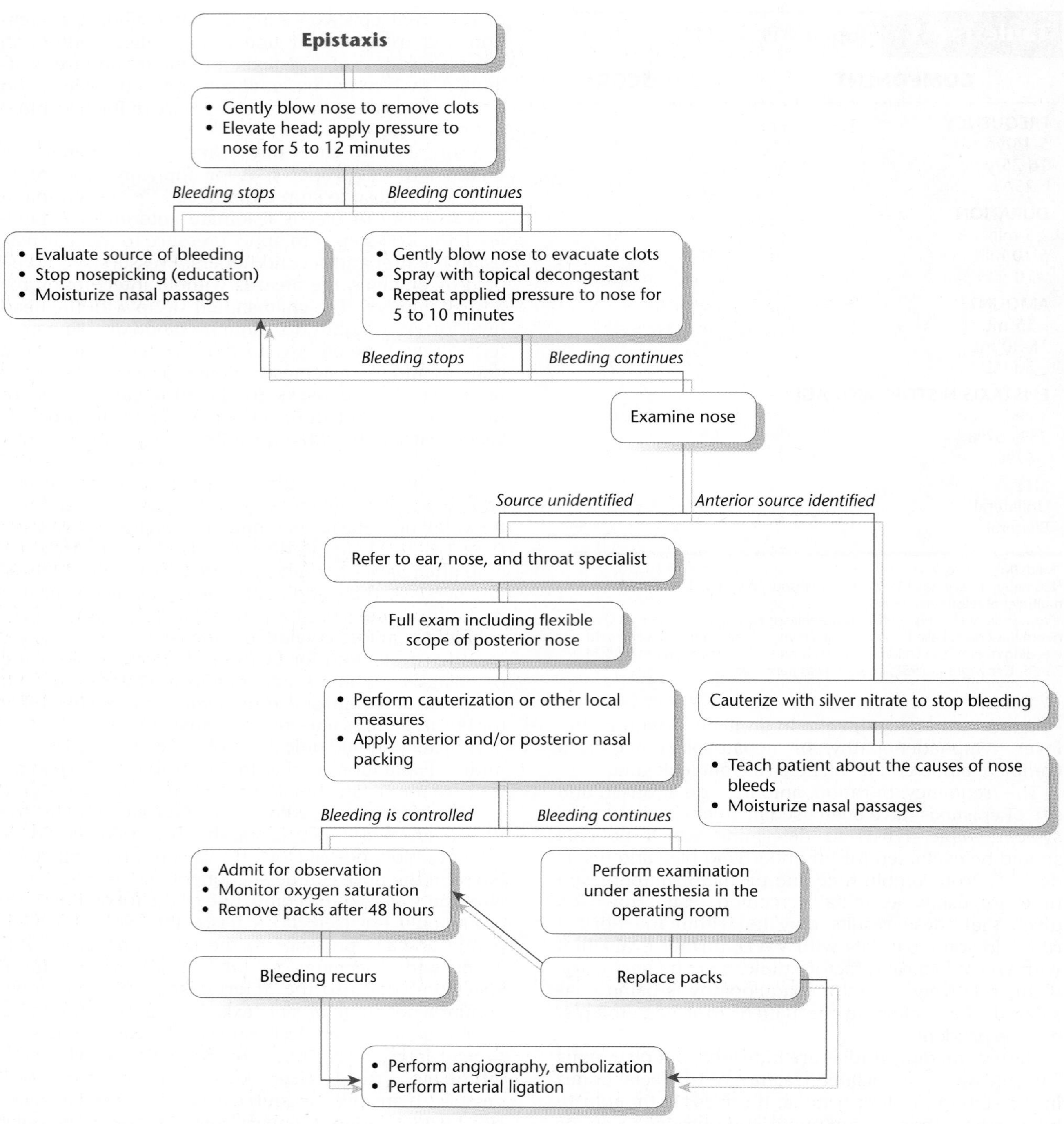

Figure 176-2 Treatment of Epistaxis. *(Rudolph AM, Rudolph CD, Hostetter MK, et al, eds.* Rudolph's Pediatrics. *21st ed. New York, NY: McGraw-Hill; 2003. Reprinted by permission of The McGraw-Hill Companies, Inc.)*

applicator sticks. First, local anesthesia with 4% lidocaine should be administered with a cotton pledget for 5 minutes to reduce the discomfort of cauterization. After inserting and opening a nasal speculum, using adequate lighting, the silver nitrate is applied to the bleeding point and can be rolled over the site for several seconds. The procedure may have to be repeated several times to achieve hemostasis.[29] Silver nitrate does not work well in pools of blood; therefore suction may be necessary to keep the area dry. A gray eschar will form at the cautery site. Excess silver nitrate should be removed with cotton or gauze to minimize dispersion by nasal secretions and resulting injury to intact mucosa.[30] Caution should be used to avoid

BOX 176-2 Equipment Used in the Initial Management of Anterior Epistaxis

EXAMINATION
Flashlight or
Otoscope with speculum or
Headlight and nasal speculum suction

VASOCONSTRICTION
oxymetazoline (Afrin) or
phenylephrine (Neo-Synephrine) or
epinephrine (1:1000)

TOPICAL ANESTHESIA
4% lidocaine or
3%-5% cocaine solution ethyl chloride

HEMOSTASIS
Silver nitrate sticks
Vaseline strip gauze
Oxycellulose sponges (Surgicel) or
Gelatin sponges (Gelfoam) or
Nasal tampons (Merocel)

ADDITIONAL ITEMS
Antibiotic ointment or cream
Cotton pledgets, gauze
Gown, gloves, mask

cauterizing too large or too deep an area and to avoid cauterizing both sides of the septum because these measures can lead to septal perforation. After cauterization, the physician should prescribe antibiotic cream or ointment to apply to the area twice a day for 5 days to prevent crusting and infection.[9] Hydration with saline or ointment should continue until healing is complete, in approximately 1 to 3 weeks. Nasal trauma and forceful nose blowing should be avoided during this time. Otolaryngologists may use electrocautery as another hemostatic measure. This type of thermal cautery however cannot be performed with topical anesthesia alone.

If an anterior bleed persists despite direct pressure or nasal cautery, then anterior nasal packing may be required. This task can be accomplished with antibiotic impregnated petroleum jelly gauze, which is layered into the anterior nose and provides a tight pack. However, packing is uncomfortable, requires subsequent removal (usually after 2 to 3 days), and can cause additional mucosal injury. Oxycellulose or gelatin sponges are absorbable and do not require later extraction. Although they do not apply a great deal of pressure to the bleeding site, these types of packing are usually adequate for most nosebleeds.[29] Commercially available nasal tampons made of a dehydrated polyvinyl polymer sponge can also be used. The tampons are inserted dry and then expand with blood or added saline partially to fill the nasal cavity. These products come in many sizes and can be cut to fit a child's nasal cavity. They must be removed, usually after 3 to 5 days, and have a tendency to adhere to the nasal lining.[27]

All types of packing and sponges should be impregnated or coated with antibiotic ointment to prevent toxic shock syndrome, which is a reported complication of anterior and posterior nasal packing.[7,9] Although no clear evidence exists to prove that prophylactic antibiotics reduce the incidence of serious infection, studies have shown that they reduce gram-negative bacterial growth and common practice is to prescribe them for any patient with nasal packing.[7,31] Antibiotics may also help prevent sinusitis that can result from stasis of nasal secretions when packing is in place.[29] Recommended antibiotics include first-generation cephalosporins or penicillins with activity against penicillinase-producing organisms.[27]

Identifying the source of a posterior bleed must be done by an otolaryngologist using a flexible fiberoptic nasopharyngoscope; sedation may be required for younger patients. In addition to locating a superior or posterior bleeding site, endoscopic visualization may also reveal causes such as foreign bodies, tumors, or sinusitis. In older more cooperative patients, a rigid endoscope may be used. Cauterization of a posterior bleeding site can be performed under general anesthesia. Posterior packing can be done with gauze or even urinary catheter balloons. Other types of packing include premade nasal tampons or balloons.[7] All patients requiring posterior packing must be admitted to the hospital and monitored in an intensive care unit for airway obstruction and respiratory compromise.[29] More invasive measures such as arterial embolization for refractory bleeds and arterial ligation for recurrent epistaxis are rarely indicated in children.[7]

Once the acute episode of epistaxis has resolved, attention can be focused on looking for predisposing factors or causes and respective preventive strategies or specific management. If a dry environment is present, then the use of normal saline nasal spray helps to humidify the nasal cavity. The spray should be used 4 to 5 times a day. A humidifier in the home may also be useful.[30] The increased moisture helps prevent the accumulation of crusts, which are often the impetus for nose picking, and keeps scabs soft, allowing them to stay in place longer and thus promoting healing of underlying mucosal injury. Local trauma should be minimized by discouraging nose picking, forceful rubbing, or blowing of the nose. Fingernails can be trimmed as well. Parents should be educated about the home management of an acute nosebleed; they should pinch the nasal tip for 5 to 10 minutes with the child sitting up, leaning slightly forward.[32]

If allergic rhinitis is a factor in epistaxis, then appropriate testing and medical management is indicated, including treatment with inhaled topical nasal steroids. For sinusitis, oral antibiotics are prescribed. If a bleeding disorder is thought to exist, then laboratory workup (see discussion under "Evaluation" earlier in this chapter) or referral to a hematologist is warranted. Otolaryngologists treat other infrequent lesions and conditions. For example, they will cauterize granulomas, monitor hemangiomas, and excise juvenile nasopharyngeal angiofibromas after hormonal therapy and embolization.[33] Patients with Osler-Weber-Rendu disease are now treated with argon laser therapy along with septal dermoplasty.[34]

A common challenge for physicians is the management of recurrent nosebleeds. A recent Cochrane review of the literature on interventions for recurrent idiopathic epistaxis in children exposed the lack of evidence for current treatments of this problem.[35] The condition was defined as repeated nasal bleeding in patients younger than 16 years without identifiable cause. Consensus does not exist on the frequency or severity of the episodes of epistaxis that warrant medical intervention. However, common interventions for less severe cases include cautery with silver nitrate, application of antibiotic nasal creams, instillation of nasal saline spray, or the coating of the interior nose with ointments such as petroleum jelly. Less frequently advocated topical agents include oxymetazoline, desmopressin, antifibrinolytics, and, most recently, fibrin sealants. No single treatment (neomycin-chlorhexidine antiseptic cream, silver nitrate cautery, petroleum jelly) was found to be superior to another or to no treatment at all. No serious adverse effects were experienced, although silver nitrate cauterization caused pain in children despite topical anesthesia.[35-38] High-quality studies are needed to ascertain which, if any, of these remedies for recurrent epistaxis in children are most effective.

Nosebleeds occur commonly in children. Although quite upsetting and worrisome to parents, most epistaxis in childhood is anterior, is controlled by simple first-aid measures, and results from benign causes. Epistaxis is therefore usually treated on an outpatient basis by general pediatricians. An understanding of all potential causes and acute and long-term management of nosebleeds will assist the pediatrician in appropriate treatment of this condition.

WHEN TO REFER

Ear, Nose, and Throat

Urgent Referral:

- Profuse, uncontrollable bleeding
- Inability to locate source of bleed
- Posterior bleeding
- Assistance with anterior packing
- Recurrence of bleed after initial emergency department measures

Nonurgent Referral:

- Removal of anterior packing
- Recurrent epistaxis
- Evaluation for structural lesions (ie, granulomas, tumors, polyps)
- Treatment of specific lesions

Hematology

- Abnormal coagulation laboratory profile
- Severe, persistent or recurrent bleeding
- Bleeding from more than 1 site, based on history or physical examination
- Bleeding that required blood transfusion or iron therapy
- Family history of coagulopathy

WHEN TO ADMIT

- Hemodynamic instability on presentation
- Posterior nasal packing in place

TOOLS FOR PRACTICE

Engaging Patients and Family

- *Nosebleeds* (fact sheet), American Academy of Pediatrics (www.aap.org/topics.html).

SUGGESTED RESOURCES

Burton MJ, Doree CJ. Interventions for recurrent idiopathic epistaxis (nosebleeds) in children. *The Cochrane Database of Systematic Reviews*. 2004; Issue 1.

Manning S, Culbertson M Jr. Epistaxis. In: Bluestone C et al, ed. *Pediatric Otolaryngology*. 4th ed. Philadelphia, Pa: Saunders; 2003: 925-931.

Sandoval C, Dong S, Visintaimer P et al. Clinical and laboratory features of 178 children with recurrent epistaxis. *J of Ped Hem/Onc*. 2002;24:47-49.

Tan LKS, Calhoun KH. Epistaxis. *Med Clin North Am*. 1999; 83:43-56.

REFERENCES

1. Kucik CJ, Clenney T. Management of Epistaxis. *Am Fam Phys*. 2005;71:305-311.
2. Quinn FB, Porter GT. Epistaxis. Grand rounds presentation. *UTMB Dept Otolaryngol*. April 2002.
3. Guarisco JL, Graham HD III. Epistaxis in children: causes, diagnosis and treatment. *Ear, Nose, Throat J*. 1989;68:522-538.
4. Nunez DA, McClymont LG, Evans RA. Epistaxis: a study of the relationship with weather. *Clinical Otolaryngol*. 1990;15:49-51.
5. Petruson B. Epistaxis in childhood. *Rhinology*. 1979;17: 83-90.
6. Pallin DJ, Chng Y, McKay MP, et al. Epidemiology of epistaxis in US emergency departments, 1992 to 2001. *Ann of Emerg Med*. 2005;46:77-81.
7. Manning S, Culbertson M Jr. Epistaxis. In: Bluestone C, Stool S, Kenna M, eds. *Pediatric Otolaryngology*. 4th ed. Philadelphia, PA: Saunders; 2003;925-931.
8. Murray AB, Milner RA. Allergic rhinitis and recurrent epistaxis in children. *Allergy Asthma Immunol*. 1995;74: 30-33.
9. Tan LKS, Calhoun KH. Epistaxis. *Med Clin North Am*. 1999;83:43-56.
10. Malik MK, Kumar A, Bhalia BP. Juvenile nasopharyngeal angiofibroma. *Indian J Med Sci*. 1991;45:336-342.
11. Komoroski EM. Nasopharyngeal carcinoma: early warning signs and symptoms. *Pediatr Emerg Care*. 1994;10: 284-286.
12. Bass IS, Haller JO, Berdon WE, et al. Nasopharyngeal carcinoma: clinical and radiographic findings in children. *Radiology*. 1985;156:651-654.
13. Zubizarreta PA, D'Antonio G, Raslawski E, et al. Nasopharyngeal carcinoma in childhood and adolescence. *Cancer*. 2000;89:690-695.
14. Buchanan GR. Thrombocytopenia during childhood: what the pediatrician needs to know. *Pediatr Rev*. 2005; 28:401-409.
15. Medeiros D, Buchanan JR. Major hemorrhage in children with idiopathic thrombocytopenic purpura: immediate response to therapy and long-term outcome. *J Pediatr*. 1998;133:334-339.

16. Lubianca Neto JF, Brito LB, Santos EF. Epistaxis as a manifestation of Bernard-Soulier syndrome. *J Pediatr (Rio J)*. 1997;73:111-114.
17. Sandoval C, Dong S, Visintaimer P, et al. Clinical and laboratory features of 178 children with recurrent epistaxis. *J of Ped Hem/Onc*. 2002;24:47-49.
18. Kiley V, Stuart JJ, Johnson CA. Coagulation studies in children with isolated recurrent epistaxis. *J Pediatr*. 1982;100:579-581.
19. Serdaroglu G, Tutuncuoglu S, Kavakli K. Coagulation abnormalities and acquired von Willebrands disease type I in children receiving valproic acid. *J Child Neurol*. 2002; 17:41-43.
20. Mei-Zahav M. Osler-Weber-Rendu—a life-threatening disease in adults and children. *Harefuah*. 2003;142: 852-856.
21. Jarjour IT, Jarjour LK. Migraine and recurrent epistaxis in children. *Ped Neurol*. 2005;33:94-97.
22. Ngo A, Ng KC, Sim TP. Otorhinolaryngeal foreign bodies in children presenting to the emergency department. *Singapore Med J*. 2005;46:172-178.
23. Katsanis E, Luke K, Hsu E, et al. Prevalence and significance of mild bleeding disorders in children with recurrent epistaxis. *J Pediatr*. 1988;113:73-76.
24. Callejo G, Velert Vila MM, Marco Algarro J. Recurrent epistaxis in children as an indicator of hemostatic disorders. *An Esp Pediatr*. 1998;49:475-480.
25. Lavy JA, Koay CB. First aid treatment of epistaxis—are patients well informed? *J Accid Emerg Med*. 1996;13: 193-195.
26. McGarry GW, Moulton C. Epistaxis first aid. *Arch Emerg Med*. 1993;10:298-300.
27. Middleton PM. Epistaxis. *Emergency Medicine Australasia*. 2004;16:428-440.
28. Dost P, Polyzoidis T. Benefit of the ice pack in the treatment of nosebleed. *HNO*. 1992;40:25-27.
29. Nadel F, Henretig F. Epistaxis. In: Fleisher G, Ludwig S, Henretig FM, eds. *Textbook of Pediatric Emergency Medicine*. 5th ed. Philadelphia, PA: Lippincott Williams & Wilkins; 2006;263-266, 1669-1671, 1893-1896.
30. Massick D, Tobin E. Epistaxis. In: Cummings C, Schuller DE, Thomas JR, et al, eds. *Otolaryngology/Head and Neck Surgery*. 4th ed. Philadelphia, PA: Elsevier Mosby 2005.
31. Derkay CS, Hirsch BE, Johnson JT, et al. Posterior nasal packing. Are intravenous antibiotics really necessary? *Arch Otolaryngol Head Neck Surg*. 1989;115: 439-441.
32. Shott SR. Epistaxis. In: Rudolph AM, Rudolph CD, Hostetter MK, et al, eds. *Rudolph's Pediatrics*. 21st ed. New York, NY: McGraw-Hill; 2002:1261-1262.
33. Mulbury P. Recurrent epistaxis. *Ped Rev*. 1991;12: 213-217.
34. Lund VJ, Howard DJ. A treatment algorithm for the management of epistaxis in hereditary hemorrhagic telangiectasis. *Am J Rhinol*. 1999;13:319-322.
35. Burton MJ, Doree CJ. Interventions for recurrent idiopathic epistaxis (nosebleeds) in children. *Cochrane Database System Rev*. 2004;(1):CD004461.
36. Kubba H, MacAndie C, Botma M, et al. A prospective, single-blind, randomized controlled trial of antiseptic cream for recurrent epistaxis in childhood. *Clin Otolaryngol*. 2001;26:465-468.
37. Loughran S, Spinou E, Clement E, et al. A prospective, single-blind, randomized controlled trial of petroleum jelly/Vaseline for recurrent paediatric epistaxis. *Clin Otolaryngol*. 2004;29:266-269.
38. Ruddy J, Proops DW, Pearman K, et al. Management of epistaxis in children. *Int J Paediatr Otorhinolaryngol*. 1991;21:139-142.

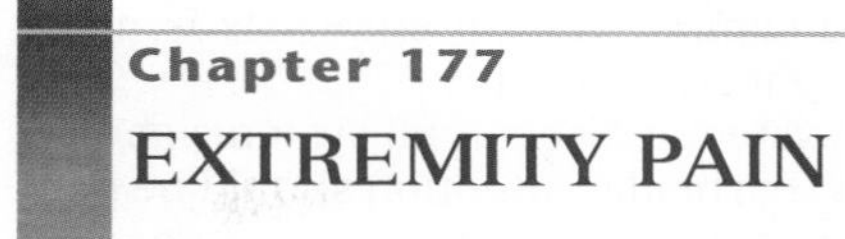

Chapter 177

EXTREMITY PAIN

Michael G. Burke, MD, MBA; David C. Hanson, MD

DEFINITION OF TERMS

Extremity pain is a common complaint in primary care pediatric practice. Up to 16% of school-aged children report at least 1 episode of activity-limiting extremity pain annually.[1] Between 6% and 7% of pediatric office visits are related to extremity pain.[2,3] Fortunately, most of these visits involve pain caused by minor trauma, overuse syndromes, and normal skeletal growth variants.[2] Occasionally, however, limb pain is the presenting complaint of a systemic illness, a neoplasm, an infectious process, a nutritional derangement, a specific orthopedic disorder, or a rheumatologic disease. The challenge for the practitioner is to determine when the pain is significant without exposing the child to excessive diagnostic studies and without delaying treatment or referral. For the most part, this determination is based on the history and physical examination alone.

EVALUATION

History

A thorough history from patients and parents often reveals the cause of extremity pain in children. Pain described as aching or cramping is likely to be muscular in origin. Bone pain is often described as deep and nerve pain as burning, tingling, or numbness. Referred pain is common in children; thus, although usually helpful, the location of pain may be deceiving. Migrating extremity pain is less likely to occur after trauma and is more typical of systemic illness such as leukemia, acute rheumatic fever, disseminated gonorrhea, and arthralgia or arthritis associated with inflammatory bowel disease. The mode of onset, variability, duration, and frequency of pain also help in determining its cause. Activities associated with worsening or relief of pain can also lead to a diagnosis. Similarly, color change associated with extremity pain may indicate inflammation (faint red), infection (intense red), or autonomic dysfunction (pallor, cyanosis, and erythema). Stiffness, especially with clinical evidence of arthritis not associated with trauma, should prompt concern about a rheumatologic process.

A history specific to trauma associated with extremity pain can be helpful. Trauma accompanied by an audible pop or snap is more likely the result of a dislocation, sprain, or fracture. Mild trauma that leads to a fracture might indicate some previous defect in the bone, as with a pathological fracture. If the physical findings of trauma are greater than would be expected from the history, then physical abuse must be considered (see Chapter 120, Child Physical Abuse and Neglect).

The child's general health history completes the picture of extremity pain. For example, the differential diagnosis changes with age. Toxic synovitis of the hip is a common diagnosis in a child younger than

10 years; a slipped capital femoral epiphysis is more likely in an overweight adolescent.

As a screen for systemic disease, all systems should be reviewed briefly. Particular attention should be paid to a history of fever, recent weight loss, sweating, rashes, and gastrointestinal symptoms. A history of recent medications is important and might reveal a serum sickness-like illness (particularly associated with cefaclor). Even a short course of systemic steroids can cause aseptic necrosis of the hip or can result in demineralization of bone. Immunizations, particularly for rubella, may cause joint or extremity pain, and a history of exposure to viral illness might explain myalgia or arthralgia. Specifically, the prodrome of hepatitis B can cause significant arthralgia.

The patient's family history may reveal a tendency toward autoimmune disease or recent exposure to infectious diseases. The family history is particularly helpful in identifying hemoglobinopathies. A family history of sickle cell anemia in a 6- to 24-month-old child whose hands and feet are painfully swollen may lead to the diagnosis of hand-foot syndrome and previously undiagnosed sickle cell disease. A sickle cell pain crisis must always be considered in a black child or one of Mediterranean origin who has a painful extremity. Human leukocyte antigen B27 is associated with Reiter syndrome, psoriatic arthritis, inflammatory bowel disease, and ankylosing spondylitis and has been described in association with enthesitis-related arthritis (inflammation of tendons, ligaments, or fascia at their attachments to bone).[4] Joint hypermobility syndrome and fibromyalgia also can be familial.

Extremity pain may be a symptom of a functional disorder and can serve as an entry to the physician's office. One large group of pediatric rheumatologists has estimated that 11% of their new patients suffer from psychosomatic musculoskeletal pain.[5] In cases of functional pain, the history may be either quite dramatic or highly understated. Pain in a nonanatomic distribution or that disturbs unpleasant but not pleasant activities (waxing on school days and waning on weekends) should raise suspicion of a functional disorder. Eliciting a history of recent events at home, recent school performance, and other social history can be essential to determining the diagnosis.

Physical Examination

At least a brief general physical examination is worthwhile, even if the history points to extremity pain from minor local trauma. Abnormalities in blood pressure, heart rate, or growth pattern can reveal an endocrine cause. An elevated resting heart rate is associated with rheumatic fever. Pallor, fever, lymphadenopathy, or organomegaly may be clues to systemic disease. A rash may be particularly helpful. Dermatomyositis occurs with muscle pain and proximal weakness associated with a vasculitic rash on the extensor surfaces of knuckles, knees, and elbows (Gottron papules). Palpable purpura and extremity pain are associated with Henoch-Schönlein purpura. A photosensitive rash in a child who has limb pain might point to systemic lupus erythematosus, dermatomyositis, or parvovirus infection. Nail pitting is associated with psoriasis.

In a child with unexplained extremity pain, a thorough eye examination by an ophthalmologist may detect uveitis, sometimes associated with juvenile idiopathic arthritis. Photophobia, eye injection, or pain with accommodation associated with extremity pain warrants a consultation with a rheumatologist and ophthalmologist. A complete physical examination can reveal generalized joint laxity and hyperextensibility, differentiating benign hypermobility syndrome from a focal ligament injury. In benign hypermobility syndrome (Ehlers-Danlos syndrome type III), the joint laxity allows chronic hyperextension, which can cause pain, typically in weight-bearing joints. The pain often is worse in the evening. Dancing and gymnastics may exacerbate arthralgia, as can any other joint-impacting activity.

Claudication is a rare cause of extremity pain in children. However, in popliteal artery entrapment syndrome, vascular calf pain that radiates to the foot is associated with an anomalous popliteal artery or anomalous placement of the gastrocnemius muscle.[6] The pain begins with activity, sometimes more with walking than with running. This syndrome is suggested if normal pedal pulses are lost with simultaneous knee extension and foot plantar flexion.

Because referred pain is common in children, the physical examination should include areas proximal and distal to the site of the complaint. A slipped capital femoral epiphysis and Legg-Calve-Perthes disease, both of which affect the hip, can produce knee or thigh pain, whereas an abscess of the psoas muscle may cause hip pain. Some intraabdominal processes, particularly if the psoas muscle is irritated, and diskitis can also cause pain that is referred to a lower extremity.

Examination of a painful extremity should include assessment of peripheral vascular status, muscle strength, soft-tissue swelling, and skeletal injury. Disruption of joint integrity may be shown by demonstration of abnormal range of motion of the joint with passive movement. Peripheral vascular status is assessed by palpating the pulses and determining the capillary refill time distal to the pain. Skin color and warmth, tenderness to palpation, and the extent of passive and active range of motion should all be assessed. Swelling, warmth, and erythema over a joint are signs of arthritis. Point tenderness over a bone raises suspicion of a fracture. Point tenderness in the absence of a clear history of trauma may indicate osteomyelitis. Comparing the opposite limb is helpful when assessing swelling, muscle wasting, or joint mobility. Observing the patient's gait or use of the painful limb when the patient is unaware of the observation helps in diagnosing a functional process. Isolated distal weakness is likely to be of neurologic origin, whereas proximal weakness is most likely from muscular disease. Finally, with chronic extremity pain, serial examinations of the patient over the course of weeks can be the key to diagnosis.

Laboratory Examination

Laboratory studies are unnecessary for most extremity pain. However, if the history and physical examination do not lead to a definitive diagnosis, if they raise suspicion of a systemic or an infectious disease, or if the pain persists longer than anticipated, then screening laboratory tests are in order. A basic evaluation should include a complete blood count, a sedimentation rate, a C-reactive protein, and a sickle cell preparation or hemoglobin electrophoresis when indicated. Appropriate serologies should be considered if features of the physical examination are consistent with rheumatologic disease. An elevated sedimentation rate raises suspicion of an infectious or inflammatory disorder or, occasionally, of a neoplastic one. A complete blood count may reveal anemia or may suggest an infectious disease. With leukemia, the white blood cell (WBC) count varies, but immature forms may be present in the differential WBC count or thrombocytopenia may be present. A creatine phosphokinase determination is occasionally indicated if muscular pain or weakness is suspected.

Imaging

Radiologic studies are often unnecessary in evaluating limb pain. However, because of the plasticity of children's bones, traumatic injury that would ordinarily cause only a sprain in an adult is more likely to result in a greenstick or buckle fracture in a child. The presence of point tenderness or gross deformity in an extremity or pain on motion of the involved limb increases the likelihood of fracture. Although a lower threshold for obtaining posttraumatic radiographs in children may therefore be justified, multiple studies have failed to establish clear clinical criteria for pursuit of radiographs.[7,8] When no clear history of trauma is revealed, when symptoms persist, and when associated systemic complaints are present, radiographs can help identify bony tumors, pathological fractures, some metabolic defects, and a significant number of orthopedic conditions.

A bone scan is a useful diagnostic tool in evaluating limb pain and should be considered when a stress fracture, osteomyelitis, or malignancy is suspected. Bone scans are more sensitive than plain-film radiography for establishing these diagnoses. The American College of Radiology has suggested a bone scan as part of the evaluation of a limping child younger than 5 years whose examination does not have a focal finding.[9,10] Increasingly, magnetic resonance imaging (MRI) is being used as a replacement for bone scans in the diagnosis of osteomyelitis. The combined use of T1, T2, and short-tau inversion-recovery images effectively rules out osteomyelitis, with a negative predictive value approaching 100%.[11] MRI offers the additional advantages of imaging of soft-tissue, as well as joint, disease.

Differential Diagnosis

The differential diagnosis of extremity pain is extremely broad (Box 177-1). However, most limb pain is benign, requires no intervention, and is self-limited. Characteristic patterns of pain and associated signs and symptoms signal the presence of certain diseases and conditions. A discussion of some of these disorders follows.

Growing Pains

Growing pains are a time-honored pediatric disorder. They are intermittent, deep extremity pains that affect the lower more often than the upper extremities. The pain is nearly always bilateral, rarely involves the joints, and is almost universally worse at night, lasts fewer than 2 hours, and resolves completely in the morning. Despite their name, growing pains do not occur most frequently during periods of rapid growth. Instead, their onset is described at 3 to 5 or 8 to 12 years of age. Most growing pains resolve in 12 to 24 months; however, they may persist into adolescence.

The cause of growing pains remains unclear. However, headache and abdominal pain, often associated with emotional illnesses, also have accompanied growing pains.

The diagnosis of growing pains is significant for its lack of associated physical signs. Thus any abnormal finding on physical examination should provoke a search for another cause. Similarly, radiographs and the results of screening laboratory tests usually prove normal. Treatment involves heat, massage, and analgesics.

Sprains

A sprain is a physical disruption of a ligament. In children, sprains occur less commonly than in adults because a child's open epiphyseal plate or plastic bony cortex tends to give way more easily than does a ligament. Therefore Salter-Harris fractures and buckle fractures should be considered when the history indicates a sprain and when physical examination reveals tenderness on palpation or pain on stretching the ligament. Joint stability should also be assessed. Sprains can be graded according to the degree of associated ligament disruption. A mild, microscopic tear that results in no laxity of the involved joint is a grade I sprain. Grade II sprains involve macroscopic but incomplete ligament tears. Joint laxity is greater, but less than a 5-mm movement differential exists between the sprained and the contralateral joint. Grade III sprains result in more than 5 mm of increased mobility of the affected joint. The primary care physician can treat grade I sprains by icing and wrapping the involved joint to minimize swelling. Early range of motion exercises should be encouraged, with a gradual return to activity. The recurrence of pain indicates too rapid a return to a given level of activity. Grade II and grade III sprains should generally be referred to an orthopedist for immobilization and consideration of surgical repair of torn ligaments.

Overuse Syndromes

Overuse injuries have become more common as organized sports for children have become popular nationwide and as the competitive level of some sports activities have increased. Localized, gradually increasing, and persistent extremity pain that worsens with weight bearing, exercise, and activity but that diminishes with rest can indicate a stress fracture. Stress fractures are rare in children younger than age 12 years. They most commonly affect the 2nd metatarsal, the proximal tibia, or the fibula. Although a radiograph may show normal findings, a bone scan can help establish the diagnosis. Treatment consists mostly of rest and treatment with nonsteroidal antiinflammatory agents. Casting or splinting is occasionally necessary.

Little League elbow is an overuse injury caused by the repetitive motion of pitching a baseball; this motion compresses the radial aspect of the elbow and stretches the ulnar aspect. The result is painful

BOX 177-1 Extremity Pain in Childhood: Differential Diagnosis

IMMUNE-MEDIATED ORIGIN
Dermatomyositis
Familial Mediterranean fever
Henoch-Schönlein purpura
Inflammatory bowel disease
Juvenile idiopathic arthritis
Kawasaki disease
Mixed connective-tissue disease
Polyarteritis nodosa
Rheumatic fever
Scleroderma
Serum sickness
Systemic lupus erythematosus

CONGENITAL ORIGIN
Caffey disease
Hemophilia
Hypermobility syndrome (Ehlers-Danlos syndrome type III)
Mucolipidosis
Mucopolysaccharidosis
Popliteal artery entrapment syndrome
Sickle cell anemia, thalassemia

ENDOCRINE ORIGIN
Hypercortisolism
Hyperparathyroidism
Hypothyroidism

IDIOPATHIC ORIGIN
Fibromyalgia
Growing pains
Guillain-Barré syndrome
Sarcoidosis

INFECTIOUS ORIGIN
Bacterial
Arthralgia or myalgia associated with streptococcal infection
Diskitis, spinal epidural abscess
Gonorrhea
Osteomyelitis
Pyogenic myositis
Septic arthritis
Enteric disease
Histoplasmosis
Immunization reaction
Lyme disease
Meningococcal disease
Syphilis: periostitis
Trichinosis
Tuberculosis
Viral
Myalgia, arthralgia
Myositis
Toxic synovitis

METABOLIC ORIGIN
Carnitine palmityltransferase deficiency
Fabry disease
McArdle syndrome
Phosphofructokinase deficiency

NEOPLASTIC ORIGIN
Histiocytosis X
Leukemia
Lymphoma
Neuroblastoma
Tumors of bone
Chondrosarcoma
Ewing sarcoma
Osteoblastoma (benign)
Osteogenic sarcoma
Osteoid osteoma (benign)
Tumors of soft tissue
Fibrosarcoma
Rhabdomyosarcoma
Synovial cell sarcoma
Tumors of the spinal cord

NUTRITIONAL ORIGIN
Gout
Hypercholesterolemia
Hypervitaminosis A
Osteoporosis
Rickets (vitamin D deficiency)
Scurvy (vitamin C deficiency)

ORTHOPEDIC ORIGIN
Chondromalacia patellae
Freiberg disease
Inflexible flat feet, tarsal coalition
Kohler disease
Legg-Calve-Perthes disease
Osgood-Schlatter disease
Osteochondritis dissecans
Osteogenesis imperfecta
Pathological fracture
Sever disease
Slipped capital femoral epiphysis

PSYCHOSOCIAL ORIGIN
Behavior disorders
Psychogenic pain
Reflex neurovascular dystrophy
School phobia

Continued

BOX 177-1 Extremity Pain in Childhood: Differential Diagnosis—cont'd

TRAUMA OR OVERUSE
Compartment syndrome
Fracture
Myohematoma
Myositis ossificans
Nerve compression syndrome
Carpal tunnel syndrome
Cervical nerve root entrapment
Other peripheral nerve root compression
Physical abuse
Shin splint
Sprain
Stress fracture
Subluxed radial head
Thoracic outlet syndrome

Modified from Bowyer SL, Hollister JR. Limb pain in childhood. *Pediatr Clin North Am.* 1984;31(5):1053-1081. Copyright © 1984, Elsevier, with permission.

inflammation of the epicondyles. The range of joint motion also may be diminished. Fragments of bone splintered into the joint may cause the joint to catch or lock. Treatment consists of resting the arm by avoiding the repetitive movement. A change in pitching technique may reduce recurrences. To prevent this problem, some Little League systems limit both the number of innings a child may pitch in 1 game and the age at which certain pitches can be thrown.

Shin splints are also caused by overuse. The term originally referred to pain along the posteromedial aspect of the tibia as a result of irritation at the origin of the posterior tibial muscle. Shin splints now refer to any of a series of painful overuse syndromes of the lower portion of the leg, including irritation of the posterior or anterior tibial muscle, inflammation of the interosseous membrane located between the tibia and fibula, and both anterior and posterior compartment syndromes. All of these abnormalities can cause pain in the lower legs. The condition, which is exacerbated by running and jumping, occurs most commonly at the beginning of a training season. Although the pain occurs initially after activity, it may occur during or before activity as the syndrome progresses. On examination, tenderness may be felt over the posteromedial aspect of the tibia, over the proximal portion of the posterior tibia, or over the anterior tibia. Differential diagnosis includes Osgood-Schlatter disease with pain localized to the tibial tuberosity. Treatment of shin splints involves rest, application of ice, and antiinflammatory drugs. For runners, training on a softer surface or with better-quality running shoes may help.

Subluxation of the Radial Head

Nursemaid's elbow is a common injury in toddlers. The injury usually follows sudden, forceful traction of the hand or forearm, which pulls the immature radial head briefly from the cuff formed by the annular ligament. Release of the force allows the radius to trap the ligament against the capitellum. A verbal patient usually localizes the pain to the elbow or, occasionally, to the wrist. More often, the child refuses to use the extremity and holds the arm with the elbow flexed, the forearm close to the chest, and the hand in pronation. The diagnosis is usually made by history alone. If the history is unclear, or if attempts to reduce the subluxation are unsuccessful, then radiographs may be obtained to rule out a fracture. Radiographic findings in subluxation of the radial head usually are negative. The practitioner can reduce the subluxation by using 1 hand to supinate the patient's forearm quickly while simultaneously exerting traction on the forearm and using the thumb of the other hand to create pressure over the patient's radial head. This maneuver is completed by placing the elbow through full extension and flexion while maintaining pressure over the radial head. Normal use of the extremity usually returns within 30 minutes. The rapid recovery is dramatic and rewarding to the parents and the physician. A prompt return to normal use of the affected arm may not occur if the subluxation has been present for some time because of swelling of the ligament. In such instances, the affected arm should be placed in a simple sling and positioned across the upper portion of the abdomen for 12 to 24 hours. Referral to an orthopedist is rarely required.

Slipped Capital Femoral Epiphysis

A slipped capital femoral epiphysis is caused by a sudden or gradual dislocation of the head of the femur from its neck and shaft at the level of the upper epiphyseal plate. The characteristic pain occurs in the affected hip or the medial aspect of the ipsilateral knee. The displacement may be sudden, in which case the pain is usually severe and associated with the inability to bear weight. Gradual displacement is associated with slowly increasing, dull pain. This condition typically affects sedentary, obese adolescent boys. The physical examination may reveal diminished abduction and internal rotation of the hip. The diagnosis is made radiographically. Management involves surgical placement of a pin through the femoral head and the epiphysis to prevent further slippage. Avascular necrosis of the femoral head is a common complication, even with early recognition and treatment.

Toxic Synovitis

Toxic synovitis, a self-limited inflammation of the hip joint, commonly occurs in children younger than age 10 years. The cause is unknown; however, because it often occurs within 2 weeks after an upper respiratory infection, a postviral inflammatory process is suspected. Typical presentation is that of a child who refuses to walk because of apparent pain in the hip. The hip is held in flexion, abduction, and external rotation.

Findings may include a slight elevation in the WBC count and the sedimentation rate, a frustrating development for the practitioner, who hopes to rule out septic arthritis. A C-reactive protein of less than 1 mg/dL has been shown to have an 87% negative predictive value for septic arthritis.[12] This study may offer reassurance. However, persistent concern for septic arthritis may lead to consultation with an orthopedist. Treatment of toxic synovitis consists of bed rest, usually for fewer than 4 days. In rare instances, avascular necrosis of the femoral head may be a late complication.

Osteochondroses

Osteochondroses (see also Chapter 302, Osteochondroses) include a group of disorders in which degeneration or aseptic necrosis of bone and overlying cartilage occurs at an ossification center and is followed by recalcification. The disorders vary in name and presentation according to their locations.

Legg-Calve-Perthes disease, or osteochondrosis of the femoral head, results from compromise of the tenuous vascular supply to the area. The condition may be idiopathic or may result from a slipped capital femoral epiphysis, trauma, steroid use, sickle cell crisis, or congenital dislocation of the hip. Toxic synovitis also is associated with subsequent Legg-Calve-Perthes disease, but, again, toxic synovitis is rare. After compromise of the vascular supply, the bone underlying the articular surface of the head of the femur becomes necrotic. Collapse of the necrotic bone flattens the femoral head and causes a poor fit with the acetabulum, even after new bone is formed. The pain associated with Legg-Calve-Perthes disease, which results from necrosis of the involved bone, is frequently referred to the medial aspect of the ipsilateral knee. A limp may be the presenting complaint. In many instances, an early diagnosis eludes the practitioner because radiographic findings may be normal or show only swelling of the joint's capsule. A bone scan may demonstrate diminished blood flow to the femoral head compared with the contralateral hip. Later, radiographs may show areas of bone resorption, irregular widening of the epiphysis, or dense new bone formation. The goal of therapy is to prevent flattening of the femoral head as it undergoes new bone formation by keeping the hip abducted so that the head of the femur is held well inside the rounded portion of the acetabulum. Either bracing or an osteotomy may accomplish this task; both require referral to an orthopedic surgeon.

Two similar processes can affect the knee joint. Osteochondritis dissecans involves degeneration of bone and cartilage at the articular surface of the knee, particularly at the lateral aspect of the medial condyle of the femur. Knee pain, crepitus, or a sensation of instability or locking caused by loose bone and cartilage fragments in the joint can result. Chondromalacia patellae occur because of a painful softening or breakdown of the inner surface of the patella. The pain is localized to the knee and increases with activities that require prolonged knee bending and even with prolonged sitting. The pain is described as grinding and can sometimes be elicited by applying pressure over the patella. Moving the patella from side to side over the knee joint may cause crepitus and apprehension. Treatment is usually limited to pain relief and reassurance that, in time, the condition will resolve. Exercise to strengthen the medial quadriceps muscles and to stretch the hamstrings may promote better alignment of the patella with the knee and thereby diminish the pain. Rarely, in severe cases, the patella may have to be realigned surgically. Osteochondrosis of the growth plate of the calcaneus (Sever disease) can produce heel pain that worsens with activity. This usually mild process requires only rest, nonsteroidal antiinflammatory agents, and padding of the heel to relieve the pain. Avascular necrosis and osteochondrosis of the tarsal navicular (Kohler disease) and of the head of the 2nd metatarsal (Freiberg disease) can cause foot pain. Treatment usually requires only pain medication and rest.

Osgood-Schlatter disease is a painful degeneration of the tibial tubercle at the site of insertion of the quadriceps ligament. It is characterized by painful swelling of the anterior aspect of the tibial tubercle, usually occurring during adolescence. The degree of swelling may be alarming, and the area is tender to palpation. Pain is exacerbated by activity that involves increased use of the quadriceps muscles. The process is self-limited and resolves toward the end of adolescence when the epiphysis at the insertion site closes and the bone becomes stronger than the inserted ligament. Until it resolves, the condition is treated with rest, analgesics, and, occasionally, supportive patellar knee straps. In rare cases, casting or surgical attachment of the quadriceps ligament is required.

Osteomyelitis

Osteomyelitis (see Chapter 303, Osteomyelitis) is a local infection of bone, usually involving one of the long bones. The highest incidence is in children 3 to 12 years of age. Although infection often occurs by hematogenous seeding, it can be caused by direct entry after local trauma. In both children and adults, the most commonly isolated organism is *Staphylococcus aureus*. In the last decade, improved diagnostic testing has allowed identification of *Kingella kingae* as one of the primary pathogens of osteomyelitis (and septic arthritis) in children younger than 6 years.[13] Effective vaccination for *Haemophilus influenza* type b has made this pathogen a rare cause of osteomyelitis in immunized children.[14] Other organisms, including *Salmonella* species and group A streptococci also infect the bone. Group B *Streptococcus* is more likely the cause of infection in newborns. Osteomyelitis caused by *Salmonella* tends to occur more often in children who have sickle cell anemia than in other children. In assessing trauma from a puncture wound to the foot, especially through a sneaker, *Pseudomonas aeruginosa* must be considered. In addition, tuberculous osteomyelitis still occurs and may become more common with the resurgence of tuberculosis.

Osteomyelitis can produce extremity pain alone or extremity pain with signs of a systemic infectious disease (fever, irritability, septic appearance). In the absence of systemic signs, distinguishing between osteomyelitis and a traumatic cause of the pain is often difficult. Two weeks or longer may be required for radiographic evidence of osteomyelitis to develop. A bone scan is usually, but not always, diagnostic. In rare cases, a reduction in perfusion caused by pressure from the exudative process may result in false-negative scans. Some experts now prefer MRI to bone scan for confirming this diagnosis. In addition, the WBC count and sedimentation rate are often elevated in osteomyelitis. The effectiveness of treatment can be monitored by repeating tests of the sedimentation rate or the C-reactive protein.

Neoplasms

Although neoplasm is not commonly the cause of limb pain, the possibility of a tumor is a common concern for parents of children who have this complaint. Even if rare, benign and malignant bone tumors and systemic malignancies can cause limb pain.

Osteoid osteoma is a benign prostaglandin-secreting bone tumor that occurs most often in adolescents and usually involves a femur, tibia, or lumbar vertebral body. Pain, the presenting complaint, is initially dull and increases in intensity to deep and boring. The pain is more intense at night and with weight bearing. Radiographic findings of sclerotic bone around a lucent center are diagnostic of this condition; tomograms are sometimes required for confirmation. Surgical excision is curative.

Systemic neoplasms in which extremity pain occurs include leukemia and metastatic neuroblastoma. One third of children who have acute lymphocytic leukemia have bone pain at the time of diagnosis, and in one fourth of children, joint or bone pain is a significant presenting complaint.[15] Unrelenting, increasing pain that worsens at night or with rest and that is not relieved by analgesics, heat, or massage may indicate the presence of a metastatic bone tumor. Systemic signs (weight loss, pallor, lymphadenopathy, hepatosplenomegaly, or fever) may accompany the pain. In leukemia, examination of the extremity may reveal strikingly little to account for the degree of pain. Radiographic studies of the extremities may show lucent leukemic lines in the subepiphyseal area.

Primary malignant tumors of bone may cause severe unilateral pain, with swelling and tenderness at the tumor site. The possibility of this diagnosis supports the use of radiographic studies when unilateral limb pain is not explained adequately by a history of trauma and when pain from trauma does not resolve as expected. The peak incidence of both osteogenic sarcoma and the less common Ewing sarcoma occurs in late childhood and during adolescence. The radiograph of an osteogenic sarcoma may reveal a tumor in the metaphysis with the presence of both radiolucent and radiopaque areas. The characteristic sunburst results from extension of calcification into the overlying soft tissue. Although periosteal elevation may be present, it is not diagnostic of the disease.

WHEN TO REFER

- Surgical procedure or subspecialist required for definitive treatment (eg, suspected anterior cruciate ligament tear, Ewing sarcoma, other associated conditions)
- Surgical procedure or subspecialist required for diagnostic evaluation (eg, suspected septic arthritis, juvenile idiopathic arthritis, systemic lupus erythematosus, other associated conditions)
- Extremity pain part of multisystemic signs and symptoms (eg, Fabry disease, Crohn disease, other associated conditions)

SUGGESTED RESOURCES

Cawkwell GD, Passo MH. Pursuing the source of musculoskeletal pain. *Contemp Pediatr.* 1994;11:72-90.

Sherry DD. Limb pain in childhood. *Pediatr Rev.* Aug 1990; 12(2):39-46.

Szer IS. Musculoskeletal pain syndromes that affect adolescents. *Arch Pediatr Adolesc Med.* 1996;150:740-747.

Tunnessen WW Jr. *Signs and Symptoms in Pediatrics.* 3rd ed. Philadelphia, PA: Lippincott Williams & Wilkins; 1999.

REFERENCES

1. Abu-Arafeh I, Russell G. Recurrent limb pain in schoolchildren. *Arch Dis Child.* 1996;74:336-339.
2. de Inocencio J. Musculoskeletal pain in primary pediatric care: analysis of 1000 consecutive general pediatric clinic visits. *Pediatrics.* 1998;102(6):e63.
3. National Center for Health Statistics. *Vital and Health Statistics: Patient's Reasons for Visiting Physicians. National Ambulatory Medical Care Survey, US, 1977-1978.* DHHS Pub No Pt 82-1717. Hyattsville, MD: US Department of Health and Human Services; 1981.
4. Olivieri I, Pasero G. Long-standing isolated juvenile onset HLA-B27-associated peripheral enthesitis. *J Rheumatol.* 1992;19:164-165.
5. Sherry DD, McGuire T, Mellins E, et al. Psychosomatic musculoskeletal pain in childhood: clinical and psychological analyses of 100 children. *Pediatrics.* 1991;88:1093-1099.
6. Cummings RJ, Webb HW, Lowell WW, et al. The popliteal artery entrapment syndrome in children. *J Pediatr Orthop.* Jul-Aug 1992;12(4):539-541.
7. Rivara FP, Parish RA, Mueller BA. Extremity injuries in children: predictive value of clinical findings. *Pediatrics.* 1986;78(5):803-807.
8. McConnochie KM, Roghmann KJ, Pasternack J, et al. Prediction rules for selective radiographic assessment of extremity injuries in children and adolescents. *Pediatrics.* 1990;86(1):45-57.
9. Englaro EE, Gelfand MJ, Paltiel HJ. Bone scintigraphy in preschool children with lower extremity pain of unknown origin. *J Nuc Med.* 1992;33(3):351-354.
10. Royal SA, Kushner DC, Babcock DS, et al. The limping child. American College of Radiology Appropriateness Criteria. *Radiology.* 2000;215(6):Supplement 801-804.
11. Tehranzadeh J, Wong E, Wang F, et al. Imaging of musculoskeletal and spinal infections: imaging of osteomyelitis in the mature skeleton. *Radiol Clin North Am.* 2001; 39(2):223-250.
12. Levine MJ, McGuire KJ, McGowan KL, et al. Assessment of the test characteristics of C-reactive protein for septic arthritis in children. *J Pediatr Orthop.* 2003;23(3):373-377.
13. Lundy DW, Kehl DK. Increasing prevalence of Kingella kingae in osteoarticular infections in young children. *J Pediatr Orthop.* 1998;18(2):262-267.
14. Howard AW, Viskontas D, Sabbagh C. Reduction in osteomyelitis and septic arthritis related to Haemophilus influenzae type B vaccination. *J Pediatr Orthop.* 1999; 19(6):705-709.
15. Leventhal BG. Neoplasms and neoplasm-like structures. In: Behrman RE, Vaughan VC, eds. *Nelson's Textbook of Pediatrics.* 14th ed. Philadelphia, PA: WB Saunders; 1992.

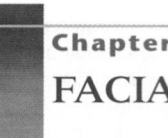

Chapter 178

FACIAL DYSMORPHISM

Robert W. Marion, MD

"It is my business to know things. Perhaps I have trained myself to see what others overlook."

SHERLOCK HOLMES
"A CASE OF IDENTITY"[1]

If someone were searching for a role model for the field of dysmorphology, the study of the recognition of patterns of congenital malformations and dysmorphic features that characterize particular syndromes, Sir Arthur Conan-Doyle's famous detective, Sherlock Holmes, would be an excellent candidate. Similar to Holmes, in evaluating a patient, the dysmorphologist, a subspecialist within the field of medical genetics, searches for clues, sometimes facts available from a carefully obtained history, sometimes facial features that are in plain site, and similar to a detective solving a crime, attempts to assemble these bits of information into a single unifying diagnosis. These clues may be obvious, or they may be so subtle that other clinicians simply overlook them. Their diagnostic significance and the information they may provide about the developmental timing of a congenital anomaly, however, may prove invaluable.

DEFINITIONS

Defined as clinically significant abnormalities in form or function, congenital *malformations* result from localized *intrinsic* defects in morphogenesis that occur in embryonic or early fetal life. These defects, which include clefting of the lip or palate, congenital heart disease such as tetralogy of Fallot, and multicystic kidney disease, may result from an unknown cause but, increasingly, can be traced to mutations in single developmental genes. Malformations usually require surgical intervention.[2]

Deformations differ from malformations in that they arise as a result of environmental forces acting on *normal tissue primordia*. For example, a fetus reared in a uterus in which a large fibroid is present may have limited space for the limbs to go through their normal range of motion; limitation of motion of the limbs leads to congenital contractures, a condition known as *arthrogryposis multiplex congenital*. Deformations occur later than malformations, usually after the 1st trimester of pregnancy is completed, and they often resolve with minimal therapy.[3]

A malformation such as a cleft lip or cleft palate or a deformation such as clubfoot deformity may occur as an isolated feature or, in instances in which multiple malformations occur together, may be part of a *malformation sequence*, a *syndrome*, or an *association*.

When a single malformation causes secondary effects on other structures later in development, a malformation sequence will result. For instance, in the Pierre Robin malformation sequence, the primary malformation, failure of the growth of the mandible during the 1st weeks of gestation, results in micrognathia (small jaw); because of the insufficient size of the jaw, the tongue, which is normal in size, is forced into an unusual position; the abnormally placed tongue blocks the fusion of the palatal shelves that normally come together in the midline, thus producing a U-shaped cleft of the palate; after delivery, the normal-sized tongue in the smaller-than-normal oral cavity leads to airway obstruction and obstructive apnea, a potentially life-threatening complication. Thus 3 anomalies result from the single malformation.[2] (See Chapter 248, Cleft Lip and Cleft Palate, for more information.)

In clinical genetics, a syndrome is defined as a group of malformations that occur together and are caused by a clearly identifiable causative agent. This agent may be a single gene mutation, such as is the case in Marfan syndrome in which a mutation in the *FBN1* gene on chromosome 15 leads to abnormally formed fibrillin, an important component of the myofibrillar array of connective tissue, resulting in a characteristic set of abnormalities of the skeletal, cardiovascular, and ophthalmologic systems. Single gene mutations account for approximately 7.5% of all multiple malformation syndromes. A 2nd cause of a syndrome can be a chromosomal abnormality, as in Down syndrome, in which an extra copy of chromosome 21 leads to craniofacial dysmorphic features, developmental disabilities, cardiac anomalies, and other abnormalities. Approximately 6% of infants with multiple malformation syndromes have a chromosomal abnormality. A 3rd underlying cause of a syndrome can be a teratogenic agent, a drug, chemical, or environmental toxin that causes damage to the developing embryo or fetus, such as valproic acid, an anticonvulsant that when given to a woman during the 1st trimester of pregnancy leads to spina bifida, a characteristic facial appearance, limb defects, and other anomalies in exposed embryos. Teratogens account for approximately 6% of cases of infants with multiple malformation syndromes. Finally, a syndrome can result from unknown factors, as is the case with Russell-Silver syndrome (intrauterine growth restriction with failure to thrive, skeletal asymmetry, a characteristic facial appearance, small, incurved fifth fingers and learning disabilities). Although a small number of individuals with Russell-Silver syndrome can be demonstrated to have maternal uniparental disomy of chromosome 7, 90% of individuals with this condition have no identifiable underlying cause.[4]

Associations differ from syndromes in that no single underlying cause has been identified to explain a recognizable pattern of anomalies that occur together more than would be expected by chance alone. For instance, the *VACTERL* association (**V**ertebral anomalies, **A**nal atresia, **C**ardiac defects, **T**racheo-**E**sophageal fistula, **R**enal anomalies, and **L**imb anomalies) is an example of a group of malformations that occur more commonly together than might be expected by chance; however, no single unifying cause has ever been identified that explains this condition. As such, it is considered an association. As the cause of an association becomes known, the disorder moves from the category of association into the category of syndrome. This change recently happened with the *CHARGE* association (***C***oloboma, ***H***eart disease, ***A***tresia choanae, ***R***etardation of growth or development, ***G***enito-urinary tract anomalies, and ***E***ar anomalies) when, in 2004, this entity was found to be related to mutations in the *CHD7* gene on chromosome 8. Identification of mutations in this gene in patients with this condition allowed CHARGE association to become CHARGE syndrome.

Between 2% and 5% of newborns are found during the neonatal period to have 1 or more congenital malformations. This percentage increases at 1 year of age to 7% to 8% because some malformations, such as congenital heart disease and renal anomalies, may remain clinically silent during the newborn period only to display later in life. In approximately one half of children with congenital malformations, only a single malformation is identifiable; in the other half, multiple malformations are present.[5]

APPROACH TO THE CHILD WITH DYSMORPHIC FEATURES: HISTORY AND PHYSICAL EXAMINATION

The birth of a child with dysmorphic features is a difficult and unsettling experience for the family, the physician, and the medical staff. In many instances, recognition of any problem in an infant will lead to a crisis for the family; the physician caring for the infant and the family may easily panic in such a situation. Therefore establishing a standardized routine is helpful for the evaluation of the child with dysmorphic features, a format that can routinely be followed when the physician is faced with such a situation. This routine should include taking the history, including a 3-generational family history, and performing a careful physical examination. Following these steps, specific diagnostic laboratory tests can be ordered to confirm a diagnosis (Box 178-1).[5]

BOX 178-1 Evaluation of the Individual Who Has Facial Dysmorphism

Review the pregnancy and medical history.
Review the family history.
Evaluate growth of the individual in height, weight, and head circumference.
Evaluate the craniofacial region for dysmorphic features, and, if present, describe these features.
Describe any other dysmorphic somatic features.
Define the development of the individual.
Develop a differential diagnosis and consider appropriate laboratory tests.
Discuss the findings with the family and, if appropriate, offer genetic counseling.

When approaching a child with dysmorphic features, health care providers should be sensitive about the terminology used to describe the infant. The terms *funny-looking kid* and *funny-looking face* are derogatory, justifiably arouse parental indignation, and should be avoided at all times. In discussing dysmorphic features with parents or describing them in written or verbal communication with colleagues, the physician should describe the abnormal features as clearly and concisely as possible.[5]

History

In taking the history, the following questions about the pregnancy should be asked:

1. *What was the birth weight?* A lower-than-expected birth weight can be associated with a chromosome anomaly or exposure to a teratogen. Babies who are large for gestational age may be infants of diabetic mothers or have an overgrowth syndrome, such as Beckwith-Wiedemann syndrome. Infants who are accurate for gestational age may have a single gene mutation, a multifactorial condition, or, most likely, no genetic disease at all.
2. *Was the baby full term, or pre- or postmature?* This information is especially important when evaluating an older child with developmental disabilities. Complications of extreme prematurity may be responsible for the patient's problems. Postmaturity is associated with some chromosome anomalies (such as trisomy 18) and anencephaly.
3. *Was the baby born by vaginal or cesarean delivery? If the latter, what was the indication?* These questions are helpful in evaluating the newborn with dysmorphic features and in older children with developmental disabilities. Cesarean delivery may be performed because of fetal distress, a risk factor for developmental disability caused by oxygen deprivation. Furthermore, babies born from breech presentation are approximately 4 times more likely than infants born from vertex presentation to have congenital malformations.
4. *How old were the parents at the time of the child's delivery?* Advanced maternal age is associated with an increased risk of nondisjunction leading to trisomies, such as Down syndrome (trisomy 21), whereas advanced paternal age may be associated with an increased risk of a new mutation leading to an autosomal-dominant trait, such as achondroplasia.
5. *Did the pregnancy have complications? Does the mother have underlying medical problems? Does she take any medications? Did she smoke cigarettes, drink alcohol, or take any drugs?* Exposure of the embryo to teratogens, medications, or environmental agents known to cause birth defects is a significant cause of congenital malformations.
6. *When did the mother feel quickening? Were fetal movements active?* Quickening, which normally occurs between 16 and 20 weeks' gestation, is delayed in hypotonic fetuses, who also have movements during fetal life that are not as vigorous as a fetus with normal muscle tone. Additionally, a mother's report of persistent hiccups in an infant found to have neonatal seizures suggests a prenatal onset of the condition.

7. *Was the amount of amniotic fluid normal?* An increased amount of amniotic fluid is associated with intestinal obstruction or a central nervous system anomaly that leads to poor swallowing, whereas a decreased amount of fluid may point to a renal or urinary tract abnormality that leads to failure to produce urine or a chronic amniotic fluid leak.

A 3-generation pedigree should be constructed, searching for similar and dissimilar abnormalities in 1st- and 2nd-degree relatives; a history of pregnancy or neonatal losses should also be documented.[5]

Physical Examination

In the process of evaluating the child with dysmorphic features, the physical examination is the most important element. Whenever possible, the patient should be examined using a standardized approach, described in the following sections.

Growth

The height (length), weight, and head circumference should be carefully measured and plotted on appropriate growth curves. Growth that is appropriate for age may be consistent with the presence of a single gene disorder, a multifactorially inherited condition, or, most commonly, no genetic disease. Small size or growth restriction may be secondary to a chromosomal abnormality, a skeletal dysplasia such as achondroplasia, or exposure to toxic or teratogenic agents. Larger-than-expected size suggests an overgrowth syndrome (eg, Sotos or Beckwith-Weidemann syndromes) or, if in the newborn period, of maternal diabetes.[5]

Proportions

Do the limbs look appropriate for the head and trunk? If not, then are the limbs too short (implying the presence of a short-limbed bone dysplasia such as achondroplasia)? A trunk and head that are too small for the extremities may suggest a disorder affecting the vertebrae, such as spondyloepiphyseal dysplasia.[5]

Craniofacial Features

Careful examination of the craniofacies is crucial for the diagnosis of many congenital malformation syndromes. Frequently, a careful observer can make a diagnosis simply by looking at the child's face.

In assessing the face, the following should be systematically observed.

HEAD SHAPE. In the newborn period, molding may cause the head to be misshapen, the result of a late prenatal deformational process (see previous discussion). The examiner will need to allow a few days for the deformation to resolve before assessing the shape. Then, the head should be described using the following terms:

Normocephaly describes a normal head shape.

Dolichocephaly or *scaphocephaly* describes a long, thin head.

Brachycephaly describes a head that is narrow in the anteroposterior diameter and broad laterally.

Plagiocephaly describes a head that is asymmetric or lopsided (see Chapter 311, Plagiocephaly).[5]

FACIAL FEATURES. A dysmorphic face may be appropriate in relation to the family's physiognomy, or it may indicate a particular syndrome. The child who has a large head who also has a parent with a large head does not prompt as much concern as the large-headed child whose parents have normal-size heads. Thus the examiner must evaluate dysmorphic facial features in light of the child's genetic background. (Table 178-1 lists examples of causes of facial malformation.)[8]

In evaluating the face, the examiner should first note the symmetry. Facial asymmetry may be due to a deformation related to intrauterine or extrauterine positioning or a malformation of 1 side of the face, as is the case with *hemifacial microsomia* (also known as Goldenhar syndrome or *facio-auriculo-vertebral syndrome*).

For purposes of evaluation, the face should be divided into 4 regions, all of which should be evaluated separately:

1. The *forehead* extends from the anterior hairline to the eyebrows.
2. The *midface* encompasses the region from the eyebrows to the upper lip and laterally from the outer canthus of each eye to the outer commissure of the lips.
3. The *malar region* extends on either side from the upper portion of the ear to the midface.

Table 178-1 Examples of Causes of Facial Malformation*

CAUSE	EXAMPLE	FACIAL DYSMORPHISM
GENETIC		
Chromosomal	Down syndrome (trisomy 21)	Midface hypoplasia, upward obliquity of palpebral fissures, epicanthal folds, flat nasal bridge, anteversion of nares
Autosomal dominant	Treacher Collins syndrome	Dysplastic ears, maxillary hypoplasia
Autosomal recessive	Hurler syndrome	Corneal clouding, coarse facies
Teratogenic: intrauterine infection	Congenital rubella	Cataracts
Drug induced	Fetal alcohol syndrome	Smooth philtrum, small eyes

**Smith's Recognizable Patterns of Human Malformation* is the most valuable resource for this purpose; it also is helpful in determining if a particular condition is genetically based.

4. The *mandible* extends from lower ear to lower ear and including the lower lip.

By analyzing each of these 4 regions and determining which is normal and which is not, a clear description of the child's dysmorphic features can be made.[5]

The forehead may show overt prominence (as is the case with achondroplasia) or deficiency (often described as a *sloping* appearance, which occurs in children with primary microcephaly).

Hypoplasia of the midface is a common component of many syndromes, including Down syndrome and fetal alcohol syndrome. In evaluating the midface, careful assessment (by both measurement and through plotting those measurements on appropriate growth curves) of both the distance between the eyes (inner and outer canthal distances) and pupils (interpupil distance) may confirm the impression of hypotelorism (eyes that are too close together), suggestive of a defect in midline brain formation (holoprosencephaly), or hypertelorism (eyes that are too far apart), suggestive of a syndrome such as *Opitz syndrome* (ocular hypertelorism, tracheal and esophageal anomalies, and hypospadias). The length of the palpebral fissure should be noted and plotted on the appropriate growth chart; palpebral fissures may be short in fetal alcohol syndrome or excessively long in Kabuki syndrome (short stature, intellectual disability, long palpebral fissures with eversion of lateral portion of lower lid).[3,4,7]

Other features of the eyes should be noted. The obliquity (slant) of the palpebral fissures may be upward (as in Down syndrome) or downward (as in Treacher Collins syndrome). The presence of epicanthal folds, flaps of skin covering the inner canthus of the eye, and usually associated with flattening of the nasal bridge may indicate Down syndrome or fetal alcohol syndrome.

Features of the nose—especially the nasal bridge that can be flattened in Down syndrome or prominent as in velocardiofacial syndrome should be noted. Are the nares oriented normally, or are they tipped back (a condition know as anteversion)? Is the body of the nose normal, or is it deficient?[5]

In evaluating the malar region, the ears should be checked for size (measured and plotted on growth charts that record length for age), shape (noting abnormal folding or flattening of the helices), position (ears are described as low set if the top of the ear is below a line drawn from the outer canthus to the occiput) and orientation (posterior rotation is present when the ear appears turned toward the rear of the head). Ears may be low set because they are small (or microtic) or because of a malformation of the mandibular region.

Finally, the examiner should evaluate the mandibular region, the area encompassing the lower portions of each ear and including the lower jaw. In most newborns, the chin is often retruded (slightly set back behind the vertical line extending from the forehead to the philtrum). If the mandible itself is small, then it is described as micrognathic, whereas an unusually prominent mandible is described as prognathic. Significant micrognathia is seen in the Pierre Robin malformation sequence.[4]

Remainder of the Body

Once facial dysmorphic features have been detected, the primary care physician must conduct a thorough examination looking for additional unusual findings. Again, findings may point to a specific diagnosis.

NECK. Examination of the neck may reveal webbing, a feature common in Turner and Noonan syndromes, or shortening, as is occasionally seen in some skeletal dysplasias and in conditions in which anomalies of the cervical spine occur, such as Klippel Feil syndrome. The position of the posterior hairline should also be evaluated, and the size of the thyroid gland should be assessed.[5]

TRUNK. The chest should be examined for shape (a shieldlike chest is found in Noonan and Turner syndromes) and symmetry (hypoplasia of the pectoralis major and minor muscles, leading to asymmetry, is a feature of the Poland malformation sequence). A pectus deformity of the chest (either pectus excavatum or pectus carinatum) is usually an isolated finding but is a cardinal feature of Marfan syndrome. Scoliosis, also usually an isolated feature, is often seen in individuals with Marfan syndrome, as well as in several other disorders.[5]

EXTREMITIES. Anomalies of the extremities are common in many congenital malformation syndromes. All joints should be examined for range of motion. The presence of single or multiple joint contractures suggests either intrinsic neuromuscular dysfunction, as in the case of some forms of muscular dystrophy, or external deforming forces that limited motion of the joint in utero. Radioulnar synostosis, an inability to pronate or supinate the elbow occurs in fetal alcohol syndrome and in some X chromosome aneuploidy syndromes (such as *48, XXXX* and *48, XXXY syndromes*).[5]

Next, the hands should be examined. Polydactyly (the presence of extra digits) occurs in isolation as an autosomal-dominant trait in up to 1% of all newborns but can also be seen as part of a malformation syndrome such as trisomy 13. Oligodactyly (a deficiency in the number of digits) is seen in Fanconi syndrome (growth retardation, aplastic anemia, development of leukemia or lymphoma and associated heart, renal and limb defects, including radial aplasia and thumb malformation or aplasia), in which it is generally part of a more severe limb reduction defect, or secondary to intrauterine amputation that may occur with *amniotic band disruption sequence*. Syndactyly (a joining of 2 or more digits) is also common to several syndromes, including Smith-Lemli-Opitz syndrome.[5]

Dermatoglyphics, especially the palmar crease pattern, are also important to note. A transverse palmar crease, indicative of hypotonia during early fetal life, is seen in approximately 50% of children with Down syndrome (and 10% of individuals in the general population). A characteristic palmar crease pattern is also seen in fetal alcohol syndrome.[5]

GENITALIA. Genitalia should be examined for abnormalities in structure. In male infants, if the penis appears short, then it should be measured and plotted on an appropriate growth chart. Ambiguous genitalia can be associated with endocrinologic disorders such as congenital adrenal hyperplasia (female infants have masculinized external genitalia, but male genital may be unaffected), chromosomal disorders such as Turner syndrome mosaicism, or part of a multiple malformation disorder such as Smith-Lemli-Opitz syndrome. Although hypospadias, which occurs in 1 in 300 male newborns, is a common congenital malformation that often occurs as an isolated defect, if it is associated with other anomalies, then the possibility of a syndrome is strong (see Chapter 279, Hypospadias, Epispadias, and Cryptorchism).[5]

Laboratory Evaluation

Following completion of the medical history, family history, and physical examination, the dysmorphologist takes the clues that have been gathered and attempts to solve the puzzle by assembling them into a diagnosis. The differential diagnosis is made up of conditions that features some or all of the clues. Once this list has been assembled, in an attempt to arrive at a definitive diagnosis, a series of laboratory and imaging tests can be performed. Typical tests used by the dysmorphologist are outlined here.

Chromosome analysis (karyotype), either metaphase or prophase (high resolution), should be routinely ordered for children with:

- Multiple congenital anomalies
- The involvement of 1 major organ system and 2 or more dysmorphic features
- The presence of intellectual disability

Chromosome analysis will identify conditions caused by too much chromosomal material (ie, trisomies) or those with too little chromosomal material (ie, monosomies).

Fluorescent in situ hybridization (FISH) uses DNA technology to identify specific regions of the genome that are either missing or duplicated. FISH uses a DNA probe that is complementary to a specific region of the genome. After a fluorescent marker is attached to this probe, it is incubated with chromosomal DNA from the patient. If the sequence is present in the patient, then the probe will hybridize, its presence announced by the appearance of the bound fluorescent marker.

A FISH study is requested when a syndrome with a known chromosomal defect is suspected. Such disorders as velocardiofacial syndrome (deletion of *22q11.2*), Prader-Willi syndrome (deletion of *15q11.2*), Angelman syndrome (deletion of *15q11.2*), and Beckwith-Wiedemann syndrome (duplication of *11p15.2*) are included in this group.

Recently, a new test called microarray comparative genomic hybridization (array CGH for short), has begun to replace, or at least complement, the standard high resolution chromosome analysis and FISH to examine subtelomeric rearrangements. Using microarray technology to compare the genetic material of the subject with a control individual, this test is 4 to 5 times more sensitive at identifying deletions and duplications than the above-named tests.

In a growing number of disorders, *direct DNA* analysis can be performed to identify specific mutations known to cause disease. Because the list of these disorders increases every day, using Web-based resources for the most recent information is necessary. An extremely helpful Web site is www.genetests.org. Frequently updated, Genetests provides information about the availability of testing for specific conditions, and identifies laboratories performing the testing.

Radiologic imaging plays an important role in the evaluation of children with dysmorphic features. Individuals found to have multiple external malformations should have a thorough evaluation to search for the presence of internal malformations. Testing might include ultrasound evaluations of the head and abdomen, the latter area to look for anomalies in the kidney, bladder, liver, and spleen. Skeletal radiographs should be taken if concern exists about a possible skeletal dysplasia. The presence of a heart murmur should trigger a cardiology consultation, and an electrocardiogram and echocardiogram may be indicated. *Magnetic resonance imaging* may be indicated in children with neurologic abnormalities or a spinal defect. The presence of craniosynosostosis triggers the need for a 3-dimensionally reconstructed *computed tomographic scan* of the head.

DIAGNOSIS

Although the presence of characteristic findings may sometimes make the definitive diagnosis of a malformation syndrome simple, in the majority of cases, no specific diagnosis is immediately evident. Some constellations of findings are rare, and finding a match may prove difficult. In many cases, all laboratory tests are normal, and confirmation relies on subjective findings. Clinical geneticists have attempted to resolve this difficulty by developing scoring systems, cross-referenced tables of anomalies that help in developing a differential diagnosis, and even computerized diagnostic programs.

An accurate diagnosis is important for 3 reasons:

1. It offers the family an explanation of why their child was born with congenital anomalies. This information may help allay feelings of guilt, given that parents frequently believe that they are responsible for their child's problem.
2. The natural history of many disorders is well described; as such, a diagnosis allows the physician to anticipate medical problems associated with a particular syndrome and can perform appropriate screening. A diagnosis may also provide reassurance that other medical problems are no more likely to occur than they might with other children who do not have the diagnosis.
3. It permits accurate recurrence risk for future progeny; only after a diagnosis is confirmed can genetic counseling and, eventually, prenatal diagnostic testing be performed.

The diagnosis also enables the clinician to provide the family with educational materials about the condition and to provide the family with the chance to meet other families who have children with the same condition. Through the years, a large network of support groups has developed for specific conditions, groups that will allow social and psychological assistance for the family of a newly diagnosed genetic disorder. The Internet has become an important source for such information, but care should be exercised because information on the Internet is not subject to editorial control, and some of the information may be inaccurate or at times inappropriate. Physicians should try to screen sites before encouraging a family to seek information from the Internet. A few good sites are the National Organization for Rare Disorders (www.rarediseases.org), which acts as a clearinghouse for information about rare diseases and their support groups. Genetic testing information is available at the Genetests Web site (www.genetests.org), which provides information on available clinical and research testing for many diseases.

Finally, once a definitive diagnosis has been made, the dysmorphologist must meet with the family in person to explain the condition and all of its ramifications. Such meetings are often difficult, often being the moment when the bad news is first delivered to the parents, and the full impact of the child's problem hits home. A sufficient amount of time should be allotted for this meeting because families may have many questions, and each question should be answered in a thoughtful and considerate way. Also often helpful is to include social support professionals as participants in these meetings; genetic counselors, social workers and psychologists can be extremely helpful in assisting the family in coming to accept the news and to begin moving on with the next phase of their lives (see Chapter 16, Disclosing a Diagnosis With Parents and Patients).

SUMMARY

The physician who is confronted with a patient who has dysmorphic facial features must decide whether the patient or family will benefit from a thorough evaluation or referral. The most important task initially is to determine whether the features are consistent with the individual's genetic background or whether they represent an abnormal phenotype. Through systematic gathering of information, the physician should attempt to establish an etiologic diagnosis and then convey the implications (including genetic counseling) to the appropriate family members.

TOOLS FOR PRACTICE

Medical Decision Support

- *Genetests* (Web page), www.genetests.org.
- *National Organization for Rare Diseases* (Web page), National Organization for Rare Diseases (NORD) (www.rarediseases.org/).
- *Online Mendelian Inheritance in Man* (Web page), National Center for Biotechnology Information (www.ncbi.nlm.nih.gov/entrez/query.fcgi?db=OMIM).
- *Genetic Alliance,* (Web page), Genetic Alliance (www.geneticalliance.org/ws_display.asp?filter=home).
- *Smith's Recognizable Patterns of Human Malformations,* (book), Jones K (www.us.elsevierhealth.com/product.jsp?isbn=9780721606156).
- *Management of Genetic Syndromes, 2nd edition* (book), Cassidy S, Allanson J (www.aap.org/bookstore).

RELATED WEB SITE

- March of Dimes (www.marchofdimes.com).

REFERENCES

1. Aase JM. *Diagnostic Dysmorphology.* New York, NY: Plenum; 1990.
2. Jones KL. *Smith's Recognizable Patterns of Human Malformation.* 6th ed. Philadelphia, PA: WB Saunders; 2005.
3. Graham JM. *Smith's Recognizable Patterns of Human Deformation.* 2nd ed. Philadelphia, PA: WB Saunders; 1988.
4. Gorlin RJ, Cohen MM, Hennakam RCM. *Syndromes of the Head and Neck.* 4th ed. New York, NY: Oxford University Press; 2001.
5. Levy PA, Marion RW. Human genetics and dysmorphology. In: Kliegman RM, Marcdante KJ, Jenson HB, et al. *Nelson Essentials of Pediatrics.* 5th ed. Philadelphia, PA: Elsevier Saunders; 2006.
6. Nuckolls GH, Shum L, Slavkin HC. Progress toward understanding craniofacial malformations. *Cleft Palate Craniofac J.* 1999;36:12-26.
7. Winter RM. What's in a face. *Nat Genet.* 1996;12(2):130-136.

Chapter 179

FAILURE TO THRIVE

Andrew D. Racine, MD, PhD

The unfortunate term *failure to thrive* has burdened generations of practitioners and their patients as an unenlightening phrase that combines a heterogeneous group of infants and young children with nothing more in common than a growth pattern irreconcilable with a predetermined standard for age. Abnormalities ranging from congestive heart failure to psychosocial deprivation can, as in a series of convergent boulevards, eventually lead to the same common plaza we call *failure to thrive.* To find a child in such a location, however, tells us little about the direction from which he or she strayed to come to our attention. Moreover, the term *failure to thrive* is as pejorative as it is devoid of content; thus recent scholarship has favored phrases such as *pediatric undernutrition* as used in the *Bright Futures in Practice* literature,[1] or *weight faltering* as adopted by our British colleagues.[2]

Given the diversity of potential causes, evaluation and management of a child who fails to gain weight adequately represents a formidable challenge that requires of the physician:

- A determination to listen attentively and examine thoroughly, given that no adequate substitute has yet been found for a complete history and physical examination
- A broad familiarity with the many pathophysiological sequences that can give rise to this condition
- An understanding of healthy infant behavior and development to identify aberrancies that may threaten weight gain at different ages
- A capacity to gather and synthesize information about the physical, psychological, emotional, familial, and social contexts of the patient's presentation
- A willingness to work with a team of other practitioners to evaluate and manage the child

- The patience to persevere for as long as required to establish adequate weight gain

DEFINITION

A diagnosis generally signals the culmination of a process of evaluation. By contrast, the diagnosis of failure to thrive merely serves to *initiate* the evaluation of a patient who has an abnormal pattern of weight gain. Deviation from normal weight gain has been defined conventionally by reference to age-adjusted nationally standardized norms of weight and rate of weight gain.[3] Infants or young children who either fall below a given percentile weight-for-age or weight-for-height or whose rate of weight gain has declined across 2 major percentiles (ie, 90th, 75th, 50th, 25th, 10th, or 5th) invite close scrutiny. The Social Security Administration, for example, defines failure to thrive as a fall in weight to below the 3rd percentile or to less than 75% of the median weight-for-height or age in children younger than 2 years.[4]

Static measurements of a child's weight-for-age or weight-for-height that document a child's *size* should be distinguished from repeated measurements over time that record a child's *growth*. Deviations from the norm in the former measurements may or may not, depending on the clinical circumstances, indicate abnormalities in the latter.

A clinical entity defined by reference to statistical norms merits some additional comment. First, although an occasional child may have obvious signs of severe malnutrition at the initial examination, a single observation of weight in a child is generally insufficient to make any diagnosis. We are concerned here, for the most part, with children who exhibit abnormal patterns of weight gain.

Second, although we aim to identify children whose weight or weight gain is abnormal, some normal children will fall into the extreme tails of the standard distributions, be it 10%, 5%, or 3%, of any cohort. The further out on the curve we observe any individual child, however, the more likely the child is to be truly abnormal with respect to weight-for-age or weight-for-height.

Third, one must understand that the national standards are constructed by using serial cross-sections of children, not longitudinal observations of cohorts as they grow. Therefore the rate at which a child gains weight individually will differ from tracks across collections of different children at different ages that appear on these charts. Over time, children's weights generally regress toward the mean, with heavier infants gaining weight at slower rates than lighter infants. To account for this pattern, British researchers developed weight charts from a cohort of 3418 full-term infants from Newcastle based on standard deviations of weight changes over time. These charts have wider percentile channels at upper weights and narrower channels at lower weights.[2]

Finally, statistical descriptions must not be allowed to obscure the salient feature common to most children who fail to gain weight adequately: They suffer from malnutrition and are therefore at risk for its attendant consequences. When acute malnutrition results in decreased weight-for-age, the condition is referred to as *wasting*. If caloric deprivation is prolonged, then it will eventually affect the child's linear growth as well, at which point the child is said to be stunted. Abnormalities in linear growth not accompanied by wasting (the child who has short stature alone) is not the subject of failure to thrive.

One common set of criteria defines failure to thrive in children younger than 2 years[5]:

- Weight consistently less than 80% of the median for age, or
- Weight on more than 1 occasion falling below the third percentile for age, or
- Weight that has fallen across 2 major percentiles on the National Center for Health Statistics standard growth charts[6]

The 2000 revised version of these charts takes into account the growth patterns of both breastfed and bottle-fed infants.

One may anticipate that these criteria will identify as many as 10% of children seen in outpatient settings[7] and 3% to 5% of hospital admissions.[8] Children who exhibit weights from 61% to 75% of the median for age are fewer but require intensive outpatient monitoring. When a child's weight falls below 60% of the median for age, the associated morbidity is severe and warrants inpatient hospitalization.[9] Children from lower socioeconomic backgrounds may be at heightened risk for malnutrition and consequent wasting.[10]

HEALTHY WEIGHT GAIN IN INFANTS

The National Center for Health Statistics growth charts have received widespread application as tools for plotting the growth patterns of healthy infants and children. (See Chapter 14, Pediatric Physical Examination.) The ease of their use makes them ideal screening instruments, but, as with all screening tools, their sensitivity and specificity are limited. They do not, for example, take into account parental size or the presence of preexisting chromosomal abnormalities, leading some researchers to argue for the use of standards that control for mean parental height or the presence of certain genetic conditions such as trisomy 21. The *Bright Futures in Practice* publication on nutrition provides references for growth charts based on specific disorders.[1]

Recent studies have examined the rate at which infants gain weight[11] and how regression to the mean reflects the tendency of some heavier infants to gain weight more slowly and some lighter infants to gain weight more quickly over time.[2] The mean weight of a newborn is approximately 3.25 kg. (±0.9 kg.). Many infants will lose between 6% and 10% of this weight in the first week as they undergo the normal diuresis associated with adaptation to the extrauterine environment. Birth weight usually is regained by the age of 10 days. Because newborn's weight at birth preferentially captures the influence of maternal characteristics and the intrauterine environment, it is an imperfect reflection of genetic growth potential. By 4 to 8 weeks of age, however, much catch-up growth in babies born light-for-dates has already occurred, thus an infant's weight at this time appears to be a more reliable predictor of weight at 12 months than is birth weight.[12] In general, infants can be expected to gain a mean of 30 g (±15 g) a day during the first 3 months of life. Infants will usually triple their birth weight by 1 year of age, at which time the mean daily weight gain has declined to approximately 10 g (±3 g).

PATHOGENESIS

Infants and children grow in the presence of adequate amounts of 4 fundamental constituents: oxygen, substrate, hormones, and love. Deficient quantities of any one or a combination of these suffice to impede normal weight gain. Oxygen deprivation at the tissue level from causes as diverse as congestive heart failure, chronic lung disease, or anemia will result in poor weight gain. Inadequate calories, protein, or micronutrients either from environmental deprivation, malabsorption, or inability to metabolize them at the tissue level also inhibit normal weight accumulation. Deficiencies in growth hormone, insulin-like growth factors, glucocorticoids, thyroid hormone, and other regulators of growth can result in failure to thrive. Finally, infants or children severely deprived of affection will often not grow despite what appears to be normal caloric intake. Chronic disease from many causes will interrupt normal weight gain through the induction of anorexia, malabsorption, an increased metabolic needs and the elaboration of inflammatory mediators, including tumor necrosis factor. Children with chromosomal or other genetic abnormalities, although they may exhibit idiosyncratic growth patterns specific to their particular condition, will also attain their full growth potential only in the presence of these critical ingredients.

In the past, patients who had inadequate weight gain have been classified as a minority whose difficulty stems from a readily identifiable *organic* cause and a majority whose problem resides in a residual *nonorganic* category.[5] Other researchers have emphasized the overlapping nature of these distinctions and have suggested a third, or *mixed*, category of failure to thrive.[13] More recent approaches have tended to depart from the organic-nonorganic dichotomy in recognition of the somewhat arbitrary nature of this distinction.

A more useful categorization of infants and children who have inadequate weight gain acknowledges an imbalance between the energy needs of the organism that does not grow and the energy at its disposition. The largest share of energy consumed, approximately 55% to 60%, is devoted to maintain a basal metabolic rate. An additional 5% to 10% of energy is lost in urine and stool, 5% is accounted for by specific dynamic action, 15% is used for normal physical activity above basal metabolic functions, and 15% is directed toward growth. To provide for all these functions, infants need approximately 100 to 110 kcal/kg/day.

An imbalance between energy needs and energy supplies can arise either from increases in the former or deficiencies in the latter. Box 179-1 lists conditions that increase the energy needs of the organism. Energy needs increase either with increases in the intensity of energy expenditure or decreases in the efficiency of energy use. Conditions that increase the intensity of energy expenditure include chronic heart disease, chronic lung disease, chronic anemia, chronic infection, certain endocrine abnormalities, malignancy, and intoxications. The efficiency of energy utilization can be compromised by chronic infection, chronic renal disease, hepatic insufficiency, inborn errors of metabolism, hormonal abnormalities, certain genetic syndromes, and deficiencies of various micronutrients, including iron, zinc, and carnitine.

BOX 179-1 Conditions that Increase Energy Needs

INCREASED INTENSITY OF ENERGY UTILIZATION

Chronic heart disease (congenital or acquired)

Chronic lung disease (bronchopulmonary dysplasia, cystic fibrosis, pulmonary lymphangiectasis)

Chronic anemia (hemaglobinopathies, enzyme deficiencies, membrane abnormalities)

Chronic infection (urinary tract infections, respiratory infections, tuberculosis)

Endocrine abnormalities (hyperthyroidism)

Malignancy (neuroblastoma, ganglioneuroma)

DRUGS OR TOXINS OR DECREASED EFFICIENCY OF ENERGY UTILIZATION

Chronic infection

Chronic renal disease

Hepatic insufficiency (cirrhosis)

Metabolic disease (disorders of amino acid or carbohydrate metabolism, idiopathic hypercalcemia of infancy)

Hormonal disturbances (hypopituitarism, hypoparathyroidism, chronic adrenocortical insufficiency, diabetes insipidus, hypothyroidism)

Genetic conditions (Down syndrome, de Lange syndrome, cri du chat syndrome, Smith-Lemli-Opitz syndrome, familial dysautonomia)

Micronutrient deficiencies (iron, zinc, carnitine)

Conditions leading to deficiency in energy supply are listed in Box 179-2. These conditions originate either because calories are withheld from or improperly presented to the child because they are refused, not ingested, vomited, or not absorbed.

In the category of caloric deprivation, nutritional deprivation in utero that may result in permanent growth retardation must be included. After delivery, a newborn may not receive sufficient calories because of parenting difficulties ranging from unfamiliarity with proper preparation of infant formula[14] or appropriate breastfeeding techniques to psychosocial dysfunction, maternal depression, and even frank abuse or neglect.[15] Other conditions that fall into this category include economic deprivation, unsound parental beliefs regarding nutrition,[16] and subtle central nervous system abnormalities in the child that make them difficult feeders.

Food refusal in children, beginning even in infancy,[17] can result from many causes, including pain (from reflux esophagitis), psychosocial adjustment disorders from emotional deprivation, anorexia from chronic infection or intoxication, and structural

BOX 179-2 Conditions that Result in Deficient Energy Supply

Calories withheld
In utero conditions
Formula preparation mistakes
Breastfeeding difficulties
Parent-child psychosocial dysfunction
Maternal depression
Intentional abuse or neglect
Poverty
Unsound parental beliefs regarding nutrition
Difficult feeders
Calories not properly ingested or digested
Anorexia (reflux esophagitis, emotional deprivation, chronic infection, dysphagia)
Structural abnormalities of the oro- or nasopharynx (cleft palate, choanal atresia, Treacher Collins syndrome, Pierre Robin syndrome, laryngeal web)
Structural abnormalities of the gastrointestinal tract (stenosis or atresia of the esophagus or duodenum, tracheoesophageal fistula, vascular ring, strictures, achalasia, malrotation, antral web, pyloric stenosis)
Neuromuscular disorders (cerebral palsy, hydrocephalus, myopathies)
Conditions leading to excessive dyspnea (congestive heart failure, chronic lung disease)
Vomiting and rumination
Malabsorption
Small bowel (celiac disease, inflammatory bowel disease, disaccharide malabsorption, intestinal lymphangiectasia, jejunal atresia, duplication cysts, chronic parasitic infections)
Pancreas (cystic fibrosis, Shwachman-Diamond syndrome, chronic pancreatitis)
Liver (cirrhosis, intrahepatic cholestatic syndromes, biliary atresia)

abnormalities resulting in dysphagia. Structural malformations of the nasal or oropharynx such as cleft palate, choanal atresia, or Treacher Collins syndrome can lead to an inability to ingest nutrients properly, as can muscular weakness, cerebral palsy or other central nervous system abnormalities, and diseases that give rise to excessive dyspnea.

Vomiting caused by structural abnormalities of the gastrointestinal tract, increased intracranial pressure from any source, chronic acidosis, rumination, and gastroesophageal reflux may all impede growth through caloric deprivation.

The principal organ of nutrient absorption is the small bowel. Malabsorption can occur from gross structural abnormalities, inflammatory conditions, infectious agents, or disorders of organs that elaborate enzymes essential for digestion.

In consideration of these potential causes for inadequate weight gain, 2 cardinal principles should be emphasized. First, the majority of cases encountered in ambulatory practice will result from inadequate caloric intake, with most of these originating in a disturbance in the parent-child feeding behavior.[18,19] At one time, maternal mental health disorders were thought to account for the majority of these cases. The particular issue of maternal depression as a risk factor for failure to gain weight in infancy has received wide attention in the literature.[20] Although case control studies have indicated a possible association between these 2 conditions,[21] more definitive population-based cohort studies have failed to confirm this finding.[22,23] Recent analysis has dissected a more subtle web of causation.[24] What has been termed a transactional model allows for the complex interplay of social conditions,[25] family interactions,[26] and individual psychodynamics[27] in creating feeding abnormalities. The 1 salient feature that distinguishes infants in this category who do not gain weight at the same rate as their peers is that they take in foods with less total energy.[28]

Second, a thorough history and physical examination is the surest route to diagnosis for the residual minority of cases not caused by caloric insufficiency. If the cause of the problem is not made clear by history and physical examination, then laboratory investigation is unlikely to reveal it.[8,29]

EVALUATION

Prompt evaluation of infants and children who do not gain weight as expected is important. The history and physical examination should be directed toward certain areas (see later discussion), and in cases in which psychosocial features predominate, most laboratory tests may be unnecessary.

HISTORY

Initial Approach

Every evaluation of an infant or child who is not gaining weight must begin with a thorough history. Although the history and physical examination will usually be conducted in the office, a home visit affords the pediatrician an opportunity to observe the family interaction around feeding in the context in which it normally occurs. A history of the present illness should assemble all data available from previous anthropometric measurements of the patient, including weight, height, and head circumference. Premature infants must have their measurements corrected for gestational age until 18 months of age for head circumference, 24 months of age for weight, and 40 months of age for height.[30] The physician should begin by asking the parent or parents, guardian or guardians, or principal caregiver or caregivers how they think the baby is doing and what they believe the problem to be. Knowledge of a parent's frame of mind may propel further evaluation toward or away from difficulty in parent-child interaction, including child neglect, as a potential explanation for a child's lack of weight gain.

Feeding

A thorough feeding history is essential. Is the baby bottle-fed or breastfed? How often does the child breastfeed, and for how long? Does the mother feel as though the child is sucking well, and does the baby appear sated after he or she feeds? If bottle-fed, how is the formula prepared and by whom? How many ounces will the baby take in a 24-hour period? Does the infant wet 6 to 8 diapers a day? For older children, when were solids introduced? Does the parent find the child to be a *picky eater* or difficult to interest in food? Does the child drink excessive amounts of juice during the day, substituting for more calorically rich nutrients? What are meal times like at home? Where does the child eat, and with whom? Are distractions, such as television, game boys, or video games, present during meals? Is food being used for discipline or in battles over control? A 24-hour dietary recall of a typical day can often help quantify the caloric intake of the patient. If this information proves difficult to elicit, then the parents can be sent home with a nutritional diary to fill out prospectively and bring in at the next visit.

Vomiting

The physician should inquire about any vomiting or spitting up, being sure to explore frequency, volume, and presence of blood or bile in the emesis. Gastric outlet obstructions (pyloric stenosis, antral web) often result in the generation of significant propulsive forces leading to projectile vomiting, whereas gastroesophageal reflux often results in less dramatic patterns of regurgitation. An obstruction distal to the ligament of Treitz will generally produce bilious vomiting, a symptom that must be taken with utmost seriousness in infancy, as it may indicate the presence of a malrotation and midgut volvulus.

Stools

The pattern and frequency of stooling must not be overlooked in the history of present illness. The child who has liquid stools may have a small-bowel pathologic condition or bulky, foul-smelling stools from fat malabsorption. If mucus or blood is in the stools, then an inflammatory condition may be present.

Medical History

Additional information should be obtained about the medical history, beginning with the parents' attitudes regarding their decision to have a baby and what their experience with the pregnancy was like. Did the mother gain a reasonable amount of weight? Did she experience any illnesses during her pregnancy? Hypertension or preeclampsia will result in an infant who is small for gestational age; gestational diabetes may produce an infant with macrosomia who fails to gain weight because of postnatal cardiac complications.

The physician should ask about specific toxic exposures in utero, particularly to tobacco, marijuana, and alcohol. Tobacco may result in a small baby who rapidly catches up in weight with her peers, whereas marijuana and alcohol exert an influence on growth that may be sustained throughout childhood.[31] Recording the child's gestational age at birth, any unusual complications of the labor and delivery, and the presence of malformations or other obvious deformities will complete this portion of the history.

Family History

A family history should document the growth patterns of siblings, record the occurrence of fetal loss or infant deaths, review the presence in the family of immune deficiencies, neurologic disorders, or metabolic derangements, and highlight any unexplained growth deficiencies in close relatives. These findings may provide clues to the cause of the growth abnormality in the child. The results of recent comprehensive longitudinal studies from England emphasize the extent to which mean parental height and parity overwhelm the influence of traditional markers of socioeconomic deprivation that includes parental education or occupational status on the weight gain of young infants.[22]

Social History

The social history should focus on the availability of social supports for the parents, the existence of economic or legal circumstances that threaten the stability of the family, the nature of the relationship between the parents, and the presence of affective disorders in the primary caregiver. Any recent disruptive events in the family's life should be explored to determine what effect they may have had on the parents' ability to care for the patient. Finally, at this point, the physician may often uncover unrealistic expectations that parents may harbor regarding feeding patterns, dietary fads, or behavior in infancy, all of which provide clues to why feeding this infant has developed into such a challenge.

PHYSICAL EXAMINATION

Repeated anthropometric measurements over time constitute the most important component of the physical evaluation of children who are not gaining weight. On the initial examination, the physician should begin with observing the child's general relatedness to the parent or parents and the examiner. Does the child appear listless, easily distractible, or irritable? Can he or she be engaged to make eye contact or to play with an age-appropriate toy? After completely undressing the child, a notation should be made of any evidence of wasting, of the presence and distribution of normal subcutaneous body fat, of muscle mass and tone, and of the presence of dysmorphic features; these observations will serve to set the stage for more detailed examination.

Particular attention should be paid to organ systems that may reflect evidence of malnutrition. The mucous membranes, hair, nails, and skin develop abnormalities in the presence of vitamin, protein, fat, and micronutrient deficiencies. The head, eyes, ears, nose, and throat may reveal conditions ranging from open fontanelles of hypothyroidism or craniotabes of nutritional rickets to the blurred disk margins of increased intracranial pressure in a child who has chronic emesis or a submucosal cleft of the hard palate in an infant who feeds poorly.

The thyroid should be palpated gently and then auscultated for evidence of hyperthyroidism before moving on to the lung and cardiac examination. Observation, palpation, and particularly auscultation of these organ systems may reveal wheezing, rales, or heart murmurs suggestive of the presence of chronic conditions. These conditions often result in substantial energy expenditures that outstrip the supply of nutrients available to the infant. Examination of the digits for clubbing in the older child should not be neglected. A thorough abdominal examination will rule out organomegaly associated with tumor, infection, or storage disease. Intestinal distention can be associated with carbohydrate malabsorption from various causes. The neurologic examination may suggest explanations for an infant's inability to ingest adequate calories. Disorders of mentation, cranial nerve abnormalities, generalized weakness, or spasticity should be carefully sought.

LABORATORY EVALUATION

In the absence of evidence from the history or physical examination indicating the need for specific laboratory testing, expectations of the yield of laboratory investigation should be modest. When charts of 185 patients who were hospitalized for failure to thrive at the Children's Hospital of Buffalo were reviewed, only 1.4% of the laboratory studies performed were found to be of diagnostic value.[29] A similar review of 122 infants who were hospitalized at the Boston Children's Hospital revealed that a mean of 40 laboratory tests were ordered, but only 0.8% revealed an abnormality that contributed to a diagnosis.[8]

Should the cause of a child's failure to gain weight adequately remain uncertain after careful history and physical examination, then a limited number of screening studies might be considered, including a complete blood count, a blood pH, serum electrolytes, blood urea nitrogen and creatinine, a urinalysis and urine culture, and an examination of the stool for reducing substances, pH, occult blood, and ova and parasites.[32] More extensive testing for malabsorption, endocrine disorders, occult infection, malignancy, and cardiac, pulmonary, or renal abnormalities should be done only when historical or physical examination evidence of these diagnoses is present.

THERAPY AND FOLLOW-UP

The therapeutic approach to children failing to gain weight adequately must be tailored to the individual needs of the family and the child. For infants and children in whom a specific diagnosis has been identified, therapy should be directed toward the underlying disease or condition. A disturbance in the parent-child interaction will more often be recognized as the cause of the patient's inability to gain weight. Regardless of the underlying etiology, the family should be approached nonjudgmentally, and the severity of the child's condition should dictate the initial approach to therapy.

Mild-to-Moderate Failure to Thrive

The primary care physician, with consultation from a nutritionist, can manage infants and children exhibiting mild degrees of malnutrition (greater than 80% of ideal body weight for age) as outpatients, with occasional consultation from subspecialist colleagues. Patients who have evidence of more severe caloric deprivation will require the involvement of a multidisciplinary team, including the primary care physician, nutritionist, mental health or behavioral therapist, and social worker.[33] Hospitalization may be necessary for a subset of these patients whose malnutrition is combined with or results from another significant medical condition. Home visitation using professionals[34] has been demonstrated to be a useful intervention in select circumstances. Others, however, have achieved less success in generating improved weight gain with this mode of intervention despite its other notable benefits.[35,36] Child protective services must be alerted about any child thought to be the victim of neglect.

The goals of management must focus on nutritional rehabilitation, parental education, and behavioral intervention. Attempts to overfeed malnourished infants at the outset of therapy should be avoided because initially they may exhibit some degree of anorexia and refeeding that is too vigorous may induce malabsorption and diarrhea. The refeeding regimen should be calculated to provide approximately 10% to 15% of calories from protein, 50% to 60% from carbohydrate, and 30% to 40% from fat.[37]

A typical 3-phase regimen[38] may begin with provision of 100% of daily age-adjusted energy and protein requirements based on the child's weight on day 1.

If this phase is well tolerated, in phase 2, intake is then increased to provide adequate nutrition to achieve catch-up growth. Multiplying the age-adjusted energy requirements (kcal/kg/day) by the ratio of the child's ideal body weight for height divided by the child's actual body weight at presentation will generate a reasonable estimate of the nutritional requirements for this stage. The same calculation can be made for protein requirements (Box 179-3). In most instances, the energy and protein requirements for these phases of infant refeeding can be accomplished with the use of a routine infant formula modified to increase its caloric density. Mixing 13 oz of concentrated formula with 10 oz of water rather than 13 oz of water will create a formula that is 24 cal/oz. Alternatively, the use of carbohydrate in the form of glucose polymers or fat in the form of medium-chain triglycerides will add calories while avoiding the complications of overhydration. For older children, the repertoire of caloric supplements will include a wide variety of solid foods as well.

BOX 179-3 Sample Nutritional Rehabilitation Schedule for Failure To Thrive

Scenario: A 6-month-old boy with poor weight gain is referred for nutritional rehabilitation. He currently weighs 5.5 kg and is 67 cm in length. The 50th percentile weight for this length is 7.7 kg, putting the infant at 71% of the ideal body weight for height.

- Normal adjustment catch-up
- Requirements factor requirements
- Calorie supplementation: 100 kcal/kg/day × 7.7/5.5 = 140 kcal/kg/day.
- Protein supplementation: 2 g/kg/day × 7.7/5.5 = 2.8 g/kg/day.
- Adding a multivitamin with iron to this child's regimen would be advisable.

In the third, or consolidation, phase of nutritional rehabilitation, a varied diet is offered ad libitum as the child gradually approaches ideal body weight. Multivitamin and iron supplementation should be part of every refeeding regimen for undernourished children.

Initiation of nutritional rehabilitation is an ideal time to engage the parents in an educational program that focuses on family interactions, psychological vulnerabilities, and social needs.[39] Emphasis should be placed on appropriate nutritional information, and concrete suggestions should be offered about how to structure mealtime at home to minimize distractions in a relaxed social environment that encourages good eating habits. For families in need, access to community resources such as the Special Supplemental Nutrition Program for Women, Infants, and Children (WIC) and food stamps must be facilitated. Pediatricians should be prepared to advocate vigorously for patients in need of supplemental nutrition or special infant formulas when families experience difficulties in obtaining these products.

Severe Failure to Thrive

Children who are less than 60% of ideal body weight for height should be hospitalized and cared for by a multidisciplinary team of nutritionists, social workers, pediatricians, and pediatric subspecialists, when appropriate. The nutritional rehabilitation of these children will be more prolonged and may entail a period of tube feedings in addition to oral supplements. In cases in which the gastrointestinal tract is temporarily inaccessible, parenteral feedings with central venous access may be necessary.

Follow-Up

Once identified, poor weight gain in infancy should be followed up assiduously. Initial weekly visits for infants may be necessary to reassure the parents and physician that the therapy undertaken is having the desired effects. Studies of hospitalized children have demonstrated that those younger than 6 months, when provided with adequate calories, begin to gain weight in a few days.[40] Older children may take longer than their younger counterparts before sustained weight gain is established. Ongoing developmental, behavioral, and social evaluations must be incorporated into any plan for follow-up. Abnormalities in these domains need to be monitored closely because they are frequently present in patients who gain weight poorly. Moreover, the lingering effects of calorie, protein, and micronutrient deprivation may show themselves in developmental and behavioral abnormalities,[41] particularly in families in which the mothers exhibit affective disorders.[42]

PROGNOSIS

Outcomes for children who have abnormal weight gain patterns in infancy and childhood should be predicted cautiously in view of the variety of conditions that may give rise to this clinical picture and the lack of high quality data on which reasonable predictions might be sustained. A systematic review of 13 long-term longitudinal studies of children with failure to thrive lamented these methodologic challenges but concluded that the growth and neurocognitive outcomes in these children probably do not differ substantially from their unaffected peers.[43] A less sanguine view was taken by an extensive review of the literature conducted by the Agency for Healthcare Research and Quality. These authors concluded that children with failure to thrive in infancy are likely to suffer immunologic, behavioral, cognitive, and psychomotor developmental deficits that persist despite interventions.[4] Such disparate findings as these suggest that most children in the mild category will experience brisk nutritional rehabilitation and, with adequate follow-up, will do quite well. More severely affected children, depending on the cause of their condition, may require more prolonged or repetitive interventions and may be left with residual cognitive, behavioral, and educational consequences of their malnutrition. Therefore all children who exhibit faltering weight gain during infancy and childhood absolutely must receive early comprehensive evaluation and prompt treatment.

WHEN TO REFER

- If a diagnosis is made of a chronic disease pertaining to an organ subspecialty discipline such as cardiac, pulmonary, renal, gastrointestinal, or endocrine
- If the psychosocial family dynamic indicates a need for psychiatric intervention for either or both parents
- If nutritional rehabilitation warrants the attention of a nutritionist

WHEN TO ADMIT

- Any child with a weight less than 60% of ideal body weight
- Any child who, despite aggressive outpatient management, continues to fail to gain weight at an acceptable rate
- Any child who presents with signs of marasmus or severe protein malnutrition (kwashiorkor)

TOOLS FOR PRACTICE

Engaging Patients and Family

- *Guide to Your Child's Nutrition* (book), American Academy of Pediatrics (www.aap.org/bookstore).

Medical Decision Support

- *Pediatric Nutrition Handbook* (policy manual), American Academy of Pediatrics (www.aap.org/bookstore).
- Growth Charts—Girls (chart), American Academy of Pediatrics (www.aap.org/bookstore).
- Growth Charts—Boys (chart), American Academy of Pediatrics (www.aap.org/bookstore).
- Growth Charts—Interactive Tutorials (Web site), Centers for Disease Control and Prevention (www.cdc.gov/growthcharts/).

AAP POLICY STATEMENT

American Academy of Pediatrics, Committee on Child Abuse and Neglect and Committee on Nutrition, Block RW, Krebs NF. Failure to thrive as a manifestation of child neglect. *Pediatrics*. 2005;116:1234-1237. (aappolicy.aappublications.org/cgi/content/full/pediatrics;116/5/1234).

SUGGESTED RESOURCES

Bithoney WG, Dubowitz H, Egan H. Failure to thrive/growth deficiency. *Pediatr Rev*. 1992;13:453-460.

Drotar D, ed. *New Directions in Failure To Thrive: Implications for Research and Practice*. New York, NY: Plenum Press; 1985.

Frank DA, Zeisel SH. Failure to thrive. *Pediatr Clin North Am*. 1988;35:1187-1206.

Gahagan S, Holmes R. A stepwise approach to evaluation of undernutrition and failure to thrive. *Pediatr Clin North Am*. 1998;45:169-187.

Zenel JA Jr. Failure to thrive: a general pediatrician's perspective. *Pediatr Rev*. 1997;18:371-378.

REFERENCES

1. Story M, Holt K, Sofka D, eds. *Bright Futures in Practice: Nutrition*. 2nd ed. Arlington, VA: National Center for Education in Maternal and Child Health; 2002.
2. Wright CM, Avery A, Epstein M, et al. New chart to evaluate weight faltering. *Arch Dis Child*. 1998;78:40-43.
3. Drotar D, et al. Early preventive intervention in failure to thrive: methods and early outcome. In: Drotar D, ed. *New Directions in Failure To Thrive: Implications for Research and Practice*. New York, NY: Plenum Press; 1985.
4. Perrin E, Frank D, Cole C, et al. *Criteria for Determining Disability in Infants and Children: Failure to Thrive. Evidence Report/Technology Assessment No. 72* (Prepared by Tufts-New England Medical center Evidence-based Practice Center under Contract No. 290-97-0019). AHRQ Publication No. 03-E026. Rockville, MD: Agency for Healthcare Research and Quality; March 2003.
5. Zenel JA Jr. Failure to thrive: a general pediatrician's perspective. *Pediatr Rev*. 1997;18:371-378.
6. Centers for Disease Control and Prevention, National Center for Health Statistics. CDC Growth Charts: United States. Available at: www.cdc.gov/growthcharts. Accessed February 29, 2008.
7. Mitchell WG, Gorrell RW, Greenberg RA. Failure-to-thrive: a study in a primary care setting epidemiology and follow-up. *Pediatrics*. 1980;65:971-977.
8. Berwick DM, Levy JC, Kleinerman R. Failure to thrive: diagnostic yield of hospitalisation. *Arch Dis Child*. 1982; 57:347-351.
9. Gomez F, Ramos GR, Frenk S, et al. Mortality in second and third degree malnutrition. *J Trop Pediatr*. 1956;2:77-83.
10. Massachusetts Department of Public Health. *The Massachusetts Growth and Nutrition Program—Summary Report FY 1996-FY 2002*. Boston, MA: Massachusetts Department of Public Health, Bureau of Family and Community Health; 2003. Available at: www.mass.gov. Accessed February 29, 2008.
11. Guo SM, Roche AF, Foman SJ, et al. Reference data on gains in weight and length during the first two years of life. *J Pediatr*. 1991;119:355-362.
12. Edwards AGK, Halse PC, Parkin JM, et al. Recognizing failure to thrive in early childhood. *Arch Dis Child*. 1990; 65:1263-1265.
13. Homer C, Ludwig S. Categorization of etiology of failure to thrive. *Am J Dis Child*. 1981;135:848-851.
14. McJunkin JE, Bithoney WG, McCormick MC. Errors in formula concentration in an outpatient population. *J Pediatr*. 1987;111:848-850.
15. Evans SL, Reinhart JB, Succop RA. Failure to thrive: a study of 45 children and their families. *J Am Acad Child Psychiatry*. 1972;11:440-457.
16. Pugliese MT, Weyman-Daum M, Moses N, et al. Parental health beliefs as a cause of nonorganic failure to thrive. *Pediatrics*. 1987;80:175-182.
17. Tolia V. Very early onset nonorganic failure to thrive in infants. *J Pediatr Gastroenterol Nutr*. 1995;20:73-80.
18. Bithoney WG, Newberger EH. Child and family attributes of failure to thrive. *J Dev Behav Pediatr*. 1987;8:32-36.
19. Hannaway PJ. Failure to thrive: a study of 100 infants and children. *Clin Pediatr*. 1970;9:96-99.
20. Drewett R, Blair P, Emmett P, et al and the ALSPAC Study Team. Failure to thrive in the term and preterm infants of mothers depressed in the postnatal period: a population-based birth cohort study. *J Child Psychol Psychiatry*. 2004; 45:359-366.
21. O'Brien LM, Heycock EG, Hanna M, et al. Postnatal depression and faltering growth: a community study. *Pediatrics*. 2004;113:1242-1247.
22. Blair PS, Drewett RF, Emmett PM, et al and the ALSPAC Study Team. Family, socioeconomic and prenatal factors associated with failure to thrive in the Avon Longitudinal Study of Parents and Children (ALSPAC). *Int J Epidemiol*. 2004;33:839-847.
23. Ramsay M, Gisel EG, McCusker J, et al. Infant sucking ability, non-organic failure to thrive, maternal characteristics, and feeding practices: a prospective cohort study. *Dev Med Child Neurol*. 2002;44:405-414.
24. Kotelchuck M, Newberger EH. Failure to thrive: a controlled study of familial characteristics. *J Am Acad Child Psychiatry*. 1983;22:322-328.
25. Frank DA, Allen D, Brown JL. Primary prevention of failure to thrive: social policy implications. In: Drotar D, ed. *New Directions in Failure To Thrive: Implications for Research and Practice*. New York, NY: Plenum Press; 1985.
26. Leonard MF, Rhymes JP, Solnit AJ. Failure to thrive in infants: a family problem. *Am J Dis Child*. 1966;111: 600-612.
27. Rosenn DW, Loeb LS, Jura MB. Differentiation of organic from nonorganic failure to thrive syndrome in infancy. *Pediatrics*. 1980;66:698-704.
28. Parkinson KN, Wright CM Drewett RF. Mealtime energy intake and feeding behavior in children who fail to thrive: a population-based case-control study. *J Child Psychol Psychiatry*. 2004;45:1030-1035.
29. Sills RJ. Failure to thrive: the role of clinical and laboratory evaluation. *Am J Dis Child*. 1978;132:967-969.
30. Brandt L. Growth dynamics of low birthweight infants with emphasis on the perinatal period. In: Falkner F, Tanner J, eds. *Human Growth: Neurobiology and Nutrition*. New York, NY: Plenum Press; 1979.
31. Cornelius MD, Goldschmidt L, Day NL, et al. Alcohol, tobacco and marijuana use among pregnant teenagers: 6-year follow-up of offspring growth effects. *Neurotoxicol Teratol*. 2002;24:703-710.
32. Schmitt BD, Mauro RD. Nonorganic failure to thrive: an outpatient approach. *Child Abuse Negl*. 1989;13:235-248.
33. Hobbs C, Hanks HG. A multidisciplinary approach for the treatment of children with failure to thrive. *Child Care Health Dev*. 1996;22:273-284.
34. Wright CM, Callum J, Birks E, et al. Effect of community based management in failure to thrive: randomized controlled trial. *BMJ*. 1998;317:571-574.
35. Black MM, Dubowitz H, Hutcheson J, et al. A randomized clinical trial of home intervention for children with failure to thrive. *Pediatrics*. 1995;95:807-814.

36. Raynor P, Rudolf MCJ, Cooper K, et al. A randomized controlled trial of specialist health visitor intervention for failure to thrive. *Arch Dis Child*. 1999;80:500-506.
37. Committee on Nutrition, American Academy of Pediatrics. *Pediatric Nutrition Handbook*. 5th ed. Elk Grove Village, Ill: American Academy of Pediatrics; 2004.
38. Adebonojo FO. Undernutrition. In: Burg FD, Ingelfinger JR, Polin RA, et al, eds. *Gellis and Kagan's Current Pediatric Therapy*. Philadelphia, PA: WB Saunders; 1996.
39. Maggioni A, Lifshitz F. Nutritional management of failure to thrive. *Pediatr Clin North Am*. 1995;42:791-810.
40. Ellerstein NS, Ostrov BE. Growth patterns in children hospitalized because of caloric-deprivation failure to thrive. *Am J Dis Child*. 1985;139:164-66.
41. Frank DA, Zeisel SH. Failure to thrive. *Pediatr Clin North Am*. 1988;35:1187-1206.
42. Hutcheson JJ, Black MM, Tally M, et al. Risk status and home intervention among children with failure-to-thrive: follow-up at age 4. *J Pediatr Psychol*. 1997;22:651-668.
43. Rudolf MCJ, Logan S. What is the long-term outcome for children who fail to thrive? A systematic review. *Arch Dis Child*. 2005;90:925-931.

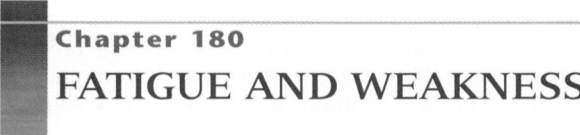

Chapter 180

FATIGUE AND WEAKNESS

Philip O. Ozuah, MD, PhD; Marina Reznik, MD, MS

DEFINITIONS

Fatigue and weakness are ubiquitous complaints that may or may not be related to medical diagnoses but are used commonly in medical and colloquial language. Both terms are difficult to define. To add to the confusion, both patients and physicians often use the 2 concepts interchangeably. Moreover, adolescents and children often use other terms to describe their perceptions of somatic weakness and fatigue. Fatigue, in fact, is very different from true body weakness. Therefore defining the 2 terms carefully is important, although the definitions must be modified for each age group.

Fatigue involves extreme and unusual tiredness, decreased physical performance, and an excessive need for rest. It often is accompanied by feelings of sleepiness, weariness, irritability, lassitude, boredom, and decreased efficiency. *Weakness*, in contrast, refers to diminished body or muscle strength. True weakness can be identified only by demonstration of abnormal neurologic or muscular function based on history, physical examination, or laboratory techniques. Practically speaking, a history of weakness, on further questioning, will often suggest hypotonia in infants and will be expressed in older children as trouble running or keeping up in gym class, clumsiness, or lack of agility.

ETIOLOGY

Fatigue

Fatigue may be a normal result of any physical or mental work in which energy expenditure exceeds the restorative processes. The temporary fatigue that follows intense exercise involves several complex mechanisms, including increased central inhibition mediated by group III and IV muscle afferents along with a decrease in muscle spindle facilitation and suboptimal cortical output.[1,2] At the level of the muscle cell, fatigue results from a reduction in adenosine triphosphate caused by high utilization rates, as well as a depletion of glycogen.[3] Normal fatigue also follows activities such as cramming for examinations and with food or sleep deprivation. In all of these instances, the degree of fatigue, even when prolonged, is usually appropriate for the amount of physical or mental exertion expended.

On the other hand, fatigue may be a pathological state with an organic or psychological foundation. The lassitude associated with somatic illness, often with definable physical or laboratory abnormalities, is well known. Fatigue has also been shown to have a strong correlation with the psychiatric diagnoses of depression and anxiety disorder.[4-7] Any acute illness or trauma may be accompanied by fatigue, but only prolonged fatigue is usually noteworthy.

Weakness

True weakness in a child should always be a cause of concern. Weakness is the result of a derangement of neuromuscular function at one of several levels, including the cerebral hemispheres, cerebellum, spinal cord, anterior horn cells, peripheral nerves, myoneuronal junction, or the muscle.

DIFFERENTIAL DIAGNOSIS

The differential diagnosis of prolonged fatigue is listed in Box 180-1. Box 180-2 lists some of the differential diagnoses for weakness in children.

Fatigue in Infants

The term *fatigue* is rarely pertinent for infants. However, parents sometimes report that their infant tires easily during feedings or seems droopy. Infants who are in heart failure often appear to tire easily and sweat excessively with feedings. Infants who have other serious conditions, including severe anemia and hypothyroidism, may also be described by their parents as being listless.

Fatigue During Childhood

Children complain only infrequently of feeling fatigued. Remarkably, even with chronic organic diseases, the child does not express fatigue itself verbally. Rather, concerned parents usually report that the child appears fatigued. Parents commonly make such statements as, "He has no energy," "She lies around all the time," "She seems bored and droopy," "He's sleeping a lot of the time," "She has no pep," "He drags around," or "I can't get her to do a thing." On questioning, younger children occasionally express a sense of lassitude and fatigue to their primary care physician. Much of the difficulty in the middle years of childhood (before adolescence), however, is children's inability to put into words what they feel. Fatigue therefore is usually exhibited in terms of a child's physical activity and performance in school, sports, and other organized activities. The younger the child is, the more likely will

BOX 180-1 Disorders Commonly Associated With Prolonged Fatigue in Different Age Groups

INFANCY
Cyanotic heart disease
Congestive heart disease
Severe anemia
Hypothyroidism

CHILDHOOD
Chronic upper respiratory tract infections
Otitis media and sinusitis
Tonsillitis
Chronic asthma
Chronic allergies
Hepatitis
Rheumatic fever
Disseminated malignancy
AIDS
Immunologic disorders
Chronic renal disease

ADOLESCENCE
Mycoplasma and other viral pneumonias
Infectious mononucleosis
Hepatitis
Rheumatoid arthritis
Lupus erythematosus
Diabetes mellitus
Malignancy
Inflammatory bowel disease
Addison disease
Drug abuse, including alcoholism
Chronic pulmonary disease
Depression
Severe obesity

BOX 180-2 Differential Diagnosis of Weakness and Hypotonia

Down syndrome
Werdnig-Hoffmann disease
Muscular dystrophies
Congenital hypothyroidism
Botulism
Myasthenia gravis
Guillain-Barré syndrome
Dermatomyositis
Polymyositis

be that the expressed or observed fatigue has a pathological basis.

Recurrent or Chronic Infection

The most common problem associated with fatigue in children is recurrent or chronic infection. Otitis media, sinusitis, and tonsillitis of a recurrent and smoldering nature are often overlooked for their systemic effects, among which fatigue may be prominent. Often mistakenly considered insignificant, upper respiratory tract allergies may cause impressive fatigue, irritability, and mild depression in children and adolescents.

Endocrine Disorders

Of the common endocrine disorders, only hypothyroidism is likely to be associated with fatigue. Certainly, a child with hypothyroidism whose rate of growth has fallen off may exhibit increasing fatigue and lassitude, at first subtle, as the only symptoms. Thyrotoxicosis, in contrast, is uncommon in young children but occasionally produces isolated fatigue in adolescents.

Diabetes Mellitus

Although any metabolic disorder can cause fatigue, only diabetes mellitus occurs with enough frequency to merit consideration. Fatigue almost always accompanies the initial or uncontrolled diabetic state.

Inflammatory Diseases

Inflammatory diseases, especially rheumatoid arthritis and other rheumatoid-like disorders, appear frequently in pediatric practice, and many children have significant fatigue, out of proportion to their musculoskeletal complaints. Lyme arthritis is a notable example (see Chapter 292, Lyme Disease).

Pulmonary Disease

Cyanotic heart disease and chronic advanced pulmonary disease, as seen with cystic fibrosis, are commonly associated with marked fatigue; in these cases, however, the underlying disease is usually readily evident before the fatigue becomes severe. The primary care physician may occasionally see an older child for the 1st time who has severe fatigue caused by a previously undiagnosed hypoxic disorder.

Anemia

Overall, the condition thought to be present most often as a cause of fatigue in both children and adults is anemia—most often, incorrectly so. Although fatigue is often ascribed to mild or moderate anemia, from whatever source, symptoms are usually not seen in children until the hemoglobin level falls to 6 or 7 g/dL; if red blood cell counts decrease gradually, then even lower hemoglobin levels may ensue without clinically evident symptoms. Irritability and attention problems may be present, with mild to moderate iron-deficiency anemia, but fatigue is usually not a common feature. Younger children especially seem to tolerate incredibly low hemoglobin levels with no symptoms at all.

Malignancy

Malignancy, particularly leukemia or lymphoma, occasionally develops insidiously, with fatigue as the major symptom. Although always feared, these diseases are seen infrequently in pediatric office practice.

Emotional Disorders

Many children who come to the primary care physician with unexplained chronic fatigue are found to have an emotionally related disorder. Before adolescence, the complaint usually centers on the parents' concern about a child's reduced activity level. A younger child will be noted to prefer sedentary activities—to "lie around the house a lot," appear tired, lack energy, and shrink from social contacts. These traits may have been longstanding, but a comment from grandparents or a teacher may arouse parental anxiety, precipitating the 1st visit to the primary care physician.

At this point, the family is often convinced that the child has a serious organic disease. Further evaluation, however, usually reveals that the child is performing very satisfactorily but not up to the family's excessive expectations. The child may be withdrawing because of failure to compete with an exceptional sibling or because of real or imagined failure in school. In other cases, a child may feel a lack of well being because of parental discord. Similarly, lack of parental involvement with a child may lead to lassitude and boredom. Stress and anxiety in children often result in either hyperactivity or withdrawal, and the more common withdrawal reaction may express itself as chronic fatigue.

Most children experience transient periods of lassitude or fatigue, but such instances are brief and usually self-limited. At the opposite extreme is the child whose chronic fatigue is a sign of true psychiatric depression. In this case, as in the adolescent, the more protracted and severe the periods of withdrawal are, the more likely that depression and fatigue are caused by a pathological process.

Fatigue in Adolescents

Complaints of chronic fatigue are encountered most often in adolescents. The normal swings in adolescent moods, from excessive exuberance to fatigue, are usually of more concern to parents and teachers than they are to the patient. In many instances, the adolescent may disagree vehemently with the parents' view and not share their concern. Adolescents, however, also initiate visits to their primary care physician because they feel fatigue. Parents may be unable or may refuse to recognize the adolescent's symptoms. Whereas a younger child who has a profound medical illness often does not experience fatigue, even minor illnesses often precipitate prolonged fatigue in adolescents.

Viral Illnesses

Mycoplasma pneumonia, often low grade and without fever, produces progressive fatigue. In addition, prolonged viral and parasitic illnesses (eg, infectious mononucleosis, hepatitis, cytomegalovirus infection, toxoplasmosis) commonly produce fatigue, especially in adolescents.

Infectious Mononucleosis

The terms *chronic infectious mononucleosis* and *chronic fatigue syndrome* have become popular with both physicians and the media. This attention has led to misuse of these terms, as well as, undoubtedly, to mild mass hysteria among young adults and adolescents who now are convinced they have one of these disorders. Most adults and many infants and children have been infected with the Epstein-Barr virus (EBV). The clinical manifestations in proved cases are extremely variable; some patients remain symptom free, whereas clinical, hematologic, and serologic findings support the diagnosis of infectious mononucleosis in others. The symptoms of infectious mononucleosis usually resolve in several weeks, but an occasional patient may have an atypical or a more prolonged course in which the initial clinical findings either persist or are intermittent over a period of months or, in rare cases, years. These unusual but documented cases of chronic infectious mononucleosis typically include complaints of chronic fatigue. Another much smaller group of patients has been described as having a serious, sometimes lethal, illness associated with EBV infection. These patients usually do not exhibit the classic findings of infectious mononucleosis; their conditions are often proved to be either acquired or genetically determined immunologic abnormalities.

Other Conditions

Always unpredictable and often insidious in its onset, inflammatory bowel disease may arouse concern initially with unexplained fatigue and a loss of sense of well being. Although eventually accompanied by fever, abdominal symptoms, or abnormal stools, this disorder can continue for months, with fatigue as the only major symptom. The possibility of Addison disease (see Chapter 233, Adrenal Dysfunction) should be considered in children or adolescents who have unexplained fatigue and associated weakness, anorexia, nausea, vomiting, or weight loss. Of more current importance in older children and adolescents are alcoholism and drug abuse—causes of chronic fatigue that are easily overlooked.

Emotional Disorders

By far, adolescents are the patients who most commonly complain of fatigue. Primary care physicians can expect to see a generous number of adolescents who characteristically appear each spring complaining of fatigue or lassitude and lack of energy and seem mildly depressed. This disorder usually appears during periods of greatest school-related stress, such as before examinations. Although the patient may have a fever, usually caused by infection (eg, infectious mononucleosis, influenza), the cause of fatigue is usually emotionally based.

In many instances, the adolescent collapses with fatigue after intense and exuberant activity involving schoolwork, extracurricular activity, sports, or social events. These individuals may also be short on sleep, may have unhealthy eating habits, and may complain of an additional variety of hypochondriacal symptoms. Burnout and fatigue are particularly common in overachieving high school and college students during late adolescence. The emotional reaction may actually be precipitated by a physical illness, particularly an infection. Most of these patients have normal findings on physical examinations and routine laboratory tests.

Chronic Fatigue Syndrome

Since 1985, adolescents, adults, and, occasionally, children have been described as having a disorder referred to as *chronic fatigue syndrome* (CFS),[8-21] which most commonly involves persistent or relapsing severe fatigue, fever, headache, sore throat, tender lymphadenitis, nausea or vomiting, myalgia, arthralgia, and abdominal pain. Neurocognitive complaints, such as an inability to concentrate, sleep disturbances, episodic confusion and memory problems, depression, anxiety, and irritability, are also especially common in CFS.[4,14,15]

The neurocognitive complaints are the most difficult to evaluate in CFS because of the extreme difference in emotional perception from person to person. Furthermore, careful physical examinations by experienced physicians often fail to document any physical abnormalities, and extensive laboratory evaluations usually produce normal results. In addition, much of the difficulty surrounding both the diagnosis and the search for a cause of CFS is attributable to confusion about the use of the terms *chronic fatigue* and *chronic fatigue syndrome*. Consequently, the Centers for Disease Control and Prevention (CDC) has formulated strict criteria for the case definition of CFS.[22,23] Unfortunately, these criteria were based mainly on observations of adult populations and may not be completely pertinent to children and adolescents.

Nevertheless, the CDC criteria for CFS stipulate that the debilitating fatigue must last at least 6 months in addition to the presence of 4 or more symptoms (see section on CFS). Individuals with at least 6 months of disabling fatigue but an insufficient number of symptoms to meet the CDC CFS criteria have been labeled as having idiopathic chronic fatigue. Although the CDC criteria exclude most past or current major psychiatric disorders, they allow some comorbid psychiatric symptoms such as anxiety and nonmelancholic depression.[23] This allowance can be problematic because both anxiety and depression have an independent and well-established relationship with fatigue.[5,17]

CFS quickly became a popular diagnosis. The syndrome was initially attributed to infection with the EBV, although few patients had documented physical findings or hematologic abnormalities consistent with the diagnosis of infectious mononucleosis. In addition, most patients had no serologic evidence of active EBV infection. Recently, however, a better understanding of the natural course of EBV antibody activity in healthy individuals months and years after an initial illness with infectious mononucleosis indicates that healthy patients who had mononucleosis years earlier could not be differentiated from fatigued patients who currently had the disease. Although few longitudinal data are available, the prognosis for adolescents with CFS is better than that for adults. Although symptoms may persist for months or several years, most adolescents with CFS have a good outcome, with approximately one half reporting complete recovery.[11,24] See Chapter 247, Chronic Fatigue Syndrome, for further discussion of this syndrome.

Weakness

Infants with weakness are often brought to their primary care physician with a complaint of being floppy. A floppy infant is usually one who has hypotonia caused by a neuromuscular disorder. (See Chapter 195, Hypotonia.) In the newborn period, some of these patients may assume a *frog-leg* position. Chromosomal anomalies such as Down syndrome, congenital hypothyroidism, and the infantile form of spinal muscular atrophy (Werdnig-Hoffmann disease) are some of the more common causes of hypotonia in infancy. Infant botulism from ingesting *Clostridium botulinum* spores in honey can cause infants to appear floppy with a weak cry caused by muscle weakness, loss of head control, lethargy, inability to feed, and constipation.

Older children and adolescents who have weakness experience difficulty walking, running, and participating in athletic activities. Myasthenia gravis and Guillain-Barré syndrome (postinfectious polyneuropathy) are perhaps the 2 most common causes of weakness in this age group. A distinguishing clinical feature is that, in myasthenia gravis, deep-tendon reflexes may be diminished but are rarely absent, whereas Guillain-Barré syndrome is remarkable for bilateral, symmetrically absent tendon stretch reflexes. Other causes of weakness in the older child include the muscular dystrophies, the juvenile form of spinal muscular atrophy, dermatomyositis, and polymyositis.

EVALUATION

Relevant History

Although the patient who is chronically fatigued may first appear to have an insignificant problem, great care must be taken to rule out underlying medical illness, to return the child to a state of well being, and to relieve parental concerns. The primary care physician must remember that either the child or the parents are worried about the child's fatigue. Because family members may disagree about the significance of the symptoms, adequate time and concern are needed to evaluate the history. The symptoms of chronic fatigue cannot be dismissed casually over the telephone or with a quick office visit.

Because most patients who come to the primary care physician complaining of fatigue have emotionally based problems, a careful history, with information from both child and parents (taken separately when appropriate), often helps narrow the differential diagnosis. Discrepancies between the child's and the parents' observations soon become evident, and the diagnosis of emotionally related fatigue emerges in most cases based on the history alone. The information derived from a longstanding physician-patient relationship contributes enormously to reducing tensions during the evaluation. Although fatigue may be the only symptom, further questioning almost always uncovers other symptoms of somatic disease. Chronic fatigue, in the absence of other physical symptoms, is usually emotionally based. Other associated complaints are somnolence, depression, anxiety, boredom, decreased activity, and inappropriate affect. In many instances, emotional stress or some disruption in the patient's life is part of the history.

Physical Examination

A physical examination, thoroughly performed, may be the only measure necessary and may reassure the anxious child or parent. The child's affect and appearance are most revealing. The impression that the child appears well invariably proves to be an accurate measure of the child's health. The condition of the adolescent, in contrast, may be more difficult to interpret. Although the physical examination may be benign, adolescents may be slovenly, uncommunicative, depressed, and unable to express their feelings; thus, at first, adolescents sometimes appear to be physically ill.

In all age groups, a search should be made for sites of chronic latent infection: adenopathy, enlargement or tenderness of the liver and spleen, and abdominal masses. Careful palpation for an enlarged or tender thyroid gland is essential. Mild scleral icterus and petechiae are easy to overlook. Similarly, a patient's pallor (a common finding, especially after long winters indoors) may evade even the most experienced clinician. On the other hand, the characteristic facies of the chronically allergic child and signs such as clubbing and cyanosis are obvious. Examination of the oropharynx may reveal hyperpigmentation of gums and buccal mucosa, which may be present in Addison disease.

An assessment of the plotted height and weight should be an essential part of every routine health visit.[25] Failure of a child to progress along the expected growth parameters should draw the clinician's attention to the possibility of an underlying systemic process affecting growth and causing unexplained fatigue. A normal linear growth velocity decreases the possibility of chronic cardiac, pulmonary, gastrointestinal, or renal disorders in children or adolescents who are excessively tired. An underlying endocrinopathy, such as hypothyroidism or Cushing syndrome, may cause fatigue in association with poor growth velocity and obesity. Poor weight gain over time may be a subtle manifestation of inflammatory bowel disease in adolescents with unexplained fatigue.

Laboratory Testing and Imaging

A limited, well-selected group of laboratory tests should be performed on most patients who are chronically fatigued. These results will reassure the family, the patient, and the primary care physician and will usually erase any lingering doubt about the diagnosis.

Other Diagnostic Tests

The laboratory evaluation should initially include a complete blood count with red blood cell indices, thyroid and liver function tests, a throat culture, and a stool examination for blood. The cold agglutinin test is often valuable as a simple initial screening test for a *Mycoplasma* infection. Radiograms are rarely necessary and should be discouraged. Critical evaluation of data collected from the history, physical examination, and laboratory tests should enable the primary care physician to detect quickly any organic causes of fatigue. Prolonged fever, however low grade, must always be viewed as significant and may suggest infection, inflammatory disease, or malignancy. Pallor points to the possibility of anemia or hypothyroidism.

Viral Disease

Cervical adenopathy, even a single enlarged node in the absence of other findings, can be a clue to the diagnosis of infectious mononucleosis. In fact, in the autumn and early winter of each year, every primary care physician begins to look for patients who have infectious mononucleosis. However, infectious mononucleosis is a protean illness, and the physical examination results are sometimes normal. Children and adolescents who have infectious mononucleosis may have no fever or signs of toxicity but may exhibit major fatigue. Furthermore, results of the heterophil antibody test for infectious mononucleosis may be negative in many young children and infants and in approximately 10% of older children and adolescents who have the disease. The reliability of EBV antibody testing has improved to the point at which the diagnosis of acute, active infectious mononucleosis can be confirmed. During the evaluation of chronic fatigue, EBV antibody titers can usually differentiate long-past infection from recent and active infection, thus eliminating EBV infection and infectious mononucleosis as causes for the fatigue and permitting a search for other likely neuropsychiatric causes. Toxoplasmosis and cytomegalovirus infections may mimic mononucleosis closely; these infections produce significant fatigue but with only minimal cervical adenopathy and fever. Positive results of a fluorescent antibody test for toxoplasmosis or cytomegalovirus with negative results of a heterophil antibody test will confirm the diagnosis. Similarly, fatigued children may have hepatitis and may be anicteric (or only slightly icteric), with little or no hepatic tenderness or enlargement. Other common viral infections, especially during convalescence, can cause a prolonged fatigue syndrome accompanied by depression.

Chronic Fatigue Syndrome

The diagnosis of CFS should be restricted to patients who meet rigid criteria, including the new onset of persistent or relapsing fatigue lasting at least 6 months with no prior history of such fatigue and the exclusion of other clinical conditions that might produce similar symptoms. In addition, symptoms must include 4 or more of the following: muscle pain, tender lymphadenopathy, headaches of new type, pattern or severity, arthralgia, impaired memory or concentration, pharyngitis, low-grade fever, postexertional malaise lasting longer than 24 hours, and sleep disturbances.[22,23] After other medical conditions are excluded, some older children and adolescents may meet these criteria for diagnosis. In any case, these patients should not be labeled with a diagnosis of chronic infectious mononucleosis syndrome or chronic EBV infection, which used to be and still is a quick fix diagnosis for patients who are chronically fatigued.

Autoimmune Disease

Children who have an autoimmune disease may have fatigue with little else at first. Mild articular or periarticular inflammation may be missed on examination. The emphasis must be on careful observation of subtle or minimal physical findings, because children usually do not display fulminant findings initially. Children with inflammatory bowel disease, arthritis, or an arthritis-like illness, and some patients with a malignancy (monocytic leukemia, in particular), may have especially prolonged symptoms, including fatigue, without any physical findings whatsoever.

Thyroid Disease

An enlarged, tender thyroid gland and fatigue may indicate thyroiditis with emerging hypothyroidism. However, the thyroid is often palpable and full in healthy adolescents. In any event, chronic fatigue from thyroid disease can usually be ruled out quickly with a thyroid-stimulating hormone and free thyroxine (free T_4) tests. Some patients who have hypothyroidism also demonstrate mild to moderate anemia, and those who have active thyroiditis may have an elevated sedimentation rate.

Anemia

To be acceptable as an explanation for fatigue, the diagnosis of pure anemia requires marked reduction of hemoglobin. Red blood cell indices and a reticulocyte count will characterize the anemia and the probable cause. Anemia accompanied by thrombocytopenia, however, suggests leukemia or aplastic anemia. The white blood cell count may be normal in infectious mononucleosis or hepatitis, but lymphocytosis with atypical lymphocytes will most likely be present in the former. The heterophil antibody screening test (the *mono test*) is diagnostic in most such circumstances.

Screening and Other Diagnostic Tests

The erythrocyte sedimentation rate is the most valuable screening test for inflammatory diseases of all varieties. A normal sedimentation rate almost always rules out autoimmune disease, inflammatory bowel disease, chronic smoldering infections, and disseminated malignancies. An elevated sedimentation rate requires further investigation. A routine urinalysis almost always reveals diabetes, and most patients who have chronic renal failure have abnormal urinalyses, as well as significant anemia. In these patients, the subsequent measurement of blood glucose in diabetes and of creatinine or blood urea nitrogen in renal disease can confirm these diagnoses. Hyperkalemia, hyponatremia, and hypoglycemia are useful diagnostic features of Addison disease, with the adrenocorticotropic hormone stimulation test being the most definitive diagnostic test.

Weakness

The evaluation of a patient who has weakness may include chromosomal studies, muscle enzyme assays, nerve conduction studies, electromyography, edrophonium (Tensilon) challenge, muscle biopsy, and a lumbar puncture, depending on the suspected diagnosis. Consultation with a pediatric neurologist is often required.

MANAGEMENT

After significant organic disease is ruled out in most patients, further management requires meaningful communication among the primary care physician, the patient, and the parents. In younger children, the variability in performance and behavior of healthy children must be put into perspective. Again, appropriate parental expectations must be emphasized. In addition, the child's and the family's daily schedule should be reviewed. A chaotic lifestyle that is frantic, with poorly structured activity and inadequate sleep patterns, is often revealed. Occasionally, true psychiatric depression is discovered, which calls for referral to a psychiatrist.

Older children and adolescents benefit from personal, warm attention. The value of a continuous relationship with 1 physician becomes self-evident. An understanding, thorough session with the patient's own primary care physician usually streamlines the evaluation and eliminates the need for excessive testing. Conversation after the physical examination should attempt to (1) reassure children or adolescents about their basic health, (2) reiterate the common and normal occurrence of fatigue, (3) examine the daily routine and stresses on patients, and (4) suggest modifications of patients' lifestyle and approaches to life's situations. This period is a time for respectful give and take. Attempting to establish the probable cause of the fatigue is the primary care physician's responsibility before the patient is referred to a specialist. If emotional fatigue is thought to exist, then the adolescent, in particular, must be comfortable with the conclusion that organic diseases have been ruled out. The patient then must be made aware of the emotional basis for the fatigue; and if psychiatric referral is needed, then the reasons must be made clear. A knowledgeable primary care physician will be reassuring but firm in approaching the child or adolescent who needs referral. Fortunately, such a referral usually is not necessary.

WHEN TO REFER

- Unexplained weight loss
- Hypotonia in infants
- Suspected major affective disorder
- Suspected malignancy

WHEN TO ADMIT

- Severe depression or suicidal ideation
- Need for evaluation of neuromuscular disorders such as Werdnig-Hoffmann disease, Guillain-Barré syndrome, and myasthenia gravis

TOOLS FOR PRACTICE

Engaging Patients and Family

- *A Parent's Guide to Building Resilience in Children and Teens* (book), American Academy of Pediatrics (www.aap.org/bookstore).
- *Children, Teens, and Resiliency* (Web page), American Academy of Pediatrics (www.aap.org/stress/).
- *Helping Your Child Cope With Life* (brochure), American Academy of Pediatrics (patiented.aap.org).
- *Stress and Your Child* (fact sheet), American Academy of Pediatrics (www.aap.org/stress).
- *Stressed? Read This* (brochure), American Academy of Pediatrics (patiented.aap.org).

SUGGESTED RESOURCES

Bright Future Guidelines for Health Supervision. Available at: www.brightfutures.org/bf2/pdf/index.html.

Farmer A, Fowler T, Scourfield J, et al. Prevalence of chronic disabling fatigue in children and adolescents. *Br J Psychiatry.* 2004;184:477-481.

Mears CJ, Taylor RR, Jordan KM, et al, and the Pediatric Practice Research Group. Sociodemographic and symptom correlates of fatigue in an adolescent primary care sample. *J Adolesc Health.* 2004;35(6):528e.21-26.

Smith MS, Martin-Herz SP, Womack WM, et al. Comparative study of anxiety, somatization, functional disability, and illness attribution in adolescents with chronic fatigue or migraine. *Pediatrics.* 2003;111(4 pt 1):e376-e381.

REFERENCES

1. Gandevia SC, Allen GM, McKenzie DK. Central fatigue. Critical issues, quantification and practical implications. *Adv Exp Med Biol.* 1995;384:281-294.
2. Gandevia SC. Spinal and supraspinal factors in human muscle fatigue. *Physiol Rev.* 2001;81(4):1725-1789.
3. Green HJ. Mechanisms of muscle fatigue in intense exercise. *J Sports Sci.* 1997;15(3):247-256.
4. Smith MS, Martin-Herz SP, Womack WM, et al. Comparative study of anxiety, somatization, functional disability, and illness attribution in adolescents with chronic fatigue or migraine. *Pediatrics.* 2003;111(4 pt 1):e376-e381.
5. Epstein KR. The chronically fatigued patient. *Med Clin North Am.* 1995;79(2):315-327.
6. Fuhrer R, Wessely S. The epidemiology of fatigue and depression: a French primary-care study. *Psychol Med.* 1995;25(5):895-905.
7. Ridsdale L, Evans A, Jerrett W, et al. Patients with fatigue in general practice: a prospective study. *BMJ.* 1993;10: 307(6896):103-106.
8. Mears CJ, Taylor RR, Jordan KM, et al, and the Pediatric Practice Research Group. Sociodemographic and symptom correlates of fatigue in an adolescent primary care sample. *J Adolesc Health.* 2004;35(6):528e.21-26.
9. Jones JF, Nisenbaum R, Solomon L, et al. Chronic fatigue syndrome and other fatiguing illnesses in adolescents: a population-based study. *J Adolesc Health.* 2004;35(1): 34-40.
10. Farmer A, Fowler T, Scourfield J, et al. Prevalence of chronic disabling fatigue in children and adolescents. *Br J Psychiatry.* 2004;184:477-481.
11. Gill AC, Dosen A, Ziegler JB. Chronic fatigue syndrome in adolescents: a follow-up study. *Arch Pediatr Adolesc Med.* 2004;158:225-229.
12. Patel MX, Smith DG, Chalder T, et al. Chronic fatigue syndrome in children: a cross sectional survey. *Arch Dis Child.* 2003;88:894-898.
13. Craig T, Kakumanu S. Chronic fatigue syndrome: evaluation and treatment. *Am Fam Physician.* 2002;65(6): 1083-1090.
14. Garralda E, Rangel L, Levin M, et al. Psychiatric adjustment in adolescents with a history of chronic fatigue syndrome. *J Am Acad Child Adolesc Psychiatry.* 1999; 38(12):1515-1521.
15. Richards J, Turk J, White S. Children and adolescents with chronic fatigue syndrome in non-specialist settings: beliefs, functional impairment and psychiatric disturbance. *Eur Child Adolesc Psychiatry.* 2005;14(6): 310-318.
16. Bou-Holaigah I, Rowe PC, Kan J, et al. The relationship between neurally mediated hypotension and the chronic fatigue syndrome. *JAMA.* 1995; 274(12):961-967.
17. Carter BD, Edwards JF, Kronenberger WG, et al. Case control study of chronic fatigue in pediatric patients. *Pediatrics.* 1995;95(2):179-186.
18. Dale JK, Straus SE. The chronic fatigue syndrome: considerations relevant to children and adolescents. *Adv Pediatr Infect Dis.* 1992;7:63-83.
19. Sigler A. Chronic fatigue syndrome: fact or fiction. *Contemp Pediatr.* 1990;7:22-50.
20. Smith MS, Mitchell J, Corey L, et al. Chronic fatigue in adolescents. *Pediatrics.* 1991;88(2):195-202.
21. Wilson A, Hickie I, Lloyd A, et al. The treatment of chronic fatigue syndrome: science and speculation. *Am J Med.* 1994;96(6):544-550.
22. Fukuda K, Straus S, Hickie I, et al. The chronic fatigue syndrome: a comprehensive approach to its definition and study. International Chronic Fatigue Syndrome Study Group. *Ann Intern Med.* 1994;121(12):953-959.
23. US Department of Health and Human Services, Centers for Disease Control and Prevention. Chronic Fatigue Syndrome: The Revised Case Definition (Abridged Version). Available at www.cdc.gov/cfs/cfsdefinitionHCP.htm. Accessed July 17, 2006.
24. Bell DS, Jordan K, Robinson M. Thirteen year follow-up of children and adolescents with chronic fatigue syndrome. *Pediatrics.* 2001;107:994-998.
25. Bright Futures Guidelines for Health Supervision. Available at www.brightfutures.org/bf2/pdf/index.html. Accessed July 14, 2006.

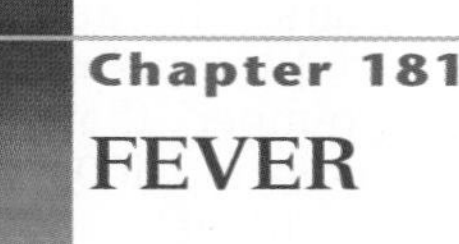

Chapter 181 FEVER

Elise W. van der Jagt, MD, MPH

For centuries, fever has been associated with illness. As many as 30% of all patients seen by primary care physicians and more than 5 million emergency department visits each year[1] have fever as their principal complaint, making it one of the most common reasons children are taken to a physician. Add to this fact the multitude of telephone calls about fever that are received day and night by health care providers, and, it becomes evident that the proper evaluation and management of fever is a basic and necessary skill for everyone caring for children.

Even though clinicians have long dealt with this common clinical sign, its mechanism, meaning, and management have remained sufficiently unclear and controversial that research on these matters continues. Although advances in neurochemistry and neurophysiology have improved the understanding of the pathophysiology of fever (see Chapter 53, Physiology and Management of Fever), clinical investigators continue to search for practical knowledge that will enhance the care of the febrile patient. Availability of such information can simplify the challenging role of the physician, who must evaluate a child quickly and effectively, arrive at a diagnosis, institute appropriate therapy, and both educate and support the parents and child during the entire process. The extent to which health care practitioners accomplish these goals depends on their knowledge of the mechanisms of disease, the various clinical manifestations of disease, and their awareness of the social context in which the disease occurs.

DEFINITION

The word *fever* is derived from the Latin *fovere,* meaning *to warm,* and commonly means an increase in body temperature. Although this general definition is acceptable in common parlance, fever is described more accurately as a disorder of thermoregulation. It must be differentiated from hyperthermia, an increased body temperature resulting from conditions that overwhelm the normal process of thermoregulation. (See Chapter 53, Physiology and Management of Fever, for a full discussion of thermoregulation.)

Normal core body temperature measured rectally ranges between 97°F and 100°F (36.1°C and 37.8°C), although on rare occasions it may be as low as 95.5°F (35.3°C) or as high as 101°F (38.3°C). The *normal* temperature of 98.6°F (37°C) was derived from an 1868 study of more than 1 million axillary temperatures taken in adults.[2] This value may have no relevance for children, not only because adults were studied, but also because axillary and rectal (core) temperatures correlate poorly. Young children appear to have higher core body temperatures than adults, with temperatures slightly higher than 37.8°C occurring frequently in those younger than 2 years. The upper limits of the normal range for a rectal temperature are 100.4°F (38.0°C) for infants younger than 1 month, 100.6°F (38.1°C) in 1 month olds, and 100.8°F (38.2°C) in 2 month olds.[3] A total of 6.2% of well babies have a rectal temperature of 100.8°F (38.2°C). Lowest body temperatures occur between 2 AM and 6 AM, and the highest ones occur between 5 PM and 7 PM, a diurnal variation that persists even during a febrile illness.

Because a range of normal body temperatures exists, knowing a child's usual body temperature can be useful so that an abnormal increase can be recognized more easily. The extent to which body temperature is increased above normal may help determine the presence and significance of fever. This circumstance may be true especially in young infants, in whom even a mild fever may be associated with serious disease. Although the variability and range of normal temperatures in children have made it difficult to define fever precisely and consistently, a consensus panel of experts[4] has recommended that the lower limit of fever be defined as a rectal temperature of 38°C (100.4°F). This definition has become standard and is used both clinically and in research studies about fever.

SIGNS AND SYMPTOMS ASSOCIATED WITH FEVER

The behavior of humans and animals is remarkably similar when fever is present.[5] When the set point in the hypothalamus is increased, patients attempt to adjust the environment to keep their bodies at this higher temperature. Young children usually seek close contact with a warm person (generally a parent), wish to be covered by a blanket, sit near a warm stove or register, and refuse cold liquids or foods. Although children may be quite comfortable at this higher body temperature, they interact less with others, have a decreased ability to concentrate, substitute quieter activities for energetic ones, and become less communicative except to indicate discomfort and distress. This adaptive withdrawal is often accompanied by loss of appetite and complaint of headache.

Such a combination of behavioral symptoms is a familiar indicator of illness to most parents and usually results first in placing the hand on the forehead, then measuring the temperature with a thermometer. Unfortunately, parents may not recognize the onset of fever in the younger child because the alterations in behavior are fewer and subtler. In a small infant, irritability and anorexia may be the sole evidence of fever and disease. If a parent is not familiar with these subtle cues, then recognition of serious illness may be significantly delayed.

In addition to the behavioral changes that may accompany fever, the general physical examination may reveal a pronounced hypermetabolic state. The child may have flushed cheeks, have an unusual glitter in the eyes, and be either sleepy and lethargic or exceptionally alert and excited (particularly 5 to 10 year olds). With rare exception, the pulse is increased by approximately 10 to 15 beats per 1°C of fever, and the respiratory rate is increased. (If the pulse rate is less than expected for the degree of fever, then typhoid fever, tularemia, mycoplasma infection, or factitious fever should be considered.) The skin may feel hot and dry ("burning up with fever"), although the distal extremities may be cold and pale (vasoconstricted), obscuring an extremely high core body temperature. Most children are not particularly uncomfortable, but some may shiver or sweat, mechanisms by which the body increases or decreases temperature. Sweating may be so excessive that dehydration may occur, particularly if the intake of fluids has been poor. Thus a dry mouth and lips may result not only from rapid mouth breathing, but also from dehydration. Finally, irritability of the central nervous system may increase, reflected in a febrile seizure.

The aforementioned signs and symptoms may be less obvious in a small infant. Shivering does not occur in the first few months of life, and diaphoresis is seen less frequently than in the older child. Because irritability and pallor may be the only suggestions of illness, a careful measurement of the temperature should be taken if the parent mentions these signs.

PRESENTATION AND EVALUATION

A febrile child may come to the attention of a primary care physician in several ways. Probably the most dramatic and frightening manifestation of fever in a child is the sudden occurrence of a seizure. A generalized tonic or tonic-clonic seizure, usually lasting less than 15 minutes and occurring within 24 hours of the onset of fever, may begin without warning. Most parents are not aware that a fever was present and often feel guilty for not having noted it. The primary care physician may be called immediately after the seizure has occurred or after the child has been transported to the emergency room. There the child is likely to be postictal and have a rectal temperature of 102° to 104°F (39° to 40°C). A thorough assessment of the patient is indicated because a seizure may be the first sign of meningitis or encephalitis.

Although some experts have suggested that every patient who has a first febrile seizure should routinely undergo a lumbar puncture (LP), the American Academy of Pediatrics recommends an approach that takes the age of the child into prime consideration.[6] Given that the younger the child is, the more difficult it is to diagnose meningitis clinically (eg, meningismus, Kernig sign, Brudzinski sign), strong consideration should be given to performing an LP in children less than 18 months. In infants less than 12 months, an LP should be strongly considered since clinical signs of meningitis may be absent. In children between 12 and 18 months, when the clinical manifestations of meningitis may be subtle, an LP should also be considered. In children older than 18 months, an LP is not routinely warranted except in the presence of signs and symptoms suggestive of meningitis or other intracranial infection. Because antibiotic treatment can mask meningitis, an LP should also be considered in a child with a febrile seizure who has received antibiotics. Reexamination of the child after the convulsive episode may also help determine whether an examination of the cerebrospinal fluid is needed.

More commonly, the patient is first examined when the fever has been present for longer than 24 hours and is associated either with nonspecific symptoms or with symptoms referable to a particular organ system. Inasmuch as many of the evaluations of the febrile child take place over the telephone (the first contact with the clinician), the physician must be able to take a pertinent history. Of particular significance are the age of the patient (the younger the child is, the more thorough the evaluation will need to be), any associated signs and symptoms, exposure to illness in the family or community, history of recent immunizations, and a history of any recurrent infections (eg, urinary tract infections, streptococcal infections, otitis media). The time of year should be considered because certain viral illnesses are more prevalent at different times of the year. For example, respiratory syncytial and influenza virus infections are more common during the winter, parainfluenza virus infections (the most common cause of croup) are more common during the spring and especially in the fall, and enterovirus infections occur primarily during the summer. In addition, questions should be asked about the duration and height of the fever. A low-grade fever that has been present for many days usually does not need to be evaluated as urgently as a temperature of 106°F (41°C) that has been present for a few hours. The former is likely to indicate a chronic or benign illness; the latter is more likely to be a potentially serious and rapidly progressive infectious disease.

A visit or telephone call for minimal fever and little evidence of disease should prompt a thorough assessment of the psychosocial factors that may be contributing to parental concern. Is the main concern about something else—a hidden agenda? What knowledge about fever and disease does the caregiver have? Has the caregiver had a previous traumatic experience with disease resulting in excessive anxiety? Might the patient be a vulnerable child? Is this family dysfunctional, in which minor illness either cannot be dealt with or is used as a means to meet other needs? Answers to these questions and others may clarify the situation.

DIFFERENTIAL DIAGNOSIS

Because many conditions may cause fever, an extensive discussion about each condition is beyond the scope of this chapter. However, classifying conditions associated with fever into broad categories is useful: (1) infection, (2) autoimmune disease, (3) neoplastic disease, (4) metabolic disease (eg, hyperthyroidism), (5) chronic inflammatory disease, (6) hematologic disease (eg, sickle cell disease, transfusion reaction), (7) drug fever and immunization reaction, (8) poisoning (eg, aspirin, atropine), (9) central nervous system abnormalities, and (10) factitious fever. In addition, dehydration, excessive muscle activity, and heat exposure may cause hyperthermia.

Although any disease in these categories may cause fever at any age, some diseases are more likely to occur at some ages than at others. Autoimmune disease and inflammatory bowel disease, for example, are unusual in infants but become progressively more frequent with increasing age. Similarly, febrile immunization reactions are much more common during the first year of life when most immunizations are administered.

Infections affecting the respiratory and gastrointestinal tracts account for the majority of fevers in all age groups. Most of these infections have a viral origin (eg, enterovirus, influenza virus, parainfluenza virus, respiratory syncytial virus, adenovirus, rhinovirus, rotavirus) and are generally self-limited. Knowledge of the seasonality of these viruses promotes correct and efficient diagnoses. In addition, knowledge of the typical physical findings in these infections and their course may help distinguish them from bacterial diseases. For example, high fever, irritability, posterior cervical adenopathy, and painful vesicles on the gums and tongue are characteristic of herpes gingivostomatitis. Failure to examine the tongue and gums may result in an unnecessary work-up in search of a possible bacterial infection. On the other hand, assuming that a high fever in a 2-month-old child is from roseola (exanthem subitum) would be erroneous because this infection (human herpesvirus type 6) usually does not occur at such an early age.

Failure to evaluate the fever further might result in missing a serious bacterial infection. Although viral infections may cause significant morbidity and mortality, the more aggressive course and serious outcomes of bacterial infections make early diagnosis especially important, particularly because effective antibiotic treatment is usually available. Bacterial infections may be especially devastating in younger children who are relatively immunocompromised because of their immature immune systems. An infection that remains localized in the older child may disseminate rapidly in the infant and toddler, particularly to the blood (bacteremia), the lungs (pneumonia), the meninges (meningitis), the bones (osteomyelitis), and the joints (arthritis).

Because these infections may be seriously debilitating or even fatal if not recognized, the physician must be able to differentiate bacterial infections from the more benign viral infections.

The younger the child is, the more difficult it is to recognize bacterial infection. Complaints cannot be verbalized, and physical signs and symptoms are more subtle and easily missed unless a high index of suspicion is maintained. Serious bacterial disease is especially difficult to diagnose in children with no obvious focus of infection. For this reason, many attempts have been made during the last 20 years to identify children in whom fever is a sign of a serious bacterial infection,[7] particularly pneumococcal disease and infections caused by *Haemophilus influenzae* type B (HiB). Children between birth and 36 months of age have been of special interest because fever is most common in this age group, and they may be difficult to assess, particularly during the first 6 months of life. Efforts to improve the ability to diagnose a serious bacterial infection have focused on 3 areas: (1) data from the history and physical examination,[8,9] (2) laboratory data,[10] and (3) response to antipyretics.[11] Of the 3 areas, the response to antipyretics has been shown most clearly to be unhelpful in distinguishing between patients who have a serious bacterial infection and those who have a more benign viral infection.[11] Children who have a serious infection respond to antipyretics no differently from those whose illness is less significant. In fact, some children who have viral illnesses do not defervesce either.

Many studies have attempted to delineate the precise combination of clinical or laboratory variables that might identify the febrile child at risk for serious disease. Defined clinical observational scales (eg, Yale Observation Scale, Young Infant Observation Scale, Severity Index) are not sufficiently discriminatory and predictive to be used alone.[12,13] Laboratory studies continue to be necessary as well.

During the early 1990s, specific practice guidelines were published to facilitate the initial management of febrile infants and children without an obvious source of infection.[14] Although these guidelines remain controversial,[15-19] as many as one third of primary care physicians have found them to be helpful and have changed the way they evaluate young children with fever.[20] Nevertheless, each patient continues to require individual assessment, with application of the recommendations as appropriate to the individual context of the patient. Considerations of the inconvenience, discomfort, and cost of laboratory testing and the increasing resistance to antibiotics in the community must be weighed carefully against the risk of missing a serious bacterial infection, with its subsequent morbidity and mortality. Therefore physicians must make the best decisions possible in an environment of incomplete certainty about the presence of serious disease. Parents need to be part of these discussions, and adequate follow-up of all patients is crucial, no matter what is decided in the initial visit.

Although the early practice guidelines were helpful during the 1990s, they were formulated before the introduction, in 2001, of the heptavalent pneumococcal vaccine for infants. This vaccine provides protection against pneumococcal serotypes 4, 6B, 9V, 14, 18C, 19F, and 23F and is administered at 2, 4, and 6 months and between 12 and 15 months of age. Since the introduction of the vaccine, a decline of 60% to 80% in pneumococcal disease has occurred in children younger than 24 months.[21] Because occult pneumococcal bacteremia and other pneumococcal infections made up most of the serious bacterial infections in young children with high fever (>102°F [>39°C]) before the vaccine, the use of this vaccine has greatly lowered the incidence of serious bacterial infections in children at greatest risk—those between 2 to 3 months and 3 years of age. A similar impact occurred when the HiB vaccine was introduced in the 1980s, nearly eliminating HiB meningitis, epiglottitis, and bacteremia. Given the marked decrease in pneumococcal and HiB serious bacterial infections, the likelihood of a serious bacterial infection when high fever (>102°F [>39°C]) is present in infants and toddlers is now even smaller, and a fairly limited assessment may be more suitable at this time.[22] In addition, with an increased ability to diagnose specific viral illnesses by rapid diagnostic testing (respiratory syncytial virus [RSV], influenza, enterovirus), even the revised, updated practice guidelines[23] (Figures 181-1 and 181-2) should be customized to the needs of the individual patient until further studies of their utility can be done.

Fever during the first 4 days of life has been associated with a high incidence of bacterial disease.[24] A temperature above 98.6°F (37°C) occurs in 1% of all newborns; of these children, 10% have a bacterial infection, usually caused by group B streptococcal or gram-negative enteric pathogens. A full work-up is indicated in these children, including a complete blood count and differential count, a urine analysis, and cultures of the blood, urine, and cerebrospinal fluid; antibiotics (usually intravenous ampicillin and gentamicin) should be administered until the results of cultures are known.

Similarly, neonates up to 28 days of age with fever have a significant risk of a bacterial infection (approximately 12% in some studies[15,25]). Pneumococcal infection is uncommon; group B *Streptococcus, Escherichia coli,* and other enteric pathogens are more usual. Urinary tract infection (UTI) and occult bacteremias are the most common types of infection; however, with group B *Streptococcus* infection, the risk of accompanying meningitis is as high as 39%.[26] Low-risk criteria, such as the Rochester criteria, may not be consistently reliable to differentiate young patients with serious bacterial infection from those who have more benign disease. Although some studies have demonstrated only a 0.2% incidence of bacteremia or meningitis in neonates satisfying the low-risk criteria,[27,28] others have found that up to 6% of neonates who satisfy low-risk criteria have a serious bacterial infection.[29,30] Of note is that neonates with RSV infection do not have a lower incidence of serious bacterial infection when they have fever.[31] Concomitant UTIs are especially common, occurring in 5% to 7% of patients.[32]

Fever greater than or equal to 100.4°F (38.0°C) in infants between 28 and 60 days of age is associated with a 5% to 10% incidence of serious bacterial

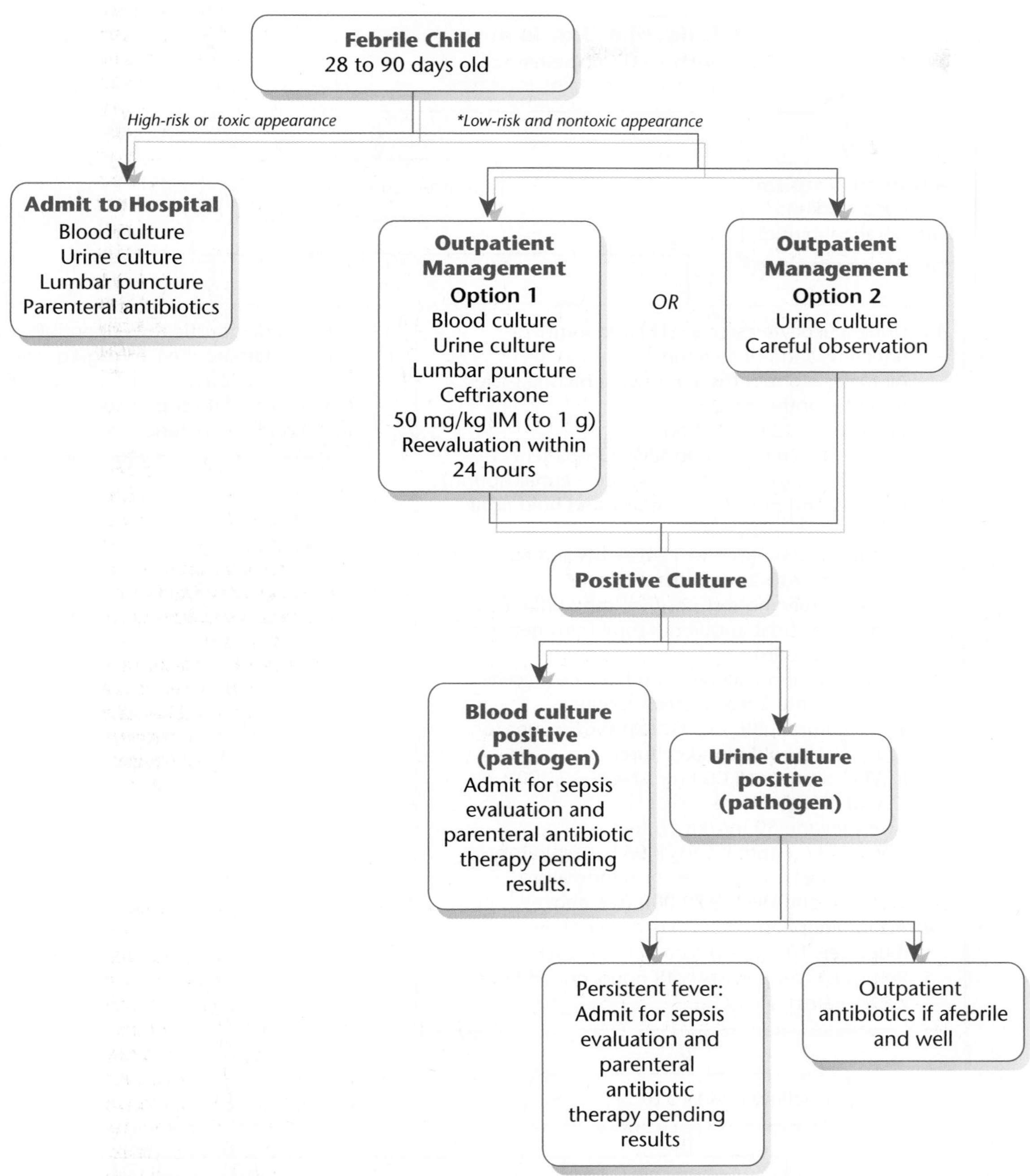

***Low-Risk Criteria for Febrile Infants**

Clinical criteria

Previously healthy
Nontoxic clinical appearance
No focal bacterial infection on examination (except otitis media)

Laboratory criteria

White blood cell (WBC) count 5000 to 15,000/mm^3, <1500 bands/mm^3
Normal urinalysis (<5 WBCs/high-powered field [hpf])
or gram-stained smear
When diarrhea is present: <5 WBCs/hpf in stool

Figure 181-1 Algorithm for the management of a previously healthy infant 28 to 90 days of age with fever without source at least 100.4°F (38°C). *(Baraff LJ. Management of fever without source in infants and children.* Ann Emerg Med. *2000;36:602-614. Copyright © 2000, Elsevier, with permission.)*

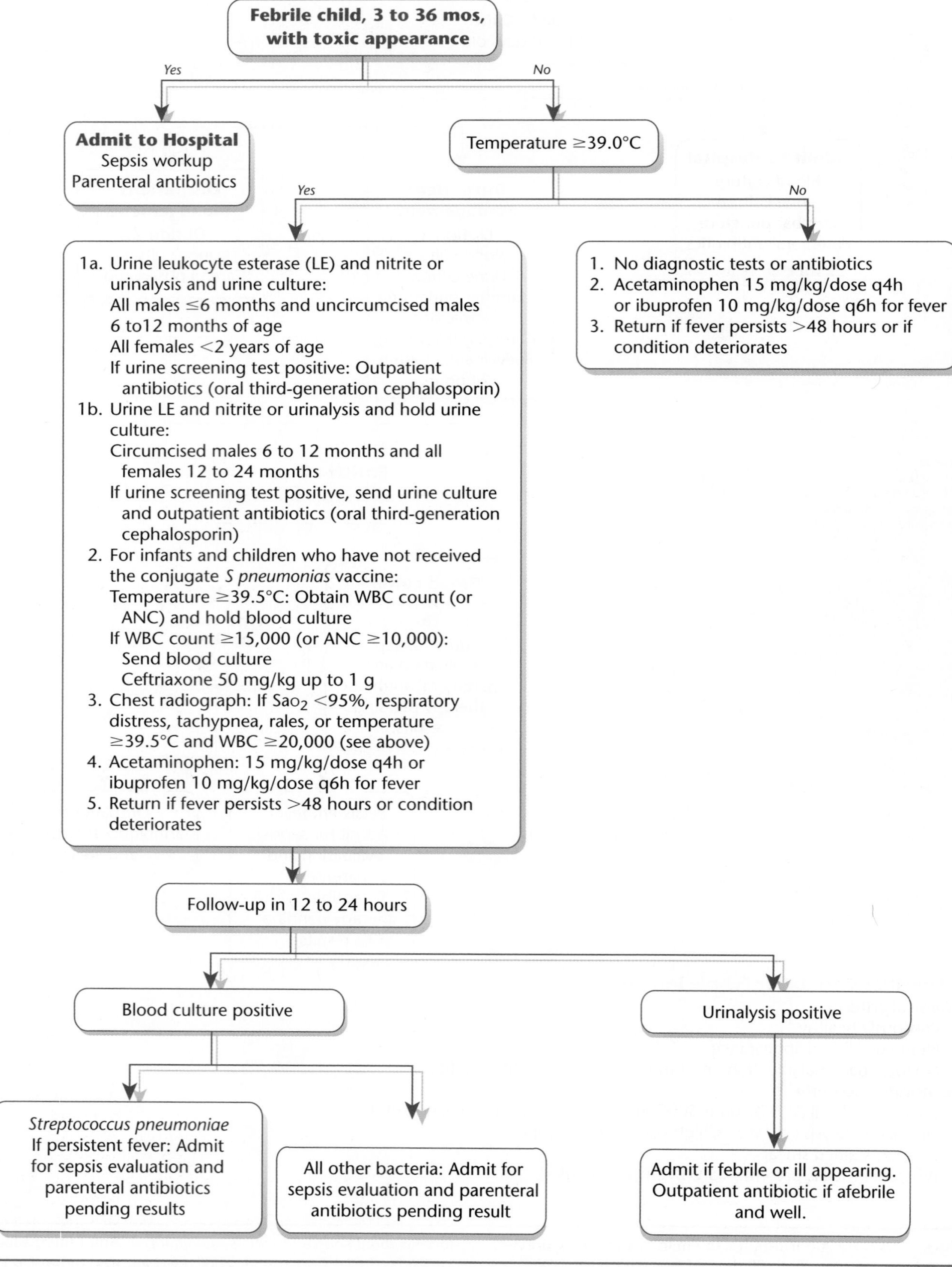

Figure 181-2 Algorithm for the management of a previously healthy child 91 days to 36 months of age with fever without source. *(Baraff LJ. Management of fever without source in infants and children.* Ann Emerg Med. *2000;36:602-614. Copyright © 2000, Elsevier, with permission.)*

Table 181-1 Rochester Criteria

1 Infant appears generally well
2 Infant has been previously healthy
  Born at term (≥37 weeks' gestation)
  Did not receive perinatal antimicrobial therapy
  Was not treated for unexplained hyperbilirubinemia
  Had not received and was not receiving antimicrobial agents
  Had not been previously hospitalized
  Was not hospitalized longer than mother
3 No evidence of skin, soft tissue, bone, joint, or ear infection
4 Laboratory values:
  Peripheral blood WBC count 5.0 to 15.0 × 10^9 cells/L (5000 to 15,000/mm^3)
  Absolute band form count ≤1.5 × 10^9 cells/L (≤1500/mm^3)
  ≤10 WBC per high-power field (×40) on microscopic examination of a spun urine sediment
  ≤5 WBC per high-power field (×40) on microscopic examination of a stool smear (only for infants with diarrhea)

From Jaskiewicz JA, McCarthy CA, Richardson AC, et al, and Febrile Infant Collaborative Study Groups. Febrile infants at low risk for serious bacterial infection—an appraisal of the Rochester criteria and implications for management. *Pediatrics.* 1994;94:390-396.

infection.[15,29,33] Unfortunately, neither height of fever nor apparent degree of toxicity has been a reliable predictor by itself of bacteremia or serious bacterial infection.[34,35] Instead of using single predictors, a combination of clinical and laboratory criteria appears to be more useful in identifying infants who are at low risk for having a bacterial infection. The most well known of these combinations are the Rochester criteria[36] (Table 181-1). The infants must satisfy all of the following conditions: previously healthy (as defined in Table 181-1), no clinical signs of toxicity (in some studies[29] defined by an infant observation score of ≤10), no focal bacterial infection found at physical examination, a white blood cell (WBC) count of 5000 to 15,000 cells/mm^3 with 1500 bands or fewer, a normal urinalysis (≤5 WBCs per high-power field [HPF] with few or no bacteria found in centrifuged urine and a Gram-stained smear of stool demonstrating fewer than 5 WBCs/HPF if diarrhea is present. If cerebrospinal fluid is obtained, then the cell count should be 8 WBCs/HPF or fewer.[36] One- to 2-month-old infants who satisfy these criteria have only a 1.1% probability of having a serious bacterial infection, and a 0.5% probability of having meningitis.[37]

Because of the difficulty in determining, based solely on the degree of fever, whether an infant younger than 2 to 3 months is at a low or high risk for bacterial disease (septicemia has occurred even in infants who have low-grade fevers[38]), evaluation should be prompt and thorough whenever a fever of at least 100.4°F (38°C) exists, paying particular attention to obtaining the data necessary for classifying the child as low or high risk. Such a comprehensive evaluation should generally include a complete physical examination, total and differential WBC count, urinalysis[39] and urine culture, a Gram-stained smear of stool if diarrhea is present, blood culture, and possibly examination and culture of cerebrospinal fluid. A urine culture is especially important because UTIs are the most common bacterial infections in this age group, even in the absence of pyuria.[27,40,41]

If the infant appears nontoxic and meets the low risk criteria, then examination and culture of the cerebrospinal fluid and blood might reasonably be avoided as long as good observation and follow-up can be made within 24 hours and antibiotics are not administered. If antibiotics are to be administered, then a full workup, including blood and cerebrospinal fluid cultures, should always be performed.

After obtaining a thorough history, including queries about illness of a similar nature in other family members and queries about whether the child has been immunized with the HiB and pneumococcal vaccines, the physician should assess the child for toxicity. If the child appears toxic (eg, lethargic or irritable, noninteractive, poor perfusion), then hospitalization should be considered along with further diagnostic tests to assess for serious bacterial infection. If the child does not appear toxic, a WBC count should be considered; if this count is greater than 15,000/mm^3, then a blood culture should be considered. (In the pre–pneumococcal vaccine era, children with WBC counts >15,000/mm^3 were 5 times as likely to experience bacteremia as those who had a WBC count <15,000/mm^3.[17] In addition, an absolute neutrophil count of at least 10,000/mm^3 correlated with an increased [8.2%] risk of pneumococcal bacteremia.) Practically, obtaining the WBC and blood culture at the same time is easiest, with the blood sent for culture only if the WBC count warrants doing so. Procalcitonin and C-reactive protein blood levels might have better sensitivity and specificity than the WBC count in predicting serious bacterial infection, but findings from various studies still vary widely with respect to the best cut-off levels to use.[42]

Given the lower incidence of pneumococcal disease now, avoiding blood tests altogether might be more cost-effective[43] and reasonable as long as the child has received at least 3 doses of the HiB and pneumococcal vaccines, does not appear toxic, has no obvious focus of infection, and has reliable health care providers with excellent follow-up capabilities.

Approximately 5% to 8% of children in the 3- to 36-month-old age group who have an undifferentiated febrile illness have a urinary tract infection (UTI).[44] Two groups of patients in this age group are especially at risk. Female infants with temperatures greater than 39°C (102.2°F) have a urinary tract infection incidence of 16% to 17%.[39,44] Uncircumcised boys in the first 12 months of life have an 8- to 9-fold higher rate of UTI than circumcised boys.[45] Because of the high rate of UTIs in this age group, a urine culture is suggested for febrile boys younger than 6 months of age (<12 months if uncircumcised) and girls younger than 12 to 24 months.[23] A urinalysis alone is not adequate as a screening tool to determine which child should have a urine culture; 20% of children who have a UTI have a normal urinalysis, including a negative test for urinary nitrites or leukocyte esterase.[41] A chest radiograph is generally necessary only if clinical symptoms or signs suggest pneumonia (eg, cough, tachypnea, dyspnea, rales, decreased breath sounds, dullness to percussion).[8] However, at least one study has suggested that up to 20% of children with fever of at least 102.2°F (39°C) and a WBC count of more than 20,000/mm^3 have pneumonia by chest radiograph, even in the absence of respiratory symptoms and signs.[46] Once the infant or child has been evaluated, a plan of management similar to those in Figures 181-1 and 181-2 should be considered. As discussed earlier in this chapter, the use of these protocols is controversial.

A further consideration in the approach to a febrile infant or child in the first 3 years of life is the increased availability of rapid diagnostic viral testing. Rapid tests are now available for influenza A and B, RSV, and enterovirus. Although sensitivity and specificity vary with individual tests, a positive test may be helpful in decreasing the number of other tests that need to be performed to rule out a bacterial infection.[47] Except for neonates younger than 28 days, the rate of serious bacterial infections in febrile patients is lower if they are infected with influenza and RSV. When this rate of infection is coupled with a generally lower incidence of serious pneumococcal and *H influenzae* infections because of the advent of vaccines given at a young age, a reasonable strategy might be to use positive viral tests as a way to reduce blood and urine tests in vaccinated children older than 2 to 3 months who do not appear toxic.

Children older than 3 years are more likely to have signs and symptoms consistent with a recognizable illness. If they have nonspecific symptoms, an urgent consultation with a physician is probably unnecessary; however, regardless of age, all febrile children with localized signs and symptoms, such as swollen joints, meningismus, labored respirations, chest pain, dysuria, petechiae, alteration of consciousness, and severe abdominal pain, should be examined immediately.

Although many febrile children do not have signs and symptoms pointing to an obvious cause, a complete physical examination may reveal important clues to the origin of the fever. Because most infections involve the respiratory tract, this area must be examined carefully. In all instances, the tympanic membranes should be examined for otitis media, the pharynx for pharyngitis, the nose for the discharge of sinusitis or a viral upper respiratory tract infection, and the lungs for evidence of pneumonia or bronchiolitis. Conjunctivitis may be a clue to adenovirus, influenza or RSV infection, conjunctivitis-otitis syndrome, or Kawasaki disease.

The skin is no less important and may demonstrate typical viral exanthems, such as those associated with rubella, roseola, or chickenpox, or it may show the erythema marginatum of rheumatic fever or the rose spots of typhoid fever.

Generalized lymphadenopathy often occurs with viral illnesses, such as infectious mononucleosis, hepatitis, or cytomegalovirus infection, but it also may be a clue to the diagnosis of leukemia or lymphoma. Localized enlargement of lymph nodes should prompt a search for a skin infection or for a tumor. Isolated cervical lymphadenopathy may be associated with tuberculosis infection or cat-scratch disease (*Bartonella* infection).

The musculoskeletal system must be examined with care. Localized bone tenderness may suggest osteomyelitis, and a restricted range of motion in a warm joint may suggest arthritis. Although the latter finding may occur in many different diseases, a meticulous examination of the heart is always indicated to detect the carditis of rheumatic fever or infective endocarditis. The spine should be palpated for any evidence of diskitis, and any costovertebral angle tenderness should prompt an examination of the urine for evidence of a UTI.

Although uncommon, factitious fever is a final consideration and a well-described entity. Children as young as 8 years have been known to increase the thermometer reading artificially by rubbing the mercury thermometer bulb on the sheets or by exposing it to warm liquids. Clues at physical examination include a pulse that is not correlated with the increase in temperature, inability to document fever when it is measured rectally, and an absence of sweating during defervescence. Investigation of psychosocial disturbances within the family is usually necessary.

A discussion of the physiology and management of fever is provided in Chapter 53, The Ill Child.

SUMMARY

Although fever can be a frightening sign that may be associated with serious illness, its treatment is much less crucial than the evaluation and treatment of the illness causing the fever. Health care professionals are responsible for educating parents about the proper management of their febrile children, emphasizing their role in the observation for signs and symptoms that are more likely to be associated with serious disease. Fever is but one sign that should be evaluated in the total context of the care of the patient.

TOOLS FOR PRACTICE

Engaging Patient and Family

- *Baby and Child Health* (book), American Academy of Pediatrics (www.aap.org/bookstore).
- *Caring for Your Baby and Young Child* (book), American Academy of Pediatrics (www.aap.org/bookstore).
- *Fever and Your Child* (brochure), American Academy of Pediatrics (patiented.aap.org).
- *What's the best way to take a child's temperature?* (Web page), American Academy of Pediatrics (www.aap.org/healthtopics/fever.cfm).

AAP POLICY STATEMENTS

American Academy of Pediatrics, Committee on Quality Improvement, Subcommittee on Urinary Tract Infection. Clinical practice guideline: practice parameter: the diagnosis, treatment, and evaluation of the initial urinary tract infection in febrile infants and young children. *Pediatrics*. 1999;103(4):843-852. (aappolicy.aappublications.org/cgi/content/full/pediatrics;103/4/843).

American Academy of Pediatrics, Provisional Committee on Quality Improvement, Subcommittee on Febrile Seizures. Practice parameter: the neurodiagnostic evaluation of the child with a first simple febrile seizure. *Pediatrics.* 1996; 97(5):769-772. (aappolicy.aappublications.org/cgi/content/abstract/pediatrics;97/5/769).

SUGGESTED RESOURCES

Cone TE. Diagnosis and treatment: children with fevers. *Pediatrics.* 1969;43:290-293.

Dagan R, Hall CB, Powel KR, et al. Epidemiology and laboratory diagnosis of infection with viral and bacterial pathogens in infants hospitalized for suspected sepsis. *J Pediatr.* 1989;115:351-356.

Dinarello CA, Cannon JG, Wolff SM. New concepts on the pathogenesis of fever. *Rev Infect Dis.* 1988;10:168-189.

Ishimine P. Fever without source in children 0-36 months of age. *Pediatr Clin North Am.* 2006;53:167-194.

Klein JO. Management of the febrile child without a focus of infection in the era of universal pneumococcal immunization. *Pediatr Infect Dis.* 2002;21:584-588.

Kluger MJ. Fever. *Pediatrics.* 1980;66:720-724.

Kramer MS, Naimark L, Leduc DG. Parental fever phobia and its correlates. *Pediatrics.* 1985;75:1110-1113.

Schmitt BD. Fever phobia. *Am J Dis Child.* 1980;134:176-181.

Vega R. Rapid viral testing in the evaluation of the febrile infant and child. *Curr Opin Pediatr.* 2005;17:363-367.

REFERENCES

1. McCaig LF, Burt CW. National hospital ambulatory medical care survey: 2002 emergency department summary. *Adv Data.* 2004;340:1-34.
2. Wunderlich C. *Das Verhalten der Eigenwarme in Krankenheiten.* Leipzig, Germany: Otto Wigard; 1868.
3. Herzog LW, Coyne JL. What is fever? Normal temperature in infants less than 3 months old. *Clin Pediatr.* 1993; 32:142-146.
4. Callanan D. Detecting fever in young infants: reliability of perceived, pacifier, and temporal temperatures in infants younger than 3 months of age. *Pediatr Emerg Care.* 2003;19:240-243.
5. Donaldson JF. Therapy of acute fever: a comparative approach. *Hosp Pract.* 1981;16:125-129, 133, 136-138.
6. American Academy of Pediatrics, Provisional Committee on Quality Improvement, Subcommittee on Febrile Seizures. Practice parameter: the neurodiagnostic evaluation of the child with a first simple febrile seizure. *Pediatrics.* 1996 May; 97(5):769-772; discussion 773-775.
7. Teele DW, Marshall R, Klein JO. Unsuspected bacteremia in young children. *Pediatr Clin North Am.* 1979;26:773-784.
8. Heulitt MJ, Ablow RC, Santos CC, et al. Febrile infants less than 3 months old: value of chest radiography. *Radiology.* 1988;167:135-137.
9. McCarthy PL, Sharpe MR, Spiesel SZ, et al. Observation scales to identify serious illness in febrile children. *Pediatrics.* 1982;70:802-809.
10. McCarthy PL. Controversies in pediatrics: what tests are indicated for the child under two with fever. *Pediatr Rev.* 1979;1:51-56.
11. Baker RC, Tiller T, Bausher JC, et al. Severity of disease correlated with fever reduction in febrile infants. *Pediatrics.* 1989;83:1016-1019.
12. Bonadio WA. The history and physical assessment of the febrile infant. *Pediatr Clin North Am.* 1998;45-65.
13. Kupperman N, Fleisher GR, Jaffe DM. Predictors of occult pneumococcal bacteremia in young febrile children. *Ann Emerg Med.* 1998;31:679-687.
14. Baraff LJ, Schriger DL, Bass JW, et al. Commentary on practice guidelines. *Pediatrics.* 1997;100:128-134.
15. Baker MD, Bell LM. Unpredictability of serious bacterial illness in febrile infants from birth to 1 month of age. *Arch Pediatr Adolesc Med.* 1999;153:508-511.
16. Bauchner H, Pelton SI. Management of the young febrile child: a continuing controversy. *Pediatrics.* 1997;100: 137-138.
17. Finkelstein JA, Christiansen CL, Platt R. Fever in pediatric primary care: occurrence, management, and outcomes. *Pediatrics.* 2000;105:260-266.
18. Kramer MS, Shapiro ED. Management of the young febrile child: a commentary on recent practice guidelines. *Pediatrics.* 1997;100:128-134.
19. Schriger DL. Clinical guidelines in the setting of incomplete evidence. *Pediatrics.* 1997;100:136.
20. Christiakis DA, Rivara FP. Pediatrician awareness of and attitudes about four clinical practice guidelines. *Pediatrics.* 1998;101:825-830.
21. Kaplan SL, Mason EO, Wald ER, et al. Decrease of invasive pneumococcal infections in children among 8 children's hospitals in the United States after the introduction of the 7-valent pneumococcal conjugate vaccine. *Pediatrics.* 2004;113(3):443-449.
22. Stoll ML, Rubin LG. Incidence of occult bacteremia among highly febrile young children in the era of the pneumococcal conjugate vaccine. *Arch Pediatr Adolesc Med.* 2004;158:671-675.
23. Baraff LJ. Management of fever without source in infants and children. *Ann Emerg Med.* 2000;36:602-614.
24. Voora S, Srinivasan G, Lilien LD, et al. Fever in full-term newborns in the first four days of life. *Pediatrics.* 1982; 69:40-44.
25. Kadish HA, Loveridge B, Tobey J, et al. Applying outpatient protocols in febrile infants 1-28 days of age: can the threshold be lowered? *Clin Pediatr (Phila).* 2000;39:81-88.
26. Pena BM, Harper MB, Fleisher GR. Occult bacteremia with group B streptococci in an outpatient setting. *Pediatrics.* 1998;102(1 pt 1):67-72.
27. Chiu CH, Lin TY. Application of the Rochester criteria in febrile neonates. *Pediatr Infect Dis J.* 1998;17:267-269.
28. Chiu CH, Lin TY, Bullard MJ. Identification of febrile neonates unlikely to have bacterial infections. *Pediatr Infect Dis J.* 1997;16:59-63.
29. Baker MD, Bell LM, Avner JR. Outpatient management without antibiotics of fever in selected infants. *N Engl J Med.* 1993;329:1437-1441.
30. Falzon A, Grech V, Caruana B, et al. How reliable is axillary temperature measurement? *Acta Paediatr.* 2003;92: 309-313.
31. Levine DA, Platt SL, Dayan PS, et al. Risk of serious bacterial infection in young febrile infants with respiratory syncytial virus infections. *Pediatrics.* 2004;113:1728-1734.
32. Pinar O, Phoenix C, St Martin D, et al. Sepsis work-up in febrile infants 0-90 days of age with respiratory syncytial virus infection. *Pediatr Emerg Care.* 2003;19:314-319.
33. Baskin MN, O'Rourke EJ, Fleisher GR. Outpatient treatment of febrile infants 28-89 days of age with intramuscular administration of ceftriaxone. *J Pediatr.* 1992;120:22-27.
34. Berkowitz CD, Uchiyama N, Tully SB, et al. Fever in infants less than two months of age: spectrum of disease and predictors of outcome. *Pediatr Emerg Care.* 1985;1: 128-135.
35. McCarthy PL, Dolan T. The serious implications of high fever in infants during their first three months. *Clin Pediatr.* 1976;15:794-796.
36. Dagan R, Powell KR, Hall CB, et al. Identification of infants unlikely to have serious bacterial infection although hospitalized for suspected sepsis. *J Pediatr.* 1985;107:855-860.

37. Jaskiewicz JA, McCarthy CA, Richardson AC, et al, and Febrile Infant Collaborative Study Groups. Febrile infants at low risk for serious bacterial infection—an appraisal of the Rochester criteria and implications for management. *Pediatrics.* 1994;94:390-396.
38. Roberts KB, Borzy MS. Fever in the first eight weeks of life. *Johns Hopkins Med J.* 1977;141:9-13.
39. Hoberman A, Wald ER, Reynolds A, et al. Pyuria and bacteriuria in urine specimens obtained by catheter from young children with fever. *J Pediatr.* 1994;124:513-519.
40. Krober MS, Bass JW, Powell JM, et al. Bacterial and viral pathogens causing fever in infants less than 3 months old. *Am J Dis Child.* 1985;139:889-892.
41. American Academy of Pediatrics, Committee on Quality Improvement, Subcommittee on Urinary Tract Infection. Practice parameter: the diagnosis, treatment, and evaluation of the initial urinary tract infection in febrile infants and young children. *Pediatrics.* 1999;103:843-852.
42. Hsiao AL, Baker MD. Fever in the new millennium: a review of recent studies of markers of serious bacterial infection in febrile children. *Curr Opin Pediatr.* 2005;17:56-61.
43. Lee GM, Fleisher GR, Harper MB. Management of febrile children in the age of the conjugate pneumococcal vaccine: a cost-effectiveness analysis. *Pediatrics.* 2001;108:835-844.
44. Hoberman A, Wald ER. Urinary tract infections in young febrile children. *Pediatr Infect Dis J.* 1997;16:11-17.
45. Shaw KN, Gorelick KL, McGowan KL, et al. Prevalence of urinary tract infection in febrile young children in the emergency department. *Pediatrics.* 1998;102:E16.
46. Bachur R, Perry H, Harper MB. Occult pneumonias: empiric chest radiographs in febrile children with leukocytosis. *Ann Emerg Med.* 1999;33:166-173.
47. Bonner AB, Monroe KW, Talley LI, et al. Impact of the rapid diagnosis of influenza on physician decision-making and patient management in the pediatric emergency department results of a randomized, prospective, controlled trial. *Pediatrics.* 2003;112:363-367.

Chapter 182

FEVER OF UNKNOWN ORIGIN

Elise W. van der Jagt, MD, MPH

Fever without a discernible cause is always difficult for clinicians because fever suggests disease. The inability to identify the cause of the fever can undermine the physician's credibility and can affect rapport with patients. The longer the fever persists, the more concern is raised by the parents. A fever of only a few days' duration that is not associated with any localizing signs or symptoms frequently does not even come to a physician's attention unless the child also appears ill. Fever that continues beyond 5 to 7 days, or one that occurs repeatedly, usually alarms parents enough to prompt a medical consultation. This discussion focuses on these prolonged fevers and their evaluation.

DEFINITION

In 1961 the classic definition for a fever of unknown origin (FUO) was proposed: fever that is higher than 38.3°C (101°F) on several occasions, that is present for more than 3 weeks, and that has a cause that is still unexplained after 1 week of evaluation in the hospital.[1] More recently, researchers have suggested that the criteria are inappropriate for immunocompromised patients and that the third criterion—evaluation—be changed either to reflect the increased emphasis on ambulatory assessment (unexplained fever after 3 days of in-hospital evaluation or 3 ambulatory visits) or to make the evaluation more qualitative by requiring specific tests that should have been performed before applying the label of an FUO.[2,3] The latter definition is closer to one accepted by most primary care physicians, who usually prefer not to delay evaluation for 3 weeks or require a week of hospitalization. An FUO in children has been defined as a daily rectal temperature greater than 38.3°C (101°F), lasting for at least 2 weeks, the cause of which has not been determined by simple diagnostic tests, including a complete history and thorough physical examination.[4] Some experts would add that 1 of the 2 weeks of fever should be documented in the hospital.

Careful documentation of fever is necessary before diagnosing FUO. A thorough explanation of the range of normal core body temperature for age, with its diurnal variation, may help to exclude patients who are not truly febrile but who instead have a high normal body temperature. The physician should instruct the parents in the technique of taking a rectal temperature and define a day of fever as a 24-hour period in which a temperature greater than 38.3°C (101°F) occurs at least once. All medications taken, the various activities in which the child has participated, and the environmental temperature during this time should be recorded because each of these may affect body temperature.

Although much importance has been attached to fever patterns in the past (ie, remittent, intermittent, sustained), detailing them may not be useful because they are rarely diagnostic of a specific disease.[5] Nevertheless, some inflammatory diseases do have recognizable fever patterns (eg, double quotidian fever of systemic idiopathic juvenile arthritis). In addition, whether even 1 or 2 days of normal temperature are interspersed between days of fever needs to be carefully determined. These children may have a series of rapidly sequenced brief febrile illnesses, which are masquerading as a single febrile illness. Careful documentation of fever should also help exclude the so-called *pseudo-FUO*.[6] Children who have a pseudo-FUO not only do not have a true fever if their body temperature is measured accurately and consistently (sometimes this needs to be done under hospital supervision), but also exhibit a specific constellation of findings that is recognizable and often diagnostic (Box 182-1). In addition to the inability to corroborate fever, and in the setting of a completely normal physical examination, the parents may relate a previous serious illness and their concerns about its possible recurrence or lasting effect on the child (vulnerable child syndrome). Their child may have missed an excessive amount of school, given the general degree of illness described; school absence is often prompted by the presence of fatigue, abdominal pain, and headache in the morning—symptoms that are conspicuously absent during the rest of the day. Others have noted a similar pattern of findings and

BOX 182-1 Characteristics of the Child Who Has Pseudo–Fever of Unknown Origin

Absence of documented, persistent fever
Lack of objective, abnormal physical findings
History of significant or near-fatal illness
Parental fear of malignant or crippling disease
Frequent environmental exposure to illness
Absence of persistent weight loss
Normal erythrocyte sedimentation rate and platelet count
Many missed school days because of subjective morning complaints
Discordance of fever and pulse rate
Medical or paramedical family background
One or more of mild self-limited diseases, behavioral problems, parents who have misconceptions concerning health and disease, or families under stress

From Kleiman MB. The complaint of persistent fever. *Pediatr Clin North Am.* 1982;29(1):201-208. Copyright © 1982, Elsevier, with permission.

called it *deconditioning syndrome,* which occurs after an acute, easily definable febrile illness and usually occurs in children who are older than 12 years and who have frequently been previously ill.[7]

In addition to the single episode of prolonged fever, some children have shorter than normal episodes of fevers that recur in a regular (periodic) fashion, along with a predictable constellation of symptoms. Patients with these types of fevers are said to have *periodic fever syndromes.*[7] Many of these periodic fevers are now known to be genetically based and can be diagnosed by sophisticated genetic testing.

DIFFERENTIAL DIAGNOSIS

Box 182-2 lists the common causes of FUO in children. The causes are subdivided into 4 categories: (1) infectious diseases, (2) autoimmune diseases, (3) malignancies, and (4) miscellaneous. This list shows that most FUOs are eventually found to be caused by common pediatric illnesses that are either self-limited or treatable.

An infectious illness is the most common cause for an FUO in children, comprising between 40% and 60% of the reported cases[4,8-10]; the second most common cause is autoimmune disease, comprising between 7% and 20% of the cases. Children younger than 6 years are most likely to have FUO resulting from an infection; autoimmune diseases start to become more common after 6 years, although infection remains the most frequent cause of FUO (Table 182-1).[9]

Although most infections that exhibit themselves as an FUO are an atypical or incomplete manifestation of a common infectious disease, several other types of infections should be considered. Epstein-Barr virus is the most common infectious cause of FUO,[8,11] followed by osteomyelitis and bartonellosis. The advent of serologic testing (indirect immunofluorescent antibodies) for Epstein-Barr virus and *Bartonella* infections has made these diagnoses easier to make. Although bartonellosis (caused by *Bartonella henselae*) usually exhibits as classic cat-scratch disease, it may also show as atypical cat-scratch disease, producing prolonged fever and hepatosplenic abscesses,[12] lymphadenopathy, or central nervous system disease.[13] Thus, when exposure to kittens and cats can be documented, serologic testing for *Bartonella* should be obtained; if positive, then an abdominal ultrasound should be considered.

Osteomyelitis, particularly of the axial skeleton (intervertebral disk space and vertebral body) and the pelvis, should also be strongly considered.

The appearance during the 1980s and subsequent increased incidence of HIV infection and AIDS should encourage primary care physicians to assess children thoroughly for the presence of the characteristic physical signs and symptoms, as well as known risk factors, including parental intravenous drug abuse, parental sexual contact with individuals who may be HIV positive, an HIV-positive mother, and hemophilia requiring transfusion of blood products. Fever is not usually the sole manifestation of HIV infection. However, HIV infection should be strongly considered and the appropriate laboratory tests performed if the fever has been present for more than 2 months and is associated with one or more of the following:

- Failure to thrive or a weight loss of more than 10% from baseline
- Hepatomegaly
- Splenomegaly
- Generalized lymphadenopathy (lymph nodes measuring at least 0.5 cm in 2 or more sites, with bilateral site involvement counting as one site)
- Parotitis
- Persistent or recurrent diarrhea[14]

Of the autoimmune diseases, systemic idiopathic juvenile arthritis (formerly known as systemic juvenile rheumatoid arthritis) is the most common. Fever is almost always associated with this illness, and it frequently precedes the joint manifestations by weeks or months. The typical double quotidian fever (2 fever spikes in 24 hours with a normal temperature in between) is a helpful clue to this diagnosis. Other common autoimmune diseases that should be considered are lupus erythematosus and chronic regional enteritis. The latter condition is more common among children older than 6 years than those in other age groups.

Malignancy, the diagnosis that provokes the most anxiety, is present in only a small percentage of patients in most studies (1.5% to 6%).[4,8,9,11] This circumstance is in contrast to adults with FUO, of whom between 7% and 16% have a neoplastic process.[3,15] The most common malignancy in children is leukemia, although solid tumors such as lymphoma, neuroblastoma, hypernephroma, and hepatoma have been reported to present as FUO. The exact reason for fever in these diseases is unclear but may be related to endogenous pyrogen and other cytokines produced by the neoplastic cells. A large spectrum of miscellaneous diseases may cause prolonged fevers (see Box 182-2). However, a clear diagnosis is never obtained in 25% to 67% of patients who have persistent fever.[8,11,16] These fevers are the genuine FUOs. Most of these patients appear to do well, and the fever eventually disappears after months or even years.[17]

Some patients have fevers that do not satisfy the classic definition of FUO. Instead, they have recurrent fevers that are associated with a well-defined constellation of symptoms each time. The most common of

BOX 182-2 Causes of Fever of Unknown Origin in Children

BACTERIAL INFECTIOUS DISEASES
Bacterial endocarditis
Bartonellosis
Brucellosis
Chlamydia
  Lymphogranuloma venereum
  Psittacosis
Leptospirosis
Liver abscess
Mastoiditis (chronic)
Osteomyelitis
Pelvic abscess
Perinephric abscess
Pyelonephritis
Salmonellosis
Sinusitis
Subdiaphragmatic abscess
Tuberculosis
Tularemia

VIRAL INFECTIOUS DISEASES
Cytomegalovirus
Epstein-Barr virus (infectious mononucleosis)
Hepatitis viruses
Q fever
Rickettsial diseases
  Q fever
  Rocky Mountain spotted fever

FUNGAL INFECTIOUS DISEASES
Blastomycosis (nonpulmonary)
Histoplasmosis (disseminated)

PARASITIC INFECTIOUS DISEASES
Malaria
Sarcoidosis
Toxoplasmosis
Visceral larva migrans
Visceral leishmaniasis

AUTOIMMUNE DISEASES
Polyarteritis nodosa
Systemic idiopathic juvenile arthritis
Systemic lupus erythematosus

MALIGNANCIES
Hodgkin disease
Leukemia or lymphoma
Neuroblastoma

PERIODIC FEVER SYNDROMES
Cyclic neutropenia
Familial Mediterranean fever
Hyperimmunoglobulinemia D and periodic fever syndrome (HIDS)
Periodic fever, aphthous stomatitis, pharyngitis, and cervical adenopathy (PFAPA)
Tumor necrosis factor receptor–associated periodic syndrome (TRAPS)
Other periodic fever syndromes

MISCELLANEOUS CAUSES
Central diabetes insipidus
Drug fever
Ectodermal dysplasia
Familial dysautonomia
Granulomatous colitis
Infantile cortical hyperostosis
Münchausen by proxy
Nephrogenic diabetes insipidus
Pancreatitis
Pseudo-fever
Sarcoidosis
Serum sickness
Thyrotoxicosis
Ulcerative colitis

Modified from Feigin RD, Cherry JD. *Textbook of Pediatric Infectious Diseases.* 5th ed. Philadelphia, PA: WB Saunders; 2004.

these periodic fever syndromes is PFAPA (periodic fever, aphthous stomatitis, pharyngitis, and cervical adenopathy).[7] This nonhereditary autoinflammatory syndrome has its onset before the age of 3 years, is associated with a sudden fever to 39°C to 40°C (102°F to 104°F) lasting 3 to 5 days. Also present are anorexia, mild oral ulcerations with pharyngitis, cervical lymphadenopathy, an increased white blood cell count, and an increased erythrocyte sedimentation rate (ESR). This constellation of symptoms returns every 3 to 6 weeks. A single dose of corticosteroids may quickly resolve the symptoms of individual episodes.[18]

Other periodic fever syndromes include cyclic neutropenia, familial Mediterranean fever, hyperimmunoglobulinemia D and periodic fever syndrome (HIDS, or mevalonate kinase deficiency) and tumor necrosis factor receptor–associated periodic syndrome (TRAPS). These syndromes are found in various populations around the world and are associated with known gene mutations.[7,19] The primary care physician should therefore know the patients' race, ethnicity, and country of origin because these factors may provide clues to a specific periodic fever syndrome.

EVALUATION

History

Whether the child has a true FUO or a pseudo-FUO cannot be determined without a precise history and

Table 182-1 Diagnoses of Prolonged Fever in Children

	AGE		
DIAGNOSIS	<6 YEARS	>6 YEARS	TOTAL
INFECTION			
Viral	14 (27%)	7 (15%)	21
Nonviral	20 (38%)	11 (23%)	31
OTHER			
Collagen	4 (8%)	16 (33%)	20
Malignancy	4 (8%)	2 (4%)	6
Miscellaneous	7 (13%)	3 (6%)	10
No diagnosis	3 (6%)	9 (19%)	12
Total	52	49	100

From Pizzo PA, Lovejoy FH, Smith DH. Prolonged fever in children: review of 100 cases. *Pediatrics.* 1975;55(4):468-473.

thorough physical examination, with the physician paying close attention to behavioral, social, familial, and environmental factors. Information regarding travel, patient residence if outside the United States, animal exposure, frequency of exposure to other persons who have common febrile illnesses, previous illness, hospitalizations, medications, family history of disease, race and ethnicity, and the precise course of the exhibiting symptoms must be obtained methodically and efficiently. Meticulous documentation of dates is especially important. To this end, having the family record on a calendar, both the daily time and height of the fever along with associated symptoms, is usually helpful.

For children older than 11 to 12 years, a separate interview should be conducted alone with the child to obtain the child's perspective on the illness and to elicit information that may be difficult to express in the presence of parents. School, peer relationships, family functioning, and sexual identity and activity should be explored.

Physical Examination

A full physical examination must be performed. Rectal temperature, respiratory rate, heart rate, and blood pressure measurements should be obtained. Any discrepancy between heart rate and temperature implies factitious fever. A thorough examination of the respiratory tract is indicated. Inspection of the pharynx for hyperemia and exudate, of the tympanic membranes for chronic otitis media, transillumination of the sinuses for sinusitis, a search for a purulent nasal discharge, and auscultation of the chest for localized wheezing are all important. In the older child, an examination of the teeth to exclude dental caries and periodontal disease should be included. A new cardiac murmur may be a clue to rheumatic fever or infective endocarditis. Lymphadenopathy, especially if generalized, may suggest a viral infection, such as infectious mononucleosis, cytomegalovirus infection, toxoplasmosis, or HIV infection. Joints must be examined meticulously for swelling, restricted range of motion, and tenderness. Skin rashes may suggest a viral disease or an autoimmune disease such as juvenile idiopathic arthritis. The absence of sweating and the presence of a smooth tongue are consistent with familial dysautonomia, a rare genetic disorder of thermoregulation. Finally, a rectal examination in the older child and a stool guaiac test are imperative; finding pararectal lymphadenopathy may suggest a pelvic infection, and a positive stool guaiac test may be consistent with inflammatory bowel disease.

Laboratory Evaluation

If the history and physical examination disclose no specific findings and growth is normal, then only simple diagnostic tests are indicated. Routine blood counts and urinalysis have not been shown to be particularly useful, although no one advocates their elimination from the work-up. A purified protein derivative tuberculin skin test should be given to detect tuberculosis, although anergy may occur in active tuberculosis infection. Negative blood, urine, and throat cultures exclude infections of these areas.

Probably the most useful laboratory tests are the ESR, C-reactive protein (CRP), and the albumin-globulin ratio. If the ESR is more than 30, the CRP is elevated, or the albumin-globulin ratio is inverted, then a higher probability of serious disease exists, particularly an autoimmune vascular disease or a malignancy. Further evaluation should be vigorously pursued.

The remainder of the evaluation should be individualized based on historical and clinical findings. Because infectious causes are the most common, pursuing specific serological tests for such diseases as hepatitis A and B, Epstein-Barr virus infection (infectious mononucleosis), bartonellosis, toxoplasmosis, and cytomegalovirus infection would be reasonable. A radioactive gallium scan may be useful in detecting occult abscesses and infections, although this scan has been found to be less useful in children than in adults.[20] Total body computed tomographic scans may help find tumors, although if the abdomen is of primary concern, then an abdominal ultrasound will also detect significant abnormalities.[16] Radiologic studies of the sinuses, the gastrointestinal tract, and the chest all may be appropriate in certain individuals but should not be routine. A bone marrow examination may occasionally help in the diagnosis of tuberculosis, leukemia, metastatic cancer, or fungal infections but should be considered only in children who either have a clinical or laboratory finding suggestive of malignancy or who are immunocompromised.[21] Finally, if the child is not visibly deteriorating, a period of observation may be necessary until new findings appear that can give more direction to the investigation.

If the ESR, CRP, and the albumin-globulin ratio are normal and no signs and symptoms are present that are specific to a particular disease, little can be gained from any of the tests previously mentioned. Observation and periodic evaluation are the only measures that are required while remaining alert for the occurrence of new symptoms or signs that might lead the investigation in a specific direction. Fortunately, most FUOs for which a cause cannot be found will resolve over time.

Since it is likely that the parents and patient will be anxious about an undiagnosable problem, the primary care physician must be ready to provide all family members with a clear explanation of the evaluative process, any normal results, and reassurance. Referrals to pediatric infectious disease specialists, rheumatologists, specialized diagnosticians, or any combination of these professionals may occasionally be necessary for additional assistance in determining a diagnosis.

SUMMARY

The evaluation of the child who has FUO must be individualized to accommodate the history, the physical examination, and the particular social environment in which the child and family live. An intensive examination of all these factors is the physician's responsibility and is the first stage of managing the patient. Whether hospitalization is part of this approach ultimately depends on the amount of parental anxiety, the necessity to document fever, and the performance of diagnostic tests that cannot be done on an outpatient basis.

The health care professional must continue to assess these children frequently to detect new findings early and to maintain the confidence of the family while the fever continues. However, children with FUO generally do well, even though the fever may last for weeks or months.

TOOLS FOR PRACTICE

Engaging Patient and Family

- *Fever and Your Child* (brochure), American Academy of Pediatrics (patiented.aap.org).

Medical Decision Support

- *Red Book: 2006 Report of the Committee on Infectious Diseases,* 27th edition (book), American Academy of Pediatrics (www.aap.org/bookstore).

SUGGESTED RESOURCE

Long SS. Fever of unknown origin. In: Long SS, Pickering LK, Prober CG, eds. *Principles and Practice of Pediatric Infectious Diseases.* 2nd ed. New York, NY: Churchill Livingstone; 2003.

REFERENCES

1. Petersdorf RG, Beeson PB. Fever of unexplained origin: report on 100 cases. *Medicine.* 1961;40:1.
2. Durack DT, Street AC. Fever of unknown origin—re-examined and redefined. *Curr Clin Top Infect Dis.* 1991;11:35-51.
3. Vanderscheuren S, Knockaert D, Adriaenssens T, et al. From prolonged febrile illness to fever of unknown origin—the challenge continues. *Arch Intern Med.* 2003; 163(9):1033-1041.
4. Feigin RD, Shearer WT. Fever of unknown origin in children. *Curr Probl Pediatr.* 1976;6:1.
5. Musher DM, Fainstein V, Young EJ, et al. Fever patterns: their lack of clinical significance. *Arch Intern Med.* 1979; 139(11):1225-1228.
6. Kleiman MB. The complaint of persistent fever. *Pediatr Clin North Am.* 1982;29(1):201-208.
7. Long SS. Distinguishing among prolonged, recurrent, and periodic fever syndromes: approach of a pediatric infectious diseases specialist. *Pediatr Clin North Am.* 2005;52(3):811-835.
8. Jacobs RF, Schutze GE. Bartonella henselae as a cause of prolonged fever and fever of unknown origin in children. *Clin Infect Dis.* 1998;26(1):80-84.
9. Pizzo PA, Lovejoy FH, Smith DH. Prolonged fever in children: review of 100 cases. *Pediatrics.* 1975;55(4):468-473.
10. Lohr JA, Hendley JO. Prolonged fever of unknown origin: a record of experiences with 54 childhood patients. *Clin Pediatr.* 1977;16(9):768-773.
11. Pasic S, Minic A, Djuric P, et al. Fever of unknown origin in 185 paediatric patients: a single-centre experience. *Acta Paediatr.* 2006;95(4):463-466.
12. Ventura A, Massei F, Not T, et al. Systemic Bartonella henselae infection with hepatosplenic involvement. *J Pediatr Gastroent Nutr.* 1999;29(1):52-56.
13. Tsujino K, Tsukahara M, Tsuneoka H, et al. Clinical implication of prolonged fever in children with cat scratch disease. *J Infect Chemother.* 2004;10(4):227-233
14. Centers for Disease Control and Prevention. Classification system for human immunodeficiency virus (HIV) infection in children under 13 years of age. *MMWR Morb Mortal Wkly Rep.* 1987;36(15):225-230, 235-236.
15. Bleeker-Rovers CP, Vos FJ, de Kleijn EM, et al. A prospective multicenter study on fever of unknown origin. *Medicine (Baltimore).* 2007;86(1):26-38.
16. Steele RW, Jones SM, Lowe BA, et al. Usefulness of scanning procedures for diagnosis of fever of unknown origin in children. *J Pediatr.* 1991;119(4):526-530.
17. Miller LE, Sisson BA, Tucker LB, et al. Prolonged fevers of unknown origin in children: patterns of presentation and outcome. *J Pediatr.* 1996;129(3):419-423.
18. Marshall GS, Edwards KM, Butler J, et al. Syndrome of periodic fever, pharyngitis, and aphthous stomatitis. *J Pediatr.* 1987;110(1):43-46.
19. Hofer M, Mahlaoui N, Prieur A. A child with a systemic febrile illness—differential diagnosis and management. *Best Pract Res Clin Rheumatol.* 2006;20(4):627-640.
20. Buonomo C, Treves ST. Gallium scanning in children with fever of unknown origin. *Pediatr Radiol.* 1993;23(4): 307-310.
21. Hayani A, Mahoney DH, Fernbach DJ. Role of bone marrow examination in the child with prolonged fever. *J Pediatr.* 1990;116(6):919-920.

Chapter 183

FOOT AND LEG PROBLEMS

Robert A. Hoekelman, MD; Maurice J. Chianese, MD

Pediatricians and family practitioners often have to make judgments concerning actual or presumed problems of the feet and legs in infants and children. The frequency and natural history of these problems is such that referral to orthopedic consultants is not always appropriate. In most instances the problems presented require no treatment, others can be managed easily without consultations, and only a few require the services of an orthopedist.

The *ped* in pediatrics and orthopedics is derived from the Greek word *paidios,* meaning child, not from the Latin *pedalis* or French *ped,* meaning foot.

Therefore pediatrics is the medicine (Greek *iatrike*) of the child, and orthopedics is the straightening or correction (Greek *orthos*) of deformities in children. Orthopedics has expanded its scope well beyond this initial thrust; nevertheless the orthopedist and the pediatrician are concerned with many problems involving the feet and legs of children.

ORTHOPEDIC TERMINOLOGY

Practitioners use certain terms to describe positional variations of the lower extremities and are often used in the nomenclature of specific orthopedic conditions.

In general, the joint that is primarily involved in the condition constitutes the first word; the subsequent word or words relate to the positioning of the extremity relative to the midline of the body. For example, coxa vara is a condition of the hip (coxa) that results in a deviation of the leg toward the midline (varus position). The orthopedic terms in Box 183-1 have special reference to abnormalities of the feet and legs.

SHOES

The foot takes the shape of the shoe, not vice versa. Improperly fitted or manufactured shoes may be the primary cause of acquired foot deformities and problems. Shoes that do not fit properly can deform an otherwise-normal foot, resulting in hammertoes, hallux valgus, bunionettes, corns, and, ultimately, the need for surgery.

BOX 183-1 Glossary of Terms That Refer to Foot and Leg Abnormalities

Abduction: deviation away from the midline of the body

Adduction: deviation toward the midline of the body

Calcaneus: foot dorsiflexed, placing the heel below the level of the toes

Cavus: medial longitudinal arch of the foot elevated

Equinus: foot plantar flexed, placing the toes below the level of the heel

Pes: the foot

Planus: medial longitudinal arch of the foot flattened

Talipes: congenital deformities of the foot that, if untreated, result in walking on the ankle (talus)

Torsion: excessive or abnormal twisting along the long axis

- *Internal torsion:* excessive or abnormal inward twisting
- *External torsion:* excessive or abnormal outward twisting

Varus: medial or inward deviation of one segment of an extremity relative to the proximal (previous) segment

Valgus: lateral or outward deviation of one segment of an extremity relative to the proximal (previous) segment

Version: physiologic or normal twisting along the long axis

- *Inversion:* physiologic or normal twist inward
- *Eversion:* physiologic or normal twist outward
- *Anteversion:* physiologic or normal twist forward
- *Retroversion:* physiologic or normal twist backward

Functions of Shoes

Parents often ask the physician when their child should begin wearing shoes and what kind of shoe should be worn. In answering these questions, the reasons for wearing shoes must be borne in mind. The shoe has two functions, the most important of which is protecting the feet from trauma and extreme temperatures. Protection implies comfort; therefore the shoe must fit properly to prevent discomfort to the foot. The 2nd function of the shoe is to provide style. Older children will often sacrifice comfort for style despite parental or medical advice to the contrary.

Support to the foot and ankle is not a function of the shoe except when a pathological condition is present. Athletes in all sports that place the feet and ankles under severe strain wear low shoes that have soft uppers. Ski boots are worn not to support the foot and ankle but to make them *one with the ski,* to ensure response to movements originating in the knee and lower leg. Babies and toddlers usually wear ankle-high shoes, not to provide support to the foot and ankle but to make removing the shoes more difficult for the child.

Style is the only reason for a baby to wear shoes at all until the child begins walking outdoors or is taken out in cold weather. Some babies may gain a certain degree of stability from hard-sole shoes when beginning to stand, but this circumstance has not been shown to enhance learning to walk. In fact, shoes that are rigid prevent foot motion and may diminish the development of the intrinsic musculature of the feet. Properly fitting shoes that have flexible, smooth soles and soft uppers should be recommended initially and subsequently. They need not be expensive. Toddlers can go barefoot in a protected environment, such as indoors. Sneakers are perfectly adequate for summer wear and for winter indoor wear for older children, but toddlers may stumble in sneakers, which can stick to the floor during the stance and step-off phases of the toe-to-heel gait that typifies this age group.[1,2]

Fitting Shoes

Determining the proper fitting of shoes involves no great science. Given that the foot widens while standing and through the day, these measurements should be made later in the day, with the child standing, and should apply only to the time the shoes are newly acquired. Both feet should be measured, given that one foot is often larger than the other, and the shoes should be fitted to the larger foot. The counter should hug the heel snugly; the length should allow a fingerbreadth (1/2 inch) between the tip of the great toe and the toe box. (Box 183-2 describes the parts of the shoe.) The foot should fit snugly into the widest part of the shoe; but the width should not crowd the ball of the foot and should allow the toes to extend without wrinkling the upper. While still in the store, parents should have the child walk in the shoes to ensure comfort. The shoes should not be expected to stretch to fit. If shoes do not fit, then they should not be purchased. Shoes in good condition can be handed down from one child to another.

The frequency with which shoes should be changed depends on the rate of growth of the feet, the quality of the shoes, and the degree of their use. Parents are

BOX 183-2 Anatomy of the Shoe

Last: the wooden or metal form on which a shoe is constructed. Shoes for regular use are built on a straight last; shoes designed to deviate the forefoot outward are built on an out-flare last; those designed to deviate the forefoot inward are built on an in-flare last. Actually, most shoes sold for general use in the United States have an adducted forefoot last rather than a truly straight last.

Sole: the part of the shoe that covers the ventral surface of the foot. It consists of the outsole, usually made of firm leather, rubber, or synthetic material that comes in contact with the surface on which the shoe is placed and the insole, made of soft leather or synthetic material that comes in contact with the plantar surface of the foot.

Heel: elevates the rear portion of the shoe. It is also made of leather, rubber, or synthetic material. It is usually absent in the shoes of infants and toddlers. The heel may be low and flat (common sense), somewhat higher (military), or more elevated and tapered (Cuban or high). The Thomas heel is of medium height and has a forward medial extension.

Shank: the part of the sole between the forward most edge of the heel and ball of the foot. A narrow flat piece of steel is sometimes placed between the inner and outer soles to prevent flexion of the shank of the shoe.

Counter: firm material placed above the heel between the outsole and insole and provides a shelf for the rear portion of the foot. It may be extended forward on the medial aspect of the shoe to provide added support to the instep.

Upper: the top of the shoe. It may be made of leather or a variety of other materials. The upper of low shoes (Oxfords) rises to a point below the malleoli; the upper of high shoes extends above the malleoli.

Toe box: the front end of the upper that accommodates the toes. It is often made of a firm material to also protect the toes.

Welt (or *vamp*)*:* the part of the upper attached to the sole.

usually able to tell when shoes become too small (or rather, feet become too large) without professional advice. The toes will be felt to press against the toe box, and getting the shoes on or having the child keep them on will be increasingly difficult.

Lightweight cotton, nylon, or wool socks that adjust to the length and width of the foot present no problem in the attainment of maximal foot comfort for children of all ages.

CLINICAL CONDITIONS

Physicians who provide primary care for children from birth through adolescence encounter a variety of positional deformities of the legs and feet. The distinction between a pathological and functional cause must be made. The former should be referred to an orthopedist for treatment. When a pathological deformity of the legs or feet is diagnosed, the physician should look for other congenital anomalies, especially those involving the skeletal system.

The lower extremity rotates medially during the 7th fetal week, bringing the great toe to midline. With growth, femoral anteversion gradually declines from 30 degrees at birth to 10 degrees at maturity, leading to lateral rotation of the lower extremity during growth (Figure 183-1). Most functional deformities of the legs and feet are self-correcting in time, through this normal developmental progression of the lower extremity, even without treatment. This characteristic must be considered in weighing the results of any treatment prescribed. Studies of functional deformities, analyzing treated versus untreated paired control patients, have demonstrated the relative ineffectiveness of various treatments for these conditions, when analyzing treated versus untreated paired control patients. Therefore most clinicians choose to observe these conditions while children grow out of them.[3-5]

Toe Deformities in Children

Hallux Valgus

Hallux valgus is a common problem. In a child with hallux valgus (Figure 183-2), the great toe is deviated laterally to overlap the second toe, and the first metatarsal bone is deviated medially, causing a prominence to form on the medial aspect of the metatarsophalangeal (MTP) joint. A bursa forms over the area as a result of the constant irritation and inflammation, forming a painful *bunion*. Some degree of foot pronation (flat feet) associated with the condition may be found.

Many factors come into play to cause the problem, including foot structure, which may or may not be hereditary, and use of narrow stylized shoes that crimp the toes. Most cases of hallux valgus are mild and asymptomatic and do not need treatment. Patients should be counseled in wearing shoes with plenty of toe room and no heels. If flatfoot is present, then a shoe insert to correct the foot pronation may help prevent progression of the disease. In the more severe cases, surgical correction may be needed.

Hammertoe

Hammertoe occurs at the proximal interphalangeal joint (PIP) (see Figure 183-2). In an infant, hammertoe is usually hereditary; in the older child, it usually results from faulty shoe wear. Most cases of hammertoe are mild, cause no pain, and can be left alone. Parents should make sure that the child has roomy shoes that allow the toes to stretch. In the more severe cases, at an older age, surgical correction may be needed.

Mallet Toe

Mallet toe occurs at the distal interphalangeal joint (DIP) (see Figure 183-2). Most cases of mallet toe are mild and need no treatment. When a corn develops over the deformity, shaving and padding will help. In the more severe cases, surgical correction can be performed.

Claw Toe

Claw toe involves all joints of the toe—hyperextension of the MTP joints and flexion at both the PIP and DIP

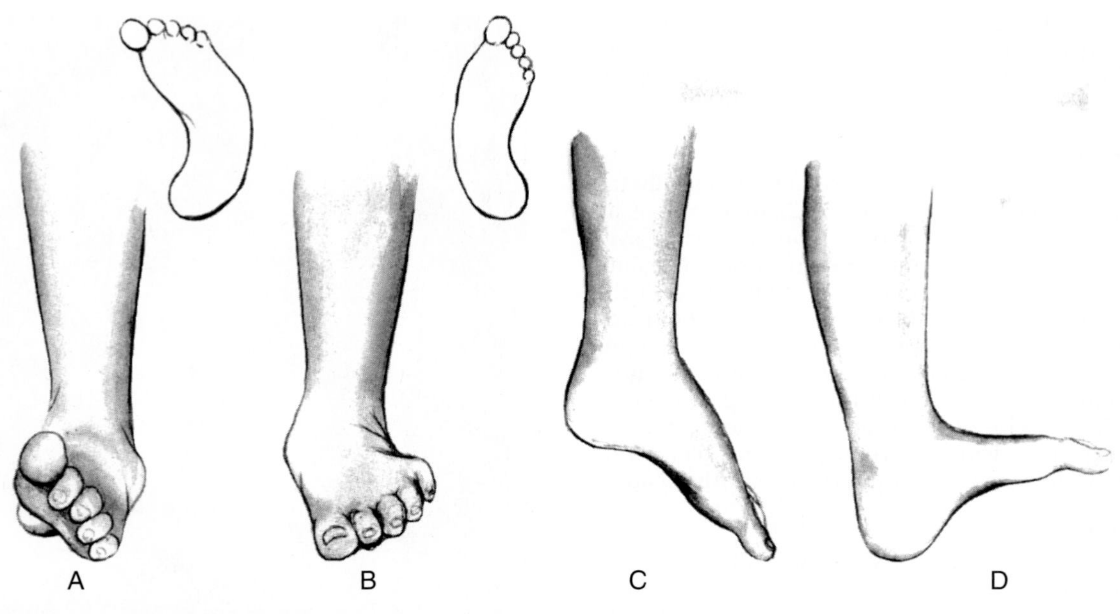

Figure 183-1 Positional deformities of the foot and ankle. **A**, Varus. **B**, Valgus. **C**, Equinus. **D**, Calcaneus. *(Tachdjian MO.* Pediatric Orthopaedics. *Philadelphia, PA: WB Saunders; 1977. Copyright © 1977, Elsevier, with permission.)*

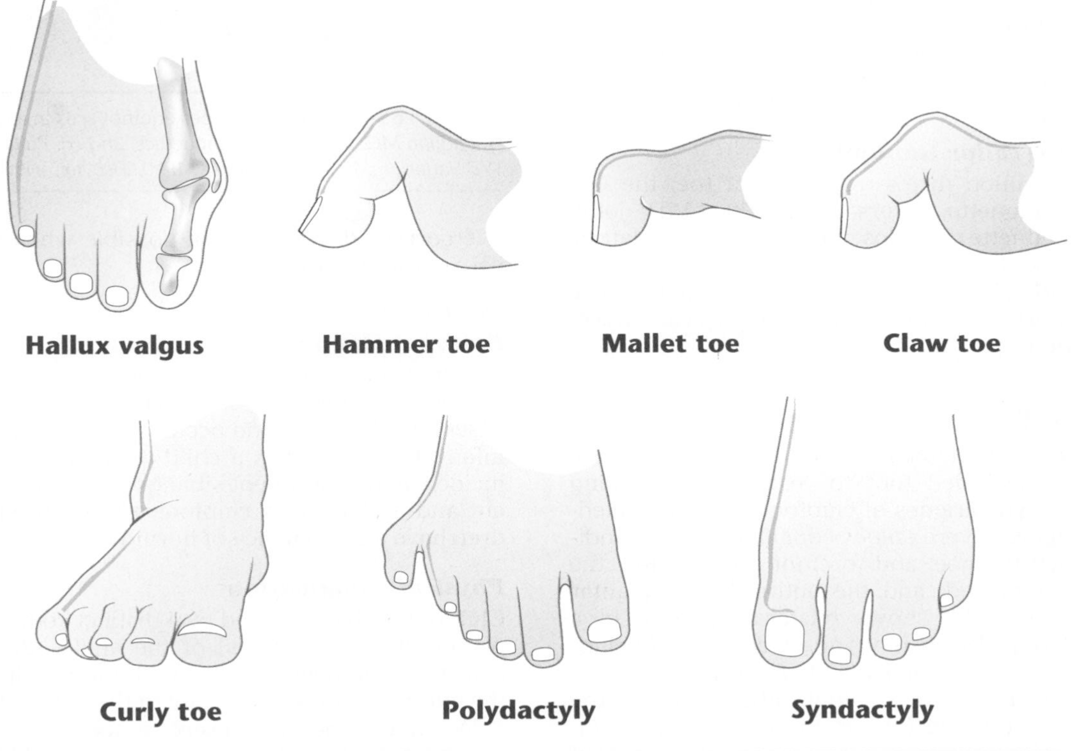

Figure 183-2 Common toe anomalies.

joints (see Figure 183-2). Claw toe is a rare condition but usually occurs in conjunction with a cavus foot, present in neuromuscular diseases such as Charcot-Marie-Tooth disease or myelomeningocele.

Curly Toe

In a child with a curly toe 4th or 5th toe is usually flexed downward and twisted underneath the adjacent toe (see Figure 183-2). Curly toe is quite common in infancy and childhood. If curly toe does not cause symptoms, then no treatment is needed; if the condition is severe and causes irritation with shoe wear, then surgical transfer of the toe flexor may correct the problem.

Polydactyly

Polydactyly, the presence of an extra digit, usually the great toe or 5th toe (see Figure 183-2), may exist as an isolated finding or as part of a more extensive syndrome of congenital anomalies (5% of cases). The family history of the same anomaly is often found. If the extra toe is not causing problems with walking and shoe wear, then no treatment is needed. Vestigial digits can be ablated by suture ligation. If the duplication occurs in the little or big toe and sticks out prominently, then difficulty with shoe wear is common. In these cases, surgical excision will remove the problem. Surgery is typically performed after 9 to 12 months of age.

Syndactyly

Syndactyly, the presence of webbed digits (toes) (see Figure 183-2), may also exist as an isolated finding or as part of a more extensive syndrome of congenital anomalies (5% of cases). A family history of the same anomaly is often found. Syndactyly is quite common and rarely causes problems. The interconnection between two or more toes can vary from thin skin to a bony attachment (synostosis) between parts of the phalanges. Unlike in the fingers, in which surgical separation is needed to obtain finer hand functions, syndactyly in the toes does not need treatment. The growth differential between the involved toes tends not to be significant.

Bunionette (Tailor Bunion)

Whereas a bunion forms on the great toe, the less common bunionette occurs at the fifth MTP joint. When a bunionette develops, the bursa over the lateral aspect of the fifth MTP joint gets prominent and inflamed and painful. If padding does not help relieve the discomfort of a bunionette, then surgical correction is needed.

CLUBFOOT

Clubfoot is a pathological deformity that causes the leg and its appended foot to resemble a clubbing instrument. Two varieties of clubfoot have been identified. The more severe *talipes equinovarus* is a condition in which the heel and forefoot are inverted, the forefoot is adducted, and the entire foot is plantar flexed. Figure 183-3 shows bilateral clubfoot in a newborn; Figure 183-4 shows an untreated right clubfoot. *Talipes calcaneovalgus* is characterized by eversion of the heel and forefoot, abduction of the forefoot, and dorsiflexion of the entire foot (Figure 183-5). Both forms occur in approximately 1 of every 200 live births, are bilateral in 50% of the cases, and affect boys almost twice as frequently as girls.

In the newborn period, functional deformities of the feet secondary to in utero positioning will often mimic both varieties of clubfoot. These functional deformities can be differentiated readily from clubfoot based on flexibility of the foot. The functionally deformed foot can be brought easily to a neutral position and even overcorrected, which is not possible when pathological deformities are present.

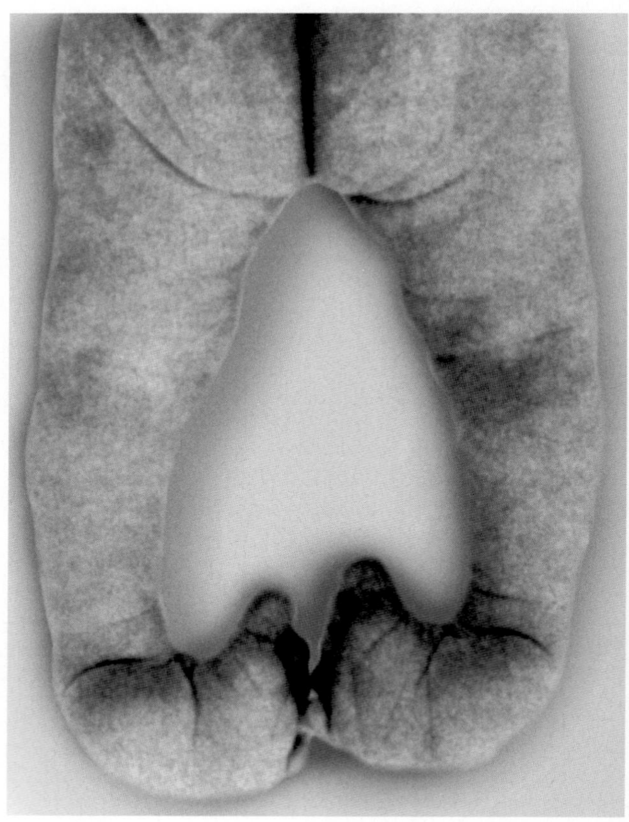

Figure 183-3 Bilateral talipes equinovarus in a newborn. *(Tachdjian MO.* Pediatric Orthopaedics. *2nd ed. Philadelphia, PA: WB Saunders; 1990. Copyright © 1990, Elsevier, with permission.)*

Evaluation

Relevant History

Although many theories have been offered about the etiology of clubfoot, none has been proved. Most cases are idiopathic and occur in an otherwise-normal infant. If a family has a child with clubfoot, then the incidence in subsequent siblings is 3% to 4%. If 1 parent and a child have clubfoot, then subsequent children have a 25% chance of having clubfoot.

Physical Examination

Clubfoot is characterized by 4 distinct components: (1) plantar flexion (equinus) of the ankle, (2) adduction (varus) of the heel (hindfoot), (3) high arch (cavus) at the midfoot, and (4) adduction of the forefoot.

When clubfoot is present, associated neurologic, muscular, or other skeletal anomalies should be sought. Neuromuscular clubfoot is a deformity associated with disorders such as arthrogryposis, meningomyelocele, and congenital constriction band syndrome.

Imaging

Radiographic examination is required at the time of diagnosis and periodically during treatment to delineate the pathological finding and to guide management.

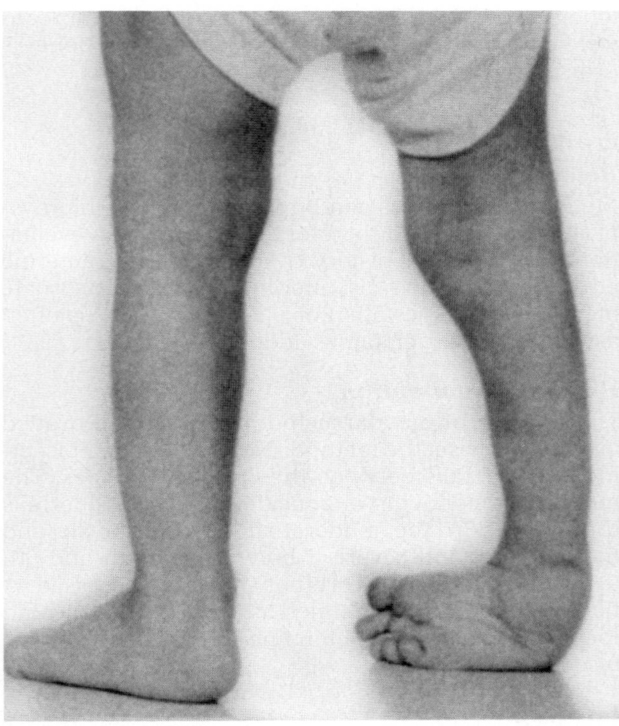

Figure 183-4 Untreated talipes equinovarus in a 3-year-old child. *(Tachdjian MO.* Pediatric Orthopaedics. *2nd ed. Philadelphia, PA: WB Saunders; 1990. Copyright © 1990, Elsevier, with permission.)*

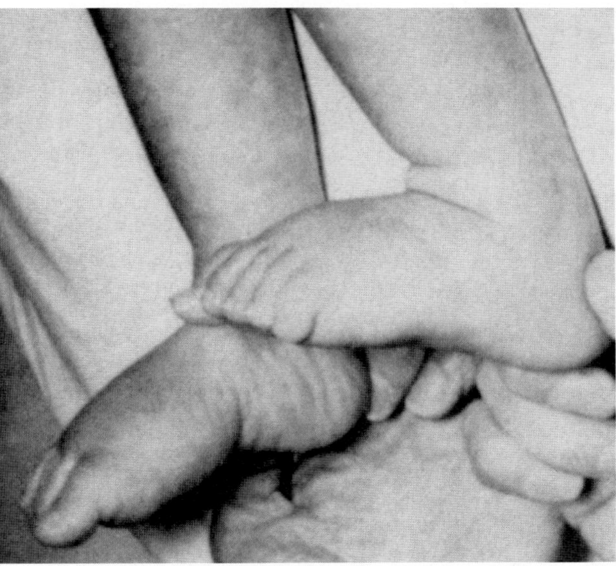

Figure 183-5 Bilateral talipes calcaneovalgus. The left foot is held dorsiflexed and the right plantar flexed to show the range of ankle movement. *(Sharrard WJW.* Paediatric Orthopaedics and Fractures. *2nd ed. Oxford, NY: Blackwell Scientific; 1979. Reprinted by permission of Blackwell Publishing Ltd.)*

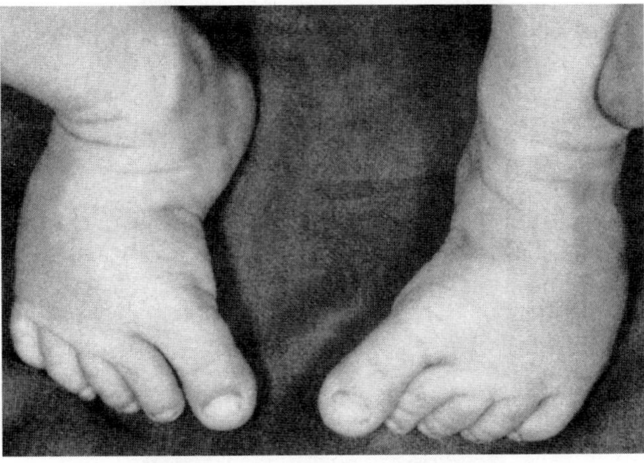

Figure 183-6 Bilateral talipes varus. The entire foot is twisted inward on its longitudinal axis, and the forefoot is adducted. *(Tachdjian MO.* Pediatric Orthopaedics. *2nd ed. Philadelphia, PA: WB Saunders; 1990. Copyright © 1990, Elsevier, with permission.)*

Management

Treatment is with casting immediately on initial diagnosis; 2 to 4 months of manipulation and casting is usually required for correction. Recurrence is common after correction by manipulation alone; therefore prolonged casting is usually required. Recurrence after casting is most common within the first 2 to 3 years but may still happen up to age 5 to 7 years. Surgical correction (tenotomies, muscle transplants, and arthrodeses) may be required in severe cases, when conservative management fails or as a result of recurrence when the child is older. Recurrence is much less likely after surgical correction. Even with successful treatment the affected foot will be smaller and less mobile than a normal foot. Early initiation of therapy will increase the success rate of manipulative or conservative management and will therefore decrease the need for surgical intervention. Functional deformities are self-correcting and require no treatment.

DEFORMITIES OF THE FOREFOOT

Definition of Terms

Much confusion surrounds the incidence and management of deformities of the forefoot because 3 different deformities are characterized by adduction of the forefoot: *talipes varus* (Figure 183-6), in which the entire foot is inverted and the forefoot is adducted; *metatarsus varus* (Figure 183-7), in which the forefoot is inverted and adducted while the hind foot and heel are in the normal position; and *metatarsus adductus* (Figure 183-8), in which the only finding is adduction of the metatarsals at the tarsometatarsal joints. The combined incidence of these 3 forefoot adductive deformities is in the neighborhood of 1 per 100 live births (the most frequent musculoskeletal congenital malformation), with metatarsus adductus being the most common and talipes varus the least common.

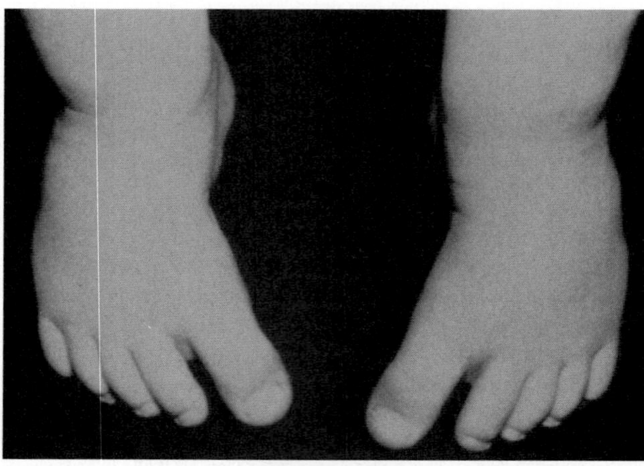

Figure 183-7 Bilateral metatarsus varus. The forefoot is inverted and adducted, the great toe is widely separated from the second toe, and the lateral border of the foot is convex. The hindfoot is in a neutral position. *(Sharrard WJW.* Paediatric Orthopaedics and Fractures. *2nd ed. Oxford, NY: Blackwell Scientific; 1979. Reprinted by permission of Blackwell Publishing Ltd.)*

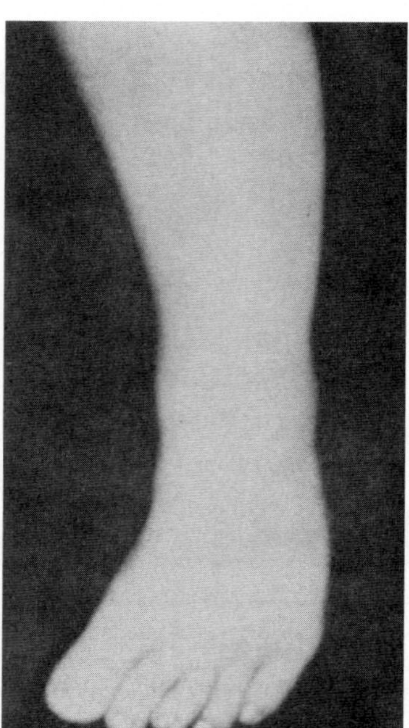

Figure 183-8 Metatarsus adductus. The forefoot is adducted but not inverted. *(Ferguson AB.* Orthopedic Surgery in Infancy and Childhood. *4th ed. Baltimore, MD: Williams & Wilkins; 1981. Reprinted by permission of Lippincott Williams & Wilkins.)*

Talipes varus and metatarsus varus have been considered lesser degrees of clubfoot and are fixed deformities of the foot that require early treatment. The medial border of the foot is concave, with a widening of the space between the 1st and 2nd toes and a high medial longitudinal arch. The lateral border of the foot is convex, and the base of the 5th metatarsal bone is prominent.

Evaluation

Relevant History

Metatarsus adductus can be associated with hip dysplasia (2% of cases); therefore a thorough hip evaluation is essential. A history of a crowded intrauterine environment, such as uterine fibroids, bicornate uterus, multiple gestation or oligohydramnios is often associated with metatarsus adductus.

Physical Examination

The severity of metatarsus adductus may be graded by the heel bisector method. Normally, a line bisecting the heel falls between the 2nd and 3rd toes. The metatarsus adductus is considered mild if line falls through the 3rd toe, moderate if between the 3rd and the 4th toes, and severe if between the 4th and 5th toes. Flexibility of the forefoot should be assessed. A flexible foot might be defined as one in which the 2nd toe can be easily brought in line with or past the heel bisector.

Imaging

In babies with limited flexibility of the forefoot, radiographic examination is necessary to rule out talipes varus and metatarsus varus.

When evaluating metatarsus adductus in the primary care physician's office, placing the child in a standing position on a copy machine and taking a photocopy of the soles of the feet is an easy way to assess the heel bisector position. Although it is somewhat subjective, this low-cost, no-risk method allows for tracking of the progression or improvement of the condition over time.

Management

Metatarsus adductus is a functional deformity and requires no treatment because it corrects spontaneously, usually during the first year. Talipes varus and metatarsus varus are fixed deformities of the foot that require early treatment. Treatment consists of serial casting, long-leg splints that abduct the forefoot, or both. Abduction stretching exercises and out-flare last shoes may be used as an adjunct to cast treatment but should not be relied on as the only therapy. Primary care physicians see metatarsus adductus frequently and observe its resolution without treatment, whereas orthopedists are more likely to see talipes varus and metatarsus varus through referrals, sometimes unfortunately in late infancy when treatment results are less satisfactory.

PRONATION

Pronation is an outward rolling of the foot with eversion of the heel and eversion and abduction of the forefoot. *Flexible foot, relaxed foot, fatfoot,* and *flatfoot (pes planus)* are other terms used to describe this condition, leading to considerable confusion.

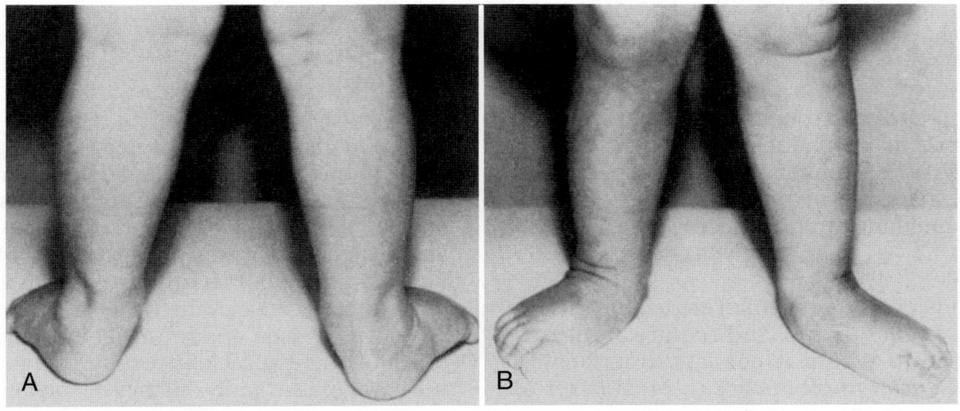

Figure 183-9 Pronation. **A**, Viewed from behind, the hindfoot is everted. **B**, Viewed from in front, the forefoot is everted and abducted. *(Sharrard WJW.* Paediatric Orthopaedics and Factures, *2nd ed. Oxford, NY: Blackwell Scientific; 1979. Reprinted by permission of Blackwell Publishing Ltd.)*

Differential Diagnosis

Certain congenital anomalies involving the bones of the foot produce flattening of the medial longitudinal arch and eversion of the forefoot *(planovalgus)*. These anomalies include *vertical talus, accessory tarsonavicular,* and fusion of one or more of the tarsal bones *(tarsal coalition)*.

Accessory tarsonavicular is a normal anatomic variant. A secondary center of ossification forms in the medial portion of the tarsonavicular at the attachment of the posterior tibialis tendon. This ossification becomes more prominent and symptomatic during adolescence, either from its size or from repetitive sprains of the fibrous attachment of the ossicle to the navicular. Tarsal conditions are not usually detected until late childhood or adolescence, when they produce pain with walking and inability to invert the foot. Two types of tarsal coalitions have been identified: (1) *calcaneonavicular coalition,* which involves the calcaneus and the navicular bones; and (2) *talocalcaneal coalition,* in which the calcaneus is coalesced to the talus.

Evaluation

Relevant History

Almost all children develop some degree of pronation during the early stages of weight bearing. Most infants have flexible flatfeet. Typically, the condition is transient, resolving with normal growth and development in 97% of children, usually before 2½ years of age. A family history may be found in children with flat foot that persists beyond the usual time of physiological resolution.

Symptoms, including aching of the feet and legs, muscle cramps in the calves at night, easy fatigability, and reluctance to participate in strenuous activity, are uncommon but may occur. Symptoms result from the strain caused by the child's continual attempt to shift weight bearing laterally toward the center of the foot, bringing about some degree of toeing-in. Persistent pronation without symptoms occurs in some children who may have a family history of pronation and often demonstrates ligamentous laxity or hyperextensibility of other joints, including the knees, elbows, wrists, and thumbs.

The incidence of pes planovalgus is unknown. Vertical talus is very rare. Accessory tarsonavicular is fairly common; 14% of adolescents experience symptoms according to 1 study. Tarsal coalitions are bilateral in 50% of patients, probably occur in 1% of the population, and are usually hereditary. They may be found in other family members who are asymptomatic but have no hindfoot motion.[6]

Physical Examination

The Achilles tendon is seen to curve inward, and the medial longitudinal arch of the foot, observed without weight bearing, disappears on standing. These changes occur because a wide-based stance is assumed for balance (accentuated by bulky diapers), causing the weight to be borne on the medial aspect of the feet (Figure 183-9). Laxity of the ligaments supporting the feet contributes to pronation. When symptoms do occur, the clinician should look for associated conditions, such as obesity, neuromuscular disorders, and structural abnormalities above the level of the ankle.

Vertical talus and accessory tarsonavicular can usually be detected in the newborn by the presence of a bony prominence on the medial and plantar aspects of the foot, with limitation of plantar flexion and inversion of the forefoot.

Tarsal coalitions are not usually detected until late childhood or adolescence, when the initially fibrous or cartilaginous bar connecting the hindfoot bones becomes ossified, producing pain with walking and an inability to invert the foot. The foot is held in a pronated position with eversion of the forefoot. The peroneal tendons stand out prominently when attempts are made to invert the foot. Calcaneonavicular coalition tends to develop between 9 and 13 years of age, whereas talocalcaneal coalition develops later, typically 13 to 16 years of age. The foot is held in a pronated position, with eversion of the forefoot. This condition, commonly called *spastic flatfoot*, is not related etiologically to simple pronation.

Imaging

Flexible flatfoot (pes planus) does not require any imaging in most cases. If pronation is persistent beyond 2½ years of age, if symptoms are present, if flexibility is limited, or if a suspicion of planovalgus exists, then radiographic examination may be necessary.

Management

Pronation is transient in most children, usually disappears before 2½ years of age, and requires no treatment. In children in whom it persists, treatment is not necessary unless symptoms occur. Most cases of physiologic, flexible pes planus only require parental reassurance.

When symptoms do occur, they may be alleviated by use of corrective shoes that have a long medial counter and a Thomas heel. Support to the medial longitudinal arch with a flexible felt, rubber, or leather pad placed beneath the inner sole may help. Wedges that are ⅛- to 3/16-inch thick applied to the medial aspect of the heel and the lateral aspect of the sole of the shoe are sometimes helpful. Steel arch supports placed within the shoe rarely are required. If neuromuscular disorders (eg, tight heel cords) are present, then heel cord–stretching exercises may be beneficial in reducing discomfort.

Treatment in most cases of pes planovalgus is symptomatic with orthopedic shoes. Surgical correction is required only for accessory tarsonavicular or tarsal coalition if symptoms cannot be relieved through conservative means (only approximately 10% of cases) and is usually performed in adulthood. Vertical talus usually requires surgical correction early in infancy.[7]

PES CAVUS

Pes cavus (cavus foot deformity) is an equinus deformity of the forefoot relative to the hindfoot, producing a high medial longitudinal arch (Figure 183-10). It is referred to as *clawfoot* when associated with flexion deformities of the toes.

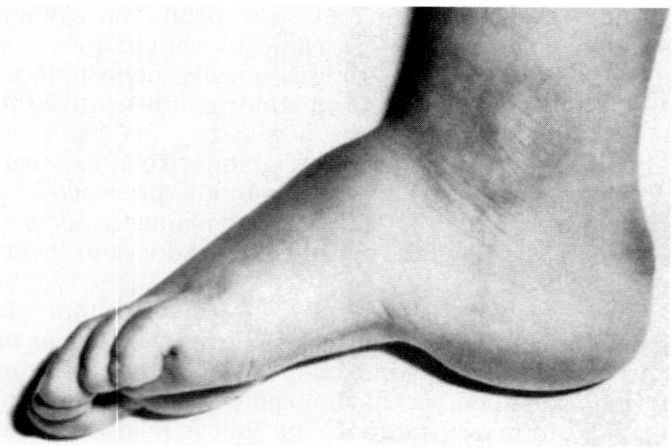

Figure 183-10 Pes cavus, viewed from the outer side. The height of the medial and lateral longitudinal arch is abnormal. *(Sharrard WJW.* Paediatric Orthopaedics and Fractures. *2nd ed. Oxford, NY: Blackwell Scientific; 1979. Reprinted by permission of Blackwell Publishing Ltd.)*

Evaluation

Pertinent History

Pes cavus is seen in muscular dystrophy, peripheral neuropathies, and disease of the spinal cord, brainstem, and cerebral cortex. Cerebral palsy, meningomyelocele, poliomyelitis, Charcot-Marie-Tooth disease, and Friedreich ataxia are examples of conditions of neurologic origin that produce pes cavus as a late manifestation. Because of the variety of conditions in which pes cavus is seen and its variability as a manifestation of some of these, incidence in the general population is not known. A family history of pes cavus should be sought because many of the conditions producing this deformity are inherited.[8]

Physical Examination

The primary pathological condition is neuromuscular rather than bony, with weakness or paralysis of the intrinsic muscles of the foot and its dorsiflexors, leading to the deformity over time. Pes cavus is therefore not seen at birth and usually does not develop clinically until late childhood or adulthood, depending on the underlying neuromuscular disease. A high-arched foot characterizes the deformity. Pes cavus takes one of two forms: (1) *cavovarus,* in which the calcaneus is inverted with tightness of the heel cord; and (2) *calcaneocavus,* in which a high arch with normal heel alignment is present, usually from weakness of the calf muscles resulting in increased ankle dorsiflexion and increased plantar flexion of the forefoot.

Imaging

Radiographic examination may be necessary, especially if surgical management is under consideration.

Management

Early treatment includes exercises designed to strengthen the affected muscles and application of metatarsal pads to the innersoles of the shoes or metatarsal bars to the outer soles. Surgical correction of the fixed deformities, including plantar fasciotomy, tendon transplants, osteotomies, and arthrodeses, may be required later.

TOE-WALKING

Walking on the toes or the ball of the foot is a variation of normal gait for many children between 10 to 18 months of age as they begin to walk. This variation usually progresses to a toe-heel gait and eventually to the normal heel-toe gait pattern within 3 to 6 months.[9]

Differential Diagnosis

Some children, when asked to walk normally, can simply put their heel down on the ground before their toes. However, as soon as no one is observing them, they revert to toe-walking because it is habitual *(idiopathic toe-walking)*. Cerebral palsy is commonly associated with toe-walking that persists beyond 2 years of age. A *congenitally short tendocalcaneus* causes persistent toe-walking even though the child can toe-heel and heel-toe walk. These latter gaits are awkward and are less comfortable for children until 6 to 8 years of age, when their toe-walking disappears.

Evaluation

Pertinent History

Children with idiopathic or habitual toe-walking have a history of normal development. A family history of persistent toe-walking may be found. As with pes cavus, certain rare muscular, peripheral, spinal, and central neurologic diseases should be ruled out when toe-walking persists beyond 2 years of age.

Physical Examination

Children with idiopathic or habitual toe-walking have a normal examination. A thorough neurologic examination is required to rule out cerebral palsy or other associated neuromusculature system disorders.

Imaging

Radiographic examination is not indicated in most cases of toe-walking. Neuroimaging is necessary if the toe-walking is acquired (develops after a period of normal gait) to rule out intracranial lesions.

Management

The only treatment required for either idiopathic or habitual toe-walking is reassurance.

However, in the child who continues to toe-walk beyond 2 years of age, a dorsiflexion-assist ankle-foot orthosis may be of benefit.[9-11]

BOWED LEGS AND KNOCK-KNEES

Genu varum (bowed legs) is an angular deformity at the knee with the tibia adducted *(varus)* in relation to the femur. *Genu valgum (knock-knees)* is characterized by alignment of the knee with the tibia abducted (valgus) in relation to the femur.

Differential Diagnosis

Genu varum (bowed legs), when extreme or unilateral, may result from a variety of underlying conditions: rickets, dyschondroplasia, osteogenesis imperfecta, osteochondritis, Blount disease (tibia vara), or injury to the medial proximal epiphysis of the tibia. Extreme degrees of physiologic bowing of the legs may occur in the young child and resolve over time without treatment (Figure 183-11).

Genu valgum (knock-knees) is often associated with pronation and is more apt to be marked in the child who is overweight. The degrees of knock-knee can be gauged by measuring the distance between the medial malleoli when the child is standing with the knees approximated (Figure 183-12). Injury to the lateral proximal tibial epiphysis can cause unilateral genu valgum (Figure 183-13). As with extreme bowing, underlying generalized diseases of the bone can cause marked bilateral genu valgum.

Evaluation

Pertinent History

A history of uterine crowding during fetal development can be associated with extreme cases of genu varum or genu valgum. Prior trauma or a variety of endocrine, metabolic, or bone abnormalities may result in pathological degrees of bowing or knock-knees.

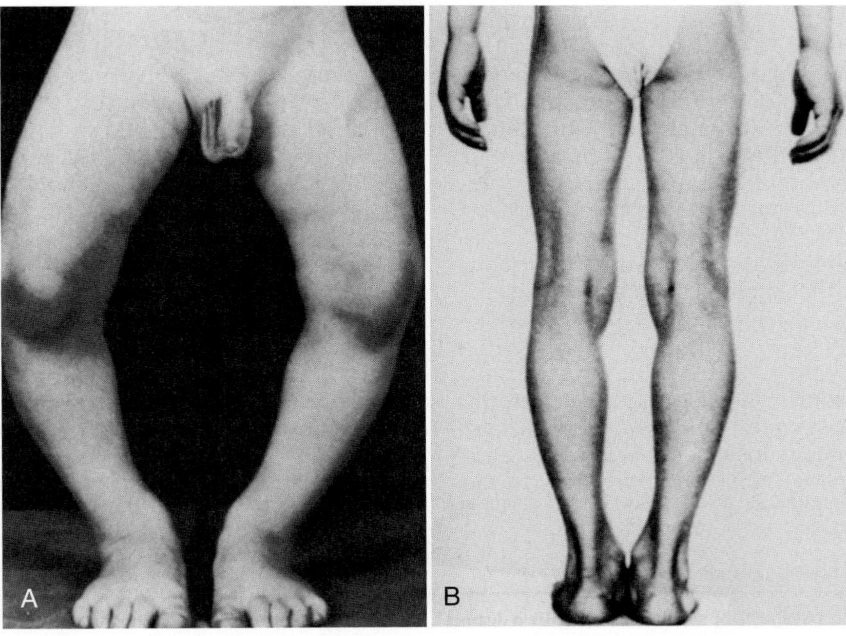

Figure 183-11 **A,** Extreme physiological bowing of the legs at age 18 months. **B,** Spontaneous resolution over time (age 7 years). *(Sharrard WJW.* Paediatric Orthopaedics and Fractures. *Oxford, NY: Blackwell Scientific; 1971. Reprinted by permission of Blackwell Publishing Ltd.)*

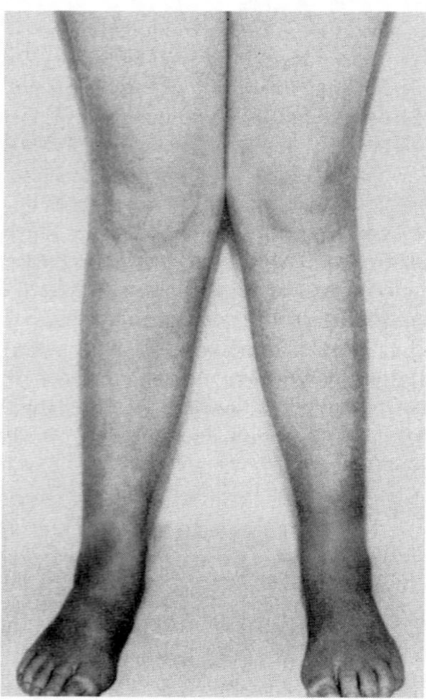

Figure 183-12 Marked degree of physiological genu valgum. At age 11 years the distance between the medial malleoli measured 4 inches. *(Sharrard WJW.* Paediatric Orthopaedics and Fractures. *2nd ed. Oxford, NY: Blackwell Scientific; 1979. Reprinted by permission of Blackwell Publishing Ltd.)*

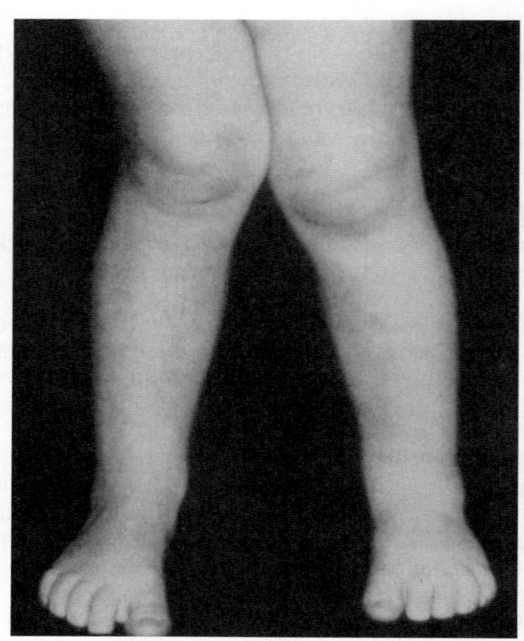

Figure 183-13 Unilateral genu valgum caused by previous injury to the lateral aspect of the right proximal tibial epiphysis. *(Sharrard WJW.* Paediatric Orthopaedics and Fractures. *2nd ed. Oxford, NY: Blackwell Scientific; 1979. Reprinted by permission of Blackwell Publishing Ltd.)*

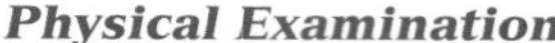

Physical Examination

From birth until 18 months of age, a distinct physiological bowing of the lower extremities of 10 to 15 degrees is normal. Bowing is followed by a transitional period over the next year or so, during which continued growth results in a knock-knee pattern of 10 to 15 degrees, which assumes prominence by age 3 to 4 years. Knock-knee persists until later childhood or early adolescence when a balancing and straightening occur spontaneously. Physicians must be aware of this normal developmental pattern to avoid unnecessary treatment of mild to moderate degrees of bowed legs and knock-knees. However, marked degrees of these conditions require investigation to rule out underlying disease that can result in permanent deformity.

Imaging

Genu varum (bowed legs), when extreme or unilateral, requires radiographic examination to exclude rickets, dyschondroplasia, osteogenesis imperfecta, osteochondritis, Blount disease (tibia vara), or injury to the medial proximal epiphysis of the tibia.

Management

Simple observation and reassurance are all that are required for physiological genu varum and genu valgum, given that these conditions spontaneously correct 99% of the time. When identified, underlying etiologies of extreme varus or valgum deformities must be effectively treated to improve angulation. Treatment of severe bowing or knocking of the knees caused by underlying disease is determined by the nature of the condition and may include wedge osteotomy or epiphyseal stapling.

IN-TOEING AND OUT-TOEING

In-toeing (pigeon toe) is a condition in which the foot turns inward more than expected during walking or running relative to the line of progression. *Out-toeing (slew foot)* occurs when the foot turns outward more than expected during walking or running relative to the line of progression.

Differential Diagnosis

Toeing-in and toeing-out are frequently seen at all ages and are caused by a variety of conditions affecting the feet, ankles, legs, knees, and hips. In-toeing is more common than out-toeing and is more likely to be caused by benign conditions. Protective or compensatory shifting of the body weight to the middle or outside of the foot in pronation and knock-knee, both normal developmental stages, is the most common cause of toeing-in and corrects itself in time. Developmental bowing of the legs, also self-correcting, may lead to temporary toeing-in. Talipes equinovarus and metatarsus varus are associated with toeing-in. Spasticity of the internal rotator muscles of the hip, as seen in cerebral palsy, produces toeing-in, as does anterior maldirection of the acetabulum.

Toeing-out is seen with calcaneovalgus and pes planovalgus. Flaccid paralysis of the internal rotator muscles of the hip results in toeing-out. Posterior maldirection of the acetabulum produces toeing-out.

The remaining causes of both conditions are related to internal or external torsion of the tibia and femur. In general, with toeing-in, if the child's patellae are noted to be rotated inward *(kissing knees)* while walking, then the underlying problem is above the knee; if they face straight forward, then the underlying problem is below the knee.[12]

Evaluation

Pertinent History

Parents often notice excessive inward or outward toeing-in infants or toddlers. Excessive in-toeing is more common than out-toeing and is more likely to be caused by benign conditions that usually represent variations of normal development from excessive rotations of the femur, the tibia, or both. In children, in-toeing does not usually cause pain or interfere with development or stability of gait. Therefore understanding the natural progression of femoral and tibial torsion, as well as the changes that occur in hip rotation, is essential for primary care physicians to reassure and advise parents about these common conditions.

Finding older family members with histories of these rotational anomalies is not uncommon. In many instances, a history of a parent who was treated as a toddler with an orthotic device for these conditions can even be found.

Physical Examination

Inward rotation of the femur at the femoral neck *(femoral anteversion)* is greatest at birth (approximately 40 degrees) and gradually declines to adult values of 10 to 15 degrees by age 8 years.

The best position in which to assess the rotation of the lower extremities is with the child in the prone position, the hips fully extended, and the knees flexed to 90 degrees. To measure hip rotation, the lower leg is used as a pointer and the legs are rotated through the axis of the hip joint (Figures 183-14 and 183-15). Until 1 or 2 years of age, the clinical measurement of hip rotation is limited by the physiological tightness of the hip joint capsule, therefore underestimating the degree of femoral anteversion. After the age of 18 to 24 months, measurement of hip rotation is a close approximation of bony femoral rotation, averaging 50 degrees of internal rotation and 40 degrees of external rotation.

The easiest way to assess tibial rotation is to measure the thigh-foot angle, the axis of the foot relative to the axis of the thigh (see Figures 183-16 and 183-17). The normal thigh-foot angle ranges from 0 to 30 degrees of external rotation; therefore an internal thigh-foot angle indicates internal tibial torsion. By age 2 years, children typically walk with the foot turned out relative to the line of progression. A thigh-foot angle of 10 to 15 degrees is normal in adults and older children.

Imaging

In-toeing and out-toeing rarely require imaging studies. Evaluation using gait analysis may help in differentiating the cause of the abnormality for individuals with extreme in-toeing or out-toeing.

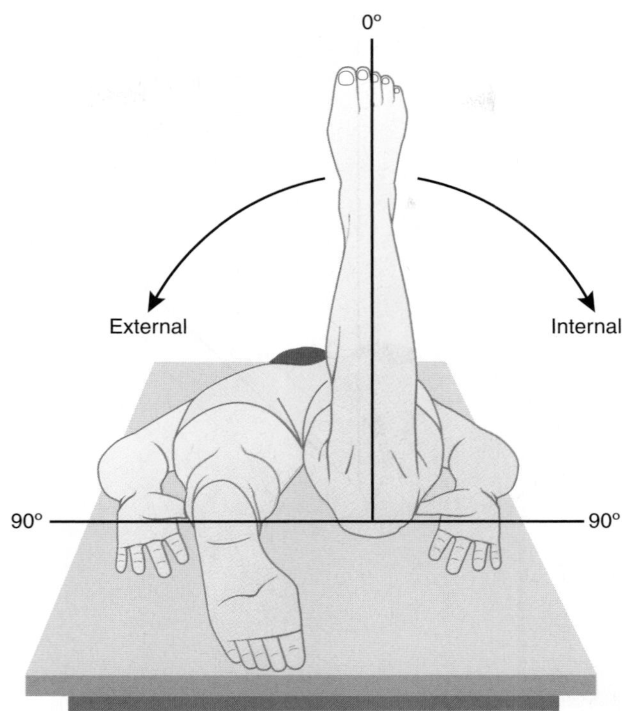

Figure 183-14 Starting position for measuring hip rotation with the hip extended while the child is in the prone position. *(Reprinted with permission from* Joint Motion Method of Measuring and Recording. *Rosemont, IL, American Academy of Orthopedic Surgeons, 1965.)*

Management

Families must be reassured about the natural history of rotational variations in the femur and tibia. Most children will simply outgrow their variant. An orthopedic or neurologic evaluation should be made if a child has severe in-toeing or an unsteady gait (especially while running), causing stumbling as the toes catch on the back of the trailing leg. A referral may also be advised if a child's condition does not follow the expected physiologic progression with growth.[13,14]

POSITIONS LEADING TO IN-TOEING AND OUT-TOEING

Infants and children often assume certain positions during sleep or while sitting for long periods (watching television) that lead to positional deformities of the femur, tibia, or feet.

Sleeping in the prone, knee-chest position with the legs internally rotated may lead to anteversion of the femoral neck, internal tibial torsion, and varus of the forefoot; having the legs externally rotated may lead to valgus of the feet; and having the legs in

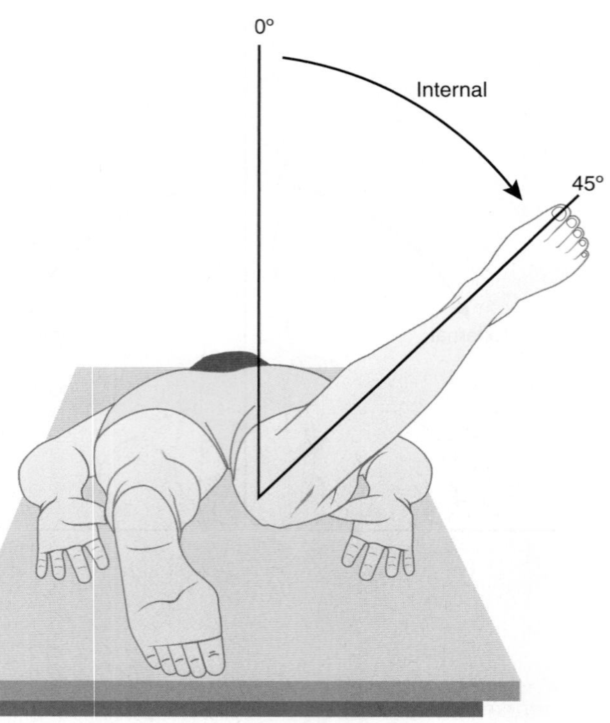

Figure 183-15 Internal rotation. *(Reprinted with permission from* Joint Motion Method of Measuring and Recording. *Rosemont, IL, American Academy of Orthopedic Surgeons, 1965.)*

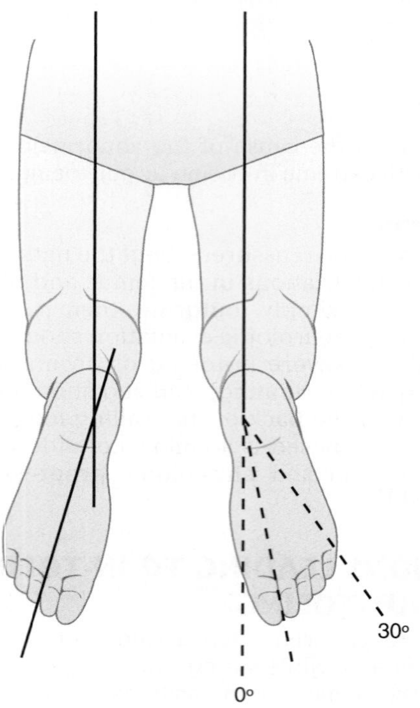

Figure 183-16 Thigh-foot angle: normal range. *(Alexander IJ.* The Foot: Examination and Diagnosis. *New York, NY: Churchill Livingstone; 1990. Copyright © 1990, Elsevier, with permission.)*

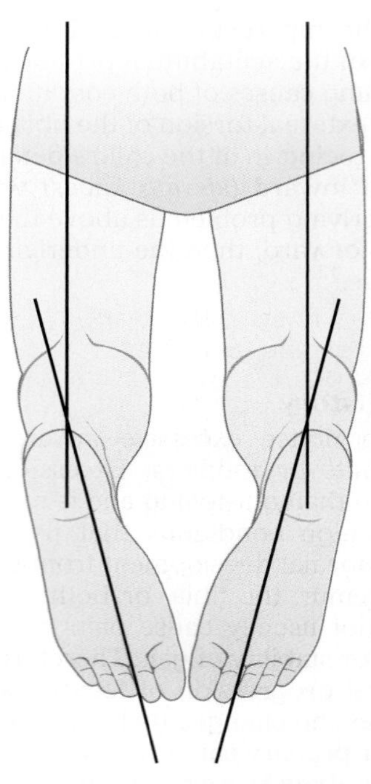

Figure 183-17 Bilateral internal tibial torsion. *(Alexander IJ.* The Foot: Examination and Diagnosis. *New York, NY: Churchill Livingstone; 1990. Copyright © 1990, Elsevier, with permission.)*

a neutral position may lead to equinus of the feet and toe-walking. Sleeping in the prone position with the legs extended and rotated inward may lead to anteversion of the femoral neck, internal tibial torsion, and varus of the forefoot; having them rotated outward may lead to retroversion of the femoral neck and valgus of the feet. Sleeping in the frog-leg position prone or supine may lead to retroversion of the femoral neck and valgus and abduction of the feet.

Sitting in the reversed tailor position with the feet internally rotated may produce anteversion of the femoral neck, internal tibial torsion, and varus of the forefoot; having the feet rotated externally may produce anteversion of the femoral neck and valgus of the feet.

When these sleeping or sitting positions occur in conjunction with the positional deformities listed, and when they raise concern, some effort can be made to change the positional sleeping or sitting habit. Success, however, is not often attained.

Although in-toeing or out-toeing may reflect a variety of underlying orthopedic diseases, no evidence has been found suggesting that in-toeing or out-toeing of developmental origin leads to any functional disabilities if left uncorrected.[15]

INTERNAL TIBIAL TORSION

Tibial torsion is a rotation of the tibia on its longitudinal axis relative to the transverse axes of the knee and ankle joints.

Differential Diagnosis

Pathological degrees of internal and external tibial torsion are found only in association with deformities of the feet, ankles, knees, and hips or as a result of improperly applied casts, braces, or Denis Browne splints.

Evaluation

Pertinent History

The incidence of internal tibial torsion is 12% at birth, gradually diminishing to near 0% at 2 years of age.

During fetal life, the tibia is rotated inward on its longitudinal axis relative to the transverse axes of the knee and ankle joints. At birth, it reaches a neutral position. External tibial torsion develops in most babies shortly after birth and is almost universal by age 2 years, reaching 20 degrees of lateral torsion by the time walking is fully established and 23 degrees by adulthood.

Physical Examination

The degree of internal and external tibial torsion can be determined by observing the relative position of the medial and lateral malleoli while the child is sitting on the edge of a table or chair with legs dangling, the patellae facing forward, and the feet in their relaxed position. The medial malleolus is placed posterior to the lateral malleolus in internal tibial torsion and anterior to it in external torsion.

Imaging

The degree of torsion can be measured exactly either radiographically or with special instruments but is not required in most cases.

Management

Treatment of primary internal tibial torsion is not required in most cases. Occasionally, if a child trips on his or her feet and falls frequently, or if parents are unduly concerned over toeing-in, then passive stretching exercises (externally rotating the foot at the ankle), corrective shoes (Thomas heel, longitudinal arch pad, inner-heel, and outsole wedges), or application of torque heels may be prescribed. Denis Browne splints should not be used without orthopedic consultation because they may create abnormal stress on the hip joint. Derotation osteotomy of the tibia rarely is required and then almost always when tibial torsion is associated with other orthopedic anomalies of the lower extremity. The primary care physician can usually observe children with tibial torsion. A referral is important if the child has extreme rotation, significant asymmetry of the torsion, a sudden proximal tibial deviation, or a condition that does not follow the typical pattern of improvement with growth.

FEMORAL ANTEVERSION

Femoral torsion is the rotation of the proximal portion of the femur on its longitudinal axis in relation to the transverse plane of the knee. *Femoral anteversion* is the extreme twisting of the femoral neck anteriorly relative to the femoral condyles. *Femoral retroversion* is the extreme twisting of the femoral neck posteriorly relative to the femoral condyles.

Evaluation

Pertinent History

In utero and postnatal positioning of the legs and hips produces stresses that bring about these rotational deformities of the femoral neck. The true incidence of anteversion and retroversion is not known, but the former is much more common and occurs twice as frequently in girls as in boys.

Physical Examination

Femoral anteversion produces *kissing knees,* toeing-in, and a clumsy gait. With the patella in neutral position, the greater trochanter of the femur lies posterior to the lateral, longitudinal midthigh line. External rotation is decreased and internal rotation of the hip in extension is increased (normally 35 to 45 degrees for both). External rotation of the hip in flexion is normal, however. The findings in retroversion are the opposite of those found in anteversion of the femoral neck. Imaging is only required in cases of extreme anteversion or retroversion.

Management

A simple measure that can be employed by the primary care physician early on for parental concern over toeing-in is to have the child learn to sit in the tailor, modified lotus, or Indian-style sitting position. The use of Denis Browne splints is contraindicated, and corrective shoes are of no value.

Most femoral torsion deformities correct themselves by 7 years of age. If they do not follow the typical pattern of improvement with growth, then an orthopedist should be consulted because the persistence of these deformities may lead to degenerative arthritis of the hip joint. Referral for evaluation should also be made if a child has extreme rotation, especially when associated with difficulty walking or running, or when significant asymmetry of the anteversion exists. Orthopedic treatment consists of the use of a bivalve lower-trunk and leg cast during sleeping hours or, in rare cases, a derotation osteotomy of the middle or lower femoral shaft.

WHEN TO REFER

Toe anomalies:

- Most toe anomalies are asymptomatic cosmetic defects and do not require referral. Referral to a podiatrist or orthopedist may be indicated if the anomaly leads to pain or uncomfortable shoe wear or ambulation and if these symptoms do not respond to conservative management.

Clubfoot:

- Immediate referral to an orthopedist should be made on diagnosis of clubfoot.

Metatarsus varus:

- Forefoot has limited flexibility.
- Condition appears to be progressing or is not improving with growth.

Pronation:
- Limited flexibility or a suspicion of planovalgus
- Persistence of pronation beyond 2½ years of age
- Symptoms are present that are not relieved through conservative management

Pes cavus:
- All individuals with pes cavus should be referred for evaluation by a neurologist, physiatrist, orthopedist, individually or in collaboration.

Toe-walking:
- Toe-walking that persists beyond 2 years of age
- A child who has an abnormal neurological history or examination

Bowed legs and knock-knees:
- Severe, asymmetric, or unilateral genu varum or genu valgus
- Condition that does not follow the expected physiologic progression with growth

Toeing-in and toeing-out:
- Severe in-toeing
- Unsteady gait (especially while running) that causes stumbling
- Condition that does not follow the expected physiologic progression with growth

Tibial torsion:
- Extreme rotation (especially when associated with difficulty walking or running)
- Significant asymmetry
- Sudden proximal tibial deviation
- Condition that does not follow the typical pattern of improvement with growth

Femoral anteversion:
- Extreme rotation (especially when associated with difficulty walking or running)
- Significant asymmetry of the femoral anteversion
- Condition that does not follow the typical pattern of improvement with growth, by 7 years of age

TOOLS FOR PRACTICE

Engaging Patient and Family

- *Orthopaedic Connections: Shoes* (fact sheet), American Academy of Orthopaedic Surgeons (orthoinfo.aaos.org/topic.cfm?topic=A00143&return_link=0).

Medical Decision Support

- *Cerebral Palsy Program—Cerebral Palsy; a guide for care* (book), Alfred I. DuPont Institute (gait.aidi.udel.edu/res695/homepage/pd_ortho/clinics/c_palsy/cpweb.htm).
- *Diagnosis and Treatment of Pediatric Flatfoot* (guideline), Harris EJ, Vanore JV, Thomas JL, et al (www.guideline.gov/summary/summary.aspx?ss=15&doc_id=6517&nbr=4086).
- *Essentials of Musculoskeletal Care, 3rd edition* (book), American Academy of Orthopaedic Surgeons and American Academy of Pediatrics (www.aap.org/bookstore).
- *Wheeless' Textbook of Orthopaedics* (book), Duke Orthopaedics (www.wheelessonline.com/).

RELATED WEB SITES

- American Academy of Orthopaedic Surgeons (orthoinfo.aaos.org/menus/children.cfm).
- American Orthopaedic Foot and Ankle Society (www.aofas.org/i4a/pages/index.cfm?pageid=1).
- National Library of Medicine and the National Institutes of Health: Medline Plus (medlineplus.gov).
- Orthoseek (www.orthoseek.com).
- Pediatric Orthopaedic Society of North America (www.posna.org).

SUGGESTED RESOURCES

Craig CL, Goldberg MJ. Foot and leg problems. *Pediatr Rev.* 1993;14(10):395-400.

Greene W. *Essentials of Musculoskeletal Care.* 3rd ed. Rosemont, IL: American Academy of Orthopedic Surgeons; 2005.

Herring JA. *Tachdjian's Pediatric Orthopaedics.* 3rd ed. Philadelphia, PA: WB Saunders; 2002.

Staheli LT. *Fundamentals of Pediatric Orthopedics.* 3rd ed. Philadelphia, PA: Lippincott Williams & Wilkins; 2003.

REFERENCES

1. American Academy of Orthopaedic Surgeons (AAOS). Shoes. Available at: orthoinfo.aaos.org/brochure/thr_report.cfm?thread_id=15&topcategory=foot. Accessed August 10, 2007.
2. Bleck EE. The shoeing of children: sham or science? *Dev Med Child Neurol.* 1971;13(2):188-195.
3. Craig CL, Goldberg MJ. Foot and leg problems. *Pediatr Rev.* 1993;14(10):395-400.
4. Sass P, Hassan G. Lower extremity abnormalities in children. *Am Fam Physician.* 2003;68(3):461-468.
5. Scherl SA. Common lower extremity problems in children. *Pediatr Rev.* 2004;25(2):52-62.
6. Pfeiffer M, Kotz R, Ledl T, et al. Prevalence of flat foot in preschool-aged children. *Pediatrics.* 2006;118(2):634-639.
7. Harris EJ, Vanore JV, Thomas JL, et al. Diagnosis and treatment of pediatric flatfoot. *J Foot Ankle Surg.* 2004;43(6):341-373. Available at: www.guideline.gov/summary/summary.aspx?ss=15&doc_id=6517&nbr=4086. Accessed August 10, 2007.
8. Duke Orthopaedics. Pes cavus: Charcot-Marie Tooth. Wheeless' Textbook of Orthopedics. Available at: www.wheelessonline.com/ortho/pes_cavus_charcot_marie_tooth. Accessed August 10, 2007.
9. Sala DA, Shulman LH, Kennedy RF, et al. Idiopathic toe-walking: a review. *Dev Med Child Neurol.* 1999;41(12):846-848.
10. Hirsch G, Wagner B. The natural history of idiopathic toe-walking: a long-term follow-up of fourteen conservatively treated children. *Acta Paediatr.* 2004;93(2):196-199.
11. Tidwell M. The child with the tip-toe gait. *Int Pediatr.* 1999;14(4):235-238.
12. Kling TF, Hensinger RN. Angular and torsional deformities of the lower limbs in children. *Clin Orthop Relat Res.* 1983;176:136-147.
13. Dietz FR. Most torsional variations of tibia, femur resolve spontaneously. *AAP News.* 2000;16(1):35.
14. Heinrich SD, Sharp CH. Lower extremity torsional deformities in children: a prospective comparison of two treatment modalities. *Orthopedics.* 1991;14(6):655-659.
15. Staheli LT, Corbett M, Wyss C, et al. Lower-extremity rotational problems in children. Normal values to guide management. *J Bone Joint Surg.* 1985;67(1):39-47.

Chapter 184

GASTROINTESTINAL HEMORRHAGE

Jeffrey R. Avner, MD

Most causes of gastrointestinal (GI) bleeding in children, unlike in adults, are relatively benign and involve small amounts of blood loss. Although rare, some GI lesions may cause severe bleeding and lead to life-threatening conditions. In addition, GI bleeding may be a symptom of systemic illness or serious underlying chronic disease.

Evaluation of GI bleeding must be systematic. The age of the child, the history, the physical examination, and associated symptoms help focus the workup and allow the clinician to identify the source of the bleeding in the majority of cases. Endoscopy and new radiologic techniques are particularly useful for diagnosis and management of many conditions.

Bleeding can occur at any point along the length of the GI tract, from the mouth to the anus. Multiple folds, coils, and villous borders of the GI mucosa provide a large surface area for secretion of enzymes and absorption of water and nutrients. A large vascular supply to the GI tract accounts for an appreciable fraction of the cardiac output, especially after eating meals. Bleeding may be arterial, venous, or both. Although most *bleeds* are slow and involve oozing from the mucosal surface, massive bleeding can result from lesions involving high-pressure arteries or a large, engorged venous plexus.

Acute GI bleeding may occur with or without symptoms and can originate in either the upper or the lower GI tract. Chronic bleeding is usually slow and intermittent and may be identified only by occult blood in the stool. The slow nature of these bleeds allows the body ample time to compensate and preserve cardiac output. Signs of chronic bleeding include compensatory tachycardia, iron-deficiency anemia, fatigue, pallor, or change in stool color.

DEFINITION OF TERMS

A variety of terms describe specific characteristics of GI bleeding that may also give clues to the nature, location, and duration of the bleeding. Hematemesis is bloody vomitus, which usually represents bleeding proximal to the ligament of Treitz. Blood, which is altered by gastric acid, becomes dark and coffee-ground in appearance. Bleeding that has little or no contact with gastric acid will be bright red. GI bleeding that occurs proximal to the ileocecal valve and is passed rectally will usually appear as melena: black, tarry, sticky stools that result from the denaturing of hemoglobin by intestinal bacteria and enzymes. Hematochezia, red bloody stools passed rectally, usually results from distal GI bleeding. Blood is usually mixed with the stool or passed just before or just after defecation. Occasionally, rapid bleeding from an upper GI source combined with the cathartic action of blood can speed transit time and cause hematochezia. Specific types of hematochezia include maroon-colored stools, seen with significant bleeding usually from the distal small bowel, and currant-jelly stools indicative of intestinal vascular congestion and hyperemia.

DIFFERENTIAL DIAGNOSIS

Identification of True Bleeding

The appearance of red color in the stool is often assumed to be blood. However, many other substances cause change in stool color. Foods that contain a high concentration of red pigments such as tomatoes, cranberries, beets, and red fruit juices and gelatin (Jell-O) can cause red stools. Similarly, red-colored medications such as acetaminophen and amoxicillin can be passed in the stools, especially if diarrhea is present. Spinach, licorice, iron, and bismuth (Pepto-Bismol) often lead to dark, black stools, which can be confused with true melena. In infants, *Serratia marcescens* can cause *red diaper syndrome* as a result of the formation of red pigment in soiled diapers stored for longer than 1 day.

Several biochemical tests are available to detect blood in the stool. The most common test, the stool guaiac, uses the peroxidase activity of hemoglobin to catalyze a color change on a test card or paper strip. This highly sensitive test is able to identify even trace amounts of blood. Foods that have peroxidase activity may cause false-positive results if eaten within 3 days of testing: red meat, liver, processed meats, and raw fruits and vegetables, especially melon, turnip, radishes, and horseradish. High vitamin C intake interferes with the peroxidase reaction and can cause false-negative results. Similarly, outdated guaiac cards and prolonged storage may affect the accuracy of the test. Stool guaiac cards are not accurate for testing emesis for the presence of blood because gastric acid can affect the reaction that causes the color change.

Nongastrointestinal Source of Bleeding

Although blood is present in the GI tract, the bleeding may originate from a peripheral source. The most common example of this phenomenon occurs in the newborn period. The infant may swallow maternal blood either during delivery or when breastfeeding if the mother has bleeding nipples. The Apt-Downey test is helpful in differentiating maternal blood from infant blood. One part of the bloody stool (or gastric aspirate) is mixed with 5 parts of water to lyse the red blood cells. After the mixture is centrifuged, 1 mL of 0.2 normal sodium hydroxide is added to the supernatant hemoglobin solution. After 2 minutes, fetal hemoglobin, which resists the alkaline reduction, remains pink, whereas maternal hemoglobin turns yellow-brown. Melena contains denatured hemoglobin and therefore cannot be used for the Apt-Downey test.

Swallowed blood by a child is usually the result of nosebleeds or bleeding mouth lesions. These nasopharyngeal bleeds can mimic hematemesis or melena. Although rare in children, pulmonary hemorrhage may exhibit acutely as hematemesis or more chronically with melena and anemia. Vaginal bleeding in a newborn with estrogen withdrawal may be mistaken for rectal bleeding. In the menstruating teenager, vaginal blood may affect the accuracy of stool guaiac testing. The possibility of blood being added to the stool by a caretaker suggests Münchausen syndrome by proxy.

Age at Presentation

Newborn

GI bleeding in newborns usually appears as rectal bleeding or blood suctioned from the stomach during routine postnatal care. In many instances, no lesion is readily discernible, and the bleeding resolves spontaneously and permanently. Common causes of GI bleeding in the first 24 hours of life include maternal blood swallowed during delivery and local trauma after nasogastric suctioning. Hemorrhagic disease of the newborn as a result of inherited deficits of coagulation factors or delay in administration of postnatal vitamin K occasionally produces GI bleeding, although it is more common for these disorders to show as diffuse bleeding from venipuncture sites.

Premature infants and newborns who have low Apgar scores are at increased risk for having gastric ulcerations and erosions that can bleed. These lesions are rarely primary, usually resulting from asphyxia associated with a difficult delivery, a cardiac lesion, or sepsis. The diagnosis is made by radiograph or upper GI endoscopy. Newborns who have persistent or severe gastroesophageal reflux can develop esophagitis. Although esophageal bleeding is upper GI bleeding, hematemesis is rare. Rather, the slow bleeding is occult and exhibits more commonly with signs of anemia or guaiac positive stools. Because a barium swallow has poor sensitivity, pH probe manometry and esophagoscopy are better tests for identifying gastroesophageal reflux. Treatment usually involves histamine H2-receptor blockers (H2-blockers).

Newborns with necrotizing enterocolitis (NEC) usually have a sudden onset of bilious vomiting, abdominal distention, lethargy, and lower GI bleeding. These symptoms usually occur after the 1st feeding but may be delayed for a few weeks. NEC is most common in premature infants but can occasionally occur in stressed full-term infants. Up to 5% of neonates in intensive care units develop NEC, and the overall mortality may be as high as 30%.[1] Complications of NEC include sepsis and shock. The diagnosis is confirmed by the presence of pneumatosis intestinalis on abdominal radiograph, but this finding is variable. These neonates remain hospitalized for bowel rest and intravenous antibiotics, and they occasionally need surgical intervention.

Intrinsic structural lesions of the GI tract are also a serious cause of lower GI bleeding in the newborn. Intestinal duplication, a tubular structure lined with normal GI mucosa adjacent to the true intestine, can be present anywhere along the GI tract. Duplications can cause lower GI bleeding, either acute or chronic, along with abdominal distention and vomiting. The diagnosis is confirmed by radiograph, computed tomography (CT) scan, or ultrasound. Unrepaired duplications may lead to obstruction, volvulus, or perforation. A volvulus or malrotation of the GI tract should be suspected in any infant who has abdominal pain, bilious vomiting, and melena. However, because these symptoms and signs are often unreliable, the diagnosis should be considered in any newborn who vomits and has guaiac-positive stools. An abdominal radiograph may show loops of small bowel overriding the liver shadow, with paucity of air in the GI tract distal to the volvulus. An upper GI series, barium enema, or both are sometimes needed to confirm the diagnosis. Midgut volvulus may also be diagnosed on CT scan or ultrasound by noting duodenal dilatation, fixed midline bowel, and the wrapping of the bowel and the superior mesenteric vein around the superior mesenteric artery (whirlpool sign). Immediate surgical repair is necessary. Vascular malformations can occur anywhere along the GI tract and produce slow or diffuse lower GI bleeding. The bleeding is usually painless, and the color of the blood in the stool will vary depending on the level of the lesion. Vascular malformations may be associated with cutaneous hemangiomas or cardiac defects.

Milk or soy protein allergy can begin as early as the 1st week of life and exhibit as severe diarrhea, gross blood in the stool, abdominal distention, and vomiting. Older infants may have occult lower GI bleeding and mucus in the stool. The diagnosis is made by clinical response to withdrawal and rechallenge with the offending protein. Infectious enteritis, although rare in the newborn, may appear later in the 1st month of life. In very young infants, bacterial gastroenteritis, especially that caused by *Salmonella*, can cause bloody diarrhea with or without fever; 8% to 13% of infants may have associated bacteremia.[2] Bright-red blood streaks on the surface of the stool suggests an anal fissure. Often associated with hard stools, anal fissures are the most common cause of rectal bleeding. Visual inspection of the anus usually confirms the diagnosis. Medications, such as indomethacin and dexamethasone, can cause mucosal erosion and GI bleeding.

Infants and Young Children

Upper GI bleeding in the young child is usually caused by mucosal lesions in the esophagus and the stomach. Infectious esophagitis is usually viral, but fungi can be the cause of disease in immunocompromised children. As infants become more mobile and dexterous, they are at higher risk for foreign body and toxic ingestions. Coins and small toys, when lodged in the esophagus, can cause drooling, vomiting, and chest pain. Persistent or unrecognized esophageal foreign bodies lead to edema and erosion of the esophagus and may cause hematemesis. Caustic ingestion severe enough to burn the esophageal mucosa can also result in painful swallowing, drooling, oral burns, and hematemesis. Children who have forceful or prolonged vomiting may develop a rent at the gastroesophageal junction known as a Mallory-Weiss tear. The emesis becomes streaked with bright-red blood and may develop into coffee-ground emesis if the tear persists. Although the bleeding is minor and usually resolves spontaneously, an H2-blocker may be needed to prevent continued irritation by stomach acid.

Gastroesophageal varices can occur at any age but usually occur in children younger than 8 years. Variceal bleeding can range from slow, persistent oozing to acute massive hematemesis. Physical examination usually reveals signs of portal hypertension, such as enlarged liver or spleen or both. Most cases result from the cavernous transformation of the extrahepatic portion of the portal vein, which has been associated with umbilical vessel catheterization, omphalitis, or neonatal conditions associated with hypoxia, prolonged jaundice, or sepsis. Intrahepatic causes of cirrhosis, leading to portal hypertension that may first show during childhood, include Wilson disease (after 6 years of age), alpha$_1$-antitrypsin deficiency, biliary cirrhosis, and metabolic, infectious, or anatomic forms of chronic liver disease. These chronic liver diseases also may be associated with coagulopathy and thrombocytopenia from the hypersplenism that usually accompanies them. If the cause of the portal hypertension is extrahepatic, then the bleeding may be tolerated remarkably well, in contrast to patients who have cirrhotic liver disease in whom rapid hepatic decompensation may occur. Fortunately, most variceal bleeding stops spontaneously, but the incidence of rebleeding is high. Endoscopy confirms the diagnosis.

Juvenile polyps are the most common cause of lower GI bleeding, reaching a peak incidence in children aged 3 to 7 years. Typically, polyps are located in the colon and are simple, solitary, benign hamartomatous lesions that may irritate the GI tract and cause intermittent, painless, bright-red rectal bleeding. Many of these polyps will autoamputate if left alone and are passed with the stool. Because most polyps are located within 25 cm of the anus, they are easily identified by digital examination, air-contrast barium enema, or sigmoidoscopy and can be removed with snare electrocautery.

Adenomatous polyps may produce rectal bleeding as early as infancy, but they are managed differently from juvenile polyps. Juvenile polyps are benign inflammatory lesions that do not cause later complications. Adenomatous polyps, conversely, are premalignant tumors, which may transform into a malignancy over an average period of 10 years.[3] Familial polyposis and Gardner syndrome are associated with adenomatous polyps. Juvenile polyposis coli (JPC) is suggested by the presence of 5 to 10 juvenile polyps; 10 or more polyps is considered diagnostic. JPC, which occurs in approximately 10% of patients who have colonic polyps, is associated with anemia, right-colon polyps, and adenomas.[3]

Meckel diverticulum, a remnant of the omphalomesenteric duct found within 2 feet of the ileocecal valve, is present in up to 2% of the population. The acid secreted by ectopic gastric mucosa, which is usually present in diverticula that bleed, causes peptic ulceration of the ileal mucosa. Meckel diverticulum typically occurs in children younger than 3 years and causes painless, maroon- or red-colored lower GI bleeding. Typically, the bleeding is severe enough to cause the hemoglobin level to fall to approximately 8 g/dL. Diagnosis is made by technetium-99 scan, which identifies the ectopic gastric mucosa. This test is fairly sensitive but only during active bleeding; thus a repeat scan is sometimes necessary when the suggestion is high. Treatment requires surgical excision.

Intussusception, the telescoping of an intestinal segment, is seen typically in children 6 to 24 months of age. The occurrence is often idiopathic and usually involves invagination of the distal ileum through the ileocecal valve into the colon. Older children who have intussusception and those who have multiple recurrences may have pathological lesions that serve as lead points (Meckel diverticulum, polyp, and tumor). The classic presentation begins with intermittent, severe, crampy abdominal pain, with vomiting following shortly thereafter. As the intussusception progresses, lethargy or paradoxical irritability develops. Guaiac-positive stools are seen as the bowel becomes ischemic and may progress to the passage of red bloody mucus, classically referred to as *currant-jelly stools*. The use of screening ultrasound has decreased unnecessary enemas for clinically suspected intussusception.[4] Diagnosis can be confirmed on ultrasound by identification of the layering of intestinal mucosa as a *bulls-eye* or *coiled spring* lesion. Confirmation of diagnosis, followed by hydrostatic reduction with barium or air enema, is successful in approximately 70% to 80% of cases, even in those with symptoms for more than 24 hours.[5] Complications include intestinal perforation, peritonitis, and significant bleeding.

Lymphonodular hyperplasia on the mucosa of the terminal ileum or colon may cause painless, blood-streaked stools. Lymphonodular hyperplasia is usually seen in children younger than 6 years and may be associated with food allergy.[6] Diagnosis is made by endoscopic examination and histologic confirmation.

Symptoms associated with infectious enterocolitis range from mild diarrhea to fever, abdominal cramping, and watery or mucoid stools (or both forms) with or without blood. *Salmonella, Shigella, Yersinia,* and *Campylobacter* are the most common bacterial causes of bloody diarrhea. Pseudomembranous colitis, caused by *Clostridium difficile,* also causes fever, diarrhea, abdominal cramping, and bloody stools. In many instances, a history of recent hospitalization and antimicrobial therapy exists, but the onset of symptoms can be delayed for weeks. A variety of parasites, such as amoebae, can cause bloody diarrhea.

Systemic disease, in particular vasculitis, may be accompanied by bloody stools. The constellation of arthritis, hematuria, purpura, intestinal cramping, and bloody stools suggests Henoch-Schönlein purpura (HSP). Children with HSP are at increased risk of intussusception, or they may have severe GI bleeding. Hemolytic-uremic syndrome (HUS) often has a prodrome of hemorrhagic colitis caused by Shiga toxin-producing *Escherichia coli* with a serotype O157:H7. The classic triad of HUS includes thrombocytopenia, hemolytic anemia, and renal disease. Milk protein allergy, anal fissures, and congenital anatomic anomalies of the GI tract can also occur in this age group.

Older Children and Adolescents

Peptic ulcer disease can occur at any age but is more common in the older child and adolescent. Symptoms usually begin with epigastric or periumbilical pain accompanied by nausea. GI bleeding is evident in approximately 50% of children either as hematemesis or as melena. *Helicobacter pylori,* bacteria found in the gastric mucous layer or adherent to the epithelial lining of the stomach, has been causally associated with ulcers. Infection is common worldwide, and in areas of high prevalence, most children are infected by 10 years of age.[7] Fortunately, infected children are usually asymptomatic and only occasionally develop disease in childhood. *H pylori* infection is diagnosed by culture of biopsy specimens from the stomach and duodenum. Serologic tests, which measure specific *H pylori* IgG antibodies, are also available. Treatment, when indicated, consists of a 7- to 14-day course of any of a variety of antibiotic regimens together with a proton-pump inhibitor.

Hemangiomas and other vascular lesions, such as hereditary hemorrhagic telangiectasia (Rendu-Osler-Weber syndrome), must be considered in the evaluation for painless rectal bleeding. Its most common form is the larger cavernous hemangioma, either polypoid or diffuse, extending several centimeters through the submucosa of the small or large intestine. The large bowel, specifically the rectum, is the area usually involved in the diffuse type. Cutaneous vascular malformations are often present but may require scrupulous searching to detect. Selective arteriography or digital subtraction angiography may aid in demonstrating the abnormal vessels if they are not visible on direct inspection.

Inflammatory bowel disease may appear in the adolescent age group as episodes of bloody diarrhea, cramping, and tenesmus. The course may be atypical in children, making the diagnosis difficult. Growth failure, weight loss, or anemia with evidence of recurrent bouts of GI bleeding should alert the clinician to the diagnosis, which colonoscopy and biopsy usually confirm.

EVALUATION OF PATIENTS WHO HAVE GASTROINTESTINAL BLEEDING

When evaluating a patient who has GI blood loss, the physician should keep 2 goals in mind. First, the severity of the blood loss must be assessed quickly to expedite appropriate resuscitative measures. Second, the physician must consider the most likely causes so that problems requiring immediate surgery can be separated from those requiring medical evaluation and management. The workup is based on the patient's age and history, clinical appearance, and on the physician's familiarity with the patient. A list of lesions commonly associated with GI bleeding is provided in Box 184-1.

Relevant History

A detailed history may help the clinician determine the location and duration of the bleeding. Particular

BOX 184-1 Causes of Gastrointestinal Bleeding

NEWBORNS

Upper GI Bleeding

- Hemorrhagic disease of the newborn
- Gastritis
- Stress ulcer
- Esophagitis

Lower GI Bleeding

- Necrotizing enterocolitis
- Duplication
- Volvulus, malrotation
- Vascular malformations
- Milk allergy
- Infectious enteritis
- Anal fissure

INFANTS AND YOUNG CHILDREN

Upper GI Bleeding

- Nasopharyngeal bleeding
- Esophagitis
- Acid reflux
- Viral, fungal, caustic sources
- Esophageal foreign body
- Mallory-Weiss tear
- Gastroesophageal varices
- Gastritis

Lower GI Bleeding

- Juvenile polyps
- Meckel diverticulum
- Intussusception
- Infectious enterocolitis
- Pseudomembranous colitis
- Vasculitis (HSP, HUS)
- Milk allergy
- Lymphonodular hyperplasia
- Anal fissure or trauma (abuse)
- Duplication
- Vascular malformation

OLDER CHILDREN AND ADOLESCENTS

Upper GI Bleeding

- Nasopharyngeal bleeding
- Esophagitis
- Mallory-Weiss tear
- Gastroesophageal varices
- Gastritis
- Aspirin, NSAIDs
- *Helicobacter pylori*
- Peptic ulcer disease

Lower GI Bleeding

- Polyps
- Infectious enterocolitis
- Inflammatory bowel disease
- Vasculitis
- Vascular malformation
- Meckel diverticulum
- Hemorrhoids
- Anal fissure

GI, Gastrointestinal; *HSP*, Henoch-Schönlein purpura; *HUS*, hemolytic-uremic syndrome; *NSAIDs*, nonsteroidal antiinflammatory drugs.

attention should be paid to the color of the stool and emesis and whether a change has occurred in the preceding days or weeks. Massive amounts of red blood from the mouth or rectum are readily apparent to the parent and the patient. However, the importance of maroon or tarry stools as a sign of GI bleeding may not be appreciated unless the clinician asks.

Antecedent symptoms are also a key to identifying many diseases. Vomiting that progresses from bile-stained to bloody is seen with intestinal obstruction (volvulus, intussusception, NEC) or with Mallory-Weiss tears. Bloody diarrhea may accompany infectious enteritis, food allergy, and inflammatory bowel disease, or it may precede HUS. Painless lower GI bleeding, if substantial, is seen with Meckel diverticulum or GI vascular anomalies, whereas a smaller amount of painless bleeding suggests polyps or lymphonodular hyperplasia. Fever is common in infectious or inflammatory disorders. Arthritis and rash are seen with HSP. Abdominal pain, fever, and weight loss suggest inflammatory bowel disease. Lower rectal disorders, such as hemorrhoids or anal fissures, produce blood-streaked stools and painful defecation. Young children who have upper GI bleeding should be questioned about foreign body or caustic ingestion. Medication use, especially of aspirin, nonsteroidal antiinflammatory drugs, steroids, and tetracycline, is a frequent cause of gastritis. A family history of polyps, bleeding disorders, or GI diseases is important. Neonatal history should focus on risk factors for NEC or varices, including umbilical vein catheters, liver disease, and birth asphyxia. Sexual activity or abuse involving anal penetration should alert the clinician to anal and rectal trauma.

Physical Examination

The physical examination should be complete and systematic because clues to the diagnosis may be present in any organ system. The general appearance and vital signs can be helpful in determining the duration of bleeding. Slow, chronic bleeding allows time for physiologic changes such as tachycardia, orthostasis, and decreased pulse pressure. Children may initially appear comfortable but tired and have some degree of pallor. Patients who have acute, rapid bleeds may be in various stages of shock depending on the amount of blood loss. The nose and mouth should be examined for bleeding lesions or burns. The abdominal examination should evaluate for tenderness, bowel sounds, masses, and hepatosplenomegaly. The physician must also look for signs of chronic liver disease, such as the presence of telangiectasias, jaundice, hepatosplenomegaly, and a prominent abdominal venous pattern. With lower GI bleeding, a thorough rectal examination should be performed, with special attention paid to: (1) the perianal region, observing for skin tags, abscesses, fissures, bleeding points, or much less commonly, hemorrhoids; (2) the character of the stool; and (3) the presence of occult blood by guaiac testing. Palpation for polyps and pelvic masses must be part of the rectal examination. Eczema may be associated with food allergy. Finally, skin lesions such as purpura and petechiae suggest a bleeding disorder, HSP, or HUS.

Laboratory Testing

In the setting of GI bleeding, laboratory testing should focus on determining the amount and duration of the bleeding, assessing for coagulopathy, and evaluating for other laboratory abnormalities that may be associated with the under-lying disease process. Hemoglobin determination can help assess the level of blood loss, with the caveat that acute bleeding may not lower the hemoglobin level until some intravascular equilibration takes place. An elevated white blood cell count may occur in infectious colitis. Coagulation studies should be obtained, including prothrombin and partial prothrombin times, as well as the platelet count. The prothrombin time may be elevated as a sign of a bleeding disorder or as a result of abnormalities in liver synthetic function. Liver function tests are useful in evaluating suspected liver disease. Serum chemistries can be used to assess renal function, although an elevation in the blood urea nitrogen may be due to increased intestinal absorption of blood with long-standing upper GI bleeding. Any patient with significant bleeding or a low hemoglobin level should have blood sent immediately for blood type and screen in the event of the need for blood transfusion. If bloody diarrhea is present, then a stool specimen should be sent for culture and, if appropriate, ova and parasites.

Imaging

Most children with GI bleeding require some type of imaging study to locate the source of the bleeding or confirm a suspected diagnosis. The type of study will depend on the age of the child, clinical presentation, and possible diagnosis. Plain radiographic films are generally nonspecific and usually require additional imaging to confirm a diagnosis. Two-view (flat and upright) abdominal radiographs may show signs of intestinal obstruction such as air-fluid levels and dilated bowel loops. Some specific radiographic findings include pneumatosis intestinalis in NEC and intestinal obstruction with absence of gas in the right colon in intussusception. Barium studies can be used to identify intestinal foreign bodies, polyps, lymphonodular hyperplasia, and inflammatory bowel disease, although, in many cases, endoscopy remains the procedure of choice for diagnosis. Color Doppler ultrasound is becoming increasingly useful as a diagnostic aid in both intussusception and malrotation, but its usefulness depends on the skill of the operator. CT scans are occasionally helpful in defining related anatomic features if the child is hemodynamically stable and either cooperative or sedated. Nuclear medicine imaging studies (Meckel scan, radioactively labeled colloid or red blood cells) or direct angiography can often identify the source of an acute, ongoing bleed.

MANAGEMENT

For a child having acute massive GI bleeding, the approach must be the same as that in any other emergency. The physician must approach the patient with an efficient, rational plan in mind that will allow obtaining the pertinent historical information, performing a brief but adequate examination, stabilizing the patient clinically, arriving at a working diagnosis, and instituting appropriate therapy or consultations. Massive upper GI bleeding may lead to vomiting, aspiration, and airway obstruction that requires stabilization of the airway with endotracheal intubation. Administration of oxygen is always indicated. Evaluation of peripheral perfusion, quality of pulses, and capillary refill time assesses the adequacy of circulation. In children, the initial response to hypovolemic shock is tachycardia. In acute bleeds, adequate blood pressure can be maintained with blood loss of up to 30% without replacement.

Tachycardia and capillary refill time are essential criteria in determining the nature of the resuscitation required. Skin turgor and the color of the mucous membranes also should be noted. If signs of shock are present (eg, orthostasis or frank hypotension, tachycardia, poorly perfused extremities, pale mucous membranes, altered mental status), then a large-bore intravenous catheter should be placed. Initial laboratory studies include complete blood count, hematocrit, reticulocyte count, coagulation times, electrolytes, and blood typing and cross matching. If percutaneous venous access is not obtained within a few minutes, then an intraosseous line should be placed and 20 mL/kg of normal saline should be given rapidly to reexpand the vascular volume. This fluid bolus may need to be repeated several times. Additional fluid should be given as needed to allow equilibration of these solutions with the extravascular space. With more than 30% to 40% acute blood loss, packed red blood cells should be given as soon as possible (see Chapter 358, Shock).

An appropriately sized nasogastric (NG) tube, preferably of the vented sump type, helps determine the source of bleeding and helps estimate the volume of ongoing blood loss. The tube should be left in place and attached either to low-pressure continuous suction, if vented, or to intermittent suction, if nonvented. The only instance in which NG tube placement may aggravate bleeding is with a patient who has varices. Nonetheless, even in this case, an NG tube may be required to quantitate blood loss adequately.

Controlling the bleeding and determining the specific diagnosis are the next steps in management. If the NG aspirate contains blood, or if the patient has hematemesis, then saline irrigation may be instituted in an attempt to decrease mucosal blood flow and thereby stop profuse bleeding. Although the efficacy of lavage in decreasing and controlling gastric bleeding has not been demonstrated conclusively, it allows easier assessment of the rate of bleeding and helps in removing clotted blood. Saline at room temperature should be used because irrigation with water can lead to hyponatremia, and iced or cold fluid may cause hypothermia. The saline is instilled through an NG tube and is withdrawn after 3 to 5 minutes. Aspirate returns that do not clear in 15 minutes suggest continued GI bleeding and should prompt additional evaluation.

If the bleeding ceases, then gastroduodenoscopy should be performed to demonstrate the bleeding source and to determine the type of lesion present. Upper GI fiber-optic endoscopy can establish the diagnosis in 75% to 90% of patients. If the bleeding is massive and cannot be controlled with saline lavage, then adequate visualization is not likely to be achieved with the fiber-optic endoscope. If the bleeding is not immediately life threatening, then arteriography, which can demonstrate bleeding that occurs at a rate of 0.5 mL/min or more, should be considered. More sensitive than arteriography, and less invasive, a sulfur-colloid isotopic study can demonstrate active bleeding at rates as low as 0.05 to 0.1 mL/min.[8] This method demonstrates active bleeding by using a tracer with a very short half-life. In small infants, a large uptake of the isotope by the liver may mask the right upper quadrant. An additional isotopic method of determining the bleeding site consists of injecting the patient with technetium-99-pertechnetate–labeled red blood cells. These labeled cells may remain in the circulation for more than a day and allow repeated imaging to locate the site of intermittent bleeding.

If the lesion is one of mucosal erosion or inflammation, then antacid therapy with or without the concomitant use of an H2-blocker may be instituted. For bleeding ulcers, intravenous therapy with a proton-pump inhibitor reduces the risk of ulcer rebleeding but does not appear to influence the overall mortality.[9] If the bleeding source is variceal, then the cause of the lesions must be determined, with appropriate treatment of the underlying disease. In particular, liver or portal venous disease should be sought. Clotting factors and platelets should be replaced as indicated.

Variceal bleeding requires special mention because of the many settings in which varices may be seen. The treatment of variceal bleeding in children has evolved over the last 2 decades. Use of balloon tamponade with a Sengstaken-Blakemore tube (an NG tube with additional lumina for a gastric balloon and an esophageal balloon in which the gastric balloon is inflated and traction is applied so that the balloon abuts the gastroesophageal junction and tamponades the variceal bleeding) was effective in controlling most cases of bleeding but had a high incidence of complications. This treatment has been replaced, in most cases, with the use of vasoactive drugs and endoscopy. Previously, the major medical therapy included the use of intravenous vasopressin as a mesenteric vasoconstrictor to reduce portal blood flow and thus decrease variceal pressure. However, vasopressin can cause peripheral vasoconstriction and malignant hypertension. Recently, somatostatin and octreotide have been found to be similarly effective in adults and in smaller studies in children.[10-12] Octreotide decreases splanchnic blood flow thereby decreasing portal pressure, has less effect on systemic blood flow and is associated with fewer side effects than vasopressin. Pediatric studies (with no control groups) have shown octreotide to be 50% to 63% effective in controlling acute variceal bleeding.[11,13] Initially, a 50-mcg bolus is infused, preferably through a central or intraosseous line, followed by an infusion of 50 mcg/hour for 5 days.

Endoscopy is the preferred intervention for variceal bleeding because it can provide both diagnosis and therapy. The 2 most commonly used techniques are endoscopic injection sclerotherapy (EIS), which uses an injection of a sclerosing solution into the varices, and endoscopic variceal band ligation (EVL), in which elastic bands are placed around the varices in the distal esophagus. Endoscopy has been found to be 80% to 100% effective in controlling variceal bleeding.[11-14]

In a randomized controlled trial in 49 children, EVL achieved variceal eradication faster than EIS, with a lower rebleeding rate and fewer complications.[13] In either case, endoscopy should be performed by an experienced gastroenterologist, with the availability of general anesthesia and endotracheal intubation, if necessary, especially when performed on small children.

Studies in adults and experience in pediatrics, although limited to date, suggest that octreotide should be used as the initial treatment for bleeding varices followed by endoscopic therapy, either EVL or EIS.[12,15] If the bleeding continues despite vasoactive and endoscopic therapies, then balloon tamponade can be attempted.

Evaluation for lower GI bleeding differs in several aspects from that for upper GI bleeding. The abdomen, perineum, and rectum are thoroughly examined. Stool must be analyzed for the presence of blood and, when appropriate, for enteric pathogens and for ova and parasites. If diarrhea is present, then the stool should be examined microscopically for polymorphonuclear leukocytes and mucus, both of which are evidence of bacterial infection. Digital rectal examination should follow in an attempt to discover the presence of anal fissures, rectal polyps, or hemorrhoids. Sigmoidoscopy may be necessary for children who have persistent rectal bleeding to identify polyps or mucosal lesions. The presence of blood originating from above the reach of the sigmoidoscope indicates the need to proceed with other diagnostic studies.

Several different imaging studies are used to evaluate persistent lower GI bleeding. An upright and supine view of the abdomen will reveal signs of obstruction or calcifications. For severe, life-threatening bleeds, angiography can be both diagnostic and therapeutic, depending on the ability to embolize the bleeding vessels. Because angiography has limited sensitivity in detecting slow or past bleeding, it is best performed when bleeding is active.

Children with persistent, active bleeding who are clinically stable should have a radionuclide scan, which identifies accumulation of an isotope at the bleeding site. With a sulfur-colloid isotopic scan, the isotope is extracted rapidly so that background radioactivity is low. Although high-contrast resolution can be found around the bleeding site, it is effective only for identifying rapid bleeding. An isotope-labeled red blood cell infusion has a lower contrast ratio but is better at detecting slower or intermittent bleeds than a sulfur-colloid isotopic scan. A Meckel scan uses technetium-99 pertechnetate, which is secreted by ectopic gastric mucosa, to identify the diverticulum. If the rate of bleeding does not permit the time necessary to perform these studies, then vasopressin or octreotide may be administered parenterally in an attempt to control the bleeding and to stabilize the patient. Air-contrast barium studies or endoscopy can identify sources of more chronic, low-grade bleeding. However, a barium enema or an upper GI series with small bowel follow-through should be the last studies performed because they make the further use of arteriography, isotope scans, and endoscopy impossible for several days thereafter. In cases in which the intestine is compromised vascularly, or when the rate of bleeding is excessive and uncontrollable by more conservative methods, prompt surgical intervention is required. Fortunately, however, conservative measures control most acute episodes of GI bleeding relatively easily; patients who eventually require surgical intervention can usually undergo surgery electively at a later time.

WHEN TO REFER

- Upper GI bleed
- Lower GI bleed that is of moderate amount, persistent, or intermittent

WHEN TO ADMIT

- Any nontrivial upper GI bleeding, such as that associated with active bleeding, moderate amount of blood, anemia, and abdominal pain
- Significant lower GI bleeding
- Hemodynamic instability
- Anemia (hematocrit <24%)
- Severe abdominal pain
- Associated systemic symptoms (eg, HUS, IBD)
- Altered mental status or lethargy
- Suggestion of surgical etiology (eg, Meckel diverticulum, intussusception, volvulus)

SUGGESTED READINGS

Balkan E, Kiristioglu I, Gurpinar A, et al. Sigmoidoscopy in minor lower gastrointestinal bleeding. *Arch Dis Child.* 1998;78:267-268.

Goggin N, Rowland M, Imrie C, et al. Effect of Helicobacter pylori eradication on the natural history of duodenal ulcer disease. *Arch Dis Child.* 1998;79:502.

Hamoui N, Docherty S, Crookes P. Gastrointestinal hemorrhage: is the surgeon obsolete? *Emerg Med Clin North Am.* 2003;21:1017-1056.

Leung A, Wong A. Lower gastrointestinal bleeding in children. *Pediatr Emerg Care.* 2002;18(4);319-323.

Park J, Wolff B, Tollefson M, et al. Meckel diverticulum: the Mayo Clinic experience with 1476 patients (1950-2002). *Ann Surg.* 2005;241(3);529-533.

Pearl RH, Irish MS, Caty MG, et al. The approach to common abdominal diagnoses in infants and children. Part II. *Pediatr Clin North Am.* 1998;45:1287.

Squires RH. Gastrointestinal bleeding. *Pediatr Rev.* 1999; 20:95.

REFERENCES

1. Caplan MS, Jilling T. New concepts in necrotizing enterocolitis. *Curr Opin Pediatr.* 2001;13(2):111-115.
2. Lin P, Huang Y, Chang L, et al. C-reactive protein in childhood non-typhi salmonella gastroenteritis with and without bacteremia. *Pediatr Infect Dis J.* 2000;19(8):754.
3. Hoffenberg EJ, Sauaia A, Maltzman T, et al. Symptomatic colonic polyps in childhood: not so benign. *J Pediatr Gastroenterol Nutr.* 1999;150:175.
4. Henrikson S, Blane C, Koujok K, et al. The effect of screening sonography on the positive rate of enemas for intussusception. *Pediatr Radiol.* 2003;33:190-193.
5. Ende E, Allema J, Hazebroek F, et al. Success with hydrostatic reduction of intussusception in relation to duration of symptoms. *Arch Dis Child.* 2005;90: 1071-1072.

6. Kokkonen J, Karttunen T. Lymphonodular hyperplasia on the mucosa of the lower gastrointestinal tract in children: an indication of enhanced immune response? *J Pediatr Gastroenterol Nutr.* 2002;34(1):42-46.
7. Malaty H. Age at acquisition of Helicobacter pylori infection: a follow-up study from infancy to adulthood. *Lancet.* 2002;359:931-935.
8. Lefkovitz Z. Radiologic diagnosis and treatment of gastrointestinal hemorrhage and ischemia. *Med Clin North Am.* 2002;86(6):1357-1399.
9. Leontiadis GI, Sharma VK, Howden CW. Systematic review and meta-analysis of proton pump inhibitor therapy in peptic ulcer bleeding. *BMJ.* 2005;330:568.
10. D'Amico G, Pagliaro LLP, Pietrosi GGPI, et al. Emergency sclerotherapy versus medical interventions for bleeding oesophageal varices in cirrhotic patients. *Cochrane Database System Rev.* 2002;1:CD002233.
11. Heikenen J, Pohl J, Werlin S, et al. Octreotide in pediatric patients. *J Pediatr Gastroenterol Nutr.* 2002;35:600-609.
12. Molleston J. Variceal bleeding in children. *J Pediatr Gastroenterol Nutr.* 2003;37:538-545.
13. Zgar S, Javid G, Khan B, et al. Endoscopic ligation compared with sclerotherapy for bleeding esophageal varices in children with extrahepatic portal venous obstruction. *Hepatology.* 2002;36:666-672.
14. McKiernan PJ, Beath SV, Davison SM. A prospective study of endoscopic esophageal variceal ligation using a multiband ligator. *J Pediatr Gastroenterol Nutr.* 2002;34:207-211.
15. Banares R, Albillos A, Rincon D, et al. Endoscopic treatment versus endoscopic plus pharmacologic treatment for acute variceal bleeding: a meta-analysis. *Hepatology.* 2002;35:609-615.

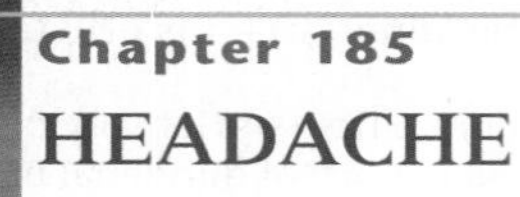

Chapter 185
HEADACHE

Andrew D. Hershey, MD, PhD

INTRODUCTION

Headache is one of the oldest known diseases, with reports in the earliest human writings, yet is frequently not recognized, diagnosed, or appropriately treated. Headaches, particularly migraine, are being increasingly recognized as a significant health problem for children and adolescents. Up to 75% of children report having a significant headache by the time they are 15 years of age,[1] and up to 28% of adolescents appear to have migraines.[2] This very common disorder can have a significant effect on a child's life, school performance, and relationship with family and peers. The disease can result in school absenteeism and lack of involvement in peer activities and may have long-term socioeconomic and biological consequences. Early recognition and correct diagnosis along with directed, appropriate treatment are essential to minimize the effect on a child's quality of life and may be important in preventing long-term disability.

DEFINITIONS

The International Classification of Headache Disorders II (ICHD-II) criteria,[3,4] which are the current foundation for the diagnosis and scientific study of headaches, classify headaches as primary or secondary. This classification system does appear as an improvement, although indications are that it remains incomplete in diagnosing primary headache disorders in children.[4] Primary headaches are directly attributed to a neurologic basis and include migraine, tension-type headaches (TTHs), cluster headaches, and other primary neuralgias (Box 185-1). Secondary headaches are attributed to a specific nonneurologic cause, which can be infectious, vascular, traumatic, toxic (including medications and overuse of medications), or a mass lesion.

BOX 185-1 Primary Headache Disorders (ICHD-II)

- Migraine (1)
  - Migraine without aura (1.1)
  - Migraine with aura (1.2)
  - Childhood periodic syndromes (1.3)
  - Retinal migraine (1.4)
  - Complications of migraine (1.5)
    - Chronic migraine (1.5.1)
    - Status migrainosus (1.5.2)
  - Probable migraine (1.6)
- Tension-type headaches (2)
  - Infrequent episodic tension-type headaches (2.1)
  - Frequent episodic tension-type headaches (2.2)
  - Chronic tension-type headaches (2.3)
  - Probable tension-type headaches (2.4)
- Cluster headache and other trigeminal autonomic cephalalgias (3)
- Other primary headaches (4)

From International Headache Society, Headache Classification Subcommittee. The International Classification of Headache Disorders. *Cephalalgia* 2004; 24(supp 1):1-160. Reprinted by permission of Blackwell Publishing Ltd.

EVALUATION

The first step in evaluating a child with headache is to rule out secondary causes, beginning with a detailed headache history, including the length of time the child has had headaches, the severity of the headaches, the quality of the headache, location of the headache, and the effect on the child's quality of life and disability. The headache history should include a detailed review of systems, medical history, and a psychosocial and family history to identify stressors that may be contributory. The parents and patient may have a preconceived idea as to the type of headache the child has, and they are often incorrect. The most sensitive indicator of the need for further assessment for a possible secondary cause is the neurologic examination.[5] If abnormalities on the neurologic examination cannot be explained by medical history, then further investigation into the cause of the headache is warranted, and neuroimaging is the most sensitive tool to detect a medically or surgically treatable cause. In addition, patients with underlying primary headaches can develop secondary headaches; thus a change in the description or pattern of the headaches or in the neurologic

BOX 185-2 Secondary Causes of Headaches (ICHD-II)

- Head or neck trauma
- Cranial or cervical vascular disorder
- Nonvascular intracranial disorder (includes high pressure and low pressure headaches)
- A substance or its withdrawal (includes medication overuse headaches)
- Infection (includes meningitis or encephalitis)
- Disorders of homeostasis (or facial pain) caused by disorders of the cranium, neck, eyes, ears, nose, sinuses, teeth, mouth, or other facial or cranial structures
- Psychiatric disorders

From International Headache Society, Headache Classification Subcommittee. The International Classification of Headache Disorders. *Cephalalgia* 2004; 24(supp 1):1-160. Reprinted by permission of Blackwell Publishing Ltd.

examination should prompt consideration of further assessment.

Once the detailed history and neurologic examination are performed, conducting a physical examination is useful and should include a thorough search for potential sources of secondary headache, including raised intracranial pressure, sinusitis, dental disease, abnormalities of the cervical spine, and temporomandibular joint disorders.[6]

After the detailed history and medical examination, the primary care physician should be able to determine whether the headaches are primary headaches or secondary headaches. Box 185-2 highlights a list of secondary causes of headache. If the headaches are secondary, then treating the secondary cause is essential. If the headaches persist after resolution of the secondary cause, then a reanalysis as to the cause of the headaches must be considered.

If secondary causes are ruled out, then the treatment of primary headaches can begin, depending on which type of primary headache the child has. The most common diagnoses include migraine without aura, probable migraine, migraine with aura, and chronic migraine.

MIGRAINE

The ICHD-II criteria subdivide migraine into migraine without aura and migraine with aura, replacing the historical terms of common and classical migraine, respectively (Box 185-3). In addition, migraine includes migraine variants, such as the periodic syndromes of childhood, and probable migraine, when not all of the features of migraine are met. The ICHD-II also added the category of chronic migraine, defined as frequent headaches—at least 15 times per month for the previous 3 months—with migraine features that cannot be attributed to a secondary cause.

In 1994, Abu-Arafeh and Russell reported that 10.6% of children between the ages of 5 and 15 had significant headaches consistent with migraine, with an increasing 1-year prevalence between the ages of 10 and 19.[7] In the meta-analysis of pediatric headache, 1.2% to 3.2% of children between the ages of 3 and 7 had migraines, with a slight male predominance.[5] From 7 to 11 years of age, the incidence of migraine increased to between 4% and 11%, with an equal male and female occurrence; and between the ages of 11 and 15, migraine increased to 18% to 23%, with a female predominance. Split and Newman examined 2353 children in the 15- to 19-year-old range using the ICHD-I criteria and found that 28% of these adolescents had migraines, with a female predominance.[2] Migraine without aura was more common than migraine with aura, and mixed headaches were seen in 6.3% with some TTHs in addition to migraines. Eighty-one percent of the adolescents with migraine had a positive family history, and nearly a quarter of the female adolescents reported a relationship between their headaches and menstruation. In addition, status migrainosus was noted in 14.8% of the girls, and 4.7% of the boys.

TENSION-TYPE HEADACHE

TTHs are generally considered mild recurrent headaches, and many features are the opposite of migraine. In the past, TTHs have been called muscle contraction headache, idiopathic headache, and tension headaches. They can be subdivided into infrequent, frequent, and chronic based on the frequency of the headaches. The headaches themselves are usually described as mild and moderate in severity, diffuse in location, and have a pressing quality and no secondary causes are identified.

TTHs have been less well studied than migraines, with estimates of their prevalence in children varying from as low as 1% to as high as 73%.[9] Studies in Sweden[10] and Finland[11] place the range between 10% and 23%, depending in part on whether recurrence and duration were included in the criteria. In the Finnish study, many of the children diagnosed with TTH had migrainous feature, whereas muscle tenderness was not a characteristic of TTH in these children, but it was for migraine.[12]

MEASURING THE EFFECT OF HEADACHES AND HEADACHE TREATMENT

Primary headaches, particularly migraines, can have a significant effect on a child's life. The 1989 National Health Interview Survey found that within a 2-week period, 975,000 children had a migraine resulting in 164,454 missed school days.[13] Measures of both disability and quality of life can be helpful in assessing the morbidity of the headaches and the effectiveness of treatment.

Disability

The Migraine Disability Assessment (MIDAS)[14-17] was created to assess disability in adults and has been used in long-term studies to demonstrate changes in disability resulting from treatment.[18,19] Because the MIDAS measures are not adequate for children, the Pediatric Migraine Disability Assessment (PedMIDAS)[20] was developed to evaluate similar domains in pediatric patients. PedMIDAS uses a patient-based disability scale[21] and has been helpful in assessing treatment strategies, showing, for example, an improvement in scores with prophylactic medication.[22] The use of MIDAS for adults and PedMIDAS for children can be

BOX 185-3 Migraine Without Aura and Migraine With Aura

MIGRAINE WITHOUT AURA (1.1)

Previously used terms: common migraine, hemicrania simplex

Description: recurrent headache disorder producing attacks lasting 4 to 72 hours. Typical characteristics of the headache are unilateral location, pulsating quality, moderate or severe intensity, aggravation by routine physical activity, and association with nausea or photophobia and phonophobia.

Diagnostic criteria:

A. At least 5 attacks fulfilling criteria B through D

B. Headache attacks lasting 4 to 72 hours (untreated or unsuccessfully treated)

  Sleep is also considered part of the headache duration.[1]

  In children, 1 to 72 hours is allowed. If between 1 and 2 hours, diary corroboration is required.[2]

C. Headache has at least 2 of the following characteristics:

  Unilateral location

  Bilateral headache is most common in children and most common in frontal.[3,4]

  Exclusive occipital location is worrisome based on meta-analysis.[4]

  Pulsating quality

  Moderate or severe pain intensity

  Aggravation by or causing avoidance of routine physical activity (eg, walking or climbing stairs)

D. During headache at least 1 of the following:

  Nausea or vomiting

  Photophobia and phonophobia

  In young children, this can be inferred by their behavior by the parents

E. Not attributed to another disorder

TYPICAL AURA WITH MIGRAINE HEADACHE (1.2.1)

Description: Typical aura consisting of visual or sensory or speech symptoms. Gradual development; duration no longer than 1 hour; a mix of positive and negative features and complete reversibility characterize the aura, which is associated with a headache fulfilling criteria for 1.1, Migraine without aura.

Diagnostic criteria:

A. At least 2 attacks fulfilling criteria B through D

B. Aura consisting of at least 1 of the following, but no motor weakness:

  Fully reversible visual symptoms including positive features (eg, flickering lights, spots, or lines) or negative features (ie, loss of vision)

  Fully reversible sensory symptoms including positive features (ie, pins and needles) or negative features (ie, numbness)

  Fully reversible dysphasic speech disturbance

C. At least 2 of the following:

  Homonymous visual symptoms or unilateral sensory symptoms

  At least 1 aura symptom develops gradually over 5 or more minutes or different aura symptoms occur in succession over 5 or more minutes

  Each symptom lasts $\geq$ 5 and $\leq$ 60 minutes

D. Headache fulfilling criteria B through D for 1.1, Migraine without aura, begins during the aura or follows aura within 60 minutes

E. Not attributed to another disorder

[1]When the patient falls asleep during migraine and wakes up without it, duration of the attack is reckoned until the time of awakening.

[2]In children, attacks may last 1-72 hours (although the evidence for untreated durations of less than 2 hours in children requires corroboration by prospective diary studies).

[3]Migraine headache is commonly bilateral in young children; an adult pattern of unilateral pain usually emerges in late adolescence or early adult life.

[4]Migraine headache is usually frontotemporal. Occipital headache in *children*, whether unilateral or bilateral, is rare and calls for diagnostic caution; many cases are attributable to structural lesions.

Modified from International Headache Society, Headache Classification Subcommittee. The International Classification of Headache Disorders. *Cephalalgia* 2004;24(supp 1):1-160. Reprinted by permission of Blackwell Publishing Ltd.

highly effective in assessing the disability caused by migraine and the effectiveness of treatment in improving outcomes.

Quality of Life

Studies have shown that headaches can have a significant negative effect on the social and psychological functioning of adults, greater even than other chronic conditions such as hypertension, diabetes, angina, and even myocardial infarction.[23,24] Similarly, the effect of headaches on the quality of life of children has been measured with the Pediatric Quality of Life Inventory version 4.0 (PedsQL 4.0) Generic Core Scales, an instrument that uses both parent and child input to evaluate health and emotional, social, and school functioning.[25,26] Although most children with migraines are able to function socially as well as healthy controls, chronic headaches have been found to have as significant an effect on emotional development and school functioning as rheumatologic, oncologic, and cardiac diseases. Treatment can also be assessed and modified according to how it improves scores on measures of quality of life.

PATHOPHYSIOLOGICAL FEATURES

The pathophysiological features of migraine headache remain undefined. Clearly, migraine has a genetic component. Twin studies and family studies have demonstrated a degree of inheritance as high as 90% in first- or second-degree relatives. For familial hemiplegic migraine, 3 genes have been identified as contributing to the disorder in several kindreds: P/Q-type calcium channel, adenosine triphosphatase, and sodium-potassium channel. Researchers have suggested a linkage with some of these genes in familial migraine with aura, but a consistent gene defect either in migraine without aura or in migraine with aura has not been identified.

The trigeminal neurovascular system's involvement with migraine has been proposed as a unifying theory to migraine. This model has been supported by several imaging studies that have demonstrated involvement of the brainstem near the trigeminal nucleus and the periaquaductal gray matter.

The pathophysiological features of TTHs in children is theoretically similar to that seen in adults. Two theories exist relating migraines and TTH. The continuum model suggests that migraine and TTH are one pathophysiological disorder, ranging from mild headaches that appear to be TTH to the most severe headaches that represent migraines associated with aura. This model is in contrast to the Spectrum model, which suggests that the 2 types are separate entities, with patients with migraine having a full spectrum of headaches, whereas patients with TTH have headaches limited to mild to moderate pain.

TTH may have a component of secondary muscle contraction, which may enhance a feedback loop to build the TTH. Recently, a role of central sensitization has been suggested and alternative theories reviewed.[27]

TREATMENT

The treatment of primary headache disorders in children is 3-fold: (1) acute therapy, (2) preventive therapy, and (3) biobehavioral therapy. The meta-analysis of the pharmacologic treatment of childhood headaches has been completed and a practice parameter developed.[28]

Acute Headache Treatment

Acute therapy is designed to ameliorate the episodic headache. The goal of this treatment is a quick return to normal activity without relapse.

Nonsteroidal Antiinflammatory Drugs and General Pain Relievers

For headache in children, medications include nonsteroidal antiinflammatory drugs (NSAIDs; ibuprofen, naproxen sodium, and for older children, aspirin) and general pain relievers (acetaminophen). Most prescriptive nonspecific medications have either not been evaluated in children or have not been proven effective. Ibuprofen has become a mainstay for the acute treatment of childhood headache and migraines because of its tolerability and its performance in clinical trials.[29,30] Proper use of ibuprofen requires the child to learn to identify the onset of the headache and initiate rapid treatment, use the proper dose based on weight, and avoid overuse typically by limiting its use to not more than 3 times per week.

Triptans

When NSAIDs are ineffective or not completely effective, migraine-specific therapy is often required. Many prescriptive medications contain sedatives or narcotics that may treat the pain, but they do not allow the child to return to normal functioning. Triptans are 5-$HT_{1B\text{-}1D}$ agonist migraine-specific medications. Currently, 7 triptans have been approved for use in the United States in adults, but none has been approved for the use of childhood migraine. Several studies in children, however, showed their effectiveness, including sumatriptan and zolmitriptan in tablet and nasal spray form and rizatriptan.[31-35]

Two treatment methods may be used when prescribing triptans.[18] One is the rescue therapy or stepwise treatment within an attack, in which the child starts with an NSAID at an appropriate dose at the onset of the headache. If this medication is not working, then a triptan is used as rescue therapy. The alternative method is the stratified care model, which requires the patient to determine the headache severity at the onset. For a mild or moderate headache, the patient takes an NSAID; and for a severe headache, the patient takes a prescribed triptan. In this way, patients stratify their headaches and the subsequent treatment. This method has not been successful in children because they often have difficulty recognizing the headache severity at its onset.

Recently, a third method—multimechanism treatment—has been found to be the most effective. In this method, NSAIDs are used for every headache within the limit of not treating more than 3 headaches per week, whereas triptans are added for moderate to severe headaches, limited to 4 to 6 times per month. This method recognizes the unique mechanisms of NSAIDs and triptans for the treatment of migraine and the synergistic nature of the combined treatment.

Dihydroergotamine

Ergot alkaloids have a long history of use dating back over 400 years. They were first recognized nearly 100 years ago for their usefulness in migraines with one of the most active forms being dihydroergotamine (DHE-45). Although DHE-45 was first found to be effective for migraine in 1945,[36] it fell out of use until Raskin reported its effectiveness in 1986.[37] Subsequently, DHE-45 has been synthesized and no longer has complications from purification. It is frequently used in the emergency management of childhood headaches.[38] Limited reports have shown the usefulness of intravenous DHE in an inpatient setting to break status migrainosus or prolonged migraines in children, possibly enhanced if patients are premedicated with dopamine antagonists such as promethazine or metoclopramide. More recently, nasal DHE has been used in adults. The extrapolation of this use in children, however, remains limited.

Dopamine Antagonists

Dopamine antagonists, which includes prochlorperazine and metoclopramide, were initially used for the nausea and vomiting effects of migraine headaches.[39] Subsequently, the dopaminergic model of migraine was developed, and these compounds have been reanalyzed for usefulness in acute therapy of the headaches themselves.[40] Because oral formulations are at best of limited effectiveness, dopamine antagonists should be given by the intravenous route. Their utility is limited, however, by extrapyramidal side effects. An open-label study in 20 children suggested prochlorperazine, when given with rehydrating fluids in the emergency room setting, can be used to break an acute episode of status migrainosus.[41]

Allodynia

Recently, cutaneous allodynia with central sensitization has been associated with migraine in adult patients.[42]

Allodynia can be considered as a painful or heightened sensation beyond the location of the headache. Patients who develop allodynia with central sensitization have decreased response to medication once the allodynia has been established.[43,44] If a patient is identified as having allodynia, then the primary care physician should stress the need for early treatment.

Analgesic Rebound Headaches

Avoiding overuse of medication is critical in acute therapy. Overuse can cause analgesic rebound headaches, which are transformed migraines, or chronic daily headaches. The process is characterized by inadequate treatment of headache with either a low-dose or a delayed treatment that then results in increase in use over time with decreased effectiveness. When rebound headaches are identified, a recovery period free of analgesic use is required.

Prophylactic Treatment

The second component of effective headache treatment is preventive therapy, or prophylactic medication. When headache or migraine becomes frequent or disabling, preventive medications must be considered, with a goal of minimizing the effect of the headache while reducing the number of headaches. A clear diminishment in severity and headache features may be observed. Although no defined threshold exists for preventive treatment, having more than 2 to 3 headaches per month typically warrants treatment. The decision to treat can be augmented by a disability instrument such as PedMIDAS.[20,21] No prophylactic medication has been approved for the prevention of childhood migraine. However, several studies have demonstrated the effectiveness of some of these medications. Prophylactic medication can be grouped into antiepileptic medications, antidepressant medications, antiserotonergic medications, and antihypertensive medications.

The antiepileptic medications used for the prevention of migraine include divalproate sodium, topiramate, gabapentin, levetiracetam, and zonisamide; however, only divalproate sodium and topiramate are currently approved for the prevention of migraines and only in adults.[45,46]

Amitriptyline, the most widely used tricyclic antidepressant for headache prevention, has been used for many decades for its antidepressive properties and was first recognized in the 1970s as an effective migraine therapy.[50-52] Most of the studies in children with amitriptyline have been open-label studies with no placebo-controlled studies.

In a crossover study by Levinstein comparing amitriptyline with propranolol and cyproheptadine, amitriptyline was found to be effective in 50% to 60% of the children.[53] In an open-label study, amitriptyline resulted in a perceived improvement in over 80% of the children, with subsequent decrease in frequency and impact of the headaches.[54] Because of side effects, especially somnolence, amitriptyline must be slowly titrated to full dose, typically over an 8- to 10-week period.

Although nortriptyline has been used instead of amitriptyline because of the concern about sleepiness as a side effect, it raises the concern of increased arrhythmia. Regular electrocardiographic evaluation may be required if nortriptyline is chosen.

Serotonin selective reuptake inhibitors have been studied for the treatment of headaches in adults but not yet in children. Their effectiveness, however, is not as notable as that of tricyclic antidepressants, suggesting that a more global decrease in neurotransmitter reuptake inhibition, rather than selective inhibition, is needed to treat childhood headache disorders.

Cyproheptadine, an antihistamine with antiserotonergic effects, has long been used for preventing childhood headaches.[55] It may also have some calcium channel–blocking properties.[56] Cyproheptadine tends to be well tolerated, with the most significant side effect being increased weight gain. Because of the significance of the weight gain, this medication tends to be limited to younger children, with less usefulness in teenagers.

Beta-blockers also have a long history of use for preventing childhood headaches.[57,58] Although one of the original studies demonstrated effectiveness, follow-up studies have been more controversial. In the recent practice parameter of the American Neurology Society,[59] propranolol was found to provide mixed responsiveness when used for childhood headaches. Furthermore, the drop in blood pressure caused by beta-blockers, as well as exercise-induced asthma, and their depressive effects limit usefulness in children. Given the availability of therapeutic alternatives, beta-blockers are generally more appropriate for adults, especially those with high blood pressure.

Calcium channel blockers have been extensively studied in adults for headache prevention. Flunarizine is a calcium channel blocker available in Europe but not in the United States, and it has been demonstrated to be an effective migraine preventive agent.[60,61] In children in a double-blinded, placebo-controlled crossover study, the baseline headache frequency was significantly reduced in the flunarizine-treated compared with the placebo group. These data cannot be extrapolated to other calcium channel blockers, which may not be as effective. For example, a double-blinded placebo-controlled crossover study using nimodipine in children showed no significant difference between the placebo and active drug groups.[62]

Additional prevention medications may include some nonpharmaceutical treatments, including both riboflavin[63,64] and coenzyme Q10.[65,66] Their effectiveness and usefulness in children has yet to be determined.

One of the keys in the use of prophylactic medications is to titrate the dose slowly to an effective level, which requires an understanding by the parent and patient that several weeks or months may be required before an effective level is achieved. The physician must identify a goal dose to achieve based on the patient's size and weight. In many instances, failure to respond to the preventive medication is caused by inadequate treatment because of either inadequate time of treatment or inadequate dosing. This failure may be based on patient's and the parents' unrealistic expectations about the rapidity of the response to the treatment protocol. Educating the patient about preventive therapy is essential to the patient's outcome.

Biobehavioral Treatment

Biobehavioral therapy for children, the third component of effective headache treatment, is essential to maintaining a lifetime response to the treatment and management of their headaches. Biobehavioral therapy can be divided into 3 components:

1. Treatment adherence entails a clear understanding by the patient and parent about the importance of the treatment. Psychological or biobehavioral intervention may be useful in assisting with adherence by identifying roadblocks to the medical plan and assist with overcoming these barriers.
2. Biobehavioral therapy also involves adjusting lifestyle habits. In many instances, unhealthy lifestyle habits, including inadequate nutrition, skipping meals, and altered sleep patterns, serve as a trigger for childhood headaches. Maintaining healthy lifestyle habits includes adequate fluid hydration with limited use of caffeine, regular exercise, adequate nutrition with regular meals and a balanced diet, and adequate sleep. The patient and parents must understand that these objectives are lifetime goals that will control the effect of migraine and minimize the use of medication. Lifestyle changes may result in an overall long-term improvement in quality of life and reverse any progressive nature of the disease.
3. Biofeedback-assisted relaxation therapy may be a useful addition.[67-70] For children, single-session biofeedback-assisted relaxation therapy has been demonstrated to be learned quickly and efficiently.

CONCLUSION

In summary, the treatment of childhood headaches requires a thorough investigation of the underlying cause, including the use of standardized diagnostic criteria and neurologic and comprehensive examinations. If secondary headaches are identified, then the headaches should resolve with treatment of the underlying cause. If the headaches persist or primary headaches are identified, then a 3-component treatment approach may need to be developed: acute therapy, preventive therapy, and biobehavioral therapy. All of these components need to be addressed in the treatment of childhood headaches and clear goals of treatment discussed with the patient and parents.

WHEN TO REFER

- Headaches that do not respond routinely to acute treatment
- Headaches that are increasing in frequency, severity, or duration
- Headaches in which the features acutely change
- Side effects of medications that limit increasing the medication to effective doses
- Psychological factors that interfere with management
- Disability that is impairing functioning

WHEN TO ADMIT

Admission or emergency department treatment should be considered when:

- Home therapies are ineffective for acute treatment.
- Headache has continued for more than 24 hours.
- Headache pain becomes intolerable.

TOOLS FOR PRACTICE

Engaging Patient and Family

- *Important Information for Teens Who Get Headaches* (brochure), American Academy of Pediatrics (patiented.aap.org).
- *What is a Pediatric Neurologist?* (fact sheet), American Academy of Pediatrics (www.aap.org/family/pedspecfact sheets.htm).

Medical Decision Support

- *American Headache Society* (Web page), American Headache Society (www.americanheadachesociety.org).

AAP POLICY STATEMENT

American Academy of Neurology, Quality Standards Subcommittee and Practice Committee of the Child Neurology Society. Pharmacological treatment of migraine headache in children and adolescents. *Pediatrics*. 2005;115(4):1107. (aappolicy.aappublications.org/cgi/content/full/pediatrics;115/4/1107). AAP endorsed.

REFERENCES

1. Bille B. Migraine in school children. *Acta Paediatrica*. 1962;51(suppl 136):16-151.
2. Split W, Neuman W. Epidemiology of migraine among students from randomly selected secondary schools in Lodz. *Headache*. 1999;39:494-501.
3. International Headache Society, Headache Classification Subcommittee. The International Classification of Headache Disorders. *Cephalalgia*. 2004;24(supp 1):1-160.
4. Hershey AD, Winner P, Kabbouche MA, et al. Use of the ICHD-II criteria in the diagnosis of pediatric migraine. *Headache*. Nov-Dec 2005;45(10):1288-1297.
5. Lewis DW, Ashwal S, Dahl G, et al. Practice parameter: evaluation of children and adolescents with recurrent headaches: report of the Quality Standards Subcommittee of the American Academy of Neurology and the Practice Committee of the Child Neurology Society. *Neurology*. 2002;59(4):490-498.
6. Linder SL. Understanding the comprehensive pediatric headache examination. *Pediatr Ann*. 2005;34(6):442-447.
7. Abu-Arafeh I, Russell G. Prevalence of headache and migraine in schoolchildren. *BMJ*. 1994;309:765-769.
8. Abu-Arafeh I. Chronic tension-type headache in children and adolescents. *Cephalalgia*. 2001;21(8):830-836.
9. Barea JM, Tannhauser M, Rotta NT. An epidemiologic study of headache among children and adolescents of southern Brazil. *Cephalalgia*. 1996;16:545-549.
10. Laurell K, Larsson B, Eeg-Olofsson O. Prevalence of headache in Swedish schoolchildren, with a focus on tension-type headache. *Cephalalgia*. 2004;24(5):380-388.
11. Anttila P, Metsahonkela L, Aromaa M, et al. Determinants of tension-type headache in children. *Cephalalgia*. 2002;22(5):401-408.
12. Anttila P, Metsahonkela L, Mikkelsson M, et al. Muscle tenderness in pericranial and neck-shoulder region in children with headache. A controlled study. *Cephalalgia*. 2002;22(5):340-344.
13. Stang PE, Osterhaus JT. Impact of migraine in the United States: data from the National Health Interview Survey. *Headache*. 1993;33:29-35.
14. Stewart WF, Lipton RB, Whyte J, et al. An international study to assess reliability of the Migraine Disability Assessment (MIDAS) score. *Neurology*. 1999;53:988-994.
15. Stewart WF, Lipton RB, Kolodner KB, et al. Validity of the Migraine Disability Assessment (MIDAS) score in comparison to a diary-based measure in a population sample of migraine sufferers. *Pain*. 2000;88:41-52.

16. Lipton RB, Stewart WF, Sawyer J, et al. Clinical utility of an instrument assessing migraine disability: the Migraine Disability Assessment (MIDAS) questionnaire. *Headache*. 2001;41(9):854-861.
17. Stewart WF, Lipton RB, Dowson AJ, et al. Development and testing of the Migraine Disability Assessment (MIDAS) questionnaire to assess headache-related disability. *Neurology*. 2001;56(6 suppl 1):S20-S28.
18. Lipton RB, Stewart WF, Stone AM, et al. Stratified care vs step care strategies for migraine: the Disability in Strategies of Care (DISC) study: a randomized trial. *JAMA*. 2000;284(20):2599-2605.
19. Lipton RB, Silberstein SD. The role of headache-related disability in migraine management: implications for headache treatment guidelines. *Neurology*. 2001; 56(6 suppl 1):S35-S42.
20. Hershey AD, Powers SW, Vockell A-LB, et al. PedMIDAS: development of a questionnaire to assess disability of migraines in children. *Neurology*. 2001;57(11):2034-2039.
21. Hershey AD, Powers SW, Vockell A-LB, et al. Development of a patient-based grading scale for PedMIDAS. *Cephalalgia*. 2004;24(10):844-849.
22. Hershey AD, Powers SW, Vockell A-LB, et al. Effectiveness of topiramate in the prevention of childhood headaches. *Headache*. 2002;42:810-818.
23. Osterhaus JT, Townsend RJ, Gandek B, et al. Measuring the functional status and well-being of patients with migraine headache. *Headache*. 1994;34:337-343.
24. Solomon GD, Skobieranda FG, Gragg LA. Quality of life and well-being of headache patients: measurement by the medical outcomes study instrument. *Headache*. 1993; 33:351-358.
25. Varni JW, Seid M, Kurtin PS. PedsQL 4.0: reliability and validity of the Pediatric Quality of Life Inventory version 4.0 generic core scales in healthy and patient populations. *Med Care*. 2001;39(8):800-812.
26. Powers SW, Patton SR, Hommel KA, et al. Quality of life in paediatric migraine: characterization of age-related effects using PedsQL 4.0. *Cephalalgia*. 2004;24(2):120-127.
27. Silberstein SD, Rosenberg J. Multispecialty consensus on diagnosis and treatment of headache. *Neurology*. 2000; 54:1553.
28. Hämäläinen ML, Hoppu K, Valkeila E, et al. Ibuprofen or acetaminophen for the acute treatment of migraine in children. *Neurology*. 1997;48:103-107.
29. Lewis DW, Kellstein D, Dahl G. Children's ibuprofen suspension for the acute treatment of pediatric migraine. *Headache*. 2002;42(8):780-786.
30. Linder SL. Subcutaneous sumatriptan in the clinical setting: the first fifty consecutive patients with acute migraine in a pediatric neurology office practice. *Headache*. 1995;35:291-292.
31. Winner PA, Prensky, Linder S. Efficacy and safety of oral sumatriptan in adolescent migraines. Presented at the American Association for the Study of Headache scientific meeting, Chicago, IL, 1996.
32. Winner P, Rothner AD, Saper J, et al. A randomized, double-blind, placebo-controlled study of sumatriptan nasal spray in the treatment of acute migraine in adolescents. *Pediatrics*. 2000;106:989-997.
33. Winner P, Hershey AD. Randomized, double-blind, placebo-controlled study of sumatriptan nasal spray in adolescent migraineurs. *Neurology*. 2004;62:A182.
34. Winner P, Lewis D, Visser WH, et al. Rizatriptan 5 mg for the acute treatment of migraine in adolescents: a randomized, double-blind, placebo-controlled study. *Headache*. 2002;42(1):49-55.
35. Linder SL, Dowson AJ. Zolmitriptan provides effective migraine relief in adolescents. *Int J Clin Pract*. 2000; 54(7):466-469.
36. Horton BT, Peters GA, Blumenthal LS. A new product in the treatment of migraine: a preliminary report. *Mayo Clin Proc*. 1945;20:241-248.
37. Raskin NH. Repetitive intravenous dihydroergotamine as therapy for intractable migraine. *Neurology*. 1986;36(7): 995-997.
38. Linder SL. Treatment of childhood headache with dihydroergotamine mesylate. *Headache*. 1994;34:578-580.
39. Jones J, Sklar D, Dougherty J, et al. Randomized double-blind trial of intravenous prochlorperazine for the treatment of acute headache. *JAMA*. 1989;261:1174-1176.
40. Peroutka SJ. Dopamine and migraine. *Neurology*. 1997; 49:650-656.
41. Kabbouche MA, Vockell AL-B, LeCates SL, et al. Tolerability and effectiveness of prochlorperazine for intractable migraine in children. *Pediatrics*. 2001;107(4):e62.
42. Burstein R, Cutrer FM. The development of cutaneous allodynia during a migraine attack: clinical evidence for the sequential recruitment of spinal and supraspinal nociceptive neurons in migraine. *Brain*. 2000;123: 1703-1709.
43. Burstein RB, Collins, Jakubowski M. Defeating migraine pain with triptans: a race against the development of cutaneous allodynia. *Ann Neurol*. 2004;55(1):19-26.
44. Burstein R, Jakubowski M. Analgesic triptan action in an animal model of intracranial pain: a race against the development of central sensitization. *Ann Neurol*. 2004;55(1):27-36.
45. Mathew NT, Saper JR, Silberstein SD, et al. Migraine prophylaxis with divalproex. *Arch Neurol*. 1995;52: 281-286.
46. Silberstein SD. Divalproex sodium in headache: literature review and clinical guidelines. *Headache*. 1996;36(9):547-555.
47. Caruso JM, Brown WD, Exil G, et al. The efficacy of divalproex sodium in the prophylactic treatment of children with migraine. *Headache*. 2000;40:672-676.
48. Serdaroglu G, Erhan E, Tekgul H, et al. Sodium valproate prophylaxis in childhood migraine. *Headache*. 2002;42(8): 819-822.
49. Winner P, Hershey AD. Topiramate for the prevention of migraines in children and adolescence: a randomized, double-blind, placebo-controlled trial. *Headache*. 2004; 44:481.
50. Couch JR, Ziegler DK, Hassanein R. Amitriptyline in the prophylaxis of migraine. Effectiveness and relationship of antimigraine and antidepressant effects. *Neurology*. 1976;26:121-127.
51. Gomersall JD, Stuart A. Amitriptyline in migraine prophylaxis. *J Neurol Neurosurg Psychiatry*. 1973;36: 684-690.
52. Couch JR, Hassanein RS. Amitriptyline in migraine prophylaxis. *Arch Neurology*. 1979;36:695-699.
53. Levinstein B. A comparative study of cyproheptadine, amitriptyline, and propranolol in the treatment of adolescent migraine. *Cephalalgia*. 1991;11:122-123.
54. Hershey AD, Powers SW, Bentti AL, et al. Effectiveness of amitriptyline in the prophylactic management of childhood headaches. *Headache*. 2000;40:539-549.
55. Bille B, Ludvigsson J, Sanner G. Prophylaxis of migraine in children. *Headache*. 1977;17:61-63.
56. Peroutka SJ, Allen GS. The calcium antagonist properties of cyproheptadine: implications for antimigraine action. *Neurology*. 1984;34(3):304-309.
57. Ludvigsson J. Propranolol used in prophylaxis of migraine in children. *Acta Neurol Scand*. 1974;50: 109-115.
58. Ziegler DK, Hurwitz A. Propranolol and amitriptyline in prophylaxis of migraine. *Arch Neurol*. 1993;50: 825-830.

59. Lewis D, Ashwal S, Hershey A, et al. Practice parameter: pharmacological treatment of migraine headache in children and adolescents: report of the American Academy of Neurology Quality Standards Subcommittee and the Practice Committee of the Child Neurology Society. *Neurology*. 2004;63(12):2215-2224.
60. Sorge F, De Simone R, Marano E, et al. Flunarizine in prophylaxis of childhood migraine. A double-blind, placebo-controlled, crossover study. *Cephalalgia*. 1988; 8(1):1-6.
61. Guidetti V, Moscato D, Ottaviano S, et al. Flunarizine and migraine in childhood. An evaluation of endocrine function. *Cephalalgia*. 1987;7(4):263-266.
62. Battistella PA, Ruffilli R, Moro R, et al. A placebo-controlled crossover trial of nimodipine in pediatric migraine. *Headache*. 1990;30(5):264-268.
63. Schoenen J, Jacquy J, Lenaerts M. Effectiveness of high-dose riboflavin in migraine prophylaxis: a randomized controlled trial. *Neurology*. 1998;50:466-470.
64. Boehnke C, Reuter U, Flach U, et al. High-dose riboflavin treatment is efficacious in migraine prophylaxis: an open study in a tertiary care centre. *Eur J Neurol*. 2004; 11(7):475-477.
65. Rozen TD, Ochinsky ML, Gebeline CA, et al. Open label trial of coenzyme Q10 as a migraine preventive. *Cephalalgia*. 2002;22(2):137-141.
66. Sandor PS, Di Clemente L, Coppola G, et al. Efficacy of coenzyme Q10 in migraine prophylaxis: a randomized controlled trial. *Neurology*. 2005;64:713-715.
67. Daly E, Donn PA, Galliher MJ, et al. Biofeedback applications to migraine and tension headaches: a double-blinded outcome study. *Biofeedback Self Reg*. 1983; 8(1):135-152.
68. Werder D, Sargent J. A study of childhood headache using biofeedback as a treatment alternative. *Headache*. 1984;24:122-126.
69. Powers SW, Spirito A. Biofeedback. In: Noshpitz JD, Harrison S, Eth S, eds. *Handbook of Child and Adolescent Psychiatry*. Vol 6. New York, NY: Wiley; 1998.
70. Powers SW, Hershey AD. Biofeedback for childhood migraine. In: Maria BL, ed. *Current Management in Child Neurology*. Hamilton, Ontario: BC Decker; 2002.

Chapter 186

HEARING LOSS

Anne Marie Tharpe, PhD; Douglas P. Sladen, PhD

Pediatricians are usually the first health care practitioners approached by parents when they have concerns about their child's hearing, and in the course of a typical practice a pediatrician will encounter approximately a dozen children with severe to profound hearing loss.[1] Although parents become concerned about their child's hearing rather early (at approximately 6 months of age) when the hearing loss is severe, milder degrees of hearing loss typically do not generate concern until the child reaches school age. As such, it is imperative that pediatricians recognize the signs, symptoms, and risk factors for hearing loss in children and become aware of appropriate referral paths. It is also important to note, that despite the widespread implementation of newborn hearing screening, such screening programs are designed to identify moderate degrees of hearing loss and greater, not mild degrees of loss. Therefore, just because a child passed a hearing screening in the newborn period does not mean that a child does not have a hearing loss. Hearing loss from otitis media, the most common type of loss encountered by pediatricians, is discussed in Chapter 39, Auditory Screening; and Chapter 304, Otitis Media and Otitis Externa. This chapter primarily addresses identifying children with permanent hearing loss.

DEMOGRAPHICS

Rubella and meningitis were once leading causes of severe to profound hearing loss in children; but the advent of vaccines for these disorders has virtually eliminated hearing loss caused by congenital rubella and has dramatically reduced hearing loss resulting from meningitis. Therefore severe to profound hearing losses are not as common as they once were, and milder degrees of hearing loss are more prevalent.[2]

Although estimates of the prevalence of severe bilateral hearing loss in newborns are 1 per 1000, estimates for very mild or minimal losses approach 1 per 20.[2] In the neonatal intensive care unit, estimates of hearing loss prevalence are approximately 20 to 40 per 1000.[1]

Figure 186-1 is the audiogram of a child with normal hearing sensitivity in both ears such that all the speech sounds fall within the range of audibility. Two of the more typical patterns of minimal to mild hearing loss are demonstrated in Figures 186-2 and 186-3. Figure 186-2 is the audiogram of a child with normal hearing sensitivity for all frequencies through 1000 Hz but exhibits a high-frequency hearing loss, a pattern typical with ototoxic drug use or perinatal anoxia. Although this child would be expected to develop speech and language in a timely manner, distortions or omissions of the high-frequency consonant sounds of speech are expected. Parents may report that the

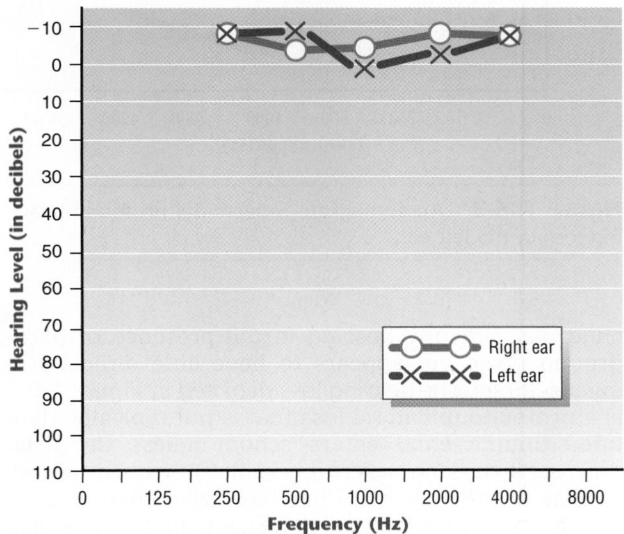

Figure 186-1 An audiogram reflecting normal hearing sensitivity in both ears.

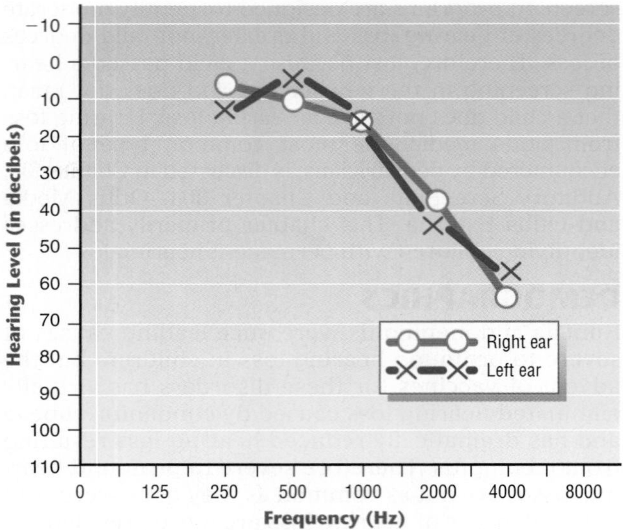

Figure 186-2 An audiogram reflecting a high-frequency hearing loss bilaterally.

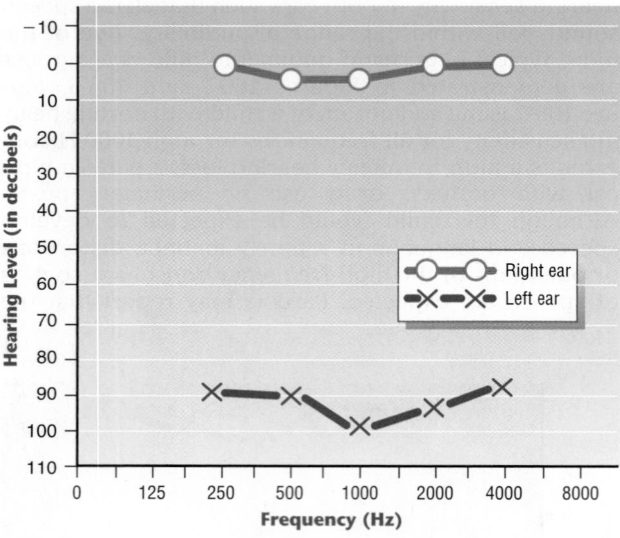

Figure 186-3 An audiogram reflecting a profound hearing loss of the left ear.

child has difficulty hearing in the presence of background noise but appears to have little difficulty in quiet settings. The hearing loss depicted in Figure 186-3 is a profound unilateral loss that is not typically identified until a child enters school unless the child receives a hearing screening in the newborn period. Similar to the child who has high-frequency hearing loss a child with unilateral hearing loss may reach age-appropriate speech and language milestones but experience difficulty hearing in the presence of background noise. In addition, children with unilateral hearing loss often demonstrate difficulty localizing sound sources.

Although these patterns of hearing loss are termed *mild* or *minimal,* recent evidence suggests that their effect is far from benign. School-aged children who have minimal and mild losses have been found to demonstrate greater academic, communicative, social, and emotional difficulty than normally hearing children. In fact, approximately 35% of children with minimal hearing losses fail at least one grade in school compared with an overall failure rate of approximately 3%.[2,3]

ASSOCIATED SIGNS AND SYMPTOMS

The Joint Committee on Infant Hearing has published a list of risk factors that provides an excellent starting place when attempting to identify hearing loss in children (see Chapter 39, Auditory Screening).[4] However, approximately 35% to 50% of children with hearing loss will not have any known risk factors,[5,6] making a complete history and keen observation accompanied by hearing screening essential if hearing loss is to be identified early. Although most congenital hearing loss is hereditary, a negative family history is common: 80% of inherited hearing loss results from autosomal-recessive transmission, 18% from autosomal-dominant transmission, and approximately 2% from X-linked recessive transmission. Furthermore, even children with dominantly inherited hearing loss may have families who demonstrate incomplete penetrance. Evidence of the gene expression can be highly variable. In addition, most children with inherited hearing loss are nonsyndromic, providing no additional clues and potentially limiting the pediatrician's level of suspicion. However, several syndromes are associated with congenital sensory hearing loss (eg, Alport syndrome, Waardenburg syndrome) or progressive loss (eg, Usher syndrome). Children with Down syndrome are at high risk for conductive hearing loss, as well as a higher-than-average risk for sensory loss.

Infants in the neonatal intensive care unit may also be at increased risk for neural conduction or auditory brainstem dysfunction, including auditory neuropathy/dyssynchrony, a recently identified disorder characterized by a unique constellation of behavioral and physiologic auditory test results.[7,8] Children with auditory neuropathy/dyssynchrony exhibit a range from normal hearing to profound hearing loss and poor speech perception. Infants who receive intensive neonatal care are at increased risk for auditory neuropathy/dyssynchrony, as are children with a family history of childhood hearing loss and infants with hyperbilirubinemia. However, some children with auditory neuropathy/dyssynchrony have no history of these risk factors. Currently, neither the prevalence of auditory neuropathy/dyssynchrony in newborns nor the natural history of the disorder is known; treatment options are not well defined. Audiologic and medical monitoring of infants at risk is recommended.

The significant speech and language delays associated with severe to profound childhood hearing loss provide a high level of suspicion to parents and physicians. However, identifying milder degrees of hearing loss may be more elusive. In addition to children who have speech and language delays or disorders, children who exhibit behavioral, social, or academic difficulties should be screened for hearing loss. Some of the concerns expressed commonly by parents of

Table 186-1 Explanations for Parental Concerns Regarding Their Child's Hearing Acuity

PARENTAL COMMENTS	EXPLANATIONS
"He can hear me when he wants to hear me. Sometimes he just ignores me."	Children who have mild hearing losses may have little or no difficulty listening in quiet settings. However, if background noise is present, then they may have more difficulty.
"When I call her, she has to look around for me. She never seems to know where I am in the house."	Children who have unilateral hearing loss often have difficulty localizing a sound source.
"When we are in crowds, I have to call his name several times before he responds."	Children who have high-frequency or other mild hearing losses often have difficulty hearing in the presence of background noise.
"My child is exhausted when she comes home from school."	Children who have minimal or mild hearing loss may be fatigued by the effort exerted to listen throughout the day.
"His speech is very difficult to understand. I don't think it's his hearing, because he always responds when I call him."	Children who have high-frequency hearing loss may have poor speech production because they are unable to hear high-frequency speech sounds (consonants) even though they can hear low- and mid-frequency sounds.
"My child is doing poorly in school, but I know she understands the material because we go over her homework at night."	Children who have minimal hearing loss may have difficulty hearing in school settings because of the background noise. When working at home in a one-on-one situation, they may demonstrate no hearing difficulties.

children who have milder forms of hearing loss are included in Table 186-1.

IDENTIFICATION APPROACHES

Despite the widespread and successful implementation of universal screening programs across the United States, significant concerns remain. First, a large percentage of infants are not brought back to the screening hospital for follow-up.[4] Many of these infants can be recaptured when they are seen in pediatricians' offices for well- or sick-baby visits. Second, even if an infant is screened for hearing loss at birth, many children diagnosed with hearing loss acquire their deficits after the newborn period. Finally, the Joint Committee on Infant Hearing recommends that universal newborn hearing screening programs target permanent, bilateral, or unilateral hearing loss averaging 40 dB or greater, a target level that will necessarily miss some minimal and mild hearing loss. The obvious implication is that, even for children who have passed their newborn hearing screens, pediatricians should be vigilant in monitoring hearing status and, with any suspicion of hearing loss, should arrange for hearing assessments by audiologists experienced in working with children.

When an infant or child fails a hearing, speech, or language screening measure in the pediatrician's office, referral for a full audiologic evaluation is recommended. Unfortunately, a recent study suggested that more than one half of children who failed hearing screenings in primary care practices did not receive rescreenings or referrals for further testing.[9] Audiologists with pediatric experience can define the degree of hearing loss and distinguish among conductive, sensory, and neural types of loss in children of all chronologic ages and developmental levels. Evaluation of hearing in infants and young children consists of a combination of physiological and behavioral measures. For infants younger than approximately 6 months, testing is typically limited to physiological measures because their behavioral responses are not yet reliable enough for defining the extent of hearing loss. A description of the procedures of choice can be found in Chapter 39, Auditory Screening.

MANAGEMENT

The early identification of hearing loss in children is of little value if intervention is not initiated in a timely manner. Many children have conductive and sensorineural hearing losses that are not amenable to medical treatment. For these children, several options remain, the most familiar being the traditional hearing aid: devices designed to pick up sounds in the child's environment and convert them to electrical signals that are amplified, filtered, and converted back to acoustic signals by a receiver. For children in noisy settings (eg, child-care centers, classrooms), frequency-modulated systems can be used alone or in combination with hearing aids. These systems use a microphone worn by the teacher to amplify only the teacher's voice while minimizing the interfering background noise. The signal is transmitted to the child via a frequency-modulated signal, which is received by a hearing aid or loudspeaker.

Most children who have hearing loss benefit from some form of amplification. However, in cases of profound hearing loss, conventional amplification may not be enough. An alternative to traditional hearing aids for these children is the cochlear implant, a surgically implanted device with electrodes that are coiled into the cochlea to stimulate the auditory nerve with electrical current. Although cochlear implants do not restore normal hearing and children vary markedly in the benefits they derive from the implant, the vast majority experience at least an awareness of sound, and some reach a high level of speech recognition enabling the development of normal speech and language skills.

As the gatekeepers for children's health care, pediatricians are responsible for recognizing the signs and symptoms of hearing loss in their young patients. Only through the vigilance of pediatricians and other health care practitioners will the age of identification of hearing loss in children be lowered, thus avoiding delays in intervention.

For infants with permanent hearing loss, communication with the state's coordinator for early hearing detection and intervention should ensure that the child and family are enrolled in appropriate early intervention services. The pediatrician should also ensure that the child has received a thorough medical evaluation to determine the cause of the hearing loss, including a genetics consultation. Children with permanent hearing loss are especially vulnerable to the effects of otitis media with effusion because additional hearing loss can negatively affect the audibility of speech through hearing aids. As such, pediatricians must closely monitor and manage children who have persistent otitis media with effusion. Furthermore, because of the high incidence of vision problems in children with hearing loss, a referral for ophthalmologic evaluation may be warranted. Finally, approximately 30% to 40% of children with hearing loss have additional disabilities. Therefore periodic developmental screening and surveillance, as recommended by the Joint Committee on Infant Hearing,[4] is an integral part of the management of these children.

WHEN TO REFER

- Family history of permanent hearing loss
- Postnatal infections associated with sensorineural hearing loss (eg, meningitis)
- History of in-utero infections (eg, syphilis, toxoplasmosis, rubella, cytomegalovirus, herpes)
- Neonatal indicators associated with progressive or late-onset hearing loss, including hyperbilirubinemia requiring exchange transfusion, persistent pulmonary hypertension of the newborn associated with mechanical ventilation, and use of extracorporeal membrane oxygenation
- Syndromes associated with progressive hearing loss (eg, Usher syndrome, neurofibromatosis)
- Neurodegenerative disorders (eg, Charcot-Marie-Tooth disease, Friedreich ataxia)
- Head trauma
- Child does not pass a hearing screen in the pediatrician's office
- Patient or caregiver concern about hearing, speech, or language development

TOOLS FOR PRACTICE

Engaging Patient and Family

- *Your Baby Needs Another Hearing Test* (brochure), Maternal Child Health Bureau, Health Resources and Services Administration and health literacy researchers at Louisiana State University (medicalhomeinfo.org/screening/Screen%20Materials/Another%20hearing%20test.pdf).

Medical Decision Support

- *NIDCD Fact Sheet: When a Newborn Doesn't Pass the Hearing Screening* (fact sheet), National Institute on Deafness and Other Communication Disorders (www.medicalhomeinfo.org/screening/Screen%20Materials/NIDCD%20Fact%20Sheet%20How%20Medical%20and%20Other%20Professionals.pdf).

RELATED WEB SITES

- Centers for Disease Control and Prevention: Developmental Disabilities—Centers for Disease Control and Prevention: Hearing Loss (www.cdc.gov/ncbddd/dd/ddhi.htm).
- Early Hearing Detection and Intervention (EHDI) Program (http://www.cdc.gov/ncbddd/ehdi/default.htm).

AAP POLICY STATEMENT

Joint Committee on Infant Hearing. Year 2007 Position Statement: Principles and Guidelines for Early Hearing Detection and Intervention Programs. *Pediatrics*. 2007;120(4):898-921. (aappolicy.aappublications.org/cgi/content/full/pediatrics;120/4/898).

REFERENCES

1. US Department of Health and Human Services, Public Health Service. *Healthy People 2000, National Health Promotion and Disease Prevention Objectives for the Nation.* (DHHS [PHS] Publication No. 91-50212). Washington, DC: US Government Printing Office; 1990.
2. Bess FH, Dodd-Murphy J, Parker RA. Children with minimal sensorineural hearing loss: prevalence, educational performance and functional status. *Ear Hear.* 1998;19(5):339-354.
3. Bess FH, Tharpe AM. Unilateral hearing impairment in children. *Pediatrics*. 1984;74:206-216.
4. Joint Committee on Infant Hearing. Year 2007 position statement. *Pediatrics*. 2007;120(4):898-921.
5. Davis A, Wood S, Healy R, et al. Risk factors for hearing disorders: epidemiologic evidence of change over time in the UK. *J Am Acad Audiol*. 1995;6(5):365-370.
6. Stein LK. Factors influencing the efficacy of universal newborn hearing screening. *Pediatr Clin North Am*. 1999;46(1):95-105.
7. Sininger YS, Hood LJ, Starr A, et al. Hearing loss due to auditory neuropathy. *Audiology Today*. 1995;7:10-13.
8. Starr A, Picton TW, Sininger Y, et al. Auditory neuropathy. *Brain*. 1996;119(3):741-753.
9. Holloran DR, Wall TC, Evans HH, et al. Hearing screening at well-child visits. *Arch Pediatr Adolesc Med*. 2005;159:949-955.

Chapter 187

HEART MURMURS

Christine Tracy, MD; Christine A. Walsh, MD

A heart murmur is a common finding during the physical examination of children. However, few children with heart murmurs will have structural cardiac disease. The challenge for the primary care physician lies in distinguishing innocent murmurs from those that indicate a cardiac abnormality.

CARDIAC CYCLE AND ASSOCIATED HEART SOUNDS

The pediatric primary care physician needs to understand the events of the cardiac cycle and its associated heart sounds when determining the significance of a heart murmur. Heart sounds as auscultated during physical examination are directly related to the hemodynamic events of systole and diastole (Figure 187-1).

The first heart sound (S1) is related to the closure of the mitral and tricuspid valves at the very end of diastole, at which time the ventricles are completely filled. The ventricles then undergo a period of isovolumic contraction, followed by opening of the aortic and pulmonary valves and the beginning of the phase of rapid systolic ejection. This phase is followed by a phase of reduced ejection later in systole.

The second heart sound (S2) is created by the closure of the aortic and pulmonary valves at the very end of systole. Physiological splitting of S2 is particularly important in the diagnosis of cardiac disease. The first component of S2 is created by the closure of the aortic valve (A2), and the second component of S2 is created by the closure of the pulmonary valve (P2).

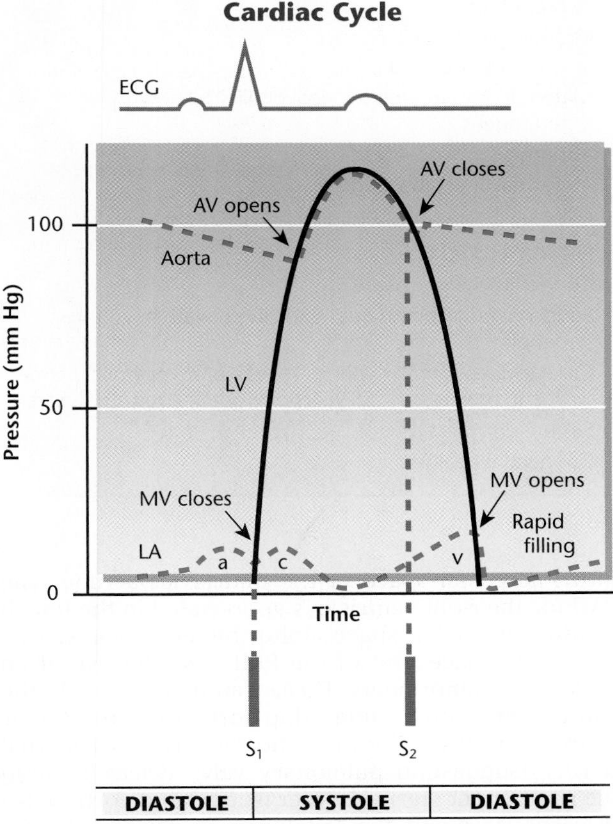

Figure 187-1 Pressure-time relationships of the left-sided heart chambers are illustrated during the normal cardiac cycle. *AV,* aortic valve; *ECG,* electrocardiogram; *LA,* left atrium; *LV,* left ventricle; *mm Hg,* millimeters of mercury; *MV,* mitral valve; S_1, first heart sound; S_2, second heart sound. (*Lilly LS.* Pathophysiology of Heart Disease, *3rd ed. Philadelphia: Lippincott Williams & Wilkins; 2003. Used by permission.*)

During inspiration P2 occurs after A2, generating an audibly split S2 (A2-P2). During exhalation, the closure of the aortic and pulmonary valves is nearly coincident, creating a single S2. Splitting of S2 can be difficult to appreciate in infants or children with accelerated heart rates, but a normal splitting pattern helps distinguish an abnormality from normalcy.

Wide splitting of S2 is associated with prolonged ejection from the right ventricle, as occurs with conditions such as an atrial septal defect (ASD), in which S2 is widely split and fixed. A narrowly split S2 is associated with pulmonary hypertension, in which closure of P2 is early, or aortic stenosis, when closure of A2 is delayed. Failure of S2 to split at all can be the result of simultaneous closure of the aortic and pulmonary valves during all phases of the respiratory cycle, found with conditions that result in high pulmonary artery pressure. A single S2 can also be associated with certain congenital cardiac anomalies, such as truncus arteriosus and tetralogy of Fallot, or with certain cardiac surgical palliations, such as the bidirectional Glenn shunt or the Fontan completion.

Third and fourth heart sounds may also be appreciated during physical examination. The third heart sound (S3) is heard early in diastole, during the initial phase of passive rapid ventricular filling. It is a low-frequency sound that can be best heard at the left lower sternal border or at the apex. An apical S3 can frequently be heard in healthy children, as well as in competitive athletes. The fourth heart sound (S4) is always pathological. S4 is also a low-frequency sound but is heard late in diastole, just before S1. It results from rapid filling of the ventricle caused by atrial contraction. An S4 gallop is associated with decreased ventricular compliance (as is seen in cardiomyopathy) and congestive heart failure. Auscultation of an S4 gallop warrants immediate evaluation by a pediatric cardiologist.

Clicks may also be audible during the cardiac cycle. Ejection clicks are heard in systole; the timing of the click in the cardiac cycle helps elucidate the cause. An early systolic click, heard just after S1, is associated with semilunar valve stenosis (aortic stenosis or pulmonary stenosis) or dilation of the great arteries (the aorta or pulmonary artery). Aortic valve clicks, best heard at the apex or right upper sternal border, do not vary in intensity with respiration. Pulmomary valve clicks increase in intensity with exhalation, and they are best heard along the left sternal border. A midsystolic apical click is heard with mitral valve prolapse and may be accompanied by a late systolic murmur.

CARDIAC ANATOMY

In evaluating a child with a heart murmur, the physician must understand the anatomy of the heart and its position in the chest. The location of the heart murmur on the chest wall can serve as an important tool in deciding whether the murmur is innocent or pathological. Figure 187-2 demonstrates the location of the valves of the heart in relation to their position on the chest wall.

PATIENT EVALUATION

History

A complete and accurate history is one of the most important aspects of evaluating a cardiac murmur in

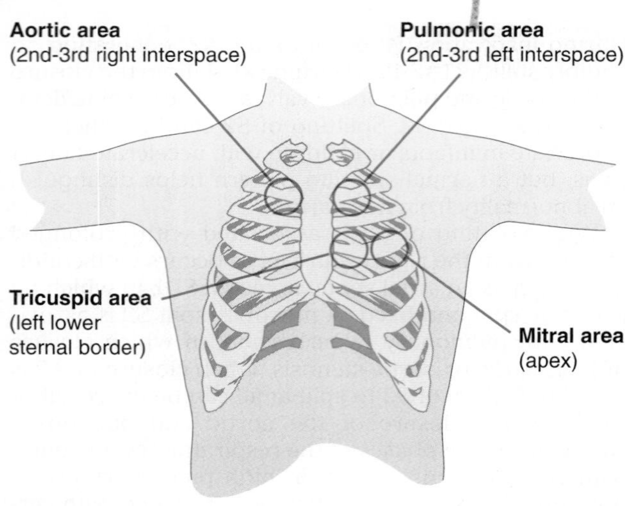

Figure 187-2 Areas of cardiac auscultation are governed by the location of the heart valves in relation to their position on the chest wall. (*Lilly LS.* Pathophysiology of Heart Disease, *3rd ed. Philadelphia: Lippincott Williams & Wilkins; 2003. Used by permission.*)

children because certain aspects of the patient's history may raise or lower the index of suspicion regarding the cause of a heart murmur. The history should include the patient's chief complaints and medical history, including the birth history and family history (Box 187-1).

Physical Examination

Evaluation of a cardiac murmur involves much more than auscultation of the heart. A complete physical examination in the child or adolescent with a heart murmur is needed to put the murmur in perspective. Pertinent aspects of the physical examination in a patient with a heart murmur are outlined in Table 187-1.

BOX 187-1 Raised Index of Suspicion for Cardiac Disease

PATIENT HISTORY

Poor weight gain or difficulty feeding
Frequent respiratory difficulties or respiratory distress
Cyanosis
Exercise intolerance
Chest pain with exercise
Unexplained syncope (especially syncope resulting in injury)
Concurrent syndromic disorder or genetic disease
Concurrent metabolic disorder or storage disease
Sickle cell anemia or blood dyscrasias resulting in anemia
History of cardiotoxic chemotherapy
Concurrent human immunodeficiency virus disease
Hypertension

BIRTH HISTORY

Maternal diabetes
Maternal TORCH (*t*oxoplasmosis, other agents, *r*ubella, *c*ytomegalovirus, *h*erpes simplex) infections during pregnancy
Multiple gestation pregnancy
In vitro fertilization pregnancy
Maternal drug use (either legal or illicit), known teratogens
Abnormal amniocentesis
Abnormal fetal ultrasound
Maternal history of congenital heart disease

FAMILY HISTORY

Congenital heart disease
Sudden cardiac death or unexplained death in young people
Cardiac disease in the young—stroke or myocardial infarction in men aged <55 years or women aged <65 years
Seizure disorders
Congenital deafness

CARDIAC EVALUATION

A detailed cardiac examination includes thorough inspection, palpation, and auscultation.

Inspection

Inspection truly begins with the overall patient: general appearance, nutritional status, genetic abnormalities, color, and comfort. The chest wall should then be inspected for abnormalities, including deformities such as a pectus excavatum, asymmetry, and surgical scars.

Palpation

Palpation usually begins with the extremities. Evaluation of overall perfusion includes assessment of pulses, capillary refill, and temperature of extremities. The precordium is then palpated to detect the point of maximal impulse (PMI) of the left and right ventricles and to detect thrills. Under normal conditions, the PMI for the left ventricle is palpated in the left fourth or fifth intercostal space in the midclavicular line. The PMI for the right ventricle is appreciated in the fourth to fifth intercostal space along the left lower sternal border. Displacement of the PMI is suggestive of an underlying abnormality. Thrills can be palpated in the suprasternal notch (suggesting aortic valve disease or coarctation of the aorta), along the left upper sternal border (suggesting pulmonary valve disease), along the right upper sternal border (suggesting aortic valve disease), or along the left lower sternal border (in association with ventricular septal defects [VSDs]). A thrill is an abnormal finding and warrants referral to a pediatric cardiologist.

Auscultation

A systematic approach to auscultation of the heart ensures that each major anatomic area of the heart is heard in systole and diastole. The major areas of

Table 187-1 Physical Examination to Evaluate a Heart Murmur

SITE	FINDING
Vital signs	Temperature, heart rate, respiratory rate, height, weight Blood pressures in the right arm, left arm, leg Pulse oximetry on room air (right hand and either foot if infant)
General	Cyanosis, pallor, dysmorphic features, overall distress Breathing pattern: retractions, grunting, nasal flaring
Head and neck	Jugular venous distension Thyromegaly, thyroid nodules
Chest	Chest wall deformity, asymmetry, surgical scars Lung aeration Rales, rhonchi, wheezes, stridor
Cardiac	Inspection Palpation Auscultation
Abdominal	Liver span Tenderness Distension, ascites
Extremities	Perfusion: capillary refill, temperature, quality of pulses Clubbing, cyanosis, edema Arachnodactyly, joint laxity (Marfan syndrome) Increased arm span/upper to lower body ratio (Marfan syndrome)

auscultation on the precordium are the apex, the left lower sternal border, the left mid or upper sternal border, and the right upper sternal border. These areas correspond to each atrioventricular and semilunar valve, as well as the outflow tracts of the right and left ventricles (see Figure 187-2). The clinician should also auscultate the left and right infraclavicular areas, the axillae, and the back. Auscultation for a continuous sound (bruit) should be performed over the liver and fontanelle. A bruit suggests an arteriovenous malformation. The patient should be examined in the supine, sitting, and left lateral decubitus positions. Other postural maneuvers, such as squatting or standing, or performing a Valsalva maneuver, may be useful during auscultation. Auscultation includes an assessment of S1 and S2, including the nature of the splitting of S2. Consideration of any S3 and S4, murmurs, clicks, and rubs completes the auscultation.

EVALUATION OF HEART MURMUR

A heart murmur is the result of turbulent blood flow. Random fluctuations in velocity and pressure during blood flow results in vibration of the surrounding tissue, which is auscultated as a murmur. A complete description of a heart murmur includes its intensity, timing, location, radiation, and quality.

Table 187-2 Intensity of Systolic Murmurs

GRADE	DESCRIPTION
I	Barely audible
II	Soft, but easily audible
III	Moderately loud without a thrill
IV	Moderately loud with a thrill
V	Loud with a thrill, heard with stethoscope barely on the chest
VI	Loud with a thrill, heard with stethoscope off the chest

Table 187-3 Intensity of Diastolic Murmurs

GRADE	DESCRIPTION
I	Barely audible
II	Soft, but immediately heard
III	Easily heard
IV	Very loud

Intensity

The intensity of a murmur is graded on a scale of I to VI for murmurs in systole (Table 187-2). Some cardiologists use a scale of I to IV for murmurs in diastole (Table 187-3). The intensity of a murmur does not necessarily reflect the severity of the abnormality. For example, a small VSD may have a very loud murmur, but critical aortic stenosis may have a very soft murmur if cardiac output is low.

Timing

Timing refers to the point in the cardiac cycle at which the murmur is heard. Murmurs are described as being systolic, diastolic, or continuous.

Systolic murmurs occur during anatomic systole, the time beginning with atrioventricular valve closure (S1) and ending with semilunar valve closure (S2). Systolic murmurs are further divided into ejection (crescendo-decrescendo) murmurs, holosystolic (pansystolic, S1 coincident) murmurs, and late systolic murmurs (Figure 187-3).

Ejection murmurs begin shortly after S1, peak in intensity, and then end at or before S2. Ejection murmurs may be innocent or pathological. Most innocent murmurs are grade I to III systolic ejection murmurs. Pathological ejection murmurs result from either obstructed blood flow across a semilunar valve (aortic or pulmonary stenosis) or excessive volume crossing a normal semilunar valve (ASD); they may be of any grade of intensity. Holosystolic murmurs start with S1 and continue to S2 at the same level of intensity, sometimes obscuring S2 during auscultation. These murmurs result from movement of blood from a higher-pressure chamber to a lower-pressure chamber, such

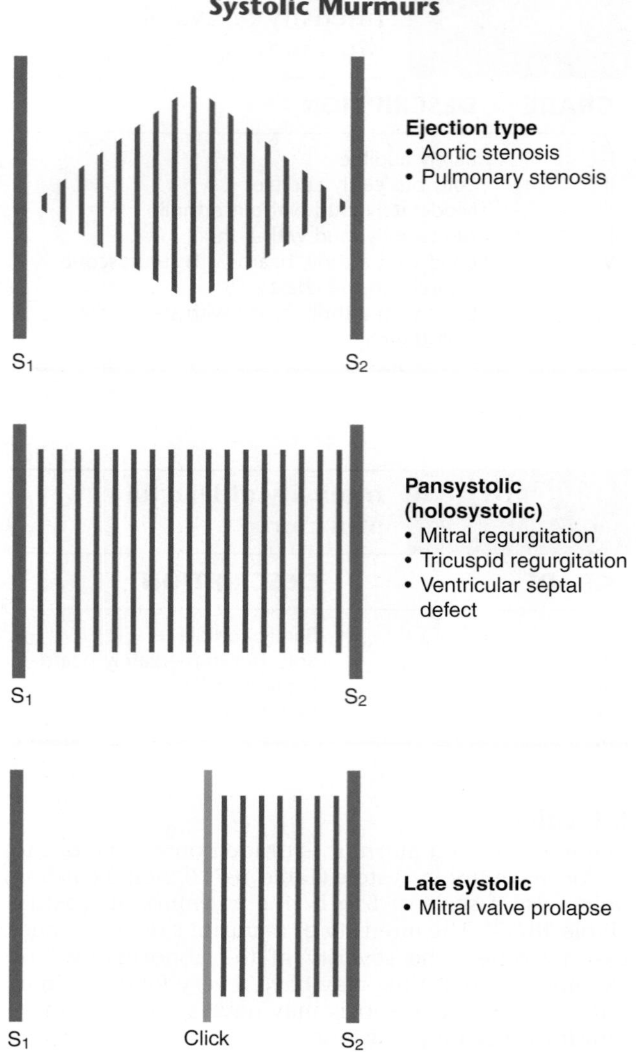

Figure 187-3 Classification of systolic murmurs. S_1, First heart sound; S_2, second heart sound. (*Lilly LS.* Pathophysiology of Heart Disease, *3rd ed. Philadelphia: Lippincott Williams & Wilkins; 2003. Used by permission.*)

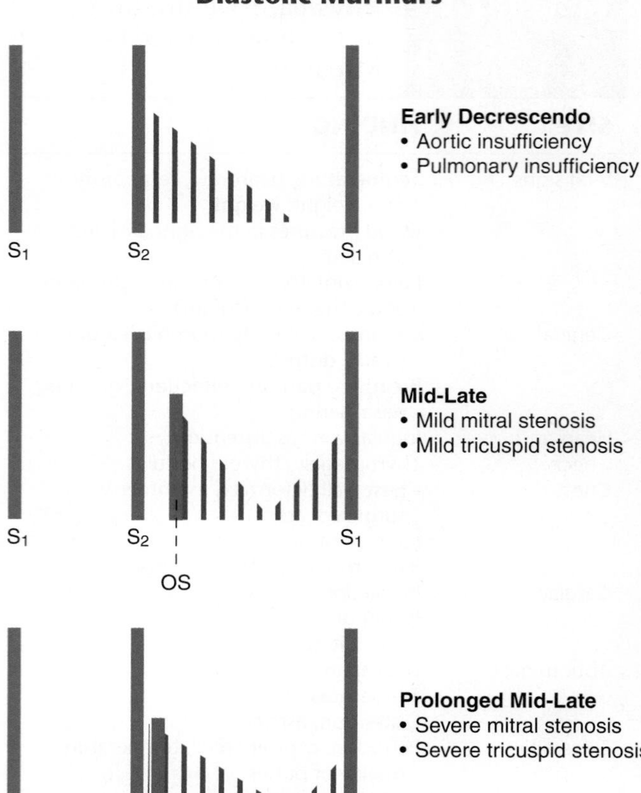

Figure 187-4 Classification of diastolic murmurs. *OS,*Opening snap; S_1, first heart sound; S_2, second heart sound. (*Lilly LS.* Pathophysiology of Heart Disease, *3rd ed. Philadelphia: Lippincott Williams & Wilkins; 2003. Used by permission.*)

as with a VSD or mitral regurgitation. Late systolic murmurs are associated with mitral valve prolapse and resultant mitral regurgitation. They are classically preceded by a midsystolic click.

Diastolic murmurs occur during anatomic diastole, the time beginning with semilunar valve closure (S2) and ending with atrioventricular valve closure (S1); they are further divided into early, mid, and late diastolic murmurs (Figure 187-4). Diastolic murmurs are all pathological by definition and require referral to a pediatric cardiologist. Early-diastolic murmurs begin immediately after S2 and are decrescendo in nature; they become less audible as the ventricle fills. Aortic insufficiency and pulmonary insufficiency are heard in early diastole. Mid-diastolic murmurs occur clearly after S2, during the rapid filling phase of the ventricle. Mitral stenosis and tricuspid stenosis murmurs are heard in mid diastole. Late-diastolic (presystolic) murmurs occur near the end of diastole, during the phase of atrial contraction. Severe mitral stenosis or tricuspid stenosis murmurs increase in late diastole.

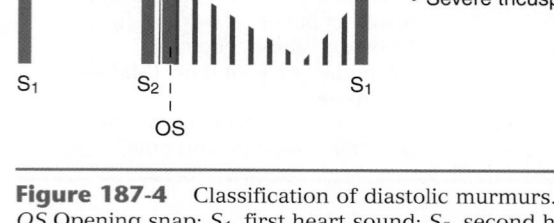

Continuous murmurs begin in systole, continue throughout systole, and end some time during diastole. These murmurs are almost always vascular in origin and are caused by aortopulmonary (eg, patent ductus arteriosus) or arteriovenous (eg, arteriovenous fistula) connections, turbulent flow in arteries (eg, coarctation of the aorta), or turbulent flow in veins (eg, venous hum). These murmurs are pathological, with the exception of the innocent venous hum (Table 187-4). Continuous murmurs sound fairly uniform until they soften in late diastole (Figure 187-5). These murmurs result from such lesions as a patent ductus arteriosus, an arteriovenous malformation, and a surgical shunt. A to-and-fro murmur describes an ejection murmur heard in systole, coupled to a decrescendo murmur early in diastole. To-and-fro murmurs

Table 187-4 Common Innocent Murmurs

MURMUR	INTENSITY	TIMING	LOCATION	QUALITY
Still	I-III/VI	Early-mid systolic	LM-LLSB or apex	Vibratory, musical
Pulmonary	I-III/VI	Early-mid systolic	LUSB	Low-pitched, ejection
Venous hum	I-III/VI	Continuous	Right or left infra- or supraclavicular	Low-pitched, disappears with head turn, supine position, jugular compression

LM-LLSB, Left mid-to-left lower sternal border; *LUSB,* left upper sternal border.

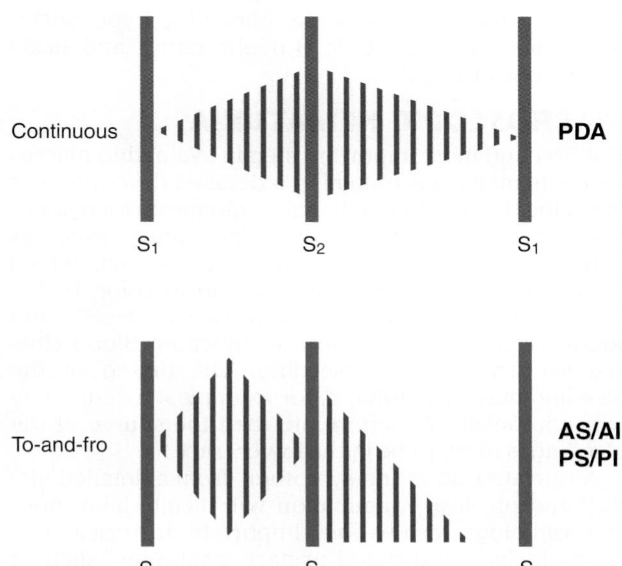

Figure 187-5 Continuous murmur versus to-and-fro murmur is illustrated. *AS/AI,* Aortic stenosis and aortic insufficiency; *PDA,* patent ductus arteriosus; *PS/PI,* pulmonary stenosis and pulmonary insufficiency; S_1, first heart sound; S_2, second heart sound. (*Lilly LS.* Pathophysiology of Heart Disease, *3rd ed. Philadelphia: Lippincott Williams & Wilkins; 2003. Used by permission.*)

are not true continuous murmurs. Combined aortic stenosis and aortic insufficiency or pulmonary stenosis and pulmonary insufficiency produce to-and-fro murmurs.

Location and Radiation

Location and radiation refer to the area where the murmur is heard the best and where it radiates. As seen in Figure 187-2, location helps narrow the differential diagnosis of the murmur. Radiation of the murmur can also aid in forming the differential diagnosis. For example, murmurs that radiate to the neck tend to be of aortic or left ventricular outflow tract origin, whereas a murmur heard best at the left upper sternal border with radiation to the axillae and back is more likely to be pulmonary in origin.

Postural maneuvers are useful in distinguishing among different types of murmurs. Innocent murmurs tend to become louder when the patient moves from an upright to a supine position. Placing the patient in the left lateral decubitus position increases the murmur of mitral stenosis. A Valsalva maneuver, by decreasing venous return, makes the murmur of aortic stenosis softer, but it makes the murmur of hypertrophic obstructive cardiomyopathy louder; it also decreases the murmurs associated with a VSD and mitral regurgitation and can nearly eliminate innocent Still murmurs (Table 187-4). Squatting increases venous return and makes the murmur of hypertrophic obstructive cardiomyopathy softer. Standing up after squatting can accentuate the murmur or click of mitral valve prolapse by moving the murmur and click closer to S1. Turning the head can eliminate the innocent continuous murmur of a venous hum.

Quality

Quality refers to the pitch and nature of a murmur. Pitch is generally described as either high or low. High-pitched murmurs occur when the pressure differential involved is large. For example, aortic insufficiency is a high-pitched murmur. Low-pitched murmurs occur when a lower pressure differential is involved. Pulmonary insufficiency is a low-pitched murmur. Systolic murmurs are described as ejection, regurgitant, harsh, blowing, musical, or vibratory. Diastolic murmurs are described as blowing, rumbling, crescendo, or decrescendo.

CONCLUSION

Primary care physicians are commonly faced with the questions of whether a heart murmur is innocent and whether the patient should be referred to a pediatric cardiologist. Most murmurs in children and adolescents are innocent. They do not reflect cardiac disease, and they do not require referral to a pediatric cardiologist, prophylaxis against endocarditis, or exercise restriction. Innocent murmurs are generally short systolic murmurs and are less than grade IV. They are often described as vibratory or musical, are best heard in the supine position, and often diminish when the patient is upright or during a Valsalva maneuver. Common innocent murmurs of childhood are described in Table 187-4. Findings that require a referral to a pediatric cardiologist are listed below.

WHEN TO REFER

- Patient, maternal, or family history raising index of suspicion for heart disease
- All diastolic murmurs
- Continuous murmurs, except venous hum
- All systolic murmurs grade IV or higher
- All systolic murmurs not clearly fitting the pattern of innocent murmur
- Cyanosis, clubbing
- Higher blood pressure in one or both arms than a leg
- Congestive heart failure—rales, respiratory distress, hepatomegaly, edema
- Abnormal electrocardiogram
- Symptoms that suggest reactive airway disease that do not improve with appropriate medical therapy

TOOLS FOR PRACTICE

Engaging Patient and Family

- *Caring for Your Baby and Young Child: Birth to Age 5* (book), American Academy of Pediatrics (www.aap.org/bookstore).

RELATED WEB SITE

- American Heart Association (www.americanheart.org/presenter.jhtml?identifier=4571).

SUGGESTED RESOURCES

Allen HD, Gutgesell HP, Clark EB, et al. *Moss and Adams' Heart Disease in Infants, Children, and Adolescents.* 6th ed. Philadelphia, PA: Lippincott Williams & Wilkins; 2001.

Berne RM, Levy MN, et al. *Physiology.* 4th ed. St Louis, MO: Mosby; 1998.

Park MK. *The Pediatric Cardiology Handbook.* 3rd ed. Philadelphia, PA: Mosby; 2003.

Chapter 188
HEMATURIA

Kimberly J. Reidy, MD; Marcela Del Rio, MD

Hematuria may manifest as a dramatic change in the color of a child's urine, with the appearance of blood on a diaper or underwear, or as a finding on a urinalysis. Red or brown (cola-colored) urine with red blood cells seen on microscopy is typical of macroscopic (or gross) hematuria. In a retrospective study of children presenting to a pediatric emergency department, gross hematuria had an incidence of 1.3 per 1000 visits.[1] In contrast, microscopic hematuria (defined as >5 red blood cells per high power field seen on microscopy of centrifuged urine) is more common. On routine screening urinalysis (as recommended by the American Academy of Pediatrics [AAP] at 5 years of age and again at 11 to 21 years of age), studies suggest up to 32 per 1000 girls and 14 per 1000 boys will have microscopic hematuria.[2,3]

The most likely causes of macroscopic and microscopic hematuria differ, infection of the upper or lower urinary tract as the most common cause of hematuria overall (Figure 188-1 and Box 188-1). Macroscopic hematuria may originate from any component of the genitourinary tract, and the differential diagnosis, in addition to infection, includes glomerular, interstitial, and tubular diseases and bleeding from trauma, stones, or coagulopathy. Many of the causes of macroscopic hematuria, such as infection, nephrolithiasis, and glomerulonephritis, may instead cause microscopic hematuria. Overall, the most common causes of asymptomatic isolated microscopic hematuria are thin basement membrane disease, idiopathic hypercalciuria, immunoglobulin A (IgA) nephropathy, and sickle cell disease or trait.[4]

MACROSCOPIC HEMATURIA

The first and most important step in evaluating macroscopic hematuria is obtaining a detailed description of the urine (Figure 188-2). Renal or glomerular causes of hematuria result in tea- or cola-colored urine, as opposed to hematuria of lower tract origin, which causes red or pink urine. In addition to color, highly turbid urine may indicate the presence of cells and suggests glomerular disease or infection. Blood clots suggest urinary tract bleeding. The timing of the bleeding may be helpful; if, for example, it occurs only with the onset of micturation, then the source of the bleeding is likely to be in the lower tract.

Associated signs and symptoms from a detailed history and physical examination will dictate laboratory and radiologic evaluation. Important historical elements include associated urinary symptoms, such as dysuria, frequency, urgency, or enuresis. A decrease in urine output should prompt particular concern and rapid evaluation and treatment. A review of systems should include associated symptoms of abdominal pain or colic, upper respiratory infection symptoms, swelling of extremities, or blurry vision or headaches suggestive of hypertension. The history should be explored for prior episodes of hematuria, preceding infections (either documented group A streptococcal throat infection or a history of sore throat or skin infection), history of trauma, or other illnesses, such as the presence of sickle cell trait or disease. Systemic illnesses may be suggested by a history of fever, malaise, weight loss, alopecia, rash, or joint pains as may be seen in rheumatologic disease. Important points on the family history include other family members with hematuria, kidney or rheumatologic disease, and any history of deafness, which may occur with Alport syndrome.

A thorough physical examination should include measurement of blood pressure, abdominal or costovertebral angle tenderness, a search for evidence of local trauma to the genitourinary tract, and inspection and palpation for periorbital, genital, or extremity edema. Hematuria in association with edema and hypertension suggests glomerulonephritis.

Laboratory evaluation begins with a urinalysis with microscopic examination of a fresh spun urine sample

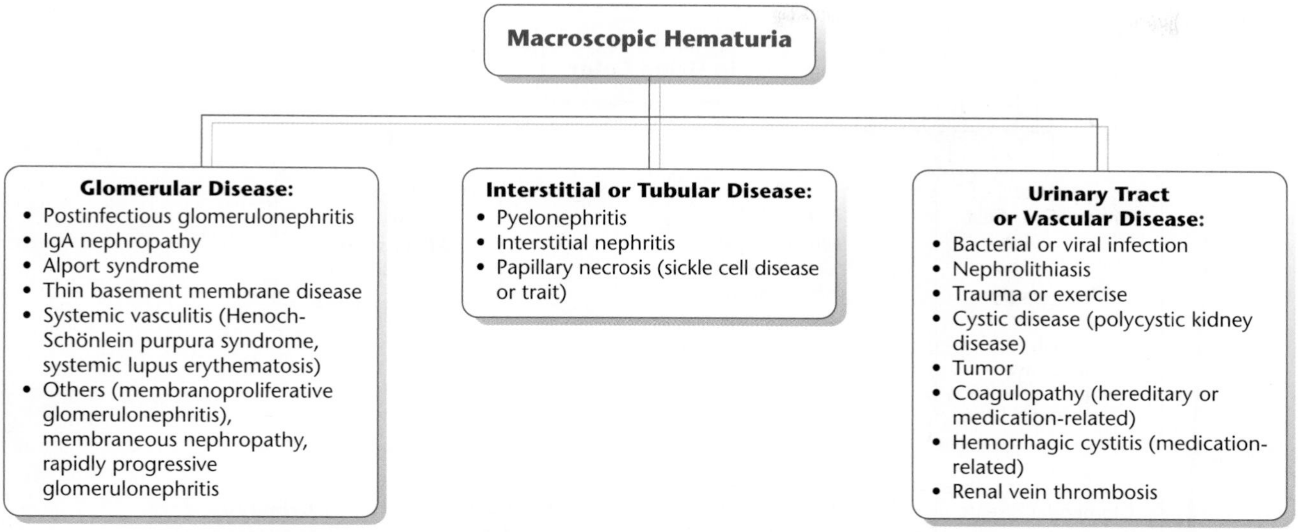

Macroscopic Hematuria

Glomerular Disease:
• Postinfectious glomerulonephritis
• IgA nephropathy
• Alport syndrome
• Thin basement membrane disease
• Systemic vasculitis (Henoch-Schönlein purpura syndrome, systemic lupus erythematosis)
• Others (membranoproliferative glomerulonephritis), membraneous nephropathy, rapidly progressive glomerulonephritis

Interstitial or Tubular Disease:
• Pyelonephritis
• Interstitial nephritis
• Papillary necrosis (sickle cell disease or trait)

Urinary Tract or Vascular Disease:
• Bacterial or viral infection
• Nephrolithiasis
• Trauma or exercise
• Cystic disease (polycystic kidney disease)
• Tumor
• Coagulopathy (hereditary or medication-related)
• Hemorrhagic cystitis (medication-related)
• Renal vein thrombosis

Figure 188-1 Differential diagnosis of macroscopic hematuria in children.

BOX 188-1 Microscopic Hematuria

Transient
Thin basement membrane disease
Idiopathic hypercalciuria
Immunoglobulin A (IgA) nephropathy or Alport syndrome
Sickle cell anemia or traits
Trauma or exercise
Postinfectious glomerulonephritis
Nephrolithiasis
Other glomerular disease or glomerulonephritis (focal and segmental glomerulosclerosis [FSGS], Henoch-Schönlein purpura [HSP] syndrome, systemic lupus erythematosis [SLE], membranoproliferative glomerulonephritis [MPGN], membraneous glomerulonephritis)
Congenital abnormality (ureteropelvic junction [UPJ] or cystic disease)
Pyelonephritis or infection
Vascular malformation
Drugs or toxins

to confirm the presence of red blood cells. Dysmorphic red blood cells and red blood cell casts are pathognomonic of hematuria of glomerular origin.[5] If the urine dipstick is positive for blood and fewer than 5 red bloods cells are found on microscopy, then the diagnosis is hemoglobinuria or myoglobinuria rather than hematuria. Several drugs, including rifampin, ibuprofen, and nitrofurantoin, as well as foods such as beets and blackberries, can discolor urine to give it the appearance of hematuria; but urinalysis will be negative for blood. The presence of calcium, uric acid, or cystine crystals in the urine is suggestive of nephrolithiasis. White blood cell casts, leukocyte esterase, or nitrate positivity on urine dipstick point to infectious causes of hematuria.

Further evaluation is determined by the most likely cause of the blood in the urine. If microscopy is not immediately available to guide the initial laboratory evaluation of a child with apparent hematuria, then a reasonable panel of tests would include serum electrolytes, blood urea nitrogen, creatinine, calcium and phosphorus, liver function tests, antinuclear antibody test, complement studies (C3, C4, and total complement), complete blood count with differential, and streptozyme (deoxyribonuclease B) and streptolysin O antibody titers. Throat culture or rapid testing for group A β-hemolytic streptococci is indicated with a history of sore throat. A urine culture should be performed on all patients with urinary symptoms or in infants with unexplained fever or sepsis, because infection is the most common cause of hematuria. Proteinuria on urinalysis should be further evaluated with a morning void for protein-to-creatinine ratio. A renal-bladder sonogram should be performed on all patients with macroscopic hematuria to evaluate for cystic disease, congenital obstruction, tumors (including Wilms tumor), nephrolithiasis, or parenchymal renal disease.

Further evaluation of glomerular hematuria may be continued as an outpatient or inpatient. Indications for admission include decreased urine output, hypertension, azotemia, or renal insufficiency. Renal biopsy is absolutely indicated in cases of hematuria with nephrotic syndrome, recurrent hematuria, azotemia, or renal insufficiency. Renal biopsy may be performed if a family history of hematuria exists or if the history or laboratory evaluation is suggestive of rheumatologic disease, such as systemic lupus erythematosus.

Management of glomerular disease will depend on the cause of the glomerulonephritis. The most

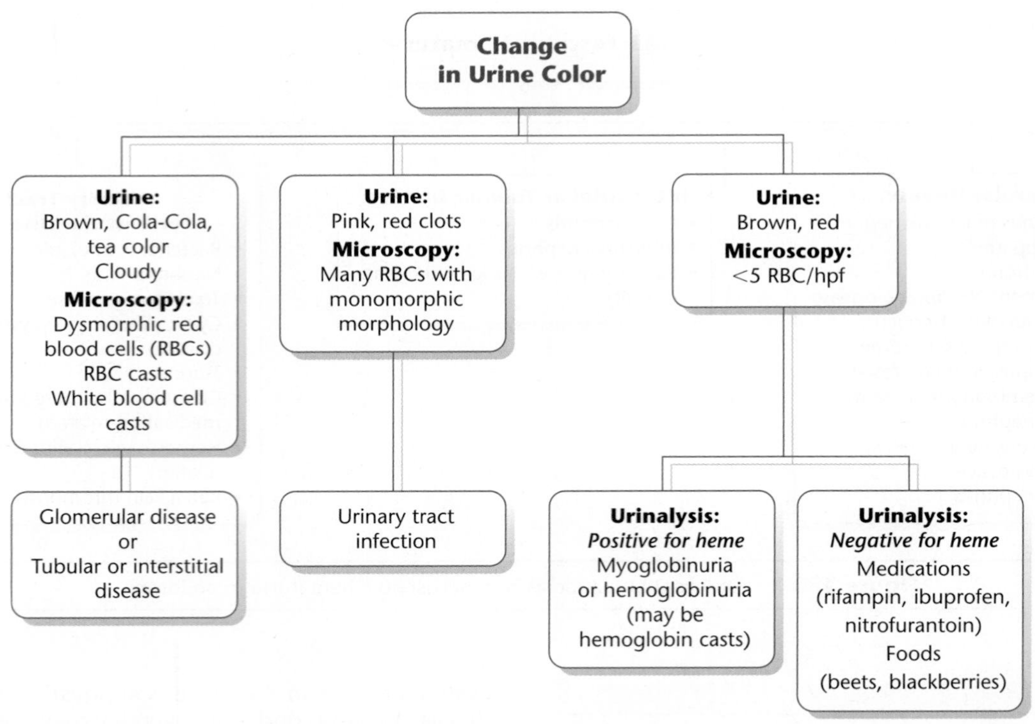

Figure 188-2 Evaluation for macroscopic hematuria begins with the examination of the urine.

common glomerulonephritis is postinfectious, an entity characterized by a prodromal infection (often a streptococcal skin or throat infection but also viral infections, such as varicella, cytomegalovirus, Epstein-Barr virus, hepatitis B and C, and parasitic infections such as toxoplasmosis) between 1 to 6 weeks before the onset of hematuria. Other causes of acute postinfectious glomerulonephritis include ventriculoperitoneal shunt infections (shunt nephritis) and acute or subacute endocarditis. Low complement (C3) and an elevated streptolysin O antibodies are characteristic of poststreptococcal glomerulonephritis. Poststreptococcal glomerulonephritis is typically self-limited with a good prognosis for long-term renal function. Admission may be required for renal insufficiency, oliguria, or acute hypertension, which requires aggressive management with fluid and salt restriction and antihypertensive medications.

Other types of glomerulonephritis often require management by a nephrologist. The most common chronic glomerulonephritis worldwide is IgA nephropathy, which characteristically results in persistent microhematuria with intermittent episodes of gross hematuria associated with upper respiratory infections. Long-term outcome is variable, with 20% to 40% of children progressing to end-stage kidney disease. Proteinuria and hypertension are poor prognostic indicators. Henoch-Schönlein purpura, a common systemic vasculitis in children, is usually associated with crampy abdominal pain, arthralgia, and palpable purpura and can produce glomerulonephritis with hematuria.[6]

Management of nonglomerular hematuria depends on the cause. Further imaging with computed tomography may be indicated. Patients with sickle cell disease or sickle cell trait and macroscopic hematuria from papillary necrosis may require admission for intravenous hydration. Trauma, tumors, cystic disease, congenital obstruction, hemorrhagic cystitis, and lower urinary tract bleeding often require urologic evaluation, which may include direct visualization by cystoscopy. Children with nephrolithiasis benefit from both nephrologic and urologic evaluation.

MICROSCOPIC HEMATURIA

The evaluation of microscopic hematuria involves a thorough history and physical examination. A family history of deafness or kidney disease and the presence of hypertension, proteinuria, or edema should prompt referral to a pediatric nephrologist for further evaluation. In the absence of any other signs and symptoms, microhematuria is often benign and in many cases resolves spontaneously (transient hematuria). Therefore, in an asymptomatic, normotensive child with isolated microhematuria, repeating a urinalysis on 1 or more occasions is often prudent before further evaluation. School-aged children may be observed in excess of 2 years before more extensive testing is undertaken. Figure 188-3 shows a proposed algorithm for the evaluation of microscopic hematuria.[7,8]

One of the most common causes of persistent microhematuria is thin basement membrane nephropathy (TBMN).[9] Persistent microhematuria distinguishes TBMN from other acute renal causes of

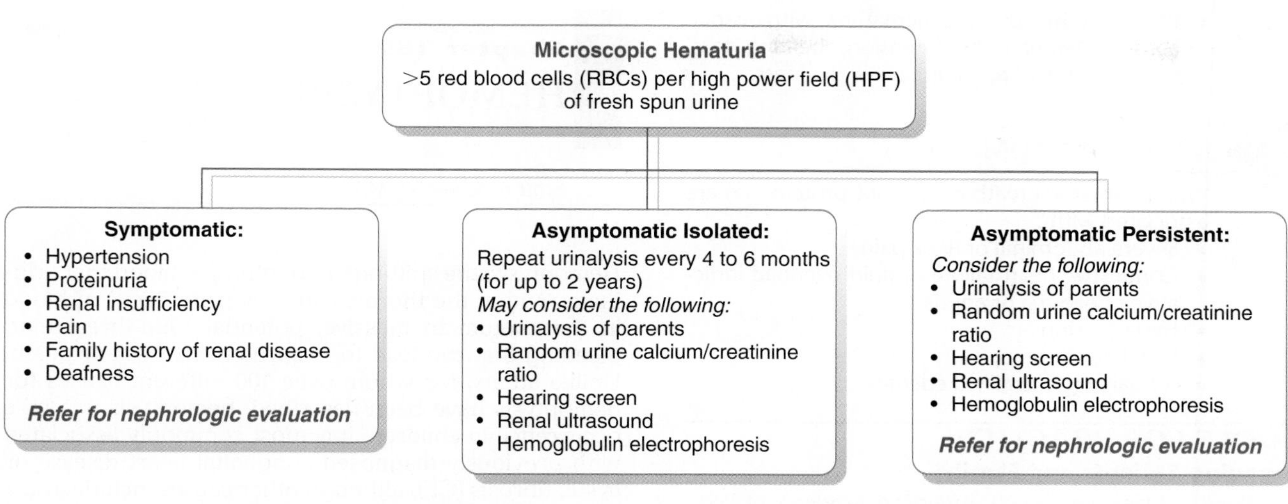

Figure 188-3 Evaluation of microscopic hematuria.

hematuria, such as postinfectious glomerulonephritis. TBMN is characterized by painless microscopic hematuria with minimal proteinuria and normal renal function. Renal biopsy reveals uniform thinning of the glomerular basement membrane. TBMN is also named thin basement membrane disease, hereditary hematuria, benign familial hematuria, and benign hereditary nephritis. Because it is transmitted in an autosomal-dominant fashion, a family history of microscopic hematuria without symptomatic renal disease, or an asymptomatic parent testing positive for hematuria, suggests the diagnosis of TBMN. The overall prevalence is estimated at 1% to 10% of the population. It is more common in females than in males and has been diagnosed in children as young as 1 year. Between 5% and 22% of affected individuals will have an episode of gross hematuria associated with an infection or exercise. No evidence has been found to support treatment of TBMN, which is typically nonprogressive. However, affected children should be monitored for hypertension, proteinuria, and renal insufficiency, which may point to the diagnosis of IgA nephropathy,[10] Alport syndrome,[11] nephrolithiasis, or glomerulonephritis, each of which has been reported in association with TBMN.

Another common cause of microscopic hematuria is hypercalciuria, defined as an urine calcium-to-creatinine ratio of greater than 0.21 or more than 4 mg/kg/day of excreted calcium on a 24-hour urine collection. Children with hematuria and underlying hypercalciuria are at risk for nephrolithiasis, the risk appearing to be greater in older children, in children with gross rather than microscopic hematuria, and when there is a family history of stone formation.[12]

Given that persistent microhematuria may represent an early presentation of a progressive glomerular disease, such as IgA nephropathy or Alport syndrome, periodic urinalysis should be done to monitor for the development of significant proteinuria. Significant proteinuria or the occurrence of gross hematuria should prompt referral to a pediatric nephrologist.

BLOOD ON A DIAPER OR UNDERWEAR

Blood on a diaper or underwear most commonly occurs with trauma to or manipulation of the genital area. Localized irritation of the meatus in boys is the most frequent cause and responds to treatment with petroleum jelly and reassurance to the parent without further evaluation. Other causes include sexual abuse and urinary tract infection with *Serratia marcescens*.

CONCLUSION

Key points for the primary care physician include:

1. Gross hematuria is a common sign of glomerular and urologic disease.
2. Hematuria of glomerular origin presents with tea-colored or cola-colored urine.
3. Hematuria arising from the urinary tract is usually red-pink with or without clots.
4. Red blood cell casts are the hallmark of hematuria of glomerular origin.
5. Proteinuria is a more important prognostic finding than gross hematuria.
6. Every child with gross hematuria should have a renal ultrasound to rule out nephrolithiasis, tumor or urologic abnormalities, such as cystic disease and obstructive uropathy.
7. Gross hematuria rarely is a cause of anemia.
8. Most children with isolated microscopic hematuria do not have a serious or treatable cause for the hematuria and do not require an extensive work-up.
9. Hematuria of glomerular origin is typically painless.

WHEN TO REFER

- Macroscopic hematuria
- Hematuria associated with pain

- Persistent microscopic hematuria with associated proteinuria, hypertension, hearing loss, family history of renal disease or deafness.

WHEN TO ADMIT

When hematuria (with or without proteinuria) are associated with:

- Severe abdominal or flank pain
- Congestive heart failure or fluid overload indicative of oliguria or anuria
- Hypertension
- Renal insufficiency
- Anasarca (generalized edema)

TOOLS FOR PRACTICE

Engaging Patients and Family

- *Blood in Urine* (fact sheet), American Academy of Pediatrics (www.aap.org/publiced/BK0_Hematuria.htm).

AAP POLICY STATEMENTS

American Academy of Pediatrics, Committee on Quality Improvement, Subcommittee on Urinary Tract Infection. The diagnosis, treatment, and evaluation of the initial urinary tract infection in febrile infants and young children. *Pediatrics*. 1999;103(4):843-852. (aappolicy.aappublications.org/cgi/content/full/pediatrics;103/4/843).

American Academy of Pediatrics, Downs SM. Technical report: urinary tract infections in febrile infants and young children. *Pediatrics*. 1999;103:e54. (aappolicy.aappublications.org/cgi/content/full/pediatrics;103/4/e54).

REFERENCES

1. Ingelfinger JR, Davis AE, Grupe WE. Frequency and etiology of gross hematuria in a general pediatric setting. *Pediatrics*. 1977;59(4):557-561.
2. Dodge WF, West EF, Smith EH, et al. Proteinuria and hematuria in schoolchildren: epidemiology and early natural history. *J Pediatr*. 1976;88(2):327-347.
3. Patel H, Bissler JJ. Hematuria in children. *Pediatr Clin North Am*. 2001;48(6);1519-1536.
4. Meyers K. Evaluation of hematuria in children. *Urologic Clin North Am*. 2004;31:559-573.
5. Crompton CH, Ward PB, Hewitt JK. The use of urinary red cell morphology to determine the source of hematuria in children. *Clin Nephrol*. 1993;39(1):44-49.
6. Lau K, Wyatt R. Glomerulonephritis. *Adol Med Clin*. 2005; 16:67-85.
7. Feld LG, Meyers KE, Kaplan BS, et al. Limited evaluation of microscopic hematuria in pediatrics. *Pediatrics*. 1998; 102(4):E42.
8. Wood EG. Asymptomatic hematuria in childhood: a practical approach to evaluation. *Indian J Pediatr*. Mar-Apr 1999;66(2):207-214.
9. Tryggvason K, Patrakka J. Thin basement membrane nephropathy. *J Am Soc Nephrol*. 2006;17:813-822.
10. Piqueras AI, White RH, Raafat F, et al. Renal biopsy diagnosis in children presenting with haematuria. *Pediatr Nephrol*. 1999;12:386-391.
11. Kashtan CE. Alport syndrome and thin glomerular basement membrane disease. *J Am Soc Nephrol*. 1998 Sep; 9(9):1736-1750.
12. Garcia CD, Miller LA, Stapleton FB. Natural history of hematuria associated with hypercalciuria in children. *Am J Dis Child*. 1991;145(10):1204-1207.

Chapter 189

HEMOPTYSIS

Scott A. Schroeder, MD

Hemoptysis, the spitting or coughing of blood that originates within the thorax, can vary from flecks of blood in the sputum to massive, potentially life-threatening bleeding that can lead to respiratory distress or death. Unlike adults, for whom over 100 different causes for hemoptysis have been described, hemoptysis is a rare occurrence in children; it is most commonly associated with previously diagnosed congenital heart disease or cystic fibrosis (CF), although other causes include infectious respiratory illnesses and, rarely, neoplasms.[1] Acute hemoptysis, respiratory failure, and cyanosis may be the result of exposure to mold growing in water-damaged homes and to environmental tobacco smoke. Affected children need to be hospitalized and placed on mechanical ventilation.[2,3]

Four important considerations should be kept in mind in evaluating children who have hemoptysis. The first consideration is to determine whether the bleeding requires an emergency resuscitative effort. Second, what appears to be hemoptysis may actually be bleeding from the upper airway or gastrointestinal tract; thus the source of the bleeding should be established. Third, children without chronic diseases who develop hemoptysis with associated symptoms of a lower respiratory tract infection usually have mild, self-limited bleeding that requires no specific treatment other than management of the underlying acute illness. Fourth, the management of hemoptysis that arises from a localized site differs from that which causes a diffuse alveolar hemorrhage because the latter may be the presenting sign of an underlying immunologic disorder.

PATHOGENESIS

Hemoptysis can result from the disruption of either arm of the dual pulmonary vascular system or from damage to the alveolar endothelial junction. The low-pressure, high-capacitance pulmonary arterial system accepts the entire cardiac output from the right ventricle and carries blood to be oxygenated at the pulmonary capillaries before returning the oxygenated blood to the left atrium via the pulmonary veins. Although the pulmonary arteries travel alongside the bronchial tree, they interact with the airways only at the level of the terminal bronchioles. The 2nd arm of the blood supply within the lungs is the high-pressure bronchial system. The bronchial arteries originate from the aorta or, less commonly, the intercostal arteries, and they receive only 1% to 2% of the cardiac output. The bronchial arteries enter the lungs at the hilum, and as they branch with the bronchi, they anastomose and penetrate the bronchial mucosa, forming an extensive submucosal plexus. The high-flow, low-pressure pulmonary capillary bed allows the exchange of gases between the alveoli and the capillaries to occur with little risk of hemorrhage in the normal state.

Localized hemoptysis, in the majority of cases, is the result of bleeding from the high-pressure bronchial circulation in inflamed airways. The pulmonary circulation is rarely to blame for hemoptysis except in necrotic infarcts and from pulmonary arterial aneurysms in tubercular cavities. Both of these conditions are extremely rare in children. Inflammation within the lungs, pulmonary vascular obstruction, and neoplasia can all cause an increase in the bronchial circulation. In chronic inflammatory conditions, such as bronchiectasis, the cardiac output to the bronchial circulation can triple and bronchopulmonary anastomoses are increased, thereby increasing the potential for erosion of vessels in the presence of superimposed infection. The pathogenesis of disease states with diffuse pulmonary hemorrhage—for example, Wegener granulomatosis—is not entirely understood, but the bleeding into the alveoli appears to result from neutrophil-mediated injury to pulmonary capillaries with interstitial and airspace fibrosis from the chronic hemorrhage.

ETIOLOGY

Hemoptysis in Children Without a Preexisting Medical Condition

In children who do not have a preexisting medical condition and who exhibit acute hemoptysis, the most common causes are acute infectious pneumonias and the aspiration of a foreign body. A child with a pneumococcal pneumonia who is old enough to expectorate is classically febrile, appears ill, and has a cough that is productive of rusty sputum. Certain other bacterial and viral lower respiratory tract infections can cause hemoptysis, and, in these cases, the hemoptysis usually occurs early in the course of the illness, is self-limited, and consists of only blood-tinged sputum. Globally, tuberculosis, echinococcus, and paragonimiasis are probably the most common causes of hemoptysis in children (Table 189-1).

After acute infectious processes, the most common cause of hemoptysis in a previously healthy child is the aspiration of a foreign body. In many children who aspirate foreign bodies, the initial choking episode is not observed or not remembered. A bout of paroxysmal coughing may occur after the initial event, but as the cough receptors in the bronchi or trachea adapt, the coughing will stop. Over time, and depending on the location and composition of the foreign object, subsequent inflammation will occur, which may result in airway obstruction, with wheezing or recurrent pneumonitis. If neovascularization of granulation tissue in the airways occurs, or if bronchiectasis develops, then hemoptysis can occur weeks to months after the initial event. Only 40% of children with a foreign-body aspiration will exhibit the classic triad of wheezing, cough, and decreased breath sounds distal to the site of obstruction.[4] The chest radiograph will be normal in 25% of children with bronchial foreign bodies and more than 50% of children with tracheal foreign bodies.[5]

Because only 10% of aspirated foreign bodies are radiopaque, a normal chest radiograph does not preclude aspiration. Inspiratory and expiratory films, decubitus films, and fluoroscopy may be necessary to confirm the diagnosis. If the evidence for aspiration is definitive, then referral to a pediatric surgeon or otolaryngologist experienced in retrieving foreign bodies for rigid bronchoscopy is indicated. If the diagnosis is uncertain, then referral to a pediatric pulmonologist or other clinician skilled in the use of the fiberoptic bronchoscopy is appropriate to determine whether a foreign body is present.

Diffuse Pulmonary Hemorrhage

Children with acute hemoptysis, cough, wheezing, or crackles, diffuse patchy infiltrates on chest radiograph, and bronchoscopic evidence of blood in all lobes or hemosiderin-laden macrophages should be assumed to have diffuse pulmonary hemorrhage or hemosiderosis. The 4 categories of diffuse hemorrhage syndromes that occur in children are (1) those associated with antiglomerular basement membrane antibodies in serum or tissue (eg, Goodpasture syndrome), (2) those associated with an autoimmune-mediated disease (eg, systemic lupus erythematosus), (3) those without any immunologic abnormalities but associated with antibodies to cow's milk, and (4) idiopathic pulmonary hemosiderosis. All of these conditions are exceedingly rare.

Goodpasture syndrome, which occurs most commonly in men in their 2nd and 3rd decades, is characterized by diffuse pulmonary hemorrhage, antiglomerular basement membrane antibodies in serum or tissue, and glomerulonephritis. The *autoimmune diseases,* which are more common in girls and women, rarely produce hemoptysis alone; more commonly, systemic manifestations occur, including fever, weight loss, malaise, anorexia, amenorrhea, rashes, or hypertension, as well as hemoptysis. Treatment for the pulmonary hemorrhage in these disorders should be directed at the underlying disease process.

In *Heiner syndrome,* or pulmonary hemosiderosis associated with cow's milk allergy, infants and children exhibit failure to thrive, vomiting, gastrointestinal bleeding, and upper respiratory tract congestion, in addition to hemoptysis.[6] Although the mechanism whereby the milk causes the multisystem damage is unclear, elimination of milk from the diet results in a dramatic improvement in the children.

In idiopathic pulmonary hemosiderosis (IPH), no evidence for an immune-mediated mechanism is found. Most children with IPH are diagnosed before the age of 7 years or after the age of 16. They usually have respiratory distress, bilateral alveolar infiltrates, and iron-deficiency anemia. The treatment of the acute exacerbations of IPH includes the use of high-dose oral or intravenous corticosteroids, as well as supportive care for the acute bleeding into the lungs. Controversy exists regarding the need for chronic immunosuppressive therapy, but most clinicians caring for children with IPH use azathioprine, chloroquine, or cyclophosphamide to help maintain normal lung function and prevent further episodes of hemoptysis.

Table 189-1 Common, Less-Common, and Uncommon Causes of Hemoptysis

POPULATION	CAUSE	DIAGNOSTIC CLUES
Common causes in children who have no preexisting medical problems	Pneumonia	Usually rusty-colored sputum early in the course of the illness
	Foreign-body aspiration	Needs a high index of suspicion; may have a normal chest radiograph; localized wheezing that does not respond to medical therapy
Less-common causes in children who have no preexisting medical problems	Pulmonary tuberculosis	Usually with systemic manifestations, such as anorexia and weight loss; may have negative purified protein derivative test
	Autoimmune disorders	Diffuse pulmonary hemorrhage, often with weight loss or other systems involved, including the kidneys and joints
	Congenital malformations	Symptoms depend on the nature of the lesion; may be associated with massive hemoptysis or respiratory distress in newborns
Rare causes in children who have no preexisting medical problem	Primary pulmonary neoplasms	Primary pulmonary cancers reported in <500 children; usually present with cough and recurrent pneumonitis
	Pulmonary embolism	Associated with pleuritic pain, cough, and dyspnea; oral contraceptive use; recent abortion; trauma to lower extremities
	Parasitic lung infections	Travel to endemic areas or sheep-raising areas; peripheral eosinophilia
	Arteriovenous malformations	Recurrent epistaxis, a positive family history for Osler-Weber-Rendu syndrome, or cutaneous telangiectasia
	Idiopathic pulmonary hemosiderosis	Cough, wheezing, iron-deficiency anemia, and diffuse pulmonary hemorrhage on chest radiograph
	Catamenial hemoptysis	Hemoptysis occurs with onset of menses
	Factitious hemoptysis	Form of Münchausen syndrome
Common causes in children who have a preexisting medical problem	Bronchiectasis	Blood-tinged sputum, clubbing, signs of increasing airway inflammation
	Congenital heart lesions	Seen with Eisenmenger complex and pulmonary venous congestion
Less-common causes in children who have a preexisting medical problem	Sickle cell anemia	Hemoptysis associated with acute chest syndrome or pulmonary infarction
	Aspergillosis	Seen in association with cystic fibrosis or asthma; peripheral eosinophilia and fungi seen on Gram stain of sputum

Primary Pulmonary Neoplasms

Unlike the situation with adults, primary pulmonary neoplasms are extremely rare in children, especially immunocompetent children. Fewer than 5% of tumors reported in the literature were associated with hemoptysis. The most frequent presentations of primary pulmonary neoplasms in children are being fever, cough, and pleural pain.[7]

Hemoptysis in Children With a Preexisting Medical Condition

The most common chronic disease associated with hemoptysis is CF. Hemoptysis in CF, which usually begins in the 2nd or 3rd decade of life, can range from the production of blood-tinged sputum with excessive coughing to massive bleeding. Mild hemoptysis can be treated with conservative medical therapy, which includes bed rest, intravenous or oral antibiotics, withholding of chest physiotherapy, and administration of vitamin K. Massive hemoptysis has an annual incidence of 1% among patients with CF and carries a high mortality rate. Massive or recurrent hemoptysis in CF and other diseases is now treated with bronchial artery embolization. Despite a moderately high rate of recurrent bleeding, embolization can relieve symptoms for a significant period. A team composed of a pulmonologist, thoracic surgeon, and interventional radiologist should evaluate these patients before bronchial artery embolization.

Although the number of children with bronchiectasis has declined because of the decline of tuberculosis and the use of effective vaccines against measles and pertussis, children with immunodeficiencies, recurrent aspiration, and ciliary dyskinesias may develop bronchiectasis and have episodes of hemoptysis. In most cases, a history of a chronic productive cough with purulent sputum and changes on the lung examination precede the hemoptysis. The diagnosis is made by

Table 189-2 Differentiation of Hemoptysis From Hematemesis and Upper Airway Hemorrhage*

CHARACTERISTIC	HEMOPTYSIS	HEMATEMESIS AND UPPER AIRWAY HEMORRHAGE
pH	Alkaline	Acidic
Color	Bright red	Dark red or brown
Consistency	Clotted, liquid, or frothy	Coffee ground
Symptoms	Cough	Nausea and vomiting
Gram stain	Macrophages	Food particles and epithelial cells

* Younger children and infants may swallow blood that originates from the lungs, which may appear to have a nonpulmonary source of bleeding.

high-resolution chest tomography, and management is similar to that for CF.

Hemoptysis is a well-recognized complication of congenital heart disease but is becoming an uncommon problem because of advances in corrective cardiac surgery. Hemoptysis in primary or secondary pulmonary hypertension occurs as a result of thromboembolic events. In right-ventricular outflow obstruction with increased bronchial arterial circulation, hemoptysis is due to hemorrhage from enlarged and tortuous bronchial arteries. Hemoptysis is seen in pulmonary vascular obstructive disease because of pulmonary hypertension, as well as thrombosis. These vascular changes take years to develop and are usually first observed in adolescents.

EVALUATION

As with any potential emergency, the 1st question to be answered is "Is the hemoptysis life threatening?" Because the expectoration of blood understandably arouses anxiety and fear, and because the blood can be mixed with saliva or phlegm and swallowed or aspirated, determining the amount of blood accurately is often difficult for children and their parents. In adults, the quantity of expectorated blood does not correlate with the seriousness of the underlying disease. In children, the gravity of the hemoptysis is determined more by the child's clinical status and ability to keep the airway clear rather than the amount of blood expectorated. The greatest danger to a child with hemoptysis is not exsanguination but rather asphyxiation from aspirated blood. The management of the child with life-threatening hemoptysis is beyond the scope of this chapter. However, if the child has evidence of cardiorespiratory distress, hypotension, orthostatic changes, poor perfusion, pallor, tachypnea, tachycardia, mental status changes, arterial hypoxemia, or hypercarbia, then the stabilization and evaluation of the child should occur simultaneously in a pediatric intensive care unit.

Before summoning the bronchoscopist, echocardiographer, and interventional radiologist and scheduling pulmonary arteriography and radionuclide scanning, the primary care physician must ascertain whether the source of bleeding is indeed from within the thorax. Thorough inspection of the oropharynx and nasal passages may identify an upper airway source of bleeding. Infants and young children with hemoptysis may not cough up blood but instead swallow the blood and vomit it later. Therefore, in infants, distinguishing hematemesis from hemoptysis is difficult. Examination of the bloodstained secretions may help differentiate the bleeding site so it can be established whether the bleeding is from the respiratory tract or not. Table 189-2 describes how to differentiate hemoptysis from bleeding from other sources.

History

As is the case for any sign or symptom with many possible causes, a detailed history of both pulmonary and nonpulmonary symptoms will often allow a tentative diagnosis to be made. The presumptive diagnosis can then be proven or disproven by the findings of specific laboratory tests and procedures. For a child or adolescent without any preexisting medical condition who displays a first episode of hemoptysis, the most common causes are acute infections of the tracheobronchial tree, pneumonias, and foreign-body aspirations.[8-10] Hemoptysis can be the presenting symptom for an autoimmune disorder or other immunologic abnormality, though this circumstance is rare. Travel to or from developing countries and areas that raise sheep may necessitate evaluation for mycobacterial, mycotic, or parasitic lung infections. Recurrent pneumonitis, sinus infections, and chronic sputum production may be indicative of bronchiectasis from CF, foreign-body aspiration, ciliary dyskinesias, or other chronic lung diseases. Other aspects of the history that will help focus the evaluation include recent trauma, easy bruising, changes in urine color, weight loss, arthralgias, previous heart disease or surgery, medication use, substance abuse, family history of bleeding disorders, surgical procedures, pica, fever, pleuritic chest pain, menstrual irregularities, and asthma not responsive to appropriate medical therapy. In adolescents with unusual or perplexing symptoms and normal findings at evaluation, factitious hemoptysis and Münchausen syndrome should also be considered. Factitious hemoptysis has been reported in children who underwent numerous invasive procedures, and, ultimately, the determination was made that these children were biting their oral mucosa to simulate hemoptysis.[9,11,12]

Physical Examination

Physical examination begins with a determination of the vital signs to decide the rapidity at which the examination should be conducted. A thorough inspection of the nasal passages and oropharynx is conducted to rule out a nonpulmonary cause of the hemoptysis. As the examination proceeds caudally, certain findings on inspection and auscultation may suggest a specific diagnosis. Cutaneous telangiectases with a murmur or bruit over the lung fields suggest hereditary hemorrhagic telangiectasia (Rendu-Osler-Weber syndrome). Clubbing with or without adventitial breath sounds suggests bronchiectasis. A saddle nose and stridor suggestive of subglottic stenosis are often seen in patients with Wegener granulomatosis. A pleuritic rub, acute pleuritic chest pain, and a history of oral contraceptive use or recent abortion suggest a pulmonary embolic event or other pleural-based lesion. Localized homophonous wheezing over a major airway or decreased breath sounds, with or without a cough, suggests an intraluminal obstruction such as an aspirated foreign body. Evidence of trauma to the thorax may be subtle and not always obvious. Thirty percent of children who experience major trauma to other organ systems will be found to have thoracic trauma as well.[13] Examination of the heart may provide evidence of pulmonary hypertension or a new murmur. Lymphadenopathy and hepatosplenomegaly should raise the possibility of a lymphoproliferative disease with an associated bleeding diathesis.

Laboratory Evaluation

Numerous laboratory tests may be helpful, but they should be focused depending on the history and physical examination. If the patient has a compromised airway, then arterial blood gas measurement may help in the decision of how quickly the intensive care unit needs to be called. Urinalysis or specific serologic markers will help determine whether the child has an immunologic disease that involves the basement membranes of both the kidneys and the lungs. A complete blood count with an eosinophil count may help differentiate a bacterial from a parasitic pneumonia. Although clotting studies are routinely ordered, they will invariably be normal because bleeding disorders do not generally cause spontaneous hemoptysis. Although skin tests for mycobacteria should always be performed, other skin tests, or serologic testing for fungi or other infectious agents, should be guided by clinical acumen. If sputum is produced or bronchoscopy is performed, then these pulmonary fluids should be cultured for bacteria, fungi, ova, parasites, and mycobacteria and stained for the presence of hemosiderin-laden macrophages. If warranted, early-morning gastric aspirates can be cultured and stained for microorganisms and macrophages.

Imaging Studies

The history and physical examination should allow a tentative diagnosis and help decide what imaging studies or procedures need to be undertaken to make a definitive diagnosis. If the child is stable, then a chest radiograph should be obtained. Any abnormality on a chest film should be considered as a potential source for the hemoptysis, but a normal radiograph does not exclude the thorax as the source of bleeding. In approximately one third of children with hemoptysis, the initial chest x-ray examination will reveal nothing abnormal.[14] Findings on the chest film that help focus the evaluation include hilar adenopathy, an air-fluid level in an abscess, a mass, a cavitary lesion, mediastinal widening, or alveolar infiltrates. Alveolar infiltrates in a child with hemoptysis are a common finding in children with autoimmune diseases that involve the lungs. Thickening of the bronchial walls with ring shadows and tramlines suggests bronchiectasis. If a foreign body is suspected to be the cause, then inspiratory and expiratory films or left and right lateral decubitus films may help localize the foreign body. If the foreign body is present and causes obstruction of an airway, then the side of the thorax that does not deflate normally on expiration or when dependent is the side with the foreign body. If the foreign body is embedded within the mucosa of the airway, or if only partial obstruction is present, then the chest x-ray examination may reveal nothing abnormal.

The next imaging studies depend on the presumptive diagnosis because not every child with hemoptysis needs special radiographic studies. If the chest x-ray examination is normal or does not add any information to that obtained from the history and physical examination, then computerized tomography (CT) or high-resolution computerized tomography (HRCT) may be contributive. CT is effective for detecting parenchymal disease, and HRCT has replaced bronchography for diagnosing bronchiectasis. CT can identify airway abnormalities, elucidate abnormalities seen on chest x-rays, define mediastinal structures, and help categorize congenital pulmonary malformations and pulmonary vasculitis syndromes. CT may also serve as a road map for subsequent bronchoscopy.

Magnetic resonance imaging (MRI) is useful for evaluating for congenital vascular malformations and for the differentiation of structures within the mediastinum and hilum. Perhaps in the future MRI will supplant CT in the evaluation of hemoptysis; but for now, the advantages of MRI do not outweigh its disadvantages, especially if excessive respiratory motion is present or the child's condition is unstable.

Bronchoscopy

The timing and need for bronchoscopy, either rigid or flexible, depends on the stability of the child's condition and the suspected cause of the hemoptysis. Not every child with hemoptysis needs to undergo bronchoscopy; research indicates that hemoptysis is rarely the primary indication for bronchoscopy.[9] If a child has rapid and complete resolution of hemoptysis after medical therapy, then bronchoscopy need not be performed. Indications for bronchoscopy include a diagnosis that is in question, massive hemoptysis, or an incomplete response to therapy.

No studies have compared the use of fiberoptic versus rigid bronchoscopy for evaluating hemoptysis in either adults or children. Both instruments can be used to administer therapeutic agents to the airways, sample bronchial fluids, and take biopsy samples. With the rigid bronchoscope, bronchoscopists have complete airway control: they can suction through a larger channel, sample suspicious lesions, and insert packing material to tamponade the bleeding. The rigid bronchoscope is the preferred instrument for removing foreign bodies from the airway. On the other hand, fiberoptic bronchoscopy does not require the use of general anesthesia; the scope is usually passed transnasally (so that the upper airways can also be examined), and it can be easily maneuvered into the upper lobes and more distal airways. If a child with hemoptysis needs bronchoscopy, then fiberoptic bronchoscopy may be used for the initial evaluation. If an anatomic lesion or foreign body is discovered, then rigid bronchoscopy will be needed.

HEMOPTYSIS IN THE NEWBORN PERIOD

Neonates who have a variety of congenital defects can develop localized hemoptysis and diffuse pulmonary hemorrhage in the newborn period. Arteriovenous malformations, extralobar sequestration, or hereditary hemorrhagic telangiectasia (Rendu-Osler-Weber syndrome) can exhibit in the nursery as respiratory distress or mild to massive hemoptysis. All of these vascular malformations cause bleeding as a result of the abnormal connections between the bronchial and pulmonary circulations. The diagnosis of these lesions is made by CT scan with contrast, and children with these defects need to be hospitalized in a center that has a pediatric surgeon and an interventional radiologist.

Diffuse pulmonary hemorrhage is not an uncommon occurrence in infants of very low birth weight. The more premature the infant is, the higher the likelihood will be of hemorrhage. The pathogenesis of the diffuse bleeding is thought to be from effects of barotrauma on an immature pulmonary capillary endothelium. The risk of pulmonary hemorrhage increases slightly with the administration of exogenous surfactant therapy. Many nonpulmonary conditions have also been associated with diffuse hemorrhage in premature newborns, including central nervous system insults and coagulation and metabolic defects.[14]

When to Refer and When to Admit

- Evidence of hemodynamic instability
- Mental status changes
- High suspicion of tuberculosis
- Known heart disease
- Chronic lung disease (eg, CF, ciliary dyskinesias, immunodeficiencies)
- High suspicion of pulmonary neoplasm
- Sickle cell anemia, vasoocclusive crisis, or acute chest syndrome
- Inability to protect airway
- Risk of pulmonary embolism
- Lung abscess
- Children younger than 1 year
- Foreign-body aspiration
- Pulmonary hypertension

REFERENCES

1. Coss-Bu J, Sachdeva RC, Bricker JT, et al. Hemoptysis: a 10 year retrospective study. *Pediatrics.* 1997;100:E7.
2. Etzel R, Montana E, Sorenson WG, et al. Acute pulmonary hemorrhage in infants associated with exposure to Stachybotrys atra and other fungi. *Arch Pediatr Adolesc Med.* 1998;152:757-762.
3. Brown CM, Redd SC, Damon SA. Acute idiopathic pulmonary hemorrhage among infants. Recommendations from the Working Group for Investigation and Surveillance. *MMWR Recomm Rep.* 2004;53(RR-2): 1-12.
4. Dore ND, Landau LI, Hallam L, et al. Haemoptysis in healthy children due to unsuspected foreign body. *J Paediatr Child Health.* 1997;33:448-450.
5. Pyman C. Inhaled foreign bodies in childhood: a review of 230 cases. *Med J Aust.* 1971;1:62-71.
6. Heiner DC, Sears JW, Kniker WT. Multiple precipitins to cow's milk in chronic respiratory disease. A syndrome including poor growth, gastrointestinal symptoms, evidence of allergy, iron deficiency anemia, and pulmonary hemosiderosis. *Am J Dis Child.* 1962;103:634-654.
7. Hancock BJ, Di Lorenzo M, Youssef S, et al. Childhood primary pulmonary neoplasms. *J Pediatr Surg.* 1993;28: 1133-1136.
8. Fabian M, Smitheringale A. Hemoptysis in children: the hospital for sick children experience. *J Otolaryngol.* 1996; 25:44-45.
9. Godfrey S. Pulmonary hemorrhage/hemoptysis in children. *Pediatr Pulmonol.* 2004;37:476-484.
10. Tom L, Weisman R, Handler S. Hemoptysis in children. *Ann Otol Rhinol Laryngol.* 1980;89:419-424.
11. Batra PS, Holinger LD. Etiology and management of pediatric hemoptysis. *Arch Otolaryngol Head Neck Surg.* 2001;127:377-382.
12. Sood M, Clarke J, Murphy M. Covert biting of the buccal mucosa masquerading as haemoptysis in children. *Acta Pediatr.* 1999;88:1038-1040.
13. Sinclair M, Moore T. Major surgery for abdominal and thoracic trauma in children and adolescence. *J Pediatr Surg.* 1974;9:155-160.
14. Pianosi P, Al-sadoon H. Hemoptysis in children. *Pediatr Rev.* 1996;17:344-352.
15. Oliveira-Santos JA, Pereira-da-Silva L, Clington A, et al. [Neonatal bronchoscopy: a retrospective analysis of 67 cases and a review of their indications.] *Acta Med Port.* 2004;17:341-348.

Chapter 190
HEPATOMEGALY

Philip O. Ozuah, MD, PhD; Marina Reznik, MD, MS

DEFINITIONS AND CLINICAL MANIFESTATIONS

Hepatomegaly is an enlargement of the liver resulting from an increase in the number or size of cells and structures within the liver. Although hepatomegaly usually exhibits clinically as a palpable liver, not all palpable livers result from hepatomegaly. In healthy children, the liver edge may be palpable up to 2 cm below the right costal margin at the midclavicular line. Clinical estimation of the liver span has a much stronger correlation with hepatomegaly than does reporting the liver projection below the costal margin as a single indicator of liver size.[1] The liver span is the distance between the upper and lower margins of the liver at the right midclavicular line. The upper margin should be determined by percussion and the lower edge by either percussion or palpation. Liver span is related curvilinearly to age, height, weight, and body surface area.[2,3] Studies have demonstrated no consistent sex differences in liver size.[4-7] A normal liver span ranges from 5.9 cm (±0.8 cm) in the 1st week of life to 6.5 to 8 cm by 15 years of age.[1-3] The upper edge of liver dullness is usually at the level of the 5th rib in the right midclavicular line. Radiographic assessment of liver size can be a helpful adjunct to the clinical examination. Ultrasonography, computed tomography (CT), and sulfur colloid scintigraphy have all been demonstrated to measure liver size reliably.[4-11]

DIFFERENTIAL DIAGNOSIS

The differential diagnoses of a palpable liver and hepatomegaly are presented in Box 190-1.

Palpable Liver Without Hepatomegaly

Several intrathoracic conditions may push the right hemidiaphragm down and thereby result in a palpable liver. For example, asthma, bronchiolitis, and pneumonitis may produce a palpable liver through hyperinflation of the lungs. Tension pneumothorax usually has other accompanying clinical features, including dyspnea, tachycardia, tracheal deviation, and hypotension. Congenital diaphragmatic hernias often manifest in the neonatal period with a scaphoid abdomen and the presence of bowel sounds in the chest. Other thoracic space–occupying lesions also can displace the diaphragm.

BOX 190-1 Differential Diagnosis of a Palpable Liver Without Hepatomegaly and With Hepatomegaly

PALPABLE LIVER WITHOUT HEPATOMEGALY

- Downward displacement of right hemidiaphragm
  - Hyperinflated lung (eg, asthma, bronchiolitis, pneumonitis)
  - Tension pneumothorax
  - Congenital diaphragmatic hernia
  - Thoracic tumors
- Subdiaphragmatic lesions (eg, abscess)
- Normal variant
- Aberrant lobe of liver (Riedel lobe)

PALPABLE LIVER WITH HEPATOMEGALY

- Inflammatory disorders
  - Viral hepatitis
  - Bacterial hepatitis (eg, abscess, sepsis)
  - Toxic hepatitis (eg, drugs)
  - Neonatal hepatitis
  - Autoimmune hepatitis (eg, systemic lupus erythematosus, sarcoidosis)
- Infiltrative disorders
  - Primary tumors
    - Hepatoblastoma
    - Hepatocellular carcinoma
    - Hemangioma
    - Focal nodular hyperplasia
  - Metastatic tumors
    - Lymphoma
    - Leukemia
    - Neuroblastoma
    - Wilms tumor
    - Histiocytosis
- Storage disorders
  - Fat accumulation
    - Obesity
    - Malnutrition
    - Reye syndrome
    - Cystic fibrosis
    - Diabetes mellitus
    - Lipid infusion
    - Metabolic liver disease
    - Lipidoses (eg, Niemann-Pick, Gaucher, Wolman diseases)
    - Glycogen excess
- Glycogen storage diseases
    - Infant of mother who has diabetes
    - Beckwith-Wiedemann syndrome
    - Total parenteral nutrition
  - Copper accumulation
    - Indian childhood cirrhosis
    - Wilson disease
  - Miscellaneous
    - Alpha$_1$-antitrypsin deficiency
    - Hypervitaminosis A
- Vascular congestion
  - Suprahepatic
    - Congestive heart failure
    - Cardiac tamponade
    - Constrictive pericarditis
  - Intrahepatic
    - Hepatic vein thrombosis (Budd-Chiari syndrome)
    - Hepatic vein web
    - Vascular malformations
      - Cavernous hemangioma
      - Capillary hemangioma
      - Hemangioendothelioma
- Biliary obstruction
  - Congenital biliary atresia
  - Congenital hepatic fibrosis
  - Caroli disease

Abdominal sepsis with a subdiaphragmatic abscess may push the liver caudally. Riedel lobe is an occasional tonguelike process extending downward from the right lobe of the liver lateral to the gall bladder. A palpable liver without hepatomegaly also may be a normal variant.

Palpable Liver With Hepatomegaly

Inflammatory Disorders

Inflammatory liver disorders frequently manifest clinically with jaundice and a liver that is firm and tender to palpation. Viral hepatitis (including hepatitis A, B, C, D, and E) may be fulminant or insidious in onset. Hepatitis A may be anicteric in 50% of infected children younger than 4 years and in more than 80% of children younger than 2 years.[12] Bacterial sepsis may result in hepatomegaly as part of a generalized process or a localized liver abscess.[13] Toxic hepatitis may result from exposure to a variety of therapeutic and other chemical agents. Idiopathic neonatal hepatitis occurs with direct hyperbilirubinemia and may be difficult to distinguish clinically from congenital biliary atresia. Liver biopsy in idiopathic neonatal hepatitis reveals marked infiltration with inflammatory cells in contrast to bile duct proliferation found in biliary atresia. Giant-cell transformation is found in both conditions. In rare instances, autoimmune diseases such as systemic lupus erythematosus and sarcoidosis may involve the liver, leading to a hepatitis with hepatomegaly.

Infiltrative Disorders

Primary or metastatic neoplasia may infiltrate the liver and is often associated with other clinical findings. Malignant hepatic tumors manifest clinically with a hard, palpable liver. Benign tumors include large hemangiomas, which occasionally lead to a platelet consumption coagulopathy (Kasabach-Merritt syndrome) as a result of excessive trapping and destruction of platelets within the vascular bed. Clinically, a bruit may be heard over the liver in patients who have hemangiomas and arteriovenous shunts.

Storage Disorders

Several genetic enzyme defects result in excessive accumulation of metabolites in the liver. These conditions produce a smooth, distended liver. Many of these syndromes are also associated with other clinical features besides hepatomegaly. Fat and glycogen accumulation are well-known causes of hepatomegaly. Less frequently, copper accumulation results in Indian childhood cirrhosis or Wilson disease.[14-18] Indian childhood cirrhosis produces jaundice and hepatomegaly predominantly in middle-income, rural Hindu children, but it also has been described in other parts of the world. Its onset is at approximately 1 to 3 years of age, usually with rapid evolution to cirrhosis and hepatic failure if left untreated. This familial disorder was previously thought to be uniformly fatal, but chelation therapy has shown promising results. Wilson disease, an autosomal-recessive inherited disorder of copper metabolism, occurs with hepatomegaly in young children but does not generally manifest clinically until after 5 years of age. Children older than 10 years often have neuropsychiatric symptoms; they may also have hemolytic anemia. Alpha$_1$-antitrypsin deficiency may occur with hepatomegaly, icterus, and acholic stools in the 1st week of life. Signs of chronic liver disease and portal hypertension are seen in older children. Excessive ingestion and accumulation of vitamin A can also result in hepatomegaly.

Vascular Congestion

Congestive heart failure, cardiac tamponade, and constrictive pericarditis all lead to impaired cardiac filling and pressure backup into the inferior vena cava and portal vein, all of which produce a smooth, distended, and tender liver. Other signs of cardiac decompensation, including dyspnea, cough, chest pain, and tachycardia, are usually present.

Budd-Chiari syndrome may be caused by a thrombus, mass, or web occluding the inferior vena cava or the hepatic veins and tributaries, resulting in an enlarged liver.

Vascular malformations produce hepatomegaly through several mechanisms, including hemorrhage into the liver or high-output cardiac failure with secondary vascular congestion or by the size of the malformation itself.

Biliary Obstruction

Biliary atresia occurs in approximately 1 of 8000 births and is the most frequent reason for liver transplantation in children. The bile duct atresia may be extrahepatic, intrahepatic, or a combination thereof. The presence of jaundice, hepatomegaly, and acholic stools beginning during the 1st months of life in otherwise healthy-appearing infants is characteristic. Extrahepatic atresia can be corrected surgically, and intrahepatic atresia can be treated using the hepatoportoenterostomy procedure of Kasai. Nevertheless, many patients develop cirrhosis and portal hypertension.

Congenital hepatic fibrosis is an autosomal-recessive disorder that occurs in childhood with hepatosplenomegaly, portal hypertension, and bleeding esophageal varices. Up to 75% of affected children have associated renal disease. Histologic analysis reveals diffuse periportal and perilobular fibrosis. Caroli disease is a congenital saccular dilation of intrahepatic bile ducts that is inherited in an autosomal-recessive fashion. Symptoms are usually those of acute cholangitis manifesting in late childhood or young adulthood, with fever, icterus, abdominal pain, and a large, tender liver.

EVALUATION

Relevant History and Physical Examination

History and physical examination remain the cornerstone of establishing a prompt diagnosis in patients with hepatomegaly. A thorough history that explores not only gastrointestinal symptoms, but also pulmonary and cardiac manifestations will often point in the right diagnostic direction. Physical examination of the liver should include an assessment of its size, consistency, texture, and tenderness. In addition, the liver should be auscultated with a stethoscope.

A firm and tender liver suggests an acute inflammatory disorder; a hard liver is often neoplastic. A smooth and exquisitely tender liver is found in conditions that cause vascular distention. Bruits are heard in arteriovenous malformations. Although a palpable liver may be a normal variant, the concomitant physical finding of an enlarged spleen usually suggests significant disease.

Laboratory Testing and Imaging

Laboratory investigations should be directed at the suspected diagnosis. Liver function studies are usually necessary. The imaging study used most widely is ultrasonography, which is cheap, portable, reliable, and quickly obtainable in most settings. Liver masses detected on ultrasonography may be defined further by CT scanning or sulfur colloid scintigraphy. Hepatic angiography may be indicated in the evaluation of suspected vascular tumors. In patients with probable metabolic or genetic disorders, a percutaneous liver biopsy may be necessary to establish a diagnosis. In addition, the definitive diagnosis of a liver abscess can be made by ultrasound or CT-guided percutaneous liver aspiration.[19]

MANAGEMENT

Treatment should be aimed at the underlying disease entity. Patients with inflammatory hepatitis require supportive care; those who have bacterial infections should receive appropriate antimicrobials. Surgical excision is the definitive treatment for liver tumors. Chemotherapy may be a helpful adjunct in reducing tumor size either pre- or postoperatively.

The treatment of metabolic-genetic disorders includes dietary modifications and chelation therapy. Frequent small feedings of a high-protein, complex-carbohydrate diet, including continuous nighttime feeding via gastrostomy tubes, have been used successfully in managing glycogen storage disorders. Early treatment with D-penicillamine can prevent the progression of Wilson disease. In many cases, the use of zinc acetate has been approved by the US Food and Drug Administration for maintenance therapy of patients with Wilson disease, even if presymptomatic.[20]

Exciting new developments have provided optimism for some disease entities for which no treatments were available in the past. For example, a recently developed synthetic enzyme, imiglucerase, has been highly effective in the treatment of Gaucher disease.[21] Previously, although Indian childhood cirrhosis was thought to be uniformly fatal, chelation therapy with penicillamine has been shown to reduce mortality significantly if administered early in the disease.[22,23]

WHEN TO REFER

- Hepatomegaly with concomitant splenomegaly
- Palpation of a hard liver
- Hepatomegaly with distended abdominal veins
- Audible bruit over the liver
- Suspicion of malignancy

WHEN TO ADMIT

- Liver failure
- Impending liver failure

SUGGESTED READINGS

Baker A, Gormally S, Saxena R, et al. Copper-associated liver disease in childhood. *J Hepatol.* 1995;23(5):538-543.

Bavdekar AR, Bhave SA, Pradhan AM, et al. Long term survival in Indian childhood cirrhosis treated with D-penicillamine. *Arch Dis Child.* 1996;74(1):32-35.

Marcellini M, Di Ciommo V, Callea F, et al. Treatment of Wilson's disease with zinc from the time of diagnosis in pediatric patients: a single-hospital, 10-year follow-up study. *J Lab Clin Med.* 2005;145(3):139-143.

Safak AA, Simsek E, Bahcebasi T. Sonographic assessment of the normal limits and percentile curves of liver, spleen, and kidney dimensions in healthy school-aged children. *J Ultrasound Med.* 2005;24(10):1359-1364.

REFERENCES

1. Reiff MI, Osborn LM. Clinical estimation of liver size in newborn infants. *Pediatrics.* 1983;71(1):46-48.
2. Carpentieri U, Gustavson LP, Leach TM, et al. Liver size in normal infants and children. *South Med J.* 1977;70(9):1096-1097.
3. Lawson EE, Grand RJ, Neff RK, et al. Clinical estimation of liver span in infants and children. *Am J Dis Child.* 1978;132(5):474-476.
4. Friis H, Hdhlovu P, Mduluza T, et al. Ultrasonographic organometry: liver and spleen dimensions among children in Zimbabwe. *Trop Med Int Health.* 1996;1(2):183-190.
5. Konus OL, Ozdemir A, Akkaya A, et al. Normal liver, spleen, and kidney dimensions in neonates, infants, and children: evaluation with sonography. *AJR Am J Roentgenol.* 1998;171(6):1693-1698.
6. Johnson TN, Tucker GT, Tanner MS, et al. Changes in liver volume from birth to adulthood: a meta-analysis. *Liver Transpl.* 2005;11(12):1481-1493.
7. Safak AA, Simsek E, Bahcebasi T. Sonographic assessment of the normal limits and percentile curves of liver, spleen, and kidney dimensions in healthy school-aged children. *J Ultrasound Med.* 2005;24(10):1359-1364.
8. Holmes JH, Sundgren C, Ikle D, et al. A simple ultrasonic method for evaluating liver size. *J Clin Ultrasound.* 1977;5(2):89-91.
9. Markisz JA, Treves ST, Davis RT. Normal hepatic and splenic size in children: scintigraphic determination. *Pediatr Radiol.* 1987;17(4):273-276.
10. Niederau C, Sonnenberg A, Muller JE, et al. Sonographic measurements of the normal liver, spleen, pancreas, and portal vein. *Radiology.* 1983;149(2):537-540.
11. Noda T, Todani T, Watanabe Y, et al. Liver volume in children measured by computed tomography. *Pediatr Radiol.* 1997;27(3):250-252.
12. Hadler SC, Webster HM, Erben JJ, et al. Hepatitis A in day-care centers. A community-wide assessment. *N Engl J Med.* 1980;302(22):1222-1227.
13. Brook I, Frazier EH. Microbiology of liver and spleen abscesses. *J Med Microbiol.* 1998;47(12):1075-1080.
14. Baker A, Gormally S, Saxena R, et al. Copper-associated liver disease in childhood. *J Hepatol.* 1995;23(5):538-543.
15. Pandit A, Bhave S. Present interpretation of the role of copper in Indian childhood cirrhosis. *Am J Clin Nutr.* 1996;63(5):830S-835S.
16. Petrukhin K, Gilliam TC. Genetic disorders of copper metabolism. *Curr Opin Pediatr.* 1994;6(6):698-701.
17. Prasad R, Kaur G, Nath R, et al. Molecular basis of pathophysiology of Indian childhood cirrhosis: role of nuclear copper accumulation in liver. *Mol Cell Biochem.* 1996;156(1):25-30.

18. Tanner MS. Role of copper in Indian childhood cirrhosis. *Am J Clin Nutr.* 1998;67(5 suppl):1074S-1081S.
19. Men S, Akhan O, Koroglu M. Percutaneous drainage of abdominal abscess. *Eur J Radiol.* 2002;43(3):204-218.
20. Marcellini M, Di Ciommo V, Callea F, et al. Treatment of Wilson's disease with zinc from the time of diagnosis in pediatric patients: a single-hospital, 10-year follow-up study. *J Lab Clin Med.* 2005;145(3):139-143.
21. Mistry P, Germain DP. Therapeutic goals in Gaucher disease. *Rev Med Interne.* 2006;27(1):S30-S38.
22. Bavdekar AR, Bhave SA, Pradhan AM, et al. Long term survival in Indian childhood cirrhosis treated with D-penicillamine. *Arch Dis Child.* 1996;74(1):32-35.
23. Pradhan AM, Bhave SA, Joshi VV, et al. Reversal of Indian childhood cirrhosis by D-penicillamine therapy. *J Pediatr Gastroenterol Nutr.* 1995;20(1):28-35.

Chapter 191

HIGH BLOOD PRESSURE IN INFANTS, CHILDREN, AND ADOLESCENTS

Kristin C. Sokol, MPH; Sarah E. Messiah, MPH, PhD; Carol J. Buzzard, MD; Steven E. Lipshultz, MD

Hypertension is a well-established cause of substantial morbidity and mortality in adults, particularly in the later years of life.[1-3] However, recent population-based studies have shown that over the last decade, mean blood pressure (BP) has increased among children and adolescents.[4] Furthermore, recent longitudinal cohort studies have revealed that elevated BP in childhood often continues into adulthood,[5,6] predicting hypertension in young adulthood, and other studies have documented the familial nature of essential hypertension.[7]

Even mild-to-moderate elevations of BP in children almost certainly warrant close attention, lifestyle modifications, and possibly therapy. Mild and moderate hypertension in childhood is generally not associated with marked symptoms, but routine screening can identify a fair number of children who have either primary or secondary hypertension. Definitive therapy can decrease later morbidity. All pediatricians should be familiar with the basic aspects of hypertension in children, including the diagnosis of normal and abnormal BP, the causes of high BP, and the therapeutic options.[8,9]

DEFINITION OF HIGH BLOOD PRESSURE IN CHILDREN

The 2nd National Heart, Lung, and Blood Institute Task Force on Blood Pressure Control in Children based operational definitions of high BP in children on a combination of values found in healthy children, clinical experience, and consensus among leaders in the field.[10] In children and adolescents, hypertension is defined as elevated BP that persists on repeated measurement at the 95th percentile or greater for age, height, and gender in a healthy population.[8] High-normal or prehypertensive BP is defined as BP greater than or equal to the 90th percentile but less than the 95th percentile (normal systolic and diastolic BPs are less than the 90th percentile). Severe hypertension (with the risk of end-organ injury) is defined as BP greater than the 99th percentile.[11]

Body size is the single most important determinant of BP in children and adolescents; thus using accurate height percentiles is critical for correctly estimating BP percentiles (Figure 191-1 and Tables 191-1 and 191-2).

FACTORS INFLUENCING BLOOD PRESSURE IN CHILDREN

Age

BP tends to increase with age throughout the first 2 decades of life.[8,12] The average systolic BP on the 1st day of life is 70 mm Hg, and it increases steadily for the first 2 months of age.[3] It tends to remain stable until 1 year of age, when it increases until adulthood. Diastolic BP increases slowly for the 1st week and then declines until 3 months of age. It then increases gradually until 1 year of age, when it reaches the level found in the 1st week. Diastolic BP remains steady for the first 5 to 6 years, after which it begins to increase, along with the systolic BP.[13] Children tend to maintain the same BP percentile rank relative to their peers as they grow, a pattern that continues through adolescence, supporting the idea that essential hypertension begins in childhood.

Body Size

Body size is a major influence on BP in children. As in adults, the relationship between BP and weight in the teenage years is particularly prominent.[12,14,15] Height is also related independently to BP at all ages[2] (see Tables 191-1 and 191-2). However, chronic hypertension is becoming increasingly common in adolescents, primarily as a result of the rise in this population of being overweight and obese. Over the last 3 decades, obesity rates have more than doubled for children ages 2 to 5 and 12 to 19, and the rates have more than tripled among children ages 6 to 11.[16] Presently in the United States, 9 million children over 6 years of age are considered obese, with a body mass index (BMI) above the 95th percentile.[17]

Metabolic Syndrome

Being overweight and having hypertension in childhood are components of the metabolic syndrome, a proposed constellation of risk factors that include elevated systolic or diastolic BP, elevated plasma triglycerides, low high-density lipoprotein cholesterol, insulin resistance, and a large waist circumference. The presence of metabolic syndrome is associated with an increased risk of type 2 diabetes and with other cardiovascular risk factors. A child might have metabolic syndrome if 3 or more risk factors are present. Although no standardized definition of metabolic syndrome currently exists, it is increasingly being recognized as a significant complication of childhood obesity. Findings from national samples estimate that roughly 10% of all 12 to 19 year olds in the United States presently have symptoms of the proposed metabolic syndrome.[1,18] Therefore the evaluation of a hypertensive child must

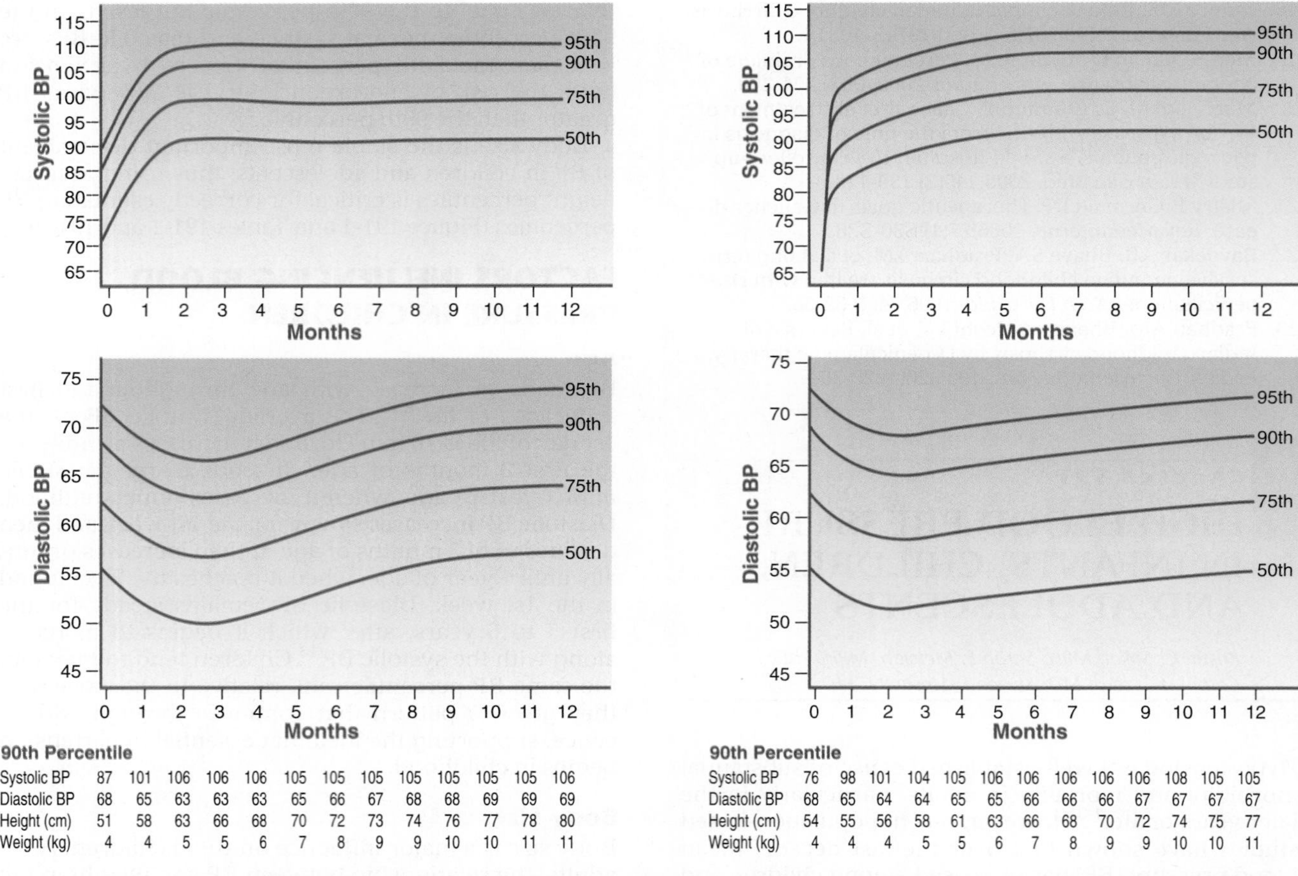

90th Percentile (boys)

	0	1	2	3	4	5	6	7	8	9	10	11	12
Systolic BP	87	101	106	106	106	105	105	105	105	105	105	105	106
Diastolic BP	68	65	63	63	63	65	66	67	68	68	69	69	69
Height (cm)	51	58	63	66	68	70	72	73	74	76	77	78	80
Weight (kg)	4	4	5	5	6	7	8	9	9	10	10	11	11

90th Percentile (girls)

	0	1	2	3	4	5	6	7	8	9	10	11	12
Systolic BP	76	98	101	104	105	106	106	106	106	106	108	105	105
Diastolic BP	68	65	64	64	65	65	66	66	66	67	67	67	67
Height (cm)	54	55	56	58	61	63	66	68	70	72	74	75	77
Weight (kg)	4	4	4	5	5	6	7	8	9	9	10	10	11

Figure 191-1 Age-, sex-, height-, and weight-specific percentiles of systolic and diastolic blood pressure in boys *(left)* and girls *(right)* from birth to 12 months of age.

include a medical history, a complete physical examination, and a laboratory evaluation to assess cardiovascular risk. In addition, although the data are limited, metabolic syndrome may also be associated with sleep-disordered breathing.[10]

Ethnicity

In the United States, the distribution of BP in adults differs among racial and ethnic groups. Non-Hispanic black adults have an increased prevalence and incidence of hypertension. However, the age at which differences in BP become apparent across racial and ethnic groups is unclear. According to the National Heart, Lung, and Blood Institute Growth and Health Study, among other reports, BP levels are significantly higher for black girls than for white girls. Although the situation for boys is less certain, studies repeatedly show that BP levels are higher among black children than among white children. In addition, Mexican-American children have a higher mean-adjusted BP than do non-Hispanic white children. In many instances, a higher BMI explains the difference in BP between different ethnic groups.[4] The increase in BMI in children in the United States has accounted for some of the increase in BP; however, other factors also likely contribute to higher BP levels.

Genetics

Children from families with a history of hypertension tend to have higher BPs than do children from normotensive families, supporting the generally accepted conclusion that genetics influence BP levels.[19,20] Other cardiovascular risk factors among parents, including disorders of lipid and glucose metabolism, hyperuricemia, poor nutrition, passive smoking, and physical inactivity, are also significantly correlated with those of their children.[21]

CAUSES OF HIGH BLOOD PRESSURE IN CHILDREN

Primary Hypertension

Primary, or essential, hypertension has long been known to be the most common cause of hypertension in adults, but it is relatively uncommon in (younger) children. However, primary hypertension is occurring more often now in children than in the past, especially in adolescents. Although primary hypertension is still considered a diagnosis of exclusion, and although the diagnosis should be made only after an extensive evaluation for secondary causes, it has become an important health issue in the young. In a recent study, approximately one half of all children seen in a

Table 191-1 Blood Pressure Levels for Boys by Age and Height Percentile

AGE (YEAR)	BP PERCENTILE *	SYSTOLIC BP (mm Hg) PERCENTILE OF HEIGHT							DIASTOLIC BP (mm Hg) PERCENTILE OF HEIGHT						
		5th	10th	25th	50th	75th	90th	95th	5th	10th	25th	50th	75th	90th	95th
1	50th	80	81	83	85	87	88	89	34	35	36	37	38	39	39
	90th	94	95	97	99	100	102	103	49	50	51	52	53	53	54
	95th	98	99	101	103	104	106	106	54	54	55	56	57	58	58
	99th	105	106	108	110	112	113	114	61	62	63	64	65	66	66
2	50th	84	85	87	88	90	92	92	39	40	41	42	43	44	44
	90th	97	99	100	102	104	105	106	54	55	56	57	58	58	59
	95th	101	102	104	106	108	109	110	59	59	60	61	62	63	63
	99th	109	110	111	113	115	117	117	66	67	68	69	70	71	71
3	50th	86	87	89	91	93	94	95	44	44	45	46	47	48	48
	90th	100	101	103	105	107	108	109	59	59	60	61	62	63	63
	95th	104	105	107	109	110	112	113	63	63	64	65	66	67	67
	99th	111	112	114	116	118	119	120	71	71	72	73	74	75	75
4	50th	88	89	91	93	95	96	97	47	48	49	50	51	51	52
	90th	102	103	105	107	109	110	111	62	63	64	65	66	66	67
	95th	106	107	109	111	112	114	115	66	67	68	69	70	71	71
	99th	113	114	116	118	120	121	122	74	75	76	77	78	78	79
5	50th	90	91	93	95	96	98	98	50	51	52	53	54	55	55
	90th	104	105	106	108	110	111	112	65	66	67	68	69	69	70
	95th	108	109	110	112	114	115	116	69	70	71	72	73	74	74
	99th	115	116	118	120	121	123	123	77	78	79	80	81	81	82
6	50th	91	92	94	96	98	99	100	53	53	54	55	56	57	57
	90th	105	106	108	110	111	113	113	68	68	69	70	71	72	72
	95th	109	110	112	114	115	117	117	72	72	73	74	75	76	76
	99th	116	117	119	121	123	124	125	80	80	81	82	83	84	84
7	50th	92	94	95	97	99	100	101	55	55	56	57	58	59	59
	90th	106	107	109	111	113	114	115	70	70	71	72	73	74	74
	95th	110	111	113	115	117	118	119	74	74	75	76	77	78	78
	99th	117	118	120	122	124	125	126	82	82	83	84	85	86	86
8	50th	94	95	97	99	100	102	102	56	57	58	59	60	60	61
	90th	107	109	110	112	114	115	116	71	72	72	73	74	75	76
	95th	111	112	114	116	118	119	120	75	76	77	78	79	79	80
	99th	119	120	122	123	125	127	127	83	84	85	86	87	87	88
9	50th	95	96	98	100	102	103	104	57	58	59	60	61	61	62
	90th	109	110	112	114	115	117	118	72	73	74	75	76	76	77
	95th	113	114	116	118	119	121	121	76	77	78	79	80	81	81
	99th	120	121	123	125	127	128	129	84	85	86	87	88	88	89
10	50th	97	98	100	102	103	105	106	58	59	60	61	61	62	63
	90th	111	112	114	115	117	119	119	73	73	74	75	76	77	78
	95th	115	116	117	119	121	122	123	77	78	79	80	81	81	82
	99th	122	123	125	127	128	130	130	85	86	86	88	88	89	90
11	50th	99	100	102	104	105	107	107	59	59	60	61	62	63	63
	90th	113	114	115	117	119	120	121	74	74	75	76	77	78	78
	95th	117	118	119	121	123	124	125	78	78	79	80	81	82	82
	99th	124	125	127	129	130	132	132	86	86	87	88	89	90	90
12	50th	101	102	104	106	108	109	110	59	60	61	62	63	63	64
	90th	115	116	118	120	121	123	123	74	75	75	76	77	78	79
	95th	119	120	122	123	125	127	127	78	79	80	81	82	82	83
	99th	126	127	129	131	133	134	135	86	87	88	89	90	90	91
13	50th	104	105	106	108	110	111	112	60	60	61	62	63	64	64
	90th	117	118	120	122	124	125	126	75	75	76	77	78	79	79
	95th	121	122	124	126	128	129	130	79	79	80	81	82	83	83
	99th	128	130	131	133	135	136	137	87	87	88	89	90	91	91

BP, Blood pressure.
*The 90th percentile is 1.28 3D, 95th percentile is 1.645 SD, and the 99th percentile is 2.326 3D over the mean.
National High Blood Pressure Education Program Working Group on High Blood Pressure in Children and Adolescents. The fourth report on the diagnosis, evaluation, and treatment of high blood pressure in children and adolescents. *Pediatrics.* 2004;114(2):555-572.

Continued

Table 191-1 Blood Pressure Levels for Boys by Age and Height Percentile—cont'd

AGE (YEAR)	BP PERCENTILE *	SYSTOLIC BP (mm Hg) PERCENTILE OF HEIGHT							DIASTOLIC BP (mm Hg) PERCENTILE OF HEIGHT						
		5th	10th	25th	50th	75th	90th	95th	5th	10th	25th	50th	75th	90th	95th
14	50th	106	107	109	111	113	114	115	60	61	62	63	64	65	65
	90th	120	121	123	125	126	128	128	75	76	77	78	79	79	80
	95th	124	125	127	128	130	132	132	80	80	81	82	83	84	84
	99th	131	132	134	136	138	139	140	87	88	89	90	91	92	92
15	50th	109	110	112	113	115	117	117	61	62	63	64	65	66	66
	90th	122	124	125	127	129	130	131	76	77	78	79	80	80	81
	95th	126	127	129	131	133	134	135	81	81	82	83	84	85	85
	99th	134	135	136	138	140	142	142	88	89	90	91	92	93	93
16	50th	111	112	114	116	118	119	120	63	63	64	65	66	67	67
	90th	125	126	128	130	131	133	134	78	78	79	80	81	82	82
	95th	129	130	132	134	135	137	137	82	83	83	84	85	86	87
	99th	136	137	139	141	143	144	145	90	90	91	92	93	94	94
17	50th	114	115	116	118	120	121	122	65	66	66	67	68	69	70
	90th	127	128	130	132	134	135	136	80	80	81	82	83	84	84
	95th	131	132	134	136	138	139	140	84	85	86	87	87	88	89
	99th	139	140	141	143	145	146	147	92	93	93	94	95	96	97

BP, Blood pressure.
*The 90th percentile is 1.28 3D, 95th percentile is 1.645 SD, and the 99th percentile is 2.326 3D over the mean.
National High Blood Pressure Education Program Working Group on High Blood Pressure in Children and Adolescents. The fourth report on the diagnosis, evaluation, and treatment of high blood pressure in children and adolescents. *Pediatrics.* 2004;114(2):555-572.

hypertension clinic, which is a selected population, had primary hypertension, leading to the conclusion that the prevalence of primary hypertension in children is increasing and that the diagnosis usually occurs in the presence of obesity and a positive family history of hypertension or cardiovascular disease.[22]

Secondary Hypertension

Secondary hypertension is more common in children than in adults, and in the majority of children, hypertension will be secondary to renal or renovascular causes[10] (Boxes 191-1 and 191-2).

Severe hypertension can be seen in the neonatal intensive care unit and has been reported in 2% to 3% of premature infants.[23] Hypertensive neonates often have evidence of congestive heart failure, respiratory distress, feeding difficulties, irritability, lethargy, coma, or seizures. In almost all cases, the hypertension is renal or renovascular in origin, most commonly from renal artery thrombi related to umbilical vessel catheterization. Another common cause of high BP, especially in the newborn period and 1st year of life, is coarctation of aorta.[21] Medical therapy is usually effective, and the long-term prognosis is surprisingly good.[23,24] High BP can also occur in infants who have bronchopulmonary dysplasia, patent ductus arteriosus, and intravascular hemorrhage.[15,25] Hypertension has been described in neonates undergoing extracorporeal membrane oxygenation, possibly caused by volume overload.[3]

Renal parenchymal disease remains the most frequent cause of hypertension in childhood, accounting for 60% to 80% of cases.[13,25,27,28] Hypertension is evident at the initial diagnosis in almost 80% of all cases of acute poststreptococcal glomerulonephritis, and of those who are normotensive at first, nearly one half will experience hypertension during the course of their illness. Hypertension is also associated with other forms of immune complex glomerulonephritis, although less commonly. It can be seen in membranoproliferative glomerulonephritis, systemic lupus erythematosus, diffuse proliferative glomerulonephritis, and immunoglobulin A nephropathy. Hemolytic uremic syndrome also is associated with hypertension, in proportion to the degree of arteriolar thrombosis. Nephrotic syndrome rarely leads to severe hypertension in childhood unless it is a manifestation of more serious renal disease. Reflux nephropathy is an important cause of hypertension in children, with a prevalence of 5% to 30%.[29] Hypertension is also seen with polycystic kidney disease and Wilms tumor but is less common with other renal structural malformations.[15,30]

Coarctation of the aorta is the most common nonrenal cause of hypertension in childhood, accounting for 5% to 15% of cases.[15,31] Hypertension can also occur immediately after repair of coarctation of the aorta and for years thereafter.[25,32] The risk for postoperative hypertension appears to be lower if the lesion is repaired before 5 years of age.[19,28] Renal artery stenosis, caused by fibromuscular dysplasia, Takayasu arteritis, Williams syndrome, or neurofibromatosis, is an uncommon cause of hypertension in childhood. Children with renal artery stenosis may have marked symptoms caused by end-organ damage (congestive heart failure, left ventricular hypertrophy, retinal changes, and renal impairment).[33,34]

Endocrinopathies must be considered as potential causes of hypertension in children. The problem may be endogenous, arising from conditions such as hyperthyroidism, hypercalcemia, adrenal cortical hyperplasia,

Table 191-2 Blood Pressure Levels for Girls by Age and Height Percentile

AGE (YEAR)	BP PERCENTILE *	SYSTOLIC BP (mm Hg) PERCENTILE OF HEIGHT							DIASTOLIC BP (mm Hg) PERCENTILE OF HEIGHT						
		5th	10th	25th	50th	75th	90th	95th	5th	10th	25th	50th	75th	90th	95th
1	50th	83	84	85	86	88	89	90	38	39	39	40	41	41	42
	90th	97	97	98	100	101	102	103	52	53	53	54	55	55	56
	95th	100	101	102	104	105	106	107	56	57	57	58	59	59	60
	99th	108	108	109	111	112	113	114	64	64	65	65	66	67	67
2	50th	85	85	87	88	89	91	91	43	44	44	45	46	46	47
	90th	98	99	100	101	103	104	105	57	58	58	59	60	61	61
	95th	102	103	104	105	107	108	109	61	62	62	63	64	65	65
	99th	109	110	111	112	114	115	116	69	69	70	70	71	72	72
3	50th	86	87	88	89	91	92	93	47	48	48	49	50	50	51
	90th	100	100	102	103	104	106	106	61	62	62	63	64	64	65
	95th	104	104	105	107	108	109	110	65	66	66	67	68	68	69
	99th	111	111	113	114	115	116	117	73	73	74	74	75	76	76
4	50th	88	88	90	91	92	94	94	50	50	51	52	52	53	54
	90th	101	102	103	104	106	107	108	64	64	65	66	67	67	68
	95th	105	106	107	108	110	111	112	68	68	69	70	71	71	72
	99th	112	113	114	115	117	118	119	76	76	76	77	78	79	79
5	50th	89	90	91	93	94	95	96	52	53	53	54	55	55	56
	90th	103	103	105	106	107	109	109	66	67	67	68	69	69	70
	95th	107	107	108	110	111	112	113	70	71	71	72	73	73	74
	99th	114	114	116	117	118	120	120	78	78	79	79	80	81	81
6	50th	91	92	93	94	96	97	98	54	54	55	56	56	57	58
	90th	104	105	106	108	109	110	111	68	68	69	70	70	71	72
	95th	108	109	110	111	113	114	115	72	72	73	74	74	75	76
	99th	115	116	117	119	120	121	122	80	80	80	81	82	83	83
7	50th	93	93	95	96	97	99	99	55	56	56	57	58	58	59
	90th	106	107	108	109	111	112	113	69	70	70	71	72	72	73
	95th	110	111	112	113	115	116	116	73	74	74	75	76	76	77
	99th	117	118	119	120	122	123	124	81	81	82	82	83	84	84
8	50th	95	95	96	98	99	100	101	57	57	57	58	59	60	60
	90th	108	109	110	111	113	114	114	71	71	71	72	73	74	74
	95th	112	112	114	115	116	118	118	75	75	75	76	77	78	78
	99th	119	120	121	122	123	125	125	82	82	83	83	84	85	86
9	50th	96	97	98	100	101	102	103	58	58	58	59	60	61	61
	90th	110	110	112	113	114	116	116	72	72	72	73	74	75	75
	95th	114	114	115	117	118	119	120	76	76	76	77	78	79	79
	99th	121	121	123	124	125	127	127	83	83	84	84	85	86	87
10	50th	98	99	100	102	103	104	105	59	59	59	60	61	62	62
	90th	112	112	114	115	116	118	118	73	73	73	74	75	76	76
	95th	116	116	117	119	120	121	122	77	77	77	78	79	80	80
	99th	123	123	125	126	127	129	129	84	84	85	86	86	87	88
11	50th	100	101	102	103	105	106	107	60	60	60	61	62	63	63
	90th	114	114	116	117	118	119	120	74	74	74	75	76	77	77
	95th	118	118	119	121	122	123	124	78	78	78	79	80	81	81
	99th	125	125	126	128	129	130	131	85	85	86	87	87	88	89
12	50th	102	103	104	105	107	108	109	61	61	61	62	63	64	64
	90th	116	116	117	119	120	121	122	75	75	75	76	77	78	78
	95th	119	120	121	123	124	125	126	79	79	79	80	81	82	82
	99th	127	127	128	130	131	132	133	86	86	87	88	88	89	90
13	50th	104	105	106	107	109	110	110	62	62	62	63	64	65	65
	90th	117	118	119	121	122	123	124	76	76	76	77	78	79	79
	95th	121	122	123	124	126	127	128	80	80	80	81	82	83	83
	99th	128	129	130	132	133	134	135	87	87	88	89	89	90	91

BP, Blood pressure.
*The 90th percentile is 1.28 3D, 95th percentile is 1.645 SD, and the 99th percentile is 2.326 3D over the mean.
National High Blood Pressure Education Program Working Group on High Blood Pressure in Children and Adolescents. The fourth report on the diagnosis, evaluation, and treatment of high blood pressure in children and adolescents. *Pediatrics*. 2004;114(2):555-572.

Continued

Table 191-2 Blood Pressure Levels for Girls by Age and Height Percentile—cont'd

AGE (YEAR)	BP PERCENTILE *	SYSTOLIC BP (mm Hg)							DIASTOLIC BP (mm Hg)						
		PERCENTILE OF HEIGHT							PERCENTILE OF HEIGHT						
		5th	10th	25th	50th	75th	90th	95th	5th	10th	25th	50th	75th	90th	95th
14	50th	106	106	107	109	110	111	112	63	63	63	64	65	66	66
	90th	119	120	121	122	124	125	125	77	77	77	78	79	80	80
	95th	123	123	125	126	127	129	129	81	81	81	82	83	84	84
	99th	130	131	132	133	135	136	136	88	88	89	90	90	91	92
15	50th	107	108	109	110	111	113	113	64	64	64	65	66	67	67
	90th	120	121	122	123	125	126	127	78	78	78	79	80	81	81
	95th	124	125	126	127	129	130	131	82	82	82	83	84	85	85
	99th	131	132	133	134	136	137	138	89	89	90	91	91	92	93
16	50th	108	108	110	111	112	114	114	64	64	65	66	66	67	68
	90th	121	122	123	124	126	127	128	78	78	79	80	81	81	82
	95th	125	126	127	128	130	131	132	82	82	83	84	85	85	86
	99th	132	133	134	135	137	138	139	90	90	90	91	92	93	93
17	50th	108	109	110	111	113	114	115	64	65	65	66	67	67	68
	90th	122	122	123	125	126	127	128	78	79	79	80	81	81	82
	95th	125	126	127	129	130	131	132	82	83	83	84	85	85	86
	99th	133	133	134	136	137	138	139	90	90	91	91	92	93	93

BP, Blood pressure.
*The 90th percentile is 1.28 3D, 95th percentile is 1.645 SD, and the 99th percentile is 2.326 3D over the mean.
National High Blood Pressure Education Program Working Group on High Blood Pressure in Children and Adolescents. The fourth report on the diagnosis, evaluation, and treatment of high blood pressure in children and adolescents. *Pediatrics.* 2004;114(2):555-572.

BOX 191-1 Common Causes of High Blood Pressure in Neonates and Infants

- Renal artery thrombosis after umbilical artery catheterization
- Coarctation of the aorta
- Congenital renal parenchymal or structural disease
- Renal artery stenosis
- Bronchopulmonary dysplasia
- Extracorporeal membrane oxygenation

or from increased catecholamine production caused by a pheochromocytoma. The problem can also be exogenous, arising from ingestion or abuse of glucocorticoids or other steroids. Because of the association of oral contraceptives with high BP, a history of contraceptive use should always be sought in adolescent girls.[15,25,34]

Various drugs can also be associated with hypertension, particularly sympathomimetics (cocaine, amphetamines, phenylephrine, and pseudoephedrine), and their use should be ruled out in older children.[15,25,34] Other drugs that can raise BP include nonsteroidal antiinflammatory drugs, erythropoietin, and cyclosporins.[21]

MEASURING BLOOD PRESSURE IN CHILDREN

Appropriate BP measurement techniques are important because false-positive readings are more likely when proper care is not taken.[2] All children older than 3 years who are seen in a medical setting should have their BP measured.[10] Children and adolescents should be seated, and infants should be supine. In addition, to obtain the best possible readings, the child should not have recently ingested stimulant drugs or food and should sit quietly for 5 minutes before the measurement, with his or her back supported and feet on the floor. The right arm should also be supported, with the antecubital fossa at heart level.[32]

An appropriately sized BP cuff should be used to take the measurement. The width of the cuff must be at least 40% of the mid-arm circumference, as measured midway between the olecranon and the acromion. The

BOX 191-2 Common Causes of High Blood Pressure in Children and Adolescents

- Renal disease
- Renal artery stenosis
- Coarctation of the aorta
- Mineralocorticoid excess
- Hyperthyroidism
- Pheochromocytoma
- Hypercalcemia
- Neurofibromatosis
- Neurogenic tumors
- Increased intracranial pressure
- Immobilization-induced essential hypertension

cuff should be long enough to cover at least 80% of the circumference of the arm.[10,32]

The cuff should be inflated to at least 30 mm Hg above the expected systolic BP, although inflating too high in young children or infants may cause agitation. The stethoscope or Doppler crystal should be placed lightly over the brachial artery in the antecubital fossa, with the arm at the level of the heart.

Systolic BP is defined as the pressure at the onset of the 1st Korotkoff (K1) sound, and diastolic BP as the pressure at the 5th Korotkoff (K5) sound or at the disappearance or muffling of the Korotkoff sounds. In some children, Korotkoff sounds can continue to be heard until 0 mm Hg, which generally excludes a diagnosis of diastolic hypertension. BP should be measured twice on each occasion, and the average systolic and diastolic pressure should be recorded.[10,32]

Automated BP devices can provide serial noninvasive BP measurements in newborns and infants, in whom auscultation is difficult, and in the intensive care unit, where frequent BP measurements are needed.[10] Automated measurements appear to correlate well with intraarterial readings.[35] Two advantages of these devices are their relative simplicity and ability to minimize observer bias and terminal digit preference.[10] However, the reliability of these instruments in the physician's office is less clear because they require frequent calibration and because reference standards have not been established.[32] Thus, in general, auscultation is the recommended method of measuring BP in children.

Ambulatory monitoring has recently been used to help establish the diagnosis of hypertension and to track diurnal variations of BP in older children. The monitors are worn on the arm for 24 hours. BP is measured periodically and the values stored for later analysis. Ambulatory BP monitoring is specifically helpful in evaluating white-coat hypertension, the risk for hypertensive end-organ injury, apparent drug resistance, and hypotensive symptoms that may occur with the use of antihypertensive drugs. In addition, ambulatory monitoring can be used to evaluate BP patterns in conditions such as episodic hypertension, chronic kidney disease, diabetes, and autonomic dysfunction. However, ambulatory BP monitoring of children and adolescents should only be used and interpreted by persons who are experienced in the field of pediatric hypertension.[10]

MECHANISMS OF BLOOD PRESSURE REGULATION

A complete discussion of the complex and intricately balanced hormonal and physical factors that regulate BP is beyond the scope of this chapter. Instead, the more important concepts are summarized.

BP is the product of cardiac output and systemic resistance; therefore anything that affects the heart rate, stroke volume, blood volume, or peripheral resistance will alter BP. Resistance is affected not only by physical changes, but also by the effect of various hormones on a given vascular bed. Angiotensin II is the major end product of the renin-angiotensin system, which exerts the major hormonal control of BP. Angiotensin II, a potent vasoconstrictor, increases intravascular volume and is closely related to renal blood flow. Renin is the enzyme that stimulates the production of angiotensin II. Renin release is stimulated by volume depletion, hypotension, and salt depletion and is inhibited by volume expansion, salt loading, and elevated electrolyte levels. Several other hormonal systems also affect renin release,[30] such as circulating catecholamines, glucagon, and adrenocorticotropic and parathyroid hormones. Angiotensin II itself provides feedback that inhibits renin release, and mineralocorticoids and antidiuretic hormone do the same.

Drugs can also affect renin release. Vasodilators and diuretics stimulate renin release, whereas mineralocorticoids and β-blockers inhibit it. Other hormonal systems also help regulate BP.[30,34] Catecholamine secretion increases BP, and in the presence of a pheochromocytoma or neuroblastoma, it can cause severe hypertension. Mineralocorticoids and glucocorticoids affect BP, and adrenal hypertrophy and tumors may lead to severe hypertension. Other, less well-known, hormonal systems may also contribute to BP regulation.

DIAGNOSTIC EVALUATION

The 1st step in evaluating a child believed to have hypertension is to conduct a thorough history and physical examination. The medical history should include questions regarding all cardiovascular risk factors, symptoms suggestive of secondary hypertension, and possible target organ damage.[21] Particular attention needs to be paid to any history suggesting the recent onset of renal disease or of chronic urinary tract infections. In adolescents, the use of exogenous steroids, oral contraceptives, illicit drugs, tobacco, or alcohol should be specifically explored. A history of prematurity, patent ductus arteriosus, or bronchopulmonary dysplasia and a positive family history, including age of onset, of essential hypertension, systemic disease, or endocrinopathy, may be valuable in directing further evaluations. A systems review that includes details regarding diet, salt intake, and exercise will be helpful in eliciting symptoms associated with specific diseases that can cause hypertension.

Critical in the physical examination is careful measurement of BP, as described earlier, with special attention to using an appropriately sized cuff and to measurement technique. BP should be measured in all 4 extremities, along with assessment of the radial, brachial, and, most important, femoral pulses. A complete examination needs to be performed to identify any abnormalities, including an examination of the optic fundi; calculation of BMI (weight in kilograms divided by the square of height in meters); auscultation for carotid, abdominal, and femoral bruits; palpation of the thyroid gland; a thorough examination of the heart and lungs; examination of the abdomen for enlarged kidneys, masses, and abnormal aortic pulsation; palpation of the legs for edema and pulses; and a neurologic assessment.[8] These findings will further direct evaluation, which should be a stepwise investigation tailored to the age of the child and to the specific findings. For example, decreased femoral pulses may indicate coarctation of the aorta.[8]

An algorithm for diagnosing and managing patients who have hypertension is given in Figure 191-2. Ideally, key BP values should be an average of at least 2 separate measurements or, even better, of

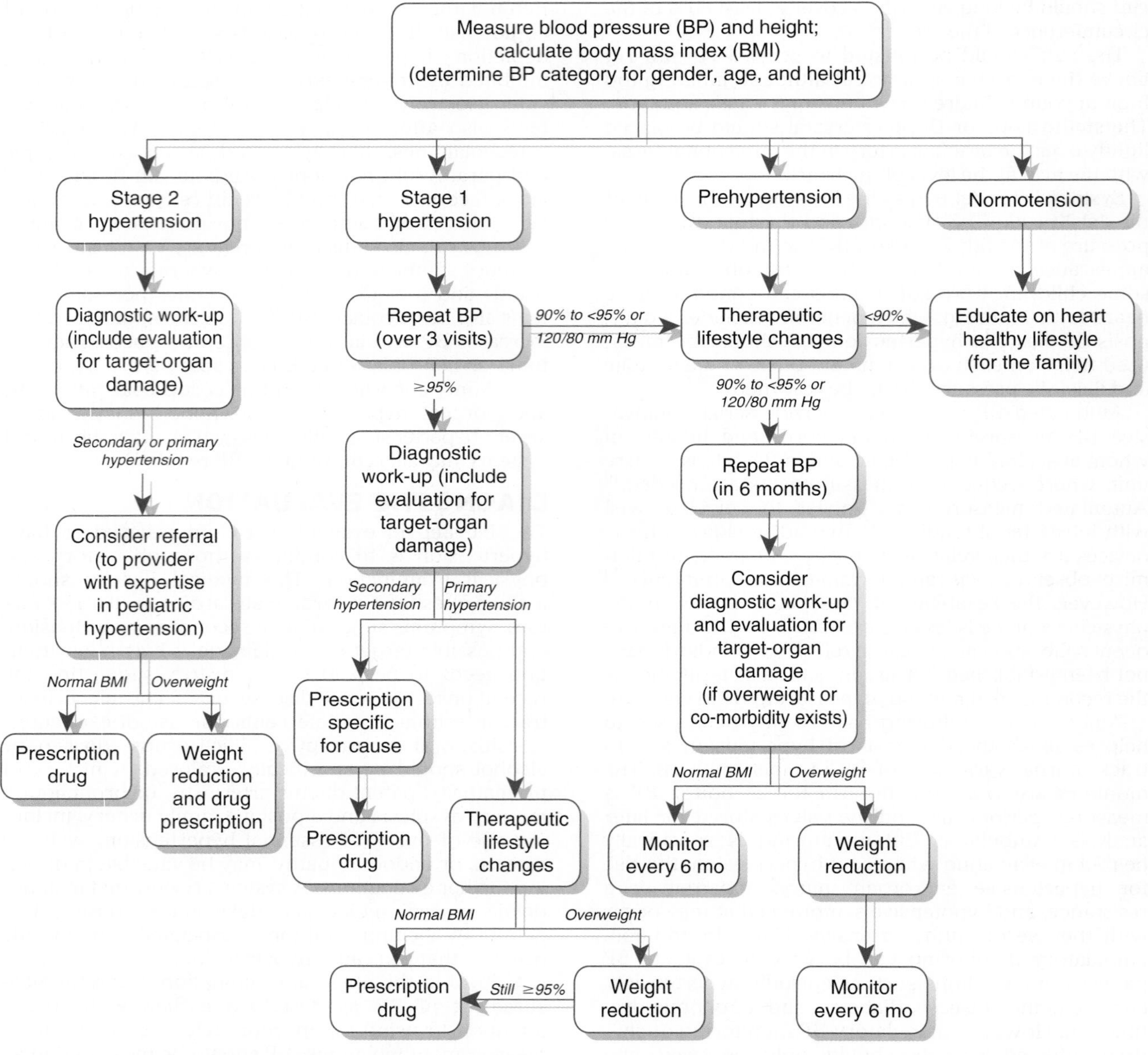

Figure 191-2 Algorithm for diagnosing high blood pressure in children. *(Modified from National High Blood Pressure Education Program Working Group on High Blood Pressure in Children and Adolescents. The fourth report on the diagnosis, evaluation, and treatment of high blood pressure in children and adolescents.* Pediatrics. *2004;114(2): 555-572.)*

measurements obtained during several visits. All patients should have a general laboratory screening for possible renal dysfunction, including urinalysis, complete blood count, serum urea nitrogen and creatinine, and serum electrolytes that includes glucose. A urine culture and a renal ultrasound may be necessary. If the family history is positive for essential hypertension, then a lipid profile that includes high-density lipoprotein cholesterol, low-density lipoprotein cholesterol, and triglycerides will help assess cardiovascular risk.[10]

If BP remains elevated after initial treatment, then more intensive investigations should follow. If a renal cause is thought to exist, then further imaging of the genitourinary system may be necessary. The recommended approaches for evaluating renovascular disease generally use older techniques such as standard intraarterial angiography, digital-subtraction angiography, or scintigraphy (with or without angiotensin-converting enzyme inhibition).[10] Plasma renin level or plasma renin activity can be used as a screening test for mineralocorticoid disease. Thyroid function tests or serum catecholamines may be helpful if hyperthyroidism or pheochromocytoma is thought to be present.

Cardiac evaluation is an important part of the examination.[10,36] In addition to a thorough physical

Table 191-3 Antihypertensive Drugs Commonly Used to Manage Chronic Hypertension in Children

DRUG	INITIAL DOSE (mg/kg/day)	MAXIMAL DOSE (mg/kg/day)	INTERVAL (TIMES/DAY)
ACE INHIBITORS			
Benazepril	0.2-10	0.6-40	4
Captopril	0.3-0.5	6	3
Enalapril	0.08-5	0.6-40	2-4
Fosinopril	5-10	40	4
Lisinopril	0.07-5	0.6-40	4
Quinapril	5-10	80	4
ANGIOTENSIN-RECEPTOR BLOCKERS			
Irbesartan			
6-12 yr	75-150	—	4
>13 yr	150-300	—	4
Losartan	0.7-50	1.4-100	4
ALPHA- AND BETA-BLOCKERS			
Labetalol	1-3	10-1200	2
Atenolol	0.5-1	2-100	2-4
Bisoprolol/HCTZ	2.5/6.25	10/6.25	4
Metoprolol	1-2	6-200	2
Propranolol	1-2	4-640	2-3
CALCIUM-CHANNEL BLOCKERS			
Amlodipine (>6 yr)	2.5-5	—	4
Felodipine	2.5	10	4
Isradipine	0.15-0.2	0.8-20	3-4
Extended-release nifedipine	0.25-0.5	3-120	2-4
CENTRAL ALPHA-AGONIST			
Clonidine (>12 yr)	0.2	2.4	2
DIURETICS			
HCTZ	1	3-50	4
Chlorthalidone	0.3	2-50	4
Furosemide	0.5-2	6	2-4
Spironolactone	1	3.3-100	2-4
Triamterene	1-2	3-300	2
Amiloride	0.4-0.625	20	4
PERIPHERAL ALPHA-AGONISTS			
Doxazosin	1	4	4
Prazosin	0.05-0.1	0.5	3
Terazosin	1	20	4
VASODILATORS			
Hydralazine	0.75	7.5-200	4
Minoxidil			
<12 yr	0.2	50	3-4
>12 yr	5	100	3-4

ACE, Angiotensin-converting enzyme; *HCTZ*, hydrochlorothiazide.

examination that includes measurement of the femoral pulse, an electrocardiogram and echocardiogram may identify coarctation of the aorta and will provide information about left ventricular mass. Left ventricular hypertrophy is the most prominent evidence of target-organ damage. Thus children with established hypertension should have echocardiographic assessment of left ventricular mass at diagnosis and periodically thereafter.[10] Formal stress testing can help assess normal and abnormal BP responses to exercise, which might be especially helpful in young athletes.[25] Ambulatory BP measurements can help detect hypertension and determine the amount of time each day that BP is elevated.

Determining if elevated BP will respond to salt restriction and whether it is sensitive to stress is also important. Isometric handgrip exercises and serial subtractions from 100 are easy to perform; if the diastolic BP increases by 20 mm Hg or more and the systolic by 30 mm Hg or more, then the patient is a stress reactor and may respond to behavioral modification techniques, diet, and exercise.

THERAPY FOR HIGH BLOOD PRESSURE

The justification for treating children who have marked hypertension comes from the results of adult trials showing that reducing BP reduces the risk of target-organ damage. Therapeutic lifestyle changes are generally recommended for children with mild or moderate hypertension. Initiating a low-salt or no-added-salt diet is reasonable because many patients will be salt sensitive. In addition, the intake of fresh vegetables, fruits, fiber, and low-fat dairy products should be increased.[37]

Body size is a major determinant of BP, and weight loss is often associated with reduction in both systolic and diastolic pressures. BP tracking and weight-reduction studies support the potential for controlling BP in children through weight reduction. Maintaining a normal weight in childhood reduces the likelihood of high BP in adulthood. Studies of overweight adolescents with high BP have repeatedly shown that weight loss is associated with a decrease in BP. Weight loss also is associated with decreased BP sensitivity to salt and decreases in other risk factors, such as dyslipidemia and insulin resistance.[10] Thus weight loss in children and adolescents can be focused on health reasons instead of aesthetic reasons.

Exercise as an adjunct to weight loss often reduces BP even more than weight loss alone. Increasing regular physical activity and decreasing sedentary activities are important in preventing hypertension in childhood and adolescents.

When children and adolescents do not respond to lifestyle modifications or have conditions such as systemic hypertension, secondary hypertension, or established hypertensive target-organ damage, pharmacologic therapy is indicated. Because data on the long-term effects of antihypertensive therapy in children are lacking, a definite indication for drug therapy is needed before it should be started.[10]

All classes of antihypertensive drugs lower BP in children; therefore the choice of therapy remains with the treating physician (Table 191-3). The basic strategy of pharmacologic therapy is to start with a single drug and assess the response. Additional drugs should be added one at a time, always attempting to target a different organ system. The drug of 1st choice is usually an angiotensin-converting enzyme inhibitor or a calcium-channel blocker. Beta-blockers can also be used, but they tend to produce more side effects and can be problematic for patients who have reactive airway disease or diabetes. The α-agonists are generally considered to be 2nd-line drugs, and diuretics are now being used less often for initial therapy of chronic hypertension. For children who have chronic primary hypertension but no hypertensive target-organ damage, the goal of pharmacologic therapy should be to reduce BP to below the 95th percentile for gender, age, and height. For children with chronic renal disease, diabetes, or hypertensive target-organ damage, the goal of therapy should be to reduce BP to below the 90th percentile for gender, age, and height.[10]

Hypertensive emergencies in children are usually accompanied by signs of hypertensive encephalopathy, typically seizures (Table 191-4). Thus initial treatment should focus on reducing BP to alleviate acute symptoms, not necessarily to make the patient normotensive. Hypertensive emergencies should be treated with an intravenous antihypertensive medication that can steadily reduce BP, decreasing the pressure by no more than 25% over the first 8 hours and then

Table 191-4 Antihypertensive Drugs Commonly Used to Manage Severe Hypertension in Children

DRUG	CLASS	DOSE	ROUTE
MOST USEFUL			
Esmolol	Beta-blocker	100-500 mcg/kg/min	IV infusion
Hydralazine	Vasodilator	0.2-0.6 mg/kg/dose	IV, IM
Labetalol	Alpha- or beta-blocker	—	—
Bolus	—	0.2-1 mg/kg/dose to 40 mg/dose	IV bolus
Infusion	—	0.25-3 mg/kg/hr	IV infusion
Nicardipine	Calcium-channel blocker	1-3 mcg/kg/min	IV infusion
Sodium nitroprusside	Vasodilator	0.53-10 mcg/kg/min	IV infusion
OCCASIONALLY USEFUL			
Clonidine	Central alpha-agonist	0.05-0.1 mg/dose (may be repeated up to 0.8 mg total dose)	Oral
Enalaprilat	ACE Inhibitor	0.05-0.1 mg/kg/dose up to 1.25 mg/dose	IV bolus
Fenoldopam	Dopamine-receptor agonist	0.2-0.8 mcg/kg/min	IV infusion
Isradipine	Calcium-channel blocker	0.05-0.1 mg/kg/dose	Oral
Minoxidil	Vasodilator	0.1-0.2 mg/kg/dose	Oral

ACE, Angiotensin-converting enzyme.
Modified from National High Blood Pressure Education Program Working Group on High Blood Pressure in Children and Adolescents. The fourth report on the diagnosis, evaluation, and treatment of high blood pressure in children and adolescents. *Pediatrics.* 2004;114(2):555-572.

gradually reducing it to normal over the next 24 to 48 hours. Hypertensive urgencies produce less-serious symptoms, such as severe headache or vomiting. Urgencies can be treated either by intravenous or by oral antihypertensives.[10]

CONCLUSION

Evidence of a link between the onset of hypertension in childhood and adult morbidity and mortality from end-organ damage is increasing. As pediatricians become more aware of the importance of monitoring BP in childhood and diagnosing hypertension earlier, they have the opportunity to decrease its long-term adverse cardiovascular effects. Even small reductions in BP can improve the health of children and their cardiovascular status later in life. Of equal importance for physicians is the need to educate parents and children about the health dangers of obesity, as this condition becomes more prevalent in today's culture.

WHEN TO REFER

- Stage-one hypertension (an average systolic or diastolic BP between the 95th and the 99th percentile plus 5 mm Hg)
- Stage-two hypertension (persistent BP above the 99th percentile plus 5 mm Hg)

Specific conditions requiring referral[38,39]:

- Abnormal BP by 2 to 3 measurements over a 1-month period
- Symptomatic essential hypertension
- Secondary hypertension
- Hypertension with diabetes
- Evidence of target-organ damage (left ventricular hypertrophy)

WHEN TO ADMIT

- Hypertensive emergencies (associated with manifestations in other organs)
- Hypertensive urgencies (severe BP elevation without other organ involvement)

Specific conditions requiring admission[39,40]:

- Hypertensive encephalopathy
- Acute glomerular diseases
- Poststreptococcal glomerulonephritis
- Hemolytic uremic syndrome
- Renal artery stenosis
- Fibromuscular dysplasia
- Previous umbilical artery catheter
- Neurofibromatosis
- Pheochromocytoma
- Coarctation of aorta
- Noncompliance with current antihypertensive medication
- Cocaine toxicity
- Dialysis patients with excessive volume expansion

AAP POLICY STATEMENT

National High Blood Pressure Education Program Working Group on High Blood Pressure in Children and Adolescents. The fourth report on the diagnosis, evaluation, and treatment of high blood pressure in children and adolescents. *Pediatrics.* 2004;114(2):555-576. (AAP endorsed).

REFERENCES

1. Cook S, Weitzman M, Auinger P, et al. Prevalence of a metabolic syndrome phenotype in adolescents: findings from the third National Health and Nutrition Examination Survey 1988-1994. *Arch Pediatr Adolesc Med.* 2003; 157:821-827.
2. National Heart, Lung, and Blood Institute. Report of the Second Task Force on Blood Pressure Control in Children—1987. *Pediatrics.* 1987;79:1-25.
3. World Health Organization. World health report 2002. Reducing risks, promoting healthy life, 2002. Geneva, Switzerland. Available at www.who.int/whr/2002.
4. Muntner P, He J, Cutler JA, et al. Trends in blood pressure among children and adolescents. *JAMA.* 2004;291: 2107-2113.
5. Chen W, Srinivasan SR, Li S, et al. Metabolic syndrome variables at low levels in childhood are beneficially associated with adulthood cardiovascular risk: the Bogalusa Heart Study. *Diabetes Care.* 2005;28:126-131.
6. Cook NR, Gillman MW, Rosner BA, et al. Combining annual blood pressure measurements in childhood to improve prediction of young adult blood pressure. *Stat Med.* 2000;19:2625-2640.
7. Zinner SH, Rosner B, Oh W, et al. Significance of blood pressure in infancy: familial aggregation and predictive effect on later blood pressure. *Hypertension.* 1985;7: 411-416.
8. Chobanian AV, Bakris GL, Black HR, et al. Seventh report of the Joint National Committee on Prevention, Detection, Evaluation, and Treatment of High Blood Pressure. *Hypertension.* 2003;42:1206-1252.
9. Sinaiko AR. Treatment of hypertension in children (review). *Pediatr Nephrol.* 1994;8:603-612.
10. National High Blood Pressure Education Program Working Group on High Blood Pressure in Children and Adolescents. The fourth report on the diagnosis, evaluation, and treatment of high blood pressure in children and adolescents. *Pediatrics.* 2004;114:555-576.
11. Sadowski RH, Falkner B. Hypertension in pediatric patients. *Am J Kidney Dis.* 1996;3:305-315.
12. Sinaiko AR. Hypertension in children. *N Engl J Med.* 1996;335:1968-1673.
13. Sealy WC. Paradoxical hypertension after repair of coarctation of the aorta: a review of its causes. *Ann Thorac Surg.* 1990;50:323-329.
14. Lauer RM, Clarke WR. Childhood risk factors for high adult blood pressure: the Muscatine Study. *Pediatrics.* 1984;84:633.
15. Sharma A, Sinaiko AR. Systemic hypertension. In: Emmanouilides GC, ed. *Moss and Adams Heart Disease in Infants, Children and Adolescents.* 5th ed. Baltimore, MD: Williams and Wilkins; 1995.
16. Institute of Medicine. *Preventing Childhood Obesity: Health in the Balance.* Washington, DC: National Academy Press; 2004.
17. Centers for Disease Control and Prevention. Overweight and Obesity 2004. Available at www.cdc.gov/nccdphp/ dnpa/obesity/index.htm.
18. de Ferranti SD, Gauvreau K, Ludwig DS, et al. Prevalence of the metabolic syndrome in American adolescents: findings from the Third National Health and Nutrition Examination Survey. *Circulation.* 2004;110:2494-2497.

19. Munger RG, Prineas RJ, Gomez-Marin O. Persistent elevation of blood pressure among children with a family history of hypertension: the Minneapolis Children's Blood Pressure Study. *J Hyperten*. 1988;6:647-653.
20. Shear CL, Burke GL, Freedman DS, et al. Values of childhood blood pressure measurements and family history in predicting future blood pressure status: results from eight years of follow-up in the Bogalusa Heart Study. *Pediatrics*. 1996;77:862-869.
21. Varda NM, Gregoric A. A diagnostic approach for the child with hypertension. *Pediatr Nephrol*. 2005;20: 499-506.
22. Flynn JT, Alderman MH. Characteristics of children with primary hypertension seen at a referral center. *Pediatr Nephrol*. 2005;20:961-969.
23. Adelman R. Neonatal hypertension. *Pediatr Clin North Am*. 1978;25:99-110.
24. Adelman RD. Long-term follow-up of neonatal renovascular hypertension. *Pediatr Nephrol*. 1987;1:35-41.
25. Peters RM, Flack JM. Diagnosis and treatment of hypertension in children and adolescents. *J Am Acad Nurse Pract*. 2003;15:56-63.
26. Boedy RF, Goldberg AK, Howell CG Jr, et al. Incidence of hypertension in infants on extracorporeal membrane oxygenation. *J Pediatr Surg*. 1990;25:258-261.
27. Gordon T, Kannel WB, eds. An epidemiological investigation of cardiovascular disease: the Framingham Study. *US DHEW* 1968-1972. 1972;1:27.
28. Shurtleff D. Some characteristics related to the incidence of cardiovascular disease and death: the Framingham Study, 18-year follow-up. *US DHEW*. September 30, 1974;74:599.
29. Lerner GR, Fleischmann LE, Perimutter AD. Reflux nephropathy. *Pediatr Clin North Am* 1987;34:747-770.
30. Ingelfinger JR. The renin-angiotensin system and other hormonal systems in the control of blood pressure. In: Ingelfinger JR. *Pediatric Hypertension*. Philadelphia, PA: WB Saunders; 1982.
31. Liberthson RR, Pennington DG, Jacobs ML, et al. Coarctation of the aorta: review of 234 patients and clarification of management problems. *Am J Cardiol*. 1979; 43:835-840.
32. National High Blood Pressure Education Program. Update on the 1987 task force report on high blood pressure in children and adolescents: a working group report from the National High Blood Pressure Education Program Working Group on Hypertension Control in Children and Adolescents. *Pediatrics*. 1996;98:649-658.
33. Deal JE, Snell MF, Barratt TM, et al. Renovascular disease in childhood. *J Pediatr*. 1992;121:378-384.
34. Hackman AM, Bricker JT. Preventive cardiology, hypertension and dyslipidemia. In: Garson A Jr, ed. *The Science and Practice of Pediatric Cardiology*. 2nd ed. Baltimore, MD: Williams and Wilkins; 1998.
35. Colan SD, Fujii A, Borow KM, et al. Noninvasive determination of systolic, diastolic and end-systolic blood pressure in neonates, infants and young children: comparison with central aortic pressure measurements. *Am J Cardiol*. 1983;52:867.
36. Frohlich ED, Apstein C, Chobanian AV, et al. The heart in hypertension. *N Engl J Med*. 1992;327:998-1008.
37. Sacks FM, Svetkey LP, Vollmer WM, et al. Effects on blood pressure of reduced dietary sodium and the Dietary Approaches to Stop Hypertension (DASH) diet. *N Engl J Med*. 2001;344:3-10.
38. Portman R, Sorof J, Ingelfinger J, eds. *Pediatric Hypertension*. Totowa, NJ: Humana Press; 2004.
39. Burg FD, Ingelfinger JR, Polin RA, et al. *Current Pediatric Therapy*. 18th ed. Philadelphia, PA: Saunders Elsevier; 2006.
40. Adelman RD. Management of hypertensive emergencies. In: Portman RJ, Sorof JM, Ingelfinger JR, eds. *Pediatric Hypertension*. Totowa, NJ: Human Press; 2004.

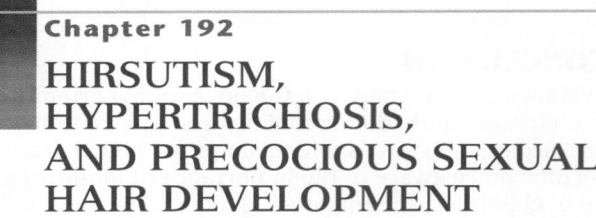

Chapter 192

HIRSUTISM, HYPERTRICHOSIS, AND PRECOCIOUS SEXUAL HAIR DEVELOPMENT

Joan DiMartino-Nardi, MD; Mala Puri, MD

BACKGROUND

The growth and distribution of body hair depends on the patient's ethnic background, age, and sex. Body hair is generally classified as either vellus or terminal.[1] Vellus hair is soft, short, fine, and less pigmented; terminal hair is coarse, long, and more pigmented. The term *sexual hair growth* refers to the presence of terminal hair on the face, chin, neck, midline chest, abdomen, upper and lower back, buttocks, axilla, pubic area, and inner aspect of the thigh. The transformation of vellus hair into terminal sexual hair is androgen dependent. Normal androgen production, in turn, depends on the gender and age of the patient. In girls, androgens are normally produced only after the age of 8 years and in boys after the age of 9 years; thus pathological hair growth refers to the timing, as well as to the amount, of sexual hair growth.

DEFINITIONS

Hirsutism refers to excessive body hair growth in the sex hormone–dependent areas, and it represents either androgen overproduction or enhanced androgen metabolism in the skin tissue. Androgen production and metabolism affect hair follicles and the sebaceous glands of the skin. Hence hirsutism may be associated with acne vulgaris, although the degree of hirsutism and acne in patients varies tremendously. *Hypertrichosis* refers to the generalized increase in fine body hair with no special preferential sites, most often not associated with pathological sex hormone production. Its presence is usually determined by genetic or ethnic background, but it may be induced by chronic ingestion of certain drugs such as oral diazoxide used for the treatment of hyperinsulinism. Hypertrichosis can be a feature of several congenital syndromes, including congenital hypertrichosis lanuginosa, generalized lipodystrophy, fetal hydantoin syndrome, mucopolysaccharidoses, trisomy 18, leprechaunism, and Cornelia de Lange syndrome. In some cases, hypertrichosis may be an early manifestation of mild androgen excess and should be monitored closely because certain children with premature adrenarche may be at risk for polycystic ovary syndrome (PCOS) and the associated metabolic syndrome. Both hirsutism and hypertrichosis can be caused by medications (Box 192-1.)

Virilization, or *masculinization,* refers to phallic or clitoral enlargement, masculine body habitus, temporal

BOX 192-1 Medications That May Cause Hirsutism or Hypertrichosis

HIRSUTISM	HYPERTRICHOSIS
Anabolic steroids	Cyclosporine (Sandimmune)
Danazol (Danocrine)	Diazoxide (Hyperstat)
Metoclopramide (Reglan)	Hydrocortisone
Methyldopa (Aldomet)	Minoxidil (Rogaine)
Phenothiazines	Penicillamine (Cuprimine)
Progestins	Phenytoin (Dilantin)
Reserpine (Serpasil)	Psoralens (Oxsoralen)
Testosterone	Streptomycin

From Leung AK, Robson WL. Hirsutism. *Int J Dermatol.* 1993;32:773-777.

hair loss, voice changes, breast atrophy, and menstrual disorders, all manifestations of pathological androgen overproduction.

Excessive androgen exposure can occur either prenatally or postnatally. Because the development of the external genitalia occurs in the first trimester, exposure of the female infant to significant androgens during this time, such as in the congenital adrenal hyperplasia syndromes, will cause genital ambiguity, including varying degrees of clitoral enlargement and labial fusion. The exposure of the female infant to excessive androgens after the first trimester results in clitoral enlargement but does not result in labial fusion. The male infant exposed to excessive androgens in utero is not born with abnormal genitalia. If the condition causing androgen overproduction is undiagnosed or inadequately treated, then the child will develop early sexual hair growth and will continue to virilize. In the growing child, excessive androgens contribute to an increased growth velocity, rapid epiphyseal maturation, excessive bone-age advancement, and short adult stature.

HYPERANDROGENISM

Hirsutism in women and early sexual hair growth in girls and boys may represent either excessive or early hyperandrogenism from either gonadal or adrenal disease.

Gonadal Androgen Production

Ovarian Androgen Production

GONADARCHE. *Gonadarche* refers to the maturation of the hypothalamic-pituitary-gonadal axis.[2] The activation of the pulsatile release of gonadotropin-releasing hormone (GnRH) from the hypothalamus results in an increase in the amplitude and frequency of pituitary gonadotropin secretion and results in gonadal maturation. Pituitary luteinizing hormone (LH) stimulates ovarian androgen synthesis, occurring mainly in the theca cells, stroma cells, and the corpus luteum. The major androgens secreted by the ovaries include Δ-4-androstenedione and testosterone, and their levels gradually increase during gonadarche. These androgens contribute to the development of pubic hair, axillary hair and odor, and acne. The ovary converts androgens to estrogen in the granulosa cell layer via stimulation from pituitary follicle-stimulating hormone (FSH). Estrogens contribute to breast development, uterine enlargement, vaginal discharge, and menarche. Recently, insulin and insulin-like growth factor (IGF-1) have been shown to have a role in normal ovarian steroidogenesis.[3] The presence of true puberty can be confirmed by detecting a rise in gonadotropins in response to a bolus dose of GnRH in the GnRH-stimulation test.[4] In addition, puberty is characterized by an increase in growth velocity (pubertal growth spurt) that results from an increase in growth hormone secretion.

TRUE PRECOCIOUS PUBERTY. The early maturation of the hypothalamic-pituitary-gonadal axis in girls before the age of 8 years is termed *true precocious puberty.* Clinically, girls have early development of pubic hair, axillary hair and odor, acne, and breast development. Most commonly, breast development occurs initially, but sexual hair growth may precede breast development. The suspicion of true precocious puberty can be confirmed by finding a pubertal gonadotropin response to a GnRH-stimulation test. In most cases, early puberty is not caused by a specific identifiable lesion. However, in some cases, especially in a child younger than 6 years, a hypothalamic or pituitary lesion may be the cause of early puberty. Hence the evaluation of the precocious child should include magnetic resonance imaging (MRI) with gadolinium of the hypothalamic-pituitary area.

Precocious puberty can be associated with astrocytomas, craniopharyngiomas, ependymomas, germinomas, and gliomas. A hypothalamic hamartoma is a congenital malformation consisting of benign neurovascular tissue containing its own GnRH pulse generator.[5] Identification of a hamartoma is important because this lesion is amenable to medical therapy with GnRH analogs. Precocious puberty can also be associated with virtually any central nervous system (CNS) insult, such as trauma, surgery, inflammation, and neurologic-mental deficits. Prolonged exposure to sex steroids can also precipitate precocious puberty. For example, in children who have poorly controlled adrenal hyperplasia or who have ovarian cysts, the chronic exposure to hyperandrogenism or estrogen can cause early maturation of the hypothalamic-pituitary-gonadal axis and secondary true precocious puberty.[6]

Pubertal progression can vary considerably in the child who is precocious. In many children, puberty is slowly progressive and may not be of major concern to the patients or their parents. However, some children can have rapid pubertal progression. In the latter group, psychosocial issues surrounding early puberty may be of particular concern. In general, a child's social maturity reflects chronologic age rather than pubertal status. Furthermore, the early production of sex steroids can cause rapid epiphyseal maturation and result in short stature. Obtaining a bone-age radiograph can help identify the child who is at risk for short stature.[7] Treatment with long-acting preparations of GnRH (GnRH analog) is available for children whose parents are particularly concerned about the psychosocial issues surrounding early sexual development or the risk for short stature.[8] The GnRH analogs are effective in halting pubertal progression and preventing menses. In addition, via a reduction in growth hormone secretion, the child's growth velocity declines.[9] The reduction in sex steroids either halts or reduces the rate of bone-age maturation. The net result is an improvement in predicted height and, ultimately, adult stature.

PERIPHERAL PRECOCIOUS PUBERTY. In girls, the production of sex steroids from the ovaries, the adrenals, or both that is independent of the activation of the hypothalamic-pituitary axis is known as peripheral precocious puberty.

Ovarian Androgen-Producing Tumors. Ovarian tumors producing androgens can cause early sexual hair growth, hirsutism, or virilization. The concurrent secretion of estrogen can result in premature breast development, vaginal discharge, or irregular uterine bleeding. Patients may have excessive weight gain, acceleration of linear growth, and an advanced bone age. Abdominal symptoms (cramps, pain, mass, distention) also may occur. In the young child, these symptoms can mimic true precocious puberty. Rapid pubertal progression suggests the presence of a tumor, but not all ovarian tumors affect pubertal progression. Virilization is never normal. Finding markedly elevated estradiol, androstenedione, or testosterone is consistent with an ovarian lesion. In contrast to true precocious puberty the peripheral precocious puberty resulting from an ovarian tumor occurs independently of the hypothalamic-pituitary axis. A GnRH-stimulation test can distinguish between the conditions because the gonadotropin response is suppressed in peripheral precocious puberty. Pelvic ultrasound can be useful in identifying cystic or solid ovarian lesions. The tumorous androgen-producing cells can occur in association with embryonal carcinomas, dysgerminomas, choriocarcinomas, gonadoblastomas, granulosa-theca cell tumors, Sertoli-Leydig cell tumors, and arrhenoblastomas.[10,11] These tumors can occur in phenotypic girls having an abnormal karyotype containing components of the Y chromosome. Because dysgenetic gonads, in which differentiation into testis or ovary is either absent or incomplete, are at risk for malignant deterioration, prophylactic gonadectomy is recommended in these girls.

Polycystic Ovary Syndrome. PCOS is a disorder with a wide spectrum of hyperandrogenic signs and symptoms, including hirsutism, acne, and chronic anovulation, with resultant irregular menses, amenorrhea, dysfunctional uterine bleeding, or infertility.[12] Virilization is not common with this condition. The precise cause of chronic ovarian hyperandrogenism is not known, but several factors have been implicated, including altered gonadotropin secretion, hyperinsulinism, IGF-1 and alterations of IGF-1–binding proteins, hyperprolactinemia, thyroid disease, and adrenal hyperandrogenism. Evidence demonstrates a link between PCOS and inappropriate gonadotropin secretion, hyperinsulinemia, and impaired glucose tolerance (IGT) independent of weight. Women who have insulin resistance are at risk of developing the complications of chronic hyperinsulinism, including hyperpigmentation in the intertriginal skin sites known as *acanthosis nigricans,* IGT, type 2 diabetes mellitus (T2DM), lipid abnormalities (low high-density lipoprotein cholesterol and high low-density lipoprotein cholesterol), atherosclerosis, and cardiovascular disease. Compared with age-matched controls, women with PCOS have an 11-fold increase in the prevalence of metabolic syndrome. The risk of metabolic syndrome is high even at a young age, highlighting the importance of early and regular screening.[13] Ovarian hyperandrogenism can also occur in certain insulin-resistant syndromes such as leprechaunism (associated with severe congenital growth retardation) and the Kahn type B insulin resistance syndrome caused by the presence of circulating antibodies for the insulin receptor.[14,15] As in adult patients with PCOS, 33% of adolescent girls with PCOS have abnormal oral glucose tolerance tests indicating IGT or T2DM.[16]

The hormonal evidence of PCOS can include an increased LH/FSH ratio greater than 2, generous levels of Δ-4-androstenedione, increased total and free testosterone with a reduced level of sex hormone–binding globulin and variable levels of estradiol. The presence of virilization or a total testosterone level greater than 150 ng/dL suggests the presence of a tumor. Insulin resistance can be confirmed by fasting hyperinsulinism and a reduced fasting glucose/insulin ratio or an increased homeostatic model assessment—a marker for insulin resistance.[17] A glucose tolerance test can detect IGT or T2DM and has been found to be the most reliable screening test for these conditions in girls with PCOS.[16]

Grossly, the ovaries in PCOS have subcapsular cysts that may be detected by ultrasound, but the absence of cysts on ultrasound does not exclude the diagnosis of PCOS. Hormonal evidence of PCOS can be discerned before the morphologic changes can be appreciated by ultrasound. However, an ultrasound should be performed if an ovarian lesion is suspected.

Although PCOS has been studied extensively in adolescents and adult women, the developmental aspects of PCOS are yet to be elucidated. Recently, premature adrenarche has been identified as a possible risk factor for PCOS (see the section on premature adrenarche).

Testicular Androgen Production

TRUE CENTRAL PRECOCIOUS PUBERTY. True central precocious puberty in boys refers to the activation of the hypothalamic-pituitary-gonadal axis before the age of 9. Levels of testosterone rise and a pubertal pattern of gonadotropin release can be detected with a GnRH-stimulation test. The rise of gonadotropins causes testicular growth and full physical pubertal development. As in girls, an MRI of the pituitary gland should be performed to identify a hypothalamic or pituitary lesion. Whereas idiopathic central precocious puberty is more frequent in girls, boys more commonly have CNS disease. Rarely, severe chronic hypothyroidism can be associated with true precocious puberty.[18] True precocious puberty in boys can be suppressed with GnRH analogs.

PERIPHERAL PRECOCIOUS PUBERTY. As in girls the production of sex steroids from either the testes or the adrenals independent of an activated hypothalamic-pituitary-gonadal axis is referred to as *peripheral precocious puberty.* Evaluation entails identifying the source of hyperandrogenism. The presence of enlarged testes suggests a gonadal source of hyperandrogenism; the presence of small (1 to 2 mL) testes is consistent with adrenal disease (see the section on adrenal hyperandrogenism).

Testicular Tumors. Leydig cell tumors and seminomas can produce testosterone. However, many testicular tumors can cause testicular enlargement without symptoms of hyperandrogenism, including the germ cell tumors (embryonal carcinoma, endodermal sinus tumor, and teratoma). Boys who have cryptorchidism and delayed orchiopexy after the age of 6 are at increased risk.[19,20] Dysgenetic gonads associated with androgen insensitivity, persistent müllerian syndrome, true hermaphroditism, and Klinefelter syndrome have a higher incidence of germ cell tumors as well.[21,22]

Familial Gonadotropin-Independent Puberty. Familial gonadotropin-independent puberty is a condition in which an autosomal-dominant, male-limited mutation of the LH receptor results in autonomous Leydig cell activity with resultant gonadotropin-independent precocity, including gonadal steroidogenesis and spermatogenesis.[23] In boys who clinically have precocious puberty, testosterone levels are high, and GnRH-stimulated gonadotropins are low. If left undiagnosed, then the chronic hyperandrogenism will eventually precipitate true precocious puberty.

Chorionic Gonadotropin-Secreting Tumors. Teratomas, embryonal tumors, hepatoblastomas, and CNS germinomas can produce human chorionic gonadotropin, which has been implicated in peripheral precocious puberty among male patients.

Adrenal Hyperandrogenism

The adrenal glands produce 3 groups of steroids: (1) glucocorticoids (cortisol), (2) mineralocorticoids (aldosterone and desoxycorticosterone), and (3) androgens (dehydroepiandrosterone, Δ-4-androstenedione, and testosterone). Glucocorticoid and androgen production are stimulated primarily by pituitary adrenocorticotropic hormone (ACTH). Exogenous glucocorticoids, by suppressing ACTH, suppress glucocorticoid and androgen production. The mineralocorticoids are regulated primarily by the renin-angiotensin enzyme system, which is stimulated and suppressed by low- and high-salt diets, respectively. Disorders of adrenal hyperandrogenism caused by enzymatic defects of steroidogenesis (congenital adrenal hyperplasia) respond to stimulation and suppression tests. On the other hand, the functional adrenal tumors are characterized by their ability to produce steroids independently of pituitary ACTH or the renin-angiotensin enzyme system. As a rule, they do not respond to the dynamic tests known to affect adrenal steroidogenesis.

Premature Adrenarche

Normal puberty is characterized by 2 generally simultaneous processes after the age of 8 in girls and 9 in boys: gonadarche and adrenarche. Gonadarche refers to the activation of the hypothalamic-pituitary-gonadal axis, and adrenarche refers to the activation of the hypothalamic-pituitary-adrenal axis, although the precise trigger for adrenarche is not known. Normal adrenarche results from the gradual increase in androgen biosynthesis that occurs as the innermost zona reticularis of the adrenal cortex matures. The increase in adrenal androgen production can be detected at approximately 6 years, and the phenotypic outcome consists of the development of axillary and pubic hair at approximately 8 years. As puberty progresses, one can detect the gradual rise in androgen levels in response to a standard test of adrenal steroidogenesis known as the ACTH-stimulation test.[24] The adrenal androgen response depends on the age, gender, and pubertal status of the child. When adrenarche occurs in girls before the age of 8 years and in boys before the age of 9 years, the condition is referred to as *premature adrenarche*. Clinically, these children display the development of early sexual hair growth usually limited to the axillary and pubic areas; the presence of facial, abdominal, or back hair is not consistent with this syndrome. Affected children may develop mildly oily skin and minimal acne, especially on the nose and forehead. Axillary odor is a frequent occurrence and generally requires deodorant. With premature adrenarche, children are never virilized; the presence of virilization suggests either a tumor or an enzymatic defect of steroidogenesis. The child's growth velocity may increase slightly, and bone-age maturation also may advance but generally within 2 years of the chronologic age. Androgen levels are in the range typical of the early Tanner II-III stages of puberty.

In the past, pubertal progression was considered to be normal in children who had premature adrenarche. However, data indicate that the pubertal outcome may not always be benign. Of 35 adolescent girls from Italy and Spain who had functional ovarian hyperandrogenism, 45% had a history of premature adrenarche.[25] In a recent study of a large cohort of black and Caribbean Hispanic girls who had premature adrenarche, approximately one third of the 72 girls who underwent testing had ACTH-stimulated androgens more than 2 standard deviations above the mean for normal Tanner II-III pubertal girls.[26] In another study, approximately 50% of the black and Hispanic girls who had premature adrenarche had mild acanthosis nigricans.[27] Because of the association among acanthosis nigricans, hyperinsulinism stemming from insulin resistance, and hyperandrogenism in adolescent and adult women who have polycystic ovarian disease, the authors assessed insulin sensitivity in 35 minority youths who had premature adrenarche.[28] Essentially, girls with marked insulin resistance had the more severe hyperandrogenism, with an exaggerated rise of Δ5 steroids to ACTH stimulation. The girls with insulin-resistance were heavier than girls whose insulin sensitivity was normal. Hyperinsulinism, possibly exacerbated by obesity, apparently has a role in the hyperandrogenism of girls with premature adrenarche just as it does in the more severe hyperandrogenism of women with PCOS. This role is of particular concern because minority children are known to be at increased risk for the complications of hyperinsulinism, including non–insulin-dependent diabetes mellitus, lipid abnormalities, PCOS, and cardiovascular disease.

Obesity is not the sole factor associated with insulin resistance. Children born with intrauterine growth retardation are at increased risk for insulin resistance, short stature, and premature adrenarche. In addition, a recent study documented that girls with functional ovarian hyperandrogenism and hyperinsulinism had the lowest birth weights of the entire group of girls who had premature adrenarche.[29] Perhaps the stress of intrauterine growth retardation induces insulin resistance and alterations in adrenal steroidgenesis. Among girls with precocious pubarche, those with low birth weight, even if they are not obese, are at high risk for progression and for developing a variant of PCOS with hyperinsulinemic hyperandrogenism, dyslipidemia, dysadipocytokinemia, central fat excess, and a deficit of lean body mass.[25,29-32] Higher leptin levels in adolescents with hyperandrogenism than in healthy girls show possible involvement of leptin in the pathogenesis of hyperandrogenism.[33]

Enzymatic Defects of Steroidogenesis

The term *adrenal hyperplasia* refers to the histologic change that occurs in the adrenal glands as a result of a deficiency of one of the several enzymes necessary for normal steroid biosynthesis.[34] Cortisol is the most important of the glucocorticoids made by the adrenal gland, and its synthesis is regulated primarily by a sensitive negative feedback system with pituitary ACTH. Any condition that causes a decrease in cortisol biosynthesis results in a compensatory rise in ACTH. In the enzymatic defects of cortisol biosynthesis, cortisol levels fall. The compensatory rise in ACTH stimulates adrenal steroidogenesis, with the resultant accumulation of steroids proximal to the enzymatic defect. These precursor steroids are then shunted to the androgen pathways, with resultant hyperandrogenism. Three autosomal-recessive disorders of adrenal steroidogenesis cause cortisol deficiency and hyperandrogenism: (1) 21-hydroxylase deficiency, (2) 11-beta-hydroxylase deficiency, and (3) 3-beta-hydroxysteroid dehydrogenase deficiency. Diagnosis is confirmed by finding elevated precursor steroids either in the basal state or in response to a bolus dose of ACTH.

The specific symptoms of the disorder depend on which class of steroids is deficient and which is overproduced. In the severe salt-wasting form of 21-hydroxylase deficiency, both cortisol and mineralocorticoid synthesis are interrupted and androgens are overproduced. The prenatal exposure of the genetic female external genitalia to the high androgens in the first trimester causes genital ambiguity. Boys do not have genital abnormalities. Children of either sex will develop salt-wasting symptoms generally within the first 3 months of life. In the simple virilizing form of 21-hydroxylase deficiency, the genetic female child is born with genital ambiguity; the genetic male child appears normal. In either form of 21-hydroxylase deficiency, delay in diagnosis or inadequate treatment results in postnatal virilization, with progressive clitoral and phallic enlargement, early development of axillary and pubic hair, axillary odor and acne, increased growth velocity, advanced bone age, precocious puberty, and, ultimately, short stature. Young women inadequately treated will develop PCOS along with its associated menstrual irregularities and infertility. The diagnosis is confirmed by finding an elevated 17-hydroxyprogesterone level.

Three alleles are associated with the 21-hydroxylase locus and can be combined in several ways in individuals who are either unaffected, heterozygote carriers or affected with classical or nonclassical disease. Variable signs and symptoms of hyperandrogenism, such as hirsutism, acne, virilization of the external genitalia or the body, short stature, menstrual irregularities, are common to both types of the disorder. Both a proven genetic linkage and a genetic linkage disequilibrium exist among the genes responsible for the synthesis of the enzyme 21-hydroxylase and the antigens of human leukocyte antigen (HLA) system. HLA-Bw47, HLA-B5, and HLA-B35 are the most common haplotypes associated with classical 21-hydroxylase deficiency, whereas the haplotype HLA-B14DR1 is the most recurrent in the nonclassical form of the disease.[35] The 21-hydroxylase gene is situated in the HLA major histocompatibility complex on the short arm of the 6th chromosome. Molecular genetic studies have identified the precise location of the gene. Currently, an affected fetus can be identified by chorionic villus sampling between the 8th and 11th week of gestation.[36] The goal of early diagnosis and treatment is to prevent genital ambiguity in the affected female fetus. However, to be effective in preventing virilization in female fetuses affected with congenital adrenal hyperplasia, prenatal treatment with dexamethasone should be instituted by 6 to 7 weeks of gestation, before prenatal diagnosis is possible.[37] Preventive therapy is controversial because many unaffected fetuses would be treated prenatally with dexamethasone. Adverse events in children treated during fetal life include isolated cases of cardiac septal hypertrophy, hydrocephalus, hydrometrocolpos, and intrauterine growth retardation.[37]

The nonclassical late-onset form of 21-hydroxylase deficiency has clinical variability and symptoms of hyperandrogenism can develop at any age. However, affected girls do not have genital ambiguity. The spectrum of symptoms includes premature pubic and axillary hair growth, premature axillary odor, acne, increased growth velocity and advanced bone age, hirsutism, male-pattern baldness in young women, and PCOS. Because the hyperandrogenism in this form of 21-hydroxylase deficiency is not as severe as the classical form, the basal unstimulated 17-hydroxyprogesterone may not be elevated; the diagnosis is confirmed by detecting an exaggerated 17-hydroxyprogesterone response to ACTH stimulation.

Treatment of 21-hydroxylase deficiency includes glucocorticoid replacement therapy as hydrocortisone at a dose of 10 to 25 mg/m^2/day to maintain normal growth and development and a normal rate of bone-age advancement. The salt-retaining steroid 9-alpha fludrocortisone acetate is used to treat children who have the salt-wasting variant and is sometimes useful with elevated plasma renin activity. Although the introduction of steroid radioimmunoassay methods has facilitated management of these children, growth and development are not always optimal. Studies are underway to determine if the addition of androgen-receptor blockers will improve growth.

Deficiency of the 11-beta-hydroxylase enzyme is characterized by sexual ambiguity in affected girls. As with 21-hydroxylase deficiency, inadequate therapy can result in early virilization. The accumulation of deoxycorticosterone, a weak mineralocorticoid, eventually leads to low renin hypertension. Milder forms of 11-beta-hydroxylase deficiency have been described and exhibit very similarly to the late-onset form of 21-hydroxylase deficiency. The diagnosis is made by finding an elevated 11-deoxycortisol that is stimulated by ACTH and suppressed by dexamethasone.

Complete 3-beta-hydroxysteroid deficiency reveals ambiguity in both sexes, as well as salt-wasting crisis. Milder forms, similar in their presentation to late-onset 21-hydroxylase deficiency, have been described.[38,39] Treatment is similar to therapy for 21-hydroxylase deficiency.

Table 192-1 Causes of Hirsutism, Associated Laboratory Findings, and Recommended Additional Testing

DIAGNOSIS	TESTOSTERONE	17-OHP	LH/FSH RATIO	PROLACTIN	DHEAS	CORTISOL	ADDITIONAL TESTING
Congenital adrenal hyperplasia	Normal to increased	Increased	Normal	Normal	Normal to increased	Normal to decreased	ACTH stimulation may be necessary to make diagnosis
Polycystic ovary syndrome	Normal to increased Increased free testosterone Decreased SHBG	Normal	Normal to increased LH and decreased to normal FSH	Normal to increased	Normal to increased	Normal	Primarily a clinical diagnosis; consider laboratory testing and ultrasonography of ovaries to rule out other disorders or tumors; consider screening for the metabolic syndrome with lipids, glucose, oral glucose tolerance test.
Ovarian tumor	Increased	Normal	Normal	Normal	Normal	Normal	Ultrasonography or CT to image tumors

ACTH, Adrenocorticotropic hormone; *CT,* computed tomography; *DHEAS,* dehydroepiandrosterone; *FSH,* follicle-stimulating hormone; *LH,* luteinizing hormone; *OHP,* hydroxyprogesterone; *SHBG,* sex-hormone binding globulin.

IDIOPATHIC HIRSUTISM OR ACNE

The term *idiopathic hirsutism* or *acne* applies to girls who have these signs without any other signs of androgen excess and who have normal circulating androgen concentrations. Menses and reproductive function should be normal. The hirsutism and acne in these women have been attributed to "increased peripheral metabolism" of androgens.[40]

EVALUATION

The evaluation of the child or adolescent who has either early sexual hair development or hirsutism begins with the history. The rapid development of sexual hair associated with symptoms of virilization (eg, severe acne, voice changes, change in body habitus, clitoral or phallic enlargement, rapid growth) suggests the presence of marked hyperandrogenism as would occur in the severe adrenal enzyme deficiencies or with either an adrenal or ovarian tumor. The presence of sexual hair growth with early breast development is consistent with either true or peripheral precocious puberty. The family history should include information regarding cardiovascular disease, atherosclerosis, obesity, and diabetes, which can be seen in the families of patients who have premature adrenarche and PCOS. A family history of early fetal demise suggests the presence of adrenal hyperplasia. Hypertension on physical examination can occur with 11-hydroxylase deficiency, an adrenal tumor, or obesity. Virilization should be noted carefully because it indicates severe hyperandrogenism. An increase in growth velocity with *crossing percentile channels* suggests precocious puberty, tumor, or adrenal hyperplasia. Labial fusion indicates exposure to hyperandrogenism during fetal life, which occurs in the congenital adrenal hyperplasia syndromes.

The hormonal evaluation should include the GnRH-stimulation test if precocious puberty is identified to distinguish true from peripheral sexual precocity. The evaluation of early sexual hair growth or hirsutism without virilization should include an ACTH-stimulation test to identify an enzymatic defect of adrenal hormone biosynthesis. The presence of virilization or high levels of testosterone (>150 ng/dL) or of dehydroepiandrosterone sulfate (>750 mcg/dL) suggests an ovarian or adrenal tumor; appropriate imaging should be done with ultrasound, computed tomography scan, or MRI. A karyotype should be obtained if an ovarian tumor is suspected because dysgenetic gonads may deteriorate to malignancy. If the ACTH testing is consistent with an enzymatic defect in the virilized patient, then the benign nature of the condition should be confirmed by suppression of hyperandrogenism with dexamethasone. Imaging studies should always be performed in equivocal cases. Table 192-1 highlights the details.

TREATMENT OPTIONS

For patients with mild hirsutism, local measures such as shaving, bleaching, depilatories, and electrolysis may suffice. Weight loss should be encouraged for obese patients, because excess weight decreases insulin resistance with a resultant increase in sex hormone–binding globulin and reduction in serum levels of androgens and LH.[41] Very few pharmacologic agents are approved by the US Food and Drug Administration for hirsutism. Response to these agents is slow; they are often used with local cosmetic options. Oral contraceptives decrease circulating androgens in patients with PCOS and synergize with the effects of antiandrogens such as spironolactone. Research has also demonstrated that adolescents with PCOS are severely insulin resistant compared with a control group matched for body composition and abdominal obesity.[42] The administration of metformin to these teens resulted in improved insulin sensitivity and a reduction of the ACTH-stimulated androgens.[43] In prepubertal and adolescent girls with premature pubarche and a history of low birth weight, metformin has been reported to prevent the development of PCOS symptoms.[44,45]

SUMMARY

Fortunately, knowledge of androgen physiology and metabolism has increased awareness of the pathophysiological features of hirsutism and early sexual hair growth. Historically, children and adolescents who had these signs were neglected and not evaluated because their abnormal hair growth was often minimized or was attributed to a familial tendency without underlying disease. Although the tools for evaluation and treatment have improved during the last 20 years, much needs to be learned about the natural history of PCOS and of idiopathic hirsutism so that prevention and treatment can be improved. Furthermore, improvement in therapy is needed. With the rising incidence of obesity comes an increased incidence of PCOS. Despite this increased incidence, every child should receive a full evaluation to rule out other potential causes of hirsutism and early sexual hair growth.

WHEN TO REFER

- Pubic hair, axillary hair, or axillary odor before 8 years of age in girls and 9 years of age in boys
- Breast development, vaginal discharge, or menses in girls before 8 years of age
- Increased facial or body hair (chest, abdomen, back) in girls with or without menstrual irregularities
- Signs of virilization in girls (clitoromegaly, masculine body habitus, voice changes) or in boys (phallic enlargement, change in body habitus, voice change) before the age of 9 years
- Rapid virilization (<1 year) in a pubertal boy

WHEN TO ADMIT

- Severe hypertension with precocious sexual development (eg, 11-hydroxylase deficiency, adrenal tumor)
- Severe anemia secondary to vaginal bleeding (eg, ovarian cyst, dysfunctional uterine bleeding)
- Any suspicion of sexual abuse
- Severe headaches, visual loss, change in mental status (increased intracranial pressure associated with CNS lesion)
- Hypotension or shock (Addison disease secondary to ACTH deficiency, pituitary apoplexy secondary to a bleed into a pituitary lesion)
- Marked hyperglycemia requiring insulin (T2DM and PCOS)
- Severe abdominal pain (torsion of ovarian cyst)

TOOLS FOR PRACTICE

Engaging Patient and Family

- *Puberty—Ready or Not, Expect Some Changes* (brochure), American Academy of Pediatrics (patiented.aap.org).
- *What is a Pediatric Endocrinologist* (fact sheet), American Academy of Pediatrics (www.aap.org/family/whatispedendo.pdf).

AAP POLICY STATEMENT

American Academy of Pediatrics, Committee on Adolescence, American College of Obstetricians and Gynecologists, Committee on Adolescent Health Care. Menstruation in girls and adolescents: using the menstrual cycle as a vital sign. *Pediatrics*. 2006;118(5):2245-2250. (aappolicy.aappublications.org/cgi/content/full/pediatrics;118/5/2245).

SUGGESTED RESOURCES

DiMartino-Nardi J. Premature adrenarche: findings in prepubertal African-American and Caribbean Hispanic girls. *Acta Paediatr Suppl*. 1999;88(433):67-72.

Dunaif A. Insulin resistance and the polycystic ovary syndrome: mechanism and implications for pathogenesis. *Endocr Rev*. 1997;18(6):774-800.

Hunter MH, Carek PJ. Evaluation and treatment of women with hirsutism. *Am Fam Physician*. 2003;67(12):2565-2572.

Lee P. Disorders of puberty. In: Lifshitz F, ed. *Pediatric Endocrinology*. New York, NY: Marcel Dekker; 1996.

Rosenfield, RL. Clinical practice. Hirsutism. *N Engl J Med*. Dec 2005;353(24):2578-2588.

Trakakis E, Laggas D, Salamalekis E, et al. 21-Hydroxylase deficiency: from molecular genetics to clinical presentation. *J Endocrinol Invest*. 2005;28(2):187-192.

REFERENCES

1. Ebling F. Hair follicles and associated glands as androgen targets in androgen metabolism in hirsute and normal females. *Clin Endocrinol Metab*. 1986;15:319-339.
2. Lee P. Disorders of puberty. In: Lifshitz F, ed. *Pediatric Endocrinology*. New York, NY: Marcel Dekker; 1996.
3. Giudice L. The insulin and insulin-like growth factor system in normal and abnormal ovarian follicle development. *Am J Med*. 1995;98(suppl 1A):48S-54S.
4. Reiter EO, Conte FA. Responsivity of pituitary gonadotropes to luteinizing hormone-releasing factor in idiopathic precocious puberty, precocious thelarche, precocious adrenarche and in patients treated with medroxyprogesterone acetate. *Pediatr Res*. 1975;(2):111-116.
5. Starceski PJ, Lee PA, Albright AL, et al. Hypothalamic hamartomas and sexual precocity: evaluation and treatment options. *Am J Dis Child*. 1990;144(2):225-228.
6. Boepple PA, Frisch LS, Wierman ME, et al. The natural history of autonomous gonadal function, adrenarche, and central puberty in gonadotropin-independent precocious puberty. *J Clin Endocrinol Metab*. 1992;**75**:1550-1555.
7. Bar A, Linder B, Sobel EH, et al. Bayley-Pinneau method of height prediction in girl with central precocious puberty: correlation with adult height. *J Pediatr*. 1995;126(6): 955-958.

8. Oerter KE, Manesco P, Barnes KM, et al. Adult height in precocious puberty after long-term treatment with deslorelin. *J Clin Endocrinol*. 1991;73:1235-1240.
9. DiMartino-Nardi J, Wu R, Varner R, et al. The effect of luteinizing hormone-releasing hormone analog for central precocious puberty on growth hormone (GH) and GH binding protein. *J Clin Endocrinol Metab*. 1994;78: 664-668.
10. Roth LM, Anderson MC, Govan ADT. Sertoli-Leydig cell tumors: a clinicopathological study of 34 cases. *Cancer*. 1981;48:187-197.
11. Young RH, Dickersin GR, Scully RE, Juvenile granulosa cell tumor of the ovary: a clinicopathological analysis of 125 cases. *Am J Surg Pathol*. 1984;8(8):575-596.
12. Dunaif A. Insulin resistance and the polycystic ovary syndrome: mechanism and implications for pathogenesis. *Endocr Rev*. 1997;18(6):774-780.
13. Dokras A, Bochner M, Hollinrake E, et al. Screening women with polycystic ovarian syndrome for metabolic syndrome. *Obstet Gynecol*. 2005;106(1):131-137.
14. Kadowaki T, Bevins CL, Cama A, et al. Two mutant alleles of the insulin receptor gene in a patient with extreme insulin resistance. *Science*. 1998;240:787-790.
15. Kahn CR, White MF. The insulin receptor and the molecular mechanism of insulin action. *J Clin Endocrinol*. 1988; 82(4):1151-1156.
16. Palmert MR, Gordon CM, Kartashov AI, et al. Screening for abnormal glucose tolerance in adolescents with polycystic ovary syndrome. *J Clin Endocrinol Metab*. 2002; 87(3):1017-1023.
17. Matthews DR, Hosker JP, Rudenski AS, et al. Homeostasis model assessment: insulin resistance and beta cell function from fasting plasma glucose and insulin concentrations in man. *Diabetologia*. 1985;28(7): 412-419.
18. Pringle PJ, Stanhope R, Hindmarsh P, et al. Abnormal pubertal development in primary hypothyroidism. *Clin Endocrinol*. 1988;28:479-486.
19. Batata MA, Whitmore WF Jr, Chu FC, et al. Cryptorchidism and testicular cancer. *J Urol*. 1980;124(3):382-387.
20. Martin DC. Germinal cell tumors of the testis after orchiopexy. *J Urol*. 1979;121(4):422-424.
21. Cassio A, Cacciari E, D'Errico A, et al. Incidence of intratubular germ cell neoplasia in androgen insensitivity syndrome. *Acta Endocrinol*. 1990;123:416-422.
22. Dexeus FH, Logothetis CJ, Chong C, et al. Genetic abnormalities in men with germ cell tumors. *J Urol*. 1988;140: 80-84.
23. Shenker A, Laue L, Kosugi S, et al. A constitutively activating mutation of the luteinizing hormone receptor in familial male precocious puberty. *Nature*. 1993;365(6557): 652-654.
24. Lashansky G, Saenger P, Fishman K, et al. Normative data for adrenal steroidogenesis in healthy pediatric population age and sex related changes after adrenocorticotropin stimulation. *J Clin Endocrinol Metab*. 1991;73: 674-686.
25. Ibáñez L, Potau N, Virdis R, et al. Postpubertal outcome in girls diagnosed of premature pubarche during childhood: increased frequency of functional ovarian hyperandrogenism. *J Clin Endocrinol Metab*. 1993;76(6): 1599-1603.
26. Banerjee S, Raghavan S, Wasserman EJ, et al. Hormonal findings in African-American and Caribbean Hispanic girls with premature adrenarche: implications for polycystic ovarian syndrome. *Pediatrics*. 1998;102(3):e36.
27. Oppenheimer E, Linder B, DiMartino-Nardi J. Decreased insulin sensitivity in prepubertal girls with premature adrenarche and acanthosis nigricans. *J Clin Endocrinol Metab*. 1995;80:614-618.
28. Vuguin P, Linder B, Rosenfeld RG, et al. The role of insulin sensitivity, insulin-like growth factor and insulin-like growth factor binding proteins 1 and 3 in the hyperandrogenism of African American and Caribbean Hispanic girls with premature adrenarche. *J Clin Endocrinol Metab*. 1999;84(6):2037-2042.
29. Ibáñez L, Potau N, Francois I, et al. Precocious pubarche, hyperinsulinism and ovarian hyperandrogenism in girls: relation to reduced fetal growth. *J Clin Endocrinol Metab*. 1998;83(10):3558-3562.
30. Ibáñez L, Potau N, de Zegher F. Precocious pubarche, dyslipidemia, and low IGF binding protein-1 in girls: relation to reduced prenatal growth. *Pediatr Res*. 1999; 46(3):320-322.
31. Ibáñez L, Ong K, de Zegher F, et al. Fat distribution in non-obese girls with and without precocious pubarche: central adiposity related to insulinemia and androgenemia from prepuberty to post-menarche. *Clin Endocrinol*. 2003;58(3):372-379.
32. DiMartino-Nardi J. Premature adrenarche: findings in prepubertal African-American and Caribbean Hispanic girls. *Acta Paediatr Suppl*. 1999;88(433):67-72.
33. Zukauskaite S, Seibokaite A, Lasas L, et al. Serum hormone levels and anthropometric characteristics in girls with hyperandrogenism. *Medicina (Kaunas)*. 2005;41(4): 305-312.
34. New MI, Speiser PW. Update on congenital adrenal hyperplasia. In: Lifshitz F, ed. *Pediatric Endocrinology*. New York, NY: Marcel Dekker; 1996.
35. Trakakis E, Laggas D, Salamalekis E, et al. 21-Hydroxylase deficiency: from molecular genetics to clinical presentation. *J Endocrinol Invest*. 2005;28(2):187-192.
36. Speiser PW, LaForgia N, Kato K, et al. First trimester prenatal treatment and molecular genetic diagnosis of congenital adrenal hyperplasia (21-hydroxylase deficiency). *J Clin Endocrinol Metab*. 1990;70:838-848.
37. Lajic S, Nordenstrom A, Ritzen EM, et al. Prenatal treatment of congenital adrenal hyperplasia. *Eur J Endocrinol*. 2004;151:U63-U69.
38. Lobo RA, Goebelsmann U, Horton R. Evidence for the importance of peripheral tissue events in the development of hirsutism in polycystic ovary syndrome. *J Clin Endocrinol Metab*. 1983;57(2):393-397.
39. Rosenfield R, Rich BH, Wolfsdorf JI, et al. Pubertal presentation of congenital Δ-5-3β-hydroxysteroid dehydrogenase deficiency. *J Clin Endocrinol Metab*. 1980;51: 345-353.
40. Pang S. Hirsutism and polycystic ovary syndrome. In: Lifshitz F, ed. *Pediatric Endocrinology*. New York, NY: Marcel Dekker; 1996.
41. Hunter M, Carek PJ. Evaluation and treatment of women with hirsutism. *Am Fam Physician*. 2003;67(12):2565-2572.
42. Lewy VD, Danadian K, Witchel SF, et al. Early metabolic abnormalities in adolescent girls with PCOS. *J Pediatr*. 2001;138(1):38-44.
43. Arslanian SA, Lewy V, Danadian K, et al. Metformin therapy in obese adolescents with polycystic ovarian syndrome and impaired glucose tolerance: amelioration of exaggerated adrenal response to adrenocorticotropin with reduction of insulinemia/insulin resistance. *J Clin Endocrinol Metab*. 2002;87(4):1555-1559.
44. Ibáñez L, Valls C, Marcos M, et al. Insulin sensitization for girls with precocious pubarche and with risk for polycystic ovary syndrome: effects of prepubertal initiation and postpubertal discontinuation of metformin treatment. *J Clin Endocrinol Metab*. 2004;89(9):4331-4337.
45. Ibáñez L, Ferrer A, Ong K, et al. Insulin sensitization early post-menarche prevents progression from precocious pubarche to polycystic ovary syndrome. *J Pediatr*. 2004;144(1):23-29.

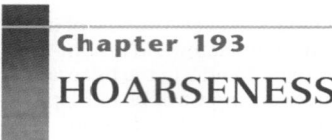

Chapter 193

HOARSENESS

Samuel T. Ostrower, MD; Sanjay R. Parikh, MD

DEFINITIONS

The result of a pathological change in the vibratory nature of the vocal folds, hoarseness is a symptom of vocal dysfunction that describes a breathy, harsh, coarse, strained, or raspy voice. In children, hoarseness can be used to describe both the quality of voice and the quality of cry. Causes vary by age group and can be attributed to infectious, anatomic, traumatic, inflammatory, neoplastic, neurologic and iatrogenic sources. The prevalence of childhood hoarseness has been described as 6% to 38%.[1-6] Although sometimes occurring concurrently, hoarseness should be discerned from stridor, which is a sign of turbulent airflow caused by obstructive lesions within the airway.

DIFFERENTIAL DIAGNOSIS

Forming a differential diagnosis (Boxes 193-1 and 193-2) for the hoarse child depends on the quality of hoarseness, progression of symptoms, related infection, history of surgery or trauma, and associated respiratory distress.[7] The age of the patient at the onset of hoarseness is a useful way to organize the potential causes.

Neonate and Infant

Hoarseness that occurs at birth or shortly thereafter is most often attributable to congenital, traumatic or iatrogenic, neoplastic, or inflammatory sources. In this

BOX 193-1 Differential Diagnosis of Pediatric Hoarseness By Category

CONGENITAL
- Laryngeal anomalies
  - Laryngomalacia
  - Glottic webs
  - Subglottic stenosis
  - Laryngeal cleft
- Cystic lesions
  - Laryngocele
  - Saccular cyst
  - Thyroglossal duct cyst
- Angiomas
  - Lymphatic malformation
  - Hemangioma
  - Arteriovenous malformation
- Cri du chat syndrome

NEUROGENIC (CONGENITAL AND ACQUIRED)
- Supranuclear (eg, hydrocephalus)
- Nuclear (eg, Arnold-Chiari malformation, Guillain-Barré syndrome)
- Peripheral (eg, myasthenia gravis, cardiovascular anomalies, recurrent laryngeal nerve trauma)
- Psychogenic hoarseness

VOCAL CORD ABUSE
- Vocal cord nodules
- Vocal cord polyps

NEOPLASIA
- Papilloma
- Squamous cell carcinoma

PHYSICAL VOICE CHANGE OF PUBERTY

INFLAMMATORY
- Infectious
  - Simple laryngitis
  - Diphtheria
  - Laryngotracheitis
  - Supraglottitis (epiglottitis)
- Noninfectious
  - Laryngopharyngeal reflux
  - Chronic laryngitis
  - Allergic laryngitis
  - Angioedema
  - Rheumatoid arthritis
  - Relapsing polychondritis
  - Smoking

TRAUMATIC
- Hematoma
- Laryngeal cartilage fracture
- Impacted foreign body
- Postintubtion
  - Arytenoid dislocation
  - Cord avulsion
  - Granuloma
  - Acquired glottic web
  - Subglottic stenosis
- Recurrent laryngeal nerve injury
  - Thyroidectomy
  - Tracheotomy
  - Cardiac surgery
  - Tracheoesophageal fistula repair
  - Tracheal resection
  - Penetrating neck wound

From Smith ME, Gray SD. Voice. In: Bluestone CD, Stool SE, Kenna MA, eds. *Pediatric Otolaryngology.* Philadelphia, PA: WB Saunders; 2003. Copyright © Elsevier, with permission.

BOX 193-2 Differential Diagnosis of Pediatric Hoarseness By Age

0 TO 6 MONTHS
Traumatic intubation
Iatrogenic: surgical
Neurogenic: central or peripheral
Neoplastic: hemangioma
Congenital: web, cleft, cyst

6 MONTHS TO 5 YEARS
Traumatic: foreign bodies, intubation
Infection: URI
Neoplastic: papillomas
Behavioral, traumatic: nodules
Inflammatory: allergy, LPR

5 TO 13 YEARS
Behavioral, traumatic: nodules
Infectious: URI
Inflammatory: allergy, LPR
Neoplastic

13 TO 18 YEARS
Infectious: URI
Inflammatory: allergy, LPR
Behavioral, traumatic:
  Male: mutational or transitional voice
  Female: nodules
Functional: muscle tension dysphonia

LPR, Laryngopharyngeal reflux; *URI*, upper respiratory infection.
From Friedberg J, El-Hakim H. Hoarseness. In: Bluestone CD, Stool SE, Kenna MA, eds. *Pediatric Otolaryngology*, Philadelphia, PA: WB Saunders; 2003. Copyright © 2003, Elsevier, with permission.

subgroup of prelingual patients, hoarseness often refers to a weak or breathy cry.

Vocal cord paralysis in the neonate is a well-known cause of hoarseness and stridor.[8] Bilateral vocal cord paralysis, which is usually congenital, frequently causes respiratory distress and stridor, whereas unilateral vocal cord paralysis is more likely to exhibit initially as hoarseness or dysphagia. Central nervous system disease such as the Arnold-Chiari malformation must be ruled out in cases of bilateral vocal cord paralysis.[9] A weak or breathy cry in a neonate after thoracic or cervical surgery should alert the clinician to the possibility of recurrent laryngeal nerve injury as a source of iatrogenic vocal cord paralysis. Additionally, traumatic intubation can cause arytenoid cartilage dislocation, with subsequent vocal cord immobility and hoarseness.

Congenital laryngeal webs form as a result of failure of the larynx to canalize fully during embryologic development.[10] Webs may occur exclusively with hoarseness, but they may be associated with aphonia, stridor, and respiratory distress. Laryngeal webs vary from thin slips of tissue between the anterior areas of the vocal cords to complete laryngeal atresia, which is incompatible with life unless recognized immediately. Atresia or near-total atresia has been referred to as congenital high airway obstruction syndrome.[11]

Laryngeal saccular cysts are characterized by symptoms of airway obstruction and dysphagia. Saccular cysts are filled with mucinous fluid and arise as a result of an abnormal dilation of the saccule of the larynx secondary to secretory outflow obstruction.

Posterior laryngeal clefts are an uncommon laryngeal anomaly resulting in an abnormal opening in the posterior larynx. Clefts can simply involve the posterior laryngeal commissure but may extend through the cricoid inferiorly through the tracheoesophageal septum. Symptoms depend on the extent of the cleft and, at birth, typically cause aspiration, stridor, respiratory distress, and weak cry.

Subglottic hemangiomas classically occur between the 1st and 6th month of life, with varying degrees of respiratory distress, stridor, cough, dysphagia, and hoarseness.[12] The natural history of hemangiomas is that of proliferation followed by involution. Subglottic hemangiomas can be unilateral, bilateral, or circumferential and are more common in girls than in boys. Cutaneous hemangiomas of the head and neck are found concurrently in approximately 50% of cases of subglottic hemangioma.[13]

A relationship may exist between pediatric and adult laryngeal disease and reflux.[14,15] Whereas gastroesophageal reflux (GER) refers to the backflow of stomach contents into the esophagus, laryngopharyngeal reflux (LPR) refers to the backflow of stomach contents into the throat, or laryngopharynx. GER disease commonly produces emesis, dysphagia, sleep disturbance, and failure to thrive.[16] The association among GER, LPR, and various neonatal laryngeal disorders such as hoarseness, posterior laryngitis, and silent aspiration, however, is an intense area of study that remains complicated and controversial.[17-19] (See Chapter 172, Dysphagia, and Chapter 264, Gastroesophageal Reflux Disease.)

Older Child

Older children and adolescents are subject to many of the same sources of hoarseness as adults. Infectious, inflammatory, traumatic, and neoplastic conditions such as laryngitis, LPR, vocal nodules, and respiratory papillomata are the leading causes of hoarseness among older children.[19]

Hoarseness of childhood from infectious disorders such as infective laryngitis, supraglottitis, and laryngotracheobronchitis rarely present a diagnostic challenge; however, concern over the airway should always take precedence. For example, hoarse voice may be an early indicator of the impending airway compromise seen in epiglottitis.

Although debate exists as to the specific role of LPR in the development of laryngeal lesions and hoarseness in children, infrequent reflux events have been shown to cause hoarseness in adults.[20] LPR has also been found in association with pediatric laryngeal manifestations such as vocal fold nodules, posterior laryngitis, false vocal cord edema, vocal cord granulomas, functional voice disorders, and hoarseness.[15,21,22] In addition, animal studies have shown that subglottic stenosis results when gastric acid is applied to the subglottic mucosa of dogs.[23]

Vocal nodules arise from phonotrauma or voice abuse and tend to occur more frequently in boys than in girls.[24] Symptoms may fluctuate based on aggravation by vocal abuse and respiratory tract infections. Sudden worsening of symptoms is sometimes seen when polyps swell from internal hemorrhage with excessive vocal trauma. Children with vocal nodules may share symptoms with other members of the immediate family who have similar vocal traits.

Airway trauma is also a potential cause of hoarseness in the older child and adolescent. Sources include blunt or penetrating injuries and intubation trauma.

Hoarseness of a progressive and unrelenting nature suggests a possible neoplastic cause. Ninety-eight percent of pediatric laryngeal neoplasms are benign, and recurrent respiratory papillomatosis (RRP) is by far the most common lesion.[18] RRP may be found on upper aerodigestive tract mucosal surfaces other than that of the larynx and have a characteristic cluster of grapes appearance. RRP may, however, be indistinguishable from the rare but ominous laryngeal squamous cell carcinoma of childhood.

Hoarseness in the adolescent years may also be of behavioral or psychogenic etiology. Mutational voice disorder occurs in male adolescents and results in hoarseness and high pitch during the stress of physiological pubertal voice change. Paradoxical vocal fold dysfunction (seen more frequently in girls) is a disorder of psychogenic origin often misdiagnosed as asthma, which can produce episodic stridor or hoarseness.[25]

EVALUATION

Relevant History

A thorough history is an essential part of the investigation of hoarseness. The age of the child is a critical factor in the development of an appropriate differential diagnosis, as is information on the quality of the voice with speech or crying, exacerbating or alleviating factors, and associated symptoms. Neurologic and congenital fixed anatomic lesions typically occur at birth, whereas inflammatory, neoplastic, traumatic, or iatrogenic causes of hoarseness occur later. The onset and course of dysphonia should be considered. Intermittent dysphonia may be related to infectious or inflammatory causes such as laryngitis, whereas persistent dysphonia may suggest a fixed anatomic lesion. A progressive, unremitting hoarse voice may suggest an enlarging neoplasm.

Patients with hoarseness who have symptoms such as regurgitation or vomiting, feeding difficulties, throat clearing, foreign body sensation, and cough may have underlying reflux.

Stridor that accompanies hoarseness should be investigated and treated in an expeditious fashion, given that turbulent airflow resulting from airway obstruction may be life threatening.

Physical Examination

A thorough physical examination, including a complete head and neck examination, should be part of the evaluation of pediatric hoarseness. Inspection of cranial nerve function and for craniofacial anomalies may reveal the underlying cause of a patient's hoarseness. Cutaneous head and neck hemangiomas, for example, may suggest a potential laryngeal hemangioma. Signs of aspiration during deglutition may be suggestive of sensorimotor causes of dysphonia such as vocal cord paralysis.

Laryngoscopy

An essential part of the otolaryngologic physical examination is visualization of the larynx. Flexible nasopharyngolaryngoscopy, indirect mirror laryngoscopy, and rigid videostroboscopy are all methods for visualizing the larynx that can provide useful, if not diagnostic, clues as to the source of a patient's hoarseness (Box 193-1).

Indirect laryngoscopy using a mirror can be performed on cooperative children and can visualize gross disease and inflammatory changes in the larynx. This technique has largely been replaced by flexible fiberoptic nasopharyngolaryngoscopy, which provides clear views of laryngeal anatomy and function. Flexible endoscopy can be performed on virtually all age groups, although toddlers and developmentally delayed patients pose the greatest challenge to the examiner. Topical anesthesia can be used with topical decongestants to facilitate the examination. The flexible endoscope is gently passed though the nose or mouth. Examination in a nonmonitored setting, however, is not advisable if the patient has a tenuous airway or severe congenital cardiac anomalies.

Videostroboscopy uses a rigid, angled telescope placed gently into the oropharynx for dynamic examination of laryngeal anatomy and function. Examination requires a cooperative child. Videostroboscopy uses rapidly pulsed light to examine the vibratory characteristics of the vocal fold mucosa. Examinations are recorded on video to allow for repeated assessments viewed at different speeds to enhance visualization of the vibratory quality of the laryngeal mucosa. Vocal nodules or other lesions on the surface of the vocal fold will dampen the mucosal wave.

Imaging

The role of diagnostic imaging in the work-up of the hoarse child is of prime importance when suspicion exists of central nervous system disease, external compression, malignancy, or external trauma.

Chest and neck plain-film radiographs may demonstrate mediastinal masses, cardiovascular anomalies, or abnormalities in the air column suggesting possible infectious or obstructive diseases.

Computed tomography and virtual bronchoscopy are excellent methods for specifically defining the caliber of the airway and for delineating the site and extent of pathologic changes in airway caliber.[26,27] Indications for laryngeal or neck computed tomography include congenital cysts, solid neoplasms, and external trauma.

Magnetic resonance imaging is helpful when suspicion exists of central nervous system disease such as the Arnold-Chiari malformation and when evaluating possible airway hemangiomas or vascular malformations.

Reflux Testing

Symptomatic or overt GER and LPR in the hoarse child may not necessitate expensive or invasive diagnostic studies. In the absence of identifiable disease in the hoarse child, however, investigation into LPR may be warranted. Although consensus on the role of LPR as it relates to various otolaryngologic manifestations is lacking, at least one study has used pH monitoring to suggest an association between pediatric reflux and hoarse voice in a cohort of children.[28,29] Several diagnostic modalities exist for the workup of LPR, including pH monitoring, impedance testing, nuclear medicine scintiscan, barium esophagoscopy, and direct laryngoscopy with or without biopsy.

Ambulatory 24-hour single-electrode pH monitoring remains the gold standard for the diagnosis of GER in infants and children.[30] The double-electrode pH probe, with distal esophageal and pharyngeal electrodes, however, is thought to be the best method for diagnosing LPR and the otolaryngologic manifestations of GER.[31,32]

Although pH-monitoring studies remain the gold standard for diagnosis of GER and LPR, they do not detect episodes of nonacidic reflux. Multichannel intraluminal impedance monitoring and nuclear medicine scintigraphy can measure both acidic and nonacidic episodes of reflux, which may play a role in such serious events as apnea, apparent life-threatening events, aspiration, and sleep disturbance.[33,34] Nuclear medicine scintiscans have specificity between 83% to 100% but have been shown to be only 15% to 59% sensitive and lack a standardized technique, making comparisons between studies of limited use.[29] Impedance monitoring evaluates the pH-independent change in intraluminal electrical resistance that occurs with the movement (anterograde or retrograde) of a bolus of food, liquid, or gas within the esophagus.[35] This technique may be a reliable tool for evaluating the association between GER-related symptoms and nonacidic reflux events, and it may ultimately replace pH monitoring as the standard tool for detecting LPR in infants and children.[27,36]

Barium esophagram has variable sensitivity and specificity for the diagnosis of LPR. It is useful mainly for detecting anatomic abnormalities such as hiatal hernia.[37]

Laryngoscopy with biopsy may be the most specific test for LPR, but at least one study has failed to show a correlation between laryngoscopy and upper pH probe findings with significant laryngeal histopathologic inflammatory findings.[38]

MANAGEMENT

Congenital Lesions

Management of hoarse voice resulting from unilateral or bilateral vocal cord paralysis is usually secondary to stabilization of the airway and management of dysphagia and aspiration. Tracheotomy is sometimes required in patients with bilateral vocal cord paralysis, but conservative management in select patients has been advocated.[39] However, patients with congenital or acquired unilateral vocal cord paralysis frequently recover normal vocal quality by spontaneous resolution of the paralysis or by compensatory movement of the unaffected cord over time. Recovery has been noted up to 11 years after paralysis.[40] In cases of persistent unilateral cord paralysis with persistent hoarseness, the treatment of choice remains speech therapy, although reports have surfaced of successful surgical vocal cord medialization techniques in the children.[39,41]

Laryngeal webs are managed surgically, either endoscopically or via more extensive open laryngotracheal reconstruction techniques. The type of operation depends primarily on the location and extent of the lesion, with thin webs being more amenable to endoscopic management.

Saccular cysts of the larynx are often managed endoscopically with excellent results via aspiration and marsupialization via sharp dissection or with the carbon dioxide (CO_2) laser. Cyst recurrence, however, is well documented following endoscopic management, and open resection of the cyst may be necessary in these cases.

Posterior laryngeal clefts vary greatly in their extent and symptoms. Extensive or symptomatic clefts must be repaired as early as possible. Although endoscopic repair is possible in small clefts limited to the larynx and upper trachea, more extensive open techniques are used for larger clefts. Tracheotomy may also be placed in cases in which staged reconstruction of the cleft is necessary, and a gastrostomy tube is often necessary to limit aspiration and protect the operative site following surgical repair of the cleft.

Neoplasia

Subglottic hemangioma is a complicated airway anomaly without a universally accepted treatment. Numerous management options exist, including close observation, systemic or intralesional steroids, laser ablation, open surgical excision, and tracheotomy.

Recurrent respiratory papilloma (RRP) represents another airway tumor with a large number of accepted primary and adjuvant therapeutic modalities. CO_2 laser excision was developed as a treatment for RRP in the 1970s and remains a popular method for removing laryngeal papilloma, although it is associated with potentially severe sequelae such as airway fire, scarring, chronic laryngeal edema with airway compromise, vocal fold scarring, and poor voice.[42] Pulsed dye laser therapy was introduced in the late 1990s as a less-traumatic alternative to the CO_2 laser that can be used safely and effectively under local anesthesia in older patients.[43] Powered instrumentation such as the microdebrider is also successfully used for excision of RRP. Several adjuvant therapies such as intralesional cidofovir, α-interferon, indole-3-carbinol, and the novel heat-shock protein E7 have been used with varying degrees of efficacy and safety.[44]

Inflammation and Infection

Behavioral and lifestyle modifications; pharmacotherapy using H2 antagonists, proton-pump inhibitors, prokinetic agents, and antacids; and surgical therapy with fundoplication are acceptable for the management of GER and LPR in infants and children.

Viral laryngitis and laryngotracheobronchitis are generally treated conservatively, but they may require airway protection or intravenous steroids in severe cases. Bacterial infections such as epiglottitis and membranous laryngotracheobronchitis, though are now rare, necessitate early airway protection and intravenous antibiotics directed against *Staphylococcus aureus* and *Haemophilus influenzae,* unless culture results direct differently.

Trauma

The management of vocal fold nodules resulting from phonotrauma primarily relies on behavioral modification and speech therapy aimed at maximizing vocal hygiene. Only in rare circumstances is surgical excision indicated because failure to correct the underlying voice misuse is likely to result in nodule recurrence.

Arytenoid dislocation resulting from intubation trauma can be adequately treated if recognized and reduced early under anesthesia with microlaryngoscopy.

Blunt laryngeal trauma resulting in hoarseness necessitates close observation and may require the use of systemic corticosteroids and tracheotomy in cases of severe laryngeal injury and edema. In adolescents with laryngeal fracture, open reduction and fixation may be required.

SUMMARY

Most cases of pediatric hoarseness result from benign, reversible, and self-limited disease; however, some causes of hoarseness are progressive, malignant, and potentially life threatening. Thorough evaluation, precise diagnosis, and appropriate intervention are therefore essential.

WHEN TO REFER

- Recognized cardiac, esophageal, or neurologic disease
- Progressive hoarseness
- Presence of cutaneous hemangioma
- Hoarseness after external trauma or uneventful intubation
- Poor speech intelligibility or psychosocial sequelae
- Hoarseness that has been present since birth

WHEN TO ADMIT

- Presence of respiratory distress, stridor, tachypnea, or tachycardia
- Hoarseness following external trauma

RELATED WEB SITES

- American Academy of Otolaryngology—Head and Neck Surgery (AAO-HNS) (www.entnet.org/index2.cfm).
- American Speech-Language-Hearing Association (ASHA) (www.asha.org/default.htm).

REFERENCES

1. Leeper HA, Leonard JE, Iverson RL. Otorhinolaryngologic screening of children with vocal quality disturbances. *Int J Pediatr Otorhinolaryngol.* 1980;2:123-131.
2. Carding PN, Roulstone S, Northstone K, ALSPAC Study Team. The prevalence of childhood dysphonia: a cross sectional study. *J Voice.* 2006;20:623-630. (E-publication ahead of print.)
3. Senturia B, Wilson F. Otorhinolaryngic findings in children with voice deviations. *Ann Otol Rhinol Laryngol.* 1968;77:1027-1041.
4. Harden JR. Voice Disorders in Children [abstract]. American Speech and Hearing Association, 1986.
5. Mutch P. Hoarseness amongst school children in proximity to a source of air pollution [Master's thesis]. University of Florida, Gainesville, FL, 1976.
6. Sauchelli K. The incidence of hoarseness amongst school-aged children in a pollution-free community [Master's thesis]. University of Florida, Gainesville, FL, 1979.
7. Friedberg J, El-Hakim H. Hoarseness. In: Bluestone CD, Stool SE, Kenna MA, eds. *Pediatric Otolaryngology.* 4th ed. Philadelphia, PA: WB Saunders; 2002.
8. De Jong AL, Kuppersmith RB, Sulek M, et al. Vocal cord paralysis in children. *Otolaryngol Clin North Am.* 2000; 33:131-149.
9. Wiatrak BJ. Congenital anomalies of the larynx and trachea. *Otolaryngol Clin North Am.* 2000;33:91-110.
10. Holinger PH, Brown WT. Congenital webs, cysts, laryngocele and other anomalies of the larynx. *Ann Otol Rhinol Laryngol.* 1967;76:744.
11. Lim FY, Crombleholme TM, Hedrick HL, et al. Congenital high airway obstruction syndrome: natural history and management. *J Pediatr Surg.* 2003;38:940-945.
12. Shikhani AH, Jones MM, Marsh BR, et al. Infantile subglottic hemangiomas, an update. *Ann Otol Rhinol Laryngol.* 1986;95:336-347.
13. Gregg CM, Wiatrak BJ, Koopman CF. Management options for infantile subglottic hemangioma. *Am J Otolaryngol.* 1995;16:409-414.
14. Kalach N, Gumpert L, Contencin P, et al. Dual-probe pH monitoring for the assessment of gastroesophageal reflux in the course of chronic hoarseness in children. *Turk J Pediatr.* 2000;42:186-191.
15. Kuhn J, Toohill RJ, Ulualp SO, et al. Pharyngeal acid reflux events in patients with vocal cord nodules. *Laryngoscope.* 1998;108:1146-1149.
16. Working Group of the European Society of Pediatric Gastroenterology and Nutrition. A standardized protocol for the methodology of esophageal pH monitoring and interpretation of the data for the diagnosis of gastroesophageal reflux. *J Pediatr Gastroenterol Nutr.* 1992; 14:467-471.
17. Mandell DL, Kay DJ, Dohar JE, et al. Lack of association between esophageal biopsy, bronchoalveolar lavage, and endoscopy findings in hoarse children. *Arch Otolaryngol Head Neck Surg.* 2004;130:1293-1297.
18. Koufman JA, Amin MR, Panetti M. Prevalence of reflux in 113 consecutive patients with laryngeal and voice disorders. *Otolaryngol Head Neck Surg.* 2000;123: 385-388.
19. Zalzal GH, Tran LP. Pediatric gastroesophageal reflux and laryngopharyngeal reflux. *Otolaryngol Clin North Am.* 2000;33:151-161.
20. Koufman JA, Sataloff RT, Toohill R. Laryngopharyngeal reflux: consensus conference report. *J Voice.* 1996;10: 215-216.
21. Bach K, McGuirt W, Postma G. Pediatric laryngopharyngeal reflux. *J Ear Nose Throat.* 2002;81:27-31.
22. Gumpert L, Kalach N, Dupont C, et al. Hoarseness and gastroesophageal reflux in children. *J Laryngol Otol.* 1998;112:49-54.
23. Little FB, Koufman JA, Kohut RI, et al. Effect of gastric acid on the pathogenesis of subglottic stenosis. *Ann Otol Rhinol Laryngol.* 1985;(5 pt 1):516-519.

24. McMurray JS. Medical and surgical treatment of pediatric dysphonia. *Otolaryngol Clin North Am.* 2000;33:1111-1126.
25. Tilles SA. Vocal cord dysfunctioning children and adolescents. *Curr Allergy Astma Rep.* 2003;3:467-472.
26. Liu P, Daneman A. Computed tomography of intrinsic laryngeal and tracheal abnormalities in children. *J Comput Assisted Tomogr.* 1984;8:662-669.
27. Burke AJ, Vining DJ, McGuirt WF Jr, et al. Evaluation of airway obstruction using virtual endoscopy. *Laryngoscope.* 2000;110:23-29.
28. Stavroulaki P. Diagnostic and management problems of laryngopharyngeal reflux disease in children. *Int J Pediatr Otorhinolaryngol.* 2006;70:579-590.
29. Gumpert L, Kalach N, Dupont C, et al. Hoarseness and gastroesophageal reflux in children. *J Laryngol Otol.* 1998;112:49.
30. Rudolph CD, Mazur LJ, Liptak GS, et al. Guidelines for evaluation and treatment of gastroesophageal reflux in infants and children: recommendations of the North American Society for Pediatric Gastroenterology and Nutrition. *J Pediatr Gastroenterol Nutr.* 2001;32(suppl 2):S1-S31.
31. Koufman JA, Aviv JE, Casiano RR, et al. Laryngopharyngeal reflux: position statement of the committee on speech, voice, and swallowing disorders of the American Academy of Otolaryngology–Head and Neck Surgery. *Otolaryngol Head Neck Surg.* 2002;127:32-35.
32. Contencin P, Narcy P. Nasopharyngeal pH monitoring in infants and children with chronic rhinopharyngitis. *Int J Pediatr Otorhinolaryngol.* 1991;22:249.
33. Ruth M, Carlsson S, Mansson I, et al. Scintigraphic detection of gastro-pulmonary aspiration in patients with respiratory disorders. *Clin Physiol.* 1993;13:19.
34. Orenstein SR. An overview of reflux-associated disorders in infants: apnea, laryngospasm, and aspiration. *Am J Med.* 2001;111(suppl 8A):60S-63S.
35. Wenzl TG, Moroder M, Trachterna M, et al. Esophageal pH monitoring and impedance measurement: a comparison of two diagnostic tests for gastroesophageal reflux. *J Pediatr Gastroenterol Nutr.* 2002;34:519-523.
36. Wenzl TG. Evaluation of gastroesophageal reflux events in children using multichannel intraluminal electrical impedance. *Am J Med.* 2003;115(suppl):161S-165S.
37. McGuirt WF. Gastroesophageal reflux and the upper airway. *Pediatr Clin North Am.* 2003;50:487-502.
38. McMurray JS, Gerber M, Stern Y, et al. Role of laryngoscopy, dual pH probe monitoring and laryngeal mucosal biopsy in the diagnosis of pharyngoesophageal reflux. *Ann Otol Rhinol Laryngol.* 2001;110:299-304.
39. Miyamoto RC, Parikh SR, Gellad W, et al. Bilateral congenital vocal cord paralysis: a 16 year institutional review. *Otolaryngol Head Neck Surg.* 2005;133:241-245.
40. Parikh SR. Pediatric unilateral vocal fold immobility. *Otolaryngol Clin North Am.* 2004;37:203-215.
41. Tucker HM. Vocal cord paralysis in small children: principles in management. *Ann Otol Rhinol Laryngol.* 1986;95:618-621.
42. Derkay CS, Darrow DH. Recurrent respiratory papillomatosis of the larynx: current diagnosis and treatment. *Otolaryngol Clin North Am.* 2000;33:1127-1141.
43. Valdez TA, McMillan K, Shapshay SM. A new laser treatment for vocal cord papilloma 585-nm pulsed dye. *Otolaryngol Head Neck Surg.* 2001;124:421-425.
44. Andrus JG, Shapshay SM. Contemporary management of laryngeal papilloma in adults and children. *Otolaryngol Clin North Am.* 2006;39:135-158.

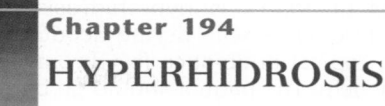

Chapter 194

HYPERHIDROSIS

Nancy K. Barnett, MD

When excessive localized sweating occurs in childhood, the child or the family usually expresses concern because the sweating is either odiferous or so intense that it interferes with hand functions (eg, holding a pencil) or foot functions. Axillary hyperhidrosis usually becomes more of a problem in adolescence because of the embarrassment of the sweat ring on clothing and the odor associated with bacterial degradation of apocrine sweat. The apocrine glands are stimulated at puberty by androgenic hormones. Palmar and plantar hyperhidrosis caused by eccrine sweat production may occur at any age. Eccrine sweat glands controlling thermoregulation are most numerous on the palms, soles, and axillae.

Palmoplantar hyperhidrosis is thought to be stimulated by anxiety, whereas axillary hyperhidrosis is probably stimulated by both heat and emotion. Researchers have postulated that emotions and the temperature of the blood perfusing the hypothalamus stimulate the secretion of the hormones that regulate the autonomic nervous system's control of perspiration.[1]

EVALUATION

Excessive sweating that is not limited to the palms, soles, and axillae may be caused by and indicate a systemic disorder, such as infection, lymphoma, thyrotoxicosis, Riley-Day syndrome, hypoglycemia, drug withdrawal, or pheochromocytoma. These disorders should be considered in the presence of generalized increased perspiring.

MANAGEMENT

Systemic anticholinergic agents may block acetylcholine, the sympathetic innervation terminal neurotransmitter to eccrine glands, and help hyperhidrosis, but the side effects of cholinergic blockage preclude their long-term use. The application of prescription 20% aluminum chloride (eg, Drysol) every other day has been an effective treatment for palmar sweating. Plantar hyperhidrosis also responds to aluminum salts, and absorbent powders (eg, Zeasorb) are used more easily here than on the palms. Some authors report successful control of palmar and plantar hyperhidrosis with tap water iontophoresis.[2]

Palmar and plantar hyperhidrosis can be controlled by inhibiting sweat production with subepidermal injections of botulinum A toxin, which purportedly blocks the presynaptic acetylcholine release and is effective for as long as 12 months. Patients as young as 14 years have been treated in this manner, but temporary or, rarely, permanent muscle and nerve injury from the injections limits its usefulness in these locations.[2,3]

For bromhidrosis (malodorous hyperhidrosis) of the soles, cleansing frequently with drying deodorant soaps and applying topical antibiotics (erythromycin or clindamycin) may help. The patient should go barefoot whenever possible.

Axillary hyperhidrosis is troublesome because continual sweating makes maintaining an effective antiperspirant in contact with the axillary skin difficult. One approach is to apply prescription 20% solution of aluminum chloride in anhydrous ethanol to the axillary vault.[4] A problematic side effect of this treatment can be an irritant contact dermatitis, uncomfortable enough to require hydrocortisone 1% cream for relief of inflammation. For individuals who have axillary hyperhidrosis and bromhidrosis, frequent clothing changes may be necessary, as well as the use of topical antibiotics and deodorant powders. Propranolol and anxiolytics are options to reduce emotional stress.

Successful axillary sweat gland chemo denervation with intradermal botulinum toxin injections is being increasingly used and is an approved indication for the toxin.[2,5] In extreme cases, when these measures fail and the patient is desperate for relief, local axillary skin can be excised or glands removed by less scarring curettage or liposuction techniques with reasonable expectation of success. Because of its attendant complications, ganglion sympathectomy cannot be recommended for most patients who have axillary hyperhidrosis.[2]

WHEN TO REFER

- Hyperhidrosis that interferes with the function of a body part (eg, hand so slippery wet that the child cannot hold a pencil)
- Generalized excessive sweating
- Socially isolating hyperhidrosis as a result of odor or excessive drenching of clothing

SUGGESTED RESOURCE

Jacobs AA, Desai A, Markus R. Don't sweat hyperhidrosis: a review of current treatment. *Cosmetic Dermatol.* 2005;18:725-731.

REFERENCES

1. Cage GW, Schwachman H, Sato K. In: Fitzpatrick TB, Eisen AZ, Wolff K, et al, eds. *Dermatology in General Medicine.* 2nd ed. New York, NY: McGraw-Hill; 1979.
2. Jacobs AA, Desai A, Markus R. Don't sweat hyperhidrosis: a review of current treatment. *Cosmetic Dermatol.* 2005;18:725-731.
3. Shelley WB, Talanin NY, Shelley ED. Botulinum toxin therapy for palmar hyperhidrosis. *J Am Acad Dermatol.* 1998; 38:227-229.
4. Shelley WB, Hurley HJ Jr. Studies on topical antiperspirant control of axillary hyperhidrosis. *Acta Derm Vener (Stockh).* 1975;55:241-260.
5. Heckmann M, Ceballos-Baumann AO, Plewig G. Botulinum toxin for axillary hyperhidrosis (excessive sweating). *N Engl J Med.* 2001;344:488-493.

Chapter 195

HYPOTONIA

Alfred J. Spiro, MD

Hypotonia indicates diminished resistance to passive movement around the range of motion of a joint. The commonly used term *floppy* refers to hypotonia, or weakness, or both. No readily administered, accurate test exists to quantitate hypotonicity. Furthermore, tone, especially in a young infant, may vary greatly during the day or even during the examination. Hypotonia is not, in itself, a diagnosis, but the origin of a neonate's floppiness may be obvious in, for example, overwhelming sepsis, meningitis, or marked hyperbilirubinemia. Central nervous system (CNS) abnormalities are commonly associated with hypotonia; generally, central hypotonia involves diminished tone without appreciably diminished strength coupled with preserved or hyperactive deep tendon reflexes. In disorders of the motor unit (lesions of the anterior horn cell, peripheral nerve, myoneural junction, and muscle), strength is usually diminished, and tone, as a result, may be reduced. Hypotonia that is not associated with a motor unit disorder is more common than hypotonia caused by an underlying motor unit disorder. Testing of strength in infants and young children is difficult, even for experienced examiners; it can usually be done by observation of how strong a baby's kicking and pushing are, for example, or by functional testing.

HYPOTONIA NOT CAUSED BY MOTOR UNIT DISORDERS

Disorders virtually anywhere in the brain may be associated with hypotonia. Global developmental delay is a common, but not a universal, accompanying feature, as is microcephaly. Magnetic resonance imaging of the brain may be helpful in documenting the lesion in some cases but is not always helpful. In many instances, a specific diagnosis cannot be made. As infants who have hypotonicity get older, the abnormal tone may evolve into spasticity, and the diagnosis of spastic quadriplegia, spastic diplegia, or other form of cerebral palsy becomes evident. A common misconception is that cerebral palsy is caused by obstetrical trauma; in most instances, the cause of cerebral palsy remains unknown.[1,2] Nevertheless, a review of birth records, drug administration, and factors surrounding prematurity is indicated. On examination, deep-tendon reflexes are usually, but not always, hyperactive. Abnormalities of tone in patients with cerebral palsy are usually global, that is, both proximal and distal. Treatment of various types of cerebral palsy is supportive and symptomatic and usually requires a multidisciplinary team effort (see Chapter 245, Cerebral Palsy).

Several genetic syndromes, Down syndrome among the most common, are associated with hypotonia; the diagnosis can be made on clinical grounds and with appropriate genetic studies. Newborns and young infants with Prader-Willi syndrome may be extremely hypotonic and obtunded. As these babies get older, tone may improve, and they may become obese. They have characteristic almond-shaped eyes, short stature, and some degree of mental retardation and hypogonadism; some have a severe eating disorder and scoliosis, but these features are usually not present until school age. The clinical features coupled with analysis showing a deletion in the chromosome 15q11-13 region can generally establish the diagnosis.

Several of the Ehlers-Danlos syndromes[3] may simulate hypotonicity, but the major feature of this group of connective tissue disorders is hyperlaxity of joints. Weakness is not a prominent feature.

Hypothyroidism and other metabolic disorders may be accompanied by hypotonia. Neonatal screening generally includes a test for hypothyroidism; if the diagnosis is not obvious on physical examination, then appropriate thyroid function studies can be done.

HYPOTONIA CAUSED BY MOTOR UNIT DISORDERS

History

In taking the history, the primary care physician should note whether hypotonia was present at birth or was recognized later. Parents of first children may have no basis for comparison and may not recognize an abnormality. Occasionally, photographs or family videotapes can be extremely useful in revealing abnormalities denied or not noted by parents. Breech presentation is common in babies who are subsequently diagnosed as having a motor unit disorder, but the reason for this has not been established. Congenital hip dislocation may be present in children who have central core disease, a congenital myopathy.[4]

Thorough questioning can usually determine if the hypotonia is improving or worsening or if weakness is periodic, as observed in hyperkalemic periodic paralysis (a rare autosomal-dominant disorder with onset usually in infancy or early childhood). The distribution of weakness, whether it is predominantly proximal, distal, or global, can also be identified with questions such as whether the baby or child moves the fingers and toes better than the large muscles of the pelvic and shoulder girdles. Details of the child's developmental milestones also can provide a clue to the nature of the lesion. For example, language development is normal in infantile progressive spinal muscular atrophy[5] and impaired in myotonic dystrophy.[6]

Facial muscle weakness, observed in some congenital myopathies, can be considered if the parents state that the child sleeps with the eyelids partially open. Extraocular muscles, in addition to facial muscles, are abnormal in myotubular myopathy.[7] Acquired autoimmune myasthenia gravis[8] and myasthenic syndromes[9] can occur in young children and may cause ptosis, extraocular muscle weakness, and, in some cases, generalized weakness and respiratory distress. Less severely affected patients may have only limited abnormal findings at the time of examination. Family videotapes taken at the times of the patient's maximal clinical involvement can be useful to document signs not seen in the examining room. Practitioners should inquire about swallowing and sucking difficulties, given that parents do not always recognize these difficulties.

Details of the family history can be helpful because many of the motor unit disorders are genetic. The presence of consanguinity suggests an autosomal-recessive entity. Examining parents and siblings can sometimes be revealing because some genetic disorders may be expressed quite subtly in family members and frequently are overlooked. Facial muscle weakness is 1 common example; patients do not seek medical attention if they cannot puff up their cheeks, whistle, or squeeze their eyelids closed completely, all features seen in certain congenital myopathies or facioscapulohumeral muscular dystrophy.[10] If early-onset myotonic dystrophy type 1 is thought to exist, then the child's mother and other family members should be examined for myotonia (slowed relaxation after a voluntary or induced muscle contraction) because neither percussion nor electrical myotonia is observed in infants or very young children.

Physical Examination

The clinician should conduct a thorough search for systemic disorders. Dysmorphic features such as high-arched palate and dental malocclusion are observed in some congenital myopathies, such as nemaline myopathy. An enlarged heart and congestive heart failure are observed in glycogen storage disease caused by acid maltase deficiency. Clubfoot deformity is commonly seen in the infantile form of myotonic dystrophy. Joint abnormalities and scoliosis are encountered frequently in several motor unit disorders.

A striking paucity of spontaneous movement is observed in infantile progressive spinal muscular atrophy[12]; paradoxical respiration, in which the chest wall moves inward during inspiration instead of expanding, is also observed frequently.

In infants and in children younger than 5 years, manual muscle testing generally cannot be accomplished reliably, making observation of spontaneous movement and functional testing, such as the ability to hold the head erect, sit, roll over, and stand, and walk on heels and toes, mandatory. Assessing cranial nerve function should emphasize identifying facial and extraocular muscle weakness, as well as fasciculation and atrophy of the tongue. Fasciculation of the tongue, observed in infantile progressive spinal muscular atrophy,[12] should be assessed with the tongue not protruded and with the child not crying. Tremulousness of the outstretched fingers (minipolymyoclonus[13]) is seen almost exclusively in spinal muscular atrophy with a protracted course. Generally, deep-tendon reflexes are reduced or absent in motor unit disorders but preserved in most cases of myasthenia gravis. With hypotonia of central origin, reflexes are preserved or hyperactive; however, many exceptions to this rule can be found. The presence or absence of extensor plantar responses is also frequently difficult to assess in young children; these responses may normally be present up to a year or more of age.

Laboratory Studies

Laboratory studies include blood testing, neurophysiological evaluation, and histologic examination of muscle. Laboratory studies should be goal directed and performed

Table 195-1 Infantile Progressive Spinal Muscular Atrophy

TYPE	AGE OF ONSET	COURSE
I	Birth to 6 mo	Never sits independently, even when placed; progressive; demise younger than 2 years
II	6–18 mo	Sits independently when placed; life expectancy into the twenties or later
III	>18 mo	Weakness after having learned to walk; normal life expectancy

in an orderly manner. Serum muscle enzyme levels, particularly creatine kinase, are always markedly elevated in Duchenne and Becker muscular dystrophy but are not always increased in congenital myopathies. They are generally normal or only minimally increased in spinal muscular atrophy. DNA studies for diagnostic purposes are readily available in many commercial and research laboratories (see Gene Tests or OMIM in Suggested Resources) for several motor unit disorders, including infantile progressive spinal muscular atrophy, myotonic dystrophy, various hereditary sensorimotor neuropathies, selected mitochondrial myopathies, and Duchenne and Becker muscular dystrophy. When these disorders are thought to exist on clinical grounds, appropriate DNA studies may be the only study needed to document the diagnosis. Thus a child who has classic infantile progressive spinal muscular atrophy can be spared many painful studies when the DNA studies are conclusive.[14] Other noninvasive studies, such as computed tomography, magnetic resonance imaging, or sonographic imaging of muscles, can assess muscle mass accurately; in the presence of very small muscles, imaging is indicated if a muscle biopsy is contemplated. Electromyographic studies can be useful in the diagnosis of motor unit disorders,[15] but because of the pain involved and the need for sedation in some cases, they should be used with discretion when DNA studies are not helpful. Nerve conduction studies can be extremely useful in distinguishing the various types of peripheral neuropathies seen in infants and children. Repetitive stimulation studies are very helpful in diagnosing disorders of the myoneural junction, including infantile botulism, but testing can be quite painful. An edrophonium test can be diagnostic when myasthenia gravis is thought to exist; clinicians who are able to interpret the results should perform this test. Clinicians who are experienced in the particular technical and other problems encountered in this age group should perform all electrodiagnostic studies in young children.

Muscle biopsies, performed either with a special needle or surgically, are most useful in myopathies such as congenital myopathies,[4] congenital muscular dystrophy, metabolic myopathies, and mitochondrial disorders.[16] Many specialized analytical studies are available when needed. In virtually all instances when a biopsy is performed, sections should be taken for histochemical, biochemical, ultrastructural, and genetic studies, although all of these studies are not always used in every case.

Selected Motor Unit Disorders

Anterior Horn Cell Disease

Given that the near elimination of paralytic poliomyelitis in the United States, the various types of infantile progressive spinal muscular atrophy constitute the major disease in this category. Eponyms have been applied to these disorders, including Werdnig-Hoffmann disease, but these terms may be misleading and confusing. Now, a much more useful operational classification of infantile progressive spinal muscular atrophy (Table 195-1) commonly is commonly used.[12]

In all types of infantile progressive spinal muscular atrophy, cognition is normal, as are extraocular muscles. Weakness and muscle wasting are proximal more than distal and are more pronounced in the legs than in the arms. Fasciculation of the tongue and minipolymyoclonus[13] (in types I and II, respectively) are observed frequently, and areflexia and normal sensation are the rule. Joint contractures and scoliosis may develop, especially in type II. All forms are autosomal recessive, with the responsible gene having been located at 5q11-q13. A deletion of the survival motor neuron gene has been identified in the vast majority of patients, making this situation useful for diagnostic purposes and for prenatal diagnosis.[17] Recent advances in understanding the molecular basis of this disorder have made phenotype-genotype correlation possible. Treatment generally is supportive and includes physical therapy and, when needed, respiratory and nutritional support and genetic counseling. Scoliosis is common in type II and must be addressed appropriately with a body jacket, molded back support, or surgery. Most children who have type II can use a motorized wheelchair at approximately 2 to 3 years of age. Life expectancy in type II can be well into adulthood.

Peripheral Nerve Disorders

Peripheral nerve disorders are rare in infancy and very early childhood. Hypomyelinating neuropathy[18] can produce severe weakness, hypotonia, and areflexia in a neonate or young infant. The diagnosis can be anticipated when extremely abnormal nerve conduction studies are encountered and can be confirmed with DNA studies or with a nerve biopsy. Hereditary sensorimotor neuropathies (many variants of Charcot-Marie-Tooth disease exist), the most common cause of childhood peripheral nerve disorders, may cause gait abnormalities from weakness of the anterior tibialis muscles or foot deformities.[19] Ankle jerks are frequently diminished or absent, but all reflexes may be preserved in the early phases of peripheral neuropathies. Nerve conduction studies can be extremely useful in separating axonal from demyelination neuropathies. DNA studies can be diagnostic in selected hereditary neuropathies, especially the demyelinating and the X-linked varieties. Treatment addresses symptoms; some children who have foot drop may require bracing.

Several CNS disorders may have a demyelinating form of peripheral nerve involvement in addition to abnormalities in the cerebral white matter; these include metachromatic leukodystrophy, Krabbe disease, and adrenoleukodystrophy.

Myoneural Junction Disorders

Several disorders of the myoneural junction[8,9] affect children and infants: (1) passively acquired autoimmune myasthenia gravis, also known as transient neonatal myasthenia; (2) acquired autoimmune myasthenia gravis, also known as juvenile or childhood myasthenia; (3) nonautoimmune myasthenic syndromes, also known as congenital myasthenia gravis; and (4) infantile botulism.[21]

Passively acquired autoimmune myasthenia gravis occurs in approximately 20% of infants born to mothers who have myasthenia gravis. All newborns of seropositive mothers have acetylcholine receptor antibodies, but only a small portion are symptomatic, most mildly, but some more severely, with hypotonia, a weak cry, swallowing and sucking difficulty, facial diapiresis, respiratory distress, external ophthalmoparesis, and ptosis. The diagnosis can be made quickly by administering intravenous edrophonium. When the newborns are symptomatic, pyridostigmine can be given orally until symptoms are no longer present. The dose is then tapered, usually over a period of 1 to 2 weeks after the treatment has commenced. These infants do not have clinical features of myasthenia gravis after the initial involvement. If weakness does not occur by 1 week of age, then it is highly unlikely to develop.

Major features of acquired autoimmune myasthenia include fatigability and fluctuating weakness of extraocular, facial, and lingual muscles, and, in some instances, mild or severe generalized weakness and hypotonicity of the limbs. An acute fulminating onset may be encountered in young children. The diagnosis can be made by using the edrophonium test and confirmed with the acetylcholine receptor antibody test, although the latter is not necessarily positive in milder cases and is less useful in children than in older individuals. Electrodiagnostic studies can be used in selected instances in children but are generally less useful than in adults. The mediastinum should be radiographed to assess thymic size, and thyroid function studies should be obtained to exclude associated hypo- or hyperthyroidism. Treatment includes judicious use of anticholinesterase drugs and, when needed, immunosuppressive treatment, intravenous gamma globulin, corticosteroids, and thymectomy.

Nonautoimmune myasthenic syndromes[9] may be associated with ocular, bulbar, or respiratory involvement and, in some instances, with progressive weakness and hypotonicity. Some disorders may be genetic; patients are seronegative. Specialized electrodiagnostic and ultrastructural studies are required to establish an exact diagnosis, which is important in selecting appropriate therapy. For the moment, genetic studies for diagnosis are available only within a research setting. Some patients respond to anticholinesterase inhibitors or corticosteroids; others require diaminopyridine or other specific medications.

Infantile botulism[21] is characterized by onset at an average age of slightly more than 3 months that produces weakness and hypotonia, poor feeding, constipation, and diminished activity. The onset may be rapid, developing over 2 to 3 days. The diagnosis is confirmed when the toxin is documented in the stool or when the organism is isolated from culture, but repetitive stimulation studies can by extremely useful in establishing the diagnosis quickly. Treatment is supportive; a possibility exists that specific immune globulin might be therapeutic.

Myopathies

Myopathies constitute a diverse group of genetic, inflammatory, and metabolic disorders that involve muscle and, in many cases, other organ systems, including the brain and heart. Inflammatory myopathies (dermatomyositis) are seen only rarely in very young children and generally produce subacute weakness, not hypotonia. Patients with Duchenne muscular dystrophy (1 of the most common muscular disorders) do not have hypotonia in infancy. In the infantile form of myotonic dystrophy–type[16] hypotonia can be severe at birth. Obtundation, difficulty with sucking and swallowing, weakness of facial muscles, clubfeet, and areflexia may be present. Myotonia will not be present either clinically or electrically until patients are older than 5 years. A neonate who survives will gain strength and tone and will eventually walk. Until strength and tone improve, assisted ventilation and gastrostomy tube feedings are often needed. Myotonic dystrophy type 1 is an autosomal-dominant disorder; however, when it occurs in the neonatal period, it is virtually always the mother who transmitted the gene. She should be examined for the characteristic features of the disease, which include reflex and percussion myotonia, weakness of the neck flexor muscles, smallness of the sternocleidomastoid muscles, weakness of the wrist extensors and anterior tibialis muscles and facial muscles, and, often, mental retardation. For children who first exhibit myotonic dystrophy beyond infancy, either parent may have transmitted the gene, which is located on 19q13. DNA studies can be done to document the diagnosis and predict the prognosis. This condition is an expanded trinucleotide repeat disorder; a correlation exists between the severity and the number of repeats. Family members should be provided with genetic counseling if they so desire, given that prenatal diagnosis is available. Treatment is supportive.

Several congenital myopathies have been identified[4] and are generally diagnosed by their characteristic morphologic mechanism on muscle biopsy. These myopathies, typified by nemaline myopathy, are frequently hereditary and are associated with varying degrees of hypotonia and weakness and sometimes with respiratory and sucking problems early in life. Some have rather characteristic clinical features. For example, in X-linked myotubular myopathy of very early onset,[7] the extraocular and facial muscles are weak, in addition to generalized hypotonia and weakness. Central core disease is associated with congenital hip dislocation and a propensity for malignant hyperpyrexia. In some congenital myopathies, the gene location has been identified, but DNA testing is not yet available for establishing the diagnosis.

The congenital muscular dystrophies comprise a diverse group of diseases in which varying degrees of weakness and hypotonia are present early in life (see

Chapter 295 Muscular Dystrophy). Muscle biopsy shows characteristic, but not specific, pathologic findings, and more refined studies are required. The serum muscle enzymes (creatine phosphokinase) are generally elevated, and, in some forms of this disorder, merosin is absent on the biopsy specimen.[22] The merosin-deficient type of congenital muscular dystrophy is often associated with mental retardation, seizures, and white matter brain abnormalities. In Japan, Fukuyama type congenital muscular dystrophy[23] is common and is also associated with severe CNS abnormalities.

Facioscapulohumeral muscular dystrophy[10] usually occurs in older children but, at times, will produce severe facial weakness in early childhood. This condition is an autosomal-dominant disorder, although some cases are sporadic. Parents of children thought to have this disorder should be examined for involvement that may be very mild and go unnoticed, such as facial muscular weakness, scapular winging, and a round-shouldered stance. This disease is genetically linked to high-frequency hearing deficits. Treatment is symptomatic; genetic advice can be offered when desired. DNA studies are available to document the diagnosis when this disorder is thought to exist, making electrodiagnostic testing and muscle biopsy unnecessary.

Glycogen storage disease caused by deficient acid maltase,[24] in addition to its neuromuscular manifestations (hypotonia and weakness), is associated with a markedly enlarged heart and congestive heart failure. The diagnosis can be made readily by specific blood tests. Enzyme replacement therapy has recently become available; without this treatment, the prognosis is dismal. This condition is an autosomal-recessive disorder with the responsible gene located at 17q23.

An increasing number of mitochondrial encephalomyopathies[16] are being reported that have varying CNS and muscle involvement. Lacticacidemia is common, but specialized genetic and other studies on muscle mitochondria are needed to provide a specific diagnosis if DNA studies are unrevealing. Treatment addresses symptoms.

Congenital hypotonia with favorable outcome[25] or benign congenital hypotonia is a retrospective diagnosis used to denote infants who have hypotonia of early onset with a benign course. This relatively unclear disorder is frequently associated with joint hyperlaxity, sometimes also noted in parents or other relatives. In many instances, by 5 years of age, the children are indistinguishable from other children their age.

WHEN TO REFER

- Persistent lack of normal motor development
- Regression of motor development
- Sudden or precipitous worsening of tone or strength
- Swallowing dysfunction
- New onset of neurologic signs

TOOLS FOR PRACTICE

Medical Decision Support

- Online Mendelian Inheritance in Man (on-line database), Johns Hopkins University (www.ncbi.nlm.nih.gov/entrez/query.fcgi?db=OMIM).
- Gene Tests (Web site), University of Washington (www.genetests.org/).

SUGGESTED RESOURCES

OMIM: Online Mendelian Inheritance in Man. Provides detailed clinical and genetic information on all genetic disorders. (www.ncbi.nlm.nih.gov/sites/entrez?db=omim).

Gene Tests. Provides detailed information on availability of genetic testing. (www.genetests.org).

REFERENCES

1. Kuban KCK, Leviton A. Cerebral palsy. *N Engl J Med*. 1994;330:188-195.
2. Perlman JM. Intrapartum hypoxic-ischemic cerebral injury and subsequent cerebral palsy: medicolegal issues. *Pediatrics*. 1997;99:851-859.
3. Grahame R. Joint hypermobility and genetic collagen disorders: are they related? *Arch Dis Child*. 1999;80:188-191.
4. Goebel HH. Congenital myopathies: the current status. *J Child Neuro*. 1999;14:30-31.
5. Anhuf D, Eggermann T, Rudnik-Dchoneborn S, et al. Determination of SMN1 and SMN2 copy number using TaqMan technology. *Hum Mutat*. 2003;22:74-78.
6. Harper PS. *Myotonic Dystrophy*. 3rd ed. London, UK: WB Saunders; 2001.
7. Barth PG, Dubowitz V. X-linked myotubular myopathy—a long-term follow-up study. *Eur J Paeditr Neurol*. 1998; 2:49-56.
8. Spiro AJ: Disorders of the myoneural junction. In: Berg BO, ed. *Principles of Child Neurology*. New York, NY: McGraw-Hill; 1996.
9. Kraner S, Laufenberg I, Strassburg HM, et al. Congenital myasthenic syndrome with episodic apnea in patients homozygous for a CHAT missense mutation. *Arch Neurol*. 2003;60:761-763.
10. Okinaga A, Matsuoka T, Umeda J, et al. Early-onset facioscapulohumeral muscular dystrophy: two case reports. *Brain Dev*. 1997;19:563-567.
11. Agrawal PB, Strickland CD, Midgett C, et al. Heterogeneity of nemaline myopathy cases with skeletal muscle alpha-actin gene mutations. *Ann Neurol*. 2004;56:86-96.
12. Prasad AS, Prasad C. The floppy infant: contribution of genetic and metabolic disorders. *Brain Dev*. 2003;27: 457-476.
13. Spiro AJ. Minipolymyoclonus: a neglected sign in childhood spinal muscular atrophy. *Neurology*. 1970;20: 1124-1126.
14. Lefebvre S, Burglen L, Reboullet S, et al. Identification and characterization of a spinal muscular atrophy-determining gene, *Cell*. 1995;80:155-165.
15. Russell JW, Afifi AK, Ross MA. Predictive value of electromyography in diagnosis and prognosis of the hypotonic infant. *J Child Neurol*. 1992;7:387-391.
16. Shoubridge EA. Mitochondrial encephalomyelopathies. *Curr Opin Neurol*. 1998;11:491-496.
17. Lefebvre S, Burglen L, Frezal J, et al. The role of the SMN gene in proximal spinal muscular atrophy. *Hum Mol Genet*. 1998;7:1531-1536.
18. Mandich P, Mancardi GL, Varese A, et al. Congenital hypomyelination due to myelin protein zero Q215X mutation. *Ann Neurol*. 1999;45:676-678.
19. Ouvrier RA. *Peripheral Neuropathy in Childhood*. 2nd ed. New York, NY: Raven Press; 2002.
20. Kaye EM, Moser H. Where has all the white matter gone? Unraveling the mysteries of leukoencephalopathies. *Neurology*. 2004;62:1464-1465.
21. McMaster P, Piper S, Schell D, et al. A taste of honey. *J Paediatr Child Health*. 2000;36:596-597.

22. Jones KJ, Morgan G, Johnston H, et al. The expanding phenotype of laminin alpha2 chain (merosin) abnormalities: case series and review. *J Med Genet.* 2001;38: 649-657.
23. Hayashi YK, Ogawa M, Tagawa K, et al. Selective deficiency of alpha-dystroglycan in Fukuyama-type congenital muscular dystrophy. *Neurology.* 2001;57: 115-121.
24. Amalfitano A, Bengur AR, Morse RP, et al. Recombinant human acid alpha-glucosidase enzyme therapy for infantile glycogen storage disease type II: results of a phase I/ II clinical trial. *Genet Med.* 2001;3:132-138.
25. Carboni P, Pisani F, Crescenzi A, et al. Congenital hypotonia with favorable outcome. *Pediatr Neurol.* 2002;26:383-386.

Chapter 196
IRRITABILITY

Diana King, MD; Waseem Hafeez, MBBS

Irritability, "a condition in which a person, organ, or a part responds excessively to a stimulus,"[1] is a common complaint in children, especially in neonates and infants. Although experienced clinicians can recognize irritability in a child, a concise definition is difficult because some subjectivity exists in the use of the term. Irritability is not a quantifiable symptom and includes episodes of crying or fussiness despite attempts at comforting the infant. Although irritability is not a symptom of any specific illness, most parents recognize that something might be wrong with the child, even though other symptoms may not yet exist.

Irritability results from lack of vital nutrients (eg, oxygen, glucose), the presence of noxious stimuli (eg, pain, toxins), or from an emotional state (eg, anger, frustration). It may have different causes and manifestations in infants, children, and adolescents. Whereas older children and adolescents may offer explanations that help clarify their complaint, an infant or preverbal child is unable to provide such information. Acute irritability may be associated with life-threatening illnesses requiring urgent intervention and stabilization before a search for the cause begins. A parent who seeks care for an infant who is fussier than usual may arrive with a child who is in shock, in respiratory distress, or having a seizure. An organized approach to the differential diagnosis minimizes unnecessary testing. If the child does not have an immediately life-threatening condition, then a complete history and thorough physical examination are the first steps in the evaluation of irritability and, in many cases, will reveal the cause of the symptom. Many common infectious, traumatic, toxic, allergic, and inflammatory conditions can be diagnosed by history and physical examination alone. Laboratory or radiologic procedures may confirm a clinical suspicion. An algorithm to differentiate some life-threatening conditions from less serious causes of irritability is outlined in Figure 196-1.

ACUTE IRRITABILITY IN THE ILL-APPEARING CHILD

Central Nervous System

Children younger than 2 years have a high risk for significant brain injury after accidental head trauma, and the overall rate of brain injury is approximately 12% in the 0- to 2-month age group, 6% in the 3- to 11-month age group, and 2% in infants older than 12 months.[1,2] The American Academy of Pediatrics has recommended guidelines for evaluation and management of head injury in this age group.[3] A history of a fall from the bed, infant-walker, stairs, or bicycle can often be found. The presence of either irritability or lethargy or of a scalp hematoma, protracted vomiting, or neurologic deficits, warrants a head computed tomographic scan, and a high index of suspicion should be maintained in infants younger than 3 months.[4]

A special concern is for children who sustain concussions from sports-related injuries. The term *postconcussive syndrome* refers to the constellation of acute symptoms, which can be somatic (headache, dizziness, blurriness), emotional (irritability, anxiety), and cognitive (concentration and memory difficulties). The American Academy of Neurology defines concussion as "a trauma-induced alteration in mental status that may or may not involve loss of consciousness." The term *second impact syndrome* has been proposed for an athlete who has sustained a concussion, sustains a second head injury before symptoms associated with the first have fully cleared, and is at risk for a catastrophic outcome such as permanent disability or death.[5] To manage these injuries, a concussion grading scale has been developed with return-to-play guidelines.[6]

Increased intracranial pressure (ICP) from a brain tumor may produce acute irritability and altered behavior without the usual preceding symptoms such as headache or loss of coordination. Primary brain tumors in the posterior fossa are the most common solid malignancies in infants and children younger than 7 years. In young children the diagnosis of a brain tumor may be delayed because their symptoms are subtle (headache, irritability, or drowsiness) or similar to those of more common illnesses, such as gastrointestinal disorders (vomiting). Hydrocephalus, another cause of raised ICP, often occurs in infancy with irritability, vomiting, a tense or bulging fontanel, and an increasing head circumference that crosses percentile lines. Older children usually complain of headaches. Neuroimaging shows congenital malformation (myelomeningocele, Chiari syndrome, Dandy Walker malformation, aqueductal stenosis, arteriovenous malformation) or germinal matrix intraventricular hemorrhage of prematurity. Hydrocephalus is treated by the introduction of ventriculoperitoneal shunts to reduce the ICP. The ventriculoperitoneal shunt may become obstructed or infected, or it may malfunction, causing overdrainage or underdrainage, initially causing irritability, headache, vomiting, or lethargy.

Undiagnosed migraine headache may occur in the preverbal child with irritability. Headaches attributable to migraine occur in 8% to 12% of children younger than 3 years.[7] Children with seizures, especially unwitnessed, may appear irritable during an aura or the

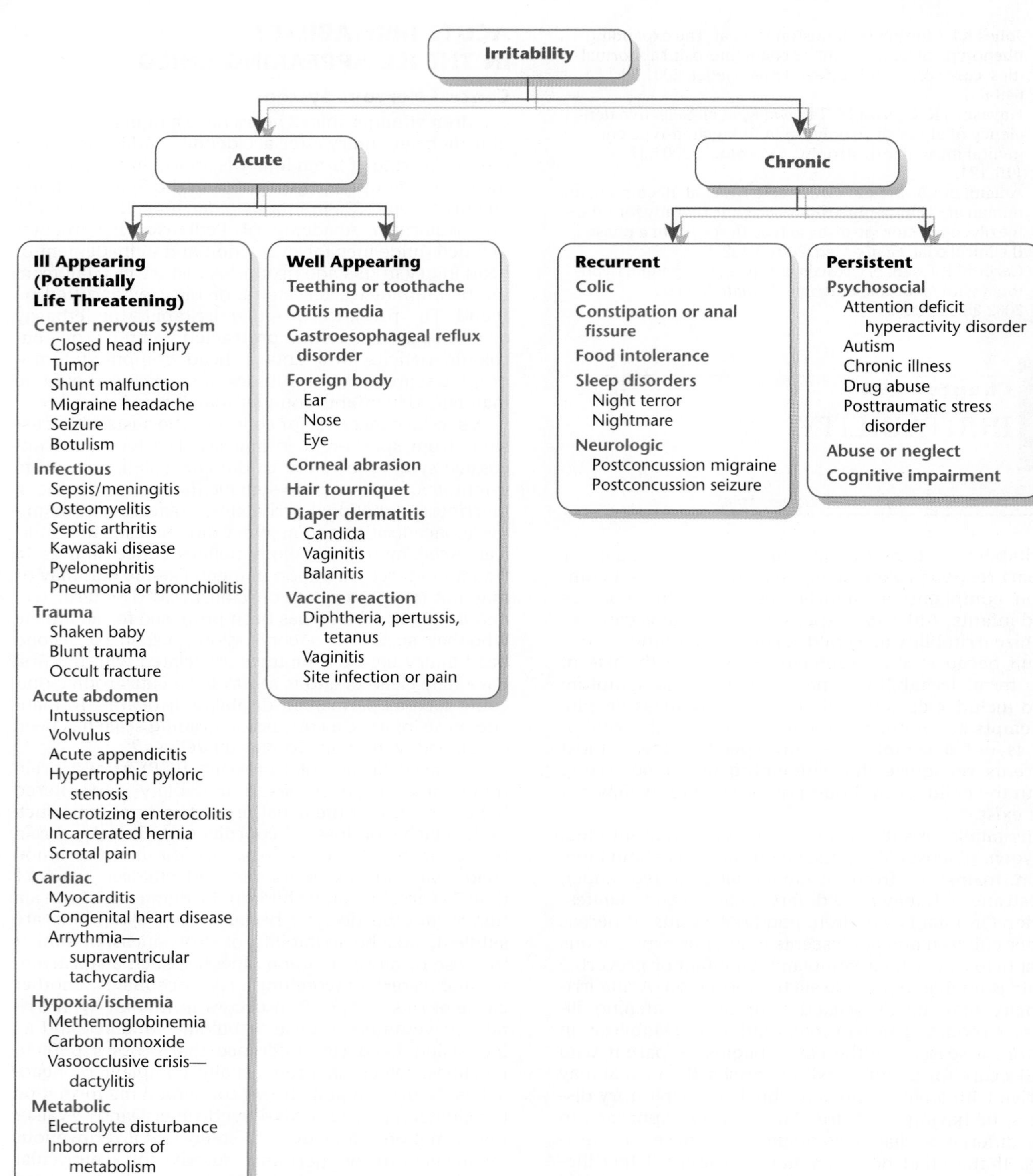

Figure 196-1 Evaluation of Irritable Infant Algorithm.

postictal phase. Neonatal seizures, more commonly seen in preterm infants than term infants, may have only subtle symptoms such as ocular or pedaling movements, lip smacking, or apnea. Nonconvulsive status epilepticus, which includes absence and partial complex seizures, is a relatively rare cause of abnormal behavior and produces continuous or intermittent seizure activity in the absence of any motor component and without a return to baseline for more than 30 minutes. The hallmark of nonconvulsive status epilepticus is a diagnostic electroencephalogram associated with irritability and a change in behavior or mental status.[8]

Infant botulism may initially cause difficulty in feeding, irritability, lethargy, weak cry, and constipation. As the disease progresses, drooling, dysphagia, loss of head control, respiratory distress, and flaccid paralysis may occur from progressive bulbar involvement.

Infections

The primary care physician should suspect a bacterial infection in a child with fever and irritability. Infants with meningitis may have irritability, lethargy, and poor feeding. If the fontanel is still open, then it may be bulging. Lumbar puncture is diagnostic, and treatment with intravenous antibiotics should not be delayed. Group B streptococci and gram-negative bacilli are the most common causes in neonates. Encephalitis from herpes simplex virus is also a consideration. In infants and children, the most common bacteria are *Streptococcus pneumoniae, Neisseria meningitidis,* and *Haemophilus influenzae* type B. (See Chapter 293, Meningitis.)

Irritability and decreased movement of a limb should raise concern for osteomyelitis. Swelling and erythema of the soft tissue overlying the bone may exist, often with a history of preceding trauma. Joint pain, fever, irritability, and a limp should raise concern for septic arthritis. Examination will reveal erythema, swelling, or warmth over the affected joint, with restricted movement. With septic arthritis of the hip, swelling and redness may not be visible, and the pain may be referred to the knee. Blood should be analyzed for culture, complete blood count, and erythrocyte sedimentation rate or C-reactive protein to help establish a diagnosis. An orthopedist should be consulted for possible surgical drainage.

Children with Kawasaki disease, a vasculitis triggered by an unknown infectious agent, are often more irritable than patients with other febrile illnesses.[9] (See Chapter 289, Kawasaki Disease.) Occult sepsis, urinary tract infections, and pneumonia can also produce irritability, along with fever and other signs that cause a patient to appear toxic.

Trauma

A systematic search for injuries should be performed on any child with a history of trauma. Inflicted injuries are more difficult to diagnose because the signs may be subtle and because the history is often misleading. Shaken baby syndrome occurs most commonly in children younger than 2 years.[10] The rotational forces sustained during shaking cause movement of the brain within the subdural space and tearing of the bridging veins.[11] Clinical signs of shaken baby syndrome may be poor feeding, vomiting, lethargy, or irritability. More severe central nervous system dysfunction can result in death.[10-12] (See Chapter 120, Child Physical Abuse and Neglect.)

In infants and young children, the pressure of the lap belt of a restraint system in a motor vehicle crash or other blunt abdominal trauma can lead to intraabdominal bleeding, initially displaying as irritability from tissue hypoperfusion and pain. Many traumatic causes of irritability that are not life threatening may be apparent on initial physical examination and include fractures or dislocations.

Acute Abdomen

Intussusception is seen most frequently between the ages of 3 months and 5 years, with a peak incidence at 6 to 11 months. The child appears colicky and cries and may draw the knees upward toward the chest; this episode may last a few minutes and then subside. The child often looks better between episodes, and the irritability gradually increases and vomiting becomes more frequent and sometimes bilious. The classic triad of intermittent colicky abdominal pain, vomiting, and bloody mucous stools is encountered in only 20% to 40% of cases, whereas at least 2 of these findings will be present in approximately 60% of patients. (See Chapter 336, Acute Surgical Abdomen.)

Malrotation with midgut volvulus peaks during the 1st month of life but can occur anytime in childhood. The neonate will be irritable initially; as bowel becomes obstructed and necrotic, bilious vomiting and shock may result from perforation.

Appendicitis is found in 2% to 3% of children with abdominal pain seen in ambulatory clinics or emergency departments. Abdominal pain in a young child may first manifest as irritability, before the appearance of nausea, vomiting, fever, and right lower quadrant tenderness. Perforation rates for appendicitis are higher in children than in adults (30% to 65%), and, given that the omentum is less developed in children, perforations are less likely to be walled off or localized.[13]

Hypertrophic pyloric stenosis may become symptomatic as early as the 1st week of life and as late as the 5th month. Symptoms begin with nonbilious vomiting after feeding, and as the disease progresses the vomiting becomes projectile. The baby may initially appear normal, but hunger makes the infant irritable, and signs of dehydration eventually become apparent. (See Chapter 315, Pyloric Stenosis.)

Necrotizing enterocolitis is typically seen in premature infants in their first few weeks of life. It may rarely be seen in full term infants, within the first 2 weeks after birth, particularly with a stressor such as infection or anoxic event.[14] Infants are ill appearing, irritable, and lethargic, with distended abdomen and bloody stools. Abdominal plain-film finding of pneumatosis intestinalis, caused by gas in the submucosal intestinal wall, is diagnostic of necrotizing enterocolitis. Because of a high mortality rate, management includes early surgical consultation and aggressive fluid resuscitation, bowel rest, and broad-spectrum antibiotic coverage.

Sixty percent of incarcerated inguinal hernias occur during the 1st year of life, with symptoms of irritability, vomiting, and pain in the groin and abdomen. A testicular examination is imperative in all male patients with irritability or abdominal pain. On examination a nonfluctuant tender mass is present in the inguinal region and may extend down into the scrotum. With the onset of ischemia of the involved bowel the pain becomes more intense and localized to the scrotum, and the infant may have bilious vomiting with the presence of bloody stools. An attempt should be made to reduce the incarcerated hernia manually by gentle compression. Sedation or analgesia, elevation of the lower torso, and an ice pack may be helpful. If reduction is unsuccessful or patient shows signs of small bowel obstruction, then operative reduction of the incarcerated hernia should be performed. Irritability with scrotal pain may also result from epididymitis, torsion of the testis, or torsion of the appendix testis.

Cardiac System

Acute myocarditis should be considered in an irritable child with tachycardia, especially if accompanied by poor perfusion. An electrocardiogram may reveal sinus tachycardia with low-voltage QRS complexes, arrhythmias, and ST changes. An elevated serum troponin level will support the diagnosis, and an echocardiogram will show reduced ventricular function.[15] The gold standard for diagnosis is an endomyocardial biopsy. Three phases have been identified in the pathogenesis: (1) viral replication, (2) autoimmune injury to myocytes, and (3) dilated cardiomyopathy. Various immunosuppressive drugs have been used (prednisolone, intravenous immunoglobulin) to decrease the autoimmune response but have not been shown to improve the outcome.[16] Treatment includes inotropic support and diuretics in a critical care setting.

Anomalous left coronary artery originating from the pulmonary artery occurs in early infancy with irritability during or soon after feedings. Associated signs may include poor weight gain, diaphoresis, a murmur, and respiratory distress. Chest x-rays and electrocardiograms are excellent screening tests. Cardiomegaly on x-ray and myocardial ischemia on electrocardiographic examination are almost universal findings.[17]

Supraventricular tachycardia may cause irritability and poor feeding. Physical examination will reveal a rapid, regular rhythm; electrocardiogram is diagnostic.

Hypoxic or Ischemic Events

Carbon monoxide (CO) poisoning and methemoglobinemia cause irritability by producing hypoxia. CO binds to hemoglobin with an affinity more than 200 times that of oxygen, whereas methemoglobin is unable to bind to oxygen. Both actions result in a leftward shift of the oxygen-hemoglobin dissociation curve and decreased oxygen delivery to the tissues. A history of smoke inhalation and exposure to an indoor gas stove or to automobile exhaust fumes is indicative. Early findings with CO poisoning are similar to influenza-like symptoms of headache, irritability, and dizziness, whereas prolonged exposure may result in altered mental status. Arterial measurement of carboxyhemoglobin is diagnostic. Methemoglobinemia in infancy may be either hereditary or related to hypoxic events, medication use (sulfonamides, topical anesthetics, metoclopropamide), products containing nitrites and nitrates (contaminated well water or foods with naturally occurring nitrates such as spinach, green beans, carrots, and squash), or to diarrhea, probably from the nitrite-forming bacteria in the gut. Hereditary methemoglobinemia is usually mild, whereas the acquired disease can be life threatening. Characteristic blue-gray cyanosis that is not improved with oxygen, despite normal arterial oxygen tension, and chocolate brown appearance of arterial blood are the hallmarks of methemoglobinemia. Treatment of the patient begins with 100% supplemental oxygen by nonrebreather mask and aggressive supportive care. In CO poisoning, hyperbaric oxygen therapy may be indicated in certain clinical conditions; methylene blue is an effective treatment for methemoglobinemia.

In children with sickle cell anemia, ischemia may cause painful vasoocclusive crisis. The 1st presentation in infants and younger children is usually irritability and dactylitis, painful swelling of the hands and feet, as a result of vascular stasis and ischemia. Treatment includes analgesia, hydration, and rest.

Metabolic System

Hypoglycemia, hypo- or hypernatremia, hypo- or hypercalcemia, hypomagnesemia, and inborn errors of metabolism can all cause irritability.[18] Hypoglycemia is defined as a glucose level of 40 mg/dL or less and can be a primary process or caused by sepsis, ingestion, or cardiac or respiratory failure.[19] Rapid detection and treatment of hypoglycemia can prevent irreversible neurologic damage. Hyponatremia can result from gastrointestinal losses or water intoxication, whereas hypernatremia is seen with diarrhea in which the water losses exceed salt loss, when replacement fluid has too high a sodium content, or with improper preparation of infant formula. Hypocalcemia in the newborn period may cause irritability, poor feeding, and lethargy; later in infancy and during childhood, hypocalcemia is seen with rickets. Hypercalcemia is a rare electrolyte disturbance resulting from hyperparathyroidism, vitamin D intoxication, or from idiopathic causes. Hypomagnesemia is found with hypocalcemia.

The inborn errors of metabolism that cause irritability are those in which a toxic intermediate accumulates. Organic and aminoacidemias and urea cycle disorders result in metabolic acidosis or hyperammonemia. They are symptomatic in the first few weeks of life, with vomiting, poor feeding, irritability, and lethargy. When a milder degree of enzyme dysfunction is present, clinical disease may be triggered by a bacterial or viral illness. (See Chapter 48, Recognition of Genetic-Metabolic Diseases by Clinical Diagnosis and Screening.)

Toxins and Drugs

Life-threatening intoxications may result from heavy metals such as lead and mercury,[20] drugs of abuse such as cocaine and alcohol, envenomations by scorpions and snakes, overdoses of or idiosyncratic reactions to medications, and contact with agricultural, industrial, or household chemicals. Thorough questioning about recent use of lawn chemicals, pesticides, and cleaning products may be the only clues to these factors as a cause of irritability because many of these chemicals will not be detected by standard toxicologic screenings of blood and urine. Prescribed or over-the-counter medications such as beta-agonists, antiepileptics, decongestants, antihistamines, antitussives, and various *cold preparations* may cause irritability even when used as directed and certainly when overused. Cocaine,[21] alcohol, phencyclidine hydrochloride,[22] inhalants, and other drugs of abuse are known to cause irritability. Infants and children may be exposed to these substances by passive means transplacentally,[23] by ingestion of breast milk,[24] or by inhalation. They may accidentally ingest alcohol or cigarettes and other substances left within reach. A positive history may be difficult to elicit, and a toxicologic screen may not always be helpful; thus a strong index of suspicion is needed. Substance use or withdrawal should be considered in the differential diagnosis when any adolescent produces chronic persistent irritability. In rare instances, intentional poisoning may be the cause of a child's distress.[25]

Many clinicians remember at least one child who has had complaints of irritability and intermittent fever in whom leukemia with bone pain was diagnosed. Malignancies of all sorts may have a component of irritability among their symptoms and must be considered carefully when no other diagnosis is forthcoming.

ACUTE IRRITABILITY IN THE WELL-APPEARING CHILD

Irritability in infants has been attributed to a variety of causes of pain or discomfort that may become obvious during the evaluation. Dental caries and teething may cause an infant to be fussy or irritable. (See Chapter 33, Prevention of Dental Caries.) In addition to irritability, teething may be accompanied by loose stools but not fever.[26] Cold teething rings may provide some relief, but numbing gels are less helpful and may be harmful.

Acute otitis media is a common cause of irritability, with or without fever, in children younger than 2 years and in those attending child care. Also common, particularly in the 1st year of life, is gastroesophageal reflux, which may be asymptomatic or reveal itself with postprandial irritability, recurrent vomiting, and inadequate weight gain.

Other sources of irritability and nonspecific crying episodes may be related to a foreign body in the ear or nose, a corneal abrasion, hair wrapped around a digit or penis, diaper rash, nonspecific vaginitis, balanitis, insect and spider bites or stings, and pain from the site of a vaccination. A thorough head-to-toe examination, including special attention to the eyes, ears, digits, and genitalia, is essential to establish a diagnosis.

A foreign body in the ear or nose, if present for a prolonged period, results in foul-smelling discharge. If visible, then the object may be removed with forceps, by gentle irrigation, or by suction; otherwise removal should be done under sedation or general anesthesia. Disk batteries need to be removed emergently because they may leak and can cause tissue destruction. An insect in the ear canal can make a child very irritable and may be removed after first killing the insect with mineral oil or lidocaine.

Foreign bodies under the eyelid, inward turned eyelashes, or a baby scratching the eyes may cause corneal abrasion. The child may be irritable, with increased tearing, conjunctival injection, and photophobia. Diagnosis is made by Wood lamp examination after instillation of fluorescein into the eye. A foreign body may be removed by a moistened cotton-tipped applicator or by irrigation.

A hair tourniquet around a child's digit or genitals can cause irritability and pain. A thorough examination in the creases of the digits is essential because prolonged constricting bands may compromise distal circulation.

In some instances the source of a child's irritability will be found only on thorough examination of the genitalia, which may reveal evidence of vaginitis, balanitis, or an anal fissure. Diaper dermatitis, common after a diarrheal illness, with *Candida* infection or as an allergic reaction to the diaper material, is another potential cause of irritability in infants.

Infants can certainly be irritable after the administration of a vaccine, with local erythema, swelling, and tenderness at the injection site. Persistent, inconsolable crying lasting 3 hours or more within 48 hours of receiving whole-cell pertussis DTP vaccine have been reported but not with the newer acellular-pertussis DTaP vaccine.[27]

CHRONIC IRRITABILITY

Chronic irritability may be recurrent or persistent in a child and challenges both the parents'[28] and the clinician's skills. Psychosocial causes may head the list, but toxic, neurologic, metabolic, and miscellaneous causes must be considered and are shown in Figure 196-1. Irritability as a chronic feature of a child's behavior may indicate significant problems with familial relationships and the ability to master the environment. Infants may be irritable because of maternal-infant temperament mismatches, maternal depression,[29] or stress within the family from, for example, the birth of a new child. Abuse and neglect of a child may provoke irritable behavior or outbursts. An older child or adolescent who has a psychiatric problem such as depression, psychosis, autism, posttraumatic stress disorder, or substance abuse may be described as irritable by parents and others. The investigation and treatment of irritability in these situations may require a multidisciplinary and long-term approach.

CHRONIC RECURRENT IRRITABILITY

Usually occurring in infants younger than 3 months, colic is characterized by paroxysms of screaming, which may persist for several hours. Criteria for the diagnosis are crying for 3 or more hours per day on 3 or more days per week lasting for more than 3 weeks. Colic typically peaks at 6 weeks and abates by 3 to 4 months.[30] The physical examination is normal and growth and development remain unchanged. (See Chapter 249, Colic.)

Constipation in the older infant or child, another common cause of recurrent irritability, is associated with inadequate fluid intake, low-fiber diet, dietary changes, and toilet training. The passage of large, hard stools can result in anal fissures, which make the situation worse as the child becomes even more reluctant to use the bathroom because of the pain.

Food allergy affects approximately 6% to 8% of infants and young children and approximately 3.5% to 4% of adults.[31] The most common food allergens include cow's milk, eggs, peanuts, wheat, and shellfish. Milk protein allergy is usually seen in the first few months of life, and children are irritable and have blood-streaked stools, although they are otherwise healthy. Treatment involves switching to hypoallergenic formulas derived from cow's milk then gradually advancing to an unrestricted diet by 9 to 12 months of age. (See Chapter 265, Gastrointestinal Allergy.)

Night terrors, typically occurring between 2 and 4 years of age during non–rapid eye movement sleep, usually begin with sudden and prolonged periods of inconsolable crying and end spontaneously, with the child rapidly returning to sleep. A nightmare occurs during rapid eye movement sleep, characterized by a frightening dream, which fully awakens the child, and return to sleep is delayed. Vivid recollection of the dream occurs that is appropriate to the child's developmental and maturational stage.

Neurologic disorders, such as brain tumors, migraine headaches, seizures, and postconcussion syndrome, are causes of chronic or recurrent irritability among older children and adolescents. Postconcussion syndrome is particularly distressing to families because the head injury may have occurred months or years before and may even have seemed minor, yet the irritability and behavior changes may be a persistent and major complaint.[32,33]

CHRONIC PERSISTENT IRRITABILITY

Psychosocial Disorders

Attention-deficit/hyperactivity disorder is the most commonly diagnosed biological-behavioral disorder of childhood, occurring in approximately 6% to 9% of school-aged children.[34] The children may have coexisting externalizing disorders (conduct disorder and oppositional defiant disorder) and internalizing disorders (depression and anxiety disorders). A common presentation in infants and young children may be irritability from frustration as a result of family and peer relationships, propensity to accidental injury, and difficulty with academic work.

Autistic disorder usually occurs in children younger than 3 years. Early symptoms include irritability, deficits in verbal and social interaction, repetitive behaviors, failure to participate within groups, and hours spent in solitary play.

Children with a chronic condition face stressors beyond their illness itself, such as altered physical development and appearance, high absenteeism, and inability of their peer groups to accept their disease.[35] The investigation and treatment of irritability in this context may require a multidisciplinary and long-term approach.

Children With Cognitive Impairments

Children with severe cognitive impairments are unable to verbalize what they are experiencing. Although their caregivers are usually adept at reading their child's body language and behaviors to know when the child is in pain, the parent is frequently unable to identify the specific cause. The children are likely to experience pain from the same sources as unimpaired children (teething, sore throat, headache, minor trauma) but are also at risk for additional sources of pain and discomfort. Constipation, muscle spasms, and irritation from feeding tubes are frequent causes of irritabilty.[36] In children with spastic quadriplegia, pathologic fractures are a common finding, related to limb rigidity, joint contractures, bone demineralization, and anticonvulsants.[37] Children with cognitive impairments often receive multiple drugs for seizures, respiratory conditions, and constipation, with a high incidence of behavioral side effects (irritability, aggression, and hyperactivity).[38]

A wide variety of chronic disorders have irritability as a prominent or sole component. Hormonal effects associated with adolescence in both boys and girls can cause moodiness and irritability.[39,40]

SUMMARY

Irritability has a variety of causes and can be indicative of life-threatening or relatively trivial or transient disorders, which is why it elicits a high degree of concern. In an ill-appearing infant or child the initial task is stabilization followed by a thorough search for a cause. In a well-appearing infant or child an organized approach is needed to determine the source of the irritability. A complete history and thorough physical examination can most often determine the cause. In puzzling cases, serial examinations and staged laboratory investigations may be necessary.

TOOLS FOR PRACTICE

Engaging Patient and Family

- *Prevent Shaken Baby Syndrome* (brochure), American Academy of Pediatrics (patiented.aap.org).

AAP POLICY STATEMENTS

American Academy of Pediatrics, Committee on Child Abuse and Neglect. Shaken baby syndrome: rotational cranial injuries—technical report. *Pediatrics.* 2001;108(1):206-210. (aappolicy.aappublications.org/cgi/content/full/pediatrics;108/1/206).

American Academy of Pediatrics, Committee on Quality Improvement. Clinical practice guideline: the management of minor closed head injury in children. *Pediatrics.* 1999; 104(6):1407-1415. (aappolicy.aappublications.org/cgi/content/full/pediatrics;104/9/1407).

REFERENCES

1. Greenes DS, Schutzman SA. Clinical indicators of intracranial injury in head injured infants. *Pediatrics.* 1999; 104:861-867.
2. Gruskin KD, Schutzman SA. Head trauma in children younger than 2 years. Are there predictors for complications? *Arch Ped Adolesc Med.* 1999;153:15-20.
3. American Academy of Pediatrics. The management of minor closed head injury in children. *Pediatrics.* 1999; 104:1407-1415.

4. Schutzman SA, Barnes P, Duhaime AC, et al. Evaluation and management of children younger than two years old with apparently minor head trauma: proposed guidelines. *Pediatrics.* 2001;107:983-993.
5. Cantu RC. Second impact syndrome *Clin Sports Med.* 1998;17:37-44.
6. McCrory P, Johnston K, Meeuwisse W, et al. Summary and agreement statement of the Second International Conference on Concussion in Sports, Prague, 2004. *Physician and Sports Med.* 2005;33:29-40.
7. Zuckerman B, Stevenson J, Bailey V. Stomachaches and headaches in a community sample of preschool children. *Pediatrics.* 1987;79:667-682.
8. Riggio S. Nonconvulsive status epilepticus: clinical features and diagnostic challenges. *Psychiatr Clin North Am.* 2005;28(3):653-664.
9. Newburger JW, Takahashi M, Gerber MA, et al. Diagnosis, treatment, and long-term management of Kawasaki disease: a statement for health professionals from the Committee on Rheumatic Fever, Endocarditis, and Kawasaki Disease, Council on Cardiovascular Disease in the Young, American Heart Association. *Pediatrics.* 2004; 114(6):1708-1733.
10. American Academy of Pediatrics, Committee on Child Abuse and Neglect. Shaken baby syndrome: rotational cranial injuries—technical report. *Pediatrics.* 2001;108(1): 206-210.
11. Blumenthal I. Shaken baby syndrome. *Postgrad Med J.* 2002;78(926):732-735.
12. Starling SP, Holden JR, Jenny C. Abusive head trauma: the relationship of perpetrators to their victims. *Pediatrics.* 1995;95(2):259-262.
13. Sharieff GQ, McCollough M. Abdominal pain in children. *Pediatr Clin North Am.* 2006;53(1):107-137.
14. Kliegman R, Walsh M. Neonatal necrotizing enterocolitis. Pathogenesis, classification, and spectrum of illness. *Curr Prob Pediatr.* 1987;27:215-288.
15. Levi D, Alejos J. Diagnosis and treatment of pediatric viral myocarditis. *Curr Opin Cardiol.* 2001;16:77-83.
16. Hia CPP, Yip WCL, Tai BC, et al. Immunosuppressive therapy in acute myocarditis: an 18 year systematic review. *Arch Dis Child.* 2004;89(6):580-584.
17. Mahle WT. A dangerous case of colic: anomalous left coronary artery presenting with paroxysms of irritability. *Pediatr Emerg Care.* 1998;24(1):24-27.
18. Claudius I, Fluharty C, Boles R. The emergency department approach to newborn and childhood metabolic crisis. *Emerg Med Clin North Am.* 2005;23(3): 843-883.
19. Losek JD. Hypoglycemia and the ABCs (sugar) of pediatric resuscitation. *Ann Emerg Med.* 2000;35(1):43-46.
20. Florentine MJ, Sanfilippo DJ: Elemental mercury poisoning (clinical conference). *Clin Pharmacol.* 1991;10: 213-221.
21. Mott SH, Packer RJ, Soldin SJ. Neurologic manifestations of cocaine exposure in childhood. *Pediatrics.* 1994; 93:557-560.
22. Schwartz RH, Einhorn A. PCP intoxication in seven young children. *Pediatr Emerg Care.* 1986; 2:238-241.
23. Levy M, Spino M. Neonatal withdrawal syndrome: associated drugs and pharmacologic management. *Pharmacotherapy.* 1993;3:202-211.
24. Chasnoff IJ, Lewis DE, Squires L. Cocaine intoxication in a breast-fed infant. *Pediatrics.* 1987; 80:836-838.
25. Woolf AD, Wynshaw-Boris A, Rinaldo P, et al. Intentional infantile ethylene glycol poisoning presenting as an inherited metabolic disorder. *J Pediatr.* 1992;120: 421-424.
26. Wake M, Hesketh K, Lucas J. Teething and tooth eruption in infants: a cohort study. *Pediatrics.* 2000;106: 1374-1379.
27. Cody CL, Baraff LJ, Cherry JD, et al. Nature and rates of adverse reactions associated with DTP and DT immunizations in infants and children. *Pediatrics.* 1981;68(5): 650-660.
28. Keefe MR, Froese-Fretz A. Living with an irritable infant: maternal perspectives. *Am J Child Nurs.* 1991;16:255-259.
29. Currie ML. The pediatrician's role in recognizing and intervening in postpartum depression. *Pediatr Clin North Am.* 2004;51(3):785-801.
30. Hiscock H, Jordan B. Problem crying in infancy. *Med J Aust.* 2004;181(9):507-512.
31. Sampson HA. Food allergy. *J Allergy Clin Immunol.* 2003; 111:540-547.
32. Evans RW. The postconcussion syndrome and the sequelae of mild head injury. *Neurol Clin.* 1992;10:815-847.
33. Goldstein J. Posttraumatic headache and the postconcussion syndrome. *Med Clin North Am.* 1991;75:641-651.
34. Green M, Wong M, Atkins D. *Diagnosis of attention deficit/hyperactivity disorder. Technical Review 3.* AHCPR publication 99–0050. Rockville, MD: US Department of Health and Human Services. Agency for Health Care Policy and Research; 1999.
35. Goldson E. The behavioral aspects of chronic illness. In: Greydanus DE, Wolraich ML, eds. *Behavioral Pediatrics.* New York, NY: Springer-Verlag; 1992.
36. Breau LM, Camfield CS, McGrath PJ, et al. The incidence of pain in children with severe cognitive impairments. *Arch Pediatr Adolesc Med.* 2003;157(12):1219-1226.
37. Bischof F, Basu D, Pettifor JM. Pathological long-bone fractures in residents with cerebral palsy in a long-term care facility in South Africa. *Dev Med Child Neurol.* 2002; 44:119-122.
38. Harbord MG. Significant anticonvulsant side-effects in children and adolescents. *J Clin Neurosci.* 2000;7(3): 213-216.
39. Buchanan CM, Eccles JS, Becker JB. Are adolescents the victims of raging hormones: evidence for activational effects of hormones on moods and behavior at adolescence. *Psychol Bull.* 1992;111:62-107.
40. Mortola JF. Issues in the diagnosis and research of premenstrual syndrome. *Clin Obstet Gynecol.* 1992;35:587-598.

Chapter 197

JAUNDICE

Debra H. Pan, MD; Yolanda Rivas, MD

Jaundice, a yellowish discoloration of the skin, sclerae, and mucous membranes, results from an increase in the serum concentration of bilirubin. Finding jaundice at clinical examination reliably indicates the presence of *hyperbilirubinemia,* which is defined as a total serum bilirubin greater than 1.5 mg/dL.[1] In general, jaundice becomes evident at serum bilirubin concentrations greater than 3 mg/dL in older children and greater than 5 mg/dL in newborns.[2]

Hyperbilirubinemia is typically characterized by the fraction of the bilirubin that is increased, unconjugated (indirect), or conjugated (direct). The normal conjugated fraction accounts for less than 5% of the total serum bilirubin. Conjugated hyperbilirubinemia refers to a direct bilirubin greater than 2 mg/dL or greater than 20% of the total bilirubin concentration. Conjugated hyperbilirubinemia should always be considered an important finding because it suggests liver or biliary tract dysfunction.

BILIRUBIN METABOLISM

To appreciate the many causes of jaundice, the primary care physician must understand the normal metabolism of bilirubin, which is the end product of heme degradation.[1,3] Heme is produced from the breakdown of hemoglobin (70% to 80%) and other hemoproteins (20% to 30%). The conversion from heme to bilirubin follows a 2-step process that occurs mainly in the reticuloendothelial cells of the spleen, liver, and bone marrow. Heme is converted to biliverdin by the microsomal enzyme heme oxygenase and then to bilirubin by the cytosolic enzyme biliverdin reductase. This unconjugated bilirubin is a hydrophobic compound that is tightly bound to serum albumin and is transported to the liver for conjugation and clearance.

In the liver, the metabolism of bilirubin follows 4 distinct steps: (1) The bilirubin is taken up across the sinusoidal (basolateral) membrane of the hepatocyte by a membrane receptor carrier.[4] (2) Once inside the hepatocyte, bilirubin binds to ligandin, an intracellular binding protein. It is then conjugated with glucuronic acid in the endoplasmic reticulum by the enzyme bilirubin uridine diphosphate-glucuronosyl transferase (BUGT) to form bilirubin mono- and diglucuronides.[5] The specific isoform *UGT1A1* is responsible for bilirubin conjugation, and different mutations in the gene for this enzyme have been found in diseases such as Gilbert syndrome and Crigler-Najjar syndrome.[6] (3) Water-soluble bilirubin glucuronides are excreted into the bile through the apical canalicular membrane. This process is mediated by an adenosine triphosphate–dependent export pump. Genetic mutations in the gene for this pump are found in cystic fibrosis and in Dubin-Johnson and Rotor syndromes.[7] Almost all the bilirubin in adult human bile is of the conjugated form, with bilirubin monoglucuronides accounting for 15% and diglucuronides accounting for 85% of the total conjugated bilirubin. In contrast, neonates have a higher concentration of bilirubin monoglucuronides in their bile because of a lower BUGT enzyme activity. The monoglucuronides are easily deconjugated and reabsorbed in the intestine. (4) The excreted bilirubin is further metabolized by intestinal bacteria to form urobilinoids, which are then eliminated in the feces, thus preventing the intestinal reabsorption of bilirubin.[8] Bilirubin glucuronides can also be deconjugated by bacterial or tissue β-glucuronidase in the intestine and then reabsorbed in the terminal ileum, a process known as *enterohepatic circulation*.[9] Newborns are more likely to absorb bilirubin from the intestine because they lack the intestinal bacterial flora to form nonabsorbable urobilinoids. Therefore conditions that delay the passage of meconium, which contains large amounts of bilirubin and β-glucuronidase, can result in neonatal hyperbilirubinemia. In addition, human milk contains high levels of β-glucuronidase, which may be a contributing factor in the development of breast milk jaundice.[10]

SERUM BILIRUBIN

Serum bilirubin is conventionally measured by spectrophotometry based on the Van den Bergh (diazo) reaction.[11] Conjugated (direct) bilirubin reacts rapidly and unconjugated (indirect) bilirubin reacts slowly with diazo reagents. Indirect bilirubin is calculated as the difference between the total bilirubin and the direct bilirubin fraction. Although the terms *direct* and *conjugated* bilirubin are used interchangeably, direct bilirubin actually consists of 2 components: (1) conjugated bilirubin and (2) δ-bilirubin. In hepatobiliary obstruction, bilirubin glucuronides are not excreted properly from the hepatocyte into the bile. Under these conditions, bilirubin glucuronides can reflux back into the systemic circulation and covalently bind to albumin. This conjugated bilirubin-albumin compound is known as δ-bilirubin,[12,13] which is not usually measured as a separate fraction. However, methods such as high-pressure liquid chromatography can measure δ-bilirubin as well as α-, β-, and γ-bilirubin, which correspond to the unconjugated, monoconjugated, and diconjugated forms, respectively.[14] δ-Bilirubin is clinically important because it is not excreted in bile or urine until albumin is degraded, which accounts for the prolonged direct hyperbilirubinemia occasionally observed after restoration of normal bile flow.

DIFFERENTIAL DIAGNOSIS

For practical purposes, the differential diagnosis of jaundice is categorized as either unconjugated or conjugated hyperbilirubinemia in 2 age groups: (1) newborns and young infants and (2) older infants and children. In general, unconjugated hyperbilirubinemia is common in neonates but relatively rare thereafter. It is typically transient and benign, but marked increases of bilirubin can be toxic to the central nervous system. On the other hand, conjugated hyperbilirubinemia is always pathological. When present in young infants, it is often related to primary hepatobiliary disorders, systemic or metabolic diseases, or genetic defects in bilirubin or bile acid metabolism or transport. Viral hepatitis and drug- or toxin-induced liver damage are more prevalent in older children.

JAUNDICE IN NEWBORNS AND YOUNG INFANTS

A brief list of the causes of jaundice in newborns and young infants is presented in Box 197-1.

UNCONJUGATED HYPERBILIRUBINEMIA

The transition from intrauterine to extrauterine life is commonly associated with hyperbilirubinemia. All newborns have a total bilirubin level greater than the adult's normal limit of 1.5 mg/dL. More than one half of newborns will develop clinical jaundice in the first week of life; most have unconjugated hyperbilirubinemia.[15] Neonatal jaundice is fully discussed in Chapter 98, Neonatal Jaundice.

Increased Production of Bilirubin

Nonphysiological jaundice should always be considered as part of the differential diagnosis of neonatal

BOX 197-1 Differential Diagnosis of Jaundice in Newborn and Young Infants

UNCONJUGATED HYPERBILIRUBINEMIA

Increased production of bilirubin

- Hemolysis (ABO-Rh incompatibility, erythrocyte defects, erythrocyte enzyme defects, disseminated intravascular coagulopathy)
- Polycythemia
- Cephalohematoma resorption

Decreased hepatocellular uptake or conjugation

- Prematurity
- Congenital hypothyroidism
- Physiological jaundice of the newborn
- Breast milk jaundice
- Drugs
- Gilbert and Crigler-Najjar syndromes

CONJUGATED HYPERBILIRUBINEMIA

Liver diseases

- Acute liver damage (ischemia, hypoxia, acidosis)
- Infection (sepsis, TORCH [toxoplasmosis, other agents, rubella, cytomegalovirus, herpes simplex])
- Viral or other hepatitis
- Total parenteral nutrition–related liver disease
- Metabolic liver disease (galactosemia, neonatal hemochromatosis, α1-antitrypsin deficiency, tyrosinemia, mitochondrial defects)
- Hormones and drugs

Obstruction of biliary system

- Congenital anomalies (biliary atresia, choledochal cyst)

Defects of bilirubin metabolism or transport

- Progressive familial intrahepatic cholestasis
- Dubin-Johnson syndrome, Rotor syndrome

jaundice. Jaundice with early onset, rapid progression, persistence beyond 2 weeks of life, and association with other signs or symptoms suggests a pathological cause. In most instances, pathological unconjugated hyperbilirubinemia results from either excessive production of bilirubin or abnormal hepatic clearance of bilirubin.

Hemolysis, the most common cause of excessive bilirubin production in neonates, is usually observed within the first 24 hours of life and rapidly progresses. Treatment often requires intensive phototherapy and exchange transfusion to prevent bilirubin encephalopathy.

Hemolysis is often seen in association with maternal-fetal blood type incompatibility. ABO and Rh incompatibility are the 2 most common types of maternal-fetal blood type incompatibility leading to hemolytic disease of the newborn. ABO incompatibility occurs in approximately 15% of all pregnancies but results in hemolytic disease in only 3% of newborns, with less than 0.1% of infants needing exchange transfusion.[27] Hemolysis caused by ABO incompatibility is usually seen in newborns with blood type A or B born to blood type O mothers. Laboratory findings include a weakly positive direct Coombs test, high reticulocyte count, spherocytes on blood smear, and high levels of unconjugated bilirubin. Hemolytic disease in Rh incompatibility usually develops when an Rh-negative mother has become sensitized after exposure to Rh-positive fetal blood during a previous pregnancy. Rh incompatibility is less common and usually more severe than ABO incompatibility.[28] In the United States, the prevalence of the Rh negative genotype is approximately 15% in whites, 5% in blacks, and less than 1% in Asians.[29] Rh incompatibility occurs in approximately 1.06 per 1000 live births.[30] Affected infants usually experience onset of jaundice in the first hours of life, and they also have anemia and hepatosplenomegaly. In severe cases, the neonate may be born with fetal hydrops from intrauterine hemolysis. Laboratory findings include a positive direct Coombs test, high reticulocyte count, anemia, and high serum unconjugated bilirubin levels. The prophylactic use of RhoGAM (anti-D γ-globulin) in Rh-negative mothers has greatly decreased the incidence of hemolytic disease of the newborn to less than 0.11% of Rh-negative pregnancies.[31,32]

Other causes of hemolysis leading to unconjugated hyperbilirubinemia in the neonate include hemoglobinopathies such as α-thalassemia, red blood cell enzyme defects, and neonatal polycythemia. α-Thalassemia should be suspected in newborns with jaundice and a moderate hypochromic, microcytic, hemolytic anemia.[33] Erythrocyte enzyme defects such as glucose-6-phosphate dehydrogenase (G6PD) or pyruvate kinase deficiency may cause hemolysis at any age.[33,34] G6PD deficiency is often benign in the newborn period; however, clinically important hemolysis and jaundice may develop in the presence of oxidant stressors such as infections. Neonatal polycythemia can cause an increase in bilirubin production as a result of an absolute increase in red blood cell mass. Polycythemia occurs in 1% to 5% of newborns, with unconjugated hyperbilirubinemia developing in 2% to 22% of affected babies.[35-37] Cephalohematomas can lead to an increased bilirubin production from rapid breakdown of red blood cells in the extravascular space.

Decreased Hepatocellular Uptake or Conjugation of Bilirubin

Drugs such as aspirin, cephalosporins, and sulfonamides can impair bilirubin transport by altering bilirubin-albumin binding.[38] Rifampin has been demonstrated to inhibit competitively hepatocellular uptake of bilirubin.[39] In several clinical conditions, such as physiological jaundice of the newborn, breast milk jaundice, and hypothyroidism, unconjugated hyperbilirubinemia is associated with impaired conjugation of bilirubin attributable to decreased activity of BUGT.[16] Unlike breastfeeding jaundice, breast milk jaundice usually occurs in a thriving breastfed newborn during the second and third weeks of life. The mechanism of breast milk jaundice is thought to be related, in part, to inhibition of BUGT activity by compounds found in human milk.[20] Unconjugated hyperbilirubinemia is seen in newborns with congenital hypothyroidism, presumably because of delayed maturation of BUGT.[40]

Gilbert and Crigler-Najjar syndromes are 2 types of familial unconjugated hyperbilirubinemia caused by several mutations in the gene encoding for BUGT.[6,41-43] *Gilbert syndrome* is a common inherited condition characterized by mild unconjugated hyperbilirubinemia. An insertional mutation of the *UGT1A1* gene results in a reduced level of expression of the gene. Gilbert syndrome is usually diagnosed during or after adolescence. *Crigler-Najjar syndrome* is a rare familial form of unconjugated hyperbilirubinemia caused by mutations in the gene encoding BUGT1, leading to either absent (type 1) or decreased (type 2) BUGT activity. Crigler-Najjar syndrome type 1 is an autosomal-recessive disease and exhibits in the first hours of life with severe nonhemolytic jaundice. Crigler-Najjar syndrome type 2 is an autosomal-dominant disease. Jaundice is usually less severe in this syndrome and may improve with phenobarbital treatment, which promotes bile flow.

Conjugated Hyperbilirubinemia

Regardless of the cause, conjugated hyperbilirubinemia, also known as *cholestatic jaundice,* is usually associated with liver dysfunction, and it is always pathological.[44] It can occur as a result of impaired bile formation by the hepatocyte or from obstruction to the flow of bile through the intrahepatic or extrahepatic biliary tree from primary hepatobiliary disorders, genetic or metabolic diseases, systemic infections, and drug toxicity.[45]

Neonatal hepatitis is a vague term that has been used to refer to infants younger than 3 months who have cholestatic jaundice with nonspecific histologic features of hepatic inflammation and no defined cause. With the advancement of the knowledge of the causes of neonatal cholestasis, and with the availability of many new advanced diagnostic techniques, the number of patients categorized as having neonatal hepatitis has been decreasing.

Systemic Illnesses

Congenital TORCH (toxoplasmosis, other agents, rubella, cytomegalovirus, herpes simplex) infections have been associated with conjugated hyperbilirubinemia.[46-48] Infants with TORCH infections often have a low birth weight, hepatosplenomegaly, and cutaneous manifestations, as well as ophthalmologic and central nervous system involvement. Common laboratory findings include anemia, thrombocytopenia, increased transaminases, and cholestasis. The diagnosis is often made by virus culture, serologic titers, imaging studies, and ophthalmologic examination. Other infections, such as HIV and hepatitis B and C, may also be associated with direct hyperbilirubinemia in newborns or young infants. However, these infections have decreased with improved prenatal screening.

Patients with sepsis may have jaundice and hepatocellular dysfunction.[49] The most frequent bacterial organisms associated with conjugated hyperbilirubinemia in neonatal sepsis are *Escherichia coli, Streptococcus* group B, and *Listeria monocytogenes.* Conjugated hyperbilirubinemia may also develop in newborns and young infants with urinary tract infections.[50]

Jaundice with other signs of hepatic dysfunction, such as hepatomegaly or increased transaminases, may develop as a result of hypoxia, sepsis, and parenteral nutrition.[51] Such jaundice is often encountered in critically ill patients, including young infants with no previous underlying liver disease. Conditions that alter the systemic circulation, such as cardiopulmonary arrest, shock, and severe metabolic acidosis, may lead to an acute ischemic insult to the liver and necrosis of hepatocytes. Affected patients will have a marked and rapid increase in serum transaminase levels and direct hyperbilirubinemia developing within 24 to 48 hours after the insult. In most cases, the liver function will normalize once the initial insult is corrected, but a small number of patients may develop acute liver failure.

Liver disease related to parenteral nutrition (PN) is common in young infants. Cholestatic jaundice is a major complication that occurs in 30% to 50% of infants and 80% of preterm babies who receive PN for more than 2 weeks.[52,53] The cause of this condition is still poorly defined, although it is considered to be multifactorial. Factors thought to contribute to PN-related liver disease include lack of enteral feeds, immaturity of the hepatobiliary system, infused nutrient composition, and sepsis. In most infants, the liver function abnormalities usually resolve within 4 to 6 months after discontinuation of PN. In severe cases, progression to end-stage liver disease may occur.

Metabolic Disorders

Metabolic liver diseases usually occur during early infancy and should always be considered in a newborn or young infant with cholestasis, especially when the child also has hypoglycemia, hyperammonemia, or lactic acidosis.[54-56]

Galactosemia is an inborn error of galactose metabolism inherited as an autosomal-recessive trait, with an estimated occurrence of 1 per 60,000. The classic transferase-deficiency galactosemia can affect many organs, including the liver, kidneys, brain, eyes, intestines, and gonads. The hepatocellular damage in galactosemia is caused by accumulation of toxic metabolites of galactose-1-phosphate and galactitol in the liver. The clinical presentation of this condition varies from mild liver disease to fulminant liver failure in the neonatal period. Jaundice and hepatomegaly can develop in association with other symptoms, such as vomiting, diarrhea, poor feeding, or *E coli* sepsis.[57] Other inborn errors of carbohydrate metabolism, such as hereditary fructose intolerance and certain types of glycogen storage diseases, can also have jaundice as part of their clinical picture. In these conditions, the onset of symptoms rarely occurs during early infancy.

Neonatal hemochromatosis is a rare idiopathic syndrome characterized by liver disease of prenatal onset and excess iron deposition in extrahepatic sites.[58,59] Infants with neonatal hemochromatosis are usually born early and have experienced intrauterine growth retardation. In most cases, signs and symptoms of acute liver failure are present at birth or develop soon thereafter. The clinical presentation includes hypoglycemia, hypoalbuminemia, profound coagulopathy, and cholestatic jaundice. Liver transaminases can be slightly increased or even normal. The diagnosis should be considered in every case of neonatal liver failure. Typical laboratory findings include increased ferritin and transferrin saturation and relatively low transferrin levels. The diagnosis of neonatal hemochromatosis is made by punch biopsy of the lower lip mucosa; the biopsy sample is analyzed for iron deposition in the salivary glands.

α1-Antitrypsin deficiency is a relatively common genetic disorder, with the homozygous *PiZZ* genotype found in 1 in 1600 to 2000 live births. Only 10% of patients with α1-antitrypsin deficiency will develop signs and symptoms of liver disease.[60,61] This condition is the most common genetic cause of neonatal liver disease.[62] It typically manifests in the first few months of life with jaundice, although the onset of the liver disease can also occur later in life. Injury to the liver is thought to be the result of the hepatotoxic effect of retained mutant *α1 ATZZ* molecule in the endoplasmic reticulum of the hepatocyte.

Tyrosinemia type 1, also known as *hepatorenal tyrosinemia,* is a rare disorder that can affect the liver, kidneys, and peripheral nerves.[63] The deficiency of fumarylacetoacetate hydrolase, an enzyme involved in tyrosine degradation, results in tissue accumulation of tyrosine and other intermediate metabolites. Clinical findings range from severe liver disease or acute liver failure in early infancy to chronic liver disease in older children. Tyrosinemia should be suspected in patients who exhibit signs and symptoms of liver disease, especially when associated with acute neurologic symptoms such as excruciating pain, weakness, and paralysis.[64] The striking laboratory finding is a markedly increased alfa-fetoprotein level. The presence of succinylacetone in urine or blood is pathognomonic for tyrosinemia. Early diagnosis is important because specific medical therapy will improve quality of life and delay disease progression.

Primary mitochondrial hepatopathies are caused by a variety of defects, including mitochondrial DNA depletion, respiratory chain defects, fatty acid oxidation defects, and mitochondrial membrane enzyme defects.[65-68] In addition to having signs and symptoms of liver disease, affected patients commonly have neuromuscular problems and may have marked lactic acidosis. Symptoms usually develop within the first few months of life.

Obstructive Jaundice

Extrahepatic biliary atresia (EHBA) is an idiopathic, destructive, inflammatory process of both the intra- and extrahepatic bile ducts.[69-72] It is one of the few causes of neonatal cholestasis that can be treated with surgery. Affected infants typically exhibit symptoms of cholestatic jaundice and acholic stools when they are approximately 2 to 4 weeks of age; however, in the early stages, the stool may still have some bile pigment. Infants with cholestatic jaundice need prompt referral and evaluation for EHBA because the prognosis can be improved by early diagnosis and timely surgery. Abdominal sonography is a useful screening tool. It can exclude other causes of cholestasis, such as choledochal cysts, gallstones, or biliary sludge. The absence of the gallbladder or the appearance of the *triangular cord* sign at the hilar region is suggestive of EHBA. However, the presence of a gallbladder on sonography does not exclude this condition because a few patients with EHBA have a gallbladder. A percutaneous liver biopsy is an essential procedure in evaluating patients with suspected EHBA. The main histopathological features observed are bile duct proliferation and fibrosis. When the suspicion of EHBA has been established, an exploratory laparotomy with intraoperative cholangiogram should be performed to confirm the diagnosis. Patients then undergo a hepatoportoenterostomy, or Kasai procedure. The highest success rate of reestablishing bile flow after surgery is seen when the procedure is performed before the child is 8 weeks of age.

Choledochal cysts are rare congenital anomalies of the biliary tract characterized by varying degrees of cystic dilation of the intra- or extrahepatic biliary tree. Choledochal cysts may be detected at any age; 18% of cases are diagnosed during the first year of life.[73-75] The classic presentation of jaundice, abdominal pain, and right epigastric mass is often not observed in infants and young children.

Alagille syndrome, also known as *arteriohepatic dysplasia,* is inherited as an autosomal-dominant condition with variable penetrance. It is characterized by paucity of the intrahepatic bile ducts, peripheral pulmonary stenosis, butterfly vertebrae, posterior embryotoxon, and peculiar faces.[76] Jaundice and pruritus are often present as the main clinical features during infancy.

Isolated Bile Acid Metabolism Defects

Progressive familial intrahepatic cholestasis has been identified as a distinct group of conditions involving intrahepatic cholestasis from bile acid transport defects leading to impairment of bile excretion.[77-79] Affected patients often develop jaundice in the first few months of life. In addition, they may also have severe pruritus, growth failure, fat-soluble vitamin deficiency, abnormal coagulation profile, and increased serum bile acids. The disease usually progresses to cirrhosis and liver failure early in life.

JAUNDICE IN OLDER INFANTS AND CHILDREN

A brief list of the differential diagnosis of jaundice in older infants and children is presented in Box 197-2. In this age group, jaundice is an unusual sign and may suggest a serious clinical condition.

Unconjugated Hyperbilirubinemia

In general, unconjugated hyperbilirubinemia is rarely seen in older infants and children. When present, it is usually associated with underlying hemolytic diseases such as sickle cell anemia, G6PD deficiency, or hereditary spherocytosis. Unconjugated hyperbilirubinemia may also result from nonhemolytic conditions such as Gilbert syndrome, a benign disorder that affects 7% of the general population. It is inherited as an autosomal-dominant trait, although an autosomal-recessive pattern has also been described.[43] Jaundice does not typically develop until after puberty and is usually intermittent and more evident with fasting. Patients usually have mild indirect hyperbilirubinemia with otherwise normal liver function tests and no evidence of ongoing hemolysis.

BOX 197-2 Differential Diagnosis of Jaundice in Older Infants and Children

UNCONJUGATED HYPERBILIRUBINEMIA

- Hemolysis: erythrocyte defects, erythrocyte enzyme defect (glucose-6-phosphate dehydrogenase), disseminated intravascular coagulopathy
- Gilbert syndrome

CONJUGATED HYPERBILIRUBINEMIA

Liver disease

- Viral hepatitis (hepatitis A, B, C, E)
- Hepatitis caused by other viruses (herpes simplex virus, Epstein-Barr virus, cytomegalovirus)
- Toxins and drugs (ethanol, acetaminophen, isoniazid, phenytoin)
- Autoimmune hepatitis
- Metabolic liver disease (α1-antitrypsin deficiency, tyrosinemia, Wilson disease, mitochondrial defects)
- Nonalcoholic fatty liver disease
- Acute liver damage: ischemia, hypoxia, acidosis
- Total parenteral nutrition related
- Pregnancy related (acute fatty liver of pregnancy, preeclampsia)
- Malignancy

Obstruction of the biliary system

- Choledochocyst
- Cholelithiasis or choledocholithiasis
- Cholecystitis
- Diseases of the bile ducts (primary sclerosing cholangitis, AIDS cholangiopathy)

Bilirubin metabolism or transport defects

- Progressive familial intrahepatic cholestasis
- Dubin-Johnson syndrome, Rotor syndrome

Conjugated Hyperbilirubinemia

Liver Disease

Compared with newborns and young infants, older children are more likely to have jaundice associated with acute or chronic viral hepatitis, autoimmune hepatitis, and drug- or toxin-induced hepatic injury. Infiltrative malignancies may occur rarely, and they can cause jaundice at any age. Acute viral hepatitis is the most common cause of jaundice in older children.[80-82] In older children and adolescents, jaundice is a common manifestation of acute viral hepatitis A infection; however, children younger than 5 years with acute hepatitis A infection tend to be anicteric. The disease rarely causes fulminant liver failure. Hepatitis E infection, which has a clinical course similar to that of hepatitis A, is endemic to Southeast Asia and India and should be suspected in children with a history of recent travel to these areas. Hepatitis B or C infection is usually anicteric and chronic in children. Other viruses (eg, Epstein-Barr virus, cytomegalovirus, adenovirus, enterovirus) can also cause acute hepatitis.[80,83-85] Jaundice is not an uncommon presenting feature in these cases.

Autoimmune hepatitis (AIH) is a condition of unknown cause that usually progresses to cirrhosis if not promptly diagnosed and treated.[86,87] AIH should always be considered in the differential diagnosis in a child with jaundice associated with increased liver transaminases. Jaundice is present in more than one half of patients with AIH. Hyperglobulinemia and autoantibodies such as antinuclear antibody, anti–smooth muscle antibody, and anti–liver kidney microsomal antibody may be found. When present, anti–liver kidney microsomal antibody categorizes the disease as AIH type 2. AIH type 1 usually has an insidious course, with patients likely to come to attention at an older age, some already with cirrhosis at the time of diagnosis. AIH type 2 may have a more fulminant course, even first exhibiting as acute liver failure.[88]

Drug-induced liver injury is initially suspected based on circumstantial evidence.[89] It can be classified into 3 types—(1) hepatitic, (2) cholestatic, or (3) mixed hepatitic-cholestatic—according to the different clinical features. Cholestasis is more prominent when damage to bile duct epithelial cells occurs, resulting in an impaired bile flow. Cholestatic jaundice can be caused by many different drugs, including estrogen or oral contraceptive pills, erythromycin, cyclosporine, and haloperidol.[90-93] Acetaminophen overdose can cause acute hepatitis with zonal hepatocyte necrosis. Jaundice develops when hepatocellular damage is sufficiently severe. Most cases of drug-induced liver damage spontaneously resolve once the drug responsible for the injury is withdrawn.

Wilson disease is an autosomal-recessive disorder of human copper metabolism[94,95] usually found in children older than 5 years. Mutations in the *ATP7B* gene lead to impaired biliary excretion of copper, which results in a progressive accumulation of copper in the liver and subsequently in other organs and tissues. Hemolytic anemia, Kayser-Fleischer rings in the eyes, and neuropsychiatric symptoms are well-reported manifestations of the disease. Copper deposition in the liver can result in acute or chronic hepatitis, cirrhosis, or fulminant liver failure. Markedly increased bilirubin is typically found in patients with Wilson disease who have fulminant liver failure.

Biliary Obstruction

Cholelithiasis, the most common cause of biliary obstruction in children, is often found in patients with an underlying hemolytic disease. Isolated gallstone disease can occur, particularly in infants. In these patients, jaundice is the most common presentation. In contrast, older children usually experience vomiting and right upper quadrant pain, with or without jaundice.[96] Primary sclerosing cholangitis is characterized by stenosis, dilatation, and fibrosis involving the intrahepatic or extrahepatic biliary tree or both. It is the most common form of chronic liver disease in children with inflammatory bowel disease. Its clinical presentation is highly variable, with cholestatic jaundice developing in less than one half of affected patients.[97,98]

Hepatic Bilirubin Transport Defects

Gilbert syndrome and Crigler-Najjar syndrome have already been discussed. Dubin-Johnson syndrome is a recessively inherited disorder caused by mutations in the gene encoding for the canalicular transporter for conjugated bilirubin, which results in an impaired secretion of conjugated bilirubin.[7,99,100] Chronic jaundice is the main clinical manifestation of Dubin-Johnson syndrome. It can be precipitated by pregnancy or the use of oral contraceptives.[101] Rotor syndrome, clinically similar to Dubin-Johnson syndrome but involving an impairment of liver storage capacity rather than a defect in bilirubin secretion, is also inherited as an autosomal-recessive disorder. In both syndromes, conjugated hyperbilirubinemia is noted without abnormalities in other liver function tests. Serum bile acids are also normal. The striking characteristic in Dubin-Johnson syndrome is a brown to black discoloration of the liver, the result of pigment deposition in the lysosomes. The liver histologic findings are otherwise normal in both syndromes.

EVALUATION

History

A detailed history is essential when evaluating a patient with jaundice because the information obtained may help the clinician identify its possible cause. Special attention should be paid to the presence of signs and symptoms of fever, viral prodrome, abdominal pain or distension, acholic stools, dark urine, or pruritus. The history in patients with neonatal jaundice should focus on prenatal history, quality of prenatal care, maternal blood test results, and birth history to identify potential risk factors. In older children, focus should be directed to the patient's age at the time of onset of jaundice, associated signs and symptoms before and during the period of jaundice, and exposure to hepatotoxic agents. A detailed family history should include information about the presence of persistent jaundice, chronic liver diseases, hemolysis, or metabolic diseases. Distinguishing among acute and chronic liver diseases, intrahepatic processes and extrahepatic biliary tract obstruction, or primary liver diseases and systemic diseases is the major goal of the initial evaluation. This approach may help in selecting appropriate laboratory tests and imaging studies that can lead to a definitive diagnosis.

Physical Examination

In general, patients with jaundice from unconjugated hyperbilirubinemia have bright yellow-colored skin, whereas patients with jaundice from conjugated hyperbilirubinemia have dark yellow-greenish–colored skin. Patients should undergo a complete physical examination with special focus on general appearance, growth, and development; signs of cardiovascular dysfunction; neurologic signs; and organomegaly. The size and the character of the liver should be carefully determined. The newborn or infant liver is a large organ relative to body size. In newborns, the mean liver span is 5.9 cm along the midclavicular line, calculated by measuring the distance between the percussed upper and palpated lower liver edge.[102] The healthy infant's liver may be palpable and is typically less than 2 cm below the right costal margin.[103] The consistency and character of the liver edge may help determine the nature of underlying liver disease. An enlarged liver resulting from an acute intrahepatic process is usually tender but soft. A cirrhotic liver may have a hard and irregular edge; however, its edge is not always palpable.

A thorough abdominal examination should be performed to identify the presence of an enlarged spleen or any other abdominal masses, areas of tenderness, and ascites, as well as the abdominal cutaneous venous pattern. The tip of the spleen can normally be palpated below the left costal margin in newborns and infants. Splenomegaly in a patient with underlying liver disease implies portal hypertension, especially in the presence of ascites and a prominent abdominal cutaneous venous pattern. Other physical findings may indicate a particular cause, such as xanthomas in primary biliary cirrhosis, Kayser-Fleischer rings in Wilson disease, and characteristic facial features and posterior embryotoxon in Alagille syndrome.

Laboratory Tests

Initial laboratory studies include a complete blood cell count, liver function tests, and a coagulation profile. Isolated hyperbilirubinemia with otherwise normal liver function suggests the possibility of hemolytic disease or bilirubin metabolism defects. A complete blood cell count is useful in detecting hemolysis, indicated by the presence of anemia with fragmented red blood cells (schistocytes) and increased reticulocytes on the smear. Thrombocytopenia is typically seen in patients with portal hypertension and hypersplenism.

Aspartate aminotransferase (AST) and alanine aminotransferase (ALT) levels are the most frequently used markers of hepatocellular injury.[104] Compared with AST, ALT is a more specific indicator of hepatocyte injury because AST may be increased with hemolysis and myocardial or skeletal muscle injury. In general, a marked increase in AST and ALT occurs in severe viral hepatitis, acute toxin- or drug-induced hepatic necrosis, or ischemia.[105] A mild increase of AST and ALT is seen in nonalcoholic fatty liver disease, chronic viral hepatitis, and drug toxicity. Declining AST and ALT levels usually indicate hepatocyte recovery. However, in the course of fulminant liver failure, if seen in association with a worsening liver synthetic function, falling AST and ALT levels may be an ominous sign of massive hepatic necrosis, with few viable hepatocytes remaining to further release these enzymes.[106] AST and ALT levels are less useful in patients with chronic end-stage liver disease because they can be normal or only slightly increased in the presence of marked fibrosis of the liver.

In a patient with jaundice, alkaline phosphatase and γ-glutamyltransferase (GGT) are 2 useful markers for intra- and extrahepatic cholestasis. In most hepatobiliary diseases, both GGT and alkaline phosphatase are increased. However, in progressive familiar intrahepatic cholestasis (types 1 and 2), a normal or low GGT is observed in the presence of a high alkaline phosphatase. Isolated increase of alkaline phosphatase may be seen in patients with nonhepatobiliary diseases such as bone disorders.[107] Normal GGT values in newborns may be 5 to 8 times greater than those in adults.[108]

Prothrombin time (PT) and albumin are used to evaluate hepatic synthetic function. An abnormal PT results from an impaired hepatic synthesis of coagulation factors I, II, V, VII, and X or deficiency of vitamin K (or both). Parenteral administration of vitamin K generally normalizes a prolonged PT in patients with vitamin K deficiency associated with cholestatic jaundice but not in patients with hepatocellular disease. In acute liver disease, a markedly increased PT suggests the possibility of fulminant liver failure. Hypoalbuminemia may be seen in patients with acute and chronic liver diseases. In the early stages of acute liver disease, the serum albumin may not be a reliable indicator of hepatic synthetic function because it has a long half-life of approximately 21 days.

Based on the gathered clinical information and results of the initial tests, further evaluation, including imaging studies, may be warranted. Additional studies may include blood and urine cultures, viral serologic studies, toxin and drug screen, autoimmune markers, α1-antitrypsin phenotype, ceruloplasmin, urine succinyl acetone, and serum bile acids. In jaundiced newborn or young infants with abnormal liver function tests, TORCH titers should also be obtained.

Imaging Studies

Ultrasonography is the most useful initial imaging modality in the assessment of the intra- and extrahepatic biliary system in patients with jaundice.[109] This simple, noninvasive study may provide information that suggests the cause of jaundice (eg, biliary atresia, choledochal cyst, hepatic cystic lesions, cholelithiasis). Computed tomographic scans may be preferred when general anatomic information of the hepatobiliary system is desired or a noncystic hepatic lesion is suspected. Nuclear scintigraphy, useful in differentiating biliary atresia from other causes of neonatal cholestasis,[110] has also been used in older children to help in the diagnosis of acute cholecystitis and chronic acalculous cholecystitis by calculating the gallbladder ejection fraction.[111] Magnetic resonance imaging cholangiopancreatography is a noninvasive study that identifies abnormalities of the intra- and extrahepatic biliary system. An endoscopic retrograde cholangiopancreatography provides information similar to that of the magnetic resonance imaging study; however, it is an invasive procedure and should be reserved for patients who need a possible therapeutic intervention such as biliary stent placement or sphincterotomy.[112]

Liver biopsy provides information on the histology and architecture of the liver and has become an invaluable diagnostic tool in the evaluation of patients with liver disease; it is also helpful in assessing disease prognosis. Percutaneous liver biopsy is most commonly used in patients with persistently abnormal liver function tests, especially when conventional laboratory and imaging studies do not lead to a firm diagnosis. The use of liver biopsy to diagnose acute hepatitis or acute cholestatic jaundice is limited because the histologic changes in these settings may be nonspecific. In fulminant liver failure, a percutaneous liver biopsy is contraindicated because of the high risk of bleeding; when needed, a transjugular liver biopsy under radiographic guidance should be performed.[113]

MANAGEMENT

The treatment of newborns with unconjugated hyperbilirubinemia is based on the revised guideline published by the American Academy of Pediatrics.[22] This guideline provides a framework in detecting neonatal hyperbilirubinemia and preventing kernicterus in term and near-term newborn infants. It also emphasizes the importance of a systematic assessment of the risk of severe hyperbilirubinemia, close follow-up, and prompt intervention when necessary.

The management of patients with direct hyperbilirubinemia should focus on correcting the underlying cause, optimizing nutrition, and controlling pruritus. Malabsorption of fat and fat-soluble vitamins is commonly seen in patients with cholestasis because they have impaired bile acid secretion. Unlike long-chain triglycerides, which require bile acid micelles for solubilization, medium-chain triglycerides (MCT) are relatively water soluble and directly absorbed into the portal system. For this reason, a diet high in MCT should be used to promote growth in children with chronic cholestasis. Infant formulas with a relatively high MCT concentration are frequently used in infants with cholestasis. Supplementation of fat-soluble vitamins A, D, E, and K is essential. Serum vitamin levels should be routinely monitored because patients may still have biochemical evidence of fat-soluble vitamin deficiency despite supplementation.

In the attempt to control cholestasis-associated pruritus, several different therapeutic agents have been used with very little success. Choleretic agents such as ursodeoxycholic acid and phenobarbital increase bile flow, which lowers the serum level of bile acid.[114] These agents have shown some beneficial effect in relieving pruritus. Other agents, such as cholestyramine, a bile acid–binding resin, and rifampin, an antibiotic used to treat tuberculosis, have been shown to reduce pruritus in some patients.[115,116]

Liver transplantation in children is now an accepted therapy for many life-threatening liver diseases.[117] Whole liver, split liver, and living donor transplantations have been successfully used to treat both infants and older children. Current survival rates for children after liver transplantation are 90% at 1 year and 85% at 3 years.[118] EHBA with a failed Kasai procedure is the most common reason children undergo liver transplantation; other indications include α1-antitrypsin deficiency, fulminant liver failure, chronic hepatitis, metabolic liver disease, and cirrhosis of unknown origin. Early referral and transfer to a liver transplant center are important to good outcome.

WHEN TO REFER

- Unexplained jaundice
- Direct hyperbilirubinemia at any age
- Abnormal liver function tests
- Hepatomegaly or splenomegaly

WHEN TO ADMIT

- Jaundice in an ill patient
- Poor feeding tolerance and intravenous hydration

- Need for intravenous antibiotics
- Inpatient management of underlying conditions
- Impending acute liver failure

TOOLS FOR PRACTICE

Engaging Patient and Family

- *Q&A: Jaundice and Your Newborn* (fact sheet), American Academy of Pediatrics (www.aap.org/family/jaundicefaq.htm).
- *Jaundice and Your Newborn* (brochure), American Academy of Pediatrics (patiented.aap.org).

Medical Decision Support

- *BilliTool* (interactive tool), Creative Commons (bilitool.org/).
- *Jaundice/Kernicterus* (Web page), Centers for Disease Control and Prevention (www.cdc.gov/ncbddd/dd/kernichome.htm).
- *Newborn Jaundice: Hot Topic* (on-line course), American Academy of Pediatric (www.pedialink.org).

AAP POLICY STATEMENTS

American Academy of Pediatrics, Subcommittee on Hyperbilirubinemia. Management of hyperbilirubinemia in the newborn infant 35 weeks or more gestation. *Pediatrics.* 2004;114(1):297-316. (aappolicy.aappublications.org/cgi/content/full/pediatrics;114/1/316).

North American Society for Pediatric, Gastroenterology, Hepatology, and Nutrition. Guideline for the evaluation of cholestatic jaundice in infants: recommendations of the North American Society for Pediatric Gastroenterology, Hepatology, and Nutrition. *J Pediatr Gastroenterol Nutr.* 2004;39:115-128. AAP endorsed.

REFERENCES

1. Berk PD. Bilirubin metabolism and the hereditary hyperbilirubinemias. *Semin Liver Dis.* 1994;14:321-322.
2. Reiser DJ. Neonatal jaundice: physiologic variation or pathologic process. *Crit Care Nurs Clin North Am.* 2004;16:257-269.
3. Ostrow JD, Jandl JH, Schmid R. The formation of bilirubin from hemoglobin in vivo. *J Clin Invest.* 1962;41:1628-1637.
4. Scharschmidt BF, Waggoner JG, Berk PD. Hepatic organic anion uptake in the rat. *J Clin Invest.* 1975;56:1280-1292.
5. Dutton G. *The Biosynthesis of Glucuronides.* London, UK: Academic Press; 1966.
6. Mackenzie PI, Owens IS, Burchell B, et al. The UDP glycosyltransferase gene superfamily: recommended nomenclature update based on evolutionary divergence. *Pharmacogenetics.* 1997;7:255-269.
7. Paulusma CC, Kool M, Bosma PJ, et al. A mutation in the human canalicular multispecific organic anion transporter gene causes the Dubin-Johnson syndrome. *Hepatology.* 1997;25:1539-1542.
8. Vitek L, Carey MC. Enterohepatic cycling of bilirubin as a cause of "black" pigment gallstones in adult life. *Eur J Clin Invest.* 2003;33:799-810.
9. Nanno M, Morotomi M, Takayama H, et al. Mutagenic activation of biliary metabolites of benzo(a)pyrene by beta-glucuronidase–positive bacteria in human feces. *J Med Microbiol.* 1986;22:351-355.
10. Gourley GR, Arend RA. beta-Glucuronidase and hyperbilirubinaemia in breast-fed and formula-fed babies. *Lancet.* 1986;1(8482):644-646.
11. Van Den Bergh HAA. Uber ein direkte und indirekte diazoreaktion auf bilirubin. *Biochem Zeitshrift.* 1916;77.
12. Brett EM, Hicks JM, Powers DM, et al. Delta bilirubin in serum of pediatric patients: correlations with age and disease. *Clin Chem.* 1984;30:1561-1564.
13. Kozaki N, Shimizu S, Higashijima H, et al. Significance of serum delta-bilirubin in patients with obstructive jaundice. *J Surg Res.* 1998;79:61-65.
14. Weiss JS, Gautam A, Lauff JJ, et al. The clinical importance of a protein-bound fraction of serum bilirubin in patients with hyperbilirubinemia. *N Engl J Med.* 1983;309:147-150.
15. Bhutani VK, Johnson LH, Keren R. Diagnosis and management of hyperbilirubinemia in the term neonate: for a safer first week. *Pediatr Clin North Am.* 2004;51:843-861, vii.
16. Hansen T. Fetal and neonatal bilirubin metabolism. In: Maisels WJ, ed. *Neonatal Jaundice.* Amsterdam, The Netherlands: Harwood Academic Publishers; 2000.
17. Levi AJ, Gatmaitan Z, Arias IM. Deficiency of hepatic organic anion-binding protein, impaired organic amnion uptake by liver and "physiologic" jaundice in newborn monkeys. *N Engl J Med.* 1970;283:1136-1139.
18. Dennery PA, Seidman DS, Stevenson DK. Neonatal hyperbilirubinemia. *N Engl J Med.* 2001;344:581-590.
19. Kramer LI. Advancement of dermal icterus in the jaundiced newborn. *Am J Dis Child.* 1969;118:454-458.
20. Schneider AP II. Breast milk jaundice in the newborn. A real entity. *JAMA.* 1986;255:3270-3274.
21. Schmorl G. Zur kenntnis des ikterus neonatorum, insbesondere der dabei auftretenden gehirnveranderungen. *Verh Dtsch Ges Pathol.* 1903;6:109.
22. American Academy of Pediatrics, Subcommittee on Hyperbilirubinemia. Management of hyperbilirubinemia in the newborn infant 35 or more weeks of gestation. *Pediatrics.* 2004;114:297-316.
23. Newman TB, Xiong B, Gonzales VM, et al. Prediction and prevention of extreme neonatal hyperbilirubinemia in a mature health maintenance organization. *Arch Pediatr Adolesc Med.* 2000;154:1140-1147.
24. Bhutani VK, Johnson LH. Jaundice technologies: prediction of hyperbilirubinemia in term and near-term newborns. *J Perinatol.* 2001;21(suppl 1):S76-S82; discussion S83-S87.
25. Bhutani VK, Donn SM, Johnson LH. Risk management of severe neonatal hyperbilirubinemia to prevent kernicterus. *Clin Perinatol.* 2005;32:125-139, vii.
26. Gartner LM, Lee KS. Jaundice in the breastfed infant. *Clin Perinatol.* 1999;26:431-445, vii.
27. Zipursky A. Isoimmune hemolytic disease. In: Nathan DG, Oski FA, eds. *Hematology of Infancy and Childhood.* 4th ed. Philadelphia, PA: WB Saunders; 1994.
28. Blanchette VS, Zipursky A. Assessment of anemia in newborn infants. *Clin Perinatol.* 1984;11:489-510.
29. Prokop UG. Rhesus blood groups. In: Prokop O, Uhlenbruck G, eds. *Human Blood and Serum Groups.* New York, NY: Wiley Interscience; 1969.
30. Chavez GF, Mulinare J, Edmonds LD. Epidemiology of Rh hemolytic disease of the newborn in the United States. *JAMA.* 1991;265:3270-3274.
31. Mayne S, Parker JH, Harden TA, et al. Rate of RhD sensitisation before and after implementation of a community based antenatal prophylaxis programme. *BMJ.* 1997;315(7122):1588.
32. Bowman JM, Lewis M, Pollock JM, et al. Rh isoimmunization during pregnancy: antenatal prophylaxis. *Can Med Assoc J.* 1978;118:623-627.
33. Luchtman-Jones L, Wilson DB. Disorders of the fetus and infant. In: Fanaroff AA, Martin RJ, eds. *Neonatal-Perinatal Medicine: Disorders of the Fetus and Infant.* 7th ed. St Louis, MO: Mosby; 2002.

34. Mentzer W. Pyruvate kinase deficiency and disorders of glycolysis. In: Nathan DG, Oski FA, eds. *Hematology of Infancy and Childhood*. 5th ed. Philadelphia, PA: WB Saunders; 1998.
35. Wirth FH, Goldberg KE, Lubchenco LO. Neonatal hyperviscosity: I. Incidence. *Pediatrics*. 1979;63:833-836.
36. Stevens K, Wirth FH. Incidence of neonatal hyperviscosity at sea level. *J Pediatr*. 1980;97:118-119.
37. Wiswell TE, Cornish JD, Northam RS. Neonatal polycythemia: frequency of clinical manifestations and other associated findings. *Pediatrics*. 1986;78:26-30.
38. Brodersen R, Robertson A. Ceftriaxone binding to human serum albumin: competition with bilirubin. *Mol Pharmacol*. 1989;36:478-483.
39. Zilly W, Breimer DD, Richter E. Pharmacokinetic interactions with rifampicin. *Clin Pharmacokinet*. 1977;2:61-70.
40. Labrune P, Myara A, Huquet P, et al. Bilirubin uridine diphosphate glucuronosyltransferase hepatic activity in jaundice associated with congenital hypothyroidism. *J Pediatr Gastroenterol Nutr*. 1992;14:79-82.
41. Kadakol A, Ghosh SS, Sappal BS, et al. Genetic lesions of bilirubin uridine-diphosphoglucuronate glucuronosyltransferase (UGT1A1) causing Crigler-Najjar and Gilbert syndromes: correlation of genotype to phenotype. *Hum Mutat*. 2000;16:297-306.
42. Sampietro M, Iolascon A. Molecular pathology of Crigler-Najjar type I and II and Gilbert's syndromes. *Haematologica*. 1999;84:150-157.
43. Bosma P, Chowdhury JR, Jansen PH. Genetic inheritance of Gilbert's syndrome. *Lancet*. 1995;346(8970): 314-315.
44. Watkins JB. Neonatal cholestasis: developmental aspects and current concepts. *Semin Liver Dis*. 1993; 13:276-288.
45. Rosenthal P, Sinatra F. Jaundice in infancy. *Pediatr Rev*. 1989;11:79-86.
46. Stern H. Cytomegalovirus and EB virus infections of the liver. *Br Med Bull*. 1972;28:180-185.
47. Hanshaw JB, Dudgeon JA. Congenital cytomegalovirus. *Major Probl Clin Pediatr*. 1978;17:97-152.
48. Jorio Benkhraba M, El Harim Roudies L, El Malki Tazi A. [Infectious jaundice of the newborn infant]. *Maroc Med*. 1983;5:150-156.
49. Kluska V, Kania V, Vachalova V. [Jaundice, sepsis, and pyuria in the newborn and in small infants]. *Cesk Pediatr*. 1968;23:678-684.
50. Seeler RA, Hahn K. Jaundice in urinary tract infection in infancy. *Am J Dis Child*. 1969;118:553-558.
51. Askin DF, Diehl-Jones WL. The neonatal liver. Part III. Pathophysiology of liver dysfunction. *Neonatal Netw*. 2003;22:5-15.
52. Bell RL, Ferry GD, Smith EO, et al. Total parenteral nutrition–related cholestasis in infants. *JPEN J Parenter Enteral Nutr*. 1986;10:356-359.
53. Kwan V, George J. Liver disease due to parenteral and enteral nutrition. *Clin Liver Dis*. 2004;8:893-913, ix-x.
54. Saudubray JM, Nassogne MC, de Lonlay P, et al. Clinical approach to inherited metabolic disorders in neonates: an overview. *Semin Neonatol*. 2002;7:3-15.
55. Moyer V, Freese DK, Whitington PF, et al. Guideline for the evaluation of cholestatic jaundice in infants: recommendations of the North American Society for Pediatric Gastroenterology, Hepatology and Nutrition. An evidence-based review of important issues concerning neonatal hyperbilirubinemia. *J Pediatr Gastroenterol Nutr*. 2004;39:115-128.
56. Odievre M. Clinical presentation of metabolic liver disease. *J Inherit Metab Dis*. 1991;14:526-530.
57. Barr PH. Association of Escherichia coli sepsis and galactosemia in neonates. *J Am Board Fam Pract*. 1992;5:89-91.
58. Knisely AS, Mieli-Vergani G, Whitington PF. Neonatal hemochromatosis. *Gastroenterol Clin North Am*. 2003; 32:877-889, vi-vii.
59. Whitington PF, Kelly S, Ekong UD. Neonatal hemochromatosis: fetal liver disease leading to liver failure in the fetus and newborn. Metabolic liver disease in the pediatric patient. *Pediatr Transplant*. 2005;9:640-645.
60. Sveger T. The natural history of liver disease in alpha 1–antitrypsin deficient children. *Acta Paediatr Scand*. 1988;77:847-851.
61. Sveger T, Eriksson S. The liver in adolescents with alpha 1–antitrypsin deficiency. *Hepatology*. 1995;22: 514-517.
62. Perlmutter DH. Alpha-1–antitrypsin deficiency: diagnosis and treatment. *Clin Liver Dis*. 2004;8:839-859, viii-ix.
63. Russo PA, Mitchell GA, Tanguay RM. Tyrosinemia: a review. *Pediatr Dev Pathol*. 2001;4:212-221.
64. Croffie JM, Gupta SK, Chong SKF, et al. Tyrosinemia type 1 should be suspected in infants with severe coagulopathy even in the absence of other signs of liver failure. *Pediatrics*. 1999;103:675-678.
65. Munnich A, Rustin P, Rotig A, et al. Clinical aspects of mitochondrial disorders. *J Inherit Metab Dis*. 1992;15: 448-455.
66. Bioulac-Sage P, Parrot-Roulaud F, Mazat JP, et al. Fatal neonatal liver failure and mitochondrial cytopathy (oxidative phosphorylation deficiency): a light and electron microscopic study of the liver. *Hepatology*. 1993; 18:839-846.
67. Morris SA, Bernstein HH. Immunizations, neonatal jaundice, and animal-induced injuries. *Curr Opin Pediatr*. 2004;16:450-460.
68. Brivet M, Boutron A, Slama A, et al. Defects in activation and transport of fatty acids. *J Inherit Metab Dis*. 1999;22:428-441.
69. Davenport M. Biliary atresia. *Semin Pediatr Surg*. 2005; 14:42-48.
70. Kobayashi H, Stringer MD. Biliary atresia. *Semin Neonatol*. 2003;8:383-391.
71. Kahn E. Biliary atresia revisited. *Pediatr Dev Pathol*. 2004;7:109-124.
72. Haber BA, Russo P. Biliary atresia. *Gastroenterol Clin North Am*. 2003;32:891-911.
73. Miyano T, Yamataka A. Choledochal cysts. *Curr Opin Pediatr*. 1997;9:283-288.
74. Shian WJ, Wang YJ, Chi CS. Choledochal cysts: a nine-year review. *Acta Paediatr*. 1993;82:383-386.
75. Olbourne NA. Choledochal cysts. A review of the cystic anomalies of the biliary tree. *Ann R Coll Surg Engl*. 1975; 56:26-32.
76. Krantz ID, Piccoli DA, Spinner NB. Clinical and molecular genetics of Alagille syndrome. *Curr Opin Pediatr*. 1999;11:558-564.
77. Cavestro GM, Frulloni L, Cerati E, et al. Progressive familial intrahepatic cholestasis. *Acta Biomed Ateneo Parmense*. 2002;73(3-4):53-56.
78. Harris MJ, Le Couteur DG, Arias IM. Progressive familial intrahepatic cholestasis: genetic disorders of biliary transporters. *J Gastroenterol Hepatol*. 2005;20: 807-817.
79. Tomer G, Shneider BL. Disorders of bile formation and biliary transport. *Gastroenterol Clin North Am*. 2003;32: 839-855, vi.
80. Reddemann H. [Acute and chronic viral hepatitis in childhood. A review]. *Kinderarztl Prax*. 1979;47:557-574.
81. Zarski JP, Leroy V, Maynard-Muet M. [Acute viral hepatitis A, B, C, D and E: epidemiology, etiology, diagnosis, course, prevention]. *Rev Prat*. 1998;48:1609-1614.
82. O'Connor JA. Acute and chronic viral hepatitis. *Adolesc Med*. 2000;11:279-292.

83. Lloyd-Still JD, Scott JP, Crussi F. The spectrum of Epstein-Barr virus hepatitis in children. *Pediatr Pathol.* 1986;5:337-351.
84. Nigro G, Mattia S, Vitolo R, et al. Hepatitis in pre-school children: prevalent role of cytomegalovirus. *Arch Virol Suppl.* 1992;4:268-272.
85. Hatch MH, Siem RA. Viruses isolated from children with infectious hepatitis. *Am J Epidemiol.* 1966;84: 495-509.
86. Oettinger R, Brunnberg A, Gerner P, et al. Clinical features and biochemical data of Caucasian children at diagnosis of autoimmune hepatitis. *J Autoimmun.* 2005; 24:79-84.
87. Saadah OI, Smith AL, Hardikar W. Long-term outcome of autoimmune hepatitis in children. *J Gastroenterol Hepatol.* 2001;16:1297-1302.
88. Squires RH Jr. Autoimmune hepatitis in children. *Curr Gastroenterol Rep.* 2004;6:225-230.
89. Maddrey WC. Drug-induced hepatotoxicity: 2005. *J Clin Gastroenterol.* 2005;39(4 suppl 2):S83-S89.
90. Plaa GL, Priestly BG. Intrahepatic cholestasis induced by drugs and chemicals. *Pharmacol Rev.* 1976;28:207-273.
91. Lucey C. Jaundice and oral contraceptive drugs. *Lancet.* 1967;1(7481):106.
92. Mirchandani LV, Joshi JM. Jaundice due to anti-tuberculous drugs—a dose related phenomenon. *J Assoc Physicians India.* 1995;43:767-769.
93. DePinho RA, Goldberg CS, Lefkowitch JH. Azathioprine and the liver. Evidence favoring idiosyncratic, mixed cholestatic-hepatocellular injury in humans. *Gastroenterology.* 1984;86:162-165.
94. Huster D, Kuhn HJ, Mossner J, et al. [Wilson disease]. *Internist (Berl).* 2005;46:731-732, 734-736, 738-740.
95. Kitzberger R, Madl C, Ferenci P. Wilson disease. *Metab Brain Dis.* 2005;20:295-302.
96. Friesen CA, Roberts CC. Cholelithiasis. Clinical characteristics in children. Case analysis and literature review. *Clin Pediatr (Phila).* 1989;28:294-298.
97. D'Albuquergue LA, Gonzalez AM, Filho HL, et al. [Primary sclerosing cholangitis in children and adolescents]. *Arq Gastroenterol.* 1998;35:267-273.
98. Wilschanski M, Chait P, Wade JA, et al. Primary sclerosing cholangitis in 32 children: clinical, laboratory, and radiographic features, with survival analysis. *Hepatology.* 1995;22:1415-1422.
99. Tazuma S, Miura H, Nakanishi T, et al. [Dubin-Johnson syndrome]. *Ryoikibetsu Shokogun Shirizu.* 1995:424-426.
100. Zimniak P. Dubin-Johnson and Rotor syndromes: molecular basis and pathogenesis. *Semin Liver Dis.* 1993;13: 248-260.
101. Schinella RA. Jaundice with Dubin-Johnson-Sprinz syndrome precipitated by oral contraceptives. *N Y State J Med.* 1972;72:2810-2813.
102. Reiff MI, Osborn LM. Clinical estimation of liver size in newborn infants. *Pediatrics.* 1983;71:46-48.
103. Walker WA, Mathis RK. Hepatomegaly. An approach to differential diagnosis. *Pediatr Clin North Am.* 1975;22: 929-942.
104. Ellis G, Goldberg DM, Spooner RJ, et al. Serum enzyme tests in diseases of the liver and biliary tree. *Am J Clin Pathol.* 1978;70:248-258.
105. De Ritis F, Coltorti M, Giusti G. Serum-transaminase activities in liver disease. *Lancet.* 1972;1(7752):685-687.
106. Chopra S, Griffin PH. Laboratory tests and diagnostic procedures in evaluation of liver disease. *Am J Med.* 1985;79:221-230.
107. Knight JA, Haymond RE. Gamma-glutamyltransferase and alkaline phosphatase activities compared in serum of normal children and children with liver disease. *Clin Chem.* 1981;27:48-51.
108. Priolisi A, Didato M, Fazio M, et al. [Changes of serum gamma-glutamyltranspeptidase activity in full-term and pre-term newborn infants during the first 2 weeks of life]. *Minerva Pediatr.* 1980;32:291-296.
109. Lai MW, Chang MH, Hsu SC, et al. Differential diagnosis of extrahepatic biliary atresia from neonatal hepatitis: a prospective study. *J Pediatr Gastroenterol Nutr.* 1994;18:121-127.
110. Johnson K, Alton HM, Chapman S. Evaluation of mebrofenin hepatoscintigraphy in neonatal-onset jaundice. *Pediatr Radiol.* 1998;28:937-941.
111. Ziessman HA. Scintigraphy in the gastrointestinal tract. *Curr Opin Radiol.* 1992;4:105-116.
112. Ohnuma N, Takahashi T, Tanabe M, et al. The role of ERCP in biliary atresia. *Gastrointest Endosc.* 1997;45: 365-370.
113. Macedo G, Maia JC, Gomes A, et al. The role of transjugular liver biopsy in a liver transplant center. *J Clin Gastroenterol.* 1999;29:155-157.
114. Alagille D. Management of chronic cholestasis in childhood. *Semin Liver Dis.* 1985;5:254-262.
115. Datta DV, Sherlock S. Cholestyramine for long term relief of the pruritus complicating intrahepatic cholestasis. *Gastroenterology.* 1966;50:323-332.
116. Cynamon HA, Andres JM, Iafrate RP. Rifampin relieves pruritus in children with cholestatic liver disease. *Gastroenterology.* 1990;98:1013-1016.
117. Tiao G, Ryckman FC. Pediatric liver transplantation. *Clin Liver Dis.* 2006;10:169-197, vii.
118. Martin SR, Atkison P, Anand R, et al, and the SPLIT Research Group. Studies of pediatric liver transplantation 2002: patient and graft survival and rejection in pediatric recipients of a first liver transplant in the United States and Canada. *Pediatr Transplant.* 2004;8:273-283.

Chapter 198
JOINT PAIN

David M. Siegel, MD, MPH; John Baum, MD

Pediatric primary care physicians are often faced with clinical situations involving musculoskeletal aches and pains, and within this group of symptoms lies the subset of joint pain. In fact, 1 of every 6 to 10 pediatric outpatient visits includes a musculoskeletal complaint.[1] Discomfort in a joint can result from a wide variety of causes, and the possibilities must be considered to allow appropriate evaluation and management. A systematic approach to patients who experience pain or swelling in one or more joints helps clinicians arrive at an accurate diagnosis and course of therapy.

DEFINITIONS

Joint pain, or *arthralgia,* is the subjective experience of pain referable to a bony articulation. In a young child, this sensation of pain might be inferred from the patient's refusal to move a particular extremity or joint, but the term *arthralgia* refers only to discomfort in a joint. On the other hand, *arthritis* (as indicated by the *-itis* suffix) should be used only when the joint can be shown to be inflamed, as evidenced by the classic signs of inflammation: redness, warmth, swelling, and tenderness, in addition to pain with motion. In the joint, this kind of inflammation can be accompanied by loss of motion. Thus all that is arthralgia is not arthritis—a critical distinction in the differential diagnosis of joint pain.

ETIOLOGY

The onset of joint pain can be sudden or indolent (over days or weeks). In cases of sudden onset, an associated history of a fall or direct blow to the joint immediately suggests a traumatic cause. The presence of fever, on the other hand, points to an infectious process (eg, septic arthritis) or a systemic inflammatory disease (eg, systemic-onset juvenile idiopathic arthritis). The complaint often expressed to the physician is loss of motion in a joint, with or without obvious swelling. Further clues are provided by the time of day the stiffness occurs and its duration. Children with juvenile idiopathic arthritis typically complain of joint stiffness when they wake up the morning. The stiffness may last from 30 minutes to several hours. However, patients with hypermobility syndrome or some other mechanical, noninflammatory condition associated with joint pain usually experience pain and stiffness at the end of a vigorous day. In systemic-onset disease, in addition to fever, other distinguishing signs can include rash, mucous membrane involvement, and lymph node inflammation or enlargement, signs and symptoms that also occur with other recognizable chronic diseases that can involve the joints.

DIFFERENTIAL DIAGNOSIS

The differential diagnosis of joint pain should begin by determining whether the disease is rheumatic or nonrheumatic. *Juvenile idiopathic arthritis* (JIA), sometimes called *Still disease*[2] and previously referred to as *juvenile rheumatoid arthritis*, is a classic rheumatic disease of childhood involving the joints. It is typically seen in children 1½ to 2 years of age, although onset can occur anytime through late adolescence. The clinical presentation can be limited to 4 or fewer joints, usually large joints (oligoarticular disease), or a greater number of joints, both large and small, might be involved (polyarticular disease). A systemic and at times initially fulminant form of JIA is known as *systemic-onset disease* and is marked by high, spiking fevers; a typical salmon-pink, maculopapular, evanescent rash; lymph node, spleen, and liver enlargement; subcutaneous nodules; anemia; and general malaise. These more systemic findings can precede the onset of any joint involvement, although arthritis should be present for at least 6 consecutive weeks to establish the diagnosis of any of the subgroups of JIA.[3] Among patients with any subtype of JIA, the clinician may glean only a history of ill-defined arthralgias and stiffness, whereas physical examination may reveal contractures of the elbows, knees, and wrists or limitation of cervical motion, all of which provide evidence of previous episodes of active inflammation in these joints. Iridocyclitis and keratopathy also may be present. Although JIA is not a common disease, it has a prevalence of 0.1 to 1 child per 1000 children worldwide.[3,4]

Rheumatic Fever

Acute rheumatic fever is another classic rheumatic disease of childhood. Although not the scourge that it once was, inclusion of acute rheumatic fever in the differential diagnosis of arthritis and arthralgia remains important. The characteristics of the disease are described at length in Chapter 317, Rheumatic Fever. The arthritis usually involves large joints, such as the knees, and is typically migratory, with the joints being tender to palpation. Although signs of marked inflammation are commonly present, arthralgia alone may also be seen.

Ankylosing Spondylitis

Ankylosing spondylitis, or spondyloarthropathy, which can involve large joints of the lower extremities during childhood and early adolescence, is typified in late adolescence by involvement of the sacroiliac joint, which can be seen on radiographs or magnetic resonance imaging, and by pain elicited on palpation or compression over the joint. In adulthood, further axial involvement can occur; the classic *bamboo spine* develops, with its diffuse paravertebral fusions and often severe limitation of back motion. The human leukocyte antigen (HLA)-B27 transplantation antigen is seen in 90% of patients with ankylosing spondylitis,[5] although the converse is not true (only 20% of those born with HLA-B27 develop arthritis).[6] Treatment begins with nonsteroidal antiinflammatory drugs (NSAIDs) and progresses to more aggressive medication (eg, biologicals) as needed.

Reactive Arthritis

Reactive arthritis, previously referred to as *Reiter syndrome*—a triad of urethritis, conjunctivitis, and arthritis—may appear in children and adolescents. In children, it is often triggered by an episode of enteritis.[7] Reactive arthritis is more common in boys than in girls, and making the diagnosis depends on excluding direct infectious causes of the inflammation. The arthritis predominantly occurs in large joints; again, it is associated with the HLA-B27 class 1 major histocompatibility locus. The disorder is treated initially with antiinflammatory drugs. Most children recover within a few months, although some follow a more chronic and relapsing course and can progress to ankylosing spondylitis.[8]

Psoriasis

Also showing a predisposition for larger joints is the arthritis sometimes seen with psoriasis. Either the characteristic involvement of the skin is present, or at least a history exists of psoriatic skin disease in the family. Affected patients do not show rheumatoid factor (see Chapter 314, Psoriasis).

Rheumatic Diseases

Systemic lupus erythematosus can cause chronic joint pain. Seen more commonly in girls than in boys, systemic lupus erythematosus is a truly multisystem disease that can involve almost every organ in the body. The joints may merely be stiff and painful, or they may show frank signs of inflammation. This disorder would be within the differential diagnosis of joint pain or arthritis in an adolescent girl. Dermatomyositis also can cause inflamed joints in addition to muscle and skin involvement. Other rheumatic diseases that can affect children and cause joint involvement are scleroderma, mixed connective-tissue disease, and Kawasaki disease (see Chapter 289). Each of these entities has its own distinguishing features, as seen at physical examination and as found by laboratory tests.

Nonrheumatic Diseases

Unlike most of the rheumatic diseases, which cause joint pain and tend to be chronic (often with waxing and waning courses), many of the nonrheumatic diseases are acute in onset and short in duration, given appropriate therapy.

Infectious Organisms

Acute bacterial infection of the joint, or *septic arthritis* (see Chapter 321), is foremost among this group and represents a medical emergency. The usual manifestation is of a child complaining of the rapid onset of pain in a joint, typically accompanied by fever. The joint itself is red, warm, swollen, and exquisitely tender to palpation or with movement. This clinical situation demands immediate arthrocentesis for diagnosis and therapy. Analysis of the fluid for appearance (opaque), viscosity (usually low), mucin clot (friable), cell count (more than 100,000 white blood cells/mm^3 with at least 80% polymorphonuclear cells), glucose (usually low, much less than serum), and protein (high) helps establish the diagnosis. Most important, a portion of the fluid must be Gram stained to assess for bacterial organisms. Cultures can direct definitive antimicrobial therapy. In the past, for a child younger than 4 years, *Haemophilus influenzae* was the most commonly responsible organism; but with the institution of regular immunization, these bacteria are no longer a major consideration in septic arthritis. *Staphylococcus aureus* and *Streptococcus* species now are more likely to be the causative organisms.[9] In addition to joint fluid cultures, blood cultures may also yield growth of the organism, occasionally in the absence of a positive joint fluid culture.

Systemic bacterial infections, notably those caused by *Neisseria gonorrhoeae* and *Neisseria meningitidis,* also can produce arthritis, although the organism is usually not isolated from the joint in these cases. After joint aspiration and establishment of at least a strong suspicion of a purulent arthritis, the child should be hospitalized and appropriate intravenous antibiotic therapy initiated. Prompt, aggressive therapy usually brings about recovery without adverse side effects, although some foci, such as the hip joint, can remain persistent problems. Because of the tenuous blood supply to the femoral capital epiphysis, purulent arthritis of the hip can lead to chronic problems despite timely intervention.

In addition to bacteria, other infectious organisms can cause joint disease. Viruses, including rubella, mumps, chickenpox, and adenovirus, as well as the Epstein-Barr virus, all can affect synovial tissue. Manifestations of the viral syndrome (rash, fever, mucous membrane involvement) usually precede joint involvement. Infectious hepatitis, on the other hand, can cause arthritis before overt hepatic involvement. Rubella immunization is associated with arthralgia and arthritis in as many as 3% of children who receive the vaccine, although rarely, if ever, with any sequelae.[10] Other infections that can involve the joints include brucellosis, leptospirosis, tularemia, Rocky Mountain spotted fever, and rat-bite fever. Mycobacteria can cause arthritis, as can various fungal agents, particularly in immunocompromised individuals.

Borrelia burgdorferi is a tick-borne spirochete responsible for Lyme disease.[7] The syndrome, which was first described in Old Lyme, Connecticut,[11] is characterized by an initial tick bite that often (but not always) causes a large, circular, spreading, erythematous lesion known as *erythema migrans*. Meningoencephalitis, neuritis, and carditis also may occur. The arthritis occurs later in the course as recurrent attacks of inflammation of the large joints (85%-90% of cases involve the knee),[12] with each recurrence usually lasting no more than 1 or 2 weeks. Occasionally, symptoms may persist for several months, and chronic, persistent arthritis of the knee has been reported.[12] A short course of high-dose amoxicillin therapy seems to shorten the course of the rash and perhaps attenuates the arthritis, and NSAID therapy relieves the symptoms. Specific antibiotic regimens are suggested for different stages of disease and ages of patients.[13] Although a vaccine against *B burgdorferi* was developed and distributed, it was taken off the market in 2002 and is no longer available (see Chapter 292, Lyme Disease).

Syphilis

Congenital syphilis (see Chapter 322, Sexually Transmitted Infections) can be seen in the infant as painful bony lesions and refusal to move the involved limb (Parrot pseudoparalysis), along with other associated stigmata. In adolescence, individuals born with this disease can develop bilateral knee effusions known as *Clutton joints.*

Osteomyelitis

Osteomyelitis is an acute infection of the bone (see Chapter 303). However, when one of the long bones next to a joint (eg, the distal femur and knee) is infected, the patient may describe pain in the joint, and a sterile effusion may even be present.[14] Although unusual, the bacterial infection can directly invade the joint space from the bone, particularly in young children.

Diskitis

Diskitis, a disorder characterized by back pain and tenderness over the spinous process contiguous to the involved disk space, causes joint pain, sometimes with low-grade fever, but often with none. *Staphylococcus aureus* have been isolated from the blood and disk space in some instances, but often no culture-proven cause can be found. The presentation can involve sensory and motor complications that occur as a result of nerve root impingement, and an epidural abscess must be considered in the differential diagnosis.

Noninfectious Causes

Noninfectious origins of arthralgia and arthritis abound. Large-joint involvement is the most common extraintestinal manifestation of inflammatory bowel disease and can produce pain alone or pain with inflammation. The joint complaints may precede the appearance of bowel disease, and the activity of the bowel disease may or may not correlate with joint flare-ups. Sarcoidosis can include arthritis, as can polyarteritis nodosa and Marfan syndrome, although arthralgia is more likely than arthritis in the latter. In the group of vasculitic disorders, Henoch-Schönlein purpura is a disease of childhood associated with fever, abdominal pain (with or without melena), purpuric lesions of the buttocks and lower extremities, and warm, swollen, painful, tender joints, usually large joints such as the knees and ankles (see Chapter 272, Henoch-Schönlein Purpura). Hematologic disorders that have articular manifestations include hemophilia and sickle cell disease. In the latter disorder, the hand-foot syndrome type of vasoocclusive crisis is a common initial presentation in children between 1 and 4 years of age. Although primary gout is exceedingly rare in children, hyperuricemia and subsequent joint disease can be seen in patients with leukemia (with chemotherapy producing sudden lysis of cells), hemolytic anemia, glycogen storage disease, and Lesch-Nyhan syndrome. In Lesch-Nyhan syndrome, a sex-linked, recessive, genetic metabolic error results in overproduction of uric acid. Polyarthritis and limb pain can be observed in children after traumatic pancreatitis. Infantile cortical hyperostosis (Caffey disease), which occurs in infants younger than 6 months of age, involves fever, irritability, increased erythrocyte sedimentation rate, and tender swellings of facial, trunk, and limb bones, with associated arthralgia. Toxic synovitis of the hip also can cause arthralgia, arthritis, or both (see Chapter 177, Extremity Pain).

Systemic Autoinflammatory Diseases

In addition to the more common diseases that have arthritis as a manifestation, a group of conditions under the general heading of systemic autoinflammatory diseases may also be associated with arthritis. These diseases include familial Mediterranean fever, the cryopyrinopathies, TRAPS (tumor necrosis factor receptor–associated periodic syndrome), and hyper–immunoglobulin D syndrome. A common feature of these disorders is periodic fever without infectious cause.[15]

Hypermobility Syndrome

A condition seen mostly in children and adolescents that can induce arthralgia without arthritis is *hypermobility syndrome*.[16] Children with this disorder have increased joint laxity, and with vigorous activity, especially when requiring extremes of joint flexion and extension, they can experience significant arthralgia. The diagnosis is made by physical examination and observation of at least 3 of the following 5 signs: (1) hyperflexion of the wrist, bringing the thumb in contact with the volar surface of the forearm; (2) hyperextension of the fingers to parallel with the forearm; (3) hyperextension of the elbow to at least −10 degrees; (4) hyperextension of the knee to at least −10 degrees; and (5) hyperflexion of the spine such that with forward flexion, the palms can be placed flat on the ground with the feet together and without flexing the knees. Arthralgia may be present in only one or two of these sites, with examination showing hypermobility only in the joints that are painful. All laboratory and radiologic studies are normal. The syndrome is treated with NSAIDs and reassurance. For some patients, exercises to increase muscle strength and tone can be beneficial.[17]

Chondromalacia Patellae

In chondromalacia patellae, or patellofemoral pain syndrome, the child has knee pain usually related to activity. The problem is irregularity of the cartilage on the underside of the patella, with resultant pain as the patella moves in the patellofemoral groove. Exercises that strengthen the quadriceps femoris and adductor muscles can produce marked improvement. NSAIDs or analgesics (or both taken together) may also be administered.

Growing Pains

Children can experience *growing pains*, an actual discomfort in the lower limbs and joints that is often worse at night. A bedtime dose of an NSAID can help alleviate this pain until it resolves by itself. Adolescent girls who have fibromyalgia syndrome can experience diffuse arthralgia, but their pain is more typically muscular or periarticular.

Physical Abuse

Physical abuse should be considered whenever signs of trauma are evident, and accidents that represent neglect on the part of parents or guardians need to be recognized and pursued. Any suspicious history or circumstance demands complete investigation (see Chapter 120, Child Physical Abuse and Neglect).

Other Causes

Fractures and dislocations are common causes of joint pain in children (see Chapter 263).

EVALUATION

A complete history is indispensable in the initial assessment of a child with joint pain. The physical examination then can substantiate or alleviate suspicions raised during the interview. Distinguishing between arthralgia and arthritis is essential.

The diagnosis can be reinforced by laboratory studies, including erythrocyte sedimentation rate, C-reactive protein, and a complete blood count, as well as by more specialized studies, which may include (1) antinuclear antibody test (among patients with JIA, children with oligoarticular are most likely to have a positive result), (2) rheumatoid factor titer (rheumatoid factor is present in only a small subset of children with polyarticular JIA), and (3) serum immunoglobulin levels.

TREATMENT

Management of joint pain focuses on subduing inflammation and preserving the normal range of joint motion and strength. In the past, salicylate therapy was a mainstay of treatment, but other NSAIDs are now used as initial therapy. Gold and D-penicillamine are no longer used in patients with JIA; instead, methotrexate has come to play a central role in the first step of medical management of children who require therapy beyond NSAIDs.[18] Other long-acting agents are also prescribed, particularly anti–tumor necrosis factor alpha agents[19] and in systemic-onset JIA anti–interleukin 1 drugs.[20] Systemic corticosteroids still have a place in therapy, although they are used less frequently than in the past and in smaller doses. For the patient who has a single persistently active joint, intraarticular corticosteroids (eg, triamcinolone hexacetonide) can be effective.[21] Surgery is used mostly in joint reconstruction or prosthetic replacement as a means of dealing with the long-term results of synovial inflammation and joint destruction (see Chapter 288, Juvenile Idiopathic Arthritis).

After arriving at a diagnosis and plan of therapy, the practitioner must also offer management for the psychological aspects of joint disease. In children with ongoing joint problems, issues related to chronic pediatric disease must be addressed. The child may be unable to keep up with peers in physical activity and may be faced with having to make many health care visits, which may result in school absences. Many clinicians think that environmental stress in addition to the stress caused by the disease can exacerbate various chronic conditions, and such may occur in children with JIA.

Children faced with hospitalization for an acute problem, such as septic arthritis, are exposed to all the complications of being taken out of their family and school environment, as well as having to deal with an institutional setting. Children with ongoing joint disease, even those with only a mild disability, should be provided with the services of a specialized social worker, counselor, or psychologist. Family resources (both emotional and financial) need to be assessed and support provided when needed. Discussion groups or support groups composed of these children and their families can be helpful because they offer an opportunity to compare experiences and coping mechanisms. Attention to the physical dimension alone does not provide adequate care in these diseases. A functionally minor disability can cause major problems of body image and feelings of lack of independence that must be dealt with appropriately. As with other chronic physical disorders of childhood and adolescence, long-term psychosocial sequelae also may develop.[22]

WHEN TO REFER

- Orthopedics
  - Fracture
  - Ligamentous or cartilage injury to joint
  - Continuous pain in a joint with deformity
- Rheumatology
  - Suspicion of juvenile arthritis or other rheumatologic disorder
- Infectious diseases
  - Septic arthritis
  - Lyme disease; other spirochetal infection
  - Osteomyelitis
- Hematology
  - Sickle cell disease
  - Hemophilia
- Gastroenterology
  - Joint symptoms associated with inflammatory bowel disease
- Occupational or physical therapy
  - Joint disease complicated by contractures, weakness, poor function
  - Hypermobility syndrome
- Mental health
  - Suspicion of somatization or conversion disorder

WHEN TO ADMIT

- Fracture requiring open fixation or traction
- Systemic onset juvenile arthritis with macrophage activation syndrome
- Septic arthritis
- Osteomyelitis
- Severe sickle cell pain crisis
- Inadequate response to outpatient occupational or physical therapy and to rehabilitation

TOOLS FOR PRACTICE

Engaging Patient and Family

- *What is a Pediatric Rheumatologist?* (fact sheet), American Academy of Pediatrics (www.aap.org/family/WhatisPedRheumatology.pdf).

Medical Decision Support

- *Red Book: 2006 Report of the Committee on Infectious Diseases,* 27th edition (book), American Academy of Pediatrics (www.aap.org/bookstore).

REFERENCES

1. De Inocencio J. Epidemiology of musculoskeletal pain in primary care. *Arch Dis Child.* 2004;89:431-434.
2. Still GF. On a form of chronic joint disease in children. *Med Chir Trans.* 1897;80:47-59.
3. Petty RE, Southwood TR, Manners P, et al. International league of associations for rheumatology classification of juvenile idiopathic arthritis: second revision, Edmonton, 2001. *J Rheumatol.* 2004;31:390-392.
4. Oen KG, Cheang M. Epidemiology of chronic arthritis in childhood. *Semin Arthritis Rheum.* 1996;26:575-591.
5. Jaakkola E, Herzberg I, Laiho K, et al. Finnish HLA studies confirm the increased risk conferred by HLA-B27 homozygosity in ankylosing spondylitis. *Ann Rheum Dis.* 2006;65:775-780.
6. van der Linden SM, Valkenburg HA, de Jongh BM, et al. The risk of developing ankylosing spondylitis in HLA-B27 positive individuals. A comparison of relatives of spondylitis patients with the general population. *Arthritis Rheum.* 1984;27:241-249.
7. Taccetti G, Trapani S, Ermini M, et al. Reactive arthritis triggered by Yersinia enterocolitica: a review of 18 pediatric cases. *Clin Exp Rheumatol.* 1994;12:681-684.
8. Khan MA. Update on spondyloarthropathies. *Ann Int Med.* 2002;136:896-907.
9. Luhmann JD, Luhmann SJ. Etiology of septic arthritis in children: an update for the 1990s. *Pediatr Emerg Care.* 1999;15:40-42.
10. Phillips P. Viral arthritis in children. *Arthritis Rheum.* 1977;20(suppl):584.
11. Steere AC, Malawista SE, Snydman DR, et al. Lyme arthritis: an epidemic of oligoarticular arthritis in children and adults in three Connecticut communities. *Arthritis Rheum.* 1977;20:7-17.
12. Gerber MA, Zemel LS, Shapiro ED. Lyme arthritis in children: clinical epidemiology and long-term outcomes. *Pediatrics.* 1998;102:905-908.
13. American Academy of Pediatrics. Lyme disease. In: Pickering LK, Baker CJ, Long SS, et al, eds. *Red Book: 2006 Report of the Committee on Infectious Diseases.* 27th ed. Elk Grove Village, IL: American Academy of Pediatrics; 2006.
14. Perlman MH, Patzakis MJ, Kumar PJ, et al. The incidence of joint involvement with adjacent osteomyelitis in pediatric patients. *J Pediatr Orthop.* 2000;20:40-43.

15. Ozen S, Hoffman HM, Frenkel J, et al. Familial Mediterranean fever (FMF) and beyond; a new horizon. *Ann Rheum Dis*. 2006;65:961-964.
16. Biro F, Gewanter HL, Baum J. The hypermobility syndrome. *Pediatrics*. 1983;72:701-706.
17. Kerr A, Macmillan CE, Uttley WS, et al. Physiotherapy for children with hypermobility syndrome. *Physiotherapy*. 2000;86:313-317.
18. Laxer RM. Pharmacology and drug therapy. In: Cassidy JT, Petty RE, Laxer RM, et al, eds. *Textbook of Pediatric Rheumatology*. 5th ed. Philadelphia, PA: Elsevier; 2005.
19. Lovell DJ, Giannini EH, Reiff A, et al. Etanercept in children with polyarticular juvenile rheumatoid arthritis. Pediatric Rheumatology Collaborative Study Group. *N Engl Med*. 2000;342:763-769.
20. Verbasky JW, White AJ. Effective use of the recombinant interleukin 1 receptor antagonist in therapy resistant systemic onset juvenile rheumatoid arthritis. *J Rheumatol*. 2004;31:2071-2075.
21. Zulian F, Martini G, Gobber D, et al. Comparison of intra-articular triamcinolone hexacetonide and triamcinolone acetamide in oligoarticular juvenile idiopathic arthritis. *Rheumatology*. 2003;42:1254-1259.
22. LeBovidge JS, Lavigne JV, Donenberg GR, et al. Psychological adjustment of children and adolescents with chronic arthritis: a meta-analytic review. *J Pediatr Psychol*. 2003:28:29-39.

Chapter 199

LIMP

Erica M. Sibinga, MD, MHS; John S. Andrews, MD

Limp, an abnormal gait pattern, is a common presenting complaint in pediatric primary care offices and emergency departments.[1] Although limp is most commonly associated with trauma, it has many possible causes, ranging from benign to life threatening.

Gait abnormalities can result from pain, mechanical problems, or neuromuscular problems. Distinguishing the type of gait abnormality is particularly helpful in guiding evaluation and management. An *antalgic* gait is characterized by a shortened stance time on the affected side caused by pain on weight bearing and has an associated shortened swing phase on the contralateral side. The *Trendelenburg* gait, seen with hip abductor weakness or hip joint instability, occurs when the hip girdle drops on the affected side and the trunk moves over the affected side to maintain balance. If the problem is bilateral, then the trunk swings from side to side. The *circumduction* (vaulting) gait is the result of straight-legged walking caused by joint pain or muscle weakness. The *steppage* (equinus) gait is seen with foot drop because of peroneal nerve injury or weakness of the tibialis anterior muscle (eg, Guillain-Barré syndrome). *Toe-walking* gait is the result of real or functional leg-length discrepancy. Contractures or muscle spasms can cause functional leg-length discrepancies. *Waddling* gaits have a wide-based stance and result from bilateral hip disease or neuromuscular disease. *Stooped* and *shuffle* gaits (symmetric or asymmetric) are the result of peritoneal inflammation, including pelvic inflammatory disease, appendicitis, salpingitis, and psoas abscess.

DIFFERENTIAL DIAGNOSIS

Despite the broad differential diagnosis of limp, approaching the diagnosis by the type of gait abnormality allows a well-organized approach to evaluation and management, as shown in Table 199-1. Additionally, several diagnoses can be made that may result in combined-type gait disturbances.

Antalgic, or painful, limps are most common. Pain is associated with causes related to mechanical difficulties, inflammatory processes, infectious processes, specific hip disorders, malignancies, and hematologic disorders. Trendelenburg limps are associated with inflammatory processes, infectious processes, and specific hip disorders. Circumduction (vaulting) limps are likely to be associated with joint stiffness, muscle weakness, or leg-length discrepancy (true or functional). Joint stiffness may be caused by inflammation, infection, or pain.

Further narrowing of the differential diagnosis depends on the time course, associated signs and symptoms, age, and physical examination. Systemic signs and symptoms, such as fever, malaise, anorexia, weight loss, and ill appearance, usually accompany limp when the cause is infectious, inflammatory, or neoplastic. The child's age may help determine the cause of a limp because some diagnoses are more common at certain ages than others (Table 199-2).

EVALUATION

History

Important historical points include the duration of limp; antecedent trauma and activity; associated or preceding symptoms that include fever, viral illness, rash, and weight loss; and changes in exercise patterns. At all ages, trauma is the most common cause of acute-onset painful limp,[2] resulting in soft-tissue or musculoskeletal injury. Although the majority of trauma is accidental, the clinician must consider whether the history and the physical examination findings correlate. If the nature or degree of the child's injury does not fit the history given, then nonaccidental injury should be considered and evaluated further.

Associated symptoms may further narrow the diagnosis. Recurrent fevers, rash, and joint pain suggest an inflammatory process, such as juvenile idiopathic arthritis (JIA). Adolescent girls who receive a rubella vaccination may develop a transient but painful reactive arthritis 1 to 2 weeks after vaccination. Lyme arthritis should be evaluated if the patient has a history of influenza-like illness and erythematous rash with central clearing.[3]

Exploring the child's or the adolescent's physical activities is important. Stress fractures, patellofemoral arthralgia syndrome, and Osgood-Schlatter disease are more common among athletes, particularly runners.[4,5] Overuse syndromes may be the result of repetitive microtrauma of the tibia (Osgood-Schlatter

Table 199-1 Differential Diagnosis of Limping by Gait Pattern

DIFFERENTIAL DIAGNOSIS BY DISEASE TYPE	GAIT PATTERN
MECHANICAL	
Soft-tissue injury, including bruising, strains, and foreign body	A
Skeletal fracture, including stress or overuse fracture	A
Toddler's fracture	A
Apophysitis of tibial tuberosity (Osgood-Schlatter disease) or calcaneum (Sever disease)	A
Chondromalacia patellae	A
Spondylolisthesis and spondylolysis	A
INFLAMMATORY	
Reactive arthritis, including transient synovitis of the hip	A, T, C*
Juvenile idiopathic arthritis	A, T, C*
Myositis	A, T
Other connective tissue disease (eg, systemic vasculitis, systemic lupus erythematosus)	A, T
Chronic recurrent multifocal osteomyelitis	A, T
INFECTION	
Skeletal, including osteomyelitis and septic arthritis	A, T, C*
Diskitis	A
Soft-tissue infection	A, T, C*
Abdominal sepsis, including psoas abscess, appendicitis, peritonitis	A, T
Inguinal lymphadenitis	A
SPECIFIC HIP DISORDERS	
Legg-Calvé-Perthes disease	A, T
Slipped capital femoral epiphysis	A, T
Idiopathic chondrolysis	A, T
CONGENITAL	
Developmental dysplasia of the hip	T
Congenital talipes equinovarus	E
Congenital short femur	C
Skeletal dysplasias	A,T,C
MALIGNANT DISEASE	
Leukemia	A
Bone neoplasia (eg, osteoid osteoma, osteoblastoma osteosarcoma, Langerhans cell histiocytosis)	A
Spinal cord tumor	A
METABOLIC	
Rickets	A
OTHERS	
Neurologic and neuromuscular disease	T, C
Hematologic disease (eg, hemophilia, sickle cell disease)	A
Tarsal coalitions	A
Chronic pain syndromes	A, C, T, S, E
Idiopathic or conversion disorder (usually bizarre gait)	A, C, T, S, E

*Depending on joints involved or site.
A, Antalgic; *C*, circumduction; *E*, equines; *S*, stepping; *T*, Trendelenburg.
Adapted from Beresford MW, Cleary AG. Evaluation of a limping child. *Current Paediatrics.* 2005;15(1):15-22. Copyright © 2005, Elsevier, with permission.

disease), the calcaneus (Sever disease), or patella (patellofemoral arthralgia syndrome).[6] A sudden increase in the amount or duration of exercise is frequently associated with injury.[7]

Underlying hematologic disorders should also be considered; hemarthrosis from hemophilia should be considered as a cause of limp in a boy who has a swollen, painful knee and a family history of bleeding problems; vasoocclusive pain crisis should be considered in a black patient with a history suggesting sickle cell disease.

Physical Examination

The extent and focus of the physical examination should be tailored to the individual based on the history obtained. If any indication of systemic illness exists, then a complete examination should be conducted. In the absence of systemic signs, most of the examination can be directed toward the back and lower extremities. Complaints of thigh or knee pain may be referred from a hip process and require thorough evaluation of the hip joint. Particularly with younger children, a great deal of useful information

Table 199-2 Common Causes of Limping According to Age

AGE	ANTALGIC	TRENDELENBURG
Toddler (1-3 yr)	Infection Septic arthritis Hip Knee Osteomyelitis Diskitis Trauma Accidental Nonaccidental Toddler's fracture Neoplasia	Hip dislocation Neuromuscular disease Cerebral palsy Poliomyelitis
Child (4-10 yr)	Infection Septic arthritis Hip Knee Osteomyelitis Diskitis Reactive arthritis, including transient synovitis of the hip Legg-Calvé-Perthes disease Tarsal coalition Rheumatologic disorder Juvenile idiopathic arthritis Acute rheumatic fever Trauma Neoplasia	Hip dislocation Neuromuscular disease Cerebral palsy Poliomyelitis
Adolescent (≥11 yr)	Slipped capital femoral epiphysis Rheumatologic disorder Juvenile idiopathic arthritis Trauma: fracture, overuse Tarsal coalition Neoplasia	Neuromuscular disease

Adapted from Thompson GH. Gait Disturbances. In: Kliegman RM, Nieder ML, Super DM, eds. *Practical Strategies of Pediatric Diagnosis and Therapy*. Philadelphia, PA: WB Saunders; 1996. Copyright © 1996, Elsevier, with permission.

may be gained by opportunistic observation of the child before entering the examination room or when engaged in other activities.

Gait Examination

Determining the gait abnormality is crucial. The clinician should observe the patient's gait with good visibility of feet, leg, and pelvis, if possible. Abnormal gait patterns are described previously.

Joints and Musculoskeletal Examination

Inspection of the lower extremities for erythema, warmth, bruising, swelling, muscle atrophy, and asymmetry may localize the cause of the limp. Erythema, warmth, and swelling suggest an infectious or inflammatory process of the underlying subcutaneous tissue, muscle, bone, or joint. Palpation along the limb from the lower spine to the toes may localize any area of pain. Pinpoint tenderness is found most often with fractures or osteomyelitis. If the hip or upper thigh appears to be involved, then the lower spine, paraspinal areas, abdomen, and inguinal areas should also be examined.

Each joint should be examined systematically for erythema, warmth, swelling, pain, and range of motion (both active and passive). Infection or inflammation are suggested by erythema, warmth, and swelling, although these signs are not likely appreciable in the hip joint. Limitation in range of motion at the joint suggests an intraarticular process. Infected or inflamed hip joints tend to be held in the position of most comfort (the affected leg held flexed, abducted, and externally rotated to decrease the pressure in the hip joint), even to the extent of *pseudoparalysis*,[6] and are painful with direct compression into the hip joint. Hip joints in particular should be assessed for both external and internal rotation (Figure 199-1). Examination of the knee joint should include evaluation for the presence of an effusion and for patellar pain with pressure and assessing the stability of the joint for ligamentous injury. Pain with active, but not passive, range of motion suggests a muscle or tendon injury.

Leg-length discrepancy (true or functional) can be detected by measuring both legs from the anterior superior spine of the ilium to the distal end of the ipsilateral medial malleolus. Developmental dysplasia of

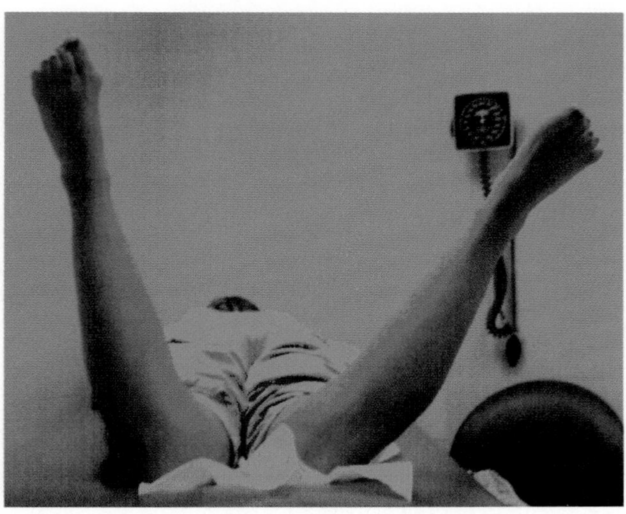

Figure 199-1 Testing of internal rotation of the hip in prone position. Note the limited internal rotation of the left hip. *(Katz DA. Slipped capital femoral epiphysis: the importance of early diagnosis.* Pediatric Ann. *2006;35[2]:102-111. Reprinted by permission of Slack Inc.)*

the hip (DDH) results in a functional leg-length discrepancy and has a significantly better prognosis if diagnosed in infancy. In infants, asymmetric skin folds suggest a leg-length discrepancy and are a characteristic finding of unilateral DDH. If DDH is not diagnosed early, then it may be characterized by a limp in an infant or toddler learning to walk. To evaluate for DDH or other leg-length discrepancy, the Galeazzi test should be performed, in which the patient lies supine, with ankles to buttocks, hips and knees flexed. The Galeazzi test is positive if the knees are at different heights (Figure 199-2).

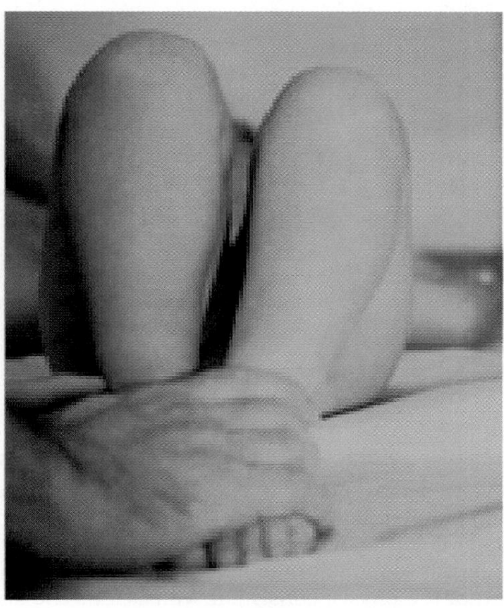

Figure 199-2 A Galeazzi test suggesting developmental dysplasia of the hip or a leg-length discrepancy. The test is positive when the knees are at different heights as the patient lies supine with ankles to buttocks and hips and knees flexed. *(Leet AI, Skaggs DL. Evaluation of the acutely limping child.* Am Fam Physician. *2000;61[4]:1011-1018. Reprinted by permission of the American Academy of Family Physicians.)*

General Examination

General examination should include attention to general appearance, temperature, and presence of a rash that may suggest a systemic cause, and bruising or scars that suggest nonaccidental injury.

Laboratory Testing

If the history and physical examination suggest an infectious, inflammatory, or neoplastic cause for the limp, then laboratory evaluation should ensue rapidly. A complete blood cell count (CBC) with differential, erythrocyte sedimentation rate (ESR), and C-reactive protein (CRP) level should be obtained. In febrile or ill-appearing patients, a blood culture sample should also be requested. Blood cultures are positive in up to 50% of cases of septic arthritis and osteomyelitis.[8] An ESR less than 20 mm/hour is unlikely to be associated with a serious infectious, inflammatory, or neoplastic cause.[9]

Distinguishing between hip septic arthritis (requiring urgent joint drainage and parenteral antibiotic treatment) and transient synovitis (treated symptomatically) can be very difficult because the potential exists for significant overlap of history, physical examination findings, laboratory results, and radiologic findings. White blood cell (WBC) counts, ESR, and CRP level all tend to be increased in septic arthritis, although none of these factors alone is entirely predictive. CRP value may be clinically useful as a negative predictor. If the CRP level is less than 1.0 mg/dL, then the probability that the patient does not have septic arthritis is 87%.[10] Although no single laboratory value is entirely effective in detecting hip septic arthritis, using the following factors together can improve the reliability: temperature greater than 37° C, ESR greater than 20 mm/hour, CRP greater than 1.0 mg/dL, WBC count greater than 11,000/mm^3, and radiographic finding of difference of more than 2 mm between affected and unaffected hips are combined. If 4 or 5 of these factors are present, then a very high likelihood (85% to 99%) of septic arthritis exists.[11]

If joint sepsis is suspected, then aspiration of the joint fluid should be performed by an orthopedic surgeon. Gram stain, culture, and cell counts should be obtained for diagnosis and treatment (culture and sensitivities). If concern exists for gonococcal arthritis, then vaginal, anal, and throat specimens should also be sent for culture.

A few diagnoses require specific laboratory tests in addition to CBC, ESR, and CRP value. Lyme titers should be obtained if the patient has a history of preceding erythema migrans rash or fever and malaise, arthritis, and travel or residence in a Lyme disease–endemic area. Recurrent fevers, rash, and joint pain should prompt a rheumatologic work-up, including antinuclear antibody levels. A child with rheumatologic disease may have elevated WBC counts, elevated platelets counts, anemia, or any combination. The

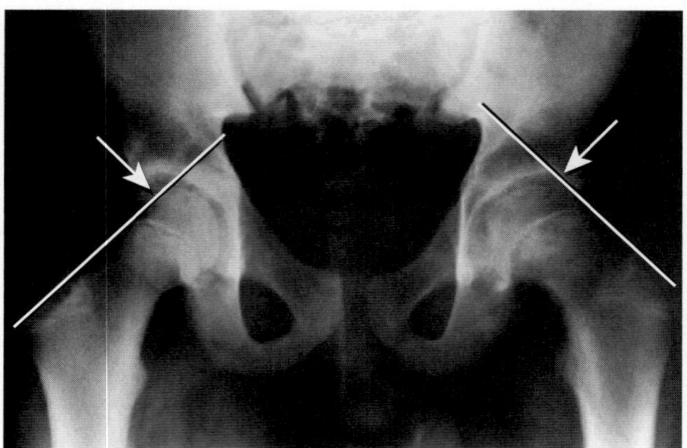

Figure 199-3 AP pelvis in a 13-year-old boy complaining of left hip pain and limp. A Klein line is drawn along the superolateral cortex of the femoral neck. The arrow shows posteromedial slippage of the left femoral epiphysis and widening of the physis, consistent with SCFE. The arrow on the right shows a normal Klein line, which dissects approximately one sixth of the femoral epiphysis. *(Barkin RM, Barkin SZ, Barkin AZ. The limping child.* J Emerg Med. *2000;18[3]:331-339. Copyright © 2000, Elsevier, with permission.)*

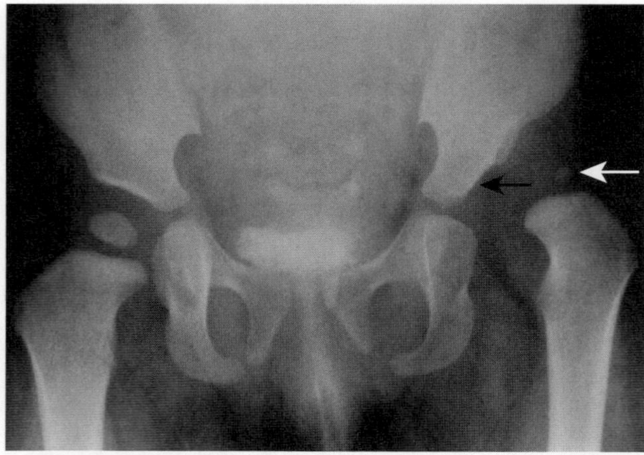

Figure 199-4 AP pelvis in a 14-month-old girl with an abnormal gait and difficulty walking. The left proximal femur is displaced superolaterally. The white arrow shows a small capital femoral epiphysis. The black arrow shows a steep acetabular roof. The patient had previously unrecognized developmental dysplasia of the left hip. Contrast in the bladder is from a voiding cystourethrogram. *(Barkin RM, Barkin SZ, Barkin AZ. The limping child.* J Emerg Med. *2000;18[3]:331-339. Copyright © 2000, Elsevier, with permission.)*

possibility of acute rheumatic fever (ARF) should be evaluated with an antistreptolysin O titer in the setting of recent pharyngitis (previous 2-4 weeks), migrating arthritis, rash, possible chest discomfort (caused by carditis). ARF is most common in children 4 to 9 years of age.

Imaging

Radiographs

Plain-film radiographs remain an important tool in the evaluation of limp,[12] particularly in diagnosing fractures, hip disease, spinal abnormalities, and foot disease (eg, tarsal coalition). Obtaining at least 2 views of the affected area is essential, with suspected hip disease requiring anteroposterior (AP) and frog-leg lateral (Lauenstein) views of the pelvis. In the diagnosis of hip disease, radiographic evidence of greater than 2 mm difference between the affected and unaffected hip are associated with septic arthritis, when combined with a fever of greater than 37° C and suggestive laboratory values, as listed previously.[11] Plain-film radiographs are diagnostic in slipped capital femoral epiphysis (SCFE), with a characteristic appearance of ice cream falling off the cone at the affected femoral head (Figure 199-3). As shown in Figure 199-4, DDH is visible on plain films, with the femoral head out of position and both sides of the joint (acetabulum and femoral head) showing abnormal development. (In infants younger than 4 months, DDH is best evaluated with hip ultrasound.) Malignancies such as Ewing sarcoma and osteosarcoma are visible on plain films, as are the multiple lesions of Langerhans cell histiocytosis, although additional imaging is needed for further assessment. However, radiographs are likely to be negative early in the course of Legg-Calvé-Perthes disease; approximately 5 months after the initial ischemia, AP radiographs of the pelvis show a dense femoral epiphysis and apparent widening of the medial joint space (Figure 199-5). Findings typical of osteomyelitis are not usually apparent on plain-film radiographs until 10 or more days after the onset of symptoms.

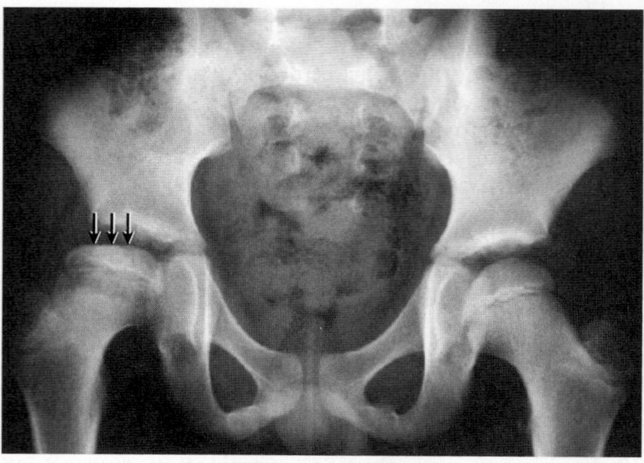

Figure 199-5 AP pelvis in an 8-year-old boy with right hip pain and limp. Right femoral head epiphysis shows loss of height and mixed sclerotic and lytic appearance *(arrows)* of Legg-Calvé-Perthes disease. *(Barkin RM, Barkin SZ, Barkin AZ. The limping child.* J Emerg Med. *2000;18[3]:331-339. Copyright © 2000, Elsevier, with permission.)*

Ultrasound

Ultrasound examination of the hip joint should be used to assess for a joint effusion. Unfortunately, if a significant effusion is detected, then ultrasound cannot differentiate among inflammation, infection, and hemorrhage, and aspiration is required for diagnosis.

Bone Scintigraphy

Uptake of technetium-99m is increased at the site of increased blood supply or bone turnover, making bone scanning useful in the diagnosis of osteomyelitis, recurrent multifocal osteomyelitis, diskitis, stress fracture, osteoid osteoma, Legg-Calvé-Perthes disease, and neoplasms.[12]

Computed Tomography

Computed tomography is most helpful in the evaluation of the bones, in particular, tarsal coalition, spondylolisthesis or spondylolysis, and osteoid osteoma.[12]

Magnetic Resonance Imaging

Magnetic resonance imaging (MRI) is useful in evaluation of intraspinal lesions, including diskitis, soft-tissue neoplasms, bone marrow disease, and early in the course of Legg-Calvé-Perthes disease.[12,13]

DIAGNOSIS AND MANAGEMENT

Mechanical or Musculoskeletal Forms

Most cases of limp seen in primary care are a result of trauma. Unless the evaluation suggests a fracture or ligament damage, rest, ice (in the initial 48-72 hours after trauma), compression, elevation, and mild analgesics are the mainstays of therapy. If symptoms are severe or persistent, then orthopedic involvement may be indicated. Fracture, ligament, and tendon injury require appropriate orthopedic referral and treatment.

Infection

If an infectious cause of limp is suspected, such as a septic arthritis or osteomyelitis, then rapid diagnosis is important because of the high morbidity of these conditions. *Septic arthritis* is more likely to be found in infants or young children who exhibit an antalgic limp. These patients are often febrile, ill appearing, have pain at the joint with limited range of motion, and have laboratory evidence of an infectious or inflammatory process. Ultrasound may show a joint effusion, but aspiration of the fluid is required to distinguish septic arthritis from transient synovitis. Septic arthritis is a surgical emergency and necessitates emergent orthopedic involvement for diagnosis and therapeutic aspiration. *Osteomyelitis* has a broad range of clinical presentations; a child may be afebrile and looking well,[14] mildly uncomfortable, or toxic in appearance. A specific area of tenderness on physical examination typically is found, and the WBC, ESR, and CRP values are usually elevated. Radiographs may be normal early in the process because periosteal elevation and osteolysis are not visible until 7 to 14 days after the onset of infection. Radionuclide bone scintigraphy is positive earlier in the disease process.[12] An effort should also be made to obtain a bacterial culture of the infected area by using needle aspiration before initiating antibiotic treatment. Septic arthritis and osteomyelitis require broad-spectrum parenteral antibiotics, including coverage for methicillin-resistant *Staphylococcus* if present in the community,[15] until significant clinical improvement takes place (decreased ESR level, WBC count, negative blood culture, afebrile). The CRP value should be monitored regularly because it decreases rapidly with effective antimicrobial treatment.[16] When clinically improved and in consultation with a pediatric infectious disease specialist, oral antibiotics can be considered for the completion of the antibiotic course (typically 3-4 weeks), if the organism is susceptible, if outpatient compliance is excellent, and if the patient is monitored closely.

Inflammatory

Transient synovitis of the hip is a common cause of limp in children, especially in those who are between 3 and 10 years of age. Although the cause is unknown, many affected children have had a viral infection preceding the onset of symptoms. The limp is caused by acute unilateral hip pain and resulting limitation in the range of motion of the hip joint. Pain may be referred to the groin, thigh, or knee, and the patient may preferentially hold the leg in flexion, abduction, and external rotation (usually less so than with a septic arthritis). In most instances a child who has transient synovitis is not ill appearing or febrile and has mild pain in the hip joint and slight limitation of adduction and internal rotation. The diagnosis can often be made by history and physical examination alone, but severe transient synovitis is difficult to distinguish from septic arthritis of the hip, and further evaluation is necessary. In transient synovitis, hip radiographs are usually normal. Ultrasound may show fluid in the joint space, and aspiration may be necessary to distinguish synovitis from septic arthritis. The treatment of transient synovitis of the hip is symptomatic, usually requiring some limitation of activity. It is a self-limited process, and full recovery should be anticipated, usually in a matter of weeks.[17]

Arthritis

JIA, ARF, Lyme arthritis, and lupus erythematosus are likely to be suggested by a history of fever, rashes, migrating arthralgias, recent pharyngitis, or tick exposure, with physical examination findings of arthritis. JIA most commonly involves arthritis of the knees, ankles, and hands.[18] Further evaluation should include a CBC and ESR evaluation, as well as antistreptolysin O titers, Lyme titers, or antinuclear antibody, as indicated by clinical suspicion. Consultation with a rheumatologist may be beneficial. Depending on the results of the laboratory tests, treatment consists of antiinflammatory agents for autoimmune processes and antibiotics for disseminated Lyme disease.

Developmental or Acquired Conditions

Unilateral DDH may exhibit as a Trendelenburg limp in an infant or toddler beginning to walk; bilateral DDH causes a *waddling* gait. Otherwise the patient is asymptomatic. With unilateral DDH, physical examination reveals an apparent leg-length discrepancy or asymmetrical skin folds or both. Because bilateral

DDH affects both hips, detecting by physical examination alone can be difficult. In the toddler or childhood years, anteroposterior and frog-leg radiographs of the pelvis are necessary (see Figure 199-4), and referral to an orthopedist is needed for treatment. Prognosis is best in children diagnosed in early infancy and with mild dysplasia.

Specific Hip Disorders

Legg-Calvé-Perthes Disease

Legg-Calvé-Perthes disease (avascular necrosis of the femoral head) is a common cause of limp in children 2 to 10 years of age. It is 5 times more likely in boys than in girls and bilateral in approximately 20% of cases. The typical presentation is an antalgic Trendelenburg limp, usually accompanied by mild pain in the thigh or knee, with mild weakness or atrophy of the hip abductor, thigh, and buttock muscles. As shown in Figure 199-5, approximately 5 months after the initial ischemia, anteroposterior radiographs of the pelvis show a dense femoral epiphysis and apparent widening of the medial joint space. Earlier diagnosis may require MRI or a bone scan,[12] given that plain radiographs are not sensitive for Legg-Calvé-Perthes disease early in the course. Legg-Calvé-Perthes disease is self-limited, with resolution in 18 to 24 months, although intermittent synovitis with discomfort may occur, requiring limitation of normal activity, bracing, or casting.[19]

Slipped Capital Femoral Epiphysis

Slipped capital femoral epiphysis (SCFE) occurs most commonly among adolescents, often during or just before the pubertal growth spurt (ages 10 to 15 years). Boys are affected more than girls (3:2), with obesity and tall stature being risk factors. Usually, acute onset of limp, a painful hip, and limitation of internal rotation occurs. However, some patients exhibit signs subtly, with dull aching in the hip or leg and pain occurring only with exercise, which may result in a delayed diagnosis.[20] Unfortunately, the diagnosis of SCFE is delayed in as many as 30% of cases, leading to increased difficulties with treatment.[21] Anteroposterior radiographs may show asymmetry and widening of the growth plate, but SCFE is seen best on Lauenstein (frog-leg) films, in which the displaced femoral head is more apparent. Because further displacement of the epiphysis is a risk, this diagnosis should prompt immediate orthopedic involvement. Treatment consists of pinning the femoral epiphysis for stabilization. Many patients who have SCFE will have bilateral involvement, usually within 18 months of the initial side.[21]

Activity-Related Limp

Overuse, as with excessive training or participation in athletics, can result in repetitive microtrauma and specific pain syndromes. Osgood-Schlatter disease is commonly seen in active adolescents, the result of repetitive microtrauma to the tibial tubercle. Tenderness on palpation is localized over the tibial tubercle; treatment requires some limitation of activity. Patients who have *patellofemoral arthralgia* syndrome have knee pain, made worse by activity, particularly stair climbing. On physical examination, compression of the patella on the femur causes pain. Rest and limited activity is the treatment of choice. Overuse syndromes can also affect the heel and foot.[6] Intense or excessive exercise may cause stress fractures of the lower extremities.

Neoplastic Disease

Limp also may be the initial symptom of a benign tumor or malignant neoplasm. Malignant conditions include leukemia, Ewing sarcoma, and osteosarcoma. Plain-film radiographs are helpful in leading to the diagnosis, but further imaging will be required for treatment planning. Multiple lesions on radiograph should raise concern of Langerhans cell histiocytosis or a metastatic process. An MRI or a bone scan may be used to define better the extent of involvement. Osteoid osteoma is a benign lesion that causes pain that is worse at night and is relieved by aspirin.[19] It may be identified on computed tomographic scan, but a bone scan is most sensitive for detection of this lesion.[12] Consultation with a pediatric oncologist is required for findings consistent with a neoplastic cause.

Unclear Diagnosis

If, despite a thorough history, physical examination, screening laboratory testing and radiographs, a diagnosis remains unclear and a condition associated with high morbidity is not a concern, then a short period of observation (perhaps 1 to 2 weeks) may be appropriate. If the limp persists, then a repeat history, physical examination, laboratory testing, and radiologic examination will likely establish the diagnosis. If the diagnosis remains unclear, then consultation with an orthopedist, rheumatologist, or neurologist is warranted.

WHEN TO REFER

Clinical, radiographic, or laboratory concern for:

- Fracture
- Septic arthritis
- Osteomyelitis
- Developmental dysplasia of the hip
- Slipped capital femoral epiphysis
- Neoplastic disease
- Appendicitis or psoas abscess
- Persistent limp of unclear cause

REFERENCES

1. Fischer SU, Beattie TF. The limping child: epidemiology, assessment and outcome. *J Bone Joint Surg Br.* 1999; 81(61):1029-1034.
2. Doughty RA, Rose C. Limp. In: Fleischer GR, Ludwig S, eds. *Textbook of Pediatric Emergency Medicine*. 3rd ed. Baltimore, MD: Williams & Wilkins; 1993.
3. Steere AC, Schoen RT, Taylor E. The clinical evolution of Lyme arthritis. *Ann Intern Med.* 1987;107(5):725-731.
4. Keller EK. Patellar management syndrome in runners. *Nurs Pract.* 1983;8(6):27, 31-32.
5. Newell SG, Bramwell ST. Overuse injuries to the knee in runners. *Phys Sportsmed.* 1984;12(3):81-92.
6. Renshaw TS. The child who has a limp. *Pediatr Rev.* 1995; 16(12):458-465.

7. Garrick JG. Knee problems in adolescents. *Pediatr Rev.* 1983;4:235-243.
8. Barkin RM, Barkin SZ, Barkin AZ. The limping child. *J Emerg Med.* 2000;18(3):331-339.
9. Huttenlocher A, Newman TB. Evaluation of the erythrocyte sedimentation rate in children presenting with limp, fever, or abdominal pain, *Clin Pediatr (Phila).* 1997;36(6): 339-344.
10. Levine MJ, McGuire KJ, McGowan KL, et al. Assessment of the test characteristics of C-reactive protein for septic arthritis in children. *J Pediatr Orthop.* 2003;23(3):373-377.
11. Jung ST, Rowe SM, Moon ES, et al. Significance of laboratory and radiologic findings for differentiating between septic arthritis and transient synovitis of the hip. *J Pediatr Orthop.* 2003;23(3):368-372.
12. Myers MT, Thompson GH. Imaging the child with a limp. *Pediatr Clin North Am.* 1997;44(3):637-658.
13. Early SD, Kay RM, Tolo VT. Childhood diskitis. *J Am Acad Orthop Surg.* 2003;11(6):413-420.
14. Ferguson LP, Beattie TF. Lesson of the week: osteomyelitis in the well looking afebrile child. *BMJ.* 2002;324(7350): 1380-1381.
15. Wang CL, Wang SM, Yang YJ, et al. Septic arthritis in children: relationship of causative pathogens, complications, and outcome. *J Microbiol Immunol Infect.* 2003; 36(1):41-46.
16. Unkila-Kallio L, Kallio MJ, Eskola J, et al. Serum C-reactive protein, erythrocyte sedimentation rate, and white blood cell count in acute hematogenous osteomyelitis of children. *Pediatrics.* 1994;93(1):59-62.
17. Waters E. Toxic synovitis of the hip in children. *Nurse Pract.* 1995;20(4):44-46, 48, 51.
18. Sharma S, Sherry DD. Joint distribution at presentation in children with pauciarticular arthritis. *J Pediatr.* 1999; 134(5):642-643.
19. Thompson GH. Gait Disturbances. In: Kliegman RM, Nieder ML, Super DM, eds. *Practical Strategies of Pediatric Diagnosis and Therapy.* Philadelphia, PA: WB Saunders; 1996.
20. Causey AL, Smith ER, Donaldson JJ, et al. Missed slipped capital femoral epiphysis: illustrative cases and a review. *J Emerg Med.* 1995;13(2):175-189.
21. Katz DA. Slipped capital femoral epiphysis: the importance of early diagnosis. *Pediatric Ann.* 2006;35(2): 102-111.

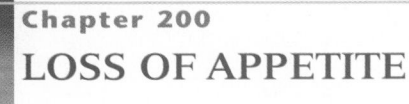

Chapter 200

LOSS OF APPETITE

Martin H. Ulshen, MD

Loss of appetite (anorexia) is a common symptom in children. Acute illness in childhood is often associated with transient loss of appetite. Prolonged loss of appetite associated with poor weight gain or loss of weight usually signifies a serious chronic illness, either organic or psychogenic.

PATHOPHYSIOLOGICAL FEATURES

The mechanisms that regulate hunger and satiety are complex and redundant, remaining incompletely understood.[1-3] Appetite is regulated by the hypothalamus, which includes the *satiety center* in the ventromedial hypothalamus and the *feeding center* in the lateral hypothalamus. Central control of appetite is influenced by anticipation of a pleasurable meal, visual and taste sensations, ambient temperature, and changes in blood levels of glucose or other nutrients, as well as by limbic signals from higher central nervous system (CNS) regions. Initiators of satiety include vagal input from gastric distention, cholecystokinin from the intestine and CNS, and other humoral factors, including insulin, glucagon, and endorphins. Each individual may have a set point for body fat content. Deviations may cause alterations in diet intake, a process apparently mediated by the interaction of the hormones leptin, produced in adipose cells, and ghrelin, produced by endocrine cells in the stomach and gastrointestinal tract, with receptors in the hypothalamus.[4,5] Leptin suppresses and ghrelin stimulates appetite. Changes in the levels of these hormones influence the release of CNS neuropeptides, including neuropeptide Y, melanocyte-stimulating hormone, and the orexins.

Cytokines are key mediators of the appetite suppression that occurs with acute and chronic illnesses.[6,7] Beta-interleukin-1 and tumor necrosis factor-α, for example, both have been shown to induce anorexia by acting directly on the hypothalamus. Effects on the peripheral nervous system and on hormone levels occur as well.

DIFFERENTIAL DIAGNOSIS

When considering anorexia, the physician must first separate complaints based on unrealistic parental dietary expectations from justified parental concern over a child's diminished nutritional intake. In the former situation, the child is typically growing well and appropriately thriving. Although significant gastrointestinal disease commonly leads to poor appetite, anorexia may be the result of disease that is distant from the bowel. In the newborn period, poor oral intake by an infant who is developmentally capable of feeding may be the first indication of a major disorder, such as sepsis, meningitis, urinary tract infection, congenital viral infection, a gastrointestinal anomaly, CNS disease, renal failure, or an inborn error of metabolism.

During infancy, a wide spectrum of causes can account for inadequate caloric intake. An acute infectious disease is a common cause of transient anorexia in infants. If no obvious explanation exists for poor feeding, then the practitioner should always consider the possibility of an oral disease (eg, thrush), gastroesophageal reflux disease, eosinophilic esophagitis, renal tubular acidosis, dietary protein intolerance, or a neurologic disorder. Occasionally, an infant will lack interest in feeding from the first days of life but in every other respect will appear normal; such an infant may well need enteral feeding supplementation.[8] Emotional deprivation is a common cause of failure to thrive; a thorough social history is essential to the evaluation. Early observation of parent-infant interaction in the hospital, including feeding techniques, may be helpful. An infant who has not received oral feedings for a prolonged period because of medical problems (eg, esophageal disease, short-bowel syndrome) may not be interested when feedings are introduced by mouth. The mother and infant may require training (typically provided by a occupational therapist, physical

BOX 200-1 Causes of Decreased Appetite in Infants and Children

ORGANIC DISEASE

- Infections (acute or chronic)
- Neurologic causes
  - Cerebral palsy (see Chapter 245)
  - Congenital degenerative disease (eg, neurodegenerative disorders, spinomuscular atrophy, muscular dystrophy)
  - Hypothalamic lesion
  - Increased intracranial pressure, including a brain tumor
  - Static encephalopathy
- Gastrointestinal causes
  - Oral or esophageal lesions (eg, thrush, herpes simplex)
  - Gastroesophageal reflux
  - Eosinophilic esophagitis
  - Dietary protein intolerance
  - Bowel obstruction (especially with gastric or intestinal distention)
  - Inflammatory bowel disease
  - Celiac disease
  - Constipation
  - Esophageal motility disorder (eg, cricopharyngeal dysfunction, achalasia, connective tissue disorder)
- Cardiac causes
  - Congestive heart failure or cyanotic heart disease
- Metabolic causes
  - Renal failure, renal tubular acidosis, or both
  - Liver failure
  - Inborn errors of metabolism
  - Lead poisoning
- Nutritional causes
  - Marasmus
  - Iron deficiency
  - Zinc deficiency
- Drugs
  - Morphine
  - Digitalis
  - Antimetabolites
  - Methylphenidate
  - Amphetamines
- Miscellaneous
  - Prolonged restriction of oral feedings, beginning in the neonatal period
  - Tumor
  - Chronic febrile conditions (eg, rheumatoid arthritis, rheumatic fever)

PSYCHOLOGICAL FACTORS

- Anxiety, fear, depression, mania (limbic influence on the hypothalamus)
- Avoidance of symptoms associated with meals (abdominal pain, nausea, diarrhea, bloating, urgency, dumping syndrome)
- Anorexia nervosa (see Chapter 135)
- Excessive weight loss and food aversion in athletes, simulating anorexia nervosa

therapist, or speech pathologist) and gradual advancement of an oral diet.

Box 200-1 presents a list of causes of loss of appetite that are applicable to both infants and children. Generally, the best approach to anorexia is to treat the underlying condition.

EVALUATION

In infants, a state of chronically inadequate caloric intake can be identified objectively by computing the total calories ingested, most of which come from formula, and comparing this total with the estimated caloric requirements for weight. Such computation is more difficult with breastfed infants compared with bottle-fed infants, although intake may be established by weighing the infant before and after feedings. If the nursing infant has a reduced intake, then the physician must establish whether maternal milk production is inadequate or the infant is too weak or disinterested to nurse.

In older children and adolescents, an adequate evaluation of nutritional intake requires careful calorie counts. If the possibility of malabsorption is a concern, then a calorie count and 72-hour stool collection for fat analysis may be ordered. Separating children who have poor appetites from children who do not eat for fear of worsening their symptoms is important from the outset. Children with abdominal pain from chronic inflammatory bowel disease or chronic constipation may not eat because doing so increases their pain. Similarly, children with chronic diarrhea may find that eating less leads to less frequent stooling. These children may actually not have anorexia, and treatment aimed at improving the other symptoms may result in rapid improvement in appetite.

TREATMENT

Enlisting the help of a dietitian to plan diets can be useful for maximizing nutritional intake in older children. Nutritional supplements may be indicated, either high-calorie milkshakes or commercial high-calorie supplements. Several medications, including cyproheptadine and megestrol acetate, have been shown to stimulate appetite. Although cyproheptadine does not seem to affect appetite in all children treated, when successful, the response is dramatic.[9] Megestrol acetate, a progesterone derivative, has been administered for cancer-related anorexia, primarily in adults.[7] Its potential side effects on the endocrine system include adrenal insufficiency. Weight gained with megestrol acetate may be, to a large extent, from increased fat mass. In some disorders, such as congenital heart disease, initial nasogastric or nasoduodenal infusion of nutrients may be necessary to promote growth.[10] If prolonged supplementation proves necessary, then a gastrostomy tube can be placed. Parenteral nutrition may be indicated in specific situations. However, expertise with this modality and close supervision are required, and caretakers need special training if the parenteral nutrition is to be provided at home. Refeeding after severe malnutrition requires careful consideration of potential cardiac and metabolic complications.[11]

WHEN TO REFER

- Loss of appetite without an obvious explanation, especially in association with weight loss or failure to thrive
- Anorexia nervosa (see Chapter 135, Anorexia and Bulimia Nervosa)

WHEN TO ADMIT

- Weight loss or lack of weight gain that is unresponsive to outpatient management
- Requirement to initiate enteral or parenteral feeding because of inadequate oral intake

REFERENCES

1. Woods SC, Seeley RJ, Porte D, et al. Signals that regulate food intake and energy homeostasis. *Science.* 1998;280: 1378-1383.
2. Plata-Salaman C. Regulation of hunger and satiety in man. *Dig Dis Sci.* 1991;9:253-568.
3. Andrews PLR. Vomiting: a gastro-intestinal defensive reflex. In: Andrews PLR, Widdicome JG, eds. *Pathophysiology of the Gut and Airways.* London, UK: Physiological Society (Portland Press);1993.
4. Auwerx J, Staels B. Leptin. *Lancet.* 1998;351:737-742.
5. Zigman JM, Elmquist JK. Minireview: from anorexia to obesity—the yin and yang of body weight control. *Endocrinology.* 2003;144(9):3749-3756.
6. Konsman JP, Dantzer R. How the immune and nervous systems interact during disease-associated anorexia. *Nutrition.* 2001;17(7-8):664-668.
7. Plata-Salaman CR. Cytokines and anorexia: a brief overview. *Semin Oncol* 1998;25(1):66.
8. Lichtman SN, Maynor A, Rhoads JM. Failure to imbibe in otherwise normal infants. *J Pediatr Gastroenterol Nutr.* 2000;30(4):467-470.
9. Homnick DN, Marks JH, Hare KL, et al. Long-term trial of cyproheptadine as an appetite stimulant in cystic fibrosis. *Pediatric Pulmonology.* 2005;40(3):251-256.
10. Vanderhoof JA, Hofschire PJ, Baluff MA, et al. Continuous enteral feedings: an important adjunct to the management of complex congenital heart disease. *Am J Dis Child.* 1982;136:825.
11. Solomon SM, Kirby DF. The refeeding syndrome: a review. *J Parenter Enteral Nutr.* 1990;14:90.

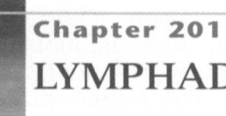

Chapter 201 LYMPHADENOPATHY

George B. Segel, MD; Caroline Breese Hall, MD

Enlargement of 1 or more lymph nodes is a common finding in childhood. Lymphadenopathy may be defined as any lymph node enlargement; all lymph nodes that are palpable are technically considered as enlarged. However, nodes in the cervical chain, occipital, and inguinal areas drain regions that are commonly infected in childhood and are often mildly enlarged (less than 1 cm in diameter) in children who are otherwise healthy.

The clinically relevant problems in assessing lymphadenopathy are (1) whether any lymph node or lymph node aggregate or chain is abnormal and requires further assessment, (2) if abnormal, whether the nodes are benign, primarily inflammatory, or malignant, and (3) what the appropriate evaluation, diagnosis, and management should be.

CHARACTERISTICS OF LYMPH NODE ENLARGEMENT

Components of the Lymphatic System

The lymphatic system includes not only lymph nodes, but also the spleen, thymus, tonsils, Waldeyer ring, appendix, and Peyer patches in the intestine. Potentially palpable lymph node groups and their drainage

Table 201-1 Correlations Between Lymph Node Locations and Disease Origin

LYMPH NODE GROUPS	AREA OF DRAINAGE
Occipital	Posterior scalp, neck
Anterior auricular, parotid	Lateral pinna, frontotemporal, eyelids
Posterior auricular	Mastoid area and pinna
Superior (anterior) cervical	Posterior scalp and neck, tongue, pharynx, larynx
Inferior (posterior) cervical	Posterior scalp, neck, pectorals, and arm
Submental	Apex of tongue and lower lip
Submaxillary	Tongue, buccal cavity, lips, and cheek
Supraclavicular	*Right:* Inferior neck and mediastinum
	Left: Inferior neck, mediastinum, and upper abdomen
Mediastinal, hilar	*Anterior:* Thymus, pericardium
	Posterior: Esophagus, pericardium, liver surface
	Hilar: Lungs
Axillary	Greater part of arm and shoulder; superficial, anterior, and lateral thoracic and upper abdominal wall
Epitrochlear	Hand, forearm, and elbow
Abdominal	Abdominal organs to various mesenteric nodes and to retroperitoneal nodes
Inguinal, femoral	Leg and genitalia

Modified from Perkins SL, et al. Work-up of lymphadenopathy in children. *Semin Diagn Pathol* 1995;12:284-287.

areas are listed in Table 201-1. The location of the lymphatics of the head and neck and lymph node drainage are shown in Figure 201-1 and may serve as a guide to palpation of these superficial nodes.

Lymph Node Features

Abnormalities of the palpable lymph nodes are assessed by noting the node's size, location, mobility, tenderness, erythema (inflammatory reaction), and consistency and whether it is matted. Nodes smaller than 1 cm are often found in the cervical chain and in the femoral areas. They are often somewhat larger in the inguinal areas. Similarly, nodes smaller than 0.5 cm may be palpated in the occipital, postauricular (mastoid), and axillary chains. Small occipital and postauricular nodes are common in infants but not older children, whereas cervical and inguinal nodes are common after age 2 years. The distribution by age is shown in Table 201-2. In the submental or submaxillary regions, intraoral or facial infections may enlarge the nodes to over 1 cm. However, finding lymph nodes of any size in the supraclavicular or epitrochlear areas is unusual. Thus lymph nodes of the same size observed in 2 different regions may have markedly different implications. For example, a 1-cm node in the cervical region of a 5-year-old child is very likely benign, whereas a 1-cm supraclavicular node requires a biopsy because it is unlikely to result from superficial inflammatory disease and may reflect intrathoracic or intraabdominal malignancy. Noninflammatory nodes greater than 2 to 2.5 cm deserve biopsy.

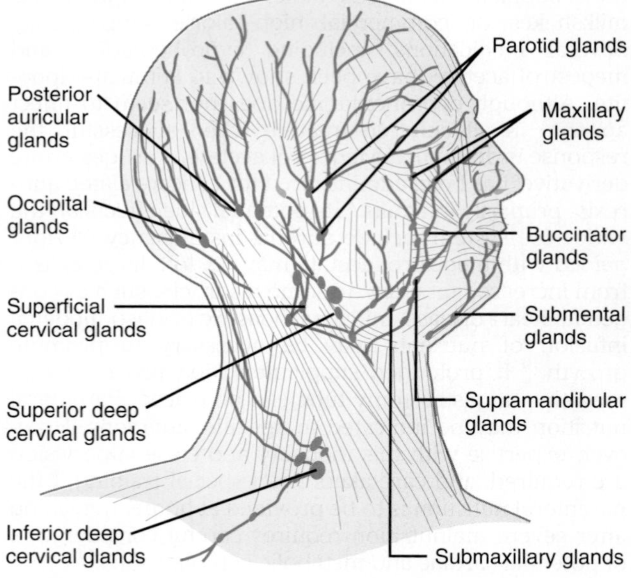

Figure 201-1 Lymph nodes and lymphatics of the head and neck. The nodes in the region below the mandible are designated *submaxillary*. (*Reproduced from* Anatomy of the Human Body by Henry Gray, *20th edition, with permission from Bartleby.com, Inc.)*

Fluctuance and signs of inflammation surrounding a group of enlarged lymph nodes are helpful in reaching a diagnosis, particularly if an infectious source is found distal to the node area. These findings strongly suggest an infectious, primarily bacterial, cause (Table 201-3), usually requiring systemic antibiotic therapy. If no inflammation is found, the consistency is firm, and the nodes are not mobile, then an underlying malignancy may be present, such as a lymphoma, sarcoma, or neuroblastoma. Hard, fixed nodes are seen more often in adults who have metastatic carcinoma. The nodes of Hodgkin disease and lymphoma are more matted than hard, although nodes associated with neuroblastoma, rhabdomyosarcoma, and other childhood malignancies may mimic the findings in adults.

Table 201-2 Prevalence of Lymphadenopathy by Age

		PALPABLE NODES									
		Occipital		Postauricular		Submandibular		Cervical		No Palpable Nodes	
AGE	NUMBER OF PATIENTS	NUMBER	(%)	NUMBER	(%)	NUMBER	(%)	NUMBER	(%)	NUMBER	(%)
0-6 mo	52	17	(32)	7	(13)	1	(2)	1	(2)	32	(62)
7-12 mo	31	8	(26)	4	(13)	1	(3)	8	(26)	16	(52)
13-23 mo	39	4	(10)	3	(7)	7	(18)	11	(28)	20	(52)
2 years	35	3	(8)	2	(6)	7	(20)	16	(45)	11	(32)
3 years	27	2	(7)	0	(0)	7	(26)	9	(33)	11	(41)
4 years	20	0	(0)	0	(0)	5	(25)	11	(55)	7	(35)
5 years	19	0	(0)	1	(5)	4	(21)	12	(63)	5	(26)
Total	223	34	(15)	17	(8)	32	(14)	68	(30)	102	(45)

Reproduced from Herzog LW. Prevalence of lymphadenopathy of the head and neck in infants and children. *Clin Pediatr.* 1983;22:485-487.

Table 201-3 Entities Associated with Lymphadenopathy

	GENERALIZED	CERVICAL	OTHER REGIONAL
INFECTIONS			
Viral			
Respiratory viruses (adenoviruses, picornaviruses, respiratory syncytial virus [RSV], parainfluenza, influenza, coronaviruses)		1–3+	
Epstein-Barr (EBV)	2–3+	3+	+
Cytomegalovirus (CMV)	2+	2+	
Primary human herpes virus type 6 (HHV-6)		+	2–3+ (postoccipital)
Parvovirus B19	1–2+		2+
Human immunodeficiency virus (HIV)	2–3+	+	+
Rubella	2+	3+	+
Rubeola	1–2+	3+	
Varicella zoster	1–2+	+	+
Herpes simplex virus (HSV)		3+	1–2+ (genital infection)
HHV-8	2–3+	2–3+	+
Hepatitis A	+	2+	
Bacterial			
Staphylococcus aureus		3+	2–3+
Streptococcal pyogenes	+	3+	2–3+
Bartonella henselae (cat-scratch disease)	+		2–3+
Bartonella bacilliformis (Oroya fever, verruga peruana)	3+	3+	3+
Yersinia enterocolitica	+		3+
Salmonella typhi	2–3+		2+
Tularemia	+	3+	2+
Brucellosis	2–3+	+	+
Anaerobic infections			
Dental, gingival infections		2–3+	2–3+
Postanginal sepsis		2–3+	
Mycobacteria			
M. tuberculosis	+	2–3+	2–3+
Atypical mycobacteria		2–3+	2–3+
Spirochetal			
Syphilis	2–3+	+	+
Lyme disease			+
Leptospirosis	3+	+	+
Rickettsia/Chlamydia			
Lymphogranuloma venereum			3+
Ehrlichiosis	2–3+		
R. tsutsugamushi	3+	2–3+	3+

Continued

Table 201-3 Entities Associated with Lymphadenopathy—cont'd

	GENERALIZED	CERVICAL	OTHER REGIONAL
Protozoan			
Toxoplasmosis	+	3+	+
Malaria	+		
Parasitic *(Toxocara canis, T. cati, Baylisascaris pyocyonis, Trichinella spiralis, filiaris)*	1–2+	+	1–2+
Myiasis		+	1–2+
Fungal			
Histoplasmosis	1–3+	+	1–2+
Coccidiomycosis	1–3+	+	1–2+
Tinea capitis			2–3+
IMMUNIZATIONS			
Viral	+		+
Typhoid	+		+
Bacille Calmette-Guérin (BCG)			1–3+
NEOPLASTIC			
Leukemia	1–2+		
Lymphoma	1–3+	2–3+	2–3+
Hodgkin's disease		2–3+	2–3+
Metastatic, solid tumors (neuroblastoma, Wilms', Ewing sarcoma, rhabdomyosarcoma)	1–2+		1–2+
HISTIOCYTOSES			
Langerhans cell histiocytosis		1–3+	
Malignant histiocytosis		1–2+	1–2+
Sinus histiocytosis (Rosai-Dorfman disease)		3+	
Hemophagocytic syndromes	1–2+	2+	
IMMUNOLOGIC			
Deficiency syndromes	1–2+	1–2+	2–3+
Autoimmune lymphoproliferative syndrome (ALPS)	2–3+		
Serum sickness	2+	+	+
Ommen's syndrome	1–2+	+	+
Juvenile rheumatoid arthritis	1–2+	+	+
Atopic disease, eczema	2–3+	2+	2–3+
Castleman's disease	1–3+	3+	2–3+
MEDICATIONS (phenytoin and others)	1–2+		
STORAGE DISEASES (Gaucher, Niemann-Pick disease)	2–3+		1–3+
GRANULOCYTE DEFECTS			
Chronic granulomatous disease	+	1–2+	2–3+
Leukocyte adhesion deficiencies		1–3+	1–3+
Chédiak-Higashi anomaly		1–3+	1–3+
OTHER			
Kawasaki disease		2–3+	
Hemoglobinopathic conditions	+	1–2+	
Hemophilia with HIV	2–3+	+	+
Sarcoidosis	2–3+	+	1–2+
Gianotti-Crosti syndrome	3+	+	+
Necrotizing lymphadenitis (Kikuchi lymphadenitis, Fujimoto necrotizing lymphadenitis)	+	2–3+	2–3+
Insect bites		+	+
Kimura		2–3+	1–2+
Addison disease	1–2+		
Hyperthyroidism	1–3+		

DIFFERENTIAL DIAGNOSIS

The major differential diagnostic categories for enlarged lymph nodes include infectious (inflammatory), neoplastic, immunologic, storage, and other diseases. Table 201-3 provides a summary of the common and unusual conditions associated with lymphadenopathy.

Infections

Infectious problems may be localized or systemic. If localized, the primary site of infection draining to the involved lymph node area should be identified (see Table 201-1). Lymph nodes enlarge most often in reaction to a localized or generalized infection, but a node

BOX 201-1 Anatomic Locations of Mediastinal Masses

ANTERIOR MEDIASTINUM	MIDDLE MEDIASTINUM
Lymphoma	Lymphoma
Thymoma	Tuberculosis
Malignant germ cell tumor	Sarcoidosis
	Histoplasmosis
Benign teratoma	Castleman disease
Substernal goiter	Bronchogenic cyst
Thymic hyperplasia	Sarcoma
Thymic cyst	
Mesenchymal tumors	
POSTERIOR MEDIASTINUM	
Neuroblastoma	Sarcoma
Ganglioneuroma	Germ cell tumor
Neurofibroma	Schwannoma
Primitive neuroectodermal tumor	Duplication cyst

From Twist CJ, Link MP. Assessment of lymphadenopathy in children. *Pediatr Clin North Am.* 2002;49(5):1019-1025. Copyright © 2002, Elsevier, with permission.

can itself become intrinsically infected, resulting in lymphadenitis.

The common pyogenic bacteria, atypical mycobacteria, anaerobic bacteria, and *Bartonella henselae* (cat-scratch disease) are most likely to cause localized adenopathy. Generalized adenopathy or regional adenopathy associated with adenopathy elsewhere is more likely caused by infections from viruses, spirochetes, or, sometimes, *Toxoplasma*. *Mycobacterium tuberculosis* may produce localized or multiple sites of adenitis. Fungal infections, such as histoplasmosis, occasionally cause generalized lymphadenopathy when disseminated, but most fungal infections, if associated with adenopathy at all, produce regional enlargement.

Neoplastic Diseases

Primary neoplastic diseases are the other major consideration in both localized and generalized adenopathy. Included in this category are lymphomas, leukemia, histiocytosis, and metastases from solid tumors such as neuroblastoma, Wilms tumor, Ewing sarcoma, and rhabdomyosarcoma. If a mediastinal mass is identified, then the diagnostic considerations vary with the anatomic location within the mediastinum (Box 201-1).

Immunologic and Inflammatory Diseases

Generalized lymphadenopathy also may be associated with chronic inflammatory conditions, such as juvenile rheumatoid arthritis, other autoimmune diseases and sarcoidosis, with reactions to certain drugs such as phenytoin and isoniazid, or with serum sickness. Unusual causes such as hyperthyroidism and Addison disease also should be included in the differential diagnosis of generalized adenopathy.

ASSESSMENT

History, Physical Examination, and Chest Imaging

The history and physical examination may reveal a source of a localized infection, such as a dental abscess, mastoiditis, scalp infection, insect bite, or cat scratch. Alternatively, systemic diseases such as infectious mononucleosis, juvenile rheumatoid arthritis, and infection with the human immunodeficiency virus, may be suggested by other characteristic historical and physical findings. The physical examination should include all the palpable nodes (see Table 201-1). Furthermore, assessment of enlarged lymph nodes that have no obvious inflammatory explanation requires a chest radiograph or computed tomographic (CT) scan to determine whether enlarged mediastinal or hilar nodes are present. The chest radiograph is the study most commonly omitted in evaluating patients who have lymphadenopathy and are referred to our center. The identification of mediastinal or hilar adenopathy would preclude trials of antibiotics, which often delay a diagnostic biopsy.

Imaging

The abdominal lymph nodes, including retroperitoneal, periportal, and celiac nodes, as well as the nodes of the splenic hilum, are difficult to evaluate without more sophisticated imaging techniques. The spleen, which is primarily lymphoid tissue, may be enlarged in infectious, immunologic, and neoplastic disorders and may be delineated by ultrasound or CT examination. Abdominal and pelvic lymph nodes may be visualized by ultrasonography or may require techniques such as CT and magnetic resonance imaging. The sensitivity and specificity of methods to define chest (mediastinal or hilar) lymphadenopathy are variable. In 1 study of patients thought to have tuberculosis, the chest x-ray was 67% sensitive and 59% specific compared with spiral chest CT with contrast. Newer techniques include positron emission tomography and scintigraphy.

Complete Blood Count and Acute Phase Reactants

The complete blood count may reveal the reactive lymphocytes of infectious mononucleosis or a granulocytosis with a shift to the left, suggesting systemic bacterial infection. Bicytopenia (eg, anemia, granulocytopenia, and/or thrombocytopenia) would be a red flag that a hematologic malignancy, such as leukemia or lymphoma, or metastatic disease involving the bone marrow such as neuroblastoma, may underlie the lymphadenopathy. The finding of nucleated erythrocytes and immature granulocytes (leukoerythroblastic blood picture) on the blood film is an ominous sign suggesting bone marrow irritation, with premature release of blood cell precursors. This finding may be seen in metastatic diseases such as neuroblastoma and rhabdomyosarcoma, with immunologic vasculitis and with granulomas (mycobacteria) in the marrow. Isolated leukopenia and neutropenia may also be seen with viral infections or severe bacterial infections (particularly in infants). Other studies may be useful in assessing lymphadenopathy, including C-reactive protein or erythrocyte sedimentation rate that detect a systemic inflammatory

Table 201-4 Evaluation of Lymphadenopathy

History	Exposures	
	Medications	
	Weight loss	
	Fevers	
	Night sweats	
	Bone pain	
Physical examination	Palpable node areas	
	Tonsils	
	Spleen and liver	
Imaging	Chest x-ray	
	Ultrasound—abdomen and pelvis	
	Possibly computed tomography, magnetic resonance imaging, nucleotide, or positron emission tomographic scanning	
Laboratory	*Neoplasia:*	
	Complete blood count with differential count and blood smear	
	Sedimentation rate, C-reactive protein	
	Uric acid, phosphate, lactate dehydrogenase	
	Catecholamines, vanillylmandelic acid, homovanillic acid	
	Infections (common):	
	General:	
	Complete blood count with differential count	
	Sedimentation rate, C-reactive protein	
	Gram stain of exudate	
	Specific:	
	Viral, respiratory:	Rapid antigen screening, polymerase chain reaction, histochemical, serology, and culture
	Epstein-Barr virus (EBV)	
	Cytomegalovirus (CMV)	
	Human immunodeficiency (HIV)	
	Cat-scratch disease	
	Bacterial:	Skin test, rapid antigen screening, histochemical, serology, and culture
	Staphylococcus aureus	
	Anaerobes	
	Streptococcus (group A)	
	Mycobacterium (purified protein derivative [PPD])	
	Atypical mycobacterium (PPD)	
	Collagen-vascular:	
	Antinuclear antibody	
	Antidouble-stranded DNA	
	Serum ferritin	
Surgery	*Biopsy*:*	
	Histology, cytochemistry, flow cytometry, DNA studies, chromosomes	
	Needle aspiration:	
	Reserved for surgically inaccessible nodes	
	Requires skilled cytopathologist	

*Requires the availability of pediatric pathology.

reaction and may reflect infection, vasculitis, or neoplasm.

Infectious Evaluation

The diagnostic workup of potential infectious lymphadenopathy is diverse and depends on the history, the patient's age, the location of the nodes whether cervical, localized or generalized, and the signs of inflammation accompanying the adenopathy. The cause of acute, inflamed, and localized adenopathy is often infectious and likely to be bacterial. Intradermal skin tests should be applied when mycobacterial infection is thought to be present. Material should be obtained for culture and histologic or pathologic examination when possible, particularly in patients who do not respond to initial therapy. In children who have acute cervical adenitis, needle aspiration of an acutely inflamed, sometimes fluctuant, node demonstrates the infecting organism in two thirds or more of cases. In certain cases, a biopsy may be required. If tuberculosis is thought to be present, then needle aspiration should be avoided to prevent spread of the infection; excisional biopsy is required. The material obtained from biopsy or aspiration should be cultured aerobically and anaerobically, examined histologically, including special stains such as that for cat-scratch disease (Worthin-Stern-Silver stain). Specific diagnosis by serologic assessment, antigen detection, by polymerase chain reaction, as well as culture is available for most of the common agents causing lymphadenopathy in children (see specific chapter for agents listed in Table 201-3). The erythrocyte sedimentation rate test or the C-reactive protein test may be useful in assessing underlying inflammation, but both are not unique to infectious diseases because they may be elevated in immunologic and neoplastic diseases as well.

After initial evaluation by history, physical examination, chest radiograph, and preliminary laboratory studies, the clinician may not yet have an obvious explanation for the node enlargement. If a bacterial source for localized adenopathy (eg, pharyngitis, cervical nodes) is suggested, then a limited course of 7 to 10 days of antibiotic therapy may be tried. However, if the nodes have not regressed significantly, then prompt further evaluation is necessary. At this time, a chest radiograph should be obtained, if it has not already been performed. Hilar or mediastinal adenopathy requires prompt assessment of neoplastic or granulomatous causes. Even in the absence of mediastinal or hilar adenopathy, significantly enlarged, unexplained lymph nodes should be biopsied promptly to permit institution of appropriate therapy.

Biopsy

Biopsy of significant adenopathy should be performed early if no evidence of infection or other cause exists and particularly if mediastinal or hilar nodes are enlarged. The biopsy should encompass the central mass of the enlarged nodes so that a misdiagnosis of reactive inflammation in adjacent nodes can be avoided. This circumstance is particularly common in Hodgkin disease in which an adjacent smaller lymph node may be more accessible and technically easier to biopsy but may not demonstrate the presence of Reed-Sternberg cells. Fine-needle aspiration is not recommended for biopsy of superficial, accessible nodes, although it might be useful for intrathoracic nodes to avoid thoracotomy. Appropriate expertise is required for interpretation, and negative findings are not definitive.

Mediastinal adenopathy may be associated with airway or vascular obstruction (superior vena cava syndrome) presenting a critical risk if anesthesia or sedation is administered and a major dilemma in establishing a diagnosis.

Any biopsy should be performed at a medical center that specializes in the care of children so that all appropriate touch preparations, cultures, special cytochemical, or immunologic stains, flow cytometry, and biochemical, cytogenetic and DNA studies are obtained. The pathology of Hodgkin disease, lymphoma, and other similar round-cell tumors may be difficult to establish and requires the assessment of a pediatric pathologist who has experience in these diseases. Immunophenotyping, cytogenetic analysis, molecular studies of gene rearrangement, and electron microscopy may be required for precise diagnosis. These studies in conjunction with the histopathologic assessment are central to the assessment and subsequent management, which may involve complex treatment with surgery, radiation, chemotherapy, or immunotherapy.

TREATMENT

Infectious Diseases (Details of Treatment—See Specific Organism)

Therapy of lymphadenitis depends on determining its cause or the most likely cause. Acute adenitis, particularly of the cervical area in young children, is frequently associated with infection from group A beta-hemolytic streptococci or *Staphylococcus aureus*. The latter is particularly likely in adenitis that progresses to fluctuance. In the neonate and rarely in older children, group B streptococci may cause localized adenitis with or without cellulitis. In children beyond the neonatal period who have acute localized adenitis, particularly cervical adenitis, therapy should be initiated with an antibiotic directed at group A streptococci and penicillinase-producing strains of *S aureus*. Recently, infections with community-acquired methicillin-resistant *S aureus* in some areas have increased dramatically in children with skin and localized infections. In such circumstances, treatment should include an antibiotic to cover methicillin-resistant *S aureus*.[1] For most patients, oral therapy is adequate.

The usual course of therapy is 10 to 14 days, but therapy should be continued for at least 5 days after the signs of acute inflammation have subsided. For patients who have suppurative adenitis from these organisms, drainage is not only diagnostic (by culturing the exudate obtained), but also therapeutic. A few patients may not respond to oral therapy, even with a drug to which the organism is sensitive. Parenteral antibiotic therapy then is required.

If an anaerobic infection is thought to be present, then therapy depends, in part, on the location of the adenitis and the type of organism. Most anaerobic infections of the cervical and submental areas are associated with mouth flora, most of which are sensitive to penicillin. Occasionally, however, such infections require alternative therapy such as clindamycin, amoxicillin-clavulanate, metronidazole, or some cephalosporins.

Both *M tuberculosis* and atypical mycobacteria can cause adenitis, with the latter being more frequent in children. Differentiating the two may be difficult but is important because many strains of atypical mycobacteria are resistant to the usual antitubercular chemotherapy, and excisional biopsy may be required. If tubercular infection is thought to be present, then appropriate therapy for *M tuberculosis* should be initiated while awaiting identification and sensitivities of the organism. Adenitis that is thought to be tubercular should not be incised or drained.

Cat-scratch adenitis is usually self-limited. The discovery of *Bartonella* species, especially *B henselae*, as the prime cause of cat-scratch disease, has raised the possibility for specific antibiotic therapy, and some antibiotics alone or combined, including azithromycin, erythromycin, rifampin, trimethoprim-sulfamethoxazole, and doxycycline, as well as with parenteral aminoglycosides may be of clinical benefit.[2-4] If nodes become markedly enlarged, tender, and fluctuant, then aspiration may help relieve symptoms; incision and drainage, however, should be avoided.[2-4]

For the unusual case of severe primary herpes simplex virus infection with localized adenitis, treatment with oral acyclovir has shortened the clinical course.[5,6]

Neoplastic Disease

The treatment of neoplastic diseases today is, in most instances, oriented toward cure, with the effectiveness of therapy for lymphocytic and myelocytic leukemia, lymphomas, and Wilms and other tumors having improved markedly. The specific treatment of childhood cancer often involves combinations of chemotherapy, radiation therapy, and surgery, all of which depend on the individual diagnosis and are beyond the scope of this presentation (see Chapter 244, Cancers in Childhood). However, prompt, accurate diagnosis is essential for instituting specific treatment and optimal care of these patients.

WHEN TO REFER

- When history and physical examination do not suggest an infectious cause
- When potentially infectious nodes have not responded to a course of antibiotics
- When mediastinal or hilar adenopathy is present
- When a biopsy is considered; biopsies should be performed only at a center specializing in the care of children

WHEN TO ADMIT

- When biopsy requires hospitalization—for example, mediastinal or hilar biopsy
- When biopsy results require inpatient treatment or further evaluation
- When an infection requires intravenous therapy

SUGGESTED RESOURCES

Journal articles

Choi TS, Doh KS, Kim SH, et al. Clinical and laboratory investigations. Clinicopathological and genotypic aspects of anticonvulsant-induced pseudolymphoma syndrome. *Br J Dermatol*. 2003:148:730-736.

Greiner T, Armitage JO, Gross TG. Atypical lymphoproliferative diseases. *Hematology*. 2000:133-146.

Hazra R, Robson CD, Perez-Atayde AR, et al. Lymphadenitis due to nontuberculous mycobacteria in children: presentation and response to therapy. *Clin Infect Dis*. 1999;28:123-129.

Leung AK, Robson WL. Childhood cervical lymphadenopathy. *J Pediatr Health Care*. 2004;18:3-7.

Nield LS, Kamat D. Lymphadenopathy in children: when and how to evaluate. *Clin Pediatr*. 2004:43:25-33.

Swingler GH, du Toit G, Andronikou S, et al. Diagnostic accuracy of chest radiography in detecting mediastinal lymphadenopathy in suspected pulmonary tuberculosis. *Arch Dis Child*. 2005;90:1153-1156.

Twist CJ, Link MP. Assessment of lymphadenopathy in children. *Pediatr Clin North Am*. 2002;49:1009-1025.

Web site

Kanwar VS. Lymphadenopathy. Available at: www.emedicine.com/PED/topic1333.htm.

REFERENCES

1. Treatment of community-associated MRSA infections. *Med Lett Drugs Ther*. Feb 2006;48(1228):13-14.
2. Batts S, Demers DM. Spectrum and treatment of cat-scratch disease. *Pediatr Infect Dis J*. 2004;23:1161-1162.
3. American Academy of Pediatrics. Cat-scratch disease. In: Pickering LK, Baker CJ, Long SS, et al, eds. *Red Book: 2006 Report of the Committee on Infectious Diseases*. 27th ed. Elk Grove Village, IL: American Academy of Pediatrics;2006:246-247.
4. Bass JW, Freitas BC, Freitas AD, et al. Prospective randomized double blind placebo-controlled evaluation of azithromycin for treatment of cat-scratch disease. *Pediatr Infect Dis J*. 1998;17:447-452.
5. Amir J, Harel L, Smetana Z, et al. Treatment of herpes simplex gingivostomatitis with acyclovir in children: a randomised double blind placebo controlled study. *BMJ*. 1997;314:1800-1803.
6. American Academy of Pediatrics. Herpes simplex. In: Pickering LK, Baker CJ, Long SS, et al, eds. *Red Book: 2006 Report of the Committee on Infectious Diseases*. 27th ed. Elk Grove Village, IL: American Academy of Pediatrics; 2006.

Chapter 202
MACROCEPHALY

Oscar H. Purugganan, MD, MPH

DEFINITION

Macrocephaly is defined as a head circumference of more than 2 standard deviations above the mean (approximately the 97th percentile) based on age and gender.

DIFFERENTIAL DIAGNOSES

Head size is influenced by the different components that make up the cranial cavity. The most common causes of a large head in children are hydrocephalus, an enlarged brain *(megalencephaly)*, a thickened skull, and space-occupying lesions. These conditions are not mutually exclusive, and some children may have more than 1 underlying factor (Box 202-1).

Hydrocephalus

Hydrocephalus, an enlargement of the ventricular system, may be congenital (present at birth) or acquired (develops after birth). The clinical presentation is influenced by the age of onset and the underlying condition causing the hydrocephalus. An enlarging head circumference is the most obvious finding in an infant whose cranial sutures have not fused. In the older child whose sutures have fused, significant head enlargement does not occur, but other signs and symptoms of increased intracranial pressure such as headaches, vomiting, and papilledema may occur.

BOX 202-1 Causes of Macrocephaly

Hydrocephalus
- Intracranial hemorrhage
- Meningomyelocele
- Dandy Walker malformation
- Aqueductal stenosis
- Malignancy
- Intrauterine infections
- Meningitis
- Space-occupying lesions
- Benign accumulation of extracranial fluid

MEGALENCEPHALY

Megalencephaly—metabolic

Mucopolysaccharidoses
Canavan disease
Alexander disease
Glutaric aciduria

Megalencephaly—anatomic

Overgrowth syndromes
Neurocutaneous syndromes
Achondroplasia
Autism
Fragile X syndrome

Megalencephaly—idiopathic (benign)

SKULL THICKENING AND SKULL ABNORMALITIES

Thalassemia
Cleidocranial dysostosis and other skeletal disorders
Space-occupying lesions
- Vascular malformations
- Intracranial tumors
- Subdural effusion
- Subdural hematoma

Conventionally, hydrocephalus has been classified as either communicating or noncommunicating, depending on whether the connection between the ventricular system and the subarachnoid space is intact. Communicating hydrocephalus results from either the impaired absorption of cerebrospinal fluid by the arachnoid villi (from meningeal irritation caused by meningitis, trauma or malignant infiltration) or less commonly with overproduction of cerebrospinal fluid from a choroid plexus papilloma. Noncommunicating or obstructive hydrocephalus is marked by enlargement of the ventricular system proximal to the site of an obstruction. The obstruction may be an anatomic defect, such as aqueductal stenosis, or the result of a tumor, infection, or infiltrate. In many cases, however, the classification of hydrocephalus as either communicating or noncommunicating may not be clear cut; common causes of hydrocephalus, such as intraventricular hemorrhage and intrauterine infections, for example, may lead to both communicating and noncommunicating hydrocephalus.

Intraventricular hemorrhage occurs in approximately 15% of premature infants with birth weights less than 1500 g.[1] The severity of hydrocephalus is graded as follows:

- Grade I: subependymal hemorrhage
- Grade II: intraventricular hemorrhage without ventricular dilatation
- Grade III: intraventricular hemorrhage with ventricular dilatation
- Grade IV: intraventricular and intraparenchymal hemorrhage[2]

Although subtle changes in head circumference may be present, macrocephaly is not always evident in an infant with intraventricular hemorrhage. Grade III and IV hemorrhages are associated with poorer neurodevelopmental outcomes than grades I and II, with an estimated 35% and 90% of affected children, respectively, showing neurologic sequelae.[1]

Hydrocephalus with Chiari type II defect is present in 80% of children with myelomenigocele.[3] Macrocephaly is commonly the 1st manifestation of the Dandy Walker malformation, a cystic dilatation of the 4th ventricle, with hypoplasia of the cerebellar vermis and a variety of other cranial malformations.[4] Head size may be normal at birth, but acceleration in head growth is noted in the majority of children by 1 year, sometimes with prominence of the posterior part of the skull.[2]

Congenital aqueductal stenosis, which may occur sporadically or be transmitted by X-linked inheritance, causes severe hydrocephalus that may complicate labor and delivery with cephalopelvic disproportion and lead to signs and symptoms of increased intracranial pressure after birth.

A condition characterized by a benign accumulation of extracranial fluid is identified in many children with macrocephaly who have an unremarkable neurologic examination. The exact nature of the extracranial collection has not been clearly established, leading to problems with nomenclature; the condition is variously referred to as benign macrocephaly, external hydrocephalus, benign extracerebral fluid collections, benign subdural collections, and benign enlargement of the subarachnoid space.[5-7] Neuroimaging reveals an extracerebral fluid collection most evident in the prefrontal area and, in some cases, mild nonprogressive dilation of the ventricular system. The size of the brain is normal. Affected children may have normal or large head circumferences at birth. In the succeeding months, the head circumference grows to greater than the 98th percentile and then generally parallels the normal growth curves. The large head size is an isolated feature, and the affected child has an otherwise normal neurologic examination and age-appropriate development, although transient early developmental delays, especially in the 1st year of life, may be observed. The condition appears to be self-limited, with normalization of computed tomographic scan findings usually by 2½ years of age.[8] The relationship of this condition to benign megalencephaly, wherein brain is large but no extracranial fluid accumulation is present in a child who is also neurologically intact, has not been established and is not fully understood.[8,9]

Megalencephaly

Another common cause of macrocephaly is an enlargement of the brain itself. Traditionally, megalencephaly is classified as metabolic or anatomic. In metabolic megalencephaly, enlargement of the brain is caused by an inborn error of metabolism that leads to the abnormal deposition of some substrate in the brain. Most such inborn errors are autosomal-recessive disorders that produce significant developmental delays, psychomotor regression, and an enlarging head that may cross percentiles over time. The mucopolysaccharidoses, Canavan disease, and Alexander disease are examples of metabolic conditions causing macrocephaly. In Hurler syndrome, the most severe form of mucopolysaccharidoses resulting from a deficiency of α-L iduronidase, an enlarging head may be noted to cross percentiles during infancy. Coarse facial features, frontal bossing, and corneal clouding are characteristic findings of the syndrome.[10] In the infantile form of Canavan disease, a leukodystrophy that predominantly affects Ashkenazi Jews from a deficiency of aspartoacylase, macrocephaly is associated with irritability, poor visual fixation, head lag, and motor delay, which are noted in the first few months of life.[11] Alexander disease is a rare, mostly sporadic condition characterized by abundant accumulation of glial fibrillary acidic protein in Rosenthal fibers. Affected infants exhibit macrocephaly, seizures, spasticity, and developmental regression[12] (refer to Chapter 48, Recognition of Genetic-Metabolic Diseases by Clinical Diagnosis and Screening).

In anatomic megalencephaly, usually associated with neurodevelopmental impairment, the brain is abnormally large because of an increase in the size and number of its cells.[2] In overgrowth syndromes, macrocephaly is usually present at birth as part of a generalized increase in body size. In Sotos syndrome, which is associated with facial dysmorphism and neurodevelopmental deficits such as poor coordination and behavioral problems, the macrocephaly may reflect a combination of megalencephaly, ventricular enlargement, and midline anomalies.[13] Neurocutaneous syndromes such as neurofibromatosis, tuberous sclerosis, and hypomelanosis of Ito, are associated with megalencephaly in addition to characteristic skin findings, intracranial conditions, and neurodevelopmental problems.[10] In achondroplasia, megalencephaly is present in a child with short stature, shortened proximal arms and legs (rhizomelia), and dysmorphic facial features. Affected individuals usually have normal intelligence but are at risk for hydrocephalus, obstructive sleep apnea or central apnea, and spine and joint problems.[14,15] Compared with the general population, a disproportionately large number of autistic children have enlarged head circumferences.[16-21] The pattern of brain growth in some autistic children appears to be abnormal, with acceleration of head growth in early childhood,[16] with hyperplasia in cerebral gray matter and cerebral and cerebellar white matter,[17] and with a slight decrease in brain volume during adolescence.[18] How this acceleration in head growth in early childhood relates to the concomitant developmental (social and language) regression that occurs in approximately a third of autistic patients remains unclear (see Chapter 136, Autism). Fragile X syndrome is associated with a constellation of physical findings, including macrocephaly, a longish face with prominent ears, joint hyperextensibility, and enlarged testes.[10] A family history on the mother's side of mental retardation, developmental and behavioral problems, and autistic behaviors suggests the possibility of this X-linked disorder.

A child with a large head who has no significant collection of extraventricular or intraventricular fluid, a normal neurologic examination and developmental history, no signs of raised intracranial pressure, and a family history of large head sizes in normal adults can be considered to have benign or idiopathic megalencephaly.[3,22,23] Although these individuals have been thought to develop normally, recent evidence suggests they may exhibit mild neurodevelopmental dysfunction such as incoordination and visual-motor weaknesses.[9]

Other Causes of Macrocephaly

Thickening of the skull is a rare cause of macrocephaly. Children with a hemolytic anemia, such as β-thalassemia, may exhibit frontal bossing attributable to extracranial hematopoieses in their skull bones. Cleidocranial dysostosis is an autosomal disorder of abnormal bone formation characterized by delayed closure of fontanelles, widening of the head circumference, and other skeletal abnormalities.[24] Space-occupying lesions, such as an arteriovenous malformation or a brain tumor, may also produce macrocephaly. Although usually asymptomatic, subdural effusion is a complication of bacterial meningitis that may produce an enlarging head circumference, bulging anterior fontanelle, and signs of increased intracranial pressure in infants.[25]

EVALUATION

Relevant History

A review of previously measured head circumferences can ascertain whether a child has had any change in the pattern or percentiles of head circumferences over time. A large head circumference at birth presupposes a cause of prenatal origin and necessitates a detailed prenatal history. Conditions that may cause congenital macrocephaly include X-linked aqueductal stenosis and the overgrowth syndromes. An abnormally enlarging head postnatally in a child with neurodevelopmental problems is a clue to an acquired condition, such as acquired hydrocephalus or a possible metabolic disorder. The history should explore delays in the developmental milestones; regression in motor, language, and social skills; seizures; and signs of increased intracranial pressure such as lethargy, vomiting, and behavioral changes. A family history of any genetic, neurologic, and developmental condition may be a red flag for similar disorders, whereas a history of otherwise normal parents and siblings with large heads can be reassuring.

Physical Examination

The physical examination of the child with macrocephaly should focus on the following:

1. Accurate measurement of the head circumference and assessment of the pattern of head growth

2. Inspection and palpation of the skull
3. Comparison of the head circumference with other growth parameters
4. Presence or absence of dysmorphic features
5. Presence or absence of congenital abnormalities involving other organ systems
6. Thorough neurologic and developmental assessment, including a check for signs of increased intracranial pressure

Monitoring of head size must be performed periodically during health care maintenance visits. In the presence of a rapid enlargement in head circumference, more frequent monitoring, at the very least, is necessary. Measurements should be plotted on the appropriate head circumference charts. A disproportionately enlarged head in relation to height and weight may indicate a primary neurologic disorder. Measuring the size of the fontanelles and palpating sutures are important. Significant hydrocephalus in infants may produce a bulging anterior fontanelle and separation of cranial sutures, which are uncommon in anatomic megalencephaly. A vein of Galen arteriovenous malformation may produce a cranial bruit on auscultation. Because macrocephaly is a feature of many genetic syndromes, dysmorphic features and other organ involvement should be noted. Examination of the skin may reveal café au lait spots, axillary freckling, ash-leaf spots, and a whorled pattern of pigmentation that may indicate a neurocutaneous disorder. Careful neurologic examination is critical and may reveal abnormalities in muscle tone and posture, asymmetries, persistence of primitive reflexes, and hyperreflexia. Developmental assessment may reveal cognitive impairment, autistic features, learning disabilities, or behavioral difficulties.

Laboratory Testing

Metabolic testing is available to identify many of the storage diseases and is recommended in a child exhibiting developmental regression. Genetic and chromosomal testing should be done for suspected cases.

Imaging

Neuroimaging is the procedure of choice in evaluating for macrocephaly. Magnetic resonance imaging is most informative, especially to identify gray and white matter disease (eg, leukodystrophy), migration defects, hydrocephalus, and posterior fossa lesions. Computed tomographic scan can identify hydrocephalus, intracranial calcifications, and hemorrhages. For infants with open fontanelles, head ultrasound is useful in identifying intraventricular hemorrhage, hydrocephalus, and intracranial tumors. A skeletal survey may reveal bone age abnormalities in the overgrowth syndromes and radiologic abnormalities that may be present in the mucopolysaccharidoses and bone dysplasias.

Management

The management of macrocephaly is dependent on its cause. Shunting procedures are the treatment of choice for significant and progressive hydrocephalus; however, shunt infection, obstruction, and malfunction are not rare and continue to be challenges in the care of these children. In premature infants, the risk of complications is even greater; medical management with pharmacologic agents (carbonic anhydrase inhibitors or other diuretics) and serial lumbar punctures may be used as initial therapy.[26] Medical management is also used in asymptomatic or minimally symptomatic patients with slowly progressive hydrocephalus. For Dandy Walker cysts, dual shunting has been recommended to drain both the hydrocephalus and the posterior fossa cyst.[2] Children suspected to have inborn errors of metabolism should be referred for genetic evaluation, treatment, and counseling. Although the treatment for these conditions is mainly supportive and symptomatic, bone marrow transplantation and enzyme replacement therapy are promising interventions for certain disorders. Although no specific treatment is available for anatomic megalencephaly, pediatricians should be aware of the association with developmental and cognitive problems, which warrant early intervention and special education services. Serial measurement of the head circumference and clinical assessments are generally all that are needed for benign accumulation of extracranial fluid and idiopathic megalencephaly.

WHEN TO REFER

- Head circumference of more than 2 standard deviations above the mean (especially 3 standard deviations above the mean)
- Head circumference that is crossing percentiles or rapidly growing
- Dysmorphic features
- Abnormal neurologic examination
- Regression in developmental skills or significant developmental delay

WHEN TO ADMIT

- Signs of increased intracranial pressure or mental status change
- Shunt infection or malfunction

SUGGESTED RESOURCES

Alvarez LA, Maytal J, Shinnar S. Idiopathic external hydrocephalus: natural history and relationship to benign familial macrocephaly. *Pediatrics*. 1986;77(6):901-907.

Centers for Disease Control and Prevention, National Center for Health Statistics. 2000 CDC Growth Charts: United States. Available at: www.cdc.gov/growthcharts.

Fenichel GM. Disorders of cranial volume and shape. In: Fenichel GM. *Clinical Pediatric Neurology: A Signs and Symptoms Approach*. Philadelphia, PA: Elsevier Saunders; 2005.

Glass RBJ, Fernbach SK, Norton KI, et al. The infant skull: a vault of information. *Radiographics*. 2004;24:507-522.

Jones KL. *Smith's Recognizable Patterns of Human Malformation*. 6th ed. Philadelphia, PA: Elsevier Saunders, 2006.

Kuczmarski RJ, Ogden CL, Grummer-Strawn LM, et al. *2000 CDC Growth Charts: United States. Advance Data From Vital and Health Statistics; no. 314*. Hyattsville, MD: National Center for Health Statistics, 2000.

OMIM—Online Mendelian Inheritance in Man. McKusick-Nathans Institute for Genetic Medicine, Johns Hopkins University (Baltimore, MD), and National Center for Biotechnology Information, National Library of Medicine (Bethesda, MD), 2000. Available at: www.ncbi.nlm.nih.gov/omim/.

REFERENCES

1. Volpe JJ. Intracranial hemorrhage: germinal matrix—intraventricular hemorrhage of the premature infant. In: Volpe JJ. *Neurology of the Newborn*. 4th ed. Philadelphia, PA: WB Saunders; 2001.
2. Fenichel GM. Disorders of cranial volume and shape. In: Fenichel GM. *Clinical Pediatric Neurology: A Signs and Symptoms Approach*. Philadelphia, PA: Elsevier Saunders; 2005.
3. DeMyer W. Microcephaly, microencephaly, megalocephaly and megalencephaly. In: Swaiman KE and Ashwal S, eds. *Pediatric Neurology: Principles and Practice*. 3rd ed. St Louis, MO: Mosby; 1999.
4. Has R, Ermis H, Yuksel A, et al. Dandy Walker malformation: a review of 78 cases diagnosed by prenatal sonography. *Fetal Diagn Ther.* 2004;19:342-347.
5. Hamza M, Bodensteiner JB, Noorani PA, et al. Benign extracerebral fluid collections: a cause of macrocrania in infancy. *Pediatr Neurol.* 1987;3(4):218-221.
6. Alper G, Ekinci G, Yilmaz Y, et al. Magnetic resonance imaging characteristics of benign macrocephaly in children. *J Child Neurol.* 1999;14(10):678-682.
7. Bodensteiner JB. Benign macrocephaly: a common cause of big heads in the first year. *J Child Neurol.* 1999;14(10): 678-682.
8. Alvarez LA, Maytal J, Shinnar S. Idiopathic external hydrocephalus: natural history and relationship to benign familial macrocephaly. *Pediatrics.* 1986;77(6):901-907.
9. Sandler AD, Knudsen MW, Brown TT, et al. Neurodevelopmental dysfunction among non-referred children with idiopathic megalencephaly. *J Pediatr.* 1997;131(2): 320-324.
10. Jones KL. *Smith's Recognizable Patterns of Human Malformation*. 6th ed. Philadelphia, PA: Elsevier Saunders, 2006.
11. Traeger EC, Rapin I. The clinical course of Canavan disease. *Pediatr Neurol.* 1998;18(3):207-212.
12. Gordon N. Alexander disease. *Eur Paediatr Neurol.* 2003;7:395-399.
13. Cohen MM. Mental deficiency, alterations in performance, and CNS abnormalities in overgrowth syndromes. *Am J Med Genet.* 2003;117(1):49-56.
14. Castiglia PT. Achondroplasia. *J Pediatr Health Care.*1996; 10:180-182.
15. Gordon N. The neurological complications of achondroplasia. *Brain Dev.* 2000;22:3-7.
16. Courchesne E, Carper R, Akshoomoff N. Evidence of brain overgrowth in the first year of life in autism. *JAMA.* 2003;290(3):337-344.
17. Courchesne E, Karns CM, Davis HR, et al. Unusual brain growth in early life in patients with autistic disorder: an MRI study. *Neurology.* 2001;57:245-254.
18. Aylward EH, Minshew NJ, Field K, et al. Effects of age on brain volume and head circumference in autism. *Neurology.* 2002;59(2):175-183.
19. Bolton PF, Roobool M, Allsopp L, et al. Association between infantile macrocephaly and autism spectrum disorders. *Lancet.* 2001;358:726-727.
20. Fidler DJ, Bailey JN, Smalley SL. Macrocephaly in autism and other pervasive developmental disorders. *Dev Med Child Neurol.* 2000;42:737-740.
21. Dementieva YA, Vance DD, Donnelly SL, et al. Accelerated head growth in early development of individuals with autism. *Pediatr Neurol.* 2005;32(2):102-108.
22. Day RE, Schutt WH. Normal children with large heads—benign familial megalencephaly. *Arch Dis Childhood.*1979;54:512-517.
23. Asch AJ, Myers GJ. Benign familial macrocephaly: report of a family and review of the literature. *Pediatrics.* 1976;57(4):535-539.
24. Glass RBJ, Fernbach SK, Norton KI, et al. The infant skull: a vault of information. *Radiographics.* 2004;24:507-522.
25. Behrman R, Kliegman R, Jenson H. eds. *Nelson Textbook of Pediatrics*. 17th ed. Philadelphia, PA: Saunders; 2000.
26. Garton HJ, Piatt JH. Hydrocephalus. *Pediatr Clin North Am.* 2004;51:305-325.

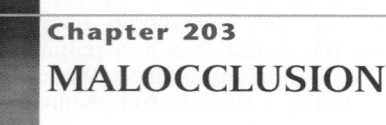

Chapter 203

MALOCCLUSION

Lindsey K. Grossman, MD

The incidence of malocclusion in school-aged children and adolescents may be as high as 90% or more, according to some reports. The 1963 to 1965 National Health and Nutrition Survey (NHANES I), which examined 7400 children 6 to 11 years of age, found 14.2% to have severe or very severe malocclusion.[1] The NHANES III survey (1988-1991) found that 15% of adults had malocclusion severe enough to affect social acceptability and function.[2] Although slightly less than 60% of all racial groups might benefit from orthodontic treatment, only 30% of white youth, 11% of Mexican Americans, and 8% of blacks report having undergone such therapy. Not surprisingly, higher-income youth are more likely to receive orthodontic care.

CLASSIFICATION

A major problem hindering objective evaluation of orthodontic treatment is the lack of a universally acceptable and quantitative classification system. The commonly used Angle classification system effectively expresses qualitative but not quantitative differences in dental occlusion; hence its use in determining the need for referral or in evaluating treatment outcome is limited.[3] Normal occlusion in the Angle system is class I, with maxillary and mandibular molars appropriately interdigitating, allowing the anterior teeth to sit in correct alignment with the maxillary incisors slightly overlapping those in the mandible, resulting in a closed bite. In a class I malocclusion, the maxillary and mandibular molars normally interdigitate, but crowding or misalignment is demonstrated in other oral positions. In a class II malocclusion, the maxillary molars are anterior to the mandibular molars, allowing the anterior teeth to appear to jut out over the lower ridge, whereas in a class III malocclusion, the reverse alignment is seen, causing the patient to have the appearance of a protruding jaw.

ETIOLOGY

Determining the cause of malocclusion is not easy, and involves both genetic and environmental factors. Only in approximately 5% of cases is a cause clearly identifiable.[4] Nasal obstruction, especially when caused by enlarged tonsils or adenoids, has been linked to the development of a high arched palate and posterior crossbite.[4,5]

Pacifiers and thumb- and finger-sucking habits[6] play a role in malocclusion problems. Most children develop such nonnutritive sucking habits during infancy. However, by 4 or 5 years of age, most have stopped the practice; and as many as 5.9% of children may continue into school age.[7] If sucking continues into the periods of mixed and permanent dentition, then the potential for developing malocclusion is increased, although a specific causal relationship may not always hold. Abnormal bites often revert to normal after the habit is stopped. Anterior open bite, excessive overjet, posterior crossbites, and other malocclusions have been reported in association with sucking habits, although other children who have such habits may show no abnormalities.[8,9] Thumb sucking may be preferable to finger sucking because fewer physical stresses are exerted on the teeth. The results of several studies of nonnutritive sucking from many countries are mixed as to the question of whether digit sucking is more or less deleterious than use of a pacifier; however, nearly all show increased incidence of malocclusion among children who have prolonged sucking habits compared with those who do not.[10] Functional exercisers such as the Nuk nipple or pacifier have no apparent advantage.[8]

REASONS TO TREAT

Significantly abnormal dental occlusion has been said to predispose individuals to many risks.[10] Dental caries, periodontal disease, increased susceptibility to trauma or root resorption, and disturbances of physiological functioning, including muscular dysfunction, speech defects, and masticatory disturbances, have been linked to malocclusion, although the data supporting such outcomes are either scanty or conflicting.[11] Temporomandibular joint (TMJ) dysfunction has been increasingly cited as a possible cause of headache and other symptoms in adolescents and school-aged children. Some studies show an amazingly high incidence of signs referable to the TMJ but usually without symptoms of TMJ dysfunction. Signs such as joint sounds with movement or condyle position do not correlate well with symptomatic TMJ dysfunction requiring treatment, especially in children. Furthermore, no convincing evidence has been found that malocclusion or orthodontic therapy has a relationship to the development of temporomandibular symptoms.[6,12,13]

ASSESSMENT

When assessing occlusion, the pediatrician should observe both the maxillary and the mandibular arches with the child's mouth open to determine if the teeth are crowded or have excess space between them.[14] Crowding almost always increases over time, whereas excess space may either improve or worsen. Excess space, especially between the upper lateral incisors and the canines and between the lower canines and the first deciduous molars, is the norm in young children who have primary dentition and allows room for the eruption of the larger, permanent teeth.

Occlusion of the posterior teeth is assessed with the teeth set in the biting position. The tongue should not be visible between the upper and lower teeth; the presence of such a space, albeit very small, or the contrasting problem of a deep bite (lower incisors biting on palatal gingiva) nearly always requires treatment. The maxillary teeth should overlap their mandibular partners slightly in the lateral plane and be placed slightly anterior (approximately one-half a tooth width) to them. Posterior crossbites where posterior maxillary teeth are either medial or lateral to the their corresponding mandibular teeth are common discrepancies that rarely self-correct. Timely treatment of such problems, during the primary or early mixed stages of dentition, is recommended for establishing optimal function to normalize dental, skeletal, and neuromuscular growth during these times of active change.[15]

Problems with the anterior dentition, readily apparent when the patient smiles, are the source of many orthodontic referrals. An open bite with space visible between the upper and lower arches, as well as underbite, are difficult to treat, whereas overbite (buck teeth) or anterior crossbite can often be corrected easily. Occasionally, 1 or more of the permanent teeth, often incisors, may erupt before the corresponding primary teeth have been shed, giving the child a double row of teeth and causing much parental concern. Extraction is rarely necessary because the primary teeth are almost always shed by age 8 years. Normal tongue movements usually ensure correct final placement of the permanent teeth.

Few data link maloccluded primary dentition with maloccluded permanent teeth. However, the presence of anterior crossbite, wherein the upper lateral incisors erupt behind the lower ones or the upper posterior teeth erupt medial to the lower ones, may interfere with ultimate maxillary growth and tooth position. The absence of normal spacing in primary dentition almost always leads to severe crowding of the permanent teeth. Children who have such conditions should be referred to an orthodontist early.[16] Considerable controversy exists over whether treatment of other abnormalities such as overbite or class III malocclusions should begin early during the period of mixed dentition or delayed until adolescence. In general, early treatment for most problems, which often requires 2 stages of treatment, increases the total amount of time the child bears braces without necessarily resulting in a superior outcome.[11,17]

Most patients seek orthodontic treatment because of malocclusion's effect on their appearance.[12] In the US, the individual's own sense of attractiveness can influence behavior and success in life. However, no direct evidence has been found that treating dental irregularities affects these outcomes positively.

Probably the most important influence pediatricians can have in promoting good dental occlusion is their advice concerning primary dentition. Congenital absence or loss of 1 or more of the primary teeth to decay or trauma can seriously affect the spacing required for normal occlusion of the permanent teeth. Thus a dental referral is advisable if any primary tooth fails to erupt or is prematurely lost.[18]

In general the decision to refer a child or young adolescent for orthodontic treatment may be difficult because objective referral guidelines are few.[19] Treatment nearly always results in an improved, although not necessarily a flawless, appearance. The pediatrician should assess the patient's and family's expectations, as well as their willingness to comply with the discomfort and cost of treatment, before arranging for referral.

WHEN TO REFER

- Posterior crossbites rarely self-correct, and treatment during the stage of primary or mixed dentition may be optimal to promote normal development of the teeth, bones, and muscular structures.
- The absence of normal dental spacing in the primary dentition requires early referral, especially if any primary tooth is lost or fails to erupt.

TOOLS FOR PRACTICE

Engaging Patient and Family

- *Thumbs, Fingers, and Pacifiers* (brochure), American Academy of Pediatrics (patiented.aap.org).

Medical Decision Support

- *A Guide to Children's Dental Health* (brochure), American Academy of Pediatrics (patiented.aap.org).
- *American Academy of Pediatric Dentistry* (Web page), American Academy of Pediatric Dentistry (www.aapd.org/).
- *American Academy of Pediatrics Oral Health Initiative* (Web page), American Academy of Pediatrics (www.aap.org/commpeds/dochs/oralhealth/pedsCare.cfm).
- *Bright Futures Oral Health Pocket Guide* (book), Bright Futures (brightfutures.aap.org/web/).
- *Oral Health Resources* (Web page), Centers for Disease Control and Prevention (www.cdc.gov/oralhealth/index.htm).

SUGGESTED RESOURCES

Dean JA, McDonald RD, Avery DR. Managing the developing occlusion. In: McDonald RE, Avery DR. *Dentistry for the Child and Adolescent*. 7th ed. St Louis, MO: Mosby; 2000.

Nowak AJ, Warren JJ. Infant oral health and oral habits. *Pediatr Clin North Am*. 2000;47:1043-1099.

Sonis A, Zaragoza S. Dental health for the pediatrician. *Curr Opin Pediatr*. 2001;13:289-295.

Vig KWL, Fields HW. Facial growth and management of orthodontic problems. *Pediatr Clin North Am*. 2000;47:1085-1125.

REFERENCES

1. Kelly JE, Sanchez M, VanKirk LE. *An Assessment of the Occlusion of Teeth of Children 6-11 Years*. NHS Series 11, No 130, Washington, DC: US Department of Health, Education and Welfare Publications, Public Health Service; 1973.
2. Profitt WR, Fields HW, Moray LJ. Prevalence of malocclusion and orthodontic treatment need in the United States: estimates from the NHANES III survey. *Int J Adult Orthod Orthognath Surg*. 1998;13:97-106.
3. Jago JD. The epidemiology of dental occlusion: a critical appraisal. *J Public Health Dent*. 1974;34:80-93.
4. Turner S, Nattrass C, Sandy JR. The role of soft tissue in the etiology of malocclusion. *Dent Update*. 1997;24:209-214.
5. Richter HJ. Obstruction of the pediatric upper airway. *Ear Nose Throat*. 1987;66:209-211.
6. McNamara JA, Seligman DA, Okeson JP. Occlusion, orthodontic treatment and temporomandibular disorders: a review. *J Orofac Pain*. 1995;9:73-90.
7. Gellin ME. Digital sucking and tongue thrusting in children. *Dent Clin North Am*. 1978;22:603-619.
8. Adair SM, Milano M, Lorenzo I, et al. Effects of current and former pacifier use on the dentition of 24- to 59-month-old children. *Pediatr Dent*. 1995;17:437-444.
9. Vanderas AP, Manetas KJ. Relationship between malocclusion and bruxism in children and adolescents: a review. *Pediatr Dent*. 1995;17:7-12.
10. Nowak AJ, Warren JJ. Infant oral health and oral habits. *Pediatr Clin North Am*. 2000;47:1043-1066.
11. Kleumper GT, Beeman CS, Hicks EP. Early orthodontic treatment: what are the imperatives? *JADA*. 2000;131:613-620.
12. Mohlin B, Kurol J. To what extent do deviations from an ideal occlusion constitute a health risk? *Swed Dent*. 2003;27:1-10.
13. Tallents RN, Catania J, Dommers B. Temporomandibular joint findings in pediatric populations and young adults: a critical review. *Angle Orthod*. 1991;61:7-16.
14. Smith RJ. Development of occlusion and malocclusion. *Ped Clin North Am*. 1982;29:475-501.
15. Zhu JF, Crevoisier R, King DL, et al. Posterior crossbites in children. *Compend Contin Educ Dent*. 1996;17:1051-1054, 1056, 1058.
16. Agapas TR. Early orthodontic treatment. *Ont Dent*. 1994;71:26-30.
17. Sonis A, Zaragoza S. Dental health for the pediatrician. *Curr Opin Pediatr*. 2001;13:289-295.
18. Schneider PB, Peterson J. Oral habits: considerations in management. *Pediatr Clin North Am*. 1982;29:523-546.
19. Currier GF. Fundamentals of orthodontics with criteria for referral. *Pediatr Ann*. 14:117, 1985.

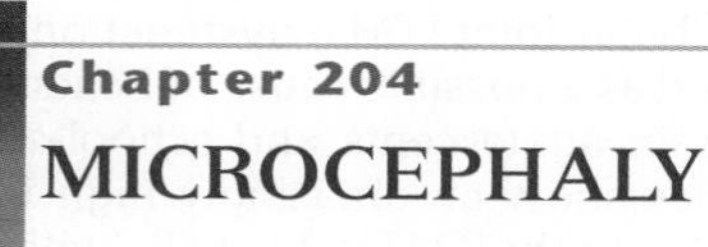

Chapter 204

MICROCEPHALY

Oscar H. Purugganan, MD, MPH

DEFINITION OF TERMS

Microcephaly refers to a head size that is 2 standard deviations below the mean (approximately the 3rd percentile) based on age and gender. In itself, microcephaly means a small head; *micrencephaly* is the accurate term for a small brain. Because the forces of brain growth generally determine ultimate cranium size, a small brain leads to a small head. Without further growth, secondary closure of the sutures of the skull will ensue before the expected time, which should be differentiated from *craniosynostosis* in which primary and premature closure of sutures occurs with a normally growing brain.[1]

Measuring the head circumference is an important element of the pediatric physical examination and should be performed at each well-child visit, especially in the 1st year of life.[2] Accurate measurements are critical and should be plotted on standardized charts. In the United States, the Centers for Disease Control and Prevention released the latest growth charts in 2000.[3,4] These charts, which include head circumference charts, were based on 5 national health surveys from 1963 to 1994 and have been updated from the 1977 growth charts. A new feature of these updated charts is the inclusion of curves for 3rd and 97th percentiles, which are important cutoffs in the measurements of head circumference. Charts are available for special populations with disturbances in growth, such as Down syndrome,[5] Williams syndrome,[6] achondroplasia,[7] and very–low-birth-weight infants.[8] Head circumferences of children older than 3 years are generally plotted on the growth curves developed by Nellhaus, which are generated from composite international standards.[9]

Head circumference is measured by using a flexible, nonstretchable tape, running along the head above the supraorbital ridges and across the most prominent part of the occiput.[10] This measurement is known as the occipitofrontal circumference and has been shown to correlate with brain volume.[11] More instructive than a single measurement is a series of measurements over time, which can identify head circumferences that may be crossing percentiles while still falling within the normal range. Brain growth is maximal during the last few weeks of gestation to the first 2 years of life. Boys possess a slightly larger head size than girls; the average head size at birth for boys in the United States is approximately 36 centimeters and for girls is approximately 35 centimeters.[3]

DIFFERENTIAL DIAGNOSIS

Microcephaly is a physical finding and not a diagnosis. A multitude of conditions exist that can lead to a small brain. A useful classification is by characterizing the cause as either genetic or environmental (Box 204-1). Some authors have termed these conditions primary microcephaly (genetic) and secondary microcephaly (environmental).[12,13] Microcephaly can also be classified as congenital (present at birth) or acquired (develops after birth), or as syndromic or nonsyndromic.

In primary microcephaly, the brain is small as a result of genetic or chromosomal factors. The brain structure may be either normal or abnormal.

In microcephaly vera, or true microcephaly, the brain is very small, usually 3 standard deviations below the mean, but the brain architecture is grossly normal.[14,15] Patients almost always have mental retardation but have an otherwise unremarkable neurologic examination. A sloping forehead and prominent ears are usually the only dysmorphic features. Transmission is mainly autosomal recessive, although autosomal-dominant and X-linked forms also exist. Three genes that cause microcephaly vera have been identified: (1) microcephalin (MCPH), (2) abnormal spindle in microcephaly[16,17] (ASPM), and (3) deoxynucleotide carrier (DNC) protein, which is implicated in Amish microcephaly.[18]

More common than microcephaly vera is a microcephalic child who has severe neurologic impairment such as seizures, spasticity, and global developmental delays. Neuroimaging may identify abnormal brain architecture such as defective prosencephalization (eg, holoprosencephaly), migration disorders (eg, lissencephaly, schizencephaly, pachygyri, polymicrogyri, heterotopias), and midline defects (eg, agenesis of corpus callosum).[14,15]

Microcephaly may be associated with other clinical findings that collectively comprise a genetic syndrome. Miller-Dieker syndrome, which is caused by a deletion in the short arm of chromosome 17, is characterized by a small smooth brain or lissencephaly (the most extreme of migration defects), facial dysmorphism, and severe mental retardation. In Seckel syndrome, a rare autosomal-recessive disorder that has been mapped to loci in chromosomes 3 and 18, central nervous system anomalies that suggest an underlying neuronal migration disorder[19] is present together with growth retardation, intellectual disability, and a *bird-headed* facial appearance.[20] Children with Rubinstein-Taybi syndrome have microcephaly, significant developmental problems, facial abnormalities, and broad thumbs and toes. Microdeletions of the cyclic adenosine monophosphate response element–binding protein gene in chromosome 16 have been implicated in this disorder.[20,21] Trisomies account for some cases of microcephaly. A classic example is Down syndrome (trisomy 21 syndrome) in which microcephaly is part of the characteristic phenotype that includes distinct facial features, congenital heart anomalies, and growth retardation. In de Lange syndrome, affected children have growth retardation, microcephaly, hirsutism, and unusual facial features such as synophrys and low anterior hairline. Most cases are

BOX 204-1 Causes of Microcephaly

GENETIC CAUSES (PRIMARY MICROCEPHALY):

- Microcephaly vera (isolated microcephaly with normal brain architecture)
- Microcephaly with abnormal brain architecture
- Genetic syndromes:
  - Miller-Dieker lissencephaly
  - Seckel syndrome
  - Rubinstein-Taybi syndrome
  - Trisomy 21 syndrome
  - Trisomy 13 syndrome
  - de Lange syndrome
  - Rett syndrome
- Asymptomatic familial

ENVIRONMENTAL CAUSES (SECONDARY MICROCEPHALY)

- Teratogens
- Intrauterine infections
- Maternal health problems
- Maternal phenylketonuria
- Intrauterine irradiation
- Hypoxic-ischemic encephalopathy
- Meningitis
- Malnutrition

sporadic, but an autosomal-dominant inheritance has been suggested. *Smith's Recognizable Patterns of Human Malformation* and the on-line reference *Online Mendelian Inheritance in Man* provide comprehensive lists of conditions that are associated with abnormalities in head size.[20,22]

Genetic microcephaly is almost always present at birth. An exception is Rett syndrome, a rare condition exhibited in girls that is associated with a deceleration in head growth leading to microcephaly, developmental regression, autistic features, and unusual hand mannerisms (hand-wringing and hand-washing movements). This genetic disorder has been mapped on the X chromosome and linked to a deletion of the *MeCP2* gene. Most cases are sporadic.[20]

Based on the definition of microcephaly, it follows that approximately 2.5% of all children would be classified as microcephalic, and, most certainly, some of these children will be neurologically normal, especially those with head sizes immediately below 2 standard deviations from the mean. (A head circumference of more than 3 standard deviations below the mean is almost always associated with some degree of neurologic impairment.) In individuals with isolated microcephaly who are neurologically intact and have normal intelligence, measuring the head circumferences of the parents and siblings is important. A family history of small head size in the context of normal development and neurologic examination describes asymptomatic familial microcephaly.[23]

Secondary microcephaly refers to a brain that had the potential to be normal but is small and abnormal as a consequence of an environmental insult; it may be present at birth or develop after birth. A small head circumference at birth often reflects a condition of early prenatal origin. Prenatal toxins[24,25] that may lead to microcephaly in the newborn are alcohol, drugs of abuse such as cocaine, and irradiation. Intrauterine infections such as cytomegalovirus, toxoplasmosis, and rubella have also been implicated in the development of microcephaly. These environmental insults affect other organ systems as well, and microcephaly may be observed as a part of a syndrome. Fetal alcohol syndrome is characterized by intrauterine growth retardation, facial features such as small palpebral fissures, smooth philtrum and thin upper lip, heart and eye defects, and behavioral and cognitive deficits. Intrauterine infections may produce intrauterine growth retardation, hepatosplenomegaly, cardiac defects, retinopathy, cataracts, and hearing loss. Untreated maternal phenylketonuria and hyperphenylalaninemia produce findings very similar to those of fetal alcohol syndrome: microcephaly (the most consistent finding), mental retardation, facial dysmorphism, and cardiac defects.[26]

Severe perinatal asphyxia is an important cause of acquired microcephaly. The asphyxiated newborn has a normal head circumference at birth, but head growth decelerates, and microcephaly and suboptimal head growth may be observed by 12 months of age.[27] Acquired microcephaly can sometimes be detected as early as 6 weeks of age in infants who have had severe asphyxia[28]; these children go on to develop significant neuromotor and cognitive deficits. Other causes of acquired microcephaly are meningitis, malnutrition, traumatic brain injury, and shaken baby syndrome.

With multiple suture craniosynostosis, primarily a problem of the skull rather than the brain, the head circumference may be small at birth or head growth may abruptly cease during infancy. The shape of the skull is asymmetric, and evidence exists of bony ridging in the area of the fused sutures. Signs of increased intracranial pressure may be present. These characteristics clearly differentiate the microcephaly associated with craniosynostosis from *micren*cephaly in which the small head is round, symmetric, smooth, and devoid of bony ridging in the area of the sutures.[1] Premature closure of sutures may be an isolated feature or a part of a syndrome. Single-suture synostoses are not likely to cause microcephaly.

EVALUATION

Relevant History

Congenital microcephaly necessitates a thorough review of the prenatal history. Any potential exposure to toxins must be explored, such as the use of alcohol or other drugs of abuse. Poor maternal health during the pregnancy, intrauterine infections, and conditions causing placental insufficiency contribute to a suboptimal uterine environment that may lead to congenital microcephaly and intrauterine growth retardation. So too do psychosocial factors, as marked by lack of prenatal care and low levels of maternal education.[29] A pedigree analysis can help identify a family history of genetic syndromes, miscarriages, or microcephaly. Taking note of the head sizes of the parents and siblings is an important component of the evaluation. A review of systems may identify medical problems such as feeding difficulties and seizures, previous infections such as meningitis, and a history of developmental regression. The history should also include a chronology of developmental milestones, as well as a description of the child's current function and behavior.

Physical Examination

The physical examination of the microcephalic child should focus on the following:

1. Accurate measurement of the head circumference and assessment of the pattern of head growth and the onset of microcephaly if previous measurements are available
2. Inspection and palpation of the skull, looking for asymmetry and bony ridging
3. Comparison of the head circumference with other growth parameters
4. Presence or absence of dysmorphic features
5. Presence or absence of congenital abnormalities involving other organ systems
6. Careful neurologic and developmental assessment

Accurate measurement and plotting on appropriate charts is critical (see earlier discussion). Head circumference of premature infants is adjusted for the degree of prematurity until approximately 2 years of age. For infants with birthweights of less than 1000 g, corrected age is often used until 3 years or when growth has caught up based on normal growth curves.[10] Inspection and palpation of the skull may reveal an asymmetric skull and face and bony ridging that are suggestive of craniosynostosis, the presence of which leads the pediatrician to a different approach in evaluation and management. A head circumference that is disproportionately small in relation to the child's weight and height is a likely indicator of a central nervous system condition. When microcephaly is part of generalized growth retardation, or when it is associated with dysmorphic facial features and multi-organ system involvement, the search for conditions that may have a more systemic effect on the child should be investigated, such as chromosomal disorders, intrauterine infections, or exposure to toxins. Children with congenital microcephaly appear to have a higher frequency of major malformations when compared with normocephalic infants.[30] A thorough neurologic examination should assess for asymmetries, abnormalities in muscle tone, posture, strength, and reflexes. A developmental assessment may reveal generalized psychomotor retardation, and motor delays, as well as speech and language and cognitive impairments.

Laboratory Testing

The laboratory evaluation should be guided by the differential diagnoses. Children who are thought to have intrauterine infections must be tested for prenatal infections (toxoplasmosis, rubella, cytomegalovirus, syphilis, HIV, herpes) and have ophthalmologic and audiologic evaluations. A microcephalic newborn with other congenital anomalies and atypical facial features should have a genetic consultation and evaluation. Genetic testing is available for many disorders, including chromosomal disorders, Miller-Dieker syndrome, and Rett syndrome.

Imaging

Several neuroimaging modalities are available to identify abnormalities in brain structure, including brain atrophy. Magnetic resonance imaging is most suitable for identifying gray and white matter disease, and migration defects such as lissencephaly, pachygyria, and polymicrogyria. However, magnetic resonance imaging is limited in its ability to study bone and calcifications. Computed tomographic scanning is useful to identify intracranial calcifications that may result from intrauterine infections, the skull abnormalities seen with premature fusion of cranial sutures, and ventricular system abnormalities. A skull radiograph can demonstrate intracranial calcifications and the characteristic bone findings in craniosynostosis but cannot detect abnormalities in brain structure. In infants with open fontanelles, ultrasonography of the head can be helpful in delineating cranial abnormalities.

MANAGEMENT

The management of microcephaly is largely symptomatic and preventive. Appropriate prenatal care, maternal education and nutrition, avoidance of teratogenic substances, screening for intrauterine infections, and management of maternal health conditions may minimize the number of preventable cases of microcephaly. Because many children with microcephaly may have other medical issues, the pediatrician should provide interventions for these conditions as needed. Children with microcephaly require close follow-up for developmental issues and the provision of early intervention and special education services as needed. Genetic counseling must be offered to parents who have offspring with genetic disorders. Children suspected to have craniosynostosis require neurosurgical consultation.

WHEN TO REFER

- Head circumference of more than 2 standard deviations below the mean (especially more than 3 standard deviations)
- Head circumference deceleration or poor head growth
- Dysmorphic features
- Abnormal neurologic examination and development
- Regression in motor, language, and social skills
- Seizures
- Suspected craniosynostosis

WHEN TO ADMIT

- Signs of increased intracranial pressure
- Mental status change

SUGGESTED RESOURCES

Centers for Disease Control and Prevention, National Center for Health Statistics. 2000 CDC Growth Charts: United States. Available at: www.cdc.gov/growthcharts.

Cohen M. Perspectives on craniosynostosis. *Am J Med Genet*. 2005;136A:313-326.

Fenichel GM. Disorders of cranial volume and shape. In: Fenichel GM. *Clinical Pediatric Neurology: A Signs and Symptoms Approach*. Philadelphia, PA: Elsevier Saunders; 2005.

Glass RBJ, Fernbach SK, Norton KI, et al. The infant skull: a vault of information. *Radiographics*. 2004;24:507-522.

Jones KL. *Smith's Recognizable Patterns of Human Malformation*. 6th ed. Philadelphia, PA: Elsevier Saunders; 2006.

Kuczmarski RJ, Ogden CL, Grummer-Strawn LM, et al. *CDC Growth Charts: United States. Advance Data From Vital and Health Statistics; no. 314*. Hyattsville, MD: National Center for Health Statistics; 2000.

Mochida GH, Walsh CA. Molecular genetics of human microcephaly. *Curr Opin Neurol*. 2001;14(2):151-156.

OMIM—Online Mendelian Inheritance in Man. McKusick-Nathans Institute for Genetic Medicine, Johns Hopkins University (Baltimore, MD), and National Center for Biotechnology Information, National Library of Medicine (Bethesda, MD), 2000. Available at: www.ncbi.nlm.nih.gov/omim/.

REFERENCES

1. Cohen MM. Perspectives on craniosynostosis. *Am J Med Genet*. 2005;136A:313-326.
2. Green M, Palfrey JS, eds. *Bright Futures: Guidelines for Health Supervision of Infants, Children, and Adolescents*. 2nd ed. rev. Arlington, VA: National Center for Education in Maternal and Child Health; 2002.
3. Kuczmarski RJ, Ogden CL, Grummer-Strawn LM, et al. *CDC Growth Charts: United States. Advance Data From Vital and Health Statistics; no. 314*. Hyattsville, MD: National Center for Health Statistics; 2000.

4. Centers for Disease Control and Prevention, National Center for Health Statistics. 2000 CDC Growth Charts: United States. Available at:www.cdc.gov/growthcharts. Accessed March 11, 2006.
5. Cronk C, Crocker AC, Pueschel SM, et al. Growth charts for children with Down syndrome: 1 month to 18 years of age. *Pediatrics*. 1988;81:102-110.
6. Williams Syndrome Association. Doctors resources for Williams syndrome. Available at: www.williams-syndrome.org. Accessed March 10, 2008.
7. Horton WA, Rotter JI, Rimoin DL, et al. Standard growth charts for achondroplasia. *J Pediatr.* 1978;93(3):435-438.
8. Sherry B, Mei Z, Grummer-Strawn L, et al. Evaluation of and recommendations for growth references for very low birth weight (<1500 grams) infants in the United States. *Pediatrics*. 2003;111(4):750-758.
9. Nellhaus G. Head circumference from birth to eighteen years: practical composite international and interracial graphs. *Pediatrics*. 1968;41:106-114.
10. US Department of Health and Human Services, Health Resources and Services Administration, Maternal and Child Health Bureau. MCHB training module: interpreting growth in head circumference. Available at: www.mchb.hrsa.gov. Accessed March 10, 2008.
11. Bray PF, Shields WD, Wolcott GJ, et al. Occipitofrontal head circumference—an accurate measure of intracranial volume. *J Pediatr.* 1969;75:303-305.
12. Fenichel GM. Disorders of cranial volume and shape. In: Fenichel GM. *Clinical Pediatric Neurology: A Signs and Symptoms Approach*. Philadelphia, PA: Elsevier Saunders; 2005.
13. Behrman R, Kliegman R, Jenson H. eds. *Nelson Textbook of Pediatrics*. 17th ed. Philadelphia, PA: Saunders; 2000.
14. Volpe J. Overview: Normal and abnormal human brain development. *Ment Retard Dev Disabil Res Rev.* 2000;6:1-5.
15. Mochida GH, Walsh CA. Molecular genetics of human microcephaly. *Curr Opin Neurol.* 2001;14(2):151-156.
16. Woods CG. Human microcephaly. *Curr Opin Neurobiol.* 2004;14:112-117.
17. Suri M. What's new in neurogenetics? Focus on "primary microcephaly". *Eur J Paediatr Neurol.* 2003;7:389-392.
18. Korf BR. What's new in neurogenetics? Amish microcephaly. *Eur J Paediatr Neurol.* 2003;7:393-394.
19. Shanske A, Caride DG, Menasse-Palmer L, et al. Central nervous system anomalies in Seckel syndrome: report of a new family and review of the literature. *Am J Med Genet.* 1997;70(2):155-158.
20. OMIM—Online Mendelian Inheritance in Man. McKusick-Nathans Institute for Genetic Medicine, Johns Hopkins University (Baltimore, MD), and National Center for Biotechnology Information, National Library of Medicine (Bethesda, MD), 2000. Available at:www.ncbi.nlm.nih.gov/omim/. Accessed January 5, 2007.
21. Breuning MH, Dauwerse HG, Fugazza G, et al. Rubinstein-Taybi syndrome caused by submicroscopic deletions within 16p13.3. *Am J Hum Genet.* 1993;52:249-254.
22. Jones KL. *Smith's Recognizable Patterns of Human Malformation*. 6th ed. Philadelphia, PA. Elsevier Saunders, 2006.
23. DeMyer W. Microcephaly, micrencephaly, megalocephaly and megalencephaly. In: Swaiman KE, Ashwal S, eds. *Pediatric Neurology: Principles and Practice*. 3rd ed. St Louis, MO: Mosby; 1999.
24. Kvigne VL, Leonardson GR, Neff-Smith M, et al. Characteristics of children who have full or incomplete fetal alcohol syndrome. *J Pediatr.* 2004;145:635-640.
25. Singer LT, Salvator A, Arendt R, et al. Effects of cocaine/polydrug exposure and maternal psychological distress of infant birth outcomes. *Neurotoxicol Teratol.* 2002;24:127-135.
26. Levy H, Ghavami M. Maternal phenylketonuria: a metabolic teratogen. *Teratology.* 1996;53:176-184.
27. Mercuri E, Ricci D, Cowan F, et al. Head growth in infants with hypoxic-ischemic encephalopathy: correlation with neonatal magnetic resonance imaging. *Pediatrics*. 2000;106:235-243.
28. Ellis M. Letter to the editor: head growth and cranial assessment at neurological examination in infancy. *Dev Med Child Neurol.* 2003;45:427.
29. Krauss MJ, Morrisey AE, Winn HN, et al. Microcephaly: an epidemiologic analysis. *Am J Obstet Gynecol.* 2003;188(6):1484-1490.
30. Vargas JE, Allred EN, Leviton A, et al. Congenital microcephaly: phenotypic features in a consecutive sample of newborn infants. *J Pediatr.* 2001;139(2):210-214.

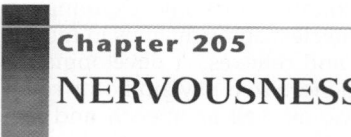

Chapter 205
NERVOUSNESS

Richard M. Sarles, MD

One vague complaint, often hard to pin down, that primary care physicians frequently encounter is *nervousness,* whether it is voiced by an older child or an adolescent or by a parent about a child—for example, the mother who describes her 12 year old as "nervous all the time," to which the 12 year old responds distractedly, "I don't know, maybe—I just feel funny." In instances such as this one an inarticulate patient may be shouting for help, and such complaints usually need the physician's attention. The physician must look beyond the chief complaint to the underlying cause: Why does this patient have this complaint? What does it mean?

With complaints of nervousness, a complete history and thorough physical examination are needed, although, because the circumstance is not life threatening, such examinations need not occur immediately. The abstraction of the term *nervousness* and the difficulty in defining it more precisely underscore the need to devote adequate time to take a complete history, conduct a thorough physical examination, and discuss the problem in depth.

What accompanies the nervousness: anorexia, restlessness at night, sluggishness, overactivity? A physical problem is implied but is often not at the root of the complaint. Nervousness, for example, is often part of the constellation of complaints in a variety of endocrine disorders (hyperthyroidism, hypoglycemia, Addison disease) and in dermatitis, pinworm infestation, and allergy. Caffeine ingestion (colas and coffee) and abuse of a variety of drugs can also cause nervousness. Mitral valve prolapse and paroxysmal tachycardia are cardiac diseases that can create symptoms of nervousness.

The primary care physician should also consider the possibility of an attention-deficit disorder with or without hyperactivity, as well as an anxiety disorder, such as separation anxiety or school phobia and somatization of depression. Many more serious problems, such as autism, childhood psychoses, obsessive-compulsive and manic-depressive disorders, panic attacks, and Tourette syndrome, can all be associated with complaints of nervousness as the parents or patient try to define perceptions and feelings. However, such problems are rarely defined as nervousness alone; the history and physical examination will quickly uncover a host of concomitant findings.

If after a conscientious search for a biopsychosocial cause, little, if anything, has been discovered, then the chief complaint of nervousness becomes even more difficult to approach. Time, caring, and sensitive understanding of the patient's needs are required. Unfortunately, little help is available in the literature. Nervousness is not usually defined or described in textbooks, and it is not listed in the American Psychiatric Association *Diagnostic and Statistical Manual of Mental Disorders* or in any standard psychiatric textbook. A discussion of its implications is not generally covered in most medical school curricula.

How, then, is the practitioner to conceptualize, diagnose, and treat nervousness, nervous stomach, or other disorders that occur as symptoms without any readily discernible underlying pathophysiological abnormality? First comes the thorough search; then comes the devotion of time and attention to sensitive exploration and, if necessary, referral to a colleague who has expertise in emotional disorders of childhood and adolescence to attempt to unravel the sometimes intricate psychosocial puzzle.

Even when the clinician knows that the patient has no physical disorder, emotional tension, restlessness, agitation, fearful apprehension, acute uneasiness, undue excitability, or excessive irritability may be evident. These manifestations, which are quite real and require care, call for individual attention to the child or for work with the family collectively. The approach needed may vary as widely as the range of complaints. A physician who is unprepared to provide the necessary time and effort should refer the patient to ease the morbidity inevitably associated with these complaints.

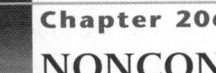

WHEN TO REFER

- Persistent, recurrent complaints unresponsive to repeated physician reassurance
- Unremitting complaints that interfere with family, school, and social functioning

Chapter 206
NONCONVULSIVE PERIODIC DISORDERS

Sarah M. Roddy, MD

A variety of paroxysmal nonepileptic disorders occur in children. These disorders have a wide range of clinical features that mimic seizures, and distinguishing them from seizures is important so that the child is not treated inappropriately with anticonvulsants. A thorough history is often all that is needed to make the diagnosis, although a few patients may require a more extensive evaluation.

BREATH-HOLDING SPELLS

Breath-holding spells, or infantile syncope, occur in approximately 5% of children.[1] Most children who have breath-holding spells begin having episodes between 6 and 18 months of age, although spells may begin in the first few weeks of life. The frequency of episodes ranges from once a year to several times daily. The history of the episode and the surrounding events is the most important part of the evaluation of a child who has such spells. Because the familial incidence of breath-holding spells is high, the parents should be questioned about episodes in other family members.

Two types of breath-holding spells occur: (1) cyanotic and (2) pallid. The cyanotic type is more common than the pallid form and is usually precipitated by frustration or anger. During such spells, children cry vigorously and then hold their breath in expiration. Apnea is followed by cyanosis, with opisthotonic posturing and loss of consciousness. Recovery is usually quick, with return of respiration and consciousness within 1 minute. Evaluation of children who have severe cyanotic breath-holding spells has shown an underlying autonomic system dysregulation that may contribute to the pathophysiological features of the episodes.[2-4] Pallid breath-holding episodes are usually provoked by sudden fright or minor injuries, especially falling and hitting the occiput. The child gasps or cries briefly and then abruptly becomes quiet, loses consciousness, has pallor, and becomes limp. The child may then develop clonic jerks. Pallid breath-holding spells are a vasovagal phenomenon. The precipitating event induces a vagally mediated asystole, leading to cerebral ischemia. Ocular compression during simultaneous electroencephalographic and electrocardiographic tracing in children who have pallid breath-holding spells has shown asystole with flattening of the electroencephalogram without electrical seizure activity.[1] The clonic jerks are caused by cerebral hypoxia rather than by epileptiform discharges from the brain.

The prognosis for children who have either type of breath holding is excellent; most outgrow the episodes by school age. Children who have pallid breath-holding spells may later develop syncope.[1] Treatment is directed mainly at reassuring the family of the benign nature of the episodes. The primary care physician should emphasize that the episodes are not seizures and that they do not lead to mental retardation or epilepsy. Because cyanotic episodes are often precipitated by temper tantrums, anger, and frustration, advice about behavior management may be helpful. Anemia has been described as a contributing factor in breath-holding spells, and treating it may reduce the incidence of the episodes.[5-7] Atropine is effective for pallid breath-holding episodes, but its use is rarely warranted. Anticonvulsants should not be used because they are not effective in treating either type of breath-holding spell (see Chapter 150, Temper Tantrums and Breath-Holding Spells).

SYNCOPE

Syncope, or fainting, is an acute and transient loss of consciousness caused by reduced cerebral perfusion. Episodes are relatively common, particularly among teenagers.[8] Postural hypotension, which may occur after a sudden change from a sitting or reclining position to a standing position, can precipitate an episode. Emotional upset, fright, and overheating are also common provoking stimuli. Cardiac disorders, including arrhythmias, aortic stenosis, and severe cyanotic heart disease, may cause syncope by reducing cardiac output and causing cerebral hypoxia. In rare cases, episodes of syncope have been reported with swallowing, coughing, urinating, and defecating.[9]

Patients have presyncopal symptoms that may include light-headedness, anxiety, sweating, nausea, generalized numbness, and visual changes described as constriction or darkening of vision. Observers notice marked pallor and clammy skin. These symptoms are followed by loss of consciousness and slumping to the floor. Once the patient is recumbent and cerebral perfusion is restored, consciousness returns within a few seconds. If the patient is held with the head above the body and cerebral perfusion is not restored, then clonic movements may occur. As with pallid breath-holding spells, these movements occur as a result of cerebral ischemia rather than epileptiform discharges from the brain. Patients are not disoriented or confused after an episode of syncope, although they may be tired.

The history is important in diagnosing syncope and should include a description of the event by the patient and an observer. Although laboratory evaluation is seldom needed, if atypical features are involved, such as absence of a precipitating factor or confusion after the episode, an electroencephalogram or a cardiac evaluation, including Holter monitoring, may be appropriate. Evaluation with tilt-table testing can be helpful for children who have unexplained syncope.[10] Treatment consists of teaching the patient and family about managing an episode. Because patients have presyncopal symptoms, they should be instructed to sit or lie down as soon as the symptoms begin, thereby preventing progression to loss of consciousness. If the patient loses consciousness, then the parent should place the child in a recumbent position with the head lower than the trunk. Parents often pick up a child who has fainted; they should be cautioned against this action because they may prolong the period of unconsciousness (see Chapter 223, Syncope, for a more detailed discussion of syncope and its causes).

BENIGN PAROXYSMAL VERTIGO

Benign paroxysmal vertigo of childhood is a disorder characterized by brief attacks of vertigo. Symptoms usually appear within the first 3 or 4 years of life, although they may begin later. Episodes are characterized by abrupt onset, with the child appearing fearful and unable to maintain normal posture and gait. The child may seek support and clutch the parent or abruptly sit down or fall. In severe cases, the child may be limp and incapable of using the extremities. Pallor and diaphoresis are usually apparent, and vomiting and nystagmus sometimes occur. An episode typically lasts less than 30 seconds or, in rare cases, a few minutes. A brief period of postural instability may follow the episode; but within a few minutes, the instability resolves. Consciousness is not altered during the episode, and only rarely does the child feel sleepy after it. The frequency of episodes varies from as many as several weekly to 1 episode every few months. Audiograms are normal. Oculovestibular testing with cold-water calorics is difficult to perform in young children, and results vary. When properly done, no abnormalities in vestibular function have been found.[11] The results of radiographic studies of the temporal bone and electroencephalographic recordings are also normal. Included in the differential diagnosis of vertigo in childhood are brain stem lesions, posterior fossa tumors, and epilepsy. The history and physical examination usually differentiate benign paroxysmal vertigo from these more serious disorders. In most cases, no treatment is necessary, and anticonvulsants are not effective. Antihistamines such as dimenhydrinate have been used in some patients who have frequent episodes, with an apparent reduction in the number of episodes. Because the frequency of attacks varies, assessing the effect of therapy accurately is difficult. Attacks of vertigo usually stop spontaneously over a period of a few years. Some children with benign paroxysmal vertigo later develop migraine headaches[12] (see Chapter 170, Dizziness and Vertigo).

SHUDDERING ATTACKS

Shuddering or shivering episodes are a benign movement disorder that probably occurs in many children at 1 time or another. The episodes are brief and characterized by paroxysmal rapid tremors involving primarily the head and arms. Some episodes may involve flexion of the head, elbow, trunk, and knees, with adduction of the elbows and knees.[13] Consciousness is not altered during the episodes. The frequency varies, with some children having more than 100 episodes daily. Emotional factors, including excitement, fear, anger, and frustration, may precipitate episodes. Shuddering episodes may start as early as a few months of age or not until later in childhood. The number of episodes usually declines gradually. The pathophysiological mechanism of the episodes is unclear, although the attacks have been postulated to be an expression of an essential tremor.[13,14] Electroencephalographic monitoring has shown that the episodes are not epileptiform in nature.[15] In most cases, no treatment is necessary. If episodes are severe and interfere with activities, then treatment with propranolol may be helpful.[16] Anticonvulsants are ineffective and should not be used.

BENIGN NEONATAL SLEEP MYOCLONUS

Sudden brief jerks of the extremities are normal in children and adults when falling asleep. Sleep-related myoclonus in neonates is called *benign neonatal sleep myoclonus*. The myoclonic jerks begin in the 1st month of life, often within the 1st day, and are present only during quiet sleep, disappearing when the infant awakens.[17] The jerking movements may start in 1 extremity and then progress to involve the other extremities, or they may begin bilaterally. The upper extremities are involved more often than the lower extremities. Jerks occur every 2 to 3 seconds for several minutes, although they have been reported to last up to 12 hours.[18] Rocking the crib has been described as a maneuver to provoke the myoclonus.[19] Development is normal, and no neurologic deficits are present. Electroencephalographic results are normal, with no epileptiform discharges associated with the myoclonus.[18] The major differential diagnosis of neonatal sleep myoclonus is a seizure disorder. A history of episodes during sleep only and a normal electroencephalogram help differentiate this benign disorder from seizures. The myoclonus usually diminishes gradually during the first 6 months of life, although it has rarely lasted until 3 years.[20] No treatment is necessary. The infants do not subsequently develop epilepsy or cognitive delay.[21]

NIGHT TERRORS

Night terrors or sleep terrors are a sleep disorder with some features that mimic partial complex seizures. They occur in up to 6% of children, with a peak incidence in late preschool and early school-aged children.[22] Affected children often have a family history of either night terrors or another sleep disorder. The episodes usually occur during the first 2 hours after falling asleep. The child sits up in bed abruptly and screams or talks unintelligibly. If the child's eyes are open, then they have a glazed look. During the episode, the child appears to be hallucinating and does not respond to the parents. Tachycardia and diaphoresis result from the response of the sympathetic nervous system. In some cases, the child may sleepwalk. Night terrors usually last approximately 10 minutes, with the child then relaxing and abruptly falling back to sleep. On awakening, the child does not remember the episode. Night terrors are caused by a rapid partial arousal from deep, slow-wave sleep. Febrile illness and sleep deprivation may trigger night terrors.[23]

Electroencephalography does not show seizure activity during the episodes. Differentiating night terrors from nightmares is important, the latter of which occur during rapid eye movement (REM) sleep and are associated with easy arousal and recall of the content, or at least the occurrence, of the nightmare. Night terrors usually occur less often as the child gets older, although episodes may continue into adolescence and adulthood. The nature of the episodes should be explained to the parents. Although parents tend to try to wake and reassure the child, they should be told that the child is not aware of their presence, and attempts to awaken the child are not helpful and may increase agitation. If the child is sleep deprived, then parents should take steps to increase the amount of sleep the child is getting. If night terrors persist despite adequate sleep, a sleep study may be needed to evaluate for obstructive sleep apnea, which can trigger night terrors.[24] In most cases, no medication is indicated; however, if episodes are frequent or severe, then benzodiazepines, imipramine, or L-5-hydroxytryptophan may be helpful.[23,25]

NARCOLEPSY

Narcolepsy is a sleep-wake disorder characterized by excessive and inappropriate periods of sleep during the day. The daytime sleepiness interrupts activities and does not diminish in response to adequate amounts of sleep at night. Naps may last from a few minutes to longer than an hour. In addition to the excessive daytime sleep, patients often have cataplexy, sleep paralysis, and hypnagogic hallucinations. Cataplexy is a transient partial or complete loss of tone, often triggered by an emotional reaction such as laughter or fright. The individual does not lose consciousness. Sleep paralysis occurs as the patient falls asleep or awakens and is characterized by the inability to move or speak. Hypnagogic hallucinations occur while falling asleep, can be auditory or visual, and may be very frightening to a child.

The estimated prevalence of narcolepsy is 0.02% to 0.05%.[26] Onset usually occurs in the 2nd decade, although it has been reported in children as young as 3 years. Sleep studies in patients who have narcolepsy show that REM sleep occurs within 15 minutes of sleep onset; in healthy patients, 90 minutes of non-REM sleep precede the 1st REM period. A strong association exists between narcolepsy and the human leukocyte class II antigen DQB1*0602.[27] Human leukocyte antigen typing may be helpful but is not diagnostic. The neuropeptides, hypocretin or orexin, which are important for maintaining wakefulness, may be absent on cerebrospinal fluid studies, especially in cases involving cataplexy.[28] Sleep studies are important in diagnosing narcolepsy. Included in the differential diagnosis of excessive daytime sleepiness are chronic illness, sleep apnea, hypothyroidism, depression, and seizures.

Narcolepsy is a lifelong condition, but central nervous system stimulants such as methylphenidate and modafinil help reduce the frequency of naps. Tricyclic medications such as imipramine are used to treat cataplexy and the other associated symptoms.[29]

WHEN TO REFER

- If a diagnosis cannot be made by history and physical examination
- If a need exists for subspecialty expertise

WHEN TO ADMIT

- If the child needs video electroencephalographic monitoring to evaluate an episode

REFERENCES

1. Lombroso CT, Lerman P. Breathholding spells (cyanotic and pallid infantile syncope). *Pediatrics.* 1967;39:563-581.
2. DiMario FJ Jr, Burleson JA. Autonomic nervous system function in severe breath holding spells. *Pediatr Neurol.* 1993;9:268-274.
3. DiMario FJ Jr, Bauer L, Baxter D. Respiratory sinus arrhythmia in children with severe cyanotic and pallid breath-holding spells. *J Child Neurol.* 1998;13:440-442.
4. Akalin F, Turan S, Guran T, et al. Increased QT dispersion in breath-holding spells. *Acta Paediatr.* 2004;93:770-774.
5. Orii KE, Kato Z, Osamu F, et al. Changes of autonomic nervous system function in patients with breath-holding spells treated with iron. *J Child Neurol.* 2002;17:337-340.
6. Colina KF, Abelson HT. Resolution of breath-holding spells with treatment of concomitant anemia. *J Pediatr.* 1995;126:395-397.
7. Daoud AS, Batieha A, al-Sheyyab M, et al. Effectiveness of iron therapy on breath-holding spells. *J Pediatr.* 1997;130:547-550.
8. Driscoll DJ, Jacobsen SJ, Porter CJ, et al. Syncope in children and adolescents. *J Am Coll Cardiol.* 1997;29:1039-1045.
9. Hannon DW, Knilas TK. Syncope in children and adolescents. *Curr Probl Pediatr.* 1993;23:358-384.
10. Samoil D, Grubb BP, Kip K, et al. Head-upright tilt table testing in children with unexplained syncope. *Pediatrics.* 1993;92:426-430.

11. Finkelhor BK, Harker LA. Benign paroxysmal vertigo of childhood. *Laryngoscope*. 1987;97:1161-1163.
12. Lanzi G, Balottin U, Fazzi E, et al. Benign paroxysmal vertigo of childhood: a long-term follow-up. *Cephalagia*. 1994;14:458-460.
13. Vanasse M, Bedard P, Andermann F. Shuddering attacks in children: an early clinical manifestation of essential tremor. *Neurology*. 1976;26:1027-1030.
14. Kanazawa O. Shuddering attacks-report of four children. *Pediatr Neurol*. 2000;23:421-424.
15. Holmes GL, Russman BS. Shuddering attacks: evaluation using electroencephalographic frequency modulation radiotelemetry and videotape monitoring. *Am J Dis Child*. 1985;140:72-73.
16. Barron TF, Younkin DP. Propranolol therapy for shuddering attacks. *Neurology*. 1992;42:258-259.
17. Di Capua M, Fusco L, Ricci S, et al. Benign neonatal sleep myoclonus: clinical features and video-polygraphic recordings. *Mov Disord*. 1993;8:191-194.
18. Turanli G, Senbil N, Altunbasak S, et al. Benign neonatal sleep myoclonus mimicking status epilepticus. *J Child Neurol*. 2004;19:62-63.
19. Alfonso I, Papazian O, Aicardi J, et al. Simple maneuver to provoke benign neonatal sleep myoclonus. *Pediatrics*. 1995;96:1161-1163.
20. Egger J, Grossman G, Auchterlonie IA. Benign sleep myoclonus in infancy mistaken for epilepsy. *BJM*. 2003; 326:975-976.
21. Vaccerio ML, Valenti MA, Carullo A, et al. Benign neonatal sleep myoclonus: case report and follow-up of four members of an affected family. *Clin Electroencephalogr*. 2003;34:15-17.
22. DiMario FJ Jr, Emery S III. The natural history of night terrors. *Clin Pediatr*. 1987;26:505-511.
23. Mason TB 2nd, Pack AI. Sleep terrors in childhood. *J Pediatr*. 2005;145:388-392.
24. Guilleminault C, Palombini L, Pelayo R, et al. Sleepwalking and sleep terrors in prepubertal children: what triggers them? *Pediatrics*. 2003;111:17-25.
25. Bruni O, Ferri R, Miano S, et al. L-5-Hydroxytryptophan treatment of sleep terrors in children. *Eur J Pediatr*. 2004; 163:402-407.
26. Hublin C, Kaprio J, Partinen M, et al. The prevalence of narcolepsy: an epidemiological study of a Finnish twin cohort. *Ann Neurol*. 1994;35:709-716.
27. Mignot E, Hayduk R, Black J, et al. HLA DQB1*0602 is associated with cataplexy in 509 narcoleptic patients. *Sleep*. 1997;20:1012-1020.
28. Mignot E, Lammers GJ, Ripley B, et al. The role of cerebrospinal fluid hypocretin measurement in the diagnosis of narcolepsy and other hypersomnias. *Arch Neurol*. 2002;59:1553-1563.
29. Dyken ME, Yamada T. Narcolepsy and disorders of excessive somnolence. *Prim Care Clin Office Pract*. 2005;32:389-413.

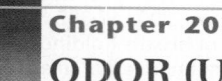

Chapter 207

ODOR (UNUSUAL URINE AND BODY)

Erik E. Langenau, DO

Unusual odors in children may be a chief complaint, symptom, or sign. The odors may emanate from the breath, urine, skin, sputum, vomitus, stool, or vagina,[1] and they can provide helpful clues in the diagnosis of many specific conditions.

DEFINITION OF TERMS

Although unusual odors can be caused by many different conditions, two terms require careful attention: (1) bromhidrosis and (2) halitosis.

A condition in which sweat is malodorous and offensive, bromhidrosis is caused by decomposition of products from the apocrine, eccrine, and sebaceous glands.[2] Apocrine bromhidrosis, which begins after puberty with a characteristic acrid or sweaty odor, results from a combination of short-chain fatty acids, ammonia, androgenic steroids, hexanoic acid, and saturated ketones and indoles.[2] Eccrine bromhidrosis results from bacterial interaction with moist keratin and is caused by hyperhidrosis, obesity, intertrigo, and diabetes mellitus; it is aggravated by hot weather and occurs primarily in the soles, palms, and intertriginous areas.[2]

Halitosis is an offensive odor emanating from the mouth or air-filled cavities such as the nose, sinuses, or pharynx[3]; it may be physiological or pathological, with numerous causes, such as xerostomia (dry mouth), periodontitis, sinusitis, tonsillitis, or gastroesophageal reflux.[4]

DIFFERENTIAL DIAGNOSIS OF UNUSUAL ODORS

The differential diagnosis of unusual odors is extensive and includes numerous systemic, metabolic, toxic, and infectious diseases. The physician may inquire about the presence or absence of an odor when evaluating a child with a particular infection, dermatologic condition, metabolic disease, or ingestion.[1,5,6] After a thorough history and physical examination is conducted, the differential diagnosis of an unusual odor can become more focused.

EVALUATION OF UNUSUAL ODORS

When approaching the differential diagnosis of unusual odors and refining a diagnostic evaluation, a thorough history and physical examination must first be conducted.

Chief Complaint

If an unusual body odor is the chief complaint, a thorough history of the present illness helps narrow the differential diagnosis. Relevant questions may include the following:

When did you first notice the odor?
What does it smell like?
Does it smell like anything familiar?
What is the quality?
What is the intensity?
Does it seem to come from a certain part of the body?
Does bathing or cleaning make it better?
Are there any other associated symptoms, such as vomiting, weight loss, lethargy?
Do other members of the family have similar odors?
Do any family members have metabolic or infectious diseases?
Have you seen any insertion of a foreign body in the nose, ear, anus, or vagina?
Has your child taken any oral or topical medications, vitamins, herbal supplements, or toxins?
How has the odor affected the child and family?

Physical Examination

In assessing an odor, the examiner should (1) note the character of the odor, (2) determine the patient's age (and stage of pubertal development), (3) check for any other signs or symptoms during a complete examination with the child unclothed, and (4) attempt to localize the odor to a particular body site.

In a routine medical encounter, the first observation when entering an examining room may be an odor. Odors have been difficult to describe because of insufficient standards for classifying, qualifying, quantifying, and teaching about odors.[7] Historically and practically, odors have been compared with others for which physicians have common experience, and odor strength is characterized by such adjectives as strong or faint. In addition, individuals differ in their ability to detect at least some odors and in their assessments of whether certain odors are offensive. Gas-liquid chromatography now allows more precise identification of odors. Artificial nose technology, which can sense a wide range of volatile chemicals and be trained in pattern recognition, may soon become a tool to supplement the clinician's own nose. Artificial noses or bioelectronic noses have already been used to detect diseases such as tuberculosis, *Helicobacter pylori* infection, urinary tract infections,[8] bacterial vaginosis,[9] and diabetes.[10]

If a patient reports an intermittent unusual odor that is never detected by others, then the possibility of temporal lobe epilepsy with olfactory manifestations should be entertained.[11] On the other hand, if the practitioner notices a clearly offensive body odor, but the patient or parent does not, then anosmia should be considered. Causes of impaired olfaction may be due to various endocrinopathies (Kallmann syndrome, diabetes, Turner syndrome, hypothyroidism), infections (rhinitis, sinusitis), autoimmune diseases (Sjögren syndrome, Wegener granulomatosis, multiple sclerosis), or medications (metronidazole, tetracycline, captopril, amphetamines).[7,12]

Physicians should also be aware that odor recognition involves complicated molecular and genetic mechanisms.[13] Genetic variation may lead to differences in abilities and thresholds for detecting odors.[7] Physicians and patients may therefore vary in their ability to detect certain odors.

CAUSES OF UNUSUAL ODOR

An array of odors can be associated with the human body and clothing, and subtle differences in odor can be found among people as well. Therefore the first task may be to decide whether a particular odor truly is peculiar and whether it emanates from the body. The odor may be simply a normal body odor that draws attention because of its intensity or because the complainant is unusually sensitive to or concerned about it.

Normal Body Odor

Normal body odors derive from secretions of the sweat and apocrine glands, vagina, cervix, respiratory tract, urine, feces, breath, and flatus.[5] Odor may be produced or modified by the action of normal or abnormal microbial flora.

In Western culture, people often minimize body odors by frequently changing their clothing, bathing, and using deodorants, antiperspirants, mouthwashes, douches, or scents applied to the skin. If one of these artificial odors is too strong, then the practitioner may wonder what the patient is trying to hide. On the other hand, if a patient does not practice these customs, then the physician may detect an odor that is offensive and then must decide why the patient is not complying with social expectations.

Body odor changes with puberty, and a characteristic adult odor may prompt a child (or the child's parents) to seek medical attention.

Axillary Odor

Axillary odor, which varies in intensity from person to person, is often the strongest odor associated with adolescents and adults.[5] Its pungency has long been attributed to the action of aerobic diphtheroids on apocrine secretions. Recent work has identified odor-binding proteins that originate in the apocrine glands. The most abundant of the smelly compounds may be (E)-3-methyl-2-hexenoic acid.[14] Bacterial decomposition of androsterone is another possible cause of axillary odor.[15] Axillary hair appears to retain or spread odor.[16]

Some adolescents and adults have axillary odor that is unusually strong, a condition called osmidrosis axillae or axillary apocrine bromhidrosis. The odor emanates from the apocrine glands. Possible explanations include specific features of apocrine androgen metabolism,[17] bacterial alteration of sweat,[18] and abnormally large and numerous apocrine glands.[19] A variety of topical interventions, as well as surgical excisions, have been used to treat this condition.

Vaginal Odor

The odor of postpubertal vaginal secretions varies among individuals and with the menstrual cycle. Vulvar secretions, vaginal wall transudates, exfoliated cells, cervical mucus, fluids from the endometrium and uterine tubes, and metabolic products of the vaginal microflora all contribute.[20] Some people characterize the resulting odor as unpleasant, even in the absence of vaginitis. Odor during menses is usually rated as the most offensive.[20] Some individuals may be concerned about these normal odors. The rotten fish smell of the vaginal discharge associated with bacterial vaginosis is caused by trimethylamine.[21]

Mouth Odor

The odor of a healthy mouth is assumed to be inoffensive in childhood; however, *bad breath* is not uncommon, even in an otherwise well child. Halitosis in the absence of disease is thought to be caused by volatile sulfur compounds (hydrogen sulfide and methyl mercaptan), which are formed when the oral flora metabolize proteins that are found in the saliva or adhering to the teeth, tongue, or gums.[4] Halitosis is exacerbated by infrequent eating and drinking, which ordinarily have a flushing action. Acutely, halitosis may accompany a variety of childhood respiratory tract and gastrointestinal infections. Persistent halitosis should prompt evaluation for dental or gingival disease, a nasal foreign body, lung disease, or gastroesophageal reflux.[4]

Simple oral hygiene can temporarily modify mouth odor. Brushing the teeth and the dorsoposterior surface of the tongue and then rinsing with water or a

Table 207-1 Metabolic Abnormalities Associated With Unusual Odor

DISEASE	DESCRIPTION OF ODOR	CLINICAL FEATURES	METABOLIC DEFECT
3-hydroxy-3-methylglutaryl-CoA lyase deficiency	Cat urine	Malaise, hypoglycemia, hepatomegaly, transaminitis, mild acidosis	3-hydroxy-3-methylglutaryl-CoA lyase
Glutaric aciduria type II (multiple acyl-CoA dehydrogenase deficiency)	Sweaty feet, acrid, stale	Hypoglycemia, hypotonia, hepatomegaly, respiratory distress, death	Electron transfer flavoprotein (ETF) or ETF: ubiquinone oxidoreductase (ETF:QO)
Hawkinsinuria	Swimming pool	Failure to thrive, hepatomegaly, anemia, irritability	4-hydroxyphenylpyruvate dioxygenase
Hypermethioninemia	Boiled cabbage	Usually asymptomatic. Some develop mental retardation, dystonia	Methionine adenosyltransferase
Isovaleric acidemia	Sweaty feet, acrid	Acidosis, vomiting, dehydration, coma, mild-to-moderate mental retardation, aversion to protein foods	Isovaleric acid CoA dehydrogenase
Ketoacidosis	Fruity, acetone-like, decomposing apples	Vomiting, dehydration, altered mental status, lethargy	Ketoacidosis (eg, from starvation or insulin deficiency)
Maple syrup urine disease	Maple syrup, burnt sugar, curry, malt, caramel, fenugreek beans	Severe form: feeding difficulty, vomiting, lethargy, acidosis, seizures, coma leading to death in 1st months of life Intermediate form: mild acidosis, mental retardation, developmental delay, ophthalmoplegia Intermittent form: episodic ataxia and lethargy that may progress to coma Thiamine-responsive form: respond to supplementation E3-deficient form: variable expression	Mitochondrial branched-chain alpha–keto dehydrogenase complex
Multiple carboxylase deficiency	Tomcat urine	Failure to thrive, hypotonia, vomiting, seizures, rash	Holocarboxylase synthetase
Oasthouse urine disease (methionine malabsorption syndrome; Smith-Strang disease)	Dried celery, malt, hops; yeast, beer	Diarrhea, mental retardation, spasticity, attacks of hyperpnea, fever, edema	Kidney and intestinal transport of methionine, branched chain amino acids, tyrosine, and phenylalanine
Phenylketonuria	Musty; similar to a mouse, horse, wolf, or barn	Vomiting, progressive mental retardation, microcephaly, eczema, decreasing pigmentation, seizures, spasticity	Phenylalanine hydroxylase
Trimethylaminuria (fish odor syndrome)	Dead or rotting fish	Usually asymptomatic with isolated finding. Fish odor of urine and body	Trimethylamine oxidase
Tyrosinemia	Boiled cabbage, rancid butter	Liver failure, death	Fumarylacetoacetate hydrolase deficiency

Data from references 1, 2, 23-39.

mouthwash supposedly reduces both the concentrations of volatile sulfur compounds and the offensive odor.[4]

Foot Odor

Eccrine bromhidrosis, tinea pedis (athlete's foot), and pitted keratolysis have been associated with increased foot odor. Each of these conditions may be exacerbated by occlusive footwear (eg, boots) and a hot, humid climate. The odor from eccrine bromhidrosis of the feet is believed to result from the breakdown of keratin and lipids by diphtheroids; fatty acid metabolites may be the agents responsible for the odor.[2] Pitted keratolysis (plantar keratolysis puncta) is characterized by white plaques and shallow pits on the plantar

Table 207-2 Inhalations, Poisonings, and Ingestions Associated With Recognizable Odors

ODOR	SITE	SUBSTANCE IMPLICATED
Bitter almond	Breath	Cyanide (chokecherry, apricot pits), jetberry bush
Burned rope	Breath	Marijuana
Camphor	Breath	Naphthalene (mothballs)
Carrots	Breath	Water hemlock (cicutoxin)
Coal gas	Breath	Coal gas (associated with odorless but toxic carbon monoxide)
Disinfectant	Breath	Phenol, creosote
Fishy	Breath	Zinc or aluminum phosphide
Fruity, acetone or decomposing apples	Breath	Lacquer, salicylates, chloroform
Fruity, alcohol	Breath	Alcohol (ethanol, isopropyl alcohol), phenol, acetone, amyl nitrites *(poppers)*
Fruity, pearlike	Breath	Chloral hydrate, paraldehyde
Garlic	Breath, vomitus, stool	Arsenic
Garlic	Breath, vomitus	Phosphorus, tellurium, parathion, malathion, dimethyl sulfoxide, selenium
Glue	Breath, vomitus	Toluene, solvents *(huffing)*
Hydrocarbon	Breath, vomitus	Hydrocarbons
Medicinal, musty	Urine	Penicillins, cephalosporins
Metallic	Breath	Iodine
	Stool	Arsenic
	Vomitus	Arsenic, phosphorus
Rotten eggs	Breath	Hydrogen sulfide mercaptans, disulfiram, dimethyl sulfate, N-acetylcysteine
Severe bad breath	Breath	Amphetamines
Shoe polish	Breath	Nitrobenzene
Stale tobacco	Breath	Nicotine
Sulfides or amines	Skin	War gases
Violets	Urine, vomitus	Turpentine
Wintergreen	Breath	Methyl salicylate

Data from references 1, 2, 6, 44, 45.

surface. Various gram-positive bacteria and dermatophytes have been identified in affected patients. The odor is believed to be related to the breakdown products (such as thiols and thioesters) of these microorganisms within the stratum corneum.[2] Conditions associated with foot odor may respond to a combination of moisture control, topical antibiotics, and antifungal agents.

Metabolic Abnormalities

Certain metabolic defects are associated with an unusual odor of the urine,[22] sweat, and other body fluids because of accumulation of odoriferous metabolic precursors or byproducts. These metabolic disorders and associated odors are listed in Table 207-1. Metabolic disorders should be suspected if an infant has an unusual body odor, especially if the patient is ill appearing, malnourished, or ketotic. Recognizing the odor in a compatible clinical situation may lead to early diagnosis, and prompt treatment may prevent progressive brain damage or death. A specialist in metabolic diseases should be consulted, and an appropriate diet should be started while a more thorough metabolic evaluation is being completed. The odor itself may lead to embarrassment, low self-esteem, and psychosocial problems. In some conditions, dietary manipulation may reduce the malodor, as well as other symptoms.[40]

Foreign Bodies

Retention of a foreign body in an orifice may lead to a focal foul smell. Retained foreign bodies within the vagina (eg, tampons, diaphragms), auditory canals, and nostrils are common causes of local foul odor. A retained foreign body may also be related to a generalized body odor because odoriferous substances are absorbed and secreted in sweat.[41] Nasal foreign bodies are the most commonly associated with this condition.[42,43]

Inhalation, Poisoning, and Ingestion

When inhalation or ingestion of a toxic substance is suspected, odor may provide a clue to the substance involved. Common associations are listed in Table 207-2. When puzzled, the practitioner should consult a poison control center.

Table 207-3 Odor as a Clue to Infection

INFECTION	ODOR
RESPIRATORY AND EAR, NOSE, AND THROAT INFECTIONS	
Candidiasis	Sweet, fruity
Diphtheria	Sweet
Intranasal foreign body	Foul and putrid
Lung abscess, empyema, bronchiectasis, fetid bronchitis	Foul, putrid breath or sputum
Pseudomonas infection, otitis externa	Foul cerumen
Rubella	Fresh-plucked feathers
Trench mouth, tonsillitis, gingivitis	Severe halitosis
Tuberculous lymphadenitis (scrofula)	Stale beer
Typhoid fever	Fresh-baked brown bread
Yellow fever	Butcher shop
SKIN INFECTIONS	
Candida (skin)	Heavily sweet
Decubitus ulcer	Foul
Diphtheria (skin)	Sweet
Erythroderma	Rancid
Hidradenitis suppurativa	Lingering, pungent
Pitted keratolysis (gram-positive bacteria and dermatophytes)	Cheesy, sweaty, rotten smell from feet
Pseudomonas skin infection (burns)	Musty, fruity, grapelike, wet corn tortillas
Syphilis (condyloma latum)	Foul
Tinea capitis	Mousy, mouse urine-like
GENITOURINARY INFECTIONS	
Bacterial vaginosis	Amine, fishy vaginal discharge
Genital warts (condyloma acuminatum)	Foul
Urinary tract infection with urea-splitting bacteria	Ammoniacal urine
Vaginal foreign body, vaginitis	Foul vaginal discharge
GASTROINTESTINAL INFECTIONS	
Rotavirus gastroenteritis	Full
Shigellosis	Rancid stool
NEUROLOGIC INFECTIONS	
Cryptococcus meningitis	Alcohol smell to cerebrospinal fluid
MISCELLANEOUS INFECTIONS	
Chorioamnionitis	Foul-smelling amniotic fluid
INFECTIOUS ETIOLOGIC AGENTS	
Anaerobic bacteria	Foul-smelling wound, rotten apples
Candida infection	Sweet, fruity, beer odor in peritoneal dialysate
Clostridium gas gangrene	Rotten apples
Proteolytic bacteria	Pus that smells similar to feces or overripe cheese
Proteus infection	Mousy
Pseudomonas aeruginosa	Musty, fruity, grapelike, wet corn tortillas

Data from references 1, 2, 4, 6, 8, 21, 49-52.

Penicillin and cephalosporins give the urine a medicinal or musty smell.[2] Topical benzoyl peroxide has been implicated in at least one case of persistent body odor.[46] Thiourea compounds give the breath a sweet smell, resembling that of decaying vegetables.[47] Newborns have smelled spicy when their mothers ate particular curries before labor.[48]

Other Diseases

Odor may suggest either the presence of an infection (Table 207-3) or other acquired medical conditions (Table 207-4).

SUMMARY

Once an odor is identified and evaluated, a proper diagnostic and treatment plan can begin. Identification of odors can be impeded by poor association between odors and names and failure to retrieve the name of an odor.[58] Physicians can be trained to improve their sense of odor recognition with the aid of educational materials (study guides), simulations with volatile samples on rounds,[59] surgical simulators,[60] and sniffing bar test tubes.[44]

Odor is imprecise. Not surprisingly, with many other diagnostic aids at hand, today's practitioners

Table 207-4 Other Conditions Associated With Specific Odors

DISEASE	ODOR
SYSTEMIC DISEASES	
Hepatic failure	Breath: musty fish, raw liver, feces, rotten eggs, or newly mown clover *(Fetor hepaticus)* (caused by mercaptans such as dimethyl sulfide)
Ketoacidosis (diabetes or starvation)	Breath: fruity; acetone-like; decomposing apples (caused by ketones)
Uremia	Urine: fishy (caused by dimethylamine and trimethylamine)
	Breath: Ammoniacal (caused by ammonia)
VITAMIN DEFICIENCIES	
Pellagra (niacin deficiency)	Sour or musty bread
Scurvy (vitamin C deficiency)	Putrid
DERMATOLOGIC CONDITIONS	
Psoriasis (pustular)	Skin: heavy
Skin diseases with protein breakdown (pemphigus)	Skin: foul, unpleasant
GASTROINTESTINAL CONDITIONS	
Malabsorption	Feces: foul
Melena (gastrointestinal bleeding)	Feces: foul
SURGICAL CONDITIONS	
Esophageal diverticulum	Breath: feculent, foul
Intestinal obstruction	Breath: feculent, foul
	Vomitus: feculent
Nasal foreign body	Skin and nasal cavity: fetid, putrid
Peritonitis	Vomitus: fecal
Portacaval shunt, portal vein thrombosis	Breath: sweet
MISCELLANEOUS	
Acute tubular necrosis	Urine: stale water
Trans-3-methyl-2-hexanoic acid, which may or may not be elevated in patients with schizophrenia[55,56]	Sweat and skin: Unpleasant, pungent, heavy[1,57]

Data from references 1, 2, 4, 6, 53-57.

have minimized olfactory cues.[41] However, odor should not be neglected; it may be the patient's primary concern, causing severe psychosocial distress. Odor identification may provide diagnostic clues that may aid in the detection and treatment of an underlying disease process.

The author would like to acknowledge the valuable contribution of Modena H. Wilson, MD, MPH, to this chapter.

SUGGESTED RESOURCES

Hayden GF. Olfactory diagnosis in medicine. *Postgrad Med J.* 1980;67:110-118.

Senol M, Fireman P. Body odor in dermatologic diagnosis. *Cutis* 1999;63:107-111.

REFERENCES

1. Hayden GF. Olfactory diagnosis in medicine. *Postgrad Med J.* 1980;67:110-118.
2. Senol M, Fireman P. Body odor in dermatologic diagnosis. *Cutis.* 1999;63:107-111.
3. Ayers KM. Calquhoun AN. Halitosis: causes, diagnosis, and treatment. *N Z Dent J.* 1998;94:156-160.
4. Messadi DV, Younai FS. Halitosis. *Dermatol Clin.* 2003;21: 147-155.
5. Liddell K. Smell as a diagnostic marker. *Postgrad Med J.* 1976;52:136-138.
6. Smith M, Smith LG, Levinson B. The use of smell in differential diagnosis. *Lancet.* 1982;2:1452-1453.
7. Stitt WZ, Goldsmith A. Scratch and sniff, the dynamic duo. *Arch Dermatol.* 1995;131:997-999.
8. Pavlou AK, Turner APF. Sniffing out the truth: clinical diagnosis using the electronic nose. *Clin Chem Lab Med.* 2000;38:99-112.
9. Chandoik S, Crawley BA, Oppenheim BA, et al. Screening for bacterial vaginosis: a novel application of artificial nose technology. *J Clin Pathol.* 1997;50: 790-791.
10. Wang P, Tan Y, Xie H, et al. A novel method for diabetes diagnosis based on electronic nose. *Biosens Bioelectron.* 1997;12:1031-1036.
11. Chen C, Shih YH, Yen DJ, et al. Olfactory auras in patients with temporal lobe epilepsy. *Epilepsia.* 2003;44: 257-260.
12. Schiffman SS. Taste and smell in disease. *N Eng J Med.* 1983;308:1275-1279.
13. Lancet D. Exclusive receptors. *Nature.* 1994;372: 321-322.

14. Spielman AI, Sunavala G, Harmony JA, et al. Identification and immunohistochemical localization of protein precursors to human axillary odors in apocrine glands and secretions. *Arch Dermatol*. 1998;134:813-818.
15. Gower DB, Mallet AI, Watkins WJ, et al. Transformations of steroid sulphates by human axillary bacteria: a mechanism for human odour formation? *Biochem Soc Trans. N Z Dent J*. 1997;25:16S.
16. Leyden JJ, McGinley KJ, Holzle E, et al. The microbiology of the human axilla and its relationships to axillary odor. *J Invest Dermatol*. 1981;77:413-416.
17. Sato T, Sonoda T, Itami S, et al. Predominance of type I 5 alpha-reductase in apocrine sweat glands of patients with excessive or abnormal odour derived from apocrine sweat (osmidrosis). *Br J Dermatol*. 1998;139:806-810.
18. Tung TC, Wei FC. Excision of subcutaneous tissue for treatment of axillary osmidrosis. *Br J Plast Surg*. 1997; 50:61-66.
19. Bang YH, Kim JH, Paik SW, et al. Histopathology of apocrine bromhidrosis. *Plast Reconstr Surg*. 1996;98:288-292.
20. Huggins GR, Preti G. Vaginal odors and secretions. *Clin Obstet Gynecol*. 1981;24:355-357.
21. Brand JM, Galask RP. Trimethylamine: the substance mainly responsible for the fishy odor often associated with bacterial vaginosis. *Obstet Gynecol*. 1986;68:682-685.
22. Burke DG, Halpern B, Malegan D, et al. Profiles of urinary volatiles from metabolic disorders characterized by unusual odors. *Clin Chem*. 1983;29:1834-1838.
23. Chhabria S, Tomasi LG, Wong PW. Ophthalmoplegia and bulbar palsy in variant form of maple syrup urine disease. *Ann Neurol*. 1979;6:71-72.
24. Morris MD, Lewis BD, Doolan PD, et al. Clinical and biochemical observations on an apparently nonfatal variant of branched-chain ketoaciduria (maple syrup urine disease). *Pediatrics*. 1961;28:918-923.
25. Sciver CR, MacKenzie S, Clow CL, et al. Thiamine-responsive maple-syrup-urine disease. *Lancet*. 1971;1: 310-312.
26. Mace JW, Goodman SI, Centerwall WR, et al. The child with an unusual odor. *Clin Pediatr*. 1976;15:57-62.
27. Robinson BH, Oei J, Sherwood WG, et al. Hydroxymethylglutaryl CoA lyase deficiency: features resembling Reye syndrome. *Neurology*. 1980;30:714-718.
28. Niederwieser A, Steinmann B, Exner U, et al. Multiple acyl-CoA dehydrogenation deficiency (MADD) in a boy with nonketotic hypoglycemia, hepatomegaly, muscle hypotonia, and cardiomyopathy: detection of N-isovalerylglutamic acid and its monoamide. *Helv Paediatr Acta*. 1983;38:9-26.
29. Dusheiko G, Kew MC, Joffe BI, et al. Recurrent hypoglycemia associated with glutaric aciduria type II in an adult. *N Engl J Med*. 1979;301:1405-1409.
30. Shevell MI, Didomenicantonio G, Sylvain M, et al. Glutaric acidemia type II: neuroimaging and spectroscopy evidence for developmental encephalomyopathy. *Pediatr Neurol*. 1995;12:350-353.
31. Monastiri K, Limame K, Kaabachi N, et al. Fenugreek odour in maple syrup urine disease. *J Inherit Metab Dis*. 1997;20:614-615.
32. Schulman JD, Lustberg TJ, Kennedy JL, et al. A new variant of maple syrup urine disease (branched chain ketoaciduria). Clinical and biochemical evaluation. *Am J Med*. 1970;49:118-124.
33. Wilcken B, Hammond JW, Howard N, et al. Hawkinsinuria: a dominantly inherited defect of tyrosine metabolism with severe effects in infancy. *N Engl J Med*. 1981;305:865-868.
34. Rezvani I. An approach to inborn errors of metabolism. In: Behrman RE, Kliegman RM, Jenson HB, eds. *Nelson Textbook of Pediatrics*. 17th ed. Philadelphia, PA: Saunders; 2004.
35. Budd MA, Tanaka K, Holmes LB, et al. Isovaleric acidemia. Clinical features of a new genetic defect of leucine metabolism. *N Engl J Med*. 1967;277: 321-327.
36. Sidbury JB Jr, Smith EK, Harlan W. An inborn error of short-chain fatty acid metabolism. The odor-of-sweaty-feet syndrome. *J Pediatr*. 1967;70:8-15.
37. Chuang DT, Shih VE. Maple syrup urine disease (branched-chain ketoaciduria). In: Scriver CR, Beaudet AL, Sly WS, et al, eds. *The Metabolic and Molecular Bases of Inherited Disease*. 8th ed. Vol II. New York, NY: McGraw-Hill; 2001.
38. McCandless SE. A primer on expanded newborn screening by tandem mass spectroscopy. Primary care. *Clin Off Pract*. 2004;31:583-604.
39. Smith AJ, Strang LB. An inborn error of metabolism with the urinary excretion of alpha-hydroxy-butyric acid and phenylpyruvic acid. *Arch Dis Child*. 1958;33: 109-113.
40. Boustead C. Fish-odour syndrome: dealing with offensive body odor. *Nurs Times*. 1996;92:30-31.
41. Feinstein RJ. Nasal foreign bodies and bromhidrosis (comment). *JAMA*. 1979;242:1031.
42. Katz HP, Katz JR, Bernstein M, et al. Unusual presentation of nasal foreign bodies in children. *JAMA*. 1979;241: 1496.
43. Moriarty RA. Nasal foreign body presenting as an unusual odor. *Am J Dis Child*. 1978;132:97-98.
44. Goldfrank L, Weisman R, Flomenbaum N. Teaching the recognition of odors. *Ann Emerg Med*. 1982;11: 684-686.
45. Anderson CE, Loomis GA. Recognition and prevention of inhalant abuse. *Am Fam Physician*. 2003;68: 869-874.
46. Molberg P. Body odor from topical benzoyl peroxide (letter). *N Engl J Med*. 1981;304:1366.
47. Stewart WK, Fleming LW. Use your nose (letter). *Lancet*. 1983;1:426.
48. Hauser GJ, Chitayat D, Berns L, et al. Peculiar odors in newborns and maternal prenatal ingestion of spicy food. *Eur J Pediatr*. 1985;144:403.
49. Kavic SM, Cohn SM. Letter to editor. *J Trauma*. 1996;41: 1077.
50. Poulton J, Tarlow MJ. Diagnosis of rotavirus gastroenteritis by smell. *Arch Dis Child*. 1987;62:851-852.
51. Newton ER. Preterm labor, preterm premature rupture of membranes and chorioamnionitis. *Clin Perinatol*. 2005;32:571-600.
52. Turney JH. Use your nose (letter). *Lancet*. 1983; 1:426.
53. Rockey DC. Gastrointestinal bleeding. *Gastroenterol Clin*. 2005;34:699-718.
54. Najarian JS. The diagnostic importance of the odor of urine (letter). *N Engl J Med*. 1980;303:1128.
55. Gordon SG, Smith K, Rabinowitz JL, et al. Studies of trans-3-methyl-2-hexenoic acid in normal and schizophrenic humans. *J Lipid Res*. 1973;14:495-503.
56. Fireman P. Response letter to the editor. *Cutis*. 2002;69: 316.
57. Smith K, Thompson GF, Koster HD. Sweat in schizophrenic patients: identification of the odorous substances. *Science*. 1969;166:398-399.
58. Cain WS. To know with the nose: keys to odor identification. *Science*. 1979;203:467-470.
59. Lukas T, Berner ES, Kanakis C. Diagnosis by smell? *J Med Educ*. 1977;52:349-350.
60. Spencer BS. Incorporating the sense of smell into haptic surgical simulators. *Stud Health Technol Inform*. 2005; 114:54-62.

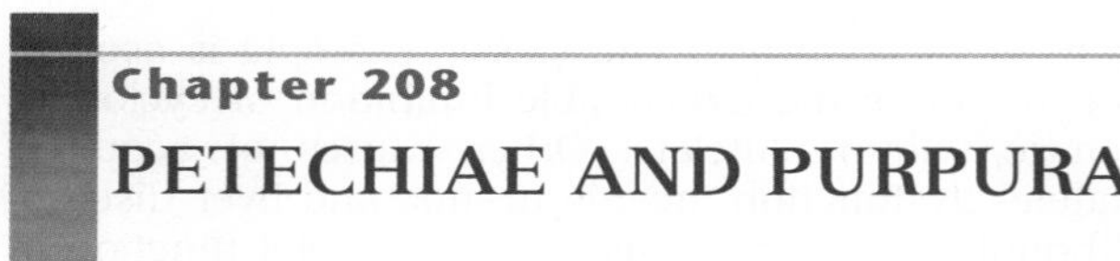

Chapter 208

PETECHIAE AND PURPURA

Adam S. Levy, MD

INTRODUCTION

Petechiae and purpura result from a wide variety of underlying disorders and may occur at any age. Petechiae are small (1-3 mm) red, nonblanching macular lesions caused by intradermal capillary bleeding. Purpura are larger, typically raised lesions resulting from bleeding within the skin. Purpura can vary somewhat in color based on the age of the lesion as the blood within the skin is metabolized and fades. Similar to petechiae, purpura do not blanch and may occur anywhere on the body.

EVALUATION

The evaluation of a patient with petechiae or purpura begins with a complete history that can readily eliminate a majority of disorders from the differential diagnosis. Special attention must be paid to recent trauma, bleeding history, medication use, and symptoms consistent with infection, malignancy, and autoimmune or rheumatologic disorders. Physical examination should determine if the skin findings are isolated or if evidence of a more generalized process is present. Particular physical findings to evaluate include hepatosplenomegaly, lymphadenopathy, arthritis, or arthralgias or findings that are consistent with an acute viral syndrome. The history and physical examination will dictate the appropriate laboratory evaluations, but at a minimum a complete blood count with platelets and differential count, as well as assessing prothrombin time and partial thromboplastin time, are typically indicated. As likely diagnoses are detailed here, the complete evaluation indicated will be discussed.

DIFFERENTIAL DIAGNOSIS—GENERAL CONSIDERATIONS

Neither petechiae nor purpura are pathognomonic of a specific disorder. The clinician must entertain a broad differential diagnosis and consider disorders of hemostasis, as well as infection, autoimmune disorders, trauma, malignancy, and other rare causes. The age at presentation, overall appearance, and the extent of the lesions may help define the underlying pathophysiological mechanism. For example, a well-appearing newborn with scant petechiae on the face would not be particularly concerning after a vaginal delivery because these lesions are likely caused by the trauma of passing through the birth canal. However, a newborn with diffuse petechiae warrants further evaluation.[1,2] (See Chapter 85, Neonatal Skin.) If the child is ill appearing, then sepsis must be strongly considered; if the child is well appearing, then a platelet disorder should be considered. Thus petechiae and purpura must be evaluated in the overall context of the patient, severity and extent of the lesions, and history and age of the patient.

With petechiae or purpura the possibility of a hemostatic defect is always a concern. For isolated petechiae, the clinician must consider a primary platelet disorder (ie, low platelet number, platelet dysfunction). Purpura may result from a platelet disorder or other coagulation defect, which can be classified as primary or as a secondary phenomenon from an underlying disease. Platelet disorders can also be classified into disorders of platelet production, disorders of platelet survival (destruction), or disorders of platelet function. In general, however, when presented with a patient with petechiae and purpura, the clinician must consider thrombocytopenia as the proximate cause.

The normal platelet count is between 150,000 and 450,000/mm^3. Patients with a platelet count greater than 80,000 will be hemostatically normal as long as platelet function is not altered. With a platelet count between 50,000 and 80,000, increased bleeding with trauma is likely, but spontaneous bleeding would be unusual. Between 20,000 and 50,000, a mild bleeding diathesis is expected. With a count less than 20,000, spontaneous mucosal bleeding can occur, and less than 10,000 is concerning for spontaneous severe bleeding.

Infectious Causes of Petechiae and Purpura

The mechanism by which a variety of viruses cause thrombocytopenia is not clear and may involve decreased platelet production or immune-mediated destruction. Live-virus vaccinations, notably varicella and measles, can cause moderate thrombocytopenia.[3] Cytomegalovirus has been implicated in thrombocytopenia, but treatment of cytomegalovirus has not affected the outcome of patients monitored for chronic thrombocytopenia.[4] Parvovirus has been associated both with isolated thrombocytopenia and with pancytopenia.[5-7] Dengue fever and other viral hemorrhagic fevers are known to cause thrombocytopenia, and patients may develop petechiae and purpura as a result.[8,9] Rickettsial diseases such as Rocky Mountain spotted fever may produce a petechial rash. Alterations of the endothelial lining of blood vessels causes thrombi formation and platelet destruction. Thrombocytopenia and disseminated intravascular coagulation (DIC) may develop.[10] Malaria can also cause either mild or profound thrombocytopenia through mechanisms that are not well defined.[11-13] HIV has been associated with thrombocytopenia resulting from bone marrow suppression (ie, poor production) and immune-mediated destruction.[14]

Platelet consumption is common in children with bacteremia and sepsis even before frank DIC has developed. In an ill-appearing child with petechiae or purpura, infectious causes must be considered and appropriate antibiotics administered based on likely pathogens. Bacterial meningitis in particular must be considered for the febrile ill child with petechiae or purpura.

Purpura fulminans has been associated with viral infections, as well as *Streptococcus* and *Meningococcus*. Microscopic thromboses in arterioles result in purpura and infarction and bleeding within the skin and subcutaneous tissue. These lesions may coalesce and become necrotic, and patients typically develop full DIC.

Disorders of Platelet Production: Malignancy and Bone Marrow Failure Syndrome

Although most patients with petechiae or purpura have a benign process, perhaps the greatest concern for the clinician and parents is malignancy. As such the history must rule out the classic signs and symptoms of malignancy, including fevers, night sweats, weight loss, lymphadenopathy or other masses, pallor, malaise, bone pain, and anorexia. Of course, many of these symptoms overlap with those seen in infectious and autoimmune processes; thus the physical examination will help the clinician greatly. Petechiae or purpura in the setting of hepatosplenomegaly or impressive lymphadenopathy would put leukemia high on the differential diagnosis. Other marrow infiltrating malignancies must also be considered. If the history or physical examination is consistent with a malignancy, then in addition to a complete blood count and screening coagulation studies, a comprehensive metabolic panel, liver function tests, lactate dehydrogenase, and uric acid should be immediately obtained. A manual differential count of the peripheral blood should be performed as well. An important point to note is that the absence of leukemic blasts on a peripheral blood smear does *not* rule out leukemia. The diagnosis of leukemia can be made if peripheral blasts are present; however, having few or no peripheral blasts seen on routine microscopy is not uncommon for patients with leukemia.

Isolated profound thrombocytopenia is not likely to result from a malignancy; however, when more than one cell line on a blood count is abnormal, a bone marrow process must be considered. Laboratory findings consistent with malignancy include elevated lactate dehydrogenase, and an elevated uric acid and abnormal serum electrolytes may result from tumor lysis even before therapy is started. A chest x-ray should be obtained immediately because patients may have occult but massive mediastinal lymphadenopathy. (For a thorough review of leukemia, see Chapter 291, Leukemias.)

Petechiae and purpura may be the presenting signs in patients with bone marrow failure secondary to nonmalignant processes. Abnormal hematopoesis usually causes alteration of more than one cell line or all cell lines (pancytopenia). Bone marrow failure may occur secondary to infectious processes (viral, bacterial with sepsis), medication use (notably a variety of antibiotics and anticonvulsants), profound nutritional deficits, or rare bone marrow failure syndromes (eg, Fanconi anemia, myelodysplastic disease, Wiskott-Aldrich syndrome). Bone marrow aspiration and biopsy are usually indicated to rule out malignancy and define the abnormal hematopoiesis.

Disorders of Platelet Function: Primary Platelet Disorders

Petechiae and purpura may result from a primary platelet disorder, either qualitative or quantitative. The qualitative disorders result from platelet dysfunction; that is, the absolute platelet number is normal, but the platelets lose normal hemostatic function. In most instances, platelet dysfunction is acquired and results from medication use. The classic example is aspirin, which causes the irreversible inhibition of cyclooxygenase within platelets. Other causes of acquired platelet dysfunction include uremia and liver disease, although the mechanisms of poor platelet function in these settings are not clear.[15]

Although von Willebrand disease typically produces mucocutaneous bleeding, it should be considered in patients who have petechiae and purpura with a normal platelet count and no other obvious systemic disease.[16] Von Willebrand disease is the most common bleeding disorder and affects approximately 1% of the population. Coagulation screening along with factor VIII and von Willebrand factor assays can establish the diagnosis.

A variety of rare platelet function disorders can be considered in patients with normal platelet number but are bleeding and have petechiae or purpura. These disorders can be diagnosed with specialized platelet aggregation studies or morphologic study of platelets. These disorders are rare and a hematology consultation should be made to define disorders such as Glanzmann thrombasthenia, Bernard-Soulier syndrome, Hermansky-Pudlak syndrome, and Chédiak-Higashi syndrome.

Disorders of Platelet Survival (Destruction)

Isolated thrombocytopenia in an otherwise well child may lead to petechiae or purpura as the chief complaint. Idiopathic (or immune) thrombocytopenic purpura is a diagnosis of exclusion that produces profound isolated thrombocytopenia and petechiae or purpura but few other findings on physical examination. The laboratory work-up should be normal except for thrombocytopenia. No other blood cell line is affected, and microscopic review of the blood reveals platelets that are too few in number but large in size, indicating that they are young. Idiopathic thrombocytopenic purpura is a disorder in which the platelet lifespan is reduced to minutes or hours rather than the normal several days. The incidence is highest in children between 2 and 8 years of age. Although clinicians performed bone marrow aspirates in the past to rule out malignancy or other bone marrow failure syndromes, most now believe that the diagnosis can be made clinically, and bone marrow studies are rarely indicated.[17-19] (See Chapter 282, Immune Thrombocytopenia Purpura, for a complete discussion.)

Typically, one third of the total body platelet mass is sequestered within the spleen at any time. Whatever the cause of increased spleen size, mild thrombocytopenia may result. Common causes of hypersplenism include liver disease, a variety of infections (including Epstein-Barr virus and malaria, among others), and metabolic diseases (eg, Gaucher disease).[20] Hypersplenism alone does not typically cause platelet counts below 50,000. Alternative explanations should be considered for patients with moderate-severe thrombocytopenia.

Henoch-Schönlein purpura produces purpura in the majority of patients diagnosed with this autoimmune vasculitic syndrome. The classic distribution of purpura is on the buttocks and legs, but purpura may be more disseminated. Other findings in Henoch-Schönlein purpura may include arthritis, arthralgias, abdominal pain, and renal impairment.[21-23] (See Chapter 272, Henoch-Schönlein Purpura.)

Hemolytic-uremic syndrome produces a constellation of findings, including thrombocytopenia, hemolytic anemia, and renal failure, and has been associated with a variety of infections, most notably *Escherichia coli* 0157:H7.[24] (See Chapter 269, Hemolytic Uremic Syndrome.)

Thrombotic thrombocytopenic purpura shares some clinical features with hemolytic-uremic syndrome but is a distinct syndrome very rarely seen in children.[25] Findings include purpura, thrombocytopenia, DIC, hemolytic anemia, and elevated lactate dehydrogenase.

Giant vascular malformations may cause intravascular destruction of platelets. Kasabach-Merritt syndrome is the classic example of a giant hemangioma causing severe thrombocytopenia secondary to platelet destruction. These lesions are generally readily apparent; however, multiple smaller vascular malformations that are more difficult to define may cause platelet destruction as well. Thrombocytopenia or altered hemostasis may be associated with rare vascular disorders and connective tissue syndromes such as the hereditary telangectasias, Ehlers-Danlos syndrome, Marfan syndrome, and osteogenesis imperfecta.[26]

SUMMARY

Petechiae and purpura may result from a variety of mechanisms requiring the clinician to obtain a complete history and perform a thorough physical examination. Both primary hematologic disorders and systemic disorders are in the differential diagnosis. Prompt referral to a pediatric hematologist may be indicated to rule out malignancy or help manage altered hemostasis.

WHEN TO REFER

- Platelet count less than 100,000/mm^3
- Diffuse petechiae or purpura
- Focal petechiae or purpura not clearly associated with trauma
- Evidence of more than one cell line abnormality on complete blood count

WHEN TO ADMIT

- Patient has toxic appearance
- Moderate to severe bleeding
- Concern for poor adherence

SUGGESTED RESOURCES

Cines DB, Bussel JB, McMillan RB, et al. Congenital and acquired thrombocytopenia. *Hematology.* 2004;2004(1):390-406.

Kaplan RN, Bussel JB. Differential diagnosis and management of thrombocytopenia in childhood. *Pediatr Clin North Am.* Aug 2004;51(4):1109-1140, xi.

REFERENCES

1. Roberts I, Murray NA. Neonatal thrombocytopenia: causes and management. *Arch Dis Child Fetal Neonatal Ed.* 2003;88(5):F359-F364.
2. Thomas AE. The bleeding child; is it NAI? *Arch Dis Child.* 2004;89(12):1163-1167.
3. Johnson CM, de Alarcon P. Evaluation of a child with thrombocytopenia in platelet dysfunction. In: Sills RH, ed. *Practical Algorithms in Pediatric Hematology and Oncology.* Basel, Switzerland: Karger; 2003.
4. Levy AS, Bussel J. Immune thrombocytopenic purpura: investigation of the role of cytomegalovirus infection. *Br J Haematol.* 2004;126(4):622-623.
5. Heegaard ED, Rosthoj S, Peterson BL, et al. Role of parvovirus B19 infection in childhood idiopathic thrombocytopenic purpura. *Acta Paediatr.* 1999;88(6): 614-617.
6. Aktepe OC, Yetgin S, Olcay L, et al. Human parvovirus B19 associated with idiopathic thrombocytopenic purpura. *Pediatr Hematol Oncol.* 2004;21(5):421-426.
7. McNeely M, Friedman J, Pope E. Generalized petechial eruption induced by parvovirus B19 infection. *J Am Acad Dermatol.* 2005;52(5 suppl 1):S109-S113.
8. Schexneider KI, Reedy EA. Thrombocytopenia in dengue fever. *Curr Hematol Rep.* 2005;4(2):145-148.
9. Halstead SB. Other viral hemorrhagic fevers. In: *Nelson's Textbook of Pediatrics.* 14th ed. Philadelphia, PA: WB Saunders; 1992.
10. Clements ML. Rickettsiae. In: *Nelson's Textbook of Pediatrics.* 14th ed. Philadelphia, PA: WB Saunders; 1992.
11. Rodriguez-Morales AJ, Sanchez E, Vargas M, et al. Occurrence of thrombocytopenia in Plasmodium vivax malaria. *Clin Infect Dis.* 2005;41(1):130-131.
12. Magill AJ. Malaria: diagnosis and treatment of falciparum malaria in travelers during and after travel. *Curr Infect Dis Rep.* 2006;8(1):35-42.
13. Rodriguez-Morales AJ, Sanchez E, Vargas M, et al. Anemia and thrombocytopenia in children with Plasmodium vivax malaria. *J Trop Pediatr.* 2006;52(1):49-51. E-publication June 24, 2005.
14. Scaradavou A. HIV-related thrombocytopenia. *Blood Rev.* 2002;16(1):73-76.
15. Dunsmore K, de Alarcon P. Platelet dysfunction. In: Sills RH, ed. *Practical Algorithms in Pediatric Hematology and Oncology.* Basel, Switzerland: Karger; 2003.
16. Favaloro EJ, Lillicrap D, Lazzari MA et al. Von Willebrand disease: laboratory aspects of diagnosis and treatment. *Haemophilia.* 2004;10(suppl 4):164-168.
17. Calpin C, Dick P, Poon A, Feldman W. Is bone marrow aspiration needed in acute childhood idiopathic thrombocytopenic purpura to rule out leukemia? *Arch Pediatr Adolesc Med.* 1998;152(4):345-347.
18. Cines DB, Blanchette VS. Immune thrombocytopenic purpura. *N Engl J Med.* 2002;346(13):995-1008.
19. Nugent DJ. Childhood immune thrombocytopenic purpura. *Blood Rev.* 2002;16(1):27-29.
20. Johnson CM, de Alarcon P. Evaluation of a child with thrombocytopenia. In: Sills RH, ed. *Practical Algorithms in Pediatric Hematology and Oncology.* Basel, Switzerland: Karger; 2003.
21. Wilson DB. Acquired platelet defects. In: *Nathan and Oski's Hematology of Infancy and Childhood.* 6th ed. Philadelphia, PA: WB Saunders; 2003.
22. Ting TV, Hashkes PJ. Update on childhood vasculitides. *Curr Opin Rheumatol.* 2004;16(5):560-565.
23. Ballinger S. Henoch-Schönlein purpura. *Curr Opin Rheumatol.* 2003;15(5):591-594.
24. Trapani S, Micheli A, Grisolia F, et al. Henoch Schönlein purpura in childhood: epidemiological and clinical analysis of 150 cases over a 5-year period and review of literature. *Semin Arthritis Rheum.* 2005;35(3):143-153.
25. Siegler R, Oakes R. Hemolytic uremic syndrome; pathogenesis, treatment, and outcome. *Curr Opin Pediatr.* 2005; 17(2):200-204.

26. Hosler GA, Cusumano AM, Hutchins GM. Thrombotic thrombocytopenic purpura and hemolytic uremic syndrome are distinct pathologic entities. A review of 56 autopsy cases. *Arch Pathol Lab Med.* 2003;127(7): 834-839.

Chapter 209

POLYURIA

Ryan S. Miller, MD; Samuel M. Libber, MD; Leslie P. Plotnick, MD

Polyuria, or excessive urinary volume, is a symptom common to many pediatric disorders. It may be defined clinically as urine production of more than 2 $L/m^2/24$ hr or functionally as inappropriately high urine output relative to circulating volume and osmolarity (Table 209-1).[1] Urine output greater than 5 mL/kg/hr in a child should raise concerns. Polyuria is often associated with polydipsia, frequent urination, and nocturia. Differentiating polyuria from other conditions depends on total urine output. In situations in which the exact daily urinary volume is unknown, a detailed history of fluid intake and urinary habits may help delineate the primary symptom.

With an older child, the parent may perceive an increase in fluid intake to be more prominent than polyuria. However, infants with polyuria, because they do not have independent access to fluids, are more likely to fall into negative water balance with weight loss, dehydration, and electrolyte disturbances. Chronic or recurrent electrolyte disturbances in unrecognized diabetes insipidus may result in growth failure and central nervous system injury.

PATHOPHYSIOLOGICAL FEATURES

Normal serum osmolality and water balance are maintained primarily by arginine vasopressin (antidiuretic hormone [ADH]) release, thirst, and kidney function. Serum osmolality is tightly regulated—an increase in osmolality as small as 1% stimulates measurable release of vasopressin from the posterior pituitary.[2] Vasopressin binds the V2 receptor of the renal tubules, resulting in insertion of aquaporin-2 protein at the apical surface of cortical cells, allowing water to enter the cell. Under normal conditions, plasma osmolality is maintained within a narrow range—approximately 285 to 290 mOsm/kg. Vasopressin levels rise as plasma osmolality increases above this range. However, maximal antidiuresis is reached at a plasma vasopressin concentration of 4 pmol/L at which point urine cannot be further concentrated (Figure 209-1).

Vasopressin alone cannot restore fluid balance and osmolality; fluid replenishment is also required. Small increases in osmolality have been shown experimentally to stimulate thirst by increasing the concentration of solutes such as sodium chloride or sucrose (solutes that do not readily cross nerve cell membranes).[3] This action results in intracellular dehydration, activating osmoreceptors in the brain that initiate neural mechanisms, resulting in generation of thirst. The osmolality at which thirst is experienced is likely higher than the point at which vasopressin production rises.

Table 209-1 Normal Urine Volume

AGE RANGE	DAILY OUTPUT (24 HR)
Newborn	150 mL/kg
Infant	110 mL/kg
Older child	40 mL/kg

DIFFERENTIAL DIAGNOSIS

Polyuria can be caused by any one of several conditions that play a role in water balance. Diabetes insipidus is characterized by polyuria, polydipsia, dilute urine, dehydration, and hypernatremia. Central diabetes insipidus results from a deficiency in vasopressin secretion, whereas nephrogenic diabetes insipidus is the result of reduced renal sensitivity to circulating vasopressin. Polyuria can also be a manifestation of excessive persistent fluid intake (primary polydipsia) or osmotic (solute) diuresis, as in uncontrolled diabetes mellitus. The overall incidence of diabetes insipidus in the general population is approximately 1 in 100,000. In reaching a diagnosis in a patient who has polyuria, the clinician must consider the systems involved in maintaining normal serum osmolality and water balance (Box 209-1).

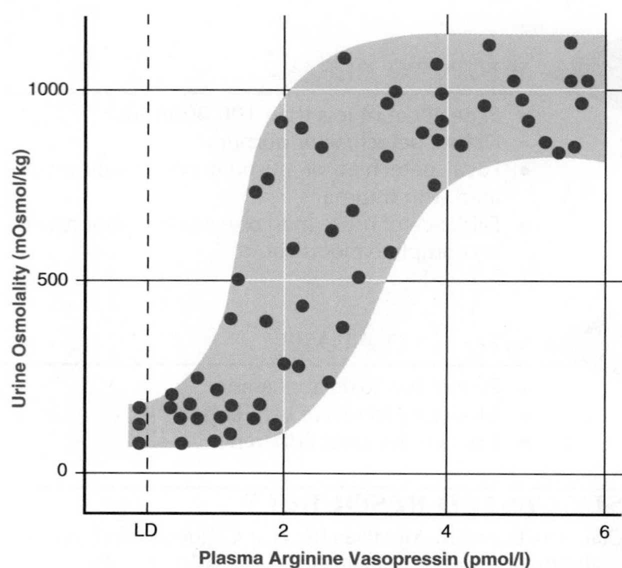

Figure 209-1 Relation between urine osmolality and plasma arginine vasopressin under various states of hydration. The stippled area is the normal reference range. *LD* represents the limit of detection of the assay (0.3 pmol/L). *(Adapted from Baylis PH and Cheetham T. Diabetes Insipidus,* Arch Dis Child. 1998;79:84-89. *Reprinted by permission of BMJ Publishing Group Ltd.)*

Central Diabetes Insipidus

Central or neurogenic diabetes insipidus is a condition in which secretion of vasopressin by the posterior lobe of the pituitary gland is inadequate to maintain normal serum osmolality, resulting in diuresis of varying degrees of severity. Of the known causes of central diabetes insipidus, nearly one half of all cases are due to a primary brain tumor, and approximately 18% are due to histiocytosis or infiltrative processes. Approximately 25% of cases are considered idiopathic. Familial vasopressin deficiency is rare, accounting for approximately 5% of all cases. The autosomal-dominant form typically does not occur until 5 to 10 years of age.[4] The syndrome consisting of diabetes insipidus, diabetes mellitus, optic atrophy, and deafness (DIDMOAD syndrome) typically presents in early childhood.[5] Vasopressin deficiency is associated with certain congenital malformations (eg, septooptic dysplasia, holoprosencephaly) and can result from central nervous system (CNS) injury or tumor resection. After head trauma or surgery, patients may have a period of antidiuresis after transient polyuria, followed by persistent central diabetes insipidus (triple phase response).[6]

In recent years, fewer cases of diabetes insipidus have been diagnosed as idiopathic, and a higher proportion has been diagnosed as occurring secondary to CNS infection or intracranial birth defects.[7] Autoantibodies to hypothalamic vasopressin cells have been detected in some children previously thought to have idiopathic diabetes insipidus. Interestingly, approximately 50% of the patients who have histiocytosis also have vasopressin cell autoantibodies.[8] In adolescents with acquired lymphocytic or granulomatous hypophysitis, hyperprolactinemia and other anterior pituitary dysfunction may accompany the diabetes insipidus.[9] The practitioner must search diligently for an underlying lesion that may not be evident at the initial evaluation.

Nephrogenic Diabetes Insipidus

Renal disorders, both congenital and acquired, may be associated with polyuria because of a complete or partial inability of the renal tubule to concentrate urine

BOX 209-1 Differential Diagnosis of Polyuria in Childhood

I. Neurogenic vasopressin deficiency
  A. Familial
  B. Idiopathic
  C. Congenital malformations (septooptic dysplasia, holoprosencephaly, encephalocele)
  D. Acquired
    1. Head trauma
    2. Vascular event (thrombosis or hemorrhage)
    3. Postinfection (meningitis, encephalitis, congenital cytomegalovirus, toxoplasmosis)
    4. Tumor (craniopharyngioma, germinoma, optic glioma)
    5. Systemic infiltrative diseases (histiocytosis, syphilis, tuberculosis, sarcoidosis)
    6. Guillain-Barré syndrome
    7. Autoimmune disorders

II. Renal vasopressin insensitivity
  A. Familial nephrogenic diabetes insipidus
    1. V2-receptor gene defect (X-linked)
    2. Aquaporin-2 gene defect (autosomal recessive)
  B. Renal tubular defects (cystinosis, distal renal tubular acidosis, Bartter's syndrome, renal Fanconi syndrome, ARC syndrome)
  C. Renal structural defect
  D. Acquired
    1. Postobstructive
    2. Drug induced (lithium, amphotericin B)
    3. Associated with systemic disease (sickle cell disease, sarcoidosis, amyloidosis)
    4. Metabolic (hypercalcemia, hypokalemia)

III. Excessive fluid intake
  A. Primary polydipsia
  B. Water intoxication

IV. Osmotic diuresis
  A. Diet induced
  B. Drug induced
  C. Diabetes mellitus (type I or II)

ARC, Arthrogryposis, renal tubular dysfunction, and cholestasis.

despite normal or elevated circulating levels of vasopressin. Inherited forms of nephrogenic diabetes insipidus are rare, and symptoms of profound polyuria—vomiting, fever, failure to thrive, and hypernatremic dehydration—typically occur within the first weeks of life. Breastfed infants may show signs later than those who are bottle fed because of the lower osmotic load in human milk. The condition can be associated with damage to the CNS or even death if the infant develops recurrent hypernatremic dehydration. Older children and adults may be able to adjust their oral fluid intake to maintain serum osmolality. Mutations in the vasopressin V2 receptors of the distal convoluted tubule and collecting duct have been reported in affected members of kindreds with nephrogenic diabetes insipidus.[10,11] A rare form of autosomal-recessive nephrogenic diabetes insipidus has been described in patients with mutations in the gene for the water-channel protein aquaporin-2.[12]

Besides the hereditary form of nephrogenic diabetes insipidus, the clinician must consider other renal tubular defects in which vasopressin resistance has been observed. Patients who have cystinosis, distal renal tubular acidosis, renal Fanconi syndrome, and Bartter syndrome may have polyuria. An association between nephrogenic diabetes insipidus and the syndrome consisting of arthrogryposis, renal tubular dysfunction, and cholestasis (ARC syndrome) has been recognized; affected children are prone to severe growth impairment, as well as to mental retardation and deafness.[13] Structural abnormalities of the kidney leading to polyuria include congenital abnormalities such as renal dysplasia, familial juvenile nephronophthisis–medullary cystic disease, and oligomeganephronia, as well as acquired lesions caused by chronic pyelonephritis or obstructive uropathy.

In a systematic review of causes of nephrogenic diabetes insipidus, the most frequently reported risk factors for reversible vasopressin insensitivity were lithium, antibiotics, antifungals, antineoplastic agents, and antivirals.[14] Longer duration of treatment with lithium correlated with increased risk of irreversible diabetes insipidus. Metabolic disturbances can also result in reversible vasopressin resistance. Hypercalcemia and hypokalemia each may be associated with a nephropathy in which tubular ability to conserve water is lost. Certain systemic disorders such as sickle cell disease, sarcoidosis, and amyloidosis also may cause renal tubular dysfunction and result in polyuria.

Excess Water Intake

Polyuria is sometimes a consequence rather than a cause of excessive fluid intake. Primary polydipsia, or compulsive water drinking, is a rare cause of polyuria in childhood.[15] It occurs most often in older children or adults who have emotional disturbances; approximately 80% of cases are believed to occur in girls and women. The ailment has a gradual onset, unlike the more abrupt onset typical of central diabetes insipidus. Although some investigators believe this disorder to be caused by a primary psychiatric disturbance, a study of adult patients with polydipsia and hyponatremia showed evidence of a defect in water excretion, osmoregulation of water intake, and vasopressin secretion.[16]

Water intoxication, seen in increasing numbers over the last 20 years, is another cause of polyuria.[17] It is particularly common among infants living in impoverished circumstances in which caretakers feed diluted formula or water when formula supplies are exhausted. Life-threatening hyponatremia may ensue if treatment is not promptly initiated.

Osmotic Diuresis

Some patients have polyuria with renal water loss resulting from an osmotic diuresis. Glycosuria is frequently found to be the cause of sudden onset of polyuria in children with uncontrolled diabetes mellitus (see Chapter 256, Diabetes Mellitus). In both type I and type II diabetes mellitus, diminished carbohydrate utilization results in hyperglycemia and glycosuria. When present in the urine at high concentrations, glucose acts as an osmotic diuretic, resulting in polyuria. Chronic hyperglycemia may also cause a form of partial nephrogenic diabetes insipidus.[18] Osmotic diuresis may also be provoked by mannitol, radiologic contrast agents, high-protein feedings (in which urea acts as the osmotic agent), or the release of bilateral urinary tract obstruction.[19] Treatment with large volumes of dextrose-containing intravenous fluids can also result in hyperglycemia and polyuria. In contrast, renal glycosuria is characterized by a defect in renal tubular reabsorption of glucose, resulting in glycosuria without hyperglycemia or polyuria.

EVALUATION

A detailed history often reveals the cause of polyuria. Age at onset, pattern of fluid intake, and rate of onset of polyuria are informative. A thorough feeding history can help identify infants who have water intoxication. New onset of nocturia is often the first manifestation of loss of concentrating ability. Young children with diabetes insipidus can have irritability as a result of hypernatremia and dehydration. Family history is important, given than familial forms of both central and nephrogenic diabetes insipidus exist. In most cases of familial nephrogenic diabetes insipidus, severe polyuria occurs within the first weeks of life. Growth failure is a feature common to both nephrogenic and central diabetes insipidus.

A 24-hour measurement of fluid intake and output is helpful to confirm polyuria before ordering laboratory tests. Urinary specific gravity on a first-voided morning specimen is helpful but can be affected by the presence of glycosuria, proteinuria, or radiocontrast material. Both types of diabetes insipidus and primary polydipsia will result in relatively dilute urine. Disorders resulting in renal tubular damage such as sickle cell disease are more likely to have isosthenuria with specific gravities in the neighborhood of 1.010. Urinalysis with microscopy performed on a first-voided morning specimen also provides valuable information. Protein, casts, or formed blood elements in the urine suggest a renal disorder. Glycosuria with ketonuria strongly suggests diabetes mellitus. Other baseline studies include serum electrolytes, glucose, urea, phosphate, creatinine, calcium, osmolality, liver function tests, and complete blood count (Table 209-2).

Table 209-2 Interpretation of Baseline Values

CLINICAL SITUATION	SERUM SODIUM (mEq/L)	SERUM OSMOLALITY (mOsm/kg)	URINE OSMOLALITY	PLASMA VASOPRESSIN
Normal	135-145	280-290	50-1200	Normal
Central diabetes insipidus	Normal or elevated	Normal or elevated	<200	Low
Nephrogenic diabetes insipidus	Normal or elevated	Normal or elevated	<300	Normal or elevated
Psychogenic polydipsia	Low normal	<280	<200	Low

Adapted from Saborio P, Tipton G, Chan J. Diabetes insipidus. *Pediatr Rev.* 2000;21:122-129.

Table 209-3 Interpretation of Water Deprivation Test and Vasopressin Administration

CLINICAL SITUATION	PLASMA VASOPRESSIN	URINE OSMOLALITY	URINE SPECIFIC GRAVITY AFTER VASOPRESSIN
Normal	Increased	>800	Increased
Central diabetes insipidus	Low	<300	Increased
Nephrogenic diabetes insipidus	High	<200	Unchanged
Psychogenic polydipsia	Unchanged	500-600	Unchanged/Increased

Adapted from Saborio P, Tipton G, Chan J. Diabetes insipidus. *Pediatr Rev.* 2000;21:122-129.

Urine osmolality is best interpreted with a concomitant serum sample. A hyperosmolar state would suggest vasopressin deficiency or insensitivity, provided the serum glucose concentration is normal. Low serum osmolality with hyponatremia suggests either primary polydipsia or water intoxication as the most likely diagnosis. Serum sodium level is usually normal in diabetes insipidus as long as free access to fluids exists and the thirst mechanism is intact. Hypernatremia is commonly seen in infants with diabetes insipidus or when a central lesion exists that also impairs thirst.[20] Blood chemistries will detect causes of nephrogenic diabetes insipidus such as hypercalcemia and renal impairment.

In polyuric children with low urine specific gravity and no glycosuria, the next step in evaluation is referral to a specialist for a formal water deprivation test to determine if a defect exists in vasopressin production or renal responsiveness.[21] In the case of patients with very low urine osmolality who are strongly suspected of having nephrogenic diabetes insipidus, the response to exogenous ADH can be determined without the need for prior fluid restriction. Water restriction testing should be undertaken with great caution in younger children and should not be performed in newborns. Because of the possibility of volume depletion, the study should be carried out during the day when supervision is optimal and should follow a 24-hour period of free access to fluids.

At baseline, the clinician should record vital signs and weight and obtain blood and urine for osmolality, urine specific gravity, serum sodium concentration, serum urea nitrogen level, and hematocrit. Blood should also be obtained at the beginning and conclusion of fluid restriction to determine plasma ADH levels, which may be helpful if the response to the water restriction test is equivocal. Fluid intake is restricted for up to 8 hours, during which the patient must be supervised closely to avoid surreptitious drinking. The patient should be weighed and have vital signs recorded every 2 hours for the first 4 hours, then hourly. Blood and urine should be collected after 4 hours, then every 2 hours for osmolality, serum sodium, and urine specific gravity measurements. The test should be terminated when one of the following endpoints is reached: (1) the patient has lost 5% or more of body weight, (2) urine specific gravity is greater than 1.020, (3) urine osmolality exceeds 600 mOsm/kg, (4) plasma osmolality exceeds 300 mOsm/kg, or (5) serum sodium exceeds 147 mEq/L. At the conclusion of the test, weight and vital signs should be recorded and blood and urine collected for osmolality, serum sodium, and urine specific gravity.

In healthy children, and in most children with primary polydipsia, the weight remains constant, the urine specific gravity rises, and the urine volume decreases. Concentrating ability is frequently impaired in primary polydipsia, resulting in a maximal urine osmolality of 500 to 600 mOsm/kg, compared with greater than 800 mOsm/kg in healthy individuals. This difference is likely due to a reduction in the osmotic gradient across the distal renal tubule, resulting in reduced renal sensitivity to vasopressin (Table 209-3).[22]

In the setting of continued diuresis, dehydration, weight loss, and hyperosmolarity, the clinician should suspect a diagnosis of diabetes insipidus. A small rise in urine osmolality may occur in both forms of diabetes insipidus from either partial vasopressin deficiency (central) or partial vasopressin resistance (nephrogenic).

Administration of exogenous ADH may help differentiate between the 2 disorders (see Table 209-3). In an older child, the test can be performed after a water deprivation test or at a subsequent visit. Extreme caution is required when performing this test on infants or small children because of the danger of fluid overload and hyponatremia.[23] The patient is given free access to water after administration of desmopressin acetate (DDAVP), a synthetic derivative of vasopressin. Subsequently, intake, output, and urine specific gravity are recorded every 30 to 60 minutes.

In a patient with complete vasopressin deficiency, the urine output will fall and urine osmolality will increase significantly. Distinguishing between patients with partial central diabetes insipidus and primary polydipsia may be difficult. Individuals with partial diabetes insipidus may have an exaggerated response to the submaximal rise in vasopressin induced by fluid restriction.[24] Urine may be maximally concentrated when plasma osmolality is greater than 295 mOsm/kg. In this situation, there may be no further response to administration of exogenous ADH, a pattern suggestive of primary polydipsia. Patients who have primary polydipsia will have an increase in urine osmolality but no response tò exogenous ADH as endogenous release is intact. Patients with complete nephrogenic diabetes insipidus do not increase urine osmolality in response to exogenous ADH administration. In patients with partial nephrogenic diabetes insipidus, urine osmolality may increase but will still be significantly lower than 300 mOsm/kg. In contrast, patients with partial vasopressin deficiency typically achieve a urine osmolality greater than 300 mOsm/kg after fluid deprivation.

Patients with vasopressin deficiency are best referred to an endocrinologist or neurologist so that the cause of the diabetes insipidus can be determined. A full investigation of other pituitary functions, visual field examination, and magnetic resonance imaging of the brain will likely be the next steps in evaluation. Patients should be allowed free access to fluids, and their serum and urine osmolality should be monitored closely. When a diagnosis of central diabetes insipidus has been made, studies must be undertaken to ascertain the cause. Although many cases are idiopathic, a thorough evaluation for an underlying organic lesion must be conducted. Tumor markers human chorionic gonadotropin and alpha-fetoprotein should be measured, and magnetic resonance imaging of the pituitary and hypothalamus should be performed to assess for pituitary masses, craniopharyngioma, pinealoma, or pituitary stalk abnormalities. Up to 70% of patients with central diabetes insipidus will lose the normal hyperintense signal of the posterior pituitary.[25]

MANAGEMENT

Management of polyuria depends largely on the underlying diagnosis and must be individualized carefully. In most cases, the results are gratifying, but patients are often found to have a chronic disease that requires close, long-term surveillance.

In a severely ill patient with central diabetes insipidus, aqueous vasopressin (0.1 to 0.2 Units/kg) may be given subcutaneously every 4 to 6 hours. Vasopressin may also be given by continuous intravenous infusion. Reported starting doses vary from 0.5 to 4.6 mU/kg/hour; these doses should be increased or decreased as needed.[26,27] Vasopressin is a potent vasoconstrictor and may cause tissue ischemia and severe lactic acidosis, particularly at high infusion rates. Once the child's condition has stabilized, management consists of desmopressin acetate. Desmopressin can be administered orally in tablet form or instilled intranasally and should be given at the lowest dose that produces antidiuretic effect. When given intranasally, the total daily dose may range from 5 mcg in infants to 40 mcg in older children divided into 2 or 3 doses as needed. Children receiving dose multiples of 10 mcg may use the nasal spray; those on smaller or intermediate doses must use the rhinal tube. Desmopressin may also be administered effectively and safely orally.[28,29] Therapeutic doses of oral desmopressin are generally 15 to 20 times larger than intranasal doses, and greater variability exists in effective dose. Consequently, response to treatment must be monitored closely if changing route of administration.

Treatment of small children and infants with central diabetes insipidus can be difficult, with rapid changes in serum osmolality potentially leading to complications. The parents must carefully monitor fluid intake and output in the younger child. Because young infants are exclusively fed liquids and have high fluid requirements, the addition of vasopressin can greatly increase the risk of severe hyponatremia. These children are best managed with fluid therapy alone. Small doses of desmopressin may be required if adequate fluid intake is difficult to maintain or if caloric intake is inadequate because of excessive fluid consumption. The risk of hyponatremia can be reduced by allowing escape from the antidiuretic effect for 1 hour before the next dose. A child with adipsia or hypodipsia is best managed by fixing the desmopressin dose and fluid intake. Daily weights and frequent sodium levels are useful in assessing fluid status at home.[30]

In patients who have primary polydipsia, once a neurogenic lesion has been ruled out, medical therapy is not indicated. Psychotherapy, however, may be useful in addressing the emotional problem causing the polydipsia.

Hyponatremia can result from several factors, including excessive ingestion of hypotonic fluids, exogenous administration of vasopressin derivatives, or both. Patients with asymptomatic hyponatremia can be safely treated with fluid restriction or with isotonic saline if a fluid deficit is present. Symptomatic or severe hyponatremia (serum sodium less than 115 mEq/L) is an emergency that should be treated with hypertonic saline to raise serum sodium at a rate of 1 mEq/L/hr for 3 to 4 hours, limiting the rise in sodium to no greater than 10 mEq/L over 24 hours. In adults, rapid increases in serum sodium may lead to central pontine myelinosis. Although children may or may not be at risk for this complication, the primary care physician should take a cautious approach and limit the initial therapeutic increase in sodium to 125 mEq/L with subsequent small incremental elevations in serum sodium concentrations.[31]

Patients who have structural renal diseases leading to polyuria should be referred to a pediatric nephrologist. Children with nephrogenic diabetes insipidus should be allowed free access to fluids; parents of infants who have this disorder need to offer frequent water feedings to allow their infants to maintain osmotic homeostasis. A low-salt diet has been helpful in reducing urine output; thiazide diuretics can reduce polyuria further by reducing the amount of urine delivered to the distal tubule. Indomethacin[32] and amiloride,[33] when given concurrently with a thiazide, have each been found effective at reducing urine output.

Osmotic diuresis induced by drugs or diet generally is self-limited. In diabetes mellitus, polyuria secondary to hyperglycemia and glycosuria resolves with treatment of the underlying condition.

WHEN TO REFER

- Hypotonic polyuria (confirmed by 24-hour urine and urine osmolality <300 mOsm)
- Need to perform water deprivation test
- Polyuria after neurosurgery
- Polyuria and polydipsia secondary to diabetes mellitus

WHEN TO ADMIT

- Polyuria and dehydration
- Diabetic ketoacidosis
- Severe hyponatremia or hypernatremia
- Suspected diabetes insipidus in an infant

REFERENCES

1. Leung A, Robson W, Halperin M. Polyuria in childhood. *Clin Pediatr.* 1991;30:634.
2. Robertson GL, Shelton RL, Athar S. The osmoregulation of vasopressin. *Kidney Int.* 1976;10:25-37.
3. McKinley MJ, Johnson AK. The physiological regulation of thirst and fluid intake. *News Physiol Sci.* 2004;19:1-6.
4. McLeod JF, Kovacs L, Gaskill MB, et al. Familial neurohypophyseal diabetes insipidus associated with signal peptide mutations. *J Clin Endocrinol Metab.* 1993;77:599A-599G.
5. Rotig A, Cormier V, Chatalain P, et al. Deletion of mitochondrial DNA in a case of early-onset diabetes mellitus, optic atrophy and deafness (DIDMOAD, Wolfram syndrome). *J Inherit Metab Dis.* 1993;16:527-530.
6. Lindsay RS, Seckl JR, Padfield PL. The triple-phase response—problems of water balance after pituitary surgery. *Postgrad Med J.* 1995;71:439-441.
7. Greger NG, Kirkland RT, Clayton GW, et al. Central diabetes insipidus: 22 years' experience. *Am J Dis Child.* 1986;140:551-554.
8. Scherbaum WA. Autoimmune hypothalamic diabetes insipidus ("autoimmune hypothalamitis"). *Prog Brain Res.* 1992;93:283-292.
9. Heinze HJ, Bercu BB. Acquired hypophysitis in adolescence. *J Pediatr Endocrinol Metab.* 1997;10:315-321.
10. Bichet DG, Birnbaumer M, Lonergan M, et al. Nature and recurrence of AVPR2 mutations in X-linked nephrogenic diabetes insipidus. *Am J Hum Genet.* 1994;55:278-286.
11. Merendino JJ, Speigel AM, Crawford JD, et al. A mutation in the vasopressin V2-receptor gene in a kindred with X-linked nephrogenic diabetes insipidus. *N Engl J Med.* 1993;328:1538-1541.
12. Deen PM, Verdijk MA, Knoers NV, et al. Requirement of human renal water channel aquaporin-2 for vasopressin-dependent concentration of urine. *Science.* 1994;264:92-95.
13. Coleman RA, Van Hove JL, Morris CR, et al. Cerebral defects and nephrogenic diabetes insipidus with the ARC syndrome: additional findings or a new syndrome (ARCC-NDI)? *Am J Med Genet.* 1997;72:335-338.
14. Garofeanu CG, Weir M, Rosas-Arellano MP, et al. Causes of reversible nephrogenic diabetes insipidus: a systematic review. *Am J Kidney Dis.* 2005;45:626-637.
15. Kohn B, Normal ME, Feldman H, et al. Hysterical polydipsia (compulsive water drinking) in children. *Am J Dis Child.* 1976;130:210-212.
16. Goldman MB, Luchins DJ, Robertson GL. Mechanisms of altered water metabolism in psychotic patients with polydipsia and hyponatremia. *N Engl J Med.* 1988;318: 397-403.
17. Keating JP, Schears GJ, Dodge PR. Oral water intoxication in infants: an American epidemic, *Am J Dis Child.* 1991;145:985-990.
18. McKenna K, Morris AD, Ryan M, et al. Renal resistance to vasopressin in poorly controlled type 1 diabetes mellitus. *Am J Physiol Endocrinol Metab.* 2000;279: E155-E160.
19. Bishop MC. Diuresis and renal functional recovery in chronic retention. *Br J Urol.* 1985;57:1-5.
20. McIver B, Connacher A, Whittle I, et al. Adipsic hypothalamic diabetes insipidus after clipping of anterior communicating artery aneurism. *Br Med J.* 1991;303: 1465-1467.
21. Dashe AM, Cramm RE, Crist CA, et al. A water deprivation test for the differential diagnosis of polyuria. *JAMA.* 1963;185:699-703.
22. Cheetham T, Baylis PH. Diabetes insipidus in children: pathophysiology, diagnosis and management. *Paediatr Drugs.* 2002;4:785-796.
23. Koskimies O, Pylkkanen J, Vilska J. Water intoxication in infants caused by the urine concentration test with vasopressin analogue (DDAVP). *Acta Paediatr Scand.* 1984;73: 131-132.
24. Miller M, Dalakos T, Moses AM, et al. Recognition of partial defects in antidiuretic hormone secretion. *Ann Intern Med.* 1970;73:721-729.
25. Sato N, Ishizaka H, Yagi H, et al. Posterior lobe of the pituitary in diabetes insipidus: dynamic MR imaging. *Radiology.* 1993;186:357-360.
26. McDonald JA, Martha PM, Kerrigan J, et al. Treatment of the young child with postoperative central diabetes insipidus. *Am J Dis Child.* 1988;143:201-204.
27. Rogers MC, Helfaer MA. *Handbook of Pediatric Intensive Care.* 2nd ed. Baltimore, MD: Williams and Wilkins; 1995.
28. Boulgourdjian EM, Martinez AS, Ropelato MG, et al. Oral desmopressin treatment of central diabetes insipidus in children. *Acta Paediatr.* 1997;6:1261-1262.
29. Fjellestad-Paulsen A, Paulson O, d'Agay-Abensour L, et al. Central diabetes insipidus: oral treatment with dDAVP. *Regul Pept.* 1993;45:303-307.
30. Ball SG, Vaidja B, Baylis PH. Hypothalamic adipsic syndrome: diagnosis and management. *Clin Endocrinol.* 1997;47:405-409.
31. Nzerue CM, Baffoe-Bonnie H, You W, et al. Predictors of outcome in hospitalized patients with severe hyponatremia. *J Natl Med Assoc.* 2003;95:335-343.
32. Libber S, Harrison H, Spector D. Treatment of nephrogenic diabetes insipidus with prostaglandin synthesis inhibitors. *J Pediatr.* 1986;108:305-311.
33. Knoers N, Monnens LA. Amiloride-hydrochlorothiazide versus indomethacin-hydrochlorothiazide in the treatment of nephrogenic diabetes insipidus. *J Pediatr.* 1990; 117:499-502.

Chapter 210

PROTEINURIA

Shefali Mahesh, MD; Robert P. Woroniecki, MD, MS

In adults, *proteinuria* is defined as a urinary protein excretion exceeding 150 mg/day. In children, protein excretion exceeding 4 mg/m^2/hour is considered abnormal.[1] Proteinuria may indicate the presence of renal injury and predict progressive renal disease[2-5]; it is also an established independent risk factor for cardiovascular disease.[6] Large losses of protein through the urine lead to hypercholesterolemia and hypertriglyceridemia, both of which, if sustained, increase cardiovascular mortality.[7] Medications that reduce proteinuria may thus provide important long-term benefits for patients with chronic kidney disease.[8]

PATHOPHYSIOLOGICAL FEATURES

Under physiological conditions, the glomerular filtration barrier, composed of podocytes and vascular endothelium separated by the glomerular basement membrane, prevents the passage of macromolecules from blood into urine based on both molecular size and electrical charge. The size barrier for filtration consists of pores with a diameter of approximately 40 Å in the slit diaphragm located between foot processes that approximate the size of albumin (69 kDa). In addition, the glomerular capillary wall contains heparan sulfate and proteoglycans, which are negatively charged and thus repel macromolecules with the same electrical charge, such as albumin. Most inflammatory glomerular diseases lead to morphologic alteration of the size barrier and loss of negative charges, leading to proteinuria. Another factor that affects protein movement across glomerular capillary walls is glomerular hemodynamics (ie, glomerular plasma flow rate, hydrostatic and oncotic forces). A reduction in the number of functioning nephrons leads to hyperfiltration in the remaining nephrons and to proteinuria.

Low–molecular-weight proteins (<40 kDa) such as β_2-microglobulin, retinol-binding protein, and α_1-microglobulin are freely filtered through the glomerulus and are subsequently reabsorbed by the proximal tubule. Tubular injury results in an inability to reabsorb these proteins and their loss in the urine.[9] Some proteins, such as the Tamm-Horsfall mucoprotein (uromodulin), a major constituent of urinary casts, are formed by the cells of the thick ascending loop of Henle.[10]

LABORATORY EVALUATION OF PROTEINURIA

The diagnosis of proteinuria depends on laboratory assessment of the level of protein in the urine. The 3 ways urine is tested are (1) the dipstick test, (2) assessment of a timed urine sample, and (3) assessment of the urine protein-creatinine (P/Cr) ratio from an untimed urine sample.

Dipstick Test

The most commonly performed urine screening method for protein is the dipstick test. Tetrabromophenol on the reagent strip reacts with the amino group of the protein and changes the color of the strip. The test reports findings as negative, trace, and 1+ (30 mg/dL), 2+ (100 mg/dL), 3+ (300 mg/dL), and 4+ (2000 mg/dL).

The dipstick test primarily detects albumin and is less sensitive to low–molecular-weight proteins and γ-globulins. Because the test measures the concentration of protein, false-negative results may occur with highly dilute urine. Conversely, false-positive results may occur with concentrated urine. Generally, a result of 1+ or more in a specimen with a specific gravity of less than 1.015 indicates abnormal protein loss.[11]

The detection of protein depends on pH; extremely alkaline urine may yield a false-positive reading. Other causes of false-positive readings are prolonged immersion of the strip; hematuria, pyuria, or bacteriuria; presence of detergents and contaminating antiseptics such as chlorhexidine and benzalkonium chloride; presence of antibiotics such as penicillins, cephalosporins, sulfonamides, and tolbutamide; or presence of radiographic contrast materials.[11,12] An alternative office procedure to measure urinary protein is precipitation with sulfosalicylic acid. This measurement is a more accurate estimate of the total urinary proteins, including those of low molecular weight.[12] False-positive results can occur in the previously mentioned conditions.

When a dipstick reads positive, the result should be confirmed by urinalysis, preferably performed on the first urine voided in the morning.

Timed Urine Sample

The traditional and most accurate way of quantifying urinary protein excretion is to measure protein in a timed sample collected over a 24-hour period. The patient is instructed to void right after waking in the morning. This first urine is discarded, and all subsequent urines are collected. The last urine sample added to the collection should be 24 hours after the first one.

In adults, a protein excretion of less than 150 mg in 24 hours is considered normal. In children, an excretion rate of less than 4 mg/m^2/hour is considered normal, 4 to 40 mg/m^2/hour is abnormal, and more than 40 mg/m^2/hour is nephrotic-range proteinuria. The adequacy of the sample can be determined by measuring the creatinine excretion in the sample. Steady-state daily creatinine excretion is 20 mg/kg/day in children from 1 to 12 years of age and 22 to 25 mg/kg in older children. However, this method is cumbersome, can be impractical in children, and is fraught with error from under- and over-collection.[13]

Urine Protein-Creatinine Ratio

Measurement of the P/Cr ratio in an untimed (spot) urine sample offers a reliable method for classification of proteinuria. This method is easier than a 24-hour urine collection.[14] Studies in adults and children have shown a strong correlation between untimed urine P/Cr ratio and 24-hour urine collection. A ratio of more than 3.5:1 indicates nephrotic-range proteinuria, and ratios of less than 0.2:1 in patients ages 2 and older and less than 0.5:1 in children aged between 6 and 24 months are considered normal.[15]

PREVALENCE

Finding proteinuria in a single urine specimen in children and adolescents is relatively common. However, the presence of persistent proteinuria, also called *fixed proteinuria,* on repeat testing indicates renal disease until proven otherwise.[16] The prevalence of proteinuria is generally between 5% and 15%.[10] Prevalence appears to rise with age, peaking in adolescence, with subsequent decline and a nadir in adulthood. For boys, prevalence peaks at age 16; for girls the peak is at 13 years.[17]

ETIOLOGY

The basic evaluation of proteinuria should address the following issues: pathological or nonpathological cause; presence or absence of symptoms; amount of protein loss; presence or absence of associated findings such as hematuria, hypertension, azotemia; and other urinary or systemic abnormalities.

Nonpathological Proteinuria

Nonpathological proteinuria results from the adjustment of the kidney to extraneous physiological conditions (ie, growth, exercise, fever, systemic illness). The level of proteinuria is generally less than 1 g/day and is not associated with edema.[18]

Postural or Orthostatic Proteinuria

Orthostatic proteinuria accounts for 60% of all cases of asymptomatic proteinuria in children, with a higher incidence in adolescents.[19] Children with this condition have normal urinary protein excretion in the supine position but spill abnormal amounts of protein in the upright position. The proteinuria decreases to normal range or disappears when they have been recumbent for a few hours, as in overnight sleep. These children are asymptomatic; proteinuria is usually found on a routine urinalysis. The cause of orthostatic proteinuria is unknown.[20] Edema, hypertension, and hematuria are absent, and creatinine clearance and complements are normal. Renal ultrasound and histopathological tests are also normal, although these tests are not usually performed in the evaluation process.

Children with low-grade asymptomatic proteinuria should be assessed for *postural proteinuria.* The orthostatic test for postural proteinuria includes 2 separate collections, one in the supine position and the other in the upright position. At bedtime, the child goes to bed without voiding. Thirty minutes later the child is asked to void. The urine is discarded, but the time is noted as the start of the collection in supine position. The child is then given a large glass of water or another fluid and allowed to sleep. All urine passed during the night, including the first specimen voided the next morning, is collected in a jar (specimen 1), and the time of the first morning voiding is recorded. Then the child goes about daily activities but collects all urine in a second jar (specimen 2) for approximately the next 12 hours. This collection is the upright collection, which ends at bedtime, when the time is again recorded. In patients with orthostatic proteinuria the sample obtained in the supine position will be free of protein or will contain a normal amount of protein; on the other hand the sample obtained in upright position will contain an abnormal amount of protein. Children with orthostatic proteinuria generally excrete less than 1 g of protein in 24 hours.[12]

The diagnosis of postural proteinuria can also be made by assessing the first-morning urine. If this sample has no protein, or if it has a P/Cr ratio less than 0.2:1, then a presumptive diagnosis of orthostatic proteinuria can be made. Long-term follow-up studies in adults have documented the benign nature of orthostatic proteinuria, although rare cases of glomerulosclerosis have been identified later in life in patients who were initially found to have proteinuria with an orthostatic component.[21-23] Therefore long-term follow-up of children is necessary unless the proteinuria resolves. Signs to anticipate include appearance of hematuria, hypertension, increase in serum creatinine concentration, or proteinuria exceeding 1 g/day.[18]

Transient Proteinuria

As many as 30% to 50% of children with proteinuria may have *transient, nonfixed proteinuria.* It can accompany fever, exercise, stress, dehydration, congestive heart failure, or seizures.[24] Transient proteinuria may be found in children having a temperature of 38.3°C or higher.[25] It usually does not exceed 2+ on the dipstick test and resolves when the fever abates.

Proteinuria associated with vigorous exercise rarely exceeds 2+ on the dipstick test. Transient proteinuria seems to be related to intensity of exercise rather than duration.[26] It may be explained by an increased glomerular filtration barrier permeability and a partial inhibition of tubular reabsorption of protein.[27] The effect of exercise increases with age.[28] Transient proteinuria is considered benign if proteinuria resolves after 48 hours of rest.

Pathological Proteinuria

Persistent or Fixed Asymptomatic Proteinuria

Patients with a positive dipstick test (1+ or greater) should undergo a more accurate test, such as P/Cr ratio or a quantitative measurement of protein excretion. Orthostatic proteinuria should be excluded by repeat measurements on a first-morning void if the initial sample was taken at random. In the absence of other abnormalities, patients with 2 or more positive semiquantitative or quantitative tests, 1 to 2 weeks apart, are diagnosed as having *fixed proteinuria.*[29] The prevalence in school-aged children may be as high as 6%.[16,30] Various causes are listed in Table 210-1.

Pathological proteinuria can be classified as either glomerular or tubular. *Glomerular proteinuria,* which is more common of the 2 forms, is associated with increased permeability of glomerular filtration barrier. Glomerular proteinuria may be selective (plasma proteins with molecular weights up to and including albumin), as in minimal change disease, or nonselective (albumin and large–molecular-weight proteins, such as immunoglobulin G), as in most forms of glomerulonephritis. *Tubular proteinuria* results from decreased tubular protein reabsorption that results from tubular dysfunction (see Table 210-1).

Table 210-1 Classification of Pathological Proteinuria

GLOMERULAR	TUBULAR
Nephrotic syndrome	Genetic
Idiopathic	Polycystic kidney disease
Minimal change	Cystinosis
Mesangial proliferation	Wilson disease
Focal segmented glomerulosclerosis	Lowe syndrome
	Galactosemia
Membranous nephropathy	Renal tubular acidosis
Glomerulonephritis	Acquired
Postinfectious	Interstitial nephritis
Immunoglobulin A nephropathy	Acute tubular necrosis
	Interstitial nephritis
Membranoproliferative glomerulonephritis	Heavy metal poisoning
Systemic disease	
Systemic lupus erythematosus	
Vasculitis	
Tumor	
Subacute bacterial endocarditis	
Infection (HIV, hepatitis)	
Other	
Drugs or toxins	
Obesity	

Symptomatic Proteinuria

Symptomatic proteinuria is often associated with gravity-dependent edema, hypoalbuminemia, and hyperlipidemia when it is defined as a nephrotic syndrome. However, some children with nephrotic-range proteinuria and hypoalbuminemia remain completely asymptomatic. Edema in nephrotic syndrome results from several factors acting in concert, including increased distal nephron sodium reabsorption, increased capillary permeability, and low plasma oncotic pressure associated with hypoalbuminemic states.

Proteinuria may be associated with other abnormalities, including hematuria, hypertension, and azotemia, as seen in glomerulonephritis. Patients with a combination of nephritis and nephrotic syndrome pose a clinical challenge even to the most experienced nephrologist.

EVALUATION

History

The first step in evaluating a child with proteinuria is obtaining a thorough history and conducting a physical examination looking for indicators of renal disease. History should include questions about recent illnesses, fever, rash, and arthralgias; change in urine output and color; symptoms of chronic disease (eg, weight loss, fatigue); and duration and severity of symptoms. History of urinary tract infections and family history of urinary reflux, hypertension, and deafness are important.

Physical Examination

Physical examination should include measurements of growth parameters, blood pressure, and identification of edema, ascites, and pallor. The presence of proteinuria should be confirmed by a urine P/Cr ratio on a first-morning urine sample. Once confirmed, the proteinuria should be quantified by a 24-hour urine collection for measurement of protein and creatinine (to determine adequacy of the sample).

BOX 210-1 Warning Signs of Proteinuria

- Persistent, fixed, nonorthostatic proteinuria
- Proteinuria associated with other urinary abnormalities, such as hematuria
- Proteinuria associated with renal insufficiency, anemia, or hypertension
- Family history of renal disease, deafness, or autoimmune conditions
- Proteinuria associated with comorbidities such as prematurity, congenital anomalies of other organ systems, hypertension, diabetes, and obesity

Laboratory Evaluation

Serum electrolytes, blood urea nitrogen, and creatinine help determine the level of kidney function. Serum albumin, cholesterol, and triglycerides guide the determination of the severity of metabolic changes that occur as a result of urine protein loss. Complement levels, antistreptolysin O titers, hepatitis serologic testing, and HIV testing may be indicated based on the child's history. Renal ultrasound should be performed to assess for structural abnormalities. The patient should be referred to a pediatric nephrologist if any abnormalities are found during the initial work-up. Some of the other warning signs of proteinuria are listed in Box 210-1.

The steps in evaluating proteinuria are illustrated in Figure 210-1.

Children should be routinely screened by a standard dipstick test on 2 occasions, once before starting school and again in early adolescence (as recommended by the American Academy of Pediatrics). Subsequent testing should be performed as needed.[12]

Assessment of total protein is appropriate in children to identify both albuminuria and low-molecular-weight proteinuria. Under most circumstances, spot urine samples should be used to detect and monitor proteinuria in children. Obtaining 24-hour timed urine collections is usually unnecessary. First-morning specimens are preferred, but random specimens are acceptable if a first-morning sample is unavailable. Patients with a positive dipstick test of 1+ or greater should undergo confirmation by assessment of the P/Cr ratio within 3 months.

Orthostatic proteinuria must be excluded by measuring P/Cr ratio in a first-morning urine sample. Patients with 2 or more positive P/Cr tests, obtained at 1- to 2-week intervals, should be diagnosed as having persistent proteinuria. Monitoring proteinuria in patients with chronic kidney disease should be performed by quantitative methods.

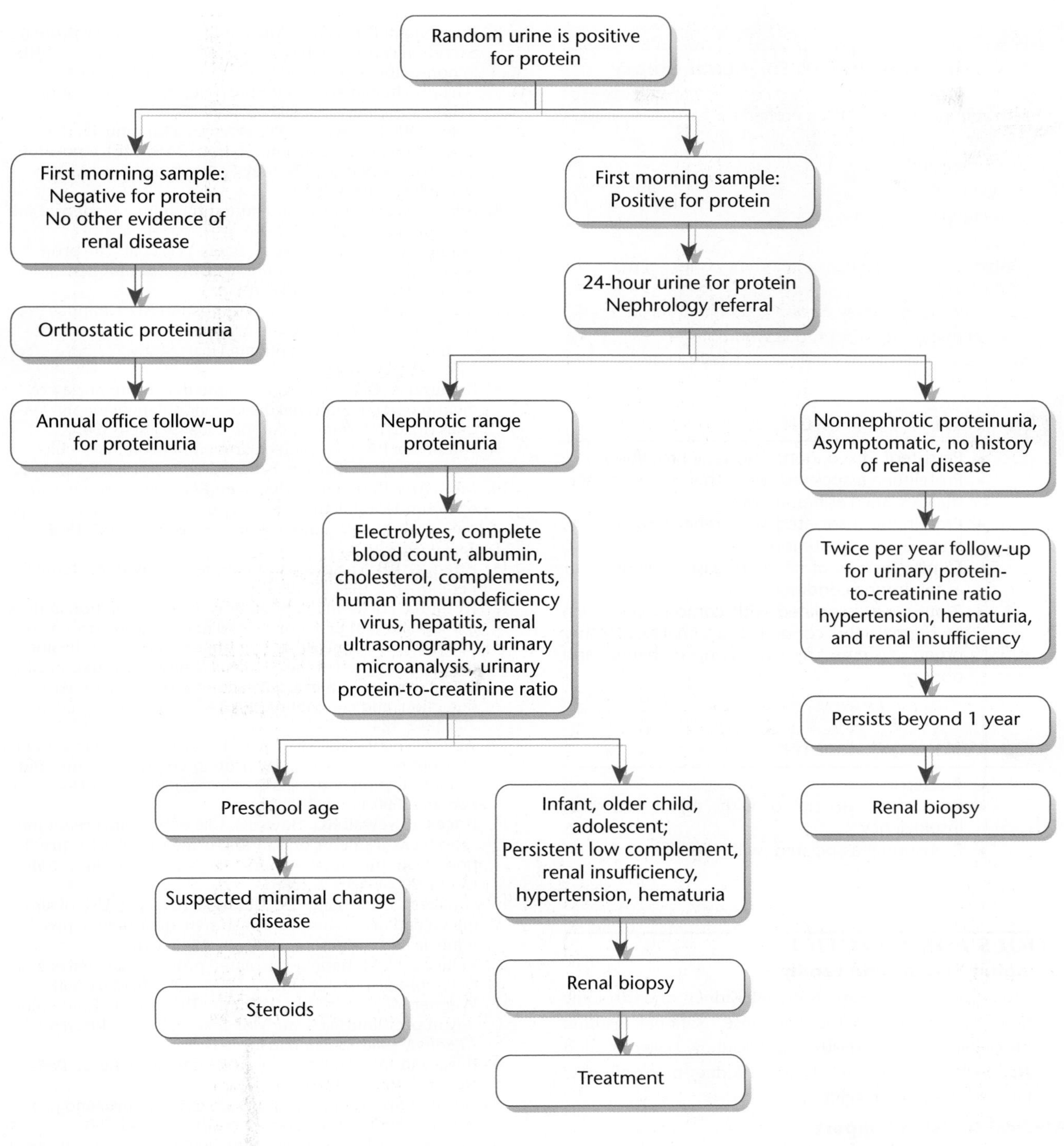

Figure 210-1 Diagnostic approach in a patient with proteinuria.

MANAGEMENT

If orthostatic proteinuria is diagnosed, then the child should be monitored with annual office visits and check of urine P/Cr ratio.

If isolated fixed proteinuria less than 1 g/day is detected (urine P/Cr ratio <1:1), then twice-yearly visits with determination of urine P/Cr ratio are sufficient. The clinician should assess for hematuria and hypertension. If proteinuria persists for more than a year, then renal biopsy should be considered (Box 210-2). Restrictions on the child's lifestyle and physical activity are not necessary. Children with proteinuria should receive the recommended daily allowance of protein for their age.[31,32]

BOX 210-2 Indications for Renal Biopsy

Fixed, asymptomatic, isolated proteinuria >1 g/day
Persistent proteinuria <1 g/day plus:
- Hematuria and casts
- Renal insufficiency
- Low complement levels
- Hypertension
- Systemic symptoms such as recurrent rashes, joint pains, or fever
- Family history of kidney disease or autoimmune disease

Corticosteroid-resistant nephrotic syndrome

WHEN TO REFER

- Persistent , fixed, nonorthostatic proteinuria
- Proteinuria associated with other urinary abnormalities, such as hematuria
- Proteinuria associated with renal insufficiency, anemia, or hypertension
- Family history of renal disease, deafness, or autoimmune condition
- Proteinuria associated with comorbidities such as prematurity, congenital anomalies of other organ systems, hypertension, diabetes, and obesity

WHEN TO ADMIT

- Anasarca
- Proteinuria associated with significant renal insufficiency
- Proteinuria associated with significant hypertension

TOOLS FOR PRACTICE

Engaging Patient and Family

- *Proteinuria* (fact sheet), National Kidney and Urologic Diseases Information Clearinghouse, National Institute of Diabetes and Digestive and Kidney Diseases, and National Institutes of Health (kidney.niddk.nih.gov/kudieseases/pub/proteinuria).

Medical Decision Support

- *Pathologic Proteinuria Calculator* (interactive tool), (www.metrohealthresearch.org/schelling).

REFERENCES

1. Nephrotic syndrome in children: a randomized trial comparing 2 prednisone regimens in steroid-responsive patients who relapse early. Report of the International Study of Kidney Disease in Children. *J Pediatr.* 1979;95:239-243.
2. Williams JD, Coles GA. Proteinuria—a direct cause of renal morbidity? *Kidney Int.* 1994;45:443-450.
3. Ruggenenti P, Perna A, Mosconi L, et al. Urinary protein excretion rate is the best independent predictor of ESRF in non-diabetic proteinuric chronic nephropathies. "Gruppo Italiano di Studi Epidemiologici in Nefrologia" (GISEN). *Kidney Int.* 1998;53:1209-1216.
4. Keane WF, Eknoyan G. Proteinuria, albuminuria, risk, assessment, detection, elimination (PARADE): a position paper of the National Kidney Foundation. *Am J Kidney Dis.* 1999;33:1004-1010.
5. Eddy AA. Proteinuria and interstitial injury. *Nephrol Dial Transplant.* 2004;19:277-281.
6. Kannel WB, Stampfer MJ, Castelli WP, et al. The prognostic significance of proteinuria: the Framingham study. *Am Heart J.* 1984;108:1347-1352.
7. Sytkowski PA, Kannel WB, D'Agostino RB. Changes in risk factors and the decline in mortality from cardiovascular disease. The Framingham Heart Study. *N Engl J Med.* 1990;322:1635-1641.
8. Remuzzi G, Chiurchiu C, Ruggenenti P. Proteinuria predicting outcome in renal disease: nondiabetic nephropathies (REIN). *Kidney Int Suppl.* 2004;(92):S90-S96.
9. Tomlinson PA. Low molecular weight proteins in children with renal disease. *Pediatr Nephrol.* 1992;6:565-571.
10. McKenzie JK, Patel R, McQueen EG. The excretion rate of Tamm-Horsfall urinary mucoprotein in normals and in patients with renal disease. *Australas Ann Med.* 1964;13:32-39.
11. Ettenger RB. The evaluation of the child with proteinuria. *Pediatr Ann.* 1994;23:486-494.
12. Hogg RJ, Portman RJ, Milliner D, et al. Evaluation and management of proteinuria and nephrotic syndrome in children: recommendations from a pediatric nephrology panel established at the National Kidney Foundation conference on proteinuria, albuminuria, risk, assessment, detection, and elimination (PARADE). *Pediatrics.* 2000;105:1242-1249.
13. Abitbol C, Zilleruelo G, Freundlich M, et al. Quantitation of proteinuria with urinary protein/creatinine ratios and random testing with dipsticks in nephrotic children. *J Pediatr.* 1990;116:243-247.
14. Price CP, Newall RG, Boyd JC. Use of protein: creatinine ratio measurements on random urine samples for prediction of significant proteinuria: a systematic review. *Clin Chem.* 2005;51:1577-1586.
15. Ginsberg JM, Chang BS, Matarese RA, et al. Use of single voided urine samples to estimate quantitative proteinuria. *N Engl J Med.* 1983;309:1543-1546.
16. Vehaskari VM, Rapola J. Isolated proteinuria: analysis of a school-age population. *J Pediatr.* 1982;101:661-668.
17. Wagner MG, Smith FG Jr, Tinglof BO Jr, et al. Epidemiology of proteinuria. A study of 4,807 schoolchildren. *J Pediatr.* 1968;73:825-832.
18. Bergstein JM. A practical approach to proteinuria. *Pediatr Nephrol.* 1999;13:697-700.
19. Norman ME. An office approach to hematuria and proteinuria. *Pediatr Clin North Am.* 1987;34:545-560.
20. Devarajan P. Mechanisms of orthostatic proteinuria: lessons from a transplant donor. *J Am Soc Nephrol.* 1993;4:36-39.
21. Springberg PD, Garrett LE Jr, Thompson AL Jr, et al. Fixed and reproducible orthostatic proteinuria: results of a 20-year follow-up study. *Ann Intern Med.* 1982;97:516-519.
22. Rytand DA, Spreiter S. Prognosis in postural (orthostatic) proteinuria: forty to fifty-year follow-up of six patients after diagnosis by Thomas Addis. *N Engl J Med.* 1981;305:618-621.
23. Berns JS, McDonald B, Gaudio KM, et al. Progression of orthostatic proteinuria to focal and segmental glomerulosclerosis. *Clin Pediatr (Phila).* 1986;25:165-166.

24. Houser M. Assessment of proteinuria using random urine samples. *J Pediatr.* 1984;104:845-848.
25. Marks MI, McLaine PN, Drummond KN. Proteinuria in children with febrile illnesses. *Arch Dis Child.* 1970;45: 250-253.
26. Poortmans JR. Postexercise proteinuria in humans. Facts and mechanisms. *JAMA.* 1985;253:236-240.
27. Poortmans JR. [Renal response to exercise in healthy and diseased patients]. *Nephrologie.* 1995;16:317-324.
28. Poortmans JR, Geudvert C, Schorokoff K, et al. Postexercise proteinuria in childhood and adolescence. *Int J Sports Med.* 1996;17:448-451.
29. National Kidney Foundation. K/DOQI clinical practice guidelines for chronic kidney disease: evaluation, classification, and stratification. *Am J Kidney Dis.* 2002;39: S1-S266.
30. Yoshikawa N, Kitagawa K, Ohta K, et al. Asymptomatic constant isolated proteinuria in children. *J Pediatr.* 1991; 119:375-379.
31. Wingen AM, Fabian-Bach C, Schaefer F, et al. Randomised multicentre study of a low-protein diet on the progression of chronic renal failure in children. European Study Group of Nutritional Treatment of Chronic Renal Failure in Childhood. *Lancet.* 1997;349:1117-1123.
32. Uauy RD, Hogg RJ, Brewer ED, et al. Dietary protein and growth in infants with chronic renal insufficiency: a report from the Southwest Pediatric Nephrology Study Group and the University of California, San Francisco. *Pediatr Nephrol.* 1994;8:45-50.

Chapter 211
PRURITUS

Nancy K. Barnett, MD

Pruritus, or itch, is the subjective perception of a cutaneous disturbance that is relieved by scratching or rubbing. It is usually not brought to the primary care physician's attention unless it is generalized, chronic, or associated with an eruption. In such instances, however, pruritus must be treated with great respect because severe itching can be physically incapacitating. In addition, scratching or rubbing the itch can produce extensive disfigurement in the form of linear excoriations or lichenified plaques and can predispose the patient to cutaneous infections. Constant scratching can even cause social isolation because, at times, people view the child with pruritus as being contagious or unclean.

DEFINITION OF TERMS

Because itch is a subjective sensation, objective evaluation to delineate its pathophysiological characteristics has been difficult. However, current thinking implicates nonspecific itch receptors. Thought to be free, fine nerve endings at the dermoepidermal junction, these receptors transmit the pruritic sensation along dedicated, slow-conduction velocity, unmyelinated C fibers.[1] The exact mediators and their release triggers are unknown. Mast cell histamine has elicited itch fairly consistently in experimental settings[2] and appears to be active in human disease, as may be other local mediators such as substance P and interleukin.[3] Other experimental triggers that have produced itch are physical pressure, heat, and electric shock. Researchers believe that the nerve impulses from the intraepithelial mechanoinsensitive C fibers ascend to the lamina I in the dorsal horn of the spinal cord and travel along the contralateral spinothalamic tract to the thalamus. They are then transferred to multiple areas of the cortex and are interpreted as itch. A subsequent desire to scratch arises in the motor cortex.[4] Area 3a in the sensorimotor cortex and the anterior cingulate cortex have been identified as activated when histamine-induced itch and scratch are traced. Itch is not a mild form of pain; the pathways are different, and aspirin alone does not relieve itch.

Certain circumstances alter the interpretation of the degree of pruritus. For example, the itch threshold in and around areas of active dermatitis can be lowered by psychic stress, decreased skin hydration, or increased skin temperature, and during the night.[2,5]

DIFFERENTIAL DIAGNOSIS

In children, local cutaneous disease rather than systemic disease is by far the most common cause of generalized pruritus. Pruritogenic itch arising in the skin is the focus of this chapter, and discussing neuropathic, neurogenic, and psychogenic itch[6] is beyond the scope. The major differential diagnoses of generalized pruritus with skin lesions in children are infestation (scabies, pediculosis, insect bites, and papular urticaria), atopic dermatitis, miliaria, contact dermatitis, and acute or chronic urticaria.

Children may also itch with cutaneous diseases such as psoriasis, lichen planus, and linear IgA bullous disease of childhood. These children should be referred to a dermatologist for evaluation and management, as should a child with pruritus who is otherwise healthy and does not have bites, eczema, heat rash, contact dermatitis or hives. The child who has pruritus, from whatever cause, is at risk for psychological damage, infection secondary to impetiginization, and scarification.

Systemic causes of pruritus in the child who has pruritus but no skin lesions are hyper- and hypothyroidism, leukemia or lymphoma, chronic renal failure, obstructive biliary disease, and xerosis (generalized dry skin).

EVALUATION AND MANAGEMENT

Most of the common cutaneous diseases associated with generalized pruritus can be diagnosed based on a thorough history and physical examination. The answers to the following questions may help diagnose infestation of one sort or another and direct therapy toward topical steroids, long clothes, and repellents:

Are any individual pruritic papules found with a central punctum?
If so, are they on exposed or nonexposed areas?
Does anyone else in the family have similar lesions?

A family history of allergy, asthma, or eczema in a child who has a chronic eczematous dermatitis over extensor surfaces in infancy and flexural areas in childhood suggests atopic dermatitis. Hydration and emollients will reduce the pruritus and should be the mainstay of therapy, although mid- and low-potency topical steroids for inflammation, antibiotics for secondary infection, and cool compresses may also be required to bring the scratch-itch cycle under control. Short courses (<8 weeks) of topical immunomodulators such as tacrolimus and pimecrolimus may be helpful in relieving atopic itch on facial skin and thin areas such as the axillae, but these medications should not be prescribed as chronic therapy. A tolerable (nonsoporific) dose of an antihistamine may relieve itch and should be given approximately 1 hour before bedtime because the itch threshold is lower at night than it is during the daytime. Hydroxyzine seems to be the most effective agent.[7] Data conflict about the use of nonsedating antihistamines for controlling itch.[8] Pinpoint crystalline or erythematous papules in areas of occlusion and sweating—that is, miliaria crystallina and miliaria rubra (heat rash)—can be controlled by simple measures such as applying dusting powders, avoiding tight clothing, and reducing exposure to high ambient temperatures.

In most instances, contact dermatitis is readily recognizable because of a linear array of papulovesicular erythematous lesions and sharp borders that conform to the shape of the contactant. The use of antihistamines, topical steroids, and compresses is discussed in detail in Chapter 252, Contact Dermatitis.

Acute urticaria, usually from exposure to a drug or other ingestant, produces intensely pruritic, erythematous, and edematous plaques and papules. (See also Chapter 259, Drug Eruptions, Erythema Multiforme, Stevens-Johnson Syndrome, and Toxic Epidermal Necrolysis.) Thorough historical and environmental sleuthing may reveal the cause of a contact allergic or contact irritant dermatitis, but the cause of 90% of acute urticaria cases remains a mystery. If the patient has not used any new drug or food, and if the hives persist despite regular use of antihistamines for several days, then a reasonable course of action would be to obtain a throat culture and a complete blood count with differential and to screen for mycoplasmal disease and infectious mononucleosis to rule out occult streptococcal, mycoplasmal, and viral infections. On rare occasions, a skin biopsy may be helpful.

For the child who has pruritus with no primary skin disorder, a complete blood count with differential count, complete chemistry panel, thyroid-stimulating hormone test, urinalysis, and chest radiograph should be obtained assessing for possible systemic causes, especially before suggesting a psychogenic cause for the itching.

To relieve itching and prevent scarring (both mental and physical), the scratch-itch cycle must be broken. Itching provokes scratching, and when the scratching stops, the itching returns. To control itching, the following steps can be helpful:

- Keep the patient's fingernails short to prevent damage from scratching.
- Keep the child fully clothed except when applying medications.
- Apply bland emollient creams frequently, especially after bathing.
- Apply cool compresses to relieve intense pruritus and to remove crusts and debris.
- Apply topical steroids for short periods (generally less than 2 weeks) to control inflammation.
- Increase the dose of antihistamine until the scratching stops or marked drowsiness occurs, and then reduce the dose to a level that controls the scratching but does not cause drowsiness.
- Advise the family to avoid stress, heat, and irritants.
- See the patient frequently to provide support.
- If the child is old enough to understand, then explain why these methods are being used.

Topical capsaicin and pramoxine may be indicated for localized use in some cases, but potential for systemic absorption limits their prolonged or widespread use.[9] Referral to the dermatologist is generally indicated in such a circumstance. Ultraviolet B light therapy may be helpful for generalized pruritus such as occurs in biliary cirrhosis or severe chronic atopic dermatitis.[10]

WHEN TO REFER

- Pruritus with uncommon disease (eg, psoriasis, bullae)
- Chronic pruritus without cutaneous disease to evaluate for systemic cause
- Pruritus uncontrolled by usual topical steroids and antihistamines

TOOLS FOR PRACTICE

Engaging Patients and Family

- *What is a Pediatric Dermatologist?* (fact sheet), American Academy of Pediatrics (www.aap.org/sections/derm/pedDermatologistfacts.pdf).

Medical Decision Support

- *Pediatric Dermatology: A Quick Reference Guide* (book), American Academy of Pediatrics (www.aap.org/bookstore).
- *PediaLink Module: Dermatology: Skin Essentials* (on-line course), American Academy of Pediatrics (www.pedialink.org/cme/_coursefinder/CMEdetail.cfm?aid=21445&area=liveCME).

SUGGESTED RESOURCES

Krishnan A, Koo J. Psyche, opioids and itch: therapeutic consequences. *Dermatol Ther.* 2005;18:314-322.

Yosipovitch G, Greaves MW, Schmelz M. Itch. *Lancet.* 2003;361:690-694.

REFERENCES

1. Yosipovitch G, Greaves MW, Schmelz M. Itch. *Lancet.* 2003;361:690-694.
2. Cormia FE. Experimental histamine pruritus. *J Invest Dermatol.* 1952;19:21.
3. Greaves MW, Wall PD. Pathophysiology of itching. *Lancet.* 1996;348:938-940.
4. Wallengren J. Neuroanatomy and neurophysiology of itch. *Dermatol Ther.* 2005;18:292-303.
5. Edwards AE, Shellow WV, Wright ET, et al. Pruritic skin disease, psychological stress and the itch sensation. *Arch Dermatol.* 1976;112:339.

6. Fazio SB. Pruritus. UpToDate Patient Information: Pruritus, 2005. Available at: patients.uptodate.com/topic.asp?file=genr_med/35767. Accessed on January 26, 2007.
7. Rhoades RB, Leifer KN, Cohan R, et al. Suppression of histamine-induced pruritus by three antihistamine drugs. *J Allergy Clin Immunol.* Mar 1975;55(3):180-185.
8. O'Donoghue M, Tharp MD. Antihistamines and their role as antipruritic. *Dermatol Ther.* 2005;18:333-340.
9. Krishnan A, Koo J. Psyche, opioids and itch: therapeutic consequences. *Dermatol Ther.* 2005;18:314-322.
10. Rivard J, Lim HW. Ultraviolet phototherapy for pruritus. *Dermatol Ther.* 2005;18:344-354.

Chapter 212

PUBERTY: NORMAL AND ABNORMAL

Dominique N. Long, MD; Robert K. Kritzler, MD; Leslie P. Plotnick, MD

Disorders of pubertal development constitute one of the most frequent referrals to pediatric endocrinology clinics. In many cases, no endocrine problem is found. A referral may be avoided by a careful evaluation, including family history, and a few simple laboratory procedures. The availability of pediatric endocrinology consultation and the primary care physician's level of comfort in diagnosing and treating disorders of puberty heavily influence the decision to refer.

NORMAL PUBERTY

At puberty, a series of complex hormonal changes takes place. The hypothalamus secretes pulses of gonadotropin-releasing hormone (GnRH), which stimulates pituitary gonadotropin production of luteinizing hormone (LH) and follicle-stimulating hormone (FSH). Concomitantly, the previously very sensitive hypothalamic-pituitary-gonadal feedback loop becomes less sensitive to the negative effect of gonadal steroids. As a result, gonadotropin levels rise, stimulating the secretion of greater amounts of sex steroids, either testosterone or estradiol, depending on the gender of the child, leading to the physical changes of puberty. This process is called gonadarche. The hypothalamic-pituitary-gonadal axis is active during fetal life and infancy until it enters an inactive state during the prepubertal years. Genetic factors determine 50% to 80% of the variation in pubertal timing.[1] Environmental influences also play a role, in particular, nutritional status. Leptin, which is secreted by adipocytes and regulates appetite and metabolism through the hypothalamus, is thought to play a permissive role in regulating the timing of puberty.[2] Adrenarche is a separate process that refers to an increase in the secretion of adrenal androgens during puberty and is associated with the development of pubic hair, axillary hair, body odor, and acne. The mechanism that triggers the maturation of the adrenal cortex at puberty remains poorly understood.

In most girls, puberty begins between 8 and 13 years of age, and breast development (thelarche) is usually the first sign of puberty. Menarche follows the onset of breast development by approximately 2 years. A growth spurt accompanies the changes, usually peaking before menarche. The range of normal variation, however, is quite wide, and differences have been reported between ethnic groups. A secular trend toward earlier puberty has taken place, and an association exists between earlier sexual maturation in girls and increasing levels of adiposity; however, from existing data, whether this relationship is causal is unclear. Recent data from the National Health and Nutrition Examination Survey (NHANES) 1999-2002 shows a decline in the overall average age at menarche to 12.34 years (12.06 years, 12.52 years, and 12.09 years in non-Hispanic black girls, non-Hispanic white girls, and Mexican American girls, respectively).[3] The average age at menarche declined by 2.3 months between NHANES III (1988-1994) and NHANES 1999-2002. Significantly, NHANES 1999-2002 had more girls with body mass index greater than the 85th or 95th percentile and had a different racial and ethnic composition.[3] Although the overall age at menarche decreased, the changes within racial and ethnic groups was much smaller, indicating that the overall decrease in age at menarche may be because of changes in the population distribution of race and ethnicity and relative weight.

The mean age for onset of breast development according to NHANES III analysis was 10.25, 11.05, and 10.70 years in non-Hispanic black girls, non-Hispanic white girls, and Mexican American girls, respectively. Similarly, the mean age for onset of sexual hair in girls was 10.25, 10.96, and 11.17 years, respectively.[4,5] Mean age of pubertal changes from NHANES 1999-2002 is not yet available.

In most boys, puberty begins between 9 and 14 years of age. Testicular enlargement is usually the first sign of puberty. NHANES III data found the mean age of genital development in boys to be 10.79, 11.08, and 11.09 years for non-Hispanic black boys, non-Hispanic white boys, and Mexican-American boys, respectively. Similarly, the mean age for onset of sexual hair was 11.48, 11.81, and 12.20 years, respectively.[5] Peak height velocity for boys is typically 2 years later than it is for girls and usually occurs during mid to late puberty (see Table 212-1 for summary of pubertal milestones by age).

The time of puberty is one of profound change, both physical and psychological. Problems of sexual identity, body image, adolescent independence, and peer acceptance are frequent. Because the ranges of age of normal puberty are wide, children of similar chronologic age may have markedly different physical maturity. When pubertal development is precocious or delayed, many of these problems are compounded.

GYNECOMASTIA

Pubertal gynecomastia occurs in approximately 40% of healthy boys and usually resolves within 2 years. Clinical presentation may include breast tenderness and asymmetry. The mean age of occurrence is between 14 and 15.5 years and usually occurs after Tanner stage 3. Pubertal gynecomastia is thought to result from an increase in the ratio of estrogen to androgen. Treatment in most cases is reassurance; however, gynecomastia that does not resolve after 2 years or that develops rapidly may require a referral.

Table 212-1 Onset of Pubertal Milestones (Years)

	NON-HISPANIC WHITES	NON-HISPANIC BLACKS	MEXICAN AMERICANS
GIRLS			
Thelarche	11.05	10.25	10.7
Sexual hair development	10.96	10.25	11.17
Menarche	12.52	12.06	12.09
BOYS			
Testicular enlargement	11.08	10.79	11.09
Sexual hair development	11.81	11.48	12.20

Note: Thelarche, testicular enlargement, and sexual hair development expressed as means, age at menarche expressed as average.
From National Health and Nutrition Examination Survey III (1988-1994) and National Health and Nutrition Examination Survey (1999-2002).

Initial screening blood work includes levels of testosterone, estradiol, LH, FSH, liver function tests, prolactin, and a β-human chorionic gonadotropin level. Medical therapy with clomiphene (antiestrogen), tamoxifen (estrogen antagonist), testolactone (peripheral aromatase inhibitor), and danazol (synthetic derivative of testosterone) has been reported to be successful; however, no randomized-controlled trials have been conducted. Surgical intervention remains the mainstay of treatment. Whereas most pubertal gynecomastia is benign, pathologic causes include Klinefelter syndrome, partial androgen insensitivity syndrome, hyperprolactinemia, liver disorders, adrenal carcinoma, biosynthetic defects in testosterone production, androgen receptor defects, increased activity of peripheral aromatase, and certain drugs. Drugs that have an estrogen-like effect (diethylstilbestrol, oral contraceptive pills, digitalis, estrogen-containing cosmetics), that increase estrogen formation (gonadotropins, clomiphene), or that inhibit testosterone action (ketoconazole, spironolactone, cimetidine, isoniazid, methyldopa, captopril, tricyclic antidepressants, diazepam, marijuana, phenothiazine) have been associated with gynecomastia.

DELAYED PUBERTY

Few matters are of greater concern to the adolescent than remaining short in stature or sexually underdeveloped. Delayed development demands the immediate attention of the practitioner.

Puberty is considered delayed in girls who have no breast development by 13 years of age or in boys who have no testicular enlargement by 14 years of age. In girls, a delay of longer than 4 to 5 years from onset of puberty to menarche is also cause for concern. Similarly, maturation arrest in boys warrants evaluation.

Constitutional delay, a slow maturation with appropriate hormonal levels and delayed bone age, accounts for the majority of cases of delayed pubertal development. This problem is identified much more frequently in boys than it is in girls, perhaps because of general societal and peer group reaction to short and sexually underdeveloped boys. The delay is frequently familial. In many instances, early signs of puberty are found on thorough examination, which permits the physician to reassure the child and the parents. Affected children should be followed up closely. The presence of chronic systemic diseases that can lead to delayed puberty (Box 212-1) may be difficult to differentiate from constitutional delay as a cause for the delay.

The remainder of the differential diagnosis of delayed development relates to failure at either the hypothalamic-pituitary level, shown by low serum gonadotropins (hypogonadotropic hypogonadism), or the gonadal level, shown by elevated gonadotropins (hypergonadotropic hypogonadism). Either of these conditions may result from genetic disorders or acquired illnesses (see Box 212-1). The workup of the patient is directed toward identifying the specific cause. Common initial screening tests are shown in Box 212-2 and include a thorough history, physical examination, and assessment of growth velocity. A bone age is often helpful. For delayed development to be the result of an undiagnosed systemic illness is relatively uncommon, but if the clinician believes a systemic illness history exists, then specific screening may include a complete blood count, electrolytes, renal and liver function tests, erythrocyte sedimentation rate and C-reactive protein analysis, inflammatory bowel disease panel, and celiac disease panel. A screen for endocrinopathies should include thyroid-stimulating hormone and thyroid hormone levels, gonadotropins (LH, FSH), testosterone, estradiol, and insulin-like growth factor 1. Other tests that a specialist may order would include insulin-like growth factor binding protein 3, prolactin, karyotype, brain magnetic resonance imaging, pelvic ultrasound, and GnRH testing assessing for signs of central puberty.

Treatment should be directed, when possible, toward the cause of the delayed development. If sex steroid secretion is deficient as a result of either gonadal failure or gonadotropin deficiency, then treatment focuses on replacing the appropriate sex steroid. In constitutional delay, waiting may be the best course. In boys, however, a short course of low-dose injectable testosterone (eg, 50 to 100 mg monthly for 4 doses) may be indicated if the delayed development is affecting the boy's psychological well being. In girls, cosmetic treatment, such as the use of a padded bra, is helpful. Estrogen therapy is necessary only occasionally. In patients who have GnRH or gonadotropin

BOX 212-1 Causes of Delayed Puberty

1. Constitutional delay
2. Deficiency of gonadotropin-releasing hormone secretion by the hypothalamus
   a. Genetic and molecular causes
      i. Isolated deficiency
      ii. Kallmann syndrome
      iii. Laurence-Moon-Bardet-Biedl syndrome
      iv. Prader-Willi syndrome
   b. Acquired causes
      i. Infection
      ii. Neoplasm
      iii. Infiltrative disease
      iv. Trauma
3. Deficiency of gonadotropin secretion by the pituitary
   a. Genetic
      i. Panhypopituitarism (including transcription factor mutations in *PROP1*, *HESX1*, and *LHX3*)
      ii. Isolated deficiency
      iii. Fertile eunuch (normal follicle-stimulating hormone, low luteinizing hormone)
      iv. Leptin or leptin-receptor deficiency
   b. Acquired
      i. Infection
      ii. Tumor
      iii. Excess prolactin secretion, adenoma
      iv. Trauma
4. Gonadal disorders
   a. Genetic and molecular
      i. Turner syndrome (45, X or structural X abnormalities or mosaicism)
      ii. Klinefelter syndrome (47, XXY)
      iii. Noonan syndrome
      iv. Syndromes of complete androgen insensitivity (no sexual hair)
      v. del Castillo syndrome (Sertoli cells only)
      vi. Pure gonadal dysgenesis
      vii. Myotonic dystrophy
      viii. Receptor mutations
   b. Acquired
      i. Infections
         (1) Gonorrhea (male)
         (2) Virus (mumps, coxsackie)
         (3) Tuberculosis (male)
      ii. After radiation or chemotherapy
      iii. Mechanical causes
         (1) Torsion
         (2) Surgery
         (3) Congenital anorchia (*vanishing testes* syndrome)
         (4) Autoimmune
5. Adrenal and gonadal steroid enzyme deficiencies
6. Excessive exercise, malnutrition
7. Chronic systemic diseases
   a. Congenital heart disease
   b. Chronic pulmonary disease
   c. Inflammatory bowel disease, celiac disease
   d. Chronic renal failure and renal tubular acidosis
   e. Hypothyroidism
   f. Poorly controlled diabetes mellitus
   g. Sickle cell anemia, thalassemia
   h. Collagen-vascular disease
   i. Anorexia nervosa
   j. HIV infection

deficiency, fertility may be induced with GnRH or gonadotropin therapy. In any case, strong psychological support must be provided to the adolescent and sometimes to the family. If the problem is difficult diagnostically, or if hormonal therapy is desired, then referral should be made to a pediatric endocrinologist.

PRECOCIOUS PUBERTY

Classically, precocious puberty is the appearance of secondary sexual characteristics before 8 years of age in girls and 9 years in boys. A substantial portion of girls have pubertal changes at 7 years of age, specifically, 27.2% of black girls and 6.7% of white girls have breast or sexual hair development by 7 years of age.[6] As a result of these data, the Drug and Therapeutics and Executive Committees of the Lawson Wilkins Pediatric Endocrine Society published recommendations proposing that the age cutoff for precocious puberty should be decreased to 7 years in white girls and 6 years in black girls unless the tempo of puberty is abnormal, the bone age is advanced more than 2 years, the predicted height is less than 150 cm (59 inches), focal neurologic deficits are present, headaches are present, or the family's or the child's emotional state is affected adversely.[7] These recommendations are controversial, and although extensive evaluation in 6- to 8-year-old girls is usually not revealing of pathological abnormality, each child must be considered individually.

Early stimulation of the hypothalamic-pituitary axis, with resultant gonadotropin secretion and sex steroid secretion, is termed central precocious puberty. Sex steroid secretion that is independent of pituitary gonadotropin secretion may be termed peripheral or pseudoprecocious puberty. Box 212-3 lists the causes of these 2 conditions. Precocity may be isosexual (appropriate for phenotype) or heterosexual (appropriate for opposite gender phenotype) and is significantly more common in girls than it is in boys. Box 212-4 lists the causes of heterosexual precocious puberty. In girls, idiopathic precocious puberty is the single most common diagnosis and accounts for 85% of central precocious puberty, whereas 60% of precocious puberty in boys is due to pathological causes.[1] Girls adopted from developing countries may be at particular risk for precocious puberty.[8] Internationally adopted girls have shown a trend toward early and rapidly progressing puberty that may be related to the increased metabolic activity exhibited if catch-up

BOX 212-2 Evaluation for Delayed Puberty

INITIAL SCREENING TESTS

Thorough history, physical examination, and calculation of growth velocity

Bone age

Luteinizing hormone, follicle-stimulating hormone

Testosterone or estrogen, depending on gender

Thyroid-stimulating hormone, thyroid hormone

If systemic disease is thought to exist:

Complete blood count

Erythrocyte sedimentation rate, C-reactive protein

Comprehensive Panel

Insulin-like growth factor 1, insulin-like growth factor binding protein 3

Urinalysis

Celiac disease panel (anti-endomesial IgA antibody or tissue transglutaminase IgA and total IgA level)

Inflammatory bowel disease panel

Prolactin

OTHER TESTS (IF INDICATED)

Karyotype

Brain magnetic resonance imaging

Pelvic ultrasound

Gonadotropin-releasing hormone (GnRH) or GnRH analog stimulation test

BOX 212-3 Causes of Isosexual Precocious Puberty

1. Central (with pituitary gonadotropin secretion)
   a. Idiopathic
   b. Central nervous system abnormalities
      i. Congenital anomalies (hydrocephalus)
      ii. Tumors (hypothalamic, pineal, other)
      iii. Hamartoma
      iv. Postinflammatory condition
      v. Trauma
      vi. Syndromes
         (1) Neurofibromatosis
         (2) Tuberous sclerosis
   c. Hypothyroidism (severe)
2. Peripheral
   a. Exogenous sex steroids
   b. Gonadal tumors or cysts
   c. Adrenal hyperplasia or tumor
   d. Ectopic gonadotropin–secreting tumors (chorioepithelioma, hepatoblastoma, teratoma)
   e. Familial Leydig cell hyperplasia, receptor mutation
   f. McCune-Albright syndrome, G-protein mutation

growth occurs after adoption.[9] Precocious puberty can significantly reduce adult height and can, in some cases, have an adverse effect on a child's and a family's emotional state.

BOX 212-4 Causes of Heterosexual Precocious Puberty

1. Girls
   a. Congenital adrenal hyperplasia
   b. Androgen-secreting tumors
      i. Adrenal
      ii. Ovarian
      iii. Teratoma
   c. Exogenous androgens
2. Boys
   a. Estrogen-producing tumors
      i. Adrenal
      ii. Teratoma
      iii. Hepatoma
      iv. Testicular
   b. Exogenous estrogens
   c. Increased peripheral conversion of androgens to estrogens

VARIATIONS OF PUBERTY

Two entities not requiring treatment are isolated premature breast development (thelarche) and isolated premature development of sexual hair (adrenarche). Premature thelarche occurs in girls between 6 months and 3 years of age. Breast development is usually moderate, often regresses, and is seen without other signs of precocious puberty. Specifically, estrogen or gonadotropic levels do not increase significantly, and statural and skeletal maturation accelerate only mildly, if at all. Premature thelarche does not progress to complete precocious puberty. Premature adrenarche usually occurs between 5 and 7 to 8 years of age. The development of sexual hair is frequently accompanied by a mild growth spurt (with slight bone age advancement) and signs of increased adrenal androgens (increased levels of plasma dehydroepiandrosterone and its sulfate to the early pubertal range). In girls, signs of increased estrogen secretion are not seen. An abnormal androgen source such as a tumor or late-onset congenital adrenal hyperplasia must be excluded. Premature adrenarche may occur in children with mild neurologic problems. In some girls, premature adrenarche may be a marker for future polycystic ovarian syndrome.[1]

With both premature thelarche and premature adrenarche, careful follow-up physical examinations are necessary to be sure they do not represent the early stages of complete sexual precocity.

Isosexual Precocious Puberty

Evaluation and treatment of precocious puberty is a matter for a pediatric endocrinologist. The diagnosis of isosexual precocious puberty is based on the physical examination and laboratory evidence of sex steroid secretion. Common initial tests (Box 212-5) include evaluation of growth velocity, bone age, LH, FSH, and estradiol or testosterone. Additional testing might include dehydroepiandrosterone sulfate, 17-hydroxyprogesterone, TSH, and thyroid hormone levels. The hormone levels should be drawn as close to 8 AM as

BOX 212-5 Evaluation for Precocious Puberty

INITIAL SCREENING TESTS

Thorough history, physical examination, and calculation of growth velocity

Bone age

Luteinizing hormone, follicle-stimulating hormone

Estradiol, testosterone

Dehydroepiandrosterone sulfate

17-Hydroxyprogesterone

Thyroid-stimulating hormone, thyroid hormone

SECONDARY TESTS (IF INDICATED)

Pelvic ultrasound

Brain magnetic resonance imaging

Serum β-human chorionic gonadotropin

Gonadotropin-releasing hormone (GnRH) or GnRH

possible because this time coincides with normal early-morning hormone level peaks. Other tests may include a pelvic ultrasound, brain magnetic resonance imaging, β-human chorionic gonadotropin, GnRH stimulation test, or an adrenocorticotrophic hormone stimulation test assessing for congenital adrenal hyperplasia. Measurement of serum gonadotropin levels before and after an injection of GnRH usually distinguishes central and peripheral precocious puberty. In central precocious puberty, further workup focuses on a search for the cause of the gonadotropin secretion. The diagnosis of idiopathic central precocious puberty can be made only after the search for a pathological cause is negative. Although onset is at an early age, the tempo and pattern of pubertal progression are normal in idiopathic central precocity. In peripheral precocious puberty, the specialist must search for the source of sex steroid, remembering that exogenous sources (eg, contraceptive pills, topical androgen creams or gels) are easily available. In boys, physical examination of the testes is particularly useful in the differential diagnosis. If both testes are of pubertal size, then the patient has gonadotropin-stimulated precocious puberty; if 1 testis is enlarged, then a testicular tumor may be present; if both testes are small, then the androgens are either exogenous or of adrenal origin.

Treatment of isosexual precocity centers on suppression or removal of the underlying cause. Idiopathic central precocious puberty is treated with GnRH analogs, which lead to pituitary desensitization and a reduction in gonadotropin secretion to prepubertal levels. Several GnRH analogs are available in intramuscular (depot), subcutaneous, and intranasal forms. Depot leuprolide is used most commonly in the United States and is usually given every 3 to 4 weeks, although longer-acting forms, which may be given every 12 weeks, are available. This treatment has been used for years, is effective, and has minimal side effects. For gonadotropin-independent precocious puberty, testolactone and other aromatase inhibitors (anastrozole, letrozole), spironolactone (androgen-receptor inhibitor), and ketoconazole (steroidogenesis inhibitor) may be used. McCune-Albright syndrome is an unusual syndrome of irregular café au lait spots, polyostotic fibrous dysplasia, and precocious puberty caused by a somatic mutation that can lead to constitutive activation of various glands, including the thyroid, parathyroid, adrenal, and gonad. Tamoxifen (estrogen-receptor inhibitor) has recently been shown to be an effective treatment for McCune-Albright syndrome.[10]

Heterosexual Precocious Puberty

Heterosexual precocious puberty is uncommon (see Box 212-4 for a list of causes). Exogenous sex steroids, including topical preparations, must be considered. The diagnostic work-up centers on the search for a sex steroid–producing tumor. These patients should be referred to a pediatric endocrinologist. Treatment is aimed at removal of the sex hormone source (exogenous or tumor) or suppression with glucocorticoid replacement therapy (congenital adrenal hyperplasia).

SUMMARY

In most cases of delayed or precocious sexual development, a thorough history and physical examination and a few basic laboratory tests identify patients who are likely to have a pathological cause requiring referral to a pediatric endocrinologist. (See Chapter 192, Hirsutism, Hypertrichosis, and Precocious Sexual Hair Development, for further discussion of various forms of precocious sexual development.)

In all cases, along with physical care, psychological care and support are extremely important, particularly when medical therapy is only partially satisfactory.

WHEN TO REFER

For delayed puberty:

- No breast development in girls by 13 years of age
- No menarche 4 to 5 years after the onset of breast development in girls
- No testicular enlargement in boys by 14 years of age
- Maturational arrest
- Hormonal abnormalities identified by initial screening tests (see Box 212-2)
- Parental or physician discomfort

For precocious puberty:

- Signs of puberty before 6 to 8 years of age in girls (see text)
- Signs of puberty before age 9 in boys
- Rapidly progressive puberty (eg, stage 3 breast when first noted)
- Heterosexual precocious puberty
- Hormonal abnormalities identified by initial screening tests (see Box 212-5)
- Parental or physician discomfort

TOOLS FOR PRACTICE

Engaging Patients and Family

- *Puberty* (brochure), American Academy of Pediatrics (patiented.aap.org).

- *What is a Pediatric Endocrinologist?* (fact sheet), American Academy of Pediatrics (www.aap.org/family/whatispedendo.pdf).

SUGGESTED RESOURCES

Books

Geffner ME, Lanes R, Nakamoto JM. Puberty and its disorders. In: Kappy MS, Allen DB, Geffner ME, eds. *Principles and Practice of Pediatric Endocrinology.* Springfield, IL: Charles C. Thomas; 2005.

Long D, Plotnick L. Puberty and gonadal disorders. In: McMillan J, Feigin RD, DeAngelis CD, et al, eds. *Oski's Pediatrics: Principles and Practice.* 4th ed. Philadelphia, PA: Lippincott, Williams, and Wilkins; 2006.

Kelch RP, Beitins IZ. Adolescent sexual development. In: Kappy MS, Blizzard RM, Migeon CJ, eds. *Wilkins the Diagnosis and Treatment of Endocrine Disorders in Childhood and Adolescence.* 4th ed. Springfield, IL: Charles C Thomas; 1994.

Tanner JM. Growth and endocrinology of the adolescent. In: Gardner LI, ed. *Endocrine and Genetic Diseases of Childhood and Adolescence.* Philadelphia, PA: WB Saunders; 1975.

Journal articles

Kulin HE. Delayed puberty in boys. *Curr Ther Endocrinol Metab.* 1997;6:346-349.

Styne D. New aspects in the diagnosis and treatment of pubertal disorders. *Pediatr Clin North Am.* 1997;44:505-529.

Thomas MA, Rebar RW. Delayed puberty in girls and primary amenorrhea. *Curr Ther Endocrinol Metab.* 1997;6:223-226.

REFERENCES

1. Nathan BM, Palmert MR. Regulation and disorders of pubertal timing. *Endocrinol Metab Clin North Am.* 2005;34:617-641.
2. Dunger DB, Ahmed ML, Ong KK. Effects of obesity on growth and puberty. *Best Pract Res Clin Endocrinol Metab.* 2005;19(3):375-390.
3. Anderson SE, Must A. Interpreting the continued decline in the average age at menarche from two nationally representative surveys of U.S. girls studied 10 years apart. *J Pediatr.* 2005;147(6):753-760.
4. Wu T, Mendola P, Buck GM. Ethnic differences in the presence of secondary sex characteristics and menarche among US girls: the third national health and nutrition examination survey, 1988-1994. *Pediatrics.* 2002;110(4):752-757.
5. Sun SS, Schubert CM, Chumlea WC, et al. National estimates of the timing of sexual maturation and racial differences among US children. *Pediatrics.* 2002;110(5):911-919.
6. Herman-Giddens ME, Slora EJ, Wasserman RC, et al. Secondary sexual characteristics and menses in young girls seen in office practice: a study from the Pediatric Research in Office Settings network. *Pediatrics.* 1997;99:505-512.
7. Kaplowitz PB, Oberfiel SE. Re-examination of the age limit for defining when puberty is precocious in girls in the United States: implications for evaluation and treatment. Drug and Therapeutics and Executive Committees of the Lawson Wilkins Pediatric Endocrine Society. *Pediatrics.* 1999;104:936-941.
8. Virdis R, Stree ME, Zampolli M, et al. Precocious puberty in girls adopted from developing countries. *Arch Dis Child.* 1998;78:152-154.
9. Mason P, Narad C. Long-term growth and puberty concerns in international adoptees. *Pediatr Clin North Am.* 2005;52(5):1351-68, vii.
10. Eugster EA, Rubin SD, Reiter EO, et al, McCune-Albright Study Group. Tamoxifen treatment for precocious puberty in McCune-Albright syndrome: a multicenter trial. *J Pediatr.* 2003;143(1):9-10.

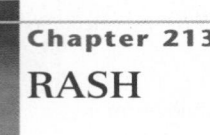

Chapter 213
RASH

Daniel P. Krowchuk, MD

Skin complaints are common in pediatrics. Surveys indicate that 10% to 20% of visits by children to outpatient facilities are associated with a dermatologic problem; it may be the primary reason for the visit, a secondary concern, or an incidental finding during physical examination. Because of the volume of skin-related problems, physicians caring for children must gain some skill in recognizing and managing the most common cutaneous disorders.

Dermatology is a visual discipline. With experience, primary care physicians can recognize most of the common problems affecting the skin, including the subtle variations in presentation. For uncommon problems, an atlas, text, consultant, or other resource can be used to aid in identification. As in most medical specialties, an organized approach to the problem is helpful in leading to the correct diagnosis.

The approach to diagnosing skin problems in children is best based on the morphology of the patient's lesions. An appropriate history and accurate description of what is seen can usually overcome any obstacle to diagnosis.

HISTORY

Although the diagnosis of skin lesions relies heavily on physical examination and the recognition of types of lesions, as with any problem, an appropriate, problem-oriented history is the first step in diagnosis. Some questions that may be useful and their rationale are presented in the following sections.

History of the Present Illness

When did the rash begin? Has it gotten better or worse? Has it occurred in the past? Conditions such as atopic dermatitis are chronic and recurrent, whereas others such as viral exanthems (eg, erythema infectiosum) are acute and self-limited.

Are there associated symptoms? A generalized erythematous macular eruption associated with fever, nasal congestion, and cough suggests the presence of a viral exanthem. Fever, petechiae, and purpura in an ill-appearing child may indicate a serious bacterial infection such as meningococcemia. Atopic or contact dermatitis and scabies characteristically produce pruritus.

Are any medications being taken? The onset of wheals in a child receiving an oral antibiotic might represent urticaria as a manifestation of drug allergy. Lithium can worsen acne, and minocycline may cause hyperpigmentation. Topical therapies also may be relevant to the patient's problem. Neomycin (used in certain topical antibiotic preparations), diphenhydramine (used to reduce pruritus), and certain anesthetics (used to reduce pain or pruritus), when applied topically, may induce a contact dermatitis.

Are there factors that worsen or precipitate the rash? The malar rash of systemic lupus erythematosus is worsened by sun exposure. For many children who have atopic dermatitis, reduced humidity during colder months is associated with an exacerbation of disease.

What treatment has been tried, and what was its effect? Knowing which therapies have been employed, if they were used appropriately, and if they were effective is helpful. Treatment for head lice infestation, for example, may fail if the product is applied incorrectly or if it is left on the scalp for an insufficient period. In addition, repeating a therapy is unwise if it was used correctly but proved ineffective.

Family History

Is there a family history of skin disease or other health problems? Children who have atopic dermatitis often have a history of atopic disease, including atopic dermatitis, allergic rhinitis, or asthma. If a child is found to have multiple café-au-lait macules and a diagnosis of neurofibromatosis type 1 is being considered, determining if the patient has any affected first-degree relatives is vital. Whether other family members are similarly affected is relevant when cutaneous infections or infestations are suspected. Impetigo, tinea capitis, scabies, and head lice are frequently transmitted within families.

Social History

For adolescents, in particular, a social history may be relevant.

Do you work after school? Occupational exposure to greases or oils (eg, in a fast-food restaurant or car repair shop) may worsen acne.

Have you ever been involved in a sexual relationship? A confidential sexual history may be important. Secondary syphilis and disseminated gonococcal infection, for example, have cutaneous manifestations. Analogously, molluscum contagiosum, infestation with pubic lice, and scabies may be transmitted through sexual contact.

PHYSICAL EXAMINATION

Recognizing and describing skin lesions accurately is essential to diagnosis. The first step is to identify the primary lesion, defined as the earliest lesion and the one most characteristic of the disease. Primary lesions, described later, include macules, papules, vesicles, and pustules, among others. Next, noting the distribution, arrangement, and color of primary lesions, along with any secondary change, such as crusting or scaling, is important.

Types of Primary Lesions

Primary lesions may be flat, elevated, or depressed. Flat lesions include macules and patches. A *macule* is a small, circumscribed area of color change without elevation or depression. An example is a café-au-lait macule (Figure 213-1). Although specific criteria for size are lacking, a *patch* is a large macule (Figure 213-2). Elevated lesions may be solid or fluid filled. Solid lesions include *papules* (<0.5 cm in diameter), *nodules* (≥0.5 cm in diameter), *wheals* (a pink, rounded, or flat-topped elevation caused by edema in the skin), and *plaques* (plateau-shaped structures often formed by the coalescence of papules) (Figures 213-3, 213-4, 213-5, and 213-6). Elevated fluid-filled lesions are

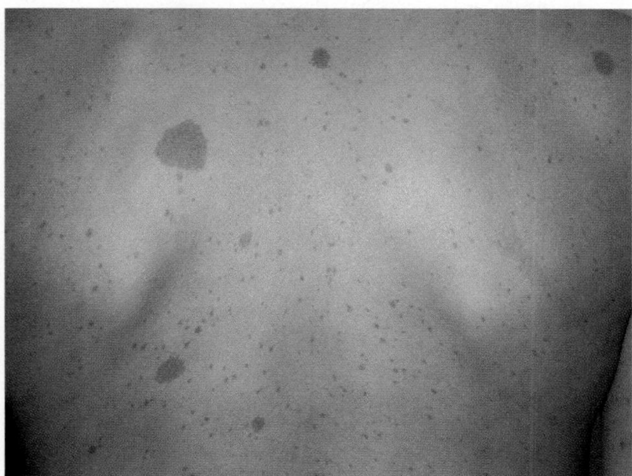

Figure 213-1 Café au lait macules in a patient who has neurofibromatosis type 1.

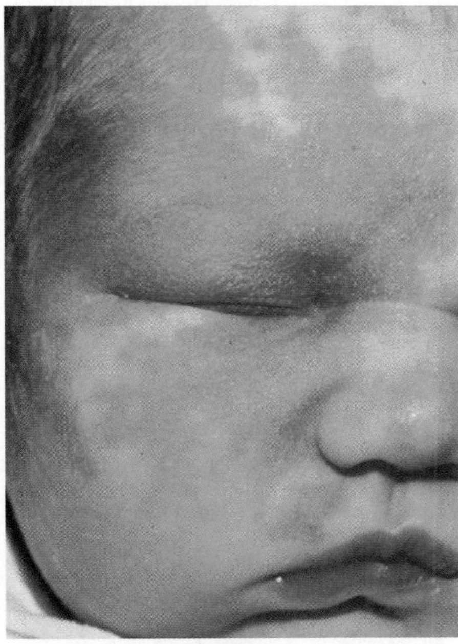

Figure 213-2 A port wine stain is an example of an erythematous patch.

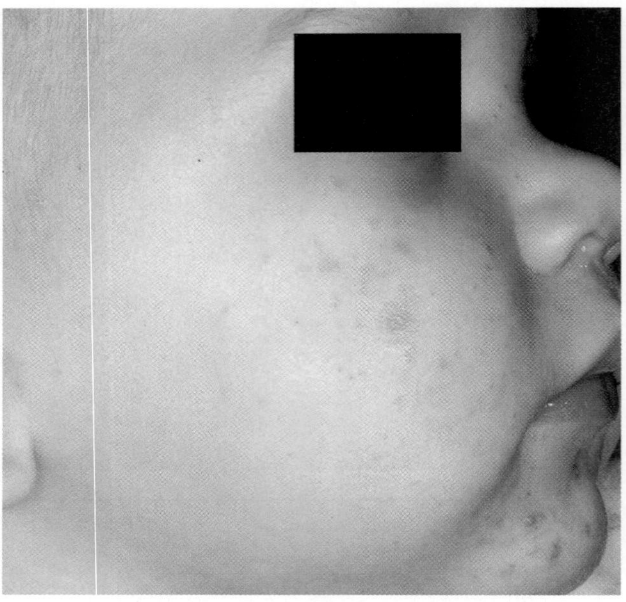

Figure 213-3 Neonatal acne is composed of erythematous papules and papulopustules.

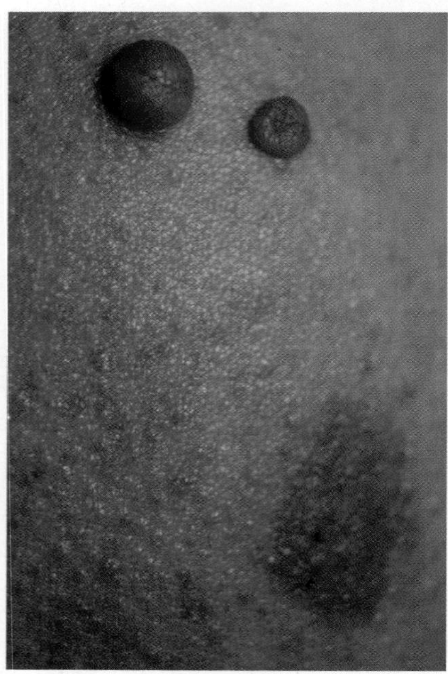

Figure 213-4 Nodules representing neurofibromas in a patient who has neurofibromatosis type 1.

vesicles (<0.5 cm in diameter and filled with serous fluid), *bullae* (≥0.5 cm in diameter and filled with serous fluid), *pustules* (<0.5 cm in diameter and filled with purulent material), and *cysts* (≥0.5 cm in diameter that represent sacs containing fluid or semisolid material) (Figures 213-7, 213-8, and 213-9).

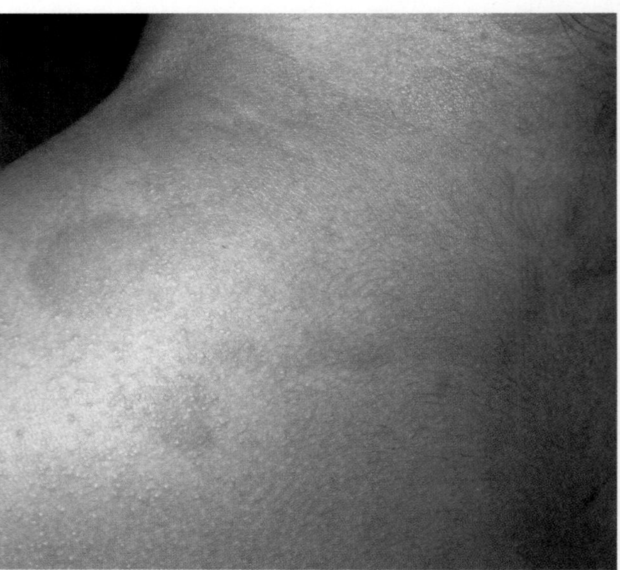

Figure 213-5 Pink wheals in a patient who has urticaria.

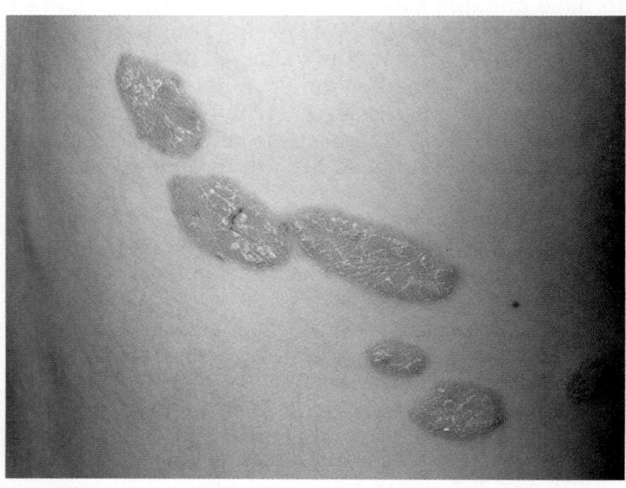

Figure 213-6 Scaling plaques, plateau-like lesions, are observed in psoriasis.

Depressed lesions include *erosions* (a superficial loss of epidermis with a moist base) or *ulcers* (a deeper lesion extending into or below the dermis) (Figure 213-10).

Distribution

Given that certain disorders have unique patterns of distribution, noting the parts of the body involved may provide an important clue to diagnosis. For example, seborrheic dermatitis commonly involves not only the scalp, but also the eyebrows and nasolabial folds. Psoriasis also affects the scalp, but lesions are often seen in areas that are traumatized, such as the elbows and knees. Acne is limited to the face, back, and chest, sites of the highest concentrations of pilosebaceous follicles.

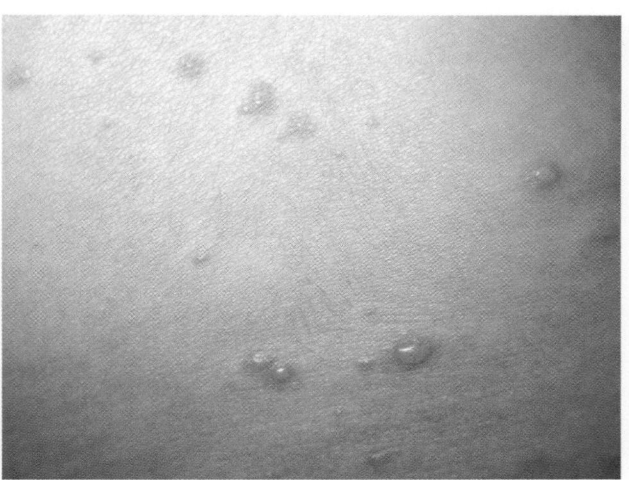

Figure 213-7 Vesicles, as seen here in varicella, are filled with clear or serous fluid.

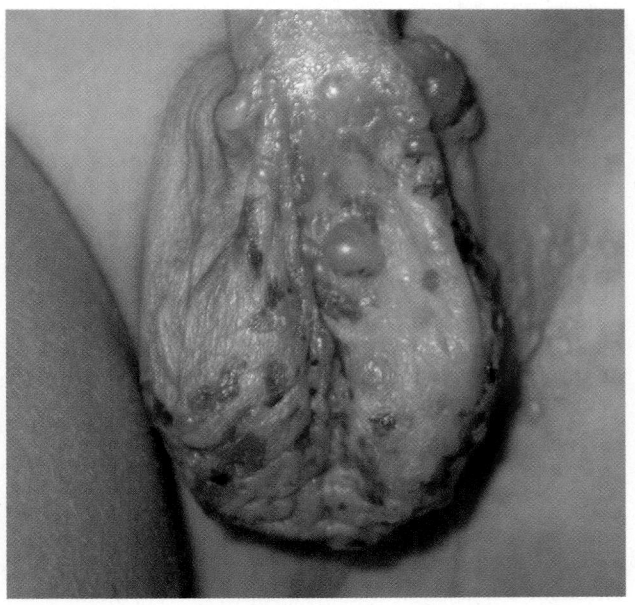

Figure 213-8 Bullae, filled with clear fluid, are observed in chronic bullous disease of childhood.

Arrangement

Lesions may appear in lines (eg, vesicles in contact dermatitis from poison ivy), be grouped or clustered (eg, vesicles in herpes simplex virus infection), follow a dermatome (eg, vesicles in herpes zoster), or form an annulus or ring (eg, papules in granuloma annulare or a patch in erythema migrans) (Figures 213-11, 213-12, 213-13, and 213-14).

Color

Although the color of a lesion may be obvious, terms that may be helpful include skin colored, erythematous

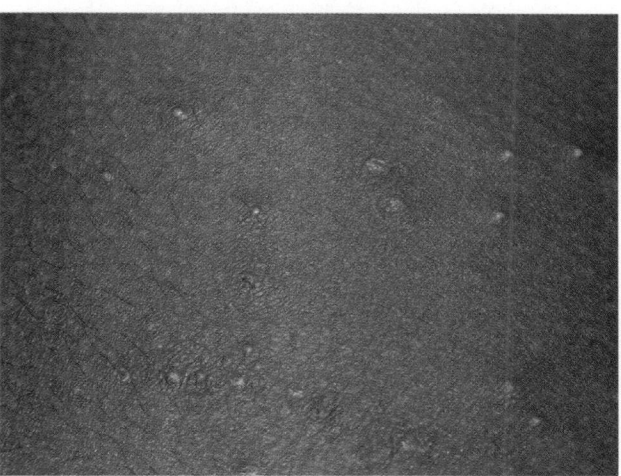

Figure 213-9 Pustules are filled with purulent material. This patient has folliculitis.

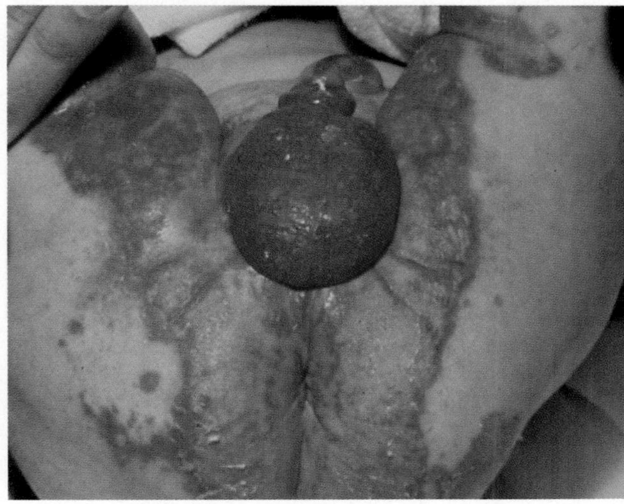

Figure 213-10 Erosions, as seen in this infant who has acrodermatitis enteropathica, represent a superficial loss of epidermis.

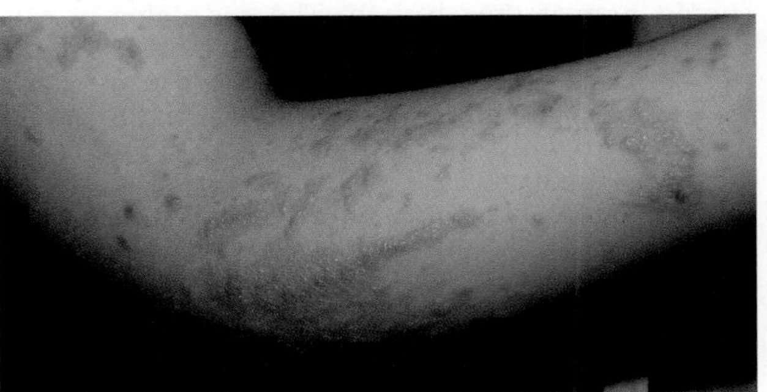

Figure 213-11 A linear arrangement of papules or vesicle often occurs in contact dermatitis caused by poison ivy.

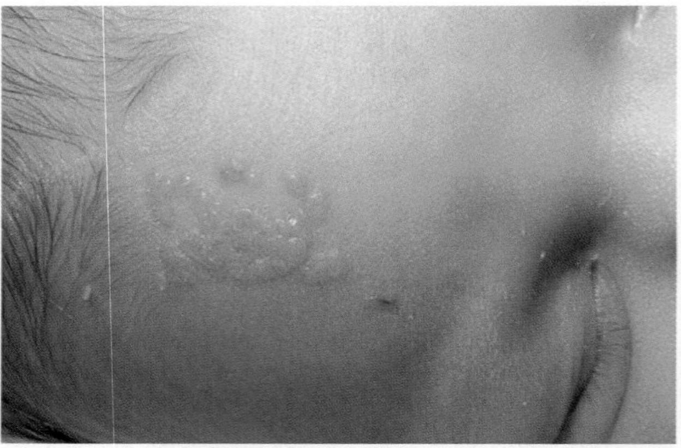

Figure 213-12 Grouped vesicles are characteristic of herpes simplex virus infection on the skin.

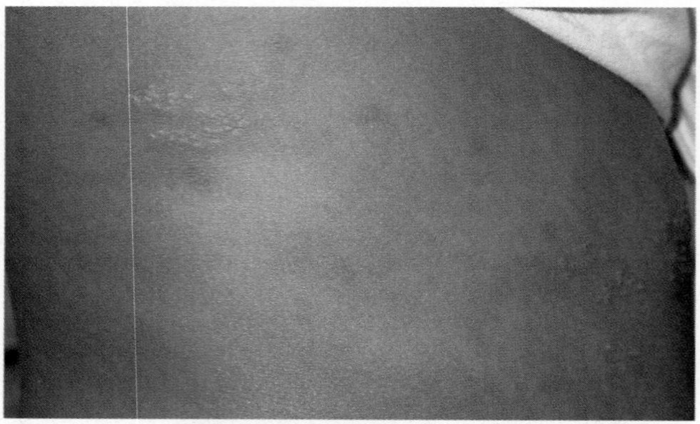

Figure 213-13 Lesions of herpes zoster appear in a dermatomal distribution.

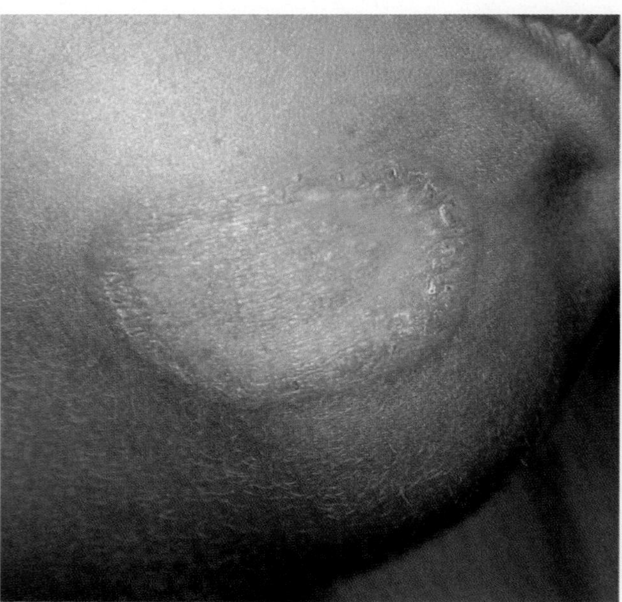

Figure 213-14 An annulus (ie, ring-shaped lesion) is typical of tinea corporis.

(pink or red), hyperpigmented (tan, brown, or black), hypopigmented (the amount of pigment is decreased but not entirely absent), depigmented (all pigment is absent, as occurs in vitiligo), or violaceous. When erythematous lesions are observed, the examiner should note if they blanch. The red color in skin depends on hemoglobin within red blood cells. If the red cells are within vessels (as occurs in urticaria, for example), compression of the skin forces the cells into deeper vessels, and blanching occurs. However, if the cells are outside vessels, as occurs in forms of vasculitis, blanching will not occur; non-blanching lesions are termed *petechiae*, *purpura*, and *ecchymoses*.

Secondary Changes

Secondary changes are alterations in the skin that may accompany primary lesions. These changes, too, can be valuable in differential diagnosis. *Crusting* represents dried fluid; it is commonly seen after the rupture of vesicles or bullae, as occurs with the honey-colored crust of impetigo. In contrast, *scaling* represents epidermal fragments that are characteristic of several disorders, among which are fungal infections (eg, tinea corporis) and psoriasis. *Atrophy* is an area of surface depression from absence of the dermis or subcutaneous fat. Atrophic skin often appears thin and wrinkled. *Lichenification* is a thickening of the skin that results from chronic rubbing or scratching (as occurs in atopic dermatitis, for example); as a result, normal creases appear more prominent.

DIAGNOSIS

Once the primary lesions are identified, along with their distribution, arrangement, color, and secondary changes, these observations should be formulated into one or two sentences. For example, "Located on the extensor surfaces of the extremities are erythematous, scaling papules, and plaques. Scaling of the scalp and pitting of the nails are evident." Such formulations assist in differential diagnosis. Identifying scaling papules and plaques, as in the previous example, places the patient's condition into the category of papulosquamous (elevated and scaling) diseases and eliminates countless other disorders from consideration. In children, the most common papulosquamous disorders are chronic atopic or contact dermatitis, tinea corporis, and pityriasis rosea; less common conditions are psoriasis, secondary syphilis, lichen planus, dermatomyositis, and lupus erythematosus. Given the location of the lesions on extensor surfaces and involvement of the scalp and nails, psoriasis becomes a primary consideration.

Boxes 213-1 and 213-2 assist in differential diagnosis based on the morphology of lesions. Notably, however, these tables are not exhaustive; rather, they list the most commonly encountered disorders and a few

BOX 213-1 Differential Diagnosis of Rashes in Neonates

ELEVATED LESIONS

Papules

Common

Erythematous
- Erythema toxicum
- Miliaria rubra
- Acne
- Candidiasis
- Scabies

White
- Milia

Yellow
- Sebaceous gland hypertrophy

Skin colored
- Epidermal nevus
- Skin tags

Uncommon

Yellow
- Juvenile xanthogranuloma
- Mastocytosis

Nodules

Common

Erythematous
- Hemangioma

Uncommon

Skin colored
- Condylomata accuminata
- Dermoid cyst

Yellow
- Mastocytosis

Plaques

Common

Skin colored or yellow
- Nevus sebaceous

Skin colored
- Epidermal nevus

Vesicles or bullae

Common

Erythema toxicum
Miliaria crystallina
Sucking blisters
Bullous impetigo
Herpes simplex virus infection

Uncommon

Incontinentia pigmenti
Aplasia cutis congenita
Varicella
Epidermolysis bullosa
Bullous ichthyosiform erythroderma

Pustules

Common

Erythema toxicum
Transient neonatal pustular melanosis
Miliaria pustulosa
Herpes simplex virus infection
Folliculitis
Acne
Candidiasis
Scabies

Uncommon

Acropustulosis of infancy

FLAT LESIONS

Macules

Common

Hypopigmented
- Prehemangioma
- Postinflammatory hypopigmentation

Hyperpigmented
- Transient neonatal pustular melanosis
- Café-au-lait macule
- Postinflammatory hyperpigmentation
- Congenital melanocytic nevus

Uncommon

Hypopigmented
- Ash leaf macule

Patches

Common

Erythematous
- Salmon patch (nevus simplex)
- Hemangioma (early)
- Port wine stain
- Atopic dermatitis
- Seborrheic dermatitis
- Diaper dermatitis (irritant or seborrheic)

Hyperpigmented
- Mongolian spot
- Lentigo

Uncommon

Erythematous
- Acrodermatitis enteropathica

Hyperpigmented
- Linear and whorled hypermelanosis

Hypopigmented
- Hypomelanosis of Ito
- Nevus depigmentosus

DEPRESSED LESIONS

Erosions

Common

Bullous impetigo
Neonatal herpes simplex virus infection
Staphylococcal scalded-skin syndrome

Uncommon

Aplasia cutis congenital
Acrodermatitis enteropathica
Epidermolysis bullosa
Bullous ichthyosiform erythroderma

BOX 213-2 Differential Diagnosis of Rashes in Older Infants, Children, and Adolescents

ELEVATED LESIONS

Papules without scaling

Common

Erythematous
- Viral exanthems (many exanthems have a papular as well as macular component)
- Scarlet fever
- Insect bites
- Scabies
- Urticaria
- Papular urticaria
- Acne
- Early lesions of guttate psoriasis
- Erythema multiforme

Skin colored
- Keratosis pilaris
- Molluscum contagiosum
- Flat warts

Hyperpigmented
- Nevus (intradermal)

Uncommon

Yellow
- Mastocytosis

Plaques without scaling

Common

Skin colored
- Nevus sebaceous
- Epidermal nevus

Hyperpigmented
- Congenital melanocytic nevus

Papules or plaques with scaling (papulosquamous diseases)

Common

Tinea corporis

Pityriasis rosea

Chronic atopic or contact dermatitis

Psoriasis

Uncommon

Dermatomyositis

Lupus erythematosus

Lichen planus

Nodules

Common

Erythematous
- Pyogenic granuloma

Skin colored
- Wart
- Callus
- Corn
- Epidermal cyst
- Granuloma annulare

Uncommon

Erythematous
- Angiofibroma

Skin colored
- Neurofibroma

Yellow
- Mastocytosis

Vesicles or bullae

Common

Contact dermatitis

Bullous impetigo

Varicella

Herpes simplex virus infection

Hand, foot, and mouth disease

Erythema multiforme

Uncommon

Polymorphous light eruption

Linear IgA dermatosis

Pustules

Common

Folliculitis

Scabies

Acne

Perioral dermatitis

Uncommon

Associated with systemic bacterial infection (eg, disseminated gonococcal infection)

FLAT LESIONS

Macules

Common

Erythematous
- Viral exanthems
- Drug eruptions

Hypopigmented
- Pityriasis alba (postinflammatory hypopigmentation)
- Tinea versicolor
- Vitiligo
- Halo nevus

Hyperpigmented
- Freckles
- Postinflammatory hyperpigmentation
- Tinea versicolor
- Café-au-lait macules
- Melanocytic nevus

Uncommon

Hypopigmented
- Lichen sclerosus et atrophicus
- Scleroderma
- Ash leaf macule
- Piebaldism

Continued

BOX 213-2 Differential Diagnosis of Rashes in Older Infants, Children, and Adolescents—cont'd

Patches

Common

Erythematous
- Salmon patch (nevus simplex)
- Port wine stain
- Atopic dermatitis

Hyperpigmented
- Mongolian spot
- Becker nevus
- Lentigo

Uncommon

Erythematous
- Toxic shock syndrome (diffuse macular erythema)

Hyperpigmented
- Linear and whorled hypermelanosis
- Incontinentia pigmenti

DEPRESSED LESIONS

Erosions

Common

Bullous impetigo
Herpes simplex virus infection
Staphylococcal scalded-skin syndrome

Uncommon

Epidermolysis bullosa

HAIR LOSS

Congenital

Localized
- Nevus sebaceous
- Epidermal nevus
- Aplasia cutis congenita

Diffuse
- Hair shaft abnormalities
- Hypothyroidism

Acquired

Localized
- Friction alopecia
- Tinea capitis
- Traction alopecia
- Trichotillomania
- Alopecia areata
- Psoriasis
- Secondary syphilis
- Scleroderma

Diffuse
- Telogen effluvium
- Chemotherapy
- Hypothyroidism
- Acrodermatitis enteropathica

IgA, Immunoglobulin A.

less common ones to consider. Formulating a dermatologic differential diagnosis rests not only on the primary lesion, but also on other information, such as the distribution, arrangement, and color of lesions and the presence of any secondary change. When the patient's physical findings are unclear, a textbook or atlas of dermatology, consultant, or other resource can provide assistance.

This chapter is reproduced from Woodhead JC. Pediatric Clerkship Guide. *Philadelphia, PA: Mosby; 2003. Copyright © 2003, Elsevier, with permission.*

TOOLS FOR PRACTICE

Medical Decision Support

- *DermAtlas* (electronic atlas), Johns Hopkins University (www.dermatlas.org/derm/).
- *Dermatologic Image Database* (electronic atlas), University of Iowa College of Medicine (tray.dermatology.uiowa.edu/DermImag.htm).
- *DermIS Dermatology Information Systems* (electronic atlas), Universities of Heidelburg and Erlangen, Germany (www.dermis.net/dermisroot/en/home/index.htm).
- *Pediatric Dermatology: Skin Essentials* (on-line course), American Academy of Pediatrics, PediaLink course (www.pedialink.org).

SUGGESTED RESOURCES

Cohen BA. *Pediatric Dermatology*. 3rd ed. London, UK: Mosby; 2005.

Krowchuk DP, Mancini AM, eds. *Pediatric Dermatology. A Quick Reference Guide*. Elk Grove Village, IL: American Academy of Pediatrics; 2007.

Paller AS, Mancini AJ. *Hurwitz Clinical Pediatric Dermatology*. 3rd ed. Philadelphia, PA: Elsevier Saunders; 2006.

Weston WL, Lane AT, Morelli JG. *Color Textbook of Pediatric Dermatology*. 4th ed. St Louis, MO: Mosby; 2007.

Chapter 214

RECURRENT INFECTIONS

David L. Goldman, MD

Pediatric primary care providers frequently encounter children who have recurrent infections, and the vast majority are otherwise healthy. For the parents of these children, reassuring them that no underlying abnormality exists is particularly important. Much less commonly, recurrent infections are a sign of an underlying, possibly immunologic, disorder. Early identification of these children is critical because prompt intervention can decrease morbidity and mortality.

NORMAL PATTERN OF INFECTIONS IN CHILDHOOD

Generally, healthy children experience 6 to 8 upper respiratory tract infections per year in the first few years of life.[1] However, up to 15 infections per year can still be within the normal range. The high frequency of infections in the first years of life results from the relative immunologic immaturity of young children and their frequent exposure to respiratory pathogens. Factors such as attendance in child care and exposure to second-hand smoke may increase the number of infections.[2-4]

In the healthy host, these infections are self-limited, occur more frequently in the winter than in other seasons, and are associated with periods of wellness in between illnesses. Considering that the average duration of a viral illness is 7 to 10 days, typically, a toddler may be sick for up to 100 days or almost one third of the year.

INFECTIONS ASSOCIATED WITH AN UNDERLYING IMMUNE DISORDER

Occasionally, a pediatrician will encounter a child who has a history of infections that number above the normal range. Certain patterns of infections should alert the clinician to the possibility of an underlying immunodeficiency. One such pattern is an increased frequency of common infections. Although an immunocompetent child can experience a single serious bacterial infection such as pneumonia, meningitis, or osteomyelitis, repeated serious bacterial infections should alert the pediatrician to the possibility of an underlying disorder. Immunodeficiency may also cause a common infection exhibiting uncommonly, with increased severity, prolonged duration, or failure to respond to appropriate treatment. Varicella, a typically benign infection in healthy, immunocompetent children, can cause overwhelming infections in children who have leukemia and prolonged illness in children who have acquired immunodeficiency syndrome (AIDS). Immunodeficiency may also be suggested by a common infection exhibiting at an uncommon age. Thrush or candidal diaper dermatitis in children older than 1 year suggests a defect in T-cell immunity. Alternatively, immunodeficiency may produce an infection with an opportunistic pathogen (ie, *Pneumocystis carinii*, *Cryptococcus neoformans*). Rarely, immunodeficiency may become apparent as an infection after the administration of a live virus vaccine.

NONIMMUNOLOGIC DISORDERS ASSOCIATED WITH ENHANCED SUSCEPTIBILITY TO INFECTIONS

Host defense against microbial pathogens involves anatomic, physiological, and inflammatory barriers. Defects in any of these systems can lead to recurrent infections. In general, recurrent bacterial infections at the same anatomic site that are not associated with other infections or other signs of an underlying syndrome should suggest the possibility of an anatomic defect that may be either congenital or acquired. This circumstance is true especially of children who have urinary tract infections and otitis media. Approximately 62% of children younger than 1 year have more than 1 episode of otitis media, and 17% have 3 or more episodes.[5] The increased susceptibility of young children to otitis media results from an age-related dysfunction of the eustachian tubes and is rarely associated with underlying immunodeficiency. Anatomic defects leading to recurrent infections may also occur in other organ systems. Recurrent meningitis may occur as the result of an occult cerebral spinal fluid leak. Recurrent pneumonia may result from various nonimmunologic causes such as alteration of the normal barrier as a result of foreign body aspiration, tracheoesophageal fistula, or gastroesophageal reflux. Impaired function of mucociliary transport, as seen in cystic fibrosis and immotile cilia syndromes, also leads to recurrent pneumonia. When repeated episodes of pneumonia are the sole presentation of recurrent infection, the clinician must also consider the possibility of reactive airway disease, which can produce recurrent respiratory symptoms in association with pulmonary infiltrates. Reactive airway disease can be distinguished from recurrent pneumonia by a thorough history and physical examination. Besides anatomic defects, recurrent or unusual infections can also occur as a result of alteration in the normal microbial flora associated with antibiotic use and circulatory disorders such as venostasis.

SECONDARY IMMUNODEFICIENCIES

Abnormalities of the immune system may be categorized as either primary or secondary. Secondary immunodeficiencies, more common than primary, are either acquired or a consequence of a nonimmunologic process, including infection, malignancy, medication (ie, cytotoxic, immunosuppressive), malnutrition, splenic dysfunction, and metabolic disorders (Table 214-1). Improvements in medical care have led to an increase in the number of children with secondary immunodeficiencies, including those with organ transplants, rheumatologic diseases, and malignancies. New therapies have also led to new risk factors for unusual infections. For example, anticytokine therapies such as antitumor necrosis factor–α for rheumatoid diseases and Crohn disease have been associated with an increased susceptibility to tuberculosis and histoplasmosis.[6,7] Similarly, the implantation of foreign materials (ie, heart valves, catheters) is associated with an increased risk of infection.

The spleen serves as a filter to remove infectious agents from the circulation and as a site for maturation of the immune response. Splenic dysfunction and associated immunodeficiency can result from a variety of disorders, including congenital absence, surgical removal, hemoglobinopathies, and infiltrative diseases. Affected patients typically experience increased susceptibility to bacterial pathogens, especially encapsulated organisms.

Human immunodeficiency virus (HIV) infection, which produces a combined deficiency in both humoral and cellular immunity (AIDS) and is an important cause of secondary immunodeficiency, may be acquired congenitally or horizontally. Children infected with HIV can develop symptoms related to a variety of infection types (ie, opportunistic, recurrent, atypical), depending on the immune status of the child.

Table 214-1 Secondary Immunodeficiencies

CAUSE	DISEASE
Infection	HIV, congenital rubella
Malignancy	Leukemia, lymphoma
Metabolic	Uremia, malnutrition, protein-losing enteropathy, diabetes, galactosemia
Chromosomal	Down syndrome, Bloom syndrome
Medications	Corticosteroids, chemotherapy, antirejection medication
Splenic dysfunction	Splenectomy, sickle cell disease, congenital asplenia

HIV, Human immunodeficiency virus.

Table 214-2 Signs Associated with Primary Immunodeficiencies

SIGN	ASSOCIATED SYNDROME
Intractable diarrhea and malabsorption	Severe combined immunodeficiency (SCID), X-linked agammaglobulinemia (XLA), common variable immunodeficiency (CVID)
Rheumatologic conditions	CIVD, IgA deficiency, XLA
Hepatosplenomegaly, lymphadenopathy	Hyper-IgM syndrome
Absence of lymph tissue	XLA
Thrombocytopenia	Wiskott-Aldrich syndrome
Eczema	Wiskott-Aldrich syndrome, chronic granulomatous disease, Job syndrome
Oculocutaneous albinism	Chédiak-Higashi syndrome

Older children, who acquire HIV infection horizontally, may develop a primary syndrome in association with the HIV infection itself, which is clinically similar to other viral illnesses (ie, influenza, infectious mononucleosis). Recent advances in HIV therapy have helped decrease the morbidity and mortality associated with this disease, making early recognition and prompt intervention essential for optimal management.

Malnutrition is an extremely important cause of secondary immunodeficiency in many areas of the world and has been linked to increased susceptibility to a variety of infections, including measles and tuberculosis.

PRIMARY IMMUNODEFICIENCY

Primary immunodeficiencies, far less common than secondary, are caused by intrinsic defects in the immune system that are genetically determined. Excluding selective IgA deficiency, primary immunodeficiencies occur at an incidence of 1 in 10,000 cases.[8,9] Because many of these syndromes are X-linked, boys are affected more commonly than girls. Most children who have primary immunodeficiencies are symptomatic within the first few years of life, with several exceptions, including common variable immunodeficiency and deficiencies of the terminal complement components. Primary immunodeficiencies are classified by the component of the immune system that is affected: humoral, cellular, complement, and phagocytic. Defects in various arms of the immune system are associated with enhanced susceptibility to infections by particular types of pathogens. Hence the type of infecting pathogen may be useful in guiding the evaluation of a child with a suggested immunodeficiency. Associated clinical findings, which can be nonspecific or syndrome specific, may also suggest a primary immunodeficiency. A child who has serious recurrent infections will often experience growth failure. However, other physical, historical, and laboratory findings associated with primary immunodeficiency syndromes can be found (Table 214-2).

Defects in Humoral Immunity

Defects in humoral immunity, the antibody-mediated arm of the immune system, comprise 50% to 70% of symptomatic primary immunodeficiencies. The defects occur at various stages of B-cell development and result in a wide variety of clinical presentations. Syndromes range in severity from a total absence of mature B cells to an isotype deficiency to a defective antibody response against polysaccharide antigens (Table 214-3). Given the protective effects of maternally acquired antibody, even the most severely affected children (eg, those who have a total absence of antibody production) do not become symptomatic until after the first few months of life. Children who have defects in the humoral immune system are characteristically susceptible to recurrent sinopulmonary infections with encapsulated bacteria, including *Streptococcus pneumonia* and *Haemophilus influenzae*. X-linked agammaglobulinemia (Bruton agammaglobulinemia), one of the first primary immunodeficiencies to be described, is associated with a complete absence of mature B cells. Affected children have poor lymph tissue development, and a physical examination may reveal the absence of lymph nodes and tonsils. Although these children are generally not more susceptible to viral illnesses, they may experience severe or persistent enterovirus and rotavirus infections. Oral vaccination with live attenuated polio (no longer available in the United States) should be

Table 214-3 Humoral Immunodeficiencies

SYNDROME	CLINICAL FEATURES	ASSOCIATED FEATURES
X-linked agammaglobulinemia	Susceptibility to encapsulated bacterial pathogens Sinopulmonary and gastrointestinal infections, sepsis, meningitis Enhanced susceptibility to enterovirus and rotavirus Symptomatic polio infection following live polio vaccination	Asymmetric arthritis, dermatomyositis, malabsorption, absence of tonsils, adenoids, and lymph nodes
Transient hypogammaglobulinemia of infancy	Recurrent sinopulmonary infections; generally improves by 3-4 yr of age	May develop IgA deficiency
Hyper-IgM syndrome	X-linked Recurrent bacterial infections including encapsulated pathogens Infections associated with T-cell defects (eg, *Pneumocystis carinii*) also seen	Low levels of IgG, IgA, and IgE Neutropenia, thrombocytopenia, T-cell defects
Common variable immunodeficiency	Sinopulmonary infections Bronchiectasis Giardiasis	Most common in second and 3rd decade Noncaseating granulomas, malabsorption, autoimmune disease
IgA deficiency	Very common (1 in 400 individuals) but usually asymptomatic Recurrent pulmonary infections leading to bronchiectasis	Systemic lupus erythematosus, rheumatoid arthritis, chronic diarrhea Allergic reactions to gamma-globulin preparations IgG subclass deficiency in some
Specific antibody deficiency with normal immunoglobulins IgG-subclass deficiency	Recurrent bacterial infections of the respiratory tract Normal immunoglobulin levels but with impaired antibody responses to polysaccharide antigens Clinical significance not well delineated	

avoided because of the risk of vaccine-associated disease. Persistent *Campylobacter* infections also may occur. Children who have defects in humoral immunity are also predisposed to autoimmune disorders, such as dermatomyositis and asymmetric arthritis. Chronic lung disease may also occur. Treatment for antibody deficiency disorders depends on the type of disorder. Lifelong replacement therapy with intravenous Ig is indicated for X-linked agammaglobulinemia.

Combined Defects in Cellular and Humoral Immunity

Combined defects in cellular immunity and humoral immunity make up the 2nd largest group of primary immunodeficiencies. Isolated defects in cellular immunity, which is mediated primarily by T lymphocytes, with preserved antibody function are very uncommon because T cells play a critical role in B-cell function and development. A deficiency in the production and response to T-cell cytokines such as interferon-gamma is a rare exception. Most children with defects in T-cell immunity have associated defects in antibody immunity. In addition to bacterial infections, affected children are characteristically more susceptible to fungal, mycobacterial, and viral infections. These children may experience recurrent or persistent candidiasis (or both) in the form of thrush and diaper candidiasis. Common viral infections of childhood, varicella for example, may cause severe or recurrent disease in affected children. Table 214-4 lists some of the more common combined immunodeficiency syndromes.

Severe combined immunodeficiency (SCID) is the prototypical combined immunodeficiency syndrome and actually represents a collection of diseases. A variety of defects may result in SCID, including those affecting the following systems: cytokine receptors, signaling pathways, enzymes of the nucleotide salvage pathway, and major histocompatibility complex. In the first few months of life, children with SCID typically experience intractable diarrhea, failure to thrive, recurrent candidiasis, and *P carinii* pneumonia. Definitive therapy depends on the type of SCID and may involve bone marrow transplantatio, or enzyme or gene therapy.

Wiskott-Aldrich syndrome is an X-linked disorder associated with the triad of thrombocytopenia, eczema, and recurrent infections. This disorder is though to be related to a deficiency in T-cell activation. Affected infants often experience bleeding in the first few years of life. These children may have low IgM levels, but normal IgG levels.

Table 214-4 Combined Immunodeficiencies

SYNDROME	CLINICAL FEATURES	ASSOCIATED FEATURES
DiGeorge syndrome	Clinically variable Increased viral and fungal infections	Hypocalcemia, hypoparathyroidism, congenital heart disease, abnormal facies
Severe combined immunodeficiency (SCID)	Both B-cell and T-cell deficiencies present Includes a variety of disorders that have multiple modes of inheritance Presents early in life (within first 3 mo of age) with recurrent or severe infections with all types of pathogens	Failure to thrive, diarrhea Most common (50%) form is X-linked Thymic hypoplasia Cartilage-hair hypoplasia with certain forms of SCID At increased risk for graft vs. host disease with red blood cell transfusions
Ataxia telangiectasia	Recurrent sinopulmonary infections	Truncal ataxia, mental retardation, thymic hypoplasia, telangiectasia of skin and conjunctiva, glucose intolerance, increased risk for malignancy
Wiskott-Aldrich syndrome	Recurrent sinopulmonary infections	Eczema, thrombocytopenia, increased risk for malignancy

Table 214-5 Phagocytic Immunodeficiencies

SYNDROME	CLINICAL FEATURES	ASSOCIATED FEATURES
Chronic granulomatous disease (CGD)	Often X-linked Recurrent infection of skin, lungs, liver, lymph nodes, and bone Infections with catalase-positive organisms (*Staphylococci* spp, *Escherichia coli*, and *Candida albicans*)	Eczema, lymphadenopathy, hepatosplenomegaly
Chédiak-Higashi syndrome	Autosomal recessive Recurrent pyogenic infections with organisms similar to those seen in CGD	Ocular albinism, lymphoreticular malignancies Neutrophils have abnormally large granules
Job syndrome	Recurrent sinopulmonary infections and skin abscesses	Eczema, red hair, coarse facies, high IgE levels
Leukocyte adhesion defect	Autosomal recessive Recurrent bacterial infections and necrotic skin lesions	Leukocytosis with absence of neutrophils at infection site Severe gingivitis, early loss of teeth Delayed separation of umbilical cord

Ataxia-telangiectasia is an autosomal-recessive disorder that produces progressive ataxia, conjunctival telangiectasias with decreased IgA levels, and altered T-cell function. Children with ataxia-telangiectasia may have thymic hypoplasia, insulin resistance, gonadal atrophy and are at increased risk for hematologic malignancies.

Defects in Phagocytic Immunity

The phagocytic arm of the immune response includes neutrophils and monocytes. Phagocytes form the first line of defense against many pathogens and are considered part of the nonspecific immune response. Defects in phagocytic immunity range from the absence of a particular cell type (ie, congenital neutropenia, cyclical neutropenia) to defects in chemotaxis (leukocyte adhesion disorder) to defects in effector function (chronic granulomatous disease) (Table 214-5). Affected children typically experience recurrent skin infections and abscesses in addition to sinopulmonary infections. Children with defects in phagocytic oxidative burst (ie, chronic granulomatous disease) are particularly susceptible to infections caused by organisms (*Staphylococcus, Nocardia,* and *Aspergillus* species) that are catalase positive and thus able to degrade hydrogen peroxide. Other clinical features associated with defects in phagocytic immunity include poor wound healing, delayed umbilical cord separation, gingivitis, and eczema.

Defects in the Complement System

Complement acts to lyse target cells and, as an opsonin, promotes the phagocytosis of microbial pathogens. Defects in the complement system are the least common among the primary immunodeficiencies. Congenital deficiencies in the late or terminal components of the complement system (C5, C6, C7, C8, and C9) are inherited as autosomal-recessive traits and result in recurrent neisserial infections. In contrast to many of the primary immunodeficiencies, terminal complement deficiencies tend to exhibit in older children and in adolescents, typically with recurrent meningococcal infection (meningitis or meningococcemia) or gonococcal arthritis. Deficiency in the C3 component results in an increased susceptibility to encapsulated bacterial pathogens and may be difficult to distinguish from antibody deficiencies except that it tends to occur at an earlier age, within the first few months of life.

EVALUATION OF THE CHILD WITH POSSIBLE PRIMARY IMMUNODEFICIENCY

History

An evaluation for a primary immunodeficiency should be performed after nonimmunologic and secondary immunodeficiency syndromes have been considered. A complete history should be obtained for all children being evaluated for recurrent infections, including a history of risk factors for HIV infection (either personal for adolescents or parental when congenital transmission is a possibility), drug use, prostitution, blood-product transfusion, multiple sexual partners, or history of sexually transmitted disease and homosexual behavior. Particular attention should be paid to documenting the characteristics of previous infections, including the types of pathogens and infections, duration of illnesses, and need for hospitalizations. Because many of the primary immunodeficiencies are hereditary, a detailed family history is important. A complete review of systems should be obtained, with attention paid to known associated features of immunodeficiency syndromes, including failure to thrive. The immunization history is important because failure to make protective antibodies in response to immunizations can be indicative of immunodeficiency.

Physical Examination

A complete physical examination should be performed. Many children who have immunodeficiency appear chronically ill. Growth parameters (height, weight, and head circumference percentiles) should be obtained to determine the presence of failure to thrive. Physical signs that may indicate underlying immunodeficiency include absence of tonsils and the presence of generalized lymphadenopathy and hepatosplenomegaly. Skin lesions (eczema, abscesses, and seborrhea) and mucous membrane involvement (telangiectasias, mucositis) are observed with some immunologic disorders. Signs of recurrent infection (eg, dull, retracted tympanic membranes) and evidence of ongoing infection (eg, thrush) may be present. Specific signs associated with a particular immunodeficiency syndrome, such as oculocutaneous albinism in Chédiak-Higashi syndrome, may be present.

Laboratory Evaluation and Referral

Laboratory evaluation for a child who is thought to have an immunodeficiency should be guided by the type of infections the child is experiencing. Initial screening tests usually include complete blood count and differential, serum Ig levels (IgG, IgA, and IgM), and lymphocyte count. Most primary immunodeficiency syndromes will be associated with abnormal serum Ig levels. HIV testing should be strongly considered, as indicated by the history and physical findings.

Table 214-6 Laboratory Examination

IMMUNODEFICIENCY	SCREENING TESTS	GENERAL COMMENTS
Humoral (B cell)	Serum immunoglobulin levels (immunoglobulin G, M, and A [IgG, IgM, IgA]) Antibody titers against protein (diphtheria, tetanus toxoid) and polysaccharide *(Haemophilus)* antigens	Antibody levels must be interpreted with respect to age-appropriate values. High or low levels can be significant.
Cellular (T cell)	Lymphocyte count anergy testing	Total lymphocyte count is obtained by multiplying total white blood cell count by the percent of lymphocytes Value $<1500/\mu L$ is considered lymphopenia. Anergy testing not reliable for children younger than 1 yr
Phagocytic (macrophage or neutrophil)	Complete blood count IgE level Nitroblue tetrazolium test (NBT), flow cytometric respiratory burst assay	Abnormal neutrophil structure may be present. IgE level elevated in Job syndrome.
Complement	CH_{50} assay	Screening assay for components of classic complement pathway. May not be sensitive for limited deficiencies in individual complement components.

In an area that has a high prevalence of HIV infection, testing should be considered even if no obvious risk factor can be identified. Other tests of humoral immunity include B-cell number, antibody levels to various antigens, and IgG subclass determinations. Tests of cellular immunity include delayed type hypersensitivity (ie, mumps, *Trichophyton* infection, tetanus toxoid), T-cell enumeration, and lymphoproliferative responses. Table 214-6 lists the initial screening tests to be considered for each component of the immune system. Radiologic studies are used primarily in the diagnosis or management of associated infections, although the absence of a thymic shadow can be indicative of DiGeorge syndrome or SCID. Regardless of the results of initial screening tests, referral to a specialist, either immunologist or infectious diseases expert, should be considered for children who have signs and symptoms suggestive of immunodeficiency (Box 214-1).

Treatment

Treatment of primary immunodeficiency is condition specific. Patients with humoral and combined immunodeficiencies may benefit from the administration of intravenous immunoglobulin (IVIg) as replacement therapy. The initial regimen is 300 to 400 mg/kg every 3 to 4 weeks and should be adjusted based on the patient's response. The trough concentration of antibody should be at least 500 mg/dL.[10] Replacement IVIg is not indicated for all types of humoral deficiency. Furthermore, patients with IgA deficiency may develop anaphylaxis to certain brands of IVIg that contain small amounts of IgA. Other therapies include bone marrow transplantation (SCID, Wiskott-Aldrich, DiGeorge syndrome), enzyme replacement (certain forms of SCID), and cytokine therapy (interleukin-2 deficiency). Recently, interferon-gamma treatment has been demonstrated to decrease the number of infections in patients with chronic granulomatous disease.[11] The genetic basis for many of the primary immunodeficiencies is now known, and prenatal screening is increasingly available.

Pending a complete immunologic evaluation, children who are thought to have immunodeficiency syndromes should not receive live attenuated vaccines, such as varicella and measles, to avoid the possibility of vaccine-associated infection. Vaccine recommendations for specific immunodeficiencies can be found in the *American Academy of Pediatrics Red Book: Report of the Committee on Infectious Diseases*.[12] Blood transfusion, when needed, should be with cytomegalovirus-negative, irradiated cells to prevent the possibility of cytomegalovirus infection and graft-versus-host disease.

BOX 214-1 Reasons for Referral to an Immunologist Suspected Immunodeficiency

Recurrent serious (ie, sepsis, pneumonia, meningitis) bacterial infection

Serious bacterial infection in the context of failure to thrive

Infection with an opportunistic pathogen (ie, pneumocystis, *Cryptococcus* infection)

Vaccine associated infection

Unusual age for infection (ie, zoster infection, thrush)

Unusual severity or chronicity for a given infection

Family history of immunodeficiency

TOOLS FOR PRACTICE

Engaging Patients and Family

- *Recurrent Infections* (fact sheet), Riley Asthma Care Center Indiana University School of Medicine Department of Pediatrics (rileychildrenshospital.com/print.jsp?locid=776).
- Recurrent Infections (Web site), American Academy of Allergy, Asthma, and Immunology (www.aaaai.org/patients/allergic_conditions/infection.stm).
- *Tips to Remember: Recurrent or Unusually Severe Infections* (fact sheet), American Academy of Allergy, Asthma, and Immunology (www.aaaai.org/patients/publicedmat/tips/recurrentinfections.stm).

Medical Decision Support

- The Clinical Presentation of the Primary Immunodeficiency Diseases (Physician's Primer) (Web site), The Immune Deficiency Foundation (www.primaryimmune.org/pubs/book_phys/book_phys.htm).

SUGGESTED RESOURCES

Immune Deficiency Foundation. Available at: www.primary immune. org/

REFERENCES

1. Wald ER, Guerra N, Byers C. Upper respiratory tract infections in young children: duration of and frequency of complications. *Pediatrics*. 1991;87(2):129-133.
2. Klein JO. Infectious diseases and day care. *Rev Infect Dis*. 1986;8(4):521-526.
3. Hurwitz ES, Gunn WJ, Pinsky PF, et al. Risk of respiratory illness associated with day-care attendance: a nationwide study. *Pediatrics*. 1991;87(1):62-69.
4. Peat JK, Keena V, Harakeh Z, et al. Parental smoking and respiratory tract infections in children. *Paediatr Respir Rev*. 2001;2(3):207-213.
5. Teele DW, Klein JO, Rosner B. Epidemiology of otitis media during the first seven years of life in children in greater Boston: a prospective, cohort study. *J Infect Dis*. 1989;160(1):83-94.
6. Nunez MO, Ripoll NC, Carneros Martin JA, et al. Reactivation tuberculosis in a patient with anti-TNF-alpha treatment. *Am J Gastroenterol*. 2001;96(5):1665-1666.
7. Wood KL, Hage CA, Knox KS, et al. Histoplasmosis after treatment with anti-tumor necrosis factor-alpha therapy. *Am J Respir Crit Care Med*. 2003;167(9):1279-1282.
8. Affentranger P, Morell A, Spath P, et al. Registry of primary immunodeficiencies in Switzerland. *Immunodeficiency*. 1993;4(1-4):193-195.
9. Stray-Pedersen A, Abrahamsen TG, Froland SS. Primary immunodeficiency diseases in Norway. *J Clin Immunol*. 2000;20(6):477-485.

10. American Academy of Pediatrics. Passive Immunization. In: Pickering LK, Baker CJ, Long SS, McMillan JA, eds. *Red Book: 2006 Report of the Committee on Infectious Diseases*. Elk Grove Village, IL: American Academy of Pediatrics; 2006:54-66.
11. Marciano BE, Wesley R, De Carlo ES, et al. Long-term interferon-gamma therapy for patients with chronic granulomatous disease. *Clin Infect Dis*. 2004;39(5): 692-699.
12. American Academy of Pediatrics. Immunization in special clinical circumstances. In: Pickering LK, Baker CJ, Long SS, McMillan JA, eds. *Red Book: 2006 Report of the Committee on Infectious Diseases*. Elk Grove Village, IL: American Academy of Pediatrics; 2006:67-103.

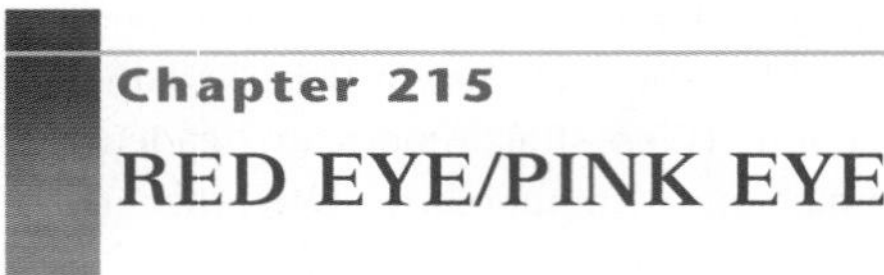

Chapter 215

RED EYE/PINK EYE

Kenneth W. Wright, MD

CONJUNCTIVITIS

Definitions

Pink eye, or conjunctivitis, is a nonspecific finding that simply indicates conjunctival inflammation. A variety of disease processes can cause conjunctival inflammation, including an extraocular foreign body, chemical toxicity, trauma, uveitis, episcleritis, allergic disease, viral or bacterial infections, and eyelid inflammation (blepharitis). Intraocular processes, including endophthalmitis (infection within the eye) and tumors associated with necrosis (eg, retinoblastoma), can also produce conjunctival inflammation, and they may produce conjunctivitis. Endophthalmitis is a devastating infection within the eye, often resulting in blindness. It is associated with vitreous inflammation that disrupts the red reflex. Endophthalmitis is extremely rare, but a neonate can develop endophthalmitis from a blood-borne infection originating in a contaminated indwelling catheter.

However, most children with pink eye have a benign, self-limiting conjunctivitis. The most common causes of pediatric conjunctivitis are listed in Box 215-1. Although determining the cause is often difficult from the eye's appearance alone, basic distinguishing features are common among the causes of pediatric conjunctivitis (Table 215-1).

BOX 215-1 Common Causes of Conjunctivitis in Children

BLEPHARITIS
Staphylococcal
Meibomian

GLAND DYSFUNCTION
Allergic conjunctivitis
Seasonal
Vernal
Atopic

BACTERIAL CONJUNCTIVITIS
Haemophilus influenzae
Streptococcus pneumoniae
Staphylococcus epidermidis
Staphylococcus aureus
Corynebacterium
Moraxella catarrhalis

VIRAL CONJUNCTIVITIS
Adenovirus
Herpesvirus
Papovavirus (conjunctival warts)
Poxvirus *(Molluscum contagiosum)*
Picornavirus
Paramyxovirus

TRAUMA
(see Chapter 301, Ocular Trauma)
Foreign body
Corneal abrasion
Chemical burn
Subconjunctival hemorrhage
Trichiasis

OCULAR INFLAMMATION
Juvenile idiopathic arthritis
Sarcoidosis
Endophthalmitis
Episcleritis

NEOPLASM
Conjunctival nevus
Lymphangioma

Evaluation and Treatment

Initial evaluation and treatment of pink eye in children should include a history and an ocular examination using the mnemonic I-ARM (inspection, acuity, red reflex, and motility; see Chapter 228, Visual Development, Amblyopia, and Vision Testing). A history of friends or family members with conjunctivitis usually indicates a contagious origin, commonly a viral infection. Itching is an important symptom because it is the hallmark of allergic conjunctivitis. Conjunctivitis associated with contact lens use may be the result of an allergy to contact lens solutions or, even more important, a vision-threatening bacterial corneal ulcer. Patients with conjunctivitis associated with contact lens use should be immediately referred to an ophthalmologist.

The red reflex test should also be performed on older children with conjunctivitis because an abnormal red reflex may indicate a serious disease process. Benign pediatric conjunctivitis almost never interferes with vision. Conjunctival cultures are not routinely obtained, and patients are treated based on their signs and symptoms. Indications for an ophthalmology referral include decreased visual acuity (worse than 20/40) or an abnormal red reflex. Fluorescein staining

Table 215-1 Distinguishing Features of Conjunctivitis in Children

FEATURE	BLEPHARITIS	ALLERGIC REACTION	BACTERIAL	VIRAL
Discharge	Minimal	Watery	Purulent	Watery
Itching	Minimal (real irritation, not itching)	Marked	Minimal	Minimal
Preauricular lymph adenopathy	Absent	Absent	Absent	Common
Laboratory test results	*Staphylococcus* on culture common	Eosinophils on conjunctival scraping	Bacteria on Gram stain; PMN response	Lymphocytes and monocytes

PMN, Polymorphonuclear neutrophil.

BOX 215-2 Initial Evaluation and Treatment of Nonspecific Pink Eye in Children

- History (trauma or foreign body, personal contacts, contact lens use, or allergy or itching)
- Mnemonic I-ARM (inspection, acuity, red reflex, motility)
- Fluorescein staining if abrasion or ulcer is suspected
- Treatment with topical antibiotic 3 times a day (eg, moxifloxacin, trimethoprim–polymyxin B, tobramycin-dexamethasone, levofloxacin, ciprofloxacin hydrochloride)
- Referral to an ophthalmologist if a corneal ulcer is suspected, conjunctivitis worsens with treatment, or no improvement is observed over 5-7 days

of the corneal epithelium is indicated if a corneal abrasion is the suspected cause of the pink eye. Fluorescein staining indicates a defect of the corneal epithelium most commonly caused by a traumatic abrasion or, less frequently, an infectious process such as a bacterial corneal ulcer or herpes simplex keratitis. Unilateral conjunctivitis may be caused by a foreign body, corneal ulcer, or herpes simplex keratitis.

Box 215-2 provides an outline of the initial evaluation and treatment of nonspecific pediatric pink eye.

NEONATAL CONJUNCTIVITIS (OPHTHALMIA NEONATORUM)

Neonatal conjunctivitis is a conjunctivitis occurring during the first month of life. Before the use of topical prophylaxis, ophthalmia neonatorum was a devastating disease associated with high morbidity. Routine topical prophylaxis with silver nitrate, tetracycline ointment, or erythromycin ointment has dramatically reduced the incidence of ophthalmia neonatorum. Infections can be acquired from vaginal microorganisms during birth or from hand-to-eye contamination from hospital workers. An infection from the birth canal is usually associated with a vaginal delivery, but it can also occur after a cesarean delivery if the amniotic membranes rupture before delivery. Infectious causes of neonatal conjunctivitis usually develop at least 48 hours after birth. Such causes include *Chlamydia trachomatis, Neisseria gonorrhoeae,* group B *Streptococcus, Staphylococcus aureus, Escherichia coli, Haemophilus influenzae,* and herpes simplex virus (HSV) type 2. The cause of the conjunctivitis can often be determined by the time of onset of the conjunctivitis (Table 215-2).

Differential Diagnosis

In addition to neonatal conjunctivitis, other causes of a red, teary eye in a newborn include congenital herpes keratitis, congenital glaucoma, and dacryocystitis. Congenital glaucoma is characterized by clear tears, large cornea, and corneal edema. Dacryocystitis is an infection of the nasolacrimal sac that causes swelling in the medial canthal area of the lower lid, and it should be distinguished from conjunctivitis (Figure 215-1).

Evaluation and Treatment

Evaluation and treatment of neonatal conjunctivitis are listed in Box 215-3. As for all newborns, the ophthalmic examination should start with the red reflex test. If the abnormality is isolated to the conjunctiva and does not involve the cornea or intraocular structures, then the red reflex should be normal. Conditions such as endophthalmitis, congenital glaucoma, and corneal infections have an abnormal red reflex test finding and require immediate consultation with an ophthalmologist. An urgent consultation is also indicated if the patient has marked lid swelling or unilateral conjunctivitis that does not improve over 1 or 2 days, because this condition may be HSV-2 keratitis. An ophthalmology consultation should be considered for any neonate with severe conjunctivitis.

The initial work-up for presumed infectious neonatal conjunctivitis includes conjunctival cultures on chocolate agar, Thayer-Martin agar, and blood agar. Conjunctival scrapings should be obtained and examined by Gram stain, Giemsa stain, and indirect immunofluorescent antibody assay for *Chlamydia*. If a herpes keratitis is suspected (unilateral conjunctivitis with corneal fluorescein staining), then a corneal scraping for herpes culture should be obtained. A serologic test for a concurrent congenital syphilis infection is advised for venereal-transmitted neonatal conjunctivitis.

Table 215-2 Causes of Neonatal Conjunctivitis

CAUSE	TIME OF ONSET	PRESENTATION	CONJUNCTIVAL SCRAPING	TREATMENT
Silver nitrate toxicity	Within 24 hr	Watery discharge	Negative gram-negative Giemsa; few PMN	None needed
Neisseria gonorrhea	2 to 4 days	Lid swelling, purulent discharge; corneal involvement can lead to corneal ulcer and perforation	Gram-negative intracellular diplococci and culture	Topical erythromycin and IV cefotaxime; treat even if asymptomatic
Other bacteria (staphylococci, streptococci)	4 to 7 days	Purulent discharge, with or without lid swelling	Gram-positive for specific bacteria and culture	Topical erythromycin or trimethoprim–polymyxin B eyedrops, or moxifloxacin
Chlamydia	4 to 10 days	Variable severity of lid swelling and serous or purulent discharge	Giemsa stain, basophilic, cytoplasmic inclusion bodies, positive direct immunofluorescent assay and culture	Initial IV erythromycin, then 50 mg/kg/day by mouth for 14 days; treat even if asymptomatic
Haemophilus	5 to 10 days	Serous or serosanguineous discharge, hemorrhagic conjunctivitis common; lid swelling with petechiae and bluish lid skin indicate preseptal cellulitis	Gram-negative *Coccobacillus* and culture	Topical trimethoprim-polymyxin B eyedrops and IV cefotaxime
Herpes simplex virus type 2	6 days to 2 wks	Usually unilateral, serous discharge with keratitis, positive corneal staining	Gram stain, multinucleated giant cells, Papanicolaou-stained intranuclear inclusion bodies, and herpes culture	Topical trifluorothymidine (Viroptic) and IV acyclovir

IV, Intravenous.

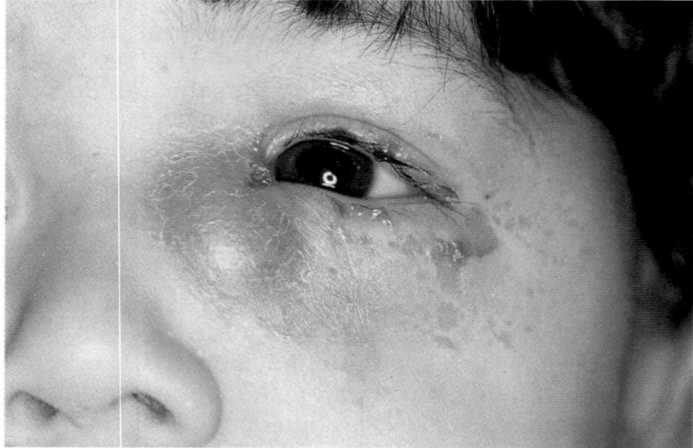

Figure 215-1 Chronically infected amniotocele with abscess in a 3-month-old infant. This patient was admitted to the hospital and treated with IV antibiotics several times but was never probed. The infection did not clear until the nasolacrimal duct (NLD) was probed. Early NLD probing in the first week of life should have been performed and would have prevented this chronic infection. Probing of the NLD opened the obstruction, drained the abscess, and cured the infection.

BOX 215-3 Initial Evaluation and Treatment of Presumed Infections Neonatal Conjunctivitis

EVALUATION

- Perform red reflex test and arrange an ophthalmology consult.
- Obtain conjunctival scrapings and test by Gram stain, Giemsa stain, and direct immunofluorescent assay for *Chlamydia*.
- Perform conjunctival culture on blood agar, chocolate agar, and Thayer-Martin agar. Virus culture should be considered, especially if only one eye is affected.

THERAPY

- Initiate initial therapy (before laboratory results) with erythromycin topical ointment and intravenous cefotaxime.
- Consider trifluorothymidine and intravenous acyclovir if herpes is suspected.
- Provide organism-specific treatment after test results come back.

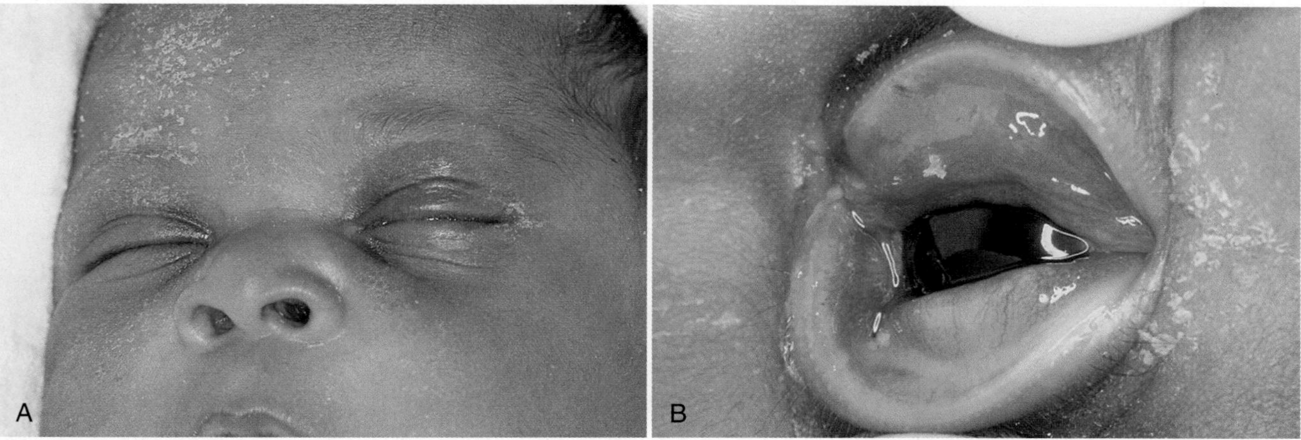

Figure 215-2 A, Two-day-old child with culture-positive gonococcal conjunctivitis. Note the bilateral lid swelling. B, With lids everted, severe conjunctivitis is disclosed.

The treatment of a presumed infectious neonatal conjunctivitis before receiving laboratory results includes the use of topical erythromycin ointment and intravenous (IV) cephalosporin such as cefotaxime. Ceftriaxone is usually avoided in neonates because it may result in hyperbilirubinemia. Antibiotic treatment should be provided immediately after samples are taken for culture. Topical trifluorothymidine (Viroptic) and IV acyclovir should be provided if herpes is suspected. Once the laboratory results are known, therapy is tailored to treat the identified organism.

INFECTIOUS CAUSES OF NEONATAL CONJUNCTIVITIS

Gonococcal Conjunctivitis

Gonococcal conjunctivitis occurs approximately 48 hours after birth. It may occur even earlier if rupture of the amniotic membranes occurs several hours before delivery. Typically, gonococcal conjunctivitis produces a bilateral, purulent conjunctivitis with copious discharge and lid edema (Figure 215-2). *N gonorrhoeae* is one of the few bacteria that can penetrate intact corneal epithelium, causing a corneal ulceration and even corneal perforation. The diagnosis is usually made by identifying gram-negative intracellular diplococci on conjunctival scrapings and verifying them by conjunctival culture. The treatment for gonococcal conjunctivitis is topical erythromycin ointment and IV cefotaxime. Parents may also need to be evaluated for possible treatment.

Chlamydial Conjunctivitis

Chlamydial conjunctivitis typically produces a bilateral, mild-to-moderate conjunctivitis approximately 4 to 10 days after birth. Eyelid swelling and a tarsal conjunctival pseudomembrane may be present (Figure 215-3). A conjunctival pseudomembrane is an accumulation of debris, not a true vascular tissue. The diagnosis of infection with *Chlamydia* is confirmed by conjunctival scrapings identifying cytoplasmic inclusion bodies in corneal epithelial cells (Giemsa stain) or by indirect immunofluorescence assay or culture. The first-line treatment is topical erythromycin ointment, along with oral erythromycin to remove *Chlamydia* organisms from the nasopharynx to decrease the risk of subsequent *Chlamydia* pneumonia at 1 to 3 months of age. Because pneumonitis can occur after neonatal conjunctivitis, parents should be warned of this possibility. Parents harbor the infection and should be treated with oral erythromycin or tetracycline even if they do not have any symptoms.

Herpes Simplex Virus Type 2

HSV-2 can cause neonatal conjunctivitis that is usually associated with a keratitis (corneal infection). Although it can occur as an isolated eye infection, herpes keratoconjunctivitis may be associated with systemic disease and encephalitis. Onset is usually between 1 and 2 weeks after birth, producing a serous discharge with moderate conjunctival injection.

In contrast to other infectious causes of neonatal conjunctivitis, herpes keratoconjunctivitis almost always occurs in only one eye. Breakdown of the normal epithelial barrier can result in a secondary bacterial corneal ulcer (Figure 215-4). Early stages of the keratitis are detected by corneal fluorescein staining with a geographic or dendritic pattern. The diagnosis is confirmed by viral cultures, which may take up to 7 to 10 days to become positive. If herpes neonatal conjunctivitis is suspected, then the treatment of choice is topical trifluorothymidine (trifluridine) combined with IV acyclovir. Topical antibiotics should be used to prevent a secondary bacterial infection.

Neonatal Conjunctivitis Prophylaxis

The best agent to use to prevent neonatal conjunctivitis is the subject of controversy. The efficacies of erythromycin ointment, tetracycline ointment, and silver nitrate are approximately the same, and the use of povidone iodine as prophylaxis has also been advocated. The advantages of povidone include effective

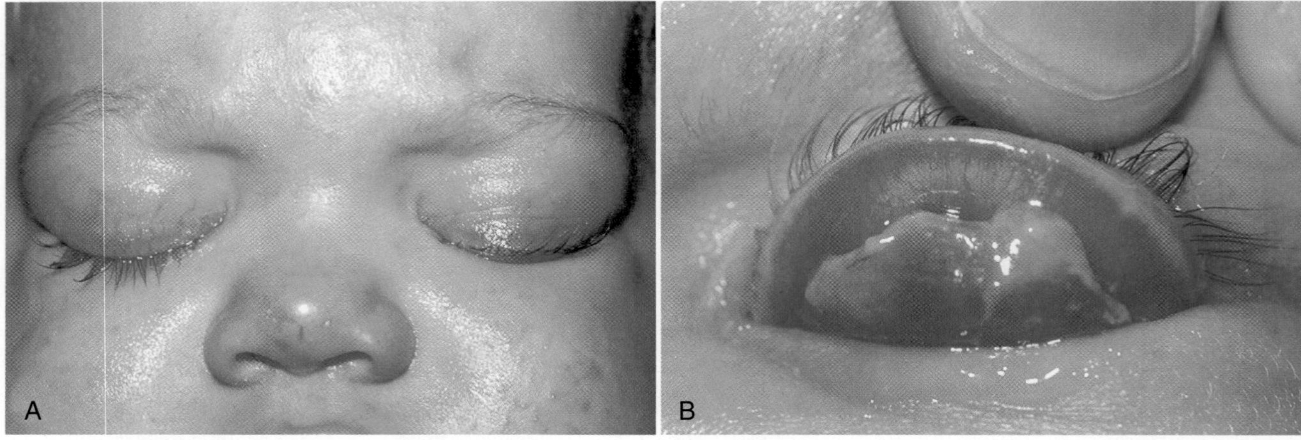

Figure 215-3 **A**, Two-week-old child with severe lid swelling caused by a *Chlamydia* conjunctivitis. **B**, Everting the upper eyelid discloses a severe conjunctivitis and a conjunctival pseudomembrane. A pseudomembrane is an accumulation of cellular debris and fibrin, not a true vascular tissue.

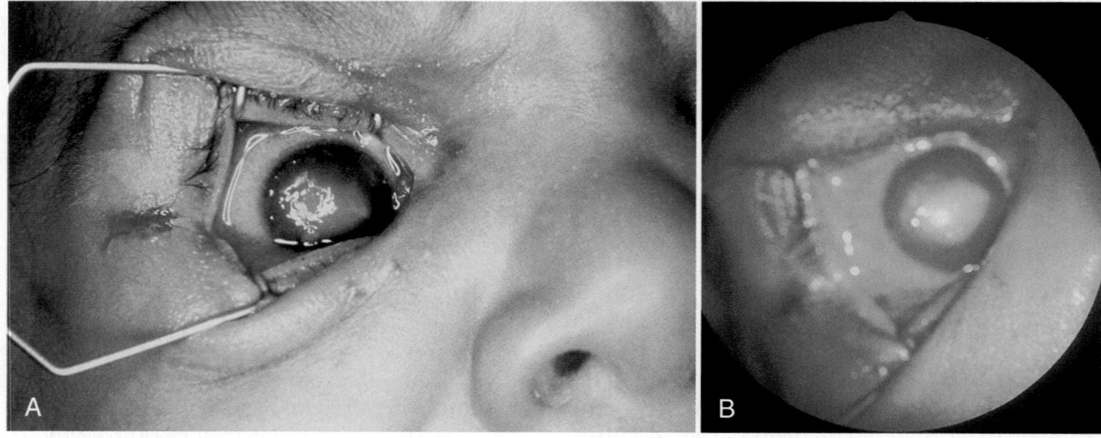

Figure 215-4 **A**, Three-week-old child with a combined bacterial corneal ulcer and HSV-2 keratitis. The white corneal lesion represents the area of infection. **B**, Fluorescein staining shows a central epithelial defect.

coverage of a broad spectrum of bacteria, coverage for viruses such as herpes simplex and HIV, and little chemical irritation reaction.[1]

Nasolacrimal Duct Obstruction

At birth, tear production by the lacrimal gland is minimal. Normal tearing develops several days to 2 weeks after birth. Tears are produced in the lacrimal gland, cross the cornea to exit via the superior and inferior puncta, then travel through the canaliculus into the lacrimal sac, to the nasal lacrimal duct, and finally through the Hasner valve into the posterior nasal pharynx (Figure 215-5). Thus the nose runs when a person cries.

Normally, the process of nasolacrimal canalization is completed by the end of the 9th month of gestation. When canalization is incomplete, the failure most often occurs at the distal end of the nasolacrimal duct (NLD) at the Hasner valve (see Figure 215-5). Outflow obstruction at the Hasner valve is the most common cause of NLD obstruction. Other, less-common anatomic variations within the nasolacrimal system can also cause obstruction of tear outflow, including agenesis of the canaliculus or crowding of the NLD opening by the inferior turbinate.

Infants with an NLD obstruction have a watery eye and an increased tear lake, eyelash matting, and mucus in the medial canthal area (Figure 215-6). Congenital NLD obstruction is common and occurs in 1% to 5% of the population, with approximately a 3rd being bilateral. If left untreated, NLD blockage spontaneously opens by 6 months of age in almost one half of cases. The incidence of spontaneous resolution after 13 months of age decreases to only 15%.[2]

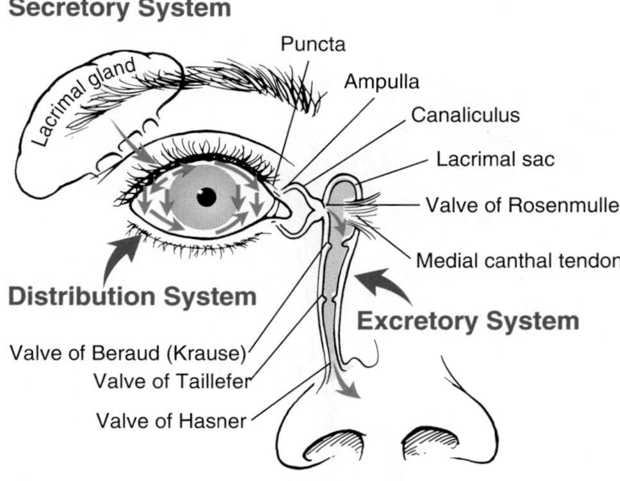

Figure 215-5 Three integral components of the lacrimal system include the secretory system (lacrimal glands), distribution system (eyelid blinking), and excretory system (puncta, canaliculus, nasolacrimal duct [NLD]). The NLD is the entire structure that connects the canaliculus to the nose (red-colored structure). Most NLD obstructions are caused by a persistent tissue membrane over Hasner valve at the distal end of the NLD.

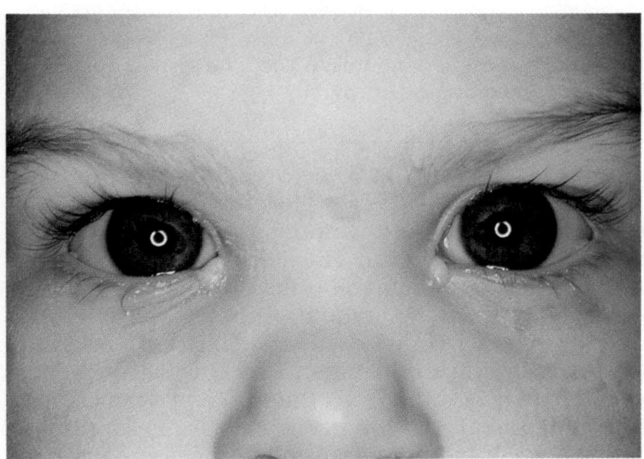

Figure 215-6 One-year-old child with bilateral nasolacrimal duct obstruction. Note the increased tear lake and mucus in the medial canthal area.

Management of Nasolacrimal Duct Obstruction

Optimal timing for initial NLD probing is controversial. Some experts advocate probing even when the patient is only a few months of age and suggest that it should be performed in the office without anesthesia. Most pediatric ophthalmologists, however, suggest waiting until the child is at least 6 months of age because almost one half the cases will have spontaneously resolved by then. Other experts suggest waiting until the child is 1 or 2 years of age for probing. Evidence indicates that delaying probing until 1½ to 2 years of age means that a single probing will be less successful. Initial probing should be performed when the patient is between 6 months and 1 year of age. This approach allows time for most cases to resolve spontaneously yet will provide the highest rate of probing success. NLD probing should be performed on an urgent basis in the case of amniotocele.

Medical management during the observational period is a combination of nasolacrimal sac massage and intermittent topical antibiotics. A 2-step massage strategy is best. The initial massage is directed inferiorly to push the tears in the normal direction, out the NLD. Subsequent massage is directed superiorly so that any tears that did not exit are at least cleared from the punctum. On occasion, inferior pressure itself will open a mild NLD obstruction. Topical antibiotic eyedrops or ointments may be provided if signs of infection are present, such as mucopurulent discharge. Antibiotic eyedrops such as moxifloxacin (Vigamox) or polymyxin B–trimethoprim sulfate work well, but they should be prescribed only when evidence of a true infection exists.

Nasolacrimal Duct Probing

NLD probing is a simple but delicate procedure. A small steel wire is passed through the nasolacrimal system, through the Hasner valve, and into the nose. In some cases, the inferior turbinate is infractured to relieve crowding. The success rate for NLD probing is more than 90% when performed before 1½ years of age. In cases in which NLD probing fails, intubation with silicone tubes is indicated to establish a patent system (Figure 215-7). In general, tubes are used only when the probing procedure fails.

Amniotocele (Dacryocystocele)

An amniotocele produces a swelling of the nasal lacrimal sac from an accumulation of fluid within the sac as a result of punctal and NLD obstruction. A few days after birth, a bluish swelling appears in the medial canthal area, representing fluid that is sequestered within a distended nasolacrimal sac (Figure 215-8). Treatment for a noninfected amniotocele is local massage. If decompression does not occur within a few days, then infection (ie, dacryocystitis) is almost certain. Because of this likelihood, probing the NLD to open the obstruction may be performed. An infected amniotocele is red, warm, and large, approximately 1 cm in diameter (Figure 215-9). Treatment of the infection consists of IV antibiotics (cephalosporin) and urgent NLD probing to relieve the obstruction and drain the abscess. Although a cutaneous incision into the sac to decompress the abscess may be performed, this procedure leaves a scar and may produce an external fistula. NLD probing does not leave a scar, avoids the fistula complication, and has the advantage of directly addressing the primary cause of the abscess by opening the NLD obstruction. If the abscess is not drained, then an infected amniotocele can result in cellulitis and even sepsis.

Congenital Glaucoma

Tearing is one of the most common signs of congenital glaucoma. Primary congenital glaucoma refers to

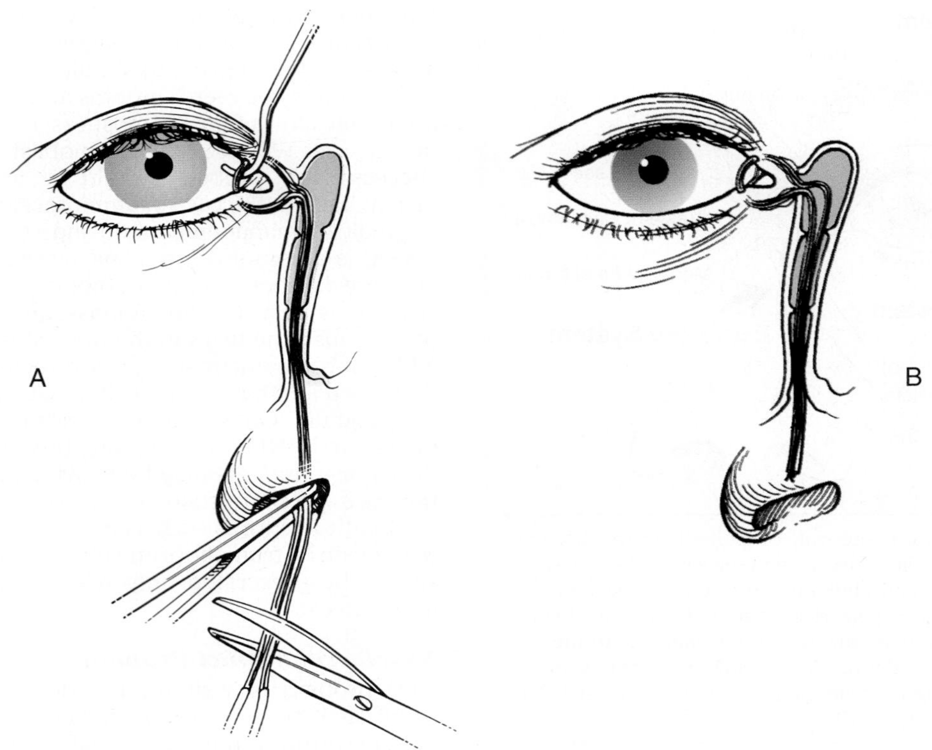

Figure 215-7 **A,** Drawing of silicone stent in the canaliculi and nasolacrimal system. The silicone tube has a probe attached to each end and a central suture inside the silicone tube. One probe is passed through the upper punctum, one probe passed through the lower punctum so the two probes meet in the nose. The probes are cut off the ends of the silicone tube to expose the central suture. **B,** The suture inside the silicone tube is tied together in the nose to join the ends of the silicone tube in a loop. The loop of tube is left in place for 1 to 3 months to keep the system open and to prevent membrane re-growth.

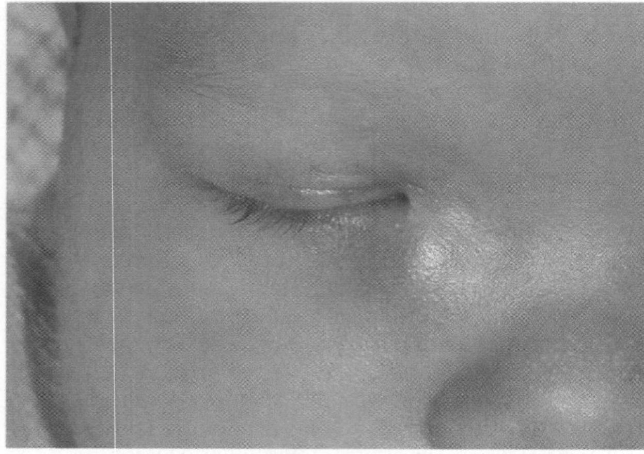

Figure 215-8 Amniotocele right lacrimal sac in 4-day-old newborn. The amniotocele is the bluish cyst just inferior to the medial canthus. The amniotocele is not infected at this time.

increased intraocular pressure occurring at birth or shortly thereafter. Normal intraocular pressure in infants is approximately 10 to 15 mm Hg, whereas intraocular pressure in infants with congenital glaucoma is often over 30 mm Hg. Congenital glaucoma differs from adult glaucoma by causing enlargement of the eye in addition to damaging the optic nerve. The eye enlarges because, in infants, the eye wall is elastic and stretches. Normal corneas at birth are approximately 10.5 mm in diameter, and corneal diameters greater than 12 mm are considered abnormally large (megalocornea). As the cornea enlarges, breaks of the basement membrane of the corneal endothelium (Haab striae) occur, resulting in corneal edema that reduces vision and can lead to amblyopia. After 3 years of age, the eye wall becomes fairly rigid, and ocular enlargement resulting from glaucoma does not occur.

Features of congenital glaucoma include tearing, photophobia, blepharospasm, large cornea, and corneal clouding (edema). Approximately 70% of cases are bilateral. The classic findings of congenital glaucoma are not always present; signs of ocular enlargement and corneal edema may be subtle (Figure 215-10). In cases with tearing, the diagnosis of congenital glaucoma may be misdiagnosed as an NLD obstruction. In contrast to NLD obstruction, however, the tearing associated with congenital glaucoma is caused by corneal edema, which can be seen as a dull red reflex with an ophthalmoscope.

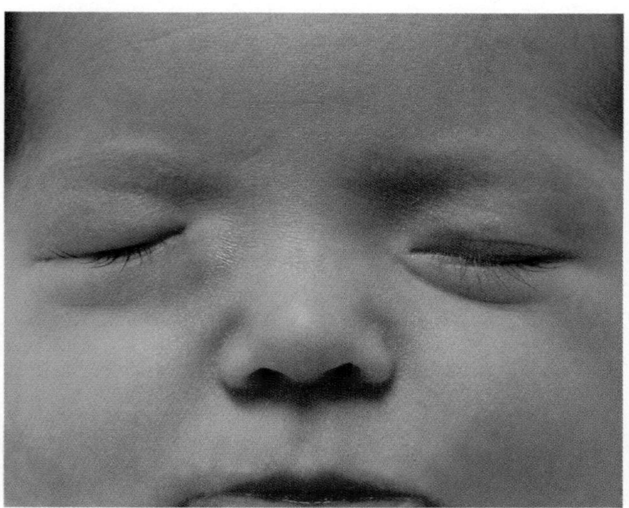

Figure 215-9 Infected amniotocele right eye at 10 days after birth. Note the redness and swelling in the medial canthal area and upper lid. Urgent probing of the nasolacrimal duct is indicated.

The pathogenesis of congenital glaucoma relates to an abnormal outflow caused by abnormal angle structures, including the trabecular meshwork. A congenital glaucoma gene *(2p21, 1p36)* and juvenile glaucoma gene *(1q23-q25)* have been found.[3-5] Juvenile glaucoma, an extremely rare condition that has onset after 2 to 3 years of age, is difficult to diagnose because virtually no signs or symptoms develop other than increased intraocular pressure and optic disk cup changes (Figure 215-11).

The treatment of congenital glaucoma is based on lowering the intraocular pressure to prevent optic nerve damage, prevent progressive expansion of the eye, and reduce corneal edema. Medications used to lower intraocular pressures include beta-adrenergic inhibitors (timolol), carbonic-anhydrase inhibitors, which can be administered topically or systemically (acetazolamide), and adrenergic agonists (apraclonidine). However, medical treatment is not effective in most cases of congenital glaucoma. It is almost always a disease treated with surgery directed at opening the outflow channels at the trabecular meshwork.

The 2 most frequently used procedures are the goniotomy and trabeculotomy ab externum. With a goniotomy, a microscopic knife is used to lyse the abnormal trabecular meshwork to open up the angle. With the trabeculotomy ab externum, a microscopic probe is placed in the Schlemm canal and then swept through the trabecular meshwork and into the anterior chamber to open up the angle. The success rate of these procedures for congenital glaucoma is approximately 60% to 70%.[6] If the 1st procedure fails, then a 2nd one may be performed.

When these procedures are not successful, a trabeculectomy is usually performed. A trabeculectomy is a filtering procedure in which aqueous fluid is filtered through a small hole in the eye to the subconjunctival space.

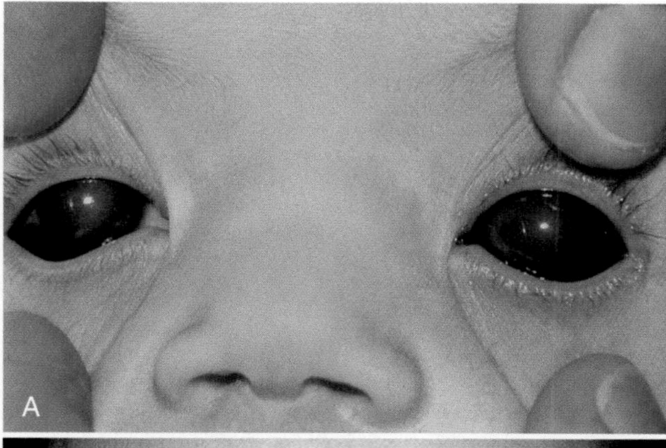

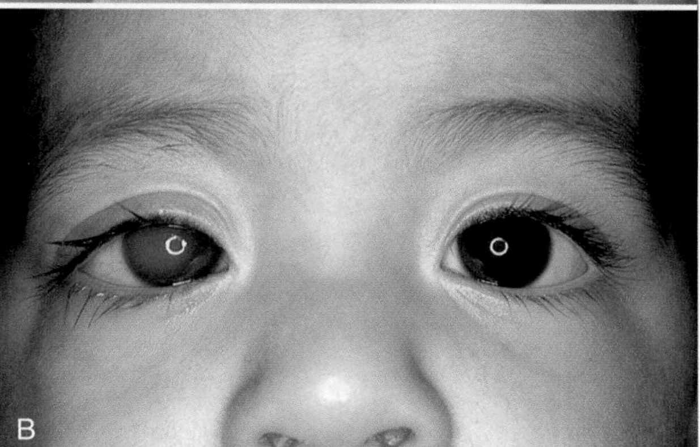

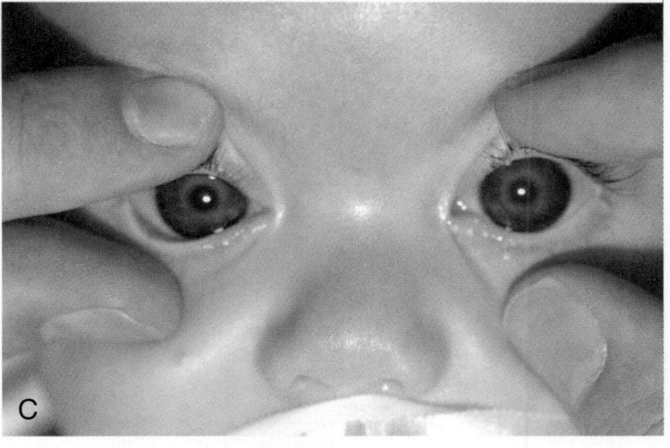

Figure 215-10 **A,** Neonate with bilateral severe congenital glaucoma. Note the extremely large corneas and corneal edema that gives the bluish appearance to the eyes indicating corneal edema. **B,** Congenital glaucoma right eye. Note the white corneal opacity, which is corneal edema secondary to increased intraocular pressure and a break in Descemet membrane (Haab striae). The corneal diameter of the right eye is 13.5 mm versus 11.5 mm in the left eye. **C,** Congenital glaucoma in a 2-month-old infant with mild bilateral corneal edema and slightly enlarged corneas. The right corneal diameter is 12 mm and the left corneal diameter is 13 mm. This child exhibited epiphora and might have been easily misdiagnosed as having an NLD obstruction. A dim red reflex caused by the corneal edema indicated to the pediatrician that this was more than a common nasolacrimal duct obstruction.

If all these procedures fail, then congenital glaucoma can sometimes be managed by ciliary body destructive procedures such as cryotherapy and laser surgery, which eliminate the ciliary body epithelium that produces aqueous fluid. These end-stage procedures have a high failure rate.

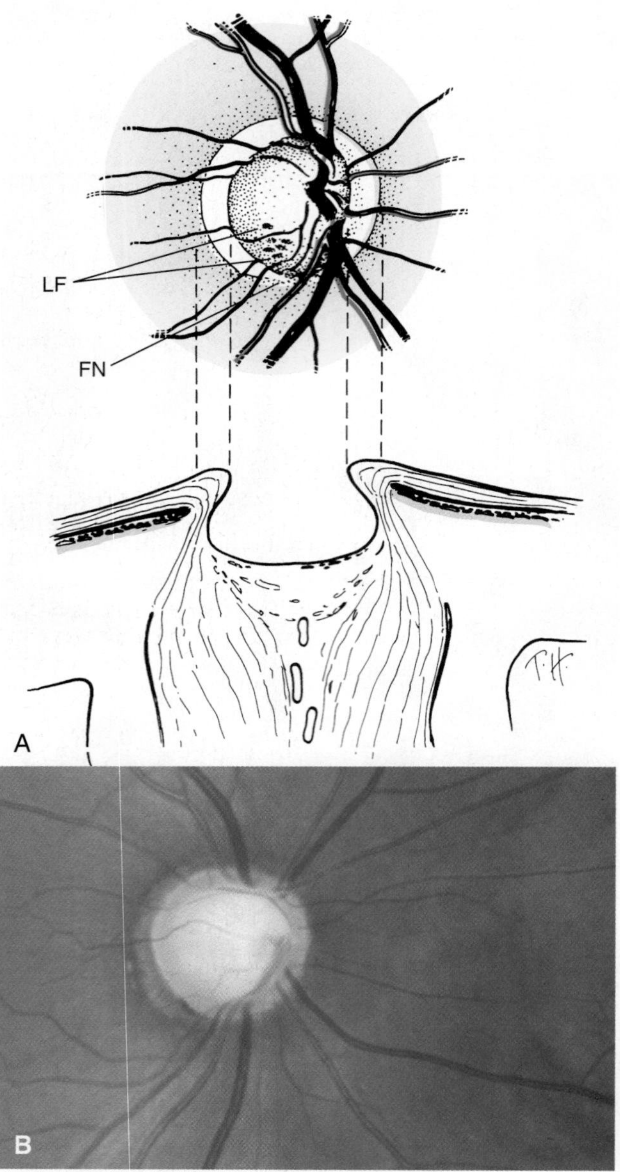

Figure 215-11 A. Glaucomatous optic nerve (anterior optic nerve head and transverse view, right eye). Note the thinning and undermining of inferior neuroretinal rim and focal notching (FN) of the inferior neuroretinal rim, the enlarged central cup with visible laminar fenestrae (LF), the nasal shift of retinal vessels, and the peripapillary atrophy. B. Glaucomatous optic nerve. Advanced cupping with diffuse thinning and undermining of the neuroretinal rim, nasalization of the retinal vessels, and loss of the normal nerve fiber layer striations (right eye).

The prognosis for congenital glaucoma is fair, with approximately 70% of patients maintaining good, long-term visual acuity.[6] Unfortunately, patients with unfavorable outcomes often become blind. The most important cause of visual loss is attributed to optic nerve damage, which is not irreversible. Other causes include chronic corneal edema with corneal scarring, refractive errors, and, importantly, dense irreversible amblyopia.

Juvenile glaucoma is more amenable to medical treatment. In many cases, however, juvenile glaucoma must also be treated with surgical techniques.

BACTERIAL CONJUNCTIVITIS

The conjunctiva is constantly exposed to bacteria, but conjunctival and tear defense mechanisms work to prevent infection. When bacterial infections do occur, they produce watery irritation of the eyes that can progress to a mucopurulent discharge (Figure 215-12). Children with a bacterial conjunctivitis often complain that their eyelids stick together in the morning. Most often, one eye is initially involved, with subsequent involvement of the other. The bulbar conjunctiva is diffusely injected, and a mucopurulent exudate is present in the inferior conjunctival fornix. The most common bacteria in children include *H influenzae, Streptococcus pneumoniae, Moraxella catarrhalis,* and *Staphylococcus* organisms. Other organisms that cause conjunctivitis are listed in Box 215-4 and are categorized as acute or chronic bacterial infections.

In general, cultures and Gram stain are not routinely performed for mild to moderate conjunctivitis, and patients are treated with antibiotic eyedrops, including the quinolones such as moxifloxacin, levofloxacin, gatifloxacin, or ofloxacin. Other antibiotic eyedrops include sulfacetamide, trimethoprim sulfate, trimethoprim–polymyxin B (Polytrim), gentamicin, and tobramycin. Erythromycin ointment may also be applied. An ophthalmology referral should be considered for severe conjunctivitis or a chronic conjunctivitis that does not improve after 7 days of treatment.

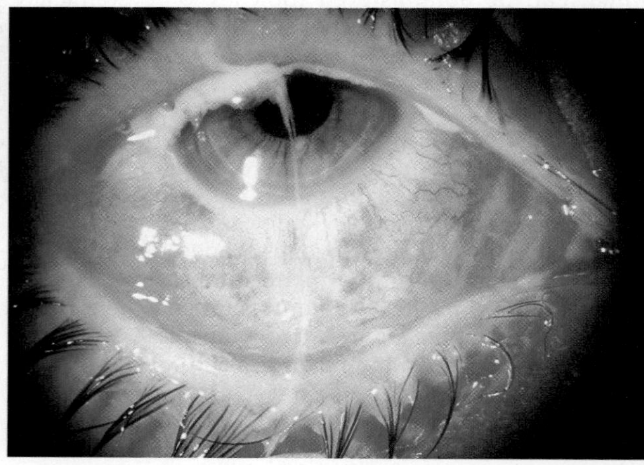

Figure 215-12 Severe bacterial conjunctivitis with mucopurulent discharge.

VIRAL CONJUNCTIVITIS

Viral conjunctivitis is usually caused by an adenovirus and is extremely contagious. Patients often begin with infection in one eye that then spreads to the other. Tearing, redness, and the sensation of having a foreign body lodged in the eye are extreme. This combination of findings is termed catarrhal conjunctivitis. In children, the eyelids may be swollen, and they may produce reactive ptosis, as well as severe conjunctival hyperemia and hemorrhagic conjunctivitis. The cornea may be involved; such patients are sensitive to light. In many instances, a history of other family members or friends having pink eye can be found.

BOX 215-4 Causes of Bacterial Conjunctivitis

ACUTE CONJUNCTIVITIS

- *Staphylococcus aureus*
- *Haemophilus aegyptius*
- *Haemophilus influenzae*
- *Streptococcus pneumoniae*
- *Streptococcus pyogenes*
- Beta-*Streptococcus*
- *Pseudomonas aeruginosa*
- *Corynebacteria diphtheriae*
- *Moraxella catarrhalis*

CHRONIC CONJUNCTIVITIS

- *S aureus*
- *Moraxella lacunata*
- *Proteus*
- *Klebsiella*
- *Serratia*
- Group B *Streptococcus*

Pharyngoconjunctival Fever

Pharyngoconjunctival fever consists of an upper respiratory infection (pharyngitis and fever) with bilateral conjunctivitis. It is most commonly associated with adenovirus type 3 and type 7. Pharyngoconjunctival fever produces a severe, watery conjunctival discharge; hyperemic conjunctivitis; chemosis (conjunctival edema); preauricular lymph adenopathy; and, quite often, a foreign-body sensation that results from corneal involvement. The disease is highly contagious and lasts approximately 2 to 3 weeks.

Epidemic Keratoconjunctivitis

Epidemic keratoconjunctivitis (EKC) is caused by adenovirus types 8, 19, and 37. It occurs most often in older children and adolescents. In contrast to pharyngoconjunctival fever, EKC is isolated to the eyes. The virus causes a severe bilateral conjunctivitis with conjunctival hyperemia, watery discharge, eyelid swelling, and a reactive ptosis (Figure 215-13). Petechial conjunctival hemorrhages are also common. In addition, a pseudomembrane may be found along the conjunctiva, and preauricular adenopathy may be present. In many instances, 1 eye is involved 1st, and the 2nd eye becomes affected several days later.

Approximately one third of patients develop corneal inflammation (keratitis), with subepithelial infiltrates 7 to 10 days after onset of the conjunctivitis (Figure 215-14).[7] The keratitis is a hypersensitive reaction to the virus, not a true viral infection. Corneal infiltrates cause severe photophobia and irritation.

The treatment of adenovirus conjunctivitis is prevention of further transmission. If a patient seems to have adenoviral conjunctivitis, then the clinician must thoroughly wash everything before seeing another patient. A patient with this disease will be contagious for up to 2 weeks and should observe isolation precautions during this time. Because of the possibility of corneal involvement, patients with adenoviral conjunctivitis should be referred to an ophthalmologist.

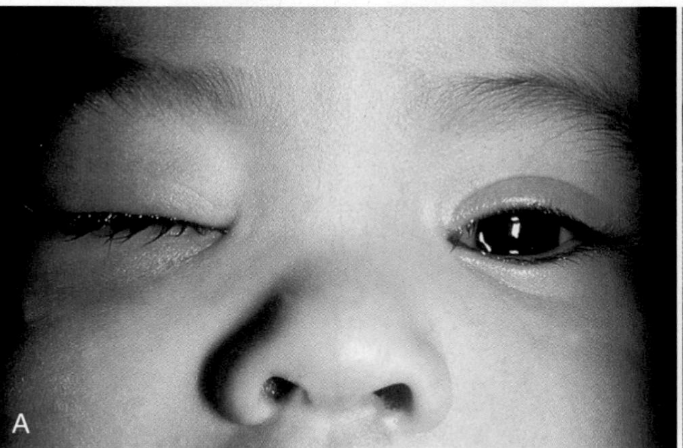

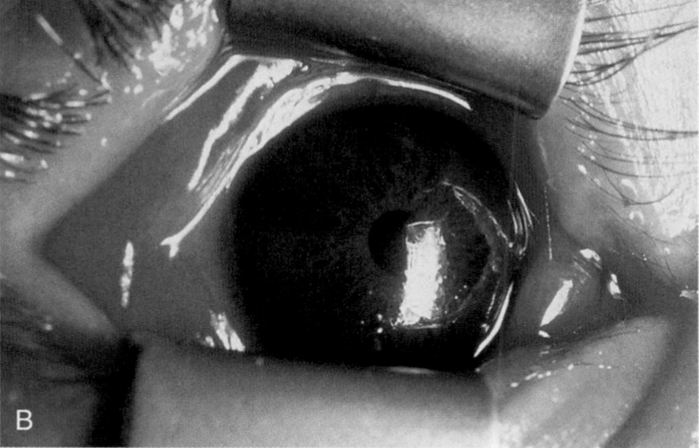

Figure 215-13 Epidemic keratoconjunctivitis bilateral involvement. **A,** Note the severe lid swelling (right eye) and tearing (left eye). The spectrum of severity is wide; some cases are mild, and other patients with a severe conjunctivitis may have severe lid swelling and the appearance of a preseptal cellulitis. **B,** A lid speculum placed to open the right eye reveals a severe hemorrhagic conjunctivitis.

No effective antiviral treatment for EKC exists. Cold compresses and topical nonsteroidal antiinflammatory drugs may reduce symptoms. Because of the contagious nature of the adenoviral conjunctivitis, a scraping for viral antigen quick preparation is indicated. If results are positive, then patients should not return to school for 1 to 2 weeks. Corticosteroids are discouraged except for the treatment of keratitis and should be administered only by an ophthalmologist.

Hemorrhagic Conjunctivitis

An alarming form of pediatric conjunctivitis is conjunctivitis with subconjunctival hemorrhage, or hemorrhagic conjunctivitis. The most common causes of hemorrhagic conjunctivitis include infection with *H influenzae*, adenovirus, or picornavirus or spontaneous subconjunctival hemorrhage without infection. *H influenzae* hemorrhagic conjunctivitis is associated with a purplish discoloration of the eyelids caused by multiple tiny subcutaneous hemorrhages (Figure 215-15).

A spontaneous subconjunctival hemorrhage is a painless rupture of a small conjunctival vessel, usually for no known reason. The conjunctiva surrounding the hemorrhage will be normal, and no tearing or exudate is present. The hemorrhage resolves without treatment, and a systemic work-up is not usually necessary unless the hemorrhage becomes recurrent or if a history of prior bleeding or bruising exists.

Primary Ocular Herpes Simplex Virus Type 1

Most adults have been exposed to HSV-1 and, unless immunocompromised, have circulating antibodies to the virus. Only 1% of the population will exhibit clinical HSV infection; most infections are asymptomatic.[8] Primary ocular herpes represents the first exposure to HSV-1, occurring initially as a skin eruption with multiple vesicular lesions (Figure 215-16). Virus can be cultured from vesicle fluid. The use of antiviral medications is controversial, but systemic or topical acyclovir may speed recovery if provided within 1 or 2 days of onset. Topical antibiotics applied to the skin may be useful for preventing secondary bacterial infection. Over several days to 2 weeks, the skin lesions heal, with or without treatment, usually without much scarring. The cornea is

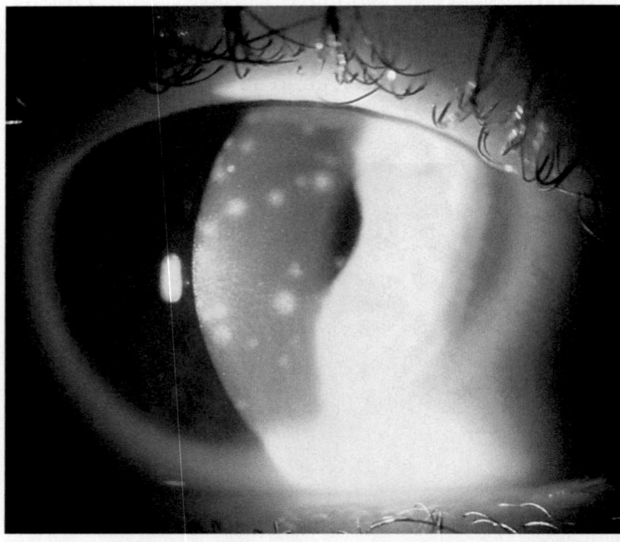

Figure 215-14 Subepithelial infiltrates of the cornea associated with epidemic keratoconjunctivitis. These infiltrates occur during the 2nd week of the infection and may persist for several months or longer. The infiltrates represent an immune response to the disorder and resolve spontaneously.

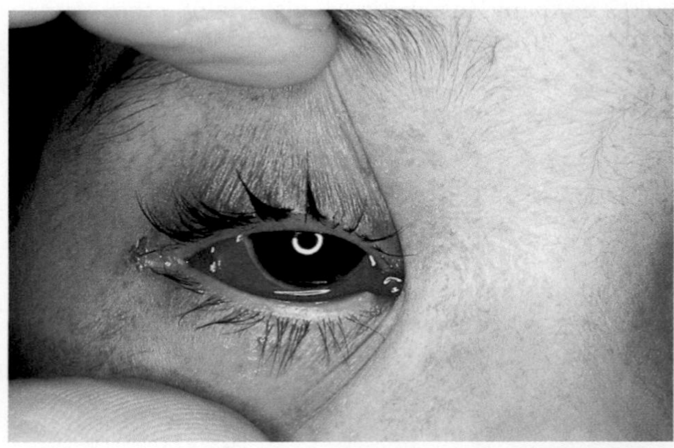

Figure 215-15 Patient with hemorrhagic conjunctivitis secondary to *Haemophilus influenzae* infection. Patient also has otitis media. Note the purplish or violaceous hue of the eyelid.

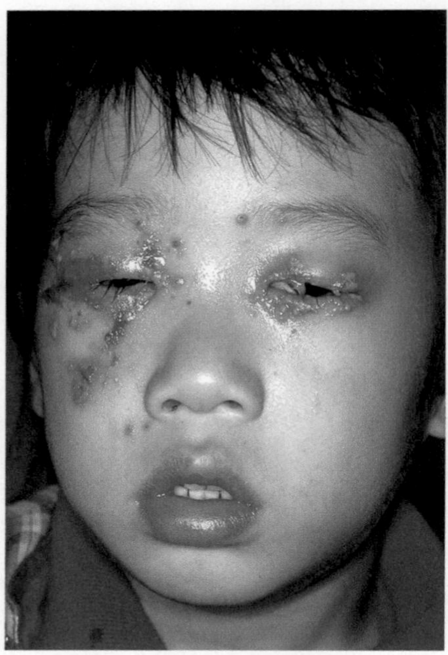

Figure 215-16 Four-year-old boy with primary herpes cutaneous eruption in both eyes and multiple vesicular lesions around the eyelid and eyelid margins. This condition resolved after 2 or 3 weeks without significant scarring.

involved in 30% of patients with primary ocular HSV-1 infection.[9] Topical ophthalmic antiviral medications, such as trifluorothymidine, may be provided to prevent secondary corneal involvement. Oral acyclovir may be used for severe skin involvement. Primary ocular HSV rarely causes intraocular inflammation or uveitis.

Recurrent Ocular Herpes Simplex Virus

After initial cutaneous facial infection or infection of the mucus membranes, the HSV gains access to the sensory nerve endings and travels up the axons to the trigeminal ganglion. The virus remains sequestered and protected within the ganglion. Recurrent ocular herpes occurs when the virus from the ganglion travels down the sensory nerve and infects the cornea or eyelids. The cutaneous eyelid disease consists of a vesicular reaction similar to primary herpes simplex. The corneal disease from recurrent HSV affects the corneal surface epithelium. Active virus replication causes punctate, dendritic, or geographic epithelial defects. The dendritic pattern is a classic sign of herpes keratitis (corneal infection) (Figure 215-17). Recurrent herpes keratitis is almost always unilateral. In addition, the cornea becomes anesthetized as a result of sensory nerve damage. With recurrent herpes, the cornea can scar, and a secondary inflammatory reaction can occur in response to the viral antigen.

The treatment for acute recurrent herpes keratitis is topical antiviral therapy, usually with trifluorothymidine (trifluridine). Systemic treatment with oral acyclovir has proven to be effective, especially in cases of multiple recurrences or in immunocompromised children. Treatment must sometimes last 6 months to a year to prevent recurrence. Topical corticosteroids are not indicated for active herpes keratitis because they will decrease the body's immune response. The clinician needs to be careful about unilateral pink eye because some of these cases may be herpes keratitis. Topical corticosteroids in conjunction with antiviral therapy may be used by ophthalmologists to reduce corneal scarring.

Herpes Zoster and Varicella-Zoster Virus

Chickenpox, or varicella-zoster virus, rarely affects the eye, even when vesicular lesions occur on the eyelid or eyelid margin. Some physicians administer topical trifluorothymidine if the conjunctiva becomes involved. In immunocompromised patients, herpes zoster can present a high risk, and these patients especially should be treated with antiviral therapy. Secondary, or recurrent, herpes zoster ophthalmicus affects patients older than 50 years or immunocompromised patients. This severe ocular inflammation can affect all layers of the eye.

Blepharitis

Blepharitis, or eyelid inflammation, is one of the most common causes of pink eye in children. The 2 most common types of blepharitis are staphylococcal blepharitis and meibomian gland dysfunction. Both types of blepharitis are treated with lid hygiene (lid scrubs with baby shampoo) and topical antibiotics.

Children with staphylococcal blepharitis complain of itching and burning and often awake with their eyelids stuck together with crusting. Their eyes are irritated, but true itching is not present, as is the case in patients with allergic conjunctivitis. Other signs of staphylococcal blepharitis include crusting and scales at the base of the eyelashes. The eyelid margins are thickened and hyperemic, with vascularization of the eyelid margin. Over time, lashes may become misdirected, broken, or absent (madarosis). Sties, or external hordeolums, are common. An external hordeolum is an abscess of the gland of Zeis on the anterior eyelid margin (Figures 215-18 and 215-19). This development is in contrast to a chalazion, which is deeper and represents an inflammation of the meibomian gland that results from breakdown of the fatty secretions. Blepharitis may be associated with corneal changes that cause severe photophobia. These corneal deposits are an immunologic response to the bacterial antigen.

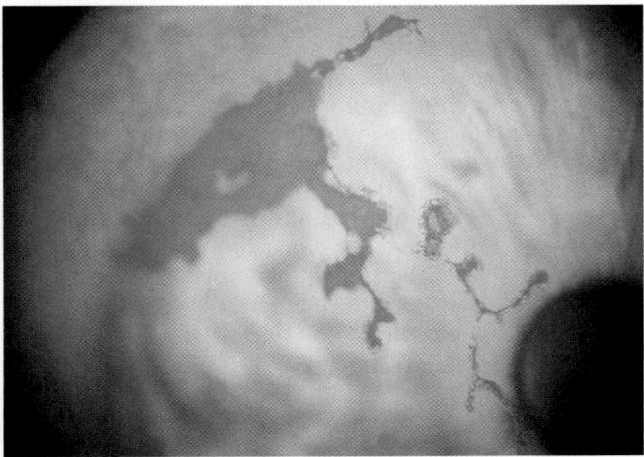

Figure 215-17 Active herpes keratitis with both dendritic and geographic patterns. Superiorly at the limbus is the confluent area of staining showing a geographic pattern; the midcornea shows the branching, dendritic pattern.

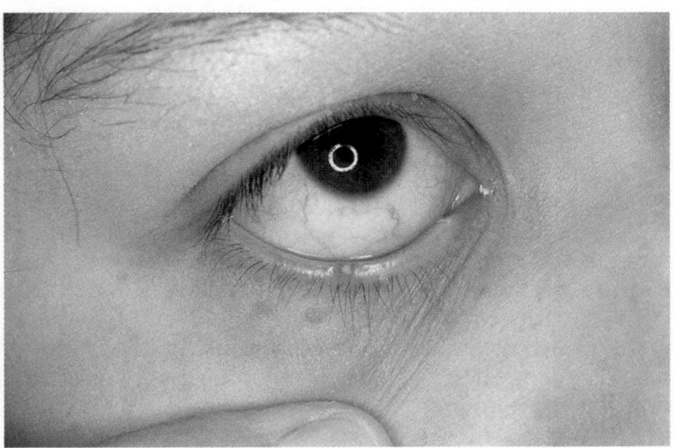

Figure 215-18 Staphylococcal blepharitis with small external hordeolum.

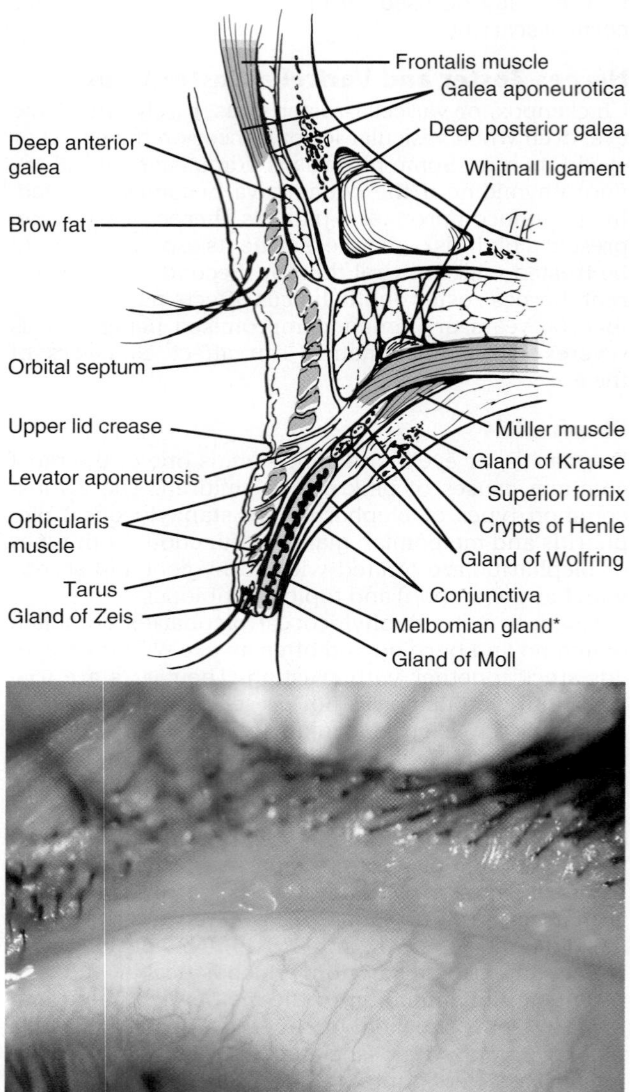

Figure 215-19 Sagittal section of the upper lid showing various tear-secreting glands *(top)*. The photograph of the eyelid margin shows droplets at the orifice of the meibomian glands *(bottom)*. *The meibomian gland opens at the lid margin.

Treatment of staphylococcal blepharitis includes eyelid hygiene and topical antibiotic ointment, usually erythromycin. In severe cases, systemic erythromycin may be indicated. Eyelid cultures are not routinely performed because most eyelids normally are colonized with *Staphylococcus* organisms. Eyelid hygiene includes lid scrubs with baby shampoo once or twice a day. Prevention of recurrent blepharitis consists of ongoing lid hygiene.

Phlyctenular Conjunctivitis

Phlyctenular conjunctivitis is a delayed hypersensitivity reaction to bacterial protein and is usually associated with staphylococcal blepharitis. The lesions are usually located at 3 and 9 o'clock around the limbus and are creamy white or yellowish-colored elevated nodules with a surrounding erythematous base (Figure 215-20). Treatment consists of treating the blepharitis (lid scrubs and topical antibiotics) and the use of topical corticosteroids. If topical corticosteroids are to be administered, then treatment should be monitored by an ophthalmologist. When tuberculosis was prevalent, it was a major cause of phlyctenulosis. Patients with phlyctenular conjunctivitis who are at risk should be evaluated for tuberculosis.

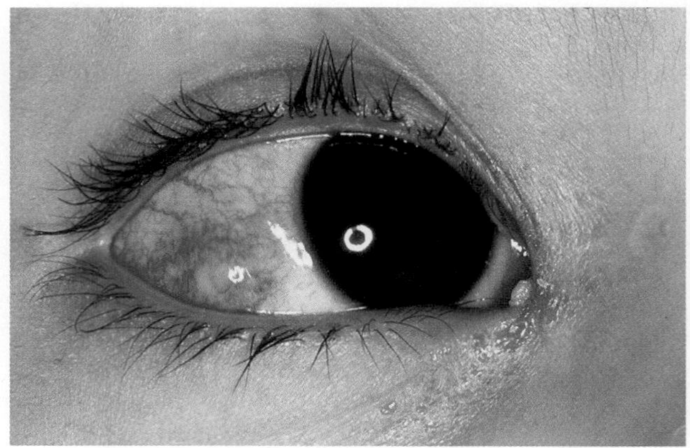

Figure 215-20 Photograph of phlyctenule in a patient with staphylococcal blepharitis. The phlyctenule is the yellow lesion at the lower lid margin surrounded by erythematous conjunctival reaction.

Meibomian Gland Dysfunction

Meibomian glands are sebaceous glands with orifices at the eyelid margins (see Figure 215-19). Meibomian gland secretions consist of sterol esters and waxes that provide a covering to the tear film, thereby preventing evaporation. Dysfunction or blockage of the meibomian gland orifice by desquamated epithelial cells results in stagnation of the lipids and causes a secondary local inflammation (see Figure 215-19, *bottom*). Microbial lipases from *Propionibacterium acnes* and other bacteria contribute to producing irritating fatty acids that increase the inflammatory response.

Obstruction of the meibomian gland orifices may result in a chalazion or sty. A chalazion appears as a lump near the eyelid margin, on either the upper or the lower lid. Because the chalazion is a swelling of a meibomian gland, the swelling can occur externally as a lump on the skin or internally as a lump underneath the conjunctiva (Figure 215-21). A chalazion is not an infection but a granulomatous inflammation that results from the irritating lipids within the meibomian gland. Chalazia may resolve without treatment; however, applying hot soaks several times a day helps the drainage of lipid material. If the chalazion does not resolve over several weeks of treatment, then incision and drainage may be necessary. An external hordeolum is an acute infection of an accessory gland, which can be treated with erythromycin ointment, hot soaks, and eyewashes with baby shampoo. Chalazia may be

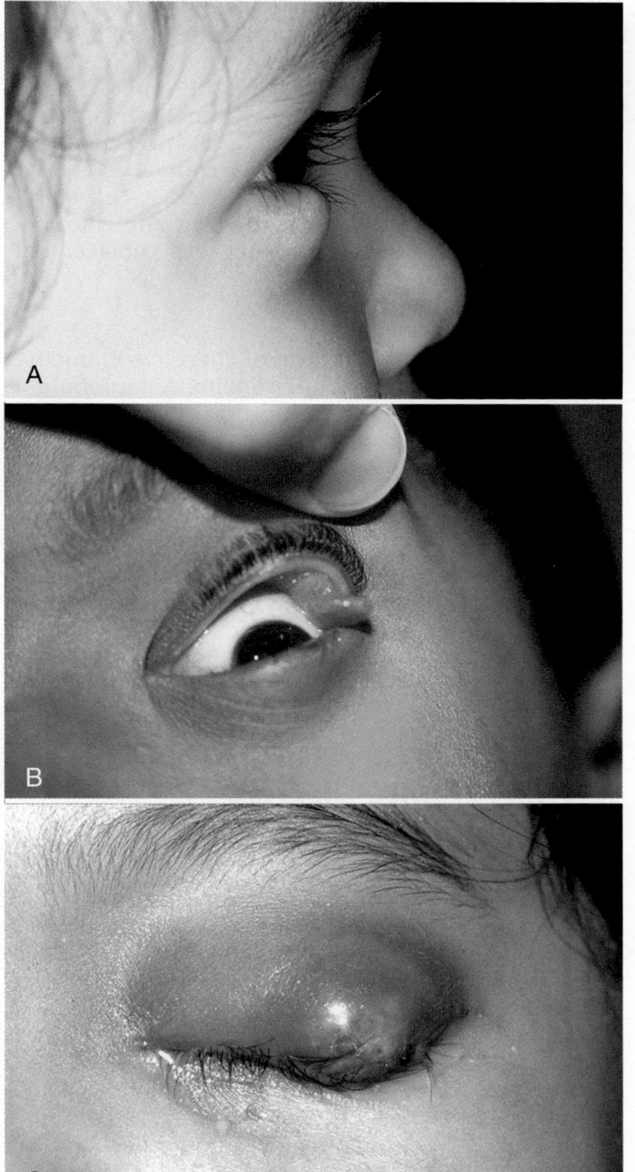

Figure 215-21 **A**, Chalazion, lower lid. Note the subcutaneous lid mass with some erythema. Over time, the overlying skin can become erythematous and inflamed. **B**, Internal chalazion in which the meibomian gland has extended posteriorly under the conjunctiva. This condition is sometimes called pyogenic granuloma. **C**, Infected chalazion.

prevented by the use of eyelid hygiene with eye wipes or a baby shampoo eyewash each day.

Molluscum Contagiosum

Molluscum contagiosum is a viral disease of the skin, often occurring on the eyelids, caused by a DNA virus of the poxvirus group. The lesions are small, round, discrete bumps with a central pit (Figure 215-22). They are presumed to be contagious and are transmitted by direct touch. When present on the eyelid margin, they can cause a conjunctival reaction and a follicular conjunctivitis. These lesions can be treated by excising the central core or, rarely, through the use of cryotherapy or application of chemical caustics such as trichloroacetic acid or aqueous phenol.

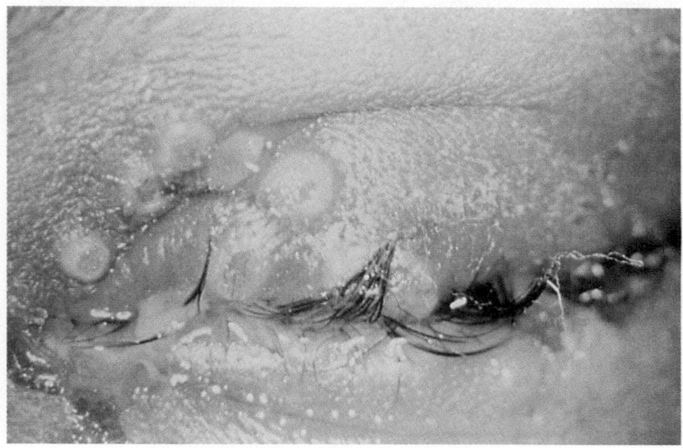

Figure 215-22 *Molluscum contagiosum.*

ALLERGIC AND INFLAMMATORY PEDIATRIC CONJUNCTIVITIS

Seasonal Allergic Conjunctivitis

Seasonal allergic (hay fever) conjunctivitis is common and affects approximately 10% of the general population. The hallmark of this allergy is itching and tearing, with the eye being relatively quiet compared with the severity of the symptoms. Seasonal allergic rhinitis often accompanies seasonal allergic conjunctivitis, which is a type-1 hypersensitivity reaction; conjunctival scrapings or biopsy samples reveal mast cells and eosinophils. Serum quantitative immunoglobulin E levels are usually high, and skin tests may be positive for environmental allergens. Allergic conjunctivitis is most common in the spring, when pollen levels are high; however, many cases occur during the winter, when forced-air heating is turned on and filters have not been cleaned or replaced. Laboratory evaluation is not usually necessary because diagnosis can be made through clinical signs and symptoms. A family history of allergies, atopic disease, or asthma may be found.

Treatment of allergic conjunctivitis has greatly improved with the advent of combination mast cell stabilizer–antihistamine eyedrops such as olopatadine. Mast cell stabilizers prevent the release of histamine but require 2 to 3 days of continued use to reduce symptoms because they do not inhibit activity of already-circulating histamines. Combination mast cell stabilizer–antihistamine eyedrops have a double effect, providing immediate relief because they directly block histamine receptors and prevent the release of histamine by mast cells. Patients with chronic allergic conjunctivitis can use the eyedrops every day, year round,

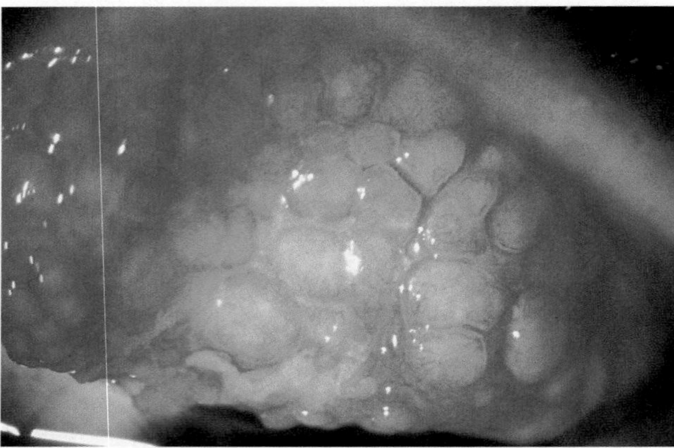

Figure 215-23 Vernal conjunctivitis; an everted upper eyelid discloses the classic giant papillary conjunctival reaction. Patients experience severe itching, burning, and mucous discharge.

because side effects are rare. In cases of severe allergic conjunctivitis, an oral antihistamine may be added to the eyedrops. Topical corticosteroids are reserved for severe allergic conjunctivitis not responsive to other treatment, and they are only used for a few days. If corticosteroids are used, then an ophthalmologist should monitor the patient for the potential side effects of glaucoma and cataracts. Fluorometholone, a mild topical corticosteroid, is a good choice because it does not penetrate the cornea, thus reducing the likelihood of glaucoma and cataracts.

Vernal Conjunctivitis

Vernal conjunctivitis is a severe allergic condition characterized by severe itching, tearing, mucus production, and giant papillae of the upper tarsal conjunctiva (Figure 215-23). It most commonly affects young boys from the Mediterranean Basin and from Central and South America. Patients often have reactive ptosis and squint in bright light, the result of secondary keratitis caused by the giant papillae scraping the cornea. Papillae may be found around the limbus (junction of the sclera and cornea) with characteristic white centers (Horner-Trantas dots) that represent an accumulation of inflammatory cells, predominantly eosinophils. Conjunctival scrapings of the papillae show many eosinophils. Full-blown vernal conjunctivitis is a vision-threatening disease. However, with the advent of topical mast cell stabilizers and antihistamines, this outcome is now rare.

Treatment is based on avoiding allergens and using combination mast cell stabilizer–antihistamine eyedrops such as olopatadine. Patients need to use the eyedrops daily during the allergy season. In temperate climates, patients with vernal conjunctivitis may need treatment year round. An oral antihistamine can be added to the use of the eye drops if necessary. In some instances, severe episodes of inflammation can be controlled only with intermittent short courses of topical corticosteroids, which should be administered and supervised by an ophthalmologist.

Giant Papillary Conjunctivitis

Giant papillary conjunctivitis is the result of wearing soft contact lenses. Similar to vernal conjunctivitis, large papillae develop underneath the superior tarsal conjunctiva. The reaction results from a sensitization of the conjunctiva to allergic materials present on the surface of the contact lens or in contact lens solutions. Treatment consists of using mast cell stabilizers, discontinuing contact lens wear, and changing to a regimen of frequent contact lens replacement. Prognosis is good.

Atopic Conjunctivitis

Atopic conjunctivitis is a form of allergic conjunctivitis associated with eczema. Serum immunoglobulin E concentrations are often high in these patients, resulting from what appears to be a deficiency in cellular immunity (deficiency of T suppressor cells). Patients with atopic dermatitis often have associated conjunctivitis, with itching, burning, and mucus discharge. Symptomatic treatment of eye complaints includes the use of cold compresses, topical vasoconstrictors, topical antihistamines, and topical mast cell stabilizers. Topical corticosteroids should be used only for short periods while being monitored by an ophthalmologist.

CONJUNCTIVITIS ASSOCIATED WITH SYSTEMIC DISEASE

Stevens-Johnson Syndrome (Erythema Multiforme Major)

Stevens-Johnson syndrome is most likely a type-III hypersensitivity reaction. It may be associated with mycoplasmal and HSV infections and with many drugs, especially antibiotics and anticonvulsants. Patients have fever, malaise, headache, loss of appetite, and nausea. A generalized erythematous papular rash can be found. The skin is friable, and traction on it can produce tears. Mucous membranes, including the nose, mouth, vagina, anus, and conjunctiva, are most severely affected. Eye involvement consists of conjunctival injection and the formation of bullae that can rupture and lead to scarring. Conjunctival scarring can distort the eyelids and turn the lashes toward the cornea, causing corneal damage.

Therapy remains controversial. Topical corticosteroids may be administered early, before advanced disease leads to conjunctival scarring; their use may prevent severe ocular sequelae. Once conjunctival scarring occurs, however, no effective treatment exists. Patients with Stevens-Johnson syndrome should be referred immediately to an ophthalmologist for consultation.

Kawasaki Disease

Kawasaki disease is a systemic vasculitis occurring in children usually younger than 8 years. It has an onset of fever, present for more than 5 days, along with 4 of the following 5 criteria: (1) nonpurulent conjunctivitis, (2) oral mucus membrane injection or swelling (or both), (3) erythema and edema of the hands and feet, (4) polymorphous rash, and (5) cervical lymphadenopathy. The vasculitis may involve the coronary arteries

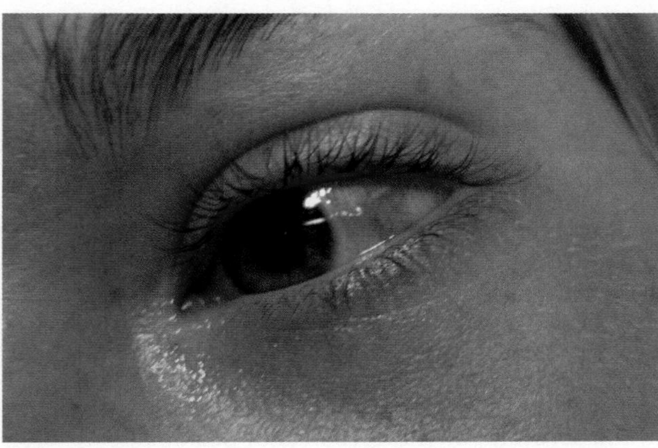

Figure 215-24 Lightly pigmented compound conjunctival nevi.

and cause a coronary aneurysm or a thrombosis that may lead to sudden death. The cause of Kawasaki disease is unknown.

Graft-Versus-Host Disease

Approximately 40% of patients who receive a bone marrow transplant will have graft-versus-host disease. Donor T lymphocytes attack the recipient cells, primarily affecting the skin, liver, intestine, oral mucosa, conjunctiva, lacrimal gland, vaginal mucosa, and esophageal mucosa. The ocular effects of graft-versus-host disease consist of conjunctivitis, dry eye, corneal epithelial erosions, and corneal ulcerations. Treatment with topical artificial tears, short courses of topical corticosteroids, and, in severe cases, cyclosporine may improve symptoms. These patients should be referred to an ophthalmologist for careful follow-up.

Conjunctival Nevi

Congenital or acquired lesions of the conjunctiva are usually located near the corneal limbus. They appear as pink or inflamed conjunctiva (Figure 215-24). Nevi come from melanocytes, but they have varying amounts of pigmentation, with 30% of patients having minimal pigmentation. The most common types include junctional, compound, and subepithelial nevi. All types have low malignant potential and usually become noticeable in the 1st decade of life through puberty. Treatment is controversial, but growth or change in pigmentation of the nevus may be an indication for surgical removal. Malignant melanoma is rare in children.

WHEN TO REFER

- Severe neonatal conjunctivitis
- Conjunctivitis with poor red reflex
- Conjunctivitis not improving after a week of treatment
- Recurrent conjunctivitis unilateral or bilateral
- Conjunctivitis with positive corneal fluorescein staining
- Conjunctivitis with decreased visual acuity (20/50 or worse)
- Unilateral conjunctivitis in a contact lens user
- Neonatal swollen nasolacrimal sac (amniotocele)
- Tearing with a poor red reflex
- Tearing with large eye (buphthalmos)

TOOLS FOR PRACTICE

Medical Decision Support

- *Pediatric Ophthalmology for Primary Care,* 3rd edition (book), Wright KW (www.aap.org/bookstore).
- *The Physician's Guide to Eye Care, 3rd edition* (book), Trobe JD (www.aap.org/bookstore).

SUGGESTED RESOURCE

Greenberg MF and Pollard ZF. The red eye in childhood. *Pediatr Clin North Am,* 2003;50(1):105-124.

REFERENCES

1. Isenberg SJ, Apt L, Wood M. A controlled trial of povidone-iodine as prophylaxis against ophthalmia neonatorum. *N Engl J Med.* 1995;332(9):562-566.
2. Paul TO, Shepherd R. Congenital nasolacrimal duct obstruction: natural history and the timing of optimal intervention. *J Pediatr Ophthalmol Strabismus.* 1994;31(6): 362-367.
3. Sarfarazi M, Akarsu AN, Hossain A, et al. Assignment of a locus (GLC3A) for primary congenital glaucoma (buphthalmos) to 2p21 and evidence for genetic heterogeneity. *Genomics.* 1995;30(2):171-177.
4. Akarsu AN, Turacli ME, Aktan SG, et al. A second locus (GLC3B) for primary congenital glaucoma (buphthalmos) maps to the 1p36 region. *Hum Mol Genet.* 1996;5(8): 1199-1203.
5. Morissette J, Côté G, Anctil JL, et al. A common gene for juvenile and adult-onset primary open-angle glaucomas confined on chromosome 1q. *Am J Hum Genet.* 1995;56(6): 1431-1432.
6. deLuise VP, Anderson DR. Primary infantile glaucoma (congenital glaucoma). *Surv Ophthalmol.* 1983;28(1):1-19.
7. Dargougar S, Grey RH, Thaker U, et al. Clinical and epidemiological features of adenovirus keratoconjunctivitis in London. *Br J Ophthalmol.* 1983;67(1):1-7.
8. Liesegang TJ, Melto LJ 3rd, Daly PJ, et al. Epidemiology of ocular herpes simplex. Incidence in Rochester, Minn, 1950 through 1982. *Arch Ophthalmol.* 1989;107(8):1155-1159.
9. Darougher S, Wishart MS, Viswalingam ND. Epidemiological and clinical features of primary herpes simplex virus ocular infection. *Br J Ophthalmol.* 1985;69(1):2-6.

Chapter 216

SCROTAL SWELLING AND PAIN

Lane S. Palmer, MD

Scrotal swelling can be particularly frightening for boys and their families, and because the differential diagnosis includes conditions that demand emergent treatment, it poses a challenge to primary care pediatricians. A helpful organizing strategy as evaluation proceeds is to classify the scrotal swelling as

BOX 216-1 Causes of Scrotal Swelling

ACUTE, PAINFUL SCROTAL SWELLING
Torsion of spermatic cord
Torsion of appendix, testis, epididymis
Acute epididymitis, orchitis
Mumps orchitis
Henoch-Schönlein purpura
Trauma
Insect bite
Thrombosis of spermatic vein
Fat necrosis
Hernia
Folliculitis
Dermatitis, acute

PAINLESS SCROTAL SWELLING
Tumor
Idiopathic scrotal edema
Hydrocele
Henoch-Schönlein purpura
Hernia

CHRONIC SCROTAL SWELLING
Hydrocele
Hernia
Varicocele
Spermatocele
Sebaceous cyst
Tumor

either painful or painless and as acute or chronic (Box 216-1). Rapid and accurate evaluation of a boy with scrotal swelling depends on a thorough history and a physical examination of the genital area and abdomen that includes both inspection and palpation. Laboratory tests may be helpful but are not usually decisive, whereas imaging studies can be helpful in confirming a diagnosis and guiding management.

EVALUATION OF THE CHILD WITH SCROTAL SWELLING

The history should be taken from both the child (when possible) and from the parent. The physician must determine if the swelling or pain is recurrent and acute or chronic. The exact timing of the onset of symptoms is vital, particularly in the presence of acute pain and swelling. The nature of the pain must be determined: sharp, dull, constant, intermittent, constant with intermittent increases in intensity, or associated with nausea or vomiting. The location of the pain needs to be ascertained (ie, in the scrotum, specifically the testis; radiation into the abdomen or from the abdomen into the scrotum; laterality of the swelling and pain). Associated factors such as activity or positions that alleviate or aggravate the pain and swelling should be elicited. The nature of the swelling is important, specifically, whether the swelling changes in size during the course of a single day or whether it is constant or, in general, increasing or decreasing with time. Other important considerations include recent trauma, sexual activity, use of medications, the presence of rashes, and weight loss.

The physical examination should include the abdomen, groin, and the scrotum. Abdominal and groin palpation is important in determining if an intraabdominal process is extending into the scrotum. Inspection of the scrotum should look for laterality of the process and scrotal erythema, and palpation will determine the presence of cremasteric reflexes, testicular position, tenderness, localization of the swelling to the scrotum, or the presence of proximal extension into the cord.

In general, laboratory tests are of limited value. The white blood cell count may be elevated in the setting of infection. Urinalysis may be helpful in distinguishing orchitis from torsion of the spermatic cord or testicular appendage when white blood cells or nitrites are present.

Imaging studies can be useful in differentiating among possible diagnoses. Ultrasound of the scrotum can be used to determine whether the scrotal swelling is fluid filled or solid, arising from the abdomen extending into the groin, limited to the scrotum, or arising from the testis or spermatic cord structures. Ultrasound with Doppler can assess the flow of blood into the testis, helping to differentiate torsion of the testis from an inflammatory process. Nuclear scintigraphy using ^{99m}Tc-pertechnetate is another way to evaluate blood flow to the testis; absence of flow results in a cold spot and suggests torsion, whereas inflammation results in increased flow to the same area. Nuclear scanning is less limited by the user variability associated with ultrasound and does not require placing a probe over a tender area. However, the study uses ionizing radiation and takes longer to perform than ultrasound, thus limiting its utility when time is of the essence. The sensitivity and specificity of the 2 modalities are similar.

ACUTE SCROTAL SWELLING WITH PAIN

The sudden onset of scrotal swelling and pain can be a surgical emergency and therefore warrants urgent evaluation and management. The primary clinical entities that constitute this constellation of signs and symptoms include torsion of the testicle, torsion of the testicular appendages, and epididymitis-orchitis (Figure 216-1).

Torsion of the Testicle

Testicular torsion is the twisting of the spermatic cord, with resulting compromise of the blood supply to the testis. This compromise and the risk it poses of testicular loss makes torsion a surgical emergency. In the neonate, the torsion occurs on the cord above the insertion of the tunica vaginalis (ie, extravaginal torsion). In the adolescent, the *bell clapper deformity* leads to torsion on the cord within the confines of the tunica vaginalis (ie, intravaginal torsion). Torsion of

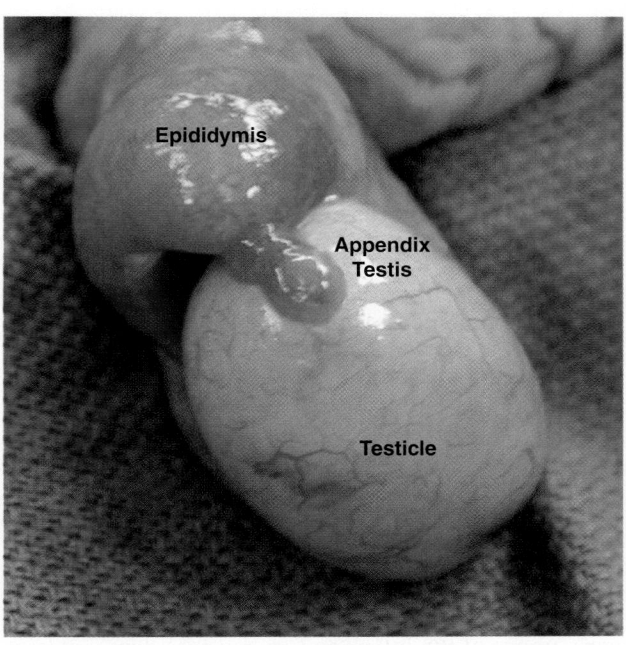

Figure 216-1 Structures of the scrotum.

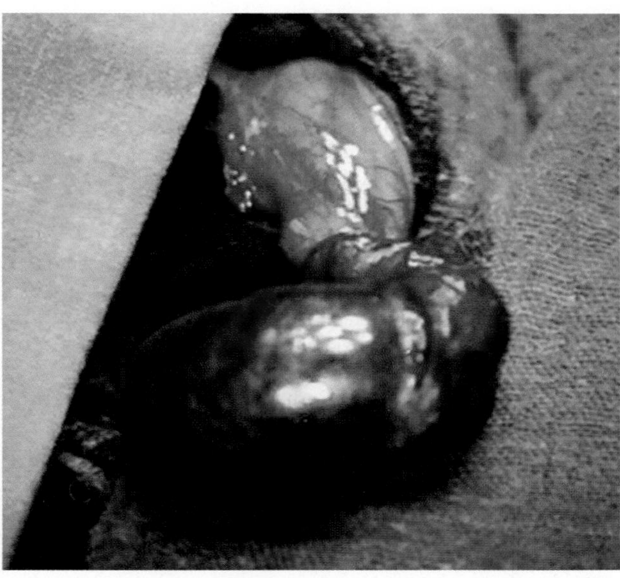

Figure 216-2 Intraoperative photograph of nonsalvageable testis after prolonged period of pain.

the spermatic cord first causes venous congestion, which is followed by compromise of arterial blood flow. Spermatogenesis may be compromised after 4 to 6 hours of ischemia.[1] Similarly, testicular salvage is time dependent, with universal loss of the testis after 24 hours of torsion.

Incidence

Testicular torsion occurs in 1:4000 boys. Although a peak in incidence occurs in the neonatal period, testicular torsion more commonly occurs between the ages of 12 to 18 years. Nevertheless, testicular torsion should not be excluded from the differential diagnosis of acute scrotal swelling and pain based on age.

Evaluation

The history typically describes acute onset of constant, severe scrotal pain aggravated by physical activity. If periods of respite from the pain occur, then intermittent torsion and detorsion should be considered. Nausea and vomiting may occur. The patient may have a history of incidental antecedent scrotal trauma, but the onset of pain usually occurs during periods of rest or sleep. Characteristic findings on physical examination include scrotal erythema and swelling of the involved hemiscrotum. Further inspection may reveal a higher-than-normal position of the testis within the scrotum, and palpation may also demonstrate a horizontal rather than the normal vertical orientation of the testicle. Evaluation of the cremasteric reflex should begin on the contralateral side, along with palpation of the apparently unaffected testis to confirm normal size and position. Unilateral loss of the cremasteric reflex on the side of the swelling and pain highly correlates with the presence of torsion.[2] The testis should then be palpated despite the pain the maneuver may cause to help differentiate torsion from epididymitis. With torsion, exquisite pain is elicited on palpation from the testis, as well as from the epididymis and distal spermatic cord. In some instances, the actual point of torsion of the spermatic cord can be palpated. An associated hydrocele may be palpated and confirmed by transillumination. A tense or large hydrocele often makes the examination difficult. Urinalysis is unremarkable, and although the white blood cell count may be mildly elevated, it is not discriminating. Imaging by nuclear scintigraphy[3,4] or Doppler ultrasound[5,6] should be performed if the diagnosis of testicular torsion is in question, but only when it will not delay surgical exploration if a torsion exists, adding to the risk of testicular loss.

Treatment

Surgical intervention is indicated not only when testicular torsion is strongly suspected, but also in equivocal cases when torsion cannot be convincingly excluded. The likelihood of salvaging the testis, the goal of surgical exploration, is highest when surgery occurs shortly after the onset of pain; the chance for a successful outcome dissipates rapidly with time (Figure 216-2). With surgery, the affected testis is explored first, and when torsion is present, the cord is detorsed. The contralateral testis, which will have the same defect in anatomy, should then be explored and fixed in place to avert a future torsion. The affected gonad is then reinspected and the possibility of salvage determined. If the testis can be saved, then it is fixed in the scrotum. Subsequent atrophy may still result because of the vascular insult,[7] and fertility may be compromised as well.[8]

When testicular torsion is diagnosed, manual detorsion can be attempted while surgery is being arranged. The testis is twisted either clockwise or counterclockwise. When twisting in 1 direction has not succeeded, an attempt in the opposite direction can be made. When the procedure is successful, the return of blood flow to the testis provides rapid relief from pain. If manual detorsion can be accomplished preoperatively, then the surgical intervention to tack down the testes can be performed electively.[9]

Neonatal Testicular Torsion

Neonatal testicular torsion can exhibit at delivery as a nontender hard scrotal mass. Salvage in these cases is rare. At exploration, the contralateral testis should be anchored and the nonviable testis removed. Torsion may also occur after delivery and then is more typical of torsion in the older patient, with a greater potential for salvage if intervention is rapid.

Torsion of the Appendix Testis

Evaluation

Torsion of the appendix testis or appendix epididymis may lead to a clinical picture similar to that of the more consequential and urgent torsion of the spermatic cord. The appendix testis is a vestige of the müllerian duct system and hangs from the upper pole of the testis. When it torses, inflammation and swelling of the testis and epididymis ensues, causing testicular pain and scrotal erythema. The onset of pain and swelling is commonly acute but can be progressive, usually occurring during periods of rest. The pain can be severe, but nausea and vomiting are less common than with testicular torsion. The physical examination may demonstrate hemiscrotal erythema and swelling. A *blue-dot* sign, the necrotic appendage visible through the scrotal skin, can help make the diagnosis.[10] A normal cremasteric reflex is present bilaterally, and the testis is normally positioned within the scrotum. Testicular discomfort, if present, is typically mild, but point tenderness may be elicited from the uppermost pole of the testis near the head of the epididymis—the location of the appendages. On palpation, the examiner may feel a 3- to 5-mm tender indurated mass on the upper pole. In some cases, the inflammatory process resulting from torsion of the appendage can lead to physical findings that make differentiating from true spermatic cord torsion impossible. In these cases, imaging may be helpful because either scrotal Doppler ultrasound or nuclear scintigraphy will demonstrate normal or increased flow to the ipsilateral testis.

Treatment

The management of the torsed appendage is nonsurgical. The patient should rest and use nonsteroidal pain relievers and cold compresses for several days to reduce the inflammation, swelling, and pain. Surgical intervention is indicated only when the diagnosis of acute testicular torsion cannot be excluded. In these cases, the infarcted appendage is removed at surgical exploration.

Acute Epididymitis-Orchitis

Evaluation

Acute inflammation of the epididymis or testis occurs in both young and older boys. Uncommon in the younger child, it usually results from an anomaly of the urinary tract, either congenital or acquired, which can often be identified by renal and bladder sonography.[11] Renal duplications and posterior urethral valves are among the more common anomalies. Traditionally, a voiding cystourethrogram has been a routine part of the evaluation, but its yield is low with a normal ultrasound and a sterile urine. In children who perform intermittent catheterization, epididymo-orchitis can occur from the retrograde passage of bacteria back from the ejaculatory ducts at the level of the prostate to the testis and epididymis.[12]

In the older child and adolescent, the history and physical examination may help distinguish epididymitis or orchitis from testicular torsion or appendix torsion, but this is not always the case. The history can reveal an acute or more protracted onset of pain. The patient may have fever or dysuria. Epididymal inflammation may arise after scrotal trauma. In the adolescent patient, a history of sexual activity or a urethral discharge helps guide antibiotic treatment. The physical examination reveals scrotal erythema and swelling and an intact cremasteric reflex. Palpation during the early phase of the inflammatory process demonstrates tenderness limited to the epididymis, whereas in the later phase, the tenderness and inflammation include both the epididymis and testis, and the distinction between the 2 structures may be difficult to appreciate. The Prehn sign (relief of pain with testicular elevation) may be positive.

Laboratory and radiologic imaging are useful in these cases. Urinalysis may prove positive for white blood cells and nitrite but is often unremarkable among adolescents. The white blood cell count is usually elevated. Ultrasound and nuclear scintigraphy studies demonstrate either normal symmetric blood flow or increased blood flow to an enlarged epididymis or testis.

Treatment

Management of epididymo-orchitis requires antibiotic therapy that is based on the results of the urine culture and sensitivities. In the sexually active adolescent, the choice of antibiotic coverage must also include coverage of gonococcal and nongonococcal sexually transmitted diseases. Additionally, antiinflammatory agents, scrotal elevation, and rest should be prescribed.

Other Causes of Acute Swelling and Pain of the Scrotum

Henoch-Schönlein Purpura

Henoch-Schönlein purpura is a systemic vasculitis that can cause abdominal pain, joint pain, renal disease, and bleeding from the gastrointestinal tract and may involve the scrotal wall in the minority of cases. (See Chapter 272, Henoch-Schönlein Purpura.) The onset may be insidious or acute, producing a variable degree of erythema and edema. In more severe cases, the process may involve the testis and epididymis mimicking testicular torsion.[13] Concurrent Henoch-Schönlein purpura and testicular torsion has been reported; therefore, if torsion is a consideration, then imaging with either Doppler ultrasound or nuclear scintigraphy is indicated to evaluate testicular blood flow. Surgical exploration may be needed in equivocal cases.

Focal Fat Necrosis

Focal fat necrosis can exhibit with scrotal pain and swelling,[14] usually after trauma in an obese boy. The examination demonstrates pain and swelling limited to the scrotum and not the testis; however, the examination can be limited by the discomfort and the degree of obesity. If properly diagnosed, then the management consists of rest and antiinflammatory agents. When spermatic cord torsion cannot be excluded clinically, either an imaging study or immediate surgical exploration is indicated.

Trauma

Injuries can vary from zipper entrapment of scrotal skin to more severe blunt or straddle trauma affecting the scrotal contents. The history can be definitive. The physical examination must include both hemiscrotums and the surrounding structures (penis, perineum), assessing for swelling, ecchymosis, and bleeding. Palpation may be limited by the degree of swelling or blood within the scrotum. The tenderness may be limited to the testis or the epididymis, depending on the extent of the trauma. Scrotal ultrasound can document the integrity of the testis and of the tunica albuginea and the adequacy of blood flow.[15] Testicular or spermatic cord contusions are managed symptomatically, whereas testicular rupture requires surgical exploration, evacuation of the hematoma, debridement, and repair (when possible).

Mumps Orchitis

Mumps orchitis can occur at any age but is more common among adolescents. Rarely occurring in isolation, the pain and swelling usually occur within a week after parotitis. The physical examination demonstrates a tender testis. Treatment is symptomatic. Infertility may occur when mumps orchitis results in atrophy of both testicles.[16]

Scrotal Skin Disease

Insect bites, folliculitis, and allergic dermatitis may cause erythema and edema of the scrotal wall. The history may be of limited utility. The examination reveals redness and edema limited to the scrotum, with a normal testicle and spermatic cord.

SCROTAL SWELLING WITHOUT PAIN

Inguinal Hernias and Hydroceles

Hernias and hydroceles, the most common causes of scrotal swelling, fall along a continuum (Figure 216-3). They are more common in premature infants and are predominately right sided. Most inguinal hernias and hydroceles are caused by persistent patency of the processus vaginalis (PPV), a peritoneal out-pouching that accompanies the testis during its abdominal-scrotal descent. The layers of the processus vaginalis condense late in gestation or early postnatally. Obliteration of the processus vaginalis only around the testis leads to an indirect inguinal hernia with the protrusion of fluid (or other contents) through the internal ring to the end of the pouch and potentially to the scrotum. A communicating hydrocele occurs when fluid travels through a PPV into the tunica vaginalis around the testis. A scrotal hydrocele occurs after complete obliteration proximally with patency distally. Hydroceles of the cord occur when the processus vaginalis obliterates proximally and distally, leaving a patent area in the midportion with retained fluid.

Idiopathic scrotal edema affects children younger than 14 years, with acute erythema, edema, and mild scrotal wall tenderness, sparing the testis and cord.[17] The process resolves spontaneously. The management includes rest and scrotal elevation.

Inguinal hernias and hydroceles may be asymptomatic or may have a spectrum of symptoms. A hernia can occur at any age as an inguinal swelling extending toward and potentially reaching the scrotum. The swelling expands with increases in intraabdominal pressure (eg, crying, bowel movements, coughing,

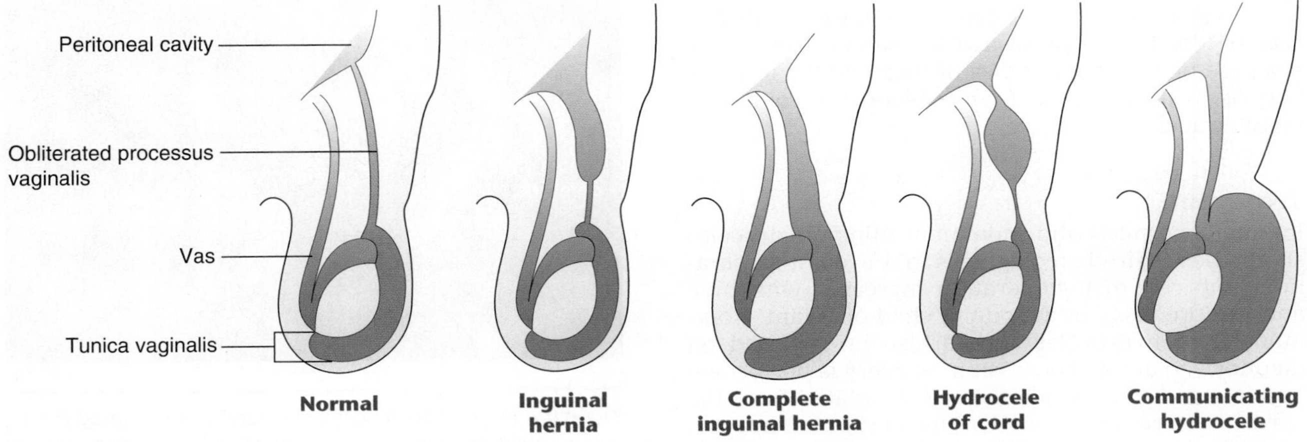

Figure 216-3 Diagram of the continuum of hernia and hydrocele.

exercise). The parent or child will often report the swelling to be smallest in the morning and largest late in the day. When omentum is in the hernia sac, the likelihood of spontaneous reduction is low, and periods of discomfort can occur. An incarcerated hernia can produce pain, fever, nausea, vomiting, and irritability. A hydrocele is usually an asymptomatic bulge in the scrotum. In many instances, whether the hydrocele is acute or whether the scrotum has been chronically enlarged is unclear. The patient may have a history of trauma to the scrotum that stimulates the production of serous fluid. When the scrotum changes sizes during the day, the physician should suspect a communicating hydrocele.

Evaluation

The physical examination is often sufficient to distinguish among these entities. The examiner should feel for the testis first and keep it in mind during the rest of the examination so as to avoid confusing it with the contents of an incarcerated hernia. A bulge in the inguinal region with fluid that can be gently reduced back into the abdomen is diagnostic of an inguinal hernia. In the cooperative child who can increase his intra-abdominal pressure, this procedure may be repeatedly demonstrated particularly with the child standing. When the fluid is limited to the testis and the spermatic cord can be palpated above the fluid, a hydrocele is present. The presence of a thickened spermatic cord or a *silk-stocking* sign (the feel of the layers of the processus vaginalis being rubbed against each other) is suggestive of a PPV or a hernia, which is helpful in distinguishing a scrotal hydrocele from a communicating hydrocele. Hydroceles transilluminate, but so can the incarcerated bowel of an infant. A hydrocele of the spermatic cord feels distinct from the testis and is round or ovoid, possibly mimicking the presence of an additional testis. Hydroceles, whether communicating, scrotal, or of the cord, are rarely associated with tenderness on palpation.

Ultrasound can be useful to delineate the scrotal contents, especially when a large or tense hydrocele limits the physical examination, and to determine the cystic or solid nature of a tense scrotal mass (eg, hydrocele, tumor) or spermatic cord mass (eg, hydrocele of the cord, paratesticular tumor). Laboratory tests are only useful in cases of incarcerated inguinal hernias, with an elevated white blood cell count and possible acidosis.

Treatment

Inguinal hernias and communicating hydroceles should be repaired on diagnosis to prevent incarceration. The risk of incarceration increases with time and is more likely in the young child or infant. Communicating hydroceles should also be repaired on diagnosis to avert progression. Surgery is performed inguinally, during which the sac is isolated from the cord structures and ligated at the level of the internal ring. The likelihood of a PPV on the contralateral side is highest in younger children, and the need for contralateral exploration remains controversial. However, diagnostic laparoscopy through the isolated ipsilateral sac allows visualization of the contralateral ring[23] (Figure 216-4). If the internal ring is open, then contralateral surgical correction proceeds. Most hydroceles resolve spontaneously by 1 year and should be repaired if they persist beyond this age. However, if the hydrocele is painful, tense, and large, then surgery should proceed sooner. In younger children, the surgical approach is inguinal; in older boys and adolescents, a scrotal approach is appropriate.

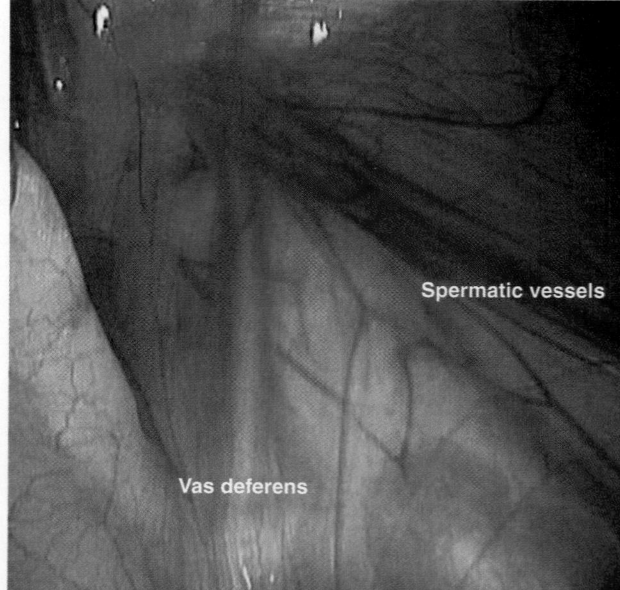

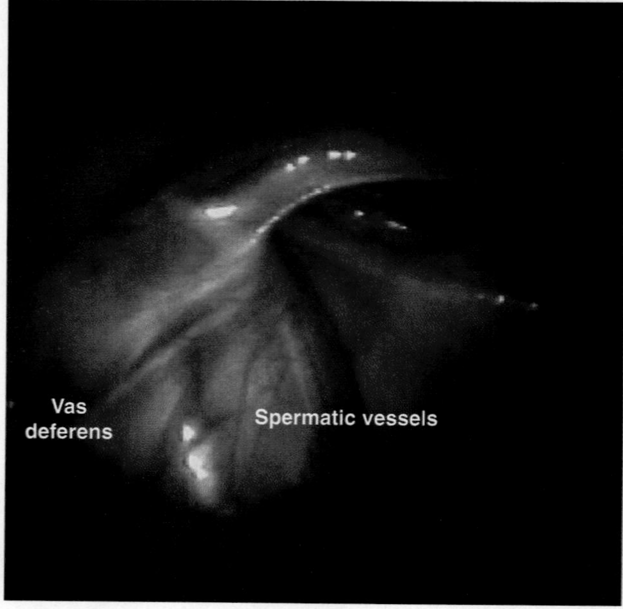

Figure 216-4 Laparoscopic appearance of a closed *(top)* and an open *(bottom)* internal inguinal ring. The ring appears at junction of the vas deferens *(V)* and the internal spermatic vessels *(SV)*.

Tumors

Testicular tumors are uncommon in children but occur in all age groups. Tumors are usually displayed as a hard, painless (or vague, heavy-feeling) mass in the testicle detected by the child, parent, or examining physician. On palpation, the mass is harder than the substance of the testis, but this distinction may be difficult to discern. The mass may bulge from the surface of the testis. Tumors do not transilluminate. Scrotal ultrasound is used to delineate the mass. Preoperative tumor markers (α-fetoprotein, β-human chorionic gonadotropin) should be drawn and used for postoperative monitoring. Radical orchiectomy is performed through an inguinal approach. If the mass is not suspicious for malignancy, then several authors have reported enucleating the mass[18,19] and proceeding with orchiectomy only if the frozen section is positive.

Varicoceles

Varicoceles, which are dilatations of the spermatic veins or pampiniform plexus, are present in 15% of male adolescents and adults and may have a negative impact on fertility. The dilated veins are usually asymptomatic and are detected either by the patient or by the physician during routine physical examination, usually between 10 to 15 years of age. On occasion, the patient may report some heaviness or a *dragging* feeling. A predilection for the left side exists, reflecting the anatomy of the left gonadal vein entering the left renal vein at a right angle. The right gonadal vein enters the vena cava directly at an angle, precluding reflux of venous blood. The presence of bilateral or right-sided varicoceles warrants an abdominal ultrasound or computed tomographic scan to evaluate for a possible mass occluding venous return. Physical examination should be performed with the patient in the supine and standing positions; the varicocele is usually decompressed in the supine position and present in the standing position. Inspection may reveal the classic *bag of worms* of dilated veins (grade 3 of 3). In other cases, increased blood pooling in the veins can be prompted by a Valsalva maneuver (grade 2 of 3). Testicular size, most accurately assesses by ultrasound, should be measured[20]; a significant loss of testicular volume is one indication for surgery. Other indications for repair include abnormal semen analysis (older adolescent patients) and pain. Corrective measures include open surgery, laparoscopic surgery, or radiologic ablative techniques—all aimed at occluding direct venous return through the internal spermatic vein to improve the likelihood of normal fertility. The majority of testes will subsequently increase in size to equal that of the contralateral testis.[21]

Spermatoceles and Epididymal Cysts

Spermatoceles and epididymal cysts represent sperm-filled cystic lesions attached to the upper pole of the testis. They are separate from the testis and can be transilluminated. Painless and round, they usually remain stable in size but can sometimes enlarge. Management consists typically of observation, but surgery may be indicated when pain or significant enlargement is present. Postoperative scarring can obstruct the epididymal ductal system and lead to infertility.[22]

WHEN TO REFER

- Acute painful scrotal swelling
- Acute hydrocele
- Hernia
- Scrotal trauma
- Cellulitis of scrotum
- Varicocele
- Testicular mass
- Paratesticular mass

TOOLS FOR PRACTICE

Engaging Patient and Family

- *Hydroceles and Inguinal Hernias* (fact sheet), American Urological Association (www.urologyhealth.org/pediatric/).
- *Neonatal Testicular Torsion* (fact sheet), American Urological Association (www.urologyhealth.org/pediatric/).
- *Testicular Trauma* (fact sheet), American Urological Association (www.urologyhealth.org/pediatric/).

REFERENCES

1. Bartsch G, Frank S, Marberger H, et al. Testicular torsion: late results with special regard to fertility and endocrine function. *J Urol.* 1980;124:375-378.
2. Rabinowitz R. The importance of the cremasteric reflex in acute scrotal swelling in children. *J Urol.* 1984;132:89-90.
3. Falkowski WS, Firlit CF. Testicular torsion: the role of radioisotopic scanning. *J Urol.* 1980;124:886-888.
4. Mendel JB, Taylor GA, Treves S, et al. Testicular torsion in children: scintigraphic assessment. *Pediatr Radiol.* 1985;15:110-115.
5. Baker LA, Sigman D, Mathews RI, et al. An analysis of clinical outcomes using color Doppler testicular ultrasound for testicular torsion. *Pediatrics.* 2000;105:604-607.
6. Nussbaum Blask AR, Bulas D, Shalaby-Rana E, et al. Color Doppler sonography and scintigraphy of the testis: a prospective, comparative analysis in children with acute scrotal pain. *Pediatr Emerg Care.* 2002;18:67-71.
7. Sessions AE, Rabinowitz R, Hulbert WC, et al. Testicular torsion: direction, degree, duration and disinformation. *J Urol.* 2003;169:663-665.
8. Nagler HM, White RD. The effect of testicular torsion on the contralateral testis. *J Urol.* 1982;128:1343-1348.
9. Cornel EB, Karthaus HF. Manual derotation of the twisted spermatic cord. *BJU Int.* 1999;83(6):672-674
10. Dresner ML. Torsed appendage: diagnosis and management blue dot sign. *Urology.* 1973;1:63-66.
11. Siegel A, Snyder H, Duckett JW. Epididymitis in infants and boys: underlying urogenital anomalies and efficacy of imaging modalities. *J Urol.* 1987;138:1100-1103.
12. Lindehall B, Abrahamsson K, Hjalmas K, et al. Complications of clean intermittent catheterization in boys and young males with neurogenic bladder dysfunction. *J Urol.* 2004;172:1686-1688.
13. Khan AU, Williams TH, Malek RS. Acute scrotal swelling in Henoch-Schönlein syndrome. *Urology.* 1977;10:139-141.
14. Hollander JB, Begun FP, Lee RD. Scrotal fat necrosis. *J Urol.* 1985;134:150-151.
15. Buckley JC, McAninch JW. Use of ultrasonography for diagnosis of testicular injuries in blunt scrotal trauma. *J Urol.* 2006;175(1):175-178.

16. Philip J, Selvan D, Desmond AD. Mumps orchitis in the non-immune postpubertal male: a resurgent threat to male fertility? *BJU Int.* 2006;97:138-141.
17. Kaplan GW. Acute idiopathic scrotal edema. *J Pediatr Surg.* 1977;12:647-649.
18. Pohl HG, Shukla AR, Metcalf PD, et al. Prepubertal testis tumors: actual prevalence rate of histological types. *J Urol.* 2004;172:2370-2372.
19. Shukla AR, Woodard C, Carr MC, et al. Experience with testis sparing surgery for testicular teratoma. *J Urol.* 2004;171:161-163.
20. Diamond DA, Paltiel HJ, DiCanzio J, et al. Comparative assessment of pediatric testicular volume: orchidometer versus ultrasound. *J Urol.* 2000;164:1111-1114.
21. Atassi O, Kass EJ, Steinert BW. Testicular growth after successful varicocele correction in adolescents: comparison of artery sparing techniques with the Palomo procedure. *J Urol.* 1995;153(2):482-483.
22. Zahalsky MP, Berman AJ, Nagler HM. Evaluating the risk of epididymal injury during hydrocelectomy and spermatocelectomy. *J Urol.* 2004;171:2291-2292.
23. Miltenburg DM, Nuchtern JG, Jaksic T, et al. Laparoscopic evaluation of the pediatric inguinal hernia—a meta-analysis. *J Pediatr Surg.* 1998;33:874-879.

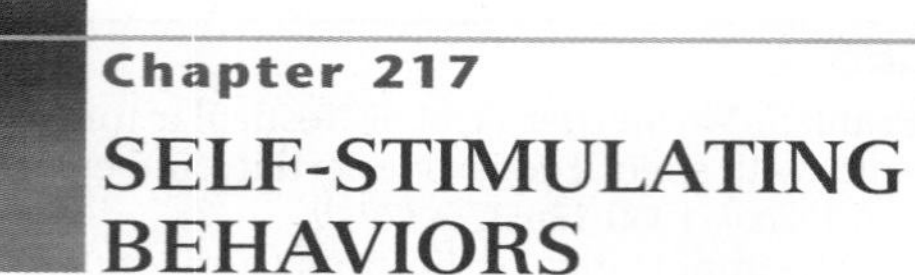

Chapter 217

SELF-STIMULATING BEHAVIORS

Richard M. Sarles, MD; Denise M. Richardson, MD

Self-stimulating behaviors, such as head banging, head rolling, rocking, thumb sucking, and masturbation, as well as habits such as hair pulling and nail biting, are of concern to both parents and pediatricians. Research has suggested that commonalties exist among such behaviors, sometimes classified as *stereotypies,* and that they represent an interaction of the stage of neuromotor development with environmental influences (eg, restrictive car seats and cribs) and are a homeostatic mechanism that serves to regulate stimulation from the environment. Many of these behaviors, such as head banging, head rolling, and rocking, typically appear before 12 months of age, peak soon thereafter, and subsequently decline rapidly.[1] Thumb sucking (25%) and nail biting (23%) are the most common behaviors described in preschool children, with only 4% developing motor stereotypies. Young children practice self-stimulation through thumb sucking and genital play, with a peak at age 2½ years.[2] In general, most of these behaviors are self-limited to the preschool period and are usually viewed as normal, common, and expected behaviors. These habits generally do not signify psychological maladjustment. They often require little intervention other than reassuring the parents and suggesting adequate interaction with their child.[3]

HEAD BANGING AND ROCKING

Head banging consists of rhythmic movements of the head against a solid object, such as the crib mattress or headboard, and is often associated with rocking the head and the entire body.[4] It is observed most commonly at bedtime or at times of fatigue or stress and may vary in duration from several minutes to hours. Head banging often continues even when the child is asleep. The age of onset shows wide variability, but the behavior is witnessed most commonly during the preschool years. The reported incidence of head-banging or rocking behavior varies between 3% and 20%, with a male-to-female ratio of approximately 3:1. Occasionally a family history of such behavior can be found, but only 20% of siblings of children who rock exhibit similar or other rhythmic pattern disturbances.[5]

Various theories have been developed to understand these self-limited but often-disturbing behaviors.[3] Rocking is thought to be a soothing, pleasurable experience that every infant encounters in utero and that most infants encounter from the neonatal period onward. The pleasure from movement is repeated throughout life, from being rocked in the mother's arms during early childhood, for example, to jumping rope and playing on swings in childhood, to dancing in adulthood. Individual constitutional patterns in childhood account for a wide variability in the amount of stimulation any particular child may require. However, in certain children, such as those who are hearing or sight impaired, emotionally disturbed, or severely mentally retarded, marked rhythmic movements are commonly found. In these cases the movements may represent a compensatory reaction for a lack of stimuli or the inability to integrate stimuli. In addition, the child who has no disability but who is inactive because of physical illness generally shows a need for motor release that is often characterized by bed rocking or other rhythmic body movements, which generally disappear once normal mobility is restored.

Physical and neurologic examinations show these children to be predominantly within normal limits, and electroencephalogram studies are not indicated because the findings are generally not helpful. These behaviors appear to be linked to maturational patterns and correlate closely with teething and other transitions of growth and development, perhaps as a mechanism for increasing or reducing arousal and maintaining homeostasis. Even though psychosocial growth and development are apparently not disturbed in these children and studies indicate no connection between rocking behavior and parental divorce or separation, the question of inadequate stimulation for the child should be raised, and the presence of family turmoil and stress should be investigated.

Treatment is generally directed toward assuring the parents that head banging cannot cause brain injury and that the child will show no adverse neurologic effects in later life; children who engage in head-banging behavior usually grow up as completely normal, coordinated children. Padding the crib and securing the bed to prevent rolling may help during the limited rocking behavior. Sedation in the form of diphenhydramine may prove effective, but psychotropic medication is generally unnecessary and is thus discouraged. Rarely, if ever, do fractures of the skull or cerebral hemorrhages result from head banging, but soft-tissue swelling and scalp contusions have been reported. A protective helmet may be advised in severe cases. Consultation with a child psychiatrist or psychologist is indicated if the head-banging or rocking behavior persists beyond 3 years of age. For children who show a lack of social interaction or a preoccupation with themselves or with self-stimulatory behavior, such as overt, compulsive masturbation, consultation is indicated.

THUMB SUCKING AND NAIL BITING

Thumb sucking occurs almost universally in infancy but varies among cultures. Infants may place virtually every object they encounter in their mouth unless parents, for safety reasons, restrict the object choice.

The pleasurable sensations associated with the double tactile experience of sucking and being sucked and the feelings of security and comfort that these experiences evoke tend to reinforce this type of behavior. Many families substitute artificial pacifiers as a more socially acceptable means of oral pleasure, and children themselves often spontaneously suck a security blanket, a doll, or a stuffed animal. Thumb sucking usually occurs during times of stress or boredom and at bedtime. Thumb sucking can also be used in young children to help them fall asleep. Social and family pressures generally limit thumb sucking to the preschool years. However, the habit may persist into adolescence. Approximately 25% to 40% of American children engage in finger sucking during the preschool years, and 10% to 20% continue beyond 6 years of age.

Nail biting is an extension or permutation of the habit of thumb sucking. Some experts consider this behavior a form of more overt self-aggression; others would define nail biting simply as a variation of thumb sucking because this behavior is also seen typically during times of stress. Approximately 25% of preschoolers and as many as 40% of all children older than 6 years bite their nails at some time or other, and 20% of college students continue to bite their nails. Thus nail biting, in contrast to thumb sucking, often continues throughout childhood and into adulthood. A family history appears to exist in most cases, but this habit is so common that such an apparent association may be of no significance. No apparent correlation has been found with the number of children in the family, the birth order, the type of feeding or feeding schedule, or the age or race of the parents. However, a significant association exists with the time of weaning, in that the later the weaning takes place, the less likely the chance is of thumb sucking.[6]

Thumb sucking, nail biting, and cuticle biting or picking increase the probability of dental malocclusion and the incidence of digital cutaneous infections. The probability of malocclusion in children who suck their thumbs appears to be directly related to the age at which the habit is discontinued. Thus children who cease the habit when they are older than 6 years generally exhibit some degree of malocclusion when examined at 12 years of age. In addition, thumb sucking that persists into school age can bring on teasing from peers and criticism from teachers and family, leaving the child with decreased self-esteem and increased psychological distress. Excessive thumb sucking, nail biting, and cuticle picking or biting should alert the clinician to investigate other possible obsessive-compulsive behaviors.[7,8]

Clarifying with parents the nature of these habits is important, as is encouraging them to avoid punishing or shaming the child for them. An underlying cause of tension should always be investigated, but simple behavioral therapy (based on positive reinforcement) is often sufficient to alleviate the habit. The parents should be advised to avoid punishment, threats, or anger. Encouragement in the place of restrictions is helpful in engaging children in their own program to decrease or eliminate the behavior.

Bitter-tasting commercial preparations applied to the fingers may be used as a reminder for the child, but these preparations are generally inadequate unless supplemented by consistent positive reinforcement. The choice of reinforcement reward should be the child's and might take the form of extra television privileges, dessert, or other special treats. A combination of aversive taste treatment and a reward system appears to be effective in treating chronic thumb sucking.[9] Weekly visits to the physician for the first month of treatment are important to reinforce the change in behavior. Hypnosis is another treatment that is often successful and poses no danger; psychotropic medications, on the other hand, are of little value. If these habits are linked to other signs of emotional distress, then referral to a specialist in behavioral disorders is warranted.

MASTURBATION

Masturbatory activity in children is almost universal and often leads to great parental concern. Masturbation typically begins at around 2 months of age and peaks at 4 years of age and again in adolescence.[2,10] Such activity may vary from direct manual genital stimulation to movements of the thighs against each other. Rhythmic swaying or thrusting motions of the child while straddling a hobby horse, pillow, stuffed animal, or other objects also are common methods of masturbation. Infants and children are capable of a physiological orgasmic response similar to that experienced by the adult, except for the absence of ejaculation in the male child, as demonstrated by the common practice in Europe in the late 1800s of masturbating an irritable child to induce relaxation and sleep. Occasionally this orgasmic response has been incorrectly thought to represent a convulsive disorder in the preschool child. Masturbatory activity is generally initiated as a response to the learned pleasure associated with touching of the genitalia that is first experienced in infancy during normal body exploration. Masturbation will continue as a lifelong pleasurable experience unless suppressed by parents or other adults.

The practitioner should counsel parents about masturbatory practices and emphasize that masturbation is a normal, harmless, and healthy practice that helps the child to derive pleasure from the child's own body. Myths must be dispelled concerning the belief that masturbation may cause mental retardation, physical deformity, blindness, poor physical and mental health, facial pimples, hair on the palms of the hand, homosexuality, and sexual perversions. Parents should be aware that masturbation occurs almost universally in children, and they should be encouraged to avoid punishing or shaming their child for a normal behavior. If parents observe masturbatory activity in their child, then they may want to suggest to the child the inappropriateness of manipulating their genitalia in public places or in front of others and inform the child that certain practices, such as using the toilet and masturbating, are best carried out in private.

Because local genital irritation, *Candida* infection, or pinworms in rare cases may cause a child to masturbate, a physical examination helps to exclude such possibilities. Compulsive, overt masturbation among children and adolescents may lead to social ridicule and condemnation, or it may signify a deeper emotional problem. Consultation with a specialist in behavioral disorders of children and adolescents is indicated if the practitioner suspects that the masturbatory activity is excessive, compulsive, or overt or may indicate the presence of a more complicated, troublesome emotional problem.

The pediatrician should be aware that even with the current trend within today's society of sexual openness and enlightenment, myths and feelings concerning masturbation often are deep seated and persistent. Thus counseling and advice given by the practitioner may be met with covert or overt resistance by parents or school authorities. The pediatrician should be well prepared to educate persons responsible for the growth and development of children.

HAIR PULLING AND TWISTING

Hair-pulling and twisting *(trichotillomania)* is an uncommon form of self-stimulating behavior that often indicates the presence of psychological stress. The scalp is the most common area affected; eyebrows and eyelashes are the next most likely sites. The obvious cosmetic damage often results in ridicule by peers and shame for the child. The formation of a hairball, or *trichobezoar,* in the stomach if the child ingests the hair is a serious problem that often results in hospitalization for surgical removal of the accumulated matted hair. This behavior, which is more common in girls than in boys, has been reported in preschoolers, school-aged children, adolescents, and adults. Classified by the *Diagnostic and Statistical Manual of Mental Disorders* as a disorder of impulse control, trichotillomania may best be grouped with the obsessive-compulsive disorder spectrum because of the common pathological compulsion of excessive grooming.[7] Two types of trichotillomania have been described in clinical practice, both of which can coexist in the same individual. In the *focused* type, which is associated with tension before and relief after the hair is pulled, time is set aside to pull the hair.[11] In the second, *sedentary* type, the patient is generally unaware of the behavior during the hair pulling or twisting itself and often recognizes the action as senseless and undesirable.

Treatment is usually indicated and varies from dynamic therapy, behavioral therapy, and psychopharmacologic measures.[12] Local irritation from a dermatologic condition is rarely the cause of this disorder, but the possibility should be investigated. Referral to a mental health professional is often warranted to investigate possible underlying causes of tension, anxiety, depression, or obsessive-compulsive disorder. Hypnosis or psychotherapy may be required in many of these cases. Clomipramine, fluoxetine, and selective serotonin reuptake inhibitors, but not desipramine, have proven useful in cases that are unresponsive to nonmedication treatment.

SPECIAL PROBLEMS IN DISTURBED CHILDREN

A broad spectrum of self-stimulating behaviors may be seen in severely retarded or emotionally disturbed children. The behaviors, including body twirling or spinning and hand or arm flapping, are often seen in cases of infantile autism or childhood schizophrenia. Excessive rocking behavior is common in severely retarded and emotionally disturbed children. In addition, severe self-mutilating behaviors, such as compulsive self-biting, severe head banging, and skin gouging, may be seen in these disorders and are characteristic of certain metabolic or genetic disorders, such as Lesch-Nyhan syndrome and Cornelia de Lange syndrome.[13] Patients who have Prader-Willi syndrome frequently demonstrate severe skin picking.[14]

These behaviors are part of a symptom complex in a severe disorder, in contrast to the generally isolated behavior discussed previously in normal children. The cause is generally linked to the basic disorder and may also reflect the lack, or disordered integration, of sensory stimuli.

All of these cases require treatment for the basic disorder and generally demand special behavioral treatment beyond the scope and expertise of the primary care physician. When severe, institutionalization is often required, and methods of treatment include the application of aversive behavior modification techniques; the use of arm and neck restraints, head helmets, and psychotropic medications; and the institution of psychotherapeutic behavioral programs.

WHEN TO REFER

- Persistence of head banging or rocking beyond the age of 3 years
- Preoccupation with self-stimulating behavior to the point that it interferes with healthy social and emotional interaction
- Presence of accompanying symptoms such as decreased socialization or other behavioral problems
- Causing tissue damage

TOOLS FOR PRACTICE

Engaging Patient and Family

- *Common Childhood Habits* (fact sheet), American Academy of Pediatrics (www.aap.org/publiced/BK5_Habits.htm).
- *How to eliminate habits like thumbsucking with simple behavior modification* (fact sheet), Edward Christophersen, PhD (www.dbpeds.org/articles/detail.cfm?TextID=%20112).

REFERENCES

1. Foster LG. Nervous habits and stereotyped behaviors in preschool children. *J Am Acad Child Adolesc Psychiatry.* 1998;37:711-717.
2. Jellinek M, Patel BP, Froehle MC. *Bright Futures in Practice: Mental Health. Volume 1. Practice Guide.* Arlington, VA: National Center for Education in Maternal and Child Health; 2002.
3. Lourie RS. Role of rhythmic patterns in childhood. *Am J Psychiatry.* 1949;105:653-650.

4. Werry JS, Carlielle J, Fitzpatrick J. Rhythmic motor activities (stereotypies) in children under five: etiology and prevalence. *J Am Acad Child Adolesc Psychiatry.* 1983; 22:329-336.
5. Kravitz H, Rosenthal V, Teplitz Z, et al. A study of head-banging in infants and children. *Dis Nerv Sys.* 1960;21: 203-208.
6. Fletcher B. Etiology of fingersucking: review of literature. *J Dent Children.* 1975;42:293-298.
7. King RA, Leonard HL, March J. Summary of practice parameters for the assessment and treatment of children and adolescents with obsessive compulsive disorder. *J Am Acad Child Adolesc Psychiatry.* 1998;37(10 suppl): 27S-45S.
8. Bohne A, Keuthen N, Wilhelm S. Pathologic hair pulling, skin picking and nail biting. *Ann Clin Psychiatry.* 2005; 17(4):227-232.
9. Friman PC, Leibowitz JM. An effective and acceptable treatment alternative for chronic thumb- and finger-sucking. *J Pediatr Psychol.* 1990;15:57-65.
10. Yang M, Fullwood E, Goldstein J, et al. Masturbation in infancy and early childhood presenting as a movement disorder: 12 cases and a review of the literature. *Pediatrics.* 2005;116:1427-1432.
11. Frey AS, McKee M, King RA, et al. Hair apparent: Rapunzel syndrome. *Am J Psychiatry.* 2005;162:242-248.
12. Bruce TO, Barwick LW, Wright HH. Diagnosis and management of trichotillomania in children and adolescents. *Paediatr Drugs.* 2005;7(6):365-376.
13. Harris JC. Destructive behavior: aggression and self injury. In: Harris JC, ed. *Developmental Neuropsychiatry: The Fundamentals,* New York, NY: Oxford University Press; 1995.
14. Donaldson MD, Chu CE, Cooke A, et al. The Prader Willi syndrome, *Arch Dis Child.* 1994;70:58-63.

Chapter 218
SHORT STATURE

Paul B. Kaplowitz, MD, PhD

The accepted medical definition of when a child is too short is often at variance with when parents worry about their child's growth. Parents may be concerned when a child is one of the shortest in the class or when a younger sibling starts to catch up to the child in question, even if the child's height clearly falls within the normal range. Statistically speaking, the normal range encompasses 2 standard deviations above and below the mean, or approximately between the 97th and the 3rd percentiles. The 3rd percentile may be difficult for primary care physicians to appreciate, given that the lowest curve on many growth charts is the 5th percentile. Furthermore, a single point on a growth chart will often not define whether a somewhat short child has a worrisome growth pattern; therefore previous growth data should be plotted whenever available, and any suggestion of growth deceleration should be carefully reviewed. An additional complication is that in boys between the ages of 12 and 14, growth charts show an upward inflection in height as boys start their growth spurts; thus a somewhat short boy who is prepubertal will appear to fall further behind, even though he is continuing to grow at a normal rate. The growth charts published by Tanner and Davis in 1985 make this point clear because they have a separate line for short, late-maturing boys and girls.[1]

DIFFERENTIAL DIAGNOSIS

Constitutional growth delay (CGD) and familial short stature (FSS) are the 2 most common causes of short stature. In the Utah Growth Study, which, through school screening, identified 555 children who were below the 3rd percentile and growing at less than 5 cm/year, 81% had CGD, FSS, or a combination of the 2 conditions.[2] In CGD, children are healthy and growing below but parallel to the 3rd percentile line. Birth weight is normal, but between 6 and 24 months' linear growth and weight track downward to the 3rd percentile or below; after age 3, children follow their own curve parallel to the low end of the growth chart. Children with CGD typically have a delayed onset of puberty and growth spurt and usually end up with heights in the lower half of the normal range. A characteristic finding is that the child has a bone age that is delayed by 2 or more years.

FSS is quite easy to recognize when the child is healthy, growing at a normal rate below the 3rd percentile, and 1 or both of the parents are quite short. Unlike CGD, children with FSS tend to have puberty at a normal age and achieve an adult height within 2 to 3 inches of their adult target height, which can be calculated by averaging the heights of the parents and adding 2.5 inches if the child is a boy and subtracting 2.5 inches if a girl. Some children may have features of both CGD and FSS.

Short Stature Associated With Syndromes and With Being Born Small for Gestational Age

Short stature associated with a syndrome should be considered when a very short child has a dysmorphic appearance, particularly if born small for gestational age (SGA) (eg, birth weight of 2500 g or less at term).

Turner syndrome should be a consideration in any girl whose height is well below the 3rd percentile, but certain features make the diagnosis more likely. Lymphedema in the newborn period or frequent ear infections well past 2 years of age are common. The most common physical findings include a narrow, high-arched palate, cubitus valgus (a large angle at the elbow when the arms are stretched out), and upturned fingernails.[3] The classic webbed neck is seen in only 40%. Approximately 15% have congenital heart disease, usually coarctation of the aorta. Mean birth weight is 2785 g; thus many patients are not born SGA.

Many less common syndromes exist in which dysmorphic features are associated with short stature. In Russell-Silver syndrome, the most characteristic features are a history of being born SGA and having a triangular face with a down-turned mouth. Noonan syndrome may be suggested by the finding of pulmonic stenosis and facial features that include a flat nasal bridge, hypertelorism, and ptosis.

Short stature associated with SGA is diagnosed when a child born SGA fails to catch up to the normal range in height by 2 years of age. Many of these children have no dysmorphic features, and no defined cause can be found for their intrauterine growth restriction.

Chronic Illness and Nutritional Disorders

A chronic illness or nutritional disorder should be considered in short children whose weight is further below the curve than their height (or whose body mass index is below the 10th percentile for age).

Inadequate calories, rarely a result of poverty in the United States because high-calorie foods are inexpensive, is sometimes seen in the setting of a child who is on a self-imposed or parent-imposed restrictive diet to avoid gaining weight or to lower cholesterol levels. The extreme example of this situation is anorexia nervosa, which is discussed in Chapter 135, Anorexia and Bulimia Nervosa.

Inflammatory bowel disease, though rarely the cause of undiagnosed short stature, may be suspected in a child whose growth has been normal but then shows a marked falloff in both height and weight, particularly in the presence of gastrointestinal (GI) symptoms such as abdominal pain, early satiety, and blood in the stools.[4] Growth attenuation may start when GI symptoms are relatively mild or even before they become apparent.

Celiac disease, or gluten enteropathy, is a not uncommon cause of short stature in Europe (up to 8% in some studies), although its frequency in the United States appears to be much lower.[5] Abdominal pain, distension, and loose stools may suggest the diagnosis, but most short children with celiac disease have few if any GI symptoms.

Renal disease can cause short stature, but only rarely is it diagnosed solely because of an abnormal growth curve. Renal tubular acidosis and chronic renal failure are the 2 renal conditions that can cause growth failure and that can be ruled out by appropriate screening tests.

Poor Growth Associated With Medications

Children treated with stimulant medications for attention-deficit disorder may have growth attenuation starting either at the time the medications are begun or between 9 and 12 years of age. One recent study, which included younger patients with a mean age of 4.4 years, found a 20% reduction in height velocity and a 50% reduction in weight gain in treated children.[6] Although the common belief asserts that decreased appetite is responsible for the slow growth, many of these children are not underweight, and the explanation for their slow linear growth is still unknown.

Chronic glucocorticoid therapy is another cause of short stature, mostly seen in children with such conditions as rheumatoid arthritis and inflammatory bowel disease treated with daily oral prednisone. The impact on the growth of children treated long-term with inhaled corticosteroids for asthma is clearly much less than for systemic glucocorticoids, though monitoring of linear growth may occasionally detect evidence of growth suppression.

Endocrine Disorders

The Utah Growth Study reported that less than 5% of short, slowly growing children had a defined endocrine disorder.[2] A major clue that an endocrine cause may exist is that height is often more affected than weight.

Growth hormone (GH) deficiency is not a common cause of short stature. In the Utah Growth Study the incidence in school aged children was estimated at 1:3480.[2] A recent study from Belgium, which ascertained all children diagnosed with GH deficiency between 1985 and 2001, estimated the incidence at 1:5600.[7] The diagnosis should be suspected in children who are well below the 3rd percentile in height and falling further below over time. One suggestive physical finding is an increase in subcutaneous fat that is greater in the trunk area than elsewhere. Most cases are congenital; birth weight is usually normal but a falloff in growth occurs starting late in the first or in the second year of life. In the much less common acquired cases, a period of normal growth is followed by deceleration; central nervous system symptoms such as severe recurrent headaches may be part of the clinical picture. Once a diagnosis of acquired GH deficiency is established, the endocrinologist will order brain imaging to look for a tumor in the area of the pituitary gland. Milder or partial forms of GH deficiency are difficult to distinguish from CGD and FSS based on growth pattern, physical findings, and laboratory tests. The apparently higher frequency of GH deficiency in recent years is, in large part, because GH testing done in the United States has many false-positive results, and many normally growing children fail the test using the accepted cut-off of 10 ng/mL.[8]

Acquired hypothyroidism, when severe, can cause slowing of growth or even complete growth arrest. Other symptoms, including fatigue and cold intolerance, are often present, and most children will have a goiter. Acquired hypothyroidism needs to be excluded as a possibility in any child with documented growth deceleration, even if height is still above the 3rd percentile.

Although iatrogenic Cushing syndrome is not uncommon, true endogenous Cushing syndrome is extremely rare. Rapid weight gain in the trunk, rather than generalized in distribution, accompanied by a slowing of linear growth are the key findings. Moon facies and purple abdominal striae are often seen, as well as increased skin pigmentation.

Idiopathic Short Stature

Idiopathic short stature (ISS) is a term used to describe moderately to severely short children who do not meet the criteria for CGD and FSS (eg, they often have a subnormal rate of growth); and after extensive testing, no cause for their poor growth is found. Studies have shown that most children with ISS respond to a variable degree to GH and see a modest average improvement in adult height.[9,10] The US Food and Drug Administration (FDA) in 2003 approved GH for children at or below the 1st percentile with an anticipated adult height (based on bone age) below the normal range.[9] However, some insurance companies refuse to cover GH to treat ISS, arguing that no medical condition causing the growth problem exists and that treatment is cosmetic.

EVALUATION

History

The most helpful information in evaluating the short child is the growth curve. If the growth rate has been normal for the previous 2 or more years, then the child most likely has CGD or FSS and is unlikely to have a defined, treatable cause. A single height point that falls off the established curve is often a measurement error and should be rechecked. A history of stimulant medications or glucocorticoid use might be a key piece of information. Many children with chronic growth-limiting illnesses have a decreased energy level and may have a poor appetite, although many short, healthy children are also described as picky eaters. An abnormal stool history should make the primary care physician think of malabsorption, celiac disease, or inflammatory bowel disease.

Heights of parents and grandparents and growth percentiles of siblings should be reviewed because they may suggest FSS in a healthy child who is short but growing at a normal rate. Approximately two thirds of children with CGD have a family history of a parent who was a late maturer (eg, mother's menarche after age 14 or a father who continued to grow after high school).

Physical Examination

Most short children do not have any physical findings that point to a specific diagnosis. A child with decreased subcutaneous fat stores and weight more affected than height may simply not be getting enough calories or may have bowel disease or another chronic illness. Conversely, a short child who is relatively pudgy (particularly if excess rippled fat is present over the trunk) may have GH deficiency. Dysmorphic features may provide a clue to a syndrome associated with short stature. In girls, the primary care physician should look for, among other things, a high-arched palate, cubitus valgus, and fingernails that bend upward, which may point to a diagnosis of Turner syndrome. An enlarged thyroid may be the only clue that a short child has hypothyroidism. Pubertal staging should be done on any short child who is 10 years or older. A short, healthy 14-year-old boy (or, less often, a short, healthy 13-year-old girl) who is still prepubertal is most likely to have a diagnosis of CGD. A child who has a flattened growth curve at 13 to 16 years of age and who, by examination, is found to be in the late stages of puberty has completed or has nearly completed growing, and nothing can be done to increase the individual's adult height.

Laboratory Evaluation

Primary care physicians should resist the temptation to order multiple laboratory tests for a child who is only mildly short (at or above the 3rd percentile) and whose growth rate appears to be normal. In this situation, a clinically significant abnormal test result is rarely found that will explain why the child is short. Most growth specialists prefer either to order a very few tests on such children or to perform no tests at all, particularly if everything points to a diagnosis of CGD or FSS.

Ordering screening tests in advance of a visit with a specialist might be appropriate if the child's height is well below the 3rd percentile or if growth deceleration that cannot be explained by medication is well-documented. However, the specialist can order any needed test at the first consultation.

Insulin-like growth factor 1 (IGF-1) is still the best screening test if GH deficiency is suspected, although many children with CGD have IGF-1 levels that are borderline low for age. IGF-binding protein 3 has not lived up to its initial promise as a better screening test for GH deficiency than IGF-1, and it is not worth ordering routinely. A random GH level is of no value because of the pulsatile nature of GH secretion.

Thyroid testing should be limited to free thyroxine (T4) and thyroid-stimulating hormone (TSH) assessment, which will pick up both primary and secondary hypothyroidism. Triiodothyronine (T3), T3 uptake, and thyroid antibodies are not helpful as screening tests for short children. A borderline increased TSH (in the 5.5- to 10-mcU/mL range) with a normal free T4 is usually a normal variation and will not explain poor growth.

Complete blood count and erythrocyte sedimentation rate are mainly useful in the occasional child in whom inflammatory bowel disease is suspected. A microcytic anemia may be a clue to occult GI blood loss. Either tissue transglutaminase immunoglobulin A (IgA) antibody or antiendomyseal antibody are good tests to screen for celiac disease. Antigliadin IgG and IgA are much less specific and are not worth the extra cost.

A comprehensive metabolic profile will rule out electrolyte disturbances, kidney disease, and liver disease, all of which are rare causes of short stature.

Imaging Studies

The only x-ray examination that should be considered is the bone age film, but this test is not a very useful diagnostic test because most children who are short for any reason (aside from genetic short stature) will have a bone age delay of a year or more. The consultant may order a bone age film in a child over 7 to make a height prediction when either CGD or FSS is suspected.

MANAGEMENT

Healthy children who are at or above the 3rd percentile and growing at a normal rate need not be referred to a specialist because the chances of finding a treatable cause for their short stature are small. If the parents insist on seeing a specialist, then they should be told that the child will not likely need or be eligible for coverage of GH therapy. Such children should have their growth carefully measured and plotted at each visit to make sure they are not dropping below the 3rd percentile in height. A few children report having poor self-esteem because they are shorter than most of their peers, and they may be subjected to teasing or bullying; referral to a psychologist may be more helpful than to an endocrinologist.

Infants or children who are maintaining linear growth at or above the 3rd percentile but whose weight is consistently below or has recently fallen below the 3rd percentile almost never have an endocrine problem. Weight gain that is fairly consistent in a child who is thin may be a normal variation; parents may say that they were thin at the same age. If weight gain is persistently poor, then referral to a GI or nutrition specialist should be considered.

The child who is still in the normal range but who is crossing percentiles may present a dilemma. Between 6 and 24 months, such percentile shifts in height and weight are common, especially in patients with CGD, and a stable growth curve is usually established between 2 and 3 years of age[11]; therefore referral may be deferred if the child is healthy.[10] If the child crosses 1 percentile channel (eg, from the 25th to the 10th percentile) over 3 or more years, and if the history and examination reveal nothing abnormal, then a cause will not likely be found. Children who cross more than 1 percentile channel in a period of less than 3 years have a greater chance of having a definable cause for their short stature. The most common cause of this growth pattern is the use of stimulant medication in children with attention-deficit disorder.

Parents of children who are short enough to be referred can be told that screening tests and a period of observation are needed before any decision can be made regarding the possible need for GH therapy. Such children are best referred between the ages of 3 and 6; children who are pubertal or on the verge of puberty are usually too old to derive much benefit from GH therapy.

WHEN TO REFER

- Any child whose height is below the 3rd percentile, particularly if the height is falling further below the normal range over time. Children who are below the 1st percentile have an even better chance of qualifying for GH therapy because they are more likely to have true GH deficiency; and if they do not have GH deficiency, then they may still meet the FDA criteria for GH treatment for idiopathic short stature.
- A child with a history of intrauterine growth retardation who was born SGA and who has not caught up to the normal range by age 2 years or older. The FDA has approved the use of GH in such children without the need for GH testing. A dysmorphic child with a history of intrauterine growth retardation should also be referred to a geneticist to try to make a specific diagnosis.
- A child who is within the normal range in height but has experienced a drop-off in linear growth of more than 1 percentile channel over a period of 3 years or less or who has shown documented growth arrest for a year.
- A child with short stature who has not started puberty by age 14. This situation occurs mostly in boys with CGD; and in many cases, when the boy is anxious to start his growth spurt sooner rather than later, treating such boys with a brief course of testosterone injections is appropriate.

SUGGESTED RESOURCE

Kaplowitz P, Baron J. *The Short Child: A Parents' Guide to the Causes, Consequences, and Treatment of Growth Problems.* New York, NY: Warner Wellness Books; 2006.

REFERENCES

1. Tanner JM, Davies PS. Clinical longitudinal standards for height and height velocity for North American children. *J Pediatr.* 1985;107:317-329.
2. Lindsay R, Feldkamp M, Harris D, et al. Utah Growth Study: growth standards and the prevalence of growth hormone deficiency. *J Pediatr.* 1994;125:29-35.
3. Frias JL, Davenport ML, and the American Academy of Pediatrics, Committee on Genetics and Section on Endocrinology. Health supervision for children with Turner syndrome. *Pediatrics.* 2003;11:692-702.
4. Savage MO, Beattie RM, Camacho-Hubner C, et al. Growth in Crohn's disease. *Acta Paediatra.* 1999;88(suppl): 89-92.
5. Rossi TM, Albini CH, Kumar V. Incidence of celiac disease identified by the presence of serum endomysial antibodies in children with chronic diarrhea, short stature, or insulin-dependent diabetes mellitus. *J Pediatr.* 1993; 123:262-264.
6. Swanson J, Greenhill L, Wigall T, et al. Stimulant-related reductions of growth rates in the Preschool ADHD Treatment Study. *J Am Acad Child Adolesc Psychiatry.* 2006;45: 1304-1313.
7. Thomas M, Massa G, Craen N, et al. Prevalence and demographic features of childhood growth hormone deficiency in Belgium during the period 1986-2001. *Eur J Endocrinol.* 2004;151:67-72.
8. Mauras N, Walton P, Nicar M, et al. Growth hormone stimulation testing in both short and normal statured children: Use of an immunofunctional assay. *Pediatr Res.* 2000;48:614-618.
9. Lescheck EW, Rose SR, Yanovski JA, et al. Effect of growth hormone treatment on adult height in peripubertal children with idiopathic short stature: a randomized, double-blind, placebo-controlled trial. *J Clin Endocrinol Metab.* 2004;89:3140-3148.
10. Wit JM, Rekers-Monbarg LT, Cutler GB, et al. Growth hormone (GH) treatment to final height in children with idiopathic short stature: evidence for a dose effect. *J Pediatr* 2005; 146:48-53.
11. Horner JM, Thorson AV, Hintz RL. Growth deceleration patterns in children with constitutional short stature: an aid to diagnosis. *Pediatrics.* 1978;62:529-534.

Chapter 219

SPLENOMEGALY

Marina Reznik, MD, MS; Philip O. Ozuah, MD, PhD

Splenomegaly is an enlargement of the spleen resulting from abnormalities of the lymphoid, reticuloendothelial, or vascular components of the spleen. Although splenomegaly is often considered to be an ominous clinical finding, certain normal variants have been found. In children, as a result of the thinness of the abdominal musculature, a palpable spleen is commonly encountered.[1] Thus a soft spleen is normally palpable in 15% to 30% of neonates. By 1 year of age, 10% of healthy children have a palpable spleen. Even after 10 years of age, 1% of children have palpable spleens.

Wide interobserver variability exists in the ability to appreciate an enlarged spleen on examination; this variability is not generally associated with clinical experience.[2] The spleen moves downward with inspiration and enlarges diagonally across the midline toward the right ileac fossa. An enlarged spleen may extend into the pelvis; thus, when examining a child with suspected splenomegaly, the physician should start palpating in the right lower quadrant and move across the abdomen toward the left upper quadrant. As the spleen enlarges, it replaces the tympany of the stomach and colon with the dullness of a solid organ. Percussion cannot confirm splenic enlargement, but it can raise suspicion of it. To assess splenomegaly, a clinician should percuss the left lower anterior chest wall between lung resonance above and the costal margin below (the Traube space).[3] The optimal clinical assessment of splenic enlargement includes the percussion of the Traube space.[4] If tympany is prominent, especially laterally, then splenomegaly is not likely. In addition, a change from tympany to dullness on inspiration when percussing at the lower interspace in the left anterior axillary line suggests splenic enlargement.[4]

Spleen length is correlated with age, height, weight, and body surface area in a nonlinear fashion, similar to the liver.[5,6] No sex-based differences in spleen size have been found.[6] Imaging of the spleen with ultrasonography, radioactive (technetium-99m) sulfur colloid scintigraphy, computed tomography, or magnetic resonance imaging can be an important adjunct to the physical examination in defining pathological changes in this organ.[7] Contrast-enhanced sonography is a novel technique that allows real-time assessment of the spleen.[8]

DIFFERENTIAL DIAGNOSIS

When assessing a child with splenomegaly, the major splenic functions should be kept in mind: its hematopoietic, phagocytic, and immunologic roles and its role as a reservoir for blood-borne elements. The spleen is a major hematopoietic organ during fetal life. However, it is capable of resuming extramedullary hematopoiesis in children and adults with bone marrow failure. The spleen removes the senescent and abnormal red blood cells, as well as particulate material, from the blood. A major lymphoreticular organ that acts as a filter for infectious organisms in the blood, the spleen also acts as a site of immunoglobulin M and properdin production. Finally, the spleen acts as a reservoir for platelets, reticulocytes, and plasma proteins, especially factor VIII. Because the spleen has so many functions, splenomegaly may be caused by systemic infections, by an increase in normal splenic process (as seen in hemolytic anemia), by infiltration of storage diseases or malignancies, by congestion from splenic or portal vein obstruction, or by inflammatory diseases. The differential diagnosis of splenomegaly is provided in Box 219-1.

BOX 219-1 Differential Diagnosis of Splenomegaly

I. Infections
   - Viral: Epstein-Barr virus, cytomegalovirus, HIV
   - Bacterial: acute bacterial infections, subacute bacterial endocarditis, congenital syphilis, tuberculosis
   - Parasitic: malaria, toxoplasmosis, leishmaniasis
   - Fungal: candidiasis, histoplasmosis, coccidioidomycosis

II. Hematologic disorders
   1. Hemolytic anemias—congenital and acquired
      - Red cell membrane defects: hereditary spherocytosis, hereditary elliptocytosis
      - Red cell hemoglobin defects: sickle cell disease and related syndromes, thalassemia
      - Red cell enzyme defects: pyruvate kinase deficiency, glucose-6-phospate dehydrogenase deficiency, others
      - Autoimmune hemolytic anemia
   2. Extramedullary hematopoiesis
      - Thalassemia major, osteopetrosis, myelofibrosis

III. Infiltrative disorders
   - Leukemias
   - Lymphomas
   - Lipidoses
   - Mucopolysaccharidosis
   - Langerhans cell histiocytosis

IV. Congestive splenomegaly
   - Portal vein thrombosis
   - Hepatic cirrhosis
   - Congestive heart failure
   - Hepatic portal or splenic vein obstruction

V. Inflammatory diseases
   - Systemic lupus erythematosus
   - Rheumatoid arthritis (Still disease)
   - Serum sickness
   - Sarcoidosis
   - Immune thrombocytopenias and neutropenias

VI. Primary splenic disorders
   - Splenoptosis (wandering spleen)
   - Cysts
   - Hemangiomas and lymphangiomas
   - Subcapsular hemorrhage
   - Accessory spleen

Infections

In infectious processes, splenomegaly results from hypertrophy of lymphatic and reticuloendothelial elements. Viral infections are the most common causes of splenomegaly in children. The splenic enlargement is usually transient and mild to moderate in severity. Infectious mononucleosis from Epstein-Barr virus, cytomegalovirus, and HIV infections lead to a greater degree of splenic enlargement. Specifically, splenomegaly occurs in 50% to 75% of cases of infectious mononucleosis. Subacute bacterial endocarditis, tuberculosis, and other chronic bacterial infections may cause splenic enlargement. Septicemia from meningococcus or pneumococcus may also be associated with splenomegaly. Malaria and visceral leishmaniasis are common causes of splenomegaly in areas endemic for these diseases.[9,10] Progressive disseminated histoplasmosis can occur in healthy children younger than 2 years who have been exposed to fungus in endemic areas of the eastern and central United States (Mississippi, Ohio, and Missouri River valleys). Early manifestations of this disease include fever, failure to thrive, and hepatosplenomegaly.

Hematologic Disorders

Splenomegaly associated with hemolytic states, such as membranopathies, hemoglobinopathies, and autoimmune hemolytic anemia, results from engorgement of the splenic sinusoids by abnormal red blood cells, as well as by increased phagocytic activity (work hypertrophy) of the reticuloendothelial elements. Splenic enlargement as a result of extramedullary hematopoiesis occurs in diseases associated with increased demand on the bone marrow for cell production (thalassemia major). In children with sickle cell anemia, a rapidly enlarging spleen with a falling hematocrit, pallor, dyspnea, weakness, and left-sided abdominal pain suggests the diagnosis of acute splenic sequestration crisis, a leading cause of death in children with sickle cell anemia and a medical emergency that requires prompt recognition and treatment.

Infiltrative Disorders

Metastatic neoplasia of the spleen is rare and is usually caused by neuroblastoma. However, the spleen is commonly infiltrated by leukemias and lymphomas. Malignant infiltration of the spleen often produces a massively enlarged, firm spleen that crosses the midline of the body. In the lipidoses and mucopolysaccharidoses, the phagocytic reticuloendothelial elements of the spleen accumulate large amounts of lipid and mucopolysaccharide, respectively. In Langerhans cell histiocytosis, the spleen is infiltrated by histiocytes.

Congestive Splenomegaly (Banti Syndrome)

Splenomegaly may occur from obstruction of the hepatic, portal, or splenic veins. The most common causes include portal-vein thrombosis, hepatic cirrhosis, and congestive heart failure. Umbilical vein catheterization or septic omphalitis in neonates may also result in obliteration of these vessels. Congestive splenomegaly is the most common cause of hypersplenism (the term used to describe patients with splenomegaly), peripheral blood cytopenias from excessive splenic function, and increased bone marrow production of the affected blood cells.

Inflammatory Diseases

Splenomegaly seen in inflammatory diseases such as systemic lupus erythematosus, rheumatoid arthritis, sarcoidosis, and serum sickness is the result of increased numbers of reticuloendothelial cells that remove antibody-coated cells and proteins. Lymphoid hyperplasia may occur as a result of accelerated antibody production in the spleen.

Primary Splenic Disorders

Splenoptosis, or wandering spleen, is a congenital fusion anomaly of dorsal mesogastrium that results in a spleen of normal size that moves freely within the peritoneal cavity.[11] A patient with splenoptosis usually has an asymptomatic abdominal mass. Splenic cysts may mimic splenomegaly. Two types of splenic cysts have been identified: those that are congenital (epidermoid) and those that are acquired (pseudocyst) from trauma or infarction. Cysts are generally asymptomatic and are confirmed by radiologic studies. Abdominal trauma may cause subcapsular hemorrhage of the spleen that results in abdominal pain and splenomegaly. Accessory spleens, which are found in 10% to 15% of individuals, may also mimic splenomegaly.

EVALUATION

History

The cause of splenomegaly can be determined by history and physical examination in addition to laboratory tests and, if necessary, radiographic studies. A thorough history, including family history, may provide valuable clues to the possible cause of splenomegaly. In a child with a history of a fever, pharyngitis, malaise, and splenomegaly, a viral cause (Epstein-Barr virus, cytomegalovirus) should be considered. Malaria or histoplasmosis may be the cause if the patient has recently traveled to areas endemic for these diseases. In the patient with fever, night sweats, malaise, weight loss, rash, arthralgia, and bone pain, an underlying inflammatory, infectious, or malignant process should be suspected. A newborn with unexplained jaundice and a family history of anemia, jaundice, splenomegaly, or splenectomy most likely has a congenital hemolytic anemia. A history of umbilical vein catheterization or omphalitis in the neonatal period may suggest a diagnosis of portal vein thrombosis.

Physical Examination

The normal palpable spleen is soft, smooth, and nontender and is less than 1 to 2 cm below the left costal margin. A pathologically enlarged spleen is usually firm, has an abnormal surface, and is often associated with signs and symptoms of an underlying disease. An enlarged spleen may be tender if it has enlarged quickly (splenic sequestration, splenic trauma with subcapsular hemorrhage). When portal hypertension causes splenomegaly, dilatation of the superficial abdominal veins can be noted at physical examination. Findings of a rash, arthritis, mucosal ulcerations, and splenomegaly may suggest an autoimmune disorder. Although a palpable spleen may be a normal variant, the concomitant finding of hepatomegaly is usually pathological and should prompt further investigation.

Laboratory Evaluation

The initial laboratory testing of a child with splenomegaly should include a complete blood count with a white blood cell differential, reticulocyte count, and examination of the peripheral blood smear. Further laboratory investigations should be directed at the suspected diagnosis, as indicated by the history, physical examination, and the results of the initial laboratory tests.

Imaging Studies

Radiologic confirmation of a mass in the left upper quadrant should be performed if any question exists about the nature of the mass. Retroperitoneal tumors such as neuroblastoma and Wilms tumor may be mistaken for an enlarged spleen. Ultrasonography is used to quantify splenic enlargement and to differentiate the spleen from other left upper-quadrant abdominal masses. Computed tomographic scanning has been used to evaluate splenic trauma and focal splenic pathology. Magnetic resonance imaging of the spleen can further clarify abnormalities in size and shape and can define parenchymal disease. Technetium-99m sulfur colloid scan is used to assess splenic function.

TREATMENT

Treatment of splenomegaly should be aimed at the underlying disease entity. Patients who have bacterial infections should receive appropriate antibiotic therapy. Viral causes of splenomegaly require supportive care. With splenomegaly from infectious mononucleosis, patients should refrain from contact or collision sports until the illness has completely resolved clinically and the spleen has returned to a normal size, generally at least 4 weeks from the onset of illness. Some experts suggest a sonographic evaluation of spleen size to help decide when the patient can resume full athletic activity.[12]

Splenectomy may be indicated to help control or stage some diseases that cause splenomegaly. Such diseases include hereditary spherocytosis, autoimmune thrombocytopenia or hemolysis, and lymphoma (Hodgkin lymphoma). Splenectomy may also be indicated for the treatment of chronic, severe hypersplenism. Laparoscopic splenectomy is being performed more commonly in children and has been found to be a safe procedure, with a shorter hospital stay, as compared with open splenectomy.[13,14] All children without spleens are at risk for fulminant bacteremia, particularly from *Streptococcus pneumoniae, Haemophilus influenzae,* and *Neisseria meningitides,* and should receive appropriate immunizations. Daily antimicrobial prophylaxis against pneumococcal infections (in addition to immunization) is recommended for these children if they are younger than 5 years and for at least 1 year after splenectomy.[15]

WHEN TO REFER

- Splenomegaly with concomitant hepatomegaly
- Palpation of a hard spleen
- Suspicion of malignancy or other infiltrative disorders
- Evidence of hemolytic anemias

WHEN TO ADMIT

- Splenic sequestration in sickle cell disease
- Injury to the spleen from abdominal trauma

SUGGESTED RESOURCES

Bates B, Bickley LS, Hoekelman RA. *A Guide to Physical Examination and History Taking.* 6th ed. Philadelphia, PA: JB Lippincott; 1995.

Buescher ES. Infections associated with pediatric sport participation. *Pediatr Clin North Am.* 2002;49:743-751.

Megremis SD, Vlachonikolis IG, Tsilimigaki AM. Spleen length in childhood with US: normal values based on age, sex, and somatometric parameters. *Radiology.* 2004;231: 129-134.

Pearson HA. The spleen and disturbances of splenic function. In: Nathan DG, Orkin SH, Lampert R, eds. *Nathan and Oski's Hematology of Infancy and Childhood.* 5th ed. Philadelphia, PA: WB Saunders; 1997.

REFERENCES

1. Pearson HA. The spleen and disturbances of splenic function. In: Nathan DG, Orkin SH, Lampert R, eds. *Nathan and Oski's Hematology of Infancy and Childhood.* 5th ed. Philadelphia, PA: WB Saunders; 1997.
2. Tamayo SG, Rickman LS, Mathews WC, et al. Examiner dependence on physical diagnostic tests for the detection of splenomegaly: a prospective study with multiple observers. *J Gen Intern Med.* 1993;8:69-75.
3. Bates B, Bickley LS, Hoekelman RA. *A Guide to Physical Examination and History Taking.* 6th ed. Philadelphia, PA: JB Lippincott; 1995.
4. Barkun AN, Camus M, Green L, et al. The bedside assessment of splenic enlargement. *Am J Med.* 1991;91:512-518.
5. Rosenberg HK, Markowitz RI, Kolberg H, et al. Normal splenic size in infants and children: sonographic measurements. *Am J Roentgenol.* 1991;157:119-121.
6. Megremis SD, Vlachonikolis IG, Tsilimigaki AM. Spleen length in childhood with US: normal values based on age, sex, and somatometric parameters. *Radiology.* 2004; 231:129-134.
7. Paterson A, Frush DP, Donnelly LF, et al. A pattern-oriented approach to splenic imaging in infants and children. *Radiographics.* 1999;19:1465-1485.
8. Catalano O, Sandomenico F, Matarazzo I, et al. Contrast-enhanced sonography of the spleen. *AJR Am J Roentgenol.* 2005;184:1150-1156.
9. Maroushek SR, Aguilar EF, Stauffer W, et al. Malaria among refugee children at arrival in the United States. *Pediatr Infect Dis J.* 2005;24:450-452.
10. Tanoli ZM, Rai ME, Gandapur AS. Clinical presentation and management of visceral leishmaniasis. *J Ayub Med Coll Abbottabad.* 2005;17:51-53.
11. Balik E, Yazici M, Taneli C, et al. Splenoptosis (wandering spleen). *Eur J Pediatr Surg.* 1993;3:174-175.
12. Buescher ES. Infections associated with pediatric sport participation. *Pediatr Clin North Am.* 2002;49:743-751.
13. Rescorla FJ, Engum SA, West KW, et al. Laparoscopic splenectomy has become the gold standard in children. *Am Surg.* 2002;68:297-301.
14. Qureshi FG, Ergun O, Sandulache VC, et al. Laparoscopic splenectomy in children. *JSLS.* 2005;9:389-392.
15. American Academy of Pediatrics. Children with asplenia. In: Pickering LK, Baker CJ, Long SS, McMillan JA, eds. *Red Book: 2006 Report of the Committee on Infectious Diseases.* 27th ed. Elk Grove Village, IL: American Academy of Pediatrics; 2006.

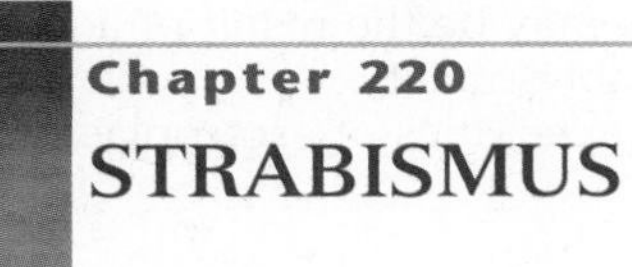

Chapter 220
STRABISMUS

Kenneth W. Wright, MD

Strabismus is the condition of ocular misalignment. It includes esotropia (eye turned in), exotropia (eye turned out), or vertical strabismus (eye turned up or down). Children with strabismus might be expected to have a difficult time dealing with confusing double vision (diplopia). Actually, if strabismus occurs before 4 to 6 years of age, the child will cortically suppress the image from the deviated eye. This defense mechanism, known as suppression, prevents bothersome double vision. Prolonged suppression of one eye, however,

BOX 220-1 Red Flags for Strabismus With a Serious Cause

Acquired strabismus
Diplopia
Limited eye movements (incomitant strabismus)
Ptosis or other neurological signs
Poor vision or abnormal red reflex

can lead to amblyopia of the suppressed eye. (See Chapter 228, Visual Development, Amblyopia, and Vision Testing.) Patients with a strong preference for one eye will constantly suppress the deviated eye, causing amblyopia and vision loss of the deviated eye. Children who alternate the use of each eye will have equal vision and will not develop amblyopia. However, the suppression eliminates binocular fusion.

Strabismus acquired after 5 to 7 years of age results in diplopia because the mature visual system cannot suppress the double image. The clinical symptom of diplopia is therefore an important clue indicating that the strabismus is acquired. Acquired strabismus often implies a more dangerous cause, such as a neurologic process or acquired visual loss. Box 220-1 lists important red flags that indicate that the strabismus may be the result of a potentially dangerous disease process. These warning signs are not pathognomonic for a neurologic process, but they should prompt urgent consultation with an ophthalmologist.

Strabismus can be classified as comitant or incomitant. In comitant strabismus, the deviation is the same in all fields of gaze. Even though the eyes are misaligned, they move normally, without restriction or muscle paresis. Most childhood strabismus is comitant, and eye movements are intact. In incomitant strabismus, eye movement is limited, and the deviation is different in different fields of gaze. Limited eye movement may be caused by a restriction (periocular scarring or tight extraocular muscles) or a muscle paresis (third, fourth, or sixth nerve paresis). Comitant strabismus is not usually associated with neurologic disease, but incomitant strabismus may be the result of a neurologic disease or muscle abnormality.

Box 220-2 lists the characteristics of esotropias and exotropias.

COMITANT STRABISMUS

Infantile Esotropia (Congenital Esotropia)

Infantile esotropia, also known as congenital esotropia, is the most common form of strabismus in infants. It is defined as a large esotropia, with onset before 6 months of age (Figure 220-1). The esotropia may be present at birth, although it is often acquired during the first 6 months of life.[1] Small, transient exodeviations are common in normal neonates, but esodeviations in newborns are rare. Persistent esotropia that is present after 2 months of age is probably pathological and will not usually resolve spontaneously, so immediate referral to an opthalmologist is necessary.

BOX 220-2 Characteristics of Esotropias and Exotropias

INFANTILE ESOTROPIA
Uncommon
Onset within first 6 months of life
Usually associated with large-angle strabismus
Best treated with early surgery
Amblyopia present in 50% of patients
Poor prognosis for high-grade stereo acuity (depth perception)

ACCOMMODATIVE ESOTROPIA
Common
Usually associated with farsightedness
Usually acquired after 6 months of age, most often at 1-5 years of age
Treatment is to prescribe spectacles; however, many will require spectacles and eye muscle surgery
Relatively good prognosis for stereo acuity and binocular fusion

SENSORY ESOTROPIA
Uncommon

INTERMITTENT EXOTROPIA
Common
Most commonly occurring between ages 2 to 8 years
Intermittent strabismus: the exotropia occurs when the child is tired or daydreaming
Patient may squint one eye
Good stereopsis and binocular fusion when the eyes are aligned
Treatment usually requires strabismus surgery if the deviation is poorly controlled

CONVERGENCE INSUFFICIENCY
Uncommon

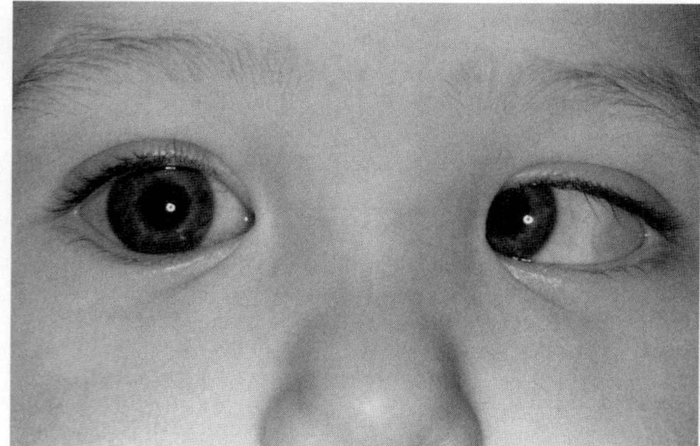

Figure 220-1 Eight-month-old child with infantile esotropia. The large-angle deviation is typical of infantile anisometropia.

No consistent inheritance pattern for infantile esotropia has been established, but it does tend to run in families. Some pedigrees appear to be autosomal recessive and others autosomal dominant; however, no family history of strabismus is found in many of these cases. The variability of inheritance patterns suggests heterogeneity for the phenotype of infantile esotropia. Thus, not surprisingly, the pathogenesis of infantile esotropia is probably multifactorial. In some cases, farsightedness (hypermetropia) is the cause, and spectacle correction is required. In other cases, infantile esotropia is associated with developmental delay, cerebral palsy, or other diseases, including Down syndrome.

Patients may show a strong fixation preference for one eye, which is an indication of amblyopia, or the patient may alternate fixation. Amblyopia occurs in approximately 50% of children with infantile esotropia. Some limitation of abduction is often found in voluntary version testing; however, the doll's head maneuver reveals normal abduction and normal lateral rectus function. Associated motor anomalies frequently related to infantile esotropia include vertical strabismus (inferior oblique overaction in 70% and dissociated vertical deviation [DVD] in 75%). Nystagmus is unusual in children with congenital esotropia, but latent nystagmus is found in approximately 50% of cases. Latent nystagmus manifests becomes evident during standard vision testing when one eye is covered. In children with latent nystagmus, the best visual potential is obtained by testing with both eyes open (binocular vision) to avoid inducing nystagmus. These associated motor anomalies develop late, at age 1 or 2 years, often several months after the esotropia has been surgically corrected.

Differential Diagnosis

The differential diagnosis of infantile esotropia includes Duane syndrome (discussed later), congenital fibrosis of extraocular muscles, congenital sixth nerve palsy, Möbius syndrome associated with sixth nerve paresis, and infantile myasthenia gravis. These disorders all have limited abduction, and they can therefore be differentiated from infantile esotropia, in which the ductions should be full. Esotropia in an infant may also be an important sign of vision loss. Disorders such as congenital cataracts and retinoblastoma often first exhibit as infantile esotropia.

Treatment

In most cases, the treatment of infantile esotropia is surgery, which will usually recess the medial rectus muscle in both eyes. In patients with farsightedness (hypermetropia of more than +3.00 diopters), spectacles should be prescribed first because spectacles alone may correct the deviation. If amblyopia is present, then it should be treated with patching before surgery. This approach is important because, after surgery, parents often think that the problem is solved, and they may not return for follow-up visits.

Surgery

Usually, surgery is performed when the patient is between 6 months and 2 years of age because peripheral fusion can be achieved if the eyes are aligned before 2 years of age.[2] However, peripheral fusion is subnormal binocular vision, and approximately one half of the children with congenital esotropia will require multiple surgeries. Poor binocular fusion may occur because even brief periods of strabismus during the early period of visual development can result in permanent loss of binocularity. Even 3 weeks of prism-induced esotropia may result in irreversible loss of binocular vision.[3] Excellent fusion with high-grade stereopsis and good alignment can be obtained when surgery is performed before the child is 6 months of age.[4] Surgery should be considered as early as 3 months of age if the following criteria are met: large-angle esotropia (40 prism diopters or more), constant or increasing deviation documented by 2 visits 1 month apart, and the infant is able to tolerate anesthesia.[5]

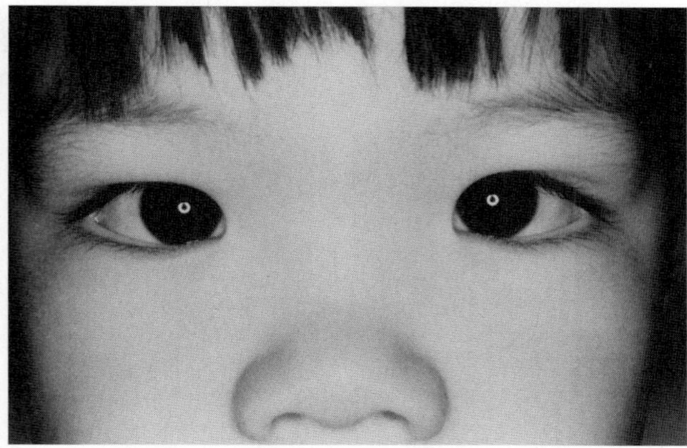

Figure 220-2 Three-year-old child with pseudoesotropia. The patient was referred for assessment of right esotropia.

Pseudoesotropia

Pseudoesotropia is a common condition that should be distinguished from infantile esotropia. With pseudoesotropia, the infant has a wide nasal bridge and wide, prominent epicanthal folds, giving the appearance of esotropia. In fact, however, the eyes are orthotropic (Figure 220-2). Documenting proper eye alignment by the Hirschberg corneal light reflex test is important. Convincing parents that the eyes are truly straight can be difficult; therefore showing the parents the normal Hirschberg corneal light reflex test may be helpful. Follow-up is important in patients with pseudoesotropia, given that a small percentage will develop true esotropia.

Accommodative Esotropia

Children who are farsighted (hypermetropic) can increase focusing effort (accommodate) to see more clearly (see Box 220-2). Because this accommodation is linked to convergence, increased accommodation will result in increased convergence. In some farsighted children, this increased convergence will result in esotropia, which is known as accommodative esotropia. Hypermetropic spectacle correction is useful in these cases to decrease accommodation, thereby reducing convergence and correcting the esotropia (Figure 220-3). The

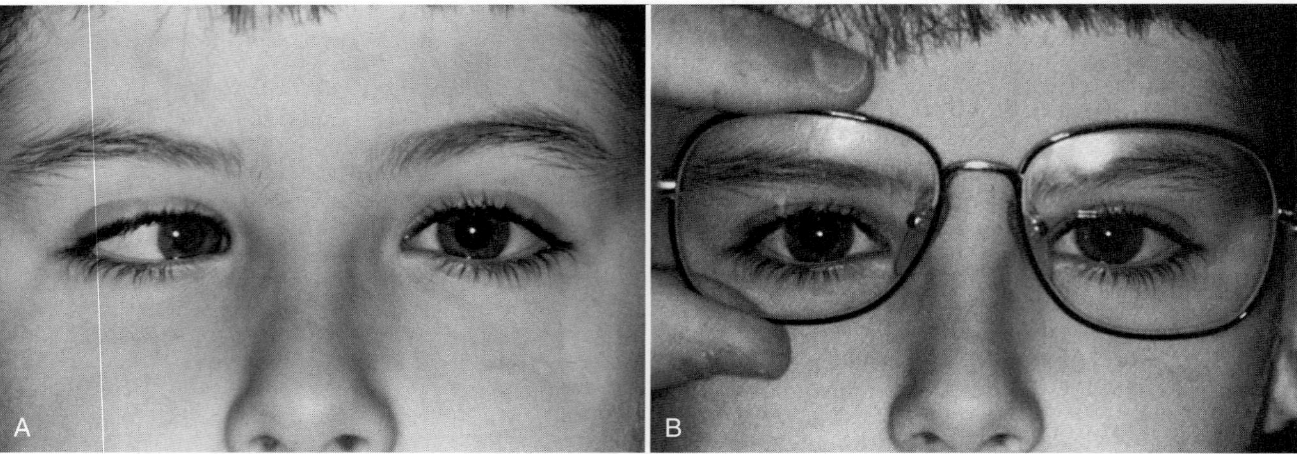

Figure 220-3 Eight-year-old child with accommodative esotropia. **A,** The large-angle esotropia is associated with accommodation for farsightedness. The patient is squinting because she is forcibly accommodating to see clearly. Increased accommodation results in increased convergence. **B,** Patient is given hypermetropic spectacle correction that focuses the retinal image without increased accommodation and convergence. With spectacle correction, accommodation and convergence diminishes, thereby allowing the eyes to straighten.

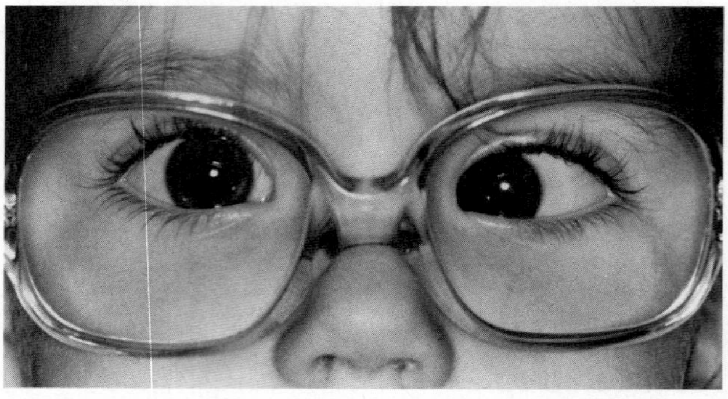

Figure 220-4 Three-year-old child with partially accommodative esotropia. The patient is wearing full hypermetropic correction of +3.00 diopters in both eyes; however, a residual esotropia persists.

presence of a combined mechanism of accommodative esotropia and a basic esotropia is termed partially accommodative esotropia. Patients with this diagnosis improve with hypermetropic spectacle correction, but they still require surgery for the residual esotropia (Figure 220-4).

Clinical Manifestations

Accommodative esotropia is acquired and can develop at any time between infancy (infantile accommodative esotropia) and late childhood, but it most often occurs in children between 12 months and 5 years of age. Initially, the deviation is small and intermittent. The esotropia is seen mostly at near fixation or when the child is tired and may be demonstrated by the child squinting or closing one eye. Over time—sometimes only a few weeks—the deviation may increase to become constant, and amblyopia may develop.

Differential Diagnosis

The differential diagnosis of acquired esotropia includes any neurologic cause of a sixth nerve palsy, including intracranial tumor, hydrocephalus, mastoiditis, virus, Arnold-Chiari malformation, and myasthenia gravis.

Treatment

Immediate referral is important in patients with acquired esotropia to provide early treatment to establish binocular vision and rule out ocular or neurologic disease. The treatment of accommodative esotropia is based on prescribing full hypermetropic correction as soon as possible by means of spectacles or contact lenses. Patients who are corrected to proper alignment with glasses for distance viewing, but whose eyes still cross at near viewing, can be prescribed bifocal glasses. If spectacles do not correct the esotropia, then surgery will be needed in addition to spectacles. In most cases, these children will need spectacles after surgery to maintain good alignment. Early treatment is critical to achieving best results.

Prognosis for Binocular Fusion

Unlike children with congenital esotropia, patients with acquired accommodative esotropia have had straight eyes during early visual development; thus they retain relatively good fusion potential. The earlier the eyes are straightened, the better the chances will be for recovering fusion. This, and the fact that acquired esotropia may have a neurologic cause, are 2 important reasons to immediately refer patients with acquired esotropia.

Sensory Esotropia

Loss of vision may cause an eye to drift. Sensory esotropia is an esodeviation caused by unilateral blindness. If the visual loss occurs before 2 years of age,

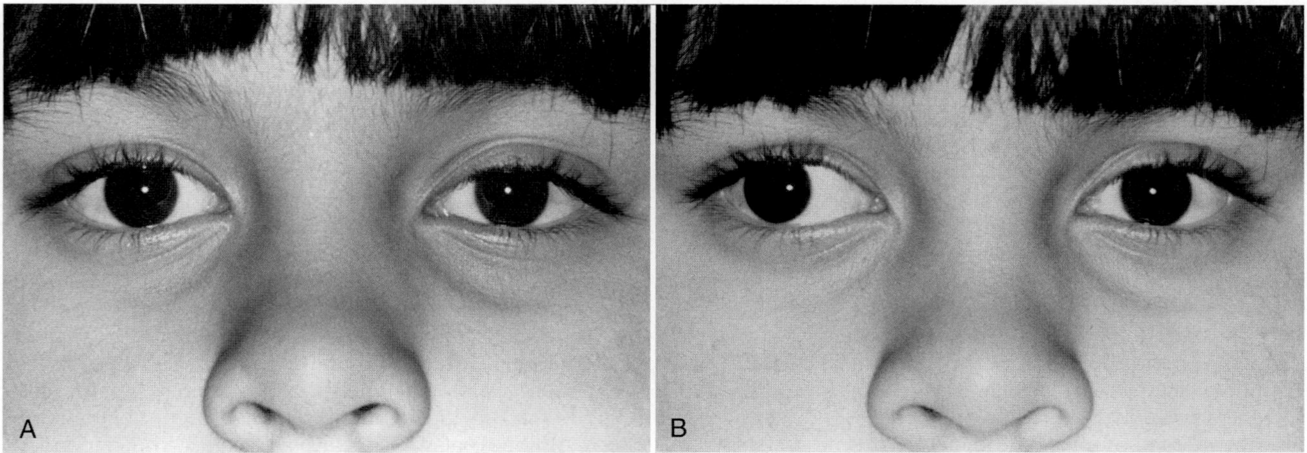

Figure 220-5 Six-year-old child with intermittent exotropia. **A,** Patient in the phoric phase with straight eyes and high-grade stereopsis. **B,** Patient in the tropic phase with large right exotropia. Patient is suppressing the right eye and does not have diplopia.

then patients develop esotropia. If the vision loss occurs after 2 years of age, then patients develop exotropia. However, this circumstance is only a general rule, with many exceptions, and the presence of an esotropia is not a good marker for the onset of blindness. The treatment of sensory esotropia is a recession-resection procedure of the blind eye; surgery is not performed on the eye with good vision.

Intermittent Exotropia

A phoria is a tendency for the eyes to drift apart, but alignment is maintained by binocular fusion (see Box 220-2). A tropia is a manifest deviation of the eyes, without binocular fusion. Small exophorias (the eye tends to drift out, but binocular fusion controls the eye alignment) are common in the general population and are easily controlled. Large exophorias, however, may become difficult to control. Intermittent exotropia is an exodeviation that is controlled part of the time by fusional convergence but that occurs some of the time (Figure 220-5). This type of exotropia is, by far, the most common type of exodeviation. The cause of intermittent exotropia is unknown.

Clinical Manifestation

Intermittent exodeviation usually occurs between 2 and 8 years of age, but it may develop at any time between infancy and adulthood. Initially, an exotropia may be present only when the patient is fatigued or ill. Covering one eye will produce the exotropia; therefore this form of strabismus is best detected by the cover test rather than the corneal light reflex test. Symptoms include blurred vision, asthenopia (vague visual discomfort, such as eyestrain or brow ache), visual fatigue, and photophobia with squinting. The photophobia and squinting is thought to be a mechanism for eliminating diplopia or confusion. The natural history of intermittent exotropia is variable. Approximately 70% of patients will show an increasing frequency of the exotropia and progressive loss of fusion, 20% will stay the same, and a small percentage will improve over time.

During the exophoric phase, patients have bifoveal fusion with excellent stereo acuity. When exotropia (developed strabismus) is present, most patients demonstrate suppression. Occasionally, patients with late-onset intermittent exotropia (after 5 or 6 years of age) will experience diplopia. Significant amblyopia is rare in patients with intermittent exotropia.

Treatment

In contrast to esotropia, which requires urgent intervention, the treatment of intermittent exotropia is elective. These children have binocular fusion and are well aligned most of the time. Eye muscle surgery is the treatment of choice for most forms of intermittent exotropia. Indications for surgery include increasing exotropia, exotropia present more than 50% of the time, and poor fusion control of the exotropia. Nonsurgical treatments include part-time occlusion of the dominant eye, correction for myopia, and eye exercises. These interventions act as temporary treatments at best, except for patients with a special type of exotropia known as convergence insufficiency.

Convergence Insufficiency

Convergence insufficiency is a type of intermittent exotropia characterized by an exotropia at near fixation but straight eyes with distance fixation (Figure 220-6). Appropriate near convergence is insufficient. Convergence insufficiency is the one form of strabismus that is best treated with eye exercises instead of surgery. It is a common cause of reading fatigue in older children and adults.

INCOMITANT STRABISMUS

Fourth Nerve Palsy

A superior oblique palsy (fourth nerve palsy) is the most common cause of a vertical deviation. The superior oblique muscle is a depressor and intortor (twists the eye nasally). A weak superior oblique muscle will cause strabismus consisting of hypertropia (vertical strabismus) and extorsion (temporal twisting of the eye). The hypertropia is worse when the patient's head tilts to the side of the weak superior oblique muscle (Figure 220-7). Patients with a superior oblique paresis usually exhibit a compensatory head tilt to the opposite side of the paresis to help keep their eyes aligned. The most common types of superior oblique palsies are congenital and traumatic.

Congenital Superior Oblique Palsy

Congenital superior oblique muscle palsy is the most common cause for a vertical strabismus in childhood. The cause of most congenital superior oblique palsies is unknown. In some cases, the superior oblique palsy is associated with a lax tendon and, rarely, an absent superior oblique tendon. The child will invariably have a compensatory head tilt, which is often misdiagnosed as a musculoskeletal problem of the neck (Figure 220-8). The family photo album should be examined to estimate the time of onset of the head tilt.

A weakness of the superior oblique muscle causes the hypertropia (vertical strabismus). The hypertropia diminishes with head tilt to the opposite side of the palsy; thus patients with a congenital superior oblique palsy tilt their head to the opposite side of the palsy to keep the eyes aligned. A compensatory head tilt is often the first sign of a congenital fourth nerve palsy. Patients with congenital superior oblique paresis typically have good stereopsis and exhibit the hyperdeviation intermittently when fatigued. Most have the ability to suppress so as not to experience diplopia when the deviation is apparent. A subtle finding in most children with a congenital superior oblique palsy is facial asymmetry. The dependent side of the face is more shallow and atrophied (Figure 220-8), which is possibly the result of the effects of gravity on facial development.

Even though the paresis is present at birth, symptoms may develop in late childhood or even adulthood. Over time, the fusional control weakens and results in a deviation that becomes apparent later in life.

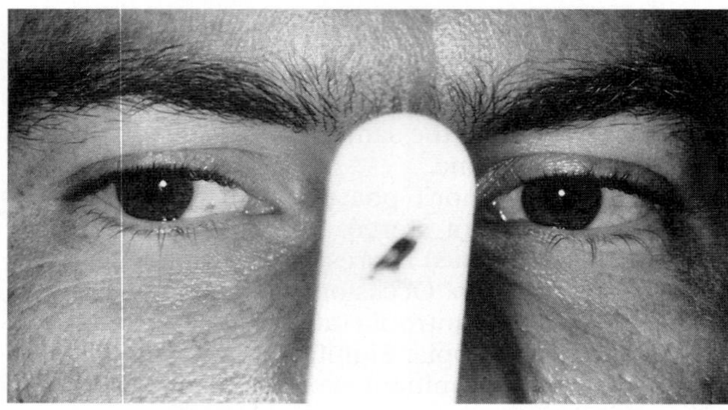

Figure 220-6 Adult with convergence insufficiency. The left eye is fixing on a target, and the right eye is exotropic. The patient had no significant deviation for the distance. Convergence insufficiency is best treated with convergence exercises.

Other Causes of Superior Oblique Paresis

Closed head trauma, even relatively mild trauma, is a common cause of superior oblique paresis. Traumatic palsies tend to be bilateral, and patients have vertical and torsional diplopia. In many cases, the palsy will spontaneously resolve; however, if diplopia persists after 6 months, then strabismus surgery is indicated. Other causes include vascular disease with brainstem lacunar infarcts, multiple sclerosis, intracranial neoplasm, herpes zoster ophthalmicus, and diabetes with an associated mononeuropathy. These disorders, however, usually occur in adults and not children. If no specific cause of an acquired superior oblique paresis can be found, then a neurologic work-up, including neuroimaging, should be performed.

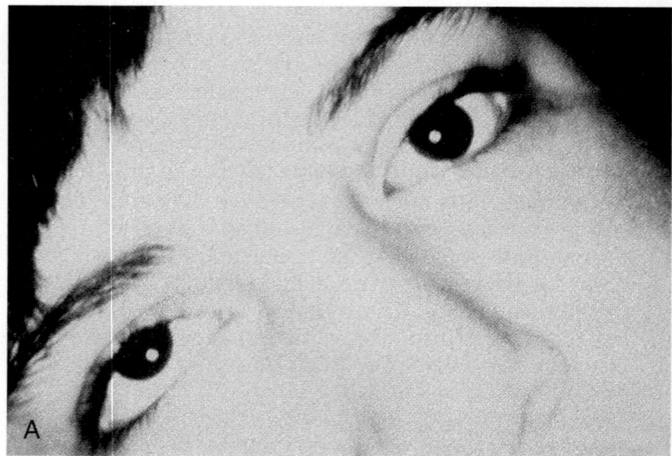

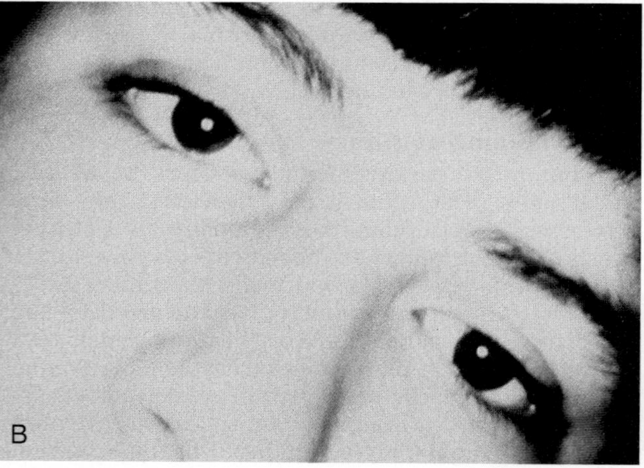

Figure 220-7 Right superior oblique muscle paresis. Right hypertropia occurs when the patient's head is tilted to the right shoulder. This patient maintained a compensatory head tilt to the left to keep his eyes aligned.

Sixth Nerve Palsy

Sixth nerve palsy, which is uncommon, results in limited abduction and an esotropia that is worse on the side of the palsy (Figure 220-9). Neonates can have a transient sixth nerve palsy often associated with a facial palsy that resolves spontaneously by 4 to 8 weeks. One of the more common causes of acquired sixth nerve palsy is postviral neuropathy, usually occurring in children between 2 and 6 years of age. Most patients in this group experience resolution of the palsy within 8 to 10 weeks. If no sign of improvement is noted, or if other neurologic signs are present, then a full neurologic evaluation is indicated. Head trauma is another common cause of a sixth nerve palsy. Approximately one half of the sixth nerve palsies will show resolution over a 6-month observational period. Other causes include intracranial tumors, meningitis, mastoiditis (Gradenigo syndrome), lumbar puncture, hydrocephalus, and migraine.

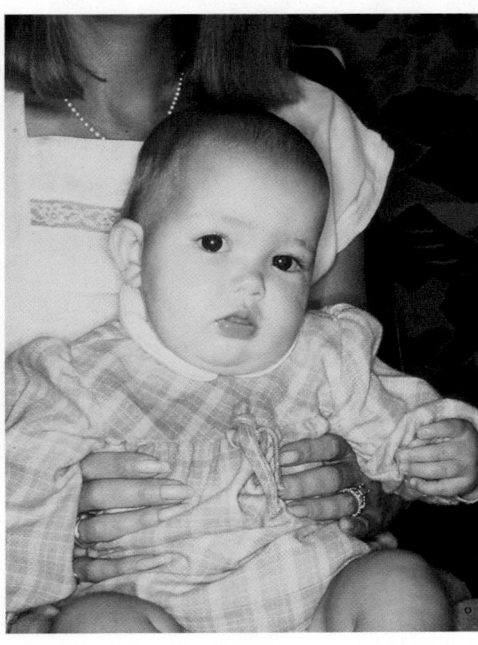

Figure 220-8 Right congenital superior oblique muscle paresis with compensatory head tilt to the left to keep the eyes aligned. Facial asymmetry is present, with the left side of the face smaller than the right.

Duane Syndrome

Duane syndrome is caused by a congenital hypoplasia of the sixth nerve nucleus with misdirection of the medial rectus nerve, innervating both the medial rectus and the lateral rectus muscles (Figure 220-10; see also Box 220-3). Because both the medial and the lateral rectus muscles are innervated by the nerve to the medial rectus muscle, both muscles fire and contract simultaneously on attempted adduction. This co-contraction of the medial and lateral rectus muscles causes globe retraction and lid fissure narrowing on

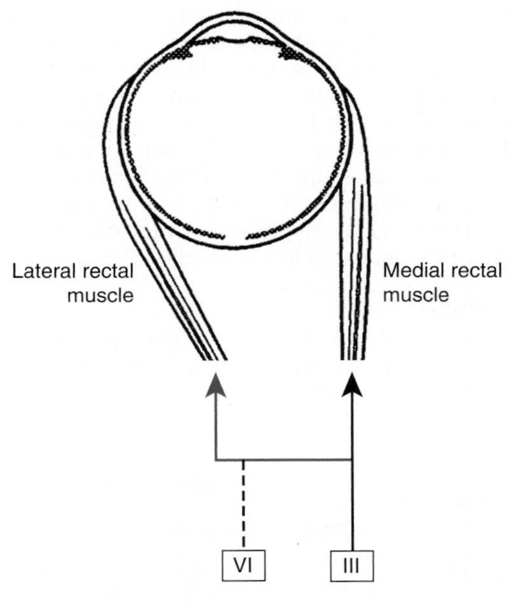

Figure 220-10 Diagrammatic representation of misdirection of nerve fibers in Duane syndrome. The aberrant nerve pathway is shown in blue, and the dotted lines represent hypoplasia or agenesis. *(Modified from Wilcox LM, Gittinger JW, Breinin GM. Congenital adduction palsy and synergistic divergence.* Am J Ophthalmol. *1981;91:1-7)*

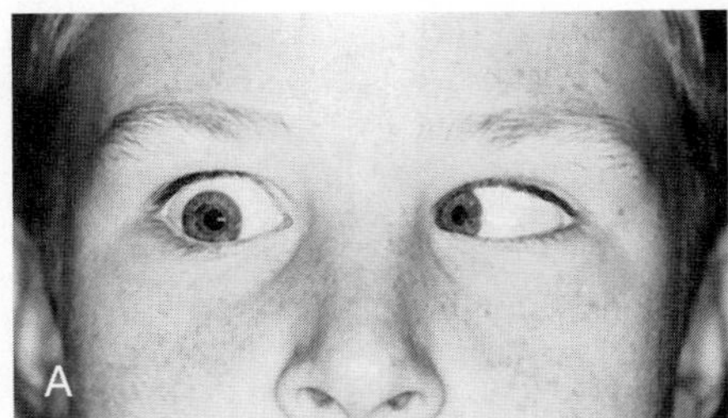

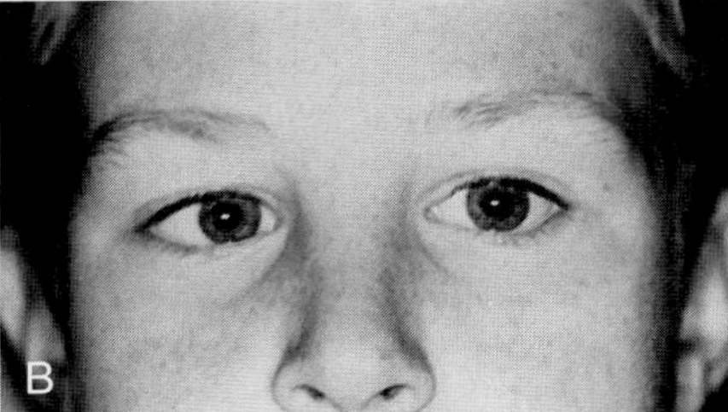

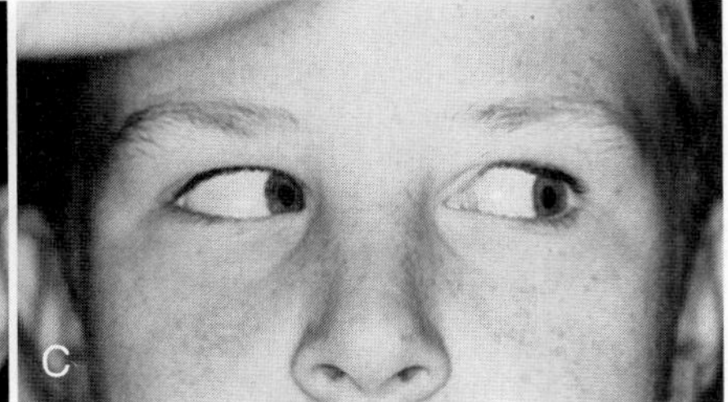

Figure 220-9 Right sixth nerve palsy. The patient demonstrates an inability to abduct the right eye. Esotropia is present in the primary position, and it increases in the right gaze because the right eye cannot abduct. In left gaze, the eyes are straight.

attempted adduction (Figure 220-11). Most children with Duane syndrome adopt a compensatory face turn to keep their eyes straight (Figure 220-12). Strabismus surgery is effective for correcting the face turn; it improves abduction slightly, but it does not result in full abduction capabilities (Figure 220-12, *C*). Duane syndrome may be associated with a variety of systemic diseases, including Goldenhar syndrome and prenatal exposure to the teratogen thalidomide. However, Duane syndrome is most often sporadic and of unknown cause.

Möbius Syndrome

Möbius syndrome, which is rare, is characterized by a combination of facial palsy, sixth nerve palsy often with a partial third nerve palsy, and distal limb abnormalities such as syndactyly or even amputation defects. Craniofacial anomalies can occur and include micrognathia, tongue abnormalities, and facial or oral clefts. Ocular motility abnormalities include failure of the eyes to abduct and the presence of lid retraction on adduction, which is also typical in some patients with Duane syndrome. The facial palsy usually spares the lower face, although orbicularis function is weak. Skeletal abnormalities also include pectoralis muscle deficits. The inheritance pattern is variable and may be familial, but most cases are sporadic.

Third Nerve Palsy

Third nerve palsy involves all the extraocular muscles (ie, medial rectus, superior rectus, inferior rectus, inferior oblique muscles) except the lateral rectus

BOX 220-3 Duane Syndrome

- Uncommon congenital absence of sixth nerve nucleus with aberrant innervation of the lateral rectus muscle by part of the medial rectus nerve
- Contralateral face turn to align eyes
- Limited abduction (rarely binocular)
- Lid fissure narrowing on adduction and lid fissure widening on abduction

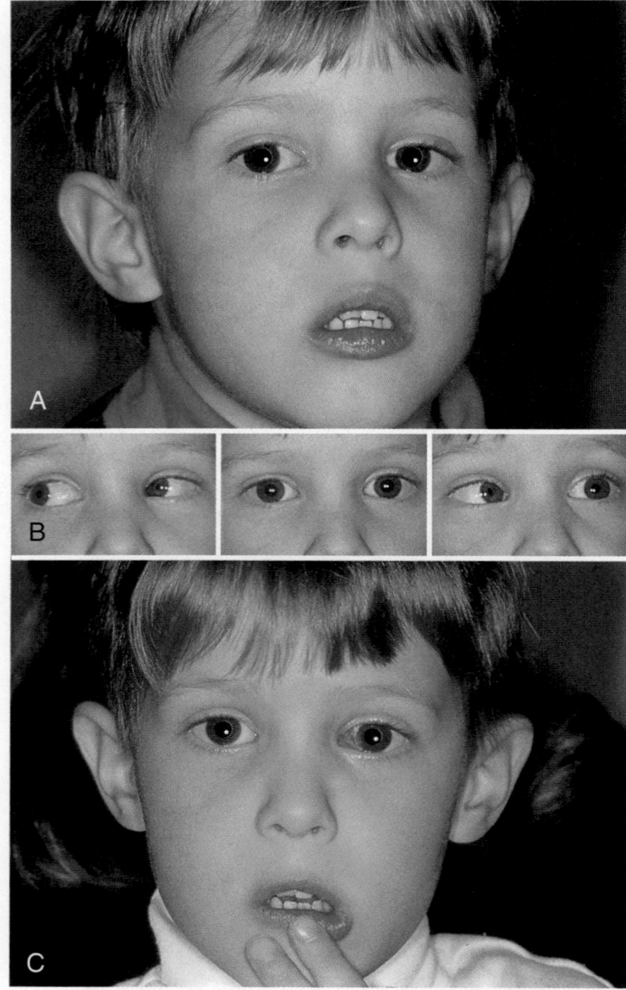

Figure 220-12 Left Duane syndrome. **A,** Compensatory face turn to the left and eyes in right gaze to place eyes into alignment. **B,** Limited abduction of the left eye and large esotropia as the patient looks to the left. At right gaze, the left eye fully adducts and eyes are aligned, but the lid fissure narrows on the left side. **C,** One day after surgery after a left medial rectus recession, the head turn has resolved, and eyes are well aligned.

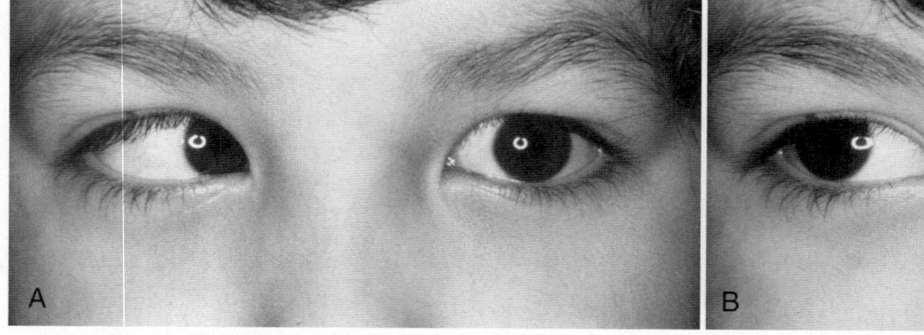

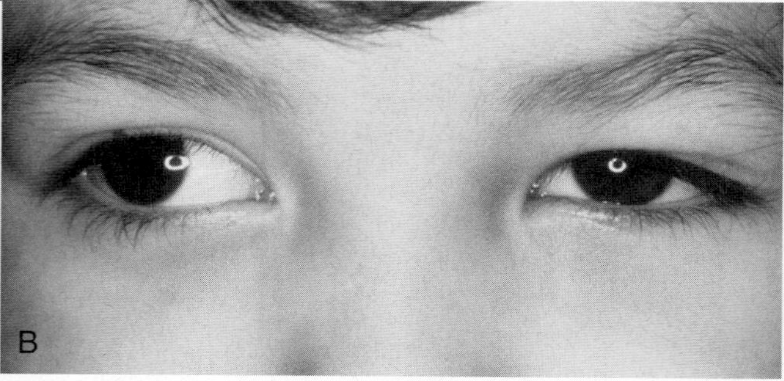

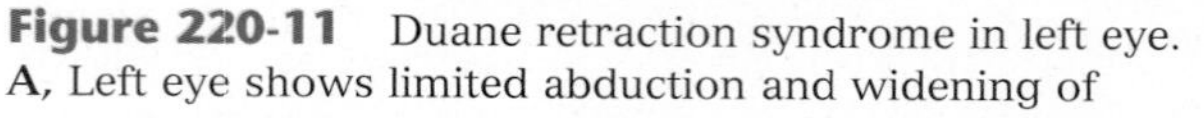

Figure 220-11 Duane retraction syndrome in left eye. **A,** Left eye shows limited abduction and widening of palpebral fissures on attempted abduction. **B,** On adduction, narrowing of palpebral fissures in the left eye is noted.

(sixth cranial nerve) and the superior oblique (fourth cranial nerve). Because both major vertical muscles are weak, the eye does not move up or down and is exotropic because of the weak medial rectus muscle. The levator muscle of the upper eyelid is also innervated by the third cranial nerve, and ptosis is usually present (Figure 220-13). The pupil will be large and nonreactive in complete third nerve palsy.

This rare disorder may be congenital (unknown cause) or the result of trauma or migraine. Other, less common, causes include intracranial tumor, viral illness, and posterior communicating aneurysm.

Brown Syndrome

Brown syndrome consists of an inability to elevate an eye when the eye is in adduction (Figure 220-14). The most common cause of this rare syndrome is a congenitally tight superior oblique muscle tendon complex, known as congenital Brown syndrome. Clinical findings include limited elevation in adduction, an exodeviation in attempted upgaze, and an ipsilateral hypotropia that increases in upgaze. Most patients with Brown syndrome have good binocular vision with a compensatory chin elevation and slight face turn away from the affected eye.

The management of true congenital Brown syndrome is conservative unless the vertical deviation in primary position is significant. In most cases, waiting until the child's vision is mature before performing surgery is advised because an induced strabismus after surgery is not uncommon and can lead to the loss of binocular vision.

Causes of acquired Brown syndrome include chronic sinusitis, trochlear inflammation (rheumatoid arthritis), glaucoma implant under superior oblique tendon in the superior nasal quadrant, or fat adherence syndrome. Virtually any periocular condition that results in limited elevation in adduction can appear as Brown syndrome. Acquired Brown syndrome is usually caused by an inflammation around the superior oblique tendon and trochlea often caused by chronic sinusitis. Pain and tenderness may be present in the superior nasal quadrant; the condition is often intermittent. Acquired Brown syndrome is treated by treating the sinusitis, if present, and providing oral nonsteroidal antiinflammatory drugs. Surgery is not usually indicated for acquired inflammatory Brown syndrome.

Double Elevator Palsy

Double elevator palsy is the rare congenital limitation of elevation of 1 eye, occurring sporadically without an inheritance pattern. The term *double elevator* implies paresis of the superior rectus muscle and inferior oblique muscle. However, this term is a misnomer; in 70% of cases, the deficient elevation is due to restriction that results from a tight inferior rectus muscle. Double elevator palsy may be mistaken for Brown syndrome, although the limited elevation in Brown syndrome is worse in adduction than in abduction.

Congenital Fibrosis Syndrome

Congenital fibrosis syndrome of the extraocular muscles is usually inherited as an autosomal-dominant trait. The cause is unknown, but this rare syndrome is associated with fibrotic replacement of extraocular muscle tissue. The clinical features may be classified

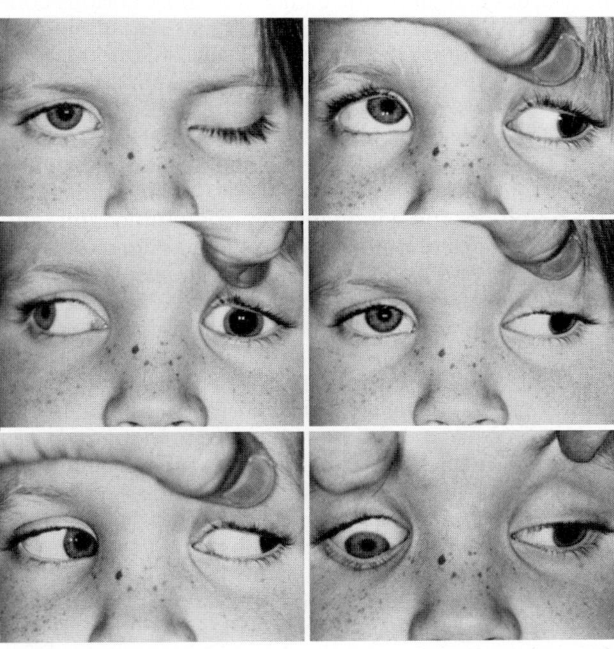

Figure 220-13 Left third nerve palsy. Patient with a left third nerve palsy illustrates the inability to adduct, elevate, or depress the left eye. Note complete ptosis and dilated pupil on the left.

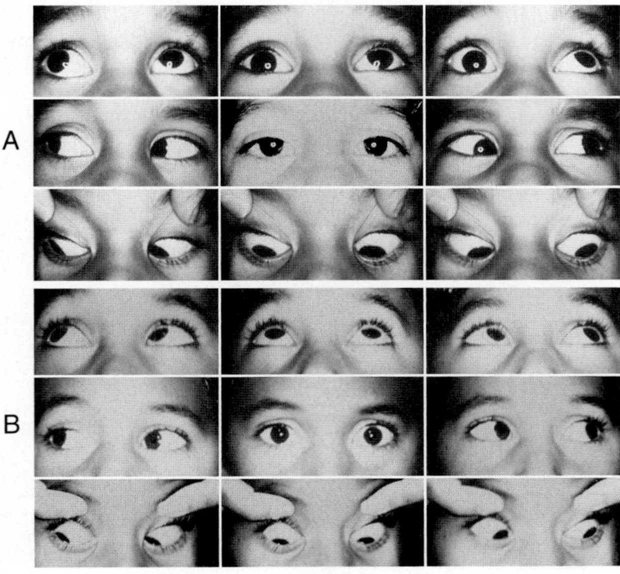

Figure 220-14 Patient with Brown syndrome in the right eye. **A,** Composite preoperative photographs show defective elevation in adduction. **B,** Postoperative photographs show normal eye movements after Wright superior oblique silicone tendon expander insertion.

into 5 groups: (1) generalized fibrosis syndrome, (2) fibrosis of inferior rectus with blepharophimosis, (3) strabismus fixus, (4) vertical retraction syndrome, and (5) unilateral fibrosis blepharoptosis and enophthalmos. Because of the tight fibrotic muscles, ductions are limited. The medial rectus muscle is most commonly affected, producing an esotropia, although the fibrosis can be generalized and can affect virtually all of the rectus muscles. Treatment is surgical recession of the fibrotic muscle. These cases can be technically difficult because exposure of the muscle is limited, especially in cases with a fibrotic medial rectus muscle.

WHEN TO REFER

- Any strabismus after 2 months of age
- Acquired strabismus
- Diplopia
- Limited eye movements (incomitant strabismus)
- Ptosis or other neurological signs
- Poor vision or abnormal red reflex

TOOLS FOR PRACTICE

Medical Decision Support

- *Pediatric Ophthalmology for Primary Care, 3rd edition* (book), Wright KW (www.aap.org/bookstore).
- *The Physician's Guide to Eye Care, 3rd edition* (book), Trobe JD (www.aap.org/bookstore).

REFERENCES

1. Archer SM, Sondhi N, Helveston EM. Strabismus in infancy. *Ophthalmology.* 1989;96:133-137.
2. Ing MR. Early surgical alignment for congenital esotropia. *Ophthalmology.* 1983;90:132-135.
3. Crawford MLJ, von Noorden GK. The effects of short-term experimental strabismus on the visual system in Macaca mulatta. *Invest Ophthalmol Vis Sci.* 1979;18:496-505.
4. Crawford MLJ, von Noorden GK. Optically induced concomitant strabismus in monkeys. *Invest Ophthalmol Vis Sci.* 1980;19:1105-1109.
5. Wright KW, Edelman PM, Terry A, et al. High grade stereo acuity after early surgery for congenital esotropia. *Arch Ophthalmol.* 1994;112:913-919.

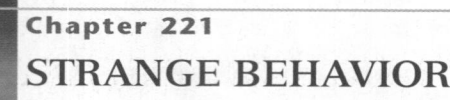

Chapter 221
STRANGE BEHAVIOR

Audrey M. Walker, MD

In the first 2 decades of life, the links among mind, body, and development are at their most complex and dynamic. Behaviors and thoughts that at one phase are entirely normal can be a harbinger of a serious pathology when they emerge in a different stage of development and with subtle differences in presentation. Furthermore, organic illness during childhood or adolescence may cause regressions or deviances in thinking and behavior, which may blur the clinician's understanding of the patient. The nuances of different cultural and belief systems can be interpreted as pathological thinking and behavior to the culturally naive observer. For all of these reasons, the successful collaboration between child psychiatry and pediatrics is crucial in the diagnosis and treatment of children.

In the past, the assessment of the child with organic illness has not been adequately informed by a sophisticated approach to the psychological issues of the patient, even though this set of diagnostic skills has been shown to improve the quality of care and decrease the pain and suffering of the child.[1,2]

INFANCY AND EARLY CHILDHOOD (BIRTH TO 5 YEARS)

The psychiatric assessment of children is unique in that the accurate evaluation of a psychopathological abnormality requires a firm grasp of the vagaries of normal development. At no time is this diagnostic endeavor more challenging than in the first 5 years of life, when keen observation must be combined with skilled and informed probing to identify abnormalities. In the assessment of infants and preschoolers, breaking down observations into the 4 categories identified by Gesell[3] is most useful: (1) motor skills; (2) language abilities; (3) personal-social abilities; and (4) adaptive functioning, which includes manipulation of objects, alertness, and hand-eye coordination. The Bayley scale,[4] which is a direct descendent of the work of Gesell, also breaks down infant assessment into useful subdivisions focusing on social communication, object constancy, and capacity for discrimination. Abnormalities in any of these areas can direct the clinician to more serious consideration of the major types of psychopathological abnormality found in infancy and early childhood.

Pervasive Developmental Disorder

Pervasive developmental disorder (PDD) is a neuropsychiatric disorder that is usually identified, when present, in the first 5 years of life. Specific deviances are noted in the language or communication and personal-social domains, with related abnormalities in stereotypic and repetitive behaviors. Approximately two thirds of children who have PDD are mentally retarded, but cognitive delay is not intrinsic to the diagnosis. The social abnormalities seen in PDD are present in the first year of life.

Children who have PDD have little interest in the human face or interactions with others. In many cases, this deficit in social interaction can be identified in the first year of life by the astute and experienced observer. The communication impairments seen in children who have PDD include abnormalities in verbal and nonverbal communication, such as delay in spoken and gestural language and the use of echolalia. Bizarre, restricted, and repetitive stereotypic behaviors such as flapping, spinning, and head banging are frequently seen. A subcategory of PDD, Asperger disorder, differs from the classical presentation of PDD in that language and cognitive functioning are preserved and social abnormalities and stereotypic behaviors are present.

Reactive Attachment Disorder of Infancy or Early Childhood

Abnormalities in the area of social relatedness are the hallmark of the child who has reactive attachment disorder; these abnormalities are rooted in grossly pathological care of the child in the earliest years of life. On the one hand, these children can display the inhibited type of reactive attachment disorder in which they appear withdrawn, hypervigilant, and resistant to all attempts to establish relatedness or to comfort. On the other hand, in the disinhibited type, children show indiscriminate, excessive, and superficial sociability. In both cases, the failure to develop developmentally appropriate attachment behaviors is obvious. In extreme cases, these children may also fail to thrive, with severe growth and cognitive delays or developmental deviances related to failure of caretaking and attachment.

Separation Anxiety Disorder

In separation anxiety disorder (SAD), the child experiences excessive anxiety of a magnitude that leads to disruptions in social or academic function when separated from home or from those to whom the child is attached. The child often refuses to go to school and is unwilling to travel independently or even to be separated from the parent for brief, developmentally appropriate activities such as play dates, sleepovers, or camping. The child with SAD will often shadow the parent and refuse to be on a different floor of the house or to sleep alone. Excessive worries, including the generation of frightening fantasies about misfortune occurring to the parent, are common. SAD must be distinguished from the developmentally appropriate anxiety of early childhood during the *rapprochement phase,* when the child, in the second year of life, shows normal separation and stranger anxiety. In addition, the cultural variations on acceptable child-from-parent separation must always be considered, as in traditional cultures in which great emphasis is placed on family interdependence.

Posttraumatic Stress Disorder

Posttraumatic stress disorder (PTSD) is one of the few entities in psychiatry in which a specific cause, the exposure to an extreme traumatic stressor involving direct personal experience of an event that involved actual or threatened death or serious injury, is necessary to the diagnosis. Although well established in adults, adolescents, and children, PTSD is a formidable challenge to diagnose in children younger than 5 years because the *Diagnostic and Statistical Manual of Mental Disorders,* 4th edition[5] (DSM-IV) criteria require verbal descriptions of thoughts and experiences that are difficult to obtain from young children whose language skills are limited. Terr[6] has made extensive clinical observations of the posttraumatic symptoms of early childhood and identified strongly visualized or repetitively perceived memories of the traumatic event, which can either take the form of the well-known *flashback* or be less intrusive in quality. Posttraumatic play, which is compulsive, repetitive, and grim and often incorporates a portion of the trauma known as *play reenactment,* differs from normal play in being much less imaginative and more rigid; it does not relieve anxiety or trauma-specific fears or change attitudes about people and life, characterized by excessive pessimism and hopelessness about the future.[7] Scheeringa et al[8] did a preliminary investigation to explore whether DSM-IV PTSD criteria accurately describe the symptoms of young, traumatized children and found that it did not. The authors suggested more objective, behaviorally anchored and developmentally sensitive criteria, including assessment of posttraumatic play and sleep disturbances and emergence of new aggressive and separation anxiety symptoms. (See Chapter 146, Posttraumatic Stress Disorder.)

Feeding and Eating Disorders of Infancy and Early Childhood

DSM-IV recognizes 3 feeding disorders in early childhood: (1) pica, (2) rumination disorder, and (3) feeding disorder of infancy or early childhood. Pica, the persistent eating of nonnutritive substances, is frequently seen in association with mental retardation and developmental disorders. The clinician should recognize that this practice is sanctioned in certain cultures and in this context would not be appropriately viewed as a pathological behavior. Rumination disorder is frequently seen in mentally retarded infants and children and is characterized by repeated regurgitation and rechewing of food. Feeding disorder of infancy or early childhood involves a persistent failure to eat adequately, judged by a failure to gain weight or significant weight loss over 1 month or more. Also known in the pediatric literature as *failure to thrive,* feeding disorder of infancy or early childhood must not result from a medical condition and is often associated with a parental psychopathological abnormality, child neglect, or abuse. Developmental disorders and extreme difficulties in temperament also may lead to feeding difficulties and must be distinguished from feeding disorders for proper management to occur. (See Chapter 179, Failure to Thrive.)

Cross-Gender Behavior and Gender Identity Disorder

A child's sense of gender identity, that is, the sense of being male or female, emerges in early childhood and is usually consolidated by age 3 or 4 years. Children who have clinically significant gender identity disorder (GID) commonly experience a persistent, pervasive desire to be of the opposite gender.[9] In DSM-IV, this disorder is defined as having 2 important components. The child with GID has a strong, persistent cross-gender identification, as well as a persistent discomfort with the child's own sex and a sense of inappropriateness in the assigned gender role. Boys with GID will assert that their genitalia are disgusting or that they wish them to disappear. Rejection of male stereotypical toys, games, and activities is common. This entity must be distinguished from developmentally normal failure to conform to stereotypical gender role behavior, such as the tomboyism of some latency age girls or cultural variants such as the effeminate style of the bohemian artist or dandy. These normal variants are usually distinguished easily from true GID by the lack of severe disgust with the individual's anatomy and assigned gender role and the absence of a strong identification with the other sex. (See Chapter 140, Children With Gender-variant Behaviors and Transgender Youth.)

Transitional Objects and Imaginary Companions

The existence of transitional objects and imaginary companions is a common experience of early childhood. In one study,[10] 65% of children between the ages of 3 and 5 years were found to have imaginary playmates, and 75% of children had transitional objects. Winnicott[11] first recognized and named the transitional object and defined it as a first possession used by the child as a defense against anxiety, which arises in the course of separation and individuation from the mother or primary caretaker. A soft object or stuffed animal, the transitional object will emerge at age 4 to 12 months and persist well into early childhood. This normal developmental element of early childhood is to be distinguished from the transitional phenomena and imaginary companions of the severely disturbed child. Children who have a history of severe physical or sexual abuse may develop symptoms of pathological dissociation or psychosis, which can include auditory hallucinations or imaginary companions. Unlike the more benign imaginary companion of the normal child, the hallucinatory experiences of the dissociative or psychotic child are threatening, frightening, and often express aggression toward others. The child feels little control over the experience and is often unable to distinguish between reality and this frightening product of the imagination. These experiences are not always easy to distinguish in early childhood and require assessment by an experienced child psychiatrist if doubt exists.

MIDDLE CHILDHOOD YEARS (5 YEARS TO PUBERTY)

The phase of middle childhood begins when the child enters elementary school and begins the stage of formal learning and participation in a structured peer group. In this developmental stage, the child emerges into the world beyond the family. Industriousness is called for in the acquisition of academic skills, social competence with peers, and a successful relationship with authority figures outside the family. One-to-one supervision by an adult gives way to the structured classroom setting, where formal rules of behavior within a distracting group of peers is the predominant experience of daily life. Several psychiatric disorders emerge or are more readily identifiable in this developmental stage and social setting. When assessing the school-aged child, the combination of a skilled interview and supporting information from parents, teachers, and other relevant reporters is necessary for an accurate understanding of symptoms. Middle childhood ushers in the period during which the disruptive behavior disorders emerge and gain clinical attention.

Attention-Deficit/Hyperactivity Disorder

Attention-deficit/hyperactivity disorder (ADHD) is one of the most prevalent and important psychiatric disorders of the middle childhood years. Current prevalence estimates for ADHD in the school-aged population are between 3% and 5%.[7] The core symptoms of ADHD according to DSM-IV require the onset of inattention and hyperactivity-impulsivity by age 7 years occurring in at least 2 settings. The symptoms must be more severe and frequent than those seen in a normal child at a comparable development level. Symptoms of ADHD tend to emerge once the child enters school, in part, because the highly structured setting, significant demands, and lack of one-to-one adult-to-child supervision all conspire to tax the limited attention and impulse control available to the child with ADHD. The most common entity that leads to a misdiagnosis of ADHD in children is the normal exuberance of early childhood. (See Chapter 137, Attention-deficit/Hyperactivity Disorder.)

Oppositional Defiant Disorder

Oppositional defiant disorder (ODD), a diagnosis that occurs frequently in children with ADHD, is characterized by a recurrent, severe pattern of negativistic, defiant, disobedient, and hostile behaviors toward authority figures lasting more than 6 months. The symptoms of ODD are seen invariably in the home and are frequently focused on one particular authority figure. The behaviors must be particularly frequent, severe, and persistent to prevent the inappropriate labeling of children exhibiting developmentally normal oppositionalism as being ODD.

Conduct Disorder

Conduct disorder is characterized by a repetitive and persistent pattern of behavior in which the basic rights of others, as well as social rules and norms, are violated.[5] Although mild antisocial behaviors can be developmentally normal in certain settings, such as the preschooler who is unable to play by the rules in structured games, in the school-aged child and adolescent, conduct disorder symptoms are grossly developmentally deviant and include aggressivity, deceitfulness, theft, serious rule violations, and property destruction. Children and adolescents who have conduct disorder are at high risk for developing antisocial personality disorder in adulthood. (See Chapter 138, Conduct Disorders.)

Dissociative Disorders

DSM-IV includes 4 diagnoses within the category of dissociative disorders, the most familiar to the nonpsychiatric clinician being dissociative identity disorder, also known as multiple personality disorder. The core of these disorders is the presence of pathological dissociation, which is defined as a disruption of the integrated functions of consciousness, memory, identity, or perception of the environment. Pathological dissociation can be transient or chronic, and its onset can be acute or gradual. The capacity for dissociation develops in childhood and is a normal process used in imaginative play. This normal process declines markedly by late adolescence. The key differences between the normal dissociation of a daydreaming child or a child in the throes of fantasy play and the pathological dissociation seen in the dissociative disorders are (1) amnesia for complex behaviors and (2) extreme forms of depersonalization, which is a subjective sense of being unreal, strange, or unfamiliar to oneself.[12] These symptoms rarely occur in healthy children or even in children who have psychiatric disorders other than the dissociative disorders. Although the prevalence of dissociative disorders in children and adolescents is unknown, clearly, childhood trauma, especially early sexual abuse, is the major risk factor for the development of pathological dissociation. Dissociation is a defensive coping mechanism that functions to protect the child against the extreme pain and vulnerability of severe childhood abuse; 85% to 100% of adults who have dissociative identity disorder have documented histories of severe childhood abuse.[13]

ADOLESCENCE

Adolescence is a developmental phase unique to human beings. In the human, hormonal and neurologic changes develop slowly over many years and culminate during puberty.[14] Adolescence is the psychological, social, and maturational process initiated by the biological event of puberty. With biological changes come several psychological and social changes, including preoccupation with the body, development of sexuality, social anxiety and increased importance of the peer group over parents and other adult figures, and the development of more abstract cognitive abilities.[15] All of these developments result in changes in thinking and behavior, which are unfamiliar and may at times be mistaken for psychopathology. Several major psychiatric disorders also occur typically in adolescence.

Major Depressive Disorder and Bipolar Disorder

Major depressive disorder is defined in the DSM-IV as the presence of a single major depressive episode, with 5 or more of the following symptoms lasting for at least 2 weeks and occurring daily: depressed mood for most of the day, markedly diminished interest or pleasure in almost all activities, significant weight loss or gain caused by a decrease or increase in appetite, insomnia or hypersomnia, psychomotor agitation or retardation, fatigue or loss of energy, feelings of excessive worthlessness or guilt, diminished ability to concentrate, and recurrent thoughts of death or suicide. Adolescents who have bipolar disorder characteristically have the occurrence of a major depressive episode before a first manic episode. A manic episode is a distinct period of abnormally and persistently elevated, expansive, or irritable mood lasting for at least 1 week and is characterized by symptoms that may include grandiosity, decreased sleep requirement, pressured speech, racing thoughts, agitation, and high-risk behaviors, including spending sprees, sexual promiscuity, and gambling. Although both major depressive disorder and bipolar disorder typically occur in adolescence, prepubertal manic and depressive disorders have been diagnosed more frequently in recent years and are associated with a more severe course.[16] In addition, milder forms of depressive and manic disorders exist and can be seen in adolescence. Finally, aspects of normal adolescent development in the psychological and cognitive area can gain clinical attention and be mistaken for an abnormality. The tendency toward egocentric, grandiose thinking and abstract theorizing is pronounced during adolescence. Obsessive, ruminative focus on the body or on the person's own thinking process can be mistaken for anxiety disorders, a hypomanic episode, or oppositional behavior. (See Chapter 143, Mood Disorders.)

Schizophrenia and Other Psychotic Disorders

Before the third edition of *Diagnostic and Statistical Manual of Mental Disorders,* published in 1980, all serious forms of childhood psychiatric disturbance were labeled schizophrenia. Over the last 20 years the label of psychosis has been significantly narrowed. The term *psychosis* currently implies a serious disturbance in an individual's reality testing, as evidenced by hallucinations, delusions, and disturbances in the form of thinking.[17] The narrowing of this diagnostic category has occurred in a climate of growing understanding that perception of reality differs in various developmental phases and, more broadly, in diverse cultural contexts. Psychotic disorders are very uncommon in prepubertal children and, when present, are harbingers of a poor prognosis.

In adolescence the frequency of schizophrenia increases dramatically, and the symptoms closely parallel those seen in adult-onset schizophrenia. DSM-IV identifies the characteristic symptoms of schizophrenia as being delusions, hallucinations, disorganized speech, grossly disorganized behavior, and the so-called negative symptoms, which include avolition, alogia, and affective flattening.[5] These symptoms are accompanied by significant occupational and social dysfunction. This severe picture is to be contrasted with the disturbances in reality testing seen in various phases of normal development. Transient hallucinatory experiences, often tactile or visual in nature, are commonly seen in early childhood and, in times of stress, in older children as well.[18] Magical, animistic thinking is common and developmentally normal in the preschool and early school-aged child. Imaginary companions and transitional objects imbued with lifelike qualities by the child are normal in early childhood. All such normal phenomena should gradually disappear by the end of middle childhood.

Eating Disorders

The 2 classic eating disorders, anorexia nervosa and bulimia nervosa, are psychiatric disorders of childhood that commonly occur in adolescence. The prevalence of eating disorders in adolescence has increased markedly over the last 50 years, and their signs and symptoms typically come to the attention of the pediatrician before any mental health intervention is sought.

In the eating disorders, both thinking and behavior are disturbed. Anorexia nervosa produces an intense fear of gaining weight or becoming fat, even when the patient is underweight, and a disturbance in the way in which body weight is experienced. The patient refuses to maintain body weight above a minimally normal level, defined in DSM-IV as 85% of expected body weight. Restricting food intake and a cycle of binge eating followed by purging are 2 forms of behavior used by patients with anorexia nervosa to inhibit weight gain. Methods of purging may include self-induced vomiting, excessive use of laxatives, excessive exercise, and use of diuretic medications and enemas. Patients with bulimia nervosa are typically within the normal weight range but often have had a prior period of anorexia nervosa. Bulimia nervosa is characterized by recurrent episodes of binge eating in which, during a discrete period, an excessive amount of food intake occurs accompanied by a feeling of total lack of control. The binge is then followed by purging behavior. Eating disorders are much more common in girls, with onset typically in later adolescence. They are seen mostly in Western industrialized nations and more typically in white, upper middle-class girls.[19] In puberty the need for the young girl to integrate the realities of menstruation, breast development, and the broadening of the hips can be a challenge that results in transient perturbations of body image and abnormal eating behaviors.[14] The distinguishing factors that identify eating disorders from the transient, developmentally normal process is the severity of the weight loss, the persistence of a disturbed body image, and in the case of anorexia nervosa, the loss of menses, which is necessary to make the diagnosis in female adolescents. (See Chapter 135, Anorexia and Bulimia Nervosa.)

SPECIAL CONSIDERATIONS

Extreme Temperament in Childhood

In the 1940s and early 1950s, Chess and Thomas[20] did their renowned work in identifying and describing the importance of temperament, or behavioral style, in the functioning of children. They identified 9 categories that defined temperament: activity level, rhythmicity or regularity, approach or withdrawal behavior, adaptability to new situations, threshold of responsiveness, intensity of reaction, quality of mood, distractibility, and attention span. Analyzing these categories, the authors identified 3 distinct temperamental styles: (1) the easy temperament, which encompasses a regular, easily adaptable child who displays a predominantly positive mood and only mild intensity; (2) the child who has the difficult temperament, behaviorally opposite of easy temperament and characterized by biological irregularity, withdrawal in reaction to novel stimuli, slow adaptability to change, predominantly negative mood, and high intensity (this group comprised 10% of Chess and Thomas's study group); and (3) the slow-to-warm-up temperament, also known as shy, which comprised 15% of the group; they were described as slow adapters who had significant withdrawal responses, low intensity, and frequent negative mood. The difficult child and the slow-to-warm-up child are developmentally and psychologically normal and yet, because of their being difficult to manage, can often be labeled as behaviorally disordered by caretakers and brought to pediatric attention. Although extremely negative temperamental features have not been found to be equivalent to psychiatric disorders in childhood,[21] they can predict poor psychiatric functioning in adolescence, particularly in the context of poor caretaker-child interaction or dysfunctional behavioral control among adult family members.

Medically Ill Child

"Where the defense mechanisms available at the time are strong enough to master the anxieties, all is well; where they have to be overstrained to integrate the experience, the child reacts to the operation with neurotic outbreaks; where the ego is unable to cope with the anxiety released, the operation becomes a trauma to the child."[22]

The pediatrician is a primary observer of the child in the sick role and is therefore in great need of an understanding of the emotional and developmental reactions to pain and illness that children exhibit. Studies and clinical observations in the areas of psychodynamic and cognitive development in children have been applied to the thinking and behavior of the medically ill child. This work has been helpful in the understanding of behavior of the child who has a medical illness and in the successful management of noncompliance in the pediatric setting.

Cognitive-developmental theory based on the work of Piaget and Inhelder defined a predictable sequence of stages by which cognitive concepts are acquired throughout childhood.[23] The sensorimotor stage of infancy through roughly the age of 2 years is when things exist only insofar as the child can act on them, and the ultimate cognitive outcome is the achievement of object permanence. From ages 2 through 7 years the child is in the preoperational stage, in which symbolic thought and representations, including language, develop. During this stage, thinking is not logical but rather egocentric and animistic. Only when the child moves into the third stage, the concrete operational stage, from ages 7 until the onset of puberty, does logical thinking take hold. Finally, in the formal operational stage, which begins at puberty, formal abstract thinking is the predominant mode of thought. Not all individuals reach the formal operational stage, even in adulthood.

In cognitive-developmental theory, a systematic and predictable sequence exists by which concepts of illness are acquired; this process is comparable to the acquisition of casual understanding described by Piaget for normal development.[23] An appreciation of the cognitive level of a child, and an understanding that children often regress to an earlier level of cognitive functioning under the stress of an illness, can be helpful to the clinician's understanding of what may appear to be very strange behavior in children who are ill. Symptoms such as enuresis, soiling, sleep difficulties, and separation anxiety, which existed previously and were overcome by the child, may recur and persist during the course of the illness. An example can be seen in the preoperational child who becomes ill with diabetes, for instance. Unable to embrace the causes of illness cognitively, the child's egocentric and magical thought processes lead to the belief that the disease is a punishment for previous *bad behavior*. The resulting feelings of guilt, shame, and anxiety pose major stumbling blocks to care, including exaggerated pain behavior and poor compliance with the medical regimen. In adolescence, when abstract thought first emerges, the reaction to illness may have a much different quality. For example, placed in a life-threatening medical situation, the adolescent may take on an obsessive, ruminative, darkly philosophical caste that may resemble clinical depression.

Other elements specific to the plight of the child with a medical illness also may predispose the child to unusual thinking and behavior. The experience of being nursed and a change in parental emotional climate, often with an uncharacteristic exclusive focus by the parents on the child, can cause great anxiety and may even be traumatic. Being forced into a passive role during hospitalization and medical procedures and being handled by the parent and medical or nursing staff as a much younger child can be upsetting to the child who only recently has acquired independent functioning and detachment of the child's body from the parents. The resulting anxiety can create a difficult, even intractable, patient.

WHEN TO REFER

When a high index of suspicion exists for a psychiatric disorder, referral to a child and adolescent psychiatrist should be made for a full diagnostic assessment.

Clinical situations in which immediate referral should be made:

- Suicidal ideation or intent
- Violence or serious recent history of violence
- Thought disorder and other psychotic symptoms
- Suspicion of serious substance abuse
- Pediatric depression
- Assessment for initiation or continuation of treatment with psychotropic medication

REFERENCES

1. Powers SW. Empirically supported treatments in pediatric psychology: procedure related pain. *J Pediatr Psychol.* 1999;24:131-145.
2. Lemanek KL, Kamps J, Chung NR. Empirically supported treatments in pediatric psychology: regimen adherence. *J Pediatr Psychol.* 2001;26:279-282.
3. Gesell A. *Mental Growth in the Preschool Child.* New York, NY: Macmillan; 1925.
4. Bayley N. *Bayley Scales of Infant Development.* New York, NY: Psychological Corporation; 1969.
5. American Psychiatric Association. *Diagnostic and Statistical Manual of Mental Disorders.* 4th ed. Washington, DC: The Association; 1994.
6. Terr L. Childhood traumas: an outline and overview. *Am J Psychiatry.* 1991;148:10-20.
7. Cantwell D. Attention deficit disorder: a review of the past 10 years. *J Am Acad Child Adolesc Psychiatry.* 1996;35:978-987.
8. Scheeringa MS, Zeanah CH, Drell MJ, et al. Two approaches to the diagnosis of posttraumatic stress disorder in infancy and early childhood. *J Am Acad Child Adolesc Psychiatry.* 1995;34:191-200.
9. Coates S. Ontogenesis of boyhood gender identity disorder. *J Am Acad Psychoanal.* 1990;18:414-438.
10. Singer JL, Singer DG. Imaginative play and pretending in early childhood: some experimental approaches. In: Davids A, ed. *Child Personality and Psychopathy, Current Topics.* New York, NY: John Wiley and Sons; 1976.
11. Winnicott D. Transitional objects and transitional phenomenon. *Int J Psychoanal.* 1953;34:89-97.
12. Lewis DO. Diagnostic evaluation of the child with dissociative identity disorder/multiple personality disorder. *Child Adolesc Psychiatr Clin North Am.* 1996;5:303-332.
13. Ross C. Epidemiology of dissociation in children and adolescents. *Child Adolescent Psychiatr Clin North Am.* 1996;5:273-284.
14. Group for the Advancement of Psychiatry, Committee on Adolescence. *Normal Adolescence.* New York, NY: Charles Scribner's Sons; 1968.
15. Anthony EJ. Normal adolescent development from a cognitive viewpoint. *J Am Acad Child Psychiatry.* 1982; 21:318-327.
16. Geller B, Luby J. Child and adolescent bipolar disorder: a review of the past 10 years. *J Am Acad Child Adolesc Psychiatry.* 1997;36:1168-1176.
17. Volkmar F. Childhood and adolescent psychosis: a review of the past 10 years. *J Am Acad Child Adolesc Psychiatry.* 1996;35:843-851.
18. Rothstein A. Hallucinatory phenomena in childhood: a critique of the literature. *J Am Acad Child Psychiatry.* 1981;20:623.
19. Steiner H, Lock J. Anorexia nervosa and bulimia nervosa in children and adolescents: a review of the past 10 years. *J Am Acad Child Adolesc Psychiatry.* 1998;37:352-359.
20. Chess S, Thomas A. Temperament. In: Lewis M, ed. *Child and Adolescent Psychiatry.* Philadelphia, PA: Williams and Wilkins; 1991.
21. Maziade M, Caron C, Côté R, et al. Psychiatric status of adolescents who had extreme temperaments at age 7. *Am J Psychiatry.* 1990;147:1531-1536.
22. Freud A. The role of bodily illness in the mental life of children. In: Eissler R, Freud A, Kris M, eds. *Physical Illness and Handicap in Childhood.* New Haven, CT: Yale University Press; 1977.
23. Schonfeld D. The child's cognitive understanding of illness. In: Lewis M, ed. *Child and Adolescent Psychiatry.* Philadelphia, PA: Williams and Wilkins; 1991.

Chapter 222
STRIDOR

Alfin G. Vicencio, MD; John P. Bent, MD

DEFINITION

Stridor is a high-pitched, monophonic noise caused by turbulent airflow through a partially obstructed extrathoracic airway, heard predominately on inspiration. Although obstruction of large intrathoracic airways (ie, main-stem bronchi, mid- and distal trachea) can produce a similar noise on expiration, these lesions are more thoroughly covered in Chapter 231, Wheezing, and will not be discussed here.

During the normal respiratory cycle, rhythmic expansion and contraction of the thorax leads to dynamic changes in thoracic pressures, allowing air to flow into and out of the lungs. (For a schematic representation, see Figure 231-1, Chapter 231, Wheezing.) During expiration the volume of the thoracic cavity decreases, thus creating positive pressures within the thorax. Airways located within the thorax are directly subjected to these positive pressures, and thus these airways are more prone to obstruction during expiration, leading to turbulent airflow and wheezing. On inspiration the thoracic cavity expands, resulting in negative intrathoracic pressures and improved patency of intrathoracic airways. However, because the intraluminal airway pressure drops to allow inflow of air, and because the extrathoracic airways (nose, nasopharynx, oropharynx, and larynx) may collapse from transmitted negative intrathoracic pressures, this portion of the airway is susceptible to obstruction, and thus stridor, during inspiration.

Because the extrathoracic airways extend from the nose to the proximal trachea, high-pitched laryngeal stridor must be differentiated from other abnormal inspiratory noises such as stertor, a noisy, rumbling-type noise similar to snoring, which can be heard with partial airway obstruction in the oropharynx or nasopharynx. Accurately recognizing stridor will facilitate the ensuing diagnostic tests, given that the offending lesion is likely to be in or around the glottic region, a relatively focused anatomic area.

DIFFERENTIAL DIAGNOSIS

Because stridor reflects obstruction of a large centralized airway and can range in severity from mild to life threatening, ensuring airway patency should precede the generation of a differential diagnosis. For the child who has signs of severe respiratory compromise—distressed appearance, severe retractions, nasal flaring, pallor or cyanosis, altered mental status—initial measures should focus on maintaining the airway and, if possible, relieving the obstruction. Only personnel skilled at airway management should attempt intubation, if required, and such a procedure should be performed in as controlled a setting as possible. In select situations for which medical intubation might prove difficult (ie, suspected epiglottitis in a patient with high fever, drooling, and severe respiratory distress), surgical support should be present before airway manipulation in the event that tracheostomy is required. Luckily, most cases of stridor that the general pediatrician encounters can be approached with a succinct, focused history and physical examination followed by directed diagnostic tests.

The most common causes of stridor in the pediatric age group, laryngomalacia and viral croup, can be easily recognized by the experienced clinician after obtaining a focused history and physical examination (see Evaluation). However, because the differential diagnosis of stridor is extensive and includes anything that obstructs the extrathoracic airway, a major challenge for the general pediatrician is identifying select patients who have less-common causes of obstruction and thus require specific diagnostic tests and different management (Table 222-1). For example, laryngomalacia, vocal cord dysfunction, subglottic stenosis, laryngeal papillomatosis, glottic cysts, laryngeal webs, subglottic hemangiomas, foreign bodies, retropharyngeal abscesses, and laryngeal fractures can all compromise the extrathoracic airway and cause stridor.[1] In most cases a careful step-wise evaluation by the astute pediatrician will lead to the correct diagnosis.

EVALUATION

History

Once airway patency has been ensured a focused history should be elicited. Age of initial presentation and a description of the events surrounding symptom onset can provide important clues to the underlying diagnosis. A commonly encountered patient is one whose stridor is preceded by fever, upper respiratory symptoms, and a *barky* or *seal-like* cough. This history, which may include repeated and similar episodes in the past, is consistent with viral croup and is easily recognized by an experienced pediatrician. Stridor beginning in the first few weeks of life that is present only during specific phases of alertness such as eating, sleeping, or excitement suggests congenital laryngomalacia as the underlying cause. Indeed, laryngomalacia is the most common cause of congenital stridor in infancy. In comparison, continuous stridor that begins soon after birth might suggest a congenital and fixed lesion such as a laryngeal web or, particularly in an infant with cutaneous hemangioma, subglottic hemangioma. Stridor that develops shortly after a prolonged intubation likely results from subglottic stenosis or granulation tissue and is often seen in premature infants who required mechanical ventilation during the neonatal period. A less-common but important patient to recognize is one with a history of Arnold-Chiari malformation or hydrocephalus. Because increasing intracranial pressure can result in bilateral vocal cord paralysis, such patients should receive appropriate and emergent care to prevent brainstem herniation. Similarly a stridulous toddler with a history of choking or placing small objects in the mouth should be evaluated for the presence of a foreign body. Recurrent respiratory papillomatosis is also usually associated with stridor or hoarseness 2 to 3 years after birth, although the infection is acquired through vertical transmission in the birth canal from maternal cervical human papillomavirus infection.

In addition to symptom onset the chronicity and progression of symptoms can help identify the underlying cause and can be particularly helpful for patients with presumed laryngomalacia or viral croup that does not follow the expected clinical course. Stridor caused by laryngomalacia is typically intermittent and worsens over the first several months of life. As the child becomes older, such episodes become less severe and less frequent. Indeed, for the majority of patients with laryngomalacia, symptoms will completely resolve by the first birthday. Similarly, stridor caused by viral croup tends to improve as the child, and thus the airway, grows. When the pediatrician is faced with a child whose stridor worsens or persists rather than improves, coexisting or alternate diagnoses should be considered, and appropriate diagnostic testing should be initiated. These children often have laryngopharyngeal acid reflux that aggravates their underlying condition. In addition, persistent symptoms may indicate different laryngeal abnormality. For example, mild stridor caused by a subglottic hemangioma may initially be attributed to a more common problem such as laryngomalacia. Similar to laryngomalacia, obstruction from a hemangioma tends to worsen after initial

Table 222-1 Causes of Stridor

	HISTORY	OBJECTIVE FINDINGS
Laryngomalacia	Develops in the first few months of life Intermittent episodes Present mostly when agitated or crying	Predominately inspiratory May be positional Obstruction of glottic space by collapsing supraglottic structures on laryngoscopy
Viral croup	Preceded by upper respiratory tract infection symptoms and fever No stridor between episodes May have history of similar episodes in past	Predominately inspiratory No change with position Steeple sign on neck radiograph
Subglottic stenosis	Develops after intubation or manipulation of airway May be continuous	Predominately inspiratory but often biphasic Flat inspiratory and expiratory loop on spirometry Subglottic narrowing on neck radiograph and direct laryngoscopy
Foreign body	Sudden onset May have a history of choking	Predominately inspiratory if obstruction is extrathoracic Foreign body may be visualized on radiograph if radio-opaque
Retropharyngeal abscess	Fever Difficulty swallowing	Often present with stertor May have drooling Retropharyngeal mass on lateral neck radiograph
Hemangioma	Worsening stridor History of cutaneous hemangiomas	May have cutaneous hemangiomas Subglottic obstruction on neck radiograph Hemangioma seen on direct laryngoscopy
Bilateral vocal cord paralysis	History of injury to both recurrent laryngeal nerves Arnold-Chiari malformation or increased intracranial pressure	No movement of vocal cords during laryngoscopy
Vocal cord cyst	Hoarse voice Chronic irritation to vocal cords or airway instrumentation	Cysts visible on laryngoscopy
Laryngeal papillomatosis	Maternal history of human papillomavirus infection Hoarse voice Can develop in the first several years of life	Papillomas visible on laryngoscopy
Laryngeal web	Develops shortly after birth (congenital) Develops after airway instrumentation (acquired)	Web visualized on laryngoscopy

presentation as the lesion enlarges. Unlike laryngomalacia, natural resolution of the hemangioma, and thus the stridor, may take several years rather than months. History of a hoarse voice or cry suggests glottic disease and might result from chronic irritation of the vocal cords. Other clues that suggest more ominous conditions include constant stridor, failure to thrive, difficulty swallowing, and severe and sudden onset of symptoms. Last, onset of stridor in an older child or adolescent with no previous history should prompt a more thorough evaluation.

Physical Examination

Laryngeal stridor represents airway obstruction at the level of the supraglottis, glottis, or subglottis. Although these anatomic regions can be difficult to examine without the use of specific diagnostic tests, several clues from thorough physical examination can

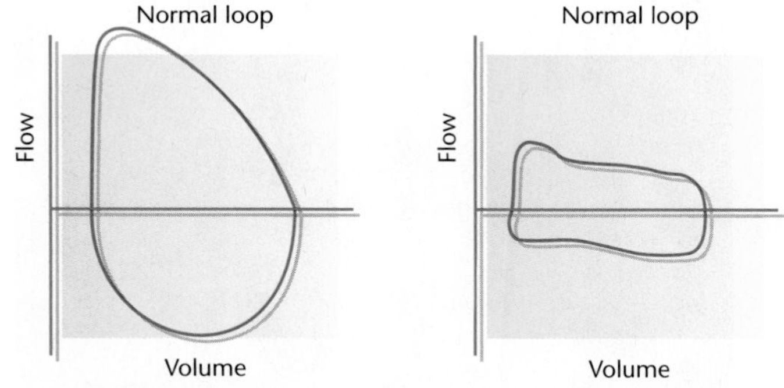

Figure 222-1 Findings on spirometry. The normal flow volume loop has a characteristic shape. In comparison, the flow volume loop in a patient with severe subglottic stenosis is flat.

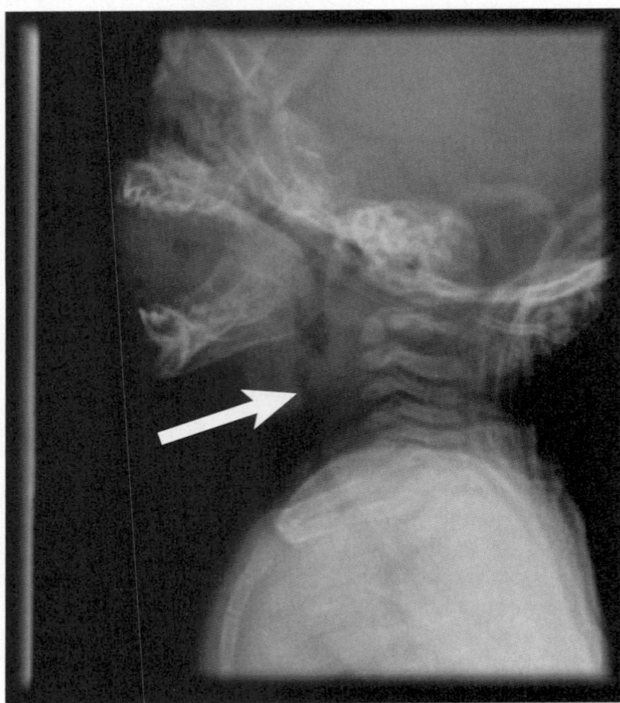

Figure 222-2 Neck radiograph. Neck radiograph demonstrates a mass causing mild obstruction of the subglottic area *(arrow)* in a child with stridor.

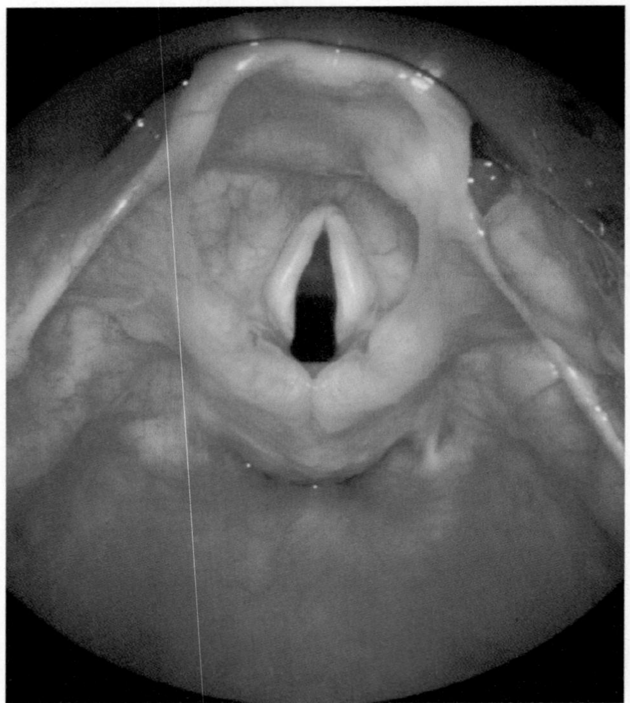

Figure 222-3 Normal larynx. Flexible and direct laryngoscopy offers a direct view of the glottis and can identify an abnormality. Shown here is a normal view of the glottis.

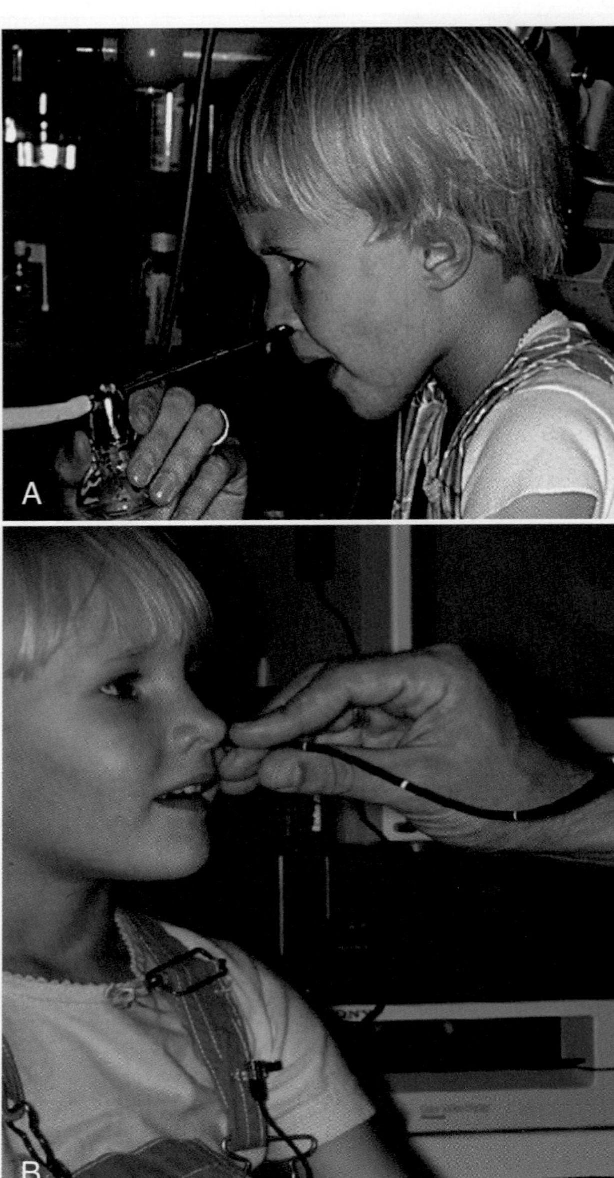

Figure 222-4 Flexible laryngoscopy. **A,** Topical anesthetic is applied before performing flexible laryngoscopy. **B,** The procedure is usually well tolerated when performed by an experienced laryngoscopist.

help confirm suspicions elicited on history. General inspection of the patient should include an assessment of position—extension of the neck is often described in patients with a serious infection such as epiglottitis or retropharyngeal abscess—as well as any drooling, which might suggest mass effect or edema in the posterior pharynx causing dysphagia in addition to the stridor (of note, these patients often exhibit stertor rather than stridor). Because such entities can be difficult or even dangerous to visualize, attention should focus on keeping the patient calm and maintaining the airway. An oropharyngeal

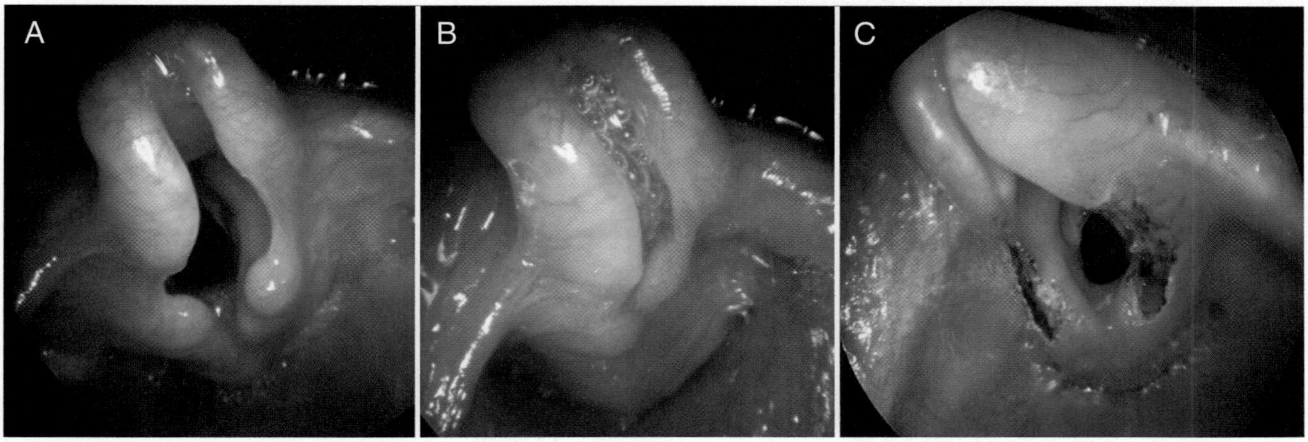

Figure 222-5 Laryngomalacia as seen by flexible laryngoscopy. **A,** During expiration the glottis is patent, and no abnormal sound is heard. **B,** During inspiration the epiglottis and arytenoids collapse and compromise the glottic opening, causing inspiratory stridor. **C,** In cases of severe laryngomalacia, surgical resection of redundant tissue can improve the glottic patency even during inspiration.

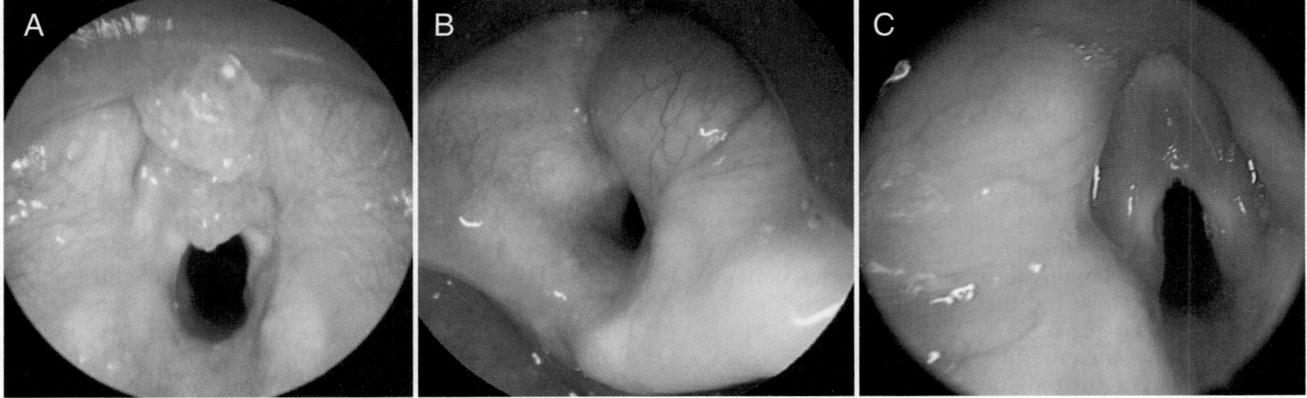

Figure 222-6 Obstructive lesions in the glottis. **A,** Laryngeal papilloma. **B,** Anterior saccular cyst. **C,** Glottic web.

examination might reveal a retropharyngeal bulge, an enlarged epiglottis or a lateral displacement of the uvula, and swelling of a tonsillar pillar from an underlying infection. External examination of the neck might show suprasternal retractions when obstruction is severe and may also reveal displacement of the larynx, a mass obstructing the airway, or signs of trauma. Finally, the quality of the voice should be noted, given that hoarseness, aphonia, or a weak cry suggests vocal cord disease.

Objective Testing

Although detailed history and physical examination are often sufficient to make a diagnosis of laryngomalacia or viral croup, additional diagnostic tests are warranted for patients whose symptoms and clinical course seem unusual or overly severe. Although laboratory testing has limited value in evaluating patients with stridor, *Bordetella pertussis* infection can sometimes cause laryngomalacia and can be diagnosed by means such as polymerase chain reaction or culture of pharyngeal secretions. Similarly, pulmonary function testing is not often necessary but can confirm suspicions of an extrathoracic obstruction (Figure 222-1). A simple radiograph of the neck can identify obstructive lesions in the retropharynx, glottis, and subglottic area (Figure 222-2). The classic *steeple sign* on anteroposterior neck radiograph depicts subglottic narrowing but does not distinguish croup from subglottic stenosis. Direct visualization of the airway by flexible laryngoscopy often provides definitive information.

Flexible laryngoscopy is a routine procedure for the practicing otolaryngologist. Because the procedure offers direct visualization of the posterior pharynx and glottis (Figure 222-3, normal glottis), numerous other lesions causing laryngeal obstruction can be visualized, leading to a correct diagnosis. In fact, before routine use of office based flexible laryngoscopy, laryngomalacia was known as *congenital laryngeal stridor,* reflecting physicians' incorrect

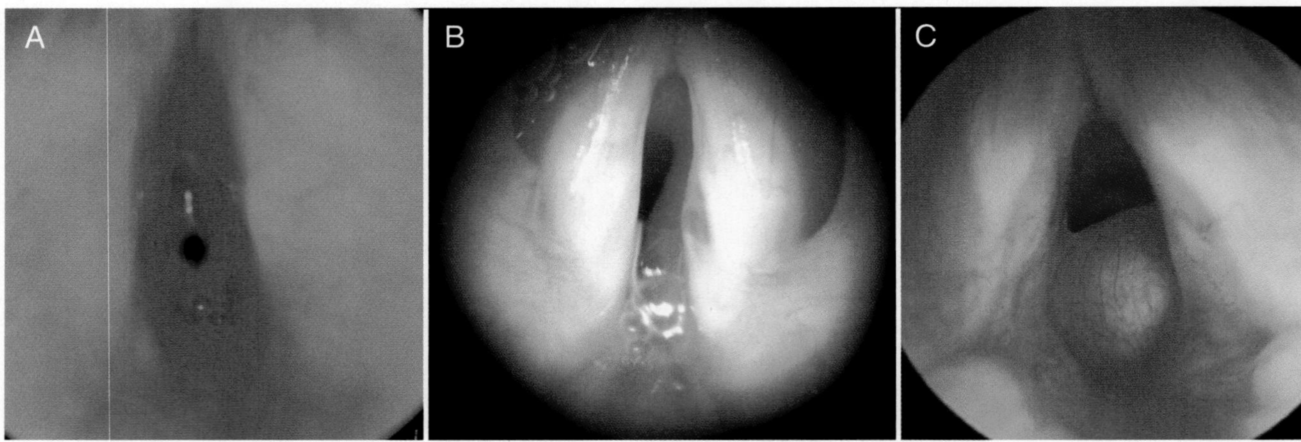

Figure 222-7 Obstructive lesions in the subglottic region. **A**, Severe subglottic stenosis. **B**, Right lateral subglottic hemangioma. **C**, Subglottic duct cyst.

assumption that all congenital laryngeal stridor might be attributed to a single cause. The procedure is usually well tolerated and can be performed most often with topical anesthesia alone (Figure 222-4). In many instances, laryngoscopy merely confirms the presence of laryngomalacia while excluding other causes of airway obstruction (Figure 222-5, *A* and 222-5, *B*). In cases of severe laryngomalacia, laryngoscopy can also identify specific structures of the larynx that are causing obstruction that might be amenable to surgical correction (Figure 222-5,*C*). Of course, direct visualization of the glottis can also identify other lesions that cause obstruction, as shown in Figure 222-6.

Importantly, successful flexible laryngoscopy is often dependent on patient cooperation, particularly with anxious, difficult-to-restrain, and younger school-aged children. Furthermore, although laryngoscopy often provides a clear view of the glottis and supraglottic structures, the subglottic area cannot be well visualized. Indeed, even with a cooperative patient, the presence of severe laryngomalacia might obscure the view of the subglottic area such that a more distal lesion would not be visible. In such cases, direct visualization of the subglottic region and proximal trachea may be indicated to exclude a second lesion. Direct laryngoscopy and bronchoscopy under sedation or general anesthesia can help diagnose and quantify the severity of subglottic stenosis or identify other subglottic lesions that cause obstruction (Figure 222-7).

MANAGEMENT

Because patients with laryngomalacia and viral croup are frequently encountered and will encompass the majority of patients with stridor the general pediatrician should be comfortable with outpatient management. Most cases of laryngomalacia can be managed with observation alone, with particular attention given to adequate caloric intake and weight gain. For patients with severe episodes of stridor causing hypoxemia or cyanosis, or if symptoms progress over time, additional diagnostic testing is indicated, and referral to a subspecialist may be warranted. In certain instances, laryngomalacia requires surgical management to relieve the obstruction caused by redundant epiglottic folds or arytenoid tissue (see Figure 222-5). Tracheostomy is rarely required. As with laryngomalacia, most patients with viral croup can be managed with close observation alone. For children with more severe obstruction (nasal flaring, retractions), racemic epinephrine and dexamethasone may temporarily relieve symptoms of obstruction and alleviate inflammation, respectively. Hospitalization is indicated for children with hypoxemia, apnea, or poor feeding or dehydration.

As discussed previously, stridor that is continuous, progressive, or severe should prompt the general pediatrician to initiate additional diagnostic tests. Referral to a pediatric otolaryngologist for further evaluation by laryngoscopy or bronchoscopy (or both) will facilitate diagnosis of other causes of glottic or subglottic obstruction, which might require surgical management. Laser therapy for a hemangioma or web can provide definitive cure, as can cricoid split and augmentation of the subglottic space for an acquired stenosis.

In summary, the pediatrician evaluating the child with stridor should (1) be aware of the various clinical entities that can present with stridor, (2) be able to recognize by history or physical examination patients who require further evaluation, (3) initiate simple diagnostic tests, and (4) refer to appropriate subspecialty physicians those children with unusual presentations or poor response to conventional therapies.

WHEN TO REFER

- Progressive or continuous stridor
- Poor weight gain or growth associated with persistent stridor
- Repeated hospitalization

- Presence of cutaneous hemangiomas in association with persistent stridor

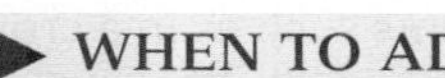

WHEN TO ADMIT

- Respiratory distress or hypoxemia
- Inability to eat or drink
- Altered mental status or signs of fatigue
- Stridor associated with signs of increased intracranial pressure

TOOLS FOR PRACTICE

Engaging Patient and Family

- *What is a Pediatric Otolaryngologist?* (fact sheet), American Academy of Pediatrics (www.aap.org/sections/sap/he3008.pdf).

SUGGESTED RESOURCES

Berkowitz RG. Neonatal airway assessment by awake flexible laryngoscopy. *Ann Otol Rhinol Laryngol.* 1998;107:75-80.

Botma M, Kishore A, Kubba H, et al. The role of fiberoptic laryngoscopy in infants with stridor. *Int J Pediatr Otorhinolaryngol.* 2000;55:17-20.

Friedman EM, Vastola AP, McGill TJ, et al. Chronic pediatric stridor: etiology and outcome. *Laryngoscope.* 1990;100:277-280.

Olney DR, Greinwald JH, Smith RJH, et al. Laryngomalacia and its treatment. *Laryngoscope.* 1999;109:1770-1775.

Vicencio AG, Parikh S. Laryngomalacia and tracheomalacia: common dynamic airway lesions. *Pediatr Rev.* 2006;27(4):e33-35.

REFERENCE

1. Bent J. Pediatric laryngotracheal obstruction: current perspectives on stridor. *Laryngoscope.* 2006;116:1059-1070.

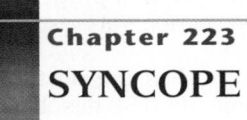

Chapter 223

SYNCOPE

Prema Ramaswamy, MD

DEFINITION

Syncope, defined as a transient sudden loss of consciousness and postural tone, is a fairly common complaint in children, particularly adolescents. Presyncope is the presence of sensory and postural impairment without the actual loss of consciousness. The origin of the word *syncope* is a Greek term meaning *to cut short* or *interrupt.* Regardless of the underlying disorder, syncope is caused by interruption of essential energy substrates to the brain, usually from a transient reduction in cerebral blood flow. In children and adolescents, syncope is most often benign; however, in rare cases, it can be a first signal of potential sudden death, and hence identifying patients at risk is critical. Even when the cause is benign, syncope can result in injury, and it certainly provokes anxiety.

Although the exact incidence of syncope in children is not known, it affects 3.5% of the general adult population. Almost one third of these adults will have recurrent syncope.[3] The corresponding numbers for children are not known, but recurrence appears to be less common in childhood.

CAUSES OF SYNCOPE

The most common cause of benign syncope is neurocardiogenic or vasovagal syncope, also termed the common faint, church faint, reflex syncope, or neurally mediated syncope (NMS). Another common cause of benign syncope is orthostatic hypotension. Together, these 2 causes are even more common in adolescents than in adults and account for almost 80% of all cases.[1] Both causes are more common in adolescence than at any other time in childhood. Syncope is also common from 6 months to 3 years, when breath-holding spells are prevalent. In particular, children with the pallid type of breath-holding spell have an increased risk of NMS as adults.[2] Syncope that is not benign can stem from cardiac, neurologic, metabolic, and psychiatric causes. Box 223-1 lists the causes of syncope.

Neurally Mediated Syncope

NMS is classified into 3 types[4]:

1. *Central syncope* occurs in response to strong emotional stimulation such as pain, anticipated pain, or the sight of blood. In susceptible individuals, emotional stimulation can activate ill-defined areas within the central nervous system that, in turn, trigger sympathetic inhibition and parasympathetic activation.
2. *Postural syncope* is associated with the upright position, typically developing while the person is standing or walking. It is the most common type of NMS, much more frequent than central or situational syncope.
3. *Situational syncope* occurs after the specific stimulation of sensory or visceral afferents, resulting in hypotension and then syncope. Examples include syncope evoked by the hypersensitivity of carotid baroreceptors, micturition syncope, defecation syncope, hair-grooming syncope, swallow syncope, cough syncope, and weight-lifter's syncope, all of which have been described in teenagers but are much less common than in adults.

Pathophysiological Features

Although the pathophysiological mechanism of NMS continues to be debated, investigators believe it occurs in persons with a predisposition when they experience peripheral venous pooling and a fall in venous return. An increase in catecholamine release follows as a compensatory mechanism. The primary abnormality in patients who faint is unclear but may include beta-adrenergic hypersensitivity, resulting in a relatively empty hypercontractile heart. Cardiac mechanoreceptors are stimulated, producing the Bezold-Jarisch reflex—a vagal response that includes sinus bradycardia, hypotension, and peripheral vasodilation. The syncope is termed *vasodepressor* if the more prominent element is hypotension, and *cardioinhibitory* if bradycardia is more prominent. In most instances, the syncope is mixed, with both hypotension and bradycardia.

Clinical Manifestations

In NMS of childhood, loss of consciousness is typically preceded by light-headedness, nausea, yawning, a feeling of being hot, and sounds appearing distant to

BOX 223-1 Causes of Syncope

NEURALLY MEDIATED SYNCOPE
Emotional
Postural
Situational:
- Deglutition syncope
- Micturition syncope
- Weight-lifter's syncope
- Defecation syncope
- Carotid sinus hypersensitivity
- Hair-grooming syncope

ORTHOSTATIC HYPOTENSION
Primary
Drugs
Pregnancy
Systemic mastocytosis
Familial dysautonomia
Postural orthostasis tachycardia syndrome

BEHAVIORAL OR PSYCHIATRIC
Hyperventilation
Hysteria, conversion reaction
Breath-holding spells
Cyanotic
Pallid infantile syncope

NEUROLOGIC
Seizure
Migraine
Trauma, concussion
Narcolepsy

CARDIAC
Structural abnormalities:
- Aortic stenosis
- Hypertrophic cardiomyopathy
- Tetralogy of Fallot
- Pulmonic stenosis
- Primary pulmonary hypertension
- Coronary artery abnormalities
- Marfan syndrome

Arrhythmia
- Bradycardia
- Sick sinus syndrome
- Atrioventricular block
- Supraventricular tachycardia
- Ventricular tachycardia, fibrillation
  - Myocarditis, pericarditis
  - Postoperative cardiac surgery
  - Prolonged QT syndrome

METABOLIC
Hypoglycemia
Anemia

the ear. Typically brief (from a few seconds to 1 or 2 minutes), the loss of consciousness is most often brought about by pain or by prolonged standing, especially in warm environments such as in a crowded room or in a hot shower. Occasionally, the cause is not identifiable. Symptoms characteristically appear after the person has been upright for at least a few minutes, in contradistinction to the patient with orthostatic hypotension whose symptoms occur within seconds of standing.

Orthostatic Hypotension

Orthostatic hypotension is the fall in blood pressure after assuming the upright position. The autonomic nervous system provides the principal responses to changes in position.[5] When a person stands, cardiac output and cerebral perfusion are maintained by a combination of pumping action of skeletal muscles, venous valves, and carotid baroreceptor–mediated arterial constriction and cerebral autoregulation. If these mechanisms are unable to maintain the blood pressure, then the decrease in the pressure in the carotid sinus leads to reduced afferent traffic in the carotid sinus and thus to an increase in the heart rate. The compensatory increase in heart rate is inadequate in patients with orthostatic hypotension, and symptoms of weakness and light-headedness develop, typically within seconds of standing. The sinus tachycardia of orthostatic hypotension sets this type of syncope apart from NMS, during which bradycardia is a prominent sign.

Volume depletion from any cause, but in children most often from vomiting and diarrhea, will exacerbate orthostatic hypotension. Drugs, which cause vasodilatation and diuretics, can also stimulate orthostasis.

Pregnancy should always be considered when a woman of childbearing age faints; pregnancy-associated fainting results from increased estrogen and progesterone levels that cause decreased peripheral vascular resistance and hypotension.

In the last few years, an entity called the postural orthostasis tachycardia syndrome (POTS) has been described.[5] The diagnosis of POTS requires orthostatic heart rate acceleration in excess of 120 bpm or an absolute increase of 30 bpm or greater in the absence of significant orthostatic hypotension. Two forms have been identified. In the more common peripheral variety, persistent tachycardia, associated with fatigue, exercise intolerance, and palpitations, is present while the patient is upright. The onset may occur after a viral illness, trauma, or surgery. The 2nd type of POTS, the beta-hypersensitivity (or central) form, is often associated with migraines, tremor, and excessive sweating. Both forms are more common in young women, and treatment can be frustrating.

Familial dysautonomia, an inherited autosomal-recessive condition with abnormalities of the autonomic nervous system, is a rare but serious cause of orthostatic syncope, with affected patients at risk for sudden death.

Behavioral or Psychiatric Causes of Syncope

Breath-holding Spells

Two types of breath-holding spells typically occur in children between 6 months and 3 years: (1) cyanotic and (2) pallid. In the former, an episode of cyanosis and apnea is precipitated after a child is upset and begins to cry. Stiffening of the body and a loss of consciousness may soon follow. Although the pathophysiological basis is unclear, crying during expiration may cause increased intrathoracic pressure, which, in turn, leads to low cardiac output. Hypoxia combined with decreased cerebral blood flow leads to the loss of consciousness. The event is brief, and afterward, the child becomes fully conscious. Pallid breath-holding spells (pallid infantile syncope) are less common and usually begin with sudden pain. The mechanism differs in that the child suddenly becomes pale and limp and loses consciousness. The pathophysiological basis is increased vagal tone, which causes an apparent asystole. The event ordinarily lasts only seconds to minutes, and the child awakens to full consciousness (also see Chapter 150, Temper Tantrums and Breath-holding Spells).

Hyperventilation

Another benign cause of syncope, hyperventilation is frequent among adolescents, especially in the presence of anxiety. The hyperventilation results in the washing out of carbon dioxide, and the resulting hypocapnia causes reduced cerebral blood flow, dizziness, and syncope. Classically, hypoventilation is also associated with numbness and parasthesias of the hands and feet.

Psychiatric Syncope

A child with hysterical syncope is likely to be unusually calm. No autonomic effects such as change in heart rate or blood pressure are noted during the episodes, which tend to be recurrent and frequent and to occur in front of an audience. Recovery of consciousness is often prolonged, and no injury is usually sustained.

Cardiac Syncope

Syncope can result from a low cardiac output secondary to either a structural problem or a dysrhythmia, and the abnormal rhythm underlying the syncope may be either too slow or too fast.

Bradyrhythmias

Sick sinus syndrome is extremely rare in a child with a normal heart and is usually seen after extensive surgery in the atria with the Senning and Mustard operations,[6] performed for transposition of the great arteries. Patients who have undergone the Fontan procedure for a single ventricle may also be at risk secondary to atriotomies and dilated atria.

Atrioventricular Block

Very slow heart rates from atrioventricular (AV) block can lead to syncopal episodes termed Stokes-Adams attacks. Congenital AV block in the presence of a structurally normal heart is most commonly associated with a history of systemic lupus erythematosus in the mother. The structural heart disease, which is most commonly associated with congenital AV block and has an ongoing risk of acquired AV block, is corrected transposition of the great arteries. AV block is also occasionally acquired after cardiac surgery or Lyme Disease.

Pacemaker Malfunction

In any child with a pacemaker, syncope should prompt immediate interrogation of the pacemaker for either a malfunction or inappropriate programming.

Tachyrhythmias

Supraventricular Tachycardia

The majority of children with supraventricular tachycardia have a structurally normal heart and in those children, palpitations and dizziness are more common symptoms of supraventricular tachycardia than syncope. However, with a structural abnormality resulting in reduced hemodynamic reserve, as with a single ventricle, syncope may be a presenting feature. In patients with congenital heart defects, Wolff-Parkinson-White syndrome is most often seen in children with disorders of the AV fibrous valve annuli such as Ebstein disease and corrected transposition of the great arteries.

Ventricular Tachycardia

Although ventricular tachycardia (VT) is rare in children, it can cause sudden death; early identification of underlying conditions that predispose to VT can be life saving. Prolonged QT syndrome is 1 such condition in which patients are at risk of sudden death secondary to a polymorphic VT termed Torsades de pointes. The prolongation of the QT interval may be part of a congenital syndrome such as Romano-Ward syndrome, which is autosomal dominant, or Jervell and Lange-Nielsen syndrome, which is autosomal recessive and associated with congenital neural deafness. Both syndromes are caused by mutations in genes encoding cardiac ion channels. Prolonged QT also may be caused by electrolyte imbalances, such as hypokalemia or hypocalcemia, and by a variety of drugs, such as tricyclic antidepressants, certain macrolide antibiotics, and antiarrhythmic medications. VT can also occur in children as a complication of myocarditis or in adolescents with Tetralogy of Fallot who have undergone surgical repair in infancy.

Structural Heart Disease

An acute reduction in cardiac output can result in reduced cerebral perfusion and syncope. With certain heart conditions, patients may be able to maintain an adequate cardiac output at rest but experience syncopal episodes with exercise.

Aortic Stenosis

An impediment to the forward flow of blood from marked left ventricular hypertrophy, stimulation of the ventricular mechanoreceptors resulting in systemic vasodilatation, and subendocardial ischemia causing a ventricular arrhythmia are all mechanisms that may contribute to syncope in children with severe aortic stenosis.

Hypertrophic Cardiomyopathy

Syncope with exercise may be an important presenting sign of hypertrophic cardiomyopathy. The majority of affected patients have no left ventricular obstruction at rest; however, with exercise, they can develop a dynamic gradient with an acute reduction in cardiac output. In addition, these patients may develop VT from subendocardial ischemia. The electrocardiogram is frequently abnormal, and an echocardiogram is diagnostic.

Tetralogy of Fallot

Children with unrepaired tetralogy of Fallot may have syncopal episodes in association with hypercyanotic *tet* spells, often precipitated by crying, straining with a bowel movement, or awakening from sleep.

Pulmonary Hypertension

With exertion, children with pulmonary hypertension may experience syncope from the inability to maintain transpulmonary flow.

Coronary Artery Abnormalities

A patient with syncope who is demonstrated to have a coronary artery aberrant either in its origin or course should be presumed at risk for sudden death. Typically, syncope occurs with exercise. Acquired abnormalities of the coronary arteries include coronary artery aneurysms and stenosis caused by Kawasaki disease in early childhood. Cocaine use can cause acute coronary vasoconstriction and ventricular arrhythmias, with consequent syncope.

Neurologic Causes of Syncope

Seizures

Typically, generalized seizures are preceded by a prodrome that includes tonic-clonic activity with loss of consciousness and a period of confusion and lethargy after recovery. However, atypical seizures can occasionally be difficult to differentiate from the benign forms of syncope. Loss of consciousness occurring in the recumbent position is more likely to be from a seizure than from syncope, especially if the heart is normal. Pallor is seen more often in benign syncope, and flushing is more common with seizures. Bowel incontinence points towards a seizure disorder.

Migraine

The primary care physician should always ask about migraine in a child who has a syncopal episode that does not fit the pattern of typical neural mediated syncope, particularly if dizziness occurs in the sitting position and no other provoking factors can be elicited. A history of flashing lights, severe headache preceding the episode of syncope, and a family history of migraines usually help clinch the diagnosis.

Head Trauma

Brief loss of consciousness with head trauma is not uncommon and is termed concussion.

Metabolic Causes

Hypoglycemia can cause syncope, most commonly in a child with diabetes on medication. Presyncopal symptoms such as weakness, a feeling of hunger, and confusion may be present, and the syncope is typically not brief. Dehydration and severe anemia also predispose the individual to syncopal episodes.

EVALUATION

History

The history is the most important tool in the diagnosis of syncope. It should include a detailed inquiry into the exact circumstances surrounding the event, including the time of the day, presence of an upper respiratory infection, time since last meal, posture during syncope and time spent in this posture before syncope, presence of prodromal symptoms, duration of loss of consciousness, bystander testimony, and any headache or prolonged disorientation after syncope.

Inquiry should also include the circumstances precipitating the event. For example, with vasovagal syncope, the child often is standing in a warm, stuffy room and is hungry, tired, or frightened. The prodrome of a seizure may consist of an aura, whereas a cardiac event often occurs without warning or is induced by exercise. The primary care physician should determine whether the child was completely unconscious or whether some degree of responsiveness was present, suggesting hysteria or malingering. A truly unconscious person will not respond if the eyelashes are lightly brushed; a hysterical person will respond, albeit often with just a mild flickering of the lids. Seizure-like movements are important; however, generalized tonic-clonic movements may be seen in any form of syncope. The duration of the episode should be estimated. In general, the conscious state is regained quickly in the case of vasovagal syncope (a few seconds to 1 or 2 minutes), whereas a seizure may last longer and the postictal state may be characterized by prolonged confusion and fatigue.

A history of congenital heart disease, seizure disorder, or endocrine abnormality such as diabetes would obviously be important. Recurrent syncopal episodes are unusual and may require more extensive testing.

The family history may be helpful. Seizure disorders and cardiac disease leading to syncope (eg, Marfan syndrome, hypertrophic cardiomyopathy, prolonged QT syndrome) may be inherited in an autosomal-dominant fashion. Breath-holding spells can also have a familial pattern.

Physical Examination

Examination of a patient with a history of syncope should begin with an assessment of the level of consciousness; a child who is not alert and oriented has not had a benign syncopal episode and needs immediate evaluation for potentially life-threatening causes. In most children who are fully alert after a syncopal episode, the findings on physical examination tend to be normal. The presence of a cardiac murmur may point to an obstructive lesion, such as aortic or pulmonic stenosis. Listening to the heart in both the supine and upright positions is important because a mild obstructive gradient in hypertrophic cardiomyopathy may become audible only when the patient is upright. The heart rate and blood pressure should also be obtained in both the supine and upright positions to ascertain the presence of orthostatic intolerance.

Evaluation

Electrocardiogram

The only test indicated in most patients with a history typical for benign syncope is an electrocardiogram, which may reveal the presence of AV block or a dysrhythmia. Abnormally large left-ventricular forces, especially with left-ventricular strain, may be the only evidence of hypertrophic cardiomyopathy in a patient with normal findings on physical examination. The corrected QT interval should be measured in all children with syncope or seizures to ensure that prolonged QT syndrome is not missed.

Holter and Event Monitor

A 24-hour electrocardiographic monitoring test is indicated only if a cardiac dysrhythmia is strongly suspected based on either prominent palpitations that occurred before the episode or the presence of cardiac surgical history that may predispose a child to abnormal rhythms. An event recorder is more practical because patients are able to keep the monitor for a month and use it at the time of their symptoms.

Echocardiogram

When a suspicion exists based either on history (eg, syncope with exercise) or on examination of a structural cardiac lesion, an echocardiogram is indicated and can usually adequately demonstrate the origin and course of the coronary arteries.

Electrophysiological Testing and Cardiac Catheterization

Electrophysiological testing and cardiac catheterization must be considered for any patient who has had syncope during active exercise in whom a physical examination, electrocardiogram, and echocardiogram have failed to demonstrate an abnormality.

Tilt-table Testing

By creating an orthostatic stress, tilt-table testing can provoke symptoms in patients with NMS and orthostatic hypotension. Patients are placed supine on a table that has a footboard. The table is then tilted up between 60 and 80 degrees for 30 to 60 minutes. Patients are monitored closely for a syncopal episode. Some centers use low-dose intravenous isoproterenol infusions to increase the sensitivity of the test, which ranges from 30% to 80%, depending on the laboratory. The specificity of a negative test without isoproterenol ranges from 80% to 100%.[7]

Although the utility of head-upright tilt-table testing in children is still controversial, it has become a means of provoking vasodepressor syncope in susceptible individuals after other more serious causes have been ruled out. Some indications[1] for the use of this test are:

1. Three or more syncopal episodes during a 12-month period with no evidence of heart disease
2. Syncope during exertion in which heart disease has been ruled out after an exhaustive workup
3. Recurrent syncopal episodes thought to be hysterical in nature

MANAGEMENT

The management of cardiac, neurologic, and psychiatric syncope depends on the cause. The management of NMS includes some of the following approaches.

Reassurance

The most important interventions for the majority of patients who have NMS or orthostatic hypotension are reassurance and education regarding the cause of the syncope and how to avoid aggravating factors (avoiding extreme heat and standing still for long periods). Patients should be instructed to sit down or lie down at the onset of any prodromal symptoms to avoid injury.

Isometric Exercises

In a small randomized trial of adults, intense gripping of hands and tensing of the arms for 2 minutes at the onset of the tilt-induced symptoms raised systolic blood pressure. Syncope occurred in 37% of these patients, compared with 89% in those who did not perform the maneuver.[8] The value of *tilt training* is still controversial, but it may be helpful to some patients; they are instructed to stand with their backs against a wall, initially for short periods, and slowly increasing the duration to approximately 30 minutes per day.

Volume Expansion

A reduced frequency of syncope in adolescents with neurocardiogenic syncope was reported after consuming 2 liters of water in the morning.[9]

Fludrocortisone is a synthetic mineralocorticoid that causes salt retention and the expansion of the central blood volume. One randomized trial in adolescents showed similar results to atenolol, but no placebo was studied.[11]

Beta-Blockers

Although beta-blockers have been used for many years as therapy for neurocardiogenic syncope, studies of their effectiveness have at best been equivocal.[10,11]

Investigational Agents

Mitodrine is a direct alpha-1 receptor agonist that has been shown to reduce episodes in adults with severely symptomatic neurocardiogenic syncope.[12] Because serotonin may have a role in regulating the sympathetic nervous system activity, selective serotonin reuptake inhibitors have also been considered for treatment of NMS. In a trial in adults, paroxetine was shown to be superior to placebo.[13]

Cardiac Pacing

Currently, cardiac pacing has a very limited role in the management of syncope. In pediatrics, cardiac pacing has been used for children in whom asystole is the prominent symptom in recurrent syncope caused by vagal hypertonia, including some patients with deglutition syncope.

WHEN TO REFER

- Patient history of cardiac disease
- Family history of sudden death, cardiac disease, or deafness
- Recurrent episodes
- Recumbent episode
- Exertional syncope
- Prolonged loss of consciousness
- Associated chest pain or palpitations
- Medications that can alter cardiac conduction

SUGGESTED RESOURCES

Grubb BP. Neurocardiogenic syncope and related disorders of orthostatic intolerance. *Circulation*. 2005; 111:2997-3006.

Kanter RJ. *Syncope and Sudden Death. The Science and Practice of Pediatric Cardiology*. 2nd ed. Baltimore, MD: Williams and Wilkins; 1998.

Krongrad E. Syncope and sudden death. In: *Moss and Adams' Heart Disease in Infants, Children and Adolescents*. 5th ed. Baltimore, MD: Williams and Wilkins; 1995.

REFERENCES

1. Kanter RJ. *Syncope and Sudden Death. The Science and Practice of Pediatric Cardiology*. 2nd ed. Baltimore, MD: Williams and Wilkins; 1998.
2. Prazar GE. Temper tantrums and breath holding spells. In: Hoekelman RA, ed. *Primary Pediatrics*. 3rd ed. Melbourne, Australia: Churchill Livingstone; 1994.
3. Savage DD, Corwin L, McGee DL, et al. Epidemiologic features of isolated syncope: the Framingham study. *Stroke*. 1985;16:626-629.
4. Mosqueda-Garcia R, Furlan R, Tank J, et al. The elusive pathophysiology of neurally mediated syncope. *Circulation*. 2000;102:2898-2906.
5. Grubb BP. Neurocardiogenic syncope and related disorders of orthostatic intolerance. *Circulation*. 2005;111: 2997-3006.
6. Krongrad E. Syncope and sudden death. In: *Moss and Adams' Heart Disease in Infants, Children and Adolescents*. 5th ed. Baltimore, MD: Williams and Wilkins; 1995.
7. Fouad FM, Sitthisook S, Vanerio G, et al. Sensitivity and specificity of the tilt test in young patients with unexplained syncope. *Pacing Clin Electrophysiol*. 1993;16:394-400.
8. Brignole M, Croci F, Menozzi C et al. Isometric arm counter-pressure maneuvers to abort impending vasovagal syncope. *J Am Coll Cardiol*. 2002;40:2053-2059.
9. Younoszai AK, Franklin WH, Chan DP, et al. Oral fluid therapy: promising treatment for vasodepressor syncope. *Arch Pediatr Adolesc Med*. 1998;152:165-168.
10. Sheldon R. The Prevention of Syncope trial (POST) results. Presented at Late-breaking Clinical Trials, Heart Rhythm 2004: 25th Annual Scientific Sessions, San Francisco, CA, May 19-22, 2004.
11. Scott WA, Pongiglione G, Bromberg BI, et al. Randomized comparison of atenolol and fludrocortisone acetate in the treatment of pediatric neurally mediated syncope. *Am J Cardiol*. 1995;76:400-402.
12. Perez-Lugones A, Schweikert R, Pavia S, et al. Usefulness of mitodrine in patients with severely symptomatic neurocardiogenic syncope: a randomized control study. *J Cardiovasc Electrophysiol*. 2001;12:935-938.
13. Di Girolamo E, Di Iorio C, Sabatini P, et al. Effects of paroxetine hydrochloride, a selective serotonin reuptake inhibitor, on refractory vasovagal syncope: a randomized, double-blind, placebo-controlled study. *J Am Coll Cardiol*. 1999;33:1227-1230.

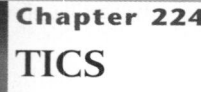

Chapter 224
TICS

Robert A. King, MD; John Scott Werry, MD

Tics, which are recurring, nonrhythmic, sudden, rapid, stereotyped, involuntary movements or vocalizations,[1] may be classified as motor or vocal and as simple or complex. The most common *simple motor tics* are eye blinking, neck twisting, shoulder shrugging, and grimacing; the most common *simple vocal tics* are coughing, throat clearing, sniffing, and grunting. *Complex motor tics* include more sustained, orchestrated, or seemingly purposeful gestures, such as touching, stomping on, or sniffing objects; jumping; sustained dystonic movements; copropraxia (obscene gestures); or echokinesis (automatic imitation of another person's movements). *Complex vocal tics* include sudden changes in volume or prosody; syllables, words, or stock phrases spoken out of context; palilalia (repeating one's own words); echolalia (repeating the words of others); and coprolalia (uttering obscenities).

The study of tics over the last 50 years is a fascinating microcosm of the history of psychiatry in that period. At first, lacking any definitive etiology or treatment, medicine considered tics to be psychological in nature. However, psychiatrists showed that tics are actually a neurobiological disorder, and as is the case with most medical disorders, they are not caused by but only worsened by psychological factors.

CLINICAL MANIFESTATIONS

The most common age at onset for tics is 6 or 7 years. The usual initial motor tics are blinking or facial grimacing, with subsequent rostral-caudal involvement. The most common initial vocal tics are sniffing, coughing, and throat clearing. Not surprisingly, these symptoms are often initially mistaken for allergies or otolaryngologic or respiratory symptoms; but with tics, the other characteristics of such disorders are absent. Characteristically, tics wax and wane in intensity and frequency, with one tic disappearing and new ones taking its place. Stress or excitement often exacerbates the tics.

Although children are generally unaware of their tics, premonitory urges[2] are often reported in more severe cases or in older children. Tics are often transiently suppressible with effort, usually resulting in an increased urge to perform the tic. Many patients describe their tics as neither fully voluntary nor involuntary[3]; some consider the effort to suppress tics in social situations as burdensome as are the tics themselves.

INCIDENCE

It once was believed that *Tourette syndrome* (TS) was rare, persistent, and disabling. That tic disorders, including TS, exist on a clinical spectrum from transient, isolated, inconsequential tics to more persistent multiple motor and vocal tics that interfere with daily functioning is now clear. Isolated and transitory tics are common (occurring in as many as 24% of first and second graders[4]) and of minimal consequence. Depending on ascertainment methods, childhood prevalence of TS is thought to be 2 to 185 per 10,000—much higher than previously believed, with many milder, uncomplicated cases not coming to clinical attention. Boys are affected more than girls, by a ratio as high as 9:1 to 14:1 in TS.[5]

ETIOLOGY

The cause of tics is unknown, but neurobiological and behavioral research shows the boundaries between psychiatry and neurology to be ill defined and increasingly obsolete.[6-8] Most of this research has been on

TS, rather than on milder forms of tic disorder. Areas of interest have been basal ganglia and cortico-striatal-thalmo-cortical circuitry,[9,10] genetics,[11,12] and immunology.[13,14] A multifactorial etiology for TS, with a convergence of genetic vulnerability, environmental and perinatal risk factors, and disturbances in the prefrontal cortex and basal ganglia, has been proposed.[10] Several factors have been shown to be associated with tics and may give clues to their cause.[6]

Developmental Stage

That tics, like all spontaneous movements, are common in middle childhood and usually begin to disappear by early adolescence points to maturation in the neuromuscular apparatus mirrored in the high frequency of all spontaneous movements, such as choreiform movements.

Sex

The preponderance of boys affected supports the motor developmental view because boys are more active in terms of motor movement than girls at all ages, but especially in middle childhood.[15] Androgens are implicated for the following reasons: postnatal exposure to androgens may elicit TS; antiandrogen therapy may improve tics; and androgen-dependent alterations in prenatal brain development may be associated with TS.[10]

Prenatal, Perinatal, and Postnatal Factors

Some association exists between severity of tics and the same risk factors that have been proposed for hyperactivity and certain other mental disorders, notably prenatal and perinatal factors (maternal smoking, vomiting and stress during pregnancy, drugs, fetal nutrition, low birth weight, and exposure to androgens).[16]

Experts have proposed that in some cases the acute onset of tics represents a form of Pediatric Autoimmune Neuropsychiatric Disorder Associated with *Streptococcus* (PANDAS).[13] This controversial hypothesis posits that group A β-hemolytic streptococcal infection can cause an autoimmune reaction that attacks the basal ganglia, resulting in tics or obsessive-compulsive disorder (OCD), or both. Despite much ongoing research, this hypothesized autoimmune condition remains unproven.[14] In the absence of a biological marker, distinguishing which cases might represent true PANDAS as opposed to the nonspecific coincidental occurrences of 2 common childhood conditions (streptococcal pharyngitis and tics or OCD) is difficult, at least at the onset. In one large study, children subsequently diagnosed with de novo tic disorder were found to have a greatly increased rate of streptococcal infections in the months before diagnosis.[2]

Pending further research to clarify this matter, the primary care physician can consider obtaining throat cultures from children with sudden onset or exacerbations of tics and from children with tics or OCD who have pharyngitis or who are exposed to *Streptococcus*. Children with positive throat cultures should receive appropriate antibiotic treatment. The role of repeat posttreatment cultures to prevent streptococcal carrier states is controversial, and the use of prophylactic antibiotic treatment has no firm basis in evidence. Plasmapheresis or intravenous immunoglobulin therapy are only suitable in intractable cases as part of an approved investigational protocol.[17]

Psychological Factors

Anxiety, stress, and excitement make existing tics worse and may even precipitate them; furthermore, children who have anxiety disorders are overrepresented in clinical samples.[15] Little is known about the psychological status of most children in the general population who have tics because they are rarely seen in clinics. However, evidence exists for increased autonomic lability in individuals with TS.[18]

Psychiatric Disorders

Defined psychiatric disorders should be distinguished from psychological or stress factors because of severity. Population and clinical studies of tics, as well as the occurrence of stimulant-induced tics in some children with hyperactivity, point to a strong relationship, most marked in TS, between tics and attention-deficit/hyperactivity disorder (ADHD).

A relationship also exists between tics (especially in TS) and OCD, with symptoms (eg, premonitory urges, intrusive thoughts, compulsive actions), putative anatomic locus (cortical, striatal, or thalamic circuits), hypothesized pathophysiological features (rogue reverberating microcircuits), and family pedigrees all showing elements in common.

Genetic Factors

Many cases of tics, especially TS, appear to be genetic in origin. Mild and transient cases of tic disorder may coexist in the same pedigree as cases of TS, suggesting that protective and risk factors also exist. Even with monozygotic twins, the concordance rate is only 77%, which suggests that environmental factors (eg, low birth weight) also play a role. The condition may well be heterogeneous and perhaps polygenic.[10-12] Penetrance increases if OCD is accepted as an alternative expression of the gene.

Drugs

Amphetamine and other dopaminergic drugs induce stereotypies in rats[19] and occasionally produce tics in children. Cocaine, other stimulants, sympathomimetics, caffeine, serotonin uptake inhibitors and other antidepressants, and anabolic steroids may also produce or exacerbate tics. Neuroleptic drugs can also produce tics or TS as a rare analog of tardive dyskinesia,[20] presumptively caused by hypersensitivity of dopamine receptors after chronic blockade.

Tics seem to appear spontaneously during middle childhood as exaggerations of spontaneous movements, which are common at this stage of development. The tics perhaps reflect manifestations of immaturity in dopaminergic or other systems. In some cases, notably TS, tics are probably the result of an as-yet-unestablished abnormality of the neuromotor system of genetic origin or, rarely, some other neurologic disorder. As with any other motor behavior, however, tics may be influenced by learning or conditioning, which may serve to prolong or shorten their course.

Tics should never be assumed to indicate another psychiatric disorder or psychological problem unless they are associated with other signs or symptoms that affect other areas of function beyond the motor system. Although tics can be controlled to some degree in public situations (eg, a physician's office), an affected child should not be expected to control them most of the time. Such control requires considerable mental energy and effort and usually cannot be sustained for long. As soon as the child relaxes, is distracted, or lets up concentration, the tics will reappear.

Referral is likely to be influenced as much by associated problems as by the tics themselves. The emphasis of treatment may thus focus less on tics per se than in mapping other areas of dysfunction.

DIFFERENTIAL DIAGNOSIS

Tics are usually distinguishable from other neurologic disorders by their stereotyped nature, variability over time, transient suppressibility, accompanying premonitory urges, and lack of other neurologic symptoms. The differential diagnosis includes dystonia, myoclonus, chorea, seizures, athetosis, and stereotypies.[21,22]

Tics are distinguishable from *chorea* (with which they are often confused) by their centripetal location, repetitive form, normal muscle tone, and lack of postural impersistence and from most other neurologically based abnormal movements by their rapidity and normal muscle tone. Even so, tics rarely reflect or portend a neurologic disorder.[21,22] Such tics are likely to be much more persistent and accompanied by signs of the disorder that causes them.

A more difficult diagnostic quandary in young children is distinguishing true tics from *stereotypies* or *self-stimulating behaviors,* such as rocking, head banging, flapping, or spinning. Tics are characterized by a later onset, lower complexity, fluctuating intensity and locus, and their intrusive, bothersome, disruptive, and involuntary nature. In contrast, stereotypies are bothersome to parents but not to the child, who finds them pleasurable and resists adult attempts to interrupt them. Self-stimulating movements mostly occur at times of boredom or excitement, but they rarely disrupt coordinated movements, and they persist without much change in form or location (see Chapter 217, Self-stimulating Behaviors).

The most recent edition of the American Psychiatric Association's *Diagnostic and Statistical Manual of Mental Disorders*[1] distinguishes 4 arbitrary subtypes of tic disorder: *transient* (duration longer than 4 weeks but less than 1 year); *chronic* (longer than 1 year); *Tourette disorder,* also known as Tourette syndrome (motor and vocal tics at least 1 year in duration with any remission <3 months); and *tic disorder not otherwise specified,* in which criteria of minimum duration of 4 weeks or frequency of many times a day and most every day are not met. Whether these 4 classifications reflect varying severity of the same disorder is unknown. Most recent research has been restricted to TS but suggests that these subtypes are probably related.

COMORBID DISORDERS

Persistent tics, even mild ones, appear to be associated with an increased risk of comorbid ADHD, which predates the tics or any accompanying OCD. This association is not simply the result of the bias toward comorbidity in clinical sample populations because it is also found in community sample populations.[23]

Individuals with TS are also at risk for other anxiety disorders, depression, fine-motor difficulties, and uneven cognitive profile (performance IQ scores lower than verbal IQ scores).[6,24] ADHD is common (present in 50% of patients with TS), and children with combined ADHD and tics have the greatest social and academic difficulties. ADHD severity is a better predictor of poor adjustment than tic severity.[25] Although the presence of ADHD with tics increases the likelihood of disruptive behavior and learning problems, chronic tics are often associated with learning impairment independent of ADHD. Investigations of both community and clinical sample populations confirm that the presence of ADHD predicts greater disability than that associated with tic disorders alone.

OCD is found in up to 50% of patients with TS, with compulsions and obsessions around symmetry, evening up, *just right* phenomena, sex, and aggression most common.[24]

TREATMENT

Most tics in children are mild and short lived and require no treatment. The possible role of any medications the child is receiving, such as stimulants, sympathomimetics, specific serotonin uptake inhibitors (SSRIs) and other antidepressants, neuroleptics, androgenic steroids, or any drug that interferes with dopamine, should be considered because their removal or reduction may be the required treatment.

Once a tic has persisted for several months, treatment may be considered, but only if the tic is conspicuous, disabling, or distressing to the child. No treatment for tics can be said to be simple, entirely effective, or free from side effects. Treatments shown to have some limited efficacy are discussed in the following sections.

Behavioral Methods

Although a variety of behavioral techniques (eg, relaxation, massed practice, avoidance learning) have been tried for tic disorders, only habit-reversal therapy appears to have good empirical support.[15,26-29] Habit-reversal therapy is best carried out by a psychologist who is experienced in the technique and who is used to working with children.

Anxiety-Reducing and Supportive Procedures

Relaxation training and biofeedback are not of proven value in treating tics. Psychotherapy (specifically focused on stressful interpersonal difficulties), work with parents, and other means of addressing environmental stresses may be helpful, not because stress causes tics, but rather because stress and high expressed emotion can exacerbate tics.[15] These procedures should not be considered specific; rather, they are ancillary and holistic in meeting therapeutic objectives.

Acceptance

In most cases, the best management is explaining to parents, teachers, and peers that the tics are a physical disability, that the child cannot help them, and that acceptance of both child and tics is the kindest, safest, and simplest way to deal with them.[15] Criticizing and belittling the child are likely to make tics worse and prolong their course. Peer problems can be a major difficulty for children with tics and TS,[25] and collaboration with school staff to reduce peer teasing and stigmatization is a major therapeutic task. In emphasizing that children cannot help their tics, the physician and parents should avoid the pitfall of concluding that the child cannot help other problematic behaviors related to impulsivity, for which firm expectations and structure may be desirable and beneficial.[24]

Pharmacotherapy

Only physicians thoroughly familiar with the drugs indicated and experienced in their use in children with tics should undertake pharmacotherapy.[6,8,30,31] The first consideration is deciding which symptom to target: the tics themselves or one of the common comorbid symptoms or conditions, such as OCD or ADHD, which are often a greater source of impairment.

Pharmacotherapy for Tics

Various medications are effective in partially suppressing tics, but they are not curative in terms of affecting the underlying course or prognosis of tics. Furthermore, because of frequent side effects (especially sedation), medication should be administered only when the tics are seriously disruptive, stigmatizing, or painful. The first mandate is to do no harm. In the case of tics, this approach means starting with low doses, titrating the dose upward only gradually, and avoiding sedation, cognitive blunting, or other distressing side effects (eg, acute dystonic reactions) that may be more burdensome than the tics themselves. Setting realistic goals in terms of reducing tics to tolerable levels is important; attempts to suppress tics completely often result in overmedication. Discontinuing anti-tic medications should be done gradually because even when medications appear ineffective, abrupt discontinuation may produce bothersome acute rebound or withdrawal-related exacerbation of tics that may persist for several weeks.

Many clinicians' first choice of anti-tic medication, especially in children with comorbid ADHD, is one of the α-adrenergic agonists, clonidine or guanfacine. Although these agents are less potent and are effective in fewer patients with severe tics than the neuroleptics, they are relatively benign, with principal dose-related side effects being sedation and hypotension. Guanfacine, when available, is the preferred first choice because it is longer acting and less sedating than clonidine, and it appears to be more effective for attentional problems.[32]

If the α-adrenergic agents are not effective or if the tics are severe, then the next line of agents is the dopamine-blocking neuroleptics, now known as antipsychotic drugs. These agents appear to be effective because tics, whatever their cause, are executed through the basal ganglia, with an apparent relative overactivity in the dopaminergic nigrostriatal systems that inhibits cholinergic basal ganglia systems. However, the neurochemistry of tic disorder is complex and probably involves several neurotransmitter systems; therefore inferring underlying deficits from the observed therapeutic effectiveness of various agents is difficult.

Of the traditional *typical* so-called *high-potency* (ie, nonatropinic) neuroleptics, haloperidol, pimozide, or fluphenazine seem to be preferred.[30,31] As with several of the other neuroleptics (eg, ziprasidone), caution must be taken with pimozide in terms of cardiotoxicity and drug interactions, especially with drugs such as erythromycin that are metabolized through the cytochrome P_{450} 3A4 isoenzyme system, because fatal drug interactions can result. Monitoring the QTc interval at baseline and with dose increases is prudent in patients receiving pimozide or ziprasidone. Even at relatively low doses, neuroleptics may produce acute dystonic reactions, sedation, cognitive blunting, medication-induced separation anxiety, parkinsonism, akathisia (restless legs), and, in the longer term, withdrawal or tardive dyskinesias, one rare type of which may be a worsening of tics caused by presumed dopamine-2 receptor hypersensitivity. If moderate doses are not effective, then higher doses are not likely to be either, and higher doses almost always increase the risk of side effects and make weaning the patient from the drug difficult without rebound exacerbation.

Although tardive dyskinesias are rare in children who receive modest doses of neuroleptics for tics, the traditional, or typical, antipsychotics are now being replaced by the newer so-called atypical antipsychotics,[26,31] which have less effect on dopamine receptors and thus appear to have a lower risk of tardive dyskinesia. However, atypical neuroleptics have the same other adverse effects as typical neuroleptics, including acute dystonic or extrapyramidal reactions. In addition, risperidone and olanzapine may cause hyperphagia and weight gain, with potentially serious metabolic consequences. Clinical trials have demonstrated the efficacy of risperidone, olanzapine, and ziprasidone for tics, but the lack of efficacy of the paradigmatic atypical neuroleptic clozapine indicates that not all atypical neuroleptics are equally effective.

When neither α-adrenergic agents nor neuroleptics are effective, a variety of second-line drugs or augmentation strategies may be tried with caution.[31] Although some neurologists use clonazepam to manage tic disorders, it should be used only in unusual instances in children. Like the other benzodiazepines, clonazepam can cause cognitive blunting, sedation, irritability, and disinhibition, and its use can lead to dependence and withdrawal symptoms.[30]

Tics should be treated pharmacotherapeutically only as a last resort and by a physician skilled in the use of the drugs concerned, ordinarily a child or adolescent psychiatrist or a pediatric neurologist. Such treatment should be carefully considered and discussed with parents, closely monitored, and undertaken only with knowledge and consideration of the risks and disadvantages involved.

Pharmacotherapy for Attention-Deficit/ Hyperactivity Disorder, Obsessive-Compulsive Disorder, Anxiety, and Depression

Pharmacotherapy for impairing comorbid ADHD, OCD, anxiety, or depression may be indicated in children with tic disorder, bearing in mind some considerations specific to tic disorder. Stimulants may increase tics or precipitate new tics; thus they should be used cautiously. Because ADHD is often more disabling than the child's tics, a cautious trial of a stimulant may be necessary, beginning with very low doses and increasing only gradually. Alternatives to the stimulants are the α-adrenergic agents (clonidine or guanfacine), atomoxetine (although this agent may also increase tics), or one of the second-line drugs such as the older tricyclic antidepressants (with appropriate electrocardiogram monitoring). Most children with tics and ADHD are able to tolerate methylphenidate, and the combination of methylphenidate and clonidine is better than either agent alone.[33]

The SSRIs appear to be effective in children with OCD and tics, although evidence suggests that monotherapy with the SSRIs is less effective in the presence of tics. In such cases, augmentation with a low dose of a neuroleptic often boosts the treatment response. In rare cases, SSRIs can exacerbate or even precipitate tics, akathisia, or other movement abnormalities, or can increase suicidal thinking.

MANAGEMENT

Most tics last only a few weeks, although they may flit from one muscle group to another or change their form at irregular intervals. Even the chronic tics of TS are likely to disappear in later adolescence, with tic severity peaking at age 10 to 12 or so.[34] Although most tics improve by late adolescence, OCD or ADHD symptoms may persist.[3,34] Because the prevalence of tics drops sharply after age 13, tics that persist into later adolescence are more likely to become chronic. Tic severity in adulthood is inversely proportional to caudate volume in childhood and to childhood performance on a dominant hand fine-motor skill test.[35,36]

Children with tics and especially TS can experience related problems of self-image when adult criticism and peer rejection result.[25] Occasionally, severe complex motor tics result in injury or self-mutilation. Finally, OCD may develop during adolescence or late in TS and can be a persistent source of distress despite the improvement in tic severity with age.[3]

Data from community surveys suggest that tic disorders, including TS, exist on a spectrum from transient to persistent multiple motor and vocal tics that in more severe forms interfere with daily living. The presence of isolated and transitory tics is common and appears to be of minimal consequence. On the other hand, persistent tics, even mild ones, appear to be associated with increased prevalence of ADHD, OCD, disruptive behavior, learning problems (although not necessarily a formal learning disability), and vulnerability to anxiety and depression.

Children should be referred to a specialist if the differential diagnosis is unclear, if a psychiatric disorder is present or is a possibility, if psychiatric drugs or treatments are needed, or if an expert opinion is required.

Criteria for referring children who have tics to a mental health specialist are the following: (1) presence of tics associated with additional evidence of psychiatric disorder, such as ADHD, generalized anxiety, or OCD; (2) presence of chronic or recurrent tics that seem to have a clear relationship to stress, particularly if a reason exists to believe that psychosocial interventions may be helpful; (3) presence of chronic, disabling, or discomforting tics for which differential diagnosis or treatment is needed; (4) when the primary physician knows little about tics and wants an expert opinion; or (5) when psychoactive drugs such as antipsychotics (neuroleptics) or clonidine may be indicated, because psychiatrists routinely use these medications and are well informed about risks, side effects, dose levels, and newer drugs.

Such referral may be only for consultation, not necessarily for continued management. In general, the preferred mental health specialist is a well-trained child or adolescent psychiatrist—one who has a broad biopsychosocial perspective, including a good grasp of neuropsychiatry and pharmacotherapy but who will not overprescribe and who has a capacity to work closely with behavioral psychologists. This kind of child psychiatrist should also be alert to the possibilities of the rare neurologically induced tics and will order any appropriate neuroimaging studies and neurologic consultations. When the tic is disabling and no further diagnostic work-up is required, or when pharmacotherapy is not an option or is already in place but further relief is necessary, referral should be made to a child psychologist experienced in behavioral types of treatment.[29]

Children should never be admitted to the hospital at the first instance for tics alone. Occasionally, for complex assessments, to initiate treatment, or to taper a child off high doses of multiple medications, children may be admitted.

WHEN TO REFER

- If the differential diagnosis is unclear
- If a psychiatric disorder is present or a possibility
- If psychiatric drugs or treatments are needed
- For expert opinion

WHEN TO ADMIT

- Never in the first instance (for tics alone)
- Occasionally, for complex assessments to initiate treatments or to taper a child from high doses of multiple medications

TOOLS FOR PRACTICE

Engaging Patient and Family

- *Tics* (book), American Academy of Pediatrics (www.aap.org/publiced/BK5_Tics.htm).

SUGGESTED RESOURCES

King RA, Scahill L. Emotional and behavioral difficulties associated with Tourette's syndrome. In: Cohen DJ, Jankovic J, Goetz C, eds. *Advances in Neurology. Vol 85: Tourette Syndrome and Associated Disorders*. Philadelphia, PA: Lippincott-Williams & Wilkins; 2001.

King RA, Scahill L, Lombroso P, et al. Psychopharmacological treatment of chronic tic disorder. In: Martin A, Scahill L, Charney D, et al, eds. *Pediatric Psychopharmacology: Principles and Practice*. New York, NY: Oxford University Press; 2003.

Kurlan R, ed. *Handbook of Tourette's Syndrome and Related Tic and Behavioral Disorders*. 2nd ed. New York, NY: Marcel Dekker; 2005.

Leckman JF, Cohen DJ, eds. *Tourette's Syndrome—Tics, Obsessions, Compulsions: Developmental Psychopathology and Clinical Care*. New York, NY: John Wiley and Sons; 1999.

Scahill L, Erenbert G, Berlin CM Jr, et al. Contemporary assessment and pharmacotherapy of Tourette syndrome. *NeuroRx*. 2006;3(2):192-206.

Spessot AL, Peterson BS. Tourette's syndrome: a multifactorial developmental psychopathology. In: Cicchetti D, Cohen DJ, eds. *Developmental Psychopathology*. 2nd ed. Vol 3. Hoboken, NJ: John Wiley & Sons; 2006.

Walkup JT, Mink JW, Hollenbeck PJ, eds. *Advances in Neurology. Vol 99: Tourette's Syndrome*. Philadelphia, PA: Lippincott Williams & Wilkins; 2006.

Woods DW, Piacentini JC, Walkup JT, eds. *Treating Tourette Syndrome and Tic Disorders: A Guide for Practitioners*. New York, NY: The Guilford Press; 2007.

REFERENCES

1. American Psychiatric Association. *Diagnostic and Statistical Manual of Mental Disorders*. 4th ed, Text Revision. Washington, DC: American Psychiatric Association; 2000.
2. Leckman JF, Walker DE, Cohen DJ. Premonitory urges in Tourette's syndrome. *Am J Psychiatry*. 1993;150:98-102.
3. Leckman JF, Bloch MH, King RA, et al. Phenomenology of tics and natural history of tic disorders. *Adv Neurol*. 2006;99:1-16.
4. Snider LA, Seligman LD, Ketchen BR, et al. Tics and problem behaviors in schoolchildren: prevalence, characterization, and associations. *Pediatrics*. 2002;110 (2 pt 1):331-336.
5. Tanner C. Epidemiology of Tourette's syndrome. In: Kurlan R, ed. *Handbook of Tourette's Syndrome and Related Tic and Behavioral Disorders*. 2nd ed. New York, NY: Marcel Dekker; 2005.
6. Leckman JF, Cohen DJ, eds. *Tourette's Syndrome—Tics, Obsessions, Compulsions: Developmental Psychopathology and Clinical Care*. New York, NY: John Wiley & Sons; 1999.
7. Walkup JT, Mink JW, Hollenbeck PJE. *Advances In Neurology; Vol. 99: Tourette's Syndrome*. Philadelphia, PA: Lippincott, Williams & Wilkins; 2006.
8. Kurlan R, ed. *Handbook of Tourette's Syndrome and Related Tic and Behavioral Disorders*. 2nd ed. New York, NY: Marcel Dekker; 2005.
9. Leckman JF, Vaccarino FM, Kalanithi PS, et al. Annotation: Tourette syndrome: a relentless drumbeat—driven by misguided brain oscillations. *J Child Psychol Psychiatry*. 2006;47:537-550.
10. Spessot AL, Peterson BS. Tourette's syndrome: a multifactorial developmental psychopathology. In: Cicchetti D, Cohen DJ, eds. *Developmental Psychopathology*. 2nd ed. Vol 3. Hoboken, NJ: John Wiley & Sons; 2006.
11. Pauls DL. An update on the genetics of Gilles de la Tourette syndrome. *J Psychosom Res*. 2003;55:7-12.
12. Abelson JF, Kwan KY, O'Roak BJ, et al. Sequence variants in SLITRK1 are associated with Tourette's syndrome. *Science*. 2005;310(5746):317-320.
13. Swedo SE, Leonard HL, Rapoport JL. The pediatric autoimmune neuropsychiatric disorders associated with streptococcal infection (PANDAS) subgroup: separating fact from fiction. *Pediatrics*. 2004;113(4):907-911.
14. Kurlan R, Kaplan EL. The pediatric autoimmune neuropsychiatric disorders associated with streptococcal infection (PANDAS) etiology for tics and obsessive-compulsive symptoms: hypothesis or entity? Practical considerations for the clinician. *Pediatrics*. 2004;113:883-886.
15. Werry JS. Physical illness, symptoms and allied disorders. In: Quay HC, Werry JS, eds. *Psychopathological Disorders of Childhood*. 3rd ed. New York, NY: John Wiley & Sons; 1986.
16. Mathews CA, Bimson B, Lowe TL, et al. Association between maternal smoking and increased symptom severity in Tourette's syndrome. *Am J Psychiatry*. 2006; 163(6):1066-1073.
17. King RA. PANDAS: to treat or not to treat? *Adv Neurol*. 2006;99:179-183.
18. Chappell P, Riddle M, Anderson G, et al. Enhanced stress responsivity of Tourette syndrome patients undergoing lumbar puncture. *Biol Psychiatry*. 1994;36:35-43.
19. Graybiel AM, Canales JJ. The neurobiology of repetitive behaviors: clues to the neurobiology of Tourette syndrome. *Adv Neurol*. 2001;85:123-131.
20. American Psychiatric Association. *Tardive Dyskinesia: A Task Force Report*. Washington, DC: American Psychiatric Association; 1992.
21. Jankovic J. Tourette's syndrome. *N Engl J Med*. 2001;345: 1184-1192.
22. Jankovic J. Differential diagnosis and etiology of tics. *Adv Neurol*. 2001;85:15-29.
23. Peterson BS, Pine DS, Cohen P, et al. Prospective, longitudinal study of tic, obsessive-compulsive, and attention-deficit/hyperactivity disorders in an epidemiological sample. *J Am Acad Child Adolesc Psychiatry*. 2001;40: 685-695.
24. King RA, Scahill L. Emotional and behavioral difficulties associated with Tourette syndrome. *Adv Neurol*. 2001; 85:79-88.
25. Bawden HN, Stokes A, Camfield CS, et al. Peer relationship problems in children with Tourette's disorder or diabetes mellitus. *J Child Psychol Psychiatry*. 1998;39(5): 663-668.
26. Piacentini J, Chang S. Habit reversal training for tic disorders in children and adolescents. *Behav Modif*. 2005; 29:803-822.
27. Piacentini JC, Chang SW. Behavioral treatments for tic suppression: habit reversal training. *Adv Neurol*. 2006; 99:227-233.
28. Wilhelm S, Deckersbach T, Coffey BJ, et al. Habit reversal versus supportive psychotherapy for Tourette's disorder: a randomized controlled trial. *Am J Psychiatry*. 2003; 160(6):1175-1177.
29. Woods DW, Miltenberger RG, eds. *Tic Disorders, Trichotillomania, and Other Repetitive Behavior Disorders: Behavioral Approaches to Analysis and Treatment*. Norwell, MA: Kluwer Academic Publishers; 2001.
30. Werry JS, Aman MG. *A Practitioner's Guide to Psychoactive Drugs for Children and Adolescents*. 2nd ed. New York, NY: Plenum Press; 1998.
31. King RA, Scahill L, Lombroso P, et al. Psychopharmacological treatment of chronic tic disorder. In: Martin A, Scahill L, Charney D, et al, eds. *Pediatric Psychopharmacology: Principles and Practice*. New York, NY: Oxford University Press; 2003.
32. Arnsten AF, Steere JC, Hunt RD. The contribution of alpha 2-noradrenergic mechanisms of prefrontal cortical cognitive function. Potential significance for attention-deficit hyperactivity disorder. *Arch Gen Psychiatry*. 1996; 53:448-455.
33. Tourette Syndrome Study Group. Treatment of ADHD in children with tics: a randomized controlled trial. *Neurology*. 2002;58:527-536.

34. Leckman JF, Zhang H, Vitale A, et al. Course of tic severity in Tourette syndrome: the first two decades. *Pediatrics*. 1998;102(1 pt 1):14-19.
35. Bloch MH, Peterson BS, Scahill L, et al. Adulthood outcome of tic and obsessive-compulsive symptom severity in children with Tourette syndrome. *Arch Pediatr Adolesc Med*. 2006;160(1):65-69.
36. Bloch MH, Sukhodolsky DG, Leckman JF, et al. Finemotor skill deficits in childhood predict adulthood tic severity and global psychosocial functioning in Tourette's syndrome. *J Child Psychol Psychiatry*. 2006;47:551-559.

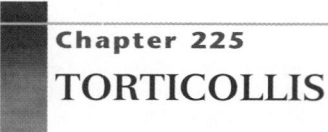

Chapter 225

TORTICOLLIS

Philip O. Ozuah, MD, PhD; Catherine C. Skae, MD

The word *torticollis* originates from 2 Latin words, *tortus*, which means *twisted*, and *collum*, meaning *neck*. The classic clinical picture of torticollis is that of the head tilted to one side and rotated in such a way that the chin and face point to the contralateral side. Torticollis can be broadly classified as either *congenital* or *acquired torticollis*. Facial asymmetry is often observed in congenital torticollis but not in acquired torticollis. This finding can thus be useful in clinically distinguishing between the 2 forms.

CLINICAL MANIFESTATIONS

Congenital Torticollis

Muscular torticollis is by far the most common form of congenital torticollis, and it occurs clinically in the first 8 weeks of life. It is frequently not obvious at birth but begins to become apparent at approximately 2 weeks of age.

Several theories have been proposed to explain the cause of this disorder. One theory suggests that stretching of the neck during a difficult delivery results in rupture and hemorrhage within the sternocleidomastoid muscle (SCM). Subsequent muscle ischemia results from increased pressure from the blood trapped within the fascial compartment, producing progressive muscle fibrosis and contracture, with eventual clinical torticollis. Support for this theory comes from the fact that approximately 40% of patients with congenital torticollis have had a difficult birth, including forceps delivery and breech presentation. However, congenital torticollis has also been reported in children after uncomplicated births. In addition, specimens of SCM in patients with torticollis have sometimes shown no evidence of trauma or hemorrhage. Another theory therefore is that torticollis results from an intrauterine position that occludes venous drainage from the SCM, leading to vascular congestion, ischemia, muscle damage, and fibrosis. This theory is supported in that 75% of congenital muscular torticollis cases are right sided because of intrauterine, left occiput–anterior positioning, and approximately 20% of patients who have congenital torticollis also have other musculoskeletal anomalies, including congenital hip dysplasias, talipes equinovarus, and metatarsus adductus.[1]

Congenital torticollis can produce some variation. Most commonly a sternomastoid tumor or pseudotumor is palpable as a characteristically nontender, soft, and mobile mass in or next to the inferior aspect of the SCM. The mass enlarges in the first few weeks of life, reaching its maximal size at 1 month of age. Thereafter, it begins to shrink until it disappears by 4 to 6 months. The mass then regresses and is replaced by a fibrous band, leading to contracture, which prevents normal growth and normal range of motion of the neck, and facial asymmetry results from the uneven growth forces. A second form of congenital torticollis involves thickening and tightness of the SCM itself.[2] Finally, *congenital postural torticollis* occurs without the presence of a palpable mass or tightness of the SCM.[3]

Acquired Torticollis

As with congenital torticollis, most cases of torticollis encountered in older children are primarily muscular in origin. Cervical muscle or ligament injury arising from trauma can cause a head tilt and unilateral neck tenderness, a condition that can also occur on awakening, presumably as a result of awkward positioning of the neck during sleep.

Benign paroxysmal torticollis is a disease of infancy with an unknown cause, although a familial pattern has been described. Manifestations of the condition begin in the first year of life with recurrent episodes of head tilt that may be associated with emesis, pallor, agitation, ataxia, malaise, and behavioral changes. Attacks may last from several hours to several days. Spontaneous and complete remission usually occurs by 5 years of age. Some patients, however, go on to develop migraines or benign paroxysmal vertigo.

DIFFERENTIAL DIAGNOSIS

The differential diagnosis of torticollis is listed in Box 225-1.

Congenital Torticollis

Several congenital cervical spine anomalies can occur in conjunction with torticollis. Most of these anomalies can be diagnosed by radiographic studies of the cervical spine. *Pterygium colli*, a congenital web of the skin of the neck extending from the acromial process to the mastoid, can be restrictive and result in torticollis. *Congenital remnant cysts* within the body of the SCM are a less common cause of torticollis. Unilateral absence of one SCM results in unopposed action of the other muscle and produces a contralateral torticollis.

Acquired Torticollis

Conditions that need to be considered in the differential diagnosis of acquired torticollis include cervical spine subluxations, infections of the head and neck (Grisel syndrome), neurologic disorders, and neoplasia. Laxity of the transverse cervical ligaments results in atlantoaxial instability in up to 15% of patients with Down syndrome.[4] Most of these children are asymptomatic, but subluxation of the cervical spine, most commonly a rotational atlantoaxial subluxation, may occur after trauma.[5] Nontraumatic subluxations of the atlantoaxial spine may arise as a result of head and neck infections or rheumatoid arthritis. The current theory is that inflammatory reactions around the spine

BOX 225-1 Differential Diagnosis of Torticollis

CONGENITAL
Muscular torticollis
Postural torticollis
Cervical spine anomalies
Hemivertebra
Atlantooccipital fusion
Klippel-Feil syndrome
Sprengel deformity
Pterygium colli
Sternocleidomastoid cysts
Cystic hygroma
Bronchial cleft cyst
Unilateral absence of sternocleidomastoid
Occipital condylar dysplasia

ACQUIRED
Muscular
Cervical muscle injury
Psychogenic torticollis
Benign paroxysmal torticollis
Vertebral
Atlantoaxial subluxation
Atlantooccipital subluxation
C2-C3 subluxation
Rotary subluxation
Cervical fractures
Cervical vertebral osteomyelitis
Rheumatoid arthritis
Acute cervical disk calcification
Eosinophilic granuloma

INFECTIOUS
Upper respiratory infection
Retropharyngeal abscess
Cervical lymphadenitis
Cervical vertebral osteomyelitis
Dental infections

NEUROLOGIC
Ocular torticollis
Spasmus nutans
Dystonic torticollis
Wilson disease
Syringomyelia
Labyrinthine torticollis
Accessory nerve palsy
Brachial plexus palsy
Arnold-Chiari malformation
Neoplastic
Cervical cord tumor
Posterior fossa tumor
Soft-tissue tumor
Histiocytosis X (Langerhans cell histiocytosis)
Infantile desmoid fibromatosis

OTHER
Sandifer syndrome
Dermatogenic torticollis
Spurious torticollis

produce hyperemia and edema, which, in turn, lead to laxity of the supporting ligaments and a predisposition to spontaneous subluxations and torticollis.

Torticollis may also arise from acute cervical disk calcification caused by trauma or an upper respiratory infection. *Ocular torticollis* may be caused by paralysis of the extraocular muscles, strabismus, nystagmus, and refractive errors. *Spasmus nutans,* also known as *nodding spasms* or *salaam spasms,* includes a triad of acquired nystagmus, head nodding, and torticollis, without a known cause. Signs and symptoms usually develop within the first 2 years of life and may persist for months to years. However, the clinical course often is benign and self-limited. A *dystonic torticollis* may follow the administration of several drugs, including phenothiazines, carbamazepine, and phenytoin. The presence of other extrapyramidal signs can often be used to distinguish between patients who have dystonic reactions.

Neoplasms associated with torticollis include cervical cord tumors and cerebellar tumors. Posterior fossa masses may exhibit similarly to spasmus nutans with nystagmus, head nodding, and torticollis. For patients with cerebellar tumors, however, ataxia is often a cardinal feature. *Sandifer syndrome* is an abnormal posturing that includes torticollis and opisthotonos. This syndrome is believed to be a protective mechanism adopted by some patients with one of several conditions, including gastroesophageal reflux, esophagitis, or hiatal hernia. *Dermatogenic torticollis* is a painful, stiff neck that results from extensive local skin lesions. Stiffness of the neck resulting from dental malformations and caries is called *spurious torticollis.*

EVALUATION

History

The first step in determining the cause of torticollis should be to obtain a thorough and detailed history. Particular attention should be given to duration of symptoms, previous trauma, presence of fever, and other systemic manifestations. In younger patients, the birth history is essential.

Physical Examination

Physical examination should not be limited to the head and neck areas but should include all organ systems. Findings such as craniofacial asymmetry suggest a congenital torticollis of long duration. The presence of webs or cysts in the neck should raise the suspicion of pterygium colli or remnant cysts. Patients with acquired torticollis as a result of trauma often have a tender SCM. Point tenderness over the cervical spine may suggest an underlying fracture or subluxation. Cervical vertebral osteomyelitis should be suspected in patients who have point tenderness in association with an unexplained fever.

Laboratory Evaluation

The presence of peripheral leukocytosis and increased sedimentation rate can be helpful adjuncts in diagnosing torticollis caused by infection or inflammation.

Imaging Studies

Imaging of the cervical spine should be obtained in all neonates with torticollis and in older children who have findings that suggest vertebral involvement or who have persistent torticollis. Ultrasound is the imaging modality of choice for initial evaluation.[6] Patients with neurologic deficits should undergo prompt computed tomography scanning or magnetic resonance imaging of the head and neck.

MANAGEMENT

Congenital muscular torticollis responds well to prompt conservative treatment during the first year of life.[7] Medical management includes passive and active stretching of the neck. *Gentle (passive) stretching* can be performed daily by the parents of the child or by a physical therapist. *Active stretching* is achieved by manipulating the infant environment in such a way that objects of interest are located on the opposite side of the room from the torticollis, inducing the infant to turn the neck in the desired direction.

Surgical correction is essential if the deformity persists beyond the first year of life, if range of motion is restricted more than 30%, or if residual craniofacial deformity exists.[8,9] Craniofacial asymmetry is best reversed at an early age when the child's growth potential is at its maximum. The surgical procedure that has the best results involves a bipolar tenotomy of the affected SCM, followed by casting or bracing to maintain the corrected posture.[10]

Acquired muscular or ligamentous torticollis is managed with local heat, massage, analgesics, muscle relaxants, and a soft cervical collar. Symptoms usually resolve in 7 to 10 days. Notably, however, patients with acquired muscular or ligamentous torticollis experience only mild discomfort. Any child with severe neck pain or tenderness over the vertebra requires immediate cervical immobilization until radiography can be performed to exclude the possibility of vertebral fracture or subluxation.

Drug-induced dystonic reactions are reversed by discontinuing the offending drug and administering intravenous diphenhydramine. The treatment of torticollis arising from other specific diseases should be directed at the cause.

WHEN TO REFER

- Presence of craniofacial asymmetry
- Radiographic evidence of cervical spine abnormality
- More than 30% restriction in range of motion
- Persistence beyond the first year of life

WHEN TO ADMIT

- Presence of neurologic deficits
- Severe neck pain
- Point tenderness over the vertebrae

TOOLS FOR PRACTICE

Engaging Patient and Family

- *Caring for Your Baby and Young Child: Birth to Age 5* (book), American Academy of Pediatrics (www.aap.org/bst).

SUGGESTED RESOURCE

Do TT. Congenital muscular torticollis: current concepts and review of treatment. *Curr Opin Pediatr.* 2006;18(1):26-29.

REFERENCES

1. Davids JR, Wenger DR, Mubarak SJ. Congenital muscular torticollis: sequela of intrauterine or perinatal compartment syndrome. *J Pediatr Orthop.* 1993;13:141-147.
2. Macdonald D. Sternomastoid tumour and muscular torticollis. *J Bone Joint Surg Br.* 1969;51:432-433.
3. Hulbert KF. Congenital torticollis. *J Bone Joint Surg Br.* 1950;32:50-59.
4. Pueschel SM, Scola FH, Pezzullo C. A longitudinal study of atlanto-dens relationships in asymptomatic individuals with Down syndrome. *Pediatrics.* 1992;89:1194-1198.
5. Msall ME, Reese ME, DiGaudio K, et al. Symptomatic atlantoaxial instability associated with medical and rehabilitative procedures in children with Down syndrome. *Pediatrics.* 1990;85:447-449.
6. Do TT. Congenital muscular torticollis: current concepts and review of treatment. *Curr Opin Pediatr.* 2006;18(1): 26-29.
7. Binder H, Eng GD, Gaiser JF, et al. Congenital muscular torticollis: results of conservative management with long-term follow-up in 85 cases. *Arch Phys Med Rehab.* 1987;68:222-225.
8. Slate RK, Posnick JC, Armstrong DC, et al. Cervical spine subluxation associated with congenital muscular torticollis and craniofacial asymmetry. *Plast Reconstr Surg.* 1993; 91:1187-1197.
9. Wolfort FG, Kanter MA, Miller LB. Torticollis. *Plast Reconstr Surg.* 1989;84:682-692.
10. Bharadwaj VK. Sternomastoid myoplasty: surgical correction of congenital torticollis. *J Otolaryngol.* 1997;26: 44-48.

Chapter 226

VAGINAL BLEEDING

Maria Trent MD, MPH; Alain Joffe MD, MPH

Assessing vaginal bleeding depends largely on the pubertal status of the patient. In prepubertal girls, vaginal bleeding probably reflects a localized problem in the vagina or uterus. In pubertal girls and young women, the differential diagnosis includes disorders affecting the hypothalamic-pituitary-ovarian (HPO) axis, complications of pregnancy, and local causes. In all cases, however, a complete history and thorough physical examination will provide important clues to the diagnosis.

PREPUBERTAL GIRLS

In utero, maternal estrogen diffuses across the placenta into the fetal circulation. After birth, estrogen levels in the infant fall, resulting in a physiological vaginal discharge that can be blood tinged or frankly bloody. No treatment, except reassurance, is necessary, and the discharge usually disappears within 10 days.

Several conditions can result in vaginal bleeding in the prepubertal child, including vulvovaginal infections, excoriations secondary to pruritus, foreign bodies, sexual abuse, trauma (eg, involving a straddle injury during bike riding), tumors, condylomata, hemangiomas, polyps, and coagulopathies.[1] If any suggestion of sexual abuse exists, such as bruises, hymenal tears, or other signs of trauma, then careful, nonthreatening questioning of the child or caretaker may reveal the necessity for a referral to child protective services for a forensic interview and examination.

Nighttime pruritus may indicate a pinworm infestation. The Scotch tape slide test, to look for pinworm eggs, can help establish *Enterobius vermicularis* infestation. If the presence of petechiae or numerous bruises is noted on physical examination, then platelet count and clotting studies are indicated to screen for a coagulopathy. A foreign body in the vagina should always be considered, even if no history of such exists. Contrary to popular belief, most girls who have bleeding from a foreign body do not have an associated foul-smelling discharge. The physician should also make sure that the bleeding is vaginal in origin, given that a prolapsed urethra can mimic vaginal bleeding.

If excoriation, erythema, or a rash in the perineal area is noted, then vaginitis is a distinct possibility. If a vaginal discharge is found and microscopic examination demonstrates large numbers of white blood cells, then vaginitis is highly likely. Concern about sexual abuse should prompt cultures for *Neisseria gonorrhoeae* and *Chlamydia trachomatis*. Other bacterial cultures may be necessary. For example, a history of diarrhea in the weeks preceding onset of the bleeding suggests vaginitis caused by *Shigella* organisms. Group A beta-hemolytic streptococcus can also cause vaginitis.

Vaginal bleeding caused by foreign bodies or vulvitis will respond to removal of the foreign body and proper perineal hygiene. Occasionally, systemic antibiotics may be necessary. Foreign bodies can often be washed out with a soft, flexible catheter; sharp objects should be removed carefully, under direct visualization. Referral to a gynecologist may be required if the patient is uncooperative. After removing a foreign body, bleeding should subside within 10 days. If it does not, then referral to a gynecologist is indicated. The entire foreign body may not have been removed, or a tumor, not readily visualized by the primary care physician, may be the actual cause of the bleeding. Similarly, if treatment of the presumed cause does not end the bleeding, then referral for a more thorough examination is indicated.

PUBERTAL GIRLS

Evaluation

Abnormal vaginal bleeding in pubertal girls can indicate a variety of disorders. Evaluation of this symptom depends on the nature of the problem: Is she bleeding between normal periods, or have her previously regular menses become more frequent or heavier? A teenager whose prior menses have been regular might possibly begin to have infrequent but heavy menstrual bleeding. In general, normal periods in adult women are 28 days apart (measured from the 1st day of one period to the 1st day of the next), with a range of 21 to 45 days and a flow of 3 to 7 days.[1] Flow greater than 1 week is considered excessive. A similar cycle pattern is observed in adolescent girls, but cycle length is more variable especially in the few years after menarche. Although the normal blood loss during menses is 30 to 40 mL, with an upper limit of 80 mL,[2] the quantity of blood loss is difficult to assess by history unless bleeding is scant.[3] Although the history should include an assessment of menstrual pattern and the quantity of pads or tampons used, laboratory assessment of hemoglobin, hematocrit, or both is useful for determining if significant blood loss resulting in anemia has occurred.

Normal menstrual function requires that the HPO axis function properly. Follicle-stimulating hormone (FSH) causes maturation of ovarian follicles, which produce estrogen. Rising levels of estrogen stimulate the endometrial lining of the uterus to proliferate and, at the same time, induce a midcycle surge of luteinizing hormone (LH) that causes the primary follicle to release an ovum, after which LH and FSH levels fall. The remnants of the follicle (termed *corpus luteum*) now produce progesterone, which converts the proliferative endometrium to a secretory phase. At the end of a normal cycle, the corpus luteum involutes, and both estrogen and progesterone levels fall. The endometrial lining is shed, and bleeding occurs.[4]

In adolescents, especially young adolescents, the HPO axis is relatively immature and highly sensitive to disturbance by several endogenous and exogenous factors; this perturbation leads to irregular bleeding. Among young adolescents (but in some older adolescents as well), the axis has not yet matured, and most cycles are anovulatory. Thus the endometrium proliferates under estrogen stimulation from the maturing follicle, but the midcycle LH surge is absent, ovulation does not occur, and the progesterone-secreting corpus luteum never forms. Toward the end of the cycle, the follicle involutes, estrogen levels fall, and bleeding occurs. Influenced by estrogen only, endometrial shedding is incomplete and irregular, accounting for the excessive bleeding of anovulatory cycles. Alternatively, fluctuating estrogen levels during an anovulatory cycle result in estrogen withdrawal bleeding. The occasional ovulatory cycle helps stabilize endometrial growth, and because the corpus luteum produces progesterone, a more organized withdrawal bleed occurs. Hence any condition that increases the frequency of anovulatory cycles is more likely to produce the kind of uterine bleeding that prompts the teenager to seek medical care.

Most teenagers who seek evaluation for genital bleeding in the first few years after menarche will have dysfunctional uterine bleeding (DUB), that is, abnormal bleeding not resulting from uterine disease, medications, systemic illness, or pregnancy. DUB is secondary to an immaturity of the HPO axis, with resultant anovulatory cycles.[3] Nonetheless, the primary care physician should search for other causes that affect the integrity of the HPO axis and can mimic DUB. Anovulatory cycles may also occur in patients with a mature HPO axis who have disorders such as polycystic ovary syndrome,[5] thyroid disease, or conditions resulting in hypothalamic amenorrhea (emotional stress, eating disorders, chronic illness, or intense athleticism). Additional causes of abnormal bleeding in this age group include disorders of pregnancy, other endocrine abnormalities, cervicitis, vaginitis, pelvic inflammatory disease, other sexually transmitted infections, foreign body, tumors, coagulopathies, drugs, and systemic disorders (Box 226-1).[2,3,6] Heavy bleeding at menarche, significant anemia, or the need to be hospitalized to control the bleeding increases the likelihood that a coagulopathy or another pathological condition is the cause of the bleeding.[4] Family history, however, has been shown to be a better predictor of coagulopathy than menstrual history.[7] DUB is considered a diagnosis of exclusion.

History

Most causes of vaginal bleeding or abnormal uterine bleeding (see Box 226-1) can be ruled out by history and physical examination. Maternal support during the initial history taking can be useful. Many mothers track the menstrual periods of their daughters in the early years and are acutely aware of quantity of bleeding based on the amount of feminine products purchased, stained laundry, evidence of fatigue, and general level of activity

BOX 226-1 Possible Causes of Abnormal Uterine Bleeding

PREGNANCY COMPLICATIONS
Spontaneous abortion
Ectopic pregnancy
Retained gestational products
Trophoblastic disease

COAGULATION DISORDERS
von Willebrand disease
Idiopathic thrombocytopenia

OTHER CAUSES OF THROMBOCYTOPENIA
Glanzmann disease
Leukemia

SYSTEMIC DISEASE
Renal failure
Hepatic failure
Malignancy

CONDITIONS OF THE REPRODUCTIVE TRACT
Vagina
Vaginitis
Trauma
Foreign body
Congenital anomaly (septum)
Neoplasia
Cervix
Cervicitis, erosion
Cervical polyp
Neoplasia
Uterus
Endometritis
Endometrial polyp
Submucosal leiomyoma
Arteriovenous malformation
Congenital anomaly
Neoplasia
Pelvis
Endometriosis

ENDOCRINE DISORDERS
Hypothalamus, pituitary
Immature hypothalamic-pituitary-ovarian axis
Hyperprolactinemia
Anorexia nervosa, malnutrition
Excessive exercise
Ovary
Polycystic ovary syndrome
Luteal phase abnormality
Premature ovarian failure
Neoplasia (hormone secreting)
Adrenal
Congenital adrenal hyperplasia
Cushing disease
Adrenal insufficiency
Neoplasm
Thyroid
Hypothyroidism
Hyperthyroidism

IATROGENIC
Hormonal medications
Anticoagulants
Neuroleptics
Intrauterine contraceptive device

From Emans SJ, Goldstein DP, Laufer MR. *Pediatric and Adolescent Gynecology.* 5th ed. Philadelphia, PA: Lippincott Williams & Wilkins; 2004. Reprinted by permission.

and behavior of the patient. They can also provide detailed family medical histories for first-degree female relatives, as well as that of their daughters.

Certain key aspects of the history may be difficult to obtain. A young woman may hesitate to reveal that she has engaged in sexual intercourse or that she has been sexually abused. The patient should be interviewed alone regarding sexual activity, sexually transmitted infections (including associated symptoms such as cramping, vaginal discharge, and dyspareunia), abuse, stress, weight changes and eating habits, participation in sports and other activities, chronic illnesses, other bleeding problems, medication use (particularly contraceptives), and substance use patterns. If a discharge is foul smelling and bloody, then a foreign body or retained tampon is likely; however, necrotic tumors can result in similar bleeding patterns. Pruritus or dysuria suggests vaginitis or cervicitis as the cause of the bleeding. Bleeding between periods is common during the first 2 or 3 cycles of oral contraceptive use and generally does not require any additional therapy; however, cervicitis secondary to *N gonorrhoeae* or *C trachomatis* infection or vaginitis secondary to *Trichomonas vaginalis* may also result in intermenstrual spotting. Young women who receive depot medroxyprogesterone acetate (Depo-Provera) injections often have frequent and irregular periods of excess bleeding, particularly in the first months after beginning use of this contraceptive method. Teenagers who forget to take 1 or 2 oral contraceptive pills may also have some bleeding.[2] Occasionally, women may have a small amount of bleeding or spotting after sexual intercourse, and some will have spotting around the time they ovulate. A complete family history is important to determine if other family members have any kind of bleeding problem. Complications of pregnancy (ectopic pregnancy or incomplete abortion) are more likely if a history of 1 or 2 missed periods exists, if the prior menstrual period was lighter than normal, if other symptoms of pregnancy are present (breast tenderness or nausea), or if the bleeding is accompanied by crampy, lower abdominal pain. A history of passing tissue or tissue present in the vaginal canal is also suggestive of complications of pregnancy. Blood dyscrasias, such as thrombocytopenia or von Willebrand disease, can cause heavy vaginal bleeding without other cutaneous manifestations of bleeding. Symptoms of endocrine disorders, such as cold intolerance, polyuria, nipple discharge, headache, acne, and increased facial hair, can be easily assessed using a comprehensive review of systems.

Physical Examination

The physical examination should include measurement of height, weight, and blood pressure, as well as thorough palpation of the thyroid gland. Visual field and funduscopic examinations are necessary to help rule out a prolactinoma. Increased facial hair is consistent with polycystic ovaries or an adrenal tumor. Striae suggest Cushing disease. An enlarged clitoris is consistent with an androgen-secreting tumor or late-onset 21-hydoxylase deficiency. Normal findings on physical examination, including pelvic examination, help rule out the many causes of vaginal bleeding or abnormal uterine bleeding listed in Box 226-1. Vulvar or vaginal bruising or lacerations suggest the probability of sexual abuse.[8,9] Lack of adnexal or cervical motion tenderness excludes pelvic inflammatory disease. If the ovaries are of normal size, then ovarian tumors or cysts are unlikely sources of the bleeding. A minimally enlarged uterus, consistent with early pregnancy, may not be noted by an inexperienced examiner. Endometrial polyps or submucous leiomyomas are distinctly unusual in women younger than 20 years, and they cannot be palpated by the examiner on the usual pelvic examination. If the patient has an intractably heavy flow, then the presence of one of these entities should be considered.

Laboratory Tests

For most cases of vaginal bleeding, relatively few laboratory tests are needed. A complete blood count with indices provides an objective measurement of the amount and duration of bleeding, and guides the treatment approach for patients with an otherwise negative evaluation. A urinalysis and urine pregnancy test should also be obtained. Bleeding associated with crampy lower abdominal pain may indicate ectopic pregnancy and a quantitative serum pregnancy test is indicated. Screening for *N gonorrhoeae, C trachomatis,* trichomonas, and bacterial vaginosis is indicated for sexually active patients. A pelvic sonogram is indicated if ectopic pregnancy is suspected, if a pelvic mass is found on bimanual examination, or if the pelvic examination is difficult.

Thyroid-stimulating hormone function tests, prolactin, LH and FSH levels, and coagulation tests should be ordered if hormonal therapy is contemplated. Any evidence of hyperandrogenism necessitates measurement of androgens, which may initially include free and total testosterone, and dehydroepiandrosterone sulfate. Coagulation tests such as a prothrombin time, partial thromboplastin time, and von Willebrand panel are indicated if the patient has profuse hemorrhage, menorrhagia at menarche, family history of bleeding disorders, or if unexplained heavy vaginal bleeding exists.

Management

Sexually transmitted infections are easily diagnosed and can usually be treated with antibiotics. The complications of pregnancy, such as threatened or spontaneous abortion, can be managed in the outpatient setting. However, a clinician experienced in the management of early pregnancy should be consulted. For patients with bleeding disorders, consultation with a hematologist may be required.

Most cases of vaginal bleeding in adolescent girls are caused by DUB. In other instances, the clinician must manage the bleeding without knowing the cause. Treatment decisions can be guided using the patient's clinical symptoms and the results of basic laboratory testing. Although some physicians may feel comfortable using hormonal therapy, others may prefer the guidance of a more experienced clinician. Because many adolescents with DUB are early adolescents accompanied by their parents, the primary care physician should include the parents in the decision to begin hormonal treatment in a non–sexually active patient. Assuring the parents that (1) combined oral contraceptives (COCs) are, in this instance, being used as treatment; (2) COCs are the most convenient way to package and deliver hormonal treatment; (3) short-term use of COCs for 3 to 6 months is anticipated; (4) and close follow-up will be provided during the treatment period, will often alleviate concerns about hormonal treatment and prevent rejection of these methods by the family. All patients with abnormal vaginal bleeding should be instructed to maintain a menstrual calendar to facilitate follow-up management.

Mild cases of bleeding that do not result in anemia and that do not greatly upset the patient and her parents can be managed expectantly with no immediate, specific therapy. Those who have mild anemia (hemoglobin value 11 to 12 g/dL) should receive iron supplementation. Some problems will resolve in 3 or 4 cycles. If the patient is sexually active, then oral contraceptive pills can be prescribed to treat the bleeding, as well as to provide contraception. Nonsteroidal anti-inflammatory agents, such as ibuprofen or naproxen, can also be used for their demonstrated antiprostaglandin effects. Patients with mild bleeding should be reevaluated in 6 to 8 weeks.

Hormonal therapy is indicated in teenagers who have moderate bleeding (enough to cause a decrease in hematocrit level to less than 34%). Girls who have menses every 1 to 3 weeks also need treatment. Treatment includes COCs or progestin alone. As previously mentioned, COCs are easier to use (one pill is taken daily every day of the month). If the patient has a condition in which COCs are contraindicated or this method is rejected by the patient or her parents, then medroxyprogesterone 10 mg orally can be given daily for 10 to 14 days, beginning on the first day of each month (calendar method) or on the fourteenth day of the menstrual cycle (day 1 being the first day of bleeding).[1] The patient with moderate bleeding should be reassessed in 4 to 6 weeks.

Patients with severe prolonged heavy bleeding accompanied by a drop in hemoglobin to 10g/dL or less need to be treated more aggressively. In this instance, adolescent medicine or gynecologic consult should be sought, clotting studies obtained, and hospitalization strongly considered.[10] For patients with severe bleeding, COCs (one tablet taken twice daily for 3 to 4 days) will generally stop the bleeding. However, prescribing a COC such as LoOvral every 4 hours may be necessary initially until the bleeding stops, then every 6 hours for 24 hours, then every 8 hours for 4 days, and then twice daily to complete 3 weeks of hormonal therapy. Antiemetic medications may be required to counteract the side effects of the high levels of estrogen contained in this regimen. A withdrawal bleed will occur 2 to 4 days after completion of this initial course of therapy. Patients with significant bleeding should avoid the placebo pills contained in the COC pill packs and continue continuous COCs until the hemoglobin and hematocrit begin to normalize. Iron and folic acid supplementation should be included as a part of the therapeutic plan.

The need for blood transfusion will depend on the hemodynamic stability of the patient. Although some clinicians prefer to use conjugated estrogens (25 mg intravenously every 4 hours) to stop the bleeding, use of LoOvral or a similar COC given 6 times a day and then gradually tapered to once a day over the next 7 to 10 days will usually stop the bleeding. Endometrial biopsy or dilation and curettage is rarely indicated. Even when these measures succeed in controlling the vaginal bleeding, these adolescents require long-term, close follow-up because an appreciable number of them will continue to have menstrual abnormalities.[10]

WHEN TO REFER

- If the patient is experiencing severe bleeding or initial attempts to control the bleeding by the primary care physician have failed
- If the vaginal bleeding appears to be secondary to a chronic illness that the primary care physician is unable to manage
- If the primary care physician feels uncomfortable performing a pelvic examination
- If long-term hormonal therapy is required
- If evidence of anatomical abnormality exists
- If evidence of a complicated endocrine disorder exists
- If evidence of a coagulopathy exists, especially if causing severe bleeding
- If evidence of a malignancy exists
- If evidence of sexual abuse exists

TOOLS FOR PRACTICE

Engaging Patient and Family

- *Puberty—Ready or Not, Expect Some Changes* (brochure), American Academy of Pediatrics (patiented.aap.org).
- *The Pelvic Exam* (brochure), American Academy of Pediatrics (patiented.aap.org).

RELATED WEB SITES

- American College of Obstetricians and Gynecologists (ACOG) (www.acog.org/).
- Young Women's Health Center, Boston Children's hospital (www.youngwomenshealth.org).

AAP POLICY STATEMENTS

Kellogg N, American Academy of Pediatrics, Committee on Child Abuse and Neglect. Clinical report: the evaluation of sexual abuse in children. *Pediatrics*. 2005;116(2):506-512. (aappolicy.aappublications.org/cgi/content/full/pediatrics;116/2/506).

American Academy of Pediatrics, Committee on Adolescence, American College of Obstetricians and Gynecologists and Committee on Adolescent Health Care. Menstruation in Girls and Adolescents: Using the Menstrual Cycle as a Vital Sign. *Pediatrics*. 2006;118(5):2245-2250. (aappolicy.aappublications.org/cgi/content/full/pediatrics;118/5/2245).

Committee on Sports Medicine and Fitness. Medical Concerns in the Female Athlete. *Pediatrics*. 2000;106(3):610-613. (aappolicy.aappublications.org/cgi/content/full/pediatrics;106/3/610).

REFERENCES

1. Treloar AE, Boynton RE, Behn BG, et al. Variation in the human menstrual cycle through preproductive life. *Int J Fertil.* 1970;12:77-126.
2. Emans SJ, Laufer MR, Goldstein DP. *Pediatric and Adolescent Gynecology.* 4th ed. Boston, MA: Lippincott-Raven; 1998.
3. Fraser IS, McCarron G, Markham R. A preliminary study of factors influencing perception of menstrual blood loss volume. *Am J Obstet Gynecol.* 1984;149: 788-793.
4. Speroff L, Fritz MA. Dysfunctional uterine bleeding. In: *Clinical Gynecologic Endocrinology and Infertility.* 7th ed. Baltimore, MD: Williams & Wilkins; 2005.
5. Franks S. Polycystic ovary syndrome. *N Engl J Med.* 1995; 333:853-861.
6. Claessens EA, Cowell CA. Dysfunctional uterine bleeding in the adolescent. *Pediatr Clin North Am.* 1981;28: 369-378.
7. Jayasingehe Y, Moore P, Donath S, et al. Bleeding disorders in teenagers presenting with menorrhagia. *Aust N Z J Obstet Gynaecol.* 2005;45:439-443.
8. Biggs M, Stermac LE, Divinsky M. Genital injuries following sexual assault of women with and without prior sexual intercourse experience. *CMAJ.* 1998;159:33-37.
9. Adams JA, Knudson S. Genital findings in adolescent girls referred for suspected sexual abuse. *Arch Pediatr Adolesc Med.* 1996;150:850-857.
10. Brawner NA, Koehler CSE. Abnormal uterine bleeding in the adolescent. *Adolesc Med.* 1994;5:157-170.

Chapter 227

VAGINAL DISCHARGE

Linda Meyer Dinerman, MD; Alain Joffe, MD, MPH

Vaginal discharge is a common complaint to pediatric practitioners. However, the presence of discharge is not necessarily abnormal; this symptom may represent the vagina's response to changes in estrogen levels, and the pediatrician need only reassure the patient and her parents. In most circumstances, the age of the patient, her pubertal status, and whether she has ever had sexual intercourse are key elements in sorting out the cause of the discharge.

NEWBORN PERIOD

In utero, the vaginal epithelium of the neonate is stimulated by maternal hormones that cross the placenta into the fetal circulation. After delivery, these hormone levels fall rapidly, and the parents may note a thick, grayish-white, mucoid discharge from the neonate's vagina. In many instances, the discharge is blood tinged or even grossly bloody. No treatment is needed, and the discharge usually resolves by 10 days of age.

PREPUBERTAL GIRLS

The genital area of prepubertal girls is more susceptible to infection than that of older, pubertal girls. The labial folds are smaller and lack pubic hair, and the distance between the vagina and the rectum is relatively short compared with adolescents and adults.[1] Low levels of circulating estrogen render the vaginal mucosa relatively thin and susceptible to irritation or infection. The alkaline pH (approximately 7.0) of the vaginal secretions affords a hospitable environment to bacteria, which together with poor perineal hygiene allows fecal flora to establish themselves more easily in the genital area. Box 227-1 lists causes of vaginal discharge in prepubertal girls.

Evaluation

When evaluating a premenarchal girl who has vaginal discharge, the physician should inquire about her hygiene. Wiping from the rectum toward the vagina brings intestinal flora to the vaginal introitus. Use of chemicals such as bubble baths, deodorants, or strong detergents to launder underwear can irritate the vulva and vagina. Occlusive nylon or rayon underwear provides a moist environment for potential pathogens, and the material itself can be an irritant. Although accounting for less than 5% of cases of vaginal discharge, the possibility that the child placed a foreign body, such as toilet paper, a coin, or a small toy, in her vagina should be considered. In such cases, the child has a discharge that can range from scant to abundant; can be white, brown, or bloody; and is frequently malodorous.[2]

BOX 227-1 Causes of Vaginal Discharge in Prepubertal Girls

Nonspecific vaginitis (the most common cause)

Irritative (bubble baths, sand); the vulva is often involved as well. Nonabsorbent, occlusive clothing such as nylon undergarments, tights, bathing suits also irritate the vulva, leading to skin breakdown and infection. Although uncommon, *Candida* infections can arise under these circumstances.

Poor perineal hygiene

Foreign body

Associated systemic illness (group A streptococci, varicella)

Other respiratory pathogens (eg, *Haemophilus influenzae*) may also cause discharge

Enteric infections

Escherichia coli with foreign body

Shigella organisms

Yersinia organisms

Enterobius vermicularis

Sexually transmitted infections (strong presumption of sexual abuse)

Neisseria gonorrhoeae

Trichomonas vaginalis

Chlamydia trachomatis (Whether this organism alone can cause discharge is unclear. *C trachomatis* is often isolated in conjunction with *N gonorrhoeae.*)

Primary vulvar skin disease

Tumor, polyps (rare)

Table 227-1 Major Causes of Vaginal Discharge in Pubertal Girls

AGENT	DISCHARGE	ODOR; PH	DYSURIA; PRURITUS
Candida albicans	Thick, white, curdlike, *cheesy*	None usually; pH 4.5 (obtained from midvagina with nitrazine paper)	Dysuria frequent; pruritus (4+)
Trichomonas vaginalis	Frothy; yellow green or gray	Foul smelling; pH 5.2-5.5	Dysuria frequent; pruritus
Bacterial vaginosis*	Homogeneous, thin, white discharge that smoothly coats the vaginal walls	A fishy odor of vaginal discharge before or after addition of 10% KOH (ie, the whiff test); pH >4.5	No dysuria; slight pruritus

Data from Amsel R et al: *Am J Med.* 1983;74:14; Brunham RC et al: *N Eng J Med.* 1984;311:1; Rein MF, Chapel TA: *Clin Obstet Gynecol.* 1975;18:73; and Sobel J: *N Engl J Med* 1997;337:1896.
*Must have 3 of these 4 criteria to make diagnosis.

The parents should be asked about recent or concomitant illness. For example, vaginal discharge is associated with *Streptococcus pyogenes* infection (with or without scarlet fever) and with *Shigella flexneri* infection, occurring coincident with or after an episode of diarrhea. Systemic illnesses such as varicella also may be associated with vaginal discharge. Rectal infestations with *Enterobius vermicularis* (pinworms) can lead to vaginitis if the eggs are deposited around or in the vagina. A history of nocturnal itching accompanying vaginal discharge suggests this diagnosis. *Candida vulvovaginitis* is an uncommon cause of vaginal discharge in prepubertal girls unless the child has recently taken antibiotics, has diabetes mellitus, or is immunocompromised.[1]

Sexually transmitted organisms, such as *Neisseria gonorrhoeae, Chlamydia trachomatis,* or *Trichomonas vaginalis,* are known to cause vaginal infections in prepubertal girls. Whereas *N gonorrhoeae* clearly causes vaginal discharge, evidence that *C trachomatis* alone does so is limited.[3,4] The possibility of sexual abuse should always be considered in the evaluation.

Although these other entities should be considered carefully as the physician evaluates the young patient, nonspecific vaginitis, in which no clear causative agent for the discharge can be established, accounts for 25% to 75% of cases of vulvovaginitis.[1] Rare causes of discharge include polyps or tumors; ectopic ureters, which drain urine into the vagina, resulting in a wetness that is mistaken for discharge; a draining pelvic abscess; or a prolapsed urethra, often associated with a bloody discharge.

The physical examination should include the entire genital and rectal area. The condition of the vulva, urethral meatus, and vaginal introitus should be noted. Infections in prepubertal girls usually involve the vulva as opposed to only the vagina. The presence of bruises, lacerations, or scrapes in the genital area is

Table 227-1 Major Causes of Vaginal Discharge in Pubertal Girls—cont'd

OTHER CLUES	DIAGNOSIS	TREATMENT*
Vulva affected; association with use of some oral contraceptives and, in some women, with antibiotic use	Hyphae on potassium hydroxide examination	A variety of effective treatments are available for vaginal candidiasis, including creams, suppositories, and intravaginal tablets. Three-, 5-, and 7-day therapies offer no advantage over single-day treatments. Fluconazole 150 mg orally as a single dose is as effective as other regimens; however, more systemic side effects may occur. Ultimately, the *best* treatment is a combination of patient preference, what treatments are covered by her insurance policy, and whether it is less expensive or more convenient for the patient to obtain a prescription medication or purchase an over-the-counter treatment.
Low abdominal pain; "strawberry" cervix; punctate vaginal hemorrhages	Motile trichomonads on wet preparation; avoid drying specimen	Metronidazole 2 g orally in a single dose. Alternatively, this medication can be given as 500 mg twice daily for 7 days. Partners of the patient must be treated. Some strains of *T vaginalis* have diminished susceptibility to metronidazole. If failure occurs with either of the indicated regimens (and reinfection is not a possibility), the patient should be treated with 500 mg twice daily for 7 days. Repeated failures should be treated with 2 g once daily for 3 to 5 days. The patient should be told to avoid alcohol until 24 hours after completion of therapy.
Occurs in association with anaerobes and *G vaginalis*	Clue cells on wet preparation (bacteria-coated epithelial cells)	Metronidazole 500 mg orally twice daily for 7 days, metronidazole gel 0.75% one full applicator (5 g) intravaginally once daily for 5 days or clindamycin cream 2%, one full applicator (5 g) intravaginally every night at bedtime for 7 days or alternative regimens that include metronidazole 2 g orally in a single dose, clindamycin 300 mg orally twice daily for 7 days, or clindamycin ovules 100 g intravaginally every night at bedtime for 3 days.

*See reference no. 12.

suggestive of sexual abuse. Excoriations around the rectum or vagina suggest itching caused by pinworms. A rash that spares skin folds is consistent with an irritative cause; one that is predominantly within the skin folds suggests candidiasis.

Having the girl sit on her mother's lap with her legs spread so that they dangle outside her mother's legs will often afford the examiner a clear view of the vulva and vaginal introitus. Alternatively, she may lie on her back in the frog-leg position or face down on the examining table in the knee-chest position. If a foreign body is thought to be present (because of a thick discharge that is often bloody and sometimes foul smelling) but not visualized, then irrigating the vagina with a soft, flexible catheter and tepid saline solution will often flush out bits of toilet paper or small objects.[1]

If sufficient vaginal discharge is present, then several drops of the secretion should be placed on 2 glass slides. If the discharge is scant, then a saline-moistened cotton swab can be introduced into the vagina to obtain samples for the glass slides. Several drops of normal saline solution should be added to 1 slide to create a wet preparation. Several drops of 10% potassium hydroxide should be added to the second slide, which should then be gently heated to dissolve epithelial cells, allowing visualization of hyphae. Slides should be examined, as indicated in Table 227-1. If indicated, cultures for *N gonorrhoeae* and *C trachomatis* should be performed.[3] A piece of cellophane tape with its sticky side applied to the perianal area and then onto a glass slide for microscopic examination may reveal the typical eggs of *E vermicularis*.

Management

If the history or physical examination suggests an irritative origin, then parents should discontinue the offending agent and have the child wear cotton underpants. Sitz baths will provide temporary relief until natural healing takes place. Removal of a foreign body will result in rapid improvement and cessation of the discharge. Pinworm infestations should be treated in the usual manner (see Chapter 305, Parasitic Infections). Infections caused by poor personal hygiene will respond to the general measures just listed, coupled with instructions about proper perineal hygiene. If the discharge is associated with another infection (such as *S pyogenes* or *Shigella* organisms), then it will disappear as the underlying infection is treated.

When the organism causing the vaginal discharge is found to be sexually transmitted, more comprehensive evaluation and treatment are required (see Chapters 122, Sexual Abuse of Children, and 322, Sexually Transmitted Infections).[1] Appropriate antibiotic treatment should be prescribed and a report to child protective services made.

Nonspecific vaginitis will usually respond to thorough perineal hygiene, sitz baths, and mild soaps. Patients should be advised to wear white cotton underpants and loose-fitting pants or skirts, to avoid nylon tights and tight pants, to avoid sitting for long periods in nylon bathing suits, and to wipe only from front to back. For persistent cases, the condition can be treated with amoxicillin, amoxicillin clavulanate, a cephalosporin, or clindamycin in standard childhood doses for 10 to 14 days.[1] Alternatively, a 1- to 2-month daily low-dose antibiotic may be helpful. If these approaches are unsuccessful, then antibiotic creams (mupirocin, gentamicin, metronidazole, or clindamycin) or estrogen creams may be used. If symptoms persist, the patient should then be referred to a pediatric gynecologist.

PUBERTAL AND POSTPUBERTAL ADOLESCENTS

With the onset of puberty, circulating estrogen and progesterone levels rise, stimulating vaginal mucus production and an increase in the turnover of vaginal epithelial cells. Bartholin and sebaceous glands are also stimulated. Generally, the clear mucoid discharge that results will not cause problems. The amount of secretion, however, can increase with sexual excitement, as well as midway through a normal menstrual cycle. Discharge is particularly prominent at the onset of puberty (physiological leukorrhea). Examination of a wet preparation will reveal vaginal epithelial cells only. The high protein content of this discharge, absorbed onto underwear, causes yellow staining. Traditionally, occlusive nylon or rayon underpants have been alleged to cause a nonspecific vaginal discharge; however, that association may be spurious.

A wide variety of organisms are normally found in the vagina. These organisms, especially the lactobacilli, help maintain the normal acidic pH of the vagina, which resists infection. Some of the organisms that cause vaginitis and vaginal discharge in this age group are sexually transmitted or associated with sexual activity.[5] Because many teenagers fear admitting to sexual intercourse, a negative response to queries about sexual activity should not rule out consideration of a sexually transmitted organism as the cause of the discharge. Sexual abuse and the presence of a foreign body (eg, a retained tampon or condom) should also be considered. If a sexually transmitted organism has caused the discharge, then the patient's sexual partner should be notified and treated. The patient should refrain from sexual intercourse until they complete treatment. Otherwise, reinfection from her partner may occur. Use of spermicides or douching can cause vaginitis.[6]

The organisms and conditions commonly responsible for vaginal infections or vaginal discharge in pubertal young women and their treatments are listed in Table 227-1. Although the characteristics of each type of infection are said to be typical, the discharge observed on examination does not always fit these classic presentations.[7,8] The laboratory methods outlined in Table 227-1 therefore are of considerable diagnostic utility. However, they are not 100% sensitive. *T vaginalis* may not be noted during microscopic examination even if the vaginal fluid is examined immediately under the microscope to avoid drying of the organisms. The vaginal wet preparation is 64% to 80% sensitive at identifying trichomonads compared with culture, depending on the presence of symptoms and the experience of the microscopist. Culture methods and newer tests such as direct fluorescent antibody, polymerase chain reaction, and enzyme immunoassay have higher detection rates but are not yet commonly used in clinical practice.[7,9] Papanicolaou tests also detect the presence of trichomonas, but the sensitivity is less than that of the wet preparation, and false positives can occur.[7,9]

The role of *N gonorrhoeae* and *C trachomatis* in causing vaginal discharge has been reassessed recently. The presence of yellow vaginal discharge on speculum examination has been associated with infection by either organism; in contrast, neither profuse vaginal discharge nor a foul or *fishy odor* predicted infection with either.[10] Nonetheless, because sexually transmitted infections often co-occur, appropriate screening tests for *N gonorrhoeae* and *C trachomatis* should be part of the evaluation of vaginitis if *T vaginalis* is found or if the patient reports a new sexual partner.

Bacterial vaginosis is a complex syndrome characterized by decreased *lactobacilli* and increased concentrations of several anaerobic microorganisms. The pathogenesis of this disorder continues to be poorly understood.[7,9] Bacterial vaginosis is associated with having multiple sex partners, douching, smoking, and the presence of sexually transmitted infections.[8,10] However, because it sometimes occurs in women who have never had sexual contact, bacterial vaginosis is not considered a sexually transmitted infection.[10] Current evidence indicates that women who have bacterial vaginosis are at increased risk for developing pelvic inflammatory disease after instrumentation of the genital tract and, if pregnant, are more likely to deliver a premature infant or experience postpartum complications. Therefore prompt treatment is essential. Treatment of sexual partners is not currently recommended because it does not affect the disease process.[7]

Occasionally, herpesvirus infections of the vulvovaginal area or cervix (or both) are associated with vaginal discharge. Typically, pain or a burning sensation is felt in the genital area. The vulva is reddened, and groups of small vesicles are noted on the vulva, in the vagina, or on the cervix. If the vesicles have ruptured, then the examiner sees only small ulcerations. Inguinal adenopathy, fever, and malaise are usually present if this attack is the first one (see Chapter 274, Herpes Infections).

A teenager who has a persistent discharge that is unresponsive to therapy may not be complying with treatment or may have become reinfected by an untreated partner. If such is not the case, and if *N gonorrhoeae, C trachomatis,* and *T vaginalis* are excluded, and if the discharge does not appear to fit any of the causes described earlier, then a trial of sitz baths, use of cotton as opposed to nylon underwear, and careful attention to perineal hygiene is warranted. If symptoms persist, then the patient should be referred to an adolescent medicine specialist or a gynecologist.

Candidal infections can be especially difficult to treat and may recur. Factors that predispose the individual to candidiasis include oral contraceptive use, broad-spectrum antibiotic use, and diabetes mellitus.[8] In cases of recurrent vulvovaginal candidiasis, either topical therapy for 7 to 14 days or oral fluconazole 150 mg repeated 72 hours after the first dose is recommended as initial treatment. If more intensive treatment is warranted, a recent study of adult women with recurrent vulvovaginal candidiasis demonstrated significant reduction of symptoms among those treated with oral fluconazole 150 mg once weekly for 6 months after initial treatment of 1 dose every 3 days for 3 doses.[11,12] A variety of month-long antifungal treatments have been successful; however, intravaginal treatment over a long period is inconvenient for most patients. Although long-term ketoconazole has been used to suppress recurrent infection, hepatotoxicity is a concern. Male sexual partners should also be treated if they have any signs or symptoms of penile candidal involvement.

WHEN TO REFER

- If the clinician is uncomfortable with evaluating genital complaints in prepubertal girls
- If the clinician lacks experience in performing pelvic examinations
- If the evaluation yields evidence of sexual abuse
- If the discharge persists despite seemingly appropriate therapy

TOOLS FOR PRACTICE

Engaging Patients and Family

- *Center for Young Women's Health* (Web page), Boston Children's Hospital (www.youngwomenshealth.org/).
- *Teenwire* (Web page), Planned Parenthood (www.teenwire.com/).
- *The Pelvic Exam* (brochure), American Academy of Pediatrics (patiented.aap.org).

AAP POLICY STATEMENT

American Academy of Pediatrics, Committee on Infectious Diseases and Committee on Fetus and Newborn. Revised guidelines for prevention of early-onset group B streptococcal (GBS) infection. *Pediatrics*. 1997;99(3):489-496. (aappolicy.aappublications.org/cgi/content/full/pediatrics;113/5/1434).

SUGGESTED WEB SITES

www.youngwomenshealth.org
www.teenwire.com/home_content.asp

REFERENCES

1. Emans SJ, Laufer MR, Goldstein DP. *Pediatric and Adolescent Gynecology*. 5th ed. Philadelphia, PA: Lippincott Williams & Wilkins; 2005.
2. Smith YR, Berman DR, Quint EH. Premenarchal vaginal discharge: findings of procedures to rule out foreign bodies. *J Pediatr Adolesc Gynecol*. 2002;13:227-230.
3. Shapiro RA, Schubert CJ, Siegel RM. Neisseria gonorrhea infections in girls younger than 12 years of age evaluated for vaginitis. *Pediatrics*. 1999;104(6):e72.
4. Stricker T, Navratil F, Sennhauser FH. Vulvovaginitis in prepubertal girls. *Arch Dis Child*. 2003;88:324-326.
5. Syed TS, Braverman PK. Vaginitis in adolescents. *Adolesc Med Clin*. 2004;15(2):235-251.
6. Jaquiery A, Stylianopoulos A, Hogg G, et al. Vulvovaginitis: clinical features, aetiology, and microbiology of the genital tract. *Arch Dis Child*. 1999;81:64-67.
7. Sobel JD. What's new in bacterial vaginosis and trichomoniasis? *Infect Dis Clini North Am*. 2005;19(2):387-406.
8. Steele RW. Prevention and management of sexually transmitted diseases in adolescents. *Adolesc Med*. 2000; 11(2):315-326.
9. Spigarelli MG, Biro FM. Sexually transmitted disease testing: evaluation of diagnostic tests and methods. *Adolesc Med Clin*. 2004;15(2):287-299.
10. Holmes KK, Stamm WE. Lower genital tract infection syndromes in women. In: Holmes KK, Mårdh PA, Sparling PF, et al, eds. *Sexually Transmitted Diseases*. 3rd ed, New York, NY: McGraw-Hill; 1999.
11. Sobel JD, Wiesenfeld HC, Martens M, et al. Maintenance fluconazole therapy for recurrent vulvovaginal candidiasis. *N Engl J Med*. 2004;351:876-883.
12. Centers for Disease Control and Prevention. 2002 Guidelines for treatment of sexually transmitted diseases. *MMWR*. 2002;51(No RR-6):1-78.

Chapter 228

VISUAL DEVELOPMENT, AMBLYOPIA, AND VISION TESTING

Kenneth W. Wright, MD

NORMAL VISUAL DEVELOPMENT

At birth, visual acuity is quite poor, probably in the range of legal blindness. For the most part, this poor visual acuity is due to immaturity of visual centers in the brain responsible for vision processing. Visual centers in the brain, including the lateral geniculate nucleus and the striate cortex, develop rapidly during the first 3 to 4 months of life. This visual development is stimulated by clear and equal in-focus retinal images and precise ocular alignment. Normal visual development therefore depends on appropriate visual stimulation during what is termed the *critical period of visual development.* Figure 228-1 shows the curve of visual acuity development in which the most rapid development occurs during the critical period, the first 4 months of life. An important point to note, however, is that development continues up to 8 to 9 years of age.

Normally we use our eyes together, integrating the retinal images from both eyes into a single three-dimensional perception. The process of fusing two separate images into one binocular image is termed *binocular fusion,* which is required to maintain proper eye alignment and provide stereopsis (depth perception).

Animal studies by Weisel and Hubel show that binocular cortical connections are present from birth. Normally, approximately 70% of striate cortex neurons are binocular neurons and respond to visual stimulation from both eyes. The minority of striate cortical cells are monocular, responding to only one eye. Even though binocular anatomy is present at birth, appropriate visual input from each eye is necessary to refine and maintain these binocular neural connections. The presence of strabismus (ocular misalignment) or a unilateral blurred retinal image (eg, congenital cataract, anisometropia) will disrupt normal monocular and binocular visual development.

Visual Developmental Milestones

Visual Fixation

A key visual developmental milestone for healthy infants is the ability to fixate and follow small objects accurately. This milestone usually occurs by 2 to 3 months of age, but even healthy infants may occasionally show delayed visual maturation. Poor fixation at 5 to 6 months of age usually indicates impaired vision, and the infant should be referred for a full evaluation.

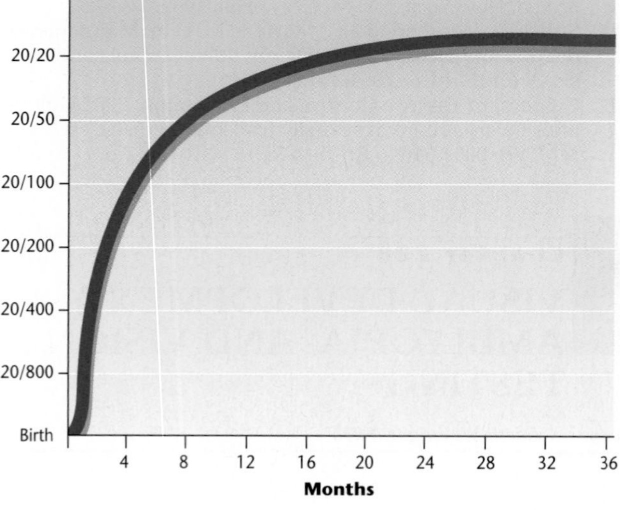

Figure 228-1 Curve represents visual acuity development with age on the horizontal axis and Snellen acuity on the vertical axis. Note the exponential improvement in visual acuity during the critical period of visual development (birth to 4 months).

Alignment

At birth, eye alignment is variable, with approximately 70% of infants showing a small variable exotropia (eye turned out), 30% have essentially straight eyes (orthotropia), and esotropia (eye turned in) is rare. By 2 months of age the majority of healthy infants will have established proper alignment. The persistence of an esotropia after 2 months of age is pathological in most cases and should be referred for ophthalmologic evaluation. Binocular vision begins in early infancy. Human studies have documented binocular vision at 2 to 3 months of age. Stereopsis (depth perception) develops later, between 3 and 6 months of age. Table 228-1 outlines the visual developmental milestones from birth to visual maturity.

Amblyopia

Normal visual development requires the stimulation provided by equally clear retinal images and proper eye alignment. Abnormal visual stimulation by a unilateral or bilateral blurred retinal image can disrupt normal visual development and cause poor vision, termed *amblyopia. Strabismus* is the condition of ocular misalignment, including esotropia (eye turned in), exotropia (eye turned out), or vertical (eye turned up or down). If strabismus occurs before 4 to 6 years of age, then the child will cortically turn off or suppress the image from the deviated eye to prevent bothersome double vision. Alternating strabismus (Figure 228-2) is associated with alternating suppression and allows for equal monocular visual development with no amblyopia. Suppression, however, disrupts binocular fusion, and if not corrected early, then the strabismus will cause a loss of binocular fusion and stereopsis. The early treatment of strabismus has improved outcomes including binocular visual function and visual acuity. (See Chapter 220, Strabismus, for descriptions of specific strabismus syndromes.)

Table 228-1 Visual Developmental Milestones

AGE	MILESTONE
Birth to 1 mo	Poor and sporadic fixation Jerky fast eye movements (saccades) Exotropia 70%, orthotropia 30% (straight eyes); esotropia is rare
2 to 6 mo	Accurate fixation (locks on target) Precise smooth pursuit eye movements Binocular fusion and stereopsis Orthotropia (straight eyes)
$2^1/_2$ to 4 yr	Visual Acuity 20/40
5 to 6 yr	Visual Acuity 20/30
7 to 9 yr	Visual Acuity 20/25 to 20/20

Amblyopia occurs in approximately 2% of the general population and is the most common cause of decreased vision in childhood. The term *amblyopia* is derived from Greek and means dull vision (amblys = dull, ops = eye). Amblyopia is caused by the disruption of neurodevelopment in visual areas of the brain because of abnormal visual stimulation during the early developmental period. If not treated early, amblyopia can result in permanent visual loss. Structural damage in visual centers in the brain, including the lateral geniculate nucleus (Figure 228-3) and visual cortex (Figure 228-4), can occur if the abnormal stimulation is severe and persists during the early period of visual development. Two basic forms of abnormal visual stimulation are (1) blurred retinal image (unilateral or bilateral) and (2) strabismus, with strong preference for one eye and constant suppression of the deviated eye. Clinically, a unilateral refractive error causing a blurred image is a common cause of amblyopia termed *anisometropic amblyopia*. An opacity in the visual axis, such as a large cataract or corneal opacity, can also blur the retinal image and cause amblyopia. A classification of amblyopia based on the type of abnormal visual stimuli is presented in Box 228-1.

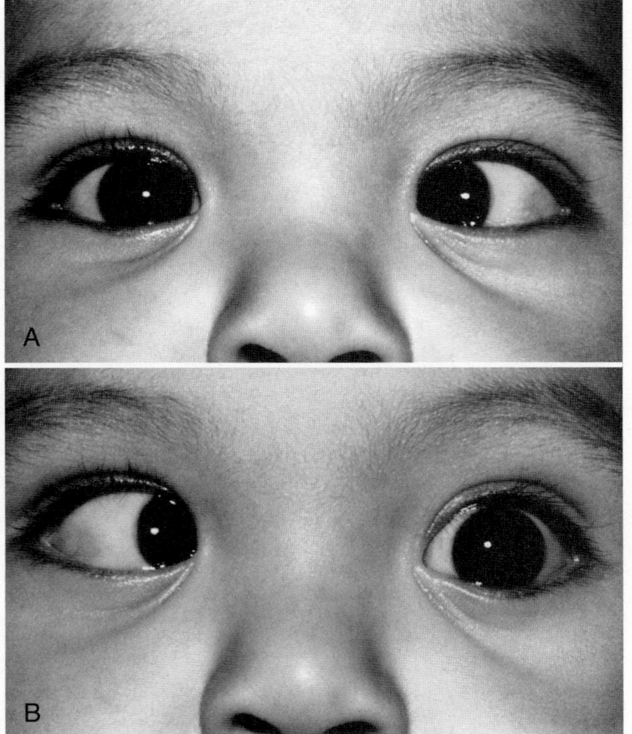

Figure 228-2 Infant with congenital esotropia and alternating fixation. **A**, The patient is fixing right eye. **B**, The patient has switched fixation to the left eye. Alternating fixation indicates equal visual preference, no amblyopia.

Amblyogenic Period

The severity of the amblyopia depends on when the abnormal stimulus begins, the length of exposure to abnormal stimulation, and the severity of the image blur. The more severe the image blur is, the earlier the onset will be; and the longer the duration of a malapropos stimulus is, the more severe the effect will be on neurodevelopment and the more severe the effect will be on visual acuity. Children are most susceptible to amblyopia during the critical period of visual development, which is the first 3 to 4 months of life. Stimulation with a severely blurred retinal image during this time results in dense, often irreversible, amblyopia. This circumstance is why visually significant congenital cataracts must be operated and visually rehabilitated within the first few weeks of life. Amblyopia can occur, however, in older children. Acquired strabismus, or an acquired media opacity such as a cataract, can cause amblyopia up to 7 or 8 years of age, albeit of

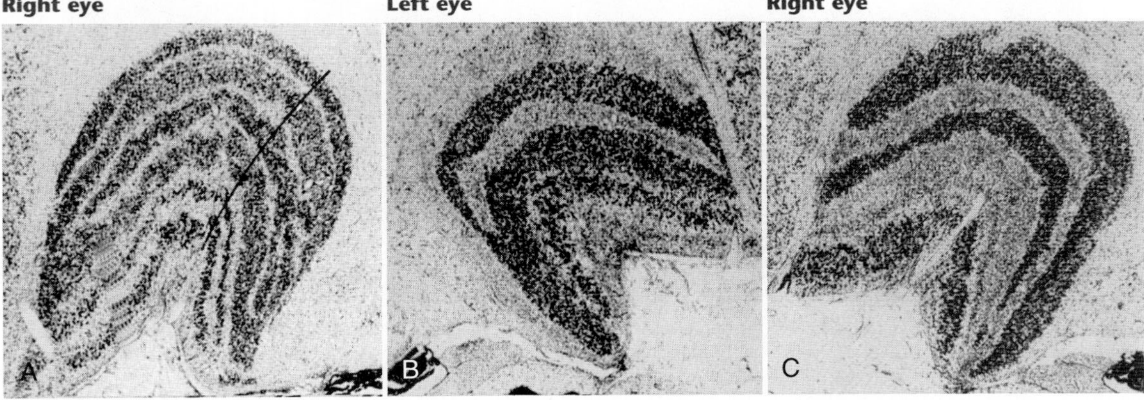

Figure 228-3 Pathological feature of amblyopia. Cross-section of lateral geniculate nucleus (LGN) from a normal monkey (**A**) versus amblyopic monkey caused by a unilateral blurred image (**B** and **C**). Note that the normal LGN (**A**) has six nuclear layers (darkly stained cell layer), and the amblyopic LGN (**B** and **C**) only has three layers and they are thicker than normal. *(Wiesel TN, Hubel DH. Ordered arrangement of orientation columns in monkeys, lacking visual experience.* J Comp Neurol. *1974;158:307-318. Reprinted by permission.)*

lesser severity. Box 228-2 lists the major periods of visual plasticity and susceptibility to amblyopia.

Treatment of Amblyopia

The strategy for treating amblyopia is (1) to provide a clear retinal image and (2) in cases of unilateral amblyopia, to force the use of the amblyopic eye by occluding the good eye. The first step to treating amblyopia is to make sure that a clear retinal image exists. Refractive errors are corrected with spectacles or contact lenses, and visually significant opacities such as cataracts must be surgically removed. Patients with strabismic amblyopia may or may not require optical correction, but virtually all require occlusion therapy to correct ocular dominance. Occluding or patching the sound eye forces the use of the amblyopic eye to stimulate visual development.

The earlier the intervention takes place, the better the prognosis will be for amblyopia. Children with visually significant congenital cataracts are best treated during the first week of life because delaying surgery until after 3 to 4 months carries a poor visual prognosis. Patients with less-severe forms of amblyopia such as anisometropic amblyopia (difference in refractive error) will have a better prognosis even when treated between 3 and 8 years of age. After 8 to 9 years of age the prognosis is poor. Even so, patients with amblyopia who are treated late can show significant improvement. Patients with presumed congenital cataracts who are identified after the critical period may show some visual improvement with aggressive amblyopia

BOX 228-1 Classification of Amblyopia

A. Strabismic amblyopia
   1. Congenital esotropia (60%)
   2. Acquired esotropia in childhood (20%)
   3. Intermittent exotropia (rare <2%)

Note: If alternating strabismus is noted, then the patient does not have amblyopia.

B. Monocular blurred image
   1. Refractive error—anisometropia (difference in refractive error)
      a. Hypermetropic
      b. Myopic
      c. Astigmatism
   2. Media opacity
      a. Unilateral cataract (>3 mm in visual axis)
      b. Unilateral corneal opacity (eg, Peter anomaly)
      c. Unilateral vitreous hemorrhage or vitreous opacity

C. Bilateral blurred image
   1. Refractive error
      a. Bilateral high hypermetropia
      b. Astigmatism
   2. Media opacity
      a. Bilateral congenital cataracts (>3 mm in visual axis)
      b. Bilateral corneal opacities (eg, Peter anomaly)
      c. Bilateral vitreous opacity (hemorrhages)

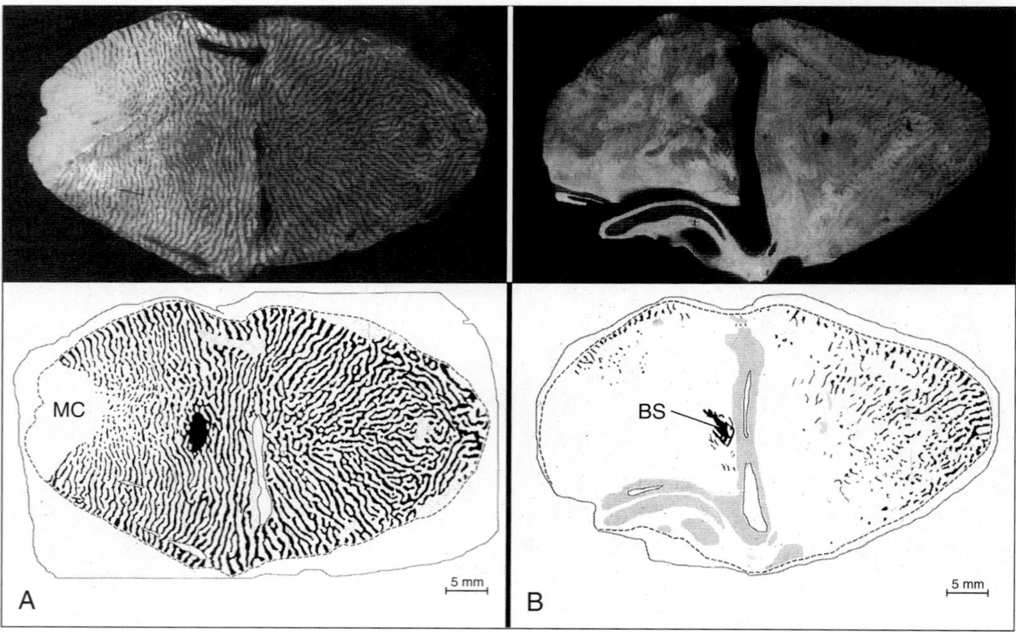

Figure 228-4 Pathological feature of amblyopia. Histopathology of monkey striate cortex (visual cortex). Well-defined cortex columns are seen in normal specimen (**A**), but cortex columns are under developed in specimen for amblyopic monkey (**B**). *MC,* Monocular crescent representation; *BS,* blind spot representation. *(Horton JC, Hocking DR. Timing of the critical period for plasticity of ocular dominance columns in macaque striate cortex.* J Neurosci. *1997;17:3684-3709. Reprinted by permission.)*

BOX 228-2 Visual Development and Amblyopia

Critical period: 1 week to 4 months (most susceptible to amblyopia)
Visual plasticity: 5 months to 8 years (susceptible to amblyopia)
Visually mature: 9 years to adulthood (persons do not develop amblyopia but may retain limited plasticity)

management. Even adults with amblyopia who lose their good eye may show limited vision improvement of the amblyopic eye.

VISION TESTING

Early detection and treatment of ocular disease and amblyopia in children is critical. Diseases such as congenital cataracts, retinoblastoma, and congenital glaucoma require early treatment during infancy. Delay in diagnosis may result in irreversible amblyopia, vision loss and, in the case of retinoblastoma, death. Providing effective vision screening of all children from newborn infants to older children is therefore imperative.

Vision screening examinations should start at birth and continue as part of routine check-ups. The acronym I-ARM (*i*nspection: *a*cuity, *r*ed reflex, and *m*otility) can be a helpful reminder of the essential parts of a pediatric screening examination. The most important test for the newborn is the *red reflex test*. If an abnormal red reflex is present, then an immediate referral to an ophthalmologist is required. Infant screening examinations take less than a minute, but this brief examination is quite powerful and, if performed properly, can detect the vast majority of eye diseases, including the important diagnoses mentioned previously. Equipment needed for the I-ARM screening examination is simple and includes the direct ophthalmoscope and a visual chart such as the E-game, Allen cards, Wright figures (Figure 228-5), or Snellen letters (for verbal children).

Inspection

Simple inspection of the eyes and lids for abnormalities of symmetry can be helpful. Figure 228-6 shows a patient with asymmetric lid fissures secondary to a superior orbital dermoid cyst. When the right eye is compared with the left eye, this patient obviously has a left ptosis and narrow lid fissure on the left. In addition, the examiner should inspect for a face turn or head tilt because they can be compensatory mechanisms to reduce strabismus or damp nystagmus. If the onset of an ocular abnormality is in question, then the examiner should seek family photographs for documentation. Box 228-3 lists the 3 major categories for ocular inspection.

Acuity

Obtaining a visual acuity on every child is important, even on infants. The following 2 sections describe how to assess visual acuity in (1) preverbal children and (2) verbal children.

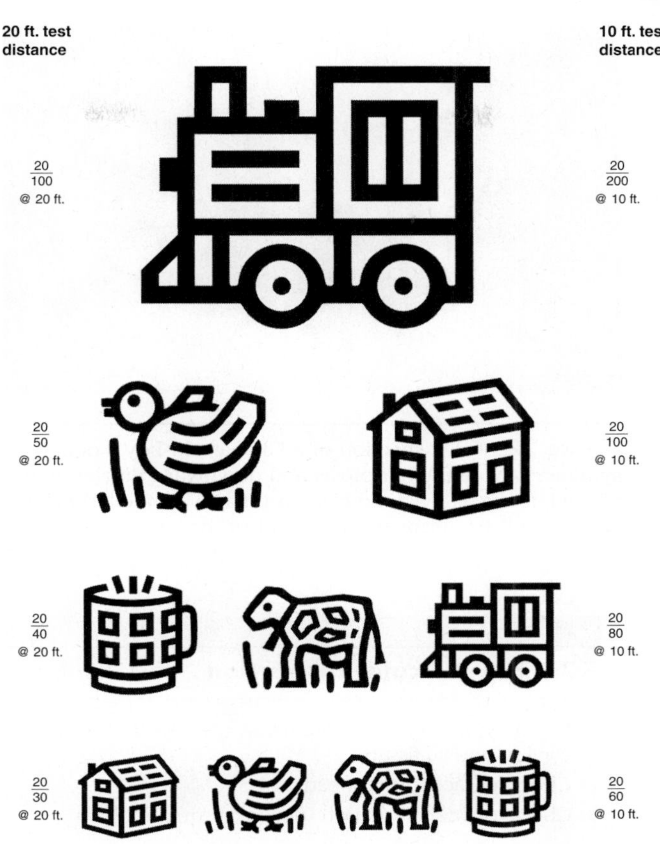

Figure 228-5 Wright figures designed to diagnose amblyopia in young children. The figures test visual two-point discrimination because the figures have similar outlines and equal contrast. *(Copyright © 2000 Dr. Kenneth W. Wright.)* Available through the AAP.org Web site.

Preverbal Children

From birth to approximately 2 months of age, infants may only sporadically fix and follow a moving target. However, this status should be documented. In addition, pupillary responses are present even in premature infants, and they should be tested and recorded. Between 2 and 6 months of age, patients should have the ability to fix and follow on a small toy or the human face. The examiner covers 1 of the patient's eyes and moves a target (eg, the examiner's face or a toy) right, left, up, and down to observe if the patient's eyes will accurately follow the motion. Each eye should be tested individually because with both eyes open the eyes will track together even if 1 eye is blind. In addition, a compelling target should be used. In infants the human face is probably the most compelling target, whereas in toddlers and young children a small toy or a finger puppet is a good target. The examiner observes for *central fixation* with the presence of accurate smooth pursuit, meaning that the child looks directly at the target, not off center, and will smoothly and accurately follow the target. If the child has trouble locking on the target and appears to be looking off center, then poor fixation and poor vision is indicated.

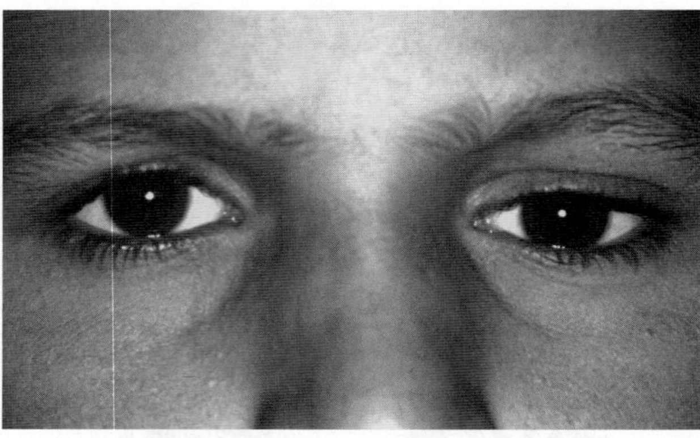

Figure 228-6 Inspection of a 13-year-old-boy. Look for symmetry. Note the left ptosis and downward displacement of the left eye. A dermoid cyst on the roof of the left orbit is causing the inferior displacement of the left eye.

BOX 228-3 Ocular Inspection

1. Check symmetry: Compare fellow eyes, look at pupils, eyelids, and lid fissures.
2. Check for face turn or head tilt.
3. Check for ocular irritation (pink-eye, squinting).

Verbal Children

By 2½ to 3 years of age, most children should be able to cooperate with optotype visual acuity testing using picture cards such as Allen cards, the E-game, Wright figures, or Snellen letters. Each eye should be tested separately, making sure that the occluded eye is truly covered. Many examiners prefer occluding one eye with an adhesive patch, rather than a paddle occluder, to prevent the child from peeking. Most vision charts are calibrated at 10 or 20 feet from the patient. Patients should be examined with their customary eyeglasses or contact lenses. If patients forget their corrective lenses, then the vision without correction is tested first and then retested using a pinhole (see later discussion). In children with very poor vision, visual acuity is measured by the ability to (1) count fingers at a distance of 1 to 2 feet, (2) see hand motions at a distance of 1 foot, or (3) perceive any light. The ability to see light is called *light perception* or *no light perception.* Most states define *legal blindness* as 20/200 or worse visual acuity.

Pinhole Test

Pinholes are commercially available; however, a pinhole test can be performed by taking a 3- × 5-inch card and placing several small pinholes close together in the card. If the patient's visual acuity improves after viewing through the pinhole, then a refractive error is probably the cause of the decreased vision. A pinhole is useful to estimate corrected visual acuity when a patient is without customary lenses. A pinhole will improve vision to approximately 20/30, even when patients have large refractive errors.

Criteria for Referral

A 3- to 5-year-old child who has a visual acuity of 20/50 or worse or greater than a two-line difference exists between fellow eyes should be referred. Children 6 years or older should be referred if visual acuity is 20/40 or worse or greater than a two-line difference exists between fellow eyes. Many young children will give inconsistent responses, and, in these cases, visual acuity should be retested, or the patient referred for a complete ophthalmic examination.

Red Reflex Test

The red reflex test is the single best vision-screening examination for infants and young children. The test is performed using the direct ophthalmoscope to view the reflex off the retina. A good method is to use the *Bruckner test,* which is simply a simultaneous bilateral red reflex. The ophthalmoscope is held at a distance of approximately 2 feet in front of the child. A broad beam is used so that both eyes are illuminated at the same time. The child is asked to look directly into the ophthalmoscope light, and the room lights are dimmed. The examiner starts with the ophthalmoscope on low illumination then slowly increases the illumination until a red reflex is seen. A red reflex will be observed that fills the pupil, and a small white light reflex appears to reflect off the cornea. The light reflex is actually a reflection coming from just behind the pupil; however, this reflection is commonly called the *corneal light reflex* or the Hirschberg reflex (see later discussion). Thus the Bruckner test will give both a red reflex and the corneal light reflex simultaneously.

An opacity in the optical media or large area of retinal disease will result in an abnormal red reflex. A cataract can either block the red reflex or reflect light to give a white reflex. Retinoblastoma has a yellowish white color and will produce a yellow reflex. Anisometropia (a difference in refractive error) will result in an unequal red reflex. Strabismus will cause a brighter red reflex in the deviated eye, and the corneal light reflex will be off center. The key sign of a normal red reflex test is symmetry. Asymmetry or an abnormality of the reflex indicates a need for an immediate ophthalmologic referral (Table 228-2).

Motility and Alignment

Ocular motility is assessed by having the patient follow a target right, left, up, and down, observing for full ocular rotation. Patients with a muscle weakness show limited eye movement. If a limitation of eye movement is identified, then an ophthalmologic consultation is indicated.

Light Reflex Test

Ocular alignment is best assessed by using the corneal light reflex, or Hirschberg, test. As described

Table 228-2 Abnormal Red Reflex Results and Their Causes

ABNORMAL RED REFLEX	RESULT (CAUSES)
Cataract	May block the red reflex (dark or dull reflex) or may appear white (leukocoria)
Vitreous hemorrhage	Blocks red reflex (dark or dull reflex)
Retinoblastoma	Appears as a yellow or white reflex (leukocoria)
Anisometropia	Results in an unequal red reflex
Strabismus	The corneal light reflex will be decentered and cause a brighter red reflex in the deviated eye.

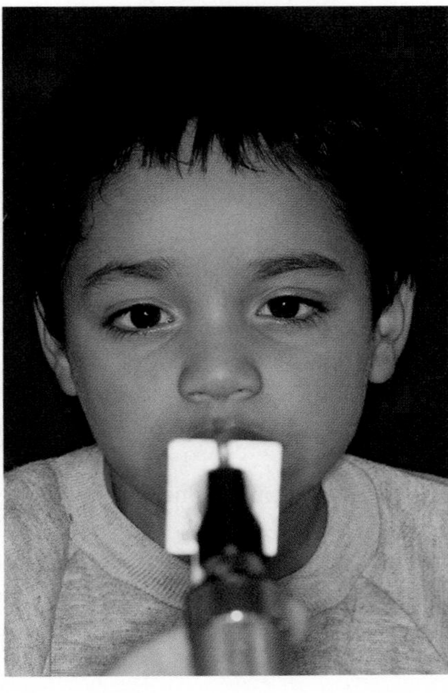

Figure 228-7 Demonstration of the corneal light reflex test (Hirschberg test). Note that the fixation target *(white square is a cartoon picture)* is in line with the light and the child is looking at the fixation target. The examiner should be situated directly behind the muscle light.

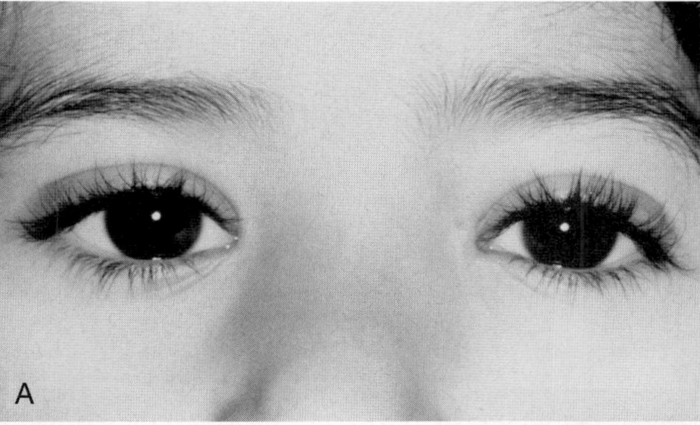

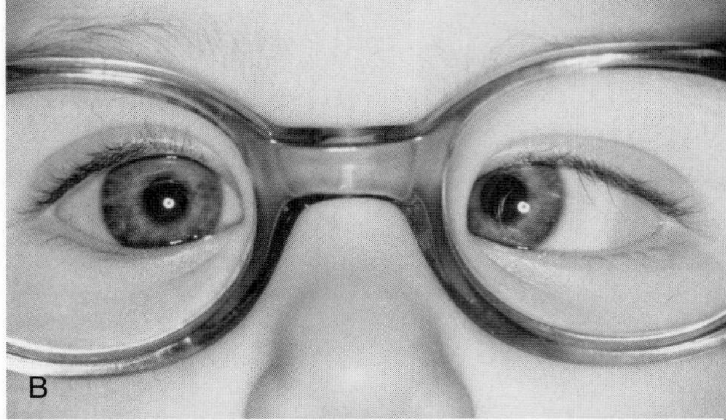

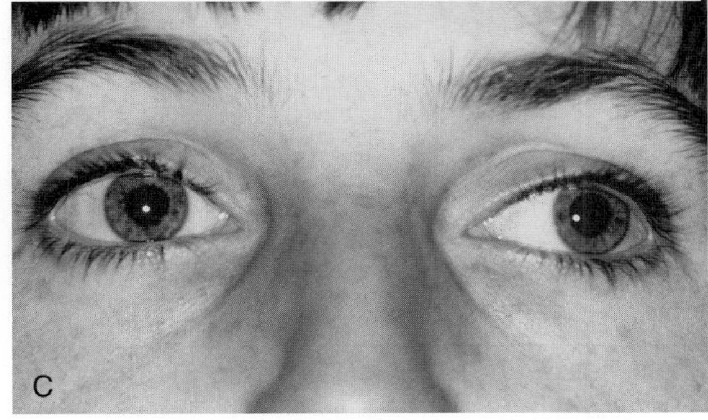

Figure 228-8 Corneal light reflex. **A**, Orthotropia (light reflexes centered). **B**, Esotropia (left light reflex temporally displaced). **C**, Exotropia (left light reflex nasally displaced).

previously the corneal light reflex can be obtained when performing the Bruckner test. Alternatively, any light source that produces a beam broad enough to illuminate both eyes can elicit a corneal light reflex. The proper procedure is to use a muscle light or flashlight held at the examiner's nose and pointed toward the patient's nose, having the child look directly at the light (Figure 228-7). The light reflex should be symmetrically centered or slightly nasally deviated. The key is that the light reflex is symmetric. Displacement of the light reflex indicates strabismus. Examples of the Hirschberg test are shown in Figure 228-8. The examiner must make sure that the patient maintains fixation on the light source; otherwise the light will appear to be off center.

Cover Test

The cover test is probably not necessary for vision screening, given that the Bruckner test (bilateral red reflex test) and the corneal light reflex test are more specific for detecting a true strabismus with a demonstrated deviation (ie, tropia). Many healthy children show an eye movement shift with alternate

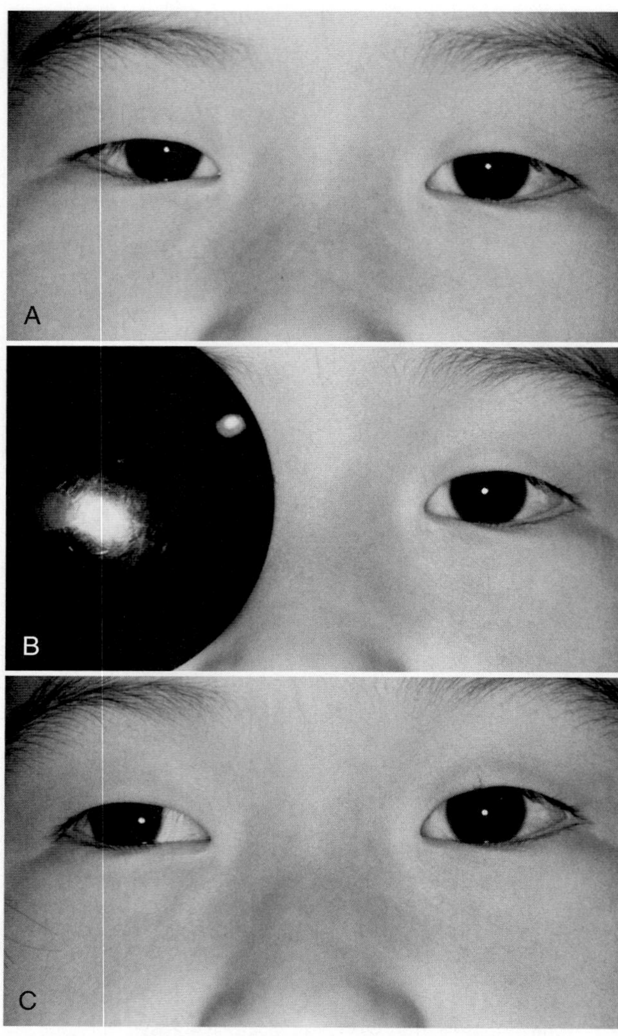

Figure 228-9 Cover test; intermittent exotropia. **A,** Straight eyes—patient fusing. **B,** Right eye covered. **C,** Right exotropia is evident after disrupting binocular fusion by covering the right eye.

cover testing, thus making the test difficult to interpret. The cover test entails covering 1 eye for 3 to 4 seconds then removing the cover. If a tendency exists for an eye to drift, then the eye under the cover will drift (Figure 228-9). If the patient has a history of intermittent strabismus (especially intermittent exotropia), yet the eyes appear well aligned, then the cover test may be helpful, although a referral to an ophthalmologist is indicated by the history alone.

WHEN TO REFER

- Poor fixation at 5 to 6 months of age
- Esotropia after 2 months of age
- Abnormal red reflex
- Visual acuity of 20/50 or worse in a 3 to 5 year old
- Greater than a two-line difference between fellow eyes
- Visual acuity of 20/40 or worse in children 6 years or older
- Lack of full ocular rotation (eye movement in a circle)
- Strabismus, including intermittent strabismus

TOOLS FOR PRACTICE

Engaging Patient and Family

- *How do I know if my child has a vision problem?* (fact sheet), American Academy of Pediatrics (www.aap.org/healthopics/visionhearing.cfm).
- *What Is a Pediatric Ophthalmologist?* (fact sheet), American Academy of Pediatrics (www.aap.org/healthopics/visionhearing.cfm).
- *When To See an Eye M.D.?* (fact sheet), American Academy of Ophthalmology (www.medem.com/search/article_display.cfm?path=\\TANQUERAY\M_ContentItem&mstr=/M_ContentItem/ZZZS1ZGZY9C.html&soc=AAO&srch_typ=NAV_SERCH).

Medical Decision Support

- *Pediatric Ophthalmology for Primary Care* (book), Kenneth W. Wright, MD, FAAP (www.aap.org/bookstore).
- *Screening for Visual Impairment in Children Younger than Age 5 Years* (report), U.S. Preventive Task Force Agency for Healthcare Research and Quality (www.ahrq.gov/clinic/uspstf/uspsvsch.htm).
- *See Red Cards (Red Reflex Testing)* (card), American Academy of Pediatrics (www.aap.org/sforms/seered.htm).
- *Snellen Eye Chart,* Hermann Snellen (www.activeforever.com).
- *Wright Eye Chart,* Kenneth W. Wright, MD, FAAP (www.aap.org/bstwww.aap.org/bst/showdetl.cfm?&DID=15&Product_ID=4375).

AAP POLICY STATEMENTS

American Academy of Pediatrics, Committee on Practice and Ambulatory Medicine, Section on Ophthalmology; American Association of Certified Orthoptists; American Association for Pediatric Ophthalmology and Strabismus; American Academy of Ophthalmology. Eye examination in infants, children, and young adults by pediatricians. *Pediatrics.* 2003;111(4):902-907. (aappolicy.aappublications.org/cgi/content/full/pediatrics;111/4/902).

American Academy of Pediatrics, Committee on Practice and Ambulatory Medicine and Section on Ophthalmology. Use of photoscreening for children's vision screening. *Pediatrics.* 2002;109(3):524-525. (aappolicy.aappublications.org/cgi/content/full/pediatrics;109/3/524).

SUGGESTED RESOURCE

Wiesel TN, Hubel DH. Ordered arrangement of orientation columns in monkeys lacking visual experience. *J Comp Neurol.* 1974;158(3):307-318.

Chapter 229

VOMITING

Martin H. Ulshen, MD

Vomiting is a common symptom of acute and chronic illness in childhood and must be distinguished from regurgitation, which is passive reflux of gastric contents into the esophagus and mouth through a relaxed lower esophageal sphincter. By contrast, vomiting is a coordinated, active process usually preceded by nausea in association with increased salivation, gastric atony, and reflux of duodenal contents into the stomach, resulting from nonperistaltic contractions of the small bowel.[1] Retching (coordinated contraction of abdominal and intercostal muscles, as well as the diaphragm, with simultaneous closure of the glottis) immediately precedes the actual vomiting. Increased intragastric pressure from contraction of the abdominal wall musculature, lowering of the diaphragm, and pyloric contraction are associated with elevation and relaxation of the cardia, and vomiting occurs.

The total process of vomiting is coordinated in the medullary vomiting center, which may be influenced directly by visceral afferent stimuli or indirectly through the chemoreceptor trigger zone. The latter region is the site of action of many of the drugs that cause nausea and vomiting, including apomorphine and digitalis. During motion sickness, stimulation of the vestibular system activates the vomiting center and perhaps the chemoreceptor trigger zone as well. Higher central nervous system centers may also influence the medullary vomiting center.

Understanding the role of neurotransmitters as mediators of the initiation of vomiting has led to a range of new antiemetics. The area postrema, which is a major lower brainstem center for coordination of drug-induced vomiting, is rich in enkephalins, 5-hydroxytryptamine (HT) receptors, and dopamine receptors. Enkephalins and 5-HT both stimulate release of dopamine. Dopamine and 5-HT antagonists have been successful in the treatment of chemotherapy-induced nausea and vomiting. Antihistamines and anticholinergics prevent motion sickness by acting at histamine (H_1) and muscarinic cholinergic receptors, respectively, in the nucleus ambiguus in the lower brainstem and in the lateral vestibular nucleus in the midpons.[2]

CAUSES AND DIFFERENTIAL DIAGNOSIS

Box 229-1 lists the most frequent causes of vomiting in infants and children. In infancy, regurgitation, or spitting up, is very common and most often a developmental event, which has no sequelae and gradually resolves. Pathological gastroesophageal reflux is defined by the association of regurgitation with severe complications, including esophagitis with or without anemia secondary to blood loss or stricture, recurrent apnea, aspiration pneumonia, or failure to thrive. Bilious vomiting, especially when associated with the first vomitus, usually occurs only with ileus or intestinal tract obstruction below the ampulla of Vater in the second portion of the duodenum. In newborns, bilious vomiting can be associated with necrotizing enterocolitis. In older children who vomit persistently, reflux of bile from the duodenum into the stomach may lead to bilious vomiting without gastrointestinal tract obstruction. Projectile vomiting commonly occurs with pyloric stenosis. When this condition persists, however, gastric atony may eliminate the projectile character. A succussion splash (the splashing sound present when a patient who has fluid in a hollow organ is shaken on physical examination) may be present, as in other causes of gastric outlet obstruction. Vomiting associated with increased intracranial pressure may be projectile and may take place in the absence of nausea or retching.

Persistent vomiting in a newborn or young infant who has no evidence of infection usually suggests a congenital gastrointestinal anomaly, inborn error of metabolism, or central nervous system abnormality such as hydrocephalus or subdural effusion. If the history and physical examination results do not suggest a cause, then evaluating all 3 possibilities simultaneously is best. When the sudden onset of bilious vomiting develops in a previously well newborn, especially within the first few days of life, the clinician must consider a malrotation with secondary midgut volvulus. A plain-film radiograph of the abdomen may show a paucity of gas distal to the upper small intestine; however, the radiograph may not be helpful. If a midgut volvulus is suspected, then an upper gastrointestinal radiographic series should be done at once, with the controlled introduction of barium through a nasogastric tube after gastric aspiration. A barium enema investigation of cecal position is a less reliable study when evaluating a patient for malrotation because of the lack of complete correlation of developmental rotation of the cecum with that of the duodenum. Midgut volvulus is a surgical emergency requiring early diagnosis and surgical intervention. In a sick newborn the diagnosis of necrotizing enterocolitis must be considered in the event of bilious vomiting, especially with blood in the stool. Beyond the first week of life but within the first 2 months, pyloric stenosis is the most common cause of persistent vomiting. In the older infant or child the entire spectrum of causes of vomiting listed in Box 229-1 should be considered. Patients who have celiac disease may occasionally have minimal or no diarrhea but prominent vomiting. When an older child exhibits acute vomiting and somnolence, the clinician should always consider drug overdose (especially aspirin toxicity), meningoencephalitis, inborn errors of mitochondrial fatty acid oxidation, and Reye syndrome in the differential diagnosis. Persistent or recurrent vomiting without other symptoms may be the major manifestation of an emotional disorder in childhood. Therefore a complete psychosocial history is an important part of the evaluation.

Cyclic vomiting is characterized by repeated episodes of vomiting (peak intensity at least 4 emeses per hour and frequency no more than 2 episodes per week), sometimes occurring in clusters and sometimes associated with abdominal pain.[3,4] Uncontrollable vomiting and retching are typical of an attack; but

BOX 229-1 Causes of Emesis (Arranged by Usual Age of Earliest Occurrence)

INFANCY/EARLY CHILDHOOD

Gastrointestinal

Congenital

- Regurgitation—gastroesophageal reflux (developmental or pathological)
- Atresia—stenosis (tracheoesophageal fistula, antral web, intestinal atresia, annular pancreas)
- Duplication
- Volvulus (secondary to an error in rotation and fixation or to Meckel diverticulum)
- Congenital bands
- Meconium ileus (cystic fibrosis), meconium plug
- Hirschsprung disease

Acquired

- Acute infectious gastroenteritis
- Pyloric stenosis
- Intussusception
- Incarcerated hernia—inguinal, internal secondary to old adhesions
- Food allergy, cow milk protein intolerance, eosinophilic gastroenteritis
- Disaccharidase deficiency
- Celiac disease—risk is inherited, but clinical manifestations occur only after introduction of gluten in diet
- Postviral gastroparesis[a]
- Adynamic ileus—the mediator for many nongastrointestinal causes of vomiting
- Neonatal necrotizing enterocolitis
- Chronic granulomatous disease with gastric outlet obstruction

Nongastrointestinal

- Infectious—otitis, urinary tract infection, pneumonia, upper respiratory tract infection, sepsis, meningitis
- Metabolic—aminoaciduria and organic aciduria, galactosemia, fructosemia, adrenogenital syndrome, renal tubular acidosis, hyperammonemia, disorders of fatty acid oxidation (eg, medium-chain acyl-coenzyme A dehydrogenase deficiency), mitochondrial disease,[b] Reye syndrome
- Central nervous system—trauma, tumor, infection, diencephalic syndrome, rumination, autonomic responses (pain, shock)
- Medications—anticholinergics, aspirin, alcohol, idiosyncratic reaction (eg, codeine)

CHILDHOOD/ADOLESCENCE

Gastrointestinal

- Appendicitis
- Food poisoning (staphylococcal, clostridial)
- Peptic disease—ulcer, gastritis, duodenitis
- Trauma—duodenal hematoma, traumatic pancreatitis, perforated bowel
- Pancreatitis—mumps, trauma, cystic fibrosis, hyperparathyroidism, hyperlipidemia, organic acidemias
- Gallbladder—cholelithiasis, choledochal cyst
- Crohn disease
- Adhesions—congenital or secondary to abdominal surgery
- Idiopathic intestinal pseudoobstruction
- Superior mesenteric artery syndrome[c]

Nongastrointestinal

- Central nervous system—cyclic vomiting, migraine, anorexia nervosa, bulimia
- Motion sickness
- Metabolic—diabetic ketoacidosis, acute intermittent porphyria
- Pregnancy

[a]Sigurdsson L, Flores A, Putnam PE, et al. Postviral gastroparesis: presentation, treatment, and outcome. *J Pediatr.* 1997;131(5):751-754.
[b]Boles RG, Williams JC. Mitochondrial disease and cyclic vomiting syndrome. *Dig Dis Sci.* 1999;44(8 suppl):103S-107S.
[c]Shandling B. The so-called superior mesenteric artery syndrome. *Am J Dis Child.* 1976;130(12):1371-1373.

between episodes, patients are well. Approximately 10% of these children have an identifiable gastrointestinal or extraintestinal (eg, renal, metabolic, or neurologic) disorder as the probable cause.[5]

Abdominal migraine is a common cause of cyclic vomiting and is characterized by the paroxysmal onset of repetitious attacks often relieved with sleep. A strong family history of migraine is common. Headache typical of migraine may occur with episodes. Cyproheptadine, amitriptyline, topiramate, and propranolol are highly effective as prophylactic treatment for abdominal migraine; treatment success helps confirm the diagnosis.[3,6] Abdominal epilepsy is a much less common cause of cyclic vomiting. A complete history of the sequence of events and electroencephalographic evaluation are useful in the evaluation, and anticonvulsants can be tried when this condition is suspected. Low-dose erythromycin has been used successfully to treat some children who have idiopathic cyclic vomiting.[7]

EVALUATION

Evaluation of the gastrointestinal tract usually includes an upper gastrointestinal contrast roentgenographic study. However, in an infant between 2 and 12 weeks of age, the 1st study is often an ultrasound of the abdomen for pyloric stenosis. Endoscopy is feasible in all children, even newborns, if performed by an experienced examiner using a pediatric instrument.[8] Esophageal pH monitoring, esophageal biopsies, and gastroesophageal scintiscan are all useful in establishing a diagnosis of gastroesophageal reflux. If brain tumor is a consideration in an infant, then magnetic resonance imaging is more sensitive than a computed tomography scan of the head. Further workup for metabolic or neurologic disease should be considered, as appropriate. With persistent vomiting, the clinician should expect to see a metabolic alkalosis; metabolic acidosis raises concerns about an underlying metabolic disorder or drug intoxication. In a postpubertal girl, pregnancy must always be considered in the differential diagnosis of vomiting.

COMPLICATIONS

The most significant complications of vomiting include dehydration and electrolyte imbalance, especially when the vomiting is persistent, as well as aspiration pneumonia, hemorrhage from prolapse gastropathy (a hemorrhagic area on the posterior wall of the proximal stomach), or, less commonly, a tear at the gastroesophageal junction (Mallory-Weiss syndrome) and rupture of the esophagus (very uncommon in children). Feeding refusal may follow persistent vomiting, especially in infants.[8]

TREATMENT

Acute intercurrent vomiting without serious underlying disease or significant dehydration should be treated by administering clear liquids by mouth (eg, in acute gastroenteritis or otitis media). The usually advisable course is to start with a period of 4 to 6 hours without oral intake and then begin with frequent small quantities of clear liquids (1 teaspoonful every few minutes for infants) and gradually increase the volume and extension of the period between oral fluids. If vomiting is associated with diarrhea and dehydration, then oral rehydration solution is indicated (see Chapter 341, Dehydration). Carbonated beverages may increase vomiting. Fluids of high osmolality, long-chain triglycerides, and anticholinergic drugs all tend to slow gastric emptying and should be avoided.

Antiemetic drugs should be avoided in infants, although they may, at times, be useful in older children.[2] The drugs used most commonly for acute symptoms are ondansetron and promethazine. Trimethobenzamide may be less effective but is also used. Rectal suppositories are preferable to oral drugs because nausea is associated with gastric atony and unpredictable absorption. Dopamine-receptor antagonists (eg, metoclopramide) are effective for chemotherapy-induced vomiting, although 5-HT_3-receptor antagonists (ondansetron) appear to have even greater efficacy without the risks of dystonic reactions associated with metoclopramide.[2] H_1-receptor antagonists (including diphenhydramine, dimenhydrinate, meclizine, and promethazine) and muscarinic cholinergic receptor antagonists (eg, scopolamine) prevent motion sickness.[2] Metoclopramide or low-dose erythromycin can help treat poor gastric emptying without mechanical obstruction. Antiemetics do not appear to have a role in the management of acute viral gastroenteritis.[9]

Patients should be monitored for signs of dehydration. For persistent vomiting, a nasoduodenal infusion may be useful. Significant vomiting that requires intravenous fluid therapy is usually associated with hypochloremic alkalosis with secondary hypokalemia. Intravenous fluids should repair the deficits (see Chapter 59, Fluids and Electrolytes in Clinical Practice).

Management of gastroesophageal reflux must be individualized. The extent of treatment depends on the volume of emesis and the presence of any of the complications of reflux (esophagitis with or without esophageal stricture or intractable anemia, failure to thrive, or respiratory manifestations). Medical management includes thickening feedings with cereal (a standard concentration is 1 tablespoonful of cereal for each 1 to 2 ounces of formula). For a sleeping infant, left lateral decubitus position may be helpful for reflux; an infant in the 1st months of life should never sleep prone. Elevating the head of the bed remains standard therapy for older children and adults.[10] Older children should also avoid snacks or liquids after dinner and agents that exacerbate esophagitis (alcohol, caffeine, and smoking). Medications can be used in an attempt to improve lower esophageal function and gastric emptying (eg, metoclopramide) and to decrease exposure of the esophageal mucosa to acid (antacids, H_1-receptor blockers, or proton pump inhibitors). A slurry of sucralfate (a cytoprotective agent) is used occasionally. When a child has severe gastroesophageal reflux, medical management may be unsatisfactory. In this case, antireflux surgery (fundoplication) should be considered. In this group of children the results of surgery are generally good when performed by an experienced surgeon, and the benefits can be long lasting. In children who have psychomotor retardation and gastroesophageal reflux, antireflux surgery may not eliminate respiratory symptoms inasmuch as other factors such as swallowing dysfunction may contribute to these findings. Among all children undergoing a Nissen fundoplication, the risk of a postoperative complication that requires further surgery may be as high as 10% and underscores the need for careful patient selection for this operation.

WHEN TO REFER

- Persistent vomiting
- Recurrent episodes of vomiting
- Vomiting associated with a significant underlying process (eg, surgical abdomen, neurologic problem)

WHEN TO ADMIT

- Intractable vomiting with dehydration
- Vomiting in association with symptoms or signs of an acute abdominal process (eg, acute appendicitis, pancreatitis, cholecystitis)

TOOLS FOR PRACTICE

Engaging Patient and Family

- *Caring for Your Baby and Young Child: Birth to Age 5* (book), American Academy of Pediatrics (www.aap.org/bookstore).

AAP POLICY STATEMENT

North American Society for Pediatric Gastroenterology and Nutrition. Guidelines for evaluation and treatment of gastroesophageal reflux in infants and children: recommendations of the North American Society for Pediatric Gastroenterology and Nutrition. *J Pediatr Gastroenterol Nutr.* 2001;32(2):S1-S31. AAP endorsed.

REFERENCES

1. Andrews PL, Richards CA, Smith JE. The neurophysiology of emesis: lessons from basic science for understanding paediatric problems. *J Pediatr Gastronnterol Nutr.* 2001; 32(suppl 1):S12-S13.
2. Allan SG. Antiemetics. *Gastroenterol Clin North Am.* 1992; 21(3):597-611.
3. Andersen JM, Sugerman KS, Lockhart JR, et al. Effective prophylactic therapy for cyclic vomiting syndrome in children using amitriptyline or cyproheptadine. *Pediatrics.* 1997;100(6):977-891.
4. Li BU, Murray RD, Heitlinger LA, et al. Heterogeneity of diagnoses presenting as cyclic vomiting. *Pediatrics.* 1998; 102(3 pt 1):583-587.
5. Pfau BT, Li BU, Murray RD, et al. Differentiating cyclic from chronic vomiting patterns in children: quantitative criteria and diagnostic implications. *Pediatrics.* 1996; 97(3): 364-368.
6. Worawattanakul M, Rhoads JM, Lichtman SN, et al. Abdominal migraine: prophylactic treatment and follow-up. *J Pediatr Gastroenterol Nutr.* 1999;28(1):37-40.
7. Vanderhoof JA, Young R, Kaufman SS, et al. Treatment of cyclic vomiting in childhood with erythromycin. *J Pediatr Gastroenterol Nutr.* 1993;17(4):387-391.
8. Richards CA, Andrews PL. Food refusal: a sign of nausea? *J Pediatr Gastroenterol Nutr.* 2004;38(2):227-228.
9. Borowitz SM. Are antiemetics helpful in young children suffering from acute viral gastroenteritis? *Arch Dis Child.* 2005;90(6):646-648.
10. Rudolph CD, Mazur LJ, Liptak GS, et al. Guidelines for evaluation and treatment of gastroesophageal reflux in infants and children: recommendations of the North American Society for Pediatric Gastroenterology and Nutrition. *J Pediatr Gastroenterol Nutr.* 2001;32(suppl 2): S1-S31.

Chapter 230

WEIGHT LOSS

Diane E. Bloomfield, MD; Elaine A. Dinolfo, MD, MS

Weight loss in an infant, child, or adolescent is an uncommon but highly significant event. As the chief complaint or as an incidental finding, weight loss should be evaluated and followed up carefully by serial measurements and documentation on standardized growth charts. Revised growth charts from the Centers for Disease Control and Prevention released January 2002 represent a broad cross-section of children in the United States. The charts are based on 5 large national samples that included breastfed and formula-fed infants, adolescents to the 20th birthday, and a racially and ethnically diverse population. With emphasis on growth parameters and body mass index, the charts include both 3rd and 97th percentile curves, which may be valuable in assessing weight loss.[1,2] The definition of significant weight loss varies by the child's age and includes acute and chronic causes.

Subjective impressions of weight loss should be verified objectively before an evaluation is undertaken. True weight loss, however, may sometimes be difficult to differentiate from factitious weight loss, even when weights are documented in the medical record. Errors in weighing children occur at frequencies ranging from 5% to 20% of all children weighed, most commonly from faulty equipment or poor technique such as weighing with the child's clothes on.

NEWBORNS AND YOUNG INFANTS

The full-term healthy newborn may lose 5% to 10% of birth weight in the 1st few days but should regain this weight by day 10 of life.[3] A loss of more than 10% to 12% of birth weight is uncommon and should be investigated. The assessment should include overall health of the infant, adequacy of oral intake, and calculation of fluid losses from vomitus, urine, or stool. In general, an infant should gain 25 to 30 g each day in the first 3 months of life.

The most common reason for the breastfed infant to lose more weight than expected or to fail to regain the lost weight by 10 days of age is inadequate intake at the breast. The parental perception that the mother's milk supply is insufficient or less nutritious than formula should not be reinforced. Inadequate weight gain occurs because of infrequent or short feedings, failure of the let-down reflex, or improper positioning of the infant for an effective suck.[4] The infant may appear well or may have signs of significant dehydration. Mothers may report less than 6 urinations a day and few bowel movements. Lack of bowel movements in the breastfed newborn is a key indicator of inadequate caloric intake.[5]

The breastfeeding mother should be observed nursing, if possible, and specific evidence of a let-down reflex should be sought, including uterine cramps, milk dripping or spraying from the opposite breast, a pins-and-needles sensation in the breast at the beginning of each nursing. The infant should be observed latching on to the breast correctly, and loud swallowing or occasional choking may be noted at the beginning of the feeding. (For more information on initiating breastfeeding, see Chapter 89, Breastfeeding the Newborn.) The mother's motivation to breastfeed and her positive or negative feelings about the experience should be discussed. Encouragement and support should be given for continuation of nursing, including specific suggestions for maternal rest, nutrition, and nursing frequency (every 2 to 3 hours in the day) to build up the milk supply. Formula or other fluids should not be recommended unless serious concerns exist about the infant's well being. Recommending discontinuing the breastfeeding prematurely is inappropriate for the physician. An appropriate weight gain in the following few days provides evidence that the infant is well and confirms the diagnosis of initial underfeeding. Infants who fail to thrive while breastfeeding require more intensive nutritional rehabilitation while still preserving breastfeeding.

The formula-fed newborn rarely loses more than 5% of birth weight in the 1st few days, inasmuch as complete nutrition is available beginning a few hours after birth.[6] Weighing less than birth weight at the age of 10 days is unusual for a formula-fed infant, and such an infant should be evaluated thoroughly. An error in feeding caused by maternal inexperience is the usual explanation, with poor caloric intake most often from

BOX 230-1 Differential Diagnosis of Weight Loss by Age Group

NEWBORNS AND YOUNG INFANTS
Difficulties in establishing breastfeeding
Inappropriate dilution or choice of formula
Inadequate intake
Infection
Metabolic abnormality
Craniofacial abnormalities
CNS dysfunction
Somnolence from maternal medications/substance abuse
Congenital heart disease
Maternal depression/inexperience/lack of knowledge
Excessive losses secondary to vomiting or diarrhea
Vomiting because of gastrointestinal malformations (duodenal atresia, others)
Polyuria (diabetes insipidus, renal disease)
Diarrhea

OLDER INFANTS, PRESCHOOLERS, AND SCHOOL-AGED CHILDREN
Pyloric stenosis
Gastroesophageal reflux
CNS tumors
Vomiting
Diarrhea
Fever and infection
Diabetes mellitus
Excessive activity
Inadequate intake
Fever and infection
Tuberculosis
Surgery
Medication effect (loss of appetite)
Malignancy
Congenital heart disease
Poor utilization
Malabsorption syndromes
Inflammatory bowel disease
Immunodeficiency disorders, especially HIV infection
Psychosocial dysfunction
Neglect; nonorganic failure to thrive
Parental depression
Childhood depression
Rumination
Childhood eating disorder

ADOLESCENTS
Dieting behavior
Adolescent eating disorders
Anorexia nervosa
Bulimia nervosa
Other eating disorders
Psychiatric affective disorders, especially depression
Malignancy
Inflammatory bowel disease
Diabetes mellitus
Hyperthyroidism
Tuberculosis

CNS, Central nervous system; *HIV*, human immunodeficiency virus.

either inadequate feedings or faulty preparation of formula. If such is not the case, then a thorough search for an organic problem and an evaluation of family dynamics, support mechanisms, and adjustment to the newborn are indicated. In rare instances a newborn will lose weight as a result of inadequate intake for other reasons, such as infection, congenital heart disease, inborn error of metabolism, somnolence from maternal medications or substance abuse, or poor suck resulting from a craniofacial or central nervous system (CNS) abnormality. Weight loss can also result from either excessive fluid loss, such as vomiting associated with congenital gastrointestinal malformations (duodenal atresia, annular pancreas, volvulus), or from diarrhea or polyuria (diabetes insipidus, renal disease) (Box 230-1).

OLDER INFANTS, PRESCHOOLERS, AND SCHOOL-AGED CHILDREN

The most common reason for weight loss in older infants and toddlers is fluid loss as a result of fever, vomiting, and diarrhea. The loss of weight typically amounts to less than 10% of premorbid body weight and is usually reversed with a few hours of oral or intravenous fluid replacement.

Infants who lose more than 10% of body weight from excessive vomiting require further investigation for pyloric stenosis and malrotation, as well as for tumors of the CNS, which may cause vomiting, anorexia, and cachexia.

Weight loss may also accompany any severe febrile illness such as pneumonia, pyelonephritis, septic arthritis, osteomyelitis, or meningitis, as well as less severe illnesses such as stomatitis and pharyngitis. Resolution of the infection is often followed by a period of catch-up growth and weight gain.

Inefficient use of caloric intake can also result in weight loss. Cystic fibrosis, the most common disease in which malabsorption occurs in childhood, may appear in infancy as poor weight gain or actual weight loss. Intestinal disorders such as celiac disease, Hirschsprung disease, inflammatory bowel disease, and other causes of malabsorption will also lead to weight loss or poor weight gain.

Weight loss from chronic diarrhea may be caused by a variety of infectious diseases, including HIV infection. A diagnosis of tuberculosis should also be considered in every child who has lost weight.

Children with new-onset insulin-dependent diabetes mellitus commonly lose weight (often 10% or more of body weight) despite polyphagia and polydipsia. Hyperthyroidism is another endocrine disorder that may lead to weight loss in childhood.

Malignancies, including leukemia, lymphoma, and neuroblastoma, may have weight loss as part of their presenting picture or even as their initial symptom.

Poverty remains the greatest single risk factor for failure to thrive in the United States; however, other psychosocial factors (poor parent-child interaction, depression, rumination) often underlie an infant's or a child's poor growth and development.[7] Actual weight loss is much less common in this setting than a slowdown or cessation of weight gain and linear growth. Psychosocial dysfunction that results in a child's weight loss requires a prompt and thorough evaluation. Eating disorders have been described in prepubertal children as young as 7 years.[8] (See Chapter 135, Anorexia and Bulimia Nervosa.)

ADOLESCENTS

Monitoring the adolescent growth curve, including body mass index, is crucial to the recognition of weight loss and should be a part of every encounter. The prevalence of obesity in children and adolescents has increased in the last decade, leading to an unhealthy emphasis on dieting and weight loss among children and adolescents.[9] Planned dieting must be distinguished from an eating disorder such as anorexia nervosa or bulimia nervosa. The 2003 American Academy of Pediatrics policy statement regarding the identification and treatment of eating disorders estimates that 0.5% of female adolescents have anorexia nervosa, that 1% to 5% meet criteria for bulimia, and that up to 5% to 10% of all cases of eating disorders occur in boys. As many as one half of adolescents with eating disorders do not meet the *Diagnostic and Statistical Manual of Mental Disorders* criteria but remain at risk for both physical and psychological complications from their altered eating habits.

Anorexia nervosa should be suspected when the adolescent is unwilling or unable to maintain body weight over a minimally normal weight for age and height and when attitudes and behaviors about eating or body image are distorted.[10] The anorectic female adolescent may experience amenorrhea associated with emaciation and overactivity. The patient may demonstrate clinical signs of malnutrition such as hypothyroidism, bradycardia, hypothermia, and growth of lanugo-like hair on the body and extremities. Nutritional rehabilitation and psychiatric treatment are indicated. (See Chapter 135, Anorexia and Bulimia Nervosa.) Adolescents who have bulimia indulge in binge eating, followed by self-induced vomiting, self-starvation, overactivity, or the use of cathartics or diuretics to reduce weight. These behaviors are practiced in secret, and the adolescent often denies them. An elevated serum bicarbonate level, hypokalemia, or high urine pH may provide evidence of chronic vomiting. The patient is often depressed and self-deprecating and may seek medical aid when the eating-vomiting pattern becomes compulsive and out of the patient's control. Psychiatric evaluation and intervention are indicated.

Young adults who participate in sports may follow unhealthy weight-control practices to seek advantage in their athletic activities, including food restriction, vomiting, overexercise, diet pills, stimulants, insulin, nicotine, and voluntary dehydration.[11] For adolescents who participate in sports in which weight loss is a goal (eg, wrestling, gymnastics, ice skating, running, swimming, diving, dancing) a thorough dietary and supplement history should be elicited.

Although significant weight loss during adolescence can often be ascribed to eating disorders, other diagnoses must be considered. These conditions include psychiatric disturbances (especially affective disorders), CNS tumors (particularly those of the hypothalamus), sella turcica or other midline areas, malignancies (especially lymphoma), or gastrointestinal problems such as inflammatory bowel disease or other malabsorption syndromes. Systemic disease such as diabetes mellitus, hyperthyroidism, collagen vascular disease, and renal disease may cause significant weight loss in adolescents. Infectious diseases such as HIV infection and tuberculosis should be considered when an adolescent patient reports weight loss.

INITIAL EVALUATION OF A COMPLAINT OF WEIGHT LOSS

The following should be included in the initial evaluation (Table 230-1):

1. A complete history and thorough physical examination, with special attention to dietary intake, family functioning, and the patient's emotional well being. The growth chart should be reviewed and updated.
2. A complete blood cell count (CBC) and erythrocyte sedimentation rate (ESR). The CBC screens for oncologic factors and provides an overview of the nutritional state. The ESR may be elevated in collagen-vascular diseases, chronic infections, certain malignancies, and inflammatory bowel disease; it may be abnormally low in anorexia nervosa.[3]
3. Serum electrolyte and kidney function tests should be conducted to evaluate for dehydration, to reveal evidence of pernicious or self-induced vomiting, and to rule out renal or adrenal disease.
4. Serum protein and albumin levels to assess liver function, to determine whether the weight loss represents malnutrition, and to rule out protein malabsorption. Reversal of the albumin/globulin ratio is often seen in collagen-vascular diseases and malignancies.[1-3]
5. Tuberculosis skin test.
6. Stool for occult blood and tests of malabsorption to diagnose gastroenteritis, inflammatory bowel disease, and the various causes of malabsorption. The serum carotene level may be low in infancy and in malabsorptive conditions but is often elevated in anorexia nervosa.[3]
7. Urinalysis and urine culture to rule out diabetes mellitus, diabetes insipidus, dehydration, urinary tract infection, and renal disease. The urine pH may be high (>8) in adolescents who have eating disorders, particularly when vomiting occurs.[4]

Table 230-1 Laboratory Studies Helpful in Weight Loss

SUGGESTED STUDIES	SUGGESTED DIAGNOSES
Complete blood cell count, smear	Anemia Infection Nutritional deficiencies Malabsorptive syndromes Malignancy
Erythrocyte sedimentation rate (ESR)	Collagen-vascular disease Infection Inflammatory bowel disease Malignancy Anorexia nervosa (very low ESR)
Serum electrolytes, kidney function tests	Dehydration Vomiting, self-induced or pernicious Renal dysfunction Adrenal disorders Metabolic disorder (with acidosis) Collagen-vascular disease
Serum protein and albumin levels	Liver dysfunction Malignancy Malnutrition Protein malabsorption Protein-losing enteropathy
Tuberculosis skin test	Tuberculosis
Stool for occult blood	Gastroenteritis Inflammatory bowel disease Enteropathies
Serum carotene; specific tests of malabsorption	Malabsorption syndromes Cystic fibrosis Anorexia nervosa (high carotene)
Urinalysis, including specific gravity; urine culture	Diabetes mellitus Diabetes insipidus Dehydration Urinary tract infection Renal disease Adolescent eating disorder (high pH)

WHEN TO REFER

Evidence or suspicion of:

- Malignancy
- Endocrinopathy (thyroid, adrenal, pituitary)
- Gastrointestinal disorder (eg, gastroesophageal reflux; malabsorption, including cystic fibrosis; inflammatory bowel disease)
- Pancreatitis
- Heart disease
- Renal disease
- Pulmonary disease
- Rheumatologic condition
- CNS abnormality
- Metabolic disorder
- Surgical abdominal problem (eg, pyloric stenosis, Hirschsprung disease, volvulus)
- Immunodeficiency
- Unusual infection
- Psychiatric diagnosis in child or caretaker
- Anorexia nervosa or bulimia nervosa in the child or adolescent

WHEN TO ADMIT

- A newborn, when:
  - Weight loss cannot be managed as outpatient
  - Weight loss of more than 12% to 15% of birth weight
  - Excessive fluid loss (vomiting, diarrhea, polyuria)
  - Evidence of infant hypernatremic dehydration
  - Suspicion of infection, metabolic abnormality, congenital heart disease, other conditions requiring evaluation
  - Extreme passivity of the infant, which may require tube feeding
  - Need for intensive maternal education and support
- At any age, when:
  - Weight loss is excessive (more than 5% to 10% of previous weight)
  - Excessive fluid loss from vomiting or diarrhea
  - New-onset diabetes mellitus (usually)
  - Evidence of severe febrile illness (pneumonia, pyelonephritis, osteomyelitis, meningitis, septic arthritis, others)
  - Evidence of dehydration
  - Physiological instability
  - Severe bradycardia
  - Hypotension
  - Hypothermia
  - Orthostatic changes
  - Electrolyte abnormalities (eg, hypernatremia, hypokalemia)
  - Evidence of significant psychosocial dysfunction
- An adolescent, when:
  - Eating disorder cannot be managed as outpatient
  - Severe malnutrition, with weight <75% of ideal body weight
  - Evidence of dehydration or electrolyte abnormalities
  - Physiological instability
  - Acute food refusal
  - Uncontrollable binge eating and purging
  - Acute medical complication of malnutrition (syncope, seizures, cardiac failure, pancreatitis)
  - Suicidal intent or ideation, or psychosis

TOOLS FOR PRACTICE

Engaging Patient and Family

- *About BMI for Children and Teens* (fact sheet), Centers for Disease Control and Prevention (www.cdc.gov/nccdphp/dnpa/bmi/childrens_BMI/about_childrens_BMI.htm).
- *Eating Disorders: What You Should Know About Anorexia and Bulimia* (brochure), American Academy of Pediatrics (patiented.aap.org).
- *New Mother's Guide to Breastfeeding* (book), American Academy of Pediatrics (www.aap.org/bookstore).

Medical Decision Support

- *BMI—Body Mass Index: Child and Teen Calculator: English* (interactive tool), Centers for Disease Control and Prevention (http://apps.nccd.cdc.gov/dnpabmi/Calculator.aspx).
- *Breastfeeding Handbook For Physician* (book), American Academy of Pediatrics (www.aap.org/bookstore).
- *Eating Behaviors of the Young Child: Prenatal and Postnatal Influences for Healthy Eating* (book), Dietz W, Birch L (www.aap.org/bookstore).
- *Growth Charts—tutorials and information* (Web page), Centers for Disease Control and Prevention (www.cdc.gov/growthcharts/).
- *Growth Charts* (chart), Centers for Disease Control and Prevention (www.cdc.gov/nchs/about/major/nhanes/growthcharts/clinical_charts.htm#Clin%201) also available at AAP bookstore (www.aap.org/bst/showprod.cfm?&DID=15&CATID=133&ObjectGroup_ID=798).
- *Pediatric Nutrition Handbook - 5th edition* (book), American Academy of Pediatrics (www.aap.org/bookstore).

AAP POLICY STATEMENTS

American Academy of Pediatrics, Section on Breastfeeding. Breastfeeding and the use of human milk. *Pediatrics.* 2005; 115(2):496-450. (aappolicy.aapublications.org/cgi/content/full/pediatrics;115/2/496).

American Academy of Pediatrics, Committee on Adolescence. Identifying and treating eating disorders. *Pediatrics.* 2003;111(1):204-211. (aappolicy.aappublications.org/cgi/content/full/pediatrics;111/1/204).

American Academy of Pediatrics, Committee on Sports Medicine and Fitness. Promotion of health weight-control practices in young athletes. *Pediatrics.* 2005;116(6):1557-1564. (aappolicy.aappublications.org/cgi/content/full/pediatrics;116/6/1557).

American Heart Association, Gidding SS, Dennison BA, Birch LL, et al. Dietary recommendations for children and adolescents: a guide for practitioners. *Pediatrics.* 2005; 117(2):554-559. AAP endorsed. (aappolicy.aappublications.org/cgi/content/full/pediatrics;117/2/544).

Block RW, Krebs NF, American Academy of Pediatrics, Committee on Child Abuse and Neglect and the Committee on Nutrition. Failure to thrive as a manifestation of child neglect. *Pediatrics.* 2005;116(5):1234-1237. (aappolicy.aappublications.org/cgi/content/full/pediatrics;116/5/1234).

REFERENCES

1. Dawson P. Normal growth and revised growth charts. *Pediatr Rev.* 2002;23(7):255-256.
2. National Center for Health Statistics. Clinical Growth Charts. Available at: www.cdc.gov/growthcharts. Accessed June 19, 2007.
3. McDonald PD, Ross Sr, Grant L, et al. Neonatal weight loss in breast and formula fed infants. *Arch Dis Child Fetal Neonatal Ed.* 2003;88(6):472-476.
4. Stashwick CA. When a breastfed infant isn't gaining weight. *Contemp Pediatr.* 1993;10:116-134.
5. Metaj M, Laroia N, Lawrence KA, et al. Comparison of breast- and formula-fed normal newborns in time to first stool and urine. *J Perinatol.* 2003;23(8):624-628.
6. Lawrence RA, Lawrence RM. *Breastfeeding: A Guide for the Medical Profession.* 5th ed. St Louis, MO: Mosby; 1999.
7. Block RW, Krebs NF, American Academy of Pediatrics, Committee on Child Abuse and Neglect, Committee on Nutrition. Failure to thrive as a manifestation of child neglect. *Pediatrics.* 2005;116(5):1234-1237.
8. Atkins DM, Silber TJ. Clinical spectrum of anorexia nervosa in children. *J Dev Behav Pediatr.* 1993;14(4):211-216.
9. American Academy of Pediatrics, Committee on Adolescence. Identifying and treating eating disorders. *Pediatrics.* 2003;111(1):204-211.
10. American Psychiatric Association: *Diagnostic and Statistical Manual of Mental Disorders (DSM-IV-TR).* 4th ed, text revision. Washington DC: The Association; 2000.
11. American Academy of Pediatrics, Committee on Sports Medicine and Fitness. Promotion of health weight-control practices in young athletes. *Pediatrics.* 2005;116(6):1557-1564.

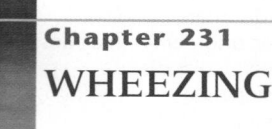

Chapter 231

WHEEZING

Alfin G. Vicencio, MD; Joshua P. Needleman, MD

DEFINITION

Wheezing is a continuous, musical sound that represents turbulent, intrathoracic airflow; it may be present in both inspiration and expiration but is usually more prominent during expiration. A history of wheezing reported by family members, however, is insensitive and nonspecific because untrained observers without appropriate equipment will often mistake many respiratory sounds for wheezing.

During the normal respiratory cycle, rhythmic expansion and contraction of the thorax leads to dynamic changes in thoracic pressures, allowing air to flow into and out of the lungs (Figure 231-1). On inspiration, the thoracic cavity expands, resulting in negative intrathoracic and airway pressures (relative to atmospheric pressure) and allowing air to flow into the lungs. Extrathoracic airway obstruction, signaled by stridor, is most likely to cause turbulent airflow during this phase of the respiratory cycle (see Figure 231-1, *A*). Expiration is accomplished by contracting the volume of the thoracic cavity, creating positive pressure in the thorax, which is transmitted to the intrathoracic airways. Thus, during expiration, the intrathoracic airways are more prone to obstruction leading to turbulent airflow (see Figure 231-1, *B*).

Although wheezing is most commonly associated with the distal airway obstruction seen in viral bronchiolitis or asthma, several other diseases can cause small airway obstruction and can be indistinguishable on physical examination. Similarly, abnormalities causing obstruction of the mid or distal trachea or mainstem bronchi, both of which reside within the thorax, can cause wheezing. Thus, although bronchiolitis and asthma will certainly account for the majority of children

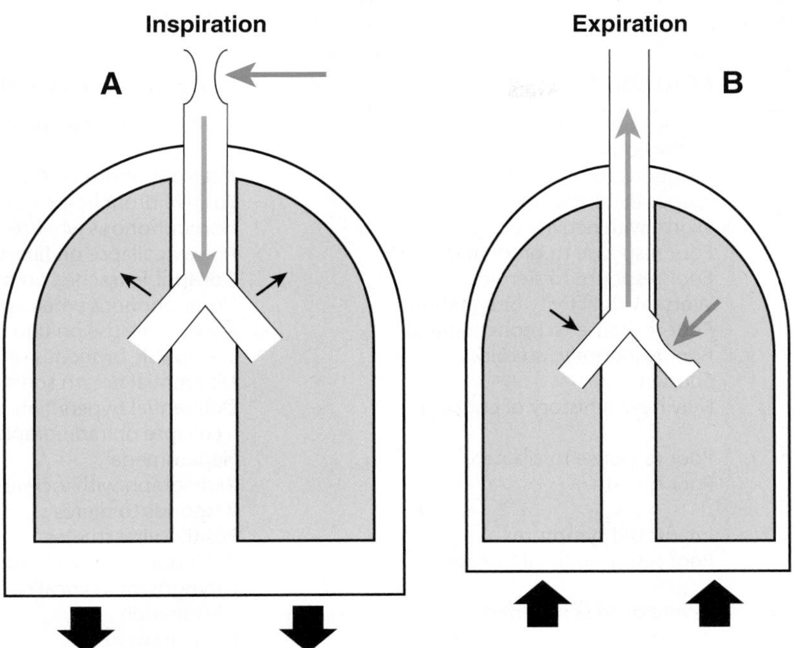

Figure 231-1 The respiratory cycle and related airway changes. **A,** During inspiration, negative intrathoracic pressures generated by thoracic expansion are likely to cause obstruction in the extrathoracic airway *(red arrow)* leading to stridor. **B,** During expiration, positive intrathoracic pressures generated by thoracic compression are likely to cause obstruction in the intrathoracic airways, including the mid and distal trachea, mainstem bronchi, and small bronchioles, leading to wheeze.

who wheeze, the general pediatrician should be prepared to initiate a more extensive evaluation for the wheezing child, particularly for patients with unusual presentations or if conventional treatment yields less-than-optimal results.

DIFFERENTIAL DIAGNOSIS

The differential diagnosis of wheezing is extensive and includes any process that can cause obstruction of intrathoracic airways. Because the intrathoracic airways include large centrally located airways and smaller peripheral bronchioles, determining the level of obstruction is often helpful before generating a list of differential diagnoses (see Evaluation).

Viral bronchiolitis and asthma account for the majority of wheezing localized to the small peripheral airways. (See Chapter 239, Asthma; and Chapter 243, Bronchiolitis.) A major challenge in evaluating the wheezing child is determining when the wheeze is not caused by asthma or bronchiolitis, but rather a different process requiring different diagnostic approaches and alternate treatment strategies. For example, cystic fibrosis, a severe genetic disease causing progressive small airway obstruction and early death, is often mistaken for poorly controlled asthma. Similarly, early congestive heart failure can produce intractable wheezing from peribronchial edema. Pulmonary hemosiderosis, a rare disorder, can cause anemia and recurrent wheezing because blood irritates the peripheral airways. In a similar manner, gastroesophageal reflux and recurrent aspiration can also result in persistent or recurrent wheezing and may also complicate large airway abnormalities.

Distinguishing large airway obstruction from peripheral obstruction is difficult because both can cause expiratory wheeze. In addition, a variety of abnormalities can cause large airway obstruction, further complicating evaluation and diagnosis. Dynamic lesions of the large airways such as tracheomalacia or bronchomalacia are fairly common causes of congenital wheezing and can also be associated with gastroesophageal reflux, tracheoesophageal fistula, or prolonged mechanical ventilation in premature infants. External compression of large airways can be seen with vascular abnormalities (rings and slings), mediastinal masses, or infectious agents, most notably lymphobronchial tuberculosis. Finally, intrinsic airway abnormalities, including complete tracheal rings and webs, and acquired obstructions, such as tracheal stenosis or granulation tissue, can cause intractable wheezing.

EVALUATION

History

A major challenge in evaluating the wheezing child is to determine when a wheeze is not from viral bronchiolitis or asthma. Wheezing caused by viral bronchiolitis is usually preceded by upper respiratory symptoms and fever, often worsens within the first few days of onset, and tends to improve slowly thereafter. Asthma exacerbations are often initiated by vigorous activity, changes

Table 231-1 Causes of Recurrent or Persistent Wheeze

	FEATURES	OBJECTIVE FINDINGS
Asthma	Worse with exercise or respiratory infections Responds to bronchodilators Responds to steroids	Reversible obstruction on PFTs Heterophonous wheeze Positive broncho-provocation
Tracheomalacia	Worse with activity or agitation Poor response to bronchodilators Poor response to steroids	Homophonous wheeze Airway collapse on fluoroscopy Collapsible trachea on bronchoscopy
Bronchomalacia	Worse with activity or agitation Poor response to bronchodilators Poor response to steroids	Homophonous wheeze Airway collapse on fluoroscopy Collapsible bronchus on bronchoscopy
Foreign body	Sudden onset May have a history of choking	Differential breath sounds Differential hyperinflation or collapse on radiograph
Heart failure or pulmonary edema	Poor response to albuterol Poor growth	Hepatomegaly Radiograph with increased fluid Responds to diuresis
Bronchiolitis	Infant: URI symptoms	Positive viral studies
Vocal cord dysfunction	Poor response to all therapies Severe distress reported	PFTs: normal or with abnormal inspiratory loop Laryngoscopy: vocal cord adduction during inspiration
Cystic fibrosis	Poor growth, GI symptoms Recurrent pneumonias	Positive sweat test
Gastroesophageal reflux and aspiration	Variable response to bronchodilators Often worse after meals	Positive reflux evaluation (upper GI, nuclear scan or pH probe)
Vascular compression	Central wheeze No bronchodilator response	Indentation on esophagram Anatomy demonstrated on thoracic MRI
Large airway abnormality (stenosis, complete rings, compression)	No response to therapy Worse with activity Stridor noted at times	Flattened or square flow–volume loop Obstruction visible on imaging or bronchoscopy

GI, Gastrointestinal; *MRI*, magnetic resonance imaging; *PFTs*, pulmonary function tests; *URI*, upper respiratory infection.

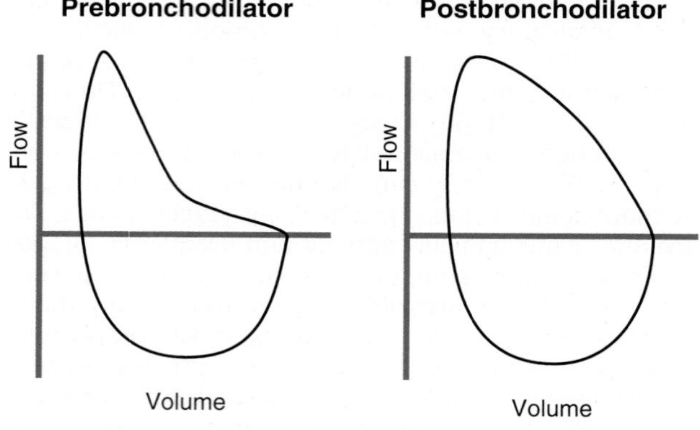

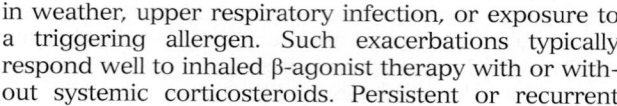

Figure 231-2 Pulmonary function test demonstrating small airway obstruction. Small airway obstruction, such as that seen in asthma, has a distinctive scooped appearance on spirometry. Normalization of the flow loop after bronchodilator treatment strongly suggests asthma as the underlying cause of recurrent wheezing.

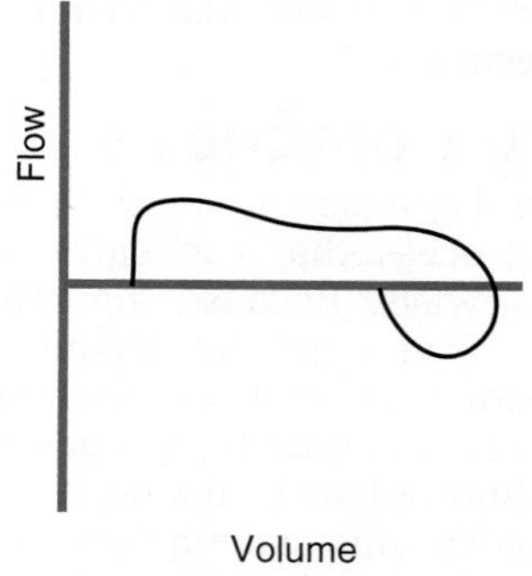

Figure 231-3 Pulmonary function test demonstrating large airway fixed obstruction. Fixed obstruction of a large airway by compression or stenosis will result in a characteristic flat expiratory loop on spirometry. No change will occur after administering bronchodilator.

in weather, upper respiratory infection, or exposure to a triggering allergen. Such exacerbations typically respond well to inhaled β-agonist therapy with or without systemic corticosteroids. Persistent or recurrent episodes of wheezing that do not fit these profiles should be evaluated more thoroughly.

A detailed and focused history can often provide clues to an accurate diagnosis. Wheezing that appears at birth or soon afterward should prompt an evaluation for congenital airway abnormalities such as tracheomalacia, complete rings, or vascular abnormalities or

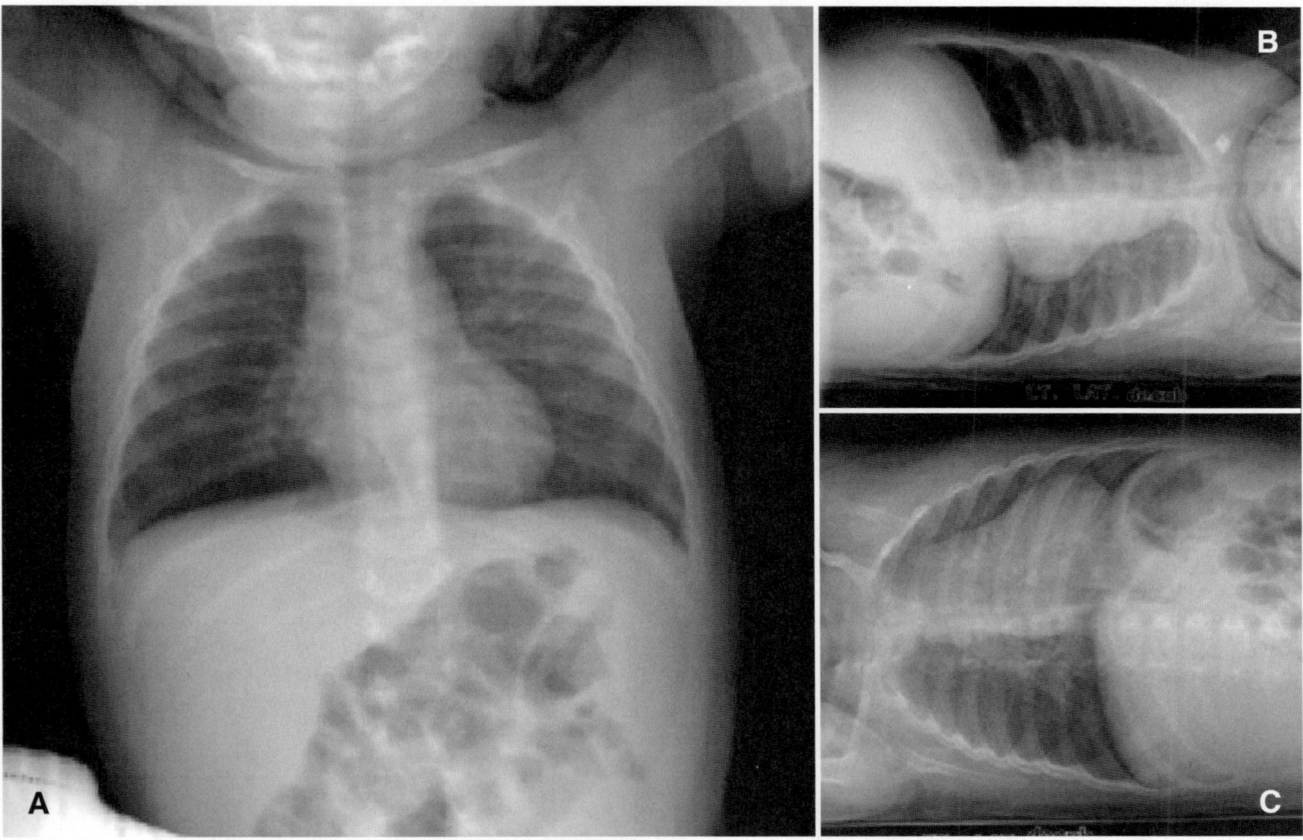

Figure 231-4 Foreign body aspiration. **A,** Chest radiograph demonstrates mild hyperaeration of the right lung and mild flattening of the right hemi-diaphragm on anterior-posterior view. **B,** On left lateral decubitus view, the hyperaeration of the right lung is accentuated. **C,** On right lateral decubitus view, the heart does not shift with gravity, and the right lung remains well inflated. A peanut was found in the right mainstem bronchus during bronchoscopy.

compression. Wheezing after a recent surgical procedure or intubation suggests acquired obstruction, whereas abrupt onset of wheezing accompanied by a history of choking should prompt an evaluation for aspiration of a foreign body. Other clues that suggest underlying illnesses or abnormalities include constant wheezing, failure to thrive, hemoptysis, difficulty swallowing, frequent vomiting, positional wheezing, worsening with agitation or crying, and poor response to conventional therapy.

Physical Examination

Location of airway obstruction can often be determined by thorough physical examination and can direct the ensuing workup. Unilateral wheezing, most often associated with aspiration of a foreign body, can also accompany unilateral bronchial compression or stenosis and should be evaluated thoroughly. In addition to determining if the wheezing is bilateral or unilateral, detailed assessment of the auditory characteristics can help determine if the obstruction is central or peripheral. For example, wheezing that varies in pitch and can be heard throughout the chest (musical, heterophonous) typically represents small airway obstruction. In contrast, central airway obstruction tends to sound more even in pitch (monophonic, homophonous) and can often be heard best in central locations such as the sternal notch, although this may be unreliable in a small infant. In addition, large airway obstruction is more likely than small to be heard throughout the entire expiratory phase.

In addition to the auditory composition of a wheeze, positional characteristics can help determine cause. For example, wheezing caused by a dynamic lesion such as tracheomalacia is often worse when a patient is supine. Mediastinal structures such as the heart and the great vessels, which lie immediately anterior to the trachea, tend to fall posteriorly in the supine position and can be obstructive. In contrast, these structures tend to fall anteriorly when the patient is prone, relieving pressure on the airway and improving the wheeze. Wheezing caused by small airway obstruction or fixed compression of a large airway does not typically change with position.

Objective Testing

Although a detailed history and physical examination can help the clinician narrow the list of potential diagnoses, additional testing is often helpful and may guide therapy. Information obtained through the

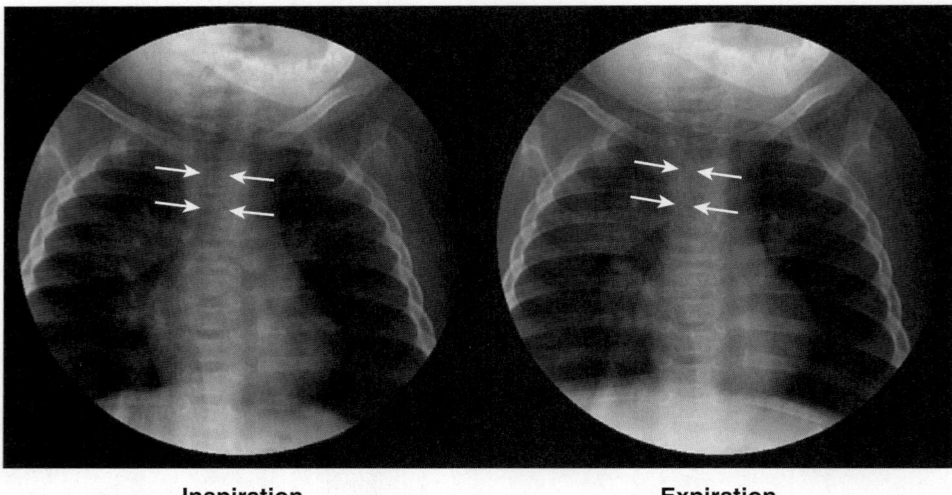

Figure 231-5 Airway fluoroscopy. Airway fluoroscopy demonstrates a normal trachea during inspiration *(arrows).* On expiration, severe collapse of the trachea is demonstrated, indicating tracheomalacia.

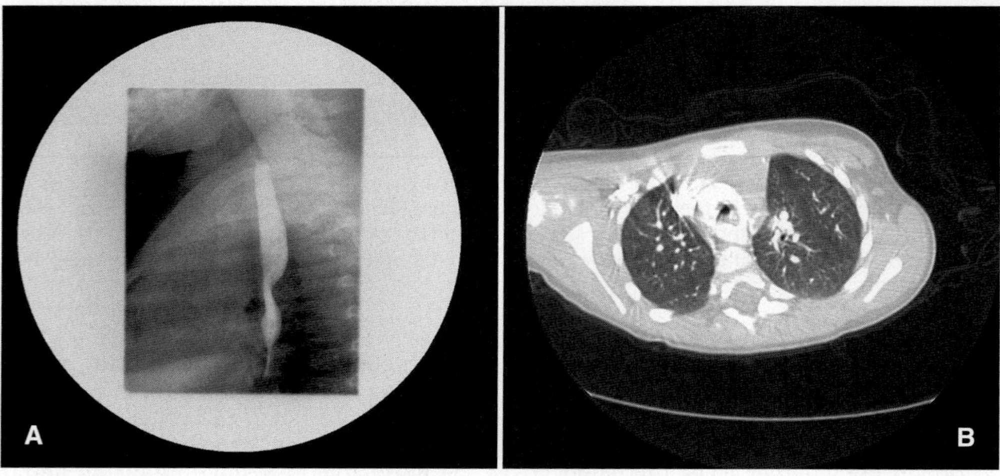

Figure 231-6 Esophagram and computed tomographic scan. **A,** Esophagram demonstrates a posterior indentation suggestive of a vascular ring. **B,** Computed tomographic scan of the chest confirms the presence of a double aortic arch.

history and physical examination should guide further evaluation. Table 231-1 highlights the features of some common abnormalities that cause wheezing.

Laboratory testing may be indicated to diagnose specific clinical entities. For example, a sweat test is required if cystic fibrosis is suspected, and viral studies can identify respiratory syncytial virus or influenza as a cause of small airway wheezing in an infant with upper respiratory symptoms.

Pulmonary function testing can help characterize a wheeze objectively. The expiratory loop shown in Figure 231-2 demonstrates small airway obstruction that improves after bronchodilator therapy, suggesting asthma as the underlying cause of recurrent wheezing. In contrast, small airway obstruction that does not demonstrate reversibility after bronchodilator therapy may require additional workup; several disease processes, including cystic fibrosis, congestive heart failure, and obliterative bronchiolitis, can cause fixed small airway obstruction. Similarly, expiratory loops suggesting fixed large airway obstruction (Figure 231-3) may require further evaluation for stenosis, rings or compression.

Radiographic studies can be helpful when evaluating a patient with persistent or recurrent wheeze, particularly when asthma or viral bronchiolitis is not likely the cause. Chest radiography can detect thoracic masses that cause obstruction of airways. In addition,

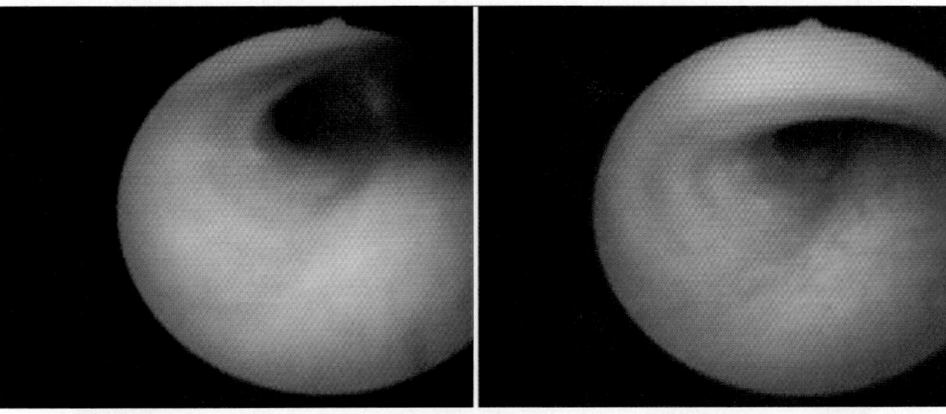

Figure 231-7 Images from fiber-optic bronchoscopy. Fiber-optic bronchoscopy demonstrates normal tracheal caliber during inspiration. During expiration, the distal trachea collapses, consistent with tracheomalacia.

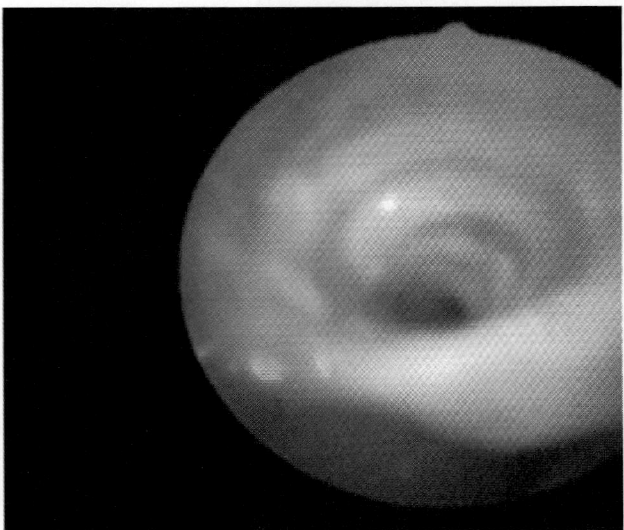

Figure 231-8 Images from fiber-optic bronchoscopy. Fiber-optic bronchoscopy demonstrates complete cartilaginous rings causing severe obstruction of the trachea.

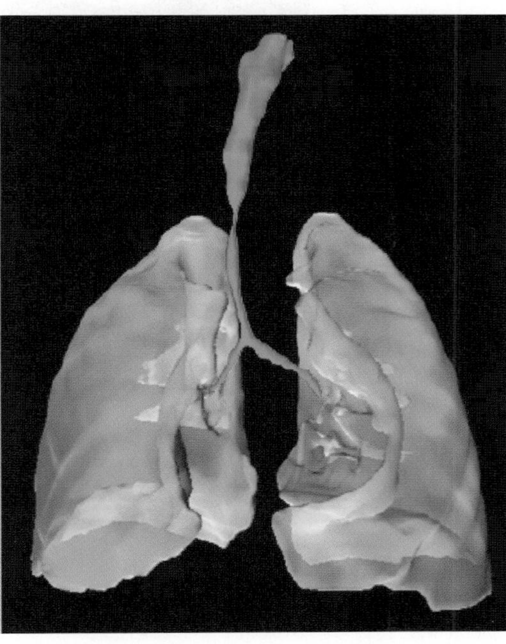

Figure 231-9 Three-dimensional reconstruction of computed tomographic image. Severe circumferential narrowing of the trachea starting at the thoracic inlet and extending to the mainstem bronchi.

chest radiography with decubitus films or inspiratory and expiratory views can be helpful in diagnosing foreign body aspiration (Figure 231-4). If history and physical examination suggest tracheobronchomalacia as an underlying diagnosis, then airway fluoroscopy (Figure 231-5) can confirm the diagnosis and help quantify the severity. An esophagram or upper gastrointestinal series is useful if a vascular abnormality is suspected. However, although a vascular abnormality can be easily identified by an esophageal notch in an esophagram, a computed tomographic scan with contrast (Figure 231-6) or magnetic resonance image is ultimately required to determine the exact anatomic variant, which may include a double aortic arch, a right aortic arch with aberrant left subclavian, or a pulmonary artery sling.

Direct visualization of the airway via flexible bronchoscopy is increasingly used to better characterize dynamic lesions such as tracheobronchomalacia better (Figure 231-7). Intrinsic airway abnormalities, such as complete cartilaginous rings, often require bronchoscopy to make a diagnosis (Figure 231-8), although improved radiologic techniques, such as 3-dimensional airway reconstruction, are valuable (Figure 231-9). Furthermore, rigid bronchoscopy can be useful in both diagnosis and treatment of tracheal stenosis (Figure 231-10). Bronchoscopy can

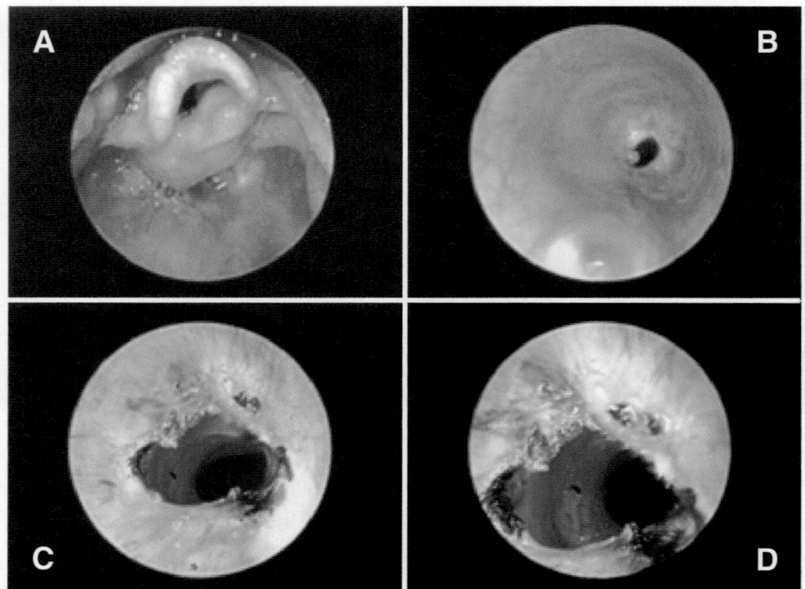

Figure 231-10 Images from rigid bronchoscopy. **A**, Epiglottis. **B**, Severe stenosis secondary to a tracheal web. **C** and **D**, After laser resection of the stenosis. *(Courtesy of Sanjay Parikh, MD.)*

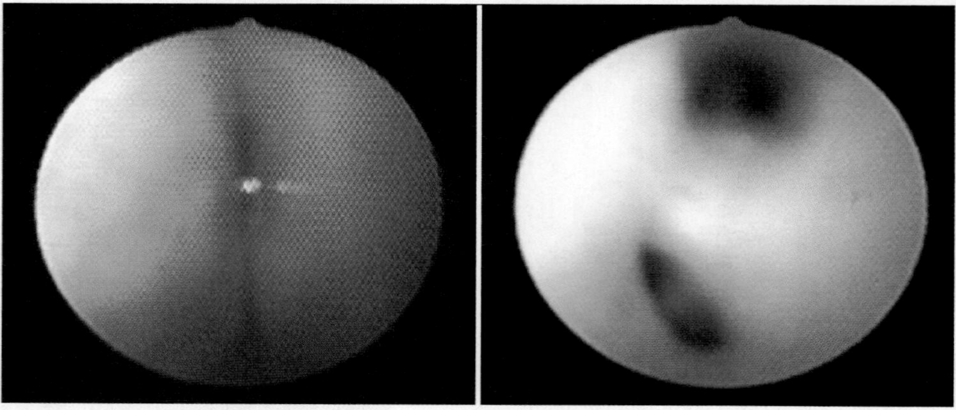

Figure 231-11 Images from fiber-optic bronchoscopy. Complete obstruction of the distal left mainstem bronchus secondary to a mediastinal mass. Immediately after resection of the mass, the segmental branch points of the left lung are easily identified.

help assess the severity of airway compression by a thoracic mass and confirm patency after resection (Figure 231-11).

MANAGEMENT

The majority of patients with wheezing have viral bronchiolitis and asthma and should be managed accordingly. Although some children with viral bronchiolitis or asthma require hospitalization for severe respiratory distress, hypoxemia, poor feeding or dehydration, the general pediatrician can care for most children in an outpatient setting. An important point to note is that, currently, no evidence exists to support the regular use of β-agonist therapy in viral bronchiolitis. Hospital admission or referral to a subspecialty physician may be indicated for chronic wheezing associated with failure to thrive, which can be a sign of a significant underlying disease. Similarly, an unusual history or physical examination should prompt more detailed evaluation and may require alternate treatment regimens, depending on the cause. In general, the pediatrician evaluating the child with wheeze should (1) be aware of the various clinical entities that can produce wheezing, (2) be able to recognize by history or physical examination patients who require further workup, (3) initiate simple diagnostic tests, and (4) refer to appropriate subspecialty physicians children with unusual presentations or poor response to conventional therapies.

WHEN TO REFER

- Persistent or recurrent wheezing in an infant younger than 1 year
- Apparent paradoxical response to bronchodilators
- Poor weight gain or growth associated with chronic or recurrent wheezing
- Repeated hospitalization or multiple courses of oral corticosteroids

WHEN TO ADMIT

- Respiratory distress unresponsive to therapy
- Hypoxemia
- Tachypnea interfering with ability to eat or drink
- Altered mental status or signs of fatigue

SUGGESTED READINGS

Callahan CW. Primary tracheomalacia and gastroesophageal reflux in infants with cough. *Clin Pediatr.* 1998;37: 725-732.

Elphick HE, Sherlock P, Foxall G, et al. Survey of respiratory sounds in infants. *Arch Dis Child.* 2001;84: 35-39.

Finder JD. Primary bronchomalacia in infants and children. *J Pediatr.* 1997;130:59-66.

Harty MP, Kramer SS. Recent advances in pediatric pulmonary imaging. *Curr Opin Pediatr.* 1998;10: 227-235.

Lowe LA, Simpson A, Woodcock A, et al. Wheeze phenotypes and lung function in preschool children. *Am J Respir Crit Care Med.* 2005;171:231-237.

Newman KB, Mason UG, Schmaling KB. Clinical features of vocal cord dysfunction. *Am J Respir Crit Care Med.* 1995;152:1382-1386.

Schellhase DE, Fawcett DD, Shutze GE, et al. Clinical utility of flexible bronchoscopy and bronchoalveolar lavage in young children with recurrent wheezing. *J Pediatr.* 1998;132:321-328.

Taylor WR, Newacheck PW. Impact of childhood asthma on health. *Pediatrics.* 1992;90:657-662.

Wood RE. The emerging role of flexible bronchoscopy in pediatrics. *Clin Chest Med.* 2001;22:311-317.

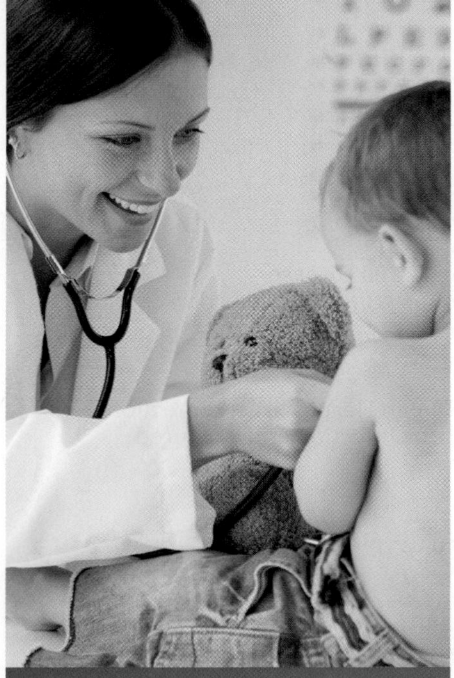

PART 9

Specific Clinical Problems

232 Acne
233 Adrenal Dysfunction
234 Allergic Rhinitis
235 Animal Bites
236 Anuria and Oliguria
237 Apparent Life-threatening Events
238 Appendicitis
239 Asthma
240 Atopic Dermatitis
241 Bacterial Skin Infections
242 Brain Tumors
243 Bronchiolitis
244 Cancers in Childhood
245 Cerebral Palsy
246 Chickenpox
247 Chronic Fatigue Syndrome
248 Cleft Lip and Cleft Palate
249 Colic
250 Common Cold
251 Congenital and Acquired Heart Disease
252 Contact Dermatitis
253 Contagious Exanthematous Diseases
254 Cystic Fibrosis
255 Cystic and Solid Masses of the Face and Neck
256 Diabetes Mellitus
257 Diaper Rash
258 Down Syndrome: Managing the Child and Family
259 Drug Eruptions, Erythema Multiforme, Stevens-Johnson Syndrome, and Toxic Epidermal Necrolysis
260 Enterovirus Infections
261 Enuresis
262 Foreign Bodies of the Ear, Nose, Airway, and Esophagus
263 Fractures and Dislocations
264 Gastroesophageal Reflux Disease
265 Gastrointestinal Allergy
266 Gastrointestinal Obstruction
267 Giardiasis

Continued

268 Gluten-sensitive Enteropathy (Celiac Sprue)
269 Hemolytic-Uremic Syndrome
270 Hemoglobinopathies and Sickle Cell Disease
271 Hemophilia and Other Hereditary Bleeding Disorders
272 Henoch-Schönlein Purpura
273 Hepatitis
274 Herpes Infections
275 Human Herpesvirus-6 and Human Herpesvirus-7 Infections
276 Human Immunodeficiency Virus Infection and Acquired Immunodeficiency Syndrome
277 Hydrocephalus
278 Hyperthyroidism
279 Hypospadias, Epispadias, and Cryptorchism
280 Hypothyroidism
281 Iatrogenic Disease
282 Immune Thrombocytopenia Purpura
283 Infectious Mononucleosis and Other Epstein-Barr Viral Infections
284 Insect Bites and Infestations
285 Intellectual Disability
286 Intersex
287 Iron-Deficiency Anemia
288 Juvenile Idiopathic Arthritis
289 Kawasaki Disease
290 Labial Adhesions
291 Leukemias
292 Lyme Disease
293 Meningitis
294 Meningoencephalitis
295 Muscular Dystrophy
296 Nephritis
297 Nephrotic Syndrome
298 Neurocutaneous Syndromes
299 Obesity and Metabolic Syndrome
300 Obstructive Uropathy and Vesicoureteral Reflux
301 Ocular Trauma
302 Osteochondroses
303 Osteomyelitis
304 Otitis Media and Otitis Externa
305 Parasitic Infections
306 Pectus Excavatum and Pectus Carinatum
307 Pertussis (Whooping Cough)
308 Pharyngitis and Tonsillitis
309 Phimosis
310 Pinworm Infestations
311 Plagiocephaly
312 Pneumonia
313 Preseptal and Orbital Cellulitis
314 Psoriasis
315 Pyloric Stenosis
316 Renal Tubule Acidosis
317 Rheumatic Fever
318 Rocky Mountain Spotted Fever
319 Seborrheic Dermatitis
320 Seizure Disorders
321 Septic Arthritis
322 Sexually Transmitted Infections
323 Sinusitis

Continued

324 Spina Bifida
325 Spinal Deformities
326 Sports Injuries
327 Staphylococcal Toxic Shock Syndrome
328 Stomatitis
329 Streptococcal Toxic Shock Syndrome
330 Sudden Infant Death Syndrome
331 Tonsillectomy and Adenoidectomy
332 Tuberculosis and Latent Tuberculosis Infection
333 Umbilical Anomalies
334 Urinary Tract Infections
335 Verrucae (Warts) and Molluscum Contagiosum

Chapter 232

ACNE

Catherine Chen, MD; Judith V. Williams, MD

Acne is so prevalent in adolescents and young adults that some people consider it a physiological event. This perspective does not take into account the effect of acne on the patient, and it may preclude therapeutic intervention. Acne is a treatable disease that deserves medical attention.

ETIOLOGY

Hormones

Acne is a disease of the pilosebaceous unit.[1-3] Androgens stimulate the sebaceous glands, which enlarge and increase their production of sebum. Before puberty, the responsible androgens are of adrenal origin.[4] After puberty, gonadal androgens further stimulate the sebaceous glands. Patients who have acne may have normal levels of circulating testosterone; therefore tissue androgen metabolism may be an important factor in the pathogenesis of acne. One of the major organs for androgen metabolism is the skin, where the enzyme 5-α-reductase metabolizes testosterone to dihydrotestosterone, which has significantly increased potent activity at the tissue level. 5-α-reductase may be more active in the skin of patients with acne than those without, increasing androgenic stimulation of the sebaceous glands, ultimately causing acne. Increased sebaceous gland activity is necessary for acne to develop; alone, it is insufficient to cause disease. Additional factors are needed.

Follicular Obstruction

If sebum is allowed to drain freely to the surface, the surface skin then becomes oily, but acne does not develop. Acne can develop only if the outlet of the follicular canal is obstructed, which occurs when adherent, keratinized cells within the canal accumulate and form an impaction that blocks the flow of sebum (Figure 232-1). Production of keratinized cells within the lining of the follicular canal is normal, but accumulation and subsequent impaction are not. This follicular obstruction, which may also be influenced by androgens, is a prerequisite for the development of acne.

Bacteria

Sebum and keratinous debris accumulate proximal to the follicular outlet obstruction. This accumulation provides an attractive environment for the growth of anaerobic bacteria, particularly *Propionibacterium acnes*, which play a role in the pathogenesis of inflammatory acne.[5] Several factors may be involved in causing the inflammation. One theory suggests that the lipase enzymes elaborated by *P acnes* hydrolyze sebaceous lipids, releasing free fatty acids, which then cause irritation when the follicle ruptures. *P acnes* also produce chemotactic factors that may attract inflammatory cells directly to a sebaceous follicle. Some evidence indicates that complement-mediated inflammation is directed against *P acnes* itself. Regardless of the mechanism of inflammation, little question remains as to the therapeutic benefit of antibiotics.

The events in the pathogenesis of acne include (1) androgenic stimulation of sebaceous glands, which increases sebum production; (2) keratinous impaction in the pilosebaceous canal, causing outlet obstruction; (3) accumulation of sebaceous and keratinous debris behind the obstruction and (4) proliferation of *P acnes*, which alters this milieu in such a way as to contribute to the rupture of the dilated pilosebaceous unit, resulting in extravasation of its contents into the surrounding dermis and inflammatory acne lesions.

CLINICAL FINDINGS

The disease process may begin at a surprisingly young age. In a study of premenarchal girls, 78% were found to have some acne.[6] The same investigators found acne to be present in 100% of adolescent boys.[7] Although the severity of the disease increases during adolescence, acne is, by no means, confined to these years. For acne activity to continue into the 3rd and 4th decades of life is not uncommon.

The pathogenic mechanisms previously described result in noninflamed open and closed comedones and inflammatory papules and pustules, as well as cystic acne in more severe cases. Cystic acne is made up of

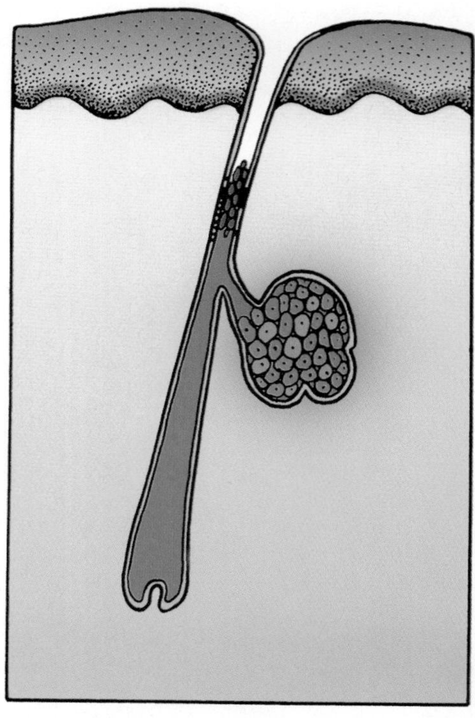

Figure 232-1 Obstruction of the pilosebaceous unit in acne.

nodules greater than 5 millimeters in diameter and true cysts, which are compressible nodules under normal-appearing skin. These nodules and cysts can result in permanent acne scars.

The acne found in prepubertal children is predominantly noninflammatory and thus may easily be overlooked. The open comedo (blackhead) and closed comedo (whitehead) are lesions caused purely by obstruction of the pilosebaceous canal, with no accompanying inflammation. Inflammatory acne is rare in young children and should suggest a possible hyperandrogenic condition, such as that associated with congenital adrenal hyperplasia or even a rare androgen-secreting tumor. Girls should be examined for virilization, and boys and girls should be checked for precocious puberty. Screening blood studies should include serum levels of testosterone, dehydroepiandrosterone sulfate (DHEA-S), and 17-hydroxyprogesterone.

Not surprisingly, acne lesions have a predilection for skin that is rich in sebaceous glands. Accordingly, the face is the prevailing site, although acne is also often found on the chest and back. The lower portions of the trunk, buttocks, and thighs are involved much less frequently, and the distal extremities are always spared.

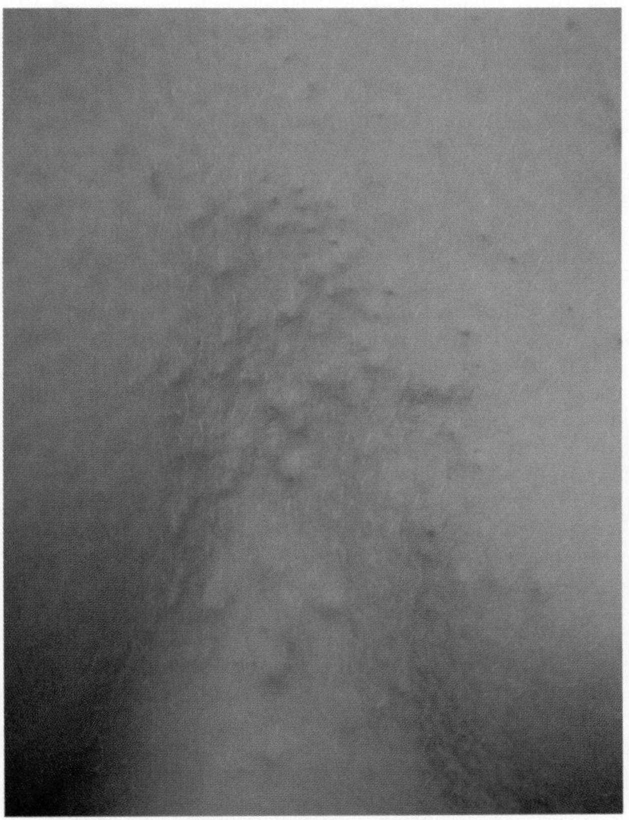

Figure 232-2 Closed comedones (whiteheads) appear as dome-shaped, flesh-colored papules that often are overlooked.

DIFFERENTIAL DIAGNOSIS

Rarely is diagnosing acne difficult. Usually, the condition can be diagnosed from across the room, although, comedonal lesions may require closer inspection (Figure 232-2). Occasionally, acne may be confused with flat warts, milia, or adenoma sebaceum; acne variants may occur.

Flat Warts

Small, flesh-colored warts may be confused clinically with closed comedones. The question can usually be resolved with close inspection. A flat wart has a sharp, right-angled edge and a finely roughened surface; a closed comedo has a dome shape and a smooth surface. Flat warts also vary in size; closed comedones are uniformly small (Figure 232-3).

Milia

Milia are small epidermal inclusion cysts that are sometimes confused with comedones and occasionally with inflammatory pustules, especially in infants who have neonatal acne.

Adenoma Sebaceum

A misnamed disorder (the lesions are actually angiofibromas), adenoma sebaceum is one of the skin manifestations in tuberous sclerosis. Clinically, the lesions appear as pink papules, which are occasionally confused with the lesions of acne. Adenoma sebaceum should be anticipated if the papules are (1) clustered primarily in the center of the face, (2) persistent, and (3) resistant to acne therapy.

Acne Rosacea

Acne rosacea[2] is an acneiform eruption that can be distinguished from acne by a background blush of erythema and telangiectasia and by the absence of comedones (Figure 232-4). In addition, rosacea occurs most often in middle-aged adults.

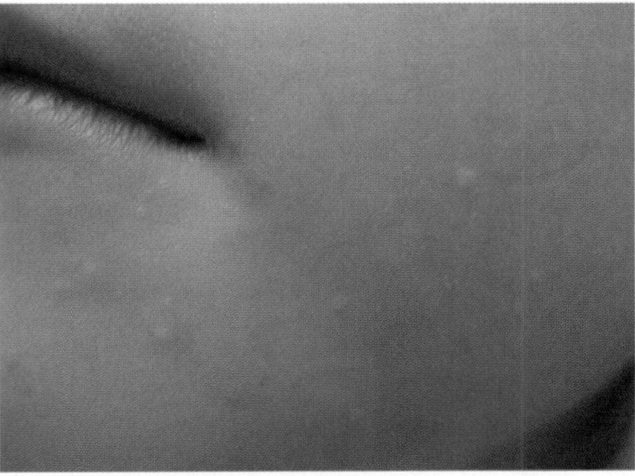

Figure 232-3 Flat warts.

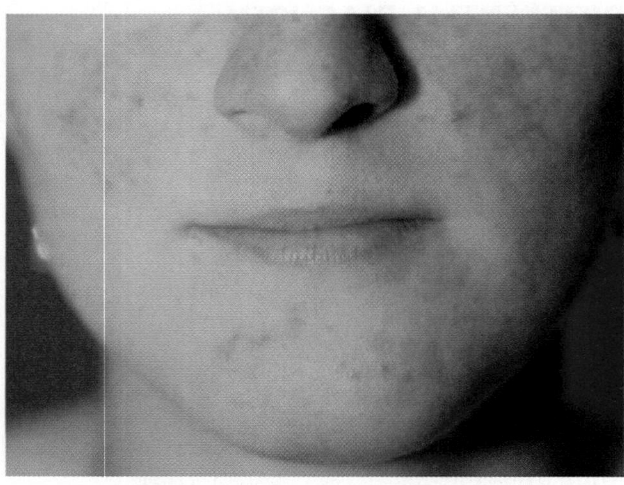

Figure 232-4 Rosacea.

Steroid Acne

Both systemic and topical steroids can induce acne.[8] Acne from systemic steroids usually appears as numerous small, uniform-sized papules and pustules that have a predilection for the upper trunk. The hallmark of steroid-induced acne is a lack of comedones. The condition involutes slowly and spontaneously after the steroids are discontinued.

Gram-Negative Folliculitis

Gram-negative organisms can occasionally produce a pustular folliculitis in patients being treated for acne with systemic antibiotics. This condition should be thought to exist in any patient whose disease flares up during therapy, especially if the flare-up produces numerous pustules. A bacterial culture with antibiotic sensitivity studies should be performed so that the diagnosis can be confirmed and the antibiotic therapy changed.

Acne Conglobata

Acne conglobata is an unusually severe acne variant that may develop as a result of a sudden deterioration of existing active acne, or it may be a recurrence of acne that has been quiet for many years. It occurs most commonly in 18- to 30-year-old men. Lesions consist of comedones, cysts with foul-smelling seropurulent material, and burrowing and interconnecting abscesses, leaving irregular and disfiguring scars. At times, acne conglobata has been associated with systemic diseases such as hidradenitis suppurativa, pyoderma gangrenosum, renal amyloidosis, and musculoskeletal syndrome. The mainstay of treatment is isotretinoin.

Acne Fulminans

Acne fulminans is a rare and severe form of acne, usually occurring in men and characterized by sudden onset of painful acne nodules and, rarely, ulcerative lesions, as well as systemic symptoms, including fever, leukocytosis, polyarthritis, splenomegaly, erythema nodosum, and lytic bone lesions in long bones, clavicle, and sternum. Treatment involves a combination of systemic corticosteroids initially followed by isotretinoin. The prognosis is good, although residual scarring and disfigurement may persist.

PSYCHOSOCIAL CONSIDERATIONS

Acne can be a devastating disease. In an ironic quirk, it occurs at a time of life when personal appearance is of prime concern and when self-consciousness is at its peak. Although some young people appear to be more affected psychologically by acne than others, no one is comfortable with it.[9,10] Patients who have severe cystic acne may be socially ostracized. Regardless of the acne's severity, the condition is important to the patient who is seeking help and deserves serious attention. Patients are not impressed with advice that trivializes their disease and reassures them that they eventually will *outgrow it.* Fortunately, a wide array of medical therapies are available that can produce effective, gratifying results.

MANAGEMENT

Four methods of treatment have proved effective for acne: topical comedolytic agents,[11] topical and systemic antibiotics,[12] systemic hormonal therapy, and systemic retinoids.[13,14] The most traditional and effective treatment regimen is a combination of comedolytics and antibiotics.

Comedolytics

Topical retinoids (tretinoin [Atralin, Avita, Retin-A, Retin-A-Micro]), adapalene Differin), tazarotene (Tazarac), bensoyl perioxide (Brevoxyl, Triz), salicylic acid, azelaic acid (Azelex, Finacea), and sodium sulfacetamide (Klaron, Plexion, Rosula, Sebizon) help disimpact the keratinous plug in the follicular canal. They are most helpful in treating superficial acne lesions, including comedones and superficial papules and pustules.[2] Although topical retinoids have been traditionally viewed as having a primarily comedolytic effect, and more so than other topical medications,[2] they also reduce inflammatory lesions and enhance penetration of other medications. In fact, consensus has now formed that, in most cases, topical retinoids (alone or in combination) should be used as 1st-line therapy for mild-to-moderate inflammatory acne in addition to comedonal acne. They are also preferred for maintenance therapy.[15]

When a topical retinoid is used in combination with another topical agent, the patient should be instructed to apply the retinoid at bedtime and the other agent (ie, benzoyl peroxide, salicylic acid, sodium sulfacetamide) each morning. Topical comedolytics are available in a variety of preparations. The strength of a given preparation reflects its irritancy and probably also its efficacy. For tretinoin, the strength of the preparation depends both on the concentration of the drug and the nature of the vehicle in which it is contained (Table 232-1). Adapalene is marketed as a gel and a cream, the gel in a concentration of 0.3% and 0.1%, and the cream in a concentration of 0.1%. Tazarotene is also available in both forms, and each is available in concentrations of 0.05% and 0.1%. Benzoyl peroxide

Table 232-1 Tretinoin Preparations				
	MILDEST	MILD	MODERATE	STRONGEST
Cream	0.025%	0.05%	0.1%	
Gel		0.01%	0.025%	0.05%
Solution				0.05%

gels are marketed in concentrations of 2.5%, 5%, and 10%. Salicylic acid is marketed in a large variety of preparations and concentrations. Sodium sulfacetamide is available as a lotion in 10% concentration. Patients are initially prescribed the mildest preparations, and the potency is increased at subsequent visits if necessary.

Skin irritation, which usually becomes less of a problem with continued use, is the major side effect of the comedolytics. In addition, approximately 1% of patients develop a true allergic contact dermatitis to benzoyl peroxide, in which case permanent discontinuation of this agent is required. Given that topical retinoids may make the skin more susceptible to the effects of sunlight, patients should be instructed to avoid excessive exposure to the sun and to use oil-free sunscreens if they need to be exposed to the sun for prolonged periods. Additionally, patients should be told that benzoyl peroxide can bleach clothing and linens.

Antibiotics

Antibiotics are indicated for patients who have inflammatory acne lesions. Topical agents such as erythromycin and clindamycin preparations can be used. Combinations of benzoyl peroxide and erythromycin or clindamycin are often prescribed before oral antibiotics. Benzamycin gel (5% benzoyl peroxide and 3% erythromycin) and Benzaclin gel (5% benzoyl peroxide and 1% clindamycin phosphate) can be applied twice daily. If acne lesions are inflammatory and are either extensive enough to make topical therapy impractical (ie, involving neck, shoulders, and upper trunk) or are unresponsive to a topical regimen, then systemic antibiotics are warranted. Tetracycline is the drug of choice because of its proven efficacy, relatively low cost, and low incidence of side effects, even when given over a long period. However, because of dental staining, tetracycline, and other antibiotics in the tetracycline class (ie, doxycycline, minocycline), should not be used in patients younger than 8 years. Food, particularly dairy products, interferes with the absorption of tetracycline; thus it needs to be taken on an empty stomach. The most convenient times are on awakening in the morning and on retiring at night. Tetracycline is usually prescribed initially at a dose of 500 mg orally twice daily. Once a sustained response is achieved, the dose can be decreased to 500 mg orally once a day. Occasionally, a patient does not respond adequately to tetracycline; erythromycin may be used as an alternative. Doxycycline and minocycline may also be substituted, but doxycycline is more likely to cause photosensitivity, and minocycline is very expensive.

Resistance to *P acnes* may affect as many as 25% of patients receiving antibiotics; therefore measures should be taken to counter this trend, such as limiting the use of oral antibiotics to shorter periods, combining topical comedolytics (especially topical retinoids) with topical antibiotics, and avoiding the use of oral antibiotics as maintenance therapy.[15]

Systemic Retinoids

Isotretinoin (Accutane, Amnesteen, Claravis, Sotret) was approved by the US Food and Drug Administration in September 1982 for use in treating severe cystic acne.[13] This drug reduces follicular keratinization, sebum production, and intrafollicular bacterial counts. The result of these (and possibly other) effects is a dramatic improvement in acne. The therapeutic effect usually takes several months to appear and often persists long after the course of therapy is discontinued. Historically, 6-month courses have been used. However, in recent years, some practitioners focus more on total dose given instead of duration, aiming for a 100 to 150 mg/kg total dose. Unfortunately, side effects are common. Almost all patients experience mucocutaneous reactions (cheilitis, conjunctivitis, and dry mucous membranes of the mouth and nose), and extracutaneous complications also occur. For example, systemic retinoids can elevate plasma lipid levels, cause asymptomatic vertebral hyperostoses and, rarely, depression and pseudotumor cerebri.[13,16] Most important is the drug's teratogenicity. Exposure to isotretinoin in pregnancy has been associated with a 25-fold increased risk of major fetal malformations.[17] Thus female patients must exercise strict birth control while taking this drug. To ensure compliance with these guidelines, and to prevent pregnancies from occurring during treatment, the US Food and Drug Administration requires that all patients being prescribed isotretinoin be enrolled in a national registry. Isotretinoin is recommended only for those who have severe cystic or scarring acne (or both) and a minority of patients who have severe noncystic acne and have not responded to therapy with topical comedolytics and oral antibiotics.

Hormonal Therapy

Hormonal therapy can be an excellent option for women with moderate to severe acne if (1) oral contraception is desired, (2) an alternative to repeated courses of isotretinoin is preferred, or (3) certain endocrine disorders are present. All combination contraceptives reduce free testosterone and have a positive effect on acne, with no single preparation being demonstrably superior. Contraceptives containing only progestins should be avoided if possible, given that some of them have intrinsic androgenic activity and may aggravate acne.[15]

Patient Compliance

Patient compliance is the single most important aspect of successful acne treatment. Without patient compliance, even the most effective medications are doomed to failure. To maximize compliance, the physician must take time at the initial visit to explain in detail the use of each medication, as well as the effects and side effects to be expected. To reinforce these instructions, giving the patient printed instructions is helpful, an example of which is shown in Box 232-1. Medications are taken twice daily. If this activity is linked to an established daily routine, such as brushing the teeth, then it too can become habitual. Given careful, specific instructions, most patients who have acne are exceptionally compliant and, given time, obtain good results for their efforts. The concept that the treatment will take time to be effective needs to be emphasized to all patients; otherwise, they may become prematurely, and inappropriately, discouraged. The acne instruction sheet can also be used to answer several other questions, often unasked, that patients or their parents frequently have. The most common of these issues pertain to diet, cleanliness, cosmetics, and picking at the lesions.

Diet

Although some evidence indicates that the usual American diet may have adverse effects on acne,[18] specific foods have not been implicated. For the vast majority of patients, remember Dr Kligman's admonition,[2] "The disease is enough of a curse without gustatory deprivations." For most people, a sensible diet is all that is suggested.

Cleanliness

The question of cleanliness is pondered more by parents than it is by patients. To help maintain peace at home, the notion that acne is a function of poor hygiene should be dispelled. It is not. In general, cleaning agents for acne need not be recommended because most irritate the skin, unnecessarily compounding the irritation caused by topical comedolytics. The use of a mild soap-free cleanser is often suggested.

Cosmetics

Because cosmetics have been implicated as possibly contributing to the acne process, it is preferable to avoid using them. If cosmetics are used, then they should be water based and used sparingly.

Picking

For many patients who have acne, much of the skin damage is self-inflicted. Although the temptation to squeeze a fresh pustule can be overwhelming, the practice must be discouraged. Picking, probing, and

BOX 232-1 Acne Instruction Sheet

TOPICAL MEDICATIONS

1. Action
   a. Help open up clogged pores.
   b. Benzoyl peroxide and sodium sulfacetamide also help kill bacteria in the pores.
2. Method of use (apply to *all* affected areas)
   a. Apply retinoid at bedtime.
   b. *Do not* use acne scrub cleaners.
   c. Apply benzoyl peroxide, salicylic acid, or sodium sulfacetamide in the morning.
3. Possible problems
   a. May make the condition look worse in first several weeks, before improvement is seen (known as *bringing acne to the surface*).
   b. May cause irritation (eg, redness, dryness, tenderness). If too much irritation occurs, then use every other night until the skin becomes accustomed to it. If irritation is severe, then medication should be stopped and a return visit scheduled.

TETRACYCLINE

1. Action: Helps kill bacteria; particularly useful for deep and inflamed lesions.
2. Method of use: Needs to be taken on an *empty* stomach. Therefore take it as soon as you get out of bed in the morning (wait a ½ hour before eating breakfast) and at bedtime (at least 1 hour after eating any evening snack).
3. Potential side effects
   a. Uncommon; most patients have no trouble.
   b. May upset stomach and cause nausea, diarrhea, or both.
   c. Occasionally causes a yeast vaginitis, particularly if you are taking birth control pills.
   d. Should not be taken if you are pregnant or trying to get pregnant.

GENERAL

1. Diet: For most patients, foods have no effect on acne. If you notice that a certain food aggravates the condition, then simply avoid that food. Otherwise, no restrictions are necessary.
2. Washing: Acne cannot be washed off. Wash your face with a mild cleanser 2 to 3 times per day, and bathe or shower daily.
3. When to expect results from medicines: *It takes time*, usually several months, to begin to see benefits. At a return visit in 2 to 3 months, some improvement should be present, but the acne will not likely be cleared. The medications and their doses will be altered at that time, depending on the response.
4. Conscientious and *regular* use of the medications is essential. They will not do any good if not used regularly.
5. Cosmetics: They may aggravate your acne. If you must use them, then do so sparingly, and use only those that are water based. You may also consider some of the newer foundations that contain salicylic acid.
6. No picking!

squeezing cause more tissue damage and sometimes produce scars. For some patients with acne, picking may become so obsessive that excoriations are the only lesions seen.

COMPLICATIONS

The major complications of acne are its psychosocial ramifications.[9,10] In addition to the cosmetic liability of active lesions, permanent scars compound and perpetuate the problem in some patients, mainly those who have inflammatory lesions. Established scars are difficult to treat. Many patients have been disappointed with the results of dermabrasion. Patients who have been treated with isotretinoin should wait for at least 1 year before having dermabrasion. Bovine collagen injections have been used in some patients, producing short-term improvement, but repeated injections are often necessary, and the long-term results are not yet known. Laser resurfacing by experienced operators has produced some promising results. Acne scars are best treated when inflammatory lesions are quiescent. Given that scars are easier to prevent than to treat, the emphasis in acne is on early, aggressive medical therapy.

PROGNOSIS

With proper treatment, the prognosis for acne is good, if not excellent. Patients should understand that most therapy controls the disease instead of curing it and that improvement does not occur overnight. However, improvement does occur, usually within 2 to 3 months of starting therapy, and this time is best for the first scheduled return visit. At this visit, the acne regimen can be adjusted as necessary. For example, the potency of the comedolytics can be increased (or reduced) and the dose of the antibiotic altered, depending on the initial response. Continued improvement is to be expected with continuation of therapy. For many patients, the dose of systemic antibiotics can be reduced gradually and eliminated after 6 to 12 months. However, most patients also require prolonged maintenance therapy (often over years) with topical agents and, in some cases, continued topical antibiotic therapy.[12]

Historically, cystic acne has been the most difficult to treat, but isotretinoin has become a powerful tool for dealing with this disease. This drug has the potential to effect prolonged remissions, sometimes lasting for years after a single course of therapy. However, as discussed previously, isotretinoin has serious side effects, and its use is usually reserved for patients who have severe cystic or scarring acne (or both) that does not respond to standard treatment.

WHEN TO REFER

- Patient who are unresponsive to oral antibiotics and topical comedolytics
- Cystic or scarring acne
- Young girl with acne or girl with acne and irregular menses
- Acne fulminans (abrupt onset of cystic acne, fever, arthralgias)

TOOLS FOR PRACTICE

Engaging Patients and Family

- *Acne: How to Treat & Control It* (brochure), American Academy of Pediatrics (patiented.aap.org).
- *Treating Acne* (fact sheet), American Academy of Pediatrics (www.aap.org/topics.html).
- *What is a Pediatric Dermatologist?* (fact sheet), American Academy of Pediatrics (www.aap.org/sections/derm/pedDermatologistfacts.pdf).

Medical Decision Support

- *Dermatology: Skin Essentials—PediaLink Learning Center* (on-line course), American Academy of Pediatrics (www.pedialink.org/cme/_coursefinder/CMEfaculty.cfm?aid=21445&area=live CME).
- *Pediatric Dermatology: A Quick Reference Guide* (book), American Academy of Pediatrics (www.aap.org/bookstore).

REFERENCES

1. Cunliffe WF. *Acne*. Chicago, IL: Mosby; 1989.
2. Plewig G, Kligman AM. *Acne and Rosacea*. New York, NY: Springer-Verlag; 1993.
3. Winston MH, Shalita AR. Acne vulgaris: pathogenesis and treatment. *Pediatr Clin North Am*. 1991;38:889-903.
4. Lookingbill DP, Horton R, Demers LM, et al. Tissue production of androgens in women with acne. *J Am Acad Dermatol*. 1985;12:481-487.
5. Webster GF. Inflammatory acne. *Int J Dermatol*. 1990;29:313.
6. Lucky AW, Biro FM, Huster GA, et al. Acne vulgaris in early adolescent boys. *Arch Dermatol*. 1991;127:210-216.
7. Lucky AW, Biro FM, Huster GA, et al. Acne vulgaris in premenarchal girls: an early sign of puberty associated with rising levels of dehydroepiandrosterone. *Arch Dermatol*. 1994;130:308-314.
8. Hurwitz RM. Steroid acne. *J Am Acad Dermatol*. 1989;21:1179-1181.
9. Koo JYM, Smith LL. Psychologic aspects of acne. *Pediatr Dermatol*. 1991;8:185-187.
10. Krowchuk DP, Stancin T, Keskinen R, et al. The psychosocial effects of acne on adolescents. *Pediatr Dermatol*. 1991;8:332-338.
11. Melski JW, Arndt KA. Topical therapy for acne. *N Engl J Med*. 1980;302:503-506.
12. Hughes BR, Murphy C, Barnett J, et al. Strategy of acne therapy with long-term antibiotics. *Br J Dermatol*. 1989;121:623-628.
13. Layton AM, Cunliffe WJ. Guidelines for optimal use of isotretinoin in acne. *J Am Acad Dermatol*. 1992;27:S2-S7.
14. Peck GL, Olsen TG, Yoder FW, et al. Prolonged remissions of cystic and conglobate acne with 13-cis-retinoic acid. *N Engl J Med*. 1979;300:329-333.
15. Gollnick H, Cunliffe W, Berson D, et al. Management of acne: a report from a global alliance to improve outcomes in acne. *J Am Acad Dermatol*. 2003;49:S1-S37.
16. Ellis CN, Pennes DR, Hermann RC, et al. Long-term radiographic follow-up after isotretinoin therapy. *J Am Acad Dermatol*. 1988;18:1252-1261.
17. Lammer EJ, Chen DT, Hoar RM, et al. Retinoic acid embryopathy. *N Engl J Med*. 1985;313:837-841.
18. Rosenberg EW. Acne diet reconsidered. *Arch Dermatol*. 1981;117:193-195.

Chapter 233

ADRENAL DYSFUNCTION

Phyllis W. Speiser, MD

Adrenal cortical disease, especially adrenal insufficiency, is far more frequent than adrenal medullary disease and often goes unrecognized for extended periods. Physicians caring for children should consider the diagnosis of adrenal insufficiency in any patient with unexplained hypoglycemia, growth failure, weight loss, vomiting, or lethargy. These nonspecific signs and symptoms may be mistaken for, and should be differentiated from, infection, malnutrition, gastrointestinal disease, inborn errors of metabolism, anorexia, chronic fatigue syndrome, and depression.

ANATOMY AND PHYSIOLOGY

The adrenal glands each weigh approximately 4 g in term neonates at birth, which is equivalent to that of adult glands; however, adrenal size decreases by approximately 50% to 60% within the 1st week of life.[1] The adrenal glands are made up of an inner medulla and an outer cortex that are linked by vascular supply and hormonal influence. Within the mature adrenal cortex are 3 functionally distinct zones: (1) the glomerulosa, comprising approximately 15% of the gland; (2) fasciculata, the largest zone, comprising approximately 75% of the gland; and (3) the reticularis, comprising approximately 10% of the gland.[2]

The adrenal medulla is regulated by the sympathetic nervous system and secretes catecholamines, whereas the 3 zones of the cortex secrete steroid hormones categorized, respectively, as mineralocorticoids, glucocorticoids, and sex steroids. Mineralocorticoid production, exemplified by aldosterone, is principally regulated by the renin-angiotensin axis and by ambient potassium levels.[3] Mineralocorticoids affect sodium and potassium homeostasis, and deficiencies in their production or action cause hyponatremia, hyperkalemia, and dehydration. Glucocorticoid and adrenal sex steroid production are primarily regulated by pituitary corticotrophin (adrenocorticotropic hormone [ACTH]) and hypothalamic corticotrophin-releasing hormone, secreted mainly in the early morning hours (0400 to 0800 hours). Cortisol is the main glucocorticoid, and dehydroepiandrosterone (DHEA) is the main adrenal sex hormone. The latter is only a weak androgen, but it may be converted via androstenedione to either estrogens or androgens. The placenta uses fetal adrenal DHEA to produce estrogens. The main gestational hormone so derived, estriol, excreted in maternal urine, is a sign of fetal viability. Rising levels of DHEA and its sulfate later in childhood signal adrenarche, which usually precedes the development of body hair and apocrine odor at puberty.

Glucocorticoids are generally catabolic, promoting protein and lipid breakdown and inhibiting protein synthesis. The effects of cortisol counterregulate those of insulin, increasing the concentration of glucose by stimulating gluconeogenesis and by decreasing glucose utilization in muscle. Amino acids and glycerol produced by catabolic actions of cortisol on protein and fat are used as gluconeogenic substrates. The net effect is increased production and conservation of glucose for use by essential tissues, such as the brain and red blood cells, at the expense of less essential tissues during times of stress or starvation.[4] Supraphysiological doses of exogenous glucocorticoids suppress growth by antagonizing the production and action of growth hormones (GHs).

Cortisol contributes to the maintenance of normal blood pressure through several mechanisms. Under normal baseline conditions, cortisol increases urine flow by stimulating glomerular filtration rate and decreasing water resorption. At high concentrations, cortisol acts as a mineralocorticoid agonist, causing sodium and water retention. Other vascular actions of cortisol include stimulating angiotensinogen synthesis by the liver and increasing vascular sensitivity to pressors. In the adrenal medulla, cortisol is required for the enzymatic activity of phenylethanolamine N-methyltransferase, which converts norepinephrine to epinephrine. Epinephrine stimulates cardiac output, as well as hepatic glucose production. Cortisol decreases capillary permeability, as well as the production and activity of nitrous oxide and the vasodilatory kinin and prostaglandin systems during stress, preventing life-threatening hypotension. Cortisol or aldosterone deficiencies, or both kinds, often result in shock if unrecognized and untreated.

ADRENAL INSUFFICIENCY

History and Physical Examination

The symptoms of cortisol deficiency include lethargy, fatigue, weakness, dizziness, and anorexia. Signs detected at physical examination include hyperpigmentation, orthostatic hypotension, tachycardia, and weight loss. These findings are nonspecific and gradual in onset, and they may be mistaken for infection, malnutrition, gastrointestinal disease, inborn errors of metabolism, anorexia, chronic fatigue syndrome, and depression. In some patients, gastrointestinal symptoms such as abdominal cramps, nausea, vomiting, and diarrhea are prominent. In adolescents and adults, sexual or reproductive dysfunction, or both, with decreased libido, potency, or amenorrhea may accompany either primary or secondary adrenal insufficiency. Orthostatic hypotension is more marked in primary than secondary adrenal insufficiency because primary adrenal insufficiency is often associated with both aldosterone and catecholamine deficiency.[5]

The most commonly recognized screening laboratory findings are hypoglycemia and low plasma cortisol. Such patients should be referred to a pediatric endocrinologist for further evaluation. Patients with chronic primary adrenal insufficiency often have hyperpigmentation of the skin and mucosal surfaces, which is the result of the high plasma corticotropin and accompanying melanocyte-stimulating hormone secretion that results from absent cortisol feedback. This hyperpigmentation may be difficult to appreciate in dark-skinned individuals. Clues to its presence may be hyperpigmentation of the creases of the palms and of the oral mucosal surfaces. In contrast, patients with secondary adrenal insufficiency tend to be pale. Another symptom of primary adrenal insufficiency is a craving for salt, which is a result of aldosterone deficiency and resultant sodium wasting. Weight loss and failure to thrive may also be observed. Loss of axillary or pubic hair is common among hypoadrenal patients, which is attributable to low levels of adrenal androgens.

Children with secondary adrenal insufficiency might have delayed growth and puberty, manifestations of GH, and gonadotropin deficiencies in addition to ACTH deficiency. Headaches, visual disturbances, polyuria and polydipsia, or any combination of these reactions indicative of diabetes insipidus may also be seen in pituitary disorders. Primary care physicians caring for children with chronic unexplained signs or symptoms such as those described previously should consult with a pediatric endocrinologist to determine whether a referral is required. Children in hypotensive crisis or shock at the time they seek care should be treated urgently in the office or transferred immediately by ambulance to the nearest emergency center.

Pathological Forms

Primary adrenal disease may be associated with either hypoplasia or hyperplasia associated with variable adrenal function. The most common forms of adrenal disease involve either deficient or excessive cortisol production. Box 233-1 lists various causes of adrenal disease. Only the most commonly encountered disorders will be reviewed in detail in this chapter. Online Mendelian Inheritance in Man (OMIM) should be consulted for a more detailed discussion of rarer diseases; OMIM catalog numbers for each adrenal disease are listed in Box 233-1.

Primary Causes of Adrenal Failure

Congenital adrenal hyperplasia (CAH) is the most common inborn error in adrenal function. It is most often caused by deficiency of steroid 21-hydroxylase.[6] In classic severe salt-wasting CAH, both cortisol and aldosterone production are impaired, and adrenal androgen production is excessive. As a result of the lack of the vital hormones cortisol and aldosterone, both boys and girls are susceptible to potentially lethal adrenal insufficiency if untreated; this susceptibility is also true of other forms of CAH that interrupt synthesis of these hormones (eg, 3-beta hydroxysteroid dehydrogenase deficiency, cholesterol desmolase deficiency[7]). Excess androgen production, a side effect of 21-hydroxylase deficiency, causes genital ambiguity in newborn girls. In contrast, however, boys affected with severe 21-hydroxylase deficiency have no overt genital anomalies, and they may not come to medical attention until they seek care while in extremis. To prevent mortality from adrenal crisis, among other reasons, the United States and many other countries perform newborn screening for this disease.[8] Prompt treatment with glucocorticoids and mineralocorticoids is life saving. Approximately a quarter of patients with classic CAH produce enough aldosterone to avoid salt-wasting crises and are termed *simple virilizers*.

A milder, nonclassic form of CAH not associated with genital ambiguity or adrenal insufficiency may be missed by newborn screening programs. Although nonclassic CAH is not always detected by random blood hormone measurements, it is much more prevalent at all ages than the classic forms of the disease. Because nonclassic CAH is characterized by less marked adrenal androgen excess, symptoms and signs do not often develop before middle childhood. These symptoms and signs often include early pubic hair and rapid advances in height in both sexes. In many cases, these individuals either go undetected or are diagnosed in adolescent girls or women with hirsutism, oligomenorrhea, or acne. The mild form of CAH may be mistaken in girls for polycystic ovarian syndrome.[9]

Not all persons with increased 17-hydroxyprogesterone typical of nonclassic 21-hydroxylase deficiency are symptomatic. Boys, in particular, are much less likely to be troubled by this mild adrenal hormone imbalance. Even some girls and women remain asymptomatic. Thus children who do not exhibit precocious pubarche and adolescents who are not troubled with symptoms of androgen excess may not require treatment, or they may discontinue treatment when symptoms have abated and growth is complete.

Laboratory Evaluation

The diagnosis of CAH rests on both the clinical manifestations and on the specific hormone measurements. Deficiency of steroid 21-hydroxylase can be identified by measuring high levels of hormones that serve as enzyme substrates. The gold standard test is a corticotropin-stimulated serum 17-hydroxyprogesterone,[10] although analysis of serum or saliva levels of this hormone taken at 0800 hours may also be diagnostic. This circumstance is true because of the natural circadian pattern of endogenous ACTH secretion, which is highest between 0400 and 0800 hours. Measuring adrenal hormones in an endocrine specialty laboratory that employs strict quality-control standards is important to avoid false-positive high levels generated by nonspecific measurement of cross-reacting hormones.

Stimulated serum 17-hydroxyprogesterone levels are usually moderately increased, usually exceeding 1500 ng/dL (approximately 45 nmol/L) in individuals affected with nonclassic 21-hydroxylase deficiency. In contrast, both basal and stimulated 17-hydroxyprogesterone levels are markedly increased, generally exceeding 10,000 ng/dL (approximately 300 nmol/L) in classic simple virilizing or salt-wasting CAH. Moreover, cortisol levels are invariably low and fail to respond robustly to stress or exogenous stimulation in classic forms of CAH. Early-morning basal serum 17-hydroxyprogesterone measurements below 200 ng/dL (approximately 6 nmol/L) usually rule out even mild forms of 21-hydroxylase deficiency.[11] Newborn screening test results from filter paper samples are measured differently and are not comparable to serum hormone levels. Each state's laboratory has its own reference range for screening tests.

Genetics

Phenotypic variability in CAH is attributable to allelic variation in the gene encoding active steroid

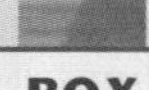

BOX 233-1 Causes of Adrenal Cortical Insufficiency

PRIMARY

Disorders associated with adrenal gland hyperplasia
- 21-Hydroxylase deficiency (gene *CYP21A2,* OMIM 210910)
- 3-Beta hydroxysteroid dehydrogenase deficiency (gene *HSD3B2,* OMIM 201810)
- Cholesterol desmolase deficiency (gene *CYP11A,* OMIM 201710, 118485)
- Lipoid hyperplasia (gene *STAR,* OMIM 201710)
- POR deficiency (gene *POR,* OMIM 201750)
- Glucocorticoid resistance (gene *GCCR,* OMIM 138040)
- Wolman disease (gene *LIPA,* OMIM 278000)

Disorders associated with adrenal gland hypoplasia
- Adrenal hypoplasia congenita (gene *NR0B1[DAX-1],* OMIM 300200)
- Adrenocortical insufficiency with or without ovarian defect (gene *NR5A1 [SF-1],* OMIM 184757)
- Familial glucocorticoid deficiency (ACTH resistance) (gene *MC2R/MRAP,* OMIM 202200)
- Triple A (ACTH resistance, achalasia, alacrima) (gene *AAAS,* OMIM 231550)
- IMAGe (intrauterine growth retardation, metaphyseal dysplasia, adrenal hypoplasia congenital and genital anomalies) syndrome (X-linked, OMIM 300290)

Metabolic diseases
- Adrenoleukodystrophy (X-linked) (gene *ABCD1,* OMIM 300100)
- Smith-Lemli-Opitz syndrome (gene *DCHR7,* OMIM 270400)
- Kearns-Sayre syndrome (gene *mitochondrial DNA deletions,* OMIM 530000)

Disorders associated with isolated aldosterone deficiency
- Pseudohypoaldosteronism, type 1 (AR) (gene *ENaC,* OMIM 264350)
- Pseudohypoaldosteronism, type 1 (AD) (gene *MR,* OMIM 177735)
- Pseudohypoaldosteronism, type 2 (AR) (gene *WNK4;WNK1,* OMIM 145260)
- Corticosterone methyl oxidase deficiency I (gene *CYP11B2,* OMIM 124080)
- Corticosterone methyl oxidase deficiency I (gene *CYP11B2,* OMIM 610600)

ACQUIRED

- Autoimmune adrenalitis, isolated
- Autoimmune polyendocrine syndrome type 1 (gene *AIRE,* OMIM 240300)
- Autoimmune polyendocrine syndrome type 2 (gene *MICA5.1* and *HLA-DR3/DQ2,* OMIM 269200)
- Hemorrhage or infarction caused by:
  - Trauma
  - Waterhouse-Friderichsen syndrome
  - Anticoagulation
  - Drug effects (aminoglutethimide, mitotane, ketoconazole, metyrapone, medroxyprogesterone, megestrol, etomidate, rifampin, phenytoin, barbiturates)
  - Infection
  - Virus (HIV, cytomegalovirus)
  - Fungus (coccidiomycosis, histoplasmosis, blastomycosis, cryptococcosis)
  - Mycobacterium (tuberculosis)
  - Amebic
  - Infiltrative
    - Hemochromatosis, histiocytosis, sarcoidosis, amyloidosis
    - Neoplasm

SECONDARY

Hypothalamus

Congenital
- Septo-optic dysplasia (gene *HESX1,* OMIM 182230)
- Corticotropin releasing hormone deficiency (gene *CRH,* OMIM 122560)
- Maternal hypercortisolemia

Acquired
- Inflammatory disorders
- Trauma
- Radiotherapy
- Surgery
- Tumors
- Infiltrative disease (sarcoidosis, histocytosis X)
- Steroid withdrawal after prolonged administration

Pituitary

Congenital
- Pituitary hormone deficiency, combined (gene *POU1F1/PIT1,* OMIM 173110, gene *PROP-1,* OMIM 601538)
- Pro-opiomelanocortin deficiency (gene *POMC,* OMIM 609734)
- Proconvertase 1 (gene *PCSK1,* OMIM 600955)
- Isolated ACTH deficiency (gene *TBX19/TPIT,* OMIM 604614)

Acquired
- Trauma
- Tumor (craniopharyngioma)
- Radiotherapy
- Lymphocytic hypophysitis
- Steroid withdrawal after prolonged administration

ACTH, Adrenocorticotropic hormone; *OMIM,* Online Mendelian Inheritance in Man.

21-hydroxylase *CYP21A2.* The disease is inherited as an autosomal-recessive trait. Approximately 100 known disease-causing mutations have been found, but approximately 10 mutations comprise 80% to 90% of alleles in most populations.[12] The spectrum of disease ranges from severe to mild, depending on which *CYP21A2* mutations a patient carries. Genotyping can be useful in verifying an equivocal hormonal

Table 233-1 Glucocorticoid Potencies

DRUG	POTENCY RELATIVE TO CORTISOL	EQUIVALENT CORTISOL DOSE	MINERALOCORTICOID ACTIVITY
Cortisol (hydrocortisone)	1	100	Present
Cortisone	0.8	125	Present
Prednisone	5	20	Absent
Prednisolone	5	20	Absent
Methylprednisolone	6	17	Absent
Dexamethasone	50	2	Absent

diagnosis; it is particularly valuable in prenatal diagnosis and genetic counseling.

Management and Long-Term Follow-Up

CAH is treatable with oral corticosteroid medications. In its classical form, CAH requires lifelong medical management. Patients with salt wasting require both glucocorticoids and mineralocorticoids; however, with older age and increasing dietary salt consumption, mineralocorticoids may be tapered and in some cases discontinued. Infants who consume very little dietary sodium, patients in tropical climates, or those who engage in intense exercise with excessive sweat sodium losses may require supplemental sodium chloride. Poorly controlled patients with simple virilizing CAH also benefit from mineralocorticoid therapy because it spares the use of high-dose glucocorticoids in some cases. Symptomatic nonclassic patients require low-dose glucocorticoids therapy only.[13,14] Some clinicians prefer to treat CAH with a higher dose of cortisol or a longer-acting glucocorticoid at night in an attempt to suppress the early-morning ACTH-mediated adrenal androgen production.

Once growth is near complete, if satisfactory control of adrenal androgens is not achieved with such a regimen, more potent and long-acting glucocorticoids, such as prednisone or dexamethasone, may be used. Table 233-1 lists approximate relative glucocorticoids potencies.

Dosing should be titrated to maintain the levels of adrenal androgen precursors in the normal to mildly increased range. The clinician should assay 17-hydroxyprogesterone, androstenedione, and testosterone; plasma renin activity is added to this profile in patients requiring mineralocorticoid replacement. Attempts to suppress 17-hydroxyprogesterone to the normal range usually require excessively high glucocorticoids doses and have the undesirable consequence of growth suppression and iatrogenic Cushing syndrome.[13] Measurement of ACTH is not helpful; this hormone seldom is completely suppressible in patients who have been treated for CAH. An important point to recognize is that testosterone is not as useful a hormonal marker of adequate therapy in adolescent boys and men, although it is helpful in managing prepubertal children of both sexes, as well as adolescent girls and women.

Other aspects of CAH treatment include ensuring that adolescent girls with severe forms of CAH undergo gynecologic examination in anticipation of sexual activity; vaginoplasty may be necessary, depending on whether and which genital surgical procedures may have been performed in the past.[15] Psychological counseling should be provided to these young women by a professional who is experienced in treating this type of disorder.[16]

Adolescent boys should undergo careful testicular palpation and sonography to rule out testicular adrenal rests that can compromise fertility. Strict control of adrenal hormone levels can shrink such benign tumors in many cases.[17]

Other Causes of Adrenal Failure

Primary adrenal insufficiency is estimated to affect approximately 100 per million people.[18] The syndrome, originally described by English physician Thomas Addison, included wasting, hyperpigmentation, and adrenal gland atrophy. In adults, over 80% of cases are caused by autoimmune adrenal destruction, which is most prevalent in women aged 25 to 45 years but which is observed in both sexes at any age. The female-to-male ratio is approximately 3:1. Autoimmune adrenalitis may be isolated or found in association with other autoimmune syndromes. Autoimmune polyendocrine syndrome type 1 is associated with mucocutaneous candidiasis, Addison disease, and autoimmune hypoparathyroidism. Other systemic problems may include autoimmune pernicious anemia, hepatitis, thyroiditis, and diabetes. The age at onset and severity of each of these problems are variable. Autoimmune polyendocrine syndrome type 2, also termed *Schmidt syndrome,* is associated with Addison disease, autoimmune thyroiditis, and diabetes. Box 233-1 lists the diseases associated with adrenal insufficiency.

Adrenal infiltration by tuberculosis is the 2nd most common cause worldwide. HIV infection is another potential infectious cause of adrenalitis; both of these infections tend to cause insidious progression to hypoadrenalism. In contrast, catastrophic adrenal hemorrhage during overwhelming bacterial sepsis causes the abrupt onset of adrenal failure.

Perhaps because of its rarity in children or its nonspecific symptoms, the diagnosis of adrenal insufficiency is frequently delayed or missed. If unrecognized, adrenal insufficiency may produce a life-threatening crisis, with acute cardiovascular collapse. The child's caregivers may have to seek the advice of more than one physician before a diagnosis will be made,[19] which may result in a lengthy delay between the onset of the 1st symptoms and the diagnosis.[20]

History and Physical Examination

As noted previously, signs and symptoms of adrenal insufficiency may include abdominal pain, headache, anorexia, weight loss, lethargy, postural hypotension or shock, proneness to dehydration, salt craving, and hyperpigmentation. Patients with adrenal insufficiency with and without GH deficiency may have hypoglycemia, but this condition is seldom severe enough to cause seizures.

Laboratory Evaluation

Primary adrenal insufficiency can be detected based on low early-morning (0800 hours) cortisol accompanied by increased ACTH. If zona glomerulosa function is affected, then hyponatremia and hyperkalemia will be accompanied by a high plasma renin activity and low serum aldosterone. In adrenal insufficiency resulting from pituitary or hypothalamic dysfunction, ACTH levels will be low. The diagnosis can be confirmed by absence of at least a 2-fold increment in serum cortisol 60 minutes after stimulation with a standard dose of intravenous cosyntropin (ACTH 1-24).[21] A low dose of cosyntropin can be used to test ACTH reserve in cases of suspected secondary adrenal insufficiency.[22]

Imaging Studies

If adrenal hemorrhage is suspected, then it can be detected by ultrasonography or computed tomographic (CT) scan.

Management

Once the diagnosis of adrenal insufficiency is established, continuing reminders to patients, families, and medical personnel regarding the need for higher doses of glucocorticoid replacement therapy during intercurrent illness and surgery are required. Failure to increase glucocorticoid supplementation during physical stress remains a significant cause of morbidity and mortality in these patients. Patients should be given letters explaining their condition and appropriate emergency management. Sample letters may be found at the Web sites of the National Adrenal Diseases Foundation for patients with Addison disease and the CARES Foundation—Congenital Adrenal Hyperplasia Research Education & Support for patients with CAH (see Suggested Resources).

In primary adrenal insufficiency in children younger than 18 years, the most common causes are CAH (72%); 13% have autoimmune adrenal insufficiency, and the remaining 15% include various rare syndromes such as adrenoleukodystrophy, Wolman disease, triple A syndrome (ACTH resistance, achalasia, alacrima), Zellweger syndrome, and unexplained adrenal insufficiency.[23] In non-CAH primary adrenal insufficiency, causes include autoimmune adrenal insufficiency, X-linked adrenoleukodystrophy, adrenal hypoplasia congenita, and the IMAGe syndrome (intrauterine growth retardation, metaphyseal dysplasia, adrenal hypoplasia congenital and genital anomalies)[20] (see Box 233-1).

Secondary Adrenal Insufficiency

Secondary adrenal insufficiency is more common than primary adrenal insufficiency. The estimated prevalence is 150 to 280 per million people.[18] Abrupt discontinuation of glucocorticoid therapy exacerbated by stress is the most frequent cause and results from the widespread use of exogenous glucocorticoids. Acute hypoglycemia has been reported after the use of inhaled glucocorticoids.[24] An important point to recognize is that normal statural growth does not preclude adrenal suppression while being treated with inhaled glucocorticoids.[25]

Administration of steroids orally, intramuscularly, intranasally, inhaled, transdermally, or intraorbitally may result in suppression of the hypothalamic-pituitary-adrenal axis.[24,26,27] In adults, as little as 2 weeks of high-dose glucocorticoid treatment may result in suppression of endogenous cortisol production for up to 1 year.[28] In children being treated for leukemia, a 4-week course of glucocorticoids may suppress the hypothalamic-pituitary axis for up to 8 weeks after discontinuation.[29] Suppression of the axis cannot be reliably predicted by either the dose or the duration of therapy.[30]

Documentation of an intact hypothalamic-pituitary-adrenal axis should be obtained before subjecting to surgery a patient who has a known history of high-dose, long-term glucocorticoid treatment. This task may be accomplished by documenting plasma cortisol level taken at 0800 hours of more than 10 mcg/dL or by performing a cosyntropin (ACTH 1-24) challenge test and observing cortisol levels above 15 to 18 mcg/dL after 30 to 60 minutes.[21] These levels have been derived mainly from adult studies and may not be relevant to infants and small children. Another robust test of ACTH reserve is insulin-induced hypoglycemia; however, many clinicians are reluctant to use this test because of the danger of potential hypoglycemic seizures. If such documentation cannot be obtained in time, then treating patients with supplemental stress corticosteroid coverage in the perioperative period within 1 year of withdrawal of therapy is safest.[31]

Most secondary adrenal insufficiency that is unrelated to withdrawal of glucocorticoid therapy occurs in association with other pituitary hormone deficiencies. *Panhypopituitarism,* or deficiency of 2 or more pituitary hormones, may be either congenital or acquired. Anatomic abnormalities in the pituitary or stalk may be evident on magnetic resonance imaging (MRI). Alternatively, the clinician may elicit a history of head trauma or cranial surgery with resulting pituitary injury.[32]

Aside from these causes of secondary adrenal insufficiency, several other rare syndromes have been found. These syndromes include ACTH resistance associated with triple A syndrome (ACTH resistance, alacrima, and achalasia). This clinical picture is caused by mutations in the *AAAS* gene encoding a protein of uncertain function.[33] In contrast, an isolated form of ACTH resistance is caused by a different genetic defect in the gene encoding the ACTH receptor *MC2R*. The latter syndrome is characterized by a familial form of glucocorticoid deficiency associated with hyperpigmentation and hypoglycemia without accompanying systemic abnormalities.[34] Granulomatous diseases such as sarcoidosis or histiocytosis can also cause pituitary failure. The risk of adrenal crisis in adults with primary adrenal insufficiency is slightly higher (3.8 admissions per 100 patient-years) compared with secondary adrenal insufficiency (2.5 per 100 patient-years).[18] Information concerning mortality in secondary adrenal insufficiency mostly comes from recent reports regarding follow-up of individuals treated with pituitary GH. An up to 4-fold increase in mortality compared with the general population in children treated with pituitary GH has been reported.[35-37] This increase is presumably because patients with 1 pituitary hormone deficiency are likely to develop other hormone deficiencies. Deaths were attributed to hypoglycemia or secondary adrenal insufficiency. These preventable deaths were observed in individuals of all ages and were associated with a variety of causes of hypopituitarism; 74% were said to occur in individuals with known multiple pituitary hormone deficiencies. The death rate resulting from secondary adrenal insufficiency remained fairly constant throughout middle childhood and with advancing age (1 per 113 to 173 person-years).

Management of secondary adrenal deficiency is similar to that of primary adrenal insufficiency. Measuring ACTH or cortisol levels in plasma to gauge the efficacy of treatment with corticosteroids is usually not helpful. Rather, the patient's growth, weight gain, and vital signs, as well as the patient's own sense of well being, should guide therapy.

RELATIVE ADRENAL INSUFFICIENCY IN THE INTENSIVE CARE UNIT

Critically ill adults with a normal baseline cortisol but inappropriately low response of serum cortisol to acute stimulation demonstrated improved survival when treated with stress doses of hydrocortisone,[38] although these findings have not been replicated.[39]

Among critically ill children, a low incremental cortisol response to ACTH does not predict mortality, although the effect of glucocorticoid treatment is not known.[40]

Much controversy still exists regarding how best to look for adrenal insufficiency in hospitalized children and adults, as well as whether and when to treat.[28,39,41] Thus the decision to treat a critically ill patient with glucocorticoids must be made on a case-by-case basis until further definitive evidence is available.

MANAGEMENT OF ACUTE ADRENAL INSUFFICIENCY

Hypotension and lethargy are common signs at presentation of acute adrenal insufficiency; patients and family members should be taught to recognize a change in energy level or demeanor as a potential warning sign. Acute adrenal insufficiency may occur during febrile illness, especially when accompanied by dehydration, vomiting, diarrhea, or any combination of these reactions. Individuals who are unable to tolerate oral maintenance or stress doses during an illness require parenteral glucocorticoid administration. Another option, especially if parenteral administration is not feasible, and provided that the patient does not have diarrhea, is to administer hydrocortisone suppositories.[42,43]

Once the patient is seen in the emergency department, a large-bore intravenous catheter should be inserted for repletion of intravascular volume with saline solutions containing 5% dextrose. More concentrated dextrose (eg, 25% dextrose in water) should be administered to treat refractory hypoglycemia. If the patient's adrenal status is unknown, then blood should be drawn for cortisol, electrolytes, glucose, ACTH, plasma renin activity, and aldosterone, preferably before exogenous steroids are administered. If acute and severe adrenal insufficiency is suspected, however, then treatment should not by delayed for diagnostic testing. Simultaneous with the administration of fluids, stress doses of glucocorticoids should be given. Hydrocortisone is the treatment of choice because of its quick onset of action and mineralocorticoid activity[18,44] Prednisone and dexamethasone are long-acting glucocorticoids with a slower onset of biological action. Table 233-1 lists the relative potencies of various steroid medications. Prednisone is not an ideal choice for treating acute adrenal crisis because it must be converted to prednisolone to be effective. Dexamethasone does not cross-react in cortisol assays; thus a diagnostic ACTH stimulation test may be performed right after its administration.

Liberal quantities of intravenous sodium chloride accompanied by large doses of hydrocortisone will usually restore normotension and correct electrolyte abnormalities, obviating mineralocorticoid treatment or pressor agents in the acute situation. As vital signs stabilize, glucocorticoids and fluid infusions are tapered over several days. Once the patient is able to eat and take oral medications, oral glucocorticoids may be substituted. Supplemental sodium chloride may be provided if dietary salt intake is inadequate.

Chronic Replacement Therapy

Maintenance glucocorticoid replacement therapy is based on estimated normal cortisol secretion rates.[45] Glucocorticoid dosing must be individually adjusted to avoid signs and symptoms of adrenal insufficiency while avoiding the growth retardation and cushingoid features that can accompany overtreament. Once growth is complete, longer-acting glucocorticoids such as dexamethasone may be considered to enhance compliance. In general, lower doses of glucocorticoids are required to treat Addison disease compared with CAH. Measuring plasma cortisol or ACTH levels in titrating the glucocorticoid dose is not usually helpful. Patients with low serum sodium, high potassium, or increased plasma renin activity should receive daily oral fludrocortisone and sodium chloride supplements, adjusted to normalize these analytes. The patient's own sense of well being, energy level, and blood pressure can help guide the adequacy of therapy in patients with Addison disease. Frequent headaches, lethargy, nausea, or abdominal pain may indicate inadequate treatment. Objective signs of inadequate replacement therapy are orthostatic pulse or blood pressure changes. If skin hyperpigmentation becomes more prominent in primary adrenal insufficiency, then plasma ACTH levels may be helpful.

DHEA has been considered an optional hormone supplement for older women with adrenal insufficiency and low energy or libido,[46] but no data on its use in adolescents have been collected.

Stress Dosing

Patients with adrenal insufficiency (primary or secondary, and patients with CAH) must be informed about the need to increase their glucocorticoid dose during stress to prevent a potentially lethal adrenal crisis. All such patients should wear a medical alert tag and carry an emergency medical information card to ensure that medical providers know about the underlying disorder.

Mild physical stresses such as immunizations, uncomplicated viral illnesses, and low-grade fever (temperature <38.5° C) do not require stress doses of glucocorticoids. Athletic activity and emotional stress also do not usually require a boost in glucocorticoid dose.[13] Adolescents with CAH who received an additional morning dose of hydrocortisone causing a 100% increase in serum cortisol level do not alter athletic performance. No changes were observed in blood glucose, lactate, free fatty acids, or epinephrine levels during short-term, high-intensity exercise compared with placebo.[47]

More severe stresses such as illness accompanied by higher fever (temperature ≥38.5° C), surgery, and major trauma should be accompanied by tripling of oral hydrocortisone maintenance doses to prevent the hypoglycemia, hypotension, and even cardiovascular collapse. Supplemental parenteral hydrocortisone is suggested before general anesthesia and surgery. Doses are empiric and are not determined by evidence-based guidelines. Intravenous or oral stress doses may be gradually tapered as the patient recovers until the maintenance dose is attained.

ADRENOCORTICAL HYPERFUNCTION

The spectrum of disorders causing adrenal hyperfunction (Box 233-2) is more limited compared with those causing hypofunction.

BOX 233-2 Causes of Adrenal Cortical Hyperfunction

- Iatrogenic
  - Glucocorticoid or mineralocorticoid treatment
  - ACTH treatment
  - Pituitary
- Pituitary tumors
- Adrenal tumors
  - Carcinoma
  - Adenoma
- Adrenal nodular hyperplasia
  - Carney complex (AD) (gene *PRKAR1A*, OMIM 160980)
  - McCune-Albright syndrome (gene *GNAS1*, OMIM 174800)
- Ectopic ACTH-producing tumors
- Apparent mineralocorticoid excess (gene *HSD11B2*, OMIM 218030)
- Glucocorticoid remediable hyperaldosteronism (AD) (gene chimeric *CYP11B1/B2*, OMIM 103900)

ACTH, Adrenocorticotropic hormone; *OMIM,* Online Mendelian Inheritance in Man.

Premature Adrenarche

Adrenal androgen excess is most commonly observed in children with early onset of pubic and body hair growth. The traditional age limit has been 8 years for the onset of pubic hair in girls and 9 years in boys. The lowest age limit for girls has been contested after a large cross-sectional study revealed the relatively common occurrence of either early pubic hair or breast enlargement in healthy black girls after age 6 years and in white girls after age 7 years.[48]

Definition

The early onset of adrenal androgen secretion accompanied by pubic hair *(pubarche)* is termed *premature adrenarche.*

Laboratory Evaluation

Premature adrenarche is heralded by mildly increased levels of DHEA and DHEA-sulfate. These hormone levels tend to be consistent with the child's Tanner stage of pubic hair. DHEA, a weak androgen, is the most abundantly produced adrenal steroid. The sulfated form has a longer half-life in the circulation and thus is not subject to circadian variability, making it a more robust screening tool. Premature adrenarche is generally considered a benign condition that does not warrant treatment with glucocorticoid suppression. Presence of isolated pubic hair or axillary hair with or without apocrine body odor does not necessarily presage early breast development and menstruation. In most cases, children with premature adrenarche do not exhibit rapid statural growth or advanced bone age.

Because premature adrenarche is most often a benign condition, telephone consultation with a pediatric endocrinologist should be considered before referring such children. Endocrine evaluation should be reserved for children who exhibit unusually early pubarche, multiple signs of early puberty, rapidly progressive pubertal development or statural growth (or both), or nonisosexual puberty (eg, a girl with hirsutism or other signs of virilization, a prepubertal boy with gynecomastia).

Overweight children secrete more adrenal sex hormones than lean children[49] and can metabolize these weak adrenal sex hormones in fat to more active sex hormones. Mean free testosterone is 6-fold higher in obese girls than nonobese girls across pubertal stages 1 to 3.[50] Consequently, they may develop secondary sexual characteristics at an earlier-than-average age. In contrast to nonobese children with premature adrenarche, obese children often do show advanced bone ages, but they are not usually short.

Most overweight and obese children who are growing in height at a normal pace do not have a causal underlying endocrine disease. Thus the primary care physician should institute dietary counseling and advise a rigorous exercise program to determine whether weight gain can be controlled. Telephone consultation with a pediatric endocrinologist is advised if in doubt. Reports have surfaced that a subset of girls with premature adrenarche go on to develop polycystic ovarian syndrome, insulin resistance, or metabolic syndrome.[51] The precise cause of this tendency is uncertain but has been related to prenatal growth restriction, especially with rapid postnatal catch-up growth.[52] In light of the role of obesity in androgen excess, intuitively, individuals with body mass indices in the overweight to obese range might be at highest risk. At present, no strong evidence has been found to warrant preventive drug treatment in anticipation of the possible occurrence of polycystic ovarian syndrome in young girls who have had premature adrenarche.[53]

The differential diagnosis of premature adrenarche includes nonclassic forms of CAH and adrenal virilizing tumors. The most common nonclassic form of CAH can be detected by measuring early-morning or ACTH-stimulated levels of 17OHP. The much rarer occurrence of tumors can be detected by finding markedly increased levels of DHEA-sulfate and frequently other hormones as well. Imaging studies are required to verify a clinical suspicion of an adrenal tumor.

Cushing Syndrome

Cushing syndrome refers to any form of glucocorticoid excess, whereas *Cushing disease* refers to glucocorticoid excess caused by ACTH hypersecretion. Although Cushing disease is rare, it is the most frequently identified noniatrogenic etiology for glucocorticoid excess in adolescents, approximately 0.5 per million persons per year.[54] Box 233-2 lists causes of glucocorticoid excess.

History and Physical Examination

Prominent clinical features of adrenocortical hyperfunction in adolescents are excess central body weight gain with stunted statural growth. An important point to emphasize is that most obese adolescents do not have Cushing syndrome and do not require screening unless growth arrest or other suspicious signs are observed. An obese child with statural growth arrest should be referred to a pediatric endocrinologist for more complete evaluation. Examination of annual school photographs can often help reveal subtle changes in physiognomy and habitus over time. Other characteristic findings are easy bruisability, broad and purplish striae, hyperglycemia, and hypertension.

Therapeutic glucocorticoids are in widespread use for a variety of inflammatory and neoplastic diseases. Exogenous administration of relatively high doses of these drugs over long periods by any route is the most common cause of Cushing syndrome, as well as secondary adrenal insufficiency. Although the relative safety of alternate-day oral and inhaled glucocorticoids has been demonstrated, individual differences in drug metabolism or sensitivity may cause an increase in bioavailable levels of these potent compounds, many of which have very long biological half-lives. Therefore obtaining a thorough medication history in children treated with these drugs is important. If possible, glucocorticoids should be tapered as soon as is practical while substituting other therapeutic agents. In some patients, attenuation of cushingoid features and improvement of statural growth may take months to years.[55]

Laboratory Evaluation

Clinical suspicion of Cushing syndrome in the absence of exogenous glucocorticoids administration should prompt appropriate screening diagnostic studies, including measurement of increased midnight salivary cortisol or high 24-hour urine-free cortisol or both.[56] The diagnosis may be confirmed by finding a nonsuppressed morning cortisol after dexamethasone administration. The latter test has been refined by the postdexamethasone administration of corticotrophin-releasing hormone. An inappropriately brisk rise in plasma ACTH after corticotrophin-releasing hormone suggests an ACTH-producing pituitary tumor, and MRI with attention to this portion of the brain is indicated. If the tumor cannot be localized by imaging, then selective catheterization of the inferior petrosal sinuses with measurement of ACTH level on either side may be done at a specialized center.[56] Ancillary laboratory studies frequently reveal impaired glucose tolerance and low bone density on radiographs or dual x-ray absorptiometry.

Adrenal carcinomas (but not typically adenomas) will secrete cortisol, as well as mineralocorticoids and androgens. Adrenal tumors are the most common cause of endogenous steroid excess in young children. The typical case appears in a round-faced, ruddy child with rapidly advancing premature pubarche, hypertension, and an abdominal mass. If adrenal carcinoma is suspected based on ACTH-independent (ie, nonsuppressible) cortisol excess, then the patient should undergo additional hormone measurements of aldosterone and plasma renin activity, as well as DHEA-sulfate and androgens.

Imaging Studies

Thin-slice CT or MRI of the abdomen including the adrenal glands should be performed. Carcinoma will often show a necrotic center or calcification and irregular borders, or both, whereas benign nonfunctioning adenomas are typically more similar in density to normal adrenal tissue and are homogeneous. Ectopic ACTH production by carcinomas is almost never seen in children.

Management

Cushing disease has traditionally been treated primarily with transsphenoidal tumor resection. Surgical success largely depends on the skill of the surgeon and the nature of the lesion. The cure rate ranges from 60% to 80%.[57] Data show that directed radiotherapy, such as gamma knife[58] and linear accelerator[59] techniques, can also induce gradual remission of ACTH hypersecretion. Once ACTH levels have decreased, the patient needs chronic glucocorticoids replacement therapy.

Patients with an adrenal tumor or nodular hyperplasia as the source for cortisol excess will most often undergo adrenalectomy. Another alternative for Cushing syndrome or Cushing disease is medical therapy with drugs such as ketoconazole. This therapy can be used either in the short term (eg, while waiting for radiotherapy to take effect) or the long term to reduce cortisol secretion; however, this type of treatment will not induce a permanent cure.

Adrenal Medullary Diseases

Neuroblastoma

In young children, the most common tumor encountered is a neuroblastoma. The incidence is approximately 1:100,000 children under age 15 per year. The average age at diagnosis in North America is 2 years; mass screening of infants is done in Japan to allow earlier diagnosis.[60]

Common presenting signs include abdominal mass, fever of unknown origin, hematuria, spinal cord compression, pathological fracture, and hypertension. Metastases to liver and bone occur in approximately 50% of cases by the time of tumor detection. Biochemical markers include plasma and urinary dopamine, vanillylmandelic acid, and homovanillic acid.

Bone scan is usually informative, revealing bone metastases, soft-tissue calcifications, or both. Other imaging modalities are discussed later in conjunction with pheochromocytoma diagnostic tests. The medical and surgical management of such tumors depends on staging risk; a possibility exists of spontaneous regression in low-grade tumors.[61]

Pheochromocytoma

In the adolescent, medullary disease is most often caused by a pheochromocytoma.

HISTORY AND PHYSICAL EXAMINATION. Pheochromocytoma, a rare tumor, may cause either episodic or chronic hypertension, usually accompanied by tachycardia, headaches, anxiety, sweating, flushing, or any combination. Weight loss may also be observed. The differential diagnosis in adolescents most saliently includes panic attacks, thyrotoxicosis, renovascular disease, and drug abuse (especially cocaine or amphetamines).

LABORATORY EVALUATION. Screening tests, besides documenting hypertension in the office, may include 24-hour ambulatory blood pressures. Chemistry profile may demonstrate hyperglycemia. Such findings should prompt referral to appropriate specialists. Extreme hypertension in a child should prompt immediate emergency referral and hospitalization.

The diagnosis of pheochromocytoma is made either by measuring increased 24-hour urine-free metanephrines (collected in an acid container) or by high-performance liquid chromatography measurement of plasma free metanephrines.[62] Blood should be obtained from an indwelling venous catheter in a patient who has been fasted overnight and at rest for at least 20 to 30 minutes; the sample tube must be iced and processed immediately. If possible, psychoactive drugs, especially tricyclic antidepressants, should be discontinued at least 2 weeks before testing.

IMAGING STUDIES. Confirmatory imaging may be done by metaiodobenzylguanidine scan.[63] Metaiodobenzylguanidine is a norepinephrine analog labeled with radioiodine that is taken up specifically by catechol-producing tumor tissue but not normal adrenal medulla. This imaging test is particularly helpful in cases in which thin-slice, contrast-enhanced CT or MRI fails to show a mass, yet biochemical tests and the clinical scenario are suggestive for pheochromocytoma. Other new imaging options include positron emission tomography and use of somatostatin analogs.[64]

A thorough family history should be obtained for endocrine tumors, especially medullary thyroid carcinoma and hyperparathyroidism, because multiple endocrine neoplasia type 2 may be associated with pheochromocytoma. Genotyping for the *RET* oncogene should be performed in the patient, and, if positive, other family members should be tested.[65] Transmission is autosomal dominant. Other syndromes prone to adrenal tumors or pheochromocytomas include von Hippel Lindau disease, neurofibromatosis type 1, paraganglioma, and tuberous sclerosis. Approximately 30% of young patients with pheochromocytoma have one of these familial disorders and should therefore be genotyped for the appropriate genes. Familial cases are more often bilateral.[66]

Children with a family history of familial tumor syndromes should be referred to the appropriate specialists for evaluation because early detection of affected genetic status may dictate intervention before tumors develop.

MANAGEMENT. Calcium channel–blocking drugs such as nifedipine are primarily used to control hypertension because calcium is needed for catechol secretion. In preparation for surgery, the patient should be treated for at least a week with a drug with both alpha-adrenergic blocking (eg, phenoxybenzamine) and beta-adrenergic blocking (eg, labetalol) properties. Unopposed alpha blockade would precipitate a hypotensive crisis at surgery, whereas unopposed beta blockade would exacerbate the hypertension from endogenous epinephrine, a potent vasoconstrictor. In addition, alpha-methyl-L-tyrosine (Demser) is also used to inhibit the rate-limiting step of catechol synthesis. Approximately 10% of pheochromocytomas are bilateral, and thus, at the time of surgery, both adrenals should be explored. If both adrenals are removed, then substitution therapy will be required as primary adrenal insufficiency. Malignancy and recurrence may occur in approximately 10% to 15% of cases. Careful long-term follow-up of patients with regular checks of blood pressure and catechol measurements is crucial.[67]

TOOLS FOR PRACTICE

Practice Management and Care Coordination

- Adrenal Crisis Emergency Letter, Cares Foundation (caresfoundation.org/acletter.html)

AAP POLICY STATEMENTS

Lee PA, Houk CP, Ahmed SF, et al. and the International Consensus Conference on Intersex. Consensus statement on management of intersex disorders. *Pediatrics* 2006;118(2): e488-e500. AAP Endorsed. (aappolicy.aappublications.org/cgi/content/full/pediatrics;118/2/e488).

American Academy of Pediatrics, Committee on Adolescence, and the American College of Obstetricians and Gynecologists, Committee on Adolescent Health Care. Menstruation in girls and adolescents: using the menstrual cycle as a vital sign. *Pediatrics*. 2006;118(5):2245-2250. (aappolicy.aappublications.org/cgi/content/full/pediatrics;118/5/2245).

American Academy of Pediatrics, Committee on Genetics, Section on Endocrinology. Technical report: congenital adrenal hyperplasia. *Pediatrics*. 2000;106(6):1511-1518. (aappolicy.aappublications.org/cgi/content/full/pediatrics;106/6/1511).

American Academy of Pediatrics, Committee on Genetics. Introduction to the newborn screening fact sheets. *Pediatrics*. 2006;118(3):1304-1312. (aappolicy.aappublications.org/cgi/content/full/pediatrics;118/3/1304).

American Academy of Pediatrics, Committee on Genetics. Newborn screening fact sheets. *Pediatrics*. 2006;118(3): e934-e963. (aappolicy.aappublications.org/cgi/content/full/pediatrics;118/3/e934).

SUGGESTED RESOURCE

National Adrenal Diseases Foundation (www.nadf.us).

REFERENCES

1. Nagata H, Hata K, Hata T, et al. Ultrasonographic measurements of fetal and neonatal adrenal glands. *Nippon Sanka Fujinka Gakkai Zasshi*. 1987;39:486-487.
2. Neville AM, O'Hare MJ. Histopathology of the human adrenal cortex. *Clin Endocrinol Metab*. 1985;14:791-820.
3. Rozansky DJ. The role of aldosterone in renal sodium transport. *Semin Nephrol*. 2006;26:173-181.
4. Tsigos C, Chrousos GP. Physiology of the hypothalamic-pituitary-adrenal axis in health and dysregulation in psychiatric and autoimmune disorders. *Endocrinol Metab Clin North Am*. 1994;23:451-466.
5. Walker BR, Connacher AA, Webb DJ, et al. Glucocorticoids and blood pressure: a role for the cortisol/cortisone shuttle in the control of vascular tone in man. *Clin Sci (Lond)*. 1992;83:171-178.
6. Speiser PW, White PC. Congenital adrenal hyperplasia. *N Engl J Med*. 2003;349:776-788.
7. White PC, Speiser PW. Congenital adrenal hyperplasia due to 21-hydroxylase deficiency. *Endocr Rev*. 2000;21: 245-291.
8. Therrell BL. Newborn screening for congenital adrenal hyperplasia. *Endocrinol Metab Clin North Am*. 2001;30: 15-30.
9. Azziz R, Dewailly D, Owerbach D. Nonclassic adrenal hyperplasia: current concepts. *J Clin Endocrinol Metab*. 1994;78:810-815.
10. New MI, Lorenzen F, Lerner AJ, et al. Genotyping steroid 21-hydroxylase deficiency: hormonal reference data. *J Clin Endocrinol Metab*. 1983;57:320-326.
11. Azziz R, Hincapie LA, Knochenhauer ES, et al. Screening for 21-hydroxylase–deficient nonclassic adrenal hyperplasia among hyperandrogenic women: a prospective study. *Fertil Steril*. 1999;72:915-925.
12. Speiser PW, Dupont J, Zhu D, et al. Disease expression and molecular genotype in congenital adrenal hyperplasia due to 21-hydroxylase deficiency. *J Clin Invest*. 1992; 90:584-595.
13. Clayton PE, Miller WL, Oberfield SE, et al. Consensus statement on 21-hydroxylase deficiency from the European Society for Paediatric Endocrinology and the Lawson Wilkins Pediatric Endocrine Society. *Horm Res*. 2002;58:188-195.
14. Charmandari E, Johnston A, Brook CG, et al. Bioavailability of oral hydrocortisone in patients with congenital adrenal hyperplasia due to 21-hydroxylase deficiency. *J Endocrinol*. 2001;169:65-70.
15. Gupta DK, Shilpa S, Amini AC, et al. Congenital adrenal hyperplasia: long-term evaluation of feminizing genitoplasty and psychosocial aspects. *Pediatr Surg Int*. 2006; 22:905-909.
16. Meyer-Bahlburg HF, Dolezal C, Baker SW, et al. Gender development in women with congenital adrenal hyperplasia as a function of disorder severity. *Arch Sex Behav*. 2006;35:667-684.
17. Stikkelbroeck NM, Otten BJ, Pasic A, et al. High prevalence of testicular adrenal rest tumors, impaired spermatogenesis, and Leydig cell failure in adolescent and adult males with congenital adrenal hyperplasia. *J Clin Endocrinol Metab*. 2001;86:5721-5728.
18. Arlt W, Allolio B. Adrenal insufficiency. *Lancet*. 2003;361: 1881-1893.
19. Ten S, New M, Maclaren N. Clinical review 130: Addison's disease 2001. *J Clin Endocrinol Metab*. 2001;86: 2909-2922.
20. Simm PJ, McDonnell CM, Zacharin MR. Primary adrenal insufficiency in childhood and adolescence: advances in diagnosis and management. *J Paediatr Child Health*. 2004;40:596-599.
21. Dorin RI, Qualls CR, Crapo LM. Diagnosis of adrenal insufficiency. *Ann Intern Med*. 2003;139:194-204.
22. Rose SR, Lustig RH, Burstein S, et al. Diagnosis of ACTH deficiency. Comparison of overnight metyrapone test to either low-dose or high-dose ACTH test. *Horm Res*. 1999;52:73-79.
23. Perry R, Kecha O, Paquette J, et al. Primary adrenal insufficiency in children: twenty years experience at the Sainte-Justine Hospital, Montreal. *J Clin Endocrinol Metab*. 2005;90:3243-3250.
24. Todd GR, Acerini CL, Ross-Russell R, et al. Survey of adrenal crisis associated with inhaled corticosteroids in the United Kingdom. *Arch Dis Child*. 2002;87: 457-461.
25. Dunlop KA, Carson DJ, Steen HJ, et al. Monitoring growth in asthmatic children treated with high dose inhaled glucocorticoids does not predict adrenal suppression. *Arch Dis Child*. 2004;89:713-716.
26. Levin C, Maibach HI. Topical corticosteroid-induced adrenocortical insufficiency: clinical implications. *Am J Clin Dermatol*. 2002;3:141-147.
27. Mortimer KJ, Tata LJ, Smith CJ, et al. Oral and inhaled corticosteroids and adrenal insufficiency: a case-control study. *Thorax*. 2006;61:405-408.
28. Lamberts SW, Bruining HA, de Jong FH. Corticosteroid therapy in severe illness. *N Engl J Med*. 1997;337:1285-1292.
29. Felner EI, Thompson MT, Ratliff AF, et al. Time course of recovery of adrenal function in children treated for leukemia. *J Pediatr*. 2000;137:21-24.
30. Schlaghecke R, Kornely E, Santen RT, et al. The effect of long-term glucocorticoid therapy on pituitary-adrenal responses to exogenous corticotropin-releasing hormone. *N Engl J Med*. 1992;326:226-230.
31. Oelkers W. Adrenal insufficiency. *N Engl J Med*. 1996; 335:1206-1212.
32. Walvoord EC, Rosenman MB, Eugster EA. Prevalence of adrenocorticotropin deficiency in children with idiopathic growth hormone deficiency. *J Clin Endocrinol Metab*. 2004;89:5030-5034.
33. Brooks BP, Kleta R, Stuart C, et al. Genotypic heterogeneity and clinical phenotype in triple A syndrome: a review of the NIH experience 2000-2005. *Clin Genet*. 2005;68:215-221.

34. Clark AJ, McLoughlin L, Grossman A. Familial glucocorticoid deficiency associated with point mutation in the adrenocorticotropin receptor. *Lancet.* 1993;341: 461-462.
35. Buchanan CR, Preece MA, Milner RD. Mortality, neoplasia, and Creutzfeldt-Jakob disease in patients treated with human pituitary growth hormone in the United Kingdom. *BMJ.* 1991;302:824-828.
36. Mills JL, Schonberger LB, Wysowski DK, et al. Long-term mortality in the United States cohort of pituitary-derived growth hormone recipients. *J Pediatr.* 2004;144: 430-436.
37. Taback SP, Dean HJ. Mortality in Canadian children with growth hormone (GH) deficiency receiving GH therapy 1967-1992. The Canadian Growth Hormone Advisory Committee. *J Clin Endocrinol Metab.* 1996;81:1693-1696.
38. Annane D, Sebille V, Charpentier C, et al. Effect of treatment with low doses of hydrocortisone and fludrocortisone on mortality in patients with septic shock. *JAMA.* 2002;288:862-871.
39. Rady MY, Johnson DJ, Patel B, et al. Cortisol levels and corticosteroid administration fail to predict mortality in critical illness: the confounding effects of organ dysfunction and sex. *Arch Surg.* 2005;140:661-668.
40. Pizarro CF, Troster EJ, Damiani D, et al. Absolute and relative adrenal insufficiency in children with septic shock. *Crit Care Med.* 2005;33:855-859.
41. Menon K, Clarson C. Adrenal function in pediatric critical illness. *Pediatr Crit Care Med.* 2002;3:112-116.
42. De Vroede M, Beukering R, Spit M, et al. Rectal hydrocortisone during stress in patients with adrenal insufficiency. *Arch Dis Child.* 1998;78:544-547.
43. Ni Chroinin M, Fallon M, Kenny D, et al. Rectal hydrocortisone during vomiting in children with adrenal insufficiency. *J Pediatr Endocrinol Metab.* 2003;16:1101-1104.
44. Charmandari E, Lichtarowicz-Krynska EJ, Hindmarsh PC, et al. Congenital adrenal hyperplasia: management during critical illness. *Arch Dis Child.* 2001;85:26-28.
45. Kerrigan JR, Veldhuis JD, Leyo SA, et al. Estimation of daily cortisol production and clearance rates in normal pubertal males by deconvolution analysis. *J Clin Endocrinol Metab.* 1993;76:1505-1510.
46. Saltzman E, Guay A. Dehydroepiandrosterone therapy as female androgen replacement. *Semin Reprod Med.* 2006;24:97-105.
47. Weise M, Drinkard B, Mehlinger SL, et al. Stress dose of hydrocortisone is not beneficial in patients with classic congenital adrenal hyperplasia undergoing short-term, high-intensity exercise. *J Clin Endocrinol Metab.* 2004; 89:3679-3684.
48. Herman-Giddens ME, Slora EJ, Wasserman RC, et al. Secondary sexual characteristics and menses in young girls seen in office practice: a study from the Pediatric Research in Office Settings Network. *Pediatrics.* 1997;99:505-512.
49. l'Allemand D, Schmidt S, Rousson V, et al. Associations between body mass, leptin, IGF-I and circulating adrenal androgens in children with obesity and premature adrenarche. *Eur J Endocrinol.* 2002;146:537-543.
50. McCartney CR, Blank SK, Prendergast KA, et al. Obesity and sex steroid changes across puberty: evidence for marked hyperandrogenemia in pre- and early pubertal obese girls. *J Clin Endocrinol Metab.* Nov 2006;92(2): 430-436.
51. Ibanez L, de Zegher F, Potau N. Premature pubarche, ovarian hyperandrogenism, hyperinsulinism and the polycystic ovary syndrome: from a complex constellation to a simple sequence of prenatal onset. *J Endocrinol Invest.* 1998;21:558-566.
52. Ibanez L, Jaramillo A, Enriquez G, et al. Polycystic ovaries after precocious pubarche: relation to prenatal growth. *Hum Reprod.* 2007;22(2):395-400.
53. Ibanez L, Valls C, Marcos MV, et al. Insulin sensitization for girls with precocious pubarche and with risk for polycystic ovary syndrome: effects of prepubertal initiation and postpubertal discontinuation of metformin treatment. *J Clin Endocrinol Metab.* 2004;89:4331-4337.
54. Lindholm J, Juul S, Jorgensen JO, et al. Incidence and late prognosis of Cushing's syndrome: a population-based study. *J Clin Endocrinol Metab.* 2001;86:117-123.
55. Lai HC, FitzSimmons SC, Allen DB, et al. Risk of persistent growth impairment after alternate-day prednisone treatment in children with cystic fibrosis. *N Engl J Med.* 2000;342:851-859.
56. Newell-Price J, Bertagna X, Grossman AB, et al. Cushing's syndrome. *Lancet.* 2006;367:1605-1617.
57. Oldfeld EH. Cushing disease. *J Neurosurg.* 2003;98: 948-951.
58. Jane JA Jr, Vance ML, Woodburn CJ, et al. Stereotactic radiosurgery for hypersecreting pituitary tumors: part of a multimodality approach. *Neurosurg Focus.* 2003; 14:e12.
59. Voges J, Kocher M, Runge M, et al. Linear accelerator radiosurgery for pituitary macroadenomas: a 7-year follow-up study. *Cancer.* 2006;107:1355-1364.
60. Nishio N, Mimaya J, Nara T, et al. Results for 79 patients with neuroblastoma detected through mass screening at 6 months of age in a single institute. *Pediatr Int.* 2006;48: 531-535.
61. Kim S, Chung DH. Pediatric solid malignancies: neuroblastoma and Wilms' tumor. *Surg Clin North Am.* 2006; 86:469-487.
62. Lenders JW, Pacak K, Walther MM, et al. Biochemical diagnosis of pheochromocytoma: which test is best? *JAMA.* 2002;287:1427-1434.
63. Guller U, Turek J, Eubanks S, et al. Detecting pheochromocytoma: defining the most sensitive test. *Ann Surg.* 2006;243:102-107.
64. Rufini V, Calcagni ML, Baum RP. Imaging of neuroendocrine tumors. *Semin Nucl Med.* 2006;36:228-247.
65. Toledo SP, dos Santos MA, Toledo RA, et al. Impact of RET proto-oncogene analysis on the clinical management of multiple endocrine neoplasia type 2. *Clinics.* 2006;61:59-70.
66. Amar L, Bertherat J, Baudin E, et al. Genetic testing in pheochromocytoma or functional paraganglioma. *J Clin Oncol.* 2005;23:8812-8818.
67. Pham TH, Moir C, Thompson GB, et al. Pheochromocytoma and paraganglioma in children: a review of medical and surgical management at a tertiary care center. *Pediatrics.* 2006;118:1109-1117.

Chapter 234

ALLERGIC RHINITIS

Robert A. Wood, MD

Allergic rhinitis is the most common of the atopic diseases. It occurs in approximately 15% of the general population and may exist alone or in combination with asthma or atopic dermatitis.[1] In children, allergic rhinitis is relatively uncommon before the age of 3 years and increases in frequency thereafter, reaching a peak prevalence in adolescence. The most easily recognized form of allergic rhinitis occurs in a typical seasonal pattern, referred to as seasonal allergic rhinitis or hay fever. Year-round, or perennial, allergic rhinitis, which is triggered by indoor allergens such as dust mites or animal dander, is more common but often less dramatic and therefore more difficult to diagnose.

ETIOLOGY

As with all atopic disease, the tendency to develop allergic rhinitis is inherited. When a child who has a genetic predisposition to atopy is exposed to an allergen, antigen-specific immunoglobulin E (IgE) molecules are produced, which bind to mast cells in the respiratory tract. Once the child has been sensitized in this way, reexposure to the same allergen causes an immediate, type I hypersensitivity reaction in which cross-linking of cell surface IgE molecules triggers the rapid release of mast cell mediators (eg, histamine, prostaglandins, leukotrienes), as well as the synthesis of cell interactive compounds called cytokines.[2] Histamine causes immediate local vasodilation, mucosal edema, and increased mucus production. Cytokines summon inflammatory cells, especially eosinophils, to the site of the allergic reaction, which leads to the slower late-phase reaction characterized by inflammation and damage to the mucosal surface that progresses to chronic nasal obstruction. The severity of the symptoms varies tremendously and depends both on the individual's level of sensitivity and on the intensity of the antigen exposure.

The allergens involved most commonly in allergic rhinitis include the following[3]:

1. Pollens. Wind-borne pollens from trees and grasses in the spring and from weeds (especially ragweed) in the fall cause well-defined seasonal symptoms, but variation is tremendous according to location. Most flower pollens are insect borne and therefore rarely cause allergic problems.
2. Molds. In colder climates, outdoor molds produce spores beginning in the early spring and peaking in the late fall. In warmer climates, outdoor molds can grow year round. Molds may grow indoors and year round in most climates, with the highest levels occurring in warmer, more humid months.
3. Animal dander. Allergens from the skin and saliva of household pets such as dogs and cats can produce severe intermittent and perennial symptoms. Rodent allergens, which are found predominantly in urine and are also potent triggers of allergic symptoms, occur both from unwanted pests, for example, rats and mice and from pets such as hamsters and guinea pigs.
4. Dust mites. These ubiquitous, microscopic arthropods are the major allergen in house dust. Mites prosper in warm, moist, indoor environments and colonize pillows, mattresses, and carpets. They are the major cause of perennial allergic rhinitis.
5. Cockroaches. Cockroach allergens are another common cause of perennial allergic rhinitis, especially in urban areas.

CLINICAL FEATURES

Allergic rhinitis is characterized clinically by a combination of nasal congestion, sneezing, rhinorrhea, and pruritus. Younger children usually have perennial symptoms, whereas pollen sensitivity becomes more common after the age of 4 years. In the acute, seasonal variety, the symptoms may be quite intense and often include severe congestion and rhinorrhea, as well as associated allergic conjunctivitis. The diagnosis typically is clearly based on the patient's history, and the specific allergens responsible for these seasonal exacerbations can usually be identified based on knowledge of the local pollen seasons (for local pollen counts, visit the American Academy of Asthma Allergy and Immunology Web site, *www.aaaai.org*). Perennial sufferers typically have less dramatic or fewer specific symptoms. Although nasal congestion is still the most prominent symptom, children often display symptoms such as frequent colds, recurrent otitis media, nasal speech, mouth breathing, snoring, and fatigue; epistaxis also is common. The nasal discharge is usually clear unless the child has a superimposed infection. Many children perform the allergic salute, a maneuver in which they sniff and sweep the palm of their hand upward across the tip of the nose in an attempt to open their nasal passages, remove secretions, or relieve nasal itching. Facial grimacing is also used to relieve nasal itching.

Although the physical examination can be very striking, especially during periods of seasonal rhinitis, it can also be quite unremarkable when symptoms are quiescent. The nasal mucosa is pale, bluish, and boggy, with a clear serous discharge. The nasal turbinates are enlarged, sometimes enough to obstruct the airway almost completely. Children who have perennial problems often have the typical allergic facies consisting of allergic shiners (a dark discoloration beneath both eyes), Dennie lines (extra folds below the lower eyelids), an allergic crease (a horizontal line across the bridge of the nose), and an elongated facies caused by chronic mouth breathing. The tonsils and adenoids often are enlarged, and evidence of middle-ear effusion may be found. Nasal polyps can occur but are uncommon in childhood allergic rhinitis.

COMPLICATIONS

Early in life, children who have allergic rhinitis may suffer from an increased incidence of respiratory infections, acute otitis media, and eustachian tube dysfunction, leading to serous otitis media. Several studies have suggested an association between allergy and chronic serous otitis media, although this association is only one of many risk factors. Abnormal facial development, a high arched palate, and orthodontic problems from chronic mouth breathing occasionally develop, especially if associated adenoid hypertrophy exists. Acute and chronic sinusitis are common, probably the result of reduced ciliary clearance and obstruction of sinus ostia.[4] Asthma is often seen in combination with allergic rhinitis but is not viewed typically as a complication of untreated allergic rhinitis.

LABORATORY FINDINGS

The nasal smear for eosinophils is a simple office procedure that can help confirm the clinical diagnosis of allergic rhinitis. The patient blows his or her nose into plastic wrap or wax paper (a cotton swab may be used to obtain secretions if the patient cannot blow), and the secretions are spread onto a glass slide and left to dry. The slide then is prepared with Hansel or Wright stain. If more than 10% of the cells seen on the smear are eosinophils, then an ongoing allergic process is probable. Strongly positive results are most likely during heavy exposure to the allergen. Concurrent nasal infection may obscure the results, and eosinophils may be absent during the off season.

Blood eosinophilia is occasionally found (more than 5% eosinophils on the differential white blood cell count or more than 250/μL eosinophils in total). An elevated total serum IgE suggests atopy, but many patients who have allergic rhinitis have a normal serum IgE. Eosinophil counts and total serum IgE levels are therefore not recommended as screening tests for allergic rhinitis.

Skin tests and radioallergosorbent tests can detect antigen-specific IgE and identify specific allergic sensitivities in patients in whom the diagnosis is in question or who are in need of more aggressive management.[5] Skin tests should be performed by a physician who is trained in their use, and they should be interpreted in the context of the clinical history. Compared with skin testing, radioallergosorbent tests have the disadvantages of higher cost and slightly lower sensitivity. However, they are accurate overall and can be used efficiently in the primary care physician's office as a limited screening test for allergy that also will identify specific allergens to be targeted for environmental control. When more extensive testing is needed, referring the patient to an allergist will usually be more cost effective.

DIFFERENTIAL DIAGNOSIS

Usually, little difficulty is encountered in diagnosing seasonal allergic rhinitis based on the clinical presentation, physical examination, and a knowledge of local pollens. On the other hand, children who have nonspecific perennial symptoms often pose a difficult diagnostic challenge. Three other conditions that are often confused with allergic rhinitis are (1) recurrent upper respiratory tract infections, (2) vasomotor rhinitis, and (3) adenoid hypertrophy.

Recurrent viral and bacterial upper respiratory tract infections can be differentiated from allergies by their intermittent course, a history of contagion, and the presence of fever, purulent nasal discharge, or erythematous, inflamed nasal mucosa. In addition, eosinophils will not be prominent on a nasal smear, and the family history for allergy is more likely to be negative.

Vasomotor rhinitis is an ill-defined condition that may begin at any age.[1] It is characterized by hyperreactivity of the nasal mucous membranes to a wide variety of irritant stimuli. The most prominent symptom is usually perennial nasal obstruction that responds poorly to environmental controls or medications. Usually, no family history of allergy is present, although other family members may report chronic nasal congestion as well. The nasal smear and skin test results are negative, the serum IgE is normal, and no eye signs or other atopic manifestations are present.

Another variant of perennial rhinitis, called nonallergic rhinitis with eosinophilia, also has been described. In this disorder, which affects adolescents and adults, the nasal smear results are positive for eosinophils, but the serum IgE is normal and skin test results are negative.

Anatomic abnormalities represent the third major cause of chronic nasal symptoms in children. By far, the most common of these is adenoid hypertrophy, which will typically exhibit as nasal obstruction with little or no rhinorrhea. Many of these children will also experience recurrent middle ear, nasal, or sinus infections. In more severe cases, the obstruction will lead to obvious changes in the structure of the face and palate caused by chronic mouth breathing. Snoring is common, and a typical nasal quality to the voice is often present.

Other less common conditions that may mimic allergic rhinitis are the presence of a nasal foreign body, choanal atresia, rhinitis medicamentosa, cystic fibrosis, and nasopharyngeal tumors.

TREATMENT

Management of allergic rhinitis incorporates the information from a thorough history and physical examination into a stepwise program that typically consists of allergen avoidance measures and pharmacotherapy.[5-7] Time must be taken to individualize each child's treatment, taking into account the patient's age, the severity of the symptoms, specific environmental issues, the presence or absence of complications, and any other medical conditions that may be present. If the symptoms are perennial, do not respond to appropriate medications, or worsen each year, then an allergist should be consulted. The allergist can confirm the diagnosis, identify specific allergens, fine tune environmental controls and pharmacotherapy, and possibly prescribe immunotherapy.

Environmental control for both allergens and nonspecific irritants should be the first line of therapy at all ages.[8] Particular attention should be directed to the child's bedroom and other settings where substantial amounts of time are spent. If an allergy to dust mites is thought to exist or has been confirmed by testing, then the first steps to reduce exposure should include dust mite–proof encasements for mattresses, box springs, and pillows; removal of stuffed animals and similar items; and hot washing of bed linens every 1 to 2 weeks. Ideally, pets should be removed if they are the cause of allergic symptoms, although some relief may be obtained by keeping the pet out of the child's bedroom, using mattress and pillow encasements, removing carpets, and using an air cleaner in the bedroom. Children who are allergic to pollens can be helped dramatically by closing windows and using an air conditioner. Forced-air heating and cooling systems can be improved by adding humidifiers and air filters, although keeping the relative humidity be kept below 50% is important so that dust mite and mold growth is not encouraged.

Oral antihistamines, which inhibit histamine-mediated symptoms by blocking histamine H1-receptors on mast cells, should be the first-line pharmacologic treatment of childhood allergic rhinitis.[6,9] They are most effective in controlling rhinorrhea, sneezing, and pruritus but are less effective in relieving symptoms of nasal congestion. The first generation antihistamines, including diphenhydramine, chlorpheniramine, and hydroxyzine, are very effective, but their use may be limited in many children by their sedative side effects. They can impair school performance significantly and should therefore be used with caution in this age group.[10] Fortunately, several second- and now third-generation antihistamines, including loratadine, desloratadine, cetirizine, and fexofenadine, have now been approved for use in children. Although not necessarily more potent, their lack of sedation is an important advantage. Alternatively, many children can be treated effectively by using a 1st-generation antihistamine as a single bedtime dose, especially if their symptoms are worse at night.

Oral decongestants, such as pseudoephedrine, may have value in treating some children, especially when nasal congestion is a major symptom.[11] They can be used either alone or in combination with an antihistamine. Oral decongestants should be used with some caution, however, because some children experience significant stimulatory effects, which may produce hyperactivity, irritability, or sleep disturbance. Although topical decongestant nasal sprays may provide transient relief, it is often followed after several days of use by rebound congestion. Because prolonged use of nasal sprays often leads to a worsening of symptoms (a condition known as rhinitis medicamentosa), their use should be discouraged.

The leukotriene antagonist montelukast has also been approved for treatment of both seasonal and perennial allergic rhinitis.[12] It is similar in efficacy to oral antihistamines and is generally well tolerated; it may also be particularly useful in children with coexistent asthma and allergic rhinitis.

A variety of topical sprays also can be helpful. Nasal corticosteroids are the most effective pharmacologic agents for allergic rhinitis, and some agents now have been approved for use in patients 3 years of age and older.[13] Available preparations include beclomethasone, budesonide, fluticasone, mometasone, and triamcinolone. Nasal steroids do have a slight potential to adversely effect growth in children; therefore, although their risk-benefit ratio generally is excellent, they should always be used at the lowest possible dose. In addition, short courses of oral steroids (eg, prednisone) may rarely be needed for severe cases that do not respond to other therapies.

Other topical preparations include the antihistamine azelastine, which is of similar potency to oral antihistamines and can also have sedative side effects.[14] Nasal cromolyn sodium is an extremely safe drug that is reasonably effective, although its usefulness is significantly limited by the need to use it 4 to 6 times a day. Finally, ipratropium nasal spray is approved for children 6 years of age and older and may be helpful in the control of rhinorrhea.[15] It may have a particular advantage in cases of nonallergic rhinitis in which excessive rhinorrhea is a major complaint.

If the symptoms do not respond to avoidance measures and reasonable doses of medication, then patients should be referred to an allergist for skin testing to identify specific allergens. If the clinical history and skin test results correlate, then immunotherapy becomes a logical part of treatment.[16,17] Usually a 3- to 5-year course of regular injections is necessary to achieve maximal benefit and to minimize the chance of relapse after discontinuing treatment. This regimen is most effective in treating seasonal allergic rhinitis, with more than 80% of patients achieving significant relief, and is also beneficial for most cases of perennial disease. As treatment progresses, patients can expect a gradual decline in symptoms and reduced reliance on medication. Because of the risk of local and generalized reactions to the material injected, and because of the inconvenience and expense associated with regular injections, immunotherapy must be used selectively, typically reserved only for patients who have failed to respond to standard medications and avoidance measures.

PROGNOSIS

Allergic rhinitis, similar to other allergic disorders, is an illness that waxes and wanes over time. Most children tend to improve with time, although very few (probably fewer than 10%) lose their symptoms completely.[18] Remission of symptoms may result from changes in environment, avoidance programs, and immunotherapy. The pediatric physician should counsel patients that allergic symptoms can be controlled but not eliminated entirely and that the success of any treatment depends on the patient's understanding of the causes of symptoms and compliance with the prescribed regimen.

WHEN TO REFER

- Perennial symptoms
- Poorly controlled disease
- Suspected complications (eg, chronic sinusitis)
- Need for immunotherapy
- Parental needs

TOOLS FOR PRACTICE

Engaging Patients and Family

- *Allergies in Children* (brochure), American Academy of Pediatrics (patiented.aap.org).
- *What is a Pediatric Allergist* (fact sheet), American Academy of Pediatrics (www.aap.org/family/WhatisPedAllergistImm.pdf).
- *Guide to Your Child's Allergies* (book), American Academy of Pediatrics (www.aap.org/bookstore).
- Allergy Medication Guide (interactive web tool), American Academy of Allergy, Asthma, and Immunology (www.aaaai.org/patients/resources/medication_guide/default.stm).
- *Allergic Rhinitis* (fact sheet), American Academy of Allergy, Asthma, and Immunology (www.aaaai.org/patients/resources/easy_reader/rhinitis.pdf).

Medical Decision Support

- Pediatric Prescribing Update (on-line course), American Academy of Pediatrics (www.pedialink.org/cme/_coursefinder/CMEdetail.cfm?aid=30368&area=liveCME).

- *When Should Students Carry and Self-Administer Emergency Medications at School* (fact sheet), National Heart, Lung, and Blood Institute, AAP endorsed (www.nhlbi.nih.gov/health/prof/lung/asthma/emer_medi.htm).

Community Coordination and Advocacy

- *Allergy Toolkit for School Nurses* (tool kit), American Academy of Allergy, Asthma, and Immunology, AAP endorsed (www.aaaai.org/members/allied%5Fhealth/tool%5Fkit/).

REFERENCES

1. National Center for Health Statistics. Summary Health Statistics for U.S. Adults: National Health Interview Survey, 2002, 2004. Available at: www.cdc.gov/nchs/fastats/allergies.htm. Accessed May 24, 2006.
2. Howarth PH. Allergic rhinitis: not purely a histamine-related disease. *Allergy*. 2000;55:7-16.
3. American Academy of Allergy, Asthma, and Immunology. *The Allergy Report*. Available at: www.theallergyreport.org. Accessed May 24, 2006.
4. American Academy of Pediatrics. Clinical practice guideline: management of sinusitis. *Pediatrics*. 2001;108:798-808.
5. Dykewicz MS, Fineman S, Skoner DP, et al. Diagnosis and management of rhinitis: complete guidelines of the Joint Task Force on Practice Parameters in Allergy, Asthma and Immunology. *Ann Allergy Asthma Immunol*. 1998;81:478-518.
6. van Cauwenberge P, Bachert C, Passalacqua G, et al. Consensus statement on the treatment of allergic rhinitis: European Academy of Allergology and Clinical Immunology. *Allergy*. 2000;55:116-134.
7. Plaut M, Valentine MD. Allergic rhinitis. *N Eng J Med*. 2005;353:1934-1935.
8. Sheikh A, Hurwitz B. House dust mite avoidance measures for perennial allergic rhinitis. *Cochrane Database Syst Rev*. 2001;4:CD001563-CD001563.
9. Simons FE. Advances in H1-antihistamines. *N Engl J Med*. 2004;351:2203-2217.
10. Bender BG, Berning S, Dudden R, et al. Sedation and performance impairment of diphenhydramine and second-generation antihistamines: a meta-analysis. *J Allergy Clin Immunol*. 2003;111:770-776.
11. Pleskow W, Grubbe R, Weiss S, et al. Efficacy and safety of an extended-release formulation of desloratadine and pseudoephedrine vs the individual components in the treatment of seasonal allergic rhinitis. *Ann Allergy Asthma Immunol*. 2005;94:348-354.
12. Wilson AM, O'Byrne PM, Parameswaran K. Leukotriene receptor antagonists for allergic rhinitis: a systematic review and meta-analysis. *Am J Med*. 2004;116:338-344.
13. Yanez A, Rodrigo GJ. Intranasal corticosteroids versus topical H1 receptor antagonists for the treatment of allergic rhinitis: a systematic review with meta-analysis. *Ann Allergy Asthma Immunol*. 2002;89:479-484.
14. Corren J, Storms W, Bernstein J, et al. Effectiveness of azelastine nasal spray compared with oral cetirizine in patients with seasonal allergic rhinitis. *Clin Ther*. 2005;27:543-553.
15. Milgrom H, Biondi R, Georgitis JW, et al. Comparison of ipratropium bromide 0.03% with beclomethasone dipropionate in the treatment of perennial rhinitis in children. *Ann Allergy Asthma Immunol*. 1999;83:105-111.
16. Till SJ, Francis JN, Nouri-Aria K, et al. Mechanisms of immunotherapy. *J Allergy Clin Immunol*. 2004;113:1025-1034.
17. Wheeler AW, Woroniecki SR. Allergy vaccines—new approaches to an old concept. *Expert Opin Biol Ther*. 2004;4:1473-1481.
18. Linna O, Kokkonen J, Lukin M. A 10-year prognosis for childhood allergic rhinitis. *Acta Pediatr*. 1992;81:100.

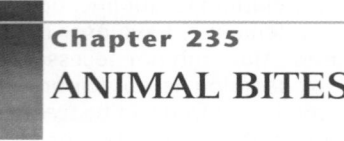

Chapter 235

ANIMAL BITES

Neil E. Herendeen, MD, MBA; Peter G. Szilagyi, MD, MPH

Estimates indicate that each year more than 2 million people across the United States are bitten by animals. Dog bites account for more than 90% of these injuries, and cat bites account for most of the remainder.[1] Although wild animal bites are rare, they are potentially more serious, given the risk of rabies and other infections. One half of all animal bites are trivial and require no medical treatment; only 10% are severe enough to require suturing, and only 2% result in hospitalization. Bite wounds account for an estimated 1% of pediatric visits to an emergency department.[1] Children experience the greatest number of animal bites (the peak age group is 5 to 14 years), with 50% of all school-aged children reporting an animal bite at some point in their life. With dog bites, adults are bitten on an extremity; children, however, are bitten primarily on the head or neck 75% of the time.[2] Boys are twice as likely to be bitten by a dog, whereas girls receive twice as many cat bites.[2] Not surprisingly, most of the animals live in the victim's neighborhood (75%) or home (15%); in most instances, the bites are provoked by humans.[1]

The major morbidity from animal bites results from direct trauma and infection. Although dog bites are more likely to cause lacerations or avulsions, these open wounds can be debrided and cleaned to prevent infection. However, puncture wounds, which usually do not require suturing, can result in deep-tissue infections.[3]

As shown in Table 235-1, the risk of infection varies according to several factors. Hand wounds are most likely to become infected, partly because of the type of

Table 235-1 Risk Factors for Infection in Animal Bites

RISK FACTOR	INFECTION RATES
Location of bite	Hand (18-36%) > arm or leg (12-16%) > face (5-11%)
Type of wound	Puncture with laceration (17-26%) > laceration alone (9-12%)
Interval between bite and medical care	If >24 hr, risk of infection increases
Type of animal	Cat bites (40-50%) Dog bites (10-30%) Human bites (13-40%)

wound (most frequently a puncture wound), the relatively poor vascular supply, and the vulnerability of the closed spaces of the hand. If more than 24 hours have elapsed before medical attention is sought, then the risk of infection is greatly increased. Cat and human bites pose a greater risk of infection than dog bites, partly because these bites more often cause puncture wounds, whereas dog bites frequently cause open lacerations.

Most bacteria associated with bite wounds are common organisms that reside in the animal's oral cavity. Bacteria on the victim's skin may also contribute to infection. Most infections involve several pathogens,[3] often both aerobes and anaerobes. *Pasteurella multocida,* a gram-negative, facultative anaerobe found in the mouths of most dogs and cats, is highly associated with cat bite infections (up to 80%) and to a lesser extent with dog bite infections (12%-50%). Although the exact prevalence of other pathogenic bacteria isolated from infected animal bites varies, gram-negative aerobes (eg, *Pseudomonas, Klebsiella,* and *Enterobacter* species) are found more often than gram-positive aerobes (eg, staphylococci, streptococci) or anaerobes (eg, *Bacteroides, Fusobacterium,* and *Peptococcus* species).[4]

Another group of gram-negative bacteria, classified by the Centers for Disease Control and Prevention as alphanumeric organisms, has frequently been isolated from dog bite wounds. Interestingly, human bites are rarely infected by *P multocida* but are often associated with gram-positive organisms, gram-negative anaerobes, or *Eikenella corrodens,* a genus almost unique to human bites that in rare cases is found in cat bites. Human bites have the potential to transmit the HIV and hepatitis B virus and should be evaluated in persons who are bitten by those at high risk for infection.

EVALUATION

History

Important points to elicit while taking the history of the wound include the length of time since injury, the type of animal (including domestic or wild), whether the attack was provoked or unprovoked, the animal's present location, immunization status and health, and the prior wound management.

Physical Examination

The physical examination entails a thorough musculoskeletal and neurologic examination to determine whether underlying structures were damaged and a thorough inspection of the wound for signs of infection. Special attention must be given to bites on the hand because, particularly in deep puncture wounds, superficial signs of infection (redness, swelling, purulent drainage) may be absent. Finally, the clinician should be aware that deep infections of tendons or bones and systemic infections can occur if animal bites go untreated. The time of the infection's onset may be a clue to *P multocida* infection. Cellulitis from this organism generally develops rapidly, within hours of the animal bite, whereas systemic signs (fever, lymphangitis) are usually absent.[3] A cellulitis that develops gradually, over days, is more likely the result of gram-positive cocci or other pathogenic bacteria.[3]

Laboratory Evaluation

Gram stain of a wound specimen is not useful because findings do not correlate with culture results. Cultures of clinically infected animal bite wounds are reported to have no growth in as many as one third of cases; conversely, cultures of clinically noninfected bite wounds grow a wide spectrum of oral flora bacteria in the same proportion of cases.[4] Moreover, such cultures do not predict the likelihood of subsequent infection, nor do results correlate with culture findings when clinical infection becomes apparent. However, cultures of clinically infected wounds may help ensure that the causative bacteria are sensitive to the antibiotic used. Radiologic studies may be necessary for deep puncture wounds to determine whether the periosteum has been penetrated. These studies include those of the calvaria of small children who experience bites to the head.

The clinician should remember that cat-scratch disease is a relatively common complication of cat bites and, less commonly, of bites by other animals. This disease often begins with the development of a red, painless papule at the site of a recent scratch or bite; within weeks, a tender, enlarged, regional lymph node appears, usually associated with fever, malaise, and other systemic symptoms. This self-limited illness, which is caused by *Bartonella henselae,* can be diagnosed clinically or confirmed by serologic testing. Antibiotics offer minimal clinical benefit, and because the disease is self-limited, their use seldom is indicated. Large, tender, fluctuant lymph nodes may require aspiration or incision and drainage.[3]

MANAGEMENT

Wound Care

The initial step in treating animal bites is meticulous wound care. This process involves gently cleaning the wound with soap and water and vigorously irrigating with saline solution. Saline irrigation of the wound with a syringe and a 19-gauge needle generates increased pressure on the tissues that facilitates cleansing of the wound and reduces the risk of infection. Devitalized tissue should be debrided. Puncture wounds should be cleaned, but irrigation is ineffective and may result in further damage to underlying structures. Elevation and immobilization are important for significant extremity injuries. The child's immunization status should be assessed and tetanus prophylaxis provided if indicated.

Primary closure of lacerations caused by animal (or human) bites is controversial.[5] Wounds that are clearly infected should not be closed. The consensus is that most noninfected lacerations can be sutured, after meticulous cleansing and irrigation, for cosmetic purposes or for hemostasis, without increasing the risk of infection. Hand wounds may be an exception because of the great likelihood of infection and the risk of serious complications from deep, closed-space infections; in these cases, suturing is suggested only for large wounds.

The use of prophylactic antibiotics in noninfected animal bite wounds is controversial. Prophylactic antibiotic therapy reduces the risk of infection after human bites or animal bites of the hand; however, no evidence has been found that it is effective for other

Table 235-2 Rabies Vaccination Guidelines

ANIMAL	MANAGEMENT
Wild carnivores	Begin HRIG/RIG and HDCV. Submit animal's head for testing.
Healthy domestic dogs and cats	Quarantine animal; treat only if animal develops symptoms.
Stray or sick dogs and cats	Submit animal's head for testing. Delay treatment until test results are known unless clinical likelihood of rabies is high. If animal is unavailable, then complete full series of HRIG/RIG and HDCV.
Rodents, rabbits	Unlikely to be rabid (except woodchucks). Treat only if animal acted strangely and cannot be tested.

HDCV, Human diploid cell vaccine; *HRIG/RIG,* human rabies immunoglobulin.
From Centers for Disease Control and Prevention. Human rabies prevention—United States, 1999. Recommendations of the Advisory Committee on Immunization Practices (ACIP). *MMWR Morb Mortal Wkly Rep.* 1999;44(RR-1):1-21.

types of cat or dog bites.[6] If infected, bite wounds brought to medical attention after 24 hours should then be treated with antibiotics. The choice of antibiotics depends on culture results or, if cultures are not available, on the likely pathogens. Although penicillin is active against *P multocida* and many oral flora, the addition of a penicillinase-resistant antibiotic provides more effective coverage. Amoxicillin/clavulanic acid (Augmentin) is an excellent choice for empirical treatment of bites from all animals.[5] Patients with infected hand bites, moderate to severe infections at other bite sites, and those who present with systemic symptoms such as high fever should be treated with intravenous antibiotics. In cases of cat bites, penicillin G for *P multocida* plus an anti-staphylococcal antibiotic such as cefazolin or trimethoprim/sulfamethoxazole (TMP/SMX) is recommended. Penicillin allergic children may be treated with azithromycin and an antistaphylococcal antibiotic. For dog bites, ampicillin/sulbactam is recommended. For children allergic to penicillin, clindamycin and TMP/SMX is recommended.

Wild Animal Bites

Animal bites from nondomestic animals require special attention. Although most primary care physicians will never treat a child who has rabies, they will evaluate children who may have been exposed to it. With the increasing spread of rabies among nondomestic animals, the number of people exposed to rabies and requiring vaccination is increasing dramatically. A full postexposure vaccination series can cost $2000 or more and requires five visits to the physician in a single month.[7] Knowing whom and when to treat requires an understanding of rabies transmission and epidemiologic mechanism. Rabies is an RNA virus present in saliva and transmitted by bites or by licking of mucosa or open wounds. In the United States, in all cases of rabies resulting from a dog or cat bite, the infected animal has been noted to become ill during the standard 10-day confinement and observation period; thus, location, confinement, and observation of the animal are important.[7,8]

In cases involving wild animal bites, consultation with the local health department is helpful in determining the risk of rabies in a specific animal for a particular geographic region. In general, bats, skunks, foxes, raccoons, and other carnivores are considered rabid until proved otherwise by laboratory tests; in the interim, or if the animal cannot be found, treatment with human rabies immunoglobulin (HRIG/RIG) and human diploid cell vaccine is suggested. Current recommendations call for most, if not all, of the HRIG/RIG dose (20 IU/kg of body weight) to be infiltrated in and around the site of the bite.[8] Rabies prophylaxis is now also suggested after exposure to bats in a confined setting, such as finding a bat in the bedroom on awakening, even when no bites are visible. Because the location of a bat bite is rarely known, the total HRIG/RIG dose may be given in the thigh. If the bat can be captured and submitted for testing, then rabies prophylaxis can be avoided in 60% of the cases[9] (Table 235-2). Rabies, which was previously considered a fatal disease, has been successfully treated with the induction of a coma.[10]

A variety of rare diseases have been described after wild animal bites; consultation with the local health department may help in establishing the diagnosis and managing treatment. Rat-bite fever, a systemic illness caused by *Streptobacillus moniliformis* or *Spirillum minus,* is one such example. The *Red Book* contains comprehensive, up-to-date descriptions of unusual diseases transmitted by various domestic and wild animals.[3]

ANTICIPATORY GUIDANCE

Although pets provide hours of delight and companionship for children, education about responsible care of a pet is important. Preschool-aged children should not be left alone with a pet, and they should be advised never to tease animals, approach strange animals, or play with pets that are eating. Families who have children should be advised not to buy wild animals or dogs bred for aggressiveness. Finally, vaccinations for pets and routine visits to a veterinarian should be encouraged (see Chapter 30, Injury Prevention, for a more detailed discussion of animal safety rules for children). Families traveling with children should be on the alert for stray animals in foreign countries, given that animal control is often poor. If families are planning to spend an extended period in a country where rabies is endemic, then prophylactic rabies vaccine should be strongly considered.

WHEN TO REFER

- Complex wounds that require surgical repair
- Bites to the face or hand that require plastic surgery
- Infected wounds not responding to initial treatment
- Children with human bites from an adult

WHEN TO ADMIT

- Infected wounds requiring intravenous antibiotics
- Extensive facial wounds requiring skilled nursing care

TOOLS FOR PRACTICE

Engaging Patient and Family

- *What You Should Know About Dog Bite Prevention* (brochure), American Medical Veterinary Association (www.aap.org/advocacy/releases/dogbiteprevention.pdf).

Medical Decision Support

- *Human Rabies Prevention—United States, 1999, Recommendations of the Advisory Committee on Immunization Practices (ACIP)* (guideline), Centers for Disease Control and Prevention (www.cdc.gov/mmwr/preview/mmwrhtml/00056176.htm).
- *Red Book 2006 Report of the Committee on Infectious Diseases* (book), American Academy of Pediatrics (www.aap.org/bookstore).

SUGGESTED RESOURCE

American Veterinary Medical Association. What You Should Know About Dog Bite Prevention. May 2006. Available at: www.aap.org/advocacy/releases/dogbiteprevention.pdf. Accessed June 13, 2007.

REFERENCES

1. Weiss HB, Friedman DI, Coben JH. Incidence of dog bite injuries treated in emergency departments. *JAMA*. 1998; 279:51-53.
2. Gandhi RR, Liebman MA, Stafford BL, et al. Dog bite injuries in children: a preliminary survey. *Am Surg*. 1999; 65;863-864.
3. American Academy of Pediatrics. Bite wounds. In: Pickering LK, Baker CJ, Long SS, et al, eds. *Red Book 2006 Report of the Committee on Infectious Diseases*. 27th ed. Elk Grove Village, IL: American Academy of Pediatrics; 2006.
4. Talan DA, Cintron DM, Abrahamian FM, et al. Bacteriologic analysis of infected dog and cat bites. *N Engl J Med*. 1999;340:85-92.
5. Cummings P. Antibiotics to prevent infection in patients with dog bite wounds: a meta-analysis of randomized trials. *Ann Emerg Med*. 1994;23:535-540.
6. Medeiros I, Saconato H. Antibiotic prophylaxis for mammalian bites. *Cochrane Database Syst Rev*. 2001;(2): CD001738.
7. Moran GJ, Talan DA, Mower W, et al. Appropriateness of rabies postexposure prophylaxis treatment for animal exposures. Emergency ID Net Study Group. *JAMA*. 2000; 284:1001-1007.
8. American Academy of Pediatrics. Rabies. In: Pickering LK, Baker CJ, Long SS, et al, eds. *Red Book 2006 Report of the Committee on Infectious Diseases*. 27th ed. Elk Grove Village, IL: American Academy of Pediatrics; 2006.
9. Willoughby RE, Hammarin AL. Prophylaxis against rabies in children exposed to bats. *Pediatr Infect Dis J*. 2005;24:1109-1110.
10. Willoughby RE, Tieves KS, Hoffman GM, et al. Survival after treatment of rabies with induction of coma. *N Engl J Med*. 2005;352:2508-2514.

Chapter 236

ANURIA AND OLIGURIA

Amrish Jain, MD; Tej K. Mattoo, MD, DCh, FRCP(UK)

A decrease in urine output is the most visible sign of acute renal failure (ARF) in all age groups, particularly younger children. *Oliguria* occurs when the urine output in an infant is less than 0.5 mL/kg per hour for 24 hours or is less than 500 mL/1.73 m^2 per day in older children. *Anuria* is defined as absence of any urine output. An important point to remember is that healthy newborns may have no urine output for 24 hours after birth.

Oliguria is much more common than anuria, and, if not treated appropriately, the patients may become anuric, which may result in serious renal damage that requires specialized care. Oliguria or anuria may be the outcome of a renal response to intravascular circulatory volume depletion or a sudden drop in the blood pressure, also called *prerenal ARF.* Oliguria or anuria may also occur as the result of intrinsic renal damage, or *renal ARF.* Rarely, obstruction to the flow of urine, or *postrenal ARF,* may result in oliguria or anuria.

INCIDENCE

The incidence of oliguria or anuria in previously healthy children is not known, particularly oliguria because many such patients have subclinical symptoms or respond promptly to appropriate management; thus they are not reported in the literature.

In hospitalized patients, oliguric ARF occurs in approximately 10% of newborns in the intensive care units, 2% to 3% of older children requiring intensive care, and 8% of patients undergoing cardiac surgery.[1,2] In newborns, the incidence of prerenal, renal, and postrenal ARF is 85%, 11%, and 3%, respectively.[3] In older children, the corresponding data extrapolated from recent studies are 66%, 33%, and less than 1%, respectively.[4-6]

ETIOLOGY

The common causes for oliguria, anuria, or ARF in children are best defined in relation to the age of the patient.

Prerenal ARF caused by dehydration is the most common cause of oliguria and anuria in younger children,

Table 236-1 Most Common Causes of Oliguria and Anuria

	PRERENAL	RENAL	POSTRENAL
Neonate	Perinatal asphyxia Respiratory distress syndrome Hemorrhage Sepsis or shock Congenital heart disease Dehydration Drugs (indomethacin, maternal use of ACE inhibitors or NSAIDs)	ATN Exogenous toxins (aminoglycosides, amphotericin B) Endogenous toxins (hemoglobin, myoglobin, uric acid) Congenital kidney diseases Vascular (renal vein thrombosis, renal artery thrombosis)	Posterior urethral valves Meatal stenosis Bilateral ureteral obstruction Neurogenic bladder
Children	Dehydration Hemorrhage Burns Third-space loss (surgery, trauma, nephrotic syndrome) Renal loss (diabetes mellitus, diabetes insipidus, diuretics) Shock Decreased cardiac output	ATN Glomerulonephritis Exogenous toxins (aminoglycosides, amphotericin B) Endogenous toxins (hemoglobin, myoglobin, uric acid) Vascular (hemolytic uremic syndrome, vasculitis)	Posterior urethral valves Meatal stenosis Bilateral ureteral obstruction Neurogenic bladder

ATN, Acute tubular necrosis; *ACE*, angiotensin-converting enzyme; *NSAIDs*, nonsteroidal antiinflammatory drugs.

accounting for 70% of community-acquired cases of ARF[7] and up to 60% of hospital-acquired cases.[8]

Renal ARF caused by intrinsic renal damage may be further categorized into 3 kinds. (1) *Acute tubular necrosis* (ATN) occurs as a result of prolonged ischemia, or drug- or toxin-mediated renal tubular injury. Oliguria reverses in most cases once repair and regeneration of tubular epithelial cell occurs. (2) *Glomerular lesions* may occur with postinfectious glomerulonephritis. (3) *Vascular lesions* may be seen in hemolytic uremic syndrome or Henoch-Schönlein purpura. Although ATN is common in children of all ages, the glomerular and vascular causes of renal ARF are more common in older children.

Postrenal ARF results from a mechanical or functional obstruction to the flow of urine. The obstruction can be in the lower urinary tract, such as posterior urethral valves, or bilaterally in the upper tract, such as bilateral ureteropelvic junction obstruction, which is rare. Unilateral obstruction can cause ARF in patients with only a single functioning kidney. Postrenal ARF is more common in newborn babies than it is in older infants.

The most common causes of oliguria and anuria in neonates and children are listed in Table 236-1.

COMORBID CONDITIONS

Although oliguria and anuria are not uncommon in previously healthy children, approximately two thirds of such patients have an underlying comorbid condition.[4] These conditions include the following: (1) neurologic conditions, when the patient has a compromised thirst mechanism or is seriously disabled and thus totally dependent on others for nutrition and hydration, as may be the case in patients with severe cerebral palsy; (2) renal diseases that impair the ability to maximally concentrate the urine, as may occur with salt-losing nephropathy or chronic renal failure; (3) gastrointestinal conditions that cause hypoalbuminemia and decreased intravascular volume as a result of a low oncotic pressure, as in celiac disease or hepatic failure; (4) endocrine disease such as diabetes insipidus and diabetes mellitus, which are associated with increased hypotonic urine output and osmolar diuresis, respectively; (5) hematologic conditions such as sickle cell disease or trait, which impair urine concentration mechanism, or oncologic emergencies such as tumor lysis syndrome, which causes renal failure, particularly if the patient is not well hydrated; and (6) therapy that may predispose the patient to renal failure (eg, nonsteroidal antiinflammatory drugs, angiotensin-converting enzyme inhibitors, aminoglycosides, contrast media), because these substances impair renal autoregulation in the presence of mild renal insufficiency or dehydration and may result in oliguria or anuria.

EVALUATION

History

A thorough history and physical examination are important in identifying the cause of oliguria or anuria, which is of particular clinical significance in prerenal and postrenal ARF cases because early diagnosis and prompt treatment often result in quick recovery. A history of vomiting, diarrhea, hemorrhage, sepsis, and decreased oral intake associated with oliguria suggests a prerenal cause. Besides symptoms related to the disease process, such children may exhibit increased thirst, palpitations, fatigue, and clinical signs of dehydration, including weight loss. A history of poor urinary stream, dribbling, or enuresis in older children may be the result of urinary tract obstruction. A history of abnormal renal findings during routine antenatal ultrasonography can help diagnose such patients.

A history of gross hematuria or edema strongly suggests intrinsic renal disease. A history of pharyngitis or impetigo a few weeks before the onset of gross hematuria can be the result of postinfectious glomerulonephritis, and bloody diarrhea often precedes hemolytic uremic syndrome. Patients with systemic vasculitis (eg, systemic lupus erythematosus) may have a history of fever, joint pains, and skin rash along with oliguria. A history of recurrent sinusitis or lower respiratory tract infections may suggest Wegener granulomatosis, and hemoptysis may indicate the presence of pulmonary-renal syndrome, as may occur with Goodpasture syndrome or microscopic polyangiitis. A detailed history of recent or ongoing chronic medications is important to exclude the possibility of interstitial nephritis. In neonates, a history of umbilical artery catheterization favors a diagnosis of renal artery thrombosis. Family history is helpful in diagnosing conditions such as diabetes insipidus and polycystic kidney disease.

Physical Examination

A comprehensive physical examination is the key to assessing the severity of the disease process and the possible cause of oliguria or anuria. The presence of tachycardia, dry mucous membranes, sunken eyes, orthostatic blood pressure changes, decreased skin turgor, or hypotension indicates hypovolemia, resulting in prerenal oliguria or anuria. A palpable bladder with a weak urine stream or dribbling suggests obstruction. A sacral tuft of hair or myelomeningocele may be associated with neurogenic bladder, which can cause obstructive uropathy with postrenal oliguria or anuria.

Children with intrinsic renal damage are likely to have a circulatory volume overload, and such children may exhibit hypertension, edema, or both. Younger children, particularly infants, may have signs of congestive heart failure, such as hepatomegaly, gallop rhythm, and pulmonary edema. Clinicians need to look closely for specific signs that point to underlying renal disease. These signs may include severe anemia in patients with hemolytic uremic syndrome, a butterfly rash on face and musculoskeletal involvement in patients with systemic lupus erythematosus, and typical purpuric rash over the buttocks and extensor surface of the lower extremity in Henoch-Schönlein purpura. Abdominal examination may reveal palpable kidney, which may be caused by renal-vein thrombosis, polycystic kidney disease, multicystic dysplastic kidney, or hydronephrosis.

Laboratory Studies

Preexisting risk factors, historical details, and the results of the physical examination will help the clinician choose appropriate laboratory tests. Urinalysis is the most important noninvasive diagnostic test. A thorough examination of a freshly voided or bladder-catheterized urine sample helps distinguish prerenal from renal causes of oliguria or anuria. A normal or near-normal urinalysis, characterized by few cells with little or no casts or proteinuria, is seen in prerenal disease, urinary tract obstruction, and some cases of ATN. A urine sample showing muddy-brown granular casts and epithelial cell casts strongly suggests ATN. The finding of red cell casts is diagnostic of glomerulonephritis, and presence of proteinuria indicates glomerular disease.

Urinary indices including urine sodium, specific gravity, creatinine, and osmolality are important diagnostic tools for oliguria. The urine sodium concentration is usually above 40 mEq/L in ATN and is below 10 mEq/L in oliguria resulting from intravascular volume depletion. Neonates have decreased ability to conserve sodium, and, as a result, prerenal disease is associated with urine sodium concentration less than 20 to 30 mEq/L. In prerenal oliguria, urine specific gravity is more than 1020, the ratio of urine to plasma creatinine is more than 40, and the ratio of urinary to plasma osmolality is more than 1.5. In renal causes of oliguria, the ratio of urine to plasma osmolality is less than 1.5, and the ratio of urine to plasma creatinine is less than 20. The effect of variations in urine volume in interpreting these urinary indices is eliminated by calculating fractional excretion of sodium (FENa). A fractional excretion of sodium of less than 1% suggests reabsorption of almost all filtered sodium in response to decreased renal perfusion (prerenal), whereas, in ATN, the excretion is more than 2%.[9,10]

The severity of renal damage or hypoperfusion is also indicated by increased blood urea nitrogen (BUN) and serum creatinine concentrations. In prerenal oliguria, increased BUN is marked, and the ratio of BUN to serum creatinine is more than 20, whereas a ratio of 10 to 15 suggests intrinsic renal damage.[9,10]

Imaging Studies

Renal ultrasonography is an important diagnostic tool in patients with oliguria or anuria and is generally not indicated in children with prerenal failure from dehydration who respond promptly to fluid resuscitation. Ultrasonography provides important information regarding kidney size and echogenicity, renal blood flow, collecting system, and urinary bladder. Children with intrinsic causes for oliguria or anuria may have echogenic and slightly enlarged kidneys. An ultrasound examination showing bilateral hydronephrosis or hydroureteronephrosis and bladder wall thickening is consistent with obstruction of bladder outlet causing postrenal oliguria or anuria. Ultrasonography can also detect congenital renal disorders such as polycystic kidney disease and multicystic dysplastic kidney. Doppler examination of the renal blood flow is helpful in diagnosing renal vascular thrombosis.

MANAGEMENT

The algorithm for managing patients with oliguria or anuria is shown in Figure 236-1.

The key to preventing oliguria or anuria is adequate hydration in at-risk patients. This group may include patients who have just undergone surgery; patients receiving nephrotoxic medications such as amphotericin B, acyclovir, or radiocontrast agent; and patients at risk of developing tumor lysis syndrome or pigment nephropathy caused by hemoglobinuria or myoglobinuria.

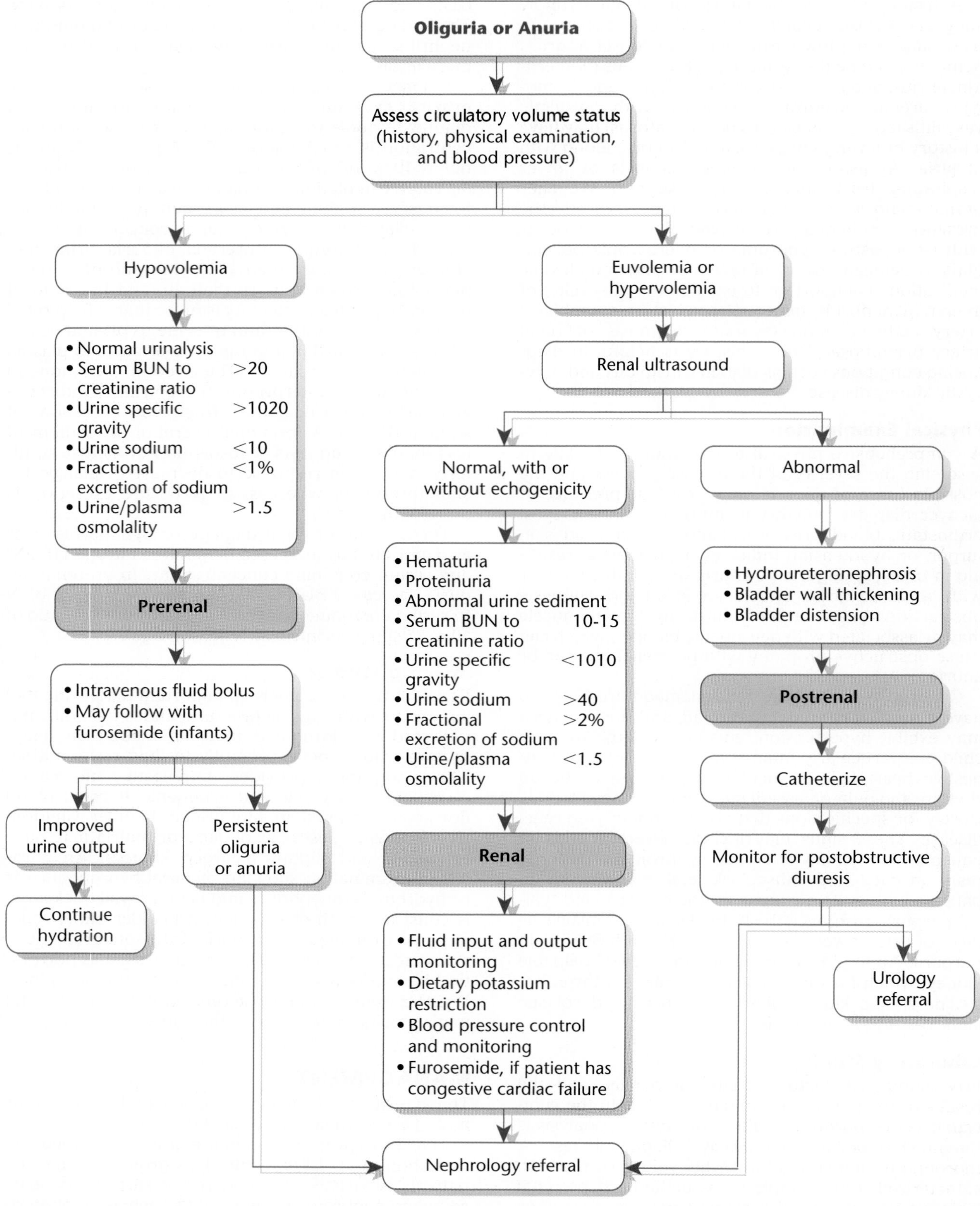

Figure 236-1 Algorithm for management of patients with oliguria or anuria. *BUN,* Blood urea nitrogen.

The major goal of treatment of prerenal oliguria or anuria is to restore intravascular volume. An estimate of volume status is needed to begin and continue fluid therapy. This amount is assessed by history and by a physical examination that includes assessment of body weight, skin turgor, capillary refill, peripheral edema, and blood pressure. A dehydrated child with oliguria or anuria should receive a fluid bolus of normal saline or Ringer's lactate at 20 mL/kg to restore fluid volume. Depending on the patient's response, another bolus may be needed.

Children with oliguria and volume overload may benefit from furosemide therapy and may require fluid restriction, as well as blood pressure and acid-base monitoring. Children with oliguria that results from obstruction may require urinary catheterization. Relief of obstruction may be followed by postobstructive diuresis and resultant hyponatremia and hypokalemia requiring fluid and electrolyte replacement.

WHEN TO REFER OR ADMIT

Children should be referred to a nephrologist or admitted to the hospital (or both) if they have any of the following:

- Persistent oliguria or anuria despite an adequate fluid challenge in a dehydrated child
- Persistent oliguria or anuria that continues after removal of the offending nephrotoxins
- Oliguria or anuria associated with swelling, hypertension, gross hematuria, abnormal blood chemistry, and severe systemic signs or symptoms
- Urology referral for oliguria or anuria caused by obstructive uropathy

REFERENCES

1. Andreoli SP. Acute renal failure. *Curr Opin Pediatr.* 2002; 14:183-188.
2. Moghal NE, Brocklebank JT, Meadow SR. A review of acute renal failure in children: incidence, etiology and outcome. *Clin Nephrol.* 1998;49:91-95.
3. Hentschel R, Lodige B, Bulla M. Renal insufficiency in the neonatal period. *Clin Nephrol.* 1996;46:54-58.
4. Hui-Stickle S, Brewer ED, Goldstein SL. Pediatric ARF epidemiology at a tertiary care center from 1999 to 2001. *Am J Kidney Dis.* 2005;45:96-101.
5. Askenazi DJ, Feig DI, Graham NM, et al. 3-5 year longitudinal follow-up of pediatric patients after acute renal failure. *Kidney Int.* 2006;69:184-189.
6. Flynn JT. Choice of dialysis modality for management of pediatric acute renal failure. *Pediatr Nephrol.* 2002;17: 61-69.
7. Kaufman J, Dhakal M, Patel B, et al. Community acquired acute renal failure. *Am J Kidney Dis.* 1991;17:191-198.
8. Nolan CR, Anderson RJ. Hospital acquired acute renal failure. *J Am Soc Nephrol.* 1998;9:710-718.
9. Albright RC Jr. Acute renal failure: a practical update. *Mayo Clin Proc.* 2001;76:67-74.
10. Andreoli SP. Clinical evaluation and management of acute renal failure. In: Avner ED, Harmon WE, Niaudet P, eds. *Pediatric Nephrology.* 5th ed. Philadelphia, PA: Lippincott Williams and Wilkins; 2004.

Chapter 237

APPARENT LIFE-THREATENING EVENTS

Keyvan Rafei, MD; Carol J. Blaisdell, MD

Apparent life-threatening events (ALTEs) are common and frequently challenging diagnostic dilemmas. Although most evaluations of these patients usually take place in a hospital, primary care physicians will be frequently asked to contribute to various stages of the management of these cases, from initial evaluation of the patient to decisions about long-term monitoring.[1]

The appropriate management of children with an ALTE requires an understanding of commonly accepted definitions, the various potential causes, and the most appropriate management strategies of these conditions. Definitions of an ALTE and other related breathing patterns were clarified in a 1986 National Institutes of Health Consensus document.[2] An ALTE has been defined as "an episode that is frightening to the observer and that is characterized by some combination of apnea, color change, marked change in muscle tone, choking, or gagging" in which, "in some cases, the observer fears that the infant has died."[2] This definition replaced aborted crib death or near-miss sudden infant death syndrome (SIDS), which misleadingly implied an association between ALTE and SIDS.[2] Other important definitions of concepts related to ALTE are listed in Table 237-1. Most notably, pathological apnea is defined as "a respiratory pause that is prolonged, lasting 20 seconds or longer, or is associated with cyanosis, pallor, hypotonia or bradycardia."[2] In contrast, periodic breathing, which is commonly noted in young infants, is "a breathing pattern in which there are 3 or more respiratory pauses of greater than 3 seconds' duration with less than 20 seconds of respiration between pauses."[2]

PREVALENCE

The exact frequency and prevalence of ALTEs are not known,[3] although rates have been estimated as 0.21% of all children and 0.6% of all patients younger than 1 year seeking care at an emergency department or as 9.4 per 1000 live births.[4-6] Recurrence rates for ALTEs vary from 0% to 24%.[7]

The median age of presentation of infants with an ALTE ranges between 7 and 8 weeks of age; sex distribution is relatively equal.[4,5,8] Approximately one third of patients with an ALTE had a history of prematurity, and 19% had a history of a previous ALTE. The morbidity and mortality resulting from an ALTE vary by the underlying diagnosis; the mortality of infants with apnea of infancy ranges between 0% and 6%.[2,7]

APPARENT LIFE-THREATENING EVENT AND SUDDEN INFANT DEATH SYNDROME

Despite popular misconception, strong evidence suggests that apnea is not predictive of or a precursor to SIDS, and ALTEs are not near-miss SIDS cases.[1,3,9] This assertion is evidenced by the fact that infants with

Table 237-1 Definitions of Breathing Patterns and Concepts Related to Apparent Life-threatening Events (ALTEs)

CONCEPT	DEFINITION
Periodic breathing	A breathing pattern in which 3 or more respiratory pauses of >3 seconds' duration with <20 seconds' respiration between pauses occur
Apnea	Cessation of respiratory airflow; apnea may be central, obstructive, or mixed
Pathological apnea	Respiratory pause that is prolonged (20 seconds) or associated with cyanosis, pallor, hypotonia, or bradycardia
Apnea of infancy	Unexplained episode of pathological apnea with onset at >37 weeks' postgestational age in infants for whom no specific cause of ALTE can be identified
Apnea of prematurity	Periodic breathing with pathological apnea in a premature infant
Sudden infant death syndrome	Sudden death of any infant or young child that is unexplained by history and by postmortem examination

From National Institutes of Health. Infantile apnea and home monitoring. *Natl Inst Health Consens Dev Conf Consens Statement.* 1986;6:1-10.

an ALTE are generally 1 to 3 months younger than infants who die of SIDS, and infants with an ALTE are more likely to be found during the daytime or while sleeping supine at the time of the event.[3] Furthermore, apnea appears to resolve when the infant is at an age before most SIDS deaths occur,[9] and less than 7% of patients with SIDS have a history of an ALTE.[2] Research has shown that although the SIDS mortality rate markedly decreased between 1986 and 1994 the mean annual admission rate for ALTEs did not change significantly.[6]

DIFFERENTIAL DIAGNOSIS

Because an ALTE describes a clinical syndrome rather than a specific diagnosis, a variety of different disorders can lead to an episode.[1,2] The most common types of problems associated with an ALTE are gastrointestinal, neurologic, respiratory, cardiovascular, metabolic, and endocrine in nature.[3] Most common specific diagnoses associated with ALTEs include gastroesophageal reflux (31%), seizures (11%), and lower respiratory tract infections (8%), although a great many different diagnoses have been recorded.[7] Up to 50% of cases of ALTE remain unexplained and are considered idiopathic.[2,3]

Although gastroesophageal reflux is the diagnosis most often associated with an ALTE, its precise role in these cases is debated. A relationship between apnea and gastroesophageal reflux disease (GERD) has been posited, but a relationship has not been found.[10,11] Although GERD can lead to an ALTE in certain infants, the frequency of GERD in the general population should caution the clinician in assuming a causal relationship when it is discovered in an infant with a history of an ALTE.[12]

Neurologic and respiratory disorders are the 2nd and 3rd most commonly associated diagnoses in patients with an ALTE. The most common specific diagnoses are seizures in the former category, and pertussis and respiratory syncytial virus infection in the latter group.[4,7] Other important but less common diagnoses in infants with an ALTE include urinary tract infections, inborn errors of metabolism, cardiac arrhythmias, brain tumor, persistent ductus arteriosus, and opioid-related apnea.[4,7]

Child abuse and factitious illness are also important to consider in the differential diagnosis of children with unexplained ALTEs. Although clinicians must be vigilant to avoid stigmatizing or adding to the distress of families, child abuse should be considered in children with a history of recurrent cyanosis, apnea, or an ALTE witnessed only by a single caretaker or in a family with previous unexplained infant deaths.[7,13,14]

EVALUATION

Because of the vast array of disorders that can lead to an ALTE and the wide spectrum of severity of its manifestations, no single accepted standard exists for evaluating these infants. A stepwise approach beginning with a detailed history and physical examination is most prudent.[4,5,7,8] Thorough clinical assessment is more likely than an array of diagnostic studies to lead to a diagnosis of the underlying problem.[8] The selection of any diagnostic studies and the extent and duration of observation should be based on the findings of the clinical assessment.

History

Seeking a detailed history and description of the infant at the time of the ALTE is particularly important because most infants appear normal by the time of the evaluation.[4,5,8] Important historical questions to address are listed in Box 237-1. A complete history should include a review of the patient's medical and family history, a description of the patient's living conditions, and descriptions of events immediately before and during the ALTE.[3]

Physical Examination

Even though most infants with an ALTE are found to be normal at the time of the initial evaluation, a detailed physical examination is essential to uncover any clues to the underlying cause. The clinician should pay particular attention to neurologic, respiratory, and cardiac abnormalities that may account for the infant's symptoms, noting any evidence for physiological compromise (eg, mental status changes, cyanosis, apnea).[3-5,8]

BOX 237-1 Essential Elements in the History of Apparent Life-threatening Events (ALTEs)

PERSONAL AND FAMILY HISTORY

- Perinatal history
  - Full-term or premature birth
  - Pregnancy or perinatal complications
- Medical and surgical history
  - Previous evaluations and treatments
  - Prior hospitalizations
  - Medications
- Sleep and feeding habits
  - Breastfeeding versus bottle feeding
  - Usual amount and frequency of feedings
  - Usual behavior and temperament
- Family history
  - Siblings with ALTE, sudden infant death syndrome, or early death
  - Family history of genetic, metabolic, cardiac, or neurologic problems
- Parental or caretaker history
  - Smoking or drinking habits
  - Recent medical problems and treatments

DAILY LIFE CONDITIONS

- Usual sleep conditions
  - Sleep position when placed down for sleep and when found
  - Sleeping attire
  - Bedding materials
- Other conditions
  - Clothing
  - Room temperature
  - Use of pacifiers

EVENTS IMMEDIATELY PRECEDING THE ALTE

- Recent fever or illness
- Medications of the infant and others in the home
- Immunizations
- Sleep deprivation
- Change in daily life routine

DESCRIPTION OF THE ALTE

- Place and time
  - Exact place in which the ALTE occurred (eg, child's bed, parent's bed, parent's arms, bathroom, sofa, car)
  - Time of event
  - Time since last feeding
  - The estimated time to recover from the ALTE
  - Estimated duration of event
- Witnesses and interventions
  - Who discovered or witnessed the ALTE
  - Reason that led to the discovery of the ALTE (noise, unusual cry)
  - Any interventions performed (gentle stimulation, shaking, cardiopulmonary resuscitation)
  - Child's response to the intervention
- Description of infant during ALTE
  - State of infant when event began—asleep or awake
  - If asleep:
    - Child's body position
    - Type of bedding
    - Face covered or free
    - If awake: Was child being fed, handled, crying, being bathed?
  - Child's appearance when found:
    - Consciousness
    - Muscle tone
    - Color
    - Respiratory effort
    - Choking
    - Gasping
    - Emesis
    - Sweating
    - Limb or eye movements
    - Pupil size
    - Skin or rectal temperature

Adapted from Kahn A, European Society for the Study and Prevention of Infant Death. Recommended clinical evaluation of infants with an apparent life-threatening event. Consensus document of the European Society for the Study and Prevention of Infant Death, 2003. *Eur J Pediatr.* 2004;163(2):108-115.

Laboratory Evaluation

No minimal standard set of diagnostic studies that are required to evaluate infants with an ALTE have been developed.[3,8] Although a detailed history of the event and the physical examination of the infant frequently result in finding a suspected cause for the ALTE, laboratory testing may be a useful adjunct to confirm the diagnosis.[8] In infants younger than 12 months the basis of the diagnosis can be found in 21% of patients by only history and physical examination.[8] With no additional information gained from laboratory testing the yield of diagnostic testing can be low (only 2.5%).[5] Therefore using the findings of the history and physical examination is important to direct appropriate diagnostic testing.[8]

A greater challenge is presented by infants without suggestive findings at the initial history and physical examination. When selecting diagnostic studies for this group, an important point to remember is that the yield of most studies is low, and even if a positive result is found, the question of a causal relationship still remains.[7,8]

To evaluate infants with an ALTE the focus must first be on identifying emergent and life-threatening causes then extending the evaluation to additional studies if no answers are found. The initial basic set of tests that might be considered in infants with no identified cause after initial clinical assessment includes a complete blood count, urinalysis, electrocardiogram, chest radiograph, blood culture, and urine culture.

Additional studies that might be considered after an initial period of observation include a pneumogram, a gastroesophageal reflux study, neuroimaging, metabolic studies, and tests for respiratory pathogens as indicated.[3,4,7,8] These studies may not be available in all hospitals, and a pediatric specialist may need to be consulted to interpret the results of the tests.

More than one half the time, when evaluating the ALTE, the result leads to the diagnosis of GERD.[8] Although the upper gastrointestinal series is not sensitive for diagnosing GERD, it may useful for identifying intestinal obstruction that contributes to GERD (eg, volvulus, gastric outlet obstruction). If GERD is the suspected cause for an ALTE, then a 24-hour pH probe or milk scan by technicum-99m is preferable; up to 89% of infants with an ALTE may have a positive milk scan, although only 41% of these infants have a correlating clinical diagnosis.[4] This circumstance highlights the problem of exhaustively testing all infants if the clinical history or physical examination are not suggestive of a diagnosis. If enough tests are performed, then the increasing likelihood of false-positive results will diminish the diagnostic use of these studies.

When the history and physical examination do not suggest a probable diagnosis for an ALTE the following studies may provide a cause for the event: white blood cell count, upper gastrointestinal series or pH probe, urinalysis and culture, brain neuroimaging, chest radiograph, and polysomnography (PSG). In up to 14% of infants the history and physical examination will not suggest an ALTE.[15] Child abuse is a potential cause for infants with ALTE; thus, if the history and physical examination do not indicate a likely cause, then a dilated funduscopic examination with brain neuroimaging, toxicology screen, and skeletal survey are indicated. Without suggestive findings in the history or physical examination the results of tests of chemistries, cerebrospinal fluid, nasopharyngeal aspirates, echocardiogram, and electrocardiogram will likely be unrevealing.[15]

MANAGEMENT

The decision to hospitalize patients with an ALTE must be guided by the findings of the initial assessment. Hospital admission may not be required if the ALTE appears to be benign and the child is normal when evaluated immediately after the event.[3] However, if the episode was significant and required intense stimulation, or when the initial physical examination reveals something abnormal, then hospitalization with continuous cardiorespiratory (CR) monitoring and further evaluation is required.[3,7] This approach is intended to ensure that additional evaluation and management are readily available for a potentially vulnerable infant. Further episodes of ALTEs may be observed by medical personnel, which will help make the diagnosis and will direct further testing (eg, an electroencephalogram in a child with witnessed seizure). Continuous CR monitoring with pulse oximetry is suggested to detect apnea, bradycardia, and hypoxemia. If the witnessed event or a review of the history suggests severe CR compromise, then the infant should be admitted to an intensive care unit. Treatment directed at the underlying diagnosis determined by the evaluation should be started—for example, antibiotics for suspected

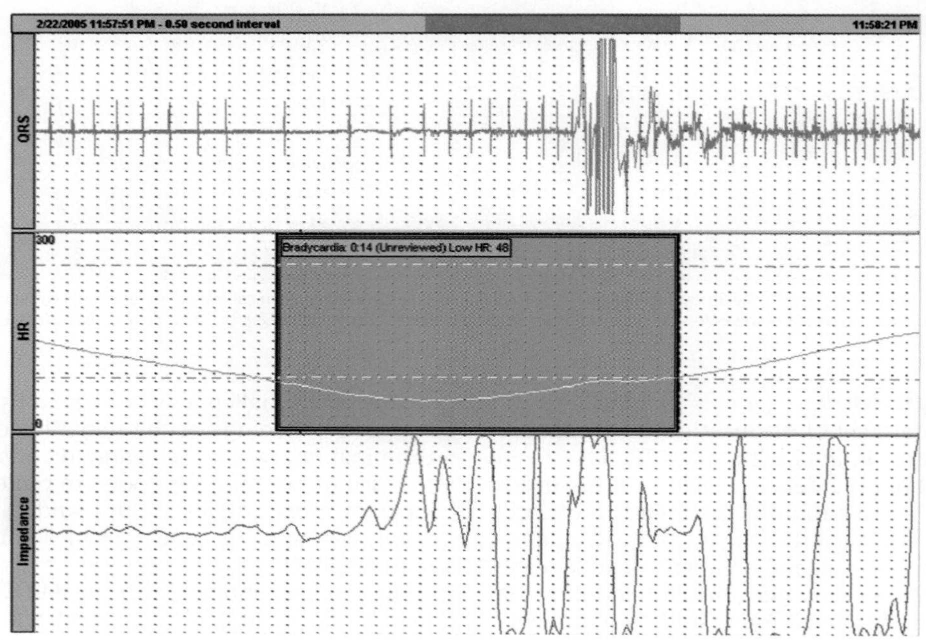

Figure 237-1 Cardiorespiratory monitor tracing from a 5-month-old premature infant with cyanosis and hypotonia born at 24 weeks' gestation. Note QRS tracing, which demonstrates slowing of the RR interval, and bradycardia of 48 beats/min on the heart rate tracing, which follows shallow breathing on the impedance tracing. This tracing suggests hypoxemia as the cause of the bradycardia, but the finding is not specific; thus a polysomnogram was requested.

bacterial infection, anticonvulsants for an infant with seizures, and medications for GERD.

As one example of the benefit of inpatient monitoring, a CR tracing of a 5-month-old infant with intermittent episodes of cyanosis and hypotonia is shown in Figure 237-1. The monitor demonstrates bradycardia, with heart rates dropping to 42 beats/min. The decreased heart rate follows an episode of decreased but continued respiratory effort. The cause of the bradycardia is not initially clear. PSG may be especially useful for infants such as this one, who are suspected of having hypoxemia or hypercarbia associated with an atypical ALTE, prolonged clinical course, or recurrent or severe episodes, and whose CR monitoring in the inpatient unit fails to provide a clear diagnosis. The infant whose CR monitor tracing is depicted in Figure 237-1 underwent PSG (Figure 237-2), which provided more information about the cause for the child's bradycardia: demonstrating mixed apneas (central and obstructive apnea) leading to hypoxemia (pulse oximeter drops to 54%) and bradycardia (rate is 42 beats/min, and the electrocardiogram shows slowing of the RR interval). Initially, no respiratory effort is noted in the thoracic and abdominal channels (central apnea), with respiratory effort following with no flow in the nasal and carbon dioxide channels (obstructive apnea). At the end of this 60-second period an adult intervenes. For this infant, hypoxemia was treated with supplemental oxygen so that oxygenation was not compromised after brief episodes of mixed and obstructive apneas.

Besides central apneas (no respiratory effort lasting 20 seconds, or shorter if associated with hypoxemia or bradycardia), obstructive apneas (respiratory effort in thoracic or abdominal impedance tracings, or both, with no airflow in nasal and end-tidal carbon dioxide tracings), mixed apneas (central and obstructive events at the same time), and episodes of periodic breathing may also be detected on PSG that might not

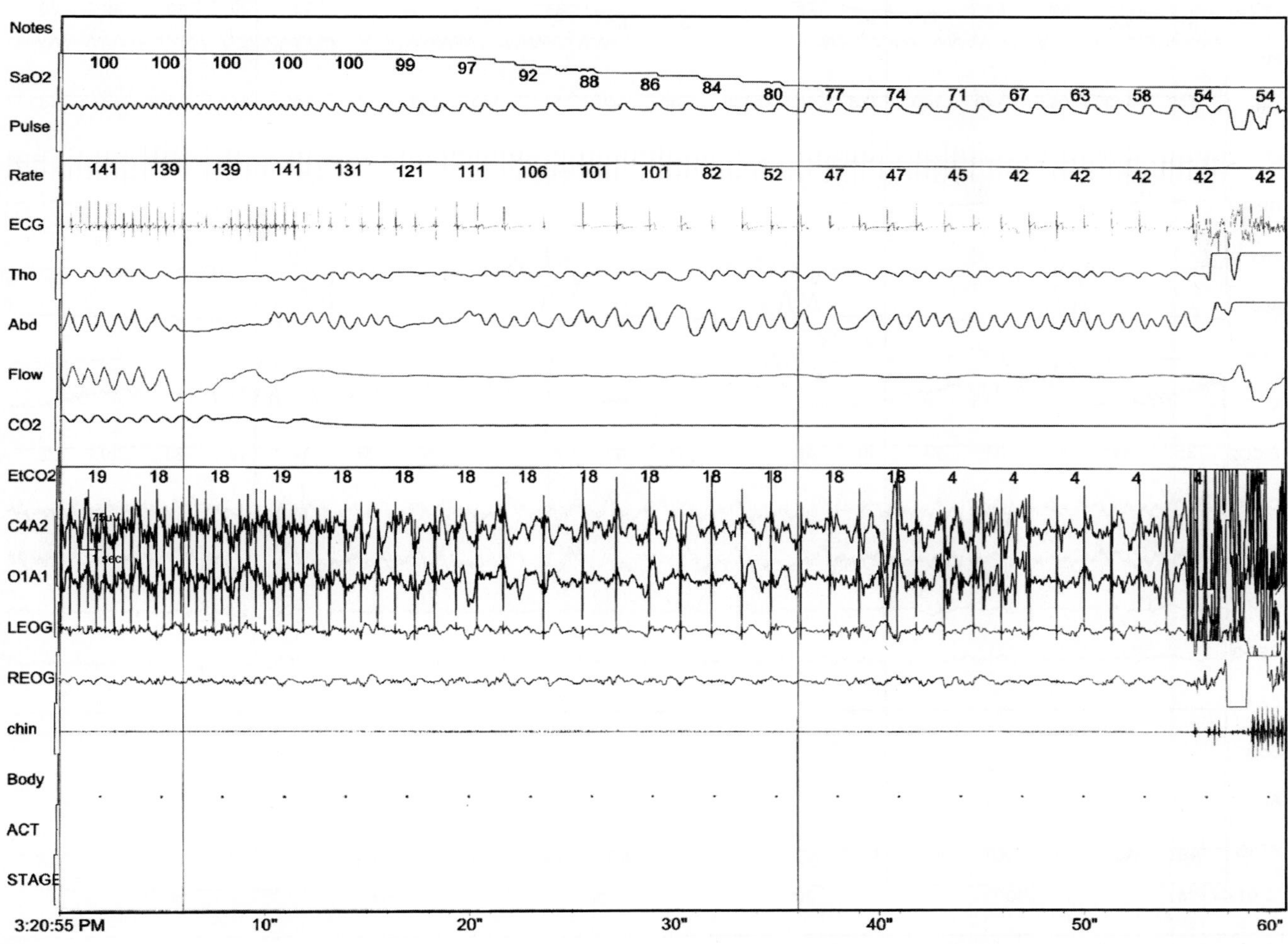

Figure 237-2 Polysomnographic tracing of the same infant as in Figure 237-1 demonstrating a mixed apnea (central for the first 5 seconds, then obstructive apnea) leading to hypoxemia (pulse oximeter drops to 54%) and bradycardia (rate is 42 beats/min, and electrocardiogram shows slowing of the RR interval). Initially, no respiratory effort in the thoracic and abdominal channels (central apnea) is noted, with respiratory effort following with no flow in the nasal and carbon dioxide channels (obstructive apnea). At the end of this 60-second period, an adult intervenes; note motion artifact particularly the electroencephalographic channels C4A2 and O1A1 and chin electromyographic channels.

be evident on hospital monitors. Periodic breathing is defined as "a breathing pattern in which there are 3 or more respiratory pauses of greater than 3 seconds' duration with less than 20 seconds of respiration between pauses"[2] (see Table 237-1). Periodic breathing that is associated with hypoxemia (Figure 237-3) is considered pathological, and stimulants such as caffeine may correct the abnormality.

At institutions where PSG is not available, home equipment companies may arrange for the data acquisition of respiratory and cardiac events by using a pneumogram, which an outside consultant reviews. Pneumograms are unattended studies that collect data on respiratory effort by using a thoracic impedance monitor, nasal flow, oxygenation, and cardiac rhythm but not sleep staging, carbon dioxide signal, or abdominal effort. More technical artifacts exist from pneumograms because no technician adjusts the leads and maintains adequate signal quality. Because the PSG is more informative, pneumograms should be limited to medical centers where PSG is unavailable.

Parents and other caregivers of the infant admitted with an ALTE should be counseled on cardiopulmonary resuscitation for infants in case further ALTEs occur after discharge. Caregivers of infants who have had an ALTE should also be taught safe sleeping tips. The American Academy of Pediatrics has made the following recommendations: Infants should be placed on their backs to sleep, redundant soft bedding and soft objects in the infant's sleeping environment should be avoided, adults and infants sleeping in the same bed is discouraged, excessive clothing and extreme

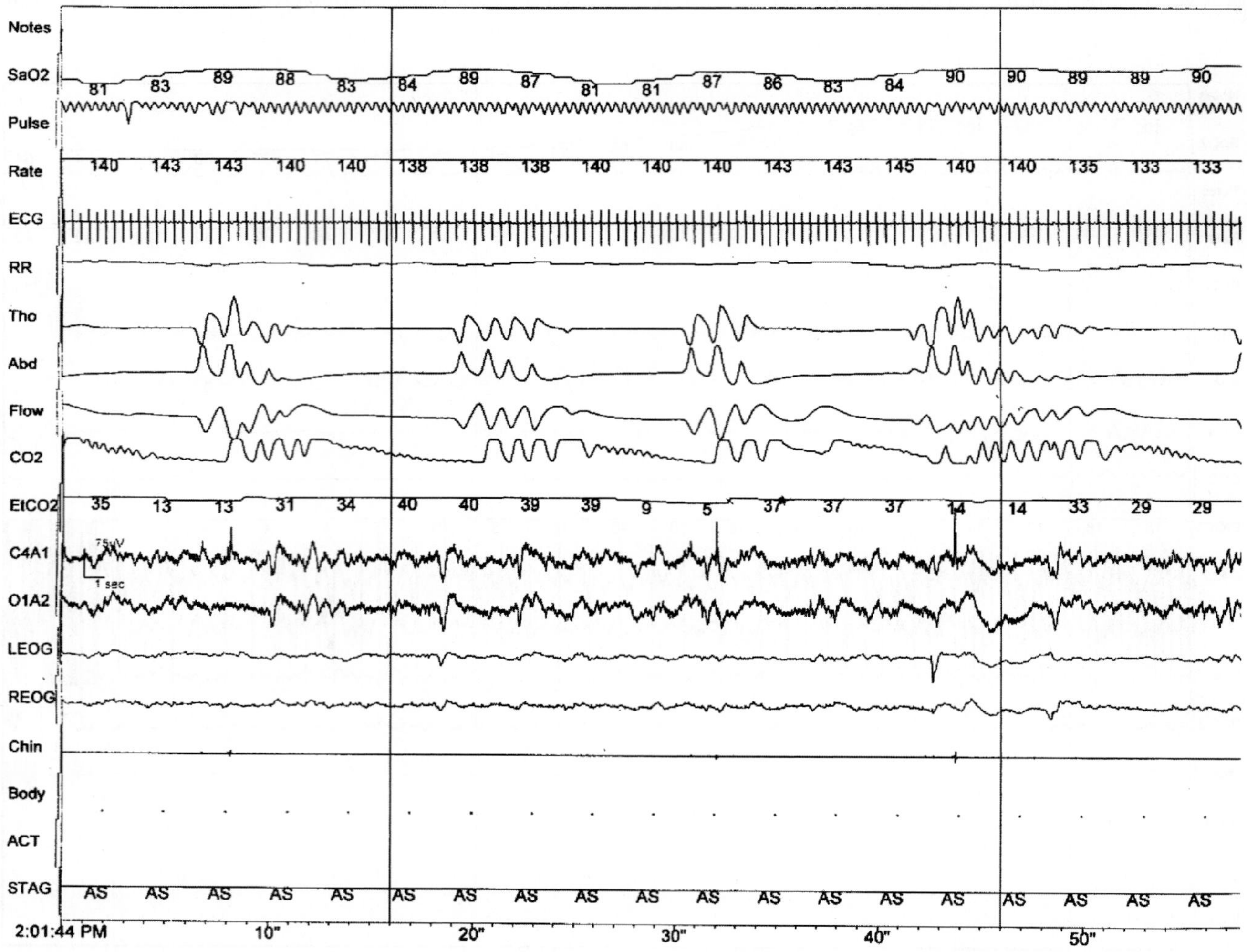

Figure 237-3 Polysomnographic tracing of a 3-month-old infant with hypoxemia noted on monitoring in hospital for an ALTE. The infant has periodic breathing, with respiratory pauses of much less than 20 seconds (see thoracic and abdominal leads with no flow when respiration stops). Cardiorespiratory monitors routinely sound an alarm only when breathing has ceased for 20 seconds or more, and they would not detect periodic breathing unless the event led to bradycardia with the heart rate below the alarm's limit. This infant has brief pauses in series that lead to hypoxemia; thus this event denotes pathological periodic breathing. Polysomnography is able to detect a cause for the hypoxemia that the hospital monitor might not. Treatment would be caffeine to stimulate breathing.

room temperatures should be avoided, and passive smoke exposure during fetal and postnatal development should be avoided.[16]

In preparation for discharge home, once the infant has been stabilized, consideration should be made for home cardiorespiratory monitoring, particularly for infants with an ALTE of unknown cause. If apneas were demonstrated, then a period of home observation on a monitor will help determine when the events have resolved and provide reassurance for the family. The American Academy of Pediatrics policy statement on apnea, SIDS, and home monitoring notes that an indication for home monitoring may include infants who have had an ALTE.[9] An important point to remember is that episodes of periodic breathing and obstructive apnea events will not be captured on home CR monitoring unless a secondary effect of these events on heart rate occurs (see Figure 237-1). The CR monitor results should be reviewed by a practitioner or specialist who is trained in their review, and the physician should establish a specific plan for periodic review. In most cases, results should be reviewed monthly if the guardian has no concerns about the baby or sooner if the guardian reports one or more significant events. The Collaborative Home Infant Monitoring Evaluation study group suggested that healthy term and premature infants may have apnea events and that these events become rare by 43 weeks' postmenstrual age.[17] Monitoring may be discontinued once no further physiologically significant events have occurred and home monitoring shows no further objective evidence of pathological events for at least 6 weeks. If obstructive apnea is identified as a cause for an ALTE, then repeat PSG may be necessary to determine when and if intervention is needed.

Long-term outcomes for infants with an unexplained ALTE are unpredictable. Infants with a severe event who require resuscitation and experience a recurrent ALTE or a seizure disorder have a more than 25% risk of death.[18] However, other studies have reported normal cognitive and behavior outcomes up to 10 years after an ALTE.[19]

SUMMARY

An ALTE is a common, nonspecific disorder of the young infant that is usually self-limited, although it is potentially serious and life threatening. By understanding the definition, and by eliciting a complete history and performing a thorough physical examination, the physician can focus on determining the best laboratory and imaging studies to diagnose the underlying cause of the event. A period of observation with CR monitoring in the hospital is necessary if a benign cause is not evident to gather additional information and direct appropriate diagnostic studies. Education and guidance should be provided to the guardian, with monitoring in the home setting after hospitalization to detect the infrequent recurrence of ALTEs.

WHEN TO REFER

- Suspected seizure disorder
- Suspected hypoxemia or hypercarbia
- Suspected cardiac dysrhythmia
- Vascular ring identified
- Congenital facial anomalies with obstructive apnea
- Evidence of child abuse
- Atypical manifestation

WHEN TO ADMIT

- When history, examination, or diagnostic studies suggest physiologic compromise

AAP POLICY STATEMENTS

American Academy of Pediatrics, Committee on Fetus and Newborn. Apnea, sudden infant death syndrome, and home monitoring. *Pediatrics*. 2003;111(4):914-991. (aap policy.aappublications.org/cgi/content/full/pediatrics;111/4/914).

Hymel KP, American Academy of Pediatrics, Committee on Child Abuse and Neglect, and National Association of Medical Examiners. Distinguishing sudden infant death syndrome from child abuse fatalities. *Pediatrics*. 2006; 118(1):421-427. (aappolicy.aappublications.org/cgi/content/full/pediatrics;118/1/421).

SUGGESTED RESOURCES

American Academy of Pediatrics, Committee on Fetus and Newborn. Apnea, sudden infant death syndrome, and home monitoring. *Pediatrics*. 2003;111(4 pt 1):914-917.

National Institutes of Health. Consensus Development Conference on Infantile Apnea and Home Monitoring, September 29 to October 1, 1986. *Pediatrics*. 1987;79(2): 292-299.

Ramanathan R, Corwin MJ, Hunt CE, et al. Cardiorespiratory events recorded on home monitors: comparison of healthy infants with those at increased risk for SIDS. *JAMA*. 2001;285(17):2199-2207.

REFERENCES

1. American Academy of Pediatrics, Task Force on Prolonged Infantile Apnea. Prolonged infantile apnea: 1985. *Pediatrics*. 1985;76(1):129-131.
2. National Institutes of Health. Infantile apnea and home monitoring. *Natl Inst Health Consens Dev Conf Consens Statement*. 1986;6(6):1-10.
3. Kahn A, European Society for the Study and Prevention of Infant Death. Recommended clinical evaluation of infants with an apparent life-threatening event. Consensus document of the European Society for the Study and Prevention of Infant Death, 2003. *Eur J Pediatr*. 2004; 163(2):108-115.
4. Davies F, Gupta R. Apparent life threatening events in infants presenting to an emergency department. *Emerg Med J*. 2002;19(1):11-16.
5. De Piero AD, Teach SJ, Chamberlain JM. ED evaluation of infants after an apparent life-threatening event. *Am J Emerg Med*. 2004;22(2):83-86.
6. Mitchell EA, Thompson JM. Parental reported apnoea, admissions to hospital and sudden infant death syndrome. *Acta Paediatr*. 2001;90(4):417-422.
7. McGovern MC, Smith MB. Causes of apparent life threatening events in infants: a systematic review. *Arch Dis Child*. 2004;89(11):1043-1048.
8. Brand DA, Altman RL, Purtill K, et al. Yield of diagnostic testing in infants who have had an apparent life-threatening event. *Pediatrics*. 2005;115(4):885-893.

9. American Academy of Pediatrics, Committee on Fetus and Newborn. Apnea, sudden infant death syndrome, and home monitoring. *Pediatrics*. 2003;111(4 pt 1): 914-917.
10. Ariagno RL, Guilleminault C, Baldwin R, et al. Movement and gastroesophageal reflux in awake term infants with "near miss" SIDS, unrelated to apnea. *J Pediatr*. 1982; 100(6):894-897.
11. Mousa H, Woodley FW, Metheney M, et al. Testing the association between gastroesophageal reflux and apnea in infants. *J Pediatr Gastroenterol Nutr*. 2005;41(2): 169-177.
12. Arad-Cohen N, Cohen A, Tirosh E. The relationship between gastroesophageal reflux and apnea in infants. *J Pediatr*. 2000;137(3):321-326.
13. American Academy of Pediatrics, Committee on Child Abuse and Neglect. Distinguishing sudden infant death syndrome from child abuse fatalities. *Pediatrics*. 2001; 107(2):437-441.
14. Altman RL, Brand DA, Forman S, et al. Abusive head injury as a cause of apparent life-threatening events in infancy. *Arch Pediatr Adolesc Med*. 2003;157(10): 1011-1015.
15. Brand DA, Altman RL, Purtill K, et al. Yield of diagnostic testing in infants who have had an apparent life-threatening event. *Pediatrics*. 2005;115(4):885-893. [Erratum in: *Pediatrics*. 2005;116(3):802-803.]
16. American Academy of Pediatrics, Task Force on Sudden Infant Death Syndrome. The changing concept of sudden infant death syndrome: diagnostic coding shifts, controversies regarding the sleeping environment, and new variables to consider in reducing risk. *Pediatrics*. 2005; 116(5):1245-1255.
17. Ramanathan R, Corwin MJ, Hunt CE, et al. Cardiorespiratory events recorded on home monitors: comparison of healthy infants with those at increased risk for SIDS. *JAMA*. 2001;285(17):2199-2207.
18. Oren J, Kelly D, Shannon DC. Identification of a high-risk group for sudden infant death syndrome among infants who were resuscitated for sleep apnea. *Pediatrics*. 1986; 77(4):495-499.
19. Kahn A, Sottiaux M, Appelboom-Fondu J, et al. Long-term development of children monitored as infants for an apparent life-threatening event during sleep: a 10-year follow-up study. *Pediatrics*. 1989;83(5):668-673.

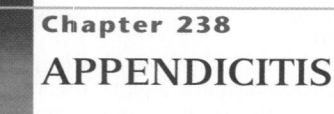

Chapter 238

APPENDICITIS

R. Scott Strahlman, MD

Although appendicitis is a surgical emergency, the pediatric primary care physician is crucial in the initial evaluation, diagnosis, and management and is often the first person to suspect appendicitis. A physician's high index of suspicion can be the driving force that leads to an appropriate, timely appendectomy. Prompt diagnosis and preoperative management help reduce the high morbidity associated with a perforated appendix.

DEFINITIONS

Appendicitis is an inflammation of the vermiform appendix, a small appendage arising from the cecum. Vermiform means *worm-shaped* and accurately describes the appearance of this structure. Appendicitis is the most common cause of an acute surgical abdomen in childhood. Although the exact incidence is unknown, appendicitis is rare in early childhood and more common after age 10. Boys and girls are affected equally before puberty, but after age 15, twice as many boys are affected as girls. An increased incidence in the spring and autumn months has also been observed. In addition, appendicitis is more common in children who have a family history of appendicitis.[1] Whether this tendency is genetic or diet related is unclear; the risk of appendicitis may be reduced with a high-fiber diet.[2]

ETIOLOGY AND PATHOPHYSIOLOGY

Appendicitis is always initiated by obstruction of the appendiceal lumen, usually by a fecalith or by lymphoid hyperplasia. In rare cases, a parasite, tumor, or foreign body may obstruct the lumen. Inspissated secretions of cystic fibrosis may also obstruct the appendiceal lumen (thus, although rare, the initial presentation of cystic fibrosis may be appendicitis).[3] As secretions accumulate within the obstructed appendix, it becomes distended, and the appendiceal wall stretches. Continued distention causes ischemia and inflammation of the appendix, leading to irritation of the adjacent somatic peritoneum.

Clinically, the initial distention of the appendix produces a dull, steady periumbilical pain. After 4 to 6 hours, this pain often shifts to the right lower quadrant as local peritoneal inflammation develops. Without surgical intervention, the appendix will eventually rupture, causing peritonitis. The incidence of rupture increases dramatically 24 to 36 hours after the onset of abdominal pain. Delaying surgery more than 36 hours results in at least a 65% incidence of perforation.[4] Organisms cultured from the peritoneal cavity after perforation include both aerobic and anaerobic bacteria.[5] The most common aerobic bacteria are *Escherichia coli, Staphylococcus aureus,* and *Enterococcus* organisms. Common anaerobes include *Bacteroides* and *Clostridium* species.

EVALUATION

History

A thorough history is invaluable in differentiating appendicitis from other disorders; an important component of this history is pain. The onset of symptoms is often heralded by a dull, steady periumbilical pain. The pain is thought to be caused by acute appendicitis if it awakens the patient from sleep. Anorexia is a consistent, but not invariable, finding. One or 2 episodes of vomiting may follow; however, these episodes essentially never precede the pain. After 4 to 6 hours, the pain commonly migrates to the right lower quadrant. Given the many variations in the location of the appendix, however, the location of abdominal pain may vary. Bowel habits usually do not change. Although the child may have a low-grade fever, the temperature is rarely above 100.3°F (37.9°C) before perforation. If the clinical picture suggests appendicitis but does not convince the physician that appendicitis is the problem, then referral for surgical evaluation would be best. Because an appendix rarely perforates within 24 hours of the onset of pain, a period of observation can safely differentiate a potential surgical condition from a nonsurgical one. It is important, however, to be aware that perforation of the appendix may be associated with an initial lessening in the pain only to be followed by a worsening of symptoms within a few hours.

Physical Examination

As always, a gentle, nonthreatening approach is most effective during the physical examination. The physician should assess for peritoneal signs such as pain on walking or coughing. If the patient can jump up on the examining table, then the patient does not usually have appendicitis. Patients may be most comfortable lying supine with their legs flexed. Abdominal tenderness is always present and is often greatest at the McBurney point (two thirds of the distance on a direct line from the umbilicus to the anterosuperior iliac spine). Rebound tenderness of the abdomen (particularly that which is referred to the right lower quadrant) is common, as is hyperesthesia of the skin overlying the painful area. (In infants, tenderness is present diffusely over the abdomen as they are rarely seen before perforation.) Pain in the right lower quadrant may be accentuated when the inflamed appendix is located retrocecally by (1) placing the patient in the left decubitus position and extending the right leg at the hip, thereby placing tension on the right psoas muscle, the origins of which underlie the appendix (psoas sign); and (2) placing the patient supine and internally rotating the flexed right hip, thereby extending the right internal obturator muscle, the origins of which also underlie the appendix (obturator sign). When the inflamed appendix is located anteriorly, pain in the right lower quadrant may be accentuated when the child is asked to sit up from the supine position while pressure is placed against the forehead. Bowel sounds may be diminished or hyperactive. A rectal examination will often facilitate making the diagnosis by revealing right-sided tenderness. Examination of the lungs is important to rule out a right lower lobe pneumonia that may generate referred pain to the right lower quadrant of the abdomen. A pelvic examination is indicated for any adolescent girl who has abdominal pain so as to rule out gynecologic conditions.

Laboratory Testing

The only essential laboratory studies are a blood count and urinalysis. Appendicitis has a characteristic blood count; the white blood cell count is most often in the range of 10,000 to 20,000/mcL, with a slight increase in the number of neutrophils, particularly young forms. The blood count may help rule out viral infection and other processes that do not increase the white blood cell count. The erythrocyte sedimentation rate is usually normal and, if elevated, may suggest such alternative diagnoses as inflammatory bowel disease. Urinalysis is performed to rule out urinary tract infection or diabetic ketoacidosis as a cause of the abdominal pain.

Imaging

If the diagnosis is in doubt, then imaging studies can provide important information. Abdominal radiographs are occasionally helpful. Radiographic features that suggest appendicitis include a calcified appendicolith or an air-filled appendix, although the absence of abnormalities does not rule out the diagnosis. Recently, ultrasonography and computed tomography have been used to establish the diagnosis in equivocal cases.[6,7] In 1 study, the selective use of computed tomography and ultrasound decreased the incidence of perforated appendicitis from 35.4% to 15.5% and decreased the rate of removing a normal appendix (a negative appendectomy) from 14.7% to 4.1%.[8] When available, consultation with a pediatric surgeon may minimize the need for imaging studies while maintaining low rates of perforation and negative appendectomy.[9]

Some clinicians use clinical decision rules to aid in the diagnosis of appendicitis and to avoid overuse of imaging studies. A white blood cell count of greater than 10,000/mcL and the presence of rebound abdominal tenderness are highly suggestive of appendicitis and warrant a prompt surgical evaluation without the need for imaging studies.[10] A white blood cell count of less than 6750/mcL with the absence of nausea and of right lower quadrant tenderness are highly associated with the absence of appendicitis.[11] Careful observation without imaging studies can be considered in such cases.

The typical progression of signs and symptoms in appendicitis may be summarized as follows: periumbilical abdominal pain followed by nausea, vomiting, and localization of the pain to the right lower quadrant. Low-grade fever, direct tenderness to palpation in the right lower quadrant and indirect tenderness referred to the right lower quadrant, right-sided tenderness on rectal examination, and a mild leukocytosis often accompany these symptoms.

DIFFERENTIAL DIAGNOSIS

The differential diagnosis of appendicitis, which is the same as the differential diagnosis of acute abdominal pain, is extensive (Box 238-1). Gastroenteritis can be differentiated from appendicitis based on a generally benign abdominal examination in the former condition. Vomiting and diarrhea usually occur before the onset of pain, not afterward, as is the case in appendicitis. Constipation can often appear to be appendicitis; however, this pain is usually diffuse, not localized to the right lower quadrant, and the patient often has a history of constipation. An abdominal flat plate radiograph can help in the diagnosis, and a small Fleet enema is often both diagnostic and therapeutic.

An appropriate initial evaluation can rule out the following nonsurgical conditions in a patient who has abdominal pain: urinary tract infection, diabetic ketoacidosis, sickle cell crisis, right lower lobe pneumonia with referred pain, nephrotic syndrome with primary peritonitis, and inflammatory bowel disease. Gynecologic disorders can be ruled out based on the history, a pelvic examination, and appropriate diagnostic studies; pelvic inflammatory disease, ovarian torsion,

BOX 238-1 Differential Diagnosis of Appendicitis

COMMON CONDITIONS
Gastroenteritis
Constipation

MEDICAL PROBLEMS
Urinary tract infection
Diabetic ketoacidosis
Sickle cell crisis
Right lower lobe pneumonia
Primary peritonitis
Inflammatory bowel disease

GYNECOLOGIC PROBLEMS
Pelvic inflammatory disease
Ovarian torsion
Ruptured ectopic pregnancy
Dysmenorrhea
Mittelschmerz
Ruptured corpus luteum cyst

UNUSUAL CONDITIONS
Henoch-Schönlein purpura
Hemolytic-uremic syndrome
Rocky Mountain Spotted Fever

SURGICAL EMERGENCIES
Meckel diverticulitis
Intestinal adhesions
Intussusception
Necrotizing enterocolitis

ectopic pregnancy, dysmenorrhea, and Mittelschmerz can all mimic appendicitis.

Unusual conditions such as Henoch-Schönlein purpura and hemolytic-uremic syndrome may be indistinguishable from appendicitis.[12] Even Rocky Mountain Spotted Fever can mimic appendicitis.[13] Surgical emergencies that mimic appendicitis (see Box 238-1) can be ruled out only in the operating room.

APPENDICITIS IN INFANTS

Appendicitis in the first 2 years of life is rare, accounting for fewer than 2% of all childhood cases.[14] The morbidity is high, however, and the incidence of perforation approaches 100%.[15] Therefore appendicitis must be considered in any infant thought to have abdominal pain. The presenting symptoms consist of vomiting and fever, and the baby may appear to be colicky. Physical examination shows abdominal distention with diffuse tenderness. Abdominal radiographs can be diagnostically helpful in a neonate by showing an appendicolith, free peritoneal fluid, bowel wall edema, or, rarely, free air. With a high index of suspicion, surgery must be performed immediately to prevent or manage perforation, with its high morbidity.

MANAGEMENT

Once the diagnosis is made, the patient must be prepared for immediate surgery. Nothing is given by mouth, and a nasogastric tube is inserted and placed on low suction if the child is vomiting. Intravenous hydration is started (eg, 10 mL/kg/hr of lactated Ringer's solution), and fever may be controlled with acetaminophen given by rectum. Broad-spectrum antibiotics (eg, ampicillin, gentamicin, and clindamycin or a cephalosporin) are administered intravenously before surgery. Antibiotics have been shown to reduce morbidity even in nonperforated cases.[16] An appendectomy is performed as soon as the patient's condition has been stabilized. Many institutions are gaining experience with laparoscopic appendectomy.[17]

For patients who have symptoms for 5 days or longer and a palpable mass consistent with an appendiceal abscess, many surgeons initially prefer nonsurgical management.[18] The patient is treated with broad-spectrum antibiotics for 14 days (initiated in the hospital and completed at home) if the child's clinical condition allows and, barring interim complications, returns in 6 to 8 weeks for an elective appendectomy. This approach lowers the incidence of diffuse peritonitis and the associated complications precipitated by surgical manipulation during the acute inflammatory stages of the disease.

PROGNOSIS

For uncomplicated appendicitis treated with prompt surgical intervention, the mortality is much less than 1%, and long-term morbidity is primarily the risk of adhesive small-bowel obstruction. The average hospital stay is approximately 2 days.[19] Although a ruptured appendix increases the risk of mortality (with most of the increase occurring in the infant age group or older children with delayed diagnosis who develop sepsis), perforation significantly extends the average hospital stay. Complications that increase morbidity include peritonitis, postoperative abscesses, and prolonged ileus. Perforation also significantly increases the risk of postoperative adhesive small-bowel obstruction. In women, although infertility was thought to be a possible long-term complication of a ruptured appendix, recent studies have shown this not to be the case.[20]

The incidence of perforated appendicitis exceeds 30%, a disconcertingly high figure, despite increasing use of radiographic imaging.[21] A higher index of suspicion on the part of families and pediatricians may lead to earlier diagnosis of the condition and reduce the incidence of appendiceal perforation and its morbid complications.

WHEN TO REFER

- Refer to surgery immediately whenever appendicitis is suspected.

WHEN TO ADMIT

- Hospitalize for inpatient observation if the diagnosis cannot be excluded and for appendectomy if the diagnosis of appendicitis is made.

SUGGESTED RESOURCES

Silen ML, Tracy TF Jr. The right lower quadrant "revisited". *Pediatr Clin North Am.* 1993;40:1201-1211.

Silen W, ed. *Cope's Early Diagnosis of the Acute Abdomen.* New York, NY: Oxford University Press; 2005.

Ziegler MM. The diagnosis of appendicitis: an evolving paradigm. *Pediatrics.* 2004;113:130-132.

REFERENCES

1. Gauderer MW, Crane MM, Green JA, et al. Acute appendicitis in children: the importance of family history. *J Pediatr Surg.* 2001;36:1214-1217.
2. Adamidis D, Roma-Giannikou E, Karamolegou K, et al. Fiber intake and childhood appendicitis. *Int J Food Sci Nutr.* 2000;51:153-157.
3. Oestreich AE, Adelstein EH. Appendicitis as the presenting complaint in cystic fibrosis. *J Pediatr Surg.* 1982;17: 191-194.
4. Brender JD, Marcuse EK, Koepsell TD, et al. Childhood appendicitis: factors associated with perforation. *Pediatrics.* 1985;76:301-306.
5. Brook I. Intra-abdominal, retroperitoneal, and visceral abscesses in children. *Eur J Pediatr Surg.* 2004;14: 265-273.
6. Garcia Peña BM, Cook EF, Mandl KD. Selective imaging strategies for the diagnosis of appendicitis in children. *Pediatrics.* 2004;113:24-28.
7. Ziegler MM. The diagnosis of appendicitis: an evolving paradigm. *Pediatrics.* 2004;113:130-132.
8. Garcia Peña BM, Taylor GA, Fishman SJ, et al. Effect of an imaging protocol on clinical outcomes among pediatric patients with appendicitis. *Pediatrics.* 2002;110: 1088-1093.
9. Kosloske AM, Love CL, Rohrer JE, et al. The diagnosis of appendicitis in children: outcomes of a strategy based on pediatric surgical evaluation. *Pediatrics.* 2004;113: 29-34.
10. van den Broek WT, van der Ende ED, Bijnen AB, et al. Which children could benefit from additional diagnostic tools in case of suspected appendicitis? *J Pediatr Surg.* 2004;39:570-574.
11. Kharbanda AB, Taylor GA, Fishman SJ, et al. A clinical decision rule to identify children at low risk for appendicitis. *Pediatrics.* 2005;116:709-716.
12. Edmonson MB, Chesney RW. Hemolytic-uremic syndrome confused with acute appendicitis. *Arch Surg.* 1978;113:754-755.
13. Davis AE Jr, Bradford WD. Abdominal pain resembling acute appendicitis in Rocky Mountain Spotted Fever. *JAMA.* 1982;247:2811-2812.
14. Grosfeld JL, Weinberger M, Clatworthy HW Jr. Acute appendicitis in the first two years of life. *J Pediatr Surg.* 1973;8:285-293.
15. Alloo J, Gerstle T, Shilyansky J, et al. Appendicitis in children less than 3 years of age: a 28-year review. *Pediatr Surg Int.* 2004;19:777-779.
16. Busuttil RW, Davidson RK, Fine M, et al. Effect of prophylactic antibiotics in acute nonperforated appendicitis: a prospective, randomized, double-blind clinical study. *Ann Surg.* 1981;194:502-509.
17. Oka T, Kurkchubasche AG, Bussey JG, et al. Open and laparoscopic appendectomy are equally safe and acceptable in children. *Surg Endosc.* 2004;18:242-245.
18. Weber TR, Keller MA, Bower RJ, et al. Is delayed operative treatment worth the trouble with perforated appendicitis in children? *Am J Surg.* 2003;186: 685-688.
19. Newman K, Ponsky T, Kittle K, et al. Appendicitis 2000: variability in practice, outcomes, and resource utilization at thirty pediatric hospitals. *J Pediatr Surg.* 2003;38: 372-379.
20. Urbach DR, Marrett LD, Kung R, et al. Association of perforation of the appendix with female tubal infertility. *Am J Epidemiol.* 2001;153:566-571.
21. Smink DS, Fishman SJ, Kleinman K, et al. Effects of race, insurance status, and hospital volume on perforated appendicitis in children. *Pediatrics.* 2005;115: 920-925.

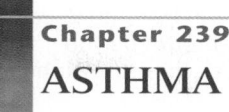

Chapter 239

ASTHMA

Robert C. Cohn, MD; James E. Martin, RRT-NPS, CPFT

EPIDEMIOLOGIC FEATURES

Asthma is the most common chronic illness of childhood. Of the 15 million people with asthma in the United States, 5 million are children or adolescents. This number represents between 3% and 7% of children in the United States. Asthma prevalence in children younger than 5 years has increased 160% from 1980 through the end of the 1990s.[1] In 80% of patients with asthma, the onset of symptoms occurred before the age of 5 years.[2] Childhood asthma is responsible for 13 million physician visits, 200,000 hospitalizations, 10 million lost school days, and over 550,000 emergency room visits per year. Over 8 million prescriptions for asthma medications are written for children. This condition is responsible for 3 times the number of missed school days when compared with children without asthma. Approximately 78% of parents have reported negative effects on their family. An estimated 36% of parents of asthmatic children have missed work in the last year, resulting in over $1 billion in lost parental productivity.[2] Most asthma care is delivered by primary care physicians. Approximately 78% of children (and 58% of adults) receive their care from primary care physicians such as pediatricians and family practitioners. Only 20% of children in the United States see a specialist for this condition (compared with 36% of adults).

Many risk factors are associated with childhood asthma. The most common cause of wheezing in infants and young children is viral upper respiratory tract infections, but the strongest predictor for wheezing continuing into asthma is atopy.[1] A significant association exists between serum immunoglobulin E (IgE) level and the development or severity of asthma. Certain allergens and irritant exposures increase the risk for asthma. In the inner city, cockroach allergy has been associated with the significant development of signs and symptoms of this condition. Irritant exposures, particularly a history of maternal smoke exposure is a risk factor as well. Prematurity is also a risk factor. Several candidate genetic loci have been proposed based on epidemiologic linkage studies. These loci include an association of chromosome *5q* with bronchial hyper-responsiveness, chromosome *11q13* with high-affinity IgE receptors, and chromosome *14q* with T-cell antigen receptor.[3,4]

Many pediatricians and primary care physicians do not realize that childhood asthma is a fatal disorder.[2] The number of deaths has more than doubled in the last 2 decades. Of great concern is that most patients who die are not seen as high risk; many are viewed to have mild disease. Certain risk factors have been associated with death from asthma, including:

1. History of sudden severe exacerbations
2. Prior admissions to an intensive care unit
3. Prior intubation for asthma

4. Two or more hospitalizations or 3 or more emergency department visits in a 12-month period
5. Use of more than 1 canister per month of inhaled short-acting β-agonist
6. Chronic use of oral corticosteroids
7. Difficulty perceiving airflow obstruction or its severity

PATHOPHYSIOLOGICAL FEATURES

Asthma is a lung disease characterized by 3 features:

1. Airway obstruction that is at least partially reversible
2. Airway hyperreactivity or hyperresponsiveness to a variety of external stimuli
3. Chronic inflammation; the inflammatory disorder in asthma is characterized by mast cell activation, inflammatory cell infiltration by eosinophils and T-helper-2 (T_H2) lymphocytes. Neutrophils may be present in sudden onset fatal asthma exacerbations.[1]

The pathological findings associated with the airway in asthma include increased mucus production, disruption of the bronchial epithelium, edema of the airways resulting from increased vascular permeability, increased thickness of the basement membrane, and smooth-muscle hypertrophy denuded.[5] Bronchial epithelium can sometimes be found in the sputum of some asthmatics. Collagen deposition beneath the basement membrane results from increased fibroblast proliferation. This deposition may cause airway remodeling, which clinically exhibits as nonreversible obstructive lung disease.[5] This feature has been described as severe in some patients. The airway histopathological feature is also notable for increased numbers of activated mast cells, inflammatory cell infiltration, and edema. Mucus hypersecretion is the result of goblet cell hyperplasia.

In many instances, an identifiable external trigger initiates the inflammatory cascade. Mediator release leads to physiological changes such as a mucus production, disruption of the bronchial epithelium, edema caused by increased vascular permeability, smooth-muscle constriction, and an increased inflammatory cell infiltration. These changes lead to airway constriction and the signs and symptoms commonly seen in asthma such as cough, wheezing, and shortness of breath. The most common types of triggers in childhood (Box 239-1) include viral respiratory infections, exercise, irritants such as tobacco smoke, allergens such as animal dander, dust, dust mites, cockroaches, and a change in the weather, particularly cold air. Emotional expression such as laughter and anger has been associated as a trigger as well. Gastroesophageal reflux disease especially has been identified as a significant contributing factor to disease and disease severity. In the presence of symptoms that seem to be worse at night or with reclining, the pediatrician should always consider gastroesophageal reflux or sinusitis.

Asthma is biphasic. The early phase or immediate response occurring within minutes of trigger exposure is characterized by bronchospasm and bronchoconstriction. This episode is followed physiologically by an immediate drop in forced expiratory volume in 1 second (FEV_1), which returns to normal between 4 and 8 hours after exposure. A 2nd more severe drop (termed a late-phase or late-asthmatic response) occurs between 8 and 24 hours after exposure to the trigger. This drop is the result of inflammatory cell infiltration.[6]

Within 5 minutes of an exposure to a trigger, IgE molecules on the surface of mast cells binds the inciting allergen, leading to degranulation and the release of histamine, prostaglandins, cytokines, and platelet activating factor from mast cells. The last 2 compounds are potent, chemotactic factors for eosinophils and lymphocytes. Within hours of the initial trigger, a significant number of eosinophils are recruited. The eosinophils are key to the chronic inflammation of the asthma cascade. After degranulation, eosinophils release tissue, damaging enzymes and proteins including major basic protein, eosinophil cationic protein, eosinophil derived neurotoxin, and eosinophil peroxidase. In addition, the release of leukotrienes (LTs) causes significant vascular permeability and bronchoconstriction.

Antigen-presenting cells influence uncommitted CD4 T_H0 lymphocytes to differentiate into either T_H1 cells or T_H2 cells. T_H1 and T_H2 cells can be distinguished from each other by the pattern of cytokine production. Thus T_H1 cells produce the cytokines interleukin-2 and interferon-gamma, and T_H2 cells produce interleukin.[4-8] Cytokines produced by T_H2 cell cause maturation and activation of B cells and cause them to produce IgE. This activity is the basis for the imbalance or hygiene hypothesis. A significant relationship exists between serum IgE levels and asthma severity. Excess synthesis of IgE in response to environmental allergens remains a major risk factor in asthma pathogenesis. Mast cells and basophils have high-affinity IgE receptors. Serum IgE binds these receptors, leading to mast-cell degranulation when an appropriate allergen cross-links the IgE molecules on mast cells.

Another important pathway in the pathophysiological features of asthma is the arachidonic acid pathway, which is responsible for the production of prostaglandins via cyclooxygenase or LTs via the 5-lipoxygenase pathway. Mast cells and eosinophils synthesize

BOX 239-1 Factors That Exacerbate Asthma

- Aerosol sprays, odors
- Aspirin, ibuprofen
- Cigarette smoke
- Cold air
- Colds
- Dust, dust mites
- Exercise
- Exposure to chemicals or other occupational sensitizers
- Foods, especially nuts, and food additives such as colorings, metabisulphite, and monosodium glutamate
- Grass, trees
- Menstrual periods (women)
- Pets
- Mold
- Rats
- Roaches
- Stress, emotions
- Weather

significant amounts of LTC4, LTD4 and LTE4. Cysteinyl LTs are responsible for significant bronchoconstriction 100 to 1000 times more potent than histamine, increased mucus secretion, decreased mucus clearance, eosinophil infiltration, and eosinophil activation.

DIAGNOSING THE CHILD WITH ASTHMA

Clinicians often miss a diagnosis of asthma; furthermore, they often misclassify the disease severity in a child diagnosed with asthma.[1] To make the diagnosis of asthma, the clinician must determine that the child has:

1. Recurrent episodic symptoms of airflow obstruction such as cough, wheezing, shortness of breath, or chest tightness
2. Airway flow obstruction or airflow limitation that is at least partially reversible; in older children and adults, spirometry before and after a bronchodilator use can determine this condition; in a younger child, a positive response to a β-agonist may be useful to determine partial reversibility.
3. Alternative diagnoses are excluded.

The clinician should suspect the diagnosis of asthma if:

1. The patient has a history of recurrent symptoms such as cough or wheezing.
2. Symptoms are made worse by triggers.
3. Symptoms that occur are worse at night.
4. Evidence exists of reversible airflow limitation clinically or on pulmonary function testing.

Warning signs and symptoms of asthma are listed in Box 239-2.

Underdiagnosis is frequent in children because clinicians commonly use terms such as reactive airway disease, recurrent bronchitis, or wheezy bronchitis. This terminology should not be used and may hinder appropriate diagnosis and therapy. Signs and symptoms that are not consistent with asthma, including failure to thrive, cyanosis, and clubbing, should alert the pediatrician to another possible diagnosis such as ciliary dyskinesia or cystic fibrosis.

To establish the diagnosis, a detailed medical history should be obtained. The clinician should assess signs and symptoms and frequency of findings and precipitating factors. The physical examination should focus on the upper respiratory tract, chest, and skin. Signs of allergic disease such as conjunctivitis, allergic shiners, pale boggy turbinates, rhinorrhea, and polyps should be noted. Nasal polyps can also be found in cystic fibrosis. A transverse nasal crease is a good tip-off for allergic disease. The chest examination is usually unremarkable in children with asthma, although dyspnea with speech, dyspnea with exertion, breath sounds, and inspiration-to-expiration ratio may be of value.

The laboratory evaluation is peripheral to the diagnosis. Testing for IgE levels and for allergies may be of use so that newer therapies can be used appropriately. Results of the complete blood cell count with differential may indicate an allergic or immunologic condition. Sputum and nasal secretions for eosinophils are rarely done. A baseline chest x-ray examination may exclude other conditions such as foreign body aspiration or vascular ring. Quantitative immunoglobulins may also be of value to rule out immune dysregulation, and a sweat chloride test for cystic fibrosis should be done if this condition is suspected.

Pre- and postbronchodilator spirometry is strongly recommended to confirm the diagnosis and classify disease severity.[1,9] Spirometry is the gold standard for measuring the severity of obstructive airway disease and should be performed on any child 5 years of age or older who is capable of performing this test. Objective measures of lung function enable the clinician to:

1. Diagnose airflow obstruction, as well as reversibility of airflow obstruction after bronchodilator treatment
2. Monitor changes over time including daily variation
3. Manage exacerbations in severe airway obstruction

For diagnosis, spirometry is generally used instead of peak flow monitoring because peak flow measurements are a measure primarily of large airway function. Spirometry should be performed before a child inhales a short-acting bronchodilator and again 15 to 20 minutes afterwards; this test determines airflow obstruction that is present, including small airway disease, and determines whether this airflow obstruction is reversible. The measurements that most specialists will assess are the FEV_1, forced vital capacity, forced midexpiratory flow rate, and an examination of the flow volume loop. Every patient with asthma should have a baseline spirometry if they are old enough and capable. A baseline spirometry should also be performed once a year.[1]

Peak flow meters are monitoring tools and lack the sensitivity for diagnostic use, and peak flow reference values vary widely and according to the brand of the peak flow meter. Peak flow monitoring can be useful because it can help determine if airway narrowing is occurring before patients become symptomatic; peak flow monitoring can also assist the clinician with the following:

1. Monitor the effect of medication addition or withdrawal
2. Determine when to seek help
3. Determine the effect of triggers
4. Determine changes in lung function

BOX 239-2 Signs and Symptoms of Asthma

Chest pain	Mood changes
Irritable, quiet, fatigue	Runny or stuffy nose
Eczema flare-up	Headaches
Fever	Wheezing
Scratchy throat	Cough
Heartburn, gastroesophageal reflux	Loss of appetite
	Hands that tremble
Heart palpitations	Watery eyes, dark circles under eyes
Decreased exercise tolerance	

Peak flow zones can be established once the child has had 1 to 2 weeks of daily or twice-a-day monitoring to establish the child's personal best.

DIFFERENTIAL DIAGNOSIS

An important point to remember is that all wheezes do not indicate asthma. The most common asthma imposters include cystic fibrosis, foreign body aspiration, vocal cord dysfunction, airway lesions such as airway stenosis, tracheal webs or tracheobronchomalacia, vascular rings, mediastinal masses, gastroesophageal reflux or recurrent aspiration, heart failure, immunodeficiency, parasitic diseases such as toxocariasis, and bronchiolitis caused by respiratory syncytial virus or other viral pathogens.

RISK FACTORS FOR ASTHMA

Can asthma in children be predicted? Wheezing in a child younger than 3 years is associated with an increased risk of asthma if the child has 1 major criterion or 2 minor criteria.[10] Major criteria include a parent with asthma or atopic dermatitis. Minor criteria include allergic rhinitis, wheezing apart from colds, and eosinophilia at or above 4%. Any wheezing in children with 1 of the 2 major criteria or 2 of the 3 minor criteria are up to 5.5 times more likely to have active asthma between 6 and 13 years of age compared with children who did not meet these criteria. Frequent wheezing in children in the first 3 years of life and 1 of the 2 major criteria or 2 of the 3 minor criteria is associated with a 9 to 10 times greater likelihood of having asthma between the ages of 6 and 13 years.[10]

BOX 239-3 Pulmonary Function Class: FEV_1 and PEFR

- Intermittent (>80% FEV_1 and PEFR before bronchodilator use and <12 and 20% change, respectively, after bronchodilator use)
- Mild persistent (>80% FEV_1 and PEFR before bronchodilator use and >12 and 20% change, respectively, after bronchodilator use)
- Moderate persistent (60-80% FEV_1 and PEFR before bronchodilator use)
- Severe persistent (<60% FEV_1 and PEFR before bronchodilator use)

FEV, Forced expiratory volume in 1 second; PEFR, peak expiratory flow rate. Modified from National Heart, Lung, and Blood Institute. *National Asthma Education Program: Guidelines for the Diagnosis and Management of Asthma, Expert Panel Report 2.* No 97-405. Bethesda, MD: National Institutes of Health; 1997.

CLASSIFYING ASTHMA SEVERITY IN CHILDREN

For any child, the severity of asthma can change over time. The clinician should classify asthma disease based on the National Heart, Lung, and Blood Institute Guidelines for Asthma Severity[9] (Box 239-3). Asthma severity is classified into 4 categories: (1) intermittent asthma, (2) mild persistent asthma, (3) moderate persistent asthma, and (4) severe persistent asthma. Persistent asthma may become more severe or less severe over time. Asthma severity is therefore continuum. Table 239-1 lists the classification for asthma severity based on daytime symptoms, nighttime symptoms, and effective activity, as well as FEV_1 or peak expiratory flow rate. Classification can occur quickly after the clinician determines 4 factors (Box 239-4).

BOX 239-4 Classifying Asthma Severity with Patients

1. _____ times per week that you have had symptoms of asthma (wheezing, coughing, shortness of breath, chest tightness, etc.)
2. _____ times per month that you have been waking up during the night because of asthma symptoms
3. Your peak flow rates have been running between ________ and ________ liters/minute.
4. Your peak flow personal best is ___________ liters/minute OR spirometry today showed an FEV_1 of ___________ liters.

Table 239-1 Symptom Class: Current Clinical Features

Intermittent	Intermittent symptoms (wheeze, cough, dyspnea) <2 times a week Brief exacerbations (from a few hours to a few days) Nighttime asthma symptoms less than 2 times a month Asymptomatic between exacerbations
Mild persistent	Symptoms more than 2 times a week but less than 1 time per day Exacerbations that may affect activity and sleep Nighttime asthma symptoms more than 2 times a month but less than 1 time per week
Moderate persistent	Symptoms daily Exacerbations more than 2 times a week; may last days and affect activity Nighttime asthma symptoms more than 1 time a week
Severe persistent	Continuous symptoms Frequent exacerbations Frequent nighttime asthma symptoms Physical activities limited by asthma symptoms

When classifying asthma severity into 1 of the 4 classifications, the presence of a single feature is sufficient to categorize the patient in the most severe category. Classification can change over time; thus constant review of symptoms and treatment every 1 to 6 months is helpful. Patients with intermittent asthma experiencing severe exacerbations requiring hospitalization should be treated as having moderate persistent asthma. Children requiring intensive care should be treated as having severe persistent asthma and should be referred to an asthma specialist.

CLASSIFYING AND MANAGING ASTHMA CONTROL

The Expert Panel Report 3 (EPR3) was published in the latter part of 2007. A key component of the new guidelines emphasizes asthma control in addition to asthma severity. Severity is emphasized for initiating therapy, whereas control, which represents the degree to which manifestations of asthma are minimized, and the goals of therapy are met, emphasizes monitoring and the adjustment of therapy. Asthma control should be used as a guide for clinical decisions to either maintain or adjust therapy once this therapy has been initiated. Assessment of asthma control should not be based solely on individual single measurements and limited interactions but rather on a combination of multiple parameters including FEV1, peak expiratory flow, daily symptom scores, beta to agonist use, nocturnal symptoms and activity limitations. The new guidelines strongly recommend assessment and monitoring of asthma using standardized questionnaires. There are several available including the asthma therapy assessment questionnaire (ATAQ); the asthma control questionnaire (ACQ); the asthma control test (ACT); and the asthma control score. Key elements include the patient's recall of symptoms, physical activity, quality of life, need for rescue medications in the past 2-4 weeks and pulmonary function. Asthma control is classified in three categories: well controlled, not well controlled and very poorly controlled using features currently described in this article.

ASTHMA MANAGEMENT STRATEGIES

Asthma therapy has 5 goals:

1. Prevent chronic and troublesome symptoms.
2. Maintain normal or near-normal pulmonary function.
3. Maintain normal activity levels, including exercise.
4. Prevent exacerbations.
5. Provide optimal medical regimen with minimal or no adverse side effects.

Appropriate asthma management includes 4 components to achieve these goals:

1. Objective measurements of lung function
2. Pharmacologic therapy
3. Environmental control of allergies and irritants
4. Patient education

Objective measurement of lung function includes spirometry and peak flow monitoring. The 2 goals of pharmacologic therapy are (1) to relieve obstruction and (2) to treat underlying inflammation. Many patients with asthma respond to removal of allergens or irritants from their environment. Patient education should be geared to empowering patients with self-management skills. Asthma action plans formally convey this information.

What influences adherence with asthma therapy? Studies have shown that medication characteristics, patient variables, and physician factors are important factors.[7] Medication characteristics such as taste, dosing schedule, side effects, and expense are critical.

Patient variables such as apathy, misperception of disease severity, and failure to obtain medication can affect the management of disease. Physician factors such as poor communication, failure to monitor patients regularly, and incorrect medication and dose level all lead to problems. Promoting open communication encourages patient adherence to therapy. The clinician should use a friendly manner and be attentive. The patient should be encouraged and praised for successes. The clinician should always elicit families concerns and allay their fears. The focus should be on what patients can do to improve adherence. The correct asthma medication regimen and technique of administration should be reinforced and evaluated. The therapy should be kept as simple as possible by limiting the number of medication and doses. If patients cannot adhere to a medication regimen, then they should be asked why (Box 239-5). The clinician should establish patient priorities on an individual basis. An asthma action plan is useful communication, and family and peer support should be enlisted. These aspects will lead to improved successful participation, and physical activity should be encouraged by using the appropriate medications to prevent exercise-induced symptoms

BOX 239-5 Asking Patients about Medication Compliance

What problems have prevented you from taking your medications? (Mark all that apply.)

- ☐ Bothered by medication taste
- ☐ Concerned about side effects
- ☐ Cost of medication
- ☐ Denial
- ☐ Difficulty remembering or organizing medications
- ☐ Difficulty tolerating side effects
- ☐ Difficulty using delivery system (ie, coordination)
- ☐ Difficulty with school
- ☐ Unable to understand how medicine works
- ☐ Inconvenient or inappropriate dosing schedule
- ☐ Embarrassment
- ☐ Fear of medication addiction
- ☐ Lack of parental supervision
- ☐ Language difficulties
- ☐ Rebellion
- ☐ Unable to refill prescription on time
- ☐ Inadequate transportation to health services
- ☐ Inadequate transportation to pharmacy

and by allowing students to carry and administer medication such as short-acting β-agonist with parental and physician approval at school. Physicians should ensure that teachers and school personnel understand the plan for each child with asthma. Families, teachers, and clinicians should be concerned if β-agonist use is greater than 1 metered dose inhaler canister per month, if controller medication refills are occurring one half as often as prescribed, or if a the patient complains that β-agonists do not seem to help as much as they had previously.

PHARMACOLOGIC THERAPY

Asthma medications are defined and categorized in 2 ways: (1) relief medication for quick relief of symptoms and (2) controller medication for long-term control of underlying the pathophysiological mechanism of asthma (Table 239-2). The quick-relief medications are used to treat acute symptoms and exacerbations. These medications include short-acting β-agonists, systemic corticosteroids, and anticholinergic agents. Long-term controller medications include long-acting β-agonists, inhaled corticosteroids, nonsteroidal antiinflammatory agents (eg, cromolyn nedocromil), LT modifiers, theophylline, and other steroid-sparing medications.

Asthma severity guides the pediatrician in selecting appropriate medication (Table 239-3). Aggressive controller therapy should be used to gain control rapidly, meaning that clinicians will often use therapy intended for a greater level of severity in attempt to accomplish quick control. In some instances, a short 3- to 5-day course of oral corticosteroid should be used with controller medication to gain control. Step-down therapy can be subsequently instituted.

A more conservative approach is to start with therapy that corresponds to the initial evaluation of the child's asthma severity and, after 2 to 4 weeks of treatments, to step up or down in terms of medical regimen. This regimen requires continuous monitoring of control, as well as choosing medications and delivery devices according to the child's ability to use them.

Controller therapy, instead of conservative therapy, should be instituted in the following situations:

- Chronic symptoms
- Exacerbations greater than once a week
- Daily use of short-acting β-agonist therapy
- Nocturnal symptoms at least twice a month
- Any evidence of airway obstruction by spirometry testing

Short-acting β2-agonists are the most well-known quick-relief medications. They bronchodilate and bronchoprotect and are indicated for the relief of acute symptoms of asthma. Notably, the long-acting β-agonists such as salmeterol or formoterol do not fit into this category. β2-Agonists also can prevent exercise-induced bronchospasm. The most well-known side effects include tachycardia, tremor, headaches, palpitations, hypokalemia, and hyperglycemia. These symptoms can be reduced with medication delivered via any aerosol delivery method and drug β-receptor selection. These drugs bind β-receptors present on smooth muscle and are known to activate adenylcyclase. Adenosine 5′-triphosphate is converted to cyclic adenosine monophosphate, leading to protein kinase A activation. The end result is smooth-muscle relaxation, decreased mediator release, increased water in secretions, and increased ciliary sweep.

Levalbuterol has gained popularity recently as an alternative to (racemic) albuterol.[11] All β-agonist medications are racemates. A racemate is composed of a 50/50 mixture of R- and S-isomers. Isomers are non–super-imposable mirror images with the same chemical structures. Albuterol is made up of the R-isomer, as well as S-isomer albuterol. Levalbuterol is 100% R-isomer albuterol. (Racemates have important implications in nature. Almost all hormones, pheromones, steroids, and mediators manufactured in the body are in single-isomer form. The human body would not be able to metabolize D-amino acids or L-sugars. Similarly, other drugs and chemicals exist whose RS-isomer leads to very different systemic effects. For example, the chemical limonene in R-isomer gives a lemon taste, and an S-isomer gives an orange taste. The drug thalidomide as an R-isomer is a narcotic and as an S-isomer is teratogenic.)

Levalbuterol at 0.31 mg demonstrated comparable efficacy in pediatric studies to 2.5 mg of racemic albuterol. This amount was also associated with less tachycardia, hyperglycemia, and hypokalemia.[11]

Anticholinergic agents in combination with albuterol have been shown to have a positive effect on acute asthma exacerbations. The most common anticholinergic agent in use is ipratropium bromide. This agent decreases vagal tone, leading to bronchodilatation, and blocks reflex bronchoconstriction to irritants; it has no effect on the early- or late-phase response, and its effect is additive to a β2-agonist.

Oral short courses of corticosteroids are considered quick-relief medications. These drugs have broad antiinflammatory effects and are usually used as a short 3- to 10-day course to gain initial control of asthma and to speed resolution of moderate or severe persistent exacerbation. Although a course of 7 days or less is usually sufficient for therapy, in some cases the exacerbation may require up to 10 days of treatment. Tapering of the dose is not necessary.

Many classes of long-term controller medications have been developed. Inhaled corticosteroids are the most important long-term controller medication. These drugs bind to the glucocorticoid receptors in cytoplasm and move into the nucleus. They regulate transcription of target genes and modify arachidonic acid metabolism, which leads to inhibition of cytokines and inflammation and augmentation β2-receptor responsiveness.

Inhaled corticosteroids are the most potent and effective long-term antiinflammatory medications currently available.[9] Depending on the drug, inhaled corticosteroids are available as a metered dose inhaler, dry powder inhaler, or nebulizer solution. They have broad actions on the inflammatory processes and have been shown to improve long-term symptoms in pulmonary function, reducing the need for quick-relief medications. The major issues and concerns with inhaled corticosteroids are growth delay, ocular problems such as cataracts and potential glaucoma, and thrush; they are contraindicated during certain infections such as herpes simplex infections.

Table 239-2 Medications Used to Treat Children With Asthma in the United States[a]

LONG-TERM CONTROL MEDICATIONS

Nonsteroidal antiinflammatory

GENERIC NAME	BRAND NAME	DOSE FORM	DOSE[b]	POTENTIAL ADVERSE EFFECTS AND THERAPEUTIC ISSUES
Cromolyn sodium	Intal	MDI: 1 mg/puff Nebulizer solution: 20 mg/2 mL (ampule)	1-2 puffs, tid-qid 1 ampule, tid-qid	• Therapeutic response to cromolyn and nedocromil often occurs within 2 weeks, but a 4- to 6-week trial may be needed to determine maximum benefit. • Dose of cromolyn MDI (1 mg/puff) may be inadequate to affect airway hyperresponsiveness. • Safety is the primary advantage of these agents.
Nedocromil sodium	Tilade	MDI: 1.75 mg/puff	1-2 puffs, bid-qid	• Unpleasant taste for some patients.

Inhaled corticosteroids

GENERIC NAME	BRAND NAME	DOSE FORM	DOSE[b] LOW	MEDIUM	HIGH
Beclomethasone dipropionate	QVAR HFA	MDI: 40 mcg/puff	1-4 puffs/day, bid	4-8 puffs/day, bid	—
		MDI: 80 mcg/puff	1-2 puffs/day, bid	2-4 puffs/day, bid	8 puffs/day, bid
Budesonide	Pulmicort Flexhaler	DPI: 90 mcg/ inhalation	2-4 inhalation/day, qd-bid	6-8 inhalation/day, (bid)	—
		180 mcg/inhalation	1-2 inhalation/day, bid	3-4 inhalation/day, bid	8 inhalation/day, bid
	Pulmicort Respules	0.5 mg/2 mL 0.25 mg/2 mL	0.5 mg/day, qd-bid	—	1.0 mg/day, qd-bid
Flunisolide	AeroBid, AeroBid-M	MDI: 250 mcg/puff	2-4 puffs/day, bid	4-6 puffs/day, bid	8 puffs/day, bid
Fluticasone propionate	Flovent	MDI: 44 mcg/puff	2-4 puffs/day, bid	—	—
		110 mcg/puff	—	2-4 puffs/day, bid	—
		220 mcg/puff	—	2 puffs/day, bid	3-8 puffs/day, bid
		DPI: 50 mcg/ inhalation	2-4 inhalation/day, bid	—	—
		100 mcg/inhalation	—	2-4 inh/day, bid	—
		250 mcg/inhalation	—	2 inhalation/day, bid	3-8 inh/day, bid
Mometasone furoate	Asmanex Twisthaler	DPI: 220 mcg/ inhalation	1 inhalation/day, once at night	2-3 inhalation/day, once at night or bid	4 inhalations/day, bid
Triamcinolone	Azmacort	MDI: 200 mcg/puff	4-8 puffs/day, tid-qid	8-12 puffs/day, bid-qid	12-16 puffs/day, bid

Long-acting β2-agonists

GENERIC NAME	BRAND NAME	DOSE FORM	DOSE[b]
Salmeterol	Serevent Diskus	DPI: 50 mcg/inhalation	1 inhalation, bid
Formoterol	Foradil Aerolizer	DPI: 12 mcg/capsule (inhaled)	1 capsule inhaled bid or 15 minutes before exercise
Sustained-release albuterol	VoSpire ER	Tablet: 4 mg, 8 mg	Maximal dose: 6-12 yr: 4 mg, bid ≥12 yr: 8 mg, bid

bid, Twice daily; *DPI,* dry powder inhaler; *MDI,* metered dose inhaler; *prn,* as needed; *qd,* every day; *qid,* 4 times daily; *tid,* 3 times daily.

[a]The most important determinant of appropriate dosing is the clinician's judgment of the child's response to therapy. The clinician must monitor several clinical parameters to assess both efficacy and adverse effect and must adjust the dose accordingly.

The stepwise approach to therapy emphasizes that, once control of asthma is achieved, the dose of medication should be carefully titrated to the minimum dose required to maintain control.

[b]These doses are suggested as guides for making clinical decisions. The clinician must use personal judgment to tailor treatment to the specific needs of the child and family.

[c]Do not use partial unit dose.

[d]Some nebulizer solutions contain benzalkonium, which may cause bronchospasm in some patients.

[e]Course of 7 days or less is usually sufficient. In some cases, the exacerbation may require up to 10 days of treatment.

Continued

Table 239-2 Medications Used to Treat Children With Asthma in the United States[a]—cont'd

Inhaled corticosteroids, long-acting β2-agonists

GENERIC NAME	BRAND NAME	DOSE FORM	DOSE[b]		
			LOW	MEDIUM	HIGH
Fluticasone propionate + salmeterol	Advair	DPI: 100 mcg/50 mcg inhalation, 250 mcg/50 mcg inhalation, 500 mcg/50 mcg inhalation	1 inhalation, 100/50, bid	1 inhalation, 250/50, bid	1 inhalation, 500/50, bid
		MDI: 45 mcg/21 mcg puff	2 puffs 45/21, bid	—	—
		115 mcg/21 mcg puff	—	2 puffs 115/21, bid	—
		230 mcg/21 mcg puff	—	—	2 puffs 230/21, bid
Budesonide +,formoterol	Symbicort	MDI: 80 mcg/4.5 mcg inhalation	2 puffs 80/4.5, bid	—	—
		160 mcg/4.5 mcg inhalation	—	—	2 puffs 160 mcg/4.5, bid

Leukotriene modifiers

GENERIC NAME	BRAND NAME	DOSE FORM	DOSE[b]
Montelukast	Singulair	Sprinkles: 4 mg for ages 12-23 mo Tablet: 4-mg chewable for ages 2-4 yr; 5-mg chewable for ages 6-14 yr; 10 mg for ages >14 yr	1 tablet or packet in evening
Zafirlukast	Accolate	Tablet: 20 mg for ages ≥12 yr; 10 mg for ages 7-11 yr	1 tablet, bid Take 1 hr before or 2 hr after meals
Zileuton	Zyflo Filmtab	Tablet: 600 mg for ages ≥12 yr	1 tablet, qid

Oral corticosteroids

GENERIC NAME	BRAND NAME	DOSE FORM	DOSE[b]
Methylprednisolone	Medrol	Tablet: 4, 6, 8, 16, 24, 32 mg	Short-course (3- to 10-day), 1-2 mg/kg/day (max: 60 mg/day)
Prednisolone	Prednisolone	Tablet: 5 mg	Short-course (3- to 10-day), 1-2 mg/kg/day (max: 60 mg/day)
	Pediapred	Liquid: 5 mg/5 mL	
	Prelone syrup	Liquid: 15 mg/5 mL	
	Orapred ODT	Chewable tablet: 10, 15, 30 mg	
Prednisone	Prednisone	Tablet: 1, 2.5, 5, 10, 20, 50 mg	Short-course (3- to 10-day), 1-2 mg/kg/day (max: 60 mg/day)
	Prednisone	Liquid: 5 mg/5 mL	
	Intensol	Liquid: 5 mg/mL	

Methylxanthines

GENERIC NAME	BRAND NAME	DOSE FORM	DOSE[b]
Theophylline	Uniphyl Theo-24	Capsules: 100, 125, 200, 300, 400, 600 mg	For all forms: Starting dose: 10 mg/kg/day
	Elixophyllin	Liquid: 80 mg/15 mL	Maximal dose (<1 yr of age): (0.2 × age in wks) + 5 = mg/kg/day
	Theo-Dur	Sprinkles: 50, 75, 125, 200 mg	Maximal dose (>1 yr of age): 16 mg/kg/day, not to exceed the adult maximum (800 mg/day)

Table 239-2 Medications Used to Treat Children With Asthma in the United States[a]—cont'd

QUICK-RELIEF MEDICATIONS

Short-acting, inhaled β2-agonists

GENERIC NAME	BRAND NAME	DOSE FORM	DOSE[b]
Albuterol	Albuterol Sulfate	Nebulizer solution: 2.5 mg/3 mL; 0.083% (unit dose[c,d])	0.05 mg/kg (min: 1.25 mg; max: 2.5 mg), tid-qid
	AccuNeb	Nebulizer solution: 1.25 mg/3 mL (unit dose), 0.63 mg/3 mL (unit dose)	0.63-1.25 mg, tid-qid
	Proair HFA Proventil HFA	MDI: 108 mcg/puff	2 puffs, 15 min before exercise; 2 puffs, tid-qid prn
	Ventolin HFA	MDI: 100 mcg/puff	
	Albuterol	Oral solution: 2 mg/5 mL	0.1 to 0.2 mg/kg 3 times daily; do not exceed 12 mg/day
Levalbuterol	Xopenex	Nebulizer solution: 0.31 mg/3 mL 0.63 mg/3 mL 1.25 mg/3 mL	0.31-0.63 mg, tid, for maintenance 1.25 mg, tid, for acute bronchospasm and for patients who are unresponsive to lower dose
	Xopenex HFA	MDI: 45 mcg/puff	1-2 puffs up to every 4 hr
Pirbuterol	Maxair	MDI: 200 mcg/puff	2 puffs tid-qid prn

Oral corticosteroids

GENERIC NAME	BRAND NAME	DOSE FORM	DOSE[b,e]
Methylprednisolone	Medrol	Tablet: 4, 6, 8, 16, 24, 32 mg	Short-course (3-10 day) 1-2 mg/kg/day (max: 60 mg/day)
Prednisolone	Prednisolone	Tablet: 5 mg	Short-course (3-10 day) 1-2 mg/kg/day (max: 60 mg/day)
	Pediapred	Liquid: 5 mg/5 mL	
	Prelone syrup	Liquid: 15 mg/5 mL	
	Orapred ODT	Chewable tablet: 10, 15, 30 mg	
Prednisone	Prednisone	Tablet: 1, 2.5, 5, 10, 20, 50 mg Liquid: 5 mg/5 mL	Short-course (3-10 day) 1-2 mg/kg/day (max: 60 mg/day)
	Prednisone Intensol	Liquid: 5 mg/5 mL	

Anticholinergics

GENERIC NAME	BRAND NAME	DOSE FORM	DOSE[b]
Ipratropium bromide	Atrovent HFA	MDI: 17 mcg/puff Nebulizer solution: 0.20 mg/mL; 0.02% (ampule)	1-2 puffs, qid 1 ampule, qid
Ipratropium bromide/ albuterol	DuoNeb	Nebulizer solution: 0.20 mg/mL/2.5 mg albuterol (ampule)	1 ampule qid

bid, Twice daily; *DPI,* dry powder inhaler; *MDI,* metered dose inhaler; *prn,* as needed; *qd,* every day; *qid,* 4 times daily; *tid,* 3 times daily.

[a]The most important determinant of appropriate dosing is the clinician's judgment of the child's response to therapy. The clinician must monitor several clinical parameters to assess both efficacy and adverse effect and must adjust the dose accordingly.

The stepwise approach to therapy emphasizes that, once control of asthma is achieved, the dose of medication should be carefully titrated to the minimum dose required to maintain control.

[b]These doses are suggested as guides for making clinical decisions. The clinician must use personal judgment to tailor treatment to the specific needs of the child and family.

[c]Do not use partial unit dose.

[d]Some nebulizer solutions contain benzalkonium, which may cause bronchospasm in some patients.

[e]Course of 7 days or less is usually sufficient. In some cases, the exacerbation may require up to 10 days of treatment.

Patients may relapse when inhaled corticosteroids are discontinued. The US Food and Drug Administration has approved many inhaled corticosteroids for maintenance treatment of asthma in children. Notably, however, approval age varies with preparation. Budesonide inhalation suspension was the 1st inhaled corticosteroid approved in the United States for nebulization; it is also the 1st inhaled corticosteroid approved for use in infants as young as 12 months. Budesonide inhalation suspension has been used in

Table 239-3	Medication Class
Intermittent	Short-acting inhaled β2-agonist as needed for symptoms but less than twice a week (reassess if needed mover than twice a week) Inhaled β2-agonist or cromolyn before exercise or exposure to allergen; no daily long-term control medication needed
Mild persistent	Daily inhaled antiinflammatory: low-dose inhaled corticosteroid of cromolyn or nedocromil or sustained-relief theophylline; or Leukotriene modifier Short-acting inhaled β2-agonist as needed for symptoms (reassess if needed daily or if use increases)
Moderate persistent	Inhaled corticosteroids: medium dose or low-medium dose and inhaled long-acting β2-agonist or sustained released theophylline; or Medium- to high-dose inhaled corticosteroids and long-acting bronchodilators Short-acting inhaled β2-agonist as needed for symptoms (reassess if needed daily or if use increases)
Severe persistent	Inhaled corticosteroids: high-dose and long-acting bronchodilators and systemic corticosteroids Short-acting inhaled β2-agonist as needed for symptoms (reassess if needed daily or if use increases)

62 countries worldwide and can be prescribed either on a daily or on a twice-daily regimen.

Several issues exist that mediate potential adverse events with inhaled corticosteroid therapy. These issues include the drug delivery device, dose level, formulation of the preparation, bioavailability, the potency of the inhaled corticosteroid, and the deposition either in the pulmonary system or in the gastrointestinal system. The choice of corticosteroid preparation prescribed depends on the adverse effects and the desired level of symptom control in individual patients.

Cromolyn sodium and nedocromil sodium have good safety profiles. Cromolyn is known to be a mast-cell stabilizer and decreases the early- and late-phase response after allergen challenge. It can be dispensed in a nebulizer solution or as a metered dose inhaler. Nedocromil is a pyranoquinoline and is also available as a metered dose inhaler, although it has not been in favor in recent years because it does not taste good. Nedocromil may be added to inhaled steroids as a possible steroid-sparing effect. Its biggest draw back is its unpleasant taste.

A relatively new class of medications includes the LT modifiers. 5-Lipoxygenase inhibitors such as zileuton block synthesis of all LTs. LT-receptor antagonists block LTD4 receptors. Examples include montelukast and zafirlukast. These medications are popular because they can be administered in oral form and have been shown in multiple studies to improve symptoms and pulmonary function; they can also be used with inhaled corticosteroids. The medications may have some drawbacks, particularly because they can, in some cases, affect the pharmacokinetics of certain medications (eg, zafirlukast affects warfarin). Rare cases of Churg-Strauss syndrome have been reported in adult patients with systemic eosinophilia and eosinophilic vasculitis.

Long-acting β2-agonists such as salmeterol and formoterol are not intended for treating acute exacerbations. These medications have lipophilic large side chains and bind tightly to β-receptors, allowing the duration of action up to 12 hours. These medications act by relaxing bronchial smooth muscle, improving symptoms, and reducing the need for quick-relief medication. Currently, long-acting β-agonists are available only as dry powder inhalers. Salmeterol has been combined with inhaled corticosteroids such as fluticasone. Preparations of formoterol combined with inhaled corticosteroids are in development. Combination therapy may be of value. The long-acting β-agonist and inhaled corticosteroid have complementary modes of action. Corticosteroids increase β-receptor synthesis, and long-acting β2-agonists prime glucocorticoid receptors for activation.

Theophylline (methylxanthine) use has diminished in the treatment of children with asthma. Although methylxanthines produce mild to moderate bronchodilation and have other potential beneficial effects, they are a challenge to use and require frequent monitoring. In addition, numerous side effects, including some that are life threatening, limit their use. Theophylline metabolism and serum levels are altered by fever, viral illnesses such as influenza, certain drugs such as cimetidine and erythromycin, and liver disease.

Currently, a relatively new asthma medication called omalizumab has been developed.[12] Omalizumab is an anti-IgE humanized monoclonal antibody that binds circulating IgE regardless of specificity and does not activate complement or cause anaphylaxis. Once bound, it forms small biologically inert anti-IgE complexes. Studies have shown that serum IgE levels directly correlate with the odds ratio for the development of asthma. In addition, total serum IgE has been shown to be directly related to asthma and wheezing in the first 5 years of life. IgE is necessary because the initial steps require binding of IgE to mast cells to begin the allergic cascade. By preventing the IgE from binding to mast cell receptors, the allergic cascade cannot be completed. Omalizumab has been shown to improve lung function, to significantly reduce sputum eosinophil counts, and to improve quality of life.[13] Currently, it is used only by asthma specialists, and dose depends on the patient's weight and serum IgE level.

For infants and children younger than 5 years, long-term controller treatment is recommended when a consistent requirement exists for symptomatic treatment greater than 2 times per week or severe exacerbations fewer than 6 weeks apart requiring inhaled β2-agonist treatment more than every 4 hours for 24 hours.

The Baylor Health Care System has recommended a Rules of Two when considering candidates for maintenance therapy.* If patients use quick-relief medication more than 2 times per week, are awakened at night from asthma symptoms more than 2 times per month, or need to refill a quick-reliever inhaler medication more than 2 times per year, then they should be on additional controller medication. Consider maintenance therapy if daytime symptoms or nighttime symptoms fulfill one of these criteria. In addition, if peak flow variability is greater than 20% or FEV_1 is less than 80%, controller therapy should be considered in children. These recommendations are based on the 2002 National Asthma Education and Prevention Program guidelines.[8]

APPROACH TO DIFFICULT-TO-MANAGE DISEASE

Five questions and issues should be assessed when dealing with a patient who does not respond to reasonable therapy.

1. Is it asthma? Anatomic lesions or other medical conditions should be ruled out.
2. Is the patient adherent to the medication regimen, and is the patient's technique for the medication delivery appropriate?
3. Did the patient run out of medication and not realize it or say so?
4. Is a continual exposure present, environmental or otherwise, that is continuing to cause problems for the patient?
5. A referral or a 2nd opinion from a specialist should be considered if the desired effect is not being achieved.

*Rules of Two™ is a registered trademark of the Baylor Health Care System, National Asthma Education and Prevention Program.

WHEN TO REFER

- The child has had a life-threatening asthma exacerbation or has been admitted to a pediatric intensive care unit.
- The goals of asthma therapy are not being met after 3 to 6 months of treatment.
- Signs and symptoms are atypical.
- The child has severe persistent asthma.
- The child requires more than 2 bursts of oral corticosteroids per year.

WHEN TO ADMIT

- Children who do not respond to β-agonists rescue therapy or who have peak flows less than 50% of personal best after β-agonist therapy
- Children who have difficulty breathing, as evidenced by:
  - Chest and neck pulling in
  - Hunched posture
  - Trouble walking or talking
  - Stopping of playing and inability to restart
  - Gray or blue lips or fingernails

TOOLS FOR PRACTICE

Community Coordination and Advocacy

- *Allergy and Asthma Tool Kit for School Nurses* (tool kit), American Academy of Allergy, Asthma and Immunology (AAAAI), AAP endorsed (www.aaaai.org/members/allied_health/tool_kit/handouts/).
- *Asthma-Friendly Schools Initiative* (tool kit), American Lung Association, AAP endorsed (www.lungusa.org).
- *Is the Action Plan Working?* (checklist), American Academy of Allergy, Asthma, and Immunology (AAAAI), AAP endorsed (www.aaaai.org/members/allied_health/tool_kit/handouts/action_plan.pdf.

Engaging Patient and Family

- *Asthma and Your Child* (brochure), American Academy of Pediatrics (patiented.app.org).
- *Guide to Your Child's Allergies and Asthma* (book), American Academy of Pediatrics (www.aap.org/bookstore).
- *What is a Pediatric Allergist/Immunologist?* (fact sheet), American Academy of Pediatrics (www.aap.org/family/WhatisPedAllergistImm.pdf).

Medical Decision Support

- *Asthma Gadgets* (on-line course), American Academy of Pediatrics (www.pedialink.org).
- *Asthma and Allergies* (Web page), Centers for Disease Control and Prevention (www.cdc.gov/health/asthma.htm).
- *eQIPP Asthma* (on-line course), American Academy of Pediatrics (www.pedialink.org).
- *My Asthma Action Plan* (form), American Academy of Allergy, Asthma, and Immunology AAAAI), AAP endorsed (www.aaaai.org/members/allied_health/tool_kit/handouts/my_action_plan.pdf).
- *Pediatric Environmental Health, 2nd edition* (book), American Academy of Pediatrics (www.aap.org/bookstore).
- *Sample Asthma Action Plan* (form), American Academy of Pediatrics Schooled in Asthma Project (www.aap.org/schooledinasthma/AsthmaActionPlan.pdf).
- *Sample Asthma Intake Form* (form), American Academy of Pediatrics Schooled in Asthma Project (www.aap.org/schooledinasthma/AsthmaForm.pdf).
- *Sample Dear Doctor Form Letter,* American Academy of Pediatrics Schooled in Asthma Project (www.aap.org/schooledinasthma/DearDoctorLetter.pdf).
- *Sample Asthma Encounter Form* (form), American Academy of Pediatrics Schooled in Asthma Project (www.aap.org/schooledinasthma/AsthmaEncounterForm.pdf).

- *When Should Students with Asthma or Allergies Carry and Self Administer Emergency Medications at School?* (fact sheet), National Heart Lung and Blood Institute, AAP endorsed (www.nhlbi.nih.gov/health/prof/lung/asthma/emer_medi.htm).

RELATED WEB SITES

- American Academy of Allergy, Asthma, and Immunology (AAAAI) (aaaai.org/).
- Asthma and Allergy Foundation of America (AAFA) (www.aafa.org/).
- National Heart, Lung, and Blood Institute (www.nhlbi.nih.gov/about/naepp/index.htm).

AAP POLICY STATEMENTS

American Academy of Pediatrics, Committee on Environmental Health. Ambient air pollution: health hazards to children. *Pediatrics*. 2004;114(6):1699-1707. (aappolicy.aappublications.org/cgi/content/full/pediatrics;114/6/1699).

American Academy of Pediatrics, Committee on Environmental Health. Environmental tobacco smoke: a hazard to children. *Pediatrics*. 1997;99(4):639-664. (aappolicy.aappublications.org/cgi/content/full/pediatrics;99/4/639).

SUGGESTED RESOURCE

National Asthma Education and Prevention Program Expert Panel Report. Guidelines for the Diagnosis and Management of Asthma. Available at: www.nhlbi.nih.gov/guidelines/asthma/index.htm. Accessed April 13, 2006.

REFERENCES

1. American Academy of Allergy, Asthma and Immunology, Incorporated [AAAAI]. *Pediatric Asthma: Promoting Best Practice. Guide for Managing Asthma in Children*. Milwaukee, WI: AAAAI; 2004.
2. Mannino DM, Homa DM, Akinbami LJ, et al. Surveillance for asthma—United States, 1980-1999. *MMWR Surveill Summ*. 2002;51:1-14.
3. Sandford A, Weir T, Pare P. The genetics of asthma. *Am J Respir Crit Care Med*. 1996;153:1749-1765.
4. Fireman P, Hoekelman RA (ed). *Asthma in Primary Care*. St Louis, MO: Mosby; 1997.
5. Bousquet J, Jeferey PK, Busie WW, et al. From bronchoconstriction to airways inflammation and remodeling. *Am J Resp Crit Care Med*. 2000;161(5):1720-1745.
6. Cockcroft DW, Ruffin RE, Frith PA, et al. Determinants of allergen induced asthma: dose of allergen, circulating IgE antibody concentration and bronchial responsiveness to inhaled histamine. *Am Rev Respir Dis*. 1979;120(5):1053-1058.
7. Cohn RC. A review of the effects of medication delivery systems on treatment adherence in children with asthma. *Curr Ther Res Clin Exp*. 2003;64:34-44.
8. National Asthma Education and Prevention Program. Expert panel report: guidelines for the diagnosis and management of asthma update on selected topics—2002. *J Allergy Clin Immunol*. 2002;110(pt2):S141-S219.
9. National Asthma Education and Prevention Program. Expert panel report. *Guidelines for the Diagnosis and Management of Asthma*. Publication No. 97-4051. Bethesda, MD: National Institutes of Health, National Heart, Lung, and Blood Institute; 1997.
10. Castro-Rodriquez JA, Holberg CJ, Wright AL, et al. A clinical index to define risk of asthma in young children with recurrent wheezing. *Am J Respir Crit Care Med*. 2000;162:1403-1406.
11. Milgrom H, Skoner DP, Bensch G, et al. Low-dose levalbuterol in children with asthma: safety and efficacy in comparison with placebo and racemic albuterol. *J Allergy Clin Immunol*. 2001;108:938-945.
12. Busse W, Corren J, Lanier BQ, et al. Omalizumab, anti-IgE recombinant humanized monoclonal antibody, for the treatment of severe allergic asthma. *J Allergy Clin Immunol*. 2001;108:184-190.
13. Brownell J, Casale TB. Anti-IgE therapy. *Immunol Allergy Clin North Am*. 2004;24:551-568.

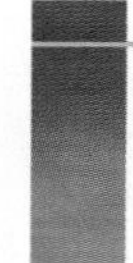

Chapter 240

ATOPIC DERMATITIS

Linda S. Nield, MD; Jonette E. Keri, MD, PhD

DEFINITION

Atopic dermatitis (AD) is a multifactorial dermatologic condition involving chronic inflammation of the skin. It is sometimes referred to as eczema, which is a general term used to describe skin that is erythematous, scaling, vesicular, and crusting. AD is common in individuals with the genetic propensity to develop immunoglobulin E (IgE)-mediated diseases. The associated IgE-mediated diseases include allergic rhinitis, asthma, and food allergies. AD may be the initial condition signaling the progression to further allergic disease, known as the *atopic march*.[1]

ETIOLOGY

The exact cause of AD in unknown, but genetic and environmental factors play a role in its development. Dysfunction of the immune system, specifically abnormal IgE-mediated type I and cell-mediated type IV reactions, and dysfunction of the epidermal barrier lead to AD.[2] The T cells responsible for atopy are mainly T_H2 subtype cells. An area of debate is the *hygiene hypothesis,* which theorizes that decreased exposure to microbes in early childhood stunts immunologic maturation of T_H1 subtype cells, thereby increasing the risk of development of atopic disease later in life caused by an imbalance in T_H2 and T_H1, with overexpression of T_H2 responses as compared with T_H1 responses.

Other cells implicated in the development of AD include macrophages, IgE-bearing Langerhans cells, eosinophils, and mast cells, which release or produce several proinflammatory agents such as histamine, leukotrienes, and prostaglandins. The resulting inflammatory reactions lead to disruption of the epidermis.

Airborne allergens (dust mites, cat and dog dander, molds, pollen), foods (especially milk, eggs, peanuts),[3,4] infectious agents, and other contact allergens have been implicated as potential antigenic triggers. Psychological stress may exacerbate AD.

EPIDEMIOLOGIC FEATURES

AD is predominantly a disease of infancy and childhood. Onset occurs in the first year of life in the majority of affected individuals. The prevalence of disease varies depending on age; more than 10% of infants and young children may be affected, whereas one half this rate occurs in adolescents.[5-7] A survey in 2007 found that almost 18 million Americans had a self-reported diagnosis of AD, and more than one third of them had diagnosis confirmed by a physician.[8] Both sexes are affected equally.[9] The yearly health care cost of AD in the United States has been projected to be as high as almost $4 billion.[10]

DIAGNOSIS

The diagnosis of AD is determined solely by history and clinical examination. The criteria for diagnosis of AD were defined by Hanifin and Lobitz.[11] These criteria are presented in Box 240-1 and are useful in identifying characteristics of patients who have AD. However, patients may have AD and not meet the criteria as originally defined.

DIFFERENTIAL DIAGNOSIS

The differential diagnosis of AD includes seborrheic dermatitis, contact dermatitis (allergic and irritant forms), psoriasis, scabies, dermatophyte infection, and systemic immunologic and metabolic disorders. Some of the systemic disorders include Wiskott-Aldrich syndrome, Leiner disease, histiocytosis X, ataxia telangiectasia, ahistidinemia, aggamaglobulinemia, Hartnup disease, Hurler syndrome, eosinophilic gastroenteritis, acrodermatitis enteropathica, and phenylketonuria. Differentiating AD from other skin conditions may be difficult in some instances, but certain characteristics will aid in the diagnosis. Seborrhea is associated with scaling, commonly on the scalp, forehead, and around the eyebrows; it can also be accompanied by pruritus. The diagnosis of contact dermatitis often requires a positive exposure history to a potential offending agent and will be limited in distribution on the body to the area of contact. Contact dermatitis is more likely to have an acute onset and localized appearance. Absence of a family history also favors a diagnosis of seborrhea or contact dermatitis.

BOX 240-1 Criteria for the Diagnosis of Atopic Dermatitis

MAJOR CRITERIA (ALL THREE MUST BE PRESENT)

1. Pruritus
2. Typical morphology and distribution
   a. Facial and extensor involvement during infancy and early childhood
   b. Flexural lichenification and linearity by adolescence
3. Chronic or recurring dermatitis

MINOR CRITERIA (TWO OR MORE MUST BE PRESENT)

1. Personal or family history of atopy (eg, asthma, allergic rhinoconjunctivitis, atopic dermatitis)
2. Immediate skin test reactivity
3. White dermatographism or delayed blanch to cholinergic agents
4. Anterior subcapsular cataracts

ASSOCIATED CONDITIONS (FOUR OR MORE MUST BE PRESENT)

1. Xerosis, ichthyosis, hyperlinear palms
2. Pityriasis alba
3. Keratosis pilaris
4. Facial pallor, infraorbital darkening *(allergic shiner)*
5. Dennie-Morgan fold
6. Elevated serum immunoglobulin E
7. Keratoconus
8. Nonspecific hand dermatitis
9. Recurring cutaneous infections

From Hanifin JM, Lobitz WC. Newer concepts of atopic dermatology. *Arch Dermatol.* 1977;113:663. Reprinted by permission of the American Medical Association.

CLINICAL MANIFESTATIONS

AD may exhibit as an acute dermatitis associated with severe pruritis, redness, vesicles, and exudation, or it may have a subacute pattern of pruritis, redness, and scaling. Chronic lesions are marked by excoriations, lichenification (thickened skin and deeper or exaggerated skin lines), and postinflammatory hypopigmentation or hyperpigmentation.

AD has 3 distinct stages: (1) infantile, (2) childhood, and (3) adult. AD in infancy is characterized by an eruption of erythematous papules on facial cheeks and extensor surfaces of arms and legs. The hair is dry, and the scalp is often scaly. The childhood stage begins at approximately age 3 years and lasts through puberty. The areas most affected include the antecubital and popliteal folds, neck, and flexor surfaces of wrists and ankles. Clinically, patients in this stage display a more subacute and chronic dermatitis. The adult stage, beginning at puberty onward, is an extension of the childhood stage. Additional clinical signs include diffuse involvement of the body, with xerosis, lichenification, and central facial pallor.

Other associated clinical manifestations include keratosis pilaris, lichen spinulosus, pityriasis alba, Dennie-Morgan folds, urticaria, hyperlinear palms, juvenile plantar dermatosis, nummular eczema, and cataracts. Keratosis pilaris is a disorder of hyperkeratosis. Its characteristic *goose flesh* appearance is secondary to multiple, small, skin-colored or mildly erythematous keratotic papules located on the upper arms, thighs, and facial cheeks. Lichen spinulosus also involves hyperkeratosis; in this condition, tiny hairlike spines top the small papules that occur in crops on various locations on the body. Juvenile plantar dermatosis mainly affects the feet, rarely the hands, and produces shiny, fissured skin on the plantar surfaces.

LABORATORY EVALUATIONS

No routine laboratory studies are needed to diagnose AD. Specific tests to rule out the disorders in the differential list may be necessary if the diagnosis is in question on a case-by-case basis. For example, if recurrent infections occur in the patient, then an immunodeficiency work-up should be considered. Bacterial cultures of encrusted or exudative skin lesions and nares to detect colonization with staphylococcal organisms are warranted in any patient in which secondary infection is suspected or improvement is not noted with standard therapy. Patch testing may be considered to pinpoint potential antigenic triggers, which may add a component of contact dermatitis to the already existing AD. Skin biopsy may be necessary when definitive diagnosis is in question.

MANAGEMENT

Uncomplicated Case

Treatment of AD is directed at relieving dryness, inflammation, and pruritus and eradicating secondary bacterial infections. Daily applications of emollients, especially after brief warm baths, in the form of creams or ointments are the most efficacious way of treating dryness. Ointments are better in more severe cases and are better than emollients. However, if discomfort (ie. stinging sensation) occurs with ointment application, or if the ointment feels too occlusive, such as in humid warm weather, then creams can be substituted. Bathing should last no longer than 5 minutes, and mild soaps or nondetergent cleansers are recommended to wash the body. The patient should be patted dry with a towel and the emollient applied immediately to all skin and the prescription topical applied to affected areas.

Inflammation is best treated with corticosteroids. Generally, ointments tend to work better than creams. However, creams are sometimes preferred for cosmetic appeal and can be used for acute weeping, erythematous lesions. Ointments remain the choice for chronic dermatitis in which dryness and lichenification predominate. A low-potency topical steroid such as 1% hydrocortisone or desonide can be used for mild disease even on the diaper area and face; twice-daily dosing should be limited to a 2-week course or less. Mid- to high-potency steroids, such as triamcinolone or fluocinonide, can be used in more severe cases of AD on the trunk and extremities. Strong, halogenated steroids should not be applied to the face, axillae, or groin, and an oral systemic steroid taper should rarely be prescribed. The adverse effects of topical steroids increase with increasing potency. The most worrisome side effects include dermal and epidermal atrophy and suppression of the pituitary-adrenal axis. Applying topical steroids to the occluded groin area of a diapered child increases the risk of systemic side effects.

Topical tacrolimus and pimecrolimus are relatively new antiinflammatory agents approved for children ages 2 years and older. Most efficacious in mild to moderate disease, these nonsteroidal immunomodulators are calcineurin inhibitors and alternatives to topical steroids that can be applied to the face. The US Food and Drug Administration has added a black-box warning to tacrolimus ointment and pimecrolimus cream based on a theoretical risk of malignancy derived from safety profiles of oral calcineurin inhibitors. In general, these topical medications are considered safe and effective.[12,13] Other topical medications for AD, such as coal tar and doxepin, are not routinely prescribed by pediatricians.

Although evidence is lacking that antihistamines help relieve the pruritis associated with AD, they are often prescribed, especially for patients with accompanying allergic rhinitis, urticaria, and sleep disturbance. Nonsedating antihistamines such as loratadine can be used daily. The sedating antihistamines, hydroxyzine and diphenhydramine, are most useful at bedtime. Behavior modification such as teaching the child to rub rather than scratch and wearing mittens or socks on the hands to bed at night will help lessen the itch-scratch cycle. Frequent trimming of the child's fingernails may decrease the amount of trauma applied to skin and reduce secondary infection.

The role of dietary management of patients with AD remains controversial. Dietary changes should be judicious. Peanuts, milk, and eggs are the most common food culprits. If food allergies are highly likely as determined by a pediatric allergist, then strict avoidance of foods that serve as antigenic triggers should be encouraged, remembering over 90% of IgE-mediated food allergies in children are caused by eight foods: cow milk, hen eggs, soy, peanuts, tree nuts (and seeds), wheat, fish, and shellfish.[4] Food allergies can produce a variety of skin reactions in addition to AD, including urticaria, anaphylaxis, and angioedema. The efficacy of alternative medicine treatments for food allergies, such as herbal or probiotic supplementation, remains unknown.

Complicated Case

If AD continues to flare despite compliance with medication and appropriate skin care, then secondary infection may be responsible. Many patients who have AD have significant colonization with *Staphylococcus aureus (S aureus)*. Along with susceptibility to recurrent bacterial infection the AD patient is also prone to herpes simplex virus, human papillomavirus (HPV), and molluscum contagiosum. Secondary bacterial infections usually respond well to topical or oral antibiotics. Cephalexin, dicloxacillin, amoxicillin-clavulanate, azithromycin, and clindamycin are reasonable choices for oral treatment, and mupirocin is the topical antibiotic of choice. If *S aureus* superinfection occurs, then hospitalization for aggressive care and intravenous antibiotics may be required. Cultures of the skin may help identify appropriate antibiotic sensitivities. Application of nasal mupirocin may be necessary to eradicate bacterial carriage. A widespread herpes infection, known as eczema herpeticum or Kaposi varicelliform eruption, will require treatment with intravenous acyclovir. Various treatment modalities are available for HPV and molluscum contagiosum infection in the patient with AD who is likely to have a more severe, persistent course of these usually self-limiting conditions. HPV treatments include vesicants, immunomodulators, cryotherapy, or ablation with carbon dioxide laser. Molluscum contagiosum can be treated with manual expression, cryotherapy, or topical application of cantharidin or imiquimod.

More aggressive interventions such as systemic immunomodulators or ultraviolet light therapy for severe cases would be prescribed at the discretion of the skin experts.

PREVENTION

AD cannot be prevented, but meticulous adherence to proper skin care can control symptoms and secondary infection. Moisturization of the skin with daily applications of emollients, especially after bathing, is crucial to keep the skin hydrated. Although some reports suggest that breastfeeding increases the risk of AD, evidence exists supporting breastfeeding as means of reducing the risk of AD.[14] Prophylactic avoidance of food allergens, both for lactating mothers and infants via exclusive breastfeeding in the first 6 months of life, may be helpful in families with a strong family history of atopy[15,16]; however, this is an area of ongoing research.

WHEN TO REFER

- Recalcitrant cases to dermatologist or an allergist
- To dermatologist for aggressive treatment of secondary HPV or molluscum contagiosum infections

WHEN TO ADMIT

- Severe cases requiring systemic immunomodulation
- Extensive secondary bacterial infection requiring intravenous antibiotics
- A widespread herpes infection (eczema herpeticum, Kaposi varicelliform eruption)

TOOLS FOR PRACTICE

Engaging Patient and Family

- *Eczema (Atopic Dermatitis)* (brochure), American Academy of Pediatrics (patiented.aap.org).

Medical Decision Support

- *Guidelines of Care for Atopic Dermatitis*, American Academy of Dermatology (www.aad.org/pm/science/_docs/ClinicalResearch_Atopic%20Dermatitis%20Part%20I.pdf).
- *Pediatric Dermatology: A Quick Reference Guide* (book), American Academy of Pediatrics (www.aap.org/bookstore).

REFERENCES

1. Hahn EL, Bacharier LB. The atopic march: the pattern of allergic disease development in childhood. *Immunol Allergy Clin North Am*. 2005;25(2):231-246.
2. Pastar Z, Lipozencic J, Ljubojevic S. Etiopathogenesis of atopic dermatitis—an overview. *Acta Dermatovenerol Croat*. 2005;13(1):54-62.
3. Garcia C, El-Qutob D, Martorell A et al. Sensitization in early age to food allergens in children with atopic dermatitis. *Allergol Immunopathol (Madr)*. 2007:35(1):15-20.
4. Allen KJ, Hill DJ, Heine RG. Food Allergy in childhood. *Med J Aust*. 2006;185(7):394-400.
5. Rodriguez Orozco AR, Nunez Tapia RM. Prevalence of atopic dermatitis in 6-14 year old children in Morelia, Michoacan, Mexico. *Rev Alerg Mex*. 2007;54(1):20-23.
6. Wuthrich B. Clinical aspects, epidemiology, and prognosis of atopic dermatitis. *Ann Allergy Asthma Immunol*. 1999;83(5):464-470.
7. Laughter D, Istvan JA, Tofte SJ, et al. The prevalence of atopic dermatitis in Oregon schoolchildren. *J Am Acad Dermatol*. 2000;43(4):649-655.
8. Hanifin JM, Reed ML. A population-based survey of eczema prevalence in the United States. *Dermatitis*. 2007; 18(2):82-91.
9. Schachner L, Ling NS, Press S. A statistical analysis of a pediatric dermatology clinic. *Pediatr Dermatol*. 1983; 1(2):157-164.
10. Ellis CN, Drake LA, Prendergast MM, et al. Cost of atopic dermatitis and eczema in the United States. *J Am Acad Dermatol*. 2002;46(3):361-370.
11. Hanifin JM, Lobitz WC. Newer concepts of atopic dermatology. *Arch Dermatol*. 1977;113:663.
12. Muzzenberger PJ, Montejo JM. Safety of topical calcineurin inhibitors for the treatment of atopic dermatitis. *Pharmacotherapy*. 2007;27(7):1020-1028.
13. Ricci G, Dondi A, Patrizi A. Role of topical calcineurin inhibitors on atopic dermatitis of children. *Curr Med Chem*. 2007;14(14):1579-1591.
14. Kilchevsky E, James E, Fong J, et al. Atopic dermatitis and breastfeeding. *Pediatrics*. 2204;114(14):1129.
15. Kajosaari M, Saarinen UM. Propyhlaxis of atopic disease by 6 months' total solid food elimination. Evaluation of 135 exclusively breast-fed infants of atopic families. *Acta Paediatr Scand*. 1983;72(3):411-414.
16. Zieger RS, Heller S, Mellon MH, et al. Effect of combined maternal and infant food-allergen avoidance on development of atopy in early infancy: a randomized study. *J Allergy Clin Immunol*. 1989;84(1):72-89.

Chapter 241

BACTERIAL SKIN INFECTIONS

Randall G. Fisher, MD; Catherine Chen, MD; Judith V. Williams, MD

Bacterial infections of the skin are common.[1] They are most often caused by gram-positive bacteria, specifically *Staphylococcus aureus* and group A streptococci.[2,3] The clinical disease that results depends on the infection's location within the skin. For example, impetigo involves only the most superficial layer of the epidermis; cellulitis is an infection deep in the dermis, even involving subcutaneous fat.

IMPETIGO

Etiology

S aureus is the major cause of impetigo in childhood. It is responsible for virtually 100% of bullous impetigo and causes approximately 75% of nonbullous impetigo; the remainder is caused by group A β-hemolytic *Streptococcus*.

In nonbullous impetigo the skin lesions may start with small vesicles or pustules, but these are often not evident by the time the physician sees the patient. Crusts, usually honey colored, are seen instead. Removing these crusts exposes a moist, glistening base, which is a superficial erosion of the epidermis; culture usually reveals *S aureus*.

History

The patient usually has no history of preceding trauma to the skin. Mild to moderate itching may be associated

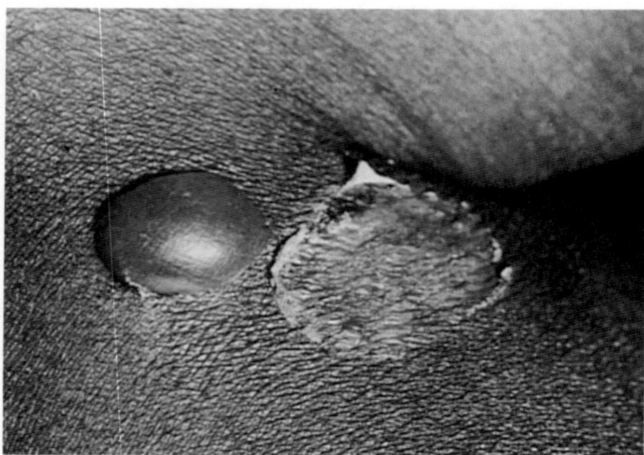

Figure 241-1 Bullous impetigo. The roof of the bulla is thin and delicate; the contents consist of some leukocytes that have settled at the inferior pole and some slightly turbid supernatant fluid. The larger adjacent bulla already has ruptured and discharged its contents. The delicate roof has collapsed onto the base. Lesions of this type may be caused by exfoliatin-producing organisms.

with the lesions. Other family members also may be affected.

Physical Findings

Impetigo is found most commonly on the face and may appear as single or multiple lesions. Lesions may be scattered elsewhere on the body as well. The usual findings are yellow- or honey-colored crusts, which when removed reveal a pink, superficially eroded, glistening base. The culture sample should be obtained from this base. With bullous impetigo, intact bullae, if present, contain deceptively clear fluid. These blisters break easily, leaving behind a superficially denuded skin surface covered with a thin, brown, varnish-like crust that is surrounded by a thin rim of loose, ragged epidermis that represents the remnants of the blister roof (Figure 241-1). Surrounding erythema is minimal, and regional lymphadenopathy is rare.

Laboratory Evaluation

A Gram stain of either the clear blister fluid or the serum underlying the crusts shows gram-positive cocci. Cultures grow *S aureus* or *S pyogenes*.

Differential Diagnosis

Herpes simplex virus (HSV) infection is the condition most often confused with impetigo. Clinical clues that suggest herpes rather than impetigo are as follows:

1. Intact vesicles are more likely to be appreciated by both the patient and the physician in HSV infection than in impetigo. In HSV infection, as the vesicles age they become cloudy and ultimately result in crusts that also may be honey colored. This crusted phase most often causes the diagnostic confusion.
2. HSV infection tends to be a recurrent condition, with the recurrences usually in the same location (usually oral and perioral lesions). Such recurrence is not the case with impetigo.
3. When an impetiginous pustule is unroofed, it is noticeably filled with pus; a herpetic lesion may appear to be pus filled, but when it is unroofed, only a scant amount of clear fluid is found. In impetigo, Gram staining shows numerous gram-positive cocci. In HSV infection, Wright staining of a scraping from the base of a crust (or preferably a vesicle) reveals multinucleated giant cells.

Exclusion From School

Given the potential infectious nature of both staphylococcal and streptococcal skin infections, school nurses are appropriately concerned with this disease, and a child may be asked to leave school until the infection is treated. The period of infectiousness of impetigo is unknown. Most child-care centers and schools recommend exclusion as long as open lesions persist. In reality, staphylococcal impetigo represents a rather low risk for spread in these settings; therefore, 24 hours after appropriate therapy has been initiated, the child can probably return to school without posing a significant risk to other children.

Management

Both topical and systemic antibiotics have been advocated for treating impetigo. Methicillin-resistant *S aureus* (MRSA) has become an increasingly common cause of skin infections in children. A recent study indicated that over 75% of community-associated *S aureus* skin infections in children are caused by MRSA, and 60% of community-onset health care–associated *S aureus* skin infections in children are caused by MRSA.[4] Mupirocin topical antibiotic ointment has been reported to equal or exceed the efficacy of oral erythromycin in the treatment of bacterial impetigo.[5] A cream form is also available. The infected area should be washed carefully and the crusts gently removed, if possible, three times daily before the antibiotic cream or ointment is applied. Traditional topical preparations that contain bacitracin or neomycin, either alone or in combination, have been used. However, because they are poorly absorbed, these preparations are not particularly effective.[6,7] Topical mupirocin should be considered whenever feasible because it can be effective in treating impetigo caused by MRSA.[8] However, notably, mupirocin resistance is increasing in the MRSA USA 300 clone, the predominant circulating strain in the United States, and similar cases have been reported in different clones in other countries.[9-12] Remarkably, mupirocin may retain the ability (albeit reduced) to decolonize patients with resistant strains.[13] However, mupirocin is not effective in treating active infection with resistant strains. To optimize its efficacy, mupirocin should be used judiciously. Some authors recommend sampling MRSA populations for mupirocin susceptibility before incorporating mupirocin into infection-control programs and avoiding extended mupirocin use where MRSA is endemic.[14,15] New topical preparations are in development. One such product, retapamulin, has some activity against MRSA in vitro,[16] but clinical data are currently lacking.

Systemic antibiotics should be used for more extensive lesions. Clindamycin might be an appropriate choice in the era of MRSA, although studies of this approach have not been published. The traditional choices in the *pre-MRSA* era were erythromycin, a penicillinase-resistant penicillin (eg, dicloxacillin), amoxicillin-clavulanic acid, or cephalexin.[4] These agents would still be appropriate for treatment of disease caused by methicillin-sensitive *S aureus* (MSSA) or *S pyogenes*. The treatment course should be 7 to 10 days. Patients with more extensive disease who fail traditional empiric antibiotic therapy should have cultures and susceptibility studies performed.

Complications and Prognosis

With appropriate antibiotic therapy, prompt healing is expected; most patients show marked improvement within several days. Bacteriologic cures occur within 7 to 10 days in nearly all cases. If the infection does not respond rapidly to therapy, then it may be caused by an antibiotic-resistant strain. In such cases the initial culture and susceptibility results serve as a guide in selecting an alternate antibiotic.

Historically, differentiating between staphylococcal and streptococcal impetigo was deemed important, given that glomerulonephritis can be a sequela of the latter form. Evidence now shows that treatment of streptococcal skin infections does not alter the risk of developing glomerulonephritis.

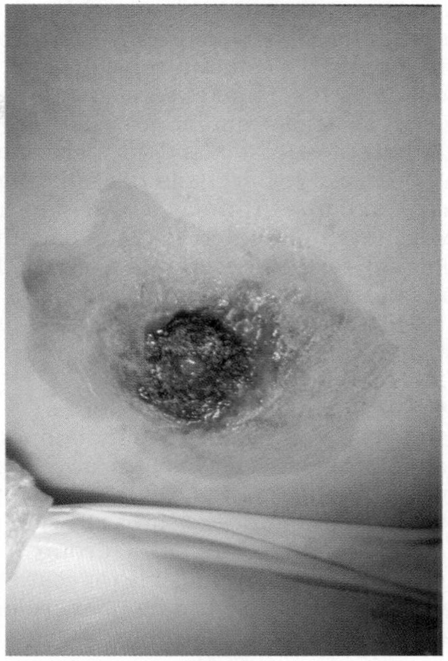

Figure 241-2 Streptococcal pyoderma (ecthyma). Lesions progress to become necrotic in appearance with deep punched-out ulcers. The surrounding erythema and the location on the lower leg are typical of this streptococcal lesion.

PYODERMA

Etiology

In contrast to the superficial nature of impetigo, which mainly involves the top layers of the epidermis, pyoderma frequently extends through the epidermal layer into the underlying dermis. The process may start with small erythematous papules and rapidly proceed through vesicular, pustular, and crusted stages, during which stage it might be clinically confused with impetigo. Streptococcal pyoderma is more common in warm, humid environments; higher humidity favors the survival of group A streptococci on normal skin. Presumably, trauma to the skin results in inoculation followed by infection.

History

Streptococcal pyoderma may occur in epidemics among children of lower socioeconomic status who live in crowded conditions in warm, humid environments. In contrast to impetigo the streptococcal skin lesions occur most commonly on the lower extremities, where they are usually preceded by trauma such as a scratch or insect bite. Family members also may be affected.

Physical Findings

The early lesion is a pustule (hence the term pyoderma) with surrounding erythema, but the more advanced lesion of ecthyma is seen more often. At first glance, this lesion appears as a thick, usually brown crust surrounded by erythema. When the crust is removed, an actual ulcer is revealed (Figure 241-2), in contrast to the superficial erosion underlying the crust of impetigo. Also in contrast to impetigo, regional adenopathy is often present with streptococcal pyoderma.

Laboratory Evaluation

A culture sample taken from the base of the denuded ulcer usually grows group A β-hemolytic streptococci. *S aureus* is occasionally recovered concomitantly, in which case it is thought to be a secondary invader.

Differential Diagnosis

Ecthyma gangrenosum is an uncommon but serious manifestation of sepsis in immune-compromised hosts. It has been most frequently associated with *Pseudomonas aeruginosa* infection but can be seen with other gram-negative organisms or even with fungi. Clinical features that help differentiate this lesion from ecthyma are (1) the location (ecthyma gangrenosum is often on the upper extremities or in the inguinal or axillary folds), (2) the lesion's appearance (a deeper ulcer covered with a tightly adherent, black [gangrenous] crust), and (3) the host (a seriously ill, usually immunocompromised patient who exhibits other signs of sepsis).

Management

Pyoderma is treated with antibiotics, although the most appropriate route of administration is still a matter of debate. Some evidence indicates that applying topical antibiotics to scratches and insect bites reduces the incidence of subsequent pyoderma[17]; thus topical antibiotics may be advocated prophylactically for traumatic skin lesions.[18] Although topical mupirocin has proven effective for impetigo caused by group A streptococci, systemic antibiotics still are recommended for streptococcal infections, particularly if the infection is extensive. Injectable benzathine penicillin G is effective, but a 7- to 10-day course of oral penicillin or erythromycin is preferred if the patient is likely to be adherent to the prescribed regimen. Penicillin treatment occasionally fails, presumably because of the persistence of coexisting penicillinase-producing *S aureus* organisms.

Complications

Complications are uncommon, although both local and systemic problems can result from streptococcal pyoderma. Cellulitis may develop if the infection extends into larger and deeper areas of skin and subcutaneous tissue. Some strains of group A streptococci produce the toxin responsible for scarlet fever.

As mentioned previously, acute glomerulonephritis may follow streptococcal infection of the skin. It is caused by only a few nephritogenic serotypes (49, 55, and 57) of pyoderma-inducing streptococci. The usual period from onset of infection to development of the glomerulonephritis is 18 to 21 days. Fortunately, skin infection with streptococci never leads to acute rheumatic fever. Systemic antibiotic therapy clears the skin infection and helps to reduce the spread of streptococcal infection to the patient's playmates and family.

Prognosis

The aforementioned complications are uncommon, and in most patients the lesions heal uneventfully. Because they are deeper, streptococcal lesions often take longer than staphylococcal lesions to heal; however, bacteriologic cures are usually accomplished within a week. If a prompt response is not achieved, then a secondary infection from a penicillinase-producing staphylococcal strain should be considered, particularly if penicillin was used for treatment. Erythromycin-resistant strains of group A streptococci also may be encountered.

FOLLICULITIS

Etiology

Bacterial folliculitis is a moderately common disorder that primarily affects older children and young adults. It is an infection of the hair follicles, caused almost exclusively by *S aureus*. In rare cases the infection is caused by gram-negative organisms, which occurs occasionally in patients whose acne is being treated with antibiotics.[19] Also, *P aeruginosa* is the usual cause of hot tub folliculitis, which causes pruritic papules and pustules on the trunk and proximal extremities. The lesions usually clear without treatment, although antipruritics can be used. Typically, however, *S aureus* causes folliculitis, and this type of infection is the subject of discussion here.

History

Staphylococcal folliculitis appears most commonly as a chronic eruption unaccompanied by symptoms, although occasionally a patient has mild discomfort or pruritus.

Physical Findings

The lesions in staphylococcal folliculitis are usually located on the buttocks and upper portion of the thighs, over which individual small papules and pustules are scattered. The key to the diagnosis is that, on close inspection, hairs can be seen growing out of the very center of many of the lesions.

Laboratory Evaluation

In the typical case, culturing is not usually necessary. If, however, the presentation is atypical and laboratory confirmation is desired, then the contents of a fresh pustule should be cultured.

Differential Diagnosis

Clinically, folliculitis caused by gram-negative organisms differs from staphylococcal folliculitis in its distribution, with lesions occurring primarily on the face (often concentrated in the perioral and perinasal areas) and shoulders. Hot tub folliculitis usually appears on the lower trunk, areas most exposed to the contaminated water in the tub.

Keratosis pilaris is another common follicular disorder that exhibits as tiny, rough, scaling papules on the back of the upper parts of the arms, the buttocks, and the thighs. Although the distribution may be similar to that of staphylococcal folliculitis the appearance of the lesions is not. In keratosis pilaris the lesions are smaller, more numerous, and scaling, but not pustular.

Management

The usual mild case of staphylococcal folliculitis can be managed by having the patient use an antiseptic cleanser (eg, chlorhexidine) or antibacterial soap containing triclosan or triclocarban daily or every other day for at least several weeks. For more extensive involvement a 7- to 10-day course of systemic antibiotics (eg, erythromycin or dicloxacillin) is suggested in addition to the topical regimen.

Complications and Prognosis

Most patients respond to treatment; if not, then a bacterial culture should be performed to rule out infection by gram-negative organisms or MRSA. Some patients are plagued with recurrences, for which a more prolonged course of antibiotic therapy is recommended. In rare cases the follicular infection extends deeply, producing a furuncle.

FURUNCLES AND ABSCESSES

Etiology

Unchecked folliculitis may result in furuncles (pus-filled nodules or boils) that are almost always caused by *S aureus*. Although most clinicians use the terms *furuncle* and *abscess* interchangeably, abscesses are collections of pus within the dermis and deeper skin tissues that do not originate from a primary folliculitis. Bacteria may be inoculated into the skin and underlying soft tissue by traumatic injury, including surgery.

Most skin abscesses are caused by *S aureus,* but gram-negative and anaerobic organisms also can be causes.[20,21]

History

A history of trauma may be elicited but often is not, especially with furuncles. Immunodeficiency states and diabetes may predispose certain patients to bacterial skin infections, but the typical patient who has a furuncle or abscess has no underlying medical disease.

Physical Findings

Furuncles and abscesses are fluctuant masses filled with pus. They often begin as hard, tender, red nodules and become more fluctuant and painful with time. Abscesses tend to be larger and deeper than furuncles, but the two lesions may sometimes be difficult to differentiate clinically.

Laboratory Evaluation

A Gram stain of the pustular material may provide a clue to the bacterial cause. However, for precise identification, cultures are required. If anaerobic cultures are desired, then material is ideally collected by aspirating the pus, sealing the syringe, and promptly delivering it to the laboratory. If insufficient material is available to aspirate, then a swab culture can be used for anaerobic, as well as aerobic, cultures. Blood culture results rarely are positive in patients with furuncles or abscesses and are not indicated unless the patient shows signs of sepsis.

Management

Very small furuncles can be treated with moist heat, which promotes drainage. For larger furuncles, incision and drainage is the mainstay of therapy. Clinical evidence suggests that, for furuncles less than 5 cm in diameter, incision and drainage alone results in complete healing in most cases.[21] For patients with abscesses larger than 5 cm, or for those with surrounding cellulitis or signs of systemic illness such as fever, systemic antibiotics should be used. If lesions are seen early in their development, then systemic antibiotics may result in involution, obviating the need for incision and drainage. In the recent past, dicloxacillin, cephalexin, and erythromycin were considered the antibiotics of choice; however, this consideration needs to be reevaluated in light of the explosion of MRSA in furunculosis. Most community-associated MRSA isolates are susceptible to trimethoprim-sulfamethoxazole, and many are sensitive to clindamycin. Clindamycin has the advantage of excellent penetration into the infected tissues; however, some erythromycin-resistant strains of MRSA have inducible resistance to clindamycin. The clinician is advised to know local susceptibility patterns. Culture results from abscesses may help in the ultimate selection of the appropriate antibiotic.

Complications

Recurrent furunculosis sometimes prompts a search for an underlying immunodeficiency, a search that almost always goes unrewarded. However, many such patients harbor *S aureus* in a sequestered mucocutaneous site, the most common of which is the anterior nares. Application of mupirocin to the external nares twice daily for 5 days and repeating the process monthly or every 2 months decreases recurrences by approximately one half. Some experts recommend an every-other-day total-body scrub with an antiseptic cleansing agent, such as chlorhexidine, or antibacterial soap containing triclosan or triclocarban, although overuse of these antiseptic soaps may dry the skin, harming skin integrity. Some clinicians are also advocating the addition of a small amount of bleach to the bath water. Anecdotally, this approach shows some promise, but as of this writing, no studies evaluating its efficacy have been conducted.

Most oral antibiotics do not eradicate nasal carriage of *S aureus,* but clindamycin is an exception. In cases that are refractory to all the previously described methods a single oral dose of clindamycin, given daily for 3 months, may be effective at eliminating recurrences.

In rare cases a staphylococcal abscess may be the focus of toxin production, resulting in staphylococcal scalded skin syndrome (most commonly seen in infants and neonates), toxic shock syndrome, or staphylococcal scarlet fever.

Prognosis

Untreated lesions often rupture and drain spontaneously. After either surgical or spontaneous drainage, uneventful healing is the rule. Larger lesions may leave scars.

CELLULITIS

Etiology

Cellulitis is a deep, locally diffuse infection of the skin that has systemic manifestations and life-threatening potential.[22] It usually involves the face, an extremity, or the perianal area.[23] On an extremity the bacteria presumably have been externally inoculated into the deep dermal tissue, although the portal of entry is often undetectable clinically. A hematogenous or lymphangitic source is also possible and may explain the development of cellulitis in some cases in which the overlying skin is unbroken. Before the introduction of protein-conjugated *Haemophilus influenzae* type b (Hib) vaccines in 1988, Hib was a frequent cause of facial cellulitis *(buccal cellulitis),* usually accompanied by bacteremia, in children. The incidence of invasive infections from this organism in the United States has declined by 95% and now occurs primarily in undervaccinated populations or in infants who have not completed the primary Hib vaccine series.[2] Almost 90% of cases of facial cellulitis in the post-Hib vaccine era are related to trauma or to dental or sinus infection. Buccal cellulitis is a disappearing disease.[24]

Other organisms figure more prominently in cellulitis at other sites. Preseptal (periorbital) cellulitis is likely to be caused by *Streptococcus pneumoniae* in younger children and by group A streptococci in older children.[25] *S aureus* and group A streptococci more commonly are responsible for cellulitis of the extremities. *S aureus* and group A streptococci are the most common cause of perianal dermatitis, with two thirds of the latter patients also having positive pharyngeal cultures. In rare cases, other aerobic and anaerobic bacterial organisms, as well as deep fungal agents such as *Cryptococcus neoformans*, can cause cellulitis. These infections usually occur in immunosuppressed individuals.

History

Children who have cellulitis often feel and appear ill. Fever is frequently present and may precede the clinical skin signs. Patients may complain of pain in the affected area. Symptoms of an accompanying otitis media may be present in buccal cellulitis. Patients who have perianal cellulitis often have pain on defecation. However, patients who have this infection are not usually systemically ill; thus the disease may persist for weeks or months before it is correctly diagnosed.

Physical Findings

Fever at the time of presentation is common. The area of involved skin shows the classic signs of inflammation: redness, swelling, heat, and tenderness.

Laboratory Evaluation

Leukocytosis is a common finding. The causative pathogen is usually assumed from the history and physical examination, given that identifying it by culture is fraught with difficulty. Blood cultures are positive in less than 5% of cases. Many experts advocate culturing the skin directly by preparing the skin with an antiseptic, introducing an 18- or 21-gauge needle into the deep dermis, and aspirating material. If no material is obtained, which is usually the case, then 0.5 to 1 mL of nonbacteriostatic saline is injected and then aspirated. All aspirates should be Gram stained and cultured. Unfortunately, this process leads to identification of the causative organism in only approximately 25% of cases. Skin aspiration is more important, and more likely to be fruitful, in special cases such as cellulitis in an immunocompromised host, cellulitis that is not responsive to empiric therapy directed at *S aureus* and beta-hemolytic streptococci, or cellulitis secondary to an unusual exposure, such as an animal bite. In neonates or undervaccinated hosts who have facial cellulitis, lumbar puncture with culture of cerebrospinal fluid may disclose unsuspected meningitis.

Differential Diagnosis

Erysipelas is a form of cellulitis caused most commonly by group A streptococci. Because infection is limited to the upper dermis, erysipelas has raised and sharply demarcated borders. Bedside differentiation of erysipelas from cellulitis, however, is sometimes difficult and clinically not particularly useful because therapeutic considerations are generally the same for both conditions.

A severe, local, confluent contact dermatitis may sometimes be confused with cellulitis in that both may show marked erythema of the skin. The important differences are that with contact dermatitis the patient complains of itch rather than pain, the skin usually is not tender, and the patient is not febrile. The presence of vesicles also favors contact dermatitis, although vesicles and bullae may sometimes occur in erysipelas or cellulitis as the condition evolves.

Perianal dermatitis, originally thought to be a cellulitis but is now known to be a more superficial infection, may be misdiagnosed as candidiasis or diaper dermatitis. Bright-pink erythema and pain or tenderness of the involved skin suggests bacterial infection, and a swab culture usually shows *S aureus* or group A streptococci. Laboratory personnel must be aware that they are to look for these organisms; otherwise, they will look for enteric flora with a culture from this site. Necrotizing fasciitis is a fulminant skin infection most often caused by group A streptococci (*flesh-eating* bacteria). It is characterized by warm, violaceous, exquisitely tender and markedly edematous (orange peel–like) skin with indiscriminate edges. Systemic toxicity with fever, leukocytosis, thrombocytopenia, hypocalcemia, and hyponatremia is often seen. Systemic antibiotics are an adjunct to prompt surgical debridement, which is the mainstay of therapy. Erythema of the cheeks occurs characteristically in erythema infectiosum (Fifth disease, caused by parvovirus B19), in which a slapped-cheek appearance is noted. Important diagnostic differences between erythema infectiosum and cellulitis are that in the former, the involvement is bilateral, the site is not usually very tender, and the patient does not appear toxic, although the patient may be mildly febrile.

Management

Systemic antibiotics are the mainstay of cellulitis therapy. Mild cases of cellulitis on an extremity may be treated with an oral antibiotic, warm soaks, and outpatient follow-up in several days. Inasmuch as cellulitis of the extremity most often is caused by gram-positive organisms, erythromycin, dicloxacillin, or cephalexin are appropriate drugs to use. More seriously ill patients, including infants and young children, patients with predisposing medical conditions such as diabetes mellitus, patients with immunodeficiencies or on immunosuppressive therapies, or those in whom sepsis is suspected should be hospitalized for parenteral antibiotic therapy.

Complications and Comorbid Conditions

In some instances, findings that are clinically diagnosed as cellulitis may actually be a clue to an underlying, deeper-seated infection. Cellulitis of the periorbital tissues may be secondary to sinusitis; abdominal wall cellulitis may hide an underlying peritonitis; redness, warmth, and swelling of tissues overlying bones or joints may indicate septic arthritis or osteomyelitis; facial cellulitis may be caused by an undiagnosed dental abscess; redness of the neck is sometimes a clue to underlying deep neck space infections; inflammation of the skin of the sacrum might be from an infected pilonidal cyst; redness of the pinna or postauricular area may point to malignant otitis externa or mastoiditis. Uncomplicated cellulitis was once a serious, life-threatening disease, but antibiotics have now reduced the fatality rate to nearly zero in otherwise healthy patients.

Prognosis

With appropriate antibiotic therapy, fever usually resolves within 24 hours. If it does not, then a change in antibiotic therapy should be considered, optimally guided by early culture and bacterial sensitivity results. The skin reaction resolves more slowly than does the fever, sometimes taking a week or longer to subside completely.

COMMUNITY-ASSOCIATED METHICILLIN-RESISTANT *STAPHYLOCOCCUS AUREUS* INFECTIONS

The prevalence of community-associated MRSA is ever increasing. In fact, these strains cause the majority of MRSA cases acquired in the community and are appearing in health care settings, traditionally the province of hospital-acquired strains.[4] The most frequently reported presentation is furunculosis, followed by skin abscesses and cellulitis. Less frequently reported are bullous and nonbullous impetigo, nodules, pustules, and scalded skin syndrome. Community-associated MRSA strains are generally more susceptible to non–β-lactam antibiotics (especially clindamycin and trimethoprim-sulfamethoxazole) than are nosocomial MRSA strains. However, some erythromycin-resistant strains develop resistance to clindamycin during treatment. The microbiology laboratory should provide results of a D-test for strains resistant to erythromycin; if the D-test is negative, then clindamycin can be used.

Community-associated MRSA is becoming a significant health concern and studies are underway to find ways to reduce the spread of MRSA in families, schools, and communities.

WHEN TO REFER

- Preseptal cellulitis
- Treatment failure
- Recurrent bacterial skin infections

WHEN TO ADMIT

- Cellulitis with suspected sepsis or suspected underlying serious infection
- Invasive infections (necrotizing fasciitis)
- Staphylococcal scalded skin syndrome
- Toxic shock syndrome

TOOLS FOR PRACTICE

Medical Decision Support

- *Community-Acquired MRSA* (on-line course), American Academy of Pediatrics (www.pedialink.org/cme/_coursefinder).
- *Pediatric Dermatology: A Quick Reference Guide* (book), American Academy of Pediatrics (www.aap.org/bookstore).
- *Pediatric Dermatology: Skin Essentials* (on-line course), American Academy of Pediatrics (www.pedialink.org/cme/_coursefinder).
- *Red Book: 2006 Report of the Committee on Infectious Diseases*, American Academy of Pediatrics (www.aap.org/bookstore).

REFERENCES

1. Hayden GF. Skin diseases encountered in a pediatric clinic. *Am J Dis Child.* 1985;139:36.
2. American Academy of Pediatrics. Haemophilus influenza infections. In: Peter G, ed. *Red Book: 1997 Report of the Committee on Infectious Diseases*. 24th ed. Elk Grove Village, IL: American Academy of Pediatrics; 1997.
3. Tunnessen WW. Practical aspects of bacterial skin infections in children. *Pediatr Dermatol.* 1985;2:255.
4. Demidovich CW, Wittler RR, Ruff ME, et al. Impetigo: current etiology and comparison of penicillin, erythromycin, and cephalexin therapies. *Am J Dis Child.* 1990; 144:1313.
5. Zetola N, Francis JS, Nuermberger EL, et al. Community-acquired methicillin-resistant Staphylococcus aureus: an emerging threat. *Lancet Infect Dis.* 2005;5:275-286.
6. Mertz PM, Marshall DA, Eaglstein WH, et al. Topical mupirocin treatment of impetigo is equal to oral erythromycin therapy. *Arch Dermatol.* 1989;125:1069.
7. Bass JW, Chan DS, Creamer KM, et al. Comparison of oral cephalexin, topical mupirocin and topical bacitracin for treatment of impetigo. *Pediatr Infect Dis J.* 1997;16: 708-710.
8. Wilkinson RD, Carey WD. Topical mupirocin versus topical Neosporin in the treatment of cutaneous infections. *Int J Dermatol.* 1988;27:514-515.
9. King MD, Humphrey BJ, Wang YF, et al. Emergence of community-acquired methicillin-resistant Staphylococcus aureus USA 300 clone as the predominant cause of skin and soft-tissue infections. *Ann Intern Med.* 2006;144: 309-317.
10. Han LL, McDougal LK, Gorwitz RJ, et al. High frequencies of clindamycin and tetracycline resistance in methicillin-resistant Staphylococcus aureus pulsed-field type USA300 isolates collected at a Boston ambulatory care center. *J Clin Microbiol.* 2007;45:1350-1352.
11. Mulvey MR, MacDougall L, Cholin B, et al. Community-associated methicillin-resistant Staphylococcus aureus, Canada. *Emerg Infect Dis.* 2005;11:844-850.
12. Upton A, Lang S, Heffernan H. Mupirocin and Staphylococcus aureus: a recent paradigm of emerging antibiotic resistance. *J Antimicrob Chemother.* 2003;51:613-617.
13. Semret M, Miller MA. Topical mupirocin for eradication of MRSA colonization with mupirocin-resistant strains. *Infect Control Hosp Epidemiol.* 2001;22:578-580.
14. Walker ES, Vasquez JE, Dula R, et al. Mupirocin-resistant, methicillin-resistant Staphylococcus aureus: does mupirocin remain effective? *Infect Control Hosp Epidemiol.* 2003; 24:342-346.
15. Vasquez JE, Walker ES, Franzus BW, et al. The epidemiology of mupirocin resistance among methicillin-resistant Staphylococcus aureus at a Veterans' Affairs hospital. *Infect Control Hosp Epidemiol.* 2000;21:459-464.
16. Champney WS, Rodgers WK. Retapamulin inhibition of translation and 50S ribosomal subunit formation in Staphylococcus aureus cells. Antimicrob Agents Chemother 2007. Electronic publication ahead of print.
17. Coskey RJ, Coskey LA. Diagnosis and treatment of impetigo. *J Am Acad Dermatol.* 1987;17:62-63.
18. Maddox JS, Ware JC, Dillon HC Jr. The natural history of streptococcal skin infection: prevention with topical antibodies. *J Am Acad Dermatol* 1985;13:207-212.
19. Leyden JJ, McGinley KJ, Mills OH. Pseudomonas aeruginosa gram-negative folliculitis. *Arch Dermatol.* 1979;115: 1203-1204.

20. Brook I, Finegold SM. Aerobic and anaerobic bacteriology of cutaneous abscesses in children. *Pediatrics.* 1981; 67:891-895.
21. Meislin HW, Lerner SA, Graves MH, et al. Cutaneous abscesses: anaerobic and aerobic bacteriology and outpatient management. *Ann Intern Med.* 1977;87:145-149.
22. Fleisher G, Ludwig S, Campos J. Cellulitis: bacterial etiology, clinical features, and laboratory findings. *J Pediatr.* 1980;97:591-593.
23. Rehder PA, Eliezer ET, Lane AT. Perianal cellulitis: cutaneous group A streptococcal disease. *Arch Dermatol.* 1988;124:702-704.
24. Fisher RG, Benjamin DK. Facial cellulitis in childhood: a changing spectrum. *South Med J.* 2002;95:672-674.
25. Schwartz GR, Wright SW. Changing bacteriology of periorbital cellulitis. *Ann Emerg Med.* 1996;28:617-620.

Chapter 242

BRAIN TUMORS

Cameron L. Nicholson, MD; Joanne M. Hilden, MD; Bruce H. Cohen, MD

The primary care physician is often the first person to evaluate children with possible brain tumors: in one half of children ultimately diagnosed with a brain tumor, the diagnostic process was initiated by the primary care physician.[1] Brain tumors, although rare, are the second most common cancer and the most common solid tumor in childhood. Therefore primary care physicians need to keep in mind the possibility of a brain tumor among the other potential explanations of the cause of a child's illness. A delayed definitive diagnosis may ultimately affect the child's outcome. Many brain tumors do not share the favorable prognosis of other common pediatric cancer diagnoses, and aside from the exceptions of medulloblastoma and nongerminomatous germ cell tumors, recent advances have only modestly affected outcomes. Survival depends on many factors, including histology; tumor behavior, size, and location; and the patient's age. Children who do survive may experience substantial morbidity.

DEFINITIONS

For the sake of this discussion, *primary brain tumors* are defined as tumors of the brain parenchyma, cranial nerves, meninges, and the pituitary gland and immediate surrounding structures. Brain tumors arise from persistence of the embryologic precursors of neurons themselves (primitive neuroectodermal tumors [PNETs]), glial elements that provide structural and nutritional support to the neurons (astrocytomas and oligodendrogliomas), the lining cells such as the arachnoid (meningioma), the nerve sheath (schwannoma), the pituitary gland (pituitary adenomas), or intracranial rests (craniopharyngiomas).[2]

INCIDENCE

In the United States the incidence of primary brain and central nervous system (CNS) tumors is approximately 4.3 cases per 100,000 person-years, with an estimated 3410 new cases diagnosed in the United States in 2005.[3] The overall incidence is inversely proportional to age, highest in children 0 to 4 years of age, with 5.0 cases per 100,000 person-years, and lowest in patients 10 to 19 years of age, with 3.9 per 100,000 person-years.[3] The incidence is slightly higher in boys than in girls probably because of the higher proportion of medulloblastoma and germ cell tumors in boys.

Reports have been issued that the incidence of both childhood cancer and, in particular, brain tumors has been rising over the last 2 decades.[4-6] The increase may be the result of improvements in diagnostic technology and reporting patterns, as well as possible environmental or other unexplained factors.[6] For example, a substantial increase was observed after 1984 and 1985 when magnetic resonance imaging became widely available. However, the incidence has continued to rise, and only a small decline has occurred in mortality associated with brain tumors during this period.[5,6]

RISK FACTORS

Only a few risk factors have been substantially proven: previous therapeutic radiotherapy, predisposing genetic syndromes, and some aspects of maternal diet. Therapeutic radiographs, such as those used in the 1950s for tinea capitis, are now linked to a long-term relative risk of meningiomas and malignant brain tumors as a result of total-dose of radiation.[7] Children who have received therapy for acute lymphoblastic leukemia, including radiotherapy, are at increased risk for 2nd malignant neoplasms, including CNS tumors.[8-10] Interestingly, children with primary CNS neoplasms without a documented genetic syndrome demonstrate an increased risk of a 2nd CNS neoplasm. A 10-year cumulative incidence of 1.4%, regardless of previous therapy with radiotherapy or chemotherapy, has been reported.[11] Inherited syndromes are also associated with a higher risk for childhood brain tumors, although they are only present in a minority of cases (Box 242-1). Certain aspects of maternal diet influence the risk of PNETs in young children, with strong protective dose-response relations observed for maternal consumption of fruit, vegetables, vitamin C, nitrate, and folate.[12]

BOX 242-1 Genetic Syndromes Associated With Increased Risk of Pediatric Brain Tumor

- Neurofibromatosis types 1 and 2
- Tuberous sclerosis types 1 and 2
- von Hippel-Landau syndrome
- Li-Fraumeni syndrome
- Nevoid basal cell carcinoma syndrome
- Turcot syndrome
- Ataxia-telangiectasia syndrome
- Gardner syndrome
- Down syndrome

From Bestak M. Epidemiology of brain tumors. In: Keating RF, Goodrich JT, Packer RJ, eds. *Tumors of the Pediatric Central Nervous System.* Washington, DC: Thieme Medical Publishers; 2001. Reprinted by permission.

Other notable associations worth mentioning include pineoblastoma in patients with retinoblastoma, pituitary tumors in multiple endocrine adenomatosis syndromes, and the high incidence of pineal germinomas in Japan.[13,14] Primary CNS lymphoma may be seen as a result of primary or secondary disorders of the immune system, as in AIDS, Wiskott-Aldrich syndrome, or ataxia-telangiectasia syndrome, and after solid organ transplantation.[15]

CLASSIFICATION

Brain tumors are classified according to their histology, but location and extent of spread are important factors that affect treatment planning and prognosis. The most widely recognized classification system is the World Health Organization classification of tumors, published in 2000, with more than 120 entries.[16] This criteria system was established with the intention of encouraging and standardizing multicenter clinical trials. The system is designed to integrate histopathologic criteria with clinical, epidemiologic, radiologic, biological, molecular genetic, and predictive factors and therefore continues to evolve, with new diagnoses continually being added.

The World Health Organization classification recognizes 4 malignancy grades or estimates of malignant potential. However, the pathological distinction between malignant and nonmalignant tumors may not always reflect the clinical course of the disease. Physicians now avoid using terms such as *benign* or *malignant* in favor of *low-grade* or *high-grade* because the former terms can be misleading. Furthermore, the prognosis for some high-grade tumors is better than for some low-grade tumors. For example, an infiltrating low-grade glioma has a less-favorable long-term prognosis than a high-grade (malignant) PNET that is low stage and completely resected. As another example, the craniopharyngioma has a benign histology, but if this tumor produces infiltration into the hypothalamic structures, then the course may be anything but benign. Finally, in some circumstances such as infiltrating brainstem gliomas, the biopsy specimen may appear to be low-grade but the disease may still have an aggressive course.

DELAY IN DIAGNOSIS

In contrast to many pediatric malignancies, especially leukemias, many weeks or months may pass for children with brain tumors between the onset of symptoms and diagnosis. Only one third of children with brain tumors are diagnosed within the 1st month after the onset of signs or symptoms.[17,18] The interval between the onset of symptoms and the time of diagnosis is approximately 9 weeks, including a parental delay of 5 weeks after noticing symptoms and a physician's delay of an additional 3 weeks.[1,19] This time to diagnosis correlates with the patient's age and the location and histologic type of the tumor. A shorter delay is common in infants, possibly because of closer supervision by their primary care physicians.[17] Older children tend to have more subtle neurologic findings and are more likely to have a longer time to diagnosis.[18]

DIFFERENTIAL DIAGNOSIS

Space-occupying lesions and causes of increased intracranial pressure (ICP) to consider are listed in Box 242-2.

EVALUATION

History

The manifestations of childhood brain tumors depend on the site of tumor origin, the child's age and developmental level, and whether accompanying hydrocephalus exists. No single clinical historical detail or physical finding is pathognomonic.[15] Children will typically have a progression of symptoms and physical findings, which may not correlate with the grade of the underlying disease. Most children will have several suggestive features at the time of diagnosis; only 12% of children have just a single symptom.[17] In infants, increased ICP may exhibit insidiously with nonspecific signs such as drowsiness or lethargy, irritability, vomiting, abnormal tilting of the head, or developmental stagnation or regression.[20] In older children, declining academic performance; fatigue; and emotional, appetite, or personality changes may occur before overt headaches and vomiting.[15]

A well-studied symptom of brain tumor is headache. Headaches may be frontal, occipital, unilateral, or diffuse in location and may be exacerbated by Valsalva maneuvers. During the first 4 months of headache complaints, children should be monitored closely for brain tumor to improve time to diagnosis.[21] Box 242-3 lists conditions that suggest a need for further evaluation in children with headaches.

Vomiting is also an established symptom of childhood brain tumors and may be the result of increased ICP or, less commonly, direct irritation of the vagal nuclei or the floor of the 4th ventricle.[22] Vomiting may be associated with morning or waking headaches and may also relieve the headaches.

In contrast to adults, seizures are not frequently observed in children with brain tumors. However, aside from some well-characterized seizure syndromes, patients of any age who have seizures with a focal onset, either simple partial (focal) seizures or partial seizures with secondary generalization, should be evaluated for a tumor by contrast-enhanced magnetic resonance imaging (MRI).[23]

BOX 242-2 Differential Diagnosis

- Arteriovenous malformations
- Subdural hematoma, effusion, or empyema
- Abscess
- Infarction
- Hemorrhage
- Demyelination
- Pseudotumor cerebri
- Hemiplegic migraine
- Todd paralysis
- Venous sinus thrombosis

From Yager JY, Hukin J. Brain tumors. In: Hoekelman RA, ed. *Primary Pediatric Care.* 4th ed. St Louis, MO: Mosby; 2001.

BOX 242-3 Symptoms Warranting Evaluation for a Brain Tumor in Patients With Headaches

- Presence or onset of neuralgic abnormality
- Ocular findings such as papilledema, decreased visual acuity, or loss of vision
- Vomiting that is persistent, increasing in frequency, or preceded by recurrent headaches
- Changes in character of headache, such as increased severity and frequency or begins awakening child from sleep
- Recurrent morning headaches or headaches that repeatedly awaken the child from sleep
- Child with short stature or deceleration of linear growth
- Diabetes insipidus
- Child 3 years of age or younger
- Child with neurofibromatosis

From Honig PJ, Charney EB. Children with brain tumor headaches. *Am J Dis Child.* 1982;136:121-124.

More specific symptoms may help localize the tumor. Infratentorial tumors commonly produce cerebellar symptoms such as clumsiness, worsening handwriting, scanning speech, or frank symptoms of ataxia and increased ICP.[15,23] The infiltrating brainstem glioma may produce typical localizing signs of ataxia, cranial nerve symptoms, particularly diplopia because of 6th-nerve palsy, and long-tract signs because this tumor invades the brainstem nuclei, the descending corticospinal tract, and the crossing cerebellar outflow tracks. The nonlocalizing signs of this tumor are headache and vomiting resulting from obstruction of cerebrospinal fluid (CSF) flow and increased ICP.[15,24]

Supratentorial tumors may result in symptoms specific to the location of the disease. Complaints of hemiparesis (muscle weakness) suggest the presence of disease in the cerebral hemispheres. Visual loss or visual field defects may be the result of disease localized anywhere along the optic tracts, and when associated with hormonal changes such as growth failure or precocious puberty, they imply the presence of tumors near the optic chiasm and hypothalamus. Tumors of the hypothalamus may also be associated with the diencephalic syndrome in infants, which is characterized by failure to thrive, emaciation, and a euphoric mood. Pineal tumors and tumors involving the midbrain tectum cause *Parinaud syndrome,* a triad of paralysis of upward gaze with associated convergence-retraction nystagmus, lid retraction, and light-near dissociation of the pupils.[25]

Physical Examination

In addition to a thorough history, a complete and thorough neurologic examination will reveal both localizing and nonlocalizing findings. These neurologic findings, with or without a complementary history, are required for further investigation and for referring the child to a specialist. Repeated neurologic examinations may be revealing because signs are frequently progressive in situations in which the diagnosis remains in question. Tumors may result in macrocephaly, generally seen when the tumor impairs the normal circulation of CSF, resulting in hydrocephalus. In an infant, this condition produces head circumference measurements that cross percentile lines on a standard chart. The findings of bulging of the fontanel, split cranial sutures, lack of upgaze, and alteration in tone are all indicative of hydrocephalus. Some infants will appear to be failing to thrive as a result of vomiting caused by the increased ICP. Papilledema is uncommon in infants because their skulls can expand; thus the ICP does not get high enough to be found clinically. In children with fused cranial sutures, hydrocephalus will result in increased ICP and cause papilledema. Focal or localizing signs can help identify the location of the tumor. Tumors of the cerebral hemisphere can result in personality changes, focal weakness, language dysfunction, visual field defects, or sensory changes. Tumors involving the visual pathway will obviously result in visual-field deficits. If the tumor involves the midline structures of the cerebellum, then truncal ataxia will be the dominant sign. Tumors involving the brainstem can result in both long-tract findings and focal brainstem signs. Tumors involving the suprasellar and hypothalamic region may be associated with signs of an endocrine disturbance such as precocious or delayed puberty, growth failure, or hypothyroidism. Symptoms and signs of spinal cord tumors depend on the location of the tumor and its extent of infiltration into surrounding tissue.

Laboratory Evaluation

Patients with tumors of the pituitary gland and tumors that involve the pituitary stalk and hypothalamus should undergo evaluation of endocrine function before surgery. If the tumor involves the pituitary stalk or the posterior portion of the gland, then electrolytes and osmolality measurements can help diagnose diabetes insipidus. Patients with nongerminomatous germ cell tumors, such as choriocarcinoma, yolk-sac tumors, embryonal cell tumors, and the mixed variety, can excrete α-fetoprotein, β-human chorionic gonadotrophin, and alkaline phosphatase. These markers, if present, are most easily found in CSF, but they may also be detected in serum. Germinomas do not typically secrete these markers. HIV serologic testing may be useful if a diagnosis of primary CNS lymphoma is suspected, although this tumor rarely occurs in children.[26]

Imaging Studies

Advancements in neuroradiology have helped clinicians make prompt and accurate diagnoses of childhood brain tumors. Computed tomography (CT) scanning is widely available, has short imaging times, and requires less sedation in young children; thus it is often the first modality to be used. The initial CT scan can provide important immediate information about the presence of hydrocephalus, cerebral edema, midline shifts, and risk of uncal herniation. However, tumors of the brainstem, posterior fossa, and mesial temporal lobe structures may not be clearly visible.

MRI is the imaging modality of choice for definitive diagnosis of CNS neoplasms. MRI is more sensitive than CT scan for most brain tumors and is the best imaging modality for tumors of the brainstem, posterior fossa, and mesial temporal lobe, as well as the spinal column. As with CT, a contrast agent will help detect many tumors because the gadolinium contrast agent accumulates in tissues that lack an intact blood-brain barrier. High-grade tumors infiltrate the surrounding tissues, inducing more surrounding edema and usually resulting in better contrast enhancement. In comparison, low-grade gliomas, the most common childhood tumor, are well demarcated and generally have little surrounding edema.[27]

MANAGEMENT

Treatment of most children with brain tumors requires a multidisciplinary team approach that includes physicians from the disciplines of neurosurgery, neurology, oncology, pathology, radiology, radiation oncology, endocrinology, and ophthalmology. In addition, these patients benefit from experienced pharmacologists; nurses; neuropsychologists; audiologists; nutritional experts; child life specialists; physical, occupational, and speech therapists; and social workers. The outcome of treatment for children with cancer has been shown to be better when care is provided at a specialized tertiary-care cancer center. In light of this circumstance, the American Academy of Pediatrics has released a statement outlining the guidelines for facilities, capabilities, and available personnel.[28]

Patients have benefited from being treated by using protocols developed by large cooperative cancer consortiums. Therefore children should be considered for enrollment into a clinical trial whenever one is available. Clinical trials are being carried out by single institutions in addition to collaborative groups such as the Children's Oncology Group and the Pediatric Brain Tumor Consortium.

The optimal therapy combination for most brain tumors is still being determined through clinical trials. However, the initial treatment of many brain tumors is often surgery. Presurgical corticosteroid therapy is essential for children with brain edema and increased ICP. Brain tumors contain tumor vessels that behave differently, favoring the formation of edema within and around the tumor as a result of disruption of the blood-brain barrier.[29] Methylprednisolone reduces capillary permeability in the tumor and adjacent brain tissue.[30] Patients treated with methylprednisolone often develop rapid and marked resolution of the edema with corresponding improvement of their symptoms, as well as a more *relaxed* brain during the operative procedure.

Excision removes the tumor and resolves the surrounding edema. Neurosurgical techniques have improved during the last 20 years, along with safer anesthesia and better intensive care management. The use of stereoscopic microscopes coupled with real-time surgical navigation systems has been the most striking advance.[31] A navigation system permits the operative burr hole to be placed with high precision, thus allowing tumor resection through small openings, and modern microscopes allow the surgeon to distinguish between healthy brain and tumor, resulting in a greater likelihood of total resection.[13] Electrophysiological monitoring during surgery has also contributed to safer and bolder approaches.[31] Intraoperative MRI has shown promise for use in select cases, but its widespread use is limited by its high cost and the often considerably longer operating times.[32]

Although surgical resection is the goal for many tumors, some tumor types are best diagnosed by neuroimaging or by histologic evaluation of biopsy material, when it can be obtained without substantial morbidity. Because of location, tumors situated in the deep gray masses, such as the thalamus and basal ganglia, are often biopsied by means of a stereotactic navigation system. Diffuse pontine gliomas and tectal plate gliomas are never biopsied because of the risk of damaging essential structures and because they have a predictable histologic appearance and clinical course.[33] The neuroimaging characteristics of visual pathway glioma and intrinsic pontine gliomas are classic; therefore seldom does an advantage exist to pathologic corroboration of a diagnosis.

For most cerebellar and hemispheric low-grade gliomas, the tumor is a pilocytic astrocytoma. The strategy of choice for a cure for these children is gross total resection. For other tumors, debulking of the primary tumor allows for more effective chemotherapy and radiotherapy.[34] Chemotherapy has been shown to improve the survival of many patients with CNS tumors, and radiotherapy is an important treatment modality for all but the youngest patients.[13] In very young patients, new treatment protocols have been developed with intensive chemotherapy with stem cell rescue in an effort to replace radiotherapy and its long-term consequences.

Current radiotherapies vary and include external-beam, 3-dimensional, and intensity-modulated radiotherapy, as well as stereotactic radiosurgery and gamma knife surgery, which allow small-volume or local irradiation while sparing surrounding tissues and essential structures.[31] Radiation is the best therapy for many tumors, but it may result in growth failure, failure of intellectual and emotional development, and an increased risk of later developing a malignancy caused by the radiation exposure.[13] Treatment planning requires balancing cure rates with such profound morbidity and late effects.

Further improvements in managing outcomes likely lie in collective clinical trials of new treatment strategies, including antiangiogenesis medications, monoclonal antibodies, immunotherapy, differentiation agents, and gene therapy.[25] Such trials are best conducted in collaboration with a network of experienced investigators working in specialized tertiary-care cancer centers.

WHEN TO REFER

Children with a history that suggests brain tumor and children with focal findings at physical examination require further evaluation. Oncologists, neurologists, and neurosurgeons prefer early referrals, hoping that if the diagnosis of a neoplasm is made, then the tumor will be smaller and easier to resect, thereby causing less damage to adjacent brain tissue. New strategies to expedite and simplify referrals in other countries, including referral guidelines and cancer referral forms, have been used with good satisfaction rates, and adopting these strategies may be beneficial in local medical networks in streamlining the care of these children.[35,36]

WHEN TO ADMIT

Patients with signs of increasing ICP should be admitted urgently for evaluation and imaging. CT scanning can provide immediate information about ventricular size, the volume of the normal cisternal spaces, shifting of normal brain structures, and degree of ICP. Progressive life-threatening symptoms may include increasing blood pressure and decreasing heart rate, 6th-nerve palsy, or occipital headaches caused by irritation of posterior roots of the cervical cord. These symptoms may quickly progress to neck stiffness and eventually opisthotonus, a spasm of the body in which the head and heels are bent backward and the body is bowed forward. In addition, patients with supratentorial mass lesions may exhibit pupillary dilatation, often unilateral initially, from uncal herniation. This manifestation may culminate in tonsillar herniation, which is also a potential sequela of an untreated posterior fossa mass lesion, obstructive hydrocephalus, or both. In all these clinical situations the neurosurgeons should be consulted urgently.

TOOLS FOR PRACTICE

Engaging Patient and Family

- *CureSearch* (www.curesearch.org/).
- *What is a Pediatric Hematologist/Oncologist?* (fact sheet), American Academy of Pediatrics (www.aap.org/family/WhatisPedHemaOncol.pdf).

Medical Decision Support

- *Central Brain Tumor Registry of the US: Pediatric Incidence Report Statistics* (database), Central Brain Tumor Registry of the United States (CBTRUS) (www.cbtrus.org/cbtrus-bin/interactive/public/2005/search_pedincidence).

AAP POLICY STATEMENT

American Academy of Pediatrics, Section on Hematology/Oncology. Guidelines for pediatric cancer centers. *Pediatrics.* 2004;113(6):1833-1835. (aappolicy.aappublications.org/cgi/content/full/pediatrics;113/6/1835).

SUGGESTED RESOURCES

Central Brain Tumor Registry of the United States (CBTRUS). Available at: www.cbtrus.org/. This Web site provides resources for gathering and disseminating current epidemiologic data on all primary brain tumors to describe accurately their incidence and survival patterns, evaluate diagnosis and treatment, facilitate etiologic studies, establish awareness of the disease, and prevent all brain tumors.

CureSearch. Available at: www.curesearch.org/. This Web site unites the world's largest childhood cancer research organization, the Children's Oncology Group, and the National Childhood Cancer Foundation through a shared mission: curing childhood cancer.

Keating RF, Goodrich JT, Packer RJ, eds. *Tumors of the Pediatric Central Nervous System.* Washington, DC: Thieme Medical Publishers; 2001.

National Cancer Institute. Available at: www.cancer.gov. This Web site provides overviews for patients and health professionals on treatment and clinical trials.

Pizzo PA, Poplack DG, eds. *Principles and Practice of Pediatric Oncology.* 5th ed. Philadelphia, PA: Lippincott Williams and Wilkins; 2005.

United Kingdom Department of Health. Referral Guidelines for Suspected Cancer, 2000. Available at: www.dh.gov.uk/policyandguidance/healthandsocialcaretopics/cancer/cancergeneralinfo/fs/en?content_id=4066665&chk=5z4d86. Accessed December 20, 2006.

REFERENCES

1. Thulesius H, Pola J, Hakansson A. Diagnostic delay in pediatric malignancies. *Acta Oncol.* 2000;39:873-876.
2. Smirniotopoulos JG. The new WHO classification of brain tumors. *Neuroimaging Clin North Am.* 1999;9:595-613.
3. Central Brain Tumor Registry of the United States. Statistical Report: Primary Brain Tumors in the United States, 1998-2002 (Years Data Collected). Available at: www.cbtrus/org. Accessed March 11, 2007.
4. Bleyer WA. Epidemiologic impact of children with brain tumors. *Childs Nerv Syst.* 1999;15:758-763.
5. Linet MS, Ries LA, Smith MA, et al. Cancer surveillance series: recent trends in childhood cancer incidence and mortality in the United States. *J Natl Cancer Inst.* 1999;19:1051-1058.
6. Smith MA, Friedlin B, Ries LA, et al. Trends in reported incidence of primary malignant brain tumors in children in the United States. *J Natl Cancer Inst.* 1998;90:1269-1277.
7. Sadetski S, Chetrit A, Freedman L, et al. Long-term follow-up of brain tumor development after childhood exposure to ionizing radiation for tinea capitis. *Radiat Res.* 2005;163:424-432.
8. Kimball Dalton VM, Gelber RD, Li F, et al. Second malignancies in patients treated for childhood acute lymphoblastic leukemia. *J Clin Oncol.* 1998;16:2848-2853.
9. Loning L, Zimmerman M, Reiter A. et al. Secondary neoplasms subsequent to Berlin-Frankfurt-Munster therapy of acute lymphoblastic leukemia in childhood: significant lower risk without cranial radiotherapy. *Blood* 2000;95:2770-2775.
10. Neglia JP, Meadows AT, Robison LL, et al. Second neoplasms after acute lymphoblastic leukemia in childhood. *N Engl J Med.* 1991;325:1330-1336.
11. Broniscer A, Weiming K, Fuller CE, et al. Second neoplasms in pediatric patients with primary central nervous system tumors. *Cancer* 100:2246-2252.
12. Bunin GR, Kuijten RR, Buckley JD, et al. Relation between maternal diet and subsequent primitive neuroectodermal brain tumors in young children. *N Engl J Med.* 1993;329:536-541.
13. Bestak M. Epidemiology of brain tumors. In: Keating RF, Goodrich JT, Packer RJ, eds. *Tumors of the Pediatric Central Nervous System.* Washington, DC: Thieme Medical Publishers; 2001.
14. Kuratsu J, Takeshima H, Ushio Y. Trends in the incidence of primary intracranial tumors in Kumamoto, Japan. *Int J Clin Oncol.* 2001;6:183-191.

15. Blarney SM, Kun LE, Hunter J, et al. Tumors of the central nervous system. In: Pizzo PA, Poplack DG, eds. *Principles and Practice of Pediatric Oncology.* 5th ed. Philadelphia, PA: Lippincott Williams and Wilkins; 2005.
16. Kleihaus P, Sobin LH. World Health Organization classification of tumours. *J Neuropathol Exp Neurol.* 2002;61: 212-225.
17. Dobrovoljac M, Hengartner H, Boltschauser E, et al. Delay in the diagnosis of paediatric brain tumours. *Eur J Pediatr.* 2002;161:663-667.
18. Flores LE, Williams DL, Bell BA, et al. Delay in the diagnosis of pediatric brain tumors. *Am J Dis Child.* 1986;140: 684-686.
19. Pollock BH, Krischer JP, Vietti TJ. Interval between symptom onset and diagnosis of pediatric brain tumors. *J Pediatr.* 1991;119:725-732.
20. Reed UC, Rosemberg S, Gherpelli JL, et al. Brain tumors in the first two years of life: a review of forty cases. *Pediatr Neurosurg.* 1993;19:180-185.
21. Honig PJ, Charney EB. Children with brain tumor headaches. *Am J Dis Child.* 1982;136:121-124.
22. Duchatelier S, Wolf SM. Diagnostic principles. In: Keating RF, Goodrich JT, Packer RJ, eds. *Tumors of the Pediatric Central Nervous System.* Washington, DC: Thieme Medical Publishers; 2001.
23. Spencer DD, Spencer SS, Mattson RH, Williamson PD. Intracerebral masses in patients with intractable partial epilepsy. *Neurology.* 1984;34:432-436.
24. Shuper A, Kornreich L, Loven D, et al. Diffuse brain stem gliomas: are we improving outcome? *Childs Nerv Syst.* 1998;14:578-581.
25. Ullrich NJ, Pomeroy SL. Pediatric brain tumors. *Neurol Clin North Am.* 2003;21:897-913.
26. Grant R. Overview: brain tumor diagnosis and management/Royal College of Physicians guidelines. *J Neurol Neurosurg Psychiatry.* 2004;75(suppl II) ii18-ii23.
27. Vezina G, Booth TN. Neuroradiology. In: Keating RF, Goodrich JT, Packer RJ, eds. *Tumors of the Pediatric Central Nervous System.* Washington, DC: Thieme Medical Publishers; 2001.
28. American Academy of Pediatrics, Section on Hematology/Oncology. Guidelines for the pediatric cancer center and role of such centers in diagnosis and treatment. *Pediatrics.* 1997;99:139-141.
29. Bingaman WE, Frank JI. Malignant cerebral edema and intracranial hypertension. *Neurol Clin.* 1995;13: 479-509.
30. Yamada K, Ushio Y, Hayakawa T, et al. Effects of methylprednisolone on peritumoral brain edema: a quantitative autoradiographic study. *J Neurosurg.* 1983;59: 612-619.
31. Messing-Junger AM, Janssen G, Pape H, et al. Interdisciplinary treatment in pediatric patients with malignant CNS tumors. *Childs Nerv Syst.* 2000;16:742-750.
32. Jolesz FA. Future perspectives for intraoperative MRI. *Neurosurg Clin North Am.* 2005;16:201-213.
33. Walter AW, Hilden JM. Brain tumors in children. *Curr Oncol Rep.* 2004;6:438-444.
34. Finlay JL, UtegR, Giese WL. Brain tumors in children. II. Advances in neurosurgery and radiation oncology. *Am J Pediatr Hematol Oncol.* 1987;9:256-263.
35. Dodds W, Morgan M, Wolfe C, et al. Implementing the 2-week wait rule for cancer referral in the UK: general practitioners' views and practices. *Eur J Cancer Care.* 2004;13:82-87.
36. United Kingdom Department of Health. Referral Guidelines for Suspected Cancer, 2000. Available at: www.dh.gov.uk/policyandguidance/healthandsocialcare topics/cancer/cancergeneralinfo/fs/en?content_id=4066665&chk=5z4d86. Accessed December 20, 2006.

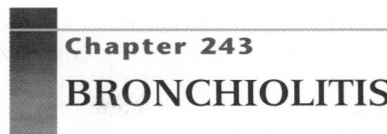

Chapter 243

BRONCHIOLITIS

Caroline Breese Hall, MD; William J. Hall, MD

DEFINITION

Bronchiolitis is a common, acute viral lower respiratory tract illness of children occurring during the first 2 years of life. Bronchiolitis is characterized by the acute onset of wheezing, hyperinflation, and tachypnea resulting from acute inflammation of the airways. Bronchiolitis, has been documented in recent years to be an increasing cause of hospitalization among infants in the United States, resulting in an appreciable and escalating economic burden to our health care system.[1-6]

The clinical picture of bronchiolitis has been described since the beginning of the 20th century, but the disease was associated with a variety of sobriquets, including *wheezy* or *asthmatic bronchitis, acute catarrhal bronchitis,* and *spastic bronchopneumonia.* The syndrome was not recognized as a separate entity until Engle and Newns[7] gave it distinction by designating the infantile disease as bronchiolitis.

Although initially, bacteria were thought to be the cause of bronchiolitis, respiratory viruses are now recognized as the major agents of bronchiolitis.[8-13] Respiratory syncytial virus (RSV) is the most frequently identified cause of bronchiolitis, accounting for approximately 50% to 85% of cases. The parainfluenza viruses, predominantly parainfluenza virus type 3, are the next most common agents.[9,11,14-16] In Monroe County, New York, RSV was isolated from 55% and parainfluenza virus type 3 from 11% of the cases of bronchiolitis examined in pediatric practices (Figure 243-1). Other

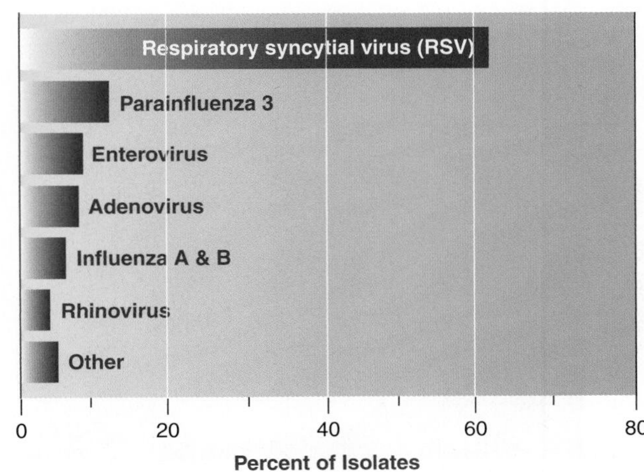

Figure 243-1 Viral origin of bronchiolitis from patients in pediatric practices participating in a community surveillance program in Monroe County, New York, ongoing since 1976. (Testing for human metapnemovirus was not included.)

viruses, including rhinoviruses, enteroviruses, influenza viruses, and adenoviruses, are less common causes of bronchiolitis. Recently, human metapneumovirus (hMPV) has been identified to be the agent of 4% to 10% of lower respiratory tract illnesses in hospitalized children and of approximately 3% of the outpatient respiratory illnesses.[17-23] The epidemiologic characteristics and clinical manifestations of bronchiolitis caused by hMPV appear to be very similar to bronchiolitis from RSV.

Children with bronchiolitis may be infected by more than 1 virus simultaneously, usually by viruses that tend to have concurrent or overlapping seasons of circulation.[24-28] Most frequently, the dual infections are caused by RSV with parainfluenza viruses type 3, hMPV 3, and influenza.

EPIDEMIOLOGIC CHARACTERISTICS

The seasonal pattern of bronchiolitis is well defined in temperate climates and reflects the activities of its viral agents, particularly RSV.[8,9,12,29] Yearly outbreaks of bronchiolitis occur during the winter to spring when RSV is epidemic in the community (Figure 243-2). In Monroe County, New York, the greatest number of cases is reported during the yearly January-to-February peak of RSV activity. Lesser peaks are observed during the fall, when parainfluenza virus type 1 is present in the community, and during the spring, concurrent with the major activity of parainfluenza virus type 3.

Bronchiolitis occurs primarily in children within the first 2 years of life. More than 80% of bronchiolitis cases occur during the 1st year of life.[1,4,5,8,11,30-34] The peak attack rate generally occurs between 1 and 10 months of age and between 2 and 6 months of age in hospitalized children. In ambulatory children, the peak attack rate occurs in the second 6 months of life.[8]

The reported rates of occurrence of bronchiolitis and of bronchiolitis-associated hospitalizations vary somewhat according to geographic location and population; but, in general, the age-specific attack rates among hospitalized infants are highest in infants younger than 6 months and among nonhospitalized infants are highest in infants between 6 and 12 months of age. The incidence rates for bronchiolitis are often reported as those associated with RSV infection because bronchiolitis is usually the major clinical manifestation of RSV, especially in hospitalized infants. The annual rates of hospitalizations attributable to RSV among infants have been reported as varying from 5 to 41 per 1000 infants. Recent population-based studies in the United States have estimated RSV-associated hospitalization rates of approximately 13 per 1000 children younger than 12 months each year, which is over 3 times that associated with parainfluenza virus or attributable to influenza.[35,36]

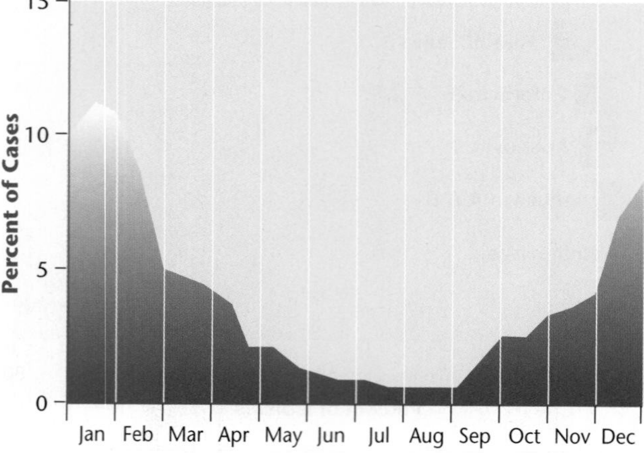

Figure 243-2 Seasonal occurrence of bronchiolitis cases obtained over a 20-year period from a community surveillance program in Monroe County, New York.

The rates of hospitalization for bronchiolitis and RSV in population-based studies from other countries have generally shown this same trend of the highest rates in infants, with estimated hospitalizations rates of 19 to 22 per 1000 children younger than 12 months each year.[24,27,31,37,38] The rates of outpatient visits attributable to bronchiolitis or RSV are less well studied, but some reports suggest these rates may be many times higher than that for hospitalized patients.[9,35] In 1 review of a private group practice, bronchiolitis caused 4% of the hospitalizations among pediatric patients of all ages.[39]

Boys are approximately 1.5 times more likely to develop bronchiolitis than girls. Anatomic and physiologic differences between boys and girls, such as airway tone, may partly explain the male preponderance.[40-42] Certain socioeconomic and environmental factors also have been correlated with a greater likelihood of developing bronchiolitis.[43-50] Among these factors are lower socioeconomic status, exposure to tobacco smoke, not being breastfed, and contact with other young children, including having 1 or more siblings, and child care attendance.

An increased risk of developing bronchiolitis that is severe or requires hospitalization has been associated with young age, particularly within the first several months of life, and the presence of certain underlying conditions, especially prematurity, low birth weight, cardiopulmonary disease, and immunodefiency.[4,5,43,51,52]

Genetic factors may predispose the infant to more severe bronchiolitis. Polymorphisms in genes coding interleukins, tumor necrosis factor, and other immune mediators have been associated with more severe disease.[53-58] An atopic family history or predisposition to hyperreactivity of the airways has been observed to be a risk factor, and Native-American children have rates of developing severe disease that are several times greater than that for the general population of children in the United States.[50,59,60]

DIFFERENTIAL DIAGNOSIS

Several conditions with wheezing and respiratory distress in the young child may appear similar to bronchiolitis. Asthma is the major consideration in the differential diagnosis of bronchiolitis.[61,62] Often in a single episode, differentiating these 2 entities is not possible. Wheezing associated with both bronchiolitis and asthma in young children is engendered by viral infections.[63] Differentiation is further confounded by the possibility that a link exists between the two, with RSV infection in infancy leading to subsequent wheezing episodes associated with asthma.[13,62] Nevertheless, previous episodes of wheezing and a family history of atopy are more suggestive of asthma than of bronchiolitis.

Another diagnostic consideration is gastroesophageal reflux, which in the infant may exhibit primarily episodes of wheezing and may produce a picture clinically identical to that of bronchiolitis. However, history of the timing in relation to feeding and frequency of the wheezing episodes, as well as the lack of upper respiratory tract signs typical of a viral infection, are helpful in differentiating gastroesophageal reflux from bronchiolitis. Other entities that may result in wheezing and respiratory distress in the bronchiolitic age group that should be considered include obstruction from an aspirated foreign body, a vascular ring, retropharyngeal abscess, and, rarely, significantly enlarged adenoids. Wheezing may also occur in congestive heart failure and in chronic lung disease, such as that associated with prematurity and cystic fibrosis.

EVALUATION

History

A carefully obtained history of wheezing in a child is integral in determining both the diagnosis and assessing the potential for developing severe or complicated illness. The diagnosis of bronchiolitis is usually based on the clinical history and physical findings.[64] Features that strongly support the diagnosis include the illness occurring during a community outbreak of 1 of the major viral agents, mainly RSV, young age (especially younger than 12 months), and no prior episode of wheezing. The risk factors, as noted in Epidemiologic Characteristics, for the development of more severe disease need to be assessed, especially the presence of prematurity, cardiopulmonary disease, immunodeficiency, and other underlying diseases.[52]

The infant with bronchiolitis typically has a recent history of signs compatible with a common cold: rhinorrhea, nasal congestion, a low-grade fever, and cough. As infection spreads to the lower respiratory tract, the cough becomes more prominent, followed by tachypnea. Fever is commonly present during the prodromal period but is usually not high. By the time the child exhibits bronchiolitis associated with RSV, only approximately 50% of children are febrile.

Clinical Manifestations and Pathogenesis of Physical Findings

On physical examination, an increased respiratory rate is almost always evident. Whether a child is tachypneic must be judged based on age. The overall respiratory rate in full-term newborns is approximately 50 breaths per minute but decreases over the 1st year of life to a mean of approximately 40 per minute at 6 months, and 30 per minute at a year of age.[64] Tachycardia commonly accompanies tachypnea. The infant may appear irritable, lethargic, or anxious. Flaring of the nasal alae and expiratory grunting signify an increased work of breathing. Retractions of the chest wall in the subcostal, intercostal, and suprasternal areas and use of the accessory muscles of respiration may also be evident.

Respiratory distress arises from inflammation of the epithelium and obstruction of the medium and small bronchi and bronchioles. The viral infection causes increased mucus production, edema, and necrosis of the bronchiolar epithelium, which is sloughed into the lumen of the small airways.[65] Because resistance to the flow of air is related inversely to the radius of the lumen, the small diameter of the bronchioles makes the infant particularly vulnerable to obstruction caused by the edema and inflammatory exudate.

Peripheral to the sites of partial obstruction, air becomes trapped by a process similar to a *ball valve* mechanism. During inspiration, the negative intrapleural pressure allows air to flow past the site of partial obstruction. On expiration, however, the positive intrathoracic pressure decreases the diameter of the bronchiolar lumen, causing an increase in the degree of obstruction, and hyperinflation of the lung ensues. If the inflammation progresses, complete obstruction can occur, and when the trapped air is absorbed, multiple areas of focal atelectasis result.

This characteristic hyperinflation is evidenced on the physical examination by an increased diameter of the chest and hyperresonance on percussion. The liver and spleen may become easily palpable from the downward placement of the overinflated lungs. The airway obstruction is further reflected by a prolonged expiration that may be difficult to detect in a young infant who has a rapid respiratory rate. The flow of air also is impeded on inspiration but to a lesser extent. Auscultation usually reveals wheezing with or without crackles, but these findings may vary from hour to hour. Indeed, fluctuating physical findings on examination is characteristic of bronchiolitis in infants. However, a decrease in the auscultatory findings accompanied by increasing respiratory distress may indicate progressive obstruction to the flow of air in the small airways and impending respiratory failure.

Additional clinical findings may develop from acute complications during the infant's course. Of major concern is apnea, which may be the 1st manifestation of the respiratory illness in 10% to 20% of infants. Most at risk for apnea are infants of premature gestation and those whose postconceptional age is under 44 weeks.[66,67] The subsequent prognosis for children with apnea associated with RSV infection is generally good and not does not appear to be associated with an increased risk of subsequent apnea, even during subsequent viral infections.[66] Otitis media is also present in 3% to 30% of infants and may be caused by the infecting virus, bacteria, or both.[68,69] The risk of dehydration complicating the course of infants with bronchiolitis arises from paroxysms of coughing that trigger vomiting and by the decreased fluid intake resulting from congested nasal passages and from the respiratory distress. In addition, tachypnea and fever may increase fluid requirements. Aspiration has been noted to occur frequently among infants hospitalized with RSV bronchiolitis and has been correlated with an increased risk of subsequently developing hyperactive airway disease.[70,71] This risk, however, has been shown to be abrogated by the prophylactic administration of therapy for aspiration.

Clinical Course

Most infants who have bronchiolitis improve appreciably within several days, and the cough and other signs resolve gradually thereafter over 1 to 2 weeks. Most hospitalized children are discharged after 3 to 7 days of hospitalization.[72] Radiographic resolution of atelectasis, however, may require several weeks. In ambulatory children, the median duration of illness has been reported to be 12 days for children younger than 24 months.[73] However, 18% remained symptomatic after 3 weeks and 9% after 4 weeks. The clinical course tends to be more prolonged in young infants, those with underlying conditions, and those who acquired the infection nosocomially.[24,72] Whether coexistence of infection with 2 viruses in children with bronchiolitis results in more severe clinical disease is unclear. A few studies suggest an increase in severity of infection when 2 viruses are present; others do not.[24,26-28,74,75]

Laboratory Testing

Laboratory diagnostic tests for healthy infants with their 1st episode of wheezing are not routinely recommended, given that the diagnosis of bronchiolitis is generally made based on the history and clinical findings.[64,76,77] Unless the child's course is atypical or abruptly changes, tests such as the white blood cell count, measurement of arterial oxygen saturation, serum chemistries, and cultures to rule out bacterial infection are generally not helpful or necessary for the management of previously healthy children who have not had prior wheezing.[39,64,78]

Pulse oximetry has now become a common part of the evaluation of children with bronchiolitis. Nevertheless, studies have not generally shown that the use of pulse oximetry has resulted in improved outcome for infants with bronchiolitis.[64] Its use in hospitalized patients has been associated with a lower threshold for hospitalization, higher rates of admission to intensive care units, and of mechanical ventilation.[64,79-81]

Tests for viral identification are also not routinely recommended because the great majority of children respond to supportive care alone. Assays to identify the specific virus may be warranted for the selected and more severely ill child in whom specific antiviral therapy for RSV or influenza is being considered. Specific viral testing may also be beneficial in determining feasible infection control procedures, such as cohorting.

The laboratory assays most commonly used to determine the viral causes are isolation in tissue culture and rapid antigen detection assays. Most of the respiratory viruses causing bronchiolitis are identifiable in cell culture within 3 to 7 days, but the sensitivity of viral isolation techniques are variable among laboratories and are highly dependent on the laboratory's expertise. A variety of rapid viral diagnostic techniques, especially for RSV and the influenza viruses, detect within hours some viruses in respiratory secretions that commonly cause cases of bronchiolitis.[82,83] However, such rapid antigen detection kits for the parainfluenza viruses are generally not available. Rapid viral antigen tests have variable sensitivities and should be used only when the virus is prevalent in the community, preferably during the period of peak activity. The positive predictive value is low when little circulation of the virus occurs in the area as the false positive rate increases as the incidence of the disease in the community falls. Recent increased use of reverse transcriptase polymerase chain reaction has demonstrated these assays to be highly sensitive and significantly better than viral isolation.[83,84]

Antibody determinations on acute and convalescent sera in the young infant are rarely helpful in clinical management because of the time required to obtain a convalescent serum, the presence of passive maternal antibody, and the diminished antibody response of young infants to the viral respiratory agents causing bronchiolitis.

Imaging

Imaging should not be used routinely in the previously healthy child in whom the diagnosis of bronchiolitis can be made based on clinical and historical finding.[64] Radiographic evaluation may be helpful when the diagnosis of bronchiolitis is not clear and if the child's course is not as expected.[77,85,86] Chest radiographs should not be used to monitor the course of an infant with bronchiolitis or to decide admission or discharge. Importantly, the findings on the chest radiograph commonly are relatively benign and do not correlate with the severity of illness. The classical findings associated with bronchiolitis on chest radiograph are increased bronchovascular markings radiating out from the hila and scattered small areas of atelectasis. Atelectasis observed on the chest radiograph may be mistakenly interpreted as areas of pneumonic infiltration and of bacterial infection. Prospective studies of children with suspected lower respiratory tract infections who were evaluated with chest radiographs were more likely to receive antibiotics, and their outcome or duration of illness was not improved.[64,86]

MANAGEMENT

Management of most infants who have bronchiolitis, whether they are outpatients or hospitalized, consists primarily of supportive care, including adequate rest, comfort, hydration, and antipyretics, if necessary.[64,77] Congestion of the nasal passages and upper airway, which may contribute to an infant's work of breathing, may be alleviated by gentle nasal suctioning and positioning of the infant. Mist therapy has not been shown to be beneficial.[87] Chest physiotherapy, including percussion and vibratory techniques, have been of no clinical value and are not recommended.[64,77,88] For the more severely affected child who is hospitalized, the need for supplemental oxygen administration should be judged by repetitive readings indicating an inadequate oxygen saturation level. Consensus does not exist as to the level of oxygen saturation that indicates the need for supplemental oxygen, but the recent bronchiolitis guidelines from the American Academy Pediatrics[64] recommend initiating supplemental oxygen when the oxyhemoglobin saturation is persistently less than 90% and consider discontinuing the supplemental oxygen when the level is persistently at or above 90%.

Beyond these measures, little agreement exists within the United States or among countries as to the value and use of therapeutic modalities.[64,89-91] Although evidence is lacking that shows benefit for most of the commonly used therapies, especially for those who are 1st-time wheezers, corticosteroids, antivirals, antibiotics, and especially bronchodilators, are frequently administered.[64,89]

Studies evaluating the use of bronchodilating agents in bronchiolitis have given variable and contrasting results.[64,92,93] Most controlled trials and reviews of the use of β-adrenergic agents have not shown consistent clinical benefit in children hospitalized with their 1st episode of wheezing.[64,92] In outpatient children, some studies have suggested transient or short-term clinical benefit when evaluated by varying clinical score systems. The American Academy of Pediatrics recommends that bronchodilators should not be used routinely in the management of bronchiolitis but that a carefully monitored trial of inhaled α- or β-adrenergic agents is an option. However, the bronchodilator should only be continued if a beneficial clinical response is clearly documented.[64,77]

Corticosteroid medications are frequently administered to infants with bronchiolitis.[4,89,91,93] In some facilities, the majority of infants with bronchiolitis are treated with systemic glucocorticosteroids.[89,93] However, meta-analyses have not shown consistent or statistically significant benefit in clinical scores, rates of hospitalization, or outcome.[64,89,93] The largest multicenter double-blind randomized trial evaluating the administration of corticosteroids to children with bronchiolitis was conducted in 20 emergency departments and completed in 2006.[94] Children 2 to 12 months of age with a 1st episode of wheezing from moderate to severe bronchiolitis received a single dose of oral dexamethasone (1 mg/kg) or placebo over 3 respiratory seasons. No significant difference between the 2 groups was observed in the requirement for hospitalization. The same lack of benefit of corticosteroid therapy was observed in the subgroups of children with asthma or with a family history of asthma. This important study supports the American Academy of Pediatrics recommendation that therapy with corticosteroid medications should not be used routinely for the care of infants with a 1st episode of bronchiolitis.[64]

Antivirals that are potentially useful for viral agents that cause bronchiolitis are few. Inhaled ribavirin, a synthetic nucleoside, is the only agent currently approved for the treatment of RSV lower respiratory tract disease in infants. Antivirals for influenza have not been approved as therapy for young infants nor evaluated in the management of bronchiolitis.

Ribavirin is not recommended routinely to treat children with bronchiolitis and generally should only be considered for use in infants with conditions that place them at high risk for developing severe disease.[64] The drug is expensive, difficult to administer to ventilated patients, and the benefits in clinical outcome controversial. Its use therefore should be decided on an individual basis after consideration of the relative benefit to cost in the child's management.

Antibiotics should not be used unless a bacterial infection is documented or evidence strongly indicates the concurrent presence of a bacterial infection, which is uncommon in bronchiolitis and RSV lower respiratory tract disease.[39,78,95]

PROGNOSIS

Despite the number of hospitalizations for bronchiolitis increasing in recent years, the mortality associated with bronchiolitis and RSV has declined.[2,4,5,51] The mortality among children younger than 5 years associated with bronchiolitis between 1979 and 1997 was estimated by the Centers for Disease Control and Prevention to be an average 95 cases, with a range of 66 to 127 cases each year for all children younger than 5 years and highest in those younger than 1 year.[5,51] Deaths in infants associated with RSV have more recently been estimated to be less than 500 per year.[4]

The most frequent sequelae of bronchiolitis, especially that caused by RSV, is recurrent wheezing, which is reported to occur in 30% to 50% of the children who were hospitalized for their bronchiolitis.[63,96-101] Episodes of recurrent wheezing tend to occur most frequently during the first 2 years after the initial episode of bronchiolitis. Most of these children subsequently improve and become asymptomatic.[100,102,103] However, lung function abnormalities may persist beyond 10 years, despite the clinical improvement. Significantly reduced mean expiratory flow rates and an increased risk of bronchial hyperreactivity during adolescence have been demonstrated.[101,104-106]

On the other hand, some follow-up studies have shown that these children, when reaching school age, have no greater risk of hyperreactive airway disease than children with no history of bronchiolitis.[100-102] One episode of bronchiolitis, and less severe bronchiolitis not requiring hospitalization also, have not been associated with later pulmonary abnormalities.[101-107] The relationship between bronchiolitis in early infancy and the subsequent development of hyperreactive airway disease is unclear and confounded by the increasing recognition that asthma or reactive airway disease is a heterogeneous group of disorders with variable pathogenesis.[54,63,108-112]

WHEN TO REFER

- When episodes of bronchiolitis or wheezing are recurrent or started at birth
- When wheezing continues despite clinical improvement

WHEN TO ADMIT

- When oral intake is inadequate
- When the child is toxic appearing or has marked tachypnea or lethargy
- When respiratory distress is rapidly progressive
- When history suggests apneic episodes

TOOLS FOR PRACTICE

Community Coordination and Advocacy

- *Managing Infectious Diseases in Child Care and Schools* (book), American Academy of Pediatrics (www.aap.org/bookstore).

Engaging Patients and Family

- *Bronchiolitis and Your Young Child* (brochure), American Academy of Pediatrics (patiented.aap.org).
- *Respiratory Syncytial Virus (RSV)* (brochure), American Academy of Pediatrics (patiented.aap.org).
- *RSV* (fact sheet), American Academy of Pediatrics (www.aap.org/publiced/BR_RSV.htm).
- *Suctioning the Nose with a Bulb Syringe* (fact sheet), Cincinnati Children's Hospital Medical Center (www.cincinnatichildrens.org/health/info/newborn/home/suction.htm).

Medical Decision Support

- *Bronchiolitis Respiratory Sheet* (form), Cincinnati Children's Hospital Medical Center (www.cincinnatichildrens.org/NR/rdonlyres/B3EC347E-65AC-490A-BC4C-55C3AF4B76D5/0/bronchiolitisrespiratory.pdf).
- *Guideline: Diagnosis and Management of Bronchiolitis* (guideline), American Academy of Pediatrics (aappolicy.aappublications.org/cgi/content/full/pediatrics;118/4/1774).
- *Highlights from guidelines for bronchiolitis in infants 1 year of age or less presenting with a first time episode* (guideline), Cincinnati Children's Hospital Medical Center (www.cincinnatichildrens.org/NR/rdonlyres/7C591A09-2F25-4CEF-832A-96BB9A5C98A7/0/bronchiolitishighlight.pdf).
- *National Respiratory and Enteric Virus Surveillance System (NREVSS)* (web page), Center for Disease Control and Prevention (www.cdc.gov/surveillance/nrvess/index.htm).
- *Respiratory Syncytial Virus* (fact sheet), Center for Disease Control and Prevention (www.cdc.gov/ncidod/dvrd/revb/respiratory/rsvfeat.htm).

Practice Management

- *Quick Reference Guide to Pediatric Coding and Documentation for Infectious Diseases* (book), American Academy of Pediatrics (www.aap.org/bookstore).

SUGGESTED RESOURCES

American Academy of Pediatrics, Subcommittee on Bronchiolitis. Guideline: diagnosis and management of bronchiolitis. *Pediatrics*. 2006;118(4):1774-1793.

Bronchiolitis Guideline Team, Cincinnati Children's Hospital Medical Center. Health Policy & Clinical Effectiveness Program—Evidence Based Clinical Practice Guideline (for medical management of bronchiolitis in infants 1 year of age or less presenting with a first time episode), 2005. Available at: www.cincinnatichildrens.org/NR/rdonlyres/FAC539F9-07B2-4FE4-A9DD-EC1013BBE64B/0/BronchGL.pdf.

Hall CB. Respiratory syncytial virus and parainfluenza virus. *N Engl J Med*. 2001;344:1917-1928.

Lemanske RF. Viruses and asthma: inception, exacerbation, and possible prevention. *J Pediatr.* 2003;142:S3-S8.

Meissner HC. Selected populations at increased risk from respiratory syncytial virus infection. *Pediatr Infect Dis J.* 2003;22:S40-S45.

REFERENCES

1. Langley JM, LeBlanc JC, Smith B, Wang EE. Increasing incidence of hospitalization for bronchiolitis among Canadian children, 1980-2000. *J Infec Dis.* 2003;188;1764-1767.
2. Leader S, Kohlhase K. Recent trends in severe respiratory syncytial virus (RSV) among US infants, 1997 to 2000. *J Pediatr.* 2003;143:s127-s132.
3. Pelletier AJ, Mansbach JM, Camargo CA Jr. Direct medical costs of bronchiolitis hospitalizations in the United States. *Pediatrics.* 2006;118;2418-2423.
4. Shay DK, Holman RC, Newman RD, et al. Bronchiolitis-associated hospitalizations among US children, 1980-1996. *JAMA.* 1999;282;1440-1446.
5. Shay DK, Holman RC, Roosevelt GE, Clarke MJ, Anderson LJ. Bronchiolitis-associated mortality and estimates of respiratory syncytial virus-associated deaths among US children, 1979-1997. *J Infect Dis.* 2001;183;16-22.
6. Stang P, Brandenburg N, Carter B. The economic burden of respiratory syncytial virus-associated bronchiolitis hospitalizations. *Arch Pediatr Adolesc Med.* 2001;155;95-96.
7. Engle S and Newns GH. Proliferative mural bronchiolitis. *Arch Dis Child.* 1940;15;219-229.
8. Denny FW and Clyde WA Jr. Acute lower respiratory tract infections in nonhospitalized children. *J Pediatr.* 1986;108;635-646.
9. Foy HM, Cooney MK, Maletzky AJ, Grayston JT. Incidence and etiology of pneumonia, croup, and bronchiolitis in preschool children belonging to a prepaid medical care group over a four-year period. *Am J Epidemiol.* 1973;97:80-92
10. Glezen WP, Denny FW. Epidemiology of acute lower respiratory disease in children. *N Engl J Med.* 1973;288;498-505.
11. Henderson FW, Clyde WA Jr., Collier AM, et al. The etiologic and epidemiologic spectrum of bronchiolitis in pediatric practice. *J Pediatr.* 1979;95:183-190
12. Mullins JA, LaMonte AC, Bresee JS, Anderson LJ. Substantial variability in community respiratory syncytial virus season timing. *Pediatr Infect Dis J.* 2003;22;857-862.
13. Smyth RL, Openshaw PJ. Bronchiolitis. *Lancet.* 2006;368;312-322.
14. Everard ML and Milner AD. The respiratory syncitial virus and its role in acute bronchiolitis. *Eur J Pediatr.* 1992;151;638-651.
15. Jartti T, Lehtinen P, Vuorinen T, et al. Respiratory picornaviruses and respiratory syncytial virus as causative agents of acute expiratory wheezing in children. *Emerg Infect Dis.* 2004;10;1095-1101.
16. Wright RB, Pomerantz WJ, Luria JW. New approaches to respiratory infections in children: Bronchiolitis and croup. *Emerg Med Clin North Am.* 2002;20;93-114.
17. Boivin G, De Serres G, Cote S, et al. Human metapneumovirus infections in hospitalized children. *Emerg Infect Dis.* 2003;9:634-640
18. Crowe JE Jr. Human metapneumovirus as a major cause of human respiratory tract disease. *Pediatr Infect Dis J.* 2004;23:S215-S221.
19. Esper F, Boucher D, Weibel C, Martinello RA, and Kahn JS. Human metapneumovirus infection in the United States: clinical manifestations associated with a newly emerging respiratory infection in children. *Pediatrics.* 2003;111;1407-1410.

20. Peiris JSM, Tang WH, Chan KH, et al. Children with respiratory disease associated with metapneumovirus in Hong Kong. *Emerg Infect Dis* 2003;9;628-633.
21. van den Hoogen BG, Osterhaus DM, Fouchier RA. Clinical impact and diagnosis of human metapneumovirus infection. *Pediatr Infect Dis J.* 2004;23:S25-S32.
22. van den Hoogen BG, van Doornum GJ, Fockens JC, et al. Prevalence and clinical symptoms of human metapneumovirus infection in hospitalized patients. *J Infec Dis.* 2003;188;1571-1577.
23. Xepapadaki P, Psarras S, Bossios A, et al. Human Metapneumovirus as a causative agent of acute bronchiolitis in infants. *J Clin Virol.* 2004;30;267-270.
24. Forster J, Ihorst G, Rieger CH, et al. Prospective population-based study of viral lower respiratory tract infections in children under 3 years of age (the PRIDE study). *Eur J Pediatr.* 2004;163;709-716.
25. Glezen WP. The changing epidemiology of respiratory syncytial virus and influenza: impetus for new control measures. *Pediatr Infect Dis J.* 2004;23:s202-s206.
26. Legg JP, Warner JA, Johnston SL, Warner JO. Frequency of detection of picornaviruses and seven other respiratory pathogens in infants. *Pediatr Infect Dis J.* 2005;24;611-616.
27. Nicholson KG, McNally T, Silverman M, et al. Rates of hospitalisation for influenza, respiratory syncytial virus and human metapneumovirus among infants and young children. *Vaccine.* 2006;24;102-108.
28. Semple MG, Cowell A, Dove W, et al. Dual infection of infants by human metapneumovirus and human respiratory syncytial virus is strongly associated with severe bronchiolitis. *J Infect Dis.* 2005;191;382-386.
29. Hall CB. Respiratory syncytial virus and parainfluenza virus. *N Engl J Med.* 2001;344;1917-1928.
30. CDC Centers for Disease Control and Prevention. National Respiratory and Enteric Virus Surveillance System (NREVSS). 2006. Available at: http://www.cdc.gov/ncidod/dvrd/revb/nrevss/index.htm.
31. Fjaerli HO, Farstad T, Bratlid D. Hospitalisations for respiratory syncytial virus bronchiolitis in Akershus, Norway, 1993-2000: a population-based retrospective study. *BMC Pediatr.* 2004;25;1-7.
32. Fleming DM, Pannell RS, and Cross KW. Mortality in children from influenza and respiratory syncytial virus. *J Epidemiol Community Health.* 2005;59;586-590.
33. Leader S, Kohlhase K. Respiratory syncytial virus-coded pediatric hospitalizations, 1997-1999. *Pediatr Infect Dis J.* 2002;21;629-632.
34. Muller-Pebody B, Edmunds WJ, Zambon MC, Gay NJ, Crowcroft NS. Contribution of RSV to bronchiolitis and pneumonia-associated hospitalizations in English children, April 1995- March 1998. *Epidemiol Infect.* 2002; 129;99-106.
35. Hall CB, Weinberg GA, Copeland J, et al. *Respiratory Syncytial Virus (RSV) Infection in Young Children: Accurate Population-Based Estimates of Hospitalizations Rates and Outpatient Medical Visits.* in *Pediatric Academic Societies Annual Meeting.* Washington, DC: 2005.
36. Iwane MK, Edwards KM, Szilagyi PG, et al. Population-based surveillance for hospitalizations associated with respiratory syncytial virus, influenza virus, and parainfluenza viruses among young children. *Pediatrics.* 2004; 113;1758-1764.
37. Eriksson M, Bennet R, Rotzen-Ostlund M, von Sydow M, Wirgart BZ. Population-based rates of severe respiratory syncytial virus infection in children with and without risk factors, and outcome in a tertiary care setting. *Acta Paediatr.* 2002;91;593-598.
38. Weigl JA, Puppe W, Schmitt HJ. Incidence of respiratory syncytial virus-positive hospitalizations in Germany. *Eur J Clin Microbiol Infect Dis.* 2001;20;452-459.
39. Hall CB, Powell KR, Schnabel KC, Gala CL, and Pincus PH. Risk of secondary bacterial infection in infants hospitalized with respiratory syncytial viral infection. *J Pediatr.* 1988;113;266-271.
40. Landau L.I., MW, McCoy KS, Taussig LM. Gender related differences in airway tone in children. *Pediatric Pulmonology.* 1993;16;31-35.
41. Landau LI. Bronchiolitis and asthma: are they related? *Thorax.* 1994;49;293-296.
42. Martinez FD, Morgan WJ, Wright AL, Holberg CJ, Taussig LM. Diminished lung function as a predisposing factor for wheezing respiratory illness in infants. *N Eng J Med.* 1988;319;1112-1117.
43. Boyce TG, Mellen BG, Mitchel EF Jr., Wright PF, Griffin MR. Rates of hospitalization for respiratory syncytial virus infection among children in Medicaid. *J Pediatr.* 2000;137;865-870.
44. Carlsen K-H, Larsen L, Bjerve O, and Leegaard J. Acute bronchiolitis: Predisposing factors and characterizations of infants at risk. *Pediatr Pulmonol.* 1987;3;153-160.
45. Henderson FW, Collier AM, Clyde WA, Denny FW. Respiratory syncytial virus infections, reinfections and immunity: A prospective, longitudinal study in young children. *N Engl J Med.* 1979;300;530-534.
46. Holberg CJ, Wright AL, Martinez FD, et al. Risk factors for respiratory syncytial virus-associated lower respiratory illnesses in the first year of life. *Am J Epidemiol.* 1991;133;1135-1151.
47. Mahabee-Gittens M. Smoking in parents of children with asthma and bronchiolitis in a pediatric emergency department. *Pediatr Emerg Care.* 2002;18;4-7.
48. Mascarenhas ML, Albernaz EP, da Silva MB, da Silveira RB. Prevalence of exclusive breastfeeding and its determiners in the first 3 months of life in the South of Brazil. *J Pediatr (Rio J).* 2006;82;289-294.
49. Reeve CA, Whitehall JS, Buettner PG, et al. Predicting respiratory syncytial virus hospitalisation in Australian children. *J Paediatr Child Health.* 2006;42;248-252.
50. Stein RT, Martinez FD. Asthma phenotypes in childhood: lessons from an epidemiological approach. *Paediatr Respir Rev.* 2004;5;155-161.
51. Holman RC, Shay DK, Curns AT, Lingappa JR, Anderson LJ. Risk factors for bronchiolitis-associated deaths among infants in the United States. *Pediatr Infect Dis J.* 2003;22;483-490.
52. Meissner HC. Selected populations at increased risk from respiratory syncytial virus infection. *Pediatr Infect Dis J.* 2003;22:S40-S45.
53. Hoebee B, Bont L, Rietveld E, et al. Influence of promoter variants of interleukin-10, interleukin-9, and tumor necrosis factor-alpha genes on respiratory syncytial virus bronchiolitis. *J Infect Dis.* 2004;189:239-247
54. Hoebee B, Rietveld E, Bont L, et al. Association of severe respiratory syncytial virus bronchiolitis with interleukin-4 and interleukin-4 receptor ??polymorphisms. *J Infect Dis.* 2003;187;2-11.
55. Hull J, Rowlands K, Lockhart E, et al. Variants of the chemokine receptor CCR5 are associated with severe bronchiolitis caused by respiratory syncytial virus. *J Infect Dis.* 2003;188;904-907.
56. Martinello RA, Chen MD, Weibel C, Kahn JS. Correlation between respiratory syncytial genotype and severity of illness. *J Infect Dis.* 2002;186;839-842.
57. Openshaw PJ, Tregoning JS. Immune responses and disease enhancement during respiratory syncytial virus infection. *Clin Microbiol Rev.* 2005;18;541-555.
58. Tal G, Mandelberg A, Dalal I, et al. Association between common Toll-like receptor 4 mutations and severe respiratory syncytial virus disease. *J Infect Dis.* 2004;189; 2057-2063.

59. Goetghebuer T, Kwiatkowski D, Thomson A, and Hull J. Familial susceptibility to severe respiratory infection in early life. *Pediatr Pulmonol.* 2004;38;321-328.
60. Lowther SA, Shay DK, Holman RC, et al. Bronchiolitis-associated hospitalizations among American Indian and Alaska Native children. *Pediatr Infect Dis J.* 2000;19; 11-17.
61. Mahesh VK, Taussig LM. When an infant wheezes: Clues to the differential. *J Respir Dis.* 1990;11;739-750.
62. Openshaw PJ, Dean GS, Culley FJ. Links between respiratory syncytial virus bronchiolitis and childhood asthma: clinical and research approaches. *Pediatr Infect Dis J.* 2003;22:s58-s65.
63. Lemanske RF. Viruses and asthma: inception, exacerbation, and possible prevention. *J Pediatr.* 2003;142:s3-s8.
64. American Academy of Pediatrics Subcommittee on Diagnosis and Management of Bronchiolitis. Diagnosis and Management of Bronchiolitis. *Pediatrics.* 2006;118; 1774-1793.
65. Visscher DW, Myers JL. Bronchiolitis: the pathologist's perspective. *Proc Am Thorac Soc.* 2006;3;41-47.
66. Church NR, Anas NG, Hall CB, Brooks JG. Respiratory syncytial virus-related apnea in infants: Demographics and outcome. *Am J Dis Child.* 1984;138;247-250.
67. Kneyber MC, Brandenburg AH, de Groot R, et al. Risk factors for respiratory syncytial virus associated apnoea. *Eur J Pediatr.* 1998;157;331-335.
68. Chonmaitree T and Henrickson KJ. Detection of respiratory viruses in the middle ear fluids of children with acute otitis media by multiplex reverse transcription: polymerase chain reaction assay. *Pediatr Infect Dis J.* 2000;19;258-260.
69. Chonmaitree T, Owen MJ, Patel JA, et al. Effect of viral respiratory tract infection on outcome of acute otitis media. *J Pediat.* 1992;120;856-862.
70. Hernandez E, Khoshoo V, Thoppil D, Edell D, and Ross G. Aspiration: a factor in rapidly deteriorating bronchiolitis in previously healthy infants? *Pediatr Pulmonol.* 2002;33;30-31.
71. Khoshoo V, Ross G, Kelly B, Edell D, and Brown S. Benefits of thickened feeds in previously healthy infants with respiratory syncytial viral bronchiolitis. *Pediatr Pulmonol.* 2001;31;301-302.
72. Purcell K, Fergie J. Driscoll Children's Hospital respiratory syncytial virus database: risk factors, treatment and hospital course in 3308 infants and young children, 1991 to 2002. *Pediatr Infect Dis J.* 2004;23;418-423.
73. Swingler GH, Hussey GD, Zwarenstein M. Duration of illness in ambulatory children diagnosed with bronchiolitis. *Arch Pediatr Adolesc Med.* 2000;154;997-1000.
74. Fuller DG, Davie G, Lamb D, Carlin JB, and Curtis N. Analysis of respiratory viral coinfection and cytomegalovirus coisolation in pediatric inpatients. *Pediatr Infect Dis J.* 2005;24;195-200.
75. Palomino MA, Larranaga C, Villagra E, Camacho J, Avendano LF. Adenovirus and respiratory syncytial virus-adenovirus mixed acute lower respiratory infections in Chilean infants. *Pediatr Infect Dis J.* 2004;23; 337-341.
76. Bordley WC, Viswanathan M, King VJ, et al. Diagnosis and testing in bronchiolitis: a systematic review. *Arch Pediatr Adolesc Med.* 2004;158:119-126
77. Bronchiolitis Guideline Team Cincinnati Children's Hospital Medical Center. Evidence based clinical practice guideline for medical management of bronchiolitis in infants 1 year of age or less presenting with a first time episode. 2005. Available at: http://www.cincinnatichildrens.org/NR/rdonlyres/FAC539F9-07B2-4FE4-A9DD-EC1013BBE64B/0/BronchGL.pdf.
78. Kuppermann N, Bank DE, Walton EA, Senac MO, McCaslin I. Risks for bacteremia and urinary tract infections in young febrile children with bronchiolitis. *Arch Pediatr Adolesc Med.* 1997;151;1207-1214.
79. Bergman AB. Pulse oximetry: good technology misapplied. *Arch Pediatr Adolesc Med.* 2004;158; 594-595.
80. Mallory MD, Shay DK, Garrett J, Bordley WC. Bronchiolitis management preferences and the influence of pulse oximetry and respiratory rate on the decision to admit. *Pediatrics.* 2003;111:e45-e51.
81. Schroeder AR, Marmor AK, Pantell RH, Newman TB. Impact of pulse oximetry and oxygen therapy on length of stay in bronchiolitis hospitalizations. *Arch Pediatr Adolesc Med.* 2004;158;527-530.
82. Kehl SC, Henrickson KJ, Hua W, Fan J. Evaluation of the Hexaplex assay for detection of respiratory viruses in children. *J Clin Microbiol.* 2001;39;1696-1701.
83. Perkins SM, Webb DL, Torrance SA, et al. Comparison of a real-time reverse transcriptase PCR assay and a culture technique for quantitative assessment of viral load in children naturally infected with respiratory syncytial virus. *J Clin Microbiol.* 2005;43;2356-2362.
84. Weinberg GA, Erdman DD, Edwards KM, et al. Superiority of reverse-transcription polymerase chain reaction to conventional viral culture in the diagnosis of acute respiratory tract infections in children. *J Infect Dis.* 2004;189;706-710.
85. El-Radhi AS, Barry W, and Patel S. Association of fever and severe clinical course in bronchiolitis. *Arch Dis Child.* 1999;81;231-234.
86. Swingler GH, Hussey GD, Zwarenstein M. Randomised controlled trial of clinical outcome after chest radiograph in ambulatory acute lower-respiratory infection in children. *Lancet.* 1998;351;404-408.
87. Gibson LE. Use of water vapor in the treatment of lower respiratory disease. *Am Rev Respir Dis.* 1974;110; 100-103.
88. Perrotta C, Ortiz Z, Roque M. Chest physiotherapy for acute bronchiolitis in paediatric patients between 0 and 24 months old. *Cochrane Database Syst Rev.* 2005:1-16.
89. Behrendt CE, Decker MD, Burch DJ, and Watson PH. International variation in the management of infants hospitalized with respiratory syncytial virus. *Eur J Pediatr.* 1998;157;215-220.
90. Wang EEL, Law BJ, Boucher FD, et al. Pediatric investigators collaborative network on infections in Canada (PICNIC) study of admission and management variation in patients hospitalized with respiratory syncytial viral lower respiratory tract infection. *J Pediatr.* 1996;129; 390-395.
91. Willson DF, Horn SD, Hendley JO, Smout R, Gassaway J. Effect of practice variation on resource utilization in infants hospitalized for viral lower respiratory illness. *Pediatr.* 2001;108;851-855.
92. Kellner JD, Ohlsson A, Gadomski AM, and Wang EEL. Bronchodilators for bronchiolitis. *Cochrane Database Syst Rev* 2005;4.
93. Patel H, Platt R, Lozano JM, Wang EEL. Glucocorticoids for acute viral bronchiolitis in infants and young children. *Cochrane Database Syst Rev.* 2005;4;1-63.
94. Corneli H, Zorc J, Majahan P, et al. A multicenter, randomized, controlled trial of dexamethasone for bronchiolitis. *N Engl J Med* 2007;357(4):331-339.
95. Levine DA, Platt SL, Dayan PS, et al. Risk of serious bacterial infection in young febrile infants with respiratory syncytial virus infections. *Pediatr.* 2004;113;1728-1734.
96. Martinez FD. Respiratory syncytial virus bronchiolitis and the pathogenesis of childhood asthma. *Pediatr Infect Dis J.* 2003;22:S76-S82.

97. Martinez FD, Wright AL, Taussig LM, et al. Asthma and wheezing in the first six years of life. *N Engl J Med.* 1995; 332;133-138.
98. McCarthy CA, Hall CB. Respiratory syncytial virus: concerns and control. *Pediatr Rev.* 2003;24;301-308.
99. Schauer U, Hoffjan S, Bittscheidt J, et al. RSV bronchiolitis and risk of wheeze and allergic sensitisation in the first year of life. *Eur Respir J.* 2002;20;1277-1283.
100. Stein RT, Sherrill D, Morgan WJ, et al. Respiratory syncytial virus in early life and risk of wheeze and allergy by age 13 years. *Lancet.* 1999;354;541-545.
101. Wennergren G, Kristjansson S. Relationship between respiratory syncytial virus bronchiolitis and future obstructive airway diseases. *Eur Respir J.* 2001;18; 1044-1058.
102. Henderson FW, Stewart PW, Burchinal MR, et al. Respiratory allergy and the relationship between early childhood lower respiratory illness and subsequent lung function. *Am Rev Respir Dis.* 1992;145;283-290.
103. ten Brinke A, Zwinderman AH, Sterk PJ, Rabe KF, Bel EH. Factors associated with persistent airflow limitation in severe asthma. *Am J Crit Care Med.* 2001;164; 744-748.
104. Kneyber MC, Moons KGM, de Groot R, Moll HA. Prediction of the duration of hospitalization in respiratory syncytial virus (RSV) infection. *Pediatr Pulmonol.* 2002; 33;453-457.
105. Kotaniemi-Syrjanen A, Reijonen TM, Korhonen K, Korppi M. Wheezing requiring hospitalization in early childhood: predictive factors for asthma in a six-year follow-up. *Pediatr Allergy Immunol.* 2002;13;418-425.
106. Sigurs N, Bjarnason R, Sigurbergsson F, Kjellman B. Respiratory syncytial virus bronchiolitis in infancy is an important risk factor for asthma and allergy at age 7. *Am J Respir Crit Care Med.* 2000;161;1501-1507.
107. McConnochie KM, Roughman KJ. Bronchiolitis as a possible cause of wheezing in childhood: New evidence. *Pediatrics.* 1984;74;1-10.
108. Hull J, Ackerman H, Isles K, et al. Unusual haplotypic structure of IL8, a susceptibility locus for a common respiratory virus. *Am J Hum Genet.* 2001;69;413-419.
109. Koeppen-Schomerus G, Stevenson J, Plomin R. Genes and environment in asthma: a study of 4 year old twins. *Arch Dis Child.* 2001;85:398-400
110. Lofgren J, Ramet M, Renko M, Marttila R, Hallman M. Association between surfactant protein A gene locus and severe respiratory syncytial virus infection in infants. *J Infect Dis.* 2002;185;283-289.
111. Martinez FD, Helms PJ. Types of asthma and wheezing. *Eur Respir J.* 1998;27:3s-8s.
112. Psarras S, Papadopoulos NG, Johnston SL. Pathogenesis of respiratory syncytial virus bronchiolitis-related wheezing. *Paediatr Respir Rev.* 2004;5(Suppl A):S170-S184.

Chapter 244
CANCERS IN CHILDHOOD

Andrea S. Hinkle, MD; Cindy L. Schwartz, MD

Advances in the treatment of solid tumors of childhood during the last 20 years have ensured the long-term survival of approximately three quarters of children with these diagnoses. The pediatrician who initially discovers a solid tumor may not—and need not—know the best treatment available. However, early referral of such a child to the appropriate specialist, a pediatric oncologist, greatly affects the likelihood and the quality of survival. Many common tumors are unique in children. For all solid tumors in children, therapies must be designed to minimize effects on growth and development. Appropriate use of the therapeutic modalities (surgery, chemotherapy, and radiation) provides maximal efficacy and minimal toxicity of therapy.

The child and parents should be encouraged to plan for the future. Educational and developmental needs must be addressed by the pediatric team, with the generalist and specialist working together. Such a team is also able to address the needs of the child, the parents, and the siblings if treatment is not successful. Fortunately, most children are cured and will return to the pediatrician for many years of general pediatric care.

This chapter describes the following solid tumors seen in children: Wilms tumor, neuroblastoma, retinoblastoma, rhabdomyosarcoma, germ cell tumors and teratomas, Ewing sarcoma, osteosarcoma, non-Hodgkin lymphoma, and Hodgkin disease. The role of the pediatrician in the care of these children is also examined.

WILMS TUMOR

Wilms tumor, or nephroblastoma, is a malignant renal tumor of childhood that occurs at an annual rate of approximately 8 per 1 million children in the United States. It is the second most common abdominal tumor of childhood. Wilms tumor comprises 5% to 6% of pediatric cancers. This number translates to approximately 600 to 700 new cases diagnosed each year in the United States.[1] Patients are usually between 2 and 5 years of age. Only rarely does the tumor occur in teenagers and adults. Bilateral disease occurs more commonly in younger patients and in girls. It is one of the few pediatric malignancies that occurs more often in black patients than in white patients.

The chemosensitivity and radiosensitivity of this tumor, in conjunction with the ability to resect most nonmetastatic tumors, have allowed a multidisciplinary approach to be highly successful. Wilms tumor has become the model for treatment of childhood cancer. The National Wilms Tumor Study (NWTS) has evaluated over the last 3 decades successive therapeutic regimens, with the goal of increasing the cure rate and decreasing the duration and toxicity of therapy. The cooperative group approach has made possible the gathering of more data than might have been obtained at single institutions. The findings, such as the superiority of multiagent chemotherapy and the importance of tumor histology, are relevant for many tumors.

Etiology

Wilms tumor has occurred in siblings, cousins, and parent-child pairs, particularly in association with specific congenital anomalies and bilateral disease.[2] Although experts have proposed that 15% to 20% of patients who have Wilms tumor have a genetic predisposition to the disease, a much lower incidence of Wilms tumor in patients who have affected relatives has been reported (approximately 1% to 2%).[3,4]

Anomalies are not infrequently reported in patients who have Wilms tumor, occurring in 13% to 28% of patients,[5] although the majority of patients who have the disease do not have anomalies.[3,4] Most of the reported anomalies involve the genitourinary tract. Hemihypertrophy is second in frequency, sometimes noted as a component of the Beckwith-Wiedemann syndrome (excessive growth of many body organs). Of children who have the sporadic form of congenital aniridia, 33% have Wilms tumor. WAGR syndrome is the association of Wilms tumor, aniridia, genitourinary abnormalities, and intellectual disability. Denys-Drash syndrome represents the association of Wilms tumor with ambiguous genitalia and diffuse glomerular disease.[6,7] These syndromes are associated with germ-line mutations of the *WT1* gene, located at 11p13.[8] *WT1* abnormalities have been identified in a small subset of patients, 6% to 10%, who have apparently sporadic Wilms tumor, usually in association with genitourinary anomalies.[9] A second Wilms tumor suppressor locus may be at 11p15, which is also the locus for the familial form of Beckwith-Wiedemann syndrome. Loss of heterozygosity at 1p and 16q has also been identified in Wilms tumors,[8] and the NWTS demonstrated a worse prognosis for patients with tumor-specific loss of heterozygosity at these chromosome regions.[10] Further investigation of chromosomal abnormalities and genetic markers in Wilms tumor and other malignancies will provide insight into tumorigenesis and potential new directions for therapy.[5,11]

Screening for Wilms tumor by ultrasound and urinalysis in patients who have aniridia, WAGR syndrome, Denys-Drash syndrome, and hemihypertrophy or Beckwith-Wiedemann syndrome is suggested every 3 months until age 7 years. Screening may also be appropriate for patients who have unexplained nephropathy and who have multiple other congenital anomaly syndromes.[6]

Clinical Manifestations

Wilms tumor in children is usually characterized as a painless mass discovered by a relative, often during bathing. The mass usually is firm, occasionally lobulated, and confined to one side of the abdomen. Rapid abdominal enlargement, anemia, and hypertension (perhaps because of a sudden subcapsular hemorrhage) are occasionally present when the child seeks care. Hypertension, malaise, abdominal pain, hematuria, and fever each occur in 20% to 30% of patients.[5] Hypertension has been attributed to hyperreninemia.[4,5]

Table 244-1 presents the differential diagnosis of abdominal and pelvic tumors of childhood that may mimic Wilms tumor.

Evaluation

The evaluation of a patient with possible Wilms tumor begins with a history and physical examination. Particular attention should be paid to the associated congenital anomalies and the family history. Laboratory studies should include a complete blood cell count, urinalysis, and renal and liver function tests. Bleeding within the tumor may cause anemia.[12] An erythropoietin-secreting Wilms tumor may cause polycythemia. Hypercalcemia may occur in patients who have congenital mesoblastic nephroma or a rhabdoid tumor of the kidney.

Table 244-1 Differential Diagnosis of Abdominal and Pelvic Tumors in Infants and Children

TUMOR*	AGE	CLINICAL SIGNS	LABORATORY FINDINGS
Wilms	Preschool	Unilateral flank mass, aniridia, hemihypertrophy	Hematuria
Neuroblastoma	Preschool	GI or GU obstruction, raccoon eyes, myoclonus-opsoclonus, diarrhea, skin nodules (infants)	Increased VMA, increased HVA, increased ferritin, stippled calcification in mass
Non-Hodgkin lymphoma	>1 yr	Intussusception in >2 yr old	Increased urate
Rhabdomyosarcoma	All	GI or GU obstruction, sarcoma botryoides, vaginal bleeding, paratesticular mass	—
Germ cell or teratoma	Preschool, teens	Girls: abdominal pain, vaginal bleeding Boys: testicular mass, new onset hydrocele Sacrococcygeal mass or dimple	Increased hCG, increased AFP
Hepatoblastoma	Birth to 3 yr	Large, firm liver	Increased AFP
Hepatoma	School age, teens	Large, firm liver; hepatitis B, cirrhosis	Increased AFP

AFP, Alfa-fetoprotein; *GI,* gastrointestinal; *GU,* genitourinary; *hCG,* human chorionic gonadotropin; *HVA,* homovanillic acid; *VMA,* vanillylmandelic acid.
*Other causes: constipation, splenomegaly, hydronephrosis, kidney cyst, full bladder.

A plain-film radiograph of the abdomen may show coarse calcifications, unlike the fine, stippled pattern commonly seen in neuroblastoma. Mass effect may be noted on the film. Ultrasonography is often performed first; this modality is particularly helpful in evaluating the renal vein, vena cava, and the right side of the heart for tumor spread.[13] An abdominal computed tomographic (CT) scan with contrast may reveal an intrarenal mass displacing and distorting the collecting system of the involved kidney. The tumors may be very large, and minimal kidney parenchyma may be identified. Six percent of patients will have bilateral disease, and in 12% multifocal involvement in a single kidney may be recognized.[5] Liver metastases may be diagnosed either by ultrasound or by CT scan. Although intravenous pyelography may indicate the presence of the tumor, with currently available imaging techniques, it is generally not indicated. Magnetic resonance imaging (MRI) may occasionally be indicated to define the extent of the tumor. A chest radiograph be obtained and may demonstrate pulmonary nodules. A CT scan of the chest to detect small pulmonary metastases should be performed before surgery because postoperative atelectasis can obscure the presence of metastatic nodules. Bone scans are indicated in patients who have clear cell sarcoma of the kidney, which often spreads to bone. At the time of surgery, the tumor is staged, as outlined in Box 244-1.[14]

Wilms tumors are pathologically designated as being of either favorable histology (FH) or unfavorable histology (UH). FH indicates the absence of unfavorable features. UH involves the presence of anaplasia, defined by the presence of gigantic polypoid nuclei within the tumor sample. Anaplasia may be focal or diffuse. Diffuse anaplasia conveys a worse prognosis, which appears to be caused by resistance to chemotherapy and radiotherapy and not to biologically more aggressive disease.[15] Anaplasia is present in 5% of patients, is more frequent in older patients than younger patients, and is more common in black patients than patients in other ethnic groups.[5] Two other renal tumors—clear cell sarcoma of the kidney and rhabdoid tumor of the kidney—were previously considered Wilms tumor variants, but they are now considered as separate entities. Only clear cell sarcoma continues to be studied as part of NWTS protocols.

BOX 244-1 Staging of Wilms Tumor

Stage I: Tumor is limited to the kidney and is completely resected.

Stage II: Tumor extends beyond the kidney but is completely resected. Isolated tumor spill may exist confined to the flank.

Stage III: Residual, nonhematogenously spread tumor is confined to the abdomen, such as lymph node involvement, peritoneal contamination before or during surgery, peritoneal implants, residual tumor postoperatively, or incomplete resection caused by local infiltration. Unresectable tumors are also stage III.

Stage IV: Hematogenous metastases are present. Sites include lung (only site in 80% of patients who have metastases), liver, lymph node, and less commonly, bone, brain, and other sites.

Stage V: Indicates bilateral renal involvement is present, although for treatment purposes each side is staged.

Management

In the United States the initial therapeutic approach is complete resection by nephrectomy. This approach requires meticulous and gentle surgical techniques to prevent tumor from spilling. A large transabdominal incision facilitates full exploration and excision. The entire ureter is removed, and lymph nodes are sampled. The practice has been examination of the contralateral kidney and abdominal cavity for evidence of disease. However, this approach may not be required with current radiologic techniques; tumors too small to be identified on CT can be expected to be treated adequately with chemotherapy.[16] For recognized bilateral disease, chemotherapy is suggested after bilateral biopsy rather than immediate resection of the most involved site (as was done in previous years). *Second-look* excision of residual disease may be accomplished by partial nephrectomies, when possible.[5,11,17] Tumors deemed unresectable by clinical and radiologic evaluation are also sampled initially, with second-look resection performed after adequate chemotherapy-induced shrinkage is achieved. Patients with underlying syndromes, such as WAGR (a chromosomal deletion giving rise to a syndrome of Wilms tumor, aniridia, genitourinary abnormalities, intellectual disability), should be considered for partial nephrectomies because of the high risk of renal failure. Because the risk of renal failure is only 0.25% to 0.6% in patients with sporadic disease, the higher surgical and potential recurrence risk does not currently justify routine use of partial nephrectomies in this population, although it may be considered in certain patients.[5,18,19]

Actinomycin D and vincristine were noted to be effective agents in the mid-1960s. The initial study revealed that radiotherapy in combination with a single agent (actinomycin D or vincristine) provided approximately 55% relapse-free survival in patients with localized disease. An 81% relapse-free survival rate was found when both agents were administered in conjunction with radiation.[20] These two drugs are now the mainstay of chemotherapy for Wilms tumor. Subsequent studies demonstrated that radiotherapy was not necessary for stage I-II FH tumors and stage I UH tumors and that the addition of doxorubicin and 10 Gy of radiation to vincristine and actinomycin D improved the prognosis for patients who had stage III-IV FH tumors, as well as for those who had stage II-IV tumors with focal anaplasia.[20,21] The addition of cyclophosphamide as a fourth agent is of benefit for patients who have stage II-IV tumors with diffuse anaplasia. Shorter-duration therapy (6 months) with single high doses of actinomycin D results in the same outcome as multiple smaller doses, with less toxicity and less cost.[22] Peritoneal seeding or a major tumor rupture necessitates radiation of the entire abdomen. In the United States, thoracic radiation is used for pulmonary metastasis visible on chest radiography or those seen on chest CT only that do not resolve with chemotherapy.[23]

Future directions for therapy potentially include shorter regimens or single-agent chemotherapy for younger patients and those with small and low-stage tumors. The role of initial surgery versus preoperative chemotherapy as used in Europe, the role of pulmonary radiation based on imaging and response to chemotherapy, and the role of first-line doxorubicin therapy are also areas for continued study.[5,11,19]

Prognosis

The prognosis of patients who have Wilms tumor is determined by the histopathologic factors of the tumor; that is, more patients with UH tumors die, compared with patients with FH tumors.[24] UH tumors, particularly diffuse anaplasia, continue to confer a worse prognosis. More intensive regimens continue to be studied for patients who have stage II-IV disease with UH features.

Prognosis also depends on the stage of disease at diagnosis. Most relapses occur within 2 years of diagnosis. Two-year relapse-free survival for stages I to III disease with FH findings is approximately 91%. The 2-year relapse-free survival rate is 84% for patients who have stage IV disease and FH features.[22] Patients who have diffuse anaplasia have a poor prognosis, with only 59% of patients with stage II, 45% of patients with stage III, and 7% of patients with stage IV disease surviving at 4 years after diagnosis.[15] Four-year event-free survival is 74.9% for patients with focal anaplasia.[11] Patients who experience relapse have a better prognosis if their initial management did not include radiotherapy or doxorubicin. Autologous transplantation procedures are being investigated in patients with high-risk, relapsed disease.[25] Future therapy will focus on improving the outcome in patients with UH tumors and incorporating prognostic tumor chromosomal analyses into treatment assignments.

Follow-Up

While patients are receiving therapy, they are monitored for disease recurrence at the primary site, usually with abdominal ultrasound, although CT may be indicated, and in the lungs, usually with chest radiography. Some patients may be followed up with CT of the chest and abdomen. Such monitoring continues at increasing intervals until approximately 5 years after diagnosis. Long-term survival is likely in patients who have Wilms tumor. Virtually all patients have had a nephrectomy. Contact sports are often discouraged, although evidence for a significant risk of renal injury is lacking. Some experts suggest a kidney guard for particularly active children, if only to serve as a reminder of the need for caution. In addition, patients should have their renal function monitored.

Scoliosis was a major problem for early survivors treated with moderate-dose radiation (30 to 40 Gy), particularly if the entire vertebrae were not included in the field, because of impaired growth of the irradiated portion of the vertebrae. The use of lower-dose radiation (10 Gy) and irradiation of the entire width of the vertebrae adjacent to the renal bed have decreased the severity, but not entirely prevented the development, of scoliosis.[26] Alterations of vertebral growth and tethering caused by hypoplasia of soft tissues may still result in some degree of curvature. Close observation of patients who received irradiation, particularly during the growth spurt during puberty, remains necessary. Hypoplasia with a decrease in adipose tissue occurs in the radiation field and is accentuated by obesity. Therefore prevention of obesity minimizes this asymmetry.

Fertility is preserved in most patients who have Wilms tumor, although a risk of ovarian failure exists with whole-abdomen radiotherapy. The average size of infants born to female survivors of irradiation is smaller than that of nonirradiated women,[27] and increased miscarriages and premature births in female survivors of Wilms tumor who received radiotherapy have been reported.[28] In addition, some of these female patients may have underlying uterine anomalies.[29] Continued follow-up of these offspring is necessary to evaluate the genetic factors involved in the occurrence of Wilms tumor.

NEUROBLASTOMA

Neuroblastoma arises from the fetal neural cells that normally develop into the sympathetic nervous system. It is a tumor that provides insight into the biological processes of malignancy. Tumors in infants may regress spontaneously or mature to benign ganglioneuromas, whereas patients older than 1 year who have disseminated disease remain difficult to cure despite aggressive use of multimodal therapy.

Neuroblastoma is the most common extracranial solid tumor in children and is the most common malignancy of infants, accounting for more than one half of cancers in infants. Neuroblastoma accounts for 7% of all children diagnosed as having cancer and 15% of childhood cancer mortality. Approximately 9.7 white children and 7.4 black children per million in the United States are diagnosed with neuroblastoma each year—approximately 800 to 900 new cases every year.[1] Ninety percent of patients who have neuroblastoma are younger than 5 years, and 97% of patients will be diagnosed before the age of 10 years.

Etiology

The high incidence of neuroblastoma in early infancy suggests that its development may be related to abnormal maturation of fetal neural crest cells. The finding of microscopic nodules of adrenal neuroblastoma in infants younger than 3 months who have died of unrelated causes suggests that spontaneous maturation or regression occurs in many children.[30]

Families have been reported in which neuroblastoma occurred in multiple siblings or occasionally in multiple generations.[31,32] Some researchers have proposed that 20% to 25% of neuroblastomas occur in patients who have a prezygotic germinal mutation.[33] Neuroblastoma has been reported to occur with an increased incidence in patients who have Hirschsprung disease. The genetic bases for these familial and Hirschsprung-related cases are being elucidated.[34] Although reported in other syndromes, no clear increased frequency has been determined. Recent studies have demonstrated that diet, particularly folic acid intake, and breastfeeding may protect against the development of neuroblastoma.[35,36]

Clinical Manifestations

Neuroblastoma[37] may arise anywhere along the sympathetic nervous system chain, including the adrenal gland (40%), the paraspinal regions of the abdomen (25%), the thorax (15%), the neck (5%), and the pelvis at the organ of Zuckerkandl (5%). The incidence of primary site varies by age, with thoracic and cervical tumors more common in infants. The presenting features largely depend on the location of the tumor. A large, firm, irregular abdominal mass that may cross the midline is often the first sign of disease. Disturbances of bowel or bladder function may be the result of compression by a pelvic mass. Thoracic masses may cause a persistent cough or respiratory distress and are detected by a CXR. Cervical masses are often initially diagnosed as lymphadenitis, but they do not respond to antibiotic therapy. Horner syndrome or heterochromia iridis suggests the possibility of neuroblastoma.

Neuroblastomas that arise in the paravertebral ganglia tend to grow into the intervertebral foramina, forming a dumbbell-shaped mass. Pain, weakness of an extremity, paralysis, or incontinence may result from spinal cord compression by the intraspinal component. Incontinence may be difficult to assess, however, because many patients will still be in diapers. Cord compression is an oncologic emergency that requires surgical decompression, radiation, or chemotherapy to prevent permanent paraplegia. Studies have shown that long-term functional outcome may be better in patients treated with chemotherapy instead of laminectomy.[38]

Most children who have neuroblastoma have metastatic disease at the time of diagnosis. The symptoms may then be related to the metastatic tumor instead of the primary tumor. Infants may have metastatic hepatic involvement. Rapid liver enlargement can cause marked abdominal distention followed by respiratory compromise. Bluish skin nodules, which may release catecholamines if palpated, are sometimes noted in infants who have neuroblastoma. Palpation causes an erythematous cutaneous flush, lasting for 2 to 3 minutes, and is followed by blanching caused by vasoconstriction.[39]

The two most common sites for metastases are bone marrow and bone; other common sites include lymph nodes, liver, and intracranial and orbital sites. Disease in the lung and central nervous system (CNS) is uncommon.[40] Infiltration of the bone marrow may cause pancytopenia. Bone involvement may produce pain, with or without palpable bone masses. Lytic bone lesions are found most often in the skull, orbit, or proximal long bones. A raccoon-like appearance caused by proptosis and eyelid ecchymosis has been described in patients who have orbital involvement. Intracranial disease is usually due to meningeal metastases.[41] In infants, this disease may show as separation of cranial sutures caused by increased intracranial pressure. Infants and children who have neuroblastoma may also have fever, malaise, and failure to thrive. Secretory products of the tumor may be the cause of the presenting features. Vasoactive intestinal polypeptide has been found in 7% to 9% of children who have neural crest tumors, most frequently ganglioneuromas or ganglioneuroblastomas.[42] Intractable diarrhea is caused by this hormone.

An unusual symptom of neuroblastoma is the syndrome of opsoclonus-myoclonus.[43] These patients have acute cerebellar ataxia and rapid, dancing-eye movements. Although these patients often have localized disease and usually are cured, residual neurologic dysfunction, including residual ataxia and intellectual disability, is common. The etiology of this syndrome is unclear, although it may have an autoimmune factor, perhaps an antibody directed against neuroblastoma that cross-reacts with the cerebellar cell antigen.[44]

Tables 244-1 to 244-3 list the differential diagnosis of abdominal, pelvic, head, neck, and mediastinal tumors that may mimic neuroblastoma.

Table 244-2 Differential Diagnosis of Head and Neck Tumors in Infants and Children

TUMOR*	AGE	CLINICAL SIGNS	LABORATORY FINDINGS
Non-Hodgkin lymphoma	>1 yr	Lymphadenopathy NR to antibiotics, immunodeficiency, EBV (in Africa)	Increased urate
Hodgkin disease	>10 yr	Lymphadenopathy NR to antibiotics; weight loss, night sweats, fever, pruritus	Increased ESR
Rhabdomyosarcoma	All	Orbital mass, hoarseness, persistent otitis, sinusitis	—
Neuroblastoma	Preschool	Heterochromia iridis, Horner syndrome, myoclonus-opsoclonus, raccoon eyes, skin nodules (infants)	Increased HVA, VMA, or both in urine; calcification
Retinoblastoma	Preschool	Cat's-eye reflex, strabismus, family history	Calcification

EBV, Epstein-Barr virus; *ESR*, erythrocyte sedimentation rate; *HVA*, homovanillic acid; *NR*, nonresponsive; *VMA*, vanillylmandelic acid.
*Other causes: infectious lymphadenopathy, histiocytosis, Caffey disease, AIDS.

Table 244-3 Differential Diagnosis of Mediastinal Tumors in Infants and Children

TUMOR*	AGE	CLINICAL SIGNS	LABORATORY FINDINGS
Non-Hodgkin lymphoma	All	Cough, respiratory distress, anterior mediastinal mass, immunodeficiency syndrome	Increased urate, malignant effusion
Hodgkin disease	>10 yr	Middle mediastinum lymphadenopathy NR to antibiotics, weight loss, night sweats, fever, pruritus	Increased ESR, increased copper
Neuroblastoma	Preschool	Posterior mediastinum, heterochromia iridis, myoclonus-opsoclonus, raccoon eyes, skin nodules (infants)	Increased HVA, increased VMA, calcification
Thymoma	>10 yr	Anterior mediastinum, myasthenia gravis, red cell aplasia, hypogammaglobulinemia	—
Germ cell or teratoma	All	Anterior mediastinum (rarely, posterior mediastinum), cough, wheeze, dyspnea	Increased AFP, increased hCG

AFP, Alfa-fetoprotein; *ESR,* erythrocyte sedimentation rate; *hCG,* human chorionic gonadotropin; *HVA,* homovanillic acid; *NR,* nonresponsive; *VMA,* vanillylmandelic acid.

*Other causes: infection, bronchogenic cysts, aneurysms, lipoid tumors, thoracic meningocele.

Evaluation

After the initial physical examination, evaluation of a patient who has neuroblastoma requires radiologic examination of the area of primary disease, as well as of areas to which neuroblastoma metastasizes. A CT scan of the abdomen, pelvis, and chest should be performed. For patients with cervical masses, the CT scan should include this area. Because paravertebral lesions may extend into the intervertebral foramina, any patient who has such a lesion should be evaluated by MRI. A skeletal survey and a bone scan should be performed to detect bony lesions.[45] Radiographs are useful for detecting small lytic lesions at the end of bones; the bone scan helps find lesions of the skull and tubular bones. Because of the frequency of metastatic involvement, bone marrow biopsy specimens should be obtained in all patients; the only exception may be patients with low-risk, resected tumors.[46] Bilateral specimens should be obtained to increase the probability of detecting metastases. The liver should be examined by contrast CT scan in all patients and by biopsy in those who have abdominal disease. Metaiodobenzylguandine (MIBG) is taken up by neuroblastomas and may be used for imaging, but it has not been universally used because it is hard to administer and the results are difficult to interpret. However, its use may offer better sensitivity and specificity.[35] Positron emission tomographic (PET) scanning may also be helpful in assessing neuroblastoma.[47]

The previously used Evans and St Jude staging systems have been synthesized into the International Neuroblastoma Staging System. Stage 1 includes tumors with complete gross resection and microscopically negative ipsilateral and contralateral lymph nodes. Stage 2 tumors are unilateral tumors with complete or incomplete gross resections but, at the most, only ipsilateral microscopically positive lymph nodes. Stage 3 includes tumors that cross the midline or unilateral tumors that have contralateral lymph node involvement. Stage 4 designates metastatic disease. Stage 4S (for special) tumors occur in infants younger than 1 year who have stage 1 or 2 primary tumors with dissemination limited to liver, skin, or bone marrow.[48]

Neuroblastoma must be diagnosed by histologic examination after biopsy. In patients who have localized disease, the biopsy specimen must be obtained from the primary tumor. For those who have metastatic disease, neuroblastoma cells can be identified in the primary tumor or in areas of metastases, including the bone, bone marrow, or liver. Neuroblastoma produces small round cells with scant cytoplasm that must be differentiated from other small round blue cell tumors of childhood, including lymphoma, leukemia, Ewing sarcoma, and retinoblastoma. Secretion of catecholamines from tumor granules results in increased levels of vanillylmandelic acid (VMA) and homovanillic acid (HVA) in 24-hour urine samples or in increased vanillylmandelic acid–creatinine or homovanillic acid–creatinine ratios in spot urine samples.[49,50] These findings can be used to confirm the diagnosis of neuroblastoma in patients who have a small round blue cell infiltrate in the bone marrow. In addition, increased urinary catecholamine levels can be used to monitor the response to therapy. Ferritin and lactic dehydrogenase levels may be obtained and have prognostic significance in that increased levels predict a poor prognosis.[51]

Amplification of the N-*myc* oncogene is an intrinsic biological property of some neuroblastomas and has been associated with poor prognosis regardless of clinical stage (although it is most commonly seen in patients who have advanced disease).[52,53] Conversely, tumors that are hyperdiploid (DNA index >1) are sensitive to chemotherapy, resulting in a good prognosis.[54,55] Specimens should be analyzed for both of these biological features, which are used to determine risk groups for treatment purposes. Additional findings, such as the association of the tyrosine kinase receptor *TRK A*, with good risk and the association of deletion of chromosomes 1p and 11q with poor risk, even in patients with low or intermediate risk features, suggest that continued study of the molecular biology of neuroblastoma may lead to additional prognostic factors and new therapeutic approaches.[34,56,57] Gene microarray technology may also contribute to identification of tumors with different biologic behavior.

Management

Neuroblastoma is sensitive to both chemotherapy and radiotherapy. Surgical therapy alone may suffice for localized disease. Minimal residual disease may regress spontaneously. Although complete removal of the tumor offers the best chance of cure in higher-risk patients,[58] often only a diagnostic biopsy is feasible. Tumor recurrence in such patients is often at the site of the primary tumor. Surgical reduction after initial cytoreductive therapy may enhance the likelihood of cure.

Chemotherapy is the major modality of therapy in neuroblastoma. Complete and partial responses have been found with several agents, including cyclophosphamide, doxorubicin, cisplatin, epipodophyllotoxin, and vincristine.[59] Ifosfamide, carboplatin, and topotecan are also effective agents. Combination therapy is used, most intensively in the more advanced stages of disease. Survival with conventional therapy remains inadequate for patients older than 1 year who have stage 3 disease with unfavorable biological features (eg, N-*myc* amplification) or stage 4 disease. However, recent studies have demonstrated that patients between 12 and 18 months with metastatic disease but nonamplified N-*myc* have a more favorable prognosis and may not require the same intensity of therapy as patients with amplified N-*myc*.[60,61]

Intensive regimens are at the limits of bone marrow tolerance. Myeloablative therapy followed by purged autologous stem cell transplantation to restore hematopoiesis improves event-free survival[62,63]; the differentiating agent, cis-retinoic acid, improves survival for high-risk patients, regardless of whether stem cell transplantation was used.[63] Other retinoids, such as fenretinide, are actively being studied. The retinoids are of particular interest because their mechanisms include both differentiation and induction of apoptosis.

Neuroblastoma is a radiation-sensitive tumor. Although rarely needed in early-stage disease, radiotherapy may facilitate surgical resection of residual disease or may reduce the risk of recurrence in surgically unresectable disease. Emergent situations, such as a large mediastinal mass resulting in respiratory compromise or a dumbbell lesion protruding into the intervertebral foramen that causes cord compression, may be treated with radiation. Total-body irradiation may also be a component of the preparative regimen used before hematopoietic stem cell transplantation. In the terminal stage of neuroblastoma, bone pain or compression of organs such as the trachea, bowel, or urinary tract may require palliative radiotherapy.

Investigations continue into other treatments to improve the outcome and potentially reduce the toxicities of therapy for children who have high-risk neuroblastoma. In addition to retinoids, these treatments include newer chemotherapy agents, radiolabeled meta-iodobenzylguanidine, and targeted immunotherapy that uses anti-GD_2 ganglioside antibodies.[64-66]

Prognosis

Age of the patient and stage of disease appear to be the most important predictors of survival. Patients who are younger than 1 year do much better than those who are older than 2 years. Patients who have stage 1, 2, or 4S neuroblastoma with favorable biological features have survival rates higher than 90%. Although some studies dispute the poor prognosis of N-*myc*–amplified tumors in infants, other studies report a significantly lower survival rate for these patients.[67,68] Long-term survival for patients who have stage 3 neuroblastoma has improved, with patients younger than 1 year and with those who have favorable biology having, respectively, survival rates of 100% and 90% at 4 years.[69] Thus intensive multiagent chemotherapy appears to result in improved cure rates for these patients. In studies of patients with stage 4 disease treated with stem cell transplants, event-free survival is 23% to 47% at 3 to 6 years.[62,70,71] Skeletal disease and persisting bone marrow involvement were predictive of a poorer outcome, and patients who have a complete response to chemotherapy benefit most from transplantation.

Follow-Up

Although late recurrences have been reported, most tumors recur while patients are receiving therapy or shortly afterward. Close follow-up with physical examination and radiologic studies should continue after completing therapy. Urinary catecholamine levels may be useful in the surveillance of patients who had increased values at diagnosis. Patients should be monitored for late toxicities of chemotherapy (eg, cyclophosphamide, doxorubicin, cisplatin) and radiotherapy. High-dose therapy associated with autologous hematopoietic stem cell procedures may result in significant late effects, including hearing loss, renal insufficiency, growth impairment, and gonadal failure.[72]

RETINOBLASTOMA

Retinoblastoma is a congenital malignant tumor of the retina that occurs in 1 per 18,000 live births.[73] Retinoblastoma develops in approximately 350 children in the United States annually. The disorder is diagnosed in 95% before age 4 years, with an incidence of 10.6 per million; the median age of diagnosis is 2 years.[1] No difference by gender, race, or left versus right eye has been found.[74] Bilateral disease represents a hereditary form of this tumor that occurs at an earlier age and is present in 30% to 40% of patients. Unilateral disease is a sporadic form of the tumor in 90% of patients with this presentation; the other 10% have familial retinoblastoma.[75]

This tumor is the model for understanding the role of genetics in the development of malignancy. The pediatrician plays an important role in initially detecting this disorder and in providing support to the family, who may carry a genetic predisposition to this malignancy.

Etiology

Two independent mutations must occur in a single retinal cell for retinoblastoma to develop.[76] The initial mutation may occur in a germinal cell (inheritable form) or in the somatic retinal cell itself (sporadic form). Patients who have an abnormality in the germinal cell have one mutation in each retinal cell. A second mutation is relatively likely to occur, causing retinoblastoma (often multiple, bilateral tumors). If the initial mutation arises in a retinal cell, then it must be followed by a second mutation in the same cell for the sporadic form of retinoblastoma to arise. The likelihood of two such events is low; hence single unilateral tumors develop. Because the germinal cell is not involved, the mutation is not inherited.

A patient who has a family history of retinoblastoma or bilateral retinoblastoma has a germinal mutation and therefore the hereditary form of the disease. Penetrance is approximately 90%[75]; thus these patients have a 45% chance of transmitting retinoblastoma to their children. The germinal mutation also may have arisen in an unaffected parent or in one who had an undiagnosed retinal lesion. Parents ought to undergo an ophthalmologic examination. If the first child of noncarrier parents has unilateral retinoblastoma, then their second child has a 1% risk of being affected, although siblings should have ophthalmologic examinations also. All families should be referred for genetic counseling.

In some families, recombinant DNA techniques may aid in determining whether the disease is hereditary and which relatives are predisposed to retinoblastoma.[74,75,77] Abnormalities of chromosome 13q14 have been detected in patients who have retinoblastoma. This retinoblastoma *(Rb)* gene has been cloned, and the *Rb* gene product is a regulator at the cell cycle checkpoint between G1 and entry into S phase. Deletion or dysfunction of the gene also has been found in nonretinal tumors such as osteosarcomas, soft-tissue sarcomas, and breast carcinomas. Testing patients and family members for mutations in the *Rb* gene requires sophisticated techniques and fails to detect the abnormality in approximately 20% of patients with bilateral disease.[74,75] Improving the ease, availability, and sensitivity of testing for families with retinoblastoma is a goal for the future. Other chromosomal abnormalities have also been identified in retinoblastoma, and as with other pediatric malignancies, they are being studied for their relationship to tumorigenesis and biologic behavior. Another area of research is the role of human papilloma virus in sporadic retinoblastoma.[74]

Clinical Manifestations

Infants who have a family history of retinoblastoma should be screened by examination under anesthesia at birth and every 2 to 4 weeks initially then again at increasing intervals to detect disease before the occurrence of clinical symptoms. Screening should continue until age 5 for these patients and for patients diagnosed with unilateral disease.[75] Pediatricians and parents usually detect the abnormality in children who have the sporadic form of disease because young children rarely complain of unilaterally decreased vision. The pediatrician plays an important role in detecting the signs and symptoms of retinoblastoma. Leukocoria, or cat's-eye reflex, describes a whiteness detected in the pupillary area caused by a large retrolental mass. It is the most commonly encountered sign of retinoblastoma. If a normal red reflex is not present in a young child, then it should be investigated. The second most common presenting feature is strabismus. Although common in childhood because of abnormalities of ocular muscle strength, strabismus rarely arises suddenly in a child who has had normal extraocular movements. In rare cases, pain in the eye may occur as a result of glaucoma. New-onset strabismus or an abnormal red reflex (leukocoria) requires prompt ophthalmologic evaluation.[78]

The differential diagnosis of retinoblastoma includes Coats disease, retrolental fibroplasia, persistent hyperplastic primary vitreous, toxoplasmosis, *Toxocara canis* infection, and other causes of severe uveitis. Although patients sometimes have nonneoplastic disorders at the time of enucleation,[79,80] this occurrence is uncommon with newer diagnostic methods, including ultrasonography and MRI. If retinoblastoma is a possibility, then referral should be directly made to an ophthalmologist experienced in ophthalmologic oncology who has a working relationship with radiation and pediatric oncologists.

Evaluation

Examination under anesthesia after dilating the pupils is necessary to evaluate fully the retina in a young child. Ultrasonography is useful to evaluate the mass, particularly if the fundal examination is obscured by hemorrhage or retinal detachment.[81] Calcification in retinoblastoma may be apparent on radiograph, ultrasound examination, or CT scan. The CT scan helps demonstrate the extent of intraocular disease and may detect possible extraocular extension. MRI can help to evaluate the tumor involvement with the optic nerve, the subarachnoid, and the brain. Biopsy is not a feasible method of diagnosis for retinoblastoma. If a family history of bilateral disease exists, then a tissue diagnosis is unnecessary. In many cases of unilateral disease, enucleation may be necessary to establish the diagnosis and to treat the tumor. For high-risk patients, bone marrow and cerebrospinal fluid specimens are obtained for evidence of dissemination. The extent of local disease (extension beyond the globe or optic nerve infiltration) is assessed at the time of enucleation. The Reese-Ellsworth classification has been used for decades as a method to describe tumors based on size, location, and multiplicity. Its original intent was to predict prognosis and vision in eyes treated with different radiation techniques, but its consistent usage has maintained its usefulness as therapy evolved. However, new classifications have been proposed to account for the emergence of new therapies, particularly chemotherapy, but none is universally accepted at this time.[74]

Management

Treatment of retinoblastoma is individualized based on the extent of disease and the possibility for the preservation of vision.[74,82] Treatments available include enucleation, external-beam radiotherapy, plaque brachytherapy, cryotherapy, photocoagulation, and chemotherapy. Most patients who have unilateral sporadic disease have large lesions and compromised vision. Enucleation is usually required, with removal of the longest segment of the optic nerve possible. Photocoagulation and cryotherapy are used for small lesions, most commonly in patients who have hereditary bilateral disease. Until recently, radiotherapy was the standard of care for patients who had massive bilateral disease; but now, chemotherapy is used to allow local therapy to preserve vision.[74,83-85] Significant tumor shrinkage can be achieved, but local therapy is required for cure. Some evidence suggests that chemotherapy also prevents pineoblastoma, a usually fatal second cancer in patients with hereditary retinoblastoma.[85] The most commonly used agents are vincristine, carboplatin, and etoposide. Radiotherapy, enucleation, or a combination of both can be avoided with the use of chemotherapy in intermediate-stage disease, and chemotherapy also plays an increasing role in the treatment of advanced-stage disease.[86] Periocular administration of carboplatin chemotherapy has also been studied and used in specific clinical situations.[85] Emerging therapy also includes the use of transpupillary thermotherapy with or without adjuvant chemotherapy.[74,85,87,88]

Cyclosporin has been used with chemotherapy to overcome multidrug resistance and has been shown to improve the long-term response to chemotherapy, although definite benefit remains to be proved.[89] Bone marrow transplantation or peripheral blood stem cell support after high-dose therapy for the treatment of recurrent disease has been reported.[90]

Prognosis

Survival of patients who have retinoblastoma is excellent; more than 85% have no recurrence of their tumor, and survival from the primary tumor is more than 95%.[85] Unfortunately, patients who have hereditary retinoblastoma have a high incidence of second malignancy. Approximately 50% occur within the radiation field; osteosarcoma or other sarcomas in particular are common. Patients irradiated when they are younger than 1 year are at increased risk.[74,85] Approximately one third of such patients have a second malignancy within 15 years. By 30 years, up to two thirds will have a second malignancy.[85,91,92] Avoiding radiotherapy may reduce but not eliminate this risk.

Follow-Up

Patients who have been treated for retinoblastoma will need close follow-up for evidence of recurrence and for second malignancies. Most recurrences happen within 3 years of diagnosis. Examinations under anesthesia should be performed every 2 to 3 months during the first year, every 3 to 4 months during the second year, and every 6 months thereafter until age 6 years. Long-term risk depends on treatment. After enucleation, a prosthesis is necessary. Radiation impairs orbital growth and increases the risk for cataract development and retinal vascular injury. Growth and pubertal development are usually unaffected by orbital radiation, but monitoring of hypothalamic-pituitary axis function is warranted. The risk of second malignancy is high in patients who have bilateral or familial disease, particularly in the radiation field. Medical care should be sought promptly for unexplained masses, pain, or other symptoms.

RHABDOMYOSARCOMA

Rhabdomyosarcoma is considered to be one of the small, round, blue cell tumors of childhood (along with neuroblastomas, Ewing sarcoma, and lymphoma). It arises from embryonal mesenchyme that can differentiate into skeletal muscle. Rhabdomyosarcoma can occur almost anywhere in the body, even in sites that do not normally contain skeletal muscle. It can be an aggressive tumor that disseminates early in the course of disease. Before the advent of chemotherapy, cure required extirpative surgery of localized disease and then radiotherapy. Marked improvement in prognosis, with survival rates increasing from less than 20% in the 1960s to more than 70% in the late 1990s, has been the result of the multidisciplinary cooperative group approach of the Intergroup Rhabdomyosarcoma Study.[93]

Rhabdomyosarcoma is the most common pediatric soft-tissue sarcoma, accounting for 2% to 4% of childhood malignancies and 5% to 15% of childhood solid tumors. Its annual incidence among children through 18 years of age in the United States is 4.5 per million. Thus approximately 400 new cases are diagnosed each year. The incidence in boys is greater than in girls, and it is more common in white patients than in black patients.[1] Forty percent of affected children are younger than 5 years, 47% are 5 to 14 years of age, and the rest are older than 15 years.

Etiology

The cause of this tumor is unknown. It has occurred in association with neurofibromatosis, Beckwith-Wiedemann syndrome, in families who have a history of multiple tumors, and in patients who have congenital abnormalities of the CNS, the heart, the gastrointestinal tract, and the urinary tract.[94,95]

Two major histopathological subtypes have been noted: (1) embryonal and (2) alveolar. Embryonal rhabdomyosarcoma, which account for over one half the cases, may have loss of heterozygosity at 11p15; the alveolar subtype is associated with a characteristic chromosomal translocation, t(2:13).[96,97] The latter subtype is more common in extremity and trunk sites and in older children. Younger children who have alveolar rhabdomyosarcoma may have t(1:13), which is associated with a somewhat better prognosis than t(2:13), particularly in patients with metastatic disease.[95] Molecular testing can be used in addition to histopathological analysis to ensure accurate diagnosis. As in other pediatric malignancies, further investigation of the cytogenetic alterations identified in the histopathological subtypes will provide insight into tumorigenesis. Undifferentiated sarcomas do not express lineage markers but have traditionally been treated by the same regimens used to treat rhabdomyosarcoma.

Clinical Manifestations

Rhabdomyosarcoma produces a painless mass with poorly defined margins.[95,96] No mass may be palpable, but patients may experience disturbance of a normal body function resulting from the presence of tumor. Pain may also be a presenting symptom. Thirty-five percent to 40% of rhabdomyosarcomas arise in the head and neck region, 25% in the genitourinary region, 20% in the extremities, and the remainder in the trunk and other sites. One common site of involvement is the orbit, in which swelling, proptosis, discoloration, and limitation of extraocular motion occur. Patients who have a tumor of the head and neck may have hoarseness, difficulty swallowing, nasopharyngeal polyps, nasopharyngeal obstruction, decreased hearing acuity, persistent otitis, sinusitis, bloody nasal discharge, parotitis, or cranial nerve palsies. In parameningeal sites, penetration to the brain may cause headache, vomiting, or diplopia. Retroperitoneal tumor may exhibit as a mass or partial or complete bowel obstruction. Vaginal bleeding, pelvic or perineal masses, hematuria, urinary frequency, and urinary retention suggest genitourinary tract involvement. Tumor may even be extruded from the bladder or female genital tract. A hydrocele, incarcerated hernia, testicular torsion, or testicular mass may be an indication of paratesticular rhabdomyosarcoma. Symptoms may be related to metastatic disease, such as pain, difficulty, or refusal to ambulate resulting from bone metastases. Patients may also have systemic symptoms, such as fever, fatigue, or weight loss.

Evaluation

Initial evaluation should include a complete history and physical examination. Radiographs CT scans or MRIs, and in some instances (eg, genitourinary tract) ultrasound examination of the involved and adjacent areas should be performed. For genitourinary disease, a cystourethrogram, barium enema, and cystoscopic and pelvic examinations may also be needed. Bone surveys, bone scan, bilateral bone marrow aspirate and biopsy, and chest and abdomen CT scan are necessary to assess for metastatic disease. Basal skull erosion may be seen by CT scan, and spinal fluid may reveal meningeal disease in patients who have parameningeal tumors. Dental films may be helpful. If spinal cord symptoms are present, then a spinal MRI is necessary. Biopsy of the lesion establishes the diagnosis and should be performed before extensive resection. Rhabdomyosarcomas are assigned a stage determined by preoperative extent and site of disease and to a clinical group based on postoperative residual disease.

Management

Rhabdomyosarcoma is a tumor that requires a multitherapeutic approach, including chemotherapy, surgery, and radiation. Aggressive surgical approaches have become less essential as chemotherapy and radiotherapy have become more efficacious.

The initial surgical procedure should be a diagnostic biopsy. A wide resection of the primary tumor, including surrounding normal tissue, is preferable if excessive functional and cosmetic morbidity can be prevented.[98] Complete resection is correlated with a better outcome but is possible in only approximately 20% of patients.[95] Extensive en bloc lymph node dissection is no longer indicated; however, biopsy should be performed on large regional nodes. Second-look surgery after chemotherapy may allow resection with reduction of surgical morbidity, provides assessment of therapeutic response by determining the presence of viable tumor, and potentially reduces the dose of radiotherapy.

All patients with rhabdomyosarcoma require chemotherapy. Regimens are determined by risk group, which is based on stage, group, histology, and age. Vincristine, actinomycin D, and cyclophosphamide are the primary agents. Although other chemotherapy agents have been studied and have activity, none has proven to be better than this combination. The dosing of these agents continues to be studied for optimal efficacy, and future studies will further investigate irinotecan in the treatment of intermediate- and high-risk patients. Other new agents continue to be developed and studied to improve the treatment of higher-risk and relapsed patients.

Rhabdomyosarcoma is an infiltrative disease, and radiation portals should include the entire extent of tumor volume. Radiation is required for patients with embryonal histology and residual disease after surgery and for all patients with alveolar histologic features.[99] Although high doses of radiation (60 to 65 Gy) control local residual disease very well, substantial late morbidity results.[100] This factor must be weighed against the use of lower doses of radiation, which result in an increased recurrence rate. Initial reports on hyperfractionated radiotherapy, which uses smaller fractions administrated twice daily, indicated that efficacy might be preserved while minimizing late toxicities[101]; however, current review does not demonstrate a benefit to this approach.[95] Brachytherapy is another investigational approach that may limit toxicity by using sealed radioisotopes placed inside or close to the tumor, thereby treating only tissues right next to the tumor and minimizing damage to the surrounding normal tissues.[102]

Prognosis

The likelihood of survival for patients who have rhabdomyosarcoma is determined by the site and the stage of disease.[103] Overall, survival is 73% at 5 years from diagnosis.[95] The prognosis is particularly good for patients who have orbital tumors, nonbladder and nonprostate genitourinary tract tumors, and localized tumors that can be resected fully (90% to 95% long-term survivors). Patients with stage IV (metastatic) disease younger than 10 years who have embryonal histology have a better prognosis than older patients who have stage IV disease. Extremity lesions are particularly difficult to treat, perhaps because many co-occur with metastatic disease. Treatment of genitourinary primary tumors has improved markedly in recent years with the use of extensive chemotherapy. Pelvic exenteration and other morbid surgeries now can be avoided in most patients, and radiotherapy may be avoided in some patients.[104] Cranial radiation and intrathecal chemotherapy were once used in all patients who had parameningeal lesions.[105] Intrathecal chemotherapy is rarely used, and early radiotherapy is reserved for patients who have basal skull lesions, CNS involvement, or spinal cord compression.

Eighty percent of recurrences occur within 2 years of treatment. Local relapse is most common, although distant spread to the lungs, CNS, lymph nodes, bone, liver, bone marrow, and soft tissues does occur.

Table 244-4 Long-Term Side Effects of Chemotherapy*

DRUG	POTENTIAL ORGAN DAMAGE	EVALUATION
Anthracyclines (eg, doxorubicin)	*Cardiac:* myocardial damage, congestive failure, arrhythmias	History: exercise intolerance, palpitations; ECG (QTc interval); echocardiogram scheduled based on age, dose, and radiation exposure; Holter monitor; exercise ECG; exercise nuclear angiography
Bleomycin	*Pulmonary:* fibrosis, impaired diffusion capacity, exacerbated by increased oxygen (eg, anesthesia)	History: shortness of breath, dyspnea on exertion, cough; chest film and pulmonary function tests (with diffusion capacity) baseline and with symptoms
Cyclophosphamide, ifosfamide	*Gonadal:* infertility, sterility, early menopause	History: menses, question of fertility; luteinizing hormone, follicle-stimulating hormone, testosterone or estradiol during pubertal development, or if a problem with fertility or amenorrhea (or both) exists; semen analysis (as required to conceive)
	Bladder: hemorrhagic cystitis	Urinalysis annually
	Marrow: secondary acute myeloblastic leukemia	Complete blood cell count annually
Lomustine (CCNU) Carmustine (BCNU)	Pulmonary, gonadal	Pulmonary, gonadal evaluation
Cisplatin	• *Kidney:* decreased glomerular filtration rate • *Ears:* hearing loss (high frequency)	• Serum creatinine baseline and per guidelines • Creatinine clearance baseline and per guidelines • Audiogram baseline and per guidelines
Methotrexate	Liver dysfunction *CNS:* learning impairment (high intravenous dose)	Liver function tests baseline and per guidelines
6-Mercaptopurine, 6-thioguanine, actinomycin D	Liver dysfunction	Liver function tests baseline and per guidelines

CNS, Central nervous system; *ECG,* electrocardiogram.
*See www.survivorguidelines.org/ for more details.

Twenty percent of patients have metastatic disease at diagnosis; these patients continue to have a low likelihood of survival.[106] Current studies indicate that 25% to 30% of these patients will survive 5 years from diagnosis. Hematopoietic stem cell transplant[107] or the use of new agents may offer hope to these patients. For patients who experience relapse, survival depends on histologic features, initial grouping, and staging. Twenty percent of patients who experienced relapse have favorable features with 50% 5-year survival; the other 80% of patients have only 10% 5-year survival.[96]

Follow-Up

Patients who have rhabdomyosarcoma should receive close follow-up for evidence of recurrent disease for at least 3 to 5 years from the time of diagnosis. CT or MRI of the primary site, chest CTs, and bone scans are frequently used for surveillance. Radiotherapy often results in unacceptable cosmetic effects in patients who have orbital tumors. For patients who have orbital or other tumors located in a region of the head or face and received radiation to the sinuses, hypothalamus, and pituitary gland, sinusitis is a common complaint, and hormone levels (eg, growth hormone, gonadotrophins) may need monitoring. Patients also should be monitored for any potential late effects of chemotherapeutic agents (Table 244-4).

GERM CELL TUMORS AND TERATOMAS

Germ cell tumors are growths arising from primordial germ cells. They account for 3% of tumors in children, with an annual incidence of approximately 4 cases per million children younger than 15 years.[1] Incidence is greatest in adolescents and very young children. The sacrococcygeal teratoma (named from the Greek *teras,* meaning *monster*) is the most common germ cell tumor of childhood and is benign in 80% of patients. It occurs in 1 per 35,000 live births and is more common in girls than in boys (2 to 4:1). Sixty percent of childhood germ cell tumors originate in other sites, including the gonads, mediastinum, intracranial region, and retroperitoneum.

Etiology

Germ cells appear in the yolk sac endoderm, migrate around the hind gut to the genital ridge on the posterior abdominal wall of the embryo, and congregate, becoming part of the developing gonad. A slightly aberrant path of migration may account for the occurrence of extragonadal germ cell tumors along the dorsal wall of the embryo in midline sites (sacrococcygeal, retroperitoneal, mediastinal, and pineal regions).[108] Children who have sacrococcygeal teratomas have an approximately 15% incidence of associated anomalies (eg, imperforate anus, rectal stenosis).[109] An association with a family history of twinning resulted in early theories suggesting that teratomas were abortive attempts at the development of twins. Of interest, the common sites of teratomas—brain, mediastinum, abdomen, and sacrococcygeal region—are all sites of twin attachment. A genetic tendency for abnormal germ cell development may exist in some families. These tumors have been reported to develop in siblings, twins, and subsequent generations. Gonadal dysgenesis has been associated with dysgerminoma or gonadoblastoma.[110] The type of germ cell tumor that forms is determined by the subsequent development of the germ cell[111]; those that maintain their total potentiality become embryonal sarcomas. The development of extraembryonic structures results in the formation of choriocarcinomas (placental tumors) or endodermal sinus tumors (yolk sac tumors). Mixed tumors are not uncommon. Seminomas or dysgerminomas arise when the gonads differentiate. Teratomas form as a result of embryonal differentiation into ectoderm, mesoderm, and endoderm.

Clinical Manifestations

The clinical manifestations of a germ cell tumor depend on the tumor's location. Sacrococcygeal tumors occur as a mass between the anus and the coccyx.[112] An abnormality of the overlying skin may be noted. An intrapelvic tumor may be associated with an external tumor or may be the only evidence of disease, noted by the onset of urinary or rectal obstruction. The incidence of intradural tumor extension is 3% to 5%. Maternal polyhydramnios may be associated with infantile sacrococcygeal teratomas.

Ovarian tumors[113] in infants occur as abdominal masses. Older girls have symptoms of abdominal pain, nausea, vomiting, constipation, or urinary tract obstruction, with palpable masses noted in 50%. Torsion or hemorrhage within the tumor may be responsible for acute abdominal pain; 5% of such children have bilateral tumors. Vaginal germ cell tumors in preschool girls (younger than 3 years) may cause bloody vaginal discharge.

Testicular tumors[114] most often occur as symptom-free scrotal masses, sometimes with a coexisting hydrocele. Torsion of the tumor in an undescended testis may result in acute abdominal pain. An undescended testis is an established risk factor for testicular germ cell tumor.[115] Because the ipsilateral or contralateral testis may be affected, an intrinsic testicular defect is likely.

Retroperitoneal teratomas that occur in children younger than 2 years are usually symptom-free abdominal masses. In older children, anorexia, vomiting, or abdominal pain may be noted. Intradural extensions may also occur, and gastric and hepatic tumors have been reported. The symptoms of patients who have germ cell tumors of the anterior mediastinum include coughing, wheezing, dyspnea, and chest pain.[116] Newborns may require immediate intubation for respiratory distress caused by mediastinal, cervical, or oropharyngeal germ cell tumors. Intrapericardial tumors can cause heart failure and cardiac tamponade. In the fetus with an oropharyngeal mass, the inability to swallow can cause maternal polyhydramnios. Cranial tumors (80% in the pineal region) cause hydrocephalus and increased intracranial pressure in infants. Teenagers have headaches, lethargy, vomiting, diabetes insipidus, seizures, and visual disturbance, especially loss of upward gaze.

The differential diagnosis of children who have germ cell tumors depends on the location of the primary tumor. For patients who have sacrococcygeal masses, meningocele is the most frequent alternative diagnosis. Abdominal or pelvic masses may be the result of neuroblastoma, Wilms tumor, rhabdomyosarcoma, or lymphomas. Nonmalignant disorders such as hydronephrosis, benign ovarian cysts, constipation, and splenomegaly must be considered. Anterior mediastinal tumors include T-cell lymphoma, leukemia, or thymoma. The differential diagnosis for an intrascrotal mass includes testicular torsion, epididymitis, and testicular infarction. (See Tables 244-1 and 244-3 for details of the differential diagnosis of germ cell tumors.)

Evaluation

As in any ill child, evaluation includes a thorough physical examination. For patients who have a sacrococcygeal mass or abdominal pain, particular attention should be paid to the abdominal and rectal examination. A pelvic examination (performed under anesthesia in young girls) will be necessary if an ovarian or a vaginal tumor is suspected.

Thorough evaluation by CT, ultrasound, or both is essential. A CT scan of benign germ cell tumors will often reveal calcifications. A teratoma frequently shows cystic and solid components, including fat, on radiologic examination. Malignant germ cell tumors often have areas of hemorrhage and necrosis.[117] A chest CT scan and bone scan should be performed to detect pulmonary and bony metastases.

Malignant germ cell tumors that have evidence of extraembryonic differentiation often produce proteins elaborated by the corresponding normal embryonic structure. Serum levels of these markers, alfa-fetoprotein (AFP) and β-human chorionic gonadotropin (B-hCG), should be assayed before surgery. AFP is found in germ cell tumors that have endodermal sinus tumor histologic features. The evaluation of AFP levels must account for their increase during fetal development; they do not return to normal levels until the child is approximately 9 months of age.[118] B-hCG, a glycoprotein normally produced by specialized placental cells, is present in increased quantity in patients who have choriocarcinomas, patients who have hydatidiform moles, and women during pregnancy. In adolescent girls who have an abdominal mass and increased B-hCG, pregnancy should not be assumed, especially if the patient denies sexual activity or symptoms are atypical. Detection of AFP or B-hCG improves the ability to monitor the disease status. The rate of disappearance after resection reflects the adequacy of the tumor removal. With response to chemotherapy, the levels of these proteins decrease. A significant increase in these levels suggests disease recurrence.

Management

Germ cell tumors may have components of teratoma, endodermal sinus tumor, embryonal carcinoma, choriocarcinoma, seminoma, or dysgerminoma. Teratomas are classified as mature, immature, or teratoma with malignant components. Mature teratomas (well-differentiated tissues) and immature teratomas (embryonic-appearing neuroglial elements and mature elements) are most commonly found in infants, although over one half of germ cell tumors that have a major component of immature teratoma are mixed tumors, all of which will contain elements of yolk sac tumor.[119] Malignant evolution may occur years after removal of an apparently benign tumor, particularly in the sacrococcygeal area. For this reason, complete excision of the coccyx is often suggested, and close follow-up is necessary.

In the past, malignant teratomas, embryonal carcinomas, endodermal sinus tumors, and choriocarcinomas were almost always fatal. Complete surgical resection was attained rarely and was only infrequently curative. Only embryonal carcinoma of the infant testis might be cured by radical orchiectomy. In the 1960s, however, the efficacy of methotrexate chemotherapy for gestational choriocarcinomas and testicular germ cell tumors was demonstrated.[120] Ovarian tumors responded to vincristine, actinomycin D, and cyclophosphamide. In the 1970s, additional agents such as vinblastine and cisplatin were found to have significant single-agent response in testicular germ cell tumors of young men. The combination of these two agents with bleomycin produced a 70% complete remission rate and a 55% long-term disease-free survival for patients who have advanced testicular carcinoma.[121] The regimens initially studied in adults also proved effective in children.[122] Chemotherapy is now the standard for significant subsets of patients with germ cell tumors.

Current studies stratify patients as follows: low risk—stage I testicular and ovarian tumors; intermediate risk—stage II-IV testicular, stage II-III ovarian, stage I-II extragonadal malignant germ cell tumors; and high risk—stage III-IV extragonadal tumors. Therapies include surgery and observation for low-risk patients, and standard therapy with cisplatin, etoposide, and bleomycin for intermediate-risk patients. Higher doses of cyclophosphamide are being studied in addition to surgery and the standard three-drug chemotherapy regimen for high-risk-patients.

Prognosis

The French Society for Pediatric Oncology has identified 3 prognostic groups for patients older than 1 year who had localized disease. Patients who had stage III disease (more than microscopic residual disease), sacrococcygeal or mediastinal primaries, and AFP more than 10,000 ng/mL had a 43% 3-year disease-free survival. Stage I disease (complete resection) or stage II disease (microscopic residual), testicular, ovarian, perineal, or retroperitoneal primary tumor, and AFP less than 10,000 ng/mL were associated with a 100% 3-year disease-free survival. The remaining patients were in an intermediate-prognosis group and had 81% disease-free survival.[123] This study also detected improved prognosis for patients treated with cisplatin versus carboplatin. The prognosis continues to improve, with event-free survivals for most patient groups better than 80% and up to 100%, with overall survival 90% to 100%.

The prognosis for a teratoma depends on its degree of maturity and age. Sacrococcygeal teratomas are usually benign in children younger than 2 months; thereafter the likelihood of malignant evolution increases rapidly. This factor may be the reason that intrapelvic teratomas that are not detected early often are found to be malignant. Mediastinal teratomas behave benignly in children and young teenagers; in older patients, they are more aggressive. Cervical and intracranial teratomas in infants are usually benign; those in adolescents and adults are often malignant.

Immature teratomas can be treated with surgery alone, with event-free survival of 97.8%, 100%, and 80% for patients who have ovarian, testicular, and extragonadal tumors, respectively. For patients who experience relapse, cisplatin-based chemotherapy offers an excellent chance of cure.[124]

Follow-Up

The response of malignant germ cell tumors to chemotherapy is encouraging, but relapse may occur as many as 10 years from the time of diagnosis.[125] Late-brain metastases have also been described. For this reason, close follow-up care is essential, including frequent physical examinations, radiologic evaluations, and monitoring of AFP and B-hCG levels, if they are found to be high at diagnosis. Salvage therapy may prolong survival or even provide a cure. Late effects of the chemotherapeutic agent administered (eg, bleomycin, cisplatin) should be monitored (see Table 244-4).

EWING FAMILY OF TUMORS

The Ewing family of tumors includes Ewing sarcoma of bone, extraosseous Ewing, and peripheral primitive neuroectodermal tumors (PNETs). These tumors are malignant tumors that usually arise in bone but may also occur in soft tissues. A PNET of the chest wall is referred to as *Askin tumor*.

The Ewing family of tumors accounts for 3% of childhood cancers and is the most common bone tumor in children younger than 10 years. In the second decade of life, it is second in incidence to osteosarcoma. The peak incidence is between the ages of 11 and 17 years, when the annual incidence is approximately 7 per million.[1] Ewing sarcoma is extremely rare in patients younger than 5 years or older than 30 years, as well as in blacks and Asians.

Etiology

The Ewing family of tumors is a primitive small, round, blue cell tumor. These tumors are of neural origin, with variable degrees of differentiation. Most of them share a common chromosomal translocation, t(11:22).[126] The resulting gene fusion rearrangements provide insight into tumorigenesis of these malignancies; specific fusion products may have prognostic significance.[127,128] No evidence suggests hereditary transmission of Ewing sarcoma, nor has it been associated with known congenital syndromes or constitutional karyotypic abnormalities. No specific environmental risk factors have been identified.[129]

Clinical Manifestations

Patients who have Ewing sarcoma most commonly consult the clinician for pain.[96,130] Swelling may also be present. Symptoms often begin insidiously, several months before diagnosis, and may initially be attributed to trauma. At the time of diagnosis, a mass is palpable in 60% of patients resulting from the propensity of this tumor to break through the bony cortex and involve the surrounding tissue.[131] This disruption of the cortex may also result in a pathological fracture. The primary tumor site is evenly distributed between central and extremity lesions. The primary lesion is most often found in the femur (22%), the fibula or tibia (21%), or the pelvis (22%). The ribs and vertebrae are other common sites of origin. Demonstrable metastatic lesions are present in 14% to 35% of patients, occurring in the lungs, bones, lymph nodes, and bone marrow.[132] CNS involvement is uncommon.

The differential diagnosis includes osteosarcoma, osteomyelitis, benign bone tumors, and bone cysts. Other tumors that occasionally involve the bone and have a similar histologic pattern of small round cells include lymphoma, leukemia, neuroblastoma, and rhabdomyosarcoma (Table 244-5).

Evaluation

A radiograph should be obtained in a patient who has a mass overlying bone or bone pain that is not characteristic of trauma (by lack of history or duration of symptoms). Radiographs of a bone that has Ewing sarcoma often show a destructive lesion in the diaphysis. An onionskin appearance arises from periosteal elevation and subperiosteal new bone formation associated with tumor extension through the cortex. A mottled pattern may be seen as a result of bone destruction, sclerosis, and cystic formation. An associated soft-tissue mass occurs in more than 50% of patients who have primary tumors of long bones. A CT scan and MRI are necessary to determine the extent of the primary lesion.

Radionuclide bone scanning detects primary and metastatic lesions, but it is not particularly useful in determining the extent of the primary disease. A CT scan of the chest is necessary to determine whether pulmonary lesions are present. The possibility of bone marrow involvement should be evaluated by bilateral bone marrow aspirates and biopsies. Identification of micrometastases in the bone marrow by polymerase chain reaction may identify high-risk patients without other evidence of metastases.[133] Cerebrospinal fluid should be examined in patients who have parameningeal tumors. PET scanning may also be used to follow the course of disease in these patients.[134]

A biopsy of the lesion is necessary to establish the diagnosis. If possible, diagnostic tissue should be obtained from soft tissue rather than from cortical bone to reduce the potential for pathological fracture.

Large tumors, primary tumors on the trunk and pelvis, and increased lactic dehydrogenase levels have been associated with worse prognosis, but they may be less important with current aggressive treatment regimens.[133] Older age is associated with worse prognosis. The most significant prognostic indicator is the presence of metastatic disease, present in 20% to 25% of patients. Isolated pulmonary metastases may be associated with a better prognosis than metastases to other sites,[135] but this association is not confirmed.[136] Histologic response also affects prognosis in that patients who have marked tissue necrosis after chemotherapy have a better prognosis.

Table 244-5 Differential Diagnosis of Malignant Tumors Involving the Extremities

TUMOR*	AGE	CLINICAL SIGNS	LABORATORY FINDINGS
Ewing sarcoma	≥5 yr	Pain, swelling; genitourinary or skeletal anomaly; weight loss, fever; malaise (metabolic)	*Onionskin* appearance on roentgenogram
Osteogenic sarcoma	Teens	Pain, swelling; familial retinoblastoma; prior radiation to bone; Paget disease	Codman triangle (cortical elevation, new bone formation); sunburst ossification of soft tissue; soft-tissue mass; increased alkaline phosphatase level
Lymphoma	All	Pain	—
Fibrosarcoma	Infants, teens	Painless mass; prior radiation; plastic implant	—
Rhabdomyosarcoma	All	Mass	—
Synovial sarcoma	Teens	Mass	Calcification (40%)

*Other causes: trauma, bone cysts, osteomyelitis.

Management

Approximately 75% of patients who have Ewing sarcoma do not have identified metastases but may have micrometastatic tumor. Therefore local therapy alone, that is, surgery or radiotherapy, is unlikely to be curative. Chemotherapy has made it possible to cure most patients who have localized Ewing sarcoma and has improved the outcome in patients with metastatic disease.

The choice of radiation or surgery for local control is made based on the likelihood of preserving function. Functionally expendable bones should be removed. Aggressive surgical procedures, including limb-sparing excisions, are frequently performed. Some evidence suggests that complete surgical resection may improve prognosis.[135] However, radiotherapy is required for local control and will improve the prognosis when resection with appropriate margins is not achieved or when the tumor is unresectable. Preoperative radiotherapy may also provide benefit. The local failure rate for patients treated with radiotherapy on more recent protocols is 22.5%, with higher failure rates in patients with central versus noncentral tumor sites.[135] Patients receiving radiotherapy are a negatively selected group with unfavorable tumor sites or size. Radiotherapy may also be helpful for treatment of pulmonary or osseous metastases.

Ewing sarcoma is extremely chemosensitive. Standard chemotherapy now includes vincristine, doxorubicin, and cyclophosphamide alternating with etoposide and ifosfamide.[137-139] Studies have demonstrated the effectiveness of these regimens for extraosseous Ewing and peripheral PNETs.[140,141]

Dose intensity of the more active agents (cyclophosphamide and doxorubicin) has played a major role in improving disease-free survival.[142,143] However, the outcome remains extremely poor for patients with metastatic disease. Additional chemotherapeutic agents, alone and in combination, and dose intensification are being studied for activity against Ewing tumors.[136] Hematopoietic stem cell transplantation has also been used to treat high-risk Ewing tumors, but the heterogenous patient population and regimens makes assessment of benefit difficult. However, benefit may occur by using high-dose busulfan and melphalan, and allogeneic transplants may provide the additional benefit of a graft-versus-tumor effect as a result of an immune response to proteins derived from the characteristic gene fusion present in these tumors.[133]

Prognosis

Before the advent of multiagent chemotherapy, 85% of children who had Ewing sarcoma died within 2 years of diagnosis.[144] Five-year, disease-free survival is approximately 75% for nonmetastatic disease,[133] with event-free survival of 12% to 24% for patients with metastatic disease.[136,142,145] The outcome for patients who experience relapse is very poor, with the small number of survivors usually among patients who experience relapse more than 2 years from initial diagnosis or those who experience relapse with lung metastases only.[146]

Follow-Up

Patients who have Ewing sarcoma require close follow-up for evidence of recurrent disease for at least 5 years from the time of diagnosis. Recurrences may occur later. Particular attention should be paid to the irradiated field of long-term survivors because second malignancies may arise (Table 244-6). Bone films should be obtained periodically. Patients who have lower-extremity lesions whose growth is incomplete should be monitored for evidence of leg-length discrepancies, which may require arresting the growth in the opposite limb. Monitoring for potential late effects of the specific chemotherapeutic agents administered (eg, cyclophosphamide, doxorubicin) is important (see Table 244-4).

OSTEOSARCOMA

Osteosarcoma is the most common bone tumor encountered in the first 3 decades of life. The incidence is 8.7 per million; approximately 400 patients are diagnosed per year in the United States. Osteosarcoma comprises 60% of malignant bone tumors. A male-to-female ratio of approximately 1.5:1 has been noted.[1] The peak incidence occurs at age 14.5 for boys and 13.5 for girls, corresponding to the age of their growth spurts, although osteosarcoma can occur before puberty and after the adolescent growth spurt. Previous evidence that taller children are at increased risk[147] has not been confirmed.[148]

Etiology

The hallmark of osteosarcoma is the production of osteoid or mature bone by proliferating malignant spindle cell sarcoma. The high incidence of this tumor in adolescents who are undergoing rapid skeletal growth, as well as individuals who have Paget disease of the bone, suggests that increased bone growth may play a role in the induction of the malignancy.[149] Although patients often report a history of trauma before the diagnosis, injuries most likely allow the recognition of an already-proliferating tumor.

Patients at increased risk of osteosarcoma include those who have received irradiation to the bone, usually for the treatment of malignancy.[150] Although radiation itself can be causative, patients who have one tumor may be at increased genetic risk for a second primary malignancy. Patients who have hereditary retinoblastoma and thus a constitutive deletion at *Rb*, the *Rb* tumor suppressor gene, have an increased incidence of osteosarcoma. Although one half of these tumors occur within the radiation field,[151] the risk of sarcoma is far greater, regardless of radiation exposure, because the abnormality at the *Rb* gene itself confers predisposition to osteosarcoma. Osteosarcoma in otherwise normal hosts also frequently involves mutation or loss of the *RB1* gene, with inactivation of the tumor suppression pathway.[148,152] Inactivation of *p53*, another tumor suppressor gene, is commonly detected in osteosarcoma. Germ-line mutations of this gene result in the Li-Fraumeni syndrome (an autosomal-dominant predisposition to multiple malignancies). Germline mutation of *p53* is present in 3% to 4% of children who have osteosarcoma.[148] Many other chromosomal abnormalities have also been detected in osteosarcoma.

Table 244-6 Long-Term Side Effects of Radiation

IRRADIATED AREA*	RISKS	MONITORING
Cranium and nasopharynx	Cataracts	Physical examination
	Growth: impaired	Growth charts (bone age, growth hormone, organ system function as appropriate)
	CNS: learning impairment	Monitoring of school function; neuropsychological evaluation
	Dentition: abnormal formation	Dental evaluation
	Thyroid: overt or compensated hypothyroidism	Free T_4, TSH levels
	High dose (>2500 Gy):	—
	Hypothalamic dysfunction (decreased growth hormone; decreased gonadotropin, hyperprolactinemia)	Growth; pubertal, menstrual, and fertility history (growth hormone, LH, testosterone, estrogen, prolactin levels)
	Hearing (especially with cisplatin)	Audiogram
Neck and mandible	Hypoplasia of bone or soft tissues	Examination of area
	Dentition: abnormal formation, abnormal salivary function	Dental evaluation
	Thyroid: hypothyroidism	Free T_4, TSH
Thorax	Hypoplasia (includes impaired chest wall growth)	Examination of area
	Thyroid: hypothyroidism	Free T_4, TSH levels
	Lungs: fibrosis, decreased capacity	History, pulmonary function tests, chest film baseline and as appropriate
	Cardiac: pericardial and valvular thickening; possibility of early myocardial infarction	History, ECG, echocardiogram scheduled based on age, dose, and radiation exposure
	Breasts: impaired growth, possibility of increased malignancy	Breast self-examination, early mammograms start 8 years after therapy or age 25
Abdomen/pelvis	Hypoplasia (including scoliosis)	Examination of area, x-ray film of spine during puberty
	Liver (if in field)	Liver function tests
	Kidneys (if in field)	Serum creatinine, urinalysis protein (24-hour collection for creatinine, protein)
	Gonads (if in field)	Pubertal, menstrual, and fertility history, LH, follicle-stimulating hormone, estradiol or testosterone levels during puberty and if fertility is doubtful, semen analysis
	Gastrointestinal tract	Nutritional history
Extremities	Hypoplasia	Examination of area

ECG, Electrocardiogram; *LH,* luteinizing hormone; *T_4,* thyroxine; *TSH,* thyroid-stimulating hormone.
*For all patients, consider radiographs of bones every 5 to 10 years after ≥35-Gy radiation (risk of secondary malignancy). Examine skin for abnormal pigmented nevi (risk of second malignancy).

As in many other malignancies in children, advances in genetic and molecular characterization are being pursued to understand tumorigenesis, to predict the behavior of disease, and to develop therapies to improve prognosis. No environmental risk factors for osteosarcoma have been identified.[129]

Clinical Manifestations

The presenting symptom of virtually all patients is pain. Palpable masses, swelling, and limited motion are common signs. Weight loss and other systemic effects such as anorexia are rarely seen; if these effects are present, then overt metastatic disease is likely. A few patients have fractures. Cough, chest pain, or dyspnea may occur with extensive pulmonary metastases, although most patients who have pulmonary metastases are symptom free.[96,148] Ninety percent of tumors occur in the extremities; the metaphyses of bones are common sites of osteosarcoma origin. The lower extremities are involved most frequently, with approximately 60% of tumors occurring around the knee, 40% in the distal femur, and 20% in the proximal tibia.[153] The sacrum, jaw, and phalanges are less commonly involved. Patients who have Paget disease of the bone or those who have undergone radiotherapy in the area of the orbit may have osteosarcoma of the cranial bones.

The presenting symptom, bone pain, is ubiquitous and is commonly associated with trauma. Prolonged symptoms, or a history inconsistent with trauma, suggest the need for further diagnostic consideration. Bone abnormalities that may be confused with osteosarcoma include benign cysts, Ewing sarcoma, lymphoma, or tumor metastases. Table 244-5 provides the differential diagnosis of osteosarcoma involving the extremities.

Evaluation

Radiographs of the involved bone show bony destruction with periosteal new bone formation. A sunburst appearance is characteristic, a result of the eruption of tumor through the cortex with subsequent formation of new bone. Soft-tissue swelling is often noted.[154] Adequate histologic examination and analysis of biopsy samples are necessary to establish the diagnosis of osteosarcoma. The biopsy site is of critical importance, and the biopsy should be performed by an orthopedic surgeon with experience in oncology.

Osteoid found within a sarcomatous tumor is the characteristic histological pattern. Osteosarcoma in the child or adolescent is usually a high-grade tumor characterized by osteoblasts that demonstrate pleomorphism and bizarre mitoses. Necrosis, fibrosis, and calcification may be noted. This classic form usually arises from the medullary cavity. A less-aggressive form of osteosarcoma arises in the parosteal area of the bone and tends to spread along the shaft of the bone without invading the cortex. Periosteal, intracortical, and extraskeletal osteosarcomas have also been described.

Baseline lactic dehydrogenase and alkaline phosphatase levels should be obtained. The extent of the primary lesion is defined further by the use of CT or, more frequently and preferentially, by MRI. Approximately 20% of patients will have metastatic disease identified at diagnosis. Metastatic disease in the lung should be sought by CT. Eighty percent of patients with metastases will have pulmonary involvement. Bone scans can be helpful both for outlining the primary tumor and for detecting multiple primary lesions and metastasis. PET scanning may also play a role in evaluation.[134]

Management

When therapy of osteosarcoma was amputation of the affected limb, the natural history of disease was notable for the rapid appearance of pulmonary metastases 6 to 12 months after diagnosis,[155] consistent with the presence of micrometastases at diagnosis. Five years after diagnosis, only 10% to 20% of patients treated with amputation alone were alive. High-dose radiotherapy was even less effective than amputation.[156] In the early 1970s, favorable responses to high-dose methotrexate with leucovorin and to doxorubicin were noted,[157-159] and survival rates improved. A report of almost 50% survival after surgery alone attributed the better outcome to improved surgical techniques rather than chemotherapy.[160] Adjuvant chemotherapy therefore was not suggested by many physicians until the 1980s, when studies confirmed the benefit of adjuvant chemotherapy.[161,162] High-dose methotrexate, doxorubicin, and cisplatin are now considered standard therapy for osteosarcoma.[154] Dose intensification and the role of other chemotherapy agents, including ifosfamide, etoposide, and carboplatin, continues to be investigated, both as front-line therapy and for patients whose disease responds poorly to initial therapy.[163-165] International studies may facilitate addressing these issues. Targeted therapies, such as the use of Herceptin (trastuzumab), a monoclonal antibody against the epidermal growth factor 2 receptor, are also being studied.[148,166]

The availability of effective chemotherapy and improved surgical technique made limb-sparing or subamputative therapies possible for many patients who have osteosarcoma.[167] Survival after limb salvage is comparable to survival after amputation. Although the complication rate is higher, function is better. The portion of bone involved with tumor is removed and replaced by a prosthesis, a bone graft, or a composite.[148,154] This procedure can be performed only if the vascular and neurologic integrity of the limb is not compromised. Preoperative chemotherapy may reduce the size of the mass enough to make such surgery possible. For patients who have lower-extremity tumors, limb-salvage procedures were previously limited to patients who have achieved most of their growth, but currently, even younger children may be candidates. For patients who have lesions of the humerus, any preservation of hand function will greatly improve the patient's quality of life.

For patients in whom pulmonary metastases develop, surgical resection of these nodules may result in long-term survival,[168-170] even if multiple surgeries are required. A similar approach has been used in patients found to have metastatic pulmonary disease at the time of diagnosis.[171]

Prognosis

Randomized studies have confirmed the role of adjuvant chemotherapy in improving the long-term, disease-free survival of patients who have nonmetastatic osteosarcoma. Approximately 65% to 75% overall disease-free survival can be achieved.[161,163,172] The initial histologic response to chemotherapy has prognostic significance, although whether subsequent tailoring of therapy achieves a better result than aggressive, early chemotherapy for all patients is unclear.[173,174] The outcome after preoperative chemotherapy is similar or better than with immediate surgical excision. Preoperative chemotherapy improves the possibility of limb-salvage procedures by decreasing tumor size, and it allows early treatment of potential or demonstrated metastases. Alkaline phosphatase level has also been shown to have independent prognostic significance.[163] Other factors that may influence prognosis are related to the size and site of the tumor (patients who have distal tumors may have better outcomes than those who have proximal or central-axis tumors) and the patient's age (outcome improves with older patients). The most significant prognostic variable is the presence of metastatic disease. The presence solely of pulmonary metastases is associated with a better prognosis than bone metastases. Among patients who have pulmonary disease, unilateral disease or fewer than eight nodules may carry a better prognosis,[171] with survival in these groups of approximately 65% to 75%, compared with 25% to 35% for other patients with pulmonary involvement at diagnosis. The prognosis for patients with bone metastases at diagnosis or relapse is grim.

Follow-Up

Adjuvant chemotherapy has resulted in an increased number of long-term survivors of osteosarcoma. Virtually all patients will have undergone either amputation or limb-salvage procedures. The hope is that less-disabling therapies will someday be feasible. Most of these patients maintain a relatively normal lifestyle, including participation in various low-impact sports, but certain activities will be restricted. Long-term follow-up care includes imaging of the primary tumor site, bone scans, and chest CTs performed semiannually for 5 years and then at least chest radiographs annually until 10 years from the time of diagnosis to monitor for recurrent disease. Orthopedic evaluations and monitoring for late effects of the chemotherapeutic agents used (eg, doxorubicin, cisplatin, methotrexate, ifosfamide, etoposide) are also necessary.

Non-Hodgkin Lymphomas

Non-Hodgkin lymphoma (NHL) of childhood comprises a heterogeneous group of malignancies arising from lymphocytes and lymphoid precursors. The migratory nature of these cells is reflected by the variable sites at which the tumors occur and to which they spread. Recognition of the systemic nature of the disease, even in patients who have only locally detectable disease, has resulted in a marked improvement in survival rates. Childhood NHL is markedly different from adult NHL both in the immunohistopathological types that occur and in the better survival rates noted in children. Formerly, 3 primary types of NHL in children were described: (1) lymphoblastic lymphoma; (2) small noncleaved lymphoma, including Burkitt; and (3) large-cell lymphoma.[175] Current classification defines 4 subtypes of childhood NHL: (1) lymphoblastic lymphoma, which comprises 30% of cases; (2) anaplastic large-cell, 10% of cases; (3) Burkitt, 40% of cases; and (4) diffuse large B-cell, 20% of cases.[176] The latter 2 subtypes are both mature B-cell immunophenotypes with surface immunoglobulin. Primary mediastinal large B-cell lymphomas are sometimes considered separately from those occurring in other sites.[177] The lymphoblastic lymphomas can be divided into precursor B-cell and T-cell immunophenotypes, the latter being the most common. Lymphoblastic lymphomas almost invariably express the enzyme terminal deoxynucleotidyl transferase. Anaplastic large-cell lymphomas generally have T-cell receptor gene rearrangements.[175] Improved diagnostic techniques have resulted in emphasis on immunophenotype in diagnosis, staging, and treatment, with more tumor-specific regimens.[178] Advances in molecular techniques and gene profiling continue to provide insights into tumorigenesis and definition.[176] These insights will affect development of therapies.

Lymphomas account for approximately 10% of childhood cancer; 60% of lymphomas are NHLs. The incidence of NHL is low in children younger than 5 years and then increases steadily throughout life.[1] It occurs more commonly in boys than in girls (2 to 3:1), with the greatest sex difference in Burkitt lymphoma, in which the male-female ratio is approximately 4.5:1. NHLs of childhood have a rapid growth rate, with the percentage of actively dividing tumor approaching 100% in some cases, and short doubling times that can be as few as 12 hours. They have a high frequency of dissemination, particularly to the bone marrow and CNS. Although the distinction between lymphoma and lymphocytic leukemia is defined by less than 25% versus more than 25% bone marrow lymphoblasts, respectively, the distinguishing biological parameters are not clear.

Etiology

Burkitt lymphoma of equatorial Africa usually harbors Epstein-Barr virus (EBV), compared with the North American variety, which does so only occasionally.[179] The presence of EBV in lymphoma specimens suggests that viral infection may play a role in the development of NHL. Immunodeficiency states are also associated with the development of lymphomas, usually of the B-cell or large-cell variety.[180] A defect of T-cell regulation that permits the expansion of EBV-affected clones of B cells has been hypothesized to result in lymphomas, particularly in immunologically abnormal hosts. Lymphomas occur with increased frequency in children receiving immunosuppressive therapy for renal, cardiac, or bone marrow allografts.

Specific chromosomal aberrations have been described in Burkitt lymphoma, which place the C-*myc* oncogene adjacent to immunoglobulin heavy or light chain constant region genes.[181,182] Cases of Burkitt lymphoma in equatorial Africa may have different breakpoints than cases outside of this area. Several specific, nonrandom chromosomal abnormalities have been reported in lymphoblastic lymphoma and large-cell lymphomas.

Clinical Manifestations

Localized lymphadenopathy is a common presentation of NHL. Common areas of involvement are supradiaphragmatic, particularly the cervical, axillary, and mediastinal areas, or the Waldeyer ring.[183] The histologic pattern of supradiaphragmatic disease is often lymphoblastic. Dissemination to the bone marrow, the CNS, or the gonads is common. Patients may also have skin or soft-tissue involvement, particularly patients who have B-lineage lymphoblastic lymphoma.[184] Patients who have mediastinal masses frequently have a history of cough and, occasionally, acute respiratory distress. Unless careful attention is paid to the state of the airway, obstruction can occur during evaluation, even in patients who have few symptoms, particularly with the administration of sedation. The obstruction may involve the lower airway, beyond the reach of an endotracheal tube, resulting in an inability to effectively ventilate the lungs.

An abdominal mass that may involve the ileocecal region, mesentery, ovaries, or retroperitoneum is seen in 30% to 40% of patients.[183,184] Such tumors often are of B-cell origin. Large-cell lymphomas may produce peripheral adenopathy, although potential primary sites include the mediastinum and extranodal sites including the tonsils, lungs, bone, testicles, and soft tissue.

Patients whose disease is localized often feel well; those who have disseminated disease experience weight loss and malaise, as well as symptoms referable to the primary site of the disease.

The differential diagnosis of cervical adenopathy includes a variety of infectious and inflammatory processes. Malignant processes that cause enlarged cervical nodes include Hodgkin disease, neuroblastoma, leukemia, nasopharyngeal carcinoma, rhabdomyosarcoma, and thyroid carcinoma. Anterior mediastinal masses may be caused by T-cell leukemia or thymoma. Abdominal masses may be caused by constipation, splenomegaly, Wilms tumor, rhabdomyosarcoma, or neuroblastoma. Lymphoma is a rare type of bone tumor. Tables 244-1 to 244-3 provide differential diagnostic aids in evaluating patients who have NHL.

Evaluation

The diagnosis of NHL should be established by surgical biopsy; if adenopathy is present, then removal of the most suspicious node is suggested. Complete resection of the diseased area is not necessary. Frozen-section and needle biopsies are to be discouraged to ensure proper diagnosis. Although the primary diagnosis is based on histologic findings, for proper determination of subtype immunophenotyping, enzyme studies (terminal deoxynucleotidyl transferase) or gene rearrangement studies may be helpful. If possible, cytogenetic studies should be performed. A sufficient number of malignant cells may be present in patients who have bone marrow involvement or pleural effusions to establish the diagnosis. In this instance, a lymph node biopsy may not be necessary. Use of polymerase chain reaction or other new techniques to identify morphologically inapparent bone marrow involvement may also be beneficial for prognosis and treatment decisions.[185] Biopsy may be contraindicated for patients who have large mediastinal masses with imminent airway obstruction unless endotracheal intubation will ensure airway patency. If the distal end of the endotracheal tube lies proximal to the mass, then localized radiation to the mediastinum may be necessary before the diagnostic specimen is obtained. Alternative sites for obtaining diagnostic specimens must then be considered.

A lumbar puncture should be performed with cytocentrifugation of cerebrospinal fluid to detect meningeal involvement. Imaging studies should include a chest radiograph and a CT scan of the chest and abdomen in all patients. Bone scans and gallium scans can be helpful in selected patients, although PET scanning is being used with increasing frequency and may replace these modalities. The role of PET scans may be limited in staging but is more important in evaluating response and monitoring for recurrence.[186-188]

A variety of staging systems are used for lymphomas. The most common, the Ann Arbor system used for Hodgkin disease, is not of prognostic significance in NHL in children because of noncontiguous patterns of spread. The Murphy staging system is the most widely applied for NHL in children.[183] Stage I disease indicates a single tumor, nodal or extranodal. Stage II indicates the involvement of 2 or more nodal or extranodal sites, both on the same side of the diaphragm. Gastrointestinal tumors with only mesenteric nodes involved are also stage II. Stage III tumors involve both sides of the diaphragm, extensive abdominal disease, paraspinal or epidural tumors, or any primary intrathoracic tumors. Stage IV designates CNS or bone marrow involvement.

Management

Most patients who have NHL have disseminated disease at the time of diagnosis. Even clinically localized disease is not curable with localized surgical or radiotherapy alone. The choice of chemotherapeutic regimens is based on the clinical stage and the immunohistologic tumor subtype.

Lymph node biopsy is usually required for diagnosis and characterization of NHL. Removal of the tumor may be indicated only for patients who have Burkitt lymphoma whose tumor can be removed en masse (90%) with minimal morbidity.[189] In general, major surgical procedures should be avoided because the healing time may delay initiation of chemotherapy, the most essential component of treatment.

The high incidence of micrometastatic disease at the time of diagnosis necessitates that all children who have NHL receive chemotherapy. Many agents are active in lymphomas. Optimal treatment regimens differ for patients who have lymphoblastic lymphoma compared with those who have nonlymphoblastic lymphoma; the histologic class of lymphoma predicts the efficacy of the regimens. Effective agents include cyclophosphamide, vincristine, prednisone, methotrexate, doxorubicin,[190] cytosine arabinoside, etoposide, and ifosfamide. Patients who have localized nonlymphoblastic lymphoma can be treated with short-course, low-intensity chemotherapy. Patients who have localized lymphoblastic lymphoma require maintenance therapy.[191] High-risk patients who have lymphoblastic lymphoma are treated with acute lymphoblastic leukemia-like protocols. Leukemia-like therapy may also be beneficial for patients with anaplastic large-cell lymphoma.[192]

Local measures of control are rarely essential in the treatment of childhood NHL.[193] Although lymphomas are radiosensitive, the use of radiotherapy does not improve survival in chemotherapy-responsive patients, and unnecessary morbidity may result. Radiotherapy is helpful in treating emergent situations, such as airway compromise or spinal cord compression, and for treating overt meningeal involvement. The exception may be patients with Stage III or IV lymphoblastic lymphoma, who may benefit from prophylactic cranial radiation.[194] Radiotherapy also plays a role in treating patients who do not achieve a complete remission after standard chemotherapy or for patients who require bone marrow transplantation or palliative therapy.

The role of targeted therapies, such as rituximab, an anti-CD20 monoclonal antibody, may improve prognosis and allow dose decrease in standard chemotherapy.[176] The monoclonal antibody may work through mechanisms of direct cytotoxicity and chemosensitization.[178] Other targeted therapies are also being developed and investigated.

Prognosis

The prognosis is excellent for most children who have NHL, with more than 95% survival for those with localized disease and 80% to 90% survival for patients who have advanced disease, although subsets of patients with worse prognosis can be found, including those with Burkitt lymphoma and bone marrow and CNS involvement, mediastinal diffuse large B-cell lymphoma, and some patients with widespread anaplastic large-cell lymphoma.[176] Histologic findings are of prognostic significance for outcome, and they provide the basis for the choice of therapeutic regimen. Clinical staging is relevant because it is determined by a combination of the primary site, tumor burden, disease extent, and primary location. Age and sex may affect prognosis, even within histologic subtypes.[177] Other prognostic factors include lactic dehydrogenase and, as with other malignancies, response to therapy.[176,178] Investigations may permit evolution of treatment strategies to lower intensity of therapy for some patients, whereas new intensive chemotherapy or bone marrow transplantation regimens should improve the likelihood of survival in patients whose prognosis is poor or who experience relapse.

Follow-Up

Patients who have NHL and are disease free 2 years from the time of diagnosis are usually cured. During this initial period, these patients should be monitored with complete blood cell counts, chest radiograph, and evaluation of the primary site of disease. The follow-up of long-term survivors of childhood lymphomas should reflect the types of therapy (eg, cyclophosphamide, doxorubicin, methotrexate) administered (see Table 244-4).

Hodgkin Disease

Hodgkin disease, or Hodgkin lymphoma, is a malignancy of the lymphoreticular system characterized by multinucleated giant cells, known as *Reed-Sternberg cells,* interspersed in an infiltration of normal-appearing cellular elements (lymphocytes, macrophages, histiocytes, plasma cells, and eosinophils).[195] The Reed-Sternberg cells are the malignant cells of Hodgkin disease.[196] Recent evidence supports a B-lymphocyte origin of the Reed Sternberg cell with a cytokine-induced cellular infiltrate.[197] Rare cases of clonal T-cell receptor gene rearrangements have been reported. The transformative steps that lead to the development of the malignant cell continue to be actively studied.[198]

Hodgkin disease comprises approximately 6% of malignancies in children; approximately 600 cases are diagnosed in children in the United States each year.[1] In developed nations, the incidence of Hodgkin disease exhibits 2 age peaks, 1 in young adults (15 to 30 years of age) and 1 in late adulthood.[199] In developing nations, the early peak occurs in preadolescence. Ten percent to 15% of the total incidence of Hodgkin disease occurs in children younger than 16 years. Hodgkin disease is extremely rare before the age of 5 years. A male predominance is present throughout the preadolescent age range; thereafter the incidence is approximately equal in both sexes. Hodgkin disease in older teenagers and young adults is most common among whites.[200]

Etiology

The role of environment or genetics in the acquisition of Hodgkin disease is suggested by national and racial differences in the epidemiologic features of the disease. First-degree relatives of patients who have Hodgkin disease have an increased risk of acquiring the disease,[199] possibly because of genetic susceptibility or similar exposures (viral, environmental). Genetic risk is supported by a study demonstrating that monozygotic twins have a much higher concordance for disease development than dizygotic twins.[201] Environmental factors that influence or delay exposure to common infection may play a role in the etiology of Hodgkin disease.[198]

Epstein-Barr viruses found in tumor DNA may reflect a causative role for the virus.[202] Alternatively, patients may have an inappropriate immune response to this virus. Evidence of EBV infection is greater in certain subtypes of Hodgkin disease, that is, mixed cellularity, and may influence response to chemotherapy.[203,204] The incidence of Hodgkin disease is known to be increased in patients who have certain underlying immunodeficiency diseases (eg, ataxia-telangiectasia, AIDS).[205,206]

Clinical Manifestations

The most common presenting feature of Hodgkin disease is painless enlargement of the lower cervical lymph nodes. Approximately 50% of the patients who have this manifestation also have mediastinal disease. The classic pattern of spread is from the cervical lymph nodes to the mediastinum and then into the spleen and abdominal lymph nodes. Spread through the thoracic duct may result in disease of the right side of the neck and of the abdomen, without mediastinal involvement. Axillary or inguinal adenopathy or extranodal primary sites (eg, bone) are occasionally seen. Mediastinal disease is present in 76% of adolescents and 33% of 1- to 10-year-old children who have Hodgkin lymphoma. Pleural involvement occurs in approximately 10% of patients. Renal, skin, or nervous system involvement is less common. Constitutional symptoms related to Hodgkin disease occur in approximately one third of patients at the time of diagnosis. The symptoms that predict a poor prognosis (*B* disease) are fever (oral temperature more than 38°C [101°F]), weight loss (more than 10% of body weight within 6 months), and drenching night sweats. Absence of these symptoms provides a better prognosis (*A* disease).[204] Hematologic abnormalities may be present in Hodgkin disease (usually in advanced stages), even in the absence of bone marrow involvement. Hemolytic disease or the anemia of chronic disease associated with impaired mobilization of iron storage may occur. Neutrophilia in the absence of infection occurs in approximately 50% of patients. Thrombocytopenia caused by immunologically mediated platelet destruction is also seen.

Lymphadenopathy occurs in children for various reasons, including infection (with bacteria, viruses, tuberculosis, atypical mycobacteria, and toxoplasmosis), malignancies (NHL, nasopharyngeal carcinoma, soft-tissue sarcoma, neuroblastoma), histiocytosis, and other inflammatory processes. A chest radiograph, a complete blood cell count, and a sedimentation rate should be obtained in any patient who has lymphadenopathy that is atypical for infection. Persistent lymphadenopathy, even after a transient response to antibiotic therapy, requires biopsy. Tables 244-2 and 244-3 provide differential diagnostic aids in evaluating patients who have Hodgkin disease.

Evaluation

Evaluation of the child who has a possible diagnosis of Hodgkin disease should begin with a complete history and thorough physical examination. Particular attention should be paid to *B* disease symptoms. Lymphatic areas to be evaluated include Waldeyer ring and the cervical, supraclavicular, axillary, and inguinal lymph nodes. The sizes of the nodes found should be recorded carefully, and whether they are tender should be noted. In addition, a thorough abdominal examination should be performed, particularly to evaluate liver and spleen size. Retroperitoneal lymph nodes are not palpable. The blood cell counts may show anemia (caused by hemolysis or chronic disease), abnormal neutrophil count, or thrombocytopenia. Increase in the sedimentation rate, serum copper level, and ferritin level resulting from activation of the reticuloendothelial system occurs in some patients and may be useful for monitoring response to therapy. Serum hepatic alkaline phosphatase isoenzyme levels may also be increased.

Radiographic evaluation of a patient who has a possible diagnosis of Hodgkin disease includes a chest radiograph and CT scans of the chest and abdomen. Gallium scanning also detects Hodgkin disease and was particularly useful in the past in detecting disease in obscure sites. PET scanning is becoming routine, although it may be most applicable for monitoring response and recurrence as opposed to staging because it has a high negative predictive value and variable positive predictive value.[186,188] Although bone involvement is rare, a bone scan should be considered in patients who have advanced disease, particularly those who have bone pain or an increased serum alkaline phosphatase level. Bone marrow biopsies should be performed in all but those with Stage IA or IIA disease.

The importance of defining subdiaphragmatic involvement is most clear when radiotherapy is the primary therapeutic modality. A staging laparotomy with splenectomy was used in earlier years to define the extent of necessary radiation. Improved imaging techniques and the use of chemotherapy in virtually all children and adolescents with Hodgkin disease obviates the need for staging laparotomy,[204,207] thus preventing the risk of overwhelming bacteremia with polysaccharide-encapsulated organisms. Survivors of earlier eras who had splenectomies during childhood should have vaccines for pneumococcus, *Haemophilus influenzae* type b, and *Neisseria meningitides* as recommended. Prophylactic antibiotics and empiric treatment for fevers are also necessary to limit risk.

The extent of disease spread is usually classified by the Ann Arbor staging system by means of either the clinical stage or the pathological stage.[208] Pathological stage implies that the most extensive degree of involvement has been confirmed pathologically:

Stage I: involvement of one lymphatic region only
Stage II: involvement of two or more lymphatic regions on the same side basis of the diaphragm
Stage III: involvement on both sides of the diaphragm, including nodal regions, the spleen, or both
Stage IV: involvement of extranodal organs such as lungs, liver, bone marrow, kidneys, bone, or skin, in addition to lymph nodes

The Cotswold modification further divides stage III based on specific subdiaphragmatic nodal sites involved. In addition to symptom designation by *A* or *B*, it also adds a subscript *X* for bulky mediastinal disease and a subscript *E* for involvement of a single nodal site that is contiguous with a known nodal site of disease.[209]

Four subtypes of Hodgkin disease are described by review of pathological specimens.[210] The nodular sclerosing subtype is distinctive because of collagenous bands that divide the lymphoid tissues into nodules and the presence of a *lacunar variant* of the Reed-Sternberg cell. It is the most common subtype in children, occurring in approximately 75% of adolescents and 40% of children younger than 10 years. The lymphocyte-predominant Hodgkin disease subtype is characterized by destruction of the lymph node architecture, with the cellular proliferation of benign-appearing lymphocytes. Reed-Sternberg cells are rarely found in the absence of fibrosis. It is more common in young children; 33% of cases are in children younger than 15 years. Disease is usually localized. In the mixed-cellularity Hodgkin disease subtype, lymph node architecture is not preserved. Approximately 10 Reed-Sternberg cells are seen per high-power field, often with interstitial fibrosis; necrosis is not pronounced. It is more common in children younger than 10 years than in adolescents and is associated with high-risk disease. The lymphocyte-depleted Hodgkin disease subtype is characterized by the presence of fibrosis, necrosis, and abnormal cells (but only a rare lymphocyte). It is rare in children.

Management

Hodgkin disease responds to radiation or chemotherapy. Protocols that use radiotherapy alone, chemotherapy alone, or both forms of therapy have all been successful, at least in some groups of patients. Choosing an appropriate therapeutic plan necessitates assessing the risk of disease recurrence and the potential risk for long-term ill effects in a particular patient.

Contiguous spread of Hodgkin disease by lymphoid organs allowed for success with radiotherapy alone.[211] Full-dose radiotherapy (35 to 45 Gy) is standard therapy for adults with low-stage (I, II, and III) disease. The involved fields, as well as 1 field beyond the area of proved disease, are treated. Skeletal and soft-tissue growth, particularly in the neck and clavicular areas, are severely compromised when these doses of radiation are used in children. Cardiac and pulmonary complications, such as coronary artery disease, valvular disease, pneumonitis, or pulmonary fibrosis, occur as well. Low-dose radiotherapy (20 to 25 Gy) to involved fields only, and not extended fields, in conjunction with chemotherapy results in fewer and less severe late effects from the radiation.[212]

Hodgkin disease is a chemotherapy-sensitive disease. The original chemotherapy agent combination that proved successful in the treatment of Hodgkin disease was MOPP (mechlorethamine, Oncovin [vincristine], procarbazine, and prednisone).[213] In 1974, 10 years after the initial application of MOPP, the regimen ABVD (Adriamycin [doxorubicin], bleomycin, vinblastine, and dacarbazine) was devised for the treatment of patients who experienced relapse.[214] The efficacy of this combination resulted in hybrid ABVD-MOPP regimens.[215] MOPP is now rarely used because of significant long-term toxicity. Current protocols use a backbone of therapy with ABVE-PC (Adriamycin [doxorubicin], bleomycin, vincristine, etoposide, prednisone, and cyclophosphamide) for treatment investigations, including the appropriate number of chemotherapy cycles for rapid and slow responders, appropriate additional chemotherapy regimens for patients who do not have a good initial response, and the role of radiotherapy for patients who respond completely and rapidly to chemotherapy.[216] Because cures with chemotherapy alone, even in higher-stage disease, have been described,[217] defining appropriate patients who can avoid even the limited side effects of lower dose–involved field radiation will be important.

In the 1980s, combined-modality therapy became the standard recommendation for younger patients who had not completed their growth and for those with advanced-stage disease, and can play a role in patients with lower-stage disease, even in mature patients.[209] The advantages of combined therapies (chemotherapy and radiation together) include improved cure rates in patients with poor prognosis and reduction in the dose of radiotherapy administered to children so that skeletal development will proceed more normally. Chemotherapy also has side effects, including infertility after MOPP chemotherapy, cardiotoxic effects of the doxorubicin of ABVD, and pulmonary toxicity caused by bleomycin.[218,219] Secondary leukemias have been described, particularly after the combination of MOPP and radiation.[220] In choosing an appropriate regimen for a given patient, the following must be considered: (1) the age and skeletal maturity of the patient (likely effects on the developing child), (2) the extent of disease present (how much therapy is necessary), and (3) symptoms that might predict a poor prognosis. The response to initial therapy is also a significant factor in treatment decisions. Because so many regimens currently appear equivalent in terms of outcome, an investigational protocol should be used (if one is available) to help delineate the best treatment for patients in the future while ensuring appropriate treatment for those under study.

Prognosis

Radiotherapy alone may cure up to 70% of patients who have stage I or IIA Hodgkin's disease and 50% of patients who have stage IIB or IIIA disease. The subsequent use of chemotherapy enables one half of patients who experience relapse after radiotherapy to be cured of the disease.[221,222] As stated, however, single-modality treatment with radiation may not be appropriate in children. Combined-modality therapy results in 5-year disease-free survival of approximately 90% to 100% for patients who have localized disease and 80% to 90% for patients who have high-risk disease.[223,224] High-risk features include advanced-stage disease, a large mediastinal mass, more than 4 sites of involvement, and *B* symptoms.[204,207,209] In patients whose disease progresses or relapses, cure may be accomplished with intensive chemotherapy and radiation or with stem cell transplantation.[225] Salvage rates of more than 60% are reported, with patients whose diseases progress while they are receiving therapy having a poorer prognosis than those who experience relapse after treatment.

Follow-Up

Patients who have Hodgkin disease should be monitored for evidence of recurrent disease for as long as 10 to 15 years after the original diagnosis. In addition to a thorough physical examination, useful tests for prolonged follow-up include a complete blood cell count, a sedimentation rate, and a chest radiograph.

After high-dose radiotherapy to the neck and mediastinum, soft-tissue and bone growth abnormalities include shortening of clavicles and underdevelopment of the soft tissues of the neck. Sitting height decreases after radiation to the axial skeleton in proportion to the growth potential remaining at the time of radiation.[226] In prepubertal girls, breast development may be impaired. The incidence of breast cancer may be increased after chemotherapy and irradiation,[227,228] particularly for girls who received radiotherapy during early adolescence during breast tissue proliferation. Patients should undergo annual mammographic examinations beginning 8 years after therapy or at age 25 years.

Overt hypothyroidism (low thyroxine and increased thyroid-stimulating hormone [TSH]) occurs in approximately 5% to 10% of patients who have undergone irradiation, whereas compensated hypothyroidism (increased TSH and normal thyroxine [T_4]) occurs in 50% to 90% of such patients.[229] Thyroid function should be assessed for at least 15 years. Thyroid replacement therapy is suggested when the TSH level is increased.

Patients who receive mediastinal irradiation may have pulmonary fibrosis with variable abnormalities detected by pulmonary function testing. Late cardiac abnormalities include pericardial thickening and, occasionally, valvular dysfunction. Early myocardial infarctions have been reported.[230] These toxicities may be exacerbated by the use of bleomycin and anthracyclines.

Fertility in women is affected by the use of radiation and chemotherapy. Pelvic irradiation of a woman causes infertility unless oophoropexy (moving ovaries to the midline) is performed. After oophoropexy, all teenaged girls treated with radiation alone and 88% of those treated with combined-modality therapy maintained normal menses.[230] Women older than 30 years experience ovarian failure after treatment with MOPP more frequently than do younger women. All women should be advised of the possibility of early menopause. A menstrual history should be elicited at each visit.

Testes are more severely affected by cytotoxic therapies than are ovaries. Fortunately, the radiation fields used in Hodgkin disease spare the gonads in male patients. Six courses of MOPP chemotherapy, however, always result in male sterility. Approximately 50% of patients treated with 3 courses of MOPP are sterile.[231] ABVD causes less impairment of spermatogenesis, and current regimens also carry less risk. Men interested in fathering a child may consider sperm banking, posttherapy monitoring of gonadotropin levels, and semen analysis. Recovery has been documented in previously sterile men.[232]

Acute myelogenous leukemia occurs in patients who have Hodgkin disease at the rate of approximately 1% per year for the first 10 years after treatment with MOPP and radiotherapy.[220] Thereafter the risk appears to decrease. The incidence is lower with single-modality therapy or after ABVD and radiation, and the risk is expected to be lower with current therapy. Other solid tumors in addition to breast cancer may occur after treatment for Hodgkin lymphoma, including thyroid cancer, bone tumors, and NHL.

Patients who have had a splenectomy are at risk for overwhelming infection, particularly by encapsulated organisms. Empirical treatment with intravenous antibiotics is recommended for fever (>38°C [101°F]) in these patients.

GENERAL ONCOLOGIC CARE

Referral to a Pediatric Oncologist

Fortunately, children who have malignancies represent a very small proportion of patients in a general pediatrics practice. The treatment of such patients is specialized. Proper care begins with referral to a pediatric oncologist, even if the initial procedure indicated is surgical. Recognition of potential malignancy in the differential of a patient's presentation is essential to ensure that inappropriate therapy will not be administered—for example, corticosteroids should not be provided to a patient whose symptoms mimic EBV infection or reactive airway disease. For many tumors, appropriate baseline studies must be obtained before surgical procedures are instituted. For example, AFP and B-hCG levels decrease rapidly after removal of the germ cell tumor, as do catecholamine levels after removal of a neuroblastoma. Delayed assays for such markers may result in an inability to recognize an important indicator of recurrent disease in a given patient. The chest CT scan should be performed before surgical procedures are performed because perioperative atelectasis may interfere with the detection of metastatic disease in the pulmonary parenchyma.

The tumors of childhood behave differently from those of adults, even when histologically identical. In addition, children tolerate radiation and chemotherapy differently than adults. Therefore all children should benefit from the care of a pediatric oncologist. Services available for children and their families at pediatric referral hospitals often ease the pain of being diagnosed with a life-threatening disease. Pediatric social workers, child life workers, and nurses experienced in dealing with children and adolescents who have cancer are available. For patients living at a distance from a center, initiating therapy at a referral medical center and administering a portion of the subsequent treatments and evaluations closer to the patient's home are often possible. At times, a local oncologist can assist in administering chemotherapy to children living at a distance from a center; however, such oncologists should not choose a therapeutic regimen or evaluate major problems that may arise without corroboration with the pediatric oncologists at the referral medical center. Several excellent resources are available for patients, families, and care physicians, including CureSearch (www.curesearch.org/), a component of the Children's Oncology Group (COG). The American Cancer Society and National Cancer Institute also have Web sites with beneficial information oriented to the care of children. Adolescents and young adults are a special group within the practice of pediatric oncology, in which the majority of patients are young children. The official COG Web resource for this population is available at www.teenslivingwithcancer.org, a component of Melissa's Living Legacy.

Several oncologic emergencies exist that general primary care physicians must recognize. Cord compression may result from neuroblastoma, Ewing sarcoma, lymphoma, or any other tumor that invades the spinal canal. Such patients experience incontinence, loss of reflexes in the lower extremities, or decreased ability to use the lower extremities. Rectal sphincter tone may be decreased. Rapid institution of therapy may reverse such findings, markedly changing the long-term functioning of the patient. Thus recognition of such findings should prompt immediate referral to a pediatric oncologist, who, in conjunction with a neurosurgeon or radiation therapist, will be able to deliver emergent therapy.

Patients whose bone marrow has been infiltrated by leukemia, Ewing sarcoma, neuroblastoma, or lymphoma may have pancytopenia and thus be at risk of infection as a result of neutropenia, bleeding caused by thrombocytopenia, and congestive heart failure as a result of anemia. Rapid lysis of cells (tumor lysis syndrome) because of the high cell turnover rate of the tumor itself (as is seen in Burkitt lymphoma) or to cytotoxic therapy is characterized by increased uric acid (risk of urate nephropathy), hyperkalemia, hypocalcemia, and hyperphosphatemia. Medical management includes allopurinol or urate oxidase, urinary alkalinization, and binders of potassium and phosphate. Dialysis may be necessary. If delayed arrival to the medical center is anticipated, allopurinol should be started by the referring physician when a tumor that has a large-cell burden (eg, leukemia, Burkitt lymphoma, and bone marrow involvement with either neuroblastoma, Ewing sarcoma, or rhabdomyosarcoma) is suspected.

Primary care physicians should recognize the signs and symptoms of superior vena cava syndrome, which may include swelling, plethora, and cyanosis of the face, neck, and upper extremities; engorged vessels; cough and wheezing; chest pain; headache; diaphoresis; and visual changes. Lymphomas and other malignancies are the leading causes of superior vena cava syndrome, which may progress rapidly enough to be life threatening. Therefore prompt recognition of the potential for mediastinal mass as the cause of the symptoms and appropriate referral is essential.

Role of the Primary Care Physician During Therapy

The most prominent toxicity that results from chemotherapy is myelosuppression. Infections in patients with neutropenia can rapidly result in septic shock, particularly if gram-negative organisms are involved. Primary care physicians who monitor these children can help by recognizing the risk of fever and immediately referring the patient to the pediatric oncologist when the patient becomes febrile. If the center is at a distance, then the primary care physician becomes the front-line caretaker, obtaining proper culture specimens and initiating antibiotic therapy (usually an aminoglycoside and semisynthetic penicillin or a 4th-generation cephalosporin). In such circumstances, the primary care physician should discuss aspects of care with the pediatric oncologist to ensure that all appropriate measures are taken. Many patients receiving intensive chemotherapy have indwelling central venous catheters that increase the risk for septicemia with gram-positive organisms. These patients, even in the absence of neutropenia, should have blood drawn for culture, and therapy with antibiotics should be considered if fever develops. Any person who is febrile and who has undergone a splenectomy should be given antibiotics empirically to treat potential infections with polysaccharide-encapsulated organisms. In the absence of splenectomy and a central line, treatment of children whose blood cell counts are normal is usually similar to that of a healthy child. The primary care physician can see such children for common pediatric complaints, including skin rashes, earaches, and respiratory and gastrointestinal infections, inasmuch as these children appear to handle such infections without undue difficulty. Varicella, however, is a major threat to all immunocompromised patients because dissemination of disease is likely even in the absence of neutropenia. Before the availability of acyclovir and the varicella vaccine, significant morbidity and mortality occurred in such patients. Immunocompromised children who are exposed to varicella by a sibling or a close playmate should receive varicella-zoster immunoglobulin within 4 days of the exposure. Should chickenpox occur, then the patient should be treated with acyclovir or related new-generation antiviral drugs, often as an inpatient. Chemotherapy is usually withheld during the treatment of varicella.

Children who are receiving treatment for a malignancy should continue to see their primary pediatrician for well-child visits. This effort is in anticipation of their ultimate successful treatment and cure. Immunizations are delayed until 1 year after therapy is terminated because live vaccines may cause disease, and inactivated vaccines rarely result in a normal immune response. An exception is made for the inactivated influenza vaccine and not the live virus influenza vaccine. This treatment may be performed by the oncologist but may also be requested of the pediatrician. In addition, the patient's family should be immunized. The pediatrician should remain involved in continuing developmental issues that are at times exacerbated by the treatment of a malignancy. With the current success rates in treating children who have cancer, pediatricians should anticipate the return of these children to their practice for most of their care. Maintenance of a relationship with the patient and family is therefore essential.

Care of Long-Term Survivors

Children treated for malignancy have, for the most part, received several extremely toxic agents, the long-term implications of which are not known in their entirety. Studies of a new treatment regimen's late toxicities are often in their early stages; and as therapy evolves, so do the potential late side effects. Children should continue to return at least annually to the treating institution or to a similar institution elsewhere to be monitored for potential side effects and to be informed of problems occurring in patients treated similarly. Many factors, including patient preference, aging out of pediatric facilities, and distance, will result in the primary care physician becoming the central figure in ensuring that patients undergo appropriate follow-up.[233] Knowledge of late effects and appropriate screening is essential,[234] as is understanding the heterogeneity of treatment, the differences in regimens from different eras, and the variability in toxicities experienced by patients treated with similar regimens. Toxicities of currently used chemotherapeutic agents and of radiation to particular areas are listed in Tables 244-4 and 244-6, respectively, and follow-up studies are described. The COG has developed long-term follow up guidelines (available at www.survivorshipguidelines.org/).

Multidisciplinary clinics, which evaluate all survivors for potential late effects, are being formed in some hospitals. Subclinical evidence of cardiac damage after anthracycline administration and of pulmonary toxicity (decreased diffusing capacity) after bleomycin administration is found in some survivors. The course of the toxicity is not clear, but evidence has been found for progression of cardiac abnormalities. The long-term effects on renal function and hearing are not yet known. Fertility has been impaired in some adolescent patients who received alkylating therapies, but the incidence of this dysfunction is lower than in adults treated similarly. Radiation to the gonads also causes infertility. Affected women need hormone replacement for feminization and to prevent the osteoporosis associated with estrogen depletion. Testosterone levels in treated male subjects usually remain in the normal range, but they should be monitored. Endocrine dysfunction after radiation may involve the thyroid, hypothalamus, and pituitary. Studies of the mechanism of impairment may help in treating other affected patients more effectively. Thyroid radiation often causes compensated (increased TSH, normal T_4) or overt (increased TSH, decreased T_4) hypothyroidism and should be treated with thyroid hormone therapy.[235]

Secondary malignancies are reported in long-term survivors. Mutagenic agents such as mechlorethamine, cyclophosphamide, etoposide, and radiotherapy play a role. A genetic predisposition to malignancy exists for patients who have certain disorders (eg, bilateral retinoblastoma).

Neurocognitive function and school performance will be affected in many children who are going through or who have undergone treatment for childhood cancer. Education specialists, pediatric oncological nurse practitioners, or persons from both fields can be extremely helpful to the child and the child's teachers by (1) explaining the child's diagnosis and treatment to school administrators and teachers, and when appropriate, to classmates; (2) defining the problems and limitations the child will have in keeping up with schoolwork during periods of intensive treatment; and (3) providing or arranging (through the school system) for lessons and special tutoring during prolonged hospitalizations and recovery periods at home.[236]

The psychosocial effects of childhood cancer also differ from patient to patient. Some patients were so young when they received treatment that they do not remember the ordeal; others were unable to participate in normal childhood experiences because of their illness. Some patients have no physical deficits; others have permanent deformities (amputations, scoliosis, hair loss, scars). Despite these issues, most survivors rate their health as good.[237] Most patients are emotionally intact people who are able to live and work normally within mainstream society, although mental health impairment is reported by survivors across the diagnostic spectrum.[237] Unfortunately, certain workplaces and insurance companies continue to discriminate based on a history of cancer. Businesses and agencies must be taught to accept people who are cured and are likely to have a normal future. Legal protection is available to survivors through the Americans With Disabilities Act, and advocacy resources exist at both the community and national level.[238,239]

Pediatricians must be advocates for these successfully treated people. Past medical conditions that will not interfere with future health should not be a barrier to success. Furthermore, pediatricians must remain aware of potential late effects of therapy. Screening for toxicities will allow for interventions that can maintain health.

TOOLS FOR PRACTICE

Medical Decision Support

- *Long-Term Follow-Up Guidelines for Survivors of Childhood, Adolescent, and Young Adult Cancers* (guideline), Cure Search (survivorshipguidelines.org).

AAP POLICY STATEMENT

American Academy of Pediatrics Section on Hematology/Oncology. Guidelines for Pediatric Cancer Centers. *Pediatrics*. 2004;113(6):1833-1835. (aappolicy.aappublications.org/cgi/content/full/pediatrics;113/6/1833).

RELATED WEB SITES

- American Cancer Society (www.cancer.org/docroot/CRI/CRI_2_6x_Children_and_Cancer.asp).
- Children's Oncology Group (www.curesearch.org).
- Melissa's Living Legacy Foundation: Teens Living with Cancer (teenslivingwithcancer.org).
- National Cancer Institute (www.cancer.gov/cancertopics/types/childhoodcancers).

REFERENCES

1. Gurney JG, Davis S, Severson RK, et al. Trends in cancer incidence among children in the US. *Cancer*. 1996; 78: 532-541.
2. Meadows AT, Lichtenfeld JL, Koop CE. Wilms' tumor in three children of a woman with congenital hemihypertrophy. *N Engl J Med*. 1974;291:23-24.
3. Breslow NE, Beckwith JB. Epidemiological features of Wilms' tumor: results of the National Wilms' Tumor Study. *J Natl Cancer Inst*. 1982;68:429-436.
4. Kobrinsky NL, Talgoy M, Shuckett B, et al. Wilms' tumor. *Pediatr Ann*. 1988;17(4):241-250.
5. Kalapurakal JA, Dome JS, Perlman EJ, et al. Management of Wilms' tumour: current practice and future goals. *Lancet Oncol*. 2004;5:37-46.
6. Clericuzio CL, Johnson C. Screening for Wilms tumor in high-risk individuals. *Hematol Oncol Clin North Am*. 1995;9:1253-1265.
7. Drash A, Sherman F, Hartman, WH, et al. A syndrome of pseudohermaphrodism, Wilms' tumor, hypertension, and degenerative renal disease. *J Pediatr*. 1970;76: 585-593.
8. Grundy P, Coppes MJ, Haber D. Molecular genetics of Wilms tumor. *Hematol Oncol Clin North Am*. 1995; 9: 1201-1215.
9. Diller L, Ghahremani M, Morgan J, et al. Constitutional WT 1 mutations in Wilms tumor patients. *J Clin Oncol*. 1998;16:3634-3640.
10. Grundy PE, Breslow NE, Li S, et al. Loss of heterozygosity for chromosomes 1p and 16q is an adverse prognostic factor in favorable-histology Wilms tumor: a report from the National Wilms Tumor Study Group. *J Clin Oncol*. 2005;23:7312-7321.
11. Metzger ML, Dome JS. Current therapy for Wilms' tumor. *Oncologist*. 2005;10:815-826.
12. Ramsey NK, Dehner LP, Coccia PF, et al. Acute hemorrhage into Wilms' tumor. *J Pediatr*. 1977;91:763-765.
13. Babyn P, Owens C, Gyepes M, et al. Imaging patients with Wilms tumor. *Hematol Oncol Clin North Am*. 1995; 9:1217-1252.
14. Farewell VT, D'Angio GJ, Breslow N, et al. Retrospective validation of a new staging system for Wilms' tumor. *Cancer Clin Trials*. 1981;4:167-171.
15. Beckwith JB. New developments in the pathology of Wilms tumor. *Cancer Invest*. 1997;15:153-162.
16. Ritchey ML, Shamberger RC, Hamilton T, et al. Fate of bilateral renal lesions missed on preoperative imaging: a report from the National Wilms Tumor Study Group. *J Urol*. 2005;174:1519-1521.
17. Kay R, Tank E. The current management of bilateral Wilms tumor. *J Urol*. 1986;135:983-985.
18. Breslow NE, Collins AJ, Ritchey ML, et al. End stage renal disease in patients with Wilms tumor: results from the National Wilms Tumor Study Group and the United States Renal Data System. *J Urol*. 2005;174: 1972-1975.
19. Wu HY, Snyder HM, D'Angio GJ. Wilms' tumor management. *Curr Opin Urol*. 2005;15:273-276.
20. D'Angio GJ, Evans AE, Breslow N, et al. The treatment of Wilms' tumor: results of the National Wilms' Tumor Study. *Cancer*. 1976;38:633-646.
21. Green DM, Thomas PR, Shochat S. The treatment of Wilms tumor. Results of the National Wilms Tumor Studies. *Hematol Oncol Clin North Am*. 1995;9:1267-1274.
22. Green DM, Brewlow NE, Beckwith JB, et al. Effect of duration of treatment on outcome and cost of treatment for Wilms' tumor: a report from the National Wilms' Tumor Study Group. *J Clin Oncol*. 1998;16: 3744-3751.

23. Green DM, Fernbach DJ, Norkool P, et al. The treatment of Wilms tumor patients with pulmonary metastases detected only with computed tomography: a report from the National Wilms' Tumor Study Group. *J Clin Oncol.* 1991;9:1776-1781.
24. Beckwith JB, Palmer NF. Histopathology and prognosis of Wilms tumors: results from the First National Wilms' Tumor Study. *Cancer.* 1978;41:1937-1948.
25. Campbell AD, Cohn SL, Reynolds M, et al. Treatment of relapsed Wilms' tumor with high-dose therapy and autologous hematopoietic stem-cell rescue: the experience at Children's Memorial Hospital. *J Clin Oncol.* 2004; 22:2885-2890.
26. Thomas PRM, Griffith KD, Fineberg BB, et al. Late effects of treatment for Wilms' tumor. *Int J Radiat Oncol Biol Phys.* 1983;9:651-657.
27. Li FP, Gimbrere K, Gelber RD, et al. Outcome of pregnancy in survivors of Wilms' tumor. *JAMA.* 1987:257: 216-219.
28. Byrne J, Mulvihill JJ, Connelly RR, et al. Reproductive problems and birth defects in survivors of Wilms' tumor and their relatives. *Med Pediatr Oncol.* 1988;16:233-240.
29. Nicholson HS, Blask AN, Markle BM, et al. Uterine anomalies in Wilms' tumor survivors. *Cancer.* 1996;78: 887-891.
30. Beckwith JB, Perrin EV. In situ neuroblastomas: a contribution to the natural history of neural crest tumors. *Am J Pathol.* 1963;43:1089-1104.
31. Chatten J, Voorhees ML. Familial neuroblastoma. *N Engl J Med.* 1967;277:1230-1236.
32. Pegelow GH, Ebben AJ, Powars D, et al. Familial neuroblastoma. *J Pediatr.* 1975;87:763-765.
33. Knudson AG, Strong LC. Mutation and cancer: neuroblastoma and pheochromocytoma. *Am J Hum Genet.* 1972;24:514-532.
34. Maris JM. The biologic basis for neuroblastoma heterogeneity and risk stratification. *Curr Opin Pediatr.* 2005; 17:7-13.
35. Henry MC, Tashjian DB, Breuer CK. Neuroblastoma update. *Curr Opin Oncol.* 2005;17:19-23.
36. Martin RM, Middleton N, Gunnell D, et al. Breastfeeding and childhood cancer: a systematic review with metaanalysis. *Int J Cancer.* 2005;117:1020-1031.
37. Kushner BH, Cheung Nai-Kong V. Neuroblastoma—from genetic profiles to clinical challenge. *N Engl J Med.* 2005;353:2215-2217.
38. DeBernardi B, Balwierz W, Bejent J, et al. Epidural compression in neuroblastoma: diagnostic and therapeutic aspects. *Cancer Lett.* 2005;228:283-299.
39. Hawthorne HC, Nelson JS, Witzleben CL, et al. Blanching subcutaneous nodules in neonatal neuroblastoma. *J Pediatr.* 1970;77:297-300.
40. DuBois S, Kalika Y, Lukens JN, et al. Metastatic sites in stage IV and IVS neuroblastoma correlate with age, tumor biology, and survival. *J Pediatr Hematol Oncol.* 1999;21:181-189.
41. Koizumi JH, Dal Canto MC. Retroperitoneal neuroblastoma metastatic to brain: report of a case and review of the literature. *Child Brain.* 1980;7:267-279.
42. Scheibel E, Rechnitzer C, Fahrenkrug J, et al. Vasoactive intestinal polypeptide (VIP) in children with neural crest tumors. *Acta Paediatr Scand.* 1982;71:721-725.
43. Russo C, Cohn SL, Petruzzi MJ, et al. Long-term neurologic outcome in children with opsoclonus-myoclonus associated with neuroblastoma: a report from the Pediatric Oncology Group. *Med Pediatr Oncol.* 1997;29:284-288.
44. Matthay KK, Blaes F, Hero B, et al. Opsoclonus myoclonus syndrome in neuroblastomas: a report from a workshop on the dancing eyes syndrome. *Cancer Lett.* 2005; 228:275-282.
45. Kauffman RA, Thrall JH, Keyes JW, et al. False negative bone scans in neuroblastoma metastatic to the ends of long bones. *Am J Roentgenol.* 1978;130:131-135.
46. Russell HV, Golding LA, Suell MN, et al. The role of bone marrow evaluation in the staging of patients with otherwise localized, low-risk neuroblastoma. *Pediatr Blood Cancer.* 2005;45:916-919.
47. Jadvar H, Alavi A, Mavi A, et al. PET in pediatric diseases. *Radiol Clin North Am.* 2005;43:135-152.
48. Brodeur G, Pritchard J, Berthold F, et al. Revisions of the international criteria for neuroblastoma diagnosis, staging, and response to treatment. *J Clin Oncol.* 1993; 11:1466-1477.
49. Gitlow SE, Bertani LM, Rausen A, et al. Diagnosis of neuroblastoma by qualitative and quantitative determination of catecholamine metabolites in urine. *Cancer.* 1970;25:1377-1383.
50. LaBrosse EH. Biochemical diagnosis of neuroblastoma: use of a urine spot test. *Proc Am Assoc Cancer Res.* 1968;9:39.
51. Matthay K. Neuroblastoma: biology and therapy. *Oncology.* 1997;11:1857-1866.
52. Rubie H, Hartmann O, Michon J, et al. N-Myc gene amplification is a major prognostic factor in localized neuroblastoma: results of the French NBL 90 Study. *J Clin Oncol.* 1997;15:1171-1182.
53. Seeger RC, Brodeur GM, Sather H, et al. Association of multiple copies of the N-*myc* oncogene with rapid progression of neuroblastomas. *N Engl J Med.* 1985;313: 1111-1116.
54. Look AT, Hayes FA, Nitschke R, et al. Cellular DNA content as a predictor of response to chemotherapy in infants with unresectable neuroblastoma. *N Engl J Med.* 1984;311:231-235.
55. Bagatell R, Runcheva P, London WB, et al. Outcomes of children with intermediate-risk neuroblastoma after treatment stratified by MYCN status and tumor cell ploidy. *J Clin Oncol.* 2005;23:8819-8827.
56. Maris J, Matthay KK. Molecular biology of neuroblastoma. *J Clin Oncol.* 1999;17:2264-2279.
57. Attiyeh EF, London WB, Mosse YP, et al. Chromosome 1p and 11q deletions and outcome in neuroblastoma. *N Engl J Med.* 2005;353:2243-2253.
58. McGregor LM, Rao BN, Davidoff AM, et al. The impact of early resection of primary neuroblastoma on the survival of children older than 1 year of age with stage 4 disease: the St. Jude Children's Research Hospital Experience. *Cancer.* 2005;104:2837-2846.
59. Carli M, Green AA, Hayes FA, et al. Therapeutic efficacy of single drugs for childhood neuroblastoma: a review. In: Raybaud C, Lebreuil G, Bernard JL, ed. *Pediatric Oncology.* Amsterdam, Netherlands: Excerpta Medica; 1982.
60. Schmidt ML, Lal A, Seger RC, et al. Favorable prognosis for patients 12 to 18 months of age with stage 4 nonamplified MYCN neuroblastoma: a Children's Cancer Group Study. *J Clin Oncol.* 2005;23:6474-6480.
61. George RE, London WB, Cohn SL, et al. Hyperdiploidy plus nonamplified MYCN confers a favorable prognosis in children 12 to 18 months old with disseminated neuroblastoma: a Pediatric Oncology Group Study. *J Clin Oncol.* 2005;23:6466-6473.
62. Matthay KK, Villablanca JG, Seeger RC, et al. Treatment of high-risk neuroblastoma with intensive chemotherapy, radiotherapy, autologous bone marrow transplantation, and 13-cis-retinoic acid. *N Engl J Med.* 1999;341: 1165-1173.
63. Berthold F, Boos J, Burdach S, et al. Myeloablative megatherapy with autologous stem-cell rescue versus oral maintenance chemotherapy as consolidation treatment in patients with high-risk neuroblastoma: a randomized controlled trial. *Lancet Oncol.* 2005;6:649-658.

64. Cheung NKV, Bushner BH, Cheung IY, et al. Anti-GD2 antibody treatment of minimal residual stage 4 neuroblastoma diagnosed at more than 1 year of age. *J Clin Oncol.* 1998;16:3053-3060.
65. Frost J, Hank JA, Reaman GH, et al. A phase I/IB trial of murine monoclonal anti-GD2 antibody 14.G2a plus interleukin-2 in children with refractory neuroblastoma. *Cancer.* 1997;80:317-333.
66. Gaze MN, Wheldon TE. Radiolabeled mIBG in the treatment of neuroblastoma. *Eur J Cancer.* 1996;32:93-96.
67. Bordow S, Norris MD, Haber PS, et al. Prognostic significance of MYCN oncogene expression in childhood neuroblastoma. *J Clin Oncol.* 1998;16:3286-3294.
68. Katzenstein H, Bowman LC, Brodeur GM, et al. Prognostic significance of age, MYCN oncogene amplification, tumor cell ploidy, and histology in 110 infants with stage D(S) neuroblastoma: the Pediatric Oncology Group experience—a Pediatric Oncology Group Study. *J Clin Oncol.* 1998;16:2007-2017.
69. Matthay K, Perez C, Seeger RC, et al. Successful treatment of stage III neuroblastoma based on prospective biologic staging: a Children's Cancer Group Study. *J Clin Oncol.* 1998;16:1256-1264.
70. Kawa K, Ohnuma N, Kaneko M, et al. Long-term survivors of advanced neuroblastoma with MYCN amplification: a report of 19 patients surviving disease-free for more than 66 months. *J Clin Oncol.* 1999;17: 3216-3220.
71. Ladenstein R, Philip T, Lasset C, et al. Multivariate analysis of risk factors in stage 4 neuroblastoma patients over the age of one year treated with megatherapy and stem-cell transplantation: a report from the European Bone Marrow Transplantation Solid Tumor Registry. *J Clin Oncol.* 1998;16:953-959.
72. Laverdiere C, Cheung NK, Kushner BH, et al. Long-term complications in survivors of advanced stage neuroblastoma. *Pediatr Blood Cancer.* 2005;45:324-332.
73. Devesa SS. The incidence of retinoblastoma. *Am J Ophthalmol.* 1975;80:263-265.
74. Abramson DH, Schefler AC. Update on retinoblastoma [review]. *Retina.* 2004;24:828-848.
75. Harbour JW. Overview of RB gene mutations in patients with retinoblastoma. Implications for clinical genetic screening. *Ophthalmology.* 1998;105:1442-1447.
76. Knudson AG. Mutation and cancer: statistical study of retinoblastoma. *Proc Natl Acad Sci U S A.* 1971;68: 820-823.
77. Wiggs J, Nordenskjold M, Yandall D, et al. Prediction of the risk of hereditary retinoblastoma using DNA polymorphisms within the retinoblastoma gene. *N Engl J Med.* 1988;318:151-157.
78. Cassady JR. Retinoblastoma: managing a childhood malignancy. *Contemp Oncol.* 1994;4:29.
79. Margo CE, Zimmerman LE. Retinoblastoma: the accuracy of clinical diagnosis in children treated by enucleation. *J Pediatr Ophthalmol Strabismus.* 1983;20:227-229.
80. Stafford WR, Yanoff M, Parnell B. Retinoblastoma initially misdiagnosed as primary ocular inflammations. *Arch Ophthalmol.* 1969;82:771-773.
81. Sterns JK, Coleman DJ, Ellsworth RM. The ultrasonographic characteristics of retinoblastoma. *Am J Ophthalmol.* 1974;78:606-611.
82. Shields CL, Shields JA. Recent developments in the management of retinoblastoma. *J Pediatr Ophthalmol Strabismus.* 1999;36:8-18.
83. Pratt CB. Use of chemotherapy for retinoblastoma. *Med Pediatr Oncol.* 1998;31:531-533.
84. Chan HSL, Gallie BL, Munier FL, et al. Chemotherapy for retinoblastoma. *Ophthalmol Clin North Am.* 2005; 18:55-63.
85. Shields CL, Meadows AT, Leahey AM, et al. Continuing challenges in the management of retinoblastoma with chemotherapy. *Retina.* 2004;24:849-862.
86. Honavar SG, Singh AS. Management of advanced retinoblastoma. *Ophthalmol Clin North Am.* 2005;18: 65-73.
87. Levy C, Doz F, Quintana E, et al. Role of chemotherapy alone or in combination with hyperthermia in the primary treatment of intraocular retinoblastoma: preliminary results. *Br J Ophthalmol.* 1998;82: 1154-1158.
88. Shields CL, Santos MCM, Dinez W, et al. Thermotherapy for retinoblastoma. *Arch Ophthalmol.* 1999;117: 885-893.
89. Chan HSL, DeBoer G, Thiessen JJ, et al. Combining cyclosporin with chemotherapy controls intraocular retinoblastoma without requiring radiation. *Clin Cancer Res.* 1996;2:1499-1508.
90. Namouni F, Doz F, Tanguy ML, et al. High dose chemotherapy with carboplatin, etoposide, and cyclophosphamide followed by a hematopoietic stem cell rescue in patients with high risk retinoblastoma: a SFOP and SFGM study. *Eur J Cancer.* 1997;33:2368-2375.
91. Abramson DH, Ellsworth RM, Grumbach N, et al. Retinoblastoma: survival, age at detection and comparison, 1914-1958, 1958-1983. *J Pediatr Ophthalmol Strabismus.* 1985;22:246-250.
92. Grabowski EF, Abramson DH. Intraocular and extraocular retinoblastoma. *Hematol Oncol Clin North Am.* 1987;1:721-735.
93. Maurer H, Beltangody M, Gehan E. The Intergroup Rhabdomyosarcoma Study—1: a final report. *Cancer.* 1988;611:209-220.
94. Ruymann F, Maddux HR, Ragab A, et al. Congenital anomalies associated with RMS: an autopsy study of 115 cases—a report from the Intergroup Rhabdomyosarcoma Study Committee. *Med Pediatr Oncol.* 1988;16: 33-39.
95. Meyer WH, Spunt SL. Soft tissue sarcomas of childhood. *Cancer Treat Rev.* 2004;30:269-280.
96. Arndt CAS, Crist WM. Medical progress: common musculoskeletal tumors of childhood and adolescence. *N Engl J Med.* 1999;341:242-252.
97. Barr FG. Molecular genetics and pathogenesis of rhabdomyosarcoma. *J Pediatr Hematol Oncol.* 1997;19: 483-491.
98. Maurer H. Rhabdomyosarcoma in childhood and adolescence. *Curr Probl Cancer.* 1977;2:1-36.
99. Wolden SL, Anderson JR, Crist WM, et al. Indications for radiotherapy and chemotherapy after complete resection in rhabdomyosarcoma: a report from the Intergroup Rhabdomyosarcoma Studies I and II. *J Clin Oncol.* 1999;17:3468-3475.
100. Tefft M, Lattin PB, Jereb B, et al. Acute and late effects on normal tissues following chemo- and radiotherapy for childhood RMS and Ewing's sarcoma. *Cancer.* 1986; 37:1201-1271.
101. Mandell L, Ghavimi F, Exelby P, et al. Preliminary results of alternating combination chemotherapy (CT) and hyperfractionated radiotherapy (HART) in advanced rhabdomyosarcoma (RMS). *Int J Radiat Oncol Biol Phys.* 1988;15:197-203.
102. Nag S, Fernandes PS, Martinez-Monge R, et al. Use of brachytherapy to preserve function in children with soft tissue sarcomas. *Oncology.* 1999;13:361-370.
103. Lawrence W, Gehan EA, Hays DM, et al. Prognostic significance of staging factors of the UICC staging system in childhood RMS: a report from the Intergroup Rhabdomyosarcoma Study (IRS-II). *J Clin Oncol.* 1987;5: 46-54.

104. Martelli H, Oberlin O, Rey A, et al. Conservative treatment for girls with nonmetastatic rhabdomyosarcoma of the genital tract: a report from the Study Committee of the International Society of Pediatric Oncology. *J Clin Oncol.* 1999;17:2117-2122.
105. Raney R, Tefft M, Newton WA, et al. Improved prognosis with intensive treatment of children with cranial soft tissue sarcomas arising in nonorbital parameningeal sites: a report from the Intergroup Rhabdomyosarcoma Study. *Cancer.* 1987;59:147-155.
106. Ruymann F, Newton WA, Ragab AH, et al. Bone marrow metastases at diagnosis in children and adolescents with RMS: a report from the Intergroup Rhabdomyosarcoma Study. *Cancer.* 1984;53:368-373.
107. Ek ET, Choong PF. The role of high-dose therapy and autologous stem cell transplantation for pediatric bone and soft tissue sarcomas [review]. *Expert Rev Anticancer Ther.* 2006;6:225-237.
108. Ashley DJB, Path FRC. Origin of teratomas. *Cancer.* 1973;32:390-394.
109. Grosfeld JL, Ballantine TV, Lowe D, et al. Benign and malignant teratomas in children: analysis of 85 patients. *Surgery.* 1976;80:297-305.
110. Hart WR, Burkons DM. Germ cell neoplasms arising in gonadoblastomas. *Cancer.* 1979;43:669-678.
111. Teilum G. Special tumors of ovary and testis and related neoplasms. In: Levine AS, ed. *Cancer in the Young.* New York, NY: Masson Publishing; 1982.
112. Whalen T, Mahour GH, Landing BH, et al. Sacrococcygeal teratomas in infants and children. *Am J Surg.* 1985; 150:373-375.
113. Mahour GH, Woolley GH, Landing BH. Ovarian tumors in children: a 33-year experience. *Am J Surg.* 1976;63: 364-367.
114. Exelby PR. Testicular cancer in children. *Cancer.* 1980; 45:1803-1809.
115. Dieckmann KP, Pichlmeier U. Clinical epidemiology of testicular germ cell tumors. *World J Urol.* 2004;22:2-14.
116. Lack EE, Weinstein HJ, Welch KJ. Mediastinal germ cell tumors in childhood: a clinical and pathologic study of 21 cases. *J Thorac Cardiovasc Surg.* 1985;89:826-835.
117. Ueno T, Tanako YO, Nagata M, et al. Spectrum of germ cell tumors: from head to toe. *Radiograph.* 2004;24: 387-404.
118. Tsuchida Y, Endo Y, Saito S, et al. Evaluation of alphafetoprotein in early infancy. *Pediatr Surg.* 1978;13: 155-162.
119. Heifetz SA, Cushing B, Giller R, et al. Immature teratomas in children: pathologic considerations: a report from the combined Pediatric Oncology Group/Children's Cancer Group. *Am J Surg Pathol.* 1998;22: 1115-1124.
120. Li MC, Hertz R, Spencer DB. Effect of methotrexate on choriocarcinoma and chorioadenoma. *Proc Soc Exp Biol Med.* 1956;96:361-366.
121. Einhorn LG, Donahue JP. Combination chemotherapy in disseminated testicular cancer. *Semin Oncol.* 1979; 6:87-93.
122. Ablin AR. Malignant germ cell tumors in childhood: an outcome analysis. *Proceedings American Society of Clinical Oncology Annual Meeting.* 1986:5:213.
123. Baranzelli MC, Kramar A, Bouffet E, et al. Prognostic factors in children with localized malignant nonseminomatous germ cell tumors. *J Clin Oncol.* 1999;17: 1212.
124. Marina NM, Cushing B, Giller R, et al. Complete surgical excision is effective treatment for children with immature teratomas with or without malignant elements: a Pediatric Oncology Group/Children's Cancer Group Intergroup Study. *J Clin Oncol.* 1999;17:2137.
125. Gerl A, Clemm C, Schmeller N, et al. Late relapse of germ cell tumors after cisplatin-based chemotherapy. *Ann Oncol.* 1997;8:41-47.
126. Delattre O, Zucman J, Melot T, et al. The Ewing family of tumors: a subgroup of small round-cell tumors defined by specific chimeric transcripts. *N Engl J Med.* 1994;331:294-299.
127. de Alava E, Kawai A, Healey JH. EWS-FLII fusion transcript structure is an independent determinant of prognosis in Ewing's sarcoma. *J Clin Oncol.* 1998;16:1248-1255.
128. Denny CT. Ewing's sarcoma: a clinical enigma coming into focus. *J Pediatr Hematol Oncol.* 1998;20:421-425.
129. Buckley JD, Pendergrass TW, Buckley CM, et al. Epidemiology of osteosarcoma and Ewing's sarcoma in childhood. *Cancer.* 1998;83:1440-1448.
130. Ewing J. Diffuse endothelioma of bone. *Proc N Y Pathol Soc.* 1921;21:17-24.
131. Mendenhall C, Marcus RB, Enneking WF, et al. The prognostic significance of soft tissue extension in Ewing's sarcoma. *Cancer.* 1983;51:913-917.
132. Vietti TJ. Multimodal therapy in metastatic Ewing's sarcoma: an intergroup study. *Natl Cancer Inst Monogr.* 1981;56:279-284.
133. Rodriguez-Galindo C, Spunt SL, Pappo AS. Treatment of Ewing sarcoma family of tumors: current status and outlook for the future. *Med Pediatr Oncol.* 2003;40: 276-287.
134. Hawkins DS, Rajendran JG, Conrad EU, et al. Evaluation of chemotherapy response in pediatric bone sarcomas by {F-18}-fluorodeoxy-D-glucose positron emission tomography. *Cancer.* 2002;94:3277-3284.
135. Schuck A, Ahrens S, Paulussen M, et al. Local therapy in localized Ewing tumors: results of 1058 patients treated in the CESS 81, CESS 86, and EICESS 92 trials. *Int J Radiat Oncol Biol Phys.* 2003;55:168-177.
136. Bernstein ML, Devidas M, Lafreniere D, et al. Intensive therapy with growth factor support for patients with Ewing tumor metastatic at diagnosis: Pediatric Oncology Group/Children's Cancer Group Phase II Study 9457—a report from the Children's Oncology Group. *J Clin Oncol.* 2006;24:152-159.
137. Craft A, Cotterill S, Malcolm A, et al. Ifosfamide-containing chemotherapy in Ewing's sarcoma: the second United Kingdom Children's Cancer Study Group and the Medical Research Council Ewing's Tumor Study. *J Clin Oncol.* 1998;16:3628-3633.
138. Rosito P, Mancini AF, Rondelli R, et al. Italian Cooperative Study for the treatment of children and young adults with localized Ewing sarcoma of bone. *Cancer.* 1999;86:421-428.
139. Grier HE, Krailo MD, Tarbell NJ, et al. Addition of ifosfamide and etoposide to standard chemotherapy for Ewing's sarcoma and primitive neuroectodermal tumor of bone. *N Engl J Med.* 2003;348:694-701.
140. Ahmad R, Mayol BR, Davis M, et al. Extraskeletal Ewing's sarcoma. *Cancer.* 1999;85:725-731.
141. Gururangan S, Marina NM, Luo X. Treatment of children with peripheral primitive neuroectodermal tumor or extraosseous Ewing's tumor with Ewing's directed therapy. *J Pediatr Hematol Oncol.* 1998;20:55-61.
142. Rosen G, Caparros B, Nirenberg A, et al. Ewing's sarcoma: ten-year experience with adjuvant chemotherapy. *Cancer.* 1981;47:2204-2213.
143. Kolb EA, Kushner BH, Gorlick R, et al. Long-term event-free survival after intensive chemotherapy for Ewing's family of tumors in children and young adults. *J Clin Oncol.* 2003;21:3423-3430.
144. Falk S, Albert M. The clinical and roentgen aspects of Ewing's sarcoma. *Am J Med Sci.* 1965;54:492-508.

145. Miser JS, Krailo MD, Tarbell NJ, et al. Treatment of metastatic Ewing's sarcoma or primitive neuroectodermal tumor of bone: evaluation of combination ifosfamide and etoposide—a Children's Cancer Group and Pediatric Oncology Group Study. *J Clin Oncol.* 2004;22:2873-2876.
146. Bacci G, Ferrari S, Longhi A, et al. Therapy and survival after recurrence of Ewing's tumors: the Rizzoli experience in 195 patients treated with adjuvant and neoadjuvant chemotherapy from 1979 to 1997. *Ann Oncol.* 2003;14:1654-1659.
147. Frauman JF. Stature and malignant tumors of bone in childhood and adolescence. *Cancer.* 1967;20:967-973.
148. Marina N, Gebhardt M, Teot L, et al. Biology and therapeutic advances for pediatric osteosarcoma. *Oncologist.* 2004;9:422-441.
149. Hems G. An etiology of bone cancer, and some other cancers, in the young. *Br J Cancer.* 1970;24:208-214.
150. Sim F, Cupps RE, Dahlin DC, et al. Postradiation sarcoma of bone. *J Bone Joint Surg.* 1972;54A:1479-1489.
151. Abramson DH, Ellsworth R, Zimmerman L. Nonocular cancer in retinoblastoma survivors. *Trans Am Acad Ophthalmol Otolaryngol.* 1976;81:454-457.
152. Gilman PA, Wang N, Fan SF, et al. Familial osteosarcoma associated with 13;14 chromosomal rearrangement. *Cancer Genet Cytogenet.* 1985;17:123-132.
153. Uribe-Botero G, Russell WO, Sutow WW, et al. Primary osteosarcoma of bone: a clinicopathologic investigation of 243 cases with necropsy studies in 54. *Am J Clin Pathol.* 1977;67:427-435.
154. Ferguson WS, Goorin AM. Current treatment of osteosarcoma. *Cancer Invest.* 2001;19:292-315.
155. Dahlin CD, Coventry MB. Osteosarcoma: a study of 600 cases. *J Bone Joint Surg (Am).* 1967;49:101-110.
156. Sweetnam R, Knowelden J, Jedden H. Bone sarcoma: treatment by irradiation, amputation, or a combination of the 2. *BMJ.* 1971;2:363-367.
157. Cortes EP, Holland JF, Wang JJ, et al. Amputation and Adriamycin in primary osteosarcoma. *N Engl J Med.* 1974;291:998-1000.
158. Jaffe N. Recent advance in the chemotherapy of metastatic osteogenic sarcoma, *Cancer.* 1972;30:1627-1631.
159. Jaffe N, Frei E, Traggis D, et al. Adjuvant methotrexate and citrovorum factor treatment of osteogenic sarcoma. *N Engl J Med.* 1974;291:994-997.
160. Taylor WF, Ivins JC, Dahlin DC, et al. Trends and variability in survival from osteosarcoma. *Mayo Clin Proc.* 1978;53:695-700.
161. Link MP. The effect of adjuvant chemotherapy on release-free survival in patients with osteosarcoma of the extremity. *N Engl J Med.* 1986;314:1600-1606.
162. Eiber F, Giuliano A, Eckhardt J, et al. Adjuvant chemotherapy for osteosarcoma: a randomized prospective trial. *J Clin Oncol.* 1987;5:21-26.
163. Bacci G, Longhi A, Fagioli F, et al. Adjuvant and neoadjuvant chemotherapy for osteosarcoma of the extremities: 27 year experience at the Rizzoli Institute, Italy. *Eur J Cancer.* 2005;41:2836-2845.
164. Ferrari S, Smeland S, Mercuri M, et al. Neoadjuvant chemotherapy with high-dose ifosfamide, high-dose methotrexate, cisplatin, and doxorubicin for patients with localized osteosarcoma of the extremity: a joint study by the Italian and Scandinavian sarcoma groups. *J Clin Oncol.* 2005;23:8845-8852.
165. Petrilli AS, de Camargo B, Filho VO, et al. Results of the Brazilian osteosarcoma treatment group studies III and IV: prognostic factors and impact on survival. *J Clin Oncol.* 2006;24:1161-1168.
166. Hayden JB, Hoang BH. Osteosarcoma: basic science and clinical implications. *Orthop Clin North Am.* 2006; 37:1-7.
167. Marcove RC, Rosen G. En bloc resections for osteogenic sarcoma. *Cancer.* 1980;45:3040-3044.
168. Martini N, Huvos AG, Mike V, et al. Multiple pulmonary resections in the treatment of osteogenic sarcoma. *Ann Thorac Surg.* 1971;12:271-280.
169. Meyer WH, Schell MJ, Kumar AP, et al. Thoracotomy for pulmonary metastatic osteosarcoma. *Cancer.* 1987; 59:374-379.
170. Briccoli A, Rocca M, Salone M, et al. Resection of recurrent pulmonary metastases in patients with osteosarcoma. *Cancer.* 2005;104:1721-1725.
171. Harris MB, Gieser P, Goorin AM, et al. Treatment of metastatic osteosarcoma at diagnosis: a Pediatric Oncology Group Study. *J Clin Oncol.* 1998;16:3641-3548.
172. Meyer WH, Pratt CB, Poquette CA, et al. Carboplatin/ifosfamide window therapy for osteosarcoma: results of the St Jude Children's Research Hospital OS-91 trial. *J Clin Oncol.* 2001;19:171-182.
173. Bacci G, Ferrari S, Delepine N, et al. Predictive factors of histologic response to primary chemotherapy in osteosarcoma of the extremity: study of 272 patients preoperatively treated with high-dose methotrexate, doxorubicin, and cisplatin. *J Clin Oncol.* 1998;16:658-663.
174. Provisor AJ, Ettinger L, Nachman JB, et al. Treatment of nonmetastatic osteosarcoma of the extremity with preoperative and postoperative chemotherapy: a report from the CCG. *J Clin Oncol.* 1997;15:76-84.
175. Leventhal BG, Kato GJ. Childhood Hodgkin's and non-Hodgkin's lymphomas. *Pediatr Rev.* 1990;12: 171-179.
176. Cairo MS, Raetz E, Lim MS, et al. Childhood and adolescent non-Hodgkin lymphoma: new insights in biology and critical challenges for the future. *Pediatr Blood Cancer.* 2005;45:753-769.
177. Burkhardt B, Zimmermann M, Oschlies I, et al. The impact of age and gender on biology, clinical features and treatment outcome of non-Hodgkin lymphoma in childhood and adolescence. *Br J Haematol.* 2005;131: 39-49.
178. Pinkerton R. Continuing challenges in childhood non-Hodgkin lymphoma. *Br J Haematol.* 2005;130:480-488.
179. Pellici PG, Knowles DM, Magrath I, et al. Chromosomal breakpoints and structural alterations of the c-myc locus differ in endemic sporadic forms of Burkitt lymphoma. *Proc Natl Acad Sci U S A.* 1986;83:2984-2988.
180. Filipovitch A, Zerbe D, Spector BD, et al. Lymphomas in persons with naturally occurring immunodeficiency disorders. In: Magrath I, O'Connor G, Ramot B, eds. *Pathogenesis of Leukemias and Lymphomas: Environmental Influences.* New York, NY: Raven Press; 1984.
181. Bernheim A, Berger R, Lenoir G. Cytogenetic studies on African Burkitt's lymphoma cell lines: t(8,14), t(2,8) and t(8,22) translocation. *Cancer Genet Cytogenet.* 1981;3:307-315.
182. Zech L, Haglund U, Nilsson K, et al. Characteristic chromosomal abnormalities in biopsies and lymphoid-cell lines from patients with Burkitt and non-Burkitt lymphomas. *Int J Cancer.* 1976;17:47-56.
183. Murphy SB. Classification, staging, and end results of treatment of childhood non-Hodgkin's lymphomas: dissimilarities from lymphomas in adults. *Semin Oncol.* 1980;1:332-339.
184. Wright D, McKeever P, Carter R. Childhood non-Hodgkin's lymphomas in the United Kingdom: findings from the UK Children's Cancer Study Group. *J Clin Pathol.* 1997;50:128-134.
185. Mussolin L, Pillon M, d'Amore ES, et al. Prevalence and clinical implication of bone marrow involvement in pediatric anaplastic large cell lymphoma. 2005;19:1643-1647.

186. Depas G, De Barsy C, Jerusalem G, et al. 18F-FDG PET in children with lymphomas. *Eur J Nucl Med Mol Imaging*. 2005;32:31-38.
187. Amthauer H, Furtg C, Denecke T, et al. FDG-PET in 10 children with non-Hodgkin's lymphoma: initial experience in staging and follow-up. *Klin Pediatr*. 2005;217: 327-333.
188. Rhodes MM, Delbeke D, Whitlock JA, et al. Utility of FDG-PET CT in follow-up of children treated for Hodgkin and non-Hodgkin lymphoma. *J Pediatr Hematol Oncol*. 2006;28:300-306.
189. Magrath IT, Lwanga S, Carswell W, et al. Surgical reduction of tumor bulk in management of abdominal Burkitt's lymphoma. *BMJ*. 1974;2:308-312.
190. Jenkin R, Anderson JR, Chilcote RR, et al. The treatment of localized non-Hodgkin's lymphoma in children: a report from the Children's Cancer Study Group. *J Clin Oncol*. 1984;2:88-97.
191. Link MP, Shuster JJ, Donaldson SS, et al. Treatment of children and young adults with early stage non-Hodgkin's lymphoma. *N Engl J Med*. 1997;337: 1259-1266.
192. Rosolen A, Pillon M, Garaventa A, et al. Anaplastic large cell lymphoma treated with a leukemia-like therapy: report of the Italian Association of Pediatric Hematology and Oncology (AIEOP) LNH-92 protocol. *Cancer*. 2005;104:2133-2140.
193. Marky I, Bjork O, Forestier E, et al. Intensive chemotherapy without radiotherapy gives more than 85% event-free survival for non-Hodgkin lymphoma without central nervous involvement. *J Pediatr Hematol Oncol*. 2004;26:555-560.
194. Burkhardt B, Woessmann W, Zimmermann M, et al. Impact of cranial radiotherapy on central nervous system prophylaxis in children and adolescents with central nervous system-negative stage III or IV lymphoblastic lymphoma. *J Clin Oncol*. 2006;24: 491-499.
195. Reed DM. On the pathological changes in Hodgkin's disease, with especial reference to its relation to tuberculosis. *Johns Hopkins Hosp Rep*. 1902;10:133-396.
196. Kanzler H, Kuppers R, Hansmann ML, et al. Hodgkin's and Reed Sternberg cells in Hodgkin's disease represent the outgrowth of a dominant tumor clone derived from germinal center B cells. *J Exp Med*. 1996;184: 1495-1505.
197. Stein H, Hummel M. Cellular origin and clonality of classic Hodgkin's lymphoma: immunophenotypic and molecular studies. *Semin Hematol*. 1999;36:233-241.
198. Thomas RK, Re D, Wolf J, et al. Part I: Hodgkin's lymphoma—molecular biology of Hodgkin and Reed-Sternberg cells. *Lancet Oncol*. 2004;5:11-18.
199. Grufferman SL, Delzell E. Epidemiology of Hodgkin's disease. *Epidemiol Rev*. 1984;6:76-106.
200. Spitz MR, Sider JG, Katz RL, et al. Ethnic patterns of Hodgkin's disease incidence among children and adolescents in the United States, 1973-1982. *J Natl Cancer Inst*. 1986;76:235-239.
201. Mack TM, Cozen W, Shibata DK, et al. Concordance for Hodgkin's disease in identical twins suggesting genetic susceptibility to the young-adult form of the disease. *N Engl J Med*. 1995;332:413-418.
202. Nonoyama M, Kawai Y, Huang CH, et al. Epstein-Barr virus DNA in Hodgkin's disease, American Burkitt's lymphoma and other human tumors. *Cancer Res*. 1974; 34:1228-1231.
203. Murray PG, Billingham LJ, Hassan HT, et al. Effect of Epstein-Barr virus infection on response to chemotherapy and survival in Hodgkin's disease. *Blood*. 1999;94: 442-447.
204. Raney RB. Hodgkin's disease in childhood: a review. *J Pediatr Hematol Oncol*. 1997;19:502-509.
205. Gatti RA, Good RA. Occurrence of malignancy in immunodeficiency disease: a literature review. *Cancer*. 1971;28:89-98.
206. Ioachim HL, Cooper MC, Hellman GC. Lymphomas in men at high risk for acquired immune deficiency syndrome (AIDS): a study of 21 cases. *Cancer*. 1985;56: 2831-2842.
207. Hudson MM, Donaldson SS. Treatment of pediatric Hodgkin's lymphoma. *Semin Hematol*. 1999;36: 313-323.
208. Carbone PP, Kaplan HS, Musshoff K, et al. Report of the Committee on Hodgkin's Disease Staging Classification. *Cancer Res*. 1971;31:1860-1861.
209. Diehl V, Thomas RK, Re D. Part II: Hodgkin's lymphoma—diagnosis and treatment. *Lancet Oncol*. 2004; 5:19-26.
210. Lukes RJ, Butler JJ. The pathology and nomenclature of Hodgkin's disease. *Cancer Res*. 1966;26:1063-1064.
211. Kaplan HS. *Hodgkin's Disease*. 2nd ed. Cambridge, MA: Harvard University Press; 1980.
212. Donaldson SS, Link MP. Combined modality treatment with low-dose radiation and MOPP chemotherapy for children with Hodgkin's disease. *J Clin Oncol*. 1987;5:742-749.
213. DeVita VT Jr, Serpick A, Carbone PP. Combination chemotherapy in the treatment of advanced Hodgkin's disease. *Ann Intern Med*. 1970;73:881-895.
214. Bonadonna G, Zucali R, Monfardini S, et al. Combination chemotherapy of Hodgkin's disease with Adriamycin, bleomycin, vinblastine, and imidazole carboxamide versus MOPP. *Cancer*. 1975;36:252-259.
215. Hutchinson RJ, Fryer CJ, Davis PC, et al. MOPP or radiation in addition to ABVD in the treatment of pathologically staged advanced Hodgkin's disease in children: results of the Children's Cancer Group phase III trial. *J Clin Oncol*. 1998;16:897-906.
216. Schwartz CL. Special issues in pediatric Hodgkin's disease. *Eur J Haematol*. 2005;(suppl 66):55-62.
217. Arya LS, Dinand V, Thavarag V, et al. Hodgkin's disease in Indian children: outcome with chemotherapy alone. *Pediatr Blood Cancer*. 2006;46:26-34.
218. Damewood MD, Grochow LB. Prospects for fertility after chemotherapy or radiation for neoplastic disease. *Fertil Steril*. 1986;45:443-459.
219. Santoro A, Bonadonna G, Valagussa P, et al. Long-term results of combined chemotherapy-radiotherapy approach in Hodgkin's disease: superiority of ABVD plus radiotherapy versus MOPP plus radiotherapy. *J Clin Oncol*. 1987;l5:27-37.
220. Coleman CN. Secondary malignancy after treatment of Hodgkin's disease: an evolving picture. *J Clin Oncol*. 1986;4:821-824.
221. Sullivan MP, Fuller LM, Chen T, et al. Intergroup Hodgkin's disease in children study of stages I and II: a preliminary report. *Cancer Treat Rep*. 1982;66: 937-947.
222. Vinciguerra V, Propert KJ, Coleman M, et al. Alternating cycles of combination chemotherapy for patients with recurrent Hodgkin's disease following radiotherapy: a prospectively randomized study by the Cancer and Leukemia Group B. *J Clin Oncol*. 1986;4:838-846.
223. Oguz A, Karadeniz C, Okur FV, et al. Prognostic factors and treatment outcome in childhood Hodgkin disease. *Pediatr Blood Cancer*. 2005;45:670-675.
224. Krasin MJ, Rai SN, Kun LE, et al. Patterns of treatment failure in pediatric and young adult patients with Hodgkin's disease: local disease control with combined-modality therapy. *J Clin Oncol*. 2005;23:8406-8413.

225. Schellong G, Dorffel W, Claviez A, et al. Salvage therapy of progressive and recurrent Hodgkin's disease: results from a multicenter study of the pediatric DAL/GPOH-HD Study Group. *J Clin Oncol.* 2005;23:6181-6189.
226. Probert JC, Parker BR, Kaplan HS. Growth retardation in children after megavoltage irradiation of the spine. *Cancer.* 1973;32:634-639.
227. Janjan NA, Wilson JF, Gillin M, et al. Mammary carcinoma developing after radiotherapy and chemotherapy for Hodgkin's disease. *Cancer.* 1988;61:252-254.
228. Bhatia S, Robison LL, Oberlin O, et al. Breast cancer and other second neoplasms after childhood Hodgkin's disease. *N Engl J Med.* 1996;334:745-751.
229. Constine LS, Donaldson SS, McDougal IR, et al. Thyroid dysfunction after radiotherapy in children with Hodgkin's disease. *Cancer.* 1984;53:878-883.
230. Donaldson SS, Kaplan HS. Complications of treatment of Hodgkin's disease in children. *Cancer Treat Rep.* 1982;66:977-989.
231. deCunha MF, Meistrich ML, Fuller LM, et al. Recovery of spermatogenesis after treatment for Hodgkin's disease: limiting dose of MOPP chemotherapy. *J Clin Oncol.* 1984;2:571-577.
232. Howell SJ, Shalet SM. Spermatogenesis after cancer treatment: damage and recovery. *J Nat Cancer Inst.* 2005;34:12-17.
233. Oeffinger KC, Mertens AC, Hudson MM, et al. Health care of young adult survivors of childhood cancer: a report from the Childhood Cancer Survivor Study. *Ann Fam Med.* 2004;2:61-70.
234. Florin TA, Hinkle AS. A guide to caring for cancer survivors. *Contemp Pediatr.* 200522:31-48.
235. Oeffinger KC, Hudson MM. Long term complications following childhood and adolescent cancer: foundations for providing risk based health care for survivors. *CA Cancer J Clin.* 2004;54:208-236.
236. Wissler KH, Proukou C. Navigating the educational system: a practical guide for nurse practitioners. *J Pediatr Oncol Nurs.* 1999;16:145-155.
237. Hudson MM, Mertens AC, Yasui Y, et al. Health status in adults treated for childhood cancer: a report from the Childhood Survivor Study. *Am J Oncol Rev.* 2004;3: 165-171.
238. Hays D, Dolgin M, Steele LL, et al. Educational achievement, employment and workplace experience of adult survivors of childhood cancer. *Int J Pediatr Hematol Oncol.* 1997;44:327-337.
239. Monaco GP, Fiduccia D, Smith G. Legal and societal issues facing survivors of childhood cancer. *Pediatr Clin North Am.* 1997;44:1043-1058.

Chapter 245

CEREBRAL PALSY

Gregory S. Liptak, MD, MPH

Cerebral palsy (CP) is a clinical descriptive term for a heterogeneous group of conditions typically classified according to the type, distribution, and severity of motor abnormality. CP describes a group of disorders of the development of movement, posture, and coordination caused by nonprogressive disturbances affecting the brain in its early development (fetal, infantile, and early childhood). The motor disorder is often accompanied by disturbances of sensation, cognition, communication, perception, behavior, or any combination or by a seizure disorder, contributing further to activity limitation and restricted participation.[1] Most children with CP develop some impairment of form or function in the musculoskeletal system. The most common impairments are contractures (eg, equinus deformity), torsional changes in long bones (eg, femoral and tibial torsion), and joint instability (eg, hip displacement).[2]

EPIDEMIOLOGIC FEATURES

The incidence of CP is approximately 2 to 2.5 cases per 1000 live births in developed countries. Although some variation has been described, the incidence has generally remained stable over the last 20 years.[3-5] CP is more common with lower birth weight and with lower gestational age. For instance, in one survey, children born weighing less than 1000 g constituted 0.2% of the survivors but accounted for 8% of the children who had CP.[6]

CP affects activities and participation, as well as body structures.[7] For example, in a national survey,[8] 59% of children who had CP attended a special school, compared with 0.5% of those who did not have CP. Use of health care services is much higher too; in the 12 months before the survey, children who had CP had 16 visits to a physician, 29 hospital admissions per 100 children, and 108 hospital days per 100 children. In comparison, children without CP had 3 visits to a physician, 4 hospitalizations per 100 children, and 20 hospital days per 100 children.

The risk of CP is higher in infants of very low birth weight and those from multiple pregnancies. CP in preterm infants is associated most commonly with periventricular leukomalacia, with or without severe periventricular bleeding or infarction. An increasing proportion of infants from both of these groups survive into childhood. The biggest challenge to the prevention of CP remains the prevention of prematurity. A recent study found that the prevalence of CP in very low–birth weight infants and those born at less than 32 weeks' gestation decreased from 6% of live births in 1980% to 4% in 1996. This improvement occurred despite an increase in live births at very low birth weight, a decrease in neonatal deaths, an increase in multiple births, and, in children with CP, a decrease in mean birth weight and gestational age.[9]

ETIOLOGY

A definite cause cannot be identified for many cases of CP, and when a cause can be identified, it is usually of prenatal origin.[10] Intrapartum events play a limited role.[11] Neither sophisticated fetal monitoring nor a higher rate of cesarean deliveries has reduced the occurrence of CP.[12] Isolated risk factors such as fetal bradycardia, neonatal acidosis, intraventricular hemorrhage in the absence of periventricular leukomalacia, and low Apgar scores taken in isolation are poor predictors of CP, especially in full-term infants. However, low birth weight (2000 g or less), periventricular leukomalacia (necrosis of white matter near the lateral ventricles), hydrocephalus, congenital malformations, and newborn encephalopathy (recurrent seizures, hypotonia, coma) are all associated with CP.[13] Prenatal maternal chorioamnionitis has been show to increase significantly the risk of CP in both term and preterm infants.[14] In approximately 10% of children who have CP, the cause of the condition is thought to be post-neonatal (after 28 days).[15] Causes include infections (eg, meningitis, encephalitis), asphyxia, and accidental injury. In some instances, CP may be prevented by reducing the occurrence of injuries during childhood and by minimizing periventricular leukomalacia in premature infants by improving circulation and countering the effects of excitatory neurotransmitters (eg, head cooling in the newborn who has had a hypoxic or ischemic event).[16] The timing of the insult to the brain may affect the manifestations of CP. For example, disturbances occurring between 24 and 28 weeks' gestation are more likely to produce spastic diplegia or tetraplegia (quadriplegia), whereas those occurring at term are more likely to produce dyskinesia (see later discussion).[17,18]

CLASSIFICATION AND DIAGNOSIS

CP may be classified according to the type, distribution, and severity of motor abnormality (Box 245-1). This classification system can be simplified into 3 categories: (1) spastic (involving the pyramidal tracts), (2) dyskinetic (involving the extrapyramidal tracts), and (3) mixed (involving both). Spasticity is defined as velocity-dependent passive resistance of muscle to stretch. It is associated with neurologic signs that include hyperreflexia, clonus, extensor plantar response, co-contractures, persistent primitive reflexes, and abnormal postural control. These abnormalities impair normal movements, such as gait and the manipulation of objects, in complex ways. Movement is often described as stiff, and patterns of movement such as fisting of the hands, retraction of the shoulders, scissoring of the legs, and toe-walking are often abnormal. Although most attention has been focused on the extremities, evaluating the trunk is important as well. Hypotonia of the trunk and neck is common, as well as impairments that affect function in a child who has spastic quadriplegia.

In diplegia, the legs are affected with general sparing of the arms. In quadriplegia all four limbs are involved. In hemiplegia, only 1 side is involved, with the arm usually more impaired than the leg. In extrapyramidal CP, the impairment is diffuse, with poor control of movement and the presence of involuntary activity. Dyskinesia includes the involuntary movements of athetosis and chorea, which are most pronounced when the child initiates a movement, as well as dystonia. Dystonia is characterized by sustained muscle contractures that lead to abnormal posture and twisting. Dysarthria commonly occurs with dyskinesia. Ataxia involves incoordination of movement and impaired balance and may be associated with an intention tremor. Because the fibers in the corticospinal tract that control the legs are closest to the ventricles, any periventricular injury is likely to lead to spastic diplegia. This condition most commonly occurs with hypoxic-ischemic injury in a preterm infant between 28 and 36 weeks' gestation, in which the periventricular area is most susceptible to injury because of poor vascularization. This injury is often characterized by subsequent enlargement of the ventricles or development of periventricular leukomalacia. Children of any gestational age with hydrocephalus are also more likely to develop spastic diplegia. Generally, children who have spastic quadriplegia have more generalized and extensive lesions, and they are more likely to be intellectually disabled (64% have an IQ below 50) and have seizures (56%) than are children who have other kinds of CP.[19] Children who have spastic quadriplegia are also more likely to have feeding difficulties, severe joint contractures, and scoliosis. Children with extrapyramidal CP frequently have problems with feeding and communication because they are unable to control the oral-motor musculature. The most common system for classifying the severity of CP is the Gross Motor Function Classification System (GMFCS).[20,21] The GMFCS is a 5-level system to classify severity of motor involvement in children with CP based on their functional abilities and their need for assistive technology and wheeled mobility.

Each form of CP can be caused by a multitude of conditions, and a single etiologic factor (eg, meningitis) can lead to different forms of CP. Therefore a direct link between the type of CP and its cause (when a cause can be found) cannot be established without using diagnostic evaluations such as cranial ultrasonography or magnetic resonance imaging (MRI).

BOX 245-1 Classification of Cerebral Palsy

SPASTIC	DYSKINETIC
Diplegic	Choreoathetotic
Quadriplegic	Dystonic
Hemiplegic	Ataxic
	MIXED

EARLY AND DIFFERENTIAL DIAGNOSIS

Although the brain lesion or anomaly, once recognized in early childhood, is no longer progressive, the clinical signs change, especially in the first several years of life. Abnormal patterns emerge as the damaged nervous system matures. For example, the child who is destined to have spastic quadriplegia will often be hypotonic in early infancy. At 6 months of age, as tone increases, the child may develop adduction of the thumb (palmar thumb) followed in a month or 2 by scissoring of the legs when held upright. By 9 months of age, the child may have diffuse spasticity and hyperactive deep-tendon reflexes. Dyskinetic patterns may not be obvious until approximately 18 months of age. Ataxia, may not be apparent until even later. In a study of 1726 children from 5 urban school districts, the mean age at which CP was diagnosed was 10 months.[22] Therefore, in addition to the formal developmental screening recommended for all children,[23] all children at risk for developing CP should have regular careful physical examinations, with special attention paid to their neurologic status.

Early diagnosis of CP is aided by a history of an abnormal pregnancy, labor, delivery, or neonatal period or by the occurrence of a serious acute illness and trauma. The diagnosis is further aided by evaluating the child's primitive reflexes (eg, the asymmetrical tonic neck response), postural responses (righting the head when tilted to the side), muscle tone, motor milestones, and neurobehavioral responsiveness.[24] Persistent or exaggerated primitive reflexes, a delay in the emergence of postural reactions, hyperreflexia, asymmetry, and abnormal muscle tone all suggest the possibility of CP. Other early signs that suggest CP include difficulty feeding because of abnormal oral-motor patterns (tongue thrusting, tonic bite, oral hypersensitivity), irritability, and delayed milestones such as head control. Children with CP may benefit from timely referral to formal early-intervention programs, which are mandated under the Individuals with Disabilities Education Act.

A diagnosis of CP implies that the neurologic process is not progressive and that the disorder is in the brain. The differential diagnosis includes neurodegenerative disorders, inborn errors of metabolism, developmental or traumatic lesions of the spinal cord, severe neuromuscular disease, movement disorders, spinocerebellar degeneration, neoplasms, hydrocephalus, and subdural hematoma. Repeated examinations are necessary to rule out a progressive degenerative condition. Recurring subclinical seizures or adverse reactions to anticonvulsants may worsen the clinical condition of children who have CP. Hypotonia in association with weak muscles and depressed tendon reflexes suggests a neuromuscular disease, although many children with both spastic and extrapyramidal CP are hypotonic in early infancy. Extrapyramidal signs in early infancy or marked worsening during periods of illness also make the diagnosis of CP a possibility. If a child diagnosed as having dyskinetic CP has symptoms that worsen significantly as the day progresses, dopa-responsive dystonia should be considered.[25] This rare but treatable form of dystonia may begin with toe-walking and difficulties with gait; it responds dramatically to administration of levodopa. In most instances, no history can be found of a preexisting condition that would be consistent with CP. Other rare inborn errors of metabolism such as arginase deficiency and glutaric aciduria may mimic CP. However, these conditions cause progressive deterioration, whereas CP does not. If a child has a parent who has CP and has late-onset spastic diplegia with no preceding history of prenatal or neonatal problems, then hereditary spastic diplegia may be the cause.[26]

ASSOCIATED DISORDERS

Table 245-1 lists disabilities and impairments associated with CP. All types of language abnormality may be encountered, from aphasia to poor articulation. Abnormal speech may be related to hearing, intelligence, experience, language development, the integration of motor mechanisms of the oropharynx, and coordination of breathing patterns. Nearly 75% of individuals who have CP are cognitively impaired. Approximately 40% are intellectually disabled (mildly so in approximately one third of cases and moderately or worse in another third).[27] In persons who function in the normal range of intelligence, specific learning disabilities such as visual-spatial impairment are common. Impaired mobility is also common and may result from spasticity with or without joint contractures and scoliosis. Self-care and hygiene may be impaired by gross-motor and fine-motor abnormalities and associated conditions such as drooling. Impairments in gastrointestinal functioning such as gastroesophageal reflux disease and in growth are common. In general, physical growth is inhibited,[28,29] and osteoporosis is common in patients with severe quadriplegia and immobility.[30] Many of these patients fail to thrive, especially those who have dyskinesia or spastic quadriplegia. Feeding difficulties caused by oropharyngeal incoordination, gastroesophageal reflux, and recurrent vomiting occur and may be associated with aspiration. Dental disease (malocclusion and dental caries) is common. Seizures are common, as are impaired vision and hearing. Roughly 40% of these children develop seizures, which most often have their onset in the first 2 years of life. Oculomotor anomalies include strabismus, refractive error, and nystagmus. Behavioral problems are 5 to 8 times more likely to occur in children who have CP than in their uninvolved peers, especially in those who have hemiplegia.[31,32] Sociocultural risk factors have a profound effect on development and interact with biological risk factors. Perinatal and other biological risk factors can lead to intellectual impairment.

EVALUATION

Neuroimaging techniques such as ultrasonography, computed tomography, and MRI have increased our understanding of the structural abnormalities associated with CP and may help clarify the timing of a lesion.[33] Neuroimaging may demonstrate periventricular leukomalacia, postischemic necrosis, cerebral dysgenesis, hydrocephalus, porencephaly, tumor, prenatal ischemic injury, or leukodystrophy. The information gained with brain imaging is rarely needed to confirm the diagnosis of CP and usually does not affect intervention strategies, but it can be useful to the physician in explaining (or demonstrating) the specific cause of a child's CP to the parents. The electroencephalogram is an important part of the diagnosis and management of associated seizures but is not helpful in the diagnosis of CP; continuous electroencephalogram monitoring with videography may help differentiate seizures from other movement disorders. The presence of dysmorphic features may trigger a search for a chromosomal abnormality or a genetic syndrome. However, an increase in minor congenital anomalies is common in patients with CP in the absence of any apparent genetic cause for them. Evaluation of complications such as altered gait and feeding disorders may require special diagnostic studies, such as gait analysis and videofluoroscopic swallowing studies. Routine screening for metabolic and genetic disorders is not recommended unless the child has atypical features, such as unusual facial features, or a progressive condition.[34]

Table 245-1 Disabilities and Impairments Associated With Cerebral Palsy in Children and Possible Interventions

DISABILITY OR IMPAIRMENT	POSSIBLE INTERVENTION	POSSIBLE CONSULTATION
Impaired communication	Augmentative communication aids	Speech therapist, audiologist
Impaired cognition	Early intervention, special education program, formal educational testing	Education specialist, psychologist, school advocate
Weakness or impaired mobility	Orthoses (braces), walker, wheeled mobility and strength training, hippotherapy	Orthopedist, orthotist, physical therapist Physical therapist specialty program, gait laboratory Equine specialist
	Constraint therapy for hemiplegia	Occupational therapist
Spasticity	Medications, selective dorsal rhizotomy, intrathecal baclofen, botulinum toxin injection	Orthopedist, neurodevelopmental specialist, physiatrist, neurologist
Joint contractures	Range of motion, orthoses, surgery	Physical therapist, orthopedist, orthotist
Scoliosis	Orthoses, surgery	Orthopedist, orthotist
Impaired self-care and hygiene	Assistive technological devices, home modifications, training	Occupational therapist, rehabilitation engineer
Drooling	Scopolamine patch, glycopyrrolate, surgery, botulinum toxin injections, acupuncture	Otolaryngologist, acupuncturist
Sexual functioning	Education, adaptive devices	Gynecologist, urologist, psychologist
Impaired nutrition or feeding	Education, monitoring, medical evaluation, medication, surgery	Nutritionist or dietitian, gastroenterologist, speech therapist, occupational therapist
Dental caries, malocclusion	Repair of dental caries, orthodonture	Dentist, pedodontist, orthodontist
Seizures	Medication, surgery	Neurologist
Impaired vision or hearing	Assistive device, surgery	Ophthalmologist, otolaryngologist
Impaired access to care	Financial counseling, care coordination, transportation	Financial counselor, care coordinator, specialty program
Adverse effects on family	Parent support group, counseling, support	Social worker, psychologist, specialty program, care coordinator
Impaired transition to adulthood	Counseling, adult-oriented health care, care coordination, transportation, recreation, vocational services, financial planning, guardianship	Internist, family physician, care coordinator, vocational specialist, independent living specialist, attorney, psychologist, financial planner

INTERVENTION

Pathophysiological abnormalities of the brain (eg, leukomalacia) lead to impairments such as spasticity. Spasticity then leads to alterations in functioning, for example, shortened stride length, which leads to disabilities (eg, difficulty ambulating independently). The disabilities may lead to adverse social consequences or worse (eg, inability to use public transportation).[35,36] Adults who have CP have identified communication skills, self-care activities, and mobility as the 3 most important issues they face. Consequently, interventions (eg, medications, surgery, braces or adaptive equipment) should focus on promoting developmental and functional outcomes that address these issues rather than on simply reducing spasticity, improving range of motion, or correcting deformity in isolation. No intervention, including therapy and surgery, will be worthwhile in the long term if it does not improve the child's ability to function. Interventions should also stress the prevention of complications.

Table 245-1 lists referrals and possible interventions to address the complications of CP. No single professional can fulfill the multiple medical, social, psychological, educational, and therapeutic needs of a child who has CP. Comprehensive management requires a multidisciplinary team, such as those found in a specialty program, the members of which instruct and support parents to enable them to achieve maximal potential for self-help and care for their child and to understand their child's ability and potential for development. The Individuals with Disabilities Education Act mandates access to early intervention services for infants at risk for disabling conditions. These services include special education; physical, occupational, and speech therapies; adaptive equipment; training for mobility and living skills; and communication. The therapies may not change the basic disorder significantly[37]; however, the therapists may help the families by teaching them how to position and handle their infant, by providing more opportunity for play and learning, and by facilitating feeding and the parent-child relationship. Whether formal early intervention services are provided or not, the family should have early professional support to help them cope with the crisis of diagnosis.[38]

The care provided should be integrated. For example, children whose legs are spastic often have dorsiflexion at the ankle, flexion at the knee, and flexion and adduction of the hip. Multiple interventions are possible, including muscle strengthening, orthotics (eg, ankle-foot orthoses), oral medication, botulinum toxin injections (with or without serial casting), intrathecal baclofen pump, selective dorsal rhizotomy, and orthopedic surgery. Deciding on the best approach requires the input of the child and family in collaboration with a team of clinicians, including therapists, orthotists, surgeons, nurses, physicians, and social workers. Even with a single choice (eg, orthopedic surgery), multiple possibilities are possible. For instance, orthopedic repair of only 1 or 2 of these problems may leave the child unimproved or worse, and therefore all 3 problems must be addressed.[39,40] Gait analysis using videography, electromyelogram, and sensors has improved the orthopedic care given to these children. After orthopedic surgery, therapy should be started to maximize range of motion and skills.

Oral medications (eg, diazepam, oral baclofen, tizanidine, dantrolene) can be used to reduce spasticity, but these drugs have potential adverse effects. No controlled studies have documented improvement in functioning from these medications. Selective dorsal rhizotomy[41,42] and intrathecal baclofen[43,44] are newer interventions that have been shown to reduce spasticity and increase range of motion. Intramuscular botulinum toxin is effective in children who have functional spasticity in transiently reducing spasticity in individual limbs.[45,46] Although spasticity can be reduced with these treatments, they cannot improve selective motor control, difficulties with balance, and weakness. Strength training has shown promise in improving function.[47] Various casting and splinting techniques that may maintain muscle length and inhibit increased tone may be helpful. In many cases, orthopedic procedures such as tenotomies, tendon releases, and transfers are necessary to address soft-tissue and bone problems. Information regarding the impact of surgery on function is limited. Constraint therapy (ie, immobilizing the better upper extremity) while providing therapy to enhance the function of the affected (or worse) arm and hand has been shown in several studies to improve function in children who have spastic hemiplegia.[48,49] Evidence suggests that constraint therapy produces anatomic changes in the brain on functional MRI.[50]

Drooling is often a significant social problem for children with CP and may be managed with scopolamine, which is available as a transdermal patch and as a tablet,[51] glycopyrrolate,[52] botulinum toxin injections into salivary glands,[53] and surgical removal of the salivary glands.[54] Because children who have CP are at increased risk for nutrition and feeding problems, careful monitoring of their physical growth is critical. Both linear growth and weight may be affected; therefore monitoring weight for length rather than weight alone is important. Reliable measures of height or length in children who have CP are often impossible to obtain because of the scoliosis, fixed joint contractures, involuntary muscle spasms, and poor cooperation stemming from cognitive deficits. Tibial length has been used as a proxy for height. Evaluating the child whose growth is impaired includes evaluation of dietary intake for calories and content and evaluation for gastroesophageal reflux (using pH probe, endoscopy with biopsy, or radionuclide gastric emptying study). A clinical feeding evaluation includes assessing the child's seating and posture during meals, as well as assessing the swallowing mechanism, which can be aided by a videofluoroscopic swallow study using foods of different consistencies.[55] The videofluoroscopic swallow study can also assess the risk of aspiration. The assistance of feeding specialists is invaluable in this evaluation. Treatment options may include providing special seating devices to maintain the child in an upright, neutral position, thickening feedings, or inserting a gastrostomy tube with or without fundoplication.[56] This therapy usually improves weight gain and general health but may not improve longitudinal growth. A controversial intervention to attenuate growth in children with severe CP (Ashley treatment) has been proposed.[57] In this treatment, girls are given estrogen to close their growth plates and their uterus and breast tissue are removed to allow their families to continue close physical contact with them and to be able to include them in family activities.

The primary care physician should act as an advocate to ensure that a child who has CP has access to optimal care in the medical home. In addition to the individual child and family, advocacy includes ensuring that the community provides access to services so that disabilities do not become worse. Primary care physicians cannot be expected to understand all the nuances of the interventions used in the treatment of their patients with CP (Are braces or wheelchair best? Should the child be treated with Botox?), but they can be active participants in the overall care of the child by monitoring the child's function (nutrition, mobility, activities of daily living, communication, and ensuring participation at the maximal level).

Because many conventional therapies are ineffective in treating the symptoms of CP and no cure exists, families often turn to alternative therapies. The primary care physician should inquire about the use of these treatments and be aware of their nature, possible interactions with medications, and potential for harm. Complementary and alternative treatments such as equine-assisted therapy (hippotherapy) and acupuncture have been shown to offer functional benefits to some children with CP. Hyperbaric oxygen has been used,[58] but it does not appear to improve function; more evidence is required before recommendations can be made supporting its use. Similarly, various forms of electrical stimulation have been used, but evidence for their effectiveness remains inconclusive.[59]

PROGNOSIS

Survival in children who have CP depends on the severity of the condition. For example, a 2 year old with severe CP would be expected to have a 40%

chance of living to age 20, whereas a child with mild CP would have a 99% chance.[60] Respiratory diseases (eg, pneumonia), epilepsy, and congenital malformation are the most commonly recorded causes of death in childhood.

Children who have intellectual disability, no independent mobility (ie, rolling), limited spontaneous movement, and can be fed only by gastronomy tube are at the greatest risk for early death.[61,62] Prognostication before the child's 2nd birthday may be difficult, except at the extremes of involvement. In general, the prognosis for functioning is related to the clinical type of CP, pace of motor development, evolution of infantile reflexes, intellectual abilities, sensory impairment, and emotional-social adjustment.[63] Patients who sit unsupported by 24 months of age and crawl by 30 months of age are more likely eventually to walk independently.[64] Most children who first sit between 3 and 4 years of age walk only with aids or braces or have restricted functional ambulation. Retention of obligatory primitive reflexes at 18 months of age makes independent ambulation unlikely. Virtually all children who have hemiplegia learn to walk, as do many who have dyskinesia or ataxia. Children who walk before 2 years of age are more likely to have a normal or borderline IQ. Individual achievement is related to many factors, such as intelligence, physical functioning, ability to communicate, and personality attributes. The availability of training, jobs, sheltered employment, and counseling is a major factor in the adjustment of affected adults. A supportive family and the availability of specialist medical care are other important factors.

Long-term planning and preparation is required to help children with CP make the transition from adolescence to adulthood, particularly when a child has multiple needs. A variety of assistive technologies, such as switches that improve the individual's ability to control the environment, computers, and small electric motors that may replace some motor activities, are available. Speech synthesizers, symbol charts, or spelling boards can enhance an individual's ability to communicate effectively. Simple environmental enhancements, such as ramps or accessible showers, and assistive devices, such as a pencil holder or mouth-activated switch, can improve the quality of life dramatically for individuals who have CP. The Individuals with Disabilities Education Act requires that school-aged children who have disabilities be assessed for the utility of assistive devices and be given the support needed to use them effectively. Gaining access to these services requires coordination of care, knowledge of the resources available in the community, referral to experts, and financial assets. The physician who cares for patients who have CP is obliged to ensure that these services are available both to the patient and to the family.

The overall goal for children with CP should be for them to be as independent as possible and to participate in family and community activities with their nonaffected peers. Opportunities for participation may be limited, but the physician should be diligent in identifying these opportunities and encouraging children to participate in any and all activities that are available.

WHEN TO REFER

- In the United States, all infants who have CP who are from birth to 3 years of age should be referred to an early intervention program.
- All children who have moderate or severe CP should be referred to an interdisciplinary clinic, if one exists. If not, then they should be referred to an orthopedist, physical therapist, and someone (developmental pediatrician, neurologist, pediatric rehabilitation specialist) who understands the needs of children with CP and can manage spasticity, other abnormalities of tone, and optimize functioning.

  Children who have CP and seizures should be referred to a neurologist. The primary care physician in the medical home should coordinate these referrals and ensure that the child is receiving coordinated, comprehensive care.

WHEN TO ADMIT

- Some children who have CP aspirate food or saliva into their lungs; others have inadequate nutrition. Therefore they demonstrate increased susceptibility to acute illnesses such as pneumonia and are likely to become more ill with these illnesses. They should be hospitalized if they are severely ill or cannot be managed at home. They should be hospitalized for most major surgeries as well, such as complex orthopedic procedures.

TOOLS FOR PRACTICE

Engaging Patients and Family

- *Cerebral Palsy* (Web page), Centers for Disease Control and Prevention (www.cdc.gov/ncbddd/dd/ddcp.htm).
- *Cerebral Palsy—Interactive Health Tutorial* (on-line course), Patient Education Institute through National Institutes of Health and Medline Plus (www.nlm.nih.gov/medlineplus/tutorials/cerebralpalsy/nr209102.pdf).

Medical Decision Support

- *Cerebral Palsy—AAP Medical Homes Initiative and Children With Special Health Care Needs* (fact sheet), American Academy of Pediatrics (www.medicalhomeinfo.org/health/cer_palsy.html).
- *Gross Motor Function Classification System for Cerebral Palsy* (fact sheet), CanChild Centre for Disability and Robert Palisano (www.canchild.ca/Portals/0/outcomes/pdf/GMFCS.pdf).
- *Identifying Infants and Young Children With Developmental Disorders in the Medical Home: An Algorithm for Developmental Surveillance and Screening* (algorithm), American Academy of Pediatrics (aappolicy.aappublications.org/cgi/content/full/pediatrics;118/1/405).
- *Neonatal Encephalopathy and Cerebral Palsy* (book), The American College of Obstetricians and Gynecologists (ACOG) (www.aap.org/bookstore).

AAP POLICY STATEMENTS

American Academy of Pediatrics, Committee on Children With Disabilities. The continued importance of supplemental security income (SSI) for children and adolescents with disabilities. *Pediatrics.* 2001;107(4):790-793. (aappolicy.aappublications.org/cgi/content/full/pediatrics;104/4/790).

American Academy of Pediatrics, Committee on Children With Disabilities. The treatment of neurologically impaired children using patterning. *Pediatrics.* 1999;104(5):1149-1151. (aappolicy.aappublications.org/cgi/content/full/pediatrics;104/5/1149).

American Academy of Pediatrics, Committee on Fetus and Newborn, American College of Obstetricians and Gynecologists, Committee on Obstetric Practice. The Apgar score. *Pediatrics.* 2006;117(4):1444-1447. (aappolicy.aappublications.org/cgi/content/full/pediatrics;117/4/1444).

American Academy of Pediatrics, Cooley WC, and the Committee on Children with Disabilities. Providing a primary care medical home for children and youth with cerebral palsy. *Pediatrics.* 2004;114(4):1106-1113. (aappolicy.aappublications.org/cgi/content/full/pediatrics;114/4/1106).

American Academy of Pediatrics, Council on Children With Disabilities, Section on Developmental and Behavioral Pediatrics, Bright Futures Steering Committee, and Medical Home Initiatives for Children With Special Needs Project Advisory Committee. Identifying infants and young children with developmental disorders in the medical home: an algorithm for developmental surveillance and screening. *Pediatrics.* 2006;118(1):405-420. (aappolicy.aappublications.org/cgi/content/full/pediatrics;118/1/405).

American Academy of Pediatrics, Michaud, LJ, and the Committee on Children With Disabilities. Prescribing therapy services for children with motor disabilities. *Pediatrics.* 2004;113(6):1836-1838. (aappolicy.aappublications.org/cgi/content/full/pediatrics;113/6/1836).

American Academy of Pediatrics, Moeschler JB, Shevell M, and the Committee on Genetics. Clinical genetic evaluation of the child with mental retardation or developmental delays. *Pediatrics.* 2006;117(6):2304-2316. (aappolicy.aappublications.org/cgi/content/full/pediatrics;117/6/2304).

American Academy of Pediatrics, Murphy NA, Elias ER, and the Council on Children with Disabilities. Sexuality of children and adolescents with developmental disabilities. *Pediatrics.* 2006;118(1):398-403. (aappolicy.aappublications.org/cgi/content/full/pediatrics;118/1/398).

REFERENCES

1. Bax M, Goldstein M, Rosenbaum P, et al, and the Executive Committee for the Definition of Cerebral Palsy. Proposed definition and classification of cerebral palsy. *Dev Med Child Neurol.* 2005;47(8):571-576.
2. Graham HK. Absence of reference to progressive musculoskeletal pathology in definition of cerebral palsy. *Dev Med Child Neurol.* 2006;48(1):78-79.
3. Meberg A, Broch H. A changing pattern of cerebral palsy. Declining trend for incidence of cerebral palsy in the 20-year period 1970-89. *J Perinat Med.* 1995;23(5):395-402.
4. O'Shea TM, Preisser JS, Klinepeter KL, et al. Trends in mortality and cerebral palsy in a geographically based cohort of very low birth weight neonates born between 1982 to 1994. *Pediatrics.* 1998;101(4 pt 1):642-647.
5. Stanley FJ, Blair E, Alberman E. *Cerebral Palsies: Epidemiology and Causal Pathways. Clinics in Developmental Medicine.* No.151. London, UK: MacKeith Press; 2000.
6. Cummins SK, Nelson KB, Grether JK, et al. Cerebral palsy in four northern California counties, births 1983 through 1985. *J Pediatr.* 1993;123(2):230-237.
7. World Health Organization. *International Classification of Functioning, Disability and Health.* Geneva, Switzerland: World Health Organization; 2001.
8. Boyle CA, Decoufle P, Yeargin-Allsopp M. Prevalence and health impact of developmental disabilities in US children. *Pediatrics.* 1994;93(3):399-403.
9. Platt MJ, Cans C, Johnson A, et al. Trends in cerebral palsy among infants of very low birthweight (<1500 g) or born prematurely (<32 weeks) in 16 European centres: a database study. *Lancet.* 2007;369(9555):43-50.
10. Nelson KB, Ellenberg JH. Antecedents of cerebral palsy. Multivariate analysis of risk. *N Engl J Med.* 1986;315(2):81-86.
11. Yudkin PL, Johnson A, Clover LM, et al. Assessing the contribution of birth asphyxia to cerebral palsy in term singletons. *Paediatr Perinat Epidemiol.* 1995;9(2):156-170.
12. Nelson KB. The neurologically impaired child and alleged malpractice at birth. *Neurol Clin.* May 1999;17(2):283-293.
13. Kuban KC, Leviton A. Cerebral palsy. *N Engl J Med.* 1994;330(3):188-195.
14. Neufeld MD, Frigon C, Graham AS, et al. Maternal infection and risk of cerebral palsy in term and preterm infants. *J Perinatol.* 2005;25(2):108-113.
15. Boyle CA, Yeargin-Allsopp M, Doernberg NS, et al. Prevalence of selected developmental disabilities in children 3-10 years of age: the Metropolitan Atlanta Developmental Disabilities Surveillance Program, 1991. *MMWR Surveill Summ.* 1996;45(2):1-14.
16. Gluckman PD, Wyatt JS, Azzopardi D, et al. Selective head cooling with mild systemic hypothermia after neonatal encephalopathy: multicentre randomised trial. *Lancet.* 2005;365(9460):663-670.
17. Wu YW, Croen LA, Shah SJ, et al. Cerebral palsy in a term population: risk factors and neuroimaging findings. *Pediatrics.* 2006;118(2):690-697.
18. Dyet LE, Kennea N, Counsell SJ, et al. Natural history of brain lesions in extremely preterm infants studied with serial magnetic resonance imaging from birth and neurodevelopmental assessment. *Pediatrics.* 2006;118(2):536-548.
19. Edebol-Tysk K, Hagberg B, Hagberg G. Epidemiology of spastic tetraplegic cerebral palsy in Sweden. II. Prevalence, birth data and origin. *Neuropediatrics.* 1989;20(1):46-52.
20. Palisano RJ, Hanna SE, Rosenbaum PL, et al. Validation of a model of gross motor function for children with cerebral palsy. *Phys Ther.* 2000;80(10):974-985.
21. Palisano RJ, Cameron D, Rosenbaum PL, et al. Stability of the gross motor function classification system. *Dev Med Child Neurol.* 2006;48(6):424-428.
22. Palfrey JS, Singer JD, Walker DK, et al. Early identification of children's special needs: a study in five metropolitan communities. *J Pediatr.* 1987;111(5):651-659.
23. Council on Children With Disabilities, Section on Developmental Behavioral Pediatrics, Bright Futures Steering Committee, and Medical Home Initiatives for Children With Special Needs Project Advisory Committee. Identifying infants and young children with developmental disorders: an algorithm for developmental surveillance and screening. *Pediatrics.* 2006;118:405-420.
24. Blasco PA. Primitive reflexes. Their contribution to the early detection of cerebral palsy. *Clin Pediatr (Phila).* 1994;33(7):388-397.
25. Jan MM. Misdiagnoses in children with dopa-responsive dystonia. *Pediatr Neurol.* 2004;31(4):298-303.
26. Fink JK. Hereditary spastic paraplegia. *Neurol Clin.* 2002;20(3):711-726.

27. Beckung E, Hagberg G. Neuroimpairments, activity limitations, and participation restrictions in children with cerebral palsy. *Dev Med Child Neurol.* 2002;44(5):309-316.
28. Samson-Fang L, Fung E, Stallings VA, et al. Relationship of nutritional status to health and societal participation in children with cerebral palsy. *J Pediatr.* 2002;141(5):637-643.
29. Liptak GS, O'Donnell M, Conaway M, et al. Health status of children with moderate to severe cerebral palsy. *Dev Med Child Neurol.* 2001;43(6):364-370.
30. Henderson RC, Gilbert SR, Clement ME, et al. Altered skeletal maturation in moderate to severe cerebral palsy. *Dev Med Child Neurol.* 2005;47(4):229-236.
31. McDermott S, Coker AL, Mani S, et al. A population-based analysis of behavior problems in children with cerebral palsy. *J Pediatr Psychol.* 1996;21(3):447-463.
32. Goodman R. The longitudinal stability of psychiatric problems in children with hemiplegia. *J Child Psychol Psychiatry.* 1998;39(3):347-354.
33. Sugimoto T, Woo M, Nishida N, et al. When do brain abnormalities in cerebral palsy occur? An MRI study. *Dev Med Child Neurol.* 1995;37(4):285-292.
34. Ashwal S, Russman BS, Blasco PA, et al, and the Quality Standards Subcommittee of the American Academy of Neurology and Practice Committee of the Child Neurology Society. Practice parameter: diagnostic assessment of the child with cerebral palsy: report of the Quality Standards Subcommittee of the American Academy of Neurology and the Practice Committee of the Child Neurology Society. *Neurology.* 2004;62(6):851-863.
35. Butler C, Chambers H, Goldstein M, et al. Evaluating research in developmental disabilities: a conceptual framework for reviewing treatment outcomes. *Dev Med Child Neurol.* 1999;41(1):55-59.
36. Goldberg MJ. Measuring outcomes in cerebral palsy. *J Pediatr Orthop.* 1991;11(5):682-685.
37. Petersen MC, Palmer FB. Advances in prevention and treatment of cerebral palsy. *Ment Retard Dev Disabil Res Rev.* 2001;7(1):30-37.
38. Raina P, O'Donnell M, Rosenbaum P, et al. The health and well-being of caregivers of children with cerebral palsy. *Pediatrics.* 2005;115(6):e626-e636.
39. Sussman MD, Aiona MD. Treatment of spastic diplegia in patients with cerebral palsy. *J Pediatr Orthop B.* Mar 2004;13(2):S1-S12.
40. Aiona MD, Sussman MD. Treatment of spastic diplegia in patients with cerebral palsy: Part II. *J Pediatr Orthop B.* 2004;13(3):S13-S38.
41. McLaughlin JF, Bjornson KF, Astley SJ, et al. Selective dorsal rhizotomy: efficacy and safety in an investigator-masked randomized clinical trial. *Dev Med Child Neurol.* 1998;40(4):220-232.
42. Wright FV, Sheil EM, Drake JM, et al. Evaluation of selective dorsal rhizotomy for the reduction of spasticity in cerebral palsy: a randomized controlled trial. *Dev Med Child Neurol.* 1998;40(4):239-247.
43. Van Schaeybroeck P, Nuttin B, Lagae L, et al. Intrathecal baclofen for intractable cerebral spasticity: a prospective placebo-controlled, double-blind study. *Neurosurgery.* 2000;46(3):603-609.
44. Fitzgerald JJ, Tsegaye M, Vloeberghs MH. Treatment of childhood spasticity of cerebral origin with intrathecal baclofen: a series of 52 cases. *Br J Neurosurg.* 2004;18(3):240-245.
45. Speth LA, Leffers P, Janssen-Potten YJ, et al. Botulinum toxin A and upper limb functional skills in hemiparetic cerebral palsy: a randomized trial in children receiving intensive therapy. *Dev Med Child Neurol.* 2005;47(7):468-473.
46. Bottos M, Benedetti MG, Salucci P, et al. Botulinum toxin with and without casting in ambulant children with spastic diplegia: a clinical and functional assessment. *Dev Med Child Neurol.* 2003;45(11):758-762.
47. Dodd KJ, Taylor NF, Damiano DL. A systematic review of the effectiveness of strength-training programs for people with cerebral palsy. *Arch Phys Med Rehabil.* 2002;83(8):1157-1164.
48. Naylor CE, Bower E. Modified constraint-induced movement therapy for young children with hemiplegic cerebral palsy: a pilot study. *Dev Med Child Neurol.* 2005;47(6):365-369.
49. Eliasson AC, Krumlinde-Sundholm L, Shaw K, et al. Effects of constraint-induced movement therapy in young children with hemiplegic cerebral palsy: an adapted model. *Dev Med Child Neurol.* 2005;47(4):266-275.
50. Levy CE, Nichols DS, Schmalbrock PM, et al. Functional MRI evidence of cortical reorganization in upper-limb stroke hemiplegia treated with constraint-induced movement therapy. *Am J Phys Med Rehabil.* 2001;80(1):4-12.
51. Lewis DW, Fontana C, Mehallick LK, et al. Transdermal scopolamine for reduction of drooling in developmentally delayed children. *Dev Med Child Neurol.* 1994;36(6):484-486.
52. Mier RJ, Bachrach SJ, Lakin RC, et al. Treatment of sialorrhea with glycopyrrolate: a double-blind, dose-ranging study. *Arch Pediatr Adolesc Med.* 2000;154(12):1214-1218.
53. Jongerius PH, van den Hoogen FJ, van Limbeek J, et al. Effect of botulinum toxin in the treatment of drooling: a controlled clinical trial. *Pediatrics.* 2004;114(3):620-627.
54. Blasco PA. Management of drooling: 10 years after the Consortium on Drooling, 1990. *Dev Med Child Neurol.* 2002;44(11):778-781.
55. Wright RE, Wright FR, Carson CA. Videofluoroscopic assessment in children with severe cerebral palsy presenting with dysphagia. *Pediatr Radiol.* 1996;26(10):720-722.
56. Samson-Fang L, Butler C, O'Donnell M; AACPDM. Effects of gastrostomy feeding in children with cerebral palsy: an AACPDM evidence report. *Dev Med Child Neurol.* 2003;45(6):415-426.
57. Gunther DF, Diekema DS. Attenuating growth in children with profound developmental disability: a new approach to an old dilemma. *Arch Pediatr Adolesc Med.* 2006;160(10):1013-1017.
58. Collet JP, Vanasse M, Marois P, et al. Hyperbaric oxygen for children with cerebral palsy: a randomised multicentre trial. HBO-CP Research Group. *Lancet.* 2001;357:582-586.
59. Liptak GS. Complementary and alternative therapies for cerebral palsy. *Ment Retard Dev Disabil Res Rev.* 2005;11(2):156-163.
60. Hutton JL. Cerebral palsy life expectancy. *Clin Perinatol.* 2006;33(2):545-555.
61. Chaney RH, Eyman RK. Patterns in mortality over 60 years among persons with mental retardation in a residential facility. *Ment Retard.* 2000;38(3):289-293.
62. Plioplys AV. Survival rates of children with severe neurologic disabilities: a review. *Semin Pediatr Neurol.* 2003;10(2):120-129.
63. Sala DA, Grant AD. Prognosis for ambulation in cerebral palsy. *Dev Med Child Neurol.* 1995;37(11):1020-1026.
64. da Paz Jr AC, Burnett SM, Braga LW. Walking prognosis in cerebral palsy: a 22-year retrospective analysis. *Dev Med Child Neurol.* 1994;36(2):130-134.

Chapter 246

CHICKENPOX

George K. Siberry, MD, MPH

Chickenpox (varicella) is a childhood viral disease characterized by a pruritic vesicular rash that appears in crops. It is highly contagious and has been regarded as a relatively benign disease, inasmuch as complications are rare in healthy children. However, the increasing number of children who are at risk for severe disease because they are immunosuppressed and the economic and social costs of days lost from school and from the work force by parents[1] have driven interest in this disease and in its prevention through immunization.

The *chicken* in *chickenpox* is believed to derive from its likeness to the chickpea *Cicer arietinum*, or from the French for chickpea, *pois chiche*.[2] Other researchers postulate that the name may come from the Old English word for itch, *gican*.[3] The word *varicella* is derived from a disease that is similar in appearance but is much more severe: variola (smallpox).

ETIOLOGY

Chickenpox is caused by the varicella-zoster virus, a DNA virus and member of the herpesvirus family. The same virus causes both chickenpox and herpes zoster, the latter being a reactivation (after a latent phase) of the initial varicella infection. Varicella-zoster virus can be isolated from the vesicles of both chickenpox and herpes zoster. It has also been isolated from blood and tissue during an infection but has proved difficult to isolate from respiratory secretions. The virus is highly labile, losing its infectivity quickly in the external environment. Inactivation can also be accomplished by heat and trypsin. Only 1 serotype of varicella-zoster virus has been isolated, but different virus strains, including vaccine strains, can be identified by means of polymerase chain reaction (PCR).[4]

TRANSMISSION

Chickenpox is one of the most contagious viral infections to cause disease in humans and is only slightly less contagious than measles and smallpox. Infection is thought to be spread by respiratory secretions because airborne particles from patients can transmit infection before onset of the rash.[5] Virus has not been cultured from these secretions, although its presence can be detected by PCR.[6] Contact with the vesicular fluid of chickenpox or herpes zoster may also result in the transmission of chickenpox infection. Indirect contact (fomite transmission) is probably rare because of the lability of the varicella-zoster virus. Chickenpox in a pregnant woman can also lead to transmission of infection to her fetus or newborn.[7] Transplacentally acquired antibody to varicella-zoster virus is partially protective to the newborn, but chickenpox can occur in young infants born to immune mothers.

EPIDEMIOLOGIC FACTORS

Humans are the only known reservoir, or natural host, of the varicella-zoster virus. The communicability period lasts from 1 or 2 days before the onset of the rash until 5 days after the onset or until all vesicles have crusted. Most vesicles have lost virus particles after 5 days. The incubation period is between 10 and 21 days, with an average of 14 to 15 days. With household exposure, clinical disease will develop in approximately 90% of susceptible contacts after 1 incubation period[8]; secondary household cases are often more severe.

In temperate climates, chickenpox is mainly a disease of childhood, with 80% to 90% of children historically having been infected by 9 to 10 years of age.[9,10] Historically, the highest incidence of varicella in the United States was among children ages 1 to 9 years of age.[11,12]

Until 1995 (before the vaccine era), approximately 4 million chickenpox cases occurred yearly in the United States, with 90% of cases occurring in children. The disease occurs throughout the year, but most cases occur during the winter and spring months. Epidemic occurrences are every 2 to 3 years, distributed worldwide. Children in tropical climates have a lower rate of infection. Up to 40% to 90% enter adulthood without having had chickenpox, creating a much larger pool of susceptible persons among older age groups in the tropics than in temperate climates.[6]

Subclinical infections with serologic conversion rarely occur. However, because varicella infects most people in temperate climates as children, most adults who report a negative or equivocal history of chickenpox are immune.[13] Infection generally confers lifelong immunity in normal hosts, but second clinical infections can occur.[14] Many such *second cases* may represent situations in which a prior nonvaricella exanthematous illness was erroneously labeled as chickenpox.[15]

Case fatality rates from chickenpox (based on data from the prevaccine era) are estimated to be 5 per 100,000 for children for infants, 1 per 100,000 for 1 to 14 year olds, 3 per 100,000 for 15 to 19 year olds, and 25 per 100,000 for 30 to 49 year olds.[16] The case fatality rates are higher for neonates, older adults, and immunocompromised patients. Before the introduction of the vaccine, varicella caused over 10,000 hospitalizations annually, predominantly in children. Annual deaths from varicella ranged from approximately 40 to 150, with a shift from most (80%) deaths occurring in children in the early 1970s to the majority (54%) occurring in adults in the early 1990s.[17] From 1990 to 1994, an average of 50 annual pediatric deaths were attributed to varicella.[17] More than 90% of the childhood deaths occurred in children who had no risk factors for severe varicella.[17,18]

The incidence of varicella in the United States has changed since the recommendation for varicella immunization of all US children older than 1 year was made in 1995.[11] By 2000 the incidence of chickenpox decreased overall by 71% to 84% in populations with varicella immunization coverage rates for 1 to 3 year olds of 74% to 84%.[12] The incidence decreased in every age group, with the greatest decrease (83% to 90%) seen in the 1- to 4-year-old age group. The highest incidence of disease, however, continued to be in children ages 1 to 4 years and those ages 5 to 9 years. By 2001 the rate of varicella-related hospitalizations (VRH) in the United States had declined by 75% overall, with fewer than 3800 such hospitalizations by 2001. This reduction in VRH was seen in all age groups but was greatest for young children, such that adults accounted for nearly one half of VRH by 2001 compared with only one third of VRH in the prevaccine period.[19] In a similar fashion, deaths in the United States caused by varicella in the vaccine era have dropped by 66% overall to an all-time low of 26 varicella deaths in 2001.[17] The drop in varicella-attributable mortality rates was most pronounced in children ages 1 to 4 years (92%) and those ages 5 to 9 years (89%) but was evident in all age groups, except for those older than 50 years.[17]

PATHOGENESIS

Varicella virus gains entry into the susceptible individual through the respiratory tract or conjunctiva via droplet or airborne transmission. It migrates to the regional lymph nodes, where primary replication occurs. Approximately 4 to 6 days later, a primary viremia spreads the virus to internal organs, where secondary replication occurs. This event is followed by a secondary viremia, which spreads the organism to the skin and is followed by clinical chickenpox. Viremia has been documented in blood-borne monocytes 9 to 12 days after exposure but 1 to 5 days before onset of the rash.[20] The appearance of the rash in crops may be the result of an intermittent secondary viremia.[21]

The rash is, at first, macular and then progresses to a papular lesion that contains a minute vacuole. Fluid accumulates in the vacuole, causing a vesicle to appear on a reddened base to produce the classic *dewdrop on a rose petal* lesion. Multinucleated giant cells and intranuclear inclusions can be identified microscopically in the base and on the edges of the vesicle. As the rash resolves, the vesicle becomes cloudy and fills with fibrinous fluid and leukocytes. A crust develops that may remain attached for 1 to 2 weeks. When a vesicle occurs on mucous membranes, its roof sloughs to leave a shallow ulcer. Evidence suggests that interferon, produced by the polymorphonuclear cells in the lesion, may contribute to resolution of the disease.[22]

CLINICAL MANIFESTATIONS

Healthy Children

Chickenpox usually begins with no noticeable prodrome or with mild malaise and low-grade fever. This phase is followed in a few hours to days by a macular rash, usually beginning on the scalp, neck, or upper portion of the trunk. The macules progress to a papular, vesicular, pruritic rash, usually within 12 to 24 hours. Vesicles appear in crops, with a new crop occurring every 1 to 2 days over the next 2 to 5 days, resulting in 2 to 4 crops during the illness. Typical childhood cases produce a total of 250 to 500 lesions.[11] The vesicles turn to pustules and then crust over. The illness usually runs its course in 5 to 10 days. At the height of the disease, lesions in all phases from early vesicles to crusts can be seen. Fever varies from none to 102°F (38.9°C) at the onset of the disease and may continue until vesicles cease to appear. The rash spreads centrifugally and involves all areas of the skin in severe cases. Vesicles are pruritic, and excoriations are frequently seen. Lesions occur more frequently in areas of irritation or dermatitis or in skin folds. Occasionally, the rash appears as a macular rash in the diaper area or on the trunk and remains for 1 day or 2 before becoming vesicular, making early diagnosis more difficult. Vesicles may occur on the mucous membranes of the mouth, conjunctiva, esophagus, trachea, rectum, or vagina. Generally, little scarring occurs, unless the lesions become superinfected or are continually traumatized. Areas where chickenpox lesions have occurred, however, may remain hypopigmented or hyperpigmented months after the rash has resolved. Occasionally, lesions are bullous as a variant of the disease itself, but these are more often caused by staphylococcal superinfection. White blood cell counts and other laboratory test results are usually normal in uncomplicated varicella.

Older Children and Adults

Chickenpox in older children and adults is usually more severe than it is in younger age groups, with a prodrome that may include irritability, listlessness, headaches, chills, anorexia, and myalgias. Fever is usually present and is higher and more prolonged than it is in the young child. The rash, too, tends to be more severe. The risk of complications is 9 to 25 times greater; for example, varicella pneumonia occurs in 15% to 50% of older patients.[23]

Breakthrough Chickenpox in Previously Immunized Children

When chickenpox occurs in children who were previously immunized against varicella, the disease is milder in most cases, typically producing milder systemic symptoms and fewer lesions (usually <50) that are less pruritic and crust over faster.[24] In some cases, the lesions may appear only as papules that never vesiculate, making diagnosis difficult.[24] In addition, children with typical, mild breakthrough varicella are also approximately one half as likely to transmit the disease to household contacts.[25]

Immunocompromised Children

Immunocompromised children usually have the most severe symptoms; they, along with neonates, are at greatest risk of death from chickenpox infection. *Progressive varicella* can be seen in children who have an immunocompromising condition or who are being treated with immunosuppressive therapy for leukemia or another malignancy.[22] After a more severe prodrome, up to 30% of such immunocompromised children develop progressive varicella, with spread of the varicella-zoster virus to the lungs, liver, pancreas, or central nervous system. Vesicles may be larger and hemorrhagic. All complications of chickenpox are increased in this population, with varicella pneumonia the most common cause of death. Even if progressive varicella does not develop, these patients still have higher fevers and more prolonged vesicular eruption than do nonimmunocompromised children.

Although severe varicella can occur in children who are infected with the human immunodeficiency virus (HIV), especially those who have very low CD4 percentages, most children infected with HIV, including those who have low CD4 percentages, do not develop severe acute varicella.[26] Many experts use high-dose oral acyclovir to manage selected children infected with HIV and who have relatively normal CD4 values, whereas others still manage *all* children infected with HIV as being at increased risk of severe disease (see Treatment).[13]

Children who receive systemic steroid therapy for diseases other than cancer also are at risk for more severe involvement and complications.[27] Some of this increased risk may be attributable to the potentially immunocompromising effect of nononcologic conditions for which steroids are prescribed.[28] Children who receive greater than 2 mg/kg or 20-mg prednisone (or equivalent) for more than 2 weeks should be considered at increased risk of severe varicella.[13] Inhaled corticosteroids do not appear to increase risk of severe varicella,[29] but definitive data are lacking.

Congenital and Neonatal Varicella

In cases of primary maternal varicella during the first 2 trimesters of pregnancy, varicella-zoster virus can cross the placenta, leading in 2% of cases to congenital varicella syndrome.[7,13,30] Skin lesions in a dermatomal distribution (76%), neurologic defects (60%), eye diseases (51%), and skeletal anomalies (49%) occur in affected infants.[7]

Maternal infection during the late third trimester of pregnancy may similarly result in transplacentally acquired varicella in the newborn. When mothers have clinical chickenpox in the 2 weeks before delivery, 24% of their infants will develop neonatal varicella. If the onset of maternal rash occurs more than 5 days before delivery, or if rash initially erupts in infants younger than 4 days, then risk of death seems to be small. This reprieve is probably attributable, at least in part, to maternally transferred immunity. If, on the other hand, the *maternal* rash emerges between 4 days before and 2 days after delivery, or if the *newborn* rash begins at 5 to 10 days of age, then an associated 20% to 30% neonatal mortality occurs.[7,13,30] The risk is uncertain for infants who are nursing when the mother contracts chickenpox.

Herpes zoster in pregnant women, on the other hand, appears to confer minimal risk of infection to the fetus. In 1 series of 366 women who had herpes zoster in pregnancy, none of the infants had evidence of intrauterine infection.[31]

COMPLICATIONS

Secondary Bacterial Infection

Secondary bacterial infection is the most common complication of chickenpox. Children younger than 5 years appear to be at increased risk.[32-34] Symptoms of secondary bacterial infection begin, on average, 4 days after the appearance of the varicella rash, often with a secondary fever. Infections are usually caused by group A streptococci or *Staphylococcus aureus* and include impetigo, cellulitis, abscess, necrotizing fasciitis, myositis, gangrene, arthritis, osteomyelitis, pneumonia, empyema, conjunctivitis, toxic shock syndrome (usually streptococcal), sepsis, and erysipelas. Bullous lesions caused by *S aureus* may begin on the 2nd or 3rd day of the rash and show as bullous impetigo. Although superficial bacterial skin infections remain most common, invasive group A streptococcal infections have become increasingly important.[32]

Reye Syndrome

Reye syndrome is an acute illness occurring almost exclusively in children and characterized by encephalopathy and fatty degeneration of the liver. Reye syndrome carries a high case-fatality rate of 30% overall, reaching rates of 43% for children younger than 5 years. In 1980 the association between Reye syndrome and use of aspirin during varicella or influenza illnesses was first reported. This report led to a advisory from the Centers for Disease Control and Prevention (CDC) in 1980, a Surgeon General advisory in 1982, and mandatory warning labels of all aspirin-containing medications in 1986 cautioning physicians and parents to avoid using salicylates in children who have varicella or influenza-like illnesses. The annual number of reported cases of Reye syndrome in the United States fell from a high of 555 cases in 1980 to no more than 36 cases per year from 1987 to 1993 and no more than 2 cases per year from 1994 to 1997.[35] Given the rare occurrence of Reye syndrome, any child suspected of Reye syndrome should be evaluated thoroughly for the presence of another metabolic disorder.

Aspirin should be avoided in any child who has chickenpox.

Neurologic Complications

Nervous system complications are the second most common complication of varicella and include acute cerebellar ataxia, encephalitis, seizures, aseptic meningitis, myelitis, and peripheral neuropathy. Many of the seizures occurring with chickenpox may be simply febrile seizures; in 1 series, 12 of 23 patients who had varicella and seizures had concomitant fever.[34] In older series, the mortality from neurologic complications reached approximately 10% overall, but most of the deaths occurred among cases of encephalitis, some of which may have represented unrecognized Reye syndrome.[36]

Acute cerebellar ataxia (ACA) is the most common neurologic complication of varicella, occurring in 1 in 4000 cases of chickenpox.[33] The average age of patients with ACA is 4 years, with the great majority of cases occurring among children younger than 5 years.[37] The onset of symptoms usually occurs 1 to 2 weeks after onset of varicella but ranges from 2 to 21 days after the appearance of the rash and, uncommonly, may even precede the rash.[36] The usual clinical features of varicella-related ACA are acute onset of vomiting and ataxic gait disturbance without major disturbance in mental status. Dysmetria (68%) and trunk ataxia (74%) also occur frequently; fever and nystagmus are much less common (5% to 10%). Laboratory studies usually reveal a normal peripheral white blood cell count, normal to mildly elevated cerebrospinal fluid protein, and, in 50% of patients, a cerebrospinal fluid pleocytosis. Between 95% and 100% of normal children who have varicella-related ACA recover completely with only supportive care.[7,45] Many cases are mild enough that hospitalization is not necessary. Recovery usually takes place within the first 3 months, although recovery may take longer for some children. Some concern exists for longer-lasting subtle behavioral and learning difficulties, but these need further study with controlled comparisons.

Varicella Pneumonia

Varicella pneumonia occurs most often among adults, adolescents, and immunocompromised children.[23] It is one of the more common causes of death resulting from varicella. In children, varicella pneumonia occurs in fewer than 1 per 10,000 cases of chickenpox.[33] In adults, it may be present in 30% to 50% of cases of varicella, although more recent studies estimate a lower incidence of 5% to 10%. Manifestations range from abnormal chest radiograph findings only to cough, rales, tachypnea, hemoptysis, chest pain, cyanosis, and respiratory failure. Onset of pneumonia typically occurs 5 to 6 days after onset of rash in immunodeficient children and adults but occurs within the first 3 days of rash onset in immunocompetent hosts (adults). Chest radiographs typically show diffuse, reticulonodular densities of various sizes, which are best viewed in the lung periphery. As the disease progresses, nodules may enlarge and coalesce into extensive infiltrates. Treatment of varicella pneumonia with intravenous acyclovir is recommended; however, mortality is still 10% to 20%, reaching higher rates among severely immunodeficient patients.[23]

Hematologic Complications

Thrombocytopenia is the most common hematologic abnormality seen with varicella. Thrombocytopenia may occur with an invasive secondary bacterial infection or sepsis, in which case it is associated with more severe illness and worse outcome.[32] In the absence of secondary bacterial infections, however, varicella may produce thrombocytopenia (or even pancytopenia) that is attributed to infection-related suppression or antibody-mediated destruction (idiopathic thrombocytopenic purpura) of platelets.[38] Onset occurs from 3 days to 3 weeks after the chickenpox rash appears. Febrile purpura, malignant chickenpox with purpura, postinfectious purpura, purpura fulminans, and Henoch-Schönlein purpura have all been described in association with varicella infection.

Hepatitis

Hepatitis has been reported during chickenpox infections and is marked by the onset of abdominal pain, vomiting, and continued fever on the second to 4th day after the rash appears.[39] Liver function tests become abnormal but return to normal with resolution of the abdominal symptoms. No progression to classic Reye syndrome occurs, and the blood ammonia level is normal. However, some experts believe that some of these cases may represent low-grade Reye syndrome. One study of 39 children who had uncomplicated chickenpox found 47% to have a mildly increased level of aspartate transaminase (serum glutamic-oxaloacetic transaminase) and 29% to have significantly increased aspartate transaminase levels.[40]

Zoster

Zoster, or shingles, is the reactivation of the varicella-zoster virus that has remained dormant after clinical chickenpox. The virus resides in the dorsal nerve ganglia and is reactivated by periods of decreased host immunity or other unknown stimuli. During reactivation, the rash covers the dermatome that corresponds to the infected nerve root. Disseminated zoster, however, also can occur, involving multiple dermatomes. Zoster has been described in all age groups, including in infancy after prenatal exposure to varicella virus resulting from maternal chickenpox.

Children who have varicella infections at younger ages, especially when the infection occurs before the child is 1 year of age, have an increased incidence of zoster later in life.[41] Children with leukemia who experience varicella develop zoster at an increased incidence of 25 cases per 1000 person-years,[42] a significantly lower rate than that for children infected with HIV. Twenty-seven percent of children infected with HIV (before anti-HIV drugs were available) and who had primary varicella after 1 year of age developed zoster 2 years (on average) after primary varicella; among children whose CD4 percentage was less than 15% at the time of varicella infection, 70% developed zoster in the same time period.[26]

Other Complications

Appendicitis, myocarditis, arthritis (viral), nephritis, orchitis, splenic hemorrhage and rupture, pancreatitis, pericarditis, and parotitis have been reported, although rarely. The most common ophthalmologic complication is papillary conjunctivitis, but keratitis, uveitis, optic neuritis, and chorioretinitis also can occur.[43]

DIAGNOSIS

Chickenpox is usually diagnosed clinically. A history of exposure in the previous 10 to 21 days may be present. White blood cell counts are usually normal. A Tzanck test (scraping of the base of a vesicle and staining with Giemsa or Wright stain) is positive for multinucleated giant cells in varicella-zoster virus infections. However, herpes simplex types 1 and 2 also produce a positive Tzanck test.[44] Varicella zoster virus–specific direct fluorescent antibody (DFA) testing of vesicle scrapings can provide specific diagnostic confirmation within hours. Vesicle fluid can also be cultured for varicella zoster virus, but growth may take weeks. PCR tests have been demonstrated to be superior to viral culture in identification of varicella virus from vesicles and can be used to distinguish eruptions due to wild-type and vaccine virus.[4,44] Viral titers during acute and convalescent stages can document a recent infection if acute titers are obtained early in the illness (preferably day 1 or 2), and higher titers are noted during convalescence 2 to 6 weeks later. Commercially available antibody tests perform well for detection of serologic responses to infection but are not as sensitive for detecting vaccine-induced antibody response.[16]

DIFFERENTIAL DIAGNOSIS

Smallpox (variola) was historically the most important disease to be differentiated from chickenpox and has once again become a concern because of its use as a bioterrorism agent. The clinical prodrome of smallpox is typically more severe than that of chickenpox. Unlike varicella in which lesions in all stages of evolution are present at once, smallpox produces an eruption in which most of the lesions are present in a uniform stage of development, *progressing together* from macules to papules to deep-seated vesicles and finally crusting.[16] Involvement of palms and soles is much more typical of smallpox. Rapid diagnostic tests such as DFA and even Tzanck test should be used to confirm varicella in all cases in which smallpox is a concern.[16]

Vaccinia (cowpox) produces a vesicular rash resulting from exposure to infected livestock or, when smallpox vaccine use was commonplace, from direct contact with a smallpox vaccination.

Disseminated herpes simplex can resemble the chickenpox rash, but the history and progression of the disease usually differentiate these 2 entities. Confusion ordinarily arises only in newborns because disseminated herpes is rare in normal children; a Tzanck test will be positive in both diseases, but DFA, culture, and PCR are specific.[4,16,44]

Rickettsialpox can resemble chickenpox, but its vesicles are deeper and are at a uniform stage of development, and prodrome is more severe.

Other viruses, especially coxsackievirus and echovirus, can produce vesicular exanthema that usually do not crust and that follow a distinctly different course. The Tzanck test is negative in these infections. Lesions of Stevens-Johnson syndrome can resemble chickenpox, but the 2 diseases follow different clinical courses, and the rashes develop differently. A Tzanck test will be negative. Contact dermatitis may produce a rash similar to that of chickenpox, including pruritus, but has a different distribution and evolution.

Insect bites and scabies occasionally cause confusion if they are vesicular. Bullous impetigo (especially staphylococcal skin infection) may produce bullae that resemble chickenpox.

TREATMENT

Treatment with acetaminophen for control of fever and relief of prodromal symptoms, along with measures to control pruritus, usually are sufficient. Concern has surfaced that use of ibuprofen during varicella infection may increase the risk of necrotizing fasciitis and other secondary bacterial (streptococcal) infections, but an association has not been firmly established, and its causal relationship may be confounded by the use of ibuprofen for the signs (eg, secondary fever) of incipient bacterial complications.[45-47] Pruritus can be controlled with oral antihistamine (eg, diphenhydramine), calamine lotion, Cetaphil lotion, or 0.25% menthol lotion. Uncommon but reported encephalopathic side effects of diphenhydramine may mimic neurologic complications of varicella.[48]

Patients should be encouraged to take daily baths to help prevent bacterial superinfection. Adding baking soda or oatmeal preparations (Aveeno) to a warm bath helps relieve the pruritus. Children's nails should be kept clean and trimmed to help discourage scratching. Occasionally, gloves or socks on the hands are required to prevent opening of lesions by scratching. If superinfection is present, then it usually is a result of group A streptococci or *S aureus*. Superinfection of a few lesions can be treated topically with mupirocin ointment; superinfection of many lesions or of lesions in difficult areas (eg, around nares or the mouth) can be treated systemically with a first-generation cephalosporin (eg, cephalexin, cefadroxil) or other antibiotics that are active against streptococci and staphylococci. In places where clindamycin-susceptible, methicillin-resistant *S aureus* commonly cause skin infections in the community, clindamycin may be an appropriate choice.[13]

The CDC recommends avoiding aspirin in the treatment of chickenpox because of its association with Reye syndrome. Physicians caring for patients who are taking aspirin chronically for juvenile rheumatoid arthritis or other diseases need to consider the risks versus the benefits of this therapy on an individual basis if such a patient contracts chickenpox.

Acyclovir has been shown to be effective in treating varicella infections in healthy children and adolescents. When instituted within 24 hours of the onset of rash, treatment has resulted in modest reductions in duration of illness, number of cutaneous lesions, fever, and systemic symptoms.[49,50] In 1 study, treatment of the index case with acyclovir did not change the transmission rate to other susceptible household contacts.[49] Use of acyclovir for varicella infection in adolescents should be considered because they are at greater risk for more severe disease[13]; however, use of acyclovir in healthy preadolescent children is not routinely recommended. Acyclovir can also be considered for other nonimmunocompromised children who are at increased risk of more severe varicella, including children with chronic lung disease, chronic skin disorders, those on salicylate therapy, those taking aerosolized or low-dose systemic corticosteroids, and those who are secondary household cases.[13,51] Valacyclovir and famciclovir have been licensed for treatment of zoster in adults, but no studies and no pediatric formulations exist on which to base recommendations for their use in children.[13,51,52]

Acyclovir, generally by the intravenous route, has been recommended for the treatment of immunocompromised children who develop varicella infection.[13] Increasingly, children infected with HIV, particularly those who have higher CD4 percentages, have been treated successfully for primary varicella with oral acyclovir.[26]

Hospitalization should be avoided whenever possible because hospital epidemics can occur even when the strictest isolation procedures are followed. Generally, spread is by infection of staff members who were thought to be immune or by airborne spread of the virus through ventilation systems. When unavoidable, hospitalization requires strict isolation. Hospitalization on an adult ward that has no immunosuppressed patients may lessen the chances of spread in hospitals where effective strict isolation is not available.[5] All health care workers should have immunity to varicella verified at the time of hire.[53]

Prevention

Isolation or exclusion of the child who has chickenpox to prevent exposure of individuals who are susceptible is the easiest prevention strategy in institutional settings such as hospitals, schools, or child care facilities. This measure is not always effective, given that the disease is contagious 1 to 2 days before the appearance of the rash. Generally, isolation is not feasible for preventing household exposures.

Until recently, varicella-zoster immunoglobulin (VZIG) has been the most common and recommended method of postexposure prophylaxis for susceptible, high-risk patients.[54] VZIG, administered to susceptible persons within 72 to 96 hours of a known or anticipated exposure, can prevent or modify disease in children and adults, though varicella occurring despite VZIG prophylaxis may occur up to 28 days after exposure, instead of the usual incubation period limit of 21 days. Because widespread vaccine use has reduced the need for VZIG, the manufacturer halted production in 2005.[55] An investigational product, VariZIG, a purified human immune globulin preparation with high antivaricella antibody titers that is similar to VZIG, has been recommended in place of VZIG; this product can be obtained through an expanded access protocol.[56,57] If VariZIG cannot be obtained, then the recommendation is for intravenous immunoglobulin (IVIg) at a dose of 400 mg/kg intravenously as the best alternative for exposed neonates, immunocompromised patients, susceptible pregnant women, and other susceptible patients as outlined later in this chapter.

A 10-day course of acyclovir at a dose of 40 to 80 mg/kg/day (divided into 4 to 5 doses) up to adult dose of 800 mg 5 times daily beginning 10 days after exposure can be used in high-risk outpatients beyond the newborn period to prevent or attenuate chickenpox; however, this use of acyclovir is not approved by the US Food and Drug Administration; it is based on small studies, and its potential effect on the immune response has not been fully evaluated.[52,55] Finally, nonpregnant, healthy adults and children at least 1 year of age (without contraindication to varicella vaccine) may be given varicella vaccine within 3 days and perhaps up to 5 days after exposure for prevention of disease.[11] Varicella vaccine is recommended for vaccine-eligible patients who received VariZIG, IVIg, or acyclovir prophylaxis unless varicella disease occurred; vaccine should be delayed by 5 months after VariZIG prophylaxis and by 8 months following 400-mg/kg IVIg prophylaxis to minimize potential interference with vaccine response by passive antibody from these products.[13]

Prophylaxis with VariZIG (or IVIg) after exposure to varicella is recommended for *susceptible* individuals who are at high risk of severe varicella, including susceptible children who are infected with HIV and other immunocompromised children, susceptible pregnant women, newborn infants whose mothers develop varicella eruption from 5 days before until 2 days after delivery, hospitalized premature infants older than 28 weeks' gestation whose mothers are susceptible, and hospitalized premature infants younger than 28 weeks or less than 1000 g, regardless of maternal susceptibility status.[13] The rationale for including all hospitalized premature infants born at less than 28 weeks' gestation *regardless* of maternal varicella susceptibility status is that infants of this degree of prematurity have been deprived of the active transport of maternal antibody that takes place in the final trimester of pregnancy. VariZIG (or IVIg) may be repeated in individuals who are reexposed to varicella more than 3 weeks after an initial dose and have not developed varicella. VariZIG (or IVIg) also may be considered for susceptible adolescents and adults exposed to varicella because these age groups are at higher risk of severe disease compared to younger children, but the alternative preventive strategies of varicella immunization or acyclovir may be more appropriate for this patient group.[55] Alternatively, susceptible adults and children (older than 1 year) who are exposed to chickenpox may be given varicella vaccine within 3 days and perhaps up to 5 days after exposure for prevention of disease.[11]

Varicella Vaccine

A live-attenuated varicella virus vaccine was licensed by the US Food and Drug Administration in 1995. This vaccine has been shown to be effective in preventing varicella infection in most recipients.[38] In 2005, varicella vaccine with the measles-mumps-rubella vaccine as a combination product (MMR-V) was licensed for use based on its safety and immunogenicity in children.[59] Two doses of varicella vaccine are recommended for all children. The second dose should routinely be given between the ages of 4 and 6 years so that most children will be able to get a single injection of MMR-V at 12 to 15 months and again at 4 to 6 years for optimal protection against all 4 of these viral exanthems. The second varicella vaccine dose can be given, however, as soon as 3 months after the initial dose (does not need toe be repeated if 2 doses given at least 28 days apart).[60] Two doses of the vaccine at least 1 month apart are recommended for susceptible adolescents who are 13 years or older.[58]

Susceptible is defined as a lack of reliable history of chickenpox. Routine serologic confirmation of susceptibility in adolescents is not likely to be cost effective, but a positive serologic result excludes the need for vaccination.[13] Modified chickenpox (shorter duration, fewer lesions, less fever) occurs at a rate of approximately 2% to 3% per year among vaccinees and is associated with low 6-week postvaccination varicella zoster virus antibody titers.[61] Studies of chickenpox outbreaks in the vaccine era have suggested an effectiveness of one dose of varicella vaccine of 44% to 88% for complete prevention of chickenpox and 86% to 90% for prevention of moderate or severe chickenpox.[62] Risk factors for breakthrough disease have included immunization at less than 15 months old, longer elapsed time since immunization, oral steroid use, and receipt of measles-mumps-rubella vaccine less than 28 days before varicella vaccine.[62,63] Limited data demonstrate persistence of humoral and cell-mediated immunity following vaccination for up to 20 years in Japan, but the contribution of boosting by continued circulation of wild-type varicella to maintaining immunity is unknown.[13]

The adverse event attributed most commonly to varivax is a mild (2 to 5 lesions on average) maculopapular or varicelliform rash at the injection site or other sites in the month following varicella vaccination.[13] Such lesions appear in 7% to 8% of vaccinated healthy children. When tested by PCR, however, the majority of rashes occurring within 2 weeks of varicella immunization[11] are determined to be due to natural infection. Other more serious but much less common adverse events—encephalitis, ataxia, erythema multiforme, pneumonia, thrombocytopenia, seizures, herpes zoster—occur at lower frequencies than would be expected following natural infection.[11]

Because immune globulin or other blood products (except washed red blood cells) may interfere with the immune response to varicella vaccination, vaccine should be deferred for 3 to 11 months after receipt of blood products, depending on the dose and type of blood product use. Salicylates should not be given for 6 weeks following vaccination because of the theoretical risk of Reye syndrome. Measles-mumps-rubella vaccine and varicella vaccine should not be given fewer than 28 days apart but they may be given simultaneously, including as the combination product MMR-V, without reducing efficacy.

Because the varicella vaccine is an attenuated-live virus vaccine, it generally is not recommended for use in pregnant women or in immunocompromised children, including those who have congenital immunodeficiencies, severely symptomatic HIV infection or HIV infection with CD4 percentages less than 15%, blood dyscrasias, leukemia, lymphoma, immunosuppressive therapy for malignancy, or high-dose steroid therapy (equivalent of prednisone 2 mg/kg/day or 20 mg/day).[11,13]

Clinical trials have demonstrated that for children whose leukemia is in remission and with a break in chemotherapy before and after vaccination, 2-dose varicella vaccine was safe, immunogenic, and completely effective in preventing severe varicella; 50% of these children developed a mild rash in the month following vaccination. They were less likely to develop zoster than were comparable leukemic children who had natural varicella infection.[63] The vaccine is not licensed or routinely recommended for susceptible children who have leukemia at this time, but these children may be eligible to receive the vaccine through a research protocol. (See *Red Book 2006* for details.[13])

Varicella vaccine should be considered for children who have asymptomatic (CDC class N), mildly symptomatic (CDC class A), or moderately symptomatic (CDC class B) infection *and* whose CD4 percentages are at least 15%.[11] Eligible children infected with HIV should receive 2 doses of varicella vaccine at least 3 months apart.

Transmission of vaccine virus to susceptible contacts has been extremely rare and has occurred only in the presence of a vaccine-associated rash; therefore vaccinees who develop a rash should avoid direct contact with susceptible, immunocompromised individuals until the rash has resolved. Presence of an immunocompromised or pregnant contact does not preclude vaccination of an otherwise eligible child.

The author gratefully acknowledges the past contributions of the previous author, Evan G. Pattishall III, MD.

WHEN TO REFER

- Chickenpox in immunodeficient child
- Chickenpox in pregnant woman

WHEN TO ADMIT

- Varicella pneumonia
- Moderately to severely immunosuppressed host
- Moderate to severe bacterial complications
- Chickenpox in neonate
- Encephalopathy

TOOLS FOR PRACTICE

Engaging Patients and Family

- *Chickenpox Information for Families* (fact sheet), American Academy of Pediatrics (www.cispimmunize.org).
- *Chickenpox Vaccine Information Statements* (fact sheet), Centers for Disease Control and Prevention and American Academy of Pediatrics (www.aap.org/bookstore).
- *Chickenpox Vaccine Information Statements—Spanish* (fact sheet), Centers for Disease Control and Prevention and American Academy of Pediatrics (www.aap.org/bookstore).
- *The Chickenpox Vaccine: What Parents Need to Know* (brochure), American Academy of Pediatrics (patiented.aap.org).
- *Varicella (Chickenpox) Vaccine—Important Information for Parents* (fact sheet), National Network for Immunization Information (www.immunizationinfo.org/assets/files/pdfs/2_VAR_facts.pdf).
- Varicella (Chickenpox) At a Glance (Web site), Centers for Disease Control and Prevention (www.cdc.gov/nip/diseases/varicella/).
- *Varicella (Chickenpox) Vaccine* (fact sheet), Vaccine Education Center Children's Hospital of Philadelphia (www.chop.edu/consumer/jsp/division/generic.jsp?iD=75731).

Medical Decision Support

- Photos of Chickenpox (Web site), American Academy of Pediatrics (www.aap.org/new/idphotos.htm).
- Varicella Vaccine Information (Web site), Immunization Action Coalition (www.immunizationinfo.org/vaccineInfo/vaccine_detail.cfv?iD=11).
- Varicella—Clinical Questions and Answers (Web site), Centers for Disease Control and Prevention (www.cdc.gov/nip/diseases/varicella/faqs-clinic-disease.htm).

- Recommendations for Postexposure Prophylaxis of Varicella of Persons at High Risk for Severe Disease (Web site), Centers for Disease Control and Prevention (http://www.cdc.gov/nip/vaccine/varicella/faqs-clinic-highrisk.htm).
- Collecting Varicella Zoster Specimens (Web site), Centers for Disease Control and Prevention (http://www.cdc.gov/nip/diseases/varicella/surv/default.htm).
- Chickenpox/Varicella (Web site), Immunization Action (www.immunize.org/genr.d/varicel.htm).

SUGGESTED RESOURCES

American Academy of Pediatrics. Varicella-zoster infections. In: Pickering LK, Baker CJ, Long SS, McMillan JA, eds: *Red Book 2006: Report of the Committee on Infectious Diseases*, 27th ed., Elk Grove Village, IL: American Academy of Pediatrics; 2006:711-725.

Enright AM, Prober C. Antiviral therapy in children with varicella zoster virus and herpes simplex virus infections [Review]. *Herpes*. 2003 Aug;10(2):32-37.

US Department of Health and Human Services. Epidemiology and Prevention of Vaccine-Preventable Diseases (The Pink Book), 10th Edition. National Immunization Program, Centers for Disease Control and Prevention, March 2008. Available at www.cdc.gov/nip/publications/pink/

Grose C. Varicella vaccination of children in the United States: assessment after the first decade 1995-2005. *J Clin Virol*. 2005 Jun;33(2):89-95.

Krause PR, Klinman DM. Efficacy, immunogenicity, safety and use of attenuated chickenpox vaccine, *J Pediatr* 1995; 127:518-525.

US Department of Health and Human Services, Centers for Disease Control and Prevention, National Immunization Program. Prevention of varicella: recommendations of the Advisory Committee on Immunization Practices (ACIP), *MMWR* 2007;56(RR-04):1-40.

Weller TH: Varicella: historical perspective and clinical overview, *J Infect Dis* 1996;174:S306-S309.

REFERENCES

1. Sullivan-Bolyai JZ, Yin EK, Cox P, et al. Impact of chickenpox on households of healthy children. *Pediatr Infect Dis J*. 1987;6:33-35.
2. Lerman SJ. Why is chickenpox called chickenpox? *Clin Pediatr*. 1981;20:111-112.
3. Scott-Wilson JH. Why "chicken" pox? *Lancet*. 1978;1: 1152.
4. Loparev VN, Argaw T, Krause PR, et al. Improved identification and differentiation of varicella-zoster virus (VZV) wild-type strains and an attenuated varicella vaccine strain using a VZV open reading frame 62-based PCR. *J Clin Microbiol*. 2000 Sep;38(9):3156-3160.
5. Gardner P, Breton S, Charles D. Hospital isolation and precaution guidelines. *Pediatrics*. 1974;53:663.
6. Weller TH. Varicella: historical perspective and clinical overview. *J Infect Dis*. 1996;174:S306-S309.
7. Sauerbrei A, Wutzler P. The congenital varicella syndrome. *J Perinatol*. 2000 Dec;20(8 Pt 1):548-554.
8. Ross AH. Modification of chickenpox in family contacts by administration of gamma globulin. *N Engl J Med*. 1962; 267:369.
9. Muench R, Nassim C, Niku S, et al. Seroepidemiology of varicella. *J Infect Dis*. 1986;153:153-155.
10. Preblud S, D'Angelo L. Chickenpox in the United States 1972-1977. *J Infect Dis*. 1979;140:257-259.
11. Centers for Disease Control and Prevention. Prevention of varicella: recommendations of the Advisory Committee on Immunization Practices (ACIP). *MMWR*. 2007; 56(RR-04):1-40.
12. Seward JF, Watson BM, Peterson CL, et al. Varicella disease after introduction of varicella vaccine in the United States, 1995-2000. *JAMA*. Feb 2002;287(5):606-611.
13. American Academy of Pediatrics. Varicella-zoster infections. In: Pickering LK, Baker CJ, Long SS, McMillan JA, eds: *Red Book 2006: Report of the Committee on Infectious Diseases*. 27th ed. Elk Grove Village, IL: American Academy of Pediatrics; 2006: 711-25.
14. Gershon AA, Steinberg SP, Gelb L. Clinical reinfection with varicella-zoster virus. *J Infect Dis*. 1984;149:137-142.
15. Wallace MR, Chamberlin CJ, Zerboni L, et al. Reliability of a history of previous varicella infection in adults. *JAMA*. 1997;278:1529-1530.
16. Atkinson W, Hamborsky J, McIntyre L, et al, eds. *Varicella in Centers for Disease Control and Prevention. Epidemiology and Prevention of Vaccine-Preventable Diseases*. 10th ed. Washington, DC: Public Health Foundation; 2008.
17. Nguyen HQ, Jumaan AO, Seward JF. Decline in mortality due to varicella after implementation of varicella vaccination in the United States. *N Engl J Med*. 2005 Feb 3;352(5): 450-458.
18. Centers for Disease Control and Prevention. Varicella-related deaths among children—United States, 1997. *MMWR*. 1998;47:365-368.
19. Davis MM, Patel MS, Gebremariam A. Decline in varicella-related hospitalizations and expenditures for children and adults after introduction of varicella vaccine in the United States. *Pediatrics*. 2004 Sep;114(3):786-792.
20. Asano Y, Itakura N, Hiroishi Y, et al. Viremia is present in incubation period in nonimmunocompromised children with varicella. *J Pediatr*. 1985;106:69-71.
21. Grose C. Variation on a theme by Fenner: the pathogenesis of chickenpox. *Pediatrics*. 1981;68:735-737.
22. Weller TH. Varicella and herpes zoster. *N Engl J Med*. 1984; 309:1362-1368.
23. Feldman S. Varicella-zoster virus pneumonitis. *Chest*. 1994; 106:22S-27S.
24. Watson BM, Piercy SA, Plotkin SA, et al. Modified chickenpox in children immunized with the Oka/Merck varicella vaccine. *Pediatrics*. 1993 Jan;91(1):17-22.
25. Seward JF, Zhang JX, Maupin TJ, et al. Contagiousness of varicella in vaccinated cases: a household contact study. *JAMA*. 2004 Aug 11;292(6):704-708.
26. Gershon AA, Mervish N, LaRussa P, et al. Varicella-zoster virus infections in children with underlying human immunodeficiency virus infection. *J Infect Dis*. 1997;176: 1496-1500.
27. Dowell SF, Bresee JS. Severe varicella associated with steroid use. *Pediatrics*. 1993;92:223-228.
28. Patel H, Macarthur C, Johnson D. Recent corticosteroid use and the risk of complicated varicella in otherwise immunocompetent children. *Arch Pediatr Adolesc Med*. 1996;150:409-413.
29. Nursoy MA, Bakir M, Barlan IB, et al. The course of chickenpox in asthmatic children receiving inhaled budesonide. *Pediatr Infect Dis J*. 1997 Jan;16(1):74-77.
30. Paryani SG, Arvin AM. Intrauterine infection with varicella-zoster virus after maternal varicella. *N Engl J Med*. 1986;314:1542-1546.
31. Enders G, Miller E, Cradock-Watson J, et al. Consequences of varicella and herpes zoster in pregnancy: prospective study of 1739 cases. *Lancet*. 1994;343:1548-1551.
32. Aebi C, Ahmed A, Ramilo O. Bacterial complications of primary varicella in children. *Clin Infect Dis*. 1996;23: 698-705.

33. Guess HA, Broughton DD, Melton LJ 3rd, et al. Population-based studies of varicella complications. *Pediatrics.* 1986;78:723-727.
34. Peterson CL, Mascola L, Chao SM, et al. Children hospitalized for varicella: a prevaccine review. *J Pediatr.* 1996; 129:529-536.
35. Belay ED, Bresee JS, Holman RC, et al. Reye's syndrome in the United States from 1981 through 1997. *New Engl J Med.* 1997;340:1377-1382.
36. Snodgrass SR. Syndromic diagnosis in para-infectious neurologic disease: varicella ataxic syndrome. *J Child Neurol.* 1998;13:83-85.
37. Connolly AM, Dodson WE, Prensky AL, et al. Course and outcome of acute cerebellar ataxia. *Ann Neurol.* 1994; 35:673-679.
38. Krause PR, Klinman DM. Efficacy, immunogenicity, safety, and use of live attenuated chickenpox vaccine. *J Pediatr.* 1995;127:518-525.
39. Ey J, Smith S, Fulginiti V. Varicella hepatitis without neurologic symptoms or findings. *Pediatrics.* 1981;67:258-263.
40. Pitel PA, McCormick KL, Fitzgerald E, et al. Subclinical hepatic changes in varicella infection. *Pediatrics.* 1980;65: 631-636.
41. Baba K, Yabuuchi H, Takahashi M, et al. Increased incidence of herpes zoster in normal children infected with varicella zoster virus during infancy: community-based follow-up study. *J Pediatr.* 1986;108:372-377.
42. Hardy IB, Gershon A, Steinberg S, et al. The incidence of zoster after immunization with live attenuated varicella vaccine: a study of children with leukemia. *N Engl J Med.* 1991;325:1545-1560.
43. Kertes PJ, Baker JD, Noel LP. Neuro-ophthalmic complications of acute varicella. *Can J Ophthalmol.* 1998;33: 324-328.
44. Nahass GT, Goldstein BA, Zhu WY, et al. Comparison of Tzanck smear, viral culture, and DNA diagnostic methods in detection of herpes simplex and varicella-zoster infections. *JAMA.* 1992;268:2541-2544.
45. Choo PW, Donahue JG, Platt R. Ibuprofen and skin and soft tissue superinfections in children with varicella. *Ann Epidemiol.* 1997;7:440-445.
46. Rosefsky JB. Varicella and necrotizing fascitis. *Pediatr Infect Dis J.* 1996;15:556-557.
47. Zerr DM, Alexander ER, Duchin JS, et al. A case-control study of necrotizing fasciitis during primary varicella. *Pediatrics.* 1999;103:783-790.
48. Tomlinson G, Helfaer M, Wiedermann BL. Diphenhydramine toxicity mimicking varicella encephalitis. *Pediatr Infect Dis J.* 1987;6:220-221.
49. Balfour HH Jr, Rotbart HA, Feldman S, et al. Acyclovir treatment of varicella in otherwise healthy adolescents. *J Pediatr.* 1992;120:627-633.
50. Dunkle LM, Arvin AM, Whitley RJ, et al. A controlled trial of acyclovir for chickenpox in normal children. *N Engl J Med.* 1991;325:1539-1544.
51. Enright AM, Prober C. Antiviral therapy in children with varicella zoster virus and herpes simplex virus infections [Review]. *Herpes.* 2003 Aug;10(2):32-37.
52. Trizna Z. Viral diseases of the skin: diagnosis and antiviral treatment. *Paediatr Drugs.* 2002;4(1):9-19.
53. Centers for Disease Control and Prevention. Immunization of health-care workers: recommendations of the Advisory Committee on Immunization Practices (ACIP) and the Hospital Infection Control Practices Advisory Committee (HICPAC). *MMWR.* Dec 1997;46(RR-18);1-45.
54. American Academy of Pediatrics. In: Pickering LK ed. *Red Book: 2003 Report of the Committee on Infectious Diseases.* 26th ed. Elk Grove Village, IL: American Academy of Pediatrics; 2003.
55. US Food and Drug Administration, Center for Biologics Evaluation and Research. Varicella Zoster Immune Globulin (VZIG) Anticipated Short Supply. September 20, 2005. Available at: www.fda.gov/cber/infosheets/mphvzig092005.htm. Accessed October 31, 2006.
56. American Academy of Pediatrics. Active immunization. In: Pickering LK, Baker CJ, Long SS, McMillan JA, eds. *Red Book: 2006 Report of the Committee on Infectious Diseases.* 27th ed. Elk Grove Village, IL: American Academy of Pediatrics; 2006.
57. Centers for Disease Control and Prevention. A new product (VariZIG) for postexposure prophylaxis of varicella available under an investigational new drug application expanded access protocol. *MMWR.* February 24, 2006;55:1-2.
58. American Academy of Pediatrics. Committee on Infectious Diseases. Prevention of Varicella: Recommendations for Use of Varicella Vaccines in Children, Including a Recommendation for a Routine 2-Dose Varicella Immunization Schedule. *Pediatrics.* 2007;120(1):221-231. Available at: aappolicy.aappublications.org/cgi/contents/full/pediatrics;120/1/221. Accessed March 21, 2008.
59. Verstraeten T, Jumaan AO, Mullooly JP, et al. Vaccine Safety Datalink Research Group. A retrospective cohort study of the association of varicella vaccine failure with asthma, steroid use, age at vaccination, and measles-mumps-rubella vaccination. *Pediatrics.* 2003 Aug;112(2): e98-e103.
60. Knuf M, Habermehl P, Zepp F, et al. Immunogenicity and safety of two doses of tetravalent measles-mumps-rubella-varicella vaccine in healthy children. *Pediatr Infect Dis J.* 2006 Jan;25(1):12-18.
61. Johnson CE, Stancin T, Fattlar D, et al. A long-term prospective study of varicella vaccine in healthy children. *Pediatrics.* 1997;100:761-766.
62. Grose C. Varicella vaccination of children in the United States: assessment after the first decade 1995-2005. *J Clin Virol.* 2005 Jun;33(2):89-95.
63. LaRussa P, Steinberg S, Gershon AA. Varicella vaccine for immunocompromised children: results of collaborative studies in the United States and Canada. *J Infect Dis.* 1996;174:S320-S323.

Chapter 247

CHRONIC FATIGUE SYNDROME

Leonard R. Krilov, MD

Chronic fatigue syndrome (CFS) describes an illness characterized by prolonged periods of debilitating fatigue for which no definitive cause is known. Although the Centers for Disease Control and Prevention (CDC) has created a working definition of CFS for study purposes,[1] CFS is not a well-defined clinical entity. No specific causative agent or agents and no characteristic pathophysiological models have been identified for CFS. Debate centers on the contributions of infectious and other medical conditions and immunologic and psychological factors to the clinical manifestations of CFS. All of these factors likely interact to produce CFS, albeit to differing degrees in each individual.

Historically, a variety of syndromes that appear similar to CFS have been described.[2] These conditions include chronic infectious mononucleosis, total allergy syndrome, chronic candidiasis, hypoglycemia, neurasthenia, myalgic encephalomyelitis, postviral syndrome, and fibromyalgia. These diagnoses are characterized by signs and symptoms similar to those of CFS and lack a definitive diagnostic test or a definitive causative agent. Cases of CFS have been reported to occur both sporadically and epidemically.

Overall, the CDC estimates a prevalence rate of approximately 200 cases of CFS-like illness per 100,000 adults over 18 years of age in the United States.[3] Dobbins and colleagues extracted data regarding adolescents from 3 CDC studies of fatiguing illness and reported a prevalence of CFS-like illness of approximately 20 per 100,000.[4]

An association between low blood pressure (postural orthostatic tachycardia syndrome (POTS) and CFS has been suggested.[5] Other investigators have proposed hormonal factors, such as depressed cortisol responses, as contributing to the signs and symptoms of CFS.

The majority of reported cases of CFS have occurred in white women—a median age of 35 to 40 years and from upper socioeconomic groups, although adolescents who have the diagnosis also have been described.[6-8] Minorities, the indigent, and people living in developing countries are strikingly underrepresented in reports of CFS. Whether this shortage reflects a bias in patient selection or predisposing factors for development of CFS remains to be determined.

BOX 247-1 Differential Diagnosis of a Patient Who Is Chronically Fatigued

- Malignancy
- Autoimmune disease
- Localized infection (eg, sinusitis, occult abscess)
- Chronic or subacute infection (eg, Lyme disease, endocarditis, tuberculosis)
- Human immunodeficiency virus infection
- Fungal disease (eg, candidiasis, histoplasmosis, coccidioidomycosis, blastomycosis)
- Parasitic disease (eg, toxoplasmosis, giardiasis)
- Chronic inflammatory disease (eg, sarcoidosis, Wegener granulomatosis)
- Endocrine disease (eg, hypothyroidism, Addison disease, diabetes)
- Neuromuscular disease (eg, myasthenia gravis, multiple sclerosis)
- Drug dependency
- Side effects of chronic medications or other toxic agents (eg, chemical solvent, heavy metal, pesticide)
- Psychiatric disorder

CLINICAL MANIFESTATIONS

The primary manifestation of CFS is severe fatigue longer than 6 months in duration that limits the individual to activity less than 50% of the premorbid level of function. Associated symptoms frequently include sore throat, low-grade fever (oral temperatures of 37.5° C to 38.6° C), painful lymph nodes, unexplained generalized weakness, myalgias or arthralgias (or both), prolonged fatigue after exercise, headaches, difficulty concentrating or memory loss, and sleep disturbances (hypersomnia or insomnia). The majority of patients describe a sudden onset of the syndrome with an initial mononucleosis or influenza-like illness, although, in some cases, a more gradual onset is related. Many patients also describe a history of atopy or multiple allergies, or both.

The initial history should include questions about the nature and duration of symptoms, as well as possible exposures to or contacts with ill persons, that might suggest an alternative diagnosis. Personal and social history to assess family dynamics, prior level of functioning, response to illness, family history of psychiatric illness, and psychological or marital problems may be helpful.

The physical examination may reveal abnormalities, including (1) mild inflammation of the pharynx, (2) cervical or axillary lymphadenopathy, or (3) low-grade temperature elevation in up to 50% of cases. However, the primary goal of the physical examination is to eliminate other causes for the patient's symptoms. Significantly elevated temperatures, enlarged lymph nodes (>2 cm), weight loss of more than 10% of body mass index without dieting, or focal neurologic abnormalities should suggest an alternative diagnosis. The differential diagnoses of illnesses associated with extensive fatigue are listed in Box 247-1.

PSYCHOLOGICAL FACTORS

Clinicians and investigators have noted a relationship of CFS to depressive symptoms, frank depression, and a family history of depression.[9] Conceptually, depression may be both part of the cause of CFS and a reaction to having CFS. We have been impressed with the family dynamics of adolescents who have CFS.[6,10] School-avoidance behaviors related to expectations for high academic performance compared with the teenager's abilities have been noted frequently. In many families, overprotection and overindulgence of the child has been observed, often associated with difficulty in mother-teen separation. A recent analysis of adolescents who have CFS compared with age-matched adolescent survivors of childhood cancer and a healthy control group showed that the CFS group had higher scores on measures of somatic complaints, depression, internalizing symptoms, and feeling different from others.[10]

The manifestations of CFS can be considered in this framework as a conversion reaction in which an infection or other stressor serves as a model for persistent symptoms that offer the individual a mechanism by which to maintain an overprotective environment or to avoid going to school (see Chapter 139, Conversion Reactions and Hysteria).

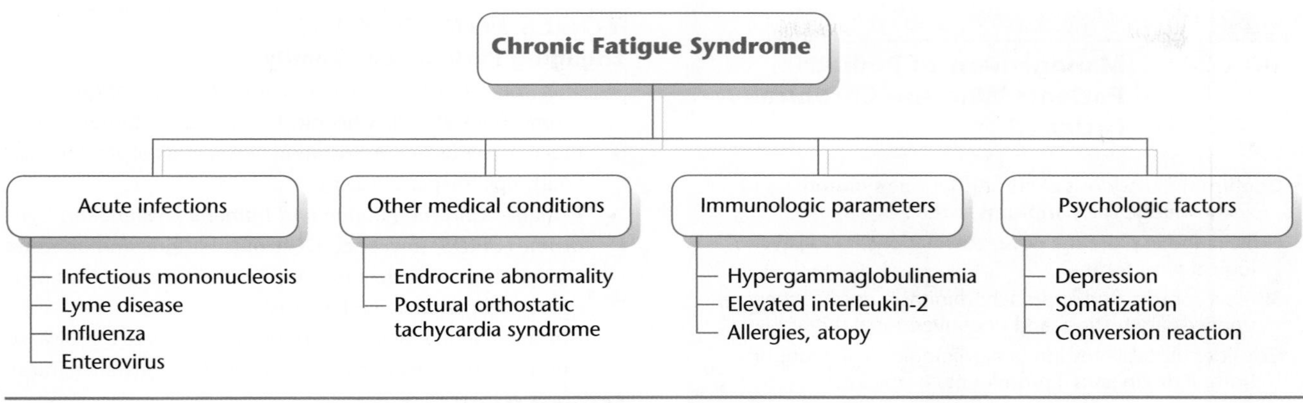

Figure 247-1 Pathogenesis of chronic fatigue syndrome.

LABORATORY DIAGNOSIS

No specific laboratory tests exist by which to diagnose CFS. As with the physical examination, the primary aim of laboratory evaluations is to eliminate other conditions that may be responsible for the patient's symptoms. A suggested battery of screening tests might include a complete blood count and differential; measurement of the erythrocyte sedimentation rate, serum electrolytes, creatinine, blood urea nitrogen, and glucose; liver enzymes and function tests; thyroid function tests; tuberculin skin test with controls; measurement of alkaline phosphatase, antinuclear antibodies, rheumatoid factor, and human immunodeficiency virus (HIV) antibody; and chest and sinus radiographs. Additional tests (eg, Lyme disease test, viral serologies) may be indicated based on history and physical examination findings. Although potential immunologic abnormalities, including altered lymphocyte subsets, qualitative defects in natural killer cell activity, hypogammaglobulinemia or hypergammaglobulinemia, elevated titers to herpes viruses (eg, Epstein-Barr virus, human herpes virus type 6), abnormal lymphokine levels, and decreased lymphocyte proliferation responses, have been described in patients who have CFS, they have not been observed consistently in different groups of patients.[11] Additionally, the magnitude of immunologic abnormalities detected in patients who have CFS has been small compared with those who have classic immunodeficiencies; the degree of immune aberrations does not correlate with the severity of symptoms, and opportunistic infections do not occur in CFS.

The role of POTS in CFS, as discussed in the introductory section of this chapter, is intriguing. Head-upright or tilt-table testing is the modality by which this abnormality is assessed. Such testing should be considered for a subset of patients in whom dizziness is a significant part of their symptom complex. Whether all patients with CFS should be evaluated for NHM is currently unknown.

Although of uncertain significance, increased white matter on T2-weighted magnetic resonance imaging scans suggestive of possible infiltration of the perivascular spaces, focal demyelination, or disease of the small blood vessels of the cerebral white matter has been reported in a number of patients with CFS.[12]

PROPOSED MODEL OF PATHOGENESIS

The exact definition of a case of CFS is difficult in that few objective findings are found in these individuals, and their most severe symptoms are difficult to quantify. To date, no specific infectious cause for CFS has been defined, and a single infectious agent is not likely responsible. A reasonable suggestion would be that it is the interaction of multiple factors that results in the development of CFS (Figure 247-1). The relative importance of each of the factors probably varies from individual to individual.

THERAPY

No specific therapy for CFS has been proven to be effective. However, management aimed at alleviating the patient's symptoms may help. If NMH is documented, then dietary (eg, increased salt intake) or pharmacologic management (or both) with drugs such as fludrocortisone, propranolol, or midorine may be beneficial. In our experience, therapy of NMH has been only of partial benefit, even in adolescents whose tilt-table tests are abnormal. An approach to the management of CFS is outlined in Box 247-2. The primary goals of this treatment are to provide counseling and symptomatic relief for depression, sleep disorders, and musculoskeletal pains; to offer emotional support with involvement of a social worker, psychologist, or psychiatrist, as needed; to identify and eliminate *secondary gain* from continuing to contribute to the illness; and to devise programs with the patient to increase school (or work) attendance and exercise capability gradually. Periodic physical examinations for possible other conditions are also important. Family therapy often helps the parents manage these issues and addresses the role of family dynamics in the evolution of a patient's symptoms. A team approach with coordination of services to avoid *doctor shopping* and fad therapy is critical to the successful management of the patient who has CFS.

Some of the unproved fad therapies described are megavitamin treatment, immune modifiers (eg, Ampligen,

BOX 247-2 Management of Pediatric Patients Who Are Chronically Fatigued

Confirm the diagnosis of chronic fatigue syndrome and acknowledge the symptoms as real.

Explain and explore the potential relationship to psychological symptoms.

Stress a coordinated approach; minimize *doctor shopping*, unnecessary testing, and unconventional therapies.

Consider tilt-table testing or cardiologic evaluation, or both, if dizziness is a prominent complaint.

Use stress-coping skills: Modify lifestyles, decrease stress, develop a realistic schedule including working with school (gradual return to classes, home tutoring, neuropsychometric testing), and develop a graduated exercise program.

Use cognitive-behavioral approaches: Pay attention to sleep patterns and nutrition; increase activity gradually.

Provide psychological support: Provide individual therapy and family therapy, and decrease secondary gain.

Maintain followup: Monitor physical symptoms and psychological issues; provide ongoing guidance and continued reassurance.

thymic extract, interleukin-2), magnesium sulfate, liver extract injections, anti-*Candida* diets, colonic irrigation, and removal of dental fillings. Immunoglobulin injections have been reported to be beneficial in 1 study of patients with CFS,[13] although 2 subsequent studies failed to confirm this observation.

PROGNOSIS AND FUTURE PROSPECTS

Despite the vagaries associated with the diagnosis of CFS and differences in each case, long-term follow-up suggests that most individuals report improvement or resolution of symptoms over a 2- to 3-year period.[6] Few patients report progressive symptoms, although symptoms may wax and wane in severity. With better definition of the nature of the neurologic, cardiovascular, endocrinologic, and immunologic alterations in CFS, additional therapeutic approaches may become available.

WHEN TO REFER

- To resolve issues relating to possibility of ongoing infection or inflammation that may be causing the patients symptoms.
- Given the often extensive and varied complaints of patients with CFS, multiple specialists may become involved and multiple laboratory tests may be ordered. A coordinated team approach to avoid redundant and/or unnecessary testing can be beneficial.
- To provide an increased level of supportive care or counseling than can be provided in the office setting, especially if the individual is not able to attend school or participate in normal activities.

TOOLS FOR PRACTICE

Engaging Patients and Family

- *Tips for Parents for Youth with Chronic Fatigue Syndrome* (fact sheet), Chronic Fatigue and Immune Dysfunction Syndrome Association (www.cfids.org/resources/youth-tips-for-parents.asp).
- *Pediatric Chronic Fatigue and Immune Dysfunction Syndrome (CFIDS)* (fact sheet), Chronic Fatigue and Immune Dysfunction Syndrome Association (www.cfids.org/resources/pediatric-CFIDS.asp).
- Chronic Fatigue Syndrome (Web site), Centers for Disease Control and Prevention (www.cdc.gov/cfs/consumers.htm).

Medical Decision Support

- Chronic Fatigue Syndrome (toolkit), Centers for Disease Control and Prevention (www.cdc.gov/cfs/toolkit.htm).
- Chronic Fatigue Syndrome (Web site), Centers for Disease Control and Prevention (www.cdc.gov/cfs/healthcareprofessionals.htm).
- Do I Have Chronic Fatigue Syndrome Assessment (questionnaire), Chronic Fatigue and Immune Dysfunction Syndrome Association (www.cfids.org/about-cfids/do-i-have-cfids.asp).

SUGGESTED RESOURCES

Journal articles

Klonoff DC. Chronic fatigue syndrome. *Clin Infect Dis.* 1992;15:812-823.

Marshall GS. Report of a workshop on the epidemiology, natural history, and pathogenesis of chronic fatigue syndrome in adolescents. *J Pediatr.* 1999;134:395-405.

Books

Dawson DM, Sabin TD, eds. *Chronic Fatigue Syndrome.* Boston, MA: Little, Brown; 1993.

Krilov LR: Chronic fatigue syndrome, In: Feigin RD, Cherry JD, eds. *Textbook of Pediatric Infectious Diseases.* Philadelphia, PA: WB Saunders; 2004.

RELATED WEB SITES

- www.cdc.gov/nicdod/diseases/cfs/.
- www.niaid.nih.gov/factsheets/cfs.
- www.cfids.org.
- www.medicineau.net.au/clinicalmedicine/CFS.html.

REFERENCES

1. Fukuda K, Straus SE, Hickie I, et al. The chronic fatigue syndrome: a comprehensive approach to its definition and study. *Ann Intern Med.* 1994;121:953-959.
2. Straus SE. History of chronic fatigue syndrome. *Rev Infect Dis.* 1991;13(suppl 1):S2-S7.
3. Centers for Disease Control and Prevention. Chronic Fatigue Syndrome. May 11, 2005. Available at: www.cdc.gov/ncidod/diseases/cfs/about/demographic.htm. Accessed 3/22/06.
4. Dobbins JG, Randall B, Reyes M, et al. CFS in adolescents. *J Chronic Fatigue Syndrome.* 1997;3:15-28.
5. Stewart JM, Gewitz MH, Weldon A, et al. Orthostatic intolerance in adolescent chronic fatigue syndrome. *Pediatrics.* 1999;103:116-121.
6. Krilov LR, Fisher M, Friedman SB, et al. Course and outcome of chronic fatigue in children and adolescents. *Pediatrics.* 1998;102:360-366.

7. Marshall GS, Gesser RM, Yamanishi K, et al. Chronic fatigue in children: clinical features of Epstein-Barr virus and human herpes virus 6 serology and long-term follow-up. *Pediatr Infect Dis J*. 1991;10:287-290.
8. Smith MS, Mitchell J, Corey L, et al. Chronic fatigue in adolescents. *Pediatrics*. 1991;88:195-202.
9. Katon WJ, Buchwald DS, Simon GE. Psychiatric assessment of patients with chronic fatigue and those with rheumatoid arthritis. *J Gen Intern Med*. 1991;6:227-285.
10. Pelcovitz D, Septimus A, Friedman SB, et al. Psychosocial correlates of chronic fatigue syndrome in adolescence. *J Dev Behav Pediatr*. 1995;16:333-338.
11. Barker E, Fujimura SF, Fadem MB, et al. Immunologic abnormalities associated with chronic fatigue syndrome. *Clin Infect Dis*. 1994;18(suppl 1):S136-S141.
12. Schwartz RB. Neuroradiologic features. In Dawson DM, Sabin TD, eds. *Chronic Fatigue Syndrome*. Boston, MA: Little, Brown; 1993.
13. Lloyd A, Hickie I, Wakefield D, et al. A double-blind, placebo-controlled trial of intravenous immunoglobulin therapy in patients with chronic fatigue syndrome. *Am J Med*. 1990;89:561-568.

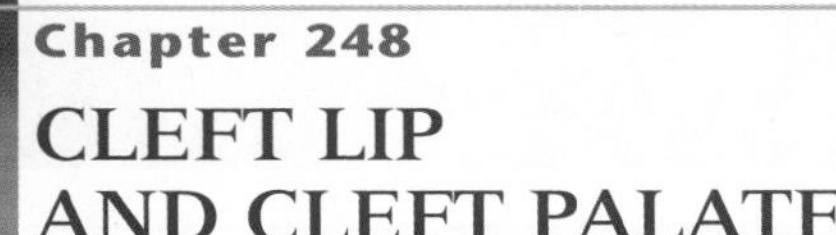

Chapter 248

CLEFT LIP AND CLEFT PALATE

Arlene A. Rozzelle, MD; Jugpal S. Arneja, MD

Clefts of the lip and palate are complicated, multifaceted problems that provide an immense challenge for treating specialists. Clefting may occur in isolation or may have several associated anomalies that represent a syndrome. As such, these problems are best addressed in a multidisciplinary team-oriented setting to maximize the child's final functional and aesthetic outcome. Aside from surgical specialists (plastic surgeons, otolaryngologists, oral and maxillofacial surgeons), cleft team members include medical specialists (pediatricians, geneticists, child psychiatrists), dental specialists (orthodontists, prosthodontists, pediatric dentists), speech and hearing specialists (speech pathologists, audiologists), and nursing specialists (pediatric or cleft-trained nurses). Results are often based on the severity of the problem, the timing of nonsurgical and surgical intervention, the experience and training of the involved specialists, and patient compliance, given that treatment is initiated at birth and is often not completed well into late adolescence. Despite the multitude of advancements in cleft care, questions remain regarding optimizing outcomes of facial growth, dental reconstruction, speech, facial form, and psychological well being. This chapter outlines the theoretical basics and practical approach to managing these challenging, although ultimately rewarding, patients.

DEFINITIONS

The primary palate consists of all structures anterior to the incisive foramen (lip and alveolus), whereas the secondary palate includes all structures posterior to the incisive foramen (hard palate and soft palate). Figure 248-1 illustrates the pertinent cleft-related anatomy of the primary and secondary palate. The development of a comprehensive and completely accepted classification method for cleft anomalies has been elusive. Most classification systems are too basic, too complex, or not comprehensive enough to include all possible clinical presentations.

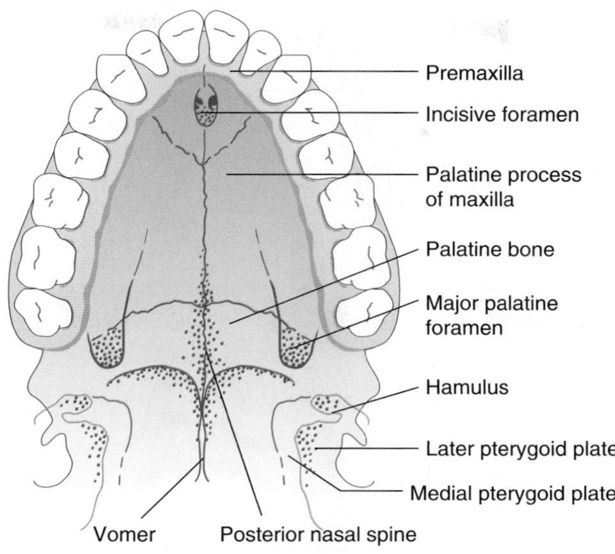

Figure 248-1 Normal palatal anatomy. (*Millard DR Jr.* Cleft Craft: The Evolution of Its Surgery. *Boston: Little, Brown & Company; 1980, p. 19.*)

An early classification system divided clefts into 4 groups[1]: (1) soft palate clefts alone, (2) clefts of both the hard and soft palate, (3) complete unilateral clefts of the lip and palate, and (4) complete bilateral clefts of the lip and palate. In 1962 the American Association for Cleft Palate Rehabilitation[2] proposed a complicated classification system that has not found universal acceptance. In 1971 a simple, yet comprehensive, diagrammatic representation of cleft classification, termed the *striped Y*, was introduced; this classification was later modified to include nasal and pharyngeal deformities.[3,4] This classification system has found acceptance at numerous cleft palate centers. In 1989 a palindromic method of classifying clefts was described; the letters LAHSHAL represent the lip (L), alveolus (A), hard palate (H), and soft palate (S).[5] In addition, a numeric recording system was proposed for the classification of clefts, termed the *RPL system*.[6] Invariably, the method that is often used to classify and describe clefts among practitioners is simply a description of the anatomic severity of the cleft of the primary or secondary palate and whether the cleft is incomplete or complete (Figure 248-2). On occasion, a complete cleft of the primary palate has a degree of skin bridging the superior aspect of the lip, termed a Simonart band.

EMBRYOLOGY

Normal facial embryonic development occurs between the third and twelfth weeks of gestation with the fusion of 5 facial prominences[7,8] (Figure 248-3). Specifically, palate development initiates at the end of the 5th week and is completed by the end of the 12th week.

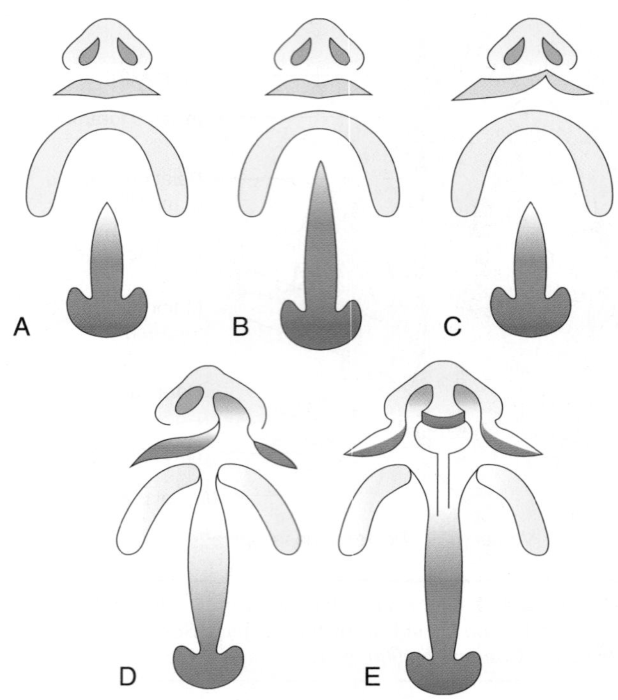

Figure 248-2 **A**, Incomplete cleft secondary palate. **B**, Complete cleft secondary palate. **C**, Left incomplete cleft primary palate and incomplete cleft secondary palate. **D**, Left complete cleft primary palate and complete cleft secondary palate. **E**, Bilateral complete cleft primary palate and complete cleft secondary palate. (*Kernahan DA, Stark RB. A new classification for cleft lip and palate.* Plast Reconstr Surg. *1958;22:435.*)

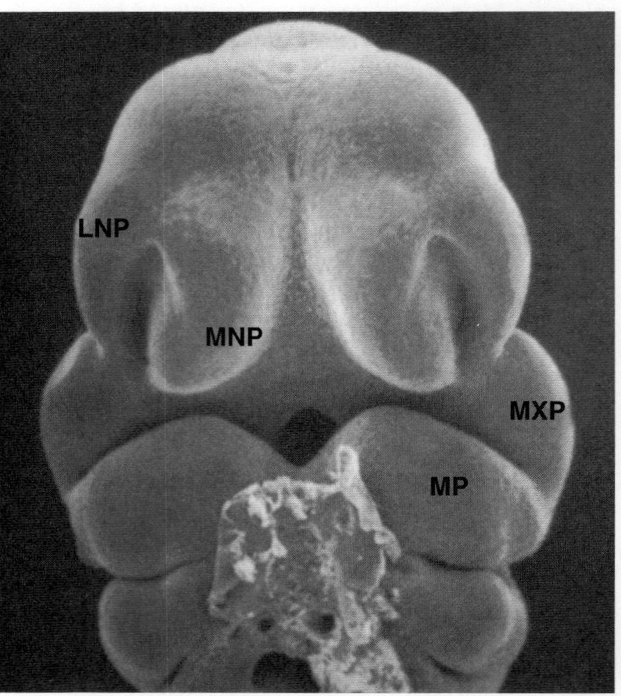

Figure 248-3 Embryological development of the primary palate. *MNP,* Medial nasal process; *LNP,* lateral nasal process; *MXP,* maxillary process; *MP,* mandibular process. (*Bronsky PT. Effects of hypoxia on facial prominence development in CL/fr mice. M.S. Thesis, University of North Carolina, 1985.*)

The primary palate is derived from the fusion of the medial nasal prominences with the maxillary prominence, whereas the secondary palate is derived from the fusion of the lateral palatine processes and the nasal septum, with closure extending from the incisive foramen posteriorly. Fusion is completed by the end of week 12 with formation of the lip, alveolus, hard palate, soft palate, and uvula.

Failure of penetration or fusion of the mesenchymal masses of the 5 facial prominences forms the embryologic basis of cleft formation. Isolated failure of fusion of the medial nasal prominence with the maxillary prominence on 1 side results in a unilateral cleft lip, whereas a bilateral cleft lip results from failure of both medial nasal prominences to fuse with the maxillary prominence.[9] Palatal clefts result from incomplete fusion of the lateral palatine processes with the nasal septum at any stage of development. As the secondary palate fuses in an anterior-to-posterior direction, soft palate clefts that occur are much more common because the fusion of the soft palate follows hard palate closure. The most accepted theory as to why secondary palatal clefts occur is delayed elevation of the palatal shelves from a vertical-to-horizontal direction.[10]

INCIDENCE

Clefting is the second most common congenital anomaly, after clubfoot, with an overall incidence of cleft lip with or without cleft palate of approximately 1 in 700 new births[11] and an overall incidence of isolated cleft palate of approximately 1 in 1000 new births. Racial differences are seen in incidence, with patients of Asian descent having a higher incidence (2.1 in 1000) and black patients having a lower incidence (0.41 in 1000) compared with white patients (1.3 in 1000).[12] Cleft lip and palate are more common in boys than girls (2:1); isolated cleft palate occurs twice as often in girls than boys, likely the result of later palatal closure in girls.[13,14] Clefts are more common on the left side and theorized to be related to earlier closure of the right side than the left, making the left side more susceptible to insult in utero. Unilateral cleft lips occur much more commonly than bilateral cleft lips (4:1). The relative frequency of orofacial clefting between cleft lip to cleft palate and cleft lip and palate is 1:1.2:2.5.

Genetics and Risk Factors

Clefting may be in isolation or associated with other conditions that meet the criteria of a syndrome. More than 300 syndromes are associated with clefting; the more common syndromes include Van der Woude syndrome, velocardiofacial syndrome, Pierre Robin sequence, Goldenhar syndrome, Treacher Collins syndrome, Down syndrome, and Stickler syndrome. Cleft lip with or without cleft palate has been suggested to be etiologically different than isolated cleft palate.[13] Syndromes are associated with approximately 29% of orofacial clefts, with an isolated cleft of the secondary palate the most common syndromic presentation.[15]

Table 248-1 Familial Risks for Nonsyndromic Cleft Lip and Palate

FAMILY HISTORY	CLEFT LIP WITH OR WITHOUT CLEFT PALATE	CLEFT PALATE
No family history of cleft lip or cleft palate	0.1%	0.04%
Unaffected parents with 1 previously affected child	4%	2%
Unaffected parents with 2 previously affected children	9%	1%
One affected parent	4%	6%
One affected parent and 1 previously affected child	17%	15%

From Kirschner RE, LaRossa D. Cleft lip and palate. Otolaryngol Clin North Am 2000;33(6):1191-1215, v-vi.

Most clefts are nonsyndromic and generally postulated to be multifactorial in nature or as a result of changes at a major single-gene locus.[15] Allelic association and linkage analysis have been related to several candidate genes. Candidate genes purported by allelic association or linkage analysis for orofacial clefts include *TGF alpha* and *beta, MSX-1,* retinoic acid receptor alpha, homeobox gene, distal-less homeobox 2, and B-cell leukemia or lymphoma 3.[16]

Risk factors for the development of clefting include family history and environmental agent exposure. Several teratogens have been found to increase the rate of clefting during the first trimester of pregnancy. Clefting has been produced in animal models with exposure to several agents, including corticosteroids, ethanol, ionizing radiation, phenytoin, isotretinoin, diazepam, and methotrexate.[17] Many of these agents have been shown to increase the risk of clefting in vivo as well; in addition, exposures to caffeine and tobacco are theorized to also increase the risk of clefting.[18] Infections, including rubella and toxoplasmosis, in the first trimester of pregnancy have also been implicated in the development of clefting.[19] Many of these agents and exposures may act in unison in patients who are biologically and genetically susceptible. A family history of clefting is a risk factor for future cleft occurrences. Table 248-1 characterizes the risk of clefting to future offspring for nonsyndromic cleft lip and palate, based on the number of parents with clefts and the number of siblings with clefts.

Prenatal Evaluation

Increasingly, a diagnosis of clefting of the lip or palate can be reliably established by prenatal ultrasound; transvaginal ultrasound can reliably detect a cleft lip by 13 to 16 weeks of gestation.[20] Clefts of the secondary palate can be diagnosed at 19 weeks of gestation using real-time magnetic resonance imaging.[21] Although these techniques offer numerous advantages to the parents, in certain societies, they may result in pregnancy termination, raising important ethical concerns.[20]

MANAGEMENT

Of primary concern in the newborn with a cleft are airway stability and feeding optimization. After these important issues are addressed, the remainder of the initial management plan in the first 3 to 4 months of age includes audiologic evaluation, ear-nose-throat evaluation for middle ear abnormalities, and possible orthodontic evaluation for the use of presurgical orthopedics. Surgical management follows with lip repair at 3 to 4 months, and palate repair at around 1 year. Speech evaluation and therapy with or without possible surgical management of velopharyngeal insufficiency are performed in children between 2 and 4 years of age. In late childhood and during the teen years, alveolar bone grafting, lip and nose revisions, orthodontics, and orthognathic surgery follow on an as-needed basis. Care is usually coordinated through a multidisciplinary cleft team (plastic surgeon, speech therapist, audiologist, otolaryngologist, oral surgeon, dentist, orthodontist, nurse, and social worker or psychologist) following the guidelines of the American Cleft Palate-Craniofacial Association. Children with clefts are evaluated annually and, in many instances, until their management plan is completed in their late teens or early twenties. The goal of management is to achieve normal function, characterized by normal occlusion, speech, and hearing with as normal growth as possible, as well as optimal form, characterized by normal lip, nose, and facial aesthetics.[22]

Fetal Surgery

Much consideration has been given to repair of diagnosed cleft lips in utero, given the potential for a scarless repair and the potential for the prevention of many of the dentoalveolar and facial growth abnormalities that follow normal cleft surgery. In scarless fetal wounds, collagen is deposited in an organized, fine reticular pattern, whereas in postnatal scarring, wounds have thick and disorganized collagen matrices.[23] However exciting this procedure may sound, it is a topic of much debate, and enthusiasm should be tempered, given the intrinsic risks of premature labor and death to the mother and fetus.[24] In addition, although an invisible scar is possible to obtain, numerous anatomic elements would remain out of position, rendering the residual lip with an unnatural appearance. Currently, fetal cleft surgery is a novel concept, with no current safety and ethical standards available for clinical utility. More important than consideration of fetal surgery, if a diagnosis of cleft lip or palate is made prenatally, then appropriate consultation should be made to specialists, including those in plastic surgery, otolaryngology, genetics, and nursing, to provide appropriate council for what is to be expected postnatally.

Early Management

Feeding

The cleft-team nurse is usually the feeding expert and will monitor the nutritional status of the infant carefully to ensure adequate caloric intake. Other feeding specialists may include occupational therapists, lactation consultants, or speech therapists. Neonates with a cleft of the primary palate (lip and alveolar ridge) can

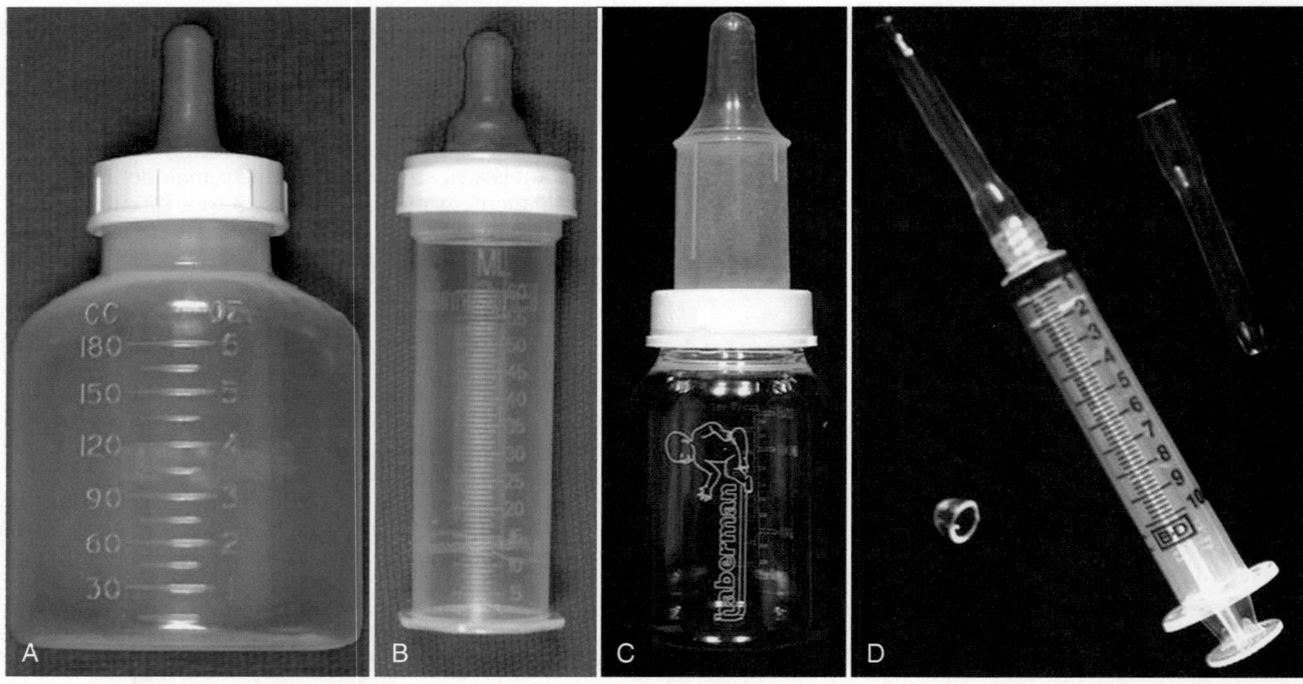

Figure 248-4 Cleft feeding bottles (from left to right: Mead-Johnson nurser, Pigeon feeder, Haberman feeder, Breck feeder [syringe]).

usually feed using a regular bottle or breastfeed without significant difficulty. Infants with a cleft of the secondary palate (hard and soft palate), however, usually require special bottles, which do not require the child to create a suction seal. These special bottles include the Haberman feeder (Medela), the Pigeon nurser (Respironics), or the Mead Johnson nurser. In some cases the infant may have to be fed with a syringe (Breck feeder) or nasogastric tube. Figure 248-4 illustrates the common cleft palate bottles used.

In addition, an infant with a cleft of the secondary palate is unlikely to be able to breastfeed because of the inability to create adequate suction. If the mother wishes to attempt breastfeeding, then a lactation consultant with experience in cleft feeding should be consulted. The infant should be monitored closely by the primary care physician, cleft-team nurse, and surgeon, with frequent weight checks. Receiving human milk is desirable for the infant, even if by bottle. To this end, supporting the mother is important, which involves a lactation consultant if necessary and providing a hospital-grade breast pump (Medela).

Many centers fit their infants with a cleft of the secondary palate with a feeding plate that is custom fabricated by the dentist or orthodontist (Figure 248-5). The feeding plate obturates the hard palate cleft, allowing infants to use their tongues to milk the nipple on the roof of the mouth and to decrease nasal regurgitation and irritation.

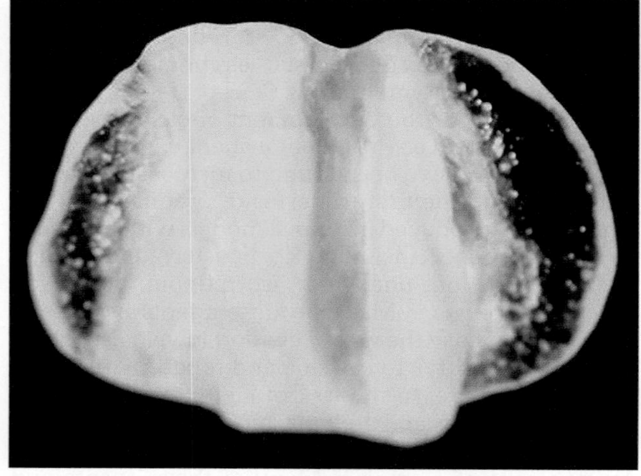

Figure 248-5 Feeding plate.

Auditory Dysfunction

Children with a cleft of the secondary palate (but not a cleft of the lip and alveolus alone) have a high incidence (90%) of middle ear disease, which is believed to be caused by eustachian tube dysfunction. This condition is due to abnormal muscular orientation, resulting in limited drainage of the middle ear through the eustachian tube and potentially causing conductive hearing loss (50%). These patients are monitored closely for middle ear effusion and hearing impairment and are almost universally treated with myringotomy tubes to prevent chronic hearing loss and cholesteatoma, which occurred with great frequency in the past. Even a mild hearing loss of

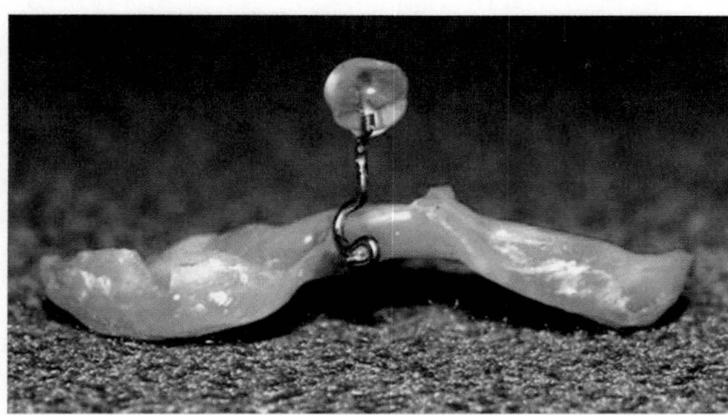

Figure 248-6 Nasoalveolar molding appliance.

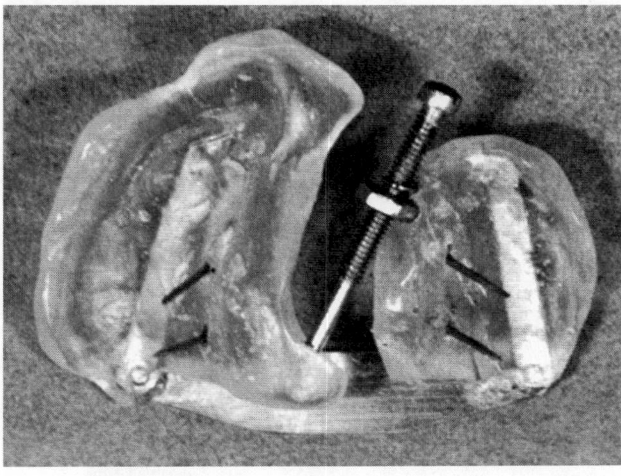

Figure 248-7 Latham appliance.

20 decibels can result in difficulty understanding the spoken word, resulting in speech impairment. Myringotomy tubes are generally placed at around 3 months of age.

Presurgical Orthopedics

Presurgical orthopedics may be passive (nasoalveolar molding appliance, Figure 248-6) or active (Latham appliance, Figure 248-7).[25] The goal of each device is to align the alveolar segments to facilitate the lip repair. Passive nasoalveolar molding has become many centers' standard of practice whereupon the cleft of the lip is narrowed, the cleft nostril is elevated into a more normal configuration, and the alveolar ridges become aligned. Presurgical orthopedics are performed by a pediatric dentist or orthodontist who monitors the child weekly, progressively modifying the appliance from birth to the time of lip repair as the child grows. Figure 248-8 illustrates the significant nonsurgical correction of the cleft deformity possible before the formal lip and nose repair performed around 3 to 4 months of age.

Cleft Lip and Palate Repair

Primary lip repair is usually performed between 3 and 4 months of age, depending on the optimization of feeding and on the results of presurgical orthopedics. The traditional teaching about the timing of lip repair was the 10-10-10 rule: 10 weeks of age, 10 g of hemoglobin, and weight of 10 pounds. Surgical techniques for lip repair include the rotation advancement repair (Millard) and the less common triangular flap repair (Tennison-Randall). Most cleft surgeons now also perform a primary cleft rhinoplasty at the time of the lip repair, which results in enhanced nasal aesthetic outcomes. In some cases the alveolus may also be repaired at the time of the lip repair (gingivoperiosteoplasty), providing the framework and potential for ossification of the cleft alveolar arch. Some surgeons perform a lip adhesion in the first few weeks of life, before the formal lip repair, which also molds the alveolar ridges, especially when used with a dental plate, in preparation for the definitive lip repair several weeks later.[22] Figures 248-9 and 248-10 illustrate respective images of unilateral and bilateral cleft lip and nose repairs.

Cleft palate repair (palatoplasty) is usually performed in children between 9 and 12 months of age, although protocols vary widely at cleft centers. Repairing the palate around 1 year of age is desirable to maximize normal speech development; however, repairing too early might result in poor maxillary growth. The 2 most common procedures to repair the soft palate are the Furlow double-opposing Z-plasty and the intravelar veloplasty technique of levator muscle reorientation. Various flaps used to repair the hard palate include the von Langenbeck and Veau-Wardill-Kilner techniques.[22]

Further Management

Cleft Palate Speech

Even after palatoplasty, some children will exhibit velopharyngeal insufficiency or incompetence, also known as cleft palate speech, because of either muscular incoordination (as is frequently the case in velocardiofacial syndrome) or a short palate.[26] Speech is formally assessed by a trained speech therapist in children between 18 and 24 months of age to establish a diagnosis of velopharyngeal insufficiency. A diagnosis of velopharyngeal insufficiency is often treated with speech therapy in conjunction with or without surgical management. Techniques most commonly performed include a pharyngeal flap or sphincter pharyngoplasty in children between 3 and 6 years of age. These surgical procedures partly obturate the oronasopharynx, resulting in decreased air escape through the nose, necessitating careful monitoring of the airway.

Lip and Nose Revisions

Intermediate lip and nose revisions are performed as necessary before the child starts school (4 to 5 years of age). A final septorhinoplasty or lip revision, or both, is performed when the children have completed growth, generally in the teen years (14 years for girls, 16 years for boys), at which time the deviated nasal septum and asymmetric nasal bones or lip (or both) are reconstructed.

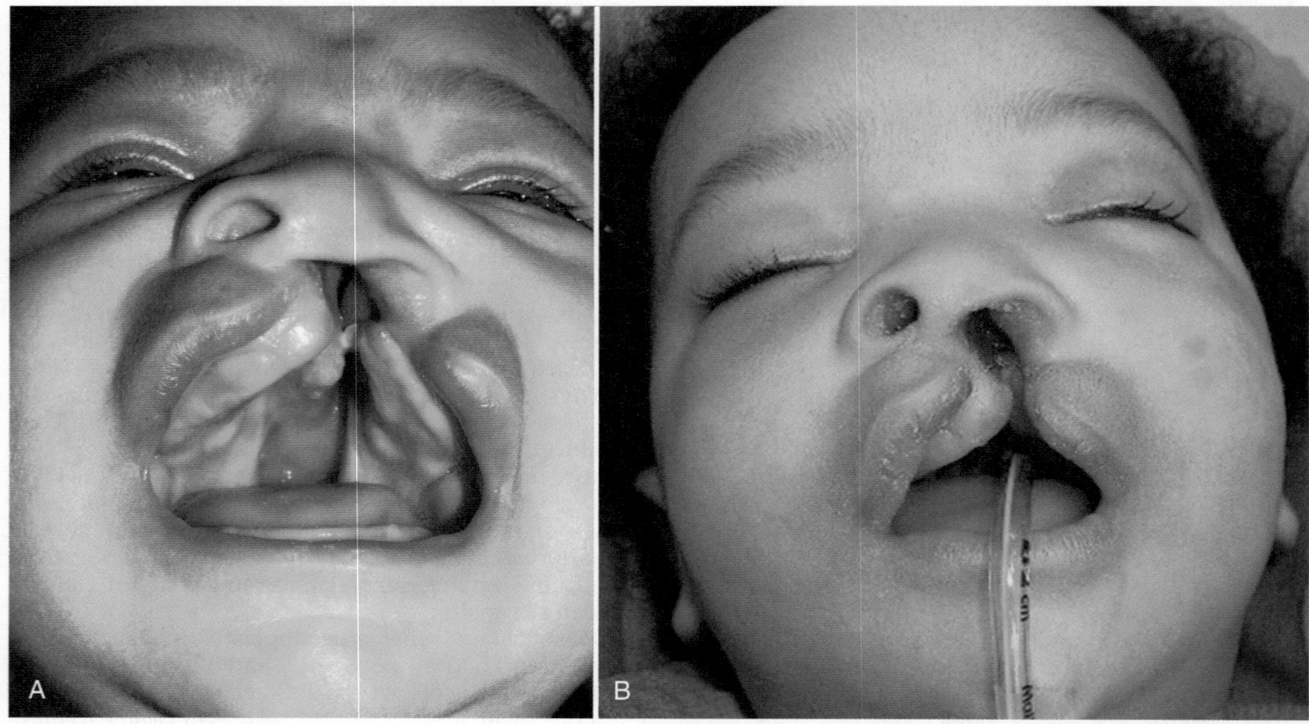

Figure 248-8 **A,** Cleft lip and nose, pre-nasoalveolar molding. **B,** Cleft lip and nose, post-nasoalveolar molding.

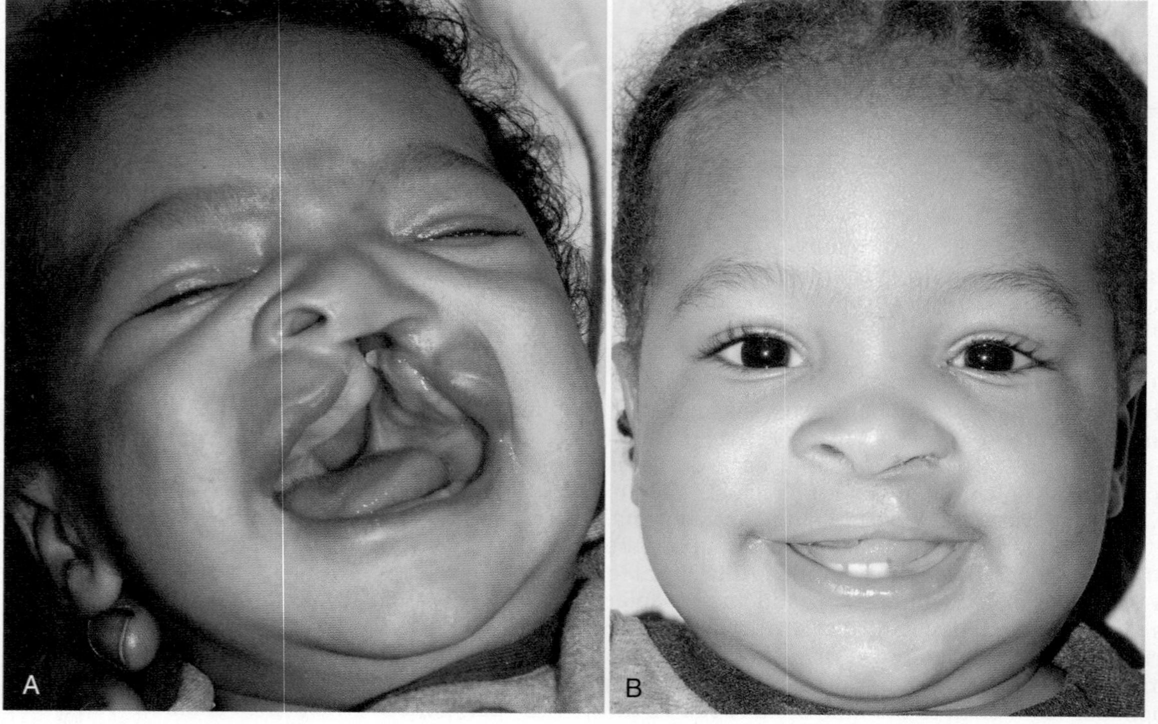

Figure 248-9 **A,** Unilateral cleft lip and nasal deformity, preoperatively. **B,** Unilateral cleft lip and nasal deformity, postoperatively.

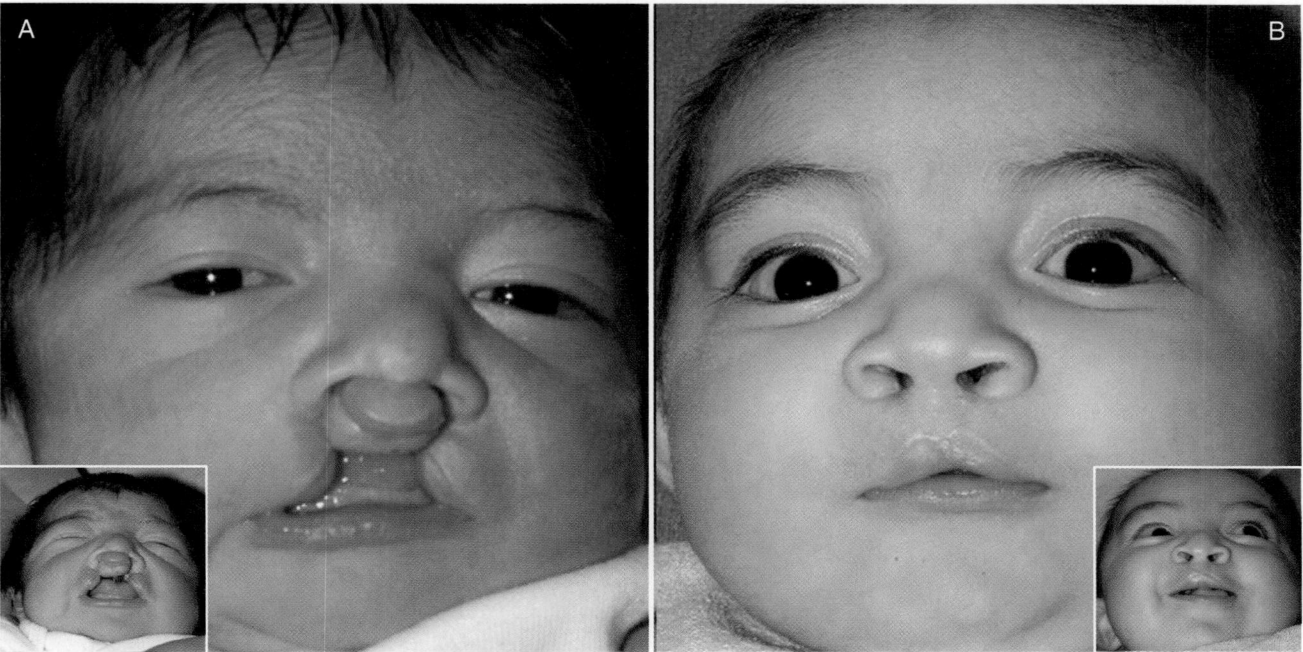

Figure 248-10 **A**, Bilateral cleft lip and nasal deformity, preoperatively. **B**, Bilateral cleft lip and nasal deformity, postoperatively.

Orthodontics/Cleft Alveolus Management

Orthodontics may be started as early as 4 years of age and continue through the teen years. The teeth adjacent to the cleft site may be missing, misshapen, or misaligned. In some cases, teeth may need to be passively molded or even extracted. For patients for whom no gingivoperiosteoplasty was performed or for whom a gingivoperiosteoplasty failed, orthodontics is performed before secondary alveolar bone grafting. This procedure involves the harvest of cancellous bone from the iliac crest and grafted into the alveolar cleft site to allow complete ossification of the alveolar arch and allow eruption of the canine tooth. Some surgeons advocate primary bone grafting in infancy (in which case a small piece of rib is used), although most surgeons perform the alveolar bone graft as needed in children between 7 and 9 years of age during the mixed dentition period.[22]

Orthognathic Surgery

Orthognathic surgery (surgery of the jaws [maxilla, mandible, or both]) is sometimes needed to align the jaws in a normal occlusal relationship. Children with clefts often have maxillary retrusion caused by intrinsic maxillary deficiency or from scarring resulting from the surgical repairs. A maxillary advancement (LeFort I osteotomy, Figure 248-11) may be performed by distraction osteogenesis in school-aged children or via the more traditional advancement osteotomy with rigid titanium plate fixation in the teenage years. In some cases the mandible is set back to meet the maxilla. Factors considered in timing orthognathic surgery include upper airway obstruction, sleep apnea, malocclusion, articulation errors, masticatory problems caused by malocclusion, and the psychosocial effects of facial disharmony. Final prosthodontic care, including dental implants or bridges, may be needed for missing or malformed teeth around the cleft site in the late teenage years.

Pierre Robin Sequence

Pierre Robin sequence (PRS) consists of micrognathia, glossoptosis, upper airway obstruction, with or without cleft palate. An infant with a small mandible and upper airway obstruction should be placed in the prone position to allow the tongue to fall forward out of the pharynx and should be kept on a pulse oximeter to assess the oxygen saturation level in the blood. If this conservative measure is not adequate to alleviate the obstruction and maintain oxygen saturations above 94%, then a nasal trumpet may be placed (12 or 14 French). If necessary, the baby may be bag ventilated with a jaw thrust, nasal trumpet, or oral airway in place and endotracheal or nasotracheal intubation carried out in a controlled environment by the medical staff. If necessary, the tongue may be pulled forward with a piece of gauze between the fingers or, rarely, a towel clamp.

Further work-up for these infants includes a 3-dimensional craniofacial computed tomographic scan to evaluate the size of the mandible and the position of the tongue in the pharynx and to rule out choanal atresia and other anomalies, nasoendoscopy to evaluate the position of the tongue in the pharynx with spontaneous respirations, and direct laryngobronchoscopy to rule out other airway anomalies (laryngomalacia or

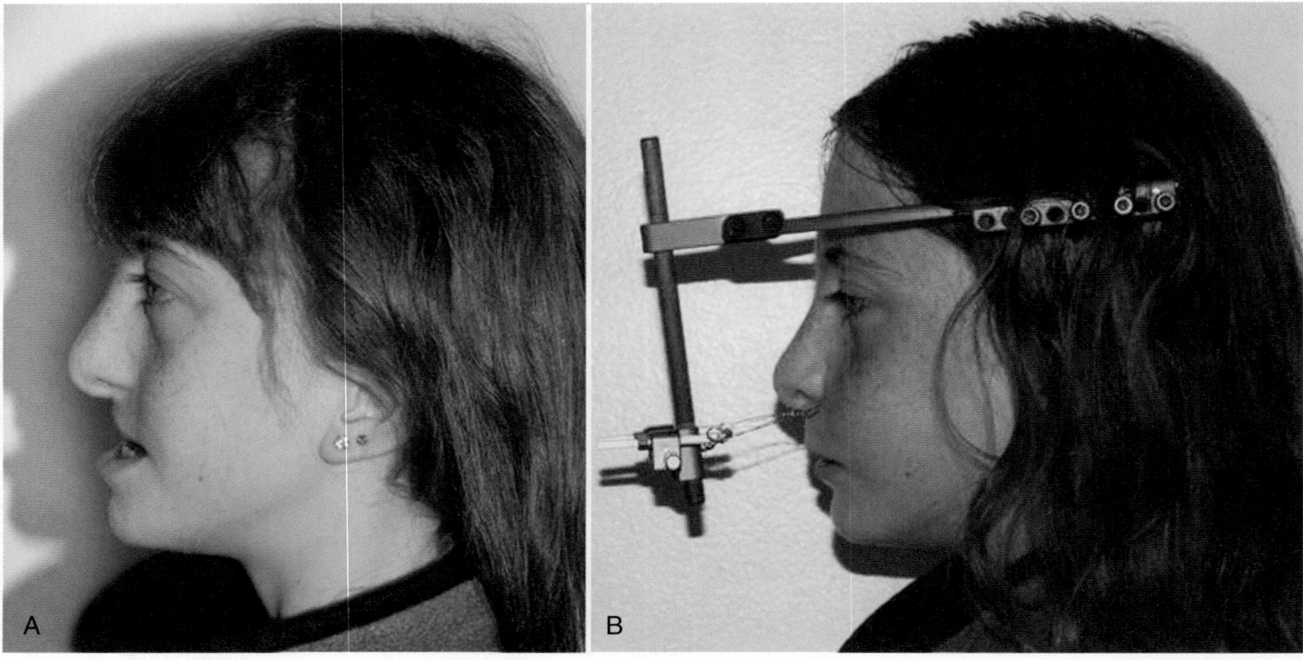

Figure 248-11 **A**, Lefort I distraction osteogenesis, preoperatively. **B**, Lefort I distraction osteogenesis, postoperatively.

tracheomalacia). Infants with PRS may also have gastroesophageal reflux disease and should be evaluated and treated as necessary. A polysomnogram may be performed if the child is stable enough. Newborns with PRS may be unable to feed adequately with a bottle because of their airway obstruction and may have to be fed via nasogastric tube or syringe until more definitive treatment is carried out.

Indications for surgical intervention include continued upper airway obstruction and oxygen desaturation such that the baby cannot be taken out of the prone position, need for nasal trumpet or intubation, an abnormal apnea-hypopnea index on sleep study, inability to be fed with a bottle, and failure to thrive. Surgical interventions include mandibular distraction osteogenesis, tongue-lip adhesion, subperiosteal release of the floor of the mouth, and tracheostomy for the most severe cases.

Mandibular distraction osteogenesis involves lengthening the mandible using either internal or external devices. The mandible is distracted 1.0 to 1.5 mm/day until the mandible is in a normal or overcorrected position and the airway obstruction and feeding difficulties are alleviated. The regenerated bone consolidates within 6 to 8 weeks, and the distractors are removed. Complications include device failure, possible tooth bud damage or inferior alveolar nerve paresis, and poor scar formation. Future growth of the mandible is unknown at this time as distraction osteogenesis does not have a sufficient long-term follow-up.[27]

Tongue-lip adhesion involves suturing a flap of muscle and mucosa from the undersurface of the tongue to a similar flap on the inner surface of the lower lip to prevent tongue base prolapse which results in airway obstruction. Complications include a dehiscence, inability to feed with a bottle, and failure to alleviate the upper airway obstruction. The tongue-lip adhesion is reversed (usually approximately 9 to 12 months of age) to allow normal oral-motor coordination for speech and swallowing, once the mandible has grown sufficiently such that the tongue base no longer obstructs the airway. The cleft palate is repaired during the tongue-lip adhesion reversal operation as well.[28]

CONCLUSIONS

The child with a cleft should be followed up closely from before birth through adulthood by a multidisciplinary team. Successful treatments result in a well-adjusted child with normal facial appearance, dental occlusion, speech, and hearing.

WHEN TO REFER

Prenatally
- Refer to plastic surgery, otolaryngology, genetics, and nursing specialists to provide appropriate council for what is to be expected postnatally

From birth until 3 to 4 months of age
- Audiologic evaluation
- Ear-nose-throat evaluation for middle ear disease
- Possible orthodontic evaluation for the use of presurgical orthopedics
- Surgical management follows with lip and nose repair

1 year of age
- Palate repair

3 to 6 years of age

- Speech evaluation and therapy with or without possible surgical management of velopharyngeal insufficiency

Late childhood and teen years

- Alveolar bone grafting as needed
- Lip and nose revisions as needed
- Orthodontics and orthognathic surgery as needed

TOOLS FOR PRACTICE

Medical Decision Support

- *Cleft Lip and Palate* (Web page), National Library of Medicine and National Institutes of Health (www.nlm.nih.gov/medlineplus/cleftlipandpalate.html).

RELATED WEB SITE

- American Cleft Palate-Craniofacial Association (ACPA) (www.acpa-cpf.org/).

REFERENCES

1. Veau V. *Division Palatine*. Paris, France: Masson; 1931.
2. Harkins CS, Berlin A, Hayding RL, et al. A classification of cleft lip and cleft palate. *Plast Reconstr Surg*. 1962;29:31-39.
3. Kernahan DA. The striped Y—a symbolic classification for cleft lips and palates. *Plast Reconstr Surg*. 1971;47:469-470.
4. Millard DR. Classification. In: Millard DR, ed. *Cleft Craft*. Boston, MA: Little, Brown; 1977.
5. Kriens O. LAHSHAL. A concise documentation system for cleft lip, alveolus, and palate diagnoses. In: Kriens O, ed. *What is a Cleft Lip and Palate? A Multidisciplinary Update*. Stuttgart, Germany: Thieme; 1989.
6. Schwartz S, Kapala JT, Rajchgot H, et al. Accurate and systematic numerical recording system for the identification of various types of lip and maxillary clefts (RPL system). *Cleft Palate Craniofac J*. 1993;30:330-332.
7. Moore KL. *The Developing Human*. 4th ed. Philadelphia, PA: WB Saunders; 1988.
8. Langman J. *Medical Embryology*. 7th ed. Baltimore, MD: Williams and Wilkins; 1995.
9. Thorne CH, Bartlett SP, Beasley RW, et al. *Grabb and Smith's Plastic Surgery*. 5th ed. Philadelphia, PA: Lippincott-Raven; 1997.
10. Ferguson MW. Palate development. *Development*. 1988;103(suppl):41-60.
11. Kaufman FL. Managing the cleft lip and palate patient. *Pediatr Clin North Am*. 1991;38:1127-1147.
12. McCarthy J. *Plastic Surgery*. Philadelphia, PA: WB Saunders; 1990.
13. Neel JV. A study of major congenital defects in Japanese infants. *Am J Hum Genet*. 1958;10:398-445.
14. Bentz MM. *Pediatric Plastic Surgery*. East Norwalk, CT: Appleton and Lange; 1998.
15. Jones MC. Facial clefting. Etiology and developmental pathogenesis. *Clin Plast Surg*. 1993;20:599-606.
16. Hibbert SA, Field JK. Molecular basis of familial cleft lip and palate. *Oral Dis*. 1996;2:238-241.
17. Houdayer C, Bahuau M. Orofacial cleft defects: inference from nature and nurture. *Ann Genet*. 1998;41:89-117.
18. Johnston MC, Millicovsky G. Normal and abnormal development of the lip and palate. *Clin Plast Surg*. 1985;12:521-532.
19. Georgiade B. *Textbook of Plastic, Maxillofacial, and Reconstructive Surgery*. 2nd ed. Philadelphia, PA: Lippincott Williams and Wilkins; 1992.
20. Blumenfeld Z, Blumenfeld I, Bronshtein M. The early prenatal diagnosis of cleft lip and the decision making process. *Cleft Palate Craniofac J*. 1999;36:105-107.
21. Kazan-Tannus JF, Levine D, McKenzie C, et al. Real-time magnetic resonance imaging aids prenatal diagnosis of isolated cleft palate. *J Ultrasound Med*. 2005;24:1533-1540.
22. Kirschner RE, LaRossa D. Cleft lip and palate. *Otolaryngol Clin North Am*. 2000;33:1191-1215.
23. Lorenz HP, Longaker MT. In utero surgery for cleft lip/palate: minimizing the "ripple effect" of scarring. *J Craniofac Surg*. 2003;14:504-511.
24. Millard DR Jr. Clefts, past, present, and future. *Clin Plast Surg*. 1993;20:597-598.
25. Grayson BH, Cutting CB. Presurgical nasoalveolar orthopedic molding in primary correction of the nose, lip, and alveolus of infants born with unilateral and bilateral clefts. *Cleft Palate Craniofac J*. 2001;38:193-198.
26. Conley SF, Gosain AK, Marks SM, et al. Identification and assessment of velopharyngeal inadequacy. *Am J Otolaryngol*. 1997;18:38-46.
27. Denny AD. Distraction osteogenesis in Pierre Robin neonates with airway obstruction. *Clin Plast Surg*. 2004;31:221-229.
28. Schaefer RB, Stadler JA 3rd, Gosain AK. To distract or not to distract: an algorithm for airway management in isolated Pierre Robin sequence. *Plast Reconstr Surg*. 2004;113:1113-1125.

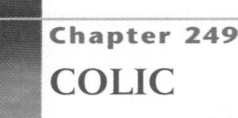

Chapter 249 COLIC

Rebecca A. Baum, MD

Few events are more overwhelming than bringing a newborn baby home from the hospital. Parents are often filled with excitement, exhaustion, and uncertainty. Imagine the parents' reaction when, once home, their infant begins to experience bouts of inconsolable crying and seemingly cannot be soothed despite their best efforts. This scenario forms the basis for the following review on colic.

DEFINITIONS

All babies cry, but what is *normal?* In 1962, Brazelton[1] surveyed mothers being cared for in a pediatric practice and showed that healthy newborns experienced a similar pattern of crying. Crying began to increase during the second week of age, peaked at 6 weeks, and decreased in frequency and duration thereafter. At their peak, these healthy babies cried for nearly 3 hours per day, and the episodes of crying often clustered in the evening. Infants with colic show a similar pattern, but their symptoms are more dramatic than in babies without colic.

The most widely used definition of colic was first put forth by Wessel et al,[2] who noted that *seriously fussy* babies cried for more than 3 hours a day, more than 3 days a week, and for longer than 3 weeks. Today this situation is referred to as the *rule of threes*. Wessel et al characterized the infants' symptoms as "unexplained paroxysms of irritability, fussing, or crying which may develop into agonized screaming. The infant may draw up his knees against his tense abdomen as if there were abdominal pain."[2] Similar to the pattern described by Brazelton, babies with colic tend to have more bouts of crying in the evening hours, when families are more stressed and pressed for time. The chronicity of symptoms follows the typical crying curve, starting in the second week, peaking at 6 weeks, and often resolving by 4 months of age.[3] The similarity in the crying patterns between babies with and without colic suggests that colic may represent the upper end of the continuum of *normal* crying.[4]

Especially frustrating for parents is the fact that babies with colic may seem inconsolable during these periods of crying. The infant may continue to cry despite various interventions such as feeding, diaper changes, and soothing techniques. Continued crying can lead to feelings of inadequacy, anxiety, and frustration for parents and caregivers. Parents often perceive their infant to be in pain and may attribute excessive gas as a potential cause of the infant's distress. Rather, gas is likely a result of swallowed air caused by excessive crying and not the primary cause of the infant's symptoms.[5]

The exact cause of colic remains elusive. A number of theories exist, including food allergy, gastrointestinal tract immaturity, parental stress, and infant temperament.[6] Whatever the cause, colic is extremely common, affecting nearly 20% of babies.[7]

DIFFERENTIAL DIAGNOSIS

One of the most salient features of the infant with colic is that the child is an otherwise healthy baby. Because crying in the newborn can be a hallmark of a myriad of other disease processes, these must be excluded before a diagnosis of colic is made.

Some common disorders can be characterized by excessive crying. The diagnosis of gastroesophageal reflux disease (GERD) may be suggested by episodes of fussiness. Fussy periods for the baby with GERD are often accompanied by emesis and typically occur soon after feeding. Milk protein intolerance can produce excessive crying but is often accompanied by diarrhea or hematochezia. Infants born to mothers who have used alcohol or other drugs during the pregnancy can be excessively fussy.

Other acute processes must be excluded. Such entities include corneal abrasion or hair tourniquet. Acute abdominal processes such as volvulus, intussusception, or an incarcerated hernia may produce irritability and constitute a medical emergency. Symptoms such as anorexia or vomiting may be present. Infectious processes such as otitis media, urinary tract infection, and meningitis are often accompanied by fever. Inflicted injuries such as fractures and intracranial bleeding must also be considered. These disorders typically exhibit persistent, rather than paroxysmal, symptoms.

EVALUATION

History

A complete history is one of the clinician's most important diagnostic tools in the evaluation of colic. The colicky baby is fussy, and parents may complain of excessive gas, crying, and concern that the infant is in pain. The clinician must understand when these symptoms began, how often they occur, during what part of the day, and for how long. The chronicity and pattern of the symptoms is important. Parents can be asked what types of methods they have tried to reduce the symptoms and what, if anything, seems to help. The clinician can use this opportunity to understand how the parent responds to the infant when the baby is in distress.

The clinician should inquire about any concerns during the pregnancy, such as maternal drug use or infections. Family history includes a focus on metabolic or allergic disorders.[6] Social factors are important. Parental anxiety regarding real or perceived health concerns can affect their tolerance for *normal* infant crying. Understanding who in the family is responsible for caregiving and the types of supports available to the family is crucial.

The review of systems should be tailored to exclude signs and symptoms of organic illness such as fever, lethargy, vomiting, diarrhea, or hematochezia. A review of feeding techniques is important. For the formula-fed infant, care must be taken to ensure that the formula is mixed properly and that the baby is not being under- or overfed. For breastfed infants, the clinician should assess the mother's supply of milk and review how often and for how long the baby is fed.

Physical Examination

The physical examination generally serves to exclude pathological abnormalities and will in most cases be normal. The clinician should perform a complete physical examination that focuses on the exclusion of organic causes of irritability. The infant will appear well, and parents may be frustrated that their overly fussy baby is quietly participating in the physical examination. Acute abdominal processes, hair tourniquet around fingers or toes, and otitis media will be excluded by a thorough physical examination. Attention must be paid to adequate growth in weight, length, and head circumference, and these parameters should be plotted on the growth chart. Poor growth suggests inadequate nutrition or other organic causes. Increasing head circumference may raise concerns for hydrocephalus, including causes resulting from child abuse.

Laboratory Evaluation

Laboratory testing is seldom indicated in the evaluation of colic. In most cases the diagnosis can be made by a complete history and thorough physical examination. Laboratory testing is most often reserved for cases in which an organic cause is suspected. Unnecessary laboratory testing should be avoided unless clinically indicated because it may convey to parents the message that the baby is ill.

MANAGEMENT

The management of colic primarily involves parental education and support. Foremost, the clinician must help the parents understand that their baby is not sick and that the baby's excessive crying is not harmful. The baby's normal growth and physical examination can be used to help illustrate this point. Parents should be reassured about their abilities as caregivers and that they are not to blame for their baby's symptoms. Clinicians should acknowledge the parents' frustration and let them know that the office will provide the family with support. Rather than informing the parents that colic may take months to resolve, clinicians should remain positive and let parents know that some simple interventions will likely help alleviate the problem.

Parents can be encouraged to respond to their baby's fussiness with a predictable set of actions; having a plan to use during these fussy periods can be particularly reassuring. After first making sure that the baby is not hungry, soiled, or tired, parents can then try to soothe the baby by encouraging nonnutritive sucking, swaddling, or gentle motions such as rocking or swinging. When crying continues despite these interventions, parents should be given permission to allow the infant to cry for a short period. This approach can allow parents to regroup and also provides the baby with some time to blow off steam. When conceptualized in these terms, parents may feel less anxious about the infant's continued crying. The pediatric office can provide families with support by offering a telephone contact in a few days to follow up on the infant's symptoms. Especially anxious parents can be offered an office visit within 1 week. Last, parents should be encouraged to take care of themselves, get adequate rest, and enlist family members or friends to take over from time to time to reduce caregiver stress.

Few medical interventions have proven helpful for colic. If indicated by history, a brief dietary change to a hypoallergenic formula or an elimination diet for breastfeeding mothers can be considered. Treatment for GERD can be instituted for infants with symptoms that suggest reflux. Pharmacologic therapies specific for colic have largely been found to be unhelpful and possibly harmful. Simethicone, a drug with few side effects, is not effective in symptom reduction.[8] Dicyclomine, an anticholinergic drug, is effective; however, the manufacturer has advised against its use in children younger than 6 months because of case reports of adverse effects in infants.[9] An herbal tea mixture of chamomile, vervain, licorice, fennel, and balm-mint has been shown to be effective, but the large volume of fluid (120 mL taken three times a day) might cause potential harm, such as hyponatremia or decreased milk intake.[5]

The prognosis for babies with colic is reassuring. For most babies, the symptoms of colic decrease dramatically by 4 months of age. Parents may be encouraged to know that the presence of colic as an infant does not necessarily predict a more difficult temperament as an older baby.[10] Despite this favorable prognosis, care must be taken to support parents until they feel more comfortable managing their child's symptoms. Excessive parental anxiety and frustration may lead to later parent-child interaction problems, such as prolonged night waking, overfeeding, or the vulnerable child syndrome.[4]

Education on infant crying is important for caregivers of all newborns. Most parents are surprised to learn that *healthy* babies cry for as long as they do. Clinicians can highlight the temperamental differences between healthy babies, with some being fussier than others. Excessive crying may be a stimulus for shaken baby syndrome.[11] The Period of PURPLE Crying program, developed by the National Center on Shaken Baby Syndrome, is aimed at parental education to help reduce the incidence of shaken baby syndrome. The mnemonic PURPLE is used to remind parents of the characteristics of infant crying: P for the peak pattern, U for the unexpected timing of episodes, R for resistance to soothing, P for pain-like look, L for long bouts, and E for the evening cluster of symptoms.

WHEN TO REFER

Babies with colic seldom require a referral to a specialist. In rare cases, referral to specialists in developmental or behavioral pediatrics or mental health may be useful when parents are extremely anxious or in need of additional reassurance. Clinicians should be alert for the parent who is overwhelmed by the infant's crying and in danger of harming the infant. In such a case, referral to children's services is necessary for the protection of the infant and support of the parent.

WHEN TO ADMIT

In most cases, colic can be successfully managed in the outpatient setting. In rare situations when the history is confusing or suggests more serious symptoms, admission might be useful for observation to exclude other causes of irritability.

SUGGESTED RESOURCES

Barr RG. Colic and crying syndromes in infants. *Pediatrics.* 1998;102:e1282.

Garrison MM, Christakis DA. A systematic review of treatments for infant colic. *Pediatrics.* 2000;106:184-190.

Levine MD, Carey WB, Crocker AC, eds. *Developmental-Behavioral Pediatrics.* 3rd ed. Philadelphia, PA: WB Saunders; 1999.

REFERENCES

1. Brazelton TB. Crying in infancy. *Pediatrics.* 1962;29: 579-588.
2. Wessel MA, Cobb JC, Jackson EB, et al. Paroxysmal fussing in infancy, sometimes called "colic." *Pediatrics.* 1954; 14:421-435.
3. Barr RG. Colic and crying syndromes in infants. *Pediatrics.* 1998;102:e1282.
4. Levine MD, Carey WB, Crocker AC, eds. *Developmental-Behavioral Pediatrics.* 3rd ed. Philadelphia, PA: WB Saunders; 1999.
5. Fireman L, Serwint J. Colic. *Pediatr Rev.* 2006;27:357-358.
6. Algranati PS, Dworkin PH. Infancy problem behaviors. *Pediatr Rev.* 1992;13:16-22.
7. Hide DW, Guyer BM. Prevalence of infant colic. *Arch Dis Child.* 1982;57:559-560.
8. Wade S, Kilgour T. Infantile colic. *BMJ.* 2001;323:437-440.

9. Garrison MM, Christakis DA. A systematic review of treatments for infant colic. *Pediatrics.* 2000;106:184-190.
10. Lehtonen L, Korhonen T, Korvenranta H. Temperament and sleeping pattern in infantile colic during the first year of life. *J Dev Behav Pediatr.* 1994;15:416-420.
11. Barr R, Trent R, Cross J. Age-related incidence curve of hospitalized shaken baby syndrome cases: convergent evidence for crying as a trigger to shaking. *Child Abuse Negl* 2006;30:7-16.

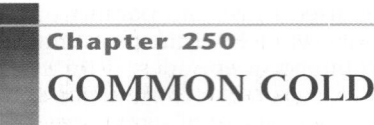

Chapter 250

COMMON COLD

Howard Fischer, MD

Colds are viral infections of the upper respiratory tract, and the mucosal surfaces that are lined with respiratory epithelium are involved. Thus nasal passages, sinuses, eustachian tubes, middle ear spaces, conjunctivae, and the nasopharynx are potentially affected. The distribution of this illness is worldwide, and adults and children of all ethnic groups are susceptible. Colds are most common in preschool children, who average 6 to 8 colds per year, a number that is approximately 4 times the number expected in adults. Children who attend child care centers or who are exposed to other school-aged children tend to have more colds than children who spend most of their time at home.[1] Frequent infection in the preschool years might lower the frequency of colds in the school years.[2]

EPIDEMIOLOGIC FEATURES

Colds have always tended to occur more frequently during the cooler months in temperate climates, probably leading to the popular myth that exposure to cold weather leads to a cold. Fortunately the common cold has been researched extensively in the last few decades, allowing primary care physicians to have a more scientific understanding of this illness. In fact, in the northern hemisphere the incidence of colds peaks in early fall, remains high during the winter, and decreases in the spring.[1] Studies have shown that exposure to a cold environment neither causes a cold nor decreases immunity that may potentially allow a viral infection to begin. Clearly, however, colds are more frequent in crowded situations, and evidence suggests that the infection begins most commonly after self-inoculation of a virus onto the individual's own nasal or conjunctival mucosa.[3]

Because the viruses of infected individuals are shed in large numbers in nasal secretions, they can be spread easily by way of fingers and hands to objects such as clothing or environmental surfaces, where fingers of other children can acquire them and then self-inoculate their respiratory tracts by picking their noses or rubbing their eyes. Inhalation of virus-containing aerosols is also an effective means of virus acquisition.[4] Studies in adult populations have shown that colds are more likely to develop after inoculation by rhinovirus in persons who are under chronic stress; whether this likelihood is the case in children is not known.[5]

ETIOLOGY

More than 100 different infectious agents can cause cold symptoms, with rhinoviruses and small RNA viruses of the picornavirus family implicated most frequently. In addition to many rhinovirus serotypes, other viruses and a few nonviral organisms are associated with the common cold (Table 250-1). Although respiratory syncytial virus and parainfluenza viruses most commonly cause a croupy cough and bronchiolitis in infants, they may cause a cold in older children and adults. Adenoviruses and enteroviruses tend to cause other symptoms in addition to those of a common cold, including pharyngitis and gastrointestinal problems.

PATHOPHYSIOLOGICAL FEATURES

Once a cold-causing virus is introduced into the host's respiratory tract, assuming no immunity exists to the particular serotype, a local infection usually begins after an incubation period, the length of which depends on the specific virus. However, not all people who have a viral respiratory tract infection (defined as evidence of viral shedding and an increase in antibody titers) develop symptoms of a cold. In one study, only 75% of

Table 250-1 Causative Agents of Colds

AGENT	RELATIVE IMPORTANCE	PEAK SEASON
Rhinovirus	Most frequent cause	Autumn
Coronavirus	Frequent cause	Winter
Influenza virus	Less frequent cause	Winter
Respiratory syncytial virus	Less frequent cause	Winter
Parainfluenza virus	Less frequent cause	Autumn and spring
Enterovirus	Occasional cause	All seasons
Mycoplasma pneumoniae	Occasional cause	All seasons
Metapneumovirus	Unknown	Autumn and winter

Modified from Heikkinen T, Järvinen A. The common cold. *Lancet* 2003; 361: 51-59; Welliver RC. The common cold. In: Long SS, Pickering LK, Prober CG, eds. *Principles and Practice of Pediatric Infectious Diseases.* New York, NY: Churchill Livingstone; 1997; Esper F, Boucher D, Weibel C, et al. Human metapneumovirus infection in the United States: clinical manifestations associated with a newly emerging respiratory infection in children. *Pediatrics* 2003;111:1407-1410.

experimentally infected adults who shed rhinovirus type 2 and developed a greater than 4-fold rise in antibody titers actually developed symptoms.[6] The symptoms of a cold are related primarily to the host's production of interleukin-8 and other vasoactive peptides in response to the viral infection,[7] resulting in increased vascular permeability and mucus hypersecretion.[8]

CLINICAL PRESENTATION

Infants may begin their illnesses with fever; an older child, however, is usually afebrile, with a stuffy nose and watery nasal discharge, followed in a few days by sneezing. Generalized symptoms such as headache, malaise, and myalgia are uncommon with a rhinovirus infection, although they are seen in adenoviral and other viral infections. Infants tend to be irritable, have changes in feeding and sleep patterns, and sometimes develop mild diarrhea. By the 3rd or 4th day of the illness, a dry cough may be present, and the nasal discharge usually becomes more purulent. Although such purulence has been interpreted in the past as indicating a secondary bacterial infection (eg, sinusitis), little evidence is available to support this impression. Of adults who had colds and sinus abnormalities on computed tomographic scan, only 2% developed bacterial sinusitis.[9] Furthermore, examination of purulent secretions has not shown increased aerobic bacterial growth or sloughing of nasal epithelial cells,[10] and biopsies in volunteers demonstrate only loss of cilia and ciliated cells.[11] Although viral sinusitis is a common finding during a cold, progression to bacterial sinusitis is probably quite rare in children.[12]

Generally the symptoms of a cold last approximately a week; however, a child may occasionally have mild rhinorrhea and a dry cough for 2 to 3 weeks. The cilia necessary for proper function of the respiratory epithelium may take as long as 3 weeks to return to their normal state,[11] thus delaying the return to a symptom-free condition.

DIFFERENTIAL DIAGNOSIS

Persistent nasal symptoms can also be caused by allergy. For allergies to be diagnosed initially as colds and later recognized as seasonal or associated with nasal eosinophilia is not uncommon.[13] Cold symptoms associated with significant pharyngitis, rashes, or other systemic symptoms are usually caused by viruses other than those causing the common cold. Streptococcal pharyngitis is not usually associated with rhinorrhea or cough.

Occasionally a persistent purulent nasal discharge in children younger than 2 years results from a beta-hemolytic streptococcal infection, although this condition is usually associated with mild excoriations around the nares. Unilateral nasal discharge must also be evaluated carefully to rule out a nasal foreign body. Finally, irritation and swelling of the nasal passages from inhalation of drugs such as cocaine or the chronic use of medicated nasal sprays should be considered in the older child who has persistent cold symptoms. The possibility of infection with *Bordetella pertussis* should be considered in a child with persistent cough.[14] Children who have been partially immunized may not have a characteristic whoop associated with *B pertussis* infection.

MANAGEMENT

Laboratory Procedures

No routine tests exist to diagnose the common cold. Viral cultures are expensive and generally unnecessary; thus the diagnosis should be made on clinical grounds. The most common concern is that an underlying bacterial infection (eg, sinusitis, acute otitis media) is missed or treated improperly. If a cold follows its expected course of causing usual symptoms for 5 to 7 days, then a concurrent bacterial infection is unlikely. When the symptoms of a cold are prolonged, a secondary infection may be present, especially if fever persists or is prominent or if ear pain or a productive cough develops. Thus ear and lung examinations are essential for a child whose cold has persisted longer than expected. The routine use of radiographs or computed tomographic scans to diagnose sinusitis is not necessary because when studied (albeit in older individuals) the radiologic finding of opacification of the sinuses has not correlated with the clinical indications of sinusitis.[15]

Treatment

The various remedies available for the common cold provide—at best—symptomatic rather than curative treatment. In children, most of the remedies give only marginal symptomatic relief, if any; in many cases, they are potentially quite harmful.[16] Over-the-counter cough and cold medications should not be used in children younger than 2 years because serious and potentially life-threatening side effects can occur from their use.[17] Furthermore, studies have shown that these medications are generally ineffective in children younger than 6 years. Most pediatricians, at most, suggest saline nose drops with the use of a bulb syringe to aspirate secretions and a cool-mist vaporizer to humidify room air.[18] The malaise and fever sometimes associated with a cold can be treated with acetaminophen or ibuprofen; aspirin should be avoided in children because of its association with Reye syndrome. Some studies suggest that ibuprofen may be more beneficial during a cold than acetaminophen because it leads to a shorter period of viral shedding and a better neutralizing antibody response.[6]

Studies conducted on preschoolers have not demonstrated a beneficial effect of decongestants or antihistamines, singly or in combination.[19,20] In older children and adolescents, an oral decongestant such as pseudoephedrine hydrochloride, either alone or with an antihistamine (probably owing to antihistamine's anticholinergic effect), provides symptomatic relief with a low possibility of side effects. The use of nasal spray or drops containing vasoconstrictors such as oxymetazoline hydrochloride should be discouraged because of the high incidence of rebound nasal congestion after only a few days of use. Although studies in adults indicate some decrease in symptoms when steroid or atropine-like nasal sprays are used, their use in children has not been evaluated.[12,21] The use of mast-cell stabilizers such as nedocromil and sodium cromoglycate given intranasally or by inhalation has shown some promise in adult studies.[22] Their place in pediatric care is not clear.

The use of zinc lozenges to reduce the duration of cold symptoms has been studied extensively in adults in recent years with conflicting results. Despite at least

8 placebo-controlled trials and several reviews of these studies, the efficacy of zinc lozenges remains controversial.[23] Studies of potential antirhinoviral drugs are still too preliminary to judge their therapeutic potential.[21] Many parents will ask about the advisability of giving vitamin C during a cold, and many will request that the physician prescribe antibiotics. Vitamin C use has not been proven efficacious, and both should be discouraged.[24] Discouraging antibiotic use is particularly important when bacterial infection is unlikely, given current evidence of the increasing drug resistance among some bacterial pathogens.

Because of the lack of effective treatment for the common cold, parents may turn to alternative treatments. A commonly used cold treatment is an extract of the plant *Echinacea*. A recent randomized clinical trial showed no benefit to the use of extract of *Echinacea purpura* in treating children 2 to 11 years of age at the onset of their colds.[25] Similarly, a randomized clinical trial in adults using *E angustifolia* extract showed no benefit in treating experimental rhinovirus infection.[26]

COMPLICATIONS

Most colds are self-limited and resolve without the help of the physician or of any medication. When a fever arises 3 to 4 days after cold symptoms begin or symptoms continue longer than expected, a complication such as otitis media or pneumonia should be suspected. A cold can apparently contribute to eustachian tube dysfunction, especially in younger children, resulting in acute otitis media. A fever, headache, and unilateral purulent nasal discharge may herald a secondary bacterial sinusitis, although this condition is probably diagnosed more frequently than it occurs. On rare occasions a lower respiratory tract infection develops and may progress to pneumonia, characterized by cough, tachypnea, and usually fever. The pneumonia may have a viral origin or may be caused by a secondary bacterial infection.[27,28] Chest radiograph can confirm the diagnosis.

The role of rhinovirus infection as a trigger of exacerbation of reactive airway disease has now been well documented[29]; thus the development of wheezing or a prolonged cough after a cold should alert the clinician to this possibility.

TOOLS FOR PRACTICE

Engaging Patient and Family

- *Get Smart: Know When Antibiotics Work* (Web page), Centers for Disease Control and Prevention (www.cdc.gov/drugresistance/community/index.htm).
- *Respiratory Syncytial Virus (RSV)* (brochure), American Academy of Pediatrics (patiented.aap.org).
- *Sinusitis and Your Child* (brochure), American Academy of Pediatrics (patiented.aap.org).

Medical Decision Support

- *Common Cold* (Web page), Centers for Disease Control and Prevention (www.cdc.gov/ncidod/dvrd/revb/respiratory/hpivfeat.htm).
- *Red Book* 2006 Report of the Committee on Infectious Diseases (book), American Academy of Pediatrics (www.aap.org/bookstore).

AAP POLICY STATEMENT

American Academy of Pediatrics, Committee on Drugs. Use of codeine- and dextromethorphan-containing cough remedies in children. *Pediatrics*. 1997;99(6):918-920. (aappolicy.aappublications.org/cgi/content/full/pediatrics;99/6/918).

SUGGESTED RESOURCES

American Academy of Pediatrics. Treating coughs and colds. Available at: (www.aap.org/new/kidscolds.htm).

Heikkinen T, Järvinen A. The common cold. *Lancet*. 2003;361:51-59.

REFERENCES

1. Heikkinen T, Järvinen A. The common cold. *Lancet*. 2003;361:51-59.
2. Vesa S, Kleemola M, Blomqvist S, et al. Epidemiology of documented viral respiratory infections and acute otitis media in a cohort of children followed from two to twenty-four months of age. *Pediatr Infect Dis J*. 2001;20:574-581.
3. Hendley JO, Wenzel RP, Gwaltney JM. Transmission of rhinovirus colds by self-innoculation. *N Engl J Med*. 1973;288:1361-1364.
4. Dick EC, Jennings LC, Mink KA, et al. Aerosol transmission of rhinovirus colds. *J Infect Dis*. 1987;156:442-488.
5. Cohen S, Tyrell DAJ, Smith AP. Psychological stress and susceptibility to the common cold. *N Engl J Med*. 1991;325:606-612.
6. Graham NM, Burell CJ, Douglas RM, et al. Adverse effects of aspirin, acetaminophen, and ibuprofen on immune function, viral shedding, and clinical status in rhinovirus-infected volunteers. *J Infect Dis*. 1990;162:1277-1282.
7. Turner RB, Weingand KW, Yeh CH, et al. Association between interleukin-8 concentration in nasal secretions and severity of symptoms of experimental rhinovirus colds. *Clin Infect Dis*. 1998;26:840-846.
8. Yuta A, Doyle WJ, Gaumond E, et al. Rhinovirus infection induces mucus hypersecretion. *Am J Physiol*. 1998;274:L1017-L1023.
9. Gwaltney JM Jr. Acute community acquired bacterial sinusitis: to treat or not to treat. *Can Respir J*. 1999;6(suppl A):46A-50A.
10. Winther B, Kawana R, Saito H. Fireside conference 11: common cold. *Rhinol Suppl*. 1992;14:228-232.
11. Rautianen M, Nuuiten J, Kiukaanniemi, et al. Ultrastructural changes in human nasal cilia caused by the common cold and recovery of ciliated epithelium. *Ann Otol Rhinol Laryngol*. 1992;101:982-987.
12. Puhakka T, Makela MJ, Alanen A, et al. Sinusitis in the common cold. *J Allergy Clin Immunol*. 1998;102:403-408.
13. Huang SW, Kimbrough JW. Mold allergy is a risk factor for persistent cold-like symptoms in children. *Clin Pediatr*. 1997;36:695-699.
14. Cherry JD. The epidemiology of pertussis: a comparison of the epidemiology of the disease pertussis with the epidemiology of Bordetella pertussis infection. *Pediatrics*. 2005;115:1422-1427.
15. Cooke LD, Hadley DM. MRI of the paranasal sinuses: incidental abnormalities and their relationship to symptoms. *J Laryngol Otol*. 1991;105:278-281.
16. Gunn VL, Taha SH, Liebelt EL, et al. Toxicity of over-the-counter cough and cold medications. *Pediatrics*. 2001;108(3):e52.
17. American Academy of Pediatrics. Treating coughs and colds. Available at: (www.aap.org/new/kidscolds.htm).
18. Gadomski A, Horton L. The need for rational therapeutics in the use of cough and cold medicine in infants. *Pediatrics*. 1992;89:774-776.

19. Hutton N, Wilson MH, Mellits ED, et al. Effectiveness of an antihistamine-decongestant combination for young children with the common cold: a randomized, controlled clinical trial. *J Pediatr.* 1991;118:125-130.
20. Smith MB, Feldman W. Over-the-counter cold medications: a critical review of clinical trials between 1950 and 1991. *JAMA.* 1993;269:2258-2263.
21. Hayden FG, Hipskind GJ, Woerner DH, et al. Intranasal pirodavir (R77, 975) treatment of rhinovirus colds. *Antimicrob Agents Chemother.* 1995;39:290-294.
22. Aberg N, Aberg B, Mestig K. The effect of inhaled and intranasal sodium cromoglycate on symptoms of upper respiratory tract infections. *Clin Exp Allergy.* 1996;26:1045-1050.
23. Marshall I. Zinc for the common cold (Cochrane Review). In: *The Cochrane Library.* Issue 2. Oxford, UK: Update Software; 2002.
24. Dowell SF, Schwartz B, Phillips WR. Appropriate use of antibiotics for URIs in children: part II. *Am Fam Physician.* 1998;58:1113-1118, 1123.
25. Taylor JA, Weber W, Standish L, et al. Efficacy and safety of echinacea in treating upper respiratory tract infections in children. *JAMA.* 2003;290:2824-2830.
26. Turner RB, Bauer R, Woelkart K, et al. An evaluation of Echinacea angustifolia in experimental rhinovirus infections. *N Engl J Med.* 2005;353:341-348.
27. Juven T, Mertsola J, Waris M, et al. Etiology of community-acquired pneumonia in 254 hospitalized children. *Pediatr Infect Dis J.* 2000;19:293-298.
28. Heiskanen-Kosma T, Korppi M, Jokinen C, et al. Etiology of childhood pneumonia. Serologic results of a prospective, population-based study. *Pediatr Infect Dis J.* 1998;17:986-991.
29. Busse WW. The role of the common cold in asthma. *J Clin Pharmacol.* 1999;39:241-245.

Chapter 251

CONGENITAL AND ACQUIRED HEART DISEASE

Michael A. McCulloch, MD; Robert J. Gajarski, MD

The initial evaluation, continued care, and timing for referral of children with congenital and acquired heart disease are aided by a basic understanding of cardiac embryology, anatomy, and physiology.

EMBRYOLOGY

Understanding fetal cardiac embryology allows insight into possible sources of error and how these imperfections can lead to clinically significant congenital heart diseases.

The primitive heart starts as a linear tube that begins pulsating in a coordinated fashion to produce forward flow at approximately 17 days postconception[1] and becomes the first functioning organ in the developing embryo. Small invaginations separate the primitive heart into five distinct regions. From caudal to cranial, they are the sinus venosus, primitive atrium, primitive ventricle, bulbus cordis (conus), and truncus arteriosus.[2] These segments ultimately form the cardiac chambers and some of the extracardiac blood vessels.

At approximately 20 to 23 days postconception, the primitive heart segments demonstrate differential rates of growth, resulting in curving or looping of the heart on itself (Figure 251-1).[3] As a result, the sinus venosus and primitive atrium are positioned dorsal and cranial to the primitive ventricle, whereas the bulbus cordis and truncus arteriosus are slightly ventral and cranial. At this stage of development, the individual cardiac segments have experienced very little differentiation. The primitive atrium is a single chamber receiving all blood from the sinus venosus, which is then propelled forward into the primitive ventricle, bulbus cordis, truncus arteriosus, and to the rest of the developing embryo (Figure 251-2).

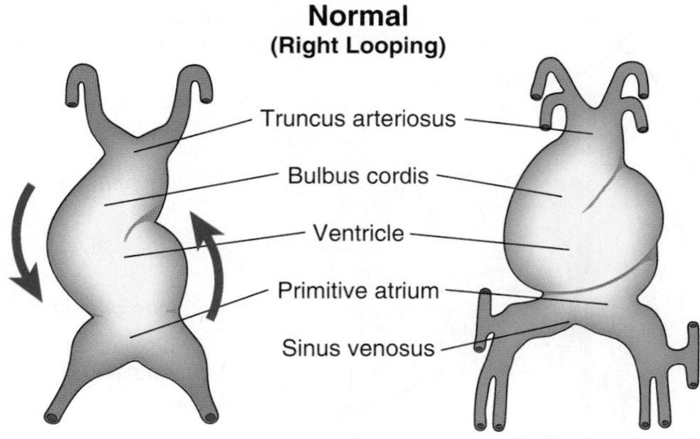

Figure 251-1 Depiction of the embryologic heart tube undergoing normal, rightward looping. The primitive atrium and sinus venosus ultimately change their location from posterior and caudal to dorsal and cephalad. (*Moore KL, Persaud TVN. The cardiovascular system. In: Moore KL, Persaud TVN, eds.* The Developing Human: Clinically Oriented Embryology. *5th ed. Philadelphia, PA: WB Saunders; 1993. Copyright © 1993, Elsevier.*)

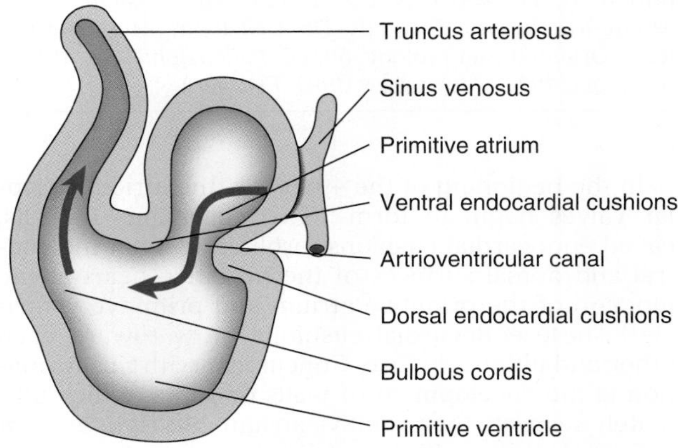

Figure 251-2 Rightward looped embryologic heart sectioned along its sagittal plane. The arrows depict the normal course of blood flow at 20 to 23 days postconception. (*Moore KL, Persaud TVN. The cardiovascular system. In: Moore KL, Persaud TVN, eds.* The Developing Human: Clinically Oriented Embryology. *5th ed. Philadelphia, PA: WB Saunders; 1993. Copyright © 1993, Elsevier.*)

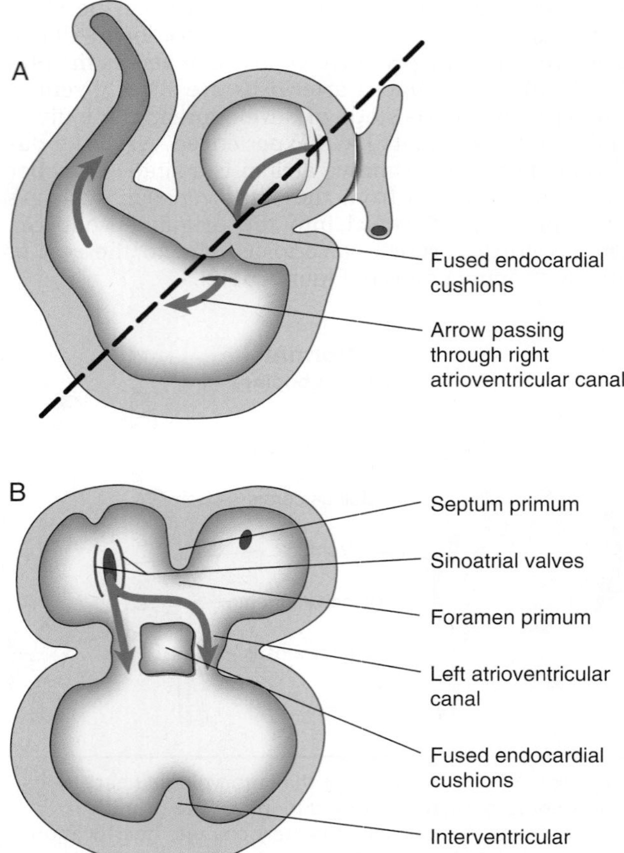

Figure 251-3 Rightward looped embryologic heart sectioned along its coronal plane. Illustration demonstrates fusion of the endocardial cushions and the resulting sites of the future mitral and tricuspid atrioventricular valves. At this stage of development, postconception days 22 to 25, the developing embryologic heart has double-inlet left-ventricle and double-outlet right-ventricle morphology. (*Moore KL, Persaud TVN. The cardiovascular system. In: Moore KL, Persaud TVN, eds.* The Developing Human: Clinically Oriented Embryology. *5th ed. Philadelphia, PA: WB Saunders; 1993. Copyright © 1993, Elsevier.*)

In the beginning of the 4th week, the atrioventricular valves begin to form.[4] Two collections of cells, called endocardial cushions, proliferate from the ventral and dorsal surfaces of the primitive heart at the junction of the primitive atrium and primitive ventricle.[5] These endocardial cushions grow toward each other and ultimately fuse. Concurrent with this formation is the development of walls or septa, which ultimately separate the primitive atrium into right and left atria and the primitive ventricle into the left ventricle and the bulbus cordis into the right ventricle (Figure 251-3). The crux of the heart is formed when the atrial and ventricular septa attach to the fused endocardial cushions, transforming the linear heart tube into four distinct chambers.

While the atrioventricular valves and cardiac septa are being formed, the truncus arteriosus is simultaneously dividing into the primitive aorta and pulmonary artery (Figure 251-4).[6] The aortopulmonary septum is formed when two ingrowths of tissue develop and proliferate toward one another. When they meet in the midline, the truncus arteriosus is divided approximately in half. The caudal end of this septum will ultimately fuse with the region of endocardial cushion and atrioventricular septal connection (Figure 251-5).

Before fusion of the endocardial cushions, aortopulmonary, and atrioventricular septa, all the blood flow from the left and right atria returns directly to the primitive ventricle (future left ventricle), through the bulbo-ventricular foramen to the bulbous cordis (future right ventricle), and ultimately to the truncus arteriosus. The truncus arteriosus then provides blood to the developing pulmonary arteries and aorta. Therefore, at this stage in development, the heart is functionally a double-inlet left ventricle and a double-outlet right ventricle.[7]

The progression from a double-inlet left ventricle and double-outlet right-ventricle heart to a four-chambered heart with separate great arteries to the body and lungs is understandably complex. This process involves migration of the developing atrioventricular valves, with their respective atria, and the truncus arteriosus, with its developing great arteries, toward one another.[7] This relocation of the major heart structures results in the atria and great arteries being positioned directly over their respective ventricles. Final cardiac anatomic form is achieved by approximately 8 weeks postconceptual age and only increases in size until birth.

CONGENITAL DEFECTS

Intracardiac Shunting Lesions

Shunting lesions are heart defects in which a proportion of the blood volume from one side of the heart is added to the blood volume on the other side. Shunting can be from the left side of the heart to the right, the right side of the heart to the left, or bidirectional. The right heart is composed of the systemic veins (inferior vena cava [IVC] and superior vena cava [SVC]), an atrium, a ventricle, and a great artery; generally, these structures are the right atrium, right ventricle, and pulmonary artery, respectively. Conversely, the left heart is composed of the pulmonary veins, an atrium, a ventricle, and a great artery; generally, these structures are the left atrium, left ventricle, and aorta, respectively.

Physiology

The process of *adding* or shunting blood from one side of the heart to the other is regulated by a few basic principles of physics. First, blood flows from a higher pressure or resistance circuit into a lower pressure or resistance circuit. In a normal heart, left-sided pressures are considerably higher than those on the right, and, if given the opportunity, blood will preferentially shunt from left to right. The volume of shunted blood also depends on the size of the defect through which it flows. A very large defect will allow considerably more flow to shunt from the left heart to the right than a small defect. However, even if the defect is large, if the

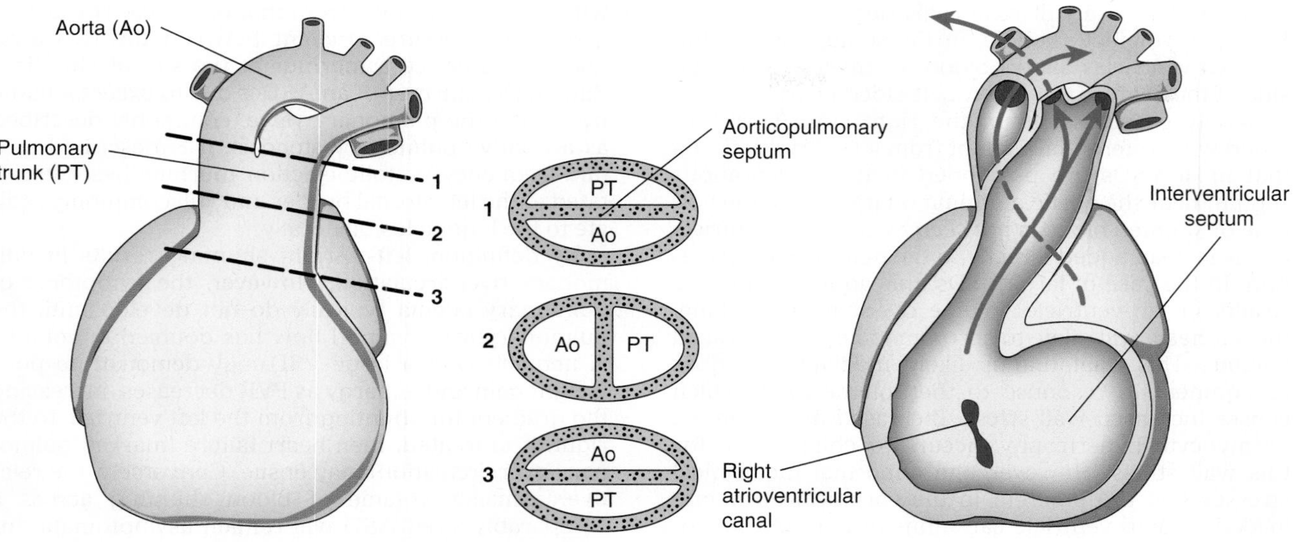

Figure 251-4 Division of the truncus arteriosus into the pulmonary artery and aorta. The aortopulmonary septum is formed by 2 opposing ingrowths of tissue and results in a spiraling of the forming great arteries around one another. (*Moore KL, Persaud TVN. The cardiovascular system. In: Moore KL, Persaud TVN, eds.* The Developing Human: Clinically Oriented Embryology. *5th ed. Philadelphia, PA: WB Saunders; 1993. Copyright © 1993, Elsevier.*)

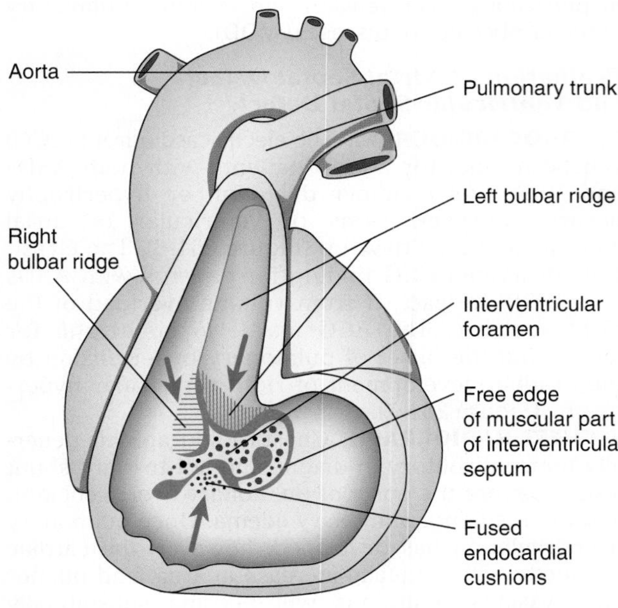

Figure 251-5 Final stages of cardiac development demonstrated in the coronal plane, removing the ventral portion of the developing right ventricle and pulmonary artery. Both the atrioventricular canal and great arteries have been formed. The superior portion of the IVS and the inferior portion of the aortopulmonary septum will meet at the region of the fused endocardial cushions. Once this step is completed, the embryologic heart will be separated into 4 distinct chambers and function as a mature heart. (*Moore KL, Persaud TVN. The cardiovascular system. In: Moore KL, Persaud TVN, eds.* The Developing Human: Clinically Oriented Embryology. *5th ed. Philadelphia, PA: WB Saunders; 1993. Copyright © 1993, Elsevier.*)

pressure difference is minimal (as with pulmonary hypertension), the volume of shunted blood will be small.

Different components of the cardiovascular system will respond uniquely to volume or pressure loading. Atria and ventricles will gradually dilate to accommodate excess blood volume (preload) being added to their respective chambers. If faced with excess pressure (or afterload), then the ventricular myofibers will hypertrophy not only to generate the required driving pressure, but also to minimize myocardial wall stress for maximal pump efficiency. The pulmonary arterioles can also hypertrophy when subjected to prolonged periods of high pressure. However, although cardiac dilatation and hypertrophy are generally reversible, the pulmonary arteriolar hypertrophy associated with longstanding pulmonary hypertension often is not and can result in increased pulmonary vascular resistance (PVR) and fixed, deadly pulmonary hypertension.

Clinical Manifestations

A cardiac murmur is audible blood flow through the heart or vascular system. A murmur can be auscultated in a normal heart resulting from hyperdynamic function or a thin chest wall. Generally, a diastolic murmur is not normal (see later discussion). A systolic murmur may be normal (functional) or it may be pathological. Regardless of the timing, location, or cause of the murmur, its frequency and pitch depend on the size of the opening through which the blood flows and the pressure gradient across it.

Left-to-Right Shunting Lesions

Ventricular Septal Defect

One of the most common types of congenital heart disease is the ventricular septal defect (VSD). Nearly 20%

of patients in heart disease registries have a solitary VSD.[8] This defect, or hole, in the septum separating the two ventricles allows blood to traverse from one side of the heart to the other. Left-sided heart pressure generally exceeds that on the right side. Therefore blood will preferentially shunt from left to right. Given that most VSDs are positioned in the membranous septum near the aortic and pulmonary valves, the volume of shunted blood is not *seen* by the right ventricle and is instead added directly to the pulmonary circulation. In the case of large VSDs, this addition of blood results in left-ventricle volume overload. Over time, the left heart will dilate to accommodate this increased volume. This dilatation is likely mediated by fiber realignment in response to the volume load, which causes increased wall stress. Increased muscle mass, or myocyte hypertrophy, occurs to compensate for this wall stress. However, the abnormal mechanical stresses that are inherent in the chronically volume-loaded, dilated ventricle can ultimately result in myocyte dysfunction and heart failure.[9] In contrast, although a small VSD will still result in left-to-right shunting, the smaller defect will allow a proportionately smaller volume of shunted blood that may never be hemodynamically significant.

Atrial Defect

Another differential lesion with left-to-right shunting is the atrial septal defect (ASD). Similar to the VSD, the volume of shunted blood depends on the size of the defect. In addition to pressure, however, a difference in chamber compliance is the dominant force directing blood from left to right. The highly compliant right atrium becomes a sink for blood draining into the smaller, less-compliant left atrium by the pulmonary veins. This additional blood volume is then routed into the right ventricle, resulting in right-heart dilatation over time.

Clinical Manifestations of Atrial Septal Defect and Ventricular Septal Defect

Despite increasing sensitivity of fetal echocardiography, smaller ASDs and VSDs may not be detected prenatally. Instead, they are usually detected by the presence of a murmur, with or without the signs of heart failure. The timing of their presentation depends on the size of the defect and whether the infant has fully transitioned from fetal circulation.

Right- and left-sided pressures are nearly equivalent shortly after birth and do not produce a substantial pressure gradient for the shunting of blood. During the transition to postnatal circulation, as the PVR falls, the left-right gradient increases along with the volume of oxygen-rich blood shunted to the right heart. A small VSD will produce a high-pitched, holosystolic murmur that continues from the onset of ventricular systole through the closure of the atrioventricular valves (obscuring the first heart sound), to the closure of the semilunar valves. A large VSD will produce a softer holosystolic murmur because the pressures of the two ventricles will more closely approximate one another. This murmur will be loudest at the left lower sternal border and may be best described as a mid-frequency blowing murmur. Auscultation of an ASD will differ significantly from that of a VSD. The lack of a marked pressure gradient between the two atria does not produce a murmur at the site of shunting. Rather, the murmur of an ASD is due to excess volume traversing the pulmonary valve, commonly described as a relative pulmonary stenosis. It is described as a mid-frequency systolic ejection murmur best auscultated at the left sternal border and will commonly radiate to the lung fields bilaterally.

By definition, left-to-right shunting results in pulmonary overcirculation. However, the symptoms of pulmonary edema typically do not develop until the pulmonary artery blood flow has doubled in volume. A neonate with a large VSD may demonstrate poor weight gain and lethargy as PVR decreases, increasing the gradient for shunting from the left ventricle to the right; if untreated, then heart failure (marked pulmonary overcirculation) may ensue. Conversely, the relatively smaller volume of blood shunting across a comparably sized ASD will remain asymptomatic for many years. Regardless of the mechanism, the PVR will reflexively increase in proportion to the degree of shunt volume (in ASD and VSD) and pressure (in VSD) to reduce stress on the arteriolar walls. Over time, these pulmonary arterioles can become quite hypertrophied and are unable to vasodilate. This irreversible state of pulmonary arteriolar vasoconstriction results in pulmonary hypertension and eventual pulmonary vascular obstructive disease (PVOD).

Evaluation of Atrial Septal Defect and Ventricular Septal Defect

ELECTROCARDIOGRAM. The electrocardiogram (ECG) can be normal for age in patients with both ASDs and VSDs. As chamber dilatation or hypertrophy occurs, however, signs of ventricular or atrial enlargement may develop (Figure 251-6). The classically described ECG finding for patients with ASDs is an RSR′ in lead V1 from volume overload of the right ventricle. The ECG may also be helpful for identifying the onset of pulmonary hypertension by the gradual development of right-ventricular hypertrophy (Figure 251-7).

CHEST RADIOGRAPH. Chest radiography is generally noncontributory in diagnosing left-to-right shunt lesions before the onset of pulmonary overcirculation and the resulting pulmonary edema. Once pulmonary overcirculation has developed, however, the cardiac silhouette will gradually increase in area, and pulmonary vascular markings will become substantially more prominent. Chest radiography can also be used to help assess effectiveness of medical management such as diuretic therapy.

ECHOCARDIOGRAM. Any child with a known congenital heart defect should be primarily managed by a pediatric cardiologist along with their primary pediatrician. When present, a two-dimensional echocardiogram will show a defect in the inter-atrial or inter-ventricular septum and allow for determination of cardiac function (Figure 251-8). Doppler flow velocities across the defect can estimate pressure differences between the respective chambers. Together, this information can help guide timing and type of surgical correction, if indicated.

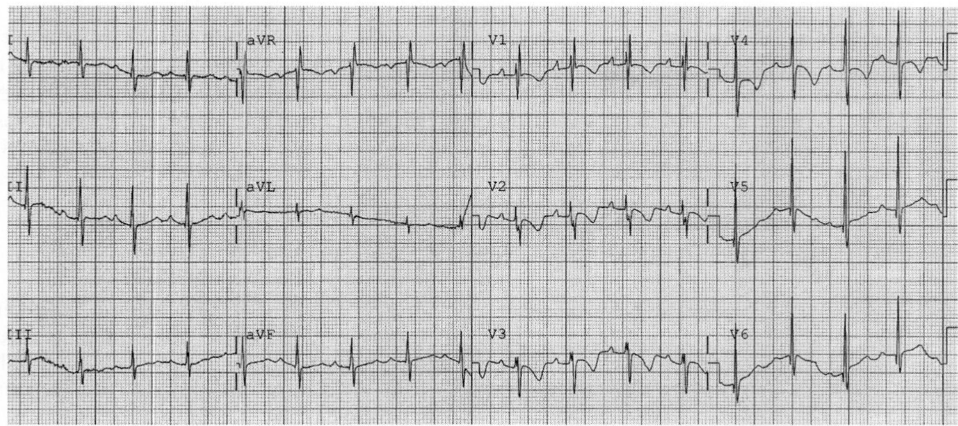

Figure 251-6 ECG of a 3-year-old boy with a large ASD. Note the RSR′ in lead V1 and mildly peaked P waves in leads V1 and II. These findings are consistent with right-ventricular and right-atrial dilatation, respectively.

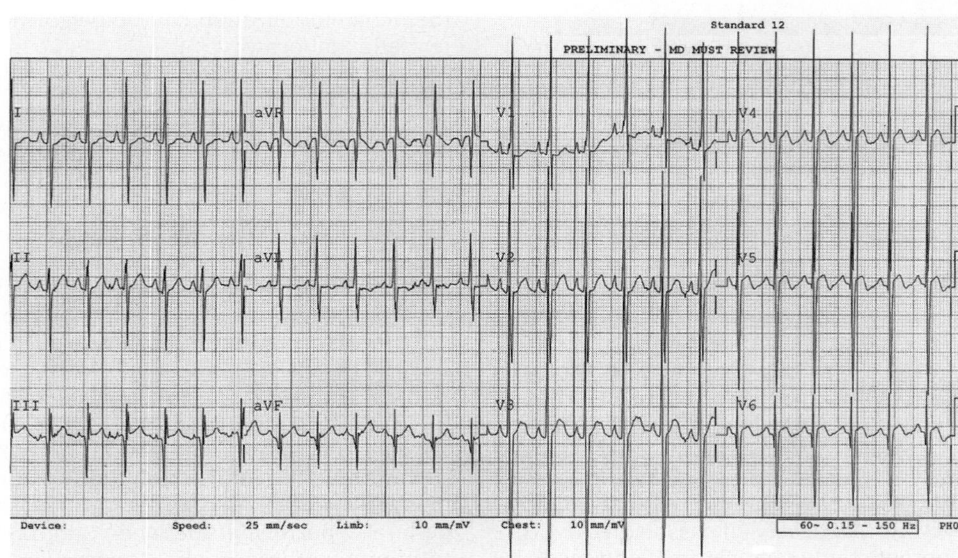

Figure 251-7 ECG of a 2-year-old child with a large VSD. Note the large voltages of both R and S waves in all of the precordial leads as well as right axis deviation of the QRS axis. These findings are consistent with biventricular hypertrophy and elevated PVR caused by longstanding exposure of the pulmonary vasculature to left-sided blood pressures.

Management of Atrial Septal Defect and Ventricular Septal Defect

Patients with known septal defects should be monitored closely for weight gain, development, and clinical status. Any signs of respiratory distress or failure to thrive will generally occur during the first 6 months of life and should prompt reevaluation by the pediatric cardiologist. Although medical management (ie, diuretics, potentially afterload reduction) can temporarily improve these complications, definitive closure of either an ASD or VSD is indicated when signs of pulmonary overcirculation develop.

Prognosis of Atrial Septal Defect and Ventricular Septal Defect

Small ASDs and VSDs can close spontaneously. Small defects in the muscular portion of the interventricular septum (IVS) are frequently closed by the trabeculated muscle growth of the right ventricle; VSDs in other regions of the IVS may also close, but this circumstance is relatively less common.[10] Researchers have suggested that the natural history of secundum-type ASDs is largely dependent on the initial defect size, with nearly 85% less than 5 mm in diameter resolving spontaneously and less than 2% resolving when more than 8 mm in diameter.[11,12] Patients in whom VSDs

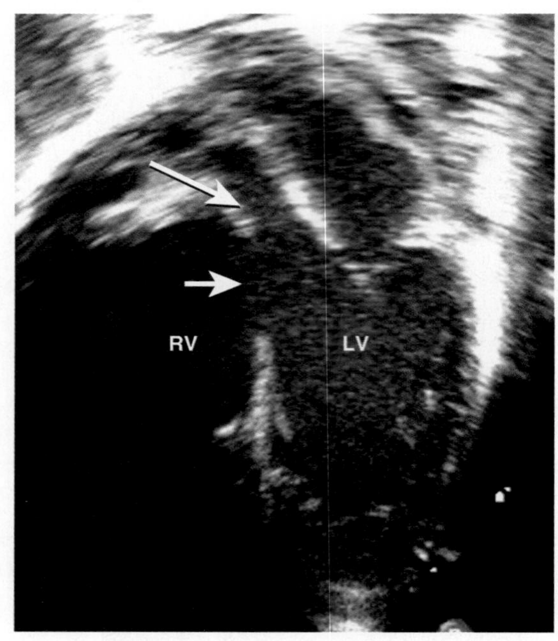

Figure 251-8 Apical 4-chamber echocardiographic view of a 4-month-old infant with a large VSD *(short arrow)*. Note the dilated left ventricle and the relationship of the defect to the aortic valve *(long arrow)*.

neither close spontaneously nor are associated with pulmonary overcirculation are at risk for developing the serious complication of PVOD. The normal, physiological decline of PVR after birth is altered when the lungs are subjected to excess volume from left-to-right shunting. In some patients, the PVR never decreases after birth or decreases at a slower rate and then increases. These patients will have few or no symptoms of pulmonary overcirculation. As a result, they may not be brought to a physician's attention. Persistently elevated PVR, especially if associated with hypoxemia, is a potent stimulus for intimal and medial thickening of the pulmonary arterioles.[13] Elevated PVR produces elevated pulmonary artery pressures and commensurate pulmonary hypertension (mean pulmonary pressures exceed 25 mm Hg at rest). If unrepaired, then patients with this physiological situation will have persistently elevated PVR that can eventually become irreversible. This state, which produces PVOD, can occur as early as 6 months of age, particularly in patients with trisomy 21 syndrome and as early as 1 year in children without Down syndrome. When pulmonary artery pressures exceed those of the left ventricle, the direction of shunted blood will become right to left, producing peripheral cyanosis (Eisenmenger syndrome). Therefore surgical correction of these defects must be accomplished in a timely fashion.

Surgical mortality rates are reported as less than 1% for both ASDs and VSDs.[14-16] Alternatively, device closure of ASDs in the cardiac catheterization laboratory is becoming more common. A recent study comparing device closure of ASD with surgical correction demonstrated a failure rate requiring surgical repair in 4% of device patients but a complication rate of only 7.2% compared with 24% in the surgical group.[17] Device closure of VSDs is currently being performed in limited situations. Success rates have been reported to be 99% but have been associated with a nearly 50% serious complication rate.[18]

Other Common Left-to-Right Shunting Lesions

Patent Ductus Arteriosus

When the ductus arteriosus does not involute shortly after birth, it is a potential source of shunting from the aorta to the pulmonary arteries once PVR decreases. A patent ductus arteriosus (PDA) is most commonly encountered in premature infants and can be associated with worsening chronic lung disease, poor renal perfusion, hemodynamic instability, intraventricular hemorrhage, and necrotizing enterocolitis. If the usual treatment with Indocin is contraindicated or unsuccessful, then the PDA can often be ligated in the neonatal intensive care unit. If persistent into childhood, then coil embolization can be performed in the catheterization laboratory.

Atrioventricular Septal Defects

Nearly 50% of all patients with trisomy 21 have congenital heart disease; nearly 50% are atrioventricular septal defects (AVSDs; also known as atrioventricular canal defects or endocardial cushion defects). Approximately 70% of all patients with AVSD have trisomy 21. This defect describes a continuum of malformations from a partial type (primum type ASD with a cleft mitral valve) to a complete type (single atrioventricular valve spanning the entire width of the heart; Figure 251-9, *A*) with variability in the attachment of the atrioventricular valve leaflets to the IVS.[19] These defects can result in a significant left-to-right shunt volume. Timing of the surgical repair for complete AVSD follows the same principles for the simple VSD described previously and is generally performed between 3 and 6 months of age to minimize the potential for irreversible pulmonary hypertension. A partial AVSD follows ASD physiological characteristics and can generally be repaired later in life (first few years) with a low risk of developing PVOD. The ECG of patients with the complete defect generally demonstrates a northwest, superior QRS axis and some element of ventricular hypertrophy (Figure 251-9, *B*).

Surgical repair of a complete AVSD includes patch closure of the ASD and VSD and the creation of two functioning atrioventricular valves from the single, frequently regurgitant common atrioventricular valve. Postoperative outcomes depend on the severity of any residual atrioventricular valve regurgitation[20,21] and the presence of pulmonary vascular disease.

Arteriovenous Malformation

Arteriovenous malformation (AVM) is a direct connection between the arterial and venous vascular systems resulting in shunting of blood to the right heart and possible high-output, left-sided heart failure. Common AVM locations in children are cerebral and abdominal.

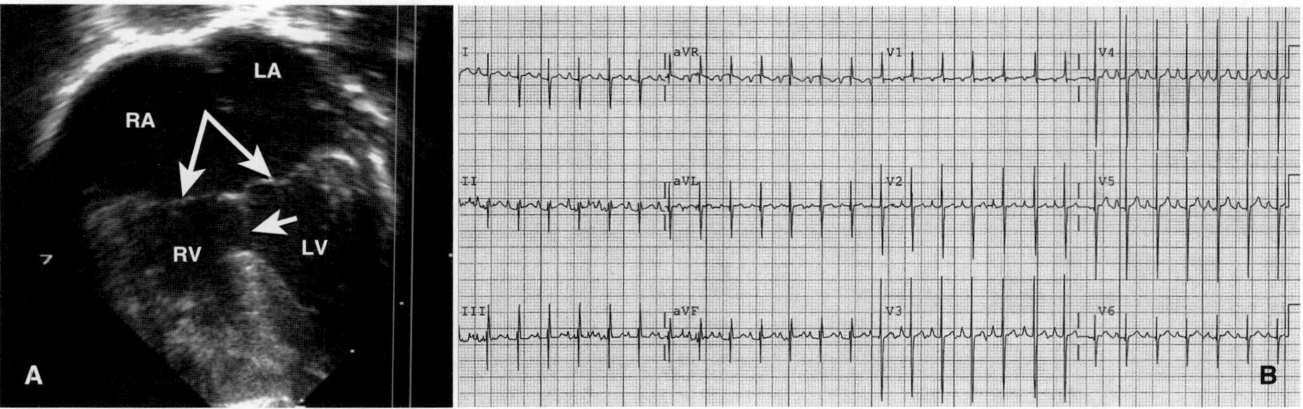

Figure 251-9 A, Apical 4-chamber echocardiographic view of a 3-month-old infant with Down syndrome and a complete AVSD. Note the large ASDs and VSDs *(top and bottom arrows, respectively)* and the dilatation of both atria and ventricles. The double arrow points to the common atrioventricular valve spanning both ventricular chambers. **B**, ECG of the same patient demonstrating a *northwest* QRS axis (QRS forces are predominantly negative in leads I and aVF) with a small Q wave in lead aVL; this finding is typical in patients with AVSDs. In addition, note the large voltages in the precordial leads and peaked P waves in leads II and aVF consistent with biventricular dilatation and right atrial enlargement, respectively.

Coil embolization may reduce or reverse heart failure in many cases.

Right-to-Left Shunting Lesions

Systemic, peripheral cyanosis is the key difference between left-to-right and right-to-left shunting lesions. By definition, a right-to-left shunting lesion is one in which oxygen-poor blood is being shunted or added to the oxygen-rich, systemic blood. As with left-to-right shunting lesions, the volume of shunted blood depends on the size of the defect and the pressure gradient across it.

Tetralogy of Fallot

Tetralogy of Fallot is one of the most commonly encountered cyanotic heart defects, occurring in 0.33 per 1000 live births and comprising approximately 7% of heart defects.[22] Although its embryologic origin remains controversial, one of the prevailing theories asserts that this defect occurs as a result of disproportionate segregation of the truncus arteriosus into the pulmonary artery and aorta.[23] This uneven distribution results in malalignment of the aortopulmonary septum with the developing IVS creating a VSD, which then underlies both the aortic and pulmonic valves. This anatomic arrangement, coupled with the stenotic pulmonary valve and narrowed right-ventricular outflow tract (RVOT), results in right-to-left shunting of right-ventricular blood through the VSD into the aorta, producing systemic, peripheral cyanosis. Not surprisingly, the volume of shunted blood can vary by altering the pressure gradient through the RVOT. The proverbial *Tet spell,* or hypercyanotic event, occurs when systemic vascular resistance (SVR) decreases, resulting in an increased right-to-left shunt. Some researchers have suggested that muscle contraction or spasms in the RVOT increase the obstruction to pulmonary flow and thereby worsen cyanosis. Direct and histologic visualization of the fibrotic, disorganized muscle tissue found in the RVOT in patients with tetralogy of Fallot makes this situation unlikely. Regardless of the cause, treatment for a hypercyanotic spell is the same. Supplemental oxygen, fluid boluses, anxiolytics, sedatives, and increased SVR (ie, knee to chest positioning, phenylephrine) work to decrease the amount of right-to-left shunting. If not treated urgently, then hypercyanotic spells can be fatal.

Eisenmenger Syndrome

Although uncommon in the current era, another potential cause for right-to-left shunting occurs in the setting of unrepaired VSDs or large ASDs with secondary pulmonary hypertension and is known as Eisenmenger syndrome. Significant shunting and progressive cyanosis with this physiological phenomenon will only occur once the pulmonary artery, and therefore right-ventricular, pressures are higher than the systemic blood pressure. In addition to the complications of systemic cyanosis and the compensatory rise in hematocrit, patients with pulmonary hypertension are at a significantly elevated risk for right-ventricular failure and sudden death.

Pulmonary Hypertension

In isolated or idiopathic pulmonary hypertension (no septal defects through which blood can shunt right to left), a pulmonary hypertensive crisis (transient, severe elevation of pulmonary artery pressures) can result in markedly decreased right-ventricular and then left-ventricular output. If not reversed, this condition can be fatal. For this reason and to prevent progression of the pulmonary hypertension, aggressive therapy with pulmonary vasodilators is indicated.

Table 251-1 Description of the Six Grades of Systolic or Diastolic Murmur Severity

MURMUR SEVERITY	DESCRIPTION
Grade I	Barely audible and may require several cardiac cycles to detect
Grade II	Soft, but easily audible
Grade III	Moderately loud murmur without a thrill
Grade IV	Loud murmur with a thrill
Grade V	Loud murmur heard with the stethoscope barely off the chest
Grade VI	Loud murmur heard without the stethoscope touching the chest

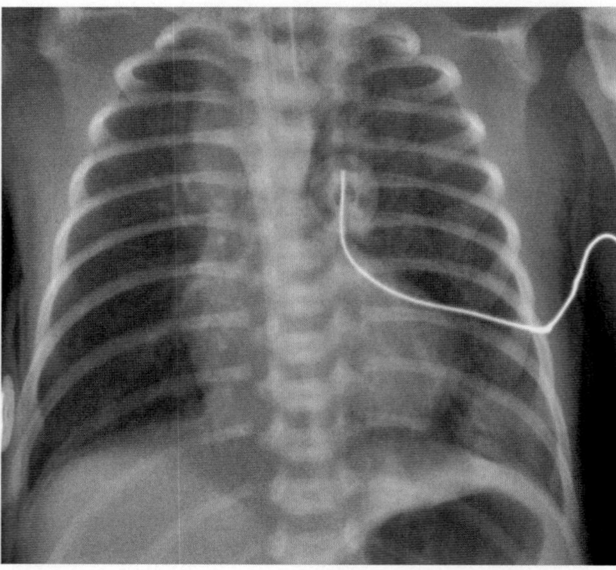

Figure 251-10 Chest radiograph of a newborn with tetralogy of Fallot demonstrating a *boot-shaped* heart. The *toe* of the boot is formed by the cardiac apex being lifted off the diaphragm from right-ventricular hypertrophy. Note the absent pulmonary artery knob expected to exist at the left sternal border between the 4th and 6th ribs.

Clinical Manifestations of Right-to-Left Shunting Lesions

Tetralogy of Fallot is a defect commonly detected by prenatal ultrasound between 18 and 22 weeks' gestation. The clinical presentation can be extremely varied depending on the degree of pulmonary stenosis or the presence of pulmonary atresia (no prograde flow across the pulmonary valve).

In addition to cyanosis, newborns with tetralogy of Fallot will commonly demonstrate an audible murmur. A systolic murmur may be appreciated at the left upper sternal border and is produced by the narrowing of the RVOT. Its grade (I-VI/VI) and quality (harsh or soft) depends on the degree of obstruction (Table 251-1). In the newborn with tetralogy of Fallot and pulmonary atresia, the RVOT murmur is replaced by a flow murmur through the ductus arteriosus, the only source of pulmonary blood flow.

With the exception of peripheral cyanosis and softer murmurs, the physical examination of a patient with pulmonary hypertension caused by an untreated septal defect (Eisenmenger syndrome) may be virtually indistinguishable from that of a simple ASD or VSD. One other subtle difference may be a loud pulmonary valve (P2) component of the second heart sound. Idiopathic pulmonary hypertension or pulmonary hypertension secondary to bronchopulmonary dysplasia may demonstrate cyanosis (from intrapulmonary or right-left atrial level cardiac shunting) and a loud P2 but should not have an associated cardiac murmur (in the absence of pulmonary or tricuspid insufficiency). Equal ventricular pressures in a patient with Eisenmenger syndrome secondary to a VSD will not produce an audible murmur.

Evaluation of Right-to-Left Shunting Lesions

ELECTROCARDIOGRAM. Tetralogy of Fallot and pulmonary hypertension often produce evidence of right-ventricular hypertrophy. Right-axis deviation and tall R waves in the early or right-sided precordial leads can be seen on ECG.

CHEST RADIOGRAPH. Right-to-left shunting, by definition, is associated with decreased pulmonary blood flow. As a result, pulmonary vascular markings may be significantly decreased in patients with either tetralogy of Fallot or secondary pulmonary hypertension. The classic radiographic finding of tetralogy of Fallot is the boot-shaped cardiac silhouette. This result is due to the superiorly displaced cardiac apex produced by right-ventricular hypertrophy and absence or reduction of the pulmonary knob (Figure 251-10). The relative right-ventricular hypertrophy in the normal newborn often results in the erroneous reading of a boot-shaped cardiac silhouette on initial chest radiographic examination.

ECHOCARDIOGRAM. Two-dimensional and Doppler echocardiogram evaluations define cardiac anatomy, function, and direction of blood flow across any cardiac defects. Doppler flow velocity across the RVOT allows estimation of outflow gradient, degree of obstruction, and any evidence of branch pulmonary artery stenosis.

Management of Right-to-Left Shunting Lesions

TETRALOGY OF FALLOT. Surgical management of tetralogy of Fallot has changed significantly over the last decade. The advent of microsurgical techniques has allowed for repair during infancy or even the newborn period. For this reason, true hypercyanotic episodes in toddlers rarely are observed in present day.

TETRALOGY OF FALLOT WITHOUT PULMONARY ATRESIA. Once diagnosed, patients with tetralogy of Fallot without pulmonary atresia are generally monitored in the intensive care unit until their ductus arteriosus (if present) closes. If these patients are able to produce enough pulmonary blood flow to maintain

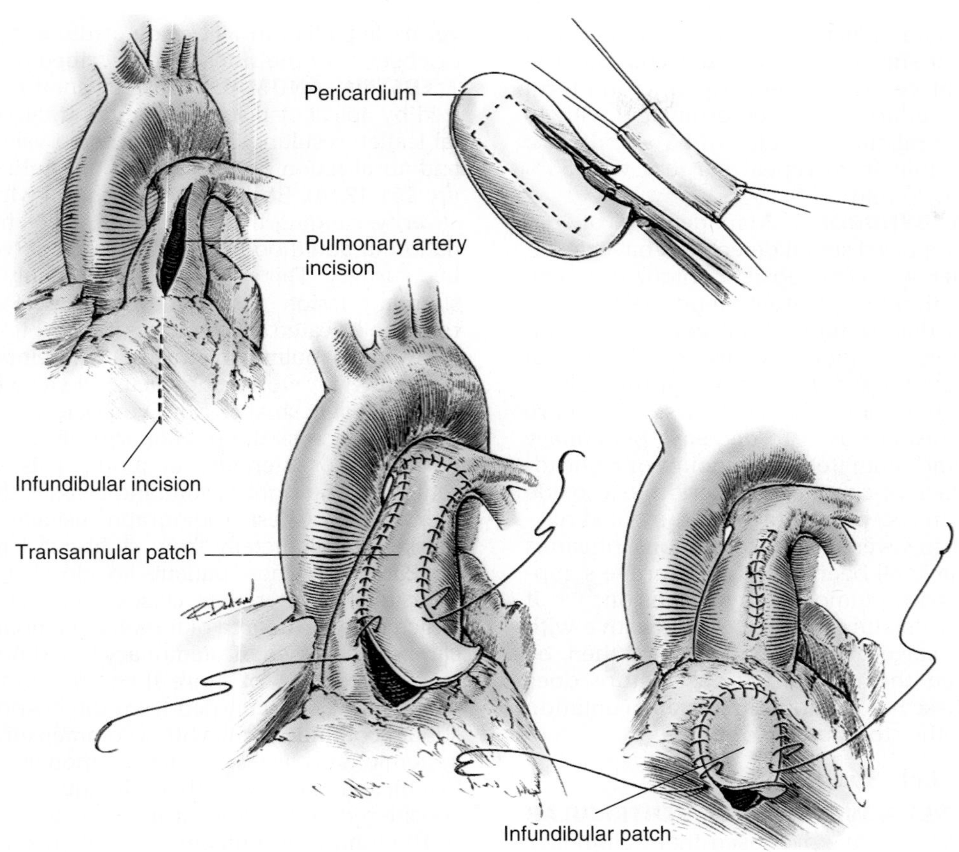

Figure 251-11 Depiction of surgical repair for tetralogy of Fallot. In the setting of a hypoplastic pulmonary valve annulus, a patch of fixed bovine pericardium is sized to fit the vertical incision site, which starts in the main pulmonary artery and traverses the pulmonary valve into the right ventricle's infundibulum. The *transannular* patch placement is depicted in the middle drawing. The bottom right drawing depicts the surgical approach to repairing a patient with tetralogy of Fallot without a hypoplastic pulmonary valve. The main pulmonary artery incision is made to allow patch augmentation of the main pulmonary artery, and the incision in the right-ventricular infundibulum is made to permit patch augmentation of the RVOT. Not shown is repair of the VSD or muscle bundle resection, which is usually performed through the tricuspid valve. (*Castanedas AR, Jonas RA.* Cardiac Surgery of the Neonate and Infant. *Philadelphia, PA: WB Saunders; 1994. Copyright © 1994, Elsevier.*)

Sao_2 levels of more than 80%, then they may be discharged from the hospital and allowed to grow. The occurrence of a tetralogy spell (Tet spell) is generally considered a semi-urgent indication for repair. Otherwise, in the absence of earlier unacceptable cyanosis (arterial saturation of oxygen [Sao_2] of <75%), elective repair is performed when the child is 4 to 6 months.

Operative correction consists of patching the VSD and correcting the obstruction to pulmonary blood flow. Resection or division (or both) of RVOT muscle bundles is performed first through the right atrium to remove this source of impedance. The VSD is then patched. Last, depending on pulmonary artery anatomy, a patch is placed in the supravalvar (main pulmonary artery), subvalvar (infundibular or outflow region), or transvalvar (across the pulmonary valve annulus and extending into the supra and subvalvar regions) regions to minimize distal outflow obstruction (Figure 251-11). In many cases, a pulmonary valvectomy is performed during these repairs, and patients are left with some degree of pulmonary insufficiency, which requires regular follow-up, given that progressive RV dilatation associated with pulmonary insufficiency is one of the sources of long-term morbidity in these patients.

TETRALOGY OF FALLOT WITH PULMONARY ATRESIA. If tetralogy of Fallot is associated with pulmonary atresia, then a prostaglandin E1 infusion will maintain ductal patency until surgical repair. If pulmonary artery size is favorable (ie, >3 mm in diameter), then complete repair can be performed in the neonate; otherwise, an aortopulmonary shunt is placed to allow pulmonary artery growth until a complete repair is performed later. In the patient without confluent pulmonary arteries who relies instead on multiple aortopulmonary collaterals, the surgical options are more difficult. The collateral arteries can be unifocalized through a single or staged procedure to a conduit arising from the right ventricle. The early and long-term results of this procedure have been promising with 10 and 20 year actuarial survival rates of 86% and 75%, respectively; freedom from repeat surgery was 55% and 29% at 10 and 20 years.[24,25]

EISENMENGER SYNDROME. Management of patients with an unrepaired septal defect that have developed Eisenmenger syndrome poses a unique problem. Right-to-left shunting in this situation occurs to maintain adequate cardiac output at the expense of systemic oxygenation. Surgical closure of the septal defect will actually worsen the outcome if the pulmonary hypertension is not addressed first. Therefore multiple approaches are used to decrease pulmonary artery pressure and ultimately the amount of right-to-left shunting. Calcium-channel blockers, nitric oxide donors, endothelin receptor antagonists, inhaled oxygen therapy, and, in severe cases, continuous infusions of prostacyclin have all been found to improve symptoms in patients with pulmonary hypertension.[26-30] If the pulmonary vasculature proves to be reactive with these measures, surgical intervention may then be considered. When the pulmonary vasculature does not respond to these medications, lung transplantation may be the only other therapeutic option.

Other Right-to-Left Shunting Lesions

PULMONARY ATRESIA WITH INTACT VENTRICULAR SEPTUM. Researchers have proposed that pulmonary atresia with intact ventricular septum occurs late in embryologic development for patients with two adequately sized ventricles. This otherwise structurally normal heart develops complete fusion of the pulmonary valve preventing any forward flow into the pulmonary artery from the right ventricle. Blood entering the right ventricle is instead regurgitated through the tricuspid valve back into the right atrium where it mixes with SVC and IVC blood. The increase in blood volume increases right atrial pressure, resulting in shunting of blood across the patent foramen ovale to the left atrium. This circuit does not change with transition from fetal circulation, and pulmonary blood flow becomes dependent on a persistently PDA. Once diagnosed, the pulmonary valve may be opened in the cardiac catheterization laboratory using balloon dilatation or radio-frequency ablation to perforate through the valve cusps.[31] This approach is controversial, and, in many institutions, surgical valvotomy is preferred.

Another subset of patients develops pulmonary atresia much earlier in cardiac development. The subsequent lack of right-heart blood flow results in hypoplasia of the right ventricle and tricuspid valve and, in some cases, can be associated with sinusoidal connections between the hypoplastic right ventricle and coronary arteries. When present, decompression of the right ventricle through a pulmonary valvotomy can result in myocardial ischemia, infarction, and death. If these right heart structures are significantly affected, the patient must instead follow the single-ventricle treatment route (see later discussion of single-ventricle physiology).[32-34] The surgical specifics of that single-ventricle palliation will be determined by the presence or absence of the sinusoids described previously.

EBSTEIN ANOMALY. Ebstein anomaly is characterized by apical displacement of the tricuspid valve's septal leaflet, resulting in both tricuspid valve insufficiency and atrialization of a section of the right ventricle (Figure 251-12, *A*). Ebstein anomaly has a wide spectrum of severity, ranging from diagnosis at postmortem examination in adulthood to requiring single-ventricle palliative surgery. This anomaly is commonly a right-to-left shunting lesion in the newborn period when PVR remains elevated. The course of blood flow is much the same as in pulmonary atresia with intact ventricular septum. With worsening tricuspid valve incompetence, the effectively smaller right ventricle is less able to propel blood across the pulmonary valve, which is usually narrowed or stenotic, or both. This blood instead returns to the right atrium and crosses the patent foramen ovale. Chest radiograph usually demonstrates marked cardiomegaly from right-atrial dilatation (Figure 251-12, *B*). These patients are closely monitored until their ductus arteriosus closes and PVR decreases at which time the degree of forward pulmonary blood flow can be reassessed. If pulmonary blood flow is adequate to produce $Sa{O_2}$ of more than 75% to 80%, then the infant may be discharged from the hospital where PVR should continue to fall with a commensurate increase in systemic $Sa{O_2}$ levels. Should pulmonary blood flow be insufficient, however, these infants will generally be considered for single-ventricle palliative surgery.

The long-term outcomes of patients diagnosed with Ebstein anomaly of the tricuspid valve are determined, in part, by the severity of disease (ie, degree of cyanosis) at presentation. When clinical symptoms are present shortly after birth and unacceptable cyanosis is unremitting ($Sa{O_2}$ of 70%), the single-ventricle treatment regimen is generally required, with outcomes similar to patients with hypoplastic left heart syndrome.[32] Conversely, fetal diagnosis with early severe tricuspid regurgitation can be associated with pulmonary hypoplasia secondary to severe right-atrial enlargement.[35,36] Severely hypoplastic lungs will preclude cardiac palliation, and most of these infants succumb shortly after birth. Newborns with acceptable saturations and adequate cardiac output can be discharged from the hospital and followed expectantly with intervention that may be necessary only during older childhood or adolescence when exercise intolerance or pronounced exercise-associated cyanosis develops.

TOTAL OR PARTIAL ANOMALOUS PULMONARY VENOUS RETURN. Embryologically, total anomalous pulmonary venous return (TAPVR) occurs when the pulmonary veins do not connect with the posterior wall of the left atrium. They, instead, form a confluence that then drains via a vertical vein indirectly to the right atrium. This vertical vein returns to either a supracardiac or infracardiac structure, generally, the innominate or hepatic veins, respectively. Although all the blood originally destined for the left heart is returning to the right, the physiological characteristics of TAPVR is consistent with a right-to-left shunting lesion, given that, within the heart, blood is shunted from the right atrium across an obligate ASD into the left atrium, providing the only source of systemic

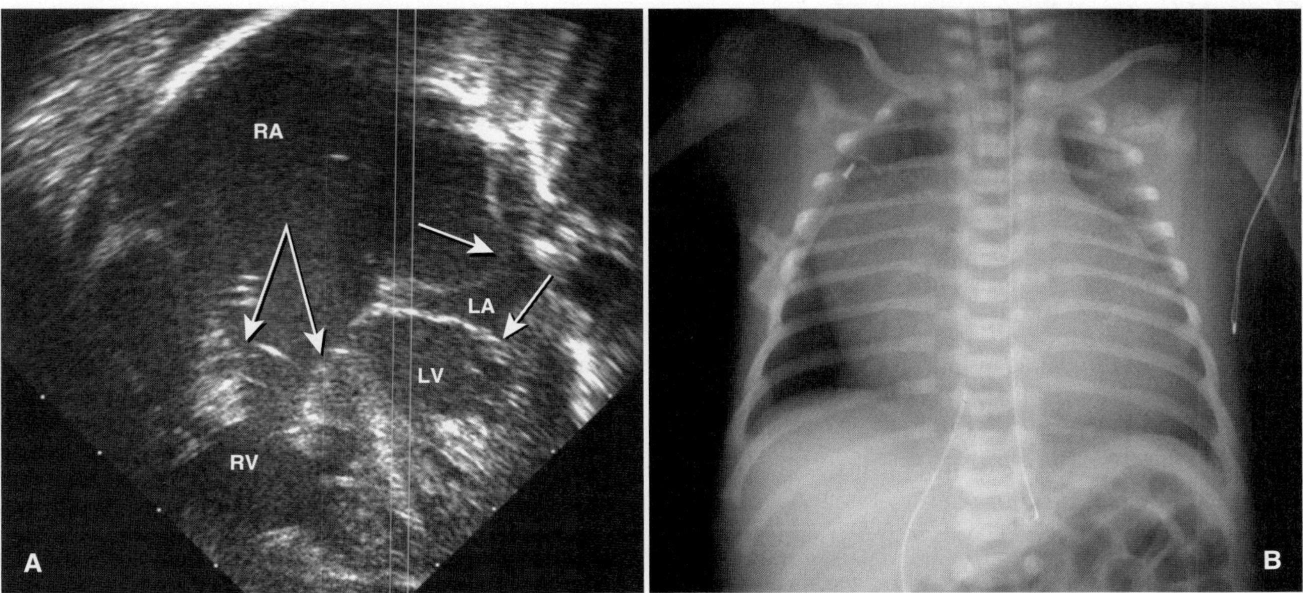

Figure 251-12 A, Apical 4-chamber echocardiographic view of a newborn with Ebstein anomaly of the tricuspid valve. The double arrow points to the apically displaced septal and posterior tricuspid valve leaflets, which result in ineffective coaptation of the tricuspid valve. The short arrow depicts right-to-left bowing of the atrial septum caused by the high right-atrial pressure from the regurgitant tricuspid valve volume. The perforated arrow demonstrates the relative size of the normal mitral valve. **B**, Chest radiograph of the same patient depicting cardiomegaly caused by severe right atrial enlargement.

cardiac output. Conversely, partial anomalous pulmonary venous return (PAPVR) is the anomalous return of one or more pulmonary veins to the right heart. Unless more than one of the pulmonary veins returns anomalously, this anomaly rarely becomes hemodynamically significant and may not require surgical correction unless symptoms develop (ie, exercise intolerance).

The diagnosis of TAPVR or PAPVR can be difficult to confirm by echocardiogram and, particularly in cases of complex anatomy, may require cardiac catheterization if clinically suspected.[37] Infracardiac drainage frequently becomes obstructed at some point along the extended, tortuous course of the vertical vein into the liver and, when present, constitutes a surgical emergency. Surgical correction for uncomplicated TAPVR consists of reanastomosis of the pulmonary venous confluence to the posterior wall of the left atrium. The most common postoperative complications are obstruction at the site of the anastomosis, pulmonary vein stenosis, and left-atrial dysrhythmias.[38-40] If unrecognized, then prolonged obstruction of the anastomosis or pulmonary veins can result in irreversible pulmonary venous obstructive disease, pulmonary vascular disease, and eventual right-heart failure.

Dextro-Rotation or Rightward Transposition of the Great Arteries

Dextro-rotation or rightward transposition of the great arteries is an embryologic defect of the conotruncus in which the aortic valve lies rightward and anterior of the pulmonary valve instead of rightward and posterior as in the normal heart. This arrangement results in the aorta receiving blood flow from the RVOT and the pulmonary artery from the left. The pulmonary and systemic circulations are subsequently in parallel rather than in series and the body relies on both intra and extracardiac shunting to provide oxygenated blood to the tissues.

The right ventricle receives oxygen-poor blood from the vena cavae and delivers it to the aorta. Left-to-right shunting of oxygenated blood across the patent foramen ovale is the only method of adding oxygenated blood to the right-ventricular cardiac output. However, if this shunting is unidirectional, then the left-sided, pulmonary circulation will become volume depleted. Therefore atrial-level shunting is bidirectional to allow exchange of blood between the two circulations. One of the main interventions to consider in the newborn period is whether a balloon septostomy (Rashkind procedure) of the atrial septum is necessary to increase blood exchange and systemic oxygen delivery. Patency of the ductus arteriosus can supplement the volume of blood exchange by increasing the blood return to the left atrium, which permits better mixing at the atrial level.

In general, oxygen-poor blood is shunted from the aorta to the pulmonary artery via the PDA, which results in equal, four-extremity cyanosis. Conversely, if persistent fetal circulation exists, with PVR greater than SVR, then oxygenated blood will shunt from the pulmonary artery to the aorta and produce paradoxical cyanosis with higher Sa_{O_2} in the legs (downstream from the ductus) compared with the arms and brain.

Clinical Signs and Symptoms

Dextro-rotation or rightward transposition of the great arteries can be diagnosed prenatally and is the most common type of cyanotic heart disease. These patients generally are cyanotic at birth without associated respiratory distress. Physical examination will therefore be remarkable for cyanosis and possibly a ductal murmur, but should otherwise be normal for a newborn. Sa_{O_2} will not increase significantly with supplemental oxygen (failed hyperoxia challenge test). Care should be taken to assess lower extremity pulses as coarctation of the aorta can be associated with dextro-looped transposition of the great arteries (d-TGA). Prostaglandin E1 infusion should be initiated once this defect is suspected.

Evaluation

ELECTROCARDIOGRAM. The ECG will generally be unremarkable for a newborn and will not offer added information unless other cardiac defects exist.

CHEST RADIOGRAPH. The classic radiographic finding for d-TGA is the *egg on a string*. The great arteries are often oriented parallel *(the string)* instead of perpendicular, removing the aortic and pulmonary nobs. This great artery orientation can also create a mesocardic orientation of the cardiac silhouette producing an egg-shaped silhouette.

ECHOCARDIOGRAM. Two-dimensional echocardiogram will confirm the diagnosis and can evaluate the extent of intra- and extracardiac shunting. ASD size, direction of ductus arteriosus shunting, and presence of a VSD are important components of intercirculatory mixing. Furthermore, coronary artery anomalies occur frequently with this congenital heart disease and can complicate the surgical repair.

Management

Transposition of the great arteries can be one of the more complex congenital heart diseases to manage in the newborn period. The single most important component of preoperative management is maintaining adequate atrial-level shunting. Although the presence of a VSD is important when considering surgical options, ventricular-level shunting does not usually contribute a significant amount of intracardiac mixing in the newborn period.

Many patients with d-TGA have already begun receiving prostaglandin E1 infusions at the time of diagnosis after failing the hyperoxia challenge. After assessing for paradoxical cyanosis (as seen with persistent fetal circulation), Sa_{O_2}, and arterial oxygen content, the pediatric cardiologist may elect to discontinue this infusion. In general, an arterial oxygen content greater than 30 mmHg (typical fetal partial pressure of oxygen in arterial blood [Pa_{O_2}]) with a corresponding Sa_{O_2} of more than 75% to 80%, in the absence of metabolic acidosis, are predictive of adequate atrial-level mixing. If these conditions are not met and the newborn demonstrates any signs of respiratory distress or pulmonary edema with marked cyanosis, then the ASD is likely restrictive and needs to be enlarged. This task can be accomplished by balloon septostomy, blade septostomy, or radio-frequency ablation of the atrial septum in the catheterization laboratory. Although these procedures are necessary life-saving interventions, they can be associated with significant risks of morbidity and mortality.

Surgical Correction

With the advent of microsurgical techniques came the ability to reimplant coronary arteries (Figure 251-13). This procedure allowed for the arterial switch (Jantene) operation, which has been the surgical option of choice for most patients with d-TGA since the 1980s. As a result, the atrial switch operation (Mustard and Senning procedures) has become obsolete. The process of switching the great arteries is conceptually intuitive but technically very complex. Once the patient is placed on cardiopulmonary bypass, the aortic and pulmonary arteries are transected above their native valves. Next, the surgeon removes the coronary arteries from the aortic root (arising from the right ventricle) by cutting small buttons of tissue surrounding the coronary artery's ostium. Similar sized buttons of tissue are removed from the pulmonary artery (arising from the left ventricle), and the coronary arteries are sutured into the native pulmonary artery root (arising from the left ventricle). The aorta is freely mobile within the thorax and is easily sutured to the exposed pulmonary artery root. The main and branch pulmonary arteries remain attached to the lungs and are subsequently more restricted in their range of motion. To minimize surgical stretch and subsequent obstruction, the Lecompte maneuver is performed, which drapes the main and branch pulmonary arteries over the ascending aorta instead of underneath.

Abnormal coronary artery anatomic configuration is relatively common and occurs in approximately 30% of all patients with d-TGA.[41,42] This abnormality can produce one of the major complications of the arterial switch operation. A single coronary artery origin necessitates *flipping* of the button before reimplantation and is often associated with kinking and compromise of coronary artery flow. Although no coronary pattern precludes a *switch*, transmural (coursing through the arterial wall) coronary artery anatomy and others may increase the risk of the procedure, necessitating alternative surgical approaches. Discordant annulus size of the great arteries can also produce difficulty but is often not a contraindication to an arterial switch. Compared with long-term atrial switch results, the outcomes data for patients with d-TGA after an arterial switch operation are substantially better, but significant morbidity persists. An overall mortality rate of 7% was reported in one study of 223 patients with d-TGA after the arterial switch operation; coronary artery pattern was not associated with an increased risk of death.[43] However, two studies with a total of 1263 patients demonstrated a rate of coronary artery events between 7% to 8% over 15 years of follow-up.[44,45] Abnormal coronary artery vasomotor function has also been demonstrated in asymptomatic children after the arterial switch operation.[46] Furthermore, a retrospective study of 119 postoperative patients with d-TGA followed for a median of 65 months found progressive aortic root dilatation without an increased prevalence of aortic insufficiency.[47] The clinical significance of these studies is

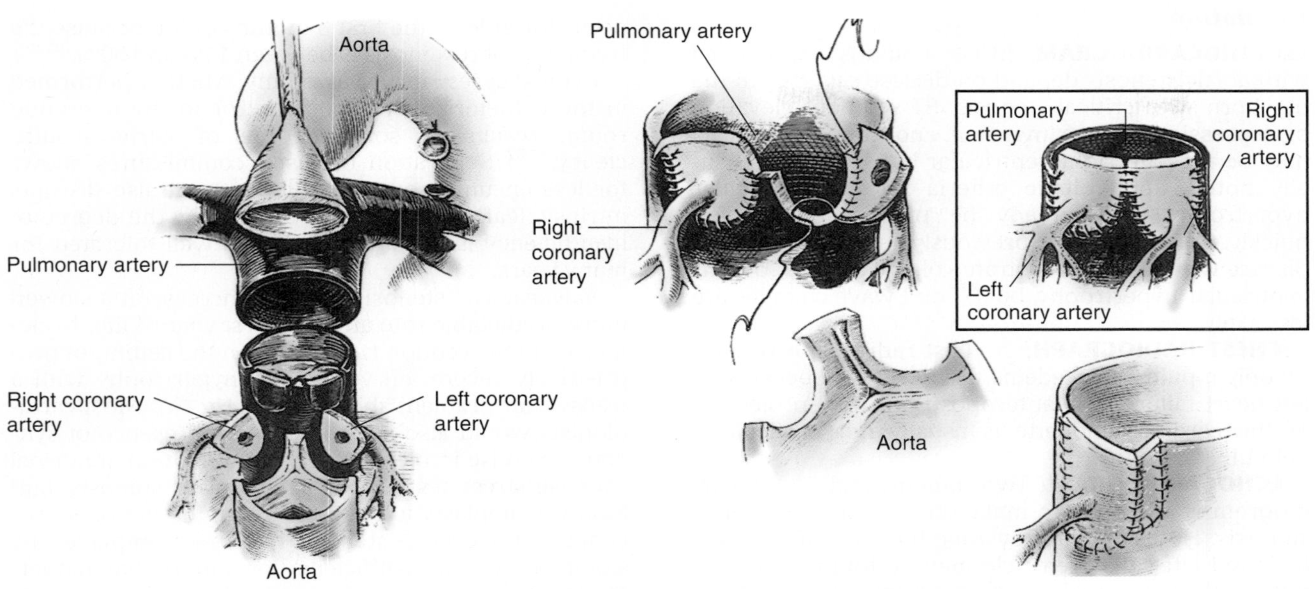

Figure 251-13 Stages of the arterial switch operation used in patients with d-TGA. The first picture demonstrates transection of the aorta and pulmonary artery just distal to their respective valves. In the middle picture, the coronary artery *buttons* are rotated from the original aortic root to the *neoaortic* root and sutured into place. (*Castanedas AR, Jonas RA.* Cardiac Surgery of the Neonate and Infant. *Philadelphia, PA: WB Saunders; 1994. Copyright © 1994, Elsevier.*)

unclear. Though the arterial switch operation remains the best surgical option available, these data suggest this patient population warrants close postoperative follow-up.

Left-Sided Obstructive Lesions

Left-sided obstructive lesions are characterized by impedance to blood flow from the systemic ventricle (generally the left) to the body. As with nearly all heart lesions, the severity of the obstruction determines the age of presentation and clinical manifestations.

Aortic Stenosis

Valvar aortic stenosis can occur in isolation or be associated with either subvalvar or supravalvar obstruction. With few exceptions, the presentation and alteration of cardiovascular physiological characteristics are very similar among the three defects. When the stenosis is mild or moderate in severity, a cardiac murmur may be the only sign of an abnormality in the newborn period. Depending on ductal dependency, a severe or critical degree of aortic stenosis, however, is associated with inadequate cardiac output and will develop in the newborn period as heart failure or clinical extremus.

A large portion of fetal cardiac output is provided by ductal flow from the pulmonary artery to the descending aorta. The transition to postnatal circulation occurs with closure of the ductus arteriosus. In the newborn with severe or critical aortic stenosis, this process is associated with a significant decrease in systemic blood flow. Although the output will be fully oxygenated, the volume will be inadequate, and signs and symptoms of congestive heart failure will ensue. Diaphoresis with feeding, irritability, lethargy, and fatigue will bring these patients to a physician's attention. The infant will be acyanotic but ashen, with a harsh cardiac murmur and diminished or absent peripheral pulses. Increasing severity of stenosis is therefore associated with increased dependence on ductal flow for systemic cardiac output, which is then associated with an earlier presentation.

Several studies[48,49] have demonstrated that aortic stenosis severity can change dramatically during the first 6 months of life and that final valvar gradients are poorly predicted by initial gradients. Most pediatric cardiologists will monitor infants with aortic stenosis on a frequent basis throughout this time to plan timely intervention on rapidly progressive stenosis before congestive heart failure and systemic shock occur. Patients not requiring intervention before 6 months of life are less likely to develop heart failure or become critically ill during the follow-up period.

Milder degrees of aortic stenosis may not develop until childhood. These patients will typically be asymptomatic, and examination will reveal an ejection click followed by a harsh systolic ejection murmur best auscultated at the right upper sternal border. ECG evaluation of these patients may or may not demonstrate signs of left-ventricular hypertrophy and is unlikely to show any signs of myocardial ischemia. Particularly in the pediatric population, mild to moderate aortic stenosis will not produce exercise intolerance, chest pain, syncope, or shock. As a result, these patients are often referred to a pediatric cardiologist after the characteristic murmur is heard during a routine physical examination.

Evaluation

ELECTROCARDIOGRAM. ECG findings associated with aortic stenosis depend on disease severity. In the newborn with critical stenosis, ST segment elevation or depression, T wave inversion, and sinus tachycardia may be present; right-ventricular hypertrophy is usually noted, and voltage criteria for left-ventricular hypertrophy may already be present or develop quickly. As mentioned previously, mild-to-moderate disease will likely demonstrate voltage criteria for left-ventricular hypertrophy, but ST or T wave changes are less likely.

CHEST RADIOGRAPH. A chest radiograph is helpful only if pulmonary edema has developed because of left heart failure. The anteroposterior (AP) projection of the cardiac silhouette is usually not particularly helpful.

ECHOCARDIOGRAM. Two-dimensional echocardiogram is adequate to make the diagnosis of aortic stenosis. Hyperdynamic systolic function of a hypertrophied left-sided ventricle may be found. A bicuspid aortic valve will be present in nearly 60% of cases. Doppler flow can approximate the systolic flow gradient across the obstructed region. In the setting of subvalvar aortic stenosis, flow acceleration begins below the valve and can be associated with aortic regurgitation. Supravalvar aortic stenosis is commonly seen with William syndrome and should prompt a search for the associated lesion of pulmonary branch stenosis. In the neonate with aortic stenosis, patency of the ductus arteriosus and its direction of flow are important to help plan an appropriate management strategy.

Management

Balloon valvuloplasty became the standard of care for valvar aortic stenosis in the 1990s, when several investigators demonstrated that this approach was equally effective with less morbidity and mortality when compared with surgical valvotomy.[50-54] However, timing of intervention is perhaps the most difficult element in the management of this disease. As discussed earlier, the progression rate of aortic stenosis during the first 6 months of life is unpredictable. If diagnosed prenatally or shortly after birth in an otherwise healthy, stable newborn, careful monitoring alone is justified. A gradient by echocardiogram of less than 50 mmHg with either a closed or left-to-right shunting ductus arteriosus is generally considered to be less than severe aortic stenosis, and the newborn can be discharged from the hospital with close follow-up. Right-to-left shunting through the ductus arteriosus suggests ductal-dependent systemic cardiac output (in the absence of persistent fetal circulation), and the patient should remain monitored in the hospital until a final decision regarding the need for intervention is reached.

Once the infant is home, most pediatric cardiologists will arrange biweekly or monthly visits for the first 6 months of life. During this rapid phase of somatic growth, changes in clinical status or aortic stenosis gradient can occur quickly. When neonatal intervention is required, frequent return visits may occur for at least the first 6 months of life because the frequency of restenosis is between 15% and 30%.[55,56]

In most cases, aortic valvotomy, whether performed in the catheterization laboratory or in the operating room, results in some degree of aortic insufficiency.[53,57] Separation of fused commissures allows for less encumbered prograde flow but also disrupts intrinsic leaflet coaptation. Fortunately, the degree of insufficiency is usually mild and is well tolerated for many years.

Valvar aortic stenosis tends to increase at a slower, more predictable rate after the first year of life. Nonemergent intervention is indicated in the setting of progressively severe left-ventricular hypertrophy with a transvalvar gradient above 50 mm Hg.[58-60] Most cardiologists would also intervene in the presence of syncope, exercise intolerance, chest pain, or an abnormal exercise stress test. For isolated valvar stenosis, balloon valvuloplasty is the preferred interventional procedure. However, if stenosis is also accompanied by significant valvar insufficiency, or if more than moderate insufficiency develops after a balloon procedure, then surgical intervention will be the only effective therapy. Surgical options include valve replacement with a prosthetic mechanical valve, cadaveric homograft, porcine xenograft, or a pulmonary valve autograft (Ross procedure). When deciding which option is best, the important considerations are patient age, size, lifestyle, and future adherence to an anticoagulation regimen.

With the exception of an absent valve click, subaortic stenosis is clinically indistinguishable from valvar stenosis. However, the pathophysiological circumstance is uniquely different in several important ways. In subvalvar aortic stenosis, the left-ventricular outflow tract (LVOT) is obstructed by a superfluous tissue membrane, hypertrophy of the IVS immediately inferior to the aortic valve, or both. The blood flow velocity becomes accelerated before reaching the aortic valve and gradually damages the leaflets over time, which can result in progressive valvar regurgitation. Surgical resection of this subaortic region is indicated to relieve obstruction and prevent progressive aortic valve damage and resultant insufficiency. A recurrence rate of 20% to 30% for subaortic obstruction[61,62] after resection coupled with an inability to predict significant valve damage accurately makes the decision to intervene extremely difficult. In general, surgical resection is performed with the onset of any degree of aortic insufficiency or gradients between 20 to 40 mm Hg.[61,62] Furthermore, the rate of progression of subaortic stenosis is insidious and is not associated with acute cardiovascular decompensation. Progressive valvar damage can ultimately require valve repair or replacement with a homograft valve, artificial valve, or autograft valve via the Ross procedure.

Supravalvar aortic stenosis is the least commonly encountered form of aortic stenosis. Its frequent association with Williams syndrome also places these patients at increased risk for supravalvar branch pulmonary stenosis and obstruction at the origin of other major vessels (ie, coronary arteries, subclavian arteries, carotid arteries, splenic arteries; Figure 251-14).[61] As with subvalvar aortic stenosis, this anatomic variant

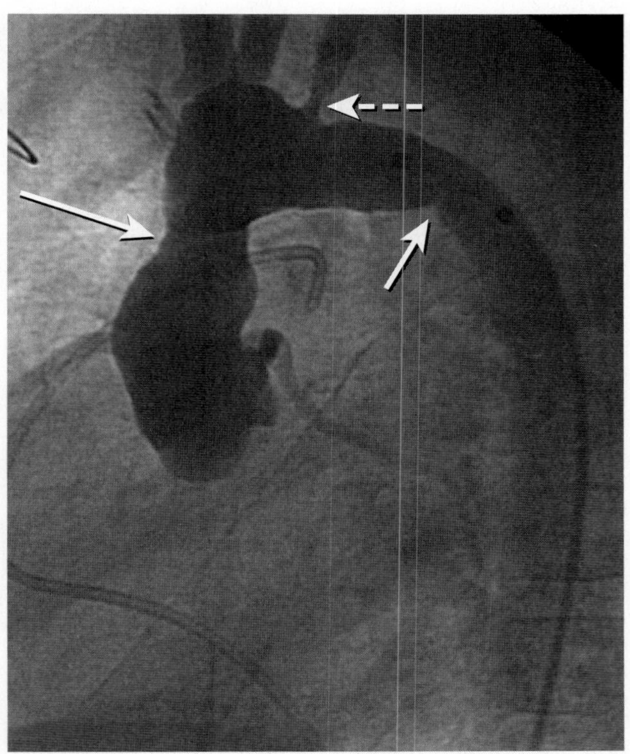

Figure 251-14 Aortogram of a 2-year-old child with non-Williams congenital supravalvar aortic stenosis *(long arrow)* with coarctation of the aorta *(short arrow)*. The perforated arrow demonstrates the narrowed origin of the left subclavian artery.

has an insidious disease progression marked by significantly elevated coronary artery perfusion pressures. Furthermore, given that the pressure gradient is located superior to the aortic root, the proximal portions of the coronary arteries are dilated in response to the persistently elevated pressures they experience. When surgery is indicated, patch aortoplasty of the narrowed region is corrective but also reduces the coronary artery perfusion pressure and can produce coronary artery ischemia if not proactively managed in the postoperative cardiac intensive care unit.

Coarctation of the Aorta

Coarctation can occur as either a discrete narrowing or a diffuse hypoplasia of the transverse and isthmic aortic arch. Although a discrete coarctation can occur in virtually any portion of the aorta, it is typically found near the insertion of the ductus arteriosus (juxtaductal). Patient presentation tends to have a bimodal distribution; those with diffuse arch hypoplasia are typically diagnosed shortly after birth and those with an isolated discrete narrowing may not be diagnosed until later in infancy or childhood (Figure 251-15).

In patients with severe coarctation, a tissue ledge protrudes from the posterior wall into the lumen of the isthmic aorta. During the transition from fetal circulation, the ductus arteriosus tissue begins to contract in response to rising oxygen concentrations. Constricting ductal tissue in combination with the adjacent posterior ledge forms an obstructive shelf. If this shelf of tissue is significantly obstructive to limit lower body flow, then systemic underperfusion and shock can ensue. Once diagnosed, infusion of

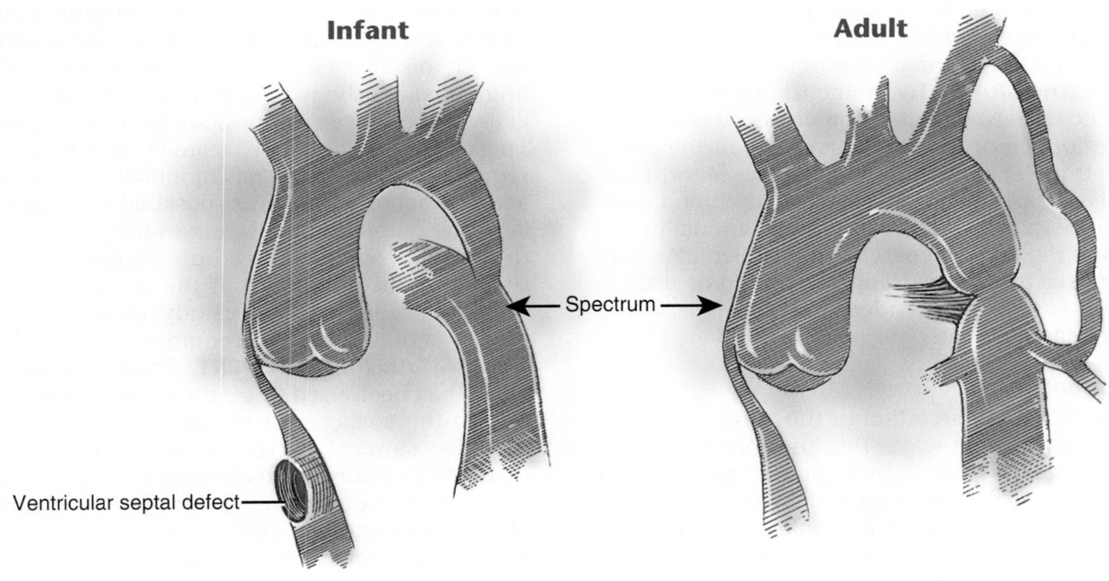

Figure 251-15 *Infantile* and *adult* types of coarctation of the aorta. The left picture demonstrates a diffusely hypoplastic aortic arch extending into the proximal descending aorta at the insertion of the ductus arteriosus. The right picture shows a more discrete area of narrowing with a large collateral vessel spanning the coarctation site. (*Castanedas AR, Jonas RA.* Cardiac Surgery of the Neonate and Infant. *Philadelphia, PA: WB Saunders; 1994. Copyright © 1994, Elsevier.*)

prostaglandin E1 can reopen the ductus. By performing this task, the physician can provide ductal flow to the lower body, eliminate the juxta-ductal obstruction to flow, or both.

Aortic coarctation diagnosed during adolescence has a distinctly different presentation. The fact that these patients survive through infancy without either detection or intervention suggests a different pathophysiological situation. The most likely difference is that a discrete, relatively undersized segment of the aorta, which was adequate for early postnatal life, did not continue to grow at a rate commensurate with the remainder of the aorta. Given that the segment never becomes acutely obstructive, the body has time to produce multiple collateral arteries connecting the aorta proximal and distal to the obstruction thus bypassing the coarctation. If undetected for many years, the intercostal arteries supplying the collateral artery system can become extensive and produce indentations or notching of the ribs. Unlike the neonatal presentation, these patients exhibit only a systolic murmur, upper extremity hypertension, or both. Upper extremity or precoarctation hypertension is the result of increased pressure proximal to the obstruction and increased renin-angiotensin activity intended to maintain normal perfusion pressure to the renal arteries. Any evaluation of pediatric hypertension should include an evaluation for coarctation of the aorta.

Evaluation

ELECTROCARDIOGRAM. As with aortic stenosis, the ECG is unlikely to contribute to the diagnosis of coarctation of the aorta unless left-ventricular hypertrophy or strain is present.

CHEST RADIOGRAPH. In the adolescent with long-standing, unrepaired coarctation of the aorta, rib notching may be seen from engorgement of the intercostal blood vessels which will provide collateral circulation around the coarctation segment.

ECHOCARDIOGRAM. Two-dimensional echocardiogram can be used to diagnose the presence of a hypoplastic aortic arch or discrete narrowing of the aorta. Although Doppler flow can estimate the blood pressure gradient, upper and lower extremity blood pressures are perhaps a more accurate modality for determining the clinical coarctation gradient. As with aortic stenosis, the echocardiogram should be used to evaluate for any other left-sided obstructive lesions to help guide management.

Management

The newborn with coarctation of the aorta may present in several different ways. Because this lesion may not be detected by prenatal ultrasound, palpation of the femoral pulses becomes a crucial part of the newborn examination. When not palpable in an otherwise healthy-appearing infant, both upper and one lower extremity blood pressure should be obtained with the infant supine and calm, if possible. Blood pressure should be checked in both arms because the left subclavian artery may arise either proximal or distal to the coarctation site. Although rare, if it arises distal to the coarctation and only the left arm was monitored, then no blood pressure gradient would be demonstrated because both the leg and left arm would have postobstruction blood pressures. However, checking only a right arm blood pressure can be misleading as well. In the case of an aberrant right subclavian artery arising distal to an aortic coarctation, both the leg and right arm would again have postobstruction blood pressures and would not demonstrate a blood pressure gradient. Other than isolated, unilateral femoral artery stenosis, no circumstances are found in which a blood pressure gradient exists between the lower extremities; therefore a single leg blood pressure should be adequate.

If a gradient is demonstrated by blood pressure cuff, then a pediatric cardiology consultation should be obtained. Although extremity blood pressures are far more accurate in determining the actual gradient across the coarctation, an echocardiogram is needed to determine if the coarctation is ductal dependent and to evaluate for other left-sided obstructive lesions. Determining the presence of a PDA is of critical importance. Additionally, because of the presence of ductal tissue in the aorta, a coarctation cannot definitively be ruled out until the ductus has closed. If the ductus is closed and a blood pressure gradient by cuff or narrowing by echocardiogram is not found, then a hemodynamically significant coarctation does not exist. Therefore, if concerns for the existence of a coarctation are present, then the patient should not be discharged until the ductus arteriosus has completely closed or close follow-up has been arranged.

Hemodynamically significant (ductal-dependent) coarctation of the aorta in the newborn period requires intensive management. The initial treatment should be initiation of a prostaglandin E1 infusion to maintain ductal patency or regain it should the ductus be closed or small. The patient should receive no enteral feeds because of possible intestinal underperfusion, and renal function should be monitored closely. For the discharged newborn whose ductus closed at home insidiously, resulting in a coarctation, shock is likely to be present from poor lower body perfusion. These patients should be treated similarly but will also require frequent blood gas monitoring for assessment and correction of acidosis, possible mechanical ventilation, and upper and lower extremity blood pressures to track the success of the prostaglandin infusion in regaining ductal patency. If the clinician is unable to reestablish adequate lower body perfusion, then emergent intervention may be required.

SURGICAL MANAGEMENT. Though balloon aortoplasty has been used in treating infant native coarctation of the aorta, most pediatric cardiologists would consider surgical correction to be the standard of care.[63,64] The surgical technique used depends on the extent of the coarctation and surgeon preference. For discrete coarctations, the two most common surgical approaches include (1) subclavian flap repair and (2) patch aortoplasty. In the former, the subclavian artery closest to the coarctation (generally the left) is ligated distally and filleted open (Figure 251-16). The coarctation region is also filleted open, and the flap of subclavian artery tissue is then rotated and sutured in place. The alternative to ligation of the subclavian artery is use of a Dacron patch to open the coarctation. Of the

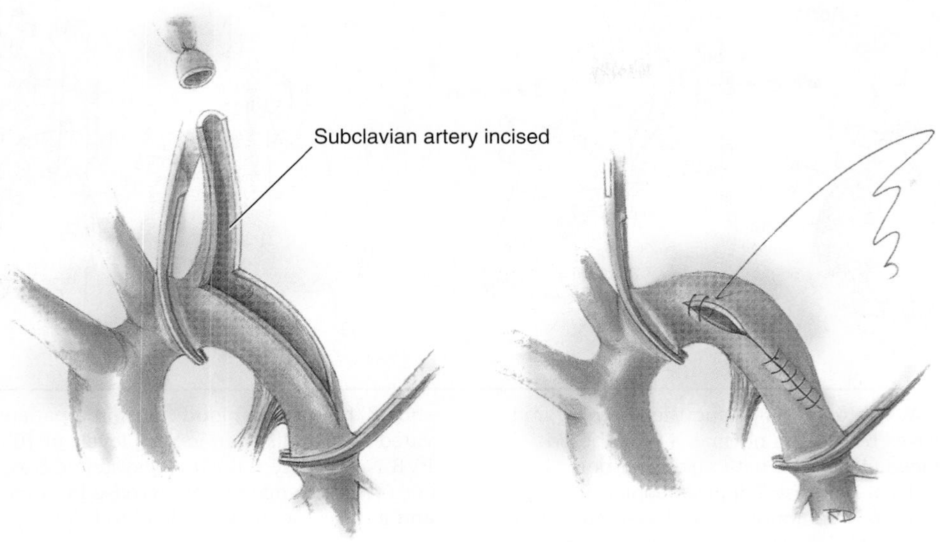

Figure 251-16 Subclavian flap repair of a discrete coarctation of the aorta. (*Jonas RA.* Comprehensive Surgical Management of Congenital Heart Disease. *London, UK: Hodder Arnold; 2004. Reprinted by permission of Edward Arnold Hodder Education Ltd.*)

two approaches, use of the subclavian flap procedure is less likely to result in aneurysmal dilatation of the segment of aorta but can be associated with a mild growth retardation and loss of strength in the respective arm.

For cases in which the coarctation is associated with some element of isthmic hypoplasia, particularly in infants, the preferred surgical approach is coarctation segment resection with *extended end-to-end* reanastomosis. By beveling the two ends before anastomosis, the circumferential sutures are distributed over a larger area and are less likely to fibrose and form a recoarctation. The rate of recoarctation varies by surgical procedure used but is reported between 5% and 25%.[65-69]

Coarctation associated with a diffuse segment of transverse arch hypoplasia is not generally amenable to an extended end-to-end reanastomosis unless the descending aorta can be fully mobilized and advanced proximally to the distal ascending aorta without disrupting cervical vessels. In these instances, arch repair will be quite extensive and usually requires arch augmentation with homograft that is sewn around the lesser curvature of the arch, from the transverse arch beyond the resected coarctation segment to the proximal descending aorta to reduce the risk of subsequent restenosis.

The actual surgical incision site may change based on the extent of the coarctation. A discrete region of affected aorta without associated intracardiac malformations will generally be repaired through a lateral thoracotomy. An intercostal incision is made in the mid-axillary line and visualization is achieved by separation of the left upper and lower lung lobes. When diffuse aortic hypoplasia or intracardiac malformations exist, a midline sternotomy approach is preferred to maximize exposure and ability to repair the defect adequately.

PROGNOSIS AFTER SURGERY. Given that the restenosis rate is up to 25% after various surgical corrections for coarctation, balloon dilatation in the cardiac catheterization laboratory is an invaluable tool for these patients. A gradient of more than 20 mm Hg is generally considered the clinical indication for intervention. Balloon dilatation results in splitting or tearing of intimal or proximal medial tissue planes and will often be repeated 2 to 3 times to ensure adequate luminal diameter. Several studies have demonstrated post-balloon dilatation restenosis rates of less than 20%, but associated transverse arch hypoplasia was associated with a higher rate of reintervention.[69,70] Stent placement during balloon dilatation has been shown to reduce the rate of restenosis and provide significant relief from obstruction in intermediate follow-up studies (3 to 6 years).[71,72] However, these studies predominantly evaluated adults. Metallic stent placement is not recommended in young children, however, because the artificial stent will not grow with the rapidly growing patient.

Postoperative or postprocedural treatment of coarctation of the aorta is frequently complicated by paradoxic hypertension or systemic blood pressure higher than preoperative measures.[73] Animal studies have shown that stimulation of sympathetic nerve fibers located between the media and the adventitia of the aorta increases norepinephrine release, which increases systemic blood pressure. The spinal reflex is a positive feedback loop, which responds to this hypertension by increasing renin secretion from the juxtaglomerular cells of the kidney. These findings have been supported by human data in patients immediately after coarctation repair.[73] A persistent hyperdynamic state of the left ventricle likely plays a causative role as well. On this basis, β-blocker medications are often employed to treat hypertension in the

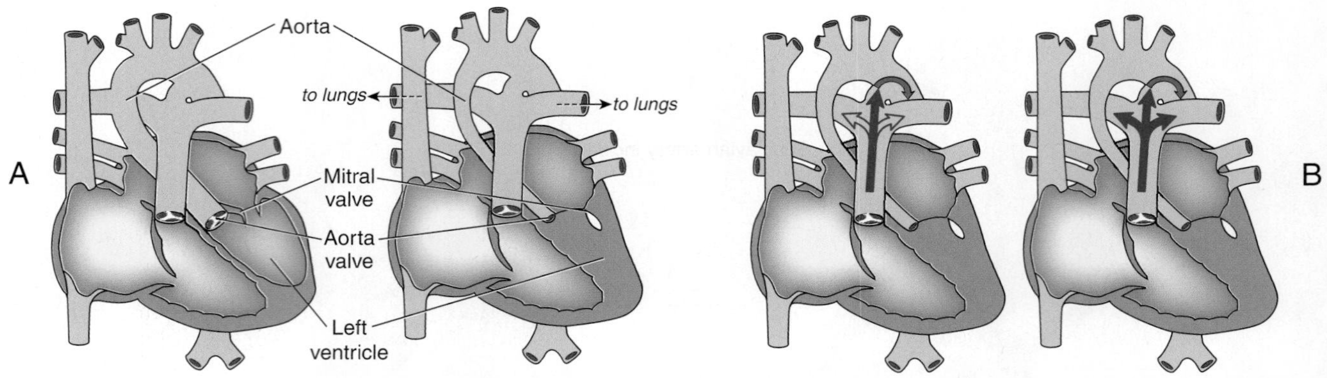

Figure 251-17 **A,** Cartoon comparing the anatomy and relative structure sizes between a normal, 4-chambered heart and a hypoplastic left heart with atresia of both the mitral and aortic valves. **B,** These 2 figures depict the relative blood flow between the pulmonary and systemic circulations in a patient with HLHS. The left-sided cartoon shows the relative blood flows in a patient with mildly elevated PVR and systemic Sao_2 levels of 70% to 80%. When PVR is decreased, however, systemic Sao_2 levels increase to 90% with a concomitant increase in pulmonary blood flow and a decrease in systemic blood flow.

immediate postoperative period. When hypertension persists beyond the first few postoperative days, most physicians will use angiotensin-converting enzyme inhibitors to offset the renin-mediated phase of hypertension. Finally, some research[74,75] suggests that dysfunctional vasodilatory mechanisms may play a large role when systemic hypertension persists after postoperative recovery. Although less likely in infants and young children, patients who undergo coarctation repair during or after adolescence have demonstrated a higher rate of persistent hypertension, which may be due to an inability to adapt to the spinal reflex described previously.[73]

Complete Mixing Lesions or the Single-Ventricle Heart

By definition, a complete mixing lesion is one in which the Sao_2 of blood is the same in both the aorta and the pulmonary artery. Systemic and pulmonary venous blood volumes drain into a single ventricle, and this combination of oxygen-rich and oxygen-poor blood produces a partially desaturated blood volume perfusing both the body and the lungs. Hypoplastic left heart syndrome will be used as the prototype for this classification of heart lesions, but the physiological mechanism and management is applicable to essentially all variations of the single-ventricle heart.

Hypoplastic Left Heart Syndrome

Hypoplastic left heart syndrome (HLHS) is a group of cardiac anomalies characterized by underdevelopment of the aortic arch, aortic valve, mitral valve, and left ventricle. Embryologically, this series of anomalies is likely propagated by inadequate blood flow through a stenotic or atretic aortic valve. Inadequate prograde flow through the left ventricle results ultimately in diminished growth. Fortunately, in utero, the fetal circulation can be adequately supplied by the right ventricle, and normal somatic growth continues. Therefore most newborns with HLHS are able to achieve normal birth weight and gestational age.

Unless diagnosed prenatally, the newborn with HLHS may not be immediately recognized. In fact, some of these patients are not diagnosed for several weeks. The timing of presentation is dependent on the delicate balance between pulmonary and systemic blood flow. All egress of blood from the single, right ventricle occurs through the pulmonary artery. Blood within the main pulmonary artery will flow to either the lungs or through the PDA into the descending aorta and retrograde into the ascending aorta (Figure 251-17). As the lungs are exposed to increasing amounts of oxygen, PVR decreases and pulmonary blood flow increases. Increased pulmonary blood flow must necessarily be associated with decreased systemic blood flow. Untreated, the oxygen-sensitive ductal tissue begins to constrict, further decreasing systemic blood flow. This condition will result in pulmonary overcirculation and systemic shock and is typically the state in which previously undiagnosed patients with HLHS present. When the condition results in end-organ damage or a delay in surgical intervention, morbidity and mortality increase significantly.[76,77]

Evaluation

CHEST RADIOGRAPH. Unless pulmonary overcirculation occurs, radiography is unlikely to contribute much to the diagnosis of HLHS except, possibly, to differentiate a cardiac from a pulmonary source of cyanosis.

ELECTROCARDIOGRAM. The healthy newborn's ECG will demonstrate right-ventricular hypertrophy with a right-axis deviation as a result of its hypertrophy relative to the left ventricle. This pattern will continue with the newborn with HLHS, but it may be more pronounced. A distinguishing feature may be a relative paucity of left-ventricular forces.

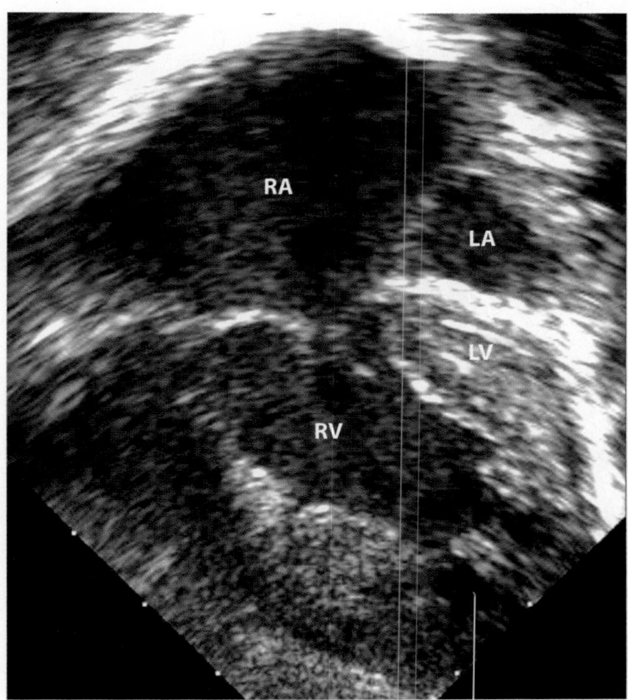

Figure 251-18 Apical 4-chamber echocardiographic view of a newborn with HLHS. Notice the severely underdeveloped left atrium and left ventricle.

ECHOCARDIOGRAM. Echocardiogram is the confirmatory study. The sonographer should document the presence or absence of the PDA and flow through both the aortic and mitral valves, estimate the left-ventricular volume, determine the size of the ascending aorta and ASD, and characterize the aortic arch and coarctation. Furthermore, size and competency of the pulmonary and tricuspid valves, and right-ventricular function are critical information to obtain to stratify surgical morbidity and mortality risks (Figure 251-18).

Management

The first step in management of HLHS is defect recognition. Early clinical manifestations can be subtle. The newborn with HLHS may not demonstrate profound systemic cyanosis until the Sa_{O_2} falls below approximately 85%, and possibly lower in dark-skinned children. A cardiac murmur is commonly not present or appreciated. Therefore palpation of femoral pulses becomes a critical step in every newborn's routine evaluation (see chapters in Part 5: Care of the Term and Late Preterm Infant). As with isolated coarctation of the aorta or aortic stenosis, the newborn with HLHS will commonly have decreased femoral pulses. These pulses will become progressively weaker as the ductus arteriosus closes. If aortic atresia exists, then all four extremity pulses will diminish with ductal closure.

Once a clinical suggestion for the diagnosis of HLHS exists, a prostaglandin E1 infusion should be started immediately. Starting doses can vary widely based on clinical status, but all can result in apnea. If a cardiac lesion is strongly suspected, beginning prostaglandin E1 infusion should not be held until a pediatric cardiology consult can be obtained.

When the diagnosis of HLHS is confirmed, arterial and venous catheters should be inserted, if possible. The preoperative medical management of these newborns varies between institutions. However, the parameters directing management are the same and include renal function (assessed by urine output and serum creatine), blood pressure, Sa_{O_2}, and arterial blood gases. When followed serially, these measurements provide a surrogate for the balance between pulmonary and systemic blood flow. If renal function and blood pressure are decreased with a concomitant rise in serum lactate, then systemic blood flow is inadequate. This circumstance generally occurs in the presence of increased Sa_{O_2} or a relative pulmonary overcirculation. Multiple strategies exist to remedy this situation, including hypoxia (ie, producing subambient oxygen by increased nitrogen infusion into the inhaled gas mixture), hypercarbia (ie, increasing carbon dioxide content of inhaled gas mixture), permissive hypercapnea (ie, when intubated, decreasing minute ventilation with resultant pulmonary vasoconstriction), or decreasing SVR via vasodilatory medications (ie, milrinone and phenoxybenzamine). Regardless of which method is used or whether the patient is intubated, the primary end points of the preoperative therapy are to provide adequate pulmonary and systemic blood flow.

The surgical intervention strategy for all single-ventricle hearts is based on two simple premises: (1) A single ventricle is not able to perform the function of two ventricles indefinitely, and (2) the PVR is elevated initially after birth and, in most cases, does not decrease completely until 2 to 6 months of age. The physiological characteristic does not change regardless of which ventricle is hypoplastic. However, the surgical options available to each patient depend on how blood flow is provided to the lungs and body.

Again, using the HLHS as the prototype for the single-ventricle heart, Figure 251-19 demonstrates the first-stage palliative surgery called the Norwood procedure. This procedure, introduced by Dr William Norwood in 1980,[78] produces a neoaorta from the main pulmonary artery and the hypoplastic ascending aorta. The main pulmonary artery is ligated at its branch bifurcation point and then attached to the ascending aortic arch, usually in a side-to-side fashion. After resection of a coarctation segment, the remainder of the hypoplastic aortic arch is augmented with homograft. As a result, the pulmonary valve becomes the systemic semilunar valve, and the coronary arteries, which arise normally from the aortic root, are perfused retrograde through the ascending aorta. The surgery is completed by providing pulmonary blood flow through either an aortopulmonary shunt (ie, Blalock-Taussig shunt from right subclavian artery to right pulmonary artery) or a right ventricle–to–pulmonary artery conduit (ie, Sano conduit[79]). The right ventricle is thus transformed into a systemic ventricle responsible for pumping blood to the body and lungs.

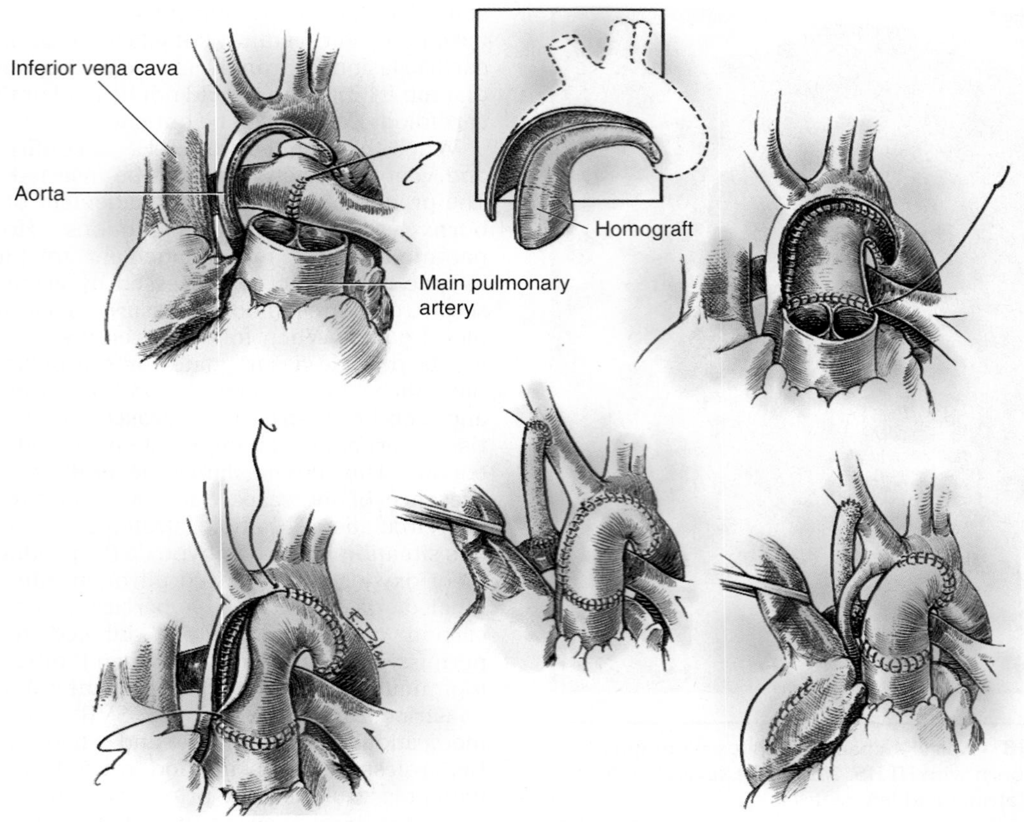

Figure 251-19 Depiction of the steps involved in the Norwood procedure. The main pulmonary artery is ligated at its insertion into the confluence of the branch pulmonary arteries. The main pulmonary artery is then connected in a side-side fashion to the hypoplastic ascending aorta. After an appropriately sized homograft patch is made by the surgeon, the new patch material is sewn to the underside of the transverse and proximal descending aortic arch augmenting the previously hypoplastic aortic arch in its entirety to a point beyond the site of native coarctation, which should eliminate any arch obstruction. This process completes the neoaortic arch reconstruction. Pulmonary blood flow is then provided through a modified Blalock-Taussig shunt, which is a Gore-Tex tube graft connecting the pulmonary arteries to the right subclavian artery. (*Castanedas AR, Jonas RA.* Cardiac Surgery of the Neonate and Infant. *Philadelphia, PA: WB Saunders; 1994. Copyright © 1994, Elsevier.*)

This initial palliation is necessary but suboptimal for the single-ventricle heart. The PVR does not fully decline for several months and requires systemic blood pressures to overcome elevated pulmonary artery pressures. The right ventricle is then obligated to perform as both a right and a left ventricle and is also volume overloaded from shunt-mediated pulmonary overcirculation. Once PVR decreases, the second stage of the palliative surgeries decreases the work of the single ventricle by removing the need for active pumping of the pulmonary blood supply. The Glenn procedure[80-82] connects the SVC to the pulmonary artery, and the previously placed shunt or conduit is ligated. By doing so, pulmonary blood flow is provided passively from the SVC into the low-resistance and low-pressure pulmonary arteries (Figure 251-20).

The systemic Sa_{O_2} in patients after the Norwood and Glenn procedures will generally remain 75% to 85%. These children will typically have a higher hemoglobin concentration than acyanotic children in response. The 3rd and final stage of these palliative surgeries is the Fontan procedure,[83-87] which baffles the IVC to the pulmonary artery, routing all systemic venous return directly into the lungs. Therefore oxygen-rich is separated from oxygen-poor blood, and the systemic Sa_{O_2} is typically near normal (>90%).

Prognosis

Cardiac dysrhythmias,[32] cerebrovascular accidents with seizures,[88] myocardial ischemia, pleural effusions, and the need for multiple cardiac catheterizations have all been described in this patient population. Improved survival after the Fontan procedure has been shown to be strongly correlated with shorter cardiopulmonary bypass and aortic cross-clamp times.[89] A spectrum of neurodevelopmental outcomes has been reported for this patient group. Recent studies have shown that a majority of postoperative 8 to 9 year olds had cognitive scores comparable to the general population,[88,90] but approximately 18% demonstrated IQ scores under 70.[88] Some of these children have also had varying degrees of

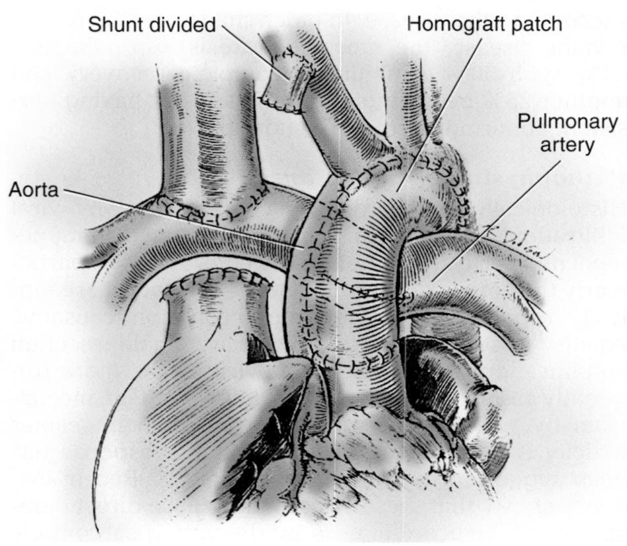

Figure 251-20 Depiction of the extracardiac anatomy after the bidirectional Glenn procedure. The Blalock-Taussig shunt is ligated, and the cardiac end of the SVC is divided and anastomosed to the pulmonary arteries becoming the sole source of pulmonary blood flow. The neoaorta created during the Norwood procedure remains unaltered. (*Castanedas AR, Jonas RA.* Cardiac Surgery of the Neonate and Infant. *Philadelphia, PA: WB Saunders; 1994. Copyright © 1994, Elsevier.*)

developmental motor delay and behavioral problems, including obsessive-compulsive disorder and attention-deficit/hyperactivity disorder. Given that this series of surgical interventions has only been routinely performed for approximately 2 decades, long-term prognostic data are lacking. Nonetheless, in many patients, this palliative approach for single-ventricle physiological arrangement may ultimately serve as an extended bridge to cardiac transplantation, given that recent studies have shown that 20% to 30% of patients after undergoing the Fontan procedure develop heart failure, resulting either in successful orthotopic heart transplantation or death.[32]

Other Complete Mixing Lesions

Tricuspid Atresia

Patients with tricuspid atresia have a physiological display comparable to those with HLHS. The major aspects of distinction are anatomic. In utero, the atretic tricuspid valve does not allow forward flow into the right ventricle or pulmonary artery, causing them to also become hypoplastic or atretic. As a result, the single ventricle is a left ventricle that is generally connected to the aorta. Although several anatomic variants exist, this type of ventriculo-arterial concordance allows for a less-complicated surgical correction because it does not require formation of a neoaorta. Instead, an aortopulmonary shunt is placed to provide pulmonary blood flow, but the Glenn and Fontan surgeries are unchanged. Although a single left ventricle is intuitively advantageous over a single right ventricle, the data have failed to demonstrate any differences in long-term survival.[91,92]

ACQUIRED HEART DISEASE—INFECTIOUS ETIOLOGIES

For a discussion on rheumatic heart disease, see Chapter 317. For a discussion on Kawasaki disease, see Chapter 289.

Endocarditis

Endocarditis is a bacterial infection of the endocardium or endothelium of the heart. Generally, endocarditis is associated with a procedural or surgical intervention. Spontaneous endocarditis does occur but is exceedingly rare without predisposing risk factors. Infective endocarditis (IE) is of clinical interest because of the significant morbidity and mortality it produces. With the increased sophistication of interventional catheterization procedures and the dramatic improvement in survival profiles for children with congenital heart disease, IE prevalence has risen substantially over the last 2 decades.[93]

Before the 1970s, fewer than one half of all children with IE had an associated congenital heart defect[94]; these children now account for approximately 90% of all cases. The remaining cases are generally associated with indwelling venous catheters without associated structural heart disease.[95]

The pathogenesis for IE is relatively well understood. Intact endocardium will not predispose the area to bacterial attachment or activation of the coagulation pathway.[96] However, cardiac endothelium can be directly damaged by venous catheters or indirectly by the turbulent flow produced with many congenital heart defects. In either situation, thrombogenesis can occur with deposition of sterile clumps of fibrin, platelets, and red blood cells.[96]

Staphylococci, streptococci, and enterococci remain the most common pathogens because of their ability to interact with platelets and resist the host's immune response.[97] The known risks of developing IE in the preoperative state of congenital heart defects are as follows: tetralogy of Fallot, above 30%; VSD, 12% to 14%; PDA, 8%; aortic stenosis, 2%; and pulmonary stenosis, 1%.

Diagnosis

The clinical course of IE is typically indolent but, in rare cases, can cause cardiogenic shock. Affected patients may have recurrent low-grade fevers (90%), arthralgias (25%), gastrointestinal discomfort (15%), fatigue, rigors, or other nonspecific findings. Physical examination may be significant for a new cardiac murmur (rare), splenomegaly (55%), and neurologic changes (20%). The classically described findings of Osler nodes (tender subcutaneous nodules on pads of fingers), Janeway lesions (nontender hemorrhagic macules on palms or soles), Roth spots (pale centered oval hemorrhages on retina), and splinter hemorrhages in the nail beds are rare in children.

In 1994 the Duke criteria[98] for diagnosis of IE were introduced. Using these lists of major and minor criteria has improved diagnostic accuracy. The Duke criteria for IE are met if a patient demonstrates both major criteria, 5 of the 6 minor criteria, or 1 major and 3 minor criteria. Because direct visualization of infected thrombi is difficult, most physicians require two distinct blood cultures with identical bacterial pathogens before considering the diagnosis of IE. Although transthoracic echocardiography (TTE) has excellent specificity, the poor sensitivity limits its role in the diagnosis of IE; transesophageal echocardiography (TEE) is the preferred visual diagnostic modality, with a sensitivity of 80% to 90%, and should be strongly considered in highly suggestive cases even if TTE is negative. Overall, the minor criteria are often used when diagnosing pediatric IE.

Treatment

The therapy for IE entails a prolonged course of intravenous antibiotics to eradicate the high concentration of organisms deeply embedded within the fibrin-platelet matrix.[96] For a complete review of the suggested regimen of antibiotic therapy, see the American Heart Association's recommendations for IE therapy in adults.[99] In brief, duration of intravenous therapy will vary between 2 and 6 weeks depending on bacterial speciation and antimicrobial sensitivity. Blood cultures should be repeated during and after antibiotic therapy to ensure proper choice and duration.

Prognosis

Before the era of antibiotics, IE was universally fatal. Today, however, survival has increased by 70% to 80%. Long-term prognosis is primarily determined by the presence of complications. If treatment is initiated early, then valvar damage, heart failure, embolic events, and heart block can be prevented. However, complete eradication becomes significantly more difficult if the endocarditis involves a prosthetic valve or is due to a *Staphylococcus* species. In these scenarios, the prognosis is more guarded.

Prevention

The complications associated with IE along with its difficult management make prevention an integral step in caring for persons at risk. Good oral hygiene and appropriate antibiotic prophylaxis constitute the primary means for achieving this goal. Inappropriate prophylaxis can pose more risk than benefit when considering hypersensitivity reactions to antibiotics. Likely, the best prevention strategy is to maintain good oral hygiene and avoid any unnecessary interventions.

Myocarditis

Myocarditis is a generalized inflammation of the cardiac muscular walls. In a 10-year study of 14,000 cardiac patients cared for at Texas Children's Hospital between 1954 and 1977, 0.5% of patients were diagnosed with myocarditis at presentation and another 2% to 5% at autopsy.[100] Nearly 20% of pediatric sudden deaths may be related to myocarditis.[100,101] Though its incidence is low in the pediatric population, an accurate and timely diagnosis is critical for improving the related morbidity and mortality. Mortality rates vary inversely with age of onset; nearly 75% of all newborns and infants who develop myocarditis will succumb to the disease. In older children with less fulminant disease, the mortality rate is approximately 25%, with 50% exhibiting a complete recovery and another 25% becoming asymptomatic but having persistent abnormal cardiac function.

Pathophysiological Features

Histologically, myocarditis is characterized by viral infiltration of myocytes and the associated immune-mediated cell lysis. Although the enteroviruses, particularly the coxsackievirus B3 and B4 serotypes, are typically reported to be the most common causative agents,[102] studies using polymerase chain reaction amplification have found adenovirus to be more frequently associated with myocarditis.[103,104] The mechanism by which these viruses produce their cellular toxicity is unclear, but an autoimmune response has been suggested by some investigators.[105] Recent evidence shows that these viruses may cause direct damage to the myocardial cells by disrupting sarcomeric linkage proteins, particularly dystrophin, which will interfere with force transduction and result in myocyte dysfunction and heart failure.[9]

Clinical Manifestations

The clinical presentation in patients with myocarditis can range from mild ECG abnormalities in an otherwise asymptomatic child to fulminant congestive heart failure.[105] Older children will typically have less fulminant presentations, occurring 7 to 10 days after a viral upper respiratory infection or gastroenteritis. Signs and symptoms may include fever, malaise, chest pain, dyspnea, pallor, and poor perfusion. Physical examination may demonstrate muffled heart sounds and a gallop rhythm, suggesting congestive heart failure. With severe, fulminant onset, cardiogenic shock may be present.

Evaluation

Laboratory values in a child with myocarditis will be nonspecific and generally consistent with a diffuse inflammatory process. Erythrocyte sedimentation rates, C-reactive protein, and white blood cell and platelet counts may all be elevated. Measures of cardiac cell damage, including troponin-I and creatinine kinase–MB fraction, can be used to establish that myocyte injury has occurred and then to follow these levels to monitor the progress of the condition. Serum viral cultures, serologic titer assays, or PCR amplification of viral genome (or all) may help verify a cause, but an endomyocardial biopsy is required for the definitive diagnosis of myocarditis.

The pathognomonic electrocardiographic finding in myocarditis is decreased precordial voltages consistent with a loss of functioning myocardium (Figure 251-21, *A*). This finding can generally be differentiated from pericarditis by the absence of diffuse ST segment elevation commonly present in pericarditis. First-, 2nd-, and 3rd-degree atrioventricular block may develop, as well as wide-complex ventricular tachycardias. A chest radiograph often demonstrates global cardiac enlargement and increased pulmonary vascularity with varying degrees of edema (Figure 251-21, *B*). Two-dimensional echocardiography commonly demonstrates global

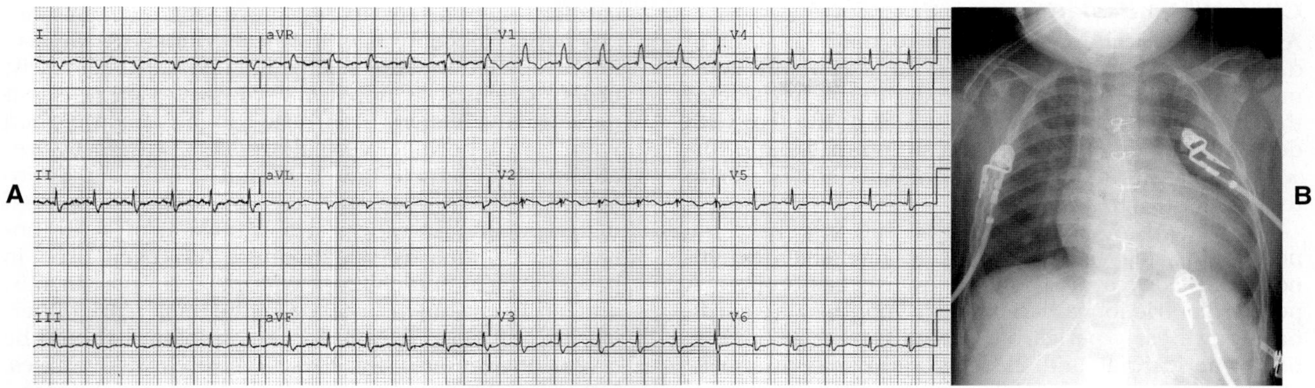

Figure 251-21 **A**, ECG of a 6 year old with myocarditis. Note the low QRS voltages throughout limb and precordial leads. Although not seen in every patient with myocarditis, this ECG finding is pathognomonic for this diagnosis. **B**, Chest radiograph of the same patient who developed myocarditis-induced DCM.

cardiac chamber enlargement with atrioventricular valve regurgitation and poorly contracting ventricles.[105]

Treatment

The treatment for myocarditis remains largely supportive. Though antiviral medications, steroids, and intravenous gamma globulin are administered, limited and somewhat controversial data exist supporting their use.[106,107] For milder cases, bed rest and hospitalization are sufficient until the patient's cardiac status returns to baseline. More severely affected children, however, commonly require aggressive diuresis, inotropy, chronotropy, afterload-reducing medications, antiarrhythmic agents, ventilator support, and even mechanical circulatory support (ie, extracorporeal membrane oxygenation, ventricular assist devices).

Management

For patients surviving the initial phase, many will require long-term medical therapy. Diuresis, afterload reduction, and, in many instances, long-term antiarrhythmia medications (and in some cases, automatic implantable cardioverter defibrillators [AICDs]) are commonly used. Adult studies examining the use of β-blockers (carvedilol, metoprolol, and bisoprolol) in the setting of heart failure have shown promise in reversing abnormal cardiac remodeling and minimizing clinical symptoms, hospitalizations, and cardiac-associated deaths.[108] Results from a similar, multicenter, randomized, controlled trial of β-blocker use in pediatric patients are soon to be published. When patients fail to respond adequately to medical or mechanical support, cardiac transplant is the only alternative for long-term survival in appropriately selected patients.

Pericarditis

Pericarditis is an inflammation of the pericardium and is often associated with effusion (fluid accumulation) within the pericardial sac. However, in conditions such as myxedema (hypothyroidism), patients may have pericardial effusion in the absence of pericarditis. Pericarditis can have both infectious and noninfectious causes. Among infectious agents, the enteroviruses (especially coxsackievirus B), influenza, cytomegalovirus, and Epstein-Barr virus, are the frequent viral causes, whereas *Staphylococcus aureus*, *Streptococcus pyogenes*, and *Streptococcus pneumoniae* are the most common bacterial pathogens.[109] Tuberculous and fungal pericarditis are unusual. Rheumatic fever, autoimmune diseases, postcardiac surgery, uremia, and malignancies such as leukemia are some of the noninfectious causes of pericarditis.

Pathophysiological Features

Both the parietal and the visceral layers of the pericardium are inflamed, and the pericardial fluid can be serous, serofibrinous, hemorrhagic, or purulent in nature. Myocarditis is frequently associated with infectious pericarditis, more so with viral than with bacterial agents.[109] However, depending on the virulence of the offending organism, pericarditis can be the more pathological component of the two processes.

The clinical features of pericarditis and the associated effusion are due to diastolic dysfunction related to abnormal, restricted filling of the heart. Therefore the symptoms and signs depend on the fluid volume within the pericardial space, the rapidity with which the fluid collects, and myocardial function. A rapid collection of fluid, as occurs in bacterial infections, may cause severe circulatory compromise (cardiac tamponade). A gradually developing pericardial effusion allows the pericardium to stretch, and therefore the increase in the pericardial pressure is slower, which is usually much more readily tolerated. However, if the myocardial function is depressed, then even this gradual increase in pericardial fluid and pressure may cause significant circulatory compromise.

With the onset of cardiac tamponade, the following compensatory mechanisms are activated:

- Tachycardia to improve the cardiac output
- Increase in SVR to raise the falling blood pressure
- Constriction of systemic and pulmonary veins to improve diastolic filling

Clinical Manifestations

A history of viral upper respiratory infection 10 to 14 days before the development of pericarditis is common. Patients typically exhibit pain in the left side of the chest, which is worse in the supine position or with deep breathing and relieved on sitting or leaning forward. The pain may radiate to the left shoulder or to the neck.

The patient may be febrile especially with bacterial pericarditis, may be pale, gray, hypotensive, tachypneic, and tachycardic (signs of low cardiac output). A pericardial friction rub (a biphasic sound) is the cardinal sign of early pericarditis. With further accumulation of pericardial fluid, the friction rub may disappear and the heart sounds may become muffled. In pericardial tamponade, because of the pressure caused by the large amount of pericardial fluid around the heart, the venous return during inspiration is compromised, resulting in a paradoxic rise in the jugular venous pressure (known as the Kussmaul sign) and a decrease in cardiac output and systolic blood pressure (known as pulses paradoxicus). These patients will also have other signs of low cardiac output such as pale, clammy skin, gray (sometimes mottled) appearance, dyspnea, and tachycardia.

Evaluation

Chest radiograph may be normal when the pericardial effusion is small. However, with a large effusion, the heart appears enlarged and has a globular appearance. The pulmonary vascular marking may be prominent in patients with tamponade. An ECG may show low-voltage QRS complexes with substantial pericardial effusion; it may also show changes caused by associated myocarditis such as diffuse ST elevation in initial stages. Gradually, the ST segment begins to normalize, with decrease in the T wave amplitude eventually leading to T wave inversion. These ECG changes may resolve completely with the exception of T wave abnormalities, which may persist for long periods.

Echocardiography is most frequently used to assess the size of a pericardial effusion, which can occur with pericarditis; it is also very useful in detecting evidence for cardiac tamponade and associated conditions (ie, myocarditis).

Computed tomography and magnetic resonance imaging are indicated when the echocardiogram is inconclusive and when pericardial effusion is suspected to be loculated or hemorrhagic.[110] When the pericardial fluid collection is large or rapidly increasing, as in the case of bacterial pericarditis or when tuberculous pericarditis is suspected, performing a diagnostic and therapeutic pericardiocentesis may be necessary. This procedure will drain the fluid to minimize the potential for clinical decompensation from tamponade and allow possible etiologic diagnosis after evaluation of cell count (total and differential), glucose, protein concentration, Gram and acid-fast stain, and appropriate cultures (with viral polymerase chain reaction as indicated) and cytologic assays.

Management

The management of pericarditis depends on the size and etiology of the effusion, as well as its effect on cardiac function. Urgent decompression by percutaneous pericardiocentesis or surgical drainage is life saving in patients with cardiac tamponade. Similarly, urgent drainage is necessary for suspected purulent pericardial effusion. This task can be accomplished with a large-bore pericardial drain or a surgically created pericardial window to permit continuous drainage of purulent material and to prevent development of tamponade. Intrapericardial infusion of a fibrinolytic agent such as streptokinase has been used in patients, including children with purulent pericarditis, and has been shown to decrease the recurrence of pericardial effusion.[111] Appropriate antibiotics should be given intravenously for 4 to 6 weeks. In many cases, after treatment of purulent effusions, a partial or total pericardiectomy will be necessary to prevent the development of constrictive pericarditis related to fibrotic scarring and adhesions within the pericardial space.

The viral form of pericarditis does not require any specific treatment other than a short course of antiinflammatory medication such as ibuprofen. In patients with pericarditis associated with other conditions, such as autoimmune disease and uremia, treatment of the underlying condition leads to the resolution of the pericardial effusion. Steroids can be considered as a treatment option for persistent or refractory viral or secondary pericarditis.

CARDIOMYOPATHIES

A cardiomyopathy refers to any structural or functional abnormality of the ventricular myocardium that is not associated with congenital heart disease or diseases of the coronary arteries, cardiac valves, or pulmonary vasculature. Four general types of cardiomyopathy exist, and in order of increasing frequency are: dilated, hypertrophic, restrictive, and miscellaneous cardiomyopathies.

Dilated Cardiomyopathy

Dilated cardiomyopathy (DCM) accounts for 60% to 70% of pediatric cardiomyopathies, with an annual incidence of between 5 and 20 cases per million children.[112-114] A viral cause is identified in 2% to 15% of cases with biopsy-proven myocarditis[115]; the remaining cases are classified as idiopathic but are likely genetic. Autosomal-dominant, autosomal-recessive, X-linked, and mitochondrial inheritance patterns have been described.[112-114] Adult studies have shown approximately 20% of patients with DCM have a familial form.[116,117] Regardless of the cause, the progressive cardiac dysfunction associated with DCM is likely related to the remodeling response of the heart after an inciting injury.

Pathophysiological Features

The remodeling cascade consists of the neurohumoral response to inadequate cardiac output. Increased levels of plasma catecholamines, renin, angiotensin II, atrial- and brain-type natriuretic peptides, and overexpression of various cytokine transcripts have been identified in this cascade. Unregulated compensation by these pathways can result in excessive vasoconstriction, intravascular volume expansion, hypertrophy of functioning myocytes, and dilatation of the cardiac chambers. If unchecked, this change in myocardial structure and function can then become irreversible.

Clinical Manifestations

The clinical presentation of DCM can vary from progressive exercise intolerance with pulmonary congestion to systemic decompensation with complete cardiovascular collapse. Regardless of severity, diagnosis typically does not occur until the cardiac reserve is exhausted or is nearly exhausted. For this reason, patients with DCM are often diagnosed after an acute viral illness that elevates their resting state metabolism enough to exceed the failing heart's compensatory mechanisms.

In symptomatic patients, the physical examination will be consistent with congestive heart failure. Tachycardia, cachexia, sallow color, and a gallop may be appreciated. Pulmonary congestion will cause tachypnea and, in older children, orthopnea. Progressive ventricular dilatation or infarction of a left-ventricular papillary muscle can cause the early systolic, regurgitant murmur of mitral regurgitation. Hepatomegaly and weakened peripheral pulses may be found with severe cardiac dysfunction. A chest radiograph will generally show cardiomegaly with or without increased pulmonary vascular markings (see Figure 251-21, *B*). An ECG may show biventricular hypertrophy by voltage criteria with ST segment and T wave abnormalities (Figure 251-22). The echocardiogram will ultimately confirm the diagnosis. Dilated cardiac chambers, atrioventricular valve regurgitation, and depressed systolic function are nearly universal findings for these patients.

Treatment

Multiple treatment modalities have been implemented to improve left-ventricular systolic function in patients with DCM. The primary intervention is pharmacologic and is directed toward treating the symptoms of congestive heart failure and blunting the neurohumoral cascade responsible for the pathological ventricular reverse remodeling. Aggressive diuresis helps reduce pulmonary edema and hepatic congestion when present and helps reduce any excessive intravascular volume expansion. Spironolactone improves outcomes in adults with congestive heart failure by inhibiting part of the neurohumoral axis.[118-120] Afterload reduction, typically using angiotensin-converting enzyme inhibitors or angiotensin receptor blockers, also decreases morbidity and mortality in this population[121,122]; its use is discouraged in the acute, decompensated period.[108] The use of β-blocker therapy, however, is one of the few medical interventions for congestive heart failure that has evidence supporting its use in both adults and children.[108,123-125] A study by Shaddy et al[125] demonstrated significant improvement in systolic ventricular function after 23 months of β-blocker therapy in 15 children with DCM and associated congestive heart failure. This class of medication is believed to reverse the maladaptive remodeling effects produced by the excessive catecholamine levels exhibited in these patients. Anticoagulation therapy (ie, aspirin, warfarin) is also commonly used to reduce the risk of thrombus formation, which is inherently elevated in the relatively low flow state associated with poor ventricular function and DCM.

Cardiac resynchronization therapy (CRT) is a novel pacing modality used in patients with DCM and heart failure that is refractory to conventional medical management. By decreasing intraventricular conduction delay and the associated uncoordinated muscle contraction, CRT can synchronize ventricular wall motion, improve both diastolic filling and systolic ejection fraction, and, ultimately, reduce patient symptoms.[126-128] Further research is needed, however, to determine its efficacy in patients without intraventricular

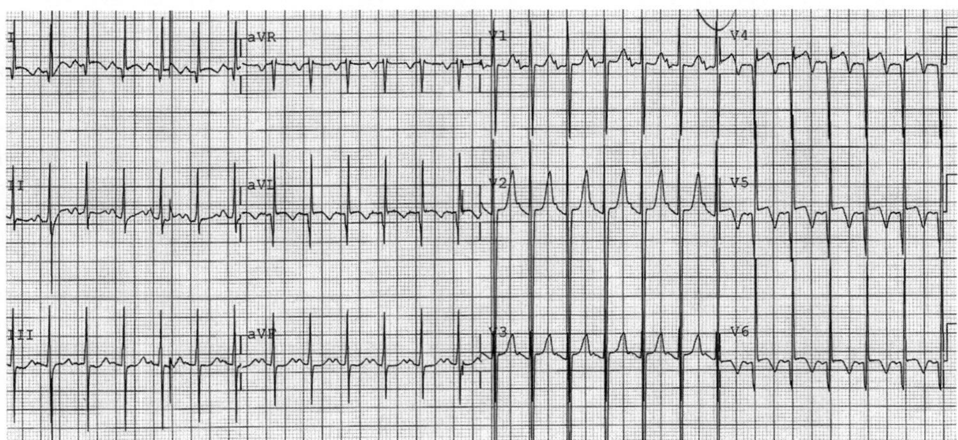

Figure 251-22 ECG of a 2-month-old infant with DCM secondary to the left coronary artery arising anomalously from the pulmonary artery. Note the large QRS voltages in the precordial leads consistent with biventricular hypertrophy and dilatation. The deep Q waves in leads I and aVL are consistent with a lateral myocardial infarction. Inverted T waves in left lateral precordial leads represent a repolarization abnormality and are consistent with left-ventricular strain.

conduction delay or with nonsinus rhythms. Its use in children is limited by the lack of controlled study data, and more research is needed before CRT can be widely prescribed in this group. In severe cases, ventricular assist devices, extracorporeal membrane oxygenation, or even cardiac transplantation may be indicated in appropriately selected patients if other treatment regimens are unsuccessful.

Hypertrophic Cardiomyopathy

Hypertrophic cardiomyopathy (HCM) is the second most common form of cardiomyopathy (20% to 30%) in children, with an annual incidence ranging between 4 and 6/1,000,000.[129] Autosomal-dominant, autosomal-recessive, and mitochondrial inheritance patterns have been described, with approximately 100 mutations mapped to 13 different cytoskeletal or sarcomeric genes.[130-138] Multiple familial forms of HCM exist, with nearly 40% to 50% demonstrating a point mutation on chromosome *14q1* (β-myosin heavy chain). HCM has also been shown to occur in association with both Noonan syndrome[130] and Friedreich ataxia.[139,140]

Pathophysiological Features

HCM is characterized by wall hypertrophy of all four heart chambers but most notably of the IVS and left-ventricular posterior wall. Hypertrophy may be concentric (50%) or asymmetric. If the IVS is disproportionately thickened, then left-ventricular outflow tract obstruction (LVOTO) can ensue in 30% of cases. Furthermore, when hypertrophy is severe, flow through the intramural coronary arteries may be decreased or even occluded, resulting in myocardial ischemia. The primary abnormality associated with HCM is diastolic dysfunction of the left ventricle, which often produces progressive exercise intolerance.[105] In the absence of LVOTO, worsening diastolic dysfunction is sufficient to produce this symptom.[141] When severe IVS thickening does occur, the increased left-ventricular outflow gradient experienced during exercise results in performance and duration limitations.

Clinical Manifestations

The clinical presentation of patients with HCM is quite variable, from infants with congestive heart failure to asymptomatic children with or without a heart murmur. Although the classic presentation is that of a syncopal patient with a loud cardiac murmur, this is rarely the case. More often, a routine examination will demonstrate a harsh systolic ejection murmur at the left sternal border with radiation to the neck. If present, this murmur of LVOTO is then accentuated when a squatting patient is asked to stand, decreasing the SVR and increasing the gradient across the LVOT. The remainder of the physical examination is typically normal. Obtaining a family history is critical because nearly one half of all patients with HCM will have a first-degree relative with the diagnosis or with a history of syncope or sudden death.

Evaluation

The ECG is abnormal in 90% to 95% of these patients,[142] with large voltages in the precordial leads, suggesting biventricular hypertrophy, ST segment elevation and depression, T wave inversion, and abnormally deep Q waves. The delta wave of Wolff-Parkinson-White syndrome is occasionally noted in association with HCM.[105] Although LVOTO is often considered the source of morbidity and mortality for these patients, ischemia-induced arrhythmias are much more likely. This finding is suggested by both the relatively low prevalence of LVOTO in patients with HCM (20% to 30%) and the tendency for frequent episodes of ventricular tachycardia and ST segment elevation on ECG during exercise. Importantly, sudden death (usually from ventricular fibrillation) is the most common cause of death in undiagnosed adolescents and young adults.[143]

Echocardiography is the method of choice for diagnosis of HCM. Attention should be focused on the type of hypertrophy (concentric versus asymmetric), ratio of IVS to left-ventricular posterior wall thickness (>1.5 is diagnostic), presence of LVOT or RVOT obstruction, and systolic anterior motion (SAM) of the anterior mitral valve leaflet. Historically, SAM is thought to be caused by the venturi effect of fluid movement in which turbulent blood flow through the ventricular outflow tract produces a pressure gradient, pulling the anterior mitral leaflet into the ventricular outflow tract, resulting in mitral regurgitation. Recent data have suggested that mid-cavitary obstruction common in HCM causes *drag* forces that may also contribute to SAM.[144]

Treatment

Once diagnosed, the primary focus of treatment for the patient with HCM is providing symptomatic relief and minimizing the risk of lethal arrhythmias. Pharmacologic intervention is indicated for patients who have symptoms or LVOTO at rest. First-line therapy for these patients is usually β-blockers.[145,146] Though its mechanism of action is unclear, β-blockade reduces heart rate and myocardial oxygen demand, allows for increased diastolic filling time, and may have some inherent antiarrhythmic properties. Furthermore, by decreasing heart rate and increasing the diastolic filling period, a larger stroke volume will be produced per heartbeat and may minimize the severity of LVOTO. If β-blockers are poorly tolerated, then calcium-channel blockers have been shown to produce similar effects. In addition, patients will generally be asked to participate in exercise stress tests and have 24-hour Holter monitoring to help stratify their risk for ventricular tachycardia and sudden death. The presence of asymptomatic, nonsustained ventricular tachycardia on Holter monitor has been shown to increase the risk of sudden death 8 to 10 times compared with HCM patients without this anomaly[147,148]; the overall risk of sudden death in patients with HCM is 1% to 2% per year (may be as high as 4% to 5% in adolescents).[143] When tachycardia is present, most experts recommend the antiarrhythmic medication Amiodarone as the drug of choice or an AICD implantation (or both) for the treatment of malignant ventricular ectopy in this patient population.[149,150] Prophylactic implantation of AICDs is being studied and has been strongly recommended under the following conditions:

left ventricle wall thickness greater than 3.0 cm, family history of death related to HCM, unexplained syncope, and nonsustained ventricular tachycardia on Holter monitor.[143,151-154] AICD placement as secondary prevention (in patients with aborted sudden death or documented ventricular tachycardia or fibrillation) is now considered standard of care in most centers.

In patients with HCM whose symptoms are related to their degree of LVOTO, reduction of flow gradient is recommended. The Brock or Morrow procedure is a surgical myomectomy reserved for symptomatic, medically refractory patients with a ventricular outflow tract gradient of more than 50 to 60 mmHg.[155] Although the 10-year survival rate after this procedure is approximately 86%,[156] the intraoperative mortality rate can approach 5%. Medical septal reduction is an alternative method of improving LVOTO by infusing desiccated alcohol into the septal perforating coronary vessels within the IVS using TEE guidance in the cardiac catheterization laboratory. As with surgical myomectomy, this procedure has been advocated for patients with HCM who are failing medical management and has been used with a resting ventricular outflow tract gradient as low as 40 mm Hg. It reduces the morbidity and mortality related to surgery, but even in experienced centers, an increased risk exists of coronary artery dissection, uncontrolled myocardial infarction and a 5% to 10% risk of complete heart block requiring pacemaker placement.

Restrictive Cardiomyopathy

Restrictive cardiomyopathy (RCM) is the rarest form of cardiomyopathy in children.[157,158] It is characterized by a loss of ventricular compliance with a subsequent increase in end diastolic filling pressures. Systolic ventricular function is preserved, but diastolic relaxation is compromised. The cause of RCM is unknown but is believed to be associated with both genetic (ie, mutations in the desmin, troponin I, transthyretin IIe genes) and nongenetic causes (sarcoid or amyloidosis, which are common causes in adult patients but reportable in pediatric cases). Care must be taken to distinguish RCM from constrictive pericarditis using echocardiogram, catheterization, magnetic resonance imaging studies, or any combination of these measures. Diagnosis is made via echocardiography, which shows normal ventricular size and function associated with dilated atria caused by the ventricular diastolic dysfunction. Elevated left-ventricle end-diastolic pressures can ultimately result in pulmonary hypertension and pulmonary vascular disease, which is one of the most common and severe complications of RCM. Pulmonary hypertension that is unresponsive to pulmonary vasodilators is the most commonly cited problem preventing heart transplantation in these patients.[159] Given that RCM is generally unresponsive to conventional medical therapy, prognosis is poor, with death occurring within 1 to 4 years of diagnosis (in symptomatic patients, usually from pulmonary hypertensive crises and sudden death).[105] Therefore these patients should be referred for heart transplantation once the diagnosis is made.[160]

Miscellaneous Cardiomyopathies

Arrhythmogenic right-ventricular dysplasia (ARVD) and mitochondrial and noncompaction cardiomyopathies comprise only 2% to 3% of pediatric cardiomyopathies. Dysplasia of the right ventricle in patients with ARVD develops from fatty deposits within the ventricular walls. As a result, these patients are at risk for life-threatening ventricular tachycardias, particularly in affected individuals younger than 30 years of age.[161] Diagnosis of ARVD is typically made from dysrhythmias, echocardiogram, or magnetic resonance imaging. Treatment is directed at preventing life-threatening arrhythmias through the use of both medications and AICDs.[161] Patients with mitochondrial cardiomyopathies often exhibit the condition early in life with a hypertrophied or, less commonly, dilated, poorly functioning heart. In general, this maternally inherited disorder can be variably associated with other muscle, liver, neurologic, and developmental abnormalities.

Last, left-ventricular noncompaction cardiomyopathy (LVNC) is characterized by deep crevices or trabeculations within the normally smooth-walled left ventricle, which reduces cardiac function. The cardiac dysfunction associated with LVNC has been demonstrated to have a varying age of onset, from the newborn period to adulthood.[162] This cardiomyopathy may also be associated with other mitochondrial, metabolic, and systemic (Barth syndrome) disorders.[163]

CARDIAC TRANSPLANTATION

Orthotopic heart transplantation (OHT) has become a standard therapy for treating both end-stage congenital and acquired heart disease. Although the indications for OHT are the same across the pediatric population, the frequency of each indication changes with age. More than 75% of all recipients younger than 1 year undergo OHT because of surgically irreparable congenital heart disease[164]; this comprises only approximately 25% of the 11- to 17-year-old OHT recipients. Conversely, cardiomyopathy-related heart failure and dysrhythmias that are unresponsive to medical therapy result in OHT in 17% and 62% of the infant and adolescent population, respectively.

Once OHT is indicated, an extensive evaluation is necessary to determine its feasibility. Cardiac catheterization is required to determine both hemodynamics and PVR. Significantly elevated PVR or elevated PVR that is unresponsive to vasodilatory therapy (ie, oxygen and nitric oxide) are absolute contraindications for OHT, as are active malignancy and hepatic cirrhosis. The presence of bacterial or viral infection is a relative contraindication, and the decision to proceed with OHT should be made based on the individual patient's clinical status. A complete antiviral antibody titer panel (for herpes simplex virus, cytomegalovirus, HIV, Epstein-Barr virus, and hepatitis A, B, and C) should be obtained to rule out infection and to help guide the use of antiviral medications in the immediate postoperative period. Panel reactive antibody testing is necessary to assess the amount of circulating preformed antibodies in the recipient's serum, which may limit acceptable donor organs or cause hyperacute rejection in the recipient if the donor has antigens to which the recipient has already made antibodies. Finally, both social and financial screening evaluates a potential recipient's emotional coping skills and verifies that the financial burden of the transplant is minimized.

Transplant status classification is the next critical step and strongly influences the expected waiting time. Potential recipients listed as UNOS (United Network for Organ Sharing) status Ia will generally wait several days to months before receiving a heart transplant, assuming survival is possible for this period. This classification, however, requires a patient to be inotrope dependent and hospitalized. Depending on weight and blood type, infants older than 6 months listed as status II can expect to wait up to several months; and adolescent children may require as long as 2 years before a suitable heart is located. Transplant status can change at any time if the clinical condition improves or worsens.

A thorough discussion of the surgical procedure involved in OHT is beyond the scope of this text. Briefly, the donor heart is harvested in its entirety, with the exception of a cuff of posterior left atrial wall, which contains the pulmonary veins. Once the recipient is placed on cardiopulmonary bypass, the heart is removed in a reciprocal fashion. Anastomosis of the donor heart to the recipient is performed by either a biatrial or a bicaval (SVC-IVC) connection. The postoperative period for OHT recipients poses the unique challenge of managing a patient with a denervated heart that has been ischemic for as long as 4 hours. Without the sympathetic and parasympathetic nerve fibers innervating the sinoatrial (SA) and atrioventricular (AV) nodes, the resulting heart rate is entirely dependent on the intrinsic SA nodal rate. Neither Valsalva nor carotid massages will influence heart rate; atropine, the cholinergic receptor antagonist, is also ineffective. Although the resting heart rate of a transplanted heart is typically higher than normal controls, it is frequently abnormally slow in the immediate postoperative period because of SA node ischemia related to harvest and transplantation. Therefore, chronotropy can be provided by the selective β_1 agonist isoproterenol and titrated to produce the desired heart rate. As the transplanted heart begins to recuperate from the surgical insult, heart rate and cardiac output will increase to meet the patient's needs.

Immunosuppressive medications are typically started soon after the transplantation is complete. Most OHT recipients receive a regimen that includes a calcineurin inhibitor (ie, tacrolimus or cyclosporine), an antimetabolite (ie, mycophenolate mofetil or azathioprine) and corticosteroids. Corticosteroids are generally weaned within the first few post-OHT months, so long as no treatable rejection is detected. These medications all carry a significant side effect profile that frequently directs dosing and choice of medication. Both cyclosporine and tacrolimus are associated with hypertension, nephrotoxicity, and derangement of the lipid profile. These adverse effects are more common with cyclosporine than with tacrolimus. Tacrolimus and cyclosporine drug levels are monitored, with the therapeutic target levels gradually decreasing with time posttransplant. Azathioprine also necessitates frequent blood monitoring because of its adverse effects of neutropenia and hepatotoxicity. Mycophenolate is known to produce lymphopenia and gastrointestinal distress and may require dose adjustments accordingly. Side effects of corticosteroids have been well described.[165]

The immunosuppressed state in which these patients live increases the risk of several potential complications. During the early phase of immunosuppression and the subsequent 6 months, patients are at the highest risk for bacterial and opportunistic infections, occurring in 52% and 15% of OHT recipients, respectively.[166] After 6 months, the predominant infectious organisms shift from bacterial to viral (83% of infections), and the specific microbes parallel those afflicting the general, nonimmunosuppressed pediatric population (ie, cytomegalovirus, Epstein-Barr virus, adenovirus, enterovirus, influenza) as the immunosuppression medications are decreased to maintenance dosing.[166] For patients still requiring routine immunizations, live viral vaccines (ie, oral poliovirus, measles-mumps-rubella, varicella, live attenuated influenza [FluMist], rotavirus) should not be given because of the risk of active infection. Furthermore, the immunosuppressed patient's response to vaccinations will be blunted, particularly during the early post-OHT period, and any systemic antigenic response may precipitate a rejection episode. Therefore recommendations are that all nonlive vaccinations be given approximately 3 months posttransplant to minimize rejection.

Although excess immunosuppression predisposes these patients to serious infectious complications, deficiency in these medications places them at significant risk for rejection. This potentially life-threatening situation occurs when immunosuppression is unable to prevent the recipient's body from recognizing and attacking the donor heart's nonself antigens. Cellular rejection is the most common subtype and is a T cell–mediated injury that can begin within the first 5 to 7 days posttransplant, with the highest incidence during the first 3 post-OHT months. Patients may exhibit complaints of malaise, anorexia, gastrointestinal distress, low-grade fever, or nonspecific changes in sleeping patterns. If significant rejection is present, then physical examination will reveal hepatomegaly, a mild elevation in heart rate from baseline, and, possibly, a new murmur or gallop. These patients require prompt evaluation and assessment, which will likely include an echocardiogram to assess cardiac function and, if indicated, an endomyocardial biopsy. If disease proves the presence of rejection, then pulse steroids are administered, and the maintenance immunosuppressive regimen will usually be augmented. Repeat biopsy is necessary to verify effective treatment for the rejection episode and any interventions (ie, scheduled vaccinations) that might upregulate the immune response should be delayed for approximately 3 months after resolution of the episode.

As pediatric heart transplantation has become increasingly successful, the medical community is learning more about the associated long-term complications. Posttransplant lymphoproliferative disease is an abnormal growth of lymphoreticular cells in immunosuppressed patients and has been linked to primary posttransplant Epstein-Barr virus infection. It occurs in approximately 5% to 10% of pediatric OHT recipients.[164] Most forms can be treated solely by a decrease in immunosuppression, but others will require chemotherapy and possibly even surgical resection. The other significant long-term complication is posttransplant coronary vasculopathy (TxCAV). This condition is described as a progressive intimal and medial thickening of the transplanted heart's coronary arteries, with loss of coronary flow reserve and eventual luminal obliteration. The risk of TxCAV increases with each episode of rejection, certain infections (ie, cytomegalovirus), original harvest time, and associated donor ischemic time; it is also increased in the presence of abnormal lipid profiles. Because of their ability to lower the cholesterol–low-density lipoprotein fraction and their antioxidant or antiproliferative effects, many physicians are recommending statins (ie, pravastatin, atorvastatin) in their OHT recipients. Freedom from TxCAV decreases with time from transplant and with each decade of life after which the transplant occurs.[164] Although newer immunosuppressant agents (ie, sirolimus) have shown initial promise as potential treatments for TxCAV, retransplantation is currently the only definitive therapy.

Actuarial survival curves currently demonstrate an overall 50% survival at 13 years' posttransplant (Figure 251-23).[164] Younger age at transplant is associated with longer survival and decreased need for retransplant. Although transplantation is a formidable treatment strategy for most patients and their parents, approximately 90% of OHT recipients surveyed at 1, 3, and 5 years' posttransplant report excellent quality of life with no activity limitations.[164] Transplantation appears to be an acceptable end-point for patients with irreparable congenital or acquired heart disease but continues to be limited by the number of available donor hearts; approximately 20% to 30% of all patients die while awaiting a suitable donor.[164] Additional research investigating novel immunosuppression or alternative biological cardiac replacement strategies may help change the fate of these end-stage patients.

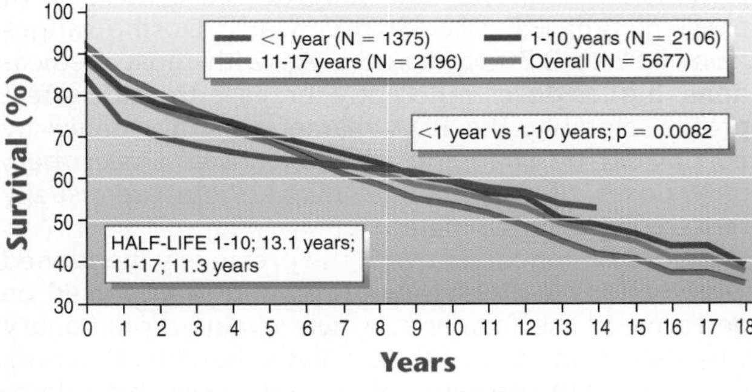

Figure 251-23 Kaplan Meier survival curve for 5677 pediatric patients after orthotopic heart transplant. (*Boucek MM, Edwards LB, Keck BM, et al. Registry of the International Society for Heart and Lung Transplantation: 8th official pediatric report-2005.* J Heart Lung Transplant. *2005; 24(8):968-982. Copyright © 2005, Elsevier.*)

WHEN TO CONSULT A PEDIATRIC CARDIOLOGIST

The question of when to refer a newborn to a pediatric cardiologist can be difficult. This issue is further complicated when practicing in rural areas where a *consult* may mean transport to another hospital or discharge home with the uncertainty of a family keeping their appointment with the pediatric cardiologist. Although some clinical findings can be pathognomonic for a cardiac anomaly, many lesions have only subtle clinical findings. The astute clinician is one who can identify abnormal from the myriad of patients they encounter in a day. The pediatric cardiologist is continuously indebted to the general pediatrician's ability to perform this function. Likely, one of the most stressful parts of a pediatrician's practice is determining when a newborn's cardiac murmur is pathological (see Chapter 100, Evaluation of the Infant With Suspected Heart Disease). Diminished or absent femoral pulses are never normal and should always be evaluated by a pediatric cardiologist. The transition from normal fetal circulation to normal postnatal circulation can produce a variety of cardiac murmurs; distinguishing physiological from pathological requires patience and experience.

A PDA is classically described as producing a *machinery* murmur because of its continuous, undulating character. The murmur is appreciated during both systole and diastole because both systolic and diastolic pressures are higher in the aorta than the pulmonary arteries. Therefore blood is continuously shunting from the aorta to the pulmonary artery (left to right). As the ductus arteriosus begins to close, the pressure gradient across this vascular conduit increases, making the murmur higher in pitch but may result in loss of the diastolic component. The ductus arteriosus arises from the proximal portion of the left pulmonary artery and generally inserts into the aorta distal to the left subclavian artery. This anatomic feature results in the murmur being best auscultated in the left, upper sternal border of the chest and may radiate to both lung fields. A pediatric cardiology consult is warranted if this murmur exists in the presence of decreased renal perfusion or pulmonary overcirculation because medical or surgical closure may be indicated. Otherwise, in a healthy infant, outpatient follow-up is recommended. Generally, PDAs close within days to months postnatally. PDAs persisting beyond the young infant period can usually be closed by coil occlusion in the catheterization laboratory.

Similar to a PDA, the systolic murmur produced by coarctation of the aorta will also be loudest at the left upper sternal border. Unlike a PDA, however, a coarctation murmur will generally radiate to the back, medial to the left scapula. In this scenario, palpable femoral artery pulses must be verified, and upper and lower extremity blood pressures must be obtained to assess for a blood pressure gradient. If pulses are absent or thready, or if lower extremity blood pressures are more than 15 mm Hg less than upper extremities, then a pediatric cardiology consult should be obtained immediately (see previous discussion section on coarctation of aorta).

Peripheral pulmonary branch stenosis, which is accompanied by a physiological murmur, does not require urgent consultation. A short, relatively high-pitched II/VI systolic ejection murmur that is auscultated equally on both sides of the sternum with diffuse radiation to both lung fields is characteristic of this natural transition period from fetal to postnatal circulation. The fact that this natural state has been declared a *diagnosis* is unfortunate because it results in undue angst for both physicians and families. Most physicians are concerned they may be missing the murmur produced by pulmonary stenosis. This murmur is distinct from that of peripheral pulmonary stenosis in both its severity and focality. A murmur produced by significant valvar pulmonary stenosis will be harsh in character, at least grade III on a severity scale of I to VI (see Table 251-1) and is often preceded by a valve click. It will be best auscultated at the left sternal border but will radiate to both lung fields. Conversely, peripheral pulmonary branch stenosis will be a softer, less intense murmur that is equally audible throughout the chest.

Another common scenario the pediatrician faces is the newborn with Down syndrome. Estimates suggest that nearly 40% to 60%[167,168] of these children are born with some form of congenital heart disease and comprise approximately 9%[169] of the pediatric cardiologist's practice. The AVSD[169,170] is the most common defect in these patients, occurring in approximately 60%, with nearly 70% of all patients with AVSD having trisomy 21. As discussed in the section on left-to-right shunting lesions, these lesions may not produce an audible murmur until PVR decreases significantly. However, because neither lesion is typically fatal in the first several weeks of life, discharging them from the hospital before seeing a pediatric cardiologist is reasonable if the patient is otherwise stable and acyanotic. Of note, the AVSD is one of the defects that can be suspected with ECG. The normal newborn ECG will meet voltage criteria for right-ventricular hypertrophy and have a concomitant right axis. The AVSD, however, will demonstrate a left axis deviation and a small Q wave in lead aVL (see Figure 251-9, *B*). Regardless of their immediate postnatal course, all patients with Down syndrome should be evaluated by a pediatric cardiologist within the first month of life.[171]

Last is the issue of managing the cyanotic newborn. In the vast majority of these situations, a cardiac lesion is not the cause. This notion is supported by the fact that only 5 to 8 of 1000 live births[169,170,172] are affected by a congenital heart lesion, and a significantly smaller number of those are cyanotic heart lesions. Pulmonary disease is more commonly the culprit. Nevertheless, the general practitioner can take several steps to help elucidate an etiology.

First, the clinician must verify that cyanosis is truly present. Acrocyanosis is a frequent occurrence in newborns, particularly in the setting of volume depletion or cool extremities. The Sa_{O_2} should be obtained on a warm, well-perfused, calm infant on both upper and at least one lower extremity. If this setting is difficult to attain, then ear lobe Sa_{O_2} offers an alternative. Once obtained, if saturations remain lower than approximately 92%, then a difference in saturation between upper and lower extremities should be evaluated. Although rare, *paradoxical cyanosis*, or lower Sa_{O_2} in the upper extremities than lower extremities, occurs in d-TGA with persistent fetal circulation. Lower-extremity cyanosis alone can occur with pulmonary hypertension, severe coarctation of the aorta, and critical aortic stenosis. Right-to-left shunting of oxygen-poor blood through a ductus arteriosus into the descending aorta is the etiology of the asymmetric cyanosis in these settings. Full-body cyanosis can occur in a number of scenarios, including respiratory distress syndrome, any of the cardiac lesions categorized as *right-to-left shunting lesions*, d-TGA (without persistent fetal circulation), or complete mixing lesions.

Paradoxically, these same lesions can produce Sa_{O_2} levels of more than 92% in the newborn period. This discrepancy can be produced by the high oxygen affinity of fetal hemoglobin. Therefore, if a cyanotic heart lesion is suspected, then obtaining arterial Pa_{O_2} values is mandatory. A hypoxemic Pa_{O_2} of 60 mm Hg produces an Sa_{O_2} of more than 90%, which alone might falsely reassure the physician. Persistent hypoxemia (<70-80 mm Hg) despite adequate oxygen therapy should increase the level of suspicion for a congenital heart defect. Failure of the *hyperoxia* challenge is often sufficient evidence for evaluation by a pediatric cardiologist and arguably for commencement of a prostaglandin E1 infusion.

This medical intervention constitutes a critical step in the management of a patient with suspected cyanotic heart disease. With the exception of the significant side effects associated with prostaglandin E1 infusion and its use in the setting of obstructed TAPVR, generally no physiologic scenario is worsened by this medication. Apnea, irritability, hyperthermia, jitteriness, and, possibly, decreased white blood cell function are the recognized complications.[173,174] The major concession the physician must make is accepting the high probability of intubation, which is often already required for patient stability. Prophylaxis with caffeine or aminophylline may decrease the risk of prostaglandin E1–associated apnea.[175] Dosing ranges from 0.02 to 0.2 mcg/kg/min. As with most medications, higher doses inherently increase the side effect profile. Notably, the PDA diameter cannot generally be titrated by changing infusion doses. Once open, only doses of 0.01 to 0.02 mcg/kg/min are usually required to maintain patency.

Before or concurrent with the previously mentioned interventions, a chest radiograph and ECG should be performed. The former can help evaluate pulmonary vasculature and size of the cardiac silhouette. Cyanosis can occur in the presence of diffusely increased pulmonary vascular markings (ie, pulmonary etiology, cardiac disease with pulmonary edema) or near absence of pulmonary vascular markings (ie, cardiac lesion with inadequate pulmonary blood flow). The cardiac silhouette is generally only helpful when extreme cardiomegaly exists, as with severe Ebstein anomaly. The classic descriptions of a *boot-shaped heart* (ie,

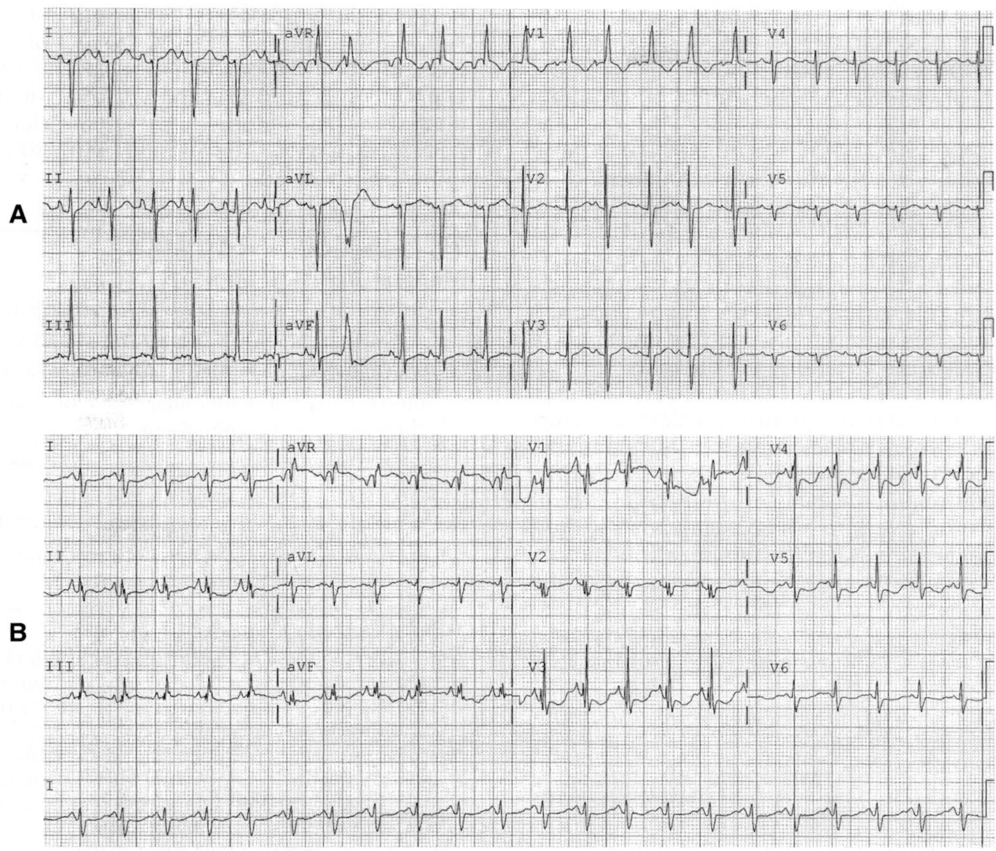

Figure 251-24 A, ECG of a newborn with HLHS. Note the left axis deviation of the QRS vector and the paucity of left-ventricular QRS forces in the precordial leads. **B**, ECG of a newborn with Ebstein anomaly of the tricuspid valve. Note the peaked P waves in leads II and V1 consistent with severe right atrial enlargement.

tetralogy of Fallot) or *egg on a string* (ie, d-TGA) are often overdiagnosed on chest radiographs because of the relative right-ventricular hypertrophy and mesocardia seen in many normal newborns. The newborn's ECG can help suggest the diagnosis of AVSDs (northwest QRS axis), hypoplastic left or right ventricles (decreased voltage in left or right precordial leads, respectively, and abnormal QRS axes), and Ebstein anomaly (right atrial enlargement) (Figure 251-24).

The pediatric cardiologist's echocardiogram can confirm a suggested diagnosis in most situations. Cardiac catheterization is required in a limited number of lesions to verify anatomy or for atrial septostomy if the existing ASD is inadequate (ie, d-TGA, single-ventricle hearts with atrioventricular valve stenosis or atresia).

The remaining management decisions entail determining whether surgical intervention is required and maintaining cardiovascular stability until that time. As described in the previous section on Complete Mixing Lesions, the major concerns during the preoperative period are end-organ perfusion and oxygen delivery. Proper preoperative management maximizes survival and minimizes morbidity and mortality. This goal is best achieved through an integrated approach involving nurses, allied health team members, family members, and physicians. Available information regarding diagnosis, prognosis, and possible morbidities should be freely exchanged to enable an informed and realistic outlook for all persons involved.

In contrast to patients needing surgical intervention, several of the children with acquired heart diseases can be primarily managed by their general pediatrician. Kawasaki disease can generally be diagnosed and treated before a pediatric cardiologist is ever consulted. An echocardiogram is needed to evaluate for coronary artery aneurysms and, in some cases, to confirm the diagnosis of atypical Kawasaki disease. However, in the absence of cardiac involvement at either presentation or a 2- to 4-week follow-up appointment, further evaluation by a pediatric cardiologist is probably unnecessary. IE is another example of heart disease that the pediatrician can both diagnose and manage with limited involvement of a pediatric cardiologist. Multiple positive blood cultures demonstrating the same organism constitutes the most accurate method for diagnosing IE. The low sensitivity of TTE for septic, valvar vegetations decreases its effectiveness in the diagnosis of IE. If IE is strongly suspected, then the more sensitive TEE can be performed if repeated TTEs have been negative. However, all types of congenital heart disease (ie, bicuspid aortic valve, VSD) must be ruled out and an adequate history of central venous catheters must be obtained to determine an etiology. Once the patient has received adequate therapy and demonstrated several negative blood cultures, the infection can generally be considered *cleared*. If no evidence exists of congenital heart disease or significant valvar derangement, then continued evaluation by a pediatric cardiologist may not be indicated. Last, patients diagnosed with rheumatic carditis should continue to be treated aggressively for all episodes of strep pharyngitis and receive appropriate procedural antibiotic prophylaxis.

The patient with cardiomyopathy typically requires long-term involvement of a pediatric cardiologist. During the first 3 or 4 years of life, however, these patients will see their general pediatrician more frequently, making this relationship crucial for the recognition of progressive disease. Weight loss or a plateau in weight gain, missed developmental milestones, fatigue, activity intolerance, or personality changes can all be subtle indicators of declining cardiac function. In the presence of a murmur, new gallop, abnormal ECG or chest radiograph, evaluation by a pediatric cardiologist is indicated.

Heart transplant recipients present another complicated situation for the general pediatrician. Their immunosuppressed status is typically the source of much concern and confusion. A febrile, immunosuppressed heart transplant recipient warrants a thorough evaluation, and, if an obvious, treatable etiology cannot be identified (ie, otitis media, viral upper respiratory infection), then their transplant cardiologist should be involved in the evaluation to minimize the chance that graft rejection will be misinterpreted as a common, benign infectious illness. New-onset fatigue, shortness of breath, exercise intolerance, low-grade fever, vomiting, or diarrhea may all be signs of rejection and require the expertise of the transplant cardiologist. Unexplained abdominal distention, pain, or vomiting should prompt evaluation for an ileus or intussusception because posttransplant lymphoproliferative disease can produce these symptoms; abdominal pain may also be a sign of intestinal angina caused by decreased cardiac output. Because the transplanted heart is denervated, C-fibers, which relay anginal-type chest pain to the brain, have been cut, and the absence of chest pain should not be comforting to the physician. Furthermore, the denervated, transplanted heart will not become significantly tachycardic in response to fever or pain. Therefore baseline heart rates in these patients become critical information for the physician, given that an increase of only 10 beats per minute may indicate imminent cardiovascular collapse. The previously mentioned scenarios are intentionally broad and nonspecific; they are intended to demonstrate the subtle clinical changes that may be harbingers of serious illness and to provide guidelines for the pediatrician to consider consultation with a pediatric transplant cardiologist.

Finally, for the previously mentioned cardiac diseases, an important point to note is that the recommendations regarding physical activity and sports participation in patients with congenital heart disease vary significantly.[176-184] The subject of exercise intensity, duration, or participation in any type of athletic event should be discussed with the health care team (including cardiologist and pediatrician), with the patient, and with the patient's family to ensure that no unnecessary or unknown risks are taken.

TOOLS FOR PRACTICE

Medical Decision Support

- S.T.A.B.L.E. *Cardiac Student Handbook* (booklet), Kristine A. Karlsen, MSN, RNC, NNP (www.aap.org/bookstore).
- McCulloch M, Middleton J, Vergales, J. Pediatric Cardiology: ECG Fundamentals. Office of Continuing Medical Education at the University of Virginia School of Medicine. http://www.cardiovillage.com (free CME website). Accessed: June 15, 2008.
- S.T.A.B.L.E. *Cardiac Slide Program* (CD-ROM), Kristine A. Karlsen, MSN, RNC, NNP (www.aap.org/bookstore).

AAP POLICY STATEMENTS

American Academy of Pediatrics, Section on Cardiology. Echocardiography in infants and children. *Pediatrics*. 1997;99(6):921. (aappolicy.aappublications.org/cgi/content/full/pediatrics;99/6/921).

American Academy of Pediatrics. ACC/AHA/AAP recommendations for training in pediatrics cardiology. *Pediatrics*. 2005;116(6):1574-1575. (aappolicy.aappublications.org/cgi/content/full/pediatrics;116/6/1574).

American Academy of Pediatrics. Guidelines for pediatric cardiovascular centers. *Pediatrics*. 2002;109(3):544-549. (aappolicy.aappublications.org/cgi/content/full/pediatrics;109/3/544).

REFERENCES

1. Srivastava D, Baldwin HS. *Molecular Determinants of Cardiac Development*. Vol I. 6th ed. Philadelphia, PA: Lippincott, Williams & Wilkins; 2001.
2. Olson EN, Srivastava D. Molecular pathways controlling heart development. *Science*. 1996;272(5262):671-676.
3. Brown N, Wolpert L. The development of handedness in left/right asymmetry. *Development*. 1990;109(1):1-9.
4. Kim J-S, Viragh S, Moorman AFM, et al. Development of the myocardium of the atrioventricular canal and the vestibular spine in the human heart. *Circ Res*. 2001;88(4):395-402.
5. Runyan R, Potts JD, Weeks DL. TGF-b3 mediated tissue interaction during embryonic heart development. *Mol Reprod Devel*. 1992;32:152-159.
6. Larsen WJ. Development of the heart. In: Larsen WJ, ed. *Human Embryology*. New York, NY: Churchill Livingston; 1997.
7. Mjaatvedt CH, Yamamura H, Wessels A, et al. Mechanisms of segmentation, septation, and remodeling of the tubular heart: endocardial cushion fate and cardiac looping. In: Harvery RP, Rosenthal N, eds. *Heart Development*. San Diego, CA: Academic; 1999.
8. McDaniel NL, Gutgesell HP. Ventricular septal defects. In: Allen LD, Gutgesell HP, Clark EB, et al, eds. *Moss and Adams' Heart Disease in Infants, Children, and Adolescents*. Vol I. 6th ed. Philadelphia, PA: Lippincott Williams & Wilkins; 2001.

9. Towbin JA, Bowles NE. The failing heart. *Nature*. 2002;415(6868):227-233.
10. Eroglu AG, Oztunc F, Saltik L, et al. Evolution of ventricular septal defect with special reference to spontaneous closure rate, subaortic ridge and aortic valve prolapse. *Pediatr Cardiol*. 2003;24(1):31-35.
11. Azhari N, Shihata MS, Al-Fatani A. Spontaneous closure of atrial septal defects within the oval fossa. *Cardiol Young*. 2004;14(2):148-155.
12. Brassard M, Fouron JC, van Doesburg NH, et al. Outcome of children with atrial septal defect considered too small for surgical closure. *Am J Cardiol*. 1999; 83(11):1552-1555.
13. Rashid A, Ivy D. Severe paediatric pulmonary hypertension: new management strategies. *Arch Dis Child*. 2005; 90(1):92-98.
14. Stark J, Gallivan S, Lovegrove J, et al. Mortality rates after surgery for congenital heart defects in children and surgeons' performance. *Lancet*. 2000;355(9208): 1004-1007.
15. Nygren A, Sunnegardh J, Berggren H. Preoperative evaluation and surgery in isolated ventricular septal defects: a 21 year perspective. *Heart*. 2000;83(2):198-204.
16. Monro JL, Alexiou C, Salmon AP, et al. Reoperations and survival after primary repair of congenital heart defects in children. *J Thorac Cardiovasc Surg*. 2003; 126(2):511-519.
17. Du Z-D, Hijazi ZM, Kleinman CS, et al. Comparison between transcatheter and surgical closure of secundum atrial septal defect in children and adults: results of a multicenter nonrandomized trial. *J Am Coll Cardiol*. 2002;39(11):1836-1844.
18. Knauth AL, Lock JE, Perry SB, et al. Transcatheter device closure of congenital and post-operative residual ventricular septal defects. *Circulation*. 2004;110(5): 501-507.
19. Geva T, Ayres NA, Pignatelli RH, et al. Echocardiographic evaluation of common atrioventricular canal defects: a study of 206 consecutive patients. *Echocardiography*. 1996;13(4):387-400.
20. Suzuki K, Tatsuno K, Kikuchi T, et al. Predisposing factors of valve regurgitation in complete atrioventricular septal defect. *J Am Coll Cardiol*. 1998;32(5):1449-1453.
21. Bonnetts PL, Goldberg SJ, Copeland JG. Frequency of left atrioventricular regurgitation post-operatively after repair of complete atrioventricular defect. *Am J Cardiol*. 1994;74(11):1157-1160.
22. Perry LW, Neill CA, Ferencz C, et al. Infants with congenital heart disease: the cases. In: Ferencz C, Rubin JD, Loffredo CA, et al, eds. *Perspectives in Pediatric Cardiology. Epidemiology of Congenital Heart Disease, the Baltimore-Washington Infant Study 1981-1989*. Armonk, NY: Futura; 1993.
23. Siwik ES, Patel CR, Zahka KG, et al. Tetralogy of Fallot. In: Allen HD, Gutgesell HP, Clark EB, et al, eds. *Moss and Adams' Heart Disease in Infants, Children, and Adolescents*. Vol II. 6th ed. Philadelphia, PA: Lippincott Williams & Wilkins; 2001.
24. Duncan BW, Mee RB, Prieto LR, et al. Staged repair of tetralogy of Fallot with pulmonary atresia and major aortopulmonary collateral arteries. *J Thorac Cardiovasc Surg*. 2003;126(3):694-702.
25. Cho JM, Puga FJ, Danielson GK, et al. Early and long-term results of the surgical treatment of tetralogy of Fallot with pulmonary atresia, with or without major aortopulmonary collateral arteries. *J Thorac Cardiovasc Surg*. 2002;124(1):70-81.
26. Fraisse A, Habib G. [Treatment of pulmonary arterial hypertension in children]. *Arch Pediatr*. 2004;11(8): 945-950.
27. Gaine S. Pulmonary hypertension. *JAMA*. 2000; 284(24):3160-3168.
28. Gaine SP, Rubin LJ. Medical and surgical treatment options for pulmonary hypertension. *Am J Med Sci*. 1998;315(3):179-184.
29. Galie N, Ghofrani HA, Torbicki A, et al. Sildenafil citrate therapy for pulmonary arterial hypertension. *N Engl J Med*. 2005;353(20):2148-2157.
30. Huffman MD, McLaughlin VV. Pulmonary arterial hypertension: new management options. *Curr Treat Options Cardiovasc Med*. 2004;6(6):451-458.
31. Lewis AB, Wells W, Lindesmith GG. Evaluation and surgical treatment of pulmonary atresia and intact ventricular septum in infancy. *Circulation*. 1983;67(6): 1318-1323.
32. Stamm C, Friehs I, Mayer JE, Jr, et al. Long-term results of the lateral tunnel Fontan operation. *J Thorac Cardiovasc Surg*. 2001;121(1):28-41.
33. Mair DD, Julsrud PR, Puga FJ, et al. The Fontan procedure for pulmonary atresia with intact ventricular septum: operative and late results. *J Am Coll Cardiol*. 1997; 29(6):1359-1364.
34. de Leval M, Bull C, Hopkins R, et al. Decision making in the definitive repair of the heart with a small right ventricle. *Circulation*. 1985;72(3 pt 2):52-60.
35. Celermajer DS, Bull C, Till JA, et al. Ebstein's anomaly: presentation and outcome from fetus to adult. *J Am Coll Cardiol*. 1994;23(1):170-176.
36. Celermajer DS, Cullen S, Sullivan ID, et al. Outcome in neonates with Ebstein's anomaly. *J Am Coll Cardiol*. 1992;19(5):1041-1046.
37. van der Velde ME, Parness IA, Colan SD, et al. Two-dimensional echocardiography in the pre- and post-operative management of totally anomalous pulmonary venous connection. *J Am Coll Cardiol*. 1991;18(7):1746-1751.
38. Yee ES, Turley K, Hsieh WR, et al. Infant total anomalous pulmonary venous connection: factors influencing timing of presentation and operative outcome. *Circulation*. 1987;76(3 Pt 2):83-87.
39. Lamb RK, Qureshi SA, Wilkinson JL, et al. Total anomalous pulmonary venous drainage. Seventeen-year surgical experience. *J Thorac Cardiovasc Surg*. 1988;96(3): 368-375.
40. Sano S, Brawn WJ, Mee RB. Total anomalous pulmonary venous drainage. *J Thorac Cardiovasc Surg*. 1989; 97(6):886-892.
41. Yacoub MH, Radley-Smith R. Anatomy of the coronary arteries in transposition of the great arteries and methods for their transfer in anatomical correction. *Thorax*. 1978;33(4):418-424.
42. Rowlatt UF. Coronary artery distribution in complete transposition. *JAMA*. 1962;179:269-278.
43. Blume ED, Altmann K, Mayer JE, et al. Evolution of risk factors influencing early mortality of the arterial switch operation. *J Am Coll Cardiol*. 1999;33(6):1702-1709.
44. Bonnet D, Bonhoeffer P, Piechaud JF, et al. Long-term fate of the coronary arteries after the arterial switch operation in newborns with transposition of the great arteries. *Heart*. 1996;76(3):274-279.
45. Legendre A, Losay J, Touchot-Kone A, et al. Coronary events after arterial switch operation for transposition of the great arteries. *Circulation*. 2003;108(suppl 1): 186-190.
46. Gagliardi MG, Adorisio R, Crea F, et al. Abnormal vasomotor function of the epicardial coronary arteries in children five to eight years after arterial switch operation: an angiographic and intracoronary Doppler flow wire study. *J Am Coll Cardiol*. 2005;46(8): 1565-1572.

47. McMahon CJ, Gauvreau K, Edwards JC, et al. Risk factors for aortic valve dysfunction in children with discrete subvalvar aortic stenosis. *Am J Cardiol.* 2004; 94(4):459-464.
48. Anand R, Mehta AV. Progressive congenital valvar aortic stenosis during infancy: five cases. *Pediatr Cardiol.* 1997;18(1):35-37.
49. Yetman AT, Rosenberg HC, Joubert GI. Progression of asymptomatic aortic stenosis identified in the neonatal period. *Am J Cardiol.* 1995;75(8):636-637.
50. Kasten-Sportes CH, Piechaud JF, Sidi D, et al. Percutaneous balloon valvuloplasty in neonates with critical aortic stenosis. *J Am Coll Cardiol.* 1989;13(5):1101-1105.
51. Meliones JN, Beekman RH, Rocchini AP, et al. Balloon valvuloplasty for recurrent aortic stenosis after surgical valvotomy in childhood: immediate and follow-up studies. *J Am Coll Cardiol.* 1989;13(5):1106-1110.
52. Peuster M, Fink C, Schoof S, et al. Anterograde balloon valvuloplasty for the treatment of neonatal critical valvar aortic stenosis. *Catheter Cardiovasc Interv.* 2002; 56(4):516-521.
53. Shaddy RE, Boucek MM, Sturtevant JE, et al. Gradient reduction, aortic valve regurgitation and prolapse after balloon aortic valvuloplasty in 32 consecutive patients with congenital aortic stenosis. *J Am Coll Cardiol.* 1990; 16(2):451-456.
54. Zeevi B, Keane JF, Castaneda AR, et al. Neonatal critical valvar aortic stenosis. A comparison of surgical and balloon dilation therapy. *Circulation.* 1989;80(4):831-839.
55. Kuhn MA, Latson LA, Cheatham JP, et al. Management of pediatric patients with isolated valvar aortic stenosis by balloon aortic valvuloplasty. *Cathet Cardiovasc Diagn.* 1996;39(1):55-61.
56. Keane J, Bernhard W, Nadas A. Aortic stenosis surgery in infancy. *Circulation.* 1975;52(6):1138-1143.
57. Sullivan ID, Wren C, Bain H, et al. Balloon dilatation of the aortic valve for congenital aortic stenosis in childhood. *Br Heart J.* 1989;61(2):186-191.
58. de Wolf D, Daniels O. Management of valvar aortic stenosis in children. *Pediatr Cardiol.* 2002;23(4):375-377.
59. Bonow RO, Carabello B, de Leon AC, et al. ACC/AHA guidelines for the management of patients with valvular heart disease. executive summary. A report of the American College of Cardiology/American Heart Association Task Force on Practice Guidelines (Committee on Management of Patients With Valvular Heart Disease). *J Heart Valve Dis.* 1998;7(6):672-707.
60. Keane JF, Driscoll DJ, Gersony WM, et al. Second natural history study of congenital heart defects. Results of treatment of patients with aortic valvar stenosis. *Circulation.* 1993;87(2):116-127.
61. Freed MD. Aortic Stenosis. In: Allen HD, Gutgesell HP, Clark EB, et al, eds. *Moss and Adams' Heart Disease in Infants, Children, and Adolescents.* Vol II. 6th ed. Philadelphia, PA: Lippincott, Williams & Wilkins; 2001.
62. Cape EG, VanAuker MD, Sigfusson G, et al. Potential role of mechanical stress in the etiology of pediatric heart disease: septal shear stress in subaortic stenosis. *J Am Coll Cardiol.* 1997;30(1):247-254.
63. Cowley CG, Orsmond GS, Feola P, et al. Long-term, randomized comparison of balloon angioplasty and surgery for native coarctation of the aorta in childhood. *Circulation.* 2005;111(25):3453-3456.
64. Ovaert C, McCrindle BW, Nykanen D, et al. Balloon angioplasty of native coarctation: clinical outcomes and predictors of success. *J Am Coll Cardiol.* 2000;35(4):988-996.
65. Fletcher SE, Nihill MR, Grifka RG, et al. Balloon angioplasty of native coarctation of the aorta: midterm follow-up and prognostic factors. *J Am Coll Cardiol.* 1995;25(3): 730-734.
66. Magee AG, Brzezinska-Rajszys G, Qureshi SA, et al. Stent implantation for aortic coarctation and recoarctation. *Heart.* 1999;82(5):600-606.
67. Rao PS, Galal O, Smith PA, et al. Five- to nine-year follow-up results of balloon angioplasty of native aortic coarctation in infants and children. *J Am Coll Cardiol.* 1996;27(2):462-470.
68. McCrindle BW, Jones TK, Morrow WR, et al. Acute results of balloon angioplasty of native coarctation versus recurrent aortic obstruction are equivalent. Valvuloplasty and Angioplasty of Congenital Anomalies (VACA) Registry Investigators. *J Am Coll Cardiol.* 1996; 28(7):1810-1817.
69. Maheshwari S, Bruckheimer E, Fahey JT, et al. Balloon angioplasty of postsurgical recoarctation in infants: the risk of restenosis and long-term follow-up. *J Am Coll Cardiol.* 2000;35(1):209-213.
70. Yetman AT, Nykanen D, McCrindle BW, et al. Balloon angioplasty of recurrent coarctation: a 12-year review. *J Am Coll Cardiol.* 1997;30(3):811-816.
71. Hamdan MA, Maheshwari S, Fahey JT, et al. Endovascular stents for coarctation of the aorta: initial results and intermediate-term follow-up. *J Am Coll Cardiol.* 2001;38(5):1518-1523.
72. Ebeid MR, Prieto LR, Latson LA. Use of balloon-expandable stents for coarctation of the aorta: initial results and intermediate-term follow-up. *J Am Coll Cardiol.* 1997; 30(7):1847-1852.
73. Fox S, Pierce WS, Waldhausen JA. Pathogenesis of paradoxical hypertension after coarctation repair. *Ann Thorac Surg.* 1980;29(2):135-141.
74. Lind L, Granstam SO, Millgard J. Endothelium-dependent vasodilation in hypertension: a review. *Blood Press.* 2000; 9(1):4-15.
75. Goetz RM, Holtz J. Enhanced angiotensin-converting enzyme activity and impaired endothelium-dependent vasodilation in aortae from hypertensive rats: evidence for a causal link. *Clin Sci.* 1999;97(2):165-174.
76. Tabbutt S, Ramamoorthy C, Montenegro LM, et al. Impact of inspired gas mixtures on preoperative infants with hypoplastic left heart syndrome during controlled ventilation. *Circulation.* 2001;104(12 suppl 1):159-164.
77. Mahle WT, Clancy RR, McGaurn SP, et al. Impact of prenatal diagnosis on survival and early neurologic morbidity in neonates with the hypoplastic left heart syndrome. *Pediatrics.* 2001;107(6):1277-1282.
78. Norwood WI, Kirklin JK, Sanders SP. Hypoplastic left heart syndrome: experience with palliative surgery. *Am J Cardiol.* 1980;45(1):87-91.
79. Sano S, Ishino K, Kawada M, et al. Right ventricle-pulmonary artery shunt in first-stage palliation of hypoplastic left heart syndrome. *Semin Thorac Cardiovasc Surg.* 2004;7:22-31.
80. Bove EL, de Leval MR, Migliavacca F, et al. Computational fluid dynamics in the evaluation of hemodynamic performance of cavopulmonary connections after the Norwood procedure for hypoplastic left heart syndrome. *J Thorac Cardiovasc Surg.* 2003;126(4):1040-1047.
81. Pridjian AK, Mendelsohn AM, Lupinetti FM, et al. Usefulness of the bidirectional Glenn procedure as staged reconstruction for the functional single ventricle. *Am J Cardiol.* 1993;71(11):959-962.
82. Lamberti JJ, Spicer RL, Waldman JD, et al. The bidirectional cavopulmonary shunt. *J Thorac Cardiovasc Surg.* 1990;100(1):22-30.
83. Mitchell ME, Ittenbach RF, Gaynor JW, et al. Intermediate outcomes after the Fontan procedure in the current era. *J Thorac Cardiovasc Surg.* 2006;131(1):172-180.

84. Kumar SP, Rubinstein CS, Simsic JM, et al. Lateral tunnel versus extracardiac conduit Fontan procedure: a concurrent comparison. *Ann Thorac Surg*. 2003;76(5): 1389-1396.
85. Azakie A, McCrindle BW, Benson LN, et al. Total cavopulmonary connections in children with a previous Norwood procedure. *Ann Thorac Surg*. 2001;71(5): 1541-1546.
86. Pearl JM, Laks H, Stein DG, et al. Total cavopulmonary anastomosis versus conventional modified Fontan procedure. *Ann Thorac Surg*. 1991;52(2):189-196.
87. Norwood WI Jr. Hypoplastic left heart syndrome. *Ann Thorac Surg*. 1991;52(3):688-695.
88. Mahle WT, Clancy RR, Moss EM, et al. Neurodevelopmental outcome and lifestyle assessment in school-aged and adolescent children with hypoplastic left heart syndrome. *Pediatrics*. 2000;105(5):1082-1089.
89. Mosca RS, Kulik TJ, Goldberg CS, et al. Early results of the Fontan procedure in one hundred consecutive patients with hypoplastic left heart syndrome. *J Thorac Cardiovasc Surg*. 2000;119(6):1110-1118.
90. Goldberg CS, Schwartz EM, Brunberg JA, et al. Neurodevelopmental outcome of patients after the Fontan operation: a comparison between children with hypoplastic left heart syndrome and other functional single ventricle lesions. *J Pediatr*. 2000;137(5):646-652.
91. Julsrud PR, Weigel TJ, Van Son JA, et al. Influence of ventricular morphology on outcome after the Fontan procedure. *Am J Cardiol*. 2000;86(3):319-323.
92. Franklin RC, Spiegelhalter DJ, Sullivan ID, et al. Tricuspid atresia presenting in infancy. Survival and suitability for the Fontan operation. *Circulation*. 1993;87(2): 427-439.
93. Baltimore RS. Infective endocarditis. In: Jenson HB, Baltimore RS, eds. *Pediatric Infectious Diseases: Principles and Practice*. Norwalk, CT: Appleton & Lange; 1995.
94. Stull TL, LiPuma JJ. Endocarditis in children. In: Kaye D, ed. *Infective Endocarditis*. 2nd ed. New York, NY: Raven Press; 1999.
95. Stockheim JA, Chadwick EG, Kessler S, et al. Are the Duke criteria superior to the Beth Israel criteria for the diagnosis of infective endocarditis in children? *Clin Infect Dis*. 1998;27(6):1451-1456.
96. Ferrieri P, Gewitz MH, Gerber MA, et al. Unique features of infective endocarditis in childhood. *Circulation*. 2002;105(17):2115-2126.
97. Yeaman MR, Bayer AS. Antimicrobial peptides from platelets. *Drug Resist Updat*. 1999;2(2):116-126.
98. Durack DT, Lukes AS, Bright DK, Duke Endocarditis Service. New criteria for diagnosis of infective endocarditis: utilization of specific echocardiographic findings. *Am J Med*. 1994;96(2):200-209.
99. Wilson WR, Karchmer AW, Dajani AS, et al. Antibiotic treatment of adults with infective endocarditis due to streptococci, enterococci, staphylococci, and HACEK microorganisms. American Heart Association. *JAMA*. 1995;274(21):1706-1713.
100. Friedman RA, Schowengerdt KO, Towbin JA. Myocarditis. In: Garson AJ, Bricker JT, Fisher DJ, et al, eds. *The Science and Practice of Pediatric Cardiology*. Vol II. 2nd ed. Baltimore, MD: Williams & Wilkins; 1998.
101. Keith JD, Rowe RD, Vlad P. *Heart Disease in Infancy and Childhood*. 2nd ed. New York, NY: Macmillan; 1967.
102. Rezkalla SH, Kloner RA. Management strategies in viral myocarditis. *Am Heart J*. 1989;117(3):706-708.
103. Griffin LD, Kearney D, Ni J, et al. Analysis of formalin-fixed and frozen myocardial autopsy samples for viral genome in childhood myocarditis and dilated cardiomyopathy with endocardial fibroelastosis using polymerase chain reaction (PCR). *Cardiovasc Pathol*. 1995;4(1):3-11.
104. Martin A, Webber S, Fricker F, et al. Acute myocarditis. Rapid diagnosis by PCR in children. *Circulation*. 1994; 90(1):330-339.
105. Gajarski RJ, Towbin JA. Recent advances in the etiology, diagnosis, and treatment of myocarditis and cardiomyopathies in children. *Curr Opin Pediatr*. 1995; 7(5):587-594.
106. Thongtang V, Chiathiraphan S, Ratanarapee S, et al. Prevalence of myocarditis in idiopathic dysrhythmias: role of endomyocardial biopsy and efficacy of steroid therapy. *J Med Assoc Thai*. 1993;76(7):368-373.
107. Drucker N, Colan S, Lewis A, et al. Gamma-globulin treatment of acute myocarditis in the pediatric population. *Circulation*. 1994;89(1):252-257.
108. Rosenthal D, Chrisant MR, Edens E, et al. International Society for Heart and Lung Transplantation: practice guidelines for management of heart failure in children. *J Heart Lung Transplant*. 2004;23(12):1313-1333.
109. Demmler GJ. Infectious pericarditis in children. *Pediatr Infect Dis J*. 2006;25(2):165-166.
110. Wang ZJ, Reddy GP, Gotway MB, et al. CT and MR imaging of pericardial disease. *Radiographics*. 2003; 23:S167-S180.
111. Ustunsoy H, Celkan MA, Sivrikoz MC, et al. Intrapericardial fibrinolytic therapy in purulent pericarditis. *Eur J Cardiothorac Surg*. 2002;22(3):373-376.
112. Scaglia F, Towbin JA, Craigen WJ, et al. Clinical spectrum, morbidity, and mortality in 113 pediatric patients with mitochondrial disease. *Pediatrics*. 2004;114(4): 925-931.
113. Martins E, Cardoso JS, Abreu-Lima C. Familial dilated cardiomyopathy. *Rev Port Cardiol*. 2002;21(12):1487-1503.
114. Towbin JA, Bowles NE. Molecular genetics of left ventricular dysfunction. *Curr Mol Med*. 2001;1(1): 81-90.
115. Kuhl U, Pauschinger M, Noutsias M, et al. High prevalence of viral genomes and multiple viral infections in the myocardium of adults with "idiopathic" left ventricular dysfunction. *Circulation*. 2005;111(7):887-893.
116. Goerss JB, Michels VV, Burnett J, et al. Frequency of familial dilated cardiomyopathy. *Eur Heart J*. 1995;16: 2-4.
117. Mestroni L, Miani D, Di Lenarda A, et al. Clinical and pathologic study of familial dilated cardiomyopathy. *Am J Cardiol*. 1990;65(22):1449-1453.
118. Jennings DL, Kalus JS, O'Dell KM. Aldosterone receptor antagonism in heart failure. *Pharmacotherapy*. 2005; 25(8):1126-1133.
119. Pitt B, Zannad F, Remme WJ, et al. The effect of spironolactone on morbidity and mortality in patients with severe heart failure. Randomized Aldactone Evaluation Study Investigators. *N Engl J Med*. 1999;341(10): 709-717.
120. Tang WH, Parameswaran AC, Maroo AP, et al. Aldosterone receptor antagonists in the medical management of chronic heart failure. *Mayo Clin Proc*. 2005;80(12): 1623-1630.
121. Cohn JN, Tognoni G. A randomized trial of the angiotensin-receptor blocker valsartan in chronic heart failure. *N Engl J Med*. 2001;345(23):1667-1675.
122. Feldman AM, Bristow MR, Parmley WW, et al. Effects of vesnarinone on morbidity and mortality in patients with heart failure. Vesnarinone Study Group. *N Engl J Med*. 1993;329(3):149-155.
123. Packer M, Bristow MR, Cohn JN, et al. The effect of carvedilol on morbidity and mortality in patients with chronic heart failure. U.S. Carvedilol Heart Failure Study Group. *N Engl J Med*. 1996;334(21): 1349-1355.

124. Bruns LA, Chrisant MK, Lamour JM, et al. Carvedilol as therapy in pediatric heart failure: an initial multicenter experience. *J Pediatr.* 2001;138(4):505-511.
125. Shaddy RE, Tani LY, Gidding SS, et al. Beta-blocker treatment of dilated cardiomyopathy with congestive heart failure in children: a multi-institutional experience. *J Heart Lung Transplant.* 1999;18(3):269-274.
126. Abraham WT, Fisher WG, Smith AL, et al. Cardiac resynchronization in chronic heart failure. *N Engl J Med.* 2002;346(24):1845-1853.
127. Leon AR, Abraham WT, Brozena S, et al. Cardiac resynchronization with sequential biventricular pacing for the treatment of moderate-to-severe heart failure. *J Am Coll Cardiol.* 2005;46(12):2298-2304.
128. Sutton MG, Plappert T, Hilpisch KE, et al. Sustained reverse left ventricular structural remodeling with cardiac resynchronization at 1 year is a function of etiology: quantitative Doppler echocardiographic evidence from the Multicenter InSync Randomized Clinical Evaluation (MIRACLE). *Circulation.* 2006;113(2): 266-272.
129. Colan SD, Lipshultz SE, Lowe AM, et al. Epidemiology and cause-specific outcome of hypertrophic cardiomyopathy in children: findings from Pediatric Cardiomyopathy Registry (PCMR). *Circulation.* 2007;115: 773-781.
130. Jamieson CR, van der Burgt I, Brady AF, et al. Mapping a gene for Noonan syndrome to the long arm of chromosome 12. *Nat Genet.* 1994;8(4):357-360.
131. Carrier L, Hengstenberg C, Beckmann JS, et al. Mapping of a novel gene for familial hypertrophic cardiomyopathy to chromosome 11. *Nat Genet.* 1993;4(3): 311-313.
132. Hejtmancik J, Brink P, Towbin J, et al. Localization of gene for familial hypertrophic cardiomyopathy to chromosome 14q1 in a diverse US population. *Circulation.* 1991;83(5):1592-1597.
133. Kelly DP, Strauss AW. Inherited cardiomyopathies. *N Engl J Med.* 1994;330(13):913-919.
134. Marian AJ, Roberts R. Molecular basis of hypertrophic and dilated cardiomyopathy. *Tex Heart Inst J.* 1994;21(1): 6-15.
135. Jarcho J, McKenna W, Pare J, et al. Mapping a gene for familial hypertrophic cardiomyopathy to chromosome 14q1. *N Engl J Med.* 1989;321(20):1372-1378.
136. Solomon SD, Geisterfer-Lowrance AA, Vosberg HP, et al. A locus for familial hypertrophic cardiomyopathy is closely linked to the cardiac myosin heavy chain genes, CRI-L436, and CRI-L329 on chromosome 14 at q11-q12. *Am J Hum Genet.* 1990;47(3):389-394.
137. Solomon SD, Wolff S, Watkins H, et al. Left ventricular hypertrophy and morphology in familial hypertrophic cardiomyopathy associated with mutations of the beta-myosin heavy chain gene. *J Am Coll Cardiol.* 1993;22(2): 498-505.
138. MacRae CA, Ghaisas N, Kass S, et al. Familial hypertrophic cardiomyopathy with Wolff-Parkinson-White syndrome maps to a locus on chromosome 7q3. *J Clin Invest.* 1995;96(3):1216-1220.
139. Van Driest SL, Gakh O, Ommen SR, et al. Molecular and functional characterization of a human frataxin mutation found in hypertrophic cardiomyopathy. *Mol Genet Metabol.* 2005;85(4):280-285.
140. Jauslin ML, Wirth T, Meier T, et al. A cellular model for Friedreich ataxia reveals small-molecule glutathione peroxidase mimetics as novel treatment strategy. *Hum Mol Genet.* 2002;11(24):3055-3063.
141. Chikamori T, Counihan PJ, Doi YL, et al. Mechanisms of exercise limitation in hypertrophic cardiomyopathy. *J Am Coll Cardiol.* 1992;19(3):507-512.
142. Lemery R, Kleinebenne A, Nihoyannopoulos P, et al. Q waves in hypertrophic cardiomyopathy in relation to the distribution and severity of right and left ventricular hypertrophy. *J Am Coll Cardiol.* 1990;16(2):368-374.
143. Yetman AT, Hamilton RM, Benson LN, et al. Long-term outcome and prognostic determinants in children with hypertrophic cardiomyopathy. *J Am Coll Cardiol.* 1998; 32(7):1943-1950.
144. Sherrid MV, Gunsburg DZ, Moldenhauer S, et al. Systolic anterior motion begins at low left ventricular outflow tract velocity in obstructive hypertrophic cardiomyopathy. *J Am Coll Cardiol.* 2000;36(4):1344-1354.
145. Doiuchi J, Hamada M, Ito T, et al. Comparative effects of calcium-channel blockers and beta-adrenergic blocker on early diastolic time intervals and A-wave ratio in patients with hypertrophic cardiomyopathy. *Clin Cardiol.* 1987;10(1):26-30.
146. Bourmayan C, Razavi A, Fournier C, et al. Effect of propranolol on left ventricular relaxation in hypertrophic cardiomyopathy: an echographic study. *Am Heart J.* 1985; 109(6):1311-1316.
147. McKenna WJ, England D, Doi YL, et al. Arrhythmia in hypertrophic cardiomyopathy. I. Influence on prognosis. *Br Heart J.* 1981;46(2):168-172.
148. Maron BJ, Savage DD, Wolfson JK, et al. Prognostic significance of 24 hour ambulatory electrocardiographic monitoring in patients with hypertrophic cardiomyopathy: a prospective study. *Am J Cardiol.* 1981;48(2): 252-257.
149. McKenna WJ, Harris L, Perez G, et al. Arrhythmia in hypertrophic cardiomyopathy. II. Comparison of amiodarone and verapamil in treatment. *Br Heart J.* 1981; 46(2):173-178.
150. McKenna WJ, Harris L, Rowland E, et al. Amiodarone for long-term management of patients with hypertrophic cardiomyopathy. *Am J Cardiol.* 1984;54(7):802-810.
151. Monserrat L, Elliott PM, Gimeno JR, et al. Non-sustained ventricular tachycardia in hypertrophic cardiomyopathy: an independent marker of sudden death risk in young patients. *J Am Coll Cardiol.* 2003;42(5): 873-879.
152. Olivotto I, Gistri R, Petrone P, et al. Maximum left ventricular thickness and risk of sudden death in patients with hypertrophic cardiomyopathy. *J Am Coll Cardiol.* 2003;41(2):315-321.
153. Maron BJ, McKenna WJ, Danielson GK, et al. American College of Cardiology/European Society of Cardiology clinical expert consensus document on hypertrophic cardiomyopathy. A report of the American College of Cardiology Foundation Task Force on Clinical Expert Consensus Documents and the European Society of Cardiology Committee for Practice Guidelines. *J Am Coll Cardiol.* 2003;42(9):1687-1713.
154. Ostman-Smith I, Wettrell G, Riesenfeld T. A cohort study of childhood hypertrophic cardiomyopathy: improved survival following high-dose beta-adrenoceptor antagonist treatment. *J Am Coll Cardiol.* 1999;34(6): 1813-1822.
155. Diodati JG, Schenke WH, Waclawiw MA, et al. Predictors of exercise benefit after operative relief of left ventricular outflow obstruction by the myotomy-myectomy procedure in hypertrophic cardiomyopathy. *Am J Cardiol.* 1992;69(19):1617-1622.
156. Cohn LH, Trehan H, Collins JJ Jr. Long-term follow-up of patients undergoing myotomy/myectomy for obstructive hypertrophic cardiomyopathy. *Am J Cardiol.* 1992;70(6):657-660.
157. Knirsch W, Mehwald P, Dittrich S, et al. Restrictive cardiomyopathy in childhood. *Z Kardiol.* 2004;93(7): 566-573.

158. Lipshultz SE, Sleeper LA, Towbin JA, et al. The incidence of pediatric cardiomyopathy in two regions of the United States. *N Engl J Med*. 2003;348(17): 1647-1655.
159. Kimberling MT, Balzer DT, Hirsch R, et al. Cardiac transplantation for pediatric restrictive cardiomyopathy: presentation, evaluation, and short-term outcome. *J Heart Lung Transplant*. 2002;21(4):455-459.
160. Denfield SW, Rosenthal G, Gajarski RJ, et al. Restrictive cardiomyopathies in childhood. Etiologies and natural history. *Tex Heart Inst J*. 1997;24(1):38-44.
161. Gemayel C, Pelliccia A, Thompson PD. Arrhythmogenic right ventricular cardiomyopathy. *J Am Coll Cardiol*. 2001;38(7):1773-1781.
162. Pignatelli RH, McMahon CJ, Dreyer WJ, et al. Clinical characterization of left ventricular noncompaction in children: a relatively common form of cardiomyopathy. *Circulation*. 2003;108:2672-2678.
163. Schlame M, Kelley RI, Feigenbaum A, et al. Phospholipid abnormalities in children with Barth syndrome. *J Am Coll Cardiol*. 2003;42(11):1994-1999.
164. Boucek MM, Edwards LB, Keck BM, et al. Registry of the International Society for Heart and Lung Transplantation: eighth official pediatric report—2005. *J Heart Lung Transplant*. 2005;24(8):968-982.
165. Taketomo CK, Hodding JH, Kraus DM. *Pediatric Dosage Handbook*. 12th ed. Hudson, OH: Lexi-Comp, Inc, 2005.
166. Gajarski RJ, Smith EO, Denfield SW, et al. Long-term results of triple-drug-based immunosuppression in nonneonatal pediatric heart transplant recipients. *Transplantation*. 1998;65(11):1470-1476.
167. Pueschel SM. Biomedical aspects in Down syndrome: cardiology. In: Pueschel SM, Rynders J, eds. *Down Syndrome: Advances in Biomedicine and the Behavioral Sciences*. Cambridge, MA: Ware Press; 1982.
168. Ghaffar S, Lemler MS, Fixler DE, et al. Trisomy 21 and congenital heart disease: effect of timing of initial echocardiogram. *Clin Pediatr*. 2005;44(1): 39-42.
169. Clark EB. Etiology of congenital cardiovascular malformations: epidemiology and genetics. In: Allen HD, Gutgesell HP, Clark EB, et al, eds. *Moss and Adams' Heart Disease in Infants, Children, and Adolescents*. Vol I. 6th ed. Philadelphia, PA: Lippincott, Williams & Wilkins; 2001.
170. Ferencz C, Neill CA, Boughman JA, et al. Congenital cardiovascular malformations associated with chromosome abnormalities: an epidemiologic study. *J Pediatr*. 1989;114(1):79-86.
171. American Academy of Pediatrics, Committee on Genetics. Health supervision for children with Down syndrome. *Pediatrics*. 1994;93(5):855-859.
172. Hoffman JI, Kaplan S. The incidence of congenital heart disease. *J Am Coll Cardiol*. 2002;39(12):1890-1900.
173. Heymann MA, Clyman RI. Evaluation of alprostadil (prostaglandin E1) in the management of congenital heart disease in infancy. *Pharmacotherapy*. 1982;2(3): 148-155.
174. Lewis AB, Freed MD, Heymann MA, et al. Side effects of therapy with prostaglandin E1 in infants with critical congenital heart disease. *Circulation*. 1981;64(5):893-898.
175. Lim DS, Kulik TJ, Kim DW, et al. Aminophylline for the prevention of apnea during prostaglandin E1 infusion. *Pediatrics*. 2003;112(1):e27-e29.
176. Mitchell JH, Haskell W, Snell P, et al. Task Force 8: classification of sports. *J Am Coll Cardiol*. 2005;45(8): 1364-1367.
177. Graham TP Jr, Driscoll DJ, Gersony WM, et al. Task Force 2: congenital heart disease. *J Am Coll Cardiol*. 2005;45(8):1326-1333.
178. Maron BJ, Douglas PS, Graham TP, et al. Task Force 1: preparticipation screening and diagnosis of cardiovascular disease in athletes. *J Am Coll Cardiol*. 2005;45(8): 1322-1326.
179. Maron BJ, Ackerman MJ, Nishimura RA, et al. Task Force 4: HCM and other cardiomyopathies, mitral valve prolapse, myocarditis, and Marfan syndrome. *J Am Coll Cardiol*. 2005;45(8):1340-1345.
180. Maron BJ, Estes NA, 3rd, Link MS. Task Force 11: commotio cordis. *J Am Coll Cardiol*. 2005;45(8): 1371-1373.
181. Mitten MJ, Maron BJ, Zipes DP. Task Force 12: legal aspects of the 36th Bethesda Conference recommendations. *J Am Coll Cardiol*. 2005;45(8):1373-1375.
182. Zipes DP, Ackerman MJ, Estes NA, et al. Task Force 7: arrhythmias. *J Am Coll Cardiol*. 2005;45(8):1354-1363.
183. Maron BJ, Chaitman BR, Ackerman MJ, et al. Recommendations for physical activity and recreational sports participation for young patients with genetic cardiovascular diseases. *Circulation*. 2004;109(22):2807-2816.
184. Pollock ML, Franklin BA, Balady GJ, et al. AHA Science Advisory. Resistance exercise in individuals with and without cardiovascular disease: benefits, rationale, safety, and prescription: an advisory from the Committee on Exercise, Rehabilitation, and Prevention, Council on Clinical Cardiology, American Heart Association; Position paper endorsed by the American College of Sports Medicine. *Circulation*. 2000;101(7):828-833.

Chapter 252
CONTACT DERMATITIS

Jonette E. Keri, MD, PhD; Linda S. Nield, MD

As the name implies, contact dermatitis is inflammation of the skin secondary to contact with an offending agent. Two broad types of contact dermatitis include *irritant contact dermatitis* and *allergic contact dermatitis*. The clinical presentation and treatment of these 2 entities are similar.

ETIOLOGY

Irritant Contact Dermatitis

Irritant contact dermatitis is the result of skin exposure to substances that cause an inflammatory reaction that is not immune mediated. An array of irritant agents may be present in the home, child care center, or school and may include harsh detergents and cleaning materials. Parents or child care providers may be aware immediately of the offending agent or may use a diary to chart symptoms and associated activities and exposures. If the irritant dermatitis is acute, then identifying the culprit is often easy, given that it may be only a single agent. In chronic cases, multiple offenders are often present. If a child has repeated episodes of irritant contact dermatitis that compromises the protective skin barrier, then a fertile environment for subsequent allergic contact dermatitis may result.

Diaper dermatitis is a common irritant dermatitis in children. Urine, feces, and persistent moisture macerate the occluded skin of the perineum. Of note, typical irritant diaper dermatitis does not involve the creases of the infant's skin. If the femoral creases or anal area are involved, then the infection is likely to be candidal. Candidiasis produces red, often macerated plaques accompanied by satellite pustules. Diaper rash that persists for greater than 3 days is likely secondarily infected with yeast.[1] (See Chapter 257, Diaper Rash.)

Irritant contact dermatitis caused by airborne agents (dust or volatile chemicals) is often missed and must be considered in all cases. Solvent sniffers, typically preteens and young adolescents who inhale aerosols to alter mental status, are susceptible to irritant contact dermatitis secondary to the airborne agent. These patients may have irritant dermatitis of the arms and chest, along with the eczematous changes found mostly around the nose and mouth.[2]

Allergic Contact Dermatitis

Allergic contact dermatitis is immune mediated and is a type IV delayed-hypersensitivity reaction. Such reactions require prior exposure to the allergen to produce the event of dermatitis. Delayed-hypersensitivity reactions are caused by primed T cells, producing a cascade of cytokines and chemotactic factors leading to dermatitis.

As with irritant dermatitis, an initial episode of allergic contact dermatitis may be easily identified because the rash usually is localized to a specific area, and the history of the offending agent can be ascertained. Poison ivy and nickel are very common causes of allergic reactions.

Commonly, poison ivy is given as an example when allergic contact dermatitis is described; it represents *Toxicodendron* (Rhus) dermatitis. This plant, along with poison oak, poison sumac, Japanese lacquer tree, the cashew nut tree (allergen in the nutshell), and mango (allergen in rind, leaves or sap), Rengas tree, and Indian marking nut tree, are members of the Anacardiaceae family of plants. The dermatitis that these plants trigger appears within 48 hours of exposure in a previously sensitized individual, often producing linear arrays of vesicles where the offending plant has come in contact with the skin. Another common site in young boys includes the genitals because, in many cases, they transfer the allergen to this area when voiding.

An allergic reaction to nickel is common and remains the most frequently positive patch test allergen in North America.[3] With the increased incidence of body piercing in the pediatric population, allergic reaction must be considered when an area at a piercing site is red, scaling, and irritated (Figure 252-1). Nickel is also located on areas of clothing such as the snaps and zippers on trousers or blouses (Figure 252-2).

Other allergens becoming more important include topical antibiotic preparations such as those containing neomycin, which have shown a notable increase in positive patch test reactions since the 1970s,[3] hair dye products that contain paraphenylenediamine,[4] and latex allergy in children who have repeated exposure to latex in the clinical settings.[5]

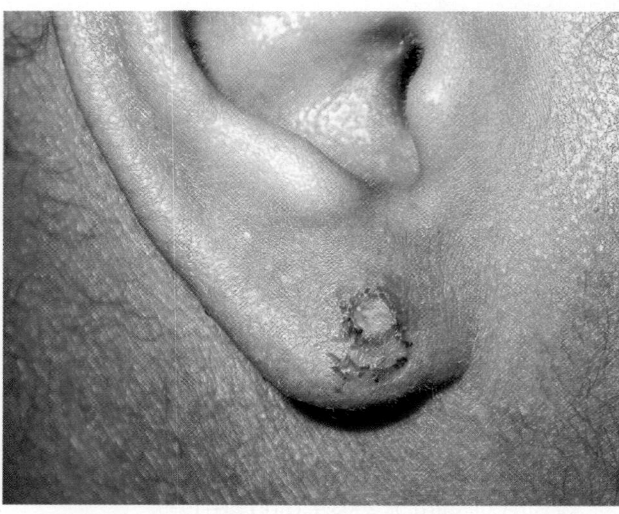

Figure 252-1 Nickel contact dermatitis at the site of an earring.

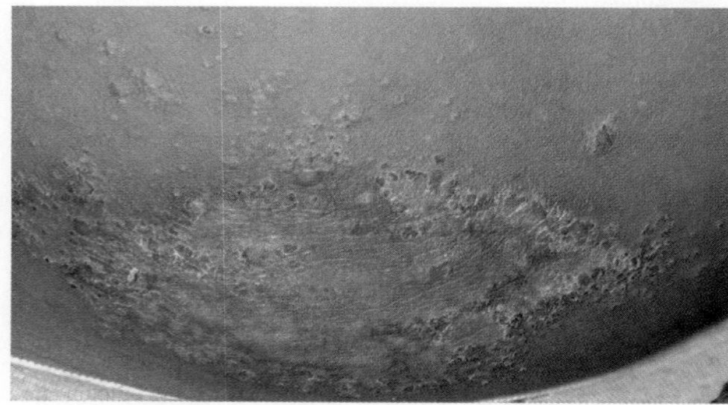

Figure 252-2 Contact dermatitis caused by nickel in a clothing snap or belt buckle affecting the lower abdomen.

EPIDEMIOLOGIC CONSIDERATIONS

Contact dermatitis affects both sexes, all ages, and all races. Differences among individuals pertain mostly to habits of exposure. In addition, regional differences can exist, depending on the allergens or irritants in the environment. Contact dermatitis represents 6% to 10% of visits to dermatologists' offices.[6]

Irritant contact dermatitis is seen more commonly than allergic contact dermatitis in very young children because they lack the repeated exposure needed for allergic contact dermatitis to develop. However, some experts suggest that allergic contact dermatitis may account for at least 20% of all childhood dermatitis.[7]

DIFFERENTIAL DIAGNOSIS

The differential diagnoses for contact dermatitides include atopic dermatitis, seborrheic dermatitis, tinea, and psoriasis. Rare conditions, such as acrodermatitis enteropathica from zinc deficiency or Letterer-Siwe disease, a serious disorder of histiocytes, can mimic diaper dermatitis and must be considered.

CLINICAL MANIFESTATIONS

The clinical presentation of both types of contact dermatitis can be similar. Allergens and irritants can produce a range of responses from eczematous changes of the skin noted by pink, scaling, irritated plaques to severe vesiculobullous eruptions characterized by blistering changes of the skin and severe pruritus.

Irritant contact dermatitis can lead to lichenification, which is characterized by accentuation of skin lines, often with hyperpigmentation, and an almost hardening of the skin. Acute irritant dermatitis can occur within minutes to hours after exposure. The intensity of the reaction is related to the nature of the chemical, the concentration, and the duration of contact. Conditions that foster a more severe reaction include wet skin and skin under friction, occlusion, or pressure. In addition, patients with a history of atopic dermatitis are likely to suffer from contact dermatitis.[8]

Allergic contact dermatitis can also produce bullous, purpuric, lichenoid,[9] papular, urticarial, pigmented, and hypopigmented[9] reactions.

MANAGEMENT

Uncomplicated Case

Treatment is similar for both irritant and allergic contact dermatitis. Topical steroids and emollients for milder disease and systemic medications including oral corticosteroids and antihistamines for more dramatic presentations are the basic treatments. Although the effectiveness of topical steroids has been well documented in allergic contact dermatitis, it is less well defined for irritant dermatitis.[10] Elimination of the offending agent and liberal application of emollients are usually curative for mild irritant contact dermatitis, given that this form of treatment will speed resolution and decrease the chance of impetiginization resulting from scratching. Identifying the causative factors so they may be avoided is accomplished by good history taking by the physician. In chronic cases, a parent or older patient may need to keep a diary. More involved cases warrant a trial of topical steroids, given that the risks are minimal when used short term. In rare severe cases of irritant, just as with allergic contact dermatitis, systemic steroids are appropriate and can be given for 2 weeks at a dose of 0.5 to 1.0 mg/kg with a rapid wean. A dermatologist may need to be consulted if the diagnosis is in question.

The treatment of diaper dermatitis requires gentle application of protective barrier ointments such as zinc oxide and petrolatum. Lowest-potency corticosteroids can be used in severe cases 2 to 3 times daily for a limited time (initially 3 days, no longer than 2 weeks), and long-term exposure should be avoided in the occluded diaper area. Care of the diaper area includes bathing the child in water with minimal use of nondetergent soaps, followed by liberal use of emollients. Barrier ointments should be used with each diaper change with care not to produce excess friction. The involved areas should be kept dry and free of urine and stool, and caregivers should be encouraged to change the diaper frequently, as often as every 2 hours or more. Commercial cleansing wipes, if used, should be fragrance free and alcohol free.[11] Topical antifungal agents work well for secondary candidal infection of the diaper area and should be considered in irritant rashes that are present for more than 3 days. Combination steroid-antifungal topical products should not be used in the diaper area.

With regard to the treatment of allergic contact dermatitis, Rhus dermatitis specifically, management includes washing the skin and other items that may have come in contact with the plant. Once the patient develops skin lesions, systemic antihistamines are usually needed. Topically, mild to moderate strength (class 7 to 4) topical steroids are appropriate. In addition, topical pramoxine, a topical antihistamine, is safe and can be used over large areas of the body 2 to 3 times a day. If the lesions are limited but very pruritic, then a more potent topical steroid cream (class 1 or 2) can be applied for no more than 2 weeks. If the lesions are more extensive, then systemic steroids for 2 weeks at a beginning dose of 0.5 to 1.0 mg/kg followed by a rapid taper over the subsequent 2 weeks is justifiable. Dermatologists do not favor quick bursts of systemic steroids because they are often associated with rebound of the rash.

Complicated Case

A suspected contact dermatitis that has not responded to treatment in a month, has involvement of a large body surface, or displays severe reactions (such as bullae) is a complicated case and may require skin biopsy. Patients who require patch testing (gold standard for identification of allergens causing allergic contact dermatitis) will require a referral to a dermatologist or pediatric allergist.

Patch testing involves the application of suspected allergens to intact uninflamed skin. The substances of interest are usually applied to the back and are left on for 48 hours. After 48 hours, the patches are removed and the coded sites evaluated for the presence of a reaction, which can be erythema or bullae formation. Some positive reactions may not show for up to 7 days; thus having the patient evaluated again at 5 and 7 days is useful. A commercially available patch testing system composed of 23 common allergens can be performed easily in the dermatologist's office. For more extensive patch testing, use of individually prepared aluminum chambers with multiple allergens can be placed and then applied with hypoallergenic tape to the back. Of note, the technique of photopatch testing that detects contact photoallergy is also available. In this test, the patch is applied, and then after 24 hours the area is exposed to ultraviolet A light; the patch is read 48 hours later.

PREVENTION

Irritant contact dermatitis can best be prevented by maintaining the skin barrier and by avoiding irritants. Parents and older children must be educated about common irritants including soaps and detergents, especially those with fragrance and dye additives. Formaldehyde, formaldehyde releasers, and other clothing treatments can aggravate the skin of children; clothing should be washed before wearing. Barrier function of the skin is preserved by maintaining a healthy stratum corneum. Skin should be well hydrated (but not overly hydrated) and well moisturized.

Allergic contact dermatitis is best prevented by identifying trigger factors and then educating the parent and older child about avoidance of triggers. Patients and their families should be taught to identify a poison ivy plant so that it can be avoided and removed, if possible. Commercial nickel spot tests are available from several sources. These user-friendly tests allow patients to detect the presence of nickel in metal items with which the patient may come in contact.

WHEN TO REFER

- A child with presumed irritant contact dermatitis (including diaper dermatitis) that has persisted for a month or longer despite aggressive topical treatment should be referred to a dermatologist.
- A child with involvement of a large body surface area or displaying severe reactions (eg, bullae) or an atypical presentation may require referral to a dermatologist for a skin biopsy.
- Patients in need of patch testing should be referred to a dermatologist or qualified pediatric allergist.

WHEN TO ADMIT

- Generalized or systemic contact dermatitis as may occur from exposure to smoke of a burning antigen (ie, Rhus family plant)
- Patient experiencing fever, chills, nausea, vomiting, or hypotension
- Secondary bacterial infection requiring intravenous antibiotics
- Secondary infection with a herpes virus requiring intravenous antivirals

TOOLS FOR PRACTICE

Engaging Patient and Family

- *What is a Pediatric Dermatologist?* (fact sheet), American Academy of Pediatrics (www.aap.org/family/PedDermatologistfacts.pdf).

Medical Decision Support

- *Pediatric Dermatology: A Quick Reference Guide* (book), American Academy of Pediatrics (www.aap.org/bookstore).

SUGGESTED RESOURCES

Gelmetti C. Skin cleansing in children. *J Eur Acad Dermatol Venereol.* 2001;15(suppl 1):S12-S15.

Kutting B, Brehler R, Traupe H. Allergic contact dermatitis in children: strategies of prevention and risk management. *Eur J Dermatol.* 2004;14:80-85.

REFERENCES

1. Gupta AK, Skinner AR. Management of diaper dermatitis. *Int J Dermatol.* 2004;43:830-834.
2. Schwartz RH, Peary P. Abuse of isobutyl nitrite inhalation (Rush) by adolescents. *Clin Pediatr.* 1986;25:308-310.
3. Cohen DE. Contact dermatitis: a quarter century perspective. *J Am Acad Dermatol.* 2004;51:S60-S63.
4. Krob HA, Fleischer AB Jr, D'Agostino R Jr, et al. Prevalence and relevance of contact dermatitis allergens: a meta-analysis of 15 years of published T.R.U.E. test data. *J Am Acad Dermatol.* 2004;51:349-353.
5. Guillet G, Guillet MH, Dagregorio G. Allergic contact dermatitis from natural rubber latex in atopic dermatitis and the risk of later Type 1 allergy. *Contact Dermatitis.* 2005;53:46-51.
6. Sherertz EF. Controversies in contact dermatitis. *Am J Contact Dermatitis.* 1994:130-135.
7. Bruckner AL, Weston WL. Allergic contact dermatitis in children: a practical approach to management. *Skin Therapy Lett.* 2002;7:3-5.
8. Akhavan A, Cohen SR. The relationship between atopic dermatitis and contact dermatitis. *Clin Dermatol.* 2003;21:158-162.
9. Schultz E, Mahler V. Prolonged lichenoid reaction and cross-sensitivity to para-substituted amino-compounds due to temporary henna tattoo. *Int J Dermatol.* 2002;41(5):301-303.
10. Cohen DE, Heidary N. Treatment of irritant and allergic contact dermatitis. *Dermatol Ther.* 2004;17(4):334-340.
11. Atherton DJ. A review of the pathophysiology, prevention and treatment of irritant diaper dermatitis. *Curr Med Res Opin.* 2004;20:645-649.

Chapter 253

CONTAGIOUS EXANTHEMATOUS DISEASES

Robert Iannone, MD

Exanthem, meaning to bloom or to break out, refers to an eruption or rash that is usually associated with fever and generally implies that the eruption is infectious in origin. These eruptions are extremely common in children and present the clinician with a major challenge in differential diagnosis, inasmuch as many contagious exanthems have similar appearances. The clinical manifestations other than the rash must often be explored to distinguish one disease from another. These factors include the incubation period, prodromal symptoms and signs, the age of the patient, immunization history, contact history, distribution and progression of the rash, evidence of other organ involvement, and pathognomonic signs, such as peeling or Koplik spots.

Exanthems may be caused by viruses, bacteria, *Rickettsia, Mycoplasma,* and fungi. Moreover, certain allergic and immune-complex diseases such as childhood arthritis can mimic infectious exanthems.

Some exanthems herald diseases for which treatment is necessary; others signal the need for quarantine or further evaluation. For example, if rubella or erythema infectiosum (infection with human parvovirus) is included in the differential diagnoses, then the primary care physician needs to investigate recent and potential exposures of the sick child to close contacts who are pregnant because fetal infection with these viruses may be devastating. Diseases that might respond to specific therapy require special consideration. These diseases include the exanthem of *Mycoplasma pneumoniae* infection, which will respond to erythromycin, or the exanthem of *Rickettsia rickettsii* (Rocky Mountain spotted fever), which requires early treatment with tetracycline or chloramphenicol. The rash of streptococcal or staphylococcal scarlet fever (scarlatina) needs specific identification so that it can be treated appropriately, and scarlatina must be differentiated from Kawasaki disease so that a patient with the latter receives careful monitoring and specific treatment (see Chapter 289, Kawasaki Disease). Some of the differentiating characteristics of these eruptions are found in Table 253-1 and in Chapter 213, Rash, Tables 213-1 and 213-2 (see also Chapter 246 for a discussion of chickenpox).

This chapter focuses on exanthems associated with contagious illness and does not discuss rashes associated with infections not transmitted person-to-person, such as Lyme disease (see Chapter 292).

ENTEROVIRAL EXANTHEMS

Enteroviral infections have now become the most common cause of exanthems in children because rubeola (measles) and rubella are controlled largely by the administration of effective vaccines. Many serotypes of echoviruses and coxsackieviruses are associated with rashes; in many instances, these rashes are generalized maculopapular types that have discrete lesions similar to those of rubella. They may appear very similar to roseola, with an initial 2 to 3 days of fever followed by the eruption. Generally, though, the prodromal fever is much lower than that of roseola. Transmission occurs via the fecal-oral route.

Although maculopapular rashes predominate, vesicular lesions have been observed in coxsackievirus-A5, -A9, and -A16 infections. Hand-foot-mouth disease commonly is seen with coxsackievirus-A16 infection and is exhibited by vesicles on the palms and soles and ulcers in the mouth. The oral ulcerations of enteroviral herpangina typically occur in the back of the mouth, which can distinguish it from the more diffuse lesions of primary herpes stomatitis.

Enteroviral exanthems typically occur in the late summer and early fall and are associated with epidemics of aseptic meningitis. A more detailed discussion of enteroviral infections and aseptic meningitis can be found in Chapters 260, Enterovirus Infections, and Chapter 293, Meningitis, respectively.

EXANTHEM SUBITUM (ROSEOLA)

Human herpesvirus-6 is the infectious agent of roseola.[1] Transmission is via secretions most likely from an asymptomatic contact. Roseola is characterized by 3 or 4 days of high fever (104° to 105°F [40° to 40.6°C]), followed by abrupt resolution of the fever and the eruption of a pink maculopapular rash that begins on the neck and then spreads to the trunk and extremities, usually sparing the face. The lesions are discrete and last only for 1 or 2 days. The child usually has no other manifestation of illness and does not appear as ill as the severity of the fever might imply.

Roseola occurs year round and is limited to children between the ages of 6 months and 3 years. See Chapter 275, Human Herpesvirus-6 and Human Herpesvirus-7 Infections, for a more complete discussion of this disease.

ERYTHEMA INFECTIOSUM (FIFTH DISEASE)

Erythema infectiosum is caused by infection with human parvovirus-B19. Susceptible persons are infected by respiratory tract droplets.

The typical clinical presentation is one of rash without fever or other systemic signs, though fever can occur in 15% to 30% of patients. The rash first erupts as a bright-red erythema of the cheeks and forehead, with circumoral pallor, 7 to 10 days after nonspecific symptoms of malaise, myalgias, and headache. This slapped-cheek appearance is the result of many large maculopapular lesions that coalesce to form a confluent red rash. These confluent lesions are hot to the touch and commonly palpable but are nontender.

After a single day, a maculopapular rash next appears on the proximal extremities. This rash then spreads gradually to the trunk and distal extremities, leaving a lacelike appearance as it clears. This second stage lasts 2 to 4 days. In a third stage the rash may reappear transiently when the skin is traumatized by pressure, sunlight, or extremes of hot and cold. Arthritis and arthralgia, which often occur in adults, are infrequent findings in children. Mild myelosuppression typically goes unnoticed in healthy individuals, whereas a life-threatening aplastic crisis may occur in patients with shortened red cell survival, such as occurs in sickle cell disease or hereditary spherocytosis.

Clinical suspicion may be confirmed, when necessary, by testing for anti-parvovirus-B19 immunoglobulin M in the immunocompetent patient or through polymerase chain reaction testing in the immunocompromised patient.[2] For patients who have HIV, dot blot hybridization of serum specimens may have adequate sensitivity. Supportive care is sufficient for most patients. Those with aplastic crises may require transfusion. In immunodeficient patients with chronic infection, intravenous immune globulin therapy should be considered. Transmission of parvovirus-B19 may be decreased through the use of routine infection control measures. [2]

RUBELLA

Rubella is also known as German measles or 3-day measles. These names served to distinguish the disease from rubeola (hard measles or 10-day measles). The virus was cultivated first in 1962[3]; its clinical spectrum was documented thoroughly in the 1965 epidemic in the United States. Transmission is through direct or droplet contact from nasopharyngeal secretions. The period of maximal communicability is just before and up to a week after onset of the rash.

The typical clinical illness is mild and brief. In most children the rash itself is the first sign of infection. It is typically a pink, maculopapular eruption beginning on the face and spreading downward to the trunk and extremities. The lesions remain discrete and pink, the

Table 253-1 Differentiating Common Childhood Exanthems

DISEASE	CHARACTER OF RASH	PRODROME	PATHOGNOMONIC SIGNS	HELPFUL SIGNS	CONTAGIOUS PERIOD
Enterovirus infection	Maculopapular; generalized to most of body; discrete	May have 3-4 days of mild fever before rash, or rash may appear with constitutional signs	Herpangina, hand-foot-mouth syndrome	Aseptic meningitis, pharyngitis, petechiae with some coxsackievirus strains; occurs in summer and early fall	Fecal virus may last several weeks after infection; respiratory limited to a week or less
Exanthem subitum (roseola)	Maculopapular and discrete; begins on trunk and spreads to face and usually spares the limbs	3-4 days of high fever and irritability with no other signs	None	Dramatic drop in fever simultaneous with onset of rash	—
Erythema infectiosum (fifth disease)	Red and flushed cheeks with circumoral pallor; subsequent proximal maculopapular rash on extremities (lacelike)	None	Slapped-cheek appearance in otherwise healthy child	Possible recurrence of eruption with irritation of skin by heat, cold, or pressure	Not contagious once rash appears
Rubella (German measles)	Pink, maculopapular, discrete; begins on face and spreads to trunk and extremities	Commonly none; adolescents may have 1-3 days of low-grade fever and malaise	None	Tender postauricular and suboccipital lymph nodes; possibly arthralgia in adolescents	A few days before to 7 days after onset of rash
Mumps	Maculopapular, discrete, concentrated on trunk; may have urticaria; may be 1st sign of illness	1-2 days of fever, headache, and malaise	None	Diffuse swelling of parotid glands, with pain and tenderness; aseptic meningitis; orchitis or pancreatitis; erythema of the Stensen duct	1-2 days before the onset of parotid swelling to 5 days after onset of parotid swelling
Infectious mononucleosis	Macular or maculopapular and discrete; when associated with ampicillin administration, is confluent (morbilliform) and more intense	2-4 days of fever, pharyngitis, malaise	None	Exudative pharyngitis, lymphadenopathy, splenomegaly, atypical lymphocytes on peripheral blood smear	Indeterminate
Mycoplasma pneumonia	Maculopapular on trunk and extremities in 10% of cases; common spectrum of urticaria, erythema multiforme, and vesicular or bullous lesions	3-5 days of progressive fever, headache, malaise, and cough	None	Pneumonia, cold agglutinins may be elevated	—

Table 253-1 Differentiating Common Childhood Exanthems—cont'd

DISEASE	CHARACTER OF RASH	PRODROME	PATHOGNOMONIC SIGNS	HELPFUL SIGNS	CONTAGIOUS PERIOD
Rubeola (measles)	Red to brown macular rash that spreads from face and neck to trunk and extremities; confluent (morbilliform), particularly on face; begins after onset of fever and fades after 6-7 days with temporary staining of skin	3-4 days of high fever, conjunctivitis, cough, and coryza	Koplik spots	Always an associated conjunctivitis and cough	1-2 days before onset of symptoms to 4 days after rash appears
Atypical measles	Rash may be maculopapular, purpuric, petechial, or vesicular; prominent at wrists and ankles	2-3 days of fever, headache, and cough	None	History of killed measles vaccine, myalgia, pneumonia	Not contagious
Scarlet fever	Erythematous papular eruption sometimes associated with generalized erythema; concentrated on trunk and proximal extremities; feels similar to fine sandpaper	Occurs within 1-4 days of onset of focal infection	None	Focal infections such as pharyngitis, vaginitis, cellulitis, erythema of palms and soles; strawberry tongue; desquamation in recovery phase; Pastia lines	Up to 24 hours after treatment is initiated
Kawasaki disease	Rash ranges from maculopapular to scarlatiniform to urticaria; marked erythema of palms and soles	At least 5 days of fever and irritability common	None	Conjunctivitis, tender lymphadenopathy, strawberry tongue, meatitis, diarrhea, prolonged fever, late desquamation, arthritis in recovery phase	No evidence showing human-to-human or common-source contagiousness

appearance of which contrasts with the raised, confluent, and deep-red lesions of rubeola. The facial rash clears as the extremity rash erupts, and all are cleared by the third to the fifth day.

Fever is very mild, ranging between 99°F and 101°F (37.2°C and 38.3°C). Lymphadenopathy is frequently impressive; the posterior auricular and suboccipital chains are most commonly involved. They are usually tender at the onset of rash, but the tenderness resolves rapidly over 2 to 3 days. Although lymphadenopathy is an important sign of rubella infection, it is not specific. Tiny reddish spots may occur on the soft palate, which are indistinguishable from those of scarlet fever or rubeola. The incubation period is 2 to 3 weeks, with a peak at 16 to 18 days.

The rubella virus can usually be grown from the pharynx within 5 days of the onset of the rash. Serological diagnosis is made by demonstrating an antibody titer rise between acute and convalescent sera 2 weeks apart. Serologic tests include the traditional hemagglutination-inhibition antibody titers, as well as newer techniques such as enzyme immunoassays.

Complications of rubella are rare in children, but a transient arthritis develops in approximately 15% of adolescents and young adults. The arthritis rarely becomes chronic.

The major serious complications of rubella virus result from fetal infection. If a pregnant woman is infected in the first trimester of gestation, then a very high probability exists that the fetus will become infected, with multiorgan involvement. See Chapter 73, Fetal Assessment, for details on congenital rubella syndrome. For this reason, the primary care physician might need to pursue objective confirmation of infection with the rubella virus by determining maternal antibody titers.

INFECTIOUS MONONUCLEOSIS

The exanthem of Epstein-Barr virus occurs in approximately 15% of children. The rash is pink to red and macular or maculopapular. The lesions are discrete and have no specific distinguishing characteristic; therefore the disease is most often diagnosed based on other signs of infectious mononucleosis and confirmed by the peripheral blood smear and serological tests.

The administration of ampicillin to persons who have infectious mononucleosis results in approximately 50% of them developing a much more intense rash, which may also occur with other penicillins. This ampicillin-associated rash is deep red and confluent, giving it a morbilliform appearance. This iatrogenic exanthem resolves spontaneously within a week. The appearance of such a rash in a patient treated for presumptive group A streptococcal pharyngitis is cause to reconsider the diagnosis. The physician should reassure parents that this rash does not represent penicillin hypersensitivity. The full spectrum of Epstein-Barr virus infection is discussed in Chapter 283, Infectious Mononucleosis and Other Epstein- Barr Viral Infections.

MEASLES (RUBEOLA)

Measles is the most serious of the childhood exanthems because of the morbidity of the acute infection and its potential for producing permanent sequelae. The virus is highly contagious and is transmitted via respiratory droplets. Typical clinical disease begins after an incubation period of 10 to 11 days. The prodromal illness is exhibited by increasing fever, cough, conjunctivitis, and coryza. By the fourth day, the fever commonly is high (104°F [40°C]) and the rash erupts. Typically a deep red macular rash begins on the face and neck and spreads down the trunk and extremities, as in rubella. The lesions on the face and upper portion of the trunk soon become confluent to produce the characteristic morbilliform rash, whereas the rash of rubella tends to remain discrete. By the sixth day, the fever subsides and the rash begins to fade; as it fades, it leaves a faint brown stain in the skin, and a fine desquamation ensues.

The exanthem of measles is pathognomonic. Koplik spots begin approximately 2 days before the rash erupts and increase in number until the first or second day of the exanthem. They are tiny bluish-white spots on an erythematous base and cluster adjacent to the molars on the buccal mucosa.

The combination of Koplik spots, fever, cough, conjunctivitis, and morbilliform rash is sufficient to make a firm clinical diagnosis of measles. Although the children are usually very ill, they recover rapidly after the eighth or ninth day and are most often back to normal in a few days, hence the moniker 10-day measles.

Measles virus induces inflammation throughout the respiratory tract; respiratory complications are common, including otitis media, pneumonia, and croup. The otitis media is treated as any acute otitis media case. The pneumonia may be either a primary measles pneumonia or a superimposed bacterial pneumonia. All children who have measles should have careful follow-up, and the examiner should have a high degree of suspicion for secondary bacterial pneumonia.

Subacute sclerosing panencephalitis, also known as Dawson encephalitis, is the major complication of persistent measles virus infection. It occurs in approximately 1 per 1000 cases and commonly results in death or permanent neurologic sequelae.[2] Subacute sclerosing panencephalitis produces headache, vomiting, drowsiness, personality changes, seizures, and coma. In most cases, the cerebrospinal fluid reveals pleocytosis and elevated protein levels. Some of these children have only a mild disease and recover in a few days; others have a fulminant course. Vitamin A supplementation should be considered for patients 6 months to 2 years of age who are hospitalized as a result of measles and its complications. Prevention of measles is discussed in Chapter 29, Immunizations.

Atypical Measles

Atypical measles syndrome occurs in some children who were exposed to wild measles virus and had been immunized with inactivated measles vaccine. Such children may have 2 to 3 days of fever and headache followed by a rash erupting on the wrists and ankles. The rash may be maculopapular, purpuric, petechial, or vesicular. Marked myalgia, with swelling of the hands and feet, may also occur; pneumonia is common.

The constitutional symptoms and the distribution of the rash are similar to that of Rocky Mountain spotted fever. Elicitation of a history of having received killed measles vaccine assists in making the diagnosis. The inactivated measles vaccine is no longer available in the United States.

Mycoplasma Pneumonia

Cutaneous signs are a minor manifestation of mycoplasmal infections. A maculopapular eruption may appear on the trunk and extremities of 10% to 15% of persons infected with *M pneumoniae*. Even more common is for these infections to be associated with allergic-type eruptions that display a spectrum of cutaneous lesions ranging from urticaria and erythema multiforme to vesicles or bullae. Such patients frequently have had a prodromal illness of fever, headache, malaise, and cough. The pneumonia may escape physical diagnosis only to crop up on the chest radiograph as an incidental finding. Macrolide antibiotics may be used to treat mycoplasma pneumoniae infections. See Chapter 312, Pneumonia.

Mumps

An exanthem will develop in fewer than 10% of persons infected with the mumps virus. The lesions are maculopapular, pale pink, discrete, and concentrated on the trunk. The virus more typically involves the salivary glands, the testicles (after puberty), the pancreas, and the meninges. After an incubation period of 16 to 18 days, clinical mumps develops in approximately 60% of infected persons. The remaining 40% have inapparent infections, without salivary gland swelling. Transmission is through direct contact via the respiratory route.

The typical illness begins with 1 or 2 days of anorexia, headache, and mild to moderate fever. This period is followed by complaints of discomfort when chewing and of pain around the ear. A diffuse but noticeable enlargement and tenderness of the parotid gland is usually present, which can be distinguished from lymph node enlargement in that it extends anterior to the ear and below the ramus of the mandible posteriorly to the mastoid bone, usually obliterating the angle of the jaw. Lymph nodes are more discrete and generally submandibular in location. Accompanying the parotitis, erythema is commonly seen around the opening of the Stensen duct. The fever usually lasts 2 to 5 days. Rarely, only 1 parotid gland is involved, or the submandibular salivary glands rather than the parotids will be swollen.

Meningoencephalitis is estimated to occur in 10% of all cases of mumps and is characterized by headache, nausea, vomiting, and mild nuchal rigidity. It may occur before, during, or after the parotitis phase of the disease. Meningoencephalitis follows a course similar to the aseptic meningitis that is caused by other viruses, and it usually has no sequelae. Some cerebrospinal fluid pleocytosis is present in most cases of mumps without clinical evidence of meningeal irritation.

Orchitis is uncommon in children, but unilateral involvement of the testes and epididymis is observed in approximately 25% of male patients who are infected with mumps virus after puberty. Patients who have orchitis are usually quite ill; however, sterility rarely occurs.[2]

The pancreas and other exocrine glands are rarely involved.

Late neurologic complications include nerve deafness and very rare postinfectious encephalitis.

Scarlet Fever

The rash of scarlet fever (scarlatina) is caused by a circulating erythrotoxin that is produced by certain strains of streptococci and staphylococci. This rash is characterized by a fine papular eruption on an erythematous base. In many instances. a generalized erythema of the skin is present, even including areas that are not yet involved with the papular rash. The eruption of scarlet fever is concentrated on the trunk and proximal extremities. It feels rough to the touch, similar to fine sandpaper. The rash is commonly associated with prominent erythema of the lips, soles, and palms. Transverse red streaks (Pastia lines) are sometimes present, usually in the antecubital spaces. Desquamation of involved skin typically occurs in the recovery phase. On the tongue, the examiner can observe prominent papillae on a very red base, giving a strawberry tongue appearance.

If streptococci are the source of the erythrogenic toxin, then the pharynx is the usual site of focal infection. Other focal infections (eg, vaginitis, cellulitis), however, may also be found. When staphylococci are the source of erythrogenic toxin, the infective focus is usually some site other than the pharynx; infected surgical or traumatic wounds have been common sites.

The treatment of scarlet fever is directed toward eradication of the focal infection. Streptococcal infections are treated with penicillin or erythromycin, whereas staphylococcal infections are treated with cephalexin, amoxicillin-clavulanate, dicloxacillin, or oxacillin.

Kawasaki disease must be carefully differentiated from scarlet fever because coronary artery disease may complicate untreated Kawasaki disease. Its cutaneous manifestations overlap remarkably with those of scarlet fever, but it can usually be distinguished by the additional signs of discrete bulbar conjunctivitis without exudate, cracking of the lips, very tender lymphadenopathy (usually solitary, unilateral, and more than 1.5 cm in diameter), changes in the extremities, including induration with erythema of palms and soles, meatitis, and diarrhea. These children are profoundly irritable, and their fever persists for more than a week in most cases (5 days of fever is necessary for diagnosis). Just as in scarlet fever, however, patients have erythema of the palms and soles, with striking desquamation during the second and third weeks of the disease. Kawasaki disease is presented in more detail in Chapter 289.

OTHER

Many other respiratory viral illnesses may result in nondescript morbilliform rashes, including respiratory syncytial virus, influenza A and B, adenovirus, and parainfluenza virus.

The author gratefully acknowledges the contribution of the author of the chapter in the previous editions, John H. Dossett.

TOOLS FOR PRACTICE

Engaging Patient and Family

- *Immunizations & Infectious Diseases: An Informed Parent's Guide* (book), American Academy of Pediatrics (www.aap.org/bookstore).

Medical Decision Support

- *Challenging Cases in Pediatric Infectious Diseases,* Volume 1 (book), American Academy of Pediatrics (www.aap.org/bookstore).
- *Pediatric Dermatology: A Quick Reference Guide* (book), American Academy of Pediatrics (www.aap.org/bookstore).
- *Red Book: 2006 Report of the Committee on Infectious Diseases,* 27th edition (book), American Academy of Pediatrics (www.aap.org/bookstore).

SUGGESTED RESOURCE

Feigin RD, Cherry JD. Viral infections. In: Feigin RD, Cherry JD, Demmler GJ, et al, eds. *Textbook of Pediatric Infectious Diseases.* 5th ed. Philadelphia, PA: WB Saunders; 2003.

REFERENCES

1. Yamanishi K, Okuno T, Shirakl K, et al. Identification of human herpesvirus-6 as a causal agent for exanthem subitum. *Lancet.* 1988;1:1065-1067.
2. Pickering LK, Baker CJ, Long SS, et al, eds. *Red Book 2006, Report of the Committee on Infectious Diseases.* 27th ed. Elk Grove Village, IL: American Academy of Pediatrics; 2006.
3. Weller TH, Neva FA. Propagation in tissue culture of cytopathic agents from patients with rubella-like illness. *Proc Soc Exp Biol Med.* 1962;111:215-225.

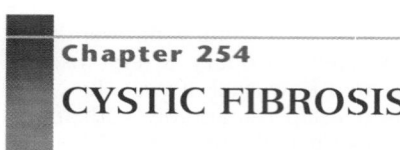

Chapter 254

CYSTIC FIBROSIS

Donna Beth Willey-Courand, MD; Bruce C. Marshall, MD

Cystic fibrosis (CF) is an autosomal-recessive disease involving multiple organs, especially the pancreas and lungs. When the disease was first described in 1938,[1] the median survival for children with CF was less than 1 year.[2] Today, the predicted median survival for people with CF in the United States is over 36 years,[3] demonstrating how dramatically the face of this disease has changed over a relatively short period.

INCIDENCE

CF occurs with a frequency of approximately 1:3600 live births in the white population in whom it is the most common inherited lethal disease. The incidence is 1:29000 in blacks and 1:6500 in Hispanics.[4] Because the carrier state is asymptomatic, the birth of a child with CF is often the 1st knowledge parents have that they carry a mutation.

PATHOPHYSIOLOGICAL FEATURES

The CF gene consists of 250 kilobase pairs located on the long arm of chromosome 7.[5-7] It codes for a 1480 amino acid glycoprotein product known as the cystic fibrosis transmembrane-conductance regulator (CFTR). Currently, more than 1000 mutations of the CFTR gene have been found that alter CFTR structure and function and result in the development of CF. The most common mutation in North America and Europe, accounting for approximately 70% of alleles in the United States,[3] is a deletion of 3 base-pairs, resulting in the deletion of phenylalanine (F) at position 508 (ΔF_{508}). Although the CFTR genotype is highly predictive of pancreatic function, it is less predictive of the pulmonary disease. Recent evidence suggests that gene modifiers, as well as environmental factors, contribute to the pulmonary phenotype.[8]

The CFTR glycoprotein is located in numerous organs throughout the body, including the lungs, the upper respiratory tract, sweat glands, pancreas, intestines, liver, and reproductive tract. CFTR is a cyclic adenosine monophosphate–regulated membrane-channel protein that secretes chloride and other ions[9,10] across the cell membrane and regulates several other proteins, including an epithelial sodium channel.[11] Reduction or absence of CFTR activity results in impaired movement of chloride across the cell membrane and increased reabsorption of sodium.[12] Because passive reabsorption of water molecules follows that of sodium, hydration of secretions is reduced in the affected organs. In CF airways, this results in a decreased periciliary fluid layer volume and height[13]; and because sufficient fluid is critical for proper ciliary function, patients with CF experience impaired mucociliary clearance.[14-16] Other cellular effects of CFTR loss, such as changes to pH[17] and fatty acid ratios,[18] have pleiotropic results at the tissue level, including altered pH of glandular secretions[19] and an exaggerated inflammatory response.[20]

CLINICAL MANIFESTATIONS

Infection

Ineffective mucociliary clearance and other changes predispose CF airways to infection. *Staphylococcus aureus* and *Haemophilus influenzae* are important bacterial pathogens, but *Pseudomonas aeruginosa* has become the primary pathogen in this disease. Initially, nonmucoid environmental strains of *P aeruginosa* are detected in the patients. However, the CF airway environment leads to a transition to mucoidy and to a biofilm mode of growth, which results in an accelerated rate of decline in lung function.[21]

Lower Respiratory Tract

Despite the chronic nature of the airway infection, ongoing neutrophilic inflammation is typical.[20,22,23] DNA released from dying neutrophils increases the viscosity of the airway secretions. Impaired ciliary function and tenacious secretions lead to stasis, and the distal airways become plugged. Bronchoscopic studies of infants with CF reveal that even if the children appear clinically well, neutrophil and proinflammatory (interleukin-8) mediator levels are increased.[22,23] Chest computed tomographic (CT) scans also show that structural changes in the lung can often be detected despite normal pulmonary function.[24] The battle in the lungs of patients with CF begins very early in life and may progress unnoticed.

A cycle of infection and inflammation (Figure 254-1) develops in the lungs of patients with CF, typically punctuated by acute exacerbations. This process eventually damages and destroys the airways, leading to bronchiectasis. Complications such as hemoptysis and pneumothorax may appear as the lung disease progresses. Death most commonly results from respiratory failure and cor pulmonale caused by recurrent or chronic pulmonary infections.[3]

Upper Respiratory Tract

The same pathophysiologic mechanism also affects the upper respiratory tract. Even a moderate loss of CFTR activity can adversely affect the sinuses,[25] and children with CF are predisposed to recurrent and chronic sinusitis despite normal nasal mucociliary clearance.[26] Hypoplasia of the sinuses is a common finding.[27] Nasal polyps are also common, especially among individuals who are homozygous for ΔF_{508} CFTR.[28] The etiology of polyposis is unknown, though it does not appear to be associated with allergies. Polyps may obstruct the nasal passages and contribute to the development of sinusitis.

Gastrointestinal Tract

CFTR is also located throughout the gastrointestinal tract in the pancreas, intestines, and liver.[29,30] In the pancreas, abnormal electrolyte secretion from the epithelial cells lining the pancreatic ducts results in dehydration of the ductal secretions and blockage of the

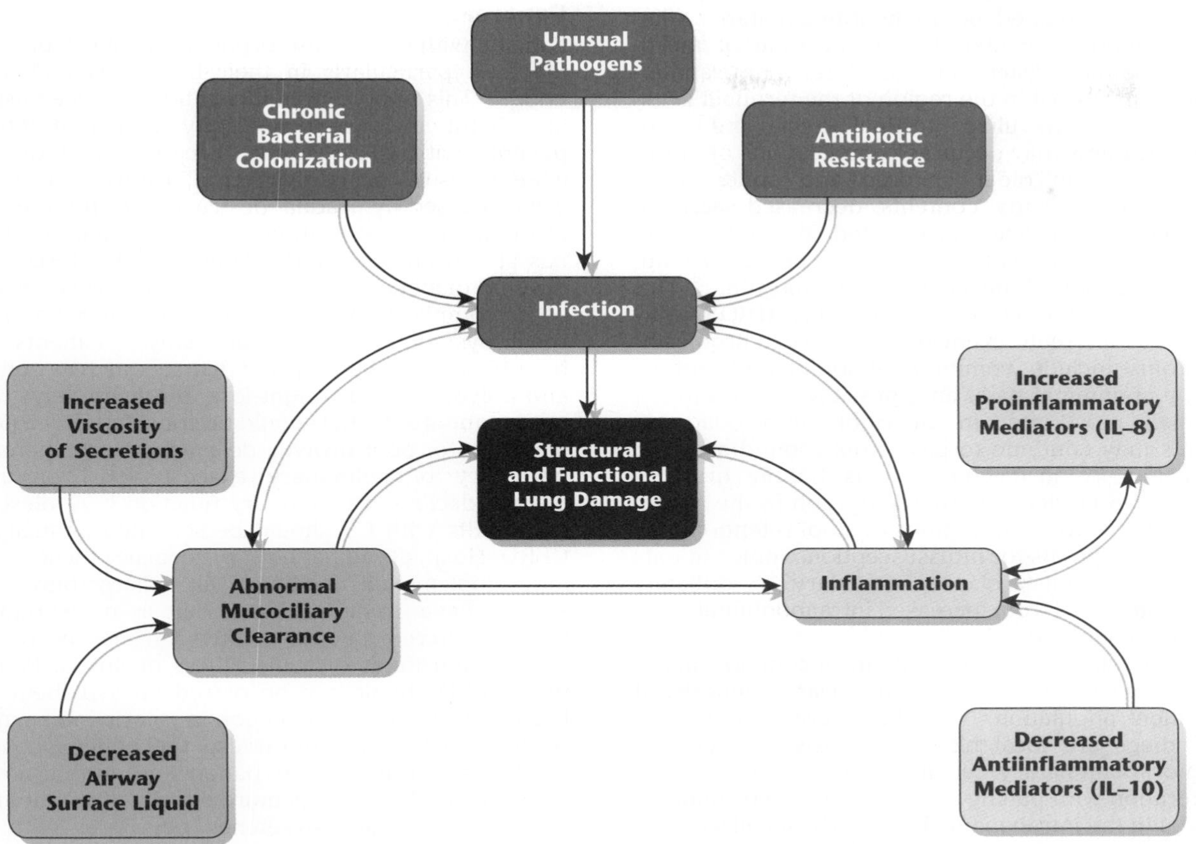

Figure 254-1 The evolution of CF-related lung disease, the end result of a multifactorial process involving abnormal mucociliary clearance, inflammation, and infection.

pancreatic ducts.[31] Destruction of the pancreatic acini occurs, and pancreatic enzyme secretion is significantly decreased. Bicarbonate secretion from the pancreatic ducts is also reduced, which further decreases the effectiveness of the pancreatic enzymes. This condition, known as pancreatic insufficiency (PI), occurs in 85% to 90% of patients with CF.[32] In general, good correlation exists between pancreatic status and genotype. Patients with 2 severe mutations such as $\Delta F_{508}/\Delta F_{508}$ have pancreatic insufficiency, and patients with 1 (or 2) mild mutations are much more likely to have pancreatic sufficiency[33] although they are at increased risk of pancreatitis.[34] Individuals who have pancreatic sufficiency generally have better clinical outcomes than patients with PI.[35] PI results in the malabsorption of fats, proteins, carbohydrates, and the fat-soluble vitamins A, D, E, and K. Children with PI have difficulty growing and gaining weight. Optimization of nutritional status is also essential to maintaining pulmonary function (Figure 254-2).[36]

Patients with PI are at risk for intestinal dysfunction. Intestinal manifestations of CF may be present even before birth. Fetal ultrasound may reveal hyperechoic bowel, suggesting retention of mucus material in the intestine. Twenty percent of infants with CF present meconium ileus,[3] an obstruction of the distal ileum

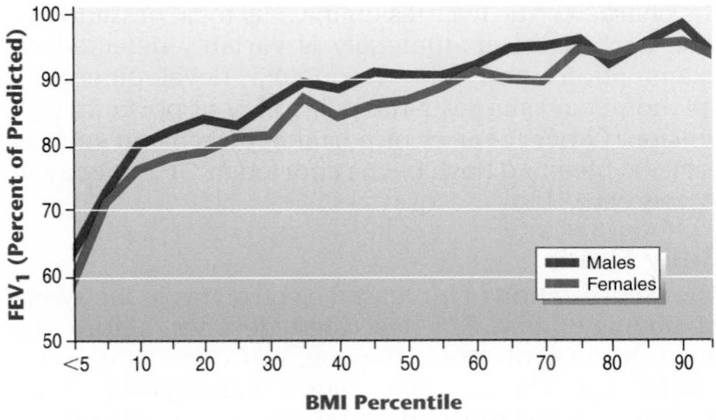

Figure 254-2 Cross-sectional analysis of the *CF Foundation Patient Registry Annual Data Report* showing the association between body mass index (BMI) percentile and pulmonary function. FEV_1 is positively correlated with BMI in pediatric patients 6 to 20 years when using the Wang & Hankinson equations. Note the decreased lung function associated with BMI less than the 50th percentile. (*Cystic Fibrosis Foundation.* Cystic Fibrosis Foundation Patient Registry, 2005 Annual Data Report to the Center Directors. *Bethesda, MD:Cystic Fibrosis Foundation; 2006. Reprinted by permission of the Cystic Fibrosis Foundation.*)

with thick, inspissated, poorly hydrated material. Clinically, newborns exhibit delayed passage of meconium, abdominal distention, and a bubbly or granular-appearing material in the region of the terminal ileum on radiograph. Volvulus, intestinal atresia, and meconium peritonitis may occur as complications of meconium ileus.[37] In older children and adults, poor hydration of intestinal contents, decreased secretion of pancreatic enzymes, inspissated intestinal secretions, and fecal stasis may produce a partial or complete obstruction of the small or large intestine.[38] This distal intestinal obstruction syndrome (DIOS) may develop as an acute event or may occur chronically. Symptoms include vomiting, abdominal distention, crampy abdominal pain, and, possibly, a mass in the abdomen, most often in the right lower quadrant. Patients may continue to pass stool around a partial obstruction. As in meconium ileus, bubbly, granular material can be detected by radiograph in the region of the obstruction, and regions of stool retention may serve as lead points for intussusception. Some patients experience rectal prolapse secondary to difficulty passing stool and from increased intraabdominal pressure from coughing.[37]

Symptomatic liver disease is an uncommon manifestation of CF but leads to death in a small minority of the patient population.[3] The characteristic pathological findings are focal biliary cirrhosis with edema, chronic inflammatory cell infiltration, and bile duct proliferation with patchy accumulation of eosinophilic material in the intrahepatic ducts.[39] The localization of CFTR to the apical membrane of the intrahepatic bile duct cells suggests that a reduction in CFTR activity in CF may result in dehydration and increased viscosity of the bile, which may be a key factor in the pathophysiological features of the hepatic disease.[40] Prolonged jaundice can occur in neonates, and some patients may develop fatty infiltration of the liver; but the characteristic liver lesion in CF is focal or multilobular cirrhosis. Hepatomegaly is variably detected on examination, and the secondary development of splenomegaly suggests the possibility of portal hypertension. Other features of portal hypertension such as variceal bleeding have been reported in CF but are relatively rare.[41]

Body Fluids

The identification of increased electrolytes in the sweat of people with CF,[42] described decades before the identification of the CF gene, provided important insights into the pathophysiological mechanism of the disease and led to the development of the diagnostic sweat test. The loss of body electrolytes caused by sweating in patients with CF can cause metabolic alkalosis either acutely or chronically.[43] Acute illness, vomiting, and thermal stress may be contributing factors. Children may initially present with to thrive, irritability, and vomiting. Salt crystals are sometimes seen caked on the skin. Laboratory tests reveal increased serum pH and bicarbonate levels, as well as decreased serum levels of sodium, chloride, and potassium. The increased consumption of salty foods in older children and the addition of salt to the formula for infants are usually adequate to prevent salt loss syndrome.[44]

Pancreas

Patients with CF are also prone to the development of diabetes, particularly in their late teens and adulthood.[45] This important complication has been associated with increased morbidity and mortality in patients with CF.[46] Cystic fibrosis related diabetes (CFRD) results primarily from a relative insulin deficiency caused by gradual destruction of the islet cells in the pancreas, but an element of insulin resistance has also been reported.[47] Patients with CFRD rarely develop diabetic ketoacidosis, but they are at risk for other complications of diabetes such as retinopathy, renal dysfunction, and neuropathy.[46] Patients may have the classic symptoms of diabetes such as polyuria and polydipsia and weight loss, but many have minimal symptoms. CFRD should be considered as a possible cause for poor growth, delayed puberty, increased frequency of pulmonary exacerbations, or unexplained decline in pulmonary function.[45] Adolescents and adults with CF should be screened annually for CFRD. Hospitalized patients, particularly those receiving supplemental feedings via gastrostomy tube, should have frequent blood sugar measurements because altered glucose metabolism may be present only during times of acute illness or stress. Patients with CFRD should *not* be placed on a diabetic diet because a significant reduction in caloric intake might result, which can compromise the patient's overall nutritional status. Instead, patients are taught how to distribute carbohydrates more equally throughout the day and to replace sweetened beverages with diet drinks.

Skeletal Complications

Osteopenia and osteoporosis are relatively common in adolescents and adults with CF for several reasons, including failure to thrive, delayed pubertal development, liver disease, physical inactivity, and malabsorption of calcium, magnesium, and vitamins D and K.[48] Steroid use may further exacerbate the problems. Patients with decreased bone mineral density are predisposed to atraumatic fractures, especially of the spine and ribs. Patients may also experience transient arthritis that may be monoarticular, pauciarticular, or polyarticular. The knees, ankles, wrists, and proximal interphalangeal joints of the hands are the most often affected.

Puberty

Pubertal development is often delayed in both boys and girls with CF.[49] Poor nutritional status and a decrease in glucose tolerance, accompanied by a delay in the rise in sex hormone levels result in delayed or blunted pubertal development. Female infants with CF demonstrate excessive cytoplasmic and extracellular mucus, which can continue into childhood; the thickened cervical secretions may reduce fertility.[50] Girls with CF may have abnormal menstrual cycles, as well as primary and secondary amenorrhea.[51] Nevertheless, increasing numbers of successful pregnancies are occurring as the CF population ages.[3,52] Boys with CF may have reduced testicular and epididymal size and reduced testosterone levels.[53,54] In the majority of boys, bilateral absence of the vas deferens occurs secondary to obstruction and subsequent resorption of the structure, resulting in infertility. However, a variety of assisted reproductive technologies have recently been developed and used to treat infertility successfully in men with CF.[55]

DIFFERENTIAL DIAGNOSIS

Patients with CF most commonly exhibit respiratory symptoms such as recurrent pulmonary infections (49% of patients at presentation), failure to thrive or malnutrition (40%), steatorrhea or abnormal stools (32%), meconium ileus or intestinal obstruction (20%), or a family history of CF (15%). Vitamin deficiency (specifically deficiencies in the fat soluble vitamins A, D, E, and K) may be seen. Other manifestations of CF that may trigger initial patient encounters include salt loss syndrome, nasal polyps, hepatobiliary disease, and impaired fertility. The mean age of diagnosis is 3.3 years, with a median age of diagnosis of 6 months. Seventy-five percent of children are diagnosed by 2 years of age.[3]

The common pulmonary symptoms at presentation include a recurrent cough that is productive of purulent sputum, difficult-to-control wheezing, nasal polyps, recurrent otitis media, sinusitis, and pneumonia. The differential diagnosis includes asthma, environmental allergies, immunodeficiency syndromes, ciliary agenesis or dyskinesia, α-1 antitrypsin deficiency, foreign body aspiration.

From the gastrointestinal standpoint, patients with CF most commonly present initially with failure to thrive (see Chapter 179, Failure to Thrive) or steatorrhea (see Chapter 169, Diarrhea and Steatorrhea).

EVALUATION

Relevant History

In the majority of cases, no known family history of CF is found.

Many children with CF initially present with respiratory symptoms, especially cough. The cough is often dry at first but becomes progressively productive of purulent sputum. Over-the-counter therapies are generally ineffective, and antibiotic treatment can produce only transient, partial improvement in the cough, which recurs with the cessation of therapy. The cough is present both day and night and may be exacerbated by physical activity and, in infants, by crying. Recurrent wheezing may also be present. Some children with CF also have asthma. Parents often report that their child has had recurrent pneumonia, sinusitis, bronchitis, and otitis media, necessitating repeated courses of antibiotics. Pneumonia and atelectasis may have occurred repeatedly in the same area of the lung. A history of nasal polyps without a concomitant history of nasal allergies is highly suggestive of CF. Finally, parents may have noted changes to the child's nail beds consistent with clubbing.

From the gastrointestinal standpoint, infants with CF are often described as voracious feeders despite having poor weight gain. The infants' stools are frequent, bulky, loose, foul smelling, and voluminous enough that parents will often complain that they overflow the diaper. Grease may be seen in the stool, absorbed in the diaper or, in the case of older children, in the toilet bowl. Abdominal cramping and bloating after eating are common complaints. Foul-smelling flatulence may be described. Any neonate born with meconium ileus or with delayed passage of meconium and any infant or child with rectal prolapse should be tested for CF.

Physical Examination

Vital Signs

Respiratory rates and heart rates should be monitored relative to age-appropriate normal values. Fever and exacerbation or progression of the underlying lung disease may elevate both values. Oxygen saturation should be assessed at each visit. The use of overnight pulse oximetry or polysomnography should be considered to evaluate for nocturnal hypoxemia and hypercarbia in patients with more advanced disease.

Growth Parameters

At all ages, particular attention should be paid to growth parameters, including weight, height, head circumference, and weight for length in children younger than 2 years and weight, height, and body mass index in children older than 2 years. The child's height percentile should be compared with the height percentile predicted from the parental height. Concern should arise whenever a child fails to gain weight, loses weight, or crosses percentiles for height or weight.

Head and Neck

Otoscopic examination should be performed at all visits to assess for otitis media. If a child has recurrent otitis media or is exposed to frequent doses of aminoglycosides, then audiometry should periodically be performed. The nasal mucosa should be inspected for discharge, swelling of the tissue, or polypoid tissue. Palpation of the sinuses should be performed. Examination of the oropharynx should include assessment of the tonsils and the posterior pharynx because children with CF have similar risk for the development of adenotonsillar hypertrophy as children without CF. The posterior pharynx should be checked for exudates emanating from the nasopharynx.

Chest and Lungs

Coughing frequency and the productivity of the cough should be assessed. The child's ability to communicate without coughing, becoming dyspneic, and without accessory muscle use is indicative of the status of the lung disease. Auscultation of the lungs may reveal clear breath sounds. With exacerbation of the underlying lung disease, wheezing, rhonchi, or crackles may be heard. As the patient's pulmonary status worsens, these findings may not change with antibiotic therapy; any clearing that does occur may be short lived. As the lung disease progresses, breath sounds may become globally decreased, and tubular breath sounds may be heard in areas of severe tissue destruction or bronchiectasis and fibrosis. Unilaterally decreased breath sounds, particularly in association with an acute onset of dyspnea, should raise concern about the development of a pneumothorax. With progression of the obstructive component of CF lung disease there is increasing hyperinflation of the lungs, and the chest may take on a barrel shape with an increased anterior-posterior diameter. Progression of the fibrotic component of the lung disease results in the development of tachypnea and decreased vital capacity.

Heart

With the progression of the lung disease and development of cor pulmonale, fixed splitting of the 1st and 2nd heart sounds with increased loudness of the 2nd heart sound may be heard.

Abdomen

Infants often present initially with protuberant abdomens. Distention of the abdomen with pain on palpation may be noted in children with acute intestinal obstructions. The frequency and distribution of bowel sounds should be assessed by auscultation. Palpation should be performed to assess for retention of stool (most commonly in the right lower quadrant), tenderness, hepatomegaly, and splenomegaly.

Genitourinary Tract

Tanner staging should be performed either by direct inspection or by having the child indicate their developmental status from a series of pictures. Girls should be questioned about the onset of menstruation, the regularity of their cycles, and associated symptoms. All sexually active girls should undergo annual pelvic examinations.

Extremities

Joints should be examined for swelling that may be caused by CF-related arthropathy. The digits and nail beds should be examined for clubbing and cyanosis. Edema may arise from hypoproteinemia especially in newly diagnosed malnourished infants and in patients with end-stage lung disease and cor pulmonale.

Laboratory Testing

Diagnostic Testing: Sweat Testing and Genotype Analysis

The diagnosis of CF requires either 2 positive sweat tests or genotype analysis revealing 2 CFTR mutations known to cause CF plus one of the following:

- Chronic sinopulmonary disease
- Gastrointestinal or nutritional abnormalities
- Obstructive azoospermia in boys
- Salt loss syndrome
- CF in a 1st-degree relative

The pilocarpine iontophoresis technique of Gibson and Cooke is the gold standard for the diagnosis of CF. Pilocarpine stimulates the secretion of sweat. The volume of sweat and concentration of chloride secreted are then measured. Sweat testing should be performed in accordance with the Clinical and Laboratory Standards Institute (formerly National Committee for Clinical Laboratory Standards) guidelines.[56] Normal chloride values in individuals older than 6 months of age are less than 40 mEq/L. Values between 40 and 60 mEq/L are considered borderline, and repeat sweat testing or genetic testing is required to make a definitive diagnosis. For some borderline cases, referral to specialized centers for an assessment of CFTR function by measuring nasal potential difference may be needed to confirm or rule out the diagnosis of CF. For example, in the case of a borderline sweat test result with identification of only 1 CFTR mutation, abnormal results on 2 nasal potential difference tests are indicative of a CF diagnosis. Chloride values greater than 60 mEq/L are considered diagnostic of CF, but many possible causes of false-positive sweat tests exist, including laboratory error, untreated adrenal insufficiency, autonomic dysfunction, ectodermal dysplasia, glucose-6-phosphate deficiency, hypothyroidism, malnutrition, mucopolysaccharidosis, glycogen storage disease (type 1), fucosidosis, hereditary nephrogenic diabetes insipidus, Mauriac syndrome, pseudohypoaldosteronism, or familial cholestasis.[57] A repeat confirmatory sweat test should be performed together with genetic mutation analysis. In asymptomatic newborns, sweat testing triggered by a positive CF newborn screening report should be performed when the infant is at least 2 weeks of age and weighs more than 2 kg. In symptomatic newborns, sweat testing may be performed as early as 48 hours of age, but the probability of inconclusive results is greater at this age. False-negative values can result from edema, malnutrition, and laboratory error. Several CFTR mutations that cause CF can also result in a false-negative sweat test.[58]

In cases in which genetic testing is done to resolve borderline sweat testing or when genetic testing alone is performed, the presence of 2 mutations known to cause CF is required to make the diagnosis. DNA from blood or buccal swabs can be used for genetic testing.

Newborn Screening

Newborn screening for CF is being widely adopted in the United States. An expert panel convened by the Centers for Disease Control and Prevention and the Cystic Fibrosis Foundation in November 2003 reviewed the data on the risks and benefits of newborn screening with the recommendation that "on the basis of evidence of moderate benefits and low risk of harm, CDC believes that newborn screening for CF is justified."[59] Evidence exists to support the efficacy of newborn screening in the areas of improved nutritional status,[60-62] cognitive development,[63,64] economic benefit[65,66] and improved survival.[67,68] The impact of newborn screening on pulmonary status is variable.[69-72] The benefit of improved height and weight on pulmonary status is well known and believed to outweigh the variability in data concerning pulmonary outcomes for newborn screening.[36,72-74]

Newborn screening for CF is typically a 2-tier test.[75] The 1st tier involves measuring serum immunoreactive trypsinogen (IRT) levels. IRT values are elevated in newborns with CF,[76] except in infants with meconium ileus, when IRT levels are low. All infants with meconium ileus should undergo sweat testing or genetic analysis. The 2nd tier of testing varies between states and may use either repeat IRT measurement or limited genetic mutation analysis. Sweat testing is performed to confirm results of newborn screening. In cases in which the child has signs and symptoms consistent with CF, sweat testing or genetic analysis should be performed regardless of newborn screening results.

Recommended Monitoring of Patients With an Established Diagnosis of Cystic Fibrosis

The Cystic Fibrosis Foundation recommends that patients with CF should have a complete blood count with differential, fat-soluble vitamin levels (retinol, α-tocopherol, 25-hydroxy vitamin D), albumin and prealbumin, prothrombin time, and measurement of liver enzymes performed annually. Patients 14 years and older should be screened for CF-related diabetes mellitus on an annual basis (Figure 254-3).[45] Patients who are on chronic inhaled aminoglycoside therapy or who receive frequent courses of intravenous aminoglycosides should have at least annual measurement of renal function.[44] All patients should receive a complete physical examination, including hearing and vision screening annually,[77] which is

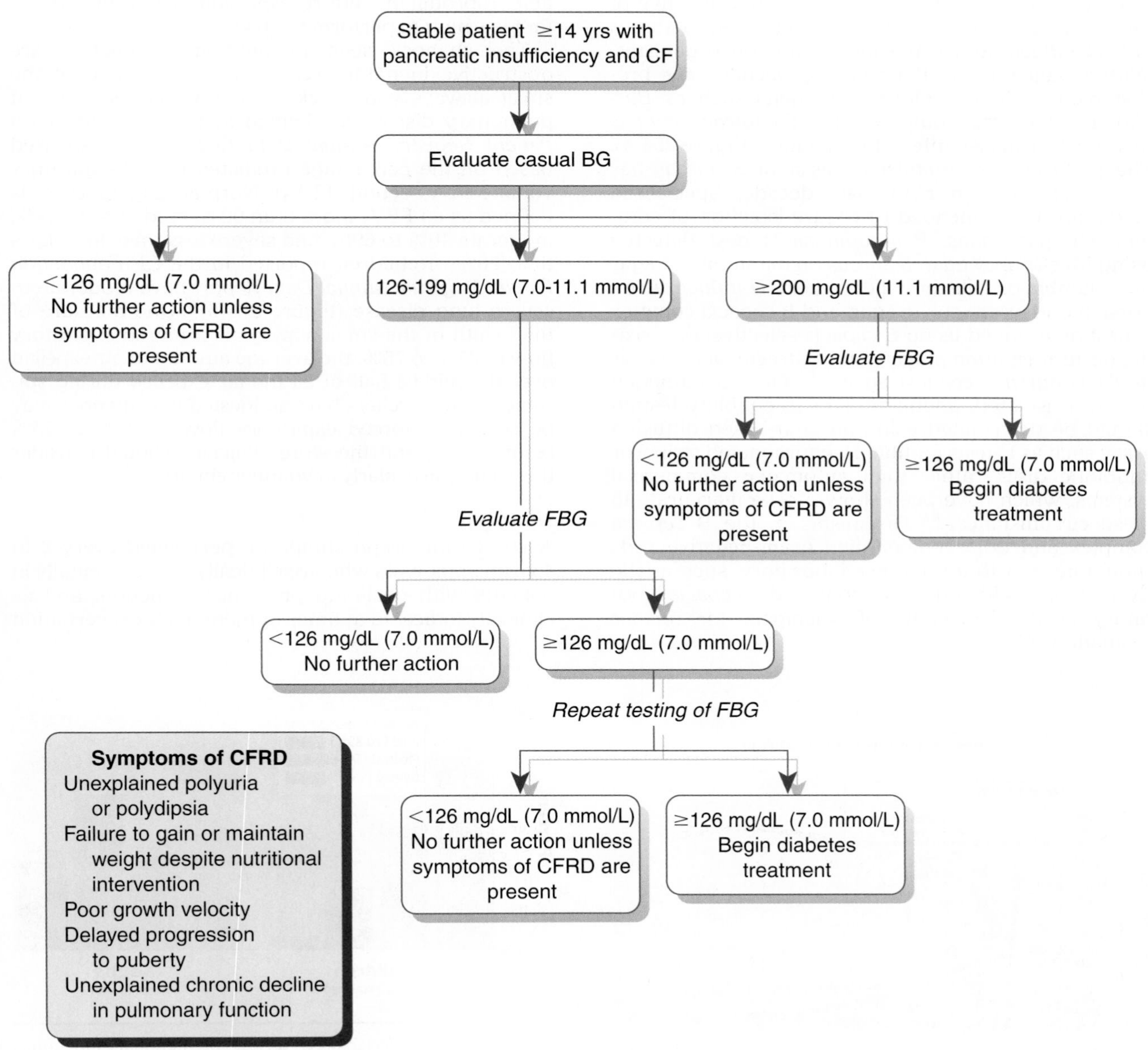

Figure 254-3 Screening algorithm for diabetes. Oral glucose tolerance test should also be considered if patient has unexplained polyuria or polydipsia, inability to gain or sustain weight, poor growth, delayed puberty, or is contemplating pregnancy. *BG,* Blood glucose; *FBG,* fasting blood glucose; *CFRD,* cystic fibrosis related diabetes.

particularly relevant for patients receiving multiple courses of aminoglycosides because of their potential ototoxicity.

Microbiological Assessment

Cultures to assess lower respiratory tract flora should be obtained at least quarterly in clinically stable patients and on any change in clinical status. An expectorated sputum sample is the usual way to obtain this culture. In infants and young children who are unable to expectorate, a throat swab or cough swab is often obtained, but it is not necessarily predictive of lower airway pathogens. In young children, *S aureus* and *H influenzae* are the most common organisms. With advancing age, *P aeruginosa* becomes the predominant pathogen. Other pathogens such as *Burkholderia cepacia* complex, and *Stenotrophomonas maltophilia* can also infect the CF lungs (Figure 254-4). The prevalence of methicillin-resistant *S aureus* has been increasing over the last decade. Specialized media are recommended to ensure isolation of common CF pathogens. *P aeruginosa* is best detected using MacConkey agar, *S aureus* on mannitol salt agar or Columbia or colistin-nalidixic acid, *H influenzae* on horse blood or chocolate agar, and *B cepacia* complex is best determined using *B cepacia* selective agar, oxidation-fermentation polymyxin bacitracin lactose agar or *Pseudomonas cepacia* agar.[78-80] Once a pathogen has been isolated, antimicrobial susceptibility testing should be determined using an agar-based diffusion assay such as E-tests (antibiotic-impregnated strips) or antibiotic discs rather than automated commercial systems, which have been shown to be inaccurate in these circumstances.[81] Organisms in the *B cepacia* complex and other unidentified gram-negative rods should be sent to a reference laboratory, such as the Cystic Fibrosis Foundation–sponsored *B cepacia* laboratory at the University of Michigan, for further evaluation.[79,80]

Spirometry

Spirometry should be performed every 3 to 6 months and as needed based on the patient's pulmonary status. Although most children younger than 6 years are unable to perform the test reliably, new approaches are being developed that may allow the extension of this test to younger patients and infant pulmonary function testing is available at many CF centers. Spirometry is best performed with the supervision of a certified respiratory therapist who is trained to work with children because it may be difficult to get a reliable, reproducible effort, especially when the child is first learning to perform the test.

The changes seen in pulmonary function are obstructive in nature secondary to plugging of the small airways with thick secretions. The severity of pulmonary disease as defined in the *CF Foundation Patient Registry Annual Data Report* is categorized based on the percentage predicted forced expiratory volume in 1 second (FEV_1). Normal lung function is defined as an FEV_1 more than 90%, mild 70% to 89%, moderate 40% to 69%, and severe less than 40%. Less than 20% of children reported in the *CF Foundation Patient Registry Annual Data Report* have moderate to severe lung disease (Figure 254-5).[3] One measure of the health of the small airways is a forced expiratory flow of 25% to 75%, the average amount of air expelled over the middle half of all the air expelled during spirometry. Researchers have suggested that changes may be seen in a forced expiratory flow of 25% to 75% before FEV_1, and therefore clinicians should consider this value, particularly in younger children.[82]

Imaging

A chest radiograph should be performed every 2 to 4 years in patients who are clinically stable, annually in patients with declining pulmonary function, and as clinically indicated at times of pulmonary exacerbation

Figure 254-4 Prevalence of pulmonary pathogens based on the age of the patient. (*Cystic Fibrosis Foundation*. Cystic Fibrosis Foundation Patient Registry 2004 Annual Data Report to the Center Directors. *Bethesda, MD: Cystic Fibrosis Foundation; 2005. Reprinted by permission of the Cystic Fibrosis Foundation.*)

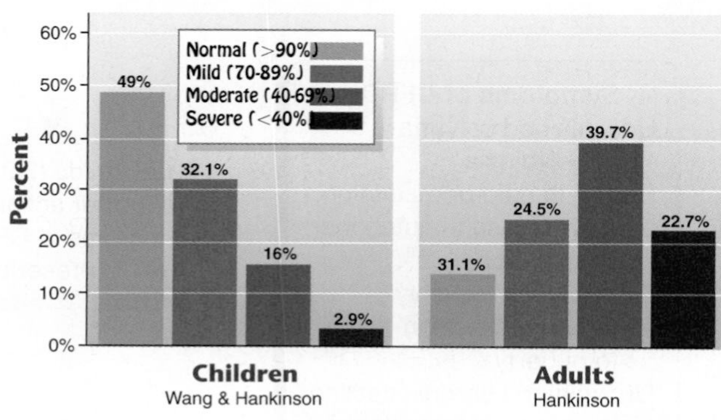

Figure 254-5 Variability in severity of pulmonary function in children and adults (≥18 years of age) classified by percentage FEV_1 predicted using Wang et al for children and Hankinson et al for adolescents (boys older than 17 years and girls older than 15 years) and adults. (*Modified from Cystic Fibrosis Foundation*. Cystic Fibrosis Foundation Patient Registry. 2004 Annual Data Report to the Center Directors. *Bethesda, MD: Cystic Fibrosis Foundation; 2005. Reprinted by permission of the Cystic Fibrosis Foundation.*)

in all patients. Bronchial wall thickening together with hyperinflation caused by small airway obstruction are the first changes noted. Bronchiectasis develops with time. Acute or chronic infiltrates may be noted depending on the clinical status of the patient. The progression of radiographic changes varies between patients and does not necessarily correlate with abnormalities in lung function tests. Pulmonary function may be relatively well maintained at the same time that radiographic changes may be fairly advanced.[24,83]

Chest CT scans also show that structural changes in the lung can often be detected before symptoms are present. Although some enthusiasm has existed for periodic chest CT scans, concerns about the radiation exposure have limited adoption of this approach. No current formal recommendations have been made for routine performance of CT scanning in patients with CF.

Patients 8 years or older with CF, who are malnourished, have severe pulmonary disease, are on chronic glucocorticoid therapy, have delayed puberty, or have low levels of 25-hydroxy vitamin D are at increased risk for bone disease. Lateral chest radiographs of these patients should be examined for fractures at least annually. Children with these risk factors who are at least 8 years of age should undergo a dual radiograph absorptiometric scan to measure bone density. All children with CF should have bone densitometry performed by their 18th birthday.[48] An abdominal ultrasound should be performed if a change is noted in liver function tests or if hepatomegaly or splenomegaly are detected.

MANAGEMENT

All children diagnosed with CF and those who have clinical stigmata of CF but equivocal diagnostic test results should be referred to a local CF care center for evaluation. At the center, children are evaluated by a pediatrician (most often a pediatric pulmonologist), a nurse, respiratory therapist, dietitian, and social worker who are highly experienced in the management of CF. These individuals are able to provide counseling and support to families of newly diagnosed children, as well as education about the disease. Pulmonary and gastrointestinal therapies can be initiated. Children should be seen at least quarterly in the CF care center where the adequacy of their therapies, as well as their growth, nutrition, and pulmonary function, can be assessed and therapies adjusted accordingly. The CF social worker is an invaluable resource for families and can help them deal with the psychological and financial aspects of raising a child with CF. The team will work with the child over the years to help them develop into an adult capable of managing their disease independently. CF centers are also able to make available to patients clinical trials of the newest cutting-edge therapies. The CF center should not be considered, however, a replacement for the primary care pediatrician. The child absolutely must continue to receive routine well-child care. CF centers generally have physicians available at all times to consult on medical management issues relating to CF. A list of accredited CF care centers in the United States can be accessed at www.cff.org.

Pulmonary Therapy

From the moment a child is diagnosed with CF, the family should be counseled to minimize environmental tobacco smoke exposure. Children, especially adolescents, should be educated about the detrimental effects of tobacco smoke and illegal inhalants on their lungs. Annual influenza vaccination is recommended for children with CF older than 6 months and their families.

The cornerstone of pulmonary therapy for children and adults with CF is chest physiotherapy (CPT). Patients are prescribed a daily regimen of CPT to help them mobilize and expectorate the thick, tenacious secretions in their airways. The frequency of therapy is generally increased during times of acute exacerbations. Numerous airway clearance modalities are available for CPT, including manual percussion with postural drainage, autogenic drainage, or a vest that inflates and vibrates the chest at different frequencies. Several different hand-held devices (eg, Flutter/Acapella) and therapies (eg, PEP [positive expiratory pressure] therapy) are also available that are designed to shear the mucus off the airways and provide backpressure to stent the airways open such that secretions may be expelled. Each modality has specific advantages, but no single modality is superior. Because CPT is a time-consuming process, the choice of therapy should be based on the method that is the most effective for that patient and that fits best into the family's lifestyle to optimize adherence. Physical activity and regular exercise should be recommended as an integral part of the regimen.

Bronchodilators are often given before CPT to maximally dilate the airways and thus help facilitate clearance of the secretions. Patients with CF have a variable response to β-agonists, and some patients exhibit a transient decline in pulmonary function most likely secondary to collapse of bronchiectatic airways.[84] Patients with CF should be assessed for bronchodilator response by pulmonary function testing and therapy adjusted accordingly. Long-acting β-agonists, however, may be beneficial in some patients with CF and asthma.[85]

The chronic inflammatory process in CF lung disease has led to considerable interest in antiinflammatory therapies. Alternate-day prednisone therapy has been shown to improve lung function in patients chronically infected with *P aeruginosa*, but an increased incidence of growth retardation, glucose abnormalities, and cataracts have dampened enthusiasm for this therapeutic approach.[86,87] Inhaled steroids and leukotriene modifiers are attractive alternatives and are widely prescribed. However, because of a lack of evidence of efficacy for CF treatment, their use should be limited to patients with concomitant asthma.[88] In patients with CF who have mild lung disease, high-dose ibuprofen has been shown to decrease the rate of decline in lung function and the need for hospitalization.[89] However, the requirements for a pharmacokinetic study to determine the optimal dose of ibuprofen and concerns about safety have limited penetration of this therapy into clinical practice.

Dornase alpha, a recombinant human deoxyribonuclease, was developed for nebulization into the airways where it cleaves the viscous DNA released by dying neutrophils as part of the exaggerated inflammatory response characteristic of CF lung disease. Deoxyribonuclease treatment improves the rheologic properties of the sputum and enables the patient to expectorate the sputum more easily. It is generally administered once a day. A multicenter study of dornase alpha revealed an improvement in lung function and a decrease in the frequency of pulmonary exacerbations with chronic use.[90] This therapy has been widely adopted in the treatment of CF. Inhaled hypertonic saline is the newest therapy in the CF armamentarium. The hypothesis is that inhaling a highly concentrated saline solution (7% saline) increases the osmotic load and stimulates water movement into the airways. The improved hydration of the secretions results in better mucociliary clearance, and patients are better able to clear their secretions. A 48-month trial of 7% saline inhaled twice daily revealed improved pulmonary function and fewer pulmonary exacerbations compared with controls who inhaled 0.9% saline twice daily.[91] Some patients may experience wheezing with the medication, which can be attenuated by pretreatment with a bronchodilator.

Chronic daily antibiotic therapy to prevent either the initial infection or to treat chronic bacterial infection is not well supported by evidence in medical literature. Antibiotic therapy is generally recommended for treating acute exacerbations when the bacterial burden increases and patients develop associated symptoms such as increased cough frequency and sputum production or declining pulmonary function with or without radiographic changes. The exceptions to this rule are the chronic use of macrolide antibiotics and inhaled tobramycin for treating *P aeruginosa*. Research has shown that 3-times-a-week administration of the macrolide antibiotic azithromycin for older children and adults with CF who are chronically colonized with *P aeruginosa* has a positive impact on lung function, weight, and the frequency of pulmonary exacerbations.[92] A high-dose preparation of tobramycin given twice a day on alternating months to patients chronically infected with *P aeruginosa* reduced the need for hospitalization and improved pulmonary function.[93] These therapies are widely used in CF.

When patients experience an exacerbation of bronchopneumonia or an apparent viral respiratory illness, antibiotic therapy directed against their most recently cultured pathogen is recommended. If the patient does not have respiratory distress or hypoxemia, then oral outpatient therapy may be initiated. When patients exhibit an acute worsening of their respiratory status, hypoxemia, or respiratory distress, hospitalization with the administration of intravenous antibiotics and aggressive chest physiotherapy is recommended. *P aeruginosa* is routinely treated with 2 antipseudomonal antibiotics. The duration of antibiotic therapy depends on the severity of the exacerbation but is generally 10 days or longer based on the response to treatment.

Hemoptysis and pneumothorax are both common complications of CF lung disease. Patients with CF may have blood-streaked sputum; however, if the volume of blood expectorated is large, then treatment with bed rest, intravenous antibiotics, and cessation of any medications with anticoagulant properties should be initiated. If the bleeding does not resolve or becomes life threatening, then bronchial artery embolization may be required. Resection of the bleeding segment is the therapeutic option of last resort. Pneumothorax occurs annually in approximately 1% of patients with CF. Patients with respiratory distress or with a pneumothorax occupying at least 20% of the pleural space will likely require a chest tube. If the pneumothorax does not resolve with chest tube placement, then pleurodesis may be required.

As the lung disease progresses, intervals of stability between exacerbations may become shorter. Patients may require supplemental oxygen therapy because of progressive hypoxemia. Noninvasive ventilation may be instituted when evidence exists of carbon dioxide retention or sleep-disordered breathing.

Lung transplantation is a final therapeutic option for the treatment of progressive, severe lung disease. It is an inherently risky procedure, with a 5-year posttransplant survival of approximately 50% to 60%. Referral for lung transplantation should be made when other therapeutic options are exhausted. Survival models have been developed that facilitate the calculation of a patient's predicted survival without a transplant to help in the selection of patients most likely to gain a survival advantage from the procedure.[94,95] Patients are informed of the advantages, risks, and potential complications of undergoing the procedure. They are made aware that the complicated medical regimen that they follow to treat their CF-related lung disease is replaced by a transplant medical regimen that is often equally as complicated. Active tuberculosis, HIV, and hepatitis B are contraindications to lung transplantation. Additionally, patients with significant psychosocial dysfunction that would preclude adherence to the posttransplant medical regimen are not good surgical candidates for transplant.[96]

Gastrointestinal Therapy

Nutritional therapy is a cornerstone of good CF therapy. Patients should be evaluated at least annually by a dietitian who is knowledgeable about CF. Infants and children with CF who have PI should receive at least 120% to 130% of the recommended daily allowance of age-appropriate calories. Fat intake should make up 35% to 40% of the daily required calories compared with less than 30% in people without CF. Caloric requirements are higher when acute illness or exacerbation of the pulmonary disease is present and when catch-up growth is needed. Lack of appetite caused by intercurrent illness and an inability to consume the increased number of calories needed to sustain normal growth, to make up for lost weight, or to achieve catch-up growth are frequent nutritional problems faced by both adults and children with CF. Modifications are initially made to increase the caloric density of the child's regular diet. High-calorie, high-fat supplements in the forms of shakes and formulas are also recommended. If the child cannot orally consume the needed daily requirement of calories, then

Table 254-1 Dosages for Vitamin Supplementation

	VITAMIN A (IU)	VITAMIN E (IU)	VITAMIN D (IU)	VITAMIN K (MG)
0-12 months	1500	40-50	400	≥0.3 mg
1-3 years	5000	80-150	400-800	≥0.3 mg
4-8 years	5000-10,000	100-200	400-800	≥0.3 mg
>8 years	10,000	200-400	400-800	≥0.3 mg

Adapted from Cystic Fibrosis Foundation. Pediatric nutrition for patients with cystic fibrosis. In: *Consensus Conferences: Concepts in CF Care, 2001*. March 28-29, 2001. Reprinted by permission of the Cystic Fibrosis Foundation.

supplementation via nasogastric or gastrostomy tube is recommended.

Pancreatic enzyme supplements are given with each fat-containing meal or snack. The recommended dose for infants is 2000 to 4000 units of lipase per 120 mL of formula or per breastfeeding.[44] Although a powdered enzyme preparation is often used for infants, it is not enteric coated; thus much of the dose may be destroyed in the stomach. In addition, infants are at risk for developing ulceration of the oral mucosa if the enzymes are not completely cleared from the oral cavity. Low-dose, enteric-coated enzyme preparations can be administered to infants with a small amount of applesauce or other nonalkaline food. Brand-name enteric-coated enzymes should be used exclusively. Enteric coating protects the enzymes from being destroyed by stomach acids. Generic preparations should be avoided because of a lack of standardization of the enzyme dose. Enzyme dosing is initially determined based on the patient's weight and subsequently adjusted based on clinical symptoms of continued malabsorption (frequency and consistency of stools, perceived greasiness of stools, and abdominal cramping). Enzyme therapy for children younger than 4 years should be initiated at a dose of 1000 units of lipase per kilogram per meal; therapy for children 4 years or older should be initiated at a dose of 500 units of lipase per kilogram per meal. Doses should generally be kept to less than 2500 units of lipase per kilogram per meal or less than 4000 units of lipase per gram-fat per day to reduce the risk of developing fibrosing colonopathy.[97,98]

Children with CF should receive a standard, age-appropriate dose of non–fat-soluble multivitamins. Children with pancreatic insufficiency should also receive supplements of vitamins A, D, E, and K (Table 254-1).[44] Vitamin K is supplemented at higher levels in patients with liver disease with abnormalities in clotting or if a patient is on prolonged antibiotic therapy. Special high-dose preparations of these vitamins are available for patients with CF.

Acid blockers should be used as needed to treat gastroesophageal reflux, which is common in patients with CF.[99,100] In addition, acid suppression may be beneficial for optimization of pancreatic enzyme function.[101,102]

DIOS is a common complication of CF, and patients with vomiting, crampy abdominal pain, and decreased stool output should be evaluated for intestinal obstruction by imaging. If DIOS is diagnosed, then oral intake should be withheld, and intravenous fluids or total parenteral nutrition should be initiated. The obstruction may be relieved with the performance of a gastrograffin enema or oral or nasogastric administration of osmotic laxatives (polyethylene glycol). If this therapy does not result in relief of the blockage, then surgical intervention may be needed. Other diagnostic considerations for these symptoms include appendicitis, pancreatitis, cholecystitis, intussusceptions, and *Clostridia difficile* colitis.

Elevated liver enzymes and abnormal liver function tests or the detection of hepatomegaly or splenomegaly (or both) during examination should raise concern about the possible development of cirrhosis. An abdominal ultrasound should be ordered. Ursodeoxycholic acid has been shown to benefit patients with cholestatic diseases such as primary biliary cirrhosis and is often administered in patients with CF who have hepatobiliary disease in an effort to improve bile flow and to limit further liver damage.[103,104] Liver transplantation is a therapeutic option when end-stage liver disease develops.

SUMMARY

The improved survival for patients with CF over the recent decades is likely to continue as more is learned about the pathobiological characteristics of the disease. The therapeutic options for patients with CF have significantly increased over the last decade. The challenge to the CF practitioner is in choosing the best, most appropriate combination of therapies for the individual patient aimed at maintaining optimal health status. Consultation with the regional CF care center and physicians who are experienced with the nuances of CF care is strongly recommended. More specific therapies aimed at the basic defect in CF are now being developed, with the ultimate goal of delivering a therapy to infants with CF that will provide them with long and healthy lives.

We gratefully acknowledge Dr Terry B. White for her assistance in the final editing and referencing of the chapter.

WHEN TO REFER

All children with CF should be referred to a local CF center for ongoing care.

WHEN TO ADMIT

Pulmonary exacerbations

- Characterized by increased cough, sputum production and a decline in pulmonary function. Associated symptoms may include fever, wheezing, dyspnea, malaise, and weight loss. Acute changes in the chest radiograph may or may not be seen. If the patient has normal oxygen saturations on room air, then efforts are made to treat the patient initially with increased pulmonary toilet and oral antibiotics based on the microbiological characteristics of the most recent sputum culture. The patient should be admitted for intravenous antibiotic therapy if response to oral antibiotic therapy is inadequate. If the patient is hypoxemic or has major hemoptysis, then the patient should be admitted to the hospital for further management.

Hemoptysis

- Hemoptysis of more than 240 mL in 24 hours or more than 100 mL per day over 3 to 7 days is defined as major hemoptysis and should lead to admission.

Pneumothorax

- Patients with respiratory distress or with a pneumothorax occupying at least 20% of the pleural space will likely require a chest tube. Other patients should be observed until the pneumothorax is clearly stable or resolving.

TOOLS FOR PRACTICE

Engaging Patients and Family

- *Cystic Fibrosis* (on-line course), Patient Education Institute through National Institutes of Health and Medline Plus (www.nlm.nih.gov/medlineplus/tutorials/cysticfibrosis/id289103.pdf).

AAP POLICY STATEMENTS

American Academy of Pediatrics, Kaye CI, Committee on Genetics. Introduction to newborn screening fact sheets. *Pediatrics*. Sep 2006;118(3):1304-1312. (aappolicy.aappublications.org/cgi/content/full/pediatrics;118/3/1304).

American Academy of Pediatrics, Kaye CI, Committee on Genetics. Newborn screening fact sheets. *Pediatrics*. Sep 2006;118(3):e934-e963. (pediatrics.aappublications.org/cgi/content/full/118/3/e934).

SUGGESTED RESOURCES

Centers for Disease Control and Prevention. Newborn screening for cystic fibrosis: evaluation of benefits and risks and recommendations for state newborn screening programs. Proceedings of a 2003 workshop. *MMWR* 2004;53(RR-13):1-36.

Cystic Fibrosis Foundation. Gastrointestinal problems in CF. In: Cystic Fibrosis Foundation Concepts in Care Consensus Conference. June 3-4; 1991; Bethesda, MD: Cystic Fibrosis Foundation; 1994.

Cystic Fibrosis Foundation. Pulmonary complications in cystic fibrosis. In: Cystic Fibrosis Foundation Concepts in Care Consensus Conference. Bethesda, MD: Cystic Fibrosis Foundation; 1994.

Cystic Fibrosis Genetic Analysis Consortium. Cystic Fibrosis Database. Available at: www.genet.sickkids.on.ca/cftr.

Cystic fibrosis newborn screening: evidence for benefit and current experience [No authors listed]. *J Pediatr* 2005; 147(3 suppl):S1-S113.

Flume PA, O'Sullivan BP, Robinson KA, et al. Cystic fibrosis pulmonary guidelines: chronic medications for maintenance of lung health. *Am J Respir Crit Care Med*. 2007; 176:957-969. First published online August 29 2007 as doi:10.1164/rccm.200705-664OC.

Hankinson JL, Odencrantz JR, Fedan KB. Spirometric reference values from a sample of the general US population. *Am J Crit Care Med*. 1999;159(1):179-187.

Orenstein D, Rosenstein B, Stern R. *Cystic Fibrosis: Medical Care*. Philadelphia, PA: Lippincott, Williams & Wilkins; 2000.

Rosenstein BJ, Cutting GR. The diagnosis of cystic fibrosis: a consensus statement. Cystic Fibrosis Foundation Consensus Panel. *J Pediatr*. 1998;132(4):589-595.

Schidlow DV, Taussig LM, Knowles MR. Cystic Fibrosis Foundation consensus conference report on pulmonary complications of cystic fibrosis. *Ped Pulmon*. 1993;15(3): 187-198.

Sokol RJ, Durie PR. Recommendations for management of liver and biliary tract disease in cystic fibrosis. Cystic Fibrosis Foundation Hepatobiliary Disease Consensus Group. *J Pediatr Gastroenterol Nutr*. 1999;28(suppl 1): S1-S13.

Stallings VA, Stark LJ, Robinson KA, et al. Clinical practice guidelines on growth and nutrition subcommittee; ad hoc working group. Evidence-based practice recommendations for nutrition-related management of children and adults with cystic fibrosis and pancreatic insufficiency: results of a systematic review. *J Am Diet Assoc*. 2008; 108:832-839.

Wang X, Dockery DW, Wypij D, et al. Pulmonary function between 6 and 18 years of age. *Pediatr Pulmonol*. 1993; 15(2):75-88.

REFERENCES

1. Anderson DH. Cystic fibrosis of the pancreas and its relation to celiac disease: a clinical and pathological study. *Am J Dis Child*. 1938;56:344.
2. FitzSimmons SC. The changing epidemiology of cystic fibrosis. *J Pediatr*. 1993;122(1):1-9.
3. Cystic Fibrosis Foundation. *Cystic Fibrosis Foundation Patient Registry, 2005 Annual Data Report to the Center Directors*. Bethesda, MD: Cystic Fibrosis Foundation; 2006.
4. Sontag MK, Hammond KB, Zielenski J, et al. Two-tiered immunoreactive trypsinogen (IRT/IRT) based newborn screening for cystic fibrosis in Colorado: screening efficacy and diagnostic outcomes. *J Pediatr*. 2005;147(suppl): S83-S88.
5. Rommens JM, Iannuzzi MC, Kerem B, et al. Identification of the cystic fibrosis gene: chromosome walking and jumping. *Science*. 1989;245(4922):1059-1065.
6. Riordan JR, Rommens JM, Kerem B, et al. Identification of the cystic fibrosis gene: cloning and characterization of complementary DNA. *Science*. 1989;245(4922):1066-1073.
7. Kerem B, Rommens JM, Buchanan JA, et al. Identification of the cystic fibrosis gene: genetic analysis. *Science*. 1989;245(4922):1073-1080.
8. Drumm ML, Konstan MW, Schluchter MD, et al. Genetic modifiers of lung disease in cystic fibrosis. *N Engl J Med*. 2005;353(14):1443-1453.
9. Gao L, Kim KJ, Yankaskas JR, et al. Abnormal glutathione transport in cystic fibrosis airway epithelia. *Am J Physiol*. 1999;277(1 pt 1):L113-L118.
10. Reddy MM, Quinton PM. Selective activation of cystic fibrosis transmembrane conductance regulator Cl^- and HCO_3^- conductances. *J Pediatr*. 2001;2(4):212-218.

11. Ismailov, II, Awayda MS, Jovov B, et al. Regulation of epithelial sodium channels by the cystic fibrosis transmembrane conductance regulator. *J Biol Chem.* 1996; 271(9):4725-4732.
12. Boucher RC, Cotton CU, Gatzy JT, et al. Evidence for reduced Cl^- and increased Na^+ permeability in cystic fibrosis human primary cell cultures. *J Physiol.* 1988; 405:77-103.
13. Blouquit S, Regnier A, Dannhoffer L, et al. Ion and fluid transport properties of small airways in cystic fibrosis. *Am J Respir Crit Care Med.* 2006;174(3):299-305.
14. Mall M, Grubb BR, Harkema JR, et al. Increased airway epithelial Na^+ absorption produces cystic fibrosis-like lung disease in mice. *Nat Med.* 2004;10(5):487-493.
15. Matsui H, Grubb BR, Tarran R, et al. Evidence for periciliary liquid layer depletion, not abnormal ion composition, in the pathogenesis of cystic fibrosis airways disease. *Cell.* 1998;95(7):1005-1015.
16. Tarran R, Grubb BR, Gatzy JT, et al. The relative roles of passive surface forces and active ion transport in the modulation of airway surface liquid volume and composition. *J Gen Physiol.* 2001;118(2):223-236.
17. Poschet J, Perkett E, Deretic V. Hyperacidification in cystic fibrosis: links with lung disease and new prospects for treatment. *Trends Mol Med.* 2002;8(11):512-519.
18. Freedman SD, Shea JC, Blanco PG, et al. Fatty acids in cystic fibrosis. *Curr Opin Pulm Med.* 2000;6(6):530-532.
19. Song Y, Salinas D, Nielson DW, et al. Hyperacidity of secreted fluid from submucosal glands in early cystic fibrosis. *Am J Physiol Cell Physiol.* 2006;290(3): C741-C749.
20. Chmiel JF, Berger M, Konstan MW. The role of inflammation in the pathophysiology of CF lung disease. *Clin Rev Allergy Immunol.* 2002;23(1):5-27.
21. Bals R, Weiner DJ, Meegalla RL, et al. Salt-independent abnormality of antimicrobial activity in cystic fibrosis airway surface fluid. *Am J Respir Cell Mol Biol.* 2001; 25(1):21-25.
22. Muhlebach MS, Stewart PW, Leigh MW, et al. Quantitation of inflammatory responses to bacteria in young cystic fibrosis and control patients. *Am J Respir Crit Care Med.* 1999;160(1):186-191.
23. Noah TL, Black HR, Cheng PW, et al. Nasal and bronchoalveolar lavage fluid cytokines in early cystic fibrosis. *J Infect Dis.* 1997;175(3):638-647.
24. de Jong PA, Lindblad A, Rubin L, et al. Progression of lung disease on computed tomography and pulmonary function tests in children and adults with cystic fibrosis. *Thorax.* 2006;61(1):80-85.
25. Wang X, Moylan B, Leopold DA, et al. Mutation in the gene responsible for cystic fibrosis and predisposition to chronic rhinosinusitis in the general population. *JAMA.* 2000;284(14):1814-1819.
26. McShane D, Davies JC, Wodehouse T, et al. Normal nasal mucociliary clearance in CF children: evidence against a CFTR-related defect. *Eur Respir J.* 2004;24(1): 95-100.
27. Yung MW, Gould J, Upton GJ. Nasal polyposis in children with cystic fibrosis: a long-term follow-up study. *Ann Otol Rhinol Laryngol.* 2002;111(12:1): 1081-1086.
28. Sakano E, Ribeiro AF, Barth L, et al. Nasal and paranasal sinus endoscopy, computed tomography and microbiology of upper airways and the correlations with genotype and severity of cystic fibrosis. *Int J Pediatr Otorhinolaryngol.* 2007;71(1):41-50.
29. Cohn JA, Strong TV, Picciotto MR, et al. Localization of the cystic fibrosis transmembrane conductance regulator in human bile duct epithelial cells. *Gastroenterology.* 1993;105(6):1857-1864.
30. Strong TV, Boehm K, Collins FS. Localization of cystic fibrosis transmembrane conductance regulator mRNA in the human gastrointestinal tract by in situ hybridization. *J Clin Invest.* 1994;93(1):347-354.
31. Durie PR. The pathophysiology of the pancreatic defect in cystic fibrosis. *Acta Paediatr Scand Suppl.* 1989;363:41-44.
32. Cystic Fibrosis Foundation. *Cystic Fibrosis Foundation Patient Registry. 2004 Annual Data Report to the Center Directors.* Bethesda, MD: Cystic Fibrosis Foundation; 2005.
33. Durie PR. Pathophysiology of the pancreas in cystic fibrosis. *Neth J Med.* 1992;41(3-4):97-100.
34. De Boeck K, Weren M, Proesmans M, et al. Pancreatitis among patients with cystic fibrosis: correlation with pancreatic status and genotype. *Pediatrics.* 2005;115(4): e463-e469.
35. Correlation between genotype and phenotype in patients with cystic fibrosis. The Cystic Fibrosis Genotype-Phenotype Consortium [No authors listed]. *N Engl J Med.* 1993;329(18):1308-1313.
36. Konstan MW, Butler SM, Wohl ME, et al. Growth and nutritional indexes in early life predict pulmonary function in cystic fibrosis. *J Pediatr.* 2003;142(6):624-630.
37. Gross K, Desanto A, Grosfeld JL, et al. Intra-abdominal complications of cystic fibrosis. *J Pediatr Surg.* 1985; 20(4):431-435.
38. Dray X, Bienvenu T, Desmazes-Dufeu N, et al. Distal intestinal obstruction syndrome in adults with cystic fibrosis. *Clin Gastroenterol Hepatol.* 2004;2(6):498-503.
39. Flora KD, Benner KG. Liver disease in cystic fibrosis. *Clin Liver Dis.* 1998;2(1):51-61.
40. Feranchak AP. Hepatobiliary complications of cystic fibrosis. *Curr Gastroenterol Rep.* 2004;6(3):231-239.
41. Noble-Jamieson G, Barnes N, Jamieson N, et al. Liver transplantation for hepatic cirrhosis in cystic fibrosis. *J R Soc Med.* 1996;89(27):31-37.
42. Di Sant'Agnese PA, Darling RC, Perera GA, et al. Abnormal electrolyte composition of sweat in cystic fibrosis of the pancreas; clinical significance and relationship to the disease. *Pediatrics.* 1953;12(5):549-563.
43. Holland AE, Wilson JW, Kotsimbos TC, et al. Metabolic alkalosis contributes to acute hypercapnic respiratory failure in adult cystic fibrosis. *Chest.* 2003;124(2):490-493.
44. Borowitz D, Baker RD, Stallings V. Consensus report on nutrition for pediatric patients with cystic fibrosis. *J Pediatr Gastroenterol Nutr.* 2002;35:246-259.
45. Moran A, Hardin D, Rodman D, et al. Diagnosis, screening and management of cystic fibrosis related diabetes mellitus: a consensus conference report. *Diabetes Res Clin Pract.* 1999;45(1):61-73.
46. Rosenecker J, Hofler R, Steinkamp G, et al. Diabetes mellitus in patients with cystic fibrosis: the impact of diabetes mellitus on pulmonary function and clinical outcome. *Eur J Med Res.* 2001;6(8):345-350.
47. Hardin DS, LeBlanc A, Lukenbough S, et al. Insulin resistance is associated with decreased clinical status in cystic fibrosis. *J Pediatr.* 1997;130(6):948-956.
48. Aris RM, Merkel PA, Bachrach LK, et al. Guide to bone health and disease in cystic fibrosis. *J Clin Endocrinol Metab.* 2005;90(3):1888-1896.
49. Aswani N, Taylor CJ, McGaw J, et al. Pubertal growth and development in cystic fibrosis: a retrospective review. *Acta Paediatr.* 2003;92(9):1029-1032.
50. Oppenheimer EA, Case AL, Esterly JR, et al. Cervical mucus in cystic fibrosis: a possible cause of infertility. *Am J Obstet Gynecol.* 1970;108(4):673-674.
51. Johannesson M, Landgren BM, Csemiczky G, et al. Female patients with cystic fibrosis suffer from reproductive endocrinological disorders despite good clinical status. *Hum Reprod.* 1998;13(8):2092-2097.

52. FitzSimmons S, Fitzpatrick S, Thompson B, et al. A longitudinal study of the effects of pregnancy on 325 women with cystic fibrosis. *Pediatr Pulmonol.* 1996;13:99-101.
53. Reiter EO, Stern RC, Root AW. The reproductive endocrine system in cystic fibrosis. I. Basal gonadotropin and sex steroid levels. *Am J Dis Child.* 1981;135(5):422-426.
54. Vanderwel M, Hardin DS. Growth hormone normalizes pubertal onset in children with cystic fibrosis. *J Pediatr Endocrinol Metab.* 2006;19(3):237-244.
55. Sokol RZ. Infertility in men with cystic fibrosis. *Curr Opin Pulm Med.* 2001;7(6):421-426.
56. LeGrys VA, Burritt MF, Gibson LE, et al. *Sweat Testing: Sample Collection and Quantitative Analysis—Approved Guideline.* Wayne, PA: National Committee for Clinical Laboratory Standards (NCCLS); 1994 (1994 NCCLS Document C34-A).
57. Hilman BC, ed. *Pediatric Respiratory Disease: Diagnosis and Treatment.* Philadelphia, PA: WB Saunders; 1993.
58. Davis PB. Cystic fibrosis since 1938. *Am J Respir Crit Care Med.* 2006;173(5):475-482.
59. Centers for Disease Control and Prevention. Newborn screening for cystic fibrosis: evaluation of benefits and risks and recommendations for state newborn screening programs. *MMWR* 2004;53(13):1-36.
60. Farrell PM, Kosorok MR, Rock MJ, et al. Early diagnosis of cystic fibrosis through neonatal screening prevents severe malnutrition and improves long-term growth. Wisconsin Cystic Fibrosis Neonatal Screening Study Group. *Pediatrics.* 2001;107:1-13.
61. Farrell PM, Kosorok MR, Laxova A, et al. Nutritional benefits of neonatal screening for cystic fibrosis. Wisconsin Cystic Fibrosis Neonatal Screening Study Group. *N Engl J Med.* 1997;337(14):963-969.
62. Farrell PM, Lai HC, Li Z, et al. Evidence on improved outcomes with early diagnosis of cystic fibrosis through neonatal screening: Enough is enough! *J Pediatr.* 2005;147:S30-S36.
63. Koscik RL, Farrell PM, Kosorok MR, et al. Cognitive function of children with cystic fibrosis: deleterious effect of early malnutrition. *Pediatrics.* 2004;113:1549-1558.
64. Koscik RL, Lai H-C, Laxova A, et al. Preventing early, prolonged vitamin E deficiency: an opportunity for better cognitive outcomes via early diagnosis through neonatal screening. *J Pediatr.* 2005;147(suppl):S51-S56.
65. Lee DS, Rosenberg MA, Peterson A, et al. Analysis of the costs of diagnosing cystic fibrosis with a newborn screening program. *J Pediatr.* 2003;142(6):617-623.
66. Rosenberg MA, Farrell PM. Assessing the cost of cystic fibrosis diagnosis and treatment. *J Pediatr.* 2005;147(3):S101-S105.
67. Doull IJ, Ryley HC, Weller P, et al. Cystic fibrosis-related deaths in infancy and the effect of newborn screening. *Pediatr Pulmonol.* 2001;31:363-366.
68. Lai H-C, Cheng Y, Cho H, et al. Association between initial disease presentation, lung disease outcomes, and survival in patients with cystic fibrosis. *Am J Epidemiol.* 2004;159:537-546.
69. McKay KO, Waters DL, Gaskin KJ. The influence of newborn screening for cystic fibrosis on pulmonary outcomes in New South Wales. *J Pediatr.* 2005;147:S47-S50.
70. Farrell PM, Li Z, Kosorok MR, et al. Longitudinal evaluation of bronchopulmonary disease in children with cystic fibrosis. *Pediatr Pulmonol.* 2003;36(3):230-240.
71. Farrell PM, Li Z, Kosorok MR, et al. Bronchopulmonary disease in children with cystic fibrosis after early or delayed Diagnosis. *Am J Respir Crit Care Med.* 2003;168(9):1100-1108.
72. Emerson J, Rosenfeld M, McNamara S, et al. *Pseudomonas aeruginosa* and other predictors of mortality and morbidity in young children with cystic fibrosis. *Pediatr Pulmonol.* 2002;34(2):91-100.
73. Zemel BS, Jawad AF, FitzSimmons S, et al. Longitudinal relationship among growth, nutritional status, and pulmonary function in children with cystic fibrosis: analysis of the CF Foundation Patient Registry. *J Pediatr.* 2000;137(3):374-380.
74. Rosenfeld M. Overview of published evidence on outcomes with early diagnosis from large US observational studies. *J Pediatr.* 2005;147:S11-S14.
75. Comeau AM, Accurso FJ, White TB, et al. Guidelines for Implementation of Cystic Fibrosis Newborn Screening Programs: Cystic Fibrosis Foundation Workshop Report. *Pediatrics.* 2007;119:495-518.
76. Davidson AG, Wong LT, Kirby LT, et al. Immunoreactive trypsin in cystic fibrosis. *J Pediatr Gastroenterol Nutr.* 1984;3(1):S79-S88.
77. Cystic Fibrosis Foundation. *Center Committee Consensus Conference on Clinical Practice Guidelines for Cystic Fibrosis, January 1995.* Bethesda, MD: Cystic Fibrosis Foundation; 1997.
78. Henry D, Campbell M, McGimpsey C, et al. Comparison of isolation media for recovery of *Burkholderia cepacia* complex from respiratory secretions of patients with cystic fibrosis. *J Clin Microbiol.* 1999;37(4):1004-1007.
79. Saiman L, Siegel J. Infection control recommendations for patients with cystic fibrosis: microbiology, important pathogens, and infection control practices to prevent patient-to-patient transmission. *Infect Control Hosp Epidemiol.* 2003;24(5):S6-S52.
80. Saiman L, Siegel J. Infection control recommendations for patients with cystic fibrosis: microbiology, important pathogens, and infection control practices to prevent patient-to-patient transmission. *Am J Infect Control.* 2003;31(3):S1-S62.
81. Burns JL, Saiman L, Whittier S, et al. Comparison of agar diffusion methodologies for antimicrobial susceptibility testing of *Pseudomonas aeruginosa* isolates from cystic fibrosis patients. *J Clin Microbiol.* 2000;38(5):1818-1822.
82. Tiddens HA. Detecting early structural lung damage in cystic fibrosis. *Pediatr Pulmonol.* 2002;34(3):228-231.
83. Brody AS, Tiddens HA, Castile RG, et al. Computed tomography in the evaluation of cystic fibrosis lung disease. *Am J Respir Crit Care Med.* 2005;172(10):1246-1252.
84. Pattishall EN. Longitudinal response of pulmonary function to bronchodilators in cystic fibrosis. *Pediatr Pulmonol.* 1990;9(2):80-85.
85. Colombo JL. Long-acting bronchodilators in cystic fibrosis. *Curr Opin Pulm Med.* 2003;9(6):504-508.
86. Eigen H, Rosenstein BJ, FitzSimmons S, et al. A multicenter study of alternate-day prednisone therapy in patients with cystic fibrosis. Cystic Fibrosis Foundation Prednisone Trial Group. *J Pediatr.* 1995;126(4):515-523.
87. Rosenstein BJ, Eigen H. Risks of alternate-day prednisone in patients with cystic fibrosis. *Pediatrics.* 1991;87(2):245-246.
88. Balfour-Lynn IM, Lees B, Hall P, et al. Multicenter randomized controlled trial of withdrawal of inhaled corticosteroids in cystic fibrosis. *Am J Respir Crit Care Med.* 2006;173(12):1356-1362.
89. Konstan MW, Byard PJ, Hoppel CL, et al. Effect of high-dose ibuprofen in patients with cystic fibrosis. *N Engl J Med.* 1995;332(13):848-854.
90. Fuchs HJ, Borowitz DS, Christiansen DH, et al. Effect of aerosolized recombinant human DNase on exacerbations of respiratory symptoms and on pulmonary function in patients with cystic fibrosis. The Pulmozyme Study Group. *N Engl J Med.* 1994;331(10):637-642.

91. Elkins MR, Robinson M, Rose BR, et al. A controlled trial of long-term inhaled hypertonic saline in patients with cystic fibrosis. *N Engl J Med.* 2006;354(3):229-240.
92. Saiman L, Marshall BC, Mayer-Hamblett N, et al. Azithromycin in patients with cystic fibrosis chronically infected with *Pseudomonas aeruginosa*: a randomized controlled trial. *JAMA.* 2003;290(13):1749-1756.
93. Ramsey BW, Pepe MS, Quan JM, et al. Intermittent administration of inhaled tobramycin in patients with cystic fibrosis. Cystic Fibrosis Inhaled Tobramycin Study Group. *N Engl J Med.* 1999;340(1):23-30.
94. Liou TG, Adler FR, Cahill BC, et al. Survival effect of lung transplantation among patients with cystic fibrosis. *JAMA.* 2001;286(21):2683-2689.
95. Liou TG, Adler FR, FitzSimmons SC, et al. Predictive 5-year survivorship model of cystic fibrosis. *Am J Epidemiol.* 2001;153(4):345-352.
96. Yankaskas JR, Mallory GB Jr. Lung transplantation in cystic fibrosis: consensus conference statement. *Chest.* 1998;113(1):217-226.
97. FitzSimmons SC, Burkhart GA, Borowitz D, et al. High-dose pancreatic-enzyme supplements and fibrosing colonopathy in children with cystic fibrosis. *N Engl J Med.* 1997;336(18):1283-1289.
98. Borowitz DS, Grand RJ, Durie PR. Use of pancreatic enzyme supplements for patients with cystic fibrosis in the context of fibrosing colonopathy. Consensus Committee. *J Pediatr.* 1995;127(5):681-684.
99. Scott RB, O'Loughlin EV, Gall DG. Gastroesophageal reflux in patients with cystic fibrosis. *J Pediatr.* 1985; 106(2):223-227.
100. Ledson MJ, Tran J, Walshaw MJ. Prevalence and mechanisms of gastro-oesophageal reflux in adult cystic fibrosis patients. *J R Soc Med.* 1998;91(1):7-9.
101. Zentler-Munro PL, Fine DR, Batten JC, et al. Effect of cimetidine on enzyme inactivation, bile acid precipitation, and lipid solubilization in pancreatic steatorrhea due to cystic fibrosis. *Gut.* 1985;26(9):892-901.
102. Heijerman HG, Lamers CB, Bakker W. Omeprazole enhances the efficacy of pancreatin (pancrease) in cystic fibrosis. *Ann Intern Med.* 1991;114(3):200-201.
103. Nousia-Arvanitakis S, Fotoulaki M, Economou H, et al. Long-term prospective study of the effect of ursodeoxycholic acid on cystic fibrosis-related liver disease. *J Clin Gastroenterol.* 2001;32(4):324-328.
104. Curry MP, Hegarty JE. The gallbladder and biliary tract in cystic fibrosis. *Curr Gastroenterol Rep.* 2005;7(2):147-153.

Chapter 255

CYSTIC AND SOLID MASSES OF THE FACE AND NECK

Neil E. Herendeen, MD, MBA; Peter G. Szilagyi, MD, MPH

The causes of neck masses range widely from common inflamed lymph nodes and cysts to rare neoplasms. An orderly approach to the work-up and management of a neck mass is therefore needed. The most practical approach involves differentiating the anatomic location of the mass into lateral neck masses versus midline neck masses and determining the exact anatomic position of the mass.[1] Localizing a lateral neck mass further into either the anterior cervical triangle (anterior to the sternocleidomastoid muscle) or the posterior cervical triangle is helpful.

DEFINITIONS

Masses in the neck can be classified into 2 broad categories: (1) cystic lesions and (2) solid masses.[2] Cystic lesions are either congenital cysts or vascular malformations; however, traumatic hematomas and abscesses may appear to be cystic. Solid neck masses usually consist of inflammatory lymph nodes or, rarely, neoplastic lesions. In general a complete history and thorough physical examination will lead to the correct diagnosis. Carefully chosen laboratory tests or radiologic studies then confirm the diagnosis.

DIFFERENTIAL DIAGNOSIS

When evaluating neck masses the primary care physician should be familiar with key anatomic structures of the neck. Because most neck masses encountered by pediatricians are lymph nodes and not cysts, understanding the location of the different groups of lymph nodes within the anterior and posterior anatomic triangles of the neck is crucial. Figure 255-1 shows the location of the major groups of lymph nodes, the sternocleidomastoid muscle, and the typical locations of the congenital cysts encountered most frequently.

EVALUATION

History

The physician should determine whether the neck mass was observed at birth, whether it has increased or decreased in size, whether it has changed color, and whether the lesion has drained or opened. Knowing the age at onset may help because lymph nodes greater than 1 cm rarely appear at birth,[3] whereas many congenital cysts are noted in the newborn period. Some congenital cysts, however, may not be

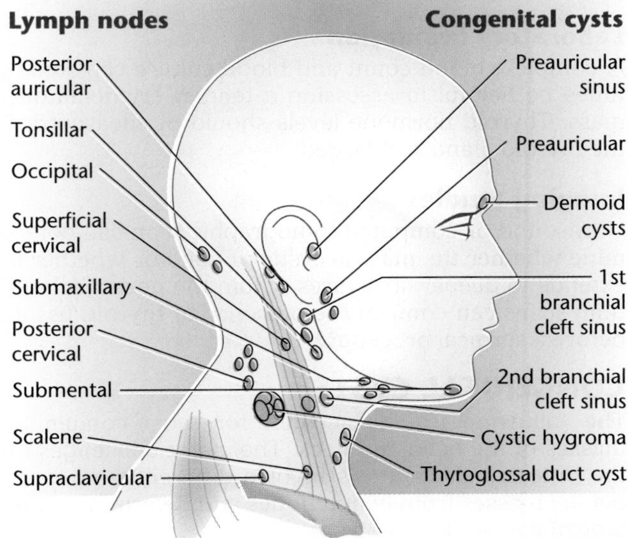

Figure 255-1 Common locations for cystic *(orange circles)* and lymph nodes *(blue circles)* of the face and neck.

noted until childhood or beyond and are detected only when they become infected.

The history of pain or tenderness is important. Congenital cysts are nontender unless they become infected. Inflamed lymph nodes are tender and painful. Pain during eating suggests parotid gland involvement. History of fever, other systemic symptoms such as loss of weight, and fatigue may need to be elicited while considering the possibilities of infectious processes and malignancies

Physical Examination

The first step in the physical examination is to determine whether abnormalities exist in other parts of the body, such as other cysts, lymphadenopathy, hepatosplenomegaly, skin lesions, or signs of infection. The exact anatomic location of the neck mass must be determined, and the clinician should note whether the mass is in the typical location of a lymph node (see Figure 255-1). The consistency, color, and firmness of the mass should be noted, as well as the presence of tenderness. The size of the mass should be measured.

Midline masses are usually associated with a thyroid abnormality. Masses that move with swallowing or with tongue protrusion suggest a thyroglossal duct cyst; these lesions may be tethered to the foramen cecum by the thyroglossal duct remnant. A mass along the anterior edge of the sternocleidomastoid muscle that moves with swallowing or that has a sinus opening to the surface of the overlying skin is likely to be a branchial cleft cyst. Both cysts and benign lymph nodes are freely mobile; malignant lesions are more likely to be fixed to underlying structures.

Rapidly growing, painless neck masses are worrisome because they might be neoplastic. Additional signs associated with a neoplastic process include fixation of the mass to subcutaneous tissue, firm consistency, size greater than 3 cm, and presence of constitutional symptoms. Supraclavicular nodes are the most likely neck mass to be malignant and should always be investigated.[3]

Laboratory Evaluation

A complete blood count and blood culture can sometimes be helpful in assessing a tender, erythematous mass. Thyroid hormone levels should be measured if the thyroid gland is enlarged.

Imaging Studies

Ultrasound or computed tomographic scan can determine whether the mass is cystic or solid or whether it extends to deeper structures within the neck. Technetium scans can confirm the presence of thyroid tissue before a surgical procedure.

CONGENITAL CYSTS

The following lesions account for most congenital masses of the head and neck. The major challenges in the differential diagnosis involve differentiating congenital masses from lymph nodes and determining the type of congenital lesion.

Thyroglossal Duct Cysts

Thyroglossal duct cysts account for more than 70% of congenital cysts of the neck, branchial cleft cysts for more than 20%, and vascular malformations and other lesions for 4% to 5%.[4]

Thyroglossal duct cysts result from failure of the embryologic thyroglossal duct to degenerate during the fifth week of gestation, leaving a fistula, sinus tract, or cyst at the midline of the neck just below the hyoid bone.[3] Thyroglossal duct cysts are not often detected at birth but are usually noted first after the age of 2 years. They may initially show as an inflamed, tender mass. When not infected, they are smooth, firm, mobile, and nontender and move upward with tongue protrusion or with swallowing. The differential diagnosis includes sebaceous cysts, epidermal cysts, submandibular lymph nodes, and lipomas. Unless normal thyroid tissue is palpable, the clinician needs to confirm the presence of the thyroid gland by ultrasonography or technetium scan because what may appear to be a thyroglossal duct cyst may actually be an ectopic thyroid gland, and its removal would leave the child dependent on thyroid hormone supplementation for life.[5] Because the likelihood of infection is high, thyroglossal duct cysts should be removed surgically.

Branchial Cleft Cysts

Branchial cleft cysts are congenital remnants of the lateral 4 branchial pouches and clefts.[2] Most branchial cleft cysts arise from the second cleft or pharyngeal pouch. They appear as a small dimple or opening anterior to the middle portion of the sternocleidomastoid muscle. The cyst is nontender, firm, and mobile and is located just under the skin. A small sinus, which occasionally drains fluid to the surface of the overlying skin, may be present, and a long fistulous tract may extend from it to the tonsil bed.[3] Branchial cleft cysts without sinuses are often unnoticed until later childhood when they become infected. Infected cysts can easily be confused with lymphadenitis. Other lesions included in the differential diagnosis are sternocleidomastoid muscle masses associated with torticollis, small cystic hygromas, epidermoid cysts, neurofibromas, lipomas, and an ectopic thyroid gland. Treatment involves surgical removal of the cyst and fistula.

Cystic Hygromas

Cystic hygromas are congenital, avascular masses derived from congenital obstruction of lymphatic vessels. They are generally multilocular, fluid filled, soft, compressible, painless masses located in the posterior triangle just behind the sternocleidomastoid muscle and in the supraclavicular fossa. Cystic hygromas can usually be transilluminated. These masses may grow rapidly because of accumulation of lymph and can reach an enormous size, compressing important structures and obstructing the airway.[1] Although the diagnosis is usually obvious during the physical examination, smaller cystic hygromas may resemble hemangiomas or other cysts. Ultrasound will reveal fluid and multiple cystic components, confirming the diagnosis. Because spontaneous regression is rare and the risk of compression of vital upper airway structures is high, surgical removal is indicated. Several procedures are often necessary to remove large lesions completely. Cystic hygromas occur infrequently in the axilla, on the trunk, or on the extremities; in older children, when they occur within the subcutaneous tissues, they may be mistaken for a lipoma or a hemangioma.[2]

Cavernous Hemangiomas

Cavernous hemangiomas are vascular lesions within the subcutaneous tissues that may appear in any part of the body and may be difficult to differentiate from congenital cysts. They are often noted in the newborn period and enlarge, sometimes rapidly, during the first year of life. Cavernous hemangiomas are less firm, more diffuse, and more easily compressible than cystic masses (except for cystic hygromas). Unlike cystic hygromas, cavernous hemangiomas do not transilluminate, and their size may increase with crying or straining. The skin overlying these vascular lesions is often bluish; cavernous hemangiomas frequently begin to increase in size during the first few months of life but usually regress spontaneously by school age.[4] Thus surgery is indicated only for masses that compress vital structures or that cause severe disfigurement.

Epidermoid Cysts

Epidermoid cysts are relatively common masses that may arise from an embryologic or fusional defect. They are usually located at midline on the face, most often at the level of the eyebrows. These small cysts feel doughy and smooth and contain sebaceous material and sometimes even hair, cartilage, or bone. One third of these cysts are present at birth; the remaining two thirds appear by school age.[6] Because these cysts may become infected and may form deep tracts, surgical excision is indicated.

Preauricular Cysts and Sinuses

Preauricular cysts and sinuses are the most common anomalies arising from an embryologic fusion failure of precursor tissues that develop into the external ear. The sinuses are pinhole-size pits that are usually located anterior to the helix (see Figure 255-1), and they may contain a short sinus tract.[3] Preauricular cysts often are bilateral. These sinuses and cysts are inherited in an autosomal-dominant manner, with incomplete penetrance, and are found more commonly in blacks than in whites. They are a far more common cause of preauricular lesions than are first branchial cleft cysts and sinuses, which are located in the same area.[6] Because preauricular cysts and sinuses may become infected, elective surgical removal is preferred. Hearing deficits may be associated with these lesions, but their prevalence is unknown.

SOLID NECK MASSES

Cervical lymph nodes are frequently palpable in healthy children and can be distinguished by their location (see Figure 255-1), size, shape, consistency, and mobility. Enlarged cervical lymph nodes (>1 cm) should be defined further by their association with surrounding nodes or generalized adenopathy, the presence of an infection of the head or pharynx, and localized signs of inflammation and erythema. Cervical adenitis typically develops in a child who has a fever as a swollen, tender, erythematous mass. *Staphylococcus aureus* and *Streptococcus pyogenes* account for 80% of acute unilateral cervical adenitis and usually respond to oral antibiotics such as a penicillin or cephalosporin. Lymph node aspiration is usually reserved for patients whose disease does not respond to initial therapy. Incision and drainage is an option for masses that become fluctuant. Some of the various causes of cervical lymphadenopathy include viral infections of the upper respiratory tract, bacterial infections, HIV infection, Kawasaki disease, and systemic disorders such as systemic lupus erythematosus, juvenile rheumatoid arthritis, sarcoidosis, and histoplasmosis. Chronic inflammation of the lymph nodes can be seen with infections such as cat-scratch disease (see Chapter 235, Animal Bites), atypical mycobacterium, and toxoplasmosis.

Malignant tumors are often found as a single supraclavicular mass or as multiple or matted masses crossing into both the anterior and the posterior triangles. More than 25% of children who have malignancies have a tumor of the head or neck.[4] The most common neck malignancies include Hodgkin and non-Hodgkin lymphoma, lymphosarcoma, rhabdomyosarcoma, fibrosarcoma, thyroid tumors, and neuroblastoma.

MANAGEMENT

All congenital cysts and masses should be monitored closely by the primary care physician. Acute bacterial infections of cysts should be treated with systemic antibiotics. Patients who have thyroglossal duct cysts, branchial cleft cysts, cystic hygromas, and epidermal cysts should be referred to a surgeon who is experienced at excising these congenital lesions. Elective surgery before an infection develops is preferable because excision of an entire sinus tract, fistula, or embryologic connection is more difficult after an infection. Many primary care physicians and surgeons prefer to delay surgery until the child is beyond infancy and can better tolerate the procedure. For patients who have thyroglossal duct cysts, a primary care physician or surgeon should confirm the presence of normal thyroid tissue by ultrasound or by a technetium scan. Hemangiomas can be observed without referral unless they begin to impinge on vital structures. Hemangiomas that interfere with physiological functions (blocking the vision, interfering with eating, among other functions) may be treated with glucocorticoid steroids or referred to a surgeon for management.

For children who have enlarged cervical lymph nodes and evidence of infection the antibiotic therapy should improve the condition within 7 days; the condition should resolve completely over the next few weeks. If the adenopathy is persistent, if inflammation is not present, and if any characteristics are worrisome (eg, size >3 cm, immobile, associated with systemic symptoms, in an abnormal location), then the child should be evaluated further and monitored closely until the enlarged node has resolved.[4]

WHEN TO REFER

- Cysts or tracts that are congenital (all congenital cysts or tracts should be removed)

- Mass that does not resolve with antibiotic therapy (≥2 weeks)
- Mass in the thyroid gland
- Mass in the parotid gland
- Rapidly enlarging mass (>3 cm)
- Mass that is fixed or lymph nodes that are matted
- Mass in a concerning area (supraclavicular)
- Abnormal chest radiograph
- When systemic signs and symptoms (eg, fever, weight loss, easy fatigability, hepatosplenomegaly) are present

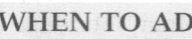

WHEN TO ADMIT

- Infected mass that is unresponsive to oral antibiotics
- Worrisome mass requiring immediate intervention and imaging
- Mass compromises the airway

SUGGESTED RESOURCES

Chesney PJ. Cervical lymphadenitis and neck infections. In: Long SS, Pickering LK, Prober CG, eds. *Principles and Practice of Pediatric Infectious Diseases.* New York, NY: Churchill Livingstone; 2003.

Hogan D, Wilkinson RD, Williams A. Congenital anomalies of the head and neck. *Int J Dermatol.* 1980;19:479.

Nield LS, Kamat, D. Lymphadenopathy in children: when and how to evaluate. *Clin Pediatr.* 2004;43:25-33.

Zitelli BJ. Evaluating the child with a neck mass. *Contemp Pediatr.* 1990;7:90.

REFERENCES

1. Zitelli BJ. Evaluating the child with a neck mass. *Contemp Pediatr.* 1990;7:90.
2. Friedberg J. Pharyngeal cleft sinuses and cysts, and other benign neck lesions. *Pediatr Clin North Am.* 1989;36:1451.
3. Nield LS, Kamat D. Lymphadenopathy in children: when and how to evaluate. *Clin Pediatr.* 2004;43:25-33.
4. Armstrong WB, Giglio MF. Is this lump in the neck anything to worry about? *Postgrad Med.* 1998;104:63.
5. Feins NR, Raffensperger JG. Cystic hygromas, lymphangioma and lymphedema. In: Raffensperger JG, ed. *Swenson's Pediatric Surgery.* 5th ed. Norwalk, CT: Appleton & Lange; 1990.
6. Raffensperger JG. Congenital cysts and sinuses of the neck. In: Raffensperger JG, ed. *Swenson's Pediatric Surgery.* 5th ed. Norwalk, Conn: Appleton & Lange; 1990.

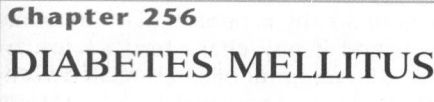

Chapter 256

DIABETES MELLITUS

Peter J. Tebben, MD; W. Frederick Schwenk II, MD

Diabetes mellitus consists of a heterogenous group of conditions with diverse underlying pathophysiological factors that result in elevated blood glucose levels. Although altered glucose metabolism is the most prominent abnormality, fatty acid and protein metabolism are also regulated by insulin. The abnormal glucose metabolism results from either an absolute or relative insulin deficiency. The 2 most common forms are called type 1 and type 2 diabetes. Type 1 diabetes (T1D) refers to conditions that result in an elevated blood glucose level caused by an absolute insulin deficiency. T1D has been further classified into type 1A and type 1B diabetes. Type 1A is the classic form caused by autoimmune destruction of the pancreatic β cells. Type 1B refers to nonimmune-mediated severe insulin deficiency caused by diseases such as cystic fibrosis or pancreatectomy.

INCIDENCE

The incidence of T1D in the United States has been estimated to be approximately 12 per 100,000 person-years for individuals younger than 20 years.[1] Certain ethnic groups such as individuals from Northern European countries have a much higher risk than individuals from most Asian countries.[2] Several authors have documented that the worldwide incidence, including the United States, of T1D has been increasing.[2,3] The cause of this global increase in T1D is not known.

ETIOLOGY

Type 1 Diabetes

Although the precise cause of T1D has remained elusive, several genetic factors play a role and likely interact with environmental factors to produce the disease. Several groups have prospectively studied the concordance rates of T1D in monozygotic and dizygotic twins. Concordance rates for monozygotic twins have ranged from 17% to 30%, which is considerably higher than the concordance rates reported in dizygotic twins or nontwin siblings of individuals with T1D.[4-8] These rates likely underestimate the lifetime risk of developing diabetes because follow-up was for a finite period. Studies using life table analysis have predicted significantly higher concordance among monozygotic twins.[8]

Genetic Factors

Many genes have been implicated in conferring genetic susceptibility to T1D, but the strongest associations have been found with the genes encoding human leukocyte antigen (HLA) molecules on chromosome 6. Individuals with T1D express the HLA DR3-DQ2/DR4-DQ8 genotype at a significantly higher rate than the general population.[9-11] Furthermore, a monozygotic twin without diabetes expressing DR3-DQ2/DR4-DQ8 whose twin has diabetes is at significantly higher risk of developing the disease than twin pairs without this genotype.[8] Other HLA molecules appear to offer protection against the development of diabetes.[12-14] The notion that offspring of fathers with T1D are more likely to develop diabetes than offspring of mothers with T1D has also been suggested.[15-17] Several other genes and chromosomal regions have been implicated in the development of T1D.[10,18] These data clearly show that the development of T1D has a genetic component. However, genetic factors do not account for all of the risk, and other factors must play a role.

Environmental Factors

Environmental exposures have been implicated in the development of T1D in genetically susceptible individuals. Viral infections have long been considered to play a role, but much of the data are conflicting.[19-24] However, congenital rubella syndrome has consistently been shown to confer added risk to the development of T1D.[25-29] A link between childhood immunizations and several autoimmune disorders, including T1D, has been postulated. This association was explored in a large study from Denmark that included almost 740,000 children and 4.7 million person-years of follow-up that found no association between T1D and immunizations status.[30]

Dietary Factors

Dietary factors such as duration and timing of breast-feeding, introduction of cow's milk, timing of introduction of cereals to the diet, gluten, and nitrate exposure have also been implicated, but definitive data are lacking.[31-44] Too little information is available regarding dietary antigen exposure to make definitive recommendations regarding introduction of certain foods to infants and children in an attempt to prevent T1D.

Antibodies

The autoimmune nature of T1D is supported by the high rate of detectible antibodies against pancreatic islet cells in patients recently diagnosed with T1D.[45] These antibodies are usually present long before the clinical onset of disease.[7] Antibodies against islet cell antigens, glutamic acid decarboxylase, and insulin have all been used to predict progression to diabetes in high-risk individuals with HLA susceptibility or a family history of diabetes.[46-49] Whether these antibodies are causal or simply a marker of disease is unclear. The sensitivity and specificity of antibody measurements are not sufficient to warrant routine clinical use.

Type 2 Diabetes

In contrast to T1D, type 2 diabetes (T2D) is caused by a relative insulin deficiency, peripheral resistance to its action, or both. Historically, T2D contributed to only a fraction of the total number of children diagnosed with the disease. However, the incidence of T2D has risen significantly in recent years,[50-52] especially among certain ethnic groups, such as African Americans, Hispanics, and Native Americans. The increase in childhood T2D has paralleled the marked rise in childhood obesity, which has prompted many communities, public health organizations, and medical societies to initiate programs to treat and prevent childhood obesity. The American Academy of Pediatrics (AAP) has published a policy statement regarding the prevention of pediatric obesity.[53] The AAP offers practical guidelines for early identification and intervention in high-risk children. Several studies have demonstrated that most children or adolescents with T2D are obese, have clinical evidence of insulin resistance (acanthosis nigricans), or have a significant family history of T2D.[52,54,55] These characteristics should prompt the primary care physician to screen a child for diabetes. The American Diabetes Association (ADA) has formed a consensus statement regarding T2D in children and adolescents, including recommendations for screening individuals from high-risk populations (Box 256-1).[51,56] The ADA recommendations focus on overweight and obese children because most cases occur in this patient population. Additionally, identification of at-risk children only requires the calculation of the body mass index, which can be performed quickly and inexpensively. However, these recommendations are based on few data, and clinical judgment may need to supersede strictly following these guidelines. Measurement of a fasting plasma glucose level is the suggested screening tool in children at high risk for developing diabetes because it is simple to perform and inexpensive, but other methods may be appropriate in establishing the diagnosis (Box 256-2).[56]

BOX 256-1 Criteria for Screening High-Risk Children for Diabetes

Overweight (BMI* >85th percentile for age and sex)

Plus any 2 risk factors:

- Family history of type 2 diabetes in a 1st- or 2nd-degree relative
- High-risk race or ethnicity (Native American, African American, Latino, Asian American, and Pacific Islander)
- Signs of insulin resistance or associated conditions:
  - Acanthosis nigricans
  - Hypertension
  - Dyslipidemia
  - Polycystic ovarian syndrome
- Maternal history of diabetes or gestational diabetes

Age to initiate screening:

- 10 years
- Onset of puberty if younger than 10 years

Frequency: every 2 years

Preferred screening test: plasma glucose after an 8-hour fast

*BMI, Body mass index (weight [kg] divided by height [meters] squared).
Adapted from American Diabetes Association. Type 2 diabetes in children and adolescents. *Pediatrics* 2000;105(3 Pt 1):671-680.

Maturity-Onset Diabetes of the Young

Monogenic forms of diabetes include a group of rare disorders known as maturity-onset diabetes of the young (MODY) (Box 256-3). These disorders likely represent less than 5% of all cases of diabetes. The clinical course can range from mild to progressive disease with the development of microvascular complications. One of the 6 forms of MODY should be considered in individuals with apparent T2D and a family history suggestive of autosomal-dominant inheritance, especially if diabetes develops at a young age in a thin individual. Because the clinical course and treatment vary considerably among the different forms of MODY, the

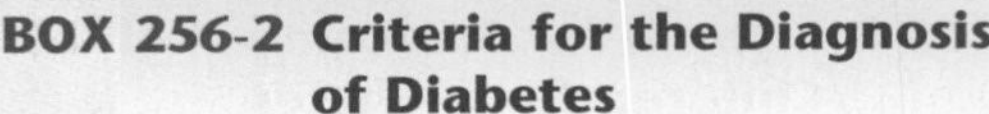

BOX 256-2 Criteria for the Diagnosis of Diabetes

- Symptoms of diabetes (polyuria, polydipsia, and unexplained weight loss) and a casual* plasma glucose of 200 mg/dL or greater **OR**
- Fasting plasma glucose of 126 mg/dL or greater (fasting for at least 8 hours) **OR**
- Plasma glucose of 200 mg/dL or greater 2 hours after an oral glucose challenge. Glucose load should contain 75 g of glucose for adults or 1.75 g/kg in children† (maximal dose of 75 g)

*Casual: any time of day without regard to time of last meal.
†1.75 g/kg of glucose has been suggested when performing an oral glucose tolerance test in children, but this dose is less well established than the 75-g dose used in adults.
Adapted from American Diabetes Association. Standards of medical care in diabetes–2007. *Diabetes Care* 2007;30(suppl 1):S4-S36. Copyright © 2007 American Diabetes Association. Reprinted with permission.

BOX 256-3 Causes of Hyperglycemia

DIABETES
Type 1A
Type 1B
Type 2
Neonatal diabetes
Gestational diabetes
Maturity-onset diabetes of the young:
- Type 1—hepatocyte nuclear factor-4-α defect
- Type 2—glucokinase defect
- Type 3—hepatocyte nuclear factor-1-α defect
- Type 4—insulin promoter factor-1 defect
- Type 5—hepatic transcription factor-2 defect
- Type 6—neurogenic differentiation factor defect

ENDOCRINOPATHIES
Cushing syndrome
Growth hormone excess
Pheochromocytoma
Glucagonoma
Somatostatinoma

DRUGS
Glucocorticoids
Diazoxide
Glucagon
Cyclosporin
Phenytoin
Niacin
Antipsychotics
Calcium channel blocker toxicity
Pentamidine
L-asparaginase
Others

OTHER
Cystic fibrosis
Pancreatitis
Pancreatectomy
Wolfram syndrome
Stiff man syndrome
Antiinsulin receptor antibodies

specific type of MODY should be characterized if the diagnosis is made or suspected. An in-depth discussion of these infrequent forms of diabetes is beyond the scope of this chapter; however, recent reviews can provide additional information.[57,58]

DIAGNOSIS

The ADA has outlined several ways to diagnose diabetes based on a patient's symptoms and their plasma glucose concentration (see Box 256-2). The diagnosis can be established in a patient who has symptoms consistent with diabetes (polyuria, polydipsia, unexplained weight loss) and a casual plasma glucose level of 200 mg/dL or greater. The ADA has defined *casual* as any time of day without regard to time since the last meal. T1D is usually diagnosed by these criteria and has a relatively acute-subacute onset of symptoms (days to weeks). T2D is more insidious than T1D in onset, and patients are typically overweight and may have signs of insulin resistance, including acanthosis nigricans and elevated lipid levels. Whereas most patients with T1D are symptomatic at the time of diagnosis, individuals with T2D can be asymptomatic, and the diagnosis may only be made as a result of screening. This fact highlights the need for identification of high-risk individuals in an effort to prevent or postpone diabetes or intervene early in the disease.

A plasma glucose level of 126 mg/dL or greater after an 8 hour fast will establish the diagnosis and is a simple test to perform in the outpatient setting. Diabetes can also be diagnosed using an oral glucose tolerance test. This method is more costly and labor intensive but may identify some individuals with diabetes who have a fasting plasma glucose level less than 126 mg/dL.

DIFFERENTIAL DIAGNOSIS

Hyperglycemia has many causes other than diabetes that should be considered when an elevated plasma glucose concentration is found (see Box 256-3). A thorough history, physical examination, and review of the patient's medications are often sufficient to determine the cause of hyperglycemia. The precise origin of hyperglycemia should be sought for each child to tailor therapy specific to the underlying pathophysiological condition.

Differentiating between T1D and T2D is usually straightforward; however, classifying diabetes in some children is difficult. Although insulin therapy may not always be necessary for children with T2D, it is a safe and effective choice if it is not initially clear whether the patient has T1D or T2D. If excess glucocorticoids or other medications cause diabetes, dose reduction or elimination of the drug (if possible) may be all that is required. However, if diabetes is due to an absolute insulin deficiency as in T1D, insulin must be a part of the treatment regimen.

EVALUATION

Pertinent History

Hyperglycemia from any cause can lead to symptoms related to an osmotic diuresis. Polyuria and polydipsia occur as a result of the loss of glucose in the urine as the plasma concentration exceeds the renal threshold for glucose reabsorption (≈180 mg/dL). This threshold is highly variable, and glucose may be seen in the urine of some normoglycemic individuals. Several other diseases may lead to glycosuria in the absence of deficient insulin production or action, and therefore glycosuria should not be used alone for the diagnosis of diabetes. In patients with diabetes (both types 1 and 2), excess glucose (and calories) is lost in the urine, and the patient may experience significant weight loss despite an increasing appetite.

As the degree of insulin deficiency or resistance (or both) worsens, additional complaints may become prominent as the body uses alternate fuel stores. When adipose tissue is broken down for energy, ketone bodies are produced, which can lead to metabolic acidosis. With ketosis, abdominal pain, headache, and nausea may develop. Diabetic ketoacidosis is a less common consequence of T2D, but it has been reported and cannot always be used to differentiate between the 2 disorders.[54,59] If severe hyperglycemia and metabolic acidosis are left uncorrected, then neurologic sequelae, including seizures and coma, may occur. Recognizing the early symptoms of diabetes may help prevent severe diabetic ketoacidosis and potentially fatal outcomes. T1D can occur at any age, including in the neonatal period. Reports of T2D have occurred in younger children as obesity becomes more common. However, children who develop T2D most commonly do so during puberty, which is a time of relative insulin resistance.[60]

Physical Examination

Patients with type 1 or 2 diabetes have no pathognomonic physical findings. Physical examination may be helpful in the case of suspected diabetes but will not substitute for laboratory confirmation of the diagnosis. A child with a recent onset of T1D will have physical findings consistent with the degree of insulin deficiency and the duration of the disorder. Typically, the child will be dehydrated and may be tachycardic. Significant weight loss caused by excretion of calories in the urine and dehydration can often be documented. If moderate or severe ketoacidosis is present, then tachypnea and a characteristic *fruity* odor to the breath may be noted. Altered mental status or seizures may occur in severe diabetic ketoacidosis.

The typical patient with T2D will often have polyuria and polydipsia. Weight loss may also be apparent, but patients are invariably obese at the time of diagnosis. Many children with T2D have acanthosis nigricans that is a result of their insulin resistance and are often hypertensive.[54,61]

Laboratory Studies

In the appropriate clinical setting, a few basic laboratory studies are usually sufficient to differentiate between T1D and T2D. Irrespective of the type, diabetes can be diagnosed using the criteria adopted by the ADA (see Box 256-2).[56] Hyperglycemia and glycosuria are the predominant features in both conditions. Significantly elevated blood and urine ketone levels are traditionally associated with T1D but are occasionally present in patients with T2D. Additional laboratory abnormalities associated with diabetic ketoacidosis are discussed in Chapter 342, Diabetic Ketoacidosis. Insulin and C-peptide concentrations are generally low in patients with established T1D compared with the elevated concentrations in patients with T2D.

Although certain HLA haplotypes are associated with an elevated risk of T1D, they play no role in the diagnosis. Most patients with T1D will have antibodies directed against insulin or pancreatic islet cell antigens at the time of diagnosis.[62] Because these antibodies can be elevated in patients who may not develop disease for many years or never develop diabetes, they should not be used to make or confirm the diagnosis.

As pancreatic β-cell function declines and endogenous insulin secretion diminishes, C-peptide concentrations fall. Plasma C-peptide concentrations that are very low or undetectable in the face of hyperglycemia are consistent with the diagnosis of T1D. However, C-peptide concentrations are often not helpful at the time of diagnosis because endogenous insulin (and thus C-peptide) production has not completely failed.

MANAGEMENT

Type 1 Diabetes

The clinical management of T1D requires an integrated multidisciplinary team consisting of physicians, nurses, diabetes educators, dietitians, social workers, and psychologists. Patients and families must be adequately educated and supported to achieve safely as near euglycemia as possible because of the unequivocal evidence that tight glucose control prevents complications of diabetes. Without adequate education, safe and successful diabetes management is difficult to attain. The education should be tailored to provide developmentally appropriate participation by the patient. Teenagers should be able to assume more responsibility for their care than toddlers. Although improved glycemic control improves outcomes with regard to micro- and macrovascular complications, these benefits do not come without risk. The main risk posed in achieving near euglycemia is increased frequency and severity of hypoglycemia. In the Diabetes Control and Complications Trial (DCCT), the rate of severe hypoglycemia in the intensive insulin group was 62 events per 100 patient-years compared with 19 events per 100 patient-years in the conventional group.[63] Most long-term trials showing improvement in chronic complication rates have been performed in adults. However, a part of the Epidemiology of Diabetes Interventions and Complications (EDIC) trial evaluated the adolescent patients who were initially enrolled in the DCCT (13-17 years of age at enrollment).[64] At the end of the DCCT, the intensive treatment group had significantly lower HbA_{1C} values, but this effect was lost during the 4-year EDIC follow-up of this cohort. Despite the patients having similar control of their diabetes by the end of the study, those previously treated intensively had a marked reduction in the progression of diabetic retinopathy,[64] which suggests that tight glycemic control is important even in this adolescent population.

Several models of successful diabetes education programs exist, but all are centered on the goal of achieving as close to euglycemia as possible while minimizing adverse events, primarily hypoglycemia. The ADA has proposed age-adjusted guidelines regarding target blood glucose values and targets for HbA_{1C} (Table 256-1).[56] Less tight control is recommended for younger children in whom the risks of hypoglycemia may be greater and the advantages of very tight control have not been proven. Postprandial glucose targets are widely used in the management of diabetes during pregnancy. However, these targets are not commonly used outside pregnancy because

Table 256-1 American Diabetes Association Guidelines for Glycemic Control Children and Adolescents

AGE (YEARS)	PLASMA GLUCOSE (mg/dL) PREMEAL	BEDTIME OR OVERNIGHT	HbA_{1c}
0-6	100-180	110-200	<8.5% (but >7.5%)
6-12	90-180	100-180	<8%
13-19	90-130	90-150	<8%
Adults	90-130	—	<7%

Adapted from American Diabetes Association. Standards of medical care in diabetes—2007. Diabetes Care 2007;30(suppl 1):S4-S36.

their value has not been studied rigorously in children. These goals are suggested, and individualized goals may be necessary. Lower HbA_{1C} values may be safely obtained in select patients in whom the risk of severe hypoglycemia is deemed low. However, the lower the HbA_{1C} level, the higher the risk of severe hypoglycemia (Figure 256-1).

Type 2 Diabetes

The treatment options available for patients with T2D are more diverse. Although many effective medications with a variety of mechanisms of action are available, few are indicated for the treatment of T2D in children. The type of therapy must be tailored to fit the clinical situation of the patient. If diabetes is discovered in an asymptomatic patient with a normal or near normal HbA_{1C} level, lifestyle modification, including medical nutrition therapy, may be the most appropriate treatment. Weight loss and exercise can significantly improve insulin sensitivity in the setting of T2D.[65] These approaches may be adequate for maintenance of glycemic goals in individuals willing to participate regularly in physical activity and modify their eating behaviors. The Diabetes Prevention Program found that lifestyle modification intervention reduced the development of T2D in adults by 58% over the 2.8 years of follow-up.[66] Although similar data are not available in children, this type of therapy for overweight children or those with impaired fasting glucose seems prudent. When a patient is experiencing symptomatic hyperglycemia or has a significantly elevated HbA_{1C} level, the clinician should consider pharmacologic intervention. Insulin is the only medication approved for the treatment of diabetes in children at all ages. When used appropriately, it is safe and effective in lowering HbA_{1C} levels. In many instances, children with T2D are able to improve their glycemic control with less-intensive programs than are needed for patients with T1D. Once- or twice-daily, intermediate- or long-acting insulin may be sufficient. However, no pharmacologic intervention is a substitute for lifestyle intervention and medical nutrition therapy. All of these tools should be used.

The United Kingdom Prospective Diabetes Study (UKPDS) showed that improvements in HbA_{1C} levels in adults with T2D improved outcomes with respect to microvascular complications, highlighting that good glycemic management is equally important for T2D as in T1D.[67] The only oral agent approved for use in children is metformin. Metformin is approved for children 10 years of age and older with T2D. It has the advantage of not inducing hypoglycemia when used as monotherapy and is also associated with weight stabilization or mild weight loss. The major side effect of metformin is gastrointestinal disturbance, which can be largely prevented by slowly titrating the dose. It should not be used in patients with significant liver disease or renal impairment.

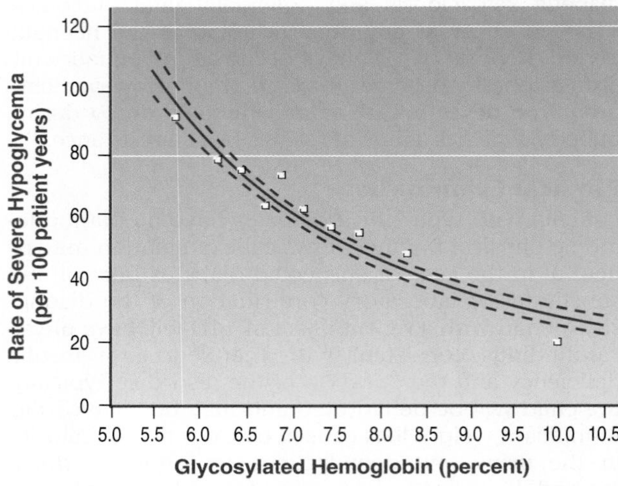

Figure 256-1 Increased risk of severe hypoglycemia with lower HbA_{1C}. (Diabetes Control and Complications Trial Research Group. The effect of intensive treatment of diabetes on the development and progression of long-term complications in insulin-dependent diabetes mellitus. N Engl J Med. 1993;329(14):977-986. *Copyright © 1993 Massachusetts Medical Society. All rights reserved.*)

INSULIN

Insulin Programs

With the availability of multiple forms of insulin (Table 256-2), many options exist for designing an insulin regimen for each patient. All patients will need to have an individualized plan with respect to the type and dose of insulin, timing of injections, and appropriate frequency of home glucose monitoring depending on their daily routine. No single program

Table 256-2 Onset, Peak, and Duration of Action of Currently Available Insulin

	ONSET	PEAK	DURATION
SHORT ACTING			
Regular	30 min	2-4 hr	4-6 hr
Lispro	<15 min	1 hr	3-4 hr
Aspart	<15 min	1 hr	3-4 hr
Glulisine	<15 min	1 hr	3-4 hr
INTERMEDIATE ACTING			
NPH	2-4 hr	4-6 hr	10-16 hr
Lente	3-4 hr	6-10 hr	10-20 hr
LONG ACTING			
Glargine	2-3 hr	None	24 hr or longer
Detemir	1-2 hr	3-9 hr*	6-23 hr*

*Higher doses result in delayed peak and longer duration of action.
From Plank J, Bodenlenz M, Sinner F, et al. A double-blind, randomized, dose-response study investigating the pharmacodynamic and pharmacokinetic properties of the long-acting insulin analog detemir. Diabetes Care. 2005;28(5):1107-1112. Copyright © 2005 American Diabetes Association. Reprinted with permission.

will be acceptable for every patient. As patient needs and technology change, programs should be updated to maintain glycemic goals. Typical doses of insulin in children rage from 0.5 to 1 unit of insulin per kilogram per day. However, during puberty, children will require higher insulin doses to achieve the same control.[68] Even in individuals without diabetes, puberty is a time of relative insulin resistance; therefore, not surprisingly, children with diabetes require higher doses during this time.[60,69]

The 3 most commonly used insulin programs are split-mixed, multiple daily injection (MDI), and continuous subcutaneous insulin injection (CSII). Each program should be designed with the same basic principles of basal and bolus insulin. In the fasting state, insulin is normally produced and secreted by the pancreas to maintain euglycemia. During a meal, additional insulin is secreted from the pancreas as the blood glucose level begins to rise when carbohydrate is absorbed from the intestinal mucosa. For patients with T1D, intermediate- or long-acting insulin is used as the basal insulin, and a short-acting insulin bolus is used to control the postmeal glucose rise (Figure 256-2).

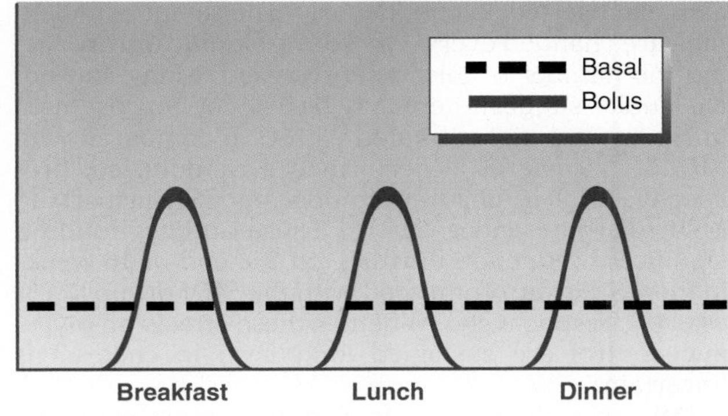

Figure 256-2 Bolus insulin is used to maintain blood glucose in the goal range after a meal. Basal insulin is used to maintain blood glucose in the goal range between meals and overnight.

Split-Mixed Program

A split-mixed program is commonly used in younger patients in whom fewer injections may be desirable. A short-acting and an intermediate-acting insulin are mixed and given as a single injection before breakfast and again before the evening meal. Considerably higher doses are generally required in the morning compared with the evening. A typical ratio would be two thirds to three fourths of the total daily dose given in the morning and the remainder in the evening. Approximately two thirds of the morning dose is intermediate-acting insulin, and the rest is short acting. Equal amounts of intermediate- and short-acting insulin are given with the evening meal. A snack at bedtime can prevent nighttime hypoglycemia because the intermediate-acting insulin will have its peak action in the early morning hours. The evening dose of intermediate-acting insulin can be given at bedtime to help prevent this complication. Although many patients like this program because only 2 shots are required daily, achieving adequate glycemic goals is sometimes not possible. A split-mixed program also requires patients to be on a fixed diet with respect to timing and nutrient content at each meal in an attempt to match consistently the insulin dose with the time and amount of food eaten. Because of these limitations, patients are often changed to or started on a more intensive insulin program (MDI or CSII).

Multiple Daily Injection Program

The MDI program consists of intermediate- or long-acting insulin as the basal insulin and short-acting as a bolus with each meal. In contrast to a split-mixed program, MDI requires 3 to 4 (or more) injections each day. This program offers more flexibility with regard to timing and content of meals than split-mixed programs. Basal insulin constitutes approximately one half of the total daily dose and is usually given in the evening. The amount of short-acting insulin given with each meal will depend on the amount of carbohydrate consumed at that meal. If the patient has been prescribed an exchange diet with a fixed amount of carbohydrate for each meal, then the dose of insulin will be the same from day to day. However, many patients will choose to vary the amount of carbohydrate at each meal within an overall meal plan and will adjust their insulin according to the amount of carbohydrate consumed.

Continuous Subcutaneous Insulin Injection Program

Insulin pumps have improved significantly since they were first introduced. The initial pumps were large and heavy, with few safety features. Today's pumps are considerably smaller and can be concealed under a person's clothing. A cartridge filled with short-acting insulin serves as both the basal and bolus insulin. Multiple basal rates can be programmed for patients whose basal insulin requirements are not constant throughout the day. This feature is not available with a split-mixed or MDI program. The insulin is delivered through tubing that is connected to a flexible plastic cannula inserted subcutaneously. The tubing and cannula are changed every 2 to 3 days, significantly reducing the number of injections required. Many, but not all, studies suggest there may be a slight improvement in HbA_{1C} in patients treated with CSII compared with MDI.[70-73] Doyle et al performed a randomized, prospective trial in children comparing CSII (aspart) to MDI (glargine and aspart).[74] These authors found a significant reduction in HbA_{1C} at the end of 16 weeks in the CSII group compared with the MDI group (7.2% vs 8.1%, respectively). Whether these effects on glycemic control are sustained long term in children is uncertain.

Data regarding the incidence of hypoglycemia and ketoacidosis between CSII and MDI are inconsistent, suggesting one is not clearly superior to the other with regard to safety.[75] Current insulin pumps contain numerous safety features that minimize the previous concerns of malfunction seen with earlier-generation pumps. No long-term data are available to suggest that microvascular or macrovascular complications are reduced with CSII compared with MDI. The goals of therapy should be the same despite the insulin program used (see Table 256-1).

Monitoring and Adjusting

Appropriate insulin dosing cannot be accomplished without adequate blood glucose monitoring. Simply checking the glucose concentration is not enough; the glucose values must be recorded in a log and reviewed on a regular basis to determine if insulin doses need to be adjusted. The data from many home glucose meters and insulin pumps can be transferred to a computer to assist in tracking glycemic control. For patients with T1D and some patients with T2D treated with insulin, blood glucose concentrations should be monitored before meals, at bedtime, and occasionally at night. For individuals with T2D treated with lifestyle modification or oral agents, less frequent monitoring is required. Additional glucose determinations may be needed during illness, exercise, or with symptoms of hyper- or hypoglycemia. Many good home glucose monitors are available. All of these monitors should be checked periodically for accuracy, and patients should receive training on proper technique.

Adjusting insulin doses is necessary to maintain good glycemic control. The glucose log serves as a guide to making appropriate changes. Because many variables exist that cannot be accounted for, patients should be informed that their blood glucose concentration will not always fall in the normal range. For some people, this circumstance can be discouraging and lead to improper insulin adjustments. For others, the lack of education or fear of hypoglycemia leads to improper dose adjusting.

When discussing insulin doses in the context of hypoglycemia or hyperglycemia, primary care physicians must be clear about the difference between insulin adjustments and supplements. Insulin doses are adjusted based on patterns of blood glucose concentrations recorded in the log. The purpose of an adjustment is to prevent future abnormal glucose levels. Primary care physicians should commonly ask patients to look for a 3-day trend of hyperglycemia before making an adjustment. For example, if a patient consistently has glucose values before their evening meal that are higher than the goal range, then an increase in the short-acting insulin before the noon meal would be made. Changes in insulin dose are generally made as a 10% increase or decrease.

Because patients will often have a glucose concentration fall outside their goal range, supplements are used to correct this situation. A supplement is used to correct a glucose concentration that is currently abnormal. For example, if a patient has a blood glucose level that is below the goal range before breakfast, then insulin would be subtracted from their morning bolus dose of short-acting insulin. If the glucose were above the goal range, then supplemental insulin may be added to the bolus dose of short-acting insulin at that meal to correct the hyperglycemia. The supplement (either adding or subtracting insulin) is used to correct the abnormal glucose, whereas the bolus dose of short-acting insulin is used to account for the food that will be eaten at a meal.

Meal Plan

One of the major determinants of blood glucose concentration is carbohydrate ingestion. Matching the amount of food intake with the appropriate amount of insulin requires knowledge of the onset, peak, and duration of action of the various types of insulin available (see Table 256-2).

Many meal plans have been used in the care of patients with diabetes to optimize glycemic control. Although a particular diabetes program may advocate one meal plan over another, comparative trials showing that one is superior to another are lacking. As children grow and vary their activity levels, caloric requirements can change significantly. Advice from a dietician experienced in the management of children with diabetes is necessary for the implementation of any successful diabetes program. The 2 most commonly used meal plans are (1) the exchange diet and (2) carbohydrate counting. Both plans require specific education to ensure that patients are able to assess the nutrient content of the foods they eat and how this factor affects the management of their disease.

An exchange diet requires a patient to eat a consistent amount of nutrients at a consistent time of day. For example, a patient may be prescribed 45 g of carbohydrate for breakfast, 60 g for lunch, and 60 g for dinner. The patient would be expected to eat according to this pattern each day. The amount of fat and protein may also be prescribed for each meal. Foods are categorized according to nutrient content, and this list is used to create a meal. Foods with equivalent nutrient content can be *exchanged* for each other to introduce variety in the diet. Snacks are usually incorporated into this diet depending on the individual patient's needs and preferences. The advantage of this diet is that nutrient intake is consistent, allowing insulin dosing to also be consistent. This diet can be used for patients on split-mixed, MDI, or CSII programs.

Carbohydrate counting is a more complex but increasingly popular option. This diet would not be appropriate for patients on a split-mixed insulin program because nutrient intake may vary substantially from meal to meal and day to day. Insulin doses in a split-mixed program cannot easily be adjusted to account for the dietary variability of carbohydrate counting. However, this diet can be used for patients on an MDI or CSII insulin regimen. For this meal plan, patients must also be familiar with the carbohydrate content of each food they eat. For each unit of carbohydrate taken, a certain amount of insulin must be given to maintain euglycemia. A typical ratio may be 1 unit of short-acting insulin for each 15 g of carbohydrate eaten. This ratio is adjusted for each patient and may even vary based on time of day for a given individual. Carbohydrate counting has the advantage of being able to vary the amount of food at a meal according to how much the patient desires to eat. Because patients are able to take more insulin to maintain glycemic control while overeating, carbohydrate counting must be a part of an overall meal plan so that overeating does not lead to obesity or contribute to hyperlipidemia. As long as healthy, well-balanced eating is maintained, carbohydrate counting offers an alternative to the exchange diet with more flexibility in the timing and content of each meal. Carbohydrate counting requires specific education and a motivated patient and family to be implemented correctly.

Exercise

Exercise can be performed safely, and children should not be discouraged from participating in sports simply because they have diabetes. Attention to the effects of activity on glucose levels can assist in preventing hypoglycemia during or after exercise. Because exercise may alter the absorption of subcutaneous insulin and can enhance insulin sensitivity,[76] hypoglycemia may occur if changes are not made in the amount of food eaten or insulin taken. Two methods have been developed for preventing hypoglycemia during planned physical activity. The dose of short-acting insulin given at the previous meal might be reduced, or a snack can be given just before or during the activity. If the activity is not planned, then a snack will be the only option. The blood glucose level should be checked before and again after exercise to determine the effect of the activity on glucose concentrations. If the activity is prolonged (longer than 45 to 60 minutes) the blood glucose level should also be checked periodically during the activity. Only by documenting the effect of exercise on an individual's glucose level can appropriate decisions be made to prevent hypoglycemia. Checking a nighttime blood glucose level is advised when prolonged activity has taken place, especially in the evening. The effect of exercise may be sustained and lead to delayed hypoglycemia.

Illness

Parents and patients need to be aware that illness can have a notable affect on blood glucose values. Hypoglycemia or hyperglycemia may result depending on the severity of the illness and the amount of food eaten. A common error made is the omission of insulin injections because the child is not eating. Regardless of food intake, insulin is necessary in health or illness. Although the dose may change, some insulin should be given even if the child is not able to eat. Some practical guidelines can assist in appropriate care during illness:

1. Never completely omit insulin. Insulin requirements may increase, and some insulin is needed even if the child is not able to eat.
2. Monitor and record blood glucose concentrations every 2 to 4 hours.
3. Monitor urine ketone concentrations frequently, even if the blood glucose level is not significantly elevated (>250 mg/dL). Some patients with T1D can develop ketosis in the absence of hyperglycemia when ill.
4. Encourage adequate hydration.

By following these simple guidelines, most children with minor illnesses can avoid hospitalization and emergency department visits. Patients will need to be seen if they have persistent moderate or large urine ketone levels, are unable to treat hypoglycemia effectively, or become significantly dehydrated.

COMPLICATIONS

Before the discovery of insulin, T1D was a fatal disease. Progressive metabolic abnormalities, including ketoacidosis, would eventually lead to death. With the availability of insulin for clinical use in the early 1920s, patients were able to survive the more immediate threat of severe acidosis. Initial goals of therapy were to prevent symptoms of hyperglycemia and ketoacidosis. With the initiation of insulin therapy, hypoglycemia and the chronic complications of diabetes became apparent.

Microvascular Complications

The DCCT was a pivotal study in understanding the importance of maintaining euglycemia. The DCCT revealed that patients with T1D who received intensive insulin therapy had significantly fewer microvascular complications. Development or progression of retinopathy was reduced by 63% and the need for laser therapy was reduced by 51%. The development of albuminuria (>300 mg/day) was reduced by 54% and clinical neuropathy by 60%. The population enrolled was relatively young at the beginning of the study (mean age = 27 years) and did not show a statistically significant decline in macrovascular events. The EDIC trial was an extension of the original DCCT cohort. After 17 years of follow-up from initial randomization, over 90% of the patients were assessed for macrovascular disease. The EDIC trial found at 17-year follow-up that patients who had previously been treated with intensive insulin therapy had a significantly lower number of macrovascular events, including acute myocardial infarction and stroke.[77] This instance was the 1st time a benefit in the reduction of macrovascular disease had been reported in patients with T1D as a result of intensive insulin therapy.

Data regarding the reduction in microvascular complications has also been demonstrated for patients with T2D.[67] Undoubtedly, diabetes (type 1 or type 2) greatly increases the risk of blindness, chronic kidney disease, neuropathy, cardiovascular disease, and stroke. The evidence is clear that these risks can be attenuated in adolescents and adults treated with intensive diabetes management. Merely treating to avoid symptoms of hyperglycemia is not acceptable. Data regarding the prevention of chronic complications of diabetes in younger children and infants with intensive glucose management are not available.

Hypoglycemia

Hypoglycemia is a common complication of intensive diabetes management. In addition to assessing the frequency of hypoglycemia, the severity of hypoglycemia should be taken into account. Mild hypoglycemia is the result of the adrenergic response to low blood glucose levels (<70 mg/dL). Patients with mild hypoglycemia have symptoms of shakiness, nervousness, tachycardia, and sweating. Older children are generally able to recognize these symptoms. However, younger children may not be able to recognize or effectively communicate these symptoms, and their primary care physicians must be responsible for identifying signs of hypoglycemia. Parents frequently report unusual behavior and irritability as signs of hypoglycemia in younger children.

Severe hypoglycemia is defined as an episode requiring assistance for treatment. With severe hypoglycemia, the patient has neurologic symptoms, which can include confusion or loss of consciousness. The DCCT clearly showed that the incidence of severe hypoglycemia markedly increased with lowering of the HbA_{1C} level (see Figure 256-1).

When a patient experiences symptoms of hypoglycemia, the blood glucose level should be checked to document that the symptoms are due to a low blood glucose level. Some symptoms of hypoglycemia are nonspecific, and unnecessary treatment should be avoided. If hypoglycemia is mild or moderate, generally, 10 to 15 g of carbohydrate will correct the situation. The glucose level should be rechecked in 15 to 20 minutes to be certain the hypoglycemia has resolved. Glucose tablets and gels are available and easy to carry. Some form of carbohydrate should always be available to the patient for the treatment of hypoglycemia.

In an unconscious patient, severe hypoglycemia may be treated with glucagon or intravenous glucose. Training on the proper use of glucagon should be provided to individuals caring for the patient, such as parents, school nurses, older siblings, and others. Glucagon is reserved for patients with severe hypoglycemia who are not able to ingest carbohydrate. Glucagon effectively raises blood glucose by stimulating glucose release from the liver. However, this response is relatively short-lived, and as soon as practical, the patient should eat (although the nausea that frequently accompanies glucagon administration makes this requirement more complicated). After an episode of hypoglycemia is successfully treated, a cause of the hypoglycemia should be considered. If no cause is readily apparent, then an adjustment in the insulin dose should be made the next day to avoid additional hypoglycemia. This advice is in contrast to monitoring glucose trends before making adjustments to prevent hyperglycemia. One episode of unexplained hypoglycemia should prompt an insulin adjustment.

Less tight glycemic control should be considered for patients with frequent severe hypoglycemia because of the possibility of long-term neurologic consequences. Children younger than 5 or 6 years at the time of diagnosis appear to be at particularly high risk of experiencing frequent hypoglycemia and cognitive impairment.[78]

Other Considerations

The successful management of diabetes is complex and requires a committed team of health care providers and significant social support for the child. Although the focus of treatment is centered on safely achieving glycemic goals in an attempt to avoid complications, these complications cannot be prevented in all patients. Screening for chronic complications must be performed to intervene early to reverse or slow disease progression. Screening for diabetic retinopathy is recommended for all individuals with diabetes. Developing retinopathy within the first 3 years of diagnosis is unusual for a child, especially if the child is younger than 10 years.[79-81] Ophthalmologic evaluation for patients with T1D should start between 3 and 5 years after the initial diagnosis.[82] This recommendation varies slightly depending on the academic society. The AAP recommends initiating screening eye examinations 3 to 5 years after diagnosis if the child is older than 9 years, with annual follow-up therafter.[83]

Diabetic nephropathy is a leading cause of chronic kidney disease and need for dialysis. Similar to retinopathy, diabetic nephropathy is uncommon in the young or newly diagnosed patient with T1D, and screening should start at age 10 in children who have had T1D for at least 5 years.[84] The ADA recommends screening with a random urine sample to determine the microalbumin-to-creatinine ratio. A ratio of 30 mg/g (albumin to creatinine) or greater is considered abnormal, and further testing may be indicated. Because other factors may contribute to albuminuria, including exercise, 2 to 3 abnormal determinations may need to be obtained to confirm the diagnosis. Screening for hyperlipidemia is also recommended at or shortly after the initial diagnosis of T1D in all patients. Depending on the lipid profile and additional risk factors, lifestyle and pharmacologic intervention may be required.[84]

Patients with T1D are at increased risk of developing other autoimmune disorders, including thyroid disease and celiac disease. One study of more than 200 patients with T1D younger than 20 years found an autoimmune thyroid disorder in 17%.[85] Screening for thyroid disease should begin at or shortly after diagnosis by measurement of sensitive thyroid-stimulating hormone and performed annually thereafter. The ADA also recommends biochemical screening of children for celiac disease because patients with T1D are at higher risk of this disease, which can significantly affect the nutritional requirements for the child.[84] Screening for celiac disease can be performed by measuring tissue transglutaminase antibodies or endomysial antibodies. Normal total immunoglobulin A (IgA) concentrations should also be documented.

CONCLUSION

Although significant advances have been made in the types of insulin available and the tools used to monitor blood glucose concentrations, the ability to replicate the function of an intact pancreas is crude at best. Because of this inability, the patient requires a significant amount of effort on a daily basis. Providing adequate, individualized education and support for patients with diabetes is imperative for successful treatment.

WHEN TO REFER

- Newly diagnosed children with T1D
- When a multidisciplinary diabetes program is needed and not available

WHEN TO ADMIT

- Considered for all patients with newly diagnosed T1D
- Diabetic ketoacidosis
- Considered for severe hypoglycemia or dehydration

TOOLS FOR PRACTICE

Community Coordination and Advocacy

- *Helping the Student with Diabetes Succeed* (book), National Institutes of Health and Centers for Disease Control and Prevention. AAP Endorsed (www.ndep.nih.gov/diabetes/pubs/Youth_NDEPSchoolGuide.pdf).
- *Issue Brief—Childhood Obesity* (fact sheet), American Academy of Pediatrics (www.aap.org/moc/displaytemp/obesity_issuebrief.pdf).

Engaging Patients and Family

- *A Parent's Guide to Childhood Obesity: A Road Map to Health* (book), American Academy of Pediatrics (www.aap.org/bookstore).
- *Diabetes & Me* (Web page), Center for Disease Control and Prevention (www.cdc.gov/diabetes/consumer/index.htm).
- *Diabetes Mellitus* (fact sheet), American Academy of Pediatrics (www.aap.org/topics.html).
- *Information about Diabetes—Parents and Kids* (Web page), American Diabetes Association (www.diabetes.org/for-parents-and-kids.jsp).
- *Tip sheets for kids with T2 Diabetes—Eat Healthy Foods* (fact sheet), National Diabetes Education Program (www.ndep.nih.gov/diabetes/youth/youthtips/youthtips_eat.htm).
- *Tip sheets for kids with T2 Diabetes—Stay at a healthy weight* (fact sheet), National Diabetes Education Program (www.ndep.nih.gov/diabetes/youth/youthtips/youthtips_weight.htm).
- *Tip sheets for kids with T2 Diabetes—Be Active!* (fact sheet), National Diabetes Education Program (www.ndep.nih.gov/diabetes/youth/youthtips/youthtips_active.htm).
- *Tip sheets for kids with T2 Diabetes—What is Diabetes?* (fact sheet), National Diabetes Education Program (www.ndep.nih.gov/diabetes/youth/youthtips/youthtips_diabetes.htm).
- *What is a Pediatric Endocrinologist?* (fact sheet), American Academy of Pediatrics (www.aap.org/family/whatispedendo.pdf).

Medical Decision Support

- *A New Spin on Childhood Obesity* (on-line course), American Academy of Pediatrics (www.pedialink.org/cme/_coursefinder/CMEdetail.cfm?aid=30256&area=live CME).
- *Pediatric Obesity: Prevention, Intervention, and Treatment Strategies for Primary Care* (book), American Academy of Pediatrics (www.aap.org/bookstore).
- *Resources for Professionals* (Web page), American Diabetes Association (www.diabetes.org/for-health-professionals-and-scientists/resources.jsp).
- *Type 2 diabetes in children and adolescents* (policy statement). American Diabetes Association. AAP Endorsed. (care.diabetesjournals.org/cgi/reprint/23/3/381.pdf).

Practice Management

- *Obesity and other Co-Morbidities Coding Fact Sheet for Primary Care Pediatricians* (fact sheet) American Academy of Pediatrics (www.aap.org/securemoc/reimburse/codingfactsheet.pdf).

AAP POLICY STATEMENTS

American Academy of Pediatrics, Council on Sports Medicine and Fitness and Council on School Health. Active healthy living: prevention of childhood obesity through increased physical activity. *Pediatrics*. 2006;117(5):1834-1842. (aappolicy.aappublications.org/cgi/content/full/pediatrics;117/5/1834).

American Academy of Pediatrics, Committee on Nutrition. Prevention of pediatric overweight and obesity. *Pediatrics*. 2003;112(2):424-430. (aappolicy.aappublications.org/cgi/content/full/pediatrics;112/2/424).

Gahagan S, Silverstein J, American Academy of Pediatrics, Committee on Native American Child Health and Section on Endocrinology. Prevention and treatment of type 2 diabetes mellitus in children, with special emphasis on American Indian and Alaska Native Children. *Pediatrics*. 2003; 112(4):e328. (aappolicy.aappublications.org/cgi/content/full/pediatrics;112/4/e328).

Lueder GT, Silverstein J, American Academy of Pediatrics, Section on Ophthalmology and Section on Endocrinology. Screening for retinopathy in the pediatric patient with type 1 diabetes mellitus. *Pediatrics*. 2005;116(1):270-273. (aappolicy.aappublications.org/cgi/content/full/pediatrics;116/1/270).

SUGGESTED RESOURCES

American Diabetes Association. Type 2 diabetes in children and adolescents. *Diabetes Care*. 2000;23(3):381-389.

American Diabetes Association. Type 2 diabetes in children and adolescents. *Pediatrics*. 2000;105(3 pt 1):671-680.

American Diabetes Association. Youth Zone. Available at: www.diabetes.org/youthzone/youth-zone.jsp.

Silverstein J, Klingensmith G, Copeland K, et al. Care of children and adolescents with type 1 diabetes: a statement of the American Diabetes Association. *Diabetes Care*. 2005; 28(1):186-212.

REFERENCES

1. Jacobson DL, Gange SJ, Rose NR, et al. Epidemiology and estimated population burden of selected autoimmune diseases in the United States. *Clin Immunol Immunopathol*. 1997;84(3):223-243.
2. Onkamo P, Vaananen S, Karvonen M, et al. Worldwide increase in incidence of type I diabetes—the analysis of the data on published incidence trends. *Diabetologia*. 1999;42(12):1395-1403.
3. Gale EA. The rise of childhood type 1 diabetes in the 20th century. *Diabetes*. 2002;51(12):3353-3361.
4. Petersen JS, Kyvik KO, Bingley PJ, et al. Population based study of prevalence of islet cell autoantibodies in monozygotic and dizygotic Danish twin pairs with insulin dependent diabetes mellitus. *BMJ*. 1997;314(7094): 1575-1579.
5. Kumar D, Gemayel NS, Deapen D, et al. North-American twins with IDDM. Genetic, etiological, and clinical significance of disease concordance according to age, zygosity, and the interval after diagnosis in first twin. *Diabetes*. 1993;42(9):1351-1363.
6. Srikanta S, Ganda OP, Jackson RA, et al. Type I diabetes mellitus in monozygotic twins: chronic progressive beta cell dysfunction. *Ann Intern Med*. 1983;99(3):320-326.
7. Verge CF, Gianani R, Yu L, et al. Late progression to diabetes and evidence for chronic beta-cell autoimmunity in identical twins of patients with type I diabetes. *Diabetes*. 1995;44(10):1176-1179.
8. Redondo MJ, Rewers M, Yu L, et al. Genetic determination of islet cell autoimmunity in monozygotic twin, dizygotic twin, and non-twin siblings of patients with type 1 diabetes: prospective twin study. *BMJ*. 1999;318(7185): 698-702.
9. Torn C, Gupta M, Nikitina Zake L, et al. Heterozygosity for MICA5.0/MICA5.1 and HLA-DR3-DQ2/DR4-DQ8 are independent genetic risk factors for latent autoimmune diabetes in adults. *Hum Immunol*. 2003;64(9):902-909.
10. Field LL. Genetic linkage and association studies of type I diabetes: challenges and rewards. *Diabetologia*. 2002; 45(1):21-35.
11. Pietropaolo M, Becker DJ, LaPorte RE, et al. Progression to insulin-requiring diabetes in seronegative prediabetic subjects: the role of two HLA-DQ high-risk haplotypes. *Diabetologia*. 2002;45(1):66-76.
12. Graham J, Kockum I, Sanjeevi CB, et al. Negative association between type 1 diabetes and HLA DQB1*0602-DQA1*0102 is attenuated with age at onset. Swedish Childhood Diabetes Study Group. *Eur J Immunogenet*. 1999;26(2-3):117-127.
13. Kockum I, Sanjeevi CB, Eastman S, et al. Population analysis of protection by HLA-DR and DQ genes from insulin-dependent diabetes mellitus in Swedish children with insulin-dependent diabetes and controls. *Eur J Immunogenet*. 1995;22(6):443-465.
14. Redondo MJ, Kawasaki E, Mulgrew CL, et al. DR- and DQ-associated protection from type 1A diabetes: comparison of DRB1*1401 and DQA1*0102-DQB1*0602*. *J Clin Endocrinol Metab*. 2000;85(10):3793-3797.
15. The Eurodiab Ace Study Group and The Eurodiab Ace Substudy 2 Study Group. Familial risk of type I diabetes in European children. *Diabetologia*. 1998;41(10): 1151-1156.
16. Warram JH, Krolewski AS, Gottlieb MS, et al. Differences in risk of insulin-dependent diabetes in offspring of diabetic mothers and diabetic fathers. *N Engl J Med*. 1984;311(3):149-152.
17. Rjasanowski I, Heinke P, Michaelis D, et al. The higher frequency of type I (insulin-dependent) diabetes in fathers than in mothers of type I-diabetic children. *Exp Clin Endocrinol*. 1990;95(1):91-96.
18. Devendra D, Liu E, Eisenbarth GS. Type 1 diabetes: recent developments. *BMJ*. 2004;328(7442):750-754.
19. Yoon JW, Austin M, Onodera T, et al. Isolation of a virus from the pancreas of a child with diabetic ketoacidosis. *N Engl J Med*. 1979;300(21):1173-1179.
20. Foulis AK, McGill M, Farquharson MA, et al. A search for evidence of viral infection in pancreases of newly diagnosed patients with IDDM. *Diabetologia*. 1997;40(1): 53-61.
21. King ML, Shaikh A, Bidwell D, et al. Coxsackie-B-virus-specific IgM responses in children with insulin-dependent (juvenile-onset; type I) diabetes mellitus. *Lancet*. 1983;1(8339):1397-1399.
22. Hyoty H, Hiltunen M, Knip M, et al. A prospective study of the role of Coxsackie B and other enterovirus infections in the pathogenesis of IDDM. Childhood Diabetes in Finland (DiMe) Study Group. *Diabetes*. 1995;44(6):652-657.
23. Hummel M, Fuchtenbusch M, Schenker M, et al. No major association of breast-feeding, vaccinations, and childhood viral diseases with early islet autoimmunity in the German BABYDIAB Study. *Diabetes Care*. 2000;23(7): 969-974.
24. Cainelli F, Manzaroli D, Renzini C, et al. Coxsackie B virus-induced autoimmunity to GAD does not lead to type 1 diabetes. *Diabetes Care*. 2000;23(7):1021-1022.
25. Menser MA, Forrest JM, Bransby RD. Rubella infection and diabetes mellitus. *Lancet*. 1978;1(8055):57-60.
26. Ginsberg-Fellner F, Witt ME, Fedun B, et al. Diabetes mellitus and autoimmunity in patients with the congenital rubella syndrome. *Rev Infect Dis*. 1985;7(suppl 1): S170-S176.
27. Forrest JM, Menser MA, Burgess JA. High frequency of diabetes mellitus in young adults with congenital rubella. *Lancet*. 1971;2(7720):332-334.
28. Plotkin SA, Kaye R, Forrest JM, et al. Diabetes mellitus and congenital rubella. *Pediatrics*. 1970;46(4):650-651.
29. Forrest JM, Menser MA, Harley JD. Diabetes mellitus and congenital rubella. *Pediatrics*. 1969;44(3):445-447.
30. Hviid A, Stellfeld M, Wohlfahrt J, et al. Childhood vaccination and type 1 diabetes. *N Engl J Med*. 2004;350(14): 1398-1404.
31. Pastore MR, Bazzigaluppi E, Belloni C, et al. Six months of gluten-free diet do not influence autoantibody titers, but improve insulin secretion in subjects at high risk for type 1 diabetes. *J Clin Endocrinol Metab*. 2003;88(1):162-165.
32. Birgisdottir BE, Hill JP, Harris DP, et al. Variation in consumption of cow milk proteins and lower incidence of type 1 diabetes in Iceland vs the other 4 Nordic countries. *Diabetes Nutr Metab*. 2002;15(4):240-245.

33. Wasmuth HE, Kolb H. Cow's milk and immune-mediated diabetes. *Proc Nutr Soc*. 2000;59(4):573-579.
34. Virtanen SM, Laara E, Hypponen E, et al. Cow's milk consumption, HLA-DQB1 genotype, and type 1 diabetes: a nested case-control study of siblings of children with diabetes. Childhood diabetes in Finland study group. *Diabetes*. 2000;49(6):912-917.
35. Virtanen SM, Saukkonen T, Savilahti E, et al. Diet, cow's milk protein antibodies and the risk of IDDM in Finnish children. Childhood Diabetes in Finland Study Group. *Diabetologia*. 1994;37(4):381-387.
36. Norris JM, Beaty B, Klingensmith G, et al. Lack of association between early exposure to cow's milk protein and beta-cell autoimmunity. Diabetes Autoimmunity Study in the Young (DAISY). *JAMA*. 1996;276(8):609-614.
37. Ziegler AG, Schmid S, Huber D, et al. Early infant feeding and risk of developing type 1 diabetes-associated autoantibodies. *JAMA*. 2003;290(13):1721-1728.
38. Moltchanova E, Rytkonen M, Kousa A, et al. Zinc and nitrate in the ground water and the incidence of type 1 diabetes in Finland. *Diabet Med*. 2004;21(3):256-261.
39. Casu A, Carlini M, Contu A, et al. Type 1 diabetes in Sardinia is not linked to nitrate levels in drinking water. *Diabetes Care*. 2000;23(7):1043-1044.
40. Parslow RC, McKinney PA, Law GR, et al. Incidence of childhood diabetes mellitus in Yorkshire, northern England, is associated with nitrate in drinking water: an ecological analysis. *Diabetologia*. 1997;40(5):550-556.
41. Samuelsson U, Johansson C, Ludvigsson J. Breast-feeding seems to play a marginal role in the prevention of insulin-dependent diabetes mellitus. *Diabetes Res Clin Pract*. 1993;19(3):203-210.
42. Kyvik KO, Green A, Svendsen A, et al. Breast feeding and the development of type 1 diabetes mellitus. *Diabet Med*. 1992;9(3):233-235.
43. Borch-Johnsen K, Joner G, Mandrup-Poulsen T, et al. Relation between breast-feeding and incidence rates of insulin-dependent diabetes mellitus. A hypothesis. *Lancet*. 1984;2(8411):1083-1086.
44. Norris JM, Barriga K, Klingensmith G, et al. Timing of initial cereal exposure in infancy and risk of islet autoimmunity. *JAMA*. 2003;290(13):1713-1720.
45. Eisenbarth GS, Gianani R, Yu L, et al. Dual-parameter model for prediction of type I diabetes mellitus. *Proc Assoc Am Physicians*. 1998;110(2):126-135.
46. Pietropaolo M, Yu S, Libman IM, et al. Cytoplasmic islet cell antibodies remain valuable in defining risk of progression to type 1 diabetes in subjects with other islet autoantibodies. *Pediatr Diabetes*. 2005;6(4):184-192.
47. Achenbach P, Ziegler AG. Diabetes-related antibodies in euglycemic subjects. *Best Pract Res Clin Endocrinol Metab*. 2005;19(1):101-117.
48. Verge CF, Gianani R, Kawasaki E, et al. Prediction of type I diabetes in first-degree relatives using a combination of insulin, GAD, and ICA512bdc/IA-2 autoantibodies. *Diabetes*. 1996;45(7):926-933.
49. LaGasse JM, Brantley MS, Leech NJ, et al. Successful prospective prediction of type 1 diabetes in schoolchildren through multiple defined autoantibodies: an 8-year follow-up of the Washington State Diabetes Prediction Study. *Diabetes Care*. 2002;25(3):505-511.
50. Ludwig DS, Ebbeling CB. Type 2 diabetes mellitus in children: primary care and public health considerations. *JAMA*. 2001;286(12):1427-1430.
51. American Diabetes Association. Type 2 diabetes in children and adolescents. *Pediatrics*. 2000;105(3 pt 1):671-680.
52. Pinhas-Hamiel O, Dolan LM, Daniels SR, et al. Increased incidence of non-insulin-dependent diabetes mellitus among adolescents. *J Pediatr*. 1996;128(5 pt 1):608-615.
53. Krebs NF, Jacobson MS, American Academy of Pediatrics, Committee on Nutrition. Prevention of pediatric overweight and obesity. *Pediatrics*. 2003;112(2):424-430.
54. Scott CR, Smith JM, Cradock MM, et al. Characteristics of youth-onset noninsulin-dependent diabetes mellitus and insulin-dependent diabetes mellitus at diagnosis. *Pediatrics*. 1997;100(1):84-91.
55. Glaser NS, Jones KL. Non-insulin dependent diabetes mellitus in Mexican-American children. *West J Med*. 1998;168(1):11-16.
56. Standards of medical care in diabetes—2007. *Diabetes Care*. Jan 2007;30(suppl 1):S4-S36.
57. Giuffrida FM, Reis AF. Genetic and clinical characteristics of maturity-onset diabetes of the young. *Diabetes Obes Metab*. 2005;7(4):318-326.
58. Timsit J, Bellanne-Chantelot C, Dubois-Laforgue D, et al. Diagnosis and management of maturity-onset diabetes of the young. *Treat Endocrinol*. 2005;4(1):9-18.
59. Newton CA, Raskin P. Diabetic ketoacidosis in type 1 and type 2 diabetes mellitus: clinical and biochemical differences. *Arch Intern Med*. 2004;164(17):1925-1931.
60. Bloch CA, Clemons P, Sperling MA. Puberty decreases insulin sensitivity. *J Pediatr*. 1987;110(3):481-487.
61. Fagot-Campagna A, Pettitt DJ, Engelgau MM, et al. Type 2 diabetes among North American children and adolescents: an epidemiologic review and a public health perspective. *J Pediatr*. 2000;136(5):664-672.
62. Glastras SJ, Craig ME, Verge CF, et al. The role of autoimmunity at diagnosis of type 1 diabetes in the development of thyroid and celiac disease and microvascular complications. *Diabetes Care*. 2005;28(9):2170-2175.
63. Diabetes Control and Complications Trial Research Group. The effect of intensive treatment of diabetes on the development and progression of long-term complications in insulin-dependent diabetes mellitus. *N Engl J Med*. 1993;329(14):977-986.
64. White NH, Cleary PA, Dahms W, et al. Beneficial effects of intensive therapy of diabetes during adolescence: outcomes after the conclusion of the Diabetes Control and Complications Trial (DCCT). *J Pediatr*. 2001;139(6):804-812.
65. Borghouts LB, Keizer HA. Exercise and insulin sensitivity: a review. *Int J Sports Med*. 2000;21(1):1-12.
66. Knowler WC, Barrett-Connor E, Fowler SE, et al. Reduction in the incidence of type 2 diabetes with lifestyle intervention or metformin. *N Engl J Med*. 2002;346(6):393-403.
67. Intensive blood-glucose control with sulphonylureas or insulin compared with conventional treatment and risk of complications in patients with type 2 diabetes (UKPDS 33). UK Prospective Diabetes Study (UKPDS) Group. *Lancet*. 1998;352(9131):837-853.
68. Kerouz N, el-Hayek R, Langhough R, et al. Insulin doses in children using conventional therapy for insulin dependent diabetes. *Diabetes Res Clin Pract*. 1995;29(2):113-120.
69. Amiel SA, Caprio S, Sherwin RS, et al. Insulin resistance of puberty: a defect restricted to peripheral glucose metabolism. *J Clin Endocrinol Metab*. 1991;72(2):277-282.
70. Tsui E, Barnie A, Ross S, et al. Intensive insulin therapy with insulin lispro: a randomized trial of continuous subcutaneous insulin infusion versus multiple daily insulin injection. *Diabetes Care*. 2001;24(10):1722-1727.
71. DeVries JH, Snoek FJ, Kostense PJ, et al, and the Dutch Insulin Pump Study Group. A randomized trial of continuous subcutaneous insulin infusion and intensive injection therapy in type 1 diabetes for patients with long-standing poor glycemic control. *Diabetes Care*. 2002;25(11):2074-2080.

72. Retnakaran R, Hochman J, DeVries JH, et al. Continuous subcutaneous insulin infusion versus multiple daily injections: the impact of baseline A1c. *Diabetes Care*. 2004;27(11):2590-2596.
73. Hanaire-Broutin H, Melki V, Bessieres-Lacombe S, et al. Comparison of continuous subcutaneous insulin infusion and multiple daily injection regimens using insulin lispro in type 1 diabetic patients on intensified treatment: a randomized study. The Study Group for the Development of Pump Therapy in Diabetes. *Diabetes Care*. 2000;23(9):1232-1235.
74. Doyle EA, Weinzimer SA, Steffen AT, et al. A randomized, prospective trial comparing the efficacy of continuous subcutaneous insulin infusion with multiple daily injections using insulin glargine. *Diabetes Care*. 2004;27(7):1554-1558.
75. Weissberg-Benchell J, Antisdel-Lomaglio J, Seshadri R. Insulin pump therapy: a meta-analysis. *Diabetes Care*. 2003;26(4):1079-1087.
76. Landt KW, Campaigne BN, James FW, et al. Effects of exercise training on insulin sensitivity in adolescents with type I diabetes. *Diabetes Care*. 1985;8(5):461-465.
77. Nathan DM, Cleary PA, Backlund JY, et al. Intensive diabetes treatment and cardiovascular disease in patients with type 1 diabetes. *N Engl J Med*. 2005;353(25):2643-2653.
78. Ryan CM, Becker DJ. Hypoglycemia in children with type 1 diabetes mellitus. Risk factors, cognitive function, and management. *Endocrinol Metab Clin North Am*. 1999; 28(4):883-900.
79. Verougstraete C, Toussaint D, De Schepper J, et al. First microangiographic abnormalities in childhood diabetes—types of lesions. *Graefes Arch Clin Exp Ophthalmol*. 1991;229(1):24-32.
80. Klein R, Klein BE, Moss SE, et al. The Wisconsin epidemiologic study of diabetic retinopathy. II. Prevalence and risk of diabetic retinopathy when age at diagnosis is less than 30 years. *Arch Ophthalmol*. 1984;102(4):520-526.
81. Klein R, Klein BE, Moss SE, et al. The Wisconsin Epidemiologic Study of Diabetic Retinopathy: XVII. The 14-year incidence and progression of diabetic retinopathy and associated risk factors in type 1 diabetes. *Ophthalmology*. 1998;105(10):1801-1815.
82. Lueder GT, Silverstein J, American Academy of Pediatrics, Section on Ophthalmology and Section on Endocrinology. Screening for retinopathy in the pediatric patient with type 1 diabetes mellitus. *Pediatrics*. 2005;116(1):270-273.
83. American Academy of Pediatrics. Sections on Endocrinology and Ophthalmology. Screening for retinopathy in the pediatric patient with type 1 diabetes mellitus. *Pediatrics*. 1998;101(2):313-314.
84. Silverstein J, Klingensmith G, Copeland K, et al. Care of children and adolescents with type 1 diabetes: a statement of the American Diabetes Association. *Diabetes Care*. 2005;28(1):186-212.
85. Roldan MB, Alonso M, Barrio R. Thyroid autoimmunity in children and adolescents with type 1 diabetes mellitus. *Diabetes Nutr Metab*. 1999;12(1):27-31.

Chapter 257

DIAPER RASH

Gregory S. Liptak, MD, MPH

Diaper rash is the most common skin disorder of infants and toddlers, occurring in 1 out of 4 infants.[1] A survey of suburban infants revealed that 25% had some diaper dermatitis, and 4% had a severe rash.[2] The greatest frequency occurs in infants between 9 and 12 months of age.[3] Diaper rash is not a single disorder, but rather a reaction of the skin to a host of factors, both local and systemic; on occasion, it may result from serious illness.

ETIOLOGY

Diaper rashes occur because infants wear diapers. In the 1940s, infants wore diapers made out of cotton; first, latex pants, then, plastic pants were used as an outer cover over the diapers. The disposable diaper became available in the 1960s. This product was followed by superabsorbent material covered by plastic. Today, diapers are made of superabsorbent material covered by a breathable cover.[4] Four factors have been associated with the occurrence of diaper rash: (1) wetness of the skin, (2) elevated pH level of the skin, (3) fecal enzymes (especially proteases and lipases), and (4) microorganisms, especially *Candida*.[5,6] Wet skin has a reduced ability to withstand frictional forces, whereas elevated pH and enzymes increase permeability. In 1 study, infants whose diapers had been changed 8 or more times during the day (and presumably were drier) had fewer rashes than those whose diapers were changed less often.[7] Diapers made with water-absorbent gel material keep skin drier and decrease the occurrence of diaper rash.[8-10] The normal pH of the skin is between 4.5 and 5.5. Elevated pH has been associated with more severe diaper rash. High pH increases the activity of fecal proteases and lipases; it also decreases normal skin microflora.[11] Although ammonia once was believed to be the primary irritant causing diaper rash,[12] it is no longer considered to be the major factor.

Fecal proteases and lipases along with moisture lead to the maceration of the skin and increase permeability to substances such as bile salts, which worsen the inflammation. Infants who have more frequent bowel movements, such as those who have gastroenteritis or who are taking antibiotics, have a higher prevalence of diaper dermatitis, presumably caused by increased enzymes, yeast, and, perhaps, pathogenic bacteria.[8] Infants who are breastfed have lower levels of enzymes in their stools, lower urinary pH, and fewer diaper rashes (Figure 257-1).

The most important microorganism found on the skin of infants who have diaper rash is *Candida albicans*. This yeast, which produces a protease that penetrates the skin, can (1) cause a primary infection, (2) be a secondary invader in systemic conditions such as seborrheic dermatitis, and (3) be found in many infants who have nonspecific diaper rash. Even a small number of *Candida* organisms can cause significant infection. In 1 survey, candidal species were isolated from one half the mouths of healthy infants.[13] Infants who routinely sucked a pacifier had a higher rate of oral candidal carriage. The use of oral or parenteral antibiotics can increase the number of *Candida* organisms on the skin, as well as the frequency of stools, and contribute to the occurrence of diaper rash.[14] *Staphylococcus aureus* also has been isolated as a secondary invader of systemic illness, such as atopic dermatitis; however, although present on the skin, it does not appear to be a common primary pathogen in other forms of diaper rashes.[15]

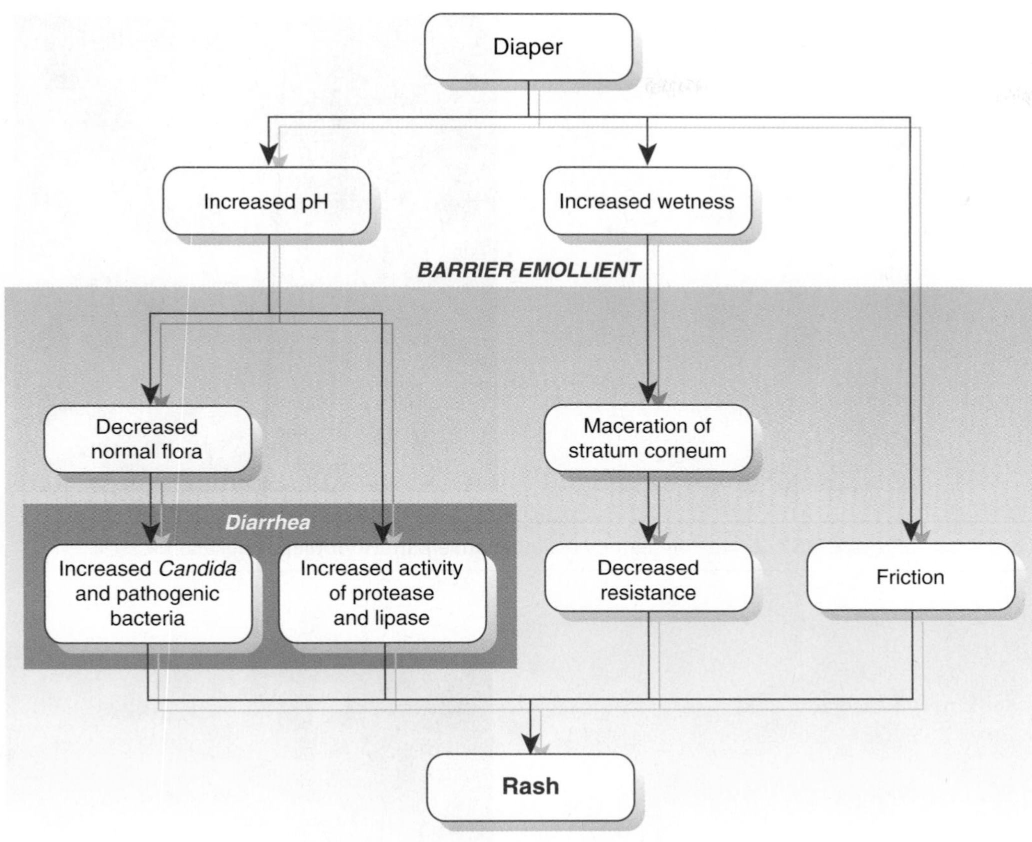

Figure 257-1 Pathogenesis of irritant diaper dermatitis, showing effects of diarrhea and barrier emollient.

PATHOLOGIC STUDIES

A few histopathologic studies of diaper rash have been described; however, most of these have dealt with unusual or chronic cases. The more common diaper rashes are believed to cause nonspecific inflammatory changes.

HISTORY

Historical factors that may help determine the factors contributing to diaper rash include duration of the rash, associated symptoms (eg, diarrhea), type of diaper, frequency of changing, method of laundering (if cloth diapers are used), use of outer coverings such as plastic or rubber pants, past illness (especially dermatologic, allergic, and infectious), medication use (eg, antibiotics) that would include the therapy for the rash, exposure to contagious disease (eg, scabies, varicella), the presence of systemic symptoms, and a family history of illness (eg, psoriasis, allergy).

PHYSICAL EXAMINATION

Although diaper rashes can be classified by presentation (appearance and location), this approach should be viewed with caution because 1 agent (eg, *C albicans*) can lead to different presentations, and a single presentation may be caused by many agents (acting either alone or in concert).

Three common distribution patterns for diaper rash occur. Chafing, or irritant dermatitis (Figure 257-2), is an erythematous desquamative rash involving the convex surfaces that touch the diaper and spare the inguinal folds. Erythema is mild, with or without papules. The skin has a shiny, glazed appearance. This rash is associated with the irritants mentioned previously. Meatitis may be seen in boys who have this type of diaper rash. Diaper rashes that have persisted for more than 72 hours are usually found to have significant *Candida* involvement.[16]

Atopic dermatitis may have the same distribution as chafing, as do zinc deficiency, Kawasaki disease, and Wiskott-Aldrich syndrome. The eczematoid appearance with lichenification (thickening), pruritus, and the occurrence of the atopic dermatitis elsewhere on the child should help substantiate this diagnosis. Diaper rash caused by atopic dermatitis is uncommon in children younger than 6 months.

The second pattern of diaper dermatitis involves skinfolds and spares convex surfaces (Figure 257-3). Rashes involving the perianal area only are common in the neonatal period and may be the result of irritation from diarrhea (and are especially common in children whose diarrhea is secondary to disaccharidase

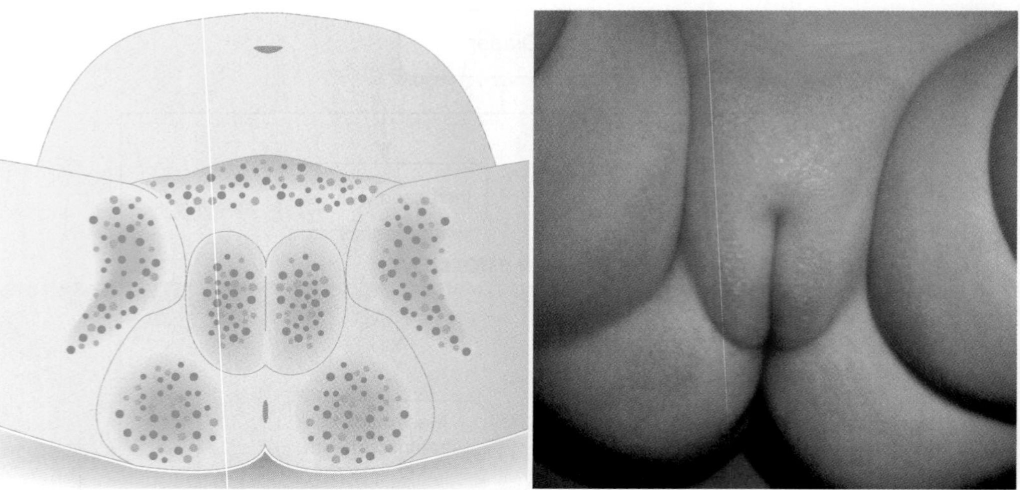

Figure 257-2 Erythematous desquamative pattern of diaper dermatitis.

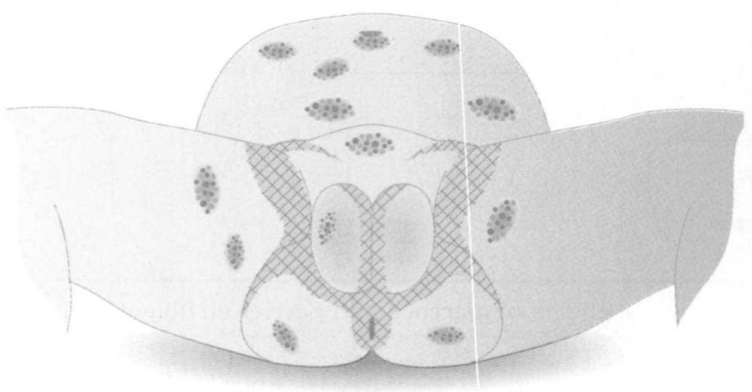

Figure 257-3 Intertriginous pattern of diaper dermatitis.

deficiency). They also may be caused by infection with *C albicans*.

Moist, macerated symmetrical eruptions in the skin-folds and creases may result from intertrigo, an ill-defined entity. It commonly becomes infected secondarily by *C albicans*, especially when satellite lesions are present. The classic primary candidal (monilial) diaper rash has this pattern, with bright red confluent lesions, often with raised borders and occasionally with pustular-vesicular satellite lesions on the trunk and legs. Other areas, such as the folds of the neck, the postauricular area, and the oral mucosa (thrush), may be involved. Dermatitis caused by *Candida* organisms usually is painful and tender. The rash of Langerhans cell histiocytosis may have the same distribution as *Candida* infection but is more papular, hemorrhagic and more likely to be eroded. It also fails to respond to conventional therapy; the child may have constitutional symptoms such as malaise and abnormal physical findings such as hepatosplenomegaly. Seborrheic dermatitis is characterized by erythematous, often salmon-colored, patches with greasy scale that involve

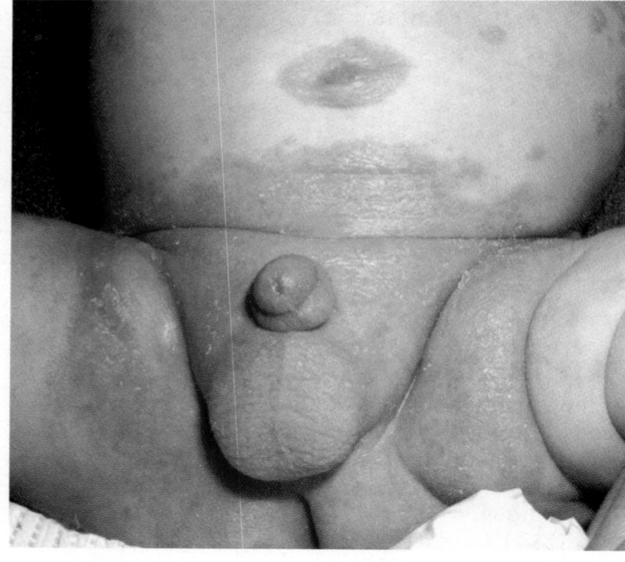

Figure 257-4 Seborrheic dermatitis is characterized by erythema that involves intertriginous and convex areas.

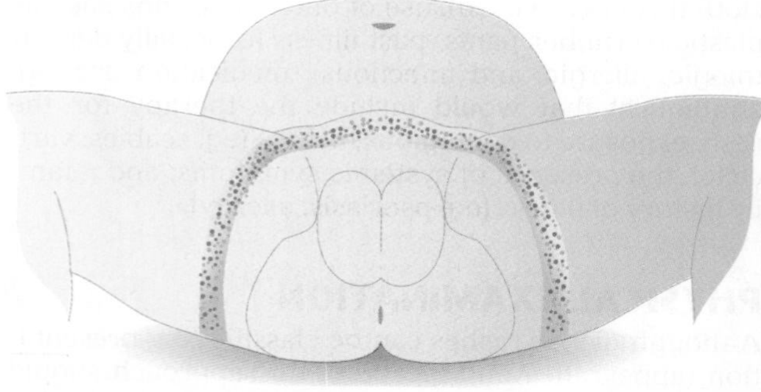

Figure 257-5 Constrictive pattern of diaper dermatitis.

Table 257-1 Less Common Conditions Associated With Diaper Rash

CONDITIONS	COMMENTS
INFECTIOUS OR PRESUMED INFECTIOUS	
Herpes simplex virus	Vesicular; may be associated with immunosuppression
Cytomegalovirus	Usually associated with immunosuppression
Kawasaki disease	Desquamating rash associated with fever
Syphilis	May have other manifestations of secondary syphilis
Trichophyton	Extremely uncommon; annular scaly patches
NEOPLASTIC	
Histiocytosis (Letterer-Siwe disease)	Resembles seborrhea plus reddish brown papules
NUTRITIONAL AND METABOLIC	
Zinc deficiency (acrodermatitis enteropathica)	Mimics monilial rash; vesicular eruptions elsewhere
PRESUMED IATROGENIC	
Granuloma gluteale infantum	May be secondary to use of halogenated steroid creams
GENETIC	
Wiskott-Aldrich syndrome	Thrombocytopenia and recurrent infections in boys

the convexities and creases (Figure 257-4). Distinguishing seborrheic dermatitis from psoriasis may be difficult, although the latter disorder is characterized by lesions that have a deeper red color.

The third major distribution pattern of diaper dermatitis is shown in Figure 257-5. Erythema in this distribution has been termed *tide mark dermatitis* and is believed to be related to frequent cycles of wetting and drying. Irritation from diapers that are too tight (constrictive) and that may have an elastic band also can lead to a similar rash.

Diaper rashes that do not fit any of these patterns, for example, from herpes simplex virus infection, also occur. In 1 study, the less a rash had the appearance of the one shown in Figure 257-3, the more likely it was to be associated with *Candida* organisms.[8] Diaper dermatitis from any cause can become secondarily infected with *Staphylococcus* or *Streptococcus* organisms, leading to impetigo, bullous impetigo, or staphylococcal scalded skin.

DIFFERENTIAL DIAGNOSIS

Systemic conditions such as seborrhea, atopic dermatitis, hand-foot-and-mouth disease, primary herpes simplex infection, psoriasis, varicella, miliaria, and scabies may begin or occur with greater intensity in the diaper area[17] and may be altered morphologically.[18] Such predilections for the diaper area probably represent the Koebner (isomorphic) response in which the skin lesions of a systemic illness concentrate on areas previously inflamed by other factors, for example, friction.

In addition to the aforementioned conditions, Langerhans cell histiocytosis, acrodermatitis enteropathica,[19] congenital syphilis, granuloma gluteale infantum,[20] and Wiskott-Aldrich syndrome may lead to rashes that are prominent in the diaper area. Table 257-1 lists some of the less common causes of diaper rash. Kawasaki disease may produce a red, desquamating perineal eruption, often during the first week after onset of the syndrome[21] (see Chapter 289, Kawasaki Disease).

Serious illness must always be considered in the child who has an atypical or a severe rash, as well as in the child who fails to respond to customary therapy. For instance, the child who has what appears to be severe seborrhea may have Langerhans cell histiocytosis or Wiskott-Aldrich syndrome. Severe, persistent, and recurrent infections with *Candida* organisms may (albeit rarely) result from immunodeficiency, including infection with human immunodeficiency virus or diabetes mellitus. Children who are immunosuppressed from human immunodeficiency virus infection or neoplasia (or its treatment) may have diaper rash from organisms such as herpes simplex virus or cytomegalovirus. If an immunosuppressed child has a serious or unresponsive diaper rash, then aggressive pursuit of an etiologic agent, including skin biopsy, should be considered.[22] The physician should suspect child (including sexual) abuse or neglect in the child who has lesions in the diaper area (especially burns) that are inconsistent with the history provided.

LABORATORY FINDINGS

Laboratory tests are generally not indicated for most diaper rashes. Tests that may be helpful in identifying the cause of a diaper rash include a potassium hydroxide preparation and a fungal culture of skin scrapings for *Candida* organisms, a bacterial culture for *Staphylococcus* organisms, a mineral oil slide preparation for scabies, a serum zinc level (to rule out acrodermatitis enteropathica), serologic tests for syphilis, and radiograms of the skull and long bones for evidence of child abuse. Rarely, a skin biopsy may be useful in cases in which the diaper rash is atypical or unresponsive to therapy.

MANAGEMENT

Because most diaper rashes, whatever the cause, are worsened by prolonged contact with wet or soiled diapers, the initial step in their management should be to minimize contact with soiled diapers. Because total abstinence from diapers is impractical, most clinicians recommend that during therapy, the diapers be changed frequently (at least 8 times a day, using breathable diapers with absorbent gel material), and stool should be wiped off the skin as soon as possible. Plastic pants that retain water should not be used, and breaks from wearing diapers should be offered as much as possible. In the past, a damp cotton washcloth was used most often. Commercial disposable baby wipes, which typically contain water, an emollient, and surfactants, are less irritating to the skin than cotton washcloths and may be better for cleaning intertriginous areas.[23] These wipes are also well tolerated by children who have atopic dermatitis.[24]

Most systemic conditions such as scabies, atopic dermatitis, and varicella can be managed for the diaper area as they are for other parts of the skin. Seborrheic dermatitis, however, is an exception. Because the diaper area is often infected secondarily with *Candida* organisms, measures to treat the yeast must be undertaken as well. For this and other diaper rashes in which *Candida* organisms are present, topical nystatin, miconazole, clotrimazole, haloprogin, or ketoconazole should be applied for 5 to 10 days. Agents such as miconazole and clotrimazole have the advantage of requiring only twice-daily application. Gentian violet also is effective but is extremely messy and is rarely if ever indicated. The simultaneous use of 1% hydrocortisone may be used to decrease inflammation. Steroids that are more potent than 1% hydrocortisone should never be used in the diaper area because diapers form an occlusive dressing. Their chronic use may lead to skin atrophy, telangiectasis, granuloma gluteale, striae, and, possibly, Cushing syndrome. The effectiveness of oral nystatin in the therapy of candidal diaper rash is uncertain. In a controlled study,[25] oral nystatin did not decrease the recurrence of candidal diaper rash significantly. In another controlled trial,[26] oral fluconazole was more effective than nystatin in eliminating oral *Candida* in infants who had oral thrush. Oral fluconazole is also effective for candida diaper rash in the absence of thrush and can be used if other therapies have failed.

For irritant diaper dermatitis, changing diapers frequently, washing the skin with plain water or with disposable baby wipes, and allowing the skin to dry between diaper changes are usually the only interventions needed. The use of diapers with absorbent gel materials has been shown to decrease wetness in the diaper area and may hasten the disappearance of a diaper dermatitis.[9] Scrubbing the rash or diaper area should be discouraged. Barrier pastes and ointments form a resistant covering over the skin surface and decrease friction. Insufficient evidence exists to choose one product over another. Rinsing cloth diapers in methylbenzethonium chloride (diaparene), a bacteriostatic agent, or in a vinegar solution (1 ounce in a gallon of water) has been shown to reduce recurrences.[7] Agents to acidify the urine (cranberry juice, vitamin C), cornstarch, and ointments that contain vitamins A and D are widely used, although no experimental evidence supports their efficacy. Eliminating fabric softeners and changing detergents may be effective in some cases, but the value of this approach also is undocumented scientifically. In cases of significant inflammation, 1% hydrocortisone may promote healing. The meatitis that occurs in this form of rash may be treated with topical antibiotics (any antibiotic solutions available in ophthalmologic containers can be used) to prevent stricture. One study showed that miconazole in a zinc oxide-petrolatum base was more effective in eliminating moderate to severe diaper rashes (even without direct evidence of candidiasis) than the base alone.[27]

Many more children have been harmed by well-intended diaper rash therapies than have ever been harmed by the rash itself. Boric acid, mercury compounds, and pentachlorophenol used in the treatment and prevention of irritative diaper rash have led to illness and death in infants. Talcum powder never should be used because it provides no protection, is abrasive, and inhalation of a large quantity can produce serious, even fatal, pulmonary damage. The dangers of topical steroids are numerous. In a nationally representative survey, 16% of diaper rashes were treated with a combination of nystatin and triamcinolone, a mid-potency steroid that should not be used in the diaper area.[1] In a survey of pediatricians,[28] 23% who prescribed clotrimazole-betamethasone diproprionate (Lotrisone) did so for diaper dermatitis. Betamethasone diproprionate is a high-potency steroid and is not indicated for the diaper area. Hair dryers should never be recommended as a means to dry the skin in the diaper area because perineal burns may result. Products containing iodochlorhydroxyquin, such as Vioform or Iodo Plain, should never be used because systemic absorption may lead to optic atrophy and neuropathy. Prudent use of therapeutic agents is necessary to avoid harm.

PREVENTION

If no diapers existed, no diaper rashes would occur. Because the complete elimination of diapers is unacceptable, alternatives to keep the skin dry, such as changing as soon as the diaper becomes wet or soiled and avoiding plastic or rubber pants, have been recommended.

Most recent studies have shown that disposable diapers that contain absorbent gel are associated with the lowest incidence of diaper rashes in otherwise healthy children and those who have atopic dermatitis.[9,10,29] Disposable diapers with covers that are breathable are associated with lower counts of *Candida* and reduced occurrence of diaper rash.[30] A recent Cochrane review concluded, however, that not enough evidence from quality randomized controlled trials exists to choose one type of disposable diapers over another.[31]

The effect of disposable diapers on the environment has received a great deal of attention.[31,32] Commercial, nonbiodegradable diapers are estimated to make up 1% to 2% of landfills. The cost of their disposal, which is borne by all citizens, should be considered when recommending their use. On the other hand, washing cloth diapers (and soiled clothes and bed linens) requires water, detergent, and energy, as well as human labor.[33] Parents who usually use cloth diapers may consider using commercial diapers that contain absorbent gel materials when their children are at increased risk for developing diaper rash, such as when they are taking antibiotics or have gastroenteritis. Commercial diapers are also convenient during travel away from home.

Breastfeeding and frequent diaper changes are associated with a lower occurrence of diaper rash; thus both should be recommended. Airing the diaper area, using barrier creams and ointments, cleansing the diaper area promptly, selecting the diaper, and educating caregivers should prevent many diaper rashes. The physician should educate parents about commonly used home remedies for diaper rash that might be harmful to children.

WHEN TO REFER

- If the rash has not responded to conventional treatment in several weeks or is worsening
- If the rash is nodular
- If abuse is suspected

WHEN TO ADMIT

If the child is systemically ill and cannot be treated safely at home or has severe illness such as septicemia

TOOLS FOR PRACTICE

Engaging Patients and Family

- *Treating Diaper Rash* (fact sheet), American Academy of Pediatrics (www.aap.org/topics.html).
- *Diaper Rash* (brochure), American Academy of Pediatrics (patiented.aap.org).

REFERENCES

1. Ward DB, Fleischer AB Jr, Feldman SR, et al. Characterization of diaper dermatitis in the United States. *Arch Pediatr Adolesc Med.* 2000;154:943-946.
2. Jacobs AH. Eruptions in the diaper area, *Pediatr Clin North Am.* 1978;25:209-224.
3. Benjamin L. Clinical correlates with diaper dermatitis. *Pediatrician.* 1987;14:21-26.
4. Richer Investment Consulting Services. Disposable Diaper History. Available at: www.richernet.com/history.htm. Accessed January 13, 2006.
5. Ferrazzini G, Kaiser RR, Hirsig Cheng SK, et al. Microbiological aspects of diaper dermatitis. *Dermatology.* 2003;206:136-141.
6. Berg RW, Buckingham KW, Stewart RL. Etiologic factors in diaper dermatitis: the role of urine. *Pediatr Dermatol.* 1986;3:102-106.
7. Grant WW, Street L, Fearnow RG. Diaper rashes in infancy: studies on the effects of various methods of laundering. *Clin Pediatr.* 1973;12:714-746.
8. Campbell RL, Bartlett AV, Sarbaugh FC, et al. Effects of diaper types on diaper dermatitis associated with diarrhea and antibiotic use in children in day-care centers. *Pediatr Dermatol.* May 1988;5(2):83-87.
9. Lane AT, Rehder PA, Helm K. Evaluations of diapers containing absorbing gelling material with conventional diapers in newborn infants. *Am J Dis Child.* 1990;144:315-318.
10. Seymour JL, Keswick BH, Hanifin JM, et al. Clinical effects of diaper types on the skin of normal infants and infants with atopic dermatitis. *J Am Acad Dermatol.* Dec 1987;17(6):988-997.
11. Atherton DJ. The aetiology and management of irritant diaper dermatitis. *J Eur Acad Dermatol Venereol.* 2001; 15(suppl 1):1-4.
12. Leyden JJ, Katz S, Stewart R, et al. Urinary ammonia and ammonia-producing microorganisms in infants with and without diaper dermatitis. *Arch Dermatol.* Dec 1977; 113(12):1678-1680.
13. Darwazeh AM, al Bashir AJ. Oral candidal flora in healthy infants. Oral Pathol Med. 1995;24:361-364.
14. Brook I. The effects of amoxicillin therapy on skin flora in infants. *Pediatr Dermatol.* Sep-Oct 2000;17(5);360-363.
15. Leyden JJ, Klingman AM. The role of microorganisms in diaper dermatitis. *Arch Dermatol.* 1978;114:56-59.
16. Benjamin L. Clinical correlates with diaper dermatitis. *Pediatrician.* 1987;14(suppl 1):21-26.
17. Jenson HB, Shapiro ED. Primary herpes simplex virus infection of a diaper rash. *Pediatr Infect Dis J.* 1987;6: 1136-1138.
18. Messner J, Miller JJ, James WD, et al. Accentuated viral exanthems in areas of inflammation. *J Am Acad Dermatol.* Feb 1999;40(2 Pt 2):345-346.
19. Munro CS, Lazaro C, Lawrence CM. Symptomatic zinc deficiency in breast fed premature infants. *Br J Dermatol.* 1989;121:773-778.
20. Bluestein J, Furner BB, Phillips SD. Granuloma gluteale infantum: case report and review of the literature. *Pediatr Dermatol.* 1990;7:196-198.
21. Friter BS, Lucky AW. The perineal eruption of Kawasaki syndrome. I. 1988;124:1805-1810.
22. Thiboutot DM, Beckford A, Mart CR, et al. Cytomegalovirus diaper dermatitis. *Arch Dermatol.* Mar 1991;127(3): 396-398.
23. Odio M, Streicher-Scott J, Hansen RC. Disposable baby wipes: efficacy and skin mildness. *Dermatol Nurs.* 2001; 13:107-108, 121.
24. Ehretsmann C, Schaefer P, Adam R. Cutaneous tolerance of baby wipes by infants with atopic dermatitis, and comparison of the mildness of baby wipe and water in infant skin. *J Eur Acad Dermatol Venereol.* 2001;15(suppl 1): 16-21.
25. Hoppe JE, Hahn H. Randomized comparison of two nystatin oral gels with miconazole oral gel for treatment of oral thrush in infants. *Infection.* 1996;24:136-139.
26. Goins RA, Ascher D, Waecker N, et al. Comparison of fluconazole and nystatin oral suspensions for treatment of oral candidiasis in infants. *Pediatr Infect Dis J.* Dec 2002;21(12):1165-1167.
27. Concannon P, Gisoldi E, Phillips S, et al. Diaper dermatitis: a therapeutic dilemma. Results of a double-blind placebo controlled trial of miconazole nitrate 0.25%. *Pediatr Dermatol.* 2001;18:149-155.
28. Railan D, Wilson JK, Feldman SR, et al. Pediatricians who prescribe clotrimazole-betamethasone diproprionate (Lotrisone) often utilize it in inappropriate settings regardless of their knowledge of the drug's potency. *Dermatol Online J.* 2002;8:3.
29. Jordan WE, Lawson KD, Berg RW, et al. Diaper dermatitis: frequency and severity among a general infant population. *Pediatr Dermatol.* Jun 1986;3(3):198-207.
30. Akin F, Spraker M, Aly R, et al. Effects of breathable disposable diapers: reduced prevalence of Candida and common diaper dermatitis. *Pediatr Dermatol.* 2001;18: 282-290.
31. Baer EL, Davies MW, Easterbrook KJ. Disposable nappies for preventing napkin dermatitis in infants. *Cochrane Database Syst Rev.* 2006 Jul 19;3:CD004262.
32. Office of Waste Reduction Services. Case Study: Nondisposal Diapers–A Cost Effective Change. Available at: es.epa.gov/techinfo/case/michigan/mich-cs5.html. Accessed January 13, 2006.

33. Smith JA, Pitts N. The Diaper Decision—Not a Clear Issue. Available at: www.mindfully.org/plastic/diaper-not-clear.htm. Accessed January 13, 2006.
34. Wong DL, Brantly D, Clutter LB, et al. Diapering choices: a critical review of the issues. *Pediatr Nurs.* Jan-Feb 1992; 18(1):41-54.

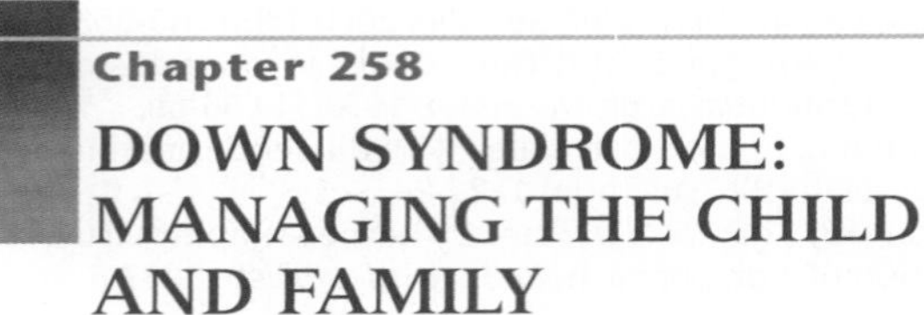

Chapter 258

DOWN SYNDROME: MANAGING THE CHILD AND FAMILY

Erawati V. Bawle, MD

INTRODUCTION

Primary care physicians are key professionals in the medical care of children with Down syndrome (DS) because they are best able to provide a medical home for the child and the family. Caring for children with DS and their families requires long-term commitment and interest on the part of the primary care physician to ensure that such children realize their full potential and families receive the support and education they need. This chapter provides current information about the special health care needs of children with DS and guidelines for meeting these needs. The guidelines also include coordination of care with medical subspecialists and early childhood educators.

INCIDENCE

By current national prevalence estimates, DS occurs in approximately 1 in every 732 births.[1] The incidence of DS is closely related to the advanced age of the mother, and the likelihood of bearing a fetus who has DS increases when maternal age is older than 35 years.[2] Recent advances have improved noninvasive techniques for identifying fetuses with DS. Regardless of maternal age, this screening should be offered to all pregnant women. Screening using a combination of maternal age and multiple serum markers, namely alpha-fetoprotein (AFP), unconjugated estriol (uE3), human chorionic gonadotropin (hCG), and dimeric inhibin A (DIA) in the second trimester of pregnancy can detect 75% of fetuses with DS with a false-positive rate of 5%.[3] Screening during the first trimester at 10 to 14 weeks using fetal nuchal translucency, maternal serum free beta human chorionic gonadotropin and pregnancy-associated plasma protein-A (PAPA) has been shown to improve the detection rate to 89% with a false-positive rate of 5%.[4] First-trimester screening may become the standard method of screening in the future.

ETIOLOGY

DS is caused by a chromosomal aberration, trisomy 21. Most individuals (95%) with trisomy 21 have 3 free copies of chromosome 21; in approximately 5% of patients, 1 copy of chromosome 21 is translocated to another chromosome, most often chromosome 14 or 21.[5] In 2% to 4% of cases with free trisomy 21, mosaicism is recognizable for a trisomic and a normal cell line.

Origin of Free Trisomy 21

Trisomy 21 occurs because of an abnormality in chromosome replication during meiosis. The abnormality, known as nondisjunction, occurs during meiosis. Normally during meiosis the process of disjunction reduces the number of chromosomes in the germ cell (sperm and ovum) from 46 to 23. At fertilization, the egg and sperm unite, giving the developing fetus the full number of 46 chromosomes in 23 pairs. Nondisjunction is the improper division of the 46 chromosomes in the egg or the sperm, resulting in 1 carrying 24 chromosomes. At fertilization, the germ cell with 24 chromosomes unites with the germ cell with 23 chromosomes, resulting in a total of 47 chromosomes. DNA testing has shown that nondisjunction of chromosomes in the 21 group takes place in the egg 95% of the time.[6] In 95% of individuals who have DS, an extra chromosome is found in the 21 group (the extra chromosome plus the normal pair), which is designated trisomy.[6] A small group of patients with DS with free trisomy 21 (2% to 3%) have a mixture of cell types (mosaicism), some cells with 46 chromosomes and some with 47. The proportion of trisomic cells to cells with normal chromosomes can vary greatly from person to person and from tissue to tissue in the same person. The mosaicism is usually detected in the lymphocytes from a peripheral blood sample; thus tests on other tissues are unnecessary. In some instances, cultured fibroblasts from a skin biopsy are analyzed when low-level mosaicism is suspected. Experts do not know if any tissues are spared of trisomy cells. This mosaicism often results from an error in maternal meiosis and only in a few cases is likely to result after fertilization owing to an error in mitosis.

Origin of Translocation Trisomy 21

Translocation refers to a chromosome rearrangement in which part of the extra chromosome attaches to yet another chromosome. In the case of DS the long arm of one of the chromosome 21 often attaches to another chromosome 21, 22, or 14. The karyotype shows the number of chromosomes as 46 and shows the abnormally attached additional chromosomal material. In one third of cases of 14:21 translocation-type DS, one of the parents is a carrier of a balanced translocation. The mother is the carrier 90% of the time. The remaining cases of 14:21 translocation type DS are de novo and the translocation occurs in the non-carrier mother's egg cell during meiosis. In DS children with a 21:21 translocation 93% of cases are de novo translocations. In de novo cases the 21:21 translocation occurs because of a meiotic error in the egg cell. In about 7% of cases the 21:21 translocation is the result of a balanced translocation in a carrier parent. In cases where the 21:21 translocation is passed from carrier parent to child the carrier is equally likely to be the mother as the father.

All of these types of DS (free trisomy 21 or translocation trisomy 21) produce the same clinical features of DS. The mosaic type of DS may have less distinct physical features and, in most cases, may show higher intellectual function, depending on the percentage of cells with trisomy 21.[7,8] Very low levels of trisomy 21 cells are reported in DS patients with higher intellectual function.

Molecular Pathological Features of Trisomy 21

The DNA sequence of chromosome 21[9] is now known, and more than 100 genes have been identified. A DS critical region on the long arm (q arm) has been identified; however, other genes outside this region of chromosome 21 also contribute to the clinical features of DS. This finding strongly suggests that DS is a contiguous gene syndrome with triplicate gene dose effects, which makes it unlikely that a single DS chromosomal region is responsible for most of the DS phenotypic features. The risk of DS in subsequent pregnancies for nondisjunction trisomy 21 is approximately 1 in 100 for women younger than 35 years and age related for older women.[2] A higher recurrence risk may exist for the translocation types of DS if the mother has a balanced translocation.

DIAGNOSIS

The birth of a child who has DS presents an abundance of clinical and family issues. The first critical task is making an accurate and prompt diagnosis, which can often be accomplished at the bedside by means of a thorough examination. When 8 of the many characteristics commonly associated with DS are present (Box 258-1), the diagnosis is relatively simple.[10] However, when the diagnosis is based on 1 or 2 findings, errors can occur. For example, 50% of children who have DS have the 4-finger sign (formerly called a simian crease), but so do 15% of children without DS. Small ears are also characteristic, but not diagnostic, of DS.

Every newborn when clinically suspected of having DS requires chromosome analysis. Confirmation of DS diagnosis by chromosome analysis helps the parents accept the clinical diagnosis. This information also forms the basis of genetic counseling for the parents regarding the risk of recurrence. Chromosomal analysis complements a detailed family history. With this information, the family can make better decisions about future pregnancies.

Many primary care physicians are reluctant to share the diagnosis of DS with the parents unless it is confirmed in the laboratory by karyotyping. Physicians delay informing the family of the diagnosis until it is definitive to avoid giving the family the wrong diagnosis. However, most families prefer that their physician share the suspected diagnosis of DS with them as soon as possible. Informing them at the time of clinical suspicion is desirable. The primary care physicians must decide which approach is best for the individual situation. In most instances, the results of the karyotype can be available in 3 to 7 days with rapid communication with the cytogenetics laboratory.

A woman who has learned that she is carrying a fetus with DS will occasionally contact the primary care physician with questions about the challenges of raising a child who has this disorder. A prenatal genetic counselor may also suggest a consultation with a pediatrician for the expectant parents. A good additional source of information is the National Down Syndrome Congress (800-232-6372). This organization can provide the names of parents who have a child with DS living in the caller's community, as well as information about DS.

BOX 258-1 Common Features of Down Syndrome That May or May Not Be Present

HEAD

Brachycephaly (flat occiput)

EYES

Inner epicanthal folds (*A*)

Upward slanting palpebral fissures (*A*)

FACE (*A*)

Flat appearing

Low nasal bridge (*A*)

Small shell-like ears with small or no earlobes

Brushfield spots (speckling of the iris) (*B*)

FINGERS AND TOES

Single-flexion crease on 5th finger and incurving of the 5th finger (*C*)

Four-finger sign (simian crease): transverse palmar lines (*D*)

Brachydactyly (short fingers) (*D*)

Wide-space between the 1st and 2nd toes (*E*)

HEART (COMMONLY, CONGENITAL DEFECTS)

Endocardial cushion defects

Ventricular septal defects

NECK

Short

Superabundant skin at nape

NEUROMUSCULAR SYSTEM

Absent or diminished Moro reflex

Muscular hypotonia

Joint hyperflexibility

TONGUE

Excessive protrusion

POTENTIAL FOR:

Increased incidence of leukemia

Increased susceptibility to infection

Increased incidence of duodenal atresia

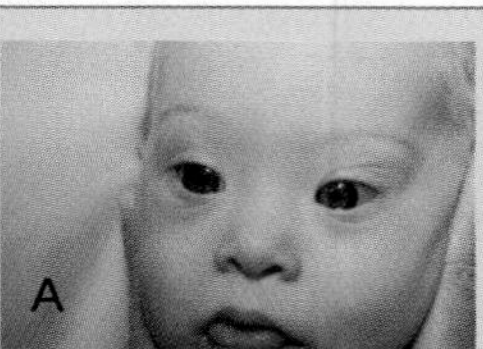
A

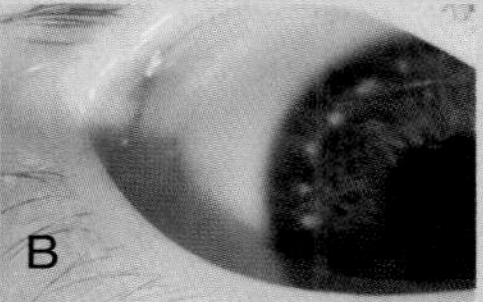
B

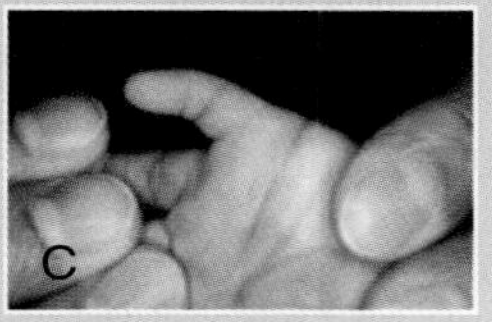
C

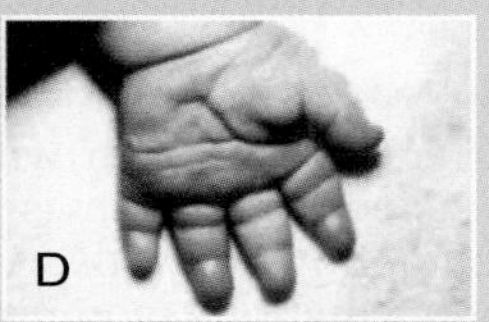
D

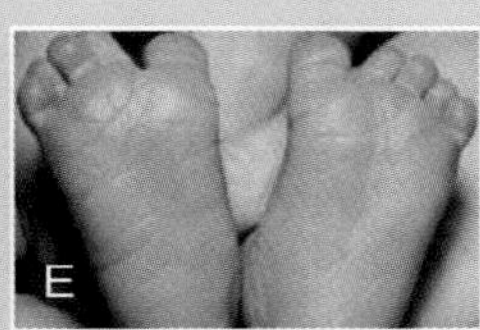
E

MANAGEMENT

Preventive management refers to early detection and correction of medical problems seen in children who have DS. Children with DS require the usual preventive interventions and anticipatory guidance given to other children and families, but the special problems of children who have DS require additional evaluation and close monitoring. The most common types of problems include the following:

1. Growth: failure to thrive and growth retardation
2. Dental: malaligned teeth and periodontal disease
3. Ophthalmologic: refractive errors, strabismus, myopia, and cataracts
4. Otologic: chronic otitis media, and hearing loss
5. Respiratory: obstructive sleep apnea
6. Cardiac: congenital heart defects
7. Endocrine: hypothyroidism and diabetes mellitus
8. Gastrointestinal: constipation and congenital intestinal obstruction
9. Neurologic: delayed development, intellectual disability, seizures, and depression
10. Immunologic disorders and leukemia

Thorough examination and testing should be performed at critical ages to detect these common problems and correct them, if possible.

Newborn to 1 Month of Age

After the newborn with DS is diagnosed clinically, a detailed evaluation is required (see Box 258-2). The child should be observed for signs of gastrointestinal malformations (vomiting, weight loss, and absence of stools), cardiac malformations (cyanosis, murmur, and irregular heart rate), and cataracts (absent red reflex). Duodenal atresia is present in 2% to 15% of cases. Laboratory testing includes karyotyping, thyroid screening, and a complete blood cell count (CBC) with a differential count. Thyroid screening is particularly important because children who have DS have a higher incidence of congenital hypothyroidism (see Chapter 280, Hypothyroidism).[11] Approximately 10% of newborns with DS show leukocytosis with presence of blast cells in the peripheral blood smear, a condition called transient leukemia (transient myeloproliferative disease).[12] Neutrophil and hemoglobin levels are normal. Most children with transient leukemia go into spontaneous remission and recover by the age of 3 months; however, close to 20% develop life-threatening complications. Of those who recover completely, approximately 20% develop acute megakaryocytic leukemia (a type of acute myelogenous leukemia) in the first 4 years of life.[13] Therefore all newborns detected with transient leukemia need follow-up with the hematologist every 3 months for review of the peripheral blood smear. The cure rate for acute megakaryocytic leukemia is more than 80%. Hearing screening is needed because 15% of children who have DS may have congenital hearing loss. A pediatric cardiologist should evaluate the infant for cardiac defects. This evaluation can be performed on an ambulatory basis after trisomy 21 is confirmed if the clinical index of suspicion is low. Once the diagnosis is made, the physician must inform the family fully; the approach must be gentle and hopeful. Some suggestions in this regard include the following:

BOX 258-2 Managing the Newborn

History
1. Evaluate the feeding pattern
2. Evaluate the stooling pattern

Physical examination
1. Perform a general physical examination and a neurologic examination.
2. Check for signs of congenital heart defects.
3. Examine the eyes for congenital cataracts.

Laboratory tests
1. Karyotype
2. Thyroid screening
3. CBC with differential count

Consultation
1. Cardiologic examination
2. Genetics for counseling regarding recurrence risk of DS in future pregnancies and prenatal diagnosis
3. Hematology consultation if CBC suggests transient myeloproliferative disorder

CBC, Complete blood cell count; *DS*, Down syndrome.

1. Avoid discussion over the telephone. Inform both parents together. Meet in a quiet and private place where the physician and parents will not be interrupted.
2. Provide current information to the family; be hopeful. Provide the name and telephone number of a local DS support group. The National Down Syndrome Congress (800-232-6372) will provide the names of local support groups, as well as educational information for the physician and family.
3. Discuss future expectations briefly. Additionally, discuss the potential medical problems, but point out that many children who have DS are healthy and participate in most of the usual childhood activities. Point out that the average life span of those who have DS is now 55 years. Discuss the plan to identify and manage medical problems.
4. Allow time for the parents to respond, to voice concerns, and to raise questions. Parents need the opportunity to express feelings of anger, guilt, or sorrow.
5. Provide written information about DS. Parents find that having something to read after their discussion with the physician is useful. Most information more than 5 years old should be considered outdated.
6. A consultation with a geneticist can help reinforce the discussion provided by the pediatrician, provide information about additional resources such as literature and support groups, and educate the family about prenatal detection and the risk of recurrence.
7. Arrange for a follow-up meeting with the family to give them time to begin adjusting to the new information and to formulate questions. Offer to meet extended family members to answer questions.

Adoption

Most families accept a child born with DS. Some families have greater initial difficulty and require more extended counseling. In rare cases, a family will not be able to accept a child who has DS. In this event, adoption should be discussed. In many instances, families are waiting to adopt children who have DS. The Down Syndrome Adoption Exchange (914-428-1236) can be called for more information.

Follow-Up

In this time of abbreviated hospital stays, the primary care physician should arrange a visit with the parents and child 1 to 2 weeks after discharge. This meeting provides time for further discussion with the family and for a follow-up medical assessment. The results of the karyotype may be unavailable at the time of discharge from the hospital. The risk of DS in future pregnancies and prenatal diagnosis should be discussed when the karyotype is available. An ophthalmologic consultation should be arranged for any abnormalities (eg, lens opacities) seen on the eye examination.

Questions

In the first few weeks of the infant's life the physician may be asked questions about the following:

1. *Oral motor problems*. Anatomic and neuromotor problems often result in a poor suck and frequent spitting. Mild feeding problems such as weak sucking, fatigue during feeding, and uncoordinated breathing while feeding usually resolve in 2 to 3 weeks. However, some measures can help simplify feeding. The parents should be instructed to (1) make sure the child is fully awake when fed at night, (2) clear mucus from the baby's nose before feeding so that breathing will be easier, and (3) support the infant's chin during feeding. The primary care physician should monitor the baby's weight and caloric intake carefully. If feeding problems are particularly severe or do not resolve with these interventions, then referral to an oral motor (swallowing) specialist should be considered.
2. *Breastfeeding problems*. Most infants who have DS can breastfeed successfully. If breastfeeding appears to be going poorly, then the primary care physician should arrange a visit to review the infant's weight gain and the mother's breastfeeding technique. After a medical examination, for particularly severe problems, referral to a lactation specialist may help, or bottle feeding may be needed.
3. *Constipation*. If an infant has constipation despite adequate intake and does not respond to stool softeners, then evaluation for Hirschsprung disease should be considered because 2% of children with DS have Hirschsprung disease (see Chapter 166, Constipation).

Infants 1 Month to 12 Months of Age

In many cases, families who have a child with DS need to see the primary care physician frequently for medical care and education (see Box 258-3). The parents' anxiety and questions decrease with time, but for the initial few months they need to be able to depend on the primary care physician to be available. Finding the extra time in a busy office, where most visits may be for routine checkups or acute care, is often difficult. Following are a few suggestions on how the primary care physician can find time for extended and frequent discussion:

1. Set aside a period each week, perhaps half a day, for consultation and family education. Keep this time free of acute-care office visits.
2. Consider the contribution of a nurse practitioner (eg, to help meet the extra educational and health care needs of the child and family).
3. Use a problem-oriented approach to the record keeping. At the start, set up the medical record with special sections for problems; procedures (date, site, and result of all special medical procedures completed); consultants involved in the child's care (with emergency telephone numbers); an updated, 1-page medical summary to be used for emergency admissions and consultations; and a flowchart of significant laboratory data and medications.
4. Provide special check-out instructions for covering or on-call physicians, especially if they are outside the office and not familiar with the patient.

Mortality

Medical care for infants in this age group who have DS involves particular diagnostic and consultative procedures, given that more than 50% have serious medical disorders. The first year of life holds the highest probability of death for children with DS when an

BOX 258-3 Managing the Infant: Ages 1 Month to 12 Months

Health concerns

History

1. Evaluate the parents' concerns.
2. Inquire about any otitis media and upper respiratory tract infection.
3. Assess the infant's nutritional intake.

Perform or refer the patient for the following tests and examinations:

Physical examination

1. Plot growth on a DS growth chart.
2. Perform a complete neurologic examination and a physical examination, looking for strabismus, cataract, and nystagmus.
3. Administer age-appropriate immunizations.

Laboratory test—thyroid screening

Consultation

1. Cardiologic examination
2. Ophthalmologic consultation at 6 months
3. Audiologic screening

Psychosocial concerns—habilitation

1. Refer the parents to an infant education program.
2. Continue educating the family about DS, and review risk of DS in future pregnancies.

DS, Down syndrome.

additional anomaly exists.[14] Approximately 78% survive with an additional anomaly, and 96% survive without an anomaly. Survival of children with cardiac malformations has improved; only 8% to 9% mortality in children with DS and heart defects is now reported.[15] Leukemia as a cause of death is present in less than 10% of cases.[16]

Physical Examination

On physical examination, the primary care physician should check thoroughly for signs of cardiac and neurologic disorders. Because frequent episodes of otitis media and upper respiratory tract infection are common in this age group, the tympanic membranes should be inspected with particular care. Hearing screening should be repeated if the newborn testing is equivocal or if signs of recurrent middle ear effusion are seen. A pediatric ophthalmologist needs to evaluate DS children at 6 months of age. The primary care physician can identify failure to thrive by plotting and monitoring the infant's weight and height on the DS growth chart.[17] Further evaluation may be indicated for pulmonary, cardiac, and gastrointestinal malformations.

Laboratory Evaluation

Celiac disease is one of the disorders that must be considered when infants who have DS exhibit failure to thrive or diarrhea.[18] Serum immunoglobulin A antigliadin antibody and anti–tissue transglutaminase antibody levels are useful for screening for celiac disease.

Thyroid function should be assessed by checking serum free thyroxine, free triiodothyronine, and thyroid-stimulating hormone levels at the age of 6 months and at the end of the first year. Because clinical signs of hypothyroidism are often subtle, routine screening should be performed. Acquired hypothyroidism is reported in approximately 9% to 35% of individuals with DS.[18-20]

Questions

During office visits for periodic health assessments, the primary care physician should ask about the infant's feeding and discuss enrollment in an early education program. Extra time should be arranged at office visits to allow families to talk about how they are adjusting. The practitioner should review with them information about DS provided earlier. The family should also be informed about Supplemental Security Income (SSI) and other government programs that help families financially with the extra costs of raising a child who has special needs.

Parents of infants who have DS often ask questions about the following issues:

1. *Tongue protrusion*. The factors that produce tongue protrusion include a small oral cavity and mouth breathing. Behavior-management techniques can be used to manage tongue protrusion. Oro-motor exercises may alleviate tongue protrusion.
2. *Controversial therapies*. Some families contemplate controversial therapies as a means of obtaining a magical cure for their child, for example, tongue resection to improve speech and silicone implants to correct micrognathia. Improvement in speech after tongue resection has not been observed.[21] The primary care physician should try to inform families about the risks and benefits of any surgical procedures. Preparations high in vitamins and minerals initially seemed to result in increased intelligence scores.[22] However, because no studies to date have replicated these results, and because side effects from megavitamin regimens have been reported,[23] unproved megavitamin and mineral therapies should be avoided. Routine nutritional screening should be performed at health assessment visits and vitamins prescribed when warranted by standard criteria.

Child 1 Year to 5 Years of Age

Children with DS need an annual health assessment (see Box 258-4). At these office visits, the primary care physician should ask about respiratory infections, constipation, hearing problems, and symptoms of sleep apnea (eg, snoring, difficulty breathing during sleep, sleep position, excessive drowsiness during the day). The studies suggested for DS children 1 to 5 years of age include thyroid, vision, and hearing screening annually.

Behavior Problems

The primary care physician also should ask about behavior problems. The personalities of many children who have DS do not fit the stereotype of being placid

BOX 258-4 Managing the Child: Ages 1 Year to 5 Years

Health concerns

History

1. Assess any parental concerns about the child's behavior and school program.
2. Ask if the child has shown any symptoms of a vision or hearing disorder.
3. Ask about snoring, restless sleep, and sleeping positions.

Perform

1. Complete physical examination
2. Height and weight plotted on a DS growth chart

Laboratory tests

1. Thyroid hormone screening each year
2. Consider a cervical spine roentgenogram

Consultation

1. Eye examination every 2 years
2. Hearing test every 6 months till age 3, annually thereafter
3. Dental examination twice a year

Psychosocial concerns—habilitation

1. Discuss behavioral management, sibling adjustments. Review the child's education program.
2. Review dietary habits and physical activity pattern.
3. Review recurrence risk of Down syndrome and prenatal diagnosis.

or compliant, and parents may not volunteer information about obstinacy or noncompliance. When the child seems to have a behavior disorder, a thorough history should be obtained, and the parents should be asked about changes in the environment or their expectations. A complete physical examination should be performed, as well as laboratory tests, if warranted, to identify medical problems that may lead to behavior disorders. A trial of behavior management should be initiated for mild problems, and the diagnoses of pervasive developmental disability or physical abuse should be considered for serious behavior disorders. For severe behavior problems or persistent mild to moderate problems that have no medical cause, the child should be referred to a behavior specialist.

Learning Problems

The primary care physician needs to review the current individual educational program (IEP) to ensure that appropriate developmental testing has been completed and that the parents have had an opportunity to provide information in the IEP process. School problems may come to the physician's attention more often when children who have DS are placed in mainstreamed or regular classes. School learning problems require further evaluation. The history should be reviewed thoroughly to ensure that the parents' and teachers' expectations are appropriate for the child's developmental age. Medical problems that can affect learning and behavior should be identified. For example, the ears should be examined for impacted cerumen that can cause moderate hearing loss. An eye examination should be done to detect cataracts.[24] Vision screening should be performed yearly or more often, if indicated.

Atlantoaxial Instability

The physical examination must include plotting of appropriate measurements on the DS growth chart. It should also include a thorough neurologic examination because atlantoaxial subluxation presents special problems for children who have DS. Atlantoaxial instability, which occurs in approximately 15% of children who have DS, refers to excess mobility of the atlantoaxial joint without neurologic complications.[25] In atlantoaxial instability, a radiogram of the cervical spine in flexion reveals an atlantoodontoid interval greater than 5 mm. Atlantoaxial subluxation, however, refers to backward movement of the odontoid process of the axis, compressing the spinal cord and resulting in the signs and symptoms of cord compression, which may include neck pain, head tilt, progressive weakness, and loss of bladder or bowel control. Neurologic examination reveals long-tract signs such as increased deep-tendon reflexes in the lower extremities, a positive Babinski sign, and ankle clonus. Atlantoaxial subluxation is a neurosurgical emergency and requires immediate referral and treatment. Although atlantoaxial subluxation occurs in only 1.5% of children who have DS, it is life threatening.

Unfortunately, the natural history of atlantoaxial instability and subluxation remains poorly understood. Whether only one set of cervical spine radiograms is necessary or whether these films need to be repeated is unclear. In addition, cervical spine radiograms may be unreliable in identifying all children at risk.[26] Until further information is available about the natural history of atlantoaxial subluxation, the diagnosis depends on a neurologic examination plus neurophysiological and imaging studies. Given incomplete understanding, the following are some general guidelines for the primary care physician:

1. Cervical radiographs in flexion and extension should be taken if the symptoms listed here are present or at the start of participation in contact sports in school or Special Olympics to identify atlantoaxial instability. The child should also have a yearly neurologic examination to identify long-tract signs. Radiographs should be interpreted by an experienced radiologist. If the child has normal neurologic examination and the radiographs are normal, then the child may participate in all sports. Radiographs should be taken again in young adulthood.
2. If the radiographs are read as being abnormal (the atlantoodontoid distance is greater than 5 mm) and the neurologic examination results are normal, then the child should be monitored yearly with repeated neurologic examinations. Avoiding certain sports that place the child's neck in extreme extension (eg, tumbling, gymnastics, and diving) is also prudent for the child. Careful monitoring during intubation for induction of anesthesia would be needed if surgery is necessary.
3. If the radiographs are normal but the neurologic examination results are abnormal, then the child should be referred to a neurosurgeon or orthopedic physician experienced with DS. Further diagnostic testing may be suggested, such as a computed tomographic scan of the cervical spine.

Other Considerations

General habilitation includes monitoring of exercise and recreational activities, good daily care of the teeth, and a dental examination twice a year beginning at the first birthday. Obesity may become a problem at approximately 5 years of age. The primary care physician should ask about the child's snacks and the amount of time the child spends watching television. The family should be asked again if they have checked into eligibility for SSI and Medicaid benefits. Parents should also investigate trust and guardian arrangements. The ARC (formerly known as The Association for Retarded Citizens) helps guide parents through these financial and custody arrangements. The local ARC chapter or the national office can be contacted for further information.

Child 5 to 13 Years of Age

The primary care physician needs to review the current individual educational program (IEP) to ensure that appropriate developmental testing has been completed and that the parents have had an opportunity to provide information in the IEP process (see Box 258-5). School problems may come to the physician's attention more often as children who have DS are placed in mainstreamed classes. School learning problems

BOX 258-5 Managing the Child: Ages 5 to 13 Years

Health concerns

History

1. Assess any parental concerns about the child's behavior and school program.
2. Ask if the child has shown any symptoms of a vision or hearing disorder.
3. Ask about snoring, restless sleep, and sleeping positions and assess for sleep apnea.
4. Ask if any skin problems such as dryness.

Perform

1. Complete physical examination
2. Height and weight plotted on a DS growth chart

Laboratory test—thyroid hormone screening each year

Consultation

1. Eye examination every year
2. Hearing test every year
3. Dental examination every year

Psychosocial concerns—habilitation

1. Review dietary habits and physical activity pattern.
2. Discuss respite and long-term care plans, guardianship, and financial arrangements with the family.
3. Review risk of Down syndrome in future pregnancies.
4. Discuss age-appropriate social skills, self-help skills, and the development of a sense of responsibility.
5. Discuss psychosexual development, menstrual hygiene, and fertility.
6. Review risk of Down syndrome in future pregnancies.

BOX 258-6 Managing the Child: Ages 13 to 21 Years

Health concerns

History

1. Answer the parents' questions.
2. Ask about any education or behavioral problems.
3. Make sure the child is up to date on immunizations.

Perform a physical examination and the following tests and examinations:

1. Look for obesity.
2. Perform a gynecologic examination and neurologic examination.

Laboratory tests—thyroid hormone screening and a CBC

Consultation

1. Eye examination every year
2. Hearing test every year
3. Dental examination twice a year

Psychosocial concerns—habilitation

1. Check to see whether the patient is obtaining vocational training.
2. Have the patient continue speech therapy.

Family concerns

1. Ask about community living plans for the patient.
2. Discuss enrolling the patient in Medicaid and Supplemental Security Income (SSI) if eligible.
3. Discuss the issue of sexuality, including preventing pregnancy.
4. Help the parents teach their child to avoid smoking and abusing drugs.
5. Facilitate transfer to the adult medical care.

CBC, Complete blood cell count.

require further evaluation. The history should be reviewed carefully to ensure that the parents' and the teachers' expectations are appropriate for the child's developmental age. Medical problems that can affect learning and behavior should be identified. For example, the ears should be examined for impacted cerumen that can cause a moderate hearing loss. An eye examination should be performed to detect cataracts. Vision screening should be performed yearly or more often, if indicated.

Questions

Parents of school-age children who have DS ask about the following issues most frequently:

1. *Obesity.* The cause of obesity in DS is multifactorial. Children who have greater hypotonia, shorter stature, and those at preschool age and in adolescence are at increased risk. A preventive approach includes monitoring the child's diet, promoting regular exercise, and screening yearly for hypothyroidism.
2. *Hyperactivity.* Parents or teachers may bring up symptoms of hyperactivity. The child should be thoroughly assessed to identify medical problems associated with inattention. After obtaining a complete history that includes information from the child's teacher, the physician should perform a complete physical and neurologic examination and evaluate the child's vision and hearing. Thyroid hormone testing should be considered when clinically suggested to rule out hyperthyroidism.[27] Behavior-management techniques and classroom adaptations should be tried before resorting to medications.

Adolescents 13 to 21 Years of Age

Adolescence is a special challenge for any family. The physical, emotional, and educational needs in adolescents who have DS, however, require a special approach (see Box 258-6). During the annual health assessment visit, the primary care physician should discuss with the family their child's health, educational program, behavior problems, and prevocational experience and training.

Physical Examination

The general physical examination should include plotting the child's height and weight and calculating body mass index to monitor for obesity. The need for a thorough neurologic examination for long-tract signs persists. A gynecologic examination of girls should be performed by at least 17 years of age. Because the examination is often not tolerated well by the adolescent, the primary care physician should consider referral to a specialist who has had experience evaluating women who have developmental disabilities. The examination can often be done less invasively with pelvic ultrasound, which requires an examiner who has appropriate experience with the procedure.

Routine studies include thyroid hormone levels and vision and hearing screening. The higher risk for periodontal disease among children who have DS highlights the need for a dental examination twice a year.

Sexuality

Although many adolescents who have DS receive some formal education about sexuality in school, primary care physicians should ensure that this education is complete and discuss this with the family. Although young men who have DS are usually sterile, a small number of girls and women have given birth to children.[28] When a young woman who has DS becomes pregnant, the father of the woman's child is usually a close relative. Families need to know about birth control options and routine procedures for safeguarding their adolescent. If the primary care physician is not experienced in answering these questions, then referral to a specialist who is experienced in these matters should be considered.

Smoking and Drug Abuse

Adolescents who have DS also need education about smoking and drug abuse. If at all possible, they should have well-balanced diets, continue regular exercise, and be involved in appropriate social activities. When possible, adolescents who have DS should also have opportunities for prevocational experiences such as doing volunteer work at a library or other facility that can provide adequate supervision. The school curriculum should make the transition to planning for a life vocation. Psychoeducational testing is often helpful in this regard to determine the individual's aptitudes and job interests.

Behavior Problems

Disruptive behavior, as well as anxiety disorders, may arise in adolescence.[29] A thorough mental status examination is helpful as part of the routine health assessment. When completing a mental status examination on an individual whose verbal skills are limited, a necessary component involves talking with the family and teachers about any changes or regression in self-care skills. In many instances, the family will report important information about withdrawal or loss of interest in recreational activities. Some emotional disorders are characterized by excessive anger, frustration, or aggressive behaviors. Other signs of a possible disorder include self-injurious behavior (hitting or biting themselves), crying spells, or refusal to participate in self-care activities.

When evaluating a patient who has a sudden increase in behavior problems, primary care physicians should look for underlying medical problems. For example, changes in vision or hearing may result in withdrawal or temper tantrums. Hypothyroidism can cause lethargy and lack of interest in activities. In rare cases, Alzheimer disease may appear in adolescence. When skills have been lost, psychological testing that includes an assessment of self-care skills should be performed to document this disease. Referral to a neurologist is suggested if loss of skills is documented and initial assessment shows no signs of a correctable problem.

Living Arrangements

The primary care physician needs to discuss with the family a long-term plan for the adolescent's living arrangements. Most communities have a spectrum of community living facilities that range from small, heavily supervised group homes to apartments that have minimal supervision. Families need to make living arrangements 2 or 3 years before they anticipate the need because a waiting list for placement in a community facility often exists.

Questions

Most families have questions about their adolescents on the following issues:

1. *Sexuality.* Families usually have many questions about a teenager's sexuality but often do not ask the primary care physician about them. For example, many parents wonder about the sexual interests of their children and the level at which they experience sexual feelings. They do not know how to deal with masturbation or questions about wanting to give birth. Management of menstrual hygiene also presents problems. Referral to community resources should be considered if the primary care physician's expertise or the school curriculum needs to be complemented.
2. *Sterilization.* Families may ask about sterilization procedures for both young men and young women. In most states, performing sterilization procedures is difficult because of the difficulty in obtaining consent. The primary care physician should counsel the family and the adolescent about preventing conception. Additional sources of counseling are available for families and professionals.[30]

Young Adult

Primary care physicians often continue to monitor adolescents into the early adult years to maintain continuity of care (see Box 258-7). Families are often attached to the primary care physician and ask about continuing care; this discussion can center on aspects of preventive medical care for the young adult. Average life expectancy in adults with DS has increased into the middle 50s; some are alive in their 60s.[31]

Adults with DS require the same annual health assessment as any other adults. Limited expressive speech may not allow accurate history, and medical problems may be seen as behavioral problems. The general physical examination includes a gynecologic and breast examination in women and testicular examination in men. The neurologic assessment must include testing for long-tract signs. Obstructive sleep apnea remains a common problem and can produce irritability, depression, or other behavioral problems. Thyroid hormone tests and vision and hearing screening should continue, and the patient should be referred to a neurologist, psychiatrist, or both if symptoms of dementia,

BOX 258-7 Managing beyond Age 21 Years

Health concerns

History

1. Evaluate the family's concerns.
2. Ask about symptoms of dementia and mental disorders.

Perform or refer the patient for the following tests and examinations:

Physical examination

1. Gynecological examination and Papanicolaou smear
2. Testicular and breast examination
3. Neurologic examination

Laboratory tests—thyroid screening

Consultation

1. Cardiologic examination and echocardiogram to check for mitral valve prolapse
2. Eye examination every 2 years
3. Hearing test every 2 years
4. Dental examination twice a year
5. Cervical spine examination at age 30 years

Psychosocial concerns—habilitation

1. Inquire about the patient's exercise and recreational activities.
2. Urge the patient and family to continue with vocational and adult education programs to allow better job placement.
3. When appropriate, check to see whether the patient has registered to vote and (for young men) has registered with the Selective Service System.

Family issues

1. Remind the family to update their estate planning and wills.
2. Evaluate the patient for community living if not already in this type of setting.
3. Check on patient's eligibility for Medicaid and Supplemental Security Income (SSI).

behavior problems, or depression arise. The dental examination continues at twice a year. Because approximately 50% of adults who have DS develop mitral valve prolapse, an echocardiographic evaluation needs to be performed when clinical findings are suggestive of mitral valve prolapse.[32] A Papanicolaou smear is necessary annually for sexually active women; in addition, a baseline mammogram is appropriate at the age of 35 years, with follow-up based on the physical examination and family history. Immunizations should be reviewed and kept current. Hepatitis B and pneumococcal vaccines should be considered for adults at special risk.

Vocational Training

Young adults should be enrolled in a vocational training program to enhance their skills for either a community job or workshop placement. The program should also include some basic educational activities for continued improvement in skills.

Community Living Arrangements

The parents and patient should be asked about family or community living arrangements. Again, the physician should discuss with the family future living arrangements if the adult with DS continues to live at home. Plans for guardianship and wills and trusts should be reviewed. Young adults also should be referred for voter registration and young men to the Selective Service System. Health education, especially about drug and alcohol abuse, smoking, and sex, should continue.

Questions

A parent of an adult who has DS usually has a compelling question: What will happen to my child after I die? Most adults who have DS will need supervision because they are not independent economically. The family should be counseled to seek community resources for information about community living options. The state office of disabilities can provide information about social insurance and medical benefits available for adults who have DS. A booklet published by ARC provides further information for the family.[33] Names and addresses of organizations that provide parent education and support in the United States, Canada, and Mexico and a suggested bibliography for parents are provided at the end of this chapter.

WHEN TO REFER A NEWBORN

All infants require cardiology and genetics consultation.

- Infants who have leukocoria require ophthalmology assessment.
- Newborns with transient myeloproliferative disease require a hematology consultation.
- Families who have serious difficulty adapting to their newborn may need a family counselor.
- Infants with severe constipation need a gastroenterology evaluation.

WHEN TO REFER INFANTS 1 MONTH TO 12 MONTHS OF AGE

- Infants who have severe constipation not responding to dietary control need a pediatric gastroenterology evaluation.
- Infants who have chronic middle ear effusions need a consultation with an ear, nose, and throat specialist.
- Ophthalmology consultation is recommended at 6 months.
- All infants should be referred to an early intervention program.

WHEN TO REFER CHILDREN 1 YEAR TO 5 YEARS OF AGE

- Children who have infantile spasms need immediate referral to a pediatric neurologist.

- Children who have neck pain, loss of bladder and bowel control, and gait disturbance need immediate pediatric neurosurgery consultation.
- Children who have disruptive behavior or excessive short attention span need an evaluation by developmental or behavioral specialists.
- Chronic middle ear effusions and symptoms of obstructive sleep apnea require a consultation with an ear, nose, and throat specialist.
- Ophthalmology evaluation is recommended every 2 years from the age of 12 months.

WHEN TO REFER CHILDREN 5 TO 13 YEARS OF AGE

- Annual audiology evaluation is recommended.
- Annual ophthalmology evaluation is recommended.
- Symptoms of obstructive sleep apnea require a consultation with an ear, nose, and throat specialist.

WHEN TO REFER ADOLESCENTS AND YOUNG ADULTS

- All girls should be evaluated by a gynecologist by 17 years for pelvic examination and birth control options.
- Neurology evaluation is recommended for all teenagers who have lost skills with no obvious medical explanation.
- All families should be directed to The ARC for guidance on financial and custody issues.
- Psychiatric evaluation is recommended for all adolescents who have severe behavior disturbances.
- Annual ophthalmologic evaluation is recommended.
- Annual audiologic evaluation is recommended.

TOOLS FOR PRACTICE

Engaging Patient and Family

- *Future Planning: Making Financial Arrangements with a Trust* (Web page), The ARC, by Rick Berkobien and Theresa Varnet (www.thearc.org/netcommunity/document.doc?&id=156).
- *Woodbine House* (Web page), (www.woodbinehouse.com/default.asp).

Medical Decision Support

- *Birth Defects* (Web page), Centers for Disease Control and Prevention (www.cdc.gov/ncbddd/bd/ds.htm).
- *Online Mendelian Inheritance in Man* (Web page), McKusick VA, et al, editors, Johns Hopkins University (www.ncbi.nlm.nih.gov/sites/entrez?db=OMIM).
- *The National Center of Medical Home Initiatives for Children With Special Needs* (Web page), American Academy of Pediatrics (www.medicalhomeinfo.org/index.html).

RELATED WEB SITES

- The ARC, Family Resource Guides (www.thearc.org/NetCommunity/Page.aspx?&pid=1400&srcid=1433).
- National Down Syndrome Congress (www.ndsccenter.org/index.php).
- National Down Syndrome Society (NDSS) (www.ndss.org/).

AAP POLICY STATEMENTS

American Academy of Pediatrics, Committee on Genetics. Health supervision for children with Down syndrome. *Pediatrics*. 2001;107(2):442-449. (aappolicy.aappublications.org/cgi/content/full/pediatrics;107/2/442).

Cunniff C, American Academy of Pediatrics Committee on Genetics. Clinical report: prenatal screening and diagnosis for pediatricians. *Pediatrics*. 2004;114(3):889-894. (aappolicy.aappublications.org/cgi/content/full/pediatrics;114/3/889).

SUGGESTED RESOURCES

Lou IT, McCoy EE. *Down Syndrome: Advances in Medical Care*. New York, NY: Wiley-Liss; 1992.

Rogers RT, Coleman M. *Medical Care in Down Syndrome*. New York, NY: Marcel Dekker; 1992.

ADDITIONAL RESOURCES

National Down Syndrome Society
666 Broadway
New York, NY 10012
Telephone: 212-460-9330 or 800-221-4602
www.ndss.org

National Down Syndrome Congress
1370 Center Drive, Suite 102
Atlanta, GA 30338
Telephone: 800-232-6372
www.ndsccenter.org

The ARC
1010 Wayne Avenue, Suite 650
Silver Spring, MD 20910
Telephone: 301-565-3842
www.thearc.org

Stray-Gundersen K, ed. *Babies with Down Syndrome: A New Parents' Guide*. 2nd ed. Bethesda, MD: Woodbine House; 1995. Spanish translation.
Woodbine House
800-843-7323
www.woodbinehouse.com

ADDITIONAL PUBLICATIONS

Cunningham C. *Down's Syndrome: An Introduction for Parents*. Brookline, MA: Brookline Books; 1987.

Hanson MJ. *Teaching Your Down's Syndrome Infant: A Guide for Parents*. Baltimore, MD: University Park Press; 1977.

Kingsley J, Levitz M. *Count Us In: Growing up with Down Syndrome*. Fort Washington, PA: Harvest Books, 1994.

Kumin L. *Communication Skills in Children with Down Syndrome: A Guide for Parents*. Bethesda, MD: Woodbine House; 1994.

Oelwein PL. *Teaching Reading to Children with Down Syndrome: A Guide for Parents & Teachers*. Bethesda, MD: Woodbine House; 1995.

Pueschel SM. *A Parent's Guide to Down Syndrome: Toward a Brighter Future*. Baltimore, MD: Paul H. Brookes Publishing; 1990.

Pueschel SM. *The Young Child With Down Syndrome*. New York, NY: Human Sciences Press: 1984.

"Welcome to Holland" an essay written in 1987 by Emily Perl Kingsley. Also available in Spanish and Chinese.

REFERENCES

1. Centers for Disease Control and Prevention. Improved national prevalence estimates for 18 selected major birth defects—United States, 1999-2001. *MMWR Morb Mortal Wkly Rep*. 2006;54:1301-1305.
2. Cuckle HS, Wald NJ, Thompson SG. Estimating a woman's risk of having a pregnancy associated with Down's syndrome using her age and serum alpha-fetoprotein level. *Br J Obstet Gynaecol*. 1987;94:387-402.
3. Palomaki GE, Bradley LA, McDowell GA, Down Syndrome Working Group, and ACMG Laboratory Quality Assurance Committee. Technical standards and guidelines: prenatal screening for Down syndrome. *Genet Med*. 2005;7:344-354.
4. O'Leary P, Breheny N, Dickinson JE, et al. First-trimester combined screening for Down syndrome and other fetal anomalies. *Obstet Gynecol*. 2006;107:869-876.
5. Down syndrome. Available at: www.ncbi.nlm.nih.gov/omim.
6. Ballesta F, Queralt R, Gomez D, et al. Parental origin and meiotic stage of non-disjunction in 139 cases of trisomy. *Ann Genet*. 1999;42:11-15.
7. Fishler K, Koch R: Mental development in Down syndrome mosaicism. *Am J Ment Retard*. 1991;96:345-351.
8. de A Moreira LM, SanJuan A, Pereira PS, et al. A case of mosaic trisomy 21 with Down's syndrome signs and normal intellectual development. *J Intellect Disabil Res*. 2000; 44:91-96.
9. Korenberg JR, Chen XN, Schipper R, et al. Down syndrome phenotypes: the consequences of chromosomal imbalance. *Proc Natl Acad Sci U S A*. 1994;24:4997-5001.
10. Hall B. Mongolism in newborn infants: an examination of the criteria for recognition and some speculation on the pathogenic activity of the chromosomal abnormality. *Clin Pediatr*. 1966;5:4-12.
11. Fort P, Lifshitz F, Bellisario R, et al. Abnormalities of thyroid function in infants with Down syndrome. *J Pediatr*. 1984;104:545-549.
12. Zipursky A. Transient leukaemia—a benign form of leukaemia in newborn infants with trisomy 21. *Br J Haematol*. 2003;120:930-938.
13. Zipursky A, Doyle J, Christensen H, et al. Leukemic cells in the transient leukemia of Down syndrome. *Blood*. 1992:80:32.
14. Bell R, Rankin J, Donaldson LJ, and the Northern Congenital Abnormality Survey Steering Group. Down's syndrome: occurrence and outcome in the north of England, 1985-1999. *Paediatr Perinat Epidemiol*. 2003;17:33-39.
15. Masuda M, Kado H, Tanoue Y, et al. Does Down syndrome affect the long-term results of complete atrioventricular septal defect when the defect is repaired during the first year of life? *Eur J Cardiothorac Surg*. 2005;27: 405-409. E-publication: December 30, 2004.
16. Yang Q, Rasmussen SA, Friedman JM. Mortality associated with Down's syndrome in the USA from 1983 to 1997: a population based study. *Lancet*. 2002;359:1019-1025.
17. Cronk C, Crocker AC, Pueschel SM, et al. Growth charts for children with Down syndrome: 1 month to 18 years of age. *Pediatrics*. 1988;81:102-110.
18. Hilhorst MI, Brink M, Wauters EA, et al. Down syndrome and coeliac disease: five new cases with a review of the literature. *Eur J Pediatr*. 1993;152:884-887.
19. Gruneiro de PL, Chiesa A, Bastida MG, et al. Thyroid dysfunction and thyroid stimulating hormone levels in children with Down's syndrome. *Pediatr Endocrinol Metab*. 2002;15:1543-1548.
20. Karlsson G, Gustafsson J, Hedov G, et al. Thyroid dysfunction in Down's syndrome: relation to age and thyroid autoimmunity. *Arch Dis Child*. 1998;79:242-245.
21. Parson CL, Lacono TA, Rozner L. Effect of tongue reduction on articulation in children with Down syndrome. *Am J Ment Deficiency*. 1987;91:328-332.
22. Harrell RF, Capp RH, Davis DR, et al. Can nutritional supplements help mentally retarded children? An exploratory study. *Proc Natl Acad Sci USA*. 1981;78:574-578.
23. Ani C, Grantham-McGregor S, Muller D. Nutritional supplementation in Down syndrome. Theoretical considerations and current status. *Dev Med Child Neurol*. 2000; 42:207-211.
24. Gaynon MW, Schimek RA. Down's syndrome: a ten-year study. *Ann Ophthalmol*. 1977;9:1493-1497.
25. Pueschel SM, Scola FH. Epidemiologic, radiographic and clinical studies of atlantoaxial instability in individuals with Down syndrome. *Pediatrics*. 1987;80:555-560.
26. Selby KA, Newton RW, Gupta S, et al. Clinical predictions and radiological reliability in atlantoaxial subluxation in Down's syndrome. *Arch Dis Child*. 1991;66: 876-878.
27. Lambyah PA, Cheah JS. Hyperthyroidism and Down syndrome. *Ann Acad Med (Singapore)*. 1993;22:603-605.
28. Sheridan R, Llerena J Jr, Matkins S, et al. Fertility in a male with trisomy. *J Med Genet*. 1989;26:294-298.
29. Myers BA, Pueschel SM. Psychiatric disorders in persons with Down syndrome. *J Nerv Ment Dis*. 1991;179: 609-613.
30. Edwards JP, Elkins TE. *Just Between Us: A Social Sexual Training Guide for Parents and Professionals Who Have Concerns for Persons With Retardation*. Portland, OR: Ednick Communications; 1988.
31. Baird PA, Sadovnick AD. Life tables for Down syndrome. *Hum Genet*. 1989;82:291-292.
32. Goldhaber S, Brown WD, Sutton MG. High frequency of mitral valve prolapse and aortic regurgitation among asymptomatic adults with Down syndrome. *JAMA*. 1987; 258:1793-1795.
33. Association for Retarded Citizens of the USA. A Family Handbook on Future Planning. Available at: www.thearc.org.

Chapter 259

DRUG ERUPTIONS, ERYTHEMA MULTIFORME, STEVENS-JOHNSON SYNDROME, AND TOXIC EPIDERMAL NECROLYSIS

Judith V. Williams, MD; Catherine Chen, MD

The clinical expression of drug eruptions varies considerably. Given that systemically administered drugs can cause almost any kind of rash, the practitioner should remember a general principle of dermatologic diagnosis: For any rash, think of drugs. The types of skin reactions caused by drugs include morbilliform eruptions, urticaria, erythema multiforme, Stevens-Johnson syndrome, toxic epidermal necrosis, erythema nodosum, vasculitis, photosensitivity reactions, acneform eruptions, alopecia, blistering disorders, fixed drug eruptions, lichenoid reactions, and drug-induced lupus erythematosus.[1-3] This chapter deals only with the types of drug eruptions seen most commonly in children—morbilliform eruptions, urticaria, and erythema multiforme—and the two most severe eruptions—Stevens-Johnson syndrome and toxic epidermal necrolysis.

MORBILLIFORM ERUPTIONS

Etiology

Morbilliform (measles-like) eruptions are the most common cutaneous expression of a drug reaction. Their pathogenesis is unknown. Although a variety of drugs can cause this reaction, the drugs that cause morbilliform or urticarial eruptions most often are listed in Table 259-1.

History

A drug-induced morbilliform eruption does not usually have an immediate onset; rather, it begins within several days of initiation of the drug. The onset is sometimes delayed up to a week but seldom longer. Because no laboratory test can identify the responsible drug, heavy reliance is placed on the history. Patients receiving more than one drug obviously present a problem. In trying to select a single drug from a list, the two variables to consider are (1) the temporal relationship between the administration of the drug and the onset of the rash and (2) the likelihood that a given medication can cause a drug eruption. For the latter variable, incidence data such as those in Table 259-1 are used. Itching is usually present, but it is not helpful as a diagnostic marker.

Eruptions have been reported in patients with Epstein-Barr virus infection taking amoxicillin. Most of these eruptions have been morbilliform in nature. Their pathogenesis remains to be elucidated.

Physical Findings

The eruption is generalized and consists of brightly erythematous macules and papules that tend to be confluent over large areas. It usually starts proximally and proceeds distally, with the legs being the last to be involved and also the last to clear. Palms and soles also are affected. Drug fever has been well described, but most drug eruptions are not accompanied by an elevation in body temperature.

Table 259-1 Allergic Skin Reactions to Drugs

DRUG	REACTION RATE (PER 100 RECIPIENTS)
Aminopenicillins	4.4-8.0
Sulfonamides	2.5-3.7
Ampicillin	3.3
Semisynthetic penicillins	2.9
Blood	2.2
Cephalosporins	2.1
Erythromycin	2.0
Penicillin G	1.6
Allopurinol	0.8
Nonsteroidal antiinflammatory drugs	0.3-0.69
Barbiturates	0.4
Diazepam	0.04

From Bigby M. Rates of cutaneous reactions to drugs. *Arch Dermatol.* 2001;137:765-770; Bigby M, Jick S, Jick H, et al. Drug-induced cutaneous reactions: a report from the Boston Collaborative Drug Surveillance Program on 15,438 consecutive inpatients, 1975 to 1982. *JAMA.* 1986;256:3358-3363. Reprinted by permission of the American Medical Association.

Differential Diagnosis

For a generalized erythematous, morbilliform eruption the major differential diagnosis is (1) a drug reaction, (2) a viral exanthem, or (3) a toxic erythema.

As the name morbilliform (measles-like) suggests, a viral exanthem and a drug eruption can be indistinguishable clinically. In many instances, a drug eruption is much more erythematous and confluent but not always. Other clinical information can help establish the diagnosis, including a drug history and the presence or absence of other signs and symptoms of a viral infection. Eosinophilia favors a drug etiology. Acute and convalescent serologic tests can be obtained for some viral infections to provide a retrospective diagnosis. In most cases, however, a presumptive diagnosis is made based on clinical data.

Examples of toxic erythema are scarlet fever, staphylococcal-induced scarlatiniform eruptions, and, possibly, Kawasaki disease. Features that help distinguish these toxic erythemas from drug eruptions include a sandpaper-like roughened texture of the rash, mucous membrane involvement (scarlet fever and Kawasaki disease), fever, a focus of infection, and lymphadenopathy. Postinflammatory desquamation from the skin of the hands and feet often follows the rash of toxic erythema, but this sign is not specific. Drug eruptions and even viral exanthems can involve the hands and feet, particularly the palms and soles in drug eruptions; if the inflammation has been sufficiently intense, then desquamation follows.

Laboratory Studies

Laboratory tests are not usually helpful. A peripheral blood eosinophilia is sometimes present and may heighten the suspicion for a drug reaction; but no laboratory test can incriminate a specific drug.

Treatment

When an offending agent is identified, its use should be discontinued. If a patient is taking several drugs and being certain of the culprit is not possible, then the number of drugs administered should be reduced to an absolute minimum; and whenever possible, any remaining possible offenders should be changed to alternative agents.

Therapy is otherwise directed toward the symptoms, with antihistamines used most commonly for the pruritus. Topical agents are usually confined to moisturizers, which are most helpful during the desquamative phase of the reaction. Although topical steroids may be of some value in controlling pruritus, systemic steroids are rarely required.

Complications

The complications of skin rashes are primarily cutaneous. When large areas of skin are inflamed, body heat increases and water is lost. If the patient is already seriously ill, then these changes might be a problem; for most patients, however, it is not.

Continuing use of an offending agent in the setting of a drug eruption can result in 2 types of consequences: (1) cutaneous and (2) renal. The cutaneous risk is that of progressive worsening of the rash, possibly resulting in Stevens-Johnson syndrome (SJS) or toxic epidermal necrolysis (TEN). Fortunately, this event is rare. In fact, in some cases a drug eruption clears even when use of the offending agent is continued. Of course, continued use of the drug is unwise if an alternative is available. The renal risk is that of allergic interstitial nephritis, an uncommon development that is usually associated with penicillins and cephalosporins and only rarely with other drugs.

Course

Drug eruptions gradually clear after the use of the responsible agent is discontinued. Usually, 1 to 2 weeks are required for the condition to clear completely, and the eruption may actually worsen for several days after use of the offending drug has been stopped. If a responsible drug has been identified, then the patient should be advised about the allergy, and the medical record should be clearly labeled to this effect. However, notably, not all of these reactions necessarily reflect true allergy.

URTICARIA (HIVES)

Etiology

Drug-induced hives can be mediated immunologically by either (1) immediate immunoglobulin E (IgE) reactions, usually within hours, or (2) delayed immune complexes that result in serum sickness-like reactions after 7 to 10 days.[4,5] The immediate reactions are more common than delayed reactions.[5]

History

A precise cause is not usually found among patients who have hives. The history can reveal the cause. The drug history is the most important but also the most difficult history to obtain, at least among outpatients. Given that many patients and their parents tend to consider over-the-counter medications unimportant, the physician should ask about specific medications to help jog their memories. Nonsteroidal antiinflammatory drugs (NSAIDs) cause hives in some patients and can aggravate them in patients who have urticaria, regardless of its cause. Aspirin can cause hives but is not widely used in children because of the risk of Reye syndrome. Whenever a drug is suspected, the physician must be aggressive and persistent in eliciting a medication history. Otherwise, some drugs are invariably overlooked.

A history of associated symptoms may also be important. Itching is almost always present. A history of an obstructed airway or urticaria with significant edema suggests anaphylaxis. Fever and arthralgia often accompany hives in serum sickness reactions, for which the 2 most common causes are drugs, especially antibiotics, and viral hepatitis.[4,6]

Physical Findings

Hives are skin lesions that are recognized more easily than described. They appear as edematous plaques, often with pale or dusky centers and red borders. Hives frequently assume geographic shapes and are sometimes confluent. The lesions may be scattered, but they are usually generalized. By definition, an individual hive is transient, lasting less than 48 hours, although new hives may develop continuously.[5,6] In serum sickness reactions, lymphadenopathy, in addition to fever and arthralgia, may be present.[4]

Differential Diagnosis

The differential diagnosis of urticaria may be approached in two ways: (1) from the causes of hives per se and (2) from consideration of the cause of lesions sometimes mistaken as hives. Usually the cause of hives cannot be determined. When a cause is found, it is usually drug-related. Other causes include infection, physical modalities (eg, cold, pressure, sunlight), emotions, and foods.

Lesions sometimes mistaken for hives include those seen in erythema multiforme and juvenile rheumatoid arthritis. The lesions in erythema multiforme are discussed later in this chapter. The individual lesions in juvenile rheumatoid arthritis behave similar to hives in that they are transient but differ in size (only 2 to 3 mm), color (typically salmon), and timing (usually appearing with fever spikes).

MANAGEMENT

Laboratory Studies

As with other drug eruptions, drug-induced hives may be accompanied by eosinophilia. To evaluate for hepatitis, the physician should obtain liver function tests in patients who have hives and fever. However, in afebrile patients, laboratory tests are rarely helpful in eliciting a cause, and they are of no help in implicating a specific drug.

Treatment

Use of any suspected medication should be discontinued. Symptomatic therapy is usually achieved with antihistamines given on a regular, rather than an as-needed schedule. Hydroxyzine is the preferred agent, given every 6 or 8 hours.

Complications

In rare cases, acute urticaria can be accompanied by anaphylactic reactions that require more immediate therapy; usually, however, hives are more of a nuisance than a morbid threat. (See Chapter 339, Anaphylaxis.)

Course

Drug-induced hives usually clear within several days after use of the responsible medication is discontinued. As with any drug reaction, if a specific agent has been identified, then the patient must be alerted to avoid that drug in the future. Because most hives are IgE mediated, a repeat challenge with the responsible drug is more likely to result in an anaphylactic response than it would in a patient who had a previous morbilliform eruption.

DRUG RASH WITH EOSINOPHILIA AND SYSTEMIC SYMPTOMS

Drug rash with eosinophilia and systemic symptoms (DRESS), formerly known as drug hypersensitivity syndrome, is characterized by the clinical triad of fever, rash, and internal organ involvement (most commonly hepatitis, nephritis, pneumonitis, or myocarditis) that occurs within 8 weeks of initiation of the medication. DRESS has been associated with the use of aromatic anticonvulsants (phenytoin, carbamazepine, phenobarbitone), sulfonamides, NSAIDs, ranitidine, calcium-channel blockers, allopurinol, and thalidomide. Cross-reactivity with structurally related drugs is common. Clinical manifestations include fever early in the course, diffuse macules, and papules or pustules that can progress to an exfoliative dermatitis mimicking SJS or TEN, eosinophilia, atypical lymphocytosis, and abnormal liver function test results. The severity of the skin involvement does not correlate with the extent of internal organ involvement.[7] The incidence of DRESS with anticonvulsants has been estimated at 1 in 10,000 exposures.[8] Treatment consists of immediate withdrawal of all suspected medications, followed by supportive care of symptoms. Systemic corticosteroids are generally used in the more severe cases involving significant exfoliative dermatitis, pneumonitis, or hepatitis.[9] Patients should be told that first-degree relatives may be predisposed to developing this syndrome.

ERYTHEMA MULTIFORME

Erythema multiforme (EM) is an acute, self-limited eruption of symmetrical erythematous macules and papules that can evolve into target lesions.[10-12] It was first described by Ferdinand von Hebra in 1860 and later divided into minor and major forms, the major form being synonymous with SJS. It also has been considered as the rather benign end of a spectrum that included SJS and TEN. However, current thinking is evolving such that, despite some clinical and histologic similarities, EM is best viewed as a separate entity from SJS and TEN.[13]

Etiology

In children and adults, EM most often occurs in association with recurrent herpes simplex virus (HSV) types I and II.[8,14-17] Circulating immune complexes have been detected in patients who have EM, a finding consistent with the concept that this distinctive cutaneous disorder is an immunologic reaction. Other infectious agents that have been rarely implicated in EM include *Histoplasma capsulatum* and viruses, possibly Epstein-Barr virus.[11] Many reported cases of presumed EM, ascribed to innumerable causes, were more likely giant urticaria.[18]

History

In approximately 50% of all cases a history of an HSV lesion in the prior few days to 2 weeks will be found, occasionally preceded by a febrile prodrome.[19] In the rest of cases a cause generally cannot be identified.

Physical Findings

As the name suggests, EM is characterized by a variety of lesions, including erythematous plaques, blisters, and targetoid lesions. Hives are sometimes confused with target lesions. The difference is that a hive has only 2 zones of color: a central pale area surrounded by an erythematous halo. The criteria for a target lesion require 3 zones: a central dark area or blister, surrounded by a pale zone, surrounded by a peripheral rim of erythema. True target lesions are diagnostic for EM. They are seen more often on the palms and soles but may occur anywhere. Typically, EM is a strikingly symmetrical eruption that most frequently favors the dorsal hands and forearms.[20] Other areas that are also often involved include the palms, neck, face, and trunk. Lesions can be quite numerous, often exceeding 100 in number, and may appear grouped on the elbows or knees. The Koebner phenomenon can be observed: after cutaneous trauma has occurred, target lesions may appear in the affected areas.[19] Mild, discrete oral erosions occur in more than one half of patients but are usually few in number and can be relatively asymptomatic.[19]

Differential Diagnosis

The skin reactions most commonly considered in the differential diagnosis are giant urticaria, subacute cutaneous lupus erythematosus, viral exanthems, vasculitis, staphylococcal scalded-skin syndrome, and other blistering eruptions.[21] Individual hives last fewer than 48 hours; the lesions in EM persist much longer. Viral exanthems are usually monomorphous and tend to be less red, more confluent, and more centrally distributed than the lesions of EM. Purpura is the distinguishing feature of vasculitic lesions. Recurrent EM caused by HSV also can be mistaken for the photosensitive disorders polymorphous light eruption and juvenile spring eruption because it too can be triggered by significant sun exposure.[22]

Laboratory Studies

For herpes simplex disease, if the responsible vesicular lesion is still present, then its base can be scraped for herpes simplex virus direct fluorescent antibody, or its fluid can be cultured for herpesvirus or examined for multinucleated giant cells (Tzanck preparation). Otherwise, laboratory evaluation usually is not helpful, although a leukocytosis can be seen.

When the diagnosis is in doubt a skin biopsy can be helpful in excluding conditions that mimic EM, such as lupus erythematosus or vasculitis.

Treatment

No convincing evidence has been found that medical therapy favorably alters the course of EM. Treating a precipitating infection seems appropriate, even though no proof exists that it alters the course of the skin reaction. Acyclovir begun after the onset of EM has not proven to be effective.[15] Symptomatic treatment also can be helpful; antihistamines may reduce the sensation of stinging and burning, and antacid suspensions applied topically may alleviate oral ulcers.

Course

Patients with mild forms of EM usually recover uneventfully within 2 to 3 weeks. EM recurs in 10% to 20% of patients and is particularly common in patients with milder disease that is precipitated by recurrent HSV infection. Children with frequently recurring EM caused by HSV may be good candidates for prophylactic acyclovir for 6 to 12 months.[23]

STEVENS-JOHNSON SYNDROME AND TOXIC EPIDERMAL NECROLYSIS

SJS and TEN, also known as Lyell syndrome, are 2 ends of a more severe process involving the acute onset of mucocutaneous necrosis.[10] SJS produces more focal skin necrosis than TEN, with 2 or more mucosal sites involved. Extensive areas of epidermal necrosis and resulting denudation are seen in TEN.[11] Although previously thought to be more severe variations of EM, they are best viewed as distinct from EM.[13]

Etiology

Medications are the most common cause of SJS and TEN. Antibiotics (especially sulfonamides), anticonvulsants, and NSAIDs have been the medications most commonly implicated; however, a history of all medications should be elicited.[24] Infections, particularly from *Mycoplasma pneumoniae,* have also been implicated in SJS.[11]

History

SJS and TEN are usually preceded by a prodrome of up to 2 weeks of influenza-like symptoms followed by the abrupt onset of skin eruption. When drug related, the eruption typically begins 7 to 21 days after initiation of the causative drug.

Physical Findings

The eruption of SJS and TEN is initially macular or morbilliform, tender, dusky, and erythematous and are widespread in distribution. The skin strips off easily with minor friction (positive Nikolsky sign). Then, lesions gradually coalesce and flaccid bullae develop. The bullae easily rupture and detach, leaving necrotic sheets of epidermis with a moist, bright red base.[10] Similar lesions are also typically seen on mucous membranes, usually involving more than 2 mucosal sites. Thick, hemorrhagic crusts may appear on the lips.[10] When up to 10% of the body surface area is involved, the eruption is termed SJS. When greater than 30% is involved, it is termed TEN. When the extent of involvement ranges from 10% to 30%, the eruption is termed *SJS-TEN overlap*.[25]

Constitutional symptoms also occur, especially fever, arthralgia, malaise, and lymphadenopathy, with occasional symptoms of an upper respiratory infection and, in rare instances, hepatitis, nephritis, and myocarditis.[11]

Differential Diagnosis

The skin in staphylococcal scalded-skin syndrome (SSSS) is diffusely red and tender and also exhibits a Nikolsky sign. A skin biopsy helps distinguish SSSS from SJS. Histologically the level of the blister is intraepidermal in SSSS, whereas in SJS and TEN the blister is subepidermal.[25]

Laboratory Findings

A chest radiograph is appropriate to screen for pulmonary involvement, including that caused by *M pneumoniae* infection, which can be confirmed further by cold agglutinins and acute and convalescent titers of IgM antibodies to *Mycoplasma*. A complete blood cell count may show leukocytosis, and urinalysis may show hematuria or proteinuria.

Treatment

Use of any drug suspected of causing the reaction should be discontinued, and any underlying infection should be treated.[26] Erythromycin is recommended for *M pneumoniae* infections, although treatment may not alter the course of the skin disease.

Supportive measures are vitally important. They are aimed mainly at (1) restoring and maintaining fluid and electrolyte balance, (2) preventing secondary infection, and (3) relieving pain. Patients who have severe oral involvement may be unable to eat and drink. When skin involvement is extensive, transcutaneous fluid loss increases and replacement volumes must be adjusted accordingly. Fluid replacement poses a unique challenge for patients with SJS and TEN: unlike burn patients, the surface area involved in SJS and TEN may change, thus altering their fluid requirements. Fluid intake may need frequent adjustment to maintain constant urine output while avoiding fluid overload, which can lead to pulmonary edema, acute respiratory distress syndrome, and death. In fact, some experts recommend inserting a nasogastric tube on admission to maximize oral intake and decrease the need for intravenous fluids or parenteral nutrition, thus decreasing risk of fluid overload should the patient's course become more complicated. In addition, parenteral nutrition requires a central venous line, with the attendant risks of sepsis and other line-associated complications. Local therapy with antiseptics and dressings may help prevent secondary infection, and patients who have severe involvement may require treatments similar to those for burn patients. In particular, silver nitrate–impregnated dressings have been shown to be particularly helpful without causing further epidermal detachment on removal.[27] Systemic analgesics are used for pain. Topical anesthetics may be used intraorally to provide temporary relief for patients who have painful mouth lesions. *Magic swizzle,* containing one part each of diphenhydramine hydrochloride elixir, aluminum and magnesium hydroxide (Maalox), and viscous lidocaine 2%, is one such agent. The clinician should be aware of the potential for systemic effects from lidocaine when ordering this agent for young children.

The use of systemic steroids is controversial. They have been used frequently in SJS and TEN but with mixed success. In fact, Rasmussen's retrospective study found that children who had SJS treated with systemic steroids required a longer hospital stay and had more complications (eg, infection, gastrointestinal bleeding) than untreated patients.[28] Nevertheless, prednisone given systemically is sometimes used early in the course of patients who have severe EM.[29]

Intravenous immunoglobulin may hasten the course of this disorder by blocking the apoptosis of epidermal cells. However, published reports have been mixed.[30-34] Well-controlled, prospective, multicenter studies are

Table 259-2 Severity-of-Illness Score for Toxic Epidermal Necrolysis (SCORTEN)

SCORTEN PARAMETER	INDIVIDUAL SCORE	SCORTEN (SUM OF INDIVIDUAL SCORES)	PREDICTED MORTALITY (%)
Age >40 years	Yes = 1, No = 0	0-1	3.2
Malignancy	Yes = 1, No = 0	2	12.1
Tachycardia (>120/min)	Yes = 1, No = 0	3	35.3
Initial surface of epidermal detachment >10%	Yes = 1, No = 0	4	58.3
Serum urea >10 mmol/L	Yes = 1, No = 0	≥5	90
Serum glucose >14 mmol/L	Yes = 1, No = 0	—	—
Bicarbonate <20 mmol/L	Yes = 1, No = 0	—	—

From Bastuji-Garin S, Fouchard N, Bertocchi M, et al. SCORTEN: a severity-of-illness score for toxic epidermal necrolysis. *J Invest Dermatol.* 2000;115:149-153.

needed to confirm its efficacy and safety and to determine optimal dosing guidelines.[13,20]

Course and Complications

The course of the disease can last as long as 4 to 6 weeks in patients with severe involvement. Oral mucous membrane involvement can produce painful erosions, restricting intake and resulting in dehydration. Similar lesions in the genital mucous membranes can cause dysuria and urinary retention.[10] Conjunctivitis can produce residual ophthalmic complications, including keratitis sicca, corneal ulceration or scarring, permanent visual impairment, and even blindness.[35] Therefore early ophthalmic evaluation is warranted. Internal organs are affected less often. TEN in particular can affect the respiratory and gastrointestinal tracts. Respiratory involvement can lead to patchy pulmonary disease, bronchiolitis obliterans, and respiratory failure. Esophageal involvement can lead to dysphasia, malnutrition, and strictures. Involvement of the small intestine can lead to abdominal pain and diarrhea.[10]

Death can occur in patients with these disorders because of extensive loss of skin integrity or complications from involvement of other organ systems. Mortality rates of up to 30% have been reported.[11] A severity-of-illness score for TEN (SCORTEN) predicts a patient's risk of death according to the presence or absence of 7 risk factors: (1) age over 40 years, (2) presence of malignancy, (3) heart rate above 120 beats per minute, (4) extent of skin involvement exceeding 10% on admission, (5) blood urea nitrogen above 28 mg/dL, (6) serum glucose above 252 mg/dL, and (7) serum bicarbonate below 20 mM (Table 259-2).[36]

Early diagnosis and management of SJS and TEN with referral to a tertiary-care center may lessen morbidity and mortality and improve the outcome of the unfortunate patient who develops this disease process.

WHEN TO REFER

- Recurrent erythema multiforme
- Drug hypersensitivity reactions with multiorgan involvement

WHEN TO ADMIT

- Stevens-Johnson syndrome
- Toxic epidermal necrolysis

TOOLS FOR PRACTICE

Medical Decision Support

- *Pediatric Dermatology: A Quick Reference Guide* (book), American Academy of Pediatrics (www.aap.org/bookstore).
- *Pediatric Dermatology: Skin Essentials* (on-line course), American Academy of Pediatrics (www.pedialink.org/cme/_coursefinder).

REFERENCES

1. Bigby M. Rates of cutaneous reactions to drugs. *Arch Dermatol.* 2001;137:765-770.
2. Blacker KL, Stern RS, Wintroub BU. Cutaneous reactions to drugs. In: Fitzpatrick TB, Arndt KA, Clarck WH, et al, eds. *Dermatology in General Medicine*. New York, NY: McGraw-Hill; 1993.
3. Dunagin WG, Millikan LE. Drug eruptions. *Med Clin North Am.* 1980;64:983-1003.
4. Jorizzo JL, ed. Symposium on urticaria and the reactive inflammatory vascular dermatomes. *Dermatol Clin.* 1985; 3:3-12.
5. Monroe EW. Urticaria: an updated review. *Int J Dermatol.* 1981;20:32-41.
6. Wintroub BU, Stern RS. Cutaneous drug reactions: pathogenesis and clinical classification. *J Am Acad Dermatol.* 1985;13:167-179.
7. Callot V, Roujeau JC, Bagot M, et al. Drug-induced pseudolymphoma and hypersensitivity syndrome: two different clinical entities. *Arch Dermatol.* 1996;132:1315-1321.
8. Sullivan JR, Shear NH. The drug hypersensitivity syndrome: what is the pathogenesis? *Arch Dermatol.* 2001; 137:357-364.
9. Wolkenstein P, Revuz J. Drug-induced severe skin reactions—incidence, management and prevention. *Drug Safety.* 1995;13(1):56-68.
10. Tidman MJ, Garzon MC. Vesiculobullous disease. In: Schachner LA, Hansen RC, eds. *Pediatric Dermatology*. New York, NY: Mosby; 2003.
11. Weston WL. Erythema multiforme and Stevens-Johnson syndrome. In: Bolognia JL, Jorizzo JL, Rapini RP, eds. *Dermatology*. New York, NY: Elsevier; 2003.

12. Weston WL, Orchard D. Vascular reactions. In: Schachner LA, Hansen RC, eds. *Pediatric Dermatology*. New York, NY: Mosby; 2003.
13. Assier H, Bastuji-Garin S, Revuz J, et al. Erythema multiforme with mucous membrane involvement and Stevens-Johnson syndrome are clinically different disorders with distinct causes. *Arch Dermatol*. 1995;131:539-543.
14. Brice SL, Stockert SS, Bunker JD, et al. The herpes-specific immune response of individuals with herpes-associated erythema multiforme compared with that of individuals with recurrent herpes labialis. *Arch Dermatol Res*. 1993;285:193-196.
15. Schofield JK, Tatnall FM, Leigh IM. Recurrent erythema multiforme: clinical features and treatment in a large series of patients. *Br J Dermatol*. 1993;128:542-545.
16. Weston WL, Stockert, SS, Jester, JD, et al. Herpes simplex virus in childhood erythema multiforme. *Pediatrics*. 1992;89:32-34.
17. Weston WL, Morelli JG. Herpes simplex virus-associated erythema multiforme in prepubertal children. *Arch Pediatr Adolesc Med*. 1997;151:1014-1018.
18. Weston JA, Weston WL. The overdiagnosis of erythema multiforme. *Pediatrics*. 1992;89:802.
19. Brice SL, Huff JC, Weston WL. Erythema multiforme. *Curr Prob Dermatol*. 1990;2:3-26.
20. Dikland WJ, Oranje AP, Stolz E, et al. Erythema multiforme in childhood and early infancy. *Pediatr Dermatol*. 1986;3:135-139.
21. Weston WL, Brice SL. Atypical forms of herpes simplex-associated erythema multiforme. *J Am Acad Dermatol*. 1998;39:124-126.
22. Wolf P, Soyer HP, Fink-Puches R, et al. Recurrent post-herpetic erythema multiforme mimicking polymorphic light and juvenile spring eruption: report of two cases in young boys. *Br J Dermatol*. 1994;131:364-367.
23. Tatnall FM, Schofield JK, Leigh IM. A double-blind, placebo-controlled trial of continuous acyclovir therapy in recurrent erythema multiforme. *Br J Dermatol*. 1995; 132:267-270.
24. Roujeau JC, Kelly JP, Naldi L, et al. Medication use and the risk of Stevens-Johnson syndrome or toxic epidermal necrolysis. *N Engl J Med*. 1995;333:1600-1607.
25. French LE, Prins C. Toxic epidermal necrolysis. In: Bolognia JL, Jorizzo JL, Rapini RP, eds. *Dermatology*. New York, NY: Elsevier; 2003.
26. Garcia-Doval I, LeCleach L, Bocquet H, et al. Toxic epidermal necrolysis and Stevens-Johnson syndrome: does early withdrawal of causative drugs decrease the risk of death? *Arch Dermatol*. 2000;136:323-327.
27. Lehrer-Bell KA, Kirsner RS, Tallman PG, et al. Treatment of the cutaneous involvement in Stevens-Johnson syndrome and toxic epidermal necrolysis with silver nitrate-impregnated dressings. *Arch Dermatol*. 1998;134: 877-879.
28. Rasmussen JE. Erythema multiforme in children: response to treatment with systemic corticosteroids. *Br J Dermatol*. 1976;95:181-186.
29. Tripathi A, Ditto AM, Grammer LC, et al. Corticosteroid therapy in an additional 13 cases of Stevens-Johnson syndrome: a total series of 67 cases. *Allergy Asthma Proc*. 2000;21:101-105.
30. Bachot N, Revuz J, Roujeau JC. Intravenous immunoglobulin treatment for Stevens-Johnson syndrome and toxic epidermal necrolysis: a prospective noncomparative study showing no benefit on mortality or progression. *Arch Dermatol*. 2003;139:33-36.
31. Metry DW, Jung P, Levy ML. Use of intravenous immunoglobulin in children with Stevens-Johnson syndrome and toxic epidermal necrolysis: seven cases and review of the literature. *Pediatrics*. 2003;112:1430-1436.
32. Prins C, Kerdel FA, Padilla RS, et al. Treatment of toxic epidermal necrolysis with high-dose intravenous immunoglobulins. *Arch Dermatol*. 2003;139:26-32.
33. Trent JT, Kirsner RS, Romanelli P, et al. Analysis of intravenous immunoglobulin for the treatment of toxic epidermal necrolysis using SCORTEN. *Arch Dermatol*. 2003; 139:39-43.
34. Tristani-Firouzi P, Petersen MJ, Saffle JR, et al. Treatment of toxic epidermal necrolysis with intravenous immunoglobulin in children. *J Am Acad Dermatol*. 2002;47: 548-552.
35. Ginsburg CM. Stevens-Johnson syndrome in children. *Pediatr Infect Dis*. 1982;1:155-158.
36. Bastuji-Garin S, Fouchard N, Bertocchi M, et al. SCORTEN: a severity-of-illness score for toxic epidermal necrolysis. *J Invest Dermatol*. 2000;115:149-153.

Chapter 260
ENTEROVIRUS INFECTIONS

Jerri Ann Jenista, MD

Every pediatrician encounters enteroviruses. The best-known serotypes are the polioviruses, but the other enterovirus serotypes also cause widespread disease. A knowledge of these viruses can save both the practitioner and the patient considerable anxiety and can reduce diagnostic and therapeutic expenses.

CLASSIFICATION

Enteroviruses are *Picornaviridae*, small RNA viruses. They are traditionally classified into 3 groups: (1) polioviruses, (2) coxsackieviruses, and (3) enteric cytopathogenic human orphan viruses (echoviruses), based on disease produced in humans and animals. Modern molecular genetic analysis has allowed a better understanding of the relationships among the various enterovirus serotypes. Thus current taxonomy divides the enteroviruses into 4 species, human enterovirus A, B, C, and D (Table 260-1). Except for those reclassified as nonenteroviral, the individual serotypes have retained their traditional names. Newly identified enteroviruses are designated by number, starting with EV68 up to the most recently identified EV101.[1]

A new picornavirus genus, *Parechovirus*, includes the former echoviruses 22 and 23 and at least one newly discovered virus, human parechovirus 3 (HPeV3). The epidemiologic mechanisms and clinical diseases associated with the *Parechovirus* genus are similar to those of the enteroviruses and will be mentioned here.[2,3]

EPIDEMIOLOGIC FEATURES

The epidemiologic features of enteroviral infection are complicated by host, virus, and environmental factors. In the United States alone, approximately 15 million cases of symptomatic enterovirus infection occur every year. Given that up to 90% of infections are silent clinically and reinfection is common, clearly a large percentage of the population must encounter enteroviruses each year. The economic impact of

Table 260-1 Classification of Enteroviruses*

TRADITIONAL TAXONOMY	CURRENT TAXONOMY
Polioviruses	Human enterovirus A (HEV-A)
PV1-3	CAV2-8, 10, 12, 14, 16; EV71, *76, 89-91*
Coxsackie A viruses	Human enterovirus B (HEV-B)
CAV1-22, 24	CAV9; CBV1-6; E1-7, 9, 11-21, 24-27, 29-33; EV69, 73-75, *77-78, 79-88, 100-101*
Coxsackie B viruses	Human enterovirus C (HEV-C)
CBV1-6	CAV1, 11, 13, 17, 19-22, 24; PV1-3
Echoviruses	Human enterovirus D (HEV-D)
E1-7, 9, 11-21, 24-27, 29-33	EV68, 70
Numbered enteroviruses	
EV68-71	

*Enterovirus 79-101, which are not yet included in the International Committee on Taxonomy of Viruses classification, are shown in italics. The gaps in numbering result from changes in classification.
From Khetsuriani N, LaMonte-Fowlkes A, Oberste MS, et al, Centers for Disease Control and Prevention. Enterovirus surveillance—United States, 1970-2005. Surveillance summaries, September 15, 2006. *MMWR.* 2006;55(No SS08):1-20.

enteroviral aseptic meningitis alone is estimated to be over $1.5 billion annually.[4]

Environment

In temperate climates, enterovirus infections show a distinct seasonality, occurring from June through October in the Northern Hemisphere, although sporadic cases are noted in all seasons. In tropical regions, however, infection is noted throughout the year, with an increased incidence during rainy periods. Crowding, poor sanitation, and low socioeconomic conditions also contribute to a high incidence of infection.

Host

Age correlates inversely with the severity of clinical disease, probably because an individual becomes immune to an increasing number of serotypes over several seasons. With certain enteroviral serotypes, neonates may develop fatal sepsis rapidly, whereas most older children and adults have mild or no symptoms. Some enteroviral syndromes (eg, poliomyelitis, acute hemorrhagic conjunctivitis, myocarditis) may be severe at any age. In childhood, boys seem to suffer both more infections and more disease than do girls.

Individuals who have humoral immunodeficiencies may suffer chronic, debilitating infection with enteroviruses.[5] Except for poliovirus, enteroviral infection does not seem to pose a particular threat to individuals who have malignancy or AIDS, although occasional reports of severe or fatal disease have surfaced in these groups. Recipients of bone marrow transplants may experience severe or prolonged infection.

Virus

Most enteroviral syndromes are not serotype specific; that is, several different types may produce the same clinical disease. For example, the coxsackieviruses were first recognized in children who had classic paralytic disease without evidence of poliovirus infection. Conversely, a single serotype may produce varying clinical syndromes in different seasons and communities and even in different individuals infected at the same time and place.

Although outbreaks of illness associated with a single serotype are often reported, the far more common pattern is endemic infection caused by several concurrently circulating enterovirus types. The predominant serotypes may vary yearly, by locality, and even within the same year. The pattern of clinical syndromes seen also tends to change over the enterovirus season. A typical sequence for 1 season might be herpangina in June, nonspecific febrile exanthem in midsummer, and aseptic meningitis by early fall. Pandemic illness is unusual but not unknown. Modern examples are the worldwide spread of acute hemorrhagic conjunctivitis caused by coxsackievirus A24[6] and enterovirus 70, which started in 1969 and affected millions of people and aseptic meningitis in 2000 and 2001 caused by echovirus 13.[7]

Transmission and Incubation

Human beings are the only known reservoir for enteroviruses in nature. These viruses are nearly always transmitted by the fecal-oral route, although infections transmitted by food, water, blood, and human milk[8] and occasionally by the perinatal route have been reported. Nosocomial transmission has resulted in several severe nursery epidemics. In the special case of acute hemorrhagic conjunctivitis, the disease is spread by hand-to-eye contact.

The incubation period for enterovirus infection is ordinarily 3 to 5 days but may range from 2 to 20 days. The period of contagion is probably greatest several days before and immediately after the onset of symptoms; however, it may be prolonged. Because infection is so commonly asymptomatic, and because virus excretion in the feces can persist for weeks after a person has recovered from the illness, identifying a patient's contact by history alone is often impossible. Transmission within households is frequent with rates of greater than 80% reported for siblings.[9,10] Scrupulous hand washing may reduce the spread of enterovirus infection but is unlikely to control it completely, given the large pool of those who shed virus asymptomatically. Reinfection is common and usually clinically inapparent.

PATHOGENESIS

Over the last decade, the technological advances in molecular biology have produced a wealth of new information and have confirmed many long-held theories about the pathogenesis of enterovirus infection. For example, the development of monoclonal antibody systems has allowed researchers to isolate and clone poliovirus receptor sites on human cells.[5] As long suspected, these receptors are different from those for echoviruses. Antibodies directed against the poliovirus receptors block infection by any of the 3 serotypes of poliovirus but not infection by echoviruses or closely related nonenteroviruses. These and many other data constitute the first steps toward understanding the specificity of enteroviruses for primates and the tissue tropism of certain serotypes. The ultimate result of these studies may be an all-enterovirus vaccine.

Enterovirus infection is initiated by viral replication in the lymphoid tissues of the oropharynx and intestines. This phase occurs over 1 to 3 days and is symptom free. A *minor viremia* follows, with spread of virions to the reticuloendothelial system at 3 to 5 days. At this point, the patient is contagious, although symptoms of disease are not yet apparent. In a subclinical infection, the process is halted at this point by host defenses. A subsequent *major viremia* results in viral dissemination to secondary organs such as the skin, heart, liver, pancreas, adrenal glands, and central nervous system. This phase is most often recognized clinically as a nonspecific febrile illness or the *minor illness* of poliomyelitis. In a very small percentage of cases, viral replication continues, producing the various clinical syndromes of enterovirus infection such as poliomyelitis, herpangina, or pleurodynia. The reason serotypes have a tropism for certain tissues, such as poliovirus for the neurons of the brain and spinal cord, is unknown.

Antibody production may be detectable as early as 1 day after exposure to an enterovirus; both serum and secretory antibody forms are induced. Although some cross-reaction occurs among antibodies to different serotypes, protection against disease is not complete. Thus a person who has suffered paralytic disease with one serotype of poliovirus may still be susceptible to a second episode with another serotype. Enterovirus antibody also is found in human milk; it may prevent enterovirus infection or may interfere with successful immunization with oral (live) poliovirus vaccine in the newborn period.

CLINICAL SYNDROMES

Large-scale epidemiologic studies of poliovirus infection indicate that probably more than 90% of enterovirus infections are inapparent. When symptoms do occur, a variety of host factors (eg, age, genetic background, antibody status) and viral factors (eg, strain virulence, inoculating dose of virions) determine the clinical disease present. Although nearly all the protean syndromes associated with enteroviruses have been noted with numerous serotypes, certain diseases are associated more frequently with specific serotypes (Table 260-2). For example, coxsackievirus A16 is the likely etiologic agent of an outbreak of hand-foot-mouth disease. In the United States, a mere 15 serotypes accounted for almost 85% of all enterovirus identification reports over the years 1970 to 2005.[1]

Nonspecific Febrile Illness

Any of the enteroviruses may cause a mild nonspecific febrile illness that lasts up to 7 or more days. Such seasonal infections account for the late summer and early fall peak of office visits noted in community surveillance studies of pediatric febrile illnesses. Because several serotypes are usually circulating within a community during any particular year, a child may suffer several episodes of enterovirus-induced febrile illness within the same season.

Nonpolio enteroviruses are the major cause of hospitalization in febrile infants younger than 3 months. In prospective studies in Rochester, New York, enterovirus infection resulted in hospitalization in 2% of infants in the first month of life and accounted for 82% of admissions for suspected sepsis. In other studies, enterovirus infection accounted for 33% of year-round admissions and 65% of summer-fall admissions for acute febrile illness in young infants.[11]

Enterovirus-associated symptoms that are serious enough to warrant laboratory evaluation in the emergency room are not uncommon in young children during the summer. Of 173 children requiring blood culture or lumbar puncture (or both) in 4 teaching hospitals over one summer season, 46% were ultimately diagnosed with enterovirus infection. Compared with enterovirus-negative children, those with enterovirus infection were hospitalized more often (82%) and had a higher risk of another hospitalization during the same illness (13%).[12] In another region, 1061 febrile infants were evaluated for enteroviral infections over a 5.5-year period; 91% of positive infants were admitted, and 2% required intensive care.[13] Concomitant bacterial infection, usually of the urinary tract, has been noted in 1% to 6% of young infants with proven enteroviral infection.[13,14]

Summer febrile illness associated with enterovirus infection is probably more common than recognized in older children also. In a prospective study of summer febrile illness in children 4 to 18 years of age in private pediatric practices, at least 33% were confirmed to have enterovirus infection. Illness lasted 7 to 9 days; caused the children to miss 2 to 3 days of summer camp, work, or school; and spread to 50% of siblings and 25% of parents.[9]

The most frequent presenting symptoms of nonspecific enteroviral illness are fever, irritability, lethargy, myalgia, malaise, and poor feeding. Diarrhea, vomiting, sore throat, or upper respiratory tract symptoms may be present but are not severe enough to be the cause of the admission. Concomitant aseptic meningitis in infants is common and is not predicted by clinical symptoms.[12,13] The illness occasionally takes a biphasic course. A relapse of fever associated with irritability within 1 or 2 days sometimes results in a second hospital admission for the same illness.

Respiratory Tract Disease

Nonexudative pharyngitis with or without lymphadenopathy is common and is probably the major cause of summertime sore throat. In a few cases, this illness may be the initial manifestation of more severe disease that appears after an apparent recovery period of 1 to 3 days. Other respiratory syndromes (eg, bronchitis, croup, pneumonia) are less common and are generally mild.

Herpangina is a disease commonly diagnosed in a young child who has fever and sore throat or pain on swallowing. An enanthem may be noted early, but it is soon succeeded by small vesicles or tiny white papules and then by ulcers on the tonsils, pharynx, and soft palate. Herpangina is differentiated from herpes simplex stomatitis by the former's milder fever, primarily posterior oropharyngeal involvement, and epidemic seasonal occurrence.

Table 260-2 Clinical Syndromes Associated With the Most Common and Other Selected Enteroviruses, United States 1970-2005

	PV 1-3	E9	E11	E30	CB V5	E6	CB V2	CA V9	E4	CB V4	E7	CB V3	E18	CB V1	E3	E5	E13	CA V16	CA V24	E68	E71	HP EV1
Endemic*							x	x		x								x			x	x
Epidemic*	x	x	x	x	x	x			x		x	x	x	x	x	x	x		x			
Aseptic meningitis	x	x	x	x	x	x	x	x	x	x	x	x	x	x	x	x	x	x			x	x
Paralysis	x	x			x						x		x		x					x	x	x
Encephalitis	x	x						x		x							x				x	x
Meningoencephalitis	x			x	x	x		x			x			x	x							
Epidemic neuropathy								x														
Neonatal sepsis		x	x		x	x	x			x	x	x	x	x				x				x
Nursery outbreak			x			x																x
AHC																			x			
Respiratory illness	x			x						x							x			x		
Pleurodynia														x								
Herpangina				x	x							x										
HFMD					x			x						x				x			x	
Myopericarditis					x					x		x										
Myocarditis	x						x							x				x				
Diabetes type 1					x																	
Rash	x					x				x		x									x	
Gastrointestinal illness						x					x						x					
Rhabdomyolysis																		x				
Death†	NA	0.2	4.6	3.2	1.5	5.9	3.8	1.7	2.8	9.8	2.5	5.4	1.8	0	NA	3.8	NA	1.1	NA	NA	NA	10.9
Chronic infection in immunodeficient persons	x	x										x					x					

*Most typical pattern of serotype circulation.
†Percentage fatality rate in cases reported with a known outcome; *NA*, cases with too few or no observations.
AHC, Acute hemorrhagic conjunctivitis; *CAV*, coxsackievirus type A; *CBV*, coxsackievirus type B; *E*, enterovirus; *HFMD*, hand, foot, and mouth disease; *HpeV*, human parechovirus; *PV*, poliovirus.
Modified from Khetsuriani N, LaMonte-Fowlkes A, Oberste MS, et al, Centers for Disease Control and Prevention. Enterovirus surveillance—United States, 1970-2005. Surveillance summaries, September 15, 2006. *MMWR*. 2006;55(No SS-8):1-20.

The coxsackievirus B serotypes are often implicated in epidemic pleurodynia, or Bornholm disease.[15] Fever with severe pain in the intercostal and abdominal muscles occurring in spasms lasting minutes to hours is characteristic. The succeeding episodes are milder than the first but may occur days and sometimes even months later. In rare cases the symptoms are severe enough to prompt an exploratory laparotomy.

Enanthem and Exanthem Diseases

Hand-foot-mouth syndrome occurs in toddlers and school-aged children. The hallmark signs are relatively painless vesicles on a red base, occasionally grouped, that appear on the buccal mucosa, tongue, hands, and feet. In rare cases the rash may spread to the extremities and buttocks. Patients usually have a low-grade fever and a sore throat and recover within a week.

A variety of exanthems may be the sole or major manifestation of enterovirus infection. Epidemics are reported with the classic macular blanching, rubella-like rash, the so-called Boston exanthem, which begins on the face and trunk and spreads to the extremities. It is distinguished from rubella by the lack of posterior auricular and suboccipital adenopathy. Unusual enterovirus rashes may be maculopapular, vesicular, roseola-like, urticarial, or petechial. When such exanthems occur in conjunction with other enterovirus syndromes, such as aseptic meningitis, the illness may be mistaken for a more serious disease, such as meningococcal meningitis.

Gastrointestinal Diseases

Despite the virus group name and the fecal-oral transmission of enteroviruses, enteric disease is not a prominent clinical syndrome. Gastrointestinal symptoms of nausea, vomiting, abdominal pain, constipation, diarrhea, or peritonitis are occasionally seen but almost always with other signs of systemic enterovirus infection, such as aseptic meningitis. Hepatitis or pancreatitis is usually part of a generalized enterovirus syndrome.

Anecdotal cases of juvenile diabetes mellitus have been related to coxsackievirus B infection.

Acute Hemorrhagic Conjunctivitis

Acute hemorrhagic conjunctivitis is an epidemic disease marked by the sudden onset of severe eye pain, photophobia, tearing, and dramatic subconjunctival hemorrhage and swelling. Recovery occurs in a week to 10 days. The illness is most often observed in middle-aged individuals, but epidemics in schools have been noted. Neurologic sequelae may be seen in adults; clinical improvement may take several months. A worldwide pandemic of this disease began in 1969 with waves of disease in Asia and Africa. The disease reached the continental United States only in the early 1980s and was confined mostly to southeastern states. The virus continues to circulate, with a major epidemic reported in Brazil in 2003.[6]

Aseptic Meningitis

Enterovirus infection is the major cause of aseptic meningitis in countries that immunize against mumps. Most cases are sporadic, although epidemic aseptic meningitis does occur, usually associated with person-to-person spread typically at summer camps or playgrounds and in child care centers.[1,16,17]

The classic disease occurs in a school-age child who has a headache, nuchal rigidity, fever, and often photophobia, pharyngitis, or a rash. Meningismus may be subtle or even absent in up to 50% of patients.[16] Infants most often have nonspecific symptoms such as fever or febrile seizures, poor feeding, cough or congestion, diarrhea, and rash.[18-20] Cerebrospinal fluid (CSF) analysis shows a moderate pleocytosis with a predominance of lymphocytes, normal glucose levels, and slightly increased protein levels. In 20% to 50% of cases of proven aseptic meningitis in infants under 30 days of age, pleocytosis is minimal or absent.[13,18]

Diagnostic dilemmas are not uncommon when a meningitis-like illness occurs in an infant younger than 1 year, in sporadic cases, during a course of antibiotic therapy, or with atypical associated findings such as a petechial rash or encephalitis. Lyme meningitis occurs in a similar age group and during the same season as enteroviral meningitis but can usually be distinguished by the presence of cranial neuropathy, papilledema, or erythema migrans, clinical findings not noted in enteroviral disease.[21] (See Chapter 292, Lyme Disease.) West Nile virus infection in children is clinically indistinguishable from enteroviral meningitis; differential diagnosis is dependent entirely on virologic evaluation.[22]

Spinal fluid obtained early in the course of enteroviral aseptic meningitis most often has a predominant polymorphonuclear cell type; cell counts greater than 1000/mm^3 have been reported. The percentage of mononuclear cells tends to increase over time; although, in some children, the polymorphonuclear predominance persists for several days.[23,24] Other laboratory studies on CSF, such as C-reactive protein level or leukocyte aggregation, show too broad an overlap to distinguish reliably from bacterial meningitis. The results of rapid virus identification techniques may reduce the empirical use of antibiotics and the length of hospitalization significantly.[25,26]

The course of enterovirus-associated meningitis is usually mild, although complications (eg, the syndrome of inappropriate secretion of antidiuretic hormone) are seen occasionally. Adults and older children may complain of headache severe enough to require narcotic analgesia. Most patients recover within 2 weeks; in rare cases, relapses occur. Early information suggested that as many as 10% of survivors of aseptic meningitis that occurred before 3 months of age suffered long-term neurologic sequelae, especially speech and language delays.[27] Recent prospective outcome studies are conflicting, with reports of subtle receptive language problems in one series but no detectable neurodevelopmental disability in others.[28,29] Older children apparently recover completely.

Paralytic Disease

Paralytic disease with wild-type poliovirus has been eradicated in the Western Hemisphere, with no cases occurring in the United States since 1979. Outbreaks continue, however, in parts of South Asia and Africa. All cases of poliovirus infection acquired in the United States since the 1990s were associated with vaccine-derived poliovirus strains and occurred in young adults or in immunodeficient or unimmunized individuals.[30] Because live polio vaccine has not been used in the United States since 2000, any case of vaccine-derived or wild-type poliovirus infection is likely to have been imported and should be reported immediately to public health authorities.

Asymmetrical weakness, paralysis, or both, without sensory loss, differentiates enteroviral paralysis from Guillain-Barré syndrome. Life-threatening disease usually involves paralysis of the primary and accessory respiratory muscles or inflammation of the bulbar respiratory center. Recovery of muscle function may continue for several months.

Infection with other enterovirus serotypes may also result in paralysis. Nonpolio enterovirus and West Nile virus–associated paralysis are more common than classic poliovirus-associated disease. In the 1980s a new syndrome of progressive weakness and fatigue was recognized in long-term survivors of paralytic poliomyelitis. This *postpolio syndrome* is seen decades after the initial infection. Apparently the previously affected muscles suffer denervation as overburdened motor neurons eventually wear out. The long-term outcome of this syndrome is unknown. Although most patients suffer only a modest decline in function even more than 50 years after infection, the associated fatigue may adversely affect the quality of life.[23,31,32]

Perinatal Infection

Enterovirus infection in neonates may occur as any of the syndromes seen in older children.[33] Enteroviruses and the closely related parechoviruses were the most commonly identified viral infections in one neonatal intensive care unit, with mortality as high as 10%.[34] Premature infants and newborns born without specific passively acquired maternal antibody may suffer a fulminant, rapidly fatal disease. Generalized neonatal infection begins as a syndrome of lethargy and poor feeding, with or without fever, indistinguishable from early bacterial sepsis. Progression is swift, with multiorgan involvement, including hepatitis, pancreatitis, coagulopathy, myocarditis, and encephalitis.[35] Mortality is high in the disseminated forms of infection, especially with the combination of hepatic necrosis, coagulopathy, and myocarditis.[36] The virus in neonates is most often transmitted from mother to infant at or near the time of delivery; however, nursery outbreaks with fatal cases have been reported.

Some evidence indicates that maternal enterovirus infection may affect the fetus, but no consistent teratogenic pattern has been recognized. Epidemiologic evidence suggests that maternal exposure to certain enteroviruses during pregnancy may increase the risk of subsequent juvenile diabetes mellitus in the offspring.

Other Diseases

Unusual enterovirus syndromes include encephalitis (often occurring in severely ill neonates), the chronic meningoencephalitis of patients who have hypogammaglobulinemia, and the *dancing eyes-dancing feet* (opsoclonus-myoclonus) syndrome. In 1998 a dramatic outbreak of enteroviral disease occurred in Taiwan. Estimates suggest that more than 1 million infections with coxsackievirus A16 and enterovirus 71 occurred. In particular, infection with enterovirus 71 was associated with an unusually high rate of severe disease that included aseptic meningitis, acute flaccid paralysis, encephalomyelitis, and death, probably caused by neurogenic pulmonary edema.[1,10] Similar but less widespread outbreaks of enterovirus 71–associated neurologic disease were noted in 1997 in Malaysia, in 1999 in Australia, and ongoing at lower levels in Southeast Asia and Pacific regions into the 2000s.

Myocarditis and pericarditis occur with a high mortality as part of the generalized disease of newborns. Fewer than 50% of older children and adults who have myocarditis die; recovery may be complete, but severe sequelae have been reported. Orchitis and parotitis occasionally occur in association with coxsackievirus B infection and are differentiated from mumps only by laboratory studies.

Parechovirus Infections

Enteroviruses 22 and 23 have been reclassified as HPeV1 and HPeV2. At least one other serotype is recognized.[2,3] The viruses continue to be included in the National Enterovirus Surveillance System at the Centers for Disease Control and Prevention; they share many clinical and epidemiologic features with the enteroviruses.[1] Disease appears in an endemic pattern with a summer-fall seasonality. Most clinical infections are reported in very young children and include necrotizing enterocolitis, nursery outbreaks, neonatal sepsis syndrome, febrile seizures, paralysis, rash, and respiratory illness.[37,38] Mortality may be up to 10% in recognized HPeV1 infection; however, asymptomatic disease must be common as over 95% of adults show serologic immunity.[2,3]

Laboratory Evaluation

Laboratory Procedures

When obtaining specimens for enterovirus identification, the clinician must keep in mind the concept of *permissive* versus *nonpermissive* sites. Permissive sites (eg, the nasopharynx and feces) are those in which enteroviruses may persist for weeks to months after infection. Identification of an enterovirus from a permissive site may be completely unrelated to the illness under investigation. Nonpermissive sites are those from which virus is identified only during periods of disease. Shedding of virus in these sites is usually brief. Thus finding an enterovirus in blood, spinal fluid, or a skin vesicle is strong evidence that the virus is related to the concurrent clinical illness.

Because almost all enterovirus serotypes can produce any enterovirus syndrome, and because no disease is associated uniquely with any enterovirus serotype, an enterovirus usually need not be identified beyond its actual presence. Enterovirus presence from a nonpermissive site is sufficient to diagnose the origin of the illness in question. In rare cases, both enteroviral and bacterial pathogens may be present in blood or spinal fluid. Invariably the symptoms associated with the bacterial agent are more severe than those with the viral agent and dictate the clinical management.

Identification of an enterovirus from a permissive site specimen, especially feces, is more problematic. Vague, nonspecific symptoms or highly unusual or rare syndromes may be completely unrelated to the finding of an enterovirus shed in the gastrointestinal tract. Many disease associations with enteroviruses are probably explained by such incidental enterovirus identification. Classic enterovirus disease during a known epidemic season is interpreted more easily; isolating an enterovirus from the stool of an infant who has fever and CSF pleocytosis in the summer, without any other pathogen isolated, is presumptive evidence of enteroviral meningitis.

Virus Isolation

Except for the coxsackievirus A serotypes, enteroviruses are isolated readily in cell cultures. A presumptive positive culture can be noted as early as 18 hours but typically requires 2 to 5 days. Specific identification of an individual serotype takes somewhat longer using either intersecting pools of antienteroviral antibodies or commercially available serotype-specific monoclonal antibodies. Suckling mouse inoculation, an expensive and difficult procedure, is the only available method of isolating most of the coxsackievirus A serotypes.

Viruses may be isolated from throat swabs, feces, CSF, blood or serum, skin vesicles, and tissues obtained at autopsy. Specimens from several sites increase the diagnostic yield because predicting the pathological stage of infection and thus the most likely source of the virus is not always possible.

Virus isolation by culture is time and labor intensive, requiring special expertise. In most clinical laboratories, it has been supplanted by more rapid diagnostic tests such as polymerase chain reaction (PCR). These newer tests, however, do not detect all enterovirus serotypes and cannot differentiate among serotypes. When a specific diagnosis is required, as in the tracing of epidemic enterovirus 71 infection, virus isolation by culture remains the technique of choice. Based on early virus isolation reports during a clinical epidemic, laboratories at the Centers for Disease Control and Prevention have been able to develop serotype-specific PCR assays rapidly.[1] These tests can then be used to promptly differentiate from other possible etiologic agents such as West Nile virus.

Rapid Virus Identification

Currently the only rapid diagnostic technique with clinical promise is PCR. When the test is available, an enterovirus can be identified directly from a specimen such as CSF in as short a time as 5 hours.[26]

Numerous studies of the use of CSF enterovirus PCR tests in clinical settings indicate that PCR is more sensitive than viral culture in identifying aseptic meningitis.[39,40] The time needed to identify a positive specimen by using PCR is considerably shorter, typically 1 day versus 3 to 4 days for viral culture, and results in briefer hospitalizations and shorter courses of empirical antibiotic therapy.[25,26] Experience with non-CSF specimens is limited. Although PCR assays are expensive, the cost is balanced by the savings in therapeutic expenses. As specific antiviral therapy directed against enteroviruses becomes available, PCR will be essential in the early identification of patients most likely to benefit from treatment.

Molecular Genetic Analysis

The genomes of the polioviruses and several of the echoviruses have been sequenced and cloned. These and other advances in genetic analysis have allowed researchers to examine precisely viral strains isolated during epidemics. Thus the epidemic of paralytic poliomyelitis in Finland in 1984 and 1985 was discovered to be caused by a typical wild-type poliovirus strain, not a new mutant, as had been suspected.[5] Ten cases of paralysis and widespread minor infection occurred in this highly immunized population because of an inadequate response to one of the inactivated vaccine components. The epidemic was terminated quickly by mass administration of a live oral polio vaccine. Similarly, molecular analysis of isolates obtained from 4 Minnesota children in 2005 indicated that the serotypes were vaccine-derived poliovirus likely imported by a person who had received oral polio vaccine in a country other than the United States or Canada.[30]

Investigations such as these may allow engineering of better vaccines to accomplish the World Health Organization's goal of eradicating polio worldwide at the beginning of the twenty-first century.

Serological Diagnosis

Obtaining serum for analysis of enterovirus antibody titers is not practical because of the numerous serotypes and the complexity of the procedure. When the clinical or pathological picture strongly suggests one enterovirus group or a limited number of serotypes (ie, myocarditis probably related to coxsackievirus B), measuring neutralizing antibody titers may be feasible.

In situations in which proving the cause of an epidemic or a particularly unusual case might be desirable, serum-neutralizing antibody titers in acute and convalescent samples may be useful. Unfortunately, because antibody production occurs early, titers may already be high during the acute phase of clinical illness, thus obscuring the diagnosis. Assays to detect enterovirus serotype–specific immunoglobulin M in serum are not available commercially.

Treatment

Intravenous immunoglobulin has been successful in eradicating chronic enterovirus infections in some patients with immunodeficiency diseases. Neonates with severe disseminated disease have been treated with infusions of intravenous immunoglobulin up to 1 g/kg and of specific serotype high antibody titer maternal plasma with no discernible benefit.[35,36]

Pleconaril, a novel oral antiviral drug with activity against picornaviruses, including enteroviruses, has been evaluated in clinical trials. Infants, older children, and adults who have enterovirus-associated aseptic meningitis treated with pleconaril suffered a shorter illness and returned to normal activity sooner. In particular, older children reported a marked decrease in headache that was apparent as early as 24 hours after the initiation of treatment.[41]

Pleconaril is available for compassionate use and is effective in stopping the replication of virus in immunodeficient individuals. Pleconaril is well tolerated, with few or no side effects attributed to the drug.[42]

Clinical enterovirus isolates resistant to pleconaril have not been detected.

PREVENTION

Attenuated live or killed poliovirus vaccines are the only preventive enterovirus preparations currently available. Enhanced-potency inactivated poliovirus vaccine is now the only choice for routine immunization in the United States.

In the prevaccine years, 0.2 mL/kg of pooled immune serum globulin given intramuscularly prevented or ameliorated poliovirus infection. In view of the severity of the disease in neonates, such injections might be indicated in nursery epidemics and for infants of mothers who develop a probable enterovirus disease within a few days of delivery.

WHEN TO REFER

- Neonates who have any evidence of disseminated or rapidly progressive enterovirus-like infection
- Immunocompromised individuals who have chronic enterovirus-like syndromes
- Normal hosts who have atypical progression of enteroviral disease, especially those who have neurologic or cardiac involvement

WHEN TO ADMIT

- Neonates and infants younger than 90 days who have suspected enteroviral syndromes in whom systemic bacterial disease is not yet ruled out
- Disease significant enough to require subspecialty expertise, especially cardiac, immunologic, or neurologic disease
- Any enteroviral syndrome that has a rapidly progressive or atypical course
- Older children who have aseptic meningitis who require symptomatic treatment for severe headache or dehydration

TOOLS FOR PRACTICE

Community Advocacy and Coordination

- *Managing Infectious Diseases in Child Care and Schools* (book), American Academy of Pediatrics (www.aap.org/bookstore).

Engaging Patient and Family

- *An Ounce of Prevention Keeps the Germs Away* (brochure), Centers for Disease Control and Prevention (www.cdc.gov/ounceofprevention/docs/oop_brochure_12-20-05.pdf).
- *Non-Polio Enterovirus Infections* (Web page), Centers for Disease Control and Prevention (www.cdc.gov/ncidod/dvrd/revb/enterovirus/non-polio_entero.htm).

Medical Decision Support

- *Enterovirus Surveillance—United States, 1970-2005* (other), Centers for Disease Control and Prevention (www.cdc.gov/mmwr/preview/mmwrhtml/ss5508a1.htm).
- *Red Book: 2006 Report of the Committee on Infectious Diseases,* 27th edition (book), American Academy of Pediatrics (www.aap.org/bookstore).

SUGGESTED RESOURCES

Khetsuriani N, LaMonte-Fowlkes A, Oberste MS, et al, Centers for Disease Control and Prevention. Enterovirus surveillance—United States, 1970-2005. Surveillance summaries, September 15, 2006. *MMWR.* 2006;55(No SS-8):1-20.

Pasquinelli L, Byington C. Enterovirus infections. *Pediatr Rev.* 2006;27:14-15.

REFERENCES

1. Khetsuriani N, LaMonte-Fowlkes A, Oberste MS, et al, Centers for Disease Control and Prevention. Enterovirus surveillance—United States, 1970-2005. Surveillance summaries, September 15, 2006. *MMWR.* 2006;55(No SS-8):1-20.
2. Joki-Korpela P, Hyypia T. Parechoviruses, a novel group of human picornaviruses. *Ann Med.* 2001;33:466-471.
3. Ito M, Yamashita T, Tsuzuki H, et al. Isolation and identification of a novel human parechovirus. *J Gen Virol.* 2004; 85(pt 2):391-398.
4. Parasuraman TV, Deverka PA, Toscani MR. Meningitis Consensus Panel. Estimating the economic impact of viral meningitis in the United States. *Infect Med.* 2000; 17:417-427.
5. Hellen CUT, Wimmer E. Enterovirus genetics. In: Rotbart HA, ed. *Human Enterovirus Infections.* Washington, DC: American Society for Microbiology; 1995.
6. Moura FE, Ribeiro DC, Gurgel N, et al. Acute haemorrhagic conjunctivitis outbreak in the city of Fortaleza, northeast Brazil. *Br J Ophthalmol.* 2006;90:1091-1093.
7. Centers for Disease Control and Prevention. Echovirus type 13-United States, 2001. *MMWR.* 2001;(No SS-50): 777-780.
8. Chang ML, Tsao KC, Huang CC, et al. Coxsackievirus B3 in human milk. *Pediatr Infect Dis J.* 2006;25:955-957.
9. Pichichero ME, McLinn S, Rotbart HA, et al. Clinical and economic impact of enterovirus illness in private pediatric practice. *Pediatrics.* 1998;102:1126-1134.
10. Chang LY, Tsao KC, Hsia SH, et al. Transmission and clinical features of enterovirus 71 infections in household contacts in Taiwan. *JAMA.* 2004;291:222-227.
11. Dagan R. Nonpolio enteroviruses and the febrile young infant: epidemiologic, clinical and diagnostic aspects. *Pediatr Infect Dis J.* 1996;15:67-71.
12. Rotbart HA, McCracken GH Jr, Whitley RJ, et al. Clinical significance of enteroviruses in serious summer febrile illnesses of children. *Pediatr Infect Dis J.* 1999;18:869-874.
13. Rittichier KR, Bryan PA, Bassett KE, et al. Diagnosis and outcomes of enterovirus infections in young infants. *Pediatr Infect Dis J.* 2005;24:546-550.
14. Finkelstein Y, Mosseri R, Garty BZ. Concomitant aseptic meningitis and bacterial urinary tract infection in young febrile infants. *Pediatr Infect Dis J.* 2001;20:630-631.
15. Ikeda RM, Kondracki SF, Drabkin PD, et al. Pleurodynia among football players at a high school: an outbreak associated with coxsackievirus B1. *JAMA.* 1993;270: 2205-2206.
16. Bottner A, Daneschnejad S, Handrick W, et al. A season of aseptic meningitis in Germany: epidemiologic, clinical and diagnostic aspects. *Pediatr Infect Dis J.* 2002;21: 1126-1132.
17. Faustini A, Fano V, Muscillo M, et al. An outbreak of aseptic meningitis due to echovirus 30 associated with attending school and swimming in pools. *Int J Infect Dis.* 2006;10:291-297.

18. Lee BE, Chawla R, Langley JM, et al. Paediatric Investigators Collaborative Network on Infections in Canada (PICNIC) study of aseptic meningitis. *BMC Infect Dis.* 2006;6:68.
19. Tee WS, Choong CT, Lin RV, et al. Aseptic meningitis in children—the Singapore experience. *Ann Aced Med (Singapore).* 2002;31:756-760.
20. Hosoya M, Sato M, Honzumi K, et al. Association of nonpolio enteroviral infection in the central nervous system of children with febrile seizures. *Pediatrics.* 2001;107:166-167. Available at: www.pediatrics.org/cgi/content/full/107/1/e12. Accessed June 13, 2007.
21. Eppes SC, Nelson DK, Lewis LL, et al. Characterization of Lyme meningitis and comparison with viral meningitis in children. *Pediatrics.* 1999;103:957-960.
22. Julian KG, Mullins JA, Olin A, et al. Aseptic meningitis epidemic during a West Nile virus avian epizootic. *Emerg Infect Dis.* 2003;9:1082-1088.
23. Negrini B, Kelleher KJ, Wald ER. Cerebrospinal fluid findings in aseptic versus bacterial meningitis. *Pediatrics.* 2000;105:316-319.
24. Shah SS, Hodinka RL, Turnquist JL, et al. Cerebrospinal fluid mononuclear cell predominance is not related to symptom duration in children with enteroviral meningitis. *J Pediatr.* 2006;148:118-121.
25. Stellrecht KA, Harding I, Woron AM, et al. The impact of an enteroviral RT-PCR assay on the diagnosis of aseptic meningitis and patient management. *J Clin Virol.* 2002; 25(suppl 1):S19-S26.
26. Robinson CC, Willis M, Meagher A, et al. Impact of rapid polymerase chain reaction results on management of pediatric patients with enteroviral meningitis. *Pediatr Infect Dis J.* 2002;21:283-286.
27. Sells CJ, Carpenter RL, Ray CG. Sequelae of central nervous system enterovirus infections. *N Engl J Med.* 1975;293:1-4.
28. Wilfert CM, Thompson RJ Jr, Sunder TR, et al. Longitudinal assessment of children with enteroviral meningitis during the first three months of life. *Pediatrics.* 1981;67:-811-815.
29. Baker RC, Kummer AW, Schultz JR, et al. Neurodevelopmental outcome of infants with viral meningitis in the first three months of life. *Clin Pediatr (Phila).* 1996;35:295-301.
30. Rorabaugh ML, Berlin LE, Heldrich F, et al. Aseptic meningitis in infants younger than 2 years of age: acute illness and neurologic complications. *Pediatrics.* 1993;92: 206-211.
31. Centers for Disease Control and Prevention. Poliovirus infections in four unvaccinated children—Minnesota, August-October 2005. *MMWR.* 2005;(No SS-54):1053-1055.
32. Sorenson EJ, Daube JR, Windebank AJ. A 15-year follow-up of neuromuscular function in patients with prior poliomyelitis. *Neurology.* 2005;64:1070-1072.
33. On AY, Oncu J, Atamaz F, et al. Impact of post-polio-related fatigue on quality of life. *J Rehabil Med.* 2006;38: 329-332.
34. Khetsuriani N, LaMonte A, Obertse M, et al. Neonatal enterovirus infections reported to the National Enterovirus Surveillance System in the United States, 1983-2003. *Pediatr Infect Dis J.* 2006;25:889-893.
35. Verboon-Maciolek MA, Krediet TG, Gerards LJ, et al. Clinical and epidemiologic characteristics of viral infections in a neonatal intensive care unit during a 12-year period. *Pediatr Infect Dis J.* 2005;24:901-904.
36. Abzug MJ. Prognosis for neonates with enterovirus hepatitis and coagulopathy. *Pediatr Infect Dis J.* 2001;20: 758-763.
37. Lin TY, Kao HT, Hsieh SH, et al. Neonatal enterovirus infections: emphasis on risk factors of severe and fatal infections. *Pediatr Infect Dis J.* 2003;22:889-894.
38. Abed Y, Boivin G. Human parechovirus types 1, 2 and 3 infections in Canada. *Emerg Infect Dis.* 2006;12:969-975.
39. Boivin G, Abed Y, Boucher FD. Human parechovirus 3 and neonatal infections. *Emerg Infect Dis.* 11;2005:103-105. Available at: www.cdc.gov/ncidod/EID/vol11no01/04-0606.htm. Accessed June 13, 2007.
40. Capaul SE, Gorgievski-Hrishoho M. Detection of enterivirus RNA in cerebrospinal fluid (CSF) using NucliSens EasyQ enterovirus assay. *J Clin Virol.* 2005;32:236-240.
41. Tsao LY, Lin CY, Yu YY, et al. Microchip, reverse transcriptase-polymerase chain reaction and culture methods to detect enterovirus infection in pediatric patients. *Pediatr Int.* 2006;48:5-10.
42. Rotbart HA. Pleconaril treatment of enterovirus and rhinovirus infections. *Infect Med.* 2000;17:488-494.

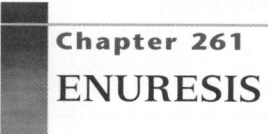

Chapter 261

ENURESIS

Franca M. Iorember, MD MPH; Andrew L. Schwaderer, MD

The acquisition of urinary continence is part of the transition from infancy to childhood. Although incontinence in a child can be an inconvenience, it is generally tolerated until a child falls behind peers. Given that parental concerns about voiding are common, primary care physicians should have an understanding of the normal acquisition of continence and departures from these normal patterns.[1] This chapter provides the basis for the primary care physician to understand the epidemiologic factors, differential diagnosis, evaluation, and management of enuresis in children.

DEFINITION OF TERMS

Definitions

Enuresis is defined as voiding in bed or on clothes that occurs at least twice per week for at least 3 consecutive months in a child who is at least 5 years of age.[2] Five years is considered the age of anticipated 24-hour-per-day bladder control. Children who are intellectually disabled should reach a mental age of 4 years before they are considered enuretic.[3] Two types of enuresis are described based on the time of occurrence of these inappropriate voiding patterns: *Diurnal* enuresis describes wetting in the daytime, whereas *nocturnal* enuresis refers to the passage of urine during the night. Enuresis is described as *primary* when it occurs in children who have never had a period of sustained dryness and *secondary* when it occurs in children who have been dry in the past for a period of at least 6 months, with nocturnal enuresis and 3 months with diurnal enuresis.[2] Nocturnal enuresis can be *monosymptomatic* when no daytime symptoms to suggest lower urinary tract disorders are present and *polysymptomatic* when it is associated with symptoms such as urgency, frequency, dribbling, or daytime enuresis.

Epidemiologic Mechanism

Nocturnal enuresis occurs in approximately 20% of children at 5 years of age, the anticipated age of

24 hour per day bladder control.[4] By age 7, the prevalence of nocturnal enuresis is between 6% and 10%.[5] The annual spontaneous resolution rate is approximately 15%,[6] with nocturnal enuresis persisting in 1% to 3% in the late teens.[6,7] The incidence of primary enuresis is twice as common as secondary enuresis. Nocturnal enuresis is 2 to 3 times more common in boys than it is in girls and is monosymptomatic in 80% of cases. Daytime wetting is more likely in girls than it is in boys. Ten percent of 5 year olds experience daytime wetting at least once every 2 weeks.

Etiology

A strong hereditary component for nocturnal enuresis has been noted. Twin studies demonstrate a concordance rate of 19% to 36% for dizygotic and 46% to 68% for monozygotic twins.[8] Children with a family history of nocturnal enuresis are more likely to experience nighttime wetting than their peers. Forty-four percent of children with 1 parent with a history of nocturnal enuresis will also have nocturnal enuresis, with the percentage of affected children increasing to 77% if the history of nocturnal enuresis is present in both parents.[9] The inheritance pattern with nocturnal enuresis is most often autosomal dominant with high penetrance.[10] In addition to genetics, developmental factors such as delayed speech, delayed walking, and early toilet training have been speculated to be associated with nocturnal enuresis; however, studies evaluating these associations have yielded conflicting results.[5]

Several factors are involved with the pathophysiologic mechanism of monosymptomatic nocturnal enuresis (MNE). Most children with MNE have relative nocturnal polyuria that exceeds the child's bladder capacity, leading to nighttime wetting.[5] Normally, the secretion of antidiuretic hormone increases during sleep; however, in some children with MNE, the secretion of antidiuretic hormone is decreased at night, resulting in increased urine production.[11] Bladder capacity has been demonstrated to vary from daytime to nighttime. In children with enuresis, bladder capacity has been found to be smaller at night compared with normal controls.[12] Normally, if children have a full bladder, whether caused by nocturnal polyuria or decreased bladder capacity, then they will awaken and void in an appropriate place. However, children with MNE are more difficult to arouse from sleep than normal controls or children with primary nocturnal enuresis.[13] Enuresis has been reported to be associated with some sleep disorders, particularly obstructive sleep apnea. Nocturnal enuresis is present in 33% of children with obstructive sleep apnea and resolves in 61% and decreases in 23% of children within 9 months after tonsillectomy and adenoidectomy.[14] Other factors such as nocturnal hypercalciuria and aquaporin-2 dysfunction have been postulated to play a role in the pathogenesis of enuresis.[5]

Anatomic abnormalities may also contribute to polysymptomatic and diurnal enuresis. Urethral obstruction may be congenital (posterior urethral valves) or acquired (foreign body). Ectopic ureters in girls may lead to continuous leaking of urine because, unlike boys, the ectopic ureter usually does not insert proximal to the external sphincter. Lesions involving the spinal cord often result in a neurogenic bladder. Vaginal reflux of urine occurs in girls who do not open the labia during voiding, leading to leakage of urine on standing. Diurnal enuresis occurs when urine is held until the last minute, a behavior common in preschoolers and older children who avoid the restroom at school or are too busy at play. Urinary tract infection contributes to enuresis when cystitis causes spontaneous detrusor contractions; urinary tract infection is also more common in children who have abnormal genitourinary anatomy.

BOX 261-1 Medical Conditions Associated With Enuresis

- Urinary tract infections
- Neurologic disorders, including neurogenic bladder or detrusor instability and spinal cord conditions
- Structural genitourinary tract defects, including ectopic ureter and posterior urethral valves
- Constipation
- Endocrine disorders, including diabetes mellitus and diabetes insipidus
- Hypercalciuria
- Sickle cell disease
- Drugs, including caffeine and methylxanthines
- Child abuse

DIFFERENTIAL DIAGNOSIS

Enuresis is most often encountered as a primary disorder, but may also be caused by other conditions. Underlying disorders that should be considered in the evaluation of enuresis are listed in Box 261-1.

EVALUATION

History

Taking a thorough history is a critical component in evaluating for enuresis. A thorough history will help the primary care physician categorize what type of enuresis is present and identify underlying conditions that might be contributing to the patient's symptoms. The International Children's Continence Society recommends using structured questionnaires for parents to complete before the evaluation. An example of a parent questionnaire may be found at the National Kidney Foundation website. Available at www.kidney.org/patients/bw/pdf/voidhist.PDF. The time of onset, frequency, time of day of occurrence, and any relationship with environmental changes should be determined. Obtaining a history on the length of time of dryness before the onset of enuresis is important because it makes the presence of a structural urinary problem unlikely, helps predict the chance of eventual dryness, and decreases the need for extensive investigation.[5] The history should include the child's fluid intake and drinking habits because some children drink large volumes of fluid in the evening, which may precipitate or exacerbate enuresis. A history of any symptoms such as urinary frequency, urgency, and dysuria should be obtained to help determine the presence of a urinary tract infection. The physician should determine the child's feelings about the enuresis and any motivation for doing something about it; this will eventually influence the decision to initiate therapy.[2] The physician should also find out what the child and parents have done about the symptom before this evaluation. A history of the child's sleeping patterns, given the association of enuresis and sleep apnea, should be obtained.[15] Box 261-2 provides a summary of questions to consider while taking a history of a patient with enuresis.

BOX 261-2 Questions to Consider When Taking a History of a Patient with Enuresis

Definition of the Enuresis: Determine between nocturnal and diurnal enuresis.

- Does the wetting occur during the day, the night or both?
- How often does the wetting occur and at what times?
- How often does the child void during the day and during the night?

Determine between primary and secondary enuresis.

- What age did the wetting start?
- Has the child ever been dry?
- Has the child had any dry spells?
- How long did dry spells last?

Identify what the social situation is regarding the enuresis.

- How does the family handle wet nights?
- Does the child wear pull ups or is a plastic sheet used?
- If sheets and clothing require laundering, then who is responsible?
- Do siblings tease the child?
- Is the child punished for wetting?
- Have any recent traumatic events or changes occurred in the child's social situation?

Identify fluid intake before bedtime: How much and when does the child drink after supper?

Define sleep habits.

- Is the child difficult to awake from sleep?
- Are signs of obstructive sleep apnea (mouth breathing, snoring, and restless sleep) present?

Evaluate for daytime symptoms.

- Is urinary frequency (the normal frequency of voiding is 4-7 times per day), urgency, or dysuria present?
- Is dribbling present between voids?
- Does the child strain with voids?
- Is constipation present?

Evaluate medical history and family medical history.

- Does the child have any psychological conditions (attention deficit disorder, depression, behavior disorders)?
- Does the family have a history of enuresis?

Medical history, including a thorough perinatal history, should be sought to determine if any neurologic explanations for enuresis exist. Specifically, a history of spina bifida or meningomyelocele is important in the pathogenesis of enuresis. Any history of delayed developmental motor milestones or spinal trauma should be obtained. Constipation in the child must be ruled out because of the strong association of constipation with enuresis. Any family history of enuresis or idiopathic hypercalciuria should be elicited. Psychological problems are known to be associated with enuresis. These factors include a poor self-esteem, chronic anxiety, and delayed development.[2]

Physical Examination

Although the results of the physical examination of a child with enuresis are often normal, the examination should be thorough and focus on signs that may indicate any of the causes of enuresis. Abnormal vital signs and growth parameters may be an indication of chronic disease. A complete neurologic examination, including an assessment of gait, muscle tone and strength, deep-tendon reflexes, sensory abnormalities, and rectal sphincter tone, is necessary to exclude central nervous system disease that may result in enuresis. An examination of the spine may reveal subtle signs of spinal dysraphism such as dimples, hair tuft, and skin discoloration. An abdominal examination should pay particular attention to the presence of a distended bladder or constipation. A rectal examination can reveal the presence of fecal impaction or decreased rectal tone. Flank examination should exclude the presence of renal masses that may indicate renal diseases. Lower abdominal tenderness may indicate a urinary tract infection. A careful genitourinary examination should be performed to evaluate for the presence of a rash, adhesions, trauma, and a foreign body in all children and vulvitis and vaginitis in girls.

Laboratory Investigations

The diagnosis of enuresis largely is dependent on a thorough history and physical examination. With MNE, a simple urinalysis can provide valuable information about the cause of enuresis. The presence of proteinuria, hematuria, and red blood cell casts may signal renal pathologic abnormality, whereas glucosuria may be an indication of diabetes mellitus. A low specific gravity on urinalysis may be associated with diabetes insipidus and psychogenic polydipsia. A urinary tract infection may be diagnosed with a urine culture. If daytime symptoms are present, or if the initial laboratory evaluation and physical examination are abnormal, then additional evaluations are indicated. Imaging studies, including a prevoid and postvoid renal and bladder ultrasound, should be obtained if daytime symptoms are present. If the result of the ultrasound is abnormal, then a voiding cystourethrogram and urodynamic studies should be considered.[2] If a spinal dysraphism is thought to exist, then a magnetic resonance imaging scan of the spine should be ordered.

MANAGEMENT

In the treatment of enuresis, any underlying organic causes of enuresis such as constipation or urinary tract infections should be treated first. If both daytime and nighttime symptoms are present, then the daytime symptoms should be treated first. Good voiding hygiene and habits should be reinforced. The treatment of MNE should be considered in a child who is between 6 and 8 years of age and must begin with careful and detailed explanation of the condition to both parents and child in language that is easily understood. The treatment of MNE is often a frustrating experience for both parents and child because relapses often occur. The combination of a motivated child and a cooperative family is the best predictor of a positive outcome.[5] Both primary and secondary nocturnal enuresis are treated similarly. The authors suggest using conservative measures including pull-ups and using absorbent plastic-lined bed sheets for children younger than 8 years. After this point, alarm therapy or pharmacotherapy may be considered if both child and parents are motivated.

Nonpharmacologic Therapy

Conservative measures that help minimize nocturnal polyuria include decreasing the amount of fluid intake several hours before bedtime. Voiding before going to bed minimizes the nocturnal bladder volume. The child may also be awakened and taken to the bathroom to urinate before the parents go to bed. During the daytime, the child should be encouraged to void often and take the time to empty the bladder completely.

Other measures that have been shown to reduce the number of wet nights include the use of charts, mainly for positive reinforcement. Children are asked to fill out a chart depicting wet and dry nights symbolically, such as stars or the sun for dry nights and a cloud for wet nights.[5] The mainstay of therapy for nocturnal enuresis is the enuresis alarm. Although the response rate is not as rapid, alarm therapy is more effective than pharmacologic therapy in treating enuresis.[16] Alarm therapy should be considered in most patients with MNE. Analysis of 25 reported studies in children with MNE suggest an average success rate of 68%, with efficacy increasing with the duration of treatment; dryness occurs in 25% in 2 months, 50% in 3 months, and 90% by 6 months.[5] Because consistent use for many months is often needed before alarm treatment is effective, patience and motivated families are required. In some families, alarms may increase parental annoyance and place the child at risk for physical or emotional abuse. Many children will not initially awaken with the alarm and need a parent to assist in awakening. Relapses occur and do not preclude future success. The percentage of children who remain dry long term after alarm therapy is stopped is 47%, suggesting that the alarm is not only a management modality, but also a cure.[5] Despite the evidence supporting the efficacy of alarm therapy, it is prescribed to less than 5% of children who are evaluated by physicians for enuresis.[1]

Dry bed training has also been shown to be effective. Dry bed training refers to comprehensive programs that include the use of enuresis alarms, positive practices, waking routines, and cleanliness and bladder training in various combinations. Studies examining dry bed training, including enuresis alarms, have shown children to have fewer wet nights compared with children not receiving any treatment.[17]

Pharmacotherapy

The pharmacologic management of enuresis depends on the cause of the condition. Historically, 3 drugs have been used to treat enuresis: desmopressin (DDAVP), imipramine, and oxybutynin. Desmopressin and alarms remain the 1st-line treatment for enuresis.[5] Desmopressin is an analogue of vasopressin (also called antidiuretic hormone). Vasopressin is a polypeptide of 9 amino acids and is produced in the hypothalamus and released from the pituitary gland. The stimulus for the release of vasopressin is hyperosmolality or intravascular volume depletion. Vasopressin acts on the collecting ducts and distal tubules to enhance water absorption. Vasopressin also has vasopressor effects. Desmopressin has significantly increased antidiuretic activity but is absent of vasopressor effects. Desmopressin is used to treat monosymptomatic nocturnal enuresis. Response to treatment might take up to 2 to 3 months. A small group of patients who do not respond to the usual dose of DDAVP may respond when the dose is doubled.[5] In the short term, desmopressin produces a more rapid improvement than alarm therapy, although in the long term, the alarms are more effective and have the highest overall cure rate in treating enuresis.[18] Relapse is common with desmopressin use with up to 80% relapsing when the desmopressin is stopped.[19] If treatment with DDAVP is successful, then a 1-week interruption every 3 months is recommended to see if enuresis has resolved. In children in whom no response to DDAVP occurs, alarm therapy should be considered, and vice versa.[5] Patients and parents should be educated on the side effects of DDAVP, some of which include nausea, vomiting, abdominal pain, headache, facial flushing, elevated blood pressure, chest pain, tachycardia, and hyponatremia from water intoxication.

Oxybutynin is an anticholinergic and smooth-muscle relaxant and has been useful in treating daytime enuresis caused by detrusor overactivity. This drug may therefore be of benefit to enuretic children who have restricted bladder capacity caused by bladder overactivity. Side effects of oxybutynin include nausea, vomiting, abdominal pain, diarrhea or constipation, urinary retention, dry mucous membranes, and blurred vision. Given alone, oxybutynin has been shown to be no more effective than placebo in the treatment of primary enuresis.[20] However, oxybutynin may be helpful if given in combination with other medications, given that combined therapy with oxybutynin and desmopressin produced more rapid results in the treatment of nocturnal enuresis than single therapy with either desmopressin or imipramine.[21] In addition to enuresis, anticholinergic medications are used to treat urge syndrome, Hinman syndrome, or the neurogenic bladder. Tricyclic antidepressants may benefit some patients with MNE potentially by increasing bladder capacity through their anticholinergic effects. The efficacy of imipramine in the treatment of MNE is low, and relapse rates are common.[4] Because of the potential for lethal effects in the setting of an accidental or intentional overdose, clinicians should be cautious with the use of tricyclic antidepressants such as imipramine. In addition, imipramine may cause nausea, vomiting, constipation, blurry vision, urinary retention, cardiac arrhythmias, and hypotension. If tricyclic antidepressants are used, then families must be aware not only of the dangerous potential of overdose, but also about safe storage and the need for supervision during administration.

WHEN TO REFER

- Abnormal urinalysis findings suggestive of a metabolic disorder
- Concerns about neurologic bladder dysfunction
- Failure to respond to appropriate therapy
- Presence of any structural urinary tract abnormality on imaging studies
- History of recurrent urinary tract infections
- History of significant constipation and encopresis

TOOLS FOR PRACTICE

Engaging Patients and Family

- *Waking Up Dry: A Guide To Help Children Overcome Bedwetting* (book), American Academy of Pediatrics (www.aap.org/bookstore).
- National Kidney Foundation Information for Parents (Web site), National Kidney Foundation (www.kidney.org/patients/bw/BWparents.cfm).
- Voiding Progress Calendar (calendar), National Kidney Foundation (www.kidney.org/patients/bw/pdf/adultscalendar.pdf).
- *Glossary for Kids* (fact sheet), National Kidney Foundation (www.kidney.org/patients/bw/BWkidsglossary.cfm).
- *Bed-Wetting* (brochure), American Academy of Pediatrics (patiented.aap.org).
- *Bed-Wetting* (fact sheet), American Academy of Pediatrics (www.aap.org/topics.html).

Medical Decision Support

- Voiding Questionnaire, National Kidney Foundation (www.kidney.org/patients/bw/BWparents.cfm).
- Voiding Diary, National Kidney Foundation (www.kidney.org/patients/bw/pdf/voiddiary.pdf).

SUGGESTED RESOURCES

Journal articles

Feehan M, McGee R, Stanton W, et al. A 6 year follow-up of childhood enuresis. Prevalence in adolescence and consequences for mental health. *J Pediatric Child Health* 1990; 26:75-79.

Foxman B, Valdez RB, Brook RH. Childhood enuresis: prevalence, perceived impact, and prescribed treatments. *Pediatrics*. 1986;77:482-487.

Fritz G, Rockney R. Practice parameter for the assessment and treatment of children and adolescents with enuresis. *J Am Acad Child Adolesc Psychiatry*. 2004;43:1540-1550.

Hjalmas K, Arnold T, Bower W, et al. Nocturnal enuresis: an international evidence based management strategy. *J Urol*. 2004;171:2545-2561.

Book

Bennett HJ. *Waking Up Dry: A Guide to Help Children Overcome Bedwetting*. Elk Grove Village, IL: American Academy of Pediatrics; 2005.

Web site

National Kidney Foundation Parent Resource Web site at: www.kidney.org/patients/bw/BWparents.cfm.

REFERENCES

1. Foxman B, RB Valdez RB, Brook RH. Childhood enuresis: prevalence, perceived impact, and prescribed treatments. *Pediatrics*. 1986;77:482-487.
2. Fritz G, Rockney R. Practice parameter for the assessment and treatment of children and adolescents with enuresis. *J Am Acad Child Adolesc Psychiatry*. 2004;43: 1540-1550.
3. Thiedke CC. Nocturnal enuresis. *Am Fam Phys*, 2003;67:1499-1506, 1509-1510.
4. Caldwell PH, Edgar D, Hodson E, et al. Bedwetting and toileting problems in children. *Med J Aust*. 2005;182: 190-195.
5. Hjalmas K, Arnold T, Bower W, et al. Nocturnal enuresis: an international evidence based management strategy. *J Urol*. 2004;171:2545-2561.
6. Forsythe WI, Redmond A. Enuresis and spontaneous cure rate. *Arch Dis Child*. 1974;49:259-263.
7. Feehan M, McGee R, Stanton W, et al. A 6 year follow-up of childhood enuresis. Prevalence in adolescence and consequences for mental health. *J Pediatric Child Health*. 1990;26:75-79.
8. Hublin C, Kaprio J, Partinen M, et al. Nocturnal enuresis in a nationwide twin cohort. *Sleep*. 1998;21:579-585.
9. Von Gontard A, Schaumburg H, Hollmann E, et al. The genetics of enuresis: a review. *J Urol*. 2001;166:2438-2443.
10. Arnell H, Hjalmas K, Jagervall M, et al. The genetics of primary nocturnal enuresis: inheritance and suggestion of a second major gene on chromosome 12q. *J Med Genet*. 1997;34:360-365.
11. Rittig S, Knudsen UB, Norgaard JP, et al. Abnormal diurnal rhythm of plasma vasopressin and urinary output in patients with enuresis. *Am J Physiol*. 1989;256:F664-F671.
12. Yeung CK, Sihoe JD, Sit FK, et al. Characteristics of primary nocturnal enuresis in adults: an epidemiological study. *BJU Int*. 2004;93:341-345.
13. Chandra M, Saharia R, Hill V, et al. Prevalence of diurnal voiding symptoms and difficult arousal from sleep in children with nocturnal enuresis. *J Urol*. 2004;172:311-316.
14. Basha S, Bialowas C, Ende K, et al. Effectiveness of adenotonsillectomy in the resolution of nocturnal enuresis secondary to obstructive sleep apnea. *Laryngoscope*. 2005;115:1101-1103.
15. Brooks LJ, Topol HI. Enuresis in children with sleep apnea. *J Pediatrics*. 2003;142:515-518.
16. Glazener CM, Evans JH, Peto RE. Alarm interventions for nocturnal enuresis in children. *Cochrane Database Sys Rev*. 2003;CD002911.
17. Lyon C, Schnall J. What is the best treatment for nocturnal enuresis in children? *J Fam Pract*. 2005;54:905-906.
18. Moffatt ME, Harlos S, Kirshen AJ, et al. Desmopressin acetate and nocturnal enuresis: how much do we know? *Pediatrics*. 1993;92:420-425.

19. Thompson S, Rey JM. Functional enuresis: is desmopressin the answer? *J Am Acad Child Adolesc Psychiatry.* 1995;34:266-271.
20. Lovering JS, Tallett SE, McKendry JB. Oxybutynin efficacy in the treatment of primary enuresis. *Pediatrics.* 1998;82:104-106.
21. Lee T, Suh HJ, Lee HJ, et al. Comparison of effects of treatment of primary nocturnal enuresis with oxybutynin plus desmopressin, desmopressin alone or imipramine alone: a randomized controlled trial. *J Urol.* 2005;174:1084-1087.

Chapter 262

FOREIGN BODIES OF THE EAR, NOSE, AIRWAY, AND ESOPHAGUS

Catherine C. Skae, MD; Sanjay R. Parikh, MD

Foreign bodies of the ear, nose, respiratory, and digestive tracts are a common problem among children, particularly those younger than 5 years. Children are at risk as soon as the pincer grasp is achieved around 9 months of age. The scope of the problem was first underscored by National Safety Council data in 1969, which showed that more children died at home from accidental foreign-body ingestion or aspiration than from any other cause.[1] By 1998, foreign-body aspiration and asphyxiation was the fourth-leading cause of accidental death in the home among children younger than 5 years.[2] National Safety Council data from 2005 to 2006 reveal that 133 deaths per 100,000 population in children from birth to 4 years were caused by choking defined as suffocation by inhalation or ingestion of food or other objects.[3]

The severity of the problems caused by the presence of a foreign body depends on the site, composition, and duration of time in the body. Removal of a foreign body is not usually an emergency, unless the airway is compromised or if the object is a battery that might cause liquefaction necrosis. Removal should be attempted only if the physician has appropriate sedation or anesthesia, proper instrumentation and illumination, and, most important, ability. Attempts to remove the foreign body without these elements may aggravate the problem and jeopardize the child's well being.

FOREIGN BODIES OF THE EAR

Foreign bodies of the external auditory canal are most common among children between 2 and 4 years of age. They can include food, insects, toys, buttons, pieces of crayons, pencil erasers, and button-shaped batteries.[4] Accidental entry of a foreign object through placement in the external auditory canal, either by the child or a companion, can occur during play. Insects also can fly or crawl into the ear canal. Some experts suggest that children who have chronic external otitis or itching are more likely than healthy children to place objects in their ear canal.[5] Earrings can become embedded in the auricle when a chronic infection of the pierced site is followed by overgrowth of granulation tissue. The use of the spring-loaded gun to pierce ears has resulted in numerous cases of embedded earrings as well.[6]

History and Physical Examination

Usually, eliciting a history of placing an object in the ear canal is difficult because most children are reluctant to admit to this activity. If insertion is not witnessed, then some foreign bodies may go undetected for extended periods. Findings depend on the depth of the foreign object within the external auditory canal, the nature and composition of the object, and its duration in the canal. Children may complain of ear pain, discomfort, bleeding, discharge, an odor, aural fullness, hearing loss, nausea, vomiting, coughing, tearing, or dizziness.

Inert substances, such as plastic, that are not obstructing the canal and are not abutting the tympanic membrane may not cause symptoms. Insects tend to incite local irritation, causing discomfort, erythema, and, occasionally, drainage. Food matter also may cause local inflammation that often leads to local pain and itching. Objects that touch the tympanic membrane cause pain, particularly with movement of the drum, as when swallowing. If the entire canal is obstructed, then hearing will likely be decreased.

Several reports have been issued of button-size alkaline batteries in the ear canal.[7-9] These objects may leak battery alkali, causing a severe local tissue reaction or destruction, with pain, swelling, and discharge. This foreign body should be handled expeditiously to prevent serious injury to the canal, tympanic membrane, or middle ear.

When the history indicates a small foreign body but it cannot be visualized on examination, it may be lodged anteriorly in the tympanic sulcus. Instillation of water to fill the medial half of the external canal may act as a concave lens, allowing visualization of the tympanic sulcus.[10] In a patient who has a small, narrow, or swollen external ear canal, microscopic evaluation will aid in visualization.

Management

Nonurgent Situations

Aural foreign bodies may be removed by irrigation, suction, or instrumentation.[11-13] Nonreactive foreign bodies that do not occlude the external canal completely or impinge on the tympanic membrane do not present an emergency. These foreign bodies can be removed with various instruments; the most useful will depend on the shape and composition of the object. In many cases, Frazier tip suction, alligator forceps, or a right-angle hook may be used to retrieve the object. The hook is used by passing it beyond the object, hooking it from behind, and pulling it out gently. Gentle irrigation also may be used on nonabsorbable substances, provided the tympanic membrane can be visualized and is intact and no evidence of inflammation of the external canal exists. Food matter tends to swell when water is applied, making removal difficult. Irrigation is accomplished using an 18-guage catheter attached to a 10- to 20-mL syringe. The flow of fluid should be directed around the retained object, allowing backpressure to force the object out of the canal. Fluids should be warmed to avoid irritation of the labyrinths.[14] A nonperforated tympanic membrane must be visualized before irrigation. Ear syringing is an effective and easy way of removing foreign bodies. The pressure generated by a 14- or 16-gauge cannula and a 20-mL syringe is well below the pressure required to burst a tympanic membrane.[15]

Urgent Situations

In older children who are cooperative, a local anesthetic injected with a small-gauge needle into the skin lining the external canal may allow complete removal of the foreign body and subsequent examination. For younger children or for those who are uncooperative, general anesthesia may be necessary and is certainly preferable to traumatic removal if a child is unable to cooperate or cannot be restrained adequately.

When the tympanic membrane cannot be visualized, or if evidence exists of inflammation or injury to the external canal, then the foreign body should be removed immediately. Expeditious removal is particularly important with an alkaline battery, because tympanic membrane perforations have been reported within only 8 hours of entry.[7] Magnets may be helpful for removing metallic objects such as batteries or metal beads.[16]

Insects

Insects should be killed before removal by instilling water, mineral oil, or topical lidocaine into the external canal. Extraction with suction or alligator forceps may then be undertaken.

Postextraction Care

After any foreign body is removed, the external canal and tympanic membrane should be thoroughly inspected. If the external auditory canal appears infected or irritated, then topical antibiotic otic drops with steroids may be instilled. The affected ear should be protected from water until it has healed completely.

Consultation with an otolaryngologist should be requested if the object cannot be removed or if perforation of the tympanic membrane is suspected. Schulze[17] studied 698 consecutive cases of pediatric external auditory canal foreign bodies. Attempts under direct visualization by emergency department physicians had lower success rates with removing spherical objects, objects touching the tympanic membrane, and objects in the canal for more than 24 hours. The physicians concluded that these cases should be referred directly to otolaryngologists for otomicroscopic removal.

Complications

Complications can be caused by the foreign body or by traumatic removal. Laceration or inflammation of the external canal is not usually serious and resolves with instillation of liquid analgesics and antibiotics. Perforations of the tympanic membrane require careful inspection to ensure that a flap of the membrane has not folded into the middle ear leading to a permanent perforation or a cholesteatoma. Similarly, when the tympanic membrane is not intact, the middle ear space can become contaminated, and otitis media can develop. Balbani et al reviewed 93 cases of foreign bodies in the ear and found that all 12 complications (11 canal lacerations and one tympanic membrane perforation) occurred in patients who had undergone previous attempts at removal.[18] Engelsma reported one case of impacted foreign body following two attempts at removal that required surgical widening of the canal before extraction.[19]

If removing a foreign object from the ear canal safely is not possible, if the tympanic membrane may have been injured by either the foreign body or its removal, or if hearing loss, nystagmus, vertigo, cranial nerve deficits, or deep-seated infection occurs,[14] then the patient must be referred to an otolaryngologist.

FOREIGN BODIES IN THE NOSE

Foreign bodies in the nose are typically soft, such as tissue paper, eraser material, or clay; however, they can also be hard, as with a bead, pebble, or piece of candy. Occasionally a foreign object enters the nose accidentally while the child is attempting to sniff or smell it. Chronic rhinitis is the most common underlying factor in children placing objects in the nose.[6] The frequency has been noted to increase during the summer and Christmas, when toy sales increase.[20]

History and Physical Examination

Children will usually not admit to placing foreign bodies in the nose. The most common symptom of a foreign body in the nose is unilateral nasal discharge that is usually foul smelling. In fact, a unilateral nasal discharge in a young child should be considered evidence of a foreign body until proved otherwise. Occasionally, epistaxis is the presenting symptom.[21] When an alkaline disk battery is lodged in the nose, the symptoms may be acute. Tissue damage can occur through 3 mechanisms: (1) electrical burn, (2) liquefaction necrosis (from sodium hydroxide), and (3) pressure necrosis.[22] If possible, the anterior nasal cavities should be examined with a nasal speculum and suction. The key to any evaluation is powerful illumination. Radiographs may be helpful if the object is radiopaque or has become calcified. An incidental finding of a nasal foreign body on a routine dental x-ray examination has been reported.[23] US toy manufacturers are required by law to make toy parts radiopaque, a regulation that proves quite valuable when a physician is looking for foreign objects in the nasal cavity or in any part of the upper aerodigestive tract. However, toys and toy parts manufactured outside the United States do not have to conform to this regulation. In their review of children who had nasal foreign bodies, Tong et al reported that 28 of 71 (39%) radiographs demonstrated a foreign body.[20]

Management

Nasal foreign bodies should be removed as quickly as possible, particularly in the case of an alkaline battery, which can cause severe local inflammation, with tissue damage occurring within 1 hour of placement.[7,24] When an alkaline disk battery is in the nasal cavity, saline irrigation should be avoided because it can cause further tissue damage.[22] Young children are averse to nasal instrumentation, and removing a nasal foreign body requires some degree of cooperation or restraint. Thus sedation or general anesthesia may be advised. Topical application of a vasoconstrictor agent (eg, oxymetazoline, phenylephrine) in conjunction with removal of secretions by a small suction tip helps visualize the foreign object, particularly one lodged in the middle or posterior nasal cavity. Use of an endoscope is recommended to visualize this region.[21] The majority of items are retrievable using grasping instruments such as straight forceps and mosquito clamps. Other methods include suction, irrigation, and adhesives.[14] A foreign body that has remained in the nose for a long time may become calcified and form a *rhinolith*. Removing a *rhinolith* is often difficult and bloody.

Foreign-body removal using pepper to induce a sneeze while the uninvolved nostril is occluded or blowing in the child's mouth while the contralateral nostril is held shut is not suggested. In a more controlled fashion, nebulized adrenaline together with nose blowing has been reported to expel nasal foreign bodies successfully.[25] Ambu-bag insufflation of the mouth with the patient in Trendelenburg position has also been described.[26] Another method of removal involves using a Fogarty or a small Foley catheter.[27,28] The catheter is placed beyond the foreign body into the posterior portion of the nasal cavity or nasopharynx and then inflated with 2 to 3 mL of saline solution. The catheter is then drawn gently forward and out of the nose, expelling the object. The danger with this technique is that the foreign object may be dislodged by pushing it posteriorly into the nasopharynx, which may lead to aspiration of the object.

Soft, friable objects can usually be removed with a Frazier tip suction device. If the foreign body is firm and flat or has an edge, then it may be removed by using a nasal bayonet or Hartmann or alligator forceps. A wire loop may be placed beyond the foreign body that is spherical and removed by pulling it forward. After removal, local inflammation exhibited by bloody or purulent oozing may be controlled with saline nose drops and an antibacterial ointment such as bacitracin or mupirocin. Sterile water should be used in place of saline if the foreign object removed was an alkaline battery.[22]

Differential Diagnosis

The differential diagnosis of foreign bodies in the nose includes suppurative rhinitis, adenoiditis, sinusitis, and nasal or nasopharyngeal tumors. Nasal polyps also may cause unilateral nasal discharge, and in a young child, the diagnosis of cystic fibrosis must be ruled out.

Complications

Complications of nasal foreign bodies include epistaxis, local infection, inflammation, and nasal septal perforation. Occasionally a scar band, or synechia, may form between the turbinate and septum. Scar bands can be prevented by placing a splint made of Gelfilm or Silastic over the raw, exposed area. Nasal septal perforation has been reported.[20] Obstruction of a sinus ostium by a foreign object may lead to the development of sinusitis, which typically causes pain and tenderness over the affected sinus or clouding and an air-fluid level on radiograph. Treatment includes oral antibiotics and nasal decongestant drops. Aspiration of a nasal foreign body can be prevented in most cases by prompt and skilled removal.

FOREIGN BODIES OF THE AIRWAY

As of 2006, foreign-body aspiration and asphyxiation account for approximately 9% of all home accidental deaths of children younger than 5 years.[3] The incidence declines rapidly among those older than age 5, until age 65, when it increases again to an even higher percentage. Increased parental awareness of the risks of leaving small objects within the reach of young children and consumer education have been important in diminishing this hazard. In addition, the development of lifesaving techniques, such as the Heimlich maneuver, that can be performed by people who are not health care workers accounts for a higher survival rate.

Complete airway obstruction is generally caused by globular foods such as hot dogs, nuts, candies, and grapes or by toys or latex balloons.[29] With regard to foreign-body impaction, the airway can be divided into three segments: (1) larynx, (2) trachea, and (3) bronchial tree. Lima[30] reviewed all airway foreign body admissions to his pediatric hospital from 1980 through 1987. Of the 91 cases, 11 involved a foreign body lodged in the larynx. Of these 11 patients, 5 died, and 3 suffered anoxic encephalopathy. Although most foreign bodies pass through the larynx, the outcome is apparently grave when one does not.

Etiology

Curiosity or boredom may lead young children to put objects in their mouth. Infants in particular will place almost anything they can handle into their mouth. A startle may cause inadvertent ingestion or aspiration. Lack of complete dentition, as well as lack of attention to chewing, allows large food particles to enter the posterior pharynx. Incomplete development of mouth and tongue coordination and the neuromuscular mechanism for swallowing in young children also may account for a greater incidence of foreign-body ingestion or aspiration.[31] A positive association between the occurrence of upper respiratory tract infections and foreign body aspiration has been noted[32] possibly stemming from the need for continuous mouth breathing. A cold interrupts a smooth breathing-swallowing pattern, leading to an increase in aspiration. Although this situation typically occurs in the younger child, some estimates indicate that 23% occurred in children older than 5 years.[31]

History and Physical Examination

When an object is aspirated into the respiratory tract, it initially produces a choking, gagging, coughing, or wheezing episode. This episode may be followed by an asymptomatic interval during which little evidence remains to suggest the presence of a foreign body.

Depending on the site of the foreign body in the airway, a patient may exhibit a spectrum of findings, ranging from an almost complete lack of symptoms to signs of complete airway obstruction. A high index of suspicion and knowledge of the many possible presentation scenarios are the best insurance against the hazards of missed or delayed diagnoses.[33]

Laryngeal foreign bodies are likely to produce the most acute and dramatic presentation. Large objects that completely obstruct the airway may result in stridor, high-pitched wheezing, cough, dysphonia, or worse—aphonia and cyanosis. Children who have small, partly obstructing, objects that allow adequate air exchange have cough, stridor, hoarseness, and pain or discomfort.

Tracheal foreign bodies are usually associated with cough and some degree of stridor or with wheezing and may produce an audible *slap* as the object moves from the carina to the glottis with respiration. Bronchial foreign bodies usually cause wheezing or coughing if they are partly obstructing, which is often misdiagnosed as asthma. With complete obstruction of a bronchus, an initial asymptomatic period is followed by a postobstructive pneumonitis or bronchiectasis.[34] Sharp objects such as pins or tacks may cause pain or hemoptysis.

Imaging

If aspiration of a foreign body into the upper airway is suspected, then plain-film radiographs may help. For objects suspected of being lodged in the laryngeal inlet, high-kilovolt, anteroposterior and lateral radiographs of the upper trachea or esophageal inlet should be obtained if the patient's condition permits. Bronchial foreign bodies may be suggested by some form of dynamic radiographic study, such as inspiratory-expiratory films, lateral decubitus films, or videofluoroscopy. These studies can demonstrate airtrapping in the affected lung.

Management

Foreign bodies that completely obstruct the laryngeal inlet create a life-threatening emergency and should be expelled immediately by using the Heimlich maneuver (abdominal thrusts). For infants younger than 1 year, the American Academy of Pediatrics recommends 5 back blows in the head-down position followed by 5 chest thrusts in the supine position, in place of the Heimlich maneuver.[35] Blind finger sweeps are dangerous and should be avoided.[35] If the foreign body cannot be expelled, then a large-bore needle or angiocatheter (14 gauge) should be inserted into the cricothyroid space to allow some degree of ventilation until the patient can be taken to the operating room for removal of the object. Alternatively, if skilled personnel are present, then an emergency tracheotomy may be necessary. Partly obstructing laryngeal foreign bodies should be treated in a manner that prevents total obstruction of the airway; therefore back blows and abdominal thrusts should not be used in these cases.

Tracheal and bronchial foreign bodies should be removed by a physician specifically trained for the task, which usually requires controlled endoscopic removal in the operating room. This situation is not usually an emergency; therefore adequate preparations can be made.

Complications

Abdominal and chest thrusts may damage intraabdominal contents (eg, liver, spleen) and ribs, respectively. Therefore these techniques should be used only in cases of complete airway obstruction that would otherwise cause certain death. Conversion of a partial airway obstruction to a complete obstruction can best be prevented by having skilled personnel retrieve the foreign body. Pneumonia was the most common complication in 127 cases of foreign body aspiration.[36]

A bronchial foreign body that remains in place for an extended period may cause air trapping and irreversible bronchiectatic changes distal to the obstruction.

Prolonged or difficult instrumentation of the airway during removal of a foreign body can lead to laryngeal edema or injury, with obstructive symptoms. This situation may require a period of intubation after surgery. As an alternative, postoperative edema can sometimes be prevented by using steroids during and after surgery.

FOREIGN BODIES INVOLVING THE ESOPHAGUS

More than one half of foreign bodies in children involve the esophagus, with the highest incidence in children 14 months to 6 years of age.[37] Young children are inquisitive and tend to explore objects orally. The objects are then intentionally swallowed or accidentally ingested as the result of a startle. Coins, food, marbles, buttons, pins, tacks, jewelry, and batteries are a few of the numerous foreign bodies children have ingested. In the United States, coins are the most common foreign body to lodge in the esophagus.[38] Coins are the most frequent esophageal foreign body in children younger than 10 years, and fish bones are the most common in children older than 10 years.[39] Developmentally delayed children are at high risk, as are children who have undergone esophageal surgery and those who have a damaged esophagus from prior caustic ingestions.

The esophagus has 4 physiological areas of narrowing: (1) the cricopharyngeal sphincter, (2) the aortic arch, (3) the region of the left main bronchus, and (4) the gastroesophageal sphincter. These areas correspond to the 4 most-common sites of foreign body obstruction. The cricopharyngeus is the most common; the arch of the aortic region is the most dangerous. If the foreign body is lodged at the lower border of the cricopharyngeus muscle, then it will be visualized at the level of the clavicles on chest radiograph.

History and Physical Examination

The history of foreign-body ingestion is often not obtained, and most foreign bodies pass through the normal esophagus undetected. A swallowed or aspirated object can cause a respiratory emergency, no symptom at all, or anything in between. Objects that do not pass freely initially stimulate the larynx and cause gagging and coughing. Subsequent symptoms depend on the size, composition, and nature of the foreign body. With young children, poor feeding or refusal to eat or drink, as well as increased salivation, are typical. When the esophagus is completely or almost completely obstructed, choking and vomiting occur. The duration of obstruction can affect the clinical presentation; that is, the longer a foreign object is present, the greater the tissue reaction and local inflammation will be. Thus, in the later stages, patients can have pain on swallowing, airway compromise, fever, and leukocytosis.

Imaging

When a foreign body is suspected, posteroanterior and lateral chest radiographs, in addition to neck radiographs, are diagnostic if the object is radiopaque, such as a coin. If the foreign body is a coin, then it will be oriented in a transverse position because the opening of the esophagus is widest in a transverse position. Contrast studies can be used when an esophageal foreign body that does not show on routine radiographs is strongly suspected.

Management

An esophageal foreign body does not usually require emergency measures, but it should be removed as soon as possible after proper evaluation and preparation.[40] In many instances, children will have eaten recently, and generally, experts recommend that an appropriate period pass before they are given general anesthesia. If the foreign body is corrosive, such as an alkaline button battery, then it should be removed as soon as possible to prevent severe inflammation and potential perforation of the esophageal wall.[41]

Endoscopic removal under anesthesia by a trained expert remains the method of choice. With rigid esophagoscopy, optical forceps are passed through the central channel for retrieval of the foreign body. This technique allows for direct visualization of the esophagus, its mucosa, and the foreign body. Removal with flexible endoscopy is also possible. Once the scope is passed, a variety of flexible graspers, forceps, baskets, and magnets can be passed through the instrument channel to retrieve the object.

Nonendoscopic techniques for removing an esophageal foreign body (ie, with a Foley or Fogarty catheter) have been described but are not recommended.[27] The child is sedated and brought to the fluoroscopy suite. While the child is in a steep Trendelenburg position, the catheter is placed beyond the foreign object, and the balloon on the catheter is inflated and withdrawn. This technique can lead to aspiration, airway obstruction, and death and is not recommended.

Complications

Perforation of the esophagus can result from the endoscopic procedure or may be caused by the foreign body itself, especially if it is sharp or caustic. Endoscopic removal is particularly dangerous with objects lodged at the level of the aortic arch. If an esophageal tear is suspected, then a radiographic gastrograffin swallow study will usually confirm or negate the suspicion.

Retropharyngeal abscess has been reported as the most frequent complication of a sharp esophageal foreign body, such as a fish bone.[39] Foreign bodies that have been in the esophagus for long periods can also cause a stricture to develop. In these cases, a contrast study, computed tomography scan, or esophagoscopy also should be performed to aid in the diagnosis.

During anticipatory guidance, parents and caregivers should be instructed not to leave small objects or inappropriate food where a young child can reach them or give them to a young infant.[42]

WHEN TO REFER

- If airway compromise exists
- Anytime a battery is involved
- If the child cannot be restrained adequately
- If an object cannot be removed
- Ear:
  - If the tympanic membrane cannot be visualized or perforation is suspected
  - If the object is touching the tympanic membrane
  - If the object is spherical or in the canal for >24 hours
  - If hearing loss, nystagmus, vertigo, central nervous system deficits, or deep-seated infection exists
- Nose: if a rhinolith has formed
- Airway: for tracheal and bronchial foreign bodies
- Esophagus: for endoscopic removal if perforation is suspected

WHEN TO ADMIT

- Airway: if prolonged or difficult instrumentation of the airway occurred during removal of the foreign body if postoperative edema develops
- Esophagus: if the object is sharp and irretrievable by endoscope

TOOLS FOR PRACTICE

Community Advocacy and Coordination

- *Prepare for Emergencies with American Red Cross First Aid, CPR and Automated External Defibrillator (AED) Courses* (Web page), American Red Cross (www.redcross.org/services/hss/courses/).

Engaging Patient and Family

- *Children and Foreign Bodies in the Ear and Nose* (fact sheet), American Academy of Otolaryngology—Head and Neck Surgery (www.entnet.org/KidsENT/Foreign_Bodies_Ear_Nose.cfm).
- *TIPP Safety Sheets* (fact sheet), American Academy of Pediatrics (www.aap.org/bookstore).

Medical Decision Support

- *3-in-1 First Aid, Choking, CPR* Chart, American Academy of Pediatrics (www.aap.org/bookstore).
- *What can I do to keep my child from choking?* (fact sheet), American Academy of Pediatrics (www.aap.org/publiced/BR_Choking.htm).

RELATED WEB SITE

- National Safety Council (www.nsc.org).

REFERENCES

1. National Safety Council. *Accident Facts*. Chicago, IL: National Safety Council; 1969.
2. National Safety Council. *Injury Facts*, Chicago, IL: National Safety Council; 1999.
3. National Safety Council. *Injury facts, 2005-6 edition*. Itasca, IL: National Safety Council; 2006.
4. The American Academy of Otolaryngology—Head and Neck Surgery. Available at: www.entnet.org/kidsent/foreign_bodies_ear_nose.cfm. Accessed July 6, 2007.
5. Das SK. Etiological evaluation of foreign bodies in the ear and nose. *J Laryngol Otol*. 1984;98:989-991.
6. Cohen HA, Nussinovitch M, Straussberg R. Embedded earrings. *Cutis*. 1994;53:82.
7. Capo JM, Lucente FE. Alkaline battery foreign bodies of the ear and nose. *Arch Otolaryngol Head Neck Surg*. 1986;112:562-563.
8. Rachlin LS. Assault with battery. *N Engl J Med*. 1984;311: 921-922.
9. Skinner DW, Chiu P. The hazards of "button-sized" batteries as foreign bodies in the nose and ear. *J Laryngol Otol*. 1986;100:1315-1318.
10. Peltola TJ, Scarento R. Water used to visualize and remove hidden foreign bodies from the external ear canal. *J Laryngol Otol*. 1992;106:157-158.
11. Mishra A, Shukla GK, Bhatia N. Aural foreign bodies. *Indian J Pediatr*. 2000;67:267-269.
12. Jones I, Moulton C. Use of an electric ear syringe in the emergency department. *J Accid Emerg Med*. 1998;15: 327-328.
13. Kadish HA, Corneli HM. Removal of nasal foreign bodies in the pediatric population. *Am J Emerg Med*. 1997;15: 54-56.
14. Belleza WG, Kalman S. Otolaryngologic emergencies in the outpatient setting. *Med Clin North Am*. 2006;90(2): 329-353.
15. Kumar S. Foreign bodies in the ear: a simple technique for removal analysed in vitro. *Emerg Med J*. 2005;22(4): 266-268.
16. Landry GL, Edmanson MB. Attractive method for battery removal. *JAMA*. 1986;256:3351.
17. Schulze SL, Kerschner J, Beste D. Pediatric external auditory canal foreign bodies: a review of 698 cases. *Otolaryngol Head Neck Surg*. 2002;127(1):73-78.
18. Balbani AP, Sanchez TG, Butugan O, et al. Ear and nose foreign body removal in children. *Int J Pediatr Otorhinolaryngol*. 1998;46:37-42.
19. Engelsma RA, Lee WC. Impacted aural foreign body requiring endaural incision and canal widening for removal. *Int J Pediatr Otorhinolaryngol*. 1998;44:169-171.
20. Tong MC, Ying SY, van Hasselt CA. Nasal foreign bodies in children. *Int J Pediatr Otorhinolaryngol*. 1996;35: 207-211.
21. Yanagisawa E, Citardi MJ. Endoscopic view of a foreign body in the nose. *Ear Nose Throat J*. 1995;74:8-9.
22. Alvi A, Bereliani A, Zahtz GD. Miniature disc battery in the nose: a dangerous foreign body. *Clin Pediatr*. 1997;36: 427-429.
23. Kittle PE, Aaron GR, Jones HL, et al. Incidental finding of an intranasal foreign body discovered on routine dental examination. *Pediatr Dent*. 1991;13:49-51.
24. Gomes CC, Sakano E, Lucchezi MC, et al. Button battery as a foreign body in the nasal cavities: special aspects. *Rhinology*. 1994;32:98-100.
25. Douglas AR. Use of nebulized adrenaline to aid expulsion of intra-nasal foreign bodies in children. *J Laryngol Otol*. 1996;110:559-560.
26. Finkelstein JA. Oral ambu-bag insufflation to remove unilateral nasal foreign bodies. *Am J Emerg Med*. 1996; 14:57-58.
27. Henry LN, Chamberlain JW. Removal of foreign bodies from the esophagus and nose with the use of a Foley catheter. *Surgery*. 1972;71:918-921.
28. Nandapalan V, McIlwain JC. Removal of nasal foreign bodies with a Fogarty biliary balloon catheter. *J Laryngol Otol*. 1994;108:758-760.
29. Tan HK, Brown K, McGill T, et al. Airway foreign bodies: a 10 year review. *Int J Pediatr Otorhinolaryngol*. 2000; 56:91.
30. Lima JA. Laryngeal foreign bodies in children: a persistent life-threatening problem. *Laryngoscope*. 1989;99: 415-420.
31. Lemberg PS, Darrow DH, Holinger LD. Aerodigestive tract foreign bodies in the older child and adolescent. *Ann Otol Rhinol Laryngol*. 1996;105:267.
32. Reichert TJ. Foreign bodies of the larynx, trachea, and bronchi. In: Bluestone CD, Stool SE, eds. *Pediatric Otolaryngology*. 2nd ed. Philadelphia, PA: WB Saunders; 1990.
33. Arnold LD. Ingested and aspirated foreign bodies: making sure that what went in comes out. *Contemp Pediatr*. 2007;23(11):32-44.
34. Mears AJ, England RM. Dissolving foreign bodies in the trachea and bronchus. *Thorax*. 1975;30:461-463.
35. American Academy of Pediatrics, Committee on Pediatric Emergency Medicine. First aid for the choking child. *Pediatrics*. 1993;92:477-479.
36. Wolach B, Raz A, Weinberg J, et al. Aspirated foreign bodies in the respiratory tract of children: eleven years experience with 127 patients. *Int J Pediatr Otorhinolaryngol*. 1994;30:1-10.
37. Witt WJ. The role of rigid endoscopy in foreign body management. *Ear Nose Throat J*. 1985;64:70-74.
38. Turtz MG, Stool SE. Foreign bodies of the pharynx and esophagus. In: Bluestone CD, Stool SE, eds. *Pediatric Otolaryngology*. 2nd ed. Philadelphia, PA: WB Saunders; 1990.
39. Singh B, Kantu M, Har-El G, et al. Complications associated with 327 foreign bodies of the pharynx, larynx, and esophagus. *Ann Otol Rhinol Laryngol*. 1997;106:301-304.
40. Giordano A, Adams G, Boies L, et al. Current management of esophageal foreign bodies. *Arch Otol*. 1981;107: 249-251.
41. Derkay CS, LeFebvre SM, St George MR. Retrieving foreign bodies from upper aerodigestive tracts of children. *AORN J*. 1994;60:53-61.
42. Skae CC. Esophageal foreign bodies. *Pediatr Rev*. 2005; 26:34-35.

Chapter 263

FRACTURES AND DISLOCATIONS

R. Scott Strahlman, MD

Physicians who care for children see scores of fractures and dislocations each year. A familiarity with the proper triage and management of injuries is essential so that the physician can feel comfortable managing an injury conservatively or referring to an orthopedic specialist. This chapter covers the pathophysiological features, clinical assessment, and classification of fractures and dislocations and discusses some of the more common fractures and dislocations encountered in primary care.

DEFINITION

A *fracture* is defined as a break or crack in a bone. The fracture may occur directly at the site of injury or indirectly when the break occurs at a site different from the applied force. Stress fractures result from recurrent trauma to a bone and often occur in athletes (eg, long-bone fractures in distance runners). Pathological fractures can occur without trauma or with minor trauma when a bone is weakened, as with osteogenesis imperfecta or a tumor.

A *dislocation* is defined as a malposition of bone ends that normally appose each other within a joint. Dislocations are far less common in children than are fractures because a child's ligaments are quite strong compared with an adult's; with an injury, a bone will more likely break or a growth plate will more likely separate than a ligament will tear.

Broad generalizations can be made about the pathophysiological features of childhood fractures. First, fractures in children heal more quickly than in adults. For example, a fractured clavicle in a 4 year old may heal in as few as 3 weeks. Second, the remodeling that occurs in the healing of pediatric fractures often corrects residual bony deformities. Third, children's bones are resilient; they bend instead of break, or they break on 1 side only (a greenstick fracture). Fourth, a phenomenon called *overgrowth* occurs in pediatric long-bone fractures. Overgrowth is an accelerated growth rate of bony fragments during healing. Long-bone fractures are therefore often corrected with overriding of the broken ends to prevent length discrepancies with the uninjured side. Finally, the growth plate must be protected when treating children's fractures because a growth plate injury can result in the loss of growth potential.

EVALUATION

Whenever a fracture or dislocation is suspected, an accurate history is essential. Historical details may provide clues about the mechanism of injury. The practitioner should find out how, where, and when the injury occurred and where any pain is located. A fall off of a skateboard or scooter increases suspicion for a forearm fracture.[1] Does the parent or child report any loss of function in the affected limb? Does the history show acute or recurrent trauma?

A complete physical examination, including vital signs and a neurovascular assessment, is key to reveal signs of serious trauma and secondary sites of injury. Pulses should be normal. Sensation should be intact and movement, even if limited by discomfort, should be present. Absence of pulses, sensation, or movement signifies a serious injury requiring immediate medical attention. The examiner should look carefully for any unnatural or deformed position of joints or limbs, pain on palpation or attempted movement, or swelling and discoloration. Crepitus can sometimes be elicited at a fracture site. Any of these findings should alert the clinician to order imaging studies.

Radiography is a mainstay in the diagnosis of fractures and dislocations. Radiographs from 2 angles are indicated to delineate subtle fractures. To rule out a dislocation, including the joint above and below the injury is sometimes helpful; in many cases, obtaining a film of the unaffected side for a comparison view is necessary. Stress fractures are often missed on radiography. If a stress fracture is suspected, then a magnetic resonance image or a radionuclide bone scan may be indicated.[2] Occasionally, when injury to the growth plate is a concern, other imaging techniques such as computed tomography can be useful.[3]

CLASSIFICATION

Fractures may be classified according to their clinical appearance. A closed fracture has no break in the skin. With an open, or compound, fracture, a bone fragment is exposed to the air, increasing the risk of infection and injury to adjacent nerves and blood vessels. A hidden fracture causes slight pain and swelling but no obvious bone deformity. Radiographs are necessary to confirm the diagnosis. An obvious fracture or dislocation is an easily seen injury, even with a cursory examination. Immediate medical attention is necessary.

Fractures also are classified by their anatomic location and according to their radiographic appearance. Breaks in the bone may be described by their appearance as transverse, oblique, or spiral. A torus or buckle fracture most commonly occurs after injury to the forearm and, radiographically shows a wrinkled appearing break of the distal radius. A fracture is comminuted when the bone has 3 or more fragments. With an impacted fracture, the bone ends are compressed into each other.

Probably the most important classification system for fractures is the Salter-Harris system of describing injury to the growth plate (Figure 263-1). Growth or epiphyseal plate injuries occur only in childhood. They must be treated with care to protect a bone's growth potential. Approximately 15% of all childhood fractures involve the growth plate.[4] In a Salter-Harris I fracture, the epiphysis is separated from the metaphysis without a true break in the bone. Radiographs are often normal, and the diagnosis is made based on the clinical picture: tenderness over the area of the growth

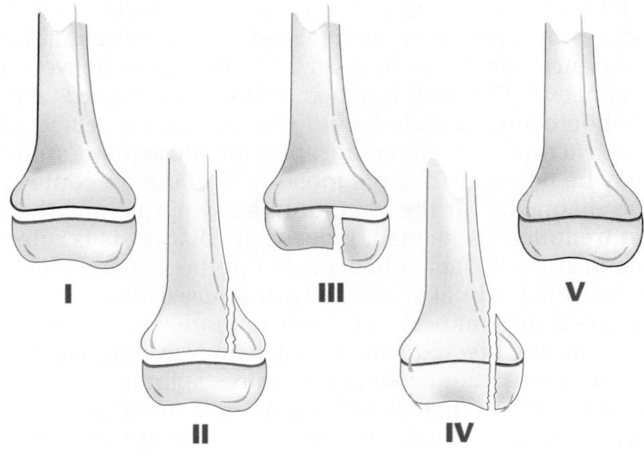

Figure 263-1 Salter-Harris classification of growth plate injuries. (See text for explanation.) (*Peterson HA. Physeal fractures: Part 3. Classification.* J Ped Orthop. *1994;14:439-448. Reprinted by permission of Lippincott Williams & Wilkins.*)

plate. Growth is usually not disturbed. The treatment is immobilization by cast for approximately 3 weeks. The most common growth plate fracture is the type II fracture, in which a fragment of metaphyseal bone separates from the epiphysis. Closed reduction of the fracture is usually possible; with proper casting, growth is not disturbed. A Salter-Harris III fracture involves a partial growth plate injury through the epiphysis. Open repair of the fracture in the operating room is indicated to align articular surfaces and preserve joint function. A Salter-Harris IV fracture extends across the growth plate, injuring both the epiphysis and the metaphysis. The fracture must be perfectly realigned to protect growth potential. In a Salter-Harris V fracture, the growth plate is compressed. The prognosis for preserving growth is poor in this case because of a crush injury to the growth plate.

Chip fractures that do not cause any direct injury to the growth plate are not usually included in the Salter-Harris classification system.

MANAGEMENT

Fractures and dislocations should be splinted and immobilized immediately. For most fractures and dislocations, consultation with an orthopedic specialist is necessary. Most pediatric fractures respond to closed reduction by the orthopedist. Even some compound fractures can be managed nonoperatively.[5] If the growth plate is affected, however, then open reduction in the operating room is performed. Close pediatric and orthopedic follow-up are always important. A child in a cast should be comfortable; if pain is persistent, or if color changes or sensory changes to the casted extremity occur, then the child needs reevaluation and possibly requires recasting.

COMMONLY ENCOUNTERED FRACTURES AND DISLOCATIONS

Fractured Clavicle

A broken clavicle, or collarbone, is the most common fracture in children. It can occur at any time during childhood as a result of trauma. This fracture often occurs at birth when vaginal delivery is difficult. The incidence can be as high as 3.5% in babies delivered vaginally.[6] Physical findings include decreased arm motion on the affected side, crepitus, and swelling at the fracture site. A radiographic or ultrasound study may be needed, if the diagnosis is in doubt, to confirm the diagnosis.[7] If the condition is asymptomatic, then no treatment is needed; indeed, the diagnosis is often made after the fact, when a callus at the fracture site is noted at a well-baby visit. If the fracture causes pain or reduced arm movement, then immobilization of the arm on the affected side for 2 to 3 weeks is indicated. In older children, treatment requires splinting for 3 to 4 weeks in a simple sling.[8] Figure-of-8 bandages have been found to be cumbersome and to work no better than a sling. Most of the fracture's healing and realignment are spontaneous.

Developmental Dysplasia of the Hip

The femoral head has a tendency to dislocate in as many as 5 of every 1000 infants.[9] This condition, formerly known as congenital hip dislocation, is termed *developmental dysplasia of the hip* (DDH). Because hip dysplasia is not always detected in the newborn period, children younger than 1 year should be examined for hip dislocation at every routine visit.

Although the exact cause is unknown, many factors contribute to DDH. The disorder may be related, in part, to abnormal intrauterine positioning and therefore is more common in breech deliveries and in infants delivered by cesarean. The condition is 6 to 8 times more common in girls than in boys. Theories suggest that female fetuses are more sensitive to maternal hormones that can induce ligamentous laxity of the hip.[10] DDH is 3 times more common on the left than the right and in approximately 20% of cases is bilateral. The tendency to occur more often on the left is believed to be the result of intrauterine positioning. Most fetuses are positioned left occiput anterior during the later stages of pregnancy. This position puts the left hip against the mother's spine, thereby putting additional pressure on the left hip to dislocate. A genetic predisposition also exists; the risk of DDH is increased when a positive family history of hip dislocation exists.[11]

Radiographs are of limited value during the neonatal period in the diagnosis of developmental dysplasia of the hip. Therefore the physical examination is of utmost importance. The Ortolani test is used to detect a dislocated hip. With the baby laying supine, the hips and knees are flexed and the knees brought together. The examiner then places a hand on each of the baby's knees, with each middle finger over the greater trochanter and each thumb over the medial thigh. With gentle abduction of the knees, the dislocated femoral head will slip back into the acetabulum, and an audible or palpable *clunk* results. Notably, a hip *click* (without a *clunk* and without any movement of the femoral head) does not indicate a hip dislocation. The Barlow test is essentially the reverse of the Ortolani test; the femoral head can be felt slipping out of the acetabulum when the knees are brought back together. Both tests are important to perform because the Ortolani test pushes a dislocated hip *back into* the hip socket, and the Barlow test pushes a dislocatable hip *out* of the hip socket. An examiner may feel unusual laxity of the hip by pushing up and down on the thigh when the hips are flexed and adducted (sometimes called the *telescoping sign*). Older infants should be examined for limited hip abduction, asymmetry of the thigh skin folds, a limp when cruising or walking, and leg length discrepancy. One way to determine leg length discrepancy is the Galeazzi sign: With the infant lying supine, the examiner flexes the infant's thighs and brings the knees together. If 1 knee is higher than the other, then the Galeazzi sign is *positive*, and the possibility of a dislocated hip exists. If the diagnosis is in doubt, then an ultrasound study, and in infants older than 4 to 6 months a radiograph, will confirm or rule out a dysplastic hip. Treatment requires referral to an orthopedist for a harness or casting. Infants diagnosed before 6 months of age can be treated with a Pavlik harness, which is worn for up to 5 months. Infants diagnosed after 6 months of age, and infants in whom the harness was not successful, require casting and sometimes

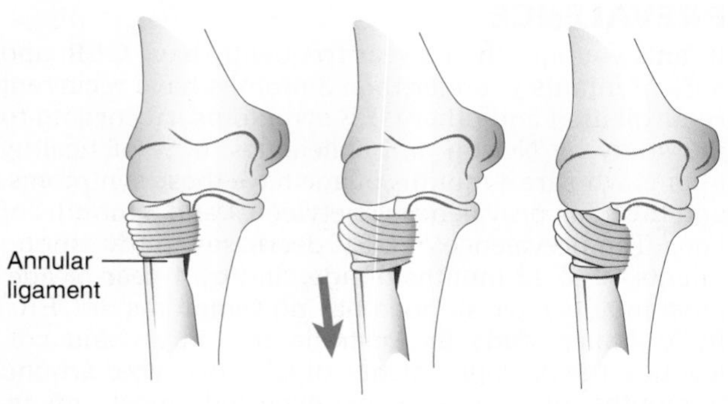

Figure 263-2 Nursemaid's elbow.

surgery. Treatment is more straightforward the earlier the diagnosis is made, which makes it imperative for the clinician to assess for DDH at every routine pediatric visit.

Nursemaid's Elbow

Nursemaid's elbow is a common dislocation in pediatrics. It is a transient subluxation of the proximal radial head (Figure 263-2) caused by pulling or *yanking*, usually inadvertently, of a child's arm, often by a parent or caretaker. The annular ligament of the radial head becomes entrapped in the radiohumeral joint (see Figure 263-2). The condition usually occurs in children between 1 and 4 years of age. The child refuses to move the arm and keeps it flexed and pronated. Radiographs are rarely necessary; the history and characteristic posture of the child's arm confirm the diagnosis. The treatment, easily performed by the pediatrician, requires rapid, forceful supination of the forearm while pressure is placed over the proximal radial head, followed by extension then flexion of the elbow. Symptoms usually resolve within 30 minutes. The condition is sometimes recurrent, in which case great care must be taken when holding hands with the affected child, lest the child suddenly tries to pull away.

Child Abuse

Unfortunately, fractures and dislocations are all too commonly suggestive of child abuse (see Chapter 120, Child Physical Abuse and Neglect). Child abuse may be suspected when an unexplained injury occurs or when an inconsistency exists between the history and the physical findings in a childhood injury. The delay between the time of injury and the time that medical attention is sought may be unusually long. Multiple bruises may be noted on physical examination. If abuse is suspected, then a radiographic bone survey should be performed in younger children. Silent fractures, or multiple fractures in varying stages of healing, may be seen.

When child abuse is suspected, the child should be hospitalized for protection and for appropriate evaluation and orthopedic care. Child protective services and social services should be involved. Pediatric care practitioners are morally and legally responsible for detecting child abuse and reporting all suspected cases.

Toddler's Fracture

Radiologists refer to a spiral fracture of the tibia as a *toddler's fracture* when the fracture occurs in a child younger than 6 years. Torsion of the foot creates a spiral break in the tibia. The trauma to the leg often is minor or unwitnessed; therefore, in many instances, no history of trauma can be found. Symptoms can be minimal; the child may be brought for medical attention only because of reluctance to bear weight on the affected leg. The physical examination is significant for tenderness over the affected area of the tibia. A diagnosis can be made with anteroposterior and lateral radiographs of the tibia-fibula, but the fracture is sometimes not evident on a radiograph for a few days. The physician therefore should not hesitate to repeat films on a child who has an unexplained limp that is not resolving spontaneously. Treatment requires immobilization in a cast for 3 to 4 weeks.

Because the signs and symptoms of a toddler's fracture can be subtle, the examiner should have a high index of suspicion in a child who has a limp or fails to bear weight. Because the cause of the fracture is often unexplained, child abuse is sometimes a consideration.[12]

WHEN TO REFER

- All fractures and dislocations not easily managed in a primary care setting

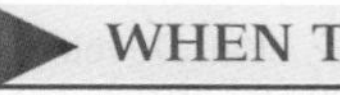

WHEN TO ADMIT

- Whenever child abuse is suspected or if the patient is not medically stable (ie, multiple injuries)

TOOLS FOR PRACTICE

Engaging Patient and Family

- *Hip Dysplasia (Developmental Dysplasia of the Hip)* (brochure), American Academy of Pediatrics (patiented.aap.org).

Medical Decision Support

- *Essentials of Musculoskeletal Care, 3rd edition* (book), American Academy of Pediatrics (www.aap.org/bookstore).
- *Sports Shorts* (fact sheet), American Academy of Pediatrics (www.aap.org/family/sportsshort.htm).

AAP POLICY STATEMENT

American Academy of Pediatrics, Committee on Quality Improvement, Subcommittee on Developmental Dysplasia of the Hip. Clinical practice guidelines: early detection of developmental dysplasia of the hip. *Pediatrics.* 2000; 105(4):896-905. (aappolicy.aappublications.org/cgi/content/full/pediatrics;105/4/896).

SUGGESTED RESOURCES

American Academy of Pediatrics. Clinical practice guideline: early detection of developmental dysplasia of the hip. *Pediatrics.* 2000;105:896-905.

American Academy of Pediatrics. Diagnostic imaging of child abuse. *Pediatrics*. 2000;105:1345-1348.

Beaty JH. Orthopedic aspects of child abuse. *Curr Opin Pediatr.* 1997;9:100-103.

England SP, Sundberg S. Management of common pediatric fractures. *Pediatr Clin North Am*. 1996;43:991-1012.

REFERENCES

1. Powell EC, Tanz RR. Incidence and description of scooter-related injuries among children. *Ambul Pediatr.* 2004;4:495-499.
2. Gaeta M, Minutoli F, Scribano E, et al. CT and MR imaging findings in athletes with early tibial stress injuries: comparison with bone scintigraphy findings and emphasis on cortical abnormalities. *Radiology*. 2005;235: 553-561.
3. Rogers LF, Poznanski AK. Imaging of epiphyseal injuries. *Radiology*. 1994;191:297-308.
4. Salter RB, Harris WR. Injuries involving the epiphyseal plate. *J Bone Joint Surg*. 1963;45A:587-622.
5. Iobst CA, Tidwell MA, King WF. Nonoperative management of pediatric type I open fractures. *J Pediatr Orthop*. 2005;25:513-517.
6. Joseph PR, Rosenfeld W. Clavicular fractures in neonates. *Am J Dis Child*. 1990;144:165-167.
7. Blab E, Geissler W, Rokitansky A. Sonographic management of infantile clavicular fractures. *Pediatr Surg Int*. 1999;15:251-254.
8. Andersen K, Jensen PO, Lauritzen J. Treatment of clavicular fractures. Figure-of-eight bandage versus a simple sling. *Acta Orthop Scand*. 1987;58:71-74.
9. Bialik V, Bialik GM, Blazer S, et al. Developmental dysplasia of the hip: a new approach to incidence. *Pediatrics*. 1999;103:93-99.
10. Aronsson DD, Goldberg MJ, Kling TF, et al. Developmental dysplasia of the hip. *Pediatrics*. 1994;94:201-212.
11. Paton RW, Hinduja K, Thomas CD. The significance of at-risk factors in ultrasound surveillance of developmental dysplasia of the hip. A ten-year prospective study. *J Bone Joint Surg Br*. 2005;87:1264-1266.
12. Coffey C, Haley K, Hayes J, et al. The risk of child abuse in infants and toddlers with lower extremity injuries. *J Pediatr Surg*. 2005;40:120-123.

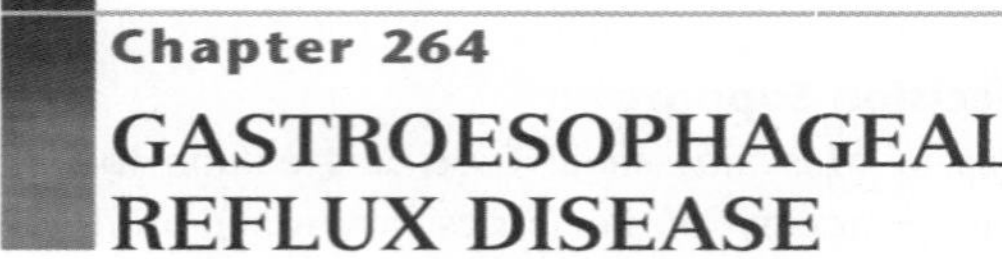

Chapter 264

GASTROESOPHAGEAL REFLUX DISEASE

Shailender Madani, MD; Harland S. Winter, MD; Mel Heyman, MD

DEFINITIONS

Gastroesophageal reflux (GER) is the passage of gastric contents into the esophagus. Most episodes are brief and unaccompanied by symptoms. In contrast, gastroesophageal reflux disease (GERD) is defined as symptoms or complications resulting from exposure of the esophagus, the oropharynx, or the airway to gastric refluxate (acid, food, bile). Regurgitation occurs when gastric contents enter into the oropharynx. Gastric contents exiting through the mouth is referred to as vomiting. Rumination is regurgitation with subsequent reswallowing of the gastric contents.

PREVALENCE

Infants younger than 1 year frequently have GER, and 50% of infants younger than 3 months have recurrent regurgitation and other GER symptoms. According to the study by Nelson and colleagues, 67% of healthy infants who are 4 months of age have these symptoms, and the peak prevalence is between 4 and 6 months of age.[1] The prevalence of GER decreases to 5% among infants 10 to 12 months of age, and by 1 year of age, most infants have stopped having symptoms of GER.[1] In a similar study in Australia by Martin and colleagues, the peak prevalence of GER occurred around 3 months of age, and, as expected, most infants had resolution of symptoms by 18 months of age[2] (Figure 264-1).

GERD, on the other hand, occurs in infants who have irritability associated with feeding or food refusal. Infants who have symptoms that last longer than 90 days are at increased risk of having symptoms of GERD 9 to 11 years later.[2] The significance of heartburn at age 10 and whether it predisposes one to complications of GERD later in life is not known. Furthermore, little is known about the natural history of children and adolescents with symptoms of GERD. Barrett syndrome, often called Barrett esophagus, is a chronic peptic ulceration of the lower esophagus acquired as a result of longstanding esophagitis. Dr. Gilger and the PedsCORI project have reported that the incidence of Barrett esophagus in children is rare and less than 1 per 1000 in children undergoing endoscopy.[3] Reports have been published of familial clustering of Barrett esophagus, and monozygotic twins have a higher concordance for GERD than dizygotic twins.[4] However, data supporting a specific genetic link are lacking.

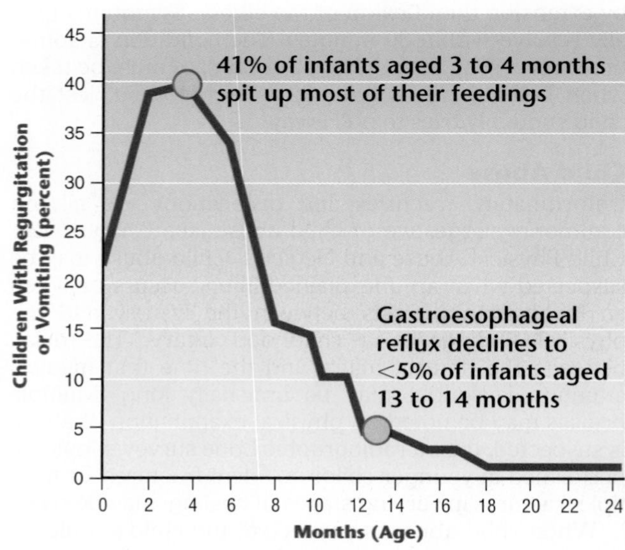

Figure 264-1 Prevalence of GER in healthy infants in the first 2 years of life. *(Martin AJ, Pratt NJ, Kennedy D, et al. Natural history and familial relationships of infant spilling to 9 years of age.* Pediatrics. *2002;109:1061-1067.)*

CLINICAL MANIFESTATIONS

Symptoms of GER depend on the age of the patient (Box 264-1). Clinical manifestations change with age and the development of language. Infants may express the discomfort from acid reflux by crying, refusing to eat, or failing to thrive. Older children may complain of abdominal pain but will not localize the pain to the epigastrium or retrosternal areas. Adolescents are more likely to report heartburn similar to symptoms reported by adults. Extraesophageal symptoms such as pneumonia, cough, hoarse voice, or dental disease may occur at any age.[5,6]

PATHOPHYSIOLOGICAL FEATURES

The causes of GERD are multifactorial and depend on anatomy, motility, and physiological factors. In an infant the normal obtuse angle of His does not occlude the hiatus when the stomach is distended postprandially and may result in regurgitation. Pathologic conditions such as malrotation, annular pancreas, or antral web may also result in symptoms of GERD. Impaired esophageal motility associated with repair of esophageal atresia or tracheoesophageal fistula or delayed gastric emptying may result in prolonged acid exposure in the esophagus and eventual complications of GERD. Impaired buffering of acid in the esophagus by saliva may lead to esophagitis in children with cystic fibrosis or adults with autoimmune disease. Lower esophageal sphincter (LES) pressure is an important antireflux barrier, but possibly because of the other factors, LES pressure by itself correlates poorly with GER.[7]

In both children and adults, the most common cause of reflux is inappropriate transient LES relaxation with inhibition of esophageal peristalsis.[8] Transient LES relaxations typically occur up to 5 times in the immediate postprandial hour with episodic movement of gastric contents into the distal esophagus. These relaxations are vagally mediated, brief in duration, and probably play a normal role in eliminating gas from the stomach. When the refluxate enters the esophagus, it is buffered by saliva and cleared by normal esophageal peristalsis. In patients with GERD, these relaxations last longer, from 5 to 35 seconds. During this period, a combination of LES hypotonia and inhibited esophageal peristalsis prolong the contact time of the gastric contents with the esophageal mucosa and contribute to tissue injury. Inappropriate LES relaxation and delayed gastric emptying has been shown to occur in 28% to 50% of children with GERD.[9] Increasing intraabdominal pressure (crying in infants, coughing, obesity) or gastric acid secretion, as well as consuming large meals, fatty foods, caffeinated beverages, candy, and certain medications (theophylline, morphine, calcium-channel blockers) that lower the LES tone, all contribute to the presence and severity of GERD. Because vagal afferents innervate both the esophagus and the bronchi, acid stimulation of receptors in the esophagus may induce reflex bronchoconstriction,[10] explaining why asthma and chronic cough are associated with GERD. Alternatively or additionally, microaspiration of gastric contents into the trachea may result in bronchoconstriction and laryngospasm.[11] Esophageal acid exposure per se has a minimal effect on pulmonary function[12] but has been shown to contribute to increased airway responsiveness in asthmatics.[13] No convincing temporal relationship exists between esophageal acidification and apnea or bradycardia in unselected groups of patients.[14]

BOX 264-1 Symptoms of Gastroesophageal Reflux

GASTROINTESTINAL	RESPIRATORY
Nausea	Chronic cough
Vomiting	Reactive airway disease
Hematemesis	Recurrent pneumonia
Melena	Stridor
Regurgitation	Chest pain
Eructation	Apnea
Heartburn	Hoarseness of voice
Dysphagia	Choking
Odynophagia	Gagging
Anorexia	**NEUROBEHAVIORAL**
Irritability during and after feedings	Apnea (ALTE)
Refusal to feed	Seizure-like events
Failure to thrive	Sandifer syndrome
Occult blood–positive stools	Rumination

ALTE, Apparent life-threatening event.
Modified from Rudolph CD, Mazur LJ, Liptak GS, et al. Pediatric GE reflux clinical practice guidelines. *J Pediatr Gastroenterol Nutr.* 2001;32(S2):1-31. Reprinted by permission of Lippincott Williams & Wilkins.

EVALUATION

No single gold standard has been developed for the diagnosis of GER, and each diagnostic test provides specific information of potential relevance to the cause and severity of acid reflux.

History and Physical Examination

In most infants with vomiting, and in most older children with regurgitation and heartburn, a history and physical examination are sufficient to diagnose GERD, recognize complications, and initiate management reliably[15] (Boxes 264-2 and 264-3). Nevertheless, generating a differential diagnosis is essential because several conditions may mimic GERD (Box 264-4).

Differential Diagnosis

A variety of conditions have clinical features that resemble GER, including eosinophilic esophagitis, food allergy, achalasia, cyclic vomiting syndrome, pill esophagitis, infectious esophagitis, and rumination syndrome. These conditions may be suspected based on characteristic features, diagnostic testing, or a failure of symptoms to respond to standard medical therapy for acid reflux.

Eosinophilic Esophagitis

Eosinophilic esophagitis occurs in young children, teenagers, and adults. The disease appears to be more

BOX 264-2 History in the Child With Suspected Gastroesophageal Reflux Disease

FEEDING HISTORY

Amount and frequency (overfeeding)
Preparation of formula
Source of dietary protein
Position and burping
Behavior during feedings (choking, gagging, coughing, arching, discomfort, feeding refusal)

PATTERN OF VOMITING

Frequency and amount
Painful
Forceful
Hematemesis
Association with fever, lethargy, diarrhea

MEDICAL HISTORY

Prematurity
Growth and development (intellectual disability, cerebral palsy, developmental delay)
Surgery
Hospitalizations
Newborn screen (galactosemia, maple sugar urine disease, congenital heart disease)
Recurrent illness (croup or stridor, pneumonia, wheeze, hoarseness, excessive fussiness or crying, hiccups)
Apnea
Inadequate weight gain

PSYCHOSOCIAL HISTORY

Stress

FAMILY HISTORY

Significant illness
Gastrointestinal disorders (familial pattern to obstructive disorders, celiac)
Other (metabolic, energy)

GROWTH CHART

Length, weight
Head circumference

WARNING SIGNS

(see Box 264-3)

Modified from Rudolph CD, Mazur LJ, Liptak GS, et al. Pediatric GE reflux clinical practice guidelines. *J Pediatr Gastroenterol Nutr.* 2001;32(S2):1-31. Reprinted by permission of Lippincott Williams & Wilkins.

common today than it was 25 years ago. The majority of patients are male, and most have dysphagia or food impaction. Younger children may have symptoms suggestive of GERD such as abdominal pain or food refusal. Dysphagia or esophageal food impaction is more commonly noted in older children. Partial or complete unresponsiveness to acid-suppression therapy suggests that GERD is not a contributing factor. A personal or family history of allergic disease can be found in 75% of cases. The diagnosis is suspected when white exudate, circular rings, or linear

BOX 264-3 Warning Signs in the Vomiting Infant

Bilious vomiting
Gastrointestinal bleeding: hematemesis, hematochezia
Forceful vomiting
Onset of vomiting after 6 months of life
Failure to thrive
Diarrhea
Constipation
Fever
Lethargy
Hepatosplenomegaly
Bulging fontanelle
Macro-, microcephaly
Seizures
Abdominal tenderness, distention
Genetic disorders (eg, trisomy 21)
Other chronic disorders (eg, HIV)

From Rudolph CD, Mazur LJ, Liptak GS, et al. Pediatric GE reflux clinical practice guidelines. *J Pediatr Gastroenterol Nutr.* 2001;32(S2):1-31. Reprinted by permission of Lippincott Williams & Wilkins.

BOX 264-4 Differential Diagnosis of Vomiting in Infants and Children

GASTROINTESTINAL OBSTRUCTION

Pyloric stenosis
Malrotation with intermittent volvulus
Intermittent intussusception
Intestinal duplication
Hirschsprung disease
Antral, duodenal web
Foreign body
Incarcerated hernia

GASTROINTESTINAL DISORDERS

Achalasia
Gastroparesis
Gastroenteritis
Peptic ulcer disease
Gastroesophageal reflux
Eosinophilic esophagitis, gastroenteritis
Food allergy or intolerance
Inflammatory bowel disease
Pancreatitis
Appendicitis

NEUROLOGIC DISORDERS

Hydrocephalus
Subdural hematoma
Intracranial hemorrhage
Mass lesion

INFECTION

Sepsis
Meningitis
Urinary tract infection
Pneumonia
Otitis media
Hepatitis

METABOLIC, ENDOCRINE DISORDERS

Galactosemia
Hereditary fructose intolerance
Urea cycle defects
Amino and organic acidemias
Congenital adrenal hyperplasia
Maple syrup urine disease

RENAL DISORDERS

Obstructive uropathy
Renal insufficiency

TOXIC

Lead
Iron
Vitamin A or D
Medications (ipecac, digoxin, theophylline, etc.)

CARDIAC DISORDERS

Congestive heart failure

From Rudolph CD, Mazur LJ, Liptak GS, et al. Pediatric GE reflux clinical practice guidelines. *J Pediatr Gastroenterol Nutr.* 2001;32(S2):1-31. Reprinted by permission of Lippincott Williams & Wilkins.

furrowing is seen during upper endoscopy. Establishing the diagnosis depends on finding more than 15 to 20 eosinophils per high-power field on an esophageal mucosal biopsy.[14]

Food Allergy

Milk protein and other food allergies in young infants may mimic symptoms of GERD, but they usually resolve with dietary restriction or time. A challenge with the suspected allergen may reproduce the symptoms but is usually not necessary for managing the patient. Eczema, skin rash, wheezing, concomitant diarrhea, or blood in the stool should alert the clinician to the possibility of allergy.

Achalasia

Achalasia is a motor disorder characterized by lack of peristalsis in the distal two thirds of the esophagus, an elevated resting pressure in the distal esophagus, and failure of the LES to relax. The result is a functional obstruction in the lower esophagus and accumulation of food in the esophagus. Children may exhibit weight loss, regurgitation of undigested food, halitosis, and cough, especially when supine or pneumonia. The most common feature on chest radiograph is absence of air in the stomach and an air-fluid level in the esophagus. With longstanding disease, one may see widening of the mediastinum. Esophageal manometry is often diagnostic and demonstrates aperistalsis in the distal two thirds of the esophagus, an elevated resting LES, and failure or incomplete relaxation of the LES. However, in young children with achalasia, sphincter relaxation and occasional peristalsis may be present. Barium esophagram often reveals a symmetrical narrowing in distal esophagus with the appearance of a bird beak.

Cyclic Vomiting Syndrome

Cyclic vomiting syndrome is a functional gastrointestinal disorder characterized by bouts of intractable nausea and vomiting lasting for hours accompanied by lethargy and pallor interspersed with complete symptom relief. Although these episodes are intense in severity, in contrast to GERD, the patient is completely asymptomatic between episodes. A bout may be triggered spontaneously, by stress, or by menstruation. No diagnostic test or identifiable neurologic, metabolic, or other gastrointestinal disease exists to explain the condition.

Pill Esophagitis

Pill esophagitis occurs when a pill is lodged in the esophagus and usually causes the acute onset of severe midchest or substernal pain and dysphagia. Minocycline, ibuprofen, iron, and potassium hydroxide are the usual suspects. The condition is suspected based on history, and endoscopy may not be necessary if symptoms improve with acid-suppression therapy or sucralfate.

Infectious Esophagitis

Most infectious causes of esophagitis present with odynophagia and not dysphagia. Herpes simplex virus, cytomegalovirus, and fungal infection such as candidiasis may occur in both the immunocompetent and the immunocompromised hosts. Upper endoscopy is beneficial in making the diagnosis both by histopathology and by culture.

Rumination Syndrome

Rumination syndrome is characterized by regurgitation of food into the mouth with subsequent reswallowing of the material. This syndrome was typically thought to occur in neurologically compromised children but is now recognized as occurring in otherwise healthy children and adolescents. Repeated masticatory movements, swallowing air, and tensing abdominal musculature help distinguish rumination from effortless GERD.

Diagnostic Procedures

Esophageal pH Monitoring

Esophageal pH is evaluated using a transnasally placed probe that records the number and duration of acid reflux episodes[15] occurring over a period of 20 hours or by clipping a Bravo pH probe to the wall of the distal esophagus and transmitting pH data to a recorder using radiofrequency signals.[16] The pH of gastric contents refluxing into the esophagus is recorded, allowing the examiner to determine the frequency and duration of acid reflux.

Percentage of total time the esophageal pH is less than 4.0, referred to as *reflux index*, is considered the most valid measure of reflux. A reflux index of 12% or greater in infants younger than 1 year and 6% or greater in children older than 1 year is considered abnormal.[14] Not all patients with GER test positive on this study, but 95% of children with esophagitis (gross and microscopic) have an abnormal reflux index. On the other hand, only 50% of patients with a positive pH study have esophagitis, and the severity of esophagitis does not correlate with the reflux index. Furthermore, daily variation in severity of acid reflux raises questions about the diagnostic utility of pH probe testing for a condition that is diagnosed by clinical criteria. Proximal esophageal and pharyngeal pH monitoring have not been proven to be useful in predicting which patients are at risk for upper airway complications of GER.[17,18]

Esophageal pH monitoring is not necessary to establish a diagnosis of GERD, but it may be beneficial to relate acid reflux with cough, apnea, bradycardia, or other extraesophageal symptoms or to determine the efficacy of therapy in a patient with persistent symptoms. Because the volume of acid that is needed to cause extraesophageal symptoms may be very small, changes in pH may not be detected by pH probe monitoring. Esophageal pH monitoring is limited because it detects only acid reflux and will not detect nonacidic, postprandial reflux.

Multiple Intraluminal Electrical Impedance Measurement

Multiple intraluminal electrical impedance measures changes in electrical resistance and conductance in the mucosa when a fluid bolus moves down the esophagus, and this resistance and conductance detects nonacid and acid reflux. The clinical value of this test is not yet determined, but preliminary studies suggest that children with pulmonary symptoms may have increased nonacid reflux. This study in conjunction with pH probe monitoring may be useful in evaluating patients who have failed to respond to acid-suppression therapy.

Endoscopy and Biopsy

Endoscopy allows direct visualization of the esophageal mucosa to detect erosions, ulceration, and reflux related complications such as peptic stricture and Barrett esophagus. Biopsies routinely obtained at endoscopy determine presence and severity of esophagitis and may help exclude conditions such as Crohn disease of the esophagus, eosinophilic esophagitis, and infection. Because endoscopy requires sedation and the diagnosis of GERD is established based on clinical evidence, the indications for performing this test are based on a suspicion of complications of GERD or the need to rule out other disorders.[19]

Scintigraphy

Scintigraphy involves the oral intake of radiolabeled technetium–containing liquid (formula or juice) or solid (often scrambled eggs) followed by scanning the esophagus, stomach, and the lungs to detect radiolabeled colloid that has been refluxed or aspirated. In addition, the gastric emptying time may be calculated and provide additional information for potential therapeutic intervention. Because the techniques of performing this test are not standardized and age specific normative data are not available, its role in evaluating GERD in children is unclear at this time; however, determining gastric emptying may contribute to management.

Upper Gastrointestinal Radiography (Barium Swallow)

The primary role of the upper gastrointestinal is to rule out anatomic causes of GERD such as malrotation, annular pancreas, and antral web. When compared with an esophageal pH study, an upper gastrointestinal is neither sensitive nor specific for the diagnosis of GER (31% to 86% and 21% to 83%, respectively) and does not reliably determine the presence or absence of GER.[14]

COMPLICATIONS OF GASTROESOPHAGEAL REFLUX DISEASE

A summary of the possible complications from GERD is listed in Box 264-5.

Esophageal Complications

Peptic strictures are a known complication of severe GERD,[20,21] especially in patients with neurologic impairment or esophageal motility disorders. Children with peptic stricture usually have dysphagia but, depending on the age of the child, may refuse to eat solids. Impaction of food may be the initial presentation. Peptic strictures are readily seen by barium swallow and are usually located in the distal third of the esophagus. Endoscopy is essential to look for Barrett epithelium, the columnar esophageal epithelium seen in Barrett syndrome. High-dose acid-suppression therapy and balloon dilation may obviate the need for fundoplication. In adults, Barrett epithelium is reported to occur in up to one half of patients with stricture,[22] but Barrett epithelium is relatively rare in children. Case reports have been issued of children with Barrett epithelium associated adenocarcinoma[23,24] and with mid-esophageal strictures,[25] but the prevalence in this population is not well known. Patients with Barrett esophagus require at least annual surveillance for dysplasia. Fundoplication may not reverse Barrett esophagus, and no consensus exists on optimal therapy.[26]

Gastrointestinal bleeding associated with hematemesis, melena, guaiac positive stools, or anemia can occur as a complication of GERD resulting from erosive esophagitis. This complication is seen primarily in children who are neurologically impaired.

Respiratory Complications

Chronic Cough, Stridor, Hoarseness

The presence of GERD in children with chronic cough, stridor, and hoarseness has been described in several studies.[27-31] Symptoms of laryngopharyngeal reflux are presented in Box 264-6. Characteristic laryngoscopic findings attributed to GERD include airway erythema, edema, nodularity, granuloma, and cobblestoning.[32,33] The differential diagnosis of hoarseness is shown in Table 264-1. Therapy with a proton pump inhibitor (PPI) is usually recommended because of its greater acid-suppression capacity. However, higher doses given for a prolonged time are often required because relapse after stopping therapy is common.

Recurrent Pneumonia

GERD may cause aspiration pneumonia and chronic pulmonary fibrosis[14] and may occur without esophagitis. Children with neurodevelopmental delay present a special diagnostic problem because oropharyngeal incoordination may result in aspiration without reflux.[34] Performing a fundoplication in such a child

BOX 264-5 Complications of Gastroesophageal Reflux

SYMPTOMS
- Recurrent vomiting
- Weight loss or poor weight gain
- Irritability in infants
- Regurgitation
- Heartburn or chest pain
- Hematemesis
- Dysphagia or feeding refusal
- Apnea or ALTE
- Wheezing or stridor
- Hoarseness
- Cough
- Abnormal neck posturing (Sandifer syndrome)

FINDINGS
- Esophagitis
- Esophageal stricture
- Barrett esophagus
- Laryngitis
- Recurrent pneumonia
- Hypoproteinemia
- Anemia

ALTE, Apparent life-threatening event.
From Rudolph CD, Mazur LJ, Liptak GS, et al. Pediatric GE reflux clinical practice guidelines. *J Pediatr Gastroenterol Nutr.* 2001;32(S2):1-31. Reprinted by permission of Lippincott Williams & Wilkins.

might potentially impair esophageal clearance and increase the risk of aspiration. Videofluoroscopic swallowing study or fiber-endoscopic swallowing evaluation with neurosensory testing may help identify patients at risk for aspiration.[35,36]

Asthma

Several studies suggest GERD may contribute to the severity of asthma.[14] Although symptoms of reflux are common in children with asthma, and a high percentage of children with persistent asthma have abnormal pH monitoring, the relationship between asthma and GERD remains a challenge for the clinician. The prevalence rates of GERD-associated asthma are reported to range from 25% to 75%. Interestingly, approximately 50% of patients with persistent asthma who test positive for GERD by pH monitoring have no or minimal symptoms of GERD. In one arm of a clinical trial of asthmatic children ages 5 to 10 years, children with normal pH monitoring were randomized to receive a PPI or no acid-suppression treatment. Approximately 25% of asthmatic children with normal pH probe studies were able to decrease their asthma medication, whereas children who were not treated with acid-suppression medication continued on the same dose of asthma medication.[37] Studies have shown improvement of asthma symptoms after a variety of medical therapies for GERD that included positional therapy, thickening of formula without medication, Cisapride, and a histamine-2 receptor antagonist (H_2RA).[14] Currently, evidence in children is insufficient to establish optimal medical therapy for GER in patients with asthma, but the best diagnostic test to determine if an association between asthma and GERD exists is an empiric trial with a PPI given twice a day for at least 3 months.

BOX 264-6 Symptoms of Laryngopharyngeal Reflux

IN INFANTS:	IN CHILDREN:
Feeding resistance or refusal, growth failure	Chronic cough
Irritability	Dysphonia
Abnormal crying	Globus, sore throat
Sleeping problems	Halitosis
Apnea	Nasal obstruction
Recurrent croup	Rhinorrhea, headache
Laryngomalacia	Regurgitation, vomiting
Excessive salivation	Abdominal pain
	Dysphagia

Adapted from Stavroulaki P. Diagnostic and management problems of laryngopharyngeal reflux disease in children. Int J Pediatr Otorhinolaryngol 2006;70(4):579-590. Copyright © 2006, Elsevier, with permission.

Apnea or Apparent Life-Threatening Event

An apparent life-threatening event (ALTE) is an episode occurring in an infant that requires intervention and is characterized by a combination of apnea, cyanosis, pallor, rubor, plethora, limpness, stiffness, choking, or gagging.[38] (See Chapter 237, Apparent Life-threatening Event.) ALTEs may be caused by cardiac, central nervous system, and infectious diseases, as well as upper airways obstruction, central apnea, and GERD.[14] Despite earlier reports of GER inducing obstructive apnea, subsequent investigations in unselected patients with ALTE have not demonstrated a convincing temporal relationship between ALTE and acid reflux, apnea, or bradycardia.[14] The most convincing relationship between GERD and episodes of obstructive or mixed apnea has been in infants in whom the episodes occurred while the patient was awake, in the supine position, and within 1 hour of a feeding. A relationship between GER and apnea was demonstrated in 8 of 15 patients undergoing pH monitoring along with simultaneous recording of heart rate, chest wall movement, and nasal airflow (polysomnographic

Table 264-1 Differential Diagnosis of Hoarseness and Laryngeal Edema

SIGNS, SYMPTOMS, OR FACTORS	LARYNGO-PHARYNGEAL REFLUX (LPR)[a]	INFECTION[b]	RHINOSINUSITIS (POSTNASAL DRIP)[c]	ALLERGY[d]	BENIGN VOCAL FOLD LESION[e]
Hoarseness	Fluctuates	Acute	Acute, chronic, or recurrent	Fluctuates	Constant
Throat pain	Common (with cough, clearing of throat)	Yes	Uncommon	No	From secondary muscle tension
Laryngeal findings	Edema, granuloma, erythema, pseudosulcus	Erythema, edema	Secretions (thick discolored), edema	Edema, clear secretions, bluish mucosa	Nodules, polyps, cysts, scars

[a]Aggravating factors are cigarette smoke, obesity, diet, or lifestyle.
[b]Aggravating factors are systemic infection, immunosuppression.
[c]Aggravating factors are LPR, allergy, cigarette smoke.
[d]Aggravating factors are environment and season.
[e]Aggravating factors are cigarette smoke, vocal trauma, LPR.
Adapted from Ford CN. Evaluation and management of laryngopharyngeal reflux. *JAMA.* 2005;294:1534. Reprinted by permission of the American Medical Association.

study).[39] At the present time, no evidence has been found that the clinical characteristics of an ALTE or a combined pH study with polysomnographic might predict risk for further episodes or sudden death. Similarly, no randomized studies have been conducted to evaluate the usefulness of esophageal pH study in infants with ALTE. The benefit of medical therapy of GERD to prevent subsequent ALTE is not known. Thickening feeds, prokinetic agents, and acid-suppression therapy are reasonable therapeutic options, whereas surgical therapy is unproven and should be considered only in infants with ALTE that is unresponsive to acid-suppression therapy and is known to be associated with GERD.

Sandifer Syndrome

Sandifer syndrome is a rare complication of GERD usually seen in otherwise neurologically normal children and is characterized by stereotypical, repetitive stretching, and arching movements thought to be related to esophageal pain. These behaviors may be mistaken for atypical seizures or dystonia.[40,41]

Additional Extraesophageal Complications

Based on uncontrolled studies and case reports, conditions such as dental erosions, recurrent sinus disease, rhinopharyngitis, hoarse voice, and otitis media have been attributed to GERD. All of these disorders have multiple causes, including infectious agents, immunoregulatory defects, and anatomic abnormalities. To attribute the cause to GERD may oversimplify what should be a more thorough evaluation to look for other underlying causes.

MANAGEMENT

The management of GERD involves lifestyle modifications, acid suppression, promotility agents, and surgical therapy. Children at different ages may respond differently to specific interventions, and consideration of issues related to growth, development, and compliance are important factors in determining the best therapeutic intervention.

Lifestyle Changes in Infants

Lifestyle changes in infants are often the first therapy that should be initiated to treat a child with GER or GERD. Normalization of feeding volume and frequency is essential to assess, given that some infants may be fed an excessive volume, and by simply reviewing the feeding history and educating the family, GER may resolve. Thickening the formula with rice cereal or purchasing a commercial formula that becomes denser when it reaches the stomach may also decrease the frequency and volume of regurgitation. The addition of 1 tablespoon of rice cereal to each ounce of formula decreases the number of vomiting episodes without reducing the reflux index.[42] When recommending this strategy to a family, increasing the hole in the nipple may be necessary, being careful to avoid increasing the flow too much so that the infant cannot swallow the volume and begins to cough. In addition, rice cereal may lead to constipation, which may decrease gastric emptying and increase GER. Thickened formula is richer in calories (providing approximately 34 cal/oz with addition of 1 tbsp/oz), and the advantage of extra calories may be beneficial for the infant with slow poor weight gain, but as GER resolves, the infant may gain excessive weight, which may pose a problem later in childhood. Close monitoring of growth during treatment for GER in the first year of life is an important aspect of clinical care.

Intolerance of dietary proteins such as cow's milk or soy may lead to symptoms identical to those of GER.[43-45] These problems are generally seen in formula-fed infants and seem to be less common in breastfed babies. Diagnostic tests are generally not helpful, but in children with GER related to dietary protein will often improve by switching to a hypoallergenic formula. A 1- to 2-week trial of hypoallergenic formula may answer the question about the role of nutrition in causing GER. For the infant with GER who is breastfed, symptoms often resolve with time, but if intervention is required, some infants will improve if the mother eliminates cow's milk and beef from her diet. Soy is more ubiquitous, and restricting cow's milk, beef, and soy is more limiting for a mother's diet.

A change in position may decrease GER in infants, and the prone position is optimal when the infant is awake; however, sleeping in the prone position has been recognized to be associated with a higher risk for sudden infant death syndrome (SIDS) when compared with the supine position. Thus, based on the new American Academy of Pediatrics recommendations, the supine position is recommended during sleep for children younger than 12 months; the reduced risk of SIDS outweighs the potential benefits of prone sleeping with respect to GERD.[46] In certain unusual situations, prone positioning during sleep may be considered when the risk of death from complications of GERD outweighs the potential increased risk of SIDS. (See Chapter 330, Sudden Infant Death Syndrome.) When prone position is a recommendation in a given case, the family should understand the rationale and be advised to avoid using soft bedding that is known to be a suffocation risk for the infant in the prone position.

Placing infants in infant seats may increase the frequency and severity of reflux. Although no evidence has been found for decreasing regurgitation by elevation of the head of the crib, many families report an improvement with this intervention. As infants begin to move around in their cribs, maintaining their head higher than their feet may become a challenge for parents. For the thriving infant with GER, feeding and positioning are important interventions that may decrease the severity of regurgitation and prevent the need for medical therapy.

Lifestyle Changes in Children and Adolescents

Although evidence-based data in children and adolescents with GERD are limited, avoiding lying down after meals and elevating the head of the bed may decrease symptoms of GERD. In addition, older children should be advised to avoid caffeine, chocolate, and spicy foods that exacerbate reflux-related symptoms. Either active or passive exposure to nicotine will exacerbate GERD, and children with GERD should be aware of the additional risks in cigarette smoking. Obesity is a known risk factor for complications of GER, and reducing body weight should be discussed with every child and family when relevant.

Drug Therapy

Several categories of drugs are effective for the management of infants, children, and adolescents with GERD. H_2RAs and PPIs suppress acid production, whereas antacids neutralize acid that has been produced. Prokinetic agents enhance gastric emptying and some may increase LES pressure. Each class of drugs has a specific role. In general, the acid suppressants reduce exposure of the esophagus to acid gastric contents and promote healing of the esophageal mucosa. The prokinetic agents have not been shown to be effective in clinical trials but theoretically may decrease the volume of reflux by raising the LES pressure, reducing the frequency of transient LES relaxations and accelerating gastric emptying. Empiric trials of medication are often used in adults to support a clinical diagnosis of GERD, but this approach, although recommended by many experts in pediatric gastroenterology, has not been validated in children.[47]

Antacids

Antacids act by buffering gastric acid and then decreasing the corrosive effect on the esophageal mucosa. They may relieve symptoms of heartburn, improve esophagitis, and prevent acid-related respiratory symptoms. Intensive high-dose antacid therapy with magnesium and aluminum hydroxide was shown to be as effective as cimetidine for the treatment of esophagitis in children, but aluminum-containing antacids may increase aluminum levels, which can potentially cause osteopenia, anemia, and neurotoxicity. Antacids are generally used for the short-term management of intermittent symptoms of GERD in children.

H_2-Receptor Antagonists

Cimetidine, nizatidine, ranitidine, and famotidine are H_2RAs that exert their antisecretory effect by blocking the histamine-2 receptors on the gastric parietal epithelial cells. All of these drugs are approved by the US Food and Drug Administration for use in children (Table 264-2). Numerous randomized controlled studies in adults have documented the efficacy of this class of medication in relieving reflux symptoms and healing esophagitis. Two randomized placebo-controlled studies in children report on the efficacy of cimetidine[48] and nizatidine[49] at improving reflux symptoms and healing of esophagitis with the medication. Concern exists about the development of tolerance or tachyphylaxis with H_2RAs. In adults, the antisecretory potency of medications in this class decreases after 3 days when compared with PPIs, suggesting that their benefit for long-term use may not be as good as other classes of medications. Nevertheless, based on case series and expert opinion, H_2RAs are considered to be efficacious and safe in infants and children with GER.[14]

Proton Pump Inhibitors

PPIs are the most potent class of acid-suppressive medications because they block the final step of acid production by covalently binding and deactivating the hydrogen-potassium-adenosine triphosphatase enzyme (pump) in the gastric parietal cell.[50] PPIs require acid in the parietal cell canaliculus to be activated and are most effective when taken after a prolonged fast, such as 30 minutes before the first meal of the day. When an evening dose is required, it should be administered 30 minutes before the evening meal. Concomitant administration of H_2RAs may, in theory, reduce the efficacy of PPI therapy by reducing the available hydrogen ions needed to activate the PPI. Pharmacokinetic parameters for PPIs in adolescents are similar to those reported in adults; however, children younger than 12 years require doses ranging from 1.5 to 2 times the adult dose of PPIs based on a per-kilogram basis to achieve adequate acid suppression.[51] This level has been attributed to a higher metabolic capacity in children, particularly those 1 to 6 years of age. Recommended dosing ranges have a large range (Table 264-3). The effective dose of omeprazole ranges from 0.3 to 3.5 mg/kg/day (maximum 80 mg/day) and for lansoprazole is from 0.73 to 1.66 mg/kg/day (maximum 30 mg/day). Efficacy data in children are mainly from open-label trials and a few controlled trials.[14] PPIs are most effective in decreasing the symptoms of reflux and healing esophagitis in children and adolescents. The benefit of PPIs alone in the treatment of GERD in children with asthma has not been well studied, but studies suggest that this class of medication is effective and is an excellent choice for an empiric trial. Over 10 years of safety data are reported with continuous use of omeprazole in

Table 264-2 FDA Approved H_2RA Therapy for Pediatric GERD

	INDICATED AGES	DOSE
Ranitidine	1 mo to 16 yr	5-10 mg/kg/day in 2 divided doses
Famotidine	1 yr to 16 yr	1 mg/kg/day in 2 divided doses up to 40 mg twice a day
Nizatidine	$\geq$12 yr	150 mg twice a day
Cimetidine	$\geq$16 yr	800 mg twice a day or 400 mg 4 times a day

FDA, US Food and Drug Administration; *GERD,* gastroesophageal reflux disease; *H_2RA,* histamine-2 receptor antagonist.
No over-the-counter H_2RAS are labeled for pediatric use.
From *Physician's Desk Reference.* 61st edition, Montvale, NJ: Thomson PDR; 2007.

Table 264-3 Proton Pump Inhibitor Therapy

	AGE	DOSE	FORMULATION
FDA APPROVED FOR CHILDREN			
Esomeprazole	12-17 yr	20 mg or 40 mg by mouth daily	Capsule Oral suspension Intravenous solution
Lansoprazole	1-17 yr	1 yr-11 yr, ≤30 kg—15 mg by mouth daily 1 yr-11 yr, >30 kg—30 mg by mouth daily 12-17 yr, nonerosive—15 mg by mouth daily 12-17 yr, erosive—30 mg by mouth daily	Capsule Oral suspension Rapidly dissolving tablet Intravenous solution
Omeprazole	1-16 yr	2-16 yr, <20 kg—10 mg by mouth daily 2-16 yr, ≥20 kg—20 mg by mouth daily	Capsule Oral suspension
NOT FDA APPROVED FOR CHILDREN			
Rabeprazole	18 yr	—	Tablet
Pantoprazole	18 yr	—	Capsule Oral suspension Intravenous solution
Zegerid (omeprazole)	18 yr	—	Tablet

FDA, US Food and Drug Administration.
From *Physician's Desk Reference*. 61st edition, Montvale, NJ: Thomson PDR; 2007.

adults, but safety data in children are more limited. However, a limited number of children receiving omeprazole have been monitored for over 8 years with good safety data,[52] and the safety of lansoprazole in children appears to be similar.[53]

Prokinetic Agents

Prokinetic agents are used in the treatment of GERD to accelerate gastric emptying. Despite this rationale, studies have not shown a decrease in acid reflux episodes, thereby raising the questions that these drugs may not reduce transient LES relaxations that are the most important pathophysiological mechanism of GERD. The only prokinetic agents that are available in the United States are metoclopramide and erythromycin. Erythromycin is rarely used in children who have only GERD unless they have significant delay in gastric emptying. Metoclopramide has limited efficacy in treating GERD and has potentially serious side effects, including dyskinesia and tardive dyskinesia that result from crossing the blood-brain barrier. Metoclopramide also results in increasing serum prolactin levels. These safety concerns limit its value in treating children with GERD.

Surgery as a Management Strategy in Gastroesophageal Reflux Disease

Surgical therapy is an option for children who remain symptomatic on chronic medical therapy or have side effects of medication. Life-threatening complications such as aspiration may lead to a recommendation of a fundoplication, but the concern that aspiration may result from swallowing and not from reflux is always present. If esophageal clearance is impaired, aspiration related to pharyngeal dysfunction may get worse after a fundoplication. The rationale to perform surgery to avoid chronic medical therapy has not been well studied in children, but approximately 30% of adults who undergo fundoplication continue to take acid-suppression therapy after surgery. Nissen fundoplication is the standard form of surgery and involves wrapping the fundus of the stomach around the LES to reinforce the antireflux barrier. Several modifications of this surgical procedure have been added, including the newer laparoscopic approach. Recent studies suggest that children who have a laparoscopic fundoplication may have fewer complications but have a higher rate of reoperation (14%) when compared with children having an open Nissen fundoplication (8%).[54]

SUMMARY

GERD is common in infants, children, and adolescents, but the prevalence appears to be increasing. GERD negatively affects health-related quality of life and has the potential for long-term complications that may begin in childhood. With the increasing nationwide trends in obesity prevalence, which is a risk factor for GERD and erosive esophagitis, pediatricians may see greater numbers of children with GERD. Familial clustering of GERD suggests that genetic or environmental factors may be relevant for some individuals. Parent and patient education is an integral part of management. Making good decisions about lifestyle choices may improve outcomes. Medical and surgical therapies are available and can be effective in treating complications of GERD.

TOOLS FOR PRACTICE

Engaging Patient and Family

- *The Infant Reflux and GERD: Distinctions and Management Video*, North American Society for Pediatric Gastroenterology and Nutrition and Children's Digestive Health and Nutrition Foundation (link4.streamhoster.com/?u=activeweb&p=/pedgerd.wmv&odaid=1579).

- *Parent's Take Home Guide to GERD* (fact sheet), North American Society for Pediatric Gastroenterology and Nutrition and Children's Digestive Health and Nutrition Foundation (gerd.cdhnf.org/User/Docs/PDF/GERDParents_Handout.pdf).

Medical Decision Support

- *Children's Digestive Health and Nutrition Foundation* (Web page), Children's Digestive Health and Nutrition Foundation (gerd.cdhnf.org/aspx/public/ContentPage.aspx?pName=MedicalProfessionals_Professional EducationResource&pType=en&menu=medical).
- *Gastroesophageal Reflux in Infants* (interactive tool), American Academy of Pediatrics (www.pedialink.org/cme/_coursefinder/CMEdetail.cfm?aid=32122&area=liveCME).

RELATED WEB SITE

- Children's Digestive Health and Nutrition Foundation (gerd.cdhnf.org/default.aspx).

SUGGESTED RESOURCE

North American Society for Pediatric Gastroenterology and Nutrition. Guidelines for evaluation and treatment of gastroesophageal reflux in infants and children. *J Pediatr Gastroenterol.* 2001;32(2):1-31.

REFERENCES

1. Nelson SP, Chen EH, Syniar GM, et al. Prevalence of symptoms of gastroesophageal reflux during infancy. A pediatric practice-based survey. Pediatric Practice Research Group. *Arch Pediatr Adolesc Med.* 1997;151(6):569-572.
2. Martin AJ, Pratt N, Kennedy D, et al. Natural history and familial relationships of infant spilling to 9 years of age. *Pediatrics.* 2002;109:1061-1067.
3. Pediatric Endoscopy Database System. Clinical Outcomes Research Initiative. Available at: www.bcm.edu/pediatrics/index.cfm?Realm=99991122&This_Template=pedi_home.cfm. Accessed January 24, 2008.
4. Cameron AJ, Lagergren J, Henricksson C, et al. Gastroesophageal reflux disease in monozygotic and dizygotic twins. *Gastroenterology.* 2002;122(1):55-59.
5. El-Serag HB, Gilger M, Kuebeler M, et al. Extraesophageal associations of gastroesophageal reflux disease in children without neurologic defects. *Gastroenterology.* 2001;121(6):1294-1299.
6. Phipps CD, Wood WE, Gibson WS, et al. Gastroesophageal reflux contributing to chronic sinus disease in children: a prospective analysis. *Arch Otolaryngol Head Neck Surg.* 2000;126:831-836.
7. Werlin SL, Dodds WJ, Hogan WJ, et al. Mechanisms of gastroesophageal reflux in children. *J Pediatr.* 1980;97(2):244-249.
8. Kawahara H, Dent J, Davidson G. Mechanisms responsible for gastroesophageal reflux in children. *Gastroenterology.* 1997;113:399-408.
9. Cucchiara S, Salvia G, Borrelli O, et al. Gastric electrical dysrhythmias and delayed gastric emptying in gastroesophageal reflux disease. *Am J Gastroenterol.* 1997;92:1103-1108.
10. Moser G, Vacariu-Granser GV, Schneider C, et al. High incidence of esophageal motor disorders in consecutive patients with globus sensation. *Gastroenterology.* 1991;101(6):1512-1521.
11. Field SK. Underlying mechanisms of respiratory symptoms with esophageal acid when there is no evidence of airway response. *Am J Med.* 2001;111(S8A):37S-40S.
12. Field SK. A critical review of the studies of the effects of simulated or real gastroesophageal reflux on pulmonary function in asthmatic adults. *Chest.* 1999;115(3):848-856.
13. Herve P, Denjean A, Jian R, et al. Intraesophageal perfusion of acid increases the bronchomotor response to methacholine and to isocapnic hyperventilation in asthmatic subjects. *Am Rev Resp Dis.* 1986;134(5):986-989.
14. North American Society for Pediatric Gastroenterology and Nutrition. Pediatric GE reflux clinical practice guidelines. *J Pediatr Gastroenterol Nutr.* 2001;32(2) S2-S31.
15. Colletti RB, Christie DL, Orenstein SR. Statement of the North American Society for Pediatric Gastroenterology and Nutrition (NASPGN). Indications for pediatric esophageal pH monitoring. *J Pediatr Gastroenterol Nutr.* 1995;21(3):253-262.
16. Pandolfino JE, Kahrilas PJ. Prolonged pH monitoring: Bravo capsule. *Gastrointest Endosc Clin North Am.* 2005;15(2):307-318.
17. Cucchiara S, Santamaria F, Minella R, et al. Simultaneous prolonged recordings of proximal and distal intraesophageal pH in children with gastroesophageal reflux disease and respiratory symptoms. *Am J Gastroenterol.* 1995;90(10):1791-1796.
18. Matthews BL, Little JP, Mcguirt WF, et al. Reflux in infants with laryngomalacia: results of 24-hour double-probe pH monitoring. *Otolaryngol Head Neck Surg.* 1999;120(6):860-864.
19. Rothbaum RJ. Complications of pediatric endoscopy. *Gastrointest Endosc Clin North Am.* 1996;6(2):445-459.
20. Ben RM, Bouche O, Zeitoun P. Study of 47 consecutive patients with peptic esophageal stricture compared with 3880 cases of reflux esophagitis. *Dig Dis Sci.* 1992;37(5):733-736.
21. Rode HJ, Miller AJ, Brown RA, et al. Reflux strictures of the esophagus in children. *J Pediatr Surg.* 1992;27:462-465.
22. Spechler SJ, Sperber H, Doos WG, et al. The prevalence of Barrett's esophagus in patients with chronic peptic esophageal strictures. *Dig Dis Sci.* 1983,28(9):769-774.
23. Hassall E, Dimmick JE, Magee JF. Adenocarcinoma in childhood Barrett's esophagus: case documentation and the need for surveillance in children. *Am J Gastroenterol.* 1993;88(2);282-288.
24. Hoeffel JC, Nihoul-Fekete C, Schmitt M. Esophageal adenocarcinoma after gastroesophageal reflux in children. *J Pediatr.* 1989;115(2):259-261.
25. Yulish BS, Rothstein FC, Halpin TC Jr. Radiographic findings in children and young adults with Barrett's esophagus. *AJR Am J of Roentgenol.* 1987;148:353-357.
26. Falk FW. Barrett's esophagus. *Gastroenterology.* 2002;122(6):1569-1591.
27. Koufman JA. The otolaryngologic manifestations of gastroesophageal reflux disease (GERD): a clinical investigation of 225 patients using ambulatory 24-hour pH monitoring and an experimental investigation of the role of acid and pepsin in the development of laryngeal injury. *Laryngoscope.* 1991,101(4 pt 2, suppl 53):1-78.
28. Fitzgerald JM, Allen CJ, Craven MA, et al. Chronic cough and gastroesophageal reflux. *CMAJ.* 1989;140(5):520-524.
29. Ing AJ, Ngu MC, Breslin AB. Chronic persistent cough and gastro-oesophageal reflux. *Thorax.* 1991;46(7):479-483.
30. Contensin P, Narcy P. Gastropharyngeal reflux in infants and children. A pharyngeal pH monitoring study. *Arch Otolaryngol Head Neck Surg.* 1992;118:1028-1030.

31. Gumpert L, Kalach N, DuPont C, et al. Horseness and gastroesophageal reflux in children. *J Laryngol Otol.* 1998;112(1):49-54.
32. Wilson JA, White A, von Haacke NP, et al. Gastroesophageal reflux and posterior laryngitis. *Ann Otol Rhinol Laryngol.* 1989;98:405-410.
33. Shaw GY, Searl JP. Laryngeal manifestations of gastroesophageal reflux before and after treatment with omeprazole. *South Med J.* 1997;90(11):1115-1122.
34. Morton RE, Wheatley R, Minford J. Respiratory tract infections due to direct and reflux aspiration in children with severe neurodisability. *Dev Med Child Neurol.* 1999; 41(5):329-334.
35. Taniguchi MH, Moyer RS. Assessment of risk factors for pneumonia in dysphagic children: significance of videofluoroscopic swallowing evaluation. *Dev Med Child Neurol.* 1994;36(6):495-502.
36. Aviv JE, Kim T, Sacco RL, et al. FEESST: a new bedside endoscopic test of the motor and sensory components of swallowing. *Ann Otol Laryngol Rhinol.* 1998;107(5): 378-387.
37. Khoshoo V, Le T, Haydel R, et al. Role of gastroesophageal reflux in older children with persistent asthma. *Chest.* 2003;123:1008-1013.
38. National Institutes of Health. Consensus statement on infantile apnea and home monitoring. *Pediatrics.* 1987; 79:292-299.
39. Spitzer AR, Boyle JT, Tuchman DN, et al. Awake apnea associated with gastroesophageal reflux: a specific clinical syndrome. *J Pediatr.* 1984;104(2):200-205.
40. Werlin SL, D'Souza BJ, Hogan WJ, et al. Sandifer syndrome: an unappreciated clinical entity. *Dev Med Child Neurol.* 1980;22(3);374-378.
41. Gorrotxategi P, Reguilon MJ, Arana J, et al. Gastroesophageal reflux in association with the Sandifer syndrome. *Eur J Pediatr Surg.* 1995;5(4):203-205.
42. Craig WR, Hanlon-Dearman A, Sinclair C, et al. Metoclopramide, thickened feedings, and positioning for gastrooesophageal reflux in children under two years. *Cochrane Data Base Syst Rev.* 2004;Oct 18(4):CD003502.
43. Forget P, Arends JW. Cow's milk protein allergy and gastro-oesophageal reflux. *Eur J Pediatr.* 1985;144(4): 298-300.
44. Iacono G, Carroccio A, Cavataio F, et al. Gastroesophageal reflux and cow's milk allergy in infants: a prospective study. *J Allergy Clin Immunol.* 1996;97(3):822-827.
45. Cavataio F, Iacono G, Montalto G, et al. Gastroesophageal reflux associated with cow's milk allergy in infants: which diagnostic examinations are useful? *Am J Gastroenterol.* 1996;91(6):1215-1220.
46. American Academy of Pediatrics, Task Force on Infant Position on SIDS. Changing concepts of sudden infant death syndrome: implications for infant sleeping environment and sleep position. *Pediatrics.* 2000;105:650-656.
47. van Pinxteren B, Numans ME, Bonis PA, et al. Short-term treatment with proton pump inhibitors, H2-receptor antagonists and prokinetics for gastro-oesophageal reflux disease-like symptoms and endoscopy negative reflux disease. *Cochrane Database Syst Rev.* 2000;(2): CD002095. Update in: *Cochrane Database Syst Rev.* 2001;(4):CD002095.
48. Cucchiara S, Gobio-Casali L, Balli F, et al. Cimetidine treatment of reflux esophagitis in children: an Italian multicentric study. *J Pediatr Gastroenterol Nutr.* 1989; 8(2):150-156.
49. Simeone D, Caria MC, Miele E, et al. Treatment of childhood peptic esophagitis: a double-blind placebo-controlled trial of nizatidine. *J Pediatr Gastroenterol Nutr.* 1997;25(1):51-55.
50. Wolfe MM, Sachs G. Acid suppression: optimizing therapy for gastroduodenal ulcer healing, gastroesophageal reflux disease, and stress-related erosive syndrome. *Gastroenterology.* 2000;118(2 supp);S9-S31.
51. Litalien C, Théorêt Y, Faure C. Pharmacokinetics of proton pump inhibitors in children. *Clin Pharmacokinet.* 2005;44(5):441-466.
52. Hassall E, Kerr W, El-Serag HB. Characteristics of children receiving proton pump inhibitors continuously for up to 11 years duration. *J Pediatr.* 2007;150(3):262-267.
53. Tolia V, Fitzgerald J, Hassall E, et al. Safety of lansoprazole in the treatment of gastroesophageal reflux disease in children. *J Pediatr Gastroenterol Nutr.* 2002;35(S4); S300-S307.
54. Diaz D, Gibbons TE, Heiss K, et al. Antireflux surgery outcomes in pediatric gastroesophageal reflux disease. *Am J Gastroenterol.* 2005;100(8):1844-1852.

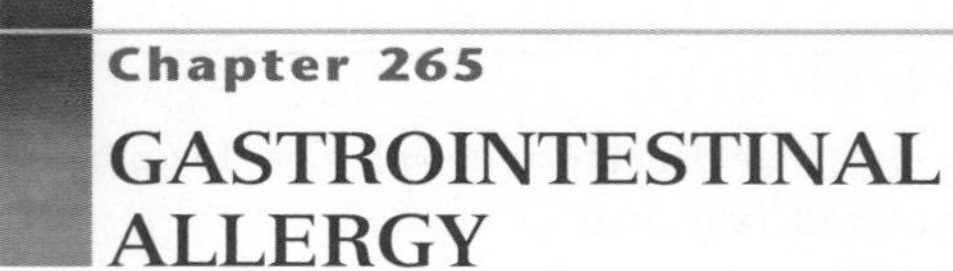

Chapter 265

GASTROINTESTINAL ALLERGY

P. Christine Nguyen, MD; John A. Kerner Jr, MD

INTRODUCTION

Food allergy is a common but often unsubstantiated diagnosis in pediatric practice. An adverse reaction to a food is any untoward reaction regardless of its cause. Such reactions can be classified under two general categories: (1) food allergy or hypersensitivity, an immunologic response, and (2) food intolerance, a non-immunologic response. Food intolerance can occur because of an underlying congenital or acquired enzyme deficiency (disaccharidase deficiency, galactosemia, hereditary fructose intolerance) in which a specific dietary nutrient cannot be metabolized properly; ingestion of a toxin in the food (*Staphylococcus*, shellfish, mushrooms); or ingestion of a pharmacologic agent (metabisulfite in wine or salad may cause bronchospasm, wine and monosodium glutamate may cause headache, and caffeine may cause arrhythmia).

The gastrointestinal (GI) tract contains lymphoid tissue capable of mounting an immunologic response to prevent the penetration of antigens across the epithelium. Lymphocytes and plasma cells are present in Peyer patches and the lamina propria of the small and large intestine; immunoglobulin A (IgA)-containing plasma cells account for only 2%. The aberrations in immunologic mechanisms that trigger GI allergic reactions are unknown.

Foods that account for 90% of allergic reactions in children are cow's milk protein, eggs, peanut, soy, tree nuts, fish, and wheat. Food allergy can cause urticaria or angioedema, anaphylaxis, atopic dermatitis, respiratory symptoms, or a GI disorder. GI allergic manifestations can be classified as immunoglobulin E (IgE)-mediated (immediate GI hypersensitivity and oral allergy syndrome) or *mixed* GI allergy syndromes (involving some IgE components and some non–IgE- or T-cell–mediated components), which include eosinophilic esophagitis and eosinophilic gastroenteritis.

Non–IgE-mediated or T-cell–mediated allergic GI disorders include dietary protein enteropathy, protein-induced enterocolitis, and proctitis. All of these conditions share a common denominator: the response of the immune system to a specific protein leading to pathological inflammatory changes in the GI tract. This immunologic response can elicit symptoms such as diarrhea, vomiting, dysphagia, constipation, or GI blood loss, symptoms consistent with a GI disorder.[1]

FOOD ALLERGY

Clinical Manifestations

In patients with specific food allergies, removing specific food allergens from the diet ameliorates symptoms. Reintroduction of the allergen leads to recurrence of symptoms. These allergies are much more common in infants than in older children because infants may be predisposed to protein allergy caused by enzymatic immaturity, increased gut permeability, and relatively low secretory IgA. Cow's milk protein allergy (CMPA) and soy protein allergy are the most clearly defined allergies in infants. Food allergy or formula sensitivity should always be considered in patients with refractory reflux because these two conditions may coexist.

Cow's Milk Protein Allergy

Early studies showed that the incidence of CMPA was between 0.5% and 7% of all infants under the age of 6 months.[2] Later studies suggested that 2.5% of newborns will have hypersensitivity to cow's milk in the first year of life.[3] β-Lactoglobulin, the main whey protein, appears to be the most antigenic component of cow's milk,[4] but some infants can be sensitive to casein or whey protein. Rarely do infants develop CMPA after the first year of age. The symptoms and signs of CMPA are listed in Box 265-1. GI symptoms predominate in many patients. In other patients, anaphylaxis or pulmonary symptoms occur.[5] Infants with severe atopic dermatitis should also be evaluated for possible CMPA and other food allergy.[6]

The GI manifestations of CMPA depend on the site of predominant inflammation in the GI tract. Esophagitis causes recurrent vomiting and reflux[7]; gastritis causes vomiting, irritability or pain, and occult GI bleeding; enteritis causes diarrhea, malabsorption, or protein-losing enteropathy[8]; and colitis causes rectal bleeding, with blood or mucus in the stool. Some infants can exhibit severe enterocolitis. Profuse vomiting and or diarrhea can lead to shock, anemia, and methemoglobinemia. Patients with milk protein–induced enterocolitis may be predisposed to a severe rare form of enterocolitis to solid food antigens later in life. These children can develop severe reactions to food proteins considered to be of low allergenicity.[9]

Although CMPA is more typically associated with colitis symptoms, other symptoms, including gastroesophageal reflux and cow's milk allergic esophagitis, are now well described. Antral gastritis is a common finding in these patients, with increased eosinophils and inflammatory cells in the antrum. Duodenal biopsy specimens reveal patchy changes, ranging from normal mucosa to *flat gut* lesions. Differentiation from celiac disease is made by the absence of antiendomysial or anti tissue transglutaminase antibodies (see Chapter 268, Gluten-sensitive Enteropathy [Celiac Sprue]). Colitis is common in these patients who have blood or mucus in the stool. Allergy is the most common cause of rectal bleeding among infants younger than 6 months. Rectal bleeding or guaiac-positive stools are probably the most common symptoms in infants with formula sensitivity. A significant number of these infants experience straining or discomfort with stools.

Previously, physicians counseled families that infants with CMPA would outgrow it by 2 years of age. Later studies revealed that allergy may persist in 72% at age 2, 44% at age 4, and 32% at age 6.[10] Other studies are less pessimistic, with 44% with persistent symptoms at 1 year, 33% at 2 years, and 23% at 3 years.[11] Patients who have longer persistence of symptoms have a higher frequency of allergic disease, multiple food allergies, and develop symptoms later after initial introduction of milk.[7,12]

BOX 265-1 Clinical Manifestations of Cow's Milk Protein Allergy

SYSTEMIC MANIFESTATIONS
Anaphylaxis
Iron-deficiency anemia (caused by GI blood loss)
Atopic dermatitis, urticaria
Peripheral eosinophilia
Poor sleep

RESPIRATORY MANIFESTATIONS
Rhinitis
Wheezing
Pulmonary hemosiderosis
Nasopharyngeal obstruction leading to cor pulmonale

GASTROINTESTINAL (GI) MANIFESTATIONS
Vomiting or gastroesophageal reflux
Diarrhea, malabsorption, protein-losing enteropathy
Enterocolitis
Constipation
GI bleeding
Failure to thrive

GI, Gastrointestinal.

Soy Protein Allergy

Thirty percent to 50% of infants allergic to cow's milk protein may also be allergic to soy protein[13]; however, soy protein allergy may occur without a concomitant allergy to cow's milk protein. The clinical features of soy protein allergy are similar to those of CMPA, including esophagitis, gastritis, enteritis, and colitis.

Human Milk Allergy

Infants who are breastfed may develop the same symptoms as patients who are formula fed, exhibiting either allergic colitis or evidence of esophagitis, gastritis, or enteritis; the most common symptom appears to be colitis.[14] These patients are commonly asymptomatic or may show significant irritability as a manifestation of their disease, with either occult blood or obvious rectal bleeding.

Laboratory Abnormalities in Gastrointestinal Food Allergies

In formula allergy the infant may not necessarily have peripheral eosinophilia. The results of IgE determinations and CAP-RAST tests (RASTs) to detect these IgE antibodies specific for milk and soy proteins usually are negative, suggesting that the immunologic mechanism occurs by means of a non-IgE (T-cell–mediated) mechanism. A significant number of these patients also have a concomitant transient hypogammaglobulinemia or hypoalbuminemia caused by protein-losing enteropathy; treatment of the milk or soy allergy or other food allergy results in normalization of serum proteins. The findings of an elevated IgE level or positive RAST result with these foods at this age in most cases would suggest long-term rather than self-limited sensitivity.

BOX 265-2 American Academy of Pediatrics 2008 Recommendations for Prevention of Allergy[17]

- Nutritional interventions are largely limited to infants at high risk of developing allergy (ie, infants with a least 1 first degree relative with allergic disease).
- There is "evidence" that compared to intact cow milk protein formula, exclusive breast feeding for at least 4 months prevents or delays the occurrence of atopic dermatitis, cow milk allergy, and wheezing.
- There is "modest evidence" that atopic disease may be delayed or prevented by the use of extensively or partially hydrolyzed formulas compared with intact cow milk formula, particularly for atopic dermatitis.
- There is "little" or "no current convincing" evidence that the timing (delaying) of introduction of complementary foods beyond 4 to 6 months of age prevents the occurrence of atopic disease.
- There is "no convincing" evidence for the use of soy formula for allergy prevention.
- Current evidence does not support maternal dietary restrictions during pregnancy or lactation.

The hallmark of GI biopsies in these patients is the increased number of eosinophils. Reports indicate that more than 20 eosinophils per high-power field on rectal biopsy specimens is indicative of an allergic cause for colitis.[15] However, any inflammatory lesion of the GI tract appears to attract eosinophils.

Management

Treatment of food allergy includes primary prevention to prevent sensitization to proteins. The American Academy of Pediatrics previous recommendations were recently revised and are listed in Box 265-2.[16] Secondary prevention involves preventing recurrence of symptoms once they occur. Secondary prevention is accomplished with either extensively hydrolyzed formulas or elemental formulas. Categories of formulas are listed in Table 265-1, and a comparison of partial versus extensive hydrolysates appears in Table 265-2.

Treatment in infants who are sensitive to mother's milk involves persuading the mothers to avoid cow's milk products, but not all infants will respond to this measure. Whether this variable is the result of accidental maternal ingestion of milk proteins or some other factor is unclear. Preventing many of the breastfeeding mothers from eliminating other foods from their diet, which can cause significant maternal weight loss, can sometimes become extremely difficult. Mothers should be told that, by far, most infants who show sensitivity to foods the mother is eating do not have severe disease. Therefore breastfeeding can be continued unless the symptoms are significant. Mothers who exclude multiple foods from their diets should consider vitamin and calcium supplementation. Sometimes using a hypoallergenic formula may be worth a trial to determine if the infant's symptoms disappear.

Cow's Milk or Soy Protein Allergy

Many choices are available for formula today (see Chapter 26, Feeding of Infants and Children). The primary care physician should be familiar with the different protein bases.

Once the infant either is suspected of having or has been diagnosed as having a specific protein allergy, the infant should initially be fed a hypoallergenic formula. The choice of formula will depend on the formula the patient is taking at the time of diagnosis. If the patient is taking a milk-based or soy-based formula, then starting with an extensively hydrolyzed casein hydrolysate formula such as Alimentum,

Table 265-1 Nonstandard Infant Formulas

PROTEIN SOURCE	ALLERGENICITY	EXAMPLES
Soy protein with L-methionine	—	Bright Beginnings Soy, Good Start Supreme Soy, Isomil Advance, Enfamil Prosobee
Partially hydrolyzed whey	—	Good Start Supreme
Partially hydrolyzed casein, partially hydrolyzed whey		Gentlease
Casein hydrolysate	Hypoallergenic	Alimentum, Nutramigen, Pregestimil
Amino acid base	Nonallergenic	Neocate, Elecare

Nutramigen, or Pregestimil is appropriate. A partially hydrolyzed whey formula may be helpful in reducing the risk of CMPA but should not be used as treatment of existing allergy symptoms. Among partially hydrolyzed formulas, Good Start has been studied extensively but Gentlease has not.

The allergy may last as little as 3 to 12 months; therefore this period is one of trial and error as the patient is gradually retried on the previously proved allergen.

Approximately 10% to 15% of infants placed on casein hydrolysate formula still have a persistent sensitivity as evidenced by continual guaiac-positive stools or overt GI bleeding. Many of these patients respond to the L-amino acid formulas such as Neocate and Elecare.[17,18] These formulas are expensive and should only be used when persistent sensitivity to all other formulas is well documented.

Milk or milk products from animals other than cows have also been used anecdotally. An example is sheep or goat milk. A risk of using such a product is the possible cross-reactivity between cow's milk and sheep or goat milk proteins. Additionally, goat milk is folate deficient.

EOSINOPHILIC GASTROINTESTINAL DISORDERS

Eosinophilic (or allergic) gastrointestinal disorders (EGIDs) are characterized by infiltration of the GI tract with eosinophils.[19] Multiple food sensitivities are often identified, and the disorders are also usually associated with other systemic allergies. EGIDs are subdivided into specific areas of the gastrointestinal tract. New focus has taken place on EGIDs because of the explosion of research into one particular subset, eosinophilic esophagitis.

Three types of disease manifestations are described, depending on the depth of GI involvement: (1) mucosal disease, (2) muscular disease, and (3) serosal disease. Depending on the site of the GI tract involved, mucosal disease causes dysphagia and heartburn if limited to the esophagus; vomiting if involving the stomach; protein-losing enteropathy, malabsorption, and diarrhea if involving the small bowel; and bloody stools if involving the colon. In submucosal or muscular disease, prominent inflammation in the stomach antrum can lead to pyloric obstruction. In serosal disease, which causes eosinophilic ascites, symptoms resemble peritonitis. The latter two types are less common in children. One half of the cases have peripheral blood eosinophilia, elevated IgE levels, and an atopic history. Hypereosinophilic syndromes are characterized by infiltration of many organs with eosinophils. Eosinophilia can also be associated with parasitic infestations, nutritional deficiencies, inflammatory bowel disease, and neoplasms.

Incidence

Although allergic gastroenteropathies were previously thought to be rare, a subset, eosinophilic esophagitis, has become well recognized. Incidence is 4 in 10,000[20] but may be underestimated because all incidence studies are based on referrals. The increased incidence appears to be the result of a combination of a higher index of suspicion and a true increase in pediatric allergy.

Etiology

Causes for EGID have included sensitization to aeroallergens,[21,22] autoimmune processes, ingested food allergies, and predisposition as a result of severe reflux or cutaneous atopy.[23] Both IgE-dependent and IgE-independent mechanisms are believed to be involved in the pathogenesis of these conditions. The presence of peripheral eosinophilia, systemic allergies, elevated IgE levels, and therapeutic response to steroids indicates an allergic basis for this disease in some patients.

Pathological Considerations

Each of the EGIDs shares a common feature of eosinophils infiltrating the GI tract, without involvement of extraintestinal organs. Eosinophilic esophagitis is the only EGID for which normal and abnormal numbers of eosinophils are established.

Research has well characterized the pathological mechanism in eosinophilic esophagitis. Although

Table 265-2 Soy vs Partial vs Extensive Hydrolysates vs L-Amino Acid Formulas

CATEGORY	SOY	PARTIALLY HYDROLYZED*	EXTENSIVELY HYDROLYZED†	L-AMINO ACID
Decreases protein sensitization	No	Yes	Yes	Yes
Treatment for established CMPA	No	No	Yes	Yes
Type of formula	Routine	Routine	Specialty	Specialty
Cost	Comparable with standard cow's milk	Comparable with standard cow's milk formula	Three to four times more costly than standard	Even more expensive than extensively hydrolyzed formula
Palatability	Comparable with standard	Comparable with standard	Less than standard	Less than standard formula

*Partially hydrolyzed whey.
†Extensively hydrolyzed casein.
CMPA, Cow's milk protein allergy.

scattered eosinophils are normal throughout the rest of the GI tract, they are pathological when seen in esophagus. In the past, eosinophils in the esophagus were attributed to reflux.[24] Current research shows the esophageal eosinophilia in reflux is mild (<15-20 eosinophils per high-power field) and is usually limited to the distal esophagus. In eosinophilic esophagitis, the eosinophilia is severe (>20 eosinophils per high-power field) and can involve most of the length of the esophagus.[25,26]

If the allergic gastroenteropathy involves the small bowel, then the lesions are in a patchy distribution, ranging from areas of normal mucosa to a flat villus lesion.[27] Eosinophilic infiltration may be mild or marked. Gastric abnormalities, found more commonly in the antrum, have been described as being consistent in the mucosal form of the disease. The stomach shows evidence of gastritis, with destruction and regeneration of gastric glands and surface epithelium. Eosinophilic infiltration usually is marked.

Clinical Manifestations

Patients with eosinophilic esophagitis will have variable manifestations. Symptoms may include a feeding disorder, abdominal pain, and vomiting. Young children may have symptoms mimicking gastroesophageal reflux, but they may have normal pH probe studies and fail to respond to antireflux medications. Older children may have dysphagia for solids or food impaction. A landmark study in 1995 involved a group of children previously diagnosed as having severe reflux that was unresponsive to medical and often surgical treatment.[28] Esophageal biopsy specimens showed up to 100 eosinophils per high-power field. Allergies to multiple foods were found using a combination of prick skin tests and food challenges. The patients' symptoms resolved on an elemental diet. Follow-up biopsy specimens showed marked reduction in symptoms and esophageal eosinophils. Follow-up studies have corroborated these findings.[29,30]

The other EGIDs have symptoms that vary with the anatomic site of eosinophilia and the depth of eosinophilic infiltration. Features are listed in Box 265-3.

BOX 265-3 Features of Eosinophilic (Allergic) Gastroenteritis

MUCOSAL FORM

Nausea, vomiting, colicky abdominal pain, diarrhea
Occult blood loss, iron deficiency anemia
Protein losing enteropathy leading to hypoalbuminemia
Failure to thrive/growth

MUSCLAR (TRANSMURAL) FORM

Obstructive symptoms, mimicking pyloric stenosis or thickening of the gastric outlet

SEROSAL FORM

Eosinophilic ascites
Approximately 75% of affected patients have peripheral eosinophilia (with all 3 types)

Because EGID has no classic symptoms, it can go undetected for several years. Furthermore, whether these entities are variants of a similar disease processes or distinctly different conditions remains to be solved. Peripheral eosinophilia can be present but is inconsistent. If the mucosa of the small intestine is involved, then patients will experience malabsorption. Growth failure is a prominent feature of mucosal disease in childhood; diarrhea is often not a feature. Iron-deficiency anemia that is caused by GI blood loss is another consistent feature, together with protein-losing enteropathy. These patients frequently have evidence of systemic allergy, especially asthma.

If the stomach is involved, then patients may have evidence of delayed gastric emptying, including nausea and bloating or vomiting, a symptom suggestive of pyloric obstructive disease. Serosal disease occurs with ascites. Numerous eosinophils are present in the ascitic fluid.

Differential Diagnosis

The diagnosis of EGID is based on clinical features and laboratory findings. Endoscopy is essential to confirm a diagnosis; therefore collaboration with a pediatric gastroenterologist is necessary. A pediatric allergist can help direct specific testing for allergy.

For eosinophilic esophagitis, diagnosis is based on a typical patient or family history of allergy, an evaluation to rule out reflux, typical eosinophilic infiltration of the esophagus on the biopsy specimen, and allergy testing. Because the mechanism of allergic gastrointestinal diseases is likely on a spectrum between immediate hypersensitivity and cell-mediated immunity, the value of any single test is variable. Allergy testing can include skin prick tests, CAP-RAST tests, and patch testing. Peripheral eosinophilia occurs and an elevated IgE level is a variable finding. Their absence does not rule out eosinophilic esophagitis or the other eosinophilic gastroenteropathies. Radiographic studies, including an esophagram, may show thickened folds or a narrowing of the esophagus. On endoscopy, the mucosa may appear grossly normal, but suggestive findings are often apparent, especially the classic ringed or furrowed esophagus and white exudates (seen exclusively in eosinophilic esophagitits). Biopsy samples help quantify eosinophilic infiltration and inflammation if mucosal disease is present.

In the other EGIDs, studies can be more confusing because no consensus of histopathological criteria has been determined. A biopsy specimen of the small intestine can reveal both normal mucosa (with or without eosinophilic infiltration) and a flat villus lesion. Laboratory studies may include hypoalbuminemia and low immunoglobulin levels caused by malabsorption and protein-losing enteropathy. In the stomach a gastric antral biopsy specimen is of diagnostic value in the mucosal form of the disease and is usually positive, revealing evidence of gastritis with marked eosinophilic infiltration.[31,32] If long-term blood loss exists, then laboratory studies may show iron-deficiency anemia. Radiographic studies, including an esophagram or upper GI tract study, may show thickened folds caused by edema in the esophagus or stomach or possibly gastric outlet obstruction. A small bowel follow-through may show nodular small bowel.[33]

Management

Because allergic gastroenteropathies have variable manifestations and lapsing and remitting courses, management must be individualized with the assistance of a pediatric gastroenterologist and allergist. Unless concomitant gastroesophageal reflux exists, patients do not usually respond to histamine-2 blockers or proton-pump inhibitors. Food diaries can be confusing; for example, if the patient experiences a delayed hypersensitivity reaction, then symptoms are not apparent when foods are ingested but occur days later. However, if foods are found positive using a combination of tests for immediate or delayed hypersensitivity and food challenges, then these foods should be eliminated from the diet. The most common foods implicated are, in order, milk, egg, soy, corn, and wheat, although several foods may be found to cause symptoms. The patients also often had symptoms of asthma, allergy, or atopy or a family history of allergy and atopy. Dietary elimination of these allergens may alleviate most of the symptoms.[27] Some patients require complete dietary elimination via an L-amino acid–based formula. The advantages of dietary management are good rates of cure. However, severely restrictive diets may be difficult for children and may create social and behavioral issues. Exclusive reliance on specialized formulas can be extremely expensive.

For patients who are unable to follow a restrictive diet, corticosteroid therapy may be required intermittently. Systemic steroids have the advantages of quick improvement of symptoms and normalization of tissue on biopsy specimens. However, they cannot be used on a long-term basis, and esophageal eosinophils and symptoms can recur after discontinuing therapy. Topical steroids, such as swallowed fluticasone propionate, improve symptoms and histologic findings. Eradication of eosinophils in the esophagus was less consistent with topical therapy, and symptoms and baseline histologic values return on discontinuation. Topical treatment is associated with esophageal candidiasis. Oral cromolyn sodium (Gastrochrome) has not been proven helpful.[29] Leukotriene receptor antagonists improve symptoms, but they do not change histologic values.[34] Symptomatic strictures resulting in food impactions or severe dysphagia may require endoscopic dilatations, and pyloric obstructive disease may require surgery. If patients have other symptoms of allergy or atopy, then these should be addressed as well.

Prognosis

Although extensive follow-up studies are lacking, evidence indicates that the EGIDs are lifelong conditions with remissions and exacerbations, often requiring careful dietary manipulation and intermittent steroid therapy. Preliminary data also suggest that younger adolescents go through a phase in which they are much better able to tolerate foods to which they were previously sensitive. If the EGID produces significant malabsorption, then osteoporosis may occur.

The natural history of eosinophilic esophagitis remains unclear. Among adults with misdiagnoses of reflux who were eventually found to have eosinophilic esophagitis, some develop strictures requiring dilation. The esophagus can be friable, tearing with the mere passage of an endoscope.[35] The possible evolution to Barrett esophagus remains to be studied.

CONCLUSION

GI food allergy can be divided into 2 types: (1) that involving a specific allergen (a self-limited condition in younger patients that resolves in most by the toddler age) and (2) that characterized by eosinophilic or allergic GI disease, with multiple food sensitivities (a more permanent condition caused by a combination of immediate hypersensitivity and non-IgE mechanisms). For both these conditions, the biopsy findings can be similar during symptomatic periods and initial treatment can be dietary management.

WHEN TO REFER

- Poor weight gain
- Immediate GI response after particular food or foods
- Incomplete response to exclusion or elemental diet
- Multiple food allergies
- Multiple allergic symptoms
- Malabsorption or protein-losing enteropathy
- Gastroesophageal reflux disease recalcitrant to appropriate therapy

WHEN TO ADMIT

- Anaphylaxis
- Severe malnutrition

TOOLS FOR PRACTICE

Medical Decision Support

- *Pediatric Nutrition Handbook, 5th edition* (book), American Academy of Pediatrics (www.aap.org/bookstore).

RELATED WEB SITES

- American Academy of Allergy, Asthma, and Immunology (www.aaaai.org/professionals/resources/rgce/guidelines.asp?group=Food+Allergy).
- American Partnership for Eosinophilic Disorders (apfed.org).
- Food Allergy and Anaphylaxis Network (www.foodallergy.org).
- Kids with Food Allergies (www.kidswithfoodallergies.org/index.html).

AAP POLICY STATEMENTS

American Academy of Pediatrics, Committee on Nutrition and Section on Allergy and Immunology. Effects of early nutritional interventions on the development of atopic disease in infants and children: the role of maternal dietary restriction, breastfeeding, timing of introduction of complementary foods, and hydrolyzed formulas. *Pediatrics* 2008;121(1):183-191.

American Academy of Pediatrics, Committee on Nutrition. The use of soy protein-based formulas in infant feeding. *Pediatrics* 2008;121(5):1062-1068.

SUGGESTED RESOURCES

Assa'ad AH, Putnam PE, Collins MH, et al. Pediatric patients with eosinophilic esophagitis: an 8-year follow-up. *J Allergy Clin Immunol.* 2007;119(3):731-738.

Blanchard C, Wang N, Rothenberg ME. Eosinophilic esophagitis: pathogenesis, genetics, and therapy. *J Allergy Clin Immunol.* 2006;118(5):1054-1059.

Garcia-Carreaga M, Kerner JA. Gastrointestinal manifestations of food allergies in pediatric patients. *Nutr Clin Pract.* 2005;20:526-535.

Liacouras CA, Spergel JM, Ruchelli E, et al. Eosinophilic esophagitis: a 10-year experience in 381 children. *Clin Gastroenterol Hepatol.* 2005;3:1198-1206.

Sampson HA. Food allergy. *J Allergy Clin Immunol.* 2003; 111(2 suppl):S540-S547.

REFERENCES

1. Garcia-Carreaga M, Kerner JA. Gastrointestinal manifestations of food allergies in pediatric patients. *Nutr Clin Pract.* 2005;20:526-535.
2. Gryboski JD. Gastrointestinal milk allergy in infants. *Pediatrics.* 1967;40:354-362.
3. Sampson HA. Food allergy. *J Allergy Clin Immunol* 2003; 111(2 suppl):S540-S547.
4. Sélo I, Clément G, Bernard H, et al. Beta lactoglobulin is a major allergen. Allergy to bovine beta-lactoglobulin: specificity of human IgE to tryptic peptides. *Clin Exp Allergy.* 1999;29(8):1055-1063.
5. Katz AJ, Twaroq FJ, Zeiger RS, et al. Milk-sensitive and eosinophilic gastroenteropathy: similar clinical features with contrasting mechanisms and clinical course. *J Allergy Clin Immunol.* 1984;74:72-78.
6. Hill DJ, Hosing CS. Food allergy and atopic dermatitis in infancy: an epidemiologic study. *Pediatr Allergy Immunol.* 2004;15:421-427.
7. Iacono G, Cavataio F, Montalto G, et al. Persistent cow's milk protein intolerance in infants: the changing faces of the same disease. *Clin Exp Allergy.* 1998;28(7):817-823.
8. Kuitenen P, Visakorpi JK, Savilahti E, et al. Malabsorption syndrome with cow's milk intolerance. *Arch Dis Child.* 1975;50:351-356.
9. Nowak-Wegrzyn, Sampson HA, Wood RA, et al. Food protein enterocolitis syndrome caused by solid food proteins. *Pediatrics.* 2003;111:829-835.
10. Bishop JM, Hill DJ, Hosking CS. Natural history of cow milk allergy: clinical outcome. *J Pediatr.* 1990;116(6): 862-867.
11. Host A, Jacobson HP, Halken S, et al. The natural history of cow's milk protein allergy/intolerance. *Eur J Clin Nutr.* 1995;49(S1):S13-S18.
12. Wood RA. The natural history of food allergy. *Pediatrics.* 2003;111(6 pt 3):1631-1637.
13. Ament ME, Rubin CE. Soy protein: another cause of the flat intestinal lesion, *Gastroenterology.* 1972;62:227-234.
14. Xanthakos SA, Schwimmer JB, Melin-Aldana H, et al. Prevalence and outcome of allergic colitis in healthy infants with rectal bleeding: a prospective cohort study. *J Pediatr Gastroenterol Nutr.* 2005;41(1):16-22.
15. Machida HM, Catto Smith AG, Gall DG, et al. Allergic colitis in infancy: clinical and pathologic aspects. *J Pediatr Gastroenterol Nutr.* 1994;19:22-26.
16. American Academy of Pediatrics, Committee on Nutrition and Section on Allergy and Immunology. Effects of early nutritional interventions on the development of atopic disease in infants and children: the role of maternal dietary restriction, breast feeding, timing of introduction of complimentary foods, and hydrolyzed formulas. *Pediatrics.* 2008;121:1062-1068.
17. Lake AM. Beyond hydrolysates: use of L-amino acid formula in resistant dietary protein-induced intestinal disease in infants. *J Pediatr.* 1997;131:658-660.
18. Vanderhoof JA, Murray ND, Kaufman SS, et al. Intolerance to protein hydrolysate infant formulas: an underrecognized cause of gastrointestinal symptoms in infants. *J Pediatr.* 1997;131:741-744.
19. Waldmann TA, Wochner RD, Laster L, et al. Allergic gastroenteropathy. *N Engl J Med.* 1967;276:762-769.
20. Noel R, Putnam PE, Rothenberg ME. Eosinophilic esophagitis (correspondence). *N Engl J Med.* 2004;351(9): 940-941.
21. Mishra A, Hogan SP, Brandt EB, et al. An etiological role for aeroallergens and eosinophils in experimental esophagitis. *J Clin Invest.* 2001;107:83-90.
22. Onbasi K, Sin AZ, Doganavsargil B, et al. Eosinophil infiltration of the esophageal mucosa in patients with pollen allergy during the season. *Clin Exp Allergy.* 2005;35: 1423-1431.
23. Akei HS, Mishra A, Blanchard C, et al. Epicutaneous antigen exposure primes for experimental eosinophilic esophagitis in mice. *Gastroenterology.* 2005;129:985-994.
24. Winter HS, Madera JL, Stafford RJ, et al. Intraepithelial eosinophils: a new diagnostic criterion for reflux esophagitis. *Gastroenterology.* 1982;83(4):812-823.
25. Ruchelli E, Wenner W, Voytek T, et al. Severity of esophageal eosinophilia predicts response to conventional gastroesophageal reflux therapy. *Pediatr Develop Pathol.* 1999;2:15-18.
26. Sant'Anna AM, Rolland S, Fournet JC, et al. Eosinophilic esophagitis in children: symptoms, histology and pH probe results. *J Pediatr Gastroenterol Nutr.* 2004;39(4): 373-377.
27. Leinbach GE, Rubin CE. Eosinophilic gastroenteritis: a simple reaction to food allergens? *Gastroenterology.* 1970;59:874-889.
28. Kelly KJ, Lazenby AJ, Row PC, et al. Eosinophilic esophagitis attributed to gastroesophageal reflux: improvement with an amino acid-based formula. *Gastroenterology.* 1995;109:1503-1512.
29. Liacouras CA, Spergel JM, Ruchelli E, et al. Eosinophilic esophagitis: a 10-year experience in 381 children. *Clin Gastroenterol Hepatol.* 2005;3:1198-1206.
30. Markowitz JE, Spergel JM, Ruchelli E, et al. Elemental diet is an effective treatment for eosinophilic esophagitis in children and adolescents. *Am J Gastroenterol.* 2003;98: 777-782.
31. Katz AJ, Goldman H, Grand RJ. Gastric mucosal biopsy in eosinophilic (allergic) gastroenteritis. *Gastroenterology.* 1977;73:705-709.
32. Lake AM. The polymorph in red is no lady. *J Pediatr Gastroenterol Nutr.* 1994;19:4-6.
33. Vitellas KM, Bennett WF, Bova JG, et al. Radiographic manifestations of eosinophilic gastroenteritis. *Abdom Imaging.* 1995;20(5):406-413.
34. Attwood SE, Lewis CJ, Bronder CS, et al. Eosinophilic oesophagitis: a novel treatment using Montelukast. *Gut.* 2003;52(2):181-185.
35. Kaplan M, Mutlu EA, Jakate S, et al. Endoscopy in eosinophilic esophagitis: "feline" esophagus and perforation risk. *Clin Gastroenterol Hepatol.* 2003;1(6):433-437.

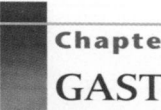

Chapter 266

GASTROINTESTINAL OBSTRUCTION

Louisa Chiu, MD; David L. Dudgeon, MD; Anthony Stallion, MD

Gastrointestinal obstruction (GIO) during infancy, childhood, and adolescence is relatively uncommon but often presents a diagnostic challenge (Table 266-1). Obstructions that occur distal to the pylorus are potential surgical emergencies, and the younger the patient is, the more ominous the probable cause is and the more urgent the required therapy will be.[1] Therefore the pediatrician must be continually alert for a GIO to facilitate early diagnosis and thus prevent tragedy.

EVALUATION

History

The symptoms and signs of a GIO (Table 266-2, Figure 266-1) vary considerably but involve the following, either singly or in combination: vomiting (often bilious), abdominal pain, abdominal distention (see Chapter 158, Abdominal Distention), change in bowel habits, fever, abdominal tenderness, or a palpable abdominal mass. The presence or absence of each of the key symptoms and signs, along with patient age, are important clues to etiology.

Vomiting

Vomiting is a ubiquitous symptom, the cause of which is most often not GIO. However, vomiting can be a sign of obstruction, particularly when marked by certain characteristics.

A small amount of nonbilious, nonprojectile vomitus by an infant is unlikely to indicate a GIO; it commonly denotes a benign, self-limited form of regurgitation or gastroesophageal reflux (chalazia). Gastroesophageal reflux can be ruled out in the majority of cases by commonly accepted diagnostic tests such as a 24-hour pH probe study or a nuclear medicine milk reflux scan.[2] However, nonbilious, nonprojectile vomitus in the newborn can also be associated with an esophageal obstruction (atresia).[3] The neonate may have copious, frothy bubbles of mucus that cause rattling respirations, coughing, choking, and cyanosis.[4,5] Respiratory distress caused by tracheal aspiration of saliva retained in the upper esophagus or aspiration through the commonly associated tracheoesophageal fistula proximal or distal to the atresia can be associated with this anomaly.[3] An esophageal block encountered during attempts to pass an 8- or 10-French transoral soft catheter approximately 17 cm into the stomach denotes esophageal atresia.[4]

Esophageal atresia and the rare entity of pediatric gastric volvulus are the two most likely neonatal conditions in which a congenital or early-acquired esophageal obstruction is likely to be encountered. Acute gastric volvulus, unlike esophageal atresia, is often accompanied by severe pain and can be associated with signs of shock, chest pain, dysphagia, dyspepsia, and acute respiratory distress.[6] Nonbilious vomiting can also be produced by the rare anomaly of a complete or incomplete gastric antral web.[7] Frequently, this diagnosis is a delayed one that occurs in late infancy and is associated with failure to thrive.

The more dramatic projectile, nonbilious vomiting of early infancy is associated with the semiurgent medical condition of dehydration and electrolyte disturbances as a result of congenital hypertrophic pyloric stenosis.[8] The electrolyte abnormalities are typically a hyponatremic, hypochloremic, hypokalemic contraction metabolic alkalosis with a possible late paradoxical aciduria.[9] (See Chapter 315, Pyloric Stenosis.)

Bilious vomiting, usually nonprojectile, is a more ominous problem and denotes GIO below the level of the ampulla of Vater. Concern arises because of the possibility of intestinal malrotation with a complicating midgut volvulus, which can produce GIO with ischemia and subsequent bowel necrosis within a few hours.[10-13] Although a premature infant who has an immature pyloric sphincter can have bilious regurgitation without obstruction, especially when it is associated with an ileus related to an underlying septic process, the threat of intestinal vascular compromise caused by an underlying volvulus requires immediate radiologic examination for diagnosis. Clinical signs of peritonitis preclude radiologic study for diagnosis, and an immediate exploratory laparotomy is necessary. Usually an upper gastrointestinal (GI) radiographic series is the diagnostic study of choice in less ill neonates, although the diagnosis may also be made by ultrasound.[14] Other causes of bilious vomiting in the neonate and infant include duodenal, jejunal, and ileal atresias; duodenal stenosis caused by an annular pancreas or Ladd bands (colonic peritoneal bands crossing the duodenum) associated with malrotation; meconium ileus; colonic atresia; congenital aganglionosis of the colon (Hirschsprung disease); and imperforate anus.[15-18]

An infant or older toddler who has bilious vomiting can have a GIO produced by an incarcerated hernia, intussusception, or previously unrecognized malrotation with associated volvulus.[19] The cause of bilious vomiting in an adolescent can include incarcerated hernias, postoperative adhesions, meconium ileus equivalent associated with cystic fibrosis, acute inflammation (appendicitis and pelvic inflammatory disease), and chronic inflammation (regional ileitis or ulcerative colitis).[20-22] At this age, malrotation is less likely. In less developed countries, masses of worms, especially *Ascaris lumbricoides*, and tuberculosis also can be a cause of obstruction.[23] A significant number of all patients who have persistent bilious emesis will have an underlying pathological abnormality requiring early diagnosis and definitive surgical treatment.

Vomitus containing small amounts of blood may be observed in infants who have congenital hypertrophic pyloric stenosis caused by gastric irritation as a result of repeated emesis.[8] In rare cases, hematemesis with larger amounts of blood is associated with GIO, as in the uncommon occurrence of an acute peptic ulcer, resulting in obstruction in a newborn or, more frequently, in an older, chronically stressed infant or

Table 266-1 Summary of Pediatric Gastrointestinal Obstruction and Surgical Intervention

DISEASE	FREQUENCY	AGE	SURGICAL TREATMENT	COMPLICATIONS	PROGNOSIS
Esophageal atresia	1/3000-1/5000	Neonates	Division of fistula, anastomosis of esophageal ends ± gastrostomy	Aspiration, leak, GERD, strictures	Associated with cardiovascular abnormalities, imperforate anus, duodenal obstruction, malrotation. If no cardiac anomaly, >95% survival.
Gastric volvulus	Rare	Any	Gastropexy and gastrostomy tube ± resection	Sepsis, leak	If no necrosis—good; with necrosis—high mortality
Antral web	Rare	Infants	Divide web modified pyloroplasty, gastrostomy	Leak	Good
Hypertrophic pyloric stenosis	1/250	Neonates, infants	Pyloromyotomy	Incomplete, mucosal leak	Good
Volvulus	1/500	Infants, but 20% >1 year of age	Detorsion of mesentery, divide Ladd bands, intestinal resection	Leak, sepsis, short-gut syndrome	If no necrosis—good; with necrosis—guarded
Intestinal atresia	1/2700	Neonates	Resection and anastomosis	Strictures, leak, poor gut motility	50% associated with other anomalies
Meconium ileus	1/2800	Neonates	Enema, intestinal cleansing through enterotomy, possible resection	Sepsis, malnutrition	Associated with cystic fibrosis immediately after surgery—good; long-term—poor
Hirschsprung disease	1/4000	Neonates	Colostomy, delayed pull-through procedure	Sepsis, incontinence	Good
Imperforate anus	1/4000	Neonates	Colostomy, delayed pull-through procedure	Sepsis, incontinence	High defects—guarded; low defects—good
Incarcerated hernia	1/1000	<1 year of age	Reduction, possible intestinal resection	Sepsis	Good to guarded
Intussusception	1/1000	3 mo-3 yr	Air-enema reduction ± resection	Ischemic bowel, leak, recurrence	May have pathological cause in older kids; good if no necrosis, with necrosis, potential short-gut syndrome
Duplication cyst	Rare	Any	Complete excision and anastomosis	Bile duct injury	Possible late malignant transformation
Meconium plug	1/500-1/1000	Neonates	Rectal stimulation, enema	Leak, acute dehydration, shock	Associated with CF, small left colon, rectal aganglionosis
Obstipation of prematurity	—	Neonates	Colostomy for severe cases	Sepsis	Good

CF, Cystic fibrosis; *GERD*, gastroesophageal reflux disease.

Table 266-2 Clinical Findings for Pediatric Gastrointestinal Obstruction

CAUSE	FINDINGS						
	VOMITING	PAIN	STOOL PATTERN	DISTENTION	BOWEL SOUNDS	TENDERNESS	MASSES
Esophageal atresia	Nonbilious (saliva)	No	Normal meconium	No	Absent to normal	No	No
Gastric obstruction	Nonbilious (curdled formula)	Severe with gastric volvulus; none with antral web	Normal meconium	Epigastric	Absent to normal	Severe with volvulus	No
Hypertrophic pyloric stenosis	Nonbilious, projectile	No	Constipation (dehydration)	Epigastric	Hyperactive (epigastric)	No	Yes (olive-size mass)
Duodenal obstruction	Bilious	Minimal	Small meconium stool	Epigastric	Absent to normal	No	No
Volvulus	Bilious	Severe	Hematochezia	Epigastric to generalized	Hyperactive	Yes (severe)	No
Jejunoileal atresia	Bilious	No	Small, hard, light-colored meconium stool	Generalized	Variable	No	No
Intussusception	Bilious	Yes (crampy)	Currant jelly stool	Generalized	Hyperactive	Yes	Yes (sausage shaped)
Meconium ileus	Bilious	No	Obstipation	Generalized	Variable	No	Yes (doughy beads)
Meconium plug	Bilious	No	Obstipation	Generalized	Variable	No	No
Congenital aganglionosis	Bilious	No	Obstipation, constipation, and intermittent diarrhea	Generalized	Hyperactive	No	Palpable stool
Obstipation of prematurity	Bilious	No	Obstipation	Generalized	Hyperactive	No	No
Incarcerated inguinal hernia	Bilious	Yes	Diarrhea or constipation	Generalized	Hyperactive	Yes	Inguinal or scrotal
Imperforate anus	Bilious	No	Obstipation	Generalized	Hyperactive	No	No

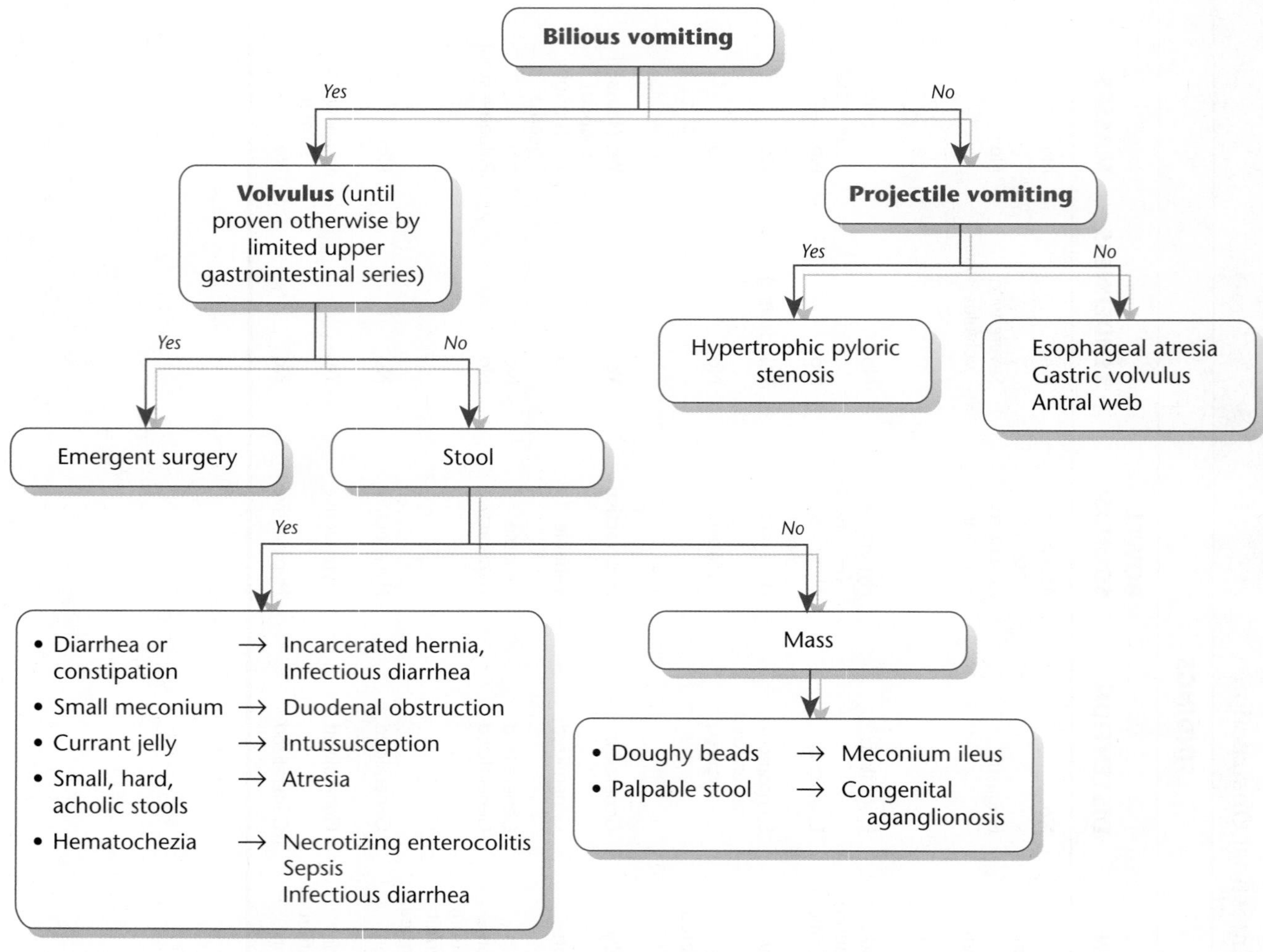

Figure 266-1 Clinical findings in pediatric gastrointestinal obstruction.

child. Infection with *Helicobacter pylori* is also a potential cause of peptic ulcer disease in children, again more so in developing countries.[24]

Abdominal Pain

Abdominal pain, which may cause inconsolable crying or irritability in an infant, usually accompanies GIO. The pain is likely to be crampy or intermittent, and it results in crying and flexion of the legs to the abdomen interspersed with periods of decreased levels or absence of distress. This sign is exemplified best by the toddler who has an intussusception.[19] However, approximately 10% of children who have intussusception will have lethargy as their only symptom.[25] A complete or partial obstruction of the intestine produces acute intermittent abdominal pain, which in a matter of hours becomes constant and is caused by intestinal distention, peritoneal inflammation, or both. Bowel wall edema ensues, increasing the degree of obstruction and causing a progression of changes that place the intussuscepted intestine at further risk for ischemic damage.

Stool

Obstipation in a newborn is an important finding. Full-term, healthy infants spontaneously pass meconium within the first 24 hours of life. With premature infants, those who are small for gestational age, and infants of mothers with diabetes, a delay of up to 72 hours may occur before the initial stool is passed.[26,27] The initial bowel movement may also be delayed if pregnancy is complicated by maternal drug abuse (narcotics such as morphine), drug therapy (eg, magnesium sulfate for toxemia), or neonatal stress (hypoxemia or sepsis).[28]

Atresias of the proximal portion of the intestinal tract do not usually cause obstipation except for those involving the most distal terminal ileum; however, the meconium passed by these infants is usually sparse and lighter in color, and it may be hard and dry. The differential diagnosis of newborn obstipation includes congenital aganglionosis of the colon, meconium ileus (with underlying cystic fibrosis), meconium plug syndrome (30% of these are associated with congenital aganglionosis of the colon or cystic fibrosis), small left colon syndrome, colonic atresia, imperforate anus, and, in rare cases, rectal atresia.[29,30]

Strictures that occur as a result of episodes of neonatal necrotizing enterocolitis or intestinal surgery, as well as extrinsic compression of the GI tract caused by congenital cysts, intestinal duplication, inflammatory masses, or malignancies, produce obstipation or constipation in an older infant or child.[31-33]

Particularly in neonates and infants, diarrhea or alternating diarrhea and constipation can occur as a sign of functional GIO or as a partial or intermittent GIO. Congenital colonic aganglionosis, intussusception, or intermittent volvulus may also be causes. The latter two conditions frequently occur along with hematochezia or melena.

Hematochezia, or grossly bloody stools, in association with GIO symptoms, indicates intestinal vascular compromise. It occurs most commonly in patients who have an intussusception or volvulus.[11,19] The so-called *currant jelly stools* of intussusception result from the admixture of blood and mucus and are a sign of superficial mucosal sloughing, but they can also accompany a full-thickness necrosis of the bowel wall. Occasionally, darker (mahogany to black), melena-type stools resulting from a more proximal intestinal bleeding site are noted, with the same potentially dire causes. In infants without grossly bloody stools, occult blood is present in up to 75% of intussusception cases. Thus a hemoccult test should be performed in all infants with altered mental status.[13]

Physical Examination

With a history of vomiting, an infant first needs to be evaluated for signs of dehydration. Inspection of the anterior fontanelle, rate and intensity of distal pulses, level of consciousness, perfusion of the extremities, and condition of the mucous membranes can aid in determining hydration status.[13] When GIO is suspected, the physical examination of the abdomen includes evaluation for distention, which is likely to be prominent if the obstruction is distal to the duodenum (see Table 266-2 and Figure 266-1). Gastric obstruction caused by a congenital antral web, hypertrophic pyloric stenosis, or duodenal atresia produces only mild to moderate epigastric distention; distal intestinal atresias or other forms of lower GIO produce generalized distention. The presence or absence of abdominal distention does not aid in the diagnosis of a potential underlying midgut volvulus because the obstruction may be at the level of the duodenum, with few air- and fluid-distended bowel loops present.

Abdominal auscultation should be performed before any other aspect of abdominal examination. An effort should be made to listen to all the abdominal quadrants. High-pitched, *tinkling* bowel sounds heard in rushes are diagnostic of a complete GIO. However, bowel sounds are often normal early, only becoming diminished or absent late in obstruction.

If the abdomen is moderately to grossly distended, then a mild amount of tenderness or discomfort with palpation is to be expected because pressure applied to gas- or fluid-filled loops of bowel causes pain. However, marked tenderness clearly indicates an accompanying peritoneal inflammation. This inflammation (or peritonitis) in the setting of GIO indicates ischemia of the bowel wall with possible necrosis and demands immediate surgical evaluation and treatment. In this situation, diagnostic radiologic studies that use contrast material are contraindicated.

The presence of multiple *doughy*, compressible, mobile, nontender abdominal masses in a newborn who has GIO is associated with meconium ileus.[34] On the other hand, a tender, palpable, immobile mass is most likely an area of cellulitis or abscess related to visceral perforation and is the result of necrotizing enterocolitis in infants or appendicitis or inflammatory bowel disease in children and adolescents. A nontender, mobile mass that produces GIO symptoms is found with congenital intestinal duplication cysts or mesenteric cysts. A sausage-like mass in the right upper quadrant with absence of bowel in the right lower quadrant is pathognomonic of intussusception and is called the *Dance sign*.[13] Malignancies in the intestinal tract are rare and do not usually produce intestinal obstruction, but lymphomas may do so in older patients. When they cause GIO, intestinal or mesenteric lymphomas in patients older than 4 years commonly present as an intussusception. An immunocompromised host who has a malignancy or AIDS may develop primary or secondary inflammatory lesions that lead to obstruction.[35]

An incarcerated inguinal hernia is an important cause of GIO in children and adolescents. Detecting an inguinal hernia in an uncooperative, chubby infant is difficult and requires considerable patience and effort. Sedation with a tranquilizer, with or without an added narcotic analgesic, while keeping the patient supine in the mild Trendelenburg position and applying an ice pack to the inguinal region may be helpful in the reduction of an incarcerated hernia. Medications must be used cautiously to prevent excessive sedation because vomiting and aspiration can occur. If possible, the hernia should be reduced gently and repaired later, when the effects of the GIO and local edema have subsided. If the hernia is reduced but left unrepaired, then recurrent incarcerations are likely, with the potential consequences of strangulation and necrosis of the bowel.

A rectal examination can often clarify the cause of GIO. In an infant who is suspected of having an incarcerated inguinal hernia, the clinician can often palpate the peritoneal side of the internal inguinal ring transanally and identify an exiting intraperitoneal structure. The rectal examination can be equally important in the diagnosis of any suspected colonic or distal GIO. Previously unsuspected perirectal or presacral pelvic masses (eg, hydrometrocolpos, appendiceal inflammatory mass, presacral teratoma) can be identified in this manner. Abnormal stool (as in the patient who has meconium plug syndrome) or blood (associated with intussusception or inflammatory bowel disease) can be detected during a rectal examination. In rare cases, an intraluminal rectal mass can be palpated, such as with a low-lying intussusception.

Imaging Studies

When deciding which radiologic tests to order, the physician must recall that estimated radiation exposure during the first 10 years of life poses a lifetime

Table 266-3 Roentgenographic Findings for Common Causes of Pediatric Gastrointestinal Obstruction

	FINDING				
CAUSE	DILATED AREA	AIR OR FLUID LEVELS	CALCIUM DEPOSITS	NONCALCIUM OPACITIES	FURTHER STUDIES THAT MAY BE INDICATED
Esophageal atresia	Esophagus and stomach	Yes (gastric)	No	No	Esophageal air instillation
Gastric obstruction	Stomach	Yes	No	No	Gastric barium instillation*
Hypertrophic pyloric stenosis	Stomach	Yes	No	No	Ultrasonography
Duodenal obstruction	Stomach, duodenum (double bubble)	Yes	No	No	None
Volvulus	Variable	Variable	No	No	Upper GI series or barium enema
Jejunoileal atresia	Stomach and small intestine	Yes	Yes (with prenatal perforation)	No	Barium enema to rule out nonrotation
Intussusception	Stomach and small intestine	Variable	No	Yes (soft-tissue densities)	Ultrasonography, barium/air enema†, or both
Meconium ileus	Stomach and small intestine	No	Yes (meconium peritonitis)	Yes (ground-glass appearance)	Water-soluble contrast enema‡
Meconium plug	Stomach to colon	Yes	No	No	Water-soluble contrast enema
Congenital aganglionosis	Stomach to colon	Yes	No	No	Barium enema
Obstipation of prematurity (short left colon syndrome)	Stomach to colon	Yes	No	No	Barium enema
Incarcerated inguinal hernia	Stomach and small intestine	Yes	No	No	None
Imperforate anus	Stomach to colon	Yes	No	No	Complete evaluation of genitourinary tract

*Should be performed cautiously to avoid aspiration.
†Should be performed cautiously to avoid bowel perforation.
‡May be therapeutic and diagnostic.

risk 3 to 4 times greater than exposure between the ages of 30 and 40 years.[5] With the widespread use of prenatal ultrasound, GIO may be diagnosed before the birth of the child. In up to 40% of cases, findings such as polyhydramnios, an inability to identify the stomach, cystic abdominal lesions, and dilated loops of bowel strongly suggest the presence of an obstructive intestinal lesion.[36] The prenatal diagnosis of GIO (ie, atresia, volvulus) alleviates the need for an emergent postnatal work-up.

Table 266-3 and Figure 266-2 list radiographic diagnostic studies required for a patient who has GIO and their expected findings; these studies are dictated by the results of the history and physical examination. A plain-film radiograph of the abdomen should be obtained for all patients suspected of having GIO. Chest radiography can demonstrate the curling of a nasogastric tube or dilated pouch in esophageal atresia (Figure 266-3). In a newborn, air localized to the stomach and duodenum (double-bubble sign) is diagnostic of a duodenal obstruction[18] (Figure 266-4). If no distal intestinal intraluminal air is seen, then the GIO is usually caused by an atresia; however, if even a small amount of air is found distally, then the diagnosis of a malrotation with possible volvulus must be suspected. Use of an upper GI series to determine the relationship among the duodenum, the jejunum, and the ligament of Treitz, or a barium enema to ascertain cecal position is necessary to rule out a malrotation or nonrotation of the intestine.[11] The presence of even a large number of air-filled loops on the plain-film radiographic study of the abdomen does not eliminate the need for a contrast study because a volvulus still is possible. In a patient with volvulus, contrast study may show a corkscrew appearance projecting forward, away from the posterior abdominal wall; and color

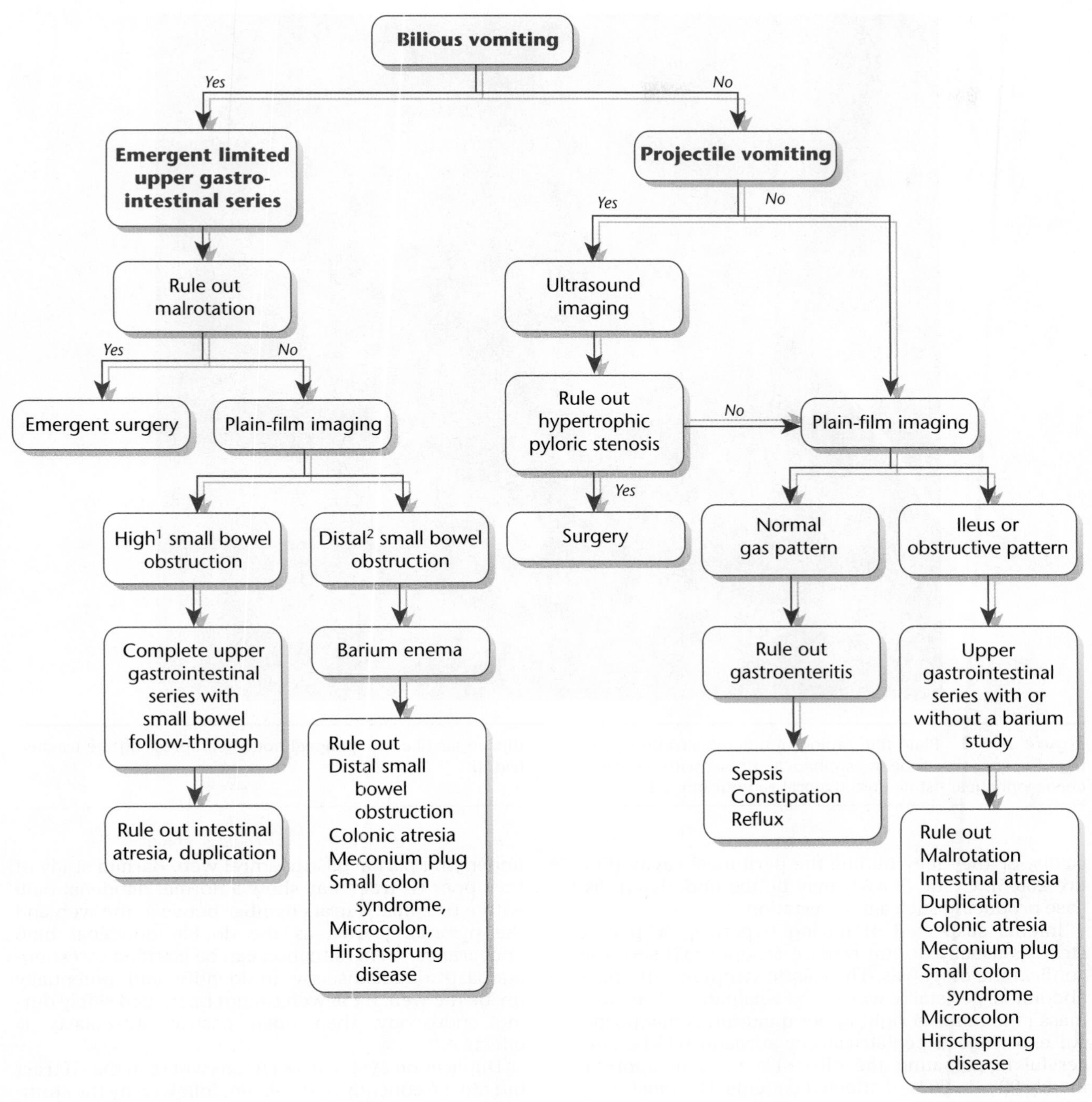

Figure 266-2 Diagnostic work-up for pediatric gastrointestinal obstruction.

Doppler ultrasound may show a distorted relationship of the superior mesenteric vessels.[37] Visualization by barium enema of an *unused,* small-caliber distal colon (microcolon) in a normal position makes the diagnosis of intestinal atresia or meconium ileus more likely than acute volvulus.

Calcifications visualized by an abdominal radiograph in a neonate with suspected GIO are evidence of an intrauterine intestinal perforation (meconium peritonitis), which is often associated with intestinal atresia. The calcifications may be small, single, or multiple and scattered throughout the entire peritoneal

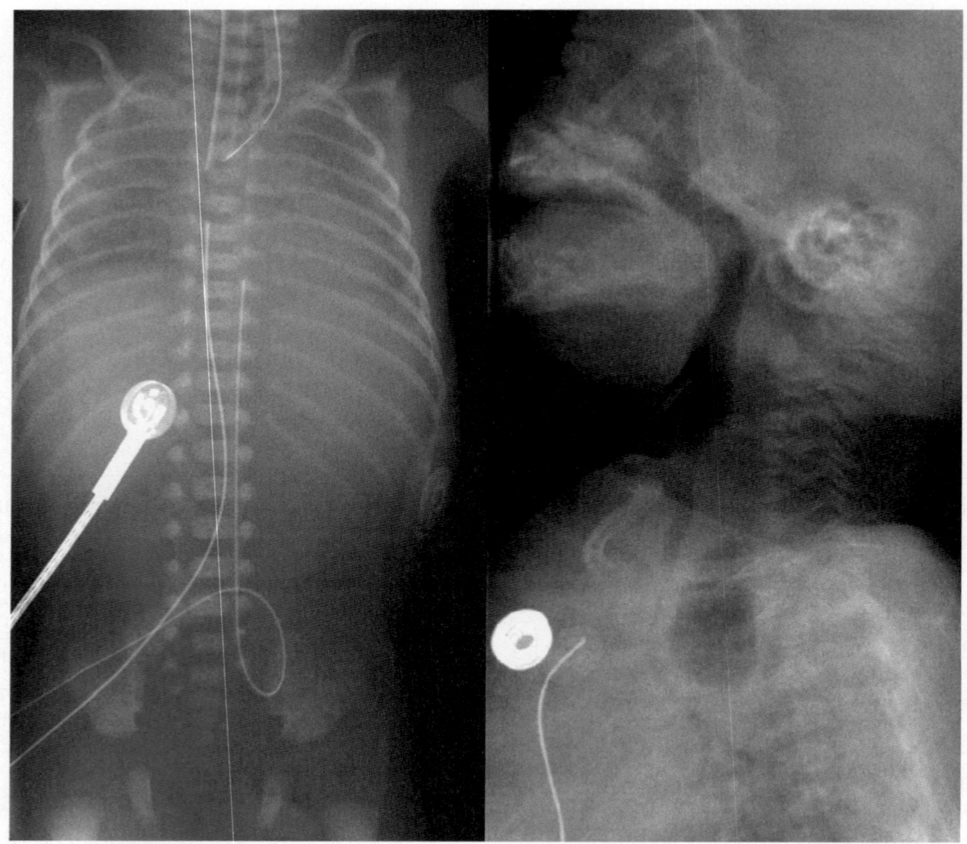

Figure 266-3 Plain-film radiograph demonstrating curling of nasogastric tube in esophageal atresia without tracheoesophageal fistula (left). Lateral radiograph with dilated air-filled esophageal pouch compressing the trachea (right).

cavity, or they may outline the peritoneal cavity (Figure 266-5). Cystic fibrosis may be the underlying disease producing such a manifestation.

Infants suspected of having hypertrophic pyloric stenosis usually do not require an upper GI series to confirm the diagnosis. The classic symptoms of upper abdominal peristaltic waves and a palpable, olive-sized mass in the mid to right upper quadrant is diagnostic. An experienced pediatrician or surgeon will be successful in palpating the olive-size mass in approximately 80% to 90% of affected patients. Diagnosis may be aided by the physical findings of a hypoplastic inferior labial frenulum or, in the near future, an abnormal mucosal reflectance of the oral mucosa.[38] An abdominal ultrasound scan can aid diagnosis in cases in which the pyloric stenosis is suspected but no palpable mass exists.[39,40] Radiographic confirmation is needless, costly, and potentially hazardous because residual barium may remain in the dilated, obstructed stomach at the time of induction of anesthesia (see Chapter 315, Pyloric Stenosis).

An unusual presentation, with nonbilious vomiting and no clinically palpable olive-size mass, a normal abdominal ultrasound examination, and a normal upper GI contrast study, is possible. This sequence of events may lead to a long delay in diagnosing an underlying partial gastric antral web. Barium study of the upper GI tract may show a normal duodenal bulb with a proximal antral chamber between the web and the pylorus, known as the double duodenal bulb appearance.[41] This situation can be clarified by esophagogastroduodenoscopy to identify and potentially divide the web. If the web cannot be treated safely during endoscopy, then open gastric antroplasty is effective.[7]

Duplication cysts can occur anywhere in the GI tract but most frequently in the ileum, followed by the stomach. Ultrasound is the most useful radiologic modality to diagnose enteric duplication cysts. The *rim* sign is composed of an echogenic inner rim of mucosa and hypoechoic outer rim of the muscle layer.[42] Peristalsis of the cyst wall and septations also aid in the diagnosis of duplication cysts.

An abdominal radiograph of GIO in association with suspected cystic fibrosis (meconium ileus) often has a peculiar hazy pattern described as a *ground glass* or *soap bubble* appearance (Figure 266-6). Gas may be absent in the right iliac fossa because of a meconium cyst.[2] This pattern is caused by the abnormal meconium mixed with air that is inspissated in the bowel lumen. Occasionally, this hard, dense stool, palpable as multiple abdominal masses, appears on the

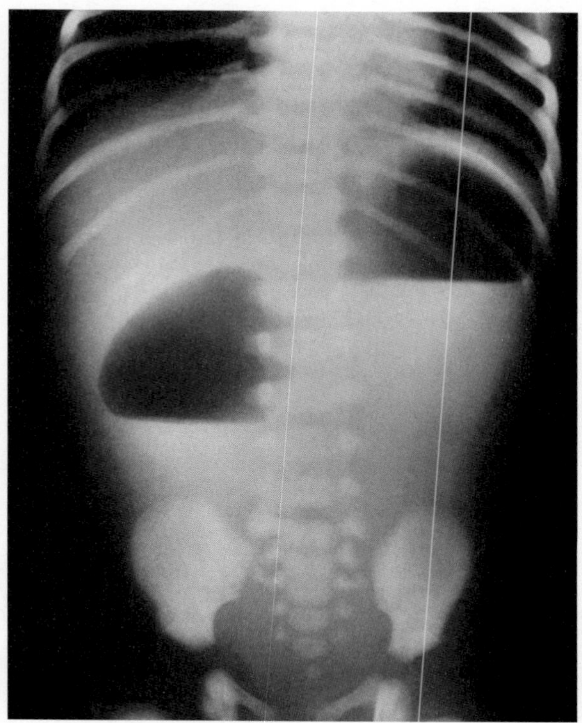

Figure 266-4 Duodenal atresia. An upright radiograph of a 4-day-old girl with persistent vomiting since birth. The double-bubble sign is classic, showing the large gastric fluid-filled air bubble on the right and the similar duodenal bubble on the left. *(From Micro X-ray Recorder, Inc, Chicago, IL.)*

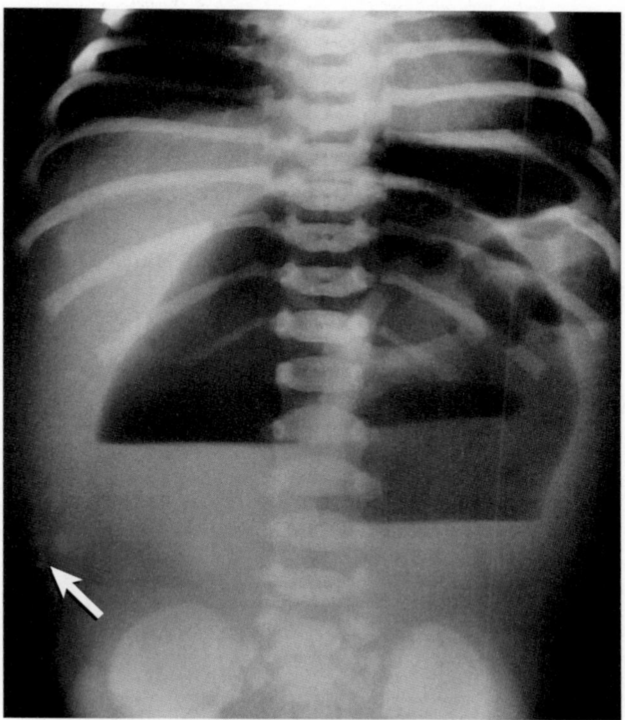

Figure 266-5 Ileal atresia with meconium peritonitis. An upright radiograph of a 36-hour-old girl with persistent vomiting since birth. The numerous dilated loops of small bowel with fluid levels indicate atresia of the ileum; the calcification *(arrow)* is diagnostic of meconium peritonitis caused by prenatal rupture of the small bowel. *(From Micro X-ray Recorder, Inc, Chicago, IL.)*

radiograph as a chain of radiolucencies, known as the *string of beads* sign.[29,34] Meconium ileus, as with ileal atresia, is associated with a complete GIO; however, air-fluid levels are rare in meconium ileus. Meconium ileus and meconium plug syndrome are two neonatal GIO conditions that can be diagnosed and frequently can be treated with a water-soluble contrast enema.

A neonate who is suspected of having meconium ileus, who has no evidence of perforation, and who is well hydrated can be given a water-soluble contrast enema cautiously by an experienced radiologist. This procedure identifies the inspissated meconium, localized to the distal ileum, and may free it from the bowel wall for spontaneous expulsion. This technique is limited in application and duration, with subsequent surgical therapy required in as many as 50% of patients treated in this way. Uncomplicated meconium plug syndrome—a lower GIO lesion infrequently associated with cystic fibrosis but occasionally associated with congenital aganglionosis—is also diagnosed and treated successfully with a barium enema.[29,43] Unlike meconium ileus, the abnormal meconium in meconium plug syndrome is localized to the distal colon. Contrast enemas in either syndrome are contraindicated when evidence exists of intestinal vascular compromise or perforation such as peritonitis, free intraperitoneal air, or intraperitoneal calcification. With meconium peritonitis, sonography may show ascites with echogenic debris, abnormal cystic masses, and thickening and dilatation of the bowel wall.[23]

Older infants and toddlers suspected of having GIO produced by intussusception can be diagnosed and often treated successfully with a barium enema.[19] The importance of an experienced radiologist for this maneuver cannot be overemphasized. The study is performed with a limited pressure (3 feet) barium column. The intussusception is slowly reduced by the hydrostatic pressure generated. Because of the potential hazard of a barium perforation, the study should always be performed with a surgical team standing by. The procedure, which can be used in approximately 75% of patients, successfully reduces the intussusception in 85% to 90% of these cases.[19,44] Surgical reduction is required in cases that are unable to be reduced radiologically. Some experts have advocated the use of laparoscopy to aid in this hydrostatic reduction.[45,46] The diagnosis can also be made effectively by ultrasound or computed tomography.[47-49] Both tests are useful in a patient whose examination is unremarkable and whose history is equivocal.

More recently, air enema reduction of the intussusception has become available. This technique consists of air insufflation of the rectum and colon by using an in-line pressure-limiting valve while maintaining fluoroscopic or sonographic observation to ensure that

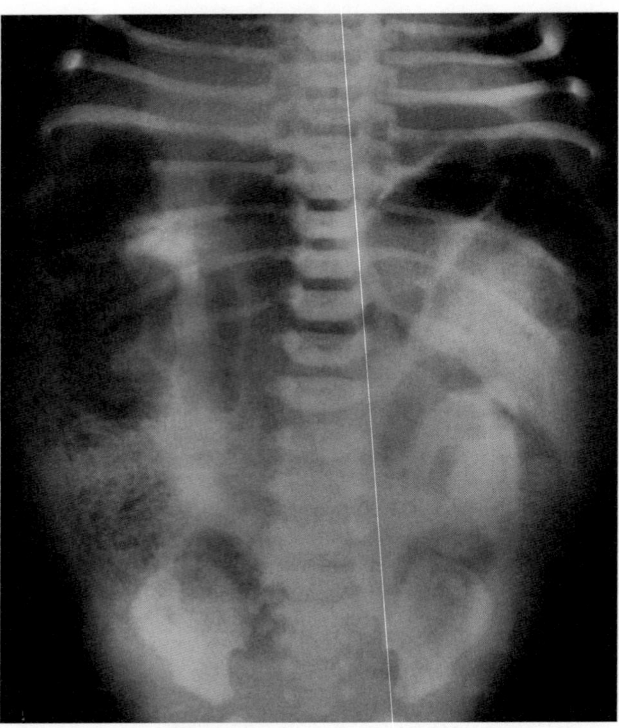

Figure 266-6 Meconium ileus. An upright radiograph of a 2-day-old boy with abdominal distention since birth. The loops of distended bowel of varying size without fluid levels are filled with meconium shadows (radiolucent soap bubbles). *(From Micro X-ray Recorder, Inc, Chicago, IL.)*

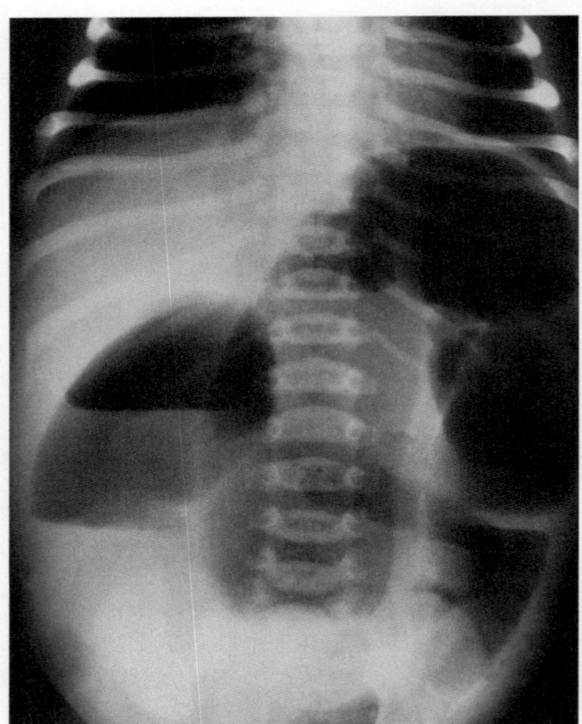

Figure 266-7 Aganglionic megacolon (Hirschsprung disease). An upright radiograph of a 2-day-old boy with distended abdomen and who failed to pass anything rectally shows extreme distention of the colon with several fluid levels. *(From Micro X-ray Recorder, Inc, Chicago, IL.)*

the reduction is under control. The advantages of this technique are, first, elimination of barium, with the threat of severe chemical peritonitis if a perforation inadvertently occurs, and second, possibly an improved mechanical advantage by using air reduction.[50-52] Investigators have stated that repeated attempts at pneumatic reduction improve the success rate without adverse outcome.[53] The patient always should be observed for 12 to 24 hours in the hospital after successful intussusception reduction.

Congenital aganglionosis of the colon (Figure 266-7), or Hirschsprung disease, in infancy can be lethal if complicated by enterocolitis. Hirschsprung disease seldom produces total GIO, which, when present, must be treated as an emergency. The initial diagnosis is made based on clinical suspicion because it cannot be verified by noninvasive diagnostic procedures. A barium enema or anorectal manometry reflecting an absent rectosphincteric reflex is often helpful in diagnosing Hirschsprung disease in older children, but either a rectal mucosal or full-thickness rectal wall biopsy specimen is required to confirm the diagnosis in infants.[30]

Colonic dysfunction of prematurity, or *small left colon syndrome* (SLCS), produces a functional mechanical obstruction that mimics Hirschsprung disease. SLCS can be related to extreme prematurity, maternal diabetes, prenatal maternal medications for eclampsia (magnesium sulfate), hypothyroidism, or maternal narcotic use. SLCS is a diagnosis of exclusion because its barium contrast appearance resembles Hirschsprung disease. Surgically, a temporary colostomy is indicated only for failure to respond to careful, small-volume, saline enema therapy or in the presence of signs of peritonitis or intestinal perforation.[27] The prognosis for uncomplicated cases is excellent.

In the infant or toddler, accidental and inflicted blunt injury to the abdomen can result in early obstruction both from bowel wall edema and from a hematoma.[54] A full-thickness bowel wall injury will often produce late sequelae such as an intestinal leak, which initially produces a normal or equivocal examination resulting in a delay in diagnosis. The diagnosis of acute bowel wall trauma requires a high index of suspicion and often thorough and repeated radiologic evaluations.

MANAGEMENT

Medical Management

A child who has GIO requires gastric decompression to prevent continued bowel distention, vomiting, and possibly aspiration. Intravenous fluid therapy is required immediately to replace third-space (ie, intraluminal and intraperitoneal) fluid loss. When replacing the fluid deficit, the clinician must remember that luminal GIO losses are high in electrolyte content, requiring administration of higher-than-maintenance concentrations of sodium, chloride, and potassium. Therefore solutions such as lactated Ringer's solution are needed to provide appropriate replacement. A urinalysis, with catheterization if necessary, as well as a complete blood count and blood chemistry studies, are needed. Because almost all children who have GIO require emergency or semi-urgent surgery, they must be well prepared for anesthesia and the surgical procedure. This approach requires correcting fluid and electrolyte, hematologic, and metabolic imbalances before surgery. Such corrective measures should begin before extensive diagnostic radiologic studies are undertaken. Medical causes of failure to pass meconium that require nonsurgical therapy include hypothyroidism, hypercalcemia, hypokalemia, sepsis, and congestive heart failure.[30]

Surgical Management

The type of surgical procedure performed and the patient's postoperative course and prognosis (see Table 266-1) depend on the type of lesion causing the GIO.[55]

Esophageal Obstruction

Esophageal atresia with associated tracheoesophageal fistula constitutes a relative emergency requiring either primary repair or a staged procedure with an initial gastrostomy for gastric decompression and prevention of aspiration. Subsequent definitive repair, including a division of the fistula and anastomosis of the esophageal ends, is carried out after treatment of any existing underlying pneumonic process. Occasionally the gastrostomy and definitive repair are performed simultaneously, and in selected patients, the esophageal repair is performed without gastrostomy. Complications of the definitive procedure include esophageal leaks, infection, and strictures. Anomalies, particularly of the cardiovascular system, as well as imperforate anus, duodenal atresia, and intestinal malrotation, are associated problems in as many as 50% of cases.[3,56] Patients who have uncomplicated atresia and tracheoesophageal fistula have a low morbidity and negligible mortality. However, associated cardiovascular anomalies and low birth weight lead to a mortality rate as high as 70%. Late complications of atresia and tracheoesophageal fistula include congenital hypertrophic pyloric stenosis and chronic gastroesophageal reflux with reactive airway symptoms.

Gastric Obstructions

Gastric volvulus is usually an acute problem that requires an immediate surgical gastropexy to prevent ischemia and necrosis and a temporary gastrostomy tube for fixation and decompression.[6] If no gastric necrosis is found, then recovery is usually uneventful. Gastric necrosis with resulting peritonitis results in high morbidity and mortality. A gastric antral web is difficult to diagnose and often requires repeated diagnostic studies, but it is not a critical problem. Surgical therapy consists of simple incision of the web and performance of a modified pyloroplasty, resulting in few postoperative complications.[57]

Hypertrophic pyloric stenosis requires surgical therapy after adequate correction of the associated, potentially life-threatening dehydration and hypochloremic alkalosis. The procedure is a muscle-splitting pyloromyotomy, leaving the mucosa intact. The procedure can be performed laparoscopically or through a right upper quadrant or supraumbilical incision with similar operative times, complications, and costs.[58] Acute complications are unusual, with the patient resuming postoperative feedings without sequelae within 8 to 24 hours, sometimes as early as in the immediate postoperative period in the recovery room. Chronic complications such as stricture related to intraoperative mucosal perforations and adhesions are rare.

Duodenal Obstructions

Duodenal atresia, stenosis, and annular pancreas constitute semiurgent problems, as long as they are not accompanied by an associated volvulus, which demands immediate abdominal exploration. Surgical therapy consists of bypassing the obstructed area by means of a duodenoduodenostomy, a duodenojejunostomy, or a gastrojejunostomy.[18] Moderate feeding problems necessitating a longer hospitalization may be encountered, particularly when a gastrojejunostomy is performed. The prognosis is good; however, with associated congenital cardiac problems, mortality can be as high as 50%. Duodenal atresia is associated with Down syndrome (trisomy 21) in as many as 10% of cases. The growth and development of patients who have uncomplicated and isolated duodenal obstructions are normal. Duodenal and other intestinal duplication cysts are treated if possible with complete excision. At the least, excision of the mucosal lining should be performed, given that cysts are associated with a late malignant transformation.[9]

Jejunal and Ileal Obstructions

Jejunal and ileal atresia are also semiurgent conditions unless they are associated with a volvulus. Surgical treatment involves excision of the atretic bowel and primary anastomosis of the dilated proximal and the narrowed distal segments.[17] When multiple atretic segments of bowel, or small-bowel atresias associated with the absence of the superior mesenteric artery, are present, the overall intestinal length and therefore the absorptive surface may be greatly reduced. Total parenteral nutrition commonly is required after surgery. Overall survival and prognosis are good unless the atresia is complicated by cystic fibrosis or the remaining small intestine is too short for adequate absorption.

Malrotation with a complicating volvulus is the most critical diagnosis in any child suspected of having GIO. The twisted bowel mesentery may lead to ischemia and bowel necrosis within 4 to 6 hours after the onset of symptoms. Untreated volvulus has a high acute mortality rate because of associated metabolic imbalance and sepsis. Even after successful surgical resection of the involved necrotic bowel, high long-term morbidity can be expected. The entire embryonically derived midgut may have to be resected, leading to reduced intestinal absorption of nutrients and the so-called *short-gut syndrome*. Thus early diagnosis, rapid correction of fluid and electrolyte imbalances, and surgical reduction of the mesenteric torsion with or without resection of potentially necrotic bowel are imperative.[11] Proximal and distal segments of involved intestine that appear ischemic but may be viable should be retained by creating abdominal enterostomas in lieu of extensive initial intestinal resection followed by a second-look operation performed in 24 hours. Postoperative complications include marked fluid and electrolyte disturbances, local and systemic infections, and malnutrition. Long-term parenteral nutrition, dietary adjustments, and repeated surgical procedures should be expected. Survival with a reasonable quality of life can be expected if the remaining viable small bowel is 30 cm or longer. Morbidity is lessened when the ileocecal valve remains intact. Long-term hospitalization and prolonged nutritional support through total parenteral nutrition are usually required.

As noted previously, meconium ileus may respond to water-soluble contrast enemas; however, evidence of an accompanying intestinal perforation or failure of a carefully managed water-soluble contrast enema necessitates surgical therapy.[34] Cystic fibrosis, which is almost always present as an underlying disease, complicates the patient's postoperative respiratory and nutritional status. Administration of cleansing solutions such as N-acetyl-cysteine by means of an enterotomy usually frees the intestinal lumen of the inspissated material. Associated atretic or necrotic intestinal segments are excised, and primary anastomoses are performed. Enterostomas are created for postoperative lavage of massively impacted meconium or in instances in which the viability of the remaining bowel segments is in question. A stoma may also be needed to protect an anastomosis. A transabdominal T tube may be left intraluminally to allow decompression and irrigation, and the appendix may be used as a conduit.[59,60] The surgical survival is good; however, the morbidity is high, and the ultimate prognosis is related to the severity of the other manifestations of cystic fibrosis.

Colonic and Rectal Obstruction

An intussusception uncomplicated by a lead point (ie, a Meckel diverticulum, a polyp, or a malignancy) can be successfully reduced hydrostatically or by air in up to 90% of appropriately selected patients.[19] Recurrences after air-hydrostatic reduction range from 5% to 7%. Surgical intervention is required if evidence of compromised bowel is found, such as a free perforation or peritoneal irritation, and in failures of air-hydrostatic reduction. Successful reduction requires retrograde reflux of contrast media or air into the terminal ileum. Most patients who have intussusceptions that are reduced intraoperatively do well postoperatively, with a low 2% to 5% recurrence rate. Bowel resection is required when an intraoperatively recognized pathological lead point is present or when an ischemic complication is found. Early diagnosis and treatment of intussusception reduces morbidity and mortality.

Rectal atresia and imperforate anus require diagnosis, initial therapy, and colostomy within 24 hours. Very low perineal lesions (anterior displaced anus and fourchet fistula) can be treated with initial dilatations only. Definitive therapy, which includes a pull-through procedure and anoplasty, is performed when the infant is 2 to 3 months of age.[15] If the lesion is not associated with any other congenital anomalies, then survival is good. The clinician should look for other anomalies, particularly those of the genitourinary tract (rectovaginal and rectovesicular fistulas, lower urinary tract obstructions with megacystis, hydroureter, and hydronephrosis). Future stool continence is related directly to the severity of the deformity, which is influenced by the degree of normal embryologic descent of the colon through the levator muscle. Definitive surgery for high lesions, in which colon descent is limited to a position above the levator muscle, results in daytime stool continence in approximately 60% of patients. The overall continence rate for high lesions is 10% to 20%. Repair of low lesions, in which the colon has descended below the levator muscle, results in an overall stool continence rate of at least 80% to 90%.

Surgical therapy for congenital aganglionosis of the colon (Hirschsprung disease) can include creating a colostomy by using a segment of proximal ganglionic colon, followed in 6 months to 1 year by excision of the affected aganglionic segment and anastomosis of the normally innervated (ganglionic) bowel to the anus (the pull-through procedure).[16] Many patients respond preoperatively to regular rectal stimulation and irrigations to evacuate the colon. This measure allows performance of a primary pull-through procedure during the immediate newborn period and up to several months of age and the avoidance of a colostomy. Infant morbidity and mortality rates are high when the disease is complicated by enterocolitis; however, patients who have no such complications usually do well, with good anal continence, growth, and development.

Minimally Invasive Surgery

The availability of minimally invasive techniques and instruments for infants and toddlers has allowed many procedures such as pyloromyotomy, fundoplication, and endorectal pull-throughs to be performed laparoscopically. Obstructions from adhesions, inflammation (inflammatory bowel disease, appendicitis, and Meckel diverticulitis), and intussusception can be successfully treated with minimally invasive techniques by the skilled laparoscopist. However, procedures such as pyloromyotomy may be performed with a modified open technique, which is less expensive and has equally acceptable cosmetic results. In addition, the use of the minimally invasive technique for the Ladd procedure may be less effective than the original open Ladd procedure, which causes desired adhesion formation that will result in natural fixation of the intestine to prevent future volvulus. As smaller-size instrumentation has improved and surgeons gain more experience, the list of procedures that can be performed laparoscopically continues to grow.[61]

Fetal Surgery

Fetal surgery is the new frontier in the treatment of many congenital anomalies. Given the risk to the mother from invasive prenatal procedures, the death of the fetus or newborn without in utero treatment has to be almost certain for fetal surgery to be considered. This assumption also applies to the newly developed endoscopic fetal procedures *(Fetendo)*. Currently, open or endoscopic fetal surgery is accepted for congenital cystic adenomatoid malformation, fetal sacrococcygeal teratoma, congenital diaphragmatic hernia, and obstructive uropathy that meet the previously mentioned criteria.[62,63] None of the prenatal GIO diagnoses or their causes pose an immediate threat to the fetus or the mother, with overall combined mortality rates of less than 5%. The benefits to the baby do not outweigh the risk to the mother; therefore these lesions are not appropriate for prenatal interventional therapy.[64-67]

The authors thank Dr Sunny Pitt for assistance with radiologic images.

WHEN TO REFER

All patients with suspected and confirmed intestinal obstruction should be referred to pediatric surgery.

WHEN TO ADMIT

All patients with intestinal obstruction should be admitted.

REFERENCES

1. Reyes HM, Meller JL, Loeff D. Neonatal intestinal obstruction. *Clin Perinatol.* 1989;16(1):85-96.
2. Maclennan AC. Investigation in vomiting children. *Semin Pediatr Surg.* 2003;12:220-228.
3. Holder TM, Ashcraft KW. Esophageal atresia and tracheoesophageal fistula: collective review. *Ann Thorac Surg.* 1970;9(5):445-467.
4. Clark DC. Esophageal atresia and tracheoesophageal fistula. *Am Fam Physician.* 1999;59:910-916.
5. Berrocal T, Torres I, Guitérrez J, et al. Congenital anomalies of the upper gastrointestinal tract. *Radiographics.* 1999;19(4):855-872.
6. Mayo A, Erez I, Lazar L, et al. Volvulus of the stomach in childhood: the spectrum of the disease. *Pediatr Emerg Care.* 2001;17:344-348.
7. Rodin D, Schwartz S, Dudgeon DL. Antral mucosal diaphragm. *Gastrointest Endosc.* 1977;24(1):33-34.
8. Scharli A, Sieber WK, Kiesewetter WB. Hypertrophic pyloric stenosis at the Children's Hospital of Pittsburgh from 1912 to 1967: a critical review of current problems. *J Pediatr Surg.* 1969;40(1):108-114.
9. Hajivassiliou CA. Intestinal obstruction in neonatal/pediatric surgery. *Semin Pediatr Surg.* 2003;12:241-253.
10. Lilien LD, Srinivasan G, Pyati SP, et al. Green vomiting in the first 72 hours in normal infants. *Am J Dis Child.* 1986; 140(7):662-664.
11. Steward DR, Colodny AL, Daggett WC. Malrotation of the bowel in infants and children: a 15-year review. *Surgery.* 1976;79(6):71-720.
12. Torres AM, Ziegler MM. Malrotation of the intestine. *World J Surg.* 1993;17(3):326-331.
13. D'Agostino J. Common abdominal emergencies in children. *Emerg Med Clin North Am.* 2002; 20:139-153.
14. Shimanuki Y, Aihara T, Takano H, et al. Clockwise whirlpool sign at color Doppler US: an objective and definite sign of midgut volvulus. *Radiology.* 1996;199(1):261-264.
15. Kiesewetter WB, Bill AH, Nixon HH, et al. Imperforate anus. *Arch Surg.* 1976;111(5):518-525.
16. Kleinhaus S, Boley SJ, Sheran M, et al. Hirschsprung's disease: a survey of the members of the surgical section of the American Academy of Pediatrics. *J Pediatr Surg.* 1979;14(5):588-597.
17. Louw JH. Resection and end to end anastomosis in the management of atresia and stenosis of the small bowel. *Surgery.* 1967;62(5):940-950.
18. Wesley JR, Majour GH. Congenital intrinsic duodenal obstruction: a 25-year review. *Surgery.* 1977;82(5): 716-720.
19. Rosenkrantz JG, Cox JA, Silverman FN, et al. Intussusception in the 1970s: indications for operation. *J Pediatr Surg.* 1977;12(3):367-373.
20. Janik JS, Firor HV. Pediatric appendicitis: a 20-year study of 1640 children at Cook County (Illinois) Hospital. *Arch Surg.* 1979;114(6):717-719.
21. Kirchmann HM, Bender SW. Intestinal obstruction in Crohn's disease in childhood. *J Pediatr Gastroenterol Nutr.* 1987; 6(1):79-83.
22. Penketh AR, Wise A, Mearns MB, et al. Cystic fibrosis in adolescents and adults. *Thorax.* 1987;42(7):526-532.
23. Chavhan GB, Masrani S, Thakkar H, et al. Sonography in the diagnosis of pediatric gastrointestinal obstruction. *J Ultrasound.* 2004; 32(4):190-199.
24. Wallis-Crespo MC, Crespo A. Helicobacter pylori infection in pediatric population: epidemiology, pathophysiology, and therapy. *Fetal Pediatr Pathol.* 2004;23:11-28.
25. Heldrich FJ. Lethargy as a presenting symptom in patients with intussusception. *Clin Pediatr (Phila).* 1986; 25(7):363-365.
26. LeQuesne GW, Reilly BJ. Functional immaturity of the large bowel in the newborn infant. *Radiol Clin North Am.* 1975;13(2):331-342.
27. Philippart AI, Reed JO, Georgeson KE. Neonatal small left colon syndrome: intramural, not intraluminal obstruction. *J Pediatr Surg.* 1975;10(5):733-740.
28. Sokal MM, Koenigsberger MR, Rose JS, et al. Neonatal hypermagnesemia and the meconium plug syndrome. *N Engl J Med.* 1972;286(15):823-825.
29. Olsen MM, Luck SR, Lloyd-Still J, et al. The spectrum of meconium disease in infancy. *J Pediatr Surg.* 1982;17(5): 479-487.
30. Loening-Baucke V, Kimura K. Failure to pass meconium: diagnosing neonatal intestinal obstruction. *Am Fam Physician.* 1999;60:2043-2050.
31. Cirino E, Vadalà G, Catania G, et al. Intestinal obstruction and incomplete obstruction from mesenteric cyst formation. *Chir Ital.* 1979;31(4):543-555.
32. Iyer CP, Mahour GH. Duplications of the alimentary tract in infants and children. *J Pediatr Surg.* 1995;30(9):1267-1270.
33. Pintér AB, Schubert W, Szemlédy F, et al. Alimentary tract duplications in infants and children. *Eur J Pediatr Surg.* 1992;2(1):8-12.
34. Mabogunjc OA, Wang CI, Mahour GH. Improved survival of neonates with meconium ileus. *Arch Surg.* 1982; 117(1):37-40.
35. Kahn E. Gastrointestinal manifestations in pediatric AIDS. *Pediatr Pathol Lab Med.* 1997;17(2):171-208.
36. Dell'Agnola CA, Tomaselli V, Teruzzi E, et al. Prenatal diagnosis of gastrointestinal obstruction: a correlation between prenatal ultrasonic findings and postnatal operative findings. *Prenat Diagn.* 1993;13(7):629-632.
37. Miller AJW, Rode H, Gywes S, et al. Malrotation and volvulus in infancy and childhood. *Semin Pediatr Surg.* 2003; 12(4):229-236.

38. Parrini S, Di Maggio G, Latini G, et al. Abnormal oral mucosal light reflectance in infantile hypertrophic pyloric stenosis. *J Pediatr Gastroenterol Nutr.* 2004; 39(1): 53-55.
39. Studen RJ, LeQuesne GW, Little KE. The improved ultrasound diagnosis of hypertrophic pyloric stenosis. *Pediatr Radiol.* 1986;16(3):200-205.
40. Weiskittel DA, Leary DL, Blane CE. Ultrasound diagnosis of evolving pyloric stenosis. *Gastrointest Radiol.* 1989; 14(1):22-24.
41. Lui KW, Wong HF, Wan YL, et al. Antral web—a rare cause of vomiting in children. *Pediatr Surg Int.* 2000; 16(5-6):424-425.
42. Khong PL, Cheung SC, Leong LL, et al. Ultrasonography of intra-abdominal cystic lesions in the newborn. *Clin Radiol.* 2003;58:449-454.
43. Clatworthy WH, Howard WH, Lloyd J. The meconium plug syndrome. *Surgery.* 1956;39(1):131-142.
44. West KW, Stephens B, Vane DW, et al. Intussusception: current management in infants and children. *Surgery.* 1987;102(4):704-710.
45. Hay SA, Kabesh AA, Soliman HA, et al. Idiopathic intussusception: the role of laparoscopy. *J Pediatr Surg.* 1999; 34(4):577-578.
46. Poddoubnyi IV, Dronov AF, Blinnikov OI, et al. Laparoscopy in the treatment of intussusception in children. *J Pediatr Surg.* 1998;33(8):1194-1197.
47. Cox TD, Winters WD, Weinberger E, et al. CT of intussusception in the pediatric patient: diagnosis and pitfalls. *Pediatr Radiol.* 1996;26(1):26-32.
48. Harrington L, Connolly B, Hu X, et al. Ultrasonographic and clinical predictors of intussusception. *J Pediatr.* 1998; 132(5):836-839.
49. Shanbhogue RL, Hussain SM, Meradji M, et al. Ultrasonography is accurate enough for the diagnosis of intussusception. *J Pediatr Surg.* 1994;29(2):324-327.
50. Jinzhe Z, Yenxia W, Linchi W. Rectal inflation reduction of intussusception in infants. *J Pediatr Surg.* 1986;21(1): 30-32.
51. Katz M, Phelan E, Carlin JB, et al. Gas enema for the reduction of intussusception: relationship between clinical signs and symptoms and outcome. *AJR Am J Roentgenol.* 1993;160(2):363-366.
52. Menor F, Cortina H, Marco A, et al. Effectiveness of pneumatic reduction of ileocolic intussusception in children. *Gastrointest Radiol.* 1992;17(4):339-343.
53. Gorenstein A, Raucher A, Serour F, et al. Intussusception in children: reduction with repeated, delayed air enema. *Radiology.* 1998;206(3):721-724.
54. Kurkchubasche AG, Fendya DG, Tracy TF, et al. Blunt intestinal injury in children: diagnostic and therapeutic considerations. *Arch Surg.* 1997;132(6):652-657.
55. Bagolan P, Nappo S, Trucchi A, et al. Neonatal intestinal obstruction: reducing short-term complications by surgical refinements. *Eur J Pediatr Surg.* 1996;6(6):354-357.
56. Cieri MV, Arnold GL, Torfs CP. Malrotation in conjunction with esophageal atresia/tracheo-esophageal fistula. *Teratology.* 1999;60:114-116.
57. Tunell WP, Smith EI. Antral web in infancy. *J Pediatr Surg.* 1980;15(2):152-155.
58. Kim SS, Lau ST, Lee SL, et al. Pyloromyotomy: a comparison of laparoscopic, circumumbilical, and right upper quadrant operative technique. *J Am Coll Surg.* 2005; 201:66-70.
59. Fitzgerald R, Conlon K. Use of the appendix stump in the treatment of meconium ileus. *J Pediatr Surg.* 1989;24(9): 899-900.
60. Steiner Z, Mongilner J, Siplovich L, et al. T-tubes in the management of meconium ileus. *Pediatr Surg Int.* 1997; 12(2/3):140-141.
61. Georgeson KE, Owings E. Advances in minimally invasive surgery in children. *Am J Surg.* 2000;180(5):362-364.
62. Flake AW. Surgery in the human fetus: the future. *J Physiol.* 2003;547:45-51.
63. Danzer E, Sydorak RM, Harrison MR, et al. Minimal access fetal surgery. *Eur J Obstet Gynecol Reprod Biol.* 2003;108(1):3-13.
64. Albanese CT, Harrison MR. Surgical treatment of fetal disease: the state of the art. *Ann N Y Acad Sci.* 1998; 847: 74-85.
65. Farmer DL. Fetal surgery: a brief review. *Pediatr Radiol.* 1998;28(6):409-413.
66. Flake AW, Harrison MR. Fetal surgery. *Annu Rev Med.* 1995;46:67-78.
67. Milner R, Adzick NS. Perinatal management of fetal malformations amenable to surgical correction. *Curr Opin Obstet Gynecol.* 1999;11(2):177-183.

Chapter 267

GIARDIASIS

Craig M. Wilson, MD

ETIOLOGY

A *Giardia*-like organism associated with gastrointestinal symptoms was described by Dutch microscopist Anton van Leeuwenhoek in 1681,[1] but only in the last few decades has the true pathogenicity of this flagellate protozoan been recognized. *Giardia intestinalis* (also known as *G lamblia* and *G duodenalis*) is one of the most common intestinal parasites in the United States and around the world,[2] and it has attained a certain notoriety as a result of diarrhea epidemics at fashionable ski resorts, in child care centers, in major metropolitan areas, among campers, and among international tourists. The prevalence of giardiasis in children is becoming widely appreciated, particularly in the child care setting.[3]

G intestinalis is an extracellular parasite that has no intermediate development outside of the intestinal lumen. This unicellular protozoan exists in 2 forms: (1) a motile, flagellated trophozoite that causes disease and (2) a dormant cyst that transmits infection. The trophozoite is 12 to 15 μm long and has 4 pairs of flagella and 2 prominent nuclei (Figure 267-1). It lacks many classical eukaryotic subcellular structures, and it has a ribosomal RNA structure, which is suggestive of a very primitive organism, although recent data question how primitive.[4] A large sucking disk, which the parasite uses to attach to the intestinal mucosa, occupies most of the flat ventral surface. Attachment is regulated by contractile proteins, including actin and myosin, which alter the structure of the disk. The mechanism by which the organism evades degradation in the intestinal lumen is not clear. The motile trophozoites divide by longitudinal binary fission in the upper small bowel and then encyst as they pass into the colon. Trophozoites are usually seen only in the stool when diarrhea is present. Cysts, the more common form seen in stool specimens, are 9 to 12 μm

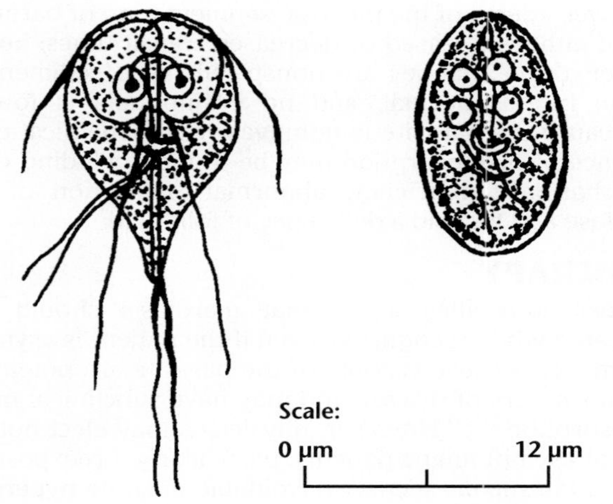

Figure 267-1 *Giardia* organisms. The trophozoite (*left*) is 12 to 15 μm long and has 4 pairs of flagella and 2 prominent nuclei. This form is not commonly seen in stools. Cysts (*right*) are 9 to 12 μm long and may have 2 to 4 nuclei.

long. Recently formed cysts have 2 nuclei; mature cysts have 4, but cysts are generally infectious on emergence in stool. The oocysts are stable for weeks to months in the environment.

EPIDEMIOLOGIC MECHANISM

G intestinalis is one of the most commonly identified pathogens in waterborne diarrheal disease in the United States, where the organism is holoendemic.[2] A seasonality to infections exists, with higher rates in late Summer and early Fall. In the United States, rates are highest among children younger than 5 years. Many large common-source outbreaks have been traced to contaminated drinking water. Epidemiologic studies have attributed these epidemics to cross-contamination of municipal drinking water supplies that have sewage, defective or deficient filtration facilities, and reliance on chlorination as the principal method of water disinfection.[5] In mountainous regions, where the prevalence of disease appears to be higher, use of surface water for drinking is the principal problem. Although zoonotic infections have been documented, recent molecular epidemiologic studies suggest it may actually be quite rare.[6] As suggested by the occurrence of epidemic giardiasis despite chlorination of municipal water supplies, routine chlorination may not be adequate for killing *G intestinalis*.[7,8] The level of chlorine necessary to kill cysts depends on many other factors, including pH, contact time, turbidity, and temperature.[9] Thus an adequate water purification system for clearing *G intestinalis* should include filtration, sedimentation, and flocculation systems. Halogen-based, small-quantity disinfection methods are also affected by water clarity and temperature.[10]

Because cysts may be shed in abundance in the stool, not surprisingly, *G intestinalis* may be transmitted by the fecal-oral route. This route is undoubtedly the main route of spread in families, in institutions, and in child care centers. With intensive exposure to stool, as in child care centers caring for infants in diapers, giardiasis quickly may become hyperendemic.[3,11-13] Foodborne giardiasis has been reported, the implicated food probably was contaminated during preparation.

PATHOGENESIS

Studies in human volunteers have demonstrated the high infectivity of *G intestinalis* cysts. Although 1 cyst rarely was infectious, infection occurred in virtually all volunteers receiving 100 to 1 million cysts orally and in 36% of those exposed to 10 to 25 cysts.[14] Molecular-based techniques suggest *G intestinalis* assemblages A and B as the predominant species infecting humans and multiple other genotypes and species infecting other hosts.[6,15]

Many mechanisms have been postulated for the diarrhea and malabsorption caused by *G intestinalis*. In all likelihood, the process is multifactorial, with the severity of symptoms dependent on the degree of focal small bowel injury. Infection is associated with injury to the mucosal brush border, with disruption of disaccharidase activity and transport mechanisms.[6,16] A basal membrane and intraepithelial inflammatory cell infiltrate have been found,[17] and evidence exists of an increased enterocyte turnover in the murine model.[18] In either case, less efficient villus function would be expected. In the extreme, the microvilli atrophy results in the severe malabsorptive diarrhea, which is a major complication of giardiasis. Recent studies suggest that parasite products play a role in the pathophysiologic mechanism of this infection.[19] Evidence also has been found that some *Giardia* strains produce more severe symptoms in humans than they do in other species,[20] and differences in phenotype and genotype have been correlated with virulence in experimental models of infection.

Host defense mechanisms appear to be relatively inefficient, given the small number of organisms required to initiate infection and the frequency of relapse and reinfection. However, intraluminal secretory antibody response, nonspecific inflammatory responses at the level of the mucosa, and antibody-dependent cell-mediated cytotoxicity appear to be important in limiting the severity of disease.[21] The role of antibody and antibody-dependent cell-mediated cytotoxicity in containing giardiasis is supported by the increased incidence and severity of disease in patients who have immunoglobulin deficiencies. Underlying immunoglobulin A deficiency and both X-linked and common variable hypogammaglobulinemia have been associated with severe or prolonged infection.

G intestinalis should be considered in the workup of diarrhea or malabsorption in patients who have human immunodeficiency infection. The role and extent of *G intestinalis* infections in children who have human immunodeficiency infection have not been established. Of course, diarrhea in patients who have acquired immunodeficiency syndrome is often multifactorial, and treatment of documented giardiasis may not result in clinical improvement if other pathogens still are present (see Chapter 276, Human Immunodeficiency Virus Infection and Acquired Immunodeficiency Syndrome).

CLINICAL MANIFESTATIONS

Based on experimental studies and point-source outbreak observational data, the incubation period of giardiasis is 7 to 14 days.[14] Most patients infected by *G intestinalis* probably remain asymptomatic, although they do shed cysts in their feces and are infectious. Children are more likely than adults to have symptomatic disease.

The principal symptoms of giardiasis are gastrointestinal. Diarrhea, abdominal cramps, and nausea are reported most often.[22] Vomiting, malodorous stools, flatulence, bloating, anorexia, and even constipation are noted less frequently. Because the colon and rectum are not involved, tenesmus should suggest another diagnosis. Blood almost never is found in the stool, and the presence of mucus is unusual. Gastrointestinal symptoms generally last 7 to 10 days, although a more protracted course is common. Because of the disaccharidase deficiency that accompanies severe infections, some patients complain of milk intolerance, which may last for weeks.

Constitutional symptoms are not prominent in giardiasis, but up to 25% of patients experience fatigue, headache, or a low-grade fever.[23] Extraintestinal syndromes, such as urticaria, erythema multiforme, and arthralgia, have occurred, but very rarely, in association with giardiasis.

Some patients, particularly children, develop chronic diarrhea, frank malabsorption, weight loss, malnutrition, and growth retardation. Thus giardiasis must be considered in the differential diagnosis of failure to thrive. Occasionally, giardiasis may be misdiagnosed as sprue, food allergy, or psychogenic abdominal pain, and its protean clinical manifestations may mimic a wide variety of gastrointestinal disturbances. Malabsorption leading to an iron deficiency anemia also has been reported with *G intestinalis*.

The physical examination is generally unremarkable unless secondary malnutrition has developed.

LABORATORY EVALUATION

The clinical laboratory diagnosis of *G duodenalis* has predominantly changed from a microscopic examination of stool to either heat-stable antigen detection in stool or detection of parasites by fluorescence. These tests are quite often combined for simultaneous detection of *Cryptosporidium* sp.[24,25] Overall, these tests compare well with standard microscopic procedures and are in most cases more sensitive although multiple samples may still be needed for optimal detection.[26]

A few patients require additional measures to have the pathogen detected. Examining the duodenal contents provides the optimum yield, and this examination can be performed either by direct duodenal aspiration or by using the Entero Test.[27] In rare patients who have chronic symptoms in whom the diagnosis must be excluded, the small bowel should be biopsied. Several sections of the biopsy specimen stained with Giemsa stain may have to be examined to find the parasite; *Giardia* organisms are detected more easily in Giemsa-stained mucosal impression smears.

Serologic tests are valuable in epidemiologic studies but are of little use diagnostically. Upper gastrointestinal radiographs may reveal mild dilation of the small bowel, edema of the mucosa, segmentation of barium, and either increased or decreased transit times; however, these changes are nonspecific. The sedimentation rate is normal, and no eosinophilia is found because the parasite is noninvasive. Biochemical evidence of malabsorption may be found, including disaccharidase deficiency, abnormal absorption of d-xylose and fat, and a deficiency of folic acid.

THERAPY

Most authorities agree that giardiasis should be treated when recognized, even if the patient is asymptomatic, because carriers of the parasite are potential transmitters of disease and may have subclinical malabsorption.[28-30] However, physicians may elect not to treat asymptomatic patients, particularly if reexposure to *G intestinalis* seems unavoidable in some hyperendemic settings.

Metronidazole (Flagyl) has been used widely to treat giardiasis in adults and children because it is well tolerated (except for the mild metallic aftertaste), has a very low incidence of serious side effects, and has an acceptable cure rate. Alcohol ingestion, including in concurrent medications, should be avoided with metronidazole because of disulfiram-like reactions. Of note, giardiasis is not an approved indication for metronidazole in the United States. Tinidazole (Tindamax), a nitroimidazole similar to metronidazole, which has been used extensively in a single-dose regimen outside of the United States, has now been approved for the treatment of giardiasis including children 3 years and older.[30] Both metronidazole and tinidazole can readily be formulated as suspensions.

Furazolidone (Furoxone) has the distinct advantages of having a pleasant taste and being available in a pediatric suspension. Side effects, which have been minimal in children, include mild gastrointestinal distress, hypersensitivity reactions, hemolysis in individuals who have glucose-6-phosphate dehydrogenase deficiency, brown discoloration of the urine, and disulfiram-like reactions. Furazolidone is contraindicated with monoamine oxidase inhibitors. The efficacy in children has been as high as 92%, which is comparable if not superior to cure rates seen with alternative agents.[31]

Nitazoxanide (Alinia) is a recently approved antiparasitic agent with specific indications for the treatment of cryptosporidiosis and giardiasis in children.[32] Cure rates in small, randomized trials were comparable to standard agents for giardiasis, and side effect rates appear comparable to placebo. On rare occasions, yellow sclera is noted, which clears with discontinuation of the drug. Nitazoxanide is the most costly of the agents discussed here.

Albendazole has been reported to be as effective as metronidazole in a study of children 5 to 10 years of age.[33] Albendazole has the advantage of being active against a broad range of intestinal parasites, including helminths, if this is a consideration. Paromomycin, a nonabsorbable aminoglycoside, has been used to treat giardiasis in pregnancy, but data regarding its efficacy are limited. Quinacrine, a previously commonly used therapy, is not commercially available in the United States but can be obtained if needed *(www.medicalletter.com)*.

Relapse is possible after using any of these regimens. If this event occurs, re-treatment with the same agent or an alternative drug is often successful. No well-documented evidence exists for actual drug resistance in *Giardia* on an individual clinical case level. In vitro sensitivity has shown variations but is assay and inoculum dependent. For cases of severe or recalcitrant infections prolonged or combination therapy may be necessary.[28,34]

PREVENTION

Because giardiasis is so prevalent, total prevention of transmission is virtually impossible. When the disease is known to be present in a household, institution, or child care center, good hand washing is essential to limit spread by the fecal-oral route. Personal hygiene is especially important when infants in diapers are affected. When an outbreak is thought to occur in child care centers that have infants in diapers, the local health department should be contacted, and an epidemiologic investigation should be undertaken to identify and treat all symptomatic children, child care workers, and family members infected with *Giardia*.

As already noted, prevention of waterborne giardiasis is contingent on adequate water purification, including filtration, sedimentation, and flocculation in addition to chlorination.[7,8] Tourists in endemic areas should avoid drinking tap water. Campers should not rely on chlorination tablets, which are ineffective against *Giardia* cysts. Boiling for at least 2 minutes, even at high altitudes, or filtration (pore size under 1 μm or with a filter rated for cyst removal) are satisfactory means for preparing drinking water free of *G intestinalis*.

TOOLS FOR PRACTICE

Engaging Patients and Family

- *Diarrhea and Dehydration* (brochure), American Academy of Pediatrics (patiented.aap.org).
- *Common Childhood Infections* (brochure), American Academy of Pediatrics (patiented.aap.org).
- *Giardiasis* (fact sheet), Centers for Disease Control and Prevention (www.cdc.gov/ncidod/dpd/parasites/giardiasis/factsht_giardia.htm).
- *Giardiasis: Recreational Water Safety* (fact sheet), Centers for Disease Control and Prevention (www.cdc.gov/healthyswimming/giardiafacts.htm).

Medical Decision Support

- Practice Guidelines for Management of Infectious Diarrhea, Infectious Disease Society of America (www.idsociety.org/content.aspx?id=9088).
- Giardiasis: Lab Assistance (Web site), Centers for Disease Control and Prevention (www.dpd.cdc.gov/dpdx/HTML/Giardiasis.htm).

REFERENCES

1. Dobell C. The discovery of the intestinal protozoa of man. *Proc R Soc Med Section Hist Med*. 1920;13:1-15.
2. Furness BW, Beach MJ, Roberts JM. Giardiasis surveillance—United States, 1992-1997. *MMWR CDC Surveill Summ*. 2000;49(7):1-13.
3. Thompson SC. *Giardia* lamblia in children and the child care setting: a review of the literature. *J Paediatr Child Health*. 1994;30:202-209.
4. Graczyk TK. Is *Giardia* a living fossil? *Trends Parasitol*. 2005;21(3):104-107.
5. Levy DA, Bens MS, Craun GF, et al. Surveillance for waterborne-disease outbreaks—United States, 1995-1996. *MMWR CDC Surveill Summ*. 1998;47(5):1-34.
6. Thompson RCA. The zoonotic significance and molecular epidemiology of *Giardia* and giardiasis. *Vet Parasitol*. 2004;126:15-35.
7. Betancourt WQ, Rose JB. Drinking water treatment processes for removal of Cryptosporidium and Giardia. *Vet Parasitol*. 2004;126:219-234.
8. Jakubowski W, Graum GF. Update on the control of *Giardia* in water supplies. In: Olson BE, Olson ME, Wallis PM, eds. *Giardia: The Cosmopolitan Parasite*. Wallingford, UK: CAB International; 2002:217-238.
9. Jarroll EL, Bingham AK, Meyer EA. Effects of chlorine on *Giardia* duodenalis cyst viability. *Appl Environ Microbiol*. 1981;41:483-487.
10. Jarroll EL, Bingham AK, Meyer EA. Cyst destruction: effectiveness of six small-quantity water disinfection methods. *Am J Trop Med Hyg*. 1980;29:8-11.
11. Keystone JS, Krajden S, Warren MR. Person-to-person transmission of *Giardia lamblia* in day-care nurseries. *CMAJ*. 1978;119(3):241-242.
12. Rauch AM, Van R, Bartlett AV, Pickering LK. Longitudinal study of *Giardia lamblia* infection in a day care center population. *Pediatr Infect Dis J*. 1990;9(3):186-189.
13. Sealy DP, Schuman SH. Endemic giardiasis and day care. *Pediatrics*. 1983;72(2):154-158.
14. Rendtorff RC. The experimental transmission of human intestinal protozoan parasites. II. *Giardia* duodenalis cysts given in capsules. *Am J Trop Med Hyg*. 1954;59:209-220.
15. Cacciò SM, Thompson RCA, McLauchlin J, et al. Unraveling Cryptosporidium and *Giardia* epidemiology. *Trends Parasitol*. 2005;21(9):430-437.
16. Hartong WA, Gourley WK, Arvanitakas C. Giardiasis: clinical spectrum and functional structural abnormalities of the small intestinal mucosa. *Gastroenterol*. 1979;77:61-69.
17. Wright SG, Tomkins AM. Quantitative histology in giardiasis. *J Clin Pathol*. 1978;31:712-716.
18. Gillon J, Thomery AL, Ferguson A. Features of small intestine pathology (epithelial cell kinetics, intraepithelial lymphocytes, disaccharidases) in primary *Giardia muris* infection. *Gut*. 1982;23:498-506.
19. Buret AG, Scott KGE, Chin AC. Giardiasis: pathophysiology and pathogenesis. In: Olson BE, Olson ME, Wallis PM, eds. *Giardia: The Cosmopolitan Parasite*. Wallingford, UK: CABI International; 2002:109-125.
20. Nash TE, Herrington DA, Losonsky GA, et al. Experimental human infections with *Giardia lamblia*. *J Infec Dis*. 1987;156(6):974-984.
21. Faubert G. Immune response to *Giardia* duodenalis. *Clin Microbiol Rev*. 2000;13(1):35-54.
22. Burke JA. Giardiasis in Childhood. *Am J Dis Child*. 1975;129:1304-1310.
23. Shaw PK, Brodsky RE, Lyman DO, et al. A community outbreak of giardiasis with evidence of transmission by a municipal water supply. *Ann Intern Med*. 1977;87:426-432.
24. Garcia LS, Shimizu RY. Evaluation of nine immunoassay kits (enzyme immunoassay and direct fluorescence) for detection of *Giardia lamblia* and *Cryptosporidium parvum* in human fecal specimens. *J Clin Microbiol*. 1997;35(6):1526-1529.

25. Johnston SP, Ballard MM, Beach MJ, et al. Evaluation of three commercial assays for detection of *Giardia* and *Cryptosporidium* organisms in fecal specimens. *J Clin Microbiol*. 2003;41(2):623-626.
26. Hanson KL, Cartwright CP. Use of an enzyme immunoassay does not eliminate the need to analyze multiple stool specimens for sensitive detection of *Giardia lamblia*. *J Clin Microbiol*. 2001;39(2):474-477.
27. Rosenthal P, Liebman WM. Comparative study of stool examinations, duodenal aspiration, and pediatric Entero-Test for giardiasis in children. *J Pediatr*. 1980;96:278-279.
28. Gardner TB, Hill DR. Treatment of giardiasis. *Clin Microbiol Rev*. 2001;14(1):114-128.
29. Zaat JOM, Mank TG, Assendelft WJJ. A systematic review on the treatment of giardiasis. *Trop Med Int Health*. 1997;2(1):63-82.
30. Tinidazole (Tindamax)—a new anti-protozoal drug [no author listed]. *Med Lett*. 2004;46(1190):70-72.
31. Craft JC, Murphy T, Nelson JD. Furazolidone and quinacrine: a comparative study of therapy for giardiasis in children. *Am J Dis Child*. 1981;135:164-166.
32. Nitazoxanide (Alinia)—a new anti-protozoal agent [no author listed]. *Med Lett*. 2003;45:29-31.
33. Hall A, Nahar Q. Albendazole as a treatment for infections with *Giardia* duodenalis in children in Bangladesh. *Trans R Soc Trop Med Hyg*. 1993;87:84-86.
34. Nash TE, Ohl CA, Thomas E, et al. Treatment of patients with refractory giardiasis. *Clin Inf Dis*. 2001;33:22-28.

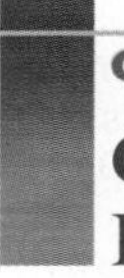

Chapter 268

GLUTEN-SENSITIVE ENTEROPATHY (CELIAC SPRUE)

Anca M. Safta, MD; John A. Kerner Jr, MD

Gluten-sensitive enteropathy (GSE), also called celiac sprue, is a condition characterized by clinical features of malabsorption and pathological changes in the jejunal mucosa, both of which improve when gluten is removed from the diet and recur when it is reintroduced. GSE is the second-most common cause of malabsorption in children, the most common being cystic fibrosis.

The classic clinical description of celiac disease was first provided in 1888.[1] In 1950 the association between the ingestion of gluten and celiac disease was noted.[2] During World War II, when grain products were in short supply, the incidence of GSE was markedly reduced, and children who had the disease improved. After the war, when cereal grain again became plentiful, the incidence of GSE quickly returned to prewar levels. In 1954 the first accurate description of intestinal lesions in patients with GSE was provided by studying surgical biopsy material.[3] Not until 1968 was the discovery made that adult nontropical sprue and celiac disease in childhood were the same disease.[4]

INCIDENCE

The precise incidence of GSE is unknown because many patients have asymptomatic disease. Screening with serologic markers has increased the estimates of prevalence of GSE in different areas. GSE has been identified in Hispanic, Indian, Chinese, Sudanese, African-Caribbean, and Middle Eastern people. Although the disorder was once thought to be more common in Europe than in the United States, such is no longer the case; in England the prevalence is 1 in 87, in Finland 1 in 99, in Spain 1 in 389, in Iran 1 in 166, in the Sahara 1 in 18, and in the United States 1 in 133. The worldwide average prevalence for GSE is estimated to be 1 in 266.[5-7]

In children the average age at the time of diagnosis is under 24 months.[8] Diagnosis occurs sooner in infants who are fed cereal at an early age. The clinical incidence declines markedly after age 2 years, and diagnosing GSE in a teenager is even less common. In adults, GSE often clinically develops after a precipitating illness, such as infectious diarrhea, or after a surgical procedure, such as gastrectomy.

Clinical diagnosis of GSE has become much more common, which has led to increased incidence.[9] This increase results from the advent of routine upper endoscopy in evaluating patients with abdominal pain and finding a flat villus lesion during routine small-bowel biopsy and from the use of serologic markers in the routine screening of family members and screening for associated diseases.

PATHOLOGICAL FEATURES

GSE primarily affects the mucosa of the small intestine. The submucosa, muscularis, and serosa are not involved. The mucosal lesion of the small intestine in GSE varies in severity and extent; lesions in the jejunum are generally more severe than those in the ileum.[10] This variability may explain the differences in the degree of malabsorption observed in some patients; those in whom more intestinal area is involved presumably have a greater degree of malabsorption. This difference in the distribution of the lesion suggests that the proximal intestine has greater exposure to undigested gluten than the distal intestine because no greater sensitivity to gluten is found in the proximal than in the distal mucosa.

Among patients with active GSE, surface epithelial-cell damage occurs, and more cells migrate from the crypt to the villus region. Compensatory crypt hypertrophy occurs, with a marked increase in mitotic activity, and gradual villus flattening develops (Figure 268-1 and Figure 268-2). The surface epithelial cells demonstrate a loss of the basal nuclei polarity and become more cuboidal. Many intraepithelial lymphocytes are noted, and the lamina propria shows a marked increase in plasma cells and lymphocytes. This flat villus lesion is not pathognomonic of GSE; it may be seen in many other diseases. With the introduction of the flexible endoscope, which permits focused biopsy rather than blind suction biopsy, investigators have found nonspecific antral gastritis in 10% of patients who have GSE, which implies the presence of some gastric sensitivity.[11] In addition, patients with chronic diarrhea and evidence of biopsy proven lymphocytic or collagenous colitis should be suspected of occult celiac disease.[12]

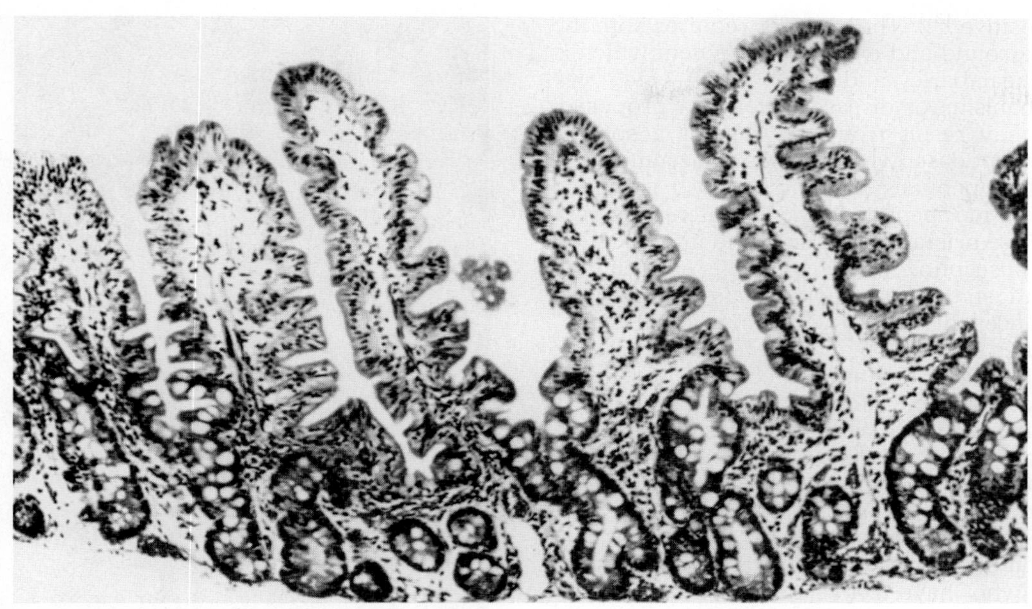

Figure 268-1 Normal jejunal mucosa. Villi are tall, crypts are relatively short, and the crypt-villus ratio is approximately 1:4. Epithelial cells are columnar, with basally oriented nuclei. Some lymphocytes and plasma cells are found in the lamina propria.

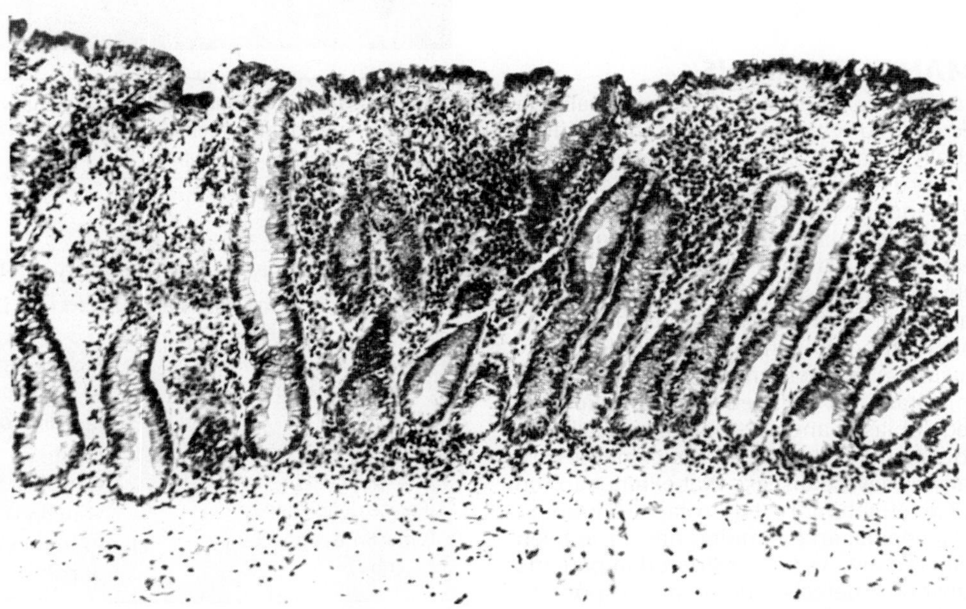

Figure 268-2 Jejunal mucosa in gluten-sensitive enteropathy (celiac sprue). Mucosa is flat, villi are absent, and crypts are deep. Epithelial cells are cuboidal, and nuclei are not basally oriented. Increased numbers of mitoses in the crypts is found. Inflammatory cells, especially plasma cells and lymphocytes, are markedly increased (×160).

PATHOGENESIS

GSE is a genetic disease, although the complete mode of inheritance remains to be fully elucidated. Several genes seem to be involved, with the most consistent genetic component being the presence of *HLA-DQ2* or *-DQ8* genes. These genes are necessary to develop disease but not sufficient by themselves; therefore patients who lack this genetic background cannot have GSE. The *HLA-DQ2* allele combination is found in 90% to 95% of patients with GSE (however, 20% to 30% of the normal population also has this combination); the remaining 5% to 10% of patients are

HLA-DQ8 positive.[13-15] The disorder requires both the genetic background and exposure to gluten, which is present in wheat, barley, and rye.

Two mechanisms of disease have been proposed. First, GSE may result from the lack of a specific enzyme, a dipeptidase, which results in accumulation of toxic gluten peptides such as a newly identified protein-rich 33-mer peptide found in gluten. This peptide may be the primary initiator of the inflammatory response in susceptible individuals. This 33-mer peptide is the antigen that reacts with tissue transglutaminase and induces the gut-derived human T-cell lines.[16] Second, gluten toxicity may be mediated through immunologic aberrations associated with genetically determined cell-surface markers.[17,18]

Various immunologic abnormalities have been described in GSE. First, increased levels of serum immunoglobulin (Ig) A and lowered levels of serum IgM are abnormalities that are reversed by a gluten-free diet (GFD). Second, intestinal mucosal immunoglobulin synthesis, notably IgA and IgM, is markedly increased in patients who have active GSE. This synthesis returns to normal with remission. Fifty percent of the increased IgA is associated with specific anti-gluten antibody.[19] Third, patients with active GSE respond to corticosteroid treatment.[20] Fourth, in-vitro duodenal mucosa and peripheral lymphocyte transformation in response to gluten has been described in patients with GSE.[21,22]

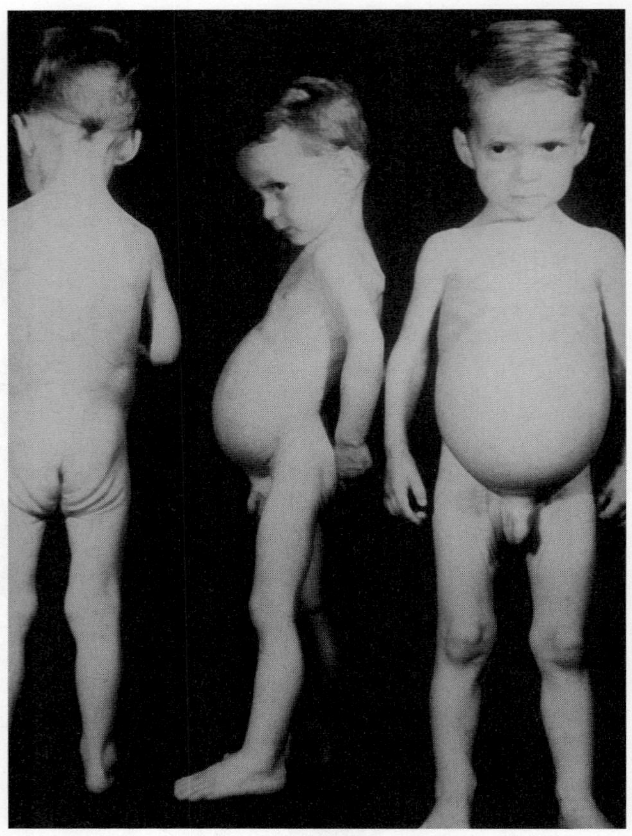

Figure 268-3 Classic profile of patient with gluten-sensitive enteropathy (celiac sprue): potbelly, thin buttocks, and proximal muscle wasting.

CLINICAL MANIFESTATIONS

A patient with an advanced case of GSE is typically an irritable, anorectic child with chronic diarrhea, failure to thrive, a potbelly, and muscle wasting, especially of the buttocks and proximal limbs.[23] These children are usually easy to diagnose (Figure 268-3). Nonetheless, many patients exhibit the disorder atypically. Box 268-1 lists atypical features of patients with GSE. Such features are usually related to selective malabsorption of various nutrients. Therefore for patients to have rickets, osteoporosis with bone pain, or pathological fractures is not unusual. Also seen are bleeding disorders that result from vitamin-K deficiency, iron-deficiency anemia, and megaloblastic anemia, which is usually the result of folate deficiency. Vitamin-B_{12} deficiency is rare and usually indicates severe disease that extends to the terminal ileum. Constipation, rectal prolapse, clubbing of the fingernails, edema, and vomiting have also been reported. GSE should always be considered in patients with specific nutritional defects who do not respond to nutrient replacement therapy.

BOX 268-1 Atypical Manifestations of Gluten-sensitive Enteropathy

- Growth failure (without gastrointestinal symptoms)
- Anemia
- Iron deficiency
- Folate deficiency
- Vitamin-B_{12} deficiency (rare)
- Rickets, osteoporosis, pathological features
- Bleeding disorders
- Edema
- Constipation
- Vomiting
- Recurrent abdominal pain

Celiac crisis is a life-threatening condition characterized by massive diarrhea, severe electrolyte imbalance, dehydration, or shock that needs to be recognized promptly. It can be triggered by severe malnutrition, an infectious process, poor compliance with the GFD, bacterial overgrowth caused by dysmotility, or hypoproteinemia. The patient needs to be admitted into the intensive care unit for further stabilization of electrolytes and fluids. Once the fluid shifts have stabilized the goal is to start parenteral nutrition with total gut rest.[20,24] Slowly, introduction of a GFD with oral supplementation of iron, folic acid, vitamin D, and calcium should be attempted. These patients might require prolonged total parenteral nutrition.[25]

DIFFERENTIAL DIAGNOSIS

In children younger than 18 months, flat villus lesions can have many causes besides GSE. Many gastrointestinal insults can damage surface epithelial cells, resulting in increased epithelial-cell turnover, crypt hypertrophy, abnormal surface epithelial cells, and eventual villus flattening. Other causes of flat villus lesion are listed in Box 268-2.

BOX 268-2 Common Causes of Flat Villus Lesion

- Food sensitivity
- Gluten-sensitive enteropathy
- Cow's milk protein allergy
- Soy protein allergy
- Eosinophilic gastroenteritis
- Infection
- Viruses (rotavirus)
- Bacteria *(Escherichia coli)*
- Parasite *(Giardia lamblia)*
- Fungi *(Candida albicans)*
- Malnutrition (kwashiorkor, not marasmus)
- Tropical sprue
- Immunodeficiency disorders (most notably AIDS)
- Familial enteropathy
- Lymphoma
- Crohn disease
- Whipple disease

For a definitive diagnosis of GSE the following criteria must be met: (1) demonstration of clinical malabsorption and abnormal intestinal lesions, (2) clinical and histologic response to gluten withdrawal, and (3) subsequent gluten challenge that may exacerbate clinical symptoms but that always produces abnormal intestinal histologic findings. The diagnosis must be made with certainty because GSE means lifelong gluten restriction, and untreated patients are at a higher risk for developing gastrointestinal cancer in late adulthood.[26]

Serologic Markers

Serologic markers have emerged as a diagnostic tool and screening test for GSE.[27] These serologic markers include anti-endomysial, anti–serum tissue transglutaminase (tTG), anti-gliadin, and anti-reticulin antibodies. tTG antibodies have been evaluated as being perhaps even more sensitive than endomysial antibodies; therefore, they are suggested as a first step in the screening process. Endomysial (IgA) antibodies have demonstrated the most specificity for the diagnosis of GSE; therefore they should be used as a confirmatory test when the findings of tTG antibody testing are equivocal. These IgA-dependent tests might produce a false-negative result in patients with GSE who are IgA deficient. Anti-gliadin antibodies seem to be less specific and less sensitive than endomysial antibodies, thus they are not suggested for screening.[28-30]

Serum tTG-IgA–based antibodies and serum IgA levels are used together to help diagnose GSE. If the serum IgA level is low or absent, then serum tTG-IgG and endomysial antibody–IgG levels should be considered.[31] Approximately 10% to 15% of patients who have GSE may have negative markers; therefore a negative serologic test does not exclude the diagnosis. False-positive endomysial and tTG antibody tests are unusual.[32] A small-bowel biopsy should be performed to confirm the diagnosis of GSE when serologic markers are positive.

Genetic Markers

The use of genetic markers such as *HLA-DQ2* and *-DQ8* in the screening process is not well clarified. These genetic tests, if negative, exclude the possibility of GSE; however, if positive, and if the patients are asymptomatic and have normal biopsy results, then it presents a diagnostic and management dilemma. These genes are necessary but not sufficient for the development of GSE.[33]

Family Screening

Because GSE is often asymptomatic, screening of family members of patients with confirmed GSE should be undertaken. Approximately 20% of family members may have GSE without being aware of it.[34] The incidence in first-degree relatives is between 1 in 18 to 22; for second-degree relatives the incidence is 1 in 24 to 39.[35,36] Parents and siblings should have serum tTG antibody screening and, if necessary, serum endomysial antibodies as a confirmatory screening test. In the IgA-deficient groups, tTG-IgG and endomysial antibody–IgG serologic markers should be assessed.[19] If these tests are positive, then small-bowel biopsies should be performed.

Associated Diseases

Several diseases associated with an increased incidence of GSE include type 1 diabetes; IgA deficiency; Down, Turner, and Williams syndromes; and autoimmune thyroiditis. These patients may be assessed for GSE with serum tTG antibody testing or *HLA-DQ2* and *-DQ8* genetic screening, or both.[36,37]

EVALUATION

Before GSE is diagnosed in childhood a sweat test should be performed to exclude cystic fibrosis, the most common cause of malabsorption in childhood. Sometimes these two disorders coexist. Tests are discussed in detail in Chapter 169, Diarrhea and Steatorrhea.

Laboratory Evaluation

Anemia is common in GSE and usually occurs as a result of iron, folate, or vitamin-B_{12} malabsorption. Hypoprothrombinemia may occur as a result of vitamin-K malabsorption. Because protein-losing enteropathy may occur in patients with GSE, serum albumin and globulin levels should be measured. Electrolyte disturbances, especially hypokalemia, are common; calcium, phosphorus, and alkaline phosphatase levels may be abnormal in patients with rickets. The radiographic findings in GSE, which are nonspecific (Figure 268-4), include distended small intestine and segmented barium as a result of hypersecretion of intestinal fluid.

Intestinal Biopsy

Biopsy of the small intestine is the best way to diagnose GSE. Previously, blind biopsies were performed with either the Crosby capsule or the Quinton-Rubin pediatric suction tube. Currently, biopsy specimens are routinely obtained by fiberoptic endoscopy to establish this diagnosis, and adequate tissue can be obtained by this technique. Endoscopy also permits visualization of the duodenum. Scalloping of the small intestinal valvulae of Kerckring has been described as pathognomonic for GSE on endoscopy (Figure 268-5).[38] In young infants this appearance may be harder to visualize, but in this patient population, edema of the duodenal mucosa is more common.

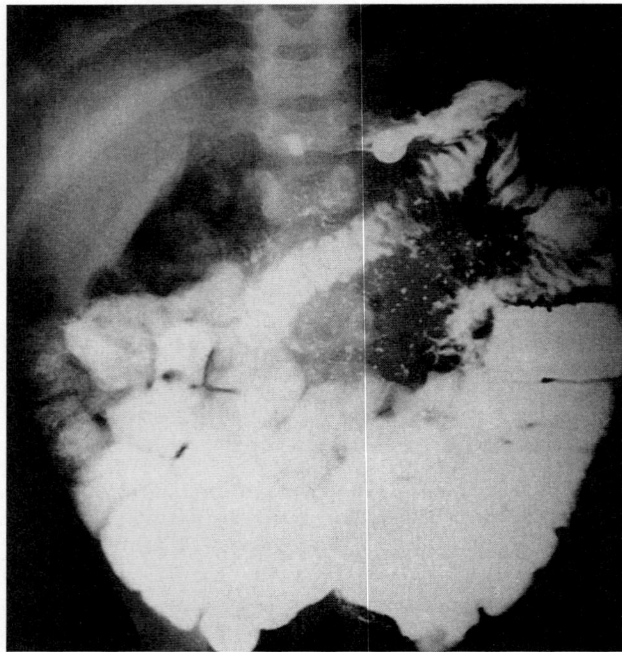

Figure 268-4 Small-bowel follow-through of child with growth failure showing mild dilation of loops of small bowel, some dilution of barium distally, and mild flocculation. Duodenal biopsy revealed typical gluten-sensitive enteropathy (celiac sprue). Patient responded to a gluten-free diet.

In the past, authorities recommended that after 1 or 2 years of a GFD, intestinal biopsies should be repeated to demonstrate complete recovery of the intestinal mucosa.[39] A rechallenge with gluten was then initiated to initiate mucosal damage, which would be reassessed by intestinal biopsy. However, the recommendations for children older than 2 years have changed.[39] Currently, repeat biopsy and rechallenge are not necessary if the child has become asymptomatic on a GFD. Instead, monitoring serum tTG or endomysial antibodies (or both) is the preferred method. In contrast, for children younger than 2 years, other conditions can lead to the same mucosal injury. Therefore they should undergo another biopsy to demonstrate healing then undergo rechallenge and another biopsy. The same approach is suggested in children with an indeterminate diagnosis.[36]

MANAGEMENT

The treatment of GSE is complete withdrawal of gluten from the diet, particularly exclusion of wheat, rye, and barley. Nutrition counseling by a qualified dietician is an important component in the treatment of such patients. GFDs and recipes should be given to all patients or their parents.[40,41] Although oats may be eaten by children with GSE because oats do not contain gluten,[42] they may be cross-contaminated with gluten during the manufacturing process.[43]

Weeks may be required for symptoms to disappear completely after gluten is withdrawn from the diet; however, subjective improvement occurs within the first few days. In children, apathy is usually the first symptom to be alleviated, followed by progressive improvement in muscle tone, a decrease in abdominal distention, and improvement of diarrhea. Disaccharidase activity is markedly depressed in GSE; thus a lactose-free diet is advocated during the initial 4 to

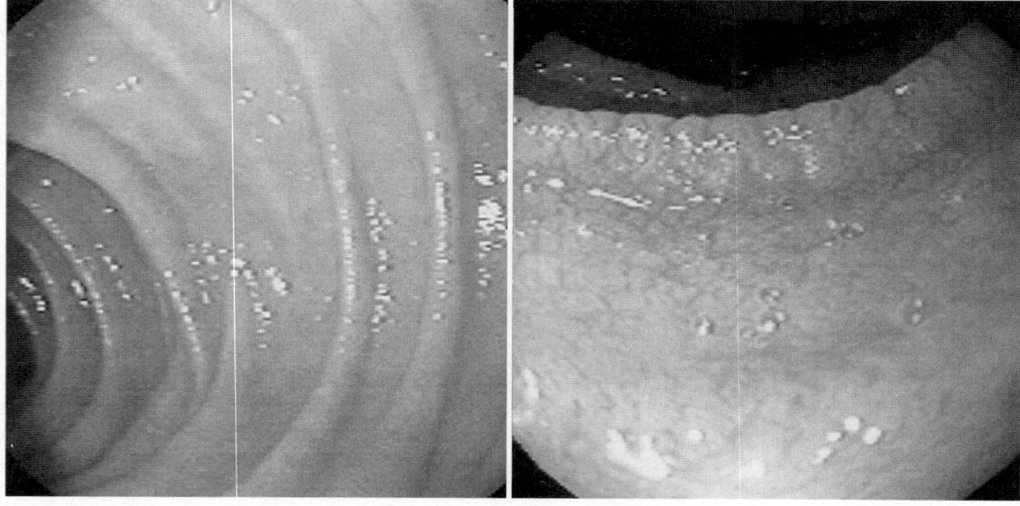

Figure 268-5 Results of endoscopy showing scalloping of the small intestinal valvulae of Kerckring, a pathognomonic finding for gluten-sensitive enteropathy (celiac sprue).

6 weeks of therapy to alleviate the diarrhea. Lactose may then be gradually reintroduced, provided no concurrent infection, severe electrolyte imbalance, dehydration, or shock (the so-called celiac crisis) occurs.

Despite good compliance with a GFD an estimated prevalence of refractory GSE between 7% and 30% of patients exists.[44] These patients are resistant to a GFD and require therapy with immunemodulators.[45] In an adult study, supplementation with pancreatic enzyme therapy has been proposed as beneficial in patients with chronic diarrhea and low fecal elastase, suggesting an exocrine pancreatic insufficiency.[46]

Replacement iron, folic acid, vitamin K, vitamin D, and calcium should be initiated when appropriate. Compliance with a GFD can now be tracked by assessing the patient's serologic markers. An increase in tTG antibody will be observed if the patient does not comply with the diet.[47]

WHEN TO REFER

Referral to a gastroenterologist needs to be made based on the clinical suspicion, the presence of positive serologic markers, first-degree relatives with GSE, syndromic presentations, and existence of other autoimmune disorders.

TOOLS FOR PRACTICE

Engaging Patient and Family

- *Celiac Disease* (fact sheet), National Digestive Diseases Information Clearinghouse (NDDIC), a service of the National Institute of Diabetes and Digestive and Kidney Diseases (NIDDK), National Institutes of Health (digestive.niddk.nih.gov/ddiseases/pubs/celiac/).

Medical Decision Support

- *Celiac Disease* (on-line course), American Academy of Pediatrics (www.pedialink.org/cme/_coursefinder).

SUGGESTED RESOURCES

Alper CA, Fleischnick E, Awdeh Z, et al. Extended major histocompatibility complex haplotypes in patients with gluten-sensitive enteropathy. *J Clin Invest.* 1987;79(1):251.

Misra S, Ament ME. Diagnosis of coeliac sprue in 1994. *Gastroenterol Clin North Am.* 1995;24(1):133-143.

Simell S, Kupila A, Hoppu S, et al. Natural history of transglutaminase autoantibodies and mucosal changes in children carrying HLA-conferred celiac disease susceptibility. *Scand J Gastroenterol.* 2005;40(10):1182-1191.

Visakorpi JK, Mäki M. Changing clinical features of coeliac disease. *Acta Paediatr Suppl.* 1994;83(395):10-13.

REFERENCES

1. Gee S. On the coeliac affection. *St Bartholomews Hosp Rep.* 1888;24:17-20.
2. Dicke WK. *Coeliakie.* [PhD thesis.] Utrecht, Netherlands: University of Utrecht; 1950.
3. Weijers HA, Lindquist B, Anderson CM, et al. Round table discussion: diagnostic criteria in coeliac disease. *Acta Paediatr Scand.* 1970;59:461-463.
4. Seah PP, Fry L, Hoffbrand AV, et al. Tissue antibodies in dermatitis herpetiformis and adult celiac disease. *Lancet.* 1971;1(7704):834-836.
5. Accomando S, Cataldo F. The global village of celiac disease. *Dig Liver Dis.* 2004;36(4):492-498.
6. Mearin ML, Ivarsson A, Dickey W. Coeliac disease: is it time for mass screening? *Best Pract Res Clin Gastroenterol.* 2005;19(3):441-452.
7. Shahbazkhani B, Malekzadeh R, Sotoudeh M, et al. High prevalence of coeliac disease in apparently healthy Iranian blood donors. *Eur J Gastroenterol Hepatol.* 2003;15(5):475-478.
8. Visakorpi JK. Changing features of celiac disease. Proceedings of Seventh International Symposium on Coeliac Disease. Coeliac Disease Study Group. Tampere, Finland: University of Tampere; 1997.
9. Visakorpi JK, Mäki M. Changing clinical features of coeliac disease. *Acta Paediatr Suppl.* 1994;83(395):10-13.
10. Katz AJ, Falchuk ZM. Current concepts in gluten-sensitive enteropathy (celiac sprue). *Pediatr Clin North Am.* 1975;22(4):767-785.
11. Drut R, Drut RM. Lymphocytic gastritis in pediatric celiac disease—immunohistochemical study of the intraepithelial lymphocytic component. *Med Sci Monit.* 2004;10(1):CR38-CR42.
12. Freeman HJ. Collagenous colitis as the presenting feature of biopsy-defined celiac disease. *J Clin Gastroenterol.* 2004;38(8):664-668.
13. Liu E, Rewers M, Eisenbarth GS. Genetic testing: who should do the testing and what is the role of genetic testing in the setting of celiac disease? *Gastroenterology.* 2005;128(4 suppl 1):S33-S37.
14. Murdock AM, Johnston SD. Diagnostic criteria for coeliac disease: time for change? *Eur J Gastroenterol Hepatol.* 2005;17(1):41-43.
15. van Heel DA, Hunt K, Greco L, et al. Genetics in coeliac disease. *Best Pract Res Clin Gastroenterol.* 2005;19(3):323-339.
16. Shan L, Molberg O, Parrot I, et al. Structural basis for gluten intolerance in celiac sprue. *Science.* 2002;297(5590):2275-2279.
17. Strober W, Falchuk ZM, Rogentine GN, et al. The pathogenesis of gluten-sensitive enteropathy. *Ann Intern Med.* 1975;83(2):242-256.
18. Unsworth DJ, Brown DL. Serological screening suggests that adult coeliac disease is underdiagnosed in the UK and increases the incidence by up to 12%. *Gut.* 1994;35(1):61-64.
19. Calabuig M, Torregosa R, Polo P, et al. Serological markers and celiac disease: a new diagnostic approach? *J Pediatr Gastroenterol Nutr.* 1990;10(4):435-442.
20. Lloyd-Still JD, Grand RJ, Khaw KT, et al. The use of corticosteroids in celiac crisis. *J Pediatr.* 1972;81(6):1074-1081.
21. Oberhuber G, Schwarzenhofer M, Vogelsang H. In vitro model of the pathogenesis of celiac disease. *Dig Dis.* 1998;16(6):341-344.
22. Gjertsen HA, Sollid LM, Ek J, et al. T cells from the peripheral blood of coeliac disease patients recognize gluten antigens when presented by HLA-DR, -DQ, or -DP molecules. *Scand J Immunol.* 1994;39(6):567-574.
23. Hamilton JR, Lynch MJ, Reilly BJ. Active celiac disease in childhood. Clinical and laboratory findings of forty-two cases. *Q J Med.* 1969;38(150):135-158.
24. Walia A, Thapa BR. Celiac crisis. *Indian Pediatr.* 2005;42(11):1169.
25. O'Mahony S, Howdle PD, Losowsky MS. Review article: management of patients with non-responsive coeliac disease. *Aliment Pharmacol Ther.* 1996;10(5):671-680.
26. Catassi C, Bearzi I, Holmes GK. Association of celiac disease and intestinal lymphomas and other cancers. *Gastroenterology.* 2005;128(4 suppl 1):S79-S86.

27. Caffrey C, Hitman GA, Niven MJ, et al. HLA-DP and celiac disease: family and population studies. *Gut.* 1990; 31(16):663-667.
28. Fraser JS, King AL, Ellis HJ, et al. An algorithm for family screening for coeliac disease. *World J Gastroenterol.* 2006;12(48):7805-7809.
29. Troncone R, Maurano F, Rossi M, et al. IgA antibodies to tissue transglutaminase: an effective diagnostic test for celiac disease. *J Pediatr.* 1999;134(2):166-171.
30. Vitoria JC, Arrieta A, Arranz C, et al. Antibodies to gliadin, endomysium, and tissue transglutaminase for the diagnosis of celiac disease. *J Pediatr Gastroenterol Nutr.* 1999;29(5):571-574.
31. Cataldo F, Marino V, Bottaro G, et al. Celiac disease and selective immunoglobulin A deficiency. *J Pediatr.* 1997; 131(2):306-308.
32. Carroccio A, Di Prima L, Pirrone G, et al. Anti-transglutaminase antibody assay of the culture medium of intestinal biopsy specimens can improve the accuracy of celiac disease diagnosis. *Clin Chem.* 2006;52(16):1175-1180.
33. Green PH, Jabri B. Celiac disease. *Annu Rev Med.* 2006; 57:207-221.
34. Polvi A, Eland C, Koskimies S, et al. HLA DQ and DP on Finnish families in celiac disease. *Eur J. Immunogenet.* 1996;23(3):221-234.
35. Korponay-Szabó I, Kovács J, Lörincz M, et al. Families with multiple cases of gluten sensitive enteropathy. *Z Gastroenterol.* 1998;36(7):553-558
36. Book L, Zone J, Neuhausen SL. Prevalence of celiac disease among relatives of sib pairs with celiac disease in U.S. families. *Am J Gastroenterol.* 2003;98(2):377-381.
37. Garcia-Careaga G, Kerner J. Malabsorptive disorders. In: Behrman RE, Kliegman RM, Jenson HB, eds. *Nelson Textbook of Pediatrics.* 17th ed. Philadelphia, PA: WB Saunders; 2004.
38. Carlsson A, Axelsson I, Borulf S, et al. Prevalence of IgA-antigliadin antibodies and IgA-antiendomysium antibodies related to celiac disease in children with Down syndrome. *Pediatrics.* 1998;101(2):272-275.
39. Brocchi E, Corazza GR, Caletti G, et al. Endoscopic demonstration of loss of duodenal folds in the diagnosis of celiac disease. *N Engl J Med.* 1988;319(12):741-744.
40. Working Group of European Society of Paediatric Gastroenterology and Nutrition. Report: revised criteria for diagnosis of celiac disease. *Arch Dis Child.* 1990;65: 909-911.
41. Sheedy CB, Keifeiz N. *Cooking for Your Celiac Child; Dietary Management in Malabsorption Disorders.* New York, NY: Dial Press; 1969.
42. Wood MN. *Gourmet Food on a Wheat-Free Diet.* Springfield, IL: Charles C Thomas; 1967.
43. Högberg L, Laurin P, Fälth-Magnusson K, et al. Oats to children with newly diagnosed coeliac disease: a randomized double blind study. *Gut.* 2004;53(5):649-654.
44. Hernando A, Mujico JR, Juanas D, et al. Confirmation of the cereal type in oat products highly contaminated with gluten. *J Am Diet Assoc.* 2006;106(5):665; discussion 665-666.
45. Ryan BM, Kelleher D. Refractory celiac disease. *Gastroenterology.* 2000;119(1):243-251.
46. Turner SM, Moorghen M, Probert CS. Refractory coeliac disease: remission with infliximab and immunomodulators. *Eur J Gastroenterol Hepatol.* 2005;17(6):667-669.
47. Leeds JS, Hopper AD, Hurlstone DP, et al. Is exocrine pancreatic insufficiency in adult coeliac disease a cause of persisting symptoms? *Aliment Pharmacol Ther.* 2007; 25(3):265-271.

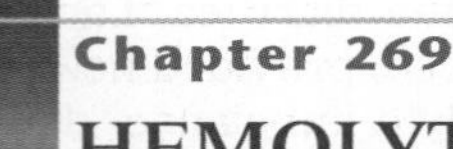

Chapter 269

HEMOLYTIC-UREMIC SYNDROME

Horacio Esteban Adrogué, MD; Horacio A. Repetto, MD

INTRODUCTION

Hemolytic-uremic syndrome (HUS) is a systemic thrombotic microangiopathy with multiple causes. It is characterized by the classic triad of microangiopathic hemolytic anemia, thrombocytopenia, and acute kidney failure. The end result of this pathological process is endothelial lesions leading to thrombosis of the microcirculation in many organ systems (Table 269-1).

HUS is divided into two types depending on whether the patient has had diarrhea. Presence of diarrhea is designated D+ HUS and absence, D− HUS. The most common type of HUS in children is D+, which is caused by toxins from a group of Enterobacteriae, enterohemorrhagic *Escherichia coli* (EHEC). HUS (both D+ and D−) is characterized by the triad of microangiopathic hemolytic anemia thrombocytopenia, and acute kidney failure. The microangiopathy lasts a short time, causing necrotic lesions in the kidney, intestine, central nervous system, pancreas, myocardium, and liver. Although organ damage may leave sequelae, the hemolytic process resolves completely after the acute event.[1]

Clinically, HUS caused by genetic mutations tends to be more severe than HUS caused by the shigatoxin (ST)-producing EHEC (STEC). It also tends to recur and have persistent activity. The long-term course is more severe, leading to chronic renal disease more frequently. In several patients with atypical familial HUS, no gene mutation has been found. Other proteins can be speculated as being involved in C activation or in the coagulation process can be genetically altered.

ETIOLOGY AND PATHOGENESIS

HUS Related to Shigatoxin

The EHECs may have a gene coding for a shigatoxin (ST), named after the toxin produced by *Shigella dysenteriae*. ST is also known as verotoxin, for its capacity to kill vero cells in culture.[2] Another protein that collaborates in the process of generating the disease is intimin (coded by the *eae* gene), which helps in the adherence of the bacteria to the intestinal epithelial cell and its receptor. The receptor named Tir, in turn, promotes the entrance of the ST into the cell, allowing its arrival into the circulation. The toxin is transported (by an unidentified vector) to the surface of endothelial and epithelial cells where it contacts its specific receptor, a lipoprotein called globotriosilceramide (GB3). The ST is then internalized by the union of the B subunit to the receptor. In the cell the A subunit interferes with protein synthesis, leading to cell death. The five B subunits contribute by stimulating apoptosis. This lesion provokes microthrombosis in the arteriolar and capillary circulation and dysfunction in the epithelial cells.[3]

Table 269-1 Hemolytic-Uremic Syndrome Clinical Entities

CLASSIFICATION	CAUSE	CLINICAL MANIFESTATION
Infectious	Bacterial cytotoxin (*E coli, Shigella, Salmonella*) pneumococcal, viral	Epidemic/*classical*/D+ enteropathic
Idiopathic	Endothelial dysfunction? Other regulatory C proteins?	Hereditary (autosomal dominant, autosomal recessive) Sporadic, atypical
Genetic	Factor H, factor I deficiency MCP (CD46) vWF protease ADAMTS 13	Recurrent Recurrent except possibly posttransplant Recurrent
Immunologic	vWF protease antibodies Factor H autoantibodies	TTP
Other	Cancer, pregnancy, malignant hypertension, transplant rejection glomerulonephritis	
Toxic	Cyclosporine, tacrolimus, sirolimus, mitomycin, radiation	

ADAMTS, A disintegrin and metalloproteinase with thrombospondin; *MCP,* membrane cofactor protein; *TTP,* thrombotic thrombocytopenic purpura; *vWF,* von Willebrand factor.

HUS Related to Gene Mutations

Multiple genetic mutations have been found in patients with atypical HUS. Mutations in the complement (C) system activation can cause atypical HUS. One of the regulatory proteins involved is factor H, an alternative pathway–activation inhibitor. This glycoprotein acts as a cofactor to factor I, which cleaves the C3 convertase of the alternative pathway: C3bBb. Its decreased activity has been shown to induce the onset of both atypical HUS and membranoproliferative glomerulonephritis.[4] Inactivation of factor H by antibodies has been described recently in children with atypical HUS.[5] Another protein involved in the complement system is membrane cofactor protein (MCP) or CD46. As opposed to factor H, which circulates in plasma, MCP is found in cell membranes. It aids factor I in the cleavage of C3b and C4b bound to host cells and consequently stops the activation of the complement cascade. MCP deficiency can lead to the onset of atypical HUS.[6]

Another pathogenetic mechanism for atypical HUS depends on the lack of the activity of ADAMTS-13 (a disintegrin and metalloproteinase with thrombospondin-1–like domains). This enzyme cleaves the large multimers of the von Willebrand factor, which can start a generalized thrombotic microangiopathy. Inactivating antibodies against the enzyme have been found in the adult form of thrombotic thrombocytopenic purpura.[7]

EPIDEMIOLOGIC FEATURES

The ST-associated HUS is prevalent in areas of the world with high incidence of gastrointestinal infections by STEC. In Argentina, ST-associated HUS is approximately 10 times more frequent than it is in other locations with high incidence, such as Canada, some Western European countries, and California and Utah in the United States.[1] The incidence of atypical genetic HUS is low; in countries with high incidence of ST HUS, the prevalence of atypical forms is less than 10%.

CLINICAL PICTURE

In the *classical* form, most patients have diarrhea (bloody in two thirds of the cases) accompanied by vomiting and fever. These symptoms usually precede the sudden onset of pallor and severe malaise by several days. At this point, caregivers may notice a decrease in urine output and edema and seek medical attention.

During the acute phase, approximately one third of patients may have involvement of the central nervous system (CNS) presenting a range of symptoms, including change in sensorium (excitement or somnolence), convulsions, and possibly severe coma. Intestinal (generally colonic) necrosis can be severe enough to require surgical intervention. Hyperglycemia caused by pancreatic insufficiency, cardiac involvement, and hepatic failure is rare.

Hypertension occurs in approximately one half of children with HUS and may have either short-term or persistent patterns. Short-term hypertension is caused by volume expansion and improves with salt restriction or dialysis when indicated. Persistent hypertension is generally associated with renal ischemia in the presence of severe lesions.[1]

Laboratory studies reveal low hemoglobin, fragmented erythrocytes (schistocytes) and thrombocytopenia, indicating acute microangiopathic anemia. If a urine sample can be obtained, then signs can be found of glomerular involvement (hematuria with erythrocyte casts) and proteinuria. Elevated levels of serum creatinine and blood urea nitrogen show a decrease in the glomerular filtration rate.[1]

DIFFERENTIAL DIAGNOSIS

The differential diagnosis of HUS is wide and includes thrombotic thrombocytopenic purpura, malignant hypertension, vasculitis, disseminated intravascular coagulation, sepsis, Reye syndrome, intussusception, and renal vein thrombosis. The best differential sign of HUS is microangiopathic anemia with schistocytes in the peripheral smear. Renal ultrasonography shows symmetrical enlargement of both kidneys as compared with patients with renal vein thrombosis in which the kidneys are generally enlarged unilaterally.

MANAGEMENT

Treatment

Treatment for HUS remains almost entirely supportive (Table 269-2). The advent of dialysis and improvements in management of acid-base, electrolyte, and volume disorders in children has significantly improved the outcome of this disease. In fact, the mortality rate has plummeted over the last 40 years from between 40% and 50% to between 3% and 5%.[8] HUS is the most frequent cause of acute kidney injury in children. Given that these patients suffer from a hypercatabolic state, they may develop several conditions requiring aggressive dialysis therapy: (1) hypervolemia leading to hypertension, cardiac failure, pulmonary edema, and encephalopathy; (2) hyperkalemia producing cardiac arrhythmias; (3) severe metabolic acidosis; and (4) hyponatremia (10% may exhibit hypernatremia), which may be associated with volume contraction caused by the preceding diarrhea or may be dilutional caused by oliguanuria.

Antimotility agents, although useful with symptomatic relief of diarrhea, have been shown to increase the risk of toxic megacolon and are contraindicated. This problem should be carefully explained to both patient and parents, thus providing clear reasons why the diarrhea is not being treated. The use of some antibiotics to treat the *E coli* bowel infection has been found to increase the risk of HUS by promoting the release of ST from the bacteria.[9]

Although still controversial, HUS associated with diarrhea does seem to respond to plasma exchange.[10,11] In patients with severe and progressive acute kidney failure and heart failure, plasma exchange might be considered. One useful regimen would be plasma exchange started within 24 hours from presentation and using one volume (40 mL/kg) exchange or more as needed. An important point to remember is that in HUS caused by *Streptococcus pneumoniae* plasma therapy is contraindicated because adult plasma contains antibodies to the Thomsen-Friedenreich antigen and thus may worsen the disease process. The use of angiotensin-converting enzyme inhibitors is recommended in those patients who exhibit persistent proteinuria. Female patients should be advised that these agents are teratogenic, and care should be taken to prevent pregnancy.

Kidney Transplant After Hemolytic-Uremic Syndrome

Kidney transplantation should be considered for patients (approximately 10%-15%) who progress to terminal renal failure after HUS associated with diarrhea. Depending on the availability of a graft, they may require dialysis, or they may get a preemptive transplantation. These children are excellent candidates because of the low likelihood of recurrence of HUS and the fact that patient and graft survival is similar or superior to children who have received transplants for other renal diseases.

For patients who are on dialysis as a result of genetic HUS and who then receive a kidney transplant, the overall 1-year graft survival is less than 30% (vs the expected 95%) because of a 50% recurrence rate of HUS. Results vary depending on the genetic defect.

Patients with factor H mutations have recurrence rates posttransplant of between 30% and 100%, in part, because factor H is made chiefly in the liver. Combined kidney and liver transplants have had mixed success and are not recommended. Factor I mutation patients have a similar circumstance and

Table 269-2 Treatment Strategies for Hemolytic-Uremic Syndrome*

CAUSE	ANTIBIOTICS	ANTIMOTILITY AGENTS	PLASMA EXCHANGE OR PLASMA INFUSION	KIDNEY TRANSPLANT
E Coli associated	Contraindicated	Contraindicated	Not effective	Recommended
S pneumonia	Not known	Not known	Contraindicated	Recommended
Factor H mutation	Not known	Not known	Variable effective Recommended	Contraindicated
Factor I mutation	Not known	Not known	Variable effective Recommended	Contraindicated
MCP mutation	Not known	Not known	Not effective	Insufficient data
ADAMTS 13 mutation	Unrelated	Unrelated	Recommended	Risk of recurrence

*Supportive care is appropriate in all types as needed.
ADAMTS, A disintegrin and metalloproteinase with thrombospondin; *MCP*, membrane cofactor protein.

outcome so they also are not recommended for kidney transplant. ADAMTS-13 deficiency HUS also can recur after transplant.[4,7]

MCP is a protein that is highly expressed in the kidney. While patients with MCP mutations (CD46) have had very good outcomes in the few patients (four) who have been transplanted, more data are required to recommend kidney transplant for patients with MCP mutations.

PROGNOSIS AND SEQUELAE

In STEC HUS, more than 95% of children recover from the acute phase of the illness. Mortality is associated with intercurrent infection or severe neurologic, intestinal, or myocardial complications associated with the more severe patterns of the systemic acute disease. With current methods of management of fluid and electrolyte disorders and hypertension, no patient should die of complications related to acute kidney injury.[1]

The long-term renal course depends on the intensity of the acute injury and the initial destruction of the nephron mass. During the acute phase, the presence and length of the anuria, the need for and duration of dialysis, the presence of persistent hypertension, and the magnitude of the extrarenal involvement (CNS, intestine) are signs associated with an increased risk of residual kidney lesions and progression to chronic renal insufficiency.[1] Children's growth and blood pressure should be closely monitored, and they should be regularly tested for glomerular filtration rate. Proteinuria may remain after all these signs normalize. Persistence of proteinuria for more than 6 months after the acute stage is a risk sign for hyperfiltration caused by the reduced renal mass, leading to progressive kidney fibrosis.[1]

Large groups of patients followed up for more than 3 years after recovery of the acute period have shown that approximately 65% may have normal function, normal blood pressure, and no proteinuria. Another 15% may have persistent proteinuria with or without hypertension but normal creatinine clearance. The remaining 20% will show chronic renal failure of different degrees.[8,12]

Much has been discovered over the last 10 to 15 years about this disease, and the medical community's knowledge can be used to guide the way patients with HUS are treated. Given that both the clinical outcomes and acute and chronic treatment of HUS vary greatly depending on the cause, the effort of searching for the causes and acting accordingly is now more important than ever. The prudent use of intensive care, nephrology, and genetic counseling can make a difference in the outcome of HUS.

WHEN TO REFER

- All patients with HUS should be referred to a nephrologist and other subspecialist as indicated.

WHEN TO ADMIT

- All patients with HUS must be admitted.

TOOLS FOR PRACTICE

Engaging Patient and Family

- *What is a Pediatric Nephrologist?* (fact sheet), American Academy of Pediatrics (www.aap.org/family/WhatisPedNephrologist.pdf).

SUGGESTED RESOURCES

Besbas N, Karpman D, Landau D, et al, from the European Pediatric Research Group for HUS. A classification of hemolytic uremic syndrome and thrombotic thrombocytopenic purpura and related disorders. *Kidney Int.* 2006;70:423-431.

Caprioli J, Peng L, Remuzzi G. The hemolytic uremic syndromes. *Curr Opin Crit Care.* 2005;11:487-492.

Noris M, Remuzzi G. Genetic abnormalities of complement regulators in hemolytic uremic syndrome: how do they affect patient management? *Nature Clin Pract Nephrol.* 2005;1:2-3.

Ruggenenti P, Noris M, Remuzzi G. Thrombotic microangiopathies. In: Brady HR, Wilcox CS, eds. *Therapy in Nephrology and Hypertension: A Companion to Brenner and Rector's The Kidney.* Philadelphia, PA: WB Saunders; 2003.

Siegler R, Oakes R. Hemolytic uremic syndrome; pathogenesis, treatment and outcome. *Curr Opin Pediatr.* 2005;17:200-204.

Siegler RL. Postdiarrheal Shiga toxin-mediated hemolytic uremic syndrome. *JAMA.* 2003;290:1379-1386.

REFERENCES

1. Repetto HA. Epidemic hemolytic-uremic syndrome in children. *Nephrol Forum Kidney Int.* 1997;52:1708-1719.
2. Karmali MA, Steele BT, Petric M, et al. Sporadic cases of hemolytic uremic syndrome associated with fecal cytotoxinand cytotoxin producing E. coli in stools. *Lancet.* 1983;1:619-620.
3. Thorpe CM. Shiga toxin-producing Escherichia coli infection. *Clin Infect Dis.* 2004;38:1298-1303.
4. Taylor CM. Complement factor H and the haemolytic uraemic syndrome. *Lancet.* 2001;358:1200-1202.
5. Dragon-Durey MA, Loirat C, Cloarec S, et al. Anti-factor H autoantibodies associated with atypical hemolytic uremic syndrome. *J Am Soc Nephrol.* 2005;16:555-563.
6. Riley-Vargas RC, Gill DB, Kemper C, et al. CD46: expanding beyond complement regulation. *Trends Immunol.* 2004; 25: 496-503.
7. Wolf G. Not known from ADAMTS-13—novel insights into the pathophysiology of thrombotic microangiopathies. *Nephrol Dial Transpl.* 2004;19:1687-1693.
8. Remuzzi G, Ruggeneti P. The hemolytic uremic syndrome. *Kidney Int.* 1995;47:2-19.
9. Wong CS, Jelacic S, Habeeb RL. The risk of the hemolytic-uremic syndrome after antibiotic treatment of Escherichia coli O157:H7 infections. *N Engl J Med.* 2000;342(26):1930-1936.
10. Lara PN, Coe TL, Zhou H, et al. Improved survival with plasma exchange in patients with thrombotic thrombocytopenic purpura-hemolytic uremic syndrome. *Am J Med.* 1999;107:573-579.
11. Magen D, Oliven A, Schechter Y, et al. Plasmapheresis in a very young infant with atypical hemolytic uremic syndrome. *Pediatr Nephrol.* 2001;16:87-90.
12. Spizzirri FD, Rahman RC, Bibiloni N, et al. Childhood hemolytic syndrome in Argentina: long-term follow up and prognostic features. *Pediatr Nephrol.* 1997;11: 156-160.

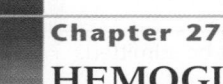

Chapter 270

HEMOGLOBINOPATHIES AND SICKLE CELL DISEASE

Sharada A. Sarnaik, MD; Meera Chitlur, MD

The inherited hemoglobin disorders comprise the most common single-gene defects in humankind. Worldwide the frequency of the carrier state has been estimated to be 270 million, with approximately 400,000 annual births a year of infants with serious hemoglobinopathies. The prevalence of hemoglobinopathies is on the rise worldwide. This prevalence is of special importance in developing countries, where it increases the burden of the health care delivery system. In the United States and other developed countries, hemoglobinopathies remain a concern, particularly among certain ethnic populations.

NORMAL HEMOGLOBIN STRUCTURE

Hemoglobin is a tetrameric protein with four peptide chains, two α or α-like chains and two non-α (or β-like) chains. The molecule is held together by interactions between peptide chains. The amino acids in the globin polypeptide chain are assembled in a long, convoluted knot; lying within the knot is the heme moiety, which carries within it a molecule of oxygen. Its iron is in the Fe^{2+} form, and it does not change its valence with release of oxygen. Abnormalities that result in a change to the ferric form (methemoglobin, or hemoglobin [Hb] M) result in a hemoglobin molecule that is unable to carry oxygen. The α1-β2 interface is an important region for the unique oxygen-carrying function of hemoglobin, and abnormalities in this area will alter its oxygen affinity. The areas of the molecule where the globin chains are in contact with each other or with the heme molecules are functionally important and are evolutionarily highly conserved.

GENETICS OF HEMOGLOBIN SYNTHESIS

The normal hemoglobins are Hb A (96% of the total content), Hb F (1%), and Hb A_2 (3%). Hemoglobin synthesis is directed by controlling genes that are switched on and off at certain stages of human life, resulting in different globin-chain synthesis at different times.

The first globin chains to be produced are the ε chains, which have similar structural sequences to β chains,[1] followed by the production of α, ζ, and γ chains. This production results in the formation of the early fetal hemoglobins such as Hb Gower-2 (α2ε2), Hb Portland (ζ2γ2), and Hb F (α2γ2). At birth, 55% to 65% of total hemoglobin synthesized is Hb F.[1] A switch from γ-chain to β-chain production starts at approximately the ninth gestational week, when Hb A ($\alpha_2\beta_2$), the predominant hemoglobin in adult red blood cells (RBCs), becomes detectable. Fetal hemoglobin synthesis declines but persists until 9 months of age, at which time the switch is complete. (This process also explains why β chain abnormalities do not occur at birth.) A small amount of fetal hemoglobin (1% or less) persists in adults in a small clone of cells called F cells. The switching from Hb F to Hb A is delayed in infants of mothers with diabetes, in infants with metabolic diseases characterized by an inability to metabolize propionic acid, and in infants with chronic bronchopulmonary dysplasia.[1]

A third minor normal hemoglobin seen in adults is Hb A_2 (α_2/δ_2). Normal A_2 levels are 1% to 3%. The importance of Hb A_2 is that it is increased in the β-thalassemias and this helps in the diagnosis.

The genes controlling α-like globin chains are located on chromosome 16, whereas genes for β-like chains are located on chromosome 11. Globin gene expression is under intense research scrutiny because of the therapeutic possibilities of preferentially stimulating Hb F synthesis (by gene manipulation) to ameliorate β-chain disorders.

SCREENING AND GENETIC DIAGNOSIS

The primary reason to screen patients for hemoglobinopathy is to identify their risk of producing offspring with a clinically important disease such as β-thalassemia major, sickle cell disease, or severe α-thalassemia (hydrops fetalis),

Screening can involve a simple test such as a complete blood count while paying attention to the RBC indices. Thalassemias are usually associated with a low mean cell volume (microcytosis) and normal or near-normal mean cell hemoglobin concentration. The hemoglobin concentration may be decreased or normal with a high RBC count. Once simple iron deficiency is ruled out and a hemoglobinopathy is suspected, the next step is to perform a hemoglobin electrophoresis evaluation for levels of Hb A_2 and F, and to assess for the presence of an abnormal hemoglobin, such as Hb C, Hb S, or Hb E.

A prenatal diagnosis of a clinically important hemoglobinopathy can be made by specific tests such as globin chain synthesis ratios or DNA analysis by sampling of fetal blood or the chorionic villus.

CLASSIFICATION OF ABNORMAL HEMOGLOBIN SYNTHESIS

Abnormal hemoglobin synthesis is the result of the production of structurally normal but decreased amounts of globin chains (the thalassemias), production of structurally abnormal globin chains (Hb S, C, E), or failure to switch globin chain synthesis (hereditary persistence of fetal hemoglobin).

Inheritance of all of these disorders is autosomal codominant. *Codominant* is the most accurate term; heterozygosity carries discernible but minor clinical findings.

THALASSEMIAS

In 1925 a severe form of anemia and splenomegaly with characteristic bone changes was described in children of Italian origin.[2] A milder form of the same condition was later described by several Italian investigators. Because all of the cases were reported in

Table 270-1 Classification of the α-Thalassemias

PHENOTYPE	NUMBER OF α GENES	α/β SYNTHETIC RATIO	HAPLOTYPE	GENOTYPE	CLINICAL FEATURES
Normal	4	1.0	α, α	αα/αα	None
Silent carrier	3	0.8	α^+, α	−α/αα	No anemia, normal red blood cell count
Two-gene deletion (α-thalassemia 1)	2	0.6	α^0, α or α^+, α^+	−−/αα or −α /−α	Mild anemia, hypochromia and microcytosis
Hemoglobin H disease	1	0.3	α^0, α^+	−−/−α	Moderate anemia, fragmented cells with hypochromia and microcytosis
Hydrops fetalis	0	0	α^0, α^0	−−/−−	Death in utero due to severe anemia

α^0, no normal α-globin
α^+, globin is reduced

children of Mediterranean origin, the disease was called *thalassemia,* from the Greek word *thalassa,* meaning *sea.*[3] Later, research apparently showed that the first description was of the homozygous or compound heterozygous state for a recessive disorder not confined to the Mediterranean, but rather occurring throughout the tropical countries.[4] The two important forms of this disorder, α- and β-thalassemia, are now recognized as the most common monogenic diseases in humans.

The thalassemias, which are all caused by mutations in the globin gene cluster, result in a genetic decrease in globin chain synthesis. Theoretically, as many types of thalassemias exist as types of globin chains. Practically, the most clinically relevant thalassemias are α- and β-thalassemia. The defects are numerous—more than 200 different mutations have been described—and include deletional or nondeletional mutations. Mutations usually have a geographic and ethnic distribution.

α-THALASSEMIAS

Definitions and Clinical Manifestations

α-Thalassemias are characterized by decreased α-chain synthesis. The most common defect is deletional, although nondeletional defects have been described. The α gene is duplicated, and two α-globin genes per haploid genome are present; thus the abnormality can result from one to four gene deletions. α-Globin gene expression occurs throughout intrauterine life. Hence serious gene mutations can have deleterious effects on fetal development, and death in utero may result. In contrast, deleterious gene mutations in the β-globin chain do not exhibit clinically until several months after birth.[5]

Recently accepted classification of the α-thalassemias is similar to the β-thalassemias: α^0 in which no normal α-globin is produced by the gene and α^+ in which globin product is reduced. When a single gene deletion and three intact genes exist, no abnormality is discernible; this state is known as the silent carrier state. The two-gene deletion results in a minor clinical condition, with mild hypochromic, microcytic anemia, similar to iron deficiency. Deletion of three genes, or Hb H (β-tetramer) disease, results in moderate anemia that is hypochromic and microcytic; hepatosplenomegaly caused by extramedullary hematopoiesis results. Deletion of all four genes is incompatible with life and results in hydrops fetalis or intrauterine death (Table 270-1).

Differential Diagnosis

Routine complete blood count shows hypochromia (mean cell Hb <27 pg), microcytosis (mean cell volume <80 fL), and mild anemia with normal Hb A_2; normal iron stores are seen in the two- and three-gene deletions. Confirmation of decreased α chains is done by globin-chain synthesis measured in reticulocytes, although this is expensive and hard to do. Restriction fragment polymorphism is reserved for prenatal diagnosis. Decreased α chains result in an excess of non-α chains, which are insoluble and form tetramers. These abnormal hemoglobin tetramers can be demonstrated by the presence of RBC inclusions on cresyl blue stain and by hemoglobin electrophoresis. They are rapid moving (faster than Hb A) and require special attention during electrophoresis testing. Hb Bart (γ-tetramers) are found in the first few weeks of life, and Hb H can be found in older patients.

Because the genes for α- and β-thalassemia are on separate chromosomes, they can be coinherited. Coinheritance of α-thalassemia can have beneficial effects on clinical severity on the phenotype of β-thalassemia, as well as the structural hemoglobinopathies, such as sickle cell disease.

Hb H Disease

Patients with Hb H disease have only one functional α-globin gene, often the result of deletion of the three other α-globin genes. Twenty percent of patients have deletion of two genes along with a nondeletional mutation of the third gene.[5] Clinically, Hb H disease is considered a mild disorder. However, a serious drop in hemoglobin can occur with infections or with ingestion of substances that induce oxidant stress.

Additionally, Hb H hydrops fetalis syndrome is a devastating complication associated with the nondeletional forms of Hb H disease.[5] It is associated with similar fetal and maternal complications as Hb Bart hydrops fetalis, including death in utero.

Hb Bart Disease

If both parents carry the α^0-thalassemia mutation in cis (−−/++), then a 25% chance with each pregnancy exists that the offspring will inherit both sets of mutations and therefore lack all four genes for production of α chains. Many of these fetuses survive into the second or third trimester of pregnancy because of persistence of the embryonic ζ chains. The fetus, however, will experience serious consequences, such as anemia and hypoxia with resultant organ and cognitive dysfunction. They invariably die in utero or shortly after birth. It is also associated with life-threatening complications to the mother such as placentomegaly, hypertension and preeclampsia, disseminated intravascular coagulation, and hemorrhage. This syndrome accounts for 90% of all hydrops fetalis in Southeast Asia.[5]

α-Thalassemia is also seen in nontropical populations in association with intellectual disability and is known as α-Thalassemia retardation or ATR. The association demonstrates two unusual features: first, it occurs in racial groups in which α-thalassemia is otherwise rare, and second, the pattern of inheritance is different from that seen in α-thalassemia.[6] This pattern occurs in association with a deletion on chromosome 16 (ATR-16) and in association with the ATR-X syndrome, which results from mutations of the *XH2* gene, located on the long arm of the X chromosome (Xq13.3). This gene regulates α-globin gene expression. The ATR-X syndrome is characterized by the presence of severe intellectual disability, minor facial anomalies, genital anomalies, and a mild form of Hb H disease.

β-Thalassemia

Definitions and Clinical Manifestations

β-Thalassemia is caused by a decrease in production of β-globin chains as a result of mutations in the β-globin gene. Approximately 200 point mutations (or, rarely, deletions) are known to cause this disease. The clinical presentation is variable because the mutations cause a variable impairment of globin synthesis. The β-thalassemias are prevalent throughout the Mediterranean region, Africa, the Middle East, the Indian subcontinent, Burma, Southeast Asia (including the Malay Peninsula), southern China, and Indonesia. The high frequency of occurrence in the tropics reflects a survival advantage of heterozygotes against *Plasmodium falciparum* malaria. Such is also true with α-thalassemia.[7]

Clinical Forms

Inheritance of one gene for β-thalassemia results in β-thalassemia trait (also called thalassemia minor). This condition can be diagnosed by simple screening to assess for microcytosis and a relatively high RBC count. The more severe forms result from homozygosity or compound heterozygosity for the mutant β-globin allele and result in thalassemia major or in thalassemia intermedia. They are characterized by early onset of anemia, characteristic blood changes, and high Hb F. Patients with thalassemia major show clinically in the first year of life and require regular transfusions for survival; those with thalassemia intermedia will exhibit symptoms later in life and will also need transfusions. The anemia in thalassemia intermedia is well compensated and may be exacerbated by infection, folate deficiency, or increasing hypersplenism.[8]

Population screening has been effectively carried out with the naked-eye single-tube RBC osmotic fragility (NESTROFF) technique. Although NESTROFF is not highly specific, it is highly sensitive, with few false-negative findings.[9,10] It is relatively inexpensive and simple and thus is suited for large-scale population screening for thalassemia trait. Information for genetic counseling for couples at risk for offspring with homozygous β-thalassemia may be aided by NESTROFF.

Pathophysiological Features and Clinical Manifestations of Thalassemia Major

Severe β-thalassemia produces clinical features in the first year of life as a result of decline in Hb F synthesis without concomitant increase in Hb A. The decreased β-chain synthesis in this condition results in an excess of α chains, some of which are used for synthesis of other hemoglobins that do not have β chains, such as Hb F ($\alpha 2\gamma 2$) or Hb A_2 ($\alpha 2\delta 2$), which are then increased. Free α chains left over form tetramers, which are insoluble; they accumulate and precipitate within the RBC, leading to increased fragility and cell death. The RBC life span is thus short, and RBCs may be destroyed within the marrow, leading to ineffective erythropoiesis, which is the hallmark of β-thalassemia. The lack of β chains leads to decreased hemoglobin content per cell, hypochromia, and microcytosis. Attempts to increase the RBC mass result in expanded marrow cavities and extramedullary erythropoiesis in the liver and spleen.

Children with thalassemia major exhibit symptoms at approximately 6 months of age with anemia that can be severe and symptomatic. Growth failure, cardiac dysfunction, pallor, jaundice, and hepatosplenomegaly are commonly seen. The bodies of these patients become loaded with iron, even when transfusions are sparingly provided, as a result of increased iron absorption from the diet. Iron toxicity affects the liver (leading to cirrhosis), pituitary (leading to hypogonadism and growth failure), heart (leading to arrhythmia and cardiomyopathy), and bone (leading to pathologic fractures) (Figure 270-1).

Management

Blood transfusions are provided to correct anemia, suppress erythropoiesis, prevent growth failure, and inhibit increased gastrointestinal absorption of iron. Splenectomy is usually performed if transfusion requirements increase caused by hypersplenism folic acid supplementation may be considered to meet its increased requirement. Iron chelation therapy is needed. Deferrioxamine as a daily 8-hour subcutaneous infusion via small portable pumps has been used since 1977 and is well tolerated and extremely effective. The oral iron chelator, deferasirox, has been approved by the US Food and Drug Administration

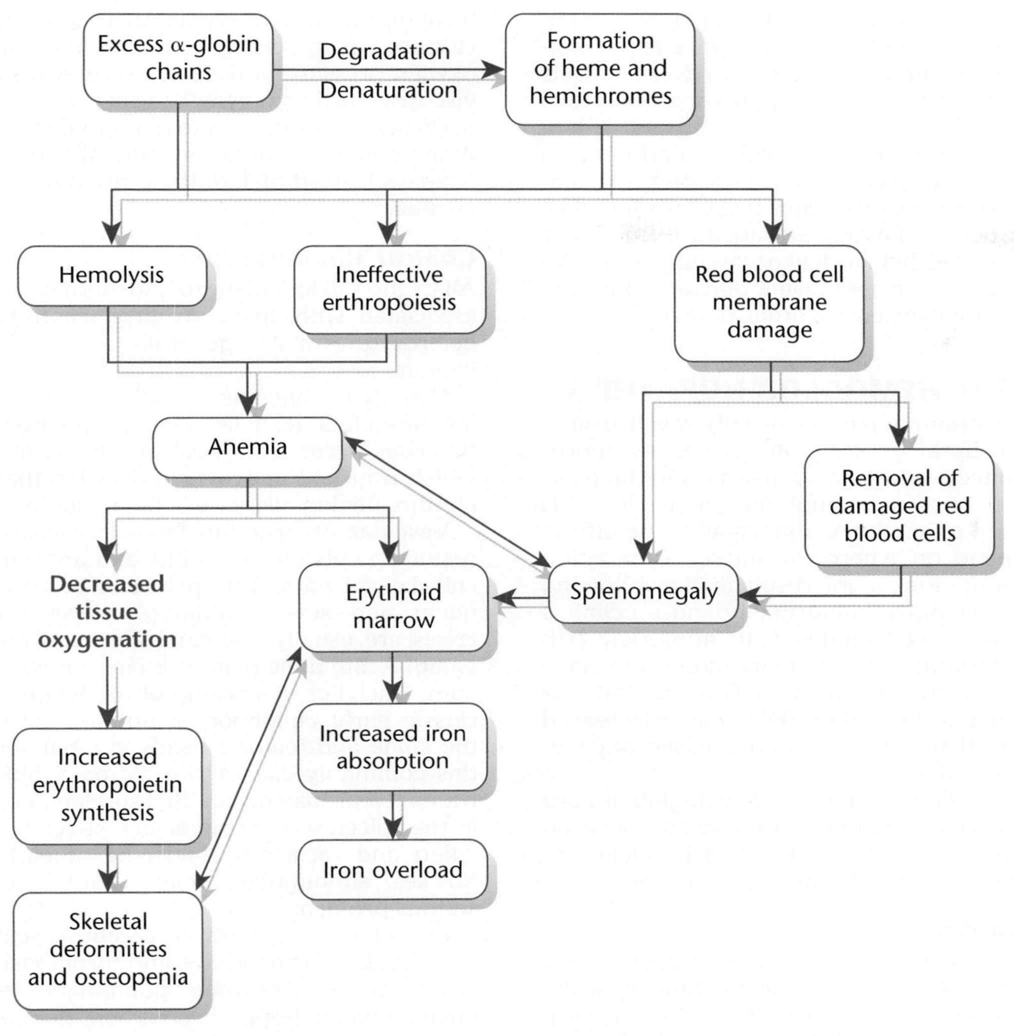

Figure 270-1 Effect of excess free α-globin chain production.

since November 2006. Deferasirox is much less cumbersome for patients and has had similar efficacy as deferrioxamine in preclinical trials. The starting dose is 20 mg/kg once daily as a dispersion in water or orange or apple juice. Highest recommended dose is 30 mg/kg/day. Toxicities affect kidneys with increases over baseline creatinine and proteinuria, and liver with chemical hepatitis or transaminase elevation over baseline. These toxicities usually respond to dose decreases to 10 mg/kg. Pediatric patients with sickle cell disease have low creatinine, and rises in serum creatinine may not reach levels above the normal for age, thus increases of 30% over baseline should prompt dose decreases for such patients. Annual audiologic and ophthalmologic examinations, as well as echocardiographic examinations, are indicated for all chelation regimens. Chelation should be interrupted for serum ferritin levels of 500 ng/mL or less because of increased drug toxicity at low ferritin levels. Another oral chelator, deferiprone, may be used for chelation, although dose-related side effects such as neutropenia, arthropathy, agranulocytosis, and possibly hepatic fibrosis have been reported. This drug is not currently licensed in the United States.[11-13]

Clinically, treatment effectiveness is measured by monitoring the serum ferritin level, even though this method is not the most accurate measure of total body iron stores. Ferritin levels lower than 2500 mg/dL are associated with improved cardiac disease–free survival.[14] Measurement of hepatic iron stores provides a quantitative, specific, and sensitive method for evaluating the body's iron burden, but this requires an invasive liver biopsy. Magnetic susceptometry provides a noninvasive method for measuring hepatic iron stores, but this test is only available in a few centers worldwide.[14]

Hematopoietic stem cell transplantation may be performed in cases in which chronic transfusions and chelation are not possible. Transplantation, if successful, reverses the need for transfusions or chelation therapy, but it carries the risk of serious adverse effects such as graft failure, rejection, graft-versus-host disease, and death. In addition, preexisting and established growth failure, endocrinopathies, and gonadal dysfunction are not reversed. The availability of supportive care after transplantation must also be taken into consideration. In the right setting, the use of either related or unrelated human leukocyte antigen (HLA)-matched donors results in excellent outcomes for low-risk patients, without extensive organ damage.[14]

STRUCTURAL HEMOGLOBINOPATHIES

Structural hemoglobinopathies usually result from a point mutation in the α- or β-globin gene, which produces an erroneous amino acid insertion in the polypeptide chain of the hemoglobin molecule. This action results in a functional abnormality, the effects of which depend on where the missense mutation occurs. The mutation might result in the following effects: no physiological abnormality and no clinical problem, an increased tendency to aggregate (Hb S, Hb C), an instability of the hemoglobin molecule resulting in a hemolytic anemia (Hb Zurich), increased oxygen affinity (Hb Bethesda), decreased oxygen affinity (Hb Kansas), and decreased oxygen-carrying capacity (Hb M).

More than 400 different abnormal hemoglobins have been described to date, but most are rare and cause no clinical disease. Sickle cell disease is a frequent and clinically relevant structural hemoglobinopathy.

Sickling Disorders

Sickling disorders depend on gene interactions. SS, known as sickle cell anemia, indicates homozygosity for the mutant Hb S, which results in no normal β alleles and therefore no Hb A. SC indicates double heterozygosity for two β-chain mutants, Hb S and Hb C, which results in no normal β alleles and therefore no Hb A. Sickle β-thalassemia results from double heterozygosity for Hb S and β-thalassemia. In this disorder, one β gene directs the synthesis of Hb S, and the other is either completely suppressed, and the patient has no Hb A (S β^0-thalassemia) or incompletely suppressed and the patient produces a small amount of Hb A (S β^+-thalassemia). Hb A_2 is increased in these conditions. Finally, SO Arab and SD indicate double heterozygosity for Hb S and Hb O or D, respectively.

In hereditary persistence of fetal Hb with Hb S, a failure to switch from γ- to β-chain synthesis is coinherited with Hb S. Patients have high levels of Hb F. Their clinical symptoms are mild because of the protective effects of Hb F.

Pathophysiological Mechanism of Sickling

In its deoxygenated state, Hb S is extremely insoluble. Polymer formation within the RBC causes a shape change to the sickled form that gives the disease its name. Sickling is accompanied by increased rigidity, loss of deformability, increased adhesiveness to endothelial cells, and RBC membrane damage, all of which adversely affect the flow properties of the RBCs through the microvasculature. This produces vasoocclusion, which sets up a vicious cycle of stasis, low oxygen pressure in tissues, tissue acidosis, increased viscosity, further polymer formation, and more vasoocclusion to complete and perpetuate the cycle. Membrane damage causes the RBC life span to be short (15 days instead of 120 days), resulting in a hemolytic anemia.

Clinical Manifestations

All of the sickling disorders mentioned previously are associated with similar clinical features; the double heterozygous states generally have a milder clinical course.

Hemolytic anemia results in pallor, jaundice, increased fatigue, gallstones, and poor growth. Aplastic crises occur after viral infections, in situations in which transient marrow suppression that results in a life-threatening decrease in hemoglobin levels occurs.

Vascular obstruction from intravascular sickling results in episodic, variable, and unpredictable musculoskeletal pain. This pain can be disabling if frequent and severe, although these so-called pain crises are usually uncomplicated and not life threatening. Acute bone pain or infarction is common at all ages. Dactylitis, a swelling of the hands and feet, is a classic early childhood symptom. Osteonecrosis of the spine and femoral heads is often seen in adults; this commonly causes chronic pain. Splenic sequestration crisis may occur. This sudden pooling of blood in the spleen with hypovolemic shock is a life-threatening and recurrent syndrome of early childhood. Strokes, although uncommon, are a recurrent and serious problem.

In addition, a variety of cerebrovascular catastrophes, such as hemorrhage and thrombosis, can occur. Acute chest syndrome—pulmonary infarction or pneumonia (or both)—is common. Beginning in early childhood, the risk of severe bacterial infections is lifelong, and commonly cause death. This circumstance is the result of a loss of splenic function (autosplenectomy) from recurrent vasoocclusion and fibrosis. Renal manifestations include the loss of urine concentration capacity caused by sickling in vessels around the loop of Henle; large volumes of dilute urine are produced even in young children, underscoring the need for copious fluid intake to avoid dehydration. Other renal problems include hematuria and glomerular nephropathy. Other manifestations of vasoocclusion include priapism, trophic leg ulcers, and blindness.

The disease is extremely variable in its severity. Factors that affect disease severity have not been clearly defined and remain the subject of research. The factors include the presence of genetic markers such as the β-gene haplotype, coinheritance of α-thalassemia (beneficial), and the amount and distribution of Hb F (higher levels are beneficial).

Sickle Cell Trait

Sickle cell trait is a benign carrier state, and most people have no clinical symptoms. The incidence of the trait in blacks varies from 6.7 to 10.1%.[15] Sickle cell trait can cause hematuria and a loss of urine-concentration capacity. Symptoms from intravascular sickling have been reported with strenuous exercise at high altitudes and with flying at high altitudes in unpressurized aircraft.

Diagnosis

The patient's clinical history and physical findings are the first steps in diagnosing sickling disorders. The presence of Hb S is evaluated by the solubility test, which is inexpensive and sensitive to the carrier state. Hemoglobin electrophoresis confirms the exact phenotype. Finally, the presence of hemolytic anemia (low hemoglobin, high reticulocyte counts, increased bilirubin, and lactic dehydrogenase) and morphologic sickling can be assessed by blood smears.

Management

Management consists of symptomatic and supportive care of complications such as treating pain episodes with analgesics (often narcotics), placing local heat packs, ensuring adequate hydration, adjusting the acid-base balance, preventing hypoxia, avoiding exposure to cold, and treating febrile episodes early and aggressively with antibiotics.

Judicious use of blood transfusions will help prevent strokes in children. Blood transfusions will also help correct severe anemia (Hb <5 g/dL, usually with aplastic crisis or splenic sequestration) and are also used for complicated pregnancies.

Management is optimized by early diagnosis with screening of newborns. Routine daily prophylactic penicillin and pneumococcal vaccine are used to prevent the high childhood mortality from infections.

Psychosocial support and self-help groups are important for improved disease adjustment, especially for adults. Pain attacks are often capricious, severe, and frequent. They can be a barrier to self-determination and independent living.

Recent advances have brought research strategies to the bedside. Agents that stimulate fetal hemoglobin production, such as hydroxyurea, may be administered. Peripheral or cord blood stem cell transplantation from an HLA-identical sibling is a high-risk procedure that can be curative. Stem cell transplantation is used for certain individuals with markers for adverse outcome, such as stroke in a young child. Finally, antisickling agents such as membrane-active drugs and gene therapy are approaches of the future.

Rare Structural Hemoglobinopathies

Table 270-2 lists the rare structural hemoglobinopathies and their prototypes.

Table 270-2 Rare Structural Hemoglobinopathies and Their Prototypes

HEMOGLOBINOPATHY	PROTOTYPE
Unstable hemoglobins	Hb Zurich
Hemoglobins with high oxygen affinity	Hb Bethesda
Hemoglobins with low oxygen affinity	Hb Kansas
Hemoglobin M prototype	Hb M Boston

Hb, Hemoglobin.

Unstable Hemoglobins

Unstable hemoglobins usually result from amino acid substitutions near the heme pocket. The instability causes a tendency of the heme to separate from the globin chain with the slightest oxidative stress. The denatured hemoglobin precipitates in the RBC and forms Heinz bodies, which cause the cells to sequester in the spleen, and a hemolytic anemia results.

Diagnosis is by demonstration of a hemolytic anemia, detection of Heinz bodies by staining, and the heat precipitation test. Hemoglobin electrophoresis is not always useful because of the tendency of the hemoglobin to rapidly denature.

Management includes avoiding oxidant drugs, providing transfusions as clinically indicated, and removing the spleen if anemia is severe.

Hemoglobins With High Oxygen Affinity

In hemoglobins with high oxygen affinity, the amino acid substitution is near the α1-β2 interface, resulting in a tight binding of oxygen. Release of oxygen to tissues is slow, resulting in inefficient tissue oxygenation. The end result is increased hemoglobin production caused by high erythropoietin levels.

Diagnosis is made by the presence of familial erythrocytosis (polycythemia), exclusion of other causes of polycythemia (eg, polycythemia vera, cyanotic heart disease), high RBC mass, high arterial oxygen saturation, and a markedly left-shifted oxygen dissociation curve.

Management consists of maintaining hematocrit levels to 70% by phlebotomy to prevent high viscosity.

Hemoglobins With Low Oxygen Affinity

In hemoglobins with low oxygen affinity, the amino acid substitution is also near the α1-β2 interface. The hemoglobin picks up oxygen poorly from the lungs, and high deoxyhemoglobin levels result, causing cyanosis.

Diagnosis is made by the oxygen-dissociation curve, which is right shifted. The hemoglobin level and RBC mass are normal.

No specific management is necessary or effective. The cyanosis is relatively well tolerated if strenuous activities are avoided.

Hb M

In Hb M, the amino acid substitution is near the heme pocket, close to the site of the iron (Fe) molecule. The mutant hemoglobin loses its ability to keep the Fe in its ferrous state, and the hemoglobin is constantly in the methemoglobin state, Fe^{3+}, and is unable to carry oxygen. Chronic cyanosis results.

Diagnosis is made by history of cyanosis since birth, with a normal oxygen saturation; by brown discoloration of freshly drawn blood, which does not change with aeration; and by spectrophotometry to confirm presence of methemoglobin. Electrophoresis also demonstrates the abnormal hemoglobin.

No management is needed because the amount of Hb M is insufficient to cause physiological derangements.

Hb C, D, and E

Structural variant hemoglobins are synthesized at a lower rate than normal β chains and comprise less than one half the total hemoglobin in heterozygotes. Heterozygous Hb C (AC) results in mild target cells but no anemia. Homozygous C (CC) produces a mild hemolytic anemia, marked RBC morphologic changes (target cells, hemoglobin crystals, and microspherocytes), and mild splenomegaly. Heterozygous E (AE) causes a mild thalassemic phenotype with mild microcytosis and hypochromia. Homozygous E (EE) results in a moderate thalassemic phenotype, with hypochromia, microcytosis, and mild anemia. A combined E- and β-thalassemia inheritance results in a transfusion-dependent thalassemic phenotype. Hb E is common in Southeast Asia and in certain areas of the Indian subcontinent.

TECHNOLOGICAL ADVANCES

Reproductive Options for Carriers of Hemoglobinopathy

Premarital screening and genetic counseling are easy and inexpensive, and they are good ways to provide reproductive options for couples at risk for having children with hemoglobinopathies. Nondirective genetic counseling should be provided and targeted to populations with a high prevalence of the hemoglobinopathy traits.

Prenatal diagnosis can be performed by chorionic villus sampling. Challenges include technical difficulties of the various methods used, as well as their expense. Furthermore, for safety and effectiveness, women with at-risk pregnancies must be assessed for prenatal diagnosis, ideally in the first trimester (8-14 weeks' gestation). This process requires awareness in communities with a high prevalence of the genetic defect. The choice of therapeutic abortion for involved pregnancies can be difficult depending on cultural and religious beliefs. Research studies report a higher acceptance of prenatal diagnosis if another child is affected.

Preconception diagnosis and implantation of normal embryos after in vitro fertilization is an alternative that is currently available in the West. It is extremely expensive and cannot be performed routinely.

In utero therapy that uses stem cell transplantation is an interesting and potentially exciting technology that would help at-risk couples that do not opt for termination. It allows for the relatively nonimmunocompetent fetus to accept the stem cell transplant more easily without experiencing graft rejection and graft-versus-host disease. This therapy is currently in early research trials.

Improvements in Transfusion Safety

The mainstay of care of patients with hemoglobinopathies continues to be blood transfusion support. Transfusion safety is thus an important consideration, particularly the prevention of transfusion-transmitted infections. Donors should be screened for hepatitis B and C, HIV, syphilis, and malaria. Donor screening may sometimes be ineffective because insensitive tests, expired kits and reagents, and improper procedures. Transfusion-transmitted infections remain a risk.[16,17]

Stem Cell Transplantation

Improved techniques of stem cell transplantation that use HLA-matched sibling donors may result in cures for the hemoglobinopathies. An interest exists in non-myeloablative or reduced intersity myeloablative stem cell transplantation, which has reduced morbidity but leads to a chimerism in the recipient. This procedure is still investigational.

Simple awareness of genetic diseases, as well as education and counseling of families at risk, although low-tech, are crucial in avoiding the burden of these diseases, both to individuals and to society.

WHEN TO REFER

- Initial and routine annual or biannual evaluation
- Serious complications such as stroke, splenic sequestration, recurrent acute chest syndrome
- Care during pregnancy

WHEN TO ADMIT

- Anemic crisis (Hb <5 g/dL)
- Sudden splenic enlargement
- Pain not responding to home and narcotics
- Difficulty in breathing, chest, pain
- High fever spikes (>38°C core)
- Any central nervous system symptoms

TOOLS FOR PRACTICE

Engaging Patient and Family

- *Sickle Cell Disease* (fact sheet), American Academy of Pediatrics (www.medicalhomeinfo.org/health/SickleCell/Fact Sheets/Gen_SCD.pdf).

Medical Decision Support

- *Sickle Cell Resource Kit* (Web page), American Academy of Pediatrics (www.medicalhomeinfo.org/health/SCD index.html).

RELATED WEB SITES

Centers for Disease Control and Prevention: Sickle Cell Disease (www.cdc.gov/ncbddd/sicklecell/).

Centers for Disease Control and Prevention: Thalassemia (www.cdc.gov/ncbddd/hbd/thalassemia.htm).

Sickle Cell Disease Association of America (www.sicklecell disease.org/index.phtml).

US Department of Health and Human Services, National Heart, Blood and Lung Institute (www.nhlbi.nih.gov/index.htm).

AAP POLICY STATEMENTS

American Academy of Pediatrics, Section on Hematology/Oncology and Committee on Genetics. Health supervision for children with sickle cell disease. *Pediatrics*. 2002;109(3):526-535. (aappolicy.aappublications.org/cgi/content/full/pediatrics;109/3/526).

Kaye CI, American Academy of Pediatrics, Committee on Genetics. Introduction to the newborn screening fact sheets. *Pediatrics*. 2006;118(3):1304-1312. (pediatrics.aappublications.org/cgi/content/full/118/3/1304).

REFERENCES

1. Nathan DG, Ginsburg D, Thomas Look A, eds. *Nathan and Oski's Hematology of Infancy and Childhood*. 6th ed. Vol 1. Philadelphia, PA: WB Saunders; 2003.
2. Cooley TB. A series of cases of splenomegaly in children with anemia and peculiar bone changes. *Trans Am Pediatr Soc*. 1925;37:29-30.
3. Whipple GH, Bradford WL. Mediterranean disease—thalassemia (erythroblastic anemia of Cooley): associated pigment abnormalities simulating hemochromatosis. *J Pediatr*. 1936;9:279-311.
4. Olivieri N. The β-thalassemias. *N Engl J Med*. 1999;341(2):99-109.
5. Chui DH. Alpha-thalassemia: Hb H disease and Hb Barts hydrops fetalis. *Ann N Y Acad Sci*. 2005;1054:25-32.
6. Gibbons RJ, Suthers GK, Wilkie AO, et al. X-linked alpha-thalassemia/mental retardation (ATR-X) syndrome: localization to Xq12-q21.31 by X inactivation and linkage analysis. *Am J Hum Genet*. 1992;51:1136-1149.
7. Williams TN. Human red blood cell polymorphisms and malaria. *Curr Opin Microbiol*. 2006;9:388-394.
8. Olivieri NF. The beta-thalassemias. *N Engl J Med*. 1999;341:99-109.
9. Mehta BC. NESTROFT: a screening test for beta thalassemia trait. *Indian J Med Sci*. 2002;11:537-545.
10. Bobhate SK, Gaikwad ST, Bhaledrao T. NESTROFF as a screening test for detection of beta-thalassemia trait. *Indian J Pathol Microbiol*. 2002;45:265-267.
11. Rund D, Rachmilewitz E. Beta-thalassemia. *N Engl J Med*. 2005;353:1135-1146.
12. Franchini M, Veneri D. Iron-chelation therapy: an update. *Hematol J*. 2004;5:287-292.
13. Olivieri NF, Brittenham GM, McLaren CE, et al. Long-term safety and effectiveness of iron-chelation therapy with deferiprone for thalassemia major. *N Engl J Med*. 1998;339:417-423.
14. Wanless IR, Sweeney G, Dhillon AP, et al. Lack of progressive hepatic fibrosis during long-term therapy with deferiprone in subjects with transfusion-dependent beta-thalassemia. *Blood*. 2002;100:1566-1569.
15. Castro O, Ranas R, Bang KM, et al. Age and prevalence of sickle cell trait in a large ambulatory population. *Genet Epidemiol*. 1987;4:307-311.
16. Singh H, Pradhan M, Singh RL, et al. High frequency of hepatitis B virus infection in patients with beta-thalassemia receiving multiple transfusions. *Vox Sang*. 2003;84:292-299.
17. Marwaha RK, Bansal D, Sharma S, et al. Seroprevalence of hepatitis C and B virus in multiply transfused beta-thalassemics: results from a thalassemic day care unit in north India. *Vox Sang*. 2003;85:119-120.

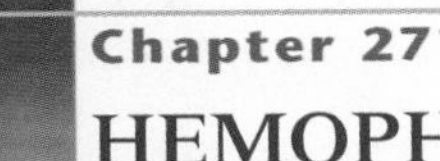

Chapter 271

HEMOPHILIA AND OTHER HEREDITARY BLEEDING DISORDERS

Eva G. Radel, MD

Hemostasis requires adhesion of platelets to an injured vascular endothelium, aggregation of additional platelets with formation of a platelet plug, activation of coagulation factors resulting in a coagulation cascade, and, finally, formation of a fibrin clot that interacts with the platelet aggregate to form a stable hemostatic seal. The coagulation factors exist in the blood mostly as precursors that become activated to become enzymes or cofactors and, in turn, activate other clotting factors. Also involved are anticoagulants, fibrinolysins, and inhibitors; all of these agents form a complex, delicate, autoregulated system.

EVALUATION TO DETECT ABNORMALITIES OF HEMOSTASIS

The most useful screening tests to study the hemostatic and coagulation mechanisms are partial thromboplastin time or activated partial thromboplastin time (aPTT), which is a modern form of this test, and prothrombin time (PT). PT alone is not adequate for screening children for coagulation disorders because it misses the most common congenital deficiencies. Falsely prolonged clotting tests may result from an insufficient amount of blood in the specimen tube or difficulty accessing the vein with release of tissue factor and consumption of coagulation factors. The tests are sensitive to clotting factor levels less than 30% to 40% of normal. A prolonged aPTT or PT must be followed by the performance of individual clotting factor assays. If both test results indicate prolonged times, then abnormal liver function or vitamin K deficiency with multiple reduced factors should be considered; a thrombin time should also be performed to look for abnormalities of fibrinogen or possible interference by heparin, and if this test is abnormal, then a reptilase time, which is not sensitive to heparin, can be performed. Disseminated intravascular coagulation or an inhibitor, such as a lupus anticoagulant, must also be considered; the latter can be ruled out by performing a *mixing aPTT* to see if the patient's plasma prolongs the clotting time of normal plasma. Lupus anticoagulant is associated with thrombosis, however, and not with bleeding. Factor XIII deficiency will not be detected with these previously mentioned tests. A much-simplified schema of the coagulation pathway and the tests that are used to study it are depicted in Figure 271-1. The normal activity (100%) of a clotting factor is defined arbitrarily as 1 unit/mL of plasma; the normal range of activity for different factors is from approximately 50% to 200%. The bleeding time, which is a useful screening test for von Willebrand disease, as well as for acquired and congenital abnormalities of platelet function, is difficult to standardize, and assessment in an uncooperative child is difficult. In many centers, the Platelet Function Analyzer (PFA)-100, a screening test using a commercially available instrument, which is more sensitive and reproducible, has replaced the test for bleeding time.[1]

HEMOPHILIA A AND B

Although factors VIII and IX are entirely different molecules that act in different ways in the coagulation cascade, their sex-linked inheritance and the clinical manifestations of their deficiencies are identical. The incidence of hemophilia is approximately 1 in 5000 male patients, with 80% to 85% being hemophilia A (classic hemophilia, congenital factor VIII deficiency) and 10% to 15% hemophilia B (Christmas disease,

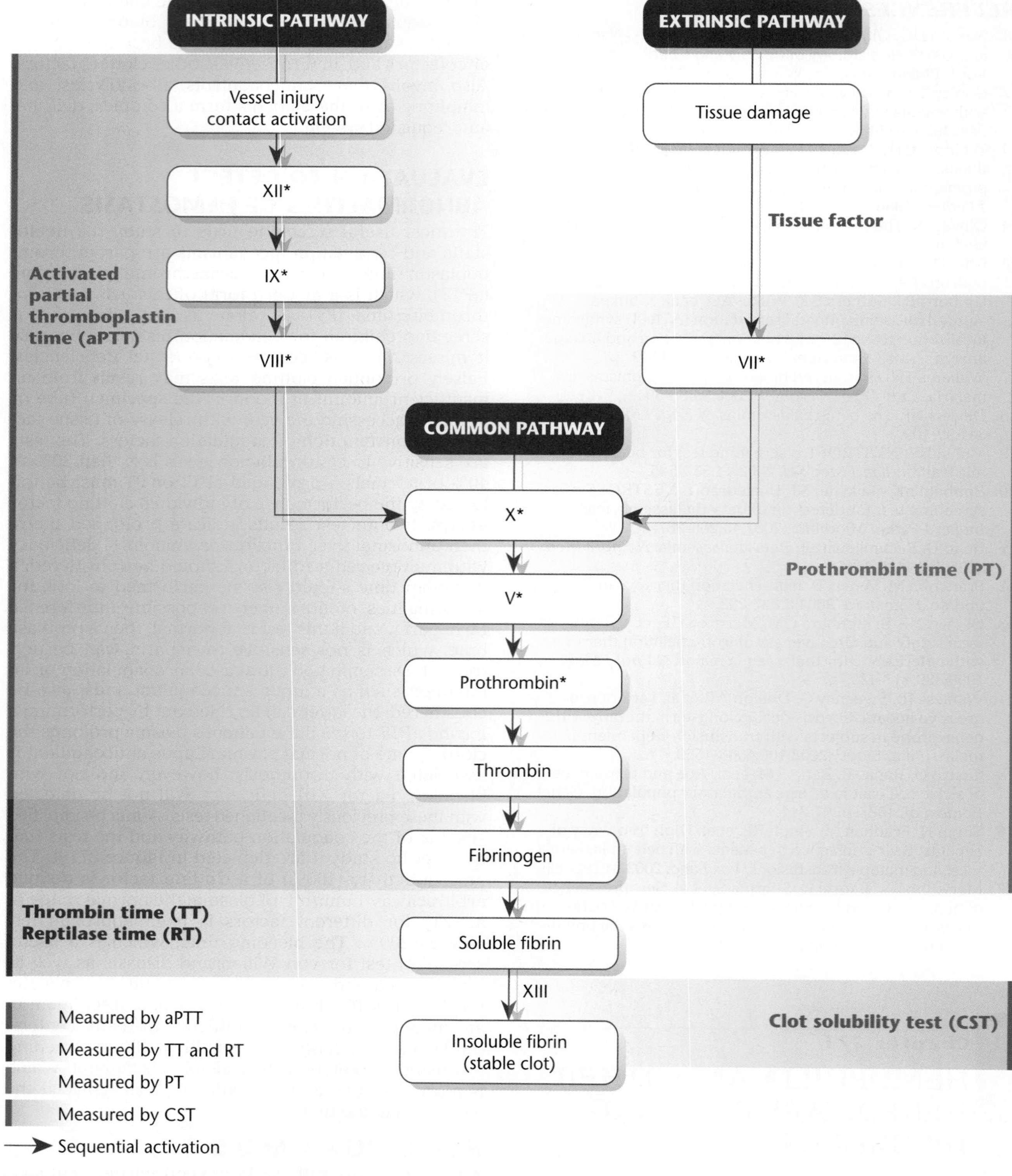

Figure 271-1 Coagulation cascade and tests to study its components. *Factors become activated and, in turn, propagate the cascade.

congenital factor IX deficiency).[2] A family history is present in approximately two thirds of cases.

DIAGNOSIS

The diagnosis can be suspected based on family and personal history, and laboratory tests will identify the deficiency. Severe hemophilia accounts for 80% of cases and is defined by a factor VIII or IX level of less than 1%. Levels above 5% are associated with mild disease, and intermediate levels are associated with moderate disease. Severe disease is characterized by hemarthroses and hematoma formation with minimal or no apparent trauma. Mild disease results in bleeding only with trauma. The factor VIII and factor IX genes have both been cloned, and many different mutations have been found in both conditions.[3,4] In most families, diagnosing hemophilia prenatally is now possible by chorionic villus biopsy or amniocentesis.

Bleeding Manifestations

Hemarthrosis

Recurrent bleeding into joints is the most frequent clinical problem for patients who have severe hemophilia. The knees, ankles, and elbows are involved most often. Many patients have one particular target joint in which recurrent episodes occur and in which chronic changes are most likely to result. Synovial thickening and vascular friability may develop, resulting in increased susceptibility to bleeding, leading to a vicious cycle. Synovitis accompanied by chronic effusion often develops and may progress to joint destruction (hemophilic arthropathy) and severe disability.[5] With prompt, adequate treatment or prevention of bleeding, the incidence of these complications is significantly decreased.

Hemarthrosis must be treated as soon as pain, tingling, or limping begins, even if evidence of swelling is not visible. If marked swelling is present, then the joint should be aspirated and immobilized after factor replacement (Table 271-1). Watchful waiting is not appropriate for the child who has hemophilia. Early synovitis should be managed by providing factor VIII or IX prophylactically for several weeks, often along with a short course of corticosteroids. Synovectomy may be effective if medical management fails, and may be accomplished by arthroscopy, even in young children.[6] Intensive physical therapy is required in conjunction with the procedure. Radiosynovectomy is a simpler procedure, requiring less factor replacement and physical therapy. Although this procedure has been performed in young children with good joint outcomes,[7] some concern exists about the possibility of inducing malignancy and interfering with growth.

Soft-Tissue Bleeding

Superficial hematomas, unless very large, do not often require treatment. However, bleeding into muscles or closed soft-tissue compartments may result in nerve or vascular compression, muscle fibrosis, and contractures; such bleeding may be difficult to diagnose because swelling is often minimal. Bleeding into the iliopsoas muscle may cause femoral nerve damage, and it must be considered whenever pain occurs in the lower abdomen, hip, or groin. Limping and flexion of the hip are often the only positive findings. Sonography or a computed tomographic (CT) scan may help in making the diagnosis. Calf bleeding may result in peroneal nerve damage. Bleeding into the thigh may cause accumulation of a large amount of blood without much external change and may result in significant anemia.

Life-Threatening Bleeding

Intracranial bleeding can occur after trauma but also appears to occur spontaneously. All but the most minor head injury must be considered to be significant and treated promptly. A CT scan should always be obtained to evaluate the presence or extent of bleeding. Airway compromise must be considered a potential threat with any hematoma of the neck or the submental or sublingual areas, as well as the retropharyngeal or parapharyngeal regions; a severe sore throat or dysphagia also suggests bleeding and should be evaluated and treated immediately. Retroperitoneal bleeding may be massive before it can be detected and must be considered when abdominal or groin pain is present. In all of these situations, CT or magnetic resonance imaging may be helpful in evaluating the patient.

Mouth Bleeding

The lip, tongue, and frenulum are areas of frequent trauma in young children. Factor replacement should be accompanied by the use of ε-aminocaproic acid or tranexamic acid to prevent fibrinolysis of the clot, although these drugs must be used cautiously in patients receiving prothrombin complex or any activated coagulation factors, because the combination can lead to thrombosis or disseminated intravascular coagulation (DIC).

Hematuria

Hematuria must be evaluated with noninvasive procedures, as in the normal individual, to rule out intrinsic renal disease. It usually resolves spontaneously with or without factor replacement, although bed rest and hydration are often suggested. Corticosteroid therapy is controversial. Fibrinolytic agents should be avoided, unless the bleeding is known to originate in the lower urinary tract, because they can result in obstruction of the renal pelvis by clot formation.[8]

GENERAL PRINCIPLES OF TREATMENT

Ideal management of patients who have hemophilia is in a comprehensive center where all the needs of the patient can be met, including medical, orthopedic, physical rehabilitation, dental, and psychosocial therapies. All elective surgical procedures must be performed in a center that has experienced personnel and immediate availability of blood clotting factor assays and a ready supply of clotting concentrates, and they should be preceded by factor inhibitor testing. Nerve blocks should be avoided. Factor replacement should always be given as promptly as possible when bleeding is suspected, before x-ray examination or other diagnostic studies. A patient who has a severe injury or life-threatening bleeding should be given an immediate dose of the appropriate clotting factor to raise its

Table 271-1 Products Available for Treatment of Coagulation Disorders

PRODUCT	CONTENT	DOSE, CONCENTRATION, SIZE OF UNITS	INDICATIONS, COMMENTS
Fresh-frozen plasma	Whole plasma	5-15 mL/kg; 1 U of each of the coagulation factors/mL; 220 or 600 mL/bag	Multiple factor deficiency; DIC; reversal of Coumadin effect; HUS or TTP; unknown coagulation defect; when no specific concentrate exists; not virus inactivated
Cryoprecipitate	Factor VIII, vWF, factor XIII, fibrinogen, fibronectin	1 U/kg raises factor VIII 2%; 75-100 U factor VIII and vWF/ bag; volume approximately 20 mL; not assayed	Factor XIII deficiency, hypofibrinogenemia; derived from single donor units; not virus inactivated
Factor VIII	Factor VIII	1 U/kg raises factor VIII 2%; preassayed; up to 100 U/mL	Hemophilia A; made by various methods, with different levels of purification; recombinant product available; virus inactivated*
Humate P	Factor VIII, vWF	Preassayed; factor VIII 20-40 U/mL; vWF 50-100 U/mL	Severe vWD; mild to moderate vWD if desmopressin ineffective or inadequate; virus inactivated*
Factor IX	Factor IX	1 U/kg (1.2-1.4 U/kg of recombinant) raises factor IX 1%; preassayed; up to 100 U/mL	Hemophilia B; recombinant product available; virus inactivated*
Prothrombin complex	Factor II, VII, IX, X	Preassayed for factor IX; content of other factors varies among products	Hemophilia B when purified factor IX cannot be used; mild bleeding in hemophilia A with inhibitor; congenital deficiency of factor II or X. Danger of thrombosis (including MI and DIC) in presence of liver disease, prolonged use; virus inactivated*
Activated prothrombin complex	Factor II, VII, IX, X; factor VIII *bypassing* activity	Preassayed for ability to shorten aPTT of plasma with high-titer factor VIII inhibitor	Hemophilia A or B with inhibitor; cannot evaluate response by measuring factor VIII activity; risk of DIC and thrombosis
Novoseven	Recombinant factor VIIa	Preassayed	Hemophilia A or B with inhibitor; factor VII deficiency; risk of thrombosis

aPTT, Activated partial thromboplastin time; *DIC,* disseminated intravascular coagulation; *HUS,* hemolytic-uremic syndrome; *MI,* myocardial infarction; *TTP,* thrombotic thrombocytopenic purpura; *vWD,* von Willebrand disease; *vWF,* von Willebrand factor.
*Virus attenuation processes may not inactivate parvovirus, hepatitis A, and possibly other viruses.

level to 100% and then be transferred to a hemophilia center (Table 271-2).

Any significant injury must be treated promptly, even without apparent evidence of active bleeding, given that bleeding is often delayed. A small, superficial laceration, if not bleeding or in need of cleaning, may be managed with a simple pressure dressing; however, if bleeding occurs or if suturing is required, then the appropriate clotting factor must be administered immediately. Casts should not be applied unless factor has been administered beforehand and is continued for several days afterward; the involved area should be watched closely for evidence of nerve or vascular compression. Treatment must be given before all surgical procedures, arterial puncture, and lumbar punctures.

Pain should be managed with acetaminophen whenever possible; however, codeine and other oral narcotics can be provided if necessary. Although aspirin must be avoided, nonacetylated salicylates (eg, choline magnesium trisalicylate, Trilisate) can be used, and nonsteroidal antiinflammatory agents such as ibuprofen can be given cautiously if the patient is not also receiving zidovudine.[9] Although cyclooxygenase-2 inhibitors showed early promise as analgesic agents for patients with hemophilia,[10] cardiovascular toxicity that led to the withdrawal of rofecoxib from the market suggests that these drugs should not be used routinely until more is known about them. Treating bleeding episodes as early as possible helps to limit severe pain so that the need for narcotics can be minimized.

Factor Replacement

Products available for the treatment of coagulation disorders are described in Table 271-1. Whole plasma can raise factor VIII levels to only 40% and factor IX to 20% because of the large volume and protein load that accompany its use. Early in the AIDS epidemic, experts suggested that plasma or cryoprecipitate be provided when possible, rather than concentrates made from large donor pools. However, the safety of

Table 271-2 Treatment of Bleeding Episodes in Hemophilia

TYPE OF BLEEDING	DESIRED LEVEL OF FACTOR VIII OR IX*	DURATION OF TREATMENT	ANCILLARY TREATMENT
Hematoma, simple	20-40%	Usually once	—
Hemarthrosis, mild muscle hematoma	30-40%	Once as soon as symptoms begin; if severe, repeat daily until better	Aspirate joint after treatment if swelling is marked. Do not use EACA.
Severe muscle hematoma	50-100%	3-7 days	—
Mouth bleeding, epistaxis, dental extractions	80-100%	Once	Start EACA 75-100 mg/kg every 6 hr or tranexamic acid 25 mg/kg every 6-8 hr by mouth for 3-7 days (until clot is gone).
Gastrointestinal bleeding	100%	3-7 days	EACA or tranexamic acid
Hematuria	Factor may not be needed	3-7 days	Bed rest; hydration; prednisone 2 mg/kg/day. Do not use EACA.
Life-threatening, central nervous system, airway obstruction, retroperitoneal	100%; do not allow drop <50%†	7-14 days	Monitor levels.
Surgery	100%; do not allow drop <50%†	7-14 days	Monitor levels.
Prophylaxis	20-40 U/kg	3 times per week for factor VIII; 2 times per week for factor IX	—

EACA, ε-aminocaproic acid.
*A total of 1 U/kg of factor VIII increases plasma level by 2%; biological half-life = 10 to 12 hours. A total of 1 U/kg of factor IX increases level by 1%; 1 U/kg of recombinant factor IX increases level by 0.8%; biological half-life = 20 to 24 hours. Slightly lower levels of factor IX than of factor VIII are effective.
†Initial dose = 50 U/kg of FVIII and 80 to 100 U/kg of factor IX; repeat one half the factor VIII dose in 8 to 12 hours and one half the factor IX dose in 12 to 24 hours, or provide a continuous infusion of 3 to 4 U/kg/hr of either factor VIII or IX after initial bolus dose.

current concentrates makes them the preferred mode of treatment in most situations. Recombinant factors VIII and IX are available and effective and appear to be free of viral contamination. Some studies have indicated an increased incidence of inhibitor development with these products,[11] although other studies have not agreed with this finding.[12] Factor IX is available in the form of prothrombin complex, as well as in purified and recombinant forms. Although mild bleeding requiring a single treatment can be managed with the complex, this approach has a danger of thrombosis or DIC from activated factors in the complex, particularly in patients with liver disease. The cost of these products increases with the degree of purification.

The desired levels of factor VIII or IX for managing different clinical problems are listed in Table 271-2. Preassayed concentrates are available in vials containing varied doses. Whole vials containing the calculated, desired dose or a higher level should be given because these products are too expensive to waste. Continuous infusion can be used for patients who are undergoing surgery or who are bleeding extensively.[13]

Health Care Maintenance

Routine immunizations, which must include hepatitis B and hepatitis A vaccines, should be given subcutaneously if possible with a 25-gauge needle; pressure should be maintained for 5 to 10 minutes. Intramuscular injections should be minimized. Routine dental evaluation, prophylaxis, and hygiene should begin by 3 years of age.[14] The most difficult part of managing the child who has hemophilia is to use appropriate caution but at the same time allow for the development of independence. Family education about the disease is essential, and support groups are beneficial. Psychosocial problems must be a major concern in managing patients and families. Not only do they have to live with a serious chronic illness associated with frequent pain and limitation of normal activities, but also the impact of AIDS on the adult population has been devastating and in many cases has eroded trust in medical caretakers.

Home Management

If a child has reasonably easy venous access and family dynamics permit it, then parents can be taught to administer treatment to children as young as 3 years, and 9 or 10 year olds can be taught to self-administer factor concentrates.[15] This approach allows for much earlier treatment of bleeding episodes, provides the satisfaction of self-sufficiency, and prevents some of the frustrations of having to get to a treatment center or emergency room. Indwelling venous access devices are being used with increasing frequency and have simplified home, as well as in-hospital, management, although infections and thrombosis have been problems.[16] Home intravenous therapy is also a convenient way to administer prophylaxis or immune tolerance induction.

Mild Hemophilia

The patient who has mild hemophilia is more likely than one with severe disease to receive inadequate treatment of bleeding episodes because neither the family nor the physicians may be aware of the need for treatment. Significant injuries require management such as that of severe disease, although smaller doses of factor concentrates may suffice to attain the desired factor levels (see Table 271-2). Desmopressin is a vasopressin analog that results in release of factor VIII from the endothelial cells where it is productive, resulting in almost a 3-fold increase of the level. It may therefore be effective if the baseline factor VIII is more than 5%, depending on the level desired. Overhydration must be prevented because water retention and hyponatremia may occur with desmopressin therapy, particularly in young children and with repeated doses. A concentrated intranasal preparation (Stimate) is available and has been used in children 6 years of age and older. A stimulation test with response assessment should be performed in each patient with both intravenous and nasal preparations before they are used therapeutically for the first time.[17] Desmopressin is ineffective in factor IX deficiency.

Prophylaxis

Prophylactic factor concentrate treatment administered several times a week is considered to be the optimal care for children who have severe hemophilia to prevent hemarthrosis and joint damage and to normalize their lives.[18] Although this form of treatment is more expensive than episodic treatment for bleeding, the additional cost saving by preventing future orthopedic complications is considerable. The psychological benefits also must be considered.

Inhibitors

Up to 50% of patients who have severe hemophilia A and 3% who have hemophilia B develop antibodies that inhibit factor VIII or factor IX activity, usually early in their treatment, although many of these antibodies are present in low titer and may subsequently disappear.[19] Such patients should be managed only by experienced practitioners. Management may include the use of large doses of factor VIII or factors that bypass factor VIII in the coagulation cascade (prothrombin complex, activated prothrombin complex, recombinant factor VIIa). Induction of immune tolerance by continuous exposure to high doses of factor over many weeks to months, with or without concomitant immunosuppression, has been found to be effective in controlling the inhibitor in most cases.[19-21] An inhibitor should be suspected if the response to appropriate therapy is inadequate, and it should be sought regularly in all patients and before all elective surgery. A Bethesda inhibitor assay will determine the presence and strength of an inhibitor. Patients who have hemophilia B with inhibitors may develop anaphylaxis or nephrotic syndrome when given factor IX.[18] Management is much more difficult than for hemophilia A, but recombinant factor VIIa has been effective.[21]

AIDS and Other Viral Infections

Most patients who had severe hemophilia in the United States in the late 1970s and early 1980s became infected with HIV. The treatment of hemophilia with clotting factor concentrates from large donor pools in the era before the virus was identified resulted in massive exposure to HIV. Chronic liver disease has also been a major problem, most often caused by hepatitis C and sometimes by hepatitis B virus infection. Currently, both donor testing and several methods to inactivate viruses in the production process make the concentrates safe with regard to HIV. Hepatitis B and C have also been largely eliminated. (See Chapter 60, Blood Products and Their Uses.) However, hepatitis A and parvovirus B19 infections may still occur with plasma products.[22,23] The increasing availability and use of recombinant factors may eliminate the problem of viral infections.

Gene Therapy

Although gene transfer of both factor VIII and factor IX genes has been accomplished in several animal models, as well as in a small number of clinical trials, the results have been disappointing. In addition, concerns about the possibility of inducing malignancy or liver disease remain. However, investigations into this modality continue to be pursued.[24]

VON WILLEBRAND DISEASE

von Willebrand disease (vWD) is the most common hereditary coagulation disorder, with estimates of an incidence as high as 1% of the population, although most of these individuals are asymptomatic.[25] von Willebrand factor (vWF) is the carrying protein for factor VIII and exists in a series of different-sized multimers of smaller subunits. Decreased vWF is associated with a corresponding decrease of factor VIII activity in most cases. The inheritance is usually autosomal dominant with variable penetrance, but autosomal-recessive variants occur. The gene is on chromosome 12 and has been cloned, and many genetic defects have been identified.[26] In addition to bleeding after surgery and trauma, the major manifestation of vWD is mucosal bleeding, which most frequently exhibits as epistaxis. Menorrhagia and, less commonly, gastrointestinal bleeding also may occur. Hemarthrosis and deep hematomas may be seen in severe (type III) vWD.

Several components of the vWF–factor VIII complex and function can be determined: factor VIII activity, vWF activity (Ristocetin cofactor, vWF:RCo), vWF antigen (vWF:Ag), and the pattern of multimers. In hemophilia the vWF is normal. Many variants of vWD exist. The most common is type I, in which all components are similarly reduced and the multimer pattern is normal. Type II has a decrease or absence of the larger multimers; type IIB exhibits increased binding to platelets. Type III represents severe homozygous deficiency with very low or absent levels of all components.

vWD may be difficult to diagnose. The bleeding time and PFA-100 test are fairly sensitive but nonspecific screening tests and are prolonged in most patients; most cases are associated with decreased levels of factor VIII. However, the aPTT may be normal if factor VIII is greater than 30% to 40%. All of the studies may be variable, both from patient to patient and in the same patient from time to time. If laboratory test results are normal, then they should be repeated if the index of suspicion is high. vWF varies with blood type and with several environmental factors. vWF levels of

35% to 50% may exist in both patients with vWD and normal individuals with blood type O, making the definitive diagnosis even more difficult.[27] A major differential diagnosis, although much more rare, is one of the disorders of platelet function (see Chapter 208, Petechiae and Purpura).

Most patients who have type I vWD will respond to desmopressin as in mild hemophilia A, and this approach can be used for most bleeding episodes. Most patients who have type IIA and all who have type III vWD do not respond to desmopressin, and its use is contraindicated in type IIB disease because it may cause platelet aggregation and DIC. Patients who have severe bleeding or those who do not respond to desmopressin should be treated with Humate P, a concentrate that contains both factor VIII and vWF. Although fresh-frozen plasma or cryoprecipitate can be used, they are not suggested because of the possibility of viral contamination. Mild epistaxis can often be controlled with ε-aminocaproic acid or tranexamic acid; these agents should also be used as adjunctive therapy for mucosal bleeding other than hematuria.

OTHER COAGULATION DEFECTS

The other coagulant deficiencies are inherited as autosomal-recessive genes, with the exception of factor XI deficiency, afibrinogenemia, and dysfibrinogenemia, which are associated with bleeding in both their heterozygous and homozygous forms. Factor XIII deficiency cannot be detected with the usual screening tests; a normal screening work-up in a patient who has a significant bleeding history should be followed with a clot solubility test. The contact factors prekallikrein, high-molecular-weight kininogen, and factor XII are necessary to initiate clotting in vitro; their absence results in a markedly prolonged aPTT but is not associated with clinical bleeding.

Although all of these deficiencies can be treated with fresh-frozen plasma, concentrates are preferable for treating factor VII deficiency because of its short half-life, as well as other deficiencies when available because they are virus depleted. Recombinant factor VIIa (Novoseven) is commercially available. Prothrombin complex products also contain factor VII, as well as factors II and X, but the content of each factor varies in different lots. These products contain activated coagulation factors that may induce thrombosis or DIC, and they must be used cautiously, particularly in patients with liver disease. Fibrinogen and factor XIII are concentrated in cryoprecipitate, and a factor XIII concentrate may be available for compassionate use. Fresh-frozen plasma can be used for patients with factor V or XI deficiency or in an emergency for patients who are bleeding but whose deficiency has not yet been identified. Factor XI concentrates are available in some European countries but not yet in the United States.

WHEN TO REFER

- All children with hemophilia should be seen at least once a year at a comprehensive hemophilia center if possible.
- All elective surgery should be performed at a hemophilia center.
- All patients with significant trauma or potentially life-threatening bleeding should be given an initial loading dose of factor (to 100%) and transferred to a hemophilia center.
- All patients with inhibitors should be managed at a hemophilia center.
- Children with vWD should have an initial evaluation by a specialized coagulation laboratory.

WHEN TO ADMIT

- Significant trauma is present.
- Bleeding is present in a potentially life-threatening area.
- Severe abdominal pain exists.
- Any surgical procedure must be performed.

TOOLS FOR PRACTICE

Engaging Patient and Family

- *Hemophilia* (fact sheet), National Heart, Lung. and Blood Institute (www.nhlbi.nih.gov/health/dci/Diseases/hemophilia/hemophilia_what.html).

Medical Decision Support

- *Hemophilia* (Web page), Centers for Disease Control and Prevention (www.cdc.gov/ncbddd/hbd/hemophilia.htm).
- *Hemophilia Treatment Centers* (Web page), Centers for Disease Control and Prevention (www.cdc.gov/ncbddd/hbd/htc_list.htm).

RELATED WEB SITE

- National Hemophilia Foundation (www.hemophilia.org).

SUGGESTED RESOURCES

Blanchette VS, Manco-Johnson M, Santagostino E, et al. Optimizing factor prophylaxis for the haemophilia population: where do we stand? *Haemophilia*. 2004;10(suppl 4): 97-104.

Cox GJ. Diagnosis and treatment of von Willebrand disease. *Hematol Oncol Clin North Am*. 2004;18(6):1277-1299.

Dunn AL, Abshire TC. Recent advances in the management of the child who has hemophilia. *Hematol Oncol Clin North Am*. 2004;18(6):1249-1276.

Hay CR, Brown S, Collins PW, et al. The diagnosis and management of factor VIII and IX inhibitors: a guideline from the United Kingdom Haemophilia Centre Doctors Organisation. *Brit J Haematol*. 2006;133(6):591-605.

Komvilaisak P, Connolly B, Naqvi A, et al. Overview of the use of implantable venous access devices in the management of children with inherited bleeding disorders. *Haemophilia* 2006;12(suppl 6):87-93.

Lethagen S. Desmopressin in mild hemophilia A: indications, limitations, efficacy, and safety. *Semin Thromb Hemost*. 2003; 29(1):101-106.

Manco-Johnson MJ, Riske B, Kasper CK. Advances in care of children with hemophilia. *Semin Thromb Hemost*. 2003; 29(6):585-594.

Teitel JM, Barnard D, Israels S, et al. Home management of haemophilia. *Haemophilia*. 2004;10(2):118-133.

REFERENCES

1. Harrison P. The role of PFA-100 testing in the investigation and management of haemostatic defects in children and adults. *Br J Haematol.* 2005;130(1):3-10.
2. Montgomery RR, Gill JC, Scott JP. Hemophilia and von Willebrand disease. In: Nathan DG, Orkin S, Ginsburg D, et al, eds. *Nathan and Oski's Hematology of Infancy and Childhood.* 6th ed. Philadelphia, PA: WB Saunders; 2003.
3. Oldenburg J, Ananyeva NM, Saenko EL. Molecular basis of haemophilia A. *Haemophilia.* 2004;10(suppl 4):133-139.
4. Lillicrap D. The molecular basis of haemophilia B. *Haemophilia.* 1998;4(4):350-357.
5. Luck JV Jr, Silva M, Rodriguez-Merchan EC, et al. Hemophilic arthropathy. *J Am Acad Orthop Surg.* 2004;12(4): 234-245.
6. Journeycake JM, Miller KL, Anderson AM, et al. Arthroscopic synovectomy in children and adolescents with hemophilia. *J Pediatr Hematol Oncol.* 2003;25(9):726-731.
7. Siegel HJ, Luck JV Jr, Siegel ME, et al. Phosphate-32 colloid radiosynovectomy in hemophilia. *Clin Orthop Relat Res.* 2001;392:409-417.
8. Pitts TO, Spero JA, Bontempo FA, et al. Acute renal failure due to high-grade obstruction following therapy with epsilon-aminocaproic acid. *Am J Kidney Dis.* 1986;8(6): 441-444.
9. Ragni MV, Miller BJ, Whalen R, et al. Bleeding tendency, platelet function, and pharmacokinetics of ibuprofen and zidovudine in HIV(+) hemophilic men. *Am J Hematol.* 1992; 40(3):176-182.
10. Rattray B, Nugent DJ, Young G. Rofecoxib as adjunctive therapy for haemophilic arthropathy. *Haemophilia.* 2005; 11(3):240-243.
11. Goudemand J, Rothschild C, Demiguel V, et al. Influence of the type of factor VIII concentrate on the incidence of factor VIII inhibitors in previously untreated patients with severe hemophilia A. *Blood* 2006;107(1):46-51.
12. Hoots WK, Lusher J. High-titer inhibitor development in hemophilia A: lack of product specificity. *J Thromb Haemost.* 2004;2(2):358-359.
13. Batorova A, Martinowitz U. Intermittent injections vs. continuous infusion of factor VIII in haemophilia patients undergoing major surgery. *Br J Haematol.* 2000;110(3): 715-720.
14. Harrington B. Primary dental care of patients with haemophilia. *Haemophilia.* 2000;6(suppl 1);7-12.
15. Teitel JM, Barnard D, Israels S, et al. Home management of haemophilia. *Haemophilia.* 2004;10(2):118-133.
16. Komvilaisak P, Connolly B, Naqvi A, et al. Overview of the use of implantable venous access devices in the management of children with inherited bleeding disorders. *Haemophilia* 2006;12(suppl 6):87-93.
17. Lethagen S. Desmopressin in mild hemophilia A: indications, limitations, efficacy, and safety. *Semin Thromb Hemost.* 2003;29(1):101-106.
18. Blanchette VS, Manco-Johnson M, Santagostino E, et al. Optimizing factor prophylaxis for the haemophilia population: where do we stand? *Haemophilia.* 2004;10(suppl 4): 97-104.
19. Lusher JM. Inhibitor antibodies to factor VIII and factor IX: management. *Semin Thromb Hemost.* 2000;26(2):179-188.
20. Hay CR, Brown S, Collins PW, et al. The diagnosis and management of factor VIII and IX inhibitors: a guideline from the United Kingdom Haemophilia Centre Doctors Organisation. *Brit J Haematol.* 2006;133(6):591-605.
21. Key NS. Inhibitors in congenital coagulation disorders. *Brit J Haematol.* 2004;127(4):379-391.
22. Jee YM, Go U, Cheon D, et al. Detection of hepatitis A virus from clotting factors implicated as a source of HAV infection among haemophilia patients in Korea. *Epidemiol Infect.* 2006;134(1):87-93.
23. Blumel J, Schmidt I, Effenberger W, et al. Parvovirus B19 transmission by heat-treated clotting factor concentrates. *Transfusion.* 2002;42(11):1473-1481.
24. Lozier J. Gene therapy of the hemophilias. *Semin Hematol.* 2004;41(4):287-296.
25. Rodeghiero F, Castaman G, Dini E. Epidemiological investigation of the prevalence of von Willebrand's disease. *Blood.* 1987;69(2):454-459.
26. Keeney S, Cumming AM. The molecular biology of von Willebrand disease. *Clin Lab Haematol.* 2001;23(4):209-230.
27. Nitu-Whalley IC, Lee CA, Griffioen A, et al. Type 1 von Willebrand disease—a clinical retrospective study of the diagnosis, the influence of the ABO blood group and the role of the bleeding history. *Br J Haematol.* 2000;108(2): 259-264.

Chapter 272

HENOCH-SCHÖNLEIN PURPURA

Horacio Esteban Adrogué, MD; Francisco Xavier Flores, MD

Henoch-Schönlein purpura (HSP) is the most common form of vasculitis in children. This small-vessel vasculitis is mediated by immunoglobulin A (IgA)-containing immune complexes and is characterized by nonthrombocytopenic purpura, abdominal pain, arthralgias, and renal disease. The diagnostic criteria published in 1990 by the American College of Rheumatology include palpable purpura, initial presentation at 20 years or younger, bowel angina, and typical biopsy findings. If 2 or more diagnostic criteria are present, then the sensitivity and specificity for the diagnosis of HSP are >87%.[1]

EPIDEMIOLOGIC FACTORS

HSP is more common in Europe and Asia than it is in the United States, with an estimated annual incidence in the United Kingdom of 20:100,000 children.[2]

HSP mainly affects young children, with a peak incidence at 4 to 6 years of age and a 1.5:1 male-to-female ratio. HSP appears to be more prevalent during the winter and spring, and in at least 30% of cases, an upper respiratory infection precedes the onset of symptoms.[3] Other infections, drug allergies, insect bites, and vaccines can also precipitate HSP. Cases also have been reported in children with C2 and C4 complement deficiencies.[4]

CLINICAL PRESENTATION

Cutaneous manifestations are the most common clinical features of patients with HSP. In 50% of patients, a macular-petechial rash is present. This rash is symmetric, sometimes purpuric, localized predominantly in the extensor surface of the lower extremities, forearms, and buttocks and tends to spare the trunk. These lesions tend to fade with time, but new lesions can recur up to 3 months after the initial presentation. Nonpitting edema of the scalp, hands, and feet may be present in 30% to 70% of young children.

Joint manifestations occur in 60% to 80% patients, with knees, ankles, wrist, and fingers most commonly affected. The joints involved are usually tender and swollen, but these symptoms resolve without any residual deformity.

Gastrointestinal manifestations develop in 50% to 70% of patients with HSP, with a higher incidence in patients with renal involvement. Intermittent colicky abdominal pain, vomiting, or gastrointestinal bleeding are most common, and up to 5% of the patients develop complications such as intestinal infarction, perforation, or intussusception.

Renal involvement occurs in 20% to 50% of cases and is responsible for the long-term morbidity in affected patients. Evidence of HSP nephritis usually coincides with or follows the cutaneous manifestations and is usually present within 4 weeks of the onset of joint or gastrointestinal manifestations.[2] The spectrum of renal involvement in HSP is broad and may include microscopic hematuria (transient or persistent), macroscopic hematuria (initial or recurrent), proteinuria, nephritic syndrome, and nephritic-nephrotic syndrome. HSP nephritis when mild tends to resolve without any particular intervention. However, 2% to 5% of patients with renal involvement progress to end-stage renal disease. Abnormal creatinine clearance at 3 years after onset, and ultrastructural abnormalities in the renal biopsy are the most consistent predictors of poor renal prognosis.

Testicular swelling and tenderness may be present in up to 35% of male patients with HSP. If this manifestation is present, then a thorough evaluation is necessary to rule out testicular torsion. Other serious complications such as pulmonary hemorrhage and central nervous system involvement have also been described.[5]

EVALUATION

The diagnosis of HSP is based on clinical findings. In general, complete blood count, platelet count, coagulation studies, and complement levels are normal. The serum albumin and renal function are normal in the majority of patients but vary according to the degree of renal involvement. IgA levels may be transiently elevated in 50% of the patients with HSP.

Urinalyses obtained at various times in the disease process may reveal hematuria and various degrees of proteinuria. A renal biopsy is not indicated in all patients with a diagnosis of HSP; however, it should be considered in patients with significant proteinuria for more than 1 month, renal insufficiency, hypertension, or nephrotic syndrome.

DIFFERENTIAL DIAGNOSIS

When pediatricians are faced with a child with acute purpuric and petechial eruptions, they must first ensure that the differential diagnosis is kept broad. These diagnoses include, but are not limited to, the following: acute bacterial infections (invasive meningococcal disease), Rocky Mountain spotted fever, toxic shock, enteroviral infections, endocarditis, idiopathic thrombocytopenic purpura, parvovirus B19, Kawasaki disease, and acute hepatitis A.[6]

Hematuria is defined as more than 5 to 10 red blood cells per high power field from a freshly voided centrifuged midstream urine sample and should persist for a month or more to merit a work-up. The differential diagnosis for hematuria is wide and can range from very benign to life threatening. Normal activities such as bike riding or snow boarding can cause benign hematuria. An important distinction is whether proteinuria is also present with hematuria. Patients without protein in the urine are more likely to have kidney cysts or other abnormalities, including hypercalciuria, kidney stones, or thin basement membrane syndrome. When proteinuria is also found, poststreptococcal acute glomerulonephritis, IgA, systemic lupus erythematosus, and Alport syndrome are more likely (see Chapter 188, Hematuria).[7]

TREATMENT AND PROGNOSIS

Once other diseases are ruled out and a diagnosis of HSP is established, supportive care will be the most important first step. A partnership between the primary care physician and nephrologist in which each patient is evaluated, treated, and monitored ensures a balance of safety and efficacy.

Careful attention to nutrition, volume status, vital signs. and laboratory data (complete blood count, kidney function, electrolytes) will be the cornerstone of treatment for most patients. Although specific therapy for HSP remains controversial, carefully selecting children who will be given more than standard supportive care is critical.

Children who do not display any urinary abnormalities within 6 months of diagnosis do not develop chronic kidney disease (CKD), and therefore steroids or other immunosuppressant are not advised for this group of children with HSP. Children who display only isolated hematuria or proteinuria have a very low risk of developing CKD (1.6%); therefore they should receive supportive care only, and not more aggressive treatment.[8] Patients who have nephritic or nephrotic syndrome have a much higher risk of CKD (10% to 19.5%) and thus merit serious consideration for aggressive therapy. Girls are especially at risk of CKD (2.5 times higher than their male counterparts) and will likely benefit most of all from therapy.[8]

Long-term follow-up of 219 patients (83 children younger than 16 years and 136 adults) with biopsy-proven HSP found that 60% of the children and 72% of the adults had been treated with steroids, and 14% of children and 22% of adults had received immunosuppressants. When kidney function outcomes (doubling of serum creatinine and eventual need for dialysis) were examined, the use of steroids or immunosuppressants failed to show any protective influence over supportive care.[9] Seven percent of these children ended up on dialysis after a mean follow-up of 6.7 years. Patients who are at higher risk of eventual dialysis were girls. Use of steroids in patients with HSP should be decided on individual bases, and cases that are considered for steroid treatment should be referred to nephrologists.

As far as the use of steroids for extrarenal manifestations, new evidence suggests that it may be of use.

Ronkainen and colleagues conducted a randomized, double-blind, placebo-controlled trial of early steroids and followed patients for 6 months. Of the 171 patients who were included and followed for 6 months, 84 were treated with prednisone and 87 received a placebo. The endpoints were renal involvement at 1, 3, and 6 months and healing of extrarenal symptoms. The analyses were performed on an intent-to-treat basis. These researchers found that the use of prednisone (1 mg/kg/day for 2 weeks, with weaning over the subsequent 2 weeks) was effective in reducing the intensity of abdominal pain (pain score, 2.5 vs 4.8; $P = .029$) and joint pain (4.6 vs 7.3; $P = .030$). Prednisone did not prevent the development of renal symptoms but was effective in treating them; renal symptoms resolved in 61% of the prednisone patients after treatment, compared with 34% of the placebo patients (difference = 27%; 95% confidence interval = 3% to 47%; $P = .024$). From this finding, the authors concluded that the general use of prednisone in HSP is not supported, but patients with disturbing symptoms may benefit from early treatment because prednisone reduces extrarenal symptoms and is effective in altering, but not preventing, the course of renal involvement.[10]

In one small but well-designed study,[11] children with HSP displaying hypertension, hematuria, and proteinuria were given 1000 mg fish oil twice daily and Enalapril 2.5 to 10 mg a day. Enalapril was subsequently stopped in all patients within 1 year. A 6-month follow-up was recorded under continued treatment with fish oil. Renal function remained the same (creatinine at a mean of 0.6 mg/dL) before and after treatment. Hypertension (135/82 vs 100/54; $P < .05$) remained better controlled and proteinuria (1041 mg/day vs 104 mg/day; $P < .05$) remained minimal at 6-month follow-up off angiotensin-converting enzyme (ACE) inhibition but on fish oil. Although this case series is very small, fish oil is a benign treatment that may provide other added benefits such as reduction of hypertriglyceridemia. Fish oils (omega-3-acid ethyl esters) have been shown to be promising in IgA nephropathy, which many researchers believe is part of the spectrum of disease related to HSP. The antiinflammatory and immune-modulating effects of fish oil have been demonstrated in other studies.[12] ACE inhibitors are also indicated for control of hypertension, especially for patients with proteinuria. ACE inhibitors are contraindicated during pregnancy.

Other options for treatment of HSP have been studied. Cyclosporine and prednisone,[13-17] plasmapheresis,[18] tonsillectomy,[19] dapsone,[20] and cyclophosphamide[21] have all been tried, with varying degrees of success. These approaches have the possibility of toxicity and lack verification from blinded, controlled, and randomized studies. Therefore, we do not recommend the use of any of these measures at this time.

In summary, the majority of patients with HSP should be managed with supportive care with close monitoring of their renal function. Patients with HSP who have persistent hematuria or proteinuria or those with abnormal renal functions or elevated blood pressure should be referred to nephrologists for management.

WHEN TO REFER

- Significant and persistent signs of kidney inflammation (nephritic or nephrotic syndrome)
- Acute kidney injury (elevation in blood, urea, nitrogen or creatinine levels) should be referred to a nephrologist.

WHEN TO ADMIT

- Toxic appearance (febrile, lethargic, hypotensive, or hypertensive, with altered mental status or not acting themselves)
- Abdominal pain may indicate acute appendicitis, intussusception, small-bowel obstruction or infarction or pain caused by HSP. Obtaining a surgical consult is advisable if abdominal pain is particularly severe or out of proportion to the physical examination.
- A significant reduction in urine output for age and weight or inability to keep fluids down.
- Any alteration from normal in the patient's kidney function (blood urea nitrogen or creatinine)
- Given that the presenting rash with HSP may be the manifestation of many other very severe diseases, a short admit in all but the most healthy looking patients may be prudent.
- Any child not able to communicate (infants or intellectually disabled patients) should be admitted for close observation.

TOOLS FOR PRACTICE

Engaging Patients and Family

- *What is a Pediatric Rheumatologist?* (fact sheet), American Academy of Pediatrics (www.aap.org/family/WhatisPedRheumatology.pdf).

REFERENCES

1. Mills JA, Michel BA, Bloch DA, et al. The American College of Rheumatology 1990 criteria for the classification of Henoch-Schönlein purpura. *Arthritis Rheum.* 1990; 33:1114-1121.
2. Kim S, Dedeoglu F. Update on pediatric vasculitis. *Curr Opin Pediatr.* 2005;17:695-702.
3. Ting TV, Hashkes P. Update on childhood vasculitides. *Curr Opin Rheumatol.* 2004;16:560-565.
4. Motoyama O, Iitaka K. Henoch Schönlein purpura and hypocomplementemia in children. *Pediatr Int.* 2005;47(1): 39-424.
5. Ballinger S. Henoch-Schönlein purpura. *Curr Opin Rheumatol.* 2003;15:591-594.
6. Ramos-e-Silvia M, Pereira AL. Life-threatening eruptions due to infectious agents. *Clin Dermatol.* 2005;23:148-156.
7. Shane Roy MD III. Consultation with the specialist. *Pediatrics Rev.* 1998;19(6):209-213.
8. Narchi H. Risk of long term impairment and duration of follow up recommended for Henoch-Schönlein purpura with normal or minimal urinary findings: a systematic review. *Arch Dis Child.* 2005;90:916-920.
9. Coppo R, Andrulli S, Amore A, et al. Predictors of outcome in Henoch-Schönlein nephritis in children and adults. *Am J Kidney Dis.* 2006;47(6):993-1003.

10. Ronkainen J, Koskimies O, Ala-Houhala M, et al. Early prednisone therapy in Henoch-Schönlein purpura: a randomized, double-blind, placebo-controlled trial. *J Pediatr.* 2006;149(2);241-247.
11. Dixit MP, Dixit NM, Scott K. Managing Henoch-Schönlein purpura in children with fish oil and ACE inhibitor therapy. *Nephrology.* 2004;9:381-386.
12. Chaudhary A, Mishra A, Sethi S. Oxidized omega-3 fatty acids inhibit pro-inflammatory responses in glomerular endothelial cells. *Nephron Exp Nephrol.* 2004;97(4): e136-e145.
13. Shin JI, Park JM, Shin YH, et al. Cyclosporin A therapy for severe Henoch-Schönlein nephritis with nephrotic syndrome. *Pediatr Nephrol.* 2005;20:1093-1097.
14. Shin JI, Park JM, Shin YH, et al. Can azathioprine and steroids alter the progression of severe Henoch-Schönlein nephritis in children? *Pediatr Nephrol.* 2005; 20:1087-1092.
15. Shin JI, Park JM, Shin YH, et al. Henoch-Schönlein purpura nephritis with nephritic-range proteinuria: histological regression possibly associated with cyclosporine A and steroid treatment. *Scand J Rheumatol.* 2005; 34:392-395.
16. Ronkainen J, Autio-Harmainen H, Nuutinen M. Cyclosporin A for the treatment of severe Henoch-Schönlein glomerulonephritis. *Pediatr Nephrol.* 2003;18:1138-1142.
17. Someya T, Kaneko K, Fujinaga S. Cyclosporine A for heavy proteinuria in a child with Henoch-Schönlein purpura nephritis. *Pediatr Int.* 2004;46:111-113.
18. Kawasaki Y, Suzuki J, Murai M, et al. Plasmapheresis therapy for rapidly progressive Henoch-Schönlein nephritis. *Pediatr Nephrol.* 2004;19:920-923.
19. Sugiyama H, Watanabe N, Onoda T, et al. Successful treatment of progressive Henoch-Schönlein purpura nephritis with tonsillectomy and steroid pulse therapy. *Intern Med.* 2005;44(6):611-615.
20. Ibal H, Evans A. Dapsone therapy for Henoch-Schönlein purpura: a case series. *Arch Dis Child.* 2005;90:985.
21. Flynn JT, Smoyer WE, Bunchman TE, et al. Treatment of Henoch-Schönlein purpura glomerulonephritis in children with high-dose corticosteroids plus oral cyclophosphamide. *Am J Nephrol.* 2001;21:128-133.

Chapter 273

HEPATITIS

Winita Hardikar, MBBS, PhD; Kathleen B. Schwarz, MD

The term *hepatitis* simply describes inflammation of the liver and does not imply a cause. The causes of hepatitis vary with age, geographic location, and the presence or absence of underlying illness. Broadly speaking, hepatitis in the pediatric age group may be viral, autoimmune, metabolic, or drug related (Table 273-1). Systemic conditions such as ischemia and trauma (including abdominal battering from child abuse) may also result in elevated serum aminotransferases. Some conditions may cause elevated enzymes that are not due to hepatitis. These conditions include the myopathies (elevated serum aminotransferases) and bone disorders (elevated alkaline phosphatase) in which the primary site of enzyme release is muscle or bone rather than liver.

VIRAL HEPATITIS

Over 16,000 cases of viral hepatitis are reported annually to the Centers for Disease Control and Prevention.[1] Not included in these figures are numerous unrecognized anicteric cases, especially in the pediatric population, in which the anicteric/icteric case ratio is thought to approach 10:1. The clinical syndromes vary from asymptomatic to fulminant hepatic failure, depending on the virus and host factors. Acute viral hepatitis may also progress to chronic liver disease, particularly with hepatitis B and C, resulting in chronic morbidity and mortality (Table 273-2).

Hepatitis A Virus

Hepatitis A virus[2] (HAV) is a 27-nm RNA virus, a member of the picornavirus group. Transmission of HAV is predominantly by the fecal-oral route, although saliva and urine are potentially important vehicles, particularly among siblings. Contaminated shellfish, polluted water, and travel to endemic areas have also been identified in the acquisition of type-A infection. HAV RNA can be detected in serum and stool as early as 2 to 3 weeks before acute illness and as much as 1 week after the onset of illness; recovery in the stool decreases as jaundice becomes evident. Parenteral transmission is possible but uncommon. Children with acute hepatitis A may be completely asymptomatic but are still infectious and therefore serve as a silent reservoir of disease. Interestingly, antibody to hepatitis A is present in 33% of the adult US population.[1] HAV immunoglobulin M (IgM) antibody is short lived, whereas HAV IgG antibody is present at least 10 years after infection and probably confers lifelong immunity to the virus.

Hepatitis B Virus

Hepatitis B virus[3] (HBV) is a common, highly infectious virus of the Hepadnaviridae family. Its double-stranded overlapping DNA codes for a surface antigen (HBsAg), a core antigen (HBcAg), e antigen (HBeAg), and DNA polymerase. HBsAg has been found in all body secretions and excretions from infected persons; however, transmission only occurs through contact with blood, vaginal and menstrual fluids, and semen. The virus is stable on environmental surfaces for at least 7 days. In hyperendemic areas (Asia, Africa, Southern Europe, Latin America), HBV infection is most often acquired perinatally or in early childhood by horizontal transmission. Aggressive immunization programs in certain areas, such as Taiwan, have substantially lowered risks.[4] Horizontal transmission is uncommon but may occur in early childhood from infectious siblings and among institutionalized patients. Improperly sterilized syringes and nosocomial transmission are also a means of acquisition in some parts of Africa and Asia.

Age of acquisition of the virus is an important prognostic determinant. Perinatal transmission from mother to infant leads to chronic hepatitis in 90% of children compared with less than 10% when the infection is acquired as adults.[5] Transmission is more likely (up to 90%) if the mother is HBeAg positive and less likely (20%) if the mother is HBeAg negative.[3] Fulminant hepatitis in the infant has been

Table 273-1 Differential Diagnosis of Hepatitis

CATEGORY	CAUSES
Infectious	Hepatitis A, B, C, D, E, G Adenovirus, Epstein-Barr virus, cytomegalovirus, varicella zoster, human herpesvirus type 6, parvovirus B19, echovirus, coxsackievirus, rubeola virus
Autoimmune	Autoimmune type 1 and 2 and seronegative autoimmune hepatitis Sclerosing cholangitis (neonatal and child forms)
Metabolic	α_1-antitrypsin deficiency; galactosemia; hereditary tyrosinemia; hereditary fructose intolerance; persistent familial intrahepatic cholestasis types 1, 2, and 3; paroxysmal diseases; mitochondrial hepatopathies; neonatal hemochromatosis; glycogen storage disease; Niemann-Pick type C disease; inborn errors of bile acid metabolism; Wilson disease; nonalcoholic steatohepatitis
Drug induced	Sodium valproate, halothane, phenytoin, herbal medications, recreational drugs (ectasy), toxins (eg, *Amanita phalloides* [wild mushrooms])
Other	Alagille syndrome, cystic fibrosis, ischemia, trauma (including child abuse)
Elevated liver enzymes without hepatitis	Myopathies, bone disorder, transient hyperphosphatasia, celiac disease

Table 273-2 Clinical Features of Acute Viral Hepatitis

	HAV	HBV	HCV
CHARACTERISTICS			
Age distribution	Children and young adults	All age groups	All age groups
Route of infection	Predominantly fecal-oral route	Parenteral	Parenteral
Incubation period (days)	15-40	50-180	20-90
Onset	Acute	Insidious	Insidious
Duration of clinical illness	Weeks	Weeks to months	Weeks to months
VIRUS PRESENCE			
Feces	Late incubation, acute	May be present	Absent
Blood	Late incubation, acute	Late incubation, acute, may persist for months	Present chronically
SIGNS AND SYMPTOMS			
Fever	High, common early	Moderate, less common	Moderate, less common
Nausea and vomiting	Common	Less common	Less common
Anorexia	Severe	Mild to moderate	Mild to moderate
Arthralgia or arthritis	Rare	Common	—
Rash or urticaria	Rare	Common	—
LABORATORY FINDINGS			
Aminotransferase elevation	1-3 weeks	Months	Fluctuates for months
Bilirubin elevation	Weeks	May be months	Unusual
HBsAg	Absent	Present	Absent
Severity	Usually mild	Often severe	Usually mild
Progression to chronic hepatitis	Rare	More common	High rate
Immunity	Homologous, lifelong	Homologous, lifelong	Unusual
Prevention	Immune serum globulin	Hyperimmune globulin; vaccine	Screen donor blood

HAV, Hepatitis A virus; *HBsAg*, hepatitis B surface antigen; *HBV*, hepatitis B virus; *HCV*, hepatitis C virus.
Modified from Krugman S, Katz SL. *Infectious diseases of children*, 8th ed. St Louis, MO: Mosby; 1985; deBelle RC, Lester R. Current concepts of acute and chronic viral hepatitis. *Pediatr Clin North Am.* 1975;22:943-961. Copyright © Elsevier, with permission.

reported in the latter group, and although the mechanism is not clear, it is not thought to be the result of selection of more potent mutant viruses.[6] Maternal antibody to HBeAg does not prevent perinatal transmission. The risk of infection to the infant appears to be markedly increased (65% to 100%) if the mother has had clinical hepatitis in the third trimester of pregnancy.[3] The principal route of infection with Hepatitis B is at the time of birth by microtransfusions or by swallowing blood and genital secretions at the time of delivery.[3]

Perinatal transmission of HBV is largely responsible for the worldwide burden of this disease. The long-term effects of acquiring HBV in infancy include cirrhosis and hepatocellular carcinoma. Although most cases of HBV-related hepatocellular carcinoma occur in adults, many cases of HBV-related liver cancer have been described in children.[7] Recent studies suggest that perinatal transmission is important in hepatocarcinogenesis perhaps related to the high dose of HBV DNA with subsequent tolerance and persistent necroinflammatory activity.[8]

Hepatitis C Virus

Hepatitis C virus[9] (HCV), recognized in 1989, is a single-stranded RNA virus of the Flaviviridae family and is responsible for the majority of posttransfusion non-A, non-B hepatitis. The seroprevalence of HCV in the general US population is estimated at 1.8%. In children the seroprevalence rate for those without known risk factors is 0.2% for those younger than 12 years and 0.4% for those 12 to 19 years of age.[10] Before screening of donor blood in 1990, most children were infected by parenteral exposure to contaminated blood and blood products. Since screening began, the risk of HCV infection has been substantially reduced to 0.004% to 0.0004% per unit transfused.[11] The major cause of new pediatric HCV infection is now perinatal, with a overall risk of transmission of 6% from HCV antibody–positive mothers.[12] The risk is minimal when the mother is HCV RNA negative and higher when mothers are coinfected with HIV. A recent European multicenter study showed no increase in transmission of HCV from HCV-HIV–coinfected mothers to their infants. One of the explanations proposed was that effective HAART (highly active antiretroviral therapy) treatment of coinfected women led to reduced immunosuppression and hence a reduced maternal viral load.[12] This study also found a doubling of the risk of HCV infection in female offspring, an observation that is novel and yet to be explained. Adolescents may acquire HCV through high-risk behaviors such as injection drug use, intranasal drug use, and body piercing. Horizontal transmission from parent to child, from sibling to sibling, and via sexual transmission is extremely low.[9]

Hepatitis D Virus

Hepatitis D virus[13] (HDV), discovered in 1977, is a defective virus that requires replication of HBV for its own replication. The epidemiologic mechanism is parallel to that for HBV infection, and prevalence has decreased significantly with better control of HBV infection. Replication occurs in the liver, and the pathological effects of the virus are limited to this organ. The hepatitis D antigen can be found in both the liver and the serum of individuals who have the disease. HDV infection may occur as a coinfection with chronic HBV or as an acute super infection of HBV; in both cases, it causes a more severe illness with significant morbidity and mortality. HDV may also be transmitted perinatally with HBV.

Hepatitis E Virus

Hepatitis E virus[14] (HEV), a 27- to 34-nm single-stranded RNA virus, is the cause of epidemic, enteric transmitted hepatitis that has occurred in India, Pakistan, Nepal, Russia, China, Algeria, central Africa, Peru, and Mexico. Only imported cases have been identified in the United States. The illness usually occurs in areas where the water supply is contaminated by feces.

Hepatitis G Virus

The hepatitis G virus[15] (HGV) identified in 1995 is an RNA virus of the Flaviviridae family and a distant relative of HCV. HGV is mainly transmitted parenterally through blood and blood products and through intravenous drug use. Its prevalence in children in the United States was estimated to be 13.8% based on a small study of blood bank samples.[16] The infection may be self-limited, resulting in the production of neutralizing antibody to the E2 envelope protein or may result in a carrier state. The virus does not replicate in the liver and does not appear to alter the course and severity of persons coinfected with HCV but may be protective in HIV infection.[15]

TT-Virus (2)

TT-virus (TTV) is a DNA virus discovered in 1997 in the sera of three out of five patients with biopsy-proven hepatitis and elevated serum alanine aminotransferase levels.[17] In North America the prevalence of TTV has been found to be 10% in volunteer blood donors, 13% of commercial blood donors, and 17% of intravenous drug users.[18] The role of TTV in the pathogenesis of acute and chronic liver disease is yet to be determined.

AUTOIMMUNE HEPATITIS

Autoimmune hepatitis[19] (AIH) is a chronic necroinflammatory hepatitis characterized by mononuclear cell infiltration of the portal tracts, hypergammaglobulinemia, and non–liver-specific autoantibodies. Two types of AIH have been classified according to the presence or absence of certain autoantibodies: AIH type 1 is characterized by the presence of antinuclear antibody (ANA) and anti–smooth-muscle antibody (anti-SMA), whereas AIH type 2 is characterized by anti–liver-kidney microsomal antibodies (anti-LKM). Approximately two thirds of affected children are girls.

DRUG-INDUCED HEPATITIS

Drug-induced liver disease[20] may occur as an unexpected idiosyncratic reaction to a drug or may be an expected consequence to a toxic dose and may cause signs of acute hepatitis and chronic hepatitis. Some forms of drug-induced liver disease are due to the presence of polymorphisms of enzymes that metabolize drugs, resulting in slower metabolism or the production of toxic intermediates by alternative pathways (eg, valproic acid–induced liver injury). Many drugs are known to cause hepatitis, including isonicotinic acid hydrazide or isoniazid (INH), α-methyldopa, and oxyphenisatin acetate.

METABOLIC LIVER DISEASE

α_1-Antitrypsin (α_1-AT) deficiency is the most common genetic cause of liver disease in children, with an incidence of 1 in 1600 to 2000 live births. It results from the retention of the mutant α_1-AT inside the endoplasmic reticulum of liver cells, which may predispose certain individuals with homozygous phenotype ZZ to significant liver injury.[21]

Wilson disease is an autosomal-recessive disorder affecting 1 in 30,000 people. It results from a mutation in the *ATP7B* gene, which encodes a copper-binding membrane protein regulating the transport of copper across cell membranes. More than 200 mutations that may produce disease in humans have been identified.[22] Accumulation of copper in the hepatocytes and other organs results in a constellation of clinical symptoms including hepatitis, neuropsychiatric disease, and Kayser-Fleischer rings in the Descemet membrane of the cornea.

Tyrosinemia (hereditary tyrosinemia type 1) is an autosomal-recessive disease that results in a deficiency in fumarylacetoacetate hydrolase, the last enzyme in the tyrosine degradation pathway. This deficiency leads to an accumulation of intermediary toxic metabolites such as maleylacetoacetate and fumarylacetoacetate, which are thought to cause hepatorenal damage and eventually hepatocellular carcinoma. The usual presentation in infants is acute liver failure with pronounced coagulopathy.[23]

Galactosemia is an autosomal-recessive disorder resulting in decreased production of galactose-1-phosphate uridyltransferase, which exhibits in the neonatal period with cholestatic jaundice, hypoglycemia, and hepatitis.[24] Hereditary fructose intolerance (HFI) is a rare condition, with an estimated prevalence of 1 in 20,000 individuals. The absence of the enzyme aldolase-B results in the build up of fructose-1-phosphate, which inhibits gluconeogenesis and glycolysis. The infant with ongoing fructose ingestion exhibits metabolic acidosis, hypoglycemia, and liver failure.[24]

Progressive familial intrahepatic cholestasis (PFIC) type 1, or Byler disease, is caused by a mutation in the gene *FIC 1* which codes for a P-type adenosine triphosphatase involved in aminophospholipid transport.[25] The mechanism by which cholestatic injury occurs in this condition is to be determined. PFIC type 2 is caused by a mutation in the gene encoding for the main adenosine triphosphate–dependent bile acid pump on the canalicular membrane.[26] PFIC-3 is caused by a mutation in the gene encoding the *MDR* protein, which is a phospholipid flippase also located on the canalicular membrane. Very few patients with this disorder have been described, although a mouse model of the disease exists.[27] PFIC types 1 and 2 cause cholestatic liver disease in infancy, whereas PFIC type 3 may occur at an older age. Inborn errors of bile acid metabolism are also rare but lead to severe cholestatic liver disease, necessitating early recognition and treatment.[28]

Alagille syndrome, or paucity of the intrahepatic bile ducts, is caused by a mutation in the human *jagged 1* gene. Approximately 50% of patients inherit the disease in an autosomal-dominant fashion, whereas the other 50% are spontaneous mutations in the index case (proband). Although multiple mutations have been identified, genotype-phenotype correlations are a little more difficult, and the pathophysiological mechanism of the gene mutation is yet to be elucidated.[29] Diagnosis in the proband still relies largely on the initial clinical criteria.

Evaluation

A complete clinical history and thorough physical examination are important in making a timely diagnosis and preventing the need for unnecessary investigations. Referral to a pediatric gastroenterologist is recommended, given that many of the conditions are uncommon and require close monitoring. The evaluation of a child with hepatitis depends primarily on the age of the child and the nature of the symptoms. Common presentations include jaundice in infancy, the child with jaundice, the incidental finding of elevated liver enzymes during routine work-up, or fulminant hepatic failure. Assessment of children in each of these categories is described in the following sections.

Jaundice in Newborns and Infants

The infant with jaundice and elevated liver enzymes may be otherwise well, have failure to thrive, or display signs of liver decompensation. The primary care physician must determine if the patient has a family history of jaundice, liver or metabolic disease, maternal exposure to drugs and toxins, and maternal serologic status for hepatitis A, B, and C. Maternal illnesses during pregnancy should also be noted particularly in an infant who is malnourished, suggesting the presence of an in utero infection. A complete dietary history to determine fructose ingestion in the infant (either through food or medication) is required if HFI is suspected.

Examination may reveal hepatosplenomegaly, icterus, and little else. The association of renal Fanconi syndrome and clotting abnormalities that are unresponsive to vitamin K therapy suggests tyrosinemia. Neonatal hemochromatosis may be present with hepatitis but often occurs with acute liver failure.

Patients with Alagille syndrome may have jaundice and hepatitis in the first 2 years of life. The diagnosis is a clinical one based on the association of bile duct paucity together with at least three of the following: typical facies, posterior embryotoxon (ophthalmologic examination), butterfly vertebrae (seen on chest x-ray examination), consistent cardiac disease (eg pulmonary stenosis), and renal disease. Other features include a markedly elevated γ-glutamyl transferase (GGT, 800 IU/L), hypercholesterolemia, growth retardation, and intracranial bleeding. Genetic testing, available in selected centers, may be useful in family studies, given that the penetrance is variable.[30] PFIC types 1 and 2 and inborn errors of bile acid synthesis should be suspected in any child with elevated serum bile acids, low GGT, and elevated aminotransferases. PFIC type 3 has a similar clinical picture except that the GGT is elevated and presentation may be delayed.

Investigations in the infant in whom a cause of hepatitis is not obvious should include serologic testing for viruses and general investigations such as a blood ammonia level, serum glucose, blood gases with pH, blood lactate level, urine metabolic screen and reducing substances, red blood cell galactose-1-phosphate uridyl transferase tests, thyroid function tests, and serum and urine bile acid tests. Other conditions that should be considered in an infant with jaundice include α_1-AT deficiency, cystic fibrosis, defects in

Table 273-3 Diagnostic Investigations for Liver Diseases

DISEASE	INVESTIGATION	INTERPRETATION
α_1-AT deficiency	Serologic Pi type	MM (normal) ZZ (α_1-AT deficiency)
	Serum α_1-AT	Less than 50 mg/dL
	Liver biopsy	PAS-positive diastase resistant granules in the hepatocytes endoplasmic reticulum
Tyrosinemia	Urinary succinyl acetone	Elevated
	Alpha-fetoprotein	Raised (indicative of immature hepatocytes) May be raised in many types of neonatal hepatitis but significantly raised in tyrosinemia
PFIC 1, 2, 3	Serum bile acids	Raised
PFIC 1, 2	GGT	Low
PFIC 3	GGT	High
Bile acid metabolic disorder	Fast atom bombardment mass spectroscopy of urine	Typical profiles
	Serum bile acids	Low
	GGT	Low
Hereditary fructose intolerance	Urine reducing substances	Positive when ingesting fructose
	Gene testing	22 Mutations for HFI, 70% of patients have two mutations in exon 5 *(A149P, A174D)*
Cystic fibrosis	Sweat chloride test	Sweat chloride >60 mEq/L
Autoimmune hepatitis		ANA; anti-SMA or anti-LKM
Neonatal hemochromatosis	Serum transferrin	Low (reflects low functioning liver cell mass)
	Serum ferritin	Markedly raised (non-specific)
	MRI	Siderosis of pancreas, myocardium
	Buccal biopsy	Siderosis of salivary glands
Niemann-Pick type C	Liver biopsy (electron microscopy)	Whirled inclusions of sphingomyelin in lysosomes
	Skin fibroblast culture	Measurement of sphingomyelinase activity

α_1-AT, α_1-Antitrypsin; *ANA,* antinuclear antibody; *anti-LKM,* anti–liver-kidney microsomal antibodies; *anti-SMA,* anti–smooth-muscle antibody; *GGT,* γ-glutamyltransferase; *HFI,* hereditary fructose intolerance; *MRI,* magnetic resonance imagine; *PAS,* periodic acid-Schiff; *PFIC,* progressive familial intrahepatic cholestasis.

amino acid synthesis, organic acid synthesis and fatty acid oxidation, glycogen storage disease, and Niemann-Pick type C disease. More sophisticated tests are required for many metabolic and inherited disorders (Table 273-3).

Child With Jaundice

Viral hepatitis, particularly HAV, HBV, HCV, and Epstein-Barr virus, should be actively sought in this age group. HAV infection is heralded by an abrupt onset associated with fever, malaise, anorexia, nausea, vomiting, and upper abdominal discomfort. Darkening of the urine and enlargement and tenderness of the liver follow. Jaundice is infrequent in young children. The bilirubin level increases in both direct and indirect fractions but does not generally exceed a total of 15 mg/dL. Generally, aminotransferase level elevation does not last more than 3 weeks. The clinical and laboratory abnormalities do not generally persist beyond 4 weeks. The disease is rarely fulminant; however, a small percentage of patients with hepatitis A may have a relapsing or protracted course.[31] The presence of IgM-class anti–hepatitis A coinciding with clinical symptoms confirms the diagnosis of acute hepatitis A infection.

In highly endemic areas, hepatitis B is acquired either perinatally or horizontally at a very young age and is generally asymptomatic. The clinical course of HBV infection depends on several viral and host factors, with the age of acquisition being the major determinant of chronicity. Approximately 90% of children who acquire HBV as neonates will develop chronic hepatitis, whereas only 20% of children and 10% of adults follow the same course.[5] In low-prevalence countries, HBV infection occurs more often in adolescents and occurs sporadically. The onset is usually insidious. Extrahepatic manifestations such as skin rash and arthralgia are common and may be prodromal. In fact, hepatitis B should be kept in mind in the differential diagnosis of serum sickness–like illness. Younger children may be asymptomatic. The duration of illness is usually 4 to 6 weeks. Aminotransferase elevation usually peaks approximately 1 month after the onset of illness. Although more than 80% to 90% of children recover without sequelae, fulminant hepatitis is seen in infants born to HBeAg-positive mothers with low levels of HBV DNA.[3]

The presence of HBsAg in the serum implies HBV infection. This occurrence is the first marker to appear and is detected 2 weeks to 6 months after exposure.

Table 273-4 Diagnostic Tests for Hepatitis B Virus (HBV) Antigens and Antibodies

FACTOR TO BE TESTED	HBV ANTIGEN OR ANTIBODY	USE
HBsAg	HBsAg	Detection of acutely or chronically infected people; antigen used in hepatitis B vaccine
Anti-HBsAg	Antibody to HBsAg	Identification of people who have resolved infections with HBV; determination of immunity after immunization
HBeAg	HBeAg	Identification of infected people at increased risk of transmitting HBV
Anti-HBeAg	Antibody to HBeAg	Identification of infected people with decreased risk of transmitting HBV
Anti-HBcAg	Antibody to HBcAg*	Identification of people with acute, resolved, or chronic HBV infection (not present after immunization)
IgM anti-HBc	IgM antibody to HBcAg	Identification of people with acute or recent HBV infections (including HBsAg-negative people during the "window" phase of infection)

HBcAg, hepatitis B core antigen; *HBsAg*, hepatitis B surface antigen; *IgM*, immunoglobulin M.
*No test is available commercially to measure HBcAg.
From American Academy of Pediatrics. Hepatitis B. In: Pickering LK, Baker CJ, Long SS, et al, eds. *2006 Red Book: Report of the Committee of Infectious Diseases.* 27th ed. Elk Grove Village, IL: American Academy of Pediatrics; 2006.

Children with HBV infection are initially HBsAg and HBeAg positive. HbeAg reflects active viral replication and infectivity. During this immunotolerant stage, which may persist for years, viral replication and serum HBV DNA levels are very high. The child is highly infectious and may serve as a source of horizontal transmission in the community. Serum aminotransferase levels fluctuate and may be in the upper limit of normal range. During childhood, conversion from HBeAg to anti-HBeAg may occur spontaneously, with a rate of 3% per year, although rates vary with the mode of acqusition.[32] Seroconversion to anti-HBeAg is often preceded by a transient elevation in serum aminotransferases. After anti-HBeAg seroconversion, HBV DNA levels remain low or undetectable. Most children remain HBsAg positive, and this chronic carrier state is not generally associated with overt disease during childhood. The annual HBsAg clearance rate in chronic carriers is low (1% to 2%) and may be associated with persistence of HBV DNA.[33] Liver cirrhosis is encountered in 3% to 5% of children with chronic HBV. These children are at risk for developing hepatocellular carcinoma before adulthood.[34] Although the best methods and frequency of surveillance have not been determined, careful follow-up that includes serial serum alpha-fetoprotein measurements and liver ultrasound examinations should be performed on these patients.

HBV DNA is detectable in serum very early in the infection, but its measurement is limited by the sensitivity of the techniques used. Target amplification techniques such as polymerase chain reaction (PCR) have a lower limit of detection of 100 to 400 copies/mL, whereas signal amplification techniques such DNA hybridization assays and branched chain DNA assays are less sensitive.[35] Interassay variation is significant, and hence viral load from different assays cannot be compared directly. Recent data suggest that the long-term outcome from HBV infection, particularly the development of hepatocellular carcinoma, is directly related to the degree of viral suppression resulting from therapy.[36] To standardize measurements, an international unit has been recently adopted, and most laboratories will report with the new unit in the near future.[35] Anti-HBsAg confers immunity and indicates resolving or past infection. Anti-HBsAg is also seen after vaccination because the vaccine contains recombinant HbsAg. The presence of anti-HBcAg, which appears 3 to 5 weeks after HBsAg, implies exposure to the native HBV and can indicate ongoing or past infection but does not appear after vaccination (Table 273-4).

Acute HCV infection is asymptomatic in the vast majority of children; however, both acute liver failure and cirrhosis have been reported in infancy.[37] Two characteristic clinical features of HCV infection are (1) fluctuation in the serum concentration of the aminotransferases and (2) progression to chronicity in 50% to 90% of patients.[10,38] Most patients remain asymptomatic without stigmata of chronic liver disease. Liver histologic test shows mild to moderate hepatitis, and fibrosis increases with duration of infection but in an unpredictable manner.[39] Patients with chronic HCV infection who become infected with HAV are at substantial risk of fulminant hepatic failure.[40] Chronic HCV infection predisposes patients to cirrhosis and hepatocellular carcinoma over 20 years in those with adult acquired infection.[41] The natural history of perinatally acquired HCV infection is still under evaluation in cohort studies.

The presence of antibodies to HCV implies exposure to native HCV virus but does not confer protective immunity. Most laboratories currently use third-generation enzyme-linked immunosorbent assay (ELISA), which have over 99% sensitivity and specificity.[42] The recombinant immunoblot assay can be used in patients whose HCV infection is suspected but the ELISA is negative or inconclusive. However, both of these tests become positive weeks after exposure to the virus. In contrast, the highly sensitive PCR assay becomes positive within days after exposure to the virus. Assays for viral detection may be quantitative or qualitative.[43] The latter two are more sensitive; however, as quantitation is an important component of guiding therapy, quantitative assays are used more often. As with HBV infection, the international unit is being adopted as a means of overcoming the variability between laboratories and different commercially available assays. Vertically acquired infection is confirmed by the persistence of anti-HCV antibody beyond 18 months of age or the presence of HCV RNA in serum after the first 3 months of life. PCR testing before this period is unreliable.[44]

Acute HDV infection in a child who is a chronic HBV carrier may produce a severe episode of hepatitis with fulminant hepatic failure or chronic hepatitis. A test for anti-HDV is commercially available.[45] Hepatitis E is similar clinically to hepatitis A. Cholestasis may be more common than with hepatitis A, and elevation of serum aminotransferases is modest. The most unusual clinical feature of the illness is its high mortality rate in pregnant women (approximately 10%).[46] Serologic identification of HBsAg is diagnostic, and real-time PCR has recently been developed.[47] HGV and TTV infections are diagnosed by detection of HGV RNA and TTV DNA by PCR methods.[48] Evaluation for acute HDV would be appropriate in a child with fulminant hepatic failure in whom HBV infection is diagnosed. Evaluation for acute HEV infection would be appropriate in a child with acute hepatitis from a developing county. Evaluation for HGV and TTV is not indicated outside of epidemiologic studies because no clear evidence exists that they are pathogens.

The mode of presentation of autoimmune hepatitis is highly variable; therefore AIH should be excluded with serologic testing in all children with signs of acute or chronic liver disease and liver failure. Hepatomegaly, splenomegaly, and jaundice are common findings.[49] Autoimmune hepatitis is strongly associated with ulcerative colitis and may precede or follow the colitis. Associated extrahepatic manifestations reported included nephrotic syndrome, autoimmune thyroiditis, Behçet disease, Crohn disease, insulin-dependent diabetes, urticaria pigmentosa, vitiligo, hypoparathyroidism, and Addison disease. Although patients with AIH type 2 have higher tendency to have acute liver failure, the overall prognosis of type-2 disease is not different from type-1 disease.[49,50]

Routine investigations reveal a hypergammaglobulinemia and raised ANA, SMA, or LKM antibodies. Histologically, portal tracts are infiltrated by lymphocytes and plasma cells. Inflammatory cells often infiltrate the parenchyma, accompanied by necrosis of cells at the periphery of the hepatic lobule (piecemeal necrosis). Fibrosis may be seen to a variable degree, or true cirrhosis may be present. In 1999 the International Auto-Immune Hepatitis Group modified a scoring system to diagnose AIH in adults. This modification was evaluated by Schreiber and colleagues and was found to be useful in children, particularly when a GGT ratio was used instead of an alanine aminotransferase/alkaline phosphatase ratio.[51]

Metabolic diseases that occur later in childhood include Wilson disease, α_1-AT deficiency, and fatty liver. Wilson disease should always be considered in the differential diagnosis of pediatric liver disease, given that it has a highly variable presentation and because effective therapy is available. Kayser-Fleischer rings and neurologic findings may be absent, and the ceruloplasmin may be normal in young children.[52] No single test is available to diagnose Wilson disease. The combination of two or more of the following is highly suggestive: decreased serum ceruloplasmin (<20 mg/dL), elevated urinary copper excretion (>100 mcg/24 hours), elevated liver copper concentration (>250 mcg/g of dry weight), and Kayser-Fleischer rings. Genetic testing is available in some centers.[53]

Non-alcoholic steatohepatitis (NASH) is fat in the liver associated with inflammation. It has a slight male predominance and generally occurs in the prepubertal age group. NASH is seen in children with a significant number of risk factors, including obesity (body mass index >30), diabetes, insulin resistance, and hypertriglyceridemia.[54] Acanthosis nigricans is a marker of insulin resistance and should be sought. Although many children are obese, only a minority of children have NASH, and hence other mechanisms are clearly involved. A fatty liver can be identified on sonography by the presence of uniform or patchy increased echogenicity. Liver biopsy, although not necessary, shows steatosis, mixed lobular inflammation, and hepatocyte ballooning.[54] Hereditary fructose intolerance can also occur in the older child with an aversion to fructose-containing products who develops vomiting and elevation of serum aminotransferases after inadvertent ingestion.

To evaluate for drug or toxin-induced hepatitis a complete medical history should be obtained for prescribed medications, herbal teas, poisons, and ingestion of wild mushrooms. Acetaminophen toxicity is the most common cause for acute liver failure in children in North America[55]; hence a serum acetaminophen level should be drawn and appropriate therapy instituted immediately. A urine toxicologic screen should also be performed when the index of suspicion is high.

Liver biopsy is required when chronic liver disease is suspected and cannot be diagnosed with the investigations discussed previously and to determine the degree of inflammation and fibrosis, both of which may influence treatment. A needle biopsy is usually adequate, and the risks are low when clotting function is normal, ultrasound guidance is used, and the biopsy is performed by an experienced physician.[56] The biopsy should be sent for histologic testing with additional stains (eg copper, iron) if necessary, and a small sample should be preserved in glutaraldehyde for electron microscopy if a metabolic liver disease is suspected. If Wilson disease is suspected, then hepatic copper should be quantified; obtaining a second biopsy core is usually necessary for this purpose.

Abnormal Liver Enzyme Levels

Many liver diseases can be silent in children, and abnormal liver function is discovered by chance. These diseases include viral hepatitis, metabolic disorders such as Wilson disease, α_1-AT deficiency, NASH, autoimmune hepatitis, and hemochromatosis. Systemic disorders may raise aminotransferases (see Table 273-1). Elevated levels of aminotransferases have been found in 32% of children with celiac disease.[57] A celiac screen should be performed in all children with unexplained elevation of serum aminotransferase levels once hepatologic causes have been excluded.

Fulminant Hepatic Failure

The broad definition of fulminant hepatic failure is hepatic encephalopathy within 8 weeks of onset of illness. This definition is problematic in children because of the difficulty in detecting encephalopathy in infants and young children and the fact that encephalopathy may arise late or not at all.[58] In children, fulminant hepatic failure can be defined as a lack of a preexisting liver disease and severe impairment of hepatic function as evidenced by the following laboratory abnormality: prolonged prothrombin time (>4 seconds over control) that is unresponsive to large doses of vitamin K.

Acetaminophen toxicity is the most common identified cause of fulminant hepatic failure in the United States.[55] In infancy, metabolic disorders such as galactosemia, HFI, tyrosinemia, and neonatal hemochromatosis may cause fulminant failure. (See Table 273-3 for appropriate investigations.) In the older child, Wilson disease, autoimmune hepatitis particularly type 2, medications, and toxins should be considered in the etiology of fulminant hepatic failure.

BOX 273-1 Indications for Hepatitis A Virus Vaccination

- All children at 1 year of age
- Catch-up immunization of unimmunized children 2-18 years of age, especially in the context of rising incidences or ongoing outbreaks among children and adolescents
- Travelers to endemic areas
- Patients with chronic liver disease
- Men who have sex with men
- Users of injection and illicit drugs
- Patients at high risk of exposure secondary to their occupation

Derived from American Academy of Pediatrics. Hepatitis B. In: Pickering LK, Baker CJ, Long SS, et al, eds. *2006 Red Book: Report of the Committee of Infectious Diseases.* 27th ed. Elk Grove Village, IL: American Academy of Pediatrics; 2006.

THERAPY AND PREVENTION

Viral Hepatitis

Hepatitis A

Two inactivated vaccines against HAV are licensed in the United States for children ages 1 to 18 years and adults (Box 273-1). In addition, Twinrix, which is the HAB-HBV combination vaccine, is licensed for adults 18 years of age or older.[59] The vaccine is given in a two- or three-dose schedule depending on the formulation. Table 273-5 shows the recommended doses for HAV vaccination. Children with underlying liver disease should receive the HAV vaccination. Either pediatric formulation induces seroconversion rates greater than 90% after the initial dose and 100% after the second dose.[60,61]

Hospitalization is generally unnecessary for the patient who has acute hepatitis A. However, the infant and young child should be hospitalized if coagulopathy or other evidence of liver decompensation is present. No particular diet or restriction of activity appears to affect the course or outcome of acute viral hepatitis because recovery of HAV in the patient's stool decreases rapidly after the onset of jaundice. Return to school 1 week after onset of illness, provided the child feels well, is recommended.[62] Although household contacts of the patient with hepatitis A are already likely to be infected by the time of diagnosis, infection-control measures should be instituted, including scrupulous hand washing and the use of disposable eating utensils in the patient's home until jaundice clears. Pooled serum immune globulin when given within 2 weeks postexposure is effective in preventing symptomatic infection, as is immunization within an 8-day window period.[63] Immune globulin should be given to household contacts; institutional contacts and to persons exposed in common source outbreaks (Table 273-6). Neonates born of infected mothers do not need special care if the mother is not jaundiced. Children traveling to endemic areas should also be immunized prophylactically. Vaccination is

Table 273-5 Recommended Doses and Schedules for Inactivated Hepatitis A Vaccines[a]

AGE (YR)	VACCINE	HEPATITIS A ANTIGEN DOSE	VOLUME PER DOSE (ML)	NUMBER OF DOSES	SCHEDULE
1-18	Havrix	720 ELU	0.5	2	Initial and 6-12 mo later
1-18	Vaqta	25 U[b]	0.5	2	Initial and 6-18 mo later
≥19	Havrix	1440 ELU	1.0	2	Initial and 6-12 mo later
≥19	Vaqta	50 U[b]	1.0	2	Initial and 6-18 mo later
≥18	Twinrix[c]	720 ELU	1.0	3	Initial and 1 and 6 mo later

ELU, Enzyme-linked immunosorbent assay units.
[a]Havrix and Twinrix are manufactured by Glaxo-Smith-Kline Biologicals; Vaqta is manufactured and distributed by Merck & Co, Inc.
[b]Antigen units (each unit is equivalent to approximately 1 mcg of viral protein).
[c]A combination of hepatitis B (Engerix-B, 20 mcg) and hepatitis A (Havrix, 720 ELU) vaccine (Twinrix) is licensed for use in people 18 years of age and older in a three-dose schedule. Havrix 360 ELU in single-dose vials is licensed in the United States but no longer available.
From American Academy of Pediatrics. Hepatitis B. In: Pickering LK, Baker CJ, Long SS, et al, eds. *2006 Red Book: Report of the Committee of Infectious Diseases.* 27th ed. Elk Grove Village, IL: American Academy of Pediatrics; 2006.

preferable; however, if travel is imminent (ie, less than 1 month), then IgG may be substituted (Table 273-7).[64]

Hepatitis B

In the United States the implementation of universal newborn infant hepatitis B immunization in 1991, followed in 1995 by routine vaccination of all adolescents aged 11 to 12 years and, in 1999, to include children younger than 18 years who had not been vaccinated previously has resulted in a significant reduction of HBV in children.[65] The rate of acute HBV infection in children and adolescents decreased 89% during the years 1990 to 2002, and racial disparities in hepatitis B incidence have narrowed.[65] Despite these recommendations, a recent study showed 70% of homeless inner-city children ages 13 to 18 years had no record of HBV vaccination.[66] Therefore HBV vaccine must be administered on any chance encounter with such children (Box 273-2). Detailed recommendations regarding doses and postexposure prophylaxis are provided in Tables 273-8 and 273-9. A neonate born to an HBsAg-positive mother or a mother who has had hepatitis B during pregnancy should be given 0.5 mL of hepatitis B immune globulin (HBIg) intramuscularly within the first 12 hours of life and 0.5 mL of HBV vaccine intramuscularly before hospital discharge but definitely within the first week of life and again at 1 and 6 months. Data linking breastfeeding to the acquisition of viremia are equivocal, but HBsAg-positive mothers whose infants have received immunoprophylaxis may breastfeed without risk of transmitting HBV to the infant.[67]

The first universal vaccination program was launched in Taiwan in 1984 and included neonates, preschool children, and adults.[4] The HBsAg carrier rate decreased from 10% to less than 1% after vaccination of children older than 10 years. Anti-HBcAg positivity decreased from 36% to 16% in children older than 10 years. These findings indicate that vaccination decreased both the vertical and horizontal transmission rates. The average annual incidence of hepatocellular carcinoma dropped from 0.70 per 100,000 children between 1981 and 1986 to 0.36 between 1990 and 1994.[68] HBV immunization also protects against HDV infection.

Two treatments for HBV in children have been approved.[69] α-Interferon, which may be given to children

Table 273-6 Recommendations for Postexposure Immunoprophylaxis of Hepatitis A

TIME SINCE EXPOSURE (WK)	FUTURE EXPOSURE LIKELY, OR IMMUNIZATION RECOMMENDED	AGE OF PATIENT (YR)	RECOMMENDED PROPHYLAXIS
≤2	No	All ages	Ig, 0.02 mL/kg[a]
	Yes	≥1	Ig, 0.02 mL/kg[a] AND Hepatitis A vaccine[b]
>2	No	All ages	No prophylaxis
	Yes	≥1	Hepatitis A vaccine[b]

Ig, Immune globulin.
[a]Immune globulin should be administered deep into a large muscle mass. Ordinarily, no more than 5 mL should be administered in one site in an adult or large child; lesser amounts (maximum 3 mL in one site) should be given to small children and infants.
[b]Dose and schedule of hepatitis A vaccine as recommended according to age in Table 273-5.
From American Academy of Pediatrics. Hepatitis B. In: Pickering LK, Baker CJ, Long SS, et al, eds. *2006 Red Book: Report of the Committee of Infectious Diseases.* 27th ed. Elk Grove Village, IL: American Academy of Pediatrics; 2006.

Table 273-7 Recommendations for Preexposure Immunoprophylaxis of Hepatitis A for Travelers

AGE (YR)	LIKELY EXPOSURE DURATION (MO)	RECOMMENDED PROPHYLAXIS
<1	<3	Ig, 0.02 mL/kg[a]
	3-5	Ig, 0.06 mL/kg[a]
	Long term	Ig 0.06 mL/kg at departure and every 5 mo if exposure to HAV continues[a]
≥1	<3[b]	Hepatitis vaccine[c,d] OR Ig, 0.02 mL/kg[a]
	3-5[b]	Hepatitis vaccine[c,d] OR Ig, 0.06 mL/kg[a]
	Long-term	Hepatitis A vaccine[c,d]

HAV, Hepatitis A virus; *Ig,* immune globulin.
[a]Immune globulin should be administered deep into a large muscle mass. Ordinarily, no more than 5 mL should be administered in one site in an adult or large child; lesser amounts (maximum 3 mL in one site) should be given to small children and infants.
[b]Vaccine is preferable, but Ig is an acceptable alternative.
[c]To ensure protection in travelers whose departure is imminent, Ig also may be given.
[d]Dose and schedule of hepatitis A vaccine as recommended according to age in Table 273-5.
From American Academy of Pediatrics. Hepatitis B. In: Pickering LK, Baker CJ, Long SS, et al, eds. *2006 Red Book: Report of the Committee of Infectious Diseases.* 27th ed. Elk Grove Village, IL: American Academy of Pediatrics; 2006.

BOX 273-2 Persons Who Should Receive Hepatitis B Virus (HBV) Immunization

All infants (infants of HBsAg-positive mothers require post-exposure immunoprophylaxis with HBIg and vaccine)
Infants and children at risk of acquisition of HBV by person-to-person (horizontal) transmission should be immunized by 6-9 months of age
Adolescents* (special efforts should be made to vaccinate those adolescents in the categories of high risk for HBV infection)
Users of intravenous drugs
Sexually active heterosexual persons with more than one sex partner in the previous 6 months or those with a sexually transmitted disease
Men who have sex with men
Health care workers at risk of exposure to blood or body fluids
Residents and staff of institutions for developmentally disabled persons
Staff of nonresidential child care and school programs for developmentally disabled persons if attended by a known HBV carrier
Patients on hemodialysis
Patients with bleeding disorders who receive certain blood products
Household contacts and sexual partners of HBV carriers
Members of households with adoptees from countries where HBV infection is endemic and who are HBsAg positive
International travelers who will live for more than 6 months in an area of high HBV endemicity and who otherwise will be at risk
Inmates of long-term correctional facilities

HBIg, Hepatitis B immune globulin; *HBsAg*, hepatitis B surface antigen.
*Implementation can be initiated before children reach adolescence.
Derived from American Academy of Pediatrics, Peter G, ed. *1997 Red Book: Report of the Committee on Infectious Diseases.* 24th ed. Elk Grove Village, IL: American Academy of Pediatrics; 1997.

1 year of age and older, results in HBeAg seroconversion in 25% to 50% of children with chronic HBV. The effect on HBsAg clearance is poor, but serum aminotransferases and liver histologic results improve.[70] Lamivudine (3 mg/kg/day up to 100 mg/day), which may be given to children 3 years of age and older, has been shown to produce HBeAg seroconversion in 22% of children versus 13% of placebo controls.[71] Response is greatest in patients with elevated alanine aminotransferase; resistance rates in the first year of therapy were 19%. Adefovir dipivoxil, the latest drug to be approved by the US Food and Drug Administration for HBV infection in adults, is currently being evaluated in pediatric trials.

An important point to remember is that seroconversion may not be permanent and that seroreversion may occur, particularly in the first year after therapy. Although newer nucleoside analogues and other families of drugs are available for treating HBV infection, resistance to each of these drugs has developed after monotherapy. For these reasons the decision to treat should be made in conjunction with a pediatric hepatologist.

Hepatitis C

Currently, no vaccine is available for the prevention of HCV infection. Natural infection does not protect from reinfection with the same or different genotypes either in patients or experimentally infected chimpanzees. The most important strategies for controlling hepatitis C include screening donor blood for anti-HCV, identifying and educating of persons at risk, and establishing risk-minimization programs for intravenous drug users.[72] Screening should include injection drug users, patients on hemodialysis, recipients of one or more units of blood or blood products before 1992, children with clinical non-A, non-B hepatitis, children (after 18 months of age) born to mothers infected with HCV, and international adoptees born to high-risk mothers.[72]

Perinatal transmission is the most common route of new infection in children, with rates in the order of 4% to 6%.[73,74] Maternal-fetal transmission has also been linked to in utero monitoring and prolonged rupture of membranes; it does not appear to be prevented by cesarean delivery.[12] Although HCV RNA has been detected in human milk, current evidence suggests that breastfeeding is not contraindicated.[73,74] However, in developed countries, perhaps mothers should consider abstaining from breastfeeding if their nipples are cracked and bleeding.[75] Patients with HCV infection should be counseled to avoid hepatotoxic medications and alcohol and should receive vaccination against HAV and HBV infections to prevent additional liver damage.[49,76] The American Association for the Study of Liver Diseases presents arguments for and against treatment of HCV infection in children. Based on treatment trials in children, the US Food and Drug Administration has approved the treatment of children with HCV ages 3 to 17 years with a combination regime of α-interferon (subcutaneously three times per week) and oral ribavirin.[77] Side effects of therapy are better tolerated in children but require close monitoring, and therapy should be supervised by persons who are experienced in treating children. More recently a single trial has evaluated pegylated interferon and ribavirin in children.[78] Sustained viral response was documented in 22 (47.8%) of 46 patients with genotype 1. A multicenter, placebo-controlled trial of pegylated interferon with or without ribavirin is currently underway.

Hepatitis E

Treatment of HEV infection is supportive. Prevention rests on improving hygiene; however, the development of recombinant peptide vaccines is well underway.[79]

Autoimmune Hepatitis

Prednisone is a potent antiinflammatory agent capable of suppressing activity in AIH. Because of its side effects particularly on growth, a second immunosuppressive agent, azathioprine, is frequently added. This treatment allows a reduction or complete weaning of the prednisone.[19] Some patients who are refractory to

Table 273-8 Recommended Doses of Hepatitis B Vaccines

PATIENTS	VACCINE[a]	
	RECOMBIVAX HB[b] DOSE (MCG/ML)	ENGERIX-B[c] DOSE (MCG/ML)
Infants of HBsAg-negative mothers and children and adolescents younger than 20 yr of age	5 (0.5)	10 (0.5)
Infants of HBsAg-positive mothers (HBIg [0.5 mL] also is recommended)	5 (0.5)	10 (0.5)
Adults 20 yr of age or older	10 (1.0)	20 (1.0)
Adults undergoing dialysis and other immunosuppressed adults	40 (1.0)[d]	40 (2.0)[e]

HBIg, Hepatitis B immune globulin; *HBsAg,* hepatitis B surface antigen.
[a]Both vaccines are administered in a three- or four-dose schedule; four doses may be administered if a birth dose is given and a combination vaccine is used to complete the series. Only single-antigen hepatitis B vaccine can be used for the birth dose. Single-antigen or combination vaccine containing hepatitis B vaccine may be used to complete the series.
[b]Available from Merck & Co., Inc.

- A two-dose schedule, administered at 0 months and then 4 to 6 months later, is available for adolescents 11 to 15 years of age using the adult formulation of Recombivax HB (10 mcg).
- A combination of hepatitis B (Recombivax, 5 mcg) and *Haemophilus influenzae* type b (PRP-OMP) vaccine is recommended for use a 2, 4, and 12 to 15 months of age (Convax). This vaccine cannot be administered at birth, before 6 weeks of age, or after 71 months of age.

[c]Available from Glaxo-Smith-Kline Biologicals. The US Food and Drug Administration has licensed this vaccine for use in an optional four-dose schedule at 0, 1, 2, and 12 months of age.

- A combination of hepatitis B (Energerix-B, 20 mcg) and hepatitis A (Havrix, 720 ELU) vaccine (Twinrix) is licensed for use in people 18 years of age and older in a three-dose schedule administered at 0, 1, and 6 or more months later.
- A combination of diphtheria and tetanus toxoids and acellular pertussis (DTaP), inactivated poliovirus (IPV), and hepatitis B (Energix-B, 10 mcg) is recommended for use at 2, 4, and 6 months of age (Pediarix). This vaccine cannot be administered at birth, before 6 weeks of age, or at ≥7 years of age.

[d]Special formulation for dialysis patients.
[e]Two 1.0-mL doses given in one site in a four-dose schedule at 0, 1, 2, and 6 months of age.
From American Academy of Pediatrics. Hepatitis B. In: Pickering LK, Baker CJ, Long SS, et al, eds. *2006 Red Book: Report of the Committee of Infectious Diseases.* 27th ed. Elk Grove Village, IL: American Academy of Pediatrics; 2006.

Table 273-9 Guide to Postexposure Immunoprophylaxis for Hepatitis B Infection

TYPE OF EXPOSURE	IMMUNOPROPHYLAXIS
Perinatal	HBIg + vaccination
Sexual—acute infection	HBIg + vaccination
Sexual—chronic carrier	Vaccination
Household contact—chronic carrier	Vaccination
Household contact—acute case with identifiable blood exposure	HBIg +vaccination
Infant (<12 mo)—acute case in primary caregiver	HBIg + vaccination
Accidental—percutaneous, perimucosal	HBIg ± vaccination

HBIg, Hepatitis B immune globulin.
Modified from American Academy of Pediatrics. Hepatitis B. In: Pickering LK, Baker CJ, Long SS, et al, ed. *2006 Red Book: Report of the Committee of Infectious Diseases.* 27th ed. Elk Grove Village, IL: American Academy of Pediatrics; 2006.

azathioprine and steroids have responded to cyclosporine[80] or tacrolimus.[81]

Prednisone is initiated at a steady dose[19]; when the patient improves the prednisone dose may be tapered at weekly intervals to a dose that achieves and maintains clinical and biochemical remission. Azathioprine may be added after symptoms improve. The patient must be monitored for azathioprine toxicity (eg, hematopoietic toxicity), particularly patients with thiopurine S-methyl-transferase deficiency.[82] Remission is defined as absence of clinical symptoms, an aminotransferase level no more than two times normal, decreasing serum γ-globulin levels, and resolution of the aggressive histologic appearance on a liver biopsy specimen. Duration of therapy once remission is achieved is controversial. Generally, once remission is achieved, steroids may be tapered gradually over 2 to 3 months. Long-term treatment with a low-dose steroid is often required.[49,50]

Clinical remission generally occurs within 3 to 6 months, biochemical remission within 6 to 12 months, and histologic remission within 12 to 24 months. During the steroid taper the patient must be monitored at 2- to 4-week intervals for approximately 3 months for evidence of early recurrence of disease. If a recurrence does not take place within this time, then the frequency of observation can be decreased. At least 80% of children appear to achieve initial remission. and although relapses are common, long-term control usually is achieved with continuous immunosuppressive therapy.[19] The child with autoimmune hepatitis and fulminant hepatic failure poses a difficult therapeutic problem. Prednisone and azathioprine have been used in this situation with success.[19] However, liver transplantation may be necessary for survival. The long-term outcome of chronic active hepatitis has been evaluated in several pediatric studies.[49,50,83] Most children are likely to have prolonged survival on minimal long-term immunosuppression.

Drug-Induced Hepatitis

The profound effects of acetaminophen toxicity can be treated with intravenous N-acetylcysteine.[84] In all other cases of suspected drug-induced hepatitis, supportive care is recommended along with discontinuation of the suspected drug.

Metabolic Liver Disease

The aim of therapy in Wilson disease is copper chelation in a controlled manner. The first-line therapy is penicillamine in the majority of cases. However, penicillamine has significant side effects, including allergies and renal disease, and the patient requires close monitoring.[85] Triethylene tetramine hydrochloride (trientine) has been effective in the same dose as penicillamine but is also associated with significant side effects.[84] Tetrathiomolybdate can be used when significant neurologic disease exists, but toxicity needs to be monitored carefully.[86] Zinc may be used as initial therapy in patients without clinical disease who are diagnosed incidentally on family screening.[85]

No specific therapy is available for α_1-AT deficiency, and liver transplantation should be considered for end-stage liver disease. Dietary restriction of galactose is the treatment of choice for galactosemia.[24] Tyrosinemia may be treated with a phenylalanine and tyrosine restricted diet together with 2-nitro 4-trifluoromethyl-benzoyl-1-1,3-cyclohexanedione (NTBC). NTBC is an inhibitor of an early enzyme in the tyrosine degradation pathway and is thought to prevent the accumulation of toxic products resulting in a clinical improvement in most patients.[23] Although costly, NTBC has been proposed as an alternative to liver transplantation. Whether it will decrease the risk of developing hepatocellular carcinoma remains to be determined. Bile acid–replacement therapy is the treatment of choice for inborn errors of bile acid synthesis.[87] Ursodeoxycholic acid may be used in the treatment of liver disease secondary to cystic fibrosis, although no data exist to support its use.[88]

Fulminant Hepatic Failure

Fulminant hepatic failure in children needs to be managed in a setting with liver transplantation expertise. The requirements of liver support must be balanced with the management of fluids, nutrition, and encephalopathy, which is a late and ominous finding in children.[58] Transferring a child with severe hepatitis early before intensive care management is required is preferable.

Liver Transplantation

Liver transplantation has improved mortality and morbidity of children who have severe liver disease. Apart from liver failure, indications may include growth failure and intractable itch from cholestasis.[89]

The management of the child pretransplantation involves aggressive nutritional therapy[90] and prevention of complications such as bacterial peritonitis and variceal hemorrhage, which may adversely affect outcome. Transplantation for chronic liver failure secondary to HBV infection is complicated by almost 100% recurrence of infection; however, the use of HBIg followed by lamivudine improves the outcome.[91] Recurrence of HCV infection after transplantation is around 90%, but transplantation is recommended because recurrent disease is mild in the majority.[92] Recurrence is related to risk factors in the donor, risk factors in the recipient, and viral and clinical factors. Recently, recurrence of HCV posttransplantation in children has been reported as mild in a small series.[93] Liver transplantation for all causes results in 5-year survival rates in children approaching 70% to 80%.[94] Focus is now directed toward improving morbidity related to immunosuppressive medications and quality-of-life issues for patients and their families.

WHEN TO REFER

- Children with fulminant liver failure of any cause should be promptly referred to a specialist affiliated with a pediatric liver transplant center.
- Children with uncomplicated hepatitis A can usually be managed by a general pediatrician. However, children with chronic hepatitis B, D, or C should be referred to a pediatric gastroenterologist or infectious disease specialist for consideration for treatment.
- Children with metabolic liver disease, drug-induced hepatitis, or AIH should be referred to a pediatric specialist in metabolic disease or gastroenterology as appropriate.
- Fulminant hepatic failure, defined as a lack of a preexisting liver disease and severe impairment of hepatic function as evidenced by the following laboratory abnormality: prolonged prothrombin time (>4 seconds over control) that is unresponsive to large doses of vitamin K
- HbsAg-positive serologic test in children 1 year of age or older
- Anti-HCV-positive serologic test in children 3 years of age or older
- Any diagnosis of drug-induced hepatitis (unexplained elevation of serum aminotransferases or bilirubin in a child who is taking or has recently taken any medication)
- Any diagnosis of metabolic liver disease (unexplained elevation of serum aminotransferases or bilirubin in a child) and a positive screening test, such as low ceruloplasmin, low galactose-1-phosphate uridyl transferase, and positive urine-reducing substances

WHEN TO ADMIT

- Prolonged prothrombin time (>4 seconds over control) in a child with severe hepatitis of any cause
- Acute encephalopathy in a child with severe hepatitis of any cause
- Dehydration requiring intravenous fluid resuscitation in a child with severe hepatitis
- Gastrointestinal bleeding in a child with acute or chronic hepatitis

TOOLS FOR PRACTICE

Medical Decision Support

- *Hepatitis A* (Web page), Centers for Disease Control and Prevention (www.cdc.gov/ncidod/diseases/hepatitis/a/index.htm).
- *Hepatitis B* (Web page), Centers for Disease Control and Prevention (www.cdc.gov/ncidod/diseases/hepatitis/b/index.htm).
- *Hepatitis C* (Web page), Centers for Disease Control and Prevention (www.cdc.gov/ncidod/diseases/hepatitis/c/index.htm).
- *Hepatitis D* (Web page), Centers for Disease Control and Prevention (www.cdc.gov/ncidod/diseases/hepatitis/d/index.htm).
- *Hepatitis E* (Web page), Centers for Disease Control and Prevention (www.cdc.gov/ncidod/diseases/hepatitis/e/index.htm).
- *Hepatitis Training Courses* (on-line course), Centers for Disease Control and Prevention (www.cdc.gov/ncidod/diseases/hepatitis/training/index.htm).
- *National Viral Hepatitis Information Center* (Web page), Centers for Disease Control and Prevention (wwwn.cdc.gov/pubs/hepa.aspx).
- *Red Book, 27th edition* (book), American Academy of Pediatrics (www.aap.org/bst/showdetl.cfm?&DID=15&Product_ID=4143&CatID=132).
- *Traveler's Health: Hepatitis, Viral, Type A* (Web page), Centers for Disease Control and Prevention (wwwn.cdc.gov/travel/yellowBookCh4-HepA.aspx).
- *Traveler's Health: Hepatitis, Viral, Type B* (Web page), Centers for Disease Control and Prevention (wwwn.cdc.gov/travel/yellowBookCh4-HepB.aspx).
- *Traveler's Health: Hepatitis, Viral, Type C* (Web page), Centers for Disease Control and Prevention (wwwn.cdc.gov/travel/yellowBookCh4-HepC.aspx).
- *Traveler's Health: Hepatitis, Viral, Type D* (Web page), Centers for Disease Control and Prevention (wwwn.cdc.gov/travel/yellowBookCh4-HepE.aspx).

RELATED WEB SITE

Centers or Disease Control and Prevention, Hepatitis (www.cdc.gov/ncidod/diseases/hepatitis/index.htm).

AAP POLICY STATEMENTS

American Academy of Pediatrics, Committee on Infectious Disease. Hepatitis A vaccine recommendations hepatitis A vaccine recommendations. *Pediatrics.* 2007;120(1):189-199.

Advisory Committee on Immunization Practices and Centers for Disease Control and Prevention. A Comprehensive Immunization Strategy to Eliminate Transmission of Hepatitis B Virus Infection in the United States. *Pediatrics* 2006;118(1):404. AAP Endorsed. (aappolicy.aappublications.org/cgi/content/full/pediatrics;118/1/404).

REFERENCES

1. Centers for Disease Control and Prevention. *Hepatitis Surveillance Report No 60.* Atlanta, GA: US Department of Health and Human Services, Centers for Disease Control and Prevention; 2005.
2. Lemon SM. Type A viral hepatitis: new developments in an old disease. *N Engl J Med.* 1985;313:1059-1067.
3. Ranger-Rogez S, Denis F. Hepatitis B mother-to-infant transmission. *Expt Rev Anti-Infective Ther.* 2004;2(1): 133-145.
4. Chang MH. Hepatitis B: long-term outcome and benefits from mass vaccination in children. *Acta Gastro-Enterologica Belgica.* 1998;61:210-213.
5. Edmunds WJ, Medley GF, Nokes DJ, et al. The influence of age on the development of the hepatitis B carrier state. *Proc Biol Sci.* 1993;253:197-201.
6. Sterneck M, Kalinina T, Otto S, et al. Neonatal fulminant hepatitis B: structural and functional analysis of complete hepatitis B virus genomes from mother and infant. *J Infect Dis.* 1998;177:1378-1381.
7. Ni Y, Chang MH, Wang KJ. et al. Clinical relevance of hepatitis B virus genotype in children with chronic infection and hepatocellular carcinoma. *Gastroenterology.* 2004;127:1733-1738.
8. Chien-Hung Chen, Yang Yuan Chen, Gran-Hum Chen, et al. Hepatitis B virus transmission and hepatocarcinogenesis: a 9 year retrospective cohort of 13,676 relatives with hepatocellular carcinoma. *J Hepatol.* 2004;40:653-659.
9. Hardikar W. Hepatitis C in childhood. *J Gastroenterol Hepatol.* 2002;17:476-481.
10. Chesney PJ, Fisher MC, Gerber MA, et al. Hepatitis C virus infection. *Pediatrics.* 1998;101:481-485.
11. Schreiber GB, Busch MP, Kleinman SH, et al. The risk of transfusion-transmitted viral infections. *N Eng J Med.* 1996;334:1685-1690.
12. European Pediatric Hepatitis C Network (Tovo A). A significant sex—but not elective cesarean section—effect on mother-to-child transmission of hepatitis C infection. *J Infect Dis.* 2005;192:1872-1879.
13. Niro GA, Rosina F, Rizzetto M. Treatment of hepatitis D. *J Viral Hepatitis.* 2005;12:2-9.
14. Krawczynski K. Hepatitis E. *Hepatology.* 1993;17: 932-947.
15. Stapleton JT. GB virus type C/hepatitis G virus. *Semin Liv Dis.* 2003;23:137-148.
16. Atsushi H, Rima FJ, Dickstein B. GB virus C/hepatitis G virus infection is frequent in American Children and young adults. *Clin Infect Dis.* 2000;30:569-571.
17. Nishizawa T, Okamoto H, Konishi K, et al. A novel DNA virus (TTV) associated with elevated transaminase levels in post transfusion hepatitis of unknown etiology. *Biochem Biophys Res Commun.* 1997;241:92-97.
18. Desai SM, Muerhoff AS, Leary TP, et al. Prevalence of TT virus infection in US blood donors and populations at risk for acquiring parenterally transmitted viruses. *J Infect Dis.* 1999;180:1748-1750.
19. Mieli-Vergani G, Vergani D. Immunological liver diseases in children. *Semin Liv Dis.* 1998;18:271-279.
20. Kaplowitz N. Idiosyncratic drug hepatotoxicity. *Nat Rev Drug Discov.* 2005;4:489-499.
21. Teckman Jh, Qu D, Perlmutter DH. Molecular pathogenesis of liver disease in a1-antitrypsin deficiency. *Hepatology.* 1996;24:1504-1516.
22. Ferenci P. Wilson disease. *Clin Gastroenterol Hepatol.* 2005;3:726-733
23. Joshi SN, Venugopalan P. Experience with NTBC therapy in hereditary tyrosinaemia type I: an alternative to liver transplantation. *Ann Trop Paediatr.* 2004;24(3): 259-65.
24. Clayton PT. Inborn errors presenting with liver dysfunction. *Semin Neonatol.* 2002;7(1):49-63.
25. Ujhazy P, Ortiz D, Misra S, et al. Familial intrahepatic cholestasis 1: studies of localization and function. *Hepatology.* 2001;34(4 pt 1):768-775.

26. Jansen PL, Strautnieks SS, Jacquemin E, et al. Hepatocanalicular bile salt export pump deficiency in patients with progressive familial intrahepatic cholestasis. *Gastroenterology*. 1999;117(6):1370-1379.
27. de Vree JM, Jacquemin E, Sturm E, et al. Mutations in the MDR3 gene cause progressive familial intrahepatic cholestasis. *Proc Natl Acad Sci U S A*. 1998;95(1):282-287.
28. Bove KE, Heubi JE, Balistreri WF, et al. Bile acid synthetic defects and liver disease: a comprehensive review. *Pediatr Dev Pathol*. 2004;7(4):315-334.
29. Boyer J, Crosnier C, Driancourt C, et al. Expression of mutant JAGGED1 alleles in patients with Alagille syndrome. *Hum Genet*. 2005;116(6):445-453.
30. Elmslie FV, Vivian AJ, Gardiner H, et al. Alagille syndrome: family studies. *Med Genet*. 1995;32(4):264-268.
31. Sagnelli E, Coppola N, Marrocco C, et al. HAV replication in acute hepatitis with typical and atypical clinical course. *Med Virol*. 2003;71(1):1-6.
32. Boxall EH, Sira J, Standish RA, et al. Natural history of hepatitis B in perinatally infected carriers. *Arch Dis Child Fetal Neonatal Ed*. 2004;89(5):F456-F460.
33. Bortolotti F, Wirth S, Crivellaro C, et al. Long term persistence of hepatitis B virus DNA in the serum of children with chronic hepatitis B after hepatitis e antigen to antibody seroconversion. *J Pediatr Gastroenterol Nutr*. 1996;22:270-274.
34. McIntosh ED. Paediatric infections: prevention of transmission and disease—implications for adults. *Vaccine*. 2005;23(17-18):2087-2089.
35. Shymala V, Arcangel P, Cottrell J, et al. Assessment of the target-capture PCR hepatitis B virus (HBV) DNA quantitative assay and comparison with commercial HBV DNA quantitative assays. *J Clin Microbiol*. 2004;42(11):5199-5204.
36. Liaw YF. Prevention and surveillance of hepatitis B virus-related hepatocellular carcinoma. *Semin Liver Dis*. 2005;25(suppl 1):40-47.
37. Jonas MM. Children with hepatitis C. *Hepatology*. 2002;36(5 suppl 1):S173-S178.
38. Resti M, Jara P, Hierro L, et al. Clinical features and progression of perinatally acquired hepatitis C virus infection. *J Med Virol*. 2003;70(3):373-377.
39. Iorio R, Giannattasio A, Sepe A, et al. Chronic hepatitis C in childhood: an 18-year experience. *Clin Infect Dis*. 2005;41(10):1431-1437.
40. Vento S, Garofano T, Renzine C, et al. Fulminant hepatitis associated with hepatitis A virus super infection in patients with chronic hepatitis C. *N Engl J Med*. 1998;338:286-290.
41. Lauer GM, Walker BD. Hepatitis C virus infection. *N Eng J Med*. 2001;345:41-52.
42. Vrielink H, Reesink HW, van den Burg PJ, et al. Performance of three generations of anti-hepatitis C virus enzyme-linked immunosorbent assays in donors and patients. *Transfusion*. 1997;37(8):845-849.
43. Desombere I, Van Vlierberghe H, Couvent S, et al. Comparison of qualitative (COBAS AMPLICOR HCV 2.0 versus VERSANT HCV RNA) and quantitative (COBAS AMPLICOR HCV monitor 2.0 versus VERSANT HCV RNA 3.0) assays for hepatitis C virus (HCV) RNA detection and quantification: impact on diagnosis and treatment of HCV infections. *J Clin Microbiol*. 2005;43(6):2590-2597.
44. Resti M, Bortolotti F, Vajro P, et al, Italian Society of Pediatric Gastroenterology and Hepatology, Committee of Hepatology. Guidelines for the screening and follow-up of infants born to anti-HCV positive mothers. *Dig Liver Dis*. 2003;35(7):453-457.
45. Gupta S, Govindarajan S, Cassidy WM, et al. Acute delta hepatitis: serological diagnosis with particular reference to hepatitis delta virus RNA. *Am J Gastroenterol*. 1991;86(9):1227-1231.
46. Kumar A, Beniwal M, Kar P, et al. Hepatitis E in pregnancy. *Int J Gynaecol Obstet*. 2004;85(3):240-244.
47. Narayanan J, Cromeans TL, Robertson BH, et al. A broadly reactive one-step real-time RT-PCR assay for rapid and sensitive detection of hepatitis E virus. *J Virol Methods*. 2006;131:65-71.
48. Allain JP, Thomas I, Sauleda S. Nucleic acid testing for emerging viral infections. *Transfus Med*. 2002;12(4):275-283.
49. Saadah OI, Smith AL, Hardikar W. Long-term outcome of autoimmune hepatitis in children. *J Gastroenterol Hepatol*. 2001;16(11):1297-1302.
50. Gregorio GV, Portmann B, Reid F, et al. Autoimmune hepatitis in childhood: a 20-year experience. *Hepatology*. 1997;25:541-547.
51. Ebbeson RL, Schreiber RA. Diagnosing autoimmune hepatitis in children: is the International Autoimmune Hepatitis Group scoring system useful? *Clin Gastroenterol Hepatol*. 2004;2(10):935-940.
52. Perman JA, Werlin SL, Grand RJ, et al. Laboratory measures of copper metabolism in the differentiation of chronic active hepatitis and Wilson disease in children. *J Pediatr*. 1979;94:564-568.
53. Cox DW, Prat L, Walshe JM, et al. Twenty-four novel mutations in Wilson disease patients of predominantly European ancestry. *Hum Mutat*. 2005;26(3):280.
54. Nanda K. Non-alcoholic steatohepatitis in children. *Pediatr Transplant*. 2004;8(6):613-618.
55. James LP, Alonso EM, Hynan LS, et al. Detection of acetaminophen protein adducts in children with acute liver failure of indeterminate cause. *Pediatrics*. 2006;118(3):e676-e681.
56. Fox VL, Cohen MB, Whitington PF, et al. Outpatient liver biopsy in children: a medical position statement of the North American Society for Pediatric Gastroenterology and Nutrition. *J Pediatr Gastroenterol Nutr*. 1996;23:213-216.
57. Farre C, Esteve M, Curcoy A, et al. Hypertransaminasemia in pediatric celiac disease patients and its prevalence as a diagnostic clue. *Am J Gastroenterol*. 2002;97(12):3176-3181.
58. Dhawan A, Cheeseman P, Mieli-Vergani G. Approaches to acute liver failure in children. *Pediatr Transplant*. 2004;8(6):584-588.
59. American Academy of Pediatrics. Summaries of infectious diseases. In: Pickering LK, Baker CJ, Long SS, et al, eds. *2006 Red Book: Report of the Committee on Infectious Diseases*. 27th ed. Elk Grove Village, IL: American Academy of Pediatrics; 2006.
60. Nalin DR, Kuter BJ, Brown L, et al. Worldwide experience with the CR326F-derived inactivated hepatitis A virus vaccine in pediatric and adult populations: an overview. *J Hepatol*. 1993;18(suppl 2):S51-S55.
61. Scheifele DW. Prevention of hepatitis A by Havrix: a review. *Expert Rev Vaccines*. 2005;4(4):459-471.
62. American Academy of Pediatrics. Summaries of infectious diseases. In: Pickering LK, Baker CJ, Long SS, et al, eds. *2006 Red Book: Report of the Committee on Infectious Diseases*. 27th ed. Elk Grove Village, IL: American Academy of Pediatrics; 2006.
63. Bianco E, De Masi S, Mele A, et al. Effectiveness of immune globulins in preventing infectious hepatitis and hepatitis A: a systematic review. *Dig Liver Dis*. 2004;36(12):834-842.
64. Centers for Disease Control and Prevention. Traveler's Health: Prevention of Infectious Diseases. Hepatitis, Viral, type A. Available at: www2.ncid.cdc.gov/travel/yb/utils/ybGet.asp?section=dis&obj=hav.htm&cssNav=browseoyb. Accessed August 9, 2007.

65. Centers for Disease Control and Prevention. Acute hepatitis B among children and adolescents—United States, 1990-2002. *MMWR Morb Mortal Wkly Rep.* 2004;53(43): 1015-1018.
66. Schwarz K, Garrett B, Lamoreux J, et al. Hepatitis B vaccination rate of homeless children in Baltimore. *J Pediatr Gastroenterol Nutr.* 2005;41(2):225-229.
67. American Academy of Pediatrics. Summaries of infectious diseases. In: Pickering LK, Baker CJ, Long SS, et al, eds. *2006 Red Book: Report of the Committee on Infectious Diseases.* 27th ed. Elk Grove Village, IL: American Academy of Pediatrics; 2006.
68. Chang MH, Chen CJ, Lai MS, et al. Universal hepatitis B vaccination in Taiwan and the incidence of hepatocellular carcinoma in children. *N Engl J Med.* 1997;336:1855-1859.
69. Lok AS, McMahon BJ, American Association for the Study of Liver Diseases (AASLD), Practice Guidelines Committee. Chronic hepatitis B: update of recommendations. *Hepatology.* 2004;39(3):857-861.
70. Vajro P, Migliaro F, Fontanella A, et al. Interferon: a meta-analysis of published studies in pediatric chronic hepatitis B. *Acta Gastro-Enterologica Belgica.* 1998;61: 219-223.
71. Jonas MM, Mizerski J, Badia IB, et al. International Pediatric Lamivudine Investigator Group. Clinical trial of lamivudine in children with chronic hepatitis B. *N Engl J Med.* 2002;346(22):1706-1713.
72. Centers for Disease Control and Prevention. Recommendations for prevention and control of hepatitis C virus (HCV) infection and HCV-related chronic disease. *MMWR Morb Mortal Wkly Rep.* 1998;47(RR19): 1-39.
73. Mast EE, Hwang LY, Seto DS, et al. Risk factors for perinatal transmission of hepatitis C virus (HCV) and the natural history of HCV infection acquired in infancy. *J Infect Dis.* 2005;192(11):1880-1889.
74. Pembreya L, Newella ML, Tovob PA, EPHN Collaborators. The management of HCV infected pregnant women and their children European paediatric HCV network. *J Hepatol.* 2005;43(3):515-525.
75. Mast EE. Mother-to-infant hepatitis C virus transmission and breastfeeding. *Adv Exp Med Biol.* 2004;554:211-216.
76. Tsai JF, Jeng JE, Ho MS, et al. Independent and additive effect modification of hepatitis C and B viruses infection on the development of chronic hepatitis. *J Hepatol.* 1996; 24(3):271-276.
77. American Association for the Study of Liver Diseases. Practice Guideline. Diagnosis, Management, and Treatment of Hepatitis C. Wiley InterScience, 2004. Available at: www.aasld.org/eweb/docs/hepatitisc.pdf. Accessed August 9, 2007.
78. Wirth S, Pieper-Boustani H, Lang T, et al. Peginterferon alfa-2b plus ribavirin treatment in children and adolescents with chronic hepatitis C. *Hepatology.* 2005;41(5): 1013-1018.
79. Li SW, Zhang J, Li YM, et al. A bacterially expressed particulate hepatitis E vaccine: antigenicity, immunogenicity and protectivity on primates. *Vaccine.* 2005;23(22):2893-2901.
80. Sciveres M, Caprai S, Palla G, et al. Effectiveness and safety of cyclosporine as therapy for autoimmune diseases of the liver in children and adolescents. *Aliment Pharmacol Ther.* 2004;19(2):209-217.
81. Czaja AJ. Treatment of autoimmune hepatitis. *Semin Liver Dis.* 2002;22(4):365-378.
82. Sanderson J, Ansari A, Marinaki T, et al. Thiopurine methyltransferase: should it be measured before commencing thiopurine drug therapy? *Ann Clin Biochem.* 2004;41(pt 4):294-302.
83. Maggiore G, Veber F, Bernard O, et al. Autoimmune hepatitis associated with anti-actin antibodies in children and adolescents. *J Pediatr Gastroenterol Nutr.* 1993;17(4): 376-381.
84. Marzullo L. An update of N-acetylcysteine treatment for acute acetaminophen toxicity in children. *Curr Opin Pediatr.* 2005;17(2):239-245.
85. Schilsky ML. Diagnosis and treatment of Wilson's disease. *Pediatr Transplant.* 2002;6(1):15-19.
86. Brewer GJ, Hedera P, Kluin JK, et al. Treatment of Wilson disease with ammonium tetrathiomolybdate: III. Initial therapy in a total of 55 neurologically affected patients and follow-up with zinc therapy. *Arch Neurol.* 2003;60(3): 379-385.
87. Clayton PT, Mills KA, Johnson AW, et al. Delta 4-3-oxosteroid 5 beta-reductase deficiency: failure of ursodeoxycholic acid treatment and response to chenodeoxycholic acid plus cholic acid. *Gut.* 1996;38(4):623-628.
88. Paumgartner G, Beuers U. Ursodeoxycholic acid in cholestatic liver disease: mechanisms of action and therapeutic use revisited. *Hepatology.* 2002;36(3):525-531.
89. McDiarmid SV, Anand R, Lindblad AS; SPLIT Research Group. Studies of Pediatric Liver Transplantation: 2002 update. An overview of demographics, indications, timing, and immunosuppressive practices in pediatric liver transplantation in the United States and Canada. *Pediatr Transplant.* 2004;8(3):284-294.
90. McDiarmid SV. Management of the pediatric liver transplant patient. *Liver Transpl.* 2001;7(11 suppl 1):S77-S86.
91. Angus PW, McCaughan GW, Gane EJ, et al. Combination low dose hepatitis B immune globulin and lamivudine therapy provides effective prophylaxis against post transplantation hepatitis B. *Liver Transplant.* 2000;6(4): 429-433.
92. Charlton M. Recurrence of hepatitis C infection: Where are we now? *Liver Transpl.* 2005;11(11 suppl 2):S57-S62.
93. Barshes NR, De Bakey ME, Udell IW, et al. The natural history of hepatitis C virus recurrence (HCV) in pediatric liver transplant recipients: an analysis of national data. *Hepatology.* 2005;42:224A.
94. Evans IVR Belle SH. U.S. Trends in Liver Transplantation, 1988 to 2001. In: Bussuttil W, Klintmalm G, eds. *Transplantation of the Liver.* 2nd ed. Philadelphia, PA: Elsevier Saunders; 2005.

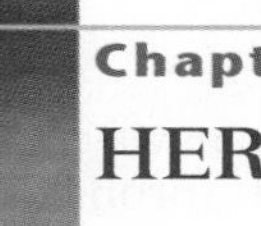

Chapter 274

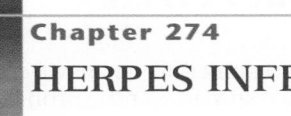

HERPES INFECTIONS

Lindsey K. Grossman, MD

DEFINITIONS

Herpesvirus hominis, or herpes simplex virus (HSV), is one of the most common agents infecting humans; although 85% to 95% of primary infections may be inapparent, in certain circumstances, the disease can be fatal. HSV is a DNA virus with a protein coat. After an incubation period of 2 to 12 days, the primary infection, if apparent, is usually heralded by constitutional symptoms such as malaise, fever, anorexia, and irritability and by the classic herpetic enanthem or exanthem. Lesions are painful vesicles, usually several millimeters in diameter, on an erythematous base. After healing and recovering from the initial infection, the host is not rid of the organism. Rather, the organism is presumed to remain in a latent phase in the ganglion cells or nerves innervating the region of localized infection. Various stimuli, including sunlight, fever, physical or emotional trauma, or menses, may induce a recurrent infection. Recurrent episodes demonstrate a similar vesicular eruption in the same general anatomic area as the primary eruption but without concomitant constitutional symptoms.

Pathologically, HSV infection is characterized by the presence of multinucleated giant cells and eosinophilic intranuclear inclusions seen in tissue scrapings taken from the base of a vesicle and stained with Giemsa (Tzanck preparation), Papanicolaou, or hematoxylin-eosin techniques. Herpes infections can be divided definitively into 2 immunologic types that correlate with clinical manifestations: herpesvirus type 1 (HSV-1), which tends to be associated with disease above the waist, and herpesvirus type 2 (HSV-2), associated with disease below the waist, with sexually related transmission, or with disease acquired neonatally.

EPIDEMIOLOGIC FACTORS

Studies have shown a sharp rise in the prevalence of antibodies to HSV-1 between 1 and 4 years of age and a slower rise of antibody acquisition between 5 and 14 years of age. From adolescence into early adulthood, coincident with the beginning of sexual activity, the presence of antibodies to HSV-2 increases significantly. Since the late 1970s, the prevalence of HSV-2 infection has increased dramatically, and HSV-2 antibody is now detectable in at least 1 of 5 persons 12 years or older nationwide.[1] Overall, 80% to 100% of adults in lower socioeconomic groups, in locations where crowding probably plays an important epidemiologic role, demonstrate antibodies to HSV-1; 30% to 40% or more may be positive for HSV-2.[2] Of persons of higher socioeconomic circumstances, 21% demonstrate antibodies to HSV-2, compared with 34% of those below the poverty level.

HERPES SIMPLEX VIRUS TYPE 1

Epidemiologic Factors

Transmission of HSV-1 is presumed to occur via person-to-person respiratory spread and probably involves close contact, such as kissing an infected person. Transmission can occur whether or not the source is symptomatic with an apparent vesicular lesion at the time. The clinical manifestation varies with site of entry, and the clinical diagnosis rarely requires laboratory confirmation.

Clinical Manifestations

Acute gingivostomatitis is the most common form of HSV-1 seen in children; the peak incidence is between 1 and 4 years of age. It is characterized by an abrupt onset of fever, irritability, poor feeding, and 1 to 2 days later by very tender, red, friable mucous membranes surrounding 2- to 3-mm white ulcerations, and severe halitosis. The vesicular stage is rarely seen, but large, tender anterior cervical and submandibular lymphadenopathy is common. The duration of the illness varies from 5 to 14 days, and the severity ranges from mild to so severe that oral intake becomes negligible, and hospitalization for intravenous hydration may be required.

Herpes labialis (or cold sores) crust and heal without scarring in 7 to 10 days. They may be found on either the upper or lower lip, and recurrence at the same site is extremely common. Traumatic herpes is the result of inoculation at the site of local trauma and includes herpetic whitlow, an extremely painful syndrome involving herpetic infection of a digit. Although the sore may resemble a bacterial paronychia, it should not be incised. This condition is common in thumb-suckers who have oral herpes.

Ocular Herpes

Ocular herpes is one of the most common causes of corneal blindness in the United States. The primary infection usually involves acute keratoconjunctivitis with intense swelling of the lids but without exudate. Frequently, typical herpetic vesicles are found on the skin surrounding the involved eye. Recurrent disease can be even more severe and may involve superficial or deep epithelial ulceration, stromal damage, or uveitis. Fortunately, treatment is available (see the discussion on treatment in this chapter), but these children should always be referred to an ophthalmologist for care. Indeed, the pediatrician should be aware that devastating results can occur with the use of topical steroid preparations in a probable case of ocular herpes. This circumstance underlines the necessity of an ophthalmologic consultation before prescribing topical corticosteroids for any use in the eye.

Herpes and Sports

Certain sport activities that result in close skin contact may increase the risk of HSV skin infection. Wrestlers may acquire herpes gladiatorum as a result of viral shedding from an infected opponent. Herpes rugbeiorum, or *scrum pox*, may result from close skin contact between rugby players.

Differential Diagnosis

The most common ulcerative enanthem to be considered in the differential diagnosis is coxsackievirus A herpangina. This infection results in lesions very similar in appearance to herpes but is located in the posterior oral cavity, as contrasted with the anterior clustering of the herpetic lesions. Other infections include varicella, cytomegalovirus and syphilis, and autoimmune diseases such as Behçet syndrome, Reiter syndrome, and inflammatory bowel disease. Systemic lupus erythematosus and cyclic neutropenia might also be considered in a broader differential. In these cases, however, the remainder of the clinical presentation would direct the diagnostician with cultures for herpes, confirming the final diagnosis if necessary.

Complications

Although HSV-1 infections are usually self-limited, certain human hosts are at more serious risk for contracting or developing severe disease with HSV-1 than are others. Individuals who have deficiencies in cell-mediated immunity, those undergoing immunosuppressive therapy for cancer or transplantation, and those who are extremely malnourished may be more likely to show serious disseminated disease. The inoculation of herpes into eczematous skin can result in eczema herpeticum, which can vary in severity from mild to fatal. Constitutional symptoms are the rule, and the temperatures of 39.4°C to 40.6°C may last for a week or more. Wide areas of skin can become denuded, with enormous fluid, protein, and electrolyte losses, which potentially may be life threatening. Secondary bacterial infection may complicate the condition. Recurrences, milder than the initial infection, occur commonly on areas of the skin affected with chronic eczema.

HSV-1 is among the most commonly reported causes of viral encephalitis in the United States, with an estimated 250 to 500 cases per year. The disease is characterized by fever and personality change and often involves seizures. A rapidly progressive encephalopathy culminates in death in 1 to 2 weeks in more than 70% of untreated cases. The infection most often localizes to a single lobe, and definitive diagnosis in the past was most often made by a biopsy of the area, demonstrating the typical morphologic picture of herpes microscopically. Early treatment has improved the prognosis of this disastrous condition among children but is most effective when begun before the onset of loss of consciousness.

HERPES SIMPLEX VIRUS TYPE 2

Epidemiologic Factors

As a result of the increase in sexual activity among young adolescents in recent years, pediatricians have been faced with the challenge of diagnosing and treating all types of sexually transmitted infections. The frequency of infection is high and underestimated by clinical history in the adolescent population.[3] The prevalence of HSV-2 infection has increased by 30% and is now detectable in roughly 1 in 5 persons 12 years or older.[1] Genital HSV-2 is of increasing concern to physicians and patients alike because of its symptomatologic issues, lack of cure, and potential for disastrous consequences to the newborn.

Clinical Manifestations

Clinically, HSV-2 is usually exhibited by typical herpetic vesicles on the penile shaft, prepuce, or glans penis in the male patient and on the labia minora or majora, mons, or nearby skin or within the vagina in the female patient. Primary infection is accompanied by significant local pain, burning, or paresthesia and constitutional symptoms of fever and malaise, dysuria, and inguinal lymphadenopathy; recurrent bouts are less severe than initial occurrences. The 5% to 10% of cases of genital herpes associated with HSV-1 are believed to result from orogenital sex.

Evaluation

Viral culture is, in general, the most sensitive method of diagnosis but requires several days, depending on the size of the inoculum, for a definitive result. Vesicles, stool, urine, and mucosal surfaces may be used as sites to obtain the culture sample. When lesions are available for scraping, direct detection methods, including fluorescent antibody and immunoperoxidase assays, give a rapid answer but with lower sensitivity; therefore a viral culture is still required for confirmation of a negative finding. Tzanck test and Papanicolaou stains are neither sufficiently specific nor sensitive to serve as a screen for HSV. Polymerase chain reaction is highly specific and sensitive and can discriminate between the HSV-1 and HSV-2 in cerebral spinal fluid; it is the diagnostic method of choice in HSV encephalitis.[4] Several point-of-care tests are available using glycoprotein-based assays for HSV-2 antibodies, with sensitivities of 80% to 98% and specificities of better than 95%.[4]

NEONATAL HERPES

Epidemiologic Factors

Although most neonatal herpes infections are caused by HSV-2, antibodies to HSV-1 are associated in 25% of cases. Transplacental transmission of HSV can occur and may induce spontaneous abortion or, in rare cases, congenital defects in newborns. However, pediatricians are more often faced with postnatal herpetic disease contracted by the newborn during the second stage of labor while moving through an infected birth canal. The incidence of neonatal herpes is estimated to vary between 1 in 3200 and 1 in 15,000 deliveries.[5,6] The prevalence of HSV-2 in healthy American women ranges from 10% to 60%.[2] As many as 50% to 60% of women from lower socioeconomic groups in the United States have antibodies to HSV-2.[2] This number results in an estimated 1500 to 2200 infants per year in the United States infected with HSV.[7] Postnatal transmission from a caregiver accounts for approximately 10% of cases.[8]

The greatest risk of neonatal HSV infection occurs when the mother has contracted primary herpes 2 to 4 weeks before delivery, although the disease may be transmitted to the infant in recurrent cases with or without a clinically detectable herpetic lesion. Transmission of HSV infection to the fetus is most frequently related to shedding of the virus at the time of delivery. The risk of neonatal herpes for a child born vaginally to a mother with primary genital herpes is 33% to 50% but less than 5% if the mother is shedding virus as a result of reactivated infection.[4,9] Distinguishing primary versus recurrent infection may be impossible because both may be asymptomatic. Indeed, approximately 75% of infants with HSV infection are born to women without a history or physical or symptomatic evidence of infection.[4] Risk factors for neonatal disease include a history of a first HSV infection during the third trimester, invasive monitoring of the fetus, delivery less than 38 weeks, and maternal age younger than 21 years.[5] Neonatal HSV disease must always be included in the differential diagnosis when a newborn or infant exhibits a skin rash ranging from vesiculopapular to vesiculoulcerative.

Clinical Manifestation

The presentation of neonatal herpes, similar to other infections in the neonatal period, is nonspecific, at least initially. The syndrome usually occurs in the first week or so of life but can uncommonly occur as late as

3 or 4 weeks of age. The infant usually experiences poor feeding, vomiting, fussiness or lethargy, and fever or hypothermia and often has increasing jaundice and hepatosplenomegaly. Seizures, cyanosis, and apnea may also occur. The majority of infants, though notably not all, who have neonatal herpes eventually demonstrate a vesicular rash with either individual lesions or clumps of vesicles.

The National Institute of Allergy and Infectious Diseases Collaborative Antiviral Study Group[10] classifies cases of neonatal HSV infection into 3 categories according to clinical manifestations. Infants who have disseminated disease involving visceral organs with or without central nervous system (CNS) involvement are most likely to die (>80% without treatment and 31% with high dose treatment).[11] Infants who have HSV type 1 disseminated infection have poorer outcomes than those who have HSV type 2 infection.[12,13] In disseminated infection, hepatoadrenal necrosis is virtually always found, and microcephaly, hydrocephalus, intellectual disability, or seizures occur in many survivors.

A second category of disease includes infants who have CNS abnormalities without involvement of viscera. In this group, mortality exceeds 50% and morbidity exceeds 90% without antiviral therapy. With appropriate antiviral therapy (see later discussion), mortality has fallen to 6%, but morbidity remains high.[11]

A third category includes infants whose skin, eyes, or mouth (SEM) are involved but not the CNS or viscera. Infants who had SEM involvement before antiviral drugs became available were not expected to die, and only 20% to 30% were left neurologically impaired; many who appeared to have SEM involvement, however, went on to develop disseminated or CNS involvement and to suffer disastrous consequences. Classically, over 50% of all neonatal HSV infections exhibited as disseminated disease, with only a minority classified as SEM involved. However, apparently as a result of earlier diagnosis and treatment, 34% now exhibit as SEM involved and 32% as disseminated disease; the remaining 34% have CNS disease.[12]

Prevention

Previously, stringent prenatal screening programs were recommended to attempt to prevent HSV infection in offspring of women who had recurrent genital herpes. Such programs proved costly, impractical to administer, and medically ineffective. A history of genital HSV alone is not an indication for caesarean delivery. Current guidelines for managing labor in women who have a history of genital herpes suggest expeditious caesarean delivery if active genital lesions are present at the time of delivery and the duration since rupture of membranes is less than 4 to 6 hours, although some would advocate caesarean delivery if the canal is visibly infected, even when the rupture of membranes has been even more prolonged.[4,14] Daily oral acyclovir has been shown to suppress subclinical shedding of HSV-2 in the genital tract[15] and to prevent clinical recurrences in pregnant women at delivery.[16] Several studies demonstrated varied results on the rate of caesarean delivery caused by genital HSV at delivery, but they were underpowered to show an effect on HSV in the infants.[5] Scalp electrodes should be avoided when the mother is suspected of having active genital HSV infection.[17]

The American Academy of Pediatrics and the American College of Obstetricians and Gynecologists have developed joint guidelines to decrease the likelihood of postpartum herpes infection in the infant.[14] These guidelines specify isolation criteria to protect healthy infants from their HSV-infected mothers, other infected infants, or infected staff.

TREATMENT

Although no universal cure exists for herpes infections, the prognosis for its many syndromes has improved greatly with currently available therapies. One of the earliest successes was with topical idoxuridine in the treatment of ocular herpetic infections. Vidarabine was the first drug shown to decrease mortality and morbidity significantly without significant drug toxicity in neonatal herpes involving the CNS; however, by the 1980s, acyclovir had become the treatment of choice, with more recent work demonstrating some improved mortality with prolonged high-dose (60 mg/kg/day divided every 8 hours) intravenous acyclovir. Unfortunately, no significant decrease in long-term developmental results among survivors has been demonstrated, allowing the morbidity of neonatal HSV to remain unacceptably high.[11] This circumstance is due at least partially to the fact that less than 10% of typical herpetic lesions appear in the first 24 hours of life, making early identification of affected infants difficult and delaying the initiation of appropriate therapy.

Oral antiviral therapy for first bouts of genital herpes shortens the duration of symptoms and viral shedding and is definitely indicated for at least a 10-day course[6] (Box 274-1). If begun within 1 day of the onset of the first lesion, then episodic therapy may limit the duration and severity of recurrences as well. The same medications have been shown to decrease recurrences by 70% to 80% when used as chronic suppressive therapy in patients with particularly severe or frequent recurrences, though the cost of such therapy may be a limiting factor in its usefulness. Therapy for immunosuppressed individuals with genital HSV may warrant hospitalization and the use of intravenous acyclovir.

Treatment for other herpetic syndromes has also been evaluated. Oral acyclovir can shorten the duration of herpetic gingivostomatitis in children by 6 days if begun within the first 72 hours of illness with the potential of significant cost savings because of the frequent need of intravenous hydration among children with this syndrome.[18] Only modest efficacy has been shown with treatment of episodic oral herpes; topical antiviral therapy for recurrences has been demonstrated to decrease the duration of symptoms by 1 day or less.[19] Topical antivirals are used to treat superficial keratitis effectively; oral acyclovir may be beneficial in situations of recurrent ocular lesions.[4]

Intravenous acyclovir remains the mainstay of treatment for herpes encephalitis. For neonates younger than 3 months, the treatment regimen should be continued for 21 days; for children older than 3 months, treatment should last 14 to 21 days. Acyclovir has

BOX 274-1 Recommended Treatment Regimens for Genital Herpes Infections

FIRST CLINICAL EPISODE OF GENITAL HERPES

Acyclovir 400 mg orally 3 times a day for 7-10 days, OR

Acyclovir 200 mg orally 5 times a day for 7-10 days, OR

Famciclovir 250 mg orally 3 times a day for 7-10 days, OR

Valacyclovir 1 g orally twice a day for 7-10 days

Note: Treatment may be extended if healing is incomplete after 10 days of therapy.

EPISODIC THERAPY FOR RECURRENT GENITAL HERPES

Acyclovir 400 mg orally 3 times a day for 5 days, OR

Acyclovir 800 mg orally 3 times a day for 2 days, OR

Acyclovir 800 mg orally twice a day for 5 days, OR

Famciclovir 125 mg orally twice a day for 5 days, OR

Valacyclovir 500 mg orally twice a day for 3 days, OR

Valacyclovir 1.0 g orally once a day for 5 days

SUPPRESSIVE THERAPY FOR RECURRENT GENITAL HERPES

Acyclovir 400 mg orally twice a day, OR

Famciclovir 250 mg orally twice a day, OR

Valacyclovir 500 mg orally once a day, OR

Valacyclovir 1.0 g orally once a day

Modified from Centers for Disease Control and Prevention. Sexually transmitted diseases treatment guidelines, 2006. *MMWR.* 2006;55:16-20.

significantly decreased mortality from this condition but only modestly affected morbidity.[13] Therapy must be initiated promptly to ensure the most favorable outcome.

WHEN TO REFER

- All infants who are thought to have neonatal herpes should be considered potentially critically ill and would benefit from subspecialty involvement to include critical care or neonatologic and infectious disease, among others, as indicated.
- Regardless of age, patients who have known or suggested immunosuppression who contact herpes may benefit from subspecialty consultation.
- Children in whom ocular steroid therapy is considered may benefit from ophthalmologic consultation to rule out any possibility of ocular herpes infection.

WHEN TO ADMIT

- Infants who have suggested or confirmed neonatal herpes must be carefully monitored and treated with intravenous acyclovir.
- All individuals thought to have herpes encephalitis must be hospitalized and treated expectantly with intravenous acyclovir.
- Immunosuppressed individuals with herpes infections may require intravenous antiviral therapy and will require hospitalization.

AAP POLICY STATEMENTS

American Academy of Pediatrics, American College of Obstetricians and Gynecologists. Guidelines for Perinatal Care. 5th ed. Elk Grove Village, IL: American Academy of Pediatrics; 2002.

American Academy of Pediatrics, Committee on Sports Medicine and Fitness. Medical conditions affecting sports participation. *Pediatrics*. 2001;107(5):1205-1209 (aappolicy.aappublications.org/cgi/content/full/pediatrics;107/5/1205).

SUGGESTED RESOURCES

Baker DA, American College of Obstetrics and Gynecology. Management of herpes in pregnancy. *Int J Gynaecol Obstet*. 2000;68:165-173.

Brady RC, Bernstein DI. Treatment of herpes simplex virus infections. *Antiviral Res*. 2004;61:73-81.

Kimberlin DW. Herpes simplex virus infections of the central nervous system. *Semin Pediatr Infect Dis*. 2003;14:83-89.

Centers for Disease Control and Prevention. Sexually transmitted diseases treatment guidelines, 2006. *MMWR*. 2006;55:16-20.

REFERENCES

1. Fleming DT, McQuillan GM, Johnson RE, et al. Herpes simplex virus type 2 in the United States, 1976 to 1994. *N Engl J Med*. 1997;337:1105-1111.
2. Smith JS, Robinson NJ. Age-specific prevalence of infection with herpes simples virus types 2 and 1: a global review. *J Inf Dis*. 2002;186(suppl 1):S3-S28.
3. Huerta K, Berkelhamer S, Klein J, et al. Epidemiology of herpes simplex virus type 2 infections in a high-risk adolescent population. *J Adolesc Health*. 1996;18:384-386
4. American Academy of Pediatrics. Herpes simplex. In: Pickering LK, Baker CJ, Long SS, et al, eds. *Red Book 2006 Report of the Committee on Infectious Diseases*. 27th ed. Elk Grove Village, IL: American Academy of Pediatrics; 2006.
5. Brown Z. Preventing herpes simplex virus transmission to the neonate. *Herpes*. 2004;11(suppl 3):175A-186A.
6. Whitely RJ, Lakeman F: Herpes simplex virus infections of the central nervous system: therapeutic and diagnostic considerations. *Clin Infect Dis*. 1995;20:4-14.
7. Jacobs RF. Neonatal herpes simplex virus infections. *Semin Perinatol*. 1998;22:64-71.
8. Connelly BL, Stanberry LR. Herpes simplex virus infections in children. *Curr Opin Pediatr*. 1995;7:19-23.
9. Brown ZA, Benedetti J, Ashley R, et al. Neonatal herpes simplex virus infection in relation to asymptomatic maternal infection at the time of labor. *N Engl J Med*. 1991;324:1247-1252.
10. Whitley RJ, Nahmias AJ, Soong SJ, et al. Changing presentation of herpes simplex virus infection in neonates. *J Infect Dis*. 1988;158:109-116.
11. Kimberlin DW, Lin CY, Jacobs RF, et al. Safety and efficacy of high-dose intravenous acyclovir in the management of neonatal herpes simplex virus infections. *Pediatrics*. 2000;108:230-238.
12. Kimberlin DW, Lin CY, Jacobs RF, et al. Natural history of neonatal herpes simplex virus infections in the acyclovir era. *Pediatrics*. 2000;108:223-229.

13. Whitley RJ, Arvin A, Prober C, et al. Predictors of morbidity and mortality in neonates with herpes simplex virus infections. *N Engl J Med.* 1991;324:450-454.
14. American Academy of Pediatrics, American College of Obstetricians and Gynecologists. *Guidelines for Perinatal Care.* 5th ed. Elk Grove Village, IL: American Academy of Pediatrics; 2002.
15. Wald A, Zeh J, Barnum G, et al. Suppression of subclinical shedding of herpes simplex virus type 2 with acyclovir. *Ann Intern Med.* 1996;124:8-15.
16. Scott LL, Hollier LM, McIntire D, et al. Acyclovir suppression to prevent clinical recurrences at delivery after first episode genital herpes in pregnancy: an open-label trial. *Infect Dis Obstet Gynecol.* 2001;9:75-80.
17. Brown ZA, Walk A, Morrow RA, et al. Effect of serologic status and cesarean delivery on transmission rates of herpes simplex virus from mother to infant. *JAMA.* 2003;289:203-209.
18. Amir J, Harel L, Smetana Z, et al. Treatment of herpes simplex gingivostomatitis with aciclovir in children: a randomised double blind placebo controlled study. *BMJ.* 1997;314:1800-1803.
19. Spruance SL, Johne TM, Blatter MM, et al. High-dose short-duration early valacyclovir therapy for episodic treatment of cold sores: results of two randomized, placebo-controlled multicenter studies. *Antimicrob Agents Chemother.* 2003;47:1072-1080.

Chapter 275

HUMAN HERPESVIRUS-6 AND HUMAN HERPESVIRUS-7 INFECTIONS

Jerri Ann Jenista, MD

Human herpesvirus (HHV)-6 and HHV-7 are two of the known causative agents of roseola,[1] a classic childhood exanthem also known as roseola infantum, exanthem subitum, 3-day fever, sixth disease, and pseudorubella. However, the spectrum of disease associated with these agents is now understood to be far broader than the benign illness of roseola.

CLASSIFICATION

HHV-6, formerly called human B-lymphotrophic virus, and HHV-7 are classified as herpesviruses based on their physical and genetic similarities to others of the group: herpes simplex virus type 1, herpes simplex virus type 2, cytomegalovirus, Epstein-Barr virus, varicella-zoster virus, and the newly discovered virus associated with Kaposi sarcoma, HHV-8.[2] HHV-6 and HHV-7 can be distinguished from these other herpesviruses by DNA hybridization or by reactions with virus-specific monoclonal antibodies.

HHV-6 exists in two forms: variant A and variant B. HHV-6B is typically associated with childhood illnesses, such as roseola, and some adult infections. The range of illnesses, if any, caused by HHV-6A is unknown.

Sophisticated antigen detection methods have demonstrated that HHV-6 and HHV-7 exist in many healthy persons, including those who have virus-specific antibody. HHV-6 has been isolated from saliva, plasma, and many cell lines.[3] HHV-7 is isolated most often from the saliva in healthy persons.[4]

As with other herpesviruses, latent or persistent asymptomatic viral infection occurs after the primary infection. The site of latency is not clear, but during reactivation these viruses may appear in oral or genital secretions, mononuclear white blood cells, human milk, or cerebrospinal fluid (CSF). HHV-6 infection may reactivate during primary HHV-7 infection, acute febrile illnesses, or periods of immunodeficiency such as treatment with steroids. Reactivation characteristics of HHV-7 are unknown.

Both viruses interfere with the function of certain classes of T lymphocytes. Evidence is emerging that HHV-6, and perhaps HHV-7, act as cofactors in the course of HIV infection. The role of these viruses in lymphoreticular malignancies, chronic fatigue syndrome, and other conditions, such as multiple sclerosis, is under investigation.

EPIDEMIOLOGIC FEATURES

Roseola was the first recognized clinical manifestation of primary HHV-6, and perhaps HHV-7, infection. This common clinical disease is diagnosed in up to 60% of children by 3 years of age. However, nonroseola illness is probably more common. Three quarters of children are infected with HHV-6 by age 2 years; most infections are symptomatic.[5] Recognition of infection is unusual, however, in children at other ages; rare cases in adults and neonates have been reported. Most HHV-6 and HHV-7 infections are sporadic, although family and institutional epidemics are occasionally noted. Cases of roseola are seen year round.

The incubation periods for HHV-6 and HHV-7 infection are apparently between 5 and 15 days; however, the modes of transmission and the period of communicability are unclear. In an extensive study of 3-generation families, DNA restriction analysis of HHV-7 isolates showed similar patterns within households.[6] HHV-6 is most frequently isolated from peripheral blood mononuclear cells. HHV-6 and HHV-7 can be isolated from the saliva of 70% to 80% of healthy persons older than 1 year of age, and saliva is thought to be the most likely mode of transmission.[5] The rate of subclinical disease is high. Most patients have no known exposure, although poverty and larger family size may be risk factors for early acquisition of HHV-6. Breastfeeding may delay the acquisition of HHV-7 and HHV-6. In spite of direct evidence of intrauterine or perinatal transmission of HHV-6,[1] no consistently recognized sequelae attributed to such infection exist.[7]

Serologic surveys show that virtually all full-term infants have passively acquired maternal antibody to both HHV-6 and HHV-7 at birth. The prevalence of antibody then falls, reaching a nadir by 6 months of age. By 1 year of age, nearly 90% of children have detectable antibody to HHV-6. Prevalence surveys of adults from various countries around the world show HHV-6 antibody detection rates of 88% to 90%.[1] The prevalence of antibody to HHV-7 also increases with age; 60% of young adolescents have detectable titers. For both viruses, these levels persist unchanged through young adulthood and then decline slightly thereafter.

DISEASE

The clinical disease associations of HHV-6 and HHV-7 are dependent on how the studied patients are selected. Thus office or emergency room samples chosen for the presence of fever or seizures cannot identify asymptomatic infections. Prospective studies of a population of children are expensive, and few have examined for the acquisition of these agents. Thus the rate of infection with minor or no signs or symptoms is likely underestimated (Table 275-1).

Nonspecific Viral Illness

As data accumulate, most HHV-7 infections appear to be asymptomatic because the rate of seropositivity is high and yet detectable viremia with clinical illness is uncommon, occurring in only 1% of children younger than 10 years. In contrast, in prospectively studied infants from birth through age 24 months, 77% acquired primary HHV-6 infection. More than 90% of the episodes were symptomatic, and 39% of the children visited a physician for the illness.[5] Primary HHV-6 infection is clearly a major cause of morbidity in infancy and early childhood.

Studies have revealed a broader role than previously recognized for febrile HHV-6 infection.[8] Primary HHV-6 infection was documented in nearly 10% of children younger than age 3 years and in 20% of children between 6 and 12 months of age exhibiting as an acute febrile illness. HHV-6 infection was the cause of one third of febrile seizures in children younger than 2 years and resulted in hospitalization of 13% of children after they sought care at an emergency room.

Although the contribution of HHV-7 infection to emergency room use, hospitalization, or physician visits is less clear, very few (1%) children younger than 10 years have demonstrated HHV-7 viremia, but of these children, 86% had fever, 40% had seizures, and 20% were hospitalized.[9]

Roseola

Roseola is so frequent an illness that fully 30% of children will experience the clinical disease between the ages of 6 months and 2 years.[10] In Japan the disease is

Table 275-1 Clinical Characteristics of Human Herpesvirus (HHV)-6 and HHV-7 Infections in Otherwise Healthy Children

SIGNS AND SYMPTOMS	ROSEOLA (1945)	FEBRILE HHV-6 (1994)	PRIMARY HHV-6 (2005)	FEBRILE HHV-7 (1997, 1998)	VIREMIC HHV-7 (2006)
Fever	100%	98-100%	58%	100%	87%
Rash at presentation	100%	6-64%	31%	13-86%	0%
Pruritus	1.2%	NR	NR	NR	NR
Desquamation	10%	0%	NR	NR	NR
Pigmentation	0%	7%	NR	NR	NR
Lymphadenopathy	97.5%	NR	NR	NR	NR
Cervical	45%	31%	NR	NR	NR
Erythematous tympanic membranes	92.5%	P	NR	NR	NR
Constipation	40%	NR	NR	NR	NR
Upper respiratory tract symptoms	25%	41%	66%	7%	13%
Nonspecific prodromal symptoms	NR	14%	NR	NR	33%
Diarrhea	15%	33-68%	26%	38%	7%
Meningismus	5%	NR	NR	NR	NR
Convulsions	3.7%	8%	0%	7-75%	40%
Bulging fontanelle	NR	26%	NR	NR	NR
Irritability	92%	P	70%	88%	NR
Edematous eyelids	NR	30%	NR	NR	NR
Nagayama spots*	87%	65%	NR	NR	NR
Anorexia	80%	NR	NR	NR	NR
Abdominal pain	25%	NR	NR	NR	NR
Cough	11.2%	P, 50%	34%	NR	NR
Headache	5%	NR	NR	NR	NR
Earache or otitis media	2.5%	30%	NR	NR	7%
Aching joints	2.5%	NR	NR	NR	NR
Vomiting	NR	NR	8%	NR	7%
Asymptomatic	NA	NA	6%	NA	0%
Roseola	100%	17%-98%	24%	NR	0%

NA, Not applicable to the study design; *NR*, not reported; *P*, reported as *present* with no numerical value.
*Erythematous streaks or spots on the soft palate and uvula.

even more common, noted in up to 60% of children in the first 3 years of life. A child's first episode of roseola is usually caused by HHV-6B and occurs when the child is an average age of 7 to 9 months.[1] Primary infection with HHV-7 accounts for approximately 10% of first and most of the second cases of roseola. HHV-7 infection occurs somewhat later than HHV-6, at a mean age of more than 12 months.[7] Approximately 15% of clinical cases of roseola cannot be attributed to either virus. Recognition of roseola is based almost entirely on the observation of a classic clinical course. Interestingly, the signs and symptoms of roseola noted before the discovery of HHV-6 are essentially the same as descriptions of disease proven to be caused by HHV-6 or HHV-7[11-13] (see Table 275-1). Typically, a fever as high as 102.2° to 105.8°F (39° to 41°C) suddenly develops in a previously well infant. Except for irritability, the child does not seem as sick as the temperature indicates. Physical findings are few and include only painless posterior auricular, suboccipital, or cervical lymphadenopathy accompanied by slight eyelid edema, giving the child a sleepy-eyed or droopy appearance. Nagayama spots are erythematous macules appearing on the soft palate and near the uvula and are observed regularly after 1 or 2 days of illness.[8,11] Rarely, mild coryza, otitis media, or a bulging fontanelle is observed.

After a 2- to 5-day course, the fever resolves dramatically while a rash simultaneously appears. With defervescence, the child seems to have recovered, despite the rash. The typical exanthem occurs as macular or maculopapular blanching patches surrounded by a lighter halo. The eruption usually begins on the neck and spreads to the trunk and extremities, sparing the face. It fades within 4 hours to 4 days and may be missed if it is faint or occurs at night. Roseola may also occur in a young infant as an afebrile exanthem.

Seizures

Seizures are not a prominent manifestation of HHV-6 infection, occurring no more frequently than with other febrile illnesses.[14] However, in childhood febrile seizures, HHV-6 infection is a major factor, accounting for up to one half of such incidents in children younger than 2 years seeking care at an emergency room.[8,15] HHV-6 DNA can be identified in CSF of up to 70% of children during primary infection and of 28% of children who have had past infection.[13] Seizures may be single or recurrent, prolonged, and partial or focal and they may be associated with postictal paralysis or acute resolving hemiplegia.[16] CSF findings are normal or negative.

Even with recurrent seizures during the same illness, complete recovery is the rule. The significance of HHV-6 in relation to recurrent seizures is not clear. At least one study detected no increase in the risk of recurrent seizures in the first year after a febrile seizure associated with primary HHV-6 infection versus first febrile seizures of other causes. Others have noted an increased incidence of subseqeunt diagnoses of epilepsy.

Febrile seizures are also noted in symptomatic primary or reactivated infection caused by HHV-7. HHV-7 DNA has been detected in the CSF of a child who had typical roseola. Some indications suggest that febrile seizures may be more common—and possibly more complicated—with primary HHV-7 than with HHV-6 infection.[13]

The pathogenesis of seizures associated with HHV-6 and HHV-7 is unknown. Although new information indicates that these viruses may have specific neurotropic qualities.[1] Other investigators claim that febrile seizures associated with these viruses are due to the underlying fever associated with the infection rather than actual central nervous system disease.[14]

Meningoencephalitis

Reports have been published of severe meningoencephalitis with neurologic sequelae or death in infants[17] and adults[18] and fatal encephalitis attributed to HHV-6B in adult recipients of bone marrow transplants.[19] The significance of HHV-6 in relation to recurrent seizures, chronic fatigue, multiple sclerosis, and other neurologic conditions is not clear. HHV-7 infection has also been described in association with encephalopathy, hemiplegia, and atypical febrile seizures. Although these neurologic conditions associated with HHV-6 and HHV-7 infections are rare, when they occur, they may be severe, requiring intensive care.[16] HHV-6 or HHV-7 (or both) infection should be looked for in order to differentiate it from encephalitis associated with vaccines.

Mononucleosis-Like Disease

HHV-6 infection in adults rarely causes a roseola-like illness. Both severe and mild infectious mononucleosis–like disease have been reported in adults who have HHV-6 infection.[20] The disease lasts several weeks and is associated with slight fatigue, headache, sore throat, cervical lymphadenopathy, and transient increase in liver enzymes. Infectious mononucleosis–like illness associated with HHV-6 has been noted in infants.

HHV-7 has been isolated from a child who had the clinical picture of chronic Epstein-Barr virus infection, characterized by pancytopenia, fever, and hepatosplenomegaly.[21]

Hepatitis

A mild hepatitis associated with HHV-6 infection is recognized in adults and children. A few cases of fulminant or fatal hepatitis (or both) have been reported, usually with an associated encephalopathy.[3] HHV-6 infection also has been implicated in mild chronic hepatitis in childhood. A single case of hepatitis has been reported in relation to HHV-7 infection.[22]

Infection in Immunocompromised Patients

HHV-6 infection may reactivate during periods of immunosuppression. A syndrome with fever and rash resembling graft-versus-host disease is recognized in children after they receive bone marrow transplants. Severe interstitial pneumonitis, disseminated infection, recurrent aseptic meningitis, and encephalitis associated with HHV-6 infection have been reported in adult recipients of bone marrow transplants.[23] Some patients have recovered after treatment with foscarnet.

The role of HHV-6 in HIV infection is unclear, although some evidence suggests that HHV-6 may potentiate the progression of HIV infection, especially in infants who have acquired HIV vertically. HHV-7 competes with HIV for CD4 receptors on T cells; theoretically, the virus may interfere with the progression of HIV infection.[23]

Other Diseases

HHV-6 has been isolated from patients who have many other conditions. Because HHV-6 is reactivated by many acute illnesses, attributing causality to the virus is difficult in most cases. Reported associations include chronic bone marrow suppression in an immunocompetent adult, idiopathic thrombocytopenic purpura, thrombocytopenia during primary HHV-6 infection, Gianotti-Crosti syndrome, hemophagocytic syndrome, fatal disseminated disease in an immunocompetent infant, lymphoproliferative disorders, and certain lymphoreticular malignancies.

The role of HHV-7 in other diseases is even less clear than its association with roseola. Several studies have purported to show evidence of reactivation of HHV-7 during relapses of adult pityriasis rosea.

DIAGNOSIS

Roseola is the only manifestation of HHV-6 or HHV-7 infection that is clinically easily recognized. The signs and symptoms of all other conditions associated with these viruses are too nonspecific to allow a definitive diagnosis at the bedside. Except in certain situations of infection in immunocompromised hosts and complicated disease in normal hosts, rarely does a clinical need exist to confirm infection with HHV-6 or HHV-7 either serologically or virologically. Identification of HHV-6 or HHV-7 in febrile infants does not obviate the need to evaluate for serious bacterial infection; approximately 10% of young infants will have concurrent viral and bacterial infections, usually bacteruria.[15,24,25] Occasionally, confirming HHV-6 or HHV-7 infection in children with complex neurologic syndromes may be helpful to rule out vaccine administration as the cause.[16]

In roseola, the only helpful laboratory finding is a leukopenia that has a nadir count as low as 2000 white blood cells per cubic millimeter by the third day of fever. A relative lymphocytosis or monocytosis is typical. Results of the CSF examination, urinalysis, and chest radiograph are normal. Because roseola is an inconsequential illness, rarely does the need exist to confirm the specific diagnosis.

Neither antibody detection methods nor virus isolation techniques are standardized for HHV-6 or HHV-7, and these assays are not available commercially. The presence of maternal antibody in the young infant and reactivation of herpesviruses during other infections confound interpretation of the results.[23] Similarly, although polymerase chain reaction identification of virus in body fluids is available as a research tool, the clinical use of this test is questionable. For example, HHV-6 can be detected in high titers in saliva specimens of infants for up to 12 months after primary infection.[5] However, the presence of virus may be irrelevant to the disease or condition being investigated.

Newly developed diagnostic methods to differentiate latent versus actively replicating virus may eventually help shed light on both the diagnosis and pathogenesis of disease associated with HHV-6 and HHV-7.[23]

DIFFERENTIAL DIAGNOSIS

Roseola is often confused with other exanthematous diseases (see Chapter 253, Contagious Exanthematous Diseases). In rubella, the rash and fever are concurrent, and enlarged lymph nodes are often tender. Coryza, respiratory symptoms, and Koplik spots distinguish rubeola. Enterovirus exanthems usually occur in epidemics, involve both older and younger children, and are more common in the late summer and fall. Erythema infectiosum, or *fifth disease,* affects the school-aged child and involves the face most prominently. Scarlet fever has a more confluent rash and is associated with marked pharyngitis. Drug eruptions, especially those resulting from sulfa-containing preparations, are not regularly preceded by fever and tend to be diffuse. In Egypt, primary infection in childhood with HHV-8, the causative agent of Kaposi sarcoma, was associated with a mild febrile exanthem indistinguishable from HHV-6 or HHV-7 related roseola.[26] The epidemiologic and clinical characteristics of HHV-8 infection in children in the United States are unknown.

MANAGEMENT

Management of roseola is based entirely on symptoms. Acetaminophen is effective in controlling the fever. Reassuring the parents that the rash is a sign of recovery often comforts them and may prevent unnecessary office visits.

Both HHV-6 and HHV-7 have antiviral agent profiles similar to cytomegalovirus, with limited susceptibility to acyclovir. In vitro studies show that either foscarnet or ganciclovir is somewhat effective, but no clinical trials have been conducted with these drugs. Because infection with either of these agents is self-limited in the immunocompetent child, antiviral therapy is reserved only for life-threatening infection.

Long-term sequelae are unusual in the healthy child with primary HHV-6 or HHV-7 infection. Neurologic damage is occasionally noted in children after complicated seizures associated with either virus.

WHEN TO REFER

- Primary HHV-6 or HHV-7 infections almost never are clinically recognized until the disease is over.
- Referral almost never is needed except to rule out an alternative diagnosis such as a seizure disorder or treatable encephalopathy or encephalitis.
- Severe clinical symptoms in immunocompromised patients should always be managed by an infectious disease consultant.

WHEN TO ADMIT

- Hospitalization is usually indicated only when an alternate disease process is suspected, such as meningitis, encephalitis, or recurrent seizures.

- Immunocompromised patients may have severe infection with HHV-6 or HHV-7, but they are typically hospitalized for their severe clinical presentation—for example, pneumonitis, encephalitis, or suspected graft-versus-host disease—rather than for suspicion of HHV-6 or HHV-7 infection.

TOOLS FOR PRACTICE

Medical Decision Support

- *Red Book: 2006 Report of the Committee on Infectious Diseases*, American Academy of Pediatrics (www.aap.org/bookstore).

SUGGESTED RESOURCE

Zerr DM. Human herpesvirus 6: a clinical update. *Herpes.* 2006;13:20-24.

REFERENCES

1. Ward KN. The natural history and laboratory diagnosis of human herpesviruses-6 and -7 infections in he immunocompetent. *J Clin Virol.* 2005;32:183-193.
2. Miyagawa H, Yamanashi K. The epidemiology and pathogenesis of infections caused by the high numbered human herpesviruses in children: HHV-6, HHV-7, and HHV-8. *Curr Opin Infect Dis.* 1999;12:251-255.
3. Levy JA. Three new human herpesviruses (HHV-6, 7 and 8). *Lancet.* 1997;349:558-563.
4. Hidaka Y, Liu Y, Yamamoto M, et al. Frequent isolation of human herpesvirus 7 from saliva samples. *J Med Virol.* 1993;40:343-346.
5. Zerr DM, Meier AS, Selke SS, et al. A population-based study of primary human herpesvirus 6 infection. *N Engl J Med.* 2005;352:768-776.
6. Takahashi Y, Yamada M, Nakamura J, et al. Transmission of human herpesvirus 7 through multigenerational families in the same household. *Pediatr Infect Dis J.* 1997;16:975-978.
7. Zerr DM. Human herpesvirus 6: a clinical update. *Herpes.* 2006;13:20-24.
8. Hall CB, Long CE, Chancel KC, et al. Human herpesvirus-6 infection in children. A prospective study of complications and reactivation. *N Engl J Med.* 1994;331:432-438.
9. Hall CB, Caserta MT, Schnabel KC, et al. Characteristics and acquisition of human herpesvirus (HHV)-7 infections in relation to infection with HHV-6. *J Infect Dis.* 2006;193:1063-1069.
10. Breese BB Jr. Roseola infantum (exanthem subitum). *N Y State J Med.* 1941;41:1854-1859.
11. Clemens HH. Exanthem subitum (roseola infantum): report of eighty cases. *J Pediatr.* 1945;26:66-77.
12. Suga S, Yoshikawa T, Nagai T, et al. Clinical features and virological findings in children with primary human herpesvirus 7 infections. *Pediatrics.* 1997;99:e4. Available at: www.pediatrics.org/cgi/content/full/99/3/e4. Accessed June 28, 2007.
13. Caserta MT, Hall CB, Schnabel K, et al. Primary human herpesvirus 7 infection: a comparison of human herpesvirus 7 and human herpesvirus 6 infection in children. *J Pediatr.* 1998;133:386-389.
14. Hukin J, Farrell K, MacWilliam LM, et al. Case-control study of primary human herpesvirus 6 infection in children with febrile seizures. *Pediatrics.* 1998;101:e3. Available at: pediatrics.aappublications.org/cgi/content/full/101/2/e3. Accessed June 28, 2007.
15. Zerr DM, Frenkel LM, Huang M, et al. Polymerase chain reaction diagnosis of primary human herpesvirus-6 infection in the acute care setting. *J Pediatr.* 2006;149:480-485.
16. Ward KN, Andrews NJ, Verity CM, et al. Human herpesviruses-6 and -7 each cause significant neurological morbidity in Britain and Ireland. *Arch Dis Child.* 2005;90:619-623. Available at: adc.bmjjournals.com/cgi/content/full/90/6/619#bibl/. Accessed June 28, 2007.
17. Yanagihara K, Tanaka-Taya K, Itagaki Y, et al. Human herpesvirus 6 meningoencephalitis with sequelae. *Pediatr Infect Dis J.* 1995;14:240-241.
18. Torre D, Speranza F, Martegani R, et al. Meningoencephalitis caused by human herpesvirus-6 in an immunocompetent adult patient: case report and review of the literature. *Infection.* 1998;26:402-404.
19. Nash PJ, Avery RK, Tang WH, et al. Encephalitis owing to human herpesvirus-6 after cardiac transplant. *Am J Transplant* 2004;4(7):1200-1203.
20. Akashi K, Eizuru Y, Sumiyoshi Y, et al. Severe infectious mononucleosis-like syndrome and primary human herpesvirus 6 infection in an adult. *N Engl J Med.* 1993;329:168-171. Available at: content.nejm.org/cgi/content/full/329/3/168/. Accessed June 28, 2007.
21. De Bolle L, Naesens L, De Clercq E. Update on human herpesvirus 6 biology, clinical features. *Clin Microbiol Rev.* 2005;18:217-245.
22. Kawa-Ha K, Tanaka K, Inoue M, et al. Isolation of human herpesvirus 7 from a child with symptoms mimicking chronic Epstein-Barr virus infection. *Br J Haematol.* 1993;84(3):545-548.
23. Hsiao AL, Chen L, Baker MD. Incidence and predictors of serious bacterial infections among 57- to 180-day-old infants. *Pediatrics.* 2006;117:1695-1701. Available at: www.pediatrics.org/cgi/content/full/117/5/1695/. Accessed June 28, 2007.
24. Hashida T, Komura E, Yoshida M. Hepatitis in association with human herpesvirus-7 infection. *Pediatrics.* 1995;96:783-785.
25. Byington CL, Zerr DM, Taggart EW, et al. Human herpesvirus 6 infection in febrile infants ninety days of age or younger. *Pediatr Infect Dis J.* 2002;21:996-999.
26. Andreoni M, Sarmati L, Nicastri E, et al. Primary human herpesvirus 8 infection in immunocompetent children. *JAMA.* 2002;287:1295-1300.

Chapter 276

HUMAN IMMUNODEFICIENCY VIRUS INFECTION AND ACQUIRED IMMUNODEFICIENCY SYNDROME

William J. Moss, MD, MPH; Deborah Persaud, MD; Michael T. Brady, MD

Children who have the acquired immunodeficiency syndrome (AIDS) were first identified in 1983, 2 years after the description of AIDS in adults.[1] By the end of 2006, approximately 10,000 children younger than 13 years were living with AIDS in the United States.[2] AIDS results from progressive immune dysfunction after infection with the human immunodeficiency virus (HIV). Two separate HIV viruses have been identified: HIV-1, which is the predominant virus responsible for disease in the United States and the rest of the world, and HIV-2, which is primarily detected in patients in West Africa. Clinical manifestations of HIV infection range from asymptomatic infection to debilitating disease and death. Prepubertal children most commonly acquire HIV infection through maternal-infant transmission, but, in rare instances, they may be infected through receipt of infected blood or blood products and through sexual abuse. At the present time, a substantial number of adolescents are contracting HIV infection through adult behaviors such as unprotected sexual activities and intravenous drug use. Before the widespread use of antiretroviral prophylaxis to prevent maternal-to-child transmission, as many as 1800 HIV-infected children were born in the United States annually. Now, fewer than 50 infants are diagnosed with AIDS in the United States each year. The great burden of pediatric HIV infection is in the resource-poor countries of Africa and Asia.

The care of HIV-infected children is complex and requires a multidisciplinary team to address the multiple medical, psychological, social, and economic issues that confront HIV-infected children and their families. Advances in the diagnosis, treatment, and prevention of pediatric HIV infection bring hope to many HIV-infected children, their families, and those who care for them, but a cure remains elusive.

TRANSMISSION OF HUMAN IMMUNODEFICIENCY VIRUS TO CHILDREN

Perinatal transmission is the most common mode of acquisition of HIV infection among children in the United States. Not all infants born to HIV-infected women acquire HIV infection; estimated perinatal transmission rates in untreated women to their infants range from 13% to 30%.[3] Perinatal HIV transmission can occur by 3 mechanisms: (1) transplacental infection in utero, (2) intrapartum infection during labor and delivery, and (3) postpartum infection through mother's milk. Before the availability of antiretroviral chemotherapy to prevent perinatal HIV transmission, intrapartum transmission was the most common mode of transmission. High maternal plasma HIV levels correlate with increased risk of transmission.[4] Thus women who have advanced HIV disease or recently acquired infection are more likely to transmit HIV to their newborns. Antiretroviral therapy administered to women during pregnancy and delivery and to infants during the first 6 weeks of life greatly reduces the rate of perinatal HIV transmission.

Routine testing of blood donors for HIV antibody began in March 1985. Children who received blood or blood products before this time were at risk of HIV infection. Children who had hemophilia were at particularly high risk because they received pooled factors from hundreds to thousands of donors. The risk of HIV infection from blood or blood products is now extremely low, estimated to be 1 in 2 million from a single unit of blood.[5]

HIV transmission through sexual contact occurs in children who are sexually abused or in sexually active adolescents. Behaviors that place adolescents at high risk of HIV infection are initiation of sexual activity at a young age, multiple sexual partners, and unprotected sexual intercourse. Given that perinatal transmission has been reduced substantially, adolescents who acquire HIV through adult behaviors represent the most common newly infected pediatric patients. Although the total number of perinatal infections have declined, the proportion caused by intrauterine transmission has increased.[6] This statistic supports a greater role of antiretroviral therapy and mode of delivery on influencing intrapartum transmission.

PATHOPHYSIOLOGICAL FEATURES OF HUMAN IMMUNODEFICIENCY VIRUS INFECTION IN CHILDREN

Perinatal HIV infection occurs during the development and maturation of the immune system. This occurrence distinguishes pediatric HIV infection from adult infection and has profound effects on the clinical course, nature, and timing of opportunistic infections and immune responses to immunizations.

HIV infects several different cell types, but the primary target for HIV replication is the $CD4^+$ T lymphocyte. In addition to the $CD4^+$ cell surface molecule, HIV requires a chemokine coreceptor to enter cells. Polymorphisms in chemokine receptors are associated with resistance to HIV infection and different rates of disease progression. Reverse transcription, in which viral DNA is synthesized from viral RNA, is carried out by the enzyme reverse transcriptase. Viral DNA is then transported to the nucleus and integrated into cellular DNA with the help of viral enzyme integrase, persisting for the life span of the cell. Subsequently, a messenger RNA is produced using human enzymes. This messenger RNA is transported outside the nucleus, and is used as a blueprint for synthesizing a large viral polypeptide (HIV proteins and enzymes) that requires cleavage by a viral protease. These newly made HIV proteins and enzymes gather along with HIV RNA to form new viral particles, which are then released from the cell. Currently available antiretroviral therapy works by interfering with the functions of these enzymes: nucleoside and nonnucleoside reverse transcriptase inhibitors, protease inhibitors, entry inhibitors, and integrase inhibitors.

The number of copies of HIV RNA in plasma can be quantified. Given that HIV, similar to other viruses, is an obligate intracellular parasite, virus in the plasma represents a replicating virus looking for a new host cell. Plasma HIV RNA levels are useful in predicting the rate of disease progression, modifying antiretroviral therapy, and understanding viral dynamics. In children who have perinatally acquired HIV infection, HIV RNA levels peak in the first few months of life and decline slowly over several years. Steady-state HIV RNA levels in children are not achieved until 2 to 6 years of age. In contrast, HIV RNA levels in adults decline rapidly to steady-state levels within several months after primary infection. Despite the decline in HIV RNA levels, intense viral replication continues to occur. Combination therapy with reverse transcriptase and protease inhibitors block HIV replication and can result in a dramatic decline in virus production and undetectable plasma HIV RNA levels. HIV persists within cellular compartments, however, and cure is not achievable with current therapies.

Infection with HIV leads to a progressive decrease in CD4$^+$ T lymphocytes. CD4$^+$ T lymphocytes are helper T cells that provide stimulatory signals to cells responsible for cellular and humoral immunity and phagocytosis. Qualitative changes in the function of CD4$^+$ T lymphocytes occur before the decline in number. Because CD4$^+$ T lymphocytes are crucial to B-lymphocyte function, humoral immunity (antibody production) can be significantly impaired in HIV-infected children, resulting in poor antibody responses to encapsulated bacteria and immunizations, despite increased levels of total immunoglobulins.

DIAGNOSIS OF HUMAN IMMUNODEFICIENCY VIRUS INFECTION IN CHILDREN

The most important factor in identifying HIV-infected women and children is that the diagnosis be considered. Several risk factors are associated with HIV infection in women of childbearing age, including history of multiple sexual partners, illicit drug use, and sexual contact with persons at high risk. However, the absence of identifiable risk factors does not exclude HIV infection.

Because maternal HIV antibody will cross the placenta and reach the fetus, detection of HIV DNA or RNA by polymerase chain reaction (PCR) is the preferred method for diagnosing HIV infection in infants. PCR amplifies HIV DNA or RNA sequences and is extremely sensitive in detecting small amounts of virus. Almost all HIV-infected infants have a positive HIV PCR by 1 month of age, and 40% of HIV-infected infants can be identified in the first 2 days of life.[7] False-positive results have occurred on rare occasions because of laboratory contamination. Positive results should be confirmed by PCR testing of a second blood specimen. Because early detection of HIV infection allows for the initiation of combination antiretroviral therapy in infancy, HIV-exposed infants should be tested by 48 hours of age. A positive PCR at 48 hours of age suggests intrauterine infection. If negative, then repeat PCR testing should be performed at 14 days of age because more than 90% of infected infants will have a positive PCR by 2 weeks of age. Infants negative for HIV by PCR at 48 hours and at 14 days should be tested at 1 to 2 months of age and, if negative, again at 3 to 6 months of age. HIV infection is diagnosed by 2 positive HIV PCR tests performed on separate blood samples. Two negative PCR results, one performed at 1 to 2 months and the other at 4 to 6 months of age, is adequate to confirm noninfection with HIV. If there are negative HIV PCR tests at either 2 and 4 weeks of age, or 8 weeks of age, then the infant is presumptively not infected. Some experts still perform HIV antibody testing at 15 to 18 months of age to assure noninfection.

The HIV enzyme-linked immunosorbent assay (ELISA) detects antibody to HIV and is the appropriate screening test for children older than 18 months of age. The HIV ELISA has high sensitivity but lacks specificity; thus false-positive results occur. Positive ELISA reactions for HIV are confirmed by Western blot analysis, which detects antibodies to several HIV proteins and is highly specific. False-negative results may occur shortly after primary infection because antibodies to HIV do not achieve detectable levels until 2 to 3 months after infection. Serologic methods should not be used to confirm HIV infection in children younger than 18 months because transplacentally derived maternal antibodies result in a positive HIV ELISA in infants born to HIV-seropositive women even if the child is not infected. These maternal antibodies can persist for 18 months.

CLINICAL MANIFESTATIONS OF HUMAN IMMUNODEFICIENCY VIRUS INFECTION IN CHILDREN

The time from infection to onset of clinical symptoms may be shorter for children who have perinatally acquired HIV infection than for children infected through blood or blood products, and it is usually shorter than for HIV-infected adults. HIV-infected infants are without symptoms in the neonatal period. Before the widespread use of prophylaxis for *Pneumocystis jirovecii* pneumonia (PCP) and early antiretroviral therapy, a subset of HIV-infected children had rapidly progressive disease and died within the first year of life, frequently from PCP. Other children remain asymptomatic or have few symptoms for many years, some into adolescence. However, most children who have perinatal HIV infection and are untreated develop symptoms by 2 years of age. High levels of plasma HIV levels and low CD4$^+$ T lymphocyte cell counts are predictive of poor prognosis.

Early clinical signs and symptoms of HIV infection are nonspecific but generally indicate a systemic illness. Children may exhibit failure to thrive, developmental delay, persistent oral candidiasis, lymphadenopathy, hepatosplenomegaly, chronic diarrhea, recurrent bacterial infections, and recurrent herpesvirus infections. PCP was a frequent illness found in affected infants before routine prophylaxis of HIV-exposed infants. Laboratory abnormalities often include anemia, thrombocytopenia, and increased immunoglobulin levels.

HIV infection and secondary opportunistic infections can involve all organ systems. Pulmonary disease is common in HIV-infected children. PCP is a fulminant pulmonary infection characterized by tachypnea, cough, hypoxemia, and, most commonly, diffuse alveolar infiltrates on chest radiograph. However, early in the course of PCP in older children, the chest radiograph may be normal or show minimal changes despite significant cough and even hypoxia. Lymphoid interstitial pneumonitis (LIP) is a chronic lung disease of HIV-infected children resulting from lymphoid hyperplasia in the lungs. Children who have LIP may be asymptomatic or may have chronic cough and wheezing. Bilateral, reticulonodular densities are seen on chest radiographs resembling miliary tuberculosis.

Table 276-1 Immunologic Categories Based on Age-Specific $CD4^+$ T-Lymphocyte Count and Percentage of Total Lymphocytes

	AGE					
	<1 YEAR		1-5 YEARS		6-12 YEARS	
SUPPRESSION	**MCL**	**%**	**MCL**	**%**	**MCL**	**%**
No evidence of suppression	≥1500	≥25	≥1000	≥25	≥500	25
Evidence of moderate suppression	750-1499	15-24	500-999	15-24	200-499	15-24
Severe suppression	<750	<15	<500	<15	<200	<15

From Centers for Disease Control and Prevention. 1994 revised classification system for HIV infection in children younger than 13 years of age. *MMWR.* 1994;43(RR-12):1.

Table 276-2 Categories of Human Immunodeficiency Virus Classification in Children

	CLINICAL CATEGORY			
	N	**A**	**B**	**C**
IMMUNOLOGICAL CATEGORY	**NO SIGNS OR SYMPTOMS**	**MILD SIGNS OR SYMPTOMS**	**MODERATE SIGNS OR SYMPTOMS**	**SEVERE SIGNS OR SYMPTOMS**
1. No evidence of suppression	N1	A1	B1	C1
2. Evidence of moderate suppression	N2	A2	B2	C2
3. Severe suppression	N3	A3	B3	C3

From Centers for Disease Control and Prevention. 1994 revised classification system for HIV infection in children younger than 13 years of age. *MMWR.* 1994;43(RR-12):1.

Children who have LIP are typically older than those who have PCP and frequently have generalized lymphadenopathy and parotid enlargement.

Central nervous system disease is also more common in HIV-infected children. Microcephaly, developmental delay, spasticity, abnormal reflexes, and gait abnormalities may be present. Characteristic findings on computed tomographic scan include cerebral atrophy and basal ganglia calcifications. Hematologic abnormalities associated with HIV infection include leukopenia, anemia, and thrombocytopenia. Thrombocytopenia may be the presenting illness. In addition, drug-induced bone marrow suppression can follow therapy with zidovudine, co-trimoxazole, and ganciclovir. Hepatomegaly and increases in hepatic transaminases are commonly seen, often in the absence of clinically apparent liver disease. HIV cardiomyopathy may lead to congestive heart failure. HIV nephropathy is a common cause of proteinuria and can progress to the nephrotic syndrome. Chronic diarrhea, resulting from several opportunistic gastrointestinal pathogens, can be debilitating.

Dermatologic conditions include recurrent herpes simplex and varicella-zoster virus infections, severe molluscum contagiosum, chronic fungal infections, atopic dermatitis, and drug-induced eruptions, particularly with co-trimoxazole. HIV-infected children in whom virus replication is not controlled by antiretroviral therapy are frequently stunted in their growth, and severe wasting may be seen in advanced disease. Malignancies are not as common in HIV-infected children, but lymphomas and leiomyosarcomas can occur.

In 1984 the CDC developed a classification system based on clinical diseases to categorize HIV infection and AIDS in children. The CDC classification was revised in 1994 to incorporate advances in the understanding of the natural history of HIV infection in children and age-specific $CD4^+$ T-lymphocyte cell counts (Table 276-1).[8] HIV-infected children are classified into 1 of 4 clinical categories (N, A, B, or C) based on clinical signs and symptoms and into 1 of 3 immunologic categories (1, 2, or 3) based on age-specific $CD4^+$ T-lymphocyte cell counts or the percentage of the $CD4^+$ T lymphocyte. However, variability in clinical status exists even within a category (Table 276-2).

COMMON CLINICAL PROBLEMS IN HUMAN IMMUNODEFICIENCY VIRUS–INFECTED CHILDREN

Most HIV-infected children who have fever and a normal clinical examination have self-limited febrile illnesses similar to those of HIV-uninfected children. However, as with other immunocompromised children, in HIV-infected children with moderate or severe immunosuppression, fever may indicate a serious infection. A detailed clinical history and thorough physical examination, with close attention to general appearance and potential areas of focal inflammation such as skin, ears, sinuses, lungs, and gastrointestinal tract, are essential in the initial assessment of the febrile HIV-infected child. However, bacteremia with *Streptococcus pneumoniae* and *Salmonella* can occur in the absence of physical findings. Additional diagnostic studies should be obtained based on the child's age, clinical appearance, degree of immunosuppression, and signs and symptoms at the time the patient seeks care. Laboratory tests to be considered include a complete blood count with differential, large-volume blood culture, chest radiograph, urinalysis and urine culture, and lumbar puncture. Administration of empirical antibiotic therapy is not always necessary and depends on the results of the clinical assessment and laboratory tests, as well as the likelihood of adequate monitoring and follow-up. A third-generation cephalosporin such as ceftriaxone or cefotaxime can be used as empirical antibiotic therapy to provide therapy against both gram-positive and gram-negative bacteria. Ill-appearing children should be hospitalized. Persistent fever in the HIV-infected child can be a diagnostic challenge, but identifiable and treatable causes include mycobacterial infection and drug-induced fever.

Pneumococcus is the most common bacterial cause of pneumonia in HIV-infected children. HIV-infected children are likely to develop severe disease as a result of infection with common respiratory pathogens such as respiratory syncytial virus, parainfluenza virus, influenza virus, and adenovirus. HIV-infected children who have advanced immunosuppression are susceptible to many opportunistic pulmonary pathogens. PCP is the most common opportunistic infection in HIV-infected infants and typically appears at 3 to 6 months of age with cough, tachypnea, and hypoxemia. Early diagnosis and treatment, usually with co-trimoxazole and corticosteroids, is critical. Physicians caring for HIV-infected children must carefully consider the diagnosis of PCP in HIV-infected children who have respiratory tract symptoms. HIV-infected children who have pulmonary disease and who fail to respond to empirical antibiotic therapy, those who are severely ill, and those who are suspected of having PCP should undergo an invasive diagnostic procedure such as bronchoscopy with bronchoalveolar lavage or lung biopsy.

Persistent diarrhea can significantly compromise the quality of life and the nutritional status of HIV-infected children. Infectious causes of diarrhea in HIV-infected children include all of the pathogens of healthy children in addition to numerous opportunistic pathogens. Common parasitic pathogens causing persistent diarrhea include *Giardia lamblia, Entamoeba histolytica, Cryptosporidium* species, and *Isospora belli*. Cytomegalovirus may cause colitis in children who have advanced immunosuppression. Diagnostic studies should include stool cultures for bacterial and viral pathogens, as well as antigen detection for *Giardia* and *Cryptosporidium* and possibly ova and parasites. Endoscopy should be considered in refractory cases.

Bacterial and viral pathogens causing meningitis and encephalitis in HIV-infected children are similar to those in nonimmunocompromised children. Opportunistic pathogens causing meningitis and encephalitis in HIV-infected children who have advanced immunosuppression include *Cryptococcus neoformans, Toxoplasma gondii,* and cytomegalovirus. Initial diagnostic studies include analysis of cerebrospinal fluid and brain imaging. In rare instances, central nervous system lymphomas can occur.

HIV-infected children are at increased risk of disseminated varicella and recurrent herpes zoster. HIV-infected children who are susceptible to varicella (no prior natural infection or age-appropriate varicella immunization) should receive a varicella-zoster immunoglobulin preparation (or intravenous immunoglobulin if varicella-zoster immunoglobulin is not available) within 96 hours of exposure to varicella. Disseminated infection can occur with herpes zoster, and oral or parenteral therapy with acyclovir is warranted.

Growth failure is common in HIV infection in children early in the course of disease. The diagnosis of HIV infection should be considered in children who fail to thrive. Frequent measurements of weight and height are important in detecting growth disturbances early and monitoring response to interventions. Effective antiretroviral therapy with suppression of viral replication, as well as nutritional supplementation, is important to maintaining growth. However, supplementation with high-calorie foods or formulas often results in increased body fat rather than lean body weight.

Delayed acquisition of developmental milestones or loss of previously acquired milestones is also a common manifestation of HIV infection in children. Effective antiretroviral therapy can minimize or reverse the neurocognitive effects of HIV infection.

PREVENTING MATERNAL-INFANT HUMAN IMMUNODEFICIENCY VIRUS TRANSMISSION

Identification of HIV-infected women before or during pregnancy is critical in preventing perinatal HIV transmission. Prenatal HIV counseling and testing should be provided to all pregnant women. Initial HIV antibody testing should be performed early in pregnancy and repeated in the third trimester for women at risk for HIV infection, for example, those with a history of multiple sexual partners, illicit drug use, or a sexual partner at risk for HIV infection. Administration of zidovudine to women during pregnancy and labor and to infants for the first 6 weeks of life has been shown to reduce perinatal HIV transmission by two thirds (26% to 8%).[9] This regimen is the standard of care for HIV-infected pregnant women and their newborns. Early identification of HIV-infected pregnant women also allows for appropriate care of the mother, avoidance of ongoing HIV exposure of the infant through human milk, and early institution of PCP prophylaxis for the infant at 4 to 6 weeks of age. Highly active antiretroviral therapy provided to the mother also reduces the risk of maternal-infant HIV transmission.

CARE OF THE HUMAN IMMUNODEFICIENCY VIRUS–INFECTED CHILD

Proper care of HIV-infected children requires a multidisciplinary team that includes pediatricians, experts in antiretroviral therapy, nutritionists, physical therapists, pharmacists, psychologists, social workers, and outreach workers. The primary care physician should rely on HIV care providers for the management of antiretroviral drugs.

Immunization of the Human Immunodeficiency Virus–Infected Child

Immunizations are generally safe for HIV-infected children, although the immune suppression caused by HIV results in less assurance of protection after immunization than in non-HIV-infected children. However, the small risk of serious complications from live viral vaccines has led to special recommendations for HIV-infected children.[10] RotaTeq should not be administered to immunocompromised children. However, HIV-exposed infants with testing that does not support HIV infection may receive their initial dose of RotaTeq before documentation that the infant is not infected (negative PCR after 4 months of age).

Toxoids, subunit vaccines, inactivated vaccines, and recombinant vaccines are not associated with increased risks of complications in HIV-infected children. Vaccines in these categories include diphtheria and tetanus toxoids, acellular pertussis vaccines, inactivated poliovirus vaccine, *Haemophilus influenzae* type b and pneumococcal conjugate vaccines, inactivated influenza vaccine, and hepatitis A and B vaccines. These vaccines should be administered to HIV-infected children according to the routine immunization schedule. Because of an increased risk of invasive infection with *S pneumoniae,* immunization of HIV-infected children with pneumococcal conjugate vaccine is particularly important. HIV-infected children may develop lower antibody titers than healthy children after immunization and are more likely to lose protective antibody earlier.

Live viral vaccines, such as varicella vaccine and measles-mumps-rubella vaccine, may result in infection and disease resulting from vaccine virus in severely immunocompromised HIV-infected children, although the risk is quite small. After the report of a death caused by measles vaccine virus after immunization, advisory groups in the United States recommended withholding measles vaccine from HIV-infected children with severe immunosuppression, defined as $CD4^+$ T lymphocytes less than 15%.[10] Measles-mumps-rubella vaccine should be administered to HIV-infected children at 12 months of age unless the children are severely immunocompromised ($CD4^+$ <15%). As with other vaccines, the immune response to measles vaccine in HIV-infected children may be poor, and vaccinated children may remain susceptible to measles virus infection. Serious complications after mumps or rubella immunization have not been reported.

Live varicella virus vaccine is also recommended for HIV-infected children based on their degree of immunosuppression and symptoms. The American Academy of Pediatrics Committee on Infectious Diseases recommends varicella vaccine for asymptomatic and mildly symptomatic HIV-infected children who have $CD4^+$ T-lymphocyte percentages of 15% or more.[10] Serious adverse events after administration of varicella vaccine to HIV-infected children are rare.

Antimicrobial Prophylaxis

Because of the high mortality rate associated with PCP in early infancy, PCP prophylaxis should be administered to HIV-exposed infants beginning at 6 weeks of age, even if HIV infection is not confirmed. Prophylaxis is not necessary for HIV-exposed infants who are not infected or who are presumptively not infected. Prophylaxis is continued until 12 months of age or until the diagnosis of HIV infection has been excluded. For children 1 to 5 years of age, PCP prophylaxis is administered if the $CD4^+$ T-lymphocyte cell count is less than 500 cells/mL and for children 6 to 12 years of age if it is less than 200 cells/mL.[11] Lifelong PCP prophylaxis is recommended for children who have a history of PCP, despite immune reconstitution. The recommended regimen is co-trimoxazole taken orally 3 days a week. Alternative regimens include dapsone or pentamidine.

HIV-infected children who have recurrent oral candidiasis may benefit from antifungal prophylaxis with oral nystatin, clotrimazole, or fluconazole. Many experts suggest weekly oral azithromycin or daily rifabutin for prophylaxis against *Mycobacterium avium-intracellulare* infection in children who have $CD4^+$ T-lymphocyte cell counts less than 100 cells/mL. Immunoglobulin should be provided to susceptible HIV-infected children within 6 days of exposure to a person who has measles, and measles immunization should be delayed 6 months after receipt of immunoglobulin.

Antiretroviral Therapy

The treatment of HIV infection with antiretroviral drugs is complex. Management of antiretroviral therapy should be directed by a specialist who has knowledge of the mechanisms of action of antiretroviral agents, potential toxicities, drug interactions, and cross-resistance patterns. Because most children acquire HIV infection during or near the time of birth, antiretroviral therapy should be initiated in infancy. Although early therapy restores immunologic function, the risks of drug toxicity and acquisition of drug-resistant virus are increased. Decisions to initiate early therapy require balancing the benefits and risks. Combination antiretroviral therapy is recommended for all infants diagnosed with HIV infection in the first year of life, regardless of clinical, immunologic, or virologic status.[12] For children diagnosed after 12 months of age, the decision to start treatment should be based on clinical symptoms, plasma HIV RNA levels, and $CD4^+$ T-lymphocyte counts.[12]

The choice of antiretroviral regimen for children is based on several factors, including the availability of pediatric formulations, potential drug interactions, the frequency of drug dosing, and potential interactions with other medications. Before therapy begins, the child's clinical, virologic, immunologic, and nutritional status should be documented. Neuropsychometric testing should be performed in children with deficits.

Baseline laboratory studies should include a complete blood count with differential, liver function tests, a $CD4^+$ T-lymphocyte cell count, and plasma HIV RNA level.

Combination antiretroviral therapy consists of a protease inhibitor or nonnucleoside reverse transcriptase inhibitor in combination with 2 or more nucleoside reverse transcriptase inhibitors. Protease inhibitors that may be used in children include lopinavir/ritonavir (preferred), nelfinavir, ritonavir (alone), amprenavir, and indinavir. Lopinavir/ritonavir, nelfinavir, ritonavir, and amprenavir are available in liquid formulations. Atazanavir, darunavir, fosamprenavir, tipranavir, and saquinavir are available protease inhibitors with insufficient data in children to recommend at this time. Preferred combinations of nucleoside reverse transcriptase inhibitors are zidovudine plus (lamivudine or emtricitabine), zidovudine plus didanose, or didanosine plus (lamivudine or emtricitabine). Alternative combinations that have been less well studied in children are abacavir plus zidovudine, abacavir plus (lamivudine or emtricitabine), and stavudine plus (lamivudine or emtricitabine). Stavudine and didanosine should not be used or used with substantial caution because of their potential synergistic toxicities. Several combinations are not recommended either because of antagonism (stavudine-zidovudine) or because of overlapping toxicities. The nonnucleoside reverse transcriptase inhibitors nevirapine, delavirdine, and efavirenz can be used in combination with the nucleoside reverse transcriptase inhibitors.

Common side effects of nucleoside reverse transcriptase inhibitors are anemia and neutropenia with zidovudine, pancreatitis with didanosine, peripheral neuropathy with didanosine and stavudine, and an influenza-like hypersensitivity reaction with abacavir. Rechallenge with abacavir can be fatal. Common side effects of the nonnucleoside reverse transcriptase inhibitors nevirapine, delavirdine, and efavirenz are rashes and hepatitis. Efavirenz can cause bad dreams, hallucinations, confusion, and impaired concentration. Gastrointestinal symptoms are the major side effects of protease inhibitors. Long-term complications of combination antiretroviral therapy include lipoatrophy, lipodystrophy, hypercholesterolemia, and bone demineralization.

Adherence to complex drug regimens can be difficult. Compliance is hindered by the large number or volume of medications, poor palatability, varied dosing schedules, and different effects of food on drug bioavailability. Mixing the drugs with foods, such as peanut butter or ice cream, may improve compliance in children. Behavioral therapy, begun before combination therapy is initiated, can be helpful in designing a routine medication schedule, teaching parents and caregivers methods to improve compliance, and teaching the child techniques for swallowing unsavory medications. Gastric tubes (g-tubes) may be necessary and helpful to ensure medication compliance in children who are not adherent because of medication taste or volume problems.

Strict adherence to the treatment regimen is essential for the prevention of drug resistance. Because of cross-resistance, resistance to one drug can limit the effectiveness of other drugs of the same class. Viral sequences obtained from plasma samples can be tested for drug resistance mutations and for susceptibility profiles to guide treatment decisions. Plasma HIV RNA levels should be measured 4 weeks after the child has started therapy to assess response. The frequency of follow-up visits depends on many factors, including the child's clinical status and expected compliance with therapy, but follow-up should include measurements of HIV RNA levels and $CD4^+$ T-lymphocyte counts every 3 months.

Drug Interactions With Antiretroviral Therapy

HIV protease inhibitors, as well as the nonnucleoside reverse transcriptase inhibitors, are metabolized in the liver by a cytochrome P450 enzyme. Protease inhibitors have the potential to inhibit this enzyme and interfere with the metabolism of many other drugs. Protease inhibitors also can act as potent inhibitors of 2 other P450 enzymes active in the metabolism of analgesics, β-blockers, and phenytoin. Ritonavir can stimulate glucuronidation, thus decreasing the concentration of drugs metabolized by this pathway, including sedatives such as lorazepam and the narcotics morphine and codeine.

Many drugs that have altered metabolism because of protease inhibitors are used in pediatric emergencies, including narcotic analgesics, anticonvulsants, antiarrhythmics, calcium-channel blockers, and corticosteroids. These drugs should be used with caution in children receiving protease inhibitors. Drugs that have narrow therapeutic margins require particularly careful monitoring for adverse effects and measurement of drug concentrations. Drugs contraindicated for use with protease inhibitors include meperidine, midazolam, astemizole, terfenadine, cisapride, and rifampin.

Several other medications frequently prescribed for HIV-infected children are inhibitors of cytochrome P450 enzymes, including ketoconazole, itraconazole, clarithromycin, and erythromycin. Inhibition of cytochrome P450 enzymes by these medications may lead to an increase in the plasma concentration of protease inhibitors. Dose reduction of the protease inhibitor may be required. Conversely, inducers of the cytochrome P450 enzyme system are also frequently prescribed for HIV-infected children. Antimycobacterial drugs (rifampin, rifabutin), anticonvulsants (phenobarbital, phenytoin, carbamazepine), and glucocorticoids (dexamethasone) are inducers of cytochrome P450 enzymes. Increased metabolism of protease inhibitors may result in subtherapeutic levels, with the potential emergence of drug resistance.

POSTEXPOSURE PROPHYLAXIS AFTER COMMUNITY NEEDLESTICK INJURIES

Parents, caretakers, and physicians often are most concerned about transmission of HIV after accidental injury from a discarded needle. However, no consensus or recommendation is available to guide management in such circumstances. The risk of HIV transmission after occupational exposure to HIV-infected blood is 0.3%. Most experts agree that the risk after community needlestick injury is lower than the risk of occupational exposure. Factors to be considered in the use of antiretroviral agents for postexposure prophylaxis after community needlestick injuries include the potential risk of HIV transmission, drug toxicities, and the ability and willingness of the family to adhere to therapy. Regimens for occupational postexposure prophylaxis may be followed.

CHILD CARE AND SCHOOL FOR THE HUMAN IMMUNODEFICIENCY VIRUS–INFECTED CHILD

Because the risk of HIV transmission appears to be negligible, HIV-infected children should not be restricted from attending child care or school. Special consideration may be warranted for children who have unusual risk factors for transmission, such as frequent biting or scratching, severe dermatitis, or bleeding disorders. In such circumstances, the pediatrician should assess the need to protect other children.

HUMAN IMMUNODEFICIENCY VIRUS–INFECTED ADOLESCENT

The number of adolescents who are infected with HIV through unprotected sex is increasing. Because the onset of AIDS occurs years after sexual transmission, AIDS in young adults reflects acquisition of HIV during adolescence. Pediatricians caring for adolescents must ensure that they have knowledge of the risks of acquiring HIV and other sexually transmitted diseases through unprotected sex and be counseled on safe sexual practices.

Primary HIV infection in adolescents and adults is frequently accompanied by a mononucleosis-like illness characterized by fever, sore throat, lethargy, and lymphadenopathy (seroconversion syndrome). Because HIV antibodies take several months to achieve detectable levels, nucleic acid–based assays (PCR) should be used to diagnose symptomatic primary HIV infection.

ROLE OF THE PRIMARY CARE PHYSICIAN IN THE CARE OF HUMAN IMMUNODEFICIENCY VIRUS–INFECTED CHILDREN

The pediatrician plays a critical role in the care of HIV-infected children and their families and can be responsible for (1) diagnosing HIV infection; (2) providing well-child care, including monitoring growth and development and administering immunizations; (3) coordinating care among the multiple specialties and services, including experts in antiretroviral therapy, developmental and psychological assessment, nutritional support, and dental care; (4) managing common medical problems; and (5) directing the family to social and financial support services.

Many parents and guardians are not willing to tell the child that he or she is infected with HIV. However, most children are made aware of their illness through frequent medical visits and medications. The primary care physician's relationship with the patient provides the best position to promote and assist with disclosure. Appropriate disclosure tailored to the child's cognitive level is helpful in alleviating guilt and allows for discussion between the child, caregivers, and health care professionals. Uninfected siblings of HIV-infected children also are emotionally affected by the diagnosis and should be included in support groups and counseling.

The primary care physician also plays a critical role in providing advice and support as the child nears death and can help the family interpret the complexities of critical care and approach a decision on the appropriateness of heroic interventions. In some circumstances, the physician may even be able to assist in the family care for the dying child at home if critical care is deemed futile. After the death of the child, the physician should continue to support the family through the grief process. Because many pediatricians invest much time and emotional energy in caring for an HIV-infected child, many of them take the opportunity to express their sympathy by attending the child's funeral.

TOOLS FOR PRACTICE

Community Advocacy and Coordination

- *Male Latex Condoms and Sexually Transmitted Diseases* (fact sheet), Centers for Disease Control and Prevention (www.cdc.gov/nchstp/od/condoms.pdf).

Engaging Patient and Family

- *Correct Use of Condoms* (fact sheet), American Academy of Pediatrics (www.aap.org/patiented/condoms.htm).
- *Deciding to Wait: Guidelines for Teens* (brochure), American Academy of Pediatrics (patiented.aap.org).
- *Making Healthy Decisions About Sex* (brochure), American Academy of Pediatrics (patiented.aap.org).

Medical Decision Support

- *Covering the Bases: Adolescent Sexual Health PediaLink* (on-line course), American Academy of Pediatrics (www.pedialink.org).
- *Red Book: 2006 Report of the Committee on Infectious Diseases*, 27th edition (book), American Academy of Pediatrics (www.aap.org/bookstore).
- *Revised Recommendations for HIV Testing of Adults, Adolescents, and Pregnant Women in Health-Care Settings* (guideline), Centers for Disease Control and Prevention (www.cdc.gov/mmwr/preview/mmwrhtml/rr5514a1.htm).

RELATED WEB SITES

US Department of Health and Human Services: AIDS Info (aidsinfo.nih.gov/default.aspx).

Centers for Disease Control and Prevention: HIV/AIDS (cdc.gov/hiv/).

AAP POLICY STATEMENTS

American Academy of Pediatrics, Committee on Adolescence. Condom use by adolescents. *Pediatrics*. 2001; 107(6):1463-1469 (aappolicy.aappublications.org/cgi/content/full/pediatrics;107/6/1463).

American Academy of Pediatrics, Committee on Adolescence. Confidentiality in adolescent health care. *AAP News* (aapnews.aappublications.org/cgi/content/full/e2005175v1).

American Academy of Pediatrics, Committee on Pediatric AIDS and Committee on Adolescence. Adolescents and human immunodeficiency virus infection: the role of the pediatrician in prevention and intervention. *Pediatrics*. 2001;107(1):188-190 (aappolicy.aappublications.org/cgi/content/full/pediatrics;107/1/188).

American Academy of Pediatrics, Committee on Psychosocial Aspects of Child and Family Health and Committee on Adolescence. Sexuality Education for Children and Adolescents. *Pediatrics*. 2001;108(2):498-502 (aappolicy.aap publications.org/cgi/content/full/pediatrics;108/2/498).

American Academy of Pediatrics, Committee on Pediatric AIDS, Section on International Child Health. Increasing antiretroviral drug access for children with HIV infection. *Pediatrics*. 2007;119(4):838-845 (aappolicy.aappublications.org/cgi/content/full/pediatrics;119/4/838).

Havens PL, American Academy of Pediatrics, Committee on Pediatric AIDS. Postexposure prophylaxis in children and adolescents for nonoccupational exposure to human immunodeficiency virus. *Pediatrics*. 2003;111(6):1475-1489 (aappolicy.aappublications.org/cgi/content/full/pediatrics;114/2/1475).

King SD, American Academy of Pediatrics, Committee on Pediatric AIDS, Canadian Paediatric Society, Infectious Diseases and Immunization Committee. Evaluation and treatment of the human immunodeficiency virus-1—exposed infant. *Pediatrics*. 2004;114(2):497-505 (aappolicy.aap publications.org/cgi/content/full/pediatrics;114/2/497).

Mofenson LM, American Academy of Pediatrics, Committee on Pediatric AIDS. Technical report: perinatal human immunodeficiency virus testing and prevention of transmission. *Pediatrics*. 2000;106(6):e88 (aappolicy.aappublica tions.org/cgi/content/full/pediatrics;106/6/e88).

Read JS, American Academy of Pediatrics, Committee on Pediatric AIDS. Diagnosis of HIV-1 infection in children younger than 18 months in the United States. *Pediatrics*. 2007;120(6):e1547-e1562 (aappolicy.aappublications.org/cgi/content/full/pediatrics;120/6/e1547).

Read JS, American Academy of Pediatrics, Committee on Pediatric AIDS. Human milk, breastfeeding, and transmission of human immunodeficiency virus type 1 in the United States. *Pediatrics*. 2003;112(5):1196-1205 (aappolicy.aap publications.org/cgi/content/abstract/pediatrics;96/5/977).

SUGGESTED RESOURCES

American Academy of Pediatrics. Human immunodeficiency virus infection. In: Pickering LK, Baker CJ, Long SS, et al, eds. *Red Book: 2006 Report of the Committee on Infectious Diseases,* 27th ed. Elk Grove Village, IL: American Academy of Pediatrics; 2006.

US Department of Health and Human Services. AIDS Info. Available at: aidsinfo.nih.gov. Accessed February 26, 2007.

REFERENCES

1. Oleske JM, Minnefor AB. Acquired immune deficiency syndrome in children. *Pediatr Infect Dis*. 1983;2:65-66.
2. World Health Organization/UNAIDS. Report on the global AIDS epidemic 2006. Available at: www.unaids.org/en/HIV_data/epi2006/default.asp. Accessed November 2, 2007.
3. Mofenson LM. Advances in the prevention of vertical transmission of human immunodeficiency virus. *Semin Pediatr Infect Dis*. 2003;14:295-308.
4. Cooper ER, Charurat M, Mofenson L, et al, and Women and Infants' Transmission Study Group. Combination antiretroviral strategies for the treatment of pregnant HIV-1-infected women and prevention of perinatal HIV-1 transmission. *J Acquir Immune Defic Syndr*. 2002;29:484-494.
5. American Academy of Pediatrics. Blood safety: reducing the risk of transfusion-transmitted infections. In Pickering LK, Baker CJ, Long SS, McMillan JA, eds. *Red Book: 2006 Report of the Committee on Infectious Diseases,* 27th ed. Elk Grove Village, IL, American Academy of Pediatrics; 2006.
6. Magder LS, Mofenson L, Paul ME, et al. Risk factors for in utero and intrapartum transmission of HIV. *J Acquir Immune Defic Syndr,* 2005;38:87-95.
7. Bremer JW, Lew JF, Cooper E, et al. Diagnosis of infection with human immunodeficiency virus type 1 by a DNA polymerase chain reaction assay among infants enrolled in the Women and Infants' Transmission Study. *J Pediatr*. 1996;129:198-207.
8. Center for Disease Control and Prevention. 1994 Revised classification system for human immunodeficiency virus infection in children less than 13 years of age. *MMWR* 1994;43(No. RR-12):1-10.
9. Connor EM, Sperling RS, Gelber R, et al. Reduction of maternal-infant transmission of human immunodeficiency virus type 1 with zidovudine treatment. Pediatric AIDS Clinical Trials Group Protocol 076 Study Group. *N Engl J Med*. 1994;331:1173-1180.
10. American Academy of Pediatrics. Human immunodeficiency virus. In Pickering LK, Baker CJ, Long SS, McMillan JA, eds. *Red Book: 2006 Report of the Committee on Infectious Diseases,* 27th ed. Elk Grove Village, IL, American Academy of Pediatrics; 2006.
11. National pediatric and Family HIV Resource Center and National Center for Infectious Diseases, Centers for Disease Control and Prevention. 1995 revised guidelines for prophylaxis against Pneumocystis carinii pneumonia for children infected with or perinatally exposed to human immunodeficiency virus. *MMWR Recomm Rep*. 1995;44(RR-4):1-11.
12. Working Group on Antiretroviral Therapy and Medical Management of HIV-Infected Children. Guidelines for the use of Antiretroviral Agents in Pediatric HIV infection. February 8, 2008 [1-141]. Available at: www.aidsinfo.nih.gov/ContentFiles/pediatricGuidelines.pdf. Accessed November 2, 2007.

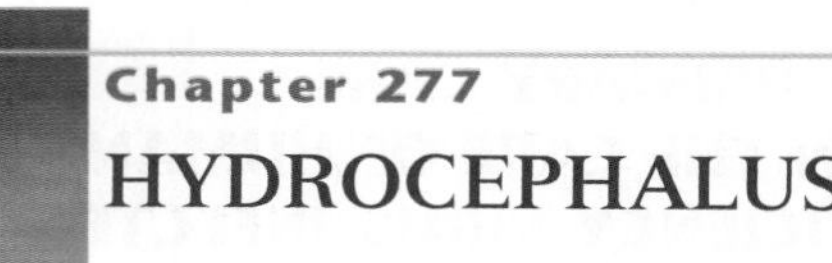

Chapter 277 HYDROCEPHALUS

Mohamad A. Khaled, MD, MSurg; Mark G. Luciano, MD, PhD

INTRODUCTION

Hydrocephalus, the most common surgically treatable neurologic disorder in children, results from a disturbance in cerebrospinal fluid (CSF) circulation and absorption (and, rarely, production) with an accumulation of CSF within the ventricles of the brain. Its diagnosis can be made *in utero,* at birth, in infancy, or in early childhood. Treating hydrocephalus with implanted shunts is life saving, resulting in most children living with hydrocephalus as a chronic surgically arrested disease and with the potential to live full lives into adulthood. However, shunt dysfunction threatens sudden crisis or insidious decline at any time. Such dysfunction risks further brain injury from pressure and requires multiple surgical procedures. Although hundreds of shunts and valves are available, the general concept of CSF shunting has not changed much over time. Unfortunately, broken and infected shunts, as well as over- and underdrainage, repeatedly bring children and young adults to primary care physicians, pediatric neurologists, and neurosurgeons. Recognizing congenital hydrocephalus, new onset–acquired hydrocephalus, and treatment failure is critical because properly treating this potentially fatal neurologic disease can often maintain full function.

DEFINITION AND EPIDEMIOLOGIC FEATURES

Hydrocephalus is the accumulation of CSF in the cerebral ventricles caused by a disorder of CSF flow dynamics. The diagnosis is often suspected in infants with abnormally rapid head growth or in children of any age with symptoms of high intracranial pressure. Hydrocephalus is verified by brain imaging that reveals a dilated ventricular system.

The incidence of congenital hydrocephalus is 3 in 1000 live births.[1] The overall incidence of pediatric hydrocephalus is greater when considering acquired forms through infection, trauma or hemorrhage, and tumors. The additional incidence of subclinical *arrested* hydrocephalus, which may result in symptoms later in childhood or in adult life, is unknown.

Hydrocephalus is listed as the principal diagnosis in approximately 27,870 admissions per year and results in 36,000 operations per year in the United States, with a medical cost of over $1 billion.[2]

PATHOPHYSIOLOGICAL FEATURES

The total volume of CSF is approximately 40 to 50 mL in neonates, 65 to 140 mL in children, 150 mL in adults, and more in older adults with atrophy. Approximately 10% of the CSF is present in the ventricles of the brain, with approximately 90% in the subarachnoid space surrounding the central nervous system. The fluid is also in continuity with the extracellular space of brain tissue and thus constitutes the fluid environment of the entire nervous system. CSF pressure also increases with age: less than 2 mm Hg in neonates, 1.5 to 6 mm Hg in infants, and up to 15 mm Hg in adolescents. Normal pressure in adults is considered to reach 18 to 20 mm Hg.

The choroid plexus in the ventricles and the brain parenchyma produce CSF at a rate of 0.3 to 0.5 mL/min or nearly 500 mL/day. As a result, a CSF turnover of approximately 2 to 3 times per day occurs. This fluid acts as a physical support and cushion for the brain, a river of communication for growth and neurohormonal factors; a system for disposing and processing toxins, metabolites, and antigens; and an area of dynamic pressure or volume exchange facilitating or restricting cerebrolvascular compliance and flow.

The traditional view of CSF circulation and hydrocephalus posits bulk flow beginning in the lateral ventricles through to the third and then fourth ventricles via the Sylvius aqueduct where it escapes to the external subarachnoid space through 2 lateral foramen of Luschka and 1 medial foramen of Magendie. From there the flow passes through the arachnoid villi into the sagittal venous sinus. In this traditional view, hydrocephalus develops with CSF obstruction of this flow that impedes absorption and dilates the ventricles, as an expanding balloon.

Clinical and experimental findings often conflict with this view, suggesting alternate absorption sites, dynamic CSF movement based on the cardiac cycle, ventricular expansion without ventricular flow obstruction, and ventricular volume stabilization even in the presence of ventricular flow obstruction. For example, the ventricle ependyma allow bulk fluid to free flow into the parenchyma; experimental evidence is growing that CSF may be absorbed at many sites, including cerebral vessels and even nasal lymphatics. In addition, investigators have suggested that chronic hydrocephalus results from a relative imbalance of cardiac-generated CSF pressure pulsation. These developing concepts may explain the problems experienced in trying to restore normal physiology with CSF drainage alone and may generate improved shunting methods, as well as treatments without shunting.

The ill effects of hydrocephalus are likely caused by decreased blood flow as a result of increased intracranial pressure (ICP) and the stretching and compressing of neural fiber and blood vessels that are consequences of ventricular expansion. Multiple studies suggest decreased blood flow and metabolism in both acute and chronic hydrocephalus. Resultant hypoxia can reduce protein production, myelination, and neuronal activity. Alteration of extracellular neurohormonal communication during development in fetal hydrocephalus may also affect neuronal migration and brain maturation. Shunting can reverse some, but not all, of these processes.

CLASSIFICATION OF HYDROCEPHALUS

Hydrocephalus is a heterogeneous set of disorders that can be classified by age of onset, time course, obstruction site, obstruction cause, associated anomalies, or syndrome (Table 277-1). One of the earliest and commonly considered classifications is obstructive versus communicating hydrocephalus, which refers to the site of obstruction within the ventricular system or the cisterns, respectively. Acute hydrocephalus exhibits differently than chronic hydrocephalus and with different pathophysiological mechanisms. Hydrocephalus in the developing neonatal brain will have different consequences for neural development than in the more mature child or adolescent brain. The degree of ventricular drainage optimal for treatment may differ based on the development stage and length of time the ventricles are dilated.

ETIOLOGY

Although all hydrocephalus may be considered an *obstruction* of CSF flow somewhere, *obstructive hydrocephalus* refers to a blockage between the ventricular system and the spinal subarachnoid space. Although an obstruction can occur in the posterior fossa with blocked fourth-ventricle outflow, it most often results from obstruction of the aqueduct of Sylvius between the third and fourth ventricles. Congenital aqueductal stenosis and myelomeningocele are both common forms of obstructive hydrocephalus in infants. Acquired obstructive hydrocephalus may develop at any time after infection, hemorrhage, or tumor growth.

Obstructive tumors of the midbrain (the tectal region), though often small, benign, and in themselves asymptomatic, may cause an acute or gradual hydrocephalus. On the other hand, intraventricular hemorrhage of prematurity, meningitis, and trauma most often result in a communicating hydrocephalus.

Hydrocephalus can be associated with diverse neurologic disorders stemming from genetic defects. One of the most common and most studied genetic hydrocephalus disorders is X-linked hydrocephalus, which occurs in 1 in 30,000 male births and represents less than 2% of all hydrocephalus.[3] This disorder results from a defect in chromosomal region X_{q28}.[4] Although hydrocephalus is a result of aqueductal stenosis, it is also characterized by developmental delay, spastic paraparesis, and clasped thumbs in approximately one half of all cases.[5]

Table 277-1 Classification of Hydrocephalus

CLASSIFICATION CRITERIA	CLASSIFICATION SUBGROUPS
Site of obstruction	Obstructive: aqueduct of fourth ventricle outlet Communicating: basal cisterns Multiloculated: atrium, foramen of Monroe, aqueduct, and other
Progression	Acute: may be caused by hemorrhage, infection, progresses to coma in hours Chronic: congenital, partial obstruction, progresses over months to years, with gradual cognitive and ambulatory decline
Course	Recurrent: with shunt failure, may be acute or chronic in onset Arrested: often congenital without symptoms; symptoms of chronic hydrocephalus can develop later Compensated: similar to arrested but with apparent mechanisms of compensation; treated
Location	Internal: in ventricular system only External: with accumulation over hemispheres (SDH, benign macrocrania)
Etiology	Congenital: myelomeningocele, aqueductal stenosis, Dandy Walker syndrome, X linked Acquired: infection, hemorrhagic, tumor
Pressure	High: acute, brain noncompliant, decreased blood flow, shunt reversible if no permanent ischemia Normal: usually chronic hydrocephalus, brain compliance abnormal with labile pressures Low: very compliant brain, ventricles remain large unless drained at very low pressure, coma may persist without aggressive drainage
Age of onset	Fetal: genetic, congenital (aqueductal stenosis, spina bifida), development affected; normal ventricular size unlikely Neonatal: congenital or acquired IVH, infection, tumor, other; comorbidity likely Child: acquired via tumor or other Adult: acquired, idiopathic

IVH, Intraventricular hemorrhage; *SDH,* subdural hematoma.

Table 277-2 Clinical Signs and Symptoms in Pediatric Hydrocephalus

AGE GROUP	SYMPTOMS	SIGNS
Premature infants	Attacks of apnea or bradycardia	Tense and nonpulsatile anterior fontanel Distended scalp veins Abnormal head contour with prominent forehead Rapid (>1 cm/wk) skull circumference increase
Full-term infants	Irritability Vomiting Drowsiness	Full or tense anterior fontanel Distended scalp veins Frontal bossing Widening of cranial sutures Cracked pot sign on percussion Macrocephaly Poor head control Sixth cranial nerve palsy Setting sun sign (appearance of sclera above iris) Impairment of upward gaze
Older children	Steady or progressive headache Vomiting Blurred vision, diplopia Lethargy Personality and behavior changes	Papilledema Spasticity, more in lower limbs Sixth cranial nerve palsy Neuroendocrinopathies

Hydrocephalus is also a component of spina bifida with myelomeningocele, requiring shunting in approximately 80% of cases. Other congenital neurologic syndromes resulting in hydrocephalus include Dandy Walker syndrome and holoprosencephaly.

CLINICAL MANIFESTATIONS

The symptoms of hydrocephalus depend on the rate of progression and the child's age. In many cases, the progression rate is rapid enough to result in symptoms of increased pressure, as listed in Table 277-2, for different age groups. In very slowly progressive chronic hydrocephalus, pressure may increase very little and only transiently. In infants this scenario may be the result of compensatory cranial expansion. Increased head growth may be the only sign in these children; however, it may be accompanied by frontal bossing of the forehead and prominent scalp veins but without apparent neurologic deficit. In older children, slow progression may result from changing *arrested* hydrocephalus or partial treatment failure. These symptoms may include gradual cognitive and motor decline without headaches or any sign of pressure.

EVALUATION

Changes in head circumference, general increased intracranial pressure, or focal neurologic deficit may signal hydrocephalus (Table 277-3). The definitive diagnosis is made with subsequent diagnostic imaging. Although a computed tomography (CT) scan is the most common form of imaging for establishing hydrocephalus, ultrasound is used in prenatal examination and in infants with open fontanels (Table 277-4). Magnetic resonance imaging (MRI) provides much more detail than CT with regard to etiology and comorbidity, as is done increasingly antenatally. Spinal taps may be used to diagnose increased pressure in communicating hydrocephalus and may be used in palliation. Special tests, such as radioactive tracer and dye studies, may be used to track fluid through ventricles and shunt systems, accumulation in loculations, and clearance.

Table 277-3 Symptoms and Their Differential Diagnosis

SYMPTOMS AND SIGNS	DIFFERENTIAL DIAGNOSIS
Enlarging head circumference	Hydrocephalus Benign familial macrocrania Arachnoid cyst Subdural hygroma or hematoma Intracranial-space-occupying lesion Hydranencephaly
Manifestations of increased intracranial pressure	Hydrocephalus Subdural hematoma Intracranial-space-occupying tumor or lesion Infections: Meningitis, brain abscess
Neurologic deficit	Hydrocephalus Space-occupying lesion Cerebrovascular disease Development/neural migration disorder

TREATMENT

Surgical treatment of hydrocephalus has changed little over the 5 decades since valved silicone shunts were introduced. CSF is diverted from a cerebral ventricle or lumbar canal to a body cavity (usually the peritoneal cavity). In the case of obstructive hydrocephalus, improved technology in the last 2 decades has led to an increase in endoscopic fenestration of the third ventricle, allowing fluid escape without a shunt.

Medical management has played a very minor role in treatment; it is usually a means of palliation before a more definitive surgical treatment. Acetazolamide is given for its effect to slow CSF production. Lasix and steroids are used in a similarly limited fashion.

Invasive nonsurgical techniques include serial lumbar or ventricular puncture via the fontanel, which can be performed in emergencies or until a premature infant can tolerate surgery (with a weight greater than 2 kg). Lumbar puncture is performed using a CT scan or an MRI after confirmation that the hydrocephalus is communicating. Lumbar puncture in obstructive hydrocephalus cannot decompress cranial CSF and can cause downward tonsillar herniation. Ventricular punctures are performed at the lateral corner of an open fontanel in infants with obstructive hydrocephalus or when lumbar puncture is not successful.

Taps may be performed serially for up to 3 to 4 weeks in premature infants with intraventricular hemorrhage (IVH) in which it is unclear if they will have a progressive hydrocephalus requiring a shunt. In these infants, an implanted ventricular catheter, either externalized or leading to a subgaleal reservoir or space, may be used to obtain more consistent drainage before permanent shunting is considered.

CEREBROSPINAL FLUID SHUNTING

An implanted shunt comprises three parts: (1) a ventricular catheter, (2) a one-way valve, and (3) a distal catheter. The catheter or valve may have a reservoir where fluid can be tapped. Some, but not all, systems have a reservoir that can be pumped by repeated compression. Although little can be learned by system palpation, a reservoir that remains depressed (dimpled) after compression is a likely sign of proximal obstruction. This system may be tapped under sterile conditions in the outpatient or emergency room setting to check for patency, pressure, or infection.

Some modern valve systems contain an adjustable portion in the valve that varies the opening pressure and thus changes the amount of drainage. Importantly, the current adjustable systems are usually affected by magnetic fields such as MRI. Children with these adjustable valves require a valve setting check and adjustment after MRI to prevent drainage changes.

Ventricular Catheter

The ventricular catheter is usually inserted through a 1-cm burr hole in the frontal or occipital cranium, usually

Table 277-4 Radiological Findings in Pediatric Hydrocephalus

MODALITY	RADIOLOGICAL FINDING
Skull x-ray	Splaying of sutures Increased gyral marking Erosion of dorsum sellae
Ultrasonography	Dilatation of lateral and third ventricles Intracerebral blood (neonatal period with open fontanel)
CT scan	Axial anatomy or size of dilated ventricles; diagnosis and follow-up Periventricular edema (in acute hydrocephalus) Decreased sulcal or subarachnoid space Identification of ventricular shunt catheter (better than MRI)
MRI	Axial, sagittal, coronal imaging and high gray matter resolution Bowing or thinning of corpus callosum Aqueductal stenosis, obstructive masses Posterior fossa abnormalities Cine phase-contrast CSF flow studies; assess blockage at aqueduct, fourth-ventricular outflow, fenestrations
Dye and tracer studies	Lumbar injection; assess lumbar shunt patency of CSF clearance rate *Shuntogram;* injection into shunt to assess patency and flow or cerebral communication

CSF, Cerebrospinal fluid; *CT,* computed tomography; *MRI,* magnetic resonance imaging.

on the nondominant side. The catheter is a soft, flexible, perforated, straight silicon tube that is inserted through the dura and stabilized at the burr hole with an angle flange or a tapping reservoir. Regardless of the entry point (frontal or occipital), the preferred site for the ventricular catheter tip is in the anterior horn of a lateral ventricle where it is away from potentially obstructing choroid plexus. Catheter insertion, however, is most often blind and based on external cranial landmarks. Attempts to visualize catheter tip location with an endoscope during surgery have not resulted in better shunt placement or survival. Currently a postoperative CT is the best way to verify catheter position. Proximal obstructions are common as a result of tissue growth, such as the vascular choroid plexus.

Valve

The valve serves 2 purposes: (1) to allow a one-way flow and (2) to regulate the amount of drainage. Although over 100 valve types are marketed, they fall into 3 major categories or *generations.* The *differential*-pressure valve is the first and simplest. This valve opens when pressure on the cranial side is greater than the distal side. In *high*-pressure valves, this pressure differential may need to be greater than 140 to 150 mm Hg, whereas in *medium-* or *low*-pressure valves, less of a gradient is needed and more fluid will be drained. An important point to realize is that the valve's differential pressure setting is not expected to be equivalent to the absolute pressure in the head; that is, a valve with an opening differential pressure of 100 mm Hg will not result in an ICP of 100 mm Hg because the distal pressure may be high with increased venous or abdominal pressure or negative, as is often the case, as a result of a siphoning effect of fluid in the vertical distal catheter when the person is standing.

Overdrainage, likely caused by this siphoning effect when standing, can result in *slit ventricles* or subdural hematomas and clinical symptoms, including headache and neurologic deficit. Overdrainage is a difficult problem often observed in patients after chronic shunting. For this reason, a second generation of shunt valves was developed that regulates flow to reduce drainage, especially in the vertical position. These devices are called *flow-controlled, antisiphon,* or *gravity-controlled* valves.

Finally, a third generation of valves provides for noninvasive CSF drainage adjustment. These valves allow drainage adjustment with changing needs, such as when an infant grows into a toddler or if hydrocephalus becomes internally compensated. It also allows for CSF drainage optimization in each patient. Importantly, overdrainage or underdrainage symptoms may be treated with adjustments alone. Inadvertent adjustment changes, as may happen if the child has an MRI, may also result in CSF drainage changes and over- or underdrainage. An external device or x-ray examination may check these systems, depending on the manufacturer.

Distal Catheter

The distal catheter extends from the valve to the drainage cavity. The most common site is the peritoneal cavity, although vascular insertion into the right atrium via the subclavian or internal jugular vein is not uncommon. Less commonly, the catheter can drain into the pleural cavity or even the gallbladder. As mentioned previously, drainage into these cavities will vary depending on the backpressure and the vertical length of the catheter. Peritoneal catheter placement can be performed through a 1-cm or less incision and has the advantage of extra catheter length insertion to allow for growth and less risk of infection problems compared with vascular shunts. Right atria catheters have the advantage of less siphoning and are often placed when the abdominal cavity must be avoided. Pleural catheters are placed only in adults because CSF drainage of the large infant cranium would too easily overwhelm the pleural space.

These CSF shunt systems are called ventriculoperitoneal, ventriculoatrial, and lumboperitoneal, depending on the collection and drainage sites. With complex or loculated hydrocephalus, 2 or more proximal catheters may be connected to drain multiple ventricles or cysts. Old ventricular catheters may be retained because pulling catheters out results in some bleeding risk (although they must be removed if a central infection develops). As a result, a shunt series may reveal a complex set of new and old shunt systems components.

Endoscopic Third Ventriculostomy

In obstructive hydrocephalus, flow is most often blocked in the aqueduct between the third and fourth ventricle or more distal in the fourth-ventricular outflow. In the last 2 decades, using endoscopic visualization, the fluid trapped in the lateral and third ventricles is released into the basal cisterns through a fenestration made in the floor of the third ventricle, just anterior to the basilar artery. This endoscopic third ventriculostomy (ETV) is performed through a right frontal burr hole similar to that used for shunt catheter placement. This procedure is successful in approximately 70% of cases and obviates the need for shunting. The advantage lies in preventing overdrainage and implanted hardware.

Successful ETV does not always decrease ventricular size, as seen with shunting, and failure must often be judged clinically as a return of symptoms. If the fenestration is reclosed, as seen in a cine phase-contrast CSF-flow MRI or on direct endoscopic inspection, then it may be reopened. Additionally, a shunt may be placed secondarily in other cases.

ETV is increasingly considered for communicating, as well as obstructive hydrocephalus, as an alternative to shunting. Such is especially the case in third-world countries where CSF shunts are considered expensive and difficult to maintain. However, ETV success in communicating hydrocephalus is still not well established.

Hydrocephalus Treatment in Specific Clinical Contexts

Although the principles of CSF drainage in hydrocephalus may be largely similar in all cases, the management of hydrocephalus associated with some common specific conditions is discussed here.

Myelomeningocele

Historically, patients with myelomeningocele constituted the largest group of children with hydrocephalus. Eighty to 90% of patients with myelomeningocele require shunting for hydrocephalus.[6] A definite correlation between the level of the lesion and the development of hydrocephalus does not exist.[7]

Although the cause of hydrocephalus is not certain, it likely relates to obstruction in the aqueduct and to posterior fossa crowding. A shunt may be placed at the time of myelomeningocele closure or, if possible, in subsequent days or weeks to reduce infection risk. ETV in myelomeningocele is controversial, although it may be considered an option even in later years in the event of shunt failure.

Intraventricular Hemorrhage of Prematurity

Twenty percent of premature infants in the United States will have an IVH; 20% to 75% of them will further develop posthemorrhagic hydrocephalus.[8] Hydrocephalus risk increases with IVH severity or grade in the premature infant. However, shunting is usually preceded by several weeks of palliative treatment. This delay allows for infant growth (preferably to greater than 2 kg) and for determining progressive hydrocephalus. Ventricular size may stabilize over weeks in infants with IVH, presumably the result of blood clearance and reestablishing the flow and absorption process. Palliative procedures include lumbar punctures (taking approximately 10 mL/kg), fontanelle tap, or surgical placement of a ventricular catheter for external or subgaleal drainage.

Posterior Fossa Tumors

Fourth-ventricular tumors commonly cause symptoms of obstructive hydrocephalus. In most cases, tumor resection allows CSF flow reestablishment and eliminates the need for shunting. Children with persisting hydrocephalus are excellent candidates for ETV treatment or standard shunt implantation.

Dandy Walker Syndrome

Dandy Walker syndrome with its cystic enlargement of the fourth ventricle has been historically treated with cyst resection or fenestration. Because of frequent treatment failure, shunting the cyst or the ventricles was adopted. In the presence of aqueductal stenosis, both the ventricles and the cyst may be shunted simultaneously. ETV may also be effective in this disorder.

Postinfectious Hydrocephalus

Postinfectious hydrocephalus is a leading cause of pediatric hydrocephalus worldwide. Hydrocephalus can follow a prenatal infection, the most common of which is cytomegalovirus and toxoplasmosis. Hydrocephalus can also follow postnatal infections, either bacterial or mycotic, and is managed by active medical treatment and an external ventricular drain if needed until the infection clears. A permanent ventriculoperitoneal shunt may be placed later.

ETV alone or in combination with choroid plexus coagulation has been attempted in postinfectious hydrocephalus in the hopes of avoiding an implanted shunt. Viral infections may especially result in minimal leptomeningeal fibrosis with a simultaneous aqueductal stenosis that an ETV may manage. Unfortunately, extensive cistern scarring may limit potential ETV efficacy in many cases.

Multiloculated Hydrocephalus

Loculations of the ventricular system may be caused from hemorrhage or infection. Loculations present a complex drainage problem, sometimes requiring multiple catheters. Open or, more recently, endoscopic cyst fenestration facilitates fluid communication, allowing simplified drainage through a single shunt catheter.

Aqueductal Stenosis

Aqueductal stenosis may result from congenital narrowing, infection, hemorrhage, or tumor. Although shunt implantation is still commonly performed, ETV

BOX 277-1 Shunt Complications

1. Infection
2. Mechanical failure: breaks, kinks, migration
3. Overdrainage—slit ventricles
4. Overdrainage—subdural hygroma or chronic subdural hematoma
5. Blockage: proximal or distal, total or partial intermittent
6. Complications specific for ventriculocardiac shunts:
   a. Thrombosis around the distal tube
   b. Cor pulmonale
   c. Shunt nephritis
   d. Septicemia and pyemic abscesses
7. Complications specific for ventriculopleural shunts:
   a. Hydrothorax: characterized by respiratory distress
   b. Pyothorax
8. Abdominal complications of ventriculoperitoneal shunts:
   a. Bowel perforation: rare with current catheter materials
   b. Pseudocyst: sterile or infected and presenting as obstruction or abdominal swelling
   c. Ascites: malabsorption of CSF; sterile or infected
   d. Hernia: at shunt insertion incisions

CSF, Cerebrospinal fluid.

is preferred. Tectum, posterior third-ventricle, or pineal region tumors can be biopsied during the same endosocopic procedure.

COMPLICATIONS OF TREATMENT

Shunting complications include bleeding at the time of insertion, infection, obstruction, and mechanical failure (Box 277-1). Working shunts may also drain too much or too little, which may cause headache and neurologic impairment.

Intracerebral Hemorrhage

Any probe insertion into the brain may result in bleeding; however, this problem occurs in less than 2% of cases. Minor bleeding may resolve on its own, with the greatest concern being an increased risk of shunt obstruction. Very rarely does bleeding require surgical evacuation. Interestingly, bleeding risk is greater in removing an old ventricular catheter that is obstructed by an in-growing choroid plexus than in inserting a new one.

Infection

As with any implanted foreign body, infection is a risk, and full treatment usually requires removing the shunt and initiating antibiotic treatment. Shunt risk increases by the existence of an inner lumen, which is away from the body's immune system and bathed in CSF—a good culture medium. The infection rate is commonly reported between 5% and 10%[9] of procedures and usually involves skin flora, such as *Staphylococcus epidermidis, Propionibacterium acnes,* and *Staphylococcus aureus.* Although most infections occur in the first 6 months, indolent infections are reported after years. Chronic infections may be difficult to diagnosis because they may produce little cellular response. Shunt infection may cause the usual signs of systemic or local infection or symptoms of meningitis. Shunt dysfunction may actually be a sign of an indolent shunt infection.

The most common management of shunt infection is to remove all hardware, place a temporary external drain if needed, administer intravenous antibiotics, and reinsert the shunt after documenting negative CSF cultures. Perioperative prophylactic antibiotics reduce shunt infection risk by 50%.[10] In addition, some institutions have found that antibiotic impregnated shunts reduce the infection rate to 1% to 2%.

Shunt Obstruction

One of the most common causes of obstruction is choroid plexus ingrowth into the proximal ventricular catheter. Distal occlusion can also occur with scar tissue or thrombus developing in vascular shunts. Hydrocephalic symptoms recurring with ventricular expansion suggest an obstruction and can be sufficient to indicate surgical exploration. A shunt tap or *shuntogram* may be diagnostic in a less clear case where ventricles are not expanded.

Mechanical Failure

Shunts can break, kink, or become displaced with activity and growth. A shunt series, including an anteroposterior and lateral view of the head, neck, chest, and abdomen, can usually detect these failures. Although shunts may last decades, they do become more brittle over time, and a calcified scar can evolve around the catheter. A break at a tethering point, such as the valve or a connector, is common. A short shunt caused by growth or migration into the preperitoneal space can also cause failure. Finally, the valve itself may become incompetent over time.

Overdrainage

Even a working noninfected shunt can cause complications, given that drainage is not physiologically regulated, and overdrainage can result in clinical symptoms, subdurals, or slit ventricles.

Subdural hygromas or hematomas develop with overdrainage in children with severe cortical thinning. Because of limited elasticity of the brain and its ability to reexpand after severe hydrocephalus, the cortical walls collapse and a subdural hematoma can develop if bridging vessels are injured. Ventricles become abnormally small or *slit like* as overdrainage proceeds in brains where elasticity is sufficient for expansion. Slit ventricles from chronic overdrainage may result in frequent shunt blockages and episodic headaches. Shunt revision to reduce CSF drainage may be required unless an adjustable valve is in place. Management may also include ICP monitoring for diagnosis and implanting antisiphon or gravity devices. An important point to note is that in the case of CSF shunting, too much drainage (acutely or chronically) can be as problematic as too little.

Complications of foreign body implantation, such as infection and nonphysiologic overdrainage seen with shunting, can be prevented with ETV. However,

ETV requires specialized experience with endoscopic procedures, and injury to the hypothalamus and basilar artery are possible. The most common complication is postoperative fever. The incidence of all complications combined ranges from 6% to 20%, most of which are reversible. With ETV, undertreatment is a concern because ventricles remain large and failure may be sudden and catastrophic or gradual and insidious. Given that ventricle size may not change after ETV as it does after shunting, success is based on clinical resolution alone. Treatment failure or underdrainage may be missed particularly if it occurs gradually.

FOLLOW-UP

Children who undergo a surgical procedure for hydrocephalus treatment are usually examined 2 weeks after surgery, every 3 months for the first year, every 6 months in the second year, and then yearly. The clinical assessment includes developmental milestones, head circumference, symptoms and signs of increased intracranial tension, symptoms and signs of infection, or other complications. Although algorithms vary, when a shunt failure is suspected, a shunt series and CT scan are generally obtained before invasive procedures, such as a shunt tap or shuntogram. ETV evaluation may include cine phase-contrast MRI flow study to evaluate fenestration patency.

OUTCOME AND PROGNOSIS

A child with isolated hydrocephalus that is well treated and monitored has the potential for a fully functional life. Of course, many factors play a role in the overall outcome, such as concomitant medical conditions, the degree of neurologic compromise at the time of surgical treatment, and the nature and etiology of the hydrocephalus. The occurrence of complications, including infection, obstruction, and intracranial hemorrhage, greatly impacts the long-term outcome.

The 5-year survival rate of children with congenital hydrocephalus is around 90%.[11] Normal intellect varies widely with each specific cause but ranges from 40% to 65%.[12] Infants with posthemorrhagic hydrocephalus (PHH) have a mortality rate of 16% to 35%, whereas low–birth-weight infants without PHH have a mortality rate of 6.5% to 13%. Additional analysis revealed that grade-I and grade-II PHH have a mortality rate of 9% versus 49% for grades III and IV.[13] A long-term study over 10 years showed that an overall shunt mortality rate after 10 years is less than 5%. Functional assessment of the children revealed a motor deficit in 80%, a visual or auditory deficit in 25%, and epilepsy in 30%. The final IQs were above 90 in 32%, between 70 and 90 in 28%, between 50 and 70 in 19%, and lower than 50 in 21% of children. Integration into the normal school system was possible for 60%, and behavioral disorders were severe in 30% of children.[14] The degree of intellectual impairment relates more to the degree of severity of underlying central nervous system anomalies and defects in the neocortex cytoarchitecture than to hydrocephalus severity.[15] Prompt recognition and treatment of hydrocephalus and treatment failure are important for a favorable outcome. Delay in surgical treatment is a risk factor for a poor outcome in hydrocephalic children.[16]

The authors gratefully acknowledge the assistance of Stephen Dombrowski, PhD, in the preparation of this chapter.

TOOLS FOR PRACTICE

Engaging Patient and Family

- *Hydrocephalus Fact Sheet* (fact sheet), National Institute of Neurological Disorders and Stroke (NINDS) (www.ninds.nih.gov/disorders/hydrocephalus/detail_hydrocephalus.htm).
- *What Is a Pediatric Neurosurgeon?* (fact sheet), American Academy of Pediatrics (www.aap.org/sections/sap/he3005.pdf).

REFERENCES

1. Milhorat TH. Hydrocephalus historical notes, etiology and clinical diagnosis. In: American Association of Neurological Surgeons, Section of Pediatric Neurosurgery, eds. *Pediatric Neurosurgery. Surgery of the Developing Nervous System*. New York, NY: Grune and Stratton; 1982.
2. Patwardhan RV, Nanda A. Implanted ventricular shunts in the United States: the billion-dollar-a-year cost of hydrocephalus treatment. *Neurosurgery*. 2005;56(1): 139-144, discussion 144-145.
3. Dirks PB. Genetics of hydrocephalus. In: Cinalli G, Maixner WJ, Sainte-Rose C, eds. *Pediatric Hydrocephalus*. New York, NY: Springer-Verlag; 2004.
4. Jouet M, Feldman E, Yates J, et al. Refining the genetic location of the gene for X linked hydrocephalus within Xq28. *J Med Genet*. 1999;64:1305-1315.
5. Halliday J, Chow CW, Wallace D, et al. X linked hydrocephalus: a survey of a 20 year period in Victoria, Australia. *J Med Genet*. 1986;23:23-31.
6. Mirzai H, Ersahin Y, Mutluer S, et al. Outcome of patients with myelomeningocele: the Ege University experience. *Childs Nerv Syst*. 1998;14:120-123.
7. Mirzai H, Ersahin Y, Mutluer S, et al. Outcome of patients with myelomeningocele: the Ege University experience. *Childs Nerv Syst*. 1998;14:120-123.
8. Van de Bor M, Verloove-Vanhorick SP, Brand R, et al. Incidence and prediction of periventricular—intraventricular hemorrhage in very preterm infants. *J Perinat Med*. 1987;15:333-339.
9. Chumas P, Tyagi A, Livingston J. Hydrocephalus—what's new? *Arch Dis Child Fetal Neonatal*. 2001;85:F149.
10. Langley JM, LeBlanc JC, Drake J, et al. Efficacy of antimicrobial prophylaxis in placement of cerebrospinal fluid shunts: metanalysis. *Clin Infect Dis* 1993;17:98-103.
11. Amacher AL, Wellington J. Infantile hydrocephalus: long-term results of surgical therapy. *Childs Brain*. 1984; 11:217-229.
12. Dennis M, Fitz CR, Netly CT, et al. The intelligence of hydrocephalic children. *Arch Neurol*. 1981;38:607-615.
13. Hanigan WC. Intracranial hemorrhage in the premature infant. In: Wilkens RH, Rengachary SS, eds. *Neurosurgery*. New York, NY: McGraw-Hill; 1996.
14. Hoppe-Hirsch E, Laroussinie F, Brunet L, et al. Late outcome of the surgical treatment of hydrocephalus. *Childs Nerv Syst*. 1998;14(3):97-99.
15. Op Heij CP, Renier WO, Gabreels FG. Intellectual sequelae of primary non-obstructive hydrocephalus in infancy: analysis of 50 cases. *Clin Neurol Neurosurg*. 1985;87: 247-253.
16. Heinsbergen I, Rotteveel J, Roeleveld N, et al. Outcome in shunted hydrocephalic children. *Eur J Paediatr Neurol*. 2002;6(2):99-107.

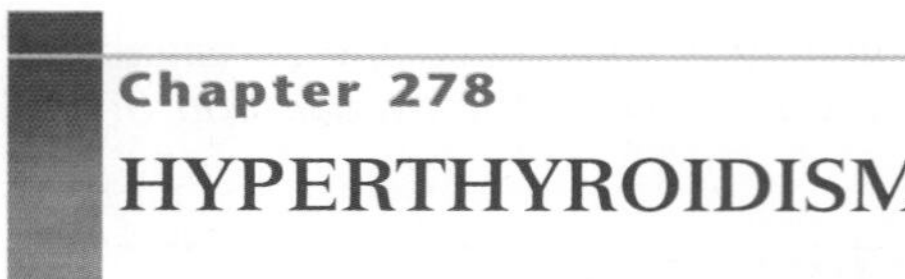

Chapter 278

HYPERTHYROIDISM

Nicholas Jospe, MD

DEFINITIONS

Hyperthyroidism is the result of excessive activity of the thyroid gland. The clinical manifestation of excessive circulating thyroid hormone is called thyrotoxicosis.

ETIOLOGY

With a few exceptions, thyrotoxicosis in children is the result of Graves disease.[1] Other causes of thyrotoxicosis include the early phase of autoimmune hypothyroidism (Hashimoto thyroiditis) before thyroid function is diminished, a hyperfunctioning thyroid nodule, pituitary resistance to thyroxine (T4) that results in excess secretion of thyrotropin, and factitious hyperthyroidism caused by administration of exogenous thyroid hormone. Graves disease occurs most frequently in early adolescence, is rare in infancy, and occurs infrequently in childhood. Affected patients frequently have a family history of thyroid disorder. The prevalence of Graves disease is 6 to 8 times greater in girls than it is in boys.

Graves disease, similar to Hashimoto thyroiditis, is an autoimmune disorder that occurs in patients who have a genetic predisposition, which is itself linked to certain human leukocyte antigen haplotypes.[2] The disease results from the interaction between environmental influences and genes, some of which are thyroid specific genetic loci while others are susceptibility or immunoregulatory genes. Hyperfunction of the thyroid gland in Graves disease is caused by autoantibodies directed against the receptor for thyrotropin.[3] These antibodies, called thyrotropin receptor antibodies (TRAbs), are characterized by an overall predominant stimulatory effect on thyroid cells leading to excessive production and release of T4. Included among the TRAbs are (1) thyroid-stimulating immunoglobulins (TSIs) that mimic thyrotropin in their stimulatory action on the production of T4, (2) thyrotropin-binding inhibitory immunoglobulins (TBIIs) that prevent thyrotropin from binding at its receptor and do not stimulate thyroid cells, and (3) thyrotropin-blocking antibodies. Other antibodies detected in patients who have Graves disease include thyroid growth-stimulating antibodies, which contribute to goiter formation, and antithyroglobulin and antiperoxidase antibodies that also are found in Hashimoto thyroiditis.[3] Graves disease can occur in conjunction with other endocrine autoimmune diseases, such as diabetes mellitus type 1, hypoparathyroidism, and Addison disease, or with other autoimmune diseases, such as myasthenia gravis, periodic paralysis, and vitiligo.

DIFFERENTIAL DIAGNOSIS

Rarely, children who have Hashimoto thyroiditis are thyrotoxic and have a high titer of TSI autoantibodies in addition to antithyroid antibodies. This condition has been called hashitoxicosis and may be differentiated from routine Graves disease in that the hyperthyroidism is usually a transient phase before progression to permanent hypothyroidism. Other causes of hyperthyroxinemia are rare, including generalized resistance to thyroid hormone that is found in association with attention-deficit/hyperactivity disorder,[4] factitious hyperthyroidism from excessive administration of thyroid hormone, thyrotropin-secreting pituitary adenomas, and binding-protein changes characterized by normal free T4 and thyrotropin levels. Finally, hyperthyroidism caused by autonomous thyroid adenomas is rare and can be seen in association with the McCune-Albright syndrome (precocious puberty, café-au-lait pigmentation, and polyostotic fibrous dysplasia).

Relevant History and Physical Examination

Table 278-1 lists the clinical signs and symptoms of children who have Graves disease. Early nonspecific findings in Graves disease include changes in behavior

Table 278-1 Clinical Signs and Symptoms of Children Who Have Graves Disease

SIGNS AND SYMPTOMS	PREVALENCE (%)		
	SAXENA ET AL.[a]	MAENPAA ET AL.[b]	BARNES ET AL.[c]
Goiter	100	100	97
Prominence of eyes	100	69	79
Exophthalmos	77	—	—
Tachycardia	91	41	88
Nervousness	80	74	92
Increased appetite	71	—	67
Weight loss	67	59	50
Emotional lability	41	—	40
Heat intolerance	40	—	25
Frequent stools	16	35	13

[a]Saxena KM, Crawford JD, Talbot NB. Childhood thyrotoxicosis: a long-term perspective. *BMJ* 1964;2:1153-1158.
[b]Maenpaa J, Hiekkala H, Lamberg BA. Childhood hyperthyroidism. *Acta Endocrinol* 1966;51:321-336.
[c]Barnes VH, Blizzard RM. Antithyroid drug therapy for toxic diffuse goiter (Graves' disease): thirty years experience in children and adolescents. *J Pediatr.* 1977; 91(2):313-320.

such as nervousness, sleeplessness, emotional lability, decreased school performance, or deteriorating handwriting; these findings largely reflect hyperactivity of the sympathetic nervous system. Graves disease often remains undiagnosed for a long time because children can continue their normal activities without complaints that are overtly suggestive of hyperthyroidism. More prominent cardiovascular signs include tachycardia, a widened pulse pressure, and an overactive precordium. Neuromuscular signs and symptoms include tremor, a shortened deep-tendon reflex relaxation phase, fatigability, and proximal muscle weakness. Despite an increased appetite, the child loses weight more frequently than gains weight and has frequent and loose bowel movements. Increased perspiration, warmth, heat intolerance, and smoothness of skin appear later. With long-standing disease, tall stature may accompany advanced skeletal maturation in childhood; curtailment of final height as a result of early closure of the epiphyses does not occur.

The size of the goiter when first examined is variable, and its presence frequently goes unnoticed. However, the thyroid gland, usually seen as diffusely enlarged, is soft and has a clearly delineated border. Thyroid gland enlargement may be difficult to discern in overweight or obese youngsters. Examination should include palpation for the presence of a thrill and auscultation for the presence of a bruit. Measurement of the size of the lobes and the isthmus is essential in monitoring disease course. Eye findings also are variable, although severe ophthalmopathy is far less common among children than adults and, if present, is more likely to resolve completely. Findings include prominence of the eyes (proptosis or exophthalmos), a conspicuous stare (caused by lid retraction and a widened palpebral fissure [Figure 278-1]), and lag of the upper lid on downward gaze. These eye findings are due to a combination of hyperactivity of the sympathetic system and of mucopolysaccharide accumulation and infiltration of the orbital fat and ocular muscle cells. The TRAbs are thought to be the cause of ophthalmopathy because orbital fibroblasts express thyrotropin receptors. Most affected children can be treated with topical ophthalmic lubrication, but orbital fat decompression may be required in patients who have advanced conditions. Management of severe ophthalmopathy can be either medical or surgical (orbital decompression, eye muscle or lid surgery). Medical management includes high-dose glucocorticoids or orbital radiotherapy, either alone or in combination. In children, mucopolysaccharide accumulation in skin and subcutaneous tissue, as with pretibial myxedema, is infrequent.

Laboratory Evaluation

The initial assessment should include measurement of serum free T4 because, in patients with binding protein increases, total T4 may be high, yet free T4 and thyrotropin will be normal, thereby ruling out hyperthyroidism. This circumstance is particularly relevant to women taking oral contraceptives, in whom the estrogen raises the binding protein levels, thus increasing the levels of total T4, and of total triiodothyronine (T3), but not affecting thyrotropin concentrations. The diagnosis of Graves disease rests on demonstrating elevated levels of T4 and depression of thyrotropin levels to below the lower limit of detectability. A comparison of the patient's levels and age-appropriate normal values of T4 must be performed before a diagnosis of hyperthyroidism can be made.[5] Measurement of T3 may help confirm the diagnosis of T3 toxicosis, although this assessment is rarely necessary. In thyrotoxicosis, the response of thyrotropin to thyroid-releasing hormone is blunted severely or absent. The thyroid-releasing hormone stimulation test is necessary only when Graves disease is thought

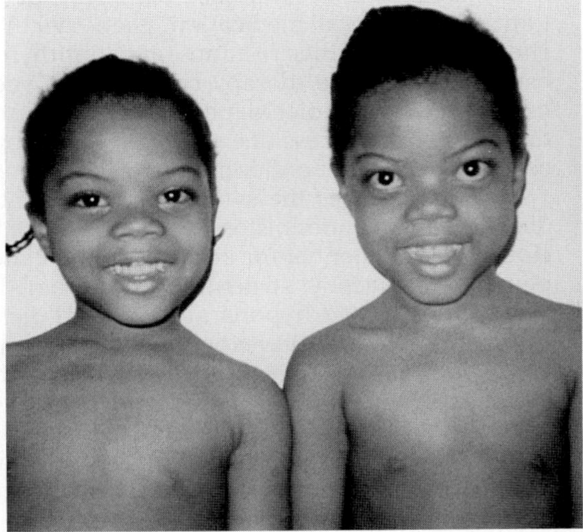

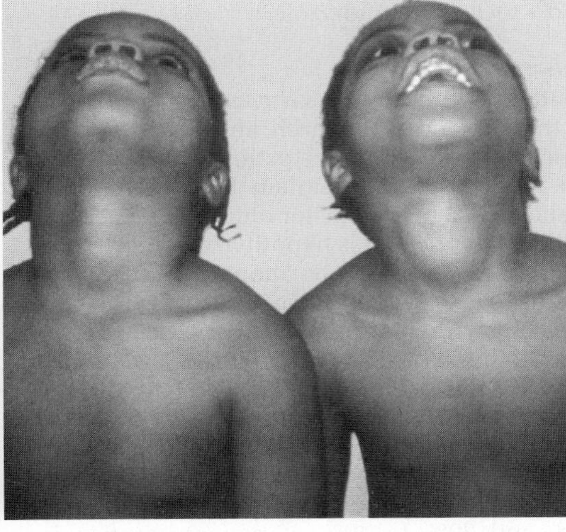

Figure 278-1 The patient on the right exhibits a widened palpebral fissure and goiter; her twin, on the left, was unaffected at the time of this photograph, although later she also developed Graves disease.

to exist but the diagnosis is unclear. In equivocal situations, measurement of TRAbs, which are present in 95% of patients who have Graves disease, may help to confirm the diagnosis. In pregnant patients, high levels of TSI are predictive of neonatal Graves disease.

The measurement of thyroid gland uptake of radioiodine (123I) or technetium (99mTc) is useful only to distinguish painless thyroiditis from Graves disease. Patients who have thyroiditis (hashitoxicosis) have a low uptake; patients who have Graves disease have a high uptake. Generally, this study is not necessary at the time of diagnosis. However, measurement of the thyroid gland uptake will be required if radioablative therapy is performed.

MANAGEMENT

Antithyroid Medications

Thioamides

The aim of treatment is to reduce thyroid hormone production and block its effect on tissue peripherally. To this end, thioamides, either methimazole (Tapazole) or propylthiouracil (PTU), are usually used first.[6,7] These antithyroid medications are equally effective in inhibiting thyroid hormone production; however, PTU also blocks the peripheral conversion of T4 to T3. The half-life is 3 to 4 hours for PTU and 6 to 13 hours for methimazole. Both drugs cross the placenta, although PTU does so less than methimazole and therefore is the preferred drug during pregnancy. Both drugs are present in small quantities in human milk, and breastfeeding may be continued. Therapy induces euthyroidism somewhat faster with methimazole than with PTU and from within weeks to a few months, depending on the size of the thyroid gland. Starting doses of PTU range from 5 to 10 mg/kg body weight, with a maximum of 300 mg/day, given in 3 to 4 divided doses; the dose of methimazole is approximately 0.5 to 1 mg/kg, with a maximum of 30 mg/day, given in 2 to 3 divided doses. Once thyroid hormone secretion is depressed, maintenance doses may be given in 2 to 3 daily doses for PTU and 1 to 2 for methimazole.

Graves Disease

Optimal long-term therapy for Graves disease continues to be the subject of research and some controversy. Some physicians prefer to titrate the dose of antithyroid medication to maintain the patient in a euthyroid state. Others administer antithyroid medication until the patient becomes hypothyroid and supplement, thereafter, with thyroid hormone. These varying approaches have no effect on rates of relapse.

Therapy with antithyroid medication is usually maintained for a minimum of 12 to 18 months, during which time monitoring the size of the thyroid gland and the TRAb levels can be useful because shrinkage of the thyroid gland and decreasing TRAb titers predict a greater likelihood of remission after discontinuation of therapy. Thereafter, treatment with antithyroid medication can be stopped, and 20% to 40% of patients remain in remission. Continued patient monitoring with thyroid function tests is indicated to detect any subclinical relapse of Graves disease.[8]

Side Effects

Potential side effects of the thioamides include minor reactions that subside spontaneously. These reactions include a purpuric and papular rash, urticaria, joint pain, stiffness, hair loss, nausea or headaches, and 1 serious reaction—agranulocytosis.[7] Agranulocytosis is an idiosyncratic reaction that occurs in 1:500 to 1:1000 cases, usually within the 1st few months of therapy after either form of antithyroid medication. White blood cell count monitoring is not useful in anticipating agranulocytosis because its onset is sudden. Patients thus need to be told about the significance of a sore throat, mouth sores, and fever as potentially heralding agranulocytosis. In addition to supportive treatment, such as antibiotic therapy, discontinuation of thioamide therapy is necessary. Agranulocytosis spontaneously reverses, and resumption of therapy with a different thioamide does not usually cause agranulocytosis to recur.[7] Finally, reactions such as drug fever, nephritis, hepatitis, or lupus-like reactions are rare.

Adjuvant Beta-Adrenergic Blockade

In addition to antithyroid medication, adjuvant β-adrenergic blockade may be accomplished with propranolol to control the sympathetic hyperactivity of severe Graves disease. This form of therapy is necessary but only transiently. It may be contraindicated in patients who have cardiac failure or asthma.

Iodide

Iodide has a minor short-term role as adjuvant therapy in patients who develop toxicity to either PTU or methimazole or as adjunctive therapy immediately before thyroidectomy and for treatment of severe thyrotoxicosis. In practice, it is seldom used. Iodide works by transient inhibitory effect on iodine organification, leading to a fall in T4 and T3.

Definitive Therapy

If a relapse of Graves disease occurs on discontinuation of antithyroid medication, then the therapeutic choices include either resumption of antithyroid medication or definitive therapy consisting of radioiodine or surgery. The choice depends on factors that affect the chances of success of each form of therapy, such as compliance, patient preference, and surgical expertise.

Surgery resolves the symptoms faster, but radioiodine is easy to administer, safer, and equally efficacious.[3,7] The potential for surgical complications from injury to adjacent structures (recurrent laryngeal nerve damage and hypoparathyroidism) dictates that referral be made to an experienced surgeon. Permanent hypothyroidism after surgery is frequent.[7] Radioiodine therapy is being used more extensively in children because fears regarding thyroid carcinoma, leukemia, and radiation and genetic damage after treatment with a radioactive substance have been alleviated.[3,9] Radioactive iodine concentrates in the thyroid gland and induces cell death over time. On average, three quarters of patients are cured of hyperthyroidism after 1 dose of radioiodine, and a small fraction may require a 2nd dose months after the

1st dose. Pregnancy is a contraindication for radioiodine therapy because the iodine crosses the placenta and destroys the fetal thyroid.

COMPLICATIONS

Thyrotoxic Crisis

Unfortunately, no reliable factors predict the natural course of Graves disease in a given patient, aside possibly from goiter size and the severity of disease at onset. The clinical course of Graves disease ranges from progression to overt hypothyroidism on one hand to progression to thyrotoxic crisis on the other. Thyrotoxic crisis is an exceptional but severe complication.[10] This diagnosis rests on finding uncontrolled hyperthyroidism and is characterized by a constellation of findings, including cardiac failure, tachycardia, hyperthermia, and central nervous system abnormalities such as confusion, apathy, or coma. Infection (even relatively minor) and trauma can be precipitating factors. Therapy must be expeditious and aggressive and should include antithyroid medication, iodide, β-blockade, antipyresis, and medications to prevent cardiac failure.

Neonatal Thyrotoxicosis

Graves disease is rare in neonates and is due to the transplacental passage of thyroid-directed immunoglobulins from the mother. Transplacental passage of maternal antibodies may occur, even if the mother no longer has active thyroid disease. In addition, stimulatory and blocking maternal thyroid antibodies may disappear at different rates, making the course of neonatal Graves disease difficult to predict. Thus its onset may be immediate or delayed for weeks, and its duration may be brief or prolonged, lasting up to 6 months.[11] Notably, transient neonatal hypothyroidism may result from the transfer of maternal TBII. Neonatal hypothyroidism may also be caused by suppression of the hypothalamic-pituitary-thyroid axis by placentally transferred maternal T4 from mothers with hyperthyroidism.

The clinical signs and symptoms of neonatal Graves disease include microcephaly, frontal bossing, tachycardia, hypertension, irritability, failure to thrive, flushing, exophthalmos, and goiter. Vomiting, diarrhea, hepatosplenomegaly, jaundice, and thrombocytopenia can also occur. Cardiac failure and arrhythmias account for a mortality that approaches 25% when the disease is severe and treated inadequately.[5] Long-term complications are severe and include hypothyroidism, premature craniosynostosis, and intellectual deficits. Until the disease resolves spontaneously, usually within 1 to 3 months as the maternal antibodies are degraded, adjunctive therapy may be necessary. In severely hyperactive neonates, propranolol, 2 mg/kg/day, and digitalis, for cardiac failure, may be required. Glucocorticoid therapy may also be beneficial.

WHEN TO REFER

New diagnosis of hyperthyroidism

WHEN TO ADMIT

Routine diagnosis and therapy of hyperthyroidism do not require hospitalization. Some severe complications of the disorder or its therapy (ocular, cardiovascular, infectious) may be managed by appropriate subspecialists and with hospitalization.

REFERENCES

1. Feldmann M, Dayan C, Grubeck-Loebenstein B, et al. Mechanism of Graves thyroiditis: implications for concepts and therapy of autoimmunity. *Int Rev Immunol.* 1992;9:91-106.
2. Davies TF. The pathogenesis of Graves' disease. In: Braverman LE, Utiger RD, eds. *Werner and Ingbar's the Thyroid: A Fundamental and Clinical Text.* Philadelphia, PA: JB Lippincott; 2005.
3. Zimmerman D, Leif AN. Thyrotoxicosis in children. *Endocrinol Metab Clin North Am.* 1998;27;109-125.
4. Hauser P, Zametkin AJ, Martinez P. Attention deficit-hyperactivity disorder in people with generalized resistance to thyroid hormone. *N Engl J Med.* 1993;328: 997-1001.
5. Fisher DA. Thyroid disorders in childhood and adolescence. In Sperling MA, ed: *Pediatric Endocrinology.* Philadelphia, PA: WB Saunders; 2002.
6. Verdainbarnes H, Blizzard RM. Antithyroid drug therapy for toxic diffuse goiter (Graves' disease): thirty years experience in children and adolescents. *J Pediatr.* 1997; 91;313-320.
7. Cooper DS. Antithyroid drugs. *N Engl J Med.* Mar 2005; 352(9):905-917.
8. Abraham P, Avenell A, Park CM, et al. A systematic review of drug therapy for Graves' hyperthyroidism. *Eur J Endocrinol.* Oct 2005;153(4):489-498.
9. Rivkees SA. The management of hyperthyroidism in children with emphasis on the use of radioactive iodine. *Pediatr Endocrinol Rev.* Dec 2003;1(suppl 2):212-221.
10. Roth RN, McAuliffe MJ. Hyperthyroidism and thyroid storm. *Emerg Med Clin North Am.* 1989;7;873-883.
11. Zakarija M, McKenzie JM, Munro DS. Immunoglobulin G inhibitor of thyroid stimulating antibody is a cause of delay in the onset of neonatal Graves' disease. *J Clin Invest.* 1983;72;1352-1356.

Chapter 279

HYPOSPADIAS, EPISPADIAS, AND CRYPTORCHISM

Amanda C. North, MD; John P. Gearhart, MD

The male genitalia are much more often a cause of parental preoccupation at the birth of a child than are the female genitalia. Untold variables govern this tendency, most of them not readily apparent. The most obvious, of course, is that they are much more accessible. Less concern usually exists about the relationship of the penis to the urinary tract than to sexual function. Nonetheless, as a part of the urinary tract, it serves its immediate purpose at birth; it must wait until puberty to begin to realize its additional potential.

GENITAL ABNORMALITY

An external genital deformity in the newborn boy is usually obvious immediately—for example, hypospadias, epispadias, injury, swelling, and, after careful palpation, undescended testes. Penile size is one cause of parental distress that is not often noted at birth but perhaps several weeks later as the baby gains weight. A retracted penis may seem to disappear despite its being 4 cm long in a suprapubic pad of fat. The parents should be assured kindly that the condition will correct itself in time. Only rarely does a real problem exist, namely a micropenis, in which the penis has a stretched length of less than 2 standard deviations below the mean or is less than 2.5 cm in length, which suggests a dysmorphic abnormality. Circumcision should be delayed in infants who have micropenis and should not be performed until a thorough evaluation has been performed by a pediatric endocrinologist and a pediatric urologist.

Hypospadias

Hypospadias is the most common penile abnormality occurring in 3 per 1000 newborn boys.[1] Some evidence exists that the incidence of hypospadias is increasing; various genetic and environmental factors have been implicated. Endocrine disruptors, such as maternal use of progestins, appear to increase the risk of hypospadias.[2] In hypospadias, the urethral meatus opens on the ventral surface of the penis, located most often on the distal half of the shaft, including the glans penis (60%), but it may be located at any proximal point along the shaft or scrotum (25%), or the perineum (15%) (Figure 279-1). The prepuce is incompletely formed, covering only the dorsal surface of the glans penis. In approximately 10% of cases, an associated unilateral or bilateral cryptorchidism is present. Any combination of hypospadias and cryptorchidism should be investigated for possible intersex anomaly.

The severity of the deformity and the position of the meatus on the undershaft of the penis will greatly influence surgical decisions. A circumcision should *not* be performed in the presence of hypospadias, however mild. None of the tissue that might be needed for repair should be sacrificed. If the hypospadias is mild and situated at or close to the corona, and if relatively little deformity is present, then the repair is quite straightforward, accomplished in same-day surgery. Occasionally a meatal stenosis is associated with hypospadias and can be corrected easily at the time of the hypospadias repair. Chordee, the downward curving of the penis as a result of abnormal ventral fibrous bands, is often present and is one of the factors that must be addressed at the time of surgical intervention. Currently, most hypospadias defects can be corrected with a single procedure. Although the frequency of an associated anomaly of the upper urinary tract is known to be low, many parents request sonography to be assured that the upper tract is normal. In any event, the pediatric urologist should be consulted as soon after birth as possible.

Even if the hypospadias defect is severe, a single-stage repair can often be performed. Multiple-stage repairs may be required when chordee is very severe and a paucity of dorsal foreskin exists. The pediatric urologist should advise the parents as to the right time for surgery and the precise approach to use. Although little research has been conducted regarding the optimal timing of hypospadias surgery, many pediatric urologists recommend the surgery as early as age 6 months. Theoretically, performing the surgery between age 6 and 15 months would avoid any of the sensitive phases of psychosocial development.[3] The pediatrician cannot relinquish responsibility for providing concomitant care; the pediatrician is needed to interpret events and, in a highly charged emotional circumstance, to provide appropriate counseling to parents (and, as the child grows older, to the child). This arrangement is especially important if sexual function is threatened or if sexual identity is of concern. On occasion, if the hypospadias is severe or accompanied by associated genital anomalies, then a referral for endocrine evaluation is indicated. In the presence of hypospadias alone, aside from a rare defect in androgen responsiveness, little likelihood exists of significant hormonal disturbance.

Epispadias

Less frequently (1 per 117,000 live male births), the meatus is formed on the dorsum of the penis at various points along the glans and shaft and, on rare occasion, so far back as to be beneath the symphysis pubis.[4] The more proximal deformity may be associated with complete urinary incontinence because of involvement of the bladder neck area along with distortion of the normal architecture of the pubic bones. Early consultation with the pediatric urologist is necessary; again, circumcision is to be avoided.

CRYPTORCHISM

The testes are generally descended in a full-term infant (depending on the birth weight), and frequently each testis is of somewhat different size. Given that the testes descend from within the abdomen to the scrotum usually by approximately week 36 of fetal life, the incidence of cryptorchism (undescended testes) is much higher in the premature infant. The incidence in male neonates weighing 2500 grams or more at birth is between 2.2% and 3.8%, but this incidence jumps to 20% to 30% in the premature infant.[5] In 10% of boys with undescended testes, the testes are nonpalpable. The testes are in the inguinal canal or in the abdomen in 50% of those boys with nonpalpable testes, and in the remaining 50%, they are absent because of intrauterine torsion and infarct. The rate of spontaneous descent is lower for full-term infants (50% to 70%) and occurs earlier (usually by age 1 to 3 months) than for the premature infants. In a premature infant the rate of spontaneous descent is as high as 80% to 90% and may occur later in the first year of life. If spontaneous descent does not happen by the first birthday, then concern is warranted. This process involves the child's potential for developing testicular cancer, for reproduction capacity, and for sexual function because with cryptorchism, testicular cellular damage is increasingly likely with each passing year, damage that is probably not reversible after the age of 4 or 5 years. On examination, the clinician must be sure that the testis truly is undescended. Occasionally an overactive

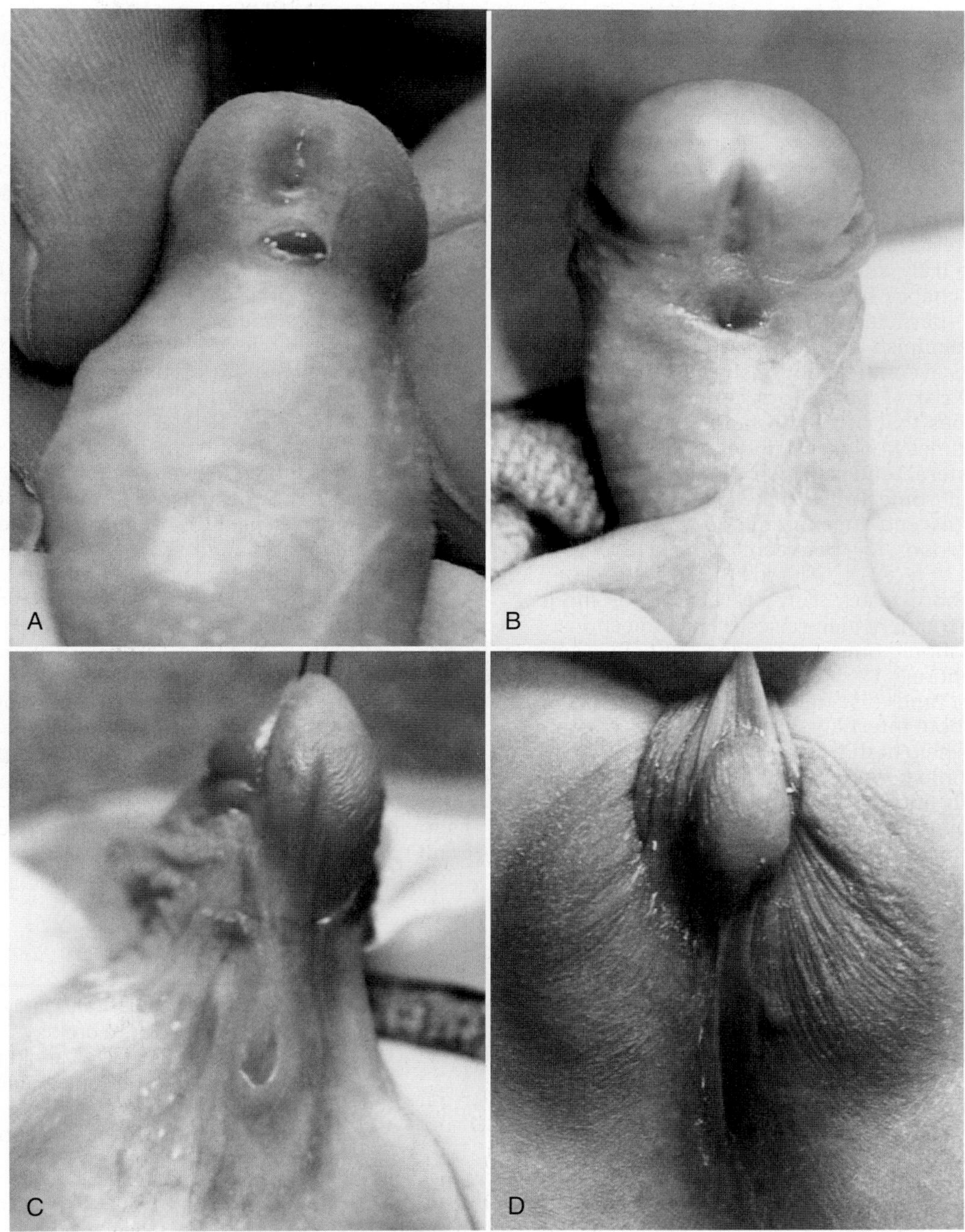

Figure 279-1 Varieties of hypospadias. **A,** Coronal. **B,** Distal shaft. **C,** Penoscrotal. **D,** Perineal.

cremasteric reflex may make palpation difficult. Moving the infant or the older child into the tailor position (sitting cross-legged) or a kneeling position can help overcome this difficulty. The examiner must feel from above downward, *milking* the testis from the inguinal canal into the scrotum. The older patient can help this process by coughing or straining. Cold hands and abrupt palpation can invoke the cremasteric reflex. If one or the other of the testes is not palpable, then the examiner should search beyond the scrotum and the inguinal canal to the femoral triangle and the inner thigh. Many undescended testes are associated with an inguinal hernia and possibly a hydrocele; these masses can make palpation of the testes even more difficult. If the testis is impalpable and a hernia is present, then the testis usually lies just inside the internal inguinal ring.

Actually, the testes, if undescended, may have stopped their descent at some point within the inguinal canal or may still be in the abdomen. If a testis has not reached the inguinal canal, then the likelihood is greater that it is abnormal; the lower the testis lies in the inguinal canal, the more likely that it is normal. Sonography has proved helpful only with the inguinal undescended testis. Computed tomography scan exposes the child to radiation, requires sedation, and has many false-positive and false-negative results. Radiation should be avoided. The patients with non-palpable testes may need endocrine or genetic evaluation.

A testis that retracts simply because of an overactive cremasteric reflex obviously should not be *repaired*. The truly undescended testis needs repair to improve the chance for fertility, to provide accessible examination (particularly in the event of malignant change), to diminish the possibility of testicular torsion, and to prevent the emotional trauma of an empty scrotum. The risk of malignancy in undescended testis is 4 to 10 times that of the normal scrotal testis, and this risk is 2 times in bilateral undescended testes than that in unilateral undescended testis. Experts have observed that some testes that appeared descended at birth may *ascend* later in childhood. Testicular ascent may account for between 2% and 20% of all orchiopexies.[5]

If one or both testes truly are ectopic or *hidden*, then the management plan raises certain questions:

- How long should one wait for descent before surgical intervention?
- Does a *best* time exist emotionally?
- Is worry about infertility warranted?
- Can repair help in this regard?

The orchiopexy does not change the incidence of malignancy in undescended testis. However, the timing of orchiopexy makes a difference in the outcome of fertility.

Certainly, no one wants an unnecessary operation. Nonetheless, a person cannot wait until puberty to see if natural descent occurs. If the testis is not down by 12 months of age, then surgery is indicated. If the parents refuse surgery or are reluctant, then the potential for descent can be explored with a therapeutic trial of human chorionic gonadotropin (hCG), 1500 IU/m^2 body surface area intramuscularly twice a week for 4 weeks. If the testis is to descend, then it will generally at this dose level and duration. Treating with hCG over a longer period has disadvantages; it can hasten the onset of puberty and can cause testicular damage and sterility. Overall success of hCG therapy is dependent on the initial location of the testis, with greater success reported with lower positioned testes. The reported success rates in randomized controlled trials range from 8% to 43%.[6] Surgery is the desirable alternative if the testis does not descend or does but retracts after the hCG trial. For persons who respond to the administration of hCG, the outlook for full sexual maturity is excellent. If the testes lie within the abdomen and are not palpable in the inguinal canal, then hCG will not bring them down into the scrotum but may bring them into the inguinal canal, where they are accessible to palpation and long-term observation, thereby avoiding immediate surgery and, if the testes subsequently descend into the scrotum, avoiding surgery altogether. Luteinizing hormone–releasing hormone and hCG treatment are equally effective in treating cryptorchism.[7]

If hormonal treatment fails, then surgery is the only other treatment that can be offered.

The optimal time for surgical correction of cryptorchism is approximately 12 months of age. If, for some reason, surgical correction is delayed until adolescence (eg, delayed diagnosis), then the possibility of the testis generating viable sperm is significantly decreased. Although bringing the testis down at this time does not diminish the potential of malignancy, it increases the likelihood of early detection. Periodic examinations are important. Finally, if the patient who has cryptorchism also has an associated inguinal hernia (with or without a hydrocele), then herniorrhaphy, along with orchiopexy, should be performed immediately. An elective herniorrhaphy is preferable to one performed in the setting of incarceration and possible strangulation.

Surgery may be done on an ambulatory basis when the testis is palpated in the inguinal canal. If it cannot be felt, then a more extensive surgical procedure with an abdominal incision probably will be necessary unless preliminary laparoscopy reveals the testis to be absent. In specialized centers, complete laparoscopic orchiopexy now is being performed. Either way, a demonstrably abnormal testis should be removed and replaced with a prosthesis. As with hypospadias or epispadias, the role of the pediatrician in the care of the patient and his family is important. The emotional support necessary when such a vital aspect of human function is threatened is enormous. Preparation for surgery requires full discussion about the child's and the parents' fears and concerns; these discussions should continue following surgery, particularly as the child grows older.

WHEN TO REFER

- All cases of hypospadias to urology
- All cases of epispadias to urology
- Undescended testis in a 1 year old to urology
- Hormonal treatment of undescended testes to endocrinology
- Hypospadias with genital abnormalities to endocrinology

WHEN TO ADMIT

- Surgical repair of hypospadias
- Surgical repair or epispadias
- Orchiopexy for intraabdominal testis or testes

TOOLS FOR PRACTICE

Engaging Patient and Family

- *Epispadias* (fact sheet), American Urological Association Education and Research (www.urologyhealth.org/pediatric/index.cfm?cat=01&topic=92).
- *Hypospadias* (fact sheet), American Urological Association Education and Research (www.urologyhealth.org/pediatric/index.cfm?cat=01&topic=96).

- *Undescended Testes* (fact sheet), American Urological Association Education and Research (www.urologyhealth.org/pediatric/index.cfm?cat=01&topic=178).
- *What is a Pediatric Urologist* (fact sheet), American Academy of Pediatrics (www.aap.org/sections/sap/he3010.pdf).

SUGGESTED RESOURCES

American Academy of Pediatrics. Timing of elective surgery on the genitalia of male children with particular reference to the risks, benefits, and psychological effects of surgery and anesthesia. *Pediatrics*. 1996:97:590.

Barthold JS, Gonzalez R. The epidemiology of congenital cryptorchidism, testicular ascent and orchiopexy. *J Urol*. 2003;170(6 pt 1):2396-2401.

Colodny AH. Undescended testes: is surgery necessary? *N Engl J Med*. 1986;314:510.

Docimo SG, Jordan GH. Laparoscopic surgery in children. In: Marshall FF, ed. *Textbook of operative urology*. Baltimore, MD: WB Saunders; 1996.

Gearhart JP, Jeffs RD. Diagnostic maneuvers in cryptorchidism. *Semin Urol*. 1988;6:79.

Manzoni G, Bracka A, Palminteri E, et al. Hypospadias surgery: when, what and by whom? *BJU Int*. 2004;94(8):1188-1195.

Neely EK, Rosenfeld RG. The undescended testicle: when and how to intervene. *Contemp Pediatr*. 1990;7:21.

Nelson CP, Park JM, Wan J, et al. The increasing incidence of congenital penile anomalies in the United States. *J Urol*. 2005;174(4 pt 2):1573-1576.

Schulze KA, Pfister RR. Evaluating the undescended testis. *Am Fam Phys*. 1988;31:133.

REFERENCES

1. Nelson DP, Park JM, Wan J, et al. The increasing incidence of congenital penile anomalies in the United States. *J Urol*. 2005;174(4 pt 2):1573-1576.
2. Carmichael SL, Shaw GM, Laurent C, et al. Maternal progestin intake and risk of hypospadias. *Arch Pediatr Adolesc Med*. 2005;159:957-962.
3. Manzoni G, Bracka A, Palminteri E, et al. Hypospadias surgery: when, what and by whom? *BJU Int*. 2004;94:1188-1195.
4. Dees J. Congenital epispadias with incontinence. *J Urol*. 1949:62:513.
5. Barthold JS, Gonzalez R. The epidemiology of congenital cryptorchidism, testicular ascent and orchiopexy. *J Urol*. 2003;170(6 pt 1):2396-2401.
6. Ong C, Hasthorpe S, Hutson JM. Germ cell development in the descended and cryptorchid testis and the effects of hormonal manipulation. *Pediatr Surg Int*. 2005;21:240-254.
7. Pyorala S, Huttunen NP, Uhari M. A review and meta-analysis of hormonal treatment of cryptorchidism. *J Clin Endocrinol Metab*. 1995;80:2795-2799.

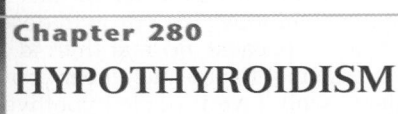

Chapter 280

HYPOTHYROIDISM

Craig C. Orlowski, MD

INTRODUCTION

Few diseases affect multiple systems so severely yet are associated with so many nonspecific symptoms and signs as hypothyroidism. The clinical manifestation of hypothyroidism during infancy differs markedly from that of childhood and adolescence; for this reason, the primary care physician must distinguish between congenital and juvenile-acquired hypothyroidism.[1] Congenital and acquired hypothyroidism occur as familial or sporadic diseases with or without enlargement of the thyroid gland (goiter, thyromegaly) and may progress as either a permanent or a transient disorder.[1]

DEFINITION

Hypothyroidism is the clinical state in which production (or incipient failure of production) of thyroid hormones is insufficient to the extent that it leads to typical clinical manifestations. Specifically, primary hypothyroidism is insufficient thyroid hormone from failure of the thyroid gland. Secondary and tertiary hypothyroidism result from insufficient production of *thyrotropin* from either pituitary or hypothalamic abnormalities, respectively.

ETIOLOGY

The causes of hypothyroidism usually differ during infancy and childhood[2] (Box 280-1). In most cases of permanent congenital hypothyroidism, the underlying mechanism of the condition is unknown.[3] Approximately 90% of patients with congenital hypothyroidism have no thyroid tissue (athyreosis), an ectopic thyroid gland, or a hypoplastic thyroid gland found in the normal anterior cervical location.[1] Mutations in genes currently known to be involved in thyroid genesis explains only a small portion of cases of congenital hypothyroidism.[4] Although evidence of maternal autoimmunity has been found in some examples of permanent congenital hypothyroidism, the etiologic role of autoimmunity in congenital hypothyroidism is controversial. Several inborn errors of thyroid hormone synthesis are inherited as autosomal-recessive traits and usually cause thyromegaly noted on physical examination.[5] Several types of transient hypothyroidism can occur. In 2% of cases, antibodies that block the thyrotropin receptor are produced by a mother who has autoimmune thyroid disease and cross the placenta and block the function of the fetal thyroid gland.[5] This form of transient hypothyroidism can persist for several weeks or months; the affected infant requires thyroxine therapy until the antibodies disappear. Another type of transient congenital hypothyroidism may occur when drugs prescribed for the mother, such as propylthiouracil, methimazole, or iodides, cross the placenta and block the fetal thyroid gland. Iodine-containing medications should not be applied to the skin or mucous membranes of neonates for more than a few days because the iodine is absorbed easily and blocks the infant's thyroid gland. Rarely, congenital secondary (pituitary) hypothyroidism is caused by mutations in the genes that code for pituitary transcription factors.[5] Milder forms of congenital hypothyroidism may be missed by newborn screening programs, with symptoms not appearing until childhood. Children with these milder symptoms usually have either familial goitrous hypothyroidism (dyshormonogenesis)[5] or thyroid dysgenesis with an ectopic thyroid gland located somewhere between the foramen cecum of the tongue and the anterior mediastinum.

BOX 280-1 Causes of Hypothyroidism

CONGENITAL HYPOTHYROIDISM

A. Thyroid dysgenesis
   1. Thyroid aplasia
   2. Thyroid hypoplasia
   3. Ectopic thyroid gland

B. Familial abnormalities of thyroid hormone synthesis and metabolism (familial dyshormonogenesis)

C. Maternal disease
   1. Therapeutic doses of iodine-131 after the 11th week of gestation
   2. Transplacental autoimmune thyroiditis
   3. Ingestion of goitrogens

D. Endemic goiter and cretinism

E. Hypothalamic-pituitary hypothyroidism
   1. Pituitary agenesis or aplasia
   2. Thyrotropin deficiency: isolated
   3. Hypothalamic hormone deficiency
      a. Isolated thyrotropin deficiency
      b. Multiple tropic hormone deficiencies
      c. Septo-optic dysplasia
      d. Anencephaly
   4. Hypothalamic-pituitary lesions

JUVENILE HYPOTHYROIDISM

A. Thyroiditis, autoimmune (Hashimoto thyroiditis)
   1. Atrophic thyroiditis of infancy
   2. Chronic lymphocytic thyroiditis of childhood
   3. Atrophic thyroiditis of childhood and adolescence
   4. Hashimoto thyroiditis (struma lymphomatosa)

B. Congenital thyroid dysgenesis
   1. Ectopic thyroid
   2. Hypoplastic

C. Congenital defects in thyroid hormone synthesis or metabolism

D. Iatrogenic thyroid ablation
   1. Surgical
   2. Radioactive iodine-131

E. Ingestion of goitrogens

F. Endemic goiter

G. Hypothalamic-pituitary disease

The most common cause of hypothyroidism in children beyond the neonatal period is autoimmune thyroiditis.[6] In rare instances, disease may begin as early as 6 months of age and progresses rapidly during infancy with few symptoms and signs of hypothyroidism.[7] Similar to other autoimmune conditions, autoimmune thyroiditis is believed to be the result of the interplay between unknown environmental factors and a genetic predisposition, which is itself associated with certain human leukocyte antigen types.[8] Occasionally, patients who have hypothalamic or pituitary disease may be seen initially with hypothyroidism. These children usually have other clinical features to suggest an abnormality of the hypothalamus or pituitary.

INCIDENCE

Congenital hypothyroidism is present at birth and has an incidence in iodine-sufficient regions of the world of approximately 1 infant for every 4000 live births.[2] The incidence is greater in iodine-deficient regions. Juvenile-acquired hypothyroidism generally occurs outside the newborn period and is almost always caused by autoimmune thyroiditis, also known as Hashimoto or chronic lymphocytic thyroiditis. The incidence of juvenile hypothyroidism in the US population, as defined by elevated serum thyrotropin concentrations, is approximately 2% of children 12 to 19 years of age.[9]

DIFFERENTIAL DIAGNOSIS

The range of nonspecific symptoms and physical findings associated with hypothyroidism (Box 280-2) may result in other diagnoses being considered initially. For example, in the newborn, prolonged jaundice may raise concerns about liver abnormalities; however, as discussed later in this chapter, most newborns with congenital hypothyroidism will be discovered not based on clinical suspicion, but via newborn screening programs. In older children, other conditions frequently cause problems that may be suggestive of hypothyroidism. These problems include chronic fatigue in children with depression, delayed growth in children with simple delayed puberty, and weight gain in children with *exogenous* obesity.

EVALUATION

Hypothyroidism can affect many different organ systems to varying degrees. Therefore a diagnosis of hypothyroidism should be considered when a patient exhibits any of the signs or symptoms listed in Box 280-2. Many of the symptoms and signs of hypothyroidism are different during infancy compared with childhood and will be considered separately.

History

During the first month of life, affected infants may have no clinical symptoms or signs of hypothyroidism. In infants who have no functioning thyroid tissue, clinical symptoms and signs are rarely present at birth but are almost always present by 6 weeks of age. The clinical symptoms and signs of older children who have acquired hypothyroidism may be nonspecific and insidious in their development.[1] If the disease has been present for more than 6 months, then growth deceleration should be evident because normal thyroid hormone secretion is essential for normal linear growth. Hence most patients who have juvenile hypothyroidism have either thyromegaly or a deceleration of growth and are usually short in stature.[1] Deceleration of linear growth should be identified by the primary care physician who routinely measures the height of the patient; an early diagnosis will prevent the development of longstanding hypothyroidism, cessation of linear growth, and the risk of a decrease in final adult height. Frank obesity, however, is an uncommon complaint in children who have hypothyroidism because

BOX 280-2 Symptoms and Signs of Hypothyroidism

HISTORY

Congenital Hypothyroidism

Decreased stooling (fewer than one stool per day)

Prolonged hyperbilirubinemia (bilirubin above 10 mg/dL after 3 days of age)

Respiratory distress in a term infant

Birth weight above 4000 g

Feeding problems

Sleepiness

Hoarse cry

Acquired Juvenile Hypothyroidism

Growth retardation (<4 cm/yr)

Delayed dental development and tooth eruption

Onset of puberty: usually delayed; rarely precocious

Menstrual disorders

Galactorrhea

Constipation

Cold intolerance

Weight gain

Fatigue

PHYSICAL FEATURES

Congenital Hypothyroidism

Facial edema

Large posterior fontanelle (>0.5 cm)

Rectal temperature below 95° F (35° C)

Umbilical hernia

Macroglossia

Bradycardia (pulse <100 beats/min)

Lethargy

Cutaneous mottling, vasomotor instability

Hirsute forehead

Acquired Juvenile Hypothyroidism

Delayed bone maturation

Short stature

Myopathy and muscular hypertrophy

Increased skin pigmentation

Physical and mental torpor

Pale, gray, cool, mottled, thickened, coarse skin

Coarse, dry brittle hair

Bradycardia

Delayed deep-tendon reflexes

reduction in physical activity, if it occurs, is usually less than the reduction in caloric intake.

Physical Examination

Diagnosing congenital hypothyroidism on clinical grounds is difficult because of the varying clinical manifestations of the disease (Figure 280-1). Some infants may have clinical features suggestive of hypothyroidism yet normal thyroid study results; others may have minimal clinical features, such as mild periorbital edema, an enlarged posterior fontanelle, decreased stooling, and abdominal distention. Children who have advanced hypothyroidism and myxedema are usually chubby and have periorbital edema. Inspection and palpation of the anterior cervical area enables the examiner to identify an enlarged thyroid gland, even in the neonate. The easiest method for examining the thyroid gland of an infant is to place the infant in the supine position with the neck hyperextended over the edge of the examining table and feel for the isthmus of the thyroid, just below the hyoid bone. After identifying the isthmus, the primary care physician should palpate laterally to delineate the lobes, which are difficult to define in a healthy infant. The thyroid examination of an older child is easier by comparison. Because the thyroid rises during swallowing, having the patient swallow water will facilitate the identification and delineation of both lobes of the thyroid gland as distinct from other adjacent tissue.

Laboratory Evaluation

Thyroid Function Tests

The most useful thyroid function tests are usually measurement of serum thyrotropin and free thyroxine (T_4), the latter of which has widely supplanted the determination of total T_4. Total T_4 values are significantly influenced by circulating protein concentrations and are therefore less clinically useful. An elevation of the serum thyrotropin value is the most sensitive test result for identifying primary hypothyroidism.[1] The combination of a low serum T_4 value and an elevated thyrotropin value is diagnostic of primary hypothyroidism.[10] A normal free T_4 level and an elevated thyrotropin level are indicative of mild hypothyroidism. In patients with low free T_4 and thyrotropin levels, hypothalamic or pituitary hypothyroidism is strongly suspected and deserves further evaluation. Male patients with normal free T_4 and thyrotropin levels but low total T_4 levels are likely to have thyroid binding–protein deficiency, a benign condition. The free T_4 determination by direct dialysis is the most accurate method and the least likely to give false-positive or false-negative results from interfering drugs or other substances in serum.[1] Occasionally a child or infant who has a coexisting and severe illness may have the nonthyroidal illness syndrome (euthyroid sick) in which the free T_4 level may be low,[1] the serum triiodothyronine (T_3) value is low, the thyrotropin value is normal, and the reverse T_3 levels are borderline or frankly elevated.

Tests other than the serum T_4 and thyrotropin determinations are not usually required for children in whom a diagnosis of hypothyroidism is suspected; however, the finding of elevated serum thyroid peroxidase or thyroglobulin antibodies confirms the presumptive diagnosis of autoimmune thyroiditis.[11,12] Transient congenital hypothyroidism may be caused by thyrotropin receptor–blocking antibodies acquired from the mother who has autoimmune thyroid disease and primary hypothyroidism.[5]

The diagnosis of congenital hypothyroidism is rarely made on clinical grounds; rather the infant is identified via a newborn hypothyroidism detection program using a dried blood spot collected in the first day or two of life, which is then analyzed at a central laboratory. In most programs, thyrotropin levels are determined either for all infants or for infants whose total T_4 level falls below a threshold value. Infants identified in these programs must have confirmatory laboratory measurements of free T_4 and thyrotropin performed as soon as possible.

Radioisotopic Studies

Although some experts suggest the use of radioisotopic studies for all infants with suspected congenital hypothyroidism, others do not, and the thyroid scan is listed as an *optional diagnostic study* in the most recent American Academy of Pediatrics guidelines.[13] If a thyroid scan is performed, then iodine-123 or technetium-99m should be used and not iodine-131, which exposes the neonatal thyroid to higher radiation doses. The thyroid scan will distinguish sporadic disease, such as thyroid dysgenesis, from familial goitrous thyroid dyshormonogenesis, a distinction important for genetic counseling.[2] With dysgenesis, the scan will be consistent with agenesis and atopic thyroid tissue. In familial dyshormonogenesis, a normally sized or enlarged thyroid gland will be found in the normal anterior cervical location of the neck.

Radioisotopic studies are rarely needed in older patients who have juvenile hypothyroidism. Thyroid uptake studies are indicated when the patient has diffuse thyromegaly and biochemical evidence of hypothyroidism not caused by autoimmune thyroiditis or goitrogen ingestion.[1,12] Although not essential, the assessment of skeletal maturation can provide additional data regarding the duration of hypothyroidism. A bone age determination consistent with that of a healthy newborn would suggest recently acquired, mild congenital hypothyroidism, whereas notation of the absence of ossification centers at the knee in addition to the presence of only the 2 ossification centers in the foot indicates that the fetus was affected by hypothyroidism during the third trimester of pregnancy.

MANAGEMENT

The treatment of choice for hypothyroidism in infancy and childhood is the daily administration of oral L-thyroxine[1,2,5,14] (Table 280-1).

Table 280-1 Doses of L-Thyroxine Used to Treat Hypothyroidism in Infancy and Childhood

AGE	T_4 DOSE/DAY (MCG)	T_4 DOSE/KG/DAY (MCG)
Full term	50	10-15
<6 mo	25-50	8-10
6-12 mo	50-75	6-8
1-5 yr	75-100	5-6
6-12 yr	100-125	4-5
>12 yr	100-200	2-3

T_4, Thyroxine.

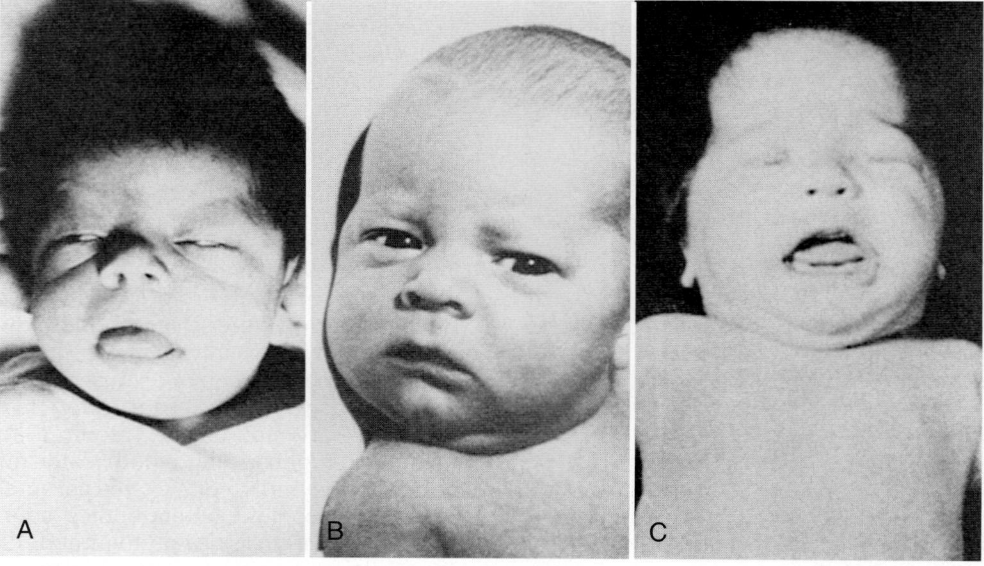

Figure 280-1 **A,** Normal infant referred at 8 months of age who had clinical signs but no clinical symptoms of congenital hypothyroidism. **B,** Infant with documented primary hypothyroidism at 4 weeks of age. Her clinical features at this age were minimal and included only mild periorbital edema, an enlarged posterior fontanelle, decreased stooling, and abdominal distention. **C,** Infant at age 6 months who has athyreosis and severe congenital hypothyroidism. *(From Foley TP Jr. Sporadic congenital hypothyroidism. In: Dussault JH, Walker P, eds.* Congenital hypothyroidism. *New York, NY: Marcel Dekker; 1983.)*

Congenital Hypothyroidism

The initial dose in a term infant is 50 mcg of L-thyroxine daily for the first 1 to 2 weeks and should be started promptly at the initial visit when screening test results are abnormal and serum samples have been sent for confirmatory tests or, if performed, whenever the scan is abnormal.[4] Infants who have hypothalamic or pituitary hypothyroidism generally have milder hypothyroidism and should be given 25 mcg/day. At the end of the second to fourth week, serum T_4 and thyrotropin values should be measured to determine that the amount of L-thyroxine is adequate but not excessive.[4] Clinical studies have indicated that the more rapid normalization of serum free T_4 and thyroid-stimulating hormone levels with initial dosing of 50 mcg L-thyroxine daily is associated with better long-term development outcomes than is using 37.5 mcg daily initially.[15,16] The American Academy of Pediatrics guidelines for monitoring free T_4 and thyrotropin values are outlined in Table 280-2.[13] After 1 or 2 weeks, the 50-mcg/day dose may need to be reduced to 37.5 g/day and infrequently to 25 mcg/day if clinical symptoms of hyperthyroidism develop or if the serum T_4 value exceeds 16 mcg/dL. In athyreotic infants who have low T_4 values, usually 50 mcg/day is adequate.

Therapy should be adjusted to maintain the serum T_4 levels during infancy in the upper half of the age-adjusted normal range to optimize developmental outcome. Concomitant administration of soy formula, iron, calcium, and high-fiber foods may interfere with absorption of the L-thyroxine and should be avoided when possible. Occasionally the thyrotropin value will not return to normal even if the T_4 dose is excessive and causes clinical thyrotoxicosis. These infants may have an abnormality in the feedback set point of thyrotropin secretion.[6] The goal of therapy in this situation should be to maintain normal serum T_4 values and clinical euthyroidism. Discontinuing L-thyroxine therapy some time after 3 years of age is a way of testing for transient congenital hypothyroidism. Serum T_4 and thyrotropin levels then are determined 2 to 4 weeks later. A trial of off therapy is not necessary for patients documented to have thyroid aplasia, ectopic thyroid dysgenesis, or elevated thyrotropin values after the initial period of therapy. Mild sensorineural hearing impairment may be fairly common in congenital hypothyroidism and should be screened for to allow early intervention.[17]

Table 280-2 American Academy of Pediatrics Policy for Monitoring Congenital Hypothyroidism*

AGE	INTERVAL
<6 mo	Every 1-2 mo
6 mo-3 yr	Every 3-4 mo
3 yr-completion of growth	Every 6-12 mo

*Recheck thyroxine and thyroid-stimulating hormone 2 to 3 weeks after starting therapy.

From American Academy of Pediatrics, Rose SR, Section on Endocrinology and Committee on Genetics, American Thyroid Association, Brown RS, Public Health Committee, Lawson Wilkins Pediatric Endocrine Society. Update of newborn screening and therapy for congenital hypothyroidism. Pediatrics 2006;117(6):2290-2303.

Acquired Hypothyroidism

Older children who have hypothyroidism do not share the same degree of urgency in achieving the euthyroid state. Although patients who have had a recent onset of mild hypothyroidism may be given a full replacement dose of L-thyroxine, children 3 years and older who have chronic hypothyroidism and clinical symptoms should be given a low dose that is gradually increased every 2 to 4 weeks to the full replacement dose.[1,12] The rapid correction of the hypothyroid state can often be associated with undesirable behavioral side effects. These children act as though they are thyrotoxic despite biochemical euthyroidism; they are often restless, have a short attention span, and are emotionally labile. In such cases a gradual increase in dose seems to minimize these problems in adjustment from the hypothyroid to the euthyroid state. Adequacy of L-thyroxine therapy is monitored by free T_4 and thyrotropin determinations every 6 to 12 months, once the patient is receiving a full replacement dose with normal values. An elevated thyrotropin level with or without a low T_4 value indicates either inadequate therapy or poor compliance; the latter is often characterized by variable serum T_4 and thyrotropin values. For example, the levels may be normal on one occasion but discordant (normal or elevated T_4 value with elevated thyrotropin value) on subsequent determinations, despite no change in therapy.

PROGNOSIS

Infants who were treated adequately for congenital hypothyroidism since the first month of age have an excellent prognosis for normal intellectual function and linear growth. However, delays in diagnosis and institution of adequate therapy are usually associated with an increased risk of intellectual disability.[18] Infants who have prolonged fetal hypothyroidism have an increased risk for impaired intellectual function because maternal hypothyroidism occurred during the first trimester or other factors blocked fetal thyroid function throughout pregnancy, such as maternal radioiodine therapy, maternal thyrotropin receptor–blocking antibodies, and prolonged use of antithyroid drugs, including iodine. Infants born with delayed skeletal maturation and low T_4 values are most likely to have neurocognitive problems.[19] In contrast, no permanent intellectual impairment is found among patients who have juvenile hypothyroidism. Adolescents who have chronic hypothyroidism and severe growth retardation may never achieve their full growth potential. In many cases, their linear growth response to therapy is not accelerated, and the height percentile achieved as an adult is lower than that predicted by their growth before the development of hypothyroidism.[20]

WHEN TO REFER

- Severe congenital hypothyroidism
- The cause of hypothyroidism is not established on the initial evaluation.

- Initial therapy does not normalize thyroid function test results within the normal range for age, which is often not necessarily the normal range provided by the laboratory. The physician must know the normal range of thyroid function test results for age for patient management during the first 2 decades of life.
- Acquired hypothyroidism is atypical or complex. The disease occurs in infancy or early childhood or is associated with other endocrine or nonendocrine autoimmune diseases.
- When the diagnosis is hypothalamic or pituitary hypothyroidism based on a low free T_4 level (by a method validated in infants and children) and normal or low thyrotropin level. Rarely is this form of hypothyroidism an isolated disease. It is expected to be associated with other hypothalamic-pituitary abnormalities; if it is isolated, then genetic evaluation is needed to define the cause and potential for recurrence in a family.

WHEN TO ADMIT

- Myxedema coma
- Parental noncompliance with treatment of the young infant who is at increased risk for permanent impairment of central nervous system function if thyroid function test results are not maintained in the normal range

TOOLS FOR PRACTICE

Engaging Patient and Family

- *Congenital Hypothyroidism* (fact sheet), Thyroid Foundation of America (www.tsh.org/disorders/pregnancy/newborns.html).

AAP POLICY STATEMENTS

Kaye CI, American Academy of Pediatrics, Committee on Genetics. Introduction to the newborn screening fact sheets. *Pediatrics.* 2006;118(3):1304-1312. (pediatrics.aappublications.org/cgi/content/full/118/3/1304).

Kaye CI, American Academy of Pediatrics, Committee on Genetics. Newborn screening fact sheets. *Pediatrics.* 2006;118(3):e934-e963. (pediatrics.aappublications.org/cgi/content/full/118/3/e934).

American Academy of Pediatrics, Rose SR, Section on Endocrinology and Committee on Genetics, American Thyroid Association, Brown RS, Public Health Committee, Lawson Wilkins Pediatric Endocrine Society. Update of newborn screening and therapy for congenital hypothyroidism. *Pediatrics.* 2006;117(6):2290-2303. (aappolicy.aappublications.org/cgi/content/full/pediatrics;117/6/2290).

SUGGESTED RESOURCES

American Academy of Pediatrics, Rose SR, and the Section on Endocrinology and Committee on Genetics, American Thyroid Association, Brown RS, and the Public Health Committee, Lawson Wilkins Pediatric Endocrine Society. Update of newborn screening and therapy for congenital hypothyroidism. *Pediatrics.* 2006;117:2290-2303.

American Academy of Pediatrics, Section on Endocrinology, Committee on Genetics, American Thyroid Association, Committee on Public Health. Newborn screening for congenital hypothyroidism: recommended guidelines. *Pediatrics.* 1993;91:1203-1209.

Brown R, Larsen PR. Thyroid gland development and disease in infants and children. In: De Groot LJ, Hennemann G, eds. *Thyroid Disease Manager* [book on line]. South Dartmouth, MA: Endocrine Education; 2005. Available at: www.thyroidmanager.org/Chapter15/15-frame.htm. Accessed June 28, 2007.

Refetoff S, Dumont JE, Vassart G. Thyroid disorders. In: Scriver CR, Beaudet AL, Sly WS, et al, eds. *The Metabolic and Molecular Bases of Inherited Disease.* 8th ed. New York, NY: McGraw-Hill; 2001.

Weetman AP, McGregor AM. Autoimmune thyroid disease: further developments in our understanding. *Endocr Rev.* 1994;15:788-830.

REFERENCES

1. Foley TP Jr, Malvaux P, Blizzard RM. Thyroid disease. In: Kappy MS, Blizzard RM, Migeon CJ, eds. *Wilkins the Diagnosis and Treatment of Endocrine Disorders in Childhood and Adolescence.* 4th ed. Springfield, IL: Charles C. Thomas; 1994.
2. Foley TP Jr. Congenital hypothyroidism. In: Braverman LE, Utiger RD, eds. *Werner and Ingbar's the Thyroid.* 8th ed. Philadelphia, PA: Lippincott, Williams & Wilkins; 2000.
3. De Felice M, Di Lauro R. Thyroid development and its disorders: genetics and molecular mechanisms. *Endocrinol Rev.* 2004;25:722-746.
4. Germak JA, Foley TP Jr. Longitudinal assessment of L-thyroxine therapy in congenital hypothyroidism. *J Pediatr.* 1990;117:211-219.
5. Matsuura N, Yamada Y, Nohara Y, et al. Familial neonatal transient hypothyroidism due to maternal TSH-binding inhibitor immunoglobulins. *N Engl J Med.* 1980;303:738-741.
6. Rallison ML, Dobyns BM, Keating FR, et al. Occurrence and natural history of thyroiditis in children. *J Pediatr.* 1975;86:675-682.
7. Foley TP Jr, Abbassi V, Copeland KC, et al. Brief report: hypothyroidism caused by chronic autoimmune thyroiditis in very young infants. *N Engl J Med.* 1994;330:466-468.
8. Tomer Y, Barbesino G, Greenberg DA, et al. Mapping the major susceptibility loci for familial Graves' and Hashimoto's diseases: evidence for genetic heterogeneity and gene interactions. *J Clin Endocrinol Metab.* 1999;84(12):4656-4664.
9. Hollowell JG, Staehling NW, Flanders WD, et al. Serum TSH, T(4), and thyroid antibodies in the United States population (1988 to 1994): National Health and Nutrition Examination Survey (NHANES III). *J Clin Endocrinol Metab.* 2002;87(2):489-499.
10. Klein AH, Foley TP Jr, Larsen PR, et al. Neonatal thyroid function in congenital hypothyroidism. *J Pediatr.* 1976;89:545-549.
11. Bachrach LK, Foley TP Jr. Thyroiditis in children. *Pediatr Rev.* 1989;11:184-191.
12. Foley TP Jr. Acquired hypothyroidism in infants, children and adolescents. In: Braverman LE, Utiger RD, eds. *Werner and Ingbar's the Thyroid.* 8th ed. Philadelphia, PA: Lippincott, Williams & Wilkins; 2000.
13. American Academy of Pediatrics, Rose SR, Section on Endocrinology and Committee on Genetics, American Thyroid Association, Brown RS, Public Health Committee, Lawson Wilkins Pediatric Endocrine Society. Update of newborn screening and therapy for congenital hypothyroidism. *Pediatrics.* 2006;117(6):2290-2303.
14. Sato T, Suzuki Y, Taketani T, et al. Age-related change in pituitary threshold for TSH release during replacement therapy for cretinism. *J Clin Endocrinol Metab.* 1977;44:553-559.

15. Selva KA, Harper A, Downs A, et al. Neurodevelopmental outcomes in congenital hypothyroidism: comparison of initial T4 dose and time to reach target T4 and TSH. *J Pediatr.* 2005;147:775-780.
16. Bongers-Schokking JJ, de Muinck Keizer-Schrama SM. Influence of timing and dose of thyroid hormone replacement on mental, psychomotor, and behavioral development in children with congenital hypothyroidism. *J Pediatr.* 2005;147:768-774.
17. Bellman SC, Davies A, Fuggle PW, et al. Mild impairment of neuro-otological function in early treated congenital hypothyroidism. *Arch Dis Child* 1996;74:215-218.
18. Klein AH, Meltzer S, Kenny FM. Improved prognosis in congenital hypothyroidism treated before age three months. *J Pediatr.* 1972;81:912-915.
19. Rovet JF. Long-term neuropsychological sequelae of early-treated congenital hypothyroidism: effects of adolescence. *Acta Paediatr Supp.* 1999;88:88-95.
20. Rivkees SA, Bode HH, Crawford JD. Long-term growth in juvenile acquired hypothyroidism. *N Engl J Med.* 1988; 318:599-602.

Chapter 281

IATROGENIC DISEASE

Ian M. Paul, MD, MSc

Iatrogenic (from the Greek word meaning *produced by the physician*) disease is the result of therapy or diagnostic procedures used to manage the health needs of a patient. Iatrogenic diseases may be caused by errors or by expected adverse outcomes of diagnostic procedures and therapies. Over the last several years, many reports have surfaced describing the frequency of iatrogenic disease in the inpatient, outpatient, and emergency department settings.[1-3]

Children are especially vulnerable to iatrogenic disease because of their size, developmental and metabolic differences that evolve with increasing age, and the use of new therapies that have not been studied or approved for use in children. Iatrogenic disease is especially significant in newborn medicine. Raju[4] surveyed a single pediatric journal and reported that 12.7% of articles published between 1965 and 1976 dealt with iatrogenic problems. In the pediatric intensive care unit, 8% of admissions had unanticipated complications of care; 42% of these cases were major. Human error was involved in 36% of cases.[5] Principi et al[6] surveyed the use of antibiotics in 9 pediatric units (765 patients) and found that nearly one third of the patients received antibiotics on an *irrational* basis (no proved infection or positive laboratory test). In 75% of the patients, the antibiotic choice was not justified by the given clinical condition. This type of therapy invites iatrogenic disease and is common, as demonstrated by the report by Holdsworth et al, which showed that adverse drug events occurred in 6% of pediatric hospitalizations at a single, metropolitan center.[2] In this study, nearly one quarter of the events resulted in severe or life-threatening complications.

CASE REPORT

Keith was referred by his family physician to an allergist at age 8 years for evaluation of continual sniffing that had been present for years and was attributed to allergies, in part, because of a positive family history and because decongestants were ineffective. From age 8 to 10 years, Keith was treated with monthly injections of triamcinolone acetate by the allergist. The parents became concerned at the onset of growth failure during this period. At age 10, he was referred to an endocrinology clinic where the evaluation revealed his height and weight to be below the 3rd percentile, with essentially no absolute gain since 8 years of age. Also noted in the history was enuresis of many years' duration. The clinic note for that visit describes the patient as "hyperactive, with constant small movements of the body and frequent repetitive sounds from the throat." Keith was evaluated with the following tests, the results of which were normal: insulin-arginine stimulation of growth hormone release, serum thyroxine, skull radiographs, bone age, and buccal smear. Conclusions of the endocrine consultation were that the growth failure was most likely caused by the administration of steroids; the family was thus advised to stop the steroids. The patient was referred to a urologist for evaluation of his enuresis and to a pediatrician for evaluation of his hyperactivity.

Keith was first seen by the urologist and hospitalized. He underwent an intravenous pyelogram with voiding cystourethrogram, cystoscopy with cystometrogram, and cystourethroscopy. The results of all these studies were normal. The patient was given 25 mg imipramine at bedtime for his enuresis.

Keith was seen next in the pediatric clinic. Tourette syndrome was diagnosed based on multiple motor and vocal tics and coprolalia. Because of the initial delight of the patient and his family in the efficacy of imipramine in controlling the enuresis, drug therapy for controlling Tourette syndrome was discussed but deferred. Six weeks later, with the patient's resumption of frequent enuresis while still receiving imipramine, this drug was stopped, and haloperidol, 1 mg twice daily, was started. Diminution of his tics was prompt and considerable, and cessation of coprolalia occurred within 2 days. After 1 week on this dose, the patient experienced acute dystonic posturing of the neck and face, which was reversed by intravenous diphenhydramine, 25 mg. The dose of haloperidol was decreased to 0.5 mg twice daily; no further side effects were noted.

Keith remained stable for the next 5 years on this regimen. After the initial diagnosis, he was placed in a special education class; subsequently, both his accomplishments and self-esteem increased; he also became a rifle marksman. The next year, Keith returned to a regular classroom and graduated 5 years later from high school with vocational training. His height was at the 20th percentile, and his weight was at the 50th percentile. At 37 years of age, he is fully employed. After 5 years of continuous haloperidol therapy at a dose of 0.5 mg twice daily, the patient began to take the medication at the same dose 2 or 3 times per year for 1 to 2 weeks when he was in stressful situations.

Iatrogenic illness in this patient occurred at several levels and for different reasons. First, Keith was misdiagnosed as being allergic because of frequent sniffing, a common symptom of Tourette syndrome. Second, the patient received a potent steroid for this symptom, which stopped his growth, leading to a lengthy, expensive, and negative endocrinologic evaluation. Third, he was referred to a specialist for evaluation of a common and usually benign developmental condition, enuresis. Keith received a lengthy, excessive evaluation that required hospitalization and the administration of an anesthetic agent. Fourth, after the patient was diagnosed correctly, initial drug therapy caused a severe dystonic drug reaction. Finally, failure to diagnose Tourette syndrome early caused serious educational problems.

ETIOLOGY

Every encounter with a patient may produce iatrogenic disease. Infants younger than 1 year are especially vulnerable to idiosyncratic central nervous system reactions to drugs (eg, extrapyramidal reaction to prochlorperazine). The risk varies from virtually zero with the insertion of a tongue depressor (the gag reflex can stimulate the vagus to produce asystole) to 100% with the use of intravenous amphotericin B. The most common, but not necessarily the most serious, possibilities for iatrogenic disease occur in 2 broad categories: (1) diagnostic procedures and (2) therapy (Table 281-1).

DATABASE

Recognizing iatrogenic disorders requires the physician's constant vigilance. The history and physical examination are most important; laboratory tests may confirm the clinical impression. Many iatrogenic disorders are obvious: ocular-gyric crisis from prochlorperazine use, sterile thigh abscesses from diphtheria-tetanus-acellular pertussis immunization, and a skin burn from touching an overhead warmer. Other disorders are more subtle: rickets in the rapidly growing premature infant from lack of sufficient vitamin D supplementation, hyponatremia from giving infants bottled mineral water, and thinning skin from long-term use of steroid cream for diaper rash. A careful review of systems coupled with specific questions concerning recent medications or other therapy (by nonphysicians and physicians) will usually uncover problem areas.

Because iatrogenic conditions may be particularly associated with therapeutic interventions, considering different scenarios in which drugs can cause these problems is particularly relevant. For example, some adverse reactions to medications may be related to the dose given, whereas others are not. A classic example of an iatrogenic state that is dose related would be the ototoxicity and nephrotoxicity caused by aminoglycoside antibiotics. In contrast, serum sickness or Stevens-Johnson syndrome may occur after antibiotic exposure regardless of the dose given. Stevens-Johnson syndrome is severe illness characterized by erythema multiforme, arthritis, nephritis, central nervous system abnormalities, and myocarditis and typically occurs after exposure to sulfonamide-containing antibiotics.

Although many drug reactions are not nearly as severe, the amount of time that they take to occur can be highly variable. The adverse effects associated with asthma therapy provide excellent examples. For the treatment of acute symptoms, β_2-adrenergic agonist agents such as albuterol are often given. Administration of this medication causes acute increases in heart rate and tremor—effects that diminish shortly after medication administration and have no long-term sequelae. Inhaled corticosteroids, the recommended maintenance medication class for children with persistent asthma, in contrast, have limited short-term adverse effects. However, with daily administration, these medications are associated with a reduced linear growth velocity for children, increased bone resorption, and the potential for osteoporosis, cataract development, and adrenal suppression.

Another potential scenario in which drugs can result in iatrogenic disease is when a drug-drug interaction occurs. A well-known class of drugs associated with numerous severe interactions is the antidepressant group known as monoamine oxidase inhibitors, which, when combined with many drugs such as tricyclic antidepressants, neuroleptics, meperidine, dextromethorphan, or clomipramine, can cause severe, potentially fatal reactions. This example highlights the need for consideration of drug interactions for patients taking more than 1 medication.

Cross-reactivity among drugs is another cause of iatrogenic diseases. Cross-reactivity can be mediated by both immunologic and nonimmunologic mechanisms. Immune-mediated cross-reactions occur as a result of shared antigens between drugs, and they can result from cell-mediated or immunoglobulin E–mediated mechanisms. The nonimmune-mediated cross-reactivity results from sharing the mechanisms of actions among different drugs (eg, cyclooxygenase-1 inhibition seen among nonsteroidal antiinflammatory drugs) or because of nonspecific release of histamine, as seen with contrast media. To assess the T cell–mediated cross-reactivity, an intradermal delayed hypersensitivity test, a patch test, or an in vitro T cell–transformation assays can be performed. Immunoglobulin E–mediated cross-reactivity may be confirmed by skin tests. The best way of establishing the tolerability of the cross-reactive drug is to perform a graded challenge with a specific drug.

DIFFERENTIAL DIAGNOSIS

The diagnosis of the condition is usually straightforward, once considered; iatrogenic causes of disease are frequently overlooked. A list of a few iatrogenic diseases with alternative causes may be illustrative (Table 281-2).

PREVENTION

Numerous strategies minimize adverse events caused by human error, including the use of computerized physician order entry.[7] The use of technology, however, cannot entirely prevent iatrogenic disease and adverse events. Other strategies to prevent medical

Table 281-1 Complications That Can Arise from Diagnostic Procedures and Subsequent Therapy

DIAGNOSTIC PROCEDURE	COMPLICATIONS
PHYSICAL EXAMINATION	
Ears (otoscope speculum)	Laceration of auditory canal; perforation of eardrum
Pharynx (tongue blade)	Laceration of soft palate
Mouth or rectum (glass thermometer)	Broken-glass laceration
Joints	Dislocation
Abdominal examination	Fractured spleen
LABORATORY TESTING	
Throat culture	Gagging; vomiting; aspiration
Venipunctures	Bruising; arterial spasm
Heel sticks	Lacerated heels; infection; osteomyelitis
RADIOGRAPHIC PROCEDURES	
Position of patient	Dislocation of joints; infiltration of intravenous lines; decubitus ulceration
Use of radiopaque dyes	Allergic reactions
Sedation	Central nervous system (CNS) depression; apnea; drug reaction; cardiac arrhythmias
Radiotherapy	Skin erythema; burns; sterility; alopecia
THERAPY	
Drug therapy	Drug reaction; drug interaction; errors in type of drug and frequency and route of administration
Fluids and electrolytes	Overhydration or underhydration; incorrect solution; incorrect route; misplacement of intravenous line; catheter infection
Nutrition (including vitamins)	Deficiency states; inadequate knowledge of formula composition; hypervitaminosis
EQUIPMENT	
Infant warmers	Burns
Electric hazards	Shocks
Transillumination (fiberoptics)	Burns
Noise (especially in incubators)	Auditory damage; sleep disturbances
Constant light	CNS dysfunction; retinal damage; hormonal dysfunction
Temperature control	Hypothermia or hyperthermia
Beds: mesh, rails, objects	Choking; falling out
Surgery	Wrong patient selected for operation; wrong part of body selected for operation
	Complications: infection, contracture, scarring, adhesions, fluid and electrolyte imbalance
Cardiopulmonary resuscitation	Fractured ribs, spleen, or liver
Instructions to patient or family	Overly restricted life at home and school; failure to appreciate impact of illness on family's and patient's life; misunderstanding of oral instructions
Immunizations	Local and systemic reactions

errors in pediatrics include (1) systems analysis, which examines time points and applications with potential for error within a particular system; (2) critical incident root-cause analysis, which dissects all events that lead up to a particular adverse event; (3) increased use of clinical pharmacists and pediatric satellite pharmacies; (4) computer-assisted decision making; and (5) global initiatives aimed at improving naming and labeling requirements of pharmaceutical products.[8]

MANAGEMENT

Management of an iatrogenic condition is no different from that of any other condition, except for the investigation. In some cases, iatrogenic events are unavoidable and expected: limb atrophy after the application of a plaster cast or postoperative scarring in a person known to form keloids. In many instances, the lesson learned is that patient-physician communication has broken down or that medical care technology contributed to confusion (eg, failure to recheck the position of a decimal point in a digoxin order, inadequate post-marketing drug surveillance). Managing iatrogenic illnesses includes the following steps:

1. *Careful explanation to parents and patient when instituting any therapy.* Preprinted handouts or brochures are helpful in anticipating and recognizing problems, for example, discussion of possible side effects of immunization, procedures, or drug therapies.
2. *Prompt investigation of any iatrogenic event.* Comments such as "Don't worry, this happens frequently," "We see this occasionally," and "Nobody knows" are not reassuring to the family. Corrective measures must be instituted immediately. Iatrogenic disease frequently occurs as a systems failure. Prompt reporting

Table 281-2 Differential Diagnosis of Iatrogenic Conditions

CONDITION (DIAGNOSIS)	CAUSES
Rickets	No vitamin D supplementation Renal disease Rapid growth in a premature infant
Seizure	Seizure disorder Tap water enemas Boiled skim milk Bottled water (no electrolytes) Fever
Fever of unknown origin	Urinary tract infection Phenytoin therapy
Hearing loss	Recurrent otitis media Aminoglycoside therapy Incubator noise with concomitant aminoglycoside therapy
Short stature	Heredity Malnutrition Steroid therapy
Loose stools	Enteritis Lactose intolerance Mineral oil and senna products
Increased intracranial pressure	Meningitis Brain tumor Vitamin A intoxication
Hair loss	Emotional Thallium poisoning Vincristine therapy

of adverse events and their immediate investigation and correction will minimize recurrence. Such investigations should not be punitive.

3. *Call for help.* This action may mean additional consultative opinions from experts within and outside of medicine. Social workers and teachers can assist in managing a chronically ill child whose medical regimen does not permit normal school attendance.

Iatrogenic disease may be cause for a medicolegal suit by a family. Such a malpractice risk will be considerably minimized if the aforementioned suggestions are followed.

REFERENCES

1. Kozer E, Scolnik D, Macpherson A, et al. Variables associated with medication errors in pediatric emergency medicine. *Pediatrics*. 2002;110:737-742.
2. Holdsworth MT, Fichtl RE, Behta M, et al. Incidence and impact of adverse drug events in pediatric inpatients. *Arch Pediatr Adolesc Med*. 2003;157:60-65.
3. Gandhi TK, Weingart SN, Borus J, et al. Adverse drug events in ambulatory care. *N Engl J Med*. 2003;348:1556-1564.
4. Raju TNK. The injured neonate of the seventies. *J Pediatr.* 1977;91:347.
5. Stambouly JJ, McLaughlin LL, Mandel FS, et al. Complications of care in a pediatric intensive care unit: a prospective study. *Intensive Care Med*. 1996;22:1098.
6. Principi N, Marchisio P, Sher D, et al. Control of antibiotic therapy in pediatric patients. *Dev Pharmacol Ther.* 1981;3:145.
7. King WJ, Paice N, Rangrej J, et al. The effect of computerized physician order entry on medication errors and adverse drug events in pediatric inpatients. *Pediatrics*. 2003;112:506S-509S.
8. Fernandez CV, Gillis-Ring J. Strategies for the prevention of medical error in pediatrics. *J Pediatr.* 2003;143:155-162.

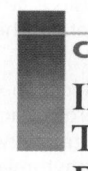

Chapter 282

IMMUNE THROMBOCYTOPENIA PURPURA

Jawhar Rawwas, MD

Immune thrombocytopenic purpura (ITP) of childhood is an acquired immune-mediated, and usually self-limiting condition of low platelet counts. ITP is caused by antibodies (mostly immunoglobulin G [IgG]) directed against antigens normally present on platelet membranes. The antibody-coated platelets are then recognized and destroyed by reticuloendothelial cells found mostly in the spleen.

INCIDENCE

The incidence of ITP is estimated to be between 4 and 8 cases per 100,000 children annually, but the rate is likely higher because of subclinical cases. ITP is most common in children ages 2 to 10 years, with a peak incidence at 2 to 4 years of age. A history of a preceding infection, subsequently resolved, is elicited in the majority of patients. In some cases, ITP is seen after measles-mumps-rubella immunization. The best estimate of absolute risk of ITP with measles-mumps-rubella vaccination is 1 in 24,000 doses and usually occurs within 6 weeks of vaccination.[1] This number is considerably less than ITP that occurs after natural infections with measles, mumps, or rubella. More than 70% of cases of ITP occur after virus infections.[2] In children, both sexes are equally affected, but female predominance over boys (2.3:1) is seen during adolescence and adulthood.[3-5]

CLINICAL PRESENTATION

A child with ITP typically has the sudden onset of petechiae, purpura, and ecchymoses in the absence of other signs of illness. A history of a recent viral illness usually exists. Mucosal (nose, mouth, and gingival surfaces) bleeding may be present. Intracranial hemorrhage (ICH), the most serious complication of ITP, is rare, occurring in 0.1% to 1% of acute ITP.[6] Other than these manifestations of thrombocytopenia, patients with ITP usually have no significant abnormalities on history and physical examination. Other systemic symptoms such as fever, weight loss, or bone or joint pain are absent. On physical examination, no significant enlargement of lymph nodes, liver, or spleen is present. If any of these symptoms or physical findings is present, then the case is not typical of ITP, and other diagnoses should be considered.

EVALUATION

For a patient with mucocutaneous signs of bleeding who is otherwise healthy, a reasonable workup includes obtaining a complete blood count, peripheral blood smear, a reticulocyte count, and blood typing. In children with ITP, thrombocytopenia is usually the only laboratory abnormality, and the platelet count is usually fewer than 20,000/mcL. A peripheral blood smear will reveal morphologically normal white blood cells and red blood cells. Large, freshly produced platelets are usually seen. These young reticulated platelets contain messenger RNA and are metabolically active, which may explain why patients with ITP do not bleed as severely as patients with bone marrow failure who have similarly low platelet counts. If other abnormalities are seen on the peripheral smear, then obtaining additional tests such as viral antibodies (human immunodeficiency virus, cytomegalovirus, Epstein-Barr virus, varicella, rubeola, mumps, or parvovirus, depending on the clinical picture) or tests for rheumatologic and other hematologic conditions (eg, leukemia, bone marrow failure) may be indicated. The reticulocyte count is a helpful test when the diagnosis of ITP is not straightforward, such as in cases in which associated mild anemia exists, which is not a rare occurrence. The purpose of blood typing is not transfusion but determination of Rh status, which determines if a patient is treatable with anti-D antibodies. Both reticulocyte count and blood typing are not strictly needed for evaluation, but blood should be drawn and kept aside for reticulocyte count and blood typing if needed instead of performing multiple traumatic blood draws on a thrombocytopenic child. Although ITP is caused by platelet antibodies, platelet antibody tests are sensitive but not specific, and therefore they are not indicated for the diagnosis of acute ITP in children.[7] In ITP, bleeding time is prolonged, but assessment of bleeding time is an unnecessary test and is traumatic and inaccurate in children. Prothrombin time and activated partial thromboplastin time are normal and are also unnecessary tests. In the past, many pediatric hematologists performed a bone marrow aspiration on patients with ITP to rule out acute lymphocytic leukemia, especially before starting a patient on steroids, for fear of partially treating and thus masking a leukemic process. Now, pediatric hematologists prefer to perform bone marrow aspiration and biopsy only on patients who have clinical or laboratory features that are atypical of ITP at presentation, suggesting an alternate diagnosis such as acute leukemia or a bone marrow failure syndrome.[8] Marrow examination also is indicated for patients who initially are diagnosed as having ITP but who do not respond to treatment. Response to intravenous immunoglobulin (IVIg) or anti-D antibodies is usually seen within 1 to 2 days and to steroids within a week. The choice as to when to perform a bone marrow evaluation is an individualized decision. The most likely time for bone marrow examination to be performed is between 7 and 14 days after treatment is begun and when response to treatment is poor. Bone marrow examination should also be considered in patients who have an atypical clinical course, in patients in whom splenectomy is contemplated for additional confirmation of the diagnosis for ITP, and to rule out any possibility of a malignant process. The bone marrow in ITP is cellular, with normal erythroid and myeloid precursors, and usually shows increased numbers of megakaryocytes.

DIFFERENTIAL DIAGNOSIS

ITP is a diagnosis of exclusion after considering the likelihood of other causes of isolated thrombocytopenia. These causes include:

a. Infections such as Epstein-Barr virus, hepatitis C, and human immunodeficiency virus type 1. These can be ruled out by history, physical examination, and, if needed, by obtaining liver function tests and viral studies.
b. Drugs such as heparin and sulfonamides. These can be ruled out by history.
c. Other autoimmune diseases such as systemic lupus erythematosus, which may be difficult to diagnose. These autoimmune diseases are more likely to affect teenagers and adults than younger children.
d. Acute leukemia or bone marrow failure. Children with leukemia usually have other symptoms along with abnormal physical findings, especially hepatosplenomegaly and lymphadenopathy, which are absent in ITP. Leukocytosis (a white blood cell count >10,000/mcL) and significant anemia (a hemoglobin count of <10/dL) are usually seen in leukemia but not ITP. In acquired aplastic anemia, a low platelet count is usually associated with other significant changes in the peripheral blood, such as macrocytic anemia, leukopenia, or neutropenia.
e. Inherited thrombocytopenia. Although thrombocytopenia in most children is either autoimmune or drug related, keeping this category in mind is important. Eliciting a family history of thrombocytopenia, especially parent-child or maternal uncle–nephew, may be important. Diagnostic features on a peripheral smear such as abnormal size of platelets (either small or giant); absence of platelet alpha granules (gray platelets); Döhle-like bodies or microcytosis may point to an inherited thrombocytopenia. Clinically, bleeding out of proportion to the platelet count, onset of thrombocytopenia early in life and associated features such as absent radii, intellectual disability, renal failure, high frequency hearing loss, cataracts and history of a stable level of thrombocytopenia for years suggest inherited thrombocytopenia.[9]

MANAGEMENT

Pediatric hematologists differ in their approach to the management of children with ITP. Approximately 85% of children with ITP will recover within a few months, with or without treatment. Patients whose platelet counts do not return to normal (>150,000/mcL) within 6 months are defined as having chronic ITP. Early treatment does not alter the natural course of ITP and does not affect the development of chronic ITP.

GENERAL ADVICE

General useful advice to families with an affected child includes (1) avoiding activities that are associated with increased likelihood of trauma such as contact sports, (2) making sure children use helmets when riding bicycles, and (3) avoiding medications that interfere with platelet function such as aspirin and nonsteroidal antiinflammatory drugs.

INTRACRANIAL HEMORRHAGE

Even though ICH is rare, it is the most likely cause of death in ITP. Recognizing which patients are more likely to develop ICH is difficult. A literature review of 62 reported pediatric and adolescent cases of ICH in the setting of ITP showed that the median time from the diagnosis of ITP to ICH was 32 days (range, 0 days to 8 years), and 72% of cases occurred within 6 months of diagnosis. The platelet count was less than 10,000/mcL in 71.4% of the cases. Treatment before the ICH was primarily steroids but also included IVIg, splenectomy, and others. A significant number of patients developed an ICH despite having already initiated steroid treatment of ITP.[10] Many patients with ICH have other risk factors, including preceding head injury, other preceding mucocutaneous bleeding, prior aspirin treatment, and arteriovenous malformations.

Management of ICH in the setting of ITP is an emergency that requires immediate imaging (computed tomographic scan) to determine the location and extent of the bleeding and immediate consultation with a pediatric intensivist, hematologist, neurosurgeon, and general surgeon. Treatment includes the administration of IVIg, steroids, continuous platelet transfusions to rapidly increase the platelet count, and surgical intervention, if needed, including craniotomy (especially with posterior fossa hemorrhages that are more likely to cause herniation or brainstem compression) and splenectomy.

MANAGING BLEEDING

Any intervention in a patient with ITP is directed at early control of symptoms, such as stopping bleeding and preventing recurrent bleeding. Most ITP cases in children can be managed on an outpatient basis. Although the consensus is that treatment is indicated for the patient with overt bleeding, the nature of the treatment and the question of management recommendations for patients with ITP who have different clinical manifestations remain a subject of debate. Therefore current therapy recommendations are not evidence based but based on expert consensus opinions.

The American Society of Hematology guidelines suggest that children with ITP who have platelet counts greater than 30,000/mcL require no treatment if they have few or no symptoms, as is usually the case. Patients with platelet counts between 10,000 and 30,000/mcL have treatment recommendations based on the presence and severity of associated bleeding symptoms or the risk of bleeding.[11] Because the severity of symptoms depends on the degree of thrombocytopenia, the lower the platelet count is, the more likely the patient is to receive treatment, even in the presence of relatively mild symptoms. Patients with extensive purpura of the mucosal membranes may have a higher bleeding risk and should be treated more often than not. Children with platelet counts below 10,000/mcL and only minor purpura should be treated. Children with any concomitant or preexisting bleeding disorder should also be treated.

Other important factors that play a role in the decision regarding treatment include the age of the child and his or her degree of activity. Social variables such as the reliability of the caregivers and ease of access to emergency medical care always play a role in the decision to treat or not to treat.

When therapy is indicated, the primary treatment options for the newly diagnosed patient with ITP are corticosteroids, IVIg, or intravenous anti-D immunoglobulin. All of these agents are effective in shortening the duration of thrombocytopenia. Platelet transfusions are ineffective because the transfused platelets are rapidly destroyed.

TREATING WITH CORTICOSTEROIDS

Corticosteroids have been used for many years for the management of ITP in all age groups. Steroids reduce the risk of symptoms in patients with ITP by different mechanisms but most likely by reducing reticuloendothelial system phagocytosis of antibody-coated platelets. Most pediatric hematologists use prednisone for 2 to 3 weeks. Shorter courses at higher doses are also effective. Intravenous or oral methylprednisolone up to 3 to 7 days and dexamethasone for 4 days every 4 weeks have been given.[12,13] Most patients with ITP respond to steroids, and the response is faster when higher doses are given; thus response can be seen after 72 hours of starting treatment. However, platelets usually decrease after the steroids are discontinued if the titer of platelet antibodies remains elevated. A second course of treatment may be necessary if bleeding develops or if the platelet count drops to fewer than 10,000/mcL. Side effects of brief courses of corticosteroids include behavioral changes, sleep disturbance, increased appetite, hyperglycemia, and weight gain. These side effects are more pronounced at higher dose levels.

TREATING WITH INTRAVENOUS IMMUNOGLOBULIN

Rapid improvement in platelet numbers in patients with ITP who are receiving IVIg, usually within 24 hours, is seen when compared with patients receiving steroids. IVIg likely interferes with Fc receptor activity, resulting in prolonged survival of antibody-coated platelets. Other mechanisms of action for IVIg include (1) regulatory properties of antiidiotypic antibodies in IVIg and (2) the IVIg effects on cytokine synthesis and on receptors for cytokines and complement. One intriguing proposal for the mechanism of action is that concentration-dependent elimination of IgG can be found from the plasma and that IVIg administration causes acceleration of the rate of IgG catabolism. Such a process would eliminate individual

IgG molecules in direct proportion to their relative concentration in plasma. Thus antiplatelet antibodies' elimination is accelerated.

Side effects of IVIg include chills, fever, headache, and nausea and vomiting. Side effects tend to be more pronounced in older patients. Neutropenia (absolute neutrophil count, <1500/mcL) develops in approximately 30% of patients. IVIg is also far more expensive than steroid therapy.

Treating With Anti-Rho (D)

Anti-Rho (D) immunoglobulin binds to the D-antigen in Rh-positive individuals and the antibody-coated red cells block the Fc receptor of reticuloendothelial cells resulting in a rapid increase in platelet count, usually in 1 to 2 days. The dose regimen commonly used is a single dose of 50 mcg/kg, although many physicians start with a 75-mcg/kg dose, which achieves a more rapid increase in platelet count that is similar to what is seen with IVIg therapy.[14] An average drop in the hemoglobin level of approximately 1.3 g is seen as a result of the mild hemolysis of the patient's Rho (D)-positive red cells. Anti-Rho (D) should be used with caution in children with preexisting anemia, and it should probably be given only to children with a hemoglobin level greater than 10 g/dL.

FOLLOW-UP

Patients should have blood counts done once or twice weekly for follow-up. In most cases, with early recovery, complete resolution of the thrombocytopenia occurs in 2 to 3 months. When the platelet count is stable, greater than 30,000/mcL, or increasing with time, blood counts should be done less frequently.

OUTCOMES

Treatment does not alter the course of ITP (ie, the incidence of patients who go on to develop chronic ITP); however, it does shorten the duration of thrombocytopenia in some patients. For typical cases of childhood ITP, 80% of patients will have the platelet counts return to normal within 2 months of presentation, with or without therapy. Another 10% will recover normal platelet levels in the next few months, and around 10% will go on to have chronic thrombocytopenia (>6 months' duration). Approximately 25% of children with ITP will have a relapse after initial treatment. The 25% of patients who will have a relapse after initial treatment consists of 10% who will have chronic ITP, 10% who will have recurrence but resolution within 6 months, and 5% who will have episodes of ITP recurrences and remissions throughout their lives.

COMPLICATIONS

Approximately 15% to 20% of pediatric patients with ITP will develop moderate or major hemorrhagic problems.[15] Life-threatening bleeding, including ICH, is rare, occurring with an incidence of 0.1% to 1%. When ICH or any other life-threatening hemorrhage occurs, immediate interventions, including IVIg and high-dose steroids, platelet transfusions, and emergency splenectomy, should be considered. For patients with ITP who are unstable or have progressive ICH, emergency craniotomy may be necessary.

Immune Thrombocytopenia in the Neonate

Most neonatal thrombocytopenia is not immune in nature but is caused by sepsis, congenital infections, drugs, asphyxia, and necrotizing enterocolitis. Two conditions occur when immune thrombocytopenia is seen in neonates. Neonatal alloimmune thrombocytopenia (NAIT) is a condition whereby the mother develops antiplatelet antibodies directed against specific antigens found on fetal platelets but lacking on hers. An associated 20% risk of ICH occurs, and treatment is usually involves administration of maternal washed platelets and IVIg. The importance of detection and accurate diagnosis of NAIT is in the ability to prevent complications in future pregnancies by treating the mother with IVIg and steroids and performing in utero blood sampling and intervening in case of thrombocytopenia. A hematologist and a high-risk fetal-maternal specialist should be involved in the management of patients with NAIT. Another less serious condition is that resulting from passive transfer of maternal platelet autoantibodies in a mother with ITP. Only 4% of babies born to mothers with ITP have platelet counts less than 20,000/mcL. The risk of ICH is low (<1%), and no proof exists that cesarian delivery alters that risk. Neonatal ITP usually resolves within a few weeks as the antibodies are used up, but physicians may choose to treat the babies with IVIg in case the platelet count drops to <30,000/mcL. Maternal ITP is not a contraindication to breastfeeding.

Chronic Immune Thrombocytopenic Purpura

Chronic ITP is defined as persistence of thrombocytopenia lasting for more than 6 months from the time of diagnosis. Approximately 10% of patients with typical ITP will develop chronic thrombocytopenia. In a prospective Dutch study,[16] variables that predicted the development of chronic disease included a platelet count greater than 10,000/mcL at the onset, the absence of infection shortly before the onset of the disease, and the 232I/T Fc gamma receptor IIB genotype. Management of children with chronic ITP should focus on minimizing the individual's risk for bleeding and maintaining a safe platelet count, knowing that many patients will require no treatment. Given sufficient time (even years), a significant proportion of such patients will improve or remit. In case treatment is needed, periodic short courses of steroids may be given. In case of chronic need for steroids, alternate day dosing may be effective in preventing bleeding while reducing side effects. IVIg or anti-Rho (D) have also been used in patients with chronic ITP, but these measures are only temporary. Some patients with chronic ITP may be good candidates for splenectomy.

SPLENECTOMY

Splenectomy is effective in improving the platelet count and reducing the associated risk of bleeding in 60% to 90% of children with chronic ITP. However, the anticipated improvement in hemostasis and platelet count must be balanced with the consideration of the small but real risk of overwhelming postsplenectomy sepsis, which may be life threatening. Splenectomy is usually delayed until the child is older than 5 years because the risk of overwhelming sepsis decreases with age. Presplenectomy immunizations and subsequent penicillin prophylaxis are necessary for all age groups. No universally accepted standards for the timing of splenectomy in chronic ITP exist, but the American Society of Hematology guidelines recommend waiting until at least 12 months after diagnosis, if possible. Platelet counts in splenectomized patients are generally monitored for an indefinite period; any drop in platelet counts or increase in symptoms should prompt an assessment for the presence of an accessory spleen. If not previously done, then recommendations are to perform a bone marrow biopsy on patients who are being considered for splenectomy.

For the treatment of refractory chronic ITP, rituximab, a chimeric murine-human anti-CD20 monoclonal antibody, has been successfully used. Rituximab acts by destroying B-lymphocytes by activating complement-dependent and an antibody-dependent cellular toxicity. Therefore the mechanism of action is a slow but effective decrease in the production of antibodies.

In a study of 24 patients (2 to 19 years of age) who received 375 mg/m^2 of rituximab in 4 weekly doses,[17] 63% achieved complete remission for 4 to 30 months (platelet count of greater than 150,000/mcL).[15] Rituximab use may be associated with infusion-related reactions and with the development of transient hypogammaglobulinemia. Although long-term remissions have been documented, the use of rituximab in the treatment of ITP is relatively recent and long-term followup may be needed for accurate prognostication. All children with refractory ITP should be referred to a pediatric hematologist.

WHEN TO REFER

- History of fevers or bone pain
- Hepatomegaly, splenomegaly, significant lymphadenopathy
- Family history of thrombocytopenia
- Platelet count less than 20,000/mcL
- Abnormal white blood cell count or peripheral smear or associated anemia
- Absence of response to initial therapy

WHEN TO ADMIT

- Significant bleeding symptoms
- Severe anemia
- Significant concern for possible traumatic injury
- Any neurologic change in the setting of thrombocytopenia

SUGGESTED RESOURCES

George JN, Woolf SH, Raskob GE, et al. Idiopathic thrombocytopenic purpura: a practice guideline developed by explicit methods for the American Society of Hematology. *Blood.* 1996;88(1):3-40.

Cines DB, Bussel JB. How I treat idiopathic thrombocytopenic purpura (ITP). *Blood.* 2005;106(7):2244-2251.

Medeiros D, Buchanan GR. Current controversies in the management of idiopathic thrombocytopenic purpura during childhood. *Pediatr Clin North Am* 1996;43(3): 757-772.

REFERENCES

1. Farmington P, Pugh S, Colville A, et al. A new method for active surveillance of adverse events from diphtheria/tetanus/pertussis and measles/mumps/rubella vaccine. *Lancet.* 1995;345:567-569.
2. Miller E, Waight P, Farrington CP, et al. Idiopathic thrombocytopenic purpura and MMR vaccine. *Arch Dis Child.* 2001;84:227-229.
3. Lusher JM, Iyer R. Idiopathic thrombocytopenic purpura in children. *Semin Thromb Hemost.* 1977;3(3): 175-199.
4. Kurtzberg J, Stockman JA 3rd. Idiopathic autoimmune thrombocytopenic purpura. *Adv Pediatr.* 1994;41: 111-134.
5. Medeiros D, Buchanan GR. Current controversies in the management of idiopathic thrombocytopenic purpura during childhood. *Pediatr Clin North Am.* 1996;43(3): 757-772.
6. Lilleyman JS. Management of childhood idiopathic thrombocytopenic purpura. *Br J Haematol.* 1999;105(4): 871-875.
7. Cines DB, Bussel JB. How I treat idiopathic thrombocytopenic purpura (ITP). *Blood.* 2005;106(7);2244-2251.
8. Vesely SK, Buchanan GR, Adix L, et al. Self-reported initial management of childhood idiopathic thrombocytopenic purpura: results of a survey of members of the American Society of Pediatric Hematology/Oncology, 2001. *J Pediatr Hematol Oncol.* 2003;25(2);130-133.
9. Cines DB, Bussel JB, McMillan RB, et al. Congenital and acquired thrombocytopenia. *Hematology (Am Soc Hematol Educ Program).* 2004;2004:390-406.
10. Butros LJ, Bussel JB. Intracranial hemorrhage in immune thrombocytopenic purpura: a retrospective analysis. *J Pediatr Hematol Oncol.* 2003;25(8);660-664.
11. George JN, Woolf SH, Raskob GE, et al. Idiopathic thrombocytopenic purpura: a practice guideline developed by explicit methods for the American Society of Hematology. *Blood.* 1996;88(1):3-40.
12. Albayrak D, Islek I, Kalayci AG, et al. Acute immune thrombocytopenic purpura: a comparative study of very high oral doses of methylprednisolone and intravenously administered immune globulin. *J Pediatr.* 1994;125(6 Pt 1): 1004-1007.
13. Borst F, Keuning JJ, van Hulsteijn H, et al. High-dose dexamethasone as a first- and second-line treatment of idiopathic thrombocytopenic purpura in adults. *Ann Hematol.* 2004;83(12):764-768.
14. Newman GC, Novoa MV, Fodero EM, et al. A dose of 75 microg/kg/d of I.V. anti-D increases the platelet count more rapidly and for a longer period of time than 50 microg/kg/d in adults with immune thrombocytopenic purpura. *Br J Haematol.* 2001;112(4);1076-1078.
15. Bolton-Maggs PH, Moon I. Assessment of UK practice for management of acute childhood idiopathic thrombocytopenic purpura against published guidelines. *Lancet.* 1997;350(9078):620-623.
16. Bruin M, Bierings M, Uiterwaal C, et al. Platelet count, previous infection and FCGR2B genotype predict development of chronic disease in newly diagnosed idiopathic thrombocytopenia in childhood: results of a prospective study. *Br J Haematol.* 2004;127(5);561-567.
17. Bennett CM, Rogers ZR, Kinnamon DD, et al. Prospective phase 1/2 study of rituximab in childhood and adolescent chronic immune thrombocytopenic purpura. *Blood.* 2006;107(7):2639-2642.

Chapter 283

INFECTIOUS MONONUCLEOSIS AND OTHER EPSTEIN-BARR VIRAL INFECTIONS

Stephen R. Barone, MD; Leonard R. Krilov, MD

EPIDEMIOLOGY

Infection with Epstein-Barr virus (EBV), a member of the herpesvirus group, is extremely common but often not apparent clinically. In Africa a strong association exists between infection with EBV and development of Burkitt lymphoma and nasopharyngeal carcinoma; this association, however, has been demonstrated less clearly in Western countries where infection with EBV occurs at a later age. In the United States, interest in EBV infection centers on the typical clinical syndrome—*infectious mononucleosis*—and on its emerging relationship with an increasing number of tumors, noted for the most part in immunocompromised patients.

In childhood, EBV infection is usually inapparent clinically or characterized by a nonspecific, uncomplicated episode of upper respiratory tract infection or pharyngitis. Although EBV antibodies are developed in 70% to 90% of children from low socioeconomic groups by age 5 years, these antibodies occur in only 40% to 50% of those from high socioeconomic groups.[1] Primary infections that do not occur until adolescence and young adulthood are much more likely, for reasons that are unclear, to produce infectious mononucleosis. Thus the annual incidence of infectious mononucleosis is highest among white high school and college students, approximately 1 in 2500 students. Infection follows entry of the EBV into the oropharynx, and its recovery from this site can be documented up to 16 months after illness. Apparently, EBV establishes latency in the epithelial cells of the oropharynx, and the virus is periodically shed from this site throughout an individual's lifetime. Transmission from one individual to another appears to occur most often through mixing of saliva (thus its description as the *kissing disease*). In the absence of such contact, transfer of infection is unlikely. In a study of families that have a childhood index case of infectious mononucleosis, seroconversion occurred in 34.6% of the susceptible siblings over a period of several months.[2] Even though the rate of transmission of the EBV infection was relatively low and slow, the development of infectious mononucleosis was quite high (55.6%) in sibling contacts who showed seroconversion. Secondary infection in typical college settings is even lower.

CLINICAL PRESENTATION

After an incubation period of 2 to 6 weeks (usually 20 to 30 days), signs of classic infectious mononucleosis are seen: fever, sore throat, and lymphadenopathy. This constellation of symptoms and signs may be preceded by vague symptoms of fatigue, malaise, and anorexia.

Because infectious mononucleosis is the result of a systemic viral infection, virtually every organ system may be involved.[3] Clinical manifestations compatible with infectious mononucleosis are listed in Figure 283-1.

The fever is usually not higher than 103°F (39.5°C), but the sore throat, frequently accompanied by tonsillar exudate (or in adolescents, more likely a grayish necrosis of the tonsillar surfaces) and a palatal enanthem, can be excruciating. Lymphadenopathy, perhaps the most striking feature of the illness, can be limited to the cervical nodes but can also be so extensive as to involve virtually all lymph node groups. Posterocervical adenopathy is noted most frequently. The lymph nodes are not tender, nor do they demonstrate other signs of inflammation.

Enlargement of the spleen and possibly the liver, together with posterocervical adenopathy, are the physical signs that usually alert the clinician to the diagnosis of infectious mononucleosis. Some patients who have this illness, however, do not have any palpable splenic enlargement; massive enlargement of the spleen should suggest an alternative diagnosis. Liver enzyme levels are elevated in virtually all patients, but the frequency of jaundice is low.

A rash, which can be erythematous, petechial, erythema multiforme–like, urticarial, or scarlatiniform, develops in approximately 20% of children who have this illness. A rash develops in 70% to 90% of young adult patients who have this illness and who are treated with ampicillin or amoxicillin. In some cases the ampicillin-related rash will appear after the medication has been discontinued.

The severity of illness is extremely variable, and some individuals may have relatively few manifestations of infection, whereas others will demonstrate virtually all the symptoms listed in Figure 283-1. In general, the clinical manifestations of the illness last approximately 2 to 3 weeks, with peak involvement during the second week. Eyelid edema occurs in approximately 25% of patients.

DIAGNOSIS AND SEROLOGIC FINDINGS

Infectious mononucleosis is diagnosed by the presence of a triad of typical clinical, hematologic, and serologic findings. In addition to the clinical profile described in the preceding section, minimal hematologic features should include a lymphocytosis of 50% or more of all leukocytes and an atypical lymphocyte count of 10% or more of all leukocytes. Other general laboratory findings usually include a decline in the number of granulocytes and platelets.

The Paul-Bunnell antibody, a heterophilic immunoglobulin M (IgM) antibody produced by humans during infection that reacts with horse, sheep, and bovine erythrocytes, but not with guinea pig kidney cells, is the cornerstone of laboratory diagnosis. This antibody will be present in 50% or fewer of children younger than 4 years.[4] Among school-aged children and young adults, Paul-Bunnell antibody is detectable 80% to 90% of the time during the second week of clinical illness.[5,6] Occasionally the heterophil response will be brief and minimal or will occur late in the illness and may therefore show negative results early in the course of the illness. Commercial diagnostic kits, which rely on differential adsorption to detect the heterophil antibody, are readily available and easy to use in a physician's office; they are 96% to 99% sensitive and give a result in 2 minutes.[7] False-positive results have been reported in cases of rubella, hepatitis, serum sickness, drug reactions, and systemic lupus erythematosus and through improper use of the kit or inaccurate interpretation of the agglutination reaction. The magnitude of the heterophil antibody titer does not correlate with clinical severity, and repeat testing, once a positive test result is obtained, provides no additional information regarding waxing or waning of the illness beyond that gained from clinical assessment of the patient.

If heterophil test results are negative and infection is strongly suspected, then confirmation of EBV infection should be sought by other serologic tests.[5] A variety of antibodies directed against various portions of EBV can be detected by numerous hospital, state health, or commercial laboratories. Patients who have negative heterophil test results will have antibodies against specific components of the virus if EBV is the cause of the clinical illness.

Four different antibodies define the EBV serologic profile: IgG antibody to the viral capsid antigen (VCA-IgG), IgM antibody to viral capsid antigen (VCA-IgM), IgG antibody to early antigen (EA), and IgG antibody to Epstein-Barr nuclear antigen (EBNA). This last antibody includes 2 patterns: (1) diffuse and (2) restricted. These antibodies usually appear in an individual who acquires a primary EBV infection. The pattern of antibody responses can help the practitioner in determining the date of onset of an individual's EBV infection. In most cases an individual develops a VCA-IgM antibody response in the acute period following an EBV infection. The same is true for the VCA-IgG antibody. Although IgG antibodies to the VCA persist for life, VCA-IgM tends to disappear in 2 to 3 months. Although the height of the VCA-IgG response decreases as the acute infection resolves, serial measurements of antibody titers are not clinically beneficial as a rule. The EA response peaks at 3 to 4 weeks into the illness and was initially thought to persist only for several months; therefore it also was considered a good marker for an acute or recent infection. However, recent evidence suggests that the EA response may persist for years in some children and may not develop at all in others.[8] Finally, the EBNA antibody response usually appears several weeks to months

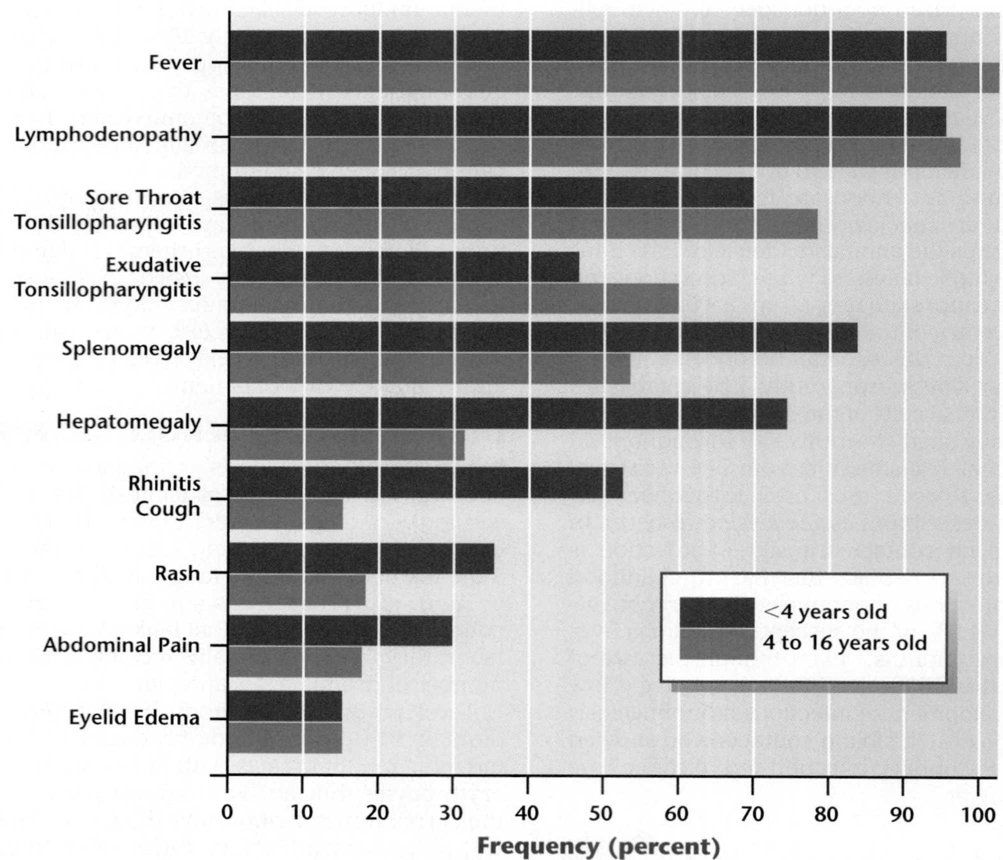

Figure 283-1 Frequency of clinical findings in 2 age groups of children with documented Epstein-Barr virus infectious mononucleosis: younger than 4 years and 4 to 16 years of age. *(Sumaya CV, Ench Y. Epstein-Barr virus infectious mononucleosis in children. I. Clinical and general laboratory findings.* Pediatrics. *1985;75:1003-1010.)*

after a primary infection and is therefore thought to be a marker for a past or convalescent infection. However, even this antibody response has to be interpreted in light of the clinical situation because a large number of children develop this response in the acute phase of their infection; 10% to 20% of individuals never develop detectable levels of antibody to EBNA.[9] In summary, children who acquire EBV infections typically develop antibodies in the same sequential pattern (Table 283-1); however, not all patients will necessarily follow the same pattern, and clinical judgment remains important in the interpretation of such findings. Additionally, interlaboratory variability in results of EBV antibody testing has been observed, making the reliability of these tests suspect in some cases. If both the heterophil test and specific serologic findings are negative, then causes for a non-EBV infectious mononucleosis–like illness should be suspected.

COMPLICATIONS AND DEATHS

Most persons who have infectious mononucleosis recover uneventfully. Serious complications, however, have resulted from this illness; death occurs in approximately 1 in 3000 cases. The true complication and death rates during this illness are uncertain because many reports do not include strict diagnostic criteria for infectious mononucleosis. The relative frequencies of more common complications associated with this illness, as documented in one large study, are listed in Table 283-2.[7] Many other complications, representing virtually every body organ, have also been reported with this disease.

Of 20 deaths clearly associated with infectious mononucleosis in one series,[10] 9 cases were of neurologic origin, 3 were caused by secondary infection, 3 by splenic rupture, 2 by hepatic failure, 1 by probable myocarditis, and 2 from an undetermined cause. Because abdominal pain is an infrequent symptom of this illness, its appearance, particularly if severe and in the left upper quadrant, should alert the clinician to the possibility of impending or actual splenic rupture. Fatal cases of Reye syndrome associated with serological evidence of EBV infection also have been reported.[11]

MANAGEMENT

Because most patients who have infectious mononucleosis recover uneventfully, physicians need do little except establish the diagnosis, explain the nature of the illness, and reassure the parents. No specific therapy is indicated. Patients should rest to the extent that they believe necessary. As long as the patient can consume adequate amounts of fluids and calories, hospitalization is unnecessary. To minimize the danger of splenic rupture, ambulatory patients should avoid strenuous physical exercise or contact sports for at least one month or until the spleen is no longer palpable. Patients who have late onset of the heterophil antibody response appear to have a prolonged convalescence.

Table 283-2 Complications Present in 113 Children With Epstein-Barr Virus Infectious Mononucleosis

COMPLICATION	NUMBER OF CHILDREN (%)
RESPIRATORY TRACT	
Pneumonia	6 (5.3)
Severe airway obstruction*	4 (3.5)
NEUROLOGIC	
Seizures	4 (3.5)
Meningitis, encephalitis	2 (1.8)
Peripheral facial nerve paralysis	1 (0.9)
Guillain-Barré syndrome	1 (0.9)
HEMATOLOGIC	
Thrombocytopenia with hemorrhages	4 (3.5)
Hemolytic anemia	1 (0.9)
INFECTIOUS	
Bacteremia	1 (0.9)
Recurrent tonsillopharyngitis	3 (2.7)
LIVER	
Jaundice	2 (1.8)
RENAL	
Glomerulonephritis	1 (0.9)
GENITAL	
Orchitis	1 (0.9)
TOTAL	31†

*Criteria consisted of nasal alar flaring, suprasternal retractions, or stridor.
†Because 4 children had more than 1 of these complications, this total is composed of 24 different children, or 21.2% of the study group.
From Sumaya CV, Ench Y. Epstein-Barr virus infectious mononucleosis in children. I. Clinical and general laboratory findings. *Pediatrics.* 1985;75:1003-1010.

Table 283-1 Interpretation of Epstein-Barr Virus Serology

	HETEROPHIL ANTIBODY	EPSTEIN-BARR VIRUS ANTIBODIES			
		VCA-IgM	VCA-IgG	EA	EBNA
No infection	–	–	–	–	–
Acute infection	+/–	+	+ (>1:320)	+/–	–
Past infection	–	–	+ (1:80-1:160)	+/–	+

Note: Other patterns may occur in an individual patient; the above profile is for a typical individual.
EA, Early antigen; *EBNA,* IgG antibody to Epstein-Barr nuclear antigen; *VAC-IgG,* IgG antibody to viral capsid antigen; *VCA-IgM,* IgM antibody to viral capsid antigen.
From Sumaya CV, Ench Y. Epstein-Barr virus infectious mononucleosis in children. I. Clinical and general laboratory findings. *Pediatrics.* 1985;75:1003-1010.

Corticosteroids are of unproved value in treating this illness.[12] They should not be used routinely merely to make the patient feel better. Most clinicians believe that their use is justified in treating severe hemolytic anemia, significant airway obstruction secondary to tonsillar hypertrophy, and thrombocytopenia. However, controlled studies documenting their efficacy for these indications are lacking. Some authorities suggest using corticosteroids if neurologic involvement is significant; but again, proof of efficacy is not available. High-dose, short-term courses of steroids (dexamethasone [0.25 mg/kg every 6 hours], methylprednisolone [1 mg/kg every 6 hours], oral prednisone [40 mg/day]) have been used with dramatic improvement typically noted over 24 to 72 hours.[13] The antiviral agent acyclovir has good activity against EBV in vitro, but it has not been shown to be beneficial in a number of clinical trials that involve patients who had infectious mononucleosis. At this time, routine use is not recommended. Several antivirals (acyclovir, ganciclovir, vidarabine) and immunomodulating agents (interferon-γ, interferon-α, interleukin-2) have been used in severe EBV infections, with varying degrees of success.[14] Novel therapeutic approaches under investigation for the treatment of EBV-associated lymphoproliferative disease include bone marrow transplantation, treatment with monoclonal antibodies, and infusions of donor peripheral leukocytes.

Inasmuch as the pharyngitis of infectious mononucleosis can be indistinguishable from that of streptococcal pharyngitis, culture specimens of the pharynx should be obtained, and patients who have positive culture findings should be treated accordingly. The clinician should avoid using ampicillin or amoxicillin this infection is suspected, given that rash develops in most young adults with EBV infection who receive this drug. The ampicillin effect has not been well demonstrated in young children who have infectious mononucleosis.

Because secondary infection in typical college settings is low, strict isolation of the patient is unnecessary. Instead, separation of drinking and eating utensils (eg, avoiding drinking from the same glass) is all that is required.

Accounts are increasing (although still rare) of infectious mononucleosis episodes that are quite severe, fatal, or result in significant long-lasting problems. Most of these patients had some form of immunological abnormality, that is, X-linked lymphoproliferative syndrome, renal or bone marrow transplant, or Chédiak-Higashi syndrome, among others. The definitive management of these patients remains unclear.

EPSTEIN-BARR VIRUS INFECTION AND CHRONIC FATIGUE SYNDROME

In the 1980s, several reports described individuals who reportedly developed a chronic EBV or mononucleosis-like syndrome following a bout of acute mononucleosis.[6,15] These patients never seemed to recover completely from their acute illnesses and complained of persistent fatigue, pharyngitis, lymphadenitis, and low-grade fevers. Subsequent studies, however, demonstrated normal immune responses to EBV and clearance of the virus in these patients. These individuals today fall under the rubric of chronic fatigue syndrome, a chronic, debilitating illness characterized by extreme fatigue, neuropsychological abnormalities, and a myriad of other problems. Although many patients who have chronic fatigue syndrome date the onset of their illness to an episode of infectious mononucleosis, virologic and clinical studies have confirmed that active EBV infection is not responsible for the illness. At present, no single infectious or other cause has been identified for chronic fatigue syndrome (see Chapter 247, Chronic Fatigue Syndrome).

EPSTEIN-BARR VIRUS–NEGATIVE INFECTIOUS MONONUCLEOSIS

Rubella, hepatitis, toxoplasmosis, cytomegalovirus, human herpesvirus-6 and adenovirus infections, systemic lupus erythematosus, and drug reactions can produce symptoms similar to those of EBV infection. Negative EBV titers and heterophil antibody responses strongly suggest one of these other agents or conditions as the cause of the illness under consideration. In hepatitis, in which the heterophil test can give a false-positive result, liver enzyme levels generally are much more elevated than those seen with infectious mononucleosis. Results of serologic tests for hepatitis will be positive, as will rubella titers in rubella infection; cytomegalovirus can be cultured from urine in those who have that infection as the cause of their illness. Illnesses that mimic infectious mononucleosis but lack serologic confirmation of EBV infection should be classified as heterophil-negative infectious mononucleosis rather than atypical mononucleosis. The cause of most of these cases remains unknown.

EPSTEIN-BARR VIRUS INFECTION AND MALIGNANCY

Lymphocytes that contain the EBV genome can divide indefinitely. The virus remains dormant in human hosts for prolonged periods. These observations, together with the known association of EBV and African Burkitt lymphoma and nasopharyngeal carcinoma, have raised speculation that EBV infection might be oncogenic in the United States as well.[16] Some cases of leukemia occurring shortly after the onset of infectious mononucleosis have been reported, but no other evidence exists to support this speculation. Although in the United States the association between EBV and classic Burkitt lymphoma is not as strong as in Africa, a significant number of lymphomas and lymphoproliferative lesions that contain EBV markers (including markers of viral replication) have been found in patients in the United States. The EBV genome can be detected in approximately 50% of Reed-Sternberg cells found in patients with the mixed cellularity form of Hodgkin lymphoma.[17] However, whether EBV is a causal agent or even a cofactor for Hodgkin disease in unknown. EBV has also been associated with several lymphoreticular malignancies in patients who have AIDS. These malignancies include malignant B-cell lymphoma and colonic lymphoid hyperplasia. Additionally, EBV has been associated with oral hairy leukoplakia and lymphoid interstitial pneumonitis in individuals with AIDS. The precise relationship between EBV and malignancies remains unknown and is the subject of intense investigation.

WHEN TO REFER

- Hospitalization may be necessary in the presence of airway compromise, splenic rupture, neurologic complications, or severe hemolytic anemia or thrombocytopenia.
- Consultation with appropriate subspecialists for the above complications would also be warranted.

TOOLS FOR PRACTICE

Medical Decision Support

- *Epstein-Barr Virus and Infectious Mononucleosis* (fact sheet), Centers for Disease Control and Prevention (www.cdc.gov/ncidod/diseases/ebv.htm).
- *Infectious Mononucleosis* (book), Medline Plus (www.nlm.nih.gov/medlineplus/infectiousmononucleosis.html).
- Red Book: 2006 Report of the Committee on Infectious Diseases, 27th edition, American Academy of Pediatrics (www.aap.org/bookstore).

SUGGESTED RESOURCES

Schuster V, Kreth HW. Epstein-Barr virus infection and associated diseases in children. I. Pathogenesis, epidemiology and clinical aspects. *Eur J Pediatr.* 1992;151:718-725.

Schuster V, Kreth HW. Epstein-Barr virus infection and associated diseases in children. II. Diagnostic and therapeutic strategies. *Eur J Pediatr.* 1992;151:794-798.

Straus SE, Cohen JI, Tosato G, et al. Epstein-Barr virus infections: biology, pathogenesis and management. *Ann Intern Med.* 1993;118:45-58.

REFERENCES

1. Andiman WA. The Epstein-Barr virus and EB virus infections in childhood. *J Pediatr.* 1979;95:171-182.
2. Sumaya CV, Ench Y. Epstein-Barr virus infections in families: the role of children with infectious mononucleosis. *J Infect Dis.* 1986;154:842-850.
3. Schooley RT. Epstein-Barr virus (infectious mononucleosis). In: Mandell GL, Bennett JE, Dolin R, eds. *Principles and Practice of Infectious Diseases.* Philadelphia, PA: Churchill Livingstone; 2000.
4. Sumaya CV, Ench Y. Epstein-Barr virus infectious mononucleosis in children. II. Heterophil antibody and viral-specific responses. *Pediatrics.* 1985;75:1011-1019.
5. Sumaya CV, Ench Y. Epstein-Barr virus infectious mononucleosis in children. I. Clinical and general laboratory findings. *Pediatrics.* 1985;75:1003-1010.
6. Jones JF, Ray CG, Minnich LL, et al. Evidence for active Epstein-Barr virus infections in patients with persistent, unexplained illness: elevated anti-early antigen antibodies. *Ann Intern Med.* 1985;102:1-7.
7. Karzon DT. Infectious mononucleosis. *Adv Pediatr.* 1976;22:231-265.
8. Centers for Disease Control and Prevention, National Center for Infectious Diseases. Epstein-Barr Virus and Infectious Mononucleosis. Available at: www.cdc.gov/ncidod/diseases/ebv.htm. Accessed July 6, 2007.
9. Vetter V, Kreutzer L, Bauer G. Differentiation of primary from secondary anti-EBNA-1 negative cases by determination of VCA-IgG. *Clin Diag Virol.* 1994;2:29-39.
10. Penman HG. Fatal infectious mononucleosis: a critical review. *J Clin Pathol.* 1970;23:765-771.
11. Fleisher G, Schwartz, Lennette E. Primary Epstein-Barr virus infection in association with Reye's syndrome. *J Pediatr.* 1980;97:935-937.
12. Collins M, Fleisher G, Kreisberg J, et al. Role of steroids in the treatment of infectious mononucleosis in the ambulatory college student. *J Am Coll Health Assoc.* 1984;33:101-105.
13. Anderson J, Ernberg I. Management of Epstein-Barr virus infections. *Am J Med.* 1988;85:107-115.
14. Okano M. Epstein-Barr virus infection and its role in the expanding spectrum of human disease. *Acta Paediatr.* 1998;87:11-18.
15. Straus SE, Tosato G, Armstrong G, et al. Persisting illness and fatigue in adults with evidence of Epstein-Barr virus infection. *Ann Intern Med.* 1985;102:7-16.
16. Giffin BE, Xue S. Epstein-Barr virus infections and their association with human malignancies: some key questions. *Ann Med.* 1998;30:249-259.
17. Pallesen G, Hamilton-Dutoit SJ, Rowe M, et al. Expression of Epstein-Barr latent gene products in tumour cells of Hodgkin's disease. *Lancet.* 1991;320:320-322.

Chapter 284

INSECT BITES AND INFESTATIONS

David H. Stein, MD, MPH, MSt; Nancy K. Barnett, MD

INSECT BITES

Insect bites and stings,[1] though a regular consequence of childhood activities, sometimes cause illness and can be life threatening in susceptible individuals. Insects and arachnids (mites, ticks, and spiders) are often vectors of serious or fatal disease, including viral encephalitis and malaria; worldwide, malaria is still one of the most common causes of serious childhood morbidity and death. Ticks are the most common insect vectors of disease in the United States, spreading Lyme disease and other infections.[2] Species of insects or arachnids causing bites or infestation vary over time and with geography. For example, bedbug infestations have increased in incidence, recently reaching epidemic proportions in several United States' cities (Figure 284-1).[3]

On examination, discrete, erythematous or flesh-colored papules, nodules, or wheals, which are usually pruritic, suggest the diagnosis of insect or arachnid bites (Figure 284-2). Bites are often grouped and are most commonly found on surfaces not covered by clothing. They may be clustered in a linear or arcuate pattern, especially when caused by a crawling insect (Figure 284-3). Some bites have central puncta or vesicles; others are capped by pustules or by hemorrhagic or serous crusts. Excoriations created by scratching are common. Larger nodules or blisters are robust reactions to insect- or arachnid-associated toxins, particularly in those with prior exposure (sensitization) to insect antigens. In an unsensitized child, discomfort varies from mild itch to pain caused by

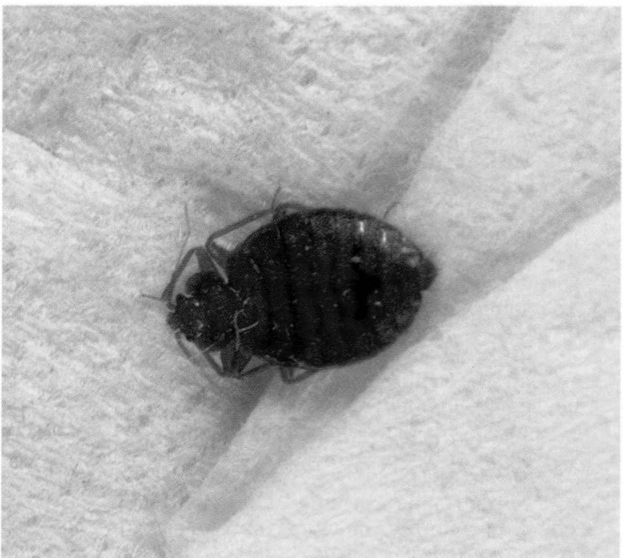

Figure 284-1 Bed bug. Note the flattened, oval body of this bug, which was brought in to the clinic by the patient's mother. *(Krowchuck DP, Mancini AJ, eds.* Pediatric Dermatology: A Quick Reference Guide. *Elk Grove Village, IL: American Academy of Pediatrics; 2007.)*

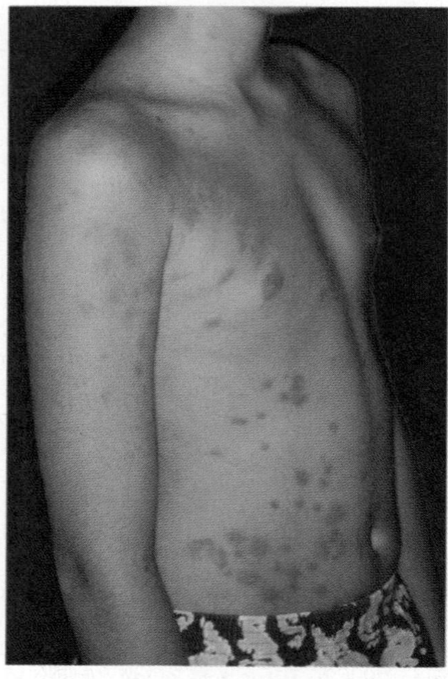

Figure 284-2 Mite bites. Multiple, clustered, edematous red papules and plaques. *(Krowchuck DP, Mancini AJ, eds.* Pediatric Dermatology: A Quick Reference Guide. *Elk Grove Village, IL: American Academy of Pediatrics; 2007.)*

toxin injection; an aggravating intense pruritus also may occur, especially in a sensitized child.

Complications of bites include infection; eczematous changes resulting in inflamed plaques; localized

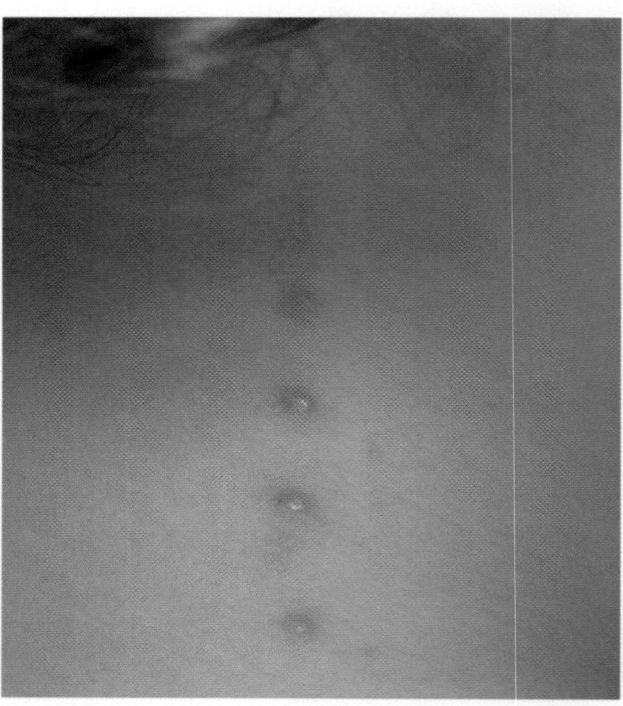

Figure 284-3 Flea bites. Note the *breakfast, lunch, and dinner* sign. *(Krowchuck DP, Mancini AJ, eds.* Pediatric Dermatology: A Quick Reference Guide. *Elk Grove Village, IL: American Academy of Pediatrics; 2007.)*

hypersensitivity reactions, including papular urticaria; and systemic reactions. Infection can vary from impetigo to cellulitis. Eczematous changes result from scratching or from topical remedies that cause irritant or allergic contact dermatitis. For example, neomycin, commonly used as a topical antibiotic, is a common topical allergen. Systemic infections, such as viral encephalitis or tickborne disease, should also be considered as potential complications, necessitating more thorough follow-up or consideration of hospital observation. Clearly, bacterial infections resulting as a complication of bites or infestations can lead to cellulitis or a multitude of toxin-induced or immune-mediated complications such as nephritis.

Papular urticaria[4] is a common hypersensitivity reaction to insect bites. These consist of recurrent crops of urticarial (hive-like) papules, nodules, or wheals on exposed surfaces that may be either new or reactivated old bites. Papular urticaria occurs in certain sensitized individuals and can last weeks or months, plaguing the patient with profound itch, especially if repeatedly scratched or otherwise traumatized. Scratching can leave scarring or postinflammatory pigment change, most often hyperpigmentation. Unlike the infestations, only one or a few family members are generally affected. Bites from insects can be controlled first by covering as much of the body as possible with clothing and then by judicious use of repellents, especially N, N-diethyl-m-toluamide (DEET) at exposed areas (avoiding children's hands, eyes, and mouth areas). Some controversy surrounds the use of DEET, which can cause central nervous system and systemic symptoms in children (see www.aap.org/healthtopics/environmentalhealth.cfm). However, DEET is usually safe to use intermittently and in moderation at concentrations of 30% or less[5] in children older than 2 months. and alternate repellents may be less effective and also toxic.[6] Mosquitoes are attracted by carbon dioxide and lactic acid from the breath and skin, but susceptibility to mosquito bites may be decreased by avoiding other potential attractants, such as bright clothing.[7] When available, the use of bed nets impregnated with repellents can be extremely effective in preventing bites.

Treatment of Insect Bites

Topical antipruritics such as calamine are sometimes soothing, as are cold soaks or ice. Topical corticosteroid creams reduce inflammation and pruritus and are usually the primary treatment along with cold packs and oral antihistamines to relieve pruritus. Topical antihistamines should be avoided; they may cause allergic contact dermatitis and are usually ineffective.

In very rare cases, for extensive bites with ensuing hypersensitivity manifesting as papular urticaria or in other ways that involve over 20% of the body, a 1-week or shorter course of oral systemic steroid at approximately 0.5 mg/kg of prednisone or equivalent might be considered. All contraindications must be excluded, and topical therapy should be started at the same time to prevent a rebound phenomenon. However, longer-term or chronic treatment is not indicated for this circumstance alone, and the risk of adverse events, though small with brief treatment courses, must be considered.

PEDICULOSIS

Lice infestation of the scalp is called pediculosis capitis (see Figure 284-1) and infestation of the eyelashes is pediculosis palpebrum. When the limbs and trunk are primarily involved, infestation is referred to as pediculosis corporis, and pubic area involvement is called pediculosis pubis.[8] Lice are obligate human ectoparasites that create pruritic dermatoses after their bites puncture the skin and inject saliva; the saliva incites inflammation and sometimes hypersensitivity. Lice can also transmit diseases, including typhus.

Lice are spread primarily by close personal contact and occasionally by fomites but the body louse is primarily spread by clothing. Outbreaks of head lice occur mainly among school-aged children (Figure 284-4). The grayish, crawling, 6-legged louse may be seen in areas of thick terminal hair growth close to the scalp. Louse eggs, called nits, may be seen as minute, white-gray fixed attachments to hair shafts. Pruritus, sometimes accompanied by erythematous papules, 1 to 2 mm in diameter and presumably caused by bites of the head louse, may be noted around the nape of the neck and the hairline, especially posteriorly. Cervical adenopathy and occasionally urticarial-like changes or involvement of other body areas may be present.

Nits or the insects themselves may be visible on the eyelashes or pubic hair. Transmission of pediculosis is frequent between individuals who sleep in the same bed or otherwise maintain close contact; therefore family members should be examined, especially if combs, towels, and other personal items are shared.[9] Pediculosis pubis is often sexually transmitted, and affected individuals may have other sexually transmitted infections.

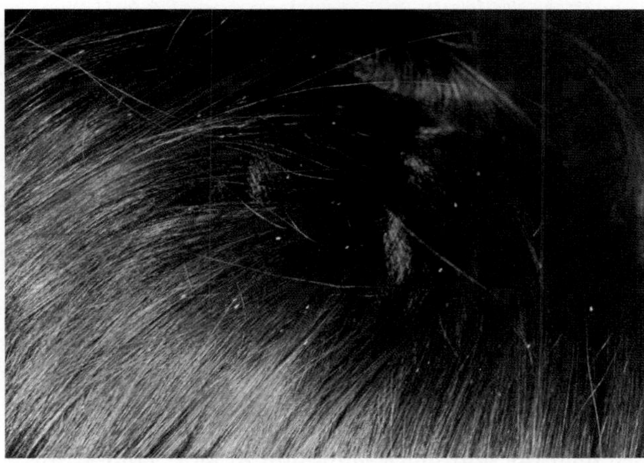

Figure 284-4 Head lice. Note numerous nits attached to hair shafts. *(Krowchuck DP, Mancini AJ, eds.* Pediatric Dermatology: A Quick Reference Guide. *Elk Grove Village, IL: American Academy of Pediatrics; 2007.)*

Pediculosis corporis should be suspected when widespread pruritus is present. In most instances, the body louse is not found on the body; rather, it and its nits are seen in the seams of clothing or bedding. The bites consist of erythematous macules and papules. Papules are often obscured by the results of scratching, including excoriation, impetiginization, eczematization, overt infection, and pigmentation.

Treatment of Pediculosis

For head lice or pubic lice, permethrin, pyrethrins, and malathion are most often the drugs of choice, but resistance to all chemical agents is increasing. Recently, careful repeated physical removal of lice and eggs using a kit for head lice has shown superior results, even compared with malathion.[10] However, this method or the use of chemical agents depends on following instructions carefully. Insecticides other than malathion or pyrethrins, especially lindane (gamma-benzene hexachloride [GBH]), are definitely more toxic and probably less effective with much resistance. Furthermore, the California legislature has banned lindane for human use because of its recognition as a water pollutant. Pyrethrins are found in several nonprescription preparations. Nix cream rinse contains 1% permethrin; it and other similar prescription products may be effective in some cases of head lice. A fine-toothed comb can be used to remove nits from hair shafts after chemical treatment. Retreatment is usually necessary about 1 week after the 1st application to kill lice that have hatched from viable nits that were not killed initially. Malathion used as a 0.5% solution must be left on for 8 to 12 hours and is a flammable preparation. Dimethicone 4% has recently been found to be effective.[11]

Two doses of oral ivermectin given 7 days apart have been shown to be effective in the treatment of several kinds of lice infestation, though this application is an off-label use.[12]

Chemical treatments for pediculosis (or for scabies) are used only with great caution by pregnant or nursing women and should be avoided by persons who have allergies to any component of the treatment. Infants should not be treated unless essential and only with very close supervision.

Clothing, bedding, combs, towels, and other items used by lice-infested persons should be washed in hot water. The most effective treatment for body lice is the total-body application of 5% permethrin cream (Elimite) for 8 to 14 hours. Simultaneously, all potentially infested clothing should be treated with wet or dry heat (or both) at a minimum of 65°C (149°F) for a minimum of 15 minutes but preferably at least 30 minutes.[1,2,6] Resistance of lice to chemical treatments has emerged; thus a limited number of treatments spaced approximately 7 days apart with various pediculicides such as permethrin, GBH, and pyrethrins may be required to eradicate lice. The application of Elimite 5% permethrin cream to the hair may be necessary. A vinegar rinse may help remove stubborn nits. All clothing, stuffed animals, comforters, and other items that cannot be washed or dry cleaned should be stored in a plastic bag and sealed for 2 weeks.

No-nit policies aimed at excluding children from school are often ineffective because overlooking nits is easy, and such policies penalize children excessively by causing missed school days. The American Academy of Pediatrics recommends avoiding such policies.[13]

Pruritus may continue for 2 weeks or more after treatment, perhaps because of continued irritancy of dead lice or because the topical pediculicides cause irritant dermatitis. Patients should be advised that they might continue to itch so that they do not overtreat themselves through excessive repeated applications. Oral antipruritics, soothing bland lotions, and topical steroids can help control pruritus. Additional current information for patients and providers is available at www.cdc.gov/ncidod/dpd/parasites/lice/default.htm.

Pediculosis palpebrum can be treated by applying plain petrolatum to the eyelashes 3 to 5 times daily. Treatment is required for approximately 8 to 10 days, and a moustache comb can be used daily to remove lice and nits from the eyelashes. Other infested body areas should be treated simultaneously. If this method fails, then physostigmine 0.25% may be similarly applied to eyelashes and is usually curative in 3 or 4 days but may interfere with vision.[6]

Pediculosis pubis is also treated with permethrin or pyrethrins, usually at 5% concentration. Nonprescription pyrethrin preparations are probably less effective, and optimal lengths of application are shortest with permethrins.

SCABIES

Infestation with the mite, *Sarcoptes scabiei hominis*, causes scabies,[14] normally a highly pruritic dermatosis with varied and protean manifestations ranging from rare scattered erythematous papules to widespread eczematous dermatitis, excoriations, and multiple areas of mite-laden crusting. This later presentation is called *Norwegian scabies*, and possibly infectious complications of any presentation.

Scabies[15,16] is generally spread by close personal contact, usually through persistent or repeated skin-to-skin contact, such as individuals sleeping in the same bed or holding a child closely. Family members, sexual partners, and other close contacts of index cases should be examined when possible but, in general, should always be treated, regardless of symptoms because they may be asymptomatic carriers. In many instances, the patient's history will reveal that several people in 1 household are itching. This contrasts with papular urticaria caused by insect bites in which frequently only the patient is affected. Fomites rarely transmit scabies, especially in temperate climates. Although humans may acquire subspecies of scabies mites that infest other mammals, such infestation is self-limiting, given that other mite subspecies do not reproduce in human skin.

The burrowing of the female mite into the stratum corneum initiates infestation. Eggs are laid within the stratum corneum, and over the next 2 to 6 weeks, itching and papules develop gradually as the eggs hatch and the host develops delayed hypersensitivity. Repeated infestation of a host with hypersensitivity to mite antigens frequently leads to more rapid development of itching and other manifestations, often within 24 to 96 hours.

The burrows created by female mites help establish the diagnosis; however, they are not always obvious and are present in fewer than one half of all patients. Burrows are most often found in the finger webs or on the wrist area but are often disguised by excoriations, eczematous reactions, or superimposed infection. Common sites of infestation, with findings of papules, nodules, eczematous changes, or excoriations, are the digital web spaces, the extensor surface of the elbows and knees, and the flexor aspect of the wrists, as well as the axillary, upper trunk, and groin area. In infants, involvement of the palms and soles, especially with vesicles, is common as are skin changes on the face and head. Confirmatory ova, mites, or feces are sometimes found by light microscopy of scrapings of burrows or papules from these locations; the burrows or papules are scraped off with a scalpel blade after a drop of mineral oil is placed on the skin and the scrapings are examined under low magnification.

The papules, pustules, vesicles, and even urticarial plaques that can occur in sarcoptic infestation justify the reputation of scabies as a great masquerader. In the setting of worsening or persistent widespread pruritus, a diagnosis of scabies must be considered, especially if close contacts are also itching. The distribution of skin changes is often the best clue to the diagnosis along with itching that is more widespread than the objective skin findings.

Treatment of Scabies

The thorough application of 5% permethrin to the entire body, except the face, is the treatment of choice as of this writing because of the efficacy and relatively low toxicity of permethrins. An alternate treatment is lindane or a similar GBH preparation. However, lindane is probably less effective, and adverse reactions from overuse of GBH preparations have raised concern about toxicity from percutaneous absorption. When used properly, lindane, GBH, and other insecticides can be safe and effective, but they should be dispensed in limited quantities. Parents should be informed about possible neurotoxicity and other complications from organophosphate exposure. Repeated treatments, especially when based only on symptoms and not clear objective demonstration of treatment failure, should be actively discouraged. Although either treatment can cause an irritant dermatitis, lindane is much more likely to do so. Current literature lacks population-based studies demonstrating the efficacy of malathion, another toxic organophosphate insecticide.

Crotamiton 10% (Eurax) is probably less efficacious, must be applied at least twice, and is used less frequently in the United States. Benzyl benzoate is used widely as an inexpensive emulsion and is sometimes recommended by the World Health Organization, although it is not available in the United States.[15]

If topical treatment fails or is not feasible, then oral ivermectin at appropriate dosing for weight is highly effective. Although not approved for this indication by the US Food and Drug Administration, ivermectin has been widely used for this indication. Published clinical data in young children are limited. Two doses, separated by approximately 1 to 2 weeks, may be necessary in some cases.[15]

Epidemiologic studies have demonstrated a high rate of spread within families and between individuals sleeping in the same bed. Therefore bed linens, clothing, and towels should always be washed in hot water immediately after the treatment of all individuals in the same household.

Although pruritus and rash often persist for at least 2 to 4 weeks or longer after successful eradication of an infestation because of continued hypersensitivity, repeat treatment should be undertaken only when continued infestation with live mites is clearly demonstrated. Pruritus alone can be treated with oral antihistamines or with mild topical agents such as emollients, pramoxine, or very minimal concentrations of menthol. Some individuals develop red to purple discrete nodules up to 2 cm in diameter on surfaces usually covered by clothing, particularly on the genitals or around the axillae, and these nodules may persist for months. These *nodular scabies* or *post-scabetic nodules* are thought to represent a hypersensitivity reaction. The nodules usually respond to topical or intralesional injections of steroids. Additional precautions regarding chemical treatments outlined previously for pediculosis apply for scabies.

Complications of scabies, pediculosis, or other infestations, such as bacterial infection with toxin producing strains or cellulitis, may necessitate systemic treatment, especially in immune-suppressed children.

WHEN TO REFER

- The patient may be referred to allergists if the patient develops severe allergic reaction to insect bites, especially repeatedly, or if hymenoptera allergy is suspected.

WHEN TO ADMIT

- If the patient has severe systemic allergic reactions to insect bites
- If the patient needs intravenous antibiotics to treat secondary bacterial infection or cellulitis
- If the patient develops noninfectious complications such as acute postinfectious glomerulonephritis and hypertension
- If the patient is suspected of having contracted viral meningitis or other severe or systemic illness through insect bites

TOOLS FOR PRACTICE

Engaging Patient and Family

- *A Parent's Guide to Insect Repellents* (brochure), American Academy of Pediatrics (patiented.aap.org).
- *Head Lice: Every Parent's Concern* (brochure), American Academy of Pediatrics (patiented.aap.org).
- *Head Lice Infestation* (fact sheet), Centers for Disease Control and Prevention (www.cdc.gov/ncidod/dpd/parasites/lice/factsht_head_lice.htm).
- *Treating Head Lice Infestation* (fact sheet), Centers for Disease Control and Prevention (www.cdc.gov/ncidod/dpd/parasites/lice/factsht_head_lice_treating.htm).
- *What You Need to Know about Mosquito Repellent* (fact sheet), Centers for Disease Control and Prevention (www.cdc.gov/ncidod/dvbid/westnile/mosquitorepellent.htm/).

Medical Decision Support

- *Head Lice—lab assistance* (Web page), Centers for Disease Control and Prevention (www.dpd.cdc.gov/dpdx/HTML/HeadLice.htm).
- *Lice Infestation* (fact sheet), Centers for Disease Control and Prevention (www.cdc.gov/ncidod/dpd/parasites/lice/default.htm).
- *Pediatric Dermatology: A Quick Reference Guide* (book), American Academy of Pediatrics (www.aap.org/bookstore).
- *Scabies—lab assistance* (Web page), Centers for Disease Control and Prevention (www.dpd.cdc.gov/dpdx/HTML/Scabies.htm).
- *West Nile Virus* (Web page), American Academy of Pediatrics (www.aap.org/family/wnv.htm).

AAP POLICY STATEMENT

Frankowski BL, Weiner LB, American Academy of Pediatrics, Committee on School Health and Committee on Infectious Diseases. Clinical report: head lice. *Pediatrics*. 2002;110(3):638-643. (aappolicy.aappublications.org/cgi/content/full/pediatrics;110/3/638).

SUGGESTED READINGS

Strong M, Johnstone PW. Interventions for treating scabies. Cochrane Database Syst Rev. 2007 Jul 18;(3):CD000320. Review. PMID: 17636630.

Chosidow O. Clinical practices. Scabies. *N Engl J Med*. 2006; 354(16):1718-1727.

Lebwohl M, Clark L, Levitt J. Therapy for head lice based on life cycle, resistance, and safety considerations. *Pediatrics*. 2007;119(5):965-974.

REFERENCES

1. Steen CJ, Carbonaro PA, Schwartz RA. Arthropods in dermatology. *J Am Acad Dermatol.* 2004;50:819-842.
2. Jones TF, Garman RL, LaFleur B, et al. Risk factors for tick exposure and suboptimal adherence to preventive recommendations. *Am J Prev Med.* 2002;23:47-50.
3. Ter Porten MC, Prose NS. The return of the common bedbug. *Pediatr Dermatol.* 2005;22:183-187.
4. Garcia E, Halpert E, Rodriquez A, et al. Immune and histologic examination of flea bite-induced papular urticaria. *Ann Allergy Asthma Immunol.* 2004;92:446-452.
5. Centers for Disease Control and Prevention. What You Need to Know About Mosquito Repellent. Available at: www.cdc.gov/ncidod/dvbid/westnile/mosquitorepellent.htm. Accessed December 31, 2005.
6. Buka RL. Sunscreens and insect repellents. *Curr Opin Pediatr.* 2004;4:378-384.
7. Fradin MS. Mosquitoes and mosquito repellents: a clinician's guide. *Ann Intern Med.* 1998;128:931.
8. Ko CJ, Elston DM. Pediculosis. *J Am Acad Dermatol.* 2004;50:1-12.
9. Hansen R. Overview: the state of head lice management and control. *Am J Manag Care.* 2004;10:S260-S264.
10. Hill N, Moor G, Cameron MM, et al. Single blind, randomised, comparative study of the bug buster kit and over the counter pediculicide treatments against head lice in the United Kingdom. *BMJ.* 2005;331:384-387.
11. Burgess IF, Brown CM, Lee PN. Treatment of head louse infestation with 4% dimethicone lotion: randomized controlled equivalence trial. *BMJ.* 2005;330:1423-1426.
12. Dourmishev AL, Dourmishev LA, Schwartz RA. Ivermectin: pharmacology and application in dermatology. *Int J Dermatol.* 2005;44:981-988.
13. Frankowski BL, Weiner LB. Head lice. *Pediatrics.* 2002; 110(3):638-643.
14. Centers for Disease Control and Prevention, National Center for Infectious Diseases, Department of Pediatric Diagnoses. Scabies. Available at: www.dpd.cdc.gov/dpdx/html/scabies.htm. Accessed December 10, 2005.
15. Johnson G, Sladden M. Scabies: diagnosis and treatment. *BMJ.* 2005;331:619-622.
16. Hengge UR, Currie BJ, Jager G, et al. Scabies: a ubiquitous neglected skin disease. *Lancet Infect Dis.* 2006;6:769-779.

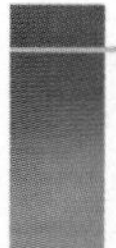

Chapter 285

INTELLECTUAL DISABILITY

Randall A. Phelps, MD, PhD; William I. Cohen, MD

DEFINITIONS

More than 50 years ago, the term *mental retardation* replaced terms such as idiot, imbecile, and moron as the descriptor of choice to describe intellectual disability. Because the term mental retardation has now acquired a pejorative connotation, the membership of the American Association on Mental Retardation has recently voted to change its name to the American Association on Intellectual and Developmental Disabilities (AAIDD).[1] Currently, however, this change in terminology does not match the current legal definition for entitlement to services for individuals with intellectual disability. For individuals who meet the diagnostic criteria, the label of mental retardation remains essential to obtaining a variety of educational and social services. Therefore primary care physicians should continue to use this term to assist their clients in obtaining appropriate supports[2] until such time as the legal and statutory language changes. However, intellectual disability is the preferred synonym for mental retardation.

In 2002 the AAIDD published 5 important elements to serve as guidelines for the accurate use of the term *intellectual disability*[3]:

1. The level of functioning of an individual should be considered within their particular social and cultural context.
2. Any assessment of cognitive and adaptive ability should take into account communication, as well as sensory, motor, and behavioral functioning.
3. An individual's strengths must be emphasized in assessments and included in support plans.
4. The purpose of assessing limitations is to guide the development of appropriate supports for the individual in question.
5. The provision of individualized supports is expected to improve functioning significantly.

Implicit in these guidelines is the understanding that, though cognitive and adaptive impairments are not reversible, intellectual disability can be ameliorated by environmental modifications and supports.

Much confusion exists about a variety of terms used to describe children who are not developing as expected. One commonly used term is *developmental delay,* which reflects functioning at less than 75% of expectations for chronologic age in a particular developmental domain (eg, gross motor, fine motor, cognition, communication). Some children experience this development in a single domain, whereas others have delays in multiple or all domains. Conceptually, this term suggests the child will at sometime make up the delay, as would the train that finally arrives at the destination. Such catch-up frequently does occur in the case of delays in isolated domains (eg, in expressive language). On the other hand, clearly, the child who is delayed in all domains, though frequently described as having *global developmental delay,* is less likely to catch up. This situation is particularly true the greater the magnitude of the delay. In general, psychologists are hesitant to describe these children as having intellectual disability until they are approximately at the age of school entry. At a practical level, this hesitation allows parents to focus on interventions that maximize the child's potential while minimizing the focus on what the child cannot accomplish. Furthermore, this term is less difficult to use by practitioners and less difficult to hear by families.

The AAIDD defines intellectual disability as impairments in cognitive functioning and in adaptive behavior, which develop before age 18 (Box 285-1). Many professionals think that any child with cognitive impairment has intellectual disability. Given that the definition of intellectual disability includes both cognitive and adaptive impairment as essential criteria, clarifying the differences here is important. *Cognitive impairment* is defined as performance in the abnormally low range on standard assessments of intelligence. The *intelligence quotient* is defined by a mean of

100, with standard deviation of 15. Cognitive impairment is also defined as an IQ two or more standard deviations below the mean. Furthermore, cognitive impairment implies significantly low scores in all domains of intelligence testing. Widely discrepant scores in various domains, for example, a verbal IQ in the normal range and a nonverbal score in the range of impairment, would be best defined as a learning disability, not as intellectual disability. Adaptive impairment is defined by functioning in the abnormally low range (more than 2 standard deviations below the mean) on formal measures of adaptive functioning, such as the Vineland Adaptive Behavior Scales. Adaptive skills include domains such as communication, self-care, home living, social or interpersonal skills, ability to use community resources, self-direction, functional academic skills, work, leisure, health, and safety.

CLASSIFICATION OF INTELLECTUAL DISABILITY

Intellectual disability is traditionally subdivided by level of functioning into mild, moderate, severe, and profound. The purpose of such subdivisions should be to identify the level of support that will help that individual function best in society. Table 285-1 summarizes these levels with respect to estimated IQ, expected academic achievement by age 18, and anticipated level of recommended support. The need for intermittent support in mild impairment reflects the fact that adults with mild intellectual disability generally function well independently and are able to work in competitive employment and to manage domestic affairs adequately. However, individuals with mild intellectual disability may have difficulty with stress, for example, following a physician's recommendations. For this reason, individuals with mild intellectual disability usually benefit from the intermittent support of a care coordinator. The need for limited support reflects the fact that most adults with moderate intellectual disability are able to work in the community but often require ongoing job coaching, particularly to cope with any changes in routine. In addition, adults with moderate intellectual disability are typically able to manage many aspects of their domestic life, such as hygiene and taking public transportation, but require some assistance with daily living. The need for pervasive support reflects that individuals with severe or profound intellectual disability are typically unable to work in the community and often require significant daily assistance with many aspects of their domestic life.

BOX 285-1 Criteria for Diagnosis of Intellectual Disability

1. Cognitive impairment (≤90) (IQ is defined by a mean of 100, with standard deviation of 15. Cognitive impairment is defined as an IQ two or more standard deviations below the mean.)
2. Adaptive impairment (adaptive skills include domains such as communication, self-care, home living, social or interpersonal skills, use of community resources, self-direction, functional academic skills, work, leisure, health, and safety). Adaptive impairment is identified by functioning in the range of impairment in these areas (more than 2 standard deviations below the mean, as measured by formal testing on measures of adaptive functioning, such as the Vineland Adaptive Behavior Scales).
3. Onset of cognitive and adaptive impairment during developmental period (<18 years of age). Onset of cognitive and adaptive impairment after the developmental period would be referred to by etiology, for example, as traumatic brain injury.

COMMUNICATING WITH FAMILIES

Communicating with families and patients about a diagnosis of intellectual disability or mental retardation is challenging. Thoughtful communication is essential in helping families acknowledge a diagnosis that is difficult to accept. This approach is crucial, given that acceptance is essential in accessing important services. Equally important to the careful and specific use of diagnostic labels is the consistent use of person-first language.[4] To state the impairment first, as in *the intellectually disabled child* implies that the disability is the most salient characteristic of the child. Using the term *child with a disability* is preferable. Sensitive use of language demonstrates respect to patients with intellectual disabilities and compassion for their families. The cases presented in this chapter demonstrate that the careful attention to these subtle language differences can promote healing in spite of the inability to cure.

Table 285-1 Levels of Intellectual Disability

LEVEL	CORRESPONDING IQ	EXPECTED ACADEMIC ACHIEVEMENT BY AGE 18	SUPPORT LEVEL
Mild	55-70	5th-grade academics	Intermittent
Moderate	40-55	2nd-grade academics	Limited
Severe	25-40	Preschool academics	Extensive
Profound	<25	—	Pervasive

DIFFERENTIAL DIAGNOSIS AND MANAGEMENT

In general, most children with intellectual disability do not have significant or atypical behavior problems. However, several behavioral symptoms that have often been associated with intellectual disability, such as irritability, aggression, and self-injury, are worthy of mention. These symptoms are also often seen in autism, which is a common comorbidity of intellectual disability. Autism does occur at a higher rate in individuals with intellectual disability, and a diagnosis of autism would prompt differences in management from intellectual disability alone. For this reason, authorities strongly recommend that the diagnosis of autism be considered, particularly in the face of characteristic symptoms. Also important to note is that such symptoms as irritability and aggression have long been seen as intrinsic features of intellectual disability, to the disservice of individuals with intellectual disability. In other words, the presence of intellectual disability has often precluded and continues to preclude more meticulous investigation into the cause of such symptoms. Frequently, irritability and aggression may be symptoms of psychiatric illness, such as depression or anxiety. Self-injury may be a sign of physical illness; for example, hitting the chest may be an indication of undiagnosed gastroesophageal reflux. Apparent hypersexuality, such as dropping the pants in public, may be a manifestation of an uncomfortable erection in the context of inadequate sexuality education. As illustrated in some of the cases presented here, avoiding diagnostic overshadowing or attributing all symptoms to intellectual disability is important.

Four cases are presented to illustrate the diagnosis and management of intellectual disability, learning disability, and global developmental delay.

Case 1

Jenny Miller, a 6-year-old girl, is accompanied by her parents to your office for a discussion about recent recommendations made by persons at Jenny's school. Jenny has a history of global developmental delay. She has been attending a developmental preschool and receiving private speech therapy through an individualized education program (IEP)[5] since she was 3 years of age. Mr and Mrs Miller are very upset about the prekindergarten assessment report that they just received. The report states that Jenny has "mild mental retardation" and recommends learning support[6] placement in kindergarten. Mr Miller explains that the school psychologist told them that he was giving Jenny this label so that she could access special education services. Mr Miller takes this statement as evidence that the psychologist is stretching the criteria for this purpose and questions whether the services are worth a label that will follow Jenny for life.

You review the evaluation report. On the WISC-III, Jenny received a verbal IQ of 67 and a performance IQ of 64. The full-scale IQ is reported as 63. On the Bracken Basic Concept Scale, a measure of early childhood academic achievement, she received a standardized score of 68. On the Adaptive Behavior Composite of the Vineland Adaptive Behavior Scales, Jenny received a standard score of 55.

On physical examination, Jenny is at the 90th percentile for height and weight. During the examination, Jenny is able to recite some of the alphabet by rote, but she has poor articulation and does not recognize her letters. She can count to 5 but incorrectly names the number of fingers you hold up. When you ask her to place the stethoscope on her heart, she places it on her belly. She is unable to dress herself after the examination and turns to her parents for help.

After the examination, Mr and Mrs Miller tell you that instead of allowing Jenny to be placed in special education, they are thinking about keeping Jenny in preschool 1 more year. This way, they hope she can catch up and enter mainstream kindergarten the following year. They ask for your advice about this plan.

Case 1 Discussion

Jenny fulfills all 3 of the diagnostic criteria for intellectual disability (see Box 285-1). First, intelligence testing estimates her cognitive abilities to be more than 2 standard deviations below the mean. Second, Jenny also has had formal assessment of adaptive skills, with a reported score on the adaptive scale of more than 2 standard deviations below the mean. In corroboration of the formal measures, the physician also has the opportunity to observe in the office pronounced delays in academic skills and communication, a notably small fund of knowledge, and significant difficulties with self-care, such as dressing. Third, of course, Jenny qualifies for the final criterion, being 6 years of age. The school psychologist's use of the term *mental retardation* is accurate and appropriate here, given that this term is the currently accepted legal term and is still essential for the provision of services as of this writing.

The questions Mr and Mrs Miller pose raise several important issues. When Jenny's parents express their concern about giving her a label, they are likely expressing their sadness about a diagnosis, which they fear and do not want. In coming to the physician for a second opinion, they are searching for a more palatable diagnosis. This delicate situation calls for a gentle, compassionate, and honest approach. Jenny will benefit from the services that can be provided by the diagnosis of mental retardation. Holding this tall, 6-year-old child back in preschool 1 more year would not address Jenny's learning needs, and the parents would face the same difficult situation the following year, with a yet taller and more conspicuous child. Therefore the best way to support Jenny's development and learning is to respectfully counsel that, as a professional opinion, Jenny will not likely make sufficient progress without adequate learning support services.

Equally important is the way in which this advice is given. Mr and Mrs Miller may seem to be naïve or to be in denial. Actually, they are afraid to accept special education and its implications and are hoping to defer the inevitable for another year. Therefore, in giving this advice, acknowledging that Mr and Mrs Miller are mourning for the loss of their idealized childis important. Nevertheless, acknowledging Jenny's educational needs now rather than deferring the inevitable for another year would be best. Although the school psychologist attempted to soften the blow by stating that the label was being used to procure services, this approach resulted in confusion for the family. In fact, the psychologist was accurately reflecting Jenny's abilities and leading the family to an appropriate educational placement.

A somewhat different approach from the psychologist would include an effort to (1) dispel myths about the meaning of mental retardation, (2) be straightforward that the diagnosis of intellectual disability is justified and that mental retardation is the currently accepted legal and educational term, and (3) actively empathize with the family's distress. To dispel myths, a helpful approach would be to start by asking "What does mental retardation mean to you?" For many families, mental retardation conjures up images of common syndromes associated with mental retardation, such as Down syndrome. Even when specific syndromes do not come to mind, most parents believe that children with mental retardation are not able to learn. This belief understandably contributes to confusion for parents such as the Millers, whose daughter has mild impairments. In such cases the professional needs to explain that individuals with mild mental retardation typically do develop functional literacy, some arithmetic proficiency, and usually obtain independent employment and living situations. Furthermore, parents may be comforted to learn that the term intellectual disability will soon officially replace mental retardation because of its negative connotations.

Case 2

Your office is the medical home[7-9] for Max Smith, a 14-year-old boy with a history of diabetes and intellectual disability. Max is accompanied by his mother today for a school physical before starting high school. On the subject of school, Mrs Smith mentions that "Max had a difficult school year, what with his grandpa passing away and his parents finalizing their divorce last fall." Max has an IEP.[6] He has been receiving learning support for all of his core academic courses and has been in mainstream classes for his electives.

Max's most recent psychoeducational assessment was performed 2 years ago. The evaluation report states that Max has a verbal IQ of 67, a performance IQ of 62, and a full-scale IQ of 66 on the WISC-III. On the WIAT-II, an academic assessment test, Max's standard scores ranged from the high 50s to the low 70s. On the Adaptive Behavior Composite of the Vineland Adaptive Behavior Scales, Max received a standard score of 68. The evaluation report notes that Max is consistently described by his teachers as "good natured" and that he "tries to follow directions and is friendly."

School reports from the last year note that Max has become increasingly withdrawn, disorganized, and irritable. Mrs Smith reports that when she asked the school counselor about Max's declining school performance, the counselor noted that, "most kids with mental retardation have the same problem when they enter high school—they start to struggle even with the learning support curriculum and often become withdrawn as they realize that they 'don't fit in.'"

During the appointment, Max is quiet and withdrawn. His answers to your questions are appropriate though somewhat concrete. Mrs Smith tells you that, citing Max's current difficulties, the school counselor recommended placing Max in a self-contained life skills classroom. She asks for your opinion about this recommendation.

Case 2 Discussion

Max has a history of mild intellectual disability, with a relatively acute onset of academic decline. His most recent psychoeducational data—with cognitive, academic, and adaptive testing 2 or more standard deviations below the mean—support the diagnosis of intellectual disability. Adolescents with intellectual disabilities often find academic work increasingly challenging in higher grades, as the demands intensify and the curriculum becomes more abstract. Nonetheless, attributing all of Max's current difficulties to his intellectual disability, as the school psychologist has done, may be misguided. Unfortunately, this tendency to assume that all functional impairments in a person with a given disability may be attributed to the disability is an error that physicians commonly make. To avoid this type of assumption, or diagnostic overshadowing,[10] a patient's functioning should be evaluated in different domains, and the physician should avoid equating a patient's functioning in any domain with a diagnosis.

Max's declining grades, in the context of significant social stressors such as his parents' divorce and his grandfather's death, may be indicative of depression, a common comorbidity of intellectual disability. At this visit, assessing or evaluating for depression with a standardized measure and considering referral for psychiatric evaluation and treatment would be prudent. Although not a factor in this particular case, another common comorbidity in adolescents with cognitive impairment is anxiety, which may be interpreted as attention-deficit/hyperactivity disorder (ADHD) or as a behavior problem. Anxiety or depression may not be obvious during an office visit, particularly in the context of cognitive impairment. Depression and anxiety disorders are at least as prevalent in individuals with intellectual disability as in the general population, and some studies have shown an increased prevalence. Therefore standardized assessment is recommended to increase detection of these common comorbid conditions.[11]

In all adolescents, particularly those with disabilities or chronic health conditions, some thought should be given to planning for the transition to adulthood. Max will likely need considerable support in managing his own diabetes care. Even if Max had no chronic health conditions, careful planning for adulthood is warranted. Between the ages of 14 and 16, all students with IEPs should be invited to the IEP meetings and begin to make substantive contributions to vocational and educational planning.[12] Max and his family should start thinking about where and with whom Max is going to live when he becomes an adult. What supports will he continue to need? What interventions are necessary now to prepare Max adequately to succeed with minimal supports?

As Max's pediatrician, some thought should be given to the transfer of Max's care to an internist. How can the primary care physician support Max in finding

Table 285-2 International Classification of Functioning to Organize Evaluation and Care Plan

DOMAINS	ELEMENTS TO INCLUDE IN EVALUATION
Learning and applying knowledge	Learning, thinking, problem solving, and decision making
General tasks and demands	Carrying out tasks, organizing routines, handling stress
Communication	Use of language, signs, and symbols; receiving and producing messages; carrying on conversation; use of communication devices and techniques
Mobility	Moving body position or location; transferring from one place to another; carrying, moving, and manipulating objects; walking running, climbing; using transportation
Self-care	Washing, dressing, grooming, eating, drinking, hygiene, health practices
Domestic life	Acquiring food, clothing, place to live; household chores; assisting others
Interpersonal interactions and relationships	Basic and complex interactions with people, including strangers, friends, relatives, immediate family members, and intimate relations in a socially appropriate manner
Major life areas	Carrying out tasks related to education, work, and economic transactions
Community, social, and civic life	Recreation and leisure, religion or spirituality, political life or citizenship

a provider for this young man with complex needs? Adolescents with disabilities should make regularly scheduled visits throughout adolescence to organize their transition process. The primary care physician can play a helpful role in pooling input from various pediatric subspecialists before transferring care to an internist and adult subspecialists. A primary care physician who has a longstanding relationship with an adolescent can also assist the adolescent and family by providing counseling related to sexuality issues or by referring to an appropriate resource for sexuality education for adolescents with intellectual disabilities.[13] A subspecialist with training in developmental and behavioral pediatrics or in neurodevelopmental disabilities can facilitate and organize transition planning. The International Classification of Functioning is a useful organizing framework. (Table 285-2)

Case 3

Hannah Ruiz is an 8-year-old new patient to your practice with a diagnosis of Coffin-Siris syndrome. She is accompanied by her mother and maternal grandmother for a follow-up of asthma and allergies. During the interview, Mrs Ruiz tells you proudly that Hannah's IQ is 88, which the geneticist said is one of the highest IQs ever reported for anyone with Coffin-Siris syndrome. She then mentions that this situation is a source of confusion for her, given that Hannah is not doing well in school in spite of the fact that she has normal intelligence.*

During the interview, Hannah requires constant redirection by her mother and grandmother. She bolts out into the hallway on several occasions. When seated, she fidgets continuously. During the examination, Hannah grabs at the stethoscope and the otoscope. Her speech is difficult to understand because of severe articulation problems. Her allergies are clearly in full force, with her nose continually running. Her mother wipes her nose frequently during the visit, to which Hannah objects strenuously. Her mother asks whether you have any thoughts about her academic difficulties.

*Very rare congenital malformation syndrome, including prenatal onset growth deficiency, mild-to-moderate intellectual disability, moderate-to-severe hypotonia, seizures, coarse facies, hirsutism, and hypoplastic to absent 5th.

Case 3 Discussion

Hannah clearly does not have a cognitive disability, with an IQ in the normal range at 88. Though most people with Coffin-Siris syndrome have mild to moderate mental retardation, she is an exception. This situation illustrates the important point that functional assessments are much more useful than diagnostic labels or genetic diagnoses in estimating abilities and in developing care plans. Although Hannah's general intelligence is technically in the normal range, it is clearly in the low-normal range, and she would be expected to be a slow learner. She may have significant discrepancies among various subscales that may be affecting her school performance, for which she would qualify for a diagnosis of learning disability. Furthermore, her adaptive skills are clearly impaired. Hannah's academic performance is being affected by inattention, hyperactivity, and impulsivity. In summary, Hannah has significant impairment of adaptive functioning but not of intellectual functioning; therefore she does not qualify for a diagnosis of intellectual disability.

The discrepancy between Hannah's IQ and her academic achievement may be the result, in part, of inattention and hyperactivity, but the explanation is likely to be more complex given the many components of IQ. Comprehensive cognitive and academic testing would help in identifying specific learning disabilities and in guiding the design of appropriate learning supports. Hannah's parents are responsible for making the request of the principal of the school for a multidisciplinary evaluation for the identification of learning disabilities; the physician can support the family by explaining this process[14] (see When to Refer).

Although IQs are generally considered to be stable over time for any given individual, seeing some change in IQs in children with learning disabilities is

Table 285-3 Minor Anomalies Associated With Specific Syndromes Associated With Intellectual Disability

SYNDROME	SIGNIFICANT FEATURES ON PHYSICAL EXAMINATION
Down syndrome	Brachycephaly, microcephaly, epicanthal folds, Brushfield spots, upslanting palpebral fissures, small ears, small nose with low nasal bridge, brachydactyly and clinodactyly, single transverse palmar crease, wide gap and plantar crease between 1st and 2nd toes, hypotonia, short stature
Fragile X syndrome	High forehead, long jaw or face, large protuberant ears, velvety palmar skin with dorsal redundancy, hyperextensible joints, peripubertal macroorchidism, early onset overgrowth, initial shyness, repetitive behaviors and stereotypies
Fetal alcohol syndrome	Microcephaly, short palpebral fissures, maxillary hypoplasia, flat philtrum, thin upper lip, small distal phalanges and small 5th fingernail, joint anomalies of position and function, short stature
Williams syndrome	Stellate iris, short palpebral fissures, medial eyebrow flare, periorbital fullness, flat nasal bridge, anteverted nares, long philtrum, prominent lips, hoarse voice, heart murmur, hyperactive deep-tendon reflexes, friendly personality, hyperactivity, short stature
Velocardiofacial syndrome	Narrow palpebral fissures, cleft palate, velopharyngeal insufficiency, prominent nose with narrow base, abundant scalp hair, long face, retruded mandible, heart murmur, slender, hypotonic limbs with hyperextensible hands and fingers
Rett syndrome	Acquired delay in head growth, acquired diminished eye contact and loss of speech, repetitive purposeless midline hand movements such as wringing or washing, apraxia, hypotonia, principally in girls

not uncommon. For example, at an early age, Hannah may have achieved an IQ in the normal range, largely owing to strong memory skills. Over time, as IQ tasks favor reasoning over rote memorization, and calculations require multiple steps, Hannah's score would then drop significantly. Notably, this situation would not represent a true regression but would be a phenomenon of standardized testing. In addition, depending on which test instrument was used, and when it was used, an erroneously elevated IQ score may have been given; as these tests are revised and upgraded, different versions of the same test do not yield comparable results.

Considering Hannah's adaptive impairments, she would likely benefit from case management for services through state or local programs for mental retardation.[15] Having psychological assessments repeated as she progresses through school would likely be to Hannah's advantage, both to guide her IEP and to identify if she might qualify for a diagnosis of intellectual disability with its accompanying service qualifications. An important point to bear in mind, however, is that Mrs Ruiz is proud of Hannah's relatively high IQ and that such a diagnostic reclassification would need to be handled sensitively despite the advantages it would bring to Hannah.

Hannah has significant symptoms of inattention, hyperactivity, and impulsivity, which may represent ADHD. Such symptoms are common comorbidities of learning disabilities and intellectual disability. Effective interventions are available for inattention, hyperactivity, and impulsivity, including school accommodations and medications.[11]

Case 4

Gavin Park, a 30-month-old boy, is accompanied by his parents in your office. This session is the first follow-up appointment since Gavin established care with you 3 months ago. At the initial visit, you noted significant delays in speech and motor development, and you referred the family to early intervention (federally funded, locally provided developmental services for children birth to 3 years of age). In the evaluation for early intervention, Gavin's developmental progress was found to be at approximately 18 months in all domains. Mr and Mrs Park are very pleased with the early intervention services they have received. They note that Gavin is making good progress in his new preschool. Today, they want your opinion about Gavin's prognosis.

Case 4 Discussion

Gavin is a toddler with moderate global developmental delays. At the chronologic age of 30 months, Gavin is functioning at a developmental age of 18 months, resulting in a developmental quotient (DQ) of approximately 60. (The DQ equals the mental age on standardized tests of intelligence divided by the chronologic age multiplied by 100.) Cognitive and adaptive skills are included together in the DQ. With a DQ between 2 and 3 standard deviations below the mean, Gavin is at high risk of having intellectual disability. For Gavin to catch up, not only would he have to make developmental progress at a rate commensurate with his peers, but he would also have to actually accelerate in his development such that he would outpace his peers. Gavin is making some nice progress in early intervention; however, considering the global nature of his delays, he will not likely accelerate in his development.

Nevertheless, making a diagnosis of intellectual disability is unnecessary at this point. A diagnosis of intellectual disability would likely be difficult for the family to hear and would not be necessary for Gavin's ability to obtain appropriate services. Therefore the

Table 285-4 Nonspecific Dysmorphic Features Associated With Anomalous Brain Development

FEATURE	ABNORMALITY	PATHOGENESIS OR POSSIBLE SIGNIFICANCE
Cranium	Microcephaly	Reduced brain growth
	Asymmetry	Premature suture fusion vs deforming external forces vs abnormal underlying brain growth
Hair	Absent or multiple (>2) parietal whorls	Abnormal brain development between 10 and 16 weeks' gestation
	Cowlick, or anterior upsweep of scalp hair	Posterior displacement of junction of parietal and frontal hair streams, resulting from reduced frontal brain development
Eyes	Short palpebral fissures	Deficient frontal brain growth
	Up-slanted palpebral fissures	Relatively deficient frontal brain growth as compared with midface
Ears	Low set (top of helix below outer canthi)	Reflects delayed morphogenesis, as ears are low set in the early fetus
	Posterior rotation (axis tilted backward >15 degrees)	Reflects delayed morphogenesis, as ears are posteriorly rotated in the early fetus
Mouth	High arched	Persistent lateral palatal ridges, indicative of oral hypotonia or other oral-motor dysfunction

Table 285-5 Neurocutaneous Findings Associated With Intellectual Disability

SYNDROME	FINDINGS ON PHYSICAL EXAMINATION	DESCRIPTION
Tuberous sclerosis complex	Hypomelanotic macules	Oval or *ash leaf* shaped, few mm to cm, mostly on trunk or extremities; may occur in infancy
	Shagreen patches	Firm yellow to red clusters of nodules, few mm to cm, on dorsum of body; particularly lumbosacral area; typically occurring at puberty (less commonly before)
	Facial angiofibroma	Pink or red shiny nodules, on face, especially on nasolabial folds, usually appearing between 2 and 5 years of age
	Forehead fibrous plaque	Yellowish-brown or flesh-colored, raised soft or hard plaque, few mm to cm, on forehead or scalp; can occur at any age
	Periungual fibroma	Reddish or flesh colored, arising from nail bed or cuticle, found on toes more often than fingers, usually occurring at puberty or later
Neurofibromatosis	Café au lait macules	Usually hyperpigmented, but also includes hypopigmented macules 5 mm or greater
	Axillary freckling	Small brown macules in axillae and perineum
	Cutaneous neurofibroma	Small, raised, soft, pigmented nodules
Sturge-Weber syndrome	Cranial port-wine stain	Light pink to deep purple birthmark, typically involving at least one upper eyelid and the forehead

most appropriate diagnosis at this point would be global developmental delay. Though the diagnosis of intellectual disability may be deferred, the opportunities for appropriate and early interventions and diagnostic work-up should not be delayed. Gavin is already receiving early intervention services. All children with similar, milder, or isolated developmental delays should be referred to early intervention.[5,16] Early intervention should be working with the family to develop an appropriate transition plan for special education services through the school district to start after the child turns 3 years of age. Even if the physician is uncertain that a significant delay exists, if the family is concerned about their child's development, then their concerns should be validated by encouraging this evaluation. Children with global developmental delay should also be evaluated for possible causes of their developmental differences. Physical examination findings that may suggest the cause of the delays are available in Tables 285-3, 285-4, and 285-5. Table 285-6 provides recommendations regarding the diagnostic work-up for children with global developmental delay.

EVALUATION

A diagnosis of intellectual disability requires documentation of impairment of cognition and of adaptive functioning acquired during development. A useful framework for organizing the collection of these data, and for organizing the care plan, is provided by the

Table 285-6 Diagnostic Work-Up for Global Developmental Delay or Intellectual Disability

TEST	INDICATIONS
Ophthalmologic assessment	Recommended in all children with moderate to severe global developmental delay or intellectual disability.
Audiologic assessment	Recommended in all children with moderate to severe global developmental delay or intellectual disability.
Karyotype	Recommended in all children with moderate to severe global developmental delay or intellectual disability.
Metabolic work-up	Not generally recommended if newborn screen is documented. Recommended with specific family history, consanguinity, regression, or episodic decompensation.
Fragile-X syndrome (DNA methylation testing)	Recommended in boys with moderate to severe global developmental delay or intellectual disability. Particularly recommended when characteristic features present (see Table 285-4).
Rett syndrome (*MECP2* gene testing)	Recommended in girls with moderate to severe global developmental delay or intellectual disability. Particularly recommended when characteristic features present (see Table 285-4).
Subtelomeric fluorescence in situ hybridization (FISH)	Before the development of complete genomic hybridization technology, this was the best test for the detection of small subtelomeric rearrangements. This test has been replaced by microarray comparative genomic hybridization.
Microarray comparative genomic hybridization	Consider in moderate to severe global developmental delay or intellectual disability. This test has higher yield when one or more of the following features are present: family history of unexplained moderate to severe intellectual disability, prenatal onset growth retardation, or postnatal growth abnormalities, including micro- or macrocephaly or short or tall stature, more than two dysmorphic facial features or nonfacial congenital anomalies.
Thyroid function testing	Recommended if no newborn screen documented or with characteristic symptoms, such as late tooth eruption or fontanelle closure, weight for age above height for age, constipation, delayed relaxation phase of deep-tendon reflexes.
Lead testing	Has been found to be elevated at higher rate in children with risk factors and global developmental delay or intellectual disability as compared with children with risk factors without, given that pica is a behavioral characteristic associated with intellectual disability.
Electroencephalogram	Recommended only if a clinical indication of seizures is present.
Brain magnetic resonance imaging	Recommended for global developmental delay, though clinical picture should be taken into account. Lower yield in mild global developmental delay, which tends to be familial. Higher yield with focal or abnormal neurological examination, in the presence of cranial anomalies (see Table 285-5) or neurocutaneous features (see Table 285-6).

Note: Many of these tests are generally ordered by subspecialists. This information is provided to give the generalist an idea of the work-up for intellectual disability.
DNA complete genomic hybridization microarray technology has replaced subtelomeric FISH.
From National Center for Biotechnical Information. Microarrays: Chipping Away At the Mysteries of Science and Medicine. Available at: www.ncbi.nlm.nih.gov/about/primer/microarrays.html. Accessed July 12, 2007.

International Classification of Functioning (ICF)[17] (see Table 285-2). The ICF was developed by the World Health Organization in 2002 in response to criticism that the 10th edition of the *International Statistical Classification of Diseases and Related Health Problems* emphasized diagnostic labels over function and consequently maintained the equation of disability with poor health. With an emphasis on function over diagnostic labels and consideration of environmental factors, the ICF provides a framework for assessment that is congruent with the guidelines put forth by the AAIDD, which were enumerated earlier. Practically speaking, for the primary care physician, the ICF can serve as a *review of functional status,* which complements the review of systems of the traditional medical model. The primary care physician may use Table 285-2 to assist with the thorough review and documentation of functioning of a comprehensive set of domains during the medical interview and during formation of the care plan.

PHYSICAL EXAMINATION AND LABORATORY TESTS

The physical examination does more than point to a possible diagnosis. In addition to determining potential causes of intellectual disability, the physical examination plays an important role in establishing a connection with the child and in assessing interpersonal interactions. Table 285-3 summarizes key features of some common syndromes associated with mental retardation and cognitive disabilities. Table 285-4 summarizes findings that, although not pathognomonic of particular syndromes, may indicate anomalous brain development.[18-26] Table 285-5 summarizes and describes the features of selected neurocutaneous syndromes.[18,19]

In most cases of mild intellectual disability, the cause is usually multifactorial; no single cause is identified, or indeed, identifiable. In contrast, in cases of moderate to severe intellectual disability, a single cause is more commonly implicated and may be identified by systematic investigation. The physical examination can provide important clues to the cause of intellectual disability. An aspect of the physical examination that deserves special mention is the formal assessment of hearing and vision; referrals for thorough evaluation of these senses should be made in the work-up of global developmental delay or intellectual disability. In the absence of clues from the physical examination, guidelines from the American Academy of Neurology may be used for the diagnostic work-up of intellectual disability and global developmental delay.[27] These guidelines are summarized in Table 285-6.

WHEN TO REFER

- Infants and toddlers failing to meet developmental milestones using standard reference instruments, such as Ages and Stages Questionnaire, the Child Development Inventory, Parents' Evaluation of Development Status, or Bright Futures guidelines, should be referred to early intervention for evaluation. In addition, a pediatrician need not conduct formal developmental screening to refer for evaluation through the early intervention program. Referrals can be based on objective criteria or clinical judgment. If the primary care physician even suspects developmental delay, erring on the side of caution would be advisable.
- Parents who express concerns about their child's development should have their concerns validated by a referral to early intervention services.
- Children who have had a new diagnosis of global developmental delay or of intellectual disability should have a medical evaluation to determine the causes of the delays. The primary care physician may wish to refer to subspecialists in genetics, developmental and behavioral pediatrics, or neurodevelopmental disabilities to assist with this evaluation.
- Children who are suspected of having intellectual disability and who have not had a formal psychological assessment should be referred for evaluation of cognitive abilities, academic achievement, and adaptive skills. Families may obtain such psychological testing free of charge through their local school district by making a formal request for a multidisciplinary evaluation. Primary care physicians can support families in this endeavor by providing references to the process of requesting an evaluation through the school district.[6] Families may also obtain an independent psychological evaluation from a private psychologist.

TOOLS FOR PRACTICE

Community Advocacy and Coordination

- *Individualized Education Programs* (fact sheet), National Dissemination Center for Children With Disabilities (www.nichcy.org/resources/IEP1.asp).
- *Mental Retardation* (fact sheet), The American Association on Intellectual and Developmental Disabilities (www.aamr.org/Policies/faq_mental_retardation.shtml).
- *People First Language* (fact sheet), Disability Is Natural (www.disabilityisnatural.com/peoplefirstlanguage.htm).

Engaging Patient and Family

- *What Is Early Intervention?* (fact sheet), National Dissemination Center for Children With Disabilities (www.nichcy.org/enews/foundations/earlyintervention.asp#overview).
- *What Is a Multidisciplinary Evaluation?* (fact sheet), The Child Advocate (www.childadvocate.net/MDE.htm).

AAP POLICY STATEMENTS

American Academy of Pediatrics Committee on Children with Disabilities. The Pediatrician's Role in Development and Implementation of an Individual Education Plan (IEP) and/or an Individual Family Service Plan (IFSP). *Pediatrics*. 1999;104(1):124-127. (aappolicy.aappublications.org/cgi/content/full/pediatrics;104/1/124).

American Academy of Pediatrics Medical Home Initiatives for Children with Special Needs Project Advisory Committee. The Medical Home. *Pediatrics*. 2002;110(1):184-186. (aappolicy.aappublications.org/cgi/content/full/pediatrics;110/1/184).

American Academy of Pediatrics Committee on Children with Disabilities. The Role of the Pediatrician in Transitioning Children and Adolescents With Developmental Disabilities and Chronic Illnesses From School to Work or College. *Pediatrics*. 2000;106(4):854-856. (aappolicy.aappublications.org/cgi/content/full/pediatrics;106/4/854).

Murphy NA, Elias EA. The American Academy of Pediatrics Council on Children With Disabilities. Clinical Report: Sexuality of Children and Adolescents With Developmental Disabilities. *Pediatrics*. 2006;118(1):398-403. (aappolicy.aappublications.org/cgi/content/full/pediatrics;118/1/398).

SUGGESTED RESOURCES

The American Association on Intellectual and Developmental Disabilities (Web page). The American Association on Intellectual and Developmental Disabilities (www.aaidd.org/index.shtml).

The ARC of the United States (Web page), The ARC of the United States (thearc.org/NetCommunity/Page.aspx?&pid=183&srcid=-2).

Batshaw ML. *Children with Disabilities*. 5th ed. Baltimore, MD: Paul Brookes; 2002.

Brown I, Percy M. *A Comprehensive Guide to Intellectual and Developmental Disabilities*. Baltimore, MD: Paul Brookes; 2007.

Capute AJ, Accardo PJ. *Developmental Disabilities in Infancy and Childhood*. 2nd ed. Baltimore, MD: Paul Brookes; 1996.

Center for Medical Home Improvement (Web page), Center for Medical Home Improvement (www.medicalhomeimprovement.org).

Evaluation of the Child with Global Developmental Delay (guideline), American Academy of Neurology (www.neurology.org/cgi/content/full/60/3/367).

Fetal Alcohol Disorders Society (Web page), Fetal Alcohol Disorders Society (www.faslink.org/).
The International Rett Syndrome Association (Web page), The International Rett Syndrome Association (rettsyndrome.org).
National Down Syndrome Society (Web page), National Down Syndrome Society (www.ndss.org).
The National Fragile X Foundation (Web page), The National Fragile X Foundation (www.fragilex.org).
National Organization on Fetal Alcohol Syndrome (Web page), National Organization on Fetal Alcohol Syndrome (www.nofas.org).
Velo-Cardio-Facial Syndrome Educational Foundation (Web page), Velo-Cardio-Facial Syndrome Educational Foundation (www.vcfsef.org).
What is a Medical Home? (Web page), American Academy of Pediatrics National Center of Medical Home Initiatives for Children with Special Needs (medicalhomeinfo.org/).
Williams Syndrome (Web page), Williams Syndrome (www.williamssyndrome.org).

REFERENCES

1. American Association on Intellectual and Developmental Disabilities. About AAIDD. Available at: www.aamr.org/about_aamr/index.shtml. Accessed July 12, 2007.
2. Personal communication, Doreen Croser, Executive Director of AAMR.
3. American Association on Intellectual and Developmental Disabilities. Policies: Definition of Metal Retardation. Available at: www.aamr.org/policies/faq_mental_retardation.shtml. Accessed July 12, 2007.
4. Disability is Natural. People First Language. Available at: www.disabilityisnatural.com/peoplefirstlanguage.htm. Accessed July 12, 2007.
5. American Academy of Pediatrics, Committee on Children With Disabilities. The pediatrician's role in development and implementation of an individual education plan (IEP) and/or an individual family service plan (IFSP). *Pediatrics.* 1992;89(2):340-342, reaffirmed May 2006.
6. National Dissemination Center for Children with Disabilities. NICHCY Connections. . .to Individualized Education Programs. Available at: www.nichcy.org/resources/iep1.asp. Accessed July 12, 2007.
7. The National Center of Medical Home Initiatives for Children with Special Needs. What is a Medical Home? Available at: www.medicalhomeinfo.org. Accessed July 12, 2007.
8. Center for Medical Home Improvement. About the Center for Medical Home Improvement. Available at: www.medicalhomeimprovement.org. Accessed July 12, 2007.
9. American Academy of Pediatrics, Medical Home Initiatives for Children with Special Needs Advisory Committee. The medical home. *Pediatrics.* 2002;110(1):184-186.
10. Reiss S. Dual diagnosis in the United States. *Aust N Z J Dev Disabil.* 1988;14(3):43-48.
11. Capone G, Goyal P, Ares W, et al. Neurobehavioral disorders in children, adolescents, and young adults with Down syndrome. *A J Med Genet.* 2006;142C(3):158-172.
12. American Academy of Pediatrics, Committee on Children With Disabilities. The role of the pediatrician in transitioning children and adolescents with developmental disabilities and chronic illnesses from school to work or college. *Pediatrics.* 2000;106(4):854-856.
13. American Academy of Pediatrics. Sexuality of children and adolescents with developmental disabilities. *Pediatrics.* 2006;118(1):398-403.
14. The Child Advocate. What is a multidisciplinary evaluation? Available at: www.childadvocate.net. Accessed July 12, 2007.
15. The Arc. Available at: www.thearc.org. Accessed July 11, 2007.
16. National Dissemination Center for Children with Disabilities. What is Early Intervention? Available at: www.nichcy.org/enews/foundations/earlyintervention.asp#overview. Accessed July 12, 2007.
17. International Classification of Functioning, Disability and Health. ICF Classification—Hypertext Version. Available at: www3.who.int/icf/onlinebrowser/icf.cfm. Accessed July 12, 2007.
18. Jones KL. *Smith's Recognizable Patterns of Human Malformation.* Philadelphia, PA: Elsevier Saunders; 2006.
19. Curatolo P. *Tuberous Sclerosis Complex.* London, UK: MacKeith Press; 2004.
20. National Down Syndrome Society. Available at: www.ndss.org/. Accessed July 12, 2007.
21. National Fragile X Foundation. Available at: www.fragilex.org/. Accessed July 12, 2007.
22. Fetal Alcohol Disorders Society. Available at: www.faslink.org/. Accessed July 12, 2007.
23. National Organization on Fetal Alcohol Syndrome. Available at: www.nofas.org/. Accessed July 12, 2007.
24. Williams Syndrome Association. Available at: www.williams-syndrome.org/index.html. Accessed July 12, 2007.
25. Velo-Cardio-Facial Syndrome Educational Foundation, Inc. Available at: www.vcfsef.org/. Accessed July 12, 2007.
26. International Rett Syndrome Association. Available at: www.rettsyndrome.org/. Accessed July 12, 2007.
27. Shevell M, Ashwal S, Donley D, et al. Practice parameter: evaluation of the child with global developmental delay. *Neurology.* 2003; 60:367-380. Available at: www.neurology.org/cgi/content/full/60/3/367. Accessed July 12, 2007.

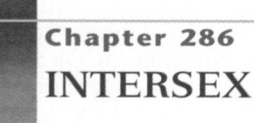

Chapter 286
INTERSEX

Lindsey A. Albrecht, MD; Dennis M. Styne, MD

EPIDEMIOLOGY

Patients with ambiguous genitalia have *disorders of sexual development* (DSD), previously termed *intersex conditions.* These conditions arise from chromosomal, gonadal, or anatomic abnormalities in the pathway of sexual differentiation. Physical findings in patients with DSD may range from an apparently normal phenotype to complete ambiguity. DSD is considered an endocrine emergency because in the majority of cases the genital findings may be accompanied by life-threatening electrolyte abnormalities, hypotension, and shock. Ninety percent of infants with ambiguous genitalia have congenital adrenal hyperplasia (CAH), and more than one half of these patients experience significant sodium loss. However, no individual patient should be assumed to have virilizing congenital adrenal hyperplasia. In addition to the potential medical emergency, the psychological stress to the family cannot be overstated.

NORMAL HUMAN SEXUAL DIFFERENTIATION

Phenotypic sex results from the culmination of many specific genetic and hormonal processes. Humans possess 23 pairs of chromosomes (22 pairs of autosomes and 1 pair of sex chromosomes), with females possessing 2 X chromosomes and males possessing an X and a Y chromosome. Early in gestation the fetus has a bipotential gonad that can develop into either ovaries or testes. Genes on the sex chromosomes, as well as on the autosomes, influence differentiation of this bipotential gonad into either ovaries or testes. Additionally, both the wolffian and müllerian ducts are present early in gestation; these have the potential to develop into either male or female nongonadal reproductive structures, respectively.

Male Sexual Differentiation

The presence of a specific gene on the Y chromosome, the sex-determining region Y *(SRY)* gene, is the initial trigger for testicular development and, eventually, the male phenotype. When the *SRY* gene is present, the bipotential gonad begins to differentiate into a testis at day 43 to 50 of gestation. Soon after, the testes begin to produce testosterone from the Leydig cells and anti–müllerian hormone (AMH) or müllerian-inhibiting substance from the Sertoli cells. AMH acts locally to repress ipsilateral development of the müllerian ducts through apoptosis. Because AMH is produced through early childhood, it can be used as a marker for Sertoli cell presence and function until 8 to 10 years of age. The wolffian ducts differentiate in the male and, with high local concentrations of testosterone from the ipsilateral testes, ultimately form the vas deferens, epididymis, seminal vesicles, and ejaculatory ducts.

Testosterone secretion early in gestation (during the critical period of sex determination) is stimulated by placental human chorionic gonadotropin (hCG); later the stimulus for testosterone secretion is luteinizing hormone (LH) released from the fetal pituitary. Testosterone is locally metabolized by the enzyme 5α-reductase in the sexual skin into dihydrotestosterone (DHT), which is responsible for masculinization of the external genitalia in the male. Thus the development of a male phenotype begins with specific genetic signals that lead to gonadal (testis) formation; the gonads then produce androgenic hormones that allow for masculinization of the genitalia. A critical window exists in which testosterone secretion must occur to lead to the normal male phenotype. If fusion of the labioscrotal folds does not occur by the 12th week of gestation, then fusion will not occur even if high levels of androgen are present later. After 12 weeks, the phallus enlarges and the testes descend into the scrotum, but most of male differentiation has already occurred by this time. A female with excessive androgen exposure from early gestation (eg, virilizing CAH) will have some degree of fusion of the labia. Virilizing CAH is incompatible with a normal female unfused vaginal opening.

Sexual Differentiation

Without the *SRY* gene, the bipotential gonad will develop into an ovary beginning between days 77 and 84 of gestation. Thus the default pathway in gonadal development is said to be female, although more recently other genes such as *Wnt4* have been identified that play a role in development of the ovary. Without the production of müllerian-inhibiting substance the müllerian ducts develop into the fallopian tubes, uterus, and upper one third of the vagina. The developing ovaries do not secrete hormones necessary for female sexual differentiation. Essentially the absence of androgenic hormones allows the normal female external genitalia to develop.

In addition to the *SRY* gene, multiple other genes play a role in human sexual differentiation. Most of these genes act downstream of the *SRY* gene to further influence testicular or ovarian differentiation. Mutations in these genes, such as *WT-1, SF-1,* and *SOX-9,* are often associated with other physical findings in the infant.

DEFINITIONS

Recently the nomenclature used to describe atypical sexual differentiation has changed, largely the result of concern on the part of patient advocacy groups that the terminology was pejorative. Historically the term *male pseudohermaphrodite* was used to describe the patient with incompletely masculinized external genitalia possessing XY chromosomes and a typical number of autosomes (*46, XY* karyotype). Incomplete masculinization of a fetus with testes may result from decreased synthesis or secretion of testosterone or DHT, peripheral tissue resistance to androgen action, or defective production or action of AMH. These conditions are now denoted as *46, XY DSD*. The term *female pseudohermaphrodite* had been used commonly to describe the patient with a *46, XX* karyotype and with masculinized external genitalia. This circumstance may result from abnormally high levels of androgen from either a fetal or exogenous source. Currently these disorders are denoted as *46, XX DSD*.

In some rare cases a patient has both ovarian and testicular tissue. These patients have been called true hermaphrodites in the past, but they may now be considered to have *ovotesticular DSD*. Rarely, disorders of either testicular or ovarian differentiation may lead to gonadal dysgenesis and thus anomalous sexual development.

DISORDERS OF SEXUAL DEVELOPMENT

46, XX Disorders of Sexual Development

Virilization of a female fetus results from excess androgen exposure from either a fetal or maternal source. Timing is important; if the female is exposed to elevated androgen levels after the 8th week of gestation but before the 13th week, then the vaginal opening may fuse posteriorly and appear slit-like. Females with CAH, for example, will have posterior fusion of the labia and some degree of clitoromegaly given their high circulating androgen levels between weeks 8 to 12 of gestation. Exposure to androgen following the 12th week of gestation (eg, exogenous administration to the mother) will result in clitoromegaly without fusion of the labioscrotal folds.

Table 286-1 Differential Diagnosis of Adrenal Enzyme Defects

DEFICIENCY	NEWBORN PHENOTYPE	POSTNATAL VIRILIZATION	OTHER
StAR (also called lipoid congenital adrenal hyperplasia)	Infantile female	–	Salt loss
3ß-Hydroxylase	Ambiguous in *XY* and *XX*	+	Salt loss
17α-Hydroxylase (P450c17)	Infantile female	–	Delayed puberty
11ß-Hydroxylase (P450c11 ß)	Male in *XY*, ambiguous in *XX*	+	Hypertension
21 Hydroxylase (P450c21)	Male in XY, ambiguous in *XX*	+	Salt loss
18 Hydroxylase (P450c11B2)	Normal	–	Salt loss

HT, Hypertension; *StAR,* steroidogenic acute regulatory protein function.
From Styne D. *Pediatric Endocrinology.* Philadelphia, PA: Lippincott Williams & Wilkins; 2004. Reprinted by permission.

Fetal Sources of Androgen Excess

CONGENITAL ADRENAL HYPERPLASIA. Overproduction of adrenal androgens by the female fetus may occur in virilizing CAH, a group of disorders in which a biochemical defect in cortisol synthesis leads to hyperplasia of the adrenal gland resulting from compensatory elevation in adrenocorticotropic hormone (ACTH). These disorders are inherited in an autosomal-recessive manner. The degree and timing of virilization, as well as the presence or absence of salt wasting, depend on the specific genetic lesion (Table 286-1).

Roughly 90% of CAH cases are caused by 21-hydroxylase deficiency, which occurs in 1 in 14,000 white births. P450c21 hydroxylase converts 17-hydroxyprogesterone (17-OHP) II-deoxycortisol; a deficiency in this enzyme leads to extreme elevation in 17-OHP levels, making serum levels of 17-OHP a useful diagnostic test. Defects in 21-hydroxylase will lead to low aldosterone and cause renal salt wasting and potassium retention in approximately 50% of patients. In its most serious form, cortisol and aldosterone deficiency are severe enough to result in hyponatremia, hyperkalemia, dehydration, hypotension, shock, or death. Male infants die more frequently than female infants, due to the lack of suspicion of the condition as a result of their visibly normal phenotype at birth, whereas female infants with virilization are usually evaluated quickly. Newborn screening should eliminate this gender discrepancy in timing of diagnosis.

Late-onset, or nonclassical, 21-hydroxylase deficiency usually occurs in childhood or the teenage years with excessive or premature acne and sexual hair. It may be associated with increased growth and bone age advancement. This condition is discussed later.

Defects in 11β-hydroxylation are rarer than defects in 21-hydroxylation, occurring in roughly 1 in 100,000 white births and more frequently in those of Middle Eastern descent. P450c11 hydroxylase deficiency typically results in (1) hypertension in either gender as a result of elevated levels of 11-deoxycorticosterone and (2) virilization of the female fetus as a result of increased adrenal androgen production. Diagnosis is usually made after the discovery of elevated levels of 11-deoxycortisol (compound S).

3β-Hydroxysteroid-dehydrogenase deficiency causes mineralocorticoid, glucocorticoid, and sex-steroid deficiency. Genetic females may be phenotypically normal or have varying levels of clitoromegaly or labial fusion. Virilization occurs in genetic females because of increased levels of dehydroepiandrosterone (DHEA) (and its sulfate DHEA-S). Additionally, peripheral conversion of DHEA to testosterone may cause virilization in females. 3β-Hydroxysteroid-dehydrogenase deficiency may be a cause of late-onset CAH. Salt loss, as a result of aldosterone deficiency, occurs to varying degrees. (Findings in males are discussed later.)

AROMATASE DEFICIENCY. In rare cases, deficiency in the enzyme aromatase caused by mutations in the *CYP19* gene may lead to virilization of the female fetus and often of the mother during pregnancy. Aromatase catalyzes the conversion of androgen to estradiol; a deficiency in this enzyme leads to elevated levels of androstenedione and testosterone and low levels of estrogens in these patients. At puberty, females often undergo progressive virilization and do not develop female secondary sexual characteristics. In addition, they have osteopenia and delayed bone age (given the estrogen deficiency). A male with aromatase deficiency will be tall and have delayed bone age and osteoporosis caused by estrogen deficiency.

Maternal or Exogenous Sources of Elevated Androgen Levels

Maternal use of androgenic steroids such as danazol or certain progesterone compounds during pregnancy may lead to virilization of the female fetus. Again, the time frame is important in the outcome, given that exposure to these compounds during weeks 8 to 12 of gestation may lead to significant ambiguity, whereas later exposure may result only in enlarged clitoral size. In rare instances, maternal CAH or a virilizing maternal tumor of ovarian or adrenal origin may lead to masculinization of the fetus. Luteomas of pregnancy have also been reported to cause genital ambiguity in the newborn, though they more commonly result only in maternal virilization.

46, XY Disorders of Sexual Development

Luteinizing Hormone–Receptor Defects

Testosterone secretion is controlled by hCG early in gestation and LH from the fetal pituitary later in gestation. Failure of hCG or LH to stimulate testosterone production at the critical times due to mutations in the

LH/hCG receptor will result in incomplete masculinization of a male fetus. This failure may result in Leydig cell agenesis or hypoplasia. Stimulation testing with hCG will result in little or no rise in androgen levels. Basal and stimulated LH levels are typically elevated.

Androgen Biosynthesis Defects

Enzyme defects in the pathways of testosterone biosynthesis may result in incomplete virilization of the male fetus; some of the defects additionally affect synthesis of corticosteroids and are thus forms of CAH.

The initial conversion of cholesterol to δ-5-pregnenolone requires the enzyme P450scc (side chain cleavage), as well as the steroidogenic acute regulatory protein, which transports cholesterol to the inner mitochondrial membrane where P450scc is located. Patients with steroidogenic acute regulatory protein or P450scc enzyme deficiencies have lipid-laden adrenal glands, adrenal insufficiency, and sexual infantilism in males as a result of low testosterone levels.

3β-Hydroxysteroid dehydrogenase deficiency may result in mineralocorticoid, glucocorticoid, and sex-steroid deficiencies. Affected males may be incompletely masculinized at birth and often experience salt loss or adrenal crisis in infancy. They may experience gynecomastia around the time of puberty. The enzyme substrates, such as DHEA and δ-5-pregnenolone, are elevated.

17-Hydroxylase deficiency caused by a defect in the *CPY17* gene results in deficiencies in cortisol and testosterone and thus can result in an incompletely masculinized *46, XY* fetus. An excess of the mineralocorticoid deoxycorticosterone leads to hypertension in both sexes (caused by increased salt and water resorption), as well as hypokalemia and suppression of aldosterone production. Females with 17-hydroxylase deficiency are phenotypically normal at birth but will not progress through pubertal changes. In some female patients, primary amenorrhea is the presenting feature.

Enzyme defects affecting testosterone biosynthesis without affecting corticosteroid production also occur. In a male fetus, 17,20 lyase (also called 17,20 desmolase) deficiency and 17β-hydroxysteroid dehydrogenase-3 deficiency will lead to an incompletely masculinized phenotype without any abnormalities related to mineralocorticoid or glucocorticoid effects. Virilization may occur at puberty in either condition. Gynecomastia may occur at puberty in those affected with 17,20 lyase deficiency.

Defects in Androgen Action

The syndrome of complete androgen resistance (androgen insensitivity syndrome or testicular feminization) results from a defect in the androgen receptor. Affected individuals are phenotypic females with a *46, XY* karyotype and bilateral testes that secrete elevated levels of testosterone. The external genitalia are phenotypically female given the inability of the tissue to respond to dihydrotestosterone. Müllerian structures such as the cervix and uterus are absent or hypoplastic, since production of AMH by the fetal Sertoli cells is normal, and thus the vagina ends in a blind pouch. At puberty, LH increases and leads to elevations in testosterone, some of which is converted peripherally to estrogens. This circumstance leads to the development of female secondary sexual characteristics. Pubic and axillary hair is sparse, if present at all, and menarche cannot occur. Diagnosis is suggested by ultrasound findings (showing absence of the corpus and cervix and the presence of testes) and elevated levels of testosterone. Removal of the testicular tissue is indicated, given the increased risk of neoplasm after puberty; the time of removal, however, is controversial. After removal of the testes, estrogen replacement is provided.

Incomplete forms of androgen resistance, also caused by mutations in the androgen receptor, have great phenotypic variability. External genitalia may range in appearance from completely ambiguous to mildly hypoplastic male genitalia with a small but normally formed phallus. Hypoplastic wolffian duct structures are typically present, and müllerian derivatives are absent because of production of AMH. At puberty, virilization is usually incomplete, and gynecomastia often becomes apparent. Axillary and pubic hair is normal in amount and distribution.

5α-Reductase-2 Deficiency

Mutations in the *SRD5A2* gene coding for 5α-reductase-2, an enzyme that converts testosterone to dihydrotestosterone, leads to deficiency of DHT. At birth, affected males may have ambiguous genitalia or be phenotypically female as a result of decreased conversion of testosterone to DHT in the sexual skin during the critical times of male genital development. These patients have well-developed wolffian ducts (since these structures are testosterone and not DHT responsive) and absent müllerian structures (given that AMH is produced from the normal testes). During puberty, virilization occurs with growth of the phallus and testes, likely secondary to expression of a different form of the 5α-reductase enzyme (type 1) in the liver and other tissues at that time with subsequent increases in circulating DHT levels. Secondary sexual characteristics such as increased muscle mass and voice deepening occur. Some patients change gender identity from female to male at the time of puberty. Laboratory testing reveals abnormally high testosterone/DHT ratios with normal to elevated testosterone and low to undetectable DHT. Confirmatory testing via mutation analysis of the 5α-reductase-2 gene is currently only available as a research tool.

Disorders of Gonadal Differentiation (Sex Chromosome Disorders of Sexual Development)

Klinefelter Syndrome

The most common form of primary hypogonadism in males is Klinefelter syndrome (*47, XXY* karyotype), with an incidence of 1 in 1000 males. Before puberty, patients have decreased upper segment to lower segment ratios, small testes, an increased incidence of developmental delay (mainly in the areas of speech and language), and behavioral problems. Onset of puberty is not usually delayed because Leydig cell function is characteristically less affected than seminiferous tubule function, and testosterone is often adequate to stimulate pubertal development. Serum gonadotropin levels rise after the onset of puberty as the testes become firm and rarely grow larger than 3.5 cm in diameter. After the onset of puberty, histologic changes of seminiferous tubule hyalinization and fibrosis, adenomatous changes of the Leydig cells, and impaired spermatogenesis occur. Gynecomastia is common (and later the risk of breast cancer is increased), and variable degrees of male secondary sexual development are found.

Turner Syndrome (Syndrome of Gonadal Dysgenesis)

Turner syndrome (*45, XO* karyotype) is associated with sexual infantilism, short stature, and a characteristic female phenotype that often includes webbing of the neck. It occurs in 1 in 2500 live-born female infants and a far greater percentage of conceived pregnancies, given that roughly 15% of first-trimester spontaneous abortions have an *XO* karyotype. Cardiac involvement is common and roughly 10% of patients have coarctation of the aorta leading to hypertension in the upper extremities. An even greater percentage of patients have bicuspid aortic valves, which increases their risk for subacute bacterial endocarditis. In some cases, though, short stature may be the sole phenotypic manifestation of the syndrome. Classic manifestations of Turner syndrome are linked to the absence of the *SHOX* gene on the X chromosome.

Patients have streak gonads consisting of fibrous tissue without germ cells. Pubic hair may appear late and is usually sparse in distribution; adrenarche progresses in Turner syndrome even in the absence of gonadarche. Serum gonadotropin concentrations in Turner syndrome are extremely high between birth and age 4 years. They decrease toward the normal range in prepubertal patients and then rise again dramatically after age 10 years. Because of decreased ovarian secretion of estrogens, puberty does not usually begin spontaneously. Patients have no pubertal growth spurt and reach a mean final height of 143 cm. Growth hormone function is usually normal in Turner syndrome, though growth hormone treatment increases growth rate and adult stature. Estrogen treatment is also initiated in adolescence in these patients to allow feminization.

Various mosaic forms of Turner syndrome have been identified, with karyotypes such as *45, X/46, XX,* or *45, X/46, XY*. These patients may have any phenotype varying from normal female to normal male to manifestations of many of the features of Turner syndrome. Some have apparently normal gonadal function; others have abnormality of one X chromosome, such as a ring X, or other abnormalities.

Other Disorders of Gonadal Development

Additional disorders of testicular development may be caused by complete *XY* gonadal dysgenesis (Swyer syndrome), partial gonadal dysgenesis or gonadal regression. In these cases, *gonadal dysgenesis* is descriptive and bears no etiologic relationship to the *syndrome of gonadal dysgenesis* or Turner syndrome. In complete gonadal dysgenesis, *46, XY* individuals fail to develop normal testes and instead have gonadal streaks, müllerian duct development and wolffian duct regression, and female external genitalia. Fifteen to 20% of these cases are caused by mutations in the *SRY* gene. Partial gonadal dysgenesis in *46, XY* individuals leads to variable amount of testosterone and AMH production; thus it is usually associated with ambiguous genitalia and partial development of both the wolffian and müllerian ducts. In gonadal regression or vanishing testes syndrome, the testes are lost after the external genitalia and internal structures have formed. Thus these *46, XY* individuals will be phenotypically male except for absence of both testes. Given this circumstance, anorchia must be considered in all phenotypic male patients with bilaterally nonpalpable testes.

Gonadal dysgenesis may occur in patients with a *46, XX* karyotype who may have streak gonads and sexual infantilism but none of the other characteristics of Turner syndrome. In addition to gonadal dysgenesis, genetic abnormalities such as translocation of the *SRY* gene can result in a *46, XX* genotypic patient developing testicular instead of ovarian tissue; these patients may phenotypically resemble Klinefelter syndrome.

Ovotesticular Disorders of Sexual Development

Patients with ovotesticular DSD (previously termed *true hermaphroditism*) have both ovarian and testicular tissue present. The majority of patients have a *46, XX* phenotype, and the remainder have a *46, XY* karyotype or *46, XX/46, XY* chimerism. Great phenotypic variability exists in both the internal and external genitalia in these patients. Although ovotesticular DSD should be considered in all patients with DSD, a *46, XX/46, XY* karyotype or a bilobate gonad in the inguinal region or labioscrotal folds should raise suspicion for the diagnosis.

EVALUATION AND DIAGNOSIS

Infants with indeterminate gender, as well as some infants with relatively subtle genital findings, should be evaluated for a disorder of sexual differentiation. (Figure 286-1 and Figure 286-2 contain diagnostic algorithms.) In males, even very mild hypospadias can be considered to represent incomplete masculinization, although most uncomplicated cases do not need diagnostic evaluation. More severe degrees of hypospadia, especially when a testis is not palpable, should awaken concern for an identifiable abnormality. Thus, in an apparently phenotypic female, mild clitoromegaly may represent severe undervirilization in a genetic male who has undescended testes or, conversely, may represent masculinization of a female fetus.

Specific recommendations exist for which genital findings should elicit concern for a sexual development disorder. In an apparent male born at term (1) bilateral nonpalpable testes, (2) micropenis, (3) perineal hypospadia, or (4) a single undescended testis with hypospadia of any degree should be further evaluated. Because the testes do not normally descend until roughly 34 weeks of gestation, significantly preterm males with nonpalpable testes alone do not necessarily require evaluation. In an apparent female, (1) clitoral hypertrophy of any degree, (2) posterior

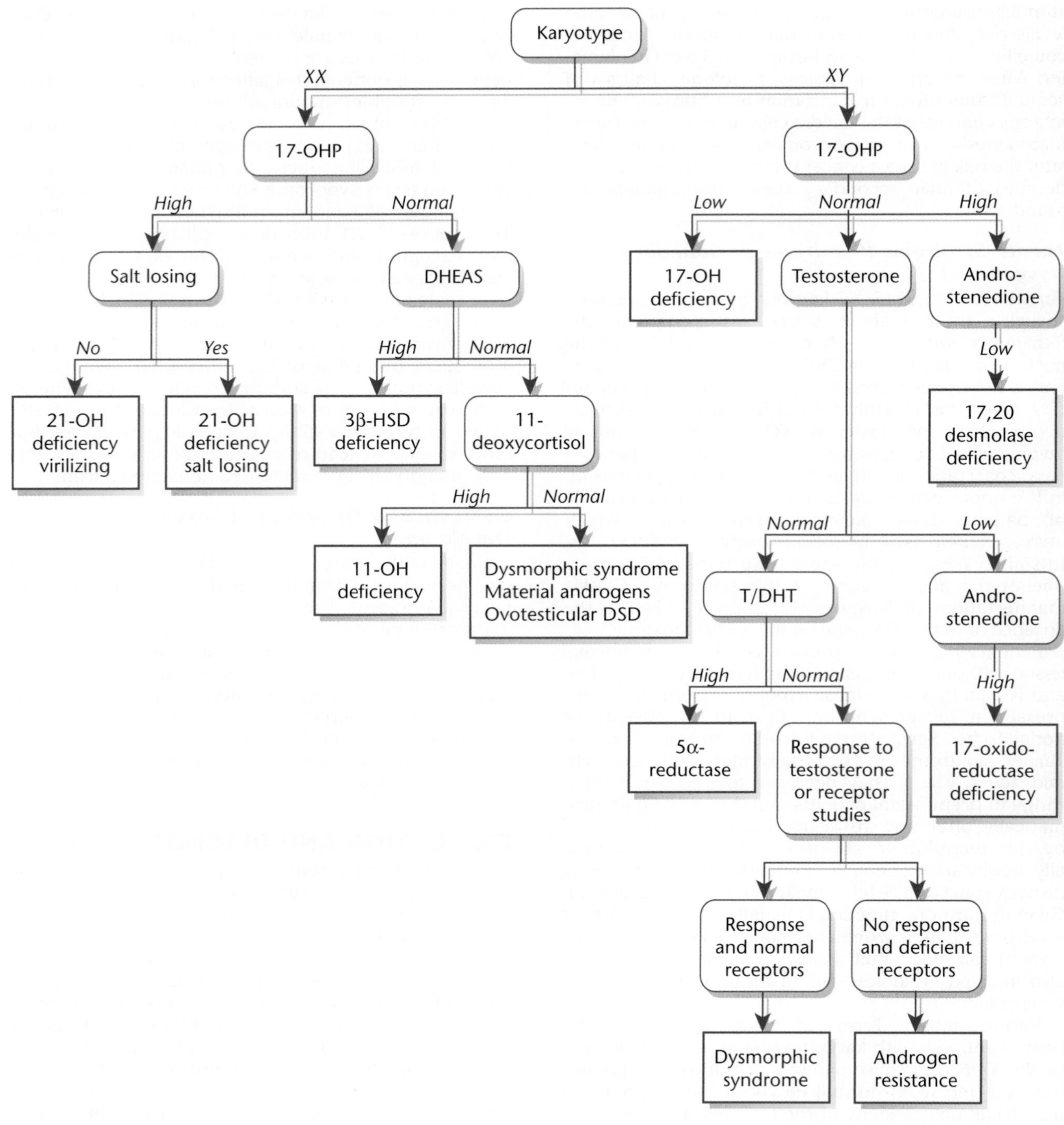

Figure 286-1 Diagnostic algorithm for a child with ambiguous genitalia without palpable gonads is presented for information only. This complex clinical situation requires the assistance of a pediatric endocrinologist for ultimate diagnosis. *(Styne D.* Pediatric Endocrinology. *Philadelphia, PA: Lippincott Williams & Wilkins; 2004. Reprinted by permission.)*

labial fusion (but not just labial adhesions), or (3) an inguinal or labial mass should alert the clinician to a possibility of a sexual differentiation disorder. Of course, all infants with truly ambiguous genitalia and thus indeterminate gender also require evaluation. In addition, if a family history of DSD is present, or if discordance exists between the apparent gender of the infant and a previously obtained prenatal karyotype, then an evaluation should ensue.

History

The evaluation of an infant with a disorder of sexual differentiation must include a detailed obstetric and family history. The patient's mother should be asked

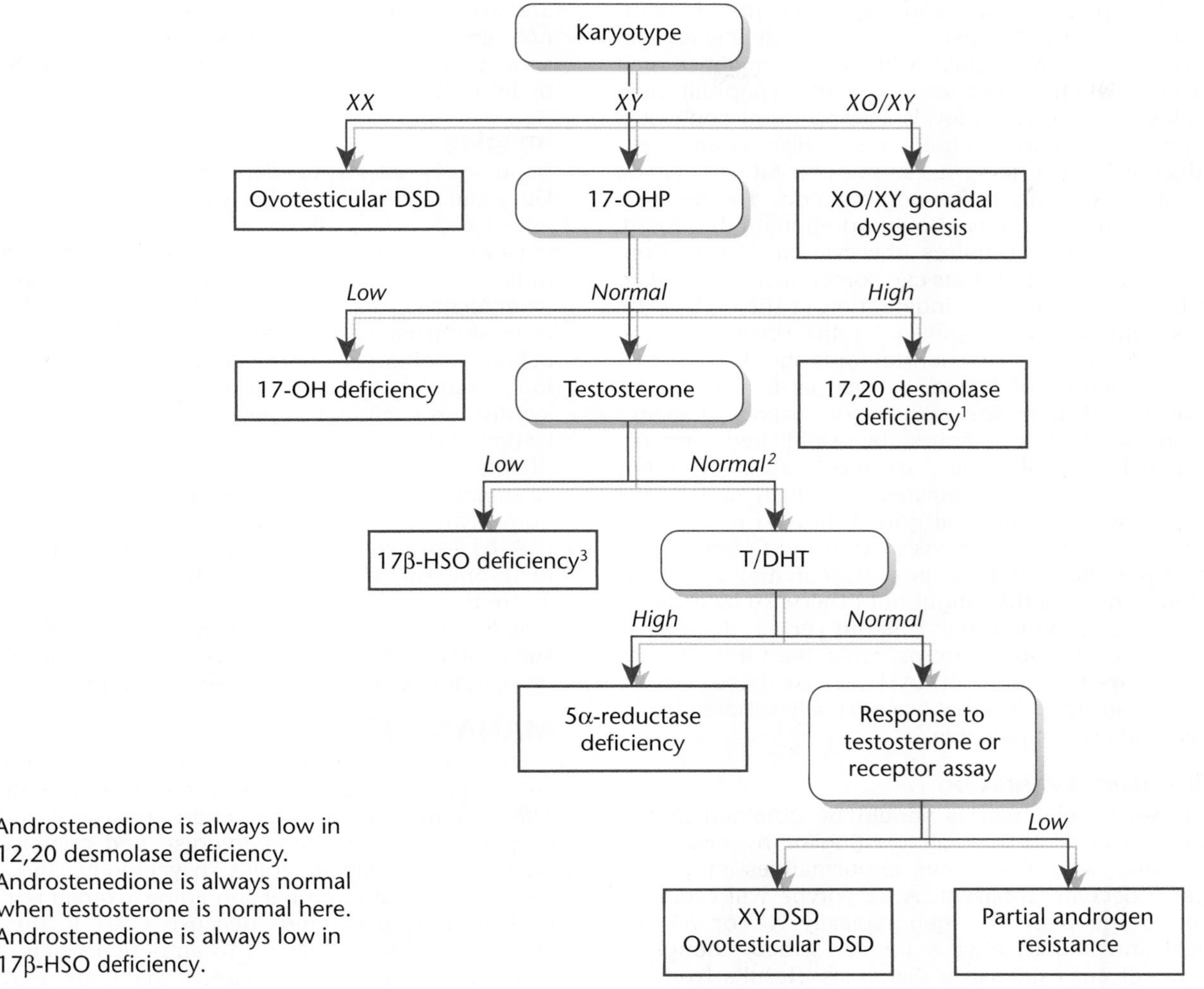

Figure 286-2 Diagnostic algorithm for a child with ambiguous genitalia with palpable gonads is presented for information only. This complex clinical situation requires the assistance of a pediatric endocrinologist for ultimate diagnosis. *(Styne D.* Pediatric Endocrinology. *Philadelphia, PA: Lippincott Williams & Wilkins; 2004. Reprinted by permission.)*

about medication use and symptoms of virilization during pregnancy, which may occur in the case of aromatase deficiency or with androgen-secreting maternal ovarian or adrenal tumors. The family history should not focus solely on genital abnormalities; a history of consanguinity, unexplained neonatal deaths especially in apparently normal phenotypic males, infertility, and disorders of puberty should also be elicited. Many of the conditions associated with ambiguous genitalia are sporadic or inherited in an autosomal-recessive manner.

Physical Examination

The initial physical examination should begin with an assessment of the general health of the patient and an evaluation for malformations or dysmorphic features. Unstable vital signs or hypoglycemia with no apparent cause should raise concern for cortisol deficiency associated with CAH. Typically the onset of shock in patients with CAH does not develop until day 4 to 5 of life, and normal electrolyte values in the few days after birth do not exclude salt losing. Patients with ambiguous genitalia may actually have the benefit of earlier diagnosis of salt loss and signs of cortisol deficiency than phenotypically normal patients. Other specific abnormalities may suggest a particular syndromic diagnosis. Increased skin pigmentation caused by elevated levels of ACTH occurs well after the newborn period and thus is not helpful in making an early diagnosis.

Stretched penile length in a term male infant should measure more than 2 cm; average length is approximately 3.5 cm. A normally formed phallus and scrotum indicates that testosterone production in the critical window of male differentiation was appropriate (around weeks 8-12 of gestation). Because further growth of the normally formed phallus is under the control of testosterone stimulated by fetal LH after midgestation (rather than hCG, which falls during this time), micropenis (penile length <2 cm) often indicates gonadotropin deficiency and may be a sign of hypopituitarism (congenital growth hormone deficiency can also cause a microphallus). Midline abnormalities such as cleft palate may be associated with hypopituitarism and low gonadotropin levels leading to microphallus. Proper examination technique is critical as an infant with chordee or a generous suprapubic fat pad may be thought mistakenly to have micropenis. The position of the urethral meatus should additionally be noted, which sometimes requires observation of urination, because a urogenital sinus can sometimes be mistaken for the urethra and the indentation at the end of the glans penis can be mistaken for the opening of the penile urethra. The labioscrotal folds should be examined for degree of fusion, as well as for symmetry, rugosity, and color. The presence or absence of a vaginal opening should of course be established. Gonads, when palpable bilaterally, are most often testes but might be ovaries or ovotestes as well. A unilaterally palpable and symmetrical gonad may be a testis, an ovotestis, or an ovary. Sweeping of the fingers down the path of the inguinal canal with soap may allow palpation of gonads that might not otherwise be located. Physical examination may rule out certain diagnoses; for example, if gonads are palpable, then the infant is *not* a virilized female with CAH because these patients have gonads (ovaries) that are normally situated in the pelvis and are not palpable.

Laboratory Evaluation

Basic serum chemistries should be obtained immediately to evaluate for salt wasting or hyperkalemia associated with CAH, but abnormalities may take days to become apparent. A karyotype will establish whether the patient is genotypically *XX* or *XY* (or other) and should always be performed, though it alone will not establish a diagnosis. Results from an urgently ordered karyotype can be available within approximately 3 days in some cytogenetics laboratories. Endocrine testing generally consists of measurement of 17-OHP, testosterone, DHT, androstenedione, follicle-stimulating hormone, LH, and AMH performed in a national specialty laboratory with pediatric standards and sample sizes, rather than the local laboratory, which is most unlikely to have pediatric standards or appropriately sensitive techniques. Based on these results, additional tests may be performed. In the first weeks after birth, measurement of testosterone may reveal the amplitude of the episodic spike of testosterone. After this period, hCG administration will help determine whether functional Leydig cells are present (given that functional cells will secrete testosterone in response to the hCG). Of course, serum testing of the steroid hormones involved in the pathways for cortisol and testosterone is indicated in many cases because the forms of CAH that are more rare than 21-hydroxylase deficiency will not cause elevations in 17-OHP levels. In some cases, stimulatory testing with ACTH is necessary to identify the defect.

Newborn screening for 21-hydroxylase deficiency (but not other forms of CAH) currently occurs in 46 states, with testing required but not yet implemented in 3 of the 4 remaining states. Results can be returned several days after the specimens are drawn and are thus available within the first week of life but not always before clinical symptoms develop. This screening test is most helpful in diagnosing the normally appearing but affected male.

Imaging

Imaging is useful to determine internal anatomy. Ultrasound examination, if performed by an experienced technician, allows determination of the presence and appearance of müllerian structures. Absent müllerian structures imply that AMH was produced from testicular tissue and that the underlying problem is an abnormality of testosterone or DHT synthesis or action. Additionally, ultrasound is valuable in evaluating associated renal problems (seen in some syndromes such as Frasier syndrome) and for visualization of the adrenal glands. The gonads may be identifiable by ultrasound examination, though magnetic resonance imaging may be required, particularly if the gonads are intraabdominal.

A trial of testosterone injections (eg, 25 mg of testosterone enanthate intramuscularly every month for 3 months) is given in some equivocal cases to assess whether phallus size responds to androgen, eliminating substantial androgen resistance. However, the effect of this cannot be assessed for several months.

MANAGEMENT

A team approach is necessary to address the multiple issues surrounding management of patients with DSD. The team may consist of an endocrinologist, urologist or plastic surgeon, neonatologist, and geneticist, as well as specialists in ethics, psychology, and social work. Gender assignment should be avoided while the evaluation is occurring. Because CAH is the most common condition leading to ambiguous genitalia, a tendency may exist to tell parents that their child most likely has CAH. Guessing should be avoided because it potentially introduces confusion and may increase distress. The infant should be referred to using gender-neutral terms such as *your baby* or *the baby* rather than *he* or *she*. The goal, of course, is to establish a diagnosis as rapidly as possible. Eventually a gender assignment is made, which should occur with the participation of the family. The underlying diagnosis may heavily influence the gender assignment, but the family must realize that not all patients with a given abnormality identify themselves in the same way. Fertility and capacity for sexual function are critically important considerations as well. Additional factors to be considered when making a gender assignment include the appearance of the genitalia and the surgical options, as well as the potential hormonal therapies available.

Surgical issues include timing and feasibility of surgery, as well as the desire to prevent the situation in which the patient is later dissatisfied with a genital reconstruction that is discordant with their gender (see below). Additionally, the potential for malignant degeneration of a gonad in certain disorders of sexual development involving Y chromosome material must be considered. In some cases, such as in the case of a streak gonad of an *XY* cell line, the gonad should be removed at the time of diagnosis. In other cases, such as they syndrome of androgen resistance, the testis may instead be brought into the scrotum where it can be observed for the development of malignant features.

Long-term psychological support is required for the majority of patients with DSD. Help should be provided to the patient by a mental health professional, preferably someone with experience in dealing with DSD. National and local support groups are also available for families and may be beneficial.

Gender identity is the personal conception of oneself as male or female and is the result of a complex interplay between both biological and environmental factors. It is distinct from sexual orientation and gender role. Hormonal effects (specifically androgen effect on the prenatal brain), brain structural differences, assigned sex of rearing, and sex-steroid effects at the time of puberty have all been shown to influence gender identity. Thus some patients who are assigned a particular gender are later dissatisfied. Some adults with this history have influenced medical practices surrounding gender assignment, particularly with respect to early surgery before the patient acquires the ability to consent to the procedure.

Unfortunately, outcome data for gender identity in DSD are relatively sparse. For example, the largest study to date showed that genetic males with active prenatal androgen effects should be raised as males, given their high rates of male gender identity. Additionally, female infants virilized as a result of CAH should be given a female gender assignment because more than 90% of these patients are content with an assigned female gender. Gender identity outcomes are more difficult to predict in other disorders.

CONCLUSION

The differential diagnosis of the infant born with developmental anomalies of the external genitalia is extensive, given the complicated process of human sexual differentiation. The birth of such patients naturally creates a stressful situation for the family of the patient, which can be attenuated by the appropriate evaluation and management by an experienced multidisciplinary team. Because fatal results may occur with improper vigilance, hospitalization and close monitoring of the infant is indicated in all cases. Given that a patient's gender identity cannot be predicted based solely on the phenotype or the biological defect, gender assignment in these infants requires several considerations. In some cases, the assigned gender may not be concordant with the patient's gender identity as the child ages. Throughout this process the general pediatrician plays an important role in helping coordinate the care of these patients.

WHEN TO REFER

Given the possibility of significant electrolyte disturbances, cortisol insufficiency, and possible shock and death, all patients with ambiguity of the external genitalia should be evaluated immediately by an experienced multidisciplinary team that includes a pediatric endocrinologist. In many cases, this process necessitates transfer of the patient to a medical center with a neonatal intensive care unit and the appropriate pediatric subspecialists. The patient should never be sent home and referred to subspecialty care as an outpatient.

Indications for referral include the following:

Male infant born at term:

- Bilateral nonpalpable testes
- Micropenis
- Perineal hypospadias
- Single undescended testes with hypospadias of any degree

Female infant:

- Clitoral hypertrophy of any degree
- Posterior labial fusion (not adhesion)
- Inguinal or labial mass

AAP POLICY STATEMENT

Lee PA, Houk CP, Ahmed SF, et al, in collaboration with the participants in the International Consensus Conference on Intersex organized by the Lawson Wilkins Pediatric Endocrine Society and the European Society for Paediatric Endocrinology. Consensus statement on management of intersex disorders. *Pediatrics*. 2006;118(2):488-500. AAP endorsed.

SUGGESTED RESOURCES

Achermann JC, Hughes IA. Disorders of Sex Development. In: Kronenberg HM, Melmed S, Polonsky KS, Larsen PR, eds. *Williams Textbook of Endocrinology*. Philadelphia, PA: WB Saunders; 2008.

American Academy of Pediatrics, Committee on Genetics. Evaluation of the newborn with developmental anomalies of the external genitalia. *Pediatrics*. 2000;106(1 pt 1):138-142.

Conte FA, Grumbach, MM. Abnormalities of sexual determination and differentiation. In: Gardner DG, Shoback D, eds. *Greenspan's Basic and Clinical Endocrinology*. 8th ed. New York, NY: McGraw-Hill Medical; 2007.

Lee PA, Houk CP, Ahmed SF, et al. Consensus statement on management of intersex disorders. Presented at the International Consensus Conference on Intersex. *Pediatrics*. 2006;118(2):e488-e500.

Reiner WG. Gender identity and sex-of-rearing in children with disorders of sexual differentiation. *J Pediatr Endocrinol*. 2005;18(6):549-553.

Styne DM. Sexual differentiation. In: Styne DM, ed. *Pediatric Endocrinology (Core Handbook Series in Pediatrics)*. Philadelphia, PA: Lippincott Williams & Wilkins; 2003.

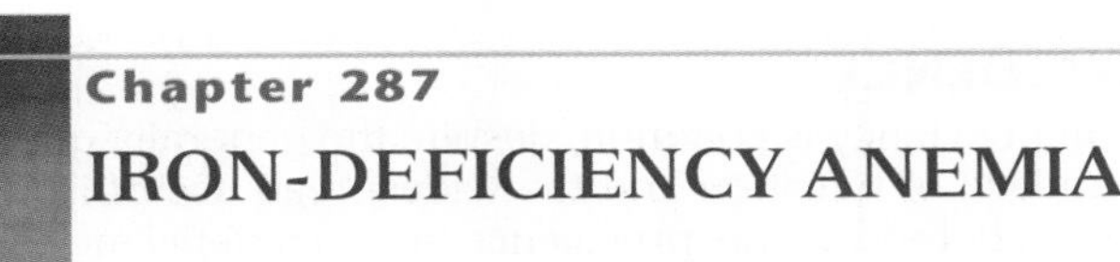

Chapter 287
IRON-DEFICIENCY ANEMIA

Lakshmanan Krishnamurti, MD

Iron-deficiency anemia (IDA) is the most common nutritional deficiency worldwide. In the United States, IDA is most common among women and young children. Iron is an important ingredient of hemoglobin and is involved in numerous cellular processes.

Children with iron deficiency in infancy continue to have poor cognition and school achievement and increased behavior problems into middle childhood.[1] Iron deficiency is also associated with deficits in work productivity, and severe anemia is associated with maternal and child mortality.[2] Prevention of iron deficiency is therefore an important public health issue.

IRON-CONTAINING COMPOUNDS IN THE BODY

Iron is the most abundant heavy metal in the body. The multiple iron-containing compounds found within the body can be grouped into two major categories: (1) those serving metabolic functions and (2) those involved with iron storage and transport.

The first category includes heme- and nonheme-containing compounds. Heme is composed of a protoporphyrin ring with noncovalently bound iron in the ferrous form (Fe^{++}). The most abundant heme-containing protein in the body is hemoglobin, which transports oxygen from the lungs to the tissues and accounts for more than 60% of total body iron. Myoglobin, which accounts for 10% of total body iron, is a heme protein that provides oxygen for use during muscle contraction. The other major heme proteins, the cytochromes, are found in the mitochondria and are necessary for the oxidative production of cellular energy. Several nonheme iron proteins are also present, such as the iron-sulfur complexes and flavoproteins. Many of these proteins are found in the mitochondria and are also involved in oxidative metabolism.

The second category of iron compounds includes molecules involved in iron transport and storage. Transferrin is a β_1-globulin capable of binding 2 atoms of iron in the ferric form. It transports iron from the intestinal epithelium to the bone marrow, where it binds to transferrin receptors on the surface of differentiating red blood cells (RBCs). The transferrin-receptor complex is then internalized and thus supplies iron for the synthesis of hemoglobin. Transferrin also plays a major role in the recycling of iron from senescent RBCs. Ferritin, an iron storage compound found in all cells of the body, is composed of a hollow protein shell encapsulating iron molecules. Hemosiderin, which also serves to store intracellular iron, is thought to be a partially degraded form of ferritin.

INCIDENCE

Iron deficiency is common, despite the generally good standard of nutrition and the widespread use of iron-fortified foods. The prevalence of iron deficiency is greatest among toddlers ages 1 to 2 years (7%) and adolescent girls and adult women ages 12 to 49 years (9%-16%). The prevalence of iron deficiency is 2 times higher among non-Hispanic black and Mexican-American women (19%-22%) than among non-Hispanic white women (10%).[3] Currently, prevalence of IDA remains higher than the goal of the national health objectives for 2010 to reduce iron deficiency in vulnerable populations by 3 to 4 percentage points.[3-5]

ETIOLOGY AND PATHOPHYSIOLOGY

The 4 most important factors in the development of iron deficiency in children are (1) the iron endowment at birth, (2) the iron needs during rapid body growth, (3) exogenous iron absorption, and (4) blood loss. The causes of iron deficiency are summarized in Table 287-1.

During gestation, the level of fetal iron stores is related to maternal iron status, and the maternal-fetal unit is dependent on exogenous iron.[6] The ratio of iron content to weight in the human fetus remains constant throughout gestation. The healthy full-term newborn has sufficient iron stores to last for 6 months, if sufficient small amounts of iron are ingested from the diet. The infant's iron endowment can be compromised by blood loss during the pregnancy or the perinatal period. Common causes of blood loss include third-trimester bleeding, such as abruptio placentae, placenta previa, fetomaternal hemorrhage, and twin-to-twin transfusions.

Gestational conditions that result in lower newborn iron stores include severe maternal iron deficiency, maternal hypertension with intrauterine growth retardation, and maternal diabetes mellitus. Stable, very low–birth-weight premature infants are also at risk for early postnatal iron deficiency because they accrete less iron during gestation, grow more rapidly after

Table 287-1 Causes of Iron Deficiency

INCREASED IRON REQUIREMENTS	INADEQUATE IRON ABSORPTION
Blood loss	Diet low in bioavailable iron
Menstruation	Formula not fortified with iron
Gastrointestinal tract	Cow's milk before the age of 6 mo
Milk enteropathy	Strict vegetarian diet
Food sensitivity	Poor dietary habits in adolescents
Inflammatory bowel disease	Impaired absorption
Meckel diverticulum	Intestinal malabsorption
Peptic ulcer disease	Gastric surgery
Reflux esophagitis	Hypochlorhydria
Hookworms	
Malignancy	
Genitourinary tract	
Respiratory tract	
Idiopathic pulmonary	
Hemosiderosis	
Cystic fibrosis	
Pulmonary tuberculosis	
Cardiac	
Hemosiderinuria due to cardiac hemolysis	
Blood donation	
Pregnancy	
Growth	
Prematurity	
Infancy	
Adolescence	

Modified from: Centers for Disease Control and Prevention. Recommendations to prevent and control iron deficiency in the United States. *MMWR Recomm Rep.* 1998;47(RR-3):1-29.

birth, are typically undertreated with enteral iron, and receive fewer RBC transfusions than term infants.[7]

Iron is needed not only for many metabolic functions and tissue replacement, but also for growth. Growth rates vary with age and are maximal during infancy and adolescence, the same periods associated with the highest frequency of iron deficiency.

Iron balance is maintained by regulation of iron absorption. The amount of iron absorbed depends both on the amount and bioavailability of dietary iron and on regulation of iron absorption by the intestinal mucosa. Most dietary iron occurs in the nonheme form and is much less bioavailable than that in heme proteins. The iron in hemoglobin and myoglobin is particularly bioavailable; up to 30% is directly absorbed by the gastrointestinal tract. Human milk and cow's milk contain small amounts of iron (0.5-1 mg/1000 mL). However, 50% of the iron in human milk is absorbed, compared with only 10% in cow's milk. Full-term infants who are exclusively breastfed for the first 6 to 9 months do not become iron deficient.[8] Nonheme iron absorption is inhibited by bran in cereals, polyphenols in many vegetables, and tannins in tea. The addition of solids to an infant's diet can greatly impair iron absorption and puts the infant at risk for developing iron deficiency. The introduced solids should therefore contain abundant amounts of iron (eg, iron-fortified cereals).

Blood loss causes iron deficiency in children less frequently than in adults. In infancy and childhood, iron deficiency caused by blood loss is most commonly associated with the ingestion of unprocessed cow's milk and with parasitic infections. Hypersensitivity to whole cow's milk causes an exudative enteropathy and frequently leads to gastrointestinal blood loss (Figure 287-1). Other less-common causes of blood loss in children include Meckel's diverticulum, intestinal duplication, peptic ulcer disease, hemorrhagic telangiectasia, and the chronic use of medications that prolong the bleeding time (eg, aspirin).

STAGES OF IRON DEFICIENCY

Iron deficiency occurs when total body iron content is diminished. When absorption exceeds losses, the iron surplus is stored in the reticuloendothelial system, principally the liver, spleen, and bone marrow. Iron is removed from the reticuloendothelial storage pool to compensate for negative iron balance. The development of iron deficiency proceeds through a series of overlapping stages.

The first stage of iron deficiency is iron storage depletion. During this stage, no deficit of iron supplied to the erythroid marrow for RBC production occurs. If the negative iron balance continues, then the second stage, iron-deficient erythropoiesis (IDE), will occur. During this stage, erythroid iron supply is diminished, but the hemoglobin concentration remains in the normal range. If the negative iron balance persists, then IDA finally develops. This third stage is characterized by a decrease in the hemoglobin concentration and a reduction in RBC size and hemoglobin content. Hematologic abnormalities in iron deficiency progress as impairment of hematopoiesis[9] progresses. Anisocytosis and an increased percentage of microcytic cells are the first hematologic abnormalities; at the second stage, the mean corpuscular volume (MCV) and mean corpuscular hemoglobin (MCH) decline; and the final stage of iron deficiency is associated with a low MCH count, a hemoglobin concentration below 9 g/dL, and a transferrin saturation of less than 16%.[9]

Functional iron deficiency is a condition that occurs primarily as a result of treatment with recombinant human erythropoietin. During the supraphysiologic burst of RBC production after a pharmacologic dose of recombinant human erythropoietin, the small circulating iron pool (0.1% of total body iron) may be insufficient to supply the stimulated erythron. Thus, even with normal iron stores, IDE may occur, with further iron repletion often required for normal erythropoiesis to resume.[10] Inflammation may also be a contributory factor.[11]

Specific laboratory findings are associated with each of the 3 stages of iron deficiency. The laboratory test findings characteristic of each stage are summarized in Table 287-2.

DIFFERENTIAL DIAGNOSIS

Diagnosis of iron deficiency is made by the combination of RBC indices and serum transferrin saturation or ferritin. Transferrin saturation and ferritin may be altered by infection, inflammation, malignancy, and starvation. Serum transferrin receptor levels help discriminate iron deficiency from the anemias of chronic disease.

Although the absence of iron stores in the bone marrow remains the gold standard for making the diagnosis of iron deficiency, this test is rarely performed for this purpose because of the obvious discomfort involved and the difficulty of standardizing bone marrow iron stain.

Once the diagnosis of IDA is made, efforts should be undertaken to establish the cause of the deficiency (see Table 287-1). In infancy (a period during which iron demands resulting from rapid growth may outstrip the supply of iron), in adolescence, and during pregnancy, iron deficiency is the result of a physiological increase in iron requirement, which is not being met by the oral supply of iron. Beyond infancy, blood loss is the most common cause of IDA.

Iron deficiency must be distinguished from other hypochromic microcytic anemias (Figure 287-2). RBC indices in infancy and childhood are described in Table 287-3.

Thalassemia Trait

IDA and thalassemia trait are the most common causes of mild microcytic anemia with hemoglobin level of 9 g/dL or more. RBC count is often increased above normal despite the presence of a mild anemia and microcytosis in thalassemia trait, whereas RBC count is reduced in IDA. The RBC distribution width (RDW) is increased in iron deficiency. The Mentzer index, defined as the MCV divided by the RBC count in millions, can help distinguish the anemia of iron deficiency from that of β-thalassemia trait.[12] In IDA the Mentzer index is often greater than 13.5; in β-thalassemia trait, it is less than 11.5 with 82% specificity. An RDW index (RDWI), which is calculated by the formula RDWI = (MCV ÷

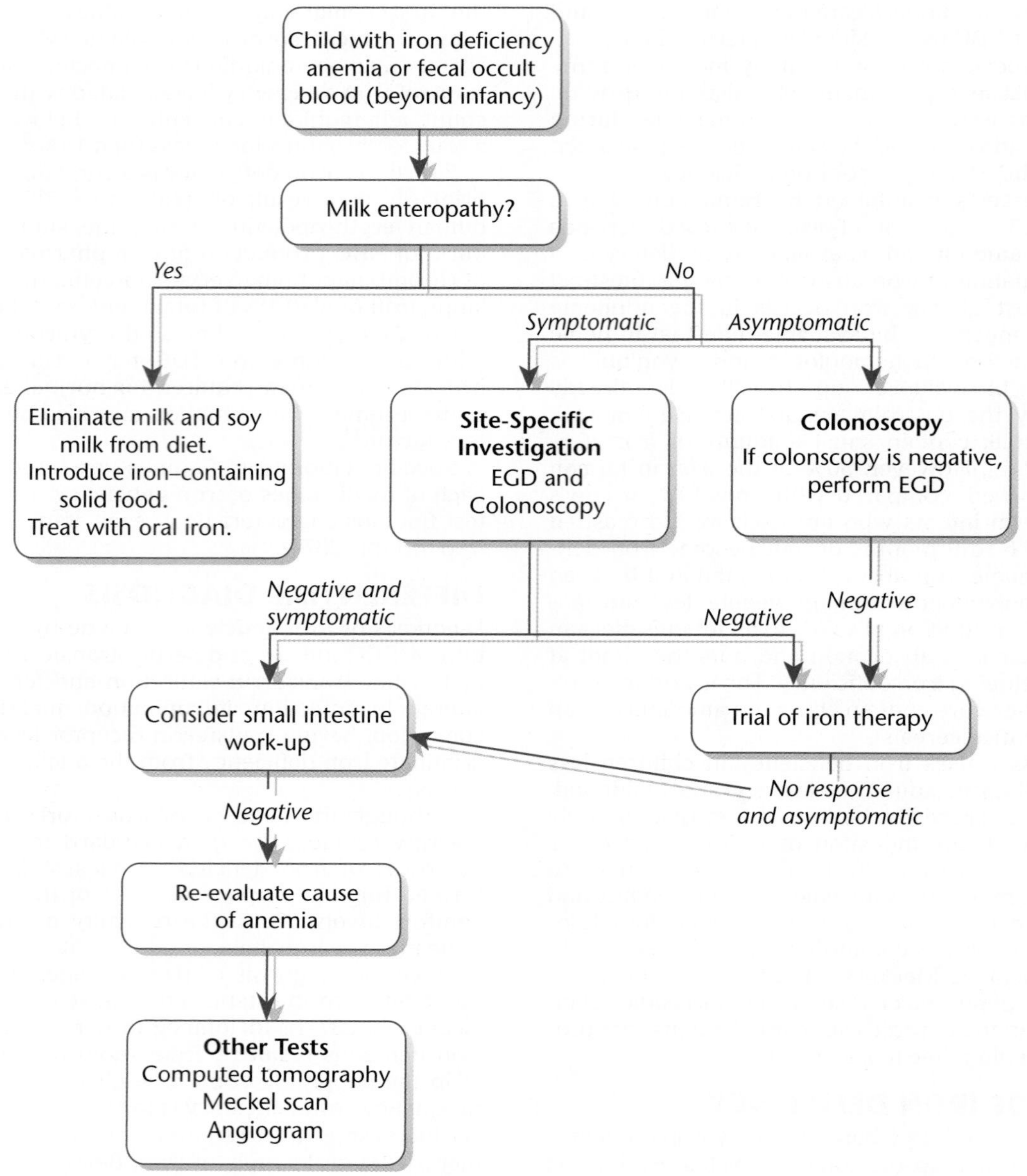

Figure 287-1 Algorithm for approach to iron deficiency with occult intestinal blood loss. EGD, esophagogastroduodenoscopy. *(Modified from Feldman M.* Sleisenger & Fordtran's Gastrointestinal and Liver Disease. *7th ed. Copyright © 2002 Saunders, An Imprint of Elsevier.)*

RBC × RDW), of at least 220 is indicative of IDA, whereas an index of less than 220 is indicative of thalassemia trait with a specificity of 92%.[13] RBC count and RDWI are the most reliable discrimination indices in differentiation between β-thalassemia trait and IDA.[14]

If α- and β-thalassemia trait or hemoglobin E disease is suspected, then the diagnosis can be established by review of the newborn screen or by obtaining a hemoglobin electrophoresis (only in cases of β-thalassemia and not α-thalassemia). Because thalassemia trait is frequently not associated with hemoglobin of less than 9 g/dL, it is not included in the differential diagnosis in severe anemia. The diagnosis of α-thalassemia trait can be assumed when a patient with a familial hypochromic microcytic anemia has normal results of iron studies (including ferritin), normal levels of hemoglobin (Hb) A2 and Hb F, and a normal hemoglobin electrophoresis. It is a diagnosis of exclusion except in the newborn period, when infants with α-thalassemia trait have 3% to 10% Hb Barts (γ_4), which may be detected in the newborn screen.

Hb H Disease

Hb H disease, another form of α-thalassemia, results from deletion of three of the four α-globin genes. It also is characterized by hypochromia and microcytosis, but

Table 287-2 Laboratory Abnormalities in the Three Stages of Iron Deficiency

STAGE	DESCRIPTION
I—Iron depletion	Serum ferritin ↓ Bone marrow iron ↓
II—Iron-deficient erythropoiesis	Serum ferritin ↓ Bone marrow iron ↓ Serum iron ↓ TIBC ↑
III—Iron-deficiency anemia	Serum ferritin ↓ Bone marrow iron ↓ Serum iron ↓ TIBC ↑ Hemoglobin ↓ Hematocrit ↓ MCV ↓ RDW ↑

↑ indicates increased; ↓, decreased.
MCV, Mean corpuscular volume; *RDW*, red blood cell distribution width; *TIBC*, total iron-binding capacity.
From Roper D, Stein S, Payne M, Coleman M. Anemias caused by impaired production of erythrocytes. In Rodak BF, ed. *Diagnostic Hematology*. Philadelphia, PA: WB Saunders; 1995. Reprinted by permission.

in addition, a mild hemolytic component is present from instability of the β-chain tetramers (Hb H) resulting from a deficiency of α-globin chains. Beyond infancy, Hb H is readily identified by hemoglobin electrophoresis. During the newborn period, the moderately severe α-globin deficiency allows for the accumulation of more γ chains, and the concentration of Hb Barts is over 20%.

Anemia of Chronic Disease and Inflammation

Inflammation impairs the supply of iron to the plasma and ultimately results in a form of anemia called anemia of chronic disease or anemia of inflammation. It is usually normocytic, although it may occasionally be slightly microcytic. Because inflammation alters screening tests for iron status in the same manner as true iron deficiency, the distinction between anemia of chronic disease and IDA requires tissue-related iron measurements. However, the usefulness of the serum ferritin in the diagnosis of IDA is compromised by the effect of inflammation on the value. Consequently, a serum ferritin concentration above 30 mg/L in an anemic patient does not exclude IDA in the presence of chronic inflammation.

C-reactive protein is generally considered to be the best laboratory marker of inflammation. If it is less than 30 mg/L, then inflammation is generally considered unlikely to be sufficient to raise the serum ferritin. A suggested ferritin level of less than 40 mg/L and less than 70 mg/L are used to diagnose IDA in anemic patients without and with inflammation, respectively. The serum transferrin receptor (STfR) measurement for identifying IDA is one in which the concentration is not affected by inflammation. Use of the STfR/ferritin ratio further improves the specificity of the diagnosis of IDA and may eliminate the need for bone marrow examination for assessment of iron stores.

Lead Poisoning and Anemia

Lead poisoning and IDA are both associated with high levels of erythrocyte zinc protoporphyrins (ZnPP). Iron deficiency and lead poisoning frequently coexist. Although the nature of their relationship is not completely elucidated, characterization of a common iron-lead transporter and epidemiologic studies among children strongly suggest that iron deficiency may increase susceptibility to lead poisoning.[15] In cases of lead poisoning associated with iron deficiency, the RBCs are morphologically similar, but coarse basophilic stippling of the RBCs is frequently prominent. Increases in blood lead, ZnPP/heme (ZnPP/H) ratio, and urinary coproporphyrin levels are seen.

EVALUATION

History

The onset and progression of iron deficiency is usually gradual, and most children will not have major symptoms. Iron deficiency in infants and children is associated with generalized weakness, irritability, easy fatigability, headaches, poor feeding, anorexia, pica, and poor weight gain.

Physical Examination

The physical examination is usually unremarkable except for marked pallor of the mucous membranes and skin. Other physical findings associated with IDA but that are rarely observed include mild hepatosplenomegaly, lymphadenopathy, glossitis, stomatitis, blue sclerae, and koilonychia (spoon-shaped nails).

Laboratory Evaluation

Laboratory tests for identifying iron deficiency include screening and definitive tests. Screening tests identify IDE by demonstrating either a reduced supply of plasma iron or poor hemoglobinization of circulating RBCs. Definitive tests identify IDA by measuring iron-related proteins derived from either the iron storage compartment in macrophages or the iron utilization compartment in RBC precursors.

Screening Measurements

Hemoglobin Concentration

Hemoglobin concentration is the most commonly used screening test for iron deficiency. Someone with normal body iron stores must lose a large portion of body iron before the hemoglobin falls below the laboratory definitions of anemia. Furthermore, low hemoglobin does not distinguish among the causes of anemia other than iron deficiency, and additional testing is required.

Serum Iron and Transferrin Saturation

Serum iron levels normally fluctuate daily, with maximal levels occurring in the morning and minimal levels in the evening. The total iron-binding capacity (TIBC) varies less than serum iron but is harder to measure accurately. The normal TIBC is 250 to 400 mg/dL, but as serum iron levels decrease, the TIBC increases to 450 mg/dL or more. Iron and TIBC measurements are useful in distinguishing IDA from anemia of chronic disease. Serum iron levels decrease with both, but the TIBC levels also decrease in chronic disease states

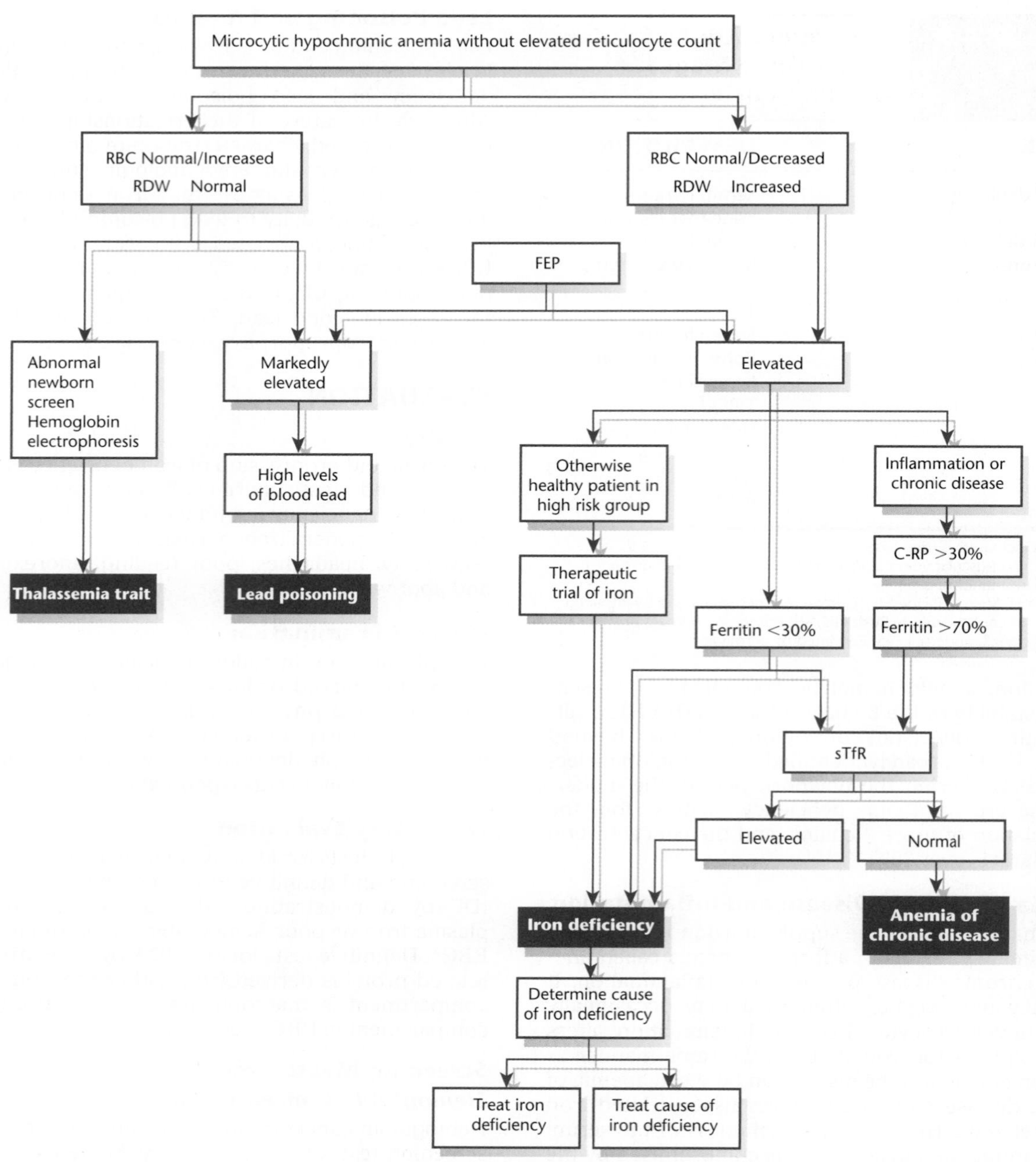

Figure 287-2 Algorithm for an approach to microcytic anemia. RBC, red blood cell; RDW, red blood cell distribution width.

(Table 287-4). The degree of iron saturation of plasma transferrin is calculated as follows: transferrin saturation = (serum iron concentration ÷ TIBC) × 100.

Serum iron and TIBC levels help confirm the diagnosis of iron deficiency, with a low serum iron and a high transferrin level resulting in a transferrin saturation of less than 10% to 15%. Transferrin levels are increased in iron-deficiency states because of increased hepatic synthesis of the protein and greater liberation of apotransferrin (the transport protein without iron) from hemoglobin-synthesizing sites. This relatively inexpensive measurement is widely available. However, marked diurnal variation in plasma iron values and the numerous clinical disorders that affect the transferrin saturation limit its use in the clinical setting. Normal or high transferrin saturation is as useful for excluding IDA as a low value is for identifying it.

Red Blood Cell Indices

The development of electronic counters has made the use of RBC indices widely available for the initial screening of infants and children for iron deficiency.

Table 287-3 Red Blood Cell Indices During Infancy and Childhood

AGE	HEMOGLOBIN (g/dL) MEAN	HEMOGLOBIN (g/dL) RANGE	HEMATOCRIT (%) MEAN	HEMATOCRIT (%) RANGE	RETICULOCYTES (%) MEAN	MCV (fL) LOWEST
CHILD						
Cord blood	16.8	13.7-20.1	55	45-65	5.0	110
2 wk	16.5	13.0-20.0	50	42-66	1.0	107
3 mo	12.0	9.5-14.5	36	31-41	1.0	80
6 mo-6 yr	12.0	10.5-14.0	37	33-42	1.0	70-74
7-12 yr	13.0	11.0-16.0	38	34-40	1.0	76-80
ADULT						
Female	14	12.0-16.0	42	37-47	1.6	80
Male	16	14.0-18.0	47	42-52	1.6	80

MCV, Mean corpuscular volume; *WBC*, white blood cells.
Modified from Behrman RE. *Nelson Text Book of Pediatrics*. 17th ed. Philadelphia: WB Saunders; 2004. Copyright © 2004, Elsevier, with permission.

Table 287-4 Laboratory Findings Associated With the Differential Diagnosis of Microcytic Anemias

FINDING	IRON DEFICIENCY	LEAD POISONING	β-THALASSEMIA TRAIT	CHRONIC DISEASE
Ferritin	↓	Normal	Normal	↑
Serum iron	↓	Normal	Normal	↓
Total iron-binding capacity	↑	Normal	Normal	↓
Erythrocyte zinc protoporphyrin	↑	↑↑	Normal	↑
Red blood cell distribution width	↑	Normal	Normal	Normal
Serum transferrin receptor	↑	Normal	↑	Normal

↑, increased; ↑↑, very increased; ↓, decreased. Iron deficiency and lead poisoning frequently co-exist.

These tests are highly reproducible and less subject to sampling error compared with hemoglobin determinations because tissue fluid dilution does not affect RBC size. The RBCs become smaller than normal with decreased MCV, and their hemoglobin content decreases with decreased MCH. The RDW approximates the standard deviation of the RBC population. Normal RDWs occur in the range of 12% to 17%. In IDA, a marked dispersion exists in cell volumes (sizes) such that the RDW increases. RBC indices in infancy and childhood are described in Table 287-3.

Zinc Protoporphyrin

A simple and reliable measurement of IDE is the erythrocyte ZnPP, a product of abnormal heme synthesis. Normally, a trace of zinc rather than iron is incorporated into protoporphyrin during the final step of heme biosynthesis. In states of IDE, ZnPP formation is enhanced.[16] An increase in the zinc protoporphyrin to heme ratio (ZnPP/H) of greater than 80 mcmol/mol is demonstrated to be a sensitive, specific, and cost-effective test for identifying preanemic iron deficiency.[16] A major advantage of this well-established assay is the ability to measure the ZnPP/H ratio directly on a drop of blood using a dedicated portable instrument called a hematofluorimeter. Initially, ZnPP was erroneously characterized as metal-free protoporphyrin or free erythrocyte protoporphyrin or erythrocyte protoporphyrin.[17] In fact, most presumed metal-free protoporphyrin in erythrocytes is now known to be largely an artifact of the analytical procedures used at the time and is still used in some laboratories that required an acid extraction that removed zinc to form metal-free or free protoporphyrin. Because approximately 95% of the nonheme protoporphyrin in erythrocytes is ZnPP, this procedure does not create a diagnostic problem in most cases. The ZnPP/H ratio is an indicator of iron available to the developing erythrocytes in the bone marrow regardless of the cause, such as iron deficiency, inflammation, or functional iron deficiency such as in chronic renal failure. Another significant limitation of ZnPP is that it increases with lead toxicity, and even the normal range varies with environmental lead exposure, infections, inflammatory diseases, and protoporphyria. However, the ZnPP/H ratio is not increased in thalassemia trait, which makes ZnPP/H ratio determinations helpful in distinguishing iron deficiency from α- or β-thalassemia trait, in addition to its role in screening for iron deficiency (see Table 287-4).

Reticulocyte Hemoglobin

The mean reticulocyte hemoglobin content (CHr) is analogous to the RBC mean corpuscular hemoglobin but with the advantage of monitoring the hemoglobinization of the most recently produced RBCs. A CHr of less than 26 pg is an early indicator of iron-restricted hematopoiesis and IDA in children.[18] The diagnostic power of CHr is limited in patients with high MCV or with RBC disorders such as thalassemia.[19]

Peripheral Blood Smear

Examination of the blood smear in IDA reveals hypochromic microcytes, poikilocytes, elliptocytes, and target cells (Figure 287-3). The presence of basophilic stippling suggests associated lead poisoning. However, the RBC changes seen on the blood smear are not specific for iron deficiency. The white blood cell count and morphology in IDA are usually normal. Both thrombocytosis and thrombocytopenia occur with iron deficiency. The latter is more common in severe iron deficiency and resolves once iron therapy is begun.

Definitive Tests

The absence of stainable iron in the bone marrow is a definitive test for IDA but is not routinely applicable for obvious reasons. The 2 key definitive measurements for diagnosing iron deficiency are the serum ferritin, which measures the size of iron stores, and the serum transferrin receptor, which measures the extent of tissue iron deficiency.[20]

Serum Ferritin

Definitive serum ferritin levels vary with age during infancy and childhood. In healthy individuals, serum ferritin levels reflect body iron stores; levels below 30 ng/L indicate iron deficiency. Ferritin is an acute-phase reactant. Serum ferritin levels are increased during infections and inflammatory processes, as well as with liver disease. Although low serum ferritin is diagnostic of iron deficiency, a high ferritin level associated with inflammation or liver disease does not rule out concomitant iron deficiency.

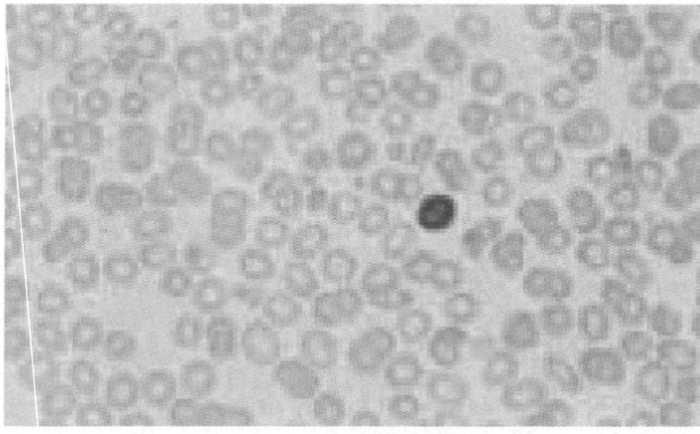

Figure 287-3 Iron-deficiency anemia. Many red blood cells are microcytic (smaller than the nucleus of the normal lymphocyte near the center of the field) and hypochromic (with central areas of pallor that exceed one half of the diameter of the cells). *(Goldman L.* Cecil Textbook of Medicine. *22nd ed. Copyright © 2004 WB Saunders, with permission.)*

Serum Transferrin Receptor

The proteolytic cleavage of transferrin receptors can be measured in the serum as sTfR. sTfR directly correlates with the total mass of erythroid precursor. The sTfR is high in iron deficiency and in conditions resulting in increased production of RBCs, including thalassemia and sickle cell disease.[21] sTfR is not affected by inflammation, and hence it is useful in distinguishing iron deficiency from chronic inflammatory states that do not have high sTfR (see Table 287-4). Infants have higher baseline sTfR levels than children and adults, indicating the need to establish age-specific references values. The ratio of sTfR to serum ferritin has been shown to have excellent performance in estimating body iron stores but is limited by the lack of standardization for sTfR assays.[22,23]

Bone Marrow Iron

The staining of a normal bone marrow aspirate sample with Prussian blue dye reveals the presence of iron in RBC precursors (normoblasts) and serves as a reliable index of body iron stores. In iron deficiency, the number of iron granules in normoblasts is decreased, and stainable iron in the marrow aspirate is almost completely absent.[3]

MANAGEMENT

Therapeutic Trial of Iron

Therapeutic trial of iron has been proposed as a convenient method to diagnose iron deficiency in patients with anemia. Although this approach is reasonable in otherwise-healthy individuals, in those at high risk of deficiency, such as infants, teenage girls, and pregnant women, making a definitive laboratory diagnosis at the outset is preferable.

Treatment of Iron Deficiency

The treatment of choice for iron deficiency is the oral administration of iron. Although various iron salts are available, ferrous sulfate is inexpensive and well tolerated, although adverse effects may occur, such as nausea, dyspepsia, constipation, and diarrhea. Adverse effects can be managed by administering the iron with or immediately after meals. If symptoms persist, then reductions in the amount of iron in each dose or reduction in frequency to a single daily dose may help control the side effects. If intolerance is persistent, then switching to ferrous gluconate may be helpful. Iron polysaccharide complex also has the advantage of availability as tablets or elixir and is well tolerated. Approximately twice as much iron is absorbed on an empty stomach as at mealtime. Consumption of milk should be limited, which will allow increased intake of iron-rich foods, and blood loss from intolerance to cow's milk proteins is reduced.

Because soy-based formulas can also lead to blood loss,[24] children with milk enteropathy should be switched to a primary diet of iron-containing solids. In the absence of ongoing blood losses, response to iron therapy is rapid and predictable (see Figure 287-1). A response of decreased irritability and increased appetite to oral iron therapy has been noted within 12 to 24 hours (Table 287-5). The reticulocyte response peaks at 5 to 7 days after the institution of iron therapy. In an otherwise-healthy individual, the recovery from anemia is approximately two-thirds complete within 1 month. The hemoglobin be measured again at 1 month to check the therapeutic progress and to emphasize compliance.

If after 4 weeks the anemia does not respond to iron treatment despite compliance with the iron supplementation regimen and the absence of acute illness, then the anemia can be further evaluated by using other laboratory tests, including MCV, RDW, and serum ferritin concentration. For example, a serum ferritin concentration of 15 mcg/L or less confirms iron deficiency, and a concentration of more than 15 mcg/L suggests that iron deficiency is not the cause of the anemia. Once the diagnosis of iron deficiency is confirmed, either by a response to a therapeutic trial or by further laboratory tests, oral therapy with elemental iron at 3 to 6 mg/kg per day should be continued for 2 to 3 months after normal hemoglobin levels have been restored. This regimen allows the repletion of body iron stores. Anemia, microcytosis, and increased free erythrocyte protoporphyrin levels are corrected completely with 3 to 5 months of treatment.

Use of intramuscular or intravenous iron is rarely warranted. Parenteral iron administration may be indicated in the face of ongoing blood loss that exceeds the body's ability to replenish iron stores through oral absorption, in the presence of iron malabsorption, or when the patient cannot tolerate or will not take oral iron preparations.[20] Intramuscular injections are painful, and skin discoloration is common. Anaphylactic reactions have occurred with both intramuscular and intravenous injection, and deaths have been reported. Parenteral treatment should therefore be used only when oral therapy is not possible—for example, in patients who have inflammatory bowel disease. Three drugs are licensed in the United States. Iron dextran has been used for several years but is associated with significant risks. Iron sucrose and iron gluconate may have a better safety profile than iron dextran.

Table 287-5 Responses to Iron Therapy in Iron-Deficiency Anemia

TIME AFTER IRON ADMINISTRATION	RESPONSE
12-24 hr	Replacement of intracellular iron enzymes; subjective improvement; decreased irritability; increased appetite
36-48 hr	Initial bone marrow response; erythroid hyperplasia
48-72 hr	Reticulocytosis, peaking at 5-7 day
4-30 day	Increase in hemoglobin level
1-3 mo	Repletion of stores

Modified from Behrman RE. *Nelson Text Book of Pediatrics.* 17th ed. Philadelphia: WB Saunders; 2004. Copyright © 2004, Elsevier, with permission.

BOX 287-1 Recommendations of the Centers for Disease Control and Prevention for the Primary Prevention of Iron Deficiency in Infants, Children, and Adolescents

BREASTFEEDING AND IRON-FORTIFIED FORMULA

- Encourage exclusive breastfeeding of infants (without supplementary liquid, formula, or food) for 4-6 months after birth.
- When exclusive breastfeeding is stopped, encourage use of an additional source of iron (approximately 1 mg/kg/day of iron), preferably from supplementary foods.
- For infants aged <12 months who are not breastfed or who are partially breastfed, recommend only iron-fortified infant formula as a substitute for human milk.
- For breastfed infants who receive insufficient iron from supplementary foods by age 6 months (ie, <1 mg/kg/day), suggest 1 mg/kg/day of iron drops.
- For breastfed infants who were preterm or who had low birth weight, recommend 2-4 mg/kg/day of iron drops (to a maximum of 15 mg/day) starting at 1 month after birth and continuing until 12 months after birth.
- Encourage use of only human milk or iron-fortified infant formula for any milk-based part of the diet (eg, in infant cereal) and discourage use of low-iron milks (eg, cow's milk, goat's milk, soy milk) until age 12 months.
- Suggest that children ages 1-5 years consume no more than 24 oz of cow's milk, goat's milk, or soy milk each day.

SOLID FOODS

- At age 4-6 months or when the extrusion reflex disappears, recommend that infants be introduced to plain, iron-fortified infant cereal. Two or more servings per day of iron-fortified infant cereal can meet an infant's requirement for iron at this age.
- By approximately age 6 months, encourage one feeding per day of foods rich in vitamin C (eg, fruits, vegetables, juice) to improve iron absorption, preferably with meals.
- Suggest introducing plain, pureed meats after age 6 months or when the infant is developmentally ready to consume such food.

ADOLESCENT GIRLS AND NONPREGNANT WOMEN

- Encourage adolescent girls and women to eat iron-rich foods and foods that enhance iron absorption and to optimize their dietary iron intake.

From Centers for Disease Control and Prevention. Recommendations to prevent and control iron deficiency in the United States. *MMWR Recomm Rep.* 1998;47:1-29.

A blood transfusion is indicated only when severe anemia leads to congestive heart failure and cardiovascular compromise. If a blood transfusion is clinically warranted, then packed RBCs should be given slowly or a partial exchange transfusion performed. Vital signs should be monitored carefully.

Failure to Respond to Therapy

When a patient fails to respond to oral iron treatment, the following factors should be considered: (1) noncompliance with oral therapy, (2) inadequate iron dose, (3) persistent or unrecognized blood loss, (4) malabsorption of iron (eg, primary gastrointestinal disease), (5) other diagnoses (eg, α- or β-thalassemia trait and Hb E disease), and (6) poor iron utilization (eg, chronic inflammatory disease, sideroblastic anemia, lead poisoning, congenital atransferrinemia).

BOX 287-2 Recommendations of the Centers for Disease Control and Prevention for the Screening for Iron Deficiency in Infants, Children, and Adolescents

- Anemia screening before age 6 months for preterm infants and low-birth-weight infants who are not fed iron-fortified infant formula
- Annual assessment of children ages 2-5 years for risk factors for iron-deficiency anemia (IDA) (eg, a low-iron diet, limited access to food because of poverty or neglect, special health care needs)
- Assessment at ages 9-12 months and 6 months later (at ages 15-18 months) for infants and young children for risk factors for anemia:
  - Preterm or low-birth-weight infants
  - Infants fed a diet of non-iron-fortified infant formula for >2 months
  - Infants introduced to cow's milk before age 12 months
  - Breastfed infants who do not consume a diet adequate in iron after age 6 months (ie, who receive insufficient iron from supplementary foods)
  - Children who consume >24 oz daily of cow's milk
  - Children who have special health care needs (eg, children who use medications that interfere with iron absorption and children who have chronic infection, inflammatory disorders, restricted diets, or extensive blood loss from a wound, an accident, or surgery)
- In populations of infants and preschool children at high risk for IDA (eg, children from low-income families, children eligible for the Special Supplemental Nutrition Program for Women, Infants, and Children,[21] migrant children, or recently arrived refugee children), screen all children for anemia between ages 9 and 12 months, 6 months later, and annually from ages 2 to 5 years
- Starting in adolescence, screen all nonpregnant women for anemia every 5-10 years throughout their childbearing years during routine health examinations
- Annually screen for anemia women having risk factors for iron deficiency (eg, extensive menstrual or other blood loss, low iron intake, a previous diagnosis of IDA)

From Centers for Disease Control and Prevention. Recommendations to prevent and control iron deficiency in the United States. *MMWR Recomm Rep.* 1998;47:1-29

PREVENTION

Increased iron intake among infants has resulted in a decline in childhood IDA in the United States. Consequently the use of screening tests for anemia has become a less efficient means of detecting iron deficiency in some populations, whereas for women of childbearing age, iron deficiency has remained prevalent. The Centers for Disease Control and Prevention has therefore developed recommendations for use by primary health care physicians for primary prevention of iron deficiency through appropriate dietary intake (Box 287-1) and secondary prevention through detecting and treating IDA (Box 287-2).[8]

WHEN TO REFER

- Cause of anemia is unknown.
- Gastrointestinal blood loss is suspected.
- Anemia is not explained by nutritional imbalance.
- Anemia is refractory to treatment.
- Patient requires intravenous iron.
- Diagnosis of iron deficiency is questionable.

WHEN TO ADMIT

- Patient exhibits signs of cardiac failure.
- Patient requires intravenous iron.
- Patient has moderate to severe blood loss.

TOOLS FOR PRACTICE

Engaging Patient and Family

- *Anemia FAQ* (fact sheet), American Academy of Pediatrics (www.aap.org/publiced/BR_Anemia.htm).
- *Anemia and Your Young Child* (brochure), American Academy of Pediatrics (patiented.aap.org).

RELATED WEB SITE

- Centers for Disease Control and Prevention: Iron Deficiency Anemia (www.cdc.gov/nccdphp/dnpa/nutrition/nutrition_for_everyone/iron_deficiency/index.htm).

SUGGESTED RESOURCES

Centers for Disease Control and Prevention. Recommendations to prevent and control iron deficiency in the United States. *MMWR Recomm Rep.* 1998;47(RR-3):1-29.

Cook JD. Diagnosis and management of iron-deficiency anaemia. *Best Pract Res Clin Haematol.* 2005;18:319-332.

Sandoval C, Jayabose S, Eden AN. Trends in diagnosis and management of iron deficiency during infancy and early childhood. *Hematol Oncol Clin North Am.* 2004;18:1423-1438.

REFERENCES

1. Grantham-McGregor S, Ani C. A review of studies on the effect of iron deficiency on cognitive development in children. *J Nutr.* 2001;131:649S-666S, discussion 666S-668S.
2. Stoltzfus RJ. Iron-deficiency anemia: reexamining the nature and magnitude of the public health problem. Summary: implications for research and programs. *J Nutr.* 2001;131:697S-700S, discussion 700S-701S.
3. Centers for Disease Control and Prevention. Iron deficiency—United States, 1999-2000. *MMWR Morb Mortal Wkly Rep.* 2002;51:897-899.
4. Looker AC, Cogswell ME, Gunter EW. Iron deficiency—United States, 1999-2000. (Reprinted from *MMWR.* 2002;51:897-899.) *JAMA.* 2002;288:2114-2116.
5. Davis RM. "Healthy people 2010": national health objectives for the United States. *BMJ.* 1998;317:1513-1517.
6. Blot I, Diallo D, Tchernia G. Iron deficiency in pregnancy: effects on the newborn. *Curr Opin Hematol.* 1999;6: 65-70.
7. Rao R, Georgieff MK. Perinatal aspects of iron metabolism. *Acta Paediatr Suppl.* 2002;91:124-129.
8. Centers for Disease Control and Prevention. Recommendations to prevent and control iron deficiency in the United States. *MMWR Recomm Rep.* 1998;47:1-29.
9. England JM, Ward SM, Down MC. Microcytosis, anisocytosis and the red cell indices in iron deficiency. *Br J Haematol.* 1976;34:589-597.
10. Schaefer RM, Bahner U. Iron metabolism in rhEPO-treated hemodialysis patients. *Clin Nephrol.* 2000;53: S65-S68.
11. Macdougall IC, Cooper AC. Hyporesponsiveness to erythropoietic therapy due to chronic inflammation. *Eur J Clin Invest.* 2005;35(suppl 3):32-35.
12. Mentzer WC Jr. Differentiation of iron deficiency from thalassaemia trait. *Lancet.* 1973;1:882.
13. Sandoval C, Jayabose S, Eden AN. Trends in diagnosis and management of iron deficiency during infancy and early childhood. *Hematol Oncol Clin North Am.* 2004;18: 1423-1438.
14. Demir A, Yarali N, Fisgin T, et al. Most reliable indices in differentiation between thalassemia trait and iron deficiency anemia. *Pediatr Int.* 2002;44:612-616.
15. Kwong WT, Friello P, Semba RD. Interactions between iron deficiency and lead poisoning: epidemiology and pathogenesis. *Sci Total Environ.* 2004;330:21-37.
16. Rettmer RL, Carlson TH, Origenes ML, et al. Zinc protoporphyrin/heme ratio for diagnosis of preanemic iron deficiency. *Pediatrics.* 1999;104:e37.
17. Labbe RF, Dewanji A. Iron assessment tests: transferrin receptor vis-a-vis zinc protoporphyrin. *Clin Biochem.* 2004;37:165-174.
18. Brugnara C, Zurakowski D, DiCanzio J, et al. Reticulocyte hemoglobin content to diagnose iron deficiency in children. *JAMA.* 1999;281:2225-2230.
19. Mast AE, Blinder MA, Lu Q, et al. Clinical utility of the reticulocyte hemoglobin content in the diagnosis of iron deficiency. *Blood.* 2002;99:1489-1491.
20. Cook JD. Diagnosis and management of iron-deficiency anaemia. *Best Pract Res Clin Haematol.* 2005;18:319-332.
21. Cook JD. The measurement of serum transferrin receptor. *Am J Med Sci.* 1999;318:269-276.
22. Brugnara C. Iron deficiency and erythropoiesis: new diagnostic approaches. *Clin Chem.* 2003;49:1573-1578.
23. Cook JD, Flowers CH, Skikne BS. The quantitative assessment of body iron. *Blood.* 2003;101:3359-3364.
24. Nickerson HJ, Silberman T, Park RW, et al. Treatment of iron deficiency anemia and associated protein-losing enteropathy in children. *J Pediatr Hematol Oncol.* 2000; 22:50-54.

Chapter 288

JUVENILE IDIOPATHIC ARTHRITIS

David M. Siegel, MD, MPH; Harry L. Gewanter, MD

Juvenile idiopathic arthritis (JIA; previously referred to as juvenile rheumatoid arthritis or juvenile chronic arthritis) is an uncommon collection of clinical syndromes that have the common feature of chronic childhood arthritis. The diagnosis is applied to any child younger than 16 years who has persistent arthritis of one or more joints lasting for more than 6 weeks in whom all other diseases have been excluded. JIA is classified further into 7 subtypes, with most patients fitting into systemic-onset, oligoarthritis, or polyarthritis based on the clinical course over the first 6 months of illness.[1]

Although JIA is the most common of the pediatric rheumatic diseases, its true incidence and prevalence are unknown. For all subtypes taken collectively, the peak age at onset is between 2 and 4 years of age, with a smaller peak later in childhood. Overall, a general female predominance is found, but not in all subtypes. The best estimate of prevalence is approximately 0.5 to 1 case per 1000 children; thus approximately 40,000 to 100,000 children in the United States have JIA at any given time.[2]

ETIOLOGY

The exact cause of JIA is unknown. Data on the frequency of certain subtypes of human leukocyte antigens (HLA) in JIA (eg, HLA-DR5 and -DR8 in younger girls who have oligoarticular JIA, HLA-DR4 in rheumatoid factor [RF]-positive polyarticular JIA, and HLA-B27 in older boys who have enthesitis-related JIA)[3] have led to the concept of a genetic predisposition for the development of an inflammatory arthritis that may be triggered by any of several events, such as trauma, infection,[4] or emotional stress.[5]

Other areas of interesting research include investigations of immunologic abnormalities involving autoantibodies,[6] cytokines, immunoregulation,[7] and the function of and communication between T and B lymphocytes and antigen-presenting cells.[3] The precise nature of these interactions and how they result in the development of JIA remain to be discovered, but the success of specific cytokine-directed therapy (eg, etanercept, anakinra) supports the central role of these proinflammatory mediators in the clinical manifestations and course of JIA.

RHEUMATOLOGIC DISORDERS WITH ARTHRITIS

Juvenile ankylosing spondylitis and the other spondyloarthropathies can present as a subtype of JIA at their onset, especially in an older child who is HLA-B27 positive. Acute rheumatic fever, although long in decline in the United States and other industrialized nations, has seen a resurgence in the last 2 decades. Patients with acute rheumatic fever can experience both arthralgia and arthritis, classically characterized as migratory.[8] Systemic lupus erythematosus has arthritis as one of its major manifestations, but it can be differentiated from JIA by its other systemic features and specific laboratory test abnormalities. Although its sex distribution is equal in younger children, female preponderance is found after puberty. Dermatomyositis is characterized more typically by inflammatory muscle involvement than by arthritis, but children can be affected with joint inflammation and contractures. Scleroderma is occasionally associated with arthritis, but it has classic dermatologic and other manifestations that distinguish it from JIA.

CLINICAL MANIFESTATION

Because the diagnosis of JIA is based on clinical findings, the history and physical examination are paramount; no unique or specific diagnostic laboratory tests yet exist. Only by considering all the data on the child's presentation and course is the physician able to diagnose JIA.

The presence of arthritis or inflammation within the joint is an absolute criterion for diagnosing JIA. Arthritis is defined as being present when intraarticular swelling or effusion is present or when 2 or more of the following occur: joint pain or tenderness with motion, limitation of joint motion, or increased warmth overlying the joint. Arthralgia (joint pain) is a relatively frequent symptom in children, but true joint inflammation, or arthritis, is much less common. Younger children rarely complain of joint pain but may instead become irritable, stop walking or using an extremity, or regress in their behavior. In fact, a recent retrospective review of presenting complaints to a pediatric rheumatology center found that pain was not a predictor of the diagnosis of juvenile arthritis.[9] Other symptoms include decreased appetite, malaise, inactivity, morning stiffness, nighttime joint pains, and failure to thrive. Features that may also be present in children who have chronic arthritis (varying with the subtype) include fever, rash, lymphadenopathy, hepatosplenomegaly, polyserositis, subcutaneous (rheumatoid) nodules, vasculitis, and growth retardation. The pattern, as well as the number of involved joints, family history and other factors are important in classifying the disease.

SYSTEMIC-ONSET JUVENILE IDIOPATHIC ARTHRITIS

Even though the hallmark of systemic-onset JIA (also known as Still disease) is its extraarticular manifestations, the eventual presence of arthritis is necessary to confirm the diagnosis. Systemic-onset JIA, which affects approximately 15% of all children who have JIA, is slightly more common among boys than girls and usually begins at an early age, although it has even been recognized in adults (adult-onset Still disease). The systemic features may persist for months and occur or recur independently of the arthritis.

Daily intermittent fevers characterize systemic-onset JIA, with rectal temperature reaching as high as 40°C to 41°C (104°F to 106°F), most often in the afternoon, and then returning to normal or subnormal levels (known as a quotidian fever pattern). An evanescent, salmon-colored rash often accompanies the fevers. The lesions are small macules or papules, frequently with central clearing, and often appear in areas of increased heat (eg, axilla). Mild abrasion of unaffected skin can precipitate appearance of the rash (Koebner phenomenon).

Polyserositis in the form of pericarditis or pleuritis is common; enlargement of the lymph nodes, liver, and spleen may be of sufficient size to suggest the presence of a malignancy. These serosal effusions, however, are rarely symptomatic or clinically significant. Although these children frequently complain of myalgias or arthralgias when they are febrile, they may have few symptoms when the fevers resolve. The arthritis may occur at any time after the onset of disease, and in some patients, it appears only days to weeks after the systemic signs occur. The arthritis tends to be polyarticular, involving both large and small joints, and can be persistent, destructive, and severe.

Laboratory studies reveal a high white blood cell count, with predominance of band forms and polymorphonuclear leukocytes. Most patients are anemic. Thrombocytosis is frequent, as are significant increases of the acute phase reactants (eg, erythrocyte sedimentation rate [ESR] and C reactive protein). RF and antinuclear antibody (ANA) tests are rarely positive. Serum immunoglobulin and complement levels are usually normal but may be elevated, reflecting the degree of inflammation, and sometimes evidence of a vasculopathy and an intravascular consumption coagulopathy is found.[10] With regard to the latter, an unusual but severe and potentially fatal complication of systemic-onset JIA is macrophage activation syndrome. This disorder can be rapidly progressive and may be difficult to distinguish from a flare in the underlying disease, but hallmarks are dramatically high ferritin levels (>10,000 ng/mL), paradoxically decreasing ESR accompanied by decreased fibrinogen, increased triglycerides, leucopenia, anemia, thrombocytopenia, and hepatic failure. Definitive diagnosis is based on bone marrow biopsy, and quick therapeutic intervention is necessary.[11]

The clinical course of systemic-onset JIA is extremely variable. Some children have a single systemic episode that lasts weeks to months and have few joint problems; others have multiple systemic episodes before developing the arthritis, which can be oligoarticular but is more commonly polyarticular in distribution. Poor prognostic signs include the continued presence of systemic features and a platelet count exceeding 600,000/mm^3 6 months after onset. At least a third of these children will develop severe arthritis.[12]

POLYARTICULAR JUVENILE IDIOPATHIC ARTHRITIS

Approximately 30% to 35% of children who have JIA have the polyarticular type, which can be subdivided into immunoglobulin (Ig) M-RF–positive (approximately 10% of the total) and IgM-RF–negative (approximately 25%) forms. So-called hidden RFs have been found in all subgroups, but their significance remains obscure.[13] Finding a meaningfully positive RF in a child younger than 7 years is rare. Systemic features in polyarticular JIA are usually mild and include low-grade fever, easy fatigability, and slowing of growth. The growth problems may be local (eg, micrognathia) or generalized and can occur regardless of whether the child receives corticosteroid treatment. Discrepancies between height and weight are seen and can help with diagnosis. For example, children who have polyarticular arthritis may be of low weight for height, whereas children who have systemic-onset JIA tend to be average in weight for height.[14] The arthritis is most often chronic and symmetrical, and it involves 5 or more joints. Any joint of the body, including the temporomandibular joint and the cervical spine, can be affected. Nearly all children have wrist involvement, and small joint involvement of the hands and feet is common. Finally, these children may develop a chronic uveitis.[15]

Rheumatoid Factor–Positive Polyarticular Juvenile Idiopathic Arthritis

Patients who have IgM RF-positive polyarticular JIA are most often older than 8 to 10 years, are more likely to be girls than boys, and are similar clinically to patients who have adult rheumatoid arthritis. Severe, rapidly progressive, erosive, crippling arthritis, subcutaneous rheumatoid nodules, and rheumatoid vasculitis can develop, just as in adults. Cyclic citrullinated protein (CCP) is a laboratory study that can be used to assess disease severity and potential for joint destruction. An elevated serum level would serve as reason to institute early and aggressive therapy.

Rheumatoid Factor–Negative Polyarticular Juvenile Idiopathic Arthritis

Children who have IgM RF-negative polyarticular JIA are usually younger. While they have a better prognosis than those are IgM RF positive, typically these children respond better to therapy and have a lower frequency of severe, early, crippling arthritis than do children who have the IgM RF-positive form and they may develop many significant problems. Because their arthritis starts earlier, it can lead to deformities and problems as a result of the tendency to develop flexion contractures and, if severe, subluxations at the involved joints. Compared with adults, hand involvement affects the interphalangeal joints more often than the metacarpophalangeal joints. Ulnar deviation of the fingers is much less common in children compared with adults, whereas flexion contractures, boutonniere (buttonhole) deformities, and radial deviation of the fingers are seen more frequently. Ulnar deviation and subluxation at the wrist may occur. Arthritis of the apophyseal joints of the cervical spine is common and can lead to rapid and significant limitation of extension and rotation. These children are at the highest risk for developing the local and generalized growth problems mentioned previously.

Oligoarticular Juvenile Idiopathic Arthritis

Oligoarticular JIA involves 4 or fewer joints, most often the large joints (eg, knee, ankle, elbow), typically in an asymmetrical distribution. The pattern and course of joint involvement are important in distinguishing this form of JIA from the others, as are the number of joints involved. Systemic features are infrequent and, if present, mild. Nearly 50% to 60% of all children who have JIA fall in this oligoarticular subgroup, and they have the best overall prognosis. Oligoarticular JIA can be subdivided further into persistent and extended oligoarticular subtypes.

Persistent Oligoarthritis

Persistent oligoarthritis (5% to 10% of all patients who have JIA) occurs classically in girls younger than 6 years of age and involves the large joints. These girls are at higher risk for developing chronic uveitis, particularly when positive for ANA.[14] Despite their obvious arthritis, these children generally function well and only rarely complain of significant pain. Little erosive joint damage typically occurs, even though these patients may have ongoing arthritis for many years. Nonetheless, they are at risk for long-term problems, including leg-length discrepancies (especially with asymmetric knee joint involvement) and muscle atrophy.[16] The growth centers around the knee with arthritis can become more active because of the inflammatory-associated hyperemia, resulting in increased growth of that leg. Similarly, as a result of changes in the child's biomechanics, decreased quadriceps mass on the affected side is frequently found.

Systemic signs and symptoms, except for uveitis, are few. The uveitis is rarely symptomatic until it has progressed to a severe stage, and it may not occur until years after the onset of the arthritis; it may even occur after the arthritis has resolved. Thus regular ophthalmologic evaluation, including slit-lamp examinations, should be instituted early, performed every 4 to 6 months, and continued indefinitely. Because the risk of uveitis decreases with time and varies by JIA subtype and age at diagnosis, the prescribed intervals between examinations vary, eventually lengthening after several years if no uveitis is present[15] (Table 288-1).

Except for ANA positivity, few laboratory abnormalities will be found. When positive, the ANA titer is typically low. Although mild increases in white blood cell count and ESR or a low-grade anemia may be observed, all of these tests are often normal. HLA-DR5 gene markers appear to confer increased susceptibility for persistent oligoarthritis, whereas HLA-DR1 and -DR4 are underrepresented in this group.

The course of children with persistent oligoarthritis can be extremely variable. Some children have a single episode; others may have recurrent exacerbations and remissions. Regardless of their individual style, this group has the fewest musculoskeletal complications and more long-term remissions.

Extended Oligoarthritis

Children with the extended oligoarthritis subtype of JIA initially have 4 or fewer joints involved within the first 6 months of their disease. However, at a variable time after the initial 6 months, they develop arthritis in more joints. This group comprises approximately 20% to 25% of all children with oligoarthritis. It differs from persistent oligoarthritis in several ways. The genetic makeup of these children appears to be different, with a higher frequency of HLA-DR1, and the children have

Table 288-1 Frequency of Ophthalmologic Examination in Patients With Juvenile Rheumatoid Arthritis

TYPE	ANA	AGE AT ONSET (yr)	DURATION OF DISEASE (yr)	RISK CATEGORY	EYE EXAMINATION FREQUENCY (mo)
Oligoarthritis or polyarthritis	+	≤6	≤4	High	3
	+	≤6	>4	Moderate	6
	+	≤6	>7	Low	12
	+	>6	≤4	Moderate	6
	+	>6	>4	Low	12
	–	≤6	≤4	Moderate	6
	–	≤6	>4	Low	12
	–	>6	NA	Low	12
Systemic disease (fever, rash)	NA	NA	NA	Low	12

ANA, Antinuclear antibodies; *NA,* not applicable.
Recommendations for follow-up continue through childhood and adolescence.
From Cassidy J, Kivlin J, Lindsley C, et al, American Academy of Pediatrics, Section on Rheumatology and Section on Ophthalmology. Ophthalmologic examinations in children with juvenile rheumatoid arthritis. *Pediatrics.* 2006;117:1843-1845.

a higher occurrence of erosive disease. The additionally involved joints are often the wrists, fingers, and other smaller joints. Although cases of chronic uveitis are fewer, it still occurs, and these children also need to be monitored closely by ophthalmologists. Although this subgroup seems to have fewer children enter a prolonged remission as compared with children with persistent oligoarthritis, they also fare better than children with a polyarthritis onset.

Enthesitis-Related Arthritis

Enthesitis-related arthritis is a newer classification that includes children who previously were classified as late-onset oligoarthritis. This subgroup includes children with arthritis and enthesitis and the presence of at least two of the following: sacroiliac joint pain or inflammatory spinal pain (or both); presence of HLA-B27; history of relatives with HLA-B27–associated disease; anterior uveitis usually associated with pain, redness, or photophobia; or onset of arthritis in a boy older than 8 years. Their arthritis is more frequently in the lower extremities, involving the knees and ankles but also occasionally the toes (resulting in so-called *sausage toe,* or dactylitis).[17]

Complaints and findings of enthesitis (ie, inflammation of the attachment of a tendon, ligament, fascia, or capsule to bone) are a hallmark of this group and may predate any joint problems. These children may progress to fulfill the criteria for ankylosing spondylitis, reactive arthritides, or arthritis associated with inflammatory bowel disease. Approximately 10% will develop an acute iritis. In contrast to the chronic uveitis seen in oligoarticular JIA, this is symptomatic, can be treated early, and is usually self-limited. As with oligoarticular JIA, mild to moderate increase in the ESR is common, but other abnormal laboratory tests are found infrequently.

Psoriatic Arthritis

Psoriatic arthritis is an additional classification subtype of JIA and bears similarity to enthesitis-related arthritis in that large joint inflammation, enthesitis, and dactylitis are often found. For this diagnostic label to be used, however, psoriasis must be present in the patient or in family members. Thus a child can have psoriatic arthritis in the absence of skin disease, although a psoriatic rash can appear at some time after the onset of joint disease. A physical finding that can be useful in identifying psoriatic arthritis in the child or adolescent with characteristic musculoskeletal findings, but no skin eruption, is pitting of the fingernails or toenails. Children are placed in the undifferentiated category if they do not meet the criteria for any of the above subtypes or if they meet criteria for more than one subtype.

DIFFERENTIAL DIAGNOSIS

Diseases to be considered in the differential diagnosis of JIA are listed in Box 288-1.

The hallmark of JIA is its chronic nature; the best initial strategy is often careful, watchful waiting. Only by meeting the criterion of sustained arthritis (>6 weeks) and excluding other possible diseases can the primary care physician avoid mislabeling other transient entities as JIA. The various osteochondroses and avascular necrosis syndromes, musculoskeletal trauma, chondromalacia patellae, Osgood-Schlatter disease, slipped femoral capital epiphysis, diskitis, psychogenic arthralgias, and nonspecific musculoskeletal aches and pains also can mimic JIA in its early stages. Hemophilia, sickle cell disease, inflammatory bowel disease, collagen disorders (eg, Ehlers-Danlos syndrome, Marfan syndrome), the autoinflammatory diseases (Familial Mediterranean Fever, tumor necrosis factor-alpha associated periodic fever syndrome (TRAPS), hyper-IgD syndrome, Muckle-Wells syndrome, neonatal-onset multisystem inflammatory disease (NOMID) [also known as chronic infantile neurologic, cutaneous and articular syndrome (CINCA)], familial cold autoinflammatory syndrome),[18] Wegener granulomatosis, and sarcoidosis may also be associated with arthritis.

If the child has a single inflamed joint, then bacterial arthritis must be considered. If any question exists as to an intraarticular septic process, then arthrocentesis must be performed to establish the diagnosis.

BOX 288-1 Differential Diagnosis of Juvenile Idiopathic Arthritis

RHEUMATIC DISEASE OF CHILDHOOD
Autoinflammatory diseases
Acute rheumatic fever
Systemic lupus erythematosus
Juvenile ankylosing spondylitis
Polymyositis and dermatomyositis
Vasculitis
Scleroderma
Mixed connective-tissue disease/overlap
Kawasaki disease
Behçet syndrome
Postinfectious reactive arthritis
Reactive arthritis
Reflex sympathetic dystrophy (complex regional pain syndrome type II)
Fibromyalgia syndrome

INFECTIOUS DISEASES
Bacterial arthritis
Viral or postviral arthritis
Fungal arthritis
Osteomyelitis
Postinfectious reactive arthritis

NEOPLASTIC DISEASES
Leukemia
Lymphoma
Neuroblastoma
Primary bone tumors

NONINFLAMMATORY DISORDERS
Trauma
Avascular necrosis syndromes
Osteochondroses
Slipped capital femoral epiphysis
Diskitis
Patellofemoral dysfunction (chondromalacia patellae)
Toxic synovitis of the hip
Overuse syndromes

HEMATOLOGIC DISORDERS
Sickle cell disease
Hemophilia

MISCELLANEOUS
Inflammatory bowel disease
Chronic recurrent multifocal osteomyelitis
Sarcoidosis
Collagen (connective tissue) disorders (eg, Ehlers-Danlos syndrome, Marfan syndrome, etc.)
Growing pains
Psychogenic arthralgias (conversion reactions)
Hypermobility syndrome
Villonodular synovitis
Foreign-body arthritis

Haemophilus influenzae type b had been the most common organism isolated in children younger than 2 years, but its incidence has markedly decreased with the advent of universal immunization against *H influenza* type b. If *Neisseria gonorrhoeae* is the cause of septic arthritis, then the most common time for this is in adolescence, whereas various strains of staphylococci may be found at any age. Other infectious agents such as fungi, viruses (including parvovirus, rubella, and hepatitis B), and *Mycoplasma* organisms must also be considered as the cause of arthritis. Lyme disease (*Borrelia burgdorferi* infection) is an etiology for childhood arthritis to consider in endemic areas, of in a child who has recently traveled to an endemic area. Osteomyelitis, involving the bone contiguous to a joint, and reactive arthritis from a gastrointestinal bacterial infection (eg, *Shigella, Salmonella, Campylobacter,* or *Yersinia* organisms) may also mimic some subgroups of JIA. Neoplasms involving the bone, either primary or metastatic (eg, leukemia, lymphoma, neuroblastoma), can be accompanied by musculoskeletal complaints. Although arthritis is uncommon and usually transient, complaints of pain that are out of proportion to physical findings and particularly nighttime pain are common and potentially important clues to heed.

Children who have various immunodeficiencies can have arthritis, either from their primary problem or as a result of infections. Serum sickness and the various vasculitides, including Kawasaki disease (see Chapter 289) and Henoch-Schönlein Purpura (see Chapter 272), can produce intermittent arthritis. Finally, several conditions may produce significant arthralgias and myalgias and may mimic an arthropathy. The complaints and disability resulting from hypermobility syndrome[19] and fibromyalgia[20] can be sufficient to make the clinician believe (although incorrectly) that a form of arthritis is present. Reflex sympathetic dystrophy (also known as complex regional pain syndrome type II) deserves diagnostic consideration in children who have a hot or cold painful extremity that they refuse to move,[21] particularly when a premorbid history of trauma (often minor) is found.

MANAGEMENT

Individualizing each patient's management in terms of the disease subtype, extent of activity, clinical course to date, and family situation is always necessary. Although most physicians are accustomed to considering pharmacologic therapy of primary importance, it is only one aspect of the treatment of children who have JIA. A multidisciplinary team approach is the most effective way to meet the needs of a child who has chronic arthritis, and of the child's family. The goal of therapy is to result in the highest possible level of physical and psychological function for the child.

Currently available drug therapy (Box 288-2), although not yet curative, can suppress the inflammatory activity in many children who have JIA. The ultimate goal is to have no detectable inflammation. Five major categories of drug therapy are available: nonsteroidal antiinflammatory drugs (NSAIDs), disease-modifying antirheumatic drugs (DMARDs), corticosteroids, immunosuppressive drugs, and agents that

BOX 288-2 Medications for Juvenile Idiopathic Arthritis

NONSTEROIDAL ANTIINFLAMMATORY DRUGS (NSAIDS)

FDA-Approved for Use in Children:

Salicylates
Indomethacin
Tolmetin sodium
Naproxen
Ibuprofen
Celecoxib
Meloxicam

Non-FDA–Approved:

Diclofenac sodium
Fenoprofen
Flurbiprofen
Ketoprofen
Phenylbutazone
Pirprofen
Piroxicam
Meclofenamate sodium
Sulindac

DISEASE-MODIFYING ANTIRHEMATIC DRUGS (DMARDS)

Intramuscular and oral gold
D-Penicillamine
Hydroxychloroquine
Sulfasalazine

CORTICOSTEROIDS

CYTOTOXIC AND IMMUNOSUPPRESSIVE DRUGS

Leflunomide
Methotrexate
Azathioprine
Chlorambucil
Cyclophosphamide
Intravenous immunoglobulin
Cyclosporin A
Thalidomide

BIOLOGIC AGENTS

Etanercept
Infliximab
Adalimumab
Anakinra
Abatacept
Rituximab

FDA, Food and Drug Administration.

possess immune- and cytokine-modulating effects (also known as biologic agents). Significant advances continue to take place, particularly in the biologic arena.

Although salicylates are historically the classic NSAIDs, they are no longer the initial NSAIDs of choice because of concerns regarding the development of Reye syndrome and because other agents have emerged that work well. Although these drugs are essentially equivalent in efficacy and toxicity, individual responses to all NSAIDs vary widely. If a child does not improve while receiving a NSAID within 4 to 6 weeks, then trying others is reasonable.[22] Naproxen, ibuprofen, indomethacin, and meloxicam are available as liquid preparations that can ease administration in younger children and in children who have trouble swallowing pills.

A relatively newer class of NSAIDs are the cyclooxygenase II (COX-2)-selective inhibitors.[23] By interfering only with COX-2, these antiinflammatory agents decrease the prostaglandin production that mediates inflammation, but in a gastroprotective manner, which reduces the risk of gastric erosion or ulcer formation, or both. However, as a result of cardiovascular safety questions, many of these preparations were removed from the market by their manufacturers. Celecoxib remains available in the United States, and is now approved for use in children with JIA. Meloxicam is predominantly COX-2 selective and is available in a generic preparation, thereby decreasing cost.

If a child does not quickly respond to NSAID therapy alone or is in a high-risk category, more aggressive interventions are clearly necessary because JIA is neither a benign condition nor one that children will typically "outgrow."[24] Moving quickly to DMARDs and/or biologic agents, as well as performing intraarticular corticosteroid injections, appears to achieve the goal of no inflammation with great effectiveness.

Although sulfasalazine has witnessed something of a resurgence,[25-27] it should not be administered to any child who is sensitive to sulfa drugs or salicylates, whose renal or hepatic function is impaired, or who has conditions such as glucose-6-phosphate dehydrogenase deficiency. Adverse effects caused by sulfasalazine include rashes, nausea, vomiting, and dyspepsia; in boys, a reversible decrease in sperm count is an adverse effect. Bone marrow depression rarely occurs.

Methotrexate has essentially replaced the other traditional DMARDs—intramuscular and oral gold, D-penicillamine and hydroxychloroquine—as the primary second-line agent in the treatment of JIA. As a competitive inhibitor of dihydrofolate reductase, it exerts both an antiinflammatory and an immunosuppressive effect on the arthritis. Its efficacy[28] and its dose-response characteristic[29] have been well established. Subcutaneous administration results in high and consistent blood levels and may provide control of the arthritis if oral dosing is ineffective.[30] Hepatic, bone marrow, gastrointestinal, pulmonary, and teratogenic adverse effects are possible. Laboratory monitoring every 4 to 8 weeks is recommended to detect any liver or hematopoetic adverse effects. The administration of folic (or folinic) acid may mitigate a number of methotrexate's adverse effects, such as nausea and oral ulcers.

Leflunomide, an immunosuppressive agent that inhibits pyridine synthesis and suppresses tumor necrosis factor–alpha (TNF-α)–induced cellular responses, has recently been shown to have beneficial effects similar to methotrexate.[31] However, leflunomide, too, has possible teratogenic effects; it requires ongoing monitoring and is not FDA-approved for use in the treatment of JIA. Other immunosuppressive agents, including azathioprine, cyclosporine, chlorambucil, cyclophosphamide, intravenous immune globulin, and thalidomide, are occasionally administered in specific patients, but they are not currently the standard.

The last decade has brought with it great advances in the understanding of the inflammatory causes of JIA. TNF-α is a major proinflammatory cytokine in both children and adults with arthritis, psoriasis, and a number of other chronic inflammatory diseases. Three biologic agents are currently available to block the activity of TNF-α: (1) etanercept, (2) infliximab, and (3) adalimumab. Etanercept and adalimumab are approved for use in children with JIA, and all three agents have demonstrated dramatic improvements in the condition of children and adults with arthritis. Because each agent is slightly different, a child who has not responded or has had an adverse effect to one agent may still respond to another. Adding a TNF-α blocker to the regimen of any child with JIA who has not responded to previously administered DMARD therapy is now considered standard therapy, as well as when tapering the dose of corticosteroids is not possible without precipitating a flare of the disease. Testing for tuberculosis is recommended before starting these agents because they can interfere with the immune response. Other adverse effects include injection site pain or reactions, an increased risk of infections, and a possible increased risk of other autoimmune conditions or neoplasms. The long-term effects of TNF-α suppression are not yet known. However, since their introduction, this class of agents has dramatically altered both the courses of these diseases and the lives of the children and adults with arthritis.

Interleukins 1 and 6 (IL-1 and IL-6) are two other proinflammatory cytokines that also play a significant role in the treatment JIA. Systemic-onset JIA is more of an IL-1– or IL-6– (or both) driven condition and often responds better to blocking these cytokines than TNF-α.[32] Anakinra, an IL-1–receptor antagonist, has been found to be effective in the treatment of JIA in many children who have not responded adequately to the TNF-α inhibitors. Anakinra should not be administered in combination with a TNF-α–inhibitor or any other biologic agent. Other agents in trials are currently showing promise in blocking IL-1 and IL-6.

Abatacept, a biologic agent recently approved for the treatment of children with JIA, works through a different mechanism. It selectively modulates the CD80/CD86:CD28 costimulatory signal required for full T-cell activation. It has demonstrated efficacy in both children and adults with arthritis who have not responded adequately to TNF-α inhibitors.

Rituximab is a monoclonal antibody directed against the CD20 marker on B-lymphocytes. Currently approved for adults who have not responded to TNF-α blockade, its use in the treatment of children has yet to be determined.

In the era of monoclonal antibodies, systemic corticosteroid use in JIA has become much less necessary. However, corticosteroids remain important and effective medications, the use of which should follow these maxims: (1) they should only be administered when other agents have failed or when the child is seriously ill or has progressive severe chronic anterior uveitis unresponsive to local or other systemic therapy; (2) as small a dose as possible should be administered; and (3) their use should be tapered and discontinued as soon as possible.

Corticosteroids are effective antiinflammatory agents but do not alter the course of the disease. They can be extremely difficult to discontinue in children who have JIA, and their long-term use is associated with many serious adverse effects, including immunosuppression, osteoporosis, and growth retardation. Small daily doses of prednisone may be effective in treating pain and stiffness; higher doses may be needed to manage systemic features such as pericarditis. High-dose intravenous pulse corticosteroid therapy can be useful in dire situations, but it is not more effective when used as chronic therapy.

Intraarticular corticosteroids have come to play a larger role in the management of JIA, especially oligoarticular JIA. They can be effective in controlling acute problems associated with one or several active joints, but they are usually used in combination with systemic, ongoing therapy. Children who have a painful or swollen joint frequently respond to arthrocentesis and instillation of a long-acting corticosteroid preparation (eg, triamcinolone hexacetonide).[33,34] This procedure should not be performed more than 3 or 4 times per year, and the physician should be absolutely certain that concomitant infectious arthritis is not the cause of the acute joint problem. Early use of intraarticular corticosteroids may even have the potential to modify the course of JIA.

Despite this progress in treatments, there are still children whose disease has proven unresponsive to all of these and other interventions. In a select group, the use of autologous stem cell transplantation has at times proven to be extraordinarily helpful. The risks are great, but for those children, the benefits can be as well.

Since children with arthritis can experience both acute and chronic pain at various times regardless of their treatments, this is an important area that needs to be considered and/or addressed. Not all pain is related to the inflammatory aspects of the arthritis. Therefore, before intervening, it is important to determine whether the pain is from the joint inflammation, joint damage or other mechanical factors, periarticular structures or other issues. Similarly, not all pain requires intervention with medications as a variety of physical or other techniques can also be effective.[35]

Pharmacologic therapy is only one aspect of the treatment required by children who have JIA. Physical therapy and occupational therapy are crucial and important adjuncts to help the child maintain strength and range of motion, to prevent contractures, and to allow the best possible quality of life. All patients should be given a home program of therapy that is reviewed and updated regularly. Heat therapy, such as taking warm baths or using a sleeping bag at night, often helps minimize morning stiffness. Swimming is an excellent exercise; affected children should be encouraged to swim and to participate in as many other activities as possible. Normal play is also a form of physical therapy and occupational therapy.

The orthopedist's contributions for patients whose disease is more extensive range from the application of splints to operative tendon releases and capsulotomies. Some children may require joint resurfacing or joint replacement surgery.[36] Even though most children will not need orthopedic intervention (particularly during childhood), the orthopedist's perspective is an important part of disease management.

In all its forms, JIA is a chronic illness, and none of the current modes of therapy is curative. Furthermore, JIA is one of the few childhood illnesses in which pain is a primary symptom. Therefore different expectations and attitudes are needed when caring for the patient and family. In addition to an attentive and understanding primary care physician, a family counselor, social worker, and psychologist or similar mental health professional are of particular value in helping the patient and family to cope with and adjust to this chronic illness. Patients, siblings, and parents may experience feelings of denial, guilt, and frustration at the time of the diagnosis and throughout the course of the disease.[37] Siblings frequently find difficulty in coping with the special and extensive treatment the affected child may receive.

Periodic depression and anger are frequent problems, especially in the early stages as the child and family realize that many changes may be necessary in their lifestyle and dreams and again as the patient enters adolescence. Despite the frequent disruptive episodes brought on by the disease, families are often able to adapt to their child's chronic illness adequately. Poor maternal function, maternal depression, and social isolation are risk factors for poor psychosocial outcomes. A sense of control and mastery are important positive factors.

Most children who have JIA can do well in school; thus all efforts should be made to keep them enrolled. Studies of children's school and family adaptations show that children who have JIA and their families develop different, albeit generally normal, styles for coping with this chronic illness.[38] Some school adjustments may be necessary, such as arranging for different transportation or physical education (or both) and allowing the child extra time between classes. Having 2 sets of books, one for school and one for home, reduces the work of carrying the books to and from school. The primary care physician or pediatric rheumatology team may have to advocate on behalf of these children within the school so that they can receive all the services they require.

Although concentrating on scholastic issues is important, these children will require preparation for adulthood. Independent living and vocational preparation must begin in childhood to reduce any potential barriers and difficulties. Anticipatory guidance about transitional issues should be provided starting in childhood and early adolescence.[39,40]

Although children whose disease is severe have several obvious problems, the child who has mild disease and a hidden disability also may have problems coping, adapting, and trying to accomplish the unrealistic goals set by a society that does not recognize the disability. Any chronic illness imposes many additional stresses on the entire family. The direct and indirect financial costs alone create significant burdens for the family of any child with JIA and for society.

COURSE AND PROGNOSIS

JIA is rarely fatal, and in general the long-term prognosis is good, particularly in the oligoarticular subtype. Approximately 60% to 75% of children will undergo a remission at some point, and many children will experience permanent remission. Most children who have JIA will complete school, be gainfully employed, and will raise families, just as their siblings and peers will.

Several patterns of disease activity are recognized: (1) persistent active arthritis and destructive arthropathy, (2) active disease, then remission, (3) polycyclic diseases characterized by acute flares of activity followed by temporary remissions, and (4) low-grade continued disease activity with little if any joint destruction.

Oligoarticular (not the extended type) JIA has the best prognosis, with 40% to 50% of children undergoing a complete remission, compared with only 25% to 30% of children who have systemic-onset and polyarticular JIA. Children who have IgM-RF positivity, systemic onset, and certain extraarticular manifestations (eg, persistent fevers, thrombocytosis, subcutaneous nodules, vasculitis), as well as younger children, usually have a poorer long-term articular outcome. Younger children who have systemic-onset and polyarticular arthritis have a poorer articular prognosis. Children who have oligoarticular arthritis and no chronic anterior uveitis have the best prognosis.

Children should be referred to an ophthalmologist at the time of diagnosis. Most clinical uveitis develops within 4 to 7 years of the diagnosis, but it can occur at any time. Therefore ophthalmologic examinations should be performed indefinitely. Table 288-1 outlines the frequency of eye examinations recommended by the American Academy of Pediatrics. If a child develops uveitis, then the child should be monitored according to the ophthalmologist's directions; uveitis can become the child's most vexing problem.

In summary, increasing awareness of the pediatric rheumatic diseases has resulted in earlier diagnosis and treatment. The rapid advances in understanding the diseases and their therapies, especially the promising biological agents, are encouraging signs that the number of children disabled by these illnesses will decrease in the future.

WHEN TO REFER

- Child has persistent oligo- or polyarticular joint inflammation.
- Child has spiking fevers and rash, but no obvious infectious cause is present.
- Child has persistent joint pain, limp, or asymmetrical use of an extremity for which no explanation has been found.

WHEN TO ADMIT

- Child has systemic-onset juvenile arthritis and develops severe chest pain with shortness of breath (suggesting pericarditis with hemodynamic compromise) or a change in voice quality and difficulty breathing (suggesting cricoarytenoid arthritis).
- Child has chronic arthritis and is receiving corticosteroid therapy, and develops signs of severe infection.
- Child has chronic arthritis and is receiving NSAIDs, and exhibits acute anemia and melanotic stools.
- Child has longstanding polyarticular arthritis complicated by multiple joint contractures and weakness and requires a period of inpatient rehabilitation (eg, physical and occupational therapy).

TOOLS FOR PRACTICE

Engaging Patient and Family

- *Juvenile Rheumatoid Arthritis* (fact sheet), Arthritis Foundation (www.arthritis.org/conditions/DiseaseCenter/jra.asp).

- *What is a Pediatric Rheumatologist?* (fact sheet), American Academy of Pediatrics (www.aap.org/family/WhatisPedRheumatology.pdf).

RELATED WEB SITES

- American College of Rheumatology (www.rheumatology.org).
- Arthritis Foundation (www.arthritis.org/index.php).
- Centers for Disease Control and Prevention: Arthritis (www.cdc.gov/arthritis/).
- Childhood Arthritis and Rheumatology Research Alliance (www.carragroup.org).
- Family Village: A Global Community of Disability-Related Resources (www.familyvillage.wisc.edu).
- National Institutes of Health (www.nih.gov).
- Pediatric Rheumatology International Trials Organization (wwww.printo.it).

AAP POLICY STATEMENT

Cassidy J, Kivlin J, Lindsley C, et al, American Academy of Pediatrics, Section on Rheumatology and Section on Ophthalmology. Ophthalmologic examinations in children with juvenile rheumatoid arthritis. *Pediatrics*. 2006;117(5):1843-1845. (aappolicy.aappublications.org/cgi/content/full/pediatrics;117/5/1843)).

SUGGESTED RESOURCES

Cassidy JT, Petty RE, Laxer M, et al. *Textbook of Pediatric Rheumatology*. 5th ed. Philadelphia, PA: Elsevier; 2005.

Isenberg DA, Miller JJ. *Adolescent Rheumatology*. London, UK: Martin Dunitz; 1999.

Szer IS, Kimura Y, Malleson PN, Southwood TR. *Arthritis in Children and Adolescents; Juvenile Idiopathic Arthritis*. Oxford University Press; 2006.

Woo P, Laxer RM, Sherry DD. *Pediatric Rheumatology in Clinical Practice*. Springer; 2007.

REFERENCES

1. Petty RE, Southwood TR, Manners, Baum J, et al. International League of Associations for Rheumatology classification of juvenile idiopathic arthritis: second revision, Edmonton 2001. *J Rheumatol*. 2004;31:390-392.
2. Oen KG, Cheang M. Epidemiology of chronic arthritis in childhood. *Semin Arthritis Rheum*. 1996;26:575-591.
3. Grom AA, Giannini EH, Glass DN. Juvenile rheumatoid arthritis and the trimolecular complex (HLA, T cell receptor, and antigen). *Arthritis Rheum*. 1994;37:601-607.
4. Taccetti G, Trapani S, Ermini M, et al. Reactive arthritis triggered by Yersinia enterocolitica: a review of 18 pediatric cases. *Clin Exp Rheumatol*. 1994;12:681-684.
5. LeBovidge JS, Lavigne JV, Donenberg GR, et al. Psychological adjustment of children and adolescents with chronic arthritis: a meta-analytic review. *J Pediatr Psychol*. 2003:28:29-39.
6. Lawrence JM, Moore TL, Osborn TG, et al. Autoantibody studies in juvenile rheumatoid arthritis. *Semin Arthritis Rheum*. 1993;22:265-274.
7. Barron KS, De Cunto CL, Montalvo JF, et al. Abnormalities of immunoregulation in juvenile rheumatoid arthritis. *J Rheumatol*. 1989;16:940-948.
8. Carapetis JR, Currie BJ. Rheumatic fever in a high incidence population; the importance of monoarthritis and low grade fever. *Arch Dis Child*. 2001;85:223-227.
9. McGhee JL, Burks FN, Sheckels JL, Jarvis JN. Identifying children with chronic arthritis based on chief complaints; absence of predictive value for musculoskeletal pain as an indicator of rheumatic disease in children. *Pediatrics* 2002;110(2 Pt 1):354-359.
10. Scott JP, Gerber P, Maryjowski MC, et al. Evidence for intravascular coagulation in systemic onset, but not polyarticular, juvenile rheumatoid arthritis. *Arthritis Rheum*. 1985;28:256-261.
11. Sawhney S, Woo P, Murray KJ. Macrophage activation syndrome: a potentially fatal complication of rheumatic disorders. *Arch Dis Child*. 2001;85:421-426.
12. Schneider R, Passo MH. Juvenile rheumatoid arthritis. *Rheum Dis Clin North Am*. 2002;28:503-530.
13. Moore TL, Dorner RW, Osborn TG, et al. Hidden 19S IgM rheumatoid factors. *Semin Arthritis Rheum*. 1988;18:72-75.
14. Bacon MC, White PH, Raiten DJ, et al. Nutritional status and growth in juvenile rheumatoid arthritis. *Semin Arthritis Rheum*. 1990;20:97-106.
15. Cassidy J, Kivlin J, Lindsley C, et al, American Academy of Pediatrics, Section on Rheumatology and Section on Ophthalmology. Ophthalmologic examinations in children with juvenile rheumatoid arthritis. *Pediatrics*. 2006;117:1843-1845.
16. Vostrejs M, Hollister JR. Muscle atrophy and leg length discrepancies in pauciarticular juvenile rheumatoid arthritis. *Am J Dis Child*. 1988;142:343-345.
17. Sheerin KA, Giannini EH, Brewer EJ, et al. HLA-B27 associated arthropathy in childhood: long term clinical and diagnostic outcome. *Arthritis Rheum*. 1988;31:1165-1170.
18. Ozen S, Hoffman HM, Frenkel J, et al. Familial Mediterranean fever (FMF) and beyond; a new horizon. *Ann Rheum Dis*. 2006;65:961-964.
19. Biro F, Gewanter HL, Baum J. The hypermobility syndrome. *Pediatrics*. 1983;72:701-706.
20. Siegel DM, Janeway D, Baum J. Fibromyalgia syndrome in children and adolescents: clinical features at presentation and status at follow-up. *Pediatrics*. 1998;101:377-382.
21. Silber TJ, Majd M. Reflex sympathetic dystrophy syndrome in children and adolescents: report of 18 cases and review of the literature. *Am J Dis Child*. 1988;142:1325-1330.
22. Lovell DJ, Giannini EH, Brewer EJ Jr. Time course of response to nonsteroidal antiinflammatory drugs in juvenile rheumatoid arthritis. *Arthritis Rheum*. 1984;27:1433-1437.
23. Fung HB, Kirschenbaum HL. Selective cyclooxygenase-2 inhibitors for the treatment of arthritis. *Clin Ther*. 1999;21:1131-1157.
24. Hashkes PJ, Laxer RM. Medical treatment of juvenile idiopathic arthritis. *JAMA*. 2005;294(13):1671-1684.
25. Ansell BM, Hall MA, Loftus JK, et al. A multicentre pilot study of sulphasalazine in juvenile chronic arthritis. *Clin Exp Rheumatol*. 1991;9:201-203.
26. Gedalia A, Barash J, Press J, et al. Sulphasalazine in the treatment of pauciarticular-onset juvenile chronic arthritis. *Clin Rheumatol*. 1993;12:511-514.
27. Hertzberger-Ten Cate R, Cats A. Toxicity of sulfasalazine in systemic juvenile chronic arthritis. *Clin Exp Rheumatol*. 1991;9:85-88.
28. Giannini EH, Brewer EJ, Kuzminan, et al. Methotrexate in resistant juvenile rheumatoid arthritis. *N Engl J Med*. 1992;326:1043-1049.
29. Takken T, Van Der Net J, Helders PJ. Methotrexate for treating juvenile idiopathic arthritis. *Cochrane Database Syst Rev*. 2001;4:CD003129.
30. Alsufyani K, Ortiz-Alverez O, Cabral DA, et al. The role of subcutaneous administration of methotrexate in children with juvenile idiopathic arthritis who have failed oral methotrexate. *J Rheumatol* 2004;31(1):179-182.

31. Silverman E, Mouy R, Spiegel L, et al. Leflunomide or methotrexate for juvenile rheumatoid arthritis. *NEJM.* 2005;352(16):1655-1666.
32. Verbasky JW, White AJ. Effective use of the recombinant interleukin 1 receptor antagonist in therapy resistant systemic onset juvenile rheumatoid arthritis. *J Rheumatol.* 2004;31:2071-2075.
33. Zulian F, Martini G, Gobber D, et al. Comparison of intra-articular triamcinolone hexacetonide and triamcinolone acetamide in oligoarticular juvenile idiopathic arthritis. *Rheumatology.* 2003;42:1254-1259.
34. Huppertz H-I, Tschammler A, Horwitz AE, et al. Intraarticular corticosteroids for chronic arthritis in children: efficacy and effects on cartilage and growth. *J Pediatr.* 1995;127:317-321.
35. Kimura Y, Walco GA. Treatment of chronic pain in pediatric rheumatic disease. *Nat Clin Pract Rheumatol* 2007; 3(4):210-218.
36. Harris CM, Baum J. Involvement of the hip in juvenile rheumatoid arthritis: a longitudinal study. *J Bone Joint Surg (Am).* 1988;70:821-833.
37. Athreya BH, McCormick MC. Impact of chronic illness on families. *Rheum Dis Clin North Am.* 1987;13:123-131.
38. Harris JA, Newcomb AF, Gewanter HL. Psychosocial effects of juvenile rheumatic disease. *Arthritis Care Res.* 1991;4:123-130.
39. White PH. Educational and vocational planning: the key to success in adulthood. In: Isenberg DA, Miller JJ, eds. *Adolescent Rheumatology.* London, UK: Martin Dunitz; 1999.
40. Rosen DS, Blum RW, Britto M, et al. Transition to adult healthcare for adolescents and young adults with chronic conditions: position paper of the Society for Adolescent Medicine *J Adolesc Health.* 2003;33:309-311.

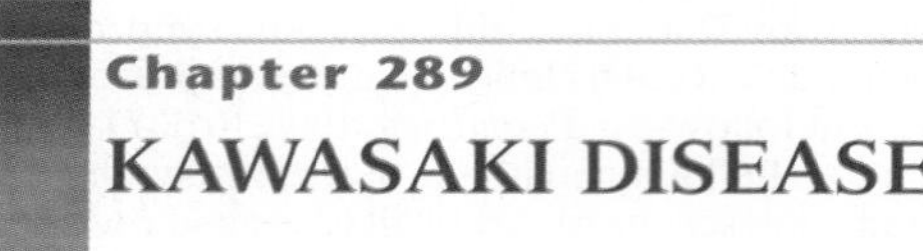

Chapter 289

KAWASAKI DISEASE

Michael E. Pichichero, MD

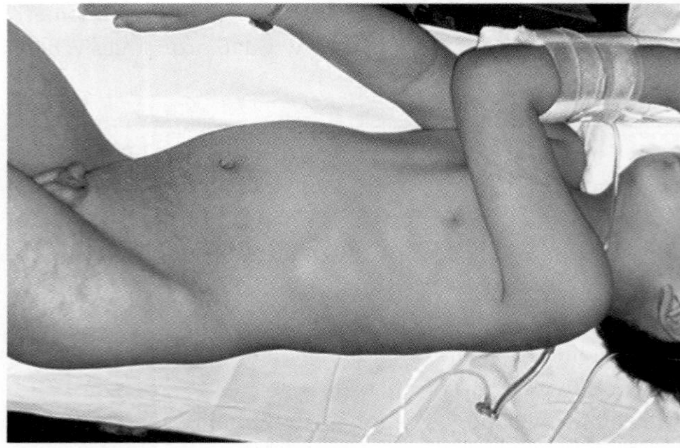

Figure 289-1 Characteristic distribution of erythroderma of Kawasaki disease. The rash is accentuated in the perineal area in approximately two thirds of patients.

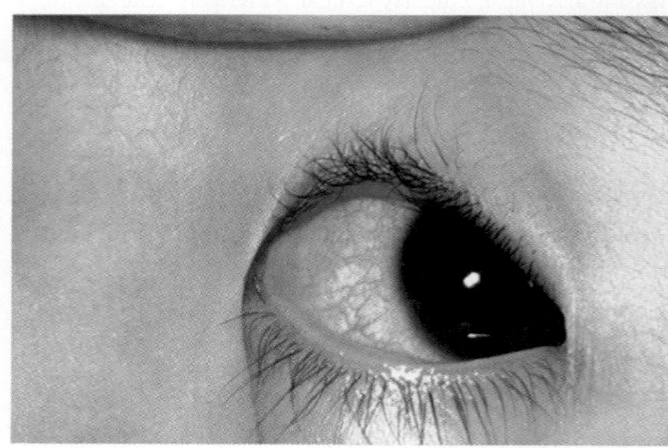

Figure 289-2 Child with Kawasaki disease with conjunctivitis. Note the absence of conjunctival discharge.

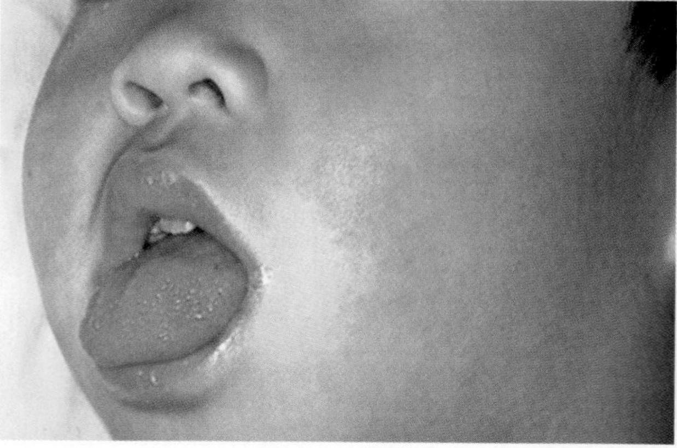

Figure 289-3 Child with Kawasaki disease with striking facial rash and erythema of the oral mucous membrane.

Kawasaki disease is an acute, multisystem vasculitis of infancy and early childhood characterized by high fever, rash (Figure 289-1), conjunctivitis (Figure 289-2), inflammation of the mucous membranes (Figure 289-3), erythematous induration of the hands and feet, and cervical adenopathy. Kawasaki disease, formerly known as mucocutaneous lymph node syndrome, is the main cause of acquired heart disease in children in the United States. It was first described in 1967 by a Japanese pediatrician, Tomisaka Kawasaki; in 1974 the 1st cases of Kawasaki disease were reported in the United States. In retrospect, illnesses that are similar to Kawasaki disease were described as early as 1871. Landing and Larson compared the features of Kawasaki disease with infantile periarteritis nodosa and found that the 2 conditions shared many clinical signs and had indistinguishable pathological findings.[1]

EPIDEMIOLOGIC FEATURES

The peak age incidence of Kawasaki disease occurs during the 2nd year of life. More than 80% of all cases occur in children younger than 5 years; the disease is quite uncommon beyond 9 years of age. Boys are more commonly affected than girls, with a male-to-female ratio of nearly 1.5:1. Now, Kawasaki disease is recognized as having a worldwide distribution, although it is most prevalent in Japan and in children of Japanese ancestry. The Centers for Disease Control and Prevention estimates the incidence for children 8 years or younger in the continental United States to be 32.5 cases per 100,000 in those of Asian or part Asian descent, 16.9 per 100,000 in blacks, 11.1 per 100,000 in Hispanics, and 9.1 per 100,000 in whites.[2] Kawasaki disease occurs more commonly in winter and spring, and numerous temporal clusters have been reported in the United States and Japan. The seasonality and temporal clustering of cases suggest an infectious cause.

Recurrent cases of Kawasaki disease have been reported in the United States and Japan, with rates ranging from 0.3% to 5% in Japan and 1% to 2% in the United States.[3] Intravenous immunoglobulin (IVIg) therapy for the 1st episode may increase the risk of recurrence within the following 12 months but not later. Kawasaki disease occurs more commonly in siblings than it does in the general population. Kawasaki disease in twins is even higher than it is in nontwin siblings but is not significantly different between monozygotic twins and dizygotic twins. The interval between sibling cases is fewer than 10 days in 54% of cases; the onset sometimes occurs on the same day. These findings suggest a common exposure to an infectious agent in a genetically predisposed population.

ETIOLOGY

No established cause for Kawasaki disease has been found, although clinical features suggest an infectious process.[4] Recently, the notion that toxin-producing staphylococcal or streptococcal bacteria are the primary cause of Kawasaki disease has received the most attention. These agents are attractive candidates because of the similarity of Kawasaki disease to illnesses such as staphylococcal toxic shock syndrome (see Chapter 327, Staphylococcal Toxic Shock Syndrome) and streptococcal toxic shock syndrome (see Chapter 329, Streptococcal Toxic Shock Syndrome).

PATHOGENESIS

Kawasaki disease is characterized by immunoregulatory abnormalities characteristic of diseases that are caused by bacterial toxins acting as superantigens.[5] Superantigens stimulate a large fraction of the T-cell population; they have dual affinity for the class II major histocompatibility complex on macrophages and monocytes and for the variable β (Vβ2) region of the T-cell receptor.[6,7] High-dose IVIg is effective in reducing coronary vasculitis (see later discussion) perhaps because it prevents immune-complex deposition on blood vessel walls or because it reverses immunoregulatory abnormalities.

Kawasaki disease is associated with increased production of cytokines by T cells and monocytes, and this feature is thought to play an important role in the pathogenesis of vascular endothelial cell injury during acute Kawasaki disease because these cytokines elicit proinflammatory and prothrombic responses in endothelial cells. Cytokines and chemokines have been detected in tissue obtained from patients in the acute stage of Kawasaki disease.[4] Selectins may also contribute to localization of leukocytes likely adding to the vascular injury of Kawasaki disease.[4]

DIFFERENTIAL DIAGNOSIS

The clinical picture of Kawasaki disease, after all major features have exhibited, is not difficult to differentiate from other mucocutaneous syndromes. In the 1st days of the illness, a whole spectrum of acute febrile diseases might be considered. Three to 5 days after the onset, certain clinical features may be singled out as compatible with other diagnoses, for example, strawberry tongue, which is suggestive of streptococcal infection. Two conditions most commonly mimic Kawasaki disease: streptococcal and staphylococcal scarlet fever. However, if all the signs and symptoms are considered carefully, then the diagnosis is readily apparent. The clinical features of Kawasaki disease and other mucocutaneous disorders are shown in Table 289-1. Other conditions that share some aspects of Kawasaki disease are ratbite fever, rubella, rubeola, infectious mononucleosis, toxoplasmosis, juvenile rheumatoid arthritis, systemic lupus erythematosus, Behçet syndrome, acrodynia (mercury poisoning), and febrile drug reactions, especially those caused by anticonvulsants. The similarities between fatal Kawasaki disease and fatal infantile polyarteritis nodosa are striking; pathologically, the 2 diseases cannot be distinguished. The exact relationship between them, however, is undetermined. The clear differentiating feature is that Kawasaki disease rarely is fatal (<1% mortality), whereas infantile polyarteritis nodosa is a pathological diagnosis made at autopsy.

CLINICAL MANIFESTATIONS

To make the diagnosis of typical Kawasaki disease, 5 of the 6 major clinical characteristics associated with the condition must be present (Box 289-1),[3] and all other illnesses having similar features must be excluded. Symptoms vary in severity, but more than 90% of patients fulfill the first 5 clinical criteria. All of the symptoms are not apparent simultaneously, but the timing of their appearance is remarkably constant.

The course of the disease can best be described as triphasic. The acute phase consists of fever, conjunctival hyperemia, oropharyngeal erythema, swelling of the hands and feet, a polymorphous erythematous rash, and cervical lymphadenopathy. Fever, rash, and lymphadenopathy fade after 10 to 12 days of the illness, marking the beginning of the subacute phase. The subacute stage is characterized by lip cracking and fissuring, desquamation of skin overlying the tips of the fingers and toes, and the onset of arthralgias or arthritis (or both), thrombocytosis, and cardiac disease. The convalescent stage usually begins approximately 25 days after onset and is characterized by the absence of clinical signs of disease but the persistence of residual inflammation, marked by an elevated erythrocyte sedimentation rate (ESR).

Fever is the most prominent symptom of the acute phase of the disease. Temperatures show a high-spiking remittent pattern in the range of 38.4°C (101.1°F) to more than 40°C (104°F). Fever persists despite the use of empirical antibiotics, corticosteroids, and

Table 289-1 Clinical Features of Kawasaki Disease and Other Mucocutaneous Diseases

	KAWASAKI DISEASE	STEVENS-JOHNSON SYNDROME	STREPTOCOCCAL SCARLET FEVER	STAPHYLOCOCCAL SCARLET FEVER	STAPHYLOCOCCAL TOXIC SHOCK SYNDROME	LEPTOSPIROSIS
Age (yr)	Usually <5	Usually 3-30	Usually 5-10	Usually 2-8	Usually adolescent	Usually >2
Fever	Prolonged	Prolonged	Variable	Variable	Usually <10 days	Variable
Eyes	Hyperemia of ocular conjunctivae; uveitis	Catarrhal conjunctivitis; chemosis; iritis; uveitis; panophthalmitis	No change	Hyperemia of ocular conjunctivae	Hyperemia of ocular conjunctivae	Hyperemia of ocular conjunctivae; uveitis
Lips	Red, dry, fissured	Erosions; crusted, fissured, bleeding	No change	No change	Red	No change
Oral cavity	Diffuse erythema; *strawberry tongue*	Erythema; bullae, ulcers, pseudomembrane formation	Pharyngitis; palatal petechiae; *strawberry tongue*	Pharyngitis	Erythema; pharyngitis	Pharyngitis
Peripheral extremities	Erythema of palms and soles; indurative edema; periungual, palmar, and plantar desquamation	No change	Periungual desquamation	No change	Swelling of hands and feet; dry gangrene	Gangrene of hands and feet (rare)
Exanthem	Erythematous, polymorphous	Erythematous, polymorphous; iris lesions, vesicles, bullae, crusts	Finely papular erythroderma; Pastia lines; circumoral pallor	Finely papular erythroderma; Pastia lines	Erythroderma	Erythematous, maculopapular, petechial, or purpuric
Cervical lymph nodes	Nonpurulent swelling; unilateral (frequent)	Nonpurulent swelling (occasional)	Nonpurulent or purulent swelling (frequent)	Nonpurulent or purulent swelling (occasional)	No change	Nonpurulent swelling (infrequent)
Other	Meatitis; diarrhea; arthralgia and arthritis; aseptic meningitis; rhinorrhea (uncommon): ECG changes	Malaise; cough, rhinorrhea, pneumonitis; vomiting; arthralgia; recurrent episodes	Malaise; vomiting; headache		Headache; confusion; hypotension; icteric hepatitis; diarrhea; coagulopathy; renal injury	Headache myalgia; abdominal pain; icteric hepatitis; meningitis

ECG, Electrocardiogram.

BOX 289-1 Diagnostic Criteria for Kawasaki Disease

PRINCIPAL SYMPTOMS

Fever of unknown cause lasting 5 days or more **AND** at least 4 of the following 5 symptoms:

- Bilateral congestion of ocular conjunctivae
- Changes of lips and oral cavity
- Dryness, redness, and fissuring of lips
- Protuberance of tongue papillae *(strawberry tongue)*
- Diffuse reddening of oral and pharyngeal mucosa

CHANGES OF PERIPHERAL EXTREMITIES

- Reddening of palms and soles (initial stage)
- Indurative edema (initial stage)
- Membranous desquamation from fingertips (convalescent stage)
- Polymorphous exanthema of body trunk without vesicles or crusts
- Acute nonpurulent swelling of cervical lymph nodes of 1.5 cm or more in diameter

OTHER SIGNIFICANT SYMPTOMS OR FINDINGS

- Carditis, especially myocarditis or pericarditis
- Diarrhea
- Arthralgia or arthritis
- Proteinuria and increase of leukocytes in urine sediment

CHANGES IN BLOOD TESTS

- Leukocytosis with shift to the left
- Slight decrease in erythrocyte and hemoglobin levels
- Increased sedimentation rate
- Elevated C-reactive protein
- Increased β_2-globulin
- Thrombocytosis
- Negative antistreptolysin titer

CHANGES OCCASIONALLY OBSERVED

- Aseptic meningitis
- Mild jaundice or slight increase of serum transaminase
- Swelling of gallbladder

standard doses of antipyretics. Fever is present on average for approximately 12 days, although prolonged courses of up to 5 weeks have been reported; defervescence occurs over 1 to 3 days. Discrete engorgement of the bulbar conjunctivae blood vessels (without associated discharge, exudate, keratitis, chemosis, or pseudomembrane formation) and an anterior uveitis develop shortly after the onset of fever. The cornea, lens, and retina are not involved. Early oropharyngeal signs include dryness and reddening of the lips and of the buccal and pharyngeal mucosa. The absence of aphthous ulceration or hemorrhagic bullae is noticeable. A *strawberry tongue* is frequently present. Later, as the intensity of the erythema subsides, the lips usually become cracked and fissured.

The most characteristic and unique feature of Kawasaki disease relates to changes that occur in the hands and feet. Early on, they become diffusely indurated and swollen, and the overlying skin develops a woody firmness suggestive of acute scleroderma. The palms and soles usually become erythematous or take on a purplish hue. Fusiform swelling of the fingers also occurs, which limits the child's ability to grasp objects. The feet are painful to the touch, and many children will refuse to stand or walk. Two to 3 weeks after the onset of illness and after the early signs involving the extremities have disappeared, an unusual desquamation of the skin beginning at the subungual and periungual regions of the fingers and toes occurs in nearly all cases (Figure 289-4). Progression to complete peeling of the palms and soles may occur, but exfoliation generally does not extend to the remainder of the body surface. During the convalescent phase, deep transverse grooves (Beau lines) may appear across the fingernails and toenails, presumably as a result of arrested growth during the illness.

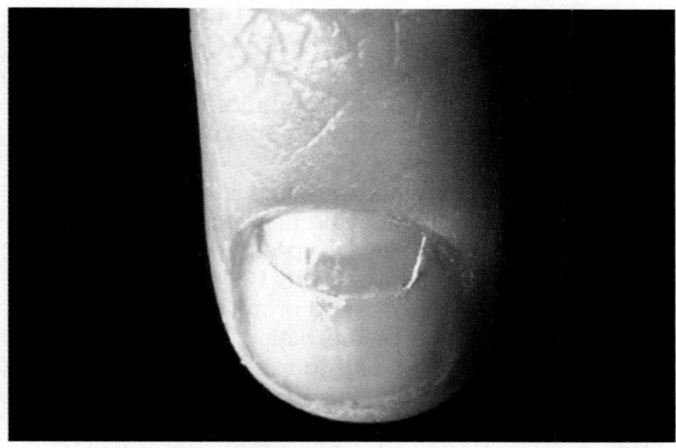

Figure 289-4 Desquamation of the skin involving the subungual and periungual regions of the fingertips. *(Kawasaki T, Kosalki F, Okawa S, et al. A new infantile acute febrile mucocutaneous lymph node syndrome (MLNS) prevailing in Japan.* Pediatrics. *1974;54:271-276.)*

A polymorphous, erythematous rash appears 1 to 5 days after the onset of fever; it usually begins on the extremities and spreads centripetally. The 3 most common patterns of rash are maculopapular (morbilliform), erythema multiforme-like with iris lesions, and scarlatiniform. The rash may be coalescent, producing large, irregular, raised plaques, and it may be pruritic. Vesicles, pustules, and bullae are not seen. The rash is not petechial or purpuric. It usually fades within 1 week but occasionally persists longer or recurs.

Lymphadenopathy typically involves a single cervical node measuring more than 1.5 cm in diameter. The node is usually not tender or warm and does not become fluctuant. Generalized lymphadenopathy does not occur. The lymph node diminishes in size with defervescence of the disease. Lymphadenopathy is least often seen of the major criteria; it occurs in only approximately 60% of patients in most US series.

In addition to the 6 major clinical signs, other features of Kawasaki disease are frequently noted. Sterile pyuria occurs more often than lymphadenopathy in most US cases; 10 to 100 white blood cells (WBCs) per high-power field may be observed on a clean-catch voided urine specimen. No WBCs will be seen on a bladder aspiration specimen because the sterile pyuria is caused by urethral inflammation or ulceration. Occasionally, a patient will demonstrate trace proteinuria or hematuria.

Irritability, mild meningismus, and lethargy are seen in nearly all of these patients, and nearly all probably have aseptic meningitis. When cerebrospinal fluid (CSF) is analyzed, it typically shows 25 to 100 WBCs/mm^3 with normal amounts of glucose and protein. Diarrhea is seen in approximately 50% of the patients. Passing 5 to 15 stools per day for 2 to 7 days during the acute or subacute phase is common. Stools do not contain polymorphonuclear cells and do not test positive for occult blood.

Either arthralgias, arthritis, or both occur in 30% to 40% of the children. Large joints, particularly the knees and ankles, are involved most often. Usually, no more than 2 or 3 joints will be affected. Joint symptoms occur 8 to 12 days after the onset of disease. Joint fluid, if analyzed, will reveal findings similar to those of rheumatoid arthritis.

Pneumonia, tympanitis, photophobia, and mild liver dysfunction are observed somewhat less commonly. Acute hydrops of the gallbladder, jaundice, convulsions, encephalopathy, Bell palsy, hearing loss, pancreatitis, orchitis, and pleural effusions are seen rarely but are clearly associated complications of Kawasaki disease.[8]

The most alarming findings of Kawasaki disease are those in the cardiovascular system. The mortality of the disease is the result of coronary artery aneurysm rupture or occlusion. During the acute phase, tachycardia and gallop rhythms may appear; however, the most serious manifestations of cardiac involvement occur during the subacute phase. These manifestations include serious arrhythmias, congestive heart failure, pericardial effusion, mitral insufficiency, and myocardial ischemia or infarction.

LABORATORY FINDINGS

Although Kawasaki disease has no pathognomonic laboratory findings, certain laboratory abnormalities are frequently seen and therefore help establish the diagnosis. In the acute phase of the disease, most patients exhibit an elevated WBC count with an associated left shift; WBC counts of 15,000 to 20,000/mm^3 are common and may remain elevated for 1 to 3 weeks. Other laboratory abnormalities in the acute phase usually include an elevated ESR (mean >55 mm/hr); increased C-reactive protein (CRP) and β_2-globulin; mild normochromic, normocytic anemia; and slight elevations of the liver enzymes. Many patients demonstrate sterile pyuria and CSF pleocytosis. In the 2nd to 3rd week of the illness, patients characteristically develop significant thrombocytosis, with platelet counts averaging in excess of 700,000/mm^3. Importantly, the results of several laboratory studies are negative. Routine cultures of blood, CSF, urine, throat, and lymph node aspirates reveal no growth or normal flora. Serologic studies for bacterial and viral agents are negative, including the antistreptolysin titer. Antinuclear antibodies, rheumatoid factor, and other autoantibodies are absent.

Sinus tachycardia, nonspecific ST segment and T wave changes, and evidence of mild left ventricular hypertrophy may be seen on an electrocardiogram in the acute phase. In the subacute phase, myocardial infarction patterns on an electrocardiogram may be observed, although infrequently.

A baseline echocardiogram should be performed as soon as the diagnosis of Kawasaki disease is suspected to evaluate cardiac function and the anatomy of the coronary arteries and to assess for the presence or absence of pericardial effusion. Coronary artery abnormalities are generally apparent by the 3rd or 4th week of the illness. The findings in atypical Kawasaki disease are listed in Box 289-2. Coronary artery disease rarely, if ever, develops after 6 to 8 weeks, although late-onset valvular disease has been reported.

BOX 289-2 Atypical Kawasaki Disease: Echocardiogram

- Useful in evaluating children with prolonged fever and some features of Kawasaki disease
- Although aneurysms rarely form before day 10 of the illness, perivascular brightness, ectasia, and lack of tapering of the coronary arteries can be seen in the acute stage of disease
- Other findings:
  - Decreased left ventricular contractility
  - Mild valvular regurgitation (mitral regurgitation)
  - Pericardial effusion

From American Academy of Pediatrics, American Heart Association. Diagnosis, treatment and long-term management of Kawasaki disease: a statement for health professionals from the Committee on Rheumatic Fever, Endocarditis, and Kawasaki Disease, Council on Cardiovascular Disease in the Young, American Heart Association. *Pediatrics.* 2004;114(6):1708-1733.

ATYPICAL KAWASAKI DISEASE

Severe or even fatal coronary abnormalities can develop after illnesses that resemble but do not fulfill the classic diagnostic features of Kawasaki disease.[9] Important aspects of atypical Kawasaki disease are listed in Box 289-3. Patients who have atypical Kawasaki disease may display prolonged high fever, nonspecific rash, arthralgia or arthritis, fissuring of the lips,

BOX 289-3 Atypical Kawasaki Disease

- Consider in infants and children with unexplained fever for more than 5 days and 2 or 3 of the principal diagnostic criteria
- Young infants may have fever only
- In children (<1 year and teens) with fever >7 days, rash with or without nonexudative conjunctivitis
- Laboratory results are similar to those of classic cases

From American Academy of Pediatrics, American Heart Association. Diagnosis, treatment and long-term management of Kawasaki disease: a statement for health professionals from the Committee on Rheumatic Fever, Endocarditis, and Kawasaki Disease, Council on Cardiovascular Disease in the Young, American Heart Association. *Pediatrics.* 2004;114(6):1708-1733.

nonexudative conjunctivitis, and extreme irritability. Atypical Kawasaki disease can occasionally produce prolonged fever for 5 or more days in the absence of other clinical criteria for the illness. In other patients, unilateral cervical adenopathy refractory to antibiotic therapy is the clue that atypical Kawasaki disease may be present. An algorithm for evaluating suspected atypical Kawasaki disease is shown in Figure 289-5. In infants younger than 6 months, atypical Kawasaki disease is likely to produce subtle manifestations

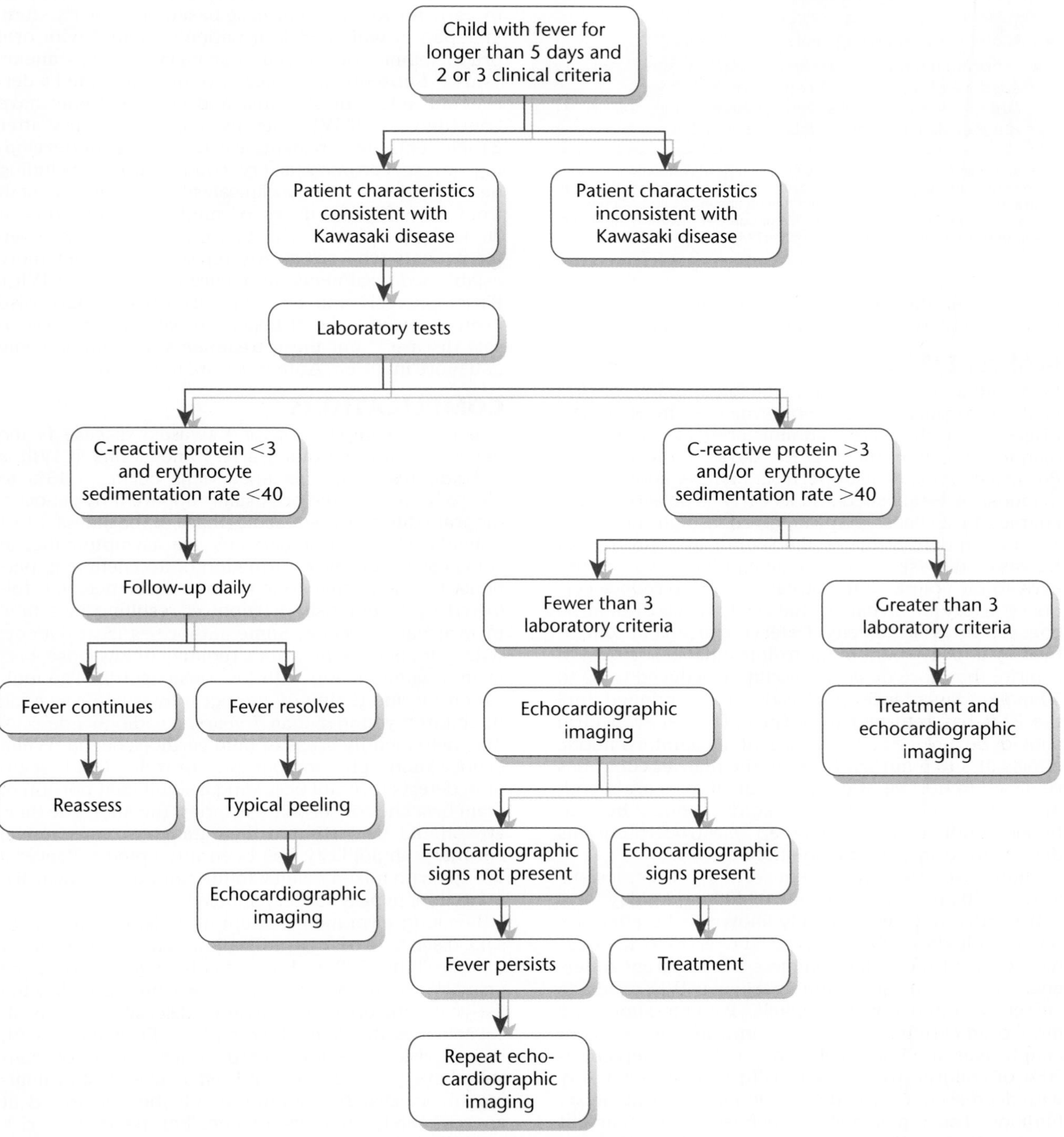

Figure 289-5 Evaluation of suspected atypical Kawasaki disease. *(American Academy of Pediatrics, American Heart Association. Diagnosis, treatment and long-term management of Kawasaki disease: a statement for health professionals from the Committee on Rheumatic Fever, Endocarditis, and Kawasaki Disease, Council on Cardiovascular Disease in the Young, American Heart Association.* Pediatrics. *2004;114(6):1708-1733.)*

BOX 289-4 Kawasaki in Infants Younger Than 6 Months

- Usually lack full diagnostic criteria
- Manifestations often subtle: fever, rash, and cerebral spinal fluid pleocytosis may be misdiagnosed as viral meningitis
- High risk for coronary abnormalities
- Echocardiography should be considered in any infant aged <6 months with fever of more than 7 days, laboratory evidence of systemic inflammation, and no other explanation for the febrile illness

From American Academy of Pediatrics, American Heart Association. Diagnosis, treatment and long-term management of Kawasaki disease: a statement for health professionals from the Committee on Rheumatic Fever, Endocarditis, and Kawasaki Disease, Council on Cardiovascular Disease in the Young, American Heart Association. *Pediatrics.* 2004;114(6):1708-1733.

(Box 289-4); this group is at highest risk (50% or greater) for coronary artery lesions if untreated.

MANAGEMENT

IVIg with aspirin is the best available therapy for preventing coronary artery abnormalities in Kawasaki disease and should be administered to all patients diagnosed within the first 10 days of the illness.[10] Physicians should institute treatment as soon as the diagnosis is established and as early as possible in the course of the illness. Aspirin, given in high doses (80-120 mg/kg/day), reduces the length and severity of Kawasaki disease during the acute phase. Aspirin use early in the course of the disease may also reduce coronary artery involvement. Salicylate levels should be checked to avoid toxicity. Defervescence is accompanied by improvement in gastrointestinal absorption of aspirin; therefore dosages should be reduced to 30 to 50 mg/kg/day after fever subsides and continued until the ESR has returned to normal. Thereafter, aspirin should be prescribed because of its antithrombotic effects at 3 to 5 mg/kg/day until the platelet count has returned to normal. If coronary aneurysms are recognized, then salicylates (3-5 mg/kg/day) should be continued until careful follow-up electrocardiograms demonstrate aneurysm resolution.

High-dose IVIg may prevent coronary artery lesions in Kawasaki disease. A dosage of 400 mg/kg/day for 4 consecutive days was initially shown to be effective, but a single dose of 2 g/kg infused over 10 to 12 hours has replaced the 4-day regimen. No apparent difference exists in efficacy among particular IVIg products currently commercially available. Patients should be monitored carefully during IVIg infusions for signs of anaphylaxis and immune hemolysis. Eighty percent to 90% of children treated with IVIg respond favorably with decreased fever and reduction in mucocutaneous findings. The remainder has persistent or recurrent fever, with or without mucocutaneous signs. If ongoing fever cannot be attributed to another cause, then the assumption should be made that Kawasaki disease is persisting or has relapsed. Because fever may be viewed as a sign of continued vasculitis, retreatment with IVIg is advocated.[10,11] The majority of patients treated again after a single dose of IVIg therapy has failed will respond to retreatment.[12-14] Patients who remain symptomatic beyond the 10th day may still benefit from IVIg. However, the decision to administer IVIg later than the 10th day of the illness must be individualized.

Corticosteroids were believed to be dangerous as therapy for Kawasaki disease based on an early study in Japan in which 65% of patients treated with oral prednisolone developed coronary artery aneurysms.[15] Subsequent studies have not confirmed a detrimental effect of steroids, and some patients have benefited.[16-18] If IVIg therapy fails (particularly after 2 treatments), then patients are at high risk for developing severe coronary artery complications, including death. Patients in this clinical situation may benefit from 1 to 3 pulse-doses of methyl prednisolone at 30 mg/kg per dose.[17] This therapy should be reserved for patients who are clearly refractory to other more established treatments (ie, failure of 2 doses of IVIg). Plasmapheresis and exchange transfusion have also been reported to be of benefit in patients with Kawasaki disease,[19] but these treatments are cumbersome and more involved. Antibiotics are not useful.

COMPLICATIONS

The major complication of Kawasaki disease is the development of coronary artery aneurysms. If IVIg is not administered, then aneurysms occur in 15% to 25% of cases[20,21] and are usually apparent by echocardiogram during the subacute phase of the illness. Most patients who have aneurysms are asymptomatic; in some cases, however, formation of an aneurysm, particularly a giant aneurysm (>8 mm in diameter), is followed by thrombosis or rupture, resulting in a fatal myocardial infarction. Some authorities treat patients with giant aneurysms with a regimen of low-dose warfarin in combination with low-dose aspirin. The indication for and timing of angiography is controversial. In children younger than 7 years, a radionuclide scan may help identify areas of mild cardioischemia. When echocardiography, angiography, or radionuclide scanning detects thrombi occluding a significant portion of main branches of coronary arteries, thrombolytic therapy should be instituted. Percutaneous transluminal coronary angioplasty has been attempted by several groups with mixed results. In the setting of myocardial infarction, bypass surgery should be undertaken.

For long-term management of patients with Kawasaki disease, a risk stratification scheme may be of benefit (Table 289-2). For patients at level-I risk, the primary care physician may fully assume care after the 1st-year anniversary of Kawasaki disease onset. Physical activities should not be restricted. For patients with level-II risk, a pediatric cardiologist should be consulted every 1 to 2 years; at least 1 stress test evaluating myocardial functioning should be performed at approximately 10 years of age. For patients in risk level III, daily low-dose aspirin therapy and annual cardiac follow-up with echocardiography and electrocardiography may be appropriate. Periodic stress tests are recommended. For patients in risk level IV, low-dose aspirin therapy should be maintained, and

Table 289-2 Levels of Risk for Determination of Methods for Management of Kawasaki Disease-Induced Coronary Artery Disease

RISK LEVEL	DESCRIPTION
I	No coronary artery abnormalities at any stage of the illness
II	Transient coronary artery ectasia followed by regression
III	Small to medium solitary coronary artery aneurysm
IV	One or more giant aneurysms or multiple aneurysms without obstruction
V	Coronary artery obstruction (thrombosis or stenosis)

From American Academy of Pediatrics, American Heart Association. Diagnosis, treatment and long-term management of Kawasaki disease: a statement for health professionals from the Committee on Rheumatic Fever, Endocarditis, and Kawasaki Disease, Council on Cardiovascular Disease in the Young, American Heart Association. *Pediatrics.* 2004;114(6):1708-1733.

low-dose warfarin should be considered. Coronary angiography may be considered 6 to 12 months after the acute disease has resolved to delineate coronary artery anatomy. Physical activities should be modified to minimize the risk of hemorrhage. Strenuous or competitive sports should be avoided. Patients at risk level V should receive daily low-dose aspirin, and warfarin should be considered. Patients should be evaluated for indications of bypass graft surgery. Mild to moderate recreational physical activities are permitted.

The coronary artery aneurysms seen in Kawasaki disease develop more frequently in boys than they do in girls, in children younger than 1 year, and in those who have a triphasic fever pattern or fever for longer than 2 weeks when a gallop rhythm or other arrhythmia is noted or when the ESR exceeds 50 mm/hr (Box 289-5). Cases of atypical Kawasaki disease followed by typical coronary artery involvement have led to the suggestion that an echocardiography examination be undertaken in children who have prolonged unexplained febrile illnesses associated with subsequent peripheral desquamation.

A rare complication of Kawasaki disease is hydrops of the gallbladder. This complication occurs in approximately 3% of cases and is seen most frequently in children who are jaundiced. It becomes evident during the acute phase of the illness and is diagnosed best by ultrasound on recognition of a right upper quadrant abdominal mass. The pathogenesis is unknown. Surgery is not indicated because the problem resolves spontaneously in convalescence.

PROGNOSIS

Kawasaki disease has a 0.3% mortality. Death occurs almost exclusively in children who have giant aneurysms, largely as a result of coronary artery thrombosis, massive myocardial infarction, and cardiogenic shock. Eighty percent of children whose aneurysms are small to moderate in size have complete resolution without apparent sequelae within 5 years.[11,22] The remaining children may experience persisting aneurysms, coronary artery stenosis or obstruction, or aortic regurgitation. Emerging evidence suggests that a portion of this last group of children may be at risk for the subsequent development of significant cardiovascular disease such as coronary arteriosclerosis or persistent aneurysms, placing some of them at risk for sudden death from aneurysm rupture or thrombosis, cardiac arrhythmias, angina, or hypertension.[11,23]

BOX 289-5 Risk Factors for Coronary Artery

ANEURYSMS IN KAWASAKI DISEASE

Risk substantially increased

- Fever lasts longer than 14 days
- Biphasic fever pattern*
- Biphasic pattern of skin rash
- Maximum WBC count of 30,000/mm^3
- Maximum ESR of 101 mm/hr
- Time until normalization of ESR or CRP of 30 days of the illness
- Biphasic elevation of ESR or CRP
- Increased Q/R ratio in leads II, III, aVF more than 0.3

SYMPTOMS OF MYOCARDIAL INFARCTION

Risk increased

- Male gender
- Age at onset younger than 1 year
- Hemoglobin less than 10 g/dL and red blood cell count less than 3.5 million
- Maximum WBC count greater than 26,000/mm^3
- Maximum ESR above 50 mm/hr
- Cardiomegaly
- Arrhythmia
- Recurrence of disease

*Separated by afebrile period of 48 hours or longer.
Causes other than Kawasaki disease must be ruled out.
CRP, C-reactive protein; *ESR,* erythrocyte sedimentation rate; *WBC,* white blood cell.

PSYCHOSOCIAL ASPECTS

Kawasaki disease is almost always a self-limited illness without complications, which should be emphasized to the parents. Even if coronary artery aneurysms do develop, they resolve spontaneously in more than 50% of cases in 2 years and 80% in 5 years. Long-term risks still remain undefined, and only as physicians gain prospective experience with the disease over several more decades will the true incidence of cardiovascular sequelae become evident.

TOOLS FOR PRACTICE

Community Coordination and Advocacy

- *Kawasaki Case Report Form* (form), Centers for Disease Control and Prevention (www.cdc.gov/ncidod/diseases/kawasaki/KSform-fillable.pdf).

Engaging Patients and Family

- *Kawasaki Disease* (fact sheet), American Academy of Pediatrics (www.aap.org/publiced/BK0_KawasakiDisease.htm).
- *Kawasaki Disease* (fact sheet), American Heart Association (www.americanheart.org/presenter.jhtml?identifier=162).
- *Kawasaki Syndrome* (fact sheet), Centers for Disease Control and Prevention (www.cdc.gov/ncidod/diseases/kawasaki/index.htm).

AAP POLICY STATEMENT

Newberger JW, Takahashi M, Gerber MA, et al, Council on Cardiovascular Disease in the Young, American Heart Association. Guide to diagnosis, treatment, and long-term management of Kawasaki disease: a statement for health professionals from the committee on rheumatic fever, endocarditis, and Kawasaki disease. *Pediatrics*. 2004; 114(6):1708-1733. AAP Endorsed.

SUGGESTED RESOURCE

Kawasaki Disease Foundation. Available at: www.kdfoundation.org. Accessed April 4, 2008.

REFERENCES

1. Landing BH, Larson EJ. Are infantile periarteritis nodosa with coronary artery involvement and fatal mucocutaneous lymph node syndrome the same? Comparison of 20 patients from North America with patients from Hawaii and Japan, *Pediatrics*. 1977;59:651-662.
2. Holman RC, Curns AT, Belay ED, et al. Kawasaki syndrome hospitalizations in the United States, 1997 and 2000. *Pediatrics*. 2003;112:495-501.
3. From American Academy of Pediatrics, American Heart Association. Diagnosis, treatment and long-term management of Kawasaki disease: a statement for health professionals from the Committee on Rheumatic Fever, Endocarditis, and Kawasaki Disease, Council on Cardiovascular Disease in the Young, American Heart Association. *Pediatrics*. 2004;114(6):1708-1733.
4. Wang CL, Wu YT, Liu CH, et al. Kawasaki disease. *Pediatr Infect Dis J*. 2005;24(11):998-1004.
5. Burns JC, Mason WH, Glode MP, et al. Clinical and epidemiologic characteristics of patients referred for evaluation of Kawasaki disease. *J Pediatr*. 1991;118:680-686.
6. Abe J, Kotzin BL, Meissner C, et al: Characterization of T cell repertoire changes in acute Kawasaki disease. *J Exp Med* 1993;177:791-796.
7. Abe J, Kotzin BL, Meissner C, et al. Selective expansion of T cells expressing T-cell receptor variable regions Vβ2 and Vβ8 in Kawasaki disease. *Proc Natl Acad Sci USA*. 1992;89:4066-4070.
8. Mason WH, Takahasi M. Kawasaki syndrome. *Clin Infect Dis*. 1999;28:169-185.
9. Rowley AH, Gonzalez-Crussi F, Gidding SS, et al. Incomplete Kawasaki disease with coronary artery involvement. *J Pediatr*. 1987;110:409-413.
10. Durongpisitkul K, Gururaj VJ, Park JM, et al. The prevention of coronary artery aneurysm in Kawasaki disease: a meta-analysis on the efficacy of aspirin and immunoglobulin treatment. *Pediatrics*. 1995;96:1057-1061.
11. Takahashi M, Mason W, Lewis AB. Regression of coronary aneurysms in patients with Kawasaki syndrome. *Circulation*. 1987;75:387-394.
12. Burns JC, Capparelli EV, Brown JA, et al. Intravenous gamma-globulin treatment and retreatment in Kawasaki disease. *Pediatr Infect Dis J*. 1998;17:1144-1148.
13. Durongpisitkul K, Soongswang J, Laohaprasitiporn D, et al. Immunoglobulin failure and retreatment in Kawasaki disease. *Pediatr Cardiol*. 2003;24:145-148.
14. Wallace CA, French JW, Kahn SJ, et al. Initial intravenous gammaglobulin treatment failure in Kawasaki disease. *Pediatrics*. 2000;105(6):e78. Available at: www.pediatrics.org/cgi/content/full/105/6/e78.
15. Kato H, Koike S, Yokoyama T. Kawasaki disease: effect of treatment on coronary artery involvement. *Pediatrics*. 1979;63:175-179.
16. Okada Y, Shinohara M, Kobayashi T, et al. Effect of corticosteroids in addition to intravenous gamma globulin therapy on serum cytokine levels in the acute phase of Kawasaki disease in children. *J Pediatr*. 2003;143:363-367.
17. Shinohara M, Sone K, Tomomasa T, et al. Corticosteroids in the treatment of the acute phase of Kawasaki disease. *J Pediatr*. 1999;135:465-469.
18. Sundel RP, Baker AL, Fulton DR, et al. Corticosteroids in the initial treatment of Kawasaki disease: report of a randomized trial. *J Pediatr*. 2003;142:611-616.
19. Imagawa T, Mori M, Miyamae T, et al. Plasma exchange for refractory Kawasaki disease. *Eur J Pediatr*. 2004;163: 263-264.
20. Dajani AS, Taubert KA, Gerber MA, et al. Diagnosis and therapy of Kawasaki disease in children. *Circulation*. 1993;87:1776-1780.
21. Kato H, Sugimura T, Akagi T, et al. Long-term consequences of Kawasaki disease. A 10- to 21-year follow-up study of 594 patients. *Circulation*. 1996;94:1379-1385.
22. Fujiwara T, Fujiwara H, Hamashima Y. Size of coronary aneurysm as a determinant factor of the prognosis in Kawasaki disease: clinicopathologic study of coronary aneurysms. *Prog Clin Biol Res*. 1987;250:519-520.
23. Burns JC, Shike H, Gordon JB, et al. Sequelae of Kawasaki disease in adolescents and young adults. *J Am Coll Cardiol*. 1996;28:253-257.

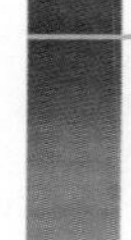

Chapter 290

LABIAL ADHESIONS

Linda S. Nield, MD

Labial adhesions, also known as labial agglutination or synechia vulvae, are membranous structures that develop as a result of fusion of the adjacent mucosal surfaces of the labia minora. The membranous structure can vary from thin and transparent to thick and fibrous. Any degree of labial involvement can occur, including covering of the urethral meatus. The condition is self-limiting, and spontaneous resolution in affected individuals has been reported to occur in 50% of cases within 6 months, 90% of cases within 12 months, and 100% of cases within 18 months.[1]

ETIOLOGY

The exact cause of labial adhesions is uncertain, but the condition is likely due to chronic irritation and inflammation of the hypoestrogenic vulva. Physical or chemical trauma, infection (*Candida albicans, Enterobius vermicularis,* and various bacteria), and poor hygiene are the triggers for the chronic inflammation. Sexual abuse may also be a source of chronic irritation,[2] but labial adhesions are generally considered a nonspecific finding. During healing of the irritated area, the medial edges of the labia minora adhere to each other, forming an adhesion.

EPIDEMIOLOGIC MECHANISM

Prepubertal girls in the first 5 years of life are most prone to this condition.[3] A rise in endogenous estrogen levels during the prepubertal period may be the reason for a decrease in the occurrence of labial adhesions in older preadolescent girls. Improved hygiene may also be a factor. Reported incidences of labial adhesions in the preadolescent in the general pediatric setting range from approximately 2% of girls who are identified by inspection alone[3] to 39% of girls identified with inspection plus magnified photographic images of the vulva.[4] Labial adhesions were found in 15.6% of girls who were referred to a gynecology clinic for various hymenal findings that were documented during well-child evaluations.[5] Labial adhesions in a neonate are a rare occurrence,[3,6-8] presumably because of the protective influence of maternal estrogen. Healthy, postpubescent young women do not develop labial adhesions, but they have been described after episiotomy, herpes infection, trauma, treatment with chemotherapy, and graft-versus-host disease.[9-11]

DIFFERENTIAL DIAGNOSIS

Ambiguous genitalia, vaginal agenesis, imperforate hymen, or septated hymen may be confused with labial adhesions, but physical examination easily differentiates these entities from one another. A line of demarcation between the clitoral hood and labial minora is seen with labial adhesions (Figure 290-1) but not with ambiguous genitalia secondary to androgen excess.[12] In vaginal agenesis and hymenal variants, the labia are normal and unfused, and the characteristic findings of these entities are located within the vaginal introitus.

CLINICAL MANIFESTATIONS

Labial adhesions are often asymptomatic and are typically discovered at routine well-child visits or brought to the attention of the pediatrician by the child's caregiver. However, the adhesions can partially dehisce, leading to spotting of a minute amount of blood and irritation as well. Uncommonly, affected girls may complain of vaginal pain, pain with ambulation or urination,[13] or suffer from a urinary tract infection, urinary retention, or an altered urinary stream.[9]

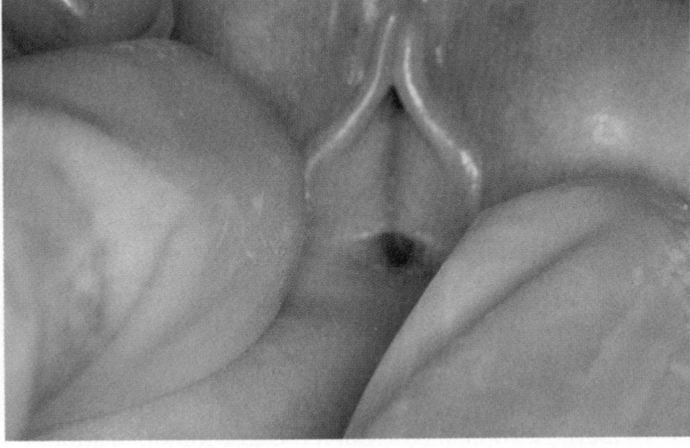

Figure 290-1 A commonly found presentation of labial adhesion in a 3 year old.

The condition is diagnosed by visual inspection of the vulva, which includes a hymenal examination in the supine frog-leg or prone knee-chest position. The labia majora should be gently stretched apart, and a membrane of variable length and thickness is seen in the midline. A small opening near the clitoris allows the outflow of urine. A line of adhesion between the 2 nonrugated labia minora or raphae can also be seen.

MANAGEMENT

Uncomplicated Case

If the child has no accompanying symptoms, then labial adhesions should not be treated. The parents should be informed of the diagnosis and an opportunity to visualize the adhesion should be provided so the parents are not surprised and concerned about the unusual appearance of the vulva. Reassurance of the benign, self-limiting nature of this condition and education about potential symptoms should be provided.

Complicated Case

If the child has accompanying symptoms such as pain on urination or ambulation, altered urinary stream, urinary retention, or a history of urinary tract infections, then a urinalysis and urine culture should be obtained. Any documented urinary tract or vulvar infection should be treated accordingly. The 1st-line treatment of the complicated labial adhesion is the application of topical estrogen.[14,15] A cream containing 0.625 mg of conjugated estrogen (Premarin Vaginal Cream, Wyeth Ayerst) can be applied to the adhesion and labial edges with a finger tip or cotton swab. Gentle traction can be placed on the opposing labia during the application of the estrogen cream. Although the optimal dosing and length of treatment is unknown, a course of twice-daily application for 2 weeks is a reasonable starting point. The goal is to use the least amount of medication that will achieve separation of the adhesion. Topical estrogen should be applied for 10 to 14 days with a cotton-tipped applicator with light pressure over the adhesion; this treatment is highly effective for the vast majority of thin, transparent adhesions but less so in others that are dense and fibrous or longstanding.[15] Even the dense adhesions should be treated initially with topical estrogens because this treatment produces thinning of the line of fusion that facilitates manual labial separation in the office.[15] The possible adverse effects of the topical estrogen include local irritation, breast budding, breast tenderness, and vulvar hyperpigmentation, all of which are reversible with discontinuation of the medication. After the estrogen therapy has separated the labia, a topical lubricant (eg, white petroleum jelly) should be applied to the affected area for several months on a daily basis to ensure complete healing and persistent separation of the opposing labial edges.

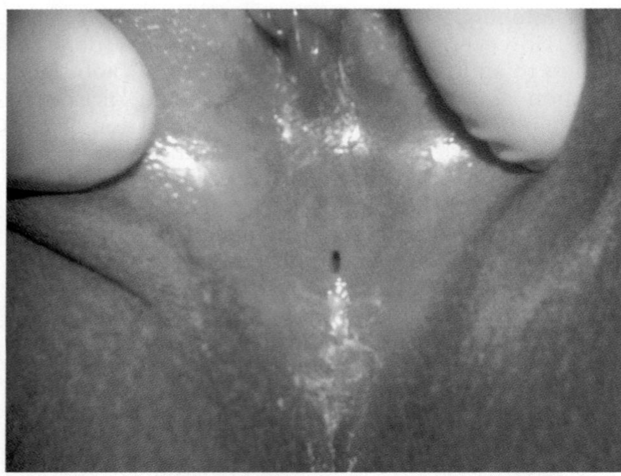

Figure 290-2 Extensive labial adhesion in a 4 year old. Hydronephrosis is a potential rare complication of an extensive labial adhesion.

Treatment with estrogen cream is considered unsuccessful if labial separation has not occurred within 8 weeks or if the child suffers untoward effects from the estrogen and cannot continue using it. If topical estrogen is unsuccessful and the girl's accompanying symptoms persist, then manual separation of adhesions can be performed. Before manual separation is performed, topical anesthetic must be applied to the affected area. After the anesthetic has taken effect, firm traction on the opposing edges of the labial minora is applied to separate the fused edges. The edges should be smoothly peeled away from each other. After separation, a lubricant should be applied to the affected area on a daily basis for several months to prevent re-adherence. Warm soaks or sitz baths in the days following separation may provide relief if the vulva is irritated from the procedure.

Rarely, in cases of thick labial adhesions that cannot be separated by the previously described treatments and those that are associated with complications, surgical lysis by a pediatric urologist or gynecologist while under general anesthesia may be required (Figure 290-2).[13] Postoperative care includes sitz baths in the immediate postoperative period and several months of application of topical lubricant. The decision to treat labial adhesions with surgery is made by weighing the significance and severity of symptoms after less aggressive treatments have failed versus the risks of general anesthesia.

PREVENTION: ADVICE TO PARENTS

The clinician should explain the value of proper hygiene of the vulva and educate the parents about practices to help their child avoid recurrent labial adhesions: (1) wiping front to back after urination or defecation, (2) wearing cotton underwear, (3) avoiding the application of detergents in the genital area, and (4) avoiding wet, tight clothing against the vulva for prolonged periods.

WHEN TO REFER

A symptomatic child with persistent or recurrent labial adhesions who has a history of urinary tract infections or complaints of urinary retention, altered urinary stream, dysuria or pain with ambulation and has failed topical estrogen therapy, should be referred to a pediatric urologist or gynecologist for surgical lysis.

SUGGESTED RESOURCES

Bacon JL. Prepubertal labial adhesions: evaluation of a referral population. *Am J Obstet Gynecol.* 2002;187:327-331.

Muram D. Treatment of prepubertal girls with labial adhesions. *J Pediatr Adolesc Gynecol.* 1999;12:67-70.

Nuzria MJ, Eickhorst KM, Ankem MK, et al. The surgical treatment of labial adhesions in pre-pubertal girls. *J Pediatr Adolesc Gynecol.* 2003;16:21-23.

Pokorny SF. Prepubertal vulvovaginopathies. *Obstet Gynecol Clin North Am.* 1992;19:39-58.

REFERENCES

1. Jenkinson SD, MacKinnon AE. Spontaneous separation of fused labia minora in prepubertal girls. *Br Med J.* 1984;289:160-161.
2. Berenson AB, Chacko MR, Wiemann CM, et al. A case-control study of anatomic changes resulting from sexual abuse. *Am J Obstet Gynecol.* 2000;182(4);820-834.
3. Leung AK, Robson WL, Tay-Uyboco J. The incidence of labial fusion in children. *J Paediatr Child Health.* 1993;29:235-236.
4. McCann J, Wells R, Simon M, et al. Genital findings in prepubertal girls selected for nonabuse: a descriptive study. *Pediatrics.* 1990;86:428-439.
5. Heger AH, Ticson L, Guerra L, et al. Appearance of the genitalia in girls selected for nonabuse: review of hymenal morphology and nonspecific findings. *J Pediatr Adolesc Gynecol.* 2002;15:27-35.
6. Bowles HE, Childs LS. Synechias of vulvu in small children. *Am J Dis Child.* 1943;66:258-263.
7. Capraro VJ, Greenberg H. Adhesions of the labia minora: a study of 50 patients. *Obstet Gynecol.* 1972;39:65-69.
8. Mesrobian HG, Balcom AH, Durkee CT. Urologic problems of the neonate. *Pediatr Clin North Am.* 2004;51:1051-1062.
9. Bacon JL. Prepubertal labial adhesions: evaluation of a referral population. *Am J Obstet Gynecol.* 2002;187:327-331.
10. DeMarco BJ, Crandall RS, Hreshchyshyn MM. Labial agglutination secondary to a herpes simplex II infection. *Am J Obstet Gyencol.* 1987;157:296-297.
11. Opipari AW Jr. Management quandary. Labial agglutination in a teenager. *J Pediatr Adolesc Gynecol.* 2003;16(1);61-62.
12. Pokorny SF. Prepubertal vulvovaginopathies. *Obstet Gynecol Clin North Am.* 1992;19:39-58.
13. Nuzria MJ, Eickhorst KM, Ankem MK, et al. The surgical treatment of labial adhesions in pre-pubertal girls. *J Pediatr Adolesc Gynecol.* 2003;16:21-23.
14. Aribarg A. Topical oestrogen therapy for labial adhesions in children. *Br J Obstet Gynaecol.* 1975;82:424-425.
15. Muram D. Treatment of prepubertal girls with labial adhesions. *J Pediatr Adolesc Gynecol.* 1999;12:67-70.

Chapter 291

LEUKEMIAS

E. Anders Kolb, MD; Richard Gorlick, MD

The incremental increase in survival among children with acute lymphoblastic leukemia over the last 50 years is often cited as the great success story in clinical oncology. In the spectrum of childhood ailments, leukemias remain quite rare; but among childhood malignancies, the leukemias are the most common. Rapid and accurate diagnosis is still the first step and, in many cases, the most important step toward cure. The role of the pediatrician in patients with leukemia will not end with the initial referral to an oncologist. Much of the treatment for acute lymphoblastic leukemia is done on an outpatient basis, and, frequently, patients should still be seen periodically by their pediatrician throughout treatment. As the number of long-term survivors among patients with leukemias continues to increase, so too will the role of the general pediatrician in their care. An understanding of the biology, treatment, prognosis, and short- and long-term side effects of childhood leukemias will be necessary for primary care physicians of children and adults in the future. This chapter reviews the epidemiologic features, pathogenesis, classification, treatment, prognosis, and outcomes in childhood leukemia.

EPIDEMIOLOGIC FEATURES

Leukemia remains the most common malignancy of childhood (Figure 291-1) with an annual incidence of 40 cases per 1,000,000 children in the United States.[1] Leukemias account for a quarter of all childhood malignancies. In the United States, more than 3000 children younger than 20 years will be diagnosed with leukemia each year, 80% of which are types of acute lymphoblastic leukemia (ALL).[2]

The peak incidence of childhood leukemia is approximately 4 years of age, although this peak is due almost entirely to patients diagnosed with ALL. Acute myelogenous leukemia (AML) is equally distributed among patients 0 to 10 years of age, with a slight increase in incidence in adolescence.[3] ALL is more common among whites than it is among blacks in the United States, but AML has an equal distribution among all ethnic groups. Early reports of worse outcomes for blacks with leukemia have been largely refuted in recent publications.[4] The incidence of leukemia is also slightly higher among boys than it is among girls. The ratio of boys with leukemia to girls with leukemia is greatest during adolescence, particularly in the subset of patients with T-cell ALL.[5,6]

LEUKEMOGENESIS

The exact cause of most leukemias is not known, although several predisposing factors and exposures exist (Box 291-1). In all likelihood, the cause or causes of most leukemias is multifactorial including genetic, immune, infectious, and environmental factors.

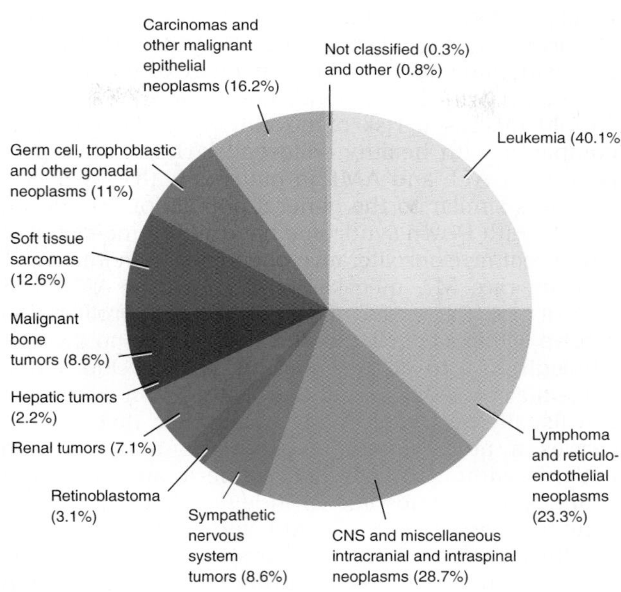

Figure 291-1 Incidence of cancer types from 1996 to 2002 in children ages 0 to 19 years. Malignancies are classified according to International Classification of Childhood Cancer. Incidence is expressed as rates per 1,000,000 and are age-adjusted to the 2000 United States standard population. (From US Cancer Statistics Working Group. United States Cancer Statistics: 1999-2002 Incidence and Mortality Web-based Report Version. Atlanta, GA: Department of Health and Human Services, Centers for Disease Control and Prevention, and National Cancer Institute; 2005.)

BOX 291-1 Factors Associated With a Higher Risk of Developing Leukemia

GENETIC PREDISPOSITION

- Siblings of patient with a childhood leukemia
- Down syndrome
- Fanconi anemia
- Bloom syndrome
- Ataxia telangiectasia
- Paroxysmal nocturnal hemoglobinuria
- Congenital hypogammaglobulinemia
- Wiskott-Aldrich syndrome
- Neurofibromatosis
- Klinefelter syndrome
- Shwachman-Diamond syndrome

ENVIRONMENTAL EXPOSURES

- Ionizing radiation (therapeutic or environmental exposure)
- Epipodophyllotoxin or alkylator-based chemotherapy

Genetic Factors

The association of leukemia with various constitutional chromosomal abnormalities, the reports of familial leukemias, and several reported karyotypic abnormalities in leukemia cells all suggest that a predisposition to childhood leukemia may be inherited.

Patients with Down syndrome (trisomy 21) have a 15-fold increased risk of developing leukemia when compared with healthy children.[7,8] The relative proportion of ALL and AML in patients with Down syndrome is similar to the general population. However, infants with Down syndrome have a high incidence of a transient myeloproliferative phenomenon in infancy[9,10] and the rare M7, megakaryocytic, form of AML.[11] A majority of the cases of transient myeloproliferation resolve within a couple months, with little or no therapy, although 25% to 33% of patients will develop a true leukemia.[12,13] AML in patients with Down syndrome can usually be treated with less-intense therapy and carries a more favorable prognosis than AML in patients without trisomy 21. Numeric and structural changes in chromosome 21 in leukemia cells are also commonly associated with ALL and AML in otherwise healthy children and adults.[14] Trisomy 21, whether it is present in the germ line or a random event occurring in a hematopoietic progenitor cell, may be the first of 2 mutations leading to an acute leukemia, the second being a random somatic event.

A well-documented high incidence of leukemia exists among children with the autosomal-recessive chromosomal fragility disorders of Bloom syndrome, ataxia telangiectasia, and Fanconi anemia.[15] In these syndromes, the propensity of dividing cells to develop random genetic mutations is likely the cause of the increased incidence of leukemias, as well as other malignancies. Although ALL is reported, both Bloom syndrome and Fanconi anemia are associated more frequently with the development of AML.

The concordance of both AML and ALL in monozygotic twins is estimated as high as 25%,[16] although more recent studies suggest the concordance rate among monozygotic twins with leukemia diagnosed in childhood to be 15% to 20%.[17,18] The risk is highest in infancy and diminishes with age. By age 7, the risk of leukemia in the unaffected twin is close to that of the general population.[19,20] Possibly, the concordance is due to a genetic predisposition or a common environmental exposure in infancy. In fact, a 1.3-fold to 4-fold greater risk of developing leukemia is found among singleton siblings of children with leukemia.[19,21,22] However, an alternative exists for the exceptionally high concordance rate among twins. By sequencing the leukemia fusion gene in 3 twin pairs, Ford and colleagues demonstrated that the leukemia in each twin pair was identical.[23] These data suggest that transplacental transfer of leukemia cells in monozygotic twins may also contribute to the concordance.

Environmental Factors

The risk of leukemia after exposure to ionizing radiation is well established. The first report of the association between ionizing radiation and leukemia came in 1944 in a publication citing a 9-fold increase in the incidence of leukemia among radiologist when compared with other physicians.[24] Subsequently, a 10- to 20-fold increased risk of leukemia is reported among the survivors of the atomic bomb detonations in Hiroshima and Nagasaki in 1944.[25] Finally, an increased incidence in leukemia is reported in patients exposed to radiation either in utero[26] or for treatment of tinea capitis, ankylosing spondylitis, or thymic hyperplasia.[27]

The speculation of the role of viruses in the pathogenesis of leukemia in children is intense (reviewed in 28 studies). Several studies have demonstrated that maternal infection during pregnancy is associated with an increased risk of childhood leukemia. In 2 recent case-controlled studies, the odds ratio of childhood leukemia after maternal Epstein-Barr virus infection is 2.9,[28] and after maternal lower genital tract infections, the odds ratio is 1.8.[29] However, 2 other recent case-controlled studies show no increased risk in children exposed in utero to recurrent maternal infections[30] and nonspecific maternal infections.[31] Similar results from before 1997 are reviewed by Little, but no consistent definitive evidence has been found for the role of maternal infections in the development of childhood leukemias.[32]

Several studies have examined the DNA derived from neonatal Guthrie cards in singleton children diagnosed with ALL. In the first report, Gale and colleagues[33] identified the t(4;11) translocation (typically associated with infant ALL) in the diagnostic specimens and Guthrie cards in patients 2, 5, and 6 years of age at diagnosis of their leukemia. Several subsequent reports analyzing dried blood spots using polymerase chain reaction–based approaches probing for specific mutations, clonal immunoglobulin rearrangements, or T-cell receptor rearrangements have confirmed these results and are thoroughly reviewed by Taub and Ge.[34] Whether the abnormal cells detected on the Guthrie cards reflect a leukemic clone or a *preleukemic* cell is unknown. In many of the cases examined, evidence of an abnormal clone was found in the Guthrie cards of patients 5 to 13 years of age.[35] This long latency period argues for the role of postnatal events in the pathogenesis of childhood leukemias. Greaves et al speculate that the mutation detected in the Guthrie cards is the first of 2 genetic hits required for a leukemic transformation. In support of this theory is the fact that a 25% concordance rate of leukemias exists among twins with *MLL* chromosome band 11q23 fusion genes but only a 5% concordance rate among twins with the *TEL/AML1* mutation.[35] These data suggest that, in certain subtypes of ALL (*TEL/AML1* and hyperdiploid ALL) and AML (associated with t(8;21)), the first preleukemic event occurs in utero, but postnatal events are necessary for the transformation to a leukemic phenotype. Supporting this hypothesis is the description of late relapse *TEL/AML1*$^+$ ALL in which the *recurrence* is actually a second de novo ALL derived from an identical premalignant stem cell.[36]

To identify the possible prenatal and postnatal insults necessary for the leukemic transformation, investigators have examined the role of toxins, electromagnetic fields, pesticides, nitrites, population mixing, seasonal and climatic variations, birth weights, socioeconomic status, breastfeeding, and maternal history of fetal loss in leukemogenesis. However, little, if any, conclusive evidence exists. Equally unclear is the role of in utero and childhood infections in the pathogenesis of childhood leukemia. In recent case-controlled studies, infections in childhood have been associated with both a protective effect against leukemia and an increased risk for leukemia.[31,37-43] Most studies evaluating childhood vaccination and leukemia demonstrated a protective effect,[37,44-46] whereas one study suggested an increased risk for childhood leukemia after measles-mumps-rubella vaccination.[47] Numerous other trials reviewed by McNally and Eden demonstrate only nonsignificant effects after childhood immunizations.[48] Using day care attendance as a surrogate for infectious exposures in children, no studies to date have demonstrated an increased risk of leukemia among children in child care. On the contrary, 5 recent case-controlled studies demonstrate a protective effect of child care attendance.[30,41,42,49,50] No study to date has identified evidence of viral genomic inclusion in leukemia cells. In fact, an apparent benefit has been found to increased social contact, suggesting that certain infections may provide a protective effect against leukemias, presumably through early development of a mature and experienced immune repertoire. The data may suggest that exposure to infections in patients with a relatively naïve immune system later in childhood may increase the risk for leukemia.

The possible environmental contributors to leukemia risk in childhood are reviewed only briefly earlier in this chapter. The agents and pathways involved in the development of childhood leukemia are not well defined, and environmental influences in leukemogenesis are likely to be complex and multifactorial. Ultimately, whether the cause is from low-level radiation, infection, toxin exposure, or an unknown carcinogen, DNA damage and inadequate DNA repair is the initial insult. Subsequently, one or more events, which may be influenced by environmental exposures, initiate the transformation to a malignant phenotype. The future of preventive medicine in childhood leukemia relies on further characterization of molecular events in leukemogenesis and the influence of environmental forces on these events.

CLINICAL MANIFESTATION

Presenting Signs and Symptoms

The presenting clinical features of childhood leukemias (Table 291-1) reflect the uncontrolled proliferation of malignant cells leading to replacement and suppression of normal hematopoietic progenitor cells and infiltration into extramedullary spaces. Symptoms frequently accumulate in days to weeks, culminating in some event that brings the child to medical attention. A frequent question of parents and practitioners alike is whether the leukemia might have been caught sooner. Many researchers would argue that the biological characteristics of the leukemia is determined at the moment the first leukemia cell transforms. Signs of advanced disease such as a high white blood cell count, extramedullary disease, or significant cytopenias may reflect the underlying biological features of the disease rather than timing of diagnosis.

The common clinical signs and symptoms of childhood leukemias are similar to common complaints among children with benign illnesses. Fever is present at diagnosis in a majority of children with leukemia.

Table 291-1 Common Clinical and Laboratory Findings Present at Diagnosis in Children With Leukemia

	ALL (%)*	AML (%)†
CLINICAL FEATURES		
Fever	61	34
Pallor	55	25
Petechiae, purpura, bleeding	48	33
Anorexia or weight loss	33	22
Fatigue, malaise	30	19
Bone, joint pain	38	18
Lymphadenopathy	50	14
Hepatosplenomegaly	68	55
Swollen gingivae	—	8
Cough, dysphagia	—	41
Recurrent infection	—	3
Neurologic symptoms	3	10
LABORATORY FEATURES		
White Blood Cell Count (per mcL)		
<10,000	53	39
10,000-49,000	30	29
>50,000	17	32
Hemoglobin (g/dL)		
<7	43	41
7-11	45	48
>11	12	11
Platelet Count (per mcL)		
<20,000	28	15
20,000-99,000	47	67
>100,000	25	18
Coagulopathy	—	17

ALL, Acute lymphoblastic leukemia; *AML,* acute myelogenous leukemia.
*Miller DR. Acute lymphoblastic leukemia. Pediatr Clin North Am, 1980;27:269-291
†Choi SR, Simone JV. Acute nonlymphocytic leukemia in 171 children. *Med Pediatr Oncol.* 1976;2:119-146.

Only subtle findings may exist on examination or in the history distinguishing fever in a child with leukemia from fever in normal children. Complaints of bone pain (manifesting as a limp in younger children), significant and diffuse lymphadenopathy, hepatosplenomegaly, pallor and petechiae, unexplained ecchymoses, and bleeding are all signs that frequently trigger further studies. More subtle and less specific complaints of fatigue and anorexia typically warrant close follow-up. Laboratory studies are typically necessary to corroborate clinical evidence.

Laboratory Findings

The white blood cell count may be normal, increased, or decreased in a newly diagnosed patient with leukemia, and blasts may or may not be present on the peripheral blood smear. Anemia and thrombocytopenia are common but not always present. In other words, although a complete blood count is certainly the first laboratory study necessary in the diagnosis of leukemia, a normal complete blood count result does not rule out leukemia. Continued close follow-up or referral to a hematologist should be guided by clinical evidence and laboratory findings.

Other abnormal laboratory findings include measures of tumor burden and cell turnover: increased potassium, increased phosphorus, decreased calcium, increased uric acid, and increased lactate dehydrogenase. These findings are hallmarks of the tumor lysis syndrome. Usually most severe after administration of chemotherapy, signs of tumor lysis may be present at diagnosis because of rapid proliferation and destruction of leukemic cells. Patients at risk for significant electrolyte abnormalities and even renal failure are those with evidence of high tumor burden: high white blood cell count, massive organomegaly, and mature B-cell leukemia (Burkitt type), especially if an extramedullary tumor mass is present. However, with appropriate preemptive management, clinically significant tumor lysis syndrome is rare in childhood leukemias.

Mediastinal masses are present in 5% to 10% of children with leukemia, especially older boys who are more likely to have a T-cell leukemia. A chest radiograph is necessary in all patients suspected of an acute leukemia and should be performed before administration of anesthesia for any procedures. Though not required in the diagnostic evaluation of childhood leukemia, radiographs of long bones will frequently demonstrate evidence of leukemic infiltration of the periosteum and bone. Patients with particularly high leukemic cell burdens may appear osteopenic; others may demonstrate signs of subperiosteal new bone formation, radiolucent bands in the metaphysis *(leukemic lines)*, discrete osteolytic lesions, and growth arrest lines.

Extramedullary Leukemia

As many as 20% of patients will have evidence of disease in the central nervous system (CNS) at diagnosis. However, fewer than 5% of children will have symptoms of disease at diagnosis, including vomiting, headache, and lethargy. Papilledema and cranial nerve palsies, which are rare as are significant signs of extensive CNS involvement, are not uncommon. Cranial nerve palsies are typically reflective of meningeal infiltration of leukemic cells rather than increased intracranial pressure. Patients at greatest risk for CNS disease are those with T-cell ALL, those younger than 2 years, and those with monoblastic forms of AML. Painless enlargement of one or both testicles has been reported in fewer than 5% of boys diagnosed with leukemia and is more common in ALL (particularly T-cell ALL) than AML.

Chloromas

Chloromas, or granulocytic sarcomas, are solid collections (tumors) of malignant cells in patients with AML. Chloromas can occur anywhere, including the skin, CNS, and bones. Rarely, chloromas can occur independent of or before evidence of bone marrow disease.

DIFFERENTIAL DIAGNOSIS

The differential diagnosis of individual or concurrent cytopenias includes several common infectious and noninfectious diseases of childhood (Box 291-2). The spectrum of signs and symptoms of childhood leukemias mirrors the spectrum of many more common illnesses. Differentiating childhood leukemia from these other illnesses frequently requires either periodic reassessment of clinical and laboratory parameters of disease or, in cases in which the index of probability is sufficient, a more definitive bone marrow aspiration and biopsy. If the leukemic cell burden is sufficient to elicit clinical symptoms, then findings on a bone marrow evaluation will not be subtle. Identifying patients with signs and symptoms severe enough to warrant a bone marrow evaluation (frequently requiring anesthesia in younger children) can be challenging. In patients with atypical findings of common diseases, the general pediatrician's best tools are a high index of probability and frequent follow-up. An acute leukemia cannot hide for long before declaring itself.

Many more common illnesses than leukemia produce fever, rash, lymphadenopathy, hepatosplenomegaly, mild cytopenias, or lymphocytosis. The appearance of atypical and variant lymphocytes on the peripheral blood smears of children with infections such as Epstein-Barr virus, pertussis, and parapertussis often bring leukemia into the differential diagnosis. Diseases such as systemic lupus erythematosus and juvenile rheumatoid arthritis may be associated with bone or joint pain and cytopenias that are indistinguishable from an acute leukemia. For many diseases, eliminating leukemia from the differential diagnosis becomes of paramount importance in specific diseases that require use of corticosteroids (systemic lupus erythematosus, juvenile rheumatoid arthritis, immune thrombocytopenia purpura, hemolytic anemia, and even infectious processes precipitating an acute asthma exacerbation). In these instances, if leukemia is possible or probable, then referral to a hematologist may be necessary. Inadvertent administration of

BOX 291-2 Differential Diagnosis of Childhood Leukemia

NONMALIGNANT DISEASES

Juvenile rheumatoid arthritis
Systemic lupus erythematosus
Infectious mononucleosis
Immune thrombocytopenia purpura
Aplastic anemia
Pertussis, parapertussis
Benign lymphocytosis
Leukemoid reaction
Sepsis
Osteomyelitis

MALIGNANCIES

Metastatic bone marrow disease in retinoblastoma
Neuroblastoma
Ewing sarcoma
Rhabdomyosarcoma
Lymphoma

corticosteroids may impair or delay the diagnosis of leukemia and may necessitate more intensive high-risk chemotherapy for patients with otherwise standard-risk disease.

CLASSIFICATION

Leukemias are a heterogeneous group of disorders classified by immunophenotype and subclassified based primarily on prognostic features. Leukemias can be classified as acute or chronic and lymphoblastic or myelogenous. In a normal marrow, blasts, which are hematopoietic progenitor cells, make up less than 5% of the total nucleated-cell population. Rarely are these cells found in the peripheral blood, except in instances of significant infection, bleeding, or a malignant process occupying the marrow space, including metastatic disease from solid tumors. The acute leukemias are defined as a clonal expansion of hematopoietic progenitor cells (blasts) such that the number of these cells exceeds 25% of the total nucleated-cell population in the marrow for ALL or 20% for AML.[51] The expansion of these cells in the confined marrow space and their impingement on normal marrow progenitors is reflected in the relatively rapid onset of symptoms in patients with acute leukemia. The natural clinical course is fulminant disease if untreated. In contrast, in chronic leukemia, a hyperproliferation of mature hematopoietic elements can be found, often in the absence of life-threatening cytopenias. Chronic leukemias have a more insidious onset than the acute leukemias. Although the initial management may not be as problematic, long-term eradication of the disease is more difficult in chronic leukemias.

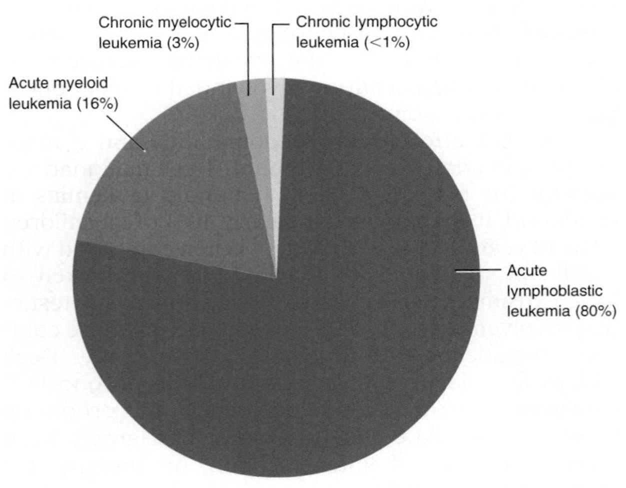

Figure 291-2 Classification and frequency of leukemias in children. *(Derived from Pui C-H. Childhood leukemias.* N Engl J Med. *1995:332:1618-1630.)*

Acute leukemia cells likely arise from a single, mutated progenitor cell that proliferates but does not differentiate into a functional mature cell. In the diagnostic bone marrow specimen, the abnormal cells predominate and determine the leukemia type. Classification into myeloid or lymphoid lineages, good or poor prognosis, is based on morphology, immunophenotype, cytogenetics, and behavior. ALL is the most common form of leukemia (Figure 291-2). Subclassification into early pre-B-cell, pre-B-cell, B-cell, and T-cell lymphoblastic leukemias is essential to treatment and prognostic stratification of patients (Table 291-2). The myeloid leukemias (Table 291-3) can be categorized based on either the cell of origin (French-American-British [FAB] system) or cytogenetic and morphologic features (World Health Organization [WHO] classification system). The FAB system is the traditional system, whereas the WHO system was developed more recently. The WHO system stratifies based on cancer cytogenetics and weighs molecular features of the disease more heavily than the morphologic features.

Immunophenotype

Classification of leukemia by immunohistochemical or immunoflow cytometric detection of lineage-specific antigens allows for a precise and biologically relevant description of the leukemia cells. From the very first

Table 291-2 Classification and Immunophenotype of Acute Lymphoblastic Leukemias

COMMON NAME	COMMON FEATURES OF IMMUNOPHENOTYPE	PATIENTS	COMMENTS
Early pre-B cell, CD10–	CD10–, CD19+, CD20+, TdT+	5.2%	Common in infants younger than 1 year, associated with t(4;11)
Early pre-B cell, CD10+	CD10+, CD19+, CD20+, TdT+	63.1%	Peak incidence in early childhood
Pre-B cell	CD10+/–, CD19+, CD20+, TdT+, Cytoplasmic immunoglobulin+	15.5%	Clinically similar to early pre-B-cell ALL
Mature B Cell	CD19+, CD20+, TdT+, surface immunoglobulin+	3.9%	Burkitt-type leukemia, treated differently than pre-B-cell ALL
Pre-T Cell	CD2+, CD3+, CD7+, TdT+	12.3%	More common in adolescents and in boys Associated with high white blood cell count and bulky extramedullary disease, particularly a mediastinal mass

bone marrow aspiration and biopsy, a crucial distinction between AML and ALL is made. ALL is often treated with a 3- or 4-drug induction regimen of limited toxicity, whereas AML is treated with much more aggressive induction regimens. Surface and cytoplasmic antigens differentially expressed on cells of myeloid or lymphoid origin can be used to reliably distinguish AML from ALL and to subclassify within each lineage.

Acute Lymphoblastic Leukemias

Many lymphoid malignancies (B and T lineage) will express terminal deoxynucleotidyl transferase. No antigen is truly lineage specific in leukemia samples, but a majority of B-cell leukemias will express CD10, CD19, CD22, or any combination, whereas T-lineage leukemias will express CD3, CD7, or both. Among 3073 patients enrolled on the ALL-BFM (Acute Lymphoblastic Leukemia, Berlin-Frankfurt-Munich) 86 and ALL-BFM 90 trials, 403 (13%) had T-cell ALL, and 2690 (87%) had B-cell ALL.[52,53] The distinction between T- and B-lineage lymphoblastic leukemia is crucial to prognosis and treatment.

Early-cell ALL arises from a precursor B cell too immature to produce cytoplasmic immunoglobulin and accounts for approximately 60% of all childhood ALL.[54] Most of these immature leukemias express CD10 (common ALL antigen-CALLA),[55-57] CD19, and CD22 but do not express cytoplasmic immunoglobulin. CD10-negative, CD19-positive, CD22-positive early pre-B-cell ALL is derived from an earlier precursor lymphoblast. When found in infants, the CD10-negative early pre-B-cell phenotype is typically associated with rearrangements involving the MLL locus (11q23) and with a poor outcome.[57]

Table 291-3 Classification of Acute Myeloid Leukemia

M1 AML without maturation - 24% of patients
M2 AML with maturation - 23% of patients
M3 Promyelocytic leukemia - 5% of patients
M4 Myelomonocytic - 27% of patients
M5 Monocytic - 10% of patients
M6 Erythroleukemia - 2% of patients
M7 Megakaryocytic - 7% of patients

WHO CLASSIFICATION AND FREQUENCY

AML with recurrent genetic abnormalities
- t(8;21)(q22;q23), *(AML/ETO)*
- AML with abnormal marrow eosinophils and inv(16) (p13q22), or t(16;16)(p13;q22), *CBFβ/MYH11*
- APML with t(15;17)(q22;q12), *(PML/RARα)* and variants
- AML with 11q23 abnormalities

AML with multilineage dysplasia
- After MDS or MPD
- No antecedent MDS or MPD, but dysplasia in 50% of cells

Therapy-related AML and MDS
- Alkylating agent, radiation related
- Topoisomerase II–inhibitor related

AML not otherwise categorized
- Apply FAB categories

AML, Acute myelogenous leukemia; *APML,* acute promyelocytic leukemia; *FAB,* French-American-British; *MDS,* myelodysplastic syndromes; *MPD,* myeloproliferative disorders.

Derived from a slightly more mature clone, the pre-B-cell ALLs express cytoplasmic (but not surface) immunoglobulin, 90% express CD10,[58] and most express CD19, CD22, or both. Pre-B-cell ALL account for approximately 15% of all cases of ALL.[55] The t(1;19)(q23;p13) translocation is found in approximately 25% of cases of pre-B-cell ALL, but only 5% of all cases of ALL.[52] This translocation results in a fusion of the *E2A* and *PBX* genes. Despite the adverse prognostic impact of this translocation in older studies, recent intensification of therapy has resulted in an improved survival for these children.[59]

Mature B cell accounts for 3% to 4% of all ALL in childhood.[60] Characteristic immunotypic features include the presence of surface immunoglobulin (usually IgM), CD20 (a mature B-cell marker), CD19, and human leukocyte antigen-DR. Cells are invariably CD10 negative. Mature B-cell leukemias are indistinguishable from Burkitt lymphoma with bone marrow involvement. Nearly all of these malignancies are associated with translocations involving the *MYC* oncogene on chromosome 8.

T-cell ALL affects boys predominantly and is more common in adolescence. Although T-cell malignancies account for only 13% of all lymphoid leukemias in childhood, it is diagnosed in nearly 40% of all children 10 to 18 years of age with ALL.[52] When compared with B-cell ALL, patients with T-cell ALL are more likely to have extramedullary disease. Mediastinal mass, testicular involvement, and CNS leukemia are all more common in patients with T-cell ALL. Historically, T-cell ALL is associated with a less-favorable prognosis.[61] However, the historical difference in prognosis between T-cell ALL and B-cell ALL has largely been erased because of intensification of therapy for patients with T-cell ALL.

Acute Myelogenous Leukemia

AML occurs in approximately 1 in 130,000 individuals under 20 years of age, accounting for only 16% of all childhood leukemias. Significant differences can be found in the surface antigen expression among the FAB subtypes of AML (see Table 291-3). The common myeloid antigens used to differential ALL from AML are CD13, CD33, CD117, CD14, CD64, glycophorin A, and CD41. CD14 and CD64 are monocytic markers, glycophorin A is an erythroid marker, and CD41 is a megakaryocytic marker.

Biphenotypic Leukemia

In 1995 the European Group for the Immunologic Classification of Leukemias developed a scoring system of lineage specificity for different markers and later revised the system in 1998.[62,63] In this system, AML is distinguished from ALL based on a scoring system (Table 291-4). Biphenotypic or mixed-lineage leukemia is defined as a score of 2 or more in 2 separate lineages. Applying the European Group's criteria to 676 patients newly diagnosed with leukemia, Owaidah et al identified biphenotypic phenotypes in 3.4% of patients. Among these patients, the Philadelphia

(Ph) chromosome (17%) and MLL (26%) abnormalities were common.[64]

Cytogenetic and Molecular Markers

Researchers have hypothesized that for an acute leukemia to develop, at least 2 relatively broad mutations must occur: class I and class II. Class I mutations offer a proliferative or survival advantage (eg, *RAS* or *FLT3* mutations), whereas class II mutations inhibit differentiation. Identification of these mutations not only offers insight into the pathogenesis of an acute leukemia, but these genetic events also significantly influence prognosis. Table 291-5 reviews the common genetic events that are hallmarks of childhood ALL and AML.

Acute Lymphoblastic Leukemia

PLOIDY. An increase in the modal number of chromosomes (>46 chromosomes) can be detected in nearly a third of newly diagnosed cases of ALL.[65]

Table 291-4 Scoring System From the European Group for the Immunological Characterization of Leukemias

POINTS	B-CELL ALL	T-CELL ALL	AML
2	cyCD79 cyCD22 cyIgM	cyCD3 or memCD3 Anti-TCR	MPO
1	CD19 CD20 CD10	CD2 CD5 CD8 CD10	CD117 CD13 CD33 CD65
0.5	TdT CD24	TdT CD7	CD14 CD15

cy, cytoplasmic; *mem*, membrane; *MPO*, myeloperoxidase; *TCR*, T-cell receptor; *TdT*, terminal deoxynucleotidyl transferase.

Hyperdiploidy is associated with increased sensitivity to chemotherapeutic agents in leukemia cells cultured in vitro.[65,66] Event-free survival in patients with hyperdiploid leukemia cells exceeds 75% to 90%, making it a reliable marker of a good prognosis.[67] Specifically, patients with simultaneous trisomies of chromosomes 4, 10, and 17 have a 7-year event-free survival in excess of 90%. Unfortunately, patients with fewer than 46 chromosomes (hypodiploidy) have a worse prognosis. The event-free survival for patients with 33 to 44 chromosomes is 40%, and for patients with fewer than 28 chromosomes, the event-free survival is 25%.[67,68]

In addition to changes in chromosome number, nearly a third of childhood leukemias will harbor chromosomal translocations, independent of ploidy. Included here is a discussion of four major translocations, each associated with a distinct biological subset.

MIXED-LINEAGE LEUKEMIA. Translocations involving the *MLL* gene at 11q23 and more than 30 potential partner chromosomes[69] can be found in 6% of childhood ALL cases.[67] The t(4;11)(q21;q23) mutation resulting in the *MLL-AF4* fusion product is commonly seen in infant ALL and is associated with an event-free survival of only 20% to 25%. In children older than 1 year, the negative impact of *MLL* gene rearrangements on survival is less.[70,71] For example, the t(11;19)(q23;q13.3) translocation fusing *MLL* with the *ENL* locus on chromosome 19 is associated with a favorable prognosis in T-cell ALL.[72]

E2A/PBX. Pre-B-Cell ALL is frequently characterized by t(1;19)(q23;q13), resulting in a fusion of the *E2A* and *PBX* genes.[59] Once thought to be associated with a poor prognosis, recent studies with more intensive therapies have shown improved survival.

BCR-ABL. The Ph chromosome[73] results from a balanced translocation between the long arms of chromosome 9 and 22 (t(9;22)[q34;q11]), resulting in the fusion of the *BCR* and *ABL* genes.[74-76] In 3% to 5% of childhood ALL and 20% of ALL cases in adults, the *BCR-ABL* fusion encodes a 185-kDa dysregulated tyrosine kinase responsible for the malignant transformation.[67,77] A 210-kDa variant is the hallmark of more than 90% of chronic myelogenous leukemias. Ph+ childhood ALL remains one of the most difficult

Table 291-5 Common Cytogenetic Abnormalities of Childhood Leukemias

	KARYOTYPE	FUSION GENE	FREQUENCY IN CHILDHOOD LEUKEMIA
ALL	t(12;21)(p13;q22)	*TEL/AML1*	25-30% of ALL
	11q23 abnormalities	Multiple *MLL* fusion genes are reported	6% of ALL
	t(1;19)(q23;q13)	*E2A/PBX*	5% of ALL
	t(12;21)(p13;q22)	*TEL/AML1*	25% of ALL
	t(9;22)(q34;q11)	*BCR/ABL*	3% to 5% of ALL
	Hyperdiploidy	—	30% of ALL
AML	t(8;21)(q22;q22)	*AML1/ETO*	10% to 15% of AML
	inv16(p13;q22)	*CBFB-MYH11*	6% to 12% of AML
	t(15;17)(q22;q21)	*APML/RARα*	8% to 10% of AML

HOX11 over expression is a common abnormality in T-cell ALL and is identified in 5% to 10% of patients.

subsets to cure, with a long-term, event-free survival of less than 50%.[77] Matched-sibling bone marrow transplant is now recommended for children in first remission, and the role of specific tyrosine kinase inhibitors such as imatinib mesylate are currently being evaluated.

TEL/AML1. The t(12;21)(p13;q22) translocation is the most common in pediatric ALL and is identified in up to 25% of B-precursor ALL.[78] Fusion of the *TEL* locus at 12p13 with the *AML1* gene at 21q22 results is a fusion transcript that serves as a co-repressor of *AML-1* target genes.[79] Patients with the *TEL/AML1* translocation do very well with conventional therapy and may be preferentially sensitive to protocols containing augmented therapy with asparaginase.[67,80,81] Patients with *TEL/AML1*–positive leukemias tend to relapse late, and salvage after relapse remains excellent.[35,82]

Acute Myelogenous Leukemia

PML/RAR. The most characteristic chromosomal abnormality in childhood AML is the t(15;17) translocation. The resulting chimeric protein, *PML/RARα* is formed by the fusion of the retinoic acid receptor-α *(RARα)* gene from chromosome 17 and the promyelocytic leukemia *(PML)* gene from chromosome 15. The *PML-RARα* fusion protein suppresses gene transcription and blocks differentiation of myeloid progenitor cells. Retinoic acid may still bind to the abnormal *RARα* portion of the protein, promoting differentiation.[83]

CORE-BINDING FACTOR. Both inv16 and t(8;21) involve subunits of the transcription factor complex core-binding factor (CBF), disrupting the normal functions of this gene. The CBF is a family of heterodimeric transcription factors containing 1 of 3 CBFα subunits (CBFα1, *AML1* [also known as RUNX1 or CBFα2], or CBFα3) and a common β subunit (CBFβ). The CBFα subunits are involved in both DNA binding and interaction with CBFβ.[84] CBFβ functions to enhance binding of CBFα and increases the affinities of the CBFα subunits for DNA.[85] Together, the CBF complex is a critical transcriptional activator of genes involved in hematopoiesis and bone development.[86,87] The *inv*16(p13;q22) abnormality results in a fusion of the *CBFβ* gene and the myosin heavy chain *(MYH11)*. The 8;21 translocation involves the *CBFα* *(AML1)* gene on chromosome 21 juxtaposed with the *ETO* gene on chromosome 8. Disruption of both the *CBFβ* gene by *CBFβ-MYH11* and the CBFα subunit by the *AML1/ETO* fusion leads to deficient transcription of *CBFA-CBFB*–controlled genes and myeloid maturation arrest.[88] As with the *TEL/AML1* mutation, these CBF-related mutations have been found in the Guthrie cards of patient who develop leukemia well into their 2nd decade. The long latency implies that class II CBF-related mutations may be only the first hit in leukemogenesis.[89,90] Class II mutations altering expression and function of *FLT3*,[91] *c-KIT*,[92] and *RAS*[93,94] may provide the second hit and a requisite proliferative advantage to preleukemic cells with already-abnormal differentiation signaling.[87] Additional, but unfavorable, abnormalities identified in AML samples include: –5/del(5q), –7/del(7q), inv(3)/t^2, +8, and complex karyotypes.[95,96]

TREATMENT OF ACUTE LYMPHOBLASTIC LEUKEMIA

Risk-Stratified Therapy

Before the 1950s, no classification system existed for childhood leukemias. However, regardless of the myeloid or lymphoid origin of the disease, childhood leukemias were uniformly fatal within months of diagnosis. Djerassi et al were the first group to attempt chemotherapy as a means to treat childhood leukemia.[97] Initial trials with folic acid only made the disease worse; thus, instead an antagonist of folate metabolism, aminopterin (a methotrexate analog) was used to induce the first temporary responses. Subsequently, 6-mercaptopurine (6-MP) and prednisone were tried, both as single agents.[98] Responses but not cures were observed. Nonetheless, from this point on, pediatric leukemia trials evolved, each sequential trial expanding from the success and failures of previous trials. Today, risk-adapted therapies, based on clinical features (age, white blood cell count, and response to induction therapies) and biological features (ploidy and mutations of known prognostic significance), are used to maximize response and cure rates while minimizing long-term side effects (Table 291-6).

Patients between 1 and 9.99 years of age with an initial white blood cell count less than or equal to 50,000/mcL are classified as standard risk according to National Cancer Institute and Rome criteria. Children younger than 1 year and older than 10 years or children with initial a white blood cell count of more than 50,000/mcL are classified as high risk.[99] In many multiinstitutional, international cooperative group studies, age and initial white blood cell count have proven to be reliable and independent predictors of prognosis. Other clinical features used to stratify therapy include gender, leukemia phenotype, and response to initial therapy. Independent of the increased incidence of T-cell ALL among boys, girls appear to do better with less therapy. Even in more recent studies that intensify therapy for boys, the differences in survival among boys and girls are still apparent, although significantly reduced.[67] The reason for these gender differences is not known.

Leukemia cells that express aberrant myeloid markers but do not meet strict criteria for biphenotypic leukemia historically yield inferior outcome. This effect is abrogated in recent trials.[100] T-cell phenotype is associated with an inferior outcome, although the clinical features of older age, male gender, and extramedullary disease frequently associated with T-cell ALL may partly account for the greater risk for relapse.[67,101] Nonetheless, the importance of T cell–directed therapy is underscored by the greater sensitivity of T-lineage malignancies to asparaginase and a new antimetabolite, ara-G (nelarabine), and by the relative resistance of these cells to low doses of methotrexate (MTX). The identification of leukemia cells in the CNS disease at diagnosis continues to be an adverse prognostic feature of childhood ALL despite attempts to intensify intrathecal therapy and CNS irradiation.[67]

Response to induction therapy is predictive of outcome and used to stratify patients for more intensified

Table 291-6 Common Prognostic Features of the Acute Leukemias[a]

	CLINICAL FEATURES	CYTOGENETICS
B-cell-precursor ALL	*Favorable* Age between 1 and 9.99 years	*Favorable* t(11;22)(p13;q22), *TEL/AML1* fusion Hyperdiploidy (>50 chromosomes) Trisomies 4, 10, and 17
	Unfavorable Age older than 10 years Initial white blood cell count >50,000/mcL Poor response to induction therapy Extramedullary disease	*Unfavorable* Philadelphia chromosome *MLL* rearrangements in infants
T-cell precursor ALL	*Favorable* Good response to steroids[b]	*Favorable* *HOX11* overexpresssion t(11;19) *MLL-ENL* fusion
	Unfavorable Poor early response to treatment Low-intensity chemotherapy regimens	*Unfavorable* —
AML	*Favorable* Acute promyelocytic leukemia AML in Down syndrome	*Favorable* t(8:21) *AML1-ETO* fusion inv(16) or t(16;16)(p13;q22) t(15;17)(q22;q21), *APML/RARα* fusion
	Unfavorable White blood cell count >100,000/mcL Secondary AML or AML after MDS	*Unfavorable* Monosomy 7 (7q-)

Adapted from [a]Pui CH, Schrappe M, Ribeiro RC, et al. Childhood and adolescent lymphoid and myeloid leukemia. *Hematology Am Soc Hematol Educ Program.* 2004;:118-145; [b]Schrappe M. Evolution of BFM trials for childhood ALL. *Ann Hematol.* 2004;83:S121-S123.
ALL, acute lumphoblastic leukemia; AML, acute myelogenous leukemia; MDS, myelodysplastic syndrome.

therapy when necessary. After 7 days of therapy, patients with less than 5% blasts in their marrow have an event-free survival of 80%, whereas those with more than 25% blasts in the marrow have an event-free survival of 68%.[102] Among patients with a slow early response to induction therapy, those who receive intensified therapy will have an improved outcome when compared with those who remain on standard therapy.[103]

Principles of Treatment

Leukemia cell infiltration in marrow space and other organ systems in patients newly diagnosed with ALL may result in pancytopenia, as well as many systemic symptoms. Resolution of symptomatic disease and recovery of normal bone marrow function can only be achieved with the administration of potentially myelosuppressive and immunosuppressive chemotherapy. Therapy is frequently divided into phases of remission induction, delayed intensification, extramedullary disease treatment or prophylaxis, and maintenance. The timing, number, and chemotherapy components of each phase may differ between protocols, but the principles of therapy are similar. Remission induction is achieved in most cases with three drugs (vincristine, asparaginase, and a corticosteroid) in standard-risk patients or four drugs in high-risk patients (the same three drugs as in standard-risk patients with the addition of daunorubicin). The goal is to induce a complete remission, defined as the reduction of the leukemia cell burden below clinical, morphologic, and molecular levels of detection after recovery of normal blood counts. With current chemotherapeutic regimens, remission induction is possible in more than 95% of children with ALL. Many protocols follow the induction phase with a consolidation phase heavy in antimetabolites to secure or consolidate the remission.

Delayed intensification is a second phase of intensified chemotherapy similar to the induction and consolidations phases. The addition of a delayed-intensification phase by the BFM group has led to significant improvement in survival in all patients with childhood ALL.[104,105] Subsequent trials in the United States and Europe have confirmed the importance of postinduction intensification in the long-term survival of patients with ALL. Survival among patients with high-risk leukemia may be further improved by augmenting the regimen with a second delayed intensification.[103]

Although the 1st successful treatment of CNS leukemia included 2400 to 3600 cGy cranial radiation, in the last 2 decades, several trials have demonstrated that CNS radiation may be reduced (to 1200 to 1800 cGy) or eliminated in patients with low-risk B-cell ALL with a rapid early response to induction therapy.[106-114] Elimination of cranial radiation in patients with T-cell ALL has not proven feasible. Reduction in cranial radiation is designed to reduce long-term endocrine and cognitive effects, as well as reduce the risk of secondary malignancies. However, the use of intensified intrathecal therapy and the use of high-dose MTX are also associated with late cognitive side effects even when administered without radiation therapy.[115] The optimal CNS treatment and prophylactic regimens in childhood ALL are not yet clearly defined, but current widely used strategies are associated with significantly fewer side effects than previous efforts.

Unlike treatment paradigms for most malignancies, successful therapy for childhood ALL includes a protracted maintenance period. Although the components of maintenance therapy vary between cooperative group studies, attempts to reduce therapy to less than 24 months have never been successful. In the current Children's Oncology Group studies, boys with standard-risk ALL receive 3 years of postremission therapy, whereas boys with high-risk disease (therapy is intensified up front) and all girls with ALL receive 2 years of postremission therapy. Maintenance consists of daily oral mercaptopurine, weekly oral MTX, monthly intravenous vincristine, monthly 5-day oral corticosteroid pulses, and intrathecal therapy once every 3 months. The therapy is adjusted to maximize the dose within a range that maximizes the antileukemic effect and minimizes toxicity, including myelosuppression and immunosuppression. Many children on maintenance chemotherapy may return to school and normal daily activities.

Infant Acute Lymphoblastic Leukemia

In the 1970s the survival among children older than 1 year with ALL approached 50%, and less than 20% of children younger than 1 year survived.[116] Currently, infants still have a higher incidence of relapse, death from toxicity, and long-term side effects when compared with older children.[117-119] Studies with intensified therapy in infants younger than 6 months demonstrated an event-free survival of less than 10%, and infants older than 6 months had an event-free survival of 40%.[120] Incremental improvement in survival with intensified chemotherapy approaches has prompted several investigators to consider bone marrow transplantation in 1st remission for infants. Transplantation poses several problems, including the facts that matched siblings are not usually available and total body radiation is associated with significant long-term side effects in young infants. Alternatively, continuous intensified multiagent chemotherapy may improve event-free survival for many infants, reserving the use of bone marrow transplantation only in the setting of a relapse or abnormalities involving 11q23 in younger infants.[121] Ongoing studies in this unique and challenging subset of patients will help further define the role of transplantation and intensified chemotherapy.

TREATMENT OF ACUTE MYELOGENOUS LEUKEMIA

Principles of Therapy

Unlike treatment strategies in ALL, the event-free survival rate in childhood AML has reached a plateau at 60% despite aggressive intensification of therapy. Individualized treatment regimens have worked to improve survival rates significantly in children with acute promyelocytic leukemia but have done little for other subsets of AML.

More than 90% of patients will obtain a complete remission with cytarabine and daunorubicin in combination with either etoposide or thioguanine.[122] Attempts to improve remission induction rates and improve long-term survival by substituting idarubicin[123] or mitoxantrone[124] for daunorubicin or by increasing the dose of cytarabine[125,126] have largely proven to be of comparable efficacy and occasionally greater toxicity. Alternative approaches currently under investigation include the introduction of monoclonal antibodies directed against CD33, a surface antigen expressed on most myeloid neoplasms.

Intensive postremission therapies have been developed using multiagent regimens cycled every 4 to 6 weeks. No randomized head-to-head comparisons have been made of the different regimens, but none have succeeded in improving long-term, event-free survival beyond 60%. Allogeneic stem cell transplantation has been extensively evaluated in childhood AML. Most studies nonrandomly assign patients with matched-sibling donors to undergo transplant and those without sibling donors to continue with conventional chemotherapy. Relapse-free survival is generally better in the patients who undergo transplantation, but overall survival is comparable because of transplant-related mortality. Among patients with t(8;21), t(9;11), t(15;17), and *inv*16, all favorable cytogenetic features, stem cell transplantation is currently not recommended in 1st remission (reviewed in 52 studies).

Acute Promyelocytic Leukemia

When treated with standard AML therapy, patients with acute promyelocytic leukemia fared poorly. Recent regimens intensifying the anthracycline dose in induction and incorporating retinoic acid, mercaptopurine, and MTX into maintenance therapy has led to 5-year survival rates exceeding 80% among children with acute promyelocytic leukemia.[127]

CHRONIC MYELOGENOUS LEUKEMIA

Chronic myelogenous leukemia (CML) accounts for approximately 3% of childhood leukemias.[128] In children and adults, CML is characterized by the presence of the Ph chromosome.[73,129] The Ph chromosome[73] results from a balanced translocation between the long arms of chromosomes 9 and 22 (t(9;22)[q34;q11]), resulting in the fusion of the *BCR* and *ABL* genes.[74-76] In CML, *BCR-ABL* encodes a 210-kDa dysregulated tyrosine kinase, which is found in more than 90% of childhood and adult CML cases.

CML in childhood typically produces leukocytosis, which is marked by the presence of myeloid progenitor cells at all levels of differentiation, and thrombocytosis. Hepatosplenomegaly is present in a majority of patients. Symptoms of fatigue, weight loss, bone pain, and low-grade fevers may be present for weeks to months.[129] Most patients are diagnosed in either the chronic phase (cytogenetic evidence of disease with fewer than 5% blasts in the marrow) or the accelerated phase (cytogenetic evidence of disease with 5% to 30% blasts in the bone marrow). Blast crisis is reflective of more advanced disease and is indistinguishable from AML, with the exception of the presence of the Ph chromosome.

Until recently, standard therapy for CML in children and adults included hydroxyurea, interferon, and low-dose cytarabine. Although clinical improvements in hematologic parameters were possible with these therapies, cytogenetic remission was infrequent. More recently, imatinib mesylate was developed as a specific inhibitor of the *BCR-ABL* tyrosine kinase. Results from recent clinical trials have rapidly established imatinib as the standard of care for CML.[130-133] Approximately 60% of patients who are refractory to interferon achieved a major cytogenetic response with imatinib, with infrequent hematologic toxicities.[132] Imatinib is reportedly most effective in patients with chronic-phase CML (76% major cytogenetic response rate reported)[133] compared with the accelerated phase,[132] or blast crisis.[132] A recent phase III prospective trial of more than 1000 patients conclusively demonstrated that imatinib is superior to interferon-α plus low-dose cytarabine in inducing cytogenetic disease remission and prolonging progression-free survival in adult patients with chronic-phase CML.[133] Limited data are available on imatinib mesylate in children, but preliminary data are promising.[134,135]

Imatinib mesylate has dramatically changed therapy for CML, but it is still not a cure. The only proven curative strategy for children with CML is allogeneic stem cell transplantation (SCT).[136-139] Survival after SCT for CML is reported to be 70% to 80% with a matched-sibling donor and 40% to 60% when unrelated donors are used. A recent editorial suggests that imatinib therapy should be administered only until an appropriate stem cell donor is identified and that imatinib therapy should not replace or delay the timing of the transplant.[140] This assertion is based, in part, on data that demonstrate inferior outcomes among patients who are in chronic phase for longer than 12 months before SCT when compared with patients who undergo SCT while in the early chronic phase of disease.[137] However, these transplants were performed before the imatinib era, at a time when residual molecular disease was not routinely measured but certainly expected. In the current era of imatinib mesylate therapy, once-unattainable cytogenetic and molecular remissions are not only possible, but also expected. Durable remissions on imatinib mesylate therapy are likely to extend beyond the 1st year after diagnosis, making the delay of transplant possible, especially in patients without an appropriate donor and in very young children.[134]

JUVENILE MYELOMONOCYTIC LEUKEMIA

Juvenile myelomonocytic leukemia (JMML) is a clonal disorder of early childhood, occurring at a median age of 1.8 years. Hallmarks of the disease at diagnosis include marked hepatosplenomegaly, peripheral blood monocyte count of more than 1×10^9/L, and myeloid precursors in the peripheral blood. Chronic infections, lymphadenopathy, rash (eczema, xanthomas, café-au-lait spots), and failure-to-thrive are also common.[141] Bone marrow aspiration will reveal hypercellularity with a predominance of all stages of granulocyte maturation and a blast count of less than 20%, similar to the findings in CML with 1 key exception: Patients with JMML do not harbor the Ph chromosome. With the exception of proving that no Ph chromosome is present, bone marrow aspiration is not diagnostic in JMML, as it is in the acute leukemias. The diagnosis of JMML can be made from clinical history and peripheral blood findings, with corroboration from bone marrow findings.

Monosomy 7 can be identified in 25% of patients with JMML, and 65% will have a normal karyotype.[141] Thirty-five percent of patients will have somatic mutations of *PTPN11*, the gene encoding SHP-2, a tyrosine kinase involved in hematopoietic cell development. *RAS*[142] and *NF-1*[141] mutations have each been identified in 25% of patients. Mutations in *PTPN11, RAS,* and *NF-I* appear to be mutually exclusive in JMML. Each one may independently activate signaling through the *RAS/MAP* kinase-signaling pathway, increasing sensitivity to cells to granulocyte monocyte colony stimulating factor (GM-CSF). The sensitivity of JMML cells to GM-CSF in culture is an important biological and diagnostic feature of the disease.[143]

The natural history of JMML, if untreated, is death within a median of approximately 1 year. At an age older than 2 years, thrombocytopenia and high hemoglobin F at diagnosis are all predictors of more aggressive disease.[141,144] The European Working Group of MDS in Childhood reported a 5-year event-free survival in approximately 50% of children with JMML transplanted from matched-related and matched-unrelated donors. Treatment failures were primarily a result of disease recurrence within the 1st year after transplant.[145] The role of conventional chemotherapy in the pretransplant setting or in patients without an appropriate donor is not clearly defined. Most European trials typically use mercaptopurine or no therapy, whereas the current Children's Oncology Group trials in the United States administer cytarabine, fludarabine, and retinoic acid. GM-CSF agonists and farnesyltransferase inhibitors are currently being studied, but their role is yet to be defined.

MYELODYSPLASIA

Myelodysplastic syndromes (MDS) are clonal disorders of ineffective or abnormal hematopoiesis that frequently precede AML or aplastic anemia. The most common chromosomal abnormality associated with MDS in children is monosomy 7 (7q-), although monosomy 5, and trisomy 8 are reported as well.[144] MDS may occur spontaneously or after exposure to radiation, epipodophyllotoxin, or alkylators. Diagnosis of the disease is based on identification of dysplastic features in the bone marrow, as well as characteristic cytogenetic abnormalities. Further classification is based on the number of blasts present in the marrow and is used primarily to predict progression to AML. AML after contracting MDS is typically more difficult to treat than de novo AML. Currently, the only available therapy for AML includes supportive care and SCT.

MYELOPROLIFERATIVE DISEASES

Current WHO classification of childhood leukemias includes JMML (discussed previously) among the myeloproliferative diseases of childhood. In addition, essential thrombocytosis and polycythemia vera are also reported in children. Newborns with Down syndrome may develop a myeloproliferation syndrome called transient abnormal myelopoiesis (TAM), with clinical features that are indistinguishable from AML, including leukocytosis, organomegaly, fevers, and cytopenias with circulating blasts. The blasts typically express megakaryocyte markers.[146] Although life-threatening complications may occur in a minority of patients, most experience spontaneous remission within a few months. Approximately 25% will develop leukemia within 1 to 3 years, and whether transient abnormal myelopoiesis is a malignant disease or a true myeloproliferative syndrome is unclear.[146,147]

RELAPSED LEUKEMIAS AND STEM CELL TRANSPLANTATION

Acute Lymphoblastic Leukemia

Despite development of successful therapies in childhood leukemias, 20% to 25% of children with ALL and 50% of children with AML will relapse after chemotherapy treatment. In fact, more children are diagnosed with relapsed leukemia than Hodgkin disease and pediatric sarcomas.[148] In most children with relapsed leukemia, long-term, event-free survival is less than 50%, even with SCT.

Two reliable predictors of survival after relapse are the duration of the 1st remission (improved survival after a longer 1st remission) and phenotype (relapse B-lineage leukemias are more curable than T-lineage leukemias). According to the BFM group, a very early relapse occurs after a first remission of less than 18 months; an early relapse occurs after a 1st remission greater that 18 months but less than 6 months after completion of therapy; and a late relapse occurs after a 1st remission of more than 18 months and more than 6 months after completion of therapy. Patient with late relapses tend to do better with both chemotherapy and SCT.[149]

In the Children's Cancer Study Group (CCG), 1900 series of clinical trials completed between 1997 and 2002, 4464 patients were treated on ALL trials. Bone marrow relapse occurred in 539 patients (12%), CNS relapse in 194 patients (4%), and testicular relapse in 56 patients (1.5%). The overall 3-year survival after marrow relapse was 28% and 60% each for CNS and testicular relapse.[148] Remission reinduction after relapse is relatively good, but overall survival remains poor owing to a deficiency in effective therapies. Most studies comparing SCT to chemotherapy approaches demonstrate an advantage to SCT. However, these studies typically include a significant selection bias (based on donor availability and response to remission reinduction). In 2005, Gaynon published a telling summary of data from the Children's Cancer Study Group 1941 study. Of a total of 214 patients with marrow relapse within 12 months of the completion of primary therapy, approximately 75% achieved second remission. Patients who achieved a second remission and who had matched-sibling donors were nonrandomly assigned to receive a SCT. The remaining patients were randomized to either an alternative donor (unrelated donor or mismatched related donor) transplant or continued chemotherapy. The disease-free survival at 3 years for the patients receiving a matched sibling transplant and an unrelated donor transplants are 40% and 30%, respectively. The 3-year event-free survival for patients with a 1st remission less than 18 months is 4%, 18 to 30 months is 10%, and longer than 30 months is 41%. Most events occur within 6 months of relapse, and less than one half of the patients assigned to unrelated-donor transplants actually made it to transplant in second remission.[114,148] These results are striking and speak strongly to the need for additional therapies for ALL.

Acute Myelogenous Leukemia

As is the case with ALL, hematologic relapse remains the most common adverse event in patients with AML. Approximately 30% to 40% of patients who achieve a remission will relapse, and 25% will have residual disease after intensive induction therapy.[52] Many patients with AML undergo SCT in 1st remission; nevertheless, as many as 40% to 50% still relapse, and their relapse therapy may be severely limited or complicated by posttransplant toxicities. Remission reinduction rates for all patients with AML in 1st relapse ranges from 50% to 80% using multiagent chemotherapy. Overall survival after relapses is a dismal 30% to 40%.[52] Although in ALL, a subset of patients may be found who relapsed late that may still be salvaged with conventional chemotherapy, the only curative alternative for patients with relapsed AML remains SCT.

PHARMACOGENETICS

Pharmacogenetics is the study of genetic differences in sensitivity of individuals to certain drugs. Genetic polymorphisms in specific genes that are responsible for regulating drug metabolism, transport, and target expression can have a profound effect on both therapeutic and toxic responses to leukemia therapies. Understanding the incidence and implication of polymorphisms affecting drug metabolism and distribution will ultimately help control for individual variability in leukemia treatment protocols, with the goal of further reducing toxicity while maximizing efficacy.

Thiopurine Metabolism

Thiopurine methyltransferase (TPMT) is a key enzyme in the metabolism of azathioprine, 6-mercaptopurine, and thioguanine. One in 300 individuals will have 2 alleles with TPMT polymorphisms, resulting in very low TPMT enzyme activity. Ten percent of individuals will have intermediate enzyme activity, resulting from 1 abnormal allele. Nearly 90% of the population is wild type and defined as having normal enzyme activity. All patients with low activity, 35% of patients with intermediate activity, and 7% of patients with wild-type activity require 6-MP dose reductions. In terms of survival, not only are higher doses of 6-MP associated with improved outcomes,[150,151] but defective TPMT metabolism is also associated with a higher incidence of topoisomerase II inhibiter–induced secondary AML and a higher risk of brain tumors in patients who receive concomitant radiation therapy.[152-154] Commercially available genotype and phenotype analysis of the TPMT enzyme helps guide current thiopurine therapy. The direct clinical applications of these relatively recent pharmacogenetic discoveries are clear.

Antifolate Metabolism

Ever since Farber gave aminopterin to a patient with childhood leukemia, antifolates (MTX eventually replaced aminopterin) have remained essential in the treatment of ALL. Polymorphisms in MTX transport, metabolism, and target expression may all effect leukemia cell sensitivity to MTX and illustrate how multiple polymorphisms may alter efficacy and toxicity of a single drug.[155] The reduced folate carrier (RFC) is an active transport system for MTX. A decrease in RFC expression will lead to a decrease in the amount of MTX that accumulates intracellularly.[155,156] Though not yet correlated to RFC function, specific RFC polymorphisms are associated with a worse outcome with standard therapy for ALL.[157] MTX is a tight-binding inhibitor of dihydrofolate reductase, and the concentration of MTX required to achieve inhibition of enzyme activity increases in direct proportion to the amount of the enzyme in the target cells. Amplification of the dihydrofolate reductase gene is seen in 30% of patients with relapsed ALL but only 10% of patients with newly diagnosed ALL.[158] Also implicated in survival in pediatric ALL are polymorphisms in other enzymes involved in MTX metabolism, including methylenetetrahydrofolate reductase (an enzyme responsible for the reduction of 5,10-methylenetrahydrofolate to 5-methlytetrahydrofolate[160]) and thymidylate synthase (a target of MTX).

In addition to the enzymes specifically involved in metabolism of MTX and thiopurines, several detoxifying enzyme systems have profound effects of a broader range of chemotherapeutic agents. The cytochrome P450 enzymes are involved in the activation or inactivation of a variety of anticancer agents. Polymorphisms in the cytochrome system have been implicated both in treatment efficacy[160] and in toxicities, including vincristine neuropathies[161] and treatment-related leukemias.[162] The implications of polymorphisms in glutathione S-transferase enzymes, glucocorticoid receptors, vitamin D receptor, and others are more controversial and not clearly defined.

LATE EFFECTS OF THERAPY

The successful treatment of childhood leukemias has not come without a significant price. Nonetheless, as one of the most curable and common malignancy in childhood, the number of survivors of childhood leukemia is ever increasing. The long-term side effects of treatment need to be monitored, anticipated, and treated effectively.

Cognitive Function

Changes in cognitive function after cranial radiation are among the most well-studied side effects of leukemia therapy. Radiation-induced white-matter changes may result in deficits in speed of information processing, potentially progressive decrements in IQ testing and poor school performance.[163] Age at the time of treatment and total dose of radiation administered are the most reliable predictors of late cognitive effects. Patients receiving cranial radiation who are younger than 5 years, and especially younger than 3 years, are more susceptible to resultant cognitive deficiencies.[164] Other significant observations include a dose-dependent effect between cognitive deficiencies after 1800, 2400, and 3600 cGy cranial radiation.[165] Accordingly, many recent treatment regimens attempt to eliminate cranial radiation for patients at lowest risk for CNS recurrence and to reduce the dose of radiation to 1200 or 1800 cGy for patients at highest risk for CNS recurrence. Intensifying intrathecal therapy has proven to be effective prophylaxis against CNS recurrence while maintaining baseline long-term cognitive function.[166]

Cardiac Effects

Anthracyclines will likely remain a crucial component of effective therapy for ALL and AML. The incidence and severity of cardiac toxicity relates to the cumulative dose of anthracycline; concomitant use of mediastinal radiation, cyclophosphamide, or ifosfamide; and younger age at diagnosis. Most current treatment regimens in childhood cancer are capped at a total cumulative anthracycline dose of 350 to 400 mg/m^2 to reduce late cardiac toxicities.[167] Most ALL treatment regimens do not approach this level. In addition to cumulative doses, bolus infusion of anthracycline (as compared with continuous infusions), female gender, and young age at diagnosis are also associated with a higher risk of late cardiac toxicities.[168,169] Cardiac toxicities may affect function or rhythm, or both, and may be asymptomatic until years after completion of therapy, usually exhibiting at times requiring rapid increases in cardiac output (eg, puberty, pregnancy, weight training).[169-171] After a median of 450 mg/m^2 of anthracycline, a reported 23% of patients have echocardiographic abnormalities 7 years after treatment.[171] Patients receiving high cumulative doses of anthracycline should maintain diligent follow-up, especially if echocardiographic abnormalities are detected before completion of therapy. Patients with no detectable abnormalities should receive an electrocardiogram and echocardiogram at least every 2 to 3 years.

Endocrine Effects

Craniospinal radiation may reduce adult standing height resulting from both deficient growth of the vertebral bodies after spinal radiation and growth hormone deficiency after cranial radiation. Reduction in the dose of cranial radiation has reduced the incidence of growth hormone deficiency in survivors of childhood leukemia.[170] For many patients, growth hormone supplementation may be necessary and effective. Referral for an endocrine evaluation should be considered for all survivors of childhood leukemia with short stature. Osteoporosis after corticosteroid administration is another significant problem that may affect growth.[172]

Infertility is a significant concern after chemotherapy (especially with alkylator-based regimens) and radiation (especially boys who required testicular radiation). Abnormal gonadal development and function may result from direct damage to the gonads after radiation or to the hypothalamic-pituitary axis after cranial radiation. In a study of 60 survivors of ALL, Sklar et al identified significant germ cell dysfunction (increased follicle-stimulating hormone and reduced testicular volume) in 55% of patients treated with testicular radiation and 17% treated with cranio-spinal radiation. Leydig cell function was relatively preserved.[173] Total alkylator dose and age at diagnosis are other predictors of fertility after treatment. With higher cumulative doses of alkylators, boys (especially those in puberty at the time of treatment) are more likely than girls to be infertile.

Second Malignant Neoplasms

The risk and development of a second malignancy is a devastating side effect of both chemotherapy and radiation therapy for childhood ALL, although the risk is significantly less than that reported for other childhood malignancies. The cumulative incidence of any second neoplasm in survivors of childhood leukemia is reportedly 1.18% at 10 years (95% confidence interval is 0.8% to 1.5%), which is a 7.2-fold increased risk above the general population.[174] Cranial radiation, relapse, and female gender have all been associated with an increased risk for developing a second malignancy. Secondary leukemias and myelodysplasia, soft-tissue sarcomas, brain tumors, and solid tumors are all reported, although secondary CNS malignancies are the most common.[170,174] Deficiencies in TPMT may predispose patients to secondary brain tumors. In protocols incorporating high doses of antimetabolites, the 8-year cumulative incidence of secondary brain tumors among TPMT-deficient children was 43%. Patients with normal TPMP activity had an 8-year cumulative incidence of secondary brain tumors of 8.3%.[175] This exceptionally high incidence of secondary brain tumors in both groups is likely reflective of the concomitant use of cranial radiation and high-dose antimetabolites.

Identification of the possible late side effects of leukemia therapy has been key in the development of risk-stratified therapy. Reducing cumulative doses of agents with significant short- and long-term side effects while maintaining excellent cure rates in children with ALL has been one of the great triumphs of oncology clinical trials. As more is learned, future therapies may take into account not only the biological feature of the leukemia that are predictive of chemoresponsiveness, but also the host factors that determine risk for acute and long-term toxicities.

CONCLUSIONS

Treatment of childhood leukemias is widely touted as a great success in oncology clinical trials, largely because of the continued incremental increases in long-term survival in children with ALL. Significant challenges still lay ahead as new strategies are defined for treating AML and relapsed leukemias, as well as the myeloproliferative and myelodysplastic disorders. Application of risk-adapted therapy to patients with ALL and AML has allowed for continued improvement in long-term, event-free survival and a reduction in long-term side effects. What has been learned about leukemia biology, host pharmacogenetics, and environmental influences on leukemia development has led to the development of effective treatment and preventive strategies for childhood leukemias. A significant amount of work still needs to be done, but the future is bright.

TOOLS FOR PRACTICE

Engaging Patients and Family

- *Leukemia—Acute Lymphocytic: Detailed Guide* (Web page), American Cancer Society (www.cancer.org/docroot/CRI/CRI_2_3x.asp?dt=57).
- *What Are the Types of Childhood Cancers?* (fact sheet), American Cancer Society (www.cancer.org/docroot/CRI/content/CRI_2_4_1X_What_are_the_types_of_childhood_cancers_7.asp?rnav=cri).
- *What Is Childhood Cancer?* (fact sheet), American Cancer Society (www.cancer.org/docroot/CRI/content/CRI_2_4_1X_Introduction_7.asp?rnav=cri).

REFERENCES

1. US Cancer Statistics Working Group. United States Cancer Statistics: 1999-2002 Incidence and Mortality Web-based Report Version. Atlanta, GA: Department of Health and Human Services, Centers of Disease Control and Prevention, and National Cancer Institute; 2005. Available at: www.cdc.gov/cancer/npcr/uscs. Accessed on January 30, 2007.
2. Pui CH. Childhood leukemias. *N Engl J Med*. 1995;332:1618-1630.
3. Alderson M. The epidemiology of leukemia. *Adv Cancer Res*. 1980;31:1-76.
4. Pui CH, Boyett J, Hancock M, et al. Outcome of treatment for childhood cancer in black as compared to white children. *JAMA*. 1995;273:633-637.
5. Fraumeni JJ, Wagoner J. Changing sex differentials in leukemia. *Public Health Rep*. 1964;79:1093-1100.
6. Neglia J, Robison L. Epidemiology of the childhood leukemias. *Pediatr Clin North Am*. 1988;35:675-692.
7. Miller R. Childhood cancer and congenital defects. A study of U.S. death certificates during the period 1960-1966. *Pediatr Res*. 1969;3:389-397.
8. Robison LL, Nesbit ME, Sather HE, et al. Down syndrome and acute leukemia in children: a 10 year retrospective survey from the Children's Cancer Study Group. *J Pediatr*. 1984;105:235-242.
9. Fong C, Brodeur GM. Down's syndrome and leukemia: epidemiology, genetics, cytogenetics and mechanisms of leukemogenesis. *Cancer Genet Cytogenet*. 1987;28:55-76.
10. Rosner F, Lee SL. Down syndrome and acute leukemia: myeloblastic or lymphoblastic? *Am J Med*. 1972;53:203-218.
11. Watson MS, Carroll A, Shuster J, et al. Trisomy 21 in childhood acute lymphoblastic leukemia: a Pediatric Oncology Group Study (8602). *Blood*. 1993;82:3098-3102.
12. Zipursky A, Poon A, Doyle A. Leukemia in Down syndrome. *Pediatr Hematol Oncol*. 1992;9:139-149.
13. Homans AC, Verissimo AM, Vlacha VI. Transient abnormal myelopoiesis of infancy associated with trisomy 21. *Am J Pediatr Hematol Oncol*. 1993;15:392-399.
14. Rowley JD. Down syndrome and acute leukemia: increased risk may be due to trisomy 21. *Lancet*. Nov 1981;2(8254):1020-1022.
15. Miller R. Relation between cancer and congenital defects: an epidemiologic evaluation. *J Natl Cancer Inst*. 1968;40:1079-1085.
16. MacMahon B, Levy M. Prenatal origin of childhood leukemia: evidence from twins. *N Engl J Med*. 1964;270:1082-1085.

17. Greaves MF, Maia AT, Wiemels JL, et al. Leukemia in twins: lessons in natural history. *Blood*. 2003;102:2321-2333.
18. Kadan-Lottick NS, Kawashima T, Tomlinson G, et al. The risk of cancer in twins: a report from the Childhood Cancer Survivor Study. *Pediatr Blood Cancer*. 2006;46: 476-481.
19. Miller R. Persons with exceptionally high risk of leukemia. *Cancer Res*. 1967;27:2420-2423.
20. Zuelzer W, Cox D. Genetic aspects of leukemia. *Semin Hematol*. 1969;6:228-249.
21. Draper G, Heaf M, Kennier-Wilson L. Occurrence of childhood cancer among sibs and estimation of familial risk. *J Med Genet*. 1977;14:81-90.
22. Friedman DL, Kadan-Lottick NS, Whitton J, et al. Increased risk of cancer among siblings of long-term childhood cancer survivors: a report from the Childhood Cancer Survivor Study. *Cancer Epidemiol Biomarkers Prev*. 2005;14:1922-1927.
23. Ford AM, Ridge SA, Cabrera ME, et al. In utero rearrangements in the trithorax-related oncogene in infant leukemia. *Nature*. 1993;363:358-360.
24. March HC. Leukemia in radiologists. *Radiology*. 1944; 43:275.
25. Bizzozero OJ, Johnson KG, Ciocco A. Radiation-related leukemia in Hiroshima and Nagasaki, 1946-1964: distribution, incidence, appearance in time. *N Engl J Med*. 1966;274:1095-1101.
26. Harvey EB, Boice JD Jr, Honeyman M, et al. Prenatal x-ray exposure and childhood cancer in twins. *N Engl J Med*. 1985;312:541-545.
27. Boice JD. Cancer following medical radiation. *Cancer*. 1981;47:1081-1090.
28. Lehtinen M, Koskela P, Ogmundsdottir HM, et al. Maternal herpes virus infections and the risk of acute lymphoblastic leukemia in the offspring. *Am J Epidemiol*. 2003; 158:207-213.
29. Naumberg E, Bellocco R, Cnattingius S, et al. Perinatal exposure to infection and risk of childhood leukaemia. *Med Pediatr Oncol*. 2002;38:391-397.
30. Infante-Rivard C, Fortier I, Olsen E. Markers of infection, breast-feeding and childhood acute lymphoblastic leukemia. *Br J Cancer*. 2000;83:1559-1564.
31. McKinney PA, Juiszczak E, Findlay E, et al. Pre- and perinatal risk factors for childhood leukaemia and other malignancies: a Scottish case control study. *Br J Cancer*. 1999;80:1844-1851.
32. Little J. *Epidemiology of Childhood Cancer*. IARC Scientific Publication No. 149, IARC, Lyon, France: WHO Press; 1999.
33. Gale KB, Ford AM, Repp R, et al. Backtracking leukemia to birth: identification of clonotypic gene fusion sequence in neonatal blood spots. *PNAS*. 1997;94: 13950-13954.
34. Taub JW, Ge Y. The prenatal origin of childhood acute lymphoblastic leukemia. *Leuk Lymph*. 2004;45:19-25.
35. Greaves M. Molecular genetics, natural history and the demise of childhood leukaemia in children. *Lancet*. 1999;354:1499-1503.
36. Konrad M, Metzler M, Panzer S, et al. Late relapses evolve from slow-responding subclones in t(12;21)-positive acute lymphoblastic leukemia: evidence for the persistence of a preleukemic clone. *Blood*. 2003;101(9): 3635-3640.
37. Schuz J, Kaletsch U, Meinert R, et al. Association of childhood leukaemia with factors related to the immune system. *Br J Cancer*. 1999;80:585-590.
38. Neglia JP, Linet MS, Shu XO, et al. Patterns of infection and day care utilization and risk of childhood acute lymphoblastic leukaemia. *Br J Cancer*. 2000;82:234-240.
39. Petridou E, Dalamaga M, Mentis A, et al. For The Childhood Haematologists-Oncologists Group: evidence on the infectious etiology of childhood leukemia: the role of low herd immunity (Greece). *Cancer Causes Control*. 2001;12:645-652.
40. Chan LC, Lam TH, Li CK, et al. Is the timing of exposure to infection a major determinant of acute lymphoblastic leukaemia in Hong Kong? *Paediatr Perinat Epidemiol*. 2002;16:154-165.
41. Perrillat F, Clavel J, Auclerc MF, et al. Day-care, early common infections and childhood acute leukaemia: a multicentre French case-control study. *Br J Cancer*. 2002;86:1064-1069.
42. Jourdan-Da Silva N, Perel Y, Mechinaud F, et al. Infectious diseases in the first year of life, perinatal characteristics and childhood acute leukaemia. *Br J Cancer*. 2004;90:139-145.
43. Dockerty JD, Skegg DC, Elwood JM, et al. Infections, vaccinations, and the risk of childhood leukaemia. *Br J Cancer*. 1999;80:1483-1489.
44. McKinney PA, Cartwright RA, Saiu JM, et al. The inter-regional epidemiological study of childhood cancer (IRESCC): a case-control study of aetiological factors in leukaemia and lymphoma. *Arch Dis Child*. 1987;62: 279-287.
45. Nishi M, Miyake H. A case-control study of non-T cell acute lymphoblastic leukaemia of children in Hokkaido, Japan. *J Epidemiol Comm Health*. 1989;43: 352-355.
46. Groves FD, Gridley G, Wacholder S, et al. Infant vaccinations and risk of childhood acute lymphoblastic leukaemia in the USA. *Br J Cancer*. 1999;81:175-178.
47. Buckley JD, Buckley CM, Ruccione K, et al. Epidemiological characteristics of childhood acute lymphocytic leukemia. Analysis by immunophenotype. The Children's Cancer Group. *Leukemia*. 1994;8:856-864.
48. McNally RJQ, Eden TOB. An infectious aetiology for childhood acute leukaemia: a review of the evidence. *Br J Haematol*. 2004;127:243-263.
49. Petridou E, Kassiomos D, Kalmanti M, et al. Age of exposure to infections and risk of childhood leukaemia. *BMJ*. 1993;307:774.
50. Ma X, Buffler PA, Selvin S, et al. Day-care attendance and risk of childhood acute lymphoblastic leukaemia. *Br J Cancer*. 2002;86:1419-1424.
51. Vardiman JW, Harris NL, Brunning RD. The World Health Organization (WHO) classification of myeloid neoplasms. *Blood*. 2002;100:2292-2302.
52. Pui CH, Schrappe M, Ribeiro RC, et al. Childhood and adolescent lymphoid and myeloid leukemia. *Hematology Am Soc Hematol Educ Program*. 2004;:118-145.
53. Schrappe M. Evolution of BFM trials for childhood ALL. *Ann Hematol*. 2004;83:S121-S123.
54. Reiter A, Schrappe M, Ludwig WD, et al. Chemotherapy in 998 unselected childhood acute lymphoblastic leukemia patients. Results and conclusions of the multicenter trial ALL-BFM 86. *Blood*. 1994;84:3122-3133.
55. Pui CH, Behm FG, Crist WM. Clinical and biologic relevance of immunologic marker studies in childhood acute lymphoblastic leukemia. *Blood*. 1993;82:343-362.
56. Ritz J, Pesando JM, Notis-McConarty J, et al. A monoclonal antibody to human acute lymphoblastic leukaemia antigen. *Nature*. 1980;283:583-585.
57. Heerema NA, Sather HN, Ge J, et al. Cytogenetic studies of infant acute lymphoblastic leukemia: poor prognosis of infants with t(4;11)—a report of the Children's Cancer Group. *Leukemia*. 1999;13:679-686.
58. Crist W, Boyett J, Roper M, et al. Pre-B cell leukemia responds poorly to treatment: a Pediatric Oncology Group study. *Blood*. 1984;63:407-414.

59. Uckun FM, Sensel MG, Sather HN, et al. Clinical significance of translocation t(1;19) in childhood acute lymphoblastic leukemia in the context of contemporary therapies: a report from the Children's Cancer Group. *J Clin Oncol.* 1998;16(2):527-535.
60. Ludwig WD, Reiter A, Loffler H, et al. Immunophenotypic features of childhood and adult acute lymphoblastic leukemia (ALL): experience of the German Multicentre Trials ALL-BFM and GMALL. *Leuk Lymphoma.* 1994;13(1):71-76.
61. Shuster JJ, Falletta JM, Pullen DJ, et al. Prognostic factors in childhood T-cell acute lymphoblastic leukemia: a Pediatric Oncology Group study. *Blood.* 1990;75:166-173.
62. Bene MC, Castoldi G, Knapp W, et al. Proposals for the immunological classification of acute leukemias. European Group for the Immunological Characterization of Leukemias (EGIL). *Leukemia.* 1995;9:1783-1786.
63. European Group for the Immunological Classification of Leukemias (EGIL). The value of c-kit in the diagnosis of biophenotypic acute leukemia. *Leukemia.* 1998;12:2038.
64. Owaidah TM, Beihany AA, Iqbal MA, et al. Cytogenetics, molecular and ultrastructural characteristics of biphenotypic acute leukemia identified by the EGIL scoring system. *Leukemia.* Nov 2006;6(11):3355-3359.
65. Trueworthy R, Shuster J, Look T, et al. Ploidy of lymphoblasts is the strongest predictor of treatment outcome in B-progenitor cell acute lymphoblastic leukemia of childhood: a Pediatric Oncology Group study. *J Clin Oncol.* 1992:10:606-613.
66. Heerema NA, Sather HN, Sensel MG, et al. Prognostic impact of trisomies of chromosomes 10, 17, and 5 among children with acute lymphoblastic leukemia and high hyperdiploidy (>50 chromosomes). *J Clin Oncol.* 2000;18:1876-1887.
67. Carroll WL, Bhojwani D, Min DJ, et al. Pediatric acute lymphoblastic leukemia. *Hematology.* 2003;1:102-131.
68. Heerema NA, Nachman JB, Sather HN, et al. Hypodiploidy with less than 45 chromosomes confers adverse risk in childhood acute lymphoblastic leukemia: a report from the Children's Cancer Group. *Blood.* 1999;94:4036-4045.
69. Huret JL, Dessen P, Bernheim A. An atlas of chromosomes in hematological malignancies example: 11q23 and MLL partners. *Leukemia.* 2001;15:987-989.
70. Pui CH, Gaynon PS, Boyett JM, et al. Outcome of treatment in childhood acute lymphoblastic leukaemia with rearrangements of the 11q23 chromosomal region. *Lancet.* 2002;359(9321):1909-1915.
71. Pui CH, Chessells JM, Camitta B, et al. Clinical heterogeneity in childhood acute lymphoblastic leukemia with 11q23 rearrangements. *Leukemia.* 2003;17:700-706.
72. Rubnitz JE, Camitta BM, Mahmoud H, et al. Childhood acute lymphoblastic leukemia with the MLL-ENL fusion and t(11;19)(q23;p13.3) translocation. *J Clin Oncol.* 1999; 17:191-196.
73. Rowley JD. A new consistent chromosomal abnormality in chronic myelogenous leukemia identified by quinacrine fluorescence and Giemsa staining. *Nature.* 1973; 243:290-293.
74. Bartram CR, de Klein A, Hagemeijer A, et al. Translocation of c-ab1 oncogene correlates with the presence of a Philadelphia chromosome in chronic myelocytic leukaemia. *Nature.* 1983;306:277-280.
75. Heisterkamp N, Stephenson JR, Groffen J, et al. Localization of the c-ab1 oncogene adjacent to a translocation break point in chronic myelocytic leukaemia. *Nature.* 1983;306:239-242.
76. Groffen J, Stephenson JR, Heisterkamp N, et al. Philadelphia chromosomal breakpoints are clustered within a limited region, bcr, on chromosome 22. *Cell.* 1984;36: 93-99.
77. Arico M, Valsecchi MG, Camitta B, et al. Outcome of treatment in children with Philadelphia chromosome-positive acute lymphoblastic leukemia. *N Engl J Med.* 2000;342(14):998-1006.
78. Romana SP, Poirel H, Leconiat M, et al. High frequency of t(12;21) in childhood B-lineage acute lymphoblastic leukemia. *Blood.* 1995;86(11):4263-4269.
79. Guidez F, Petrie K, Ford AM, et al. Recruitment of the nuclear receptor corepressor N-CoR by the TEL moiety of the childhood leukemia-associated TEL-AML1 oncoprotein. *Blood.* 2000;96(7):2557-2561.
80. Loh ML, Silverman LB, Young ML, et al. Incidence of TEL/AML1 fusion in children with relapsed acute lymphoblastic leukemia. *Blood.* 1998;92(12):4792-4797.
81. Ramakers-van Woerden NL, Pieters R, et al. TEL/AML1 gene fusion is related to in vitro drug sensitivity for L-asparaginase in childhood acute lymphoblastic leukemia. *Blood.* 2000;96(3):1094-1099.
82. Seeger K, Buchwald D, Peter A, et al. TEL-AML1 fusion in relapsed childhood acute lymphoblastic leukemia. *Blood.* 1999;94(1):374-376.
83. Konoplev S, Bueso-Ramos CE. Advances in the pathologic diagnosis and biology of acute myeloid leukemia. *Ann Diag Path.* 2006;10:39-65.
84. Meyers S, Downing JR, Hiebert SW. Identification of AML1 and the (8;21) translocation protein AML1-ETO as sequence specific DNA binding proteins: the runt domain is required for DNA binding and protein-protein interactions. *Mol Cell Biol.* 1993;13; 6336-6345.
85. Wang Q, Stacy T, Miller JD, et al. The CBFbeta subunit is essential for CBFalpha2 (AML1) function in vivo. *Cell.* 1996;87:697-708.
86. Takahashi A, Satake M, Yamaguchi-Iwai Y, et al. Positive and negative regulation of granulocytic-macrophage colony-stimulating factor promoter activity by AML-1 related transcription factor, PEBP2. *Blood.* 1995;86: 607-616.
87. Komori T, Yagi H, Nomura S, et al. Targeted disruption of Cbfa1 results in a complete lack of bone formation owing to maturational arrest of osteoblasts. *Cell.* 1997; 89:755-764
88. Reilly JT. Pathogenesis of acute myeloid leukaemia and inv(16)(p13;q22): a paradigm for understanding leukaemogenesis? *Br J Haematol.* 2005;128:18-34.
89. McHale CM, Wiernels JL, Zhang L, et al. Prenatal origin of childhood acute myeloid leukemias harbouring chromosomal rearrangements t(15;17) and inv(16). *Blood.* 2003;101:4640-4641.
90. Wiemels JL, Xiao Z, Buffler PA, et al. In utero origin of t(8;21) AML1-ETO translocations in childhood acute myeloid leukaemia. *Blood.* 2002;99:3801-3805.
91. Nakao M, Yokota S, Iwai T, et al. Internal tandem duplication of the flt3 gene found in acute myeloid leukemia. *Leukemia.* 1996;10:1911-1918.
92. Beghini A, Cairoli R, Morra E, et al. In vivo differentiation of mast cells from acute myeloid leukemia blasts carrying a novel activating ligand-independent c-kit mutation. *Blood Cells Mol Dis.* 1998;24:262-270.
93. Beaupre DM, Kurzrock R. RAS and leukemia: from basic mechanisms to gene-directed therapy. *J Clin Oncol.* 1999;17:1071-1079.
94. Reuter CW, Morgan MA, Bergmann L. Targeting the Ras signaling pathway: a rational, mechanism-based treatment for hematologic malignancies? *Blood.* 2000; 96:1655-1669.
95. Grimwade D, Walker H, Oliver F, et al. The importance of diagnostic cytogenetics on outcome in AML: analysis of 1,612 patients enrolled into the MRC AML 10 trial. *Blood.* 1998;92:2322-2333.

96. Downing JR, Shannon KM. Acute leukemia: a pediatric perspective. *Cancer Cell.* 2002;2:437-445.
97. Djerassi I, Farber S, Abir E, et al. Continuous infusion of methotrexate in children with acute leukemia. *Cancer.* 1967;20:233-242.
98. Skipper HE, Thomson JR, Elion GB, et al. Observations of the anticancer activity of 6-mercaptopurine. *Cancer Res.* 1954;14:294-298.
99. Smith M, Bleyer A, Crist W, et al. Uniform criteria for childhood acute lymphoblastic leukemia risk classification. *J Clin Oncol.* 1996;14:680-681.
100. Uckun FM, Sather HN, Gaynon PS, et al. Clinical features and treatment outcome of children with myeloid antigen positive acute lymphoblastic leukemia: a report from the Children's Cancer Group. *Blood.* 1997:90(1): 28-35.
101. Uckun FM, Gaynon PS, Sensel MG, et al. Clinical features and treatment outcome of childhood T-lineage acute lymphoblastic leukemia according to the apparent maturational stage of T-lineage leukemic blasts: a Children's Cancer Group study. *J Clin Oncol.* 1997:15:2214-2221.
102. Gaynon PS, Desai AA, Bostrom BC, et al. Early response to therapy and outcome in childhood acute lymphoblastic leukemia: a review. *Cancer.* 1997;80:1717-1726.
103. Nachman JB, Sather HN, Sensel MG, et al. Augmented post-induction therapy for children with high-risk acute lymphoblastic leukemia and a slow response to initial therapy. *N Engl J Med.* 1998;338:1663-1671.
104. Riehm H, Langermann HJ, Gadner H, et al. The Berlin Childhood Acute Lymphoblastic Leukemia Therapy study, 1970-1976. *Am J Pediatr Hematol Oncol.* 1980;2: 299-306.
105. Henze G, Langermann HJ, Bramswig J, et al. The BFM 76/79 acute lymphoblastic leukemia therapy study. *Klinische Padiatrie.* 1981;193:145-154.
106. Conter V, Arico M, Valsecchi MG, et al. Long-term results of the Italian Association of Pediatric Hematology and Oncology (AIEOP) acute lymphoblastic leukemia studies, 1982-1995. *Leukemia.* 2000;14:2196-2204.
107. Eden OB, Harrison G, Richards S, et al. Long-term follow-up of the United Kingdom Medical Research Council protocols for childhood acute lymphoblastic leukaemia, 1980-1997. Medical Research Council Childhood Leukaemia Working Party. *Leukemia.* 2000;14:2307-2320.
108. Tsuchida M, Ikuta K, Hanada R, et al. Long-term follow-up of childhood acute lymphoblastic leukemia in Tokyo Children's Cancer Study Group 1981-1995. *Leukemia.* 2000;14:2295-2306.
109. Pui CH, Boyett JM, Rivera GK, et al. Long-term results of total therapy studies 11, 12 and 13A for childhood acute lymphoblastic leukemia at St Jude Children's Research Hospital. *Leukemia.* 2000;14:2286-2294.
110. Vilmer E, Suciu S, Ferster A, et al. Long-term results of three randomized trials (58831, 58832, 58881) in childhood acute lymphoblastic leukemia: a CLCG-EORTC report. Children Leukemia Cooperative Group. *Leukemia.* 2000;14:2257-2266.
111. Silverman LB, Declerck L, Gelber RD, et al. Results of Dana-Farber Cancer Institute Consortium protocols for children with newly diagnosed acute lymphoblastic leukemia (1981-1995). *Leukemia.* 2000;14:2247-2256.
112. Kamps WA, Veerman AJ, van Wering ER, et al. Long-term follow-up of Dutch Childhood Leukemia Study Group (DCLSG) protocols for children with acute lymphoblastic leukemia, 1984-1991. *Leukemia.* 2000;14: 2240-2246.
113. Harms DO, Janka-Schaub GE. Co-operative Study Group for Childhood Acute Lymphoblastic Leukemia (COALL): long-term follow-up of trials 82, 85, 89 and 92. *Leukemia.* 2000;14:2234-2239.
114. Gaynon PS, Trigg ME, Heerema NA, et al. Children's Cancer Group trials in childhood acute lymphoblastic leukemia: 1983-1995. *Leukemia.* 2000;14:2223-2233.
115. Mahoney DH Jr, Shuster JJ, Nitschke R, et al. Acute neurotoxicity in children with B-precursor acute lymphoid leukemia: an association with intermediate-dose intravenous methotrexate and intrathecal triple therapy—a Pediatric Oncology Group study. *J Clin Oncol.* 1998;16:1712-1722.
116. Reaman G, Zeltzer P, Bleyer WA, et al. Acute lymphoblastic leukemia in infants less than one year of age: a cumulative experience of the Children's Cancer Study Group. *J Clin Oncol.* 1985;3:1513-1521.
117. Chessells JM, Eden OB, Bailey CC, et al. Acute lymphoblastic leukaemia in infancy: experience in MRC UKALL trials. Report from the Medical Research Council Working Party on Childhood Leukaemia. *Leukemia.* 1994;8: 1275-1279.
118. Reaman G, Sposto R, Sensel M, et al. Treatment outcome and prognostic factors for infants with acute lymphoblastic leukemia treated on two consecutive trials of the Children's Cancer Group. *J Clin Oncol.* 1999;17:445-455.
119. Pui C-H, Ribeiro RC, Campana D, et al. Prognostic factors in the acute lymphoid and myeloid leukemias of infants. *Leukemia.* 1996;10:952-956.
120. Chessells Richards SM, Bailey CC, Lilleyman JS, et al. Gender and treatment outcome in childhood lymphoblastic leukaemia: report from the MRC UKALL trials. *Br J Haematol.* 1995;89:364-372.
121. Dreyer ZE, Steuber CP, Bowman WP, et al. Induction intensification for infant acute lymphoid leukemia (ALL). *Proc Am Soc Clin Oncol.* 1996;15:1094a.
122. Hann IM, Stevens RF, Goldstone AH, et al. Randomized comparison of DAT versus ADE as induction chemotherapy in children and younger adults with acute myeloid leukemia. Results of the Medical Research Council's 10th AML trial (MRC AML10). Adult and Childhood Leukaemia Working Parties of the Medical Research Council. *Blood.* 1997;89:2311-2318.
123. Creutzig U, Ritter J, Zimmermann M, et al. Improved treatment results in high-risk pediatric acute myeloid leukemia patients after intensification with high-dose cytarabine and mitoxantrone: results of Study Acute Myeloid Leukemia-Berlin-Frankfurt-Munster 93. *J Clin Oncol.* 2001;19:2705-2713.
124. Perel Y, Auvrignon A, Leblanc T, et al, and the Group LAME of the French Society of Pediatric Hematology and Immunology. Impact of addition of maintenance therapy to intensive induction and consolidation chemotherapy for childhood acute myeloblastic leukemia: results of a prospective randomized trial, LAME 89/91. Leucamie Aique Myeloide Enfant. *J Clin Oncol.* 2002;20: 2774-2782.
125. O'Brien TA, Russell SJ, Vowels MR, et al, and the Australian and New Zealand Children's Cancer Study Group. Results of consecutive trials for children newly diagnosed with acute myeloid leukemia from the Australian and New Zealand Children's Cancer Study Group. *Blood.* 2002;100:2708-2716.
126. Ravindranath Y, Yeager AM, Chang MN, et al. Autologous bone marrow transplantation versus intensive consolidation chemotherapy for acute myeloid leukemia in childhood. Pediatric Oncology Group. *N Engl J Med.* 1996;334:1428-1434.
127. de Botton S, Coiteux V, Chevret S, et al. Outcome of childhood acute promyelocytic leukemia with all-trans-retinoic acid and chemotherapy. *J Clin Oncol.* Apr 2004;22(8):1404-1412.

128. Castro-Malaspina H, Schaison G, Briere J, et al. Philadelphia chromosome-positive chronic myelocytic leukemia in children. Survival and prognostic factors. *Cancer.* 1983;52:721-727.
129. Nowell PC. A minute chromosome in human granulocytic leukemia. *Blut.* 1962;8:65-66.
130. Druker BJ, Sawyers CL, Kantarjian H, et al. Activity of a specific inhibitor of the BCR-ABL tyrosine kinase in the blast crisis of chronic myeloid leukemia and acute lymphoblastic leukemia with the Philadelphia chromosome. *N Engl J Med.* 2001;344:1038-1042.
131. Druker BJ, Talpaz M, Resta DJ, et al. Efficacy and safety of a specific inhibitor of the BCR-ABL tyrosine kinase in chronic myeloid leukemia. *N Engl J Med.* 2001;344: 1031-1037.
132. Kantarjian H, Sawyers C, Hochhaus A, et al, and the International STI571 CML Study Group. Hematologic and cytogenetic responses to imatinib mesylate in chronic myelogenous leukemia. *N Engl J Med.* 2002; 346:645-652.
133. O'Brien SG, Guilhot F, Larson RA, et al, and the IRIS Investigators. Imatinib compared with interferon and low-dose cytarabine for newly diagnosed chronic-phase chronic myeloid leukemia. *N Engl J Med.* 2003; 348:994-1004.
134. Kolb EA, Pan Q, Ladanyi M, et al. Imatinib mesylate in Philadelphia chromosome-positive leukemia of childhood. *Cancer.* 2003;98:2643-2650.
135. Champagne MA, Therrien M, Krailo M, et al. STI571 in the treatment of children with Philadelphia chromosome-positive leukemia: results from a Children's Oncology Group (COG) Phase I study [abstract 578]. *Blood.* 2001;98:137a.
136. Dini G, Rondelli R, Miano M, et al. Unrelated-donor bone marrow transplantation for Philadelphia chromosome-positive chronic myelogenous leukemia in children: experience of eight European Countries. The EBMT Paediatric Diseases Working Party. *Bone Marrow Transplant.* 1996;18(2):80-85.
137. Davies SM, DeFor TE, McGlave PB, et al. Equivalent outcomes in patients with chronic myelogenous leukemia after early transplantation of phenotypically matched bone marrow from related or unrelated donors. *Am J Med.* 2001;110:339-346.
138. Cwynarski K, Roberts IA, Iacobelli S, et al, and the Paediatric and Chronic Leukaemia Working Parties of the European Group for Blood and Marrow Transplantation. Stem cell transplantation for chronic myeloid leukemia in children. *Blood.* 2003;102:1224-1231.
139. Gamis AS, Haake R, McGlave P, et al. Unrelated-donor bone marrow transplantation for Philadelphia chromosome-positive chronic myelogenous leukemia in children. *J Clin Oncol.* 1993;11:834-838.
140. Thornley I, Perentesis JP, Davies SM, et al. Treating children with chronic myeloid leukemia in the imatinib era: a therapeutic dilemma? [editorial] *Med Pediatr Oncol.* 2003;41:115-117.
141. Niemeyer CM, Arico M, Basso G, et al. Chronic myelomonocytic leukemia in childhood: a retrospective analysis of 110 cases. European Working Group on Myelodysplastic Syndromes in Childhood (EWOG-MDS). *Blood.* 1997;89:3534-3543.
142. Tartaglia M, Niemeyer CM, Fragale A, et al. Somatic mutations in PTPN11 in juvenile myelomonocytic leukemia, myelodysplastic syndromes and acute myeloid leukemia. *Nat Genet.* 2003;34:148-150.
143. Emanuel PD. Myelodysplasia and myeloproliferative disorders in childhood: an update. *Br J Haematol.* Jun 1999;105(4):852-863.
144. Passmore SJ, Chessells JM, Kempski H, et al. Paediatric myelodysplastic syndromes and juvenile myelomonocytic leukaemia in the UK: a population-based study of incidence and survival. *Br J Haematol.* 2003;121:758-767.
145. Locatelli F, Nollke P, Zecca M, et al. Hematopoietic stem cell transplantation (HSCT) in children with juvenile myelomonocytic leukemia (JMML): results of the EWOG-MDS/EBMT trial. *Blood.* 2005;105:410-419.
146. Zipursky A, Brown E, Christensen H, et al. Leukemia and/or myeloproliferative syndrome in neonates with Down syndrome. *Semin Perinatol.* 1997;21:97-101.
147. Hasle H, Niemeyer CM, Chessells JM, et al. A pediatric approach to the WHO classification of myelodysplastic and myeloproliferative diseases. *Leukemia.* 2003;17: 277-282.
148. Gaynon PS. Childhood acute lymphoblastic leukaemia and relapse. *Br J Haematol.* 2005;131:579-587.
149. Borgmann A, von Stackelberg A, Hartmann R, et al. Unrelated donor stem cell transplantation compared with chemotherapy for children with acute lymphoblastic leukemia in a second remission: a matched-pair analysis. *Blood.* 2003;101:3835-3839.
150. Relling MV, Hancock ML, Rivera GK, et al. Mercaptopurine therapy intolerance and heterozygocity at the thiopurine S-methyltransferase gene locus. *J Natl Cancer Inst.* 1999;91:2001-2008.
151. Relling MV, Hancock ML, Boyett JM, et al. Prognostic importance of 6-mercaptopurine dose intensity in acute lymphoblastic leukemia. *Blood.* 1999;93:2817-2823.
152. Relling MV, Yanishevski Y, Nemec J, et al. Etoposide and antimetabolite pharmacology in patients who develop secondary acute myeloid leukemia. *Leukemia.* 1998;12:346-352.
153. Bo J, Schroder H, Kristinsson J, et al. Possible carcinogenic effect of 6-mercaptopurine on bone marrow stem cells. *Cancer.* 1999;86:1080-1086.
154. Relling MV, Rubnitz JE, Rivera GK, et al. High incidence of secondary brain tumors after radiotherapy and antimetabolites. *Lancet.* 1999;354:34-39.
155. Gorlick R, Goker E, Trippett T, et al. Intrinsic and acquired resistance to methotrexate in acute leukemia. *N Engl J Med.* 1996;335:1041-1048.
156. Gorlick R, Goker E, Trippett T, et al. Defective transport is a common mechanism of acquired methotrexate resistance in acute lymphocytic leukemia and is associated with decreased reduced folate carrier expression. *Blood.* 1997;89:1013-1018.
157. Belkov VM, Krynetski EY, Schuetz JD, et al. Reduced folate carrier expression in acute lymphoblastic leukemia: a mechanism for ploidy but not lineage differences in methotrexate accumulation. *Blood.* 1999;93:1643-1650.
158. Laverdiere C, Chiasson S, Costeal I, et al. Polymorphisms in the reduced folate carrier gene and its relationship to methotrexate plasma levels and outcome of childhood acute lymphoblastic leukemia. *Blood.* 2002; 100:3832-3834.
159. Goker E, Waltham M, Kheradpour A, et al. Amplification of the dihydrofolate reductase gene is a mechanism of acquired resistance to methotrexate in patients with acute lymphocytic leukemia and is correlated with p53 gene mutations. *Blood.* 1995;86:677-684.
160. Krajinovic M, Lemieux-Blanchard E, Chiasson S, et al. Role of polymorphisms in the MTHFR and MTHFD1 genes in the outcome of childhood acute lymphoblastic leukemia. *Pharmacogenomics J.* 2004;4:66-72.
161. Aplenc R, Glatfelter W, Han P, et al. CYP3A genotype and treatment response in paediatric acute lymphoblastic leukemia. *Br J Haematology.* 2003;122: 240-244.

162. Felix, CA, Walker AH, Lange BH, et al. Association of CYP3A genotypes with treatment related leukemias. *Proc Nat Acad Sci.* 1998;95:13176-13181.
163. Hill JM, Kornblith AB, Jones D, et al. A comparative study of the long term psychosocial functioning of childhood acute lymphoblastic leukemia survivors treated by intrathecal methotrexate with or without cranial radiation. *Cancer.* 1998;82:208-218.
164. Smibert E, Anderson V, Godber T, et al. Risk factors for intellectual and educational sequelae of cranial irradiation in childhood acute lymphoblastic leukaemia. *Br J Cancer.* 1996;73:825-830.
165. Silber JH, Radcliffe J, Peckham V, et al. Whole-brain irradiation and decline in intelligence: the influence of dose and age on IQ score. *J Clin Oncol.* 1992;10: 1390-1396.
166. Kaleita TA, Reaman GH, MacLean WE, et al. Neurodevelopmental outcome of infants with acute lymphoblastic leukemia: a Children's Cancer Group report. *Cancer.* 1999;85:1859-1865.
167. Jakacki RI, Goldwein JW, Larsen RL, et al. Cardiac dysfunction following spinal irradiation during childhood. *J Clin Oncol.* 1993;11:1033-1038.
168. Silber JH, Jakacki RI, Larsen RL, et al. Increased risk of cardiac dysfunction after anthracyclines in girls. *Med Pediatr Oncol.* 1993;21:477-479.
169. Lipshultz SE, Lipsitz SR, Mone SM, et al. Female sex and drug dose as risk factors for late cardiotoxic effects of doxorubicin therapy for childhood cancer. *N Engl J Med.* 1995;332:1738-1743.
170. Shusterman S, Meadows AT. Long term survivors of childhood leukemia. *Cur Opin Hemat.* 2000;17:217-222.
171. Steinherz LJ, Steinherz PG, Tan CT, et al. Cardiac toxicity 4 to 20 years after completing anthracycline therapy. *JAMA.* 1991;266:1672-1677.
172. Nysom K, Holm K, Michaelsen KF, et al. Bone mass after treatment for acute lymphoblastic leukemia in childhood. *J Clin Oncol.* 1998;16:3752-3760.
173. Sklar CA, Robison LL, Nesbit ME, et al. Effects of radiation on testicular function in long term survivors of childhood acute lymphoblastic leukemia: a report from the Children's Cancer Study Group. *J Clin Oncol.* 1990; 8:1981-1987.
174. Bhatia S, Sather HN, Pabustan OB, et al. Low incidence of second neoplasms among children diagnosed with acute lymphoblastic leukemia after 1983. *Blood.* 2002; 99:4257-4264.
175. Relling MV, Rubnitz JE, Rivera GK, et al. High incidence of secondary brain tumours after radiotherapy and antimetabolites. *Lancet.* 1999;354:34-39.

Chapter 292
LYME DISEASE

H. Cody Meissner, MD

EPIDEMIOLOGY, ETIOLOGY, AND PATHOGENESIS

Lyme disease was first recognized in 1975 after an investigation of a cluster of arthritis cases among children in Lyme, Connecticut, and soon thereafter the black legged deer tick *Ixodes scapularis* was implicated as the vector of this disease.[1] In 1982 a spirochete, *Borrelia burgdorferi*, was detected in the midgut of the tick and identified as the etiologic agent.[2] In 2005, 23,305 cases of Lyme disease were reported to the Centers for Disease Control and Prevention, making this condition the most common tickborne infectious disease in the United States. Although Lyme disease has been reported in almost every state, 95% of all cases are concentrated in 11 states from 3 geographic regions: (1) the Northeast from Maine to Maryland, (2) the Midwest in Wisconsin and Minnesota, and (3) the West in Northern California and Oregon.[3] The occurrence of disease corresponds with the distribution of the tick vectors *I scapularis* in the East and Midwest and *I pacificus* in the West.

B burgdorferi live in mice, squirrels, and other small animals and are transmitted among these animals and to humans by the bite of the tick. The tick lives for 2 years and has 3 stages: larvae, nymph, and adult. A blood meal is required at each stage of development. When the tick feeds on an infected animal, the spirochete is acquired, and when the tick feeds again the spirochete can be transmitted to a new host. Most cases of human Lyme disease are acquired in June, July, or August when the nymphal stage is most active and human outdoor activity is greatest. Although deer are important for maintaining the tick population, deer do not become infected by the spirochete.

CLINICAL MANIFESTATIONS

Because the clinical manifestations of Lyme disease vary with the time that elapses after inoculation by the tick, the infection has been divided into early localized, early disseminated, and late phases.

Early Localized Phase

Erythema migrans (EM) is the most common manifestation of early Lyme disease. Approximately 70% to 80% of patients exhibit or have a history of a skin lesion at the site of the tick bite. The macule gradually expands over several days to a large erythematous lesion that may increase in size to 5 cm or greater, sometimes with central clearing. Early lesions may not have central clearing or the characteristic target-like appearance. The rash may be warm but is not painful. Influenza-like symptoms that include malaise, fatigue, headache, arthralgia, myalgia, fever, or regional lymphadenopathy may accompany the skin lesion.[3] Cough, rhinorrhea, vomiting, or diarrhea are not typical. The rash typically appears within 7 to 14 days (range 3 to 30 days) of the tick bite and, if untreated, resolves within 3 to 4 weeks.

Early Disseminated Phase

In the absence of antimicrobial therapy, spread of the spirochete may occur, producing the disseminated phase of early Lyme disease. Within days or weeks, in an untreated person, early disseminated disease may produce multiple secondary EM lesions, Bell palsy, lymphocytic meningitis, or conjunctivitis. Systemic symptoms that include arthralgia, myalgia, headache, and fatigue are common.[4] Serum antibody to *B burgdorferi* is usually not present during this stage of early disease, requiring 3 to 4 weeks before antibody is detectable. However, the spirochete is cultured from the skin more easily during early infection than at any other time in the illness.

Approximately 60% of untreated patients will develop monoarticular or oligoarticular arthritis, which generally involves the knees.[5] Approximately 5% to 10% of untreated patients will develop neurologic manifestations.[5] Nervous system involvement may include cranial neuropathy (especially unilateral or bilateral facial palsy) and radiculopathy. Central nervous system involvement may include lymphocytic meningitis. Encephalopathy associated with late-stage Lyme disease consisting of mild abnormalities of memory and cognitive function is poorly understood and is a rare occurrence. Less than 5% of untreated patients will develop cardiac disease.[5] Cardiac involvement is characterized most commonly by varying degrees of atrioventricular block but may include myopericarditis. Hospitalization is appropriate for patients with syncope, dyspnea, or chest pain. Complete heart block is usually brief, and only temporary cardiac pacing is needed.[5] In untreated persons, symptoms involving the joints, central nervous system, or heart reflecting spread of the spirochete to other parts of the body may occur months after the tick bite.

Late-Stage Disease

Late-stage disease most commonly produces recurrent pauciarticular arthritis that involves the knees. Peripheral or central nervous system involvement is rare. Late-stage disease is uncommon in children who receive antimicrobial therapy early in the disease.

Congenital Infection

Although other spirochetal infections during pregnancy (eg, syphilis) can cause congenital infection, no causal relationship between maternal Lyme disease and congenital disease has been documented. No evidence exists to support transmission of *B burgdorferi* via human milk. Doxycycline should not be used to treat Lyme disease in pregnant or lactating patients.[6,7]

Coinfections

The same tick that transmits *B burgdorferi* also can transmit *Anaplasma phagocytophilum* (the agent of ehrlichiosis) and *Babesia microta* (the agent of babesiosis) either as a mixed infection or as a single infection.[5] Ehrlichiosis or anaplasmosis should be suspected in the appropriate epidemiologic setting in a patient with fever, chills, and headache in association with thrombocytopenia, leukopenia, or increased liver enzyme levels. Babesiosis in symptomatic patients may produce fever, malaise, chills, and sweats.

DIFFERENTIAL DIAGNOSIS

In children who have what appears to be Lyme arthritis, the differential diagnosis includes pauciarticular juvenile arthritis, septic arthritis, acute rheumatic fever, and fibromyalgia syndrome. Other considerations in the differential diagnosis may include aseptic meningitis caused by enterovirus infection, Bell palsy, a peripheral neuropathy not caused by *B burgdorferi*, or multiple sclerosis. Although such diagnoses are less likely after a history of a tick bite and EM, some patients with Lyme disease may offer no history of these events. Especially during summer months in an endemic area, Lyme disease should be considered in a patient who has lymphocytic meningitis or arthritis involving the knee.

SEROLOGIC TESTING

EM can be diagnosed in a person who lives in or has traveled to an endemic area and generally is a sufficient basis for a clinical diagnosis without laboratory confirmation. Serologic testing in a person with typical EM is generally discouraged because of the lack of sensitivity at this early stage of disease. As many as 60% of cases will have a false-negative test result at this stage. However, not all patients with Lyme disease will develop EM, and many may not recall a tick bite.

Serologic testing may be useful in the few patients in whom a diagnosis is uncertain, particularly when symptoms have been present for more than several weeks. A 2-tier approach to serologic testing for Lyme disease should be used with both acute- and convalescent-phase serum specimens.[8,9] Initial testing is most often conducted using an enzyme immunoassay. If positive or equivocal results are obtained, then a standardized Western immunoblot for both Lyme-specific immunoglobulin M (IgM) and IgG should be performed, using the same serum specimen for tier 1 and tier 2 testing. Based on Centers for Disease Control and Prevention guidelines, an IgM immunoblot is considered positive if 2 of 3 bands are present. An IgG immunoblot is defined as positive if 5 of 10 bands are detected. In endemic areas, a positive immunoblot result is not always due to an active *B burgdorferi* infection and may reflect previous infection. Two-tier testing should be used because of the high sensitivity but low specificity of the commercial enzyme immunoassays used in the 1st step. Testing by immunoblot should not be performed without first performing an enzyme immunoassay. Laboratory testing should not be performed for people who do not have symptoms of Lyme disease. Testing of individual ticks is not useful for deciding whether antibiotic therapy should be initiated after a tick bite. Early antibiotic therapy may prevent seroconversion. Other laboratory tests such as urine antigen assays, immunofluorescence staining for cell wall deficient forms of *B burgdorferi*, and lymphocyte transformation assays should not be used.

MANAGEMENT

Pharmacotherapy

Patients with early localized or disseminated disease who do not have neurologic or cardiac involvement should be treated for 14 to 21 days with doxycycline (for children 8 years and older) except for pregnant or lactating women.[5,6] An advantage of doxycycline is efficacy against the agent of human granulocytic ehrlichiosis, which may be a coinfecting microbe. Amoxicillin should be used for children younger than 8 years and in pregnant women. In patients who are unable to take doxycycline or Amoxicillin, cefuroxime axetil is a third drug of choice. Clinical trials of patients with EM show resolution of symptoms in more than 90% of patients treated with doxycycline, amoxicillin,

Table 292-1 Treatment Regimens for Lyme Disease

MANIFESTATION	REGIMEN
EARLY INFECTION	
Children (>8 yr) and adults (except pregnant or lactating women)	Doxycycline, 100 mg orally twice a day for 14-21 days Amoxicillin, 500 mg orally 3 times a day for 14-21 days Cefuroxime axetil, 500 mg orally twice a day daily for 14-21 days
Children (<8 yr) and pregnant or lactating women	Amoxicillin 50 mg/kg body weight/day in 3 divided doses for 14-21 days Cefuroxime axetil, 30 mg/kg/day in 2 divided doses for 14-21 days (max 1 g/day)
NEUROLOGICAL ABNORMALITIES (EARLY OR LATE)*	
General	Ceftriaxone, 75-100 mg/kg/day intravenously or intramuscularly once a day for 14-28 days (max 2 g/day) Penicillin G, 300,000 U/kg/day intravenously, 6 divided doses daily for 14-28 days (max 20 million U/day) In case of ceftriaxone or penicillin allergy, consult with expert in Lyme disease
Facial palsy alone	Oral antibiotic regimens, as above, may be adequate
CARDIAC ABNORMALITIES	
First-degree atrioventricular block (PR interval <0.3 sec)	Oral antibiotic regimens, as for early infection
High-degree atrioventricular block	Ceftriaxone, 75-100 mg/kg/day intravenously in 1 or 2 divided doses for 14 days Penicillin, 300,000 U/kg/day intravenously, 6 divided doses daily for 14 days
Arthritis (persistent or recurrent)	Same regimen as that for early disease or ceftriaxone, 75-100 mg/kg/day intravenously in 1 or 2 divided doses (max 2 gm/day) for 14-28 days, or Penicillin, 300,000 U/kg/day intravenously, 6 divided doses daily (max 20 million Units/day) for 14-28 days

Modified from American Academy of Pediatrics. Lyme disease. In : Pickering LK, Baker CJ, Long SS, McMillan JA, eds. *Red Book: 2006 Report of the Committee on Infectious Diseases.* 27th ed. Elk Grove Village, IL: American Academy of Pediatrics; 2006.

or cefuroxime axetil. Macrolide antibiotics are less effective than other antimicrobial agents and should be reserved for patients who are unable to take preferred agents. Intravenous ceftriaxone is not superior to oral agents except in patients with neurologic or cardiac involvement.

Oral antimicrobial agents are effective for treating multiple EM and uncomplicated Lyme arthritis. Oral agents can be used to treat most people with facial nerve palsy, but central nervous system involvement such as meningitis should be treated with parenteral antibiotic therapy. Although 1st-degree atrioventricular block usually responds to oral therapy, higher-grade blocks are usually treated with parenteral therapy with ceftriaxone or penicillin. Persistent or recurrent arthritis should be treated with either parenteral ceftriaxone or penicillin. Specific dosages and durations are given in Table 292-1.

Vaccine

In December 1998 the US Food and Drug Administration approved a vaccine against Lyme disease (LYMErix) for individuals 15 to 70 years of age, but the vaccine was withdrawn in 2002 and is no longer available.

Prophylaxis After a Tick Bite

Clinical practice guidelines developed by the Infectious Diseases Society of America for prevention of Lyme disease after a tick bite suggest that the following conditions be satisfied: (1) The biting tick is identified as *I scapularis,* with an estimated attachment time of more than 36 hours based on the size of the engorged tick, (2) prophylaxis can be started within 72 hours of tick removal, (3) local rates of tick infection by *B burgdorferi* exceed 20%, and (4) the use of doxycycline is not contraindicated.[5] Doxycycline is the only antibiotic shown to be effective for postexposure prophylaxis.[10] No data are available to support amoxicillin use in this setting.

PREVENTION OF TICK BITES

Ticks are most likely to be located in wooded and bushy areas with high grass. When walking in a tick-infested area, people should walk in the center of the path to avoid contact with grass and brush. Insect repellent containing DEET should be applied to skin and clothing. DEET-containing compounds can be used for children older than 2 months, should not be applied to the face or hands, and should be removed from skin with soap and water once the risk of exposure is over. Permethrin kills ticks on contact and can be applied to clothing but should not be applied directly to skin because it is inactivated by skin lipids. Long pants and sleeves will help keep ticks off skin, and light-colored clothing makes the task of spotting ticks easier. Daily tick checks should be performed. If a tick is attached for less than 24 hours, then the risk of acquiring Lyme disease is extremely small. Attached ticks should be removed as soon as possible using fine-tip forceps.

WHEN TO REFER

- Cardiac involvement (heart block, pericarditis, myocarditis)

- Neurologic involvement (except isolated facial palsy in patient with definite Lyme disease diagnosis)
- Nonspecific clinical history but positive or equivocal laboratory testing
- Persistent arthritis

WHEN TO ADMIT

- Cardiac involvement
- Meningitis or encephalopathy

TOOLS FOR PRACTICE

Engaging Patients and Family

- *A Parent's Guide to Insect Repellents* (brochure), American Academy of Pediatrics (patiented.aap.org).
- *Learn about Lyme Disease* (Web page), Centers for Disease Control and Prevention (www.cdc.gov/ncidod/dvbid/lyme/index.htm).
- *Lyme Disease* (on-line course), National Library of Medicine, Patient Education Institute (www.nlm.nih.gov/medlineplus/tutorials/lymedisease/htm/index.htm).
- *Lyme Disease and Animals* (fact sheet), Centers for Disease Control and Prevention (www.cdc.gov/healthypets/diseases/lyme.htm).

Medical Decision Support

- Red Book: 2006 Report of the Committee on Infectious Diseases, American Academy of Pediatrics (www.aap.org/bookstore).

REFERENCES

1. Steere AC, Malawista SE, Snydman DR, et al. Lyme arthritis: an epidemic of oligoarticular arthritis in children and adults in three Connecticut communities. *Arthritis Rheum*. 1977;20:7.
2. Burgdorfer W, Barbour AG, Hayes SF, et al. Lyme disease: a tick-borne spirochetosis? *Science*. 1982;216:1317.
3. Steere AC. Lyme disease. *N Engl J Med*. 2001;345:115-125.
4. Wormser GP. Early Lyme disease. *N Engl J Med*. 2006; 354:2794-2801.
5. Wormser GP, Dattwyler RJ, Shapiro ED, et al. The clinical assessment, treatment and prevention of Lyme disease, human granulocytic anaplasmosis, and babesiosis: clinical practice guidelines by the Infectious Diseases Society of America. *Clin Infect Dis*. 2006;43:1089-1134.
6. American Academy of Pediatrics. Lyme disease. In : Pickering LK, Baker CJ, Long SS, et al, eds. *Red Book: 2006 Report of the Committee on Infectious Diseases*. 27th ed. Elk Grove Village, IL: American Academy of Pediatrics; 2006.
7. Strobine BA, Williams CL, Abid S, et al. Lyme disease and pregnancy outcome: a prospective study of two thousand prenatal patients, *Am J Obstet Gynecol*. 1993; 169(2 pt 1):367-374.
8. Centers for Disease Control and Prevention. Notice to readers: recommendations for test performance and interpretation from the Second National Conference on Serologic Diagnosis of Lyme Disease. *MMWR*. 1995; 44:590-591.
9. Centers for Disease Control and Prevention. Notice to readers: caution regarding testing for Lyme disease. *MMWR*. 2005;54:125-126.
10. Nadelman RB, Nowakowski J, Fish D, et al, and the Tick Bite Study Group. Prophylaxis with single dose doxycycline for the prevention of Lyme disease after an Ixodes scapularis tick bite. *N Engl J Med*. 2001;345:79-84.

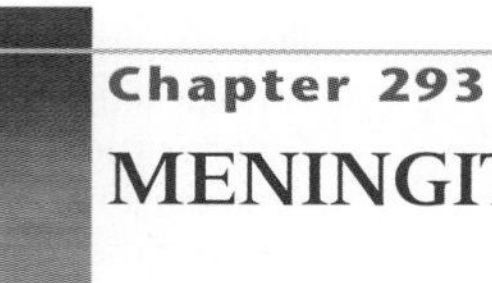

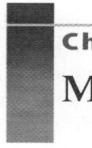

Chapter 293

MENINGITIS

Geoffrey A. Weinberg, MD; Ann M. Buchanan, MD, MPH

The meninges of the central nervous system (CNS) include 3 membranes that support, protect, and nourish the brain and spinal cord. The outermost layer, the dura mater, is a tough, inelastic, connective tissue layer that sheaths the brain and spinal cord and terminates caudally at the first coccygeal vertebra. The middle and innermost layers, the arachnoid and the pia mater, respectively, are similar in structure and are often referred to singly as the leptomeninges. The arachnoid and pia are partly separated, leaving a subarachnoid space containing cerebrospinal fluid (CSF). The CSF is formed in the choroid plexuses within the ventricles of the brain, which communicate with the subarachnoid space through the foramina of the fourth ventricle (via the medial aperture of Magendie and the lateral apertures of Luschka).[1] The CSF slowly circulates in both directions around the brain and spinal cord; it is reabsorbed predominantly by the arachnoid villi of the superior sagittal sinus.[1]

Meningitis, or inflammation of the meninges, is most often caused by an infectious agent and less commonly by a chemical (medication) or malignancy. Bacterial meningitis, also known as pyogenic meningitis, is often quickly fatal, making early diagnosis and treatment essential.

Aseptic meningitis refers to inflammation of the meninges, as demonstrated by CSF pleocytosis, without the presence of visible microorganisms on routine Gram staining. Nonpolio enteroviruses cause 85% of cases of aseptic meningitis in the United States. However, fungi, parasites, reactions to medications, and atypical bacteria not well seen on Gram staining may also cause aseptic meningitis. Thus the term is not synonymous with *viral meningitis*, although the 2 terms are often used interchangeably. The CSF findings characteristic of both pyogenic and aseptic meningitis are listed in Table 293-1. When encephalitis accompanies aseptic meningitis, the cause may be distinct, and the clinical course may be much more severe (see Chapter 294, Meningoencephalitis).

In partially treated meningitis, antibiotics have been provided before lumbar puncture is performed, rendering Gram staining and bacterial culture less useful (because of the possibility of temporary bacterial sterilization). Distinguishing partially treated bacterial meningitis with false-negative CSF cultures from aseptic meningitis can be difficult, although the accompanying CSF laboratory studies (white blood cell [WBC] count and differential, CSF protein and glucose concentrations) may often be of assistance.[2-4]

Table 293-1 Characteristic Cerebrospinal Fluid (CSF) Findings in Children With and Without Meningitis*

CSF FINDINGS	NORMAL	BACTERIAL	VIRAL	FUNGAL OR TUBERCULOUS
LEUKOCYTES/mcL				
Usual	<5	>500	<500	50-750
Range	0-10	10-20,000	0-1000	10-1500
POLYMORPHONUCLEAR NEUTROPHILS (% OF LEUKOCYTES)				
Usual	2	>80	<50	<50
Range	0-20	20-100	0-100	0-80
GLUCOSE, mg/dL				
Usual	60	<40	>40	<40
Range	45-65	0-65	30-65	5-50
Usual CSF/blood (%)	≥60	<30	30-60	<40
PROTEIN, mg/dL				
Usual	≤30	>100	<100	50-200
Range	0-40	40-500	20-200	40-1500
OTHER POSITIVE TESTS	None	Gram stain, antigen detection	Polymerase chain reaction	Cryptococcal antigen, acid-fast stain

*See Table 293-5 for CSF findings of neonates.

EPIDEMIOLOGIC FEATURES

The incidence of bacterial meningitis is related closely to age. In the United States, during the first month of life, the age-specific incidence is as high as 300 to 400 cases per 100,000 live births[5]; it decreases to 141 per 100,000 during the second month of life and to less than 50 per 100,000 in the second year of life. Until recent years, a second peak occurred at 6 to 8 months, with an incidence of nearly 180 per 100,000 infants.[5] This second peak, which was due to *Haemophilus influenzae* type b (Hib) meningitis, has declined dramatically since 1988, when Hib conjugate vaccines were approved for use.[6-9] As illustrated in Figure 293-1, between 1987 and 1997 the incidence of Hib meningitis fell from 40 cases per 100,000 children younger than 5 years to 1 case per 100,000, and current annual estimates are as low as 0.1 cases per 100,000.[10,11] This remarkable decline in Hib meningitis has converted bacterial meningitis to a disease predominantly of adults rather than of infants and young children, with the median age at diagnosis of 25 years in 1995 as opposed to 15 months in 1985 (Figure 293-2).[12]

In addition to age-related changes in incidence, the spectrum of etiologic agents of bacterial meningitis changed remarkably with age—at least before the routine implementation of antibiotic prophylaxis for group B β-hemolytic streptococci and the licensure of conjugate vaccines (Figure 293-3). Until recently, during the first month of life, more than two thirds of the cases of neonatal bacterial meningitis were caused by group B β-hemolytic streptococci *(Streptococcus agalactiae)* or gram-negative enteric organisms, primarily *Escherichia coli, Klebsiella,* and *Enterobacter* species. With antibiotic prophylaxis, the contribution of group B β-hemolytic streptococci to early-onset meningitis is decreasing (although late-onset disease has not decreased).[13-16] In some regions, another fairly common cause of neonatal meningitis is *Listeria monocytogenes.*[3,4,17] After the first month of life, *Listeria* organisms are found as the cause of meningitis only in debilitated or elderly persons.

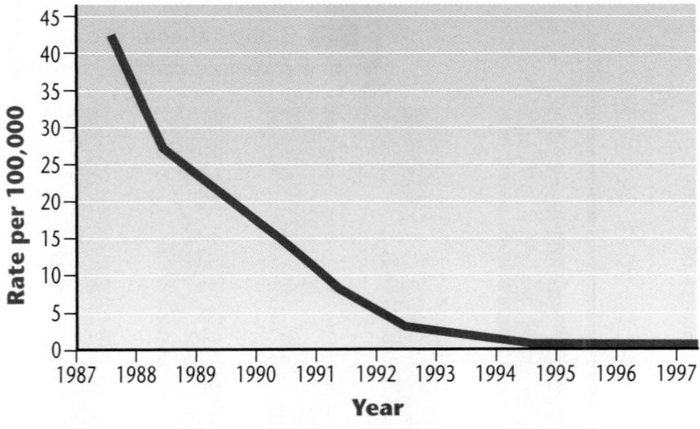

Figure 293-1 Incidence of *Haemophilus influenzae* type b meningitis per 100,000 children younger than 5 years of age in the United States, 1987-1997. *(Redrawn from Centers for Disease Control and Prevention. Progress toward eliminating Haemophilus influenzae type b disease among infants and children—United States, 1987-1997.* MMWR Morb Mortal Wkly Rep. *1998;47:993.)*

The cause of pediatric bacterial meningitis in the United States is again changing, with the implementation of *S pneumoniae* (pneumococcal) conjugate vaccination in infancy.[4] The heptavalent pneumococcal conjugate vaccine was licensed in 2000,[18,19] and just 4 years later a 70% to 90% decline was documented in cases of invasive pneumococcal disease, including

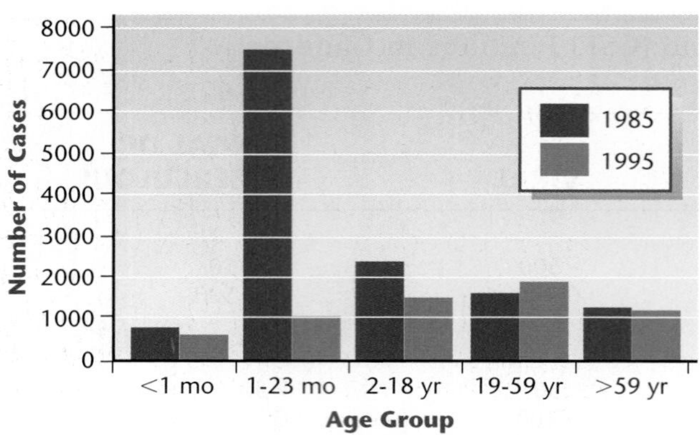

Figure 293-2 Number of cases of bacterial meningitis caused by the 5 major pathogens in the United States during 1985 and 1995 according to age group. *(Redrawn from Schuchat A, Robinson K, Wenger JD, et al. Bacterial meningitis in the United States in 1995.* N Engl J Med. *1997;337: 970-976. Used by permission.)*

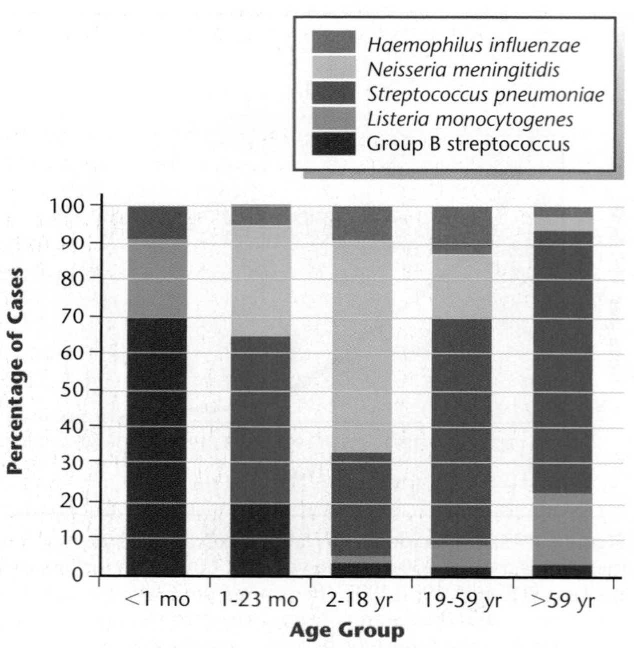

Figure 293-3 Distribution of 248 cases of bacterial meningitis according to age group and causative organism, from an active, population-based, surveillance project performed in 22 counties across 4 states during 1995. Meningitis caused by enteric pathogens in infants younger than 1 month of age was not included in the surveillance. *(Redrawn from Schuchat A, Robinson K, Wenger JD, et al. Bacterial meningitis in the United States in 1995.* N Engl J Med. *1997;337:970-976. Used by permission.)*

meningitis (Table 293-2).[11,20,21] Current annual incidence rates of invasive pneumococcal disease in children ages 5 years or younger are 21 per 100,000 per year, as opposed to 100 per 100,000 per year before routine conjugate vaccination began.[11] A tetravalent *Neisseria meningitidis* (meningococcal) conjugate vaccine was licensed in 2005 for use in adolescents[22,23]; similar monovalent and bivalent conjugate vaccines provided to infants and younger children have reduced meningococcal meningitis rates in Europe (see Table 293-2).[24] However, because the fraction of meningococcal disease in young children in the United States caused by the nonconjugate vaccine serogroup B is greater than that in Europe, use of the current tetravalent conjugate vaccine (serogroups ACYW135) will not eliminate meningococcal infection in infants.[22-25]

The incidence of aseptic meningitis (predominantly caused by enteroviruses) ranges, in different years, from 1.5 to 4 cases per 100,000 population. The incidence in children is actually much higher because aseptic meningitis is still a disease of the young, with few reported cases occurring in persons over 30 years of age; however, age-adjusted incidence rates are not available.

BACTERIAL MENINGITIS AFTER THE NEONATAL PERIOD

After the age of 1 month, most cases of bacterial meningitis are caused by *N meningitidis* or, increasingly less often, *S pneumoniae* or Hib in regions where pneumococcal and Hib conjugate vaccines are widely used (see Figure 293-3 and Table 293-2).[4,10,12,21] Mortality varies with the pathogen and has been reported to be 21% for *S pneumoniae*, 3% for *N meningitidis*, and 6% for Hib.[12]

All 3 of these pathogens can be isolated from the throat or nasopharynx of healthy individuals. Most studies of microorganism carrier states suggest that children at highest risk for disease are also the most likely to be colonized. In the pre-Hib conjugate vaccine era, approximately 70% of toddlers and 48% of the preschool-aged children in some child care centers were colonized with Hib,[26] but no invasive Hib disease was observed. Thus colonization with Hib, as well as that with *S pneumoniae* and *N meningitidis*, does not always cause meningitis. Indeed, nasopharyngeal colonization may be a partially immunizing event that contributes to future host defense. However, when microbial virulence factors overcome host defense, bacterial meningitis ensues.

The successful meningeal pathogen must follow several sequential steps.[3,27,28] Nasopharyngeal mucosal colonization is facilitated by various microbial-binding adhesins and secreted enzymes such as immunoglobulin A protease, which cleaves host secretory immunoglobulin A. Next, invasion across the epithelium, followed by survival of bacteria in the bloodstream (by evading the action of the alternative complement pathway) are required. Finally, the bacteria must invade the CSF by crossing the blood-brain barrier.

Meningitis may occasionally occur after head trauma, particularly with fractures of the paranasal sinuses or middle ear.[29] The pathogens most often associated with meningitis after trauma are *S pneumoniae* (often less pathogenic capsular serotypes) and *H*

Table 293-2 Changes in Incidence of Invasive Bacterial Disease (Including Meningitis) With Universal Implementation of Immunization With Conjugate Vaccines

			INCIDENCE PER 100,000 POPULATION PER YEAR		
INFECTION	STUDY POPULATION	AGE GROUP, Y	PRECONJUGATE VACCINE USE	POSTCONJUGATE VACCINE USE	PERCENTAGE CHANGE
Haemophilus influenzae b	US children[a]	<5	23	0.3	–99
Streptococcus pneumoniae (all serotypes)*	US children[b]	<2	188	59	–69
	US children[c]	<2	112	10	–91
Neisseria meningitidis serogroup C	UK children and adolescents[d]	<17	74	1.4	–81

[a]Centers for Disease Control and Prevention. Progress toward eliminating *Haemophilus influenzae* type b disease among infants and children—United States, 1988-2000. *MMWR.* 2002;51:234-237.
[b]Whitney CG, Farley MM, Hadler J, et al. Decline in invasive pneumococcal disease after the introduction of protein-polysaccharide conjugate vaccine. *N Engl J Med.* 2003;348:1737-1746.
[c]Black S, Shinefield H, Baxter R, et al. Postlicensure surveillance for pneumococcal invasive disease after use of heptavalent pneumococcal conjugate vaccine in Northern California Kaiser Permanente. *Pediatr Infect Dis J.* 2004;23:485-489.
[d]Miller E, Salisbury D, Ramsay M. Planning, registration, and implementation of an immunization campaign against meningococcal serogroup C disease in the UK: a success story. *Vaccine.* 2002;20(suppl 1):S58-S67.
*Both studies demonstrated herd effects of lowered rates of pneumococcal invasive disease in adults after initiation of conjugate immunization in children.[a,b] Decreases in outpatient pneumonia and otitis reported to be 10- to 100-fold greater than that of the invasive disease in other studies of US children.
From Weinberg GA, Granoff DM. Polysaccharide-protein conjugate vaccines for the prevention of *Haemophilus influenzae* type b disease. *J Pediatr.* 1988; 113:621-631.

influenzae (often nontypable or encapsulated but non-type b strains). Posttraumatic meningitis can recur if CSF leakage persists. Meningitis can also occur by direct spread from a congenital dermal sinus that communicates with the CNS. Any time meningitis is caused by bacteria that normally reside on the skin or in the gastrointestinal tract, a diligent search of the craniospinal axis should be made. Meningitis can develop after neurosurgery and is not uncommon after procedures performed to shunt ventricular fluid. Coagulase-negative staphylococci are the organisms most often associated with shunt infections. Cochlear implantation has been recognized as an additional risk factor for bacterial meningitis.[30,31]

Once bacteria establish growth in the CSF, cell wall products, such as lipopolysaccharide (endotoxin), teichoic acid, and peptidoglycans, are liberated, which, in turn, induce the local production and secretion of inflammatory cytokines (especially interleukin-1 and -6 and tumor necrosis factor).[32] The action of these cytokines results in activation of leukocytes and vascular metabolism, which leads to leukocyte migration (diapedesis), endothelial injury, and blood-brain barrier breakdown. The injury to the cerebral microvasculature, along with increasing inflammation, culminate in brain edema, reduction of cerebral blood flow, thrombosis, and impairment of oxygen and glucose delivery.[3,5,27,28,33]

Differential Diagnosis

Signs and symptoms suggesting meningeal inflammation or increased intracranial pressure can be seen with other infections of the CNS besides pyogenic meningitis. The most common cause of meningeal inflammation is enteroviral aseptic meningitis, which is discussed later in this chapter. Aseptic meningitis can also be caused by Lyme disease spirochetes *(Borrelia burgdorferi), Mycobacterium tuberculosis,* fungi, parasites, or inflammatory conditions. Meningitis or meningoencephalitis may also be present in patients who have Rocky Mountain spotted fever, Kawasaki disease (see Chapter 289, Kawasaki Disease), cat-scratch disease, or toxic shock syndrome, and it often is associated with or occurs after mumps, rubeola, rubella, varicella, infectious mononucleosis, roseola, and erythema infectiosum (Table 293-3). A brain abscess, epidural abscess, primary amebic meningoencephalitis, embolic diseases (eg, endocarditis, thrombophlebitis), venous sinus thrombosis, space-occupying lesions, reactions to medications (eg, intravenous immunoglobulin, intravenous monoclonal antilymphocyte antibody, oral trimethoprim-sulfamethoxazole, some oral nonsteroidal antiinflammatory drugs), ingestion of toxins (eg, lead), spider bites, pemphigus, and Behçet syndrome can mimic bacterial meningitis. However, interpretation of the CSF findings in the context of the clinical manifestations usually differentiates bacterial meningitis from other diseases. Eosinophilic meningitis is rarely seen; the differential diagnosis includes reactions to ventriculoperitoneal shunts, unusual presentations of bacterial or *Toxoplasma* infection, or parasitic roundworms.[34-38] Conditions that can simulate a clinical picture of meningitis but that usually have normal CSF findings include pharyngitis, retropharyngeal abscess, cervical adenitis, cervical spine arthritis or osteomyelitis, pyelonephritis, pneumonia, torticollis, tetanus, and oculogyric crisis.[39,40]

Clinical Manifestations

Children who have bacterial meningitis usually have a fever; however, the absence of fever in a child who has signs of meningeal irritation does not preclude the diagnosis.[5,33,41] Inflammation of the meninges can be

Table 293-3 Selected Causes of Aseptic Meningitis*

CAUSE	COMMON	UNCOMMON	RARE
Viruses	Enteroviruses	HIV-1	Adenovirus
	Arboviruses	Epstein-Barr virus	Varicella zoster virus
	Herpes simplex type 2	Lymphocytic choriomeningitis virus	Cytomegalovirus
	Human herpesvirus 6	Mumps	Measles
			Rubella
			Parvovirus B19
			Influenza A and B
Bacteria	Pyogenic (partially treated)	*Treponema pallidum*	*Chlamydophila psittaci*
	Mycobacterium tuberculosis	*Borrelia* species	*Chlamydophila pneumoniae*
	Borrelia burgdorferi	*Bartonella henselae*	*Rickettsia prowazekii*
	Mycoplasma pneumoniae	*Rickettsia rickettsii*	*Coxiella burnetii*
	Leptospira species	*Ehrlichia canis*	*Brucella abortus*
			Streptobacillus moniliformis
Fungi	*Candida* species	*Blastomyces dermatitidis*	Various molds
	Cryptococcus neoformans		
	Histoplasma capsulatum		
	Coccidioides immitis		
Parasites	—	*Toxoplasma gondii*	*Angiostrongylus cantonensis*
		Neurocysticercosis	*Baylisascaris procyonis*
			Strongyloides stercoralis
			Free-living amoebae
Miscellaneous	Parameningeal infections	Medications (TMP-SMX, IgIV, ibuprofen)	Sarcoidosis
	Kawasaki disease	Systemic lupus erythematosus	Behçet syndrome
	Foreign bodies (CSF shunts)		Heavy metal poisoning
	CNS leukemia, tumors		—
	ADEM		—

*Common, uncommon, and rare refer to relative frequencies within each broad category of etiologic agents (eg, viruses, bacteria). Overall, enteroviruses cause at least 85% of the aseptic meningitis diagnosed in children in the United States, and arboviruses cause approximately 5%; all other causes combined account for the remaining 10% or less of cases.
ADEM, Acute disseminated encephalomyelitis; *CNS,* central nervous system; *CSF,* cerebrospinal fluid; *HIV,* human immunodeficiency virus; *IgIV,* intravenous immunoglobulin; *TMP-SMX,* trimethoprim-sulfamethoxazole.

characterized by irritability, anorexia, headache, nausea, vomiting, confusion, back pain, nuchal rigidity, and photophobia. Kernig and Brudzinski signs can be assessed during the physical examination to demonstrate meningeal inflammation (Figure 293-4).[42] Kernig sign is elicited in the supine patient by extending the leg at the knee while the hip is flexed at 90 degrees. When positive, this maneuver causes extensor spasm of the knee and pain in the hamstrings of a person who has meningitis when the lower leg is extended to approximately 135 degrees. Brudzinski sign is elicited by flexing the neck of a patient in the supine position; in a positive test, the patient will involuntarily flex the hips and knees.[42] Stiffness of the neck is a sensitive (80%-98%) indicator of true bacterial meningitis in children, adolescents, and adults.[43-47]

In a young infant, however, signs of meningeal inflammation can be minimal or absent.[5,33,48] Thus, in patients younger than 12 months, the absence of nuchal rigidity must not be used to exclude meningitis. Distinguishing nuchal rigidity from voluntary movement and guarding can also be difficult in a sick infant with irritability. In this case, the additional signs of lethargy, poor feeding, and restlessness may be helpful. Additionally, laying the infant near the edge of the examining table with the head supported by the examiner's hand but gently extended off the edge of the table may be useful. The natural tendency for the infant in this position will be to try to lift the head, at which time the examiner can feel whether nuchal rigidity, rather than voluntary guarding or noncooperation, is preventing flexion of the neck.

The patient with meningitis may also have signs of increased intracranial pressure, such as a headache or a bulging fontanelle. Papilledema is uncommon with bacterial meningitis, and when it is present, other causes should be sought; bacterial meningitis progresses so quickly that the time needed for papilledema to develop may not be sufficient. Cranial nerve involvement occurs with bacterial meningitis, and although it is often transient, it can be permanent.[5,33] The auditory nerve is often affected, as demonstrated by deafness or disturbances of vestibular function. Blindness has been reported but is rare. Children may also have paralysis of extraocular or facial nerves. The degree of CNS derangement observed with bacterial meningitis ranges from irritability to coma. Approximately 15% of children who have bacterial meningitis are comatose or semicomatose at the time of hospitalization.[33] This circumstance occurs more often with *S pneumoniae* or *N meningitidis* than with Hib. Seizures occur before or within 1 to 2 days after admission in

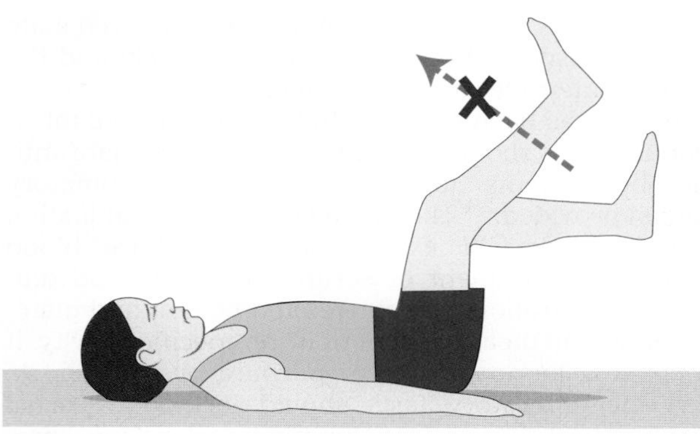

Kernig Sign
When the hips are flexed at 90 degrees, attempting to extend the leg at the knee past 135 degrees causes pain and/or extensor spasm.

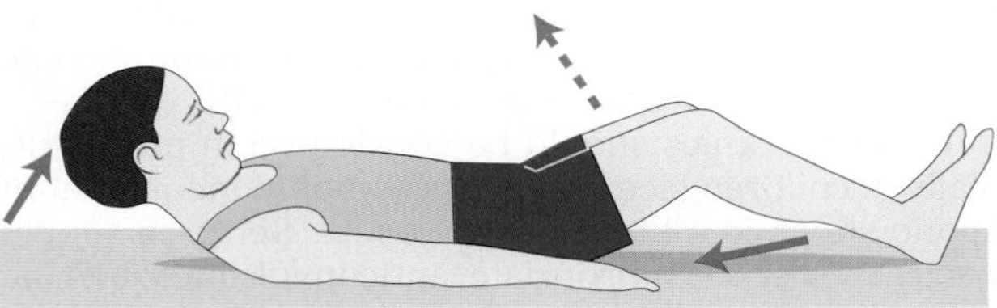

Brudzinski Sign
Flexion of the neck while laying supine causes involuntary hip and knee flexion.

Figure 293-4 Kernig sign and Brudzinski sign, signs of meningitis at physical examination in addition to nuchal rigidity.

approximately 30% of patients. Focal neurologic signs, which are present in approximately 16% of the patients, correlate with persistent abnormal neurologic and developmental examinations 1 year after discharge.

Subdural effusions occur in approximately 50% of children who have bacterial meningitis, but they are seldom clinically significant.[5,33] Therefore, unless focal neurologic signs or signs of increased intracranial pressure develop, the presence of such effusions need not be sought through the performance of subdural taps or computed tomographic (CT) scans. Infection of subdural effusions is extremely rare.

Arthralgia and myalgia often occur in patients who have meningitis, particularly those who have meningococcemia.[5,33] Vasculitis can be seen in children who have any type of bacterial meningitis, but petechiae and purpura are more commonly associated with meningococcal disease. Children who have such rashes should be considered in imminent danger of developing septic shock and should be treated accordingly (see Chapter 353, Meningococcemia).

Laboratory Testing and Findings

When meningitis is suspected in a patient who does not have papilledema, a lumbar puncture should be performed, the opening pressure measured, and the CSF examined immediately.[2] The clinical situation should influence the amount of data required before a therapeutic decision is made. If the CSF from an ill, febrile child is turbid or purulent, then antimicrobial therapy should be initiated as treatment for bacterial meningitis before further laboratory results are available. In any case, the CSF should be examined as soon as possible. If the nucleated blood cell count of the CSF is not above 6/mcL, then the only other tests likely to be useful in diagnosing bacterial meningitis are Gram stain and a culture.[49] However, most experts suggest that a Gram stain, bacterial culture, cell count, differential cell count, and CSF concentrations of total protein and glucose should be performed on CSF from all samples drawn by lumbar puncture.[2,5] If possible, the blood glucose should be measured just before the lumbar puncture is performed so that the ratio of CSF to blood glucose can be determined. (Measuring the blood glucose level before the lumbar puncture is best because the stress of the procedure can temporarily increase it.) If only a small amount of CSF is obtained, then the most important tests to perform are a Gram stain and bacterial culture. Characteristic CSF findings are listed in Table 293-1. A useful review and Internet-accessible video on the performance of lumbar puncture has been published recently.[50]

The CSF should be cultured on chocolate and blood agar plates and in broth. Generally, bacterial cultures will be positive within a few days if pathogens are present. The causative agent may also be identified by latex agglutination reactions or counterimmunoelectrophoresis to detect soluble capsular antigens in CSF and, if needed, in serum or concentrated urine. Although these tests are rapid, they should not be viewed as essential because their negative predictive value does not approach 100%, and they are not that useful in directing patient care.[51] Rapid diagnostic tests are likely to be only truly valuable in patients who have received a significant amount of antibiotics 24 hours or more before lumbar puncture.[5,51]

Blood cultures should be obtained for all children suspected of having bacterial meningitis; blood cultures are positive in 80% to 90% of children who have not previously received antimicrobial agents and who have meningitis caused by Hib, *S pneumoniae*, or *N meningitidis*.[33]

A common clinical concern is how to distinguish the CSF abnormalities caused by infection from those associated with traumatic lumbar puncture. Common clinical practice is to use the ratio of red blood cells to WBCs to correct the observed CSF WBC count, either by subtraction or by examination of the ratio of observed to *expected* cells.[1] Despite the apparently sound theoretical basis for these calculations, in practice, they are generally not helpful to the clinician in deciding whether to proceed with antibiotic therapy, and bacterial or viral cultures will yield a more definitive answer relatively quickly.

Two additional common clinical concerns regard (1) the timing of a diagnostic lumbar puncture and (2) when it may be performed safely; a third related concern is the need to perform cranial CT scans before lumbar puncture.[2] In general, lumbar puncture should be performed whenever the diagnosis of meningitis is known or suspected.[5] In most cases, children younger than 12 months, and perhaps those younger than 18 months, with a first febrile seizure (or any atypical febrile seizure) should also undergo a lumbar puncture to exclude meningitis.[5,52]

Four reasons for delaying lumbar puncture exist: (1) clinically important cardiorespiratory compromise, most often observed in the neonate; (2) signs of significantly increased intracranial pressure (eg, retinal changes, altered pupillary responses, increased blood pressure with associated bradycardia and hyperpnea [Cushing triad], focal neurologic signs during the physical examination); (3) infection in the skin, soft tissues, or epidural area at the site of lumbar puncture; or (4) suspicion or history of bleeding disorders (eg, hemophilia, severe thrombocytopenia).[2,3] In these circumstances, blood cultures should be obtained, and antibiotics are provided empirically without performing a lumbar puncture. In cases of suspected increased intracranial pressure, arrangements should be made for a neuroimaging study (eg, cranial CT scan with and without contrast enhancement) during or immediately after antibiotic administration, and if the imaging study suggests that it would be safe to proceed, then lumbar puncture may follow. However, performing CT scans routinely before lumbar puncture is not necessary in patients with suspected meningitis, even though all patients with meningitis have some degree of increased intracranial pressure by virtue of the disease process.[2] Herniation of the brain on removal of a small amount of CSF is rare in meningitis, especially in infants with open fontanelles. Herniation associated with meningitis has also been observed before lumbar puncture and in the presence of normal cranial CT scans. Nevertheless, lumbar puncture should be performed cautiously if significantly increased intracranial pressure is suspected, and obtaining CT scans before lumbar puncture in selected patients is reasonable, especially in children or adults with a history of immunosuppression, hydrocephalus, ventricular shunts, or head trauma, as well as in those who have focal neurologic signs or who have signs of greatly increased intracranial pressure.[2]

If the lumbar puncture was not initially able to be performed or was contraindicated, then the procedure may be reconsidered after the patient has been stabilized and contraindications to the procedure have been resolved. Lumbar puncture may be performed even 12 to 24 hours after initiation of antimicrobial therapy.[1,33] In this situation, the interpretation of CSF WBC counts, and protein and glucose concentrations may still be helpful in discerning the likelihood of true bacterial meningitis.

Management

General Care

At the initial examination, children who have meningitis may appear only mildly ill with fever and irritability, or they may be profoundly ill with an altered state of consciousness and hypotension. The severity of illness at the time the patient seeks care can predict morbidity and should dictate immediate management. Acute bacterial meningitis is always a medical emergency, and all infants and children who have an altered state of consciousness should be observed closely and the need for intensive care anticipated.[5,39,41]

As soon as bacterial meningitis is diagnosed, intravenous access should be secured and appropriate antimicrobial agents (and possibly antiinflammatory agents) provided.[2,4] The initial laboratory examination should include CSF examination and culture, blood culture, measurement of serum electrolyte and glucose concentrations, complete blood count and platelet count, and measurement of urine specific gravity. If the patient has petechiae or purpura or is in shock, then the laboratory tests should include a partial thromboplastin time, prothrombin time, and measurement of fibrinogen- or fibrin-breakdown products. Management of the child who is awake and has stable cardiorespiratory vital signs consists primarily of administering antimicrobial agents and fluids and careful monitoring for changes in level of consciousness, development of seizures, changes in vital signs, and development of the syndrome of inappropriate secretion of antidiuretic hormone (SIADH).

Other therapies should be considered in more critically ill children (see the discussion of management of septic shock in Chapter 358, Shock). Seizures should be treated with appropriate anticonvulsants, and an open airway that provides good oxygenation should be ensured. Patients who are in profound coma or whose level of consciousness deteriorates while receiving therapy should be evaluated for complications such as a cerebral abscess, obstructive hydrocephalus, or high intracranial pressure. A CT scan of the brain with and without contrast is helpful in determining the diagnosis in such cases.

Radiographs may help in identifying suspected bone or joint infection in selected patients. Radionuclide and CT studies play a role in complicated cases of meningitis and may be helpful for decisions on management later during the course of therapy, as well as, for example, evaluating selected cases of prolonged (primary) or recurrent (secondary) fever. However, CT scans should not be routinely obtained as a result of prolonged or secondary fever because such scans are unlikely to affect clinical management.[33,53]

If high intracranial pressure is a major clinical concern and treatment has been initiated or is anticipated, then a neurosurgeon should be consulted and an intracranial pressure monitoring device placed, although, notably, all children with bacterial meningitis have some increase in intracranial pressure, and monitoring devices are not required for most patients. If an intraventricular catheter can be placed, then increased intracranial pressure can often be treated by removing CSF. The placement of a pressure transducer affords continuous intracranial monitoring so that mannitol and hyperventilation can be used as necessary to decrease pressure and maintain cerebral perfusion. Decreased inflammation and increased cerebral perfusion likely account for the benefits reported by some investigators with dexamethasone therapy.[54,55]

Fluid management, possible antiinflammatory adjunctive treatments, and antimicrobial therapy are crucial for all patients who have bacterial meningitis. Even today, controversy remains about mechanisms of action, usefulness, and choice of these interventions that would at first glance seem beyond question.[2,4]

Fluid Therapy

Traditionally, fluids were restricted to two thirds of the total daily maintenance amount in patients who had bacterial meningitis to minimize brain edema and prevent SIADH, which has been reported to occur in 29% to 88% of cases of bacterial meningitis.[5,33] However, some studies have found that plasma antidiuretic hormone concentrations return to normal in patients with bacterial meningitis who receive replacement plus maintenance fluids for 24 hours, whereas concentrations remain high in patients restricted to two thirds of maintenance requirements.[56]

How should the clinician interpret these contradictory data? Dehydration likely produces an appropriate increase of antidiuretic hormone, but SIADH may still occur in nondehydrated or fluid-replete children.[33] Maintenance fluids are believed to be necessary to perfuse, oxygenate, and deliver host defenses to the CNS, and although SIADH occurs in bacterial meningitis, no firm evidence has been found that fluid restriction prevents it. Obvious fluid deficits should be rapidly corrected, and serum sodium concentrations should be closely monitored several times during the first 24 hours of therapy, along with measurements of urine specific gravity. If the serum sodium concentration drops below 125 mEq/L, then the test should be repeated as soon as possible. If the serum sodium is still below 125 mEq/L, then fluids should be restricted to keep the vein open until the serum electrolyte concentrations have been corrected. Otherwise, for the child with bacterial meningitis, providing routine maintenance fluids (such as 0.2% saline with added potassium and dextrose) at approximately 80% of the maintenance rate after fluid repletion and advancing to full maintenance rates as the serum sodium increases beyond 135 mEq/L would appear to be appropriate. The period of fluid restriction may only need to be 1 day or less.[4,33]

Antiinflammatory Therapy

The use of glucocorticoids as adjunctive therapy in patients who have bacterial meningitis has been studied for decades yet continues to be controversial.[4,54,57-59] Dexamethasone most likely improves the hearing and neurologic outcomes of children who have bacterial meningitis caused by Hib,[2,33,41,58] but the usefulness of dexamethasone therapy in children with bacterial meningitis in children and adults caused by *S pneumoniae* or *N meningitidis* is less certain.[2,4,28,41,58,60] Glucocorticoids and other antiinflammatory compounds produce definite salutary changes in experimental meningitis models that ought to imply better outcomes for children. However, such therapy may also cause gastrointestinal bleeding, decreased penetration of antimicrobial agents into the CSF, and obfuscation of the clinical assessment of children's response to therapy.[4,61,62] Dexamethasone may be beneficial when administered before or within 1 hour of the first dose of antimicrobial agents to children 6 weeks of age or older who have Hib meningitis.[61] Dexamethasone therapy should be considered for children who have pneumococcal meningitis, although uncertainty exists regarding its benefits and risks.[61]

Antimicrobial Therapy

Because knowing which causative agent is present at the time of diagnosis of bacterial meningitis is difficult, empirical guides to therapy are primarily based on age, which, in turn, predicts the most likely cause; adjustment to therapy can later be made as conjugate vaccination history and results of the CSF Gram stain and culture are confirmed (Table 293-4). In addition, some organism-specific points must be noted.

Until the early 1990s, all *N meningitidis,* Hib, and most *S pneumoniae* strains were susceptible to very low concentrations of the third-generation cephalosporins—ceftriaxone and cefotaxime.[60] Since then, numerous reports have been issued of infections in infants and children caused by resistant strains of pneumococci.[62-64] Up to 40% of pneumococcal isolates may be resistant to penicillin at some level, and many also are resistant to the third-generation cephalosporins.[19,61] Therefore infants and children suspected of having bacterial meningitis caused by pneumococci (ie, gram-positive cocci in pairs seen on a Gram stain of the CSF) should receive vancomycin in addition to either ceftriaxone or cefotaxime. Because dexamethasone can decrease the CSF penetrance (and thus the activity) of vancomycin, some experts advise that either dexamethasone should be omitted altogether or rifampin plus vancomycin plus a third-generation cephalosporin should be used when dexamethasone is provided.[41,44,61,67] As soon as the antimicrobial susceptibility of an isolate is known, vancomycin should be discontinued if the isolate is susceptible to penicillin or if it is nonsusceptible to penicillin but still susceptible to the third-generation cephalosporins.[61] Vancomycin is continued with ceftriaxone or cefotaxime for those isolates found nonsusceptible to both penicillin and the third-generation cephalosporins (and rifampin is added to the combination in some circumstances). Consultation with an infectious diseases subspecialist is suggested.[61]

In areas with low prevalence of penicillin-nonsusceptible pneumococci, especially when examination of the CSF Gram stain shows the absence of gram-positive cocci, providing a third-generation cephalosporin alone (without vancomycin) for empiric therapy is reasonable. Suspected or proven Hib disease may be treated reliably with either ceftriaxone or cefotaxime; ampicillin may be used only if the isolate is known to be susceptible. Disease caused by *N meningitidis* is treated reliably with penicillin G at high doses or alternatively by ampicillin or a third-generation cephalosporin.

Meningitis caused by *N meningitidis* is usually treated for 7 days, that caused by Hib for 10 days, and that caused by *S pneumoniae* for 10 to 14 days, although a 7-day course of antimicrobial therapy for uncomplicated Hib and *S pneumoniae* meningitis may be effective.[4,60,61,65,66] Chloramphenicol is now rarely used for therapy in the industrialized world; if an alternative agent beyond ampicillin or third-generation cephalosporins is required, then meropenem may be administered, although consultation with an infectious

Table 293-4 Antimicrobial Therapy of Bacterial Meningitis

PART A. EMPIRICAL THERAPY PENDING CULTURE AND SUSCEPTIBILITY DATA

AGE	LIKELY PATHOGENS	ANTIMICROBIAL AGENT
0-1 mo	*Streptococcus agalactiae, Escherichia coli, Listeria monocytogenes*	Ampicillin + cefotaxime *or* Ampicillin + aminoglycoside
1-3 mo	*S agalactiae, L monocytogenes, Streptococcus pneumoniae, Neisseria meningitidis, Haemophilus influenzae* b	Ampicillin + (cefotaxime or ceftriaxone) *plus* Vancomycin (see text)
3 mo-21 yr	*S pneumoniae, N meningitidis* (*H influenzae* b if not vaccinated)	(Ceftriaxone or cefotaxime) *plus* Vancomycin (see text)

PART B. SPECIFIC THERAPY

PATHOGEN	THERAPY
Streptococcus agalactiae	Ampicillin or penicillin G for 14-21 day; first 3 days, add gentamicin
Listeria monocytogenes	Ampicillin for 14-21 day; first 3 days, add gentamicin
Streptococcus pneumoniae	Penicillin MIC <0.1 mcg/mL and ceftriaxone or cefotaxime MIC ≤0.5 mcg/mL: penicillin G or ampicillin for 10-14 days
	Penicillin MIC ≥0.1 mcg/mL and ceftriaxone or cefotaxime MIC ≤0.5 mcg/mL: ceftriaxone or cefotaxime for 10-14 days
	Penicillin MIC ≥0.1 mcg/mL and ceftriaxone or cefotaxime MIC 1.0 mcg/mL: (ceftriaxone or cefotaxime) + vancomycin for 10-14 days
	Penicillin MIC ≥0.1 mcg/mL and ceftriaxone or cefotaxime MIC ≥2.0 mcg/mL: (ceftriaxone or cefotaxime) + vancomycin ± rifampin for 10-14 days
Neisseria meningitidis	Penicillin G for 7 days; alternatives: ampicillin, ceftriaxone, cefotaxime
Haemophilus influenzae b	Ceftriaxone or cefotaxime for 10 days; alternative: ampicillin if isolate is susceptible

PART C. ANTIMICROBIAL DOSAGE

	DOSE (mg/kg/day)		
AGENT	AGE 0-7 DAYS	AGE 8-28 DAYS	INFANTS AND CHILDREN
Ampicillin	150-200 divided every 8 hr	200-300 divided every 6 hr	200-300 divided every 6 hr
Cefotaxime	100 divided every 12 hr	200 divided every 8 hr	200-300 divided every 6 hr
Ceftriaxone	Not recommended	80-100 divided every 12-24 hr	80-100 divided every 12-24 hr
Gentamicin	5 divided every 12 hr	7.5 divided every 8 hr	7.5 divided every 8 hr
Penicillin G	100,000-150,000 Units divided every 12 hr	150,000-200,000 Units divided every 6 hr	300,000-400,000 Units divided every 4-6 hr
Rifampin	10 divided every 12 hr	20 divided every 12 hr	20 divided every 12 hr
Vancomycin	20 divided every 12 hr	30 divided every 8 hr	40-60 divided every 6 hr

MIC, Minimum inhibitory concentration.

diseases specialist is suggested.[4,61] Although these three organisms cause most cases of bacterial meningitis beyond the neonatal period, other bacteria can cause meningitis. In such cases, antimicrobial therapy must be individualized.

Most therapeutic failures can be related to inadequate therapy with the correct antimicrobial agent, resistant organisms, or a long delay in diagnosis. A repeat lumbar puncture performed after therapy is completed does not reflect the adequacy of therapy or predict the likelihood of recurrence, and such a procedure is usually not indicated. However, a delay in sterilizing the CSF beyond 24 to 36 hours has been associated with adverse outcomes; therefore another lumbar puncture may be performed at that time. Repeat lumbar puncture at 24 to 48 hours of therapy is also indicated if drug-resistant *S pneumoniae* is present, especially if dexamethasone therapy is provided.[60,62,67]

Some contacts of patients who have *N meningitidis* or Hib meningitis are at increased risk for the disease and should therefore receive prophylaxis.[61] Prophylactic regimens for those at risk for *N meningitidis* are described in Chapter 353, Meningococcemia. Whether all contacts of patients who have Hib disease should receive prophylaxis remains controversial. The American Academy of Pediatrics recommends that rifampin be provided to all household contacts, including adults, in households that have at least 1 contact under age 4 years whose immunization status against Hib is incomplete.[61] The definition of complete immunization depends on the age of the individual involved.[61] A household contact is anyone who resides with the index patient or a nonresident who has spent 4 or more hours a day with the index patient for 5 of the 7 days before the index patient was hospitalized. Prophylaxis for all household contacts, regardless of age, is provided in households that have a child younger than 12 months. Prophylaxis for nonhousehold contacts of Hib disease does not appear to be necessary. The index patient should also receive rifampin either during or at the completion of treatment for Hib or meningococcal meningitis, unless ceftriaxone was used for treatment (ceftriaxone itself may clear meningococcal and likely Hib carriage; nevertheless, many authorities still recommend that the index patient should receive rifampin either during or at the completion of treatment for Hib or meningococcal meningitis).

Complications

Early in the course of bacterial meningitis, increased intracranial pressure, septic shock, disseminated intravascular coagulation, and even cardiorespiratory arrest may occur. Subdural effusions occasionally cause seizures or focal neurologic deficits; in such cases, the fluid should be removed by subdural taps. Such effusions are rarely infected directly, but subdural empyemas are occasionally reported. SIADH can also complicate bacterial meningitis; thus the patient should be monitored carefully for this complication. If it occurs, then fluid should be sharply restricted. A brain abscess is extremely rare after bacterial meningitis except in neonates who have meningitis caused by *Citrobacter* or certain *Enterobacter* species.

Sequelae

Despite the appropriate use of bactericidal antibiotics, the mortality rate for bacterial meningitis remains at 5% to 10%.[5] Approximately 15% to 25% of survivors will have long-term morbidity, including developmental delay, seizure disorder, spasticity, and hearing loss.[3,5,68-72]

Predicting long-term sequelae for an individual child is difficult at the time of discharge from the hospital. Some children who are apparently normal are later found to have hearing or learning deficits or will develop a seizure disorder. Conversely, some children expected to have a dismal prognosis based on abnormal neurologic examinations at discharge make remarkable gains. The practitioner should therefore be guardedly optimistic with the family while remaining sensitive to possible sequelae and observing these children closely for attainment of developmental milestones. Hearing should be tested formally before discharge from the hospital because most sensorineural hearing loss can be detected at this time. The rate of persistent bilateral or unilateral sensorineural hearing loss is 31% after pneumococcal meningitis, 10.5% after meningococcal meningitis, and 6% after Hib meningitis.[69] In young infants, auditory brainstem response or otoacoustic emissions testing is necessary for screening; in older toddlers and children, conditioned response, play, or conventional audiometry may be performed.[73]

Current thinking asserts that much of the hearing loss in meningitis occurs soon after infection.[5,33,58] This circumstance may explain why not all studies have shown reduction of hearing loss by dexamethasone therapy. The timing of other neurologic sequelae is even less certain. Some cases of bacterial meningitis exhibit fulminantly; outcome in these cases may be poor, no matter how quickly therapy is rendered.[74-76] In many cases, the exact onset of disease is difficult to pinpoint, and thus the length of prodromal symptoms before therapy does not correlate well with outcome.[74-76]

Prevention

In 1985 a purified capsular polysaccharide vaccine against Hib was licensed for use in the United States in children older than 2 years (in whom the risk of Hib disease was albeit substantially lower than that of the highest-risk group, infants younger than 1 year).[77] Subsequently, several conjugate vaccines were made by coupling the Hib capsular polysaccharide to various protein carriers to boost immunogenicity in infants.[77,78] These conjugate vaccines were also more immunogenic in older children with conditions associated with impaired responses to capsular polysaccharide vaccine.[79] The early to mid-1990s marked the beginning of the conjugate vaccine era, with the widespread use of these vaccines resulting in a dramatic decline in the incidence of invasive Hib disease (see Figure 293-1).[6-12,61] Similarly, use of pneumococcal and meningococcal polysaccharide-protein conjugate vaccine promises to lead to a marked decline in invasive pneumococcal and meningococcal infection. Such changes have been noted in the United States with pneumococcal conjugates and in the United Kingdom with meningococcal serogroup C conjugates (see Table 293-2).[18-22,24,25,61,80,81]

One of 3 Hib conjugate vaccines or 1 of 3 Hib conjugate–containing combination vaccine products is routinely provided to US infants beginning at 2 months of age.[61] Pneumococcal conjugate vaccine is recommended for routine universal administration to infants and children younger than 2 years of age, in a similar fashion to Hib conjugate vaccines.[18,19,61] The pneumococcal conjugate vaccine is also suggested for high-risk children 2 to 5 years of age, including children who have sickle cell disease, functional or anatomic asplenia, immunosuppression, cancer, chronic renal disease, chronic cardiopulmonary disease, CSF leaks, and diabetes.[18,19,61]

At present, the tetravalent meningococcal polysaccharide conjugate vaccine is routinely used only for children and adults at higher risk of disease, including young adolescents 11 to 12 years of age or on entry to high school (15 years), college freshmen (especially those living in dormitories), certain travelers, and in those with sickle cell disease, functional or anatomic asplenia, immunosuppression, and CSF leaks.[22,23,61] Meningococcal conjugate vaccine is also used as an adjunct to chemoprophylaxis in outbreak control.[23,61] Additionally, it is undergoing clinical trials for safety and immunogenicity in US children as young as 2 years.

NEONATAL MENINGITIS

Neonatal meningitis merits separate consideration because the incidence is high, the agents that cause it are unique, and it is more often fatal than is meningitis in the older child. The incidence of neonatal meningitis varies with the reporting institution, from 0.2 to 1 case per 1000 live births.[82] The age-specific incidence of bacterial meningitis in the first month of life in the United States between 1978 and 1981 was 366 per 100,000 neonates. Case fatality rates generally range from 20% to 25% in the modern era.[13,82] In general, mortality is lower for full-term infants than for infants of low birth weight (<2500 g). Early recognition and treatment are critical because the case fatality rate falls to approximately 5% for neonates who survive the first 24 hours of the disease.[13]

The cause of neonatal meningitis has changed since 1970, and clinicians should be alert to the possibility of future shifts.[82] During the 1960s, most cases were caused by gram-negative enteric organisms, primarily *E coli;* gram-positive isolates were likely to be *L monocytogenes.* During the 1970s, group B β-hemolytic streptococci *(S agalactiae)* became prevalent; currently this organism and *E coli* account for 50% to 66% of cases of neonatal meningitis and *L monocytogenes* for approximately 1% to 5%.[82,83] Neonatal sepsis and meningitis caused by non–group D α-hemolytic streptococci and coagulase-negative staphylococci also have been reported. Group B β-hemolytic streptococci can cause sepsis or meningitis (or both) in the first hours of life; by definition, such infection at an age younger than 7 days is termed early onset. Late-onset disease—that is, group B β-hemolytic streptococcal infection at age older than 7 days—is characteristically meningitis rather than sepsis, and it tends to be associated with capsular serotype III organisms.[13,82] Antimicrobial prophylaxis of pregnant women found to be carrying group B β-hemolytic streptococci at term or those with fever, premature labor, or prolonged rupture of membranes is now performed in the United States, which has led to a decrease in the incidence of early-onset sepsis and meningitis.[13,14,61,82] However, late-onset meningitis rates remain unchanged, reflecting unique differences between these syndromes that remain not well understood.[13,14]

The clinical signs associated with neonatal meningitis are nonspecific and therefore not very helpful. Neonates with meningitis often have apneic episodes or feed poorly, and they can be hyperthermic or hypothermic, irritable or lethargic, and have respiratory distress or diarrhea (or both); only rarely do they have nuchal rigidity. They may exhibit a bulging fontanelle. The neonate has a limited repertoire of clinical responses to disease or insult; most sick neonates therefore receive a diagnostic evaluation for sepsis, including a lumbar puncture, and antimicrobial agents are initiated pending culture results. The cytology and chemistry of the CSF in neonates have a much broader normal range than children in other age groups, especially during the first week of life (Table 293-5); thus any single test result may not appear abnormal.[84,85] However, infants who have bacterial meningitis rarely have completely normal CSF at examination. During the first 24 hours of life, isolated meningitis without sepsis occurs rarely enough that lumbar puncture has sometimes been omitted for infants appearing septic on the day of birth. However, this practice may lead to missed cases of both early-onset and late-onset meningitis because as many as 25% of neonates with meningitis have been found to have sterile blood cultures despite positive CSF cultures,[86,87] and the proportion of such cases might rise as antibiotic prophylaxis is given to mothers and babies in the peripartum period. In general, if possible, any infant thought to have sepsis or meningitis should undergo lumbar puncture.[82]

Management of Neonatal Meningitis

Antimicrobial Therapy

The principles of antimicrobial therapy for neonatal meningitis are the same as those for infants and children, but because the organisms are different, the antimicrobial selection must be adjusted. Based on the most common organisms that cause neonatal meningitis, the ideal antimicrobial agent would be effective against *E coli* and other enteric organisms, as well as against group B

Table 293-5 Representative Cerebrospinal Fluid (CSF) Findings in Neonates Without Meningitis*

	FULL-TERM NEONATES MEAN (RANGE)		PRETERM NEONATES MEAN (RANGE)	
CSF FINDING	**0-7 DAYS**	**8-28 DAYS**	**0-7 DAYS**	**8-28 DAYS**
Leukocytes/mcL	8 (1-30)	6 (0-18)	4 (1-10)	7 (0-44)
Polymorphonuclear neutrophils (% of leukocytes)	5	3	7	9
Protein (mg/dL)	81	64	150 (85-222)	148 (54-370)
Glucose (mg/dL)	46	51	72 (4-96)	64 (33-217)
CSF/blood glucose (%)	0.73	0.62	Not reported	Not reported

*Data from Ahmed A, Hickey SM, Ehrett S, et al. Cerebrospinal fluid values in the term neonate. *Pediatr Infect Dis J.* 1996;15:298-303; Rodriguez AF, Kaplan SL, Mason EO Jr. Cerebrospinal fluid values in the very low birth weight infant. *J Pediatr.* 1990;116:971-974.

β-hemolytic streptococci and other gram-positive organisms. Two third-generation cephalosporins—cefotaxime and ceftriaxone—are extremely active against the organisms that usually cause neonatal meningitis, except for poor activity against *L monocytogenes*. The major difference between these drugs is their pharmacokinetic profile; ceftriaxone exhibits a much longer serum half-life than cefotaxime. In addition, because ceftriaxone is highly protein bound and can displace unconjugated bilirubin from albumin, it is generally not used in premature infants at risk for kernicterus or in term infants who have hyperbilirubinemia.

No formal comparison of these newer agents with the historical regimen of ampicillin plus an aminoglycoside such as gentamicin has taken place. However, because the third-generation cephalosporins are safe, are very active against the common pathogens, and enter the CSF relatively well, cefotaxime plus ampicillin (the latter to empirically treat *Listeria*) should be used to treat suspected neonatal meningitis (suspected disease plus abnormal CSF). Some authorities would add gentamicin as a third agent if gram-negative enteric meningitis were thought likely. Because some enteric pathogens such as *Pseudomonas aeruginosa* and Enterobacteriaceae readily become resistant to the third-generation cephalosporins, these antibiotics should not be used empirically for all cases of suspected sepsis in neonates (the choice of empiric ampicillin with gentamicin remains appropriate in this situation when the CSF appears normal). Dosages and characteristics of the antimicrobials used most often to treat neonatal meningitis are listed in Table 293-4.

Fluid and Antiinflammatory Therapy, and Supportive Care

The role of intraventricular antimicrobial therapy remains uncertain and may even be harmful.[82] Other therapeutic considerations (eg, fluid management, close serial monitoring) are the same for neonates as for infants and children who have bacterial meningitis, except that no data support the use of dexamethasone in infants younger than 6 weeks.[61] The head circumference should be measured serially to detect early signs of hydrocephalus. Conflicting data have been reported regarding whether intravenous immunoglobulin is helpful; at present, it does not have a defined role in the therapy of neonatal bacterial meningitis.

Prognosis

The complications of neonatal meningitis, which are similar to those seen among older infants but are perhaps more common, include hydrocephalus, deafness, and blindness. The case fatality rate is 20% to 25% in general but may approach 50% in low–birth-weight infants with gram-negative enteric meningitis. Approximately 65% of survivors of coliform meningitis are normal 3 to 7 years after the illness, approximately 15% to 30% have mild to moderate neurologic sequelae, and 5% to 10% have major sequelae.[17,83,88,89] Approximately 50% of cases of group B β-hemolytic streptococcal meningitis survivors are normal, 20% have mild to moderate sequelae, and 15% to 30% have major sequelae (ie, hydrocephalus, seizures, profound retardation).[17,82,88,89]

For unknown reasons, as many as 80% of neonates who have gram-negative enteric meningitis caused by either *Citrobacter* or certain *Enterobacter* species will develop single or multiple brain abscesses. This complication is distinctly unusual in meningitis caused by any other organism. Routine follow-up with cranial CT scans is indicated for neonates with meningitis or sepsis caused by *Citrobacter* species or *Enterobacter sakazakii*. As with older infants and children, all infants recovering from meningitis should have careful audiologic testing and close evaluation for attainment of developmental milestones.

PARTIALLY TREATED MENINGITIS

Values for WBC counts in CSF, percentage of polymorphonuclear cells, and glucose and protein concentrations in patients who have partially treated bacterial meningitis do not greatly differ from those in patients who were not previously treated.[1,33] Even children who have received intravenous antibiotics for 44 to 68 hours have CSF findings still characteristic of bacterial meningitis.[1,33] Cultures of CSF from pretreated children with bacterial meningitis frequently grow Hib, although pneumococci and meningococci grow less often after pretreatment.[1,33] However, some patients who have partially treated bacterial meningitis will have CSF findings indistinguishable from the classic findings of aseptic meningitis. Unless clear evidence of a nonbacterial cause exists (eg, isolation of virus from CSF or blood), antibiotics should be administered to partially treated patients for 7 to 10 days at doses appropriate for bacterial meningitis.[1,33]

ASEPTIC MENINGITIS

The syndrome of aseptic meningitis consists of a clinical picture of meningitis with CSF pleocytosis and the absence of bacteria on gram stain or culture. The CSF findings characteristic of aseptic meningitis are shown in Table 293-1. Although aseptic meningitis is usually caused by a virus, treatable causes of this syndrome should be considered in the differential diagnosis. Table 293-3 lists a wide variety of infectious and noninfectious agents and diseases that have been associated with aseptic meningitis. Nonpolio enteroviruses cause 85% of cases of aseptic meningitis in the United States, but mumps and polio should be considered in other areas of the world where they are still endemic. A longer duration of symptoms, especially if accompanied by erythema migrans or cranial neuropathies, has been associated with Lyme disease meningitis.[90] West Nile virus infection may cause aseptic meningitis, meningoencephalitis, or acute flaccid paralysis.[91,92] In general, when encephalitis accompanies aseptic meningitis, the clinical course is more severe, and the chance of sequelae increases (see Chapter 294, Meningoencephalitis).

Clinical Manifestations

Infants and children who have aseptic meningitis caused by enteroviruses are often acutely febrile, irritable, and lethargic. Their temperature is usually 38.0°C to 40.5°C (100.4°F to 105°F) for 4 to 5 days. Upper respiratory tract symptoms, headache, photophobia, nausea, and vomiting also are commonly present; rashes may be seen as well. In general, a child who has viral meningitis does not appear as critically ill as a child who has bacterial meningitis and is less likely to have meningeal signs.[5,33,48,93]

The diagnosis of aseptic meningitis is likely when CSF pleocytosis ranges from 10 to 500 cells/mcL that are predominantly lymphocytes; the CSF protein is mildly high, at 50 to 150 mg/dL; and the CSF glucose concentration is normal. Early in the course of viral meningitis, polymorphonuclear neutrophils can predominate in the CSF. A transition from a predominance of polymorphonuclear neutrophils to lymphocytes usually occurs rapidly, and a repeat lumbar puncture after 8 to 12 hours may show this transition.[94,95] Tuberculous and fungal meningitis generally have gradual onsets of illness over days to weeks.

Hypoglycorrhachia (low CSF glucose level) rarely occurs with viral meningitis caused by enteroviruses, mumps, herpes simplex, and Eastern equine encephalitis viruses. Hypoglycorrhachia caused by these viruses tends to result in CSF glucose concentrations that equal approximately 30% of the simultaneous blood glucose concentration, whereas bacterial meningitis usually results in CSF glucose concentrations of less than 30% of the blood glucose. The CSF glucose concentration can also be low with tuberculous and fungal meningitis.

Many physicians are reluctant to obtain specimens for viral culture because they believe that isolating viruses takes too long to affect patient management. Almost one half of the patients with aseptic meningitis, whose CSF specimens were sent promptly at admission for viral culture, had enteroviral meningitis.[96] Approximately 4 days are required for CSF cultures to show a typical enterovirus cytopathic effect. The diagnosis of enteroviral meningitis frequently results in discontinuation of antimicrobial therapy and early discharge from the hospital. Therefore, when viral meningitis is a possibility, the CSF should be cultured for viruses, as should nasopharyngeal or throat and rectal swab specimens. Although isolation of a virus from a site other than the CSF can be misleading, if taken in the context of other clinical and laboratory findings, then a presumptive diagnosis can often be made when a virus is isolated from one or more of these sites.

The polymerase chain reaction (PCR) holds much promise as a rapid and sensitive method of diagnosing meningitis caused by enteroviruses, herpesviruses, and perhaps other viruses as well. PCR amplification of enteroviral RNA from CSF and serum appears to have good sensitivity, specificity, and predictive value.[97-99] The technique will likely continue to be studied for the diagnosis of several other causes of aseptic meningitis.[100-102] Where PCR for enterovirus is available, it may substitute for viral culture in many cases.[103]

Management

The management of aseptic meningitis is directed mainly to supportive care. An antienteroviral agent, pleconaril, has been evaluated in both adults and children with enteroviral meningitis[104]; this or other similar drugs may be useful in the future, but the clinical development of pleconaril has been halted at present. Meningoencephalitis caused by herpes simplex or varicella-zoster viruses should be treated with acyclovir. Aseptic meningitis caused by one of the other less common causes noted in Table 293-3 may also require specific therapy.

Outcome

The outcome of aseptic meningitis relates to both the causative agent and the child's age. Patients who have the most common known cause of viral meningitis—enteroviral meningitis—usually recover completely.[105,106] However, some studies[107-109] have reported low intelligence and delayed speech development after enteroviral meningitis in very young infants. In light of these findings, the prognosis for an infant younger than 3 months of age is somewhat guarded, and the child's development should be monitored carefully.

WHEN TO REFER

- All patients with bacterial meningitis should be treated in consultation with pediatric infectious diseases subspecialists, and pediatric neurologic, critical care, and neurosurgical subspecialists should be available if required.
- Patients with viral meningitis may be managed by the primary care physician, unless unusual features or complications are present (eg, immune compromise, unexpected severity, slow resolution of illness, possibility of nonviral aseptic meningitis, etc.).
- Patients with neonatal meningitis should be referred to pediatric infectious diseases, newborn medicine, and neurologic subspecialists.

WHEN TO ADMIT

All patients with suspected or proven meningitis should be hospitalized for evaluation and management.

- Patients with bacterial meningitis initially hospitalized at the referral hospital should be transferred to a facility experienced in the management of critically ill children, with availability of consultation by pediatric critical care, infectious diseases, neurologic, and neurosurgical subspecialists, which is especially important for newborns with neonatal meningitis. Treatment must begin at the referral hospital, however.
- Infants and toddlers with viral meningitis may continue to be hospitalized at the primary care level hospital; transfer to a referral facility may be required for complicated cases (eg, uncertainty in diagnosis, slow resolution, presence of immune compromise, etc.).
- Older children and adolescents with viral meningitis do not always require hospitalization if the CSF evaluation strongly suggests that bacterial disease is not present, if adequate hydration and pain control can be undertaken at home, and if follow-up with the physician can be assured.

REFERENCES

1. Bonadio WA. The cerebrospinal fluid: physiologic aspects and alterations associated with bacterial meningitis. *Pediatr Infect Dis J.* 1992;11:423-431.
2. Tunkel AR, Hartman BJ, Kaplan SL, et al. Practice guidelines for the management of bacterial meningitis. *Clin Infect Dis.* 2004;39:1267-1284.
3. Sáez-Llorens X, McCracken GH Jr. Bacterial meningitis in children. *Lancet.* 2003;361:2139-2148.
4. Yogev R, Guzman-Cottrill J. Bacterial meningitis in children: critical review of current concepts. *Drugs.* 2005; 65:1097-1112.
5. Feigin RD, McCracken GH Jr, Klein JO. Diagnosis and management of meningitis. *Pediatr Infect Dis J.* 1992; 11:785-814.
6. Adams WG, Deaver KA, Cochi SL, et al. Decline of childhood *Haemophilus influenzae* type b (Hib) disease in the Hib vaccine era. *JAMA.* 1993;269:221-226.
7. Bisgard KM, Kao A, Leake J, et al. *Haemophilus influenzae* invasive disease in the United States, 1994-1995: near disappearance of a vaccine-preventable childhood disease. *Emerg Infect Dis.* 1998;4:229-237.
8. Murphy TV, White KE, Pastor P, et al. Declining incidence of *Haemophilus influenzae* type b disease since introduction of vaccination. *JAMA.* 1993;269:246-248.
9. Peltola H. Worldwide *Haemophilus influenzae* type b disease at the beginning of the 21st century: global analysis of the disease burden 25 years after the use of the polysaccharide vaccine and a decade after the advent of conjugates. *Clin Microbiol Rev.* 2000;12:302-317.
10. Centers for Disease Control and Prevention. Progress toward eliminating *Haemophilus influenzae* type b disease among infants and children—United States, 1988-2000. *MMWR Morb Mortal Wkly Rep.* 2002;51: 234-237.
11. Centers for Disease Control and Prevention. Active Bacterial Core Surveillance Reports, Emerging Infections Program Network, 2005. Available at: www.cdc.gov/ncidod/dbmd/abcs/survreports.htm. Accessed October 11, 2007.
12. Schuchat A, Robinson K, Wenger JD, et al. Bacterial meningitis in the United States in 1995. *N Engl J Med.* 1997;337:970-976.
13. Centers for Disease Control and Prevention. Prevention of perinatal group B streptococcal disease. *MMWR Morb Mortal Wkly Rep.* 2002;51(RR-11):1-22.
14. Centers for Disease Control and Prevention. Diminishing racial disparities in early-onset neonatal group B streptococcal disease—United States, 2000-2003. *MMWR Morb Mortal Wkly Rep.* 2004;53:502-505.
15. Centers for Disease Control and Prevention. Early-onset and late-onset neonatal group B streptococcal disease—United States, 1996-2004. *MMWR Morb Mortal Wkly Rep.* 2005;54:1205-1208.
16. Schrag SJ, Zywicki S, Farley MM, et al. Group B streptococcal disease in the era of intrapartum antibiotic prophylaxis. *N Engl J Med.* 2000;342:15-20.
17. Sáez-Llorens X, McCracken GH Jr. Perinatal bacterial diseases. In: Feigin RD, Cherry JD, Demmler GJ, et al, eds. *Textbook of Pediatric Infectious Diseases.* 5th ed. Philadelphia, PA: WB Saunders; 2004.
18. American Academy of Pediatrics, Committee on Infectious Diseases. Policy statement: recommendations for the prevention of pneumococcal infections, including the use of pneumococcal conjugate vaccine (Prevnar), pneumococcal polysaccharide vaccine, and antibiotic prophylaxis. *Pediatrics.* 2000;106(pt 2):362-366.
19. Centers for Disease Control and Prevention. Preventing pneumococcal disease among infants and young children: recommendations of the Advisory Committee on Immunization Practices (ACIP). *MMWR Morb Mortal Wkly Rep.* 2000;49(RR-9):1-35.
20. Black S, Shinefield H, Baxter R, et al. Postlicensure surveillance for pneumococcal invasive disease after use of heptavalent pneumococcal conjugate vaccine in Northern California—Kaiser Permanente. *Pediatr Infect Dis J.* 2004;23:485-489.
21. Whitney CG, Farley MM, Hadler J, et al. Decline in invasive pneumococcal disease after the introduction of protein-polysaccharide conjugate vaccine. *N Engl J Med.* 2003;348:1737-1746.
22. American Academy of Pediatrics. Prevention and control of meningococcal disease: recommendations for use of meningococcal vaccines in pediatric patients. *Pediatrics.* 2005;116:496-505.
23. Centers for Disease Control and Prevention. Prevention and control of meningococcal disease: recommendations of the Advisory Committee on Immunization Practices (ACIP). *MMWR Morb Mortal Wkly Rep.* 2005; 54(RR-7):1-21.
24. Miller E, Salisbury D, Ramsay M. Planning, registration, and implementation of an immunization campaign against meningococcal serogroup C disease in the UK: a success story. *Vaccine.* 2002;20(suppl 1): S58-S67.
25. MacLennan JM, Shackley F, Heath PT, et al. Safety, immunogenicity, and induction of immunologic memory by a serogroup C meningococcal conjugate vaccine in infants: a randomized controlled trial. *JAMA.* 2000; 283:2795-2801.
26. Murphy TV, Granoff D, Chrane DF, et al. Pharyngeal colonization with *Haemophilus influenzae* type b in children in a day care center without invasive disease. *J Pediatr.* 1985;106:712-716.
27. Quagliarello VJ, Scheld WM. Bacterial meningitis: pathogenesis, pathophysiology, and progress. *N Engl J Med.* 1992;327:864-872.
28. Quagliarello VJ, Scheld WM. New perspectives on bacterial meningitis. *Clin Infect Dis.* 1993;17:603-608.
29. [No author listed]. Case Records of the Massachusetts General Hospital. Case 40-2001. *N Engl J Med.* 2001; 345:1901-1907.
30. Biernath KR, Reefhuis J, Whitney CG, et al. Bacterial meningitis among children with cochlear implants beyond 24 months after implantation. *Pediatrics.* 2006; 117:284-289.
31. Reefhuis J, Honein MA, Whitney CG, et al. Bacterial meningitis in children with cochlear implants. *N Engl J Med.* 2003;349:435-445.
32. Tauber MG, Moser B. Cytokines and chemokines in meningeal inflammation: biological and clinical implications. *Clin Infect Dis.* 1999;28:1-11.
33. Feigin RD, Pearlman E. Bacterial meningitis beyond the neonatal period. In: Feigin RD, Cherry JD, Demmler GJ, et al, eds. *Textbook of Pediatric Infectious Diseases.* 5th ed. Philadelphia, PA: WB Saunders; 2004.
34. Gavin PJ, Kazacos KR, Shulman ST. Baylisascariasis. *Clin Microbiol Rev.* 2005;18:703-718.
35. Hsu W-Y, Chen JY, Chien CT, et al. Eosinophilic meningitis caused by *Angiostrongylus cantonensis. Pediatr Infect Dis J.* 1990;9:443-445.
36. Miron D, Snelling LK, Josephson SL, et al. Eosinophilic meningitis in a newborn with group B streptococcal infection. *Pediatr Infect Dis J.* 1993;12:966-967.
37. Slom TJ, Cortese MM, Gerber SI, et al. An outbreak of eosinophilic meningitis caused by *Angiostrongylus cantonensis. N Engl J Med.* 2002;346:668-675.

38. Woods CR, Englund J. Congenital toxoplasmosis presenting with eosinophilic meningitis. *Pediatr Infect Dis J*. 1993;12:347-348.
39. Lipton JD, Schafermeyer RW. Evolving concepts in pediatric bacterial meningitis. I. Pathophysiology and diagnosis. II. Current management and therapeutic research. *Ann Emerg Med*. 1993;22:1602-1615, 1616-1629.
40. Stein MT, Trauner D. The child with a stiff neck. *Clin Pediatr*. 1982;21:559.
41. Tunkel AR, Scheld WM. Acute bacterial meningitis. *Lancet*. 1995;346:1675-1680.
42. Verghese A, Gallemore G. Kernig's and Brudzinski's signs revisited. *Rev Infect Dis*. 1987;9:1187-1192.
43. Thomas KE, Hasbun R, Jekel J, et al. The diagnostic accuracy of Kernig's sign, Brudzinski's sign, and nuchal rigidity in adults with suspected meningitis. *Clin Infect Dis*. 2002;35:46-52.
44. van de Beek D, de Gans J, Tunkel AR, et al. Community-acquired bacterial meningitis in adults. *N Engl J Med*. 2006;354:44-53.
45. Geisler PJ, Nelson KE. Bacterial meningitis in children without clinical signs of meningeal irritation. *South Med J*. 1982;75:448-450.
46. Durand ML, Calderwood SB, Weber DJ, et al. Acute bacterial meningitis in adults. A review of 493 episodes. *N Engl J Med*. 1993;328:21-28.
47. Sigurdardottir B, Bjornsson OM, Jonsdottir KE, et al. Acute bacterial meningitis in adults: a 20-year overview. *Arch Intern Med*. 1997;157:425-430.
48. Walsh-Kelly C, Nelson DB, Smith DS, et al. Clinical predictors of bacterial versus aseptic meningitis in childhood. *Ann Emerg Med*. 1992;21:910-914.
49. Rodewald LE, Woodin KA, Szilagyi PG, et al. Relevance of common tests of cerebrospinal fluid in screening for bacterial meningitis. *J Pediatr*. 1991;119:363-369.
50. Ellenby MS, Tegtmeyer K, Lai S, et al. Lumbar puncture. *N Engl J Med*. 2006;355:e12-e15.
51. Perkins MD, Mirrett S, Reller LB. Rapid bacterial antigen detection is not clinically useful. *J Clin Microbiol*. 1995;33:1486-1491.
52. American Academy of Pediatrics. Practice parameter: the neurodiagnostic evaluation of the child with a first simple febrile seizure. *Pediatrics*. 1996;97:769-775.
53. Friedland IR, Paris MM, Rinderknecht S, et al. Cranial computed tomographic scans have little impact on management of bacterial meningitis. *Am J Dis Child*. 1992; 146:1484-1487.
54. Odio CM, Faingezicht I, Paris M, et al. The beneficial effects of early dexamethasone administration in infants and children with bacterial meningitis. *N Engl J Med*. 1991;324:1525-1531.
55. Schaad UB, Lips U, Gnehm HE, et al. Dexamethasone therapy for bacterial meningitis in children. *Lancet*. 1993;342:457-461.
56. Powell KR, Sugarman LI, Eskenazi AI, et al. Normalization of plasma arginine vasopressin concentrations when children with meningitis are given maintenance plus replacement fluid therapy. *J Pediatr*. 1990;117: 515-522.
57. Lebel MH, Freij BJ, Syrogiannopoulos GA. Dexamethasone therapy for bacterial meningitis: results of two double-blind, placebo-controlled trials. *N Engl J Med*. 1988;319:964-971.
58. Wald ER, Kaplan SL, Mason EO Jr, et al. Dexamethasone therapy for children with bacterial meningitis. *Pediatrics*. 1995;95:21-28.
59. Molyneux EM, Walsh AL, Forsyth H, et al. Dexamethasone treatment in bacterial meningitis in Malawi: a randomized controlled trial. *Lancet*. 2002;360:211-218.
60. Quagliarello VJ, Scheld WM. Treatment of bacterial meningitis. *N Engl J Med*. 1997;336:708-716.
61. American Academy of Pediatrics. In: Pickering LK, Baker CJ, Long SS, ed. *Red Book 2006: Report of the Committee on Infectious Diseases*, 27th ed. Elk Grove Village, IL: American Academy of Pediatrics; 2006.
62. Kleiman MB, Weinberg GA, Reynolds JK, et al. Meningitis with beta-lactam-resistant *Streptococcus pneumoniae:* the need for early repeat lumbar puncture. *Pediatr Infect Dis J*. 1993;12:782-784.
63. Bradley JS, Connor JD. Ceftriaxone failure in meningitis caused by *Streptococcus pneumoniae* with reduced susceptibility to beta-lactam antibiotics. *Pediatr Infect Dis J*. 1991;10:871-873.
64. Tan TQ, Mason EO Jr, Kaplan SL. Systemic infections due to *Streptococcus pneumoniae* relatively resistant to penicillin in a children's hospital: clinical management and outcome. *Pediatrics*. 1992;90:928-933.
65. Jadavji T, Bigger WD, Gold R, et al. Sequelae of acute bacterial meningitis in children treated for seven days. *Pediatrics*. 1986;78:21-25.
66. Lin TY, Chrane DF, Nelson JD. Seven days of ceftriaxone therapy is as effective as 10 days' treatment for bacterial meningitis. *JAMA*. 1985;253:3559-3563.
67. Kaplan SL, Mason EO Jr. Management of infections due to antibiotic-resistant *Streptococcus pneumoniae*. *Clin Microbiol Rev*. 1998;11:628-644.
68. D'Angio CT, Froehlke RG, Plank GA, et al. Long-term outcome of *Haemophilus influenzae* meningitis in Navajo Indian children. *Arch Pediatr Adolesc Med*. 1995;149: 1001-1008.
69. Dodge PR, Davis H, Feigin RD, et al. Prospective evaluation of hearing impairment as a sequelae of acute bacterial meningitis. *N Engl J Med*. 1984;311:869-874.
70. Grimwood K, Anderson VA, Bond L. Adverse outcomes of bacterial meningitis in school-age survivors. *Pediatrics*. 1995;95:646-656.
71. Pomeroy SL, Holmes SJ, Dodge PR, et al. Seizures and other neurologic sequelae of bacterial meningitis in children. *N Engl J Med*. 1990;323:1651-1657.
72. Taylor HG, Mills EL, Ciampi A, et al. The sequelae of *Haemophilus influenzae* meningitis in school-age children. *N Engl J Med*. 1990;323:1657-1663.
73. Richardson MP, Williamson TJ, Reid A, et al. Otoacoustic emissions as a screening test for hearing impairment in children recovering from acute bacterial meningitis. *Pediatrics*. 1998;102:1364-1368.
74. Kallio MJ, Kilpi T, Anttila M, et al. The effect of a recent previous visit to a physician on outcome after childhood bacterial meningitis. *JAMA*. 1994;272:787-791.
75. Kilpi T, Attila M, Kallio MJ, et al. Length of prediagnostic history related to the course and sequelae of childhood bacterial meningitis. *Pediatr Infect Dis J*. 1993;12:184-188.
76. Radetsky M. Duration of symptoms and outcome in bacterial meningitis: an analysis of causation and the implications of a delay in diagnosis. *Pediatr Infect Dis J*. 1992;11:694-698.
77. Robbins JB, Schneerson R, Anderson P, et al. Prevention of systemic infections, especially meningitis, caused by *Haemophilus influenzae* type b: impact on public health and implications for other polysaccharide-based vaccines. *JAMA*. 1996;276:1181-1185.
78. Weinberg GA, Granoff DM. Polysaccharide-protein conjugate vaccines for the prevention of *Haemophilus influenzae* type b disease. *J Pediatr*. 1988;113:621-631.
79. Weinberg GA, Granoff DM. Immunogenicity of *Haemophilus influenzae* type b polysaccharide-protein conjugate vaccines in children with conditions associated with impaired antibody responses to type b polysaccharide vaccine. *Pediatrics*. 1990; 85:654-661.

80. Black S, Shinefield H, Fireman B, et al. Efficacy, safety, and immunogenicity of heptavalent pneumococcal conjugate vaccine in children. *Pediatr Infect Dis J.* 2000; 19:187-195.
81. Poehling KA, Lafleur BJ, Szilagyi PG, et al. Population-based impact of pneumococcal conjugate vaccine in young children. *Pediatrics.* 2004;114:755-761.
82. Palazzi DL, Klein JO, Baker CJ. Bacterial sepsis and meningitis. In: Remington JS, Klein JO, Wilson CB, et al, eds. *Infectious Diseases of the Fetus and Newborn Infant.* 5th ed. Philadelphia, PA: Elsevier WB Saunders; 2006.
83. Unhanand M, Mustafa MM, McCracken GH Jr, et al. Gram-negative enteric bacillary meningitis: a twenty-one-year experience. *J Pediatr.* 1993;122:15-21.
84. Ahmed A, Hickey SM, Ehrett S, et al. Cerebrospinal fluid values in the term neonate. *Pediatr Infect Dis J.* 1996;15:298-303.
85. Rodriguez AF, Kaplan SL, Mason EO Jr. Cerebrospinal fluid values in the very low birth weight infant. *J Pediatr.* 1990;116:971-974.
86. Stoll BJ, Hansen N, Fanaroff AA, et al. To tap or not to tap: high likelihood of meningitis without sepsis among very low birth weight infants. *Pediatrics.* 2004;113: 1181-1186.
87. Wiswell TE, Baumgart S, Gannon CM, et al. No lumbar puncture for early neonatal sepsis: will meningitis be missed? *Pediatrics.* 1995;95:803-806.
88. Franco SM, Cornelius VE, Andrews BF. Long-term outcome of neonatal meningitis. *Am J Dis Child.* 1992; 146:567-571.
89. Stevens JP, Eames M, Kent A, et al. Long term outcome of neonatal meningitis. *Arch Dis Child Fetal Neonatal Ed.* 2003;88:F179-F184.
90. Eppes SC, Nelson DK, Lewis LL, et al. Characterization of Lyme meningitis and comparison with viral meningitis in children. *Pediatrics.* 1999;103:957-960.
91. Cunha B. Differential diagnosis of West Nile encephalitis. *Curr Opin Infect Dis.* 2004:17;413-420.
92. Gea-Banacloche J, Johnson RT, Bagic A, et al. West Nile virus: pathogenesis and therapeutic options (NIH Conference). *Ann Intern Med.* 2004;140;545-553.
93. Cherry JD, Nielsen KA. Aseptic meningitis and viral meningitis. In: Feigin RD, Cherry JD, Demmler GJ, Kaplan SL, eds. *Textbook of Pediatric Infectious Diseases.* 5th ed. Philadelphia, PA: WB Saunders; 2004.
94. Amir J, Harel L, Frydman M, et al. Shift of cerebrospinal polymorphonuclear cell percentage in the early stage of aseptic meningitis. *J Pediatr.* 1991:119:938-941.
95. Feigin RD, Shackelford PG. Value of repeat lumbar puncture in the differential diagnosis of meningitis. *N Engl J Med.* 1973;289:571-574.
96. Chonmaitree T, Menegus MA, Powell KR. The clinical relevance of CSF viral culture: a 2-year experience with aseptic meningitis in Rochester, NY. *JAMA.* 1982:247: 1843-1847.
97. Ahmed A, Brito F, Goto C, et al. Clinical utility of the polymerase chain reaction for diagnosis of enteroviral meningitis in infancy. *J Pediatr.* 1997;131:393-397.
98. Rotbart HA. Diagnosis of enteroviral meningitis with the polymerase chain reaction. *J Pediatr.* 1990;117: 85-89.
99. Schlesinger Y, Sawyer MH, Storch GA. Enteroviral meningitis in infancy: potential role for polymerase chain reaction in patient management. *Pediatrics.* 1994; 94:157-162.
100. Huang C, Chatterjee NK, Grady LJ. Diagnosis of viral infections of the central nervous system. *N Engl J Med.* 1999;340:483-484.
101. Jeffery KJM, Read SJ, Peto TE, et al. Diagnosis of viral infections of the central nervous system: clinical interpretation of PCR results. *Lancet.* 1997;349: 313-317.
102. Read SJ, Jeffery KJM, Bangham CRM. Aseptic meningitis and encephalitis: the role of PCR in the diagnostic laboratory. *J Clin Microbiol.* 1997;35:691-696.
103. Ramers C, Billman G, Hartin M, et al. Impact of a diagnostic cerebrospinal fluid enterovirus polymerase chain reaction test on patient management. *JAMA.* 2000;283: 2680-2685.
104. Desmond RA, Accortt NA, Talley L, et al. Enteroviral meningitis: natural history and outcome of pleconaril therapy. *Antimicrob Agents Chemother.* 2006;50: 2409-2414.
105. Rorabaugh ML, Berlin LE, Heldrich F, et al. Aseptic meningitis in infants younger than 2 years of age: acute illness and neurologic complications. *Pediatrics.* 1993; 92:206-211.
106. Rotbart HA. Enteroviral infections of the central nervous system. *Clin Infect Dis.* 1995;20:971-981.
107. Farmer K, MacArthur BA, Clay MM. A follow-up study of 15 cases of neonatal meningoencephalitis due to Coxsackie virus B5. *J Pediatr.* 1975; 87:568-571.
108. Sells CJ, Carpenter RL, Ray CG. Sequelae of central nervous system enterovirus infections. *N Engl J Med.* 1975;293:1-4.
109. Wilfert CM, Thompson RJ Jr, Sunder TR, et al. Longitudinal assessment of children with enteroviral meningitis during the first 3 months of life. *Pediatrics.* 1981;67: 811-815.

Chapter 294

MENINGOENCEPHALITIS

Richard S. K. Young, MD, MPH

Infections of the meninges and underlying brain parenchyma can be differentiated into septic and aseptic categories. The former is traditionally termed *bacterial meningitis* and is characterized by high fever, coma, and purulent cerebrospinal fluid (CSF). The latter category consists of aseptic meningitis and encephalitis. These infections are most often caused by viruses; but they are occasionally caused by parasites, spirochetes, rickettsia, and prions.

Depending on the extent of the infection, the patient may have signs and symptoms of meningitis, encephalitis, or myelitis. A patient who has meningitis characteristically experiences intense headache, pain on flexion of the neck, and photophobia. Physical findings include fever and meningismus, with positive Kernig and Brudzinski signs (see Chapter 293, Meningitis). In patients with encephalitis, mental status changes such as lethargy, delirium, or hallucinations may be mistakenly attributed to intoxication or psychosis. A central nervous system (CNS) infection should be presumed in any child with a fever who has an acute change in mental status.

VIRUSES

Enteroviruses

Enteroviruses are a common cause of aseptic meningitis in infants and may also cause encephalitis.[1,2] Enteroviral infection is usually heralded by the development of malaise and gastroenteritis, and it occurs most often during the summer (see Chapter 260, Enterovirus Infections). Nonpolio enteroviruses include coxsackieviruses A and B and echoviruses. Progression to meningoencephalitis is uncommon with most enteroviral infections. When meningoencephalitis does occur, it is usually a mild, self-limited disease. Echovirus infections commonly begin with a petechial rash. Coxsackievirus infections may be heralded by lesions of the palms, soles, and mouth (hand, foot, and mouth disease) (Figure 294-1). An enterovirus may infect a fetus transplacentally.

Cases of polio in the United States now occur primarily in immigrant children, immunodeficient children, or among small communities of unimmunized children.[3] Polio continues to cause epidemics in developing countries where clean water and sewage treatment facilities are lacking.[4]

Herpesvirus

Herpes simplex virus (HSV) encephalitis has a bimodal age distribution, with one third of cases occurring in childhood. In the neonate, HSV may produce cutaneous disease, meningoencephalitis, or disseminated disease. Neonatal infection results from passage through an infected birth canal. HSV commonly produces a necrotizing encephalitis, and 50% to 70% of untreated cases are fatal. Two thirds of patients who survive will have neurologic sequelae. Mothers of infected infants often have no symptoms of herpes infection during or before gestation, which makes the diagnosis of a neonatal infection more difficult.

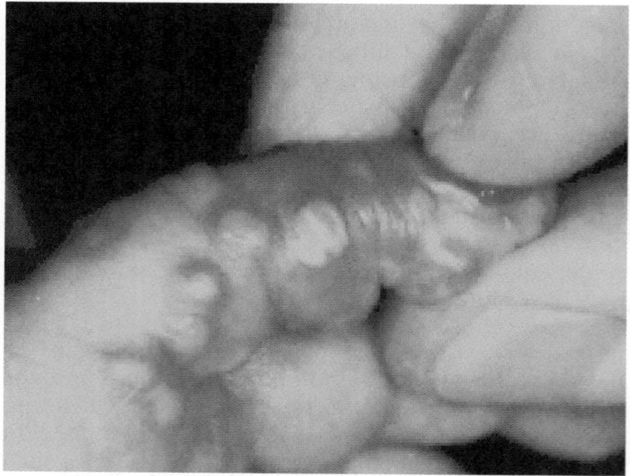

Figure 294-1 Coxsackievirus infections may be heralded by lesions of the palms, soles, and mouth (hand, foot, and mouth disease).

Treatment with acyclovir for a minimum of 15 days is suggested to prevent relapses of HSV encephalitis.[5] The polymerase chain reaction (PCR) test may be falsely negative in 25% of infants with neonatal HSV.[6] For more information, see Chapter 274, Herpes Infections.

Infections with human herpesvirus (HHV)-6 and -7 are accompanied by fever and rash, and occur primarily in children. The seropositivity rate of 6-year-old children is 80%. HHV-6 may occasionally cause meningitis in infants.[7] HHV-6 DNA has been detected in CSF in a minority of children with recurrent febrile seizure.

Nervous system infection with the Epstein-Barr virus may result in involvement of the cortex, cerebellum, or cranial nerves. Neurologic manifestations include combative behavior, seizures, and headache.[8]

Arboviruses

Arboviral infections caused by *Bunyavirus* species and togavirus are transmitted to humans by arthropods. Arbovirus meningoencephalitis typically occurs in epidemics during the summer and early fall. California virus encephalitis should be suspected in any child in a known endemic region who has signs of fever and cerebrocortical dysfunction. The course is usually mild, with a fatality rate of less than 5%. Western equine encephalitis, an arboviral disease primarily of infancy, causes a more severe syndrome. Eastern equine encephalitis has a predilection for infants and young children and is usually fatal. St Louis encephalitis occurs most often in epidemic form and produces illness in adults more often than in children.

Other viral diseases may be transmitted by vectors. The virus that causes Colorado tick fever, a reovirus transmitted by rodent arthropods, produces a dengue-like illness in humans. Viral disease transmitted directly to humans from animals includes lymphocytic choriomeningitis (arenavirus), which is transmitted by infected laboratory or domestic rodents.

West Nile virus (WNV) is principally transmitted by *Culex* mosquitoes. It occurs mostly in older adults, but cases of intrauterine transmission and possible transmission through breastfeeding have occurred.[9] Mothers should continue breastfeeding even in areas with WNV transmission. A total of 2866 West Nile neuroinvasive cases were reported in 2003,[10] 8% of which were fatal. Cases of WNV encephalitis have been reported in children.[11] Although most women infected with WNV during pregnancy have delivered apparently healthy infants, an infant born to a mother infected at 27 weeks' gestation developed chorioretinitis and cystic encephalomalacia.[12] The risk for encephalitis increases with age and immunosuppression.

Congenital lymphocytic choriomeningitis mimics congenital toxoplasmosis or cytomegalovirus (CMV) infection with chorioretinopathy, hydrocephaly, or microcephaly.

Rabies

Rabies is transmitted by a bite, scratch, or droplet from an infected wild animal (eg, raccoon, bat) or an unimmunized domestic animal. Rabies has the highest case fatality of any infection and causes an estimated 50,000 deaths worldwide, frequently in children who are bitten by rabid dogs. In the United States, however, rabies infections in children have been attributed most often to rabid bats, raccoons, and cats.

Rabies characteristically has a long incubation period and invariably produces meningoencephalitis. All but 1 reported cases of rabies encephalitis have been fatal. The single survivor was a 15-year-old girl who received antiviral therapy while in an induced coma.[13] Rabies has been documented after transplants, as was the case when multiple individuals contracted rabies when tissue was transplanted from a teenager who had unknowingly been bitten by a rabid bat.[14]

Viruses Associated With Childhood Exanthems

Common childhood viral infections such as rubella, adenovirus, influenza, CMV, and Epstein-Barr virus (infectious mononucleosis) can occasionally cause meningoencephalitis. Measles viruses cause meningoencephalitis in approximately 1 in 1000 cases and within 4 to 7 days after onset of the rash. The severity of the neurologic illness (including irritability, drowsiness, and ataxia) does not appear to be related to the intensity of the systemic illness. In 2003, 56 confirmed measles cases were reported in the United States.[10] Mortality in patients with measles meningoencephalitis approximates 10%, and as many as one half of survivors may have neurologic sequelae.

An unusual syndrome of dementia and myoclonic seizures can develop in children of school age many years after measles infection or immunization. This disorder results from a persistent measles infection known as *subacute sclerosing panencephalitis* (SSPE) (Figure 294-2). A syndrome of subacute measles encephalitis has also been reported in immunosuppressed individuals.

Varicella-zoster virus (VZV) is a herpesvirus that causes chickenpox or herpes zoster (shingles) (Figure 294-3). Varicella may cause mild encephalitis or a focal cerebellitis with prominent ataxia. In the United States, more deaths occur as a complication of varicella infection than from all other disorders for which immunizations exist.

Rubella is a mild febrile exanthem of childhood with prominent arthralgia. As many as one half of individuals are asymptomatic. Infection during the 1st trimester of pregnancy may result in congenital rubella syndrome. Cases have declined from 57,686 in 1969 to 271 in 1999. Rubella in the United States now primarily affects infants born to foreign-born women.[15] A child affected with rubella in utero may be infectious for 12 months or more. Mumps meningoencephalitis is a mild illness that generally has a good prognosis. Mumps meningoencephalitis may occur without parotitis, before the appearance of parotitis, or after it has resolved.

AIDS

AIDS is caused by a retrovirus known as *human immunodeficiency virus*. AIDS is noteworthy for meningoencephalitides caused both by HIV and by unusual organisms such as *Toxoplasma gondii* or *Candida albicans* and Epstein-Barr virus. An estimated 1687 cases of HIV infection (not AIDS) in 33 states were reported in 2003.[10] The prevalence of AIDS is estimated at 9419 in children younger than 13 years.[16] More than 1 kind of organism, whether viral or bacterial, can be recovered in immunosuppressed patients who have AIDS.

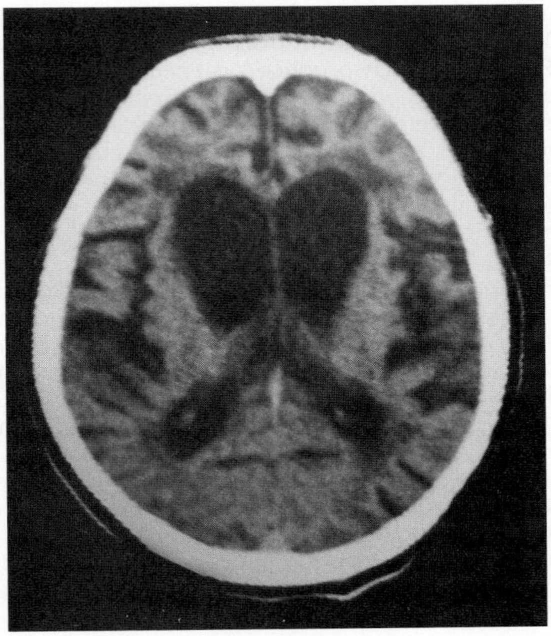

Figure 294-2 Subacute sclerosing panencephalitis (SSPE). Marked atrophy of both the cerebral cortex and the deep gray nuclei has occurred in this child, who has long-standing SSPE.

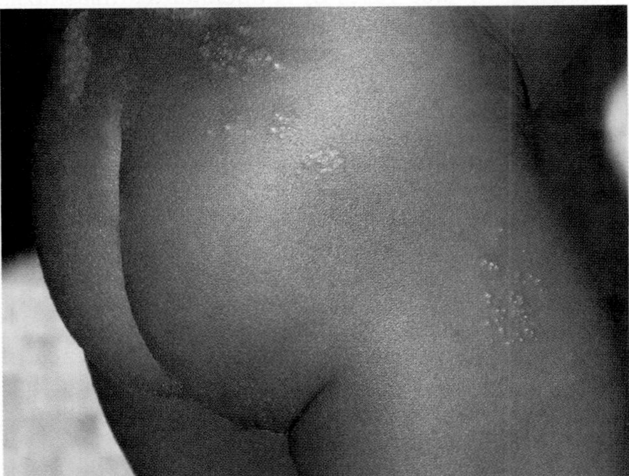

Figure 294-3 Varicella-zoster virus (VZV) is a herpesvirus that causes chickenpox or herpes zoster (shingles). This child received a VZV vaccination 2 months before eruption of herpes zoster.

Table 294-1 Typical Cerebrospinal Fluid Findings in Meningoencephalitis and Bacterial Meningitis

FINDING	VIRAL MENINGOENCEPHALITIS	BACTERIAL MENINGITIS
Leukocytes	Initial predominance of polymorphonuclear neutrophils, followed by shift to mononuclear cells	Predominantly neutrophils
	Range, 0-2000/mm³	Range, 0-200,000/mm³
Glucose	>50% of serum concentration	<30% of serum concentration
Protein	Mild-to-moderate increase	Marked increase
	Range, usually <200 mg/dL	Range, usually >150 mg/dL
Gram stain	Negative	Usually reveals bacteria

Fungi, Spirochetes, and Parasites

Nonviral causes of meningoencephalitis include infectious (fungi, spirochetes, and parasites) and noninfectious conditions associated with CSF pleocytosis (Table 294-1). Amebic meningoencephalitis may result from swimming in infected freshwater rivers or lakes infected with *Naegleria*. (See Chapter 305, Parasitic Infections.)

In 2003, 413 cases of congenital syphilis related to absent or late prenatal care were reported.[10] In many patients, a rash develops on the palms and soles. The rate has sharply declined in recent years. Congenital syphilis is more common in the southern United States, possibly because of the greater number of women with inadequate prenatal care.

The case fatality rate of Rocky Mountain spotted fever (RMSF) may be as high as 30%. RMSF is transmitted by *Dermacentor* species ticks. Notably, 81% of 16 patients with RMSF were children. In the summer of 2003, 3 fatal cases of RMSF were reported in children.[17]

Toxoplasmosis causes cerebral calcifications, microcephaly, and seizures resulting from transplacental infection by the protozoa *T gondii* to the fetus. An estimated 400 to 4000 cases of congenital toxoplasmosis occur each year transmitted to humans through ingestion of inadequately cooked meat or ingestion of oocysts from cat feces.[18]

Prions

The transmissible spongiform encephalopathies include kuru (children of the Fore tribe of New Guinea), bovine spongiform encephalopathy (BSE) (cattle), and Creutzfeldt-Jakob (CJ) disease (humans). New-variant CJ disease is related to BSE, which is endemic in the United Kingdom. Susceptibility to new-variant CJ disease may be highest in teenagers. Prohibition of beef products in cattle feed has reduced the incidence of both new-variant CJ disease and BSE. CJ disease has been transmitted to children through administration of cadaveric growth hormone.[19]

INCIDENCE

The actual incidence of meningoencephalitis is unknown. The Centers for Disease Control and Prevention tallied 2840 cases of arboviral encephalitis (367 children) in 2004.[10] An estimated 75,000 cases of aseptic meningitis occur annually.[20] The difficulty in identifying the specific agent in each suspected case makes precision impossible.

CLINICAL FEATURES

Most viruses spread via the bloodstream to the choroid plexus and from there to the brain parenchyma. Rabies and HSV travel in a retrograde manner via the peripheral nerves. The course of meningoencephalitis depends on the virulence of the organism. Typically, children with aseptic meningitis have intense headache, meningismus, and photophobia but a clear sensorium. In contrast, amoebae, fungi, and the viruses causing Eastern equine encephalitis, HSV, or rabies may cause cerebral or brain stem dysfunction, seizures, increased intracranial pressure, and death.

The presenting signs and symptoms produced by viruses are often protean and include fever, chills, myalgia, and headache. However, differences in seasonal occurrence, clinical course, and outcome allow differentiation of some disorders.

Encephalitis may produce focal neurologic findings. Herpes simplex encephalitis, for example, is classically heralded by temporal lobe seizures and olfactory hallucinations. VZV and Epstein-Barr virus may infect the cerebellum, producing an acute ataxia.[8] If spinal cord involvement is present, then the patient may have symmetrical limb paralysis, transverse sensory symptoms, and bowel and bladder dysfunction.

An important point to note is that viral infection of the CNS may be occult. CSF pleocytosis may or may not be present in meningoencephalitis. Only 50% of patients positive by PCR for enterovirus infection in CNS had pleocytosis in the CSF.[1] Conversely, 90% of children with facial nerve palsy caused by *Borrelia burgdorferi* had CSF pleocytosis or increased CSF protein, although none of them had meningeal signs.[21] In contrast, other children with Lyme disease may develop pseudotumor, radiculopathy, diplopia, headache, or meningismus. For every patient who is paralyzed by polio, 200 infected individuals may be excreting poliovirus in their stool.

DIFFERENTIAL DIAGNOSIS

Because laboratory tests require time to establish the diagnosis of meningoencephalitis, the clinician must consider the differential diagnosis carefully. Metabolic encephalopathy resulting from Reye syndrome or from lead, alcohol, or other toxins can be ruled out by appropriate laboratory investigations. The clinical course of a brain abscess is usually slower, and focal findings may be prominent; a history of sinus infection, bronchiectasis, or congenital heart disease may be elicited. A myelitic form of viral nervous system infection may be mimicked by a mass lesion or Guillain-Barré syndrome.

LABORATORY EVALUATION

Every attempt should be made to identify the offending organism to help determine the prognosis and to document potential epidemic outbreaks. Typical CSF alterations among patients who have meningoencephalitis consist of mild pleocytosis, a slight increase in protein level, and no alteration in glucose concentration (see Table 294-1). Red blood cells in the CSF may indicate hemorrhagic brain necrosis, commonly seen with herpesvirus infections and Eastern equine encephalitis. A predominance of mononuclear cells in the CSF is the exception in acute bacterial meningoencephalitis but may be present with syphilis, Lyme disease, listeriosis, or tuberculosis.

PCR is a powerful tool in identifying enterovirus, mumps virus, CMV, VZV, and other viruses. PCR of CSF in patients with herpes simplex encephalitis is 98% specific and 94% sensitive.[2] A rapid screening test for Epstein-Barr virus (Monospot) is available at most hospitals.

Magnetic resonance imaging of viral encephalitis shows "diffuse scattered or confluent areas of T2-weighted hyperintensities that are isointense or hypointense on T1-weighted imaging."[2] In more severe cases, increased intracranial pressure (ventricular compression) or cerebral cortical enhancement occurs. Temporal lobe enhancement or necrosis may be evidence of herpesvirus infection. An electroencephalogram showing a periodic pattern in an infant who has partial motor seizures and signs of meningoencephalitis is diagnostic of HSV encephalitis.

Newborns who have cutaneous vesicles and who are thought to have herpes simplex meningoencephalitis need not undergo brain biopsy for the diagnosis to be established. Rather, attempts should be made to isolate the virus from the throat, eye, or cutaneous lesions or from blood, urine, stool, and CSF.

TREATMENT

Treatment of a patient who has meningoencephalitis is supportive and includes reducing high intracranial pressure (see Chapter 352, Increased Intracranial Pressure), providing respiratory support, and treating seizures. Maintaining the fluid and electrolyte balance is essential because two thirds of infants who have aseptic meningitis develop inappropriate secretion of antidiuretic hormone. Corticosteroids have not proved useful in treating meningoencephalitis and may blunt host defenses.

Specific treatment of acute viral infections of the nervous system is indicated in herpes simplex infections of the CNS. Although nephrotoxic, acyclovir is the drug of choice and is generally well tolerated by neonates and by children with renal dysfunction. Ganciclovir has been approved for use in CMV infections.

Seventeen HIV drugs are currently available, including nucleoside and nonnucleoside reverse transcriptase inhibitors, protease inhibitors, and fusion inhibitors.[22] Another drug treatment that may be of benefit is intravenous immunoglobulin, which is known to contain viral antibodies for specific viral infections. These nonspecific immunoglobulin preparations have been used as replacement therapy or as adjuncts to treatment of meningoencephalitis in immunodeficient patients. However, immunoglobulin therapy for overwhelming viral sepsis remains controversial. α-Interferon has been used as prophylaxis against CMV and VZV in immunocompromised children but not as adjunct therapy in meningoencephalitis.

Prevention is the most cost-effective method of reducing the morbidity and mortality caused by viral meningoencephalitis. Immunization has reduced, but not eliminated, poliomyelitis and has made rubella, mumps, and measles meningoencephalitis uncommon. Repeat measles immunizations of older children should reduce the incidence of measles encephalitis and SSPE further. The use of varicella vaccine may reduce incidence of VZV infections.

PROGNOSIS

The developing nervous system may be more susceptible to viral infection and more likely to sustain serious sequelae. Patients who survive Eastern equine encephalitis are severely impaired. Western equine encephalitis is associated with complete recovery in virtually all adults but causes death in 20% of children and has a high prevalence of neurologic sequelae among the survivors. HSV commonly produces a destructive encephalitis in neonates, infants, and children. The sole survivor of rabies encephalitis is neurologically impaired.

Even the more benign meningoencephalitides of infancy, such as those caused by enteroviruses, may result in substantial reductions in head circumference, intelligence, and learning ability. California encephalitis, a relatively mild arbovirus infection, causes emotional or learning disorders in 15% of affected children. Focal epilepsy may be a sequel of a *mild* encephalitis caused by Epstein-Barr virus. Every child who has a documented or suspected viral nervous system infection must be carefully monitored for auditory, visual, and cognitive aftereffects because these children are at risk for cerebral cortical dysfunction.

TOOLS FOR PRACTICE

Engaging Patient and Family

- *A Parent's Guide to Insect Repellents* (brochure), American Academy of Pediatrics (patiented.aap.org).
- *Fact Sheet: Variant Creutzfeldt-Jakob Disease* (fact sheet), Centers for Disease Control and Prevention (www.cdc.gov/ncidod/dvrd/vcjd/factsheet_nvcjd.htm).
- *How do I choose an insect repellent?* (other), Centers for Disease Control and Prevention (www.cdc.gov/ncidod/diseases/index.htm).
- *Rabies Information for Kids* (Web page), Centers for Disease Control and Prevention (www.cdc.gov/ncidod/dvrd/kidsrabies).

Medical Decision Support

- *About Prion Diseases* (Web page), Centers for Disease Control and Prevention (www.cdc.gov/ncidod/dvrd/prions/index.htm).
- *Arboviral Encephalitides* (Web page), Centers for Disease Control and Prevention (www.cdc.gov/ncidod/dvbid/arbor/index.htm).
- *Bovine Spongiform Encephalopathy, or Mad Cow Disease* (Web page), Centers for Disease Control and Prevention (www.cdc.gov/ncidod/dvrd/bse).
- *Epstein-Barr Virus and Infectious Mononucleosis* (Web page), Centers for Disease Control and Prevention (www.cdc.gov/ncidod/diseases/ebv.htm).
- *Herpes Simplex Virus* (Web page), Centers for Disease Control and Prevention (www.cdc.gov/std/Herpes/STDFactHerpes.htm).
- *HIV/AIDS* (Web page), Centers for Disease Control and Prevention (www.cdc.gov/hiv).
- *Japanese Encephalitis* (Web page), Centers for Disease Control and Prevention (wwwn.cdc.gov/travel/contentYellowBook.aspx).
- *Rabies* (Web page), Centers for Disease Control and Prevention (www.cdc.gov/ncidod/dvrd/rabies).
- *Red Book: 2006 Report of the Committee on Infectious Diseases*, American Academy of Pediatrics (www.aap.org/bookstore).
- *Rocky Mountain Spotted Fever* (Web page), Centers for Disease Control and Prevention (www.cdc.gov/ncidod/dvrd/rmsf/index.htm).
- *Tickborne Encephalitis (TBE)* (Web page), Centers for Disease Control and Prevention (wwwn.cdc.gov/travel/contentYellowBook.aspx).
- *Variant Creutzfeldt-Jakob Disease* (Web page), Centers for Disease Control and Prevention (www.cdc.gov/ncidod/dvrd/vcjd/index.htm).
- *West Nile Virus Information* (Web page), American Academy of Pediatrics (www.aap.org/family/wnv.htm).
- *West Nile Virus* (Web page), Centers for Disease Control and Prevention (www.cdc.gov/ncidod/dvbid/westnile/index.htm).

AAP POLICY STATEMENT

Whitley RJ, MacDonald N, Asher DM, American Academy of Pediatrics, Committee on Infectious Diseases. Technical report: transmissible spongiform encephalopathies: a review for pediatricians. *Pediatrics.* 2000;106(5):1160-1165. (aappolicy.aappublications.org/cgi/content/full/pediatrics;106/5/1160).

REFERENCES

1. Rittichier KR, Bryan PA, Bassett KE, et al. Diagnosis and outcomes of enterovirus infections in young infants. *Pediatr Infect Dis J.* 2005;24:546-550.
2. Silvia MT, Licht DJ. Pediatric central nervous system infections and inflammatory white matter disease. *Pediatr Clin North Am.* 2005;52:1107-1126.
3. Harris G. Five cases of polio in Amish group raises new fears. *New York Times.* November 8, 2005:1.
4. Young RSK, Eccles T, Gangiulio L, et al. Army pediatricians in Iraq. *Clin Pediatr.* 2005;44:189-192.
5. DeTiege N, Rozenberg F, DesPortes V, et al. Herpes simplex encephalitis relapses in children. *Neurology.* 2003;61:241-243.
6. Whitley RJ, Kimberlin DW. Herpes simplex encephalitis: children and adolescents. *Semin Pediatr Infect Dis.* 2005;16:17-23.
7. Ansari A, Shaobing L, Abzug MJ, et al. Human herpesviruses 6 and 7 and central nervous system infection in children. *Emerg Infect Dis.* 2004;10:1-12. Available at: www.cdc.gov/ncidod/EID/vol1no8/03-0788.htm. Accessed March 20, 2007.
8. Domachowske JB, Cunningham CK, Cummings DL. Acute manifestations and neurologic sequelae of Epstein-Barr virus encephalitis in children. *Pediatr Infect Dis J.* 1996;15:871-875.
9. Hayes EB, Komar N, Nasci RS, et al. Epidemiology and transmission dynamics of West Nile virus disease. *Emerg Infect Dis.* 2005;11:1167-1173.
10. Hopkins RS, Jajosky RA, Hall PA, et al. Centers for Disease Control and Prevention: summary of notifiable diseases—United States, 2003. *MMWR Morb Mortal Wkly Rep.* 2005:52:1-85.
11. Arnold JC, Revivo GA, Senac MO, et al. West Nile virus encephalitis with thalamic involvement in an immunocompromised child. *Pediatr Infect Dis J.* 2005;24:932-934.
12. Centers for Disease Control and Prevention, Division of Vector Borne Infectious Diseases. Intrauterine West Nile virus infection. *MMWR.* Dec 2002;51(5):1135-1136.
13. Willoughby R, Tieves KS, Hoffman GM, et al. Survival after treatment of rabies with induction of coma. *N Engl J Med.* 2005;352:2508-2514.
14. Burton EC, Burns DK, Opatowsky MJ, et al. Rabies encephalomyelitis: clinical, neuroradiological, and pathological findings in 4 transplant patients. *Arch Neurol.* 2005;62:873-882.
15. Centers for Disease Control and Prevention. Control and prevention of rubella: evaluation and management of suspected outbreaks, rubella in pregnant women, and surveillance for congenital rubella syndrome. *MMWR Morb Mortal Wkly Rep.* 2001;50(RR12):1-23. Available at: www.cdc.gov/mmwr/preview/mmwrhtml/rr5012a1.htm. Accessed March 20, 2007.
16. Centers for Disease Control and Prevention and the National Center for HIV, STD and TB Prevention, Division of HIV/AIDS Prevention. *HIV/AIDS Surveillance Report: HIV Infection and AIDS in the United States.* Atlanta, GA: Centers for Disease Control and Prevention; 2003.
17. Centers for Disease Control and Prevention. Fatal cases of Rocky Mountain spotted fever in family clusters—three states. *MMWR Morb Mortal Wkly Rep.* May 2004;53(19):407-410.
18. Hughes JM, Colley DG. Preventing congenital toxoplasmosis. *MMWR Morb Mortal Wkly Rep.* 2000;49(RR02):57-75.
19. Whitley RJ, MacDonald N, Asher DM. Technical report: transmissible spongiform encephalopathies: a review for pediatricians. *Pediatrics.* 2000;106:1160-1165.
20. Faust S. Aseptic meningitis. October 4, 2004. Available at: www.emedicine.com/PED/topic3004.htm/. Accessed March 19, 2007.
21. Belman AL, Reynolds L, Preston T, et al. Cerebrospinal fluid findings in children with Lyme disease–associated facial nerve palsy. *Arch Pediatr Adolesc Med.* 1997; 151:1224-1228.
22. Kimberlin DW. Antiviral therapies in children: has their time arrived? *Pediatr Clin North Am.* 2005;52:837-867.

Chapter 295

MUSCULAR DYSTROPHY

Richard T. Moxley III, MD; Emma Ciafaloni, MD

The muscular dystrophies are a group of slowly progressive inherited diseases with specific patterns of muscle wasting and weakness. These disorders occur infrequently in childhood; a busy pediatrician may care for only a few patients during a career. However, breakthroughs in molecular biology have provided direct genetic tests for these diseases and have created opportunities to suggest and coordinate family counseling and prenatal testing. Primary care physicians play important roles by coordinating care with specialists in neuromuscular disease, helping with genetic testing, and monitoring patients for the complications of these muscular dystrophies. Duchenne dystrophy is the most common muscular dystrophy in childhood, and major advances have been made in its diagnosis and treatment. For these reasons, this chapter focuses on Duchenne dystrophy, although other muscular dystrophies that occur in childhood are also addressed.

DUCHENNE DYSTROPHY

Definition

Duchenne dystrophy is a slowly progressive muscle-wasting disease marked by symptoms that develop before age 5 years. Early in its course, Duchenne dystrophy affects the proximal hip and shoulder girdle muscles, as well as the anterior neck and abdominal muscles.[1-8] The symptoms arise from an absence or extreme deficiency of a large cytoskeletal protein, dystrophin, that attaches to the inner surface of the muscle fiber membrane as a part of a complex of glycoproteins.[1-15] Dystrophin is also part of the inner membrane structure of smooth and cardiac muscle and of certain cells in the central nervous system and in specialized connective tissues, such as the myotendinous junctions.[9] This distribution of dystrophin corresponds closely to tissues that have major clinical manifestations in Duchenne dystrophy.

The mechanism by which dystrophin deficiency causes dysfunction in some muscle groups while sparing others is a puzzle. Some experts have speculated that dystrophin protects and strengthens the muscle membrane to withstand the stresses of repeated muscle contractions and that it helps prevent excessive influx of calcium to speed the effective repair of tears in the muscle membrane that occur with vigorous exercise.[5,7,9,15] However, this puzzle still remains: Why do heavily used muscles, such as the extraocular and laryngeal muscles or the gastrocnemius muscles, maintain their strength despite the lack of dystrophin? Some experts speculate that another large cytoskeletal protein, such as utrophin, can take the place of dystrophin and help maintain muscle function.[5,10,13-15] Further research is in progress to clarify the role that such alternative proteins may play in rescuing muscle fibers from destruction in diseases involving dystrophin deficiency. The findings will help in developing new strategies for treatment.

Genetics

The gene for dystrophin in the *Xp21* region is among the largest known, occupying 1% of the entire X chromosome.[5,9,10,12,15] It contains 79 exons and 5 different promoters control production of isoforms that are cell-type specific (eg, muscle, cerebral cortex, Purkinje, glial, Schwann cells).[5,9,10,12,15] Large deletions occur in approximately two thirds of cases of Duchenne dystrophy and in an even higher percentage of cases of Becker dystrophy (a later-onset X-linked dystrophy also caused by a deficiency of dystrophin).[5,9,10,12,15] In addition to large deletions, smaller point mutations occur in approximately 30% of patients who have Duchenne dystrophy and 15% of those who have Becker dystrophy.[5,7] No consistent relationship has been established between clinical severity (Duchenne dystrophy versus the milder Becker dystrophy) and the size of the gene mutation. However, deletion of the first muscle exon and the adjoining muscle promoter region appears to produce 2 phenotypes that have either mild muscle involvement or that have mild muscle involvement but severe cardiomyopathy.[5,16]

Clinical Presentation and Differential Diagnosis

As outlined in Table 295-1, Duchenne dystrophy typically occurs in patients aged between 2 and 4 years. Parents notice weakness of forward head flexion that persists beyond infancy, accompanied by slowed motor development. Patients demonstrate progressive gluteal and shoulder girdle muscular weakness, leading to a widened stance, lumbar lordosis, forward thrusting of the abdomen, and winging of the scapulae. Patients never run normally and usually put their hands on their knees to rise from the floor (Figure 295-1) and to assist in climbing steps. These patients have difficulty keeping up with their peers, a difficulty that becomes more apparent as they enter nursery school and kindergarten. The teacher often observes a problem and helps the parents decide to bring the child to the pediatrician. The situation becomes clear that their child has a real problem. The child is not just normally clumsy, and poor motivation is not the cause for the child's tendency to fall easily and for complaints of tiredness and calf cramps. Primary care physicians must be sensitive to the protean nature of these early complaints in Duchenne dystrophy.

Because patients with Duchenne dystrophy usually have mild cognitive deficits,[5,7] the patient may appear to be intellectually disabled, and the pediatrician may not consider Duchenne dystrophy. Because of the gradual development of hip and knee extensor weakness in middle childhood, patients often toe-walk to use the power of the gastrocnemius to help stabilize knee extension. Reliance on the calf muscles during ambulation contributes to the typical hypertrophy of the calf muscles. However, the pattern of walking in these patients and the presence of mild cognitive

Table 295-1 Symptoms, Genetics, and Diagnostic Tests for Muscular Dystrophies in Childhood

CHARACTERISTIC	DUCHENNE DYSTROPHY	BECKER DYSTROPHY	MYOTONIC DYSTROPHY
Age at onset	Before age 5 yr, typically at 2-4 yr	After age 5; can begin in adult life	Infancy, childhood, or adult life
Initial symptoms	Cannot run or keep up with peers; can take only one step at a time	Fatigue or marked thigh weakness; trouble climbing steps; occasional calf or thigh cramps; patients can ambulate beyond age 15 yr	Congenital form—floppy infant, poor suck, weak respiratory effort, talipes; childhood form—bifacial weakness, slurred speech, impaired hearing, intellectual disability
Incidence	1:3500 of male births	1:35,000 of male births	1:8000 of all births
Genetics	X-linked recessive/*XP21* region of gene for dystrophin	X-linked recessive/*XP21* region of gene for dystrophin	Autosomal-dominant chromosome 19
Gene lesion	Absence of dystrophin	Marked deficiency of dystrophin	Abnormal expansion of CTG trinucleotide repeat in 3′ nontranslated region of a gene coding for a serine/threonine kinase
Serum creatine phosphokinase	10× above normal	5-10× above normal	Normal or 2-5× above normal
Electrodiagnostic testing	Normal nerve conductions	Normal nerve conductions; mildly myopathic EMG	Normal nerve conductions; myotonic discharges present in children and adults, but often absent in infants (EMG should be performed on the mother)
Muscle biopsy	Active myopathy, absence of dystrophin, severe reduction in dystrophin-associated proteins	Moderately active myopathy, absence or deficiency of dystrophin, reduction in dystrophin-associated proteins	Increased central nuclei atrophy of type I fibers, ringbinden, and subsarcolemma masses
Leukocyte DNA testing	If suspicion is high, perform DNA screening first. If leukocyte DNA testing is negative, perform muscle biopsy. DNA is screened for deletions (60-70% have them); if deletion is found, deletion tests are performed in at-risk family members; if no deletion is found, DNA sequencing for point mutation should be performed	Same as Duchenne dystrophy	If this diagnosis is suspected, a Southern blot analysis is performed to identify an abnormally large expansion of CTG repeats in the gene; if the Southern blot test is normal, a polymerase chain reaction test is done to search for smaller expansion of the repeat; most childhood cases show abnormal CTG repeat enlargements (eg, 500-4000 repeats), whereas normal alleles have 5-30 repeats

FACIOSCAPULOHUMERAL DYSTROPHY	FUKUYAMA-TYPE CONGENITAL MUSCULAR DYSTROPHY	CONGENITAL MUSCULAR DYSTROPHY: PRIMARY DEFICIENCY OF MEROSIN	EMERY-DREIFUSS MUSCULAR DYSTROPHY
Rare cases in infancy, occasionally in childhood, usually in adult life	Infancy	Infancy	Middle to late childhood
Congenital form (rare)—bifacial weakness, sometimes ophthalmoparesis, occasionally floppy, deafness; childhood form (more common)—mild facial weakness and weakness of scapular fixator muscles	Floppy infant, slow improvement up to 6-8 yr, then a decline	Floppy, contractures	Mild elbow contractures and mild weakness of triceps, biceps, and scapular fixator muscles; occasionally as isolated cardiomyopathy
1:20,000 of all births	1:18,000 of all births	Unknown	1:100,000 of all births
Autosomal dominant; most cases localize to chromosome 4	Autosomal recessive, chromosome 9, *q31-33* region for most cases	Autosomal recessive, chromosome *6q22-23* region, laminin $\alpha 2$ gene	X-linked recessive form *Xq28* and autosomal-dominant form *1q21.3*
Deletion of a variable quantity of 3.3-kb tandem repeats at *4q35*	3-kb insertion of 3′ noncoding region of gene encoding fukutin; mutation caused instability of mRNA for fukutin. Fukutin probably helps stabilize the muscle membrane.	Complete (or partial) loss of merosin (laminin $\alpha 2$) in both muscle and skin	X-linked form involves gene for emerin and dominant form gene for lamins A and C. Emerin and lamins A and C are attached to nuclear membrane. Their functions are not yet known.
2-5× above normal	>10× above normal	>10× above normal	5-10× above normal
Normal nerve conductions; EMG occasionally myopathic, often within normal limits	Normal nerve conductions; myopathic EMG	Normal nerve conductions; myopathic EMG	Normal nerve conductions; EMG often normal in early stages
Nonspecific myopathy, up to 30% have mononuclear inflammation	Mixture of necrotic and regenerating fibers, fibrosis, and an increased number of small fibers	Dystrophic changes with adipose and connective tissue replacement, and often prominent inflammatory infiltrates	Mild to moderate active myopathy with occasional atrophic type 1 fibers
DNA analysis available to identify the 3.3-kb deletions noted above; should perform before obtaining muscle biopsy if clinical suspicion is high	Not yet commercially available	Not yet commercially available	Not yet commercially available

EMG, Electromyography.

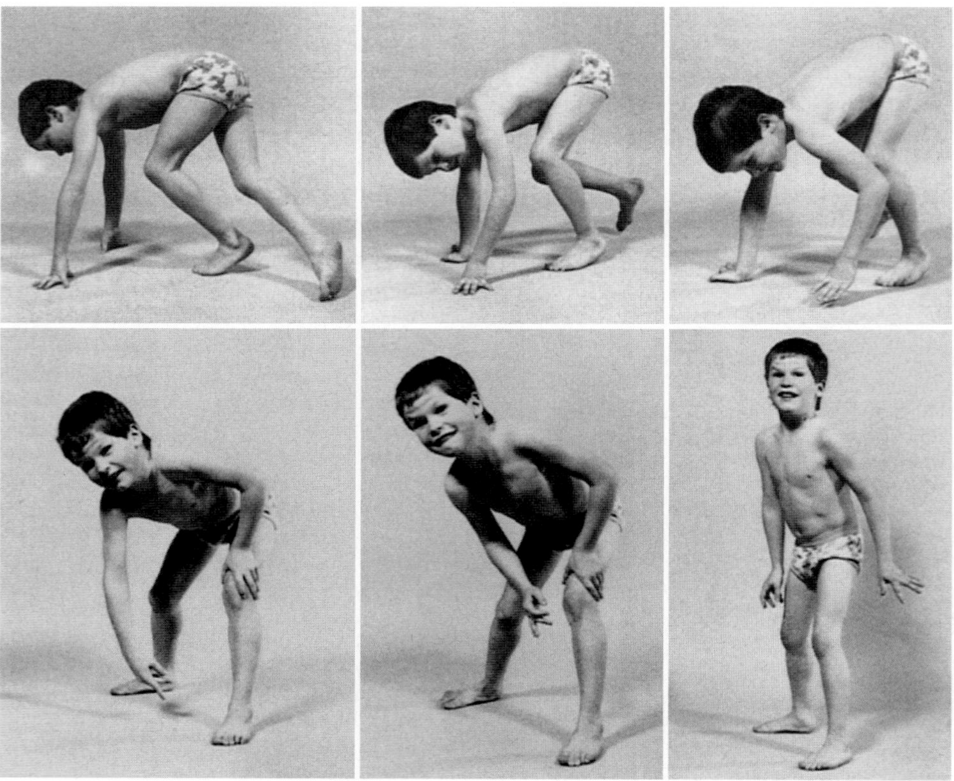

Figure 295-1 Boy who has Duchenne muscular dystrophy demonstrating the sequence of maneuvers that constitutes Gowers sign. The child pushes off the floor with all 4 extremities, then prepares to push up by moving the hands along the floor closer to the feet, and finally places the hands on the thighs and pushes up to the erect position. The maneuver is necessary because of the marked weakness of the hip extension. *(Swaiman KF. Pediatric Neurology: Principles and Practice. 2nd ed. St Louis, MO: CV Mosby; 1994. Copyright © 1994, Elsevier, with permission.)*

deficits can sometimes lead to the incorrect diagnosis of cerebral palsy, delaying effective treatment.

A complete history almost always distinguishes patients who have Duchenne dystrophy from those who have other conditions that cause proximal weakness without sensory findings in childhood. Hypothyroidism usually has more generalized symptoms, as does carnitine deficiency. Blood tests can exclude these two conditions from the differential diagnosis. Neither of these conditions causes the high creatine kinase (CK) levels that occur in Duchenne dystrophy. Variants of spinal muscular atrophy and early-onset cases of facioscapulohumeral dystrophy (FSHD) may resemble Duchenne dystrophy. Hypertrophy of the calf muscles may be a feature of either condition. Spinal muscular atrophy produces no increase or only a mild increase in creatine phosphokinase; FSHD causes only a mild to moderate increase. As outlined in Table 295-1 and Figure 295-2, DNA analyses and, if necessary, muscle biopsy are the appropriate diagnostic tests to establish the diagnosis of Duchenne dystrophy. If muscle biopsy is needed, then the findings will help distinguish among many of the autosomal-dominant and autosomal-recessive forms of limb girdle muscular dystrophy (LGMD) that sometimes have a close clinical similarity to Duchenne dystrophy.[16-20]

Other, more acute, conditions such as childhood myasthenia gravis and inflammatory myopathy are not usually confused with Duchenne dystrophy. The more rapid evolution of weakness, along with the presence of ptosis, ophthalmoparesis, and facial weakness, distinguish myasthenia gravis from Duchenne dystrophy. The more generalized weakness that occurs in inflammatory myopathy, along with a skin rash, helps separate these patients from those who have Duchenne dystrophy. In rare cases, chronic demyelinating polyneuropathy may be confused with Duchenne dystrophy, but the absence of ankle reflexes, more generalized weakness, a more rapid course, the lack of marked increase of CK, and abnormally slowed nerve conduction identify these patients.

The combination of a complete history and judicious use of the tests outlined in Table 295-1 will establish the diagnosis of Duchenne dystrophy in virtually all cases. In rare cases, a floppy infant will have a markedly increased serum CK level, and physicians will wonder whether the baby has a variant of Duchenne dystrophy. Newborns or infants who have Duchenne dystrophy also have a marked increase in CK, but they are not floppy. Some other problem must be present as well if a patient with Duchenne dystrophy is floppy. Floppy infants who have high CK levels usually do not

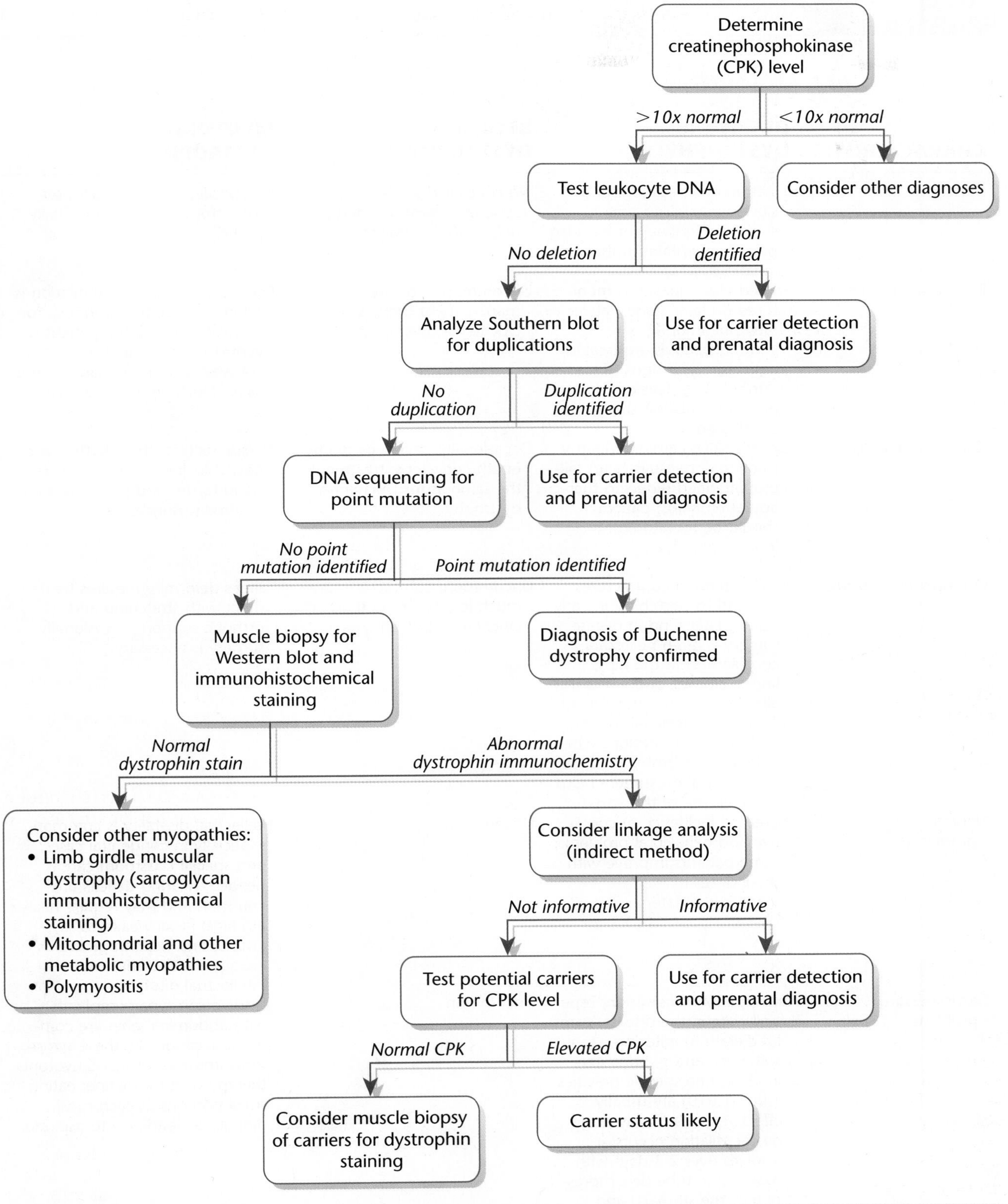

Figure 295-2 Flow chart outlining diagnostic tests for a boy suspected of having Duchenne muscular dystrophy (DMD) without a family history of this disorder.

Table 295-2 Complications and Treatment of Muscular Dystrophies in Childhood

CHARACTERISTIC	DUCHENNE DYSTROPHY	BECKER DYSTROPHY	MYOTONIC DYSTROPHY
Muscle weakness	Treatment with prednisone slows or stabilizes muscle strength; lightweight long-leg bracing maintains ambulation in later stages	No controlled studies of prednisone treatment; bracing is helpful in late stages	No specific therapy; braces for foot drop; children can usually participate in gym in school
Respiratory problems	Forced vital capacity is monitored (in later stages, atelectatic pneumonitis is common); colds are treated aggressively; if signs of respiratory failure develop, nasal or oral ventilation should be considered.	Uncommon until late stages; management then as with Duchenne dystrophy	For congenital cases, ventilation is often needed; the prognosis for survival is poor if the patient is ventilator dependent at >4 weeks; other management is as for Duchenne dystrophy.
Cardiac problems	Occasionally, cardiomyopathy leads to congestive heart failure; afterload-reducing therapy often helps; patient should be monitored for intracardiac clots.	Occasionally, severe cardiomyopathy develops; treatment is the same as for Duchenne dystrophy	Occasionally, tachyarrhythmias or heart block develops in childhood forms, and pacemaker treatment is indicated.
Orthopedic problems	Achilles tendon contractures respond to stretching in early stages; later tendon release surgery is often necessary; contractures at the hips, knees, elbows, and wrists usually develop after the patient becomes wheelchair bound; scoliosis often develops when patients stop ambulating; spinal stabilization surgery helps maintain use of the arms.	Uncommon; contractures are much less common than in Duchenne dystrophy	Talipes deformity requires treatment with stretching and orthotic support; occasionally, surgery is necessary.
Nervous system problems	Increased incidence of cognitive and behavioral problems; some patients improve with small doses of methylphenidate.	Uncommon	Intellectual disability is common, especially in congenital cases, and special classroom care is needed; hearing deficits are common and may require hearing aids; facial weakness, dysarthria, and hearing problems exaggerate the impression of intellectual disability.
Gastrointestinal problems	Constipation is common, especially late in the disease; careful dietary monitoring, stool softeners, and good water intake (urine specific gravities 1.007-1.010) are usually effective; occasionally acute gastric dilation occurs; it resolves over 2-3 days with nasogastric tube decompression of the stomach and intravenous hydration.	Uncommon	Spastic colon-type complaints with abdominal pain are common; occasionally, these symptoms improve with antimyotonia therapy with mexiletine; eating small portions at each meal diminishes tendency to aspirate.

FACIOSCAPULOHUMERAL DYSTROPHY	FUKUYAMA-TYPE CONGENITAL MUSCULAR DYSTROPHY	CONGENITAL MUSCULAR DYSTROPHY: PRIMARY DEFICIENCY OF MEROSIN	EMERY-DREIFUSS MUSCULAR DYSTROPHY
No specific treatment; patients should avoid lifting with arms fully extended and abducted; braces are sometimes needed.	No specific treatment; bracing and physical therapy are useful in some patients.	Same as Fukuyama-type congenital muscular dystrophy	No specific treatment; skeletal muscle weakness often is relatively mild compared with cardiac problems and does not limit function.
Uncommon	As with Duchenne dystrophy; patients often die of respiratory failure late in childhood or in early teens.	Same as Fukuyama-type congenital muscular atrophy	Mild other than symptoms related to cardiac dysfunction
Uncommon	Uncommon	Uncommon	Frequent cardiac conduction defects; atrial paralysis, cardiac arrest, and sudden death are common; pacemaker treatment and preventive therapy for cardiac emboli are often necessary
Occasionally, knee effusion and low back pain develop as a result of weakness; conservative care measures are effective; in late stages, surgery to stabilize the scapula may be performed, but surgery is uncommon.	Contractures develop in 70% of patients by 3 months of age at the ankles, knees, and hips.	Contractures, especially feet and hips	Contractures, especially in the elbows and ankles, occur early and respond somewhat to physical therapy; surgical release of Achilles tendon may be necessary; some patients develop a rigid spine syndrome, for which no effective therapy is available.
Uncommon; in rare cases, the infant-onset form of the disease occurs in association with hearing loss, retinal disease, or both.	Generalized or focal seizures occur in most patients; anticonvulsant therapy is necessary; intellectual disability is common; most patients have microcephaly, polymicrogyria, pachygyria, and heterotopias.	Intellectual disability common; magnetic resonance imaging of head shows increased signal from white matter on T2-weighted images; occipital agyria	Caused only by stroke from heart block or cardiac emboli
Uncommon	Uncommon	Uncommon	Uncommon

have Duchenne dystrophy. If such a patient does not have an infectious, toxic, or metabolic disorder that causes muscle destruction to account for the marked increase of serum CK level, then the child usually has one of the two relatively rare childhood muscular dystrophies noted in Tables 295-1 and 295-2. These diseases are the severe childhood autosomal-recessive forms of congenital muscular dystrophy. The work-up and treatment of these disorders are summarized in Tables 295-1 and 295-2.[21-28] Certain congenital myopathies may be marked by floppiness, but these infants do not have significantly increased CK levels.[25]

Evaluation

Once the physician suspects the diagnosis of Duchenne (or Becker) dystrophy, the serum CK should be measured. A marked increase (10-fold or more above normal) excludes most other disorders and strongly suggests the diagnosis of Duchenne dystrophy. At this point, discussing the possibility that the child has a muscular dystrophy with the parents would be appropriate. However, the clinician should refer the patient for further evaluation to a neurologist skilled in the care of patients with neuromuscular disease. Also useful is to mention that the neuromuscular specialist may want to perform other diagnostic tests, such as whole blood DNA testing and muscle biopsy. A detailed discussion of the natural history of Duchenne dystrophy or a discussion of the procedures for screening the mother and other at-risk family members for carrier status at this time is premature and can be postponed. This discussion is best initiated after the neurologic consultation and after specific diagnostic information is available (see Table 295-1 and Figure 295-2). The neuromuscular specialist should take responsibility for the initial description of the course of Duchenne dystrophy and should discuss the treatment options. Figure 295-2 provides a flow chart that neurologists typically follow to arrive at a diagnosis of Duchenne dystrophy.

A continuously updated list of laboratories and tests available for the genetic diagnosis of Duchenne muscular dystrophy can be found at GeneTests (www.geneclinics.org).

Management

Supportive Care

The overall goals in managing patients who have Duchenne dystrophy are to maintain ambulation for as long as possible, to optimize the development of the patient's cognitive abilities, and to anticipate the occurrence of complications such as excessive weight gain, joint contractures (especially of the Achilles tendons), respiratory insufficiency, scoliosis, gastrointestinal hypomotility, and cardiomyopathy.[8,29-43] Table 295-2 summarizes the principal problems and treatment options.

The patient and family need to work closely with the physicians, schoolteachers, physical educators, and physical and occupational therapists to develop an individualized care plan for the patient for each stage of the disease. Early in the illness, the patient can usually play with peers in most activities; however, by the first or second grade, some adaptation of physical education requirements becomes necessary. The natural history of Duchenne dystrophy in the absence of treatment with prednisone predicts that the patient will become wheelchair bound between 10 and 12 years of age.[2] Lightweight long-leg bracing is often helpful at this stage to prolong weight bearing and ambulation, both of which delay the development of joint contractures and scoliosis. Contractures and scoliosis both develop when the patient becomes wheelchair bound. They do not appear at a specific age but depend on the patient's functional status.

Once contractures begin to develop, usually at the ankles and elbows (flexion), physical therapy (PT) and occupational therapy (OT) consultations should be obtained. Follow-up care can be coordinated with PT and OT, and patients can usually receive this care in their schools. Once significant heel cord contractures develop, obtaining an orthopedic consultation is also useful. The orthopedist can help guide the timing of the use of long-leg bracing and can discuss the possible need for surgery to lengthen the Achilles tendons. Since the use of prednisone began, the need for tendon release surgery, long-leg bracing, and spinal stabilization surgery for scoliosis has decreased. The orthopedist can monitor the severity of contractures, as well as the degree of spinal curvature. Orthopedic consultation becomes a particular need in the early nonambulatory stage of Duchenne dystrophy because this time is when contractures and spinal curvature become prominent. The orthopedic care, PT, OT, and neurologic care are often coordinated by the neuromuscular specialist and are typically provided in a clinic financed partly by the Muscular Dystrophy Association.

Although Muscular Dystrophy Association clinics provide an excellent opportunity to offer multiple services to patients, the role of the primary care physician remains critical. The pediatrician usually provides routine care of upper respiratory infections, as well as treatment for other common medical problems. In the middle and late nonambulatory stages of Duchenne dystrophy, minor medical problems can provoke major complications. A mild cold may lead to atelectatic pneumonitis and acute respiratory insufficiency. Such a problem, if treated aggressively, is fully reversible. Even chronic constipation can produce respiratory compromise in the later stages of Duchenne dystrophy because of abdominal distention and upward pressure on the diaphragm. An effective regimen to maintain regular bowel movements becomes important in routine care. Respiratory insufficiency often develops in the late stages of Duchenne dystrophy. Forced vital capacity declines, usually into the range of 600 to 1000 mL. Management options include nasal ventilation, rather than positive pressure ventilation via tracheostomy.[32,34,40,43] The use of assistive cough devices (insufflator-exsufflator) is helpful in speeding recovery from episodes of bronchitis and pneumonia. Ventilatory care is usually coordinated among the pediatrician, neuromuscular specialist, pediatric pulmonologist, and the patient and family. All have to participate if the treatment plan is to be effective. Considerable discussion is necessary to educate the patient and family at this stage and to help decide which options are most appropriate. Physicians and nurses who have special training in neuromuscular diseases are often the ones who educate the family, and the roles of the pediatric pulmonologist and pediatrician have to be tailored to each medical care setting.

Periodic consultation with a pulmonologist is important once a patient with Duchenne dystrophy becomes wheelchair bound. Pulmonary consultation before and after general anesthesia is an integral part of any elective surgery. This preoperative consultation needs to include training of the patient and the home care providers in the use of assisted coughing techniques and in the use of nasal bilevel positive airway pressure (BIPAP). The use of nasal BIPAP and assisted coughing hastens recovery after general anesthesia and decreases the likelihood of postoperative pneumonia.[32,34,36]

In the late stages of Duchenne dystrophy, patients occasionally develop cardiomyopathy.[5,7,14,44,45] A chest radiograph reveals a dilated heart, and the cardiac ejection fraction decreases to 10% to 20% of normal. Heart failure is often exacerbated by coexisting respiratory insufficiency. In all of these cases, simultaneous ventilatory support must be considered if the patient and family have decided to pursue a vigorous course of treatment. Heart failure is difficult to manage, and afterload reduction therapy is often more effective than digoxin. An initial trial with an angiotensin-converting enzyme inhibitor, such as lisinopril, is often undertaken. If left-ventricular function worsens, then treatment with β-blocker therapy, such as carvedilol, is initiated with the goal of keeping the heart rate between 55 and 70 beats/min. Cardiology consultation needs to guide the care plan. Occasionally, ventricular or atrial clots (or both) are present, and long-term anticoagulant therapy is necessary.

Acute gastric dilation is another infrequent complication in the late stages of Duchenne dystrophy. This condition typically occurs in association with an idiopathic metabolic acidosis and responds rapidly to nasogastric tube decompression of the stomach and intravenous hydration. Caution must be used with intravenous repletion of potassium because in the late stages of the disease, the patient's muscle mass is considerably diminished and is not available to buffer an acute rise in extracellular potassium.

Although the cause of the gastric dilation is unknown, this problem, as well as the chronic intestinal hypomotility (constipation), probably results from the deficiency of dystrophin in the smooth muscle of the gastrointestinal tract. Good hydration, a balanced dietary intake, and regular bowel habits are the mainstays of treatment for these problems.

Prednisone Treatment

The only effective therapy for Duchenne dystrophy is prednisone, which is administered daily to maintain muscle strength and function.[29,30] The mechanism responsible for the beneficial effect of prednisone is unknown. However, several clues exist about the process involved. The increase in strength begins to develop after only 10 days of treatment[29,30] and reaches a maximal response after 3 months of therapy.[29,30] Muscle mass increases 10% after 3 months of prednisone treatment,[3,4,29,30] and the rate of muscle breakdown declines in association with maintenance of a normal rate of muscle protein synthesis.[46] Although azathioprine immunosuppressive therapy has been used, it confers no beneficial effect,[3] which argues against the possibility that an immunosuppressive effect accounts for the improvement in muscle strength with the use of prednisone.

Patients have been treated with prednisone at only a small number of specialized neuromuscular centers.[29,30] Prednisone treatment is preferably monitored by or coordinated with one of these centers. The protocols for monitoring side effects and for assessing muscle strength and function have been discussed elsewhere.[3,4] The most common side effects are excessive weight gain, mood disturbances (more aggressive, more tearful), and cushingoid facial appearance.[29,30] More serious side effects (compression fractures of the spine, high blood pressure, gastrointestinal bleeding, severe infections, or diabetes) are uncommon. Some patients have developed small, dot-shaped cataracts; others, as expected, have experienced decreased linear growth, which has probably helped maintain ambulation.

To allow monitoring for the development of side effects, patients are seen every 3 months for weight, blood pressure, pulse, and forced vital capacity checks, urinalysis, and assessment of neuromuscular functioning. At each visit, the patient undergoes timed function tests (time needed to travel 30 feet, to arise from supine to standing position, and to climb 4 standard steps) and a muscle strength evaluation (shoulder abductors, elbow flexors and extensors, knee extensors, hip flexors and extensors). These measures help guide the physicians in adjusting the dose of prednisone. The blood count and serum electrolyte levels are measured at 6-month intervals.

With close follow-up, patients have been kept stable or showed only mild progression of muscle weakness for periods exceeding 5 years.[29,30] Even in the late stages, prednisone appears to maintain respiratory muscle power and has reduced the number of patients who develop respiratory failure.

The discovery of the gene in Duchenne dystrophy and the ability to manufacture small segments of DNA containing the normal gene for dystrophin has raised hopes that direct gene therapy, either by local injection or by viral vector,[47-49] will prove feasible. Research is in progress. Other advances in research include stem cell therapy[50] and treatments to *read through* certain types of mutations.[51]

OTHER MUSCULAR DYSTROPHIES IN CHILDHOOD

Myotonic dystrophy type 1 (DM1), or dystrophica myotonia (Steinert disease), is due to an abnormal enlargement of a trinucleotide repeat in the third nontranslated region of the *DM* gene on chromosome 19.[52-54] Discovery of the gene has led to the development of gene probes to identify both symptomatic and asymptomatic carriers.[54] Genetic counseling and prenatal testing can now be performed with a high degree of accuracy, an important advance in preventive

Table 295-3 Autosomal-Dominant Forms of Limb Girdle Muscular Dystrophy (LGMD 1A-D)*

CHARACTERISTIC	LGMD 1A	LGMD 1B	LGMD 1C	LGMD 1D
Age at onset	18-35 yr	4-38 yr (half of the cases in childhood)	~5 yr	<25 yr
Gene location (chromosome)	*5q31*	*1q21.2*	*3p25*†	*6q23*
Protein	Myotilin	Lamin A/C	Caveolin 3	Unknown
Serum creatine kinase	Normal or 2-5× normal	Normal or 2-5× normal	Often >10× normal	22-5× normal
Muscle biopsy	Fiber size variation; moth-eaten fibers; increased internal nuclei; occasional necrotic and regenerating fibers	Fiber size variation; increased internal nuclei; mild endomysial fibrosis; occasional necrotic and regenerating fibers	Similar findings to 1A and 1B; absence or deficiency of caveolin 3 on immunocytochemistry	Similar findings to 1A and 1B
Clinical features	Proximal weakness: occasional dysarthria; slow progression; Achilles tendon contractures; may show anticipation	Cardiac disturbances prominent; proximal weakness; slow progression; may be allelic to autosomal dominant locus for Emery-Dreifuss dystrophy	Proximal weakness; calf hypertrophy; muscle pain on exertion; variable progression; muscle cramps	Cardiac conduction disturbances prominent; proximal weakness; problems worse in boys

*Each of these has been described in a single family. Linkage analysis has excluded other known LGMD loci, but new causative genes have not yet been identified.
†Mutations alter the scaffolding domain of the protein.

Table 295-4 Autosomal-Recessive Forms of Limb Girdle Muscular Dystrophy (LGMD 2G-I)

CHARACTERISTIC	LGMD 2G	LGMD 2H	LGMD 2I
Age at onset	9-15 yr	1-27 yr	Early childhood to 27 yr (61% <5 yr)
Genetics	Chromosome 17q12; mutation found in the gene encoding the sarcomeric protein telethonin	D487N homozygous mutation in the *TRIM 32* gene, *9q31-0.34-1* coding for a E3 ubiquitin ligase responsible for posttranslational regulation of protein levels	Chromosome 19q13.3 fukutin-related protein gene *(FKRP)*
Serum creatine kinase	Usually <5× normal; may be >10× normal early in the disease	From near normal to 20× normal	Markedly increased, 5-70× normal
Muscle biopsy	Rimmed vacuoles in some patients	Mild dystrophic changes (fiber size variation, degeneration/regeneration); fiber splitting, internal nuclei; endomysial fibrosis	Dystrophic changes; type I fiber predominance; reduced staining for merosin (α2 chain of lamin)
Clinical features	Anterior tibialis weakness early in the course in some patients	Proximal lower limb weakness; weakness of facial muscles with flat smile; slow progression (patients remain ambulatory through midadulthood)	Severe limb girdle weakness; cardiac failure (30%-50%) and respiratory failure (30%)

therapy.[54,55] Myotonic dystrophy type 2 (DM2) is a disorder similar to but distinct from DM1 and is also a multisystem autosomal-dominant disorder associated with myotonia, weakness, and cataracts.[52-59] However, DM2 does not occur in infancy or childhood.[52,59] Complications can occur when patients receive anesthetics and during pregnancy and delivery.[54,55]

FSHD is not common in childhood. The severe cases that uncommonly occur in infancy and early childhood may result in considerable weakness of facial and bulbar muscles, and affected patients can develop respiratory insufficiency along with generalized weakness.[60-64] The affected gene responsible for this disease may soon be isolated from its localization on chromosome 4.q35. DNA testing is now available.[65]

The infant-onset congenital muscular dystrophies are rare disorders and have already been mentioned in the discussion of the differential diagnosis of Duchenne dystrophy.[6,21-24]

Emery-Dreifuss muscular dystrophy is a rare, X-linked, autosomal-dominant disorder[66,67] that is clinically and genetically distinct from, but occasionally confused with, Becker dystrophy. It can produce severe cardiac complications that require urgent treatment. These cardiac symptoms may prompt medical evaluation before the muscle weakness or contractures occur.[66]

Table 295-3 and Table 295-4 outline the forms of autosomal-dominant and autosomal-recessive[17-20] forms of LGMD. These disorders can occur during childhood or in the teens, and on superficial evaluation, they resemble Duchenne dystrophy. Unlike Duchenne dystrophy, most of the forms of LGMD progress more slowly, and the prognosis differs. The autosomal-dominant forms (LGMD 1A-D)[17,18] are especially uncommon, as are some of the autosomal-recessive forms of LGMD 2A and LGMD 2B.[17-20] However, the sarcoglycanopathies (especially LGMD 2I) probably account for more than 10% of patients who have a limb-girdle pattern of muscle weakness whose muscle biopsy samples stain normally for dystrophin.[11,19,20] The sarcoglycans are glycoproteins associated with dystrophin and other muscle membrane–associated proteins with relationships to specific forms of LGMD, and these different disorders have different causes.[17-20]

The various forms of LGMD are important to consider in referring children to the neurologist. Simply being aware that a variety of uncommon muscular dystrophies with different prognoses exists will help parents and patients understand that different tests may be necessary to establish a specific diagnosis, a prognosis, and a plan of treatment.

WHEN TO REFER

Neuromuscular clinic or specialist
- When the diagnosis of Duchenne dystrophy is strongly suspected (ie, symptoms and high creatine kinase levels)
- To facilitate the work-up
- Once the diagnosis is confirmed

Genetic counselor
- After the diagnosis of Duchenne dystrophy is established
- Offered to family members of patients, especially at-risk carrier women

Cardiologist
- After the patient with Duchenne dystrophy becomes wheelchair bound
- To obtain a baseline cardiologic evaluation
- In the late stages of the disease for monitoring of cardiac function and management of cardiomyopathy
- Before surgery

Pulmonologist
- After the patient with Duchenne dystrophy becomes wheelchair bound
- To obtain a baseline pulmonary evaluation
- In the late nonambulatory stage of the disease to monitor and manage respiratory failure
- Before surgery

Orthopedic surgeon
- After the patient with Duchenne dystrophy becomes wheelchair bound
- To obtain a baseline orthopedic consultation
- When the nonambulatory patient shows signs of spinal curvature or progressive heel cord contractures
- For consideration of scoliosis surgery
- For release of heel cord contractures

Physical therapist, occupational therapist, or both
- During the ambulatory stage of Duchenne dystrophy, to develop a heel cord stretching program and an individualized exercise program
- In the late ambulatory stage of Duchenne dystrophy, when the patient may appear to be close to becoming wheelchair limited
- To be fitted with adaptive equipment and long-leg braces
- To evaluate and manage contractures

Dietitian
- During the ambulatory stage of Duchenne dystrophy, particularly in patients receiving corticosteroid treatment
- To help manage weight gain
- To establish a healthy eating pattern for the future

Neuropsychologist
- During the ambulatory and nonambulatory stages of Duchenne dystrophy because these patients are at risk of having emotional, cognitive, and behavioral problems
- In patients with borderline intellectual abilities
- In patients with cognitive or behavioral abnormalities
- In patients and family members who need end-of-life counseling

WHEN TO ADMIT

- Before surgery for medical, cardiology, and pulmonary consultations
- After surgery for 24 hours (or longer, depending on the type of surgery) to monitor cardiac and pulmonary function
- For evaluation and management of pneumonia or respiratory insufficiency, especially in nonambulatory patients with Duchenne dystrophy and in patients with advanced cardiomyopathy with cardiac failure

TOOLS FOR PRACTICE

Medical Decision Support

- *Neuromuscular Diseases* (Web page), Muscular Dystrophy Association (www.mdausa.org/disease/40list.html).

- GeneTests (Web page). University of Washington (www.geneclinics.org).
- Neuromuscular Disease Center (Web page). Washington University (neuromuscular.wustl.edu/).

RELATED WEB SITE

- Muscular Dystrophy Association (www.mdausa.org/).

AAP POLICY STATEMENTS

American Academy of Pediatrics, Council on Children With Disabilities. Care coordination in the medical home: integrating health and related systems of care for children with special health care needs. *Pediatrics*. 2005;116(5): 1238-1244. (aappolicy.aappublications.org/cgi/content/full/pediatrics;116/5/1238).

American Academy of Pediatrics, Medical Home Initiatives for Children With Special Needs Project Advisory Committee. The medical home. *Pediatrics*. 2002;110(1):184-186. (aappolicy.aappublications.org/cgi/content/full/pediatrics;110/1/184).

American Academy of Pediatrics, Section on Cardiology and Cardiac Surgery. Cardiovascular health supervision for individuals affected by Duchenne or Becker muscular dystrophy. *Pediatrics*. 2005;116(6):1569-1573. (aappolicy.aappublications.org/cgi/content/full/pediatrics;116/6/1569).

SUGGESTED RESOURCES

Bonnemann C. Limb-girdle muscular dystrophies. In: Jones H, De Vivo D, Darras B, eds. *Neuromuscular Disorders of Infancy, Childhood, and Adolescence: A Clinician's Approach*. Philadelphia, PA: Butterworth Heinemann; 2003.

Engel A, Ozawa E. Dystrophinopathies. In: Engel A, Franzini-Armstrong C, eds. *Myology*. 3rd ed. New York, NY: McGraw-Hill; 2004.

Finder JCCP. Respirator care of the patient with Duchenne muscular dystrophy: an official ATS consensus statement. *Am J Respir Crit Care Med*. 2004;170:456-465.

Moxley RT III, Ashwal S, Pandya S, et al. Practice parameter: corticosteroid treatment of the Duchenne dystrophy: report of the Quality Standards Subcommittee of the American Academy of Neurology and the Practice Committee of the Child Neurology Society. *Neurology*. 2005; 64:13-20.

Moxley RT III, Tawil R. Channelopathies: myotonic disorder and periodic paralysis. In: Swaiman KF, Ashwal S, Fierriero DM, eds. *Pediatric Neurology: Principles and Practice*. Vol 2. 4th ed. Philadelphia, PA: Mosby Elsevier; 2006:2085-2110.

Muntoni F, Voit T. The congenital muscular dystrophies in. 2004: a century of exciting progress. *Neuromuscul Disord*. 2004;14:635-649.

North K. Congenital myopathies. In: Engel A, Franzini-Armstrong C, eds. *Myology*. 3rd ed. New York, NY: McGraw-Hill; 2004.

REFERENCES

1. Brooke MH, Feinchel GM, Griggs RC, et al. Clinical investigation in Duchenne dystrophy. II. Determination of the "power" of therapeutic trials based on the natural history. *Muscle Nerve*. 1983;6:91-103.
2. Brooke MH, Fenichel GM, Griggs RC, et al. Duchenne muscular dystrophy: patterns of clinical progression and effects of supportive therapy. *Neurology*. 1989;39:475-481.
3. Griggs RC, Patterson MC, Horowitz M, et al. Duchenne dystrophy: randomized, controlled trial of prednisone (18 months) and azathioprine (12 months). *Neurology*. 1993;43:520-527.
4. Mendell JR, Moxley RT, Griggs RC, et al. Randomized, double-blind six-month trial of prednisone in Duchenne's muscular dystrophy. *N Engl J Med*. 1989;320:1592-1597.
5. Engel A, Ozawa E. Dystrophinopathies. In: Engel A, Franzini-Armstrong C, eds. *Myology*. 3rd ed. New York, NY: McGraw-Hill; 2004.
6. Escolar D, Leshner R. Muscular dystrophies. In: Swaiman K, Ashwal S, Ferriero D, eds. *Diseases of the Neuromuscular Junction*. Philadelphia, PA: Elsevier; 2006.
7. Darras B, Menache C, Kunkel L. Dystrophinopathies. In: Jones H, De Vivo D, Darras B, eds. *Neuromuscular Disorders of Infancy, Childhood, and Adolescence: A Clinician's Approach*. Philadelphia, PA: Butterworth Heinemann; 2003.
8. Moxley RT. Clinical overview of Duchenne muscular dystrophy. In: Chamberlain JS, Rando TA, eds. *Duchenne Muscular Dystrophy: Advances in Therapeutics*. New York, NY: Taylor and Francis; 2006.
9. Ahn AH, Kunkel LM. The structural and functional diversity of dystrophin. *Nat Genet*. 1993;3:283-291.
10. Brown RH Jr. Dystrophin-associated proteins and the muscular dystrophies. *Ann Rev Med*. 1997;48:457-466.
11. Duggan DJ, Gorospe JR, Fanin M, et al. Mutations in sarcoglycan genes in patients with myopathy. *N Engl J Med*. 1997;336:618-624.
12. Nobile C, Marchi J, Nigrov V, et al. Exon-intron organization of the human dystrophin gene. *Genomics*. 1997;45: 421-424.
13. Deconinck N, et al. Expression of truncated utrophin leads to major functional improvements in dystrophin-deficient muscles of mice. *Nat Med*. 1997;3:1216-1221.
14. Fanin M, et al. Could utrophin rescue the myocardium of patients with dystrophin gene mutations? *J Mol Cell Cardiol*. 1999;31:1501-1508.
15. Ozawa E. The functional biology of dystrophin: structural components and the pathogenesis of Duchenne muscular dystrophy. In: Chamberlain JS, Rando TA, eds. *Duchenne Muscular Dystrophy: Advances in Therapeutics*. New York, NY: Taylor and Francis; 2006.
16. Muntoni F, Gobbi P, Sewry C, et al. Deletions in the 5 region of dystrophin and resulting phenotypes. *J Med Genet*. 1994;31:843-847.
17. Laval SH, Bushby KM. Limb-girdle muscular dystrophies—from genetics to molecular pathology. *Neuropathol Appl Neurobiol*. 2004;30:91-105.
18. Bushby KM, Beckmann JS. The 105th ENMC sponsored workshop: pathogenesis in the non-sarcoglycan limb-girdle muscular dystrophies, Naarden, April 12-14, 2002. *Neuromuscul Disord*. 2003;13:80-90.
19. Mathews KD, Moore SA. Limb-girdle muscular dystrophy. *Curr Neurol Neurosci Rep*. 2003;3:78-85.
20. Bonnemann C. Limb-girdle muscular dystrophies. In: Jones H, De Vivo D, Darras B, eds. *Neuromuscular Disorders of Infancy, Childhood, and Adolescence: A Clinician's Approach*. Philadelphia, PA: Butterworth Heinemann; 2003.
21. Yoshioka M, Kuroki S. Clinical spectrum and genetic studies of Fukuyama congenital muscular dystrophy. *Am J Med Genet*. 1994;53:245-250.
22. Di Blasi C, et al. LAMA2 gene analysis in congenital muscular dystrophy: new mutations, prenatal diagnosis, and founder effect. *Arch Neurol*. 2005;62:1582-1586.
23. Jimenez-Mallebrera C, Brown SC, Sewry CA, et al. Congenital muscular dystrophy: molecular and cellular aspects. *Cell Mol Life Sci*. 2005;62:809-823.

24. Muntoni F, Voit T. The congenital muscular dystrophies in 2004: a century of exciting progress. *Neuromuscul Disord.* 2004;14:635-649.
25. North K. Congenital myopathies. In: Engel A, Franzini-Armstrong C, eds. *Myology.* 3rd ed. New York, NY: McGraw-Hill; 2004.
26. Flanigan KM, von Niederhausern A, Dun DM, et al. Rapid direct sequence analysis of the dystrophin gene. *Am J Hum Genet.* 2003;72:931-939.
27. Dent KM, Dunn DM, von Niederhausern AC, et al. Improved molecular diagnosis of dystrophinopathies in an unselected clinical cohort. *Am J Med Genet A.* 2005;134:295-298.
28. White S, Kalf M, Liu Q, et al. Comprehensive detection of genomic duplications and deletions in the DMD gene, by use of multiplex amplifiable probe hybridization. *Am J Hum Genet.* 2002;71:365-374.
29. Manzur AY, Kuntzer T, Pike M, et al. Glucocorticoid corticosteroids for Duchenne muscular dystrophy. *Cochrane Database Syst Rev.* 2004;(2)CD003725.
30. Moxley RT III, Ashwal S, Pandya S, et al. Practice parameter: corticosteroid treatment of the Duchenne dystrophy: report of the Quality Standards Subcommittee of the American Academy of Neurology and the Practice Committee of the Child Neurology Society. *Neurology.* 2005;64:13-20.
31. Finder JCCP. Respirator care of the patient with Duchene muscular dystrophy: an official ATS consensus statement. *Am J Respir Crit Care Med.* 2004;170:456-465.
32. American Academy of Pediatrics, Section on Cardiology and Cardiac Surgery. Cardiovascular health supervision for individuals affected by Duchenne or Becker muscular dystrohy. *Pediatrics.* 2005;116:1569-1573.
33. Phillips MF, Quinlivan RC, Edwards RH, et al. Changes in spirometery over time as a prognostic marker in patients with Duchenne muscular dystrophy. *Am J Respir Crit Care Med.* 2001;164:2191-2194.
34. Simonds AK, Muntoni F, Heather S, et al. Impact of nasal ventilation on survival in hypercapnic Duchenne muscular dystrophy. *Thorax.* 1998;53:949-952.
35. Ishikawa Y, Bach JR. Nocturnal oxygenation and prognosis in Duchenne muscular dystrophy. *Am J Respir Crit Care Med.* 2000;161:675-676.
36. Gomez-Merino E, Sancho J, Marin J, et al. Mechanical insufflation-exsufflation: pressure, volume and flow relationships and the adequacy of the manufacturer's guidelines. *Am J Phys Med Rehabil.* 2002;81:579-583.
37. McDonald DG. Fracture prevalence in Duchenne muscular dystrophy. *Dev Med Child Neurol.* 2002;44:695-698.
38. Liu M, Mineo K, Hanayama K, et al. Practical problems and management of seating through the clinical stages of Duchenne's muscular dystrophy. *Arch Phys Med Rehabil.* 2003;84:818-824.
39. Jaffe KM, McDonald CM, Ingman E, et al. Symptoms of upper gastrointestinal dysfunction in Duchenne muscular dystrophy: case-control study. *Arch Phys Med Rehabil.* 1990;71:742-744.
40. Bach JR, Campagnolo DI, Hoeman S. Life satisfaction of individuals with Duchenne muscular dystrophy using long-term mechanical ventilatory support. *Am J Phys Med Rehabil.* 1991;70:129-135.
41. Iannaccone ST, Owens H, Scott J, et al. Postoperative malnutrition in Duchenne muscular dystrophy. *J Child Neurol.* 2003;18:17-20.
42. MacLeod M, Kelly R, Robb SA, et al. Bladder dysfunction in Duchenne muscular dystrophy. *Arch Dis Child.* 2003; 88:347-349.
43. Eagle M, Baudouin S, Chandler C, et al. Survival in Duchenne muscular dystrophy: improvements in life expectancy since 1967 and the impact of home nocturnal ventilation. *Neuromuscul Disord.* 2002;12:926-929.
44. Jefferies JL, Eidem BW, Belmont JW, et al. Genetic predictors and remodeling of dilated cardiomyopathy in muscular dystrophy. *Circulation.* 2005;112:2756-2758.
45. Markham LW, Spicer RL, Khoury PR, et al. Steroid therapy and cardiac function in Duchenne muscular dystrophy. *Pediatr Cardiol.* 2005;26:768-771.
46. Rifai Z, Welle S, Moxley RT III. Effect of prednisone on protein metabolism in Duchenne dystrophy. *Am J Physiol.* 1995;268:(1 pt 1):E67-E74.
47. Goldberg L, Clemens PR. Adenoviral-mediated gene therapy. In: Chamberlain JS, Rando TA, eds. *Duchenne Muscular Dystrophy: Advances in Therapeutics.* New York, NY: Taylor and Francis; 2006.
48. Blankinship M, Gregorevic P, Chamberlain JS. Gene therapy of muscular dystrophy using adeno-associated viral vectors: promises and limitations. In: Chamberlain JS, Rando TA, eds. *Duchenne Muscular Dystrophy: Advances in Therapeutics.* New York, NY: Taylor and Francis; 2006.
49. Su LT, Stedman HH. Regional and systemic gene delivery using viral vectors. In: Chamberlain JS, Rando TA, eds. *Duchenne Muscular Dystrophy: Advances in Therapeutics.* New York, NY: Taylor and Francis; 2006.
50. Liadaki K, Montanaro F, Kunkel LM. Cellular mediated delivery: the intersection between regenerative medicine and genetic therapy. In: Chamberlain JS, Rando TA, eds. *Duchenne Muscular Dystrophy: Advances in Therapeutics.* New York, NY: Taylor and Francis; 2006.
51. Bertoni C, Rando T. Oligonucleotide-mediated exon skipping and gene editing for Duchenne muscular dystrophy. In: Chamberlain JS, Rando TA, eds. *Duchenne Muscular Dystrophy: Advances in Therapeutics.* New York, NY: Taylor and Francis; 2006.
52. Moxley RT, Meola G. The myotonic dystrophies. In: Rosenberg R, Prusiner S, DiMauro S, Barchi R, Nestler E, eds. *The Molecular and Genetic Basis of Neurologic and Psychiatric Disease.* 3rd ed. Philadelphia, PA: Butterworth Heinemann; 2003.
53. Moxley RT III, Tawil R. Channelopathies: myotonic disorder and periodic paralysis. In: Swaiman KF, Ashwal S, Fierriero DM, eds. *Pediatric Neurology: Principles and Practice.* Vol 2. 4th ed. Philadelphia, PA: Mosby Elsevier; 2006.
54. Harper PS. *Myotonic Dystrophy.* 3rd ed. London, UK: WB Saunders; 2001.
55. Harper PS, Bunner HG. Genetic counseling and genetic testing in myotonic dystrophy. In: Harper PS, van Engelen BGM, Eymard B, et al, eds. *Myotonic Dystrophy: Present Management, Future Therapy.* Oxford, UK: Oxford University Press; 2004.
56. Thornton CA, Griggs RC, Moxley RT. Myotonic dystrophy with no trinucleotide repeat expansion. *Ann Neurol.* 1994;34:269-274.
57. Ricker Kkoch MC, Lehmann-Horn F, Pongratz D, et al. Proximal myotonic myopathy: a new dominant disorder with myotonia, muscle weakness, and cataracts. *Neurology.* 1994;44:1448-1454.
58. Liquori CL, Ricker K, Moseley ML, et al. Myotonic dystrophy type 2 caused by a CCTG expansion in intron 1 of ZNF9. *Science.* 2001;293:864-866.
59. Day J, Ricker K, Jacobsen J. Fetal myotonic dystrophy type 2: molecular, diagnostic and clinical spectrum. *Neurology.* 2003;60:657-667.
60. Orrell RW, Darras BT, Griggs RC. Facioscapulohumeral dystrophy, scapuloperoneal syndromes, and distal myopathies. In: Jones H, De Vivo D, Darras B, eds. *Neuromuscular Disorders of Infancy, Childhood, and Adolescence: A Clinician's Approach.* Philadelphia, PA: Butterworth Heinemann; 2003.

61. Tawil R, Griggs RC. Facioscapulohumeral muscular dystrophy. In: Karpati G, Hilton-Jones D, Griggs RC, eds. *Disorders of Voluntary Muscle*. Cambridge, UK: Cambridge University Press; 2001.
62. Felice KJ, Jones JM, Conway SR. Facioscapulohumeral dystrophy presenting as infantile facial diplegia and late-onset limb-girdle myopathy in members of the same family. *Muscle Nerve*. 2005;32:368-372.
63. Brouwer OF, Padberg GW, Wijmenga C, et al. Facioscapulohumeral muscular dystrophy in early childhood. *Arch Neurol*. 1994;51:387-394.
64. Shapiro F, Specht L, Korf BR. Locomotor problems in infantile facioscapulohumeral muscular dystrophy: retrospective study of 9 patients. *Acta Orthop Scand*. 1991;62:367-371.
65. Tawil R, Van Der Maarel SM. Facioscapulohumeral muscular dystrophy. *Muscle Nerve*. 2006;34:1-15
66. Maraldi N, Merlini L. Emery-Dreifuss muscular dystrophy. In: Engel A, Franzini-Armstrong C, eds. *Myology*. 3rd ed. New York, NY: McGraw-Hill; 2004.
67. Mercuri E, Brown SC, Nihoyannopoulos P, et al. Extreme variability of skeletal and cardiac muscle involvement in patients with mutations in exon 11 of the lamin A/C gene. *Muscle Nerve*. 2005;31:602-609.

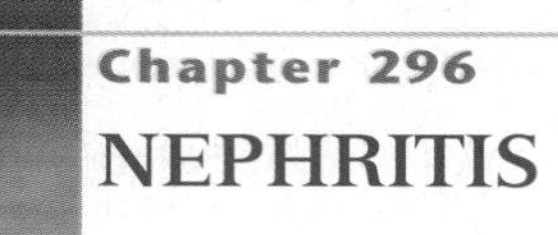

Chapter 296

NEPHRITIS

William S. Varade, MD

DEFINITION

Nephritis is the general term for noninfectious inflammation of the kidney parenchyma. This inflammation may involve primarily the glomerulus (glomerulonephritis), the interstitium (interstitial nephritis), or both. Because glomerulonephritis historically has been the subject of more intense interest, when the term nephritis is used, many practitioners think only of glomerular lesions.

CLINICAL MANIFESTATION

The components of a classic nephritic syndrome are hematuria, proteinuria, the presence of red blood cell casts in the urine, oliguria, hypertension, and uremia. Some or all of these parameters may be evident initially. The finding of hematuria and proteinuria together strongly suggests underlying glomerular inflammation. Hematuria may be microscopic or macroscopic. Proteinuria can range from mild to nephrotic range. Presentation can range from acute, with sudden onset of gross hematuria, edema, and oliguria, to subacute or chronic, with a more protracted course in which symptoms may be lacking and urine abnormalities detected on routine urinalysis are the only findings.

INCIDENCE

The true incidence of nephritis in children is difficult to ascertain. Many cases of acute glomerulonephritis may be mild and self-limited and thus go undetected or not lead to biopsy. Of 487 children younger than 15 years who underwent renal biopsy, 43% had a diagnosis of glomerulonephritis. Only 8.4% of these had a classical nephritic picture with hematuria, hypertension, oliguria, edema, and reduced glomerular filtration rate.[1] Thus incomplete nephritic syndrome presentations are more common in children who are ultimately diagnosed with nephritis. Incidence reports of nephritis may be skewed by differing criteria for biopsy in different parts of the world and differences in the frequency of specific nephritides in different regions.

GENERAL EVALUATION OF SUSPECTED NEPHRITIS

Blood pressure should be monitored carefully and frequently in any patient with suspected nephritis, and it should be compared with normal values for gender, age, and height percentile.[2] Weight should be measured. Significant weight gain compared with values from prior visits might suggest fluid retention. Similarly, poor growth with crossing height percentiles with inappropriate weight gain or loss might suggest a chronic renal disorder. Children with nephritis may have the following findings on physical examination: periorbital or pretibial edema, changes in eye grounds, a uremic odor to the breath, pleural or pericardial friction rubs, ascites, costovertebral angle tenderness, joint swelling or tenderness, and vasculitic rashes.

Laboratory evaluation should include urinalysis with microscopy, serum electrolytes, blood urea nitrogen, creatinine, calcium, phosphorous, albumin, liver enzymes, and complete blood count with platelets. Decreased levels of the third component of complement (C3) and on occasion that of the fourth component (C4), can help narrow the differential diagnosis by distinguishing the hypocomplementemic nephritides from those with normal complement levels (Box 296-1). Antinuclear antibody and antistreptolysin O or other antibodies to streptococcal antigens should be obtained. Anti–double-stranded DNA, antineutrophil cytoplasmic antibodies, and hepatitis B and C serologic tests may be useful in cases of lupus nephritis, Wegener granulomatosis, microscopic polyangiitis, and some cases of membranoproliferative glomerulonephritis or membranous nephropathy. Although pyelonephritis can usually be distinguished from glomerulonephritis on clinical grounds, urine culture should be obtained in unclear cases. Imaging studies, in general, are

BOX 296-1 Glomerulonephritides With Low Complement Levels

Acute poststreptococcal glomerulonephritis
Lupus nephritis
Membranoproliferative glomerulonephritis
Nephritis of chronic infection
Cryoglobulinemia

nonspecific and not helpful in evaluating patients with nephritis.

ACUTE GLOMERULONEPHRITIS

Acute glomerulonephritis is characterized by the abrupt onset of hematuria, proteinuria, hypertension, and edema. The hematuria is often grossly visible as tea-colored or cola-colored urine. In some children, however, the hematuria may be microscopic only. Red blood cell casts and dysmorphic red blood cells are present, although several urine samples may have to be examined to demonstrate them (Figure 296-1).[3] White blood cells on microscopy and a positive test for leukocyte esterase are often found but suggest inflammation and not bacterial infection. Acute glomerulonephritis is often the initial presentation of the renal diseases listed in Box 296-2.

This clinical syndrome can have 2 presentations: (1) acute glomerulonephritis with no or mild renal failure and (2) acute glomerulonephritis with rapidly progressive renal failure.

ACUTE GLOMERULONEPHRITIS WITH NO OR MILD RENAL FAILURE

Acute Poststreptococcal Glomerulonephritis

Acute poststreptococcal glomerulonephritis (APSGN) is a common form of glomerulonephritis in childhood. The true incidence is unknown because many cases are subclinical.[4] Although poststreptococcal nephritis may happen at any age the peak incidence occurs at age 7 years, with a slight predominance among boys. It is less common before age 3 years and in adults. Sporadic cases of APSGN are most common, though epidemics may occur. Cases of nephritis after streptococcal pharyngo-tonsillitis are more common in temperate regions, whereas those after streptococcal skin infections are more common in tropical and subtropical climates.[5]

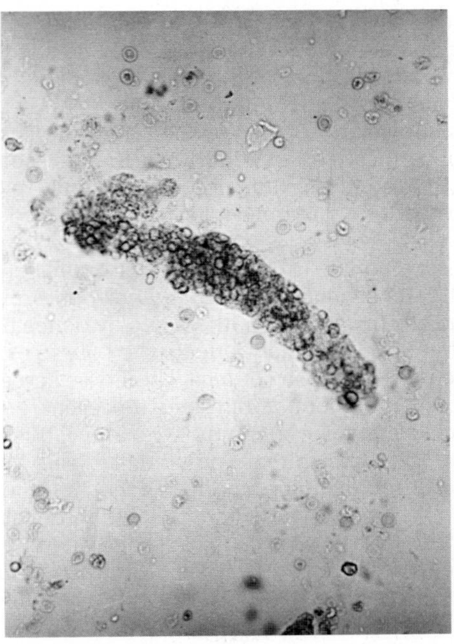

Figure 296-1 Red blood cell cast (unstained).

Etiology

Poststreptococcal glomerulonephritis is the consequence of the host's immune response to a nonrenal infection with group A β-hemolytic streptococci (GABHS). Not all GABHS strains are nephritogenic. Nephritogenic strains include types 1, 2, 4, 12, 18, 25, 49, 55, 57, and 60 and possibly some nontypable strains.[5] Types 12 and 49 are the strains most commonly associated with nephritis.[5-7] The pathogenesis of APSGN remains uncertain. One possibility is that streptococcal proteins are released and lodge in the glomerulus where they form nephritogenic immune complexes leading to complement activation. Bacterial components suspected of comprising these immune complexes are the streptococcal preabsorbing antigen, nephritis strain–associated protein, endostreptosin, and nephritis-associated plasmin receptor.[4,8,9] These proteins induce an antibody response, can be found in the glomeruli of patients with APSGN, and can activate complement. Approximately 15% of patients infected with a nephritogenic strain of streptococci subsequently develop nephritis.[5] The risk of developing nephritis may differ according to site of infection (skin vs throat) and the particular M-type.

Pathological Features

The typical glomerular findings are proliferation of mesangial and endothelial cells, as well as the influx of polymorphonuclear leukocytes and mononuclear cells. The glomeruli are larger than normal, and the capillary lumens are compromised by the cellular proliferation within the glomeruli. By immunofluorescence microscopy, granular deposits of immunoglobulin and complement can be seen, corresponding to the subepithelial electron-dense humps seen on electron microscopy. With healing, the increased cellularity and immune deposits become limited to the mesangial region and then gradually resolve.

BOX 296-2 Acute Glomerulonephritides That Are Usually Characterized By No or Mild Renal Failure

MORE COMMON

- Acute poststreptococcal glomerulonephritis
- Henoch-Schönlein purpura with nephritis
- Postinfectious (nonstreptococcal) glomerulonephritis
- Interstitial glomerulonephritis
- Radiation nephritis

LESS COMMON

- Acute episodes in patients with chronic glomerulonephritis
- Hemolytic-uremic syndrome (milder cases)
- Membranoproliferative glomerulonephritis (some)
- Nephritis of systemic lupus erythematosus (some)

Clinical Presentation

Mild and subclinical cases of APSGN are common. Renal involvement characteristically occurs 8 to 14 days after a pharyngeal infection or 14 to 21 days after a skin infection caused by the nephritogenic streptococci. Two thirds of patients with APSGN exhibit macroscopic hematuria.[10] Patients will usually have oliguria and, in rare cases, anuria. Fluid retention leads to edema that is usually periorbital and, rarely, severe. Intravascular overload caused by salt and water retention can lead to signs of congestive heart failure. Approximately 60% to 70% of the patients have hypertension also related to salt and water retention.[11] Patients who have severe hypertension may have symptoms of headache, drowsiness, vomiting, personality and visual changes, and convulsions. Anorexia and pain in the abdomen or flank are common, although palpation of the abdomen usually does not reveal significant findings. Costovertebral angle tenderness often is present. Although a history of preceding skin or pharyngeal infection supports the diagnosis, such a history cannot be elicited in many cases.

Laboratory Findings

The urine of children with APSGN usually is tea colored and opaque. The specific gravity is generally increased, and hemoglobin can be detected by dipstick testing. Proteinuria usually parallels the degree of hematuria and rarely reaches the nephrotic range (>40 mg/m^2/hr or >3.5 g/day in older children and adults). Microscopic examination usually reveals red and white blood cells, and granular or cellular casts. Because identifiable erythrocyte casts and dysmorphic erythrocytes may or may not be present, serial urine specimens may need to be examined.

Serum complement levels show a reduction of C3 in 80% of patients with APSGN and, early in the course, a reduction of C4 in 50%. The erythrocyte sedimentation rate (ESR) is usually elevated. With severe oliguria, azotemia and acidosis may be seen. The plasma volume is usually expanded, causing a decline in serum protein, hemoglobin, and hematocrit levels by dilution. Hemolysis, a shortened erythrocyte half-life, and reduced erythrocyte production may contribute to these hematologic changes. Salt retention with a decreased fractional excretion of sodium is often seen even in the setting of increased intravascular volume.

Evidence of a preceding streptococcal infection is important to support the diagnosis. The antistreptolysin O titer is elevated in 80% of patients, although increases in titer are less common in patients who have skin infection and in those who receive early treatment with antibiotics.[12] When other streptococcal antibodies (antihyaluronidase, antideoxyribonuclease B) are measured, 80% to 90% of patients will have serologic evidence of preceding streptococcal infection.[12] Cultures often are negative for GABHS by the time nephritis develops particularly if antibiotics were prescribed.

The chest radiograph in patients who have significant fluid retention and hypertension may reveal a large heart with prominent pulmonary vasculature, pulmonary edema, or, in rare cases, pleural effusions.[11] Ultrasound examination is nonspecific, usually revealing bilaterally enlarged echogenic kidneys.

Course

The acute phase of APSGN will usually resolve after 1 week, heralded by diuresis. Creatinine levels should normalize by 3 to 4 weeks. Gross hematuria resolves within 1 or 2 weeks, although microscopic hematuria may persist for more than 1 year. Proteinuria should resolve by 3 months, and complement levels should normalize by 6 to 8 weeks. The presence of nephrotic-range proteinuria or extensive crescents by biopsy portends a poor prognosis. The failure of complement levels to normalize by 8 weeks suggests the presence of a form of nephritis other than ASPGN, such as membranoproliferative glomerulonephritis, the nephritis of chronic infection, or lupus nephritis.

Treatment

Acute poststreptococcal glomerulonephritis most often resolves spontaneously and is not affected by corticosteroids or immunosuppressive agents. Even so, the practitioner must be aggressive in treating hypertension, oliguria, and the resulting vascular overload, pulmonary edema, and encephalopathy that may occur in the acute phase of the illness because these can be associated with significant morbidity and mortality.

Although mild hypertension may resolve spontaneously, more severe degrees of hypertension should be controlled with antihypertensive agents that act quickly. Because increased intravascular volume is theorized to be the main determinant of hypertension in acute glomerulonephritis, diuretics are a mainstay of therapy.[11] Control of severe hypertension will often require the use of intravenous sodium nitroprusside, labetalol, nicardipine, or fenoldopam. Oral minoxidil may be effective. Slower-acting, less-potent antihypertensive drugs are not good initial choices but can be substituted once blood pressure has been acutely stabilized.

Oliguria results from decreased glomerular filtration and salt and water retention. In the absence of evidence of dehydration, administration of fluid boluses will not hasten the resolution of oliguria, and excessive fluid administration will worsen hypertension. The signs of congestive heart failure usually resolve with control of the hypertension. Occasionally a patient develops acute renal failure severe enough to require dialysis.

A 10-day course of antibiotics is usually given to eradicate any remaining GABHS and thus prevent the spread of the organism to others. No evidence has been found that such treatment affects the course of nephritis in the patient. Close contacts should be screened for streptococcal infection and treated if present.

Hospitalization for patients who have this disease needs to be determined individually (see When to Admit). Although many children who have mild episodes do well as outpatients, the sudden development of hypertension and oliguria may produce life-threatening symptoms quite rapidly, necessitating hospitalization. After the acute phase the child may be allowed to resume normal activities gradually. Every child should be monitored regularly until the hypertension, electrolyte and creatinine abnormalities, and serum complement values return to normal. To be certain of the diagnosis, a renal biopsy may be indicated for a child whose clinical or laboratory findings are atypical. Any child whose C3 value does not return to normal within 8 weeks should be considered for kidney biopsy.

Prognosis

Studies have shown that more than 95% of children who have APSGN recover from their illness.[13] For most children the critical period is early in the illness when potentially fatal hypertension or fluid overload presents a danger. Occasionally, patients who have severe involvement, as evidenced by nephrotic-range proteinuria or the presence of extensive glomerular crescents on biopsy, have some residual damage or may even progress to end-stage renal failure. In general, however, the kidneys have an outstanding recovery potential in this disease.[13,14] Recurrences of APSGN are rare.

Postinfectious (Nonstreptococcal) Glomerulonephritis

A variety of viruses are suspected of causing acute glomerulonephritis, including varicella, echovirus 10, coxsackieviruses, the viruses that cause infectious mononucleosis, measles, and mumps.[15] However, significant renal involvement is unusual in infections caused by these viruses. Children who have such involvement have no serologic evidence of recent streptococcal infection. In most cases the acute nephritis resolves spontaneously and gradually, and renal function returns completely. No effective way has been discovered to differentiate the nonstreptococcal postinfectious glomerulonephritides from other nephritides that progress to renal failure, except by observing the clinical course.

Henoch-Schönlein Purpura Nephritis

Henoch-Schönlein purpura (HSP) is a small-vessel vasculitis most often affecting children, with a peak between 4 and 6 years of age.[15] It is characterized by palpable purpuric lesions, arthritis, abdominal pain and gastrointestinal bleeding, and nephritis. Not all manifestations need be present at the same time. Renal involvement is the most significant complication of HSP. Its presentation can vary considerably from minimal abnormalities on urinalysis to an aggressive rapidly progressive glomerulonephritis with nephrotic syndrome and renal failure. The true incidence of renal involvement in HSP is difficult to ascertain and has been reported to range from 20% to 90%, depending on the definition of renal involvement used and whether the report is from a referral center or not. (See Chapter 272, Henoch-Schönlein Purpura.)

Rapidly Progressive Glomerulonephritis

Rapidly progressive glomerulonephritis (RPGN) is a variant of acute glomerulonephritis characterized by symptoms of acute nephritis associated with relentless progression to renal failure over days or weeks.[16] Although acute interstitial nephritis stemming from pyelonephritis or hypersensitivity to certain drugs may develop in this way, most cases are the result of glomerular disease. Almost any of the acute or chronic glomerulonephritides may at times exhibit a rapidly progressive course. This group includes rare cases of poststreptococcal glomerulonephritis, indicating the need to monitor renal function and the general clinical course closely even in seemingly routine cases. As shown in Box 296-2, RPGN can be classified into three categories based on immunopathological findings as seen in kidney biopsies.[17]

Systemic lupus erythematosus (SLE) not infrequently may result in an acute glomerulonephritis with a rapidly deteriorating course. Of the primary renal disease group, IgA nephropathy and membranoproliferative glomerulonephritis may result in this presentation as well.

Occasionally, patients who have undiscovered chronic renal failure suffer a sudden deterioration that may be interpreted as acute glomerulonephritis (Box 296-3). Evaluation of these patients often reveals evidence of preexisting chronic renal failure, such as osteodystrophy or hyperphosphatemia.

Idiopathic RPGN without immune deposits is much less common among children and includes Wegener granulomatosis, associated with upper and lower respiratory findings, and microscopic polyangiitis. The

BOX 296-3 Classification of Acute Glomerulonephritis With Rapidly Progressive Renal Failure

IMMUNE COMPLEX

- Postinfectious reaction
  - Streptococcal infection
  - Visceral abscess
  - Other
- Collagen-vascular disease
  - Systemic lupus erythematosus
  - Henoch-Schönlein purpura
  - Mixed cryoglobulinemia
- Primary renal disease
  - IgA nephropathy
  - Membranoproliferative glomerulonephritis
  - Unknown cases (ie, idiopathic)

NO IMMUNE DEPOSIT

- Unknown cause
- Vasculitis
  - Microscopic polyangiitis
  - Wegener granulomatosis
  - Hypersensitivity vasculitides
- Hemolytic-uremic syndrome

ANTI-GLOMERULAR BASEMENT MEMBRANE ANTIBODY

- With lung hemorrhage (Goodpasture syndrome)
- Without lung hemorrhage
- Complicating membranous nephropathy

Modified from Couser WG. Rapidly progressive glomerulonephritis: classification, pathogenetic mechanisms, and therapy. *Am J Kidney Dis.* 1988; 11(6):449-464.

presence of anti–neutrophil cytoplasmic antibodies (ANCA) in the serum may help distinguish these disorders from each other and from other causes of rapid deterioration of renal function. In particular, antimyeloperoxidase with a perinuclear or P-ANCA pattern of antibody staining is often associated with microscopic polyangiitis, whereas antiproteinase 3 with a cytoplasmic or C-ANCA pattern of antibody staining is often associated with Wegener granulomatosis. Of note, some of these patients will be negative for ANCA, and other patients with microscopic polyangiitis may be positive for antiproteinase 3, and some patients with Wegener granulomatosis are positive for antimyeloperoxidase. Anti–glomerular basement membrane (GBM) antibody–mediated RPGN is even more rare in children.

The hemolytic-uremic syndrome (see Chapter 269, Hemolytic-Uremic Syndrome) is a triad of renal failure, hemolytic anemia, and thrombocytopenia, which in children is most frequently related to infection by shigatoxin-producing *Escherichia coli* O157:H7. It is the most common cause of community acquired acute renal failure in pediatric patients. This entity frequently follows a prodrome of hemorrhagic colitis. Nondiarrheal forms of hemolytic-uremic syndrome (HUS), including inherited forms, thrombotic thrombocytopenic purpura, and disseminated intravascular coagulation are less common but have a poorer prognosis and must be included in the differential diagnosis.

Although the characteristic clinical and laboratory features of a particular RPGN presentation may suggest specific causative factors, a renal biopsy often is indicated to make the diagnosis and to determine the extent of the disease.[17]

Treatment of RPGN depends on the particular diagnosis, often determined by kidney biopsy. Methylprednisolone pulses are frequently given initially for fulminant cases of SLE nephritis, membranoproliferative glomerulonephritis, IgA nephropathy, HSP nephritis, Wegener granulomatosis, and polyarteritis nodosa. These pulses are frequently followed by oral or intravenous alkylating agents. Plasmapheresis may be helpful in anti-GBM-antibody disease, atypical forms of HUS, thrombotic-thrombocytopenic purpura, and some other resistant forms of RPGN. Typical diarrhea-associated HUS is treated supportively.

CHRONIC GLOMERULONEPHRITIS

The glomerulonephritides that follow a prolonged, chronic course may be associated with an acute or subacute nephritis or, more insidiously, with only an abnormal urinalysis in an asymptomatic patient. Advanced cases may be discovered during investigation of nonspecific complaints such as anorexia, intermittent vomiting, and malaise that are found to result from undiagnosed chronic renal failure. IgA nephropathy, Alport syndrome, the nephritis of SLE, and membranoproliferative glomerulonephritis commonly follow a chronic course. Nonnephritic causes of chronic kidney failure, such as renal dysplasia and obstructive uropathies with significant unrecognized parenchymal damage, should be considered in the differential diagnosis.

IgA Nephropathy

IgA nephropathy was first described by Berger and Hinglais in 1969 and has also been called IgA-IgG nephropathy, or Berger disease.

Etiology

The cause of IgA nephropathy is unknown. Abnormal glycosylation of the hinge region of the IgA antibody molecule has been observed and has been suggested as a possible mechanism of disease. Mesangial IgA deposition and complement activation may play a role in damaging the kidneys. Secondary forms of IgA nephropathy can be seen with inflammatory bowel disease and liver disease.

Pathological Features

The sine qua non for the diagnosis of IgA nephropathy is the finding of dominant or codominant IgA staining of the glomerular mesangium by immunofluorescence microscopy. IgG and C3 generally are seen as well. Histologically, a wide variety of glomerular lesions can be seen from essentially normal glomeruli to mesangial hypercellularity with an increase in mesangial matrix or focal segmental proliferative, necrotizing, or sclerosing lesions. IgA nephropathy is difficult to differentiate morphologically from HSP, which has led to speculation that HSP is a form of IgA nephropathy with systemic findings.

Clinical Presentation

IgA nephropathy typically occurs in the second or third decade of life but can affect all ages.[18] Male children are affected more often than female children, and it appears to occur less frequently in blacks than in whites. Characteristically, children with IgA nephropathy have a sudden onset of painless gross hematuria concomitant with an infection, usually of the respiratory tract,[18] which may be associated with flank pain. The gross hematuria usually clears within a few days to a week as the infection resolves. Frequently, gross hematuria recurs with subsequent infections. Microscopic hematuria may persist with or without proteinuria between episodes, or the urine may clear totally. The simultaneous onset of an upper respiratory tract infection with the gross hematuria helps differentiate this disease from APSGN, in which a delay between infection and hematuria is the rule. The absence of a rash, abdominal pain, and arthritis helps differentiate IgA nephropathy from the nephritis of HSP. Approximately 10% of patients with IgA nephropathy may have nephrotic syndrome or acute renal failure at presentation.

Laboratory Findings

Other than an abnormal urinalysis, laboratory studies, at least in milder cases, are often normal. In particular, hypocomplementemia and serologic evidence of recent streptococcal infection usually are absent. Azotemia or heavy proteinuria, when they do occur, are poor prognostic signs. A renal biopsy may be indicated in patients with renal insufficiency, nephrotic-range proteinuria, or persistent hematuria and proteinuria to confirm the diagnosis and to clarify the prognosis.

Treatment

Treatment of IgA nephropathy remains controversial. Suggested regimens for patients with poor prognostic indicators include long-term, alternate-day prednisone, with or without methylprednisolone pulses, and mycophenolate mofetil.[19-22] Control of hypertension, as for other renal diseases, is essential.

Prognosis

Although IgA nephropathy was originally considered to be a benign disorder in children, from 10% to 30% of pediatric patients are anticipated to progress to renal failure over the course of several decades. Progression has been related to higher amounts of proteinuria, the presence of hypertension, renal insufficiency at presentation, and the severity of the histologic changes found on the kidney biopsy.[18-21,23-25]

Benign Familial Hematuria

Although not a chronic glomerulonephritis per se, benign familial hematuria is characterized by persistent hematuria among similarly affected, otherwise-healthy family members.[26] As such, it is an important disorder in the differential diagnoses of both IgA nephropathy and Alport syndrome (see previous and following sections) and hypercalciuria. Benign familial hematuria is a benign condition inherited as an autosomal-dominant trait. Undoubtedly, many of the early reports included patients who had IgA nephropathy because of the similarities of clinical presentation and because renal biopsy specimens often were not obtained. This condition has also been called benign recurrent hematuria.

Etiology

Mutations in the type-IV collagen α-3 and α-4 genes have been associated with benign familial hematuria.[27,28] However, linkage to this chromosomal region was not detected in other studies, suggesting that the cause of benign familial hematuria is heterogeneous.[29,30]

Pathological Features

Light and fluorescence microscopy of renal biopsy specimens are generally normal. Widespread thinning of the GBM is present by electron microscopy, and, consequently, benign familial hematuria is also often referred to as thin basement membrane disease. These pathological findings may be similar to those seen early in the course of Alport syndrome. Only the family history of lack of progressive renal impairment, deafness, and eye findings distinguishes it from early Alport syndrome.

Clinical Presentation

Persistent asymptomatic microscopic hematuria in the absence of hearing loss, proteinuria, or progressive renal impairment is the usual presentation.

Laboratory Findings

All laboratory test results are usually normal except for the urinalysis. The presence of hematuria in otherwise-asymptomatic family members suggests this diagnosis.

Course

Most cases are discovered by finding microscopic hematuria on urinalysis during a routine evaluation. Benign familial hematuria may be similar to IgA nephropathy. It was found to be the cause of isolated asymptomatic microscopic hematuria in approximately one third of adults, whereas IgA nephropathy was responsible for another third of the cases.[31] The hematuria is persistent, but renal failure, deafness, and eye findings do not develop, in contrast to Alport syndrome. No treatment is indicated for benign familial hematuria, and the prognosis is excellent.

Alport Syndrome

Alport syndrome, or hereditary nephritis, is an inherited renal disease associated with sensorineural deafness and ocular abnormalities. Alport syndrome is inherited as an X-linked–dominant trait in 80% to 85% of cases.[32] Families with Alport syndrome with autosomal-recessive inheritance (15% of cases) or, very rarely, autosomal-dominant inheritance have also been described.[33] The combination of Alport features and macrothrombocytopenia is known as Epstein syndrome. Rarely, X-linked Alport syndrome can also be associated with leiomyomatosis.

Etiology

X-linked Alport syndrome is caused by a mutation of the gene encoding the α-5 chain of type-IV collagen.[33] Mutations range from point mutations, leading to an amino acid substitution or a premature stop codon, to small or large deletions. The particular type of mutation may influence the severity of the clinical expression of the disease. Ten percent to 15% of cases represent new mutations.[32] X-linked Alport syndrome with leiomyomatosis appears to arise from deletions involving the contiguous genes encoding the α-5 and α-6 chains of type-IV collagen.[33] Autosomal-recessive Alport syndrome has been related to mutations in the genes encoding the α-3 and α-4 chains of type-IV collagen on chromosome 2.[33] Autosomal-dominant Alport syndrome also has been linked to the region of chromosome 2 containing the genes encoding the α-3 and α-4 chains of type-IV collagen.[33]

Pathological Features

The characteristic findings of Alport syndrome are seen by electron microscopy of renal biopsy specimen. These findings include variations in the thickness of the GBM, with splitting and lamellation of the lamina densa of the GBM, giving it a basket-weave appearance. However, early on in the course of the disease the only ultrastructural abnormality may be diffuse attenuation of the GBM. Thus, in these cases, distinguishing patients with Alport syndrome from those with thin basement membrane nephropathy may be difficult based on biopsy findings alone. In these indeterminate cases, special stains for the individual type-IV collagen chains may prove of value for making the correct diagnosis.

Clinical Presentation

Renal disease is severe and progressive in male patients with X-linked Alport syndrome, with approximately

90% developing end-stage renal failure by age 40 years.[32] Female patients are generally less severely affected, with approximately 12% reaching end-stage renal failure by age 40 and 30% by age 60. Age at the development of renal failure tends to run true within families, although exceptions are well documented. Persistent microscopic hematuria is found early on in all affected male patients. Most female patients have intermittent microscopic hematuria. Macroscopic hematuria occurs in up to 70% of male patients and 33% of female patients, often at the time of a respiratory infection. Proteinuria develops in male patients with age and reaches nephrotic range in approximately 30%. Sensorineural hearing loss is progressive starting with high frequencies and affects male patients more than female patients. It is not, however, present in all families with Alport syndrome. Eye abnormalities are found in approximately 50% of patients with Alport syndrome. These abnormalities include anterior lenticonus, retinal abnormalities, and corneal ulcerations.

Male and female patients are equally affected in autosomal-recessive Alport syndrome. The course is similar to that of male patients with X-linked Alport syndrome. Approximately two thirds of patients with the autosomal-recessive form will develop hearing loss.[32] Approximately one half the carriers of the abnormal gene will also have microscopic hematuria.

Laboratory Findings

Laboratory findings reflect the degree of renal impairment and may vary from normal early on to advanced renal failure as the disease progresses. Blood urea nitrogen and creatinine levels become elevated with advancing disease. Serum electrolytes may become abnormal, and hypoalbuminemia may develop in select patients who develop nephrotic syndrome. Serum complement values usually are normal. A renal biopsy may help establish the diagnosis in patients in whom the family history is unclear or who has a new mutation.

Course

The disease is progressive in male patients and some female patients with X-linked Alport syndrome and in patients of both sexes with autosomal-recessive and autosomal-dominant forms of Alport syndrome. Proteinuria is not present initially but usually develops later in the course of the disease. The course is usually similar for members of an affected family, although variations in the progression have been reported.

Treatment

Treatment is supportive, with medical management of hypertension and the complications of renal insufficiency. Dialysis or transplantation is instituted when medical management is no longer sufficient. Audiologic screening can identify hearing impairment early and allow for the timely implementation of hearing-augmentation services.

Prognosis

In affected individuals, renal disease and hearing loss are progressive. Families carrying mutations consisting of large deletions or stop codons leading to truncated proteins may be at risk for more severe disease than those with mutations leading to an amino acid substitution.[32] Dialysis and transplantation are offered when end-stage renal failure occurs. Three percent to 4% of patients with Alport syndrome receiving a kidney transplant develop anti-GBM nephritis, leading to loss of the transplanted kidney in 75% of these cases.[33]

Nephritis of Systemic Lupus Erythematosus

SLE is an autoimmune disease that affects multiple organ systems and is seen mainly in young women during the childbearing years. Twenty percent of cases, however, involve children.[34]

Etiology

The cause of SLE is unknown. Dysregulation of the cellular and humoral branches of the immune system occurs and results in an autoimmune state, with autoantibody production and the deposition of circulating immune complexes or the formation of immune complexes in situ. Complement proteins are activated and lead to damage to the glomeruli. Clearly, however, other factors are involved in disease production as well. Female sex clearly predisposes the patient to the development of SLE. A genetic predisposition to the development of SLE also appears to exist, with increased evidence of autoimmune phenomena within these families. Blacks and Asians seem to be disproportionately affected. Some cases are related to inherited deficiencies of early components of the complement cascade.[35]

Pathological Features

Renal histologic findings vary greatly in patients with lupus nephritis. The World Health Organization (WHO) classification of renal disease in lupus nephritis is widely used for interpreting the renal biopsy findings and guiding therapy in this disease. Focal proliferative (WHO class III) and diffuse proliferative (WHO class IV) lesions indicate severe disease and are found in the kidney biopsies of more than one half the children with lupus nephritis.[36] Immunofluorescence microscopy demonstrates deposition of immunoglobulins and complement components in the mesangium and along the capillary loops. Dense deposits, corresponding to the immune complexes detected by immunofluorescence, are seen by electron microscopy. Cellular proliferation and basement membrane thickening are also seen.

Clinical Presentation

Children with SLE may initially have constitutional, cutaneous, or musculoskeletal symptoms such as fever, malaise, rash, or arthritis.[37] Initial complaints may be vague, and a high index of suspicion is warranted. However, childhood SLE tends to be more severe at presentation than adult-onset SLE. Up to 75% of children will have some evidence of renal involvement on presentation. Renal involvement usually evolves with time in most children with SLE and is an important cause of morbidity and mortality. When present, renal involvement may be characterized by isolated hematuria, hematuria with proteinuria, nephrotic syndrome, hypertension, or rapidly progressive renal failure. In a retrospective study, 17% of children with SLE developed renal failure, and approximately 90% developed renal involvement within the first year.[34,35] One half the children with kidney involvement will have the more severe and aggressive diffuse proliferative glomerulonephritis (WHO class IV) on biopsy.[34,38]

Laboratory Findings

Antinuclear antibodies are positive in most children with SLE. Anti–double-stranded DNA is positive in many patients with renal involvement as well. Serum complement components are frequently decreased and tend to correlate with disease activity. Evidence of renal disease may be characterized by elevation of serum urea and creatinine levels and decrease in serum albumin levels in the setting of nephrotic-range proteinuria. Findings on urinalysis vary greatly and range from isolated hematuria, hematuria with proteinuria, to nephrotic-range proteinuria. Pyuria is common and reflects the underlying glomerular inflammation. Red blood cell, white blood cell, and renal tubular epithelial cell casts frequently are seen.

Hematologic abnormalities include Coombs-positive anemia, leukopenia, and thrombocytopenia. Antiphospholipid antibodies are found in as many as 67% of children with SLE and are a risk factor for thrombotic complications.

Course

The course of SLE varies considerably. Renal manifestations can wax and wane with changes in disease activity, intercurrent illness, and type of therapy. In addition to the risk for morbidity and mortality from the underlying disease, children with SLE are at risk for complications related to treatment and are at increased risk of infectious complications.

Treatment

High-dose corticosteroid therapy has been the mainstay of treatment of lupus nephritis, although it is accompanied by considerable morbidity. Pulse methylprednisolone is used for the treatment of rapidly progressive lupus glomerulonephritis. Oral or pulse-intravenous cyclophosphamide frequently is recommended for the treatment of WHO class-III, -IV, and, sometimes, class-V renal disease. Azathioprine and, more recently, mycophenolic acid have been used as steroid-sparing agents.[39] Mycophenolic acid has even shown promise in decreasing exposure to, or even as a substitute for, cyclophosphamide, thus preventing the significant side effects of this agent, particularly its effects on fertility.[40,41] This circumstance is especially important given the predilection of SLE for young women of childbearing age. Cyclosporine has been used with variable results. A renal biopsy should be performed before therapy is begun. The danger of overwhelming sepsis among these immunosuppressed patients is constant. The effectiveness of therapy is indicated by changes in serologic parameters, blood chemistries, and complement levels. Care of the patient who has SLE is a highly specialized endeavor that requires knowledge of current treatment modalities, the availability of highly specialized tests, and the willingness to deal with a patient who has a chronic, severe, life-threatening illness for which treatment with steroids often is disfiguring. These patients are managed best by a team trained in dealing with all aspects of this disease.

Prognosis

Overall survival of children with SLE appears to have improved over the last several decades, with many, but not all, reports citing survival rates of 70% to 80% and higher at 15 to 20 years.[31,34,42,43] Reported renal survival in childhood lupus nephritis ranges from 29% to 71% at 10 years. Patients with WHO class-IV diffuse proliferative glomerulonephritis have the poorest renal outcome. In addition, sclerosis on biopsy specimens, hypocomplementemia, decreased renal function, nephrotic range proteinuria, and persistent hypertension portend a poor renal prognosis.

Membranoproliferative Glomerulonephritis

Membranoproliferative glomerulonephritis (MPGN), also referred to as mesangiocapillary glomerulonephritis, is a chronic inflammatory disease of the kidney with a poor prognosis.

Etiology

The cause of MPGN is unknown in most instances; some forms are associated with immune complex deposition in the glomeruli. Complement activation is prominent in all three types of MPGN, and the pattern of complement consumption suggests different mechanisms involved in each type.[44] Type-1 MPGN is thought to be mediated by immune complex formation and deposition, with activation of the classical pathway of complement as indicated by immunofluorescence and the pattern of serum complement depression. Complement consumption in MPGN types 2 and 3 is thought to be the result of the presence of circulating autoantibodies called nephritic factors (NFs) that stabilize the C3 convertases activating the alternative (NF_a) and terminal (NF_t) pathways of complement activation, respectively.[45] These can also be found in the serum of some patients with type-1 MPGN. Although thought at one time to be epiphenomena, the various NFs and their resulting complement activation and consumption have more recently been considered to be of potential pathological significance.[45]

Pathological Features

Three types of MPGN have been described based on ultrastructural abnormalities of the GBM. MPGN types 1, 2, and 3 account for 44%, 20%, and 36% of cases, respectively.[46] All 3 types appear similar by light microscopy and have increased mesangial cellularity and matrix expansion. By electron microscopy, type 1 shows normal-appearing GBM, with subendothelial electron-dense deposits. MPGN type 2, also known as dense-deposit disease, appears to be a distinct disease and has thickening and increased electron density of the lamina densa of the GBM. In MPGN type 3, deposits are present on both the subepithelial and the subendothelial sides of the GBM, as well as within the GBM. With special stains the GBM appears fenestrated, and deposits are covered by layers of new GBM.[46]

Deposition of complement components in the glomeruli is seen by immunofluorescence microscopy.[47,48]

Clinical Presentation

The average age of onset of primary MPGN is approximately 9 years.[49] Hematuria is present in 60% to 100%, hypertension in 42% to 67%, and decreased renal function in 17% to 50% on presentation.[50-52] Between 50% and 67% of patients have a nephrotic syndrome, and some of these patients may not have significant hematuria.[53,54]

Laboratory Findings

The serum C3 level is depressed in 67% to 75% of patients on presentation. Blood urea nitrogen and creatinine values may be elevated and albumin may be low in severe cases. Anemia is common. Electrolyte disturbances reflect the presence of renal insufficiency. Urinalysis most commonly has both hematuria and proteinuria present. Proteinuria may reach the nephrotic range. Hematuria may be macroscopic. Cellular casts are a common finding.

Course and Prognosis

Fifty percent of patients reach end-stage renal failure within approximately 11 years of diagnosis, and 90% do so within 20 years.[51] Nephrotic-range proteinuria, renal insufficiency, hypertension, and sclerosis on biopsy examination are poor prognostic indicators. Type-1 MPGN has a better prognosis than the other two types. Secondary forms of MPGN type 1 may be associated with chronic bacterial infections or with hepatitis B or C infection, and serologic evidence for these entities should be sought before initiating therapy.[55]

Treatment

The treatment of MPGN is controversial. Rigorous controlled studies are lacking. Treatment with cytotoxic agents, anticoagulants, platelet function inhibitors, and nonsteroidal antiinflammatory agents has not shown clear evidence of efficacy. The most experience reported regarding treatment of this disorder has been with high-dose, long-term, alternate-day prednisone therapy.[46,49,51,56] Cumulative renal survival of 82% at 10 years and 56% at 20 years have been reported with this therapeutic approach. Some differences in the clinical course and response to treatment may be seen according to the type of MPGN.[57]

INTERSTITIAL NEPHRITIS

Inflammation of the interstitium is much less common than glomerular inflammation. Acute interstitial nephritis is often caused by an immune reaction to drugs and may present with acute renal failure in the absence of a clear inciting event. Peripheral eosinophilia may or may not be seen. If present, urinary eosinophils, demonstrated on Hansel stain, may suggest this diagnosis. A high index of suspicion must be maintained and the most likely offending agent discontinued. Renal biopsy is often necessary to confirm the diagnosis. Prominent lymphocytic interstitial infiltrates are seen with interstitial fibrosis in more severe cases. The role of corticosteroids in treatment of acute interstitial nephritis is controversial. Interstitial nephritis may be seen on renal biopsies concomitantly with severe glomerulonephritis, in which case it is the consequence of degeneration of the tubules of the most severely affected glomeruli. This combination has a much more guarded prognosis because the combined glomerular and interstitial involvement reflects the greater severity of the renal disease. In this circumstance the interstitial inflammation tends to heal by fibrosis, thereby damaging segments of the remaining kidney. The finding of glomerulonephritis associated with tubular dysfunction should be evaluated by kidney biopsy.

WHEN TO REFER

- Acute glomerulonephritis with significant complications
- Acute glomerulonephritis that is not following a typical course expected of poststreptococcal glomerulonephritis
- Failure of complement level to normalize within 6 to 8 weeks in suspected acute glomerulonephritis
- Rapidly progressive course
- Glomerulonephritis with the development of nephrotic syndrome
- Persistent hematuria and proteinuria
- Persistent hypertension
- Elevated creatinine level for age
- Family history of renal failure or deafness
- Any chronic glomerulonephritis

WHEN TO ADMIT

- Severe hypertension
- Renal failure with significant electrolyte disturbances
- Congestive heart failure from volume overload
- Oliguria or anuria
- Rapidly progressive renal failure

RELATED WEB SITE

- National Kidney Foundation (www.kidney.org/).

SUGGESTED RESOURCES

Galla JH. IgA nephropathy. *Kidney Int.* 1995;47:377-387.

Goldstein AR, White RHR, Akuse R, et al. Long-term follow-up of childhood Henoch-Schönlein nephritis. *Lancet.* 1992;339:280-282.

Jardim HM, Leake J, Risdon RA, et al. Crescentic glomerulonephritis in children. *Pediatr Nephrol.* 1992;6:231-235.

Kashtan C. Alport syndrome and thin glomerular basement membrane disease. *J Am Soc Nephrol.* 1998;9:1736-1750.

Klein-Gitelman M, Reiff A, Silverman ED. Systemic lupus erythematosus in childhood. *Rheum Dis Clin North Am.* 2002;28:561-577.

Pozzi C, Andrulli S, Del Vecchio L, et al. Corticosteroid effectiveness in IgA nephropathy: long-term results of a randomized, controlled trial. *J Am Soc Nephrol.* 2004; 15:157-163.

Savige J, Rana K, Tonna S, et al. Thin basement membrane nephropathy. *Kidney Int.* 2003;64:1169-1178.

Tejani A, Ingulli E. Poststreptococcal glomerulonephritis: current clinical and pathologic concepts. *Nephron.* 1990; 55:1-5.

Ting RV, Hashkes PJ. Update on childhood vasculitides. *Curr Opin Rheumatol.* 2004;16:560-565.

West CD. Idiopathic membranoproliferative glomerulonephritis in childhood. *Pediatr Nephrol.* 1992;6:96-103.

REFERENCES

1. Rivera F, Lopez-Gomez JM, Perez-Garcia R. Frequency of renal pathology in Spain 1994-1999. *Nephrol Dial Transplant.* 2002;17:1954-1602.
2. National High Blood Pressure Education Program Working Group on High Blood Pressure in Children and Adolescents. The 4th report on the diagnosis, evaluation and treatment of high blood pressure in children and adolescents. *Pediatrics.* 2004;114:555-576.
3. Birch DF, Fairley KF, Whitworth JA, et al. Urinary erythrocyte morphology in the diagnosis of glomerular hematuria. *Clin Nephrol.* 1983;20:78-84.
4. Yoshizawa N, Suzuki Y, Oshima S, et al. Asymptomatic acute poststreptococcal glomerulonephritis following upper respiratory tract infections caused by group A streptococci. *Clin Nephrol.* 1996;46:296-301.
5. Yoshizawa N. Acute glomerulonephritis. *Int Med.* 2000; 39:687-694.
6. Markowitz M. Changing epidemiology of group A streptococcal infections. *Pediatr Infect Dis J.* 1994;13:557-560.
7. Tejani A, Ingulli E. Poststreptococcal glomerulonephritis: current clinical and pathologic concepts. *Nephron.* 1990; 55:1-5.
8. Peake PW, Pussell BA, Karplus TE, et al. Post-streptococcal glomerulonephritis: studies on the interaction between nephritis strain-associated protein (NSAP), complement and the glomerulus. *APMIS.* 1991;99:460-466.
9. Yoshizawa N, Oshima S, Sagel I, et al. Role of streptococcal antigen in the pathogenesis of acute poststreptococcal glomerulonephritis: characterization of the antigen and a proposed mechanism for the disease. *J Immunol.* 1992;148:3110-3116.
10. Lewy JE, Salinas-Madrigal L, Herdson PB, et al. Clinicopathological correlations in acute poststreptococcal glomerulonephritis: a correlation between renal functions, morphologic damage and clinical course of 46 children with acute poststreptococcal glomerulonephritis. *Medicine.* 1971;50:453-501.
11. Fleisher DS, Voci G, Garfunkel J, et al. Hemodynamic findings in acute glomerulonephritis. *J Pediatr.* 1966; 69:1054-1062.
12. Sulyok E. Acute proliferative glomerulonephritis. In: Avner ED, Harmon WE, Niaudet P, eds. *Pediatric Nephrology.* 5th ed. Philadelphia, PA: Lippincott Williams and Wilkins; 2004.
13. Potter EV, Lipschultz SA, Abidh S, et al. Twelve to seventeen-year follow-up of patients with poststreptococcal acute glomerulonephritis in Trinidad. *N Engl J Med.* 1982;307:725-729.
14. Buzio C, Allegri L, Mutti A, et al. Significance of albuminuria in the follow-up of acute poststreptococcal glomerulonephritis. *Clin Nephrol.* 1994;41:259-264.
15. Jordan SC, Lemire JM. Acute glomerulonephritis: diagnosis and treatment. *Pediatr Clin N Am.* 1982;29:857-873.
16. Jardim HM, Leake J, Risdon RA, et al. Crescentic glomerulonephritis in children. *Pediatr Nephrol.* 1992;6:231-235.
17. Couser WG. Rapidly progressive glomerulonephritis: classification, pathogenetic mechanisms, and therapy. *Am J Kidney Dis.* 1988;11:449-464.
18. Galla JH. IgA nephropathy. *Kidney Int.* 1995;47:377-387.
19. Wyatt RJ, Hogg RJ. Evidence-based assessment of treatment options for children with IgA nephropathies. *Pediatr Nephrol.* 2001;16:156-167.
20. Pozzi C, Bolasco PG, Fogazzi GB, et al. Coricosteroids in IgA nephropathy: a randomized controlled trial. *Lancet.* 1999;353:883-887.
21. Pozzi C, Andrulli S, Del Vecchio L, et al. Corticosteroid effectiveness in IgA nephropathy: long-term results of a randomized, controlled trial. *J Am Soc Nephrol.* 2004; 15: 157-163.
22. Tang S, Leung JCK, Chan LYY, et al. Mycophenolate mofetil alleviates persistent proteinuria in IgA nephropathy. *Kidney Int.* 2005;68:802-812.
23. Berg UB. Long-term follow-up of renal function in IgA nephropathy. *Arch Dis Child.* 1991;66:588-592.
24. Gallo GR, Katafuchi R, Neelakantappa K, et al. Prognostic pathologic markers in IgA nephropathy. *Am J Kidney Dis.* 1988;12:362-365.
25. Niaudet P, Beaufils MI, Broyer M, et al. Primary IgA nephropathies in children: prognosis and treatment. *Adv Nephrol.* 1993;2:121-140.
26. Savige J, Rana K, Tonna S, et al. Thin basement membrane nephropathy. *Kidney Int.* 2003;64:1169-1178.
27. Lemmink HH, Nillesen WN, Mochizuki T, et al. Benign familial hematuria due to mutation of the type IV collagen alpha 4 gene. *J Clin Invest.* 1996;98:1114-1118.
28. Badenas C, Praga M, Tazon, et al. Mutations in the COL4A3 and COL4A4 genes cause familial benign hematuria. *J Am Soc Nephrol.* 2002;13:1248-1254.
29. Piccini M, Casari G, Zhou J, et al. Evidence for genetic heterogeneity in benign familial hematuria. *Am J Nephrol.* 1999;19:460-467.
30. Yamazaki J, Nakagawa Y, Saito A, et al. No linkage to the COL4A3 gene locus in Japanese thin basement membrane disease families. *Nephrol.* 1996;1:315-321.
31. Tiebosch A, Frederik PM, van Breda Vriesman PJ, et al. Thin basement membrane nephropathy in adults with persistent hematuria. *N Engl J Med.* 1989;320:14-18.
32. Pirson Y. Making the diagnosis of Alport's syndrome. *Kidney Int.* 1999;56:760-775.
33. Kashtan C. Alport syndrome and thin glomerular basement membrane disease. *J Am Soc Nephrol.* 1998;9:1736-1750.
34. Klein-Gitelman M, Reiff A, Silverman ED. Systemic lupus erythematosis in childhood. *Rheum Dis Clin North Am.* 2002;28:561-577.
35. Bakkalogly A. Lupus nephropathy in children. *Nephrol Dial Transplant.* 2001;16(suppl 6):126-128.
36. Weening JJ, D'Agati VD, Schwartz MM, et al. The classification of glomerulonephritis in systemic lupus erythematosus revisited. *Kidney Int.* 2004;65;521-530.
37. Iqbal S, Sher MR, Good RA, et al. Diversity in presenting manifestations of systemic lupus erythematosus in children. *J Pediatr.* 1999;135:500-505.
38. Cameron JS. Lupus and lupus nephritis in children. *Adv Nephrol.* 1993;2:59-119.
39. Ginzler EM, Dooley MA, Aranow C, et al. Mycophenolate mofetil or intravenous cyclophosphamide for lupus nephritis. *N Engl J Med.* 2005;353:2219-2228.
40. Contreras G, Pardo V, Leclercq B, et al. Sequential therapies for proliferative lupus nephritis. *N Engl J Med.* 2004; 350:971-980.
41. Burchardi C, Schlondorff D. Induction therapy for active lupus nephritis: mycophenolate mofetil versus cyclophosphamide. *Nature Clin Prac Nephrol.* 2006;2:314-315.
42. Gloor JM. Lupus nephritis in children. *Lupus.* 1998;7:639-643.
43. McCurdy DK, Lehman TJ, Bernstein B, et al. Lupus nephritis: prognostic factors in children. *Pediatr.* 1992;89: 240-246.

44. Varade WS, Forristal J, West CD. Patterns of complement activation in membranoproliferative glomerulonephritis types I, II, and III. *Am J Kidney Dis.* 1990;16:196-206.
45. West CD, McAdams AJ. The alternative pathway C3 convertase and glomerular deposits. *Pediatr Nephrol.* 1999;13:448-453.
46. West CD. Idiopathic membranoproliferative glomerulonephritis in childhood. *Pediatr Nephrol.* 1992;6:96-103.
47. Donadio JV, Holley KE. Membranoproliferative glomerulonephritis. *Semin Nephrol.* 1982;2:214-227.
48. Strife CF, Jackson EC, McAdams AJ. Type III membranoproliferative glomerulonephritis: long-term clinical and morphological evaluation. *Clin Nephrol.* 1984;21:323-334.
49. McEnery PT. Membranoproliferative glomerulonephritis: the Cincinnati experience: cumulative renal survival from 1957 to 1989. *J Pediatr.* 1990;116:S109-114.
50. International Study of Kidney Disease in Childhood. Nephrotic syndrome in children: prediction of histopathology from clinical and laboratory characteristics at the time of diagnosis. *J Pediatr.* 1981;98:561-564.
51. Tarshish P, Bernstein J, Tobin JN, et al. Treatment of mesangiocapillary glomerulonephritis with alternate-day prednisone: a report of the International Study of Kidney Disease in Children. *Pediatr Nephrol.* 1992;6:123-130.
52. White RHR, Glasgow EF, Mills RJ. Clinicopathological study of nephrotic syndrome in childhood. *Lancet.* 1970;1:1353-1359.
53. Cameron JS, Turner DR, Heaton J, et al. Idiopathic mesangiocapillary glomerulonephritis: comparison of types I and II in children and adults and long-term prognosis. *Am J Med.* 1983;74:175-192.
54. Habib R, Kleinknecht C, Gubler MC, et al. Idiopathic membranoproliferative glomerulonephritis in children: report of 105 cases. *Clin Nephrol.* 1973;1:194-214.
55. Rennke HG. Secondary membranoproliferative glomerulonephritis. *Kidney Int.* 1995;47:643-656.
56. Warady BA, Guggenheim SJ, Sedman A, et al. Prednisone therapy of membranoproliferative glomerulonephritis in children. *J Pediatr.* 1985;107:702-707.
57. Braun MC, West CD, Strife CF. Differences between membranoproliferative glomerulonephritis types I and III in long-term response to an alternate-day prednisone regimen. *Am J Kidney Dis.* 1999;34:1022-1032.

Chapter 297

NEPHROTIC SYNDROME

William S. Varade, MD

Nephrotic syndrome is defined by the clinical findings of heavy proteinuria, hypoalbuminemia, edema (often to the point of frank anasarca), and hyperlipidemia. Many causes of nephrotic syndrome exist, and the most likely cause varies by age. Nephrotic syndrome may be the result of an underlying systemic disease, or it may manifest as a primary idiopathic renal disorder. Examples of causes of primary and secondary nephrotic syndrome in children are listed in Box 297-1. The overall outcome of nephrotic syndrome depends on the etiology and ranges from complete remission with no long-term sequelae to inexorable progression to end-stage renal failure. Newer treatments offer alternatives for patients with resistant forms of nephrotic syndrome or who experience significant side effects from first-line treatments, although such treatments themselves carry the potential for significant side effects.

BOX 297-1 Examples of Primary and Secondary Causes of Nephrotic Syndrome in Children

PRIMARY NEPHROTIC SYNDROME
- Minimal change nephrotic syndrome
- Focal segmental glomerulosclerosis
- Mesangial hypercellularity
- Membranoproliferative glomerulonephritis
- Membranous nephropathy

SECONDARY NEPHROTIC SYNDROME
- Inherited diseases (congenital nephrotic syndrome, diffuse mesangial sclerosis, Alport syndrome, nail-patella syndrome, Lowe syndrome)
- Vasculitides (lupus nephritis, Henoch-Schönlein purpura nephritis, Wegener granulomatosis, Goodpasture syndrome)
- Postinfectious (poststreptococcal, human immunodeficiency virus, hepatitis B and C, malaria, syphilis, intrauterine infections, other viruses and bacteria)
- Drugs and toxins (nonsteroidal antiinflammatory drugs, gold)
- Diabetes mellitus (rare in children)

EPIDEMIOLOGIC FEATURES

The annual incidence of idiopathic nephrotic syndrome in children is estimated to be 2 to 7 cases per 100,000 children.[1] The incidence is 10-fold lower in adults.[2] The male-to-female ratio is reported to be 2:1 for children and 1:1 in adolescents and adults. In nephrotic children 3 months to 16 years of age, 76% have minimal change nephrotic syndrome (MCNS), 7% have focal segmental glomerulosclerosis (FSGS), 2% to 5% have diffuse mesangial hypercellularity or mesangial proliferation, and 7% have membranoproliferative glomerulonephritis (MPGN).[3-5] Only 1% of nephrotic children have membranous nephropathy, which is in contrast to adults with nephrotic syndrome, in whom 22% have MCNS, 12% have FSGS, 20% have membranous nephropathy, and 25% have proliferative lesions.[3]

Occurrence of MCNS peaks between 2 and 5 years of age.[5] Eighty-seven percent of nephrotic children between the ages of 3 months and 6 years have MCNS, and 92% of these will experience remission of their disease when treated with a course of prednisone.[6] However, more recently, a trend has been recognized for a higher incidence of FSGS in children and adults, with FSGS accounting for up to 25% of diagnoses in children who undergo biopsy for nephrotic syndrome.[7-9] Adolescents are more likely to have a more aggressive cause of the nephrotic syndrome, such as FSGS, MPGN, or membranous nephropathy, than younger children.[10]

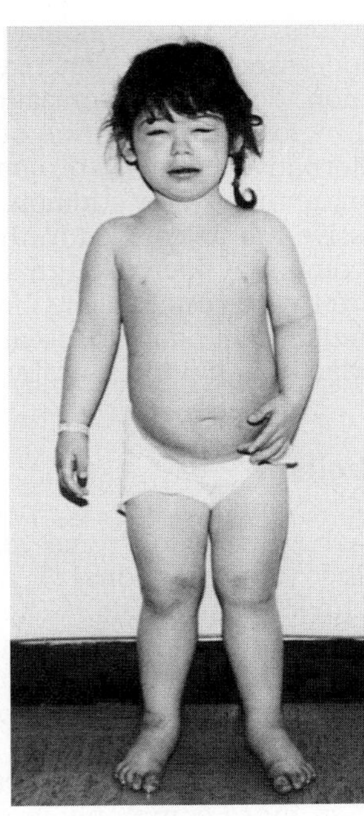

Figure 297-1 A 2-year-old girl with nephrotic syndrome.

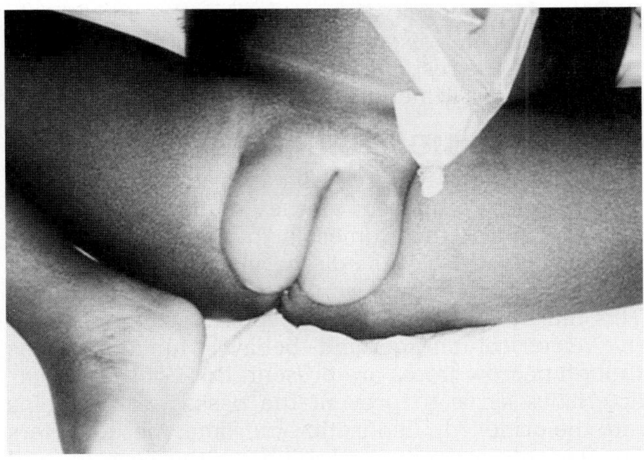

Figure 297-2 Severe labial edema in a 3-year-old girl with nephrotic syndrome.

Racial differences affect the incidence of underlying histopathological mechanism and prognosis in nephrotic patients. Black and Hispanic adolescents are more likely than white adolescents to have FSGS and to progress to end-stage renal disease.[11,12] In a predominantly black and Hispanic population of nephrotic adolescents, 55% had FSGS, 20% had MCNS, and 7% had MPGN.[13]

EVALUATION

Clinical Presentation

Typically, children with nephrotic syndrome (Figure 297-1) gradually develop edema and an inappropriate weight gain, although cases associated with glomerulonephritis may have a more acute onset, with signs and symptoms of nephritis predominating. The presence of periorbital edema when arising in the morning that resolves during the course of the day is often mistaken for allergy. Clothing may be tight, and socks may leave indentations in the skin of the shins and ankles. The abdomen may be distended, and a fluid wave may be discernible on examination. Breath sounds may be decreased at the lung bases because of accumulation of pleural fluid. Although intravascular volume is low in most children with nephrotic syndrome, in some children, it may be increased. These children may have a gallop on auscultation of the heart, rales over the lung fields, and hepatomegaly. Boys may develop significant scrotal swelling, and girls may develop labial swelling (Figure 297-2). The child or parents may report decreased frequency of urination and the passage of dark, amber-colored, concentrated-appearing urine that appears to foam when voided. Overall, 16% of children with nephrotic syndrome have hypertension at presentation.[4] The presence of marked hypertension should suggest the possibility of underlying glomerulonephritis.

Laboratory Evaluation

Laboratory evaluation begins with a urinalysis in the child with edema. This evaluation will demonstrate significant proteinuria in cases of nephrotic syndrome. Up to approximately 25% of children who have primary nephrotic syndrome will also have 3 to 5 red blood cells per high-power field on urinalysis.[14] The presence of significant microscopic hematuria or gross hematuria suggests that nephrotic syndrome might be the result of an underlying nephritic process. The presence of glycosuria in untreated children with nephrotic syndrome suggests underlying tubular injury that may be seen with FSGS. Blood urea nitrogen and creatinine values are generally normal or only slightly increased in primary nephrotic syndrome. Serum total protein and albumin levels are low. Mild hyponatremia may be present because of water retention. Total calcium levels are low because of the low serum albumin level, but ionized calcium levels are usually normal. The serum cholesterol level is usually increased. The third component of complement (C3) is generally normal. A lowered level suggests MPGN, poststreptococcal glomerulonephritis, or lupus nephritis. Chest radiographs will usually show a small cardiac silhouette and, in severe cases, the presence of pleural fluid. Cardiomegaly may be seen in patients with increased intravascular volume.

Urinary protein losses can be quantified with a 24-hour urine collection or, in incontinent children, estimated with a urine protein-to-creatinine ratio on a random urine sample. Nephrotic-range proteinuria is defined as (1) urinary protein excretion on a timed urine collection of more than 3.5 g/day in adults or more than 40 mg/m^2/hr or 1 g/m^2/day in children or (2) a urine protein-to-creatinine ratio (mg/mg) of more than 2:1 on a random urine sample.[1] Urinary protein quantification is not critical in the management of nephrotic syndrome with heavy proteinuria demonstrated by dipstick determination and with a typical clinical presentation. It is more helpful for monitoring the response to treatment of children with resistant forms of nephrotic syndrome.

PATHOPHYSIOLOGICAL FEATURES

The glomerular capillary wall acts as a selective filtration barrier composed of the glomerular capillary endothelial cell, the glomerular basement membrane, and the podocytes of the glomerular visceral epithelial cells. Slit diaphragms connect adjacent podocytes. This filtration barrier normally possesses a net negative electrical charge and behaves functionally as though narrow pores are present. Both of these characteristics serve to prevent the passage of proteins into the urine.[15] In nephrotic syndrome, these barriers are variably altered, depending on the severity and nature of the underlying disease process. Examples of alterations in the filtration barrier include the loss of negative charge seen in MCNS, the altered organization of glomerular basement membrane components in Alport syndrome, or mutations of genes encoding proteins associated with glomerular podocytes, leading to alterations in podocyte structure and function.[1] The changes in the barriers allow the passage of large quantities of plasma proteins into the urine[16] which, in turn, may lead to a decrease in the level of proteins in the blood.

Classically, the development of edema has been explained by massive losses of plasma proteins, in particular albumin, in the urine, with the consequent development of hypoalbuminemia,[17,18] which leads to decreased plasma oncotic pressure and leakage of fluid from the vascular space into the interstitium. The subsequent drop in the circulating blood volume stimulates the renin-angiotensin-aldosterone system, leading to avid sodium retention, and it produces a nonosmotic stimulus for vasopressin secretion and free-water reabsorption. The result of these responses is the development of massive tissue edema with the excretion of a decreased volume of concentrated urine. However, this scenario does not explain the edema formation in all nephrotic patients.[17-20] Studies have demonstrated that in patients who experience remission, diuresis often begins as the proteinuria is resolving but before normalization of plasma albumin levels. In addition, primary sodium retention has been demonstrated with the onset of proteinuria (but before the development of hypoproteinemia) in at least some patients experiencing a relapse of nephrotic syndrome. This circumstance would then lead to expansion of vascular volume and the development of edema.

COMPLICATIONS

Infection

Morbidity and mortality were high in nephrotic syndrome before the introduction of corticosteroid and antibiotic therapy. Infection was the leading cause of death in children with nephrotic syndrome. Infectious complications include spontaneous bacterial peritonitis, sepsis, cellulitis, and pneumonia. *Staphylococcus pneumoniae* and gram-negative bacteria are responsible for most infections in nephrotic syndrome.[21]

Predisposing factors for the development of bacterial infections include tissue edema that may facilitate the spread of infection, defective opsonization of invading bacteria caused by loss into the urine of small components of the alternative pathway of complement, and impaired cellular immunity. In addition, the effects of immunosuppressive therapies used in the treatment of nephrotic syndrome may increase the susceptibility to infection. Children with recurrent nephrotic syndrome should receive multivalent pneumococcal vaccination. A role for prophylactic antibiotic therapy has not been established.

Thromboembolism

Thromboembolic events such as deep-vein thrombosis, pulmonary embolism, and renal-vein thrombosis are well-described complications of nephrotic syndrome in both children and adults.[22] They are reported to occur less frequently in children than in adults, although the documentation of subclinical pulmonary embolism by radionuclide ventilation-perfusion lung scanning in 28% of nephrotic children suggests that the true incidence may be underreported.[23] Arterial thrombosis occurs more commonly in nephrotic children than in nephrotic adults.[24] Contributory factors include increased plasma levels of procoagulant factors, urinary loss of inhibitors of coagulation, and thrombocytosis.[25] The predisposition to thrombus formation may be exacerbated by decreased intravascular volume, especially in the face of vigorous forced diuresis.

Hyperlipidemia

Elevation of plasma lipids in nephrotic syndrome has classically been said to result from increased hepatic lipoprotein synthesis caused by generalized increased hepatic protein synthesis in response to a lowered plasma albumin level.[26] The mechanism behind the increase in plasma lipids is probably more complex than this and may involve production of inflammatory cytokines leading to, or at least associated with, alterations in lipid synthesis, catabolism, and recycling.[27-29] In severe disease with heavy proteinuria, lipoprotein lipase activity may be decreased, leading to decreased lipolysis and resulting in high triglyceride levels.[26,28,29] The return of high cholesterol levels to normal at remission of nephrotic syndrome often lags behind the normalization of serum albumin levels. In unremitting nephrotic syndrome, increased plasma lipids may contribute to cardiovascular morbidity, and treatment of lipid abnormalities should be considered.

SPECIFIC HISTOPATHOLOGICAL ENTITIES ASSOCIATED WITH PRIMARY NEPHROTIC SYNDROME OF CHILDHOOD

Minimal Change Nephrotic Syndrome

MCNS, also known as *lipoid nephrosis* and *nil* (nothing in light microscopy) *disease,* is the most common pathological diagnosis in nephrotic children; 92% will experience remission with a course of corticosteroids.[6] Hematuria is found in approximately 13% and hypertension in 10% to 20% of cases.[4,5] Relapses are common, but the long-term prognosis is excellent. Relapses tend to become less frequent with age, and the disorder usually resolves around the time of puberty without permanent renal impairment. In many instances, the diagnosis is assumed in most children because biopsy is generally not performed in those who follow a typical course and who respond to corticosteroid therapy. These children should more correctly be considered to have the clinical diagnosis of steroid-responsive idiopathic nephrotic syndrome of childhood, which encompasses a variety of histopathological diagnoses.

Investigators have proposed that MCNS may be an immune-mediated disease. Evidence supporting this theory includes the response of MCNS to immunosuppressive therapy, an association with allergens, an association with lymphomas, the presence of altered T-lymphocyte function, and the description of various circulating cationic proteins, immunomodulatory substances, permeability factors, and lymphokines.[16]

The histopathology of MCNS shows minimal abnormalities by light microscopy. Most pathologists allow for a small amount of mesangial hypercellularity within this classification. Immunofluorescence is negative for immunoglobulin and complement. Electron microscopy shows diffuse fusion of the glomerular epithelial cell foot processes.

Focal Segmental Glomerulosclerosis

FSGS is found as both a primary and secondary pathological diagnosis. Secondary forms are thought to represent a final common pathway to glomerular epithelial cell injury, glomerular adaptation to significant nephron loss with glomerular hypertension or hyperfiltration, inherited abnormalities of the glomerular basement membrane, or severe glomerulonephritis.[30] Disease processes that can be associated with FSGS lesions include diabetic nephropathy, sickle cell disease, HIV nephropathy, and glomerulonephritides such as IgA nephropathy, MPGN, and lupus nephritis.

Children with primary FSGS tend to be older and black.[11] Many are steroid resistant or dependent from the time of initial treatment, or they become steroid resistant over time. Hematuria may be found in 50% or more and hypertension in approximately 50% of cases.[4,5] The prognosis of FSGS is more guarded; 42% of children may experience complete remission without progression to end-stage renal disease,[31] but up to 50% may progress to end-stage renal disease with time, and a subgroup will progress rapidly within 3 years of presentation. FSGS recurs in 20% to 50% of patients reaching end-stage renal failure who receive a renal transplant.[32,33]

Primary FSGS may actually be the manifestation of a systemic disorder. Evidence for this view includes the following: (1) disease may recur in transplanted kidneys, (2) proteinuria can be induced in animals by infusion of serum from a patient with recurrent FSGS, (3) recurrent FSGS in transplanted kidneys may respond to plasmapheresis, and (4) a circulating factor capable of increasing the permeability of isolated glomeruli to albumin has been demonstrated in the serum of some patients with recurrent FSGS.[34-36]

The histopathology of FSGS is characterized by the presence of scars affecting portions or segments of some, but not all, glomeruli.[28] Mesangial hypercellularity, tubular atrophy, and interstitial fibrosis are often present. Weak mesangial and segmental deposits of C3 and IgM can be seen by immunofluorescence but probably represent nonspecific trapping of these proteins. Electron microscopy may show widespread effacement of foot processes and separation of glomerular epithelial cells from the underlying basement membrane. Different subtypes of FSGS have been described that may reflect different stages of disease development, pathogenesis, and prognosis.[30]

Membranoproliferative Glomerulonephritis

MPGN is a chronic inflammatory disease of the kidney with a poor prognosis. It is discussed in more detail in Chapter 296, Nephritis. The average age at onset of primary MPGN is approximately 9 years.[37] Between 50% and 67% of patients develop nephrotic syndrome, and some of these patients may not have significant hematuria.[38,39] The serum C3 level is low in 67% to 75% of patients.

Membranous Nephropathy

Membranous nephropathy is a chronic glomerular disease that can also be idiopathic or the result of a systemic disorder. It can affect any age group but is rare in children and adolescents; it is responsible for only approximately 1% of children with nephrotic syndrome.[4] At presentation, 73% of children with membranous nephropathy have nephrotic syndrome, 80% have microscopic hematuria, and 37% have hypertension. Six percent of children develop gross hematuria at the time they seek care, and 20% will develop it sometime during the course of their illness.[40] Complement protein levels are usually normal. Spontaneous remissions occur in most patients, but remission may not occur for several years after onset.[40,41] Approximately 13% of affected children progress to end-stage renal failure.[42] Poor prognostic factors include persistent heavy proteinuria (>8 g/day for more than 6 months), hypertension, increased creatinine, and significant scarring on biopsy.[43,44]

By light microscopy, membranous lesions are seen as diffuse thickening of the glomerular capillary walls.[42,45] Capillary lumens are patent, and little mesangial proliferation is found. Silver-stained biopsy specimens show spikes of basement membrane material projecting from the subepithelial side of the glomerular basement membrane. By electron microscopy, glomerular capillary walls are thickened by subepithelial electron-dense deposits and projections (spikes) of the lamina densa. The extent of these projections with relation to the deposits forms the basis for classifying the stages of membranous nephropathy. Immunofluorescence studies show granular deposits of IgG along the glomerular basement membrane. C3 usually is seen in a similar distribution.

Genetic Causes of the Nephrotic Syndrome

Mutations of certain genes, especially those intimately associated with glomerular epithelial podocytes or the glomerular basement membrane, have been implicated in the development of hereditary forms of the nephrotic syndrome.

Congenital nephrotic syndrome refers to nephrotic syndrome presenting in the first 3 months of life. Pathologically, it may be a Finnish-type congenital nephrotic syndrome, diffuse mesangial sclerosis, FSGS, minimal change disease, or membranous nephropathy. Secondary forms may be caused by congenital infections, heavy metal exposure, or genetic syndromes, among other more uncommon associations. Congenital nephrotic syndrome of the Finnish type is an autosomal-recessive disorder caused by mutations in the *NPHS1* gene encoding nephrin, a protein forming the slit diaphragms between adjacent podocytes, or the *NPHS2* gene encoding podocin, a podocyte membrane protein.[46-48] Infants are often premature and small for gestational age. The placenta is markedly enlarged, and amniotic levels of alpha-fetoprotein are high. Edema often becomes evident within days of birth. Prognosis of congenital nephrotic syndrome depends on the underlying cause. It is guarded for congenital nephrotic syndrome of the Finnish type with significant morbidity and mortality from complications, particularly malnutrition, infection, and thrombotic events caused by the massive protein losses. Treatment is supportive but must be aggressive, and it may include intensive nutritional support and nephrectomies to stem the protein losses and maintain the patient on dialysis until kidney transplantation can be performed.[49]

Diffuse mesangial sclerosis may be part of Denys-Drash syndrome, consisting of onset of nephrotic syndrome in the first months of life with rapid progression to end-stage kidney failure, male pseudohermaphroditism, and Wilms tumor. It is associated with mutations of the *WT1* gene. Support until kidney transplantation is required for the renal disease while the risk or actual presence of Wilms tumor is addressed.[48] Mutations in *WT1* may also be seen in patients with Frasier syndrome, consisting of male pseudohermaphroditism and FSGS.[48]

Podocin mutations have also been associated with a steroid-resistant, autosomal-recessive form of FSGS in older children with a rapid progression to renal failure. Mutations in the *ACTN4* gene encoding α-actinin, a podocyte protein that associates with actin filaments of the cytoskeleton and slit diaphragms, results in an autosomal-dominant form of FSGS with onset during early childhood and slow progression to renal failure.[50]

MANAGEMENT

Although a great deal of attention has been paid to the underlying pathological diagnoses in idiopathic childhood nephrotic syndrome, the clinical response to a course of corticosteroids seems to be as informative in determining long-term outcome as the underlying histopathology.[51] Initially, eighty-five percent of nephrotic children will respond to a trial of prednisone. Seventy-five percent of patients who will respond do so within 2 weeks of initiating therapy, and 94% will have responded by 4 weeks.[6] Most corticosteroid-responsive patients have MCNS. However, up to 25% of corticosteroid-resistant nephrotic children are found by biopsy to have MCNS, whereas 5% to 10% of the corticosteroid-responsive patients have FSGS.[6,51] Biopsy findings do not predict which children who have MCNS will be corticosteroid resistant or which children who have FSGS will be corticosteroid responsive. In general, nephrotic patients who achieve a remission on steroids, whether they have MCNS or FSGS, do not progress to renal failure if they remain responsive to corticosteroid therapy.

Children between the ages of 1 and 6 years are most likely to have MCNS as determined by renal biopsy and respond clinically to a trial of corticosteroids by experiencing remission.[6] Therefore treating a child in this age range (or even up to age 10) who has the new onset of typical, pure nephrotic syndrome with a trial of corticosteroids is now customary. Treatment consists of prednisone at 2 mg/kg/day or 60 mg/m^2/day (maximum, 60 to 80 mg/day) for 4 to 6 weeks[6,52] usually given in divided doses, though some studies suggest that it can be given as a single morning dose with a similar rate of response.[53] This treatment is followed by a single dose of 1.3 mg/kg or 40 mg/m^2 for an additional 4 to 6 weeks given in the morning on alternate days.[6,52,54] Daily prednisone was initially recommended for 4 weeks followed by 4 weeks of alternate day dosing, with the medication gradually tapered off afterward.[6] More recently, studies have shown a decreased frequency of relapses in the first year and a lower total steroid dose if daily prednisone is given initially for 6 weeks, followed by 6 weeks of alternate-day prednisone and then tapered off over an additional 4 weeks.[52,55] Depending on the treatment regimen employed, 36% to 61% of children will have a relapse of nephrotic syndrome within the first year of the initial episode.[52] A relapse is diagnosed if the urine tests 2+ or greater for protein for 3 consecutive days. Relapses are usually triggered by intercurrent illnesses or allergies, and parents can be taught to use albumin test sticks or sulfosalicylic acid at home to monitor urinary protein excretion. Relapses are treated with prednisone 2 mg/kg/day or 60 mg/m^2/day until the urine is free of protein for 3 consecutive days. The prednisone dose then is changed to 40 mg/m^2 on alternate days for 4 weeks and then tapered off over an additional 4 weeks.[52]

Approximately 25% of children who experience relapse will follow a frequently relapsing course, defined as two relapses occurring within 6 months of completing a course of corticosteroids or three relapses within 1 year. Children who experience relapse while corticosteroids are being tapered or within 2 weeks of completing a course of corticosteroids are considered to be corticosteroid dependent. Both children who have frequently relapsing and corticosteroid-dependent nephrotic syndrome are more likely to develop corticosteroid toxicity. Second-tier therapies for difficult cases of nephrotic syndrome are listed in Box 297-2. Consideration for treatment with these agents should be made in consultation with a pediatric nephrologist. Alkylating agents, either cyclophosphamide or chlorambucil, can induce a prolonged remission in patients with frequently relapsing and some patients with corticosteroid-dependent nephrotic syndrome.[1,55] Use of chlorambucil can be associated with seizures; therefore cyclophosphamide tends to be used more frequently. Intravenous nitrogen mustard can be considered in noncompliant patients.[56]

BOX 297-2 Secondary, Tertiary, and Complementary Therapies for Difficult Cases of Nephrotic Syndrome

- Cyclophosphamide
- Chlorambucil
- Cyclosporine
- Tacrolimus
- Methylprednisolone infusions
- Levamisole
- Mycophenolate mofetil
- Angiotensin-converting enzyme inhibitors
- Angiotensin-receptor blockers
- Nonsteroidal antiinflammatory drugs

Levamisole has been used to decrease corticosteroid doses in patients who experience frequent relapse.[57] Nonsteroidal antiinflammatory drugs have been used to decrease proteinuria in resistant nephrotic syndrome but can lead to acute renal failure in the child who has significantly decreased intravascular volume. Cyclosporine or tacrolimus can be used as a corticosteroid-sparing agent in patients who do not respond to an alkylating agent.[1,55] Mycophenolate mofetil has also shown some success as a corticosteroid-sparing agent.[1]

Children whose disease fails to respond to the initial or subsequent courses of corticosteroids have corticosteroid-resistant nephrotic syndrome and a more guarded prognosis. Many of these children will have focal segmental glomerulosclerosis as the cause of their nephrotic syndrome. Consultation with a pediatric nephrologist should be made for consideration of a renal biopsy and more aggressive treatment. Similarly, children who are outside the usual age range for typical idiopathic nephrotic syndrome of childhood, who have refractory edema, or who have complicated nephrotic syndrome should be referred to a pediatric nephrologist for help with establishing the diagnosis and choosing a treatment plan. Current treatment regimens for corticosteroid-resistant nephrotic syndrome are given in Box 297-2 and include high-dose, long-term intravenous methylprednisolone, cyclosporine, or tacrolimus.[58-60] Cytotoxic agents such as cyclophosphamide have not been as successful in the setting of corticosteroid resistance as the other therapies noted previously.[58]

Complications of corticosteroid therapy include the development of cushingoid features, cataract formation, glaucoma, gastritis, peptic ulcer disease, pancreatitis, hypokalemia, hypertension, increased risk of infection, behavioral changes, and growth delay if treatment is prolonged. Cytotoxic agents (eg, cyclophosphamide, chlorambucil, nitrogen mustard) can be associated with increased risk of infection, malignancy, and sterility but usually only with higher doses than those typically used for nephrotic syndrome or after repeated or prolonged courses. Cyclophosphamide can cause hemorrhagic cystitis. Therefore a large fluid intake and frequent voiding should be encouraged. Chlorambucil therapy has been associated with induction of seizure activity. Nonsteroidal antiinflammatory drugs can cause salt retention and edema. A risk of renal failure exists, especially in patients with decreased intravascular volume. Cyclosporine and tacrolimus both have nephrotoxic potential and can cause acute and chronic renal injury. Acute renal failure can occur in severely nephrotic patients who are treated with cyclosporine and who have markedly decreased intravascular volume. Mycophenolate mofetil can cause bone marrow suppression and gastrointestinal upset.

Angiotensin-converting enzyme (ACE) inhibitors or angiotensin-receptor blockers can be tried in resistant nephrotic syndrome, even in the presence of normotension, to decrease urinary protein excretion. ACE inhibitors act by decreasing glomerular capillary pressure and can cause a reversible increase in serum creatinine and hyperkalemia that must be monitored. High doses of ACE inhibitors may decrease progressive sclerosis.

Salt intake should be restricted in edematous children because of their avid sodium retention. Water intake does not usually need to be restricted, especially if sodium intake is adequately limited, unless significant hyponatremia develops or edema is intractable. Diuretics are used judiciously, given the already reduced intravascular volume in most nephrotic patients and the attendant risk of thromboembolism. Furosemide alone or in combination with a thiazide diuretic is used to treat clinically significant edema. Severe edema interfering with ambulation, compromising respiratory status, or causing tissue breakdown can be treated with intravenous albumin followed by intravenous furosemide if renal function and urine output are fairly well maintained. Patients must be monitored closely during infusion for the development of signs of intravascular overload such as rales, cardiac gallop, and hepatomegaly. This therapy can also be used in the severely edematous, corticosteroid-resistant nephrotic patient in whom cyclosporine therapy is being considered in an attempt to improve renal perfusion and prevent the precipitation of acute renal failure.

Hospital admission should be considered for children during their first episode of nephrotic syndrome, especially if complications are present, for teaching the parents home management and monitoring. Children who have severe edema compromising their ventilatory status, causing cardiovascular congestion, or interfering with ambulation should be admitted for forced diuresis. Infectious complications of nephrotic syndrome may require treatment with parenteral antibiotics. Hypertension, renal insufficiency, and electrolyte disturbances may also require hospitalization for stabilization. Children with significant renal insufficiency may require dialysis to manage edema, electrolyte disturbances, and uremia.

The treatment of membranous nephropathy is controversial with regard to the choice of agent and the timing of intervention. Investigators have suggested that therapy need not be provided in most patients, given the high rate of spontaneous remission. Patients who have evidence of renal insufficiency, persistent heavy proteinuria, hypertension, or sclerosis on biopsy should be considered for treatment. Agents that have been used for the treatment of membranous nephropathy include high-dose corticosteroids provided orally or intravenously alone or in combination with cytotoxic agents.[40,43]

WHEN TO REFER

- Complicated nephrotic syndrome
- Outside the expected age range (<1 year or >10 years of age)
- Accompanied by signs of glomerulonephritis (renal insufficiency, hypertension, hematuria, hypocomplementemia)
- Refractory edema
- Frequently relapsing nephrotic syndrome
- Corticosteroid-dependent nephrotic syndrome
- Corticosteroid-resistant nephrotic syndrome

WHEN TO ADMIT

- Initial episode for teaching of parents
- Anasarca interfering with ambulation or compromising ventilation
- Pleural effusions or ascites interfering with ventilation
- Signs of volume overload (congestive heart failure)
- Infection (eg, severe cellulitis, peritonitis)
- Significant hypertension
- Significant electrolyte abnormalities
- Compromised renal function

TOOLS FOR PRACTICE

Engaging Patient and Family

- *What is a Pediatric Nephrologist?* (fact sheet), American Academy of Pediatrics (www.aap.org/family/WhatisPedNephrologist.pdf).

SUGGESTED RESOURCES

Benchimol C. Focal segmental glomerulosclerosis: pathogenesis and treatment. *Curr Opin Pediatr.* 2003;15:171-180.

Eddy AA, Symons JM. Nephrotic syndrome in childhood. *Lancet.* 2003;362:629-639.

Habashy D, Hodson EM, Craig JC. Interventions for steroid-resistant nephrotic syndrome: a systematic review. *Pediatr Nephrol.* 2003;18:906-912.

Hodson EM, Craig JC, Willis NS. Evidence-based management of steroid-sensitive nephrotic syndrome. *Pediatr Nephrol.* 2005;20:1523-1530.

Papez KE, Smoyer WE. Recent advances in congenital nephrotic syndrome. *Curr Opin Pediatr.* 2004;16:165-170.

REFERENCES

1. Eddy AA, Symons JM. Nephrotic syndrome in childhood. *Lancet.* 2003;362:629-639.
2. Ritz E. Pathogenesis of "idiopathic" nephrotic syndrome. *N Engl J Med.* 1994;330:61-62.
3. Cameron JS. Nephrotic syndrome and its complications. *Am J Kidney Dis.* 1987;10:157-171.
4. [No author listed]. Nephrotic syndrome in children: prediction of histopathology from clinical and laboratory characteristics at time of diagnosis. A report of the International Study of Kidney Disease in Children. *Kidney Int.* 1978;13:159-165.
5. White RHR, Glasgow EF, Mills RJ. Clinicopathological study of nephrotic syndrome in childhood. *Lancet.* 1970;1:1353-1359.
6. [No author listed]. The primary nephrotic syndrome in children: identification of patients with minimal change nephrotic syndrome from initial responders. A report of the International Study of Kidney Disease in Children. *J Pediatr.* 1981;98:561-564.
7. Bonilla-Felix M, Parra C, Dajani T, et al. Changing patterns in the histopathology of idiopathic nephrotic syndrome in children. *Kidney Int.* 1999;55:1885-1890.
8. Haas M, Spargo BH, Coventry S. Increasing incidence of focal-segmental glomerulosclerosis among adult nephropathies: a 20-year renal biopsy study. *Am J Kidney Dis.* 1995;26:740-750.
9. Filler G, Young E, Geier P, et al. Is there really an increase in non-minimal change nephrotic syndrome in children? *Am J Kidney Dis.* 2003;42:1107-1113.
10. Hogg RJ. Adolescents with proteinuria and/or the nephrotic syndrome. *Adolesc Med.* 2005;16:163-172.
11. Ngulli E, Tejani A. Racial differences in the incidence and renal outcome of idiopathic focal segmental glomerulosclerosis in children. *Pediatr Nephrol.* 1991;5:393-397.
12. McAdams AJ, Valentini RP, Welch TR. The nonspecificity of focal segmental glomerulosclerosis: the defining characteristics of primary focal glomerulosclerosis, mesangial proliferation, and minimal change. *Medicine.* 1997;76:42-52.
13. Baqi N, Singh A, Balachandra S, et al. The paucity of minimal change disease in adolescents with primary nephrotic syndrome. *Pediatr Nephrol.* 1998;12:105-107.
14. Strauss J, Zilleruelo G, Freundlich M, et al. Less commonly recognized features of childhood nephrotic syndrome. *Pediatr Clin North Am.* 1987;34:591-607.
15. Myers BD, Guasch A. Mechanisms of proteinuria in nephrotic humans. *Pediatr Nephrol.* 1994;8:107-112.
16. Savin VJ. Mechanisms of proteinuria in noninflammatory glomerular diseases. *Am J Kidney Dis.* 1993;21:347-362.
17. Hisano S, Hahn S, Kuemmerle NB, et al. Edema in childhood. *Kidney Int.* 1997;51(suppl 59):S100-S104.
18. Humphreys MH. Mechanisms and management of nephrotic edema. *Kidney Int.* 1994;45:266-281.
19. Donckerwolcke RA, Vande Walle JG. Pathogenesis of edema formation in nephrotic syndrome. *Kidney Int.* 1997;51(suppl 58):S72-S74.
20. Vande Walle JGJ, Donkerwolcke RA, Koomans HA. Pathophysiology of edema formation in children with nephrotic syndrome not due to minimal change disease. *J Am Soc Nephrol.* 1999;10:323-331.
21. McIntyre P, Craig JC. Prevention of serious bacterial infection in children with nephrotic syndrome. *J Paediatr Child Health.* 1998;34:314-317.
22. Harris RC, Ismail N. Extrarenal complications of nephrotic syndrome. *Am J Kidney Dis.* 1994;23:477-497.
23. Hoyer PF, Gonda S, Barthels M, et al. Thromboembolic complications in children with nephrotic syndrome: risk and incidence. *Acta Paediatr Scand.* 1986;75:804-810.
24. Mehls O, Andrassy K, Koderisch J, et al. Hemostasis and thromboembolism in children with nephrotic syndrome: differences from adults. *J Pediatr.* 1987;110:862-867.
25. Schlegel N. Thromboembolic risks and complications in nephrotic children. *Semin Thrombosis Hemostasis.* 1997;23:271-280.
26. Querfeld U. Should hyperlipidemia in children with nephrotic syndrome be treated? *Pediatr Nephrol.* 1999;13:77-84.

27. Saland JM, Ginsberg H, Fisher EA. Dyslipidemia in pediatric renal disease: epidemiology, pathophysiology, and management. *Curr Opin Pediatr.* 2002;14:197-204.
28. Delvin EE, Merouania A, Levy E. Dyslipidemia in pediatric nephrotic syndrome: causes revisited. *Clin Biochem.* 2003;36:95-101.
29. Prescott QA, Streetman DD, Streetman DS. The potential role of HMG-CoA reductase inhibitors in pediatric nephrotic syndrome. *Ann Pharmacother.* 2004;38:105-114.
30. Schwartz MM, Korbet SM. Primary focal segmental glomerulosclerosis: pathology, histological variants, and pathogenesis. *Am J Kidney Dis.* 1993;22:874-883.
31. Cattran DC, Rao P. Long-term outcome in children and adults with classic focal segmental glomerulosclerosis. *Am J Kidney Dis.* 1998;32:72-79.
32. Senggutuvan P, Cameron JS, Hartley RB, et al. Recurrence of focal segmental glomerulosclerosis in transplanted kidneys: analysis of incidence and risk factors in 59 allografts. *Pediatr Nephrol.* 1990;4:21-28.
33. Tejani A, Stablein DH. Recurrence of focal segmental glomerulosclerosis posttransplantation: a special report of the North American Pediatric Renal Transplant Cooperative Study. *J Am Soc Nephrol.* 1992;2(suppl 3):S258-S263.
34. Artero ML, Sharma R, Savin VJ, et al. Plasmapheresis reduces proteinuria and serum capacity to injure glomeruli in patients with recurrent focal glomerulosclerosis. *Am J Kidney Dis.* 1994;23:574-581.
35. Savin VJ, Sharma R, Sharma M, et al. Circulating factor associated with increased glomerular permeability to albumin in recurrent focal segmental glomerulosclerosis. *N Engl J Med.* 1996;34:878-883.
36. Zimmerman SW. Increased urinary protein excretion in the rat produced by serum from a patient with recurrent focal glomerular sclerosis after renal transplantation. *Clin Nephrol.* 1984;22:32-38.
37. McEnery PT. Membranoproliferative glomerulonephritis: the Cincinnati experience: cumulative renal survival from 1957 to 1989. *J Pediatr.* 1990;116:S109-S114.
38. Cameron JS, Turner DR, Heaton J, et al. Idiopathic mesangiocapillary glomerulonephritis: comparison of types I and II in children and adults and long-term prognosis. *Am J Med.* 1983;74:175-192.
39. McEnery PT, McAdams AJ, West CD. Membranoproliferative glomerulonephritis: improved survival with alternate day prednisone therapy. *Clin Nephrol.* 1980; 13:117-124.
40. Cameron JS. Membranous nephropathy in childhood and its treatment. *Pediatr Nephrol.* 1990;4:193-198.
41. Schieppati A, Mosconi L, Perna A, et al. Prognosis of untreated patients with idiopathic membranous nephropathy. *N Engl J Med.* 1993;329:85-89.
42. Habib R, Kleinknecht C, Gubler M-C. Extramembranous glomerulonephritis in children: report of 50 cases. *J Pediatr.* 1973;82:754-766.
43. Hebert LA. Therapy of membranous nephropathy: what to do after the after (meta) analysis. *J Am Soc Nephrol.* 1995;5:1543-1545.
44. Pei Y, Cattran D, Greenwood C. Predicting chronic renal insufficiency in idiopathic membranous glomerulonephritis. *Kidney Int.* 1992;42:960-966.
45. Ehrenreich J, Churg J. Pathology of membranous nephropathy. *Pathol Annu.* 1968;3:145-186.
46. Koziell A, Grech V, Jussain S, et al. Genotype/phenotype correlations of NPHS1 and NPHS2 mutations in nephrotic syndrome advocate a functional inter-relationship in glomerular filtration. *Hum Mol Genet.* 2002;11:379-388.
47. Papez KE, Smoyer WE. Recent advances in congenital nephrotic syndrome. *Curr Opin Pediatr.* 2004;16: 165-170.
48. Niaudet P. Genetic forms of nephrotic syndrome. *Pediatr Nephrol.* 2004;19:1313-1318.
49. Holmberg C, Antikainen M, Ronnholm K, et al. Management of congenital nephrotic syndrome of the Finnish type. *Pediatr Nephrol.* 1995;9:87-93.
50. Benchimol C. Focal segmental glomerulosclerosis: pathogenesis and treatment. *Curr Opin Pediatr.* 2003;15: 171-180.
51. Niaudet P. Nephrotic syndrome in children. *Curr Opin Pediatr.* 1993;5:174-179.
52. Brodehl J. The treatment of minimal change nephrotic syndrome: lessons learned from multicentre co-operative studies. *Eur J Pediatr.* 1991;150:380-387.
53. Warshaw BL, Hymes LC. Daily single-dose and daily reduced-dose prednisone therapy for children with nephrotic syndrome. *Pediatrics.* 1989;83:694-699.
54. Alternate-day versus intermittent prednisone in frequently relapsing nephrotic syndrome. A report of "Arbeitsgemeinschaft für Padiatrische Nephrologie." *Lancet.* 1979;1:401-403.
55. Hodson EM, Craig JC, Willis NS. Evidence-based management of steroid-sensitive nephrotic syndrome. *Pediatr Nephrol.* 2005;20:1523-1530.
56. Broyer M, Meziane A, Kleinknecht C, et al. Nitrogen mustard therapy in idiopathic nephrotic syndrome of childhood. *Int J Pediatr Nephrol.* 1985;6:29-34.
57. Niaudet P, Drachman R, Gagnadoux MF, et al. Treatment of idiopathic nephrotic syndrome with levamisole. *Acta Paeditr Scand.* 1984;73:637-641.
58. Habashy D, Hodson EM, Craig JC. Interventions for steroid-resistant nephrotic syndrome: a systematic review. *Pediatr Nephrol.* 2003;18:906-912.
59. Mendoza SA, Tune BM. Treatment of childhood nephrotic syndrome. *J Am Soc Nephrol.* 1992;3:889-894.
60. Niaudet P, Gagnadoux MF, Broyer M. Treatment of childhood steroid-resistant idiopathic nephrotic syndrome. *Adv Nephrol.* 1998;28:43-61.

Chapter 298

NEUROCUTANEOUS SYNDROMES

Michael L. Smith, MD

The neurocutaneous disorders consist of a heterogeneous group of conditions in which abnormalities of skin and nervous system predominate. Classically, neurofibromatosis, tuberous sclerosis, and von Hippel-Lindau disease are considered the prototypical neurocutaneous conditions. However, several other genetic or developmental anomaly syndromes share the phenotypic association of cutaneous and neurologic abnormalities, such as Sturge-Weber syndrome, ataxia-telangiectasia, incontinentia pigmenti, hypomelanosis of Ito, and the epidermal nevus syndromes. In addition, many genetic disorders with neurodevelopmental features may exhibit skin lesions, but these myriad conditions are beyond the scope of this chapter. The current discussion focuses on neurofibromatosis, tuberous sclerosis, Sturge-Weber syndrome, von Hippel-Lindau disease, and ataxia-telangiectasia.

NEUROFIBROMATOSIS

Definition

Neurofibromatosis (NF) is classically divided into NF type 1 (NF-1) and NF type 2 (NF-2), although these are different conditions with only minimal overlap. Both are autosomal-dominant disorders with high penetrance but variable phenotypic expression. NF-1 is more common, occurring in approximately 1 in 3500, whereas the prevalence of NF-2 is approximately 1 in 40,000. No race or sex predilection has been found. Approximately one half of the cases with each condition represent new mutations.[1] Further recognition of variants has led to expanded classification into 7 subtypes (Table 298-1).

Neurofibromatosis Type 1

NF-1, or von Recklinghausen disease, is a complex disorder with neurologic, cutaneous, skeletal, vascular, and endocrinologic abnormalities. A loss of function mutation in the neurofibromin tumor suppressor gene is thought to be responsible for most of the clinical features. The characteristic lesion is the neurofibroma, a proliferation of Schwann cells and fibroblasts, from which the condition derives its name. Neurofibromas are benign tumors that appear in late childhood, grow in response to hormonal changes, proliferate with age, and may compromise local function by mass effect. Small neurofibromas appear as pink to flesh color to brown papules with a soft, spongy texture (Figure 298-1). On occasion, gentle downward pressure can cause these lesions to sink through the underlying dermis, creating a dimple (Figure 298-2). Size and number vary greatly. A slight predilection for trunk involvement seems to exist, although neurofibromas can occur anywhere on the body.[2-4]

A variant of neurofibroma, the plexiform type, can be large and can cause considerable disfigurement. Plexiform neurofibromas (Figure 298-3) are highly variable masses that may have surface hyperpigmentation

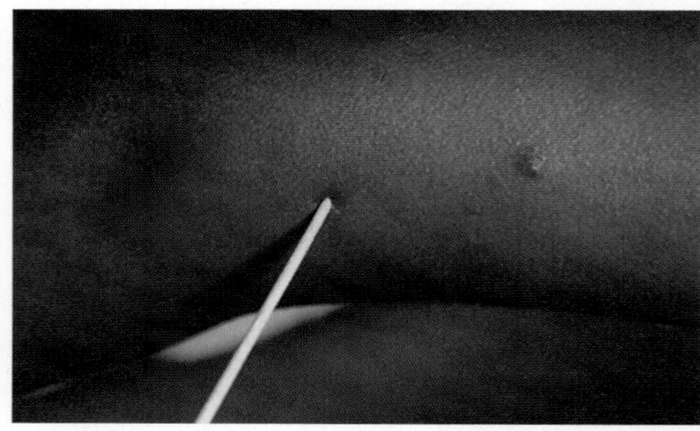

Figure 298-2 Neurofibroma dimpling through underlying dermis.

Table 298-1 Neurofibromatosis Spectrum

CLASSIFICATION	CHARACTERISTICS
Type 1	See text
Type 2	See text
Type 3 (mixed), type 4 (variant)	Autosomal dominant; resemble type 2; more cutaneous NFs; greater risk of optic gliomas, neurilemmoma, meningiomas
Type 5 (segmental)	Skin lesions all on 1 body segment (eg, leg); somatic mosaicism
Type 6 (CALMs)	Only has CALM; must have 2 generations to diagnose
Type 7 (late onset)	Symptoms manifest in the 20s; uncertain whether heritable

CALM, Multiple café au lait macules; *NF,* neurofibromatosis.
From Jabbour SA, Davidovici BB, Wolf R. Rare syndromes. *Clin Dermatol.* 2006;24:299-316. Copyright © 2006, Elsevier, with permission.

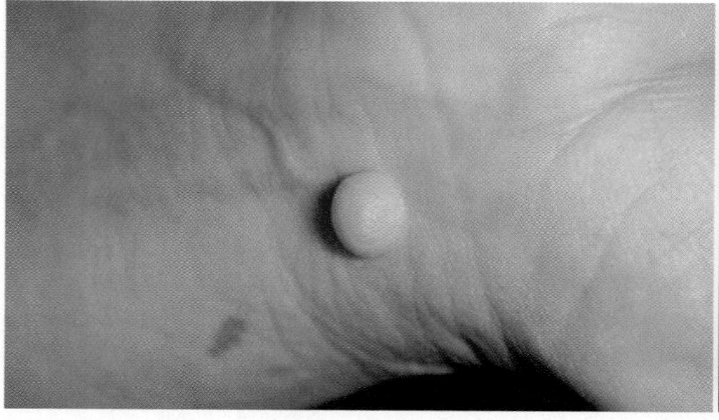

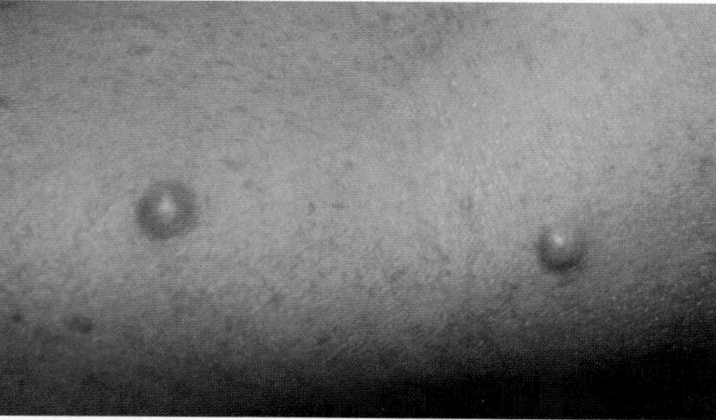

Figure 298-1 Cutaneous neurofibromas in neurofibromatosis type 1.

or may remain flesh colored. Overlying skin may be somewhat thickened and may exhibit increased hair growth. Plexiform neurofibromas often produce soft tissue masses, sometimes feeling soft and spongy in texture, other times feeling similar to a bag of rope. Plexiform lesions are seen in approximately 50% of patients with NF-1.[2,4]

The earliest features are often café au lait macules (CALM), which are tan, oval macules with smooth margins and no surface texture change (Figure 298-4). They remain flat and do not exhibit increased hair growth. They may vary in size and shape, and they may increase in number and size with age.[4,5]

Diagnosis

NF-1 is a highly variable condition, with age-specific expression of its clinical features. Although minor evidence occurs often in infancy with only CALMs, NF-1 cannot be diagnosed clinically until 2 or more of the major diagnostic criteria are met (Box 298-1). This feature is particularly important in view of the many other disorders in which CALMs are a presenting feature (Table 298-2).

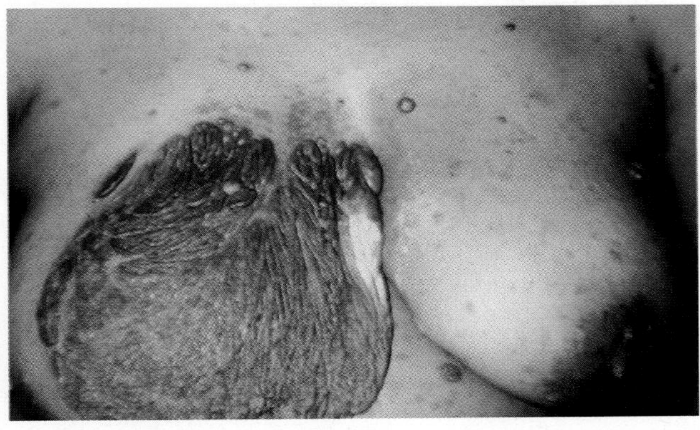

Figure 298-3 Plexiform neurofibroma on a breast.

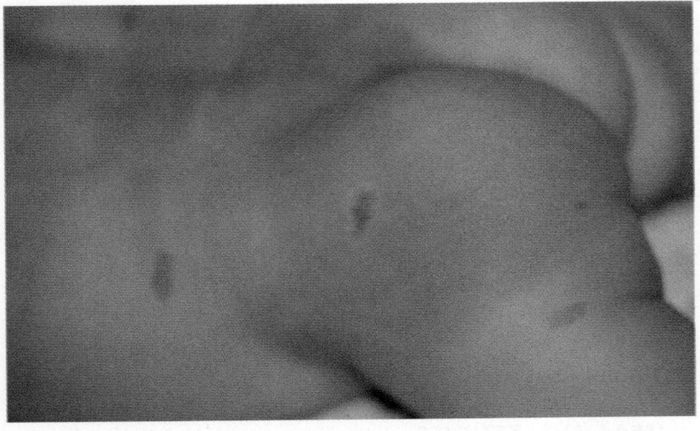

Figure 298-4 Multiple café au lait macules on an infant, with coincidental gray Mongolian spot.

Evaluation

The evaluation of patients for possible NF-1 depends on age; many of the features develop over time. For example, CALMs are present at birth but will increase in size and number for the first 5 to 7 years. Bowing of the long bones (especially tibia) and cutaneous plexiform neurofibromas typically are visible within the 1st year of life, whereas axillary (Figure 298-5) and inguinal freckling, optic gliomas, and scoliosis may not be apparent until age 7 years. Cutaneous neurofibromas and iris Lisch nodules usually appear during or after the teenage years.[4]

HISTORY. Relevant history should include questions about development, language and learning, socialization, and self-esteem as age appropriate. Family history is of paramount importance in the initial evaluation of a child with only CALMs because the presence of NF-1 in a 1st-degree relative secures the diagnosis.[4]

PHYSICAL EXAMINATION. Initial examination of any child for NF-1 should start with a thorough skin survey for CALMs. Six or more CALMs should raise the index of suspicion. Thorough examination of the entire skin surface should also reveal the presence of plexiform neurofibromas. Plexiform neurofibromas may be present at birth or may develop in the 1st few years of life.[2,4] Careful attention should also be paid to the long bones of the lower leg because congenital tibial dysplasia is an early finding in up to 5% of children with NF-1.[1,5,6] Any curvature or nodularity of the tibia is worrisome, as is any length discrepancy. Head circumference should be monitored at each visit because approximately 50% of children with NF-1 have macrocephaly.[1] Thorough developmental evaluation should be undertaken at each visit and repeated at regular intervals, with preschool attention to language, visual motor skills, and learning.[4,7]

Examination of the back for evidence of scoliosis should start by age 2 years because scoliosis appears

BOX 298-1 Diagnostic Criteria for Neurofibromatosis Type 1 (NF-1)

NF-1 is present when a patient has 2 or more of the following:

- Six or more café au lait spots larger than 5 mm in prepubertal child and 15 mm after puberty
- Axillary or inguinal freckling
- At least 2 neurofibromas of any type or at least 1 plexiform neurofibroma
- Optic pathway glioma
- At least 2 Lisch nodules
- Characteristic bony lesion (sphenoid wing dysplasia, or thinning of the cortex of long bones—with or without pseudoarthrosis)
- First-degree relative with NF-1

Adapted from Yohay K. Neurofibromatosis types 1 and 2. *Neurologist.* 2006;12:86-93; Tonsgard JH. Clinical manifestations and management of neurofibromatosis type 1. *Semin Pediatr Neurol.* 2006;13:2-7.

Table 298-2 Differential Diagnosis of Multiple CALMs*

CONDITION	OTHER CLINICAL FEATURES	COMMENT
Normal	—	Up to 25% of normal individuals may have 1-3 CALMs. Up to 40% of people with >6 CALMs and no other symptoms never progress to NF-1.
NF-1	Axillary freckling, cutaneous NFs, plexiform NFs, Lisch nodules, optic glioma, bony abnormalities, positive FH	Present in 95% of patients with NF-1; must have >6 CALMs (>5 mm before puberty; >15 mm after puberty).
Watson syndrome	Pulmonic stenosis, MR, axillary freckling	Axillary freckling only in NF-1 and Watson syndrome type 1.
McCune-Albright syndrome	Polyostotic fibrous bony dysplasia, precocious puberty, hyperthyroid, Cushing syndrome	Usually large-segment CALM with irregular border *(coast of Maine).*
Russell-Silver syndrome	Short stature, skeletal asymmetry, abnormal pubertal development	—
Bloom syndrome	Malar facial erythema and telangiectasia; photosensitivity; long, narrow face with prominent nose; short stature; hypogonadism; malignancy risk	Facial photosensitivity with multiple CALMs triggers evaluation.
Tuberous sclerosis	Hypopigmented macules, facial and periungual angiofibromas, seizures, MR, renal and cardiac hamartomas	Hypopigmented macules more common; mixture very concerning for tuberous sclerosis complex.
Noonan syndrome	Hypertelorism, webbed neck, short stature, leg lymphedema, pulmonic stenosis, hypogonadism	—

CALM, Multiple café au lait macules; *FH,* family history; *MR,* mental retardation; *NF,* neurofibromatosis; *NF-1,* neurofibromatosis type 1.
Adapted from Krowchuk DP, Mancini AJ, eds. *Pediatric Dermatology: A Quick Reference Guide.* Elk Grove Village, Ill: American Academy of Pediatrics; 2007; Spitz JL. *Genodermatoses: A Full-Color Clinical Guide to Genetic Skin Disorders.* New York, NY: Williams & Wilkins; 1996.

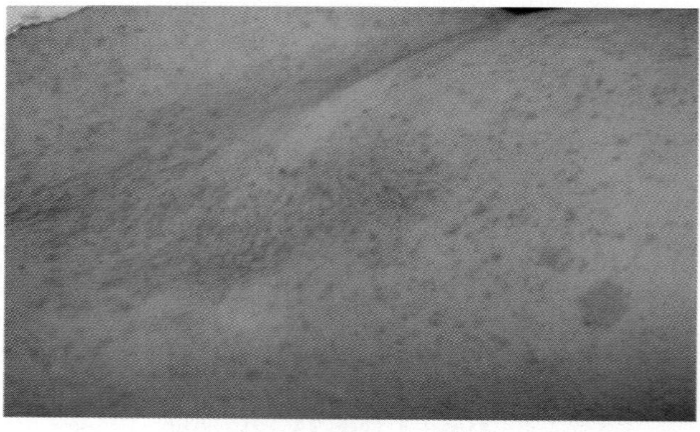

Figure 298-5 Axillary freckling in neurofibromatosis type 1.

at an earlier age in NF-1, and a severe dystrophic form of kyphoscoliosis can appear between 3 and 5 years of age. Regular blood pressure assessment should also begin by age 2 years. Ophthalmologic evaluation should be obtained annually to age 10 years to assess for the presence of optic pathway glioma. These grade-1 pilocytic astrocytomas, which are present in approximately 15% of children with NF-1 under age 10, may produce proptosis, strabismus, papilledema, or vision loss. If the optic chiasm is involved, then hypothalamic extension can produce an endocrinopathy, resulting in precocious or delayed puberty. The development of precocious puberty should prompt evaluation for an optic glioma. Other ocular findings may include congenital ptosis or orbital asymmetry (the latter the result of sphenoid wing dysplasia).[4,5,8]

School-aged children should be assessed for limb asymmetry, long bone bowing, scoliosis, and cutaneous neurofibromas. School performance should be addressed with particular attention to learning disabilities, attention-deficit/hyperactivity disorder (ADHD), self-esteem, and socialization.[4,7,9]

Teens should be assessed for limb asymmetry, scoliosis, neurofibromas, and hypertension. Ophthalmologic evaluation, including slit-lamp examination, should be obtained to look for iris hamartomas (Lisch nodules). These tan to brown papules usually appear in the teenaged years, but they have minimal impact other than support of diagnosis. Any complaint of pain, particularly pain associated with focal neurologic deficit or arising from a plexiform tumor, should be thoroughly evaluated by examination and imaging studies. School performance, socialization, and self-esteem should be addressed as well.[4,7]

LABORATORY EVALUATION. Routine laboratory testing is unnecessary in NF-1. However, if reason exists to test for gene mutations (in cases of uncertain diagnosis), then a complementary series of analyses—including premature truncation test, heteroduplex analysis, and fluorescent in situ hybridization assay—is available. This tiered analysis provides a sensitivity of 95%.[1,10]

IMAGING STUDIES. Imaging in NF-1 should be directed toward evaluation of symptoms. Routine neuroimaging is generally not undertaken. However, head magnetic resonance imaging (MRI) is indicated for evaluation of focal neurologic changes, new-onset seizures, severe headaches, vision changes, proptosis, short stature, rapid change in head circumference, plexiform lesions, severe cognitive deficits, and precocious or delayed puberty.[1,3] Any evidence of scoliosis or any long bone anomaly should merit plain-film radiography. Scoliosis may also require MRI or computed tomography (CT) to define the extent and help map surgical intervention.[6] MRI is also useful to assess for radiculopathy because neurofibromas have a propensity to develop along or within the spine, often impinging on nerve roots. The development of pain, or any focal neurologic deficit, also warrants a thorough evaluation, including MRI. This evaluation is particularly important if pain develops in a plexiform neurofibroma because pain may herald malignant change. Although MRI is the mainstay of evaluation of plexiform neurofibromas, positron emission tomographic scanning may be of more value in distinguishing benign from malignant lesions. Cranial MRI is indicated to evaluate for possible optic pathway glioma once symptoms have developed. Routine imaging before symptom onset is not indicated. Once optic gliomas are diagnosed, MRI should be obtained every 2 years and with any symptom change to age 10 years. Imaging is also useful in evaluation of cerebrovascular disease and renal artery stenosis.[1,4,5,11]

One unusual finding in NF-1 is the presence of unidentified bright objects on T2-weighted sequences of cranial MRI. These lesions, which are present in 60% to 90% of children but only approximately 30% of adults, are of uncertain significance. Controversial evidence suggests that some learning disabilities seem to correlate with the presence and specific locations of unidentified bright objects.[7,11]

Management

Management of NF-1 should focus on the organ system involved, given the wide variability of expression. As a rule, genetic counseling should be provided for all NF-1 families because affected individuals have a 50% chance of transmission with each pregnancy.

Neurofibromas present unique management issues of their own. Smaller lesions may become painful or may interfere with activities as a result of location. Plexiform lesions can be disfiguring, especially when they are present on the head or neck. The presence of numerous or large lesions may exert a profound effect on self-esteem and socialization. Surgical excision may be necessary for problematic tumors. Sudden development of pain or focal neurologic deficit in plexiform tumors may represent malignant degeneration. Malignant peripheral nerve sheath tumors (formerly called neurofibrosarcoma) develop in 5% to 13% of patients with NF-1 with devastating effect. These aggressive tumors are often multicentric, and they metastasize quickly. Despite aggressive therapy, they are usually fatal within a year.[1,4] Other malignant tumors are seen in NF-1 with an overall incidence 3% higher than the general population. These tumors include leukemia (especially juvenile myelomonocytic leukemia), rhabdomyosarcoma, pheochromocytoma, and carcinoid. The last 2 tumors are predominantly adult-onset tumors.[4,10]

Optic pathway gliomas develop in 15% to 20% of patients with NF-1 at a mean age of 4.2 years.[5] Careful ophthalmologic monitoring for vision change, afferent pupillary defect, or change in funduscopic examination findings should begin in the 1st year of life and continue annually to age 10 years. Progression of the gliomas beyond age 10 is rare. Other ocular findings may include congenital ptosis, congenital glaucoma, and pulsating exophthalmos.[1,4,5] If optic pathway glioma is present, MRI evaluation should be repeated every 2 years until age 10 in addition to annual ophthalmologic examination.[8] Precocious or delayed puberty may be a later clinical sign of optic glioma extending from the chiasm into the hypothalamus and should prompt reevaluation and MRI.[1,4]

Hormonal surges may affect NF-1 and should be discussed with preteens and teens. Oral contraceptives, puberty, and pregnancy are likely to cause increases in both size and number of neurofibromas.[4]

Neurodevelopmental issues are of paramount importance in the management of patients with NF-1. Headaches occur in 20% of patients; these are usually migraines that respond well to standard therapy such as amitriptyline or topiramate.[4] Seizures occur in 4% to 10% of patients with NF-1 and may include partial or generalized variants or even infantile spasms.[1,4] Management should be directed toward the specific seizure type (see Chapter 320, Seizure Disorders). Hearing loss, usually unilateral, occurs in approximately 10% of patients with NF-1.[4] Learning disabilities are observed in 35% to 65% of children with NF-1, compared with less than 20% of the general population. A slight downward shift often occurs in IQ compared with age-matched controls, but the incidence of intellectual disability is only 4% to 8% (approximately twice that of the general population).[1,7,9] Learning disabilities are variable but may include math and reading comprehension problems. In addition, visual perception deficits and delays in both gross- and fine-motor skills are common. Speech and language delays are seen in approximately one half of these children.[7,9] ADHD is also common, occurring in approximately one half of NF-1 children. A variety of behavioral problems is seen with increased frequency in NF-1 and may include anxiety, depression, social problems, aggression, and unusual behaviors. These issues seem to correlate more with the comorbid diagnosis of ADHD than with academic achievement.[12]

Vascular disease is more common in patients with NF-1, which may include congenital heart defects, hypertension, occlusive arterial disease, aneurysms, or arteriovenous fistulae. Hypertension in young children may result from renal artery stenosis (1% of patients with NF-1). Hypertension in adults may be primary or associated with pheochromocytoma (rarely renal artery stenosis in adults). Workup should include renal angiography in children and urine catecholamine levels in adults.[1,4]

Bone abnormalities are common in NF-1, ranging from skeletal dysplasia to nonossifying fibroma to short stature to kyphoscoliosis. Long bone dysplasia (especially tibia) may be seen during the 1st year of life and may present as bowing or, rarely, pseudoarthrosis (nodule at the site of a healing pathological fracture).

Pseudoarthrosis occurs in only 3% of children with NF-1. Nonossifying fibromas occur in late childhood to the teen years and may lead to pathological fracture, particularly in the femur, tibia, and humerus. Scoliosis is seen in 10% of children with NF-1 and may develop earlier than in the general population. An aggressive dystrophic form may develop between 3 and 7 years of age.[1,4-6]

Life expectancy is approximately 10 to 15 years shorter in NF-1 compared with the general population, with malignancy and vascular disease as the leading causes of death.[1,4]

Neurofibromatosis Type 2

NF-2 is a tumor syndrome defined by the presence of bilateral vestibular schwannomas; it is also known as multiple inherited schwannomas, meningiomas, and ependymomas syndrome because of the occurrence of numerous central and peripheral nervous system tumors. The NF-2 gene encodes merlin, or schwannomin, a cytoskeletal protein that may have regulatory and signaling functions. The precise mechanism of tumor formation is uncertain.[1,13,14] In addition to the characteristic vestibular schwannomas that lead to progressive deterioration of hearing, patients with NF-2 may develop intracranial or spinal meningiomas; ependymomas; astrocytomas; neurofibromas; schwannomas of the cranial, spinal, and peripheral nerves; and cutaneous schwannomas (the latter with minimal clinical impact).[1,13,15] Ependymomas and astrocytomas are seen in up to 33% of patients. Peripheral schwannomas may arise from any nerve and may produce pain or sensory or motor dysfunction. Patients with NF-2 may also develop peripheral neuropathy that is not related to tumor growth. Seizure disorders are uncommon in NF-2. Similarly, cognitive impairment is not a feature of NF-2.[1,13] Ocular findings in NF-2 include juvenile posterior subcapsular lens opacities, retinal hamartomas, and cortical wedge opacities.[1,14] The average age at onset of symptoms is approximately 20 years, with average age at diagnosis 28 years. However, 18% of patients show symptoms before age 15 years.[1,13,15]

Evaluation

HISTORY. Relevant history for NF-2 should include any vision or hearing changes, tinnitus, vertigo, gait disturbances, decreased facial sensation, facial weakness or twitching, hoarseness, dysphagia, or headaches. Family history of NF-2 is crucial for diagnosis (Box 298-2).[13,15]

PHYSICAL EXAMINATION. Examination of a patient for NF-2 should focus on vision, hearing, and cranial and peripheral nerve function. Younger patients often have headache, tinnitus, cranial nerve symptoms, or skin or spinal tumors before the onset of hearing loss. Eye examination should assess the presence of lens opacities. Cranial nerve examination should specifically address the trigeminal, facial, and auditory nerves. Neurologic examination should assess balance, gait, and deep tendon reflexes. At the skin examination, the physician should note the presence of neurofibromas, CALMs, or cutaneous schwannomas. Cutaneous schwannomas are present in approximately one half of patients with NF-2; they may be subcutaneous nodules or plaques with thickened texture and occasional hair growth, or surface pink to flesh-colored papules (Figure 298-6).[1,13,15]

LABORATORY EVALUATION. Laboratory testing for possible NF-2 should always include formal audiologic testing for sensorineural hearing loss. Once the diagnosis of NF-2 is established, audiometry should be

BOX 298-2 Diagnostic Criteria for Neurofibromatosis Type 2 (NF-2)

DEFINITE NF-2

Bilateral vestibular schwannomas

or

First-degree relative with NF-2

plus

Unilateral vestibular schwannomas

or

Any 2 of the following: meningioma, schwannoma, glioma, neurofibroma, juvenile posterior subcapsular cataract

PROBABLE NF-2

Unilateral vestibular schwannoma

plus

Any 2 of the following: meningioma, schwannoma, glioma, neurofibroma, juvenile posterior subcapsular cataract

or

Multiple meningiomas

plus

Unilateral vestibular schwannoma

or

Any 2 of the following: schwannoma, glioma, neurofibroma, juvenile posterior subcapsular cataract

Adapted from Yohay K. Neurofibromatosis types 1 and 2. *Neurologist.* 2006;12:86-93; Neff BA, Welling DB. Current concepts in the evaluation and treatment of neurofibromatosis type II. *Otolaryngol Clin North Am.* 2005;38:671-684.

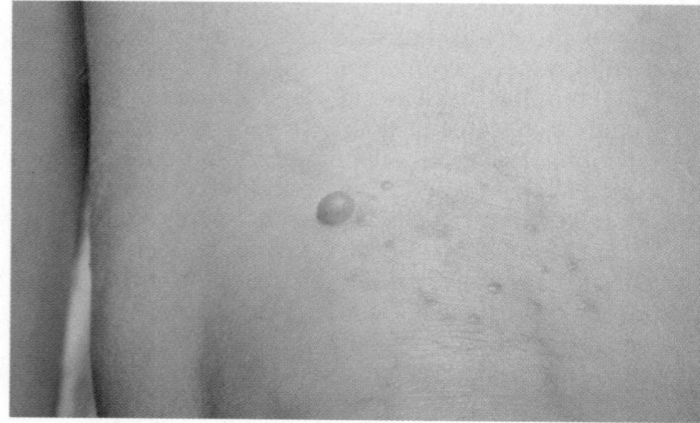

Figure 298-6 Multiple schwannomas in neurofibromatosis type 2.

repeated every 6 to 12 months. Genetic testing for the mutations is available on a clinical basis, but the sensitivity is low (34% in sporadic mutations, 54% if familial). With this high false-negative rate, children at risk would still require annual screening, as would any asymptomatic child with a detected mutation.[1,13]

IMAGING STUDIES. The most useful imaging modality for assessment of vestibular schwannomas is gadolinium-enhanced MRI with thin cuts through the internal auditory canals. Routine screening MRI of the brain is required for any patient with unilateral vestibular schwannoma, multiple intracranial or spinal tumors, 1st-degree relative with NF-2, or a child with meningioma. As with audiometric testing, any child at risk for NF-2 should have a screening brain MRI annually beginning at age 7 years. Spinal MRI should be considered if any symptoms or neurologic deficits are noted.[1,11,13]

Management

The most important aspect of management in NF-2 is early diagnosis so that surgery to preserve the hearing can be performed. Advanced tumors may prevent the preservation of hearing, leading to need for either cochlear or auditory brainstem implants or may lead to complete deafness. At present, cochlear implants seem to be better than auditory brainstem implants for patients with NF-2. Once a diagnosis of NF-2 is made, the child should be evaluated by ophthalmologic, otolaryngologic, audiologic, and imaging studies. Screening examinations, audiometry, and imaging should then be repeated at least annually starting at age 7 years. Children of a parent with NF-2 should have annual ophthalmologic examinations starting in infancy and neurologic and audiometric examinations annually from age 7 years. Most patients with NF-2 should be encouraged to learn sign language to prepare for possible future complete hearing loss.[1,13]

WHEN TO REFER

NF-1
- Pediatric ophthalmologic evaluation beginning in the 1st year
- Neurologic evaluation if seizures are difficult to manage
- Neurodevelopmental testing if evidence of learning disability, ADHD, and speech delay
- Surgical referral for symptomatic neurofibromas, renovascular hypertension

NF-2
- Hearing loss, gait or balance difficulty, headache, and tinnitus

WHEN TO ADMIT

- Sudden neurologic decline or uncontrollable seizures

TUBEROUS SCLEROSIS COMPLEX

Definitions

Tuberous sclerosis complex (TSC), or Bourneville disease, is an autosomal-dominant multisystem disorder characterized by perturbed cellular growth and differentiation in the brain, heart, kidneys, skin, eyes, and other tissues. Although a dominant disorder, approximately 70% of cases arise as spontaneous new mutations. The prevalence of TSC is approximately 1 in 6000. TSC results from mutations in 1 of 2 genes: *TSC1,* which encodes hamartin, or *TSC2,* which encodes tuberin.[15,16] Hamartin and tuberin bind together as a heterodimeric protein involved in regulation of cell growth. The intact protein suppresses the protranslational effects of mammalian target of rapamycin. When either hamartin or tuberin is defective, mammalian target of rapamycin starts uncontrolled promotion of protein synthesis and cell growth, leading to tumor formation.[17-20] Mutations of *TSC1* are more common in familial cases and seem to result in less severe disease.[16]

The classic triad of seizures, intellectual disability, and facial angiofibromas is far from a complete picture of this complex but highly variable condition. Seizures and facial lesions do indeed occur frequently, but mental function is often normal or only slightly impaired. Approximately one half of patients with TSC have normal intelligence, whereas approximately 30% have profound intellectual disability. The hallmark of TSC is the development of hamartomas in the various organ systems involved. An international consensus conference in 1998 developed revised diagnostic criteria for TSC based on newer understanding of the disease and its underlying pathophysiological features.[21] A summary of these criteria is found in Box 298-3. An important point to note is that TSC has no pathognomonic feature. Because an individual feature may occur as an isolated finding, the primary care physician must consider the diagnosis of TSC only if more than 1 organ system is involved or if different lesion types occur in a single system.[22]

Central Nervous System Manifestations

Central nervous system (CNS) disease is the most common and often most disabling aspect of TSC. The neurologic features of TSC include seizures, cognitive disability, and behavioral disturbances. Seizures occur in 80% to 90% of patients with TSC. All types of seizures except classic absence seizures have been reported in TSC. One of the more common forms is infantile spasms, seen in approximately one third of infants with TSC. Infantile spasms are the presenting feature in 70% of infants with TSC.[15,16,23] A thorough description of the clinical and electroencephalographic findings in infantile spasms is found in Chapter 320, Seizure Disorders. Children with infantile spasms are likely to have cognitive disability.[22,24]

Seizure onset and severity are also closely associated with severity of cognitive impairment. Early onset of seizures or infantile spasms is associated with poor cognitive outcome. Although most patients with TSC and cognitive disability have epilepsy, many patients with TSC and seizures have normal intellect. However, children with infantile spasms are often cognitively impaired, corresponding to increased cortical hamartoma (tuber) burden in both circumstances.[12,16] Furthermore, the presence of at least 7 cortical tubers on MRI confers a 5-fold increase in risk of moderate to profound cognitive impairment, although a few patients with multiple tubers and normal intellect have been reported.[12,25]

Autism spectrum disorder is also more common in TSC, with prevalence estimates ranging from 17% to 68%.[25] Autism spectrum disorder is much more common in children with global cognitive impairment in TSC (>60%), compared with only 6% among TSC children with normal cognitive function. Almost all children with autism spectrum disorder and TSC have epilepsy.[26,27] Patients with autism and TSC do not exhibit the male preponderance seen in autism without TSC.[12] Among children with autism spectrum disorder, TSC is found in up to 4%. Similarly, among children with autism and seizures, TSC is the underlying genetic condition in 14%.[25]

A variety of behavioral abnormalities may be seen in children with TSC, including severe temper tantrums, restlessness, impulsivity, attention deficit with hyperactivity, self-injury, anxiety, and depression.[27] Among children with TSC and a history of infantile spasms and autism, 69% exhibit behaviors disruptive to the family by age 5 years.[25] Anxiety disorder is seen in up to 59% and depression in 35% of adults with TSC.[27]

Learning disabilities have been noted frequently in TSC, although no systematic studies are available to date.[27]

The neuropathologic findings responsible for many of the symptoms of TSC include tubers, subependymal nodules, and subependymal giant cell astrocytomas. The cortical tubers are nodular areas of gray and white matter dysplasia, often seen on the apex of a gyrus.[15,22] Tubers are present in over 95% of patients with TSC. Tubers have been noted as early as 20 weeks' gestation and are known to persist throughout life. No risk of malignant degeneration exists. Large numbers of tubers are associated with worse overall prognosis (infantile spasms, cognitive impairment, and difficult seizure control). The tubers also function as epileptogenic foci. Subependymal nodules are present in up to 80% of patients with TSC. They arise from the lateral and 3rd ventricle walls and often protrude into the lumen. They can be present before birth and may sometimes be noted on imaging studies during infancy. The presence and number of subependymal nodules do not seem to correlate with severity of neurologic symptoms, in contrast to tubers.[15,16,22] Subependymal giant cell astrocytomas, on the other hand, may be symptomatic. They occur in up to 14% of patients with TSC and seem to arise from subependymal nodules. They continue to grow during childhood and may produce focal neurologic deficits or obstructive hydrocephalus.[15,22]

BOX 298-3 Diagnostic Criteria for Tuberous Sclerosis Complex (TSC)*

MAJOR CRITERIA

Facial angiofibroma or forehead plaque
Ungual or subungual fibroma
More than 3 hypomelanotic macules
Connective tissue nevus (Shagreen patch)
Cortical tuber
Subependymal nodule
Subependymal giant-cell astrocytoma
Multiple retinal hamartomas
Cardiac rhabdomyoma
Renal angiomyolipoma
Lymphangiomyomatosis

MINOR CRITERIA

Dental enamel pits
Hamartomatous rectal polyps
Bone cysts (radiographic evidence sufficient)
Cerebral white matter migration lines
Gingival fibromas
Retinal achromic patch
Nonrenal hamartomas
Multiple renal cysts
Confetti skin lesions

DIAGNOSIS FOR TSC

Definitive: 2 major or 1 major and 2 minor criteria
Probable: 1 major criterion plus 1 minor criterion
Possible: 1 major or 2 or more minor criteria

*When cortical dysplasia (tuber) and cerebral white matter migration tracks are both present, they count as 1 criterion rather than 2 criteria.
Adapted from Rosser T, Panigrahy A, McClintock W. The diverse clinical manifestations of tuberous sclerosis complex: a review. *Semin Pediatr Neurol.* 2006;13:27-36; Roach ES, Sparagana SP. Diagnosis of tuberous sclerosis complex. *J Child Neurol.* 2004;19:643-649; Crino PB, Nathanson KL, Henske EP. The tuberous sclerosis complex. *N Engl J Med.* 2006;355:1345.

Cutaneous Manifestations

Skin findings are the most consistent features of TSC. Hypomelanotic macules (formerly known as *ash leaf spots*) are found in more than 90% of patients with TSC and may be present at birth (Figure 298-7). In lighter-skinned individuals, they may be visible only with a Wood lamp. They are usually larger than 1 cm and have a characteristic leaf shape: oval with 1 blunt end and

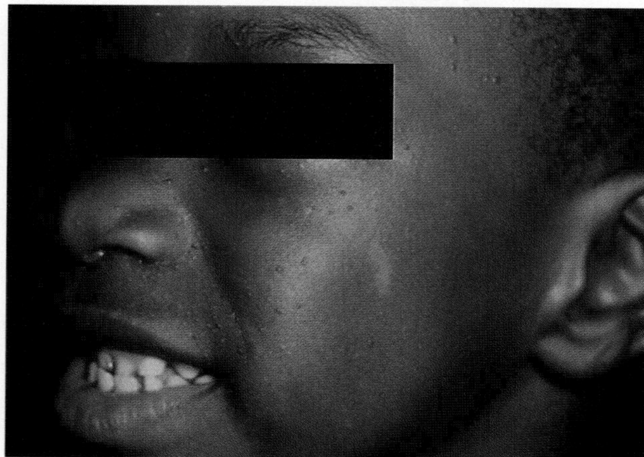

Figure 298-7 Facial angiofibromas and hypomelanotic macules in tuberous sclerosis complex.

1 pointed end. At least 3 lesions must be visible for diagnostic significance. Hypomelanotic macules are seen most commonly on the trunk, but they may occur anywhere. Fine, stippled hypopigmentation on the extremities is known as *confetti lesions*. When hypomelanotic macules occur on hair-bearing surfaces, associated poliosis (white hair) may be found.[15,16,22,23]

Facial angiofibromas (formerly known as *adenoma sebaceum*) are noted in 70% to 75% of individuals with TSC. These small, discrete, shiny pink to reddish papules develop by approximately age 5 years, but they increase in number and size into the teenage or early adult years (see Figure 298-7). Although they are initially distributed over the malar areas, they often spread to chin and nasolabial folds during puberty.[15,16,22] Forehead plaques are flesh-colored to erythematous fibrotic plaques on the forehead or frontal scalp in approximately 19% of patients with TSC. They appear later than angiofibromas.[16]

Shagreen patches are connective tissue nevi seen in 20% to 50% of patients with TSC. These patches are flesh-colored, slightly raised, irregularly shaped plaques with prominent follicles and cobblestone texture seen most often on the lower back (Figure 298-8). They are usually noted in later childhood.[15,16,22]

Ungual and subungual fibromas are firm flesh-colored to red papules that develop beside or beneath the nails. Lesions under the nail may appear as a longitudinal ridge or groove. Toenail involvement is more common. These typically appear during puberty.[15,16,22]

Cardiac Manifestations

Cardiac rhabdomyomas are present in one half to two thirds of infants with TSC, but they usually remain asymptomatic. These tumors, which are often multiple, decrease in size over time. They are often diagnosed on prenatal ultrasound. Complications may include heart failure in infancy and various dysrhythmias, including Wolff-Parkinson-White syndrome.[15,16,22,23]

Ocular Manifestations

Retinal hamartomas are seen in 50% to 87% of patients with TSC, although most remain asymptomatic. They may be bilateral in up to one half of patients. Three clinical types include (1) the raised mulberry-like calcified nodule, (2) the flat translucent gray patch, and (3) a transitional lesion with mixed features. Involvement of the macula, enlargement of the hamartoma, vitreous hemorrhage, or retinal detachment may lead to loss of vision.[15,16,22,28] Other ocular findings in TSC may include retinal pigment anomalies, strabismus, cataracts, colobomas, iris depigmentation, and eyelid angiofibromas.[16]

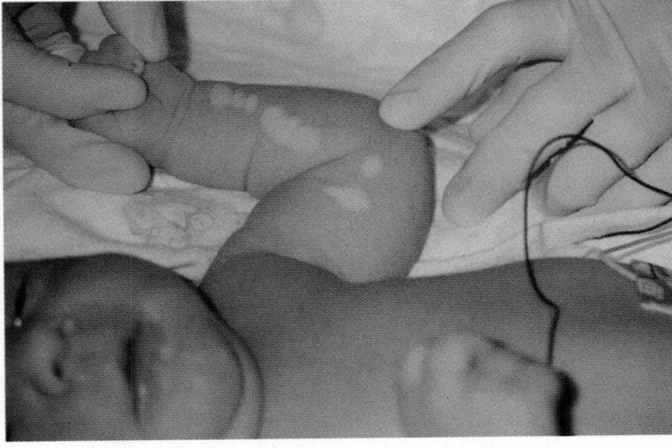

Figure 298-8 Shagreen patch on the arm of an infant with tuberous sclerosis complex.

Renal Manifestations

Renal lesions occur in 80% of patients with TSC and may include angiomyolipoma, cysts, and renal cell carcinoma (RCC). The prevalence increases with age. Angiomyolipomas develop in 55% to 75% of patients with TSC who are older than 10 years. Bilateral and multiple tumors are common. Small lesions may remain asymptomatic, but lesions over 4 cm pose risks of severe hemorrhage, hypertension, or renal insufficiency.[22,23,28] Renal cysts occur in approximately 17% of children and 47% of adults with TSC. Solitary epithelial cysts are the most common. However, approximately 3% to 5% of patients with TSC will develop polycystic kidney disease as a contiguous gene deletion syndrome because the *TSC2* gene is adjacent to the adult polycystic kidney disease gene *PKD1* on chromosome 16. Polycystic kidney disease may lead to renal insufficiency in late adolescence. RCC is a less common but potentially severe complication of TSC. Although the lifetime risk of RCC is the same in TSC as in the general population, it typically occurs at a much earlier age in TSC (average age 28 years in TSC; 52 years in general population). The overall morbidity of renal lesions in TSC is predominantly related to angiomyolipomas.[16,23,28,29]

Pulmonary Manifestations

Symptomatic lymphangiomyomatosis occurs in 1% to 2% of patients with TSC, almost exclusively in young women. Radiographic evidence of lymphangiomyomatosis may be seen in 26% to 39% of women with TSC. Spontaneous pneumothorax, dyspnea, cough, and hemoptysis are the main clinical findings. This condition is often progressive and is a leading cause of death among women with TSC.[15,16,22,23]

Vascular Manifestations

Arterial dysplasia is seen most often in renal angiomyolipomas, but it has also been reported with basilar artery and aortic aneurysms.[28]

Dental Manifestations

Gingival fibromas occur in approximately 50% of adults with TSC. Almost all patients with TSC have dental enamel pits in permanent teeth. The dental pits rarely cause problems, although extensive fibromas may result in malocclusion or abnormal tooth eruption.[28]

Differential Diagnosis

TSC does not have a pathognomonic lesion; thus fulfillment of diagnostic criteria is of paramount importance (see Box 298-3). Facial angiofibromas were once considered diagnostic but are now known to occur in multiple endocrine neoplasia syndrome type 1.[22]

Evaluation

History

In infants, seizures are often the 1st symptom. Any infant with new-onset seizures should have a detailed history, including skin lesions, developmental milestones, and family history. Initial examination should include Wood lamp examination of the entire skin surface, funduscopic examination for hamartomas, and a thorough neurologic examination. Older children should be screened for seizure disorder, developmental delay, and autism spectrum disorders.[16,23]

Laboratory Evaluation

Laboratory testing should include an electrocardiogram, especially in infants or children with radiographic evidence of cardiac rhabdomyomas. Once diagnostic criteria are fulfilled for a diagnosis of TSC, molecular testing can be performed to determine the specific mutation. However, 15% to 20% of patients who fulfill TSC diagnostic criteria have no identifiable mutations. Clinical gene testing is available by using combined techniques such as denaturing high-performance liquid chromatography and heteroduplex analysis. Even with combined methods, the mutation detection rate is only 85%.[17,22,23]

Imaging Studies

Imaging studies are valuable for initial evaluation and long-term management of patients with TSC. Initial imaging studies for an infant with TSC includes brain studies (MRI or CT), echocardiography, and renal ultrasound. Cortical tubers are best evaluated by MRI. Subependymal nodules may be seen in infancy on MRI as T1-weighted hyperintense nodules. By age 1 year, the subependymal nodules contain calcium and may be visualized with CT scanning. MRI may be useful to identify subependymal giant cell astrocytomas, but radiologic distinction from subependymal nodules is difficult.[11,30] Renal lesions in older children and adults may be evaluated by ultrasound, CT, or MRI. Chest CT is indicated for all women with TSC to evaluate for possible lymphangiomyomatosis.[23,28]

Management

The 2 basic principles of management in TSC are (1) establishing the correct diagnosis and (2) long-term follow-up for the later manifestations.[23] The treatment of epilepsy in TSC is the same as in other forms of epilepsy (see Chapter 320, Seizure Disorders) with 1 exception. Infantile spasms in TSC do not respond as well to adrenocorticotropic hormone as infantile spasms without TSC. The irreversible gamma-aminobutyric acid transaminase inhibitor vigabatrin is much more effective, with response rates up to 96% in infants with TSC and infantile spasms. Vigabatrin is not currently approved by the US Food and Drug Administration because of potential severe ophthalmic toxicity. However, because of the potentially devastating cognitive impact of uncontrolled infantile spasms, vigabatrin may be considered despite its toxicity.[24] With any type of seizures in TSC, better control seems to improve prognosis. Seizures become refractory to treatment in up to 50% of children with TSC.[22,24]

Neurobehavioral assessment and monitoring are integral to the management of TSC. Routine formal testing should be performed at age-appropriate levels in infancy, preschool, early school age, and periodically into adulthood to identify cognitive and behavioral issues as early as possible. In addition, any regressive behavior or new cognitive dysfunction should prompt urgent reevaluation.[27]

Brain and abdominal imaging should be performed at least every 3 years, more often if lesions exhibit progressive growth or if any acute change in symptoms occurs (sudden neurologic or cognitive decline, hypertension, hematuria). Annual brain MRI is suggested to age 21 years. Annual renal imaging is suggested for monitoring of angiomyolipomas. Serial renal ultrasound is adequate if maximal lesion size is less than 4 cm. Larger renal lesions should be assessed by Doppler or MRI or magnetic resonance angiography for abnormal vasculature. Screening chest CT for lymphangiomyomatosis is suggested for all women with TSC. Women with lung lesions should have annual pulmonary function tests.[23,28]

Genetic counseling is mandatory for families and patients with TSC. Because the disorder is autosomal dominant, affected individuals have a 50% risk of affected offspring. Germ-line mutations occur in approximately 2% of patients; thus seemingly unaffected parents with a single affected child still have approximately a 2% risk of having another affected child.[22,23]

WHEN TO REFER

- Ophthalmologic screening: infancy if TSC is suspected
- Neurologic screening: when seizures are hard to manage or progressive
- Surgery: symptomatic or progressive renal lesions larger than 4 cm
- Neurodevelopmental testing: at diagnosis

WHEN TO ADMIT

- Sudden neurologic deterioration
- Intractable seizures
- Gross hematuria
- Heart failure or dysrhythmia

STURGE-WEBER SYNDROME

Sturge-Weber syndrome (SWS), or encephalotrigeminal angiomatosis, is a rare sporadic disorder characterized by the presence of upper facial port wine stain (PWS), ipsilateral ocular abnormalities, and ipsilateral leptomeningeal angiomatosis. Although the syndrome may consist of only 1 or 2 of the triad features, the defining entity is leptomeningeal involvement.[31] SWS has an estimated frequency of approximately 1 in 50,000 live births. It is thought to result from failed regression of the cephalic venous plexus. By the 6th week of embryologic development, a vascular plexus forms around the cephalic part of the neural tube and under the facial skin ectoderm. This plexus usually regresses by the 9th week. In SWS, the plexus persists, with the extent of involvement correlating with the extent of facial and leptomeningeal lesions.[32,33] No sex predilection has been found. Although a few case reports have suggested familial occurrence, the disorder is thought to result from somatic mosaicism. This concept is supported by discordance between monozygotic twins.[34]

SWS exhibits at birth with an upper facial capillary malformation (PWS), involving the area of skin innervated by the ophthalmic (V1) division of the trigeminal nerve. This area includes the forehead, brow ridge, upper eyelid, and perhaps the lower eyelid as well.[34] Lower areas of the face (V2 or V3 distributions) may also be involved, but no apparent significant risk of SWS exists in the absence of V1 involvement. Unilateral PWS is the rule, with only 10% to 30% having bilateral PWS. With unilateral facial PWS, the risk of having SWS is approximately 8%, but the risk is much higher if bilateral PWS is present.[31,34] One of the more useful clinical clues seems to be eyelid involvement, a significant predictor of disease. PWSs are pink to red blanching macules to patches with variable irregularity of the borders (Figure 298-9). They are capillary malformations that remain fixed in location and show no tendency to evolve or involute over time. Growth should be commensurate with the child's growth. With age, the PWS may thicken and darken, becoming somewhat cobblestoned by adulthood.[31,35]

Ocular manifestations of SWS may include glaucoma, vascular anomalies of the globe (conjunctiva, episclera, retina, or choroid), buphthalmos, iris heterochromia, retinal detachment, retinal pigment degeneration, cataract, and optic disc coloboma. Glaucoma is the most common ocular problem in SWS, occurring in up to 70% of patients.[31,34] Glaucoma is usually ipsilateral to the PWS, but it may be bilateral, even if the PWS is unilateral.[34] Although glaucoma may develop from birth to the 5th decade, the median age at onset is 5 years, with 60% developing in infancy to early childhood. Glaucoma developing in infancy, when the globe is more sensitive to increased intraocular pressure, may lead to increased corneal diameter, buphthalmos, or iris heterochromia. Choroidal hemangioma ipsilateral to the PWS is seen in up to 71% of patients with SWS. Choroidal hemangioma is almost always associated with leptomeningeal lesions, making CNS imaging mandatory. Over time, the retinal changes can lead to visual field defects and vision loss.[34]

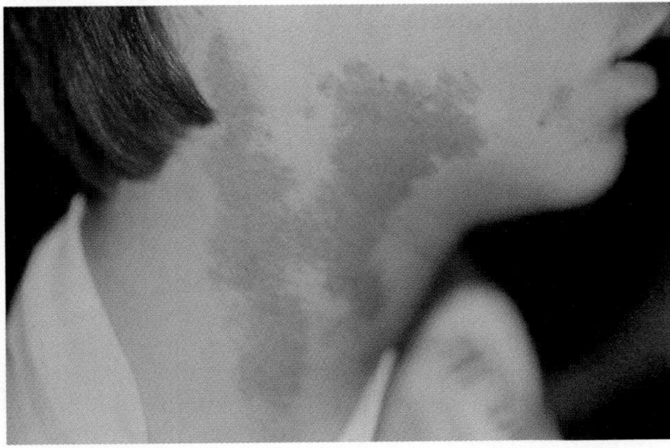

Figure 298-9 Port wine stain on the neck (not associated with Sturge-Weber syndrome).

Neurologic features of SWS may include seizures, focal neurologic deficits, developmental delay, progressive intellectual disability, or headaches. Seizures are the most common neurologic problem, occurring in 75% to 83% of patients with SWS. Approximately 75% of seizure disorders develop in the first 2 years of life.[34,36] Partial motor seizures are the most common type (40%), but generalized tonic-clonic, atonic, and absence seizures may also occur.[15,34] Infantile spasms may be the presenting seizure type. Seizures tend to worsen with age, becoming more frequent, severe, and complex. Seizures may be provoked by febrile episodes. Status epilepticus may occur in up to one half of these children.[37] Earlier onset may predict worse outcome, with poor seizure prognosis, more difficult seizure control, and higher risk of cognitive impairment,[15,34] although no definite link exists between age at onset and neurologic outcome.[31] Bilateral leptomeningeal angiomatosis (7% to 26% of patients) has a poor neurologic prognosis.[34] Some patients may develop sudden episodes of weakness, even in the absence of seizures. These episodes are strokelike and may be transient or may leave permanent hemiplegia. Hemianopsia may develop in up to one half of SWS patients.[15]

Developmental delays are seen in up to one half of patients with SWS. Early milestones are often normal, with decline in function noted over time. At least some of the cognitive decline occurs during periods of encephalopathy after prolonged or severe seizures, whereas other patients experience decline in function as a result of recurrent strokelike episodes.[15,31,37] Factors that seem to correlate best with developmental delay and its severity are presence of bilateral cerebral lesions, degree of cerebral atrophy, presence of intractable seizures or multiple seizure types, and possibly early onset of seizures, although the last of these factors remains controversial.[12,31,34,36] In the absence of seizures, cognitive development is normal. Furthermore, 85% of patients with seizure onset after age 4 years have normal intelligence.[12]

Psychological manifestations of SWS may include ADHD, irritability, and social problems. Inattentive and oppositional behaviors may be noted. Approximately 85% of patients with SWS who have cognitive disability exhibit emotional or behavioral problems, including aggressive behavior toward others and self-abuse.[12,31]

Headache, including migraine, is seen in 30% to 45% of individuals with SWS. The median age at onset is 8 years. Migraines may be associated with visual aura and visual field defects.[31,36]

Differential Diagnosis

The differential diagnosis of SWS includes isolated (ie, nonsyndromic) facial PWS and Wyburn-Mason syndrome. Unilateral forehead PWS has no underlying syndrome in 92% of patients. Bilateral PWS, in contrast, has a much higher likelihood of association with SWS.[34] Wyburn-Mason syndrome is a rare disorder consisting of retinal and CNS arteriovenous malformations associated with upper facial PWS. Headaches, seizures, focal neurologic deficits, retinal hemorrhage, and subarachnoid hemorrhage may occur.[35]

Evaluation

History

The earliest manifestation of SWS is the PWS present at birth. Relevant history in a child with facial PWS should include history of seizures, history of eye or vision problems, and any concerns about development. Older children should be asked about headaches, vision changes, episodes of weakness, and school progress.

Physical Examination

Examination of any child with facial PWS should include a thorough eye examination. Any difference in sizes of cornea or globe, or any iris heterochromia, may be clues to early glaucoma. Presence of PWS on eyelids should be noted. Auscultation of the orbits, fontanelles, and temples should be performed to detect bruits. Funduscopic examination might reveal the characteristic *ketchup stains* of choroidal angiomas. Tortuous vessels or colobomas should be noted.[34] Neurologic examination should search for focal deficits. Developmental evaluation is important, particularly if the child has a seizure history. Observation of an infant should specifically address the presence of a head turn or early handedness, which are potential clues to visual field cuts.

Laboratory Evaluation

Routine laboratory testing is not useful in SWS. Evaluation of seizures should include electroencephalography. The typical findings include asymmetry, with background slowing and reduced voltage in the affected hemisphere. The asymmetry becomes more prominent with the progressive cerebral atrophy.[36]

Imaging Studies

The most sensitive imaging modality to evaluate for leptomeningeal angiomatosis is gadolinium-enhanced MRI. Leptomeningeal enhancement, with or without cortical atrophy, is the radiologic hallmark of SWS. The leptomeningeal involvement is ipsilateral to the PWS. It may be seen before calcifications develop. Calcification of adjacent gyri may give the classic *tram track* appearance seen on CT and even plain-film radiographs (although the latter rarely are used). Involvement of the parietal and occipital lobes is often noted before frontal or temporal findings. Positron emission tomography and single-photon emission CT may reveal areas of altered metabolism and hypoperfusion. Chronic venous engorgement leading to reduced perfusion is thought to be the mechanism underlying progressive cerebral atrophy in SWS. Choroidal angiomas are best visualized with MRI.[11,31,34,36]

Management

Infants with facial PWS on the forehead and eyelids should be evaluated for the possibility of SWS. Evaluation should include ophthalmologic examination. If eye findings or any other typical clinical features such as seizures are present, then neuroimaging is mandatory. Routine MRI may be performed even in the absence of seizures because prophylactic anticonvulsant therapy may be useful for infants with extensive intracranial disease.[34] Seizure control is the most important aspect of management because seizure activity may further compromise cerebrovascular function and lead to worse neurologic decline. Carbamazepine and oxcarbazepine are useful 1st-line anticonvulsants for SWS. Valproic acid, topiramate, phenobarbital, phenytoin, and vigabatrin have also been suggested.[31,34,36] (For a thorough discussion of anticonvulsant therapy, see Chapter 320, Seizure Disorders.) Refractory seizures in SWS may lead to consideration of seizure surgery. Hemispherectomy has been found to be effective in reducing refractory seizures.[38] Fevers should be treated aggressively to prevent the triggering of seizures. Hydration status should be monitored, especially during gastrointestinal illness, because dehydration may create intravascular sludging and further compromise the cerebral circulation. Antipyretic agents should be given prophylactically with immunizations. Iron-deficiency anemia should be corrected. Low-dose aspirin is suggested for prevention of the strokelike episodes.[31,34,36] Avoiding fatigue, sleep deprivation, stress, and minor head trauma may help prevent headaches.[36] Ibuprofen is useful in management of common headaches; migraines may require sumatriptan.[31,36] Glaucoma may be managed medically in most patients with β-adrenergic blockers or carbonic anhydrase inhibitors. Surgical approaches are not usually required.[31,34] PWSs may be treated effectively with pulsed dye laser.[34]

WHEN TO REFER

- Ophthalmologic evaluation: any infant with forehead and eyelid PWS
- Neurologic evaluation: difficult seizure management

WHEN TO ADMIT

- Refractory seizures

VON HIPPEL-LINDAU DISEASE

Von Hippel-Lindau disease (VHL) is an autosomal-dominant multiorgan familial cancer syndrome. Prevalence is estimated at about 1 in 40,000 live births. The disease is inherited in 80% of patients, with the remainder representing new mutations. The disease is more than 90% penetrant by age 65 years.[15,17,39] The VHL gene is a tumor suppressor gene found on chromosome 3. The normal gene product is part of a protein complex responsible for ubiquitination of

Table 298-3 Classification of von Hippel-Lindau Disease

SUBTYPE	HEMANGIO-BLASTOMA†	RENAL CELL CARCINOMA	PHEOCHROMO-CYTOMA	PANCREATIC CYST OR TUMOR
1	+	+	–	+
2a	+	–	+	–
2b	+	+	+	+
2c	–	–	+	–

+, High risk; –, low risk.
†Retinal, central nervous system.
Adapted from Joerger M, Koeberle D, Neumann HP, et al. Von Hippel-Lindau disease: a rare disease important to recognize. *Onkologie.* 2005;28:159-163; Shuin T, Yamasaki I, Tamura K, et al. Von Hippel-Lindau disease: molecular pathological basis, clinical criteria, genetic testing, clinical features of tumors and treatment. *Jpn J Clin Oncol.* 2006;36:337-343.

hypoxia-inducible factors, leading to their degradation. With functional loss of the VHL protein, these hypoxia-inducible factors trigger transcription of vascular proliferation mediators, including vascular endothelial growth factor, platelet-derived growth factor, transforming growth factor alpha, and erythropoietin. These growth factors then lead to unregulated endothelial and vascular proliferation to produce vascular neoplasms. Erythropoietin production may lead to development of polycythemia.[39] The mechanism of nonvascular tumorigenesis remains uncertain. Almost all patients with VHL have germ-line mutations in the VHL gene, as well as secondary somatic mutations (Knudson's 2-hit hypothesis).[17,39-41] VHL is subdivided into 2 major categories that are based on the type of mutation. Type 1 disease mutations are premature termination mutations or deletions, whereas type 2 disease is characterized by missense mutations.[39] Phenotypically, type 1 disease is not associated with significant risk for pheochromocytoma, whereas pheochromocytoma is a predominant tumor in type 2 disease. Further subdivision is listed in Table 298-3.[17,39] The diagnosis of VHL is established in a patient who has 1 characteristic tumor and positive family history, or hemangioblastoma plus 1 other tumor when the family history is negative.[40] The most common tumors in VHL are cerebellar, spinal, and retinal hemangioblastomas. The other associated tumors include renal cysts, RCC, pheochromocytoma, pancreatic cysts or neuroendocrine tumors, endolymphatic sac tumors of the inner ear, and cystadenomas of the epididymis or broad ligament.[15,39,40,42] The major causes of death are RCC and complications from CNS hemangioblastomas.[15,39]

CNS hemangioblastomas are the most common tumors in VHL (21% to 72%). They occur most commonly in the cerebellum (63%), followed by the spinal cord (32%) and brainstem (5%).[15,43] The mean age at presentation is 33 years, but tumors may develop in childhood through the 4th decade of life. These slow-growing benign tumors produce symptoms largely by mass effect or obstructive hydrocephaly. Cerebellar tumors may present with headache, nausea, vomiting, vertigo, slurred speech, and broad-based gait. Clinical signs may include papilledema, nystagmus, ataxia, and dysmetria.[15,43] Spinal hemangioblastomas may produce back pain, numbness, pain or weakness in arms or legs, posterior column proprioceptive defects, or bowel and bladder dysfunction.[15,39,40] CNS hemangioblastomas tend to exhibit alternating periods of growth and stability so that low-level chronic symptoms may worsen acutely during a critical growth phase.[43]

Retinal hemangioblastomas (capillary hemangiomas) develop in more than one half of patients with VHL. Although most of these patients have solitary tumors, approximately one third will have multiple lesions, and one half will have bilateral retinal tumors. Most of these lesions develop in the 2nd to 3rd decade of life, with mean age at diagnosis of 25 years. However, retinal tumors may develop at any time from infancy to the 9th decade.[15,42] Patients may experience painless loss of visual acuity or visual field defects, although they may remain asymptomatic.[8,15] Exudation or hemorrhage from the hemangiomas may lead to macular edema or retinal detachment. Secondary changes in the anterior chamber may lead to glaucoma or cataract.[15,39,42]

Renal cysts are seen in approximately one half of patients with VHL. Often multiple and bilateral, they may remain asymptomatic. Stable lesions may not require intervention. RCC develops in 75% of patients with VHL by age 60.[15,39] RCC is seen in patients with types 1 or 2b disease. It usually develops after 20 years of age, though often earlier than with sporadic renal carcinoma. Lesions are frequently multiple and bilateral. The tumors may be associated with cysts and may have a better 10-year survival than sporadic RCC. However, metastatic RCC is a leading cause of death in VHL. Symptoms may include hematuria, flank pain, or flank mass. By the time symptoms develop, metastases are present in 30% to 50% of patients.[15,39,40]

Pheochromocytoma occurs in type 2 disease with a frequency of 10% to 24%, which may be the only manifestation of VHL (type 2c). VHL accounts for approximately 20% of all pheochromocytomas. Mean age at presentation is 27 years, but tumors may be present even before age 10 years.[40,44] Pheochromocytoma in VHL differs from sporadic tumors by occurring at an earlier age and by developing multiple, bilateral, and extraadrenal tumors in VHL. Only 5% of VHL pheochromocytomas are malignant.[15,39,40] Clinical features may include hypertension (paroxysmal or sustained), palpitations, sweating, flushing, headache, tachycardia, pallor, and nausea.[15,39] Pancreatic cysts or tumors occur in approximately 90% of patients with VHL but rarely cause disease. Benign adenomas occur in approximately 12% of patients with VHL.[41] Approximately 5% to 10% of patients with VHL will develop neuroendocrine islet cell tumors. The latter may be multifocal and may metastasize in 10% to 20%. The average age at diagnosis of pancreatic lesions is 41 years, although islet cell tumors may be seen as early as 10 years of age.[15,41,44] Most pancreatic lesions are asymptomatic and are found during routine imaging surveillance.

Approximately 10% of patients with VHL will develop endolymphatic sac tumors. These cystadenomas arising from the inner ear labyrinth ectoderm may cause deafness, tinnitus, or vertigo. Facial nerve and vocal paralysis may result from progressive tumor growth.[14,15]

Finally, cystadenomas may develop in the epididymis in men and the uterine broad ligament in women. These are usually asymptomatic.[39,42]

Differential Diagnosis

CNS hemangioblastomas create symptoms by mass effect, as with many other tumors, cysts, and obstructive hydrocephalus. Evaluation of mass effect with neurologic symptoms should reveal the characteristic radiologic findings of hemangioblastomas. The differential diagnosis of retinal capillary hemangiomas is provided in Table 298-4. The differential diagnosis of renal cysts includes the diagnosis of polycystic kidney disease. Pheochromocytoma may occur sporadically or may occur in the setting of VHL, multiple endocrine neoplasia 2a or 2b with associated medullary thyroid carcinoma, or neurofibromatosis, or with succinate dehydrogenase subunit mutations.[41,44]

Evaluation

History

The most important historical information is family history because 80% of cases are familial. Other relevant history might include changes in vision; development of neurologic symptoms such as clumsiness, broad-based gait, hearing loss, slurring of speech, pain, numbness or weakness in limbs, or loss of bowel or bladder control after complete toilet training; hematuria or flank pain; heart palpitations, flushing, or sweating spells; or episodic nausea and vomiting.

Physical Examination

Physical examination should include regular blood pressure evaluation, thorough eye examination, and thorough neurologic examination with particular attention to cerebellar and spinal functions. Observation of gait, test of balance, deep tendon reflexes, and test for sensation should be included in the examination.

Laboratory Evaluation

Laboratory testing in VHL should begin with molecular testing for the specific mutation because the phenotypic profile and tumor risk are directly related to the types of mutation.[39,40] Subsequent laboratory evaluation for patients with type 2 disease should consist of annual screening for plasma or urine catecholamines and metanephrines beginning at age 10 years.[39]

Imaging Studies

MRI with gadolinium contrast is the modality of choice for most of the features of VHL. Hemangioblastomas of the cerebellum are usually subpial in location. They may appear as a solid enhancing mass with or without surrounding fluid space or as a more complex tissue or fluid mass.[11,30] Spinal hemangioblastomas are solid enhancing intramedullary masses frequently associated with a surrounding fluid filled syrinx that enlarges and displaces the cord.[30] Renal cysts may be found on MRI, ultrasound, or CT.[15,40]

Management

The most important aspect of management in VHL is regular screening for the various tumors. First-degree relatives should also be screened for tumors. Once a

Table 298-4 Differential Diagnosis of Retinal Capillary Hemangioma in von Hippel-Lindau Disease

CONDITION	FEATURE	PRESENCE OF RETINAL OR SUBRETINAL EXUDATES
Von Hippel-Lindau disease	Orange-red circumscribed tumors Pair of prominent vessels Stellate macular exudates	Yes
Coat disease	Diffuse retinal vascular anomaly	Yes
Wyburn-Mason syndrome	Dilation and tortuosity of retinal arteries and veins, but no intervening hemangioma.	No
Retinal cavernous hemangioma	Cluster of small dilated vessels around central vein Lacks prominent feeder vessels	No
Vasoproliferative tumor of the retina	Pink to yellow retinal tumor Lacks dilated feeder vessels Lacks stellate macular exudates	Yes (nonstellate)

From Magee MA, Kroll AJ, Lou PL, et al. Retinal capillary hemangiomas and von Hippel-Lindau disease. *Semin Ophthalmol.* 2006;21:143-150. Reprinted by permission of Taylor & Francis.

diagnosis is established, regular imaging and ophthalmologic examinations are indicated. Eye examinations including dilated funduscopy should begin by age 6 years and should be repeated annually. Annual cranial and spinal MRI should begin by age 10 to 11 years. Abdominal imaging for kidneys and possible pheochromocytoma should begin by age 15 to 18 years and may consist of ultrasound, CT, or MRI, with MRI being the best modality for finding all the possible intraabdominal tumors (renal, pheochromocytomic, and pancreatic). Hearing loss or tinnitus should be evaluated by MRI with thin sections through the ear structures, as well as formal audiologic examination.[39,40]

Surgical excision is generally considered the best treatment for most symptomatic VHL tumors. CNS hemangioblastomas that remain stable and asymptomatic may be followed by serial imaging. Proper management for asymptomatic but radiologically progressive lesions is a matter of debate. Spinal hemangioblastomas and large or symptomatic intracranial tumors are generally resected.[43] Small retinal lesions are often treated with laser photocoagulation; larger lesions may require cryotherapy, brachytherapy, or vitreoretinal surgery.[8,42] Screening for eye lesions is of critical importance because the visual prognosis is better when ocular lesions are detected before development of symptoms.[42] Small renal tumors (<3 cm) are often followed by serial imaging. Larger lesions may be addressed by partial nephrectomy. Radical nephrectomy is rarely indicated.[39,40] Symptomatic pheochromocytomas require excision.[15]

WHEN TO REFER

- Ophthalmologic examination—by age 6 years
- Neurologic examination or neurosurgery—on detection of CNS tumors
- General surgery—on detection of intraabdominal tumors

WHEN TO ADMIT

- Hypertension crisis with pheochromocytoma
- Sudden neurologic deterioration

ATAXIA-TELANGIECTASIA

Ataxia-telangiectasia (A-T), or Louis-Bar syndrome, is an autosomal-recessive progressive neurodegenerative disorder with a frequency of 1 in 40,000 in the United States to 1 in 300,000 in the United Kingdom. Consanguinity is a common finding. The characteristic features are progressive decline in cerebellar function, oculocutaneous telangiectasia, immunodeficiency, susceptibility to cancer, and sensitivity to ionizing radiation.[45-47] A-T is caused by mutations in the *ATM* (ataxia-telangiectasia, mutated) gene. The ATM protein is a nuclear serine-threonine protein kinase that acts as a regulator of many cellular control pathways. Its primary function appears to be mobilization of cellular responses to breaks in double-stranded DNA. Once a DNA break occurs, *ATM* activates numerous proteins involved in DNA repair, apoptosis, and control of cell cycling. Loss of *ATM* function leads to accumulation of defective DNA and inability to repair or eliminate genetically defective cells.[45,47,48] Defective DNA repair explains the sensitivity to ionizing radiation, whereas inability to remove damaged cells has been postulated as a cause of many of the diverse abnormalities in A-T.[47,48] Similarly, cancer has been linked to genomic instability, helping explain the cancer risks in A-T.[48]

Infants with A-T are normal; they begin to walk at approximately age 12 months. However, by age 2 to 3 years, they develop unsteady gait and staggering. By age 10 years, most children require wheelchairs for mobility because they have slow reflexes and tend to fall. Ocular apraxia (difficulty with voluntary eye movement), which may be confused with absence seizures in infants, develops in early childhood. Similarly, dysarthric speech is often present early in childhood but can be difficult to assess.[45,46]

Telangiectasias (tortuous dilated capillaries) develop several years after the onset of neurologic symptoms. They are found on the bulbar conjunctiva, nasal bridge, ears, neck, knuckles, and both antecubital and popliteal fossae.[45]

Immunodeficiency varies but may be severe in approximately one third of patients with A-T. Many patients have reduced numbers of T lymphocytes with poor mitogen response. Low serum levels of immunoglobulin (Ig) E (80% of patients), IgG_2 (80%), and IgA (60%) are noted despite normal to high numbers of B cells. In addition, IgM levels vary widely, at times rising enough to create a hyperviscous state. Some patients exhibit poor immune response to pneumococcal polysaccharides. Patients with severe immunodeficiency may develop recurrent sinopulmonary infections. However, opportunistic organisms are not a problem in patients with A-T.[45,46] Patients with A-T are at higher risk (one third) for developing cancer. In children, acute lymphoblastic leukemia predominates, followed by other lymphoid tumors such as B-cell non-Hodgkin lymphoma, T-cell lymphoma, and Hodgkin disease. Older children sometimes develop T-prolymphocytic leukemia. Adults tend toward nonlymphoid cancers such as breast, stomach, ovarian, liver, and uterus, melanoma, and basal cell skin cancer. Women who are *ATM* mutation carriers have a 5-fold increase in risk of breast cancer compared with the noncarrier population.[46,47] Approximately 15% of patients with A-T die of lymphoid malignancies during childhood.[47]

Because of the inability to repair defective DNA, patients with A-T are also susceptible to injury by ionizing radiation and radiomimetic chemotherapeutic drugs. This susceptibility complicates therapy for the various malignancies and poses a life-threatening risk to patients with A-T exposed to these agents.[46,47]

Differential Diagnosis

The differential diagnosis of A-T is provided in Table 298-5.

Table 298-5 Differential Diagnosis of Ataxia-Telangiectasia

CONDITION	NEUROLOGIC FEATURES	PRESENCE OF TELANGIECTASIA	INCREASED ALPHA-FETOPROTEIN	CANCER RISK	IMMUNE DEFICIENCY	SENSITIVITY TO RADIATION
Ataxia-telangiectasia	Early ataxia, oculomotor apraxia, progressive neurologic decline	Yes	Yes	Yes	Yes	Yes
Ataxia-telangiectasia–like disorder (*hMRE11* mutation)	Ataxia early	No	No	No	No	Yes
Nijmegen breakage syndrome	Microcephaly, intellectual disability	No	No	Yes	Yes	Yes
Ataxia oculomotor apraxia I	Early ataxia, progressive neurologic decline	No	No	No	No	No
Ataxia oculomotor apraxia II	Late-onset ataxia	No	Yes	No	No	No

Adapted from Chun HH, Gatti RA. Ataxia-telangiectasia, an evolving phenotype. *DNA Repair (Amst).* 2004;3:1187-1196; Perlman S, Becker-Catania S, Gatti RA. Ataxia-telangiectasia: diagnosis and treatment. *Semin Pediatr Neurol.* 2003;10:173-182; Taylor AM, Byrd PJ. Molecular pathology of ataxia telangiectasia. *J Clin Pathol.* 2005;58:1009-1015.

Evaluation

The earliest manifestation of A-T is the ataxia, beginning as broad-based gait or staggering by age 2 to 3 years. Any other history should focus on additional neurologic symptoms and developmental milestones. Additional history should include the presence of similar neurologic problems or consanguinity in the family.

Examination should focus on neurologic findings including cerebellar function. Although difficult to assess in young children, voluntary visual tracking of objects will often reveal the early development of oculomotor apraxia. In older children, telangiectasia may be noted on the bulbar conjunctiva and on the skin of the neck, face, ears, and extremity flexures. The examination should include thorough lymph node examination and abdominal evaluation for hepatosplenomegaly.

Laboratory testing in suspected A-T should include serum alpha-fetoprotein, which is increased in more than 95% of patients with A-T. Serum alpha-fetoprotein increase is only useful beyond age 2 years because some children have persistent mild increases beyond the neonatal period.[46] Karyotyping is rarely normal in A-T, often showing translocations between chromosomes 7 and 14. Quantitative immunoglobulins may show low levels of IgE, IgA, and IgG2. IgM is normal or high. Quantitative T- and B-cell numbers will reveal low levels of T cells, but normal to slightly high levels of B cells. The only radiosensitivity test currently available is the colony survival assay, which uses the patients' transformed lymphocytes. It requires approximately 3 months to complete. Gene testing is not useful unless the family mutation is known because *ATM* is a huge gene with 66 exons and over 400 known mutations (none with a frequency more than 3%). Measurements of the ATM protein from the transformed lymphocyte cell line is also possible (by immunoblotting).[45-47]

Imaging in A-T is limited. Cranial MRI will reveal gradual cerebellar atrophy, almost always noted by age 10 years. Imaging with radiation should be considered carefully because of these patients' extreme radiosensitivity. Adult female patients and carriers should be screened for breast cancer with regular examinations and ultrasound, but not mammograms.[45,46]

Management

The most important aspects of therapy in this degenerative condition are family and patient counseling and support, followed by rehabilitation and assistance with the progressive ataxia. Speech, physical, and occupational therapy should be obtained early to help the child and family with the problems that arise over time. Speech therapy may help with the communication and swallowing difficulties, whereas mobility, safety, and daily living skills can be supported by physical and occupational therapy. Careful monitoring is crucial for the recurrent infection and cancer risks. Recurrent sinopulmonary infections should be treated aggressively, and aspiration should be anticipated. Emotional support is crucial, with depression, anger, and isolation occurring frequently. Life expectancy varies, but survival into the 6th decade is likely. The leading causes of death are malignancy, infection, and pulmonary failure (the latter from combined recurrent infection and recurrent aspiration).[46]

WHEN TO REFER

- Neurologic examination—on development of ataxia
- Speech therapy—on development of speech or swallowing difficulty
- Physical and occupational therapy—before ataxia becomes severe

WHEN TO ADMIT

- Severe pulmonary infection, especially if respiratory distress is present
- Severe aspiration event

TOOLS FOR PRACTICE

Engaging Patient and Family

- *Let's Face It* (Web page), University of Michigan (www.faceit.org/).

RELATED WEB SITES

- British Columbia Neurofibromatosis Foundation (www.bcnf.bc.ca).
- Children's Tumor Foundation (www.ctf.org/).
- Let's Face It (www.faceit.org).
- National NF Foundation (support and information). (www.nf.org).
- National Institute of Neurological Disorders and Stroke (www.ninds.nih.gov/).
- National Organization of Vascular Anomalies (www.novanews.org).
- Neurofibromatosis, Inc. (NF, Inc.) (www.nfinc.org).
- Sturge-Weber Foundation (www.sturge-weber.com).
- Tuberous Sclerosis Alliance (www.tsalliance.org).
- Tuberous Sclerosis Alliance, UK (www.tuberous-sclerosis.org).
- Tuberous Sclerosis International (www.stsn.nl/tsi/tsi.htm).
- Vascular Birthmarks Foundation (www.birthmark.org).
- VHL Family Alliance (von Hippel-Lindau) (www.vhl.org).

SUGGESTED RESOURCES

Baselga E. Sturge-Weber syndrome. *Semin Cutan Med Surg.* 2004;23:87-98.

Comi AM. Advances in Sturge-Weber syndrome. *Curr Opin Neurol.* 2006;19:124-128.

Crino PB, Nathanson KL, Henske EP. The tuberous sclerosis complex. *N Engl J Med.* 2006;355:1345-1356.

Joerger M, Koeberle D, Neumann HP, et al. Von Hippel-Lindau disease: a rare disease important to recognize. *Onkologie.* 2005;28:159-163.

Levine TM, Materek A, Abel J, et al. Cognitive profile of neurofibromatosis type 1. *Semin Pediatr Neurol.* 2006;13:8-20.

Neff BA, Welling DB. Current concepts in the evaluation and treatment of neurofibromatosis type II. *Otolaryngol Clin North Am.* 2005;38:671-684.

Perlman S, Becker-Catania S, Gatti RA. Ataxia-telangiectasia: diagnosis and treatment. *Semin Pediatr Neurol.* 2003;10:173-182.

Prather P, de Vries PJ. Behavoral and cognitive aspects of tuberous sclerosis complex. *J Child Neurol.* 2004;19:666-674.

Roach ES, Sparagana SP. Diagnosis of tuberous sclerosis complex. *J Child Neurol.* 2004;19:643-649.

Rosser T, Panigrahy A, McClintock W. The diverse clinical manifestations of tuberous sclerosis complex: a review. *Semin Pediatr Neurol.* 2006;13:27-36.

Shuin T, Yamasaki I, Tamura K, et al. Von Hippel-Lindau disease: molecular pathological basis, clinical criteria, genetic testing, clinical features of tumors and treatment. *Jpn J Clin Oncol.* 2006;36:337-343.

Thomas-Sohl KA, Vaslow DF, Maria BL. Sturge-Weber syndrome: a review. *Pediatr Neurol.* 2004;30: 303-310.

Tonsgard JH. Clinical manifestations and management of neurofibromatosis type 1. *Semin Pediatr Neurol.* 2006;13:2-7.

Yohay K. Neurofibromatosis types 1 and 2. *Neurologist.* 2006;12:86-93.

REFERENCES

1. Yohay K. Neurofibromatosis types 1 and 2. *Neurologist.* 2006;12:86-93.
2. Jabbour SA, Davidovici BB, Wolf R. Rare syndromes. *Clin Dermatol.* 2006;24:299-316.
3. Rose VM. Neurocutaneous syndromes. *Missouri Med.* 2004;101:112-116.
4. Tonsgard JH. Clinical manifestations and management of neurofibromatosis type 1. *Semin Pediatr Neurol.* 2006; 13:2-7.
5. Ward BA, Gutmann DH. Neurofibromatosis 1: from lab bench to clinic. *Pediatr Neurol.* 2005;32:221-228.
6. Crawford AH, Schorry EK. Neurofibromatosis update. *J Pediatr Orthop.* 2006;26:413-423.
7. Levine TM, Materek A, Abel J, et al. Cognitive profile of neurofibromatosis type 1. *Semin Pediatr Neurol.* 2006;13: 8-20.
8. Kreusel KM. Ophthalmological manifestations in VHL and NF 1: pathological and diagnostic implications. *Fam Cancer.* 2005;4:43-47.
9. Acosta MT, Gioia GA, Silva AJ. Neurofibromatosis type 1: new insights into neurocognitive issues. *Curr Neurol Neurosci Rep.* 2006;6:136-143.
10. Theos A, Korf BR. Pathophysiology of neurofibromatosis type 1. *Ann Intern Med.* 2006;144:842-849.
11. Lin DD, Barker PB. Neuroimaging of phakomatoses. *Semin Pediatr Neurol.* 2006;13:48-62.
12. Zaroff CM, Isaacs K. Neurocutaneous syndromes: behavioral features. *Epilepsy Behav.* 2005;7:133-142.
13. Neff BA, Welling DB. Current concepts in the evaluation and treatment of neurofibromatosis type II. *Otolaryngol Clin North Am.* 2005;38:671-684.
14. Korf BR. The phakomatoses. *Clin Dermatol.* 2005;23: 78-84.
15. Dahan D, Fenichel GM, El-Said R. Neurocutaneous syndromes. *Adolesc Med.* 2002;13:495-509.
16. Rosser T, Panigrahy A, McClintock W. The diverse clinical manifestations of tuberous sclerosis complex: a review. *Semin Pediatr Neurol.* 2006;13:27-36.
17. Jentarra G, Snyder SL, Narayanan V. Genetic aspects of neurocutaneous disorders. *Semin Pediatr Neurol.* 2006; 13:43-47.
18. Jozwiak J. Hamartin and tuberin: working together for tumour suppression. *Int J Cancer.* 2006;118:1-5.
19. McCall T, Chin SS, Salzman KL, et al. Tuberous sclerosis: a syndrome of incomplete tumor suppression. *Neurosurg Focus.* 2006;20:E3.
20. Mak BC, Yeung RS. The tuberous sclerosis complex genes in tumor development. *Cancer Invest.* 2004;22: 588-603.

21. Roach ES, Gomez MR, Northrup H. Tuberous sclerosis complex consensus conference: revised clinical diagnostic criteria. *J Child Neurol.* 1998;13:624-628.
22. Roach ES, Sparagana SP. Diagnosis of tuberous sclerosis complex. *J Child Neurol.* 2004;19:643-649.
23. Crino PB, Nathanson KL, Henske EP. The tuberous sclerosis complex. *N Engl J Med.* 2006;355:1345-1356.
24. Thiele EA. Managing epilepsy in tuberous sclerosis complex. *J Child Neurol.* 2004;19:680-686.
25. Asato MR, Hardan AY. Neuropsychiatric problems in tuberous sclerosis complex. *J Child Neurol.* 2004;19:241-249.
26. Wiznitzer M. Autism and tuberous sclerosis. *J Child Neurol.* 2004;19:675-679.
27. Prather P, de Vries PJ. Behavoral and cognitive aspects of tuberous sclerosis complex. *J Child Neurol.* 2004;19:666-674.
28. Franz DN. Non-neurologic manifestations of tuberous sclerosis complex. *J Child Neurol.* 2004;19:690-698.
29. Henske EP. The genetic basis of kidney cancer: why is tuberous sclerosis complex often overlooked? *Curr Mol Med.* 2004;4:825-831.
30. Smirniotopoulos JG. Neuroimaging of phakomatoses: Sturge-Weber syndrome, tuberous sclerosis, von Hippel-Lindau syndrome. *Neuroimaging Clin N Am.* 2004;14:171-183.
31. Thomas-Sohl KA, Vaslow DF, Maria BL. Sturge-Weber syndrome: a review. *Pediatr Neurol.* 2004;30:303-310.
32. Cohen MM Jr. Vascular update: morphogenesis, tumors, malformations, and molecular dimension. *Am J Med Genet A.* 2006;140:2013-2038.
33. Comi AM. Pathophysiology of Sturge-Weber syndrome. *J Child Neurol.* 2003;18:509-516.
34. Baselga E. Sturge-Weber syndrome. *Semin Cutan Med Surg.* 2004;23:87-98.
35. Elluru RG, Azizkhan RG. Cervicofacial vascular anomalies II. Vascular malformations. *Semin Pediatr Neurol.* 2006;15:133-139.
36. Comi AM. Advances in Sturge-Weber syndrome. *Curr Opin Neurol.* 2006;19:124-128.
37. Cross JH. Neurocutaneous syndromes and epilepsy: issues in diagnosis and management. *Epilepsia.* 2005;46(suppl 10):17-23.
38. Kossoff EH, Buck C, Freeman JM. Outcomes of 32 hemispherectomies for Sturge-Weber syndrome worldwide. *Neurology.* 2002;59:1735-1738.
39. Joerger M, Koeberle D, Neumann HP, et al. Von Hippel-Lindau disease: a rare disease important to recognize. *Onkologie.* 2005;28:159-163.
40. Shuin T, Yamasaki I, Tamura K, et al. Von Hippel-Lindau disease: molecular pathological basis, clinical criteria, genetic testing, clinical features of tumors and treatment. *Jpn J Clin Oncol.* 2006;36:337-343.
41. Woodward ER, Maher ER. Von Hippel-Lindau disease and endocrine tumour susceptibility. *Endocr Relat Cancer.* 2006;13:415-425.
42. Magee MA, Kroll AJ, Lou PL, et al. Retinal capillary hemangiomas and von Hippel-Lindau disease. *Semin Ophthalmol.* 2006;21:143-150.
43. Glasker S. Central nervous system manifestations in VHL: genetics, pathology and clinical phenotypic features. *Fam Cancer.* 2005;4:37-42.
44. de Krijger RR. Endocrine tumor syndromes in infancy and childhood. *Endocr Pathol.* 2004;15:223-226.
45. Chun HH, Gatti RA. Ataxia-telangiectasia, an evolving phenotype. *DNA Repair (Amst).* 2004;3:1187-1196.
46. Perlman S, Becker-Catania S, Gatti RA. Ataxia-telangiectasia: diagnosis and treatment. *Semin Pediatr Neurol.* 2003;10:173-182.
47. Taylor AM, Byrd PJ. Molecular pathology of ataxia telangiectasia. *J Clin Pathol.* 2005;58:1009-1015.
48. McKinnon PJ. *ATM* and ataxia telangiectasia. *EMBO Rep.* 2004;5:772-776.

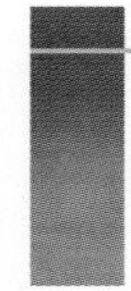

Chapter 299

OBESITY AND METABOLIC SYNDROME

Heather A. Van Mater, MD; Sheila Gahagan, MD, MPH

INTRODUCTION

Childhood obesity has reached epidemic proportions in the United States and worldwide. The US trend toward an increasing prevalence of obesity continues, with one third of all adults and one sixth of all children aged 6 to 19 years now classified as obese.[1,2] The medical complications associated with obesity, including non–insulin-dependent diabetes mellitus, hypertension, and dyslipidemia, are rising at a similar pace, with estimates that the medical costs from obesity will overtake those of cigarette smoking.[3,4] The cause of this epidemic is multifactorial, including biological, psychological, environmental, and social factors. Despite tremendous research efforts, inadequate understanding of risk factors and protective factors still exists. Furthermore, strategies to prevent and treat childhood obesity need to be developed and evaluated. Child health professionals will play a crucial role in preventing further escalation of this epidemic and in treating people who are already affected.

DEFINITIONS

The terms *overweight* and *obese* commonly are used to describe adiposity in the adult population. The currently accepted definitions of overweight and obesity in children and adults are based on body mass index (BMI). BMI is weight in kilograms divided by height in meters squared. This calculation has been validated as an approximation of a person's body fat and correlates well with medical complications associated with obesity[5]; it is also easily calculated from standard measurements obtained during health care visits. The Centers for Disease Control and Prevention provides age- and sex-specific growth curves for BMI. Electronic medical records allow for routine calculation and plotting of BMI when height and weight data are entered into the record.[6]

In adults, a BMI of 25 or greater is considered overweight, whereas a BMI of 30 or greater is obese.[7] In children, body fat changes throughout development. Therefore BMI percentile must be used. Normal BMI trajectories include a decrease during the preschool years followed by an increase beginning at 5 to 6 years and continuing through adolescence, stabilizing in early adulthood. For children and adolescents, the terms *at risk for overweight* and *overweight* have been used in the United States instead of overweight and obese, with the at-risk group having a BMI between the 85th and the 95th percentiles for age and sex and the overweight group having a BMI at or above the 95th percentile.[8] In this chapter, the terms *overweight* and *obese* will be used interchangeably for children. Furthermore, the focus is not on children in the *at risk for overweight* group.

EPIDEMIOLOGY

The prevalence of obesity has dramatically increased worldwide in developed and underdeveloped countries. Only the very poorest geographic areas where food scarcity is widespread such as Haiti and sub-Saharan Africa have yet to be affected.[9]

Currently, 30% of US adults are obese, and an additional 35% are overweight.[10] A 3-fold increase in childhood obesity has occurred over the last 2 decades among children aged 12 to 19 years and a doubling of obesity in children between 6 and 11 years[11] (Figure 299-1). Estimates indicate that 16% of children and adolescents aged 6 to 19 years and more than 10% of children younger than 5 years have a BMI greater than the 95th percentile. Although these increases are seen across all age groups, ethnicities, and socioeconomic classes, some minority groups have shown more rapid increases.[12,13]

Black and Hispanic youth showed increases in obesity prevalence more than double that of non-Hispanic white youth between 1986 and 1998.[14] Children living in southern states showed greater increases in obesity prevalence than those in northern and western states. Although adult studies show an inverse relationship between socioeconomic status (SES) and obesity, the relationship between SES and obesity in children is more complicated.[15] Poverty appears to be a risk factor for obesity in non-Hispanic white adolescents. However, no SES-obesity relationship has been found in Hispanic children. Conversely, higher SES is associated with higher rates of overweight and obesity in blacks.[14] Further research is needed to understand the role played by family income in determining nutrition and physical activity patterns. The risk for obesity imparted by gender differs by ethnicity. Hispanic boys are more likely to be overweight than Hispanic girls, whereas black girls are more likely to be overweight than black boys.[16]

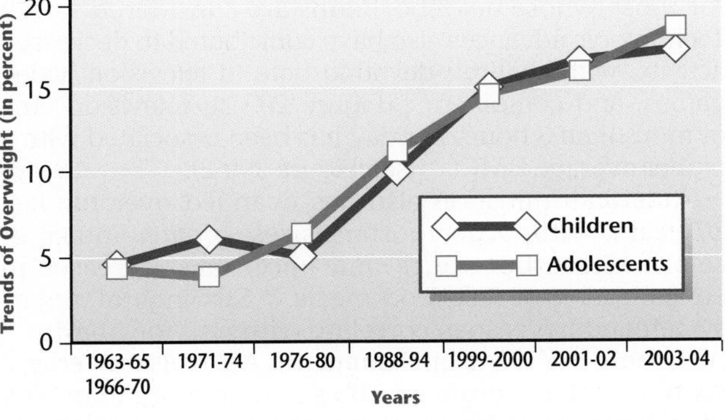

Figure 299-1 Prevalence of overweight status among children ages 6 to 11 years and adolescents ages 12 to 19 years for selected years 1963-1965 through 1999-2002. Based on data from the National Health and Nutrition Examination Surveys.

The age at which a child becomes obese is related to how likely the child is to be obese in adulthood. Of children who are obese from 6 to 11 years, 50% of girls and 30% of boys will be obese as adults compared with 18% of age-matched peers. Obesity during adolescence poses greater risk; over 60% will maintain obesity into adulthood. Obese adults who became obese during childhood are more likely to have severe obesity (BMI over 40) than those who become obese during adulthood.[17-19]

Childhood obesity is associated with smaller family size, single-parent families, parental neglect, and overparenting. However, parental obesity imparts greater risk than any other identified risk factor for developing obesity before young adulthood.[20,21] For children younger than 3 years, parental weight is a better predictor of adult obesity than the child's actual weight. This effect lessens as children age, with the child's weight becoming an equal predictor at school age and a more important predictor as they reach adolescence.[22] Both overweight and normal-weight children who have one obese parent are at twice the risk of adult obesity compared with children who do not have an overweight parent. Of overweight 10- to 14-year-olds with at least one obese parent, 80% remain obese as adults.[22] Although genetic influences may be important, the rapid rise in obesity over the last 20 years demonstrates that lifestyle and societal influences clearly play a significant role.[23] The fact that children and parents share neighborhood and family environmental conditions further supports the importance of causal environmental factors. Understanding genetic contributions to childhood obesity will allow more targeted prevention and intervention efforts.

PATHOPHYSIOLOGICAL FEATURES

Weight gain is caused by a positive energy imbalance resulting from increased caloric intake, decreased energy expenditure, or a combination of the two. Even small surpluses in energy balance over time can have important effects. Estimates suggest that a sustained positive balance of 100 calories per day leads to a weight gain of 10 pounds per year.[24] A common myth is that a slow metabolism causes obesity. However, overweight and normal-weight children do not differ by metabolic rate. Furthermore, overweight adolescents have higher total daily energy expenditures and resting energy expenditures than adolescents who are not overweight.[25] Therefore overweight children need to eat more to maintain their higher body weight.

Infancy, the time of adiposity rebound (typically 5 to 6 years), and adolescence are considered sensitive periods, times during which children are at increased risk of becoming overweight. High prepregnancy maternal BMI is associated with rapid growth in the child. Higher birth weight also correlates with later obesity.[26,27] Infant BMI is high at birth and increases slightly for the 1st months of infancy and then declines for 5 to 6 years before gradually increasing toward adult levels. The nadir between 5 and 6 years has been called adiposity rebound. Early adiposity rebound is associated with increased risk for childhood obesity.[28] However, the mechanism is unclear. Finally, adolescence is a time of significant growth, with notable changes in fat distribution and body composition. In girls, body fat increases by approximately 40%, whereas body fat in boys decreases over this same period by approximately 40%.[29,30] These normal developmental changes in adiposity may relate to increased risk for adult obesity in overweight female adolescents. Although almost 70% of overweight male adolescents develop normal adult BMI, only 20% of overweight girls normalize their weight.[31]

Many food preferences are established by 2 to 3 years of age, and family environment plays a role in the development of food choices. These food preferences and feeding behaviors are believed to result from food availability, role modeling by caregivers, and positive and negative reinforcement of the child's choices. This fact may explain why children of overweight parents are more likely to prefer high-fat foods compared with children of normal-weight parents.[32] Children with higher BMI consume less at breakfast and more at dinner than their normal-weight peers. Skipping breakfast is also associated with poorer food choices and increased risk for obesity. Families who eat meals together consume less fried food and carbonated beverages and more fruits and vegetables.[33-35] Healthy eating in families may come as a package: eating 3 meals a day, preferably together, and choosing nutritional foods.

Eating behaviors and appetite regulation—the response to hunger and satiety—are, at least, partially conditioned. Overeating can develop in response to environments that interfere with normal regulatory mechanisms, as is seen with extremes of parental behavior, including neglect and overinvolvement.[36,37] Overprotective parents have been shown to use food to comfort their children. Parents who prompt their children to finish what is on their plate may actually impair children's ability to self-regulate appetite and satiety. Overweight children have been found to eat faster and slow their eating less at the end of meals, suggesting a decreased sensation of satiety.[38] These feeding habits, which may be learned from caregivers early in life, can have a lasting effect on a child's eating habits and preferences.

Food insecurity may also place individuals at higher risk for obesity. Malnutrition during gestation and early infancy is associated with both stunting and obesity.[39] Possible mechanisms include excess deposition of fat in subsequent times of nourishment or perhaps preference for high-fat foods and overeating when food is plentiful.[40-46] Another hypothesis is that individuals develop increased sensitivity to hunger- and satiety-related hormones and neurotransmitters, resulting in fat deposition in response to early life stress. Further research is needed to determine whether development of signaling pathways, entrainment of adipocytes, or other factors during the prenatal period and early infancy might explain long-term regulation of adiposity.

Leptin, a hormone that acts on the hypothalamus to regulate hunger and satiety, is secreted by adipocytes.[47-49] Serum leptin levels correlate with adiposity in both children and adults.[50] Whether increased adiposity results in decreased leptin production or whether primary leptin deficiency is followed by weight gain is unclear. Leptin resistance or deficiency results in increased food intake in animal models. The role of hormones and neurotransmitters in human energy regulation remains poorly understood.

BOX 299-1 Activity and Nutrition Changes Over the Last Two Decades

ACTIVITY

Increased screen time (television, video game, computer)
Decreased physical education in schools
Decreased walking to school
Decreased outdoor play time

NUTRITION

Increase in sugar-sweetened beverages (including juice)
Increase in fast-food consumption
Increase in fat in school lunches
Increase in portion size
Decrease in family meals

ETIOLOGY

Environmental changes over the last few decades, including urbanization, technologic advances, and easy access to calorie-dense foods, may be related to population-level increases in obesity. Urbanization and urban sprawl have contributed to more sedentary lifestyles because of increased reliance on motorized transportation. Fewer children walk to school today than they did in the past[51-55] (Box 299-1). Furthermore, many families perceive their neighborhoods as unsafe and therefore limit their children's outdoor playtime. Outdoor playtime has decreased for US children, even for those whose neighborhoods are considered safe.[51] Technologic advances also have contributed to decreased activity, with children devoting time to television, video games, and computers[56] (Figure 299-2). Television time of more than 3 hours per day has been associated with a higher average BMI[52,53] (see Figure 299-2).

American nutrition also has changed over the last 20 years, with larger portion sizes, greater intake of calorie-dense beverages and juice, and increases in consumption of fast-food meals.[54] Servings of sugar-sweetened beverages correlate with risk for obesity.[54] Although the US Department of Agriculture federal school lunch program specifies that no more than 30% of calories may be from fat, many schools provide foods from fast-food contractors, resulting in availability of more high-fat foods. Consequently, school lunches usually contain more than 30% of calories from fat. Vending machines in schools have also increased children's access to sugar-sweetened beverages and snack foods[53,57] (see Box 299-1).

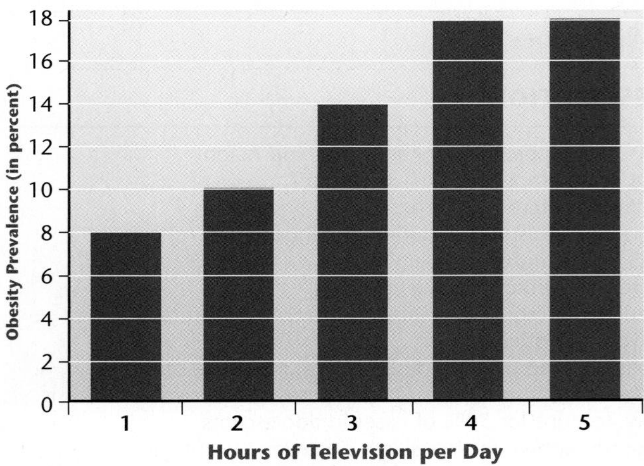

Figure 299-2 Television viewing and obesity prevalence.

MEDICAL COMORBIDITY

Obesity is associated with medical comorbidities in many organ systems. Although some problems are apparent after a relatively short duration of excess body fat, other complications do not arise for decades. Nonetheless, obesity is responsible for the childhood appearance of diseases previously seen only during adulthood, most notably type 2 diabetes mellitus.

Cardiovascular complications of obesity include hypertension and dyslipidemia. Hypertension is defined as systolic or diastolic blood pressure at or above the 95th percentile for age, sex, and height. The prevalence of diastolic hypertension increases with BMI, and the prevalence of hypertension is 3 times greater in overweight children compared with their normal-weight peers.[58,59] Blood pressure can decrease with as little as 5 to 10 pounds of weight loss.[60] Disturbances in autonomic function and abnormalities in vasculature may play important mediating roles in the development of hypertension in obese children. Hypertension continues to be underdiagnosed in children, in part, because blood pressure norms change with height age and gender. Furthermore, technical difficulties including the use of the wrong-size blood pressure cuff can cause errors.[55,61,62] (See Chapter 191, High Blood Pressure in Infants, Children, and Adolescents.) Obesity in adults and children leads to increased concentrations of triglycerides and decreased high-density lipoprotein (HDL) cholesterol.[63,64] Obese individuals have increased hepatic production of triglyceride-bearing very–low-density lipoprotein (VLDL) particles. Hyperlipidemia in youth is a potentially atherogenic condition as is family history of hyperlipidemia.[65] Therefore family history and fasting lipid levels are recommended for obese children. Intervention is indicated if total cholesterol, low-density lipoprotein (LDL) cholesterol, or triglycerides are at or above the 95th percentile. Initial treatment begins with reductions in dietary cholesterol and calories and increases in activity. Lipid-lowering medication is considered if behavioral modifications are unsuccessful.[62] Obese youth may exhibit impaired glucose tolerance with insulin resistance and postprandial hyperinsulinemia. In female adolescents, this tendency correlates with visceral fat rather than subcutaneous fat. Impaired glucose tolerance is most common in children with a family history of type 2 diabetes mellitus.[66-69] Insulin resistance is associated with acanthosis nigricans and menstrual irregularities. Insulin resistance is considered an independent risk factor for cardiovascular disease through effects on lipid metabolism and vascular changes. Development of type 2 diabetes poses further health risks including renal, ophthalmologic, and vascular disease.[70]

BOX 299-2 Metabolic Syndrome—Clinical Manifestations

OBESITY
Excess body fat
Increased visceral fat
Central fat distribution

INSULIN RESISTANCE
Decreased beta-cell number
Elevated fasting insulin levels
Fasting insulin level >15 mg/dL
Peak insulin level >150 mg/dL

DYSLIPEDIMA
Hypertriglyceridemia (very–low-density lipoprotein)
Low high-density lipoprotein
Increased free fatty acids

HYPERTENSION
Elevated systolic or diastolic blood pressure (or both)

GLUCOSE INTOLERANCE ON NON-INSULIN-DEPENDENT DIABETES MELLILTUS
Fasting plasma glucose level >126 mg/dL
2-hour plasma glucose level >200 mg/dL (oral glucose tolerance test)

Metabolic syndrome, also called syndrome X, is a cluster of metabolic abnormalities that lead to cardiovascular disease and increased mortality (Box 299-2).[71] Obesity, insulin resistance or hyperinsulinemia, dyslipidemia, and hypertension are the most commonly noted features. In adults, patients with 3 of the following 5 findings qualify for the diagnosis of metabolic syndrome: (1) elevated blood pressure, (2) high triglyceride level, (3) low HDL-cholesterol level, (4) high fasting glucose, and (5) central obesity.[72] This entity is increasingly recognized in children and adolescents as the prevalence of overweight rises in this age group. Data from the National Health and Examination Survey (1988-1994) estimates the prevalence of metabolic syndrome to be as high as 30% in obese adolescents (12 to 19 years of age).[73,74] BMI, waist circumference, and subscapular skin fold thickness are good predictors of metabolic syndrome.[75] Therefore profoundly obese youth are most likely to be affected (see Box 299-2).

Table 299-1 Medical Conditions Associated With Obesity

CONDITION	DISEASE	DESCRIPTION
Cardiovascular	Hypertension	SBP >95th percentile for sex, age, and height
	Dyslipidemia	HDL <40 mmol/L, LDL >130 mmol/L Total cholesterol >200 mmol/L
	Cardiovascular disease	Atherosclerosis begins during childhood
Endocrine	Type 2 diabetes mellitus	FBG >110 mg/dL
	Insulin resistance	Increased serum insulin levels
	Polycystic ovarian syndrome	Menstrual irregularities, hirsutism, acne, insulin resistance, hyperandrogenemia
	Metabolic syndrome	Obesity, hypertension, dyslipidemia, insulin resistance
Gastrointestinal	Nonalcoholic steatohepatitis	Increased transaminases; may progress to fibrosis or cirrhosis
	Gallbladder disease	May account for 50% of cases in adolescents
Pulmonary	Obstructive sleep apnea	Snoring, apnea, restless sleep, behavioral problems
Orthopedic	Slipped capital femoral epiphysis	Hip or knee pain, decreased mobility of hip
	Blount disease (tibia vara)	Severe bowing of the tibia
	Osteoarthritis	May present in adolescence
Neurologic	Pseudotumor cerebri	
Psychiatric	Anxiety	Sometimes difficult to assess if the depression or low self-esteem is the cause of the weight gain or if the weight gain is the cause of the depression
	Low self-esteem	Headaches, vision changes, papilledema
	Depression	
Oncologic	Endometrial cancer	Increased prevalence with adult obesity
	Breast cancer	
	Colon cancer	

FBG, Fasting blood glucose; *HDL,* high-density lipoprotein; *LDL,* low-density lipoprotein; *SBP,* systolic blood pressure.

Insulin resistance is thought to play a major role in the pathophysiologic mechanism of metabolic syndrome, with independent effects on lipid metabolism and cardiovascular health. Obese adolescents have higher plasma insulin levels than adolescents who are not obese. This comparison is true for fasting insulin levels and summed insulin levels during the glucose tolerance test.[76] Overweight school children are more likely to have elevated total cholesterol, LDL-cholesterol, triglycerides, and hyperinsulinemia than normal-weight children.[77] Elevated insulin acts in the liver and in peripheral tissues to increase plasma triglyceride and LDL-cholesterol levels. Controlling glucose metabolism is an important intervention for reducing cardiovascular risk.

Mounting evidence associates obesity with chronic inflammation.[78-81] Adipose tissue itself serves as a secretory organ, releasing peptides and cytokines into the circulation. Adiponectin, an antiinflammatory peptide, is abundant in lean, insulin-sensitive individuals and is reduced in obese individuals. Low adiponectin levels correlate with high BMI, as well as elevated levels of plasma triglycerides and free fatty acids. High adiponectin levels correlate with peripheral insulin sensitivity across age groups.[78] In contrast, proinflammatory peptides, such as tumor necrosis factor-α and interleukin (IL)-6, are elevated in obese patients. IL-6 stimulates the liver to produce C-reactive protein (CRP), a marker of inflammation and may be the link among obesity, subclinical inflammation, and coronary disease.[79] Obese children have elevated CRP. Furthermore, a linear relationship exists among BMI and CRP and IL-6 levels.[80,81] These markers have also been shown to correlate with other components of metabolic syndrome in children.[82] Treatment of metabolic syndrome is aimed primarily at weight reduction and treating the component diagnoses: hypertension, diabetes, and hyperlipidemia. Evidence for short- and long-term efficacy of pharmacologic treatment of metabolic syndrome in youth remains sparse. Although studies of oral hypoglycemics (specifically metformin) in adolescents have demonstrated reductions in blood glucose, they have shown little effect on insulin resistance or lipid abnormalities. Although this medication may be helpful as an adjuvant therapy, behavioral and dietary modifications remain 1st line.[83]

Other associated conditions include polycystic ovarian syndrome (PCOS) and nonalcoholic steatohepatitis (Table 299-1).[59,62,72,84-91] PCOS is characterized by oligomenorrhea, insulin resistance, and hyperandrogenemia and may produce hirsutism or acne. PCOS is associated with increased risk for cardiovascular disease and infertility.[92] Nonalcoholic steatohepatitis, which is increasingly recognized in overweight youth, is most often asymptomatic and is characterized by mildly to moderately elevated transaminase levels. Because nonalcoholic steatohepatitis may progress to fibrosis and cirrhosis, screening in overweight youth is recommended.[93] (See Table 299-1 for conditions associated with obesity.)

MENTAL HEALTH COMORBIDITY

"Mental health conditions are often comorbid with obesity."[94] Nonetheless, the effects of obesity on child and adolescent mental health are still not well understood. During early childhood, body weight is not

Table 299-2 Endocrine and Genetic Causes of Obesity

DIAGNOSIS	ASSOCIATED SYMPTOM	SIGNS AND SYMPTOMS	TESTING
Hypothyroidism	Short stature	Weight gain, fatigue, constipation, cold intolerance, myxedema	TSH, FT4
Cushing syndrome	Short stature	Central obesity, hirsutism, moon face, plethora, hypertension	Dexamethasone suppression test
Pseudohypoparathyroidism	Short stature	Short metacarpals, subcutaneous calcifications, dysmorphic facies, intellectual disability, hypocalcemia, hyperphosphatemia	Urine cAMP after synthetic PTH infusion
Growth hormone deficiency	Short stature	Fatigue	Evoked GH response, IGF-1
Down syndrome	Short stature	Dysmorphic facies, intellectual disability	Karyotype
Turner syndrome	Short stature	Web neck	Karyotype
Prader-Willi	Cognitive impairment	Hypogonadism, small hands and feet	FISH *15q11* microdeletion (70% of cases)
Bardet-Biedl syndrome	Cognitive impairment	Retinitis pigmentosa, renal abnormalities, polydactyly, hypogonadism	*BBS1* gene
Biemond syndrome	Cognitive impairment	Iris coloboma, hypogonadism, polydactyly	Clinical
Alstrom syndrome	Cognitive impairment	Retinitis pigmentosa, diabetes mellitus, and hearing loss	*ALMS1* gene

cAMP, Cyclic adenosine monophosphate; *FISH,* fluorescent in situ hybridization; *FT4,* free thyroxine; *GH,* growth hormone; *IGF,* insulin-like growth factor; *PTH,* parathyroid hormone; *TSH,* thyroid-stimulating hormone.

associated with self-esteem.[95] However, as children approach adolescence, self-esteem is lower in overweight children than it is their normal-weight peers. Poor emotional and social functioning is self-reported by 12- to 14-year-old overweight girls. Adolescent girls who are concerned about their weight also report more depressive symptoms.[96,97] Furthermore, depressed adolescents are at increased risk for developing persistent obesity. Otherwise, overweight youth are likely to report physical but not emotional problems, even though some studies show that they may be socially excluded.[95,98] When caring for overweight and obese children, assessing affect and mental health status is advisable.

COSTS

The current epidemic of obesity poses a significant threat to health care systems already struggling with escalating costs. The US Surgeon General predicted that the costs related to obesity will overtake those of tobacco, based on the alarming increased expenses associated with obesity and related conditions. Current costs for obese patients exceed those of patients who are not obese by 36%. Similar figures show that costs for smokers exceed those of nonsmokers by 21%. Furthermore, medication expenses are 77% higher for obese compared to individuals who are not obese. Obesity is associated with increased numbers of medical diagnoses and medications, leading to increased medical costs comparable to 20 years of aging.[99] These figures do not attempt to capture psychological morbidity.

DIFFERENTIAL DIAGNOSIS

Primary medical causes of obesity are rare. Endocrine and genetic causes of obesity often cause short stature or cognitive impairment[100-105] (see Box 299-2). Children who consume excess calories are likely to experience accelerated linear growth. Therefore short stature in an overweight child warrants further evaluation. Similarly, syndromes associated with intellectual disability and obesity should be considered in obese children with developmental delay. Table 299-2 lists endocrine and genetic causes of obesity.

LABORATORY EVALUATION

The Centers for Disease Control and Prevention and the American Academy of Pediatrics recommend a cholesterol panel (including LDL, HDL, and triglycerides) and fasting plasma glucose for evaluating overweight children (BMI over 95%).[53,106] The American Diabetes Association recommends a fasting glucose test for children whose BMI is between the 85th and the 95th percentile if they have a family history of diabetes mellitus or obesity or signs of insulin resistance, including acanthosis nigricans, PCOS, or hirsutism[106] (Box 299-3). Hemoglobin A_{1c} is sometimes used to screen patients who are unable to comply with fasting before the laboratory test. Insulin levels are not currently recommended for evaluating obesity because they can be elevated, low, or normal at the time of presentation of type 2 diabetes. Furthermore, insulin levels do not alter medical management. Insulin levels are helpful when uncertainty exists as to whether the patient has type 1 or type 2 diabetes mellitus. The clinician should check liver function tests at baseline and should do so before pharmacologic management for type 2 diabetes or surgical intervention for obesity.[53] Other studies are ordered only as indicated by history or physical examination (Table 299-3; see also Box 299-3).

PRIMARY PREVENTION

Prevention of childhood obesity is crucial to the public health.[107] This endeavor will require concerted effort of public health officials, government at all levels, schools, and the health care system.

Clinicians who care for children have the opportunity to educate families about the importance of healthy nutrition and physical activity from the earliest years. Much confusion exists about good nutrition. Healthful nutrition begins with breastfeeding, which is associated with lower childhood obesity risk. Exclusive breastfeeding is recommended for the first 4 to 6 months of life. (See Chapter 26, Feeding of Infants and Children.) Consideration of nutrient quality and caloric content is the basis of a healthy diet. Calorie-laden foods with little nutritional value are reserved for occasional treats. Families can begin by planning meals and snacks based on fruits, vegetables, and grains. Healthy diets include appropriate portion sizes of meat and dairy products. These foods should supply fewer calories than fruits, vegetables, and grains. Milk supplies important nutrients during childhood, and low-fat milk is recommended for most children after age 2 years. Children should be encouraged to drink water to quench thirst, reserving highly sugared beverages for occasional treats. Even fruit juice should be consumed in moderation. Healthy desserts that include fruit, yogurt, cookies made with oatmeal, occasional puddings made with milk and eggs, and ice cream are satisfying components of a healthy diet. Using lower-fat alternatives is suggested for cardiovascular health. Attention to portion size is important. Children learn food preferences early in life and may also develop habits associated with appetite and satiety.

Physical activity habits similarly begin early in life. Children whose parents are physically active are more likely to be physically active. Clinicians can encourage families to consider planning opportunities for physical activity as a parental responsibility. Children should engage in at least 60 minutes of physical activity on most, preferably all, days of the week. Children who participate in organized sports should be encouraged to be physically active on the days they do not have these organized activities as well. Pediatricians can reinforce with parents the importance of daily physical activity and to resist the reliance on organized sports for all of their child's physical activity needs. Older children and adolescents may benefit from strength training. Overweight children often find this form of physical activity the most rewarding because, given their increased body mass, they may be stronger than their peers, and strength training does not require aerobic endurance or agility. Overweight children can therefore benefit both psychologically and physically from these activities.[108] This increase in physical activity should be accompanied by decreases in sedentary activities. Limiting television and other recreational screen time to less than 2 hours per day is recommended. The American Academy of Pediatrics recommends no television for children younger than 2 years. Parents should strive to be role models for their children in their eating and activity habits. Child health professionals can begin to talk to parents about healthy nutrition and activity during the 1st year of life. These themes can be revisited at annual health care maintenance visits.

The other key role for child health professionals is monitoring. BMI should be calculated and plotted at each health are maintenance visit. Computerized systems that automatically calculate and plot these percentiles make this feasible. Tracking growth trajectories and explaining these patterns to parents is an essential component of primary prevention. Children

BOX 299-3 Indications for Diabetes Testing (Fasting Blood Glucose)

- Patient is overweight, with BMI >95th percentile
- BMI is between the 85th-95th percentile with any of the following:
  - Family history of type 2 diabetes
  - Native American, black, Hispanic, Asian and Pacific Islander
  - Signs of insulin resistance, acanthosis nigricans, hypertension, dyslipidemia, PCOS

BMI, Body mass index; *PCOS*, polycystic ovary syndrome.
From American Academy of Pediatrics, Consensus Panel of American Diabetes Association. Type 2 diabetes in children and adolescents. *Pediatrics.* 2000;105(3:1):671-680.

Table 299-3 Laboratory Testing as Indicated by History or Physical Examination

TEST	INDICATIONS
Thyroid function tests	When symptoms of hypothyroidism are present
Plain-film radiographs	For deformity, hip or knee pain (SCFE or Blount disease)
Head computed tomographic scan, lumbar puncture	Headache, visual changes, papilledema (pseudotumor cerebri)
LH, FSH, total and free testosterone; consider pelvic ultrasound	Menstrual irregularity, acne, hirsutism (PCOS)
Genetic consultation, karyotype	Short stature, dysmorphic features, cognitive impairment

FSH, Follicle-stimulating hormone; *LH*, luteinizing hormone; *PCOS*, polycystic ovary syndrome; *SCFE*, slipped capital femoral epiphysis.

with increasing BMI percentiles may be at risk for developing obesity. Health care professionals can help families evaluate nutritional and activity patterns and make adjustments. Child heath professionals need to identify parental obesity as a risk factor for the child. Given that early childhood obesity often resolves, optimism is warranted in the early years. By adolescence, nutritional and activity patterns are more difficult to change, and families have less influence. Strategies to engage the parent in preventive efforts are needed. Obesity remains an emotionally charged issue, creating more difficulties for the family and the clinician as compared to more purely medical problems.

INTERVENTION—PREVENTION OF SECONDARY COMORBIDITY

Preventing secondary comorbidity and disability is the principle goal in treating overweight children and adolescents. The primary care physician is faced with the challenge of educating the child and family about lifetime health risks imparted by excess body weight. These risks may seem abstract to the family because they are unlikely to occur for many years. Obesity should be approached as a chronic condition that requires permanent lifestyle change to achieve optimal body weight. Recent work with obese children and their families supports the utility of using a stages of change model for assessment of readiness to change followed by motivational interviewing.[109] (See Chapter 24, Communication Strategies.) Prescribing a treatment plan without engaging the child and family can lead to frustration and feelings of futility, impairing future attempts at weight control. Enhancing the therapeutic relationship can begin with a question to the parent, "Have you ever struggled with your weight?" The answer to this question will reveal a great deal about the family's perception of body weight as an indicator of health and well being and the parent's empathy for the child. Readiness to change can be assessed by asking the child and parent 3 questions:

- How concerned are you about your weight (your child's weight)?
- Do you think that you can improve your body fitness (your child's body fitness)?
- Do you think that your family can change eating and physical activity patterns?

If the child is seriously overweight (above the 99th percentile) or has medical complications, then counseling may be necessary for the family to progress to a state of readiness to change.[84]

Once the patient and family are ready to begin a treatment plan, the clinician should assist them in setting realistic goals[84] (Box 299-4). Weight maintenance

BOX 299-4 Role of the Pediatrician

Intervene early.
Assess family's readiness to change.
Educate family about medical complications of obesity.
Involve family and caregivers in the treatment program.
Aim for permanent dietary and activity change.
Avoid short-term diets or exercise programs aimed at rapid weight loss.
Teach family to monitor eating and activity.
Assist family in making small, gradual changes.
Encourage and empathize.
Avoid criticism.

BOX 299-5 Parenting Skills for Weight Loss

Find reasons to praise child's behavior.
Avoid using food as a reward.
Establish daily family meal and snack times, as well as physically active family time.
Determine what food is offered and when.
Allow child to decide whether to eat.
Offer only healthy options.
Remove temptations (snack food in home).
Walk instead of driving, take the stairs; decrease television-viewing time.
Be a role model in diet and physical activity.
Be consistent.

BOX 299-6 Dietary Modifications

Drink water, sugar-free beverages, or milk with no more than 1% fat.
Use cooking spray instead of frying.
Make cut-up fruits and vegetables accessible.
Limit seconds to fruits and vegetables.
Serve appropriate portions: meat-size of your palm, starch (1/2 cup).
Review school lunch menu with child to pick healthy options.
Pack lunch with 4 oz lean meat, whole grain bread, fruit or vegetable, and milk.
Limit restaurant dining to once per week or less.
Limit fast food to rarely.
Eat meals together, and turn off the television while eating.
Schedule at least 20 minutes for each meal. Eating slowly helps to avoid overeating.
Eat regular meals. Skipping meals can lead to overeating.
Remove snack foods, chips, cookies, and desserts from the house.
Allow occasional treats.
Make salads with vegetables, not eggs, meat, bacon, or cheese.
Toss family salad to decrease amount of dressing.

Adapted from Baker S, Barlow S, Cochran W, et al. Overweight children and adolescents: a clinical report of the North American Society of Pediatric Gastroenterology, Hepatology and Nutrition. *J Pediatric Gastro Nutr.* 2005;40(5):533-543.

rather than weight loss is usually the 1st step for growing youth. The objective is to decrease the rate of weight gain and allow the child to achieve a healthier body mass[84] (Box 299-5). Learning healthy eating and activity habits improves the child's health over time[53] (Box 299-6 and Box 299-7). Focusing on health and healthy behavior changes allows for gradual and long-term change. Fad diets and very–low-calorie regimens are not recommended for children because these diets cannot be maintained.[84] Children who suffer from acute comorbidity such as sleep apnea may be managed medically (usually in an inpatient treatment program) on a very–low-calorie diet. Recommendations for weight maintenance or weight loss are based on level of overweight, age, and existence of complications[84] (Figure 299-3). Setting goals for weight maintenance or weight loss may be based on BMI, age, and complications[84] (see Figure 299-3 and Boxes 299-4 through 299-7).

No evidence has been found that pharmacologic agents for weight loss are safe and effective for children. Bariatric surgery may be considered in severely overweight adolescents (BMI above 40) with nearly complete skeletal maturity and significant medical complications and who have not been able to change their weight or obesity comorbidities despite dietary and exercise modifications for 6 months. After evaluation by a multidisciplinary team, surgery can be performed by surgeons who are experienced in gastric bypass surgery. A major dilemma for care of adolescents is how to give informed consent or assent about the consequences of both obesity and the alternative of bariatric surgery. The procedure will change their ability to eat and may have unforeseen long-term consequences.[53] On the other hand, obesity may threaten their lives.

BOX 299-7 Increasing Physical Activity

Limit television and video games to no more than 1-2 hours per day.

Engage in active family activities: Ride a bike, walk after dinner, swim, go to zoo or museum.

Dance to your favorite music.

Walk with a friend rather than talking on the telephone.

Walk while you talk on the telephone.

Engage in team sports.

Take classes—dance, martial arts, or swimming.

Strategies for toddlers and preschool-age children:

- Engage in outdoor play every day.
- Engage in active indoor play, soft balls, jumping, or bouncy balls.
- Buy active toys rather than computer games or videos.

Adapted from Baker S, Barlow S, Cochran W, et al. Overweight children and adolescents: a clinical report of the North American Society of Pediatric Gastroenterology, Hepatology and Nutrition. *J Pediatric Gastro Nutr.* 2005; 40(5):533-543.

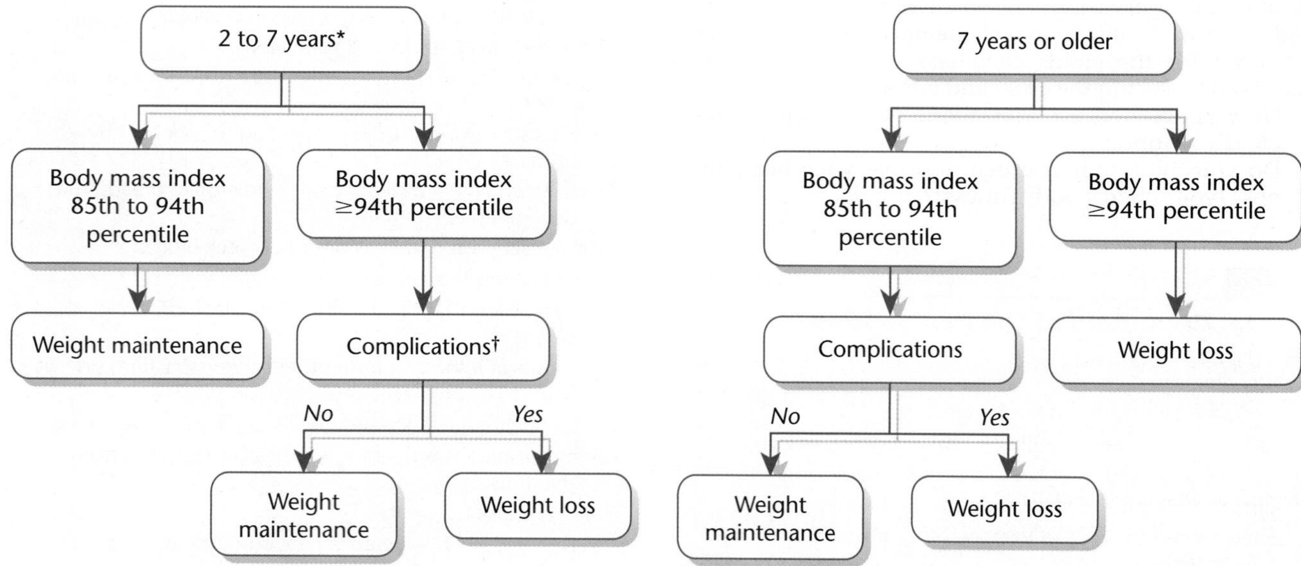

Figure 299-3 Recommendations for weight goals. Asterisk (*) indicates that children younger than 2 years should be referred to a pediatric obesity center for treatment. Dagger (†) indicates complications such as mild hypertension, dyslipidemias, and insulin resistance. Patients with acute complications, such as pseudotumor cerebri, sleep apnea, obesity hypoventilation syndrome, or orthopedic problems, should be referred to a pediatric obesity center.

TOOLS FOR PRACTICE

Community Coordination and Advocacy

- *Action for Healthy Kids* (Web page), Action for Healthy Kids (www.actionforhealthykids.org/).
- *Issue Brief—Childhood Obesity* (fact sheet), American Academy of Pediatrics (www.aap.org/moc/displaytemp/obesity_issuebrief.pdf).

Practice Management and Care Coordination

- *Obesity and Other Co-Morbidities Coding Fact Sheet* (fact sheet), American Academy of Pediatrics (www.aap.org/securemoc/reimburse/codingfactsheet.pdf).

Engaging Patient and Family

- *A Parent's Guide to Childhood Obesity: A Road Map to Health* (book), American Academy of Pediatrics (www.aap.org/bookstore).
- *About BMI for Children and Teens* (fact sheet), Centers for Disease Control and Prevention (www.cdc.gov/nccdphp/dnpa/bmi/childrens_BMI/about_childrens_BMI.htm).
- *BAM site* (Web page), Centers for Disease Control and Prevention (www.bam.gov/).
- *Better Health and Fitness Through Physical Activity* (brochure), American Academy of Pediatrics (patiented.aap.org).
- *Encourage Your Child to Be Physically Active* (brochure), American Academy of Pediatrics (patiented.aap.org).
- *Feeding Guide for Children* (other), American Academy of Pediatrics, Hassink S (practice.aap.org/content.aspx?aid=2001).
- *Feeding Kids Right Isn't Always Easy* (brochure), American Academy of Pediatrics (patiented.aap.org).
- *Growing Up Healthy* (brochure), American Academy of Pediatrics (patiented.aap.org).
- *My Pyramid—Steps to a Healthier You* (Web page), US Department of Agriculture (www.mypyramid.gov/).
- *Right From the Start: ABCs of Good Nutrition for Young Children* (brochure), American Academy of Pediatrics (patiented.aap.org).
- *Sports and Your Child* (brochure), American Academy of Pediatrics (patiented.aap.org).
- *Television and the Family* (brochure), American Academy of Pediatrics (patiented.aap.org).
- *VERB* (Web page), Centers for Disease Control and Prevention (www.verbnow.com/).
- *What's to Eat? Healthy Foods for Hungry Children* (brochure), American Academy of Pediatrics (patiented.aap.org).

Medical Decision Support

- *A New Spin on Childhood Obesity* (on-line course), American Academy of Pediatrics (www.pedialink.org/cme/_coursefinder/CMEdetail.cfm?aid=30256&area=liveCME).
- *BMI—Body Mass Index: Child and Teen Calculator: English* (interactive tool), Centers for Disease Control and Prevention (apps.nccd.cdc.gov/dnpabmi/Calculator.aspx).
- *Bright Futures: Guidelines for Health Supervision of Infants, Children, and Adolescents* (book), Bright Futures (brightfutures.aap.org/web).
- *Environmental Assessment, Appendix A.4, Pediatric Obesity: Prevention, Intervention, and Treatment Strategies for Primary Care* (questionnaire), American Academy of Pediatrics (practice.aap.org/content.aspx?aid=2001).
- *Family History: Your Child's Genetics and Family History, Appendix A.4, Pediatric Obesity: Prevention, Intervention, and Treatment Strategies for Primary Care* (questionnaire), American Academy of Pediatrics (practice.aap.org/content.aspx?aid=2001).
- *Food Diary: What Is Your Child Eating Now? Appendix A.4, Pediatric Obesity: Prevention, Intervention, and Treatment Strategies for Primary Care* (questionnaire), American Academy of Pediatrics (practice.aap.org/content.aspx?aid=2001).
- *Goal Assessment, Appendix A.4, Pediatric Obesity: Prevention, Intervention, and Treatment Strategies for Primary Care* (questionnaire), American Academy of Pediatrics (practice.aap.org/content.aspx?aid=2001).
- *Goal Achievement Plan Appendix A.4, Pediatric Obesity: Prevention, Intervention, and Treatment Strategies for Primary Care* (questionnaire), American Academy of Pediatrics (practice.aap.org/content.aspx?aid=2001).
- *Growth Charts—Tutorials and Information* (Web page), Centers for Disease Control and Prevention (www.cdc.gov/growthcharts/).
- *Growth Charts* (chart), Centers for Disease Control and Prevention, (www.cdc.gov/nchs/about/major/nhanes/growthcharts/clinical_charts.htm#Clin%201); also available at AAP bookstore (www.aap.org/bookstore).
- *Home Environment Assessment, Appendix A.4, Pediatric Obesity: Prevention, Intervention, and Treatment Strategies for Primary Care* (questionnaire), American Academy of Pediatrics (practice.aap.org/content.aspx?aid=2001).
- *Introducing Patients to Healthy Family Lifestyles* (fact sheet), R. Joe Jopling, MD (practice.aap.org/content.aspx?aid=2001).
- *Parental Concerns Assessment, Appendix A.4, Pediatric Obesity: Prevention, Intervention, and Treatment Strategies for Primary Care* (questionnaire), American Academy of Pediatrics (practice.aap.org/content.aspx?aid=2001).
- *Pediatric Obesity: Prevention, Intervention, and Treatment Strategies for Primary Care* (book), American Academy of Pediatrics (www.aap.org/bookstore).
- *Physical Activity Assessment, Appendix A.4, Pediatric Obesity: Prevention, Intervention, and Treatment Strategies for Primary Care* (questionnaire), American Academy of Pediatrics (practice.aap.org/content.aspx?aid=2001).
- *Physician Tracking Form for Pediatric Obesity, Appendix A.4, Pediatric Obesity: Prevention, Intervention, and Treatment Strategies for Primary Care* (form), American Academy of Pediatrics (practice.aap.org/content.aspx?aid=2001).

- *Set Backs Worksheet, Appendix A.4, Pediatric Obesity: Prevention, Intervention, and Treatment Strategies for Primary Care* (questionnaire), American Academy of Pediatrics (practice.aap.org/content.aspx?aid=2001).
- *Snacking Worksheet, Appendix A.4, Pediatric Obesity: Prevention, Intervention, and Treatment Strategies for Primary Care* (questionnaire), American Academy of Pediatrics (practice.aap.org/content.aspx?aid=2001).
- *VERB Campaign* (Web page), Centers for Disease Control and Prevention (www.cdc.gov/youthcampaign/index.htm).

AAP POLICY STATEMENTS

American Academy of Pediatrics Council on Sports Medicine and Fitness and Council on School Health. Active healthy living: Prevention of childhood obesity through increased physical activity. *Pediatrics.* 2006;117(5)1834-1842. (aappolicy.aappublications.org/cgi/content/full/pediatrics;117/5/1834).

American Academy of Pediatrics, Committee on Communications. Children, adolescents, and advertising. *Pediatrics.* 2006;118(6):2563-2569. (aappolicy.aappublications.org/cgi/content/full/pediatrics;118/6/2563).

American Academy of Pediatrics, Committee on Public Education. Children, adolescents, and television. *Pediatrics.* 2001;107(2):423-426. (aappolicy.aappublications.org/cgi/content/full/pediatrics;107/2/423).

American Academy of Pediatrics, Committee on Adolescence. Identifying and treating eating disorders. *Pediatrics.* 2003;111(1):204-211. (aappolicy.aappublications.org/cgi/content/full/pediatrics;111/1/204).

American Academy of Pediatrics, Committee on Nutrition. Prevention of pediatric overweight and obesity. *Pediatrics.* 2003;112(2):424-430. (aappolicy.aappublications.org/cgi/content/full/pediatrics;112/2/424).

American Academy of Pediatrics, Committee on School Health. Soft drinks in schools. *Pediatrics.* 2004;113(1):152-154. (aappolicy.aappublications.org/cgi/content/full/pediatrics;113/1/152).

American Academy of Pediatrics, Committee on Sports Medicine and Fitness. Strength training by children and adolescents. *Pediatrics.* 2008;121(4):835-840. (aappolicy.aappublications.org/cgi/content/full/pediatrics;107/6/1470).

National High Blood Pressure Education Program Working Group on High Blood Pressure in Children and Adolescents. The fourth report on the diagnosis, evaluation, and treatment of high blood pressure in children and adolescents. *Pediatrics.* 2004;114(2/S2):555-576. AAP endorsed.

American Academy of Pediatrics, Committee on Nutrition. The use and misuse of fruit juice in pediatrics. *Pediatrics.* 2001;107(5):1210-1213. (aappolicy.aappublications.org/cgi/content/full/pediatrics;107/5/1210).

American Diabetes Association. Type 2 diabetes in children and adolescents. *Diabetes Care.* 2000;23(3):381-389. AAP endorsed.

Gahagan S, Silverstein J, American Academy of Pediatrics, Committee on Native American Child Health and Section on Endocrinology. Prevention and treatment of type 2 diabetes mellitus in children, with special emphasis on American Indian and Alaska Native children. *Pediatrics.* 2003;112(4):e328. AAP endorsed.

REFERENCES

1. Troiano RP, Flegal KM. Overweight children and adolescents: description, epidemiology, and demographics. *Pediatrics.* 1998;101:497-504.
2. Troiano RP, Flegal KM. Overweight prevalence: why so many different numbers? *Int J Obes Relat Metab Disord.* 1999;23(1):S22-S27.
3. US Department Health and Human Services. *The Surgeon General's Call to Action to Prevent and Decrease Overweight and Obesity.* Rockville, MD: US Department of Health and Human Services, Public Health Service, Office of the Surgeon General; 2001.
4. Wolf AM, Colditz GA. Current estimates of the economic cost of obesity in the United States. *Obes Res.* Mar 1998;6(2):97-106.
5. Pietrobelli A, Faith MS, Allison DB, et al. Body mass index as a measure of adiposity among children and adolescents. *J Pediatr.* 1998;132:204-210.
6. Centers for Disease Control and Prevention, National Center for Health Statistics. Clinical Growth Charts. Available at: www.cdc.gov/nchs/about/major/nhanes/growthcharts/clinical_charts.htm. Accessed June 21, 2006.
7. World Health Organization. *Obesity: Preventing and Managing the Global Epidemic. Report of a WHO Consultation on Obesity, Geneva, June 3-5, 1997.* Geneva, Switzerland: World Health Organization; 1998.
8. Centers for Disease Control and Prevention. Overweight and Obesity: Defining Overweight and Obesity. Available at: www.cdc.gov/nccdphp/dnpa/obesity/defining.htm. Accessed June 21, 2006.
9. York DA, Rossner S, Caterson I, et al. American Heart Association. Prevention Conference VII: obesity, a worldwide epidemic related to heart disease and stroke: Group I: worldwide demographics of obesity. *Circulation.* Nov 2004;110(18):e463-e470.
10. Centers for Disease Control and Prevention, National Center for Health Statistics. Prevalence of Overweight and Obesity Among Adults: United States, 1999-2002. Available at: www.cdc.gov/nchs/products/pubs/pubd/hestats/obese/obse99.htm. Accessed June 21, 2006.
11. Centers for Disease Control and Prevention, National Center for Health Statistics. Prevalence of Overweight Among Children and Adolescents: United States, 2003-2004. Available at: www.cdc.gov/nchs/products/pubs/pubd/hestats/obese03_04/overwght_child_03.htm. Accessed July 10, 2006.
12. Mei Z, Scanlon KS, Grummer-Strawn LM, et al. Increasing prevalence of overweight among US low-income preschool children: the Centers for Disease Control and Prevention Pediatric Nutrition Surveillance, 1983 to 1995. *Pediatrics.* 1998;101:e12.
13. Ogden CL, Troiano RP, Breifel RR, et al. Prevalence of overweight among preschool children in the United States, 1971 through 1995. *Pediatrics.* 1997;99:e1.
14. Strauss RS, Pollack HA. Epidemic increase in childhood overweight, 1986-1998. *JAMA.* 2001;286(22):2845-2848.
15. Sobal J, Stunkard AJ. Socioeconomic status and obesity: a review of the literature 1989. *Psychol Bull.* 1989;105(2):260-275.
16. Ogden CL, Carroll MD, Curtin LR, et al. Prevalence of overweight and obesity in the United States 1999-2004. *JAMA.* 2006;295(13):1549-1555.
17. Charney M, Goodman HC, McBride M, et al. Childhood antecedents of adult obesity: do chubby infants become obese adults? *N Engl J Med.* 1976;295:6-9.
18. Stark D, Atkins E, Wolff DH, et al. Longitudinal study of obesity in the National Survey of Health and Development. *BMJ.* 1981;283:12-17.
19. Guo SS, Chumlea WC. Tracking of body mass index in children in relation to overweight in adulthood. *Am J Clin Nutr.* 1999;70:145S-148S.
20. Gahagan S. Kindergarten children from single parent families more likely to be overweight. *Pediatr Res.* 2003;41:6-43.

21. Strauss RS, Knight K. Influence of the home environment on the development of obesity in children. *Pediatrics*. 1999;103:85.
22. Whitaker RC, Wright JA, Pepe MS, et al. Predicting obesity in young adulthood from childhood and parental obesity. *N Engl J Med*. 1997;337(13):869-873.
23. Gregory S, Barash I, Sadaf F, et al. Genetics of bodyweight regulation. *Nature*. 2000;404:644-651.
24. Hill JO, Wyatt HR, Reed GW, et al. Obesity and the environment: where do we go from here? *Science*. 2003; 299(5608:7):853-855.
25. Bandini LG, Schoeller DA, Dietz WH. Energy expenditure in obese and non-obese adolescents. *Pediatr Res*. 1990;27:198-203.
26. Jung E, Czajka-Narins DM. Birth weight doubling and tripling times: an updated look at the effects of birth weight, sex, race and type of feeding. *Am J Clin Nutr*. 1985;42:182-189.
27. Eriksson J, Forsen T, Osmond C, et al. Obesity from cradle to grave. *Int J Obes Relat Metab Disord*. 2003;27(6): 722-727.
28. Dietz WH. Critical periods in childhood for the development of obesity. *Am J Clin Nutr*. 1994;59(5):955-959.
29. Dietz WH. Periods of risk in childhood for the development of adult obesity—what do we learn? *J Nutrition*. 1997;127(9):1884S-1885S.
30. Melits ED, Cheek DB. The assessment of body water and fatness from infancy to adulthood. *Monogr Soc Res Child Dev*. 1970;35:12-26.
31. Garn SM, Cole PE. Do the obese remain obese and the lean remain lean? *Am J Public Health*. 1980;70:351-353.
32. Fisher JO, Birch LL. Fat preferences and fat consumption of 3- to 5-year-old children are related to parental adiposity. *J Am Dietet Assoc*. 1995;95:759-764.
33. Neumark-Sztainer D, Story M, Resnick MD, et al. Correlates of inadequate fruit and vegetable consumption among adolescents. *Prev Med*. 1996;25:497-505.
34. Krebs-Smith SM, Cook A, Subar AF, et al. Fruit and vegetable intakes of children and adolescents in the United States. *Arch Pediatr Adolesc Med*. 1996;150: 81-99.
35. Kennedy E, Powell R. Changing eating patterns of American children: a view from 1996. *J Am Coll Nutr*. 1997;16:524-529.
36. Lissau I, Sorensen TIA. Parental neglect during childhood and increased risk of obesity in young adulthood. *Lancet*. 1994;343:324-327.
37. Johnson SL, Birch LL. Parents' and children's adiposity and eating style. *Pediatrics*. 1994;94:653-661.
38. Berkeling B, Ekman S, Rossner S. Eating behaviour in obese and normal weight 11-year-old children. *Int J Obes Relat Metab Disord*. 1992;16:355.
39. Sorensen HT, Sabroe S, Rothman KJ, et al. Relation between weight and length at birth and body mass index in young adulthood: cohort study. *BMJ*. 1997;315: 1137.
40. Widdowson EM. Changes in pigs due to undernutrition before birth, and for one, two, and three years afterwards, and the effects of rehabilitation. In: Roche AF, Falkner F, editors. *Nutrition and Malnutrition, Identification and Measurement. Advances in Experimental Medicine and Biology*. Vol. 49. New York, NY, and London, UK: Plenum Press; 1974.
41. Popkin BM, Richards MK, Montiero CA. Stunting is associated with overweight in children of four nations that are undergoing the nutrition transition. *J Nutr*. 1996;126:3009.
42. Cameron N. Changing prevalence of childhood obesity in developing countries. *Int J Obes Relat Metab Disord*. 1998;22(4):S1.
43. Pasquet P, Meleman F, Koppert G, et al. *Growth, Maturation and Nutrition Transition: With Special Reference to Urban Populations in Central Africa* [abstract]. 14th International Anthropological Congress of Ales Hrdlicka "World Anthropology at the Turn of Centuries." August 31-September 4, 1999: Prague-Humpolec.
44. Popkin BM, Richards MK, Adair LS. Stunting is associated with childhood obesity: dynamic relationships. In: Johnston FE, Zemel B, Eveleth PB, eds. *Human Growth in Context*. London, UK: Smith-Gordon/Nishimura; 1999.
45. Keys A, Brozek J. Body fat in adult man. *Physiol Rev*. 1953; 33:245.
46. Alaimo K, Olson CM, Frongillo EAJ. Low family income and food insufficiency in relation to overweight in US children: is there a paradox? *Arch Pediatr Adolesc Med*. 2001;155:1161-1167.
47. Juge-Aubry CE, Meier CA. Immunomodulatory actions of leptin. *Mol Cell Endocrinol*. 2002;194(1-2):1-7.
48. Hwang CS, Loftus TM, Mandrup S, et al. Adipocyte differentiation and leptin expression. *Annu Rev Cell Dev Biol*. 1997;13:231-259.
49. Zakrzewska KE, Cusin I, Sainsbury A, et al. Glucocorticoids as counter regulatory hormones of leptin: toward an understanding of leptin resistance. *Diabetes*. 1997; 46(4):717-719.
50. Danadian K, Suprasongsin C, Janosky JE, et al. Leptin in African-American children. *J Pediatr Endocrinol Metab*. 1999;12(5):639-644.
51. Burdette HL, Whitaker RC. A national study of neighborhood safety, outdoor play, television viewing, and obesity in preschool children. *Pediatrics*. 2005;116(3): 657-662.
52. Andersen RE, Crespo CJ, Bartlett SJ, et al. Relationship of physical activity and television watching with body weight and level of fatness among children: results from the Third National Health and Nutrition Examination Survey. *JAMA*. 1998;279:938-942.
53. Baker S, Barlow S, Cochran W, et al. Overweight children and adolescents: a clinical report of the North American Society of Pediatric Gastroenterology, Hepatology and Nutrition. *J Pediatric Gastro Nutr*. 2005;40(5): 533-543.
54. Ludwig DS, Peterson KE, Gortmaker SL. Relation between consumption of sugar-sweetened drinks and childhood obesity: a prospective, observational analysis. *Lancet*. 2001;357:505-508.
55. Whincup PH, Cook DG, Shaper AG. Blood pressure measurement in children: the importance of cuff bladder size. *J Hypertens*. 1989;7:845-850.
56. Crespo CJ, Smit E, Troiano RP, et al. Television watching, energy intake, and obesity in US children: results from the Third National Health and Nutrition Examination Survey, 1988-1994. *Arch Pediatr Adolesc Med*. 2001; 155(3):360-365.
57. Dwyer J. The school nutrition dietary assessment study. *Am J Clin Nutr*. 1995;61:173S-257S.
58. Sorof JM, Poffenbarger T, Franco K, et al. Isolated systolic hypertension, obesity, and hyperkinetic hemodynamic states in children. *J Pediatr*. 2002;140:660-666.
59. Rosner B, Prineas R, Daniels SR, et al. Blood pressure differences between blacks and whites in relation to body size among US children and adolescents. *Am J Epidemiol*. 2000;151:1007-1019.
60. Williams CL, Hayman LL, Daniels SR, et al. Cardiovascular health in childhood: a statement for health professionals from the Committee on Atherosclerosis, Hypertension, and Obesity in the Young (AHOY) of the Council on Cardiovascular Disease in the Young, American Heart Association. *Circulation*. 2002;106(1):143-160.

61. Gomez-Marin O, Prineas RJ, Rastam L. Cuff bladder width and blood pressure measurement in children and adolescents. *J Hypertens*. 1992;10:1235-1241.
62. Sinaiko AR, Donahue RP, Jacob DR, et al. Relation of weight and rate of increase in weight during childhood and adolescent to body size, blood pressure, fasting insulin, and lipids in young adults. The Minneapolis Children's Blood Pressure Study. *Circulation*. 1999;99(11): 1471-1476.
63. Zwiauer KFM, Pakosta R, Mueller T, et al. Cardiovascular risk factors in obese children in relation to weight and body fat distribution. *J Am Coll Nutr*. 1992;11:41S-50S.
64. Freedman DS, Srinivasan SR, Harsha DW, et al. Relation of body fat patterning to lipid and lipoprotein concentrations in children and adolescents: the Bogalusa Heart Study. *Am J Clin Nutr*. 1989;50:930-939.
65. Slyper AH. Childhood obesity, adipose tissue distribution, and the pediatric practitioner. *Pediatrics*. 1998; 102(1):e4.
66. Le Stunff C, Bougneres P. Early changes in postprandial insulin secretion, not in insulin sensitivity, characterize juvenile obesity. *Diabetes*. 1994;43:696-702.
67. Monti LD, Brambilla P, Stefani I, et al. Insulin regulation of glucose turnover and lipid levels in obese children with fasting normoinsulinemia. *Diabetologia*. 1995;38(6): 739-747.
68. Caprio S, Hyman LD, Limb C, et al. Central adiposity and its metabolic correlates in obese adolescent girls. *Am J Physiol*. 1995;269:E118-E126.
69. Sinha R, Fisch G, Teague B, et al. Prevalence of impaired glucose tolerance among children and adolescents with marked obesity. *New Eng J Med*. 2002;346(11):802-810.
70. Nathan DM. Long-term complications of diabetes mellitus. *N Engl J Med*. 1993;328(23):1676-1685.
71. Hansen B. The metabolic syndrome X. *Ann NY Acad Sci*. 1999;892:1-24.
72. Weiss R, Caprio S. The metabolic consequences of childhood obesity. *Best Pract Res Clin Endocrinol Metab*. 2005;19(3):405-419.
73. Cook S, Weitzman M, Auinger P, et al. Prevalence of a metabolic syndrome phenotype in adolescents: findings from the Third National Health and Nutrition Examination Survey, 1988-1994. *Arch Pediatr Adolesc Med*. 2003;157(8):821-827.
74. Cruz ML, Weigensberg MJ, Huang TT, et al. The metabolic syndrome in overweight Hispanic youth and the role of insulin sensitivity. *J Clin Endocrinol Metab*. 2004; 89(1):108-113.
75. Moreno LA, Pineda I, Rodriguez G, et al. Waist circumference for the screening of the metabolic syndrome in children. *Acta Paediatr*. 2002;91(12):1307-1312.
76. Steinberger J, Moorehead C, Katch V, et al. Relationship between insulin resistance and abnormal lipid profile in obese adolescents. *J Pediatr*. 1995;126:690-695.
77. Freedman DS, Dietz WH, Srinivasan SR, et al. The relation of overweight to cardiovascular risk factors among children and adolescents: The Bogalusa Heart Study. *Pediatrics*. 1999;103:1175-1182.
78. Weiss R, Dufour S, Groszmann A, et al. Low adiponectin levels in adolescent obesity: a marker of increased intramyocellular lipid accumulation. *J Clin Endocrinol Metab*. 2003;88(5):2014-2018.
79. Yudkin JS, Kumari M, Humphries SE, et al. Inflammation, obesity, stress and coronary heart disease: is interleukin-6 the link? *Atherosclerosis*. 2000;148(2):209-214.
80. Ford ES, Galuska DA, Gillespie C, et al. C-reactive protein and body mass index in children: Findings from the Third National Health and Nutrition Examination Survey, 1988-1994. *J Pediatr*. 2001;138(4):486-492.
81. Reaven GM. Banting lecture 1988. Role of insulin resistance in human disease. *Diabetes*. 1988;37:1595-1607.
82. Cook DG, Mendall MA, Whincup PH, et al. C-reactive protein concentration in children: relationship to adiposity and other cardiovascular risk factors. *Atherosclerosis*. 2000;149(1):139-150.
83. Freemark M, Bursey D. The effects of Metformin on body mass index and glucose tolerance in obese adolescents with fasting hyperinsulineamia and a family history of type 2 diabetes. *Pediatrics*. 2001;107(4):e55.
84. Barlow SE, Dietz WH. Obesity evaluation and treatment: Expert Committee recommendations. The Maternal and Child Health Bureau, Health Resources and Services Administration and the Department of Health and Human Services. *Pediatrics*. 1998;102(3):E29.
85. Marcus CL, Curtis S, Koerner CB, et al. Evaluation of pulmonary function and polysomnography in obese children and adolescents. *Pediatr Pulmonol*. 1996;21: 176-183.
86. Wieckowska A, Feldstein AE. Nonalcoholic fatty liver disease in the pediatric population: a review. *Curr Opin Pediatr*. 2005;17(5):636-641.
87. Swallen KC, Reither EN, Haas SA, et al. Overweight, obesity, and health-related quality of life among adolescents: The National Longitudinal Study of Adolescent Health. *Pediatrics*. 2005;115(2):340-347.
88. Crichlow RW, Seltzer MH, Jannetta PJ. Cholecystitis in adolescents. *Dig Dis*. 1972;17:68-72.
89. Lauer RM, Connor WE, Leaverton PE. Coronary heart disease risk factors in school children: The Muscatine Study. *J Pediatr*. 1975;86:697-706.
90. Calle EE, Kaaks R. Overweight, obesity and cancer: epidemiological evidence and proposed mechanisms. *Nat Rev Cancer*. 2004;4(8):579-591.
91. Loder RT. The demographics of slipped capital femoral epiphysis. An international multicenter study. *Clin Orthop Relat Res*. Jan 1996322:8-27.
92. Buggs C, Rosenfield RL. Polycystic ovary syndrome in adolescence. *Endocrinol Metab Clin North Am*. 2005; 34(3):677-705.
93. Baldridge AD, Perez-Atayde AR, Graeme-Cook F, et al. Idiopathic steatohepatitis in childhood: A multicenter retrospective study. *J Pediatr*. 1995;127(5):700-704.
94. Whitaker RC. Mental health and obesity in pediatric primary care: a gap between importance and action. *Arch Pediatr Adolesc Med*. 2004;158(8):826-828.
95. Strauss RS, Pollack H. Social marginalization of overweight children. *Arch Pediatr Adolesc Med*. 2003;157: 746-752.
96. Goodman E, Whitaker RC. A prospective study of the role of depression in the development and persistence of adolescent obesity. *Pediatrics*. 2002;110(3):497-504.
97. Erickson SJ, Robinson TN, Haydel KF, et al. Are overweight children unhappy? *Arch Pediatr Adolesc Med*. 2000;154(3):931-935.
98. Eisenberg ME, Neumark-Sztainer D, Story M. Association of weight-based teasing and emotional well being among adolescents. *Arch Pediatr Adolesc Med*. 2003; 157(8):733-738.
99. Sturm R. The effects of obesity, smoking, and drinking on medical problems and costs. *Health Affairs*. 2002; 21(2):245-253.
100. Larsen PR, Kronenberg HM, Melmed S, et al, eds. *Williams Textbook of Endocrinology*. 10th ed. Philadelphia, PA: WB Saunders; 2003.
101. National Center for Biotechnology Information (NCBI). Online Mendelian Inheritance in Man (OMIM). Available at: www.ncbi.nlm.nih.gov/entrez/query.fcgi?db=omim. Accessed June 30, 2006.

102. National Center for Biotechnology Information (NCBI). Online Mendelian Inheritance in Man (OMIM). #176270 Prader-Willi Syndrome; PWS. Available at: www.ncbi.nlm.nih.gov/entrez/dispomim.cgi?id=176270. Accessed June 20, 2006.
103. National Center for Biotechnology Information (NCBI). Online Mendelian Inheritance in Man (OMIM). #209900 Bardet-Biedl Syndrome; BBS. Available at: www.ncbi.nlm.nih.gov/entrez/dispomim.cgi?id=209900. Accessed June 30, 2006.
104. National Center for Biotechnology Information (NCBI). Online Mendelian Inheritance in Man (OMIM). #210350 Biemond Syndrome II. Available at: www.ncbi.nlm.nih.gov/entrez/dispomim.cgi?id=210350. Accessed June 30, 2006.
105. National Center for Biotechnology Information (NCBI). Online Mendelian Inheritance in Man (OMIM). #203800 Alstrom Syndrome; ALMS. Available at: www.ncbi.nlm.nih.gov/entrez/dispomim.cgi?id=203800. Accessed June 30, 2006.
106. Consensus Panel of American Diabetes Association and American Academy of Pediatrics. Type 2 diabetes in children and adolescents. *Pediatrics*. 2000;105(3:1):671-680.
107. Koplan JP, Liverman CT, Kraak VA, eds. *Preventing Childhood Obesity: Health in the Balance*. Washington, DC: National Academies Press; 2005.
108. Council on Sports Medicine and Fitness and Council on School Health. Active healthy living: prevention of childhood obesity through increased physical activity. *Pediatrics*. 2006;117:1834-1842.
109. Rollnick S, Butler CC, McCambridge J, et al. Consultations about changing behaviour. *BMJ*. 2005;331(7522):961-963.

Chapter 300

OBSTRUCTIVE UROPATHY AND VESICOURETERAL REFLUX

Hiep T. Nguyen, MD

Impairment of urinary flow results in characteristic biological changes in the kidney, collectively known as *obstructive uropathy.* These changes include proliferation and myofibroblastic transformation of interstitial fibroblasts, expansion of extracellular matrix, loss of renal tubular cells, and decreased numbers of nephrons.[1,2] They may have a wide range of effects on the kidney, from sodium wasting, hyperkalemic acidosis, and nephrogenic diabetes insipidus to renal insufficiency or failure. Their impact on renal growth, development, and function depends on the timing, severity, and duration of the urinary obstruction. Obstruction that occurs early during renal development will lead to dysplasia and an arrest of renal development with the persistence of fetal architecture. In contrast, obstruction at the later stages of development may result only in dilatation of the collecting system (ie, hydronephrosis). Complete obstruction, such as from urethral atresia, has more detrimental effects on renal development and function than partial obstruction.

Children with obstructive uropathy usually exhibit urinary tract infections (UTIs). Less common modes of presentation included abdominal mass, hematuria, urinary stone, poor urinary stream, incontinence, failure to thrive, and renal insufficiency or failure. With the advent of routine 2nd-trimester ultrasound (US) screening, most children with obstructive uropathy are now being detected prenatally. The incidence of prenatal hydronephrosis ranges from 1:100 to 1:500,[3] representing one half of all abnormalities detected by prenatal US. However, clinical experience has shown that the presence of hydronephrosis does not necessarily indicate the presence of urinary obstruction. The dilemma lies in determining which patients have dilatation that has the potential for compromising renal function. The ability to diagnose clinically important obstruction properly is essential because obstructive uropathy is the leading cause of renal failure in children younger than 2 years and accounts for 17% of the cases of kidney transplants in children.[4]

DIFFERENTIAL DIAGNOSIS

Obstruction can develop at various locations, resulting in dilatation of urinary tract (ie, hydronephrosis). The differential diagnosis for hydronephrosis is listed in Box 300-1. Ureteropelvic junction (UPJ) obstruction occurs when an impairment of urine flow occurs from the renal pelvis into the proximal ureter, causing progressive dilatation of the renal pelvis and calyces and potential renal injury. Its anatomic basis is from either an intrinsic or an extrinsic cause. The intrinsic obstruction results from luminal narrowing of the UPJ, with or without kinking, and usually characterized by excessive connective tissue and decreased smooth muscle content in the ureteral wall[5] (Figure 300-1, *A*). In contrast, extrinsic obstruction is caused by compression of the ureter by anomalous

BOX 300-1 Differential Diagnosis for Hydronephrosis

UNILATERAL
- Ureteropelvic junction obstruction
- Ureterovesical junction obstruction
- Ureterocele
- Ectopic ureter
- Polycystic kidney disease
- Extrarenal pelvis
- Unilateral vesicoureteral reflux
- Transient physiologic-nonpathological

BILATERAL
- Posterior urethral valves
- Urethral atresia
- Prune belly syndrome
- Megacystis-megaureter syndrome
- Vesicoureteral reflux
- Polycystic kidney disease

UNCOMMON CAUSES
- Megacalycosis
- Renal cyst
- Urachal cyst
- Ovarian cyst
- Hydrocolpos
- Sacrococcygeal teratoma
- Bowel duplication
- Duodenal atresia
- Anterior meningocele

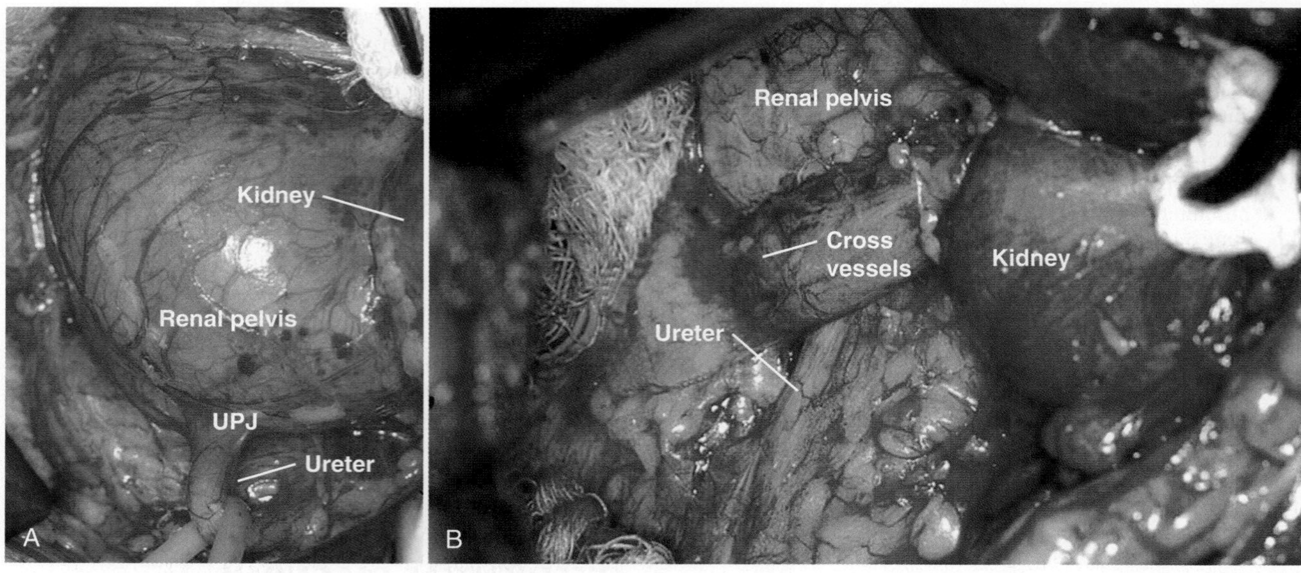

Figure 300-1 **A**, Intrinsic ureteropelvic junction obstruction. **B**, Extrinsic ureteropelvic junction obstruction cause by crossing vessels.

Table 300-1 Etiology of Prenatal Hydronephrosis

ETIOLOGY	REPORTED INCIDENCE
Transient physiologic-nonpathological	50-70%
Ureteropelvic junction obstruction	10-40%
Vesicoureteral reflux	10-30%
Ureterovesical junction obstruction	5-20%
Multicystic dysplastic kidney	2-5%
Posterior urethral valves	1-5%
Other*	<1%

*Other causes include ureterocele, ectopic ureter, duplex system, urethral atresia, prune belly, polycystic kidney disease, and renal cysts.

(eg, lower pole) renal vasculature (Figure 300-1, *B*). This type of UPJ obstruction is more commonly found in older children and adults.[6] UPJ obstruction is the most common cause of obstructive uropathy in children and is second only to transient, physiologic nonpathologic hydronephrosis as the most common cause of antenatal hydronephrosis[7] (Table 300-1). The incidence of UPJ obstruction is estimated to be 1 in 1500, with a male-to-female ratio of 2:1.[8] The left side is more commonly affected than the right side (left-right ratio of 1.5:1).[9] Bilateral UPJ obstruction is present in 10% to 40% of the cases of neonatal hydronephrosis.[7]

Ureterovesical junction (UVJ) obstruction, also referred to as *obstructed megaureter*, occurs when an impairment of urinary flow occurs from the distal ureter into the bladder, resulting in dilatation of the entire collecting system from the distal ureter to calyces. UVJ obstruction may be primary or secondary.

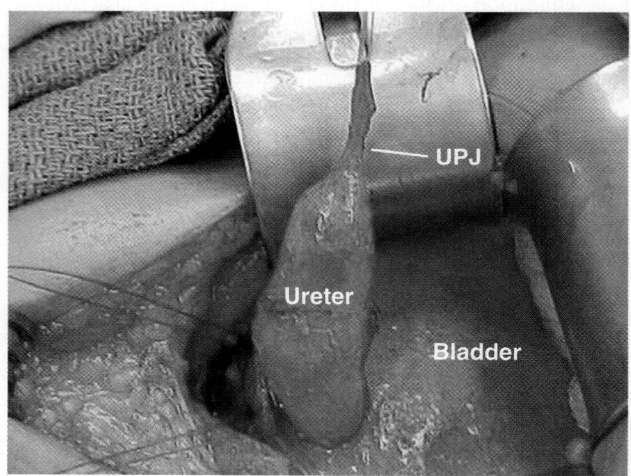

Figure 300-2 Primary ureterovesical junction obstruction.

Primary obstruction is due to a deficiency of smooth muscle in the intravesical ureter, resulting in an adynamic distal segment that impedes normal peristalsis of urine through the ureter[10] (Figure 300-2). Secondary obstruction results from extrinsic compression of the ureter by a thick bladder wall in pathological states such as posterior urethral valves (PUVs) or neurogenic bladder. Clinically significant UVJ obstruction accounts for approximately 8% of children who had symptoms such as infection, hematuria, or pain and who were found to have hydroureteronephrosis by imaging studies.[11] However, it accounts for 23% of newborns with prenatally diagnosed hydronephrosis and is the 3rd most common cause of prenatal

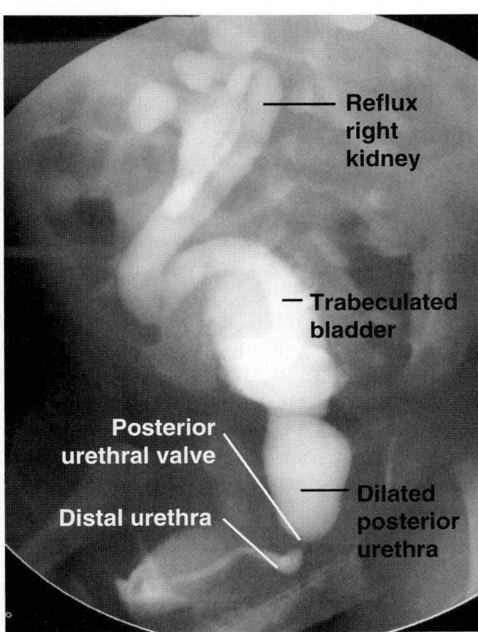

Figure 300-3 Voiding cystourethrogram demonstrating posterior urethral valves as a cause for bladder outlet obstruction.

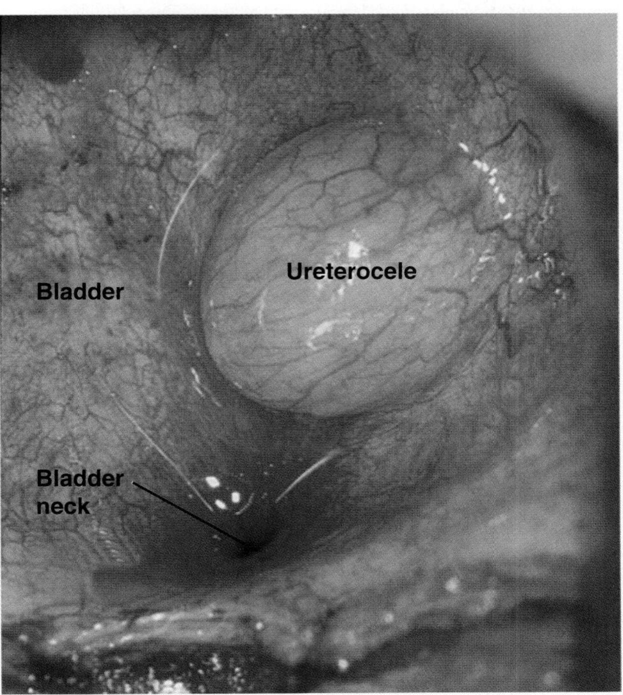

Figure 300-4 Ureterocele.

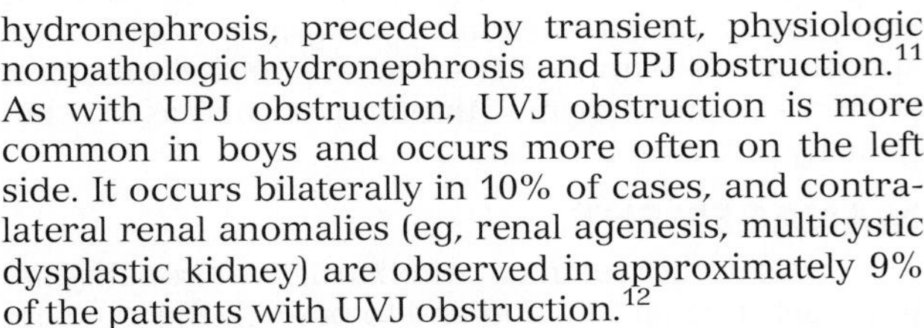

hydronephrosis, preceded by transient, physiologic nonpathologic hydronephrosis and UPJ obstruction.[11] As with UPJ obstruction, UVJ obstruction is more common in boys and occurs more often on the left side. It occurs bilaterally in 10% of cases, and contralateral renal anomalies (eg, renal agenesis, multicystic dysplastic kidney) are observed in approximately 9% of the patients with UVJ obstruction.[12]

Lower urinary tract obstructions are a less common cause of obstructive uropathy. The most common cause of infravesical obstruction is PUV. One hypothesis suggests that the terminal ends of the wolffian ducts mismigrate and are abnormally integrated into the urethral wall. This action results in obliquely oriented ridges that act as a one-way valve, impeding urine flow from the bladder[13] (Figure 300-3). The incidence of PUV is estimated to be 1 in 5000 to 1 in 8000 boys.[14]

Other notable but uncommon causes of obstructive uropathy include ureterocele and ectopic ureter. A ureterocele is a cystic dilatation of the intravesical submucosal ureter, usually associated with a stenotic orifice that impairs urinary flow into the bladder (Figure 300-4). The cause of the ureterocele remains unknown, but investigators hypothesize that it results either from an incomplete breakdown of the ureteral (Chwalla) membrane present at the time of ureteral bud arising from the mesonephric duct[15] or from a delay in the establishment of the lumen of the ureteral bud.[16,17] The incidence of ureteroceles is approximately 1 in 500 to 1 in 4000 children. Ureteroceles are found more commonly in girls (female-male ratio of 7:1)[18] and are bilateral in 10% of the cases.[18] In 80% of the cases, they are associated with the upper pole ureter of a duplex kidney.[19] An ectopic ureter is one that inserts into an abnormal site (ie, a site other than the bladder trigone), which results from a ureteral bud with an abnormally high origin from the mesonephric duct. In boys, the possible insertion sites for the ectopic ureter are always above the urinary sphincter, whereas in girls, they can be above or below the sphincter. Consequently, ectopic ureters in boys are often obstructive, whereas those in girls may not be. The incidence of ectopic ureter is approximately 1 in 1900.[13] Only 15% of the ectopic ureter occur in boys,[20] and in 80% of the cases, the ectopic ureter is associated with the upper pole of a duplex kidney. It occurs bilaterally in approximately 10% of cases.[21] Hypoplasia or dysplasia of the associated renal unit is commonly associated with the ectopic ureter.

RADIOLOGIC EVALUATION

Before the advent of routine maternal US, children with obstructive uropathy primarily displayed symptoms such as febrile UTI, abdominal mass, pyuria, pain, hematuria, and gastrointestinal symptoms. Less common presenting symptoms include failure to thrive, anemia, sudden onset of hypertension, and renal insufficiency or failure.

A renal and bladder US should be performed first. In children with obstructive uropathy, hydronephrosis is almost always present. However, its presence should not be interpreted as a sign of clinically significant obstruction because US cannot adequately assess renal function and drainage of the upper urinary tract. Although increased echogenicity and marked parenchymal thinning may portend poor renal function,

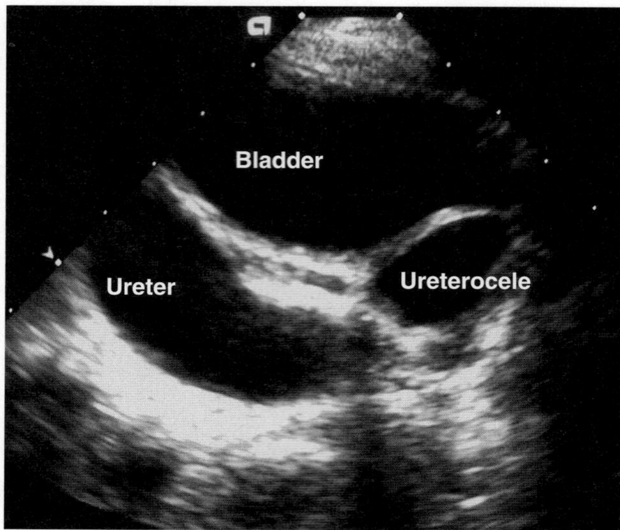

Figure 300-5 Ultrasound demonstrating dilated ureter seen behind bladder caused by ureterocele.

these findings are not sensitive or specific.[22] Aside from the presence of hydronephrosis, the US may help differentiate the cause of obstructive uropathy. The presence of a dilated ureter on US suggests that the level of obstruction occurs distal to the UPJ, such as from UVJ obstruction, ectopic ureter, ureterocele, or PUV (Figure 300-5). A ureterocele can be visualized as a cystic mass inside the bladder, whereas the presence of a thick wall bladder and a dilated posterior urethra suggests the diagnosis of PUV.

To identify the cause of the obstructive uropathy and to assess renal function accurately, additional imaging studies are often required. A voiding cystourethrogram (VCUG) will identify the presence of vesicoureteral reflux (VUR), a condition that may cause hydronephrosis itself but is found in association with other diagnoses of obstructive uropathy, including UPJ obstruction, ureterocele, and PUV. In addition, a VCUG will help delineate bladder and urethral anomalies such as ureterocele and PUV, respectively. Renal function can be assessed with radionuclide renography. ^{99m}Tc dimercaptosuccinic acid (DMSA) provides the most accurate assessment of renal function and the presence of renal scarring. ^{99m}Tc diethylenetriaminepentaacetic acid and ^{99m}Tc mercuroacetyltriglycine diuretic renography are less accurate in determining renal function[23] but do provide an assessment of drainage and a quantitative measurement of the degree of obstruction (ie, $t_{1/2}$, the time required to achieve 50% clearance of pyelocaliceal activity in the region of interest). However, debate remains about the accuracy of using $t_{1/2}$ in diagnosing obstruction.[24] Diuretic renography should only be obtained in children at least 2 months of age (because of tubular function maturation) who have moderate or severe hydronephrosis; in these cases, the studies are the most informative. Intravenous pyelogram is an alternative study that can provide assessment of both renal function and anatomy. However, its use in children is limited because of the amount of radiation exposure and the presence of bowel gas, which interferes with the visualization of the urinary tract.

With the advent of routine prenatal US, many children with obstructive uropathy are now detected in utero with hydronephrosis before they develop symptoms. However, not all children with prenatal hydronephrosis have obstructive uropathy; most have transient or physiological hydronephrosis that often resolves during pregnancy or after birth and do not have any clinical sequelae. Consequently, not all children with prenatal hydronephrosis require extensive radiologic evaluation. If the hydronephrosis persists during pregnancy, then a postnatal US after 48 hours is indicated. In severe cases, such as bilateral moderate to severe hydronephrosis, solitary kidney, oligohydramnios, or giant hydronephrosis, the postnatal US should be done sooner. Because patients with high-grade VUR can have normal US without any hydronephrosis, whether patients with prenatal hydronephrosis should undergo a VCUG regardless the degree of hydronephrosis is a point of debate; the incidence of VUR in children with mild prenatal hydronephrosis was only 4.4% and was 14% in the moderate group.[25] Consequently, a VCUG in patients with mild prenatal hydronephrosis is not needed. However, a VCUG may be indicated if a dilated ureter is seen on US or other clinically significant obstructive uropathies such as UPJ obstruction or PUV are suspected. Additional radiographic evaluation with diuretic renography or intravenous pyelogram is limited to specific cases with moderate to severe hydronephrosis, marked parenchymal, thinning, or increased echogenicity noted on US.

MANAGEMENT

The goals in the treatment of obstructive uropathy are to preserve renal function and to prevent the development of associated complications such as UTI, pain, and stone formation. Although, in some cases, the hydronephrosis can spontaneously resolve as the child grows, in other cases, it persists, leading to progressive renal compromise. Consequently, the primary care physician must determine which patients will benefit from surgical intervention and which should be observed, with the expectation that hydronephrosis will resolve without compromising renal function. In many instances, making this determination is difficult, leading to controversies in the management of obstructive uropathy.

In the management of UPJ obstruction, patients with a severely dilated renal pelvis (anteroposterior >2 cm on US), decreased renal function (relative renal function >40%), and marked obstructed pattern on renography ($t_{1/2}$ >20 minutes) should undergo surgical correction.[26] Surgical correction is accomplished by either removing the stenotic or adynamic UPJ or transposing the ureter anterior to the lower pole-crossing vessels. Other indications for surgery include UTI, renal colic, or pulmonary compromise from giant hydronephrosis. Patients with moderate to severe hydronephrosis but preserved renal function may be managed without surgery. The hydronephrosis will resolve in many cases, although it may take several years. In a minority of cases, declining renal function may occur, necessitating surgery. However, in most cases, renal function is recovered after surgery, suggesting that the risk to the obstructed kidney from conservative management is small.

In the management of UVJ obstruction, removal of the distal adynamic segment of the ureter with or without ureteral tapering is indicated in patients with symptoms who seek care for UTI, pain, or nausea and vomiting.[12] In patients who are asymptomatic (ie, diagnosed by evaluation of prenatal hydronephrosis), observation and prophylactic antibiotics have been shown to be safe, allowing for spontaneous regression of the obstruction without a compromise in renal function and minimizing the risk of UTI. Most symptoms will resolve spontaneously.[27] Occasionally, infants with UVJ obstruction diagnosed in the evaluation for prenatal hydronephrosis have greatly decreased renal function at the onset. In these patients, surgical correction is indicated. Although renal function after the procedure is preserved, it is never normalized.

Lower urinary tract obstruction, such as from PUV, usually requires more urgent intervention because both kidneys are at risk. In patients with suspected PUV, catheter drainage is needed until the diagnosis is confirmed and surgical correction can be performed. Stabilization of the patient's pulmonary status (particularly in newborns diagnosed in utero with oligohydramnios), correction of associated metabolic abnormalities, and treatment of UTI should be performed before any surgical intervention. In most patients, endoscopic fulguration of the PUV relieves the bladder outlet obstruction. However, a vesicostomy or alternative treatment such as ablation with a Fogarty balloon may be required in very small or premature infants when endoscopic procedure cannot be performed because of the size of the instruments.

Long-term therapy is directed toward the identification and treatment of associated metabolic abnormalities and bladder dysfunction. After the PUV are treated, the patients may develop postobstructive diuresis with urine output as high as 15 mL/kg/hour; careful attention to the patient's fluid balance is therefore essential after the relief of distal obstruction. Renal insufficiency and failure can occur in up to 50% of patients with PUV. Children with PUV who have a nadir creatinine of more than 0.8 mg/dL at 1 year of age are at high risk of developing renal insufficiency or failure.[28] Not uncommonly, children with PUV and renal insufficiency lack the ability to concentrate their urine to a specific gravity of more than 1.015, leading to excessive fluid loss. These patients may also develop renal salt wasting and metabolic acidosis with hyperkalemia. In these patients, minor gastrointestinal illness can result in severe dehydration and cardiovascular compromise. In addition to the associated metabolic complications, bladder dysfunction is often associated with PUV despite adequate relief of the obstruction. VUR occurs in approximately 30% to 75% of children with PUV.[29,30] Antibiotic prophylaxis is indicated in children with PUV and VUR because improvement in the grade of the reflux occurs with time in most patients. The valve bladder is often poorly compliant and functionally lacks normal sensation. Consequently, many patients with PUV are able to hold large urine volumes at high intravesical pressures. With time, this circumstance can lead to increased upper tract dilatation and pressure and progressive renal compromise. Early treatment of the valve bladder with anticholinergic medications, intermittent catheterization, and nighttime drainage appear to reduce the incidence of bladder and renal dysfunction.[31]

In the management of ureterocele and ectopic ureter, surgical correction is usually needed. As in the management of the other types of the obstructive uropathy, urgent surgical correction is indicated in patients who are symptomatic. In children diagnosed during the evaluation for prenatal hydronephrosis, the type and timing of surgical correction are controversial. Long-term follow-up is needed to evaluate renal function and to look for recurrent obstruction. Hypertension and proteinuria can develop in patients with renal insufficiency or dysplasia. Consequently, yearly blood pressure and urinalysis are indicated in all patients with obstructive uropathy.

Fetal intervention for obstructive uropathy is indicated only in specific cases. The goal of fetal intervention is to prevent pulmonary hypoplasia and to preserve renal function. Open fetal surgery, percutaneous vesicoamniotic shunt placement, and fetoscopic surgery have been used with varying success in the treatment of obstructive uropathy such as PUV. Because of the inherent risks of the procedure for the fetus and the mother, fetal intervention should be considered only in cases in which pulmonary or renal dysfunction can be identified and cases in which the treatment of obstructive uropathy will improve pulmonary and renal function. In most cases, obstruction occurs unilaterally; thus overall renal function and hence pulmonary function are normal, and fetal intervention is not indicated. In cases of lower urinary tract obstruction or bilateral obstruction, assessment of renal function should be performed to determine whether fetal intervention is warranted. Serial measurements of urine electrolytes are helpful in assessing fetal renal function.[32] Healthy fetal kidneys produce hypotonic urine, whereas those that are impaired produce isotonic urine. Consequently, increased urine sodium, chloride, and osmolality suggest the presence of renal damage or dysplasia. Favorable prognosis for good renal function is associated with sodium concentration less than 100 mEq/L, chloride less than 90 mEq/L, osmolality less than 210 mOsm/kg, and β_2-microglobulin less than 508 mmol/L.[33] Analysis of the urine obtained from serial bladder taps at 48- to 72-hour intervals better reflects renal function because the initial sample may be stagnant.[34]

The success of fetal intervention has been variable. Typically, normal amniotic fluid volume is restored, and an associated improvement in lung development is seen. Unfortunately, renal outcome is not significantly improved.[35-37] A high complication rate is associated with fetal intervention, including premature labor, inadequate drainage or migration of the shunt, perforation of fetal bowel or bladder, chorioamnionitis, iatrogenic gastroschisis, and bleeding. Currently, fetal intervention is primarily reserved for cases in which severe oligohydramnios occurs without associated renal dysplasia, poor renal function, or associated chromosomal anomalies.[38]

VESICOURETERAL REFLUX

Definition and Epidemiologic Features

VUR occurs when urine in the bladder flows in a retrograde manner into the upper urinary tracts. Under normal condition, the ureter passes obliquely through the bladder wall with an appropriate submucosal tunnel length and opens onto the trigone of the bladder in a correct location. VUR is prevented by the compression of the intravesical ureter against the bladder wall, which can be accomplished only with the appropriate UVJ anatomy. VUR may develop from maldevelopment or delayed maturity of the UVJ (primary reflux) or may result from distortion of the UVJ by changes in the bladder that are caused by other conditions, such as PUVs or neurogenic bladder (secondary reflux). Researchers have long recognized that an association exists between the presence of VUR and renal abnormalities, termed *reflux nephropathy*. The 3 forms of reflux nephropathy are (1) renal scarring associated with intrarenal reflux of infected urine (commonly seen in older children with primary reflux), (2) congenital nephropathy associated with VUR but in the absence of infection (commonly seen in infants with primary reflux) and (3) nephropathy associated with VUR and impairment of urinary flow (commonly seen in children with secondary reflux).

VUR is most often identified after investigation for other urinary tract problems such as UTI and prenatal hydronephrosis or in evaluation of a family history of VUR. The prevalence of VUR in children without any UTI or urologic anomalies is believed to be from 0.4% to 1.8% of the pediatric population.[39] In children with UTI, the prevalence ranges from 30% to 50%,[40-42] whereas in children with prenatal hydronephrosis, it is approximately 25%.[43] VUR appears to be heritable; 50% to 67% of the children of parents with VUR[44] and 33% to 50% of the siblings of children with VUR[45] will have the condition. The incidence of VUR is significantly lower in blacks than it is in whites.[46] Similarly, the incidence of VUR is much lower in boys than it is in girls.[47] However, in infants younger than 1 year, the proportions of boys and girls with VUR are more equivalent.[48] In children with UTI, the ratio of girls to boys with VUR is approximately 4:1, whereas in infants evaluated for prenatal hydronephrosis, the ratio is the reverse.

Differential Diagnosis

VUR is diagnosed after evaluation for UTI, prenatal hydronephrosis, or family history of reflux. Less common modes of presentation include hypertension, renal insufficiency or failure, or incidental findings of a small or scarred kidney or hydronephrosis observed on radiologic imaging tests such as US, computed tomography, or magnetic resonance imaging. Young children with UTIs frequently have generalized signs and symptoms such as fever, vomiting, and failure to thrive. Older children may exhibit more specific signs and symptoms for UTI, such as flank pain, dysuria, and gross hematuria. Differentiating between UTI and other causes of sepsis may be difficult, particularly in young infants. Considerable debate exists as to which children with UTI require a VCUG to rule out VUR. In general, young children, especially boys with a febrile UTI, should be evaluated by VCUG because the incidence of VUR in this group ranges from 30% to 50%.[40-42,49] In contrast, older girls with cystitis, nonfebrile UTI, or asymptomatic bacteriuria are less likely to have VUR[49] and consequently do not always require a VCUG for evaluation. Similarly, whether all children with prenatally diagnosed hydronephrosis require a VCUG to rule out reflux is controversial. The incidence of VUR is low in children with mild hydronephrosis detected on prenatal US, but it increases with the moderate and severe grades.[25] Consequently, a VCUG should be performed in children with a history of moderate or severe hydronephrosis observed on prenatal US. Additional indications for a VCUG include findings on prenatal US of a dilated ureter, abnormal bladder wall thickness, renal echogenicity, renal parenchymal thinning, or decreased amniotic fluid volume.

As indicated previously, a strong genetic component exists in the development of VUR. Consequently, screening for reflux in families with VUR is indicated, with the goal of identifying these children early and decreasing their risk of developing long-term complications from VUR. Screening with a radionuclide cystogram (RNC) should be performed in siblings or offspring who are younger than 5 years. They are the ones with the highest likelihood of having VUR and have the greatest risk of developing renal scarring from pyelonephritis. In older siblings or offspring who have never had any UTIs, a screening US would be sufficient. If a history of UTI or hydronephrosis were present, or if evidence of parenchymal thinning were present on the screening US, then a RNC would be indicated.

Evaluation

In the evaluation for UTI or prenatal hydronephrosis, an US is usually first obtained. However, US cannot confirm the presence or absence of reflux because severe reflux may be present in the absence of any significant hydronephrosis (Figure 300-6). In children, the VCUG remains the principal method of detecting and quantifying the degree of VUR. A VCUG is performed by placing a urethral catheter into the bladder, instilling a contrast agent, and obtaining images of the bladder and kidneys during filling and voiding. VUR is diagnosed when contrast instilled into the bladder is detected in the ureter or upper urinary tract (Figure 300-7). The degree of VUR is quantified by the International Reflux Study Group classification system (Table 300-2). In addition to detecting and quantifying the degree of VUR, the VCUG also helps identify other bladder and urethral anomalies, such as PUVs, ureterocele, bladder diverticula, and neurogenic bladder, that may cause secondary reflux.

With the conventional fluoroscopic VCUG, images are captured at fixed time points, and episodic reflux might thus be missed. Consequently, especially in infants, a fill-void cycle should be repeated at least

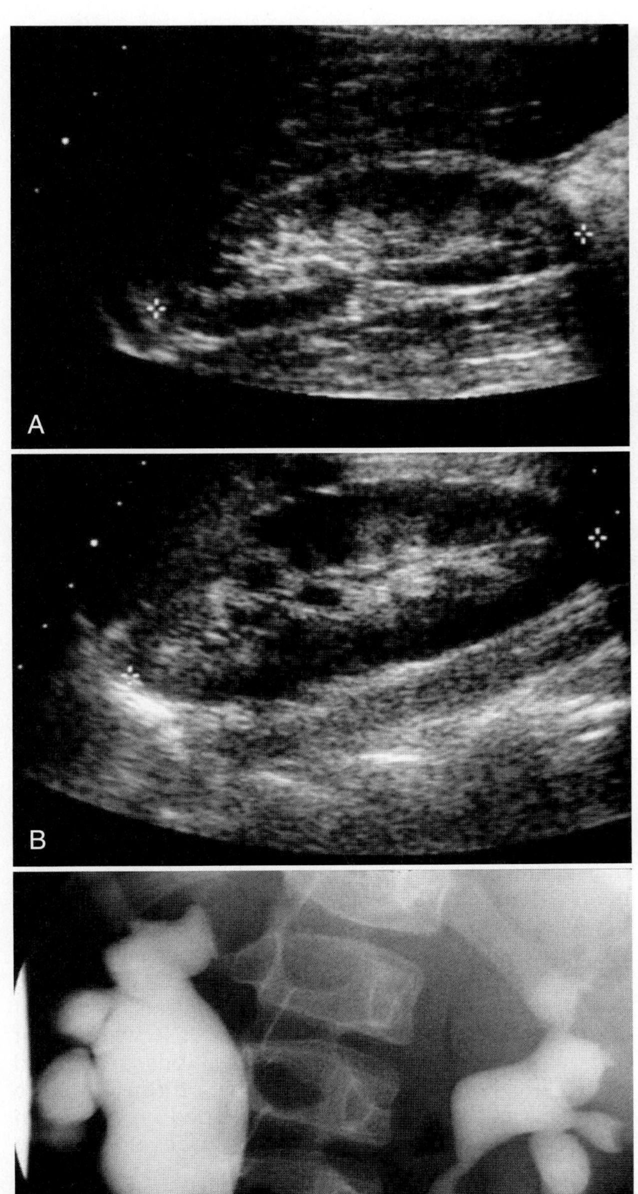

Figure 300-6 Normal ultrasound of the right and left kidneys despite the presence of high-grade vesicoureteral reflux as seen on voiding cystourethrogram.

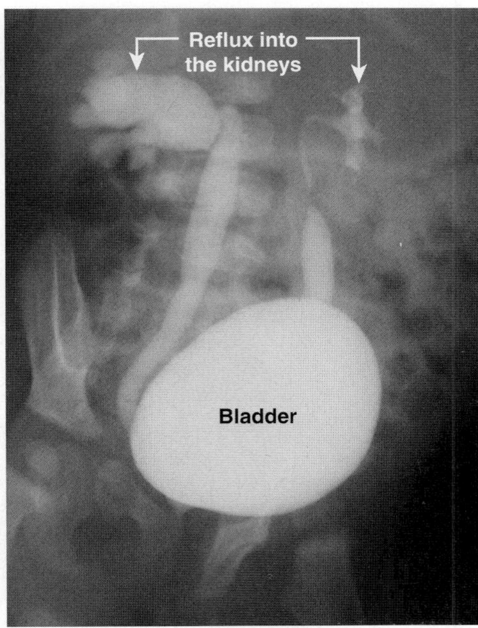

Figure 300-7 Vesicoureteral reflux seen on voiding cystourethrogram.

Table 300-2 International Reflux Study Classification System for Vesicoureteral Reflux

GRADE	REFLUX INTO URETER	REFLUX INTO CALICES
I	Distal segment only	None
II	Without tortuosity	Without distention
III	With minimal tortuosity	With mild distention
IV	With moderate tortuosity	With moderate distention
V	With severe tortuosity	With severe distention

once during the test to improve the sensitivity of the VCUG in detecting VUR. An alternative imaging test is the RNC. A radioisotope (eg, DTPA) is placed in the bladder, and the bladder, kidneys and ureters are continuously monitored (Figure 300-8). Because the imaging is continuous, the sensitivity in detecting reflux with a RNC is increased compared with fluoroscopic VCUG. In addition, the use of the RNC exposes the patient to less radiation compared with conventional VCUG. However, the anatomic details (eg, grade of reflux and associated urethra, bladder abnormalities) cannot be resolved well with RNC. VCUG should thus be used as the initial study to identify and characterize the reflux; RNC should then be used for follow-up studies.[50] The VCUG should be performed after the infection has resolved and a repeat urine culture is negative. Instrumentation while the infection is still active may lead to sepsis.

Because renal parenchymal abnormalities are found in association with VUR, proper functional imaging of the kidneys is indicated in patients with reflux. Although US is not invasive or costly, its ability to detect renal abnormalities such as dysplasia and scarring is limited.[51] Renal scanning by DMSA provides an accurate assessment of renal development and permits evaluation for the presence of renal scarring resulting from UTI[52,53] (Figure 300-9). In the past, intravenous pyelogram has been used to assess renal

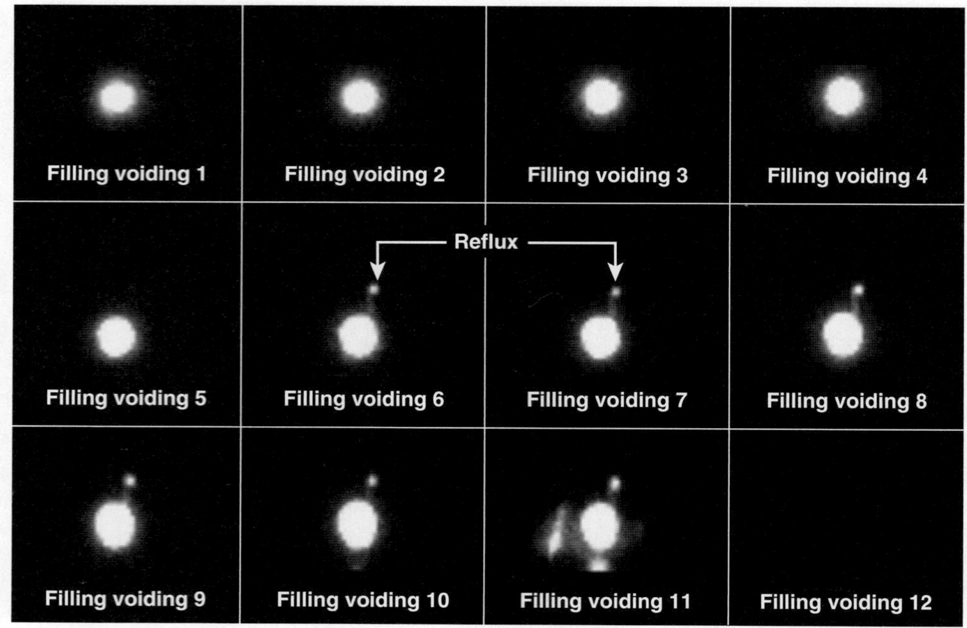

Figure 300-8 Vesicoureteral reflux seen on nuclear cystogram.

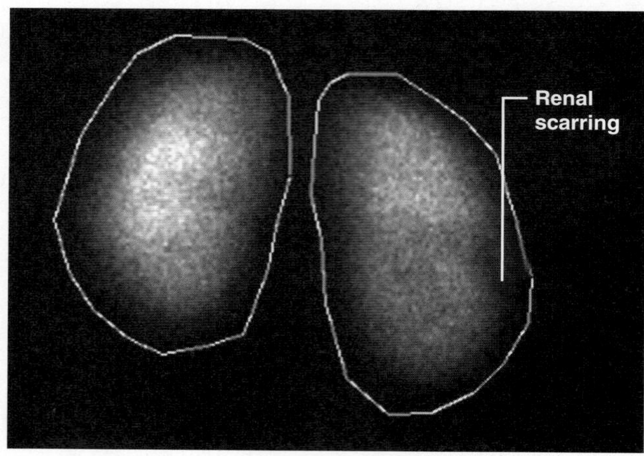

Figure 300-9 ^{99m}Tc dimercaptosuccinic acid renal scan demonstrating renal scarring in a patient with vesicoureteral reflux.

parenchymal abnormalities. However, it has been replaced by renal scintigraphy as the gold standard because of the increased sensitivity of DMSA scans in detecting renal scarring.[52,54] Not all children with VUR require imaging with renal scintigraphy. Renal abnormalities such as scarring and dysplasia are more often found in children with at least 1 UTI[55] and in those with higher grades of reflux (grade III and above)[56]; therefore renal scintigraphy is indicated for children with VUR who have at least 1 episode of UTI and those with at least grade III VUR.

Management

In most patients, VUR will resolve spontaneously without requiring surgical intervention. Consequently, medical therapy should be instituted, with the goal of preventing the long-term complications associated with VUR such as renal scarring, hypertension, and renal insufficiency or failure by the prevention of UTI. The generally accepted theory asserts that the use of chronic low-dose antibiotic prophylaxis can prevent UTI and thus prevent the complications associated with VUR. In children with VUR who did not receive prophylactic antibiotics, 21% developed new scars in previously normal kidneys, and 66% developed new scars in previously scarred kidneys.[57] More importantly, predicting which children would and would not develop renal scarring is impossible. In children with similar grades of reflux but receiving antibiotic prophylaxis, no progression of renal scars occurs unless a breakthrough UTI is present. The current suggestions for antibiotic prophylaxis are summarized in Table 300-3. Antibiotic prophylaxis should be maintained until VUR has resolved spontaneously or after surgical correction. In children older than 7 to 8 years who have persistent low-grade VUR but have not had any recent UTIs, observation while they are no longer receiving antibiotic prophylaxis may be tried because the risk of renal scarring in these children is low.[58] Antibiotic prophylaxis can be used as long as no breakthrough UTIs or compliance issues occur. Length of therapy varies depending on parental preference and the likelihood of reflux resolution. When reflux resolution seems unlikely, stopping the antibiotics and correcting the reflux should be considered. Debate is ongoing about whether to use alternating antibiotic prophylaxis versus monotherapy. Most providers use monotherapy, and very little evidence has

Table 300-3 Antibiotic Prophylaxis Suggestions

AGE	MEDICATION	DOSAGE
<3 mo	Amoxicillin	25 mg/kg once a day
	Cephalexin	25 mg/kg once a day
>3 mo	Trimethoprim alone or in combination with sulfa	2 mg/kg once a day
	Nitrofurantoin	1-2 mg/kg once a day (not to exceed 100 mg/day)

been found in the literature that suggests alternating antibiotic prophylaxis is more effective than monotherapy. In teenagers with reflux, a trial of antibiotic is reasonable; however, their chance of resolution is believed to be somewhat lower.

The spontaneous resolution rate of VUR depends on several factors, including the grade of the reflux, laterality, sex, and mode of presentation. In general, low-grade VUR is more likely to resolve than high-grade reflux (grades I and II, 70% to 80% resolution rate; grade III, 50%; grades IV and V, >30%).[59] Bilateral high-grade VUR tends to resolve less often than unilateral high-grade VUR.[60] VUR in girls tend to resolve at a slower rate than in boys.[60] High-grade VUR detected after evaluation for prenatal hydronephrosis tends to resolve more quickly than that detected after evaluation for UTIs. In patients with sibling reflux, the rate of resolution is similar to the probands, with grade as the primary determining factor.[61]

Voiding dysfunction can greatly affect the resolution rate of VUR. Voiding abnormalities such as detrusor instability or detrusor-sphincter dyssynergy can impede the resolution of reflux, and in some patients, it can worsen its severity with time. Consequently, in the medical management of reflux, symptoms for dysfunctional voiding such as urinary urgency and incontinence must be ascertained, and treatment of dysfunctional voiding with timed voiding, anticholinergic therapy, or both needs to be instituted. Similarly, constipation can increase the risk of UTI and delay the resolution of VUR. Aggressive treatment of constipation will help to decrease the risk of UTI and improve voiding function.

In some patients, surgical correction for VUR may be required. Recurrent UTI while receiving prophylactic antibiotic therapy is an indication for surgical correction because protection from renal scarring cannot be adequately achieved with medical management. Additional indications for surgery include lack of compliance with a medical regimen, low probability of spontaneous resolution of reflux (eg, in older children with higher-grade reflux), new renal scar formation while receiving prophylaxis, and anatomic abnormalities such as a paraureteral diverticulum. The overall rate of surgical correction in a general population of children with all grades of VUR ranges from 13% to 20%.[62-64] The types of surgical correction include transurethral (endoscopic), laparoscopic, and open techniques. The open antireflux procedures have a high success rate (98%) but often require a few days of hospitalization and subsequent recovery time. In contrast, the endoscopic techniques have much lower associated morbidity and shorter recovery time; however, its success rates are not as good as that of open surgery.[65,66]

In the management of reflux, the goal is not merely to prevent UTIs and to determine whether VUR has resolved. The primary care physician should monitor children for long-term complications such as reflux nephropathy. Approximately 10% of children and 50% of adults with renal scarring will develop hypertension.[67] In addition, estimates suggest that approximately 10% of children with reflux nephropathy will develop end-stage renal disease, and 90% will have diminished glomerular filtration rate.[68] Consequently, blood pressure and urinary protein levels should be measured periodically if renal scarring is present. Women with a history of VUR and in particular with reflux nephropathy should be monitored closely during pregnancy because of the increased rates of pyelonephritis, toxemia, preterm delivery, fetal growth retardation, fetal loss, and decreased maternal renal function.[69-71]

TOOLS FOR PRACTICE

Engaging Patient and Family

- *What is a Pediatric Nephrologist?* (fact sheet), American Academy of Pediatrics (www.aap.org/family/WhatisPedNephrologist.pdf).
- *What is a Pediatric Urologist?* (fact sheet), American Academy of Pediatrics (www.aap.org/sections/sap/he3010.pdf).

AAP POLICY STATEMENT

American Urological Association, Vesicoureteral Reflux Clinical Guidelines Panel. The report on the management of vesicoureteral reflux in children. *American Urological Association Clinical Guidelines*. 1997;1-91. AAP Endorsed. (aappolicy.aappublications.org/misc/Management_of_Primary_Vesicoureteral_Reflux_in_Children.dtl).

REFERENCES

1. Chevalier RL. Pathogenesis of renal injury in obstructive uropathy. *Curr Opin Pediatr.* 2006;18:153-160.
2. Nguyen HT, Kogan BA. Upper urinary tract obstruction: experimental and clinical aspects. *Br J Urol.* 1998;81(2):13-21.
3. Roth JA, Diamond DA. Prenatal hydronephrosis. *Curr Opin Pediatr.* 2001;13:138-141.
4. Seikaly MG, Ho PL, Emmett L, et al. Chronic renal insufficiency in children: the 2001 annual report of the NAPRTCS. *Pediatr Nephrol.* 2003;18:796-804.
5. Zhang PL, Peters CA, Rosen S. Ureteropelvic junction obstruction: morphological and clinical studies. *Pediatr Nephrol.* 2000;14:820-826.
6. Lowe FC, Marshall FF. Ureteropelvic junction obstruction in adults. *Urology.* 1984;23:331-335.
7. Lebowitz RL, Griscom NT. Neonatal hydronephrosis: 146 cases. *Radiol Clin North Am.* 1977;15:49-59.
8. Flashner SC, King LR. Ureteropelvic junction. In: Kelalis PP, King LR, Belman AB, eds. *Clinical Pediatric Urology.* Philadelphia, PA: WB Saunders; 1992.

9. Johnston JH, Evans JP, Glassberg KI, et al. Pelvic hydronephrosis in children: a review of 219 personal cases. *J Urol.* 1977;117:97-101.
10. Mackinnon KJ, Foote JW, Wiglesworth FW, et al. The pathology of the adynamic distal ureteral segment. *J Urol.* 1970;103:134-137.
11. Brown T, Mandell J, Lebowitz RL. Neonatal hydronephrosis in the era of sonography. *Am J Roentgenol.* 1987; 148:959-963.
12. Kass EJ. Megaureter. In: Kelalis PP, King LR, Belman AB, eds. *Clinical Pediatric Urology.* 3rd ed. Philadelphia, PA: WB Saunders; 1992.
13. Campbell MF. Anomalies of the ureters. In: Campbell MF, Harrison JH, eds. *Urology.* 3rd ed. Philadelphia, PA: WB Saunders; 1970.
14. Becker N, Avner ED. Congenital nephropathies and uropathies. *Pediatr Clin North Am.* 1995;42:1319-1341.
15. Chwalla R. The process of formation of cystic dilatations of the vesical end of the ureter and of diverticula at the ureteral ostium. *Urol Cutan Rev.* 1927;31:499-504.
16. Stephens D. Caecoureterocele and concepts on the embryology and aetiology of ureteroceles. *Aust N Z J Surg.* 1971;40:239-248.
17. Tanagho EA. Embryologic basis for lower ureteral anomalies: a hypothesis. *Urology.* 1976;7:451-464.
18. Eklof O, Lohr G, Ringertz H, et al. Ectopic ureterocele in the male infant. *Acta Radiol Diagn (Stockh).* 1978;19:145-153.
19. Brock WA, Kaplan GW. Ectopic ureteroceles in children. *J Urol.* 1978;119:800-803.
20. Schulman CC. [Ectopic implantations of the ureter]. *Acta Urol Belg.* 1972;40:201-478.
21. Ellerker AG. The extravesical ectopic ureter. *Br J Surg.* 1958;45:344-353.
22. Chi T, Feldstein VA, Nguyen HT. Increased echogenicity as a predictor of poor renal function in children with grade 3 to 4 hydronephrosis. *J Urol.* 2006;175:1898-1901.
23. Domingues FC, Fujikawa GY, Decker H, et al. Comparison of relative renal function measured with either ^{99m}Tc-DTPA or ^{99m}Tc-EC dynamic scintigraphies with that measured with ^{99m}Tc-DMSA static scintigraphy. *Int Braz J Urol.* 2006;32:405-409.
24. Conway JJ. "Well-tempered" diuresis renography: its historical development, physiological and technical pitfalls, and standardized technique protocol. *Semin Nucl Med.* 1992;22:74-84.
25. Lee RS, Cendron M, Kinnamon DD, et al. Antenatal hydronephrosis as a predictor of postnatal outcome: a meta-analysis. *Pediatrics.* 2006;118:586-593.
26. Ransley PG, Dhillon HK, Gordon I, et al. The postnatal management of hydronephrosis diagnosed by prenatal ultrasound. *J Urol.* 1990;144(2:2):584-587.
27. Baskin LS, Zderic SA, Snyder HM, et al. Primary dilated megaureter: long-term followup. *J Urol.* 1994;152(2:2): 618-621.
28. Ylinen E, Ala-Houhala M, Wikstrom S. Prognostic factors of posterior urethral valves and the role of antenatal detection. *Pediatr Nephrol.* 2004;19:874-879.
29. Close CE, Carr MC, Burns MW, et al. Lower urinary tract changes after early valve ablation in neonates and infants: is early diversion warranted? *J Urol.* 1997;157: 984-988.
30. Johnston JH. Vesicoureteric reflux with urethral valves. *Br J Urol.* 1979;51:100-104.
31. Glassberg KI. The valve bladder syndrome: 20 years later. *J Urol.* 2001;166:1406-1414.
32. Miguelez J, Bunduki V, Yoshizaki CT, et al. Fetal obstructive uropathy: is urine sampling useful for prenatal counseling? *Prenat Diagn.* 2006;26:81-84.
33. Vanderheyden T, Kumar S, Fisk NM. Fetal renal impairment. *Semin Neonatol.* 2003;8:279-289.
34. Nicolini U, Tannirandorn Y, Vaughan J, et al. Further predictors of renal dysplasia in fetal obstructive uropathy: bladder pressure and biochemistry of "fresh" urine. *Prenat Diagn.* 1991;11:159-166.
35. Biard JM, Johnson MP, Carr MC, et al. Long-term outcomes in children treated by prenatal vesicoamniotic shunting for lower urinary tract obstruction. *Obstet Gynecol.* 2005;106:503-508.
36. McLorie G, Farhat W, Khoury A, et al. Outcome analysis of vesicoamniotic shunting in a comprehensive population. *J Urol.* 2001;166:1036-1040.
37. Holmes N, Harrison MR, Baskin LS. Fetal surgery for posterior urethral valves: long-term postnatal outcomes. *Pediatrics.* 2001;108:E7.
38. Freedman AL, Johnson MP, Gonzalez R. Fetal therapy for obstructive uropathy: past, present, future? *Pediatr Nephrol.* 2000;14:167-176.
39. Bailey RR. Vesicoureteric reflux in healthy infants and children. In: Hodson J, Kincaid-Smith P, eds. *Reflux Nephropathy.* New York, NY: Masson; 1979.
40. Abbott GD. Neonatal bacteriuria: a prospective study in 1,460 infants. *Br Med J.* 1972;1(5795):267-269.
41. Smellie JM, Normand IC. [Clinical features and significance of urinary tract infection in children.]. *Proc R Soc Med.* 1966;59:415-416.
42. Winberg J, Andersen HJ, Bergstrom T, et al. Epidemiology of symptomatic urinary tract infection in childhood. *Acta Paediatr Scand Suppl.* 1974:1-20.
43. Thomas DF. Prenatally detected uropathy: epidemiological considerations. *Br J Urol.* 1998;81(2):8-12.
44. Noe HN, Wyatt RJ, Peeden JN Jr, et al. The transmission of vesicoureteral reflux from parent to child. *J Urol.* 1992; 148:1869-1871.
45. Noe HN. The long-term results of prospective sibling reflux screening. *J Urol.* 1992;148(5 pt 2):1739-1742.
46. Askari A, Belman AB. Vesicoureteral reflux in black girls. *J Urol.* 1982;127:747-748.
47. Smellie JM, Prescod NP, Shaw PJ, et al. Childhood reflux and urinary infection: a follow-up of 10-41 years in 226 adults. *Pediatr Nephrol.* 1998;12:727-736.
48. Clarke SE, Smellie JM, Prescod N, et al. Technetium-99m-DMSA studies in pediatric urinary infection. *J Nucl Med.* 1996;37:823-828.
49. Wein AJ, Schoenberg HW. A review of 402 girls with recurrent urinary tract infection. *J Urol.* 1972;107:329-331.
50. Belman AB. Vesicoureteral reflux. *Pediatr Clin North Am.* 1997;44:1171-1190.
51. Merguerian PA, Jamal MA, Agarwal SK, et al. Utility of SPECT DMSA renal scanning in the evaluation of children with primary vesicoureteral reflux. *Urology.* 1999; 53:1024-1028.
52. Goldraich NP, Ramos OL, Goldraich IH. Urography versus DMSA scan in children with vesicoureteric reflux. *Pediatr Nephrol.* 1989;3:1-5.
53. Rushton HG, Majd M, Jantausch B, et al. Renal scarring following reflux and nonreflux pyelonephritis in children: evaluation with ^{99m}technetium-dimercaptosuccinic acid scintigraphy. *J Urol.* 1992;147:1327-1332.
54. Elison BS, Taylor D, Van der Wall H, et al. Comparison of DMSA scintigraphy with intravenous urography for the detection of renal scarring and its correlation with vesicoureteric reflux. *Br J Urol.* 1992;69:294-302.
55. Orellana P, Baquedano P, Rangarajan V, et al. Relationship between acute pyelonephritis, renal scarring, and vesicoureteral reflux. Results of a coordinated research project. *Pediatr Nephrol.* 2004;19:1122-1126.
56. Nguyen HT, Bauer SB, Peters CA, et al. ^{99m}Technetium dimercapto-succinic acid renal scintigraphy abnormalities in infants with sterile high grade vesicoureteral reflux. *J Urol.* 2000;164:1674-1678.

57. Lenaghan D. Results of conservative treatment of vesicoureteric reflux in children. *Br J Urol.* 1970;42:736.
58. Thompson RH, Chen JJ, Pugach J, et al. Cessation of prophylactic antibiotics for managing persistent vesicoureteral reflux. *J Urol.* 2001;166:1465-1469.
59. Elder JS, Peters CA, Arant BS Jr, et al. Pediatric Vesicoureteral Reflux Guidelines Panel summary report on the management of primary vesicoureteral reflux in children. *J Urol.* 1997;157:1846-1851.
60. Wennerstrom M, Hansson S, Jodal U, et al. Disappearance of vesicoureteral reflux in children. *Arch Pediatr Adolesc Med.* 1998;152:879-883.
61. Kenda RB, Zupancic Z, Fettich JJ, et al. A follow-up study of vesico-ureteric reflux and renal scars in asymptomatic siblings of children with reflux. *Nucl Med Commun.* 1997;18:827-831.
62. Belman AB, Skoog SJ. Nonsurgical approach to the management of vesicoureteral reflux in children. *Pediatr Infect Dis J.* 1989;8:556-559.
63. Greenfield SP, Ng M, Wan J. Experience with vesicoureteral reflux in children: clinical characteristics. *J Urol.* 1997;158:574-577.
64. Koff SA, Wagner TT, Jayanthi VR. The relationship among dysfunctional elimination syndromes, primary vesicoureteral reflux and urinary tract infections in children. *J Urol.* 1998;160(3 pt 2):1019-1022.
65. Elder JS, Diaz M, Caldamone AA, et al. Endoscopic therapy for vesicoureteral reflux: a meta-analysis. I. Reflux resolution and urinary tract infection. *J Urol.* 2006;175:716-722.
66. Harrell WB, Snow BW. Endoscopic treatment of vesicoureteral reflux. *Curr Opin Pediatr.* 2005;17:409-411.
67. Dillon MJ, Goonasekera CD. Reflux nephropathy. *J Am Soc Nephrol.* 1998;9:2377-2383.
68. Jacobson SH, Eklof O, Lins LE, et al. Long-term prognosis of post-infectious renal scarring in relation to radiological findings in childhood—a 27-year follow-up. *Pediatr Nephrol.* 1992;6:19-24.
69. El-Khatib M, Packham DK, Becker GJ, et al. Pregnancy-related complications in women with reflux nephropathy. *Clin Nephrol.* 1994;41:50-55.
70. Jungers P, Houillier P, Chauveau D, et al. Pregnancy in women with reflux nephropathy. *Kidney Int.* 1996;50:593-599.
71. Weaver E, Craswell P. Pregnancy outcome in women with reflux nephropathy—a review of experience at the Royal Women's Hospital Brisbane, 1977-1986. *Aust N Z J Obstet Gynaecol.* 1987;27:106-111.

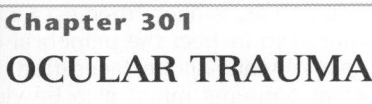

Chapter 301

OCULAR TRAUMA

Lisa I. Bohra, MD; Rajesh C. Rao, MD

INTRODUCTION

Accidental ocular trauma represents a major public health issue. Although only 5% of all eye injuries are serious enough to result in permanent visual loss, trauma still accounts for 40% of all cases of monocular blindness in the general population.[1] In addition to the obvious visual consequences, severe trauma in children can also present significant developmental and emotional challenges, especially if a cosmetic defect is present. Amblyopia can develop after injury in children younger than 8 years, placing an additional physical and psychological burden.[2]

Demographic data from several studies has demonstrated that boys are more susceptible to injury than girls, with a ratio of approximately 3 to 1.[3,4] Common sources of injury include sports, motor vehicle crashes, falls, projectiles, and other children. Among sports-related injuries, baseball was most common, followed by basketball, tennis, and hockey.[3] In children who had visual outcome of 20/200 or worse, BB guns, knives, and rocks were commonly implicated. Mandatory eye protection in organized sports such as hockey has significantly reduced eye injuries, but common sense precautions are not always exercised on the playground or at home. Most severe injuries occur in children with no eye protection, whereas only 5% occurred in those who were wearing safety glasses or regular glasses.[1] Primary care physicians and eye-care providers should actively educate parents and children regarding the importance of eye protection to prevent ocular injuries.

ANATOMIC CONSIDERATIONS

The orbit is a pear-shaped cavity in the skull that protects the globe from lateral injury. The orbital rim tends to absorb the impact of most blunt injury with large objects such as a ball or fist. The medial wall and orbital floor are thinner and susceptible to fracture, whereas the lateral wall is the thickest and strongest. The orbital roof is also the floor of the anterior cranial fossa; therefore an orbital roof fracture requires neurosurgical evaluation.[5] Any child with an orbital fracture must undergo a careful eye examination to rule out globe injury.

The eyelids protect the globe from debris and direct trauma involving smaller objects. The eyelids are also vital in maintaining a normal smooth tear film over the cornea. Injury to the eyelid, particularly if it involves the lid margin, can result in exposure of the cornea and lead to scarring or infection. Deeper injury to the lids can be associated with globe injury or injury to the levator muscle if the orbital septum has been violated. The lacrimal drainage system starts in the medial aspect of the upper and lower lid at the punctal opening and connects to the lacrimal sac and bony nasolacrimal duct via canaliculi. An eyelid injury medial to the punctal opening frequently results in a canalicular laceration, which requires surgical repair.

The globe rests in the orbit, cushioned by orbital fat and suspended by its attachment to extraocular muscles and surrounding elastic tissues. The exposed structures in the interpalpebral fissures are the cornea and conjunctiva, which are frequently involved in eye injuries. The cornea is 0.5 mm thick centrally and 1 mm thick at the periphery. A corneal injury that is limited to the epithelium often resolves without sequelae, whereas an injury that penetrates the epithelial basement membrane into the stroma can result in permanent scarring and vision loss. The bulbar conjunctiva extends from the corneal limbus and covers the sclera. It then forms the cul-de-sac or fornix and reflects over the inner surface of the eyelids as the palpebral conjunctiva. Hemorrhages in the subconjunctival space are usually benign but can hide deeper injuries to the sclera or extraocular muscles. The sclera covers the posterior four fifths of the globe and is largely avascular. It is 0.5 mm thick at the equator and 1.0 mm in thickness posteriorly. The sclera is thinnest (0.3 mm) just behind the insertion of the rectus muscles, making this area a common site for globe rupture after blunt trauma. The iris is the most anterior portion of the uveal tract, the vascular coat of the eye. Trauma can result in bleeding or tears in the iris, especially at its root where it is thinnest. The lens is located just behind the iris and is entirely covered by a capsule. Disruption of the capsule as a result of sharp or blunt trauma can compromise the clarity of the lens, resulting in a traumatic cataract.

The posterior segment of the eye comprises the posterior sclera, choroid, retina, and vitreous. The macula represents the critical central portion of the retina, which is responsible for fine visual acuity. Severe trauma can result in vitreous hemorrhage and retinal edema, as well as retinal tears and retinal detachment. Injury affecting the macula can result in severe central vision loss, whereas damage to the peripheral retina can be asymptomatic. In general, trauma affecting the posterior segment structures usually carries a worse prognosis for recovery than injury limited to the anterior segment.

EVALUATION

History

An accurate and detailed history is helpful in evaluating a trauma patient because it can suggest the mechanism and nature of injuries. This history can be difficult to obtain in circumstances in which an adult or other reliable observer did not witness the injury, and details obtained from smaller children may not always be reliable. In such instances, the primary care physician must verify that the physical findings are consistent with the history obtained.

Certain historical details are particularly helpful:

1. Does a potential exist of chemical injury? If so, then treatment must be delivered immediately before obtaining a full history and performing an examination to minimize damage from an acid or alkali burn.
2. Has a severe head injury or other nonocular injury occurred that may require attention? Significant head trauma can been associated with globe rupture, traumatic optic neuropathy, cranial nerve palsies, and orbital fractures, as well as cortical visual damage.[6-8]
3. Is the injury blunt or sharp in nature? A sharp injury is more likely to be penetrating, resulting in a full-thickness laceration through the cornea or sclera. A severe blunt impact can also lead to globe rupture through an inside-out mechanism as a result of globe compression and increased intraocular pressure.
4. Does the possibility exist of a foreign body? A foreign body can be superficial (in the eyelid, cornea, or conjunctiva), intraocular, or intraorbital. An injury associated with flying debris, metallic fragments, projectiles, or any broken object is high risk for a retained foreign body.

Once details surrounding the mechanism of injury have been obtained, additional history taking should focus on prior ocular history (eg, the presence of amblyopia), medical history, medications and allergies, and the date of the last tetanus immunization.

Physical Examination

A thorough and complete examination ensures proper diagnosis and treatment, particularly when historical details are lacking. If the history is clear and reliable, such as being poked in the eye with a finger, then a more directed examination is possible. This circumstance can be quite challenging in a child who is in discomfort or who is otherwise uncooperative. If a full-thickness injury through the eyeball is apparent, then further examination is best left to an ophthalmologist. If the index of suspicion for a serious injury or foreign body is high in an uncooperative patient, then examination under sedation or anesthesia is occasionally necessary.

Vision Testing

The examination should begin with an age-appropriate assessment of vision. Verbal children should have acuity measured with letter charts or with letter matching (such as the HOTV chart) if they cannot name the letters. Acuity testing should be performed with proper optical correction, if applicable, and care should be taken to ensure that the normal eye is fully occluded when testing the injured eye. If the child is unable to see the largest target on the chart (usually 20/200 or 20/400), then alternative methods such as their ability to count fingers (recorded as "count fingers at *x* feet"), perceive hand motion (recorded as "hand motion at *x* feet"), or perceive light (recorded as "light perception" or "no light perception") is helpful. Preverbal children are assessed by their ability to *fix and follow* a small object or toy. Once again, each eye should be tested separately. An inability to follow smoothly with one eye when compared with the other or attempts to look around the occlusion of the normal eye are suggestive of decreased vision in the injured eye.

External Examination—Ocular Motility

External inspection and observation is helpful to characterize the severity of the injury. Important signs include swelling or bruising of the lids, lacerations of the lids or face, proptosis or enophthalmos, foreign bodies and possible entrance sites, and conjunctival hemorrhage. If a foreign body is likely, then eversion of the upper lid is required to inspect the palpebral conjunctiva properly. An obvious globe laceration with prolapse of intraocular contents might also be visible by inspection alone. If the globe appears intact, then palpation of the orbital rim can be performed to check for fracture of orbital or facial bones. Ocular motility should be evaluated to ensure full range of motion in all gaze positions. Limited movement can result from orbital hemorrhage or swelling, orbital fractures, cranial nerve palsies, or direct muscle trauma. Diplopia generally results from limited motility, although young children may not verbalize this symptom.

Pupils

The presence of round and equally reactive pupils greatly reduces (but does not eliminate) the likelihood of a severe, vision-threatening injury. An irregularity in the size or shape of the pupil can result from blunt trauma with damage to the pupillary sphincter or from a full thickness laceration of the cornea or sclera. Ideally, the reaction of each pupil to light (direct and consensual) is checked with the child fixating at a distant target. The swinging flashlight test is then performed to check for the presence of an afferent pupillary defect, or Marcus Gunn pupil. This test is performed by alternately shining the light source into each eye. Both pupils should normally stay constricted as a result of the direct and consensual response to light. Paradoxical dilatation of the illuminated pupil indicates the presence of an afferent pupillary defect, which results from optic nerve or extensive retinal injury.

Anterior Segment

Initial assessment of the anterior chamber can be performed simply with a penlight examination or with a direct ophthalmoscope. Conjunctival hemorrhages, corneal or conjunctival lacerations, foreign bodies, anterior chamber depth, and iris and pupillary irregularities can be diagnosed without the aid of the slit-lamp. If a slit-lamp is available, then a more detailed and accurate examination is possible in a cooperative child. The primary care physician can use the slit-lamp to evaluate for smaller conjunctival or corneal lacerations, foreign bodies that might not be visible with a penlight, the presence of red or white blood cells in the anterior chamber, and cataract formation or dislocation of the lens. Once penlight or slit-lamp or both types of examination has been completed, fluorescein solution or strips and a cobalt-blue filter or lamp should be used to check for abrasions, lacerations, or foreign bodies that might otherwise go undetected.

Fundus

Detailed fundus examination can be difficult in a child without pupillary dilatation. However, the red reflex should be observed, looking for asymmetry. An absence or asymmetry of the red reflex can indicate the presence of vitreous hemorrhage, cataract formation, or hyphema. In addition, other findings such as corneal abrasion or irregularity and corneal foreign body can also be appreciated as an opacity in the red reflex. Although visualization of the optic nerve and macula is possible with the direct ophthalmoscope, the view is generally limited. Any child who is thought to have posterior segment injury or unexplained vision loss should have a dilated fundus examination by an ophthalmologist with the aid of the indirect ophthalmoscope.

SPECIFIC OCULAR INJURIES

Eyelid and Lacrimal Injury

Superficial lacerations to the eyelid can be closed with a 6-0 nylon suture, which are removed in 5 to 7 days, or a 6-0 plain suture if the child might be uncooperative for suture removal. A thorough examination of the anterior segment is required to exclude globe injury. Three special categories of eyelid injuries require special attention: (1) lacerations involving the lid margin, (2) lacerations medial to the lacrimal puncta, and (3) deep lacerations of the upper lid, which expose orbital fat. Lacerations involving the lid margin should be repaired by an experienced surgeon to ensure that the smooth contour of the lid margin is maintained. Poor closure or reapproximation can result in a notch along the lid margin, leading to both cosmetic and functional consequences. Laceration or injury medial to the punctum carries a high risk of disrupting the lacrimal drainage system, given that the canaliculus is quite superficial just under the surface of the lid margin (Figure 301-1). Failure to recognize and treat a canalicular laceration can result in chronic tearing, particularly if the lower canaliculus is involved. A canalicular injury requires referral and surgical repair with tube placement in the lacrimal drainage system, followed by removal of the tube several months later. Dog bite injuries have an uncanny predilection for involving the lacrimal system. Upper lid lacerations deep enough to expose orbital fat carry the risk of damage to the levator muscle. Surgical exploration is required to repair any involvement of the levator muscle and to close the laceration itself. Failure to recognize levator involvement can result in posttraumatic ptosis, which might require additional surgery.

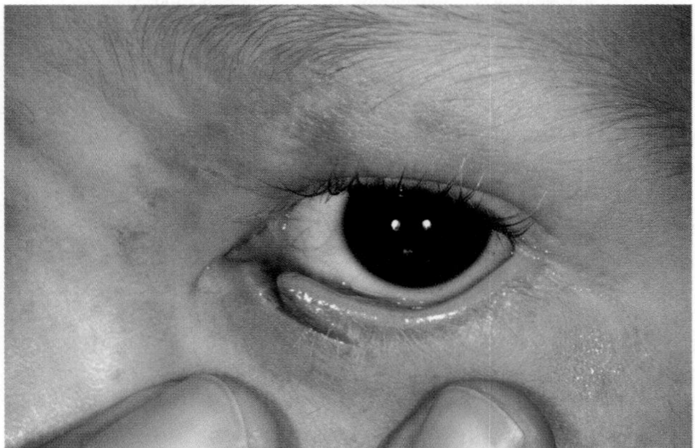

Figure 301-1 Full-thickness injury involving the lid margin and lower canaliculus. The laceration is medial to the lacrimal punctum.

Anterior Segment Trauma

Chemical Injury

Chemical injuries are acute emergencies and require immediate management to help prevent serious complications. When a child reaches the pediatrician's office or emergency care setting after a chemical injury, the history should be limited to the estimated time of injury and nature of the offending agent (eg, household cleaning product); any treatment should be administered before arrival, either by the caregiver or by emergency medical services.

A helpful 1st step is to use pH indicator paper to determine the nature and extent of acid or alkali injury. A small strip can be quickly placed in the conjunctival sac; normal pH of the eye is between 6.8 and 7.4. The point must be emphasized, however, that if pH paper is not readily available, however, time should not be wasted in obtaining it. The eye or eyes should then be irrigated with up to 2 liters of a pH-neutral solution, such as buffered saline.[9] A lid speculum may be used to keep the lids open if necessary. Alternatively, an irrigating contact lens can be used. Care must be taken to ensure the flow of saline is adequate; a steady drip will not be sufficient. Once irrigation is completed, pH indicator paper can again be used to determine that the pH of the eye has returned to normal. The conjunctival fornices should be examined to check for any residual chemical agent. If present, then a cotton tip applicator may be used to gently remove this precipitate and the area should be reirrigated.

After irrigation, a more detailed examination should be performed. First, the examiner should note the degree of conjunctival injection. A lack of hyperemia, particularly in the perilimbal area, may be an ominous sign of ischemia. Permanent damage to stem cells located in this area can significantly impair the patient's ability to regenerate any corneal epithelial loss.[10] Second, the cornea should be examined for clarity. A hazy or edematous cornea is a sign of serious injury. Finally, the examiner should instill fluorescein to check for corneal abrasions.

Treatment should be tailored to the injury but will often include an antibiotic drop or ointment and artificial lubricants. Corneal abrasions associated with chemical injuries should not be patched so that tears and natural blinking may eliminate any residual chemical. Referral to an ophthalmologist within 24 hours is indicated, particularly with moderate to severe injuries, which can result in permanent vision loss from corneal scarring, corneal vascularization, and other sequelae.

Ocular involvement from thermal injury can be isolated, but is often seen in the setting of severe facial burns. Although globe injury is typically mild because of the protective blink reflex, it can be severe if the blink reflex is impaired or if loss of consciousness occurs. As with chemical injuries, immediate irrigation is important, given that it serves to cool the ocular surface. Corneal and conjunctival abrasions are treated with artificial lubricants and topical antibiotics. Severe lid involvement can lead to contracture and cicatricial changes resulting in corneal exposure and ulceration. Initial treatment of lid injury consists of topical antibiotic ointment, and severe injury may require subsequent skin grafting to prevent lid malposition and exposure.[11]

Subconjunctival Hemorrhages

Significant discoloration is associated with subconjunctival hemorrhages; this condition may be quite alarming to patients and their families (Figure 301-2). They are harmless, however, and require no treatment. Patients need only be aware that various color changes may occur while the blood is being resorbed and that several days to weeks may elapse before the hemorrhage has completely disappeared.

Surrounding blood often masks a conjunctival laceration. A small, superficial laceration often does not require repair, but a thorough ophthalmic examination may be necessary to ensure that no underlying laceration of the sclera or other trauma to the eye has occurred.

Nontraumatic causes of subconjunctival hemorrhage also exist. Newborns often have small, bilateral hemorrhages, presumably from the pressure of uterine contractions.[12] Severe coughing such as that caused from pertussis or forceful vomiting can cause small hemorrhages. Some forms of viral conjunctivitis can be hemorrhagic and are usually associated with chemosis (edema of the conjunctiva) and symptoms of irritation and mild discharge. Rarely, certain blood dyscrasias such as leukemia can also be associated with subconjunctival hemorrhage, usually bilateral.[13]

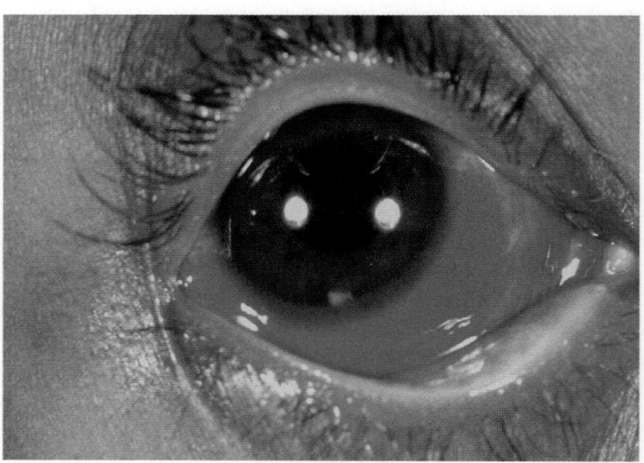

Figure 301-2 Subconjunctival hemorrhage after blunt injury.

Corneal Abrasion

Corneal abrasions are areas of disruption of the corneal epithelium. The epithelium is laced with numerous fine sensory nerve endings of the 1st branch of the trigeminal nerve, and abrasions result in extreme pain and sensitivity. Only in rare situations of neurotrophic disease are corneal abrasions relatively asymptomatic. Typically, photophobia and blepharospasm accompany the pain. Associated signs usually include conjunctival injection and mild lid swelling.

Diagnosis of a corneal abrasion may be facilitated by the instillation of a topical anesthetic followed by fluorescein (Figure 301-3). Use of a cobalt blue filter will then easily highlight areas of epithelial loss. Abrasions may be linear or patchy and can be of any size. Care must be taken to open the lids well enough to gain view of the entire cornea. Fine, linear abrasions in the superior cornea, for example, may be easily missed and are often a sign of an associated conjunctival foreign body lodged in the superior tarsal conjunctiva.

Most abrasions heal quickly, particularly in children. Treatment is aimed at keeping the patient comfortable and preventing infection. Typically, an antibiotic ointment or drop is used 2 to 4 times a day until the abrasion has healed. Nonsteroidal antiinflammatory drops may be used as an adjunct to reduce pain, particularly in older children. The use of a pressure patch is somewhat controversial. When a patch is used, an antibiotic ointment in instilled with soft oval gauze taped over the eye to keep it shut. The patch and antibiotic are then replaced after 24 hours, or the decision is made to discontinue its use. Prolonged patching is

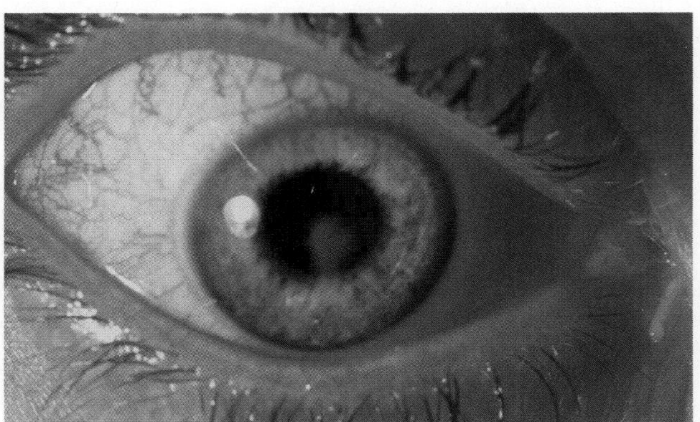

Figure 301-3 Central corneal abrasion is highlighted with fluorescein dye.

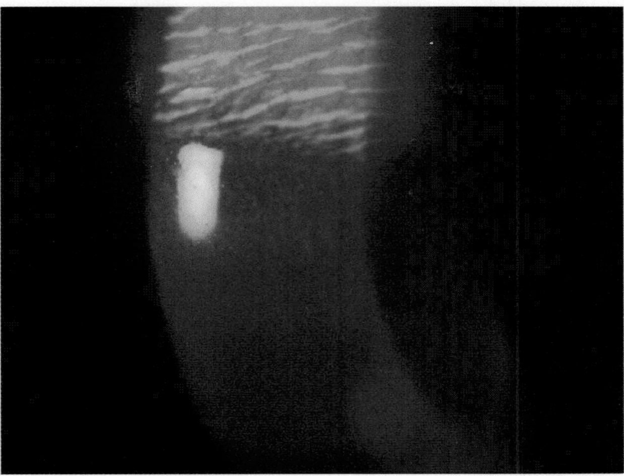

Figure 301-4 Fine, linear abrasions of the superior cornea are luminated with fluorescein dye and the use of a cobalt blue filter.

discouraged for young children because of the possibility of developing amblyopia or strabismus. The placement of a patch may provide additional patient comfort and may be particularly useful if a child tends to rub the eye excessively. However, no evidence has been found to suggest the abrasion will heal more quickly.[14] Some ophthalmologists believe that allowing natural tears, which contain immunoglobulin A, lysozyme, and other antiinfective properties, to stream over the cornea with normal blinking may result in improved healing and decreased risk of infection. Whichever method is used, the patient should be monitored closely, usually within 1 to 2 days. Delayed healing may suggest the presence of a foreign body, an ulcer, or even a different pathological process (eg, herpes keratitis).

Conjunctival and Corneal Foreign Bodies

The sources of most surface, or nonpenetrating, foreign bodies in children are small objects that can be thrown or carried by the wind, such as dirt, sand, gravel, grass, or leaves. In many instances, the foreign body will be readily eliminated from the eye with rubbing and secondary tearing. In some cases, however, medical attention will be necessary to help dislodge the foreign material.

Conjunctival foreign bodies will typically produce irritation and discomfort, and the child will have a mild to moderate amount of conjunctival injection. The lids should be forcefully opened, if necessary, and the bulbar conjunctiva should be directly examined. If this area appears normal, attention is then turned to the tarsal conjunctival surfaces. Eversion of the lower lid can be accomplished readily with gentle inferior traction. Upper lid eversion can be much more difficult, especially if the child is very young or uncooperative. The lashes are grasped and the lid stretched minimally; next, the shaft of a cotton tip applicator is placed horizontally along the superior margin of the tarsal plate. The lid is then reflected over the applicator for inspection. Once a conjunctival foreign body has been identified, a drop of topical anesthetic should be administered and a cotton tip used to remove it gently. If a conjunctival foreign body is not easily identified, then a cotton tip may still be used to sweep the upper and lower conjunctival fornices to ensure that a very small foreign particle has not been missed. Finally, fluorescein should be administered to check for associated corneal abrasions. Multiple, fine vertical abrasions of the superior aspect of the cornea are highly suggestive of a foreign body of the upper tarsal conjunctiva (Figure 301-4 and Figure 301-5).

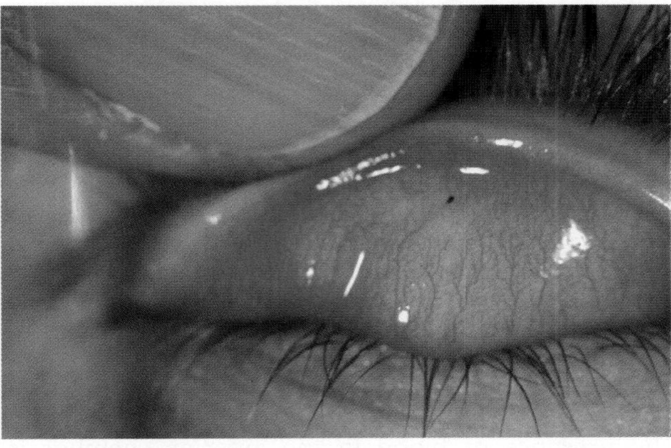

Figure 301-5 Eversion of the upper lid reveals a small particle resting in the superior tarsal conjunctiva.

Corneal foreign bodies usually represent particles that are resting on the surface of the epithelium or have penetrated the epithelium and are embedded in the anterior stroma. The latter types are more common as the normal blink, and secondary movement of the tears will usually either expel a nonembedded particle or move it to a conjunctival surface. Again, the lids should be opened to gain full view of the cornea and a light source used to help identify a possible foreign body. A topical anesthetic and cotton tip applicator can be used to dislodge the particle gently, with

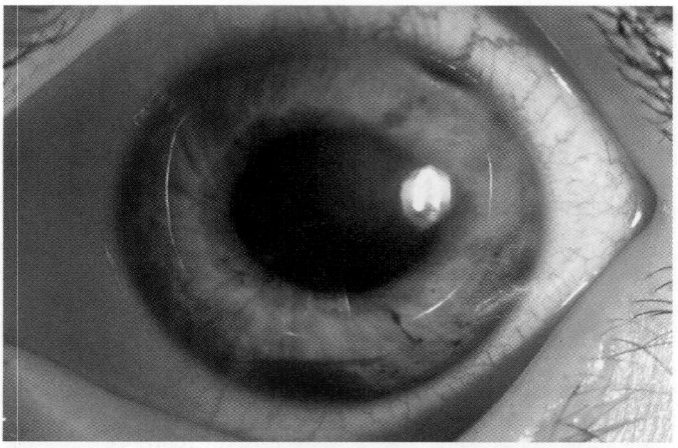

Figure 301-6 Small hyphema is associated with an iris root tear at the 2 o'clock position.

care not to debride a greater area of epithelium in the process. In many instances, however, this method will not be successful in removing an embedded object, and referral to an ophthalmologist will be necessary. If the child is able to sit at a slit-lamp, then the ophthalmologist may be able to use a fine needle, forceps, or burr to remove the foreign body. Younger or uncooperative children will usually require sedation or general anesthesia.

An antibiotic drop or ointment is typically prescribed for a few days after removing a surface foreign body, particularly if the source was organic or if any disturbance occurred in the corneal epithelium. Follow-up is not necessarily indicated for a simple conjunctival foreign body but is required in cases of corneal involvement.

Hyphema

The presence of blood in the anterior chamber is termed a hyphema (Figure 301-6). In the setting of blunt trauma, blood in this area results when enough force is transmitted to the globe to cause rupture of the blood vessels located within the iris root and ciliary body. Hyphemas can be of varying severity, from what is labeled as a micro hyphema (floating red blood cells in the aqueous fluid without layering) to an 8-ball hyphema (blood filling the entire anterior chamber). Most cases are in between and described based on the percentage of the anterior chamber occupied by the layered blood. Hyphemas are readily identified with a light source and good exposure of the anterior segment. Once diagnosed, initial management involves placing a protective shield over the eye to avoid the possibility of further injury. Patients should also be instructed to limit their activities until seen by a specialist. Because of their potential vision threatening complications, all hyphemas, regardless of size, should be referred to an ophthalmologist.

Most ophthalmologists will treat hyphemas with a topical steroid drop to reduce the associated inflammation, as well as a topical cycloplegic agent. A shield is usually continued and bed rest often advised. If the hyphema is worrisome and the child is too young to cooperate with restricted activity, then hospitalization may be indicated. This circumstance is of particular importance in the first 2 to 5 days after injury, at which time the clotted blood may start to resorb and cause a rebleed of injured vessels.[15] In many instances, this rebleed can be more visually devastating than the original injury. Other direct complications of hyphemas include corneal bloodstaining, glaucoma, and amblyopia. Glaucoma is perhaps the most common of the aforementioned complications. It is often controlled with topical medications but, in certain situations, requires timely surgical evacuation of the hyphema to prevent irreversible optic nerve damage. Patients with sickle cell anemia or trait are at greater risk for having visual compromise from optic neuropathy or central artery occlusion at lower pressures than is the general population and therefore require the surgeon to have a lower threshold for intervention.[16]

Traumatic Iritis

Iritis, or anterior uveitis, refers to inflammation of the iris and ciliary body. This inflammation can occur in a nontraumatic setting, such as in association with autoimmune disorders; it may also occur in the setting of trauma and will cause the patient to experience blurry vision, pain, and significant photophobia. The eye is usually quite injected, and the pupil may not constrict briskly. If the diagnosis is suspected, then referral to an ophthalmologist is indicated. Floating white blood cells in the anterior chamber are visualized under the high magnification of a slit-lamp, confirming the diagnosis. Similar to a hyphema, potential complications include iris synechiae, glaucoma, and cataract formation. Treatment includes a topical steroid and cycloplegic agent if the inflammation is severe.

Traumatic Mydriasis

A mid-dilated pupil noted on examination of a patient after a blunt, traumatic event can be a result of small ruptures or tears of the iris sphincter muscle. The pupil is therefore unable to constrict normally. The injury may involve only part of the sphincter muscle, giving a slightly irregular appearance to the pupil. Care must be taken to rule out the possibility of a ruptured globe, which can also cause an irregularly shaped pupil.

The ophthalmologist will often be able to identify free pigment cells released into the anterior chamber. However, unless true associated inflammation exists, or iritis, treatment is usually not indicated.

Ruptured Globe

Open-globe injuries occur primarily in adults.[17,18] Penetrating injuries are most common in boys. Blunt trauma is the primary cause of ruptured globe in girls. Pediatric open-globe injuries are caused by penetrating injury (79%), blunt trauma (13%), and perforating injury (8%).[19] Pediatric penetrating injuries are caused by many different objects, including household knives and sticks. Blunt trauma includes motor vehicle crashes, as well as air bag, paint ball, and fist injuries.[20,21]

Anterior segment penetration may exhibit as lid laceration, conjunctiva laceration, subconjunctival hemorrhage, scleral laceration with uveal prolapse, corneal laceration with iris prolapse, and cataract. Blunt trauma may rupture the sclera. With blunt trauma, external signs may consist of an irregular pupil, a deep anterior chamber, a subconjunctival hemorrhage, or conjunctival chemosis. The most common rupture locations are at the limbus and posterior to the eye muscle insertion. Associated clinical findings in an open-globe injury include vision loss, an afferent pupillary defect, retinal detachment, and optic disc edema.

In many cases, the diagnosis is evident from initial inspection with a penlight. Otherwise, further assessment can include a dilated ophthalmic examination and intraocular pressure measurement. In most instances, the intraocular pressure is less than 8 mm Hg. Intraocular pressure measurement is safest with applanation tonometer or Tono-Pen. A Schiotz tonometer should not be used because the weight of the tonometer may cause an expulsive hemorrhage.

If a rupture is suspected, then the patient should be placed at bed rest, given antiemetics, if required, and the eye shielded. An ophthalmology consultation is required for operative repair.

An intraocular foreign body should be considered based on the mechanism of injury. The presence of a hyphema or vitreous hemorrhage may preclude visualizing an intraocular foreign body. Ultrasound or computed tomographic evaluation for orbital or intraocular foreign body should performed. A retinal tear or detachment is commonly associated with intraocular penetration. Copper or iron are toxic to the retina and require urgent removal. Plastic, graphite, lead, and aluminum are better tolerated in the eye than either copper or iron. Removal by a retina specialist with a vitrectomy is the treatment.

Serious complications of ruptured globe include spontaneous or induced expulsive hemorrhage, retinal detachment, and endophthalmitis. The incidence of associated endophthalmitis after an open-globe injury has been reported at 6.8%.[22] The visual prognosis is worse with blunt compared to penetrating trauma.

Orbital Trauma

Blunt or penetrating trauma may cause an intraorbital hemorrhage. Iatrogenic hemorrhage is well reported with preoperative peribulbar and retrobulbar anesthetic injections. Traumatic orbital hemorrhage in a child is unusual. Hemorrhage causes anterior displacement of the globe. Blindness may be caused by a marked elevation of the intraocular pressure or tension on the optic nerve. To relieve the tension on the globe, a lateral canthotomy of the upper and lower lids may be performed at the bedside.

Blunt trauma to the midface and orbital rim may cause a fracture of the orbital wall. The inferior floor is the most common site, with the medial wall second. Associated facial fractures are frequent, most commonly a zygoma-malar fracture.[23] Diplopia is a common finding. A defect in the orbital floor may allow prolapse of orbital fat leading to enophthalmos. Vertical restrictive strabismus may be caused by prolapse of the inferior rectus into the floor defect or bony impingement on the muscle. Reduced vision can occur secondary to retrobulbar hemorrhage, optic neuropathy, optic nerve impingement, retinal detachment, or a rupture of the globe.[24]

Primary care evaluation includes assessment of visual acuity, motility, the pupils, the anterior segment, and intraocular pressure. Obvious proptosis or enophthalmos should also be noted. A marked decrease in vision, a relative afferent pupillary defect, or an elevation of intraocular pressure warrants an emergent ophthalmologic evaluation. Decreased facial sensation inferior to the orbital rim may indicate damage to the infraorbital nerve. Midfacial trauma may be associated with a traumatic optic neuropathy.[25] Radiologic evaluation of the orbit will delineate the size of the floor defect. A large defect or bony muscle impingement may require early surgical treatment, but treatment of a globe injury is primary.

Most floor fractures do not require immediate surgery. Lid edema, proptosis, and diplopia may resolve in the 1st week. If diplopia persists or enophthalmos is significant, then repair of the orbital floor defect can be done safely up to 4 weeks after the injury.

Neurologic findings with facial trauma may include cranial nerve palsies and optic neuropathy. Examination of traumatic optic neuropathy may demonstrate decreased vision, an afferent pupillary defect, and decreased color vision. The optic nerve may appear normal or edematous. Radiologic evaluation of the optic canal for a displaced fracture is paramount. Bone impingement into the optic nerve requires urgent neurosurgical intervention. Standard treatment of traumatic optic neuropathy is intravenous steroids for 1 to 3 days after injury. However, the dose, time, and efficacy are controversial.

Abusive Trauma

Abusive injury in a child with unexplained fractures on x-ray examination was described first in 1946.[26] The incidence of inflicted injury has been reported as high as 1% of all childhood injuries. Eye injuries may be present in up to 40% of pediatric abusive injury.[27] Retinal hemorrhage associated with a shaking injury is a primary concern, but many other signs of trauma may involve the eyes. These signs include cranial nerve palsies, external lid trauma, anterior and posterior segment injuries, orbital injury, and sexually transmitted infections.[28,29] Infections such as *Chlamydia* and gonorrhea conjunctivitis, as well as phthiris pubis on the lashes, have been reported. Munchausen syndrome by proxy has been reported in a case of recurrent conjunctivitis.[30]

Retinal hemorrhages, retinal schisis, retinal folds, and cranial nerve palsy have been related to violent, repetitive, abusive acceleration-deceleration injury (Figure 301-7, *A*). This type of injury typically occurs in children younger than 3 years. However, an 8-year-old boy developed bilateral retinal hemorrhage and cerebral edema after severe, abusive shaking injury.[31] Retinal hemorrhages occur at multiple layers of the retina, which includes vitreous, preretinal, nerve fiber layer, and intra- and subretinal layers (Figure 301-7, *B*). Nerve fiber layer heme is the most common type. The hemorrhages are distributed primarily around the optic nerve and macula but are often distributed to the periphery of the retina. A severe shaking injury may be associated with cerebral edema only, subdural bleeding, or a normal brain on computed tomography.[32]

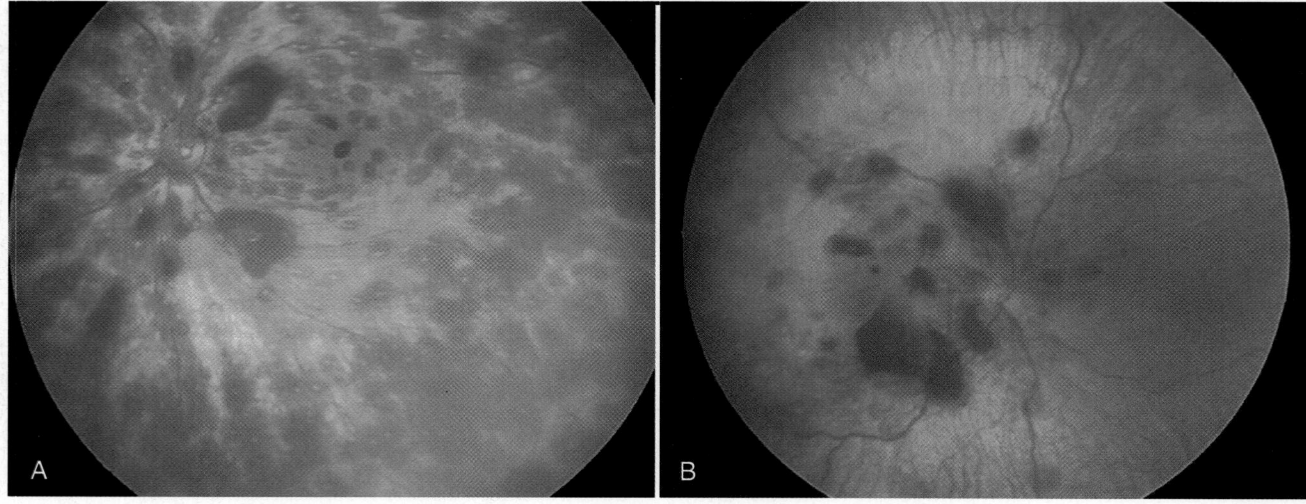

Figure 301-7 **A**, Severe retinal hemorrhages as the result of a shaking injury. **B**, Moderate retinal hemorrhages as a result of a shaking injury. Preretinal hemorrhages, which obscure the retinal vessels, and intraretinal hemorrhages, which are beneath the retinal vessels, are both visualized.

Retinal hemorrhages occur associated with abusive head trauma. Brain findings include subdural (93%), cerebral edema (44%), subarachnoid (16%), and parenchymal bleeds (8%).[33] Reported retinal heme occurred in 60% to 72% of abusive head trauma and 0% to 20% of nonabusive cases.[34,35] Bilateral involvement was more common in abusive injury, but unilateral hemorrhages is well reported in known shaking injuries.[36] Abusive head trauma is associated with much more severe retinal hemorrhages.

Forceful vomiting does not commonly cause retinal hemorrhaging. One study found no retinal heme in 100 infants with excessive vomiting as a result of pyloric stenosis.[37] A febrile seizure caused mild unilateral retinal heme in one of 153 patients between the ages of 2 months to 2 years.[38] Cardiopulmonary resuscitation has been reported to cause rarely few retinal hemorrhages around the optic nerve. No retinal findings were seen in 43 children undergoing cardiopulmonary resuscitation in a pediatric intensive care unit setting.[39] Falls from less than 1.5 meters are not likely to call serious neurologic trauma.[40]

Retinal folds associated with a severe shaking injury are perimacular along the vascular arcades. The presence of perimacular folds most likely indicates a shaking injury, although there are reports of retinal folds with known severe accidental injury.[41,42] Macular holes and peripheral retinoschisis (separation of the layers of the retina) have also been noted. The vitreous gel of the eye is tightly adherent to the retina at the macula, optic nerve, and periphery in a child. This adherence creates tractional forces on the retina with a repetitive acceleration-deceleration injury. Retinal folds and peripheral retinoschisis are predictive of severe neurologic trauma.[43]

In shaken baby syndrome (SBS), hemorrhages resolve within 4 weeks but have been reported to last up to 4 months.[44] Retinal hemorrhages often resolve without serious visual effects unless the macula is involved. Macular holes and macular scar tissue may result in visual loss.[45] Severe visual impairment or blindness may occur with significant neurologic trauma and cortical damage, optic atrophy, or retinal detachment.[46]

Abusive head trauma combined with retinal heme offers a poor neurologic prognosis. One study reported 71% of deaths and 90% of severe disability occurred in the 38% of children in pediatric intensive care units with an abusive etiology of head trauma and retinal heme.[47]

The history and associated physical findings will aid in establishing the etiology of the trauma. Patients exhibit physical findings inconsistent with the history or variable caregiver histories. The perpetrator is found to be the father (45%) or boyfriend (25%) most commonly.[48] If abuse is suspected, then a dilated fundus examination by an ophthalmologist is mandatory. In a study of suspected cases of SBS, reports indicate that 36% of nonophthalmologists did not attempt to examine the retina, and 19% were unable. If the nonophthalmologist attempted the examination, then 87% were accurate. False-negative examinations occurred in 13%.[49] A thorough history and examination will prevent inappropriate accusations. Preseptal edema caused by an orbital hemangioma, preseptal ecchymosis caused by neuroblastoma, and a ruptured vascular malformation have been mistakenly reported as abuse.[50] Other causes of retinal hemorrhage confused with SBS include Zellweger syndrome, glutaric aciduria type 1, and Hermansky-Pudlak syndrome.[51,52]

WHEN TO REFER

- In the case of lacerations involving the lid margin, those medial to the lacrimal puncta, and deep lacerations of the upper lid

- Canalicular injury
- Levator muscle injury
- Corneal abrasion
- Removal of corneal foreign bodies
- Hyphema treatment
- Traumatic iritis
- Traumatic mydriasis
- Ruptured globe
- Abusive trauma

WHEN TO ADMIT

- To treat hyphemas in certain patients
- Ruptured globe
- Abusive trauma

TOOLS FOR PRACTICE

Engaging Patient and Family

- *What is a Pediatric Ophthalmologist?* (fact sheet), American Academy of Pediatrics (www.aap.org/sections/he3006.pdf).

Medical Decision Support

- *Pediatric Ophthalmology for Primary Care, 3rd edition* (book), American Academy of Pediatrics (www.aap.org/bookstore).
- *The Physician's Guide to Eye Care, 3rd edition* (book), American Academy of Ophthalmology (www.aap.org/bookstore).

REFERENCES

1. May DR, Kuhn FP, Morris RE, et al. The epidemiology of serious eye injuries from the United States Eye Injury Registry. *Graefe's Arch Clin Exp Ophthalmol.* 2000;238: 153-157.
2. Good WV. Accidental trauma in children. In: Taylor D, Hoyt CS, eds. *Pediatric Ophthalmology and Strabismus.* Edinburgh, Scotland: Elsevier Saunders; 2005.
3. Nelson LB, Wilson TW, Jeffers JB. Eye injuries in childhood: demography, etiology, and prevention. *Pediatrics.* 1989;84:438-441.
4. Cascairo MA, Mazow ML, Prager TC. Pediatric ocular trauma: a retrospective survey. *J Pediatr Ophthalmol Strabismus.* 1994;31:312-317.
5. Kardon RH: Anatomy. In: Van Bueren J, Denny M, eds. *Fundamentals and Principles of Ophthalmology.* San Francisco, CA: American Academy of Ophthalmology; 1994-1995.
6. Garcia TA, McGetrick BA, Janik JS. Ocular injuries in children after major trauma. *J Pediatr Ophthalmol Strabismus.* 2005;42:349-354.
7. Poon A, McCluskey PJ, Hill DA. Eye injuries in patients with major trauma. *J Trauma.* 1999:4603:494-499.
8. Odebode TO, Ademola-Popoola DS, Ojo TA, et al. Ocular complications of head injury. *Eye.* 2005;19:561-566.
9. Saidinejad M, Burns MM. Ocular irrigant alternatives in pediatric emergency medicine. *Pediatr Emerg Care.* 2005; 21(1):23-26.
10. No author. Corneal trauma. In: Arffa RC, ed. *Grayson's Diseases of the Cornea,* St Louis, MO: Mosby; 1997.
11. Kuckelkorn R, Schrage N, Keller G, et al. Emergency treatment of chemical and thermal eye burns. *Acta Ophthalmol Scand.* 2002;80(1):4-10.
12. Clarke M. Red eye in infancy. In: Taylor D, Hoyt CS, eds. *Pediatric Ophthalmology and Strabismus.* Edinburgh, Scotland: Elsevier Saunders; 2005.
13. Parsa CF. Conjunctiva and subconjunctival tissue. In: Taylor D, Hoyt CS, eds. *Pediatric Ophthalmology and Strabismus.* Edinburgh, Scotland: Elsevier Saunders; 2005.
14. Kaiser P and Corneal Abrasion Patching Study Group. A comparison of pressure patchng versus no patching for corneal abrasions due to trauma or foreign body removal. *Ophthalmology.* 1995;102:1936-1942.
15. Bloom J. Traumatic hyphema in children. *Pediatr Ann.* 1990;19(6): 368-375.
16. Cohen SB, Fletcher ME, Goldberg MF, et al. Diagnosis and management of ocular complications of sickle hemoglobinopathies: part V. *Ophthal Surg.* 1986;17(6):369-374.
17. Koo L, Kapadia MK, Singh RP, et al. Gender differences in etiology and outcome of open globe injuries. *J Trauma.* 2005;59:175-178.
18. Casson RJ, Walker JC, Newland HS. Four-year review of open eye injuries at the Royal Adelaide Hospital. *Clin Experiment Ophthalmol.* 2002;30:15-18.
19. Jandeck C, Kellner U, Bornfeld N, et al. Open globe injuries in children. *Graefes Arch Clin Experiment Ophthalmol.* 2000:238:420-426.
20. Stein JD, Jaeger EA, Jeffers JB. Air bags and ocular injuries. *Trans Am Ophthalmol Soc.* 1999;97:59-82.
21. Thach AB, Ward TP, Hollifield RD, et al. Ocular injuries from paint ball pellets. *Ophthalmology.* 1999;106:533-537.
22. Essex RW, Yi Q, Charles PG, et al. Post-traumatic endophthalmitis. *Ophthalmology.* 2004;111:2015-2022.
23. Tong L, Bauer RJ, Buchman SR. A current 10 year retrospective survey of 199 surgically treated orbital floor fractures in a nonurban tertiary center. *Plast Reconstruct Surg.* 2001;108:612-621.
24. Lee HJ, Jilani M, Frohman L, et al. CT of orbital trauma. *Emerg Radiol.* 2004;10:168-172.
25. Ashar A, Kovacs A, Khan S, et al. Blindness associate with midfacial fractures. *J Oral Maxillofac Surg.* 1998; 56(10):1146-1150.
26. Caffey J. Multiple fractures in long bones of children suffering from chronic subdural hematomata. *Am J Radiol.* 1964;56:163-173.
27. Cavanagh N. Non-accidental injury. In: Taylor D. ed. *Pediatric Ophthalmology.* London, UK: Blackwell Scientific Publications; 1990.
28. Cackett P, Fleck B, Mulhivill A. Bilateral fourth nerve palsy occurring after shaking injury in infancy. *J Am Assoc Pediatr Ophthalmol Strabismus.* 2004;8:280-281.
29. Spitzer SG, Luorno J, Noel LP. Isolated subconjunctival hemorrhages in nonaccidental trauma. *J Am Assoc Pediatr Ophthalmol Strabismus.* 2005;9:53-56.
30. Baskin DE, Stein F, Coats DL, et al. Recurrent conjunctivitis as a presentation of Munchausen syndrome by proxy. *Ophthalmology.* 2003;110:1582-1584.
31. Mierisch RF, Frasier LD, Braddock SR, et al. Retinal hemorrhages in an 8-year-old child: an uncommon presentation of abusive injury. *Pediatr Emerg Care.* 2004;20:118-120.
32. Morad Y, Avni I, Capra L, et al. Shaken baby syndrome without intracranial hemorrhage on initial computed tomography. *J Am Assoc Pediatr Ophthalmol Strabismus.* 2004;8:521-527.
33. Morad Y, Kim YM, Armstrong DC, et al. Correlation between retinal abnormalities and intracranial abnormalities in the shaken baby syndrome. *Am J Ophthalmol.* 2002;134:354-359.
34. Dashti SR, Decker DD, Razzaq A, et al. Current patterns of inflicted head injury in children. *Pediatr Neurosurg.* 1999;31:302-306.
35. Bechtel K, Stoessel K, Leventhal JM, et al. Characteristics that distinguish accidental from abusive injury in hospitalized young children with head trauma. *Pediatrics.* 2004; 114:165-168.

36. Drack AM, Petronio J, Capone A. Unilateral retinal hemorrhages in documented cases of child abuse. *Am J Ophthalmol.* 1999;128:340-344.
37. Herr S, Pierce MC, Berger RP, et al. Does valsalva retinopathy occur in infants? An initial investigation in infants with vomiting by pyloric stenosis. *Pediatrics.* 2004;113:1658-1661.
38. Mei-Zahav M, Useil Y, Raz J, et al. Convulsion and retinal haemorrhage: should we look further? *Arch Dis Child.* 2002;86:334-335.
39. Odom A, Christ E, Kerr N, et al. Prevalence of retinal hemorrhages in pediatric patients after in-hospital cardiopulmonary resuscitation: a prospective study. *Pediatrics.* Jun 1997;99(6):E3.
40. Oehmichen M, Meisssner C, Saternus KS. Fall or shaken: traumatic brain injury in children caused by falls or abuse at home—a review on biomechanics and diagnosis. *Neuropediatrics.* 2005;36(4):240-245.
41. Lantz PE, Sinal SH, Stanton CA, et al. Perimacular retinal folds from childhood head trauma. *BMJ.* 2004;328:754-756.
42. Lueder GT, Turner JW, Paschall R. Perimacular retinal folds simulating nonaccidental injury in an infant. *Arch Ophthalmol.* 2006;124:1782-1783.
43. Mills M. Funduscopic lesions associated with mortality in shaken baby syndrome. *J Am Assoc Pediatr Ophthalmol Strabismus.* 1998;2:67-71.
44. McCabe CF, Donahue SP. Prognostic indicators for vision and mortality in shaken baby syndrome. *Arch Ophthalmol.* 2000;118:373-377.
45. Ells AL, Kherani A, Lee D. Epiretinal membrane formation is a late manifestation of shaken baby syndrome. *J Am Assoc Pediatr Ophthalmol Strabismus.* 2003;7:223-225.
46. Gonzales CA, Scott IU, Chaudry NA, et al. Bilateral rhegmatogenous retinal detachments with unilateral vitreous base avulsion as the presenting signs of child abuse. *Am J Ophthalmol.* 1999;127:475-477.
47. Vinchon M, Defoort-Dhellemmes S, Desurmont M, et al. Accidental and nonaccidental head injuries in infants: a prospective study. *J Neurosurg.* 2005;102:380-384.
48. Starling SP, Holden JR. Perpetrators of abusive head trauma: a comparison of two geographic populations. *South Med J.* 2000;93:463-465.
49. Morad Y, Kim YM, Mian M, et al. Nonophthalmologist accuracy in diagnosing retinal hemorrhages in the shaken baby syndrome. *J Pediatrics.* 2003;142:431-434.
50. Weissgold DJ, Budenz DL, Hood I, et al. Ruptured vascular malformation masquerading as battered/shaken baby syndrome. *Surv Ophthalmol.* 1995;39:509-512.
51. Fledelius HC. Retinal haemorrhages in premature infants: a pathogenetic alternative to child abuse. *Acta Ophthalmol Scand.* 2005;83:424-427.
52. Russell-Eggitt IM, Thompson DA, Khair K, et al. Hermansky-Pudlak syndrome presenting with subdural haematoma and retinal haemorrhages in infancy. *J R Soc Med.* 2000;93:591-592.

Chapter 302
OSTEOCHONDROSES

Edward M. Sills, MD

The ossification centers of growing bones may develop irregular mineralization during childhood, leading to varying degrees of discomfort, dysfunction, and deformity. This irregular mineralization is the result of necrosis followed by regeneration of bone tissue. Known as juvenile osteochondroses, the disorders occur in bones preformed in cartilage and ossified from a central nucleus and are categorized according to anatomic location (Table 302-1). Because damage to cartilage is not an instigating factor in these disorders, the root *chondro* is inaccurate.

Table 302-1 Osteochondroses

SITE	PEAK AGE AT APPEARANCE (YEARS)
UPPER EXTREMITY	
Humeral head	2-8
Humeral capitulum	4-10
Lower ulna	13-20
Carpal navicular	16-24
Carpal semilunar	16-20
Bilateral entire carpus	10-14
Metacarpal heads	9-15
Basal phalanges	8-14
LOWER EXTREMITY	
Femoral epiphysis	3-12*
Greater trochanter	6-11
Primary patellar center	8-15
Secondary patellar center	8-10
Shaft of tibia	1-5† 6-12‡
Tibial tubercle	10-15
Distal tibial epiphysis	4
Calcaneal epiphysis	3-18
Astragalus	2-8
Tarsal navicular	3-7
Second metatarsal	8-17
Fifth metatarsal	8-16
SPINE AND PELVIS	
Vertebral epiphysis	13-20
Vertebral disk	Over 16
Symphysis pubis	12-18
Iliac crest	12-19
Ischial apophysis	13-18
Ischiopubic synchondrosis	12-19

*Maximum is 6-8 years.
†Form of disease in infants.
‡Form of disease in adolescents.

The exact causes and mechanisms are not known. However, endogenous stress, ischemia, and heredity are possible factors. Excessive endogenous mechanical stress appears to play an important role in each disorder, and the degree of deformity and disability depends on the duration and degree of stress to which the softened fibrous parts are subjected. Excessive stress can lead to disordered cellular or local microvascular growth. Inherited tendencies to hypercoagulability may cause vascular thromboses in the osteochondroses. In a study of Legg-Calve-Perthes disease, for example, the prevalence of factor V Leiden mutation was found to be higher in patients than in controls (4.9% vs 0.7%; p=.03).[1] Similar studies with antithrombin III, protein-C, and protein-S deficiency and

BOX 302-1 Clinically Significant Sites of Osteochondroses

- Femoral head (Legg-Calve-Perthes disease)
- Tibial tuberosity (Osgood-Schlatter disease)
- Tibial shaft (adolescent tibia vara or adolescent Blount disease)
- Proximal tibial physis (infantile and juvenile Blount disease, rickets)
- Tarsal navicular (Köhler bone disease)
- Metatarsal heads 2, 3, or 4 (Freiberg disease)
- Carpal semilunar
- Lower thoracic vertebral end plates (Scheuermann disease)
- Distal radial epiphysis (Madelung disease)
- Osteochondrosis of the lunate (Kienbock malacia)

activated protein C resistance have shown significant relationship to thrombotic venous occlusion in the femoral head in a few instances.[2] Box 302-1 lists clinically significant sites of osteochondroses.

FEMORAL HEAD

In Legg-Calve-Perthes disease, the blood supply to the ossification center of the femoral head is interrupted, resulting in aseptic necrosis of the center. The femoral head, neck, and acetabulum become deformed and, in time, extensively reconstructed. Legg-Calve-Perthes disease has its onset in the early school-aged years and occurs in boys 4 times more frequently than in girls. In the vast majority of instances the disorder is unilateral. In rare instances (less than 10%) when both hip joints are involved, the 2 joints are involved successively rather than simultaneously.

The earliest sign is an intermittent limp, noticed especially after exertion. This limp may be associated with hip and ipsilateral knee pain. The quadriceps muscles and adjacent thigh soft-tissues atrophy and the hip may develop adduction flexion contracture. The child experiences discomfort in the hip or knee when attempts are made to rotate the hip internally. Associated quadriceps muscle spasm and associated quadriceps tendon distraction may cause distal thigh or knee tenderness. A radiograph taken early in the course of the disease shows widening of the hip joint and, occasionally, metaphyseal demineralization. This *acute phase* generally lasts for 1 or 2 weeks and is followed by the *active phase,* which can last for 12 to 40 months, during which time no clinical signs or symptoms are evident; however, the process of reparative revascularization causes an increased radiodensity in the femoral head ossification center (seen on radiographs), which is caused by resorption of dead trabecular bone. During this remolding phase, orthopedic care should be directed to maintaining the femoral head abducted and internally rotated in relation to the acetabulum. Surgery or orthotic devices encourage the regaining of a spherical femoral head and prevent irregular contour, flattening, or mushrooming of the head, shortening and broadening of the neck, and flattening of the vertical wall of the acetabulum. If these changes occur, then osteoarthritis develops at an early age.

TIBIA

Tibial Tuberosity

Osgood-Schlatter disease results from avulsion of part of the patellar ligament and attached bony and cartilaginous fragments from the tuberosity. Its incidence is higher in boys than in girls, but the age of onset is earlier in girls than in boys (see Table 302-1) because ossification of the tibial tuberosity occurs earlier in girls. Approximately 25% of cases have bilateral involvement. The child's complaint is that of local pain and tenderness in the region of the knee, particularly the tuberosity. The pain is most severe at the end of active flexion or extension of the knee. If the condition has been present for several months, then the tuberosity is enlarged, and a bony prominence may be found on its anterior aspect. The radiographic changes vary, depending on the size of the avulsed fragments (cartilage, and bone) and on the duration of the condition. The best view is one with the knee rotated inward, giving a tangential view of the tibial tuberosity. Soft-tissue swelling, an opaque patellar ligament, and a fragmented tuberosity are seen. Treatment is directed at decreasing the stress on the tubercle until the tuberosity fuses with the tibial metaphysis. This bony fusion occurs at approximately 15 years of age in girls and 17 years in boys. Depending on the degree of pain, strenuous activities involving deep-knee bending and jumping may have to be restricted, or casting may be required to immobilize the knee totally. The former approach is usually sufficient.

TIBIAL SHAFT

Infants usually have some leg bowing until 18 months of age, after which time the legs straighten and then progress to a slight degree of knock-knee. Bowing of the legs that persists or progresses beyond 2 years of age should be evaluated. The differential diagnosis lies between tibia vara (Blount disease) and renal or nutritional rickets. In Blount disease, cartilage has failed to transform to bone at the medial aspect of the epiphysis. The metaphysis beneath the epiphyseal ossification center becomes demineralized, and the medial aspect of the proximal tibia fails to grow as rapidly as the lateral aspect, resulting in a bowleg deformity.

Trauma to the proximal tibial physis medially can be characterized as unilateral tibia vara in the adolescent. Obesity appears to be a factor in adolescent-onset tibia vara, which is most common in male black teens. Dynamic gait deviations to compensate for increased thigh girth associated with obesity (fat-thigh gait) have been shown to result in increased loading of the medial compartment of the knee during the gait cycle and resultant adolescent tibia vara.

In rickets, calcification and growth of the epiphyseal cartilage of the long bones are suppressed, their metaphyses become softened, and they flare at both ends with resultant bowing. Appropriate treatment with vitamin D will produce radiographic evidence of healing within a few weeks and eventual straightening of the bones. Most children whose Blount disease persists or develops beyond 6 years of age require an osteotomy to correct the bowing.

TARSAL NAVICULAR

Kohler bone disease of the tarsal navicular bone results from an interruption of the blood supply to the developing navicular bone, causing necrosis of its ossification center. The navicular is in a crucial position in the arch of the foot; thus symptoms can be alarming. The condition is self-limited, and the ossification center becomes revascularized and completely reconstructed. The disorder is seen primarily in boys between 3 and 7 years of age but predominantly in younger children.

Pain is localized to the inner aspect of the midtarsal part of the foot. The foot is held in a slight varus position, and the child walks on the outer side of the foot or in a flat-footed manner. The skin over the navicular may be warm, red, and swollen, and palpation of the bone elicits tenderness. Lateral radiographs of the feet show a very narrowed, wafer-like, irregular navicular ossification center, with increased radiopacity and loss of trabecular markings. The process of revascularization and reconstruction takes from 1 to 3 years. Various orthotic pads can be used to absorb weight and pressure forces until the healing occurs. Surgical intervention is to be avoided.

METATARSAL HEADS

Freiberg disease is a condition in which a part of the head of a metatarsal bone undergoes aseptic necrosis and becomes sufficiently weakened to be susceptible to functional trauma (running, jumping), which may cause compressional collapse of the metatarsal head. The second metatarsal bone is most often involved; the third metatarsal bone is the next most likely to be so. Girls are affected more often than boys.

While walking, pain occurs in the region of the affected metatarsal. Plantar pressure elicits tenderness, as does abrupt release of this pressure. Swelling occurs over the dorsum of the involved metatarsophalangeal joint, plantar flexion becomes limited, and the transverse arch of the involved foot becomes flattened. A callus develops on the plantar surface of the foot, overlying the involved metatarsal head. A deformed, broadened metatarsal head is seen on radiograph. High heels should not be worn, and long walks should be avoided until symptoms subside. Symptomatic use of nonsteroidal antiinflammatory agents is recommended.

CARPAL SEMILUNAR

Aseptic necrosis of the lunate bone (Kienbock disease) weakens the bony structure and usually leads to a compression fracture. The lunate bone of the right hand (the usual working hand) is involved more frequently than that of the left, and boys are affected more frequently than girls.

Pain is experienced on movement of the wrist, and in longstanding cases the pain may be present at rest. Swelling over the dorsum of the wrist and tenderness over the affected bone often are exhibited. The radiograph shows a flattened fragmented lunate bone with variations in its radiodensity. The lunate, lying adjacent to the radius, is subjected to great forces and pressures; hence treatment includes wrist immobilization. On occasion, fusion of the lunate with the wrist bones of the wrist that surround it is required for stabilization and relief of pain.

LOWER THORACIC VERTEBRAE

Scheuermann disease is a common cause of kyphosis in teenagers, occurring in approximately 5% of the teen population. The lower thoracic vertebrae are affected most often. The pathological condition involves a swelling of the intervertebral disks that exerts pressure on the cartilage plates covering the vertebral bodies; this pressure causes the plates to thin and interferes with endochondral bone formation. The disk spaces become narrowed (more anteriorly than posteriorly), and pressure is exerted on the anterior portions of the contiguous vertebral bodies, which impedes their longitudinal growth and thus leads to kyphosis. An aching pain aggravated by physical exertion is present in the affected portion of the vertebral column. The affected area is tender to palpation. Assuming a stooping position often will cause the pain to increase. Within a year or so, the kyphosis easily is apparent as a round back deformity. In many instances the pain is so minor that the patient's complaint is that of poor posture rather than backache. Radiographs reveal narrowing of the anterior disk spaces and defects on the surfaces of adjacent vertebrae. In some children the condition progresses to cause severe deformity and dysfunction; in others the condition stabilizes, and the deformity disappears. Treatment is aimed at preventing further deformity, occasionally with the use of casting or bracing. In rare instances of rapid progression or of persistent, severe pain, spinal fusion is necessary. The majority of youngsters, however, require only careful observation. Rare instances of myopathy associated with Scheuermann disease have occurred.

WHEN TO REFER

- Whenever uncertain of diagnosis or when treatment requires orthopedic assessment or intervention

WHEN TO ADMIT

- Only for surgical intervention

TOOLS FOR PRACTICE

Engaging Patient and Family

- *What is a Pediatric Orthopedic Surgeon?* (fact sheet), American Academy of Pediatrics (www.aap.org/sections/he3007.pdf).

SUGGESTED RESOURCES

Bowen JR, Abrams JS. Legg-Calve-Perthes disease. *Contemp Orthop*. 1985;10:27.

Davids JR, Huskamp M, Bagley AM. A dynamic biomechanical analysis of the etiology of adolescent tibia vara. *J Pediatr Orthop.* 1996;16(4):461-468.

Fitzsimons RB. Idiopathic scoliosis, Scheuermann's disease and myopathy: two case reports. *Clin Exp Neurol.* 1979; 16:303-307.

Gallistl S, Reitinger T, Linhard W, et al. The role of inherited thrombotic disorders in the etiology of Legg-Calve-Perthes disease. *J Pediatr Orthop.* 1999;19(1)82-83.

Glueck CJ, Freiberg R, Tracy T, et al. Thrombophilia and hypofibrinolysis: pathophysiologies of osteonecrosis. *Clin Orthop.* 1997;334:43-56.

Lonstein JE, Bradford D, Winter R, et al. *Textbook of Scoliosis and Other Spinal Deformities.* 3rd ed. Philadelphia, PA: WB Saunders; 1995.

Stulberg SD, Cooperman DR, Wallenstein R. The natural history of Legg-Calve-Perthes disease. *J Bone Joint Surg (Am).* 1981;63(7):1095-1108.

Tachdjian MO. *Clinical Pediatric Orthopedics: The Art of Diagnosis and Principles of Management.* Stamford, CT: Appleton & Lange; 1997.

REFERENCES

1. Balasa VV. Legg-Calve-Perthes disease and thrombophilia. *J Bone Joint Surg Am.* 2004;86-A(12):2642-2647.
2. Arruda VR, Belangero WD, Ozelo MD, et al. Inherited risk factors for thrombophilia among children with Legg-Calve-Perthes disease. *J Pediatr Orthop.* 1999;19(1):84-87.

Chapter 303

OSTEOMYELITIS

Stephanie Yee-Guardino, DO; Johanna Goldfarb, MD

Osteomyelitis, or infection of the bone, in children is most often the result of hematogenous spread of bacteria to bone. Osteomyelitis can also occur after an open fracture or operative procedure or by direct extension from an adjacent soft-tissue infection.[1-8] Chronic osteomyelitis can occur if the infection is indolent and the diagnosis is delayed or if treatment does not completely eradicate infection. Acute osteomyelitis should be diagnosed and aggressively treated to decrease the risk of osteomyelitis becoming chronic; chronic infection requires surgical drainage and is more difficult to eradicate than acute cases. Chronic osteomyelitis can result in lifelong disability related to recurrences and, rarely, to cancer.[9] Regardless of age, osteomyelitis is most often caused by infection with *Staphylococcus aureus*; however, other pathogens can cause osteomyelitis in certain age groups or hosts, or they can be related to the type of contamination (dirt, water, and other sources). Establishing the diagnosis of osteomyelitis can be difficult, especially when the illness begins insidiously. Physicians who care for children must have a high index of suspicion to avoid missing or delaying the diagnosis.

DEFINITION OF TERMS

Acute Osteomyelitis

In children, osteomyelitis caused by hematogenous seeding usually begins in the metaphyses of the long bones,[10] reflecting the rich blood supply in this area throughout childhood. Often, but not always, a history of trauma to the area can be found. Occult transient bacteremia likely seeds a traumatized area more easily than a healthier site.

In infants, osteomyelitis is often accompanied by rapid spread into the adjacent joint, especially the hip. Infection appears to spread rapidly across the metaphysis into the epiphysis and then into the adjacent joint.[11] The presence of penetrating vessels that pass through the growth plate to connect the metaphysis with the epiphysis is thought to allow the rapid spread.[10] These vessels are only present in infancy, most commonly before 6 months of age. Infection may also cross the growth plate directly (see Table 326-1 in Chapter 326, Sports Injuries, for the components of the growth plate).[10] Infants with signs and symptoms of septic arthritis of the hip must always be evaluated for an accompanying osteomyelitis of the femur. In children older than 1 year, infection tends to be held in place by the metaphysis. Infection after infancy is most likely to spread into the diaphysis and down the bone. However, infection of the hip, shoulder, or elbow joints can also be the result of infection of the bone breaking out of the cortex located within the joint capsule. Much more rare is infection that begins in the epiphyseal or metaepiphyseal area.[12] *S aureus* is the organism most likely to be responsible for hematogenous osteomyelitis in all age groups. In newborns, other frequent pathogens include group B streptococcus *(Streptococcus agalactiae)* and Gram-negative bacteria such as *Escherichia coli*. Fungal pathogens, especially *Candida* species, occur in infants who have been in the neonatal intensive care unit and who have had vascular lines in place. In older infants and children, *S aureus* followed by the group A *Streptococcus (S pyogenes)* are the most common pathogens. Because an effective vaccine has been developed, *Haemophilus influenzae* type b infection has become very rare but was previously a frequent pathogen in preschool-age children. *S pneumoniae* occurs mostly in children younger than 2 years,[13] and *Kingella kingae* occurs in young children.[14] Children with hemoglobinopathies are at risk for osteomyelitis, perhaps related to bone infarcts that occur with sickle cell crisis. In this population, *Salmonella* species and *S aureus* are the most common pathogens. *Salmonella* infections in this population occur at rates much higher than in other children who only rarely have this pathogen as a cause of osteomyelitis.[15,16] Organisms that cause a bacteremia can result in an osteomyelitis in the child.

Osteomyelitis following direct invasion of the joint is also most often due to *S aureus*, but other pathogens and sometimes multiple pathogens can be present. In children, trauma is most often the cause, especially after an open fracture, but this circumstance can also occur after orthopedic surgery, especially in the setting of placement of a foreign body such as the insertion of pins or screws into bone. In addition to

S aureus, coagulase-negative staphylococci, Gram-negative organisms, and other unusual organisms can become pathogens. Unusual pathogens reflect the source of contamination. For instance, *Pseudomonas aeruginosa* commonly follows puncture wounds of the foot through a sneaker; *Aeromonas* infections may occur after trauma to bare feet while walking in river water. Multiple pathogens, including anaerobes, may be present, especially if the wound has been contaminated with dirt.

Chronic Osteomyelitis

Chronic osteomyelitis refers to infection in the bone that has become long-standing (usually months of untreated infection), often related to a delay in the diagnosis or to incomplete eradication of an acute infection.[5] Chronic infection is most often indolent and much harder to cure than acute osteomyelitis.[17] Infection can spread insidiously throughout the diaphysis of the affected bone. This spread can occur even with a staphylococcal species when an infection begins around a foreign body such as a pin to stabilize a bone after orthopedic surgery. Infection in chronic osteomyelitis can track outward to result in a spontaneously draining sinus. A sinus tract that closes can result in more acute symptoms and signs. Chronic osteomyelitis results in bone loss and areas of devascularized bone, which separate and results in the creation of sequestrum or pieces of dead bone in the shaft of the long bones. Once this situation occurs, surgery will be required to treat the infection.[3] A *Brodie abscess* is an abscess with a capsule that can develop in the bone and appears to be the result of walled-off chronic infection, often with no active organisms recoverable when drained.

DIFFERENTIAL DIAGNOSIS

Osteomyelitis should always be considered in a child who has localized bone pain, especially if fever is present, which may be low grade. Trauma can be confused with bone infection, especially if fever is minimal. In many instances, osteomyelitis does follow a fracture or trauma; thus even in the presence of a fracture, the possibility of osteomyelitis must be considered if fever is present or pain persists after casting. Fever may be minimal and can be overlooked by both parent and physician. Careful examination, seeking focal areas of tenderness, is necessary in the young child who may not be able to describe pain adequately. Hip or femur pain can be confused with intraabdominal infection, especially infection in the area of the psoas muscle. An example is a missed appendicitis that can result in a phlegmon in this area, causing a limp that can be confused with osteomyelitis of the femur. Careful abdominal examination is therefore necessary in the child who limps so as to avoid missing intraabdominal abnormalities. Back pain and diskitis can also be confused with osteomyelitis. The differential diagnosis of a child with back pain must include vertebral body infection,[18] with or without nearby epidural abscess and diskitis. Bone pain can also be a presenting symptom of leukemia. An abnormal blood count with anemia, a low white blood count, or thrombocytopenia will often be a clue. Cat-scratch disease can cause osteomyelitis and be confused with lymphoma or other malignancy,[19-21] but this condition resolves untreated over time. Some bone tumors can cause nonspecific bone pain and lytic bone lesions on radiograph that must also be differentiated from chronic osteomyelitis by biopsy for pathologic abnormalities and by culture of the bone. When fever is not a prominent sign, osteomyelitis is more likely to be confused with a condition not caused by infection. The differential diagnosis of a limp also includes septic arthritis and juvenile idiopathic arthritis. The manifestations of septic arthritis may be similar to those of acute osteomyelitis, and, especially in the infant, the two entities may coexist. When septic arthritis is present, the urgency for prompt treatment is acute (see Chapter 321, Septic Arthritis). When erythema over the infected bone is present, distinguishing between cellulitis and osteomyelitis may be difficult. Chronic multifocal osteomyelitis is a recurring inflammatory disease that most often is not associated with infection but can mimic bacterial osteomyelitis. In many cases, it can only be diagnosed over time by observing the pattern of recurring disease, usually with cultures negative for acute infection.[22,23]

EVALUATION

Relevant History

A history of localized bone pain and fever is the history most typically given in acute osteomyelitis, at times with prior trauma to the area. In infants and young children, the caretaker may have noticed that the child has pain with movement of the affected limb, has stopped using the limb, or has begun to limp. When the infection causes a bacteremia, a history of a high fever spike before the onset of pain may be described, or, if ongoing, signs of bacteremia may be present, such as chills and high fever, malaise, and acute illness. In older children, one bone is usually involved, whereas, in newborns, more than one site may be infected with a bacteremia.[24] Nonspecific malaise and poor appetite may occur in the child with chronic osteomyelitis, but only nonspecific complaints of pain may be elicited in the area of the bone. Specific pathogens may have unique histories, such as the child with gastroenteritis and *Salmonella* infection who later has new fever and bone pain or the child with an open fracture or bone surgery who later develops fever and new pain or drainage at the same site. A child with a fracture, either open or closed, who has new or worsening pain under a cast should have the cast removed and the area evaluated for infection.

The history may be acute, especially if the child is bacteremic, or more subacute or chronic in cases in which the bacteremia has resolved or the pathogen is less virulent. In chronic osteomyelitis, symptoms may have been present for months.

Physical Examination

Vital signs of the child with osteomyelitis may be normal, especially with chronic infection, or abnormal if the child is bacteremic at presentation. Fever will often be present when measured, even in the absence of a history of fever. Localized pain will almost always be present. Tenderness is often exquisite, but in younger children, only a new limp or absence of movement of an arm or leg may be noted. Other local signs may be associated with inflammation, including swelling, redness, and warmth over the involved bone, which can be confused with a cellulitis. Characteristically, the child is reluctant to move the adjacent joint and, when a lower extremity is involved, may refuse to bear weight. In the young infant, the loss of active movement in an extremity may be confused with a neurologic problem. Erythema is often present over the infected bone, in addition to tenderness to palpation or movement. If associated arthritis occurs, then pain on movement of the joint may be prominent.

Laboratory Testing

The diagnostic evaluation for possible osteomyelitis includes a complete blood cell count and smear review, erythrocyte sedimentation rate, C-reactive protein, blood cultures, and radiographs. However, all of these tests can produce normal findings, especially early in the infection. The white blood cell count can be elevated in acutely ill children with bacteremia, though very low counts occur with sepsis. The presence of anemia, low white blood cell count, or thrombocytopenia in the absence of disseminated intravascular coagulation should raise concern for leukemia or other malignancy. The sedimentation rate may be normal at first but almost always becomes elevated in acute osteomyelitis. The C-reactive protein is usually elevated early. These clinical markers are helpful in following the course and response to treatment. The C-reactive protein rises more quickly and normalizes more rapidly than the sedimentation rate, which eventually is most useful in following long-term therapy.

Imaging

Early in the clinical course, no bony changes are seen radiographically; the earliest detectable signs are those of blurred soft-tissue planes secondary to edema spreading into fatty tissues. Bone changes are not apparent until at least 7 to 10 days or longer after the onset of symptoms. The first signs consist of nonspecific periosteal reaction.[25] Lytic lesions occur later. Bony radiographs should always be obtained, however, to exclude other pathologic abnormalities such as fracture or a malignant lesion. Although skeletal scintigraphy (technetium bone scan) was recommended in the past for evaluating children with possible osteomyelitis,[26] the advantage of using magnetic resonance imaging (MRI) initially have recently become clear.[27] MRI provides excellent views of the bony and soft-tissue anatomy, revealing subperiosteal abscesses that require surgical intervention.[27-31] The presence of a subperiosteal abscess is diagnostic for an acute osteomyelitis that has broken through the metaphyseal cortex. MRI is also the image of choice when pelvic or spine osteomyelitis is suspected.[28,32,33] Technetium bone scans are sensitive, though less sensitive than MRI, are also less specific, and are often difficult to interpret,[34] with frequent false negative results.[35-37] Bone scans are not useful in the neonate because of low bone mineralization.[38] Bone scans provide limited information regarding soft-tissue involvement, subperiosteal space, and bone marrow edema, and the results may be normal in up to 20% of children in the first days of illness. In addition, malignancy, cellulitis, trauma, and bone infarction can affect the specificity of a bone scan, though 3-stage scans improve sensitivity. Finally, bone scans require large amounts of radiation. However, the bone scan does not ordinarily require sedation or general anesthesia, which frequently are needed for a young child to lie still for an MRI. Bone scans can be useful in cases in which multiple sites of osteomyelitis are suspected.

Ultrasonography can detect a subperiosteal abscess and may be helpful in guiding needle aspiration of an infected bone. The finding of such a collection distinguishes osteomyelitis from cellulitis in an inflamed extremity, but the failure to visualize an abscess does not rule out early osteomyelitis still contained within the bone. Ultrasound also can help evaluate a nearby joint for an effusion that is present with an associated arthritis.

In chronic osteomyelitis, the radiograph will show extensive disease, usually along the diaphysis of the bone, with bone changes that may need to be differentiated from malignancy by history and ultimately by cultures and biopsy.

MANAGEMENT

A blood culture and a needle aspirate of the site of infection are the most helpful procedures for diagnosing osteomyelitis. Aspiration confirms the diagnosis and can determine the necessity for operative decompression if frank pus is obtained, may alleviate pain caused by pressure from an abscess, and provides a specimen for pathogen identification by culture and material for immediate Gram stain. Blood cultures are also helpful in identifying the presence of bacteremia and the cause of the infection, and they are frequently positive in 40% to 50% of cases. If the history and examination fit with the diagnosis and a blood culture is positive, then therapy can be started without a bone aspiration. If response to therapy is prompt, then aspiration may not be required.[9] Needle aspiration of the subperiosteal space and of the metaphysis for culture is indicated to obtain culture identification of the pathogen when blood cultures are pending and whenever a collection of pus exists. When surgery is indicated, it should be prompt and antibiotics started as soon as culture material is obtained. In indolent cases and in cases with unusual presentations, aspirating the bone is especially important to obtain the pathogen and to guide therapy. Evaluation for related arthritis also is crucial, given that joint infections can progress rapidly and need adequate drainage to avoid damage to the joint (see Chapter 321, Septic Arthritis). If infection with tuberculosis is suggested because of history or setting, then cultures for acid-fast bacteria should be included and a tuberculin skin testing added to the evaluation.[39]

Once blood cultures and needle aspiration have been performed, antibiotics should be given empirically and by the intravenous route. After the newborn period, in a previously well child thought to have hematogenous osteomyelitis, a penicillinase-resistant penicillin or 1st-generation cephalosporin is sufficient unless the child is severely ill or has signs of bacteremia and sepsis. In a child with sepsis, vancomycin should be considered because of the rising incidence of methicillin-resistant *S aureus* (MRSA) in community-associated infection. In each case, therapy should be individualized to include other likely pathogens. For example, in the newborn, *S aureus* remains the most common cause, but *S agalactiae*, coagulase negative staphylococcus, Gram-negative enterics, and *Candida* species are encountered in neonates in the intensive care unit. Initial therapy in the newborn should always include coverage against Gram-negative enterics and might include oxacillin and gentamicin, or vancomycin and ceftazidime, when concern for MRSA infection exists or for coagulase-negative staphylococci. Neonates who have been in a neonatal intensive care unit and who have been on antibiotics should be treated most broadly, pending culture results. Fungal coverage is usually not empiric therapy, unless a blood culture or other epidemiologic data suggest the presence of a fungal infection. Children with sickle cell hemoglobinopathies who are at special risk for infection with *Salmonella* species in addition to *S aureus* might be treated with cefuroxime or with vancomycin and ceftriaxone or cefotaxime, pending culture results. If a pseudomonal infection is suspected, such as in the child with infection after puncture wound of the foot, then the initial treatment should be ceftazidime or a carboxypenicillin or acylureidopenicillin combined with an aminoglycoside such as piperacillin-tazobactam and gentamicin or ceftazidime and gentamicin. Piperacillin-tazobactam will also treat *S aureus* while cultures are pending.

If infection is the result of open wounds, then the setting should guide empiric therapy. Wounds contaminated by dirt should include broad coverage of Gram negatives and anaerobes, such as piperacillin-tazobactam with an aminoglycoside.

Antibiotics should be adjusted once cultures and sensitivities are available, narrowing the spectrum to cover the pathogen. Clindamycin has good bone penetration and is often used in cases of allergy to β-lactams or to treat MRSA isolates that are sensitive. It has been recommended as empiric therapy if MRSA is suggested, though some isolates may be resistant. The role of the antibiotic linezolid in treating osteomyelitis in children remains to be determined. It should not be used empirically but may be helpful in patients with β-lactam allergies and as a drug that can be used orally to treat a serious infection, though the side effect of thrombocytopenia limits its long-term use. Antibiotics should be continued for 4 to 8 weeks, using clinical response and sedimentation rate to guide length of therapy.

Oral antibiotics can be considered to finish the course of therapy, if an oral agent is available that has good bone penetration, has excellent activity against the pathogen, is palatable, and if the child has a social situation that will guarantee compliance. The switch to oral therapy should not occur before clinical response to intravenous therapy, including absence of fever, return to normal function, and a decrease or normalization of inflammatory markers. Oral antibiotics often require 2 to 3 times the usual dose to achieve adequate bone penetration, making gastrointestinal tolerance of high doses of the antibiotic a requirement.

An abscess must be drained surgically when detected or suspected. The lack of pus on aspiration should suggest that the site of aspiration may have been inaccurate, or pus may be present but too thick to pass through even a large-bore needle. Care must be taken not to miss infection. A clinical suspicion or failure of the patient to respond to nonoperative therapy is an indication for operative decompression. The risks of unnecessary surgery in the child who has an acute infection are far less than those of necessary surgery not performed. MRI can help locate and define the anatomy of the infection in children failing conservative therapy. Chronic osteomyelitis always requires surgical debridement and prolonged antimicrobial therapy for up to 1 year.

WHEN TO REFER

The diagnosis of possible osteomyelitis requires thorough evaluation and usually includes consultation with radiology and orthopedic surgery. Discussing the specifics of the case with the radiologist can help focus the radiologic evaluation effectively. Consulting early with the orthopedic surgeon helps expedite aspiration of the bone or open drainage. Infectious diseases specialists help organize the evaluation, begin therapy, and follow-up with children who are discharged on home intravenous therapy and who have chronic disease.

WHEN TO ADMIT

Children with acute osteomyelitis require admission to the hospital for rapid evaluation and to initiate treatment. The initial evaluation can begin as an outpatient, when the diagnosis of osteomyelitis is not yet established, perhaps with complete blood count, blood culture, and radiograph. However, the physician must follow up closely and consider hospitalization as soon as the diagnosis becomes likely.

TOOLS FOR PRACTICE

Engaging Patients and Family

- *Osteomyelitis* (fact sheet), National Foundation-Kids Health (www.kidshealth.org/teen/diseases_conditions/bones/osteomyelitis.html).

SUGGESTED RESOURCES

Dich VQ, Nelson JD, Haltalin KC. Osteomyelitis in infants and children. A review of 163 cases. *Am J Dis Child*. Nov 1975;129(11):1273-1278.

Frank G, Mahoney HM, Eppes SC. Musculoskeletal infections in children. *Pediatr Clin North Am*. 2005;52:1083-1106.

Kaplan SL. Osteomyelitis in children. *Infect Dis Clin North Am*. Dec 2005;19(4):787-797, vii.

Nelson JD. Acute osteomyelitis in children. *Infect Dis Clin North Am* Sep 1990;4(3):513-522.

Waldvogel FA, Medoff G, Swartz MN. Osteomyelitis: a review of clinical features, therapeutic considerations and unusual aspects (second of three parts). *N Engl J Med*. Jan 1970;282(5):260-266.

Waldvogel FA, Papageorgiou PS. Osteomyelitis: the past decade. *N Engl J Med*. Aug 1980;303(7):360-370.

REFERENCES

1. Waldvogel FA, Medoff G, Swartz MN. Osteomyelitis: a review of clinical features, therapeutic considerations and unusual aspects (second of three parts). *N Engl J Med*. Jan 1970;282(5):260-266.
2. Waldvogel FA, Medoff G, Swartz MN. Osteomyelitis: a review of clinical features, therapeutic considerations and unusual aspects. *N Engl J Med*. Jan 1970;282(4): 198-206.
3. Waldvogel FA, Papageorgiou PS. Osteomyelitis: the past decade. *N Engl J Med*. Aug 1980;303(7):360-370.
4. Kaplan SL. Osteomyelitis in children. *Infect Dis Clin North Am*. Dec 2005;19(4):787-797, vii.
5. Dich VQ, Nelson JD, Haltalin KC. Osteomyelitis in infants and children. A review of 163 cases. *Am J Dis Child*. Nov 1975;129(11):1273-1278.
6. Green NE, Edwards K. Bone and joint infections in children. *Orthop Clin North Am*. Oct 1987;18(4):555-576.
7. Nelson JD. Acute osteomyelitis in children. *Infect Dis Clin North Am*. Sep 1990;4(3):513-522.
8. Mahoney FG, Eppes HM, Stephen C. Musculoskeletal infections in children. *Pediatric Clin North Am*. 2005;52: 1083-1106.
9. Fitzgerald RH Jr, Brewer NS, Dahlin DC. Squamous-cell carcinoma complicating chronic osteomyelitis. *J Bone Joint Surg Am*. Dec 1976;58(8):1146-1148.
10. Trueta J, Morgan JD. Late results in the treatment of one hundred cases of acute haematogenous osteomyelitis. *Br J Surg*. Mar 1954;41(169):449-457.
11. Ogden JA, Lister G. The pathology of neonatal osteomyelitis. *Pediatrics*. Apr 1975;55(4):474-478.
12. Hempfing A, Placzek R, Gottsche T, et al. Primary subacute epiphyseal and metaepiphyseal osteomyelitis in children. Diagnosis and treatment guided by MRI. *J Bone Joint Surg Br*. May 2003;85(4):559-564.
13. Jacobs NM. Pneumococcal osteomyelitis and arthritis in children. A hospital series and literature review. *Am J Dis Child*. Jan 1991;145(1):70-74.
14. Yagupsky P, Dagan R, Howard CB, et al. Clinical features and epidemiology of invasive Kingella kingae infections in southern Israel. *Pediatrics*. Dec 1993;92(6):800-804.
15. Syrogiannopoulos GA, McCracken GH Jr, Nelson JD. Osteoarticular infections in children with sickle cell disease. *Pediatrics*. Dec 1986;78(6):1090-1096.
16. Givner LB, Luddy RE, Schwartz AD. Etiology of osteomyelitis in patients with major sickle hemoglobinopathies. *J Pediatr*. Sep 1981;99(3):411-413.
17. Ramos OM. Chronic osteomyelitis in children. *Pediatr Infect Dis J*. May 2002;21(5):431-432.
18. Bolivar R, Kohl S, Pickering LK. Vertebral osteomyelitis in children: report of four cases. *Pediatrics*. Oct 1978; 62(4):549-553.
19. Sakellaris G, Kampitakis E, Karamitopoulou E, et al. Cat scratch disease simulating a malignant process of the chest wall with coexistent osteomyelitis. *Scand J Infect Dis*. 2003;35(6-7):433-435.
20. Hipp SJ, O'Shields A, Fordham LA, et al. Multifocal bone marrow involvement in cat-scratch disease. *Pediatr Infect Dis J*. May 2005;24(5):472-474.
21. Prybis BG, Eady JL, Kotchmar GS Jr. Chronic osteomyelitis associated with cat-scratch disease. *J South Orthop Assoc*. Summer 2002;11(2):119-123.
22. Chun CS. Chronic recurrent multifocal osteomyelitis of the spine and mandible: case report and review of the literature. *Pediatrics*. Apr 2004;113(4):e380-e384.
23. King SM, Laxer RM, Manson D, et al. Chronic recurrent multifocal osteomyelitis: a noninfectious inflammatory process. *Pediatr Infect Dis J*. Oct 1987;6(10):907-911.
24. Weissberg ED, Smith AL, Smith DH. Clinical features of neonatal osteomyelitis. *Pediatrics*. Apr 1974 1974;53(4): 505-510.
25. Wenaden AE, Szyszko TA, Saifuddin A. Imaging of periosteal reactions associated with focal lesions of bone. *Clin Radiol*. Apr 2005;60(4):439-456.
26. Darville T, Jacobs RF. Management of acute hematogenous osteomyelitis in children. *Pediatr Infect Dis J*. Mar 2004;23(3):255-257.
27. Mazur JM, Ross G, Cummings J, et al. Usefulness of magnetic resonance imaging for the diagnosis of acute musculoskeletal infections in children. *J Pediatr Orthoped*. 1995;15(2):144-147.
28. Marin C, Sanchez-Alegre ML, Gallego C, et al. Magnetic resonance imaging of osteoarticular infections in children. *Curr Prob Diagn Radiol*. 2004;33(2):43-59.
29. Kaiser S, Jorulf H, Hirsch G. Clinical value of imaging techniques in childhood osteomyelitis. *Acta Radiologica*. 1998;39(5):523-531.
30. Dangman BC, Hoffer FA, Rand FF, et al. Osteomyelitis in children: gadolinium-enhanced MR imaging. *Radiology*. 1992;182(3):743-747.
31. Poyhia T, Azouz EM. MR imaging evaluation of subacute and chronic bone abscesses in children. *Pediatr Radiol*. 2000;30(11):763-768.
32. Connolly LP, Connolly SA, Drubach LA, et al. Acute hematogenous osteomyelitis of children: assessment of skeletal scintigraphy-based diagnosis in the era of MRI. *J Nucl Med*. 2002;43(10):1310-1316.
33. Jaramillo D, Treves ST, Kasser JR, et al. Osteomyelitis and septic arthritis in children: appropriate use of imaging to guide treatment. *AJR Am J Roentgenol*. 1995; 165(2):399-403.
34. Sullivan DC, Rosenfield NS, Ogden J, et al. Problems in the scintigraphic detection of osteomyelitis in children. *Radiology*. 1980;135(3):731-736.
35. Wald ER, Mirro R, Gartner JC. Pitfalls on the diagnosis of acute osteomyelitis by bone scan. *Clin Pediatr*. 1980; 19(9):597-601.
36. Berkowitz ID, Wenzel W. 'Normal' technetium bone scans in patients with acute osteomyelitis. *Am J Dis Child*. 1980;134(9):828-830.
37. Fleisher GR, Paradise JE, Plotkin SA, et al. Falsely normal radionuclide scans for osteomyelitis. *Am J Dis Child*. 1980;134(5):499-502.
38. Ish-Horowicz MR, McIntyre P, Nade S. Bone and joint infections caused by multiply resistant Staphylococcus aureus in a neonatal intensive care unit. *Pediatr Infect Dis J*. 1992;11(2):82-87.
39. Teo HE, Peh WC. Skeletal tuberculosis in children. *Pediatr Radiol*. Nov 2004;34(11):853-860.

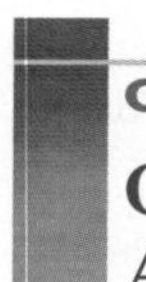

Chapter 304

OTITIS MEDIA AND OTITIS EXTERNA

Tina Q. Tan, MD

OTITIS MEDIA

Otitis media is the most common reason that children in the United States receive a prescription for an antibiotic. More than 90% of all antibiotic use in the first 2 years of life is attributable to the treatment of otitis media.[1] By the age of 7 years, between 65% and 95% of children will have been treated for at least one episode of otitis media.[2] Because it is such a prevalent condition, much attention is focused on the consequences of otitis media and its treatment. Rare suppurative complications, such as intracranial abscess, can be serious. Conductive hearing loss resulting from chronic middle-ear effusions associated with otitis media may contribute to speech and language delay in some children. The overuse of antibiotics to treat otitis media is thought to contribute significantly to the emergence of antibiotic-resistant bacteria.[3] Each year in the United States, more than $3.5 billion is spent on the treatment of otitis media.[4] In response to growing concerns over the increasing rates of antibacterial resistance and the escalating costs of antibacterial prescriptions for the treatment of this disease, in 2004 the American Academy of Pediatrics and the American Academy of Family Physicians published an evidence-based clinical practice guideline on the diagnosis and management of acute otitis media. The major aim of this guideline is to focus attention on the need for the judicious use of antibacterial agents in the treatment of acute otitis media.[5] Despite this attention the management of otitis media remains a source of debate in the medical literature.

Classification

Otitis media literally means inflammation of the middle ear. It encompasses several clinical entities. *Acute otitis media* (AOM) describes the presence of inflammatory fluid in the middle-ear space accompanied by the acute onset of local findings such as ear pain, otorrhea, or distortion of the tympanic membrane (eg, bulging, erythema, opacity, limited or absence of mobility). Systemic findings such as fever and irritability may also be present. *Otitis media with effusion* (OME), or serous otitis media, describes the presence of inflammatory fluid in the middle-ear space in an asymptomatic child or in a child with mild upper respiratory tract symptoms, a common reason for examining the ears in the first place. The term *recurrent otitis media* has generally been used to refer to the occurrence of 3 or more episodes of AOM in 6 months or 4 episodes in 1 year. Recurrent otitis media should not be confused with chronic otitis media, which may be used to describe OME that lasts for greater than 3 months or a suppurative middle-ear process that fails to respond to initial antibiotic therapy. Specificity in diagnosis is important because of its significant implications for management.

Epidemiologic Features

By the age of 1 year, 62% of children have experienced at least 1 episode of AOM.[6] Otitis media is more common in boys and in children of low socioeconomic status. Incidence rates in white and black children are similar. Several environmental factors increase the risk for developing otitis media, including exposure to tobacco smoke,[7] use of a pacifier,[8] and attendance at child care centers, particularly those serving large numbers of children.[9] Exclusive breastfeeding early in life has a protective effect.[10] Children at high risk for developing AOM include those with craniofacial anomalies (eg, cleft palate) that alter the normal air and fluid dynamics of the middle-ear space, those with immunodeficiencies, and those of certain ethnic groups such as Native Americans and Alaskan Natives. A mild hereditary predisposition to develop recurrent otitis media appears to exist, with some of the variation in presentation and incidence explained by genetic factors; familial and individual environmental factors account for the remainder.[11]

Pathogenesis

Otitis media is an inflammatory process of the upper respiratory tract and usually results from a viral infection. As viruses infect the respiratory mucosa, edema can lead to eustachian tube dysfunction. Inflammatory fluid and pathogenic respiratory bacteria that reflux into the middle-ear space do not drain normally. This process effectively leads to the formation of an abscess in the middle ear. Otitis media is usually self-limited; as the viral illness resolves, eustachian tube function is restored, and the middle-ear space drains normally. Although acute symptoms generally resolve spontaneously within a few days, middle-ear effusions can persist for weeks after an episode of AOM. Sixty percent of middle-ear effusions resolve spontaneously within 3 months, 85% within 6 months.[12] The persistence of middle-ear effusions (or OME) after an episode of AOM has raised concern about the conductive hearing loss that accompanies these effusions and its impact on speech and language development, especially in younger children. These effusions are sterile and in the absence of other acute signs and symptoms do not require antibacterial therapy.

In studies of children with AOM, specimens of middle-ear fluid obtained by tympanocentesis have been used to clarify the microbiological mechanism of this disease. These specimens are positive for bacteria approximately 70% of the time.[13] The most frequently identified pathogens are *Streptococcus pneumoniae, Haemophilus influenzae,* and *Moraxella catarrhalis.* Group A β-hemolytic streptococcus and *Staphylococcus aureus* (including methicillin-resistant strains) are much less common. Rarely, *Mycoplasma pneumoniae* is detected but not often enough to affect the empirical selection of an antibiotic for treatment of AOM. Respiratory viruses such as respiratory syncytial virus (RSV), influenza viruses, and parainfluenza viruses are also recovered often from middle-ear aspirates, either in addition to bacteria or in isolation. RSV, in particular, has a tendency to infect the mucosa of the middle ear and probably contributes substantially to the development of otitis media in children.[14]

Diagnosis

Concern is growing that overdiagnosis of otitis media and liberal use of antibiotics for its treatment have contributed to the rapid emergence of antibiotic-resistant bacteria, particularly penicillin-resistant *S pneumoniae*.[15] Therefore accurate diagnosis is critical to the appropriate management of otitis media. Diagnosis is based on recognition of the characteristic clinical context and physical findings on pneumatic otoscopic examination.

In the classic case of AOM a young child with a history of a recent upper respiratory tract infection suddenly develops the acute onset of a new fever and ear discomfort. In children old enough to localize pain the affected ear is often obvious. In younger children, discomfort may be more generalized, and they may exhibit unexplained crying or irritability. Examination may reveal other signs of upper respiratory infection such as rhinorrhea, cough, or conjunctival injection.

The diagnosis of AOM is confirmed using pneumatic otoscopy. To perform this technique, the child must either cooperate or be restrained in a comfortable position that allows the examiner to manipulate the pinna and insert the otoscope into the external auditory canal without difficulty. Cleansing the external auditory canal must be accomplished to free it of obstructions so as to visualize of the tympanic membrane; cerumen or foreign bodies should be removed using a cerumen spoon or gentle irrigation with warm water. The largest speculum that will fit into the external auditory canal at a depth of 1/3-inch to 1/2-inch should be attached to the pneumatic otoscope. This tool permits visualization of the largest possible area and ensures a relatively airtight seal for effective insufflation.

AOM is present when distortion (usually bulging) of the tympanic membrane is noted on direct visualization and when restricted movement of the tympanic membrane, indicative of fluid in the middle ear, is noted with gentle insufflation and exsufflation of air using a squeeze bulb attached to the otoscope. Erythema of the tympanic membrane alone is not sufficient to make the diagnosis of AOM and may be the incidental result of fever or crying. In some cases of AOM the tympanic membrane may be retracted rather than bulging.

Occasionally a child with AOM experiences spontaneous rupture of the tympanic membrane. This event leads to marked improvement in ear pain and the presence of otorrhea on examination.

OME may be an incidental finding on physical examination and is characterized by decreased mobility of the tympanic membrane without the signs of acute inflammation seen in AOM.

In AOM, some experts advocate making a specific bacteriologic diagnosis by obtaining middle-ear fluid for culture and sensitivities using the technique of tympanocentesis or carbon dioxide laser-assisted myringotomy. These techniques are not necessary for the routine diagnosis of AOM but are useful in specific clinical situations in which identification of an organism to guide therapeutic decisions is a high priority. These situations include: (1) episodes of AOM that do not respond to empirical antibiotic therapy, (2) the child who experiences frequent recurrences of AOM despite what seems to be appropriate therapy, and (3) the child who is young and particularly toxic in appearance.

Cultures of other areas of the upper respiratory tract are useful for research purposes but do not assist in the management of individual episodes of AOM. Organisms recovered from tympanocentesis or laser-assisted myringotomy specimens are usually recovered from the nasopharynx also, but the presence of an organism on a nasopharyngeal culture does not prove that it is present in the middle-ear fluid.

Tympanometry is a technique for documenting tympanic membrane compliance. It can be used to document objectively the presence of fluid in the middle-ear space but does not add to the information obtained on carefully performed pneumatic otoscopy. Tympanometry measurements can be useful to monitor the course of an episode of OME over time.

MANAGEMENT OF ACUTE OTITIS MEDIA

Whether an episode of AOM should be treated with antibiotics is a matter of ongoing discussion. The 2004 American Academy of Pediatrics and American Academy of Family Physicians practice guidelines delineate very specific criteria for which patients should receive antibiotic therapy and which patients are candidates for observation. However, patients whose condition do not quite fit the criteria have been noted; in these cases, clinical experience should be used to determine which course of therapy is most appropriate. Some of the acute symptoms of AOM such as fever and ear pain may resolve more quickly with antibiotic therapy. Early empirical antibiotic therapy may also obviate the need for follow-up office visits to evaluate the patient with otitis media who is not responding to expectant management. However, most episodes of AOM resolve spontaneously, middle-ear effusions may persist despite effective antibiotic therapy, and rare suppurative complications are generally easily treated with antibiotics and surgical techniques. The modest benefits of antibiotic therapy also must be weighed against the negative impact of widespread antibiotic use and its effect on producing antibiotic-resistant species of organisms such as *S pneumoniae*.[3] In some areas of the United States, 40% of strains of this organism are resistant to penicillin.[16]

Several guiding principles should be observed when selecting patients with AOM to be treated with antibiotics. First, the diagnosis of AOM should be clear. The presence of fever, upper respiratory symptoms, or a middle-ear effusion may be consistent with AOM, but without objective findings on pneumatic otoscopy these criteria are not sufficient and should not lead to prescription of antibiotics. Second, younger patients may benefit more from empirical antibiotic therapy than older children. The positive effects of antibiotic administration have been more prevalent in children younger than 2 years. This circumstance is due, perhaps, to their more limited immune response to encapsulated organisms. Third, uniquely susceptible individuals such as those with immunodeficiencies or those with craniofacial anomalies are at increased risk of developing complications or a protracted course of illness and therefore warrant a lower threshold for treatment. Observation of a patient off antibiotic therapy for 48 to 72 hours is now considered an acceptable management option in low-risk patients older than 6 months with early AOM.[5] If symptoms have not resolved spontaneously with 48 to 72 hours, then reexamination is indicated with prescription of antibiotics if objective findings of AOM are still present.

When a decision is made to treat a child with AOM, an effective antibiotic with the narrowest spectrum should be chosen. Many antibiotics are marketed for the treatment of this common condition including penicillins; first-, second-, and third-generation cephalosporins; macrolides; and carbacephems. In the absence of specific microbiological information, the selection of empirical antibiotic therapy should be guided by both the knowledge of the most common bacterial pathogens identified in middle-ear aspirates of children and by the efficacy of the antibacterial agent (based on minimal inhibitory concentration and pharmacokinetic and pharmacodynamic data) against these organisms. In population-based studies of children with AOM the most common organisms isolated were *S pneumoniae, H influenzae,* and *M catarrhalis.*[17-19]

High-dose amoxicillin is inexpensive; has a good spectrum of activity against these organisms, including strains of *S pneumoniae* with intermediate resistance to penicillin; and is the recommended first-line choice. Studies of amoxicillin treatment of AOM show cure rates of 85% to 94% based on clinical criteria, an acceptable figure given the high rate of spontaneous resolution. Treatment should be administered for 10 days, although shorter courses of 5 to 7 days may be acceptable in low-risk patients, such as older children with uncomplicated histories.[20]

If fever, ear pain, and the objective findings of AOM persist despite at least 72 hours of therapy, then a change of antibiotic may be warranted. Second-line agents such as second- or third-generation cephalosporins or amoxicillin plus clavulanate may be used to broaden the antimicrobial spectrum to cover β-lactamase-producing strains of *H influenzae* and *M catarrhalis,* as well as penicillin-resistant *S pneumoniae*. Clindamycin only provides coverage for resistant gram-positive organisms and may be used as an alternative agent if the otitis is proven to be secondary to a resistant strain of *S pneumoniae*. For patients who develop hives or anaphylaxis to the β-lactam antibiotics, azithromycin may be used for therapy; however, this drug has decreased activity against penicillin-resistant strains of *S pneumoniae* and β-lactamase-producing strains of *H influenzae*.

No proven benefit has been found to the use of antihistamine or decongestant preparations, steroids, or nonsteroidal antiinflammatory medications in the treatment of AOM. Topical Auralgan otic solution is somewhat effective in reducing the acute ear pain associated with AOM.[21]

FOLLOW-UP AFTER ACUTE OTITIS MEDIA TREATMENT

Most children who respond satisfactorily to treatment of an episode of AOM do not require specific follow-up. As long as a child is asymptomatic the main reason for follow-up is to document resolution of a middle-ear effusion that may contribute to conductive hearing loss. Only 50% of middle-ear effusions resolve by 6 weeks after initial presentation. Therefore follow-up for the otherwise-healthy and asymptomatic child should be scheduled no sooner than 6 weeks post-diagnosis, if at all. An effusion that is persistent at 6 weeks does not warrant specific intervention other than perhaps checking for resolution again in 6 more weeks. Further management of an effusion that persists beyond this point is described in the treatment of OME later.

MANAGEMENT OF OTITIS MEDIA WITH EFFUSION

OME presents a different therapeutic challenge than AOM. The goal of therapy for this disorder is to limit any potential long-term detrimental effects on speech and language development that may be caused by conductive hearing loss associated with the presence of a chronic middle-ear effusion. Weak associations have been found between OME and abnormal speech and language development in children younger than 4 years and problems with attention and expressive language delay in older children.[22-24] However, these associations may be the result of environmental influences that predispose the patient to both OME and developmental delays. The effects of treating OME on these outcomes are not well established.

Medical therapies for OME have produced largely unsatisfactory results. Although very limited scientific evidence exists, a few experts believe that empirical antibiotic therapy either early in the course of OME or later, when the effusion has persisted for 3 months or more, may hasten resolution of the effusion. Most experts strongly discourage this practice, given the increasing rates of antibacterial resistance that is being seen. No role exists for steroid medications, antihistamine or decongestant preparations, or for tonsillectomy or adenoidectomy in the management of OME. The most effective therapy for OME is the surgical insertion of tympanostomy tubes. Placement of tympanostomy tubes evacuates a middle-ear effusion and restores near-normal hearing, but the effect of this procedure on long-term speech and language outcomes is unclear.[25] Laser-assisted myringotomy may soon replace tympanostomy tube placement for the treatment of OME.[15]

When OME is documented in a child, follow-up at 3 months is reasonable, assuming acute symptoms have not intervened. If, at 3 months, middle-ear effusions are persistent and are bilateral, then referral for audiologic testing is indicated. If hearing is normal, then further observation to allow spontaneous resolution is appropriate. If a conductive hearing loss at a threshold of 20 dB or greater is documented at the 3-month follow-up, then consideration should be given to tympanostomy tube placement or laser-assisted myringotomy to drain the effusions and restore hearing. The use of these procedures for OME in otherwise-healthy children with normal hearing is not recommended.

Adenoidectomy is used in the management of patients with OME and may be effective in a select group of children.[26] Chronically infected adenoids is thought to serve as a reservoir of pathogenic organisms that leads to tubal edema and malfunction, which may clinically produce persistent OME. The removal of enlarged adenoids has been shown to improve effusion resolution.[27,28] In the otolaryngology literature, adenoidectomy and myringotomy plus ventilation tube insertion is recommended therapy for children with severe ear disease and those undergoing replacement of a second set of ventilation tubes.[29,30]

MANAGEMENT OF RECURRENT OTITIS MEDIA

The occurrence of 3 or more episodes of AOM within 6 months or of 4 episodes within a year satisfies many experts' definition of recurrent or chronic otitis media. The therapy of recurrent otitis media is also controversial. Studies have shown that long-term administration of prophylactic antibiotics (usually either amoxicillin or trimethoprim plus sulfamethoxazole) can reduce the incidence of subsequent episodes of AOM in these children. However, the effect is modest; to improve outcome in 1 child, 9 must be treated with daily medication, and prophylactic antibiotics contribute to the development of resistant organisms.[31] Therefore the use of prophylactic antibiotics is currently not recommended for management of recurrent otitis media.[32] Controlling environmental risk factors such as exposure to tobacco smoke and attendance at large child care centers is a more desirable approach to this problem.

Tympanostomy tube placement or laser-assisted myringotomy should be considered in the management of recurrent otitis media. This approach may be justified when recurrent AOM complicates OME and is accompanied by hearing loss, as described previously. However, frequent episodes of AOM (without OME) that respond to appropriate antibiotic therapy are not an indication for these procedures. Although AOM does tend to occur less frequently in children who have had tympanostomy tubes placed, this approach is a surgical procedure requiring administration of anesthesia, and tubes may not remain in place for a sufficient duration to have a measurable impact on the health of an individual child.

Use of a conjugated vaccine against *S pneumoniae*, widespread use of the influenza vaccine in healthy children, and development of an effective vaccine against RSV are all strategies that show promise for prevention of future episodes of otitis media.

CARE OF THE CHILD WITH TYMPANOSTOMY TUBES

Tympanostomy tube placement is the most common surgical procedure performed in children.[33] All physicians who care for children will encounter tympanostomy tubes in their practice. Examination of the child with tympanostomy tubes should show a patent tube traversing the pars flaccida. Because the tympanic membrane that contains a tympanostomy tube is not intact, its mobility is affected, and pneumatic otoscopy cannot be used as a reliable indicator of the presence of AOM.

Tympanostomy tubes are usually extruded naturally sometime after insertion. Some otolaryngologists recommend actively removing tympanostomy tubes that have been in place for 2 or more years to prevent complications such as chronic perforation or tympanosclerosis. If a tympanostomy tube is visualized in the external canal and is no longer seated within the tympanic membrane, then it may be removed with a cerumen spoon under direct visualization.

Occasionally a granuloma may develop at the site of tympanostomy tube insertion, which can lead to bleeding from the external auditory canal. When this event occurs, these patients should be referred to an otolaryngologist for intervention.

Otorrhea is common in children with tympanostomy tubes. Otorrhea associated with other symptoms of upper respiratory infection may indicate the presence of AOM and should be treated accordingly. When otorrhea occurs in isolation, it may respond to topical application of an otic solution containing neomycin, polymyxin B, and hydrocortisone. Otorrhea is no more common in children with tympanostomy tubes who swim or submerge their heads in a bathtub than it is in those who do not engage in these activities.[34] The use of topical antibiotics or earplugs does not reduce the incidence of swimming-related otorrhea. Children with tympanostomy tubes who do not dive to depths of greater than 6 feet nor swim in potentially contaminated water (such as a pond) require no special precautions to swim, and the use of earplugs or molds may actually increase drainage from the ears.

COMPLICATIONS

The possible effects of otitis media on speech and language development are discussed in Chapter 45, Language and Speech Assessment.

Suppurative complications of otitis media include mastoiditis, intracranial extension of infection, and lateral sinus thrombosis.[35] These complications are rare and occur much less frequently than in the era before routine antibiotic treatment of AOM. However, the incidence of these complications has also declined in areas of the world where routine antibiotic treatment of AOM is less common, suggesting that factors other than early antibiotic treatment have contributed to this trend.[36]

Recognizing the early signs and symptoms associated with suppurative complications of otitis media is important so that effective medical or surgical therapy can be instituted promptly. These signs and symptoms include mastoid tenderness, persistent fever associated with chronic tympanic membrane perforation, persistent and severe headache, severe otalgia, retro-orbital pain on the side of the affected ear, vertigo, mental status changes, and nystagmus. Other focal neurologic signs such as facial paralysis, meningismus, and papilledema can also signal intracranial extension of suppurative otitis media.[37]

OTITIS EXTERNA

Otitis externa (OE) is an inflammatory process that involves the structures of the outer ear, specifically the external auditory canal, and is a common finding in children, especially during the warm-weather months of the year. The site of the inflammation is different from otitis media, and the signs and symptoms associated with OE reflect this condition.

OE is multifactorial in etiology and involves an interaction between the host and environmental factors. Some of these factors include trauma to the external auditory canal; the presence of a foreign body; repeated ear cleansing; prolonged exposure to standing water in the canal; which occurs following swimming or bathing *(swimmer's ear);* high environmental temperature and humidity; increased sweating, allergy, and stress. Inflammation may be focal, at the site of trauma or an infected hair follicle, or diffuse, as is the case with swimmer's ear. When inflammation is focal and associated with infection the organism is often *S aureus,* which can lead to furuncle formation at the site of the inflammation. The most common organism associated with diffuse inflammation is *Pseudomonas aeruginosa,* a hydrophilic bacterial species. Infection is often polymicrobial.[38] Enteric bacilli and fungi are less common causes of OE.

Children with OE complain of ear pain and may also report pain with chewing (because of the proximity of the temporomandibular joint to the external auditory canal) and difficulty hearing (as a result of swelling within the external auditory canal and conductive hearing loss).

Examination reveals tenderness with manipulation of the pinna or pressure on the tragus. Insertion of an otoscope into the external auditory canal can be painful and should be undertaken carefully. Within the canal, focal erythema and swelling may be seen at a site of trauma or folliculitis. If the inflammation is diffuse, then swelling of the entire canal renders a boggy appearance. Edema and the presence of inflammatory debris may prevent complete visualization of the tympanic membrane. The tympanic membrane should appear normal in cases of OE unless coexistent otitis media is present.

MANAGEMENT

When OE is accompanied by furuncle formation, incision and drainage may be necessary. Diffuse OE usually responds to application of a topical otic solution containing neomycin, polymyxin B, and hydrocortisone 4 times a day. With the patient lying on the unaffected side, 5 drops of this solution are instilled into the affected ear. The patient should remain in this position for 5 to 10 minutes after instillation to ensure that the medication has come in contact with affected skin. Insertion of a cotton wick can prolong this contact.

OE can be prevented by keeping the external auditory canal dry and by avoiding vigorous cleaning of the canal that can lead to superficial trauma.

MALIGNANT OTITIS EXTERNA

Malignant OE is a complicated form of OE that can develop in immunocompromised children or those with severe malnutrition. It is a necrotizing infection of the external auditory canal, often beginning as minor trauma to the canal, usually caused by *P aeruginosa,* which rapidly spreads to involve the soft tissue, cartilage, nerves, and the temporal bone, leading to osteomyelitis of the base of the skull.[33] Pain is severe, and discharge from the external canal is copious. Patients may develop facial paralysis, which is a poor prognostic sign. Treatment requires administration of intravenous antibiotics and, occasionally, surgical intervention. Complications of malignant OE include stenosis of the external auditory canal, auricular cartilage deformity, tympanic membrane necrosis, and sensorineural hearing loss.[39]

WHEN TO REFER

Patients with recurrent or chronic otitis media and persistent otitis media with effusion (present for at least 3 months) should be referred for ear, nose, and throat evaluation. Infectious diseases consultation should be obtained in patients with the following conditions:

- Suppurative complications of otitis media
- Recurrent or chronic episodes of otitis media unresponsive to standard therapy
- Patients with unusual or multiple antibiotic-resistant organisms isolated from middle ear fluid
- Patients with chronic suppurative otitis media unresponsive to conventional therapy
- Patients with malignant otitis externa

In many of the these conditions mentioned, a team approach with both ear, nose, and throat and infectious diseases referrals should be used for optimal management of the patient's condition.

WHEN TO ADMIT

Any patient with severe otitis media who is toxic in appearance, patients with malignant otitis externa, and patients with suppurative complications of otitis media should be admitted to the hospital, which allows for the institution of prompt, effective intravenous antibiotic therapy and evaluation for possible surgical intervention.

TOOLS FOR PRACTICE

Community Advocacy and Coordination

- *Get Smart: Know When Antibiotics Work* (Web page), Centers for Disease Control and Prevention (www.cdc.gov/drugresistance/community/index.htm).

Engaging Patient and Family

- *Ear Infections and Children* (brochure), American Academy of Pediatrics (patiented.aap.org).

Medical Decision Support

- *Otitis Media Online Learning—Case Studies* (on-line course), American Academy of Pediatrics (www.aap.org/otitismedia/www/).
- *A View Through the Otoscope: Distinguishing Acute Otitis Media from Otitis Media with Effusion* (on-line video), American Academy of Pediatrics (www.aap.org/sections/infectdis/video.cfm).

RELATED WEB SITE

- Centers for Disease and Prevention: Ear Infection (Otitis Media) (www.cdc.gov/ncidod/diseases/submenus/sub_ear_Infection.htm).

AAP POLICY STATEMENTS

American Academy of Family Physicians, American Academy of Otolaryngology-Head and Neck Surgery; American Academy of Pediatrics, Subcommittee on Otitis Media With Effusion. Otitis media with effusion. *Pediatrics*. 2004; 113(5):1412-1429. (aappolicy.aappublications.org/cgi/content/full/pediatrics;113/5/1412).

American Academy of Pediatrics, Subcommittee on Management of Acute Otitis Media. Diagnosis and management of acute otitis media. *Pediatrics*. 2004;113(5):1451-1465. (aappolicy.aappublications.org/cgi/content/full/pediatrics; 113/5/1451).

REFERENCES

1. Paradise JL, Rockette HE, Colborn DK, et al. Otitis media in 2253 Pittsburgh-area infants: prevalence and risk factors during the first two years of life. *Pediatrics*. 1997; 99(3):318-333.
2. Klein JO, Teele DW, Rosner BA. Epidemiology of acute otitis media in Boston children from birth to seven years of age. In: Lim DJ, Bluestone CD, Klein JO, et al, eds. *Recent Advances in Otitis Media With Effusion*. Proceedings of the Fourth International Symposium. Toronto, Canada: BC Decker; 1988.
3. Chartrand SA, Pong A. Acute otitis media in the 1990s: the impact of antibiotic resistance. *Pediatr Ann*. 1998;27(2): 86-95.
4. Stool SE, Field MJ. The impact of otitis media. *Pediatr Infect Dis J*. 1997;8:S11.
5. American Academy of Family Physicians, American Academy of Otolaryngology—Head and Neck Surgery, American Academy of Pediatrics, Subcommittee on Otitis Media With Effusion. Otitis media with effusion. *Pediatrics*. 2004;113(5):1412-1429.
6. Teele DW, Klein JO, Rosner B. Epidemiology of otitis media during the first seven years of life in children in greater Boston: a prospective, cohort study. *J Infect Dis*. 1989;160(5):83-94.
7. Ey JL, Holberg CJ, Aldous MB, et al. Passive smoke exposure and otitis media in the first year of life. *Pediatrics*. 1995;95(5):670-677.
8. Niemala M, Uhari M, Möttönen M. A pacifier increases the risk of recurrent acute otitis media in children in day care centers. *Pediatrics*. 1995;96(5 pt 1):884-888.
9. Uhari M, Mäntysaari K, Niemelä M. A meta-analytic review of the risk factors for acute otitis media. *Clin Infect Dis*. 1996;22(6):1079-1083.
10. Duncan B, Ey J, Holberg CJ, et al. Exclusive breastfeeding for at least 4 months protects against otitis media. *Pediatrics*. 1993;91(5):867-872.
11. Kvaerner KJ, Tambs K, Harris JR, et al. Distribution and heritability of recurrent ear infections. *Ann Otol Rhinol Laryngol*. 1997;106(8):624-632.
12. Zielhaus GA, Rach GH, van den Broek P. The natural history of otitis media with effusion in preschool children. *Eur Arch Otorhinolaryngol*. 1990;247(4):215-221.
13. Klein JO. Otitis media. *Clin Infect Dis*. 1994;19(5):823-833.
14. Heikkinen T, Thint M, Chonmaitree T. Prevalence of various respiratory viruses in the middle ear during acute otitis media. *N Engl J Med*. 1999;340(4):260-264.
15. Bauer C, Waner M. Laser-assisted myringotomy. *Curr Opin Otolaryngol Head Neck Surg*. 1999;7:335.
16. Stein CR, Weber DJ, Kelley M. *Emerg Infect Dis*. 2003; 9:211-216.
17. Dowell SF, Butler JC, Giebink GS, et al. Acute otitis media: management and surveillance in an era of pneumococcal resistance—a report from the Drug-resistant Streptococcus pneumoniae Therapeutic Working Group. *Pediatr Infect Dis J*. 1999;18(1):1-9.
18. Block SL, Hedrick J, Harrison CJ, et al. Community-wide vaccination with the heptavalent pneumococcal conjugate significantly alters the microbiology of acute otitis media. *Pediatr Infect Dis J*. 2004;23(9):829-833.
19. Casey JR, Pichichero ME. Changes in frequency and pathogens causing acute otitis media in 1995-2003. *Pediatr Infect Dis J*. 2004;23(9):824-828.
20. Paradise JL. Short-course antimicrobial treatment for acute otitis media: not best for infants and young children. *JAMA*. 1997;278(20):1640-1642.
21. Hoberman A, Paradise JL, Reynolds EA, et al. Efficacy of Auralgan for treating ear pain in children with acute otitis media. *Arch Pediatr Adolesc Med*. 1997;151(7):675-678.
22. Roberts J, Hunter L, Gravel J, et al. Otitis media, hearing loss, and language learning: controversies and current research. *J Dev Behav Pediatr*. 2004;25(2):110-122.
23. Burton LJ, Felding JU, Ovesen T, et al. Grommets (ventilation tubes) for hearing loss associated with otitis media with effusion in children. *Cochrane Database Sys Rev*. 2007;3:1-49.
24. Roberts JE, Rosenfeld RM, Zeisel SA. Otitis media and speech and language: a meta-analysis of prospective studies. *Pediatrics*. 2004;113:e238-e248.
25. Kadhim AL, Spilsbury K, Semmens JB, et al. Adenoidectomy for middle ear effusion: a study of 50,000 children over 24 years. *Laryngoscope*. 2007;117(3):427-433.
26. Maw AR, Parker A. Surgery of the tonsils and adenoids in relation to secretory otitis media in children. *Acta Otolaryngol Suppl*. 1988;454:202-207.
27. Gates GA. Adenoidectomy for otitis media with effusion. *Ann Otol Rhinol Laryngol Suppl*. 1994;163:54-58.
28. Mattila PS. Adenoidectomy and tympanostomy tubes in the management of otitis media. *Curr Allergy Asthma Rep*. 2006;6(4):321-326.
29. Paradise JL. Tonsillectomy and adenoidectomy. In: Bluestone CD, Stool SE, Kenna MA, eds. *Paediatric Otolaryngology*. Philadelphia, PA: WB Saunders; 1996.
30. Williams RL, Chalmers TC, Stange KC, et al. Use of antibiotics in preventing recurrent acute otitis media and in treating otitis media with effusion: a meta-analytic attempt to resolve the brouhaha. *JAMA*. 1993;270:1344.
31. Rosenfeld RM, Culpepper L, Doyle KJ, et al. Clinical practice guideline: otitis media with effusion. *Otolaryngol Head Neck Surg*. 2004;130(5 suppl):S95-S118.
32. Hern JD, Almeyda J, Thomas DM, et al. Malignant otitis externa in HIV and AIDS. *J Laryngol Otol*. 11(8):770-775.
33. Salata JA, Derkay CS. Water precautions in children with tympanostomy tubes. *Arch Otolaryngol Head Neck Surg*. 1996;122(3):276-280.
34. Bluestone CD, Klein JO. Intracranial suppurative complications of otitis media and mastoiditis. In: Bluestone CD, Stool SE, Kenna MA, eds. *Pediatric Otolaryngology*. 3rd ed. Philadelphia, PA: WB Saunders; 1996.
35. Fliss DM, Leiberman A, Dagen R. Medical sequelae and complications of acute otitis media. *Pediatr Infect Dis J*. 1994;13(1):34-40.
36. Elidan J, Saah D, Gomori M. Intracranial complications of otitis media. *Ann Otol Rhinol Laryngol*. 1997;106:873-874.
37. Clark WB, Brook I, Bianki D, et al. Microbiology of otitis externa. *Otolaryngol Head Neck Surg*. 1997;116(1):23-25.
38. Hirsch B. Infections of the external ear. *Am J Otholaryngol*. 1992;13(3):145-155.

Chapter 305

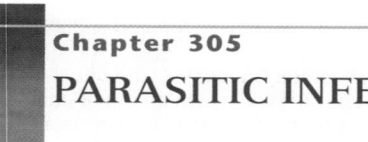

PARASITIC INFECTIONS

Nahed Abdel-Haq, MD; Pimpanada Chearskul, MD; Yaseen Rafee, MD; Basim I. Asmar, MD

PROTOZOAL INFECTIONS

Leishmaniasis

Leishmaniasis is caused by protozoa that belong to the genus *Leishmania,* an obligate intracellular parasite of macrophages. The disease is transmitted by the sandfly: *Phlebotomus* species in the Old World and *Lutzomyia* in the New World. Depending on the geographic distribution, the disease is classified into the Old and the New World disease. Clinically, the disease is classified into the cutaneous, mucocutaneous, and the visceral forms.[1]

Pathogenesis and Life Cycle

Leishmaniasis is a zoonosis. Dogs and rodents are considered reservoir hosts.[2,3] *Leishmania* species exist in 2 morphologic types. The amastigote form appears within macrophages in human tissue and has a nucleus and kinetoplast. The other type is the promastigote form that occurs in the sandfly or in cultures; it has a kinetoplast, a nucleus, and a flagellum.[4]

The disease is transmitted by bite of the female sandfly. When blood is sucked by the fly, amastigotes residing in macrophages in peripheral blood and soft tissues are taken up. Inside the fly, the amastigote is transformed to a promastigote, which migrates from the gut to the pharynx and proboscis in 1 week.[5] When the sandfly bites a host for a blood meal, the promastigotes are inoculated into the host and are almost immediately engulfed by tissue macrophages and transformed to amastigotes. The parasite multiplies by binary fission. When cells rupture, amastigotes are taken up by other macrophages, and the cycle continues.

Infected macrophages either remain in the skin, causing localized cutaneous disease, or disseminate to the reticuloendothelial system, causing disseminated disease. Infected tissue macrophages induce a host cell–mediated immune response characterized by infiltration of lymphocytes, plasma cells, and monocytes, with subsequent formation of granulomas, histiocytes, and multinucleated giant cells.[6]

Epidemiologic Features

The cutaneous form is typically a sporadic disease in endemic areas, which include the Mediterranean Basin, the Middle East, Southern Asia, and parts of Africa.[7] The cutaneous disease is mainly caused by *Leishmania tropica* and *Leishmania major* in the Old World. The former causes the moist (ulcerative) form in rural areas, and the latter causes the dry (nonulcerative) form in urban areas.[8] The third species that causes cutaneous disease in the Old World is *Leishmania aethiopica,* which is endemic in Ethiopia, Yemen, and Kenya.[8]

The other endemic areas of cutaneous leishmaniasis are Central and South America. In these areas the disease is caused by New World species such as *Leishmania mexicana* and *Leishmania braziliensis.*[9] Mucosal leishmaniasis is a subtype of cutaneous leishmaniasis and is seen after infections with *L braziliensis.*[10] An anergic form of cutaneous leishmaniasis is called diffuse cutaneous leishmaniasis. The disease is characterized by disseminated skin lesions and usually occurs in patients with cell-mediated immunodeficiency.[4] In the United States, cutaneous disease has been reported in Texas.[11] The disease has also been reported in military personnel, especially among those stationed in Iraq.[12]

Visceral leishmaniasis is seen mainly in Asia, the Middle East, the Mediterranean Basin, and Africa. The disease is caused mainly by *Leishmania donovani* in India and Africa and by *Leishmania infantum* in the Middle East, Southern Europe, and North Africa.[13] Relatively few patients with the viscerotropic disease may be found in Latin America, where it is mainly caused by *Leishmania chagasi.* Rarely, visceral disease may be caused by species that typically cause cutaneous lesions, such as *L mexicana* and *L major.*[14] In the early 1990s a viscerotropic disease caused by *L tropica* was found in a small number of American soldiers who returned from the Operation Desert Storm in the Arabian Gulf.[15]

Other than bite by the sandfly, leishmaniasis may rarely be transmitted by blood transfusion or transplanted organs.[16,17]

The incubation period of leishmaniasis varies from several days to years or even decades. The incubation period of the cutaneous form is usually several weeks after the sandfly bite and several months for the visceral form.[18]

Clinical Manifestations

The 3 major clinical manifestations of leishmaniasis are: (1) cutaneous, (2) mucosal, and (3) visceral.

CUTANEOUS LEISHMANIASIS. After an incubation period of 2 to 8 weeks, a skin lesion appears on an exposed area of the body, mostly on the face and extremities. The lesion begins as an itchy papule surrounded by erythema and induration, and it progresses to become a nodule. The primary lesion may have accompanying satellite lesions and adjacent adenopathy resembling sporothroid nodules. In the moist cutaneous form, a shallow ulcer with raised borders may develop. The lesion may progress slowly, leading to an open sore as large as 5 cm in diameter with a granular center. The lesion takes 3 to 12 months to heal and leaves a depressed scar. Secondary bacterial infection commonly occurs. However, in the dry form, no ulcers form, and the papule instead heals to a scar over a longer time period, which may extend to a year or more.[19-21]

Diffuse cutaneous leishmaniasis is seen in patients with underlying immune disorders, particularly cellular immunodeficiency. The primary lesion is a localized papule with surrounding satellite lesions. The amastigotes then disseminates, forming multiple nodules on the face and extremities. The lesions slowly progress and may last for years. The lesions do not ulcerate. This form is seen most commonly with *L aethiopica* in the Old World and *L mexicana* in the New World.[22]

MUCOSAL LEISHMANIASIS (ESPUNDIA). Mucosal leishmaniasis occurs in a small number of patients who are infected with *L mexicana*. The lesions occur months to years after the primary cutaneous lesion heals.[23] The lesions commonly involve the nose, mouth, soft palate, and larynx. The disease usually begins with nasal congestion and ulceration. The cartilage of the nose is commonly involved, leading to nasal septal perforation.[24] The lesions do not heal spontaneously and may not respond well to treatment. Formation of granulomas and secondary bacterial infections are common. Considerable morbidity and disfigurement may result from these lesions.[25]

VISCERAL LEISHMANIASIS (KALA-AZAR). In the visceral form of leishmaniasis, the amastigotes spread from macrophages at the site of inoculation to the liver, spleen, bone marrow, and sometimes lymph nodes. The disease involves different age groups depending on the species and the geographic distribution. In the Mediterranean Basin and northern China, visceral leishmaniasis affects infants and young children; the disease is caused by *L infantum* and *L donovani*, respectively. Epidemic cases of kala-azar have been reported in India and mostly occur in adolescents and young adults.[26] No animal reservoir exists, and the etiologic species is *L donovani*. In Sudan and East Africa, kala-azar is usually seen in adult men. The disease is caused by *L donovani* and one of its variants.[27] In contrast, kala-azar cases in Latin America are caused by *L chagasi*. The disease is seen primarily in infants and young children.[28,29]

The typical manifestations of visceral leishmaniasis are fever, anorexia, malaise, and weight loss. The symptoms progress over weeks to months. Physical findings typically include hepatomegaly and splenomegaly. The spleen is massively enlarged.[30] In Mediterranean areas, in East Africa, and in China, patients may also have lymphadenopathy. Skin hyperpigmentation occurs commonly in Indian patients; kala-azar means *black fever* in Hindi. Less common findings include jaundice that results from severe liver involvement, and Guillain-Barré syndrome.[28,31,32]

Laboratory findings include leukopenia, anemia and thrombocytopenia, hypoalbuminemia, and hypergammaglobulinemia. Reversal of the albumin-globulin ratio may be seen.[4]

Complications of visceral leishmaniasis are secondary bacterial and mycobacterial infections, including tuberculosis. Untreated symptomatic infections are almost always fatal. Epistaxis, gingival bleeding, and other hemorrhagic manifestations may occur as a result of thrombocytopenia. Disseminated intravascular coagulation and pulmonary or intestinal superinfections are common causes of death in untreated patients.

Patients infected with HIV, as well as stem cell and solid organ transplant recipients, are at risk of reactivation of latent infection and disseminated disease.[33]

Post–kala-azar dermal leishmaniasis follows recovery of patients from visceral disease and indicates the reversal of the agent to the dermal form. The lesions are polymorphic and occur predominantly on the face, extremities, and upper trunk.[34]

Diagnosis

The diagnosis is made by identification of the parasites in tissue biopsy samples or in aspirate.[25] Wright, Giemsa, or even hematoxylin and eosin staining can be used to demonstrate the characteristic intracellular amastigotes (Leishman-Donovan bodies). Skin samples can be obtained by punch biopsy or alternatively by scraping or needle aspiration of the nonnecrotic edge.[35] Specimens can also be obtained from bone marrow aspirate and biopsy or from needle aspirate and biopsy of lymph node, liver, or spleen. The highest yield for diagnosis is the splenic aspirates, but this procedure is considered too invasive. Amastigotes characteristically have kinetoplasts and remain inside macrophages without invading surrounding parenchyma. These features are distinctive and help differentiate *Leishmania* from other intracellular parasitic infection.[29]

Culture of tissue or peripheral blood on special media (Novy-MacNeal-Nicolle medium) should be attempted if available. However, a few days to several weeks may be needed for cultures to become positive.[36]

The leishmanin skin test (Montenegro test) can be used in the diagnosis of cutaneous leishmaniasis. However, the test usually turns positive in the ulcerative phase, which occurs 1 to 3 months after infection. The Montenegro test is not helpful for diagnosing visceral disease because of decreased cellular immune responses.[37] A positive skin test may also indicate an old rather than an acute infection.[37] The leishmanin skin test is not approved for use in the United States.

Serologic tests may be helpful in diagnosing visceral and mucosal leishmaniasis but not cutaneous disease.[38] However, false-positive results may occur with other diseases, such as trypanosomiasis, tuberculosis, leprosy, and malaria.[38]

Nucleic acid-based techniques such as DNA hybridization and polymerase chain reaction (PCR) can be used to identify parasite sequence in tissue samples and peripheral blood.[39] They are especially useful in the diagnosis of visceral leishmaniasis and in aspirates that are negative for parasites by microscopy.[40] Although PCR is highly sensitive, it is not routinely available.

Treatment

Treatment decisions should be individualized. In general, all patients with visceral and mucosal leishmaniasis should be treated. Patients with cutaneous leishmaniasis, particularly those acquired in the Old World, may not need treatment because most of them will heal spontaneously.[19] However, if the lesion is cosmetically important (eg, on the face), or if the lesions are multiple, are enlarging, or overlie joints, then treatment should be considered.[1] In addition, cutaneous lesions that may be caused by *L braziliensis* or other species that may disseminate to nasopharyngeal mucosa should be considered for treatment.[24]

The drugs of choice for treatment of leishmaniasis are the pentavalent antimonials.[24,41] Two forms are available: (1) sodium stibogluconate (Pentostam) and

(2) meglumine antimonate (Glucantime). Common side effects of these medications include nausea, vomiting, myalgia, headache, and malaise. High hepatic and pancreatic enzymes may also occur. More severe and dose-dependent side effects include leukopenia, thrombocytopenia, and behavioral changes. Electrocardiographic abnormalities may include S-T segment changes, Q-T prolongation, and arrhythmias. Cardiac toxicity and sudden death may occur in patients who receive higher-than-recommended doses.[42] Patients who receive antimonials should have complete blood counts and electrocardiographic monitoring at baseline and weekly thereafter.

Amphotericin B is increasingly being used in cases of visceral leishmaniasis because of its efficacy and the availability of less toxic lipid formulations.[43] The side effects of amphotericin B include infusion-related reactions and nephrotoxicity. Liposomal amphotericin B (AmBisome) is better tolerated than amphotericin B and distributes well to the reticuloendothelial system, but it is expensive.[43,44]

Alternative medications for treatment of leishmaniasis include pentamidine isothionate.[41,44] Pentamidine has significant side effects, including hypotension, hypoglycemia, nausea, vomiting, and headache, as well as electrolyte disturbances such as hyperkalemia, hypomagnesemia, and hypocalcemia.[41,45]

Topical paromomycin is a partially effective in treatment of Old World cutaneous leishmaniasis when the risk of mucosal spread is low.[46] Parenteral paromomycin has been used as adjunctive therapy with antimonial therapy in the treatment of visceral leishmaniasis. However, the response to treatment is variable when used alone.[47]

A newer drug, miltefosine, can be provided orally and shows promise in treating cutaneous and visceral leishmaniasis.[48] Oral fluconazole may speed healing of cutaneous lesions caused by *L major*.[49] Other drugs that have been used with limited efficacy are itraconazole, allopurinol, and dapsone; immunomodulation has been provided with interferon gamma.

Local treatments such as thermotherapy and cryotherapy have been used in selected patients with cutaneous leishmaniasis. However, such therapies are unreliable in patients with New World lesions as a result of the risk of mucosal dissemination.

Prevention

No approved vaccines or drugs have been developed for preventing leishmaniasis in travelers. Travelers to endemic areas should use personal-protection measures to prevent bites by the sandfly. However, such measures are not practical for residents in endemic areas. To prevent the bites, travelers should wear long-sleeve shirts, pants, and socks; use insect repellants; limit exposure to the fly from dusk to dawn; and use bed nets.[50] Early diagnosis and treatment may prevent complications.

Chagas Disease (American Trypanosomiasis) (*Trypanosome cruzi*)

Chagas disease is a zoonotic multisystemic disease caused by the flagellated protozoan parasite *Trypanosoma cruzi*. Infection is transmitted to human by blood-sucking insect vectors of the family Reduviidae. Chagas disease affects people throughout the Americas, predominantly Central and South America. Clinical manifestations can be divided into 3 phases: (1) acute phase, (2) asymptomatic latent or indeterminate phase, and (3) chronic phase.

Epidemiologic Features and Life Cycle

Infection caused by *T cruzi* is limited to the Western Hemisphere. Eighteen countries in North, Central, and South America from the southern United States to southern Argentina are affected.[51] Most infections occur in poor remote rural areas or areas with poor sanitation.[52] Estimates indicate that approximately 16 to 18 million people in endemic areas are infected, with the highest prevalence of infection in Brazil, Argentina, and Venezuela.[52,53] In the United States, infection is common in immigrants from Central and South America, with an estimated 100,000 chagasic Latin American immigrants living in the United States.[52]

Humans are accidental hosts for *T cruzi*. Parasites are transmitted through feces of the insect vectors of the Triatominae family (cone-nose, kissing, or assassin bug). The infected Triatominae insect vectors defecate and release trypomastigote on the host during or after taking a blood meal. Trypomastigotes enter the host at the site of bite wound or through intact mucous membranes of the eye or the mouth, usually when infected fecal material is inadvertently rubbed in. The bite wounds are frequently found at the lateral canthus of the eye, mucocutaneous border of the lips, and exposed areas of the face and upper extremities. The parasite can also be transmitted by blood transfusion, by organ transplantation, transplacentally, by ingestion of the vector, by the vector's excretion, and in the laboratory from handling blood from infected people or laboratory animals. Blood transfusion is the second-most common mode of transmission for Chagas disease.[53]

Inside the host, trypomastigote penetrates various cells at the inoculation site and later transforms into intracellular amastigotes. The amastigotes multiply by binary fission and differentiate into trypomastigotes, which enter the bloodstream after infected cells burst. These bloodstream trypomastigotes can infect various types of cells at the new infection sites and transform into intracellular amastigotes, resulting in clinical manifestation of Chagas disease as this infective cycle continues. The Triatominae insect becomes infected after taking a blood meal from a person with circulating parasites. The parasites transform into epimastigotes, multiply, and undergo metamorphosis into infective trypomastigotes inside the insect before being passed in its feces.[54]

Clinical Manifestations

ACUTE PHASE. The usual incubation period is 4 days to 2 weeks after percutaneous infection. A local inflammatory reaction commonly occurs at the site of parasite inoculation. A chagoma (an erythematous, firm, nodular swelling at the bite site) or Romaña sign (a unilateral periorbital edema associated with conjunctivitis and ipsilateral preauricular lymphadenopathy) may be present when the portal of entry is at the lateral canthus of the eye. As the parasites disseminate in the bloodstream, the patient experiences manifestation of generalized infection with fever, malaise, and headache. The infection usually goes unrecognized at this stage and is diagnosed only 1% or 2% of all patients.[53] Generalized lymphadenopathy, hepatosplenomegaly, and edema are usually observed. Some degree of acute myocarditis is generally present in all symptomatic cases of Chagas disease, and it is responsible for most deaths during the acute phase in severe cases. Meningoencephalitis may follow and is usually associated with a high mortality rate. In the acute phase, patients who are infected congenitally may be asymptomatic or may have hepatosplenomegaly, jaundice, skin hemorrhage, and neurologic signs, especially in premature infants.

LATENT OR INDETERMINATE PHASE. Individuals who survive the acute phase enter the indeterminate phase after 1 to 3 months of acute disease. In this phase, patients are asymptomatic but still have low levels of parasitemia that can be detected by xenodiagnosis, blood culture, or PCR.[55] The indeterminate latent phase can persist for years, even for life. Information is limited about this phase of disease, but generally, investigators believe that tissue destruction from the infection has already occurred.

CHRONIC PHASE. The most common manifestation of the chronic phase is chagasic heart disease.[56] Chronic heart failure, severe cardiomegaly, ventricular conduction defects, and various types of arrhythmia can occur. Patients may experience palpitations, dizziness, syncope, dyspnea, or chest pain. More than one half of all cases will develop right bundle branch block, which is the most common conduction defect observed.[57] A pathognomonic apex aneurysm, typically at the left ventricle, is present in many cases. Sudden death may occur as a result of ventricular fibrillation or systemic and pulmonary embolism.[58]

The hollow viscera are usually involved with the loss of autonomic control or damage to the smooth muscle, or both. Approximately 8% to 10% of all patients have a variable degree of changes in motility or severe dilatation of the digestive tract.[53] Extreme enlargement of the colon is slightly more common than esophagus. Patients may experience difficulty in swallowing, as well as regurgitation, severe constipation, and abdominal pain. Esophagitis and cancer of the esophagus are common complications of the megaesophagus, whereas fecaloma, volvulus, rupture of the bowel accompanied by peritonitis can complicate the megacolon.

Neurologic symptoms can occur in a minority of patients. The central, peripheral, or autonomic nervous system can all be involved.[52] Neuritis with paresthesia or anesthesia, convulsion, and alteration of homeostatic equilibrium have been observed.

The prognosis depends on the stage of the disease and its complications. In the acute phase, children younger than 2 years who develop heart failure or meningoencephalitis have the highest mortality rate.[53] Patients in the chronic phase with digestive tract involvement generally have a good prognosis. The prognosis is usually poor among chronic-phase patients with heart failure.

DIAGNOSIS. The diagnostic test of choice during the acute phase of Chagas disease is detection of the parasites in blood specimen. This test is relatively easy and almost always yields positive results.[52] Thin and thick blood smears stained with Giemsa or direct wet mount of the fresh blood sample or the buffy coat can be examined for the parasites. In the chronic phase, which is generally characterized by low level of parasitemia, diagnosis is usually made by immunodiagnostic tests or isolation of the parasite. Several immunodiagnostic methods, such as the indirect fluorescent antibody (IFA) test, complement fixation, and enzyme immunoassay (EIA), are available commercially. In the United States, IFA and complement fixation tests are available at the Centers for Disease Control and Prevention (CDC). Sensitivity and specificity of these serologic tests are highly variable; therefore 2 different, independently performed methods should be used to confirm the diagnosis of Chagas disease.[59] These serologic tests may cross-react with other conditions, such as leishmaniasis, malaria, syphilis, infectious mononucleosis, tuberculosis, leprosy, and collagen vascular diseases.[56] Isolation of the parasite can be accomplished by culture in special media, by mice inoculation, or by xenodiagnosis (reduviid insects are fed the infected patient's blood, and their gut contents are examined 4 weeks later for the parasites). The animal inoculation method is unreliable and should be performed only after repeated culture attempts have failed to isolate the organism.[53] A molecular method such as PCR is available as an investigational diagnostic tool.

TREATMENT. Treatment of Chagas disease consists of both specific and symptomatic treatment. In children, specific treatment should be provided during the acute and indeterminate phases of infection.[53] Other forms of infection that may benefit from specific treatment include congenital infection, reactivation of infection associated with immunosuppression, and infection associated with transfusion or organ transplantation. The drugs of choice are benznidazole and nifurtimox.[54] Benznidazole is not available generally in the United States but may be obtained through a compounding pharmacy. Nifurtimox is available in the United States under an investigational new drug protocol from the CDC drug service. Treatment with benznidazole or nifurtimox is usually associated with a high rate of adverse drug reactions that sometimes leads to suspension of treatment. These side effects are dose dependent and generally include hypersensitivity reactions, bone marrow suppression, and peripheral neuropathy.[53] In children, treatment is usually effective and well tolerated.[60] Management of patients with the chronic phase of Chagas disease is mainly symptomatic and supportive. Pacemakers are implanted in patients with symptomatic heart block. Balloon dilation of the esophagogastric junction may be performed in patients with megaesophagus. Fecaloma and atonic segment of megacolon can be removed surgically. Primary chemoprophylaxis is still controversial.[52]

African Trypanosomiasis *(Trypanosoma brucei)*

Epidemiologic Features

African trypanosomiasis is caused by the extracellular protozoan hemoflagellates *Trypanosoma brucei*. Two subspecies infect humans; they are different in morphology and distribution. *Trypanosoma brucei gambiense* is the cause of West African sleeping sickness, and *Trypanosoma brucei rhodesiense* is the cause of East African sleeping sickness. The organisms are transmitted to human by the bite of tsetse fly *(Glossina)*. Transmission occurs in areas between the latitudes of 15 degrees North and 20 degrees South, with temperatures between 20°C and 30°C corresponding to the distribution of the tsetse fly vector.[61] Disease can affect humans of all ages, but it occurs rarely in children because of limited exposure.[53] Infection with *T b rhodesiense* is found most commonly in East Africa, whereas infection with *T b rhodesiense* is found mainly in West and Central Africa. Humans are the only important reservoir of *T b gambiense*. For *T b rhodesiense*, natural infection also occurs in various types of domestic and wild animals, which thus makes them a major reservoir for disease transmission to humans.[62]

Life Cycle

Disease is transmitted to human by the tsetse fly, which injects metacyclic trypomastigotes into tissue of the human skin while taking a blood meal. The metacyclic trypomastigotes penetrate tissue into lymphatic system and enter blood circulation, where they transform into bloodstream trypomastigotes. In the bloodstream, trypomastigotes multiply by binary fission and are carried to various sites and other fluid spaces throughout the body. The tsetse flies become infected after taking a blood meal from an infected person with circulating trypomastigotes. Inside the tsetse fly's midgut, the bloodstream trypomastigotes transform into procyclic trypomastigotes and continue to multiply by binary fission. The procyclic trypomastigotes leave the midgut, transform into epimastigotes, and migrate to the salivary gland of the tsetse fly. The multiplication by binary fission continues in the tsetse fly's salivary gland, and later the epimastigotes transform into metacyclic trypomastigotes, an infective stage for humans. The cycle inside the tsetse fly takes approximately 3 weeks. The cycle becomes complete after the tsetse fly takes a blood meal and transmits the infection to the human.[62]

Clinical Manifestations

The clinical course is different between the 2 forms of African trypanosomiasis. The East African form *(T b rhodesiense)* is characterized by acute, severe, rapidly fatal disease with minimal central nervous system (CNS) symptoms, whereas the West African type *(T b gambiense)* has a milder chronic course associated with lymph node and CNS invasion. In general, infection can be divided into 3 stages. The first stage, or trypanochancre stage, is characterized by local proliferation of the parasites. The second phase, or hemolymphatic stage, occurs when the parasites multiply rapidly and disseminate throughout the body. Finally, the third phase, or meningoencephalitic stage, occurs when lesions develop in the CNS.

The trypanosomal chancre, which usually develops a few days after inoculation, is characterized by an indurated, erythematous, painful lesion that develops at the bite site. The trypanosomal chancre usually resolves within 3 weeks. During the dissemination of the parasite in the parasitemic or hemolymphatic stage, patients may develop fever, headache, and generalized malaise. As infection progresses, the patient may experience papular skin lesion, generalized lymphadenopathy, especially in the posterior cervical triangle (Winterbottom sign), and mild hepatosplenomegaly. Generalized weakness, dyspnea, chest pain, anemia, arthralgia, cachexia, and local swelling of the joints, hands, or feet may develop. As the parasites invade the CNS, the meningoencephalitic stage or sleeping sickness stage is initiated. Symptoms include severe headache, irritability, and personality and behavioral change. Gradual loss of cognitive function, alteration in motor function, and psychiatric manifestations may occur. The common manifestation during the meningoencephalitic stage is sleep disorders. Patients usually experience somnolence, inappropriate episodes of sleeping, and nocturnal insomnia.[63] Signs and symptoms of congestive heart failure may develop as the parasites invade the heart. Mortality is usually from meningitis, heart failure, and other complications.

Diagnosis

Diagnosis can be made by microscopic detection of the trypomastigotes in specimens from various sites such as chancre fluid, blood, bone marrow, lymph node aspirates, and cerebrospinal fluid (CSF).[62] The best techniques to demonstrate the motile trypanosomes are Giemsa stain and wet preparation.[63] Concentration technique may be used with body fluid specimen examination to increase sensitivity of detection. Serologic studies are generally not helpful because of inconsistent sensitivity and specificity.[62] Isolation of the parasite by rat or mice inoculation is a sensitive test, but the use is limited only for *T b rhodesiense*.[62]

Treatment

The treatment regimen depends on the infecting species and stage of infection. In West African trypanosomiasis, the drug of choice during the hemolymphatic stage is pentamidine isethionate.[44,61] In late-stage disease with CNS involvement of West African trypanosomiasis, the drug of choice is melarsoprol or eflornithine.[44,61] For East African trypanosomiasis, suramin is the drug of choice during the hemolymphatic stage, and melarsoprol is the drug of choice during late disease with CNS involvement.[44,61] Suramin and eflornithine are available only as investigational new drugs from the CDC's drug service.[44] While receiving the therapy, patients should be monitored closely for possible adverse reactions.

Giardiasis

Giardia intestinalis (syn *Giardia duodenalis* or *Giardia lamblia*) is a flagellated binucleated protozoan that is considered to be one of the most common intestinal parasites worldwide. It was first described in 1681 and was found to infect mammals, reptiles, and birds. The incidence of giardiasis in humans ranges from 20% to

30% in developing countries to 2% to 7% in the developed world.[64,65] It exists in trophozoite and cysts forms; the cyst is the infectious form of the parasite.[66,67] *G intestinalis* causes both endemic and epidemic cases of gastroenteritis among children. It causes outbreaks in child-care centers and may also cause chronic diarrhea in children.

Epidemiologic Features

Approximately 2.5 million new cases of giardiasis occur annually in the United States.[67] Most cases occur in children in the first 5 years of life. The peak incidence is in late summer and early fall.[67] Among children, 2 groups have been identified as being at high risk of acquiring giardiasis. The first group includes children attending child-care centers. The prevalence among children who attend child-care centers can be as high as 35%.[67] The other risk group for giardiasis includes internationally adopted children.[68] These children tend to be older than those in child-care centers and tend to have additional parasitic infections. The stools of these children should be screened for ova and parasites to ensure the long-term well being of these children and their adopting families.[68]

Humans acquire giardiasis directly by ingesting cysts by hand-to-mouth transfer of fecally contaminated material from an infected person or indirectly by ingesting contaminated water or food.[69] As few as 10 cysts may cause infection in humans.[70] Asymptomatic cyst carriage may last more than 6 months, and infected persons will continue to be infective as long as they excrete cysts. The most common source of epidemics is contaminated surface water, such as municipal reservoirs and mountain streams.[71] Giardia cysts are resistant to the usual chlorination levels and are not easily killed in cold water. *Giardia* cysts are killed by boiling water or cooking; thus food-borne outbreaks occur infrequently. Animals may transmit *Giardia* to humans by their cyst-containing feces.[72] However, molecular typing studies of *G intestinalis* suggest that most animal parasites are not associated with human disease.[73] Person-to-person transmission accounts for the high transmission and endemic rates of giardiasis in child-care centers and chronic-care facilities, including workers in these facilities. The risk of infection and transmission is highest among children aged 12 to 36 months and those who are not toilet trained.[74,75] In young adults, homosexual activity has been demonstrated to be a risk factor for giardiasis because of direct contact with infectious cysts.[76,77]

G intestinalis is a common cause of traveler's diarrhea. Travelers at highest risk are those traveling in the former Soviet Union, South and Southeast Asia, tropical Africa, western South America, and Mexico.[77]

Risk factors for acquisition of giardiasis include hypochlorhydria, previous gastric surgery, reduced gastric acidity, cystic fibrosis, and chronic pancreatitis.[78-81]

Pathogenesis and Life Cycle

The trophozoites of *G intestinalis* are the replicating form of the parasite. They are pear shaped and measure 10 to 20 mcm long and 5 to 15 mcm wide. In the middle are 2 axostyles with 2 parabasal bodies across. The trophozoites also contain 2 nuclei, 4 pairs of flagellae, and 2 ventral sucking disks serving as tissue attachment organs.[82]

The cysts are the infective stage. Excystment occurs in the upper small intestine after digestion by the gastric and duodenal secretions.[83] Trophozoite multiplication occurs in the upper portions of the small intestine. However, encystment occurs again in the lower small intestine and in the colon. Encystment is a periodic phenomenon, explaining the absence of cysts in the stools of patients when the trophozoites are present in the duodenum.[82]

The pathogenesis of giardiasis is unclear. Many hypotheses have been proposed, including bile salt deconjugation, mechanical barrier mechanism, and toxin production.[84] The damage caused by *Giardia* to the microvilli may also cause a decrease in enzymes, particularly the disaccharidases, leading to osmotic diarrhea and symptoms of malabsorption. Decreased secretion of pancreatic enzymes has been found. Although patients with giardiasis have steatorrhea, a higher degree exists of carbohydrate malabsorption than fat malabsorption.[85] Children with humoral immunodeficiencies such as X-linked agammaglobulinemia and common variable immunodeficiency are predisposed for chronic symptomatic infections.[86] Although secretory immunoglobulin (Ig) A deficiency has been suggested as a risk factor of giardiasis, the association has not yet been well established.

Clinical Manifestations

G intestinalis infections are associated with a wide range of clinical severity. Most infections are asymptomatic.[87] The incubation period is 1 to 4 weeks. Symptomatic children may have acute self-limited infection or chronic infection associated with malabsorption.[88] Acute symptoms are commonly encountered in travelers from nonendemic or low endemic infections to highly endemic areas. Acute giardiasis is characterized by acute watery diarrhea and is frequently associated with malaise, abdominal pain, and cramps and bloating. Flatulence, foul-smelling and fatty stools, nausea, and fatigue also occur frequently during the course of giardiasis. Blood, mucus, and pus are not usually present in stools. Symptoms may be intermittent. The duration of illness is usually over 1 week and may last 2 to 4 weeks.[89] Chronic giardiasis may develop after the acute phase of the illness or may occur without preceding acute symptoms. During the chronic phase, patients frequently develop chronic diarrhea with steatorrhea and marked weight loss.[88,90] Vitamin deficiencies, including A, B_{12}, and folate, as well as secondary lactase deficiency and hypoalbuminemia, have also been reported. Failure to thrive and growth retardation are common complications of chronic giardiasis in children, particularly those in developing countries.[91]

In addition to gastrointestinal manifestation, hypersensitivity phenomena such as rash, urticaria, aphthous ulcers, reactive arthritis, iridocyclitis, and retinal arteritis may rarely occur during the course of giardiasis.[92-95]

G intestinalis uncommonly spreads from the duodenum to other organs through the biliary and pancreatic ducts, causing hepatitis, cholangitis, and pancreatitis.[96,97]

Diagnosis

Routine blood tests are not helpful in diagnosing giardiasis. Peripheral leukocytosis and eosinophilia are typically absent, as well as fecal leukocytes. Fecal fat and other tests of malabsorption may be positive. The mainstay of diagnosis is demonstrating cysts or trophozoites by direct stool examination for ova and parasites. Cysts are more likely to be seen in formed stools because of the encystment that occurs in the colon. Conversely, frequent loose stools increase the yield of identifying trophozoites. Because of the intermittent presence of cysts in stool samples, 3 stool samples should be collected and examined for *Giardia* every other day.[98] To help identification, fresh stools should be examined; alternatively, samples may be preserved with polyvinyl alcohol or merthiolate-formalin. Both the cysts and trophozoites are identified in saline wet mount. Different staining procedures, including iodine, trichrome, Giemsa, or iron hematoxylin, have been used to help identification in stool and duodenal fluid samples. Different radiopaque materials and medications such as antacids, antibiotics, and mineral oil may mask identification of *Giardia* in stools.

If the organism is not found on direct examination of 3 stool specimens, then the feces should be checked for *Giardia* antigens. Several commercial kits are available that use either enzyme-linked immunosorbent assay (ELISA) or the IFA test. The sensitivity is 95% to 99% and specificity is 95% to 100% when compared with stool microscopy.[99,100]

If the clinical suspicion is high and the stool studies by various techniques are negative, then duodenal fluid sampling may be warranted.[101] Duodenal fluid can be examined by the Entero-Test®, in which the patient swallows a gelatin capsule that contains a string (string test).[102] Examination of fresh specimens for motile trophozoites is diagnostic. Duodenal biopsy is considered the last resort for diagnosis of giardiasis and is rarely required.[84]

Serologic testing for *Giardia* is not helpful for diagnostic purposes. Both IgM and IgG can be demonstrated and can persist for a long time. Serologic tests are reserved for epidemiologic studies.[64]

Giardia can also be identified by RNA and DNA gene probes or by the PCR.[103] Although these tests are highly sensitive and specific, they are not commercially available.

Treatment

Generally, treatment is not warranted for asymptomatic patients. However, to prevent spread, therapy may be provided to children attending child-care centers and to carriers who are in close contact with patients who have hypogammaglobulinemia or cystic fibrosis.[104]

The drugs of choice for treating giardiasis are metronidazole, tinidazole, and nitazoxanide.[104] Although not approved by the US Food and Drug Administration (FDA), metronidazole is the principal drug used for treatment of giardiasis and has a cure rate of 80% to 95%.[105,106] Common side effects include metallic mouth taste, nausea, headache, and dizziness. Tinidazole, a nitroimidazole, has been used for giardiasis with a cure rate of 90%, but it is not available for use in the United States.[105] A shorter course of nitazoxanide is as effective as a longer course of metronidazole and has the advantage of treating other intestinal parasites, such as *Cryptosporidium*.[107]

Alternative medications for giardiasis are furazolidone and quinacrine.[104] Furazolidone is well tolerated and results in a cure rate of 72% to 100%. Quinacrine has an excellent cure rate (90%-95%), but it has adverse effects, including gastrointestinal upset, nausea, vomiting, and abdominal pain.[105] Rarely, quinacrine may cause dermatitis, jaundice, and toxic psychosis.[106] The drug is no longer available in the United States. Paromomycin is a nonabsorbable aminoglycoside that acts locally on the gut and is used for treating symptomatic giardiasis in pregnant women.[105]

Prevention

Personal hygiene is the most important way to prevent spread of giardiasis. In child-care centers, strict hand washing and appropriate diaper disposal are essential. Symptomatic children should be excluded from child-care centers. However, exclusion of carriers is not suggested.[104] *Giardia* cysts can be killed by boiling or heating water to at least 70° C for 10 minutes.[108] Travelers, hikers, and campers should be advised to ensure that their drinking water is safe; they should heat or boil water, chemically disinfect it, or filter it.[108] High-quality filtration units are available and are effective in removing *Giardia* and *Cryptosporidium* cysts.[109]

Amebiasis (*Entamoeba histolytica*)

Epidemiologic Features

Amebiasis is caused by the protozoan *Entamoeba histolytica,* which also causes amoebic liver abscesses and other rare extraintestinal diseases. Worldwide, approximately 40 to 50 million people develop colitis or extraintestinal disease annually, with 40,000 deaths.[110] Amebiasis is a worldwide disease, but developing countries have far higher prevalence rates—as high as 50% in certain developing areas. These high rates are related to poor hygiene, inadequate water sanitation, and human waste that is used to fertilize crops.[111]

In developed countries such as the United States, amebiasis is mainly seen in migrants from and travelers to endemic countries. Infection with pathogenic *E histolytica* is not a common cause of traveler's diarrhea, and gastrointestinal infection with *E histolytica* is uncommon in travelers who have spent less than 1 month in endemic areas.[112]

Three species of *Entamoeba* have been identified, a pathogenic one (*E histolytica*) and 2 nonpathogenic ones (*Entamoeba dispar* and *Entamoeba moshkovskii*). For this reason, finding the cysts does not provide evidence of having invasive disease.[111]

Pathogenesis and Life Cycle

E histolytica has 2 forms: (1) the cysts (the infective forms of the parasite) and (2) the trophozoite. The cysts, when ingested along with contaminated food or drink, each liberate 4 metacystic trophozoites. The ingested cysts, but not trophozoites, can survive the gastric barrier in normal humans. The trophozoites continue to divide by binary fission. The actively motile trophozoites lodge in the submucous layer of the cecum and rectosigmoid, their normal habitat. After a period, trophozoites transform into cysts, which are passed in the stool. Trophozoites may be passed in the stool as well, but only the cysts are infective.[113]

Under certain circumstances, the trophozoites invade the bowel wall, producing ulcers and causing destruction and tissue necrosis. The organism then gradually moves from the dead tissue toward healthy tissue. Trophozoites may disseminate to the liver, lungs, pericardium, or the brain through the bloodstream.[113]

Clinical Manifestations

All *E dispar* and *E moshkovskii* infections and 90% of *E histolytica* infections are asymptomatic.[111] In general, intestinal amebiasis has a subacute onset, usually over 1 to 3 weeks. Symptoms range from mild diarrhea to severe dysentery, producing abdominal pain, diarrhea, and bloody stools. Weight loss is present in just under 50% of patients.[114] Eight percent to 38% of the patients may experience fever.[115] Fulminant colitis with bowel necrosis leading to perforation and peritonitis occurs rarely but is associated with a mortality rate of more than 40%.[116] Ameboma (a nodular, tumorlike focus of proliferate inflammation in the wall of the colon), toxic megacolon, local perforation, peritonitis, and extraintestinal extension are other rare complications.[117,118]

Amoebic liver abscess is the most common extraintestinal manifestation of amebiasis. The infection occurs by the trophozoites ascending the portal venous system.[119] Amoebic liver abscess (and other extraintestinal disease) is less common in children than in adults.[120] Most patients diagnosed with amoebic liver abscess in the United States will either be from a country where amebiasis is endemic or will have traveled there. Pain in the right upper quadrant, fever, anorexia, and fatigue are the symptoms of abscess formation. Concurrent diarrhea is present in less than one third of patients, although some patients will note that they had dysentery in the previous few months. Jaundice is uncommon. For travelers returning from an endemic area, manifestation of symptoms usually occurs within 8 to 20 weeks (within 5 months of their return in 95% of patients), although longer lags—sometimes of years—have been reported.[111] Extension or rupture into the lung, pleural space, peritoneum, or pericardium may complicate the course of the amoebic hepatic abscess.[115]

Diagnosis

Stool examination is less sensitive than antigen testing, and it is a poor method of making the diagnosis of intestinal amebiasis. Three fresh stool samples from separate days should be sent to improve the sensitivity.[111,121] Moreover, the demonstration of cysts or trophozoites in the stool suggests an intestinal amoebic infection, but microscopy cannot differentiate between *E histolytica* and *E dispar* or *E moshkovskii* strains. Therefore other methods have been developed to differentiate between the different species and to diagnose the invasive disease.

Serologic testing is useful to differentiate between infections with *E histolytica* from infection with *E dispar* because infection with *E histolytica* results in the development of antibodies, whereas *E dispar* infection does not. Because 10% to 35% of uninfected individuals in endemic areas have antiamoebic antibodies as a result of previous, often undiagnosed, infection with *E histolytica*, a negative serologic result in these populations helps exclude disease, but a positive serologic finding is not particularly helpful because it does not distinguish between acute infection and past exposure to the parasite.[111]

In endemic areas, agar gel diffusion and counterimmunophoresis are more useful than indirect hemagglutination (IHA) because they usually become negative after 6 to 12 months. However, they are less sensitive than the IHA.[122]

Fecal and serum antigen detection assays have many advantages, including quick and easy tests, the ability to differentiate between strains, greater sensitivity than microscopy, and potential for diagnosis in early infection and in endemic areas where serologic testing is less useful. These assays use monoclonal antibodies to bind to epitopes present on pathogenic *E histolytica* strains but not on nonpathogenic *E dispar* or *E moshkovskii* strains. They are being used commercially to detect *E histolytica* infection by ELISA, radioimmunoassay, or immunofluorescence.[111,123-126]

Diagnosing amoebic infection and differentiating between the 3 different strains can be accomplished by detecting parasitic DNA or RNA in feces via probes, but these methods are currently reserved as research tools.[127,128] PCR techniques can detect *E histolytica* in stool specimens. These PCR-based techniques are the most sensitive and specific methods, but they are not widely available.[129]

Liver amoebic abscesses are usually diagnosed based on clinical presentation, recognition of epidemiologic risk factors, serologic testing, and noninvasive imaging studies.

Treatment

The goals of antibiotic therapy of intestinal amebiasis are both to eliminate the invading trophozoites and to eradicate intestinal carriage of the organism. The treatment for intestinal amebiasis is metronidazole.[110] This initial step should be followed by treatment that targets the cyst stage by administering the intraluminal agents iodoquinol or diloxanide furoate. The most commonly used tissue agent for amoebic liver abscess is metronidazole. If the patient's disease is slow to respond to metronidazole therapy, or if the patient has a relapse after therapy, then aspiration or a prolonged course of metronidazole, or both, should be considered.

Asymptomatic *E histolytica* infection should be treated with an intraluminal agent because of the potential risk of developing invasive disease and the risk of spread to household members.

E dispar and *E moshkovskii* infections do not require treatment.[111]

Amoebic Meningoencephalitis (*Naegleria fowleri, Entamoeba histolytica, Acanthamoeba, Leptomyxa, Gephyramoeba,* and *Balamuthia*)

Knowledge that free-living amoebas are capable of causing human disease dates back some 50 years, before which time they were regarded as harmless soil organisms or, at most, commensals of mammals. Later, however, many different amoebic organisms were found to cause significant clinical disease in humans. These organisms are *Naegleria, Acanthamoeba, Balamuthia,* and *Prototheca.*[130]

These free-living amoebas cause 2 distinct clinical manifestations: (1) an acute, fulminant disease known as primary amoebic meningoencephalitis (PAM) that is caused by *N fowleri* in previously healthy children and young adults; and (2) granulomatous amoebic encephalitis (GAE) in immunocompromised patients caused by *Acanthamoeba* and *Balamuthia* species that is usually chronic and slowly progressive.[130,131]

E histolytica causes CNS abscesses that are distinct from CNS lesions caused by free-living amoebas that usually cause meningitis. Cerebral amebiasis results from hematogenous dissemination. Symptoms are usually of abrupt onset, and rapid progression to death occurs if treatment is delayed. Lesions may be seen on computed tomographic (CT) scan as irregular foci without a capsule or surrounding enhancement. Treatment should be prompt; it includes metronidazole and surgical intervention if required for decompression.[132]

Epidemiologic Features

Warm bodies of water such as human-made lakes and ponds, hot springs, and thermally polluted streams, rivers, and healing swimming pool waters are where *Naegleria* can be found. They are not found in seawater.[130] The olfactory neuroepithelium and the nasal passage are the ports of entry. Disease typically occurs in previously healthy children and young adults. Affected individuals characteristically have a recent history of water-sports activities in lakes, ponds, or inadequately chlorinated swimming pools. The organism has been isolated from nasal passages and throats of healthy individuals. The reason that disease occurs in only a small proportion of exposed individuals is unclear.[131] *N fowleri* exists in the environment in 3 forms: (1) the trophozoite, which is the invasive form that penetrates the cribriform plate and invades the brain; (2) resistant cysts; and (3) transient flagellates.

Several species of *Acanthamoeba* can cause granulomatous meningoencephalitis disease in humans. *Acanthamoeba* species have a trophozoite and a resistant cyst stage but no flagellate stage. They have been identified in soil, various water sources, air conditioners, and contact lens fluid, and from the nose and throats of healthy individuals.[130,131] The hematogenous route is how *Acanthamoeba* species are believed to gain access into the brain, after entering the human host through the respiratory tract or the skin and then traveling via the circulation to the brain. They may cause a chronic infection in immunocompromised hosts (*Acanthamoeba* encephalitides). *Acanthamoeba* keratitis has been reported in immunocompetent hosts who wore contact lenses exposed to contaminated water.[130]

Clinical Manifestations

The symptoms of PAM resemble those of fulminant bacterial meningitis and other meningoencephalitides. The incubation period is usually 2 to 15 days. After that, symptoms start as bifrontal headaches that do not respond to analgesia and fever (38°C-41°C). Alteration in the senses of taste or smell, with or without rhinitis, may also be noted early. Patients then develop emesis, seizures, and lethargy. The findings at physical examination include nuchal rigidity; cerebellar ataxia; and dysfunction of the third, fourth, and sixth cranial nerves. Death usually occurs within 3 to 7 days after onset of initial signs and symptoms.[133]

GAE is a disease of the immunocompromised and debilitated individuals. These patients include those with AIDS, neoplasms, and liver disease or patients who have received a liver transplant. As the name reflects, this infection is characterized by the host's granulomatous response to the presence of the amoeba. This infection is typically chronic and insidious; weeks to years may be required to become clinically apparent. The symptoms include hemiparesis, personality changes, seizures, neck stiffness, headaches, and fever. These symptoms are the result of the single or multiple space-occupying intracranial lesions. In addition to the GAE, *Acanthamoeba* is known to cause sinusitis, otitis media, cutaneous lesions, and corneal ulcers.[134]

Diagnosis

In general, infections caused by the free-living amoebas are difficult to diagnose, and most are recognized at autopsy or necropsy.

In PAM, neuroimaging studies may be normal early in the disease but may show signs of increased intracranial pressure later. Meningeal enhancement of the basilar region is frequently reported. Severe brain edema is a late finding and is indicative of poor outcome. Laboratory studies often reveal increased leukocyte count, hyperglycemia, and glycosuria. CSF examination shows a pleocytosis with polymorphonuclear neutrophil predominance, increased CSF protein, and normal or decreased glucose. Routine Gram stain and bacterial culture will be negative. The motile amoebas may be seen on a wet mount of the CSF, preferably unrefrigerated CSF collected within 30 minutes of the evaluation. Culturing the amoebas on nonnutrient agar plated with *Escherichia coli* is a definitive way to make the diagnosis. Because most cases are fatal, staining of brain tissue with hematoxylin and eosin or an IFA test can help confirm a diagnosis of PAM, but this assessment is usually done after death. Little or no antibody response exists to the presence of the amoebas, again because of the short duration of this fatal infection; thus serologic procedures are of little or no help. PCR has been used to detect amoeba DNA in tissue and CSF samples, but the technique is still in its early developmental stages and requires more testing before its reliability can be certified.[133,134]

In GAE, neuroimaging may reveal space-occupying lesions resembling abscesses, tumors, or hemorrhagic infarction. CSF examination findings are similar to those of aseptic meningitis. Diagnosis is made by finding the amoebas in tissue sections stained with hematoxylin and eosin or by IFA staining with rabbit antiamoeba sera. Cysts of infecting amoebas can be recognized in corneal scrapings that have been stained with calcofluor white, a fluorescent stain that binds to polysaccharide polymers in the *Acanthamoeba* cyst wall. The *Acanthamoeba* can also be cultured onto nonnutrient agar with bacteria for identification.[134]

Treatment

The mainstay in therapy for PAM is intravenous or intrathecal amphotericin B.[133-135] Even with combined therapy, survival has been the exception.

No optimal antimicrobial therapy has been developed for the encephalitides caused by *Acanthamoeba*. Multiple drugs have been used in both of these infections with varying degrees of success, including amphotericin B, azithromycin, fluconazole, flucytosine, pentamidine isethionate, and sulfa drugs.[134] In vitro, miltefosine and voriconazole are potentially useful drugs for treating patients with free-living amoebic infections, although sensitivities differ between genera, species, and strains.[136]

Amoebic keratitis is treatable with 1 or more drugs topically. Chlorhexidine gluconate (a component of germicidal soaps) and polyhexamethylene biguanide (a disinfectant and swimming pool cleaner) have become the drugs of choice in treating keratitis cases.[137]

Treatment of cases of amoebic CNS infections should be in centers where neurologic, neurosurgical, and infectious disease experts are available. Consultation with the CDC is advisable.

Prevention

Natural or artificially warm waters, if they are not properly chlorinated, might harbor *Naegleria amoeba*. Maintaining effective levels of chlorine in water used for recreation is achievable in swimming pools and spas, but less so in lakes and ponds. However, even maintaining a level of chlorine between 0.5 and 1.5 parts per million is not protective all the time.[138] In general, swimming in warm, stagnant, and possibly feces-contaminated waters should be avoided. Compliance with procedures for contact lens care should protect wearers against infection.[139]

Cryptosporidiosis

Cryptosporidium is an intracellular coccidian protozoan parasite that causes gastrointestinal disease among humans, as well as different animals such as mammals, reptiles, and fish.[140] The organism is 2 to 6 mcm in diameter. Ten species of this protozoan have been named. However, *Cryptosporidium parvum* is the main species that causes disease in humans.[140,141] *C parvum* is further divided into 2 separate species: (1) *Cryptosporidium hominis* (previously *C parvum* genotype 1) that only infects humans, and (2) *C parvum* (previously *C parvum* genotype 2) that infects both humans and animals.[141,142]

Cryptosporidium is one of the most common parasitic intestinal pathogens in humans. It has been increasingly recognized as a cause of diarrhea in healthy individuals, as well as severe gastrointestinal disease and life-threatening illness in patients with AIDS.[141]

Epidemiologic Features

Cryptosporidium is associated with both sporadic cases and outbreaks of diarrheal illness worldwide. Cryptosporidiosis is particularly common in developing countries that have increased crowding and poor sanitation. Patients with underlying cellular and humoral immunodeficiencies are at increased risk of prolonged and severe clinical course. These patients include those with AIDS, IgA deficiency, and hypogammaglobulinemia, as well as those receiving immunosuppressive treatment and those who have undergone organ transplantation.[141]

Cryptosporidiosis is present in 1% to 3% of immunocompetent patients with diarrhea in developed countries, compared with 7% to 10% in developing countries.[143,144] The annual incidence is reported as 3.0 cases per 100,000 persons in the United States and 6.0 per 100,000 persons in Canada.[145,146] The incidence is higher in children than in adults. Reported seroprevalence rates are 25% to 60% in the United States and as high as 65% to 90% in developing countries.[147,148]

Cryptosporidium is transmitted to humans by person-to-person spread or by an infected animal.[149,150] Because autoinfection can occur, ingestion of only 10 to 50 oocysts may cause infection. The 50%-infectious dose in healthy persons is 132 oocysts.[151] Extensive outbreaks of cryptosporidiosis have occurred from fecally contaminated environments such as municipal drinking water and swimming pools.[152,153] The transmission and spread of cryptosporidiosis is facilitated by the resistance of the oocysts to disinfectants, the ineffective removal of oocysts by many filtration systems, and their ability to survive in the environment for months. The oocysts are resistant to chlorine; thus appropriately functioning filtration systems are critical to prevent their spread. Most swimming pool sand filters are ineffective in oocyst removal.[154] Several outbreaks of cryptosporidiosis have been reported, most of which are the result of contamination of drinking water, but also as the result of drinking contaminated apple cider or playing in contaminated water at a water park.[153,155,156] Outbreaks involving consumption of contaminated food are less frequent than waterborne outbreaks.[157]

Person-to-person transmission of *Cryptosporidium* can also cause outbreaks at child-care centers, with reported attack rates of 30% to 60%.[158,159] Transmission is also common among household members, homosexuals, and health care workers.[160-162] *Cryptosporidium* can also be a cause of traveler's diarrhea from contaminated drinking and swimming water.[163] The incubation period of cryptosporidiosis is 2 to 14 days.[164] Oocyst excretion may continue for 1 week after resolution of symptoms.[164]

Pathogenesis and Life Cycle

The complete life cycle of *Cryptosporidium* requires only 1 host. Humans acquire the infection by ingesting thick-walled oocysts. The oocyst sporulates in the host and is infective immediately after excretion in the stools. Excystation in the gastrointestinal tract occurs in the upper small intestine via the action of proteolytic enzymes and bile salts and causes the release of 4 infectious sporozoites that invade the epithelial cells.[165] The first intracellular stage is the trophozoite, which subsequently undergoes 3 nuclear divisions to form a group of 8 merozoites; these merozoites become the first-generation schizont. The merozoites released from the schizont invade other epithelial cells, forming the second-generation schizont, which is composed of only 4 merozoites. The second-generation merozoites invade other epithelial cells and enter the sexual stage, forming microgametocytes and macrogametocytes. Each microgametocyte produces 12 to 16 microgametocytes, and each macrogametocyte transforms into 1 macrogametocyte.[165] The two sexual stages combine to form the zygote, which later develops into an oocyst, thus completing the life cycle. Oocysts exist in 2 forms: (1) thin-walled oocysts and (2) thick-walled oocysts. Thin-walled oocysts sporulate and cause infection in the same person (autoinfection), whereas thick-walled oocysts are excreted in feces and infect new hosts.[166] Infection is generally limited to the superficial parts of the small intestine, but in immunocompromised patients the infection may spread to involve the biliary tree and the pancreas or may disseminate to extraintestinal sites, mainly the respiratory tract.[167,168]

The mechanism by which *Cryptosporidium* causes diarrhea is not well understood. *Cryptosporidium* causes secretory diarrhea that is associated with malabsorption. No specific toxin associated with *Cryptosporidium* has been identified yet. However, increased proinflammatory cytokine release has been demonstrated during the course of infection.[169] The pathogenesis is probably mulifactorial. Loss of vacuolated villous tip epithelium causes reduction in the absorption area.[170] Reduced lactase activity may cause lactose intolerance and malabsorption. Accumulation of abnormal metabolites in the intestinal lumen may stimulate bacterial overgrowth.

In addition, the host immune response to the infection, both cellular and humoral, may contribute to the inflammatory changes in the gastrointestinal tract. The T-lymphocyte immune responses are essential to control the infection. Although specific IgA, IgG, and IgM are produced during the course of illness, they are not associated with clearance of infection, especially in HIV-infected patients.[171] However, the production of interferon gamma seems to be involved in clearing the infection.[172]

Clinical Manifestations

Cryptosporidiosis varies from an asymptomatic infection to severe enteritis and dehydration that leads to death. In children, up to 30% of infections may be asymptomatic.[173] The most common manifestation of cryptosporidiosis is acute diarrhea, characterized by frequent, watery, foul-smelling, nonbloody stools. Diarrhea is commonly associated with malaise, nausea, anorexia, fatigue, abdominal cramps, and weight loss. Fever and vomiting are commonly seen in children who may be misdiagnosed as having viral gastroenteritis.[174] In immunocompetent patients, including healthy children, the diarrhea is self-limited and resolves spontaneously in 1 to 20 days, although resolved diarrhea may recur.[153] Occasionally, healthy infants with cryptosporidiosis may develop chronic and persistent diarrhea, leading to malnutrition and growth retardation.[175,176]

In immunocompromised patients, particularly those infected with HIV, cryptosporidiosis frequently takes a severe and protracted course and can lead to significant malnutrition and wasting, dehydration, and death. The disease is particularly severe in patients with extremely low CD4 counts (<180 cells/mcL).[177] Other clinical manifestations of cryptosporidiosis in patients with AIDS include cholecystitis, cholangitis, hepatitis, pancreatitis, and respiratory tract involvement. The biliary tract is affected in 10% to 30% of HIV-infected patients and can lead to sclerosing or acalculous cholangitis. Biliary cryptosporidiosis is exclusively seen in patients with AIDS.[178] Symptoms include right upper quadrant pain, fever, and nausea and vomiting with or without diarrhea. Serum alkaline phosphatase and gamma glutamyl transpeptidase levels are high. Radiologic investigations may show dilatation of the intra- and extrahepatic bile ducts, as well as a dilated, thick-walled gallbladder. Rarely, pancreatitis may result from involvement of the pancreatic duct.

Respiratory cryptosporidiosis is seen mainly in patients with AIDS. Whether *Cryptosporidium* is a true pathogen or merely colonizes the respiratory tract is not clear because *Cryptosporidium* is frequently coexistent with other pathogens such as cytomegalovirus, *Mycobacterium* species, and *Pneumocystis jirovecii*. Clinical symptoms include cough, dyspnea, fever, expectoration, and chest pain.[179,180]

Diagnosis

Diagnosis of cryptosporidiosis depends on microscopic identification of the oocysts in stools, aspirated fluid, or tissue samples. Routine laboratory examination of the stools for ova and parasites will not detect *Cryptosporidium*. The laboratory should be alerted to the potential diagnosis of cryptosporidiosis to perform specific staining of the samples. A modified Kinyoun acid-fast stain is used to identify *Cryptosporidium*. The stool samples are usually concentrated by either the sucrose flotation or the formalin acetate methods before staining. The oocysts of *Cryptosporidium* are small (4-6 mcm) and can be missed by careless scanning of slides. At least three stool samples should be tested before considering a negative result. Immunofluorescent staining that uses monoclonal antibodies, and ELISA kits can be used to detect oocysts in stool and tissue specimens.[181,182]

Serologic testing is available by different methods, but testing is useful only for epidemiologic studies. PCR can be performed on stool samples and has been shown to be more sensitive than immunofluorescent staining and acid-fast stain.[183] The test is not commercially available, but it is particularly useful in detecting common-source outbreaks by differentiating among different *Cryptosporidium* genotypes.[184]

Treatment

In immunocompetent patients, cryptosporidiosis is a self-limited disease. Supportive care, including hydration and nutritional support, may be adequate.[166] The recovery from cryptosporidiosis largely depends on the immune status of the host. The FDA has approved nitazoxanide (Alinia), a nitrothiazole benzamide, for treatment of children one year of age and older, as well as adults with diarrhea caused by cryptosporidiosis or giardiasis.[185] Paromomycin, a nonabsorbable aminoglycoside, provided with or without azithromycin has been used in HIV-infected patients with cryptosporidiosis, although reliable efficacy data are lacking.[186] The most important part of treating HIV-infected patients is immune reconstitution by providing highly active antiretroviral therapy.[187] Immune therapy such as oral administration of human immunoglobulin, hyperimmune bovine colostrum, and bovine transfer factor has demonstrated some benefit.[188]

Diarrhea in cryptosporidiosis is copious, and attention to fluid and electrolyte management of affected patients is essential. Chronic diarrhea is frequently associated with malnutrition. Nutritional supplements containing medium-chain triglycerides may be helpful. Because of lactase deficiency, milk and dairy products should be avoided. Total parenteral nutrition may be needed in HIV-infected patients with chronic diarrhea and weight loss.[166]

Prevention

The most important preventive measures are good hygiene practices, such as effective hand washing and appropriate disposal of infected material. Contact precautions are suggested for diapered and incontinent children. People with cryptosporidiosis should not use public recreational water when they have diarrhea and for at least 2 weeks after resolution of symptoms.[189] Although not universally suggested for immunocompromised patients, boiling water intended for drinking for 1 minute is the most reliable method of killing *Cryptosporidium*.[190] Alternatively, filtration devices with particle-size ratings of 1 to 5 mcm will remove *Cryptosporidium*.[191]

Isosporiasis (*Isospora belli*)

Isospora belli, similar to *Cryptosporidium* and *Cyclospora,* is a coccidian protozoan. Humans are the only reservoir for this parasite. Infections are mainly gastrointestinal.[192]

Epidemiologic Features

Isosporiasis is common in tropical and subtropical regions of Central and South America, Africa, and Southeast Asia.[163] In the past, isosporiasis was rarely seen in the United States. However, more cases have been identified after the outbreak of AIDS, especially among homosexual men. Oral-anal contact may play an important role in this group of patients. *I belli* has also been identified as a causative agent of traveler's diarrhea in returned travelers from endemic areas.[163,193]

Humans acquire infection by ingestion of sporulated oocysts in contaminated food or water. The incubation period is 8 to 10 days. After ingesting a sporulated oocyst, 8 sporozoites are released from the 2 sporocysts in the small intestine. These sporozoites invade epithelial cells and go into a cycle of asexual maturation followed by sexual reproduction, resulting in formation of oocysts that are released into the intestinal lumen.[194] The oocysts that are passed in stools are not infectious; they require exposure to oxygen and temperatures lower than body temperature before becoming infectious.[194]

Clinical Manifestations

Most immunocompetent individuals develop diarrhea that is self-limited and resolves spontaneously in days to weeks.[163] Diarrhea is typically watery and resembles that caused by *Cryptosporidium*. Malabsorption may be present.[163,194] Other commonly associated symptoms include fever, malaise, vomiting, headache, abdominal pain, and weight loss.[163] Mild to moderate eosinophilia may be present.[195]

In immunocompromised patients, particularly those with AIDS, the disease can be associated with a devastating, protracted course lasting months or even years.[196,197]

Diagnosis

The diagnosis of isosporiasis is made by finding oocysts in the stools. As with *Cryptosporidium* and *Cyclospora, Isospora* oocysts are easily missed on routine ova and parasite testing, and special stains should be used. The staining technique of choice is the Kinyoun acid-fast or modified acid-fast stain.[198] Alternatively, specific fluorescent techniques may be used.[198,199] Oocysts may also be detected in duodenal fluid aspirates.[200] Parasites may also be found in biopsy specimens from the small intestine.[201]

Treatment

The drug of choice is trimethoprim-sulfamethoxazole (TMP-SMX) for 10 days.[202] TMP-SMX should not be provided to infants younger than 2 months because of the risk of kernicterus.[202] For patients who cannot tolerate TMP-SMX, pyrimethamine may be provided.[203] Ciprofloxacin may also be effective,[204] although it should not be provided to people younger than 18 years. Patients with AIDS may require maintenance courses with TMP-SMX or pyrimethamine-sulfadoxine to prevent relapses.[197]

Cyclosporiasis (*Cyclospora cayetanensis*)

Cyclosporiasis is caused by the coccidian protozoan parasite *Cyclospora cayetanensis*.[205]

Epidemiologic Features

Cyclosporiasis is distributed worldwide. Cases have been reported in the United States, Germany, the United Kingdom, Latin America, the Caribbean, and Asia.[205-210] Humans acquire cyclosporiasis by ingesting contaminated food or water.[210,211] Outbreaks have been reported to be caused by drinking water from an infected water tank and eating infected fruit, herbs, and vegetables.[205,211-214] Most sporadic cases and disease outbreaks in developing countries are due to contaminated water sources.[210]

Secreted oocysts in stools are not infectious; thus person-to-person transmission is unlikely. After several days or sometime weeks, the oocysts will become infectious after sporulation.[215] Each oocyst releases 4 sporozoites in the gastrointestinal tract. The sporozoites invade the enterocytes and undergo asexual and sexual cycles of reproduction culminating in the formation of oocysts.[212] The complete life cycle of *Cyclospora* may be similar to *Cryptosporidium* and *Isospora*. The incubation period is 1 to 14 days.[215]

Clinical Manifestations

The symptoms are similar to cryptosporidiosis and isosporiasis. Most infections in immunocompetent patients are self-limited.[205,216] The most common symptom is profuse, watery diarrhea. The diarrhea is intermittent and prolonged. Other common associated symptoms are prolonged fatigue and anorexia. Abdominal cramps and bloating, nausea, vomiting, fever, myalgia, and weight loss are other common findings.[205] Prolonged diarrhea occurs in immunocompromised patients, especially those with AIDS.[209] Asymptomatic patients may continue to excrete oocysts.[217]

Diagnosis

Diagnosis of cyclosporiasis is made by microscopic examination of stool specimens.[218] The laboratory should be alerted to the potential diagnosis of cyclosporiasis because, as with *Cryptosporidium* and *Isospora,* special stains are needed.[218] The best stains are the modified Ziehl-Nelson or Kinyoun acid-fast staining. The oocysts of *Cyclospora* (8-10 mcm) are larger than those of *Cryptosporidium* (4-5 mcm). In addition, fluorescent microscopy is another distinguishing feature. It reveals the autofluorescence of the cell wall of *Cyclospora* oocysts. In contrast, *Cryptosporidium* shows no autofluorescence, and *Isospora* shows bright autofluorescence of the entire oocyst.[198,212] PCR can be used for diagnosis but is not commercially available.[219]

Treatment

The drug of choice is TMP-SMX.[220] In patients infected with HIV, a prolonged course may be needed; secondary prophylaxis with TMP-SMX for months may also be needed in these patients.[209]

Toxoplasmosis *(Toxoplasma gondii)*

Toxoplasma gondii is an obligate intracellular coccidian parasite that belongs to the class Sporozoa. *Toxoplasma* infects several animal species as well as humans. Members of the cat family are considered the definite hosts; humans and other mammals are considered intermediate hosts.[221]

Epidemiologic Features

Toxoplasma infections are distributed worldwide. The highest incidence of infection is in countries where consumption of raw meat by people is common, such as France, the United States, and other Western countries.[222,223] Infections are also common in regions with warm, humid climates, including tropical areas. The presence of a domestic cat is an important risk factor associated with disease transmission in different parts of the world.

Humans acquire infection by ingesting cysts that are present in raw or undercooked meat or oocysts in material contaminated by cat feces.[222,224]

Outbreaks of disease have occurred after contamination of drinking water supplies.[225] Infection may occur after blood transfusion.[226] It may also follow stem cell or solid organ transplantation.[227,228] Congenital infection occurs after acquisition of primary maternal infection during pregnancy. Newborns are most frequently infected when maternal infection is acquired in the third trimester. However, the clinical manifestations of congenital toxoplasmosis are most severe when maternal infection occurs in the first trimester, during fetal organ development.[229]

Pathogenesis and Life Cycle

Cats acquire infection by eating rodents or uncooked kitchen meat that contains *Toxoplasma* cysts. The sexual phase takes place in the intestinal epithelial cells of cats. This phase is followed by appearance of oocysts in the feces in 3 to 18 days.[221] Shedding of oocysts may persist for approximately 2 to 3 weeks. Shedding is more likely to occur in kittens than in older cats. First infection in a cat is associated with shedding of millions of oocysts per day. The oocyst becomes infectious in 1 to 3 days after it sporulates.[230]

The asexual phase occurs in the intermediate host including humans and mammals. After ingestion, the sporozoites are released in the intestine and become free trophozoites.[221] From there, trophozoites are taken up by macrophages and transported via the bloodstream to different organs.[231] The most commonly involved organs are the skeletal muscles, brain, cardiac muscle, lymph nodes, eyes, and lungs. They proliferate by budding and form clusters consisting of vacuoles of macrophages called pseudocysts. Because of their rapid proliferation and invasion, they are called tachyzoites. After establishment of the host immune response, as occurs in immunocompetent patients, the cysts are formed.[221] The wall of the cyst will form, and the organisms within the organisms will no longer actively multiply. The organisms in these cysts are thus called bradyzoites. Morphologically, the tachyzoites and bradyzoites are similar except for the rate of proliferation. Both measure 2 to 6 mcm.[21,231,232] Oocysts are not shed in intermediate hosts. Only cats shed oocysts.[230]

Infection in immunocompetent patients is limited, and cellular necrosis is controlled. The incubation period is 4 to 21 days. Both cellular and humoral immune responses develop to *Toxoplasma*. However, not all organisms are killed, and cysts may remain in any organ without causing any symptoms or significant damage.[221,232] Under certain conditions, such as immune dysfunction or in patients with the HIV infection, multiplication of organisms causes rupture of the cysts and release of bradyzoites. An inflammatory response characterized by infiltration of lymphocyte, monocytes, and plasma cells and formation of granulomas will develop. This response may lead to significant dysfunction in affected organs, especially the brain and the eye; it may also lead to disseminated toxoplasmosis.[233]

Clinical Manifestations

CONGENITAL DISEASE. Congenital toxoplasmosis follows a primary infection in the mother during pregnancy. In rare instances the fetus may be infected after *Toxoplasma* reactivation in immunocompromised mothers, including those with HIV. After a primary maternal infection the risk of transmission of *Toxoplasma* infection to the fetus is 15% to 20% in the first trimester and 60% to 65% in the third trimester.[234] The incidence of congenital toxoplasmosis in the United States is 1 in 1000 live births.[235] Severely affected fetuses may result in stillbirth, miscarriage, or early neonatal death. However, most (70%-90%) congenitally infected infants are asymptomatic.[236] If untreated, a large proportion of these infants may develop late-onset sequelae such as chorioretinitis, learning disabilities, and intellectual disability months to years later.[237,238] Clinical manifestations of congenital toxoplasmosis at birth can include hepatosplenomegaly, lymphadenopathy, hydrocephalus, or microcephaly. Clinical signs of meningoencephalitis such as seizures and neurologic deficits may also be present. Other manifestations include chorioretinitis, rash, jaundice, thrombocytopenia, and anemia.[239] Radiologic studies such as ultrasound or CT may show calcifications or dilated ventricles.[239] The calcifications in toxoplasmosis are scattered throughout the brain, in contrast to the periventricular calcifications of cytomegalovirus infection.[240]

ACQUIRED DISEASE. Most *Toxoplasma* infections acquired after birth are asymptomatic.[241] In symptomatic patients the most frequent clinical manifestation is cervical lymphadenopathy.[225] Concomitant nonspecific signs and symptoms such as fever, myalgia, and fatigue may be present.[241] The lymphadenopathy may less frequently occur in other regions or may be generalized. In some patients, infectious mononucleosis–like manifestations such as sore throat, fever, malaise, adenopathy, splenomegaly, rash, and atypical lymphocytes may be present.[233,242] Rare complications of primary infection include hepatitis, pneumonitis, myocarditis, pericarditis, and encephalitis.

DISEASE IN IMMUNODEFICIENT PATIENTS. Disease in immunocompromised patients, including those infected with HIV, is more severe than infection in a normal host.[243] Disseminated toxoplasmosis and death may rarely occur. More frequently, these patients develop localized infections in different organs; these infections include encephalitis, meningoencephalitis, pneumonitis, myocarditis, pericarditis, and hepatitis. Encephalitis in patients with AIDS usually follows reactivation of chronic disease, especially in those with CD4 counts of less than 100 cells/mcL.[244] *Toxoplasma* is the most frequent cause of focal brain lesions in this group of patients. Brain involvement can be localized or diffuse. Patients experience fever, headache, deterioration in mental status, seizures, and focal neurologic deficits.[245] Hemiparesis and abnormal speech are the most typical focal findings. CT scans typically show brain abscesses or ring-enhancing lesions.[244] *Toxoplasma* pneumonitis in patients with AIDS may mimic *P jirovecii* pneumonia.[246,247]

OCULAR DISEASE. *Toxoplasma* is the most common recognized cause of chorioretinitis in the United States.[248] Isolated ocular toxoplasmosis most frequently follows congenital infection but may follow an acquired infection, though rarely.[249,250] Chorioretinitis is bilateral in the congenital form and unilateral in the acquired form of toxoplasmosis.[251] Most affected patients are young adults. Chorioretinitis is unusual as the sole manifestation of acquired toxoplasmosis. Nystagmus is a common manifestation of congenital ocular toxoplasmosis.[252] Acute chorioretinitis is characterized by blurred vision, photophobia, and central vision loss that results from the involvement of the macula. Funduscopy shows yellow-white cotton-like patches with indistinct borders.[248] During the healing stage, black pigment will be seen at the margins. The lesions heal in few weeks to several months. Relapses are frequent, and vision loss may occur.[233,249] Other complications of congenital ocular involvement include chorioretinal scars, microphthalmia, cataract, and retinal detachment.[248,253]

Diagnosis

The most definite test for diagnosis of toxoplasmosis is isolation of the organism from infected tissue or body fluids by either inoculation into laboratory animals or by tissue culture. However, these techniques are not routinely available. Thus the primary method currently used for diagnosis is based on detecting specific antibodies and monitoring the immune response. Molecular methods involving PCR for detecting *Toxoplasma* DNA in tissue and fluid samples have been used.[246,254] Clinical and laboratory data should be carefully correlated during patient evaluation and management.

The most commonly used serologic tests are ELISA tests. Serum IgG usually becomes positive 4 to 8 weeks after infection and remains positive indefinitely. Paired sera should be tested simultaneously 3 weeks apart to document rise in antibody titers of at least 4-fold. Serum IgM levels should also be tested simultaneously with IgG.[255] The ELISA IgM tests are more sensitive than the IFA test. The IgM test may remain positive for 6 months, and false-positive results can occur.[255] In newborns and pregnant women, the serum levels of IgA and IgE for *Toxoplasma* can also be tested.[256] These tests become negative sooner than the IgM test, thus giving more precise information about the timing of infection. However, anti-*Toxoplasma* IgA and IgE tests are only available at *Toxoplasma* referral laboratories.

IgG avidity testing is used to predict the timing of *Toxoplasma* infection.[257] The presence of these high-avidity antibodies reflects infection at least 3 to 5 months earlier. Testing of high-avidity antibodies is most useful in assessing the risk of transmission of *Toxoplasma* from the mother to the fetus or when only one sample is available at time of decision making. Low-avidity antibodies are unreliable in predicting a recent infection.[257,258]

Pregnant women should ideally have a serologic status for *Toxoplasma* before conception. If positive, then no further testing is needed. However, if the mother was found to have a positive *Toxoplasma* IgG antibody during pregnancy, then the serum titers should be repeated for both IgM and IgG after 3 weeks to determine whether she has a primary infection.[259] A definitive diagnosis of congenital toxoplasmosis during pregnancy can be made by testing amniotic fluid. Detecting *Toxoplasma* in amniotic fluid by either DNA PCR or tissue culture or mouse inoculation is considered diagnostic.[260,261] Similarly, fetal blood sampling to isolate *Toxoplasma* from fetal white blood cells and to test for IgM antibody may also be used. Serial ultrasound examinations to assess brain ventricular size or other signs of infection can also be performed.[262]

After delivery, infants should be evaluated for congenital toxoplasmosis if the mother has a primary infection or if she is HIV infected and has serologic findings suggestive of past infection.[236] If the diagnosis is suspected, then the patient should undergo complete clinical evaluation, including ophthalmologic, neurologic, and auditory examination.[239,259] CT scan of the brain should be performed to rule out brain calcification or hydrocephalus. Serum samples should be evaluated for IgG, IgM, IgA, and IgE antibodies for *Toxoplasma*.[263] CSF should be analyzed for cells, protein, glucose, *Toxoplasma* antibodies, and PCR. Diagnosis is confirmed serologically by demonstrating a positive IgM or IgA, a higher infant IgG titer than the mother, or a persistently positive IgG beyond 1 year of age.[259]

The diagnosis of toxoplasmosis in older children and adults who are immunocompetent relies on identification of a positive IgM titer or a 4-fold rise in IgG titers after 3 weeks.[241] Demonstrating classic histopathological findings in tissue samples such as lymph nodes strongly supports the diagnosis.[264] Identification of proliferating organisms on histology provides a definite diagnosis. Similarly, isolation of *Toxoplasma* from tissue or body fluid by culture or identification of nucleic acid material by DNA PCR is definitive.[246,254,265]

In immunocompromised patients, including those with HIV infection, serologic testing may not be reliable. A 4-fold rise in titer may not occur in these patients when they acquire a primary infection; those who had an old infection are diagnosed on the basis of a positive IgG titer.[233] The diagnosis of *Toxoplasma* encephalitis in patients with AIDS relies on characteristic clinical and radiologic findings.[244,245] Patients with positive *Toxoplasma* IgG titers are treated presumptively. If treatment produces no response, then identification of *Toxoplasma* in blood or CSF by DNA PCR may be needed.[265]

Patients with ocular involvement are diagnosed based on classical eye findings and serologic testing.[249,266]

Treatment

Treatment is not indicated in immunocompetent patients unless clinical symptoms are severe or complications occur.[233] Immunocompromised patients, especially those with HIV or AIDS, with acute infection should be treated even if they are asymptomatic.[233] Infected pregnant women and neonates, whether symptomatic or not, should also be treated as soon as the diagnosis is established.[259] Patients with chorioretinitis are treated when symptoms are present or progressive.[266]

The best treatment for most cases is pyrimethamine-sulfadiazine.[267] These drugs act on the tachyzoites, and the cysts forms are not affected. Thus lifelong daily maintenance therapy is needed in patients with AIDS.[268] Because pyrimethamine is a folic acid antagonist, supplemental leucovorin (folinic acid) is provided to prevent bone marrow toxic effects. In pregnant women, pyrimethamine is not provided because of its teratogenic effects, especially during the first trimester.[259] Instead, sulfadiazine alone or spiramycin can be used. However, pyrimethamine and sulfadiazine may be considered for treatment of infections acquired in the third trimester. Patients who are allergic to sulfa drugs can be provided a combination of clindamycin and pyremethamine.[267,269]

For congenital toxoplasmosis, pyrimethamine and sulfadiazine (with folinic acid supplements) should be continued for a prolonged period, often for 1 year.[267]

Corticosteroids are provided in addition to pyrimethamine and sulfadiazine in patients with ocular toxoplasmosis and selected patients with CNS disease.[233,267]

Prophylactic therapy is provided for prevention of toxoplasmosis in children with HIV or AIDS with severe immunosuppression and positive *Toxoplasma* IgG antibodies.[270] The drug of choice is TMP-SMX. Alternative therapies are dapsone plus pyrimethamine (with supplemental folinic acid) or atovaquone. Prophylaxis is also provided to prevent recurrence of toxoplasmosis in immunosuppressed patients with prior *Toxoplasma* encephalitis.[270] The best regimen is pyrimethamine plus sulfadiazine plus folinic acid. Alternatively, clindamycin plus pyrimethamine plus folinic acid may be used for patients who cannot tolerate sulfa drugs.[267,271]

Prevention

Preventive measures are aimed at hygienic practices during cat contact and prevention of consuming raw meat.[272] Pregnant women with negative or unknown serostatus for *Toxoplasma*, as well as immunocompromised individuals, should avoid contact with cats, cat litter, or soil that have been contaminated by cat feces. Hygienic practices such as wearing gloves and hand washing should be stressed in such settings.[272] Deep freezing and cooking meat, particularly ham and lamb, to an internal temperature of 65.5°C to 76.6°C or until no longer pink will kill cysts. All fruits and vegetables should be washed thoroughly. Cats may be prevented from acquiring infection by restricting their outdoor activities and feeding them commercially prepared cat food. Because the oocysts are not infective until at least 36 to 48 hours after passage, daily cleaning of cat litter boxes is a simple and effective control measure.[267,272]

Malaria (*Plasmodium falciparum, Plasmodium vivax, Plasmodium ovale, Plasmodium malariae*)

Epidemiologic Features

Malaria is a global problem and a leading cause of death and illness worldwide. Between 350 and 500 million clinical episodes of malaria occur every year, resulting in at least 1 million deaths. Most of the cases and deaths are in sub-Saharan Africa; most occur in African children younger than 5 years.[273,274]

Four species of the plasmodia infect humans: *Plasmodium falciparum, Plasmodium vivax, Plasmodium ovale*, and *Plasmodium malariae*. They are transmitted from person to person by the bite of the female *Anopheles* mosquito. *P falciparum* causes the most severe disease and is the predominant malarial parasite in tropical Africa, Southeast Asia, and Oceania. *P vivax*, which is predominant in Southeast Asia, causes most malaria infections worldwide, along with *P falciparum*. *P malariae*, the least common, produces long-lasting infections. *P ovale* is uncommon and is found mostly in Africa.

Life Cycle

The malaria parasites have 2 different life cycles in 2 hosts, the female *Anopheles* mosquito and the human. When certain forms of blood-stage parasites (gametocytes) are picked up by a female *Anopheles* mosquito during a blood meal, they start the sexual stage of life inside the mosquito, which results in forming the infective-stage sporozoites that reside in the mosquito's salivary gland and that can access the bloodstream of a human when the mosquito feeds again.[275]

In humans, the parasites grow and multiply first in the liver cells (extraerythrocytic stage) and then in the red blood cells (RBCs; erythrocytic stage). In the blood, successive broods of parasites grow inside the RBCs and destroy them, releasing daughter parasites (merozoites) that continue the cycle by invading other RBCs. Thus the mosquito carries the disease from 1 human to another. Unlike the human host, the mosquito vector does not experience any adverse reactions from the presence of the parasites.[275]

Pathogenesis

All the typical clinical symptoms and severe disease pathological features associated with malaria are caused by the asexual erythrocytic, or blood-stage, parasites. When the parasite develops in the erythrocyte, numerous waste substances such as hemozoin pigment and other toxic factors accumulate in the infected RBC. When the infected cells lyse and release invasive merozoites, these waste products are dumped into the bloodstream. The hemozoin and other toxic factors such as glucose phosphate isomerase stimulate macrophages and other cells to produce cytokines and other soluble factors, which act to produce fever and rigor, and probably influence other severe pathophysiological mechanism associated with malaria.[276,277]

In *P falciparum* infections, consciousness can be impaired by various mechanisms that interact with each other.[278] One of these mechanisms is obstruction of the cerebral microvascular flow by parasite-induced sequestration of the infected and uninfected erythrocytes. Parasite binding is mediated by a group of variant surface antigens expressed at the RBC surface during development. The best-described antigen is *P falciparum* erythrocyte membrane protein 1, which is encoded by a family of approximately 60 variant genes associated with different binding phenotypes.[279-282] Interleukin-6 and -10, nitric oxide, tumor necrosis factor, and various other inflammatory factors may play a role in the pathogenesis of cerebral malaria.[283-285]

Clinical Manifestations

The incubation period in most cases varies from 7 to 30 days, with *P falciparum* on the shorter end of the spectrum and *P malariae* on the longer end.[286] Antimalarial drugs taken for prophylaxis by travelers can delay the appearance of malaria symptoms by weeks or months, especially after infection with *P vivax* and *P ovale,* long after the traveler has left the malaria-endemic area. Because both *P vivax* and *P ovale* might have dormant liver-stage parasites that may reactivate and cause disease months after the infective mosquito bite, returned travelers should always remind their health care providers of any travel in malaria-risk areas during the previous 12 months.[286]

The attacks occur every second day with the tertian parasites (*P falciparum, P vivax,* and *P ovale*) and every third day with the quartan parasite *(P malariae)*; but these classic patterns are rarely observed. More commonly, the patient displays a combination of the following influenza-like symptoms: fever, chills, sweats, headaches, nausea and vomiting, body aches, and general malaise. Anemia and enlarged spleen may be seen at physical examination.[286]

Severe malaria occurs when *P falciparum* infections are complicated by serious organ failure or abnormalities in the patient's blood or metabolism. The manifestations of severe malaria that might be confused with severe bacterial sepsis include cerebral malaria, with abnormal behavior, impairment of consciousness, seizures, coma, or other neurologic abnormalities; severe anemia caused by hemolysis; hemoglobinuria; pulmonary edema; acute respiratory distress syndrome, which may occur even after the parasite counts have decreased in response to treatment; abnormalities in blood coagulation; and thrombocytopenia, cardiovascular collapse, and shock.[287]

Cerebral malaria is a clinical syndrome characterized by coma at least 1 hour after termination of a seizure or correction of hypoglycemia, detection of asexual forms of *P falciparum* malaria parasites on peripheral blood smears, and exclusion of other causes of encephalopathy.[287] The main neurologic features are coma, seizures, and brainstem signs. The mortality rate in adults and children is approximately 20%, and most deaths happen within 24 hours of admission, before antimalarial drugs may have had time to work.[288] In African children, neurologic deficits have been reported.[289] Some deficits are transient (eg, ataxia), whereas others (eg, hemiparesis) improve over months but may not resolve completely.

Congenital malaria may occur in babies born to infected mothers. Symptoms include fever, severe anemia, and hepatosplenomegaly.[290,291]

Diagnosis

Prompt and accurate diagnosis of malaria is part of effective disease management. The most commonly used diagnostic tools are microscopic diagnosis and rapid diagnostic tests that are based on immunochromatographic techniques. Microscopic examination remains the gold standard for laboratory confirmation of malaria. Thick smears are more sensitive, but they cannot be used to differentiate between the different species of malaria.[292] Diagnosis of malaria can be difficult in nonendemic areas. Health care providers may not be familiar with the disease, and laboratory workers may fail to detect parasites when examining blood smears under the microscope because they have never seen them before.[293] In endemic areas, finding malaria parasites in blood might represent solely a carrier state because these individuals developed enough immunity to protect them from the illness but not from the infection. In such individuals, finding the parasites in their blood should not stop the clinician from looking for other diagnoses.

Quantitative buffy coat technique is useful for screening populations for malaria and for detecting asymptomatic carriers to control further transmission of the disease in the community. However, the diagnosis has to be confirmed by peripheral smears.[294]

Serologic testing, either the IFA test or ELISA, does not detect current infection but rather measures past experience; thus it may be useful for epidemiologic surveys.[295]

Other new tests—including detection of the parasite nucleic acid by PCR, DNA probe, and rapid diagnostic tests that use different methods, such as immunochromatography—are available but are not approved by the FDA.[296-300]

Treatment

CHEMOTHERAPY. Malaria must be recognized promptly to treat the patient in time, to prevent cerebral malaria, and to prevent further spread of infection in the community. Malaria is a nationally notifiable disease, and all cases should be reported to the state health department, which forwards them to the CDC. Three main factors should be considered when treating malaria: (1) the infecting *Plasmodium* species, (2) the clinical status of the patient, and (3) the drug susceptibility of the infecting parasites, as determined by the geographic area where the infection was acquired. For treatment of *P vivax* and *P ovale,* because these 2 species continue to release new crops of merozoites from the liver cells, antimalarial drug that target the liver stage (eg, primaquine) should be added to prevent recurrence. Patients should be checked for glucose-6-phosphate dehydrogenase deficiency before they are provided primaquine. In general, if the diagnosis of malaria is suspected and cannot be confirmed, or if the diagnosis of malaria is confirmed but species determination is not possible, then antimalarial treatment effective against *P falciparum* must be initiated immediately. Detailed information about the treatment of malaria is available (www.cdc.gov/malaria/diagnosis_treatment). The standard drug treatment for uncomplicated (not severe) malaria is summarized in Table 305-1. The treatment of severe malaria should be parenteral administration of quinidine gluconate, with

Table 305-1 Chemotherapy of Uncomplicated Malaria

ROUTE	DRUG	DOSAGE
ALL *PLASMODIUM* SPECIES EXCEPT CHLOROQUINE-RESISTANT SPECIES		
Oral drug of choice	Chloroquine phosphate	10-mg base/kg (max 600-mg base), then 5-mg base/kg 6 hr later, then 5-mg base/kg at 24 and 48 hr
Parenteral drug of choice	Quinidine gluconate	10-mg/kg loading dose (max 600 mg) in normal saline over 1-2 hr, followed by continuous infusion of 0.02 mg/kg/min until oral therapy can be started
OR		
	Quinine dihydrochloride for *P falciparum* acquired in areas of chloroquine-resistance	20-mg/kg loading dose in 5% dextrose over 4 hr, followed by 10 mg/kg over 2-4 hr every 8 hr (max 1800 mg/day) until oral therapy can be started
Oral drug of choice	Atovaquone-proguanil	• <5 kg: not indicated • 5-8 kg: 2 pediatric tablet once a day × 3 days • 9-10 kg: 3 pediatric tablet once a day × 3 days • 11-20 kg: 1 adult tablet once a day × 3 days • 21-30 kg: 2 adult tablet once a day × 3 days • 31-40 kg: 3 adult tablet once a day × 3 days • >40 kg: 4 adult tablet once a day × 3 days
OR		
	Quinine sulfate	30 mg/kg/day in 3 doses × 3-7 days
PLUS		
	Doxycycline	4 mg/kg/day in 2 doses × 7 days
OR		
	Quinine sulfate	30 mg/kg/day in 3 doses × 3-7 days
PLUS		
Alternatives	Clindamycin	20 mg/kg/day in 3 doses × 7 days
	Mefloquine	15 mg/kg followed 12 hr later by 10 mg/kg
OR		
	Artesunate	4 mg/kg/day × 3 days
PLUS		
	Mefloquine prevention of relapses: *P vivax* and *P ovale* only	15 mg/kg followed 12 hr later by 10 mg/kg
	Primaquine phosphate	0.6-mg base/kg × 14 days

Modified in part from Pickering LK, Baker CJ, Long SS, et al, eds. *Red Book: 2006 Report of the Committee on Infectious Diseases.* 27th ed. Elk Grove Village, IL: American Academy of Pediatrics; 2006.

continuous infusion provided until the patient can take oral medication and the parasite density is less than 1%. Therapy should be combined with doxycycline, tetracycline, or clindamycin. A patient with severe malaria or cerebral malaria who is being treated should be monitored closely in an intensive care unit setting; side effects of the medications, such as hypoglycemia, should also be monitored. The CDC should be consulted regarding the treatment of such severe cases.[301,302]

In China and Southeast Asia, artemisinin derivatives such as artemether and artesunate are replacing quinine. These agents can be administered orally or rectally. However, some concerns about possible neurotoxicity and a high rate of recurrence have been raised; thus the drug should be used when malaria resistance to the quinine is suspected. It should be administered for a minimum of 3 days and followed up with mefloquine to assure a cure rate of greater than 90%.[303-307]

Finally, a self-treatment course of atovaquone-proguanil can be provided to travelers who do not receive antimalarial drugs for prophylaxis, who are on a less-than-effective regimen, or who may be in remote areas, when they develop fever. Travelers should be advised that self-treatment is not considered a replacement for seeking prompt medical help.[293]

SUPPORTIVE TREATMENT. Various supportive measures should be taken to optimize the management of patients. These measures include closely monitoring the fluid and electrolytes status of the patient, treating the convulsions with phenobarbital or diazepam, and being vigilant about hypoglycemia, a common complication of severe malaria. Anemia should be corrected with packed RBC transfusions. The CDC recommends that exchange transfusion be considered for persons with a parasite density of more than 10% or severe complications. Gram-negative sepsis must be suspected whenever patients experience shock. Appropriate antibiotic therapy should be initiated after blood cultures are obtained. No added benefits have been shown from providing corticosteroids, dextran, heparin, or osmotic diuretics.[301,302,308,309]

Prevention

Prevention of malaria is achieved by preventing infection, by reducing the population of the *Anopheles* mosquitoes, by avoiding bites by parasite-carrying mosquitoes (vector control), or by providing antimalarial drugs prophylactically.

Travelers from nonendemic countries should take precautions against acquiring malaria when they visit a malaria risk area. These precautions include chemoprophylaxis in addition to following measures to prevent contact with mosquitoes. Detailed guidelines about the chemoprophylaxis of malaria for travelers to endemic areas are available (www.cdc.gov/travel/). Table 305-2 summarizes the chemoprophylaxis for travelers. Chemoprophylaxis should begin 1 week

Table 305-2 Chemoprophylaxis for Malaria*

AREA	DRUG	DOSE
Areas with chloroquine-sensitive *Plasmodium* species	Chloroquine phosphate	5-mg base/kg once a week, up to adult dose of 300-mg base
Areas with chloroquine-resistant *Plasmodium* species	Atovaquone-proguanil	5-10 kg: 1-8 tablets once a week 11-20 kg: 1 pediatric tablet/day 21-30 kg: 2 pediatric tablet/day 31-40 kg: 3 pediatric table/day >40 kg: 1 adult tablet/day
OR	Mefloquine	11-20 kg: ¼ tablet once a week 21-30 kg: ½ tablet once a week 31-45 kg: ¾ tablet once a week 45 kg: 1 tablet once a week
OR	Doxycycline	2 mg/kg/day, up to 100 mg/day
ALTERNATIVES	Primaquine	0.6-mg base/kg daily
OR	Chloroquine phosphate	5-mg base/kg once/week, up to 300-mg base
PLUS	Proguanil	2-6 yr: 100 mg once a day 7-10 yr: 150 mg once a day >10 yr: 200 mg once a day

*Chemoprophylaxis should begin 1 week before arrival in the area with endemic infection (except doxycycline and atovaquone-proguanil, which should be started 1-2 days before arrival). These medications should be continued for 1 week when receiving atovaquone-proguanil and 4 weeks when receiving the other medications after the departure from the endemic area.

Modified in part from Pickering LK, Baker CJ, Long SS, et al, eds. *Red Book: 2006 Report of the Committee on Infectious Diseases.* 27th ed. Elk Grove Village, IL: American Academy of Pediatrics; 2006.

before arrival in the area with endemic infection (except doxycycline and atovaquone-proguanil, which should be started 1 to 2 days before arrival), which will allow time for the traveler to develop blood concentrations of the drug and which will permit evaluation for adverse reactions. These medications should be continued after departure from the endemic areas. In endemic areas, chemoprophylaxis is used for selected high-risk groups, such as pregnant women and young children.[310]

Vector control aims to decrease contacts between humans and vectors of human disease. Vector control for the prevention of malaria includes insecticide-treated bed nets, indoor residual spraying, and source reduction (larval control).[311] Dichlorodiphenyltrichloroethane (DDT) meets most of the World Health Organization criteria for indoor insecticide.[311] However, resistance to DDT and dieldrin and concern over their environmental impact led to the introduction of other, more-expensive insecticides, such as pyrethroids.[312] Pyrethroids are safer to apply than most other insecticides. Resistance to them is presently limited, and they are easier to store and transport.[311] Source reduction (larval control) is the method of choice for mosquito control when the breeding sites of the mosquito species are easy to find and treat.[311]

Insecticide-treated bed nets are an important method for controlling malaria. However, to maintain their efficacy, the bed nets must be retreated at intervals of 6 to 12 months, or more frequently if the nets are washed. Screening the house to prevent entry of mosquitoes and using other repellents such as meta-N,N-diethyltoluamide (DEET) are other effective methods to prevent contact with mosquitoes.[311]

Developing vaccines against malaria is difficult because of the inaccessibility of the malarial parasites to immune attack by replicating inside RBCs, the generally poor immune response to key antigens compared with the level required for effective immunity, and the high levels of polymorphisms in antigens that are targets of protective responses.[313] Vaccines are currently in development; some are in phase-3 trials.[314]

Babesiosis

Babesiosis is a malaria-like illness that is mostly caused by a tick bite. It is a zoonotic disease; the main animal reservoirs are rodents and cattle. More than 100 species of *Babesia* have been discovered, with different animal reservoirs. However, human disease is mostly caused by the bovine species (*Babesia bovis* and *Babesia divergens*), particularly in Europe, and by the rodent (*Babesia microti*) species, particularly in the United States. New emerging species have been identified.[315-317]

Epidemiologic Features

The disease is caused by the bite of the *Ixodes* tick, the same that transmits Lyme disease and human granulocytic anaplasmosis.[318,319] The tick has 3 stages (larva, nymph, adult) and requires a blood meal to mature between stages. The dead end of babesiosis is humans, who get the infection by bite at the nymph stage.[319] Rare cases of babesiosis have resulted from blood transfusion.[320] The possibility of perinatal and transplacental transmission has also been considered.[321]

Two major geographic areas of *Babesia* transmission have been identified, with distinct forms of disease in Europe and the United States. In Europe, the disease is mostly due to bovine species, particularly *B divergens*. Patients affected with this species are mostly those who have undergone splenectomy. The disease is transmitted by the tick *Ixodes ricinus*. The disease is typically severe, with a high mortality rate.[322] European cases have been reported from Yugoslavia, France, Germany, Spain, Sweden, Ireland, Great Britain, and the former Soviet Union.[323]

However, in the United States, most cases are caused by *B microti*. The white-footed mouse (*Peromyscus leucopus*) is the reservoir of infection.[324] The vector of transmission is the tick *Ixodes scapularis*.[319] Most cases occur in the northeastern part of the country. This area includes islands and coastal areas near Massachusetts, New York, New Jersey, and Rhode Island, as well as areas in Connecticut.[325] Cases from other states have also been reported. Most tick bites go unnoticed, and only 10% to 20% of patients recall a tick bite. Most cases occur between May and August, the time of nymph abundance and peak outdoor activity.[326] The tick should attach for at least 24 hours to transmit infection. Most infected patients in the United States are immunocompetent, and most infections are asymptomatic. The incubation period is 1 week to several months.[327,328]

Babesiosis cases have also been reported in other parts of the world, including Taiwan, Canary Islands, Egypt, South Africa, Mexico, and China.[322,329]

Risk factors for severe disease and mortality caused by babesiosis include age older than 40 years, asplenia, HIV infection, and immunosuppressive therapy, including corticosteroids. The disease is particularly overwhelming in patients without spleens.[326,330]

Pathogenesis and Life Cycle

The life cycle of *Babesia* is somewhat similar to malaria. The parasite multiplies in the vector sexually and in the infected mammal or human asexually.[331] During transmission, humans acquire sporozoites from the salivary gland of the *Ixodes* vector. The sporozoites invade the RBCs and differentiate into trophozoites, which replicate asexually by budding, and then release merozoites. This event will lead to lysis of RBCs and hemolytic anemia.[330] Released merozoites subsequently attack other RBCs, and the cycle continues. Autoimmune mechanisms may also be implicated in hemolysis, as evidenced by positive Coombs test in some patients with babesiosis.[332]

In addition to hemolysis, intraerythrocytic multiplication leads to vascular stasis that results from increased adherence to endothelial cells, which results in ischemic damage in different organs, including the liver, spleen, heart, and brain.[333] Hemolysis and vascular injury may also cause renal insufficiency. Increase proinflammatory cytokine release has also been demonstrated in patients.[334] All of these factors may contribute to the pulmonary edema- and sepsis-like picture that may eventually develop.[330]

The spleen plays an essential role in limiting babesiosis by removing deformed erythrocytes, which explains the high levels of parasitemia and severe disease that occurs in patients without spleens. Both cell-mediated and humoral immunity are demonstrated during infection. However, the cell-mediated immune responses via CD4 cells and interferon-γ are known to play a critical role in controlling babesiosis.[335]

Clinical Manifestations

Most babesiosis cases are subclinical or mild.[336] In symptomatic patients, the clinical manifestations range from nonspecific symptoms to severe hemolysis. The typical symptoms are characterized by a influenza-like illness, with gradual onset of malaise fatigue and anorexia, followed by episodes of fever associated with chills, sweats, myalgia, headache, and vomiting.[336] Less commonly, conjunctival injection, meningismus, altered sensorium, and nonproductive cough may be present.[337] The nonspecific symptoms may cause delay in diagnosis. Symptoms may last for several weeks or sometimes months. Patients who are coinfected with *Borrelia burgdorferi,* the agent of Lyme disease, or *Anaplasma phagocytophila,* the agent of human granulocytic anaplasmosis, tend to develop more prolonged symptoms.[338] HIV-infected patients have also been reported to have a prolonged clinical course.[339]

Immunodeficient patients and those without spleens develop severe infection characterized by hemolytic anemia, jaundice, and dark urine.[326,340] Severe babesiosis may also occur in posttransfusion cases.[340,341] Many signs and symptoms are similar to those of malaria. Lactate dehydrogenase levels will be high. The hemolysis in babesiosis is milder than that of malaria.[337] As a result of hemolysis, renal insufficiency, anuria, and azotemia may develop. Other possible complications of babesiosis in this group of patients include hypotension, shock, disseminated intravascular coagulation, heart failure, and acute respiratory distress syndrome.[330]

Diagnosis

The diagnosis of babesiosis is made by demonstrating the organism in blood smears. Similar to malaria diagnosis, thick and thin smears should be prepared for Wright and Giemsa staining.[342] *Babesia* species may sometimes be difficult to differentiate from *Plasmodium* species. However, differentiating features of *Babesia* species include the presence of a cluster of 4 small merozoites, called the tetrads, in RBCs.[342] Because the RBCs tend to be infected repeatedly, multiple parasites may be present in a single cell. The occasional presence of 3 chromatin dots in a single parasite is another differentiating feature. In addition, in *Babesia* smears, no pigment is seen. Schizonts and gametocytes are also absent.[342]

Serologic testing should be considered when blood smears are nondiagnostic, such as in cases with low parasitemia. The most sensitive test is the IFA test, which is available in reference laboratories.[338,343] PCR has also become available for diagnosis of babesiosis. The test is more sensitive than blood smear. It may also be used for monitoring therapy and for epidemiologic surveillance.[344]

Treatment

The regimens for treatment of symptomatic infection are clindamycin plus oral quinine or atovaquone plus azithromycin.[345] Fulminant cases with severe hemolysis and high-grade parasitemia (>10%) should be considered for exchange transfusion.[340,341]

Prevention

Suggestions for prevention of tick-borne infections should be followed.[345] Tick-infested areas, particularly May to September, should be avoided if possible. Wearing clothing that covers the arms, legs, and other exposed areas and tucking pants into socks or boots should be considered. Tick and insect repellants that contain DEET may be considered, but repeat applications may be needed. Tick-toxic agents such as permethrin may be sprayed on clothes and shoes but not the skin. In addition, people should inspect themselves and the bodies of their children, as well as all clothing, for ticks after possible exposure. Exposed hairy areas, including the scalp and behind the ears, should be thoroughly inspected. If a tick is found, it should then be grasped with a tweezers close to the skin and gently pulled out straight. Pets should also be inspected for ticks daily.

NEMATODE INFECTIONS

Trichinellosis *(Trichinella spiralis)*

Trichinellosis is caused by the roundworm of the genus *Trichinella.* Six species can infect humans and animals, but the most common is *Trichinella spiralis.*[346] In contrast to other parasitic infections, trichinellosis (or trichinosis) is more common in Europe and America than in Asia and Africa.[347]

Epidemiologic Features

Trichinella can infect different carnivorous animals, particularly scavengers. Humans acquire infection by eating raw, inadequately cooked meat containing *Trichinella* cysts. Domestic pigs are the most common source of infection in America and Europe. The incidence of trichinellosis has been declining steadily in the United States.[348] This decline is believed to be the result of new laws governing production and processing of pork meat, including food provided to swine, routine slaughterhouse surveillance, and improved public awareness.[348] Undercooked wild game, especially bear, seal, and walrus meat, has emerged in recent years as the most common cause of trichinellosis.[349] *Trichinella nativa* is the subspecies associated most frequently with arctic sources.[350] Consumption of horse meat has also been associated with trichinellosis.[351] The incubation period is 1 to 2 weeks.

Pathogenesis and Life Cycle

After humans eat infected meat, the larvae are liberated from the cysts in the intestine and mature into adults in epithelial cells.[352] The male adult dies after mating. The fertilized female adult produces embryos at a rate of 1 every 30 minutes during her life span of 4 to 16 weeks. The larvae then enter the bloodstream via the intestinal lymphatics and disseminate to different organs.[353] *Trichinella* larvae survive only in the skeletal muscles and become encysted in 2 to 3 weeks.[354] The most frequently affected muscles are those of the limbs and the diaphragm, followed by the tongue, intercostals, extrinsic muscles of the eye, and laryngeal and paravertebral muscles.[355]

Clinical Manifestations

Most infections are asymptomatic. The severity of infection correlates with the number of ingested larvae.[356] Infection occurs in 2 stages. The first is the intestinal stage, which begins 24 hours after infection and lasts for 1 to 7 days. During this phase, patients may be asymptomatic or may experience gastrointestinal symptoms such as nausea, vomiting, diarrhea, constipation, and abdominal pain.[350] The muscle stage starts after the first week and correlates with dissemination of larvae from the intestine to the bloodstream. The typical symptoms consist of the triad of myalgia, eyelid edema, and eosinophilia. This phase may last 1 to 5 weeks or longer. The myalgias may be prominent and may mimic rheumatic pain. Muscle pain, tenderness, swelling, and weakness can occur.[354,357] The larvae may remain viable in muscles for years. Calcification may occur after several months and may be detected on radiography.[355] The edema often involves the face, eyelids, and conjunctiva. Other common associated findings are high and prolonged fever, which is rarely seen in parasitic infections, weakness, and malaise. Other less-frequent findings include headache, subconjunctival hemorrhages, retinal hemorrhages, splinter hemorrhages under fingernails, facial flushing, urticarial or macular rashes, hoarseness, dyspnea, and dysphagia.[354,355] The clinical manifestations of trichinellosis are caused by either larval invasion or host immune response to the parasite.

The most common cause of death in cases of severe trichinellosis is myocarditis with subsequent heart failure and cardiac arrhythmias.[358] Cardiac involvement usually occurs in the second to third week of infection. Severe trichinellosis may also be associated with encephalitis, meningitis, focal neurologic deficits, bronchopneumonia, and nephritis.[354,359,360]

Diagnosis

The diagnosis of trichinellosis should be suspected in patients with suggestive clinical history, including consumption of inadequately cooked meat, particularly pork, and eosinophilia. The presence of clinical symptoms in other patients who shared the same food makes the diagnosis stronger. Eosinophilia usually appears during the second week of the muscle phase and may be as high as 70%. Muscle enzymes such as creatine kinase and lactate dehydrogenase may be high, as will immunoglobulin levels.[357]

Serologic tests are usually used to make the diagnosis of trichinellosis. Different assays are used, including ELISA, IFA test, and latex agglutination. ELISA is the most sensitive.[361] Serologic tests are only helpful after the second week of infection, when antibody titers start to rise. Testing of paired acute and convalescent serum samples is diagnostic. Antibody levels may remain positive for more than 1 year after clinical improvement.[357]

The most definitive diagnostic test is finding larvae in muscle biopsy samples. However, this event only occurs after the first week after ingestion. The number of larvae per gram of muscle may be used as a guide of severity of infection.[362] When tested, specimens should be fresh and compressed between 2 microscope slides or should be digested by artificial gastric juice to increase yield. Suspected infected meat sources may also be tested for larvae.[357] PCR testing to detect *Trichinella*-specific DNA in muscle biopsy specimens has been used.[363] The test is sensitive and specific, but it is not readily available.

Treatment

Mebendazole and albendazole treat trichinellosis with comparable efficacy.[364] Both drugs are ineffective for larvae already in the muscles.[365] Coadministration of corticosteroids such as prednisone is indicated in severe cases, especially with cardiac and CNS involvement.[354,357] People who have recently eaten *Trichinella*-contaminated meat should be treated with mebendazole or albendazole.[364]

Prevention

Control can be achieved by thorough cooking of pork and game meat. Freezing is also effective in killing larvae in meat.[355] The encysted larvae of *Trichinella* are killed by heating at a temperature of 77°C or freezing at −15°C for 3 weeks, which is available in home freezers. Freezing pork meat at −23°C for 10 days is also effective, although *Trichinella* species in arctic areas may be resistant and may remain viable.[366] Transmission to pigs can be decreased by not feeding them garbage and by effective control of rats.

Trichuriasis *(Trichuris trichiura)*

Trichuriasis is caused by *Trichuris trichiura*. The adult worm is 30 to 50 mm in length. It is commonly called the whipworm because it has a whiplike anterior portion and a handle-like posterior portion.[367]

Epidemiologic Features

Trichuriasis is one the most common intestinal helminthic infections worldwide, but it is most frequently found in tropical and subtropical areas and in areas of poor sanitation.[368] Most cases are seen in Asian countries.[369] Infection is common in warm, humid areas. In the United States, trichuriasis is most common in Latin immigrant children in rural areas of the southeastern states.[370] Eggs must remain in soil for 3 to 4 weeks to become infectious.[371] Children are more likely to be infected than adults. No person-to-person transmission has been noted.

Humans acquire infection by ingesting eggs. The larvae are released in the intestine and develop into adult worms over 2 to 3 weeks. Adult worms live in the intestine with the thin end embedded in the mucosa and the thick end visible in the intestinal lumen. The life span of adult worms is 1 to 5 years.[372] The worms are found in the cecum and ascending colon in cases with light infection. However, they may also be found in the rectum and distal colon in cases with heavy infection. Eggs may not be shed in the stools until 3 months after infection.[373]

Clinical Manifestations

Patients who develop mild infection are usually asymptomatic, and this is true for most children.[367]

Trichuriasis is often present with other helminthic and protozoal infections. This combination results in an overlap of clinical features of these infections. However, in contrast to other helminthic infections, diarrhea is a common manifestation of trichuriasis. Heavy infestation is associated with a dysentery syndrome characterized by mucoid bloody stools associated with abdominal pain and tenesmus, which is referred to as trichuris dysentery syndrome.[367] Colitis results from chronic infection, and symptoms may mimic inflammatory bowel disease.[367] Rectal prolapse is a characteristic finding of trichuriasis and mainly seen in heavily infected patients.[372] Colonic obstruction and perforation may occur.[374] Finger clubbing is also seen in heavily infected children who have chronic diarrhea and may be a helpful clue for diagnosis.[374,375] Clubbing can be reversed after treatment of trichuriasis. Chronic infection in children may also be associated with malnutrition, growth retardation, and cognitive abnormalities.[376,377]

Diagnosis

Trichuriasis is diagnosed by detecting the typical ova on direct stool examination. The egg has a typical barrel shape, 3-layer eggshell, and transparent bipolar plugs.[373] In addition, the presence of Charcot-Leyden crystals in stools is suggestive of trichuriasis.[371] The eggs can be quantified by the Kato-Katz smear, and the number of eggs per gram of stools can be used to assess worm burden.

Treatment

The drug of choice for treatment of trichuriasis is mebendazole. Alternative treatments are albendazole or ivermectin.[378] Nitazoxanide has been shown to be effective against trichuriasis, but it is not yet FDA approved for this indication.[379]

Prevention

A single dose of either mebendazole or albendazole has been used in mass treatment programs to reduce worm burden and transmission in some developing countries.[380] The targets of these programs are preschool- and school-aged children. However, reinfection is common. Proper disposal of human fecal material may be the most effective control measure.[378]

Strongyloidiasis

Strongyloidiasis is caused by the nematode (roundworm) *Strongyloides stercoralis*. The disease may range from asymptomatic eosinophilia in healthy people to life-threatening disseminated infection with septic shock in immunocompromised patients.[170,381] Strongyloidiasis is less frequently caused by *Strongyloides fulleborni*, which causes infantile protein-losing enteropathy with high mortality rates.[382]

Epidemiologic Features and Life Cycle

Strongyloidiasis is widely distributed all over the world but is particularly common in the tropical and subtropical regions. In the United States the infection is most common in the southeastern states.[383] The disease is also found in immigrants from endemic areas.[384] Unlike other helminthic infections, the disease is most frequent among white men.[385] *S fulleborni* is endemic in Papua New Guinea and parts of sub-Saharan Africa.[382]

Humans are the principal host. However, animals such as cats and dogs can be reservoirs. Humans acquire infection by skin contact with infective (filariform) larvae that are present in the soil or other material contaminated with human feces. The larvae reach the lungs via the venous circulation. From the tracheobronchial tree, the larvae are coughed and swallowed; thus they enter the gastrointestinal tract.[371] In contrast to other helminths, *S stercoralis* can complete its life cycle in its host; therefore autoinfection can also occur in humans.[386] During autoinfection, immature (rhabditiform) larvae mature into filariform larvae in the gastrointestinal tract and then penetrate the perianal skin or the mucosa of the colon to complete the life cycle. This process may be accelerated by constipation or by other medical conditions associated with decreased bowel motility. The larvae mature into adult worms in the gut and can burrow in the mucosa of the duodenum and jejunum. Worms live for up to 5 years. Rhabditiform larvae appear in the stools approximately 1 month after infection. When they reach the soil, these larvae either mature into infective filariform larvae or into free-living adult forms that produce larvae. Because of autoinfection in humans, patients may remain infected for decades. In patients with immunodeficiency, autoinfection may lead to hyperinfection and disseminated disease.[387,388]

Clinical Manifestations

Most infected patients are asymptomatic; peripheral eosinophilia may be the only clue for diagnosis.[384] The presentation correlates with the stage of infection: cutaneous, pulmonary, or gastrointestinal. Cutaneous reactions may develop when larvae penetrate the skin, especially on the feet. These reactions include edema, rashes, and severe pruritus. Migration of the larvae under the skin may cause a distinctive eruption called larva currens.[389] The pulmonary migration of larvae may cause dry cough, wheezing, tachypnea, and hemoptysis. Pneumonitis or a Loeffler-like syndrome (acute transient pneumonitis) may be seen.[390] Adult worms in the gastrointestinal tract may cause abdominal pain, vomiting, and diarrhea. Malabsorption and failure to thrive may be seen in children with high worm burden.[391] Larvae that migrate to the perianal skin may cause pruritic lesions, including larva currens in the perianal area, the buttocks, and the upper thighs. Infants with *S fulleborni* infection may develop swollen belly syndrome, which is characterized by marked abdominal distension, ascites, and pleural effusions. Mortality rates are high in affected infants.[382]

Hyperinfection occurs in patients who are immunocompromised, including those with the human T-lymphotropic virus type 1 infection.[392] Corticosteroids use appears to be major risk factor for dissemination of *S stercoralis*.[387] During hyperinfection, filariform larvae penetrate the intestinal mucosa to the bloodstream. This event is followed by massive dissemination of filariform larvae to different organs including the lungs, liver, heart, and the CNS.[388,393] In hyperinfection, translocation of bowel flora by filariform larvae can cause gram-negative bacteremia and sepsis, which is seen in one third of affected patients.[388] Eosinophilia is often absent when major complications such as sepsis occur, as well as in patients who are receiving corticosteroids.[387,388]

Diagnosis

The diagnosis is made by detecting rhabditiform larvae in stool specimens. The detection rate is low because of the low parasitic burden and the periodic excretion of larvae. Examining multiple specimens and using stool concentration procedures may increase the yield.[394]

In highly suspected cases and when the stool samples are not diagnostic, examination of duodenal fluid for larvae should be considered. Duodenal fluid can be obtained by the string test (Entero-Test) or by endoscope.[395]

Serologic testing is available at reference laboratories, including the CDC. The test is highly sensitive and specific. However, false-negative results occur in immunocompromised patients.[396] Treatment may cause negative serologic results after 6 to 12 months.[397]

In disseminated infection, rhabditiform larvae may be recovered from stools, sputum, or bronchoalveolar lavage, as well as from pleural, peritoneal, or spinal fluid.[398,399]

Treatment

The drug of choice is ivermectin.[400] Thiabendazole and albendazole are alternative treatments.[400] In the past, thiabendazole was the preferred medication. However, lower cure rates have been reported with the use of either thiabendazole or albendazole compared with ivermectin.[401] In immunocompromised patients with hyperinfection or disseminated disease, prolonged or repeat courses of treatment (or both) may be needed.[402]

Prevention

Proper disposal of human fecal material is essential. Screening patients with immunodeficiency, especially those receiving corticosteroids or with human T-lymphotropic virus type 1 infection, should be considered if the patient has a history of living in or traveling to endemic areas. Screening of immigrants or returned travelers from endemic areas should also be considered before initiating immunosuppressive therapy.

Hookworm Infections (*Ancylostoma duodenale* and *Necator americanus*)

Hookworm infections are widely prevalent in tropical and subtropical regions. Factors that favor spread of hookworm in these regions include warm climate, abundance of rain, soil contaminated with human feces, and people walking barefooted.[403] The 2 most common hookworms are *Ancylostoma duodenale* and *Necator americanus.*

Epidemiologic Features

The prevalence of hookworm species varies in different geographic areas. *A duodenale* is prevalent in the Mediterranean countries, India, Pakistan, Iran, and the Far East. *N americanus* is prevalent in North and South America, Central Africa, Indonesia, and islands of the South Pacific.[404] Humans are the only reservoir of infection. Hookworm eggs excreted in stool hatch in soil within 1 to 2 days, forming larvae that mature within approximately 1 week into infective larvae. These larvae may persist for weeks or even months in soil if appropriate temperature (23°C-33°C) and conditions such as moisture are found.[405]

Humans acquire infection after percutaneous penetration of larvae. However, *A duodenale* may also be acquired by the oral route or by human milk. As few as 3 larvae are enough to cause infection.[406] From the skin, larvae reach the lungs and then the tracheobronchial tree. Then the larvae are coughed and swallowed, and they reach the small intestine and develop into adult worms.[403] Eggs appear in the stools 1 to 3 months after infection.[404]

Clinical Manifestations

Persistent eosinophilia is a common finding.[407] The symptoms and signs correlate with the stage of infection. The earliest findings result from larval penetration of the skin. Itching, focal eruptions with or without edema, or enlargement of adjacent lymph nodes is referred to as ground itch.[403] Pulmonary migration is associated with mild respiratory symptoms such as cough. However, in severe cases, Loeffler syndrome may develop.[403]

In the intestinal phase, patients may complain of abdominal pain, nausea, vomiting, increased flatulence, diarrhea, and constipation.[408] However, the main symptoms of hookworm infection are related to iron-deficiency anemia and loss of plasma protein.[409-411] A single worm of *A duodenale* sucks 0.01 to 0.04 mL of blood per day, whereas *N americanus* sucks 0.05 to 0.3 mL of blood per day. Greater blood losses occur around the worm-attachment site.[404] Malnutrition, blood loss, and iron-deficiency anemia are the most significant complications of heavy infection in normal hosts. The severity of anemia and malnutrition is higher in children infected with *A duodenale* than those infected with *N americanus.*[411] Antihelminthic therapy causes improvement in nutritional status and hemoglobin levels in these patients.[412]

Diagnosis

Hookworm infection is diagnosed by identifying eggs in stools. The eggs of *A duodenale* and *N americanus* are morphologically indistinguishable.[403] However, species identification can be accomplished by PCR.[413] Adult worms are rarely seen. Larvae are rarely seen in stool samples when stools are left at room temperature for 24 hours or in constipated patients. Stool smears are often negative in early stages of infection because of delayed egg excretion.[404] Stool concentration techniques may be needed in patients with light infection. Repeat stool examinations may also be needed.

Treatment

Malnutrition and anemia may need correction, including iron supplementation. Albendazole, mebendazole, and pyrantel pamoate are the drugs of choice for treating hookworms in children and adults.[414] Repeat stool examination should be performed 2 weeks after treatment; if positive, then additional treatment should be considered.[414]

Prevention

Proper disposal of human feces is essential. Patients at risk, including children from endemic areas, should be screened and appropriately treated. Education of the population regarding footwear may reduce transmission of hookworm infection.[415]

Cutaneous Larva Migrans *(Ancylostoma braziliense)*

Cutaneous larva migrans is caused by the infective larvae of the cat and dog hookworms *Ancylostoma braziliense* and *Ancylostoma caninum*.[416]

Epidemiologic Features

Infection occurs among individuals with direct skin contact to infective larvae. Contact with soil contaminated with canine or feline feces is the main risk factor.[417] Commonly affected people are children, travelers, swimmers, and gardeners.[418] Most cases occur in tropical and subtropical areas of Africa, Southeast Asia, the Caribbean, and Central and South America.[22,419,420] In the United States, most cases occur in the southeastern parts of the country.[421]

Clinical Manifestations

The larva produces an erythematous pruritic papule at site of skin entry. Lesions most commonly involve the lower extremities.[422] The number of lesions correlates with the number of penetrating larvae. Days or sometimes weeks later, and as the larva migrates, a dermal skin rash develops along the larval tract (creeping eruption). It characteristically appears as a pruritic, elevated serpiginous tract that elongates several millimeters a day.[423] The skin lesion may become vesiculated and secondarily infected by bacteria. On rare occasions, when the parasite load is high, pulmonary symptoms may develop as a result of larval migration in the lungs. The most common symptom is dry cough. A Loeffler-like syndrome characterized by peripheral eosinophilia and migratory lung infiltrates may also develop.[424]

Diagnosis

Most cases of cutaneous larva migrans are diagnosed clinically, and no further diagnostic evaluation is needed. Peripheral eosinophilia may be present in some cases.[425] In cases with pulmonary involvement, eosinophils and sometimes larvae can be demonstrated.[426] If biopsy is performed, then eosinophils will be demonstrated in tissue samples, but the parasite can rarely be seen.[421]

Treatment

The disease is usually self-limited, but specific treatment may be needed.[422] Therapy with topical thiabendazole should be provided if available, or albendazole or ivermectin should be administered.[421]

Pinworm *(Enterobius vermicularis)*

Pinworm infections are distributed worldwide. The disease is caused by the nematode (roundworm) *Enterobius vermicularis*. Humans are the only hosts.[389]

Epidemiologic Features

Unlike other parasitic diseases, pinworm infection is most common in developed countries.[427] Infections are more prevalent in temperate and cold climate regions than in the tropics. Enterobiasis is the most common parasitic disease in the United States and Europe.[372,428] Infections occur among people of all socioeconomic levels but are more common in closed crowded conditions.

The eggs of *E vermicularis* are highly infectious. This infectious nature is due to the ability of eggs to survive in cool and humid environments for long periods. Humans acquire infection by ingesting eggs from the same host (autoinfection) or from another person. Infection occurs by direct anus-mouth contact, by eating contaminated food, or from contaminated hands and fomites. Contaminated clothing, linen, toilet seats, and baths contribute to spread among families and close contacts.[389]

Eggs hatch in the intestine into larvae, and adult worms develop over several weeks. No egg shedding occurs inside the intestinal lumen. Instead, female adult worms travel at night from the gastrointestinal tract and migrate through the rectum to lay eggs onto the perianal skin. Female pinworms usually die after egg deposition.[429]

Clinical Manifestations

Most infections are asymptomatic. However, the most common symptom is perianal itching (pruritus ani), which occurs mainly at night.[428] Itching is due to local irritation by adult worms and laid eggs. Bacterial superinfection may develop.[430] Autoinfection is facilitated by trapping of eggs under the fingernails of the child. Less frequently, pinworms may also cause pruritus vulvae as a result of aberrant migration to the female genital tract.[431] Other rare manifestations of apparent worm migrations include salpingitis, urethritis, vaginitis, and pelvic peritonitis.[432]

Patients with heavy worm burden may develop gastrointestinal symptoms such as abdominal pain, nausea, and vomiting. Pinworms have been found in the lumens of inflamed appendices after surgical removal.[433] However, a causal relationship between appendicitis and pinworm has not been found.[434]

Diagnosis

Stool examination for ova and parasites is not helpful in establishing the diagnosis. The test of choice is the use of cellophane tape swab.[389] A higher diagnostic yield is achieved if the specimen is taken at night or early morning. The adhesive part of the tape is applied to the skin and then onto a glass slide and examined by light microscopy. Alternatively, commercially available sterile pinworm collector kits that are based on the same principle may be used. Examination of multiple samples may be needed.

Treatment and Prevention

Mebendazole, pyrantel pamoate, or albendazole are the drugs of choice for enterobiasis.[435] Reinfection rates are high, and subsequent treatment may be needed. Preventive measures should be discussed at the onset of treatment, especially in patients with recurrent infection. Hand hygiene is essential. Morning bathing is suggested for all infected persons. Autoinfection may be decreased by avoiding scratching the perianal area, washing the hands before eating, and keeping the fingernails short. Frequently changing and washing of underwear, bed linen, and clothing may decrease the egg burden and transmission. Shaking of bed linen should be avoided. Treating all family contacts should be considered with repeated symptomatic infections.[389,435]

Ascariasis (*Ascaris lumbricoides*)

Ascariasis is the most prevalent helminthic infection worldwide. Estimates suggest that more than 1.4 billion people are infected with ascariasis. It is most common in the tropics and areas with poor sanitation practices, such as using human feces for fertilization.[436] In the United States, ascariasis is the third-most common helminthic infection after hookworm and *T trichiura* infection. It is caused by *Ascaris lumbricoides,* the largest roundworm that infects humans.[371]

Epidemiologic Features

The female adult worm measures 22 to 35 cm in length and 3 to 6 mm in diameter and resides in the lumen of the jejunum and ileum. Female adults produce 200,000 eggs per day, which are excreted in stools. Fertilized eggs become infective in soil 3 to 4 weeks after they are excreted.[437] Human infection occurs by ingesting eggs from contaminated soil. Larvae hatch in the intestine, penetrate the intestinal wall, and migrate to the right side of the heart, lungs, and bronchial tree. From there the larvae ascend to the pharynx and are subsequently swallowed to mature into adult worms in the small intestine.[371] Female worms begin laying eggs 2 to 3 months after exposure. The life span of the parasite is 6 months to 1 year.

Clinical Manifestations

Most infections are asymptomatic. However, the burden of the disease is high because of the widespread prevalence. Symptoms are caused by either the larval migration or the presence of the adult worm in the small intestine. Clinical features and complications are caused by direct tissue damage, the immune response of the host, obstruction, and malnutrition.[438,439]

During larval migration, Loeffler syndrome tends to occur 1 to 2 weeks after ingestion of the eggs. This syndrome is often associated with fever, marked eosinophilia, and other symptoms related to hypersensitivity such as urticaria.[440,441] Nonspecific gastrointestinal symptoms occur in patients with ascariasis, such as abdominal discomfort, nausea, vomiting, and diarrhea. Moderate to heavy infections in children may be associated with malnutrition and malabsorption of proteins, lactose, and vitamins.[441] Heavy infection may also lead to acute intestinal obstruction caused by a mass of worms in the bowel lumen. The obstruction most frequently occurs at the ileocecal valve. Most affected patient are young children 1 to 5 years of age.[442] Other intestinal complications in endemic areas may occur, such as ileocecal intussuscept, which is the primary cause of death in ascariasis.[438]

Worm migration into the biliary tree can cause biliary colic, cholecystitis, and ascending cholangitis.[443] Biliary strictures and hepatic abscesses are other, less-frequent complications.[444,445] Pancreatitis may also result from migration of the adult worm into the pancreatic duct.[443] Worm migration to the appendix may lead to appendicitis.[446] Migration may occur through body orifices such as the mouth, nose, anus, and lacrimal duct.[447] Worm migration is stimulated by stress factors such as fever, intercurrent illness, diarrhea, spicy foods, and anesthesia. Some anthelmintic may also stimulate worm migration.[448]

Diagnosis

Diagnosis of ascariasis is made by demonstrating characteristic eggs in stools by direct microscopy. Eggs may not appear in the stools until after at least 40 days of infection. Usually a single stool sample is sufficient to confirm the diagnosis.[371] Adult worms are sometimes passed in the stool and provide a clue to the diagnosis. Peripheral eosinophilia occurs during the pulmonary phase of infection.[449] In addition, eosinophils and occasionally *Ascaris* larvae may be demonstrated in sputum samples. Imaging studies may demonstrate worms in cases of intestinal obstruction, as well as in cases of hepatobiliary or pancreatic ascariasis.[450,451] Serologic testing is not helpful in diagnosis but can be used in epidemiologic studies.[452] Serum IgG antibodies are not protective.[453]

Treatment

The treatment for symptomatic and asymptomatic infections is albendazole, mebendazole, or ivermectin.[454] Experience with these drugs is limited in children younger than 2 years. Limited data suggest that these drugs are safe. However, the risk and benefits of treating ascariasis should be considered in this age group.[454] Pyrantel pamoate and nitazoxanide are also effective in treating ascariasis.[379,455]

Cases with suspected intestinal or biliary obstruction should be treated with piperazine solution (75 mg/kg/day, maximum 3 g/day), which may be provided by a nasogastric tube. Piperazine paralyzes the worm and prevents migration during passage through the intestine. If piperazine is not available, as in the United States, then conservative management to alleviate obstruction followed by albendazole, mebendazole, or ivermectin may be considered.[456] Pyrantel pamoate and piperazine are antagonistic and should not be provided together.

Surgery should be performed if medical therapy is not successful in relieving obstruction or if complications exist, such as volvulus peritonitis or perforation. During laparotomy for obstructive cases, the small bowel should be milked down to the cecum, avoiding incision of the bowel wall.[457] Endoscopic retrograde cholangiopancreatography is used to extract worms in hepatobiliary cases.[443]

Prevention

Prevention of reinfection is a challenging problem because of the abundance of ascaris eggs in soil.[458] Sanitary disposal of human feces is essential to prevent soil contamination, particularly near children's play areas. In some areas, educational programs aimed at stopping the use of human feces as a fertilizer may be needed. In such areas, people should also be educated about proper food washing and cooking.[459]

Mass deworming programs with a single dose of mebendazole or albendazole have been used in some communities endemic for ascariasis. Schoolchildren are the target in most programs. These programs are used every 3 to 4 months and are aimed at treating and preventing morbidity in children, as well as decreasing the worm burden in the community.[460] In highly endemic areas where more than 50% of the population is infected, the whole population may be targeted for mass treatment.[439]

Toxocariasis

Toxocariasis, or visceral larva migrans, is caused by migration of *Toxocara* larvae in the viscera of the host. This syndrome is caused by the dog ascarid, *Toxocara canis,* and less frequently by the cat ascarid, *Toxocara cati.*[461] Other nematodes such as *Baylisascaris procyonis,* the common raccoon roundworm, rarely cause toxocariasis.[462] The life cycle of *T canis* and *T cati* in their respective animal species is similar to that of *A lumbricoides* in humans. Humans are considered unusual hosts for *T canis* and *T cati.* Thus, infection with these parasites causes failure to complete the life cycle or aberrant migration of larvae. Because the parasite fails to mature in humans, it remains alive in the body for months to years.[461]

Epidemiologic Features

Humans acquire infection by ingesting soil contaminated with infective eggs of the parasites.[463] The disease is endemic in areas where dogs are present.[464] Most reported cases of toxocariasis occur in the United States.[465] Many pets, especially puppies, are infected and routinely contaminate yards, school playgrounds, and sandboxes. Most affected patients are children 1 to 4 years of age. History of pica is common.[466] The eggs are not immediately infective after shedding by dogs. However, after approximately 3 weeks in soil, they can cause infection to humans. Hot, humid regions are associated with persistence of eggs in soil and increased risk of infection.[461] The disease may be found anywhere dogs are present. The highest rates of transmission are in the southern United States, particularly in rural areas. However, infection can also be acquired in urban areas. Estimates suggest that 20% of dogs and 98% of puppies are infected.[465]

Pathogenesis and Life Cycle

The reservoir of *T canis* infection is the female dog.[467] The disease is reactivated during pregnancy and then transmitted to the puppies via placenta or breast milk.[461] The puppies shed eggs in the surrounding environment. When humans ingest eggs, the larvae hatch in the intestine and spread via the portal circulation to the liver and then to the systemic circulation. Because the parasite cannot mature, it passes through different organs and tissues before it overwhelms the immune system. The most commonly involved organ in the liver.[468] However, the lungs, heart, kidneys, eye, skeletal muscles, and brain may also be involved.[469-474] During tissue migration, granulomas are formed, and significant host immune response occurs, demonstrated by peripheral eosinophilia and high IgE levels.[461] The manifestations and severity of infection depend on the immune status of the host, the burden of infection, and the site of involvement.

Clinical Manifestations

Most patients who are lightly infected are asymptomatic.[475] Incidental findings or eosinophilia and hepatomegaly in these patients may prompt a search for the diagnosis of toxocariasis. Symptomatic children with toxocariasis usually experience fever, leukocytosis with eosinophilia, hypergammaglobulinemia, and hepatomegaly. Splenomegaly and lymphadenopathy are other associated findings. Patients may also have allergic manifestations such as urticaria, rhinorrhea, and asthma.[476] Pulmonary infiltrates may be evident on radiographs. Constitutional symptoms such as anorexia, weakness, failure to gain weight, myalgia, arthralgia, and nighttime sweats may also be present. Neurologic symptoms include irritability and seizures, but these symptoms are less frequent.[477] Other reported findings include myocarditis, congestive heart failure, pleural effusion, eosinophilic ascitics, and meningoencephalitis.[475,478]

Ocular involvement usually affects patients older than 4 years, and when it occurs, usually no other systemic involvement occurs, which suggests that the ocular and visceral forms of toxocariasis are 2 distinct entities. This form of disease, which is seen in older children with no history of pica, is called ocular larva migrans (OLM).[479] Patients often have unilateral solitary posterior retinal lesion. A granulomatous mass or multiple lesions may be seen. Lesions are painless; some are asymptomatic and are found incidentally during routine retinal examination.[480] Common symptoms include strabismus, visual impairment, unilateral loss of vision, and lukocoria.[481] Complications of OLM include chronic endophthalmitis, retinal detachment, keratitis, uveitis, iritis, vitreous abscess, optic neuritis, and retinal tracks with larvae.[482] Some cases in the past were misdiagnosed and managed as intraocular tumors such as retinoblastoma.[483] Patients with OLM typically have other organ-systemic involvement.

Diagnosis

A definitive diagnosis of toxocariasis requires demonstration of the larvae in tissue sections, but this is rarely needed. In most cases, the diagnosis is based on clinical findings and serologic testing.[475] In systemic toxocariasis, eosinophilia is a consistent finding. The total white blood cell count may be as high as 30,000/mm,[3] with up to 80% eosinophils.[484] Other consistent and nonspecific laboratory findings include hypergammaglobulinemia with high IgE levels—sometimes 10 to 15 times the normal levels—as well as increased isohemagglutinins to the A and B blood groups.[461] During the pulmonary phase of involvement, eosinophils may be detected in respiratory secretions.[485] With CNS involvement, CSF may also show eosinophils.

Serologic testing is used to confirm the diagnosis of toxocariasis. ELISA is the most frequently used test, with high sensitivity and specificity. Western blot and immunofluorescence tests have also been used. In OLM, serologic tests are often negative.[486]

Treatment

Infections in most patients are self-limited and require no specific treatment. Treatment is suggested for symptomatic patients and those with systemic forms of the disease. The drugs for treatment in children are albendazole and mebendazole.[487] Corticosteroids are indicated for patients with severe cardiac and CNS involvement.[488,489] Ocular involvement is treated with anthelmintic therapy, surgery, corticosteroids, or a combination of these modalities.[490,491] Diethylcarbazine is another alternative.[492]

Prevention

Underlying causes of pica in children should be corrected. Cat and dog feces should be properly disposed. Sandboxes that are not in use should be covered. Antihelmintic therapy for puppies and kittens at 2, 4, 6, and 8 weeks may prevent secretion of eggs in feces and subsequent potential transmission to toxocariasis.[487]

Lymphatic Filariasis

The disease is caused by the 3 species of filarial nematodes: *Wuchereria bancrofti, Brugia malayi,* and *Brugia timori*. The most common nematode is *W bancrofti,* which accounts for 90% of lymphatic filariasis cases.[493]

Epidemiologic Features and Life Cycle

Lymphatic filariasis is most prevalent in hot humid climates. *W bancrofti* is endemic in tropical regions of Asia, Africa, and the Americas, as well as the Pacific regions. *B malayi* is found in India, China, Indonesia, Malaysia, Korea, Vietnam, and the Philippines. *B timori* is found only in parts of Indonesia.[494,495] Most cases worldwide occur in sub-Saharan Africa, China, India, and Indonesia. Most affected patients are 15 to 44 years of age. Humans are the only definitive host.

Humans acquire infection by bites of mosquito of the genera *Anopheles, Culex,* and *Aedes*.[496] The infective larvae travel to the lymphatic vessels, where they mature into adult worms. The worms are threadlike and measure 40 to 100 mm in length; they may live for years.[497] After fertilization, the female adult worm releases microfilariae in the bloodstream. Microfilaremia is characterized by nocturnal periodicity. The greatest numbers of microfilariae in peripheral blood appear between 10 PM and 2 AM.[497] When a mosquito vector bites an infected person for a blood meal, the microfilariae are ingested and undergo maturation into infective larvae, and the cycle continues. The incubation period from the mosquito bite to the onset of filaremia is usually 2 to 12 months, depending on the parasite; the longest period is seen with *W bancrofti*.[497]

Clinical Manifestations

Most infected patients are asymptomatic, including those with microfilaremia.[498] Subclinical lymphatic dysfunction or dilatation is common. Symptoms are usually elicited by the inflammatory response to the microfilariae or ova in the lymph nodes.[499] The most common acute symptoms in the early stages are lymphangitis and lymphadenitis. Fever, headache, myalgia, and pain in the affected extremities are common. The male genital area is commonly involved, leading to acute epididymitis, orchitis, and funiculitis. Microfilaremia and eosinophilia occur commonly in this stage.

During the chronic stage, obstruction of the lymphatic system occurs, leading to elephantiasis (lymphedema). Recurrent superimposed bacterial infections contribute to progression to this stage.[500] The skin over the affected extremity becomes thick and warty. Hydrocele and chyluria result from obstructed lymph drainage in the genital area and urinary bladder, respectively. Other complications of lymphatic obstruction include chylothorax and chylous ascitis.[501,502]

Tropical eosinophilia or tropical pulmonary eosinophilia develops in a small proportion of patients. This entity is characterized by eosinophilia, high IgE titers, high titers of microfilarial antibodies, and nocturnal paroxysmal respiratory symptoms such as cough and wheezing. Affected patients develop pulmonary infiltrates. Response to diethylcarbamazine (DEC) is favorable.[503]

Diagnosis

The diagnosis of lymphatic filariasis is made by demonstrating microfilaria on peripheral blood smears obtained between 10 PM and 2 AM.[504] If blood cannot be obtained at night, then a dose of DEC can be provided to stimulate filaria release, followed by a blood draw an hour later. If microfilariae cannot be demonstrated on blood smears, then fine-needle aspirate or biopsy of the involved lymph node or epididymis may demonstrate adult worms or microfilariae.[505,506] However, lymph node biopsies may worsen the obstructive manifestations of filariasis and should not be routinely done.

Serologic tests are helpful in diagnosis during the chronic stage, when microfilariae are no longer detectable. The enzyme immunoassays may cross-react with other helminthic infections. However, antifilarial IgG4 antibody detection has been found to be a good index of the intensity and duration of filarial exposure in endemic areas.[507] Filarial antigen can be detected by monoclonal antibodies; filaremic patients are more likely to have positive results than those who are not.[508] The diagnosis of chronic filariasis (lymphedema) is made on clinical grounds in most cases. DNA probes and PCR assays have been developed.[509] However, these tests are not routinely available.

Treatment

The drug of choice for treatment of lymphatic filariasis is DEC. It kills adult worms of the 3 filarial species.[510] Systemic and local reactions have been reported with DEC. Systemic side effects include headache, anorexia, nausea, and vomiting. Lymphadenitis and transient lymphedema have been reported during treatment. Patients with heavy infections may develop systemic reactions that result from the rapid killing of parasites; therefore some experts suggest initiating low-dose treatment at first.[511] A single oral dose of ivermectin has been shown to be effective in treating microfilaremia.[512] However, recurrence of filaremia has been reported. Combination therapy of single doses of DEC and ivermectin may be more effective than single doses alone.[513]

Surgical and cosmetic therapy may be needed in some patients with chronic filariasis.[514] Decongestive physiotherapy may be helpful in some cases of lymphedema.[514] Bacterial superinfections are most commonly caused by *Staphylococcus* and group A *Streptococcus* and should be treated appropriately.

Control

Mosquito control and chemotherapy are the main control measures used in areas endemic with lymphatic filariasis. Annual campaigns that use a combination of either DEC and albendazole or albendazole and ivermectin have been used in community infection-control programs.[515,516]

Onchocerciasis *(Onchocerca volvulus)*

Onchocerciasis is caused by the filarial nematode, *Onchocerca volvulus.*

The disease is transmitted by various species of the blackfly of the genus *Simulium.* The blackfly is distributed along high-flow, turbulent waters, including rivers, and thus the disease is distributed along these areas, giving it the name *river blindness.*[517]

Epidemiologic Features and Life Cycle

Blackflies serve as the insect vector.[518] They are not bloodsuckers but tissue breeders. When a blackfly bites, it sucks microfilariae from human skin and subcutaneous tissue. *O volvulus* is a strict human parasite. No animal reservoirs have been found. Infective larvae develop inside the blackfly and are released in the skin when a human host is bitten. Adult worms develop from larvae inside the skin, subcutaneous tissue, or fascia over approximately 1 year. They may live for 14 years.[519] Both male and female adult worms live curled up in nodules under the skin and subcutaneous tissue. The female worms produce microfilariae in the skin. The migration of microfilariae is responsible for skin lesions. The microfilariae are subsequently picked by the blackfly after biting an infected host. If not ingested by a blackfly, then the microfilaria die after 2 years.[518]

Onchocerciasis is endemic mainly in tropical Africa. However, other areas are endemic, including Central and South America. Most recent foci of infection have been reported in the Arabian Peninsula, mainly in Yemen.[520,521]

Clinical Manifestations

The clinical features are related to the presence of microfilariae or adult worms in skin, lymph vessels, and eyes. These features include dermatitis, subcutaneous nodules, lymphadenitis, and ocular lesions.[522,523] Dermatitis is intensely pruritic and may develop into an erythematous papular rash. Subcutaneous nodules are the result of the presence of adult worms under the skin. In Africa, they are present in the lower part of the body; in Central and South America, they occur in the upper part of the body. The skin nodules vary from few millimeters to several centimeters and can be discrete or clustered. They tend to occur over bony prominences.[518,524] Secondary bacterial infection of these nodules may cause acute inflammation or abscess formation. Lymphedema, regional lymphadenopathy, skin papules, and depigmentation of the skin occur in chronic infections.[524-526] Hydroceles and elephantiasis have also been reported. Adenolymphoceles may develop in the groin and femoral area, leading to hanging groins.[527]

Ocular involvement occurs as a result of the presence of microfilariae. Lesions may develop in any part of the eye. The most common and typical lesion is punctuate keratitis.[528] Other lesions such as sclerosing keratitis, iridocyclitis, chorioretinitis, and optic neuritis may also occur.[528] If untreated, patients with these lesions may develop blindness.

Diagnosis

The diagnosis of onchocerciasis is made by identifying microfilariae in direct histologic examination of skin snips or biopsy samples or by a lymph node biopsy sample.[529] Surgical excision of a skin nodule can be diagnostic and therapeutic. Adult worms are found in these nodules. Microfilariae are not usually present in peripheral blood smears. Ocular lesions are diagnosed by slit-lamp examination, which may reveal microfilariae in the cornea or anterior chamber of the eye.[530] When the diagnosis of onchocerciasis is suspected but the parasites cannot be demonstrated, DEC can cause worsening of the skin lesions after few hours; this situation is known as the Mazzotti reaction.[531] Peripheral eosinophilia is common among patients with onchocerciasis.

Treatment

The drug of choice for treating onchocerciasis is ivermectin. Treatment does not kill adult worms; thus therapy is considered noncurative.[532] However, ivermectin is a microfilaricidal agent that improves dermatitis and prevents ocular lesions.[533] Surgical excision of the lesions (nodulectomy), particularly on the head, can reduce the microfilarial load and decrease the risk of ocular complications. DEC is no longer the drug of choice because of the high incidence of severe Mazzotti reactions.

Wolbachia endosymbiotic bacteria have emerged as a target for treatment. Doxycycline leads to long-term sterilization of female filaria and may be used as an adjunct treatment.[534,535] Doxycycline should not be provided to children younger than 8 years.

Control

Individuals should be educated on how to prevent blackfly bites in endemic areas. The blackfly bites during the day. Insect repellants and protective clothing are suggested. Mass community campaigns that provide ivermectin to endemic areas have been effective in preventing severe morbidity from onchocerciasis.[536]

TREMATODE INFECTIONS

Schistosomiasis

Schistosomiasis or bilharziasis was first described in 1851. The disease is caused by the trematode *Schistosoma.* It affects more than 200 million people in at least 74 countries and continues to spread to new geographic areas.[537,538] Five species cause the disease in different countries. Human disease is caused by *Schistosoma mansoni, Schistosoma japonicum,* and *Schistosoma haematobium* and to a lesser extent by *Schistosoma mekongi* and *Schistosoma intercalatum.*[537]

Epidemiologic Features

Humans are the principal host of infection. Each species of *Schistosoma* has a specific geographic distribution. For example, *S haematobium, S mansoni,* and *S intercalatum* are endemic in sub-Saharan Africa. *S mansoni* remains also endemic in parts of Brazil, Venezuela, the Caribbean, and the Arabian Peninsula. *S haematobium* also occurs in the Eastern Mediterranean. *S japonicum* infections occur in China, Indonesia, and the Philippines. Infections with *S mekongi* occur in Cambodia and Laos along the Mekong River Basin.[537]

Most human cases involve school-aged children, women, and persons involved in water-related occupations such as irrigation, fishing, and farming. Infected humans remain communicable as long as they secrete eggs in stools or urine. Because children have the habit of uncontrolled defecation and urination, they are considered a major reservoir of infection in endemic areas. Travelers may acquire infection. Most cases are among those traveling to Africa, particularly in those who swim in Lake Malawi and the Zambezi River.[539] The average life span of the schistosome is 5 years. Adult worms may live for decades; therefore immigrants from endemic areas may remain infected for 30 to 40 years.[540]

Pathogenesis and Life Cycle

The life cycle of *Schistosoma* requires the presence of an intermediate host, the snail. Different schistosome species have different snail hosts.[541,542] Infected humans excrete eggs in the stools (*S mansoni* and *S japonicum*) or in the urine *(S haematobium).* In water the eggs hatch into miracidia that infect the snails. After undergoing asexual multiplication in snails, cercariae are released and penetrate the skin of humans who are exposed in fresh water.[543] After skin penetration, cercariae lose their tails and become schistosomulae. From the skin, the schistosomulae travel via the blood vessels and lymphatics to the right side of the heart and pulmonary circulation and from there to the arterial circulation. They are then carried to the mesenteric arteries, splanchnic arteries, and finally the portal circulation, where they mature to adult forms. The mature worms migrate to their final habitat in the mesenteric vein (*S mansoni* and *S japonicum*) or the vesical veins *(S haematobium).*[544]

The female worms will start laying their eggs 1 to 3 months after infection. The eggs are either transported hematogenously to other organs or traverse the circulation through adjacent tissue to the lumen of the intestine or the urinary bladder.[545]

The penetration of skin by cercariae induces a delayed-type hypersensitivity reaction leading to dermatitis.[545] Acute schistosomiasis, which is characterized by fever and systemic symptoms, is caused by an immune complex–mediated reaction related to early infection and oviposistion.[546] Otherwise, most of the clinical manifestations of schistosomiasis are caused by the host response to the eggs by formation of granulomas and by infiltration of cells around the eggs.[547] Granulomas are gradually replaced by fibrosis and subsequent scar formation. In the final stages the eggs are destroyed and calcified. This chronic inflammatory process of granuloma formation and fibrosis causes the clinical manifestations in different organs. For example, in the intestine the process leads to ulceration and fibrosis of the intestinal wall. In the liver, it leads to hepatosplenomegaly and portal hypertension. In the urinary bladder, it may lead to dysuria, hematuria, and obstructive uropathy.[547-549]

Clinical Manifestations

A maculopapular eruption may develop at site of cercarial penetration of the skin. This reaction occurs a few hours after infection, but it may develop up to 1 week later. It is similar but less severe than swimmer's itch, a reaction that occurs in sensitized individuals who are exposed to nonhuman schistosomes. Swimmer's itch may be caused by various mammalian and avian schistosomes. No systemic complications develop after swimmer's itch because the cycle is not completed in humans.[550]

Acute schistosomiasis or Katayama fever is an immune complex–mediated reaction caused by egg deposition in tissues. All affected patients have eosinophilia. The illness occurs 4 to 8 weeks after exposure and is characterized by fever, headache, and generalized myalgia. Less commonly, tender hepatomegaly and bloody diarrhea may occur. Splenomegaly develops in 30% of patients. Respiratory symptoms such as cough, headache, and aseptic meningitis are other associated findings.[546,551]

The clinical manifestations of chronic schistosomiasis depend on the schistosome species, the organs involved, and the intensity of the fibroobstructive disease. *S mansoni* and *S japonicum* mostly involve the intestine and the liver. *S haematobium* involves the genitourinary tract. The inflammatory process assists in the migration of the eggs to the lumen of the intestine and the urinary bladder. Involvement of the gut wall leads to inflammation, hyperplasia, ulcers, microabscesses, and polyposis.[547] Symptoms may include colicky pain, diarrhea, and, occasionally, constipation. Blood, either gross or occult, may appear in stools. Chronic inflammation may lead to colonic or rectal stenosis. Chronic intestinal polyposis may lead to protein-losing enteropathy.[552,553]

Liver involvement occurs as a result of egg embolization from the portal circulation to the liver with subsequent inflammatory changes. Most cases are due to *S mansoni* and *S japonicum.*[554] In early stages of involvement, patients may develop hepatomegaly, indicating granulomatous inflammation.[549] In late stages, pathological findings include presinusoidal inflammation and periportal fibrosis, which occur in 4% to 8% of affected patients. These changes may take years to develop and indicate a heavy infection.[554] In schistosomiasis, liver synthetic function is preserved until late in the course of illness. The liver architecture is also retained. However, deposition of periportal collagen will lead to obstruction of blood flow and portal hypertension, which eventually may lead to esophageal varices, bleeding, and splenomegaly.[538]

Genitourinary involvement is most commonly caused by *S haematobium*. Microscopic hematuria is the most common finding in early stages of involvement. Affected children frequently develop moderate to severe lesions in the urinary tract. These lesions include obstructive lesions that may eventually lead to chronic renal failure.[548] Bladder carcinoma is a serious late complication of urinary schistosomiais.[555]

Schistosome eggs may occasionally embolize to other organs with subsequent granuloma formation. These organs include the skin, lungs, brain, adrenal glands, and skeletal muscles.[538]

Neurologic complications have also been reported during the course of schistosomiasis. The most common neurologic complication is transverse myelitis, which occurs with either *S mansoni* or *S japonicum* infection.[538] Seizures, either focal or generalized, have been reported in patients infected with *S japonicum*. Focal neurologic deficits may rarely occur.[556] These complications occur either because of aberrant migration of the worms or egg embolization to the CNS.[556,557]

Diagnosis

Nonspecific laboratory tests may demonstrate peripheral eosinophilia, anemia, hypoalbuminemia, and hypergammaglobulinemia.[538] The diagnosis of schistosomiasis is made by demonstrating eggs in stool or urine samples. Because of the intermittent shedding of eggs, 3 specimens may be needed.[558] Egg excretion peaks at noon to 3 PM. Morphologic features of the eggs help in differentiating different schistosome species. The eggs of *S mansoni* are characterized by a lateral spine, whereas the *S haematobium* egg has a prominent terminal spine. *S japonicum* eggs are round with obscured lateral spine.[559]

If the diagnosis of schistosomiasis is suspected and the stool or urine smears are negative, then a rectal or bladder biopsy may be needed. Analysis of tissue biopsy samples is considered the most sensitive way to test for schistosomiasis.[539,560]

Serologic tests are available at reference laboratories. These tests are only helpful in patients with either light infection or early infection (Katayama fever), when eggs are not present in the stools.[561] The tests remain positive for years and may persist after parasitologic cure.[562] Serologic testing is therefore not useful in differentiating old infection from reinfection.

Treatment

The drug of choice is praziquantel.[563] The drug causes tetanic contractions in the adult worm, causing its detachment and death. However, because praziquantel does not kill developing worms, patients provided treatment in the first 4 to 8 weeks of exposure should be retreated in 1 or 2 months. Reexamination of the stool or urine 1 month after treatment should be performed to assess efficacy of treatment.[538] If patients continue to shed eggs, then they should be treated again. A single dose of praziquantel has been used in community-based control programs in endemic areas.[564,565]

Alternative treatments include oxamniquine for *S mansoni* and metrifonate for *S haematobium*. These medications may play a role in the emerging resistance to praziquantel.[566,567]

Prevention

Sanitary disposal of human waste and education of the population in endemic areas are essential control measures. Large-scale population-based chemotherapy programs that use praziquantel have been administered.[563]

Travelers should be advised to avoid contact with fresh water in lakes or streams. Providing environmental control measures directed against snail habitats and delivering molluscicide are difficult and costly to sustain in endemic areas.[542,568]

Artemether, an antimalarial agent, has been suggested for use as a prophylactic agent for schistosomiasis.[569] This agent kills schistosomula (the migrating larvae) in the first 21 days in the body. When administered every 2 weeks, artemether kills all immature schistosomes. The use of artemether for schistosomiasis prophylaxis should be avoided in malaria-endemic areas because of the risk of emergence of resistance.

CESTODE INFECTIONS

Taeniasis and Cysticercosis (*Taenia solium* and *Taenia saginata*)

Epidemiologic Features

Two *Taenia* species have been found for which humans are the only definitive host, *Taenia solium* and *Taenia saginata*. Taeniasis is caused by the adult worm of both species, whereas cysticercosis is caused by the larval stage of only *T solium* (not *T saginata*). Both species have worldwide distribution, with a higher prevalence in areas with the customary culinary habit of eating undercooked beef or pork. *T saginata* is found most commonly in some new independent states of the former Soviet Union, the Near East, and Central and Eastern Africa. It is less commonly found in Europe, Southeast Asia, and South America.[570] *T solium* is prevalent in Mexico, Central and South America, Africa, and Southeast Asia; it is rare in Muslim countries.[570] In the United States, human infections are usually found in immigrants from areas with high disease prevalence or travelers to endemic areas who consume undercooked meats.[570] Although most cases of human cysticercosis in the United States have been imported, cysticercosis can be acquired in the United States from patients or immigrants from endemic area who have adult-stage *T solium* infection in the intestine.[571]

Life Cycle

Taeniasis is a human infection caused by the adult stage of *T solium* or *T saginata*. People are infected by eating undercooked beef (for *T saginata*) or pork (for *T solium*) that contains cysticerci in the muscle. Inside the human intestine, proctoscopics are released from the cysticerci and attach to the intestinal wall with suckers and hooks. The proctoscopics become the head of the tapeworm, which later develop by forming proglottids and maturing into adult tapeworms over 2 months. This maturation occurs inside the human small intestine, where the tapeworms can survive for years. As the adult tapeworm develops, mature proglottids are produced and later become gravid. The gravid proglottids that contain egg-filled uterus detach from the tapeworm, migrate to the anus, and are passed in the stool. The eggs inside the gravid proglottids are released in the stool after the proglottids are passed with the feces. In the environment, eggs can survive for days or months. The intermediate host, cattle for *T saginata* and pigs for *T solium*, becomes infected after ingesting vegetation contaminated by eggs or gravid proglottids. The oncospheres hatch inside the animal intestine, invade the intestinal wall, and later migrate through hematogenous or lymphatic system to the straight muscles. The oncospheres develop into cysticerci in the animal muscle. The cycle is completed when a human ingests undercooked meats that contained cysticerci in the muscle. The cysticerci can survive in the muscle of the animal for years.[572]

Cysticercosis in humans is an infection that occurs when the person becomes infected with the larval stage of *T solium*. Infection occurs after embryonated eggs are ingested, which can be either from eating food contaminated with human feces or by autoinfection. In the case of autoinfection, the human will become infected after ingesting eggs produced by that tapeworm by oral-fecal contamination or possibly from proglottids that are carried backward into the stomach by the reverse peristalsis. Inside the human intestine, the oncosphere hatch, penetrate intestinal wall, and migrate via circulation or lymphatic channels to various tissue sites.[573] Cysticerci may develop in any organ, most commonly in the brain, subcutaneous tissue, eye, and liver, resulting in cysticercosis.[571,573]

Clinical Manifestations

Taeniasis is often asymptomatic.[571] Patients may experience minimal gastrointestinal tract symptoms such as nausea, diarrhea, and abdominal pain or discomfort. The main symptom is usually the intermittent passage of the proglottids, either with the stool or spontaneously.[572] The proglottids may enter the appendix, common bile duct, or pancreatic duct and cause obstruction. A large amount of worms can also cause intestinal obstruction.[570]

Cysticercosis can affect humans at any age.[570] Most of the infections occur during the third or fourth decades of life; only approximately 10% of cases occur in children.[570] Cysts can be found anywhere in the body but are most commonly found in the CNS.[571] Clinical manifestations usually depend on the location, stage, and number of cysts, as well as the host immune reaction. Symptoms frequently become evident when an inflammatory response develops around a degenerating cyst after a variable period.

Cysticercosis in children occurs differently than in adults.[570] The most serious manifestation of cysticercosis is neurocysticercosis or cysticercosis of the CNS. In infants the initial clinical manifestation of neurocysticercosis is generalized seizures.[574] In most cases, cysts resolve spontaneously, but in approximately one third of cases, cysts may remain as granulomas that later become calcified.[570] Children with calcified granulomas in the CNS have a high risk of developing chronic seizures. In adolescents and young adults, neurocysticercosis may remain clinically silent through out the multiple stages of infection until they become calcified granulomas, which eventually serve as foci that cause epilepsy, frequently after 25 years of age.[575]

Neurocysticercosis in adults occurs differently than in children and is generally asymptomatic. Patients frequently have cysts in more than 1 location. Cysts can be in various stages, and some patients may have both active and inactive cysts at the same time.[576] Symptoms, if present, are mainly the result of mass effect, inflammatory response, or obstruction of the ventricular system of the brain.[577] The most common form of neurocysticercosis in adults is the active parenchymal cyst. Patients may experience severe headache and focal or generalized seizures. Physical examination usually reveals nothing abnormal; the patient will not have neurologic deficits or symptoms. Calcified parenchymal cysts are found less commonly and are usually asymptomatic. However, clinical symptoms such as focal neurologic deficit and seizure may develop as perilesional edema occurs. The other, less-common forms of neurocysticercosis are subarachnoid cysts, ventricular cysts, and spinal cysticercosis. Patients with subarachnoid cyst may experience visual field defect or cranial nerve palsies as a result of cranial nerve entrapment from meningeal inflammation and irritation. Hydrocephalus or signs and symptoms of increased intracranial pressure are the common manifestations in patients with ventricular cysticercosis. Spinal cysticercosis is rare, found in only approximately 1% to 3% of all neurocysticercosis cases.[578] Symptoms depend on the location of the cyst and may not be distinguishable from other spinal cord lesions.

Cysticercal encephalitis is characterized by encephalitis and generalized brain edema that occurs as a result of a severe immune response of the human host to massive amount of cysts in the brain parenchyma. Symptoms include fever, headache, vomiting, impaired consciousness, reduced visual acuity, and seizures. This reaction may develop spontaneously or after medication treatment that leads to degeneration of large numbers of cysts at the same time. Cysticercal encephalitis occurs most commonly in children and young girls.[579]

Extraneural cysticercosis typically involves the eyes, muscles, and subcutaneous tissue. Ocular cysticercosis is found in approximately 1% to 3% of all cases.[580] Generally, patients are asymptomatic, but symptoms may become apparent as the cyst degenerates with surrounding inflammatory reaction. In patients with neurocysticercosis, ocular cysticercosis should be excluded before treatment begins. Patients with subcutaneous or intramuscular cysticercosis are usually asymptomatic. Some patients may notice small palpable nodules that may become inflamed or may experience muscle pain. Subcutaneous and muscular cysticercosis are found more commonly in patients from Asia and Africa than those in Latin America.[570]

Diagnosis

Diagnosis of taeniasis is made by microscopic identification of eggs or proglottids in the stool. Diagnosis may not be possible during the first 3 months of infection before maturation of the adult worm and production of gravid proglottids.[572] The egg of *T solium* is indistinguishable microscopically from the egg of *T saginata*, as well as the egg of other tapeworm species, especially *Echinococcus*. Species determination can be made by microscopic examination of the gravid proglottids and rarely the scolex, if available.

The definitive diagnosis of cysticercosis is made by demonstrating the cysticercus in the involved tissue. Demonstration of eggs or proglottids in the stool specimen may help support the diagnosis but does not essentially prove the presence of cysticercosis. For neurocysticercosis, CT scan and magnetic resonance imaging (MRI) are the most reliable imaging techniques.[570] MRI has an advantage of better visualization of ocular, ventricular, and subarachnoid cysts. It also clearly demonstrates the degree of edema and inflammation, as well as the viability of the cysticercus. The advantage of CT scan over MRI is a better detection of a granuloma or calcification, which can be missed by an MRI.[581] Several serologic studies have been developed to diagnose cysticercosis. The serologic test of choice for confirming the diagnosis and that has been acknowledged by World Health Organization and the Pan America Health Organization is the CDC immunoblot assay with purified *T solium* antigens.[573] It has 100% specificity and 50% to 97% sensitivity, depending on the number and stage of the cysticerci. The other available serologic study is the EIA technique. Compared with the immunoblot, the EIA test has lower sensitivity and specificity. In addition, the EIA test can also cross-react with other helminthic infections such as echinococcosis and filariasis, thus making the EIA test less preferable than the immunoblot technique.[573] To date, no available serologic test that can distinguish between active and inactive infection are available.[573] Both cysticercosis immunoblot tests and EIA kits are commercially available in the United States.

Treatment

Praziquantel is the drug of choice for the treatment of taeniasis from both *T solium* and *T saginata* and is highly effective in eradicating the adult stage (intestinal stage) of the tapeworm.[571] Niclosamide is an alternative agent, but the drug is not available commercially in the United States.[44]

Treatment of cysticercosis is complicated, especially for ocular and neurocysticercosis. The appropriate management of a patient depends on the location of the cyst, viability of the cyst, the host immune response, and the presence or absence of symptoms. In general, the widely accepted cysticidal agents are albendazole and praziquantel.[571] For neurocysticercosis, treatment is not generally provided to an asymptomatic patient with a nonviable single parenchymal cyst that is evidently destroyed by the host immune response.[570] In children with viable cysticercus with minimal or no surrounding inflammatory response, a cysticidal agent should be provided to prevent further perilesional damage and to reduce the risk of developing chronic seizures.[582] After treatment initiation, patients may develop treatment reaction as a result of the sudden destruction of the cysticerci. This reaction is usually accompanied by an inflammatory reaction in the surrounding tissue. Clinical manifestations include severe headache and vomiting. The treatment reaction can be minimized by administration of corticosteroid (dexamethasone) 2 to 3 days before treatment initiation and during the treatment with cysticidal agent. Praziquantel is an alternative cysticidal agent.[44] In general, albendazole is preferred over praziquantel because of its higher cysticidal activity and lower cost.[570]

An anticonvulsant agent is usually provided to patients with seizures, as well as to patients with multiple cysts but no history of seizure because of their risk of developing seizures after treatment starts. For cysticercal encephalitis, the initial goal of treatment is to reduce inflammation and cerebral edema with a corticosteroid or an immunosuppressive agent. In these patients, treatment with a cysticidal agent should be deferred until clinical signs of encephalitis have subsided and the imaging studies demonstrate improvement of brain edema.[583] A small cyst located in the lateral ventricle can be treated effectively with antihelminthic agent. A ventriculoperitoneal shunt should be placed before treatment begins in patients with hydrocephalus.[570] In a patient with a cyst in the fourth ventricle, a cyst attached to the middle cerebral artery, or a cyst compressing the optic chiasm, surgery should be performed before the cysticidal agent is administered. Patients with subarachnoid cysts or a large cyst in the fissures should be treated for at least 30 days.[584] For intraocular subretinal cyst, treatment with albendazole combined with corticosteroid is effective; an intraocular cyst located in the vitreous chamber should be removed surgically.[585] An ophthalmologic examination should be performed in all cases to rule out intraocular cyst before initiating treatment.[44,571] For patients with symptomatic subcutaneous or muscular lesions, treatment with antiinflammatory medication may be provided. Surgical excision of a solitary subcutaneous or intramuscular cyst may be considered for patients with persistent symptoms. Patients with neurocysticercosis should be monitored with a brain imaging study after completion of treatment.

Hydatid Disease, Human Echinococcosis, Hydatidosis (*Echinococcus granulosus, Echinococcus multilocularis, Echinococcus vogeli,* and *Echinococcus oligarthrus*)

Echinococcal disease is caused by the cestode tapeworm of the genus *Echinococcus*. Infection occurs when humans serve as inadvertent intermediate host for the larval stage (metacestode stage) of the parasite. Four species in the genus *Echinococcus* infect humans. *Echinococcus granulosus* causes cystic echinococcosis, *Echinococcus multilocularis* causes alveolar echinococcosis, and *Echinococcus vogeli* and *Echinococcus oligarthrus* cause polycystic echinococcosis. *E oligarthrus* is an extremely rare cause of human echinococcosis.

Epidemiologic Features

Each cestode in the genus *Echinococcus* has a different geographic distribution and different host affinity.

E granulosus is the most common species infecting humans and is seen practically worldwide.[586] Prevalence of human infection by *E granulosus* varies widely in different areas of the world but is seen predominantly in rural livestock-raising areas. The rural practice of feeding dogs with home-slaughtered animal viscera facilitates disease transmission. Areas with high disease prevalence where cystic echinococcosis is the major public health problem include South and Central America, the Middle East, some sub-Saharan countries, Central Asia, Southern Europe, and the former Soviet Union.[587,588] In the United States, most human infections are seen in immigrants from areas with high disease prevalence; however, sporadic transmission has been recognized in some certain states, including California, Arizona, New Mexico, Utah, and Alaska.[589] *E multilocularis* is seen only in the Northern Hemisphere, particularly in Northern and Central Europe, Russia, Western China, certain areas of North America, and Northern Africa.[590] The precise disease prevalence is not known but is significantly less common than *E granulosus*. *E vogeli* and *E oligarthrus* are seen in Central and South America and have only rarely been associated with human infection.[586]

Life Cycle

The life cycle of the *Echinococcus* cestode requires a definitive host and an intermediate host. Humans are only an incidental intermediate host and do not play any role in the biological life cycle. Each of the 4 *Echinococcus* species has its specific definitive and intermediate hosts that vary among different geographic distributions.[590] The adult worm resides in the small intestine of the definitive host. Eggs are released from the worm's proglottids and are passed with the stool to the external environment. Eggs are ingested by the intermediate host, and under appropriate conditions, they hatch and release oncospheres in the intermediate host's small intestine. The oncosphere penetrates intestinal mucosa and migrates through circulatory or lymphatic system into various visceral organs, mainly lungs and liver. In the visceral organ the oncosphere develops into a fluid-filled cyst, gradually enlarges, and subsequently differentiates into the metacestode or hydatid cyst. Each of the different species of the *Echinococcus* has different pattern of cyst development, daughter cyst formation, and protoscolices (adult form) formation.

The definitive host becomes infected after ingesting a cyst-containing organ from the infected intermediate host. Inside the definitive host's small intestine, protoscolices evaginate and attach to the intestinal mucosa. The worm develops into mature adult stage within 4 to 7 weeks and completes the life cycle. Humans become infected after ingesting the parasite's eggs. Infection is usually from contamination of the environment such as water or cultivated vegetables and direct contact with infected pet dogs through the fecal-oral route. Fecal-oral transmission occurs mostly in children.[589] Because 2 mammalian animals are required to complete the life cycle, direct human-to-human transmission does not occur. The adult worm of *E granulosus* is found mainly in the dog or another canid and occasionally cats. Intermediate hosts include sheep, horse, camel, and goat. Different strain of *E granulosus* require different intermediate hosts, with the sheep strain being the most prevalent and pathogenic in humans.[589]

The life cycle of *E multilocularis* involves wild canids (mainly foxes) and to a lesser extent dogs and cats as the definitive host and rodents as the natural intermediate host.[586] Unlike *E granulosus*, larvae of *E multilocularis* remain in the proliferative stage inside the liver indefinitely,[586] which results in invasion and destruction of the surrounding tissue, similar to a malignancy. The incubation period of *E multilocularis* cyst is estimated to be 5 to 15 years, and the average age at its manifestation is 55 years.

The definitive hosts for *E vogeli* are bush dogs and domestic dogs, and the principal intermediate hosts are pacas and rodents.[586] The larval stage inside visceral organ develops internally and externally, resulting in a large cyst with multiple vesicles separated by septae. The life cycle of *E oligarthrus* involves wild felids such as puma and jaguar as definitive hosts and rodents and rabbits as intermediate hosts.[586] The larval form of *E oligarthrus* tends to be localized in muscles or other extrahepatic sites in the intermediate host animal, which may be the same as in human infection.

Clinical Manifestations

The clinical manifestations of echinococcal disease are different among *Echinococcus* species. Factors contributing to clinical manifestation are location, size, and condition of the cyst.[591]

ECHINOCOCCUS GRANULOSUS. The initial phase of primary infection is usually asymptomatic. Although most infections are acquired during childhood, clinical manifestations do not develop until adulthood because of the slow-growing nature of the cyst. Echinococcal cysts can be found in almost any organ in the human body from either primary inoculation or secondary dissemination of the protoscolices. Most human infections consist of a single cyst, but multiple cysts or multiple-organ involvement can occur up to 20% to 40% of cases.[591] The liver is the most common visceral organ involved (>65%) followed by the lungs (25%). Spleen, kidneys, heart, bone, and CNS are less frequently involved.[589] Cysts located in or near vital organs such as the brain or an eye, even when small, usually occurs early in the course; therefore most cerebral echinococcal infections are diagnosed in children.[589]

A hydatid cyst located in the liver usually produces no symptoms until it reaches at least 10 cm in diameter. The right lobe of the liver is affected in approximately 60% to 85% of cases. Clinical manifestations are hepatic enlargement with or without a palpable mass at the right upper quadrant, nausea, vomiting, and right upper quadrant pain. Cyst rupture into the biliary system and can cause biliary colic, obstructive jaundice, cholangitis, or pancreatitis. Pressure effect from the cyst on the biliary system can produce cholestasis or portal hypertension. Cysts can also rupture into the pleural cavity or peritoneal cavity, causing pulmonary hydatidosis or peritonitis. Liver abscess can be a result of secondary bacterial infection of a liver cyst. Release of cyst content after rupture or leakage of a cyst may cause fever and hypersensitivity reaction that can range from mild reaction to anaphylaxis.

Signs and symptoms of pulmonary hydatidosis include chronic cough, chest pain, pleuritis, or dyspnea. Some patients may experience hemoptysis or cough up the cyst material. Pleural effusion or lung abscess can also develop. Involvement of other visceral organs is uncommon but can also lead to significant morbidity and mortality.

ECHINOCOCCUS MULTILOCULARIS. Infections caused by *E multilocularis* are more likely to be symptomatic than infections caused by *E granulosus*. Clinical signs and symptoms, frequently nonspecific, include malaise, weight loss, right upper quadrant discomfort, and hepatomegaly. Primary disease involving visceral organs other than liver is rare. More than 90% of patients, if untreated, will die within 10 years after the onset of clinical manifestation.[592]

ECHINOCOCCUS VOGELI. *E vogeli* is the cause of polycystic echinococcosis. Clinical manifestations are intermediate in severity between cystic echinococcosis *(E granulosus)* and alveolar echinococcosis *(E multilocularis)*. Liver is the most common visceral organ involved during primary inoculation.[593] The polycystic echinococcal cyst in the liver is usually large and extensive. Progressive invasion of the liver and biliary tree may result in liver failure, portal hypertension, and biliary cirrhosis. The cyst is in the lungs in approximately 15% of cases.

ECHINOCOCCUS OLIGARTHRUS. *E oligarthrus* is an extremely rare cause of human echinococcosis. Clinical manifestations are similar to those of polycystic echinococcal disease caused by *E vogeli*.

Diagnosis

Diagnosis is usually made by a combination of imaging studies and serologic testing.[586,594] A history of exposure to possible animal hosts in an endemic area in a patient with a cystic, masslike lesion may help support the diagnosis. The most commonly used imaging techniques include ultrasound, CT, and MRI. In general, ultrasound is the most widely used imaging study because of its wide availability. Sensitivity of ultrasound is 90% to 95%.[595,596] In addition, ultrasound also allows cyst classification based on biological activity (active, transitional, or inactive), which helps guide the choice of treatment. CT scan has higher sensitivity than ultrasound.[595,596] CT is also better than ultrasound in detecting extrahepatic cysts and cyst complications. MRI does not have any major advantages over CT scan for detecting abdominal or pulmonary cysts and is usually not required.[597]

Eosinophilia is seen in less than 25% of cases.[589] Serologic testing, in general, is reliable in diagnosing *E multilocularis* infection than *E granulosus* infection.[598] The commonly used serologic tests include EIA and IHA as a screening test and immunoelectrophoresis or immunoblot assay as a specific confirmatory test.[586] Both false-positive and false-negative serologic test results can occur. False-positive results may occur with other helminthic infections, cancer, or a chronic immunologic disorder. False-negative serologic tests can vary in frequency depending on location, integrity, and vitality of the cyst, and tests are almost always negative with an intact calcified or nonviable cyst. Children and pregnant women usually have less antibody response and more frequently have a negative serologic test.[599] A cyst in the liver also elicits more antibody response than a cyst in the lung.[600] A cyst located in the brain, eye, or spleen almost always yields negative serologic findings, whereas a cyst in bone typically elicits serologic response.

Antibody titer usually remains positive after medical treatment but may become negative after a complete surgical resection of the cyst. Serologic tests can also be used to monitor treatment result because they remain negative after a successful surgical resection, and a reappearance of the antibody titer may indicate recurrence of disease. Cyst aspiration or biopsy is usually reserved for cases with uncertain diagnosis because of the potential anaphylaxis reaction or the spread of the infection after the procedure.[601] If needed, aspiration is usually performed under ultrasound or CT guidance along with benzimidazole treatment to minimize the risk of spreading. The commercial EIA kit is available in the United States.

Treatment

The most common treatment modality for hydatid cyst is surgery. The goal is complete removal of the cyst, which may lead to a cure.[589] For nonresectable cysts, medical treatment with an antihelminthic agent such as albendazole or mebendazole usually provides improvement and sometimes cures the infection.[602] Albendazole is the preferred agent because of its greater oral bioavailability and higher plasma concentration.[603] The response to medical treatment depends on the size and location of the cyst. Cysts inside the bone generally respond less well to drug therapy.[604]

Another treatment modality for nonresectable intraabdominal cyst that has been developed is the puncture, aspiration, injection, and reaspiration (PAIR) treatment.[605,606] PAIR is percutaneous drainage of the cyst with a needle or catheter, followed by instillation of the protoscolicide agent and reaspiration of the cyst content. PAIR has been demonstrated to be safe and effective worldwide; however, in children, it should be provided only to those older than 3 years. The possible complications from surgical procedures or PAIR are spreading of the infection and allergic or anaphylaxis reaction. These risks can be minimized by perioperative administration of antihelminthic agents affective against *Echinococcal* cyst.[601] In alveolar echinococcosis caused by *E multilocularis,* the lesion is usually extensive and left undiagnosed until the disease is advanced and inoperable. However, surgical resection is the only reliable means of cure. Long-term treatment with albendazole and mebendazole have been demonstrated to inhibit growth of the cyst, reduce metastasization, and sometimes may lead to a cure.[607]

Diphyllobothriasis *(Diphyllobothrium latum)*

Epidemiologic Features

Diphyllobothriasis is caused by the cestode *Diphyllobothrium*. *Diphyllobothrium latum* (fish tapeworm or broad tapeworm) is the most common *Diphyllobothrium* species infecting people worldwide. Other

Diphyllobothrium tapeworms that have been reported to cause disease in human include *Diphyllobothrium pacificum, Diphyllobothrium cordatum, Diphyllobothrium ursi, Diphyllobothrium dendriticum, Diphyllobothrium lanceolatum, Diphyllobothrium dalliae,* and *Diphyllobothrium yonagoensis*. Infestation occurs worldwide, with a high prevalence in population with the common culinary habit of eating undercooked or raw fish. Areas with high disease prevalence include Scandinavia, the newly independent states of the former Soviet Union, North America, Latin America, and Asia.[608] Infestation in the United States occurs mostly in the southeast.[609]

Life Cycle

All *Diphyllobothrium* cestodes have the same life cycle. Infestation in humans is acquired by ingesting raw or undercooked infected freshwater fish that contains the plerocercoid larvae, the infective stage for humans. In the human small intestine, the plerocercoids develop into mature adult worm and later release immature eggs from the worm's proglottids. The eggs are passed to the environment, and under appropriate conditions, they mature and develop into coracidia. Coracidia are ingested by the crustaceans, the copepod first intermediate host, and develop into procercoid larvae inside the crustacean body cavity. The infected crustaceans are ingested by small freshwater fish and later release procercoid larvae into the fish flesh. Inside small fish, the procercoid larvae develop into plerocercoid larvae. The big predator fish become infected after eating small fish that contained the plerocercoid larvae. The plerocercoid larvae migrate to the musculature of the large predator fish, and humans can acquire the disease by eating these fish raw or undercooked. The big predator fish represent a significant source of human infection because they generally do not eat minnows or small freshwater fish.

Clinical Manifestations

Infections occur primarily in older children and adults. Most infections are asymptomatic, especially in the younger age group.[610] Clinical manifestations include abdominal pain, nausea, vomiting, diarrhea, and weight loss. Other nonspecific symptoms that have been described with the infestation include fatigue, numbness, dizziness, and allergic symptoms. Because of the ability of *D latum* to compete for vitamin B_{12} absorption with the human host, chronically infected people may develop pernicious anemia as a result of vitamin B_{12} deficiency.[609] Infestation with massive amounts of worms may result in intestinal obstruction.

Diagnosis

Diagnosis is made by microscopic identification of eggs or proglottids in the stool. An infected person usually passes a large number of eggs and can be demonstrated without concentration technique.[608] Pernicious anemia and vitamin B_{12} deficiency provide clues to the diagnosis of diphyllobothriasis.

Treatment

Praziquantel is the treatment of choice.[44,587] An alternative agent, niclosamide, is no longer available in the United States. Patients with clinical or laboratory evidence of vitamin B_{12} deficiency should be treated with cobalamin injections and oral folic acid.

Hymenolepiasis *(Hymenolepis nana)*

Epidemiologic Features

Hymenolepis nana (dwarf tapeworm) is the most common cestode tapeworm infecting humans worldwide.[611] Transmission is associated with poor sanitation and hygiene. Infection is usually acquired by ingesting food or water contaminated with human or rodent feces. Infections occur most commonly in children because they are prone to fecal-oral contamination. The highest disease prevalence is among institutionalized school-aged children in the developing areas of the world.[612] In the United States, a 4% infection rate has been reported among schoolchildren in the rural Southeast.[613]

Life Cycle

H nana differs from all other cestodes because of its ability to complete its entire life cycle in a single host. The embryonated eggs are passed in the stools of an infected person and become infective immediately. Eggs are ingested by intermediate arthropod host and develop into cysticercoids inside the insect. Humans can acquire infection by ingesting embryonated eggs through contaminated food, water, hands, or cysticercoids-infected arthropods. In the human small intestine the oncospheres (hexacanth larvae) are released from the eggs and penetrate into intestinal villus. The oncospheres develop into cysticercoids inside the intestinal villus and later migrate back into the intestinal lumen. The cysticercoids evaginate their scoleces, attach themselves to the ileal part of intestinal mucosa, and mature into adult worms. Eggs are released from the gravid proglottids of the adult worm and are passed in the stool. Internal autoinfection can occur when eggs remain in the intestine. The eggs release their oncospheres, which penetrate the intestinal villus and continue the cycle without being passed to the external environment. The adult worms mature within 4 to 6 weeks.[611]

Clinical Manifestations

Most infections are asymptomatic. Patients with heavy infection may experience abdominal pain, nausea, vomiting, diarrhea, anorexia, weakness, irritability, and headache.

Diagnosis

Diagnosis is made by demonstrating eggs in the stool specimens.[611] Proglottids are rarely observed in stools. Detection of light infection may require a concentration technique and repeated examination. Peripheral blood eosinophilia may be present.

Treatment

Praziquantel is the drug of choice.[44,587] Close family members, especially siblings, should have their stools examined. Simultaneous treatment of family members may be indicated. Stool examination should be repeated at 2 to 4 weeks after treatment to document cure, especially in patients with many worms.[609]

WHEN TO REFER

If the physician is not well versed with taking care of children with parasitic infections, referring the patient to a infectious disease specialist would be prudent.

WHEN TO ADMIT

All the patients with systemic symptoms either caused by primary infection or as a complication of parasitic infection should be hospitalized.

TOOLS FOR PRACTICE

Medical Decision Support

- *Amebiasis* (Web page), Centers for Disease Control and Prevention (www.cdc.gov/ncidod/dpd/parasites/amebiasis/default.htm).
- *Ascaris Infection* (Web page), Centers for Disease Control and Prevention (www.cdc.gov/ncidod/dpd/parasites/ascaris/default.htm).
- *Babesia Infection* (Web page), Centers for Disease Control and Infection (www.cdc.gov/ncidod/dpd/parasites/babesia/default.htm).
- *Chagas Disease* (Trypanosoma cruzi infection) (Web page), Centers for Disease Control and Prevention (www.cdc.gov/ncidod/dpd/parasites/chagasdisease/index.htm).
- *Cryptosporidium Infection* (Web page), Centers for Disease Control and Prevention (www.cdc.gov/ncidod/dpd/parasites/cryptosporidiosis/default.htm).
- *Cyclospora Infection* (Web page), Centers for Disease Control and Prevention (www.cdc.gov/ncidod/dpd/parasites/cyclospora/default.htm).
- *Diphyllobothrium Infection* (Web page), Centers for Disease Control and Prevention (www.cdc.gov/ncidod/dpd/parasites/diphyllobothrium/default.htm).
- *DPDx Laboratory Identification of Parasites of Public Health Concern* (Web page), Centers for Disease Control and Prevention (www.dpd.cdc.gov/dpdx/Default.htm).
- *Giardiasis* (Web page), Centers for Disease Control and Prevention (www.cdc.gov/ncidod/dpd/parasites/giardiasis/default.htm).
- *Hookworm Infection* (Web page), Centers for Disease Control and Prevention (www.cdc.gov/ncidod/dpd/parasites/hookworm/default.htm).
- *Hymenolepis Infection* (Web page), Centers for Disease Control and Prevention (www.cdc.gov/ncidod/dpd/parasites/hymenolepis/default.htm).
- *Isospora Infection* (Web page), Centers for Disease Control and Prevention (www.cdc.gov/ncidod/dpd/parasites/isospora/default.htm).
- *Leishmania Infection* (Leishmaniasis) (Web page), Centers for Disease Control and Prevention (www.cdc.gov/ncidod/dpd/parasites/leishmania/default.htm).
- *Lymphatic Filariasis* (Web page), Centers for Disease Control and Prevention (www.cdc.gov/ncidod/dpd/parasites/lymphaticfilariasis/index.htm).
- *Malaria* (Web page), Centers for Disease Control and Prevention (www.cdc.gov/malaria).
- *Onchocerciasis/River Blindness* (Web page), Centers for Disease Control and Prevention (www.cdc.gov/ncidod/dpd/parasites/onchocerciasis/default.htm).
- *Pinworm Infection* (Web page), Centers for Disease Control and Prevention (www.cdc.gov/ncidod/dpd/parasites/pinworm/default.htm).
- *Red Book: 2006 Report of the Committee on Infectious Diseases, 27th edition*, American Academy of Pediatrics (www.aap.org/bookstore).
- *Schistosomiasis* (Web page), Centers for Disease Control and Prevention (www.cdc.gov/ncidod/dpd/parasites/schistosomiasis/default.htm).
- *Strongyloides Infection* (Web page), Centers for Disease Control and Prevention (www.cdc.gov/ncidod/dpd/parasites/strongyloides/default.htm).
- *Toxoplasmosis* (Web page), Centers for Disease Control and Prevention (www.cdc.gov/ncidod/dpd/parasites/toxoplasmosis/default.htm).
- *Trichinellosis* (Web page), Centers for Disease Control and Prevention (www.cdc.gov/ncidod/dpd/parasites/trichinellosis/default.htm).
- *Whipworm Infection* (Web page), Centers for Disease Control and Prevention (www.cdc.gov/ncidod/dpd/parasites/whipworm/default.htm).

REFERENCES

1. Murray HW, Berman JD, Davies CR, et al. Advances in leishmaniasis. *Lancet.* Oct-Nov 2005;366(9496):1561-1577.
2. Reithinger R, Espinoza JC, Davies CR. The transmission dynamics of canine American cutaneous leishmaniasis in Huanuco, Peru. *Am J Trop Med Hyg.* Nov 2003;69(5):473-480.
3. McHugh CP, Melby PC, LaFon SG. Leishmaniasis in Texas: epidemiology and clinical aspects of human cases. *Am J Trop Med Hyg.* Nov 1996;55(5):547-555.
4. Wilson ME, Streit JA. Visceral leishmaniasis. *Gastroenterol Clin North Am.* Sep 1996;25(3):535-551.
5. Rogers ME, Ilg T, Nikolaev AV, et al. Transmission of cutaneous leishmaniasis by sand flies is enhanced by regurgitation of fPPG. *Nature.* Jul 2004;430(6998):463-467.
6. Louzir H, Melby PC, Ben Salah A, et al. Immunologic determinants of disease evolution in localized cutaneous leishmaniasis due to Leishmania major. *J Infect Dis.* Jun 1998;177(6):1687-1695.
7. Desjeux P. Leishmaniasis: current situation and new perspectives. *Comp Immunol Microbiol Infect Dis.* Sep 2004;27(5):305-318.
8. Evans TG. Leishmaniasis. *Infect Dis Clin North Am.* Sep 1993;7(3):527-546.
9. Schwartz E, Hatz C, Blum J. New world cutaneous leishmaniasis in travelers. *Lancet Infect Dis.* Jun 2006;6(6):342-349.
10. Couppie P, Clyti E, Sobesky M, et al. Comparative study of cutaneous leishmaniasis in human immunodeficiency virus (HIV)-infected patients and non-HIV-infected patients in French Guiana. *Br J Dermatol.* Dec 2004;151(6):1165-1171.

11. Shaw PK, Quigg LT, Allain DS, et al. Autochthonous dermal leishmaniasis in Texas. *Am J Trop Med Hyg.* Nov 1976;25(6):788-796.
12. Centers for Disease Control and Prevention. Cutaneous leishmaniasis in US military personnel—Southwest/Central Asia, 2002-2003. *MMWR Morb Mortal Wkly Rep.* Oct 2003;52(42):1009-1012.
13. Marsden PD. Current concepts in parasitology. Leishmaniasis. *N Engl J Med.* Feb 1979;300(7):350-352.
14. Monroy-Ostria A, Hernandez-Montes O, Barker DC. Aetiology of visceral leishmaniasis in Mexico. *Acta Trop.* Mar 2000;75(2):155-161.
15. Magill AJ, Grogl M, Gasser RA Jr, et al. Visceral infection caused by Leishmania tropica in veterans of Operation Desert Storm. *N Engl J Med.* May 1993;328(19):1383-1387.
16. Magill AJ. Epidemiology of the leishmaniases. *Dermatol Clin.* Jul 1995;13(3):505-523.
17. Cruz I, Morales MA, Noguer I, et al. Leishmania in discarded syringes from intravenous drug users. *Lancet.* Mar 2002;359(9312):1124-1125.
18. Melby PC. Experimental leishmaniasis in humans: review. *Rev Infect Dis.* Sep-Oct 1991;13(5):1009-1017.
19. Dowlati Y. Cutaneous leishmaniasis: clinical aspect. *Clin Dermatol.* Sep-Oct 1996;14(5):425-431.
20. Machado P, Araujo C, Da Silva AT, et al. Failure of early treatment of cutaneous leishmaniasis in preventing the development of an ulcer. *Clin Infect Dis.* Jun 2002;34(12):E69-E73.
21. Magill AJ. Cutaneous leishmaniasis in the returning traveler. *Infect Dis Clin North Am.* Mar 2005;19(1):241-266, x-xi.
22. Wilson ME, Chen LH. Dermatologic infectious diseases in international travelers. *Curr Infect Dis Rep.* Feb 2004;6(1):54-62.
23. Machado-Coelho GL, Caiaffa WT, Genaro O, et al. Risk factors for mucosal manifestation of American cutaneous leishmaniasis. *Trans R Soc Trop Med Hyg.* Jan 2005;99(1):55-61.
24. Franke ED, Wignall FS, Cruz ME, et al. Efficacy and toxicity of sodium stibogluconate for mucosal leishmaniasis. *Ann Intern Med.* Dec 1990;113(12):934-940.
25. Herwaldt BL. Leishmaniasis. *Lancet.* Oct 1999;354(9185):1191-1199.
26. Bern C, Chowdhury R. The epidemiology of visceral leishmaniasis in Bangladesh: prospects for improved control. *Indian J Med Res.* Mar 2006;123(3):275-288.
27. Jamjoom MB, Ashford RW, Bates PA, et al. Leishmania donovani is the only cause of visceral leishmaniasis in East Africa; previous descriptions of L infantum and "L archibaldi" from this region are a consequence of convergent evolution in the isoenzyme data. *Parasitology.* Oct 2004;129(pt 4):399-409.
28. Rey LC, Martins CV, Ribeiro HB, et al. American visceral leishmaniasis (kala-azar) in hospitalized children from an endemic area. *J Pediatr (Rio J).* Jan-Feb 2005;81(1):73-78.
29. Leishmaniasis. In: Sun T, ed. *Parasitic Disorders: Pathology, Diagnosis, and Management.* 2nd ed. Baltimore, MD: Williams & Wilkins; 1999.
30. Kafetzis DA, Maltezou HC. Visceral leishmaniasis in paediatrics. *Curr Opin Infect Dis.* Jun 2002;15(3):289-294.
31. Pahwa R, Gupta SK, Singh T, et al. Acute fulminant visceral leishmaniasis in children—a report of two cases. *Indian J Pathol Microbiol.* Jul 2004;47(3):428-430.
32. Fasanaro AM, Scoleri G, Pizza V, et al. Guillain-Barré syndrome as presenting manifestation of visceral leishmaniasis. *Lancet.* Nov 1991;338(8775):1142.
33. Pintado V, Martin-Rabadan P, Rivera ML, et al. Visceral leishmaniasis in human immunodeficiency virus (HIV)-infected and non-HIV-infected patients. A comparative study. *Medicine (Baltimore).* Jan 2001;80(1):54-73.
34. Zijlstra EE, Musa AM, Khalil EA, et al. Post-kala-azar dermal leishmaniasis. *Lancet Infect Dis.* Feb 2003;3(2):87-98.
35. Ramirez JR, Agudelo S, Muskus C, et al. Diagnosis of cutaneous leishmaniasis in Colombia: the sampling site within lesions influences the sensitivity of parasitologic diagnosis. *J Clin Microbiol.* Oct 2000;38(10):3768-3773.
36. Vega-Lopez F. Diagnosis of cutaneous leishmaniasis. *Curr Opin Infect Dis.* Apr 2003;16(2):97-101.
37. Evans TG, Teixeira MJ, McAuliffe IT, et al. Epidemiology of visceral leishmaniasis in northeast Brazil. *J Infect Dis.* Nov 1992;166(5):1124-1132.
38. Kar K. Serodiagnosis of leishmaniasis. *Crit Rev Microbiol.* 1995;21(2):123-152.
39. de Oliveira CI, Bafica A, Oliveira F, et al. Clinical utility of polymerase chain reaction-based detection of Leishmania in the diagnosis of American cutaneous leishmaniasis. *Clin Infect Dis.* Dec 2003;37(11):e149-e153.
40. Oliveira JG, Novais FO, de Oliveira CI, et al. Polymerase chain reaction (PCR) is highly sensitive for diagnosis of mucosal leishmaniasis. *Acta Trop.* Apr 2005;94(1):55-59.
41. Andersen EM, Cruz-Saldarriaga M, Llanos-Cuentas A, et al. Comparison of meglumine antimoniate and pentamidine for peruvian cutaneous leishmaniasis. *Am J Trop Med Hyg.* Feb 2005;72(2):133-137.
42. Herwaldt BL, Berman JD. Recommendations for treating leishmaniasis with sodium stibogluconate (Pentostam) and review of pertinent clinical studies. *Am J Trop Med Hyg.* Mar 1992;46(3):296-306.
43. Sundar S, Mehta H, Suresh AV, et al. Amphotericin B treatment for Indian visceral leishmaniasis: conventional versus lipid formulations. *Clin Infect Dis.* Feb 2004;38(3):377-383.
44. [No author listed]. Drugs for parasitic infections [editorial]. *Med Lett Drugs Ther.* 2004;46(1189):e1-e12.
45. Sands M, Kron MA, Brown RB. Pentamidine: a review. *Rev Infect Dis.* Sep-Oct 1985;7(5):625-634.
46. el-On J, Halevy S, Grunwald MH, et al. Topical treatment of Old World cutaneous leishmaniasis caused by Leishmania major: a double-blind control study. *J Am Acad Dermatol.* Aug 1992;27(2 pt 1):227-231.
47. Aggarwal P, Handa R, Singh S, et al. Kala-azar—new developments in diagnosis and treatment. *Indian J Pediatr.* Jan-Feb 1999;66(1):63-71.
48. Sundar S, Jha TK, Thakur CP, et al. Oral miltefosine for Indian visceral leishmaniasis. *N Engl J Med.* Nov 2002;347(22):1739-1746.
49. Alrajhi AA, Ibrahim EA, De Vol EB, et al. Fluconazole for the treatment of cutaneous leishmaniasis caused by Leishmania major. *N Engl J Med.* Mar 2002;346(12):891-895.
50. Davies CR, Kaye P, Croft SL, et al. Leishmaniasis: new approaches to disease control. *BMJ.* Feb 2003;326(7385):377-382.
51. Centers for Disease Control and Prevention, National Center for Infectious Diseases, Division of Parasitic Diseases. Laboratory Identification of Parasites of Public Health Concern: Trypanosomiasis, American. Available at: www.dpd.cdc.gov/dpdx/html/trypanosomiasisamerican.htm. Accessed April 6, 2007.
52. Prata A. Clinical and epidemiological aspects of Chagas' disease. *Lancet Infect Dis.* Sep 2001;1(2):92-100.
53. Ortega-Bari E. Trypanosoma species (trypanosomiasis). In: Long SS, Pickering LK, Prober CG, eds. *Principles and Practice of Pediatric Infectious Diseases.* 2nd ed. New York, NY: Churchill Livingstone; 2003.

54. American Academy of Pediatrics. American trypanosomiasis (Chagas' disease). In: Pickering LK, Baker CJ, Long SS, et al, eds. *Red Book: 2006 Report of the Committee on Infectious Diseases*. 27th ed. Elk Grove Village, IL: American Academy of Pediatrics; 2006.
55. World Health Organization. Control of Chagas' disease. Report of a WHO Expert Committee. *World Health Organ Tech Rep Ser.* 1991;811:1-95.
56. Kirchhoff LV. American trypanosomiasis (Chagas' disease)—a tropical disease now in the United States. *N Engl J Med.* Aug 1993;329(9):639-644.
57. Maguire JH, Hoff R, Sherlock I, et al. Cardiac morbidity and mortality due to Chagas' disease: prospective electrocardiographic study of a Brazilian community. *Circulation.* Jun 1987;75(6):1140-1145.
58. Hagar JM, Rahimtoola SH. Chagas' heart disease in the United States. *N Engl J Med.* Sep 1991;325(11):763-768.
59. World Health Organization. Parasite antigens. *Bull World Health Organ.* 1975;52(3):237-249.
60. Sosa Estani S, Segura EL, Ruiz AM, et al. Efficacy of chemotherapy with benznidazole in children in the indeterminate phase of Chagas' disease. *Am J Trop Med Hyg.* Oct 1998;59(4):526-529.
61. American Academy of Pediatrics. African trypanosomiasis (African sleeping sickness). In: Pickering LK, Baker CJ, Long SS, et al, eds. *Red Book: 2006 Report of the Committee on Infectious Diseases*. 27th ed. Elk Grove Village, IL: American Academy of Pediatrics; 2006.
62. Centers for Disease Control and Prevention, National Center for Infectious Diseases, Division of Parasitic Diseases. Laboratory Identification of Parasites of Public Health Concern: Trypanosomiasis, African. Available at: www.dpd.cdc.gov/dpdx/html/trypanosomiasisafrican.htm. Accessed April 6, 2007.
63. World Health Organization. Epidemiology and control of African trypanosomiasis. Report of a WHO Expert Committee. *World Health Organ Tech Rep Ser.* 1986; 739:1-127.
64. Gilman RH, Brown KH, Visvesvara GS, et al. Epidemiology and serology of Giardia lamblia in a developing country: Bangladesh. *Trans R Soc Trop Med Hyg.* 1985; 79(4):469-473.
65. Mason PR, Patterson BA. Epidemiology of Giardia lamblia infection in children: cross-sectional and longitudinal studies in urban and rural communities in Zimbabwe. *Am J Trop Med Hyg.* Sep 1987;37(2): 277-282.
66. Curtale F, Nabil M, el Wakeel A, et al. Anaemia and intestinal parasitic infections among school age children in Behera Governorate, Egypt. Behera Survey Team. *J Trop Pediatr.* Dec 1998;44(6):323-328.
67. Furness BW, Beach MJ, Roberts JM. Giardiasis surveillance—United States, 1992-1997. *MMWR CDC Surveill Summ.* Aug 2000;49(7):1-13.
68. Saiman L, Aronson J, Zhou J, et al. Prevalence of infectious diseases among internationally adopted children. *Pediatrics.* Sep 2001;108(3):608-612.
69. Mintz ED, Hudson-Wragg M, Mshar P, et al. Foodborne giardiasis in a corporate office setting. *J Infect Dis.* Jan 1993;167(1):250-253.
70. Rendtorff RC. The experimental transmission of human intestinal protozoan parasites. II. Giardia lamblia cysts given in capsules. *Am J Hyg.* Mar 1954;59(2):209-220.
71. Welch TP. Risk of giardiasis from consumption of wilderness water in North America: a systematic review of epidemiologic data. *Int J Infect Dis.* 2000;4(2):100-103.
72. Dykes AC, Juranek DD, Lorenz RA, et al. Municipal waterborne giardiasis: an epidemilogic investigation. Beavers implicated as a possible reservoir. *Ann Intern Med.* Feb 1980;92(2 pt 1):165-170.
73. Hunter PR, Thompson RC. The zoonotic transmission of Giardia and Cryptosporidium. *Int J Parasitol.* Oct 2005; 35(11-12):1181-1190.
74. Overturf GD. Endemic giardiasis in the United States—role of the daycare center. *Clin Infect Dis.* May 1994;18(5): 764-765.
75. Pickering LK, Woodward WE, DuPont HL, et al. Occurrence of Giardia lamblia in children in day care centers. *J Pediatr.* Apr 1984;104(4):522-526.
76. Keystone JS, Keystone DL, Proctor EM. Intestinal parasitic infections in homosexual men: prevalence, symptoms and factors in transmission. *Can Med Assoc J.* Sep 1980;123(6):512-514.
77. Black RE. Epidemiology of travelers' diarrhea and relative importance of various pathogens. *Rev Infect Dis.* Jan-Feb 1990;12(suppl 1):S73-S79.
78. Slonim JM, Ireton HJ, Smallwood RA. Giardiasis following gastric surgery. *Aust N Z J Med.* Oct 1976;6(5): 479-480.
79. Berney DM, Rampton D, van der Walt JD. Giardiasis of the stomach. *Postgrad Med J.* Mar 1994;70(821): 237-238.
80. Roberts DM, Craft JC, Mather FJ, et al. Prevalence of giardiasis in patients with cystic fibrosis. *J Pediatr.* Apr 1988;112(4):555-559.
81. Sheehy TW, Holley HP Jr. Giardia-induced malabsorption in pancreatitis. *JAMA.* Sep 1975;233(13):1373-1375.
82. Lewis DJ, Freedman AR. Giardia lamblia as an intestinal pathogen. *Dig Dis.* 1992;10(2):102-111.
83. Ward W, Alvarado L, Rawlings ND, et al. A primitive enzyme for a primitive cell: the protease required for excystation of Giardia. *Cell.* May 1997;89(3):437-444.
84. Wolfe MS. Giardiasis. *Clin Microbiol Rev.* Jan 1992;5(1): 93-100.
85. Eckmann L, Gillin FD. Microbes and microbial toxins: paradigms for microbial-mucosal interactions I. Pathophysiological aspects of enteric infections with the lumen-dwelling protozoan pathogen Giardia lamblia. *Am J Physiol Gastrointest Liver Physiol.* Jan 2001;280(1): G1-G6.
86. Boyd WP Jr, Bachman BA. Gastrointestinal infections in the compromised host. *Med Clin North Am.* May 1982; 66(3):743-753.
87. Nash TE, Herrington DA, Losonsky GA, et al. Experimental human infections with Giardia lamblia. *J Infect Dis.* Dec 1987;156(6):974-984.
88. Caeiro JP, Mathewson JJ, Smith MA, et al. Etiology of outpatient pediatric nondysenteric diarrhea: a multicenter study in the United States. *Pediatr Infect Dis J.* Feb 1999;18(2):94-97.
89. Hopkins RS, Juranek DD. Acute giardiasis: an improved clinical case definition for epidemiologic studies. *Am J Epidemiol.* Feb 1991;133(4):402-407.
90. Bai JC. Malabsorption syndromes. *Digestion.* Aug 1998; 59(5):530-546.
91. Ortega YR, Adam RD. Giardia: overview and update. *Clin Infect Dis.* Sep 1997;25(3):545-549; quiz 550.
92. Grant SC, Harrington CI, Harris SC. Aphthous ulceration as a presentation of Giardia lamblia infection. *Br Dent J.* Jun 1989;166(12):457.
93. Tupchong M, Simor A, Dewar C. Beaver fever—a rare cause of reactive arthritis. *J Rheumatol.* Dec 1999;26(12): 2701-2702.
94. Erel F, Sener O, Erdil A, et al. Impact of Helicobacter pylori and Giardia lamblia infections on chronic urticaria. *J Investig Allergol Clin Immunol.* Mar-Apr 2000; 10(2):94-97.
95. Knox DL, King J Jr. Retinal arteritis, iridocyclitis, and giardiasis. *Ophthalmology.* Dec 1982;89(12):1303-1308.

96. Roberts-Thomson IC, Anders RF, Bhathal PS. Granulomatous hepatitis and cholangitis associated with giardiasis. *Gastroenterology.* Aug 1982;83(2):480-483.
97. Chapoutot C, Verdier E, Bismuth M, et al. [Recurrent acute Giardia intestinalis pancreatitis]. *Gastroenterol Clin Biol.* 1997;21(5):438-439.
98. Hiatt RA, Markell EK, Ng E. How many stool examinations are necessary to detect pathogenic intestinal protozoa? *Am J Trop Med Hyg.* Jul 1995;53(1):36-39.
99. Aldeen WE, Hale D, Robison AJ, et al. Evaluation of a commercially available ELISA assay for detection of Giardia lamblia in fecal specimens. *Diagn Microbiol Infect Dis.* Feb 1995;21(2):77-79.
100. Winiecka-Krusnell J, Linder E. Detection of Giardia lamblia cysts in stool samples by immunofluorescence using monoclonal antibody. *Eur J Clin Microbiol Infect Dis.* Mar 1995;14(3):218-222.
101. Goka AK, Rolston DD, Mathan VI, et al. The relative merits of faecal and duodenal juice microscopy in the diagnosis of giardiasis. *Trans R Soc Trop Med Hyg.* Jan-Feb 1990;84(1):66-67.
102. Jones JE. String test for diagnosing giardiasis. *Am Fam Physician.* Aug 1986;34(2):123-126.
103. Guy RA, Xiao C, Horgen PA. Real-time PCR assay for detection and genotype differentiation of Giardia lamblia in stool specimens. *J Clin Microbiol.* Jul 2004;42(7): 3317-3320.
104. American Academy of Pediatrics. Giardia intestinalis infections (giardiasis). In: Pickering LK, Baker CJ, Long SS, et al, eds. *Red Book: 2006 Report of the Committee on Infectious Diseases.* 27th ed. Elk Grove Village, IL: American Academy of Pediatrics; 2006.
105. Gardner TB, Hill DR. Treatment of giardiasis. *Clin Microbiol Rev.* Jan 2001;14(1):114-128.
106. Nash TE. Treatment of Giardia lamblia infections. *Pediatr Infect Dis J.* Feb 2001;20(2):193-195.
107. Ortiz JJ, Ayoub A, Gargala G, et al. Randomized clinical study of nitazoxanide compared to metronidazole in the treatment of symptomatic giardiasis in children from Northern Peru. *Aliment Pharmacol Ther.* Sep 2001;15(9): 1409-1415.
108. Ongerth JE, Johnson RL, Macdonald SC, et al. Backcountry water treatment to prevent giardiasis. *Am J Public Health.* Dec 1989;79(12):1633-1637.
109. Ferguson C, Kaucner C, Krogh M, et al. Comparison of methods for the concentration of Cryptosporidium oocysts and Giardia cysts from raw waters. *Can J Microbiol.* Sep 2004;50(9):675-682.
110. Li E, Stanley SL. Protozoa. Amebiasis. *Gastroenterol Clin North Am.* Sep 1996;25(3):471-492.
111. Haque R, Petri WA Jr. Diagnosis of amebiasis in Bangladesh. *Arch Med Res.* Feb 2006;37(2):273-276.
112. Weinke T, Friedrich-Janicke B, Hopp P, et al. Prevalence and clinical importance of Entamoeba histolytica in two high-risk groups: travelers returning from the tropics and male homosexuals. *J Infect Dis.* May 1990;161(5):1029-1031.
113. Marshall MM, Naumovitz D, Ortega Y, et al. Waterborne protozoan pathogens. *Clinical Microbiology Reviews.* 1997;10(1):67-85.
114. Petri WA Jr. Recent advances in amebiasis. *Crit Rev Clin Lab Sci.* Jan 1996;33(1):1-37.
115. Adams EB, MacLeod IN. Invasive amebiasis. II. Amebic liver abscess and its complications. *Medicine (Baltimore).* Jul 1977;56(4):325-334.
116. Aristizabal H, Acevedo J, Botero M. Fulminant amebic colitis. *World J Surg.* Mar-Apr 1991;15(2):216-221.
117. Misra SP, Misra V, Dwivedi M. Ileocecal masses in patients with amebic liver abscess: etiology and management. *World J Gastroenterol.* Mar 2006;12(12): 1933-1936.
118. Stockinger ZT. Colonic ameboma: its appearance on CT: report of a case. *Dis Colon Rectum.* Apr 2004;47(4): 527-529.
119. Aikat BK, Bhusnurmath SR, Pal AK, et al. The pathology and pathogenesis of fatal hepatic amoebiasis—A study based on 79 autopsy cases. *Trans R Soc Trop Med Hyg.* 1979;73(2):188-192.
120. Maltz G, Knauer CM. Amebic liver abscess: a 15-year experience. *Am J Gastroenterol.* Jun 1991;86(6):704-710.
121. Haque R, Kress K, Wood S, et al. Diagnosis of pathogenic Entamoeba histolytica infection using a stool ELISA based on monoclonal antibodies to the galactose-specific adhesin. *J Infect Dis.* Jan 1993;167(1): 247-249.
122. Patterson M, Healy GR, Shabot JM. Serologic testing for amoebiasis. *Gastroenterology.* Jan 1980;78(1): 136-141.
123. Haque R, Neville LM, Hahn P, et al. Rapid diagnosis of Entamoeba infection by using Entamoeba and Entamoeba histolytica stool antigen detection kits. *J Clin Microbiol.* Oct 1995;33(10):2558-2561.
124. Gonzalez-Ruiz A, Haque R, Rehman T, et al. Diagnosis of amebic dysentery by detection of Entamoeba histolytica fecal antigen by an invasive strain-specific, monoclonal antibody-based enzyme-linked immunosorbent assay. *J Clin Microbiol.* Apr 1994;32(4):964-970.
125. Haque R, Ali IK, Akther S, et al. Comparison of PCR, isoenzyme analysis, and antigen detection for diagnosis of Entamoeba histolytica infection. *J Clin Microbiol.* Feb 1998;36(2):449-452.
126. Petri WA Jr, Singh U. Diagnosis and management of amebiasis. *Clin Infect Dis.* Nov 1999;29(5):1117-1125.
127. Garfinkel LI, Giladi M, Huber M, et al. DNA probes specific for Entamoeba histolytica possessing pathogenic and nonpathogenic zymodemes. *Infect Immun.* Mar 1989; 57(3):926-931.
128. Bracha R, Diamond LS, Ackers JP, et al. Differentiation of clinical isolates of Entamoeba histolytica by using specific DNA probes. *J Clin Microbiol.* Apr 1990;28(4): 680-684.
129. Blessmann J, Buss H, Nu PA, et al. Real-time PCR for detection and differentiation of Entamoeba histolytica and Entamoeba dispar in fecal samples. *J Clin Microbiol.* Dec 2002;40(12):4413-4417.
130. Schuster FL, Visvesvara GS. Free-living amoebae as opportunistic and non-opportunistic pathogens of humans and animals. *Int J Parasitol.* Aug 2004;34(9): 1001-1027.
131. Ma P, Visvesvara GS, Martinez AJ, et al. Naegleria and Acanthamoeba infections: review. *Rev Infect Dis.* May-Jun 1990;12(3):490-513.
132. Schmutzhard E, Mayr U, Rumpl E, et al. Secondary cerebral amebiasis due to infection with Entamoeba histolytica. A case report with computer tomographic findings. *Eur Neurol.* 1986;25(3):161-165.
133. Barnett ND, Kaplan AM, Hopkin RJ, et al. Primary amoebic meningoencephalitis with Naegleria fowleri: clinical review. *Pediatr Neurol.* Oct 1996;15(3):230-234.
134. Schuster FL, Visvesvara GS. Amebae and ciliated protozoa as causal agents of waterborne zoonotic disease. *Vet Parasitol.* Dec 2004;126(1-2):91-120.
135. Wang A, Kay R, Poon WS, et al. Successful treatment of amoebic meningoencephalitis in a Chinese living in Hong Kong. *Clin Neurol Neurosurg.* Sep 1993;95(3): 249-252.
136. Schuster FL, Guglielmo BJ, Visvesvara GS. In-vitro activity of miltefosine and voriconazole on clinical isolates of free-living amebas: Balamuthia mandrillaris, Acanthamoeba spp., and Naegleria fowleri. *J Eukaryot Microbiol.* Mar-Apr 2006;53(2):121-126.

137. Kumar R, Lloyd D. Recent advances in the treatment of Acanthamoeba keratitis. *Clin Infect Dis.* Aug 2002;35(4): 434-441.
138. Rivera F, Ramirez E, Bonilla P, et al. Pathogenic and free-living amoebae isolated from swimming pools and physiotherapy tubs in Mexico. *Environ Res.* Jul 1993; 62(1):43-52.
139. Ledee DR, Hay J, Byers TJ, et al. Acanthamoeba griffini. Molecular characterization of a new corneal pathogen. *Invest Ophthalmol Vis Sci.* Mar 1996;37(4): 544-550.
140. Chen XM, Keithly JS, Paya CV, et al. Cryptosporidiosis. *N Engl J Med.* May 2002;346(22):1723-1731.
141. Fayer R, Ungar BL. Cryptosporidium spp and cryptosporidiosis. *Microbiol Rev.* Dec 1986;50(4):458-483.
142. Peng MM, Xiao L, Freeman AR, et al. Genetic polymorphism among Cryptosporidium parvum isolates: evidence of two distinct human transmission cycles. *Emerg Infect Dis.* Oct-Dec 1997;3(4):567-573.
143. Kuhls TL, Mosier DA, Crawford DL, et al. Seroprevalence of cryptosporidial antibodies during infancy, childhood, and adolescence. *Clin Infect Dis.* May 1994; 18(5):731-735.
144. Jelinek T, Lotze M, Eichenlaub S, et al. Prevalence of infection with Cryptosporidium parvum and Cyclospora cayetanensis among international travellers. *Gut.* Dec 1997;41(6):801-804.
145. Laupland KB, Church DL. Population-based laboratory surveillance for Giardia sp and Cryptosporidium sp infections in a large Canadian health region. *BMC Infect Dis.* 2005;5:72.
146. Centers for Disease Control and Prevention. Preliminary FoodNet data on the incidence of infection with pathogens transmitted commonly through food—10 States, United States, 2005. *MMWR Morb Mortal Wkly Rep.* Apr 2006;55(14):392-395.
147. Ungar BL, Mulligan M, Nutman TB. Serologic evidence of Cryptosporidium infection in US volunteers before and during Peace Corps service in Africa. *Arch Intern Med.* Apr 1989;149(4):894-897.
148. Ungar BL, Gilman RH, Lanata CF, et al. Seroepidemiology of Cryptosporidium infection in two Latin American populations. *J Infect Dis.* Mar 1988;157(3):551-556.
149. Casemore DP, Sands RL, Curry A. Cryptosporidium species: a "new" human pathogen. *J Clin Pathol.* Dec 1985;38(12):1321-1336.
150. Meinhardt PL, Casemore DP, Miller KB. Epidemiologic aspects of human cryptosporidiosis and the role of waterborne transmission. *Epidemiol Rev.* 1996;18(2): 118-136.
151. DuPont HL, Chappell CL, Sterling CR, et al. The infectivity of Cryptosporidium parvum in healthy volunteers. *N Engl J Med.* Mar 1995;332(13):855-859.
152. Levy DA, Bens MS, Craun GF, et al. Surveillance for waterborne-disease outbreaks—United States, 1995-1996. *MMWR CDC Surveill Summ.* Dec 1998;47(5):1-34.
153. MacKenzie WR, Schell WL, Blair KA, et al. Massive outbreak of waterborne Cryptosporidium infection in Milwaukee, Wisconsin: recurrence of illness and risk of secondary transmission. *Clin Infect Dis.* Jul 1995;21(1): 57-62.
154. Juranek DD. Cryptosporidiosis: sources of infection and guidelines for prevention. *Clin Infect Dis.* Aug 1995; 21(suppl 1):S57-S61.
155. Centers for Disease Control and Prevention. Outbreaks of Escherichia coli O157:H7 infection and cryptosporidiosis associated with drinking unpasteurized apple cider—Connecticut and New York, October 1996. *MMWR Morb Mortal Wkly Rep.* Jan 1997;46(01):4-8.
156. Causer LM, Handzel T, Welch P, et al. An outbreak of Cryptosporidium hominis infection at an Illinois recreational waterpark. *Epidemiol Infect.* Feb 2006;134(1): 147-156.
157. Quiroz ES, Bern C, MacArthur JR, et al. An outbreak of cryptosporidiosis linked to a foodhandler. *J Infect Dis.* Feb 2000;181(2):695-700.
158. Cordell RL, Addiss DG. Cryptosporidiosis in child care settings: a review of the literature and recommendations for prevention and control. *Pediatr Infect Dis J.* Apr 1994;13(4):310-317.
159. Hannah J, Riordan T. Case to case spread of cryptosporidiosis; evidence from a day nursery outbreak. *Public Health.* Nov 1988;102(6):539-544.
160. Current WL. Cryptosporidium parvum: household transmission. *Ann Intern Med.* Mar 1994;120(6): 518-519.
161. Hellard M, Hocking J, Willis J, et al. Risk factors leading to Cryptosporidium infection in men who have sex with men. *Sex Transm Infect.* Oct 2003;79(5):412-414.
162. Squier C, Yu VL, Stout JE. Waterborne nosocomial infections. *Curr Infect Dis Rep.* Dec 2000;2(6):490-496.
163. Goodgame R. Emerging causes of traveler's diarrhea: Cryptosporidium, Cyclospora, Isospora, and Microsporidia. *Curr Infect Dis Rep.* Feb 2003;5(1):66-73.
164. Jokipii L, Jokipii AM. Timing of symptoms and oocyst excretion in human cryptosporidiosis. *N Engl J Med.* Dec 1986;315(26):1643-1647.
165. Smith HV, Nichols RA, Grimason AM. Cryptosporidium excystation and invasion: getting to the guts of the matter. *Trends Parasitol.* Mar 2005;21(3):133-142.
166. Kosek M, Alcantara C, Lima AA, et al. Cryptosporidiosis: an update. *Lancet Infect Dis.* Nov 2001;1(4): 262-269.
167. Manabe YC, Clark DP, Moore RD, et al. Cryptosporidiosis in patients with AIDS: correlates of disease and survival. *Clin Infect Dis.* Sep 1998;27(3):536-542.
168. Vakil NB, Schwartz SM, Buggy BP, et al. Biliary cryptosporidiosis in HIV-infected people after the waterborne outbreak of cryptosporidiosis in Milwaukee. *N Engl J Med.* Jan 1996;334(1):19-23.
169. Kirkpatrick BD, Noel F, Rouzier PD, et al. Childhood cryptosporidiosis is associated with a persistent systemic inflammatory response. *Clin Infect Dis.* Sep 2006; 43(5):604-608.
170. Heyworth MF. Parasitic diseases in immunocompromised hosts. Cryptosporidiosis, isosporiasis, and strongyloidiasis. *Gastroenterol Clin North Am.* Sep 1996;25(3):691-707.
171. Benhamou Y, Kapel N, Hoang C, et al. Inefficacy of intestinal secretory immune response to Cryptosporidium in acquired immunodeficiency syndrome. *Gastroenterology.* Mar 1995;108(3):627-635.
172. Rehg JE. Effect of interferon-gamma in experimental Cryptosporidium parvum infection. *J Infect Dis.* Jul 1996; 174(1):229-232.
173. Crawford FG, Vermund SH, Ma JY, et al. Asymptomatic cryptosporidiosis in a New York City day care center. *Pediatr Infect Dis J.* Nov 1988;7(11):806-807.
174. Isaacs D. Cryptosporidium and diarrhoea. *Arch Dis Child.* Jul 1985;60(7):608-609.
175. Newman RD, Sears CL, Moore SR, et al. Longitudinal study of Cryptosporidium infection in children in northeastern Brazil. *J Infect Dis.* Jul 1999;180(1):167-175.
176. Hart CA, Baxby D, Blundell N. Gastro-enteritis due to Cryptosporidium: a prospective survey in a children's hospital. *J Infect.* Nov 1984;9(3):264-270.
177. Flanigan T, Whalen C, Turner J, et al. Cryptosporidium infection and CD4 counts. *Ann Intern Med.* May 1992; 116(10):840-842.

178. Gross TL, Wheat J, Bartlett M, et al. AIDS and multiple system involvement with cryptosporidium. *Am J Gastroenterol.* Jun 1986;81(6):456-458.
179. Moore JA, Frenkel JK. Respiratory and enteric cryptosporidiosis in humans. *Arch Pathol Lab Med.* Nov 1991; 115(11):1160-1162.
180. Meynard JL, Meyohas MC, Binet D, et al. Pulmonary cryptosporidiosis in the acquired immunodeficiency syndrome. *Infection.* Jul-Aug 1996;24(4):328-331.
181. Garcia LS, Brewer TC, Bruckner DA. Fluorescence detection of Cryptosporidium oocysts in human fecal specimens by using monoclonal antibodies. *J Clin Microbiol.* Jan 1987;25(1):119-121.
182. Parisi MT, Tierno PM Jr. Evaluation of new rapid commercial enzyme immunoassay for detection of Cryptosporidium oocysts in untreated stool specimens. *J Clin Microbiol.* Jul 1995;33(7):1963-1965.
183. Zhu G, Marchewka MJ, Ennis JG, et al. Direct isolation of DNA from patient stools for polymerase chain reaction detection of Cryptosporidium parvum. *J Infect Dis.* May 1998;177(5):1443-1446.
184. Morgan UM, Pallant L, Dwyer BW, et al. Comparison of PCR and microscopy for detection of Cryptosporidium parvum in human fecal specimens: clinical trial. *J Clin Microbiol.* Apr 1998;36(4):995-998.
185. Bobak DA. Use of nitazoxanide for gastrointestinal tract infections: treatment of protozoan parasitic infection and beyond. *Curr Infect Dis Rep.* Mar 2006;8(2): 91-95.
186. Hewitt RG, Yiannoutsos CT, Higgs ES, et al. Paromomycin: no more effective than placebo for treatment of cryptosporidiosis in patients with advanced human immunodeficiency virus infection. AIDS Clinical Trial Group. *Clin Infect Dis.* Oct 2000;31(4):1084-1092.
187. Carr A, Marriott D, Field A, et al. Treatment of HIV-1-associated microsporidiosis and cryptosporidiosis with combination antiretroviral therapy. *Lancet.* Jan 1998; 351(9098):256-261.
188. Louie E, Borkowsky W, Klesius PH, et al. Treatment of cryptosporidiosis with oral bovine transfer factor. *Clin Immunol Immunopathol.* Sep 1987;44(3):329-334.
189. American Academy of Pediatrics. Cryptosporidiosis. In: Pickering LK, Baker CJ, Long SS, et al, eds. *Red Book: 2006 Report of the Committee on Infectious Diseases.* 27th ed. Elk Grove Village, IL: American Academy of Pediatrics; 2006.
190. Hoepelman AI. Current therapeutic approaches to cryptosporidiosis in immunocompromised patients. *J Antimicrob Chemother.* May 1996;37(5):871-880.
191. Centers for Disease Control and Prevention. Assessing the public health threat associated with waterborne cryptosporidiosis: report of a workshop. *MMWR Recomm Rep.* Jun 1995;44(RR-6):1-19.
192. Goodgame RW. Understanding intestinal spore-forming protozoa: cryptosporidia, microsporidia, isospora, and cyclospora. *Ann Intern Med.* Feb 1996;124(4): 429-441.
193. Shaffer N, Moore L. Chronic travelers' diarrhea in a normal host due to Isospora belli. *J Infect Dis.* Mar 1989;159(3):596-597.
194. Lindsay DS, Dubey JP, Blagburn BL. Biology of Isospora spp. from humans, nonhuman primates, and domestic animals. *Clin Microbiol Rev.* Jan 1997;10(1): 19-34.
195. ABT WB. Eosinophilia in Isospora infections. *Parasitol Today.* Jan 1986;2(1):22.
196. DeHovitz JA, Pape JW, Boncy M, et al. Clinical manifestations and therapy of Isospora belli infection in patients with the acquired immunodeficiency syndrome. *N Engl J Med.* Jul 1986;315(2):87-90.
197. Pape JW, Verdier RI, Johnson WD Jr. Treatment and prophylaxis of Isospora belli infection in patients with the acquired immunodeficiency syndrome. *N Engl J Med.* Apr 1989;320(16):1044-1047.
198. Varea M, Clavel A, Doiz O, et al. Fuchsin fluorescence and autofluorescence in Cryptosporidium, Isospora and Cyclospora oocysts. *Int J Parasitol.* Dec 1998;28(12):1881-1883.
199. Berlin OG, Conteas CN, Sowerby TM. Detection of Isospora in the stools of AIDS patients using a new rapid autofluorescence technique. *AIDS.* Apr 1996;10(4):442-443.
200. Centers for Disease Control and Prevention, National Center for Infectious Diseases, Division of Parasitic Diseases. Laboratory Identification of Parasites of Public Health Concern: Isosporiasis. Available at: http://www.dpd.cdc.gov/dpdx/html/isosporiasis.htm. Accessed April 6, 2007.
201. Colebunders R, Lusakumuni K, Nelson AM, et al. Persistent diarrhoea in Zairian AIDS patients: an endoscopic and histological study. *Gut.* Dec 1988;29(12): 1687-1691.
202. American Academy of Pediatrics. Isosporiasis. In: Pickering LK, Baker CJ, Long SS, et al, eds. *Red Book: 2006 Report of the Committee on Infectious Diseases.* 27th ed. Elk Grove Village, IL: American Academy of Pediatrics; 2006.
203. Weiss LM, Perlman DC, Sherman J, et al. Isospora belli infection: treatment with pyrimethamine. *Ann Intern Med.* Sep 1988;109(6):474-475.
204. Verdier RI, Fitzgerald DW, Johnson WD Jr, et al. Trimethoprim-sulfamethoxazole compared with ciprofloxacin for treatment and prophylaxis of Isospora belli and Cyclospora cayetanensis infection in HIV-infected patients. A randomized, controlled trial. *Ann Intern Med.* Jun 2000;132(11):885-888.
205. Huang P, Weber JT, Sosin DM, et al. The first reported outbreak of diarrheal illness associated with Cyclospora in the United States. *Ann Intern Med.* Sep 1995;123(6): 409-414.
206. Doller PC, Dietrich K, Filipp N, et al. Cyclosporiasis outbreak in Germany associated with the consumption of salad. *Emerg Infect Dis.* Sep 2002;8(9):992-994.
207. Cann KJ, Chalmers RM, Nichols G, et al. Cyclospora infections in England and Wales: 1993 to 1998. *Commun Dis Public Health.* Mar 2000;3(1):46-49.
208. Madico G, McDonald J, Gilman RH, et al. Epidemiology and treatment of Cyclospora cayetanensis infection in Peruvian children. *Clin Infect Dis.* May 1997;24(5): 977-981.
209. Pape JW, Verdier RI, Boncy M, et al. Cyclospora infection in adults infected with HIV. Clinical manifestations, treatment, and prophylaxis. *Ann Intern Med.* Nov 1994; 121(9):654-657.
210. Hoge CW, Shlim DR, Rajah R, et al. Epidemiology of diarrhoeal illness associated with coccidian-like organism among travellers and foreign residents in Nepal. *Lancet.* May 1993;341(8854):1175-1179.
211. Ho AY, Lopez AS, Eberhart MG, et al. Outbreak of cyclosporiasis associated with imported raspberries, Philadelphia, Pennsylvania, 2000. *Emerg Infect Dis.* Aug 2002;8(8):783-788.
212. Herwaldt BL. Cyclospora cayetanensis: a review, focusing on the outbreaks of cyclosporiasis in the 1990s. *Clin Infect Dis.* Oct 2000;31(4):1040-1057.
213. Lopez AS, Dodson DR, Arrowood MJ, et al. Outbreak of cyclosporiasis associated with basil in Missouri in 1999. *Clin Infect Dis.* Apr 2001;32(7):1010-1017.
214. Centers for Disease Control and Prevention. Outbreak of cyclosporiasis associated with snow peas—Pennsylvania, 2004. *MMWR Morb Mortal Wkly Rep.* Sep 2004; 53(37):876-878.

215. Soave R. Cyclospora: an overview. *Clin Infect Dis.* Sep 1996;23(3):429-435, quiz 436-427.
216. Hoge CW, Shlim DR, Ghimire M, et al. Placebo-controlled trial of co-trimoxazole for Cyclospora infections among travellers and foreign residents in Nepal. *Lancet.* Mar 1995;345(8951):691-693.
217. Ortega YR, Sterling CR, Gilman RH, et al. Cyclospora species—a new protozoan pathogen of humans. *N Engl J Med.* May 1993;328(18):1308-1312.
218. Eberhard ML, Pieniazek NJ, Arrowood MJ. Laboratory diagnosis of Cyclospora infections. *Arch Pathol Lab Med.* Aug 1997;121(8):792-797.
219. Varma M, Hester JD, Schaefer FW 3rd, et al. Detection of Cyclospora cayetanensis using a quantitative real-time PCR assay. *J Microbiol Methods.* Apr 2003;53(1):27-36.
220. American Academy of Pediatrics. Cyclosporiasis. In: Pickering LK, Baker CJ, Long SS, et al, eds. *Red Book: 2006 Report of the Committee on Infectious Diseases.* 27th ed. Elk Grove Village, IL: American Academy of Pediatrics; 2006.
221. Dubey JP, Lindsay DS, Speer CA. Structures of Toxoplasma gondii tachyzoites, bradyzoites, and sporozoites and biology and development of tissue cysts. *Clin Microbiol Rev.* Apr 1998;11(2):267-299.
222. Tenter AM, Heckeroth AR, Weiss LM. Toxoplasma gondii: from animals to humans. *Int J Parasitol.* Nov 2000; 30(12-13):1217-1258.
223. Jones JL, Kruszon-Moran D, Wilson M, et al. Toxoplasma gondii infection in the United States: seroprevalence and risk factors. *Am J Epidemiol.* Aug 2001;154(4): 357-365.
224. Cook AJ, Gilbert RE, Buffolano W, et al. Sources of toxoplasma infection in pregnant women: European multicentre case-control study. European Research Network on Congenital Toxoplasmosis. *BMJ.* Jul 2000;321(7254):142-147.
225. Bowie WR, King AS, Werker DH, et al. Outbreak of toxoplasmosis associated with municipal drinking water. The BC Toxoplasma Investigation Team. *Lancet.* Jul 1997;350(9072):173-177.
226. Raisanen S. Toxoplasmosis transmitted by blood transfusions. *Transfusion.* May-Jun 1978;18(3):329-332.
227. Saad R, Vincent JF, Cimon B, et al. Pulmonary toxoplasmosis after allogeneic bone marrow transplantation: case report and review. *Bone Marrow Transplant.* Jul 1996;18(1):211-212.
228. Barsoum RS. Parasitic infections in transplant recipients. *Nat Clin Pract Nephrol.* Sep 2006;2(9):490-503.
229. Desmonts G, Couvreur J. Congenital toxoplasmosis. A prospective study of 378 pregnancies. *N Engl J Med.* May 1974;290(20):1110-1116.
230. Dubey JP, Miller NL, Frenkel JK. The Toxoplasma gondii oocyst from cat feces. *J Exp Med.* Oct 1970;132(4):636-662.
231. Black MW, Boothroyd JC. Lytic cycle of Toxoplasma gondii. *Microbiol Mol Biol Rev.* Sep 2000;64(3):607-623.
232. Lyons RE, McLeod R, Roberts CW. Toxoplasma gondii tachyzoite-bradyzoite interconversion. *Trends Parasitol.* May 2002;18(5):198-201.
233. Montoya JG, Liesenfeld O. Toxoplasmosis. *Lancet.* Jun 2004;363(9425):1965-1976.
234. Lynfield R, Guerina NG. Toxoplasmosis. *Pediatr Rev.* Mar 1997;18(3):75-83.
235. Guerina NG. Congenital infection with Toxoplasma gondii. *Pediatr Ann.* Mar 1994;23(3):138-142, 147-151.
236. Lebech M, Joynson DH, Seitz HM, et al. Classification system and case definitions of Toxoplasma gondii infection in immunocompetent pregnant women and their congenitally infected offspring. European Research Network on Congenital Toxoplasmosis. *Eur J Clin Microbiol Infect Dis.* Oct 1996;15(10):799-805.
237. Vutova K, Peicheva Z, Popova A, et al. Congenital toxoplasmosis: eye manifestations in infants and children. *Ann Trop Paediatr.* Sep 2002;22(3):213-218.
238. Safadi MA, Berezin EN, Farhat CK, et al. Clinical presentation and follow up of children with congenital toxoplasmosis in Brazil. *Braz J Infect Dis.* Oct 2003;7(5): 325-331.
239. Swisher CN, Boyer K, McLeod R. Congenital toxoplasmosis. The Toxoplasmosis Study Group. *Semin Pediatr Neurol.* Sep 1994;1(1):4-25.
240. Martin S. Congenital toxoplasmosis. *Neonatal Netw.* Jun 2001;20(4):23-30.
241. Hill D, Dubey JP. Toxoplasma gondii: transmission, diagnosis and prevention. *Clin Microbiol Infect.* Oct 2002;8(10):634-640.
242. Evans AS. Infectious mononucleosis and related syndromes. *Am J Med Sci.* Nov-Dec 1978;276(3):325-339.
243. Holliman RE. Toxoplasmosis and the acquired immune deficiency syndrome. *J Infect.* Mar 1988;16(2):121-128.
244. Porter SB, Sande MA. Toxoplasmosis of the central nervous system in the acquired immunodeficiency syndrome. *N Engl J Med.* Dec 1992;327(23):1643-1648.
245. Luft BJ, Hafner R, Korzun AH, et al. Toxoplasmic encephalitis in patients with the acquired immunodeficiency syndrome. Members of the ACTG 077p/ANRS 009 Study Team. *N Engl J Med.* Sep 1993;329(14):995-1000.
246. Charles PE, Doise JM, Quenot JP, et al. An unusual cause of acute respiratory distress in a patient with AIDS: primary infection with Toxoplasma gondii. *Scand J Infect Dis.* 2003;35(11-12):901-902.
247. Bergin C, Murphy M, Lyons D, et al. Toxoplasma pneumonitis: fatal presentation of disseminated toxoplasmosis in a patient with AIDS. *Eur Respir J.* Sep 1992;5(8): 1018-1020.
248. Bonfioli AA, Orefice F. Toxoplasmosis. *Semin Ophthalmol.* Jul-Sep 2005;20(3):129-141.
249. Montoya JG, Remington JS. Toxoplasmic chorioretinitis in the setting of acute acquired toxoplasmosis. *Clin Infect Dis.* Aug 1996;23(2):277-282.
250. Holland GN. Reconsidering the pathogenesis of ocular toxoplasmosis. *Am J Ophthalmol.* Oct 1999;128(4): 502-505.
251. Perkins ES. Ocular toxoplasmosis. *Br J Ophthalmol.* Jan 1973;57(1):1-17.
252. Perry DD, Merritt JC. Congenital ocular toxoplasmosis. *J Natl Med Assoc.* Feb 1983;75(2):169-174.
253. Mets MB, Holfels E, Boyer KM, et al. Eye manifestations of congenital toxoplasmosis. *Am J Ophthalmol.* Jan 1997; 123(1):1-16.
254. Vidal JE, Colombo FA, de Oliveira AC, et al. PCR assay using cerebrospinal fluid for diagnosis of cerebral toxoplasmosis in Brazilian AIDS patients. *J Clin Microbiol.* Oct 2004;42(10):4765-4768.
255. Roberts A, Hedman K, Luyasu V, et al. Multicenter evaluation of strategies for serodiagnosis of primary infection with Toxoplasma gondii. *Eur J Clin Microbiol Infect Dis.* Jul 2001;20(7):467-474.
256. Pinon JM, Toubas D, Marx C, et al. Detection of specific immunoglobulin E in patients with toxoplasmosis. *J Clin Microbiol.* Aug 1990;28(8):1739-1743.
257. Montoya JG, Liesenfeld O, Kinney S, et al. VIDAS test for avidity of Toxoplasma-specific immunoglobulin G for confirmatory testing of pregnant women. *J Clin Microbiol.* Jul 2002;40(7):2504-2508.
258. Remington JS, Thulliez P, Montoya JG. Recent developments for diagnosis of toxoplasmosis. *J Clin Microbiol.* Mar 2004;42(3):941-945.
259. Rorman E, Zamir CS, Rilkis I, et al. Congenital toxoplasmosis—prenatal aspects of Toxoplasma gondii infection. *Reprod Toxicol.* May 2006;21(4):458-472.

260. Hohlfeld P, Daffos F, Costa JM, et al. Prenatal diagnosis of congenital toxoplasmosis with a polymerase-chain-reaction test on amniotic fluid. *N Engl J Med.* Sep 1994; 331(11):695-699.
261. Derouin F, Thulliez P, Candolfi E, et al. Early prenatal diagnosis of congenital toxoplasmosis using amniotic fluid samples and tissue culture. *Eur J Clin Microbiol Infect Dis.* Jun 1988;7(3):423-425.
262. Crino JP. Ultrasound and fetal diagnosis of perinatal infection. *Clin Obstet Gynecol.* Mar 1999;42(1):71-80, quiz 174-175.
263. Pinon JM, Dumon H, Chemla C, et al. Strategy for diagnosis of congenital toxoplasmosis: evaluation of methods comparing mothers and newborns and standard methods for postnatal detection of immunoglobulin G, M, and A antibodies. *J Clin Microbiol.* Jun 2001;39(6): 2267-2271.
264. Gupta RK. Fine needle aspiration cytodiagnosis of toxoplasmic lymphadenitis. *Acta Cytol.* Jul-Aug 1997;41(4): 1031-1034.
265. Julander I, Martin C, Lappalainen M, et al. Polymerase chain reaction for diagnosis of cerebral toxoplasmosis in cerebrospinal fluid in HIV-positive patients. *Scand J Infect Dis.* 2001;33(7):538-541.
266. Holland GN, Lewis KG. An update on current practices in the management of ocular toxoplasmosis. *Am J Ophthalmol.* Jul 2002;134(1):102-114.
267. American Academy of Pediatrics. Toxoplasma gondii infections (toxoplasmosis). In: Pickering LK, Baker CJ, Long SS, et al, eds. *Red Book: 2006 Report of the Committee on Infectious Diseases.* 27th ed. Elk Grove Village, IL: American Academy of Pediatrics; 2006.
268. Decker CF, Tuazon CU. Toxoplasmosis: an update on clinical and therapeutic aspects. *Prog Clin Parasitol.* 1993;3:21-41.
269. Dannemann B, McCutchan JA, Israelski D, et al. Treatment of toxoplasmic encephalitis in patients with AIDS. A randomized trial comparing pyrimethamine plus clindamycin to pyrimethamine plus sulfadiazine. The California Collaborative Treatment Group. *Ann Intern Med.* Jan 1992;116(1):33-43.
270. Kaplan JE, Masur H, Holmes KK. Guidelines for preventing opportunistic infections among HIV-infected persons—2002. Recommendations of the US Public Health Service and the Infectious Diseases Society of America. *MMWR Recomm Rep.* Jun 2002;51(RR-8): 1-52.
271. Chirgwin K, Hafner R, Leport C, et al. Randomized phase II trial of atovaquone with pyrimethamine or sulfadiazine for treatment of toxoplasmic encephalitis in patients with acquired immunodeficiency syndrome: ACTG 237/ANRS 039 study. AIDS Clinical Trials Group 237/Agence Nationale de Recherche sur le SIDA, Essai 039. *Clin Infect Dis.* May 2002;34(9):1243-1250.
272. Lopez A, Dietz VJ, Wilson M, et al. Preventing congenital toxoplasmosis. *MMWR Recomm Rep.* Mar 2000; 49(RR-2):59-68.
273. Snow RW, Craig MH, Newton CRJC, et al. *The Public Health Burden of Plasmodium falciparum Malaria in Africa: Deriving the Numbers.* Bethesda, MD: Fogarthy International Center, National Institues of Health; 2003. Working Paper No. 11, Disease Control Priorities Project.
274. Snow RW, Korenromp EL, Gouws E. Pediatric mortality in Africa: plasmodium falciparum malaria as a cause or risk? *Am J Trop Med Hyg.* Aug 2004;71 (2 suppl):16-24.
275. Suh KN, Keystone JS. Malaria and babesiosis. In: Gorbach SL, Bartlett JG, Blacklow NR, eds. *Infectious Diseases.* 3rd ed: Philadelphia, PA: WB Saunders; 2004.
276. Keller CC, Davenport GC, Dickman KR, et al. Suppression of prostaglandin E2 by malaria parasite products and antipyretics promotes overproduction of tumor necrosis factor-alpha: association with the pathogenesis of childhood malarial anemia. *J Infect Dis.* May 2006; 193(10):1384-1393.
277. Keller CC, Yamo O, Ouma C, et al. Acquisition of hemozoin by monocytes down-regulates interleukin-12 p40 (IL-12p40) transcripts and circulating IL-12p70 through an IL-10-dependent mechanism: in vivo and in vitro findings in severe malarial anemia. *Infect Immun.* Sep 2006;74(9):5249-5260.
278. Newton CR, Hien TT, White N. Cerebral malaria. *J Neurol Neurosurg Psychiatry.* Oct 2000;69(4):433-441.
279. Bull PC, Kortok M, Kai O, et al. Plasmodium falciparum-infected erythrocytes: agglutination by diverse Kenyan plasma is associated with severe disease and young host age. *J Infect Dis.* Jul 2000;182(1):252-259.
280. Craig A, Scherf A. Molecules on the surface of the Plasmodium falciparum infected erythrocyte and their role in malaria pathogenesis and immune evasion. *Mol Biochem Parasitol.* Jul 2001;115(2):129-143.
281. Lindenthal C, Kremsner PG, Klinkert MQ. Commonly recognised Plasmodium falciparum parasites cause cerebral malaria. *Parasitol Res.* Nov 2003;91(5):363-368.
282. Newbold C, Warn P, Black G, et al. Receptor-specific adhesion and clinical disease in Plasmodium falciparum. *Am J Trop Med Hyg.* Oct 1997;57(4):389-398.
283. Clark IA, Awburn MM, Whitten RO, et al. Tissue distribution of migration inhibitory factor and inducible nitric oxide synthase in falciparum malaria and sepsis in African children. *Malar J.* Apr 2003;2:6.
284. Clark IA, Rockett KA, Cowden WB. Possible central role of nitric oxide in conditions clinically similar to cerebral malaria. *Lancet.* Oct 1992;340(8824):894-896.
285. Cramer JP, Nussler AK, Ehrhardt S, et al. Age-dependent effect of plasma nitric oxide on parasite density in Ghanaian children with severe malaria. *Trop Med Int Health.* Jul 2005;10(7):672-680.
286. Svenson JE, MacLean JD, Gyorkos TW, et al. Imported malaria. Clinical presentation and examination of symptomatic travelers. *Arch Intern Med.* Apr 1995;155(8): 861-868.
287. World Health Organization, Communicable Diseases Cluster. Severe falciparum malaria. *Trans R Soc Trop Med Hyg.* Apr 2000;94(suppl 1):S1-S90.
288. Idro R, Jenkins NE, Newton CR. Pathogenesis, clinical features, and neurological outcome of cerebral malaria. *Lancet Neurol.* Dec 2005;4(12):827-840.
289. Newton CR, Krishna S. Severe falciparum malaria in children: current understanding of pathophysiology and supportive treatment. *Pharmacol Ther.* Jul 1998; 79(1):1-53.
290. Marques HH, Vallada MG, Sakane PT, et al. [Congenital Malaria. Case reports and a brief review of literature]. *J Pediatr (Rio J).* Mar-Apr 1996;72(2):103-105.
291. Wiwanitkit V. Congenital malaria in Thailand, an appraisal of previous cases. *Pediatr Int.* Dec 2006;48(6): 562-565.
292. World Health Organization. *Malaria Diagnosis—New Perspectives. Report of a Joint WHO/USAID Informal Consultation.* Geneva, Switzerland: World Health Organization; 1999.
293. American Academy of Pediatrics. Malaria. In: Pickering LK, Baker CJ, Long SS, et al, eds. *Red Book: 2006 Report of the Committee on Infectious Diseases.* 27th ed. Elk Grove Village, IL: American Academy of Pediatrics; 2006.
294. Mirdha BR, Samantray JC, Burman D, et al. Quantitative buffy coat: a special adjunct for diagnosis of malaria. *J Commun Dis.* Mar 1999;31(1):19-22.

295. Noedl H, Yingyuen K, Laoboonchai A, et al. Sensitivity and specificity of an antigen detection ELISA for malaria diagnosis. *Am J Trop Med Hyg.* Dec 2006;75(6): 1205-1208.
296. Forney JR, Magill AJ, Wongsrichanalai C, et al. Malaria rapid diagnostic devices: performance characteristics of the ParaSight F device determined in a multisite field study. *J Clin Microbiol.* Aug 2001;39(8):2884-2890.
297. Forney JR, Wongsrichanalai C, Magill AJ, et al. Devices for rapid diagnosis of malaria: evaluation of prototype assays that detect Plasmodium falciparum histidine-rich protein 2 and a Plasmodium vivax-specific antigen. *J Clin Microbiol.* Jun 2003;41(6):2358-2366.
298. Iqbal J, Khalid N, Hira PR. Comparison of two commercial assays with expert microscopy for confirmation of symptomatically diagnosed malaria. *J Clin Microbiol.* Dec 2002;40(12):4675-4678.
299. Iqbal J, Sher A, Hira PR, et al. Comparison of the OptiMAL test with PCR for diagnosis of malaria in immigrants. *J Clin Microbiol.* Nov 1999;37(11):3644-3646.
300. Johnston SP, Pieniazek NJ, Xayavong MV, et al. PCR as a confirmatory technique for laboratory diagnosis of malaria. *J Clin Microbiol.* Mar 2006;44(3): 1087-1089.
301. World Health Organization. Guidelines for the Treatment of Malaria/World Health Organization. Available at: http://www.who.int/malaria/docs/treatmentguidelines2006.pdf. Accessed April 6, 2007.
302. US Department of Health and Human Services, Centers for Diseases Control and Prevention. Treatment of Malaria (Guidelines for Clinicians). March 7, 2006. Available at: www.cdc.gov/malaria/diagnosis_treatment/tx_clinicians.htm. Accessed April 6, 2007.
303. Jiao X, Liu GY, Shan CO, et al. Phase II trial in China of a new, rapidly-acting and effective oral antimalarial, CGP 56697, for the treatment of Plasmodium falciparum malaria. *Southeast Asian J Trop Med Public Health.* Sep 1997;28(3):476-481.
304. Lefevre G, Looareesuwan S, Treeprasertsuk S, et al. A clinical and pharmacokinetic trial of six doses of artemether-lumefantrine for multidrug-resistant Plasmodium falciparum malaria in Thailand. *Am J Trop Med Hyg.* May-Jun 2001;64(5-6):247-256.
305. Piola P, Fogg C, Bajunirwe F, et al. Supervised versus unsupervised intake of six-dose artemether-lumefantrine for treatment of acute, uncomplicated Plasmodium falciparum malaria in Mbarara, Uganda: a randomised trial. *Lancet.* Apr 2005;365(9469):1467-1473.
306. van Vugt M, Looareesuwan S, Wilairatana P, et al. Artemether-lumefantrine for the treatment of multi-drug-resistant falciparum malaria. *Trans R Soc Trop Med Hyg.* Sep-Oct 2000;94(5):545-548.
307. Vugt MV, Wilairatana P, Gemperli B, et al. Efficacy of six doses of artemether-lumefantrine (benflumetol) in multidrug-resistant Plasmodium falciparum malaria. *Am J Trop Med Hyg.* Jun 1999;60(6):936-942.
308. Rampengan TH. Cerebral malaria in children. Comparative study between heparin, dexamethasone and placebo. *Paediatr Indones.* Jan-Feb 1991;31(1-2):59-66.
309. Warrell DA, Looareesuwan S, Warrell MJ, et al. Dexamethasone proves deleterious in cerebral malaria. A double-blind trial in 100 comatose patients. *N Engl J Med.* Feb 1982;306(6):313-319.
310. US Department of Health and Human Services, Centers of Disease Control and Prevention. Traveller's Health-Yellow Book: Health Information for International Travel, 2005-2006, Prevention of Specific Infectious Diseases [Malaria]. Available at: www2.ncid.cdc.gov/travel/yb/utils/ybget.asp?section=dis&obj=index.htm&cssnav=browseoyb. Accessed April 10, 2007.
311. World Health Organization. Strategic Orientation Paper on Prevention and Control of Malaria, for National and International Programme Officers Involved in Malaria Control at Country Level. Available at: www.who.int/malaria/docs/trainingcourses/nporeport.pdf. Accessed April 1, 2007.
312. Brogdon WG, McAllister JC. Insecticide resistance and vector control. *Emerg Infect Dis.* Oct-Dec 1998;4(4): 605-613.
313. Good MF. Vaccine-induced immunity to malaria parasites and the need for novel strategies. *Trends Parasitol.* Jan 2005;21(1):29-34.
314. US Department of Health and Human Services, National Institutes of Health. The Jordan Report, 20th Anniversary, Accelerated Development of Vaccines 2002. Available at: www.niaid.nih.gov/dmid/vaccines/jordan20/jordan20_2002.pdf. Accessed April 1, 2007.
315. Quick RE, Herwaldt BL, Thomford JW, et al. Babesiosis in Washington State: a new species of Babesia? *Ann Intern Med.* Aug 1993;119(4):284-290.
316. Herwaldt B, Persing DH, Precigout EA, et al. A fatal case of babesiosis in Missouri: identification of another piroplasm that infects humans. *Ann Intern Med.* Apr 1996;124(7):643-650.
317. Persing DH, Herwaldt BL, Glaser C, et al. Infection with a babesia-like organism in northern California. *N Engl J Med.* Feb 1995;332(5):298-303.
318. Piesman J, Mather TN, Donahue JG, et al. Comparative prevalence of Babesia microti and Borrelia burgdorferi in four populations of Ixodes dammini in eastern Massachusetts. *Acta Trop.* Sep 1986;43(3):263-270.
319. Spielman A. Human babesiosis on Nantucket Island: transmission by nymphal Ixodes ticks. *Am J Trop Med Hyg.* Nov 1976;25(6):784-787.
320. Herwaldt BL, Neitzel DF, Gorlin JB, et al. Transmission of Babesia microti in Minnesota through four blood donations from the same donor over a 6-month period. *Transfusion.* Sep 2002;42(9):1154-1158.
321. New DL, Quinn JB, Qureshi MZ, et al. Vertically transmitted babesiosis. *J Pediatr.* Jul 1997;131(1 pt 1): 163-164.
322. Gorenflot A, Moubri K, Precigout E, et al. Human babesiosis. *Ann Trop Med Parasitol.* Jun 1998;92(4):489-501.
323. Boustani MR, Gelfand JA. Babesiosis. *Clin Infect Dis.* Apr 1996;22(4):611-615.
324. Healy GR, Speilman A, Gleason N. Human babesiosis: reservoir in infection on Nantucket Island. *Science.* Apr 1976;192(4238):479-480.
325. Eskow ES, Krause PJ, Spielman A, et al. Southern extension of the range of human babesiosis in the eastern United States. *J Clin Microbiol.* Jun 1999;37(6):2051-2052.
326. Meldrum SC, Birkhead GS, White DJ, et al. Human babesiosis in New York State: an epidemiological description of 136 cases. *Clin Infect Dis.* Dec 1992;15(6): 1019-1023.
327. Villar BF, White DJ, Benach JL. Human babesiosis. *Prog Clin Parasitol.* 1991;2:129-143.
328. Ruebush TK 2nd, Juranek DD, Spielman A, et al. Epidemiology of human babesiosis on Nantucket Island. *Am J Trop Med Hyg.* Sep 1981;30(5):937-941.
329. Olmeda AS, Armstrong PM, Rosenthal BM, et al. A subtropical case of human babesiosis. *Acta Trop.* Sep 1997; 67(3):229-234.
330. Sun T, Tenenbaum MJ, Greenspan J, et al. Morphologic and clinical observations in human infection with Babesia microti. *J Infect Dis.* Aug 1983;148(2):239-248.
331. Anderson AE, Cassaday PB, Healy GR. Babesiosis in man. Sixth documented case. *Am J Clin Pathol.* Nov 1974;62(5):612-618.

332. Wright IG, Goodger BV, Buffington GD, et al. Immunopathophysiology of babesial infections. *Trans R Soc Trop Med Hyg.* 1989;83(suppl):11-13.
333. Hemmer RM, Wozniak EJ, Lowenstine LJ, et al. Endothelial cell changes are associated with pulmonary edema and respiratory distress in mice infected with the WA1 human Babesia parasite. *J Parasitol.* Jun 1999; 85(3):479-489.
334. Shaio MF, Lin PR. A case study of cytokine profiles in acute human babesiosis. *Am J Trop Med Hyg.* Mar 1998;58(3):335-337.
335. Igarashi I, Suzuki R, Waki S, et al. Roles of CD4(+) T cells and gamma interferon in protective immunity against Babesia microti infection in mice. *Infect Immun.* Aug 1999;67(8):4143-4148.
336. Ruebush TK 2nd, Juranek DD, Chisholm ES, et al. Human babesiosis on Nantucket Island. Evidence for self-limited and subclinical infections. *N Engl J Med.* Oct 1977;297(15):825-827.
337. Ruebush TK 2nd. Human babesiosis in North America. *Trans R Soc Trop Med Hyg.* 1980;74(2):149-152.
338. Krause PJ, Telford SR 3rd, Spielman A, et al. Concurrent Lyme disease and babesiosis. Evidence for increased severity and duration of illness. *JAMA.* Jun 1996;275(21): 1657-1660.
339. Falagas ME, Klempner MS. Babesiosis in patients with AIDS: a chronic infection presenting as fever of unknown origin. *Clin Infect Dis.* May 1996;22(5):809-812.
340. Jacoby GA, Hunt JV, Kosinski KS, et al. Treatment of transfusion-transmitted babesiosis by exchange transfusion. *N Engl J Med.* Nov 1980;303(19):1098-1100.
341. Cahill KM, Benach JL, Reich LM, et al. Red cell exchange: treatment of babesiosis in a splenectomized patient. *Transfusion.* Mar-Apr 1981;21(2):193-198.
342. Healy GR, Ruebush TK 2nd. Morphology of Babesia microti in human blood smears. *Am J Clin Pathol.* Jan 1980;73(1):107-109.
343. Chisholm ES, Ruebush TK 2nd, Sulzer AJ, et al. Babesia microti infection in man: evaluation of an indirect immunofluorescent antibody test. *Am J Trop Med Hyg.* Jan 1978;27(1 pt 1):14-19.
344. Krause PJ, Telford S 3rd, Spielman A, et al. Comparison of PCR with blood smear and inoculation of small animals for diagnosis of Babesia microti parasitemia. *J Clin Microbiol.* Nov 1996;34(11):2791-2794.
345. American Academy of Pediatrics. Babesiosis. In: Pickering LK, Baker CJ, Long SS, et al, eds. *Red Book: 2006 Report of the Committee on Infectious Diseases.* 27th ed. Elk Grove Village, IL: American Academy of Pediatrics; 2006.
346. Murrell KD, Pozio E. Trichinellosis: the zoonosis that won't go quietly. *Int J Parasitol.* Nov 2000;30(12-13): 1339-1349.
347. Murrell KD, Bruschi F. Clinical trichinellosis. *Prog Clin Parasitol.* 1994;4:117-150.
348. Moorhead A, Grunenwald PE, Dietz VJ, et al. Trichinellosis in the United States, 1991-1996: declining but not gone. *Am J Trop Med Hyg.* Jan 1999;60(1):66-69.
349. Centers for Disease Control and Prevention. Trichinellosis associated with bear meat—New York and Tennessee, 2003. *MMWR Morb Mortal Wkly Rep.* Jul 2004; 53(27):606-610.
350. MacLean JD, Poirier L, Gyorkos TW, et al. Epidemiologic and serologic definition of primary and secondary trichinosis in the Arctic. *J Infect Dis.* May 1992;165(5): 908-912.
351. Ancelle T, Dupouy-Camet J, Desenclos JC, et al. A multifocal outbreak of trichinellosis linked to horse meat imported from North America to France in 1993. *Am J Trop Med Hyg.* Oct 1998;59(4):615-619.
352. Stewart GL, Despommier DD, Burnham J, et al. Trichinella spiralis: behavior, structure, and biochemistry of larvae following exposure to components of the host enteric environment. *Exp Parasitol.* Apr 1987;63(2): 195-204.
353. Wright KA. Trichinella spiralis: an intracellular parasite in the intestinal phase. *J Parasitol.* Jun 1979;65(3): 441-445.
354. Capo V, Despommier DD. Clinical aspects of infection with Trichinella spp. *Clin Microbiol Rev.* Jan 1996;9(1): 47-54.
355. Bruschi F, Murrell KD. New aspects of human trichinellosis: the impact of new Trichinella species. *Postgrad Med J.* Jan 2002;78(915):15-22.
356. Kociecka W. Trichinellosis: human disease, diagnosis and treatment. *Vet Parasitol.* Dec 2000;93(3-4): 365-383.
357. Pozio E, Gomez Morales MA, Dupouy-Camet J. Clinical aspects, diagnosis and treatment of trichinellosis. *Expert Rev Anti Infect Ther.* Oct 2003;1(3):471-482.
358. Compton SJ, Celum CL, Lee C, et al. Trichinosis with ventilatory failure and persistent myocarditis. *Clin Infect Dis.* Apr 1993;16(4):500-504.
359. Mawhorter SD, Kazura JW. Trichinosis of the central nervous system. *Semin Neurol.* Jun 1993;13(2):148-152.
360. Taratuto AL, Venturiello SM. Trichinosis. *Brain Pathol.* Jan 1997;7(1):663-672.
361. Gomez-Priego A, Crecencio-Rosales L, de-La-Rosa JL. Serological evaluation of thin-layer immunoassay-enzyme-linked immunosorbent assay for antibody detection in human trichinellosis. *Clin Diagn Lab Immunol.* Sep 2000;7(5):810-812.
362. Clausen MR, Meyer CN, Krantz T, et al. Trichinella infection and clinical disease. *Qjm.* Aug 1996;89(8): 631-636.
363. Wu Z, Nagano I, Pozio E, et al. Polymerase chain reaction-restriction fragment length polymorphism (PCR-RFLP) for the identification of Trichinella isolates. *Parasitology.* Feb 1999;118 (pt 2):211-218.
364. American Academy of Pediatrics. Trichinellosis (Trichinella spiralis). In: Pickering LK, Baker CJ, Long SS, et al, eds. *Red Book: 2006 Report of the Committee on Infectious Diseases.* 27th ed. Elk Grove Village, IL: American Academy of Pediatrics; 2006.
365. Pozio E, Sacchini D, Sacchi L, et al. Failure of mebendazole in the treatment of humans with Trichinella spiralis infection at the stage of encapsulating larvae. *Clin Infect Dis.* Feb 2001;32(4):638-642.
366. Pozio E, La Rosa G, Rossi P, et al. Biological characterization of Trichinella isolates from various host species and geographical regions. *J Parasitol.* Aug 1992;78(4): 647-653.
367. Bundy DA, Cooper ES. Trichuris and trichuriasis in humans. *Adv Parasitol.* 1989;28:107-173.
368. Bundy DA. Epidemiological aspects of Trichuris and trichuriasis in Caribbean communities. *Trans R Soc Trop Med Hyg.* 1986;80(5):706-718.
369. Stephenson LS, Holland CV, Cooper ES. The public health significance of Trichuris trichiura. *Parasitology.* 2000;121(suppl):S73-S95.
370. Hargus EP, Lepow M, Lau T, et al. Intestinal parasitosis in childhood populations of Latin origin. Lessons from a survey of 129 such children in Hartford Connecticut. *Clin Pediatr (Phila).* Oct 1976;15(10):927-929.
371. Cappello M, Hotez PJ. Intestinal nematodes. In: Long SS, Pickering LK, Prober CG, eds. *Principles and Practice of Pediatric Infectious Diseases.* 2nd ed. New York, NY: Churchill Livingstone; 2003.
372. Wolfe MS. Oxyuris, Trichostrongylus and trichuris. *Clin Gastroenterol.* Jan 1978;7(1):201-217.

373. Trichuriasis. In: Sun T, ed. *Parasitic Disorders: Pathology, Diagnosis, and Management.* 2nd ed. Baltimore, MD: Williams & Wilkins; 1999.
374. Bahon J, Poirriez J, Creusy C, et al. Colonic obstruction and perforation related to heavy Trichuris trichiura infestation. *J Clin Pathol.* Jul 1997;50(7):615-616.
375. Bowie MD, Morison A, Ireland JD, et al. Clubbing and whipworm infestation. *Arch Dis Child.* May 1978;53(5): 411-413.
376. Nokes C, Grantham-McGregor SM, Sawyer AW, et al. Moderate to heavy infections of Trichuris trichiura affect cognitive function in Jamaican school children. *Parasitology.* Jun 1992;104 (pt 3):539-547.
377. Forrester JE, Bailar JC III, Esrey SA, et al. Randomised trial of albendazole and pyrantel in symptomless trichuriasis in children. *Lancet.* Oct 1998;352(9134): 1103-1108.
378. American Academy of Pediatrics. Trichuriasis (whipworm infection). In: Pickering LK, Baker CJ, Long SS, et al, eds. *Red Book: 2006 Report of the Committee on Infectious Diseases.* 27th ed. Elk Grove Village, IL: American Academy of Pediatrics; 2006.
379. Juan JO, Lopez Chegne N, Gargala G, et al. Comparative clinical studies of nitazoxanide, albendazole and praziquantel in the treatment of ascariasis, trichuriasis and hymenolepiasis in children from Peru. *Trans R Soc Trop Med Hyg.* Mar-Apr 2002;96(2):193-196.
380. Bundy DA, de Silva NR. Can we deworm this wormy world? *Br Med Bull.* 1998;54(2):421-432.
381. Scowden EB, Schaffner W, Stone WJ. Overwhelming strongyloidiasis: an unappreciated opportunistic infection. *Medicine (Baltimore).* Nov 1978;57(6):527-544.
382. Barnish G, Ashford RW. Strongyloides cf. fuelleborni and hookworm in Papua New Guinea: patterns of infection within the community. *Trans R Soc Trop Med Hyg.* Sep-Oct 1989;83(5):684-688.
383. Kitchen LW, Tu KK, Kerns FT. Strongyloides-infected patients at Charleston area medical center, West Virginia, 1997-1998. *Clin Infect Dis.* Sep 2000;31(3):E5-E6.
384. Seybolt LM, Christiansen D, Barnett ED. Diagnostic evaluation of newly arrived asymptomatic refugees with eosinophilia. *Clin Infect Dis.* Feb 2006;42(3):363-367.
385. Walzer PD, Milder JE, Banwell JG, et al. Epidemiologic features of Strongyloides stercoralis infection in an endemic area of the United States. *Am J Trop Med Hyg.* Mar 1982;31(2):313-319.
386. Chu E, Whitlock WL, Dietrich RA. Pulmonary hyperinfection syndrome with Strongyloides stercoralis. *Chest.* Jun 1990;97(6):1475-1477.
387. Fardet L, Genereau T, Cabane J, et al. Severe strongyloidiasis in corticosteroid-treated patients. *Clin Microbiol Infect.* Oct 2006;12(10):945-947.
388. Lam CS, Tong MK, Chan KM, et al. Disseminated strongyloidiasis: a retrospective study of clinical course and outcome. *Eur J Clin Microbiol Infect Dis.* Jan 2006; 25(1):14-18.
389. Meinking TL, Burkhart CN, Burkhart CG. Changing paradigms in parasitic infections: common dermatological helminthic infections and cutaneous myiasis. *Clin Dermatol.* Sep-Oct 2003;21(5):407-416.
390. Velasco A, Sanchez F, de la Coba C, et al. [Malabsorption syndrome due to Strongyloides stercoralis associated with Loeffler syndrome in a 29-year-old woman]. *Gastroenterol Hepatol.* Jun-Jul 2006;29(6):341-344.
391. Burke JA. Strongyloidiasis in childhood. *Am J Dis Child.* Nov 1978;132(11):1130-1136.
392. Gotuzzo E, Terashima A, Alvarez H, et al. Strongyloides stercoralis hyperinfection associated with human T cell lymphotropic virus type-1 infection in Peru. *Am J Trop Med Hyg.* Jan 1999;60(1):146-149.
393. Cappello M, Hotez PJ. Disseminated strongyloidiasis. *Semin Neurol.* Jun 1993;13(2):169-174.
394. Dreyer G, Fernandes-Silva E, Alves S, et al. Patterns of detection of Strongyloides stercoralis in stool specimens: implications for diagnosis and clinical trials. *J Clin Microbiol.* Oct 1996;34(10):2569-2571.
395. Thompson BF, Fry LC, Wells CD, et al. The spectrum of GI strongyloidiasis: an endoscopic-pathologic study. *Gastrointest Endosc.* Jun 2004;59(7):906-910.
396. Neva FA, Gam AA, Burke J. Comparison of larval antigens in an enzyme-linked immunosorbent assay for strongyloidiasis in humans. *J Infect Dis.* Nov 1981;144(5): 427-432.
397. Loutfy MR, Wilson M, Keystone JS, et al. Serology and eosinophil count in the diagnosis and management of strongyloidiasis in a non-endemic area. *Am J Trop Med Hyg.* Jun 2002;66(6):749-752.
398. Igra-Siegman Y, Kapila R, Sen P, et al. Syndrome of hyperinfection with Strongyloides stercoralis. *Rev Infect Dis.* May-Jun 1981;3(3):397-407.
399. Takayanagui OM, Lofrano MM, Araugo MB, et al. Detection of Strongyloides stercoralis in the cerebrospinal fluid of a patient with acquired immunodeficiency syndrome. *Neurology.* Jan 1995;45(1):193-194.
400. American Academy of Pediatrics. Strongyloidiasis (strongyloides stercoralis). In: Pickering LK, Baker CJ, Long SS, et al, eds. *Red Book: 2006 Report of the Committee on Infectious Diseases.* 27th ed. Elk Grove Village, IL: American Academy of Pediatrics; 2006.
401. Igual-Adell R, Oltra-Alcaraz C, Soler-Company E, et al. Efficacy and safety of ivermectin and thiabendazole in the treatment of strongyloidiasis. *Expert Opin Pharmacother.* Dec 2004;5(12):2615-2619.
402. Torres JR, Isturiz R, Murillo J, et al. Efficacy of ivermectin in the treatment of strongyloidiasis complicating AIDS. *Clin Infect Dis.* Nov 1993;17(5):900-902.
403. Hotez PJ, Brooker S, Bethony JM, et al. Hookworm infection. *N Engl J Med.* Aug 2004;351(8):799-807.
404. Hookworm disease. In: Sun T, ed. *Parasitic Disorders: Pathology, Diagnosis, and Management.* 2nd ed. Baltimore, MD: Williams & Wilkins; 1990.
405. Hawdon JM, Hotez PJ. Hookworm: developmental biology of the infectious process. *Curr Opin Genet Dev.* Oct 1996;6(5):618-623.
406. Beaver PC. Light, long-lasting Necator infection in a volunteer. *Am J Trop Med Hyg.* Oct 1988;39(4):369-372.
407. Nutman TB, Ottesen EA, Ieng S, et al. Eosinophilia in Southeast Asian refugees: evaluation at a referral center. *J Infect Dis.* Feb 1987;155(2):309-313.
408. Maxwell C, Hussain R, Nutman TB, et al. The clinical and immunologic responses of normal human volunteers to low dose hookworm (Necator americanus) infection. *Am J Trop Med Hyg.* Jul 1987;37(1):126-134.
409. Hotez PJ, Pritchard DI. Hookworm infection. *Sci Am.* Jun 1995;272(6):68-74.
410. Stoltzfus RJ, Dreyfuss ML, Chwaya HM, et al. Hookworm control as a strategy to prevent iron deficiency. *Nutr Rev.* Jun 1997;55(6):223-232.
411. Albonico M, Stoltzfus RJ, Savioli L, et al. Epidemiological evidence for a differential effect of hookworm species, Ancylostoma duodenale or Necator americanus, on iron status of children. *Int J Epidemiol.* Jun 1998; 27(3):530-537.
412. Friis H, Mwaniki D, Omondi B, et al. Effects on haemoglobin of multi-micronutrient supplementation and multi-helminth chemotherapy: a randomized, controlled trial in Kenyan school children. *Eur J Clin Nutr.* Apr 2003;57(4):573-579.

413. Hawdon JM. Differentiation between the human hookworms Ancylostoma duodenale and Necator americanus using PCR-RFLP. *J Parasitol.* Aug 1996;82(4):642-647.
414. American Academy of Pediatrics. Hookworm infection (Ancylostoma duodenale and Necator americanus). In: Pickering LK, Baker CJ, Long SS, et al, eds. *Red Book: 2006 Report of the Committee on Infectious Diseases.* 27th ed. Elk Grove Village, IL: American Academy of Pediatrics; 2006.
415. Udonsi JK, Ogan VN. Assessment of the effectiveness of primary health care interventions in the control of three intestinal nematode infections in rural communities. *Public Health.* Jan 1993;107(1):53-60.
416. Brenner MA, Patel MB. Cutaneous larva migrans: the creeping eruption. *Cutis.* Aug 2003;72(2):111-115.
417. Sherman SC, Radford N. Severe infestation of cutaneous larva migrans. *J Emerg Med.* Apr 2004;26(3):347-349.
418. Santarem VA, Giuffrida R, Zanin GA. [Cutaneous larva migrans: reports of pediatric cases and contamination by Ancylostoma spp larvae in public parks in Taciba, Sao Paulo State]. *Rev Soc Bras Med Trop.* Mar-Apr 2004;37(2):179-181.
419. French SJ, Lindo JF. Severe cutaneous larva migrans in a traveler to Jamaica, West Indies. *J Travel Med.* Jul-Aug 2003;10(4):249-250.
420. Caumes E, Carriere J, Guermonprez G, et al. Dermatoses associated with travel to tropical countries: a prospective study of the diagnosis and management of 269 patients presenting to a tropical disease unit. *Clin Infect Dis.* Mar 1995;20(3):542-548.
421. American Academy of Pediatrics. Cutaneous larva migrans. In: Pickering LK, Baker CJ, Long SS, et al, eds. *Red Book: 2006 Report of the Committee on Infectious Diseases.* 27th ed. Elk Grove Village, IL: American Academy of Pediatrics; 2006.
422. Jelinek T, Maiwald H, Nothdurft HD, et al. Cutaneous larva migrans in travelers: synopsis of histories, symptoms, and treatment of 98 patients. *Clin Infect Dis.* Dec 1994;19(6):1062-1066.
423. Caumes E, Danis M. From creeping eruption to hookworm-related cutaneous larva migrans. *Lancet Infect Dis.* Nov 2004;4(11):659-660.
424. Del Giudice P, Desalvador F, Bernard E, et al. Loeffler's syndrome and cutaneous larva migrans: a rare association. *Br J Dermatol.* Aug 2002;147(2):386-388.
425. Leicht SS, Youngberg GA. Cutaneous larva migrans. *Am Fam Physician.* Jun 1987;35(6):163-168.
426. Chitkara RK, Krishna G. Parasitic pulmonary eosinophilia. *Semin Respir Crit Care Med.* Apr 2006;27(2):171-184.
427. Cook GC. Enterobius vermicularis infection. *Gut.* Sep 1994;35(9):1159-1162.
428. Kucik CJ, Martin GL, Sortor BV. Common intestinal parasites. *Am Fam Physician.* Mar 2004;69(5):1161-1168.
429. Enterobiasis. In: Sun T, ed. *Parasitic Disorders: Pathology, Diagnosis, and Management.* 2nd ed. Baltimore, MD: Williams & Wilkins; 1999.
430. Mattia AR. Perianal mass and recurrent cellulitis due to Enterobius vermicularis. *Am J Trop Med Hyg.* Dec 1992; 47(6):811-815.
431. MacPherson DW. Intestinal parasites in returned travelers. *Med Clin North Am.* Jul 1999;83(4):1053-1075.
432. Knuth KR, Fraiz J, Fisch JA, et al. Pinworm infestation of the genital tract. *Am Fam Physician.* Nov 1988;38(5): 127-130.
433. Wiebe BM. Appendicitis and Enterobius vermicularis. *Scand J Gastroenterol.* Mar 1991;26(3):336-338.
434. Arca MJ, Gates RL, Groner JI, et al. Clinical manifestations of appendiceal pinworms in children: an institutional experience and a review of the literature. *Pediatr Surg Int.* May 2004;20(5):372-375.
435. American Academy of Pediatrics. Pinworm infection (Enterobius vermicularis). In: Pickering LK, Baker CJ, Long SS, et al, eds. *Red Book: 2006 Report of the Committee on Infectious Diseases.* 27th ed. Elk Grove Village, IL: American Academy of Pediatrics; 2006.
436. Khuroo MS. Ascariasis. *Gastroenterol Clin North Am.* Sep 1996;25(3):553-577.
437. Ascariasis. In: Sun T, ed. *Parasitic Disorders: Pathology, Diagnosis, and Management.* 2nd ed. Baltimore, MD: Williams & Wilkins; 1999.
438. de Silva NR, Guyatt HL, Bundy DA. Morbidity and mortality due to Ascaris-induced intestinal obstruction. *Trans R Soc Trop Med Hyg.* Jan-Feb 1997;91(1):31-36.
439. Crompton DW. Ascariasis and childhood malnutrition. *Trans R Soc Trop Med Hyg.* Nov-Dec 1992;86(6):577-579.
440. Spillmann RK. Pulmonary ascariasis in tropical communities. *Am J Trop Med Hyg.* Sep 1975;24(5):791-800.
441. Hlaing T. Ascariasis and childhood malnutrition. *Parasitology.* 1993;107(suppl):S125-S136.
442. de Silva NR, Guyatt HL, Bundy DA. Worm burden in intestinal obstruction caused by Ascaris lumbricoides. *Trop Med Int Health.* Feb 1997;2(2):189-190.
443. Sandouk F, Haffar S, Zada MM, et al. Pancreatic-biliary ascariasis: experience of 300 cases. *Am J Gastroenterol.* Dec 1997;92(12):2264-2267.
444. al-Karawi M, Sanai FM, Yasawy MI, et al. Biliary strictures and cholangitis secondary to ascariasis: endoscopic management. *Gastrointest Endosc.* Nov 1999; 50(5):695-697.
445. Javid G, Wani NA, Gulzar GM, et al. Ascaris-induced liver abscess. *World J Surg.* Nov 1999;23(11):1191-1194.
446. Pandit SK, Zarger HU. Surgical ascariasis in children in Kashmir. *Trop Doct.* Jan 1997;27(1):13-14.
447. Cunha MC, Veloudios A, Dantas PE, et al. Obstruction of the nasolacrimal duct by Ascaris lumbricoides. *Ophthal Plast Reconstr Surg.* 1989;5(2):141-143.
448. Tietze PE, Tietze PH. The roundworm, Ascaris lumbricoides. *Prim Care.* Mar 1991;18(1):25-41.
449. Weller PF. Eosinophilia in travelers. *Med Clin North Am.* Nov 1992;76(6):1413-1432.
450. Deeg KH. Sonographic diagnosis of biliary ascariasis. *Eur J Pediatr.* Dec 1990;150(2):95-96.
451. Beitia AO, Haller JO, Kantor A. CT findings in pediatric gastrointestinal ascariasis. *Comput Med Imaging Graph.* Jan-Feb 1997;21(1):47-49.
452. Santra A, Bhattacharya T, Chowdhury A, et al. Serodiagnosis of ascariasis with specific IgG4 antibody and its use in an epidemiological study. *Trans R Soc Trop Med Hyg.* May-Jun 2001;95(3):289-292.
453. McSharry C, Xia Y, Holland CV, et al. Natural immunity to Ascaris lumbricoides associated with immunoglobulin E antibody to ABA-1 allergen and inflammation indicators in children. *Infect Immun.* Feb 1999;67(2):484-489.
454. American Academy of Pediatrics. Ascaris lumbricoides infections. In: Pickering LK, Baker CJ, Long SS, et al, eds. *Red Book: 2006 Report of the Committee on Infectious Diseases.* 27th ed. Elk Grove Village, IL: American Academy of Pediatrics; 2006.
455. Warren KS, Mahmoud AA. Algorithms in the diagnosis and management of exotic diseases. xxii. ascariasis and toxocariasis. *J Infect Dis.* May 1977;135(5):868-872.
456. Crompton DW. Ascaris and ascariasis. *Adv Parasitol.* 2001;48:285-375.
457. Villamizar E, Mendez M, Bonilla E, et al. Ascaris lumbricoides infestation as a cause of intestinal obstruction in children: experience with 87 cases. *J Pediatr Surg.* Jan 1996;31(1):201-204, discussion 204-205.
458. Massara CL, Enk MJ. Treatment options in the management of Ascaris lumbricoides. *Expert Opin Pharmacother.* Mar 2004;5(3):529-539.

459. Gunawardena GS, Karunaweera ND, Ismail MM. Socio-economic and behavioural factors affecting the prevalence of Ascaris infection in a low-country tea plantation in Sri Lanka. *Ann Trop Med Parasitol.* Sep 2004;98(6):615-621.
460. Albonico M, Stoltzfus RJ, Savioli L, et al. A controlled evaluation of two school-based anthelminthic chemotherapy regimens on intensity of intestinal helminth infections. *Int J Epidemiol.* Jun 1999;28(3):591-596.
461. Despommier D. Toxocariasis: clinical aspects, epidemiology, medical ecology, and molecular aspects. *Clin Microbiol Rev.* Apr 2003;16(2):265-272.
462. Gavin PJ, Kazacos KR, Shulman ST. Baylisascariasis. *Clin Microbiol Rev.* Oct 2005;18(4):703-718.
463. Glickman LT, Cypess RH. Toxocara infection in animal hospital employees. *Am J Public Health.* Dec 1977;67(12): 1193-1195.
464. Marmor M, Glickman L, Shofer F, et al. Toxocara canis infection of children: epidemiologic and neuropsychologic findings. *Am J Public Health.* May 1987;77(5): 554-559.
465. Schantz PM, Glickman LT. Toxocaral visceral larva migrans. *N Engl J Med.* Feb 1978;298(8):436-439.
466. Worley G, Green JA, Frothingham TE, et al. Toxocara canis infection: clinical and epidemiological associations with seropositivity in kindergarten children. *J Infect Dis.* Apr 1984;149(4):591-597.
467. Overgaauw PA. Aspects of Toxocara epidemiology: human toxocarosis. *Crit Rev Microbiol.* 1997;23(3): 215-231.
468. Hartleb M, Januszewski K. Severe hepatic involvement in visceral larva migrans. *Eur J Gastroenterol Hepatol.* Oct 2001;13(10):1245-1249.
469. Sane AC, Barber BA. Pulmonary nodules due to Toxocara canis infection in an immunocompetent adult. *South Med J.* Jan 1997;90(1):78-79.
470. Haralambidou S, Vlachaki E, Ioannidou E, et al. Pulmonary and myocardial manifestations due to Toxocara canis infection. *Eur J Intern Med.* Dec 2005;16(8): 601-602.
471. Sabrosa NA, de Souza EC. Nematode infections of the eye: toxocariasis and diffuse unilateral subacute neuroretinitis. *Curr Opin Ophthalmol.* Dec 2001;12(6):450-454.
472. Griffiths RW. Human toxocariasis (visceral larva migrans) causing an abscess of the rectus sheath in an infant. *Br J Surg.* Dec 1973;60(12):977-979.
473. Shetty AK, Aviles DH. Nephrotic syndrome associated with Toxocara canis infection. *Ann Trop Paediatr.* Sep 1999;19(3):297-300.
474. Magnaval JF, Galindo V, Glickman LT, et al. Human Toxocara infection of the central nervous system and neurological disorders: a case-control study. *Parasitology.* Nov 1997;115(pt 5):537-543.
475. Taylor MR, Keane CT, O'Connor P, et al. The expanded spectrum of toxocaral disease. *Lancet.* Mar 1988;1(8587): 692-695.
476. Buijs J, Borsboom G, van Gemund JJ, et al. Toxocara seroprevalence in 5-year-old elementary schoolchildren: relation with allergic asthma. *Am J Epidemiol.* Nov 1994;140(9):839-847.
477. Critchley EM, Vakil SD, Hutchinson DN, et al. Toxoplasma, Toxocara, and epilepsy. *Epilepsia.* Jun 1982; 23(3):315-321.
478. Vidal JE, Sztajnbok J, Seguro AC. Eosinophilic meningoencephalitis due to Toxocara canis: case report and review of the literature. *Am J Trop Med Hyg.* Sep 2003; 69(3):341-343.
479. Dinning WJ, Gillespie SH, Cooling RJ, et al. Toxocariasis: a practical approach to management of ocular disease. *Eye.* 1988;2(pt 5):580-582.
480. Molk R. Ocular toxocariasis: a review of the literature. *Ann Ophthalmol.* Mar 1983;15(3):216-219, 222-217, 230-211.
481. Gillespie SH, Dinning WJ, Voller A, et al. The spectrum of ocular toxocariasis. *Eye.* 1993;7(pt 3):415-418.
482. Small KW, McCuen BW II, de Juan E Jr, et al. Surgical management of retinal traction caused by toxocariasis. *Am J Ophthalmol.* Jul 1989;108(1):10-14.
483. Wolach B, Sinnreich Z, Uziel Y, et al. Toxocariasis: a diagnostic dilemma. *Isr J Med Sci.* Nov 1995;31(11): 689-692.
484. Aur RJ, Pratt CB, Johnson WW. Thiabendazole in visceral larva migrans. *Am J Dis Child.* Mar 1971;121(3): 226-229.
485. Roig J, Romeu J, Riera C, et al. Acute eosinophilic pneumonia due to toxocariasis with bronchoalveolar lavage findings. *Chest.* Jul 1992;102(1):294-296.
486. Schantz PM. Toxocara larva migrans now. *Am J Trop Med Hyg.* Sep 1989;41(3 suppl):S21-S34.
487. American Academy of Pediatrics. Toxocariasis (visceral larva migrans, ocular larva migrans). In: Pickering LK, Baker CJ, Long SS, et al, eds. *Red Book: 2006 Report of the Committee on Infectious Diseases.* 27th ed. Elk Grove Village, IL: American Academy of Pediatrics; 2006.
488. Mrissa R, Battikh R, Ben Abdelhafidh N, et al. [Toxocara canis encephalitis: case report]. *Rev Med Interne.* Oct 2005; 26(10):829-832.
489. Abe K, Shimokawa H, Kubota T, et al. Myocarditis associated with visceral larva migrans due to Toxocara canis. *Intern Med.* Sep 2002;41(9):706-708.
490. Barisani-Asenbauer T, Maca SM, Hauff W, et al. Treatment of ocular toxocariasis with albendazole. *J Ocul Pharmacol Ther.* Jun 2001;17(3):287-294.
491. Shields JA. Ocular toxocariasis. A review. *Surv Ophthalmol.* Mar-Apr 1984;28(5):361-381.
492. Magnaval JF. Comparative efficacy of diethylcarbamazine and mebendazole for the treatment of human toxocariasis. *Parasitology.* Jun 1995;110 (pt 5):529-533.
493. Melrose WD. Lymphatic filariasis: new insights into an old disease. *Int J Parasitol.* Jul 2002;32(8):947-960.
494. Ottesen EA. The global programme to eliminate lymphatic filariasis. *Trop Med Int Health.* Sep 2000;5(9): 591-594.
495. Supali T, Wibowo H, Ruckert P, et al. High prevalence of Brugia timori infection in the highland of Alor Island, Indonesia. *Am J Trop Med Hyg.* May 2002;66(5):560-565.
496. Atmosoedjono S, Partono F, Dennis DT, et al. Anopheles barbirostris (Diptera: Culicidae) as a vector of the timor filaria on Flores Island: preliminary observations. *J Med Entomol.* Jan 1977;13(4-5):611-613.
497. Lymphatic filariasis. In: Sun T, ed. *Parasitic Disorders: Pathology, Diagnosis, and Management.* 2nd ed. Baltimore, MD: Williams & Wilkins; 1999.
498. Ottesen EA. The Wellcome Trust Lecture. Infection and disease in lymphatic filariasis: an immunological perspective. *Parasitology.* 1992;104(suppl):S71-S79.
499. Piessens WF, McGreevy PB, Piessens PW, et al. Immune responses in human infections with Brugia malayi: specific cellular unresponsiveness to filarial antigens. *J Clin Invest.* Jan 1980;65(1):172-179.
500. Dreyer G, Noroes J, Figueredo-Silva J, et al. Pathogenesis of lymphatic disease in bancroftian filariasis: a clinical perspective. *Parasitol Today.* Dec 2000;16(12): 544-548.
501. Kitchen ND, Hocken DB, Greenhalgh RM, et al. Use of the Denver pleuroperitoneal shunt in the treatment of chylothorax secondary to filariasis. *Thorax.* Feb 1991; 46(2):144-145.

502. Sen SB, Chatterjee H, Pillai NK. Chylous ascites precipitated by rupture of a pathological thoracic duct. A rare complication of filarial chyle reflux. *J Indian Med Assoc.* Jan 1971;56(2):44-46.
503. Neva FA, Ottesen EA. Tropical (filarial) eosinophilia. *N Engl J Med.* May 1978;298(20):1129-1131.
504. Fontes G, Rocha EM, Brito AC, et al. The microfilarial periodicity of Wuchereria bancrofti in north-eastern Brazil. *Ann Trop Med Parasitol.* Jun 2000;94(4):373-379.
505. Arora VK, Singh N, Bhatia A. Cytomorphologic profile of lymphatic filariasis. *Acta Cytol.* Sep-Oct 1996;40(5): 948-952.
506. Jungmann P, Figueredo-Silva J, Dreyer G. Bancroftian lymphadenopathy: a histopathologic study of fifty-eight cases from northeastern Brazil. *Am J Trop Med Hyg.* Sep 1991;45(3):325-331.
507. Maizels RM, Sartono E, Kurniawan A, et al. T-cell activation and the balance of antibody isotypes in human lymphatic filariasis. *Parasitol Today.* Feb 1995;11(2): 50-56.
508. Weil GJ, Lammie PJ, Weiss N. The ICT filariasis test: a rapid-format antigen test for diagnosis of bancroftian filariasis. *Parasitol Today.* Oct 1997;13(10):401-404.
509. Walther M, Muller R. Diagnosis of human filariases (except onchocerciasis). *Adv Parasitol.* 2003;53:149-193.
510. American Academy of Pediatrics. Lymphatic filariasis (bancroftian, malayan, and timorian). In: Pickering LK, Baker CJ, Long SS, et al, eds. *Red Book: 2006 Report of the Committee on Infectious Diseases.* 27th ed. Elk Grove Village, IL: American Academy of Pediatrics; 2006.
511. Fan PC. Diethylcarbamazine treatment of bancroftian and malayan filariasis with emphasis on side effects. *Ann Trop Med Parasitol.* Aug 1992;86(4):399-405.
512. Soboslay PT, Newland HS, White AT, et al. Ivermectin effect on microfilariae of Onchocerca volvulus after a single oral dose in humans. *Trop Med Parasitol.* Mar 1987;38(1):8-10.
513. Mak JW. Antifilarial compounds in the treatment and control of lymphatic filariasis. *Trop Biomed.* Dec 2004; 21(2):27-38.
514. Shenoy RK. Management of disability in lymphatic filariasis—an update. *J Commun Dis.* Mar 2002;34(1):1-14.
515. Richard-Lenoble D, Chandenier J, Gaxotte P. Ivermectin and filariasis. *Fundam Clin Pharmacol.* Apr 2003;17(2): 199-203.
516. de Kraker ME, Stolk WA, van Oortmarssen GJ, et al. Model-based analysis of trial data: microfilaria and worm-productivity loss after diethylcarbamazine-albendazole or ivermectin-albendazole combination therapy against Wuchereria bancrofti. *Trop Med Int Health.* May 2006;11(5):718-728.
517. Murdoch ME, Asuzu MC, Hagan M, et al. Onchocerciasis: the clinical and epidemiological burden of skin disease in Africa. *Ann Trop Med Parasitol.* Apr 2002;96(3): 283-296.
518. Onchocerciasis. In: Sun T, ed. *Parasitic Disorders: Pathology, Diagnosis, and Management.* 2nd ed. Baltimore, MD: Williams & Wilkins; 1999.
519. Plaisier AP, van Oortmarssen GJ, Remme J, et al. The reproductive lifespan of Onchocerca volvulus in West African savanna. *Acta Trop.* Feb 1991;48(4):271-284.
520. Taylor HR. Onchocerciasis. *Int Ophthalmol.* May 1990; 14(3):189-194.
521. World Health Organization. Epidemiology of onchocerciasis. Report of a WHO Expert Committee. *World Health Organ Tech Rep Ser.* 1976;(597):1-94.
522. Berger IB, Nnadozie J. Onchocerciasis and other eye problems in developing countries: a challenge for optometrists. *J Am Optom Assoc.* Oct 1993;64(10): 699-702.
523. Burnham G. Onchocerciasis. *Lancet.* May 1998; 351(9112):1341-1346.
524. Murdoch ME, Hay RJ, Mackenzie CD, et al. A clinical classification and grading system of the cutaneous changes in onchocerciasis. *Br J Dermatol.* Sep 1993; 129(3):260-269.
525. Gibson DW, Connor DH. Onchocercal lymphadenitis: clinicopathologic study of 34 patients. *Trans R Soc Trop Med Hyg.* 1978;72(2):137-154.
526. Anderson J, Fuglsang H, al-Zubaidy A. Onchocerciasis in Yemen with special reference to sowda. *Trans R Soc Trop Med Hyg.* 1973;67(1):30-31.
527. Connor DH, George GH, Gibson DW. Pathologic changes of human onchocerciasis: implications for future research. *Rev Infect Dis.* Nov-Dec 1985;7(6): 809-819.
528. Mackenzie CD, Williams JF, O'Day J, et al. Onchocerciasis in southwestern Sudan: parasitological and clinical characteristics. *Am J Trop Med Hyg.* Mar 1987;36(2): 371-382.
529. Boatin BA, Toe L, Alley ES, et al. Diagnostics in onchocerciasis: future challenges. *Ann Trop Med Parasitol.* Apr 1998;92(suppl 1):S41-S45.
530. Enk CD. Onchocerciasis—river blindness. *Clin Dermatol.* May-Jun 2006;24(3):176-180.
531. Francis H, Awadzi K, Ottesen EA. The Mazzotti reaction following treatment of onchocerciasis with diethylcarbamazine: clinical severity as a function of infection intensity. *Am J Trop Med Hyg.* May 1985;34(3): 529-536.
532. Awadzi K, Addy ET, Opoku NO, et al. The chemotherapy of onchocerciasis XX: ivermectin in combination with albendazole. *Trop Med Parasitol.* Dec 1995;46(4): 213-220.
533. Brieger WR, Awedoba AK, Eneanya CI, et al. The effects of ivermectin on onchocercal skin disease and severe itching: results of a multicentre trial. *Trop Med Int Health.* Dec 1998;3(12):951-961.
534. Hoerauf A, Buttner DW, Adjei O, et al. Onchocerciasis. *BMJ.* Jan 2003;326(7382):207-210.
535. American Academy of Pediatrics. Onchocerciasis (river blindness, filariasis). In: Pickering LK, Baker CJ, Long SS, et al, eds. *Red Book: 2006 Report of the Committee on Infectious Diseases.* 27th ed. Elk Grove Village, IL: American Academy of Pediatrics; 2006.
536. Richards FO Jr, Boatin B, Sauerbrey M, et al. Control of onchocerciasis today: status and challenges. *Trends Parasitol.* Dec 2001;17(12):558-563.
537. Chitsulo L, Engels D, Montresor A, et al. The global status of schistosomiasis and its control. *Acta Trop.* Oct 2000;77(1):41-51.
538. Ross AG, Bartley PB, Sleigh AC, et al. Schistosomiasis. *N Engl J Med.* Apr 2002;346(16):1212-1220.
539. Harries AD, Fryatt R, Walker J, et al. Schistosomiasis in expatriates returning to Britain from the tropics: a controlled study. *Lancet.* Jan 1986;1(8472):86-88.
540. Whitty CJ, Mabey DC, Armstrong M, et al. Presentation and outcome of 1107 cases of schistosomiasis from Africa diagnosed in a non-endemic country. *Trans R Soc Trop Med Hyg.* Sep-Oct 2000;94(5):531-534.
541. El-Ansary A, Al-Daihan S. Important aspects of Biomphalaria snail-schistosome interactions as targets for antischistosome drug. *Med Sci Monit.* Dec 2006;12(12):RA282-RA292.
542. Ohmae H, Sinuon M, Kirinoki M, et al. Schistosomiasis mekongi: from discovery to control. *Parasitol Int.* Jun 2004;53(2):135-142.
543. Ruppel A, Chlichlia K, Bahgat M. Invasion by schistosome cercariae: neglected aspects in Schistosoma japonicum. *Trends Parasitol.* Sep 2004;20(9):397-400.

544. Strickland GT. Gastrointestinal manifestations of schistosomiasis. *Gut.* Oct 1994;35(10):1334-1337.
545. Elliott DE. Schistosomiasis. Pathophysiology, diagnosis, and treatment. *Gastroenterol Clin North Am.* Sep 1996; 25(3):599-625.
546. Doherty JF, Moody AH, Wright SG. Katayama fever: an acute manifestation of schistosomiasis. *BMJ.* Oct 1996; 313(7064):1071-1072.
547. Chen MC, Wang SC, Chang PY, et al. Granulomatous disease of the large intestine secondary to schistosome infestation. A study of 229 cases. *Chin Med J (Engl).* Sep 1978;4(5):371-378.
548. Hatz CF, Vennervald BJ, Nkulila T, et al. Evolution of Schistosoma haematobium-related pathology over 24 months after treatment with praziquantel among school children in southeastern Tanzania. *Am J Trop Med Hyg.* Nov 1998;59(5):775-781.
549. Olds GR, Olveda R, Wu G, et al. Immunity and morbidity in schistosomiasis japonicum infection. *Am J Trop Med Hyg.* Nov 1996;55(5 suppl):121-126.
550. Warren KS, Mahmoud AA. Algorithms in the diagnosis and management of exotic diseases. I. Schistosomiasis. *J Infect Dis.* May 1975;131(5):614-620.
551. Bethlem EP, Schettino Gde P, Carvalho CR. Pulmonary schistosomiasis. *Curr Opin Pulm Med.* Sep 1997;3(5): 361-365.
552. Hussein AM, Medany S, Abou el Magd AM, et al. Multiple endoscopic polypectomies for schistosomal polyposis of the colon. *Lancet.* Mar 1983;1(8326, pt 1): 673-674.
553. Zhou H, Ross AG, Hartel GF, et al. Diagnosis of schistosomiasis japonica in Chinese schoolchildren by administration of a questionnaire. *Trans R Soc Trop Med Hyg.* May-Jun 1998;92(3):245-250.
554. Da Silva LC, Carrilho FJ. Hepatosplenic schistosomiasis. Pathophysiology and treatment. *Gastroenterol Clin North Am.* Mar 1992;21(1):163-177.
555. Bedwani R, Renganathan E, El Kwhsky F, et al. Schistosomiasis and the risk of bladder cancer in Alexandria, Egypt. *Br J Cancer.* Apr 1998;77(7):1186-1189.
556. Fowler R, Lee C, Keystone JS. The role of corticosteroids in the treatment of cerebral schistosomiasis caused by Schistosoma mansoni: case report and discussion. *Am J Trop Med Hyg.* Jul 1999;61(1):47-50.
557. Pittella JE. The relation between involvement of the central nervous system in schistosomiasis mansoni and the clinical forms of the parasitosis. A review. *J Trop Med Hyg.* Feb 1991;94(1):15-21.
558. Katz N, Chaves A, Pellegrino J. A simple device for quantitative stool thick-smear technique in Schistosomiasis mansoni. *Rev Inst Med Trop Sao Paulo.* Nov-Dec 1972;14(6):397-400.
559. Schistosomiasis. In: Sun T, ed. *Parasitic Disorders: Pathology, Diagnosis, and Management.* 2nd ed. Baltimore, MD: Williams & Wilkins; 1999.
560. Lucey DR, Maguire JH. Schistosomiasis. *Infect Dis Clin North Am.* Sep 1993;7(3):635-653.
561. Tsang VC, Wilkins PP. Immunodiagnosis of schistosomiasis. *Immunol Invest.* Jan-Feb 1997;26(1-2): 175-188.
562. Al-Sherbiny MM, Osman AM, Hancock K, et al. Application of immunodiagnostic assays: detection of antibodies and circulating antigens in human schistosomiasis and correlation with clinical findings. *Am J Trop Med Hyg.* Jun 1999;60(6):960-966.
563. American Academy of Pediatrics. Schistosomiasis. In: Pickering LK, Baker CJ, Long SS, et al, eds. *Red Book: 2006 Report of the Committee on Infectious Diseases.* 27th ed. Elk Grove Village, IL: American Academy of Pediatrics; 2006.
564. Lin D, Zhang S, Murakami H, et al. Impact mass chemotherapy with praziquantel on schistosomiasis control in Fanhu village, People's Republic of China. *Southeast Asian J Trop Med Public Health.* Jun 1997; 28(2):274-279.
565. Talaat M, Miller FD. A mass chemotherapy trial of praziquantel on Schistosoma haematobium endemicity in Upper Egypt. *Am J Trop Med Hyg.* Oct 1998;59(4): 546-550.
566. Gryseels B, Stelma FF, Talla I, et al. Epidemiology, immunology and chemotherapy of Schistosoma mansoni infections in a recently exposed community in Senegal. *Trop Geogr Med.* 1994;46(4 spec no): 209-219.
567. Ismail M, Botros S, Metwally A, et al. Resistance to praziquantel: direct evidence from Schistosoma mansoni isolated from Egyptian villagers. *Am J Trop Med Hyg.* Jun 1999;60(6):932-935.
568. Yuan Y, Xu XJ, Dong HF, et al. Transmission control of schistosomiasis japonica: implementation and evaluation of different snail control interventions. *Acta Trop.* Nov-Dec 2005;96(2-3):191-197.
569. Xiao SH, Booth M, Tanner M. The prophylactic effects of artemether against Schistosoma japonicum infections. *Parasitol Today.* Mar 2000;16(3):122-126.
570. Sotelo J. Taenia solium and Taenia saginata (taeniasis and cysticercosis). In: Long SS, Pickering LK, Prober CG, eds. *Principles and Practice of Pediatric Infectious Diseases.* 2nd ed. New York, NY: Churchill Livingstone; 2003.
571. American Academy of Pediatrics. Tapeworm diseases (taeniasis and cysticercosis). In: Pickering LK, Baker CJ, Long SS, et al, eds. *Red Book: 2006 Report of the Committee on Infectious Diseases.* 27th ed. Elk Grove Village, IL: American Academy of Pediatrics; 2006.
572. Centers for Disease Control and Prevention, National Center for Infectious Diseases, Division of Parasitic Diseases. Laboratory Identification of Parasites of Public Health Concern: Taeniasis. Available at: www.dpd.cdc.gov/dpdx/html/taeniasis.asp?body=Frames/s-z/taeniasis/body_taeniasis_page1.htm. Accessed April 6, 2007.
573. Centers for Disease Control and Prevention, National Center for Infectious Diseases, Division of Parasitic Diseases. Laboratory Identification of Parasites of Public Health Concern: Cysticercosis. Available at: www.dpd.cdc.gov/dpdx/html/cysticercosis.htm. Accessed April 6, 2007.
574. Mitchell WG, Crawford TO. Intraparenchymal cerebral cysticercosis in children: diagnosis and treatment. *Pediatrics.* Jul 1988;82(1):76-82.
575. Medina MT, Rosas E, Rubio-Donnadieu F, et al. Neurocysticercosis as the main cause of late-onset epilepsy in Mexico. *Arch Intern Med.* Feb 1990;150(2):325-327.
576. Botero D, Tanowitz HB, Weiss LM, et al. Taeniasis and cysticercosis. *Infect Dis Clin North Am.* Sep 1993;7(3): 683-697.
577. Gordon E, Cartwright M, Avasarala J. Ventricular obstruction from neurocysticercosis. *Arch Neurol.* Jun 2005;62(6):1018.
578. Alsina GA, Johnson JP, McBride DQ, et al. Spinal neurocysticercosis. *Neurosurg Focus.* Jun 2002;12(6):e8.
579. Rangel R, Torres B, Del Bruto O, et al. Cysticercotic encephalitis: a severe form in young females. *Am J Trop Med Hyg.* Mar 1987;36(2):387-392.
580. Garcia HH, Gonzalez AE, Evans CA, et al. Taenia solium cysticercosis. *Lancet.* Aug 2003;362(9383):547-556.
581. Rodriguez-Carbajal J, Boleaga-Duran B, Dorfsman J. The role of computed tomography (CT) in the diagnosis of neurocysticercosis. *Childs Nerv Syst.* 1987;3(4): 199-202.

582. Sotelo J, Del Brutto OH. Brain cysticercosis. *Arch Med Res.* Jan-Feb 2000;31(1):3-14.
583. Sotelo J, Jung H. Pharmacokinetic optimisation of the treatment of neurocysticercosis. *Clin Pharmacokinet.* Jun 1998;34(6):503-515.
584. Proano JV, Madrazo I, Avelar F, et al. Medical treatment for neurocysticercosis characterized by giant subarachnoid cysts. *N Engl J Med.* Sep 2001;345(12): 879-885.
585. Wood TR, Binder PS. Intravitreal and intracameral cysticercosis. *Ann Ophthalmol.* Jul 1979;11(7):1033-1036.
586. Centers for Disease Control and Prevention, National Center for Infectious Diseases, Division of Parasitic Diseases. Laboratory Identification of Parasites of Public Health Concern: Echinococcosis. Available at: www.dpd.cdc.gov/dpdx/html/echinococcosis.htm. Accessed April 6, 2007.
587. American Academy of Pediatrics. Other tapeworm infections (including hydatid disease). In: Pickering LK, Baker CJ, Long SS, et al, eds. *Red Book: 2006 Report of the Committee on Infectious Diseases.* 27th ed. Elk Grove Village, IL: American Academy of Pediatrics; 2006.
588. Sadjjadi SM. Present situation of echinococcosis in the Middle East and Arabic North Africa. *Parasitol Int.* 2006; 55(suppl):S197-S202.
589. Schantz PM. Echinococcus species (agents of cystic, alveolar, and polycystic echinococcosis). In: Long SS, Pickering LK, Prober CG, eds. *Principles and Practice of Pediatric Infectious Diseases.* 2nd ed. New York, NY: Churchill Livingstone; 2003.
590. Eckert J, Deplazes P. Biological, epidemiological, and clinical aspects of echinococcosis, a zoonosis of increasing concern. *Clin Microbiol Rev.* Jan 2004;17(1):107-135.
591. Kammerer WS, Schantz PM. Echinococcal disease. *Infect Dis Clin North Am.* Sep 1993;7(3):605-618.
592. Ammann RW, Eckert J. Cestodes. Echinococcus. *Gastroenterol Clin North Am.* Sep 1996;25(3):655-689.
593. D'Alessandro A. Polycystic echinococcosis in tropical America: Echinococcus vogeli and E oligarthrus. *Acta Trop.* Sep 1997;67(1-2):43-65.
594. Morar R, Feldman C. Pulmonary echinococcosis. *Eur Respir J.* Jun 2003;21(6):1069-1077.
595. Dhar P, Chaudhary A, Desai R, et al. Current trends in the diagnosis and management of cystic hydatid disease of the liver. *J Commun Dis.* Dec 1996;28(4):221-230.
596. Safioleas M, Misiakos E, Manti C, et al. Diagnostic evaluation and surgical management of hydatid disease of the liver. *World J Surg.* Nov-Dec 1994;18(6):859-865.
597. Taourel P, Marty-Ane B, Charasset S, et al. Hydatid cyst of the liver: comparison of CT and MRI. *J Comput Assist Tomogr.* Jan-Feb 1993;17(1):80-85.
598. Lanier AP, Trujillo DE, Schantz PM, et al. Comparison of serologic tests for the diagnosis and follow-up of alveolar hydatid disease. *Am J Trop Med Hyg.* Nov 1987; 37(3):609-615.
599. Bhatia G. Echinococcus. *Semin Respir Infect.* Jun 1997; 12(2):171-186.
600. Biava MF, Dao A, Fortier B. Laboratory diagnosis of cystic hydatic disease. *World J Surg.* Jan 2001;25(1): 10-14.
601. Khuroo MS, Dar MY, Yattoo GN, et al. Percutaneous drainage versus albendazole therapy in hepatic hydatidosis: a prospective, randomized study. *Gastroenterology.* May 1993;104(5):1452-1459.
602. Davis A, Dixon H, Pawlowski ZS. Multicentre clinical trials of benzimidazole-carbamates in human cystic echinococcosis (phase 2). *Bull World Health Organ.* 1989;67(5):503-508.
603. Horton RJ. Chemotherapy of Echinococcus infection in man with albendazole. *Trans R Soc Trop Med Hyg.* Jan-Feb 1989;83(1):97-102.
604. Kammerer WS, Schantz PM. Long term follow-up of human hydatid disease (Echinococcus granulosus) treated with a high-dose mebendazole regimen. *Am J Trop Med Hyg.* Jan 1984;33(1):132-137.
605. Filice C, Strosselli M, Brunetti E, et al. Percutaneous drainage of hydatid liver cysts. *Radiology.* Aug 1992; 184(2):579-580.
606. Filice C, Brunetti E. Percutaneous drainage of hydatid cysts. *N Engl J Med.* Feb 1998;338(6):392, author reply 392-393.
607. Wilson JF, Rausch RL, McMahon BJ, et al. Parasiticidal effect of chemotherapy in alveolar hydatid disease: review of experience with mebendazole and albendazole in Alaskan Eskimos. *Clin Infect Dis.* Aug 1992; 15(2):234-249.
608. Centers for Disease Control and Prevention, National Center for Infectious Diseases, Division of Parasitic Diseases. Laboratory Identification of Parasites of Public Health Concern: Diphyllobothriasis. Available at: www.dpd.cdc.gov/dpdx/html/diphyllobothriasis.htm. Accessed April 6, 2007.
609. Richards FO. Diphyllobothrium, Dipylidium, and Hymenolepis species. In: Long SS, Pickering LK, Prober CG, eds. *Principles and Practice of Pediatric Infectious Diseases.* 2nd ed. New York, NY: Churchill Livingstone; 2003.
610. Saarni M, Nyberg W, Grasbeck R, von B. Symptoms in carriers of Diphyllobothrium latum and in non-infected controls. *Acta Med Scand.* Feb 1963;173:147-154.
611. Centers for Disease Control and Prevention, National Center for Infectious Diseases, Division of Parasitic Diseases. Laboratory Identification of Parasites of Public Health Concern: Hymenolepiasis. Available at: www.dpd.cdc.gov/dpdx/html/hymenolepiasis.htm. Accessed April 6, 2007.
612. Buscher HN, Haley AJ. Epidemiology of Hymenolepis nana infections of Punjabi villagers in West Pakistan. *Am J Trop Med Hyg.* Jan 1972;21(2):42-49.
613. Flores EC, Plumb SC, McNeese MC. Intestinal parasitosis in an urban pediatric clinic population. *Am J Dis Child.* Aug 1983;137(8):754-756.

Chapter 306

PECTUS EXCAVATUM AND PECTUS CARINATUM

Ikenna C. Okereke, MD; Anthony Stallion, MD

PECTUS EXCAVATUM

Pectus excavatum is a syndrome characterized by a concave depression of the sternum. It is the most common congenital chest wall deformity, affecting approximately 1 in 400 live births.[1] Eighty percent of persons affected are boys. Family history is a risk factor for development of pectus excavatum. Phenotypically the appearance resembles a funnel chest. The concavity is often asymmetric, with the right side usually more depressed than the left side. The severity of the defect can range from a mild depression to a profound indentation. This congenital defect occurs from excessive growth of the costal cartilage, which displaces the sternum posteriorly.[2]

CLINICAL FEATURES

Pectus excavatum typically becomes problematic as children reach early adolescence, both as a result of embarrassment over the cosmetic appearance of the chest and of respiratory impairment from the defect. A pectus excavatum defect can proceed from barely noticeable to extremely prominent in the span of a few years. Rapid skeletal growth during this period tends to exaggerate the defect. The severity of the defect usually does not increase after the age of 18, by which time most of the skeletal growth has occurred. Although most patients do not exhibit symptoms, some may have decreased exercise tolerance, easy fatigability, and frequent respiratory tract infections from decreased chest excursion and diminished inspirations.[3] Nonetheless, other patients have chest pain related to the defect.

Pectus excavatum has a known association with many disorders (Box 306-1). Scoliosis is present in approximately 15% of patients, and mitral valve prolapse may be seen up to 30% of the time.[4] Pectus excavatum also has a strong association with Marfan syndrome and represents the most common chest wall abnormality seen in these patients.[5]

Patients with pectus excavatum tend to have rounded shoulders and a protuberant abdomen, which is referred to as the *pectus posture*. Rapid growth during the adolescent years tends to make the deformity more pronounced. This disfigurement can have serious psychological ramifications. Many patients with pectus excavatum describe having social anxiety, problems with body image, and depression.[6]

EVALUATION

Examination of the patient with pectus excavatum should include a thorough history and physical examination, with an attempt to rule out any associated disorders that may have been previously undiagnosed. Auscultation of the chest may reveal diminished inspiration or a cardiac murmur, especially in the presence of mitral valve prolapse. Pulmonary function tests tend to demonstrate a restrictive pattern. A transthoracic echocardiogram may reveal diminished cardiac output from decreased stroke volume and mitral valve prolapse.

The severity of the defect is measured by the Haller index, which is the computed tomographic scan–measured transthoracic diameter divided by the sternovertebral diameter. An index of more than 3.5 is considered to be a severe defect, but even indices that are less than 2.5 can cause significant cardiopulmonary impairment.[7] Defects with an index of more than 1.5 to 1.7 are usually considered for repair.

BOX 306-1 Disorders Associated With Pectus Excavatum

Asthma	Poland syndrome
Bronchial atresia	Rett syndrome
Bronchomalacia	Rickets
Down syndrome	Scoliosis
Marfan syndrome	Turner syndrome
Mitral valve prolapse	Wolff-Parkinson-White syndrome
Noonan syndrome	
Osteogenesis imperfecta	

TREATMENT

Some nonoperative measures exist that are aimed at decreasing the patient's symptoms, but they are generally only minimally effective. Patients can be taught to increase breathing efforts to increase diaphragmatic excursion, allowing for increased oxygen exchange. Improvement in posture, either through conscious efforts to straighten posture or with the help of support vests, can improve air exchange. External braces can help correct posture, but these have been largely associated with only minimal correction of the deformity. Some authorities have advocated the use of continuous external vacuum as another alternative to surgical therapy.[8,9]

Repair of pectus excavatum should be performed in patients with cardiopulmonary impairment, pain, or concerns about cosmesis resulting in poor body image. Although the best time for repair is uncertain, children should ideally undergo surgical repair between the ages of 12 and 18 years, when they are old enough to understand the nature, consequences, and magnitude of the surgery. This awareness includes knowing of the level of pain that might be experienced postoperatively and temporary limitation of activity. Although the surgery can be performed when the patient is older than 18 years, it should not be delayed too long so as to take advantage of the pliable chest wall of the growing adolescent and effect the greatest change on chest contour.

Two methods of surgical repair exist for pectus excavatum. Previously, the standard repair method had been the Ravitch repair method, introduced by Ravitch in 1949.[10] To perform this repair, a transverse incision is made over the middle portion of the sternal defect, and the dissection is performed below the level of the pectoralis fascia and muscles. The costal cartilage of ribs 1 through 8, on each side of the sternum, is resected, proceeding from the costochondral junction to the costosternal junction. A transverse osteotomy of the sternum is performed at the level of the third costal cartilage. The lower sternum is then repositioned to correct the deformity, and the pectoralis muscles are reattached to the midline. Despite its extensive nature, this repair has been associated with good long-term outcome.

A less-invasive procedure, the Nuss repair method, was developed in 1987.[11] The Nuss repair method elevates the sternal depression without cartilage resection. The Nuss repair method involves making bilateral incisions at the anterior axillary line at the level of the greatest depression of the pectus defect. Then an incision is made in the fourth intercostal space, and a thoracoscope is introduced. Under direct vision, a pectus bar is passed across the chest. This bar then is flipped anteriorly so as to raise the sternum. The Nuss repair method has been associated with equivalent cosmetic results, and the procedure may be more cost effective because it has a shorter operating time than the Ravitch repair method. The bar remains in place for 2 to 3 years to allow for proper remodeling of the costal cartilage. This process is slower in the older patient because of the decrease in growth. The bar is removed as an outpatient procedure.

Adequate analgesia is typically the most troublesome problem in the postoperative period. Use of an epidural patient-controlled analgesia catheter greatly reduces pain after the procedure. Generally the epidural catheter is required for several days, and it represents the main reason the patient remains in the hospital.

PROGNOSIS

Long-term outcomes have shown both types of repair to be effective. Almost all patients report satisfaction with the cosmetic results of the surgery. Symptoms of pain and decreased exercise intolerance that are present before surgery generally improve after surgery.[9] Many asymptomatic patients who have a normal preoperative pulmonary function test and cardiac echo report significant improvement in their exercise tolerance and endurance, although they had not realized they had had any limitations before surgery. Complications with the Ravitch repair method include impairment of growth of the chest wall, with possible constriction of the thorax, from inability of the thorax to develop after surgery. The most common complication with the Nuss repair method is displacement of the bar, but modifications in the technique and increased surgeon experience have led to low rates of bar migration.[12] Only one case of cardiac perforation has been reported, but this occurred with blind passage of the pectus bar across the chest.[13] No cases of cardiac perforation have occurred with the use of thoracoscopy during the procedure.

The advent of a minimally invasive technique to repair pectus excavatum has changed the approach to a patient with this deformity. Children who previously lived with psychological issues because of poor body image or physical limitations (or both) can now undergo a safe and effective operation with minimal morbidity. The breadth of patients who are referred for surgical repair is likely to widen, and more patients should be able to undergo a secure and dependable elimination of the defect.

PECTUS CARINATUM

Pectus carinatum (PC) is the second-most common chest wall abnormality. Although excavatum deformities account for approximately 90% of chest wall defects, PC makes up less than 5%.[14] PC is characterized by a protuberance of the sternum that mimics a pigeon's chest. It is usually a symmetric, midline deformity and is only infrequently associated with cardiovascular compromise. Most commonly, the open Ravitch repair method for pectus excavatum is performed to correct deformity. Thoracoscopic techniques are also are used to repair this defect.[15,16] Some investigators have advocated the use of conservative measures, such as external braces applying constant pressure, as an alternative to surgical repair.[17,18] In addition, minimal open repair has been described for both the excavatum and carinatum deformities.[19]

TOOLS FOR PRACTICE

Engaging Patient and Family

- *Chest Wall Deformities* (fact sheet), Children's Hospital of Boston (www.childrenshospital.org/az/Site698/mainpage S698P0.html).

REFERENCES

1. McGuigan R, Azarow K. Congenital chest wall defects. *Surg Clin North Am.* 2006;86:353-370.
2. Goretsky M, Kelly R, Croitoru D, et al. Chest wall anomalies: pectus excavatum and pectus carinatum. *Adolesc Med Clin.* 2004;15:455-471.
3. Quigley P, Haller J, Jelus K, et al. Cardiorespiratory function before and after corrective surgery in pectus excavatum. *J Pediatr.* 1996;128:638-643.
4. Sawin R. Pediatric chest lesions. *Pediatr Clin North Am.* 1998;45:861-874.
5. Tsipouras P, Silverman D. The genetic basis of aortic disease: Marfan syndrome and beyond. *Cardiol Clin.* 1999; 17:683-696.
6. Einsiedel E, Clausner A. Funnel chest: psychological and psychosomatic aspects in children, youngsters, and young adults. *J Thorac Cardiovasc Surg.* 1999;40: 733-762.
7. Ravitch M. The operative treatment of pectus excavatum. *Ann Surg.* 1949;129:429-444.
8. Haecker FM, Mayr J. The vacuum bell for treatment of pectus excavatum: an alternative to surgical correction? *Eur J Cardiothorac Surg.* 2006;29:557-561.
9. Schier F, Bahr M, Klobe E. The vacuum chest wall lifter: an innovative, nonsurgical addition to the management of pectus excavatum. *J Pediatr Surg.* 2005;40:496-500.
10. Nuss D, Kelly R, Croitoru D, et al. A 10-year review of a minimally invasive technique for the correction of pectus excavatum. *J Pediatr Surg.* 1998;33:545-552.
11. Schaarschmidt K, Kolberg-Schwerdt A, Dimitrov G, et al. Submuscular bar, multiple pericostal bar fixation, bilateral thoracoscopy: a modified Nuss repair in adolescents. *J Pediatr Surg.* 2002;37:1276-1280.
12. Robicsek F, Cook J, Daugherty H, et al. Pectus carinatum. *J Thorac Cardiovasc Surg.* 1979;78:52-61.
13. Moss RL, Albanese CT, Reynolds M. Major complications after minimally invasive repair of pectus excavatum: case reports. *J Pediatr Surg.* 2001;36:155.
14. Williams AM, Crabbe DC. Pectus deformities of the anterior chest wall. *Paediatr Respir Rev.* 2003;4:237-242.
15. Schaarschmidt K, Kolberg-Schwerdt A, Lempe M, et al. New endoscopic minimal access pectus carinatum repair using subpectoral carbon dioxide. *Ann Thorac Surg.* 2006; 81:1099-1103.
16. Kobayashi S, Yoza S, Komuro Y, et al. Correction of pectus excavatum and pectus carinatum assisted by the endoscope. *Plast Reconstr Surg.* 1997;99:1037-1045.
17. Frey AS, Garcia VF, Brown RL, et al. Nonoperative management of pectus carinatum. *J Pediatr Surg.* 2006;41: 40-45.
18. Banever GT, Konefal SH Jr, Gettens K, et al. Nonoperative correction of pectus carinatum with orthotic bracing. *J Laparoendosc Adv Surg Tech A.* 2006;16:164-167.
19. Fonkalsrud EW, Mendoza J. Open repair of pectus excavatum and carinatum deformities with minimal cartilage resection. *Am J Surg.* 2006;191:779-784.

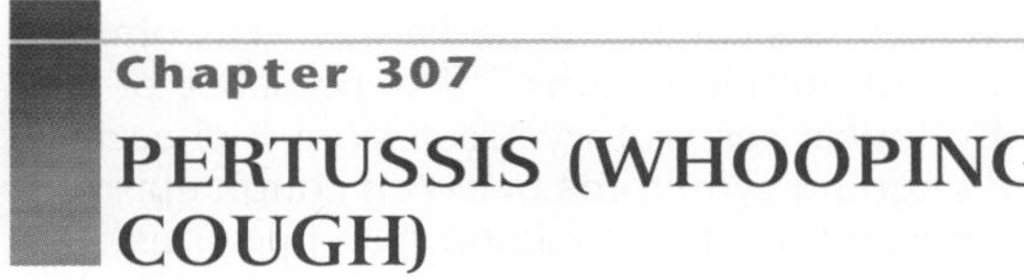

Chapter 307

PERTUSSIS (WHOOPING COUGH)

Camille Sabella, MD

DEFINITIONS

Pertussis (whooping cough) is a highly contagious, bacterial respiratory infection caused by *Bordetella pertussis,* an aerobic gram-negative coccobacillus. The illness is characterized by spasms of intense coughing and a protracted clinical course lasting several weeks. A characteristic severe paroxysmal cough ending in the inspiratory *whoop* is most often seen in infants and young children, who experience the most severe manifestations of this illness.

EPIDEMIOLOGIC FEATURES

Worldwide, pertussis is an important killer of children, with an estimated 300,000 pertussis-related deaths annually.[1] Before the availability of whole-cell pertussis vaccines in the late 1940s, pertussis was a major cause of morbidity and mortality in the United States, accounting for almost 300,000 cases and 10,000 deaths annually.[2] After introduction of an effective vaccine, a significant decrease in cases ensued, and by the early 1970s, the incidence had declined by 99% compared with the prevaccine era, with a record low number of 1010 cases reported in 1976[3] (Figure 307-1). Since the early 1980s, however, the incidence of pertussis in this country has steadily increased (Figure 307-2). Although the disease is endemic, with all 50 states reporting cases annually, epidemic peaks occur every 3 to 5 years, and several large outbreaks in North America have been reported in the last several years.[4-6] These outbreaks have occurred both in highly immunized populations and in infants who had not received three doses of vaccine. In 2003, 11,647 cases were reported in the United States, marking the highest number of cases reported since the early 1960s, with an annual incidence of 4.0 cases per 100,000 population.[7] Provisional data from 2004 and 2005 confirm this continuing increase in incidence (see Figures 307-1 and 307-2).[8]

During the last several decades, the age distribution of pertussis has changed significantly. In the prevaccine era, the peak incidence of disease occurred in children aged 1 to 5 years. With widespread vaccination and by the late 1980s, infants younger than one year had the highest age-specific incidence, which declined with increasing age.[3] Since the early 1990s, however, a marked increase has occurred in reported cases in children 10 years and older. Data from the National Notifiable Diseases Surveillance System between 2001 and 2003 reveal that children aged 10 to 19 years comprised 33% of all reported cases, whereas 23% of cases occurred in individuals 20 years and older.[7] During the same period, infants younger than one year comprised 23% of all cases (Figure 307-3). Infants younger than one year, however, continue to have the highest average annual incidence (55.2 per 100,000 population compared with 7.7 for persons aged 10 to 19 years and 1.1 for adults). The overall number of cases of pertussis, however, is likely underestimated because the infection is often underdiagnosed in adolescents and adults.[8]

B pertussis is a highly contagious organism, as demonstrated by 80% to 90% secondary attack rates among susceptible household contacts.[8] The organism is acquired through direct transmission from close respiratory contact. Most cases in the United States occur between the months of June and October.[9,10] Although chronic carriage of the organism does not occur, clearly, subclinical or mild illness commonly occurs in fully or partially immunized, as well as naturally immune, individuals.[11,12] This proclivity occurs because immunity wanes within 3 to 5 years of vaccination or natural infection and is often undetectable at 12 years.[13] Thus neither vaccination nor natural disease provides long-lasting immunity, and adults in this

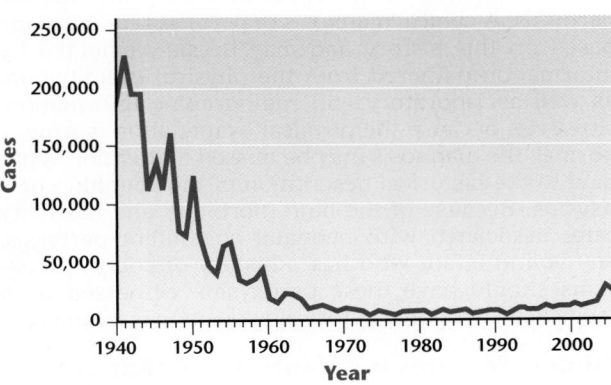

Figure 307-1 Pertussis—United States, 1940-2005. *(Centers for Disease Control and Prevention.* Epidemiology and Prevention of Vaccine-Preventable Diseases. January 2006. *Available at: www.cdc.gov/nip/publications/pink/pert.pdf.)*

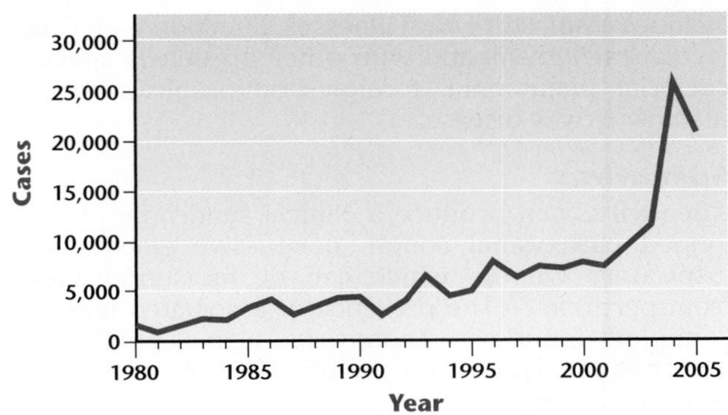

Figure 307-2 Pertussis—United States, 1980-2005. *(Centers for Disease Control and Prevention.* Epidemiology and Prevention of Vaccine-Preventable Diseases. January 2006. *Available at: www.cdc.gov/nip/publications/pink/pert.pdf.)*

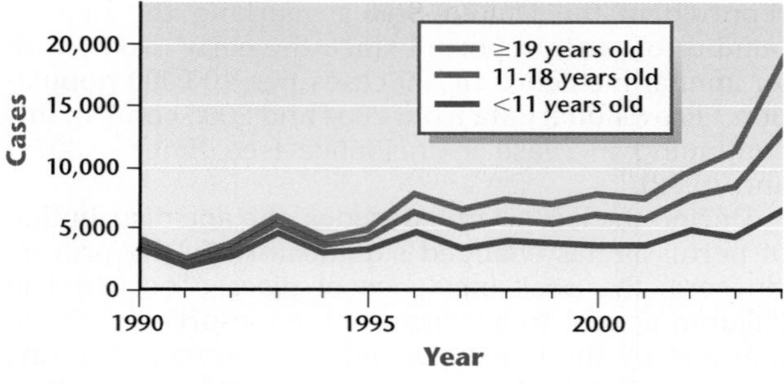

Figure 307-3 Reported pertussis by age group, 1990-2004. *(Centers for Disease Control and Prevention.* Epidemiology and Prevention of Vaccine-Preventable Diseases. January 2006. *Available at: www.cdc.gov/nip/publications/pink/pert.pdf.)*

country do not have adequate protection against pertussis.[12] Importantly, adults and adolescents with pertussis serve as important reservoirs for infection and often serve as the index cases for younger infants and children.[4,12,14] An example of this circumstance occurred during the Chicago outbreak of 1993, where mothers served as an important source of pertussis for their infants.[4]

Many studies have proven that pertussis is a very common cause of prolonged cough in adolescents and adults, accounting for 12% to 32% of cases of cough lasting 2 weeks or longer. A prospective, US population–based study with active surveillance has revealed that 13% of study participants between the ages of 10 and 49 years who visited their community clinic with an acute paroxysmal cough or a persistent cough illness of more than 2 weeks' duration had evidence of an acute pertussis infection.[15] A recent Canadian study, the largest prospective study examining the rates of pertussis disease in adolescents and adults, demonstrated that 20% of 442 adolescents and adults with cough illness lasting 7 to 56 days' duration were diagnosed with pertussis.[16]

DIFFERENTIAL DIAGNOSIS

In infants, the differential diagnosis of pertussis includes respiratory viral illnesses, infection with *Chlamydia trachomatis* and with other *Bordetella* species, bacterial pneumonia, foreign body aspiration, and reactive airway disease.

Adenovirus

Adenovirus can produce a clinical syndrome of prolonged paroxysmal cough, posttussive emesis, and inspiratory whoop, which can be indistinguishable from pertussis.[17] The presence of associated features commonly found with adenovirus, such as pharyngitis and conjunctivitis, can help distinguish clinically among these entities.

Respiratory Syncytial Virus

Respiratory syncytial virus (RSV) is a common cause of upper and lower respiratory tract infection in neonates and infants and can occasionally be difficult to distinguish from pertussis. In addition, dual infection with RSV and *B pertussis* can occur, and apnea is a common complication of both infections.[18] The presence of predominantly lower respiratory tract signs (wheezing), fever, and ongoing symptoms between cough episodes is more suggestive of RSV infection than pertussis.

Chlamydia trachomatis

Chlamydia trachomatis, which is a common cause of afebrile pneumonia in young infants, can mimic pertussis. However, infants with chlamydial infection usually have a staccato rather than paroxysmal cough, lower respiratory tract signs such as tachypnea and rales, and, frequently, a history of conjunctivitis in the neonatal period.

Other *Bordetella* Species

Bordetella parapertussis and rarely *Bordetella bronchiseptica* have been associated with a pertussis-like illness but characteristically cause a less protracted illness.

Bacterial pneumonia

Bacterial pneumonia caused by *Staphylococcus aureus* and *Streptococcus pneumoniae* is not difficult to distinguish from pertussis based on the clinical manifestations (high temperature, ill appearance, respiratory distress). However, these agents can secondarily complicate pertussis infection.

The differential diagnosis of pertussis in the older child, adolescent, and adult includes adenoviral infection, infection with *Mycoplasma pneumoniae* and *Chlamydophila pneumoniae,*[19] reactive airway disease, and upper respiratory tract infection. *M pneumoniae* is a common cause of prolonged cough and may be difficult to distinguish from pertussis.[20] Concurrent outbreaks have been reported. The presence of systemic symptoms such as headache, sore throat, rales on auscultation of the chest, and the presence of a chest radiograph, which characteristically appears worse than the appearance of the patient, all favor the diagnosis of *M pneumoniae.*

EVALUATION

A complete history is by far the most important aspect of the evaluation of the infant or child with possible pertussis. A clinical diagnosis of pertussis can be made based on this history and may be supplemented by information gathered from the physical examination, as well as laboratory and radiographic information. However, because the physical examination is usually normal, the diagnosis may be missed if attention is not paid to the historical description of the coughing paroxysms. Because of the high morbidity and mortality rates associated with neonatal and infant pertussis, any young infant who has a history of cough paroxysms should have these paroxysms witnessed by a medical professional before a disposition is planned.

Clinical Features in Infants and Children

Three stages of illness are classically described, each lasting at least 2 weeks. The classic stages are evident mostly in unimmunized infected young children. Thus, in partially or totally immunized children, the stages are shortened and may be atypical. Neonates do not have an apparent catarrhal phase.

After an incubation period of 7 to 10 days, the *catarrhal* phase consists of nonspecific upper respiratory tract symptoms with rhinorrhea, lacrimation, mild cough, and conjunctival injection. This phase is followed by the *paroxysmal* stage, which is characterized by an intermittent dry hacking cough. In this stage, a repetitive series of forceful coughs within a single expiration occur. A sudden massive inspiratory respiratory effort often occurs at the end of the cough paroxysm, resulting in a high-pitched *whoop*. Between the attacks, the patient appears comfortable without apparent distress. The paroxysmal stage in very young infants often lacks the characteristic *whoop* and is characterized by episodes of gagging, gasping, apnea, bradycardia, and cyanosis.[21] The *convalescent* stage is characterized by diminishing severity and frequency of paroxysms. However, patients with pertussis commonly continue experiencing intermittent coughing for weeks to months, which are often exacerbated by subsequent intercurrent respiratory illness.

Physical examination of patients with pertussis is usually normal, except that they may have conjunctival hemorrhage and upper body petechial lesions, evidence of the forcefulness of their cough and posttussive emesis. Fever is characteristically absent at all stages and, if present, should immediately suggest secondary bacterial infection.[22] Leukocytosis caused by absolute lymphocytosis is a common finding in unimmunized infants and children who are in the paroxysmal or late catarrhal stage of pertussis. The degree of lymphocytosis parallels the severity of disease. Chest radiography is commonly normal but may reveal perihilar infiltrates, pneumothorax, or pneumomediastinum.

Clinical Features in Adolescents and Adults

Pertussis in adolescents and adults does not usually have distinct phases. A persistent (>21 days) cough, which is indistinguishable from other respiratory infections, can be the only symptom. However, a paroxysmal nature to the cough is present in approximately 70% to 99% of infected individuals.[23] Other features include inspiratory whoop, posttussive emesis, choking, and sleep disturbed by cough.[23,24] Positive predictors of confirmed pertussis infection include a history of prolonged duration of violent cough (median, 43 days), a longer duration of cough illness (median, 56 days), and posttussive emesis.[16] Posttussive emesis is common at all ages and serves as a clue to the diagnosis in older children and adults.

Similar to infants and children, adults with pertussis do not have fever. Unlike in infants, leukocytosis and lymphocytosis are not common in adults and in partially immunized children with pertussis.

Diagnosis

Definitive diagnosis of pertussis is problematic. Culture and polymerase chain reaction testing of nasopharyngeal secretions are insensitive modes of diagnosis, whereas serologic testing is sensitive but impractical.

Culture

Isolation of the organism by culture remains the diagnostic standard but because of the fastidious nature of the organism is highly dependent on appropriate specimen collection, specimen transport, and isolation technique. Appropriate culture is obtained from the posterior nasopharynx using a calcium alginate or Dacron-tipped (not cotton) swab. The specimen should then be immediately inoculated onto Regan-Lowe medium and incubated for 7 days. A semisolid transport media is available if the specimen cannot be immediately inoculated onto solid media. Even when ideal conditions are met, the sensitivity of culture is suboptimal because cultures are most likely to be positive early in the illness (catarrhal and early paroxysmal phase) in unimmunized children. The sensitivity of culture is greatly diminished when obtained late in the illness, in immunized individuals, and in those who have received macrolides or sulfonamides.[25]

Polymerase Chain Reaction Testing

Polymerase chain reaction (PCR) testing of nasopharyngeal specimens has been developed and has become more widely available. The PCR test appears to be more sensitive than culture, including in individuals who are mildly symptomatic and in those who have been treated with macrolides.[26,27] The sensitivity of PCR when compared with serologic tests that are used for research purposes is highly dependent on the age of the patient (60% to 70% sensitive in infants and young children but less than 10% sensitive in older children and adults),[28] which is likely a reflection of past immunization and immune responses. PCR can detect *B parapertussis* as well.

Direct Fluorescent Antibody Testing

Direct fluorescent antibody testing of nasopharyngeal specimens for pertussis antigens has been used in the past but was plagued by poor sensitivity when compared with culture and required experienced laboratories for accurate results. This test is rarely used today.

Serologic Testing

Serologic testing for the detection of antibodies to components of *B pertussis* in acute and convalescent samples is the most sensitive mode of diagnosis. These tests have been used extensively in epidemiologic studies and vaccine trials and have enabled an understanding of the role of pertussis in adolescents and adults with prolonged cough illness.[29] Unfortunately, these tests are not readily available, the results are difficult to interpret in immunized individuals, and the tests are not helpful for the diagnosis of pertussis.

Complications of Pertussis

Young infants have the highest incidence of morbidity and mortality, with 91% of pertussis-related deaths occurring in children younger than 6 months.[7] Secondary bacterial pneumonia is the most common complication, occurring in approximately 5% of all reported cases, and the cause of most pertussis-related deaths. Infants younger than 6 months have the highest rate of hospitalization (69%), secondary bacterial pneumonia (13%), and seizures (2%).[7] Other important complications include apnea, bradycardia, dehydration, pulmonary hypertension, pneumothorax, central nervous system changes, and retinal hemorrhages. Although complications are much more common in infants, pertussis causes significant morbidity in adults, including pneumonia, otitis media, sinusitis, rib fracture, pneumothorax, pneumomediastinum, weight loss, and urinary incontinence.[23,24]

MANAGEMENT

Supportive Care

Supportive care continues to be the mainstay of management of pertussis infections. Hospitalization is indicated for most infants younger than 6 months to assess for life-threatening events associated with paroxysms, such as apnea, bradycardia, and hypoxia. Hospitalization also provides continuous cardiorespiratory monitoring, vigilant suctioning of the nasopharynx, oxygen therapy if needed, careful attention to feeding and hydration, and monitoring and treatment of acute complications.

Antibiotics

A macrolide antibiotic is indicated for proven or suspected pertussis to eliminate the organism from the nasopharynx and thus limit the spread to others.[30] If administered early in the illness, this therapy can reduce the duration and severity of symptoms. However, these agents have little influence on the clinical course of pertussis unless their use is started early in the catarrhal phase of the illness.[31]

Erythromycin has traditionally been the antibiotic of choice for the treatment of pertussis. However, data have shown that the newer macrolide agents—clarithromycin and azithromycin—are as effective as erythromycin for treating pertussis in persons 6 months and older, are better tolerated, and are associated with fewer and milder adverse effects than erythromycin.[32-36] Based on these data, the Centers for Disease Control and Prevention developed guidelines recommending that erythromycin, clarithromycin, and azithromycin be used for the treatment of pertussis in persons one month and older (Table 307-1). Although studies evaluating the safety and efficacy of the newer macrolides for infants younger than 6 months are limited, their use is encouraged based on their in vitro effectiveness, demonstrated safety in older infants and children, and more convenient dosing schedule. Because erythromycin therapy is associated with infantile hypertrophic pyloric stenosis,[37] azithromycin is the preferred macrolide in infants younger than one month. Limited data to date have not documented this association between azithromycin and infantile hypertrophic pyloric stenosis.

Care of Household and Other Close Contacts

Because of the high transmission rate from infected to susceptible individuals and proven efficacy of chemoprophylaxis, a macrolide should be given promptly to all household and close contacts (eg, those in child care) of infected individuals.[38] Chemoprophylaxis significantly reduces but does not eliminate the risk of pertussis. Because immunization may not always prevent infection, chemoprophylaxis should be given to close contacts regardless of age and immunization status.[39,40] Health care workers who have a definite or likely exposure to pertussis should also receive chemoprophylaxis.[41] The antimicrobial agents that should be used for postexposure prophylaxis are the same as for treatment of pertussis (see Table 307-1). Trimethoprim-sulfamethoxazole is an alternative treatment or prophylactic option for patients who cannot tolerate macrolides; however, this antibiotic is contraindicated in infants younger than 2 months. Treatment of parapertussis is the same as for pertussis.

Prevention

Universal immunization with pertussis vaccines for children younger than 7 years is recommended by the American Academy of Pediatrics (AAP) and is the mainstay of prevention.[42] Vaccination of all children starting in infancy has resulted in a greater than 97% decrease in the incidence of pertussis in the United States as compared with the prevaccine era. The currently available acellular vaccines, which are purified subunit vaccines and combination vaccines with diphtheria and tetanus toxoids (diphtheria-tetanus-acellular pertussis [DTaP]), have been shown to be 75% to 90% effective and are well tolerated. The AAP recommends that a total of five doses of pertussis vaccine be administered to every child before school entry, unless

Table 307-1 Antimicrobial Treatment and Postexposure Prophylaxis for Pertussis by Age Group

AGE GROUP	RECOMMENDED AGENT
<1 mo	Azithromycin 10 mg/kg/day as single daily dose for 5 days
1-5 mo	Azithromycin 10 mg/kg/day as single daily dose for 5 days, OR erythromycin 40-50 mg/kg/day in four divided doses for 14 days, OR clarithromycin 15 mg/kg/day in two divided doses for 7 days
Infants ≥ 6 mo and children	Azithromycin 10 mg/kg/day as single dose on day 1 then 5 mg/kg/day (maximum 500 mg) on days 2-5, OR erythromycin 40-50 mg/kg/day (maximum 2 g/day) in four divided doses for 14 days, OR clarithromycin 15 mg/kg/day in two divided doses (maximum 1 g/day) for 7 days
Adults	Azithromycin 500 mg as single daily dose on day 1 then 250 mg/day on days 2-5, OR erythromycin 2 g/day in four divided doses for 14 days, OR clarithromycin 1 g/day in two divided doses for 7 days

Adapted from Centers for Disease Control and Prevention. Recommended antimicrobial agents for the treatment and postexposure prophylaxis of pertussis. 2005 CDC guidelines. *MMWR*. 2005;54(RR14):1-16.

contraindicated.[42] The first dose is given at 2 months of age followed by two subsequent doses at intervals of 2 months. A fourth and fifth dose are recommended at 15 to 18 months of age and at 4 to 6 years of age, respectively.

Despite the successes of universal immunization, reported cases of pertussis in this country are steadily increasing, with resultant significant morbidity and mortality. This increase appears to be because waning immunity occurs after vaccination and natural infection, mild disease is underdiagnosed, and infants who have not completed their primary immunization series remain susceptible to infection.

Because of the role that adolescents and adults play in the transmission of pertussis, much interest has been generated in studies evaluating the efficacy and safety of pertussis vaccination in these age groups. Traditionally, pertussis vaccine has not been recommended for persons 7 years and older because of past concerns about the safety of the previously used whole-cell vaccines in this age group.[43,44] However, with the advent of the less reactogenic acellular vaccines during the last decade, studying these vaccines in adolescents and adults is of great interest. Adverse reactions to these vaccines among adolescents and adults have been mild, with local swelling and redness as the most commonly reported events. A National Institutes of Health–sponsored prospective multicenter trial, in which 2781 healthy subjects aged 15 to 65 years were randomized to receive acellular pertussis vaccine or hepatitis A vaccine, found that the acellular pertussis vaccine is safe, immunogenic, and effective in preventing clinical pertussis.[45] Although these pertussis vaccines appear to be well tolerated in the trials performed to date, concern exists about the possibility of more severe limb swelling in individuals vaccinated with booster doses of acellular vaccines after primary immunization with the same acellular vaccines.

BOX 307-1 American Academy of Pediatrics Recommendations for Use of Tetanus and Diphtheria Toxoids and Acellular Pertussis (Tdap) Vaccines in Adolescents

- Single dose of Tdap instead of tetanus and diphtheria toxoids (Td) vaccine for booster immunization for adolescents 11 to 18 years of age.
- The preferred age for Tdap immunization is 11-12 years.
- Adolescents 11 to 18 years of age who have received Td but not Tdap are encouraged to receive a single dose of Tdap. An interval of at least 5 years between Td and Tdap is suggested; however, intervals less than 5 years can be used, particularly in settings of increased risk of acquiring pertussis, having complicated disease, or transmitting infection to vulnerable contacts.

Adapted from American Academy of Pediatrics, Committee on Infectious Diseases. Prevention of pertussis among adolescents: recommendations for use of tetanus toxoid, reduced diphtheria toxoid, and acellular pertussis (Tdap) vaccine. *Pediatrics.* 2006;117:965-978.

Such swelling has been shown to occur in children who are given booster doses of acellular pertussis vaccines after primary immunization with acellular vaccine.[46] However, limb swelling does not appear to be a problem in individuals who received whole-cell pertussis vaccine as their primary immunization. Thus adolescents and adults who previously received acellular vaccines will need to be observed closely when they are given booster doses of pertussis vaccines to determine the frequency and severity of such reactions.

Given the immunogenicity and safety of these vaccines in adolescents and adults, the AAP recommends that adolescents aged 11 to 18 years receive acellular pertussis vaccine combined with tetanus and reduced diphtheria toxoid (Tdap) (Box 307-1).

WHEN TO REFER OR ADMIT

- Strongly consider in any young infant younger than 6 months suspected of having pertussis
- When complications such as apnea, bacterial pneumonia, bradycardia, or pulmonary hypertension exist
- When the infant has an oxygen requirement or when the infection is interfering with feeding

TOOLS FOR PRACTICE

Engaging Patient and Family

- *Pertussis* (fact sheet), Centers for Disease Control and Prevention (www.cdc.gov/ncidod/dbmd/diseaseinfo/pertussis_t.htm).
- *Vaccine Information Statement: DTP/DTaP Vaccine* (fact sheet), Centers for Disease Control and Prevention (www.aap.org/bst).

Medical Decision Support

- *Epidemiology and Prevention of Vaccine-Preventable Diseases: Pertussis* (booklet), Centers for Disease Control and Prevention (www.cdc.gov/vaccines/pubs/pinkbook/downloads/pert.pdf).
- *Recommended Antimicrobial Agents for the Treatment and Postexposure Prophylaxis of Pertussis* (guideline), Centers for Disease Control and Prevention (www.cdc.gov/mmwr/preview/mmwrhtml/rr5414a1.htm).
- Red Book: 2006 Report of the Committee on Infectious Diseases, American Academy of Pediatrics (www.aap.org/bookstore).

RELATED WEB SITE

- Centers for Disease Control and Prevention: Pertussis Vaccination (www.cdc.gov/vaccines/vpd-vac/pertussis/default.htm#disease).

AAP POLICY STATEMENT

American Academy of Pediatrics, Committee on Infectious Diseases. Prevention of pertussis among adolescents: recommendations for use of tetanus toxoid, reduced diphtheria toxoid, and acellular pertussis (Tdap) vaccine. *Pediatrics* 2006;117(3):965-978. (aappolicy.aappublications.org/cgi/content/full/pediatrics;117/3/965).

SUGGESTED RESOURCES

Centers for Disease Control and Prevention. Pertussis—United States, 2001-2003. *MMWR.* 2005;54(50):1283-1286.

Centers for Disease Control and Prevention. Recommended antimicrobial agents for the treatment and postexposure prophylaxis of pertussis. 2005 CDC guidelines. *MMWR.* 2005;54(RR14):1-16.

Edwards KM. Is pertussis a frequent cause of cough in adolescents and adults? Should routine pertussis immunization be recommended? *Clin Infect Dis.* 2001;32:1698-1699.

Heininger U, Klich K, Stehr K, et al. Clinical findings in Bordetella pertussis infections: results of a prospective multicenter surveillance study. *Pediatrics.* 1997;100:E10.

Langley JM, Halpering SA, Boucher FD, et al. Azithromycin is as effective as and better tolerated than erythromycin estolate for the treatment of pertussis. *Pediatrics.* 2004; 114:e96-e101.

Long SS, Welkon CJ, Clark JL. Widespread silent transmission of pertussis in families: antibody correlates of infection and symptomatology. *J Infect Dis.* 1990;161:480-486.

Rosenthal S, Strebel S, Cassiday P, et al. Pertussis infection among adults during the 1993 outbreak in Chicago. *J Infect Dis.* 1995;171:1650-1652.

Ward JI, Cherry JD, Chang SJ, et al. Efficacy of an acellular pertussis vaccine among adolescents and adults. *N Engl J Med.* 2005;353:1555-1563.

REFERENCES

1. World Health Organization. *WHO Vaccine-Preventable Diseases: Monitoring System. 2003 Global Summary.* Geneva, Switzerland: World Health Organization; 2003. Available at: www.who.int/vaccines-documents/Global Summary/GlobalSummary.pdf Accessed June 8, 2007.
2. Cherry JD, Brunell PA, Golden GS, et al. Report of the Task Force on Pertussis and Pertussis immunization—1988. *Pediatrics.* 1988; 81(suppl):933-984.
3. Centers for Disease Control and Prevention. Pertussis Surveillance—United States, 1989-1991. *MMWR.* 1992; 41(SS-8):11-19.
4. Rosenthal S, Strebel S, Cassiday P, et al. Pertussis infection among adults during the 1993 outbreak in Chicago. *J Infect Dis.* 1995;171:1650-1652.
5. Christie CD, Marx ML, Marchant C, et al. The 1993 epidemic of pertussis in Cincinnati: resurgence of disease in a highly immunized population of children. *N Engl J Med.* 1994;331:16-21.
6. Halperin SA, Bortulossi R, MacLean D, et al. Persistence of pertussis in an immunized population: results of the Nova Scotia enhanced pertussis surveillance program. *J Pediatr.* 1989;115:686-693.
7. Centers for Disease Control and Prevention. Pertussis—United States, 2001-2003. *MMWR.* 2005;54(50):1283-1286.
8. Centers for Disease Control and Prevention. Epidemiology and Prevention of Vaccine-Preventable Diseases. January 2006. Available at: www.cdc.gov/nip/publications/pink/pert.pdf. Accessed June 8, 2007.
9. Guris D, Strebel PM, Bardenheier B, et al. Changing epidemiology of pertussis in the United States: increasing reported incidence among adolescents and adults, 1990-1996. *Clin Infect Dis.* 1999;28:1230-1237.
10. Farizo KM, Cochi SL, Zell ER, et al. Epidemiologic features of pertussis in the United States, 1980-1989. *Clin Infect Dis.* 1992;14:708-719.
11. Tozzi AE, Rava L, Ciofi degli Atti ML, et al. Clinical presentation of pertussis in unvaccinated and vaccinated children in the first six years of life. *Pediatrics.* 2003; 112:1069-1075.
12. Long SS, Welkon CJ, Clark JL. Widespread silent transmission of pertussis in families: antibody correlates of infection and symptomatology. *J Infect Dis.* 1990;161: 480-486.
13. He Q, Viljanen MK, Nikkari S, et al. Outcomes of Bordetella pertussis infection in different age groups of an immunized population. *J Infect Dis.* 1994;170:873-877.
14. Deen JL, Mink CM, Cherry JD, et al. Household contact study of Bordetella pertussis infections. *Clin Infect Dis.* 1995;21:1211-1219.
15. Strebel P, Nordin J, Edwards K, et al. Population-based incidence of pertussis among adolescents and adults, Minnesota, 1995-1996. *J Infect Dis.* 2001;183:1353-1359.
16. Senzilet LD, Halperin SA, Spika JS, et al. Pertussis is a frequent cause of prolonged cough illness in adults and adolescents. *Clin Infect Dis.* 2001;32:1691-1697.
17. Von Konig CH, Rott H, Bogaerts H, et al. A serologic study of organisms possibly associated with pertussis-like coughing. *Pediatr Infect Dis J.* 1998;17:645-649.
18. Nelson WL, Hopkins RS, Roe MH, et al. Simultaneous infection with Bordetella pertussis and respiratory syncytial virus in hospitalized children. *Pediatr Infect Dis.* 1986;5:540-544.
19. Hagiwara K, Ouchi K, Tashiro N, et al. An epidemic of a pertussis-like illness caused by Chlamydia pneumoniae. *Pediatr Infect Dis J.* 1999;18:271-275.
20. Davis SF, Sutter RW, Strebel PM, et al. Concurrent outbreaks of pertussis and Mycoplasma pneumoniae infection: clinical and epidemiologic characteristics of illnesses manifested by cough. *Clin Infect Dis.* 1995;20: 621-628.
21. Long SS, Edwards KM. Bordetella pertussis (pertussis) and other species. In: Long SS, Pickering LK, Prober CG, eds. *Principles and Practices of Pediatric Infectious Diseases.* Philadelphia, PA: Lippincott Williams & Wilkins; 2003.
22. Heininger U, Klich K, Stehr K, et al. Clinical findings in Bordetella pertussis infections: results of a prospective multicenter surveillance study. *Pediatrics.* 1997;100:E10.
23. De Serres G, Shadmani R, Duval B, et al. Morbidity of pertussis in adolescents and adults. *J Infect Dis.* 2000; 182:174-179.
24. Cherry JD. Epidemiologic, clinical, and laboratory aspects of pertussis in adults. *Clin Inf Dis.* 1999;28(suppl 2): S112-S117.
25. Hallander HO. Microbiologic and serological diagnosis of pertussis. *Clin Infect Dis.* 1999;28(suppl 2):S99-S106.
26. Edelman K, Nikkari S, Ruuskanen O, et al. Detection of Bordetella pertussis by polymerase chain reaction and culture in the nasopharynx of erythromycin-treated infants with pertussis. *Pediatr Infect Dis J.* 1996;15:54-57.
27. Heininger U, Schmidt-Schlapfer G, Cherry JD, et al. Clinical validation of a polymerase chain reaction assay for the diagnosis of pertussis by comparison with serology, culture, and symptoms during a large pertussis vaccine efficacy trial. *Pediatrics.* 2000;105:e31.
28. van der Zee A, Agterberg C, Peeters M, et al. A clinical validation of Bordetella pertussis and Bordetella parapertussis polymerase chain reaction: comparison with culture and serology using samples from patients with suspected whooping cough from a highly immunized population. *J Infect Dis.* 1996;174:89-96.
29. Edwards KM. Is pertussis a frequent cause of cough in adolescents and adults? Should routine pertussis immunization be recommended? *Clin Infect Dis.* 2001;32: 1698-1699.
30. Bortolussi R, Miller B, Ledwith M, et al. Clinical course of pertussis in immunized children. *Pediatr Infect Dis J.* 1995; 14:870-874.

31. Bergquist SO, Bernander S, Dahnsjo H, et al. Erythromycin in the treatment of pertussis: a study of bacteriologic and clinical effects. *Pediatr Infect Dis J.* 1987;6:458-461.
32. Langley JM, Halpering SA, Boucher FD, et al. Azithromycin is as effective as and better tolerated than erythromycin estolate for the treatment of pertussis. *Pediatrics.* 2004;114:e96-e101.
33. Aoyama T, Sunakawa K, Iwata S, et al. Efficacy of short-term treatment of pertussis with clarithromycin and azithromycin. *J Pediatr.* 1996;129:761-764.
34. Bace A, Zrnic J, Begovac J, et al. Short-term treatment of pertussis with azithromycin in infants and young children. *Eur J Clin Microbiology Infect Dis.* 1999;18:296-298.
35. Lebel MH, Mehra S. Efficacy and safety of clarithromycin versus erythromycin for the treatment of pertussis: a prospective, randomized, single blind trial. *Pediatr Infect Dis J.* 2001;20:1149-1154.
36. Pichichero ME, Hoeger WJ, Casey JR. Azithromycin for the treatment of pertussis. *Pediatr Infect Dis J.* 2003;22:847-849.
37. Honein MA, Paulozzi LJ, Himelright IM, et al. Infantile hypertrophic pyloric stenosis after pertussis prophylaxis with erythromycin: a case review and cohort study. *Lancet.* 1999;354:2101-2105.
38. American Academy of Pediatrics. Pertussis. In: Pickering LK, ed. *2003 Red Book: Report of the Committee on Infectious Diseases,* 26th ed. Elk Grove Village, IL: American Academy of Pediatrics; 2003.
39. Halperin SA, Bortolussi R, Langley JM, et al. A randomized, placebo-controlled trial of erythromycin estolate chemoprophylaxis for household contacts of children with culture-positive Bordetella pertussis infection. *Pediatrics.* 1999;104:E42.
40. De Serres G, Boulianne N, Duval B. Field effectiveness of erythromycin prophylaxis to prevent pertussis within families. *Pediatr Infect Dis J.* 1995;14:969-975.
41. Weber DJ, Rutala WA. Management of healthcare workers exposed to pertussis. *Infect Control Hosp Epidemiol.* 1994;15:411-415.
42. American Academy of Pediatrics. Pertussis. In: Pickering LK, Baker CJ, Long SS, et al, eds. *Red Book: 2006 Report of the Committee on Infectious Diseases,* 27th ed. Elk Grove Village, IL: American Academy of Pediatrics; 2006.
43. Volk VK, Gottshall RY, Anderson HD, et al. Antibody response to booster dose diphtheria and tetanus toxoids and pertussis vaccine: thirteen years after inoculation of institutional subjects. *Public Health Rep.* 1964;79:424-434.
44. Linneman CC, Ramundo N, Perlstein PH, et al. Use of pertussis vaccine in an epidemic involving hospital staff. *Lancet.* 1975;2:540-544.
45. Ward JI, Cherry JD, Chang SJ, et al. Efficacy of an acellular pertussis vaccine among adolescents and adults. *N Engl J Med.* 2005;353:1555-1563.
46. Rennels MB, Deloria MA, Pichichero ME, et al. Extensive swelling after booster doses of acellular pertussis-tetanus-diphtheria vaccines. *Pediatrics.* 2000;105:e12.

Chapter 308

PHARYNGITIS AND TONSILLITIS

Russell W. Steele, MD

INTRODUCTION

Acute pharyngitis is one of the more common diagnoses made in pediatric practice, exceeded only by otitis media and viral upper respiratory tract infections. It is also the most common diagnosis requiring treatment with antibiotics in school-aged children.

DEFINITIONS

The term *pharyngitis* implies inflammation of the throat with or without the presence of exudate; when the tonsils are affected, the terms *tonsillitis, tonsillopharyngitis,* and *pharyngotonsillitis* are more commonly used. Pharyngitis may be associated with other inflammatory conditions of the mucous membranes (eg, herpes gingivostomatitis, herpangina, Stevens-Johnson syndrome, Kawasaki disease), or it may be the sole finding in an illness. Generally, a clinical complaint of sore throat indicates some degree of pharyngitis.

ETIOLOGY

Although pharyngitis is most commonly caused by viral agents, the major management step is to establish whether group A beta-hemolytic *Streptococcus* (GABHS) is the responsible pathogen. The presence of GABHS mandates early antimicrobial therapy within 9 days of onset of symptoms to eradicate this bacterium and thereby prevent acute rheumatic fever. In children younger than 3 years, GABHS is the cause of tonsillopharyngitis in less than 3% of cases, whereas in children older than 3 years, estimates suggest that 15% to 20% of pharyngitis episodes are caused by GABHS. The cause of pharyngitis varies somewhat, depending on the geographic location and season, particularly during recognized outbreaks of GABHS, influenza, respiratory syncytial virus, and mycoplasma. In addition to these causes, many other infectious agents have been associated with pharyngitis (Box 308-1).

Viruses

Although many primary care physicians associate pharyngitis and tonsillitis with bacterial origins, viruses play a major role in the cause of these illnesses. Moreover, when pharyngitis is associated with upper

BOX 308-1 Causes of Pharyngitis

BACTERIA
Streptococcus pyogenes
Corynebacterium diphtheriae
Arcanobacterium haemolyticum
Neisseria gonorrhoeae
Group C streptococci
Group G streptococci
Chlamydia pneumoniae
Chlamydia trachomatis
Mycoplasma pneumoniae
Yersinia enterocolitica
Francisella tularensis
Coxiella burnetii

VIRUSES
Epstein-Barr virus
Adenovirus
Enteroviruses
Herpes simplex viruses
Influenza
Parainfluenza
Rhinoviruses
Coronavirus
Respiratory syncytial virus

From Tanz RT, Shulman ST. Pharyngitis. In: Long SS, Pickering LK, Prober CG, eds. *Principles and Practice of Pediatric Infectious Diseases.* New York, NY: Churchill Livingstone; 1997.

respiratory tract symptoms, such as conjunctivitis, nasal congestion, and rhinorrhea, GABHS and other bacterial agents are highly unlikely causes.

Adenoviruses

At least 12 different types of adenoviruses have been found to cause pharyngitis in children and adolescents, accounting for up to 23% of cases in some reports.[1] These viruses cause both a nasopharyngitis and a tonsillitis that can be exudative. Outbreaks of a unique clinical illness caused by adenovirus type 3, called pharyngoconjunctival fever because of these consistent features, occur frequently. Affected patients may also have cough, myalgias, and conjunctivitis.

Enteroviruses

Two prominent members of the enterovirus class of viruses, coxsackievirus A and echovirus, have been shown to cause pharyngitis, often accompanied by respiratory symptoms, commonly in the late summer or early fall. Herpangina is a specific entity caused by various strains of coxsackievirus A and B, typified by pharyngitis associated with small, shallow, ulcerated areas on the soft palate and peritonsillar area.

Epstein-Barr Virus

Epstein-Barr virus (EBV) is an etiologic agent of infectious mononucleosis that frequently causes a severe exudative pharyngitis with a characteristic white, *shaggy* membrane on the tonsils and palatal petechiae. In older children, EBV infection is accompanied by fever, adenopathy, malaise, swelling of the eyelids, and hepatosplenomegaly. EBV is a copathogen of GABHS in 5% to 10% of cases.

Herpes Simplex Virus

Although most oral colonization and covert infection with herpes simplex virus type 1 is asymptomatic, this virus can cause painful gingivostomatitis and pharyngitis in approximately 1% of infected children. Studies in a college-aged population have also documented that herpes simplex virus type 1 and 2 account for 5.7% of pharyngitis cases.[2]

Other Viruses

Many other viruses cause pharyngitis, although pharyngitis is usually not the primary manifestation of the illness. These viruses include influenza, parainfluenza, respiratory syncytial virus, human metapneumovirus, measles, coronavirus, and rhinoviruses.[3]

Bacteria

One of the main considerations in evaluating a child who has pharyngitis and tonsillitis is to determine whether the cause is bacterial, thus requiring specific antibiotic therapy. GABHS infections are the major bacterial cause, but other organisms should be considered in certain situations.

Streptococcus pyogenes

S pyogenes causes complete (beta) hemolysis when grown on blood agar and hence has been called beta-hemolytic *Streptococcus*. Streptococci have been subdivided into groups based on the C-substance in the cell wall, and most human pathological disease has been found to be caused by the A group. GABHS was not fully recognized as a frequent cause of pharyngitis with the possibility of subsequent rheumatic fever until the 1940s. Whereas other groups of *Streptococcus* (B, C, F, and G) have been associated at times with pharyngitis,[4] GABHS is by far the most frequent bacterial cause. GABHS can be divided into M and T serotypes, and a certain number of these serotypes have been associated with both the rash of scarlet fever (GABHS T4)[5] and the development of rheumatic fever (GABHS M3 and M18).[6]

The pharyngitis caused by GABHS characteristically begins after a 2- to 5-day incubation period, usually after exposure to another individual who has the infection. Spread is thought to occur by way of respiratory secretions, although fomites, such as shared silverware or household cats (but not dogs), have occasionally been shown to be vectors. The ingestion of GABHS-contaminated food also has led to outbreaks of pharyngitis. The illness is heralded by sudden onset of fever, sore throat, and dysphagia, often associated with headache and abdominal pain. Examination of the throat reveals an erythematous pharynx and tonsillar area, often with exudate present. Small petechiae (enanthem) are sometimes seen on the uvula and soft palate. Cervical lymph nodes are usually enlarged and tender. These symptoms can last for 4 to 5 days, gradually subsiding when no antibiotic therapy is instituted. Penicillin therapy shortens the duration of fever and sore throat by 1 to 1½ days and, if given within 9 days of onset, prevents rheumatic fever.

Key Findings:

1. Red throat or tonsils and or exudative tonsils
2. Swollen and usually tender anterior cervical nodes
3. Fever
4. Scarlet fever rash

Neisseria gonorrhoeae

Pharyngitis in sexually active adolescents or sexually abused children can be caused by *N gonorrhoeae* acquired from oral sex, and the organism should be sought when appropriate. Exudative tonsillitis is rarely seen with pharyngitis caused by *N gonorrhoeae*.

Hemophilus influenzae type b

The possible involvement of the *H influenzae* type b (Hib) organism in pharyngitis and tonsillitis has been controversial, but evidence suggests that it may contribute to infection in some children, especially those with recurrent tonsillitis. Fine-needle aspiration of tonsils during acute tonsillitis and pathological specimens from tonsillectomy have documented that as many as 20% of sampled tonsils have Hib infection.[7,8] However, with Hib immunization of most infants in the United States in recent years, this organism may be less likely to play a role in the pathogenesis of acute tonsillitis and pharyngitis.

Arcanobacterium hemolyticum

Approximately 7% of tonsillopharyngitis in adolescents and young adults is caused by *Arcanobacterium hemolyticum*.[9] Physical findings are identical to those seen with GABHS infection, including a scarlatiniform rash present in approximately 20% of cases. The sore throat may persist until patients are treated with erythromycin, azithromycin, or clarithromycin.

Other Bacteria

A century ago, *Corynebacterium diphtheria* was a frequent and deadly cause of pharyngitis, with a characteristic gray pseudomembranous exudate over the posterior pharynx and tonsils. Fortunately, *C diphtheriae* now is rare in North America, although it is still being reported in some developing countries. Various reports have been published of other bacteria causing pharyngitis and tonsillitis, including *Actinomyces, Chlamydia trachomatis* and *Chlamydia pneumoniae, Yersinia enterocolitica, Coxiella burnetii,* and *Francisella tularensis* (oropharyngeal tularemia).

Other Causes

Mycoplasma pneumoniae

Two types of *Mycoplasma pneumoniae* have been shown to cause pharyngitis, namely *Mycoplasma pneumoniae* and *M hominis*. In children, the former causes a mild pharyngitis, often associated with a laryngotracheitis or progressing to bronchitis or pneumonia. In school-aged children, as much as 5% of pharyngitis may be caused by this organism.

Fungi

Candida infection is an uncommon cause of pharyngitis in the healthy host but can be certainly seen in immunocompromised patients or those taking steroids. With oral thrush in otherwise healthy children, severe mouth pain can occur, which may be interpreted as a sore throat.

Kawasaki Disease

Of unknown cause, Kawasaki disease occurs mostly in preschool children who have pharyngitis associated with erythema and fissuring of the lips, as well as palmar and pedal edema and erythema. An association with staphylococcal toxin has been postulated,[10] as have other viral and bacterial etiologies. (See Chapter 289, Kawasaki Disease.)

Exposure to Cigarette Smoke

Although smoke itself has not been reported to cause pharyngitis or tonsillitis, a highly significant association has been found between the incidence of tonsillectomy in children and parental smoking.[11] Children of smokers also had a much higher frequency of attacks of acute tonsillitis compared with children in a smoke-free environment. Whether this association will be confirmed in other studies remains to be seen, but among children seeking treatment for frequent tonsillitis, a history of parental smoking should be sought. If such a history exists, advising measures to reduce the child's exposure to cigarette smoke would be prudent.

DIFFERENTIAL DIAGNOSIS

Sore throats are common in children, and almost all children older than 3 years need to be examined to rule out GABHS as the cause. If GABHS is the documented cause, then antibiotic therapy should be instituted in an effort to prevent rheumatic fever. Unfortunately, multiple studies have shown that streptococcal pharyngitis cannot be distinguished purely on clinical grounds.[12-14] Streptococcal infections should be considered in children older than 3 years who have pharyngitis, even if no exudate is present. However, pharyngitis associated with nasal, chest, or *cold* symptoms is much more likely to be a viral illness.

When pharyngitis is atypical, either in its duration or its severity, the clinician should suspect infectious mononucleosis or one of the rarer bacterial causes, including those that are sexually transmitted. A peritonsillar abscess or cellulitis also may cause a sore throat, but thorough examination will reveal swelling extending into the soft palate, with deviation of the uvula and a change in the tonal quality of the voice. Allergies may lead to chronic inflammation of the mucous membranes, which might include the pharynx, but pharyngitis would be infrequent as a sole manifestation. Postnasal drip from a viral respiratory tract infection or allergies has been thought to irritate the posterior pharynx, but this finding is not well documented.

Acute tonsillopharyngitis may progress to a peritonsillar abscess. Researchers have observed that 41% to 70% of peritonsillar abscesses occur in the superior pole. This infection begins with the typical signs and symptoms of pharyngitis such as sore throat, dysphagia, and fever, usually in an older child who often has a history of recurrent tonsillitis. Systemic symptoms such as malaise, poor appetite, and chills appear early and mild dehydration may develop. These symptoms progress rapidly to more severe pharyngeal symptoms, such as difficulty in swallowing and speaking. The child has a toxic appearance and trismus almost always occurs. Characteristic signs are a muffled *(hot potato)* voice, trismus, and major leukocytosis. Needle aspiration can be performed only if the abscess is within the superior pole and the success rate with needle aspiration compares favorably with that of incision and drainage in these type cases. Computed tomography scanning and intraoral ultrasonography are quite reliable in distinguishing abscesses from cellulitis alone. Initial antimicrobial therapy is clindamycin plus a third-generation cephalosporin such as ceftriaxone, cefotaxime, or ceftazidime. Routine tonsillectomy along with or after medical management is recommended by some experts.[15]

The one entity in the differential diagnosis not to be missed is epiglottitis, which can be life threatening. Generally, the child who has epiglottitis has severe throat pain, rapidly becomes ill, appears to have a toxic condition, and experiences respiratory distress accompanied by stridor or a croupy cough.

MANAGEMENT

Laboratory Procedures

Rapid Streptococcal Test and Cultures

The traditional method for determining whether pharyngitis or tonsillitis was caused by a virus or GABHS was to obtain a throat swab and perform a culture. Fortunately, with the availability of rapid streptococcal tests, this process was made simpler, allowing a result to be obtained in minutes rather than waiting 1 to 2 days. Unfortunately, with the advent of strict federal guidelines for office laboratories, even the use of these rapid tests requires certification. Despite such encumbrances, most clinicians now perform a rapid streptococcal diagnostic test on all patients whose pharyngitis is suggestive of GABHS.

The various rapid streptococcal tests claim differing levels of specificity and sensitivity. They appear to be specific (95% to 98%), but their sensitivity can be as low as 70% to 85%; thus some cases of GABHS are not detected. For this reason, a positive rapid streptococcal test result is sufficient indication to treat the patient; however, if the test result is negative but a high index of suspicion exists that GABHS is the causative agent, then a culture should be sent. If little clinical evidence of pharyngitis or tonsillitis can be found in a child who complains of sore throat or for those with manifestations highly suggestive of viral infection (coryza, conjunctivitis, cough, hoarseness, herpangina, stomatitis Sindbis virus), then a throat culture is not necessary. The physician also needs to be aware that some individuals are *Streptococcus* carriers, and they may well be found to be positive for *Streptococcus* infection during a viral illness. An asymptomatic *Streptococcus* carrier does not need to be treated but when symptoms are present, most physicians treat these individuals, given the difficulty of being certain that GABHS is not the cause of the illness. Because performing pre- and post-illness rapid streptococcal tests or cultures on every child who presumably has GABHS pharyngitis are impractical, all those who test positive are treated.

Serologic Tests

In cases in which EBV infection is suspected, a heterophile antibody or specific EBV test can be ordered. The physician needs to ascertain with the reference laboratory whether an immunoglobulin G (IgG) or IgM test has been performed because a positive heterophile test result may confirm only that children were exposed sometime in their life to EBV. Tests of specific IgG and IgM levels of antibody to various components of EBV are available but are usually expensive and slow to produce results, making it a less-than-ideal test to determine the cause of an acute pharyngitis (see Chapter 283, Infectious Mononucleosis and Other Epstein-Barr Viral Infections).

Although serologic tests exist to determine recent streptococcal infections, they are rarely helpful in evaluating for acute pharyngitis. An antistreptolysin-O titer is used more commonly in diagnosing rheumatic fever by documenting a recent exposure to streptolysin with production of antibody.

White Blood Cell Count

The only real value in performing a white blood cell count is if infectious mononucleosis is suspected. Patients who have an acute EBV infection tend to have relative lymphocytosis, with 10% to 20% atypical lymphocytes. Thus a white blood cell count may be a helpful diagnostic study, together with a heterophile or specific EBV antibody test, in a child who has a severe pharyngitis and is culture negative for GABHS.

Treatment

Pharyngitis caused by viruses generally is treated symptomatically with saline gargles, throat lozenges, and analgesics such as acetaminophen. When GABHS has been documented, either by a positive rapid *Streptococcus* test or by culture, antibiotics are indicated primarily to prevent the subsequent development of rheumatic fever. Various antibiotic regimens have been used for GABHS pharyngitis or tonsillitis, but the standard therapy has been a 10-day oral course of potassium penicillin or amoxicillin given 2 or 3 times a day. Alternatively, intramuscular benzathine penicillin G may be given as a single injection, although these injections are often painful not only initially, but also for a few days afterward. Patients allergic to penicillin may be given erythromycin or a cephalosporin for 10 days or azithromycin for 5 days. Although shorter courses of newer antibiotics have been studied and shown to be effective in eradicating GABHS from the pharynx,[16,17] their efficacy in preventing rheumatic fever is not clear although presumed.

Controversy exists over whether to begin antibiotics for presumptive GABHS pharyngitis while waiting for culture results. Because rheumatic fever can be prevented even if treatment is started as late as the 9th day of symptoms, the decision to begin therapy immediately rests with the individual physician who knows the circumstances of the patients. Early antibiotic treatment will shorten the duration and severity of symptoms by 24 to 36 hours. Patients should only be kept out of school and avoid close contact with family and friends for 24 hours, given that numerous studies have shown that they become culture negative after just 24 hours of antibiotic therapy.[18]

Cephalosporins have been shown to be superior to penicillin in eradicating GABHS from pharynx.[19] In cases of gonococcal pharyngitis, one intramuscular injection of ceftriaxone is recommended. In young children who have this diagnosis, sexual abuse must be investigated. Other possible bacterial causes of pharyngitis are treated with appropriate antibiotics, once the causative organism has been determined.

Parents often raise the question of tonsillectomy after a child has multiple episodes of pharyngitis or tonsillitis. Except in cases of documented recurrent, frequent streptococcal infection or the development of a peritonsillar abscess, tonsillectomy is not indicated in children who have recurrent pharyngitis. (See Chapter 331, Tonsillectomy and Adenoidectomy.)

Although the administration of steroids to decrease pain in acute exudative pharyngitis has been studied in adults and found to provide some benefit,[20] their use in children is not recommended except in rare situations such as infectious mononucleosis infection with imminent airway obstruction.[21]

COMPLICATIONS

Most cases of pharyngitis present no unusual complications because so many of them are viral and resolve with or without therapy. However, the physician must be aware of the possibility of a peritonsillar or retropharyngeal abscess or cellulitis developing and should reexamine the throat of any patient who is not improving. Other suppurative complications can also develop, such as cervical adenitis, acute otitis media, sinusitis, and pneumonia. In addition, hematogenous spread of a bacterial organism is possible and can result in bacteremia, as well as joint, bone, or meningeal infection.

Rheumatic fever (see Chapter 317) is the major complication of streptococcal pharyngitis that can be life threatening, although it occurs some time after the acute throat infection. Although the incidence of rheumatic fever is low in North America, it still occurs and has been seen in increasing numbers at some centers.[22] Although acute glomerulonephritis is possible after streptococcal throat infections, it is much more likely after streptococcal skin infections.

Some evidence has shown an association between GABHS infection and obsessive-compulsive disorders and tic behavior in children. This clinical entity is termed pediatric autoimmune neuropsychiatric disorder associated with group A streptococcal infection (PANDAS). Documentation is largely anecdotal but includes the observation that these children have high concentrations of antibody to streptococcal antigens. Small series have noted improvement in obsessive-compulsive disorder behavior or tics when these children are GABHS positive and treated with penicillin.[23,24] However, many still question the authenticity of PANDAS.

WHEN TO REFER

- Suspected peritonsillar abscess
- Suspected retropharyngeal abscess
- Recurrent GABHS (5 episodes in 1 year) for tonsillectomy

WHEN TO ADMIT

- Toxic appearance (suspected toxic shock syndrome)
- Peritonsillar abscess
- Retropharyngeal abscess
- Acute rheumatic fever

TOOLS FOR PRACTICE

Engaging Patient and Family

- *Sore Throat* (fact sheet), American Academy of Pediatrics (www.aap.org/publiced/BK0_SoreThroat.htm).

Medical Decision Support

- *Pharyngitis in Children* (Web page), Centers for Disease Control and Prevention (www.cdc.gov/drugresistance/community/files/ads/pharyn_children.htm).
- Red Book: 2006 Report of the Committee on Infectious Diseases, American Academy of Pediatrics (www.aap.org/bookstore).

REFERENCES

1. Moffet HL, Seigel AC, Doyle HK. Non-streptococcal pharyngitis. *J Pediatr.* 1985;73:51-57.
2. McMillan JA, Weiner LB, Higgins AM, et al. Pharyngitis associated with herpes simplex virus in college students. *Pediatr Infect Dis J.* 1993;12:280-284.
3. Tanz RR, Shulman ST. Pharyngitis. In Long SS, Pickering LK, Prober CG, eds. *Principles and Practice of Pediatric Infectious Diseases.* New York, NY: Churchill Livingstone; 1997.
4. Dudley JP, Sercarz J. Pharyngeal and tonsil infections caused by non-group A Streptococcus. *Am J Otol.* 1991; 12:292-298.
5. Ohga S, Okada K, Mitsui K, et al. Outbreaks of group A beta-hemolytic streptococcal pharyngitis in children: correlation of serotype T4 with scarlet fever. *Scand J Infect Dis.* 1992;24:599-605.
6. Johnson DR, Stevens DL, Kaplan EL. Epidemiologic analysis of group A streptococcal serotypes associated with severe systemic infections, rheumatic fever, or uncomplicated pharyngitis. *J Infect Dis.* 1992;166:374-379.
7. Gaffney RJ, Cafferkey MT. Bacteriology of normal and diseased tonsils assessed by fine-needle aspiration: Haemophilus influenzae and the pathogenesis of recurrent acute tonsillitis. *Clin Otolaryngol Allied Sci.* 1998;23: 181-185.
8. Stjernquist-Desatnik A, Preller K, Schalen C. High recovery of Haemophilus influenzae and group A streptococci in recurrent tonsillar infection or hypertrophy as compared with normal tonsils. *J Laryngol Otol.* 1991;105: 439-444.
9. Waagner DC. Arcanobacterium hemolyticum: biology of the organism and diseases in man. *Pediatr Infect Dis J.* 1991;10:933-939.
10. Leung DYM. Toxic shock syndrome toxin-secreting Staphylococcus aureus in Kawasaki syndrome. *Lancet.* 1993;342:1385-1388.
11. Hinton AE, Herdman RC, Martin-Hirsch D, et al. Parental cigarette smoking and tonsillectomy in children. *Clin Otolaryngol Allied Sci.* 1993;18(3):178-180.
12. Alpert AM, Pickering MR, Warren RJ. Failure to isolate streptococci from children under the age of 3 years with exudative tonsillitis. *Pediatrics.* 1966;38:663-666.
13. Wannamaker LW. Diagnosis of pharyngitis: clinical and epidemiologic features. In: Shulman S, ed. *Management of Pharyngitis in an Era of Declining Rheumatic Fever.* Columbus, OH: Ross Conference on Pediatric Research; 1984.
14. Bisno AL. Acute pharyngitis: etiology and diagnosis. *Pediatrics.* 1996;97:949-954.
15. Steele RW. Could your patient have Quincy? Defining peritonsillar abscess. *J Resp Dis Pediatr.* 2002;4:89-92.
16. Mehra S, Van Moerkerke M, Welck J, et al. Short course therapy with cefuroxime axetil for group A streptococcal tonsillopharyngitis in children. *Pediatr Infect Dis J.* 1998; 17:252-258.
17. Venuta A, Laudizi L, Beverelli A, et al. Azithromycin compared with clarithromycin for the treatment of streptococcal pharyngitis in children. *Int Med Res.* 1998;26: 152-158.
18. Kaplan EL. Benzathine penicillin G for treatment of group A streptococcal pharyngitis: a reappraisal in 1985. *Pediatr Infect Dis J.* 1985;4:592-596.
19. Casey JR, Pichichero ME. The evidence base for cephalosporin superiority over penicillin in streptococcal pharyngitis. *Diagn Microbiol Infect Dis.* 2007;57(suppl 3): S39-S45.
20. Marvez-Valls EG, Ernst AA, Gray J, et al. The role of betamethasone in the treatment of acute exudative pharyngitis. *Acad Emerg Med.* 1998;5:567-572.
21. Boglioli LR, Taff ML. Sudden asphyxial death complicating infectious mononucleosis. *Am J Forensic Med Pathol.* 1998;19:174-179.
22. Kaplan EL. Return of rheumatic fever: consequences, implications, and needs. *J Pediatr.* 1987;111:244-249.
23. Murphy ML, Pichichero ME. Prospective identification and treatment of children with pediatric autoimmune neuropsychiatric disorder associated with group A streptococcal infection (PANDAS). *Arch Pediatr Adolesc Med.* 2002;156:356-361.

24. Swedo SE, Leonard HL, Garvey M, et al: Pediatric autoimmune neuropsychiatric disorders associated with streptococcal infections: clinical description of the first 50 cases. *Am J Psychiatry*. 1998;155:264-271.

Chapter 309

PHIMOSIS

A. Barbara Oettgen, MD, MPH

Problems and questions related to the foreskin of young boys are relatively frequent among families in pediatric practices. Understanding the diagnosis and treatment of boys with foreskin problems such as phimosis, paraphimosis, and balanoposthitis is therefore important for physicians caring for children.

DEFINITION

Phimosis, or unretractile foreskin, can be both physiologic and pathologic. At birth, most boys have physiologic phimosis—the inner surface of the foreskin is developmentally fused to the glans penis.[1] Over time, desquamation and glanular secretions allow gradual separation of the foreskin. Accumulation of smegma (the epithelial debris generated during desquamation) can sometimes be seen under the foreskin as pearls and requires no intervention. When these accumulations are eventually released, as the foreskin becomes more retractile, they may be mistaken for infection.[1] Retractability increases yearly. By 1 year of age, 50% of uncircumcised boys have retractile foreskins, 90% by age 3, 92% by age 6 to 7, and 99% by adolescence.[2,3] Distinguishing pathologic phimosis from physiologic phimosis can be difficult because of the lack of clear diagnostic criteria.[2] Probably most of the referrals made to urologists are for boys with physiologic phimosis that will resolve spontaneously over time.[2]

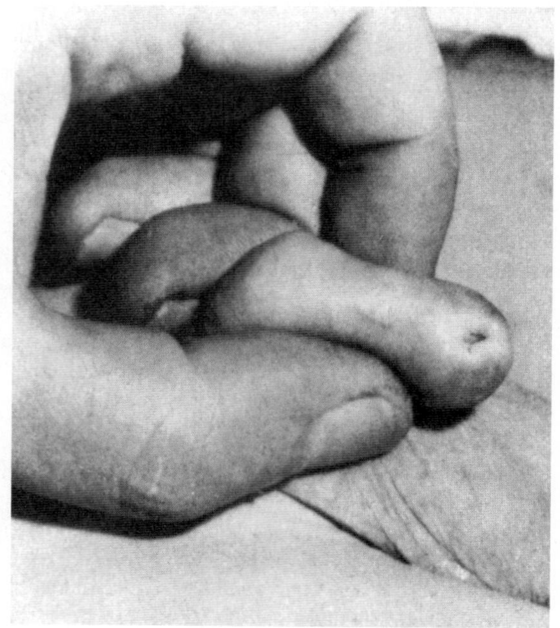

Figure 309-1 Physiologic phimosis. *(From Rickwood AMK. Medical indications for circumcision.* BJU Int. *1999;83[suppl 1]:45-51. Used with permission.)*

Physiologic phimosis is described as an unretractile foreskin that is supple and unscarred. On attempted retraction, the foreskin lies flat against the penis and is effaced, and the tip opens as a flower (Figure 309-1). Young boys may also exhibit preputial adhesions where part of the foreskin does not completely retract, but no constricting ring is seen—this also is not pathologic and largely resolves on its own.[4] With pathologic phimosis, the margin between the foreskin and the glans is rolled and thickened.

INCIDENCE

The incidence of true phimosis is probably fairly infrequent. Smith and colleagues reported 1 case per 1000 boys; a study in France reported a rate of 2.6% and in England 0.9%.[2] These rates were obtained after looking at pathologic specimens after circumcision. Individuals with evidence of inflammation were counted as true phimosis.

ETIOLOGY

Pathologic phimosis is believed to have a few different causes. It can be the result of a chronic nonspecific inflammatory process or repeated infections that cause scarring and stricture. It can also be caused by forcible premature retraction of the foreskin, causing scarring and adhesions. Balanitis xerotica obliterans (BXO) is a chronic dermatitis of unknown cause, histologically resembles lichen sclerosus et atrophicus, and causes pathologic phimosis.[4]

MANAGEMENT

Treatment of phimosis depends on whether it is thought to be physiologic or pathologic. Watchful waiting will result in resolution of most cases of physiologic phimosis. However, if the child is believed to have pathologic phimosis, then the treatment alternatives include topical steroid cream or surgery.

Steroid creams

Multiple studies have investigated the use of topical steroid creams for treatment. A recent review of the literature showed at least 12 studies (2 randomized controlled) in children 1 to 15 years of age. A 4- to 8-week course of therapy was found to be, on average, 85% effective.[5] High-potency steroid creams such as 0.05% betamethasone have been studied the most frequently. However, a medium-potency topical steroid (clobetasone butyrate 0.05%) has been shown to have similar resolution rates, suggesting that a lower-strength steroid may be an option.[6] The creams are applied to the tip of the prepuce and down to the junction with the glans twice a day for 4 to 8 weeks. Steroid creams were even used in a much younger population (1- to 31-month-old boys) who had urinary tract infections, balanitis, or genitourinary tract anomalies and were found to be successful in relieving phimosis in 92% of children.[7] Steroids are believed to be therapeutic by decreasing any potential inflammation between the foreskin and glans and by thinning the skin, making it more supple.[6]

Topical steroid therapy has multiple advantages over more traditional surgical management; it is less invasive and avoids the risks of surgery (bleeding, deformity, meatal stenosis) and anesthesia.[2] It is much more cost effective—only 25% the cost of surgery.[2,5] The prepuce also may deserve preservation for social and cultural reasons, as well as the fact that it is a neurologically complex and erogenous tissue. Finally, medical therapy can prevent severe emotional problems in some boys who undergo circumcision at an older age.[2,8]

Surgery

The surgical alternatives for phimosis include dorsal slit surgery or circumcision. The dorsal slit procedure involves making a single slit dorsally in the foreskin, which mostly preserves the prepuce but allows easy retraction of the foreskin.[9] Although the surgery is less involved and preserves the prepuce, the cosmetic result is not as satisfactory as with circumcision and can also be complicated by scarring.[10] Circumcision is the much more commonly practiced surgery for phimosis. Forced premature retraction of the foreskin is *never* recommended and may lead to significant adhesions and scarring, as well as being painful and traumatic.

WHEN TO TREAT

Given that true phimosis can be a difficult diagnosis to establish, the choice as to which patients should be referred and receive therapy may be unclear. There are some instances for which uniform agreement exists that treatment, in the form of circumcision, should be undertaken, and these instances include BXO, phimosis that is resistant to steroid therapy, and voiding problems.[10] Recurrent balanitis and urinary tract infections may be other indications if topical steroid therapy is unsuccessful. Ballooning of the foreskin during micturition is, by itself, not necessarily a reason for circumcision. Using noninvasive urodynamic studies, no evidence of obstruction could be found in children with physiologic phimosis, even with ballooning of the foreskin.[3]

Given that most cases of phimosis are probably physiologic and will resolve spontaneously over time, the question remains which children to treat either medically or surgically. Little agreement exists in the literature. Some urologists would question whether true phimosis can exist before age 5[11] and therefore whether any treatment need be initiated. Others use the age of 3 years as an upper limit and would at least initiate a trial of steroid creams (if no indication for surgery) at that time.[4] An argument in favor of treating children who are younger (older than 3 but younger than 5 or 6) is that the most noninvasive therapy (topical steroids) is more successful in younger children than older children. Compliance is greater with the treatment at that age because the parents are still able to apply the cream. When older children become responsible for cream application, compliance—and therefore success—of therapy decreases.[6]

PARAPHIMOSIS

Definition

Paraphimosis, unlike phimosis, is a urologic emergency. It occurs when the foreskin is retracted and is not replaced immediately and becomes trapped behind the corona.[9] Paraphimosis may happen during cleaning or during a procedure such as catheterization. The fibrous ring at the base of the corona causes venous congestion, leading to extreme penile pain and swelling of the glans with a collar of swollen foreskin at the coronal sulcus. If no treatment is initiated, then ischemia and necrosis of the glans can result.

Management

The goal of treatment is to replace the foreskin in its normal position. If the condition is in its early stages, the foreskin may then be replaceable manually without sedation. As the condition progresses, anesthesia in the form of penile block, sedation, or general anesthesia may be required.[9] Gentle persistent pressure is the goal of treatment to decrease edema and allow reduction of the foreskin. Ice packs or a compressive elastic dressing are 2 techniques used to decrease swelling.[12] Sometimes an incision must be made in the fibrous ring or multiple punctures must be made in the glans to relieve swelling.[9]

BALANOPOSTHITIS

Definition

Balanitis, or balanoposthitis, is characterized by erythema and edema of the prepuce that produces purulent discharge from the preputial orifice. Occasionally, edema can involve some of the penile shaft as well, and patients may complain of dysuria. The condition usually occurs when the prepuce is wholly or partially retractable. In children, balanitis occurs most frequently between the ages of 2 and 5 and is more commonly nonspecific balanitis, caused by poor hygiene, trauma, or irritation from soaps or detergents.

Management

The treatment for nonspecific balanoposthitis includes local hygienic measures such as sitz baths, gentle cleaning, and 1% hydrocortisone cream. If irritation does not resolve, then treatment with antimicrobials may be necessary, with the most common causative organisms being *Staphylococcus*, coliforms, *Pseudomonas*, and *Candida*. Another potential cause is *Streptococcus*, which can cause a thin purulent discharge in the preputial-glanular sulcus (but not from the urethra) associated with a red, glistening glans. Finally, sexually transmitted infections (gonorrhea and chlamydia) must also be considered when purulent discharge from the urethra is present, and therefore appropriate diagnostic tests (eg, DNA probes) should be obtained. The presence of sexually transmitted infections in the absence of purulent discharge is extremely unlikely in a prepubertal boy.

Surgical treatment, that is, circumcision, is usually considered only for recurrent episodes of balanoposthitis.[10,13]

WHEN TO REFER

Phimosis:

- Failure of topical steroids
- Balanitis xerotica obliterans (BXO)
- Parents desire circumcision
- Association with urinary tract abnormalities/obstructive uropathy

Paraphimosis: failure of manual reduction
Balanoposthitis: recurrent episodes

WHEN TO ADMIT

Paraphimosis: Failure of manual reduction with vascular compromise of the glans
Balanoposthitis:

- Systemic infection or sepsis
- Inability to urinate
- Vascular compromise of the glans

REFERENCES

1. Brown MR, Cartwright PC, Snow BW. Common office problems in pediatric urology and gynecology. *Pediatr Clin North Am.* Oct 1997;44(5):1091-1115.
2. Howe RS. Cost-effective treatment of phimosis. *Pediatrics.* 1998;102(4):E43.
3. Babu R, Harrison SK, Hutton KA. Ballooning of the foreskin and physiological phimosis: is there any objective evidence of obstructed voiding? *BJU Int.* Aug 2004;94(3); 384-387.
4. Monsour MA, Rabinovitch HH, Dean GE. Medical management of phimosis in children: our experience with topical steroids. *J Urol.* 1999 Sep;162(3 Pt2):1162-1164.
5. Berdeu D, Sauze L, Ha-Vinh P, et al. Cost-effectiveness analysis of treatments for phimosis: a comparison of surgical and medicinal approaches and their economic effect. *BJU Int.* Feb 2001;87(3):239-244.
6. Yang SS, Tsai YC, Wu CC, et al. Highly potent and moderately potent topical steroids are effective in treating phimosis: a prospective randomized study. *J Urol.* April 2005; 173:1361-1363.
7. Elmore JM, Baker LA, Snodgrass WT. Topical steroid therapy as an alternative to circumcision for phimosis in boys younger than 3 years. *J Urol.* Oct 2002;168(4Pt 2): 1746-1747.
8. Yilmaz E, Batislam E, Basar MM, et al. Psychological trauma of circumcision in the phallic period could be avoided by using topical steroids. *Int J Urol.* Dec 2003; 10(12);651-656.
9. Langer JC, Coplen DE. Circumcision and pediatric disorders of the penis. *Pediatr Clin North Am.* Aug 1998;45(4): 801-812.
10. Rickwood AMK. Medical indications for circumcision. *BJU Int.* 1999;83(suppl 1):45-51.
11. Rickwood AM, Walker J. Is phimosis overdiagnosed in boys and are too many circumcisions performed as a consequence? *Ann R Coll Surg Engl.* Sep 1989;71(5): 275-277.
12. Choe JM. Paraphimosis: Current treatment options. *Am Fam Phys.* 2000;62:2623-2626.
13. Schwartz RH, Rushton HG. Acute balanoposthitis in young boys. *Pediatr Infect Dis J.* 1996;15(2):176-177.

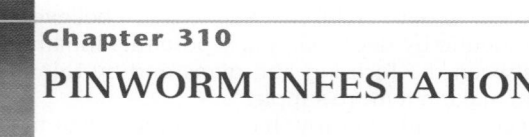

Chapter 310

PINWORM INFESTATIONS

Craig M. Wilson, MD

ETIOLOGY

Pinworm *(Enterobius vermicularis)* infestation is exceptionally common. When sought carefully, the parasite can be found in at least 30% of children worldwide, and infestation rates may approach 100% in child care centers, boarding schools, and institutions.[1-3] Good sanitation and advanced socioeconomic status are feeble deterrents to pinworms. Adults are often infested, and finding pinworms in all members of a family is not uncommon. The discovery of *Enterobius* eggs in 10,000-year-old human coprolites from the Hogup and Danger caves in Utah proves that the parasite was no stranger to our ancestors.[4,5]

E vermicularis is a white, threadlike worm that lives primarily in the cecum and adjacent bowel.[1,6] The gravid female worm, which is approximately 1 cm long, migrates to the perianal area to deposit up to 10,000 eggs and dies shortly thereafter. Thus the infestation would be self-limited were it not for reinfestation. Unfortunately, the eggs, which are approximately 50 × 30 mcm, oval, flat on 1 side, and thin shelled, become infective in approximately 6 hours.

Autoinfestation occurs readily through ingestion of eggs if the host scratches the perianal area or does not wash the hands thoroughly after defecating. Moreover, *Enterobius* eggs are rather hardy and may survive for weeks in dirt, house dust, clothing, and bed sheets. Survival is enhanced by lower temperature and if inhaled and swallowed. Pets may carry eggs in their fur. Once ingested, the eggs hatch in the upper small intestine, and the worms mature while migrating to the lower ileum and ascending colon. The cycle from ingestion to deposition of eggs is approximately 4 to 6 weeks, although the adult worms may live up to 13 weeks. The worm burden within an individual may reach the hundreds; but within an infested population, most individuals would be harboring few parasites.

CLINICAL MANIFESTATIONS

Localized perianal pruritus is the most commonly reported symptom, but one third or more of infestations are asymptomatic.[1,6] Restlessness and fitful sleep are common complaints, as well as secondary excoriation and dermatitis. Migrating pinworms entering the vagina or urinary tract in female patients may lead to genitourinary symptoms.[7] The general lack of abdominal complaints supports the notion of minimal gastrointestinal abnormality with this parasite.

In rare cases, pinworms invade tissue and cause a granulomatous reaction, and granulomas-containing worms have been an incidental finding in the gut, vulva, cervix, fallopian tubes, peritoneum, and bladder. Inflammation associated with the parasite has been found in cases of appendicitis and eosinophilic colitis, suggesting causality with *E vermicularis*.

LABORATORY EVALUATION

Diagnosis is dependent on identifying either the adult worms or the eggs. Occasionally, adult pinworms may be noted near the anus, particularly in the morning. Eggs are seldom found in the patient's feces even if concentration techniques are used. The best way to make a diagnosis is to use the cellophane tape technique. When the child awakens in the morning, the adhesive side of a 2-inch strip of clear cellophane tape should be pressed against the perianal skin; this task is most easily done using a tongue depressor (commercially produced kits are available for this purpose). The tape should then be placed on a microscope slide with the adhesive side down and scanned for eggs. The eggs are naturally transparent, and staining with lactophenol cotton blue enhances detection. A single test should detect at least 50% of infestations, 3 tests will detect 90%, and 5 tests will detect virtually 100%.

PREVENTION AND THERAPY

Zealous physicians who believe elimination of pinworm from their patients is easily accomplished are doomed to frustration and failure. The ubiquity and infectivity of the parasite, the high level of infestation in symptomatic patients, and its persistence in the environment make eradication extremely difficult. Moreover, vigorous pursuit of a permanent cure may provoke needless turmoil and anxiety in the family. When the diagnosis is confirmed in a patient who has symptoms, the following approach seems reasonable.

Although initial treatment of only a confirmed individual patient is reasonable, initial therapy for the entire family is similarly reasonable. A single dose of either mebendazole (100 mg for all ages) or albendazole (400 mg for all ages) is extremely effective and has virtually no side effects.[8] Pyrantel pamoate, administered as a single dose of 11 mg/kg (maximum 1 g), is also effective; a transient headache and abdominal complaints have been reported with this therapy. All of these treatments are effective against the adult worms only, and therefore therapy is usually repeated in 2 weeks to eradicate any emerging parasites.

Other simple, prudent measures can be followed, such as clipping the fingernails (a favorite repository for eggs), washing the hands frequently, and showering daily in the morning. Wearing tight-fitting cotton underpants and applying a bland ointment (eg, petroleum jelly) to the perianal region may limit dispersal of the eggs. The floors in sleeping areas should be cleaned thoroughly, particularly in cases of recurrence. Clothing and bedding should be washed at the time of treatment. The most important aspects of treatment, however, are humility on the part of the physician and reassurance of the family.

TOOLS FOR PRACTICE

Engaging Patients and Family

- *Pinworm Infection* (fact sheet), Centers for Disease Control and Prevention (www.cdc.gov/ncidod/dpd/parasites/pinworm/factsht_pinworm.htm).

Medical Decision Support

- *Enterobius vermicularis—Lab Identification* (Web page), Centers for Disease Control and Prevention (www.dpd.cdc.gov/dpdx/HTML/Enterobiasis.htm).

REFERENCES

1. Cook GC. Enterobius vermicularis infection. *Gut*. 1994;35:1159-1162.
2. Cram EB, Jones MF, Reardon L. The incidence of pinworm (Enterobius vermicularis) in various population groups. *Revista De Medicina Tropical Y Parasitoologia*, 1941;7(1-2):4.
3. Burkhart CN, Burkhart CG. Assessment of frequency, transmission, and genitourinary complications of enterobiasis (pinworms). *Intl J Derm*. 2005;44(10):837-840.
4. Libbus MK. Enterobiasis. *Nurse Pract*. 1983;8(8):17-18.
5. Hugot JP, Reinhard KJ, Gardner SL, et al. Human enterobiasis in evolution: origin, specificity and transmission. *Parasite*. 1999;6(3):201-208.
6. Russell LJ. The pinworm, Enterobius vermicularis. *Prim Care*. 1991;18:13.
7. Ok UZ, Ertan P, Limoncu E, et al. Relationship between pinworm and urinary tract infections in young girls. *APMIS*. 1999;107(5):474-476.
8. Drugs for parasitic infections [no authors listed]. *Med Lett*. 2004.

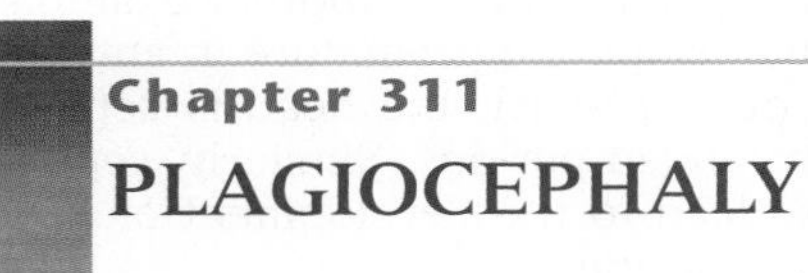

Chapter 311

PLAGIOCEPHALY

Ahdi Amer, MD; Deepak M. Kamat, MD, PhD

Plagiocephaly, a term with a Greek origin, means *oblique head*. It is used to describe any abnormality in the shape of the head, irrespective of its cause. Posterior deformational plagiocephaly (PDP) is a phenomenon in which flattening of the occiput occurs as a result of mechanical factors that affect the malleable growing skull in utero or during early infancy. It is also referred to as *benign positional molding*, *posterior plagiocephaly*, and *occipital plagiocephaly*. In most patients, the head shape improves with changes in head position or helmet therapy.[1-3] Early recognition and intervention is crucial because early intervention improves outcome.[4] If not treated appropriately, then quality of life may be reduced.[5]

PATHOGENESIS

During development, genetic makeup and environmental factors determine the shape of the head. Abnormalities in skull shapes may develop prenatally or postnatally during the first 2 years of life. Whether PDP begins prenatally or is an acquired phenomenon remains controversial. Some investigators believe that many infants who develop PDP are born with a mild flattening of the occiput that goes unnoticed in the neonatal period and worsens as the infant continues to sleep on the flat side.[6] Because the infant sleeps in the position of comfort (ie, on the flat side), this condition is termed *positional plagiocephaly*.

A deformity present from birth is usually the result of in utero conditions such as small maternal pelvis, uterine abnormalities, large baby, multiple gestations, and oligohydromnios or polyhydromnios.[7,8] Controversy exists regarding the reason that leads to the development of PDP in these conditions. Some researchers believe that the constrictive and restrictive uterine environment leads to conformational changes in the skull, which includes fusion of the sutures, whereas others believe that this environment simply causes severe molding and leads to flattening.[6,9]

Mechanical pressure on the malleable skull caused by static supine positioning leads to the flattening of the occiput in patients with PDP. Therefore supine sleeping position, congenital torticollis, prolonged periods in car seats and infant carriers, prematurity, and neurologic conditions such as hydrocephalus are frequently associated with PDP. The correlation between PDP and supine sleeping positioning is explained by the fact that by the time most infants reach 2 months of age, they have slept for almost 700 hours.[10]

Congenital torticollis is a prime example of the static position of the head in which limited neck motion leads to an asymmetrical flattened occiput involving the torticollis side. However, theories suggest that torticollis develops as a result of PDP.[6] Another example of static head position is among premature infants on ventilator support during which the head is kept in one position for prolonged periods. Similarly, cephalhematoma can also lead to the development of PDP on the opposite occipital side.[6]

Hydrocephalus is another risk factor for the development of PDP because of the movement of bones and sutures as a result of volume changes in the cranium and because of the limitations imposed by the draining devices and shunts that result in the infant's head being placed in one position for prolonged periods.

Another possible mechanism that may promote favoring one side of the head and the development of PDP is the position of the baby's crib in relation to the room's major light source. Infants usually spend much time looking toward the source of light in the room when the baby is in the supine position. Therefore PDP may develop if the crib is kept in the same location (particularly if it is placed in a corner of the room) and the baby is placed in the same position in relation to the light source.

EPIDEMIOLOGIC FEATURES

Before 1992, when more than 70% of infants were placed in the prone position during sleep, the incidence of PDP was estimated to be 1 in 300 live births.[11] However, after the *Back to Sleep* campaign was initiated by the American Academy of Pediatrics (AAP) in 1992,[12] the incidence of PDP has been on the rise,[7,13,14] with a 2004 study showing that almost 1 in 68 infants may have PDP.[15]

PDP is more common on the right side than it is on the left side because of the right-sided sleep position preference of most infants.[16,17] Almost 85% of neonates have left occipital anterior presentation during birth, which causes pressure on the infant's right occiput and left forehead by the mother's pelvis and lumbosacral spine, respectively.[6]

PDP is more common in boys than it is in girls,[6,18,19] probably because male infants have larger heads than female infants and because boys tend to be less flexible than girls. PDP is also common with primiparity, prolonged labor, and assisted delivery.[6]

PDP is first noticed by parents and health care providers when the infants are 2 to 3 months of age. The severity of PDP peaks at 4 months and then resolves gradually over time. In two thirds of the cases, PDP resolves by 2 to 3 years of age.[20] The resolution is observed to be slow in children with limited head rotation and low activity level.[21]

DIFFERENTIAL DIAGNOSIS

Distinguishing lambdoid synostosis from PDP in infants with flat posterior plagiocephaly is critical because the management of these 2 conditions is different. Lambdoid synostosis is a rare condition that occurs in approximately 2% of all cases of craniosynostosis.[22] In patients with lambdoid synostosis, the head is trapezoid shaped; in PDP, conversely, the head is shaped as a parallelogram, with significantly greater protrusion of the forehead on the same side of the occipital flattening as compared with lambdoid synostosis. In PDP, the ear on the flattened side is displaced anteriorly, whereas in lambdoid synostosis, it is displaced inferiorly and posteriorly. In lambdoid synostosis, the posterior basal skull is tilted, with the prominence of mastoid process present on the same side. In addition, the facial deformity seen in patients with PDP is absent or minimal in patients with lambdoid synostosis. Rarely, however, clinically differentiating between PDP and lambdoid synostosis may be difficult.

DIAGNOSIS OF POSTERIOR DEFORMATIONAL PLAGIOCEPHALY

The diagnosis of PDP in infancy is made primarily based on history and physical examination. Imaging studies are not indicated in most situations. If the infant has a normal, rounded head at birth and after a few weeks or months develops an occipital flattening, then the most likely diagnosis is PDP.

Infants with PDP exhibit preferential head position—that is, the infant turns the head only to one side. When the head is viewed from above, a frontal prominence on the same side as the occipital flattening may be observed, and the ear on that side is anterior as compared with the other ear (Figure 311-1). Other craniofacial abnormalities that may be observed on the affected side of infants with PDP are prominent mandibular sulcus with mandibular tilt, uplifted lower helix, smaller ear, and unilateral epicanthal fold. Most infants with PDP have one-sided occipital bald spots.

The presence of torticollis has to be ruled out in every case of flattened occiput because of its greater association with PDP. Therefore the primary care physician should perform both passive and active head rotations and to check for the tightness of the sternocleidomastoid muscle. The eye on the side of torticollis

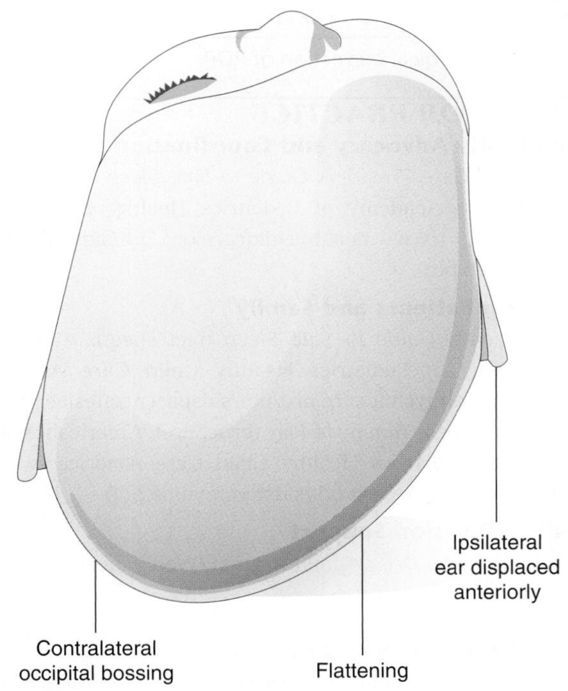

Figure 311-1 This figure shows typical clinical findings in a scalp of an infant with deformational plagiocephaly namely flattening of occiput on right side with anterior displacement of ear and frontal bossing on the same side and occipital bossing on the opposite side. *(Adapted from Lin KY, Ogle RC, Jane JA, eds.* Craniofacial Surgery: Science and Surgical Technique. *Philadelphia, PA: WB Saunders; 2002. Copyright © 2002, Elsevier, with permission.)*

appears to be incompletely open as a result of the vertical displacement of soft tissues of the cheek. In addition, the mothers of infants with torticollis note that they have difficulty feeding the infant from both breasts because the infants have trouble turning their head.

Laboratory or imaging studies are not routinely required to confirm the diagnosis of PDP. In the past, skull radiographs were used to rule out lambdoid suture synostosis. However, ultrasound examination of the lambdoid suture has also been shown to be useful in ruling out lambdoid suture synostosis.[21,23] Three-dimensional computed tomographic scans have been shown to be sensitive in diagnosing common and rare cases of posterior plagiocephaly.[24]

PREVENTION

In most infants, PDP can be prevented by alternating the supine head position during sleep and by periodically changing the position of the crib in the room to require the child to look away from the flattened side to see parents and others in the room or to look at the source of light in the room.

The AAP has recommended a certain amount of prone positioning, or *tummy time,* while the infant is awake and being observed.[25] This positioning may help prevent the development of a flat occiput and may also facilitate development of the upper shoulder girdle strength necessary for timely attainment of certain motor milestones. Theories suggest that prone position prevents PDP by correcting or preventing infants' positional preferences.[26]

Parents and health care professionals, such as those working in newborn care units, should be educated on different techniques to reduce the risk for development of PDP in infants. Nursing staff and other caregivers should be encouraged to change the head position of a sick newborn whenever possible. Because most caregivers are right handed, much of the care to the baby is provided from the right side of the bed, and thus the baby is placed facing the right side. Caregivers should be encouraged to provide care from the left side of the crib whenever possible and to reposition the infant from head to foot from time to time.

Infants who are breastfed are less likely to develop PDP because, during breastfeeding, alternate head positioning is promoted. However, during bottle feeding, babies are often held in the left arm, promoting right occipital flattening. Parents should be advised to use alternate arms during each bottle feeding.

TREATMENT

Definitive guidelines for the management of PDP have not been developed. However, early treatment is successful in most cases of mild to moderate PDP. Investigators have observed that treatment started after 12 months does not produce significant benefits.[18,19,27] Therefore treating PDP early and effectively is important because uncorrected or improperly treated PDP can lead to marked psychosocial developmental sequelae.[5]

The initial management of PDP is the same as the prevention measures, which consists of educating parents about changing the infant's head position frequently. If the infant is found to have torticollis, then parents should be taught to use neck motion exercises for the baby. The first exercise is used to stretch the sternocleidomastoid muscle and consists of placing one hand on the infant's upper chest and rotating the infant's neck with the other hand so the chin touches the shoulder. The head should be held in this position for 10 seconds. The head is then rotated to the other side and held for an additional 10 seconds. In the second exercise, the infant's head is tilted so that the ear touches the shoulder and is held in that position for 10 seconds. The same process is followed on the other side. This exercise stretches the trapezius muscle. The parents should be asked to perform these neck exercises with every diaper change, with three repetitions of each exercise. Estimates suggest that an additional two minutes are required for these exercises per diaper change. In most cases, with early implementation of repositioning and neck exercises, considerable response is seen over a 2- to 3-month period. The infant should be referred for physical therapy for stretching exercises if these excises fail to improve torticollis within 2 to 3 months. If no improvement is evident, or if plagiocephaly worsens after 2 months of repositioning and physical therapy, then the infant should be referred to a pediatric neurosurgeon or a craniofacial surgeon for further management.

Skull-molding helmets have been used for reshaping the affected skull. To achieve the desired response, helmets have to be used in the age range of 4 to 12 months because of the malleability of the young infant's skull during this period. Ideally, therapy is begun at 4 to 6 months of age and may be continued until 12 to 14 months of age.[1,2] Head growth remains normal during helmet therapy and works by symmetrically shaping the cranial growth.[19] The use of helmets is more beneficial for patients with severe deformity and in infants with mild to moderate severity who are resistant to position changes and physical therapy.

No consensus exists on the use of helmets in infants with positional plagiocephaly. Far better improvement in the skull shape has been observed in infants treated with helmets as compared with that achieved by repositioning alone.[18] On the other hand, research has shown that repositioning infants may produce improvement in mild to moderate cases similar to that reported with external orthotic devices.[28] Disagreement also exists on the cost effectiveness of helmets in the treatment of PDP.[1,29] The AAP states that helmets are beneficial in the treatment of PDP after the position changes and exercise have failed.[3] Helmets used for treating PDP are considered to be class II neurologic devices and are regulated by the US Food and Drug Administration.[30] Information on the approved orthotics can be obtained at www.fda.gov.

Although surgery is rarely needed to treat PDP, it may be indicated in severe cases in which infants have been presented late for management, thus missing the window of opportunity for success with repositioning, physical therapy, or helmet therapy. Craniotomy does not provide superior results in comparison with physical or helmet therapy as far as a cosmetic outcome is considered. Surgery is also associated with significant morbidity.

SEQUELAE

The ipsilateral temporomandibular joint is pushed anteriorly in patients with PDP, and therefore the mandible develops asymmetrically. The positional and helmet therapy improve the head shape but not the position of the temporomandibular joint or the asymmetry of the mandible.[31] PDP also causes forehead and facial shifts that may lead to asymmetric positioning of the eyes and causes bilateral astigmatism.[32] Fitting corrective glasses on an asymmetric head is also difficult.

Cognitive and psychomotor development has been observed to be mildly delayed in patients with PDP. Whether these delays can be corrected with therapy or whether they are the cause or the effect of PDP is not known.[33] Long-term follow-up of patients with PDP also has shown persistence of developmental delay.[34]

WHEN TO REFER

- After position change and physical therapy have failed to correct PDP
- In severe cases
- When the patient who has PDP is older than 12 months
- When lambdoidal craniosynostosis is a possibility

WHEN TO ADMIT

- Surgical correction of PDP

TOOLS FOR PRACTICE

Community Advocacy and Coordination

- *A Child Care Providers Guide to Safe Sleep* (fact sheet), American Academy of Pediatrics Healthy Child Care America (www.healthychildcare.org/pdf/sidschildcaresafesleep.pdf).

Engaging Patients and Family

- *A Parent's Guide to Safe Sleep* (fact sheet), American Academy of Pediatrics Healthy Child Care America (www.healthychildcare.org/pdf/sidsparentsafesleep.pdf).
- *Back to Sleep, Tummy to Play* (brochure), American Academy of Pediatrics Healthy Child Care America (www.healthychildcare.org/pdf/sidstummytime.pdf).

Medical Decision Support

- *US Food and Drug Administration* (Web page) (www.fda.gov/).

AAP POLICY STATEMENTS

American Academy of Pediatrics, Committee on Practice and Ambulatory Medicine, Section on Plastic Surgery, Section on Neurological Surgery. Prevention and management of positional skull deformities in infants. *Pediatrics*. 2003;112(1):199-202. (aappolicy.aappublications.org/cgi/content/full/pediatrics;112/1/199).

American Academy of Pediatrics, Task Force on Sudden Infant Death Syndrome. The changing concept of sudden infant death syndrome: diagnostic coding shifts, controversies regarding the sleeping environment, and new variables to consider in reducing risk. *Pediatrics*. 2005;116(5):1245-1255. (aappolicy.aappublications.org/cgi/content/full/pediatrics;116/5/1245).

REFERENCES

1. Brunner TW, David LR, Gage HD, et al. Objective outcome analysis of soft shell helmet therapy in the treatment of deformational plagiocephaly. *J Craniofac Surg*. 2004;15:643-650.
2. Teichgraeber JF, Seymour-Dempsey K, Baumgartner JE, et al. Molding helmet therapy in the treatment of brachycepahly and plagiocephaly. *J Craniofac Surg*. 2004;15:118-123.
3. Persing J, James H, Swanson J, et al. American Academy of Pediatrics, Committee on Practice and Ambulatory Medicine, Section on Plastic Surgery and Section on Neurological Surgery. Prevention and management of positional skull deformities in infants. *Pediatrics*. 2003;112:199-202.
4. Kelly KM, Littlefield TR, Pomatto JK, et al. Importance of early recognition and treatment of deformational plagiocephaly with orthotic cranioplasty. *Cleft Palate Craniofac J*. 1999;36:127-130.
5. Huang MH, Mouradian WE, Cohen SR, et al. The differential diagnosis of abnormal head shapes: separating craniosynostosis from positional deformities and normal variants. *Cleft Palate Craniofac J*. 1998;35:204-211.
6. Peitsch WK, Keefer CH, Labrie RA, et al. Incidence of cranial asymmetry in healthy newborns. *Pediatrics*. 2002;110:1-8.
7. Kane AA, Mitchell LE, Craven KP, et al. Observations on a recent increase of plagiocephaly without synostosis. *Pediatrics*. 1996;97:877-885.

8. Littlefield TR, Kelly KM, Pomatto JK, et al. Multiple-birth infants at higher risk for development of deformational of deformational plagiocephaly. *Pediatrics.* 1999;103: 565-569.
9. Dias MS, Klein DM. Occipital plagiocephaly: deformation or lambdoid synostosis. A unifying theory regarding pathogenesis. *Pediatr Neurosurg.* 1996;24:69-73.
10. Cartwright CC. Assessing asymmetrical infant head shapes. *Nurse Pract.* 2002;27:33-39.
11. Dunn PM. Congenital sternomastoid torticollis: an intrauterine postural deformity. *Dis Child.* 1974;824-825.
12. American Academy of Pediatrics, Task Force on Positioning and Sudden Infant Death Syndrome. Positioning and SIDS. *Pediatrics.* 1992;89:1120-1126.
13. Turk AE, McCarthy JG, Thorne CH, et al. The "Back to Sleep Campaign" and deformational plagiocephaly: is there cause for concern? *J Craniofac Surg.* 1996;7:12-18.
14. Argenta LC, David LR, Wilson JA, Bell WO. An increase in infant cranial deformity with supine sleeping position. *J Craniofac Surg.* 1996;7:5-11.
15. Littlefield TR, Saba NM, Kelly KM. On the current incidence of deformational plagiocephaly: an estimation based on prospective registration at a single center. *Semin Pediatr Neurol.* 2004;114:301-304.
16. Volpe JJ. *Neurology of the Newborn.* Philadelphia, PA: WB Saunders; 1995.
17. Bruneteau RJ, Mulliken JB, Frontal plagiocephaly: synostotic, compensational, or deformational. *Plast Reconstr Surg.* 1992;89:21-33.
18. Mulliken JB, Vander Woude DL, Hansen M, et al. Analysis of posterior plagiocephaly: deformational versus synostotic. *Plast Reconstr Surg.* 1999;103:371-380.
19. Kelly KM, Littlefield TR, Pomatto JK, et al. Cranial growth unrestricted during treatment of deformational plagiocephaly. *Pediatr Neurosurg.* 1999;30:193-199.
20. Boere-BooneKamp MMM, van der Linden-Kuiper LT. Positional preference: prevalence in infants and follow up after 2 years. *Pediatrics.* 2001;107:339-343.
21. Hutchinson BL, Hutchinson LA, Thompson JA, et al. Plagiocephaly and brachycephaly in the first 2 years of life: a prospective cohort study. *Pediatrics.* 2004;114:970-980.
22. Ridgeway EB, Weiner HL. Skull deformities. *Pediatr Clin North Am.* 2004;51:359-387.
23. Sze RW, Parisi MT, Sidhu M, et al. Ultrasound screening of the lambdoid suture in the child with posterior plagiocephaly. *Pediatr Radiol.* 2003;33:630-636.
24. Sze RW, Hopper RA, Ghioni V, et al. MDCT diagnosis of the child with posterior plagiocephaly. *Am J Radiol.* 2005; 185:1342-1346.
25. American Academy of Pediatrics, Task Force on Infant Sleep Position and Sudden Infant Death Syndrome. Changing concepts of sudden infant death syndrome: implications for infant sleeping environment and sleep position. *Pediatrics.* 2000;105:650-656.
26. Palmen K. Prevention of congenital dislocation of the hip: the Swedish experience of neonatal treatment of hip joint instability. *Acta Orthop Scand.* 1984;55:58-67.
27. Pollack I, Losken H, Fasick P. Diagnosis and management of posterior plagiocephaly. *Pediatrics.* 1997;99:180-185.
28. Moss SD. Nonsurgical, nonorthotic treatment of occipital plagiocephaly. What is the natural history of the misshapen neonatal head? *J Neurosurg.* 1997;87:667-670.
29. Bridges SJ, Chambers TL, Pople IK. Plagiocephaly and head binding. *Arch Dis Child.* 2002;86:144-145.
30. Littlefield TR. Food and Drug Administration regulation of orthotic cranioplasty. *Cleft Palate Craniofac J.* 2001;38: 337-340.
31. St John D, Mulliken JB, Kaban LB, et al. Anthropometric analysis of mandibular asymmetry in infants with deformational posterior plagiocephaly. *J Oral Maxilofac Surg.* 2002;60:873-877.
32. Gupta PC, Foster J, Crowe S, et al. Ophthalmologic findings in patients with nonsyndromic plagiocephaly. *J Craniofac Surg.* 2003;14:529-532.
33. Panchal J, Amirsheybani H, Gurwitch R, et al. Neurodevelopment in children with single-suture craniosynostosis and plagiocephaly without synostosis. *Plast Reconstr Surg.* 2001;108:1492-1500.
34. Miller RI, Clarren SK. Long-term developmental outcomes in patients with deformational plagiocephaly. *Pediatrics.* 2000;105:e26. Available at: pediatrics.aappublications.org/cgi/content/abstract/105/2/e26. Accessed March 1, 2007.

Chapter 312

PNEUMONIA

Christopher Harris, MD

Pneumonia has been defined in several ways throughout the world. In less-developed parts of the world, evidence of retractions along with tachypnea leads to a clinical diagnosis of pneumonia. In areas that have more technology available, the presence of infiltrates on a chest radiograph is needed to diagnose pneumonia formally.[1] Regardless of how diagnosed, however, pneumonia in infants and children is a common cause for families to seek medical attention. In addition, infections of the lower respiratory tract have varying morbidity and mortality when comparing illness in developed and developing countries. The combined effects of malnutrition and inadequate immunization may cause much more severe respiratory disease for children who also may not have the benefits of advanced therapy to treat the underlying infection and subsequent complications. This circumstance, then, leads to many more deaths caused by pneumonia in the developing world. However, the general concepts regarding pneumonia are the same and are reviewed here.

The incidence of acute pneumonia varies by age. Infants and toddlers are more commonly infected by respiratory pathogens than older children. Children in the first 5 years of life have an incidence of 30 to 45 episodes of acute lower respiratory illness per 1000 children per year. This figure drops to approximately 16 to 20 cases in the 5- to 9-year-old age group. In older children and adolescents the incidence of pneumonia is estimated to be 6 to 12 cases per 1000 patients.[2] Many risk factors have been investigated that may alter the risk for developing pneumonia. Importantly, exposure to environmental tobacco smoke and air pollutants has been shown to be associated with more than 190,000 cases of pneumonia per year in the United States among persons in the youngest age groups. Other factors that may increase the risk of pneumonia include malnutrition, immune deficiency, or severe developmental delay. Infants who have a history of prematurity and chronic lung disease may also be at risk for acute lower respiratory infection.

Infection of the lower airways occurs as a result of introduction of an overwhelming load of pathogenic organisms or a breach of host defense mechanisms. Certainly well known is the fact that particular organisms can invade the lower airways, causing a significant lower respiratory tract infection. Mechanisms of host defense that provide protection to the lung include the ciliary elevator, which serves to trap foreign material that is inhaled and then removed on a continuously produced thin layer of mucus. Ciliary dysfunction or loss is part of viral infection and may allow colonizing bacteria to gain entry to the lung parenchyma, allowing pneumonia to develop. Loss of the normal cellular components of the immune system (polymorphonuclear leukocytes and alveolar macrophages) caused by either acquired or congenital immune deficits are well known to place patients at risk for lung infection. Immunoglobulin is also vital in protection against pneumonia. Aspiration of foreign material, either from the oral cavity in the form of excess saliva or food contents, may lead to pneumonia. Pathologically, increased numbers of inflammatory cells, organisms, and alveolar fluid are seen during the course of illness. Early on, high numbers of pathogens are seen; during the resolution phase, inflammatory cells abound as the infectious process is contained and cleared.[3]

ETIOLOGY

The cause of pneumonia in infants and children greatly depends on the age of the patient. However, research into etiologies has often used indirect evidence to prove causation because of the difficulty of obtaining sputum from children. Some investigators have evaluated acute and convalescent serologic testing, whereas others have used antigen tests of nasopharyngeal secretions or urine to indirectly determine pathogens in the lower respiratory tract. Some researchers have used lung puncture to obtain specimens for culture. In addition, blood has been cultured to provide etiologic information, but blood cultures are infrequently positive.

In the neonatal period, acute pneumonia is caused by bacteria that may cause sepsis and meningitis. Most importantly, group B *Streptococcus* (GBS) causes a severe lower respiratory tract infection with major morbidity and mortality. Infections from GBS have been found in infants up to 8 months of age, but approximately three quarters develop infection by 2 months of age.[4] Other organisms that cause pneumonia in the first few months of life include *Escherichia coli, Klebsiella pneumoniae,* and other enteric gram-negative bacteria. *Listeria monocytogenes* must also be considered as a cause of pneumonia in newborns. Less frequently, nontypeable *Haemophilus influenzae,* other strains of *Streptococcus,* and *Enterococcus* may be implicated in episodes of lower pulmonary infections. Rarely, anaerobic bacteria may be found infecting the respiratory tract of neonates. Infants may also be infected with *Chlamydia trachomatis,* leading to pneumonia with significant auscultatory findings.[1,5] Frequently, conjunctivitis may precede or accompany the respiratory infection in infants who become colonized during delivery.

With regard to bacterial causes of acute lower respiratory tract illness in children beyond the neonatal period, *Streptococcus pneumoniae* is the most important pathogen, in terms of both the numbers of cases and the potential for complications.[1,2,5] Pneumococcus may be the etiologic agent in 25% to 38% of pneumonia cases. Patients may be gravely ill, and complications such as sepsis and meningitis may be seen. The overuse of antibiotics in treating young children has led to the development of pneumococci with reduced antibiotic susceptibility, and *S pneumoniae* resistant to penicillins and advanced-generation cephalosporins may be seen. Resistance to other antibiotics may also occur because resistance genes are frequently plasmid borne and may be transferred between bacteria. Routine use of conjugated pneumococcal vaccine has lessened the incidence of *S pneumoniae* infections, including those of the lung parenchyma.[6]

Other bacterial pathogens associated with acute lower respiratory infections in toddlers and young children include *H influenzae* type B and other nontypeable strains of *H influenzae, C trachomatis, Mycoplasma pneumoniae,* and *Moraxella catarrhalis.* Cases of severe group A β-hemolytic streptococcal pneumonia have been reported, often with marked comorbidity (eg, pleural effusion, empyema, shock).

Among school-aged children and adolescents, *M pneumoniae* is the major treatable cause of pneumonia. *Chlamydia pneumoniae* may also cause pneumonia in this age group.[7,8] As with younger children, *S pneumoniae* may also be the cause for significant lower respiratory tract infections. *Legionella pneumophila* may also be a rare cause of lower respiratory tract infection in older children and adolescents.

Children younger than 5 years are also at risk for viral pneumonias. Respiratory syncytial virus (RSV) infects almost all toddlers by the age of 3 years, with 1% being ill enough to require hospitalization. (See Chapter 243, Bronchiolitis.) Other viral etiologies that may be seen in the first years of life include parainfluenza virus, influenza, and adenovirus. Human metapneumovirus has also been shown to cause bronchiolitis that may be similar to that caused by RSV.[9] Influenza may also cause significant respiratory illness within all pediatric age groups and infants are at risk during yearly influenza outbreaks. An important point to remember is that multiple pathogens may be found in the same patient. In addition, viral infections, with consequent epithelial loss and inflammation, may lead to secondary bacterial infections; 16% to 50% of patients may harbor more than one pathogen.

EVALUATION

History and Physical Examination

During the neonatal period, signs and symptoms may be nonspecific; infants may have fever, irritability, altered feeding patterns, cough, and either tachypnea or apnea.[1] Findings on examination may include retractions, nasal flaring, and grunting. Auscultation may reveal crackles, decreased breath sounds, and occasionally wheezing, especially if the cause is viral.

Among older children, tachypnea, cough, fever, crackles, and respiratory distress also indicate the presence of pneumonia. Complaints of pleuritic chest pain may accompany pneumonia and will help localize attention to the chest. Abdominal pain may be associated with acute lower respiratory tract infections. Milder cases of pneumonia may be associated with findings in the upper respiratory tract, usually pharyngitis and hoarseness. Such is especially the case for illnesses caused by *Mycoplasma* and *Chlamydia* organisms.

Laboratory Evaluation

As is true in adult pneumonia, sputum samples should be obtained if the patient is able to provide a good specimen.[6] However, producing sputum samples is often difficult for children. Clinical guidelines for childhood pneumonia have been published by the Canadian Medical Association and the British Thoracic Society.[2,5] Neither set of guidelines supports the use of nasopharyngeal or throat culture specimens for the diagnosis of lower respiratory tract disease. Blood cultures may be useful in the diagnosis of pneumonia, but they are positive only approximately 10% of the time.[2] Serologic testing may be useful but will often yield results (based on acute and convalescent titers) after the patient has recovered from the acute illness. To assist in determining viral etiologies, direct antigen testing is currently available for influenza A, influenza B, and RSV. Because of the availability of effective therapies against influenza, consideration should be given to obtaining nasal or respiratory secretions for testing.

In patients with significant respiratory distress and a clinical picture that fails to fall into a readily recognized category, bronchoalveolar lavage may yield important diagnostic information that may help define therapeutic choices[8]; it may also allow the discontinuation of certain antimicrobial drugs, thereby alleviating risks of adverse reactions and cost associated with these agents. Bronchoscopy with lavage is particularly valuable in patients with immune defects. This procedure may be performed quickly with minimal morbidity in almost any child. This important diagnostic test should be considered early in the illness, before therapy with multiple antibiotics has been initiated, so as to increase the yield of the test. However, bronchoscopy may not be available to every practitioner.

Imaging Studies

If pneumonia is suspected, then radiographs of the chest are indicated. Radiographic patterns may be helpful in suggesting whether the infection is bacterial or viral, but often no further characterization is possible. Lobar involvement, pleural effusions, pneumatoceles, and pulmonary abscess often point to a bacterial process; bilateral perihilar infiltrates and increased interstitial markings may be associated with a viral etiology. Focal or interstitial infiltrates suggest a mycoplasmal infection. Radiographic evaluation also aids in decision making about the need for antimicrobial therapy. Repeat chest radiographs are important for documenting resolution of the pneumonic process and should be obtained in 3 to 6 weeks after diagnosis. Lack of radiologic resolution may suggest the presence of a congenital lung malformation, foreign body, or neoplastic process.[2]

MANAGEMENT

In devising a treatment plan for the patient with pneumonia, a primary consideration must be the need for hospitalization.[5] Clinical assessment is most important in making this decision. Attention must be paid to hydration status, degree of respiratory distress, presence of hypoxemia, and the existence of other medical conditions. The ability of the family to assess the patient for clinical deterioration or to bring the child back for further care may also influence whether a child is discharged. If the clinician thinks that a patient requires admission to the hospital, then parenteral antibiotics should be provided. For patients with less severe illness, oral antibiotics may be prescribed.

For young infants in the first several weeks of life with bacterial pneumonia, hospitalization is usually necessary. In these cases, ampicillin along with either an aminoglycoside or a third-generation cephalosporin are suggested. This combination provides good coverage for specific organisms frequently seen in the neonatal period—GBS, gram-negative enteric bacteria, and *Listeria* organisms. Older infants and toddlers requiring hospitalization may be treated with intravenous cefuroxime or cefotaxime. Many of these illnesses will be caused by pneumococci, which are increasingly resistant to β-lactam antibiotics. Therefore, if the illness worsens significantly while the patient is receiving either of these antibiotics, then consideration should be given to the institution of therapy with vancomycin. Fortunately, treatment failures are uncommon in spite of penicillin-nonsusceptible strains of *S pneumoniae*. For children with severe illness, additional antibiotic coverage with erythromycin or a newer macrolide may be considered. These antibiotics may also be first-line choices for the treatment of pneumonia in school-aged children and adolescents, thereby covering *M pneumoniae* and *C pneumoniae*.[6,7]

Patients with less severe illness may be treated with the same antibiotics mentioned previously, again providing adequate antibiotic coverage for the same organisms.

Occasionally, in spite of appropriate antimicrobial therapy, complications of pneumonia are seen. Parapneumonic effusions may occur in close to 40% to 60% of pneumonia cases.[10] These effusions initially result from inflamed pleural surfaces caused by underlying infection; later, fibrin levels increase along with increased numbers of inflammatory cells. This circumstance may then allow the previously thin fluid to organize and become a thick rind, compromising lung function. Management of complicated parapneumonia effusions entails either video-assisted thoracoscopic drainage or thoracostomy tube placement.[11] Lung abscesses are also intermittently seen during the evolution of pediatric pneumonia. In spite of worrisome imaging studies showing an irregularly shaped cavity with an air-fluid level inside, prolonged antibiotic therapy will lead to resolution of this complication.[3]

SUMMARY

Many infants and children will experience episodes of respiratory distress as a result of infection with a common bacterium or virus. Clinical assessment and radiographs are necessary in establishing a diagnosis of pneumonia. Careful consideration must be given about the need for antimicrobial therapy and a general assessment of illness. Clinicians should ensure that patients recover fully from an acute lower respiratory tract infection.

WHEN TO REFER

- The child continues to have fever 48 hours after starting appropriate antibiotic therapy.
- The child develops a pleural effusion.
- The child develops a lung abscess.

WHEN TO ADMIT

- The child is younger than 8 weeks.
- The child is in significant respiratory distress (presence of grunting, nasal flaring, or retractions).
- Hypoxia is present.
- The child appears toxic.
- The family cannot adequately assess and care for the child.
- Normal hydration status cannot be maintained.
- The child cannot be brought back for reassessment after outpatient therapy.
- Other medical conditions are present that might influence the child's response to treatment.
- The pneumonia is recurrent.

REFERENCES

1. McIntosh K. Community-acquired pneumonia in children. *N Engl J Med* 2002;346(6):429-437.
2. Jadavji T, Law B, Lebel MH, et al. A practical guide for the diagnosis and treatment of pediatric pneumonia. *CMAJ.* 1997;156(5):S703-S711.
3. Sandora TJ, Harper MB. Pneumonia in hospitalized children. *Pediatr Clin North Am.* 2005;52:1059-1081.
4. Bonadio WA, Jeruc W, Anderson Y, et al. Systemic infection due to group B beta-hemolytic Streptococcus in children. *Clin Pediatr.* 1991;31:230-233.
5. British Thoracic Society of Standards of Care Committee. BTS guidelines for the management of community acquired pneumonia in childhood. *Thorax.* 2002;57:1-24.
6. Bradley JS. Management of community-acquired pediatric pneumonia in an era of increasing antibiotic resistance and conjugate vaccines. *Pediatr Infect Dis J.* 2002; 21(6):592-598.
7. McCracken GH. Etiology and treatment of pneumonia *Pediatr Infect Dis J.* 2000;19(4):373-377.
8. McCracken GH. Diagnosis and management of pneumonia in children. *Pediatr Infect Dis J.* 2000;19(9):924-928.
9. Williams JV, Harris PA, Tollefson SJ, et al. Human metapneumovirus and lower respiratory tract disease in otherwise healthy infant and children. *N Engl J Med.* 2004; 350(5):443-450.
10. Kunyoshi V, Cataneo DC, Cataneo AJ. Complicated pneumonias with empyema and/or pneumatocele in children. *Pediatr Surg Int.* 2006;22:186-190.
11. Kurt BA, Winterhalter KM, Connors RH, et al. Therapy of parapneumonic effusions in children: video-assisted thoracoscopic surgery versus conventional thoracostomy drainage. *Pediatrics.* 2006;118(3):e547-e553.

Chapter 313

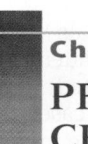

PRESEPTAL AND ORBITAL CELLULITIS

Ellen R. Wald, MD

The practitioner frequently has the opportunity to manage the child for whom the chief complaint is a swollen eye. Some children have trivial or self-limited disorders, but others can have sight- or life-threatening problems.

DIFFERENTIAL DIAGNOSIS

The noninfectious causes of swelling of or around the eye include (1) blunt trauma (leading to the proverbial *black* eye), (2) tumor, (3) local edema, and (4) allergy. In cases of blunt trauma, history provides the key to the diagnosis. Eyelid swelling continues to increase for 48 hours and then resolves over several days. Tumors that characteristically involve the eye include hemangioma of the lid, ocular tumors such as retinoblastoma and choroidal melanoma, and orbital neoplasms such as neuroblastoma, rhabdomyosarcoma, and Langerhans cell histiocytosis.[1] Tumors usually cause gradual onset of proptosis in the absence of inflammation. Orbital pseudotumor, an autoimmune inflammation of the orbital tissues, exhibits eyelid swelling, red eye, pain, and decreased ocular motility.[2] Hypoproteinemia and congestive heart failure cause eyelid swelling as a result of local edema. Characteristic findings are bilateral, boggy, nontender, nondiscolored, soft-tissue swelling. Allergic inflammation includes angioneurotic edema or contact hypersensitivity.[3] Superficially, these problems can resemble the findings in acute infection. However, the presence of pruritus and the absence of tenderness are helpful distinguishing characteristics of allergic inflammation.

PATHOGENESIS OF INFECTIOUS CELLULITIS

Infections can spread to the eye from contiguous structures. Veins that drain the orbit, the ethmoid and maxillary sinuses, and the skin of the eye and periorbital tissues (Figure 313-1) constitute an anastomosing and valveless network.[1] This venous system provides opportunities for spread of infection from 1 anatomic site to another and predisposes the patient to involvement of the cavernous sinus, meninges, and brain.

The relationship between the eye and the paranasal sinuses is shown in Figure 313-2. The roof of the orbit is the floor of the frontal sinus, and the floor of the orbit is the roof of the maxillary sinus. The medial wall of the orbit is formed by the frontal maxillary process, the lacrimal bone, the lamina papyracea of the ethmoid bone, and a small part of the sphenoid bone.[4] Infection originating in the mucosa of the paranasal sinuses can spread to involve the bone (osteitis with or without subperiosteal abscess) and the intraorbital contents. Orbital infection can occur through natural bony dehiscences in the lamina papyracea of the ethmoid

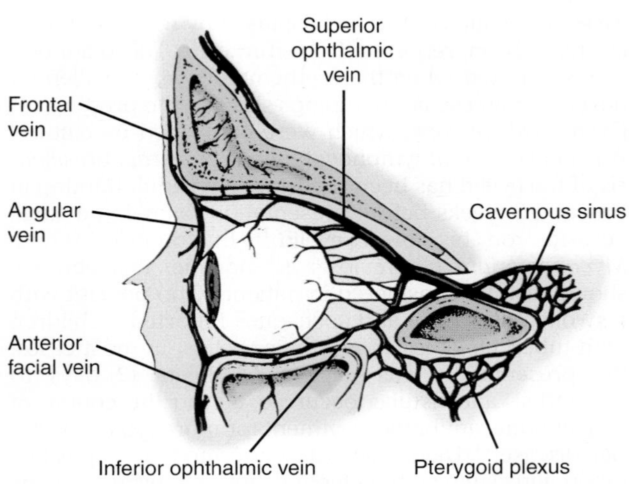

Figure 313-1 The valveless venous system of the orbit and its many anastomoses. *(Harris GJ. Subperiosteal abscess of the orbit.* Arch Ophthalmol. *1983;101:753-754. Reprinted by permission of the American Medical Association.)*

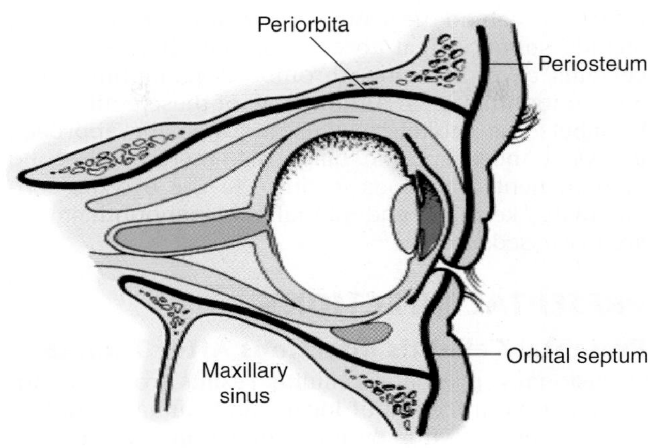

Figure 313-3 The orbital septum is a connective tissue extension of the periosteum that is reflected into the upper and lower lid. *(Shapiro ED, Wald ER, Brozanski BA. Periorbital cellulitis and paranasal sinusitis: a reappraisal.* Pediatr Infect Dis J. *1982;1:91-94. Reprinted by permission of Lippincott Williams & Wilkins.)*

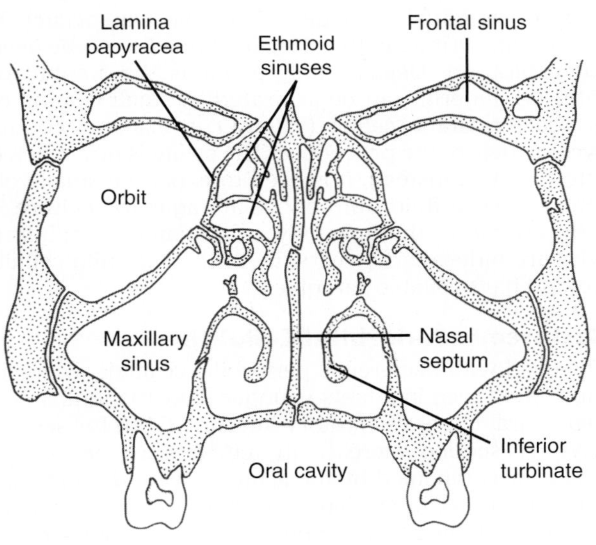

Figure 313-2 The relationship between the eye and the paranasal sinuses is shown schematically. The roof of the orbit, the medial wall, and the floor are shared by the frontal, ethmoid, and maxillary sinuses, respectively. *(Shapiro ED, Wald ER, Brozanski BA. Periorbital cellulitis and paranasal sinusitis: a reappraisal.* Pediatr Infect Dis J. *1982;1:91-94. Reprinted by permission of Lippincott Williams & Wilkins.)*

or frontal bones or via foramina through which the ethmoidal arteries pass.[3]

The orbital septum is a connective-tissue extension of the periosteum (or periorbita) that is reflected into the upper and lower eyelids (Figure 313-3). Infection of tissues anterior to the orbital septum is described as a *periorbital* or *preseptal* infection.[5] The septum provides a nearly impervious barrier to spread of infection to the orbit. Although preseptal cellulitis, or periorbital cellulitis (the terms may be used interchangeably), is often considered as a diagnosis, the term is an inadequate diagnostic label unless accompanied by a modifier that indicates likely pathogenesis.

BOX 313-1 Infectious Causes of Preseptal and Orbital Cellulitis

PRESEPTAL CELLULITIS	ORBITAL CELLULITIS (POSTSEPTAL)
Localized infection of the eyelid or adjacent structure	Subperiosteal abscess
Conjunctivitis	Orbital abscess
Hordeolum	Orbital cellulitis
Dacryoadenitis	Cavernous sinus thrombosis
Dacryocystitis	Hematogenous dissemination
Bacterial cellulitis (trauma)	Endophthalmitis
Hematogenous dissemination	Traumatic inoculation
Bacteremic periorbital cellulitis	Panophthalmitis
Acute sinusitis	
Inflammatory edema	

Infectious causes of preseptal cellulitis occur in the following 3 settings:

1. Secondary to a localized infection or inflammation of the conjunctiva, eyelids, or adjacent structures (eg, conjunctivitis, hordeolum, acute chalazion, dacryocystitis, dacryoadenitis, impetigo, traumatic bacterial cellulitis)
2. Secondary to hematogenous dissemination of nasopharyngeal pathogens to the periorbital tissue
3. As a manifestation of inflammatory edema in patients with acute sinusitis (Box 313-1)[5]

Infections behind the septum that cause eyelid swelling include subperiosteal abscess, orbital abscess, orbital cellulitis, cavernous sinus thrombosis, panophthalmitis, and endophthalmitis. Although all of these entities can be labeled as orbital cellulitis, a systematic approach allows a more specific diagnosis, thereby directing management. Infections intrinsic to the eye (ie, conjunctivitis, keratitis, endophthalmitis, panophthalmitis) are discussed elsewhere.

PRESEPTAL INFECTIONS

Preseptal Cellulitis Infections After Trauma

Occasionally, preseptal cellulitis results from secondary bacterial infection of local skin trauma, including insect bites, or with spread of infection from a focus of impetigo. The traumatic injury may be extremely modest or completely inapparent. Loosely bound periorbital soft tissues permit impressive swelling to accompany minor infection. The overlying skin can be bright red with subtle textural changes, or intense swelling can lead to shininess (Figure 313-4). Some patients have fever, but many are afebrile despite dramatic local findings. The peripheral white blood cell count is variable. In these cases, cellulitis, similar to that on any other cutaneous area, is caused by *Staphylococcus aureus* or *Streptococcus pyogenes*.[6]

Several less common causes of lid cellulitis have been reported. Periocular cellulitis and abscess formation has resulted from infection with *Pasteurella multocida* in a healthy child who sustained a cat bite and cat scratch to the eyelid.[7] Ringworm (caused by *Trichophyton* species) has also been recognized as a cause of lid infection (leading to preseptal cellulitis) characterized by redness, swelling, and ulceration and vesicle formation.[8,9] Palpebral myiasis (larval infection) involving the eyelid of a 6-year-old child was reported from the Massachusetts Eye and Ear Infirmary.[10] A small draining fistula through which the larvae was extracted was noted at the site of the erythematous and edematous lid. Several cases of cellulitis of the eyelid caused by *Bacillus anthracis* have been reported from Turkey.[11] The diagnosis was suggested when the erythematous and swollen lid developed an eschar. Scrapings showed the presence of Gram-positive rods, which were confirmed by culture. A primary case of lymphocutaneous *Nocardia brasiliensis* of the eyelid has been reported in an adult hunting in England 2 weeks before presentation following a small abrasion on his lower eyelid.[12] In countries where *Mycobacterium tuberculosis* is endemic, this etiology should also be considered in patients who present with a swollen lid. Raina and colleagues reported 7 children with tuberculous lesions of their eyelids. In most cases, the presentation was relatively indolent (2 days to 2 months), and fistulas occurred during the course of conventional antibiotic treatment for more typical bacterial disease.[13] Diagnosis was confirmed by a positive tuberculin skin test, the identification of a primary focus of tuberculosis in lung or bone, and the response to antituberculous therapy.

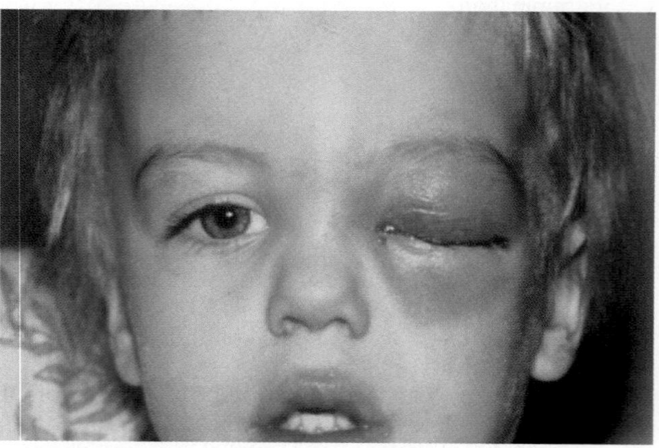

Figure 313-4 A 3-year-old boy with rapid onset of left eyelid swelling and erythema after he incurred a small laceration at the lateral margin of the left eye. He had had an upper respiratory tract infection for 10 days. Group A *Streptococcus* was recovered from the wound.

Patients with bacterial cellulitis of traumatized areas rarely have bacteremia. Precise bacteriologic diagnosis is made through culture of exudate from the wound. If there is no drainage, then a careful attempt at tissue aspiration is undertaken if it can be done safely (ie, at a distance far enough from the orbit that no potential damage to the eye can occur). A tuberculin syringe with a 25-gauge needle can be used for aspiration. Usually, only a minuscule amount of infected material can be aspirated. A small volume of nonbacteriostatic saline (0.2 mL) is drawn into the syringe before the procedure. The saline is not injected into the skin; instead, it is used to expel the small volume of tissue fluid onto chocolate agar for culture.[14] Oral antibiotic therapy may be initiated in children who are older than 5 years, afebrile, with mild cellulitis, and have reliable caregivers.

Bacteremic Periorbital Cellulitis

The child with bacteremic periorbital cellulitis, which is most often seen in infants younger than 18 months, has had a viral upper respiratory infection (URI) for several days. A sudden increase in temperature occurs (to >39°C) accompanied by the acute onset and rapid progression of eyelid swelling. Swelling usually begins in the inner canthus of the upper and lower eyelid and can obscure the eyeball within 12 hours. Periorbital tissues are markedly discolored and usually erythematous, although if the swelling has been rapidly progressive, then the area may have a violaceous discoloration.[15,16] The child's resistance to examination commonly leads to the erroneous impression of tenderness. Retraction or separation of the lids reveals that the globe is normally placed and extraocular eye movements are intact. If retraction of the lids is not possible, then orbital computed tomography scan may be necessary.[17] The young age, high fever, and rapid progression of findings differentiate bacteremic preseptal cellulitis from other causes of swelling around the eye (Figure 313-5).

In the era before universal *Haemophilus influenzae* type b (Hib) immunization, this organism was the most common cause of bacteremic periorbital cellulitis accounting for approximately 80% of cases. *S pneumoniae* accounted for the remaining 20%. The substantial decline in the total number of cases of bacteremic periorbital cellulitis is attributable to the widespread use of the Hib vaccine since 1991 and the introduction of pneumococcal conjugate vaccine in 2000.[18] A precise bacteriologic diagnosis is made by recovery of the organism from blood culture. If tissue aspiration is performed, culture of the specimen may have a positive result.

The pathogenesis of most of these infections, which usually occur during the course of a viral URI, is hematogenous dissemination from a portal of entry in the nasopharynx. This process is akin to the mechanism of most infections caused by Hib and some infections caused by *S pneumoniae*.

In patients with bacteremic periorbital cellulitis, radiographs of the paranasal sinuses are often abnormal. However, the abnormalities almost certainly reflect the viral respiratory syndrome that precedes and probably predisposes the patient to the bacteremic event rather than a clinically significant sinusitis.[5] Bacteremic cellulitis rarely arises from the paranasal sinus cavities, as evidenced by the finding that typeable *H influenzae* organisms are almost never recovered from maxillary sinus aspirates and, similarly, are rarely recovered from abscess material in patients who have serious local complications of paranasal sinus disease, such as subperiosteal abscess. Although *S pneumoniae* can cause subperiosteal abscess in patients with acute sinusitis, such patients are not usually bacteremic.

Treatment for suspected bacteremic periorbital cellulitis requires parenteral therapy. *S pneumoniae* is the most likely cause in a child who has received both the Hib and pneumococcal conjugate vaccine series. Because this infection is usually bacteremic in the age group in whom the meninges are susceptible to inoculation, using an advanced-generation cephalosporin such as cefotaxime or ceftriaxone (150 or 100 mg/kg/day, respectively, divided into 8- or 12-hour doses, respectively) may be prudent. Lumbar puncture should be performed unless the clinical picture precludes meningitis. Addition of vancomycin (60 mg/kg/day divided into doses every 6 hours) or rifampin (20 mg/kg once daily, not to exceed 600 mg/day) is appropriate if cerebrospinal fluid pleocytosis is present. When evidence of local infection has resolved and no meningitis is present, oral antimicrobial therapy is prescribed to complete a 10-day course.

Preseptal (Periorbital) Cellulitis Caused by Inflammatory Edema of Sinusitis

Several complications of paranasal sinusitis can result in swelling around the eye. The most common and least serious complication is often referred to as *inflammatory edema* or a *sympathetic effusion*.[4] This entity is a form of preseptal cellulitis, although infection is confined to the sinuses.

Typically, a child at least 2 years of age has had a viral URI for several days when swelling is noted. A history of intermittent early-morning periorbital swelling that resolves after a few hours is often present. On the day of presentation, the eyelid swelling does not typically resolve but progresses gradually (Figure 313-6).

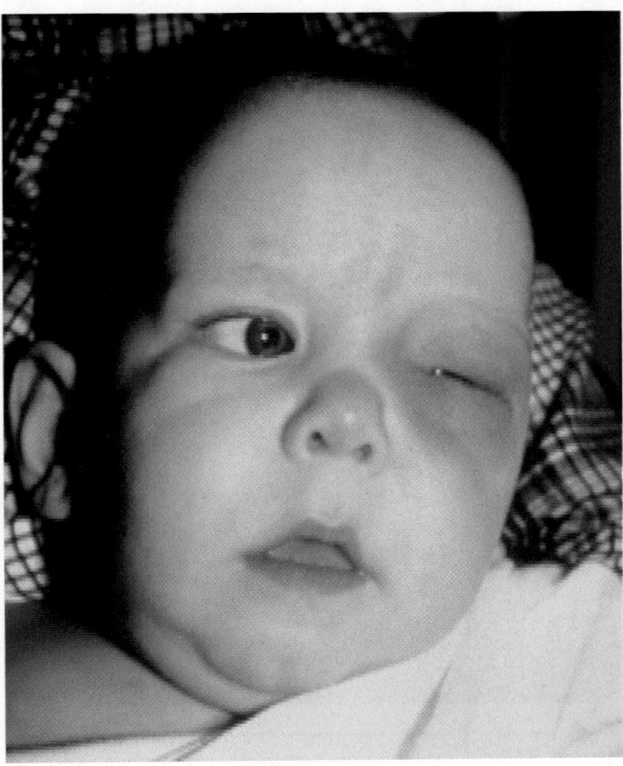

Figure 313-5 A 10-month-old with bacteremic periorbital cellulitis due to *Haemophilus influenzae* type b.

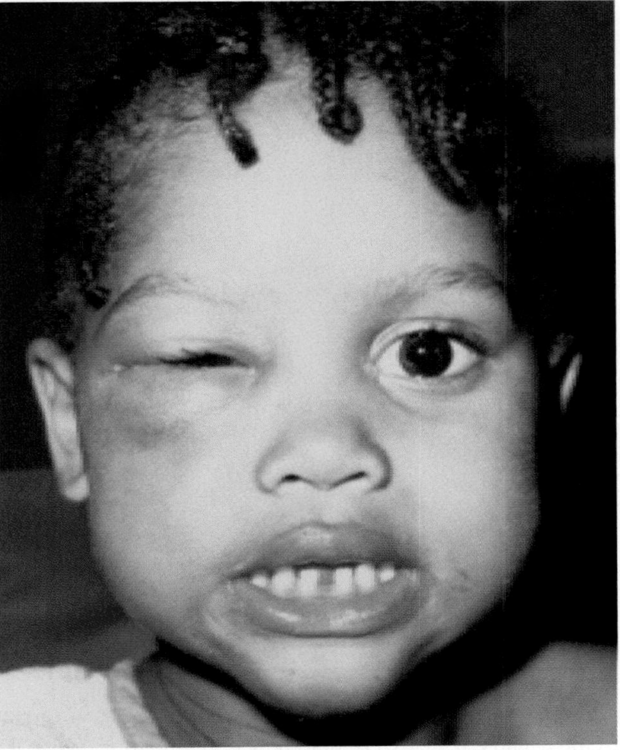

Figure 313-6 A 3-year-old child with inflammatory edema caused by ethmoiditis.

Surprisingly, striking degrees of erythema can also be present. Eye pain and tenderness are variable. Eyelids can be very swollen and difficult to evert, requiring the assistance of an ophthalmologist. However, no displacement of the globe or impairment of extraocular eye movements occurs. Fever, if present, is usually low grade.

The peripheral white blood cell count is unremarkable. Blood culture results are always negative. If a tissue aspiration is performed, then culture of the specimen has a negative result. Sinus radiographs show ipsilateral ethmoiditis or pansinusitis. The age of the child, gradual evolution of lid swelling, and modest temperature elevation differentiate inflammatory edema from bacteremic periorbital cellulitis.

The pathogenesis of sympathetic effusion or inflammatory edema is attributable to the venous drainage of the eyelid and surrounding structures. The inferior and superior ophthalmic veins, which drain the lower lid and upper lid, respectively, pass through or just next to the ethmoid sinus. When the ethmoid sinuses are completely congested, physical impedance of venous drainage occurs, resulting in soft-tissue swelling of the eyelids, maximal at the medial aspect of the lids. In this instance, infection is confined within the paranasal sinuses. The globe is not displaced, and no impairment of the extraocular muscle movements occurs. However, inflammatory edema is part of a continuum, with more serious complications resulting from the spread of infection outside the paranasal sinuses into the orbit.[19] Rarely, infection progresses despite initial optimal management of sympathetic effusions.

The infecting organisms in cases of inflammatory edema are the same as those that cause uncomplicated acute sinusitis (ie, *S pneumoniae*, nontypeable *H influenzae, Moraxella catarrhalis*). Antibiotic therapy can be given orally if, at the time of the first examination, the eyelid swelling is modest, the child does not appear toxic, and the parents will adhere to management. Otherwise, admission to the hospital and parenteral treatment should be undertaken.

The only source of bacteriologic information is that obtainable by maxillary sinus aspiration, which is usually not performed. Appropriate agents for outpatient therapy have activity against β-lactamase–producing organisms (eg, amoxicillin–potassium clavulanate, cefuroxime axetil, cefpodoxime proxetil). Parenteral agents include cefuroxime and ampicillin-sulbactam. The latter combination, although not approved for

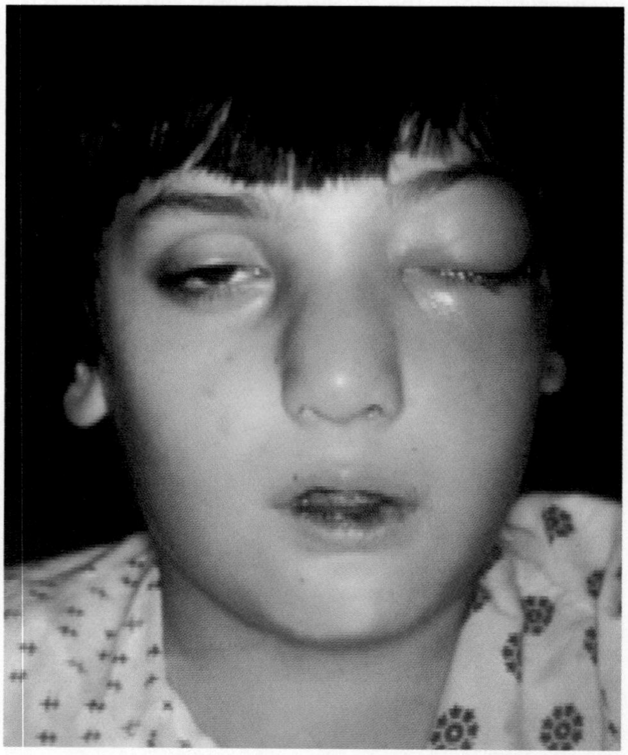

Figure 313-7 A 12-year-old boy with orbital cellulitis. He had a 5-day history of eye pain and progressive swelling of the eyelids, which were markedly erythematous. When his eyelids were retracted, anterior and lateral displacement of the globe and impairment of upward gaze were noted.

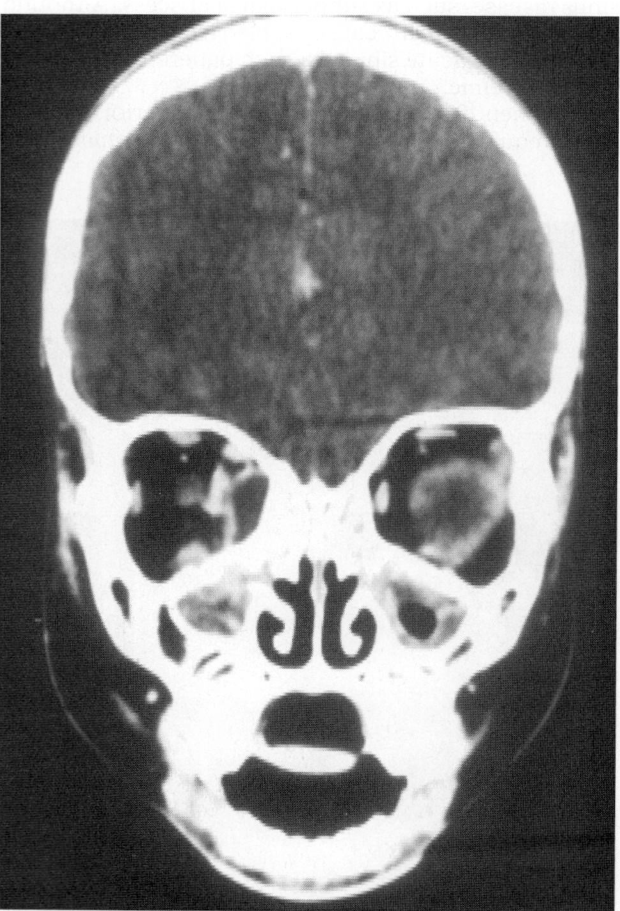

Figure 313-8 Axial computed tomography scans show a subperiosteal abscess extending from the left ethmoid sinus.

children younger than 12 years, is an attractive choice. Although the use of topically applied intranasal decongestants such as oxymetazoline has not been systematically evaluated, such agents may be helpful during the first 48 hours. After several days, once the affected eye has returned to near normal, an oral antimicrobial agent is substituted to complete a 14-day course of therapy.

ORBITAL INFECTIONS

The child or adolescent with true orbital disease secondary to sinusitis usually has sudden onset of erythema and swelling about the eye after several days of a viral URI (Figure 313-7). Eye pain can precede swelling and is often dramatic. The presence of fever, systemic signs, and toxicity is variable. Orbital infection is suggested by proptosis (with the globe displaced usually anteriorly and downward), impairment of extraocular eye movements (most often upward gaze), chemosis (edema of the bulbar conjunctiva), or, late in the evolution of the infection, loss of visual acuity or decreased pupillary reaction. Fortunately, orbital infection is the least common cause of the swollen eye.

Most orbital infections involve the formation of a subperiosteal abscess that, in young children, results from ethmoiditis and ethmoid osteitis. In the adolescent, subperiosteal abscess can be a complication of frontal sinusitis and osteitis. Rarely, orbital cellulitis evolves, without formation of subperiosteal abscess, by direct spread from the ethmoid sinus to the orbit via natural bony dehiscences in the bones that form the medial wall of the orbit.

Imaging studies are usually performed if orbital disease is suspected. They help determine if subperiosteal abscess, orbital abscess, or orbital cellulitis is the cause of the clinical findings (Figure 313-8). In the presence of a large, well-defined abscess, complete ophthalmoplegia or impairment of vision prompt operative drainage of the paranasal sinuses and the abscess is commonly performed.[20-22] Several studies have reported on the successful drainage of a subperiosteal abscess via endoscopy. This method, performed through an intranasal approach, has been successful, thereby avoiding an external incision.[23,24] In many cases, a well-defined abscess is not seen. Instead, inflammatory tissue is observed interposed between the lateral border of the ethmoid sinus and the swollen medial rectus muscle. Usually, patients with these symptoms are managed successfully with antimicrobial therapy alone.[22,25-27] On occasion, the computed tomography scan can be misleading, suggesting abscess when inflammatory edema is present[19,28]; accordingly, the clinical course is the ultimate guide to management.

Empirical antimicrobial therapy should be chosen to provide activity against *S aureus*, *S pyogenes*, and anaerobic bacteria of the upper respiratory tract (anaerobic cocci, *Bacteroides* species, *Prevotella* species, *Fusobacterium* species, and *Veillonella* species) in addition to the usual pathogens associated with acute sinusitis (ie, *S pneumoniae*, *H influenzae*, and *M catarrhalis*).[29-31] Appropriate selections include cefuroxime (150 mg/kg/day divided into doses every 8 hours) or ampicillin-sulbactam (200 mg/kg/day divided into

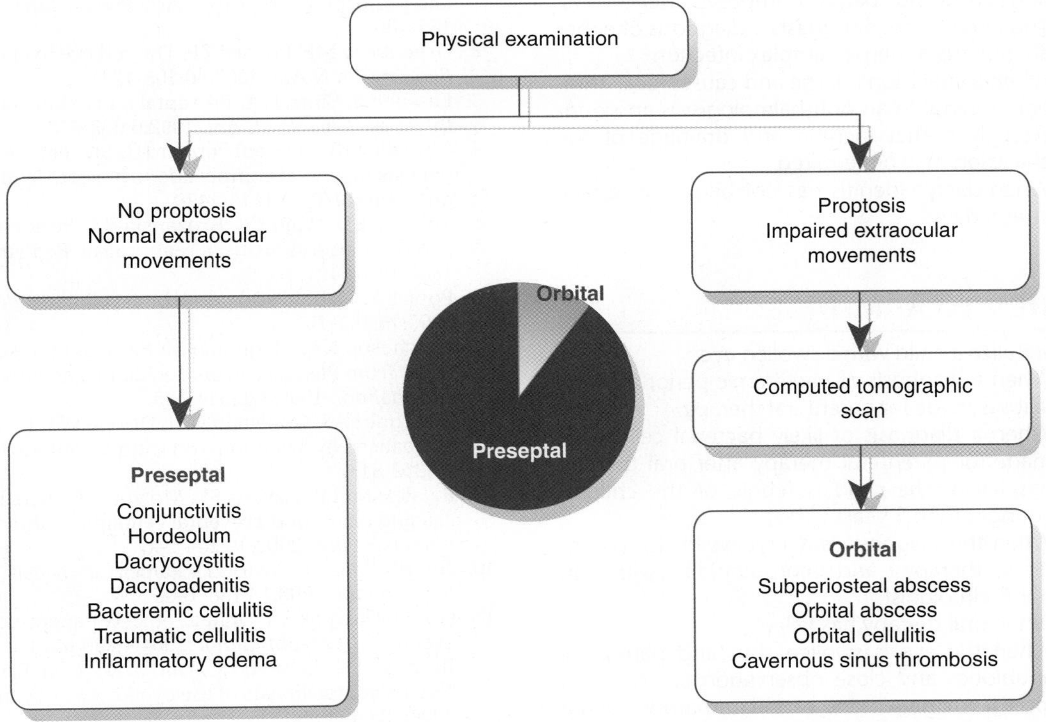

Figure 313-9 Algorithm for the differential diagnosis of the swollen eye.

doses every 6 hours). Clindamycin (40 mg/kg/day divided into doses every 6 hours) or metronidazole (30 to 35 mg/kg/day divided into doses every 8 to 12 hours) can be added if cefuroxime is used and anaerobic infection is likely. Patients with diabetes and immunocompromised children are at higher risk of fungal orbital cellulitis (especially *Mucor* species). If surgery is performed, then a Gram stain of material drained from the sinuses or the abscess guides consideration of additional drugs or an altered regimen. When final results of culture are available, antibiotic therapy may be changed, if appropriate. Intravenous therapy is maintained until the infected eye appears nearly normal. At that time, oral antibiotic therapy can be substituted to complete a 3-week course of treatment.

SUMMARY

The child with a swollen eye is commonly seen in primary care. Figure 313-9 depicts an approach to diagnosis depending on physical examination. By far, children with preseptal infections are most common.

WHEN TO REFER

Refer a child with a swollen eye to an ophthalmologist in the following instances:

- When visual acuity is lost
- When any eyelid swelling occurs in an immunocompromised child or child with diabetes, referral should be immediate because this situation may require urgent treatment
- If conjunctivitis is the diagnosis, then referral to an ophthalmologist is appropriate if the clinical findings do not begin to improve after 5 days. This circumstance suggests a diagnosis of either adenovirus or herpes simplex infection
- When a chalazion is large and causes local irritation, referral to an ophthalmologist is appropriate, given that incision and drainage of the chalazion may be required
- When dacryoadenitis has not begun to resolve after 5 days

WHEN TO ADMIT

Hospitalize a child with a swollen eye:

- When a diagnosis of bacteremic periorbital cellulitis is made for parenteral therapy
- When a diagnosis of likely bacterial cellulitis is made for parenteral therapy after oral therapy has failed, the child is febrile or the child is younger than 5 years
- When the diagnosis is dacryocystitis for parenteral therapy and consultation with an ophthalmologist
- When oral therapy has failed
- When the eye is swollen shut and parenteral antibiotics and close observation are required for the management of inflammatory edema (sympathetic effusion)
- When proptosis, impairment of extraocular movements or diminished pupil reaction, or loss of visual acuity occurs. These situations are the herald signs of subperiosteal abscess, orbital abscess, orbital cellulitis, and cavernous sinus thrombosis. Their presence indicates the need for parenteral antibiotics and the likely need for surgical intervention.

TOOLS FOR PRACTICE

Engaging Patients and Family

- *Children's Eye Health and Safety* (fact sheet), Medem-American Academy of Ophthalmology (www.medem.com).
- *What is a Pediatric Ophthalmologist?* (fact sheet), American Academy of Pediatrics (www.aap.org/sections/he3006.pdf).

Medical Decision Support

- *Pediatric Ophthalmology for Primary Care,* 3rd edition (book), American Academy of Pediatrics (www.aap.org/bookstore).
- *The Physician's Guide to Eye Care,* 2nd edition (book), American Academy of Pediatrics (www.aap.org/bookstore).

AAP POLICY STATEMENTS

American Academy of Pediatrics. Eye examination in infants, children, and young adults by pediatricians. *Pediatrics.* 2003;111(4):902-907. (aappolicy.aappublications.org/cgi/content/full/pediatrics;111/4/902).

American Academy of Pediatrics. Protective eyewear for young athletes. *Pediatrics.* 2004;113(3):619-622. (aappolicy.aappublications.org/cgi/content/full/pediatrics;113/3/619).

REFERENCES

1. VanDyke RB, Desky AB, Daum RS. Infections of the eye and periorbital structures. *Adv Pediatr Infect Dis.* 1988;3:125-180.
2. Greenberg MF, Pollard ZF. The red eye in childhood. *Pediatr Clin N Am.* 2003;50:105-124.
3. Lessner A, Stern GA. Preseptal and orbital cellulitis. *Infect Dis Clin North Am.* 1992;6:933-952.
4. Chandler JR, Langenbrunner DJ, Stevens ER. The pathogenesis of orbital complications in acute sinusitis. *Laryngoscope.* 1970;80:1414-1428.
5. Shapiro ED, Wald ER, Brozanski BA. Periorbital cellulitis and paranasal sinusitis: a reappraisal. *Pediatr Infect Dis.* 1982;1:91-94.
6. Powell K. Orbital and periorbital cellulites. *Pediatr Rev,* 1995;16:163-167.
7. Hutcheson KA, Magbalon M. Periocular abscess and cellulitis from Pasteurella multocida in a healthy child. *Am J Ophthalmol.* 1999;128:514-515.
8. Velazquez AJ, Goldstein MH, Driebe WT. Preseptal cellulitis caused by Trichophyton (ringworm). *Cornea.* 2002;21:312-314.
9. Rajalekshmi PS, Evans SL, Morton CE, et al. Ringworm causing childhood preseptal cellulitis. *Ophthal Plast Reconstr Surg.* 2003;19:244-246.
10. Jun BK, Shin JC, Woog JJ. Palpebral myiasis. *Korean J Ophthalmol.* 1999;13:138-140.
11. Caca I, Cakmak SS, Unlu K, et al. Cutaneous anthrax on eyelids. *Jpn J Ophthalmol.* 2004;48:268-271.
12. Brannan PA, Kersten RC, Hudak DT, et al. Primary Nocardia brasiliensis of the eyelid. *Am J Ophthalmol.* 2004;138:498-499.
13. Raina UK, Jain S, Monga S, et al. Tubercular preseptal cellulitis in children—a presenting feature of underlying systemic tuberculosis. *Ophthalmol.* 2004;111:291-296.

14. Todd JK. Office laboratory diagnosis of skin and soft tissue infections. *Pediatr Infect Dis J*. 1985;4:84-87.
15. Smith TF, O'Day D, Wright PF. Clinical implication of preseptal (periorbital) cellulitis. *Pediatrics*. 1978;62:1006-1009.
16. Thirumoorthi MB, Asmar BI, Dajani AS. Violaceous discoloration in pneumococcal cellulitis. *Pediatrics*. 1978;62:492-493.
17. Goldberg F, Berne AS, Oski FA. Differentiation of orbital cellulitis from preseptal cellulitis by computed tomography. *Pediatrics*. 1978;62:1000-1005.
18. Donahue SP, Schwartz G. Preseptal and orbital cellulitis in childhood—a changing microbiologic spectrum. *Ophthalmology*. 1998;105:1902-1906.
19. Skedros DG, Haddad J Jr, Bluestone CD, et al. Subperiosteal orbital abscess in children: diagnosis, microbiology and management. *Laryngoscope*. 1993;103:28-32.
20. Eustis HS, Armstrong DC, Buncic JR, et al. Staging of orbital cellulitis in children: computerized tomography characteristics and treatment guidelines. *J Pediatr Ophthalmol Strabismus*. 1986;23:246-251.
21. Wong VYM, Duncan NO, Edwards MS. Medical management of orbital infection. *Pediatr Infect Dis J*. 1994;13:1012-1013.
22. Sobol SE, Marchand J, Tewfik TL, et al. Orbital complications of sinusitis in children. *J Otolaryngol*. 2002;31:131-136.
23. Pereira KD, Mitchell RB, Younis RT, et al. Management of medial subperiosteal abscess of the orbit in children—a five year experience. *Int J Pediatr Otorhinolaryngol*. 1997;38:247-254.
24. Deutsch E, Eilon A, Herron I, et al. Functional endoscopic sinus surgery of orbital subperiosteal abscess in children. *Int J Otorhinolaryngol*. 1996;34:181-190.
25. Rubin SE, Rubin LG, Zito J, et al. Medical management of orbital subperiosteal abscess in children. *J Pediatr Ophthalmol Strabismus*. 1989;26:21-27.
26. Noel LP, Clarke WN, MacDonald N. Clinical management of orbital cellulitis in children. *Can J Ophthalmol*. 1990;25:11-16.
27. Souliere CR Jr, Antoine GA, Martin M, et al. Selective non-surgical management of subperiosteal abscess of the orbit: computerized tomography and clinical course as indication for surgical drainage. *Int J Pediatr Otorhinolaryngol*. 19: 1990;109-119.
28. Andres TM, Myers CM III. The role of computed tomography in the diagnosis of subperiosteal abscess of the orbit. *Clin Pediatr*. 1992;31:37-43.
29. Harris GJ. Subperiosteal inflammation of the orbit: a bacteriologic analysis of 17 cases. *Arch Ophthalmol*. 1988;106:947-952.
30. Harris GJ. Subperiosteal abscess of the orbit age as a factor in the bacteriology and response to treatment. *Ophthalmology*. 1994;101:585-595.
31. Harris GJ. Subperiosteal abscess of the orbit. *Arch Ophthalmol*. 1983;101:753-754.

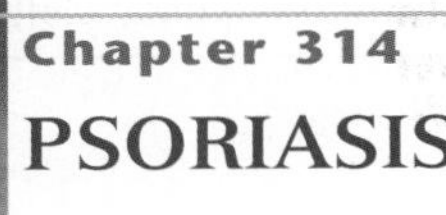

Chapter 314

PSORIASIS

Ginette A. Hinds, MD; Richard J. Antaya, MD

Psoriasis is a T cell–mediated chronic inflammatory disease that is clinically characterized by well-demarcated, erythematous plaques with overlying silvery-white scale. Although the true incidence of childhood psoriasis is unknown, it is not an uncommon disorder in children. A total of 31% to 45% of adult patients developed psoriasis during childhood,[1] with 10% of affected children experiencing onset of disease before the age of 10 years and 2% before the age of 2 years.[2] Psoriasis can also occur during infancy.[2,3]

Psoriasis has been reported to be more common in girls than boys, with a female-male ratio approaching 2:1,[2,4] although in some studies, no sex predilection was found.[5] Childhood- and adult-onset psoriasis occur more frequently in the white population compared with the black, Asian, and Native-American populations.

Both genetic and environmental factors play a role in the development of psoriasis. Childhood psoriasis has been associated with a family history of psoriasis in first-degree relatives,[1] as well as with certain human leukocyte antigen (HLA) subtypes such as HLA-Cw6, -A3, -Cw1, -DR-7, and -DR-8.[4,6] Chromosome 6, the site of HLA I and II complexes, is thought to carry a gene important in determining genetic susceptibility to psoriasis.[6] Environmental triggers that likely precipitate or exacerbate childhood psoriasis include streptococcal infections, upper respiratory infections, trauma, and psychological stress.[1,2]

CLINICAL VARIANTS OF PSORIASIS

Psoriasis can occur as one of several types (see summary in Table 314-1). *Plaque-type psoriasis* is the most common type of psoriasis in both adults and children.[2,6] Plaque psoriasis usually produces large, erythematous, well-circumscribed plaques covered by the characteristic silvery-white psoriatic scale (Figures 314-1 and 314-2). Presentations vary from solitary lesions to widely distributed plaques. The scalp, elbows, knees, and lumbosacral regions are the most commonly affected areas, often with bilateral symmetry (Figures 314-3, 314-4, and 314-5). The scalp is the most frequently involved site in children[2,7] and may be misdiagnosed as seborrheic dermatitis or tinea capitis (Figure 314-6). Facial psoriatic lesions, especially around the eyes, are more common in affected children and may be the only involved site.[2,6]

Inverse psoriasis—psoriasis that involves intertriginous areas such as the postauricular area, axillae, groin, and the genital and perianal areas—is also common in children. Inverse psoriasis tends to produce a glazed, bright-red erythema, sometimes with fissuring, and the characteristic psoriatic scale is usually absent (Figure 314-7). Psoriatic diaper rash can be the initial presentation of psoriasis in children younger than 2 years[2] and can be difficult to differentiate from other causes of diaper dermatitis.

Guttate psoriasis is more commonly seen in children and adolescents than in adults, and it can be the first manifestation of psoriasis. In guttate psoriasis, the lesions tend to be 2 to 10 mm in size, widespread, and symmetrically distributed. They are round or oval erythematous papules and plaques with silvery-white scale, often with a predilection for the trunk and proximal extremities (Figures 314-8 and 314-9). Guttate psoriasis can be triggered by group A streptococcal infection of the oropharynx or perianal skin, but in some cases, an inciting infection is never found.

Table 314-1 Psoriasis Variants

VARIANT OF PSORIASIS	MORPHOLOGY	DISTRIBUTION
Plaque psoriasis	Large erythematous plaques with overlying silvery-white or grayish scale	Scalp, face, elbows, knees, lumbosacral area, gluteal cleft, umbilicus
Inverse psoriasis	Bright-red glazed erythema with no scale	Diaper area, axillae, groin, postauricular area
Pustular psoriasis	Widespread bright-red erythema studded with 1-2-mm pustules; deep-seated 2-4-mm pustules in areas of erythema and scaling	Widespread; especially flexural areas, genitals, finger web spaces, palms, and soles
Erythrodermic psoriasis	Bright-red erythema with massive exfoliation	Widespread

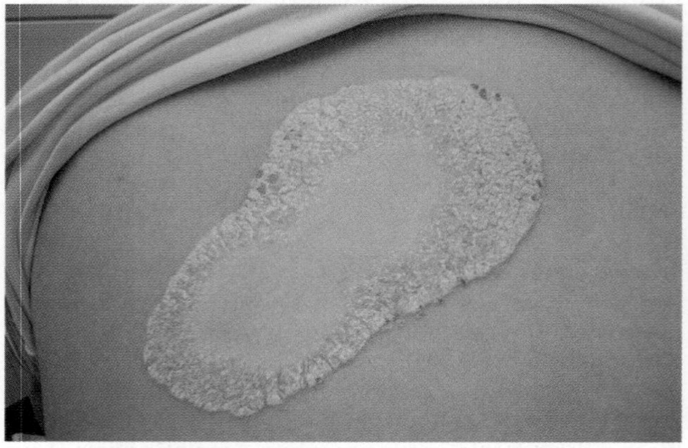

Figure 314-1 Plaque psoriasis. Large, well-circumscribed plaque covered by silvery-white scale.

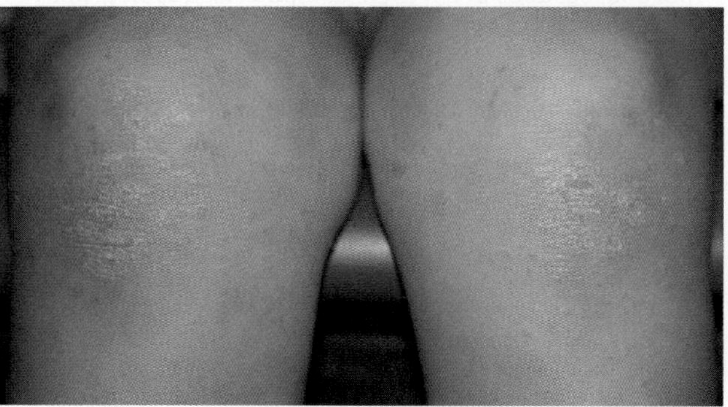

Figure 314-3 Thin psoriatic plaques on the knees.

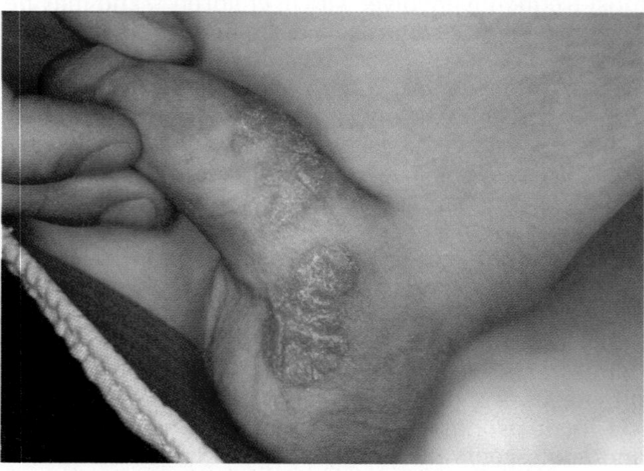

Figure 314-2 Plaque psoriasis on the penis and scrotum.

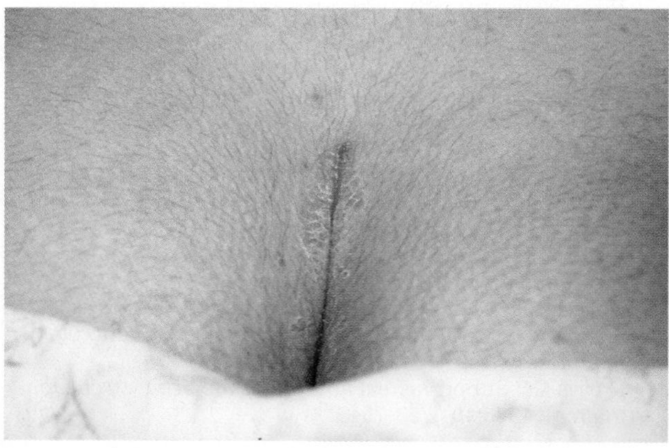

Figure 314-4 Psoriasis involving the gluteal cleft.

Childhood *pustular psoriasis* is rare, but it can be the first manifestation of psoriasis in infants and children. The cause of pustular psoriasis in children is unknown, but several triggers have been implicated, including dental and upper respiratory tract infections,[8] streptococcal infection, withdrawal of systemic corticosteroids, and vaccinations.[9] In addition, experts have postulated that a relationship exists between a history of severe seborrheic dermatitis and the development of pustular psoriasis.[9] Pustular psoriasis can be limited to the palms and soles (palmoplantar pustular psoriasis), but it more commonly occurs as an

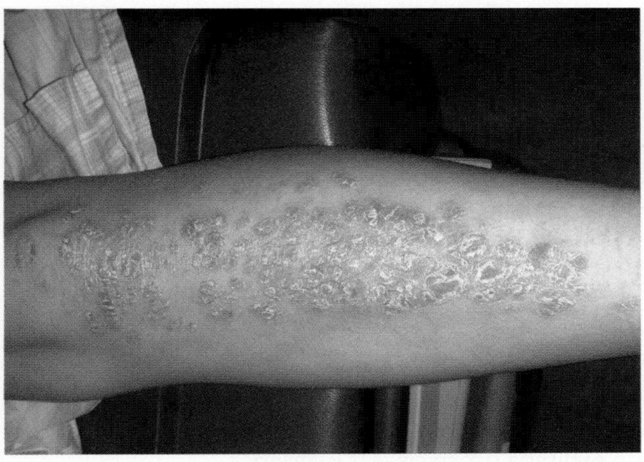

Figure 314-5 Plaques of linear psoriasis on the shin.

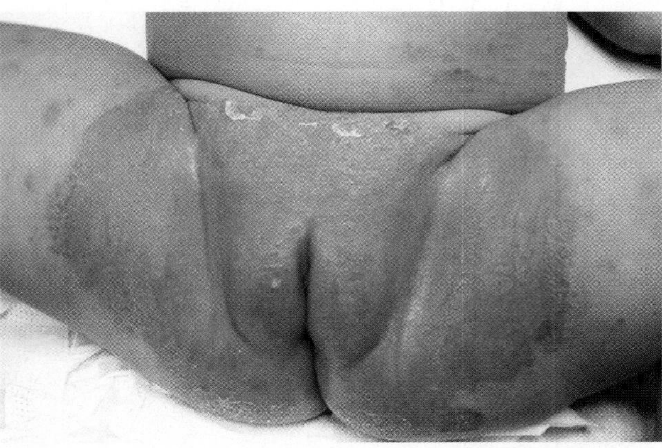

Figure 314-7 Diaper area psoriasis (inverse psoriasis) with bright-red, glazed erythema. Note the absence of the characteristic scale.

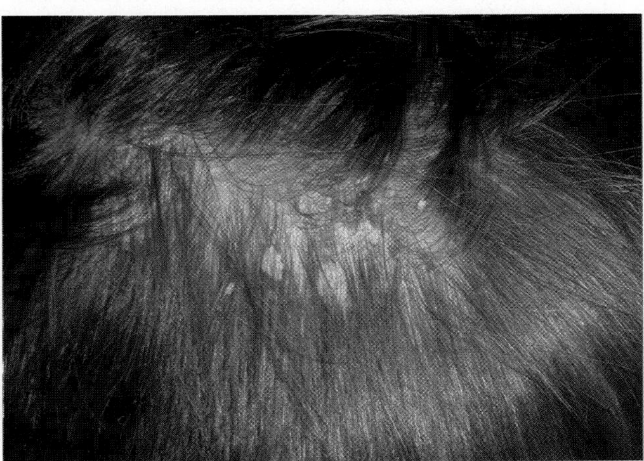

Figure 314-6 Tinea amiantacea. Scales are thick and strongly adherent, encasing the underlying hair, producing an asbestos-like appearance. This can be a feature of seborrheic or atopic dermatitis but is most commonly associated with psoriasis in the scalp.

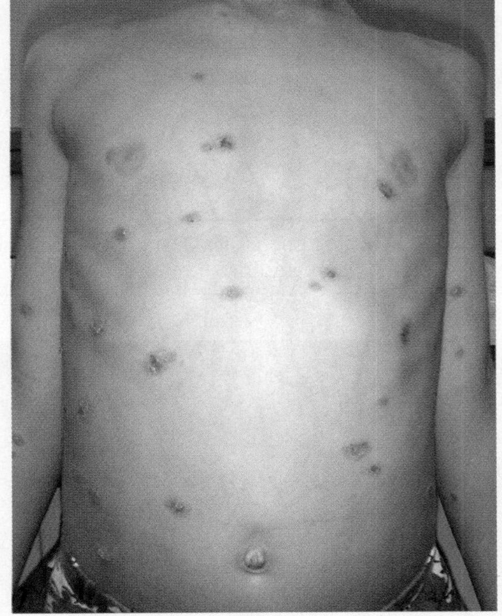

Figure 314-8 Guttate psoriasis. Note the small, droplike plaques.

explosive generalized eruption of pustules on psoriatic plaques or on previously normal skin (generalized pustular psoriasis). These patients develop extensive areas of bright erythema studded with sterile pustules, sometimes associated with fever and malaise. The pustules coalesce into lakes, followed by extensive desquamation. Mucous membrane and nail involvement occasionally occurs. Palmoplantar pustular psoriasis and generalized pustular psoriasis tend to follow a chronic, cyclic course, with unexplained exacerbations and remissions, but are generally benign.

Erythrodermic psoriasis is rare in children. It is characterized by diffuse erythema, exfoliation, and decreased ability to regulate body temperature. This type of psoriasis can be complicated by electrolyte imbalances, cardiovascular compromise, and sepsis, and it is considered a dermatologic emergency.

Many children with psoriasis have nail involvement (Figure 314-10). Nail pitting, the most characteristic finding, is best described as multiple, small, irregularly spaced depressions in the nail plate. Other nail findings in psoriasis include discoloration, onycholysis (separation of the nail from the nail bed), longitudinal striations, and subungual hyperkeratosis. Evaluation for characteristic nail changes can help make the diagnosis of psoriasis be made when it is otherwise not apparent.

PSORIATIC ARTHRITIS

Psoriatic arthritis is uncommon in children. It can occur with either plaque or guttate psoriasis, and in

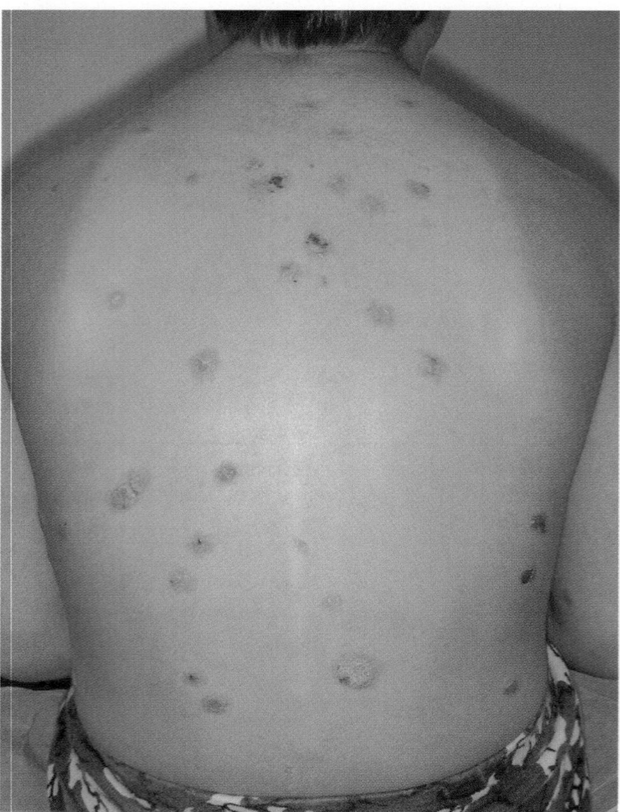

Figure 314-9 Guttate psoriasis. Guttate psoriasis has a predilection for the trunk and proximal extremities.

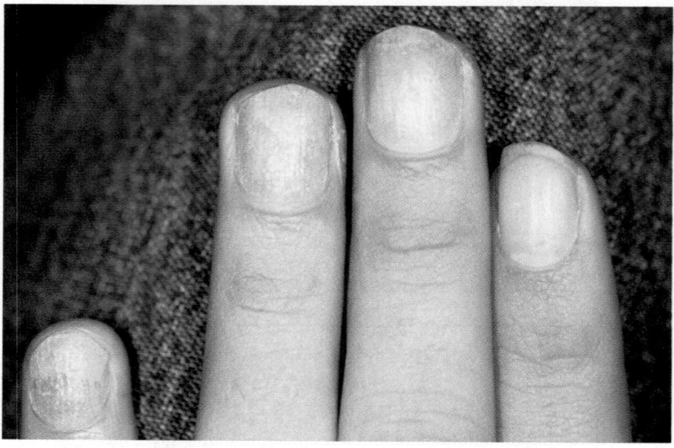

Figure 314-10 Nail psoriasis. Mild involvement with discoloration, onycholysis, and pitting.

80% of patients, skin lesions precede the onset of psoriatic arthritis.[10] The clinical presentation of psoriatic arthritis in children is similar to that seen in rheumatoid arthritis, but the absence of the rheumatoid factor and systemic symptoms, and the presence of a bluish discoloration over affected joints in psoriatic arthritis can help differentiate between these two entities.[10] Psoriatic arthritis tends to preferentially affect the distal interphalangeal and proximal interphalangeal joints of the hands and feet but can also affect the knees and ankles. The most severe form of psoriatic arthritis, arthritis mutilans, is exceedingly rare in children.

DIFFERENTIAL DIAGNOSIS

The differential diagnosis for plaque psoriasis includes other papulosquamous disorders, such as atopic dermatitis (AD) and pityriasis rubra pilaris (PRP). Compared with the lesions of AD, psoriatic plaques tend to be more clearly demarcated from the surrounding uninvolved skin and are usually less pruritic than AD lesions. In addition, AD lesions lack the characteristic silvery-white scale of psoriasis. Psoriasis generally tends to localize to the extensors, whereas AD preferentially affects flexural areas. However, some children do exhibit a psoriasis-AD overlap.

Juvenile PRP can be the most difficult condition to differentiate from psoriasis. However, in addition to biopsy findings, the classic salmon color of PRP lesions, the focal areas of sparing, and follicular accentuation help clinically distinguish this condition from psoriasis.

Pustular psoriasis may be confused with infectious pustular eruptions, such as disseminated candidiasis or staphylococcal scalded-skin syndrome. A skin biopsy, Gram stain, and culture of the contents of several pustules can help differentiate these conditions from pustular psoriasis. Noninfectious pustular eruptions, such as pustular drug eruptions, may also mimic pustular psoriasis. The history of a recently started medication and a skin biopsy can sometimes help differentiate between pustular psoriasis and a pustular drug eruption.

The differential diagnosis of psoriatic diaper rash and other forms of inverse psoriasis includes seborrheic dermatitis and Langerhans cell histiocytosis, candidal intertrigo, and contact dermatitis.

Scalp psoriasis may be mistaken for tinea capitis or seborrheic dermatitis. Performing a potassium-hydroxide preparation and a fungal culture of the scale is important to rule out tinea capitis because the treatment for scalp psoriasis (topical corticosteroids) can exacerbate tinea capitis.

In guttate psoriasis, the differential diagnosis includes pityriasis rosea and pityriasis lichenoides.

The nail changes seen in psoriasis can also be seen in other conditions. For example, nail pitting can also be seen in alopecia areata, and nail discoloration, onycholysis, and subungual hyperkeratosis are also features of onychomycosis.

Box 314-1 lists issues to address when evaluating a child suspected of having psoriasis. Laboratory tests important in diagnosing psoriasis are summarized in Table 314-2.

MANAGEMENT

One of the most important considerations in the management of psoriasis in children is the psychosocial impact of the disease on the affected child and the child's family. The fact that psoriasis can have an adverse effect on the quality of life in children is well known.[3] Emphasis must be placed on educating the child, siblings, and parents, as well as teachers and classmates, about the nature of psoriasis. Affected families should be provided with information about

BOX 314-1 Issues to Address When Evaluating a Child Suspected of Having Psoriasis

- Family history of psoriasis
- Recent history of streptococcal throat or perianal infection
- Frequency and duration of eruptions
- Tendency for lesions to appear on traumatized skin (eg, sunburned, scratched, tattooed) (Koebner phenomenon)
- Nail changes (eg, nail pitting)
- Behavior of lesions in response to ultraviolet light (natural sunlight or tanning beds).
- Joint pains
- Previous treatment modalities and their efficacy

Table 314-2 Laboratory Testing in Diagnosing Psoriasis

LABORATORY TEST	REASON
Bacterial culture of oropharynx and perianal area; antistreptolysin titer	Rule out streptococcal infection, especially in guttate psoriasis; may play a role in pustular psoriasis
Potassium hydroxide preparation of scale	Rule out fungal infection, especially in scalp psoriasis and annular lesions
Skin biopsy	Confirm clinical diagnosis of psoriasis, especially in atypical presentations

available psoriasis support groups. In addition, psychological counseling should be sought so as to equip these patients with effective coping skills for this chronic and potentially disfiguring disease.

Another important consideration in the management of psoriasis is the identification and elimination of potential triggers. Streptococcal infection, medications (eg, lithium, β-blockers, interferon, systemic corticosteroids), stress, and skin trauma are known triggering or exacerbating factors in psoriasis. Patients and their parents must be educated about the so-called Koebner phenomenon, or the development of psoriasis lesions in areas of trauma to the skin such as piercings, tattoos, or sunburns.

Topical Therapy

The topical agents most commonly used to treat psoriasis in children include topical corticosteroids, calcipotriol, tar preparations, and anthralin. Less commonly used topical therapies include keratolytic agents, such as salicylic acid, topical retinoids, and topical calcineurin inhibitors. Bland emollients, such as petrolatum, are an essential part of the skin care regimen in affected patients. Moisturization and application of emollients lessens the dryness and scaling associated with psoriasis, and, in some cases, emollients alone may be sufficient to improve mild psoriasis. However, in most patients, emollients should be used as adjunctive therapy to antiinflammatory topical medications. Table 314-3 summarizes treatment for children with psoriasis.

Topical Corticosteroids

Medium- to high-potency (class II - IV) corticosteroid ointments are effective as monotherapy in many cases of childhood psoriasis. Ultrapotent (class I) corticosteroid ointments are reserved for unresponsive, thick psoriatic plaques. Continuous treatment should not last for more than 2 weeks. Long-term use of topical corticosteroids can lead to side effects such as striae, atrophy, telangiectasia, tachyphylaxis, and acne. When used over a large body surface area, topical corticosteroids may rarely cause pituitary-adrenal axis suppression and other systemic side effects.

Hydrocortisone 2.5% can be used for facial psoriasis, but this may be ineffective in many children. For lesions on the trunk and extremities, medium- to high-potency corticosteroids tend to be more effective. The continuous use of corticosteroids in the groin or other intertriginous areas should be avoided.

For lesions on the scalp, liquid or foam corticosteroid preparations (eg, clobetasol foam, clobetasol solution, fluocinonide solution) work well, as do corticosteroid, tar, zinc, or salicylic acid shampoos (eg, Clobex shampoo [clobetasol], T-Sal shampoo). However, parents should be warned that these products might cause dryness of the hair and scalp. The alcohol base in foam and gel preparations may also cause stinging, especially on already excoriated or otherwise irritated lesions.

The nighttime application of oils, such as Derma-Smoothe Oil (fluocinolone), or nonsteroid oils, such as olive, mineral, or soybean oil, can be a useful adjunct in treating scalp psoriasis in older children. These preparations can be applied to the scalp at night to loosen adherent scale and then shampooed out in the morning. Some black patients prefer oilier scalp preparations, such as lotions, ointments, or oils, rather than the foams or gels because the former preparations also lubricate the hair, preventing brittleness and breakage.

Calcipotriol

Calcipotriol is a vitamin-D analog that has been shown to be safe and effective in treating psoriasis in children.[11] It can be used twice a day as monotherapy in limited disease or as an adjunct to topical corticosteroids in more severe disease. The ointment form is suitable for use on any affected area, but it is more likely to cause burning and irritation on the face or groin. Calcipotriol is also available in liquid form for use on the scalp.

Tar Preparations

Tar preparations can be used in an emollient base (eg, liquor carbonis detergens 5% in petrolatum) or in combination with topical corticosteroids. However, the undesirable odor and potential for staining make it difficult for children and adolescents to accept.

Table 314-3 Treatment of Psoriasis in Children

AGENT	USE	SIDE EFFECTS AND COMMENTS	EXAMPLES
TOPICAL AGENTS			
Emollients	Decreases dryness and scaling; useful in mild psoriasis; use as adjunctive therapy in more severe disease	None Should not replace medicated topicals in patients with significant disease	Petroleum jelly Aquaphor Theraplex emollient
Topical corticosteroids	First-line therapy for all types of psoriasis	Possible cutaneous side effects: atrophy, striae, telangiectasia Possible systemic side effects: hypothalamic-pituitary-adrenal axis suppression, growth impairment, cataracts, glaucoma Avoid use of high-potency preparations on face and intertriginous areas Ointment is the preferred vehicle when treating psoriasis because of occlusive effect and increased potency; useful for dry, scaly lesions Gels readily absorbed; useful in hairy areas, but can cause dryness and irritation Creams rub in well and are aesthetically pleasing; may be less potent than ointment form of same drug Foams, solutions, and oils can be used in the scalp	Class 1 (ultrapotent) Clobetasol propionate 0.05% Betamethasone dipropionate 0.05% Class 2 and 3 (medium to high potency) Fluocinonide 0.05% Betamethasone valerate 0.1% Triamcinolone ointment 0.1% Class 4/5 (medium potency) Hydrocortisone valerate 0.2% Mometasone cream Class 6/7 (low potency) Hydrocortisone (all concentrations) Desonide 0.05%
Calcipotriol	Useful alone in limited disease; useful adjunct to corticosteroids	Irritation	Dovonex
Coal tar preparations	Useful for thicker plaques	Irritation, staining, unpleasant odor, folliculitis Increased risk of irritation on face and intertriginous areas	Liquor carbonis detergens in combination with emollients or corticosteroids Liquid form in bath
Anthralin	Short-contact therapy; large, thick plaques	Irritation, staining	—
Topical calcineurin inhibitors	Useful for lesions of face, intertriginous areas	Occasional burning or itching with first few applications US Food and Drug Administration black-box warning (theoretical malignancy risk based on oral forms)	Tacrolimus ointment (Protopic) 0.03% or 0.1% Pimecrolimus cream (Elidel) 1%
Topical retinoids	Useful in limited, mild to moderate disease	Dryness, local irritation Pregnancy category X	Tazarotene cream or gel (Tazorac)
PHOTOTHERAPY			
Psoralens plus ultraviolet A	Rarely used in children	Cataracts, skin aging, skin cancer, expensive, inconvenient	—
Ultraviolet B	Widespread psoriasis	Expensive, inconvenient, skin aging and skin cancer; very difficult for younger patients	—
SYSTEMIC AGENTS			
Methotrexate	Recalcitrant widespread psoriasis; erythrodermic psoriasis, pustular psoriasis, psoriatic arthritis	Bone marrow toxicity, hepatotoxicity	—

Table 314-3 Treatment of Psoriasis in Children—cont'd

AGENT	USE	SIDE EFFECTS AND COMMENTS	EXAMPLES
Cyclosporine	Recalcitrant widespread psoriasis; erythrodermic psoriasis, pustular psoriasis	Renal, hepatic toxicity, hypertension, hypertrichosis, immunosuppression	Neoral
Oral retinoids	Erythrodermic psoriasis, pustular psoriasis	Cheilitis, xerosis, skin fragility, hypertriglyceridemia, skeletal abnormalities Avoid in adolescent girls (teratogenicity)	Acitretin (Soriatane)
Etanercept	Severe generalized, recalcitrant psoriasis in older children; psoriatic arthritis	Injection site reactions Live vaccination should be avoided; caution in patients with congestive heart failure, multiple sclerosis, tuberculosis risk factors	Enbrel

Anthralin

Short-contact anthralin therapy can be a useful adjunct in treating thick, stubborn plaques. In short-contact therapy, anthralin 1% is applied for 5 minutes, with increasing contact time with subsequent treatments as tolerated. Side effects include local irritation and brownish staining of the skin, bathtubs, and sinks.

Topical Calcineurin Inhibitors

Topical calcineurin inhibitors (tacrolimus and pimecrolimus) are preferred to topical corticosteroids for both facial and intertriginous psoriasis in children. Because the substance does not penetrate thicker plaques well, it is not particularly efficacious in other body sites. The most common adverse effect is burning with initial application, but the topical calcineurin inhibitors are generally well tolerated. Parents must be informed of the US Food and Drug Administration (FDA) black-box warning about a theoretical risk of skin cancer and lymphoma that can occur with oral forms of this medication class.

Topical Retinoids

The topical retinoid tazarotene can be useful in treating limited (<20% body surface area), mild to moderate psoriasis.[7] It is FDA approved for use in adults, but no data have been collected about its efficacy and safety in children. The most common side effect is local irritation. Tazarotene is a potential teratogen and should be used with caution in adolescent girls.

Phototherapy

In older children, ultraviolet (UV) B phototherapy may be used in conjunction with topical or systemic therapy. However, it has been shown to be well tolerated and efficacious in treating psoriasis in children as young as 14 months.[7] The most significant short-term adverse effect associated with UVB is temporary erythema. Narrow-band UVB (311-313 nm) can clear plaques with lower amounts of UV light.[10] The long-term safety of UVB is unclear, but the risk of photoaging and skin cancer may be slightly increased.[3] As a rule, oral psoralen plus UVA should not be administered in preadolescent children.

Systemic Therapy

Systemic treatment of psoriasis is indicated for severe forms of psoriasis, such as extensive plaque psoriasis, generalized pustular psoriasis, erythrodermic psoriasis, and psoriatic arthritis. However, because these forms of psoriasis are uncommon in children, clinical experience is limited in the use of systemic agents in treating childhood psoriasis. Methotrexate, oral retinoids, cyclosporine, and etanercept have all been used in children with varying degrees of success. Oral retinoids, such as acitretin, should be the first-line systemic agent for severe, recalcitrant cases of childhood psoriasis.

Methotrexate

Although methotrexate has been extensively used in treating psoriasis in adults, its use in children is uncommon, though its efficacy and safety in this population have been demonstrated in short-term use.[12,13] The side effects of methotrexate include nausea, vomiting, bone marrow toxicity, and hepatic fibrosis, and its use necessitates monitoring the patient's complete blood count and liver function tests. A liver biopsy is often performed after a cumulative dose of 1.5 to 2 g.

Systemic Retinoids

Systemic retinoids (eg, acitretin, etretinate, isotretinoin) have been studied in children with keratinization disorders but have not been studied in childhood psoriasis. Children with generalized pustular psoriasis have been successfully treated with etretinate.[7,14,15] The most frequently encountered side effects are pruritus, cheilitis, and skin fragility. Chronic use of systemic retinoids has been associated with ossification of interosseous ligaments and tendons, skeletal hyperostosis, and premature epiphyseal closure, leading to concerns that retinoids might affect growth in children.[10]

Cyclosporine (Neoral, Sandimmune)

Cyclosporine is FDA approved for treating severe plaque psoriasis in adults. It is not commonly used in children primarily because of its immunosuppressive effects. Cyclosporine has been used in children with psoriasis with mixed results.[16-18] The adverse effects associated with cyclosporine include hypertension, hypertrichosis, hyperlipidemia, and nephropathy.

Etanercept (Enbrel)

Etanercept is a dimeric fusion protein that competitively inhibits the binding of tumor necrosis factor (TNF) molecules to TNF receptor sites, resulting in a marked reduction in inflammatory activity. It is FDA approved for treating psoriasis, psoriatic arthritis, and rheumatoid arthritis in adults, and for treating juvenile rheumatoid arthritis. Etanercept has been used to treat psoriasis successfully and safely in children,[19,20] although more clinical studies are needed to evaluate its role in treating psoriasis and psoriatic arthritis in children.

WHEN TO REFER

- Unresponsive to first- or second-line therapy
- Widespread disease
- Pustular psoriasis
- Erythrodermic psoriasis
- Worsening joint pains (refer to rheumatologist)

WHEN TO ADMIT

- Widespread pustular psoriasis
- Erythrodermic psoriasis

TOOLS FOR PRACTICE

Engaging Patient and Family

- *National Psoriasis Foundation* (Web page), National Psoriasis Foundation (www.psoriasis.org/home/).
- *What is a Pediatric Dermatologist?* (fact sheet), American Academy of Pediatrics (www.aap.org/family/peddermatologistfacts.pdf).

SUGGESTED RESOURCES

Burden AD. Management of psoriasis in childhood. *Clin Exp Dermatol.* 1999;24:341-345.

Lewkowicz D, Gottlieb A. Pediatric psoriasis and psoriatic arthritis. *Dermatol Ther.* 2004;17:364-375.

Paller AS, Mancini AJ, eds. *Hurwitz Clinical Pediatric Dermatology.* 3rd ed. Philadelphia, PA: WB Saunders; 2006.

OTHER RESOURCES

National Psoriasis Foundation
6600 SW 92nd St., Suite 300, Portland, OR 97223
800-723-9166
www.psoriasis.org

PsoriasisNet
American Academy of Dermatology
www.skincarephysicians.com

REFERENCES

1. Raychaudhuri SP, Gross J. A comparative study of pediatric onset psoriasis with adult onset psoriasis. *Pediatr Dermatol.* 2000;17:174-178.
2. Seyhan M, Coskun BK, Saglam H, et al. Psoriasis in childhood and adolescence: evaluation of demographic and clinical features. *Pediatr Int.* 2006;48:525-530.
3. Burden AD. Management of psoriasis in childhood. *Clin Exp Dermatol.* 1999;24:341-345.
4. Nanda A, Al-Fouzan AS, El-Kashlan M, et al. Salient features and HLA markers of childhood psoriasis in Kuwait. *Clin Exp Dermatol* 2000;25:147-151.
5. Morris A, Rogers M, Fischer G, et al. Childhood psoriasis: a clinical review of 1262 cases. *Pediatr Dermatol.* 2001;18:188-198.
6. Rogers M. Childhood psoriasis. *Curr Opin Pediatr.* 2002; 14:404-409.
7. Howard R, Tsuchiya A. Adult skin disease in the pediatric patient. *Dermatol Clin.* 1998;16:593-608.
8. Nanda A, Kaur S, Kaur I, et al. Childhood psoriasis: an epidemiologic survey of 112 patients. *Pediatr Dermatol.* 1990;7:19-21.
9. Cassandra M, Conte E, Cortez B. Childhood pustular psoriasis elicited by the streptococcal antigen: a case report and review of the literature. *Pediatr Dermatol.* 2003;20:506-510.
10. Lewkowicz D, Gottlieb A. Pediatric psoriasis and psoriatic arthritis. *Dermatol Ther.* 2004;17:364-375.
11. Darley CR, Cunliffe WJ, Green CM, et al. Safety and efficacy of calcipotriol ointment (Dovonex) in treating children with psoriasis vulgaris. *Br J Dermatol.* 1996;135: 390-393.
12. Dogra S, Handa S, Kanwar AJ. Methotrexate in severe childhood psoriasis. *Pediatr Dermatol.* 2004;21:283-284.
13. Kumar B, Dhar S, Handa S, et al. Methotrexate in childhood psoriasis. *Pediatr Dermatol.* 1994;11:271-273.
14. Kopp T, Karlhofer F, Szepfalusi Z, et al. Successful use of acitretin in conjunction with narrowband ultraviolet B phototherapy in a child with severe pustular psoriasis, von Zumbusch type. *Br J Dermatol.* 2004;151:912-916.
15. Kim HS, Kim GM, Kim SY. Two-stage therapy for childhood generalized pustular psoriasis: low-dose cyclosporine for induction and maintenance with acitretin/narrowband ultraviolet B phototherapy. *Pediatr Dermatol.* 2006;23:306-308.
16. Mahe E, Bodemer C, Pruszkowski A, et al. Cyclosporine in childhood psoriasis. *Arch Dermatol.* 2001;137: 1532-1533.
17. Perrett CM, Ilchyshyn A, Berth-Jones J. Cyclosporin in childhood psoriasis. *J Dermatol Treat.* 2003;14:113-118.
18. Pereira TM, Vieira AP, Fernandes JC, et al. Cyclosporin A treatment in severe childhood psoriasis. *J Eur Acad Dermatol Venereol.* 2006; 20:651-656.
19. Hawrot AC, Metry DW, Theos AJ, et al. Etanercept for psoriasis in the pediatric population: experience in nine patients. *Pharmacol Therapeut.* 2006;23:67-71.
20. Papoutsaki M, Costanzo A, Mazzota A, et al. Etanercept for the treatment of severe childhood psoriasis. *Br J Dermatol.* 2006;154:181-183.

Chapter 315

PYLORIC STENOSIS

Sushma Reddy, MD; Deepak M. Kamat, MD, PhD

Pyloric stenosis (PS) is one of the most common conditions requiring surgery in infants. It is characterized by abnormal thickening of the antropyloric muscles. The intervening lumen of the pyloric channel is obstructed, which causes progressively worsening vomiting and results in dehydration. Management of PS consists of hydration and pyloromyotomy.

EPIDEMIOLOGICAL FEATURES

PS was recognized as a clinical entity by Hezekiah Beardsley and Harald Hirschsprung in 1887.[1] The incidence of PS ranges from 1 to 3 per 1000 live births.[2,3] Early population-based studies reported a rise in the incidence of PS,[4,5] but more recent reports indicate that the incidence appears to have leveled.[2,4] Boys are affected 4 times as frequently as girls. However, the commonly held belief that PS primarily afflicts 1st-born male infants has not been confirmed. The incidence in white infants exceeds that in black, Native-American, and Asian infants. Nonetheless, whether PS is an acquired or congenital disorder is still unclear. The onset of clinical symptoms between 2 and 8 weeks of life supports an acquired condition,[5] whereas male predilection, familial cases, PS among twins, and an increased frequency of coexisting malformations support a genetic basis for PS.[6] PS is believed to be associated with the variable transmission of an inheritable trait. Transmission of the PS trait is more frequent from the mother compared with the father. PS develops in 5% of boys and 2.5% of girls whose fathers had PS and in 19% of boys and 7% of girls whose mothers were affected.[7] Concordance is 0.25 to 0.44 in monozygotic twins and 0.05 to 0.1 in dizygotic twins.[7]

ETIOLOGY

The mechanism for hypertrophied pyloric muscle and gastric outlet obstruction is not known. Uncoordinated gastric peristalsis and pyloric relaxation have been speculated to lead to gastric contractions against a closed pylorus, resulting in work hypertrophy of the pyloric muscle. Alterations in gastrin production,[8] changes in breastfeeding practices,[9] and variations in infant milk formulas[10] are among other theories that have been proposed to explain hypertrophy of the pyloric muscle. Impaired neuronal function has been implicated in the development of PS caused by reduction in smooth-muscle vasoactive amines,[11] neurons and nerve fibers,[12] and interstitial *pacemaker* cells of Cajal.[13] Investigators have proposed that deficiency of nitric oxide, a ubiquitous mediator of smooth-muscle relaxation, may be associated with the development of PS because nitric oxide synthase is selectively depleted in the pyloric muscle of patients with PS.[14,15] Studies of neuronal nitric oxide synthase gene polymorphisms suggest that this gene represents a susceptibility locus for PS.[14]

Children with prenatal exposure to macrolides or postnatal exposure to systemic erythromycin, particularly within the first 2 weeks of life, have been observed to be at increased risk for developing PS.[16,17] Postnatal prostaglandins have also been implicated in a case report.[18]

DIAGNOSIS

History

Projectile, nonbilious vomiting in a full-term male infant between 3 and 6 weeks of age is a typical history associated with PS. Although the common age of symptom manifestation is 3 to 6 weeks, PS has been reported in newborns and older infants. Initially, an infant vomits a small amount of food immediately after feeding and continues to gain weight. After a few weeks, the vomiting becomes more frequent and projectile and, eventually, occurs after every feeding. The infant continues to be hungry immediately after vomiting. Infants with PS are usually active and alert, with lethargy ensuing only after significant dehydration. Initially, the vomitus is nonbilious, but the infant may subsequently develop gastritis, and the vomitus may become brownish in color.

Physical Examination

Physical examination reveals weight loss and dehydration. The enlarged pylorus may be felt as a firm, mobile, ovoid-shaped mass—the so-called olive. If the infant is relaxed, then the mass can be felt in approximately 80% to 90% of cases. For this examination, the infant's feet should be elevated and the knees placed in the flexed position to relax the abdominal muscles. Two or 3 fingertips are placed in the right upper quadrant, gently advanced into the deeper tissues below the liver edge, and then slowly swept toward the umbilicus. The mass can be felt to roll under the fingertips during this sweeping motion and is usually felt to deep abdominal palpation in a quiet, cooperative infant and is almost never palpable in an agitated, crying infant with a contracted abdominal wall. The mass can be best felt immediately after an episode of projectile emesis because, at this time, the pylorus is fully contracted and is at its firmest consistency. If the mass is not felt with the infant in the supine position, then palpation while the infant is lying prone may be successful. Occasionally, the primary care physician may need to pass a nasogastric tube, empty the stomach, and feed the infant small quantities of dextrose in water to help relax the abdominal wall. Once the mass is felt unequivocally, the diagnosis of PS is established, and no further diagnostic maneuvers are necessary. A large volume of fluid aspirated from the stomach of a fasting infant who has a history of projectile vomiting strengthens a possibility of PS.[19] Gastric contractions, which move across the upper abdomen from left to right, may be seen in some infants. These contractions are best observed with a bright light directed across the abdomen from the patient's side, with the examiner standing at the foot of the examining table.

Although most infants with PS are otherwise healthy and genetically normal, PS has been reported with a greater frequency in infants with hiatal and inguinal hernias.[20] Associations with malrotation, junctional epidermolysis bullosa, Hirschsprung disease, ovarian cysts, ichthyosis, Smith-Lemli-Opitz syndrome, and deletions of the long arm of chromosome 11 have also been reported.[21-23]

Laboratory Studies

Persistent vomiting caused by gastric outlet obstruction results in the continuous loss of gastric hydrochloric acid. Dehydration causes an increase in aldosterone production, leading to increased renal excretion of potassium. The potassium excretion results

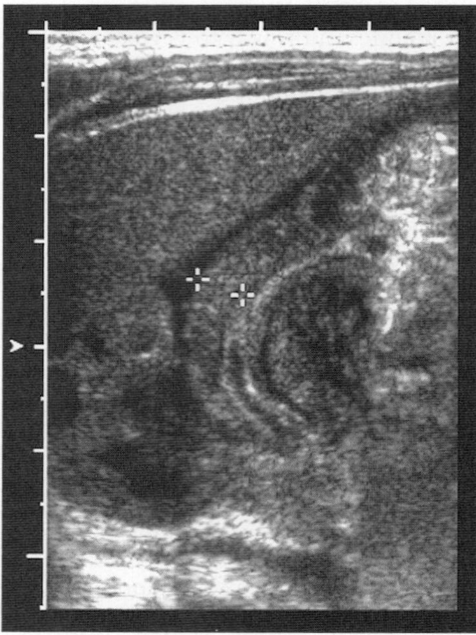

Figure 315-1 Ultrasound of the abdomen shows abnormal thickening (4.5 mm) of pyloric wall, which is consistent with pyloric stenosis.

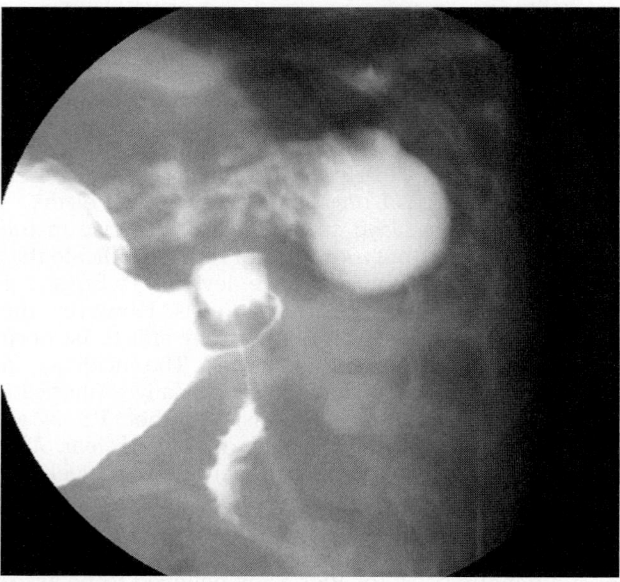

Figure 315-2 Upper gastrointestinal study shows that the pyloric channel is narrowed and elongated with a double-track appearance. This finding is consistent with pyloric stenosis.

in a hypochloremic, hypokalemic metabolic alkalosis. The depletion of chloride in the blood leads to an exchange of hydrogen and potassium for sodium in the distal tubule, resulting in a paradoxic aciduria.[24] However, a spectrum of electrolyte abnormalities may be seen.[25] Hypoglycemia may be present and may cause seizures. Unconjugated hyperbilirubinemia is common and correlates with a decrease in hepatic glucuronosyl transferase activity, which resolves after treatment.

Imaging Studies

With a sensitivity approaching 100%, an ultrasound scan is the most useful modality to confirm the diagnosis in cases in which PS is suspected clinically but the hypertrophied pylorus cannot be palpated.[26] Measurement of pyloric wall thickness, diameter, and pyloric channel length accurately establishes the diagnosis of PS. A pyloric muscle wall thickness of 3.7 mm or greater and a channel length of 17 mm or greater have been shown to have a more than 90% positive predictive value[27] (Figure 315-1). Diagnostic criteria for wall thickness may be reduced to 3 mm in infants younger than 30 days.[28,29] An upper gastrointestinal (GI) tract contrast study may be performed in infants in whom the ultrasound is not diagnostic. Characteristic upper GI tract findings in infants with PS include an elongated and narrowed pyloric channel (string sign) with the shoulders of the hypertrophied pylorus bulging into the intestinal lumen (Figure 315-2). The palpation of a mass on physical examination alone should aid in making an accurate diagnosis in most patients. However, increasing reliance is now placed on noninvasive, highly accurate, and relatively inexpensive radiologic tests such as the ultrasound.[30-32]

DIFFERENTIAL DIAGNOSIS

Other causes of gastric outlet obstruction such as foregut stenosis, gastric duplications, antral webs, pylorospasm, annular pancreas, and malrotation should be considered in the differential diagnosis of an infant with nonbilious emesis. Many of these causes can be excluded by ultrasound and upper GI tract series. When a diagnosis of PS cannot be established in an infant with persistent emesis and normal ultrasound examination and upper GI tract series, the possibilities of a poor feeding regimen, gastroesophageal reflux, sepsis, intracranial disease, renal disorder, or adrenal insufficiency should be considered. Prompt diagnosis and immediate therapy are crucial in an infant with salt-losing congenital adrenal hyperplasia. This condition should be suspected in an infant with abnormal genitalia, hyponatremia, and hyperkalemia. When the workup is inconclusive, reevaluating the infant in a week to 10 days is reasonable when the pyloric mass may become palpable or the ultrasound examination or upper GI tract series may become diagnostic.[33]

MANAGEMENT

Preoperative Management

In the past, infants often had overwhelming malnutrition and electrolyte abnormalities. In the current era of early diagnosis, infants infrequently progress to this severe state.[34] The anatomic correction of PS is not a surgical emergency because, although PS is a form of intestinal obstruction, gangrene and intestinal perforation do not occur with this condition. Infants should not undergo surgery until the fluid and electrolyte deficits have been corrected. If infants undergo surgery with uncorrected alkalosis, then the profound effect that surgical stress has on the urinary excretion of sodium may intensify the electrolyte abnormalities.

Fluid replacement should include deficit correction, daily maintenance fluids, and ongoing losses. Replacement therapy includes continuous maintenance infusion of 5% dextrose in 0.45 normal saline with the addition of 20 mEq/L potassium chloride once urine output is established. In addition, repeated boluses of isotonic sodium chloride at 20 mL/kg can be given until a serum chloride level of 100 mEq/L is achieved. Given that gastric decompression is necessary for surgery and induction of anesthesia, nasogastric decompression should be performed during fluid and electrolyte resuscitation.

Surgical Management

Once the volume and electrolyte status is corrected, the infant is ready for surgery. Ramstedt pyloromyotomy through a right upper quadrant transverse incision has been the traditional treatment for hypertrophic PS. Laparoscopic and circumumbilical approaches have now been introduced as alternative methods. Earlier data suggested that the circumumbilical approach is associated with greater mean operative time and cost, and the laparoscopic method offers shorter mean operative time with no increase in complications or costs.[35] The only randomized trial conducted by Ostlie et al shows no difference between the two approaches.[36]

Medical Management

Because surgical myotomy is a reliable and safe procedure, medical therapy alone has been largely discarded during the last several decades. However, medical therapy may be considered an alternative to pyloromyotomy, particularly in children with major concurrent primary disease. Medical therapy with the anticholinergic agent atropine sulfate has been used with success, although the duration of hospital stay was prolonged.[37,38] Studies comparing predominantly oral atropine sulfate regimen to surgical myotomy have reported similar success rates.[37]

Postoperative Management

Postoperative vomiting occurs is most infants and will usually subside by the 2nd to 5th feeding. Parental education regarding postoperative vomiting is important before surgery. Infants should be fed full-strength formula or human milk every 3 to 4 hours starting 6 hours after surgery. In case of emesis, infants can be refed the amount vomited one hour later with resumption of the feeding schedule thereafter. This early refeeding has resulted in a reduction in the postoperative hospital stay.[39]

Discharge Criteria

Infants are usually discharged 24 to 48 hours after surgery. Feeding tolerance must be reassessed before discharge criteria.

COMPLICATIONS

Intraoperative and Early Postoperative Complications

Morbidity and mortality from surgical repair have decreased from 50% to less than 1% in the current era. The risk of complications such as intestinal perforation, hemorrhage, wound dehiscence, and postoperative infection is negligible.[40,41]

Hypoglycemia

Reactive hypoglycemia has been reported in infants who have a wide variety of medical and surgical conditions and may cause respiratory arrest and death. A constant infusion of dextrose results in hyperinsulinemia and can result in severe hypoglycemia if the infusion is suddenly terminated before adequate oral feeding is established. This reaction is particularly likely if liver glycogen stores have been depleted, as has been shown in infants with PS.

Death

The mortality rate in infants with PS is less than 0.1%.[42] Improvement in anesthetic techniques and monitoring has contributed to these improved results.[43] Delayed diagnosis, inadequate preoperative rehydration, pulmonary aspiration, unrecognized perforation, hypoglycemia, persistent obstruction, hemorrhage, and the presence of other associated congenital anomalies are potential causes of death.

Late Complications

Postoperative obstruction

Radiographic evaluation is necessary if vomiting persists beyond 5 to 7 days. Excessive vomiting may be caused by persistent stenosis, gastroesophageal reflux, gastric outlet obstruction, or small-bowel obstruction attributable to adhesions. An upper GI tract contrast series may be helpful but is also difficult to interpret. Narrowing and elongation of the pyloric channel usually persist for weeks to months after a successful operation, even in infants who have minimal or no postoperative vomiting.[37,45] Subsequent operation may be indicated in the rare event of persistent pyloric obstruction.

Long-Term Outcome

The long-term outcome for patients treated for PS is excellent. Rapid gastric emptying and duodenogastric reflux have been identified in some patients who had undergone pyloromyotomy 5 to 7 years earlier.[45] However, other studies have shown no differences between previous patients with PS and controls after a long-term follow-up.[46-49]

WHEN TO REFER

- All infants with PS should be referred to a surgeon for surgery.

WHEN TO ADMIT

- All infants need to be hospitalized to correct the electrolyte imbalance and for the surgery.

SUGGESTED RESOURCES

Rollins MD, Sheilds MD, Quinn RJ, et al. Pyloric stenosis: congenital or acquired? *Arch Dis Child*. Jan 1989;64(1): 138-139.

Shafagh H, Soltani MA, Douvoyiannis M, et al. Index of suspicion. *Pediatr Rev*. Dec 2005;26(12):461-466.

Sretenovic A, Smoljanic Z, Korac G, et al. Conservative treatment of hypertrophic pyloric stenosis in children. *Srp Arh Celok Lek*. Oct 2004;132(1):93-96.

REFERENCES

1. Touloukian RJ. Pediatric surgery between 1860 and 1900. *J Pediatr Surg*. 1995;30(7):911-916.
2. Schechter R, Torfs C, Bateson T. The epidemiology of infantile hypertrophic pyloric stenosis. *Paediatr Perinat Epidemiol*. 1997;11(4):407-427.
3. Lammer EJ, Edmonds LD. Trends in pyloric stenosis incidence, Atlanta, 1968 to 1982. *J Med Genet*. 1987;24(8): 482-487.
4. Applegate M, Druschel C. The epidemiology of infantile hypertrophic pyloric stenosis in New York State, 1983 to 1990. *Arch Pediatr Adolesc Med*. 1995;149(10):1123-1129.
5. Rollins MD, Shields MD, Quinn RJ, et al. Pyloric stenosis: congenital or acquired? *Arch Dis Child*. 1989;64(1): 138-139.
6. Velaoras K, Bitsori M, Galanakis E, et al. Hypertrophic pyloric stenosis in twins: same genes or same environments. *Pediatr Surg Int*. 2005;21(8):669-671.
7. Carter C, Evans K. Inheritance of congenital pyloric stenosis. *J Med Genet*. 1969;6(3):233-254.
8. Rogers IM, Drainer IK, Moore MR, et al. Plasma gastrin in congenital hypertrophic pyloric stenosis. A hypothesis disproved. *Arch Dis Child*. 1975;50(6):671.
9. Knox EG, Armstrong E, Haynes R. Changing incidence of infantile hypertrophic pyloric stenosis. *Arch Dis Child*. 1983;58(8):582-585.
10. Webb AR, Lari J, Dodge JA. Infantile hypertrophic pyloric stenosis in South Glamorgan 1970-9. Effects of changes in feeding practice. *Arch Dis Child*. 1983;58(8): 586-590.
11. Malmfors G, Sundler F. Peptidergic innervation in infantile hypertrophic pyloric stenosis. *J Pediatr Surg*. 1986; 21(4):303-306.
12. Langer JC, Berezin I, Daniel EE. Hypertrophic pyloric stenosis: ultrastructural abnormalities of enteric nerves and the interstitial cells of Cajal. *J Pediatr Surg*. 1995; 30(11):1535-1543.
13. Vanderwinden J-M, Liu H, Menu R, et al. The pathology of infantile hypertrophic pyloric stenosis after healing. *J Pediatr Surg*. 1996;31(11):1530-1534.
14. Kusafuka T PP. Altered messenger RNA expression of the neuronal nitric oxide synthase gene in infantile hypertrophic pyloric stenosis. *Pediatr Surg Int*. 1997; 12(8):576-579.
15. Chung E, Curtis D, Chen G, et al. Genetic evidence for the neuronal nitric oxide synthase gene (NOS1) as a susceptibility locus for infantile pyloric stenosis. *Am J Hum Genet*. 1996;58(2):363-370.
16. Mahon B, Rosenman M, Kleiman M. Maternal and infant use of erythromycin and other macrolide antibiotics as risk factors for infantile hypertrophic pyloric stenosis. *J Pediatr*. 2001;139(3):380-384.
17. Sorensen H, Skriver M, Pedersen L, et al. Risk of infantile hypertrophic pyloric stenosis after maternal postnatal use of macrolides. *Scand J Infect Dis*. 2003;35(2):104-106.
18. Callahan M, McCauley R, Patel H, et al. The development of hypertrophic pyloric stenosis in a patient with prostaglandin-induced foveolar hyperplasia. *Pediatr Radiol*. 1999;29(10):748-751.
19. Mandell GA, Wolfson PJ, Adkins ES, et al. Cost-effective imaging approach to the nonbilious vomiting infant. *Pediatrics*. 1999;103(6):1198-1202.
20. Iijima T, Okamatsu T, Matsumura M, et al. Hypertrophic pyloric stenosis associated with hiatal hernia. *J Pediatr Surg*. 1996;31(2):277-279.
21. Muller H, Bode H, Krone C, et al. Herlitz syndrome and "pyloric atresia." *Helv Paediatr Acta*. 1989:43(5-6):457-466.
22. O'Hare AE, Grace E, Edmunds AT. Deletion of the long arm of chromosome 11 [46,XX,del(11)(q24.1—qter)]. *Clin Genet*. 1984;25(4):373-377.
23. Stoll C, Grosshans E, Binder P, et al. Hypertrophic pyloric stenosis associated with X-linked ichthyosis in two brothers. *Clin Exp Dermatol*. 1983;8(1):61-64.
24. Shafagh H, Soltani MA, Douvoyiannis M, et al. Index of suspicion. *Pediatrics in Review*. 2005;26(12):461-466.
25. Touloukian RJ, Higgins E. The spectrum of serum electrolytes in hypertrophic pyloric stenosis. *J Pediatr Surg*. 1983;18(4):394-397.
26. Macdessi J, Oates RK. Clinical diagnosis of pyloric stenosis: a declining art. *BMJ*. 1993;306(6884):1065-1066.
27. Haider N, Spicer R, Grier D. Ultrasound diagnosis of infantile hypertrophic pyloric stenosis: determinants of pyloric length and the effect of prematurity. *Clinical Radiology*. 2002;57(2):136-139.
28. Lamki N, Athey PA, Round ME, et al. Hypertrophic pyloric stenosis in the neonate—diagnostic criteria revisited. *Can Assoc Radiol J*. 1993;44(1):21-24.
29. Shkolnik A. Applications of ultrasound in the neonatal abdomen. *Radiol Clin North Am*. 1985;23(1):141-156.
30. Macdessi J, Oates RK. Clinical diagnosis of pyloric stenosis: a declining art. *BMJ*. 1993;306(6884):1065-1066.
31. Breaux CW, Georgeson KE, Royal SA. Changing patterns in the diagnosis of hypertrophic pyloric stenosis. *Pediatrics*. 1988;81(2):213-217.
32. Poon TSC, Zhang A-L, Cartmill T, et al. Changing patterns of diagnosis and treatment of infantile hypertrophic pyloric stenosis: A clinical audit of 303 patients. *J Ped Surg*. 1996;31(12):1611-1615.
33. Geer LL, Gaisie G, Mandell VS, et al. Evolution of pyloric stenosis in the first week of life. *Pediatr Radiol*. 1985; 15(3):205-206.
34. Papadakis K, Chen E, Luks F, et al. The changing presentation of pyloric stenosis. *Am J Emerg Med*. 1999;17(1): 67-69.
35. Kim SS, Lau ST, Lee SL, et al. Pyloromyotomy: a comparison of laparoscopic, circumumbilical, and right upper quadrant operative techniques. *Journal of the American College of Surgeons*. 2005;201(1):66-70.
36. St. Peter SD, Holcomb GWI, Calkins CM, et al. Open versus laparoscopic pyloromyotomy for pyloric stenosis: a prospective, randomized trial. *Ann Surg*. 2006;244(3): 363-370.
37. Yamataka A, Tsukada K, Yokoyama-Laws Y, et al. Pyloromyotomy versus atropine sulfate for infantile hypertrophic pyloric stenosis. *J Pediatr Surg*. 2000;35(2): 338-342.
38. Sretennovic A, Smoljanic Z, Korac G, et al. Conservative treatment of hypertrophic pyloric stenosis in children. *Srp Arh Celok Lek*. 2004;132(Suppl 1):93-96.
39. Michalsky MP, Pratt D, Caniano DA, et al. Streamlining the care of patients with hypertrophic pyloric stenosis: application of a clinical pathway. *J Pediatr Surg*. 2002; 37(7):1072-1075.
40. Ly DP, Liao JG, Burd RS. Effect of surgeon and hospital characteristics on outcome after pyloromyotomy. *Arch Surg*. 2005;140(12):1191-1197.
41. Langer JC, To T. Does pediatric surgical specialty training affect outcome after Ramstedt pyloromyotomy? A population-based study. *Pediatrics*. 2004;113:1342-1347.

42. Zeidan B, Wyatt J, Mackersie A, et al. Recent results of treatment of infantile hypertrophic pyloric stenosis. *Arch Dis Child*. 1988;63(9):1060-1064.
43. MacDonald NJ, Fitzpatrick GJ, Moore KP, et al. Anaesthesia for congenital hypertrophic pyloric stenosis: A review of 350 patients. *Br J Anaesth*. 1987;59(6):672-677.
44. Sauerbrei EE PG. The ultrasonic features of hypetrophic pyloric stenosis, with emphasis on the postoperative appearance. *Radiology*. 1983;147(2):503-506.
45. Tam PK, Saing H, Koo J, et al. Pyloric function five to eleven years after Ramstedt's pyloromyotomy. *J Pediatr Surg*. 1985;20(3):236-239.
46. Asai A TH, Harada M, Tashiro S. Ultrasonographic evaluation of gastric emptying in normal children and children after pyloromyotomy. *Pediatr Surg Int*. 1997;12(5-6): 344-347.
47. Ludtke FE, Bertus M, Voth E, et al. Gastric emptying 16 to 26 years after treatment of infantile hypertrophic pyloric stenosis. *J Pedia Surg*. 1994;29(4):523-526.
48. Ludtke FE, Bertus M, Michalski S, et al. Long-term analysis of ultrasonic features of the antropyloric region 17-27 years after treatment of infantile hypertrophic pyloric stenosis. *J Clin Ultrasound*. 1994;22(5):299-305.
49. Vilmann P, Hjortrup A, Altmann P, et al. A long-term gastrointestinal follow-up in patients operated on for congenital hypertrophic pyloric stenosis. *Acta Paediatr Scand*. 1986;75(1):156-158.

Chapter 316

RENAL TUBULAR ACIDOSIS

Ronald J. Kallen, MD

DEFINITION

Renal tubular acidosis (RTA) is the principal cause of hyperchloremic metabolic acidosis in an infant or child ingesting a typical diet and who does not have gastroenteritis or chronic kidney disease. The term *tubular* means that metabolic acidosis is a consequence of a defect affecting tubular mechanisms for acid excretion, with intact glomerular filtration, rather than being caused by underexcretion of acid caused by kidney failure or an increase in acid production, as might occur in diabetic ketoacidosis, lactic acidosis, or total parenteral nutrition. RTA is an impaired capacity of the kidney to excrete the usual daily load of acid arising from metabolism. Renal excretory function, as estimated by creatinine clearance, is relatively intact.

The diagnosis of RTA should be considered in any infant or young child with failure to thrive, recurrent vomiting, short stature, rickets, nephrocalcinosis, hypotonia, muscle weakness, sensorineural hearing loss, recurrent episodes of dehydration, kidney stones, gastroenteritis with incomplete recovery from metabolic acidosis, or a family member already known to have RTA. The serum potassium may be normal, low, or high. RTA associated with episodic hypokalemia may be accompanied by profound muscle weakness and, in some instances, recurrent paralysis. In the absence of a blood gas analysis confirming acidemia, a venous blood carbon dioxide (CO_2) content less than 20 mEq/L in an infant or young child, accompanied by hyperchloremia and a normal anion gap, should raise the possibility of RTA, especially if the urine pH is not less than 5.5.

RTA, in association with hyponatremia and hyperkalemia, can also present as an acute life-threatening event in some infants with a profound salt-losing condition and hypovolemia, such as pseudohypoaldosteronism (PHA) type 1 or congenital adrenal hyperplasia with insufficient mineralocorticoid production.

RTA rarely presents as isolated idiopathic hypercalciuria or by passage of a kidney stone in a child with incomplete RTA, which may be accompanied by a family history of nephrolithiasis in association with hypocitraturia. For some children in an at-risk family, hypocitraturia may be the only indication of so-called incomplete RTA.[1]

The family history should be explored with questions regarding other affected family members in preceding generations or affected siblings of an individual with suspected RTA. In the instance of an apparent de novo occurrence of RTA, consanguinity may play a role. The occurrence of apparent isolated nephrolithiasis in other family members may be significant. A history of a sudden unexplained demise in a neonate suggests the possibility of a salt-losing condition that may be associated with RTA.

Heredofamilial RTA syndromes (Table 316-1) in children are due to mutations of genes encoding ion transporters or channels that play a key role in the kidney's contribution to acid-base balance.[2,3] These rare conditions are primary monogenic disorders and have classical Mendelian patterns of inheritance. However, the clinician is more likely to encounter secondary forms of RTA that result from drugs, toxins, or acquired medullary tubulointerstitial disease. Other instances of RTA are associated with another heredofamilial disorder, such as cystinosis, or from other causes of the Fanconi syndrome. Moreover, a transient form of RTA may occur in young infants with delayed maturity of renal tubular function. RTA in adults may be associated with autoimmune disease and other conditions not generally encountered in children. These disorders will not be considered further in this chapter.

Failure to thrive during infancy is often the presenting feature of RTA. Growth is a complex process, and the molecular mechanisms of impaired growth in children with RTA are not completely understood, but research in animal models suggests several possible explanations.[4] Metabolic acidosis suppresses the pulse amplitude of growth hormone secretion in rats. The principle mediator on target organs of growth hormone is insulinlike growth factor 1 (IGF-1), which is also suppressed by acidosis. The consequent antianabolic effect results in decreased net protein synthesis. The expression of an IGF-1 receptor in the epiphyseal growth plate of long bones and of hepatic growth hormone receptor is also suppressed by acidosis. Metabolic acidosis impairs the conversion of 25-hydroxy vitamin D_3 to the biologically active form, 1,25-dihydroxy vitamin D_3. Studies in humans have shown

Table 316-1 Heredofamilial Renal Tubular Acidosis Syndromes

RTA DISORDER	OMIM	MODE OF INHERITANCE	LOCUS	ALLELE	GENE PRODUCT
Primary reclamation defect, ocular abnormalities	604278	AR	4q21	*SLC4A4*	NBC1
Primary regeneration defect	179800, 109270	AD	17q21-22	*SLC4A1*	AE1
Primary regeneration defect with deafness	267300	AR	2p13	*ATP6V1B1*	B1 subunit of H^+-ATPase
Primary regeneration defect, later-onset hearing impairment	602722	AR	7q33-34	*ATP6V0A4*	a4 subunit of H^+-ATPase
Hybrid RTA with osteopetrosis	+259730	AR	8q22	*CA2*	Cytosolic CA II CA II, osteoclasts
REGENERATION DEFECTS WITH HYPERKALEMIA					
PHA type 1a (renal)	177735, 600983	AD	4q31.1	*MLR*	Mineralocorticoid receptor
PHA type 1b (systemic)	264350	AR	16p12	*SCNN1B*	Beta subunit of ENaC
				SCNN1G	Gamma subunit of ENaC
			12p13	*SCNN1A*	Alpha subunit of ENaC
PHA type 2 (familial hyperkalemic hypertension)	145260	AD AD	12p13 17q21-q22	*WNK1* *WNK4*	WNK1 kinase WNK4 kinase

AD, Autosomal dominant; *AE1,* Cl^-, HCO_3^- exchanger; *AR,* autosomal recessive; *ATPase,* adenosine triphosphatase; *CA,* carbonic anhydrase; *ENaC,* epithelial sodium channel; *NBC1,* Na^+, $3HCO_3^-$ cotransporter, proximal tubule; *OMIM,* Online Mendelian Inheritance in Man; *PHA,* pseudohypoaldosteronism; *RTA,* renal tubular acidosis.

that the increase in 1,25-dihydroxy vitamin D_3 by dietary phosphorous restriction is reversed by metabolic acidosis. The impaired phosphate reabsorption of the Fanconi syndrome contributes to rickets and short stature. Moreover, the buffering of hydrogen ion (H^+) by bone causes the release of calcium (Ca^{2+}) and consequent hypercalciuria, which may contribute to osteopenia and short stature in certain forms of RTA. Metabolic acidosis inhibits osteoblasts and bone turnover. However, growth impairment is multifactorial, and some children with Fanconi syndrome continue to lag in growth despite correction of metabolic acidosis.[5]

RTA is a consequence of a mismatch between the usual rate of acid production and renal acid excretion. The daily production of endogenous acid mainly arises from dietary protein, primarily sulfur-containing amino acids (methionine, cystine) that are not subsequently resynthesized into protein, ultimately yielding the strong mineral acid, sulfuric acid (H_2SO_4). The accession of protons derived from H_2SO_4 into the extracellular fluid is promptly buffered by bicarbonate (HCO_3^-), which only accounts for approximately one half of the disposition of an acid load. In more chronic forms of metabolic acidosis, buffering of H^+ by bone mineral is accompanied by the release of Ca^{2+}, hydroxyl ion (OH^-), and phosphate (PO_4^{3-}) from the hydroxyapatite crystal surface. During the rapid growth phase of infancy and early childhood, the accretion of calcium, phosphate, and hydroxyl ion into the hydroxyapatite crystal structure of bone also contributes to the endogenous acid load by the release of approximately 1 mEq of H^+ for each milliequivalent of Ca^{2+} retained in bone.[6] Quantitatively, the accretion of approximately 200 mg of Ca^{2+} per day in an infant weighing 10 kg contributes approximately 1 mEq/kg/day of H^+ of the total endogenous acid load of 2 to 3 mEq/kg/day.

The rate of endogenous acid production in infants and children, 2 to 3 mEq/kg/day, must be matched, milliequivalent for milliequivalent, by the excretion of H^+ bound to the two principal urinary buffers, ammonia (NH_3) and monohydrogen phosphate (HPO_4^{2-}). The major adaptive response to an increasing acid load is an increase in ammonium (NH_4^+) production and excretion in contrast to phosphate, which has a relatively fixed rate of excretion. NH_4^+ production is elastic and can expand up to 10-fold in acute metabolic acidosis, such as diabetic ketoacidosis. The essential defect in all forms of RTA is a diminished ability to excrete NH_4^+.

RENAL MECHANISMS FOR EXCRETION OF ACID

RTA is not a single entity but a collection of complex disorders that are better understood after some background discussion of the role of the kidney in maintaining acid-base balance. One principal aspect is the

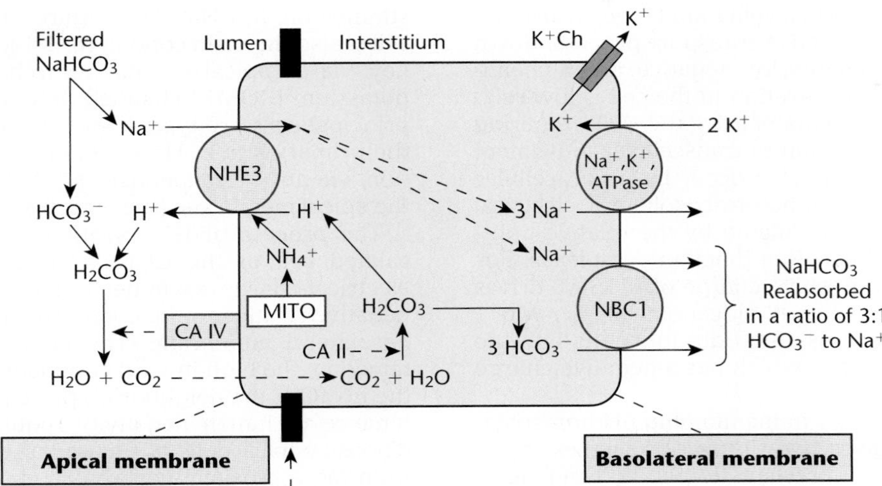

Figure 316-1 Approximately 80% to 90% of filtered HCO_3^- is absorbed in the proximal tubule. The basolateral Na^+,K^+-ATPase maintains transmembrane gradients of Na^+ and K^+ that drive the apical Na^+,H^+-exchanger (NHE3) and the basolateral $Na^+,3HCO_3^-$-cotransporter (NBC1). Not depicted in the figure is an apical proton (H^+-ATPase) pump, which is responsible for a smaller proportion of H^+ secretion and HCO_3^- absorption. NH_4^+ is generated within mitochondria and secreted after binding to the H^+ site of the NHE3 exchanger. The production of NH_4^+ is inhibited by hyperkalemia. Although not depicted, the apical membrane is arranged as a brush border with many infoldings, which provide a large surface area for absorption. *CA II,* Carbonic anhydrase II (cytosolic); *CA IV,* carbonic anhydrase IV (apical membrane); *MITO,* mitochondrion.

segmental topology of the nephron for the absorption and secretion of particular solutes and, in the context of RTA, especially the absorption of sodium bicarbonate and H^+ secretion.

The epithelial cells of the proximal tubule, thick ascending limb of the loop of Henle (TAL), distal tubule, connecting tubule, and the cortical and medullary segments of the collecting duct are specialized for ion translocation against a gradient and ultimately require the expenditure of energy. These epithelia separate two fluid compartments: (1) the lumen of the tubule and (2) the interstitial fluid compartment of the kidney. The epithelial cells are polarized and have a distinct apical membrane facing the lumen and a distinct basolateral membrane interfacing the interstitial fluid compartment (Figure 316-1). The apical and basolateral membranes meet at the tight-junction complexes between adjacent cells. Each membrane has a unique complement of ion-translocating mechanisms, either transporters anchored to the lipid bilayer of the cell membrane or ion-specific channels. A transporter is a complex molecule, largely a protein, with a binding site for the specific ion to be translocated. The rate of translocation is regulated by the cycling of transporters, or channels, between the membrane and specialized structures in the cytosol. Some transporters perform primary active transport against an electrochemical gradient and have a catalytic site for the hydrolysis of adenosine triphosphate (ATP).

The energy released from the high-energy phosphate bond is used to translocate an ion against an electrochemical gradient. These translocation *motors* affect the distribution of electrical charges on either side of the membrane. If a transported ion is accompanied by an ion with an equivalent but opposite charge, then the transport activity is electroneutral. Other ion transport activities are electrogenic, resulting in an asymmetrical transepithelial distribution of charges. One notable example of the latter relevant to this discussion of RTA is sodium (Na^+) absorption via the apical epithelial sodium channel (ENaC) in the aldosterone-sensitive distal nephron, which generates a lumen-negative potential and is a precondition for H^+ secretion in the distal nephron. The failure to generate this lumen-negative electrical gradient is referred to as a voltage defect.

All Na^+-transporting epithelial cells of the nephron have a basolateral sodium-potassium-adenosine triphosphatase (Na^+,K^+-ATPase), which maintains a high intracellular concentration of K^+ and a low intracellular concentration of Na^+. During each transport cycle, for every three Na^+ ions extruded from the cell, two K^+ ions are translocated into the cell. This process results in the electrical polarization of the cell membrane—negative inside relative to the opposite side of the membrane. In the instance of Na^+ and K^+, each of these ions is transported across the basolateral membrane against its concentration gradient by Na^+,K^+-ATPase. The latter is the principal means by which Na^+

ions absorbed at the apical membrane are then extruded across the basolateral membrane, ultimately leaving the kidney via renal vein blood. The absorption of Na^+ is a secondary active transport process, down both an electrical (cell interior, negative) and a chemical gradient (Na^+ concentration in the cell is low relative to the lumen), maintained by the ATP-requiring Na^+,K^+-ATPase. In addition to transcellular movement of ions, absorption may also occur by a paracellular pathway, driven by a lumen-to-basolateral electrical gradient and further modulated by the relative tightness of the intercellular tight junction complexes. For example, the lumen-positive charge of the TAL drives the paracellular movement of cations (NH_4^+, Mg^{2+}, Ca^{2+}, Na^+, and K^+) across the tight junctions into the interstitial compartment, which has a negative charge relative to the lumen.

The role of the kidney in maintaining pH homeostasis principally involves two discrete processes in the handling of HCO_3^-: (1) reclamation and (2) regeneration of HCO_3^-. The first is to absorb filtered HCO_3^- in proximal segments of the nephron, and the second is to excrete H^+ in the form of NH_4^+ and dihydrogen-phosphate ($H_2PO_4^-$) in the collecting duct and, in the process, generate new HCO_3^-. The task of absorbing filtered HCO_3^- is referred to as reclamation and is mediated by H^+ secretion in exchange for absorbed Na^+ (see Figure 316-1). The secreted H^+ is generated by the action of cytosolic carbonic anhydrase type 2 (CA II) on CO_2 and water (H_2O), yielding carbonic acid (H_2CO_3), which dissociates to H^+ and HCO_3^-. The secreted H^+ reacts with luminal HCO_3^-, yielding H_2CO_3, which is rapidly broken down to CO_2 and H_2O by luminal brush border carbonic anhydrase type 4 (CA IV). The luminal CO_2 diffuses back into the cell for another cycle of H_2CO_3 generation. The intracellular HCO_3^- generated by CA II is transported across the basolateral membrane by the $Na^+,3HCO_3^-$ cotransporter (NBC1; see Figure 316-1). The net effect is that the HCO_3^- ion returned to the blood is not actually the same HCO_3^- that was filtered; nevertheless, it is effectively reclaimed. This process of reclamation conserves filtered, preformed HCO_3^-; it does not replace HCO_3^- consumed by endogenous acid.

In the more distal segments of the nephron, mainly the cortical collecting duct (CCD), the bulk of filtered HCO_3^-, approximately 80% to 90%, has already been reabsorbed by the reclamation process in more proximal segments. The remaining filtered HCO_3^- is reabsorbed, mainly in the TAL. The task now is to generate new HCO_3^- to replenish the pool of HCO_3^- and nonbicarbonate buffers that has had its stock depleted at a rate of 2 to 3 mEq/kg/day as buffer is consumed by H^+ arising from metabolism. This process of HCO_3^- regeneration is depicted in Figure 316-2, which shows that for every new HCO_3^- generated, a H^+ is also generated *pari passu* and available for secretion.

The salient segment of the nephron ultimately responsible for H^+ excretion, the CCD, lies between the connecting tubule terminating the distal convoluted tubule and the medullary portion of the collecting duct. The epithelium of the CCD is a mosaic of specialized cells. The most abundant cell type, the principal cell, has mineralocorticoid receptors and is aldosterone responsive. The apical membrane has a variable density, depending on the state of aldosterone stimulation, of ENaC (see Figure 316-2). The principal cell is also the main conduit for K^+ secretion by the kidney, via an apical K^+ channel (renal outer medullary potassium [ROMK] channel). Interspersed among the principal cells are type A intercalated cells, which are the primary site of H^+ secretion for urinary acidification, via an ATP-dependent H^+-ATPase transporter in the apical membrane (see Figure 316-2).

The process of H^+ secretion by the type-A intercalated cell of the CCD is critically dependent on electrical-charge asymmetry such that the lumen is negative relative to the compartment surrounding the basolateral membrane. The negative charge is sustained by the high inward conductivity of Na^+ through the ENaC of the neighboring principal cells. The maintenance of lumen negativity requires that two conditions be fulfilled: (1) adequate Na^+ delivery to the CCD from more proximal nephron segments and (2) a sufficient rate of inward Na^+ movement via the ENaC. The number of ENaCs is dependent on aldosterone, which regulates the cycling of channels in and out of the apical membrane. The lumen-negative charge also favors K^+ efflux from the principal cell into the lumen via the ROMK channel. This is the primary mechanism for aldosterone-dependent K^+ excretion.

H^+ secretion must be distinguished from H^+ excretion and the respective demands of each on energy. The apical Na^+-H^+ exchanger in the proximal tubule is the main mechanism for HCO_3^- reclamation, and indirectly depends on the expenditure of ATP by the basolateral Na^+-K^+-ATPase, which maintains a favorable Na^+ gradient across the apical membrane. This mechanism is effective because H^+ is translocated against a modest gradient in the proximal tubule. At a luminal pH of 6.5, the H^+ gradient is 8:1 (pH 6.5 versus pH 7.4 in the interstitial compartment). Most H^+ secretion is used for HCO_3^- reclamation. A 10-kg infant with a glomerular filtration rate of 45 mL/min filters 1560 mEq of HCO_3^- each day, practically all of which is reclaimed by the secretion of a comparable amount of H^+. This same infant may have a rate of endogenous acid production of 3 mEq/kg/day, or 30 mEq/day. The excretion of 30 mEq of acid is equivalent to the regeneration of 30 mEq of HCO_3^-, which entails the secretion of 30 mEq of H^+ in the collecting duct. The secretion of this relatively small amount requires only 2% of the total H^+ secretory capacity (30 mEq excreted versus 1560 + 30, or 1590 mEq secreted). Thus only a small proportion of the total of H^+ secretion is destined for excretion, mainly as $H_2PO_4^-$ and NH_4^+. H^+ secretion in the collecting duct proceeds against a steep H^+ gradient: 80:1 at a luminal pH of 5.5 and 800:1 at a luminal pH of 4.5 (versus pH 7.4). The translocation of H^+ against a steep gradient in the collecting duct requires active ATP-dependent transport, by the apical proton pumps of the type A intercalated cell, mainly H^+-ATPase and, to a lesser extent, H^+,K^+-ATPase. Hence the acidification mechanism of the collecting duct has been referred to as a low-capacity, steep-gradient system.

These two basic processes of HCO_3^- absorption serve as the basis for a physiological classification of RTA into two main types: (1) a reclamation defect type

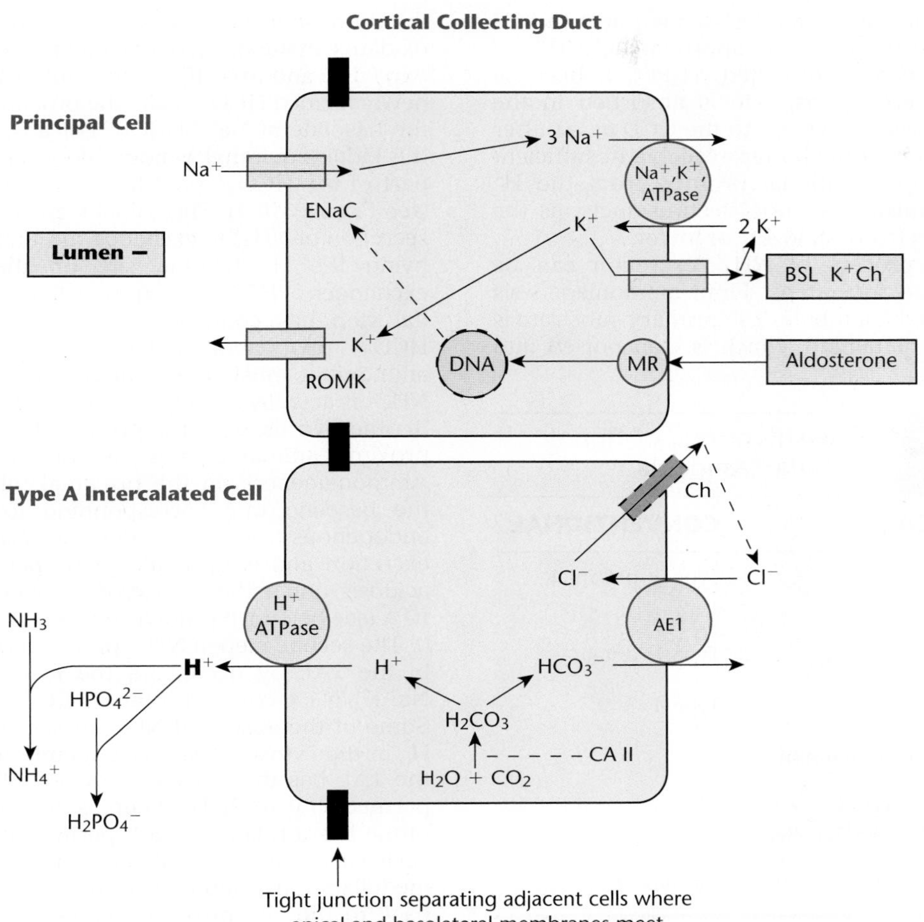

Figure 316-2 The epithelium of the cortical collecting duct is a mosaic of Na^+-absorbing and K^+-secreting principal cells and H^+-secreting type-A intercalated cells. The lumen-negative transepithelial potential difference is maintained by the aldosterone-stimulated apical epithelial Na^+ channel (ENaC) of the principal cell. The lumen negativity facilitates K^+ secretion by the apical K^+-channel (ROMK) of the principal cells and H^+ secretion by the type-A intercalated cells. The absence of a lumen-negative electrical gradient is referred to as a *voltage defect*. The apical H^+-ATPase and the basolateral Cl^-,HCO_3^--exchanger (AE1) of the type-A intercalated cell are affected by loss-of-function mutations causing primary secretory RTA. Aldosterone interacts with the mineralocorticoid receptor (MR), which then translocates to the nucleus and after binding to a promoter region triggers upregulation of ENaC and Na^+-K^+-ATPase. Hyperkalemic RTA arises secondary to aldosterone deficiency or unresponsiveness of the mineralocorticoid receptor. The consequent hyperkalemia inhibits NH_4^+ production by the proximal tubule. *BSL K^+ ch,* Basolateral K^+ channel; *ROMK,* renal outer medullary (apical) K^+ channel; *RTA,* renal tubular acidosis.

and (2) a regeneration defect type (Table 316-2). The reclamation defect type is traditionally referred to as proximal RTA or type 2 RTA. Although the bulk of HCO_3^- absorption, 80% to 90%, occurs in the proximal tubule, reclamation is completed in more distal segments, and the term *proximal* is not physiologically accurate. Most reclamation-type RTA disorders in children are also accompanied by other defects localized to the proximal tubule, including impaired absorption of amino acids, glucose, and phosphate (Fanconi syndrome). However, it may also be an isolated defect and, in some infants, simply a transient immaturity of function that eventually resolves.

RTA arising from an impairment of the distal mechanism for generating new HCO_3^- will be referred to as a regeneration defect type, but it is conventionally classified as distal RTA or type 1 RTA (see Table 316-2). The two subtypes of regeneration defect RTA are (1) a nonhyperkalemic and (2) a hyperkalemic subtype.

AMMONIUM EXCRETION MECHANISM

All forms of RTA are ultimately due to the inability of the kidney to maintain plasma HCO_3^- concentration at its physiologic level in the face of the usual rate of acid production. The common feature of this inability is a low rate of NH_4^+ excretion. The process of NH_4^+ excretion is complex and involves both proximal and distal segments of the nephron.

The primacy of NH_4^+ for the excretion of H^+ is a direct consequence of the limitation of phosphate as a urinary buffer after only a modest reduction in the pH of tubular fluid. At a pH of 5.8, approximately 91% of phosphate is already protonated ($H_2PO_4^-$). Because much of the filtered phosphate is absorbed in the proximal tubule, its availability to the CCD as a buffer is limited. NH_3 is the only buffer available in sufficient quantity to accept additional protons from the H^+ secretory mechanisms in the collecting ducts, as the urine pH declines from 5.8 to 4.8, or lower.

The complex process of NH_4^+ excretion can be broken down into four steps. First, ammoniagenesis occurs in the proximal tubule. The primary substrate is the amino acid, glutamine, which is transported into the mitochondria of cells of the proximal tubule. The oxidative metabolism of one glutamine ultimately yields two NH_4^+ and two HCO_3^- in equimolar quantities. This newly formed HCO_3^- exits the proximal tubular cell via the basolateral Na^+-$3HCO_3^-$ cotransporter and leaves the kidney in renal venous blood and then becomes part of the HCO_3^- pool that is filtered and reclaimed (see Figure 316-1). This initial step is completed by the secretion of NH_4^+ in exchange for luminal Na^+ by occupying the H^+ binding site on the apical Na^+,H^+ exchanger (NHE1; see Figure 316-1). Although this initial step has contributed to the restoration of the HCO_3^- pool, additional steps in the processing of ammonium must unfold before acid, in the form of NH_4^+, is actually excreted and new HCO_3^- is generated. In other words, the NH_4^+ produced in this initial step of proximal ammoniagenesis is not yet out of the body. Ammoniagenesis in the proximal tubule proceeds at the baseline rate corresponding to the portion of endogenous acid production not balanced by $H_2PO_4^-$ excretion and is upregulated by persistent metabolic acidosis, and in the context of the hyperkalemic form of RTA (see below), it is downregulated by hyperkalemia.

The second step in NH_4^+ processing is its absorption in the TAL by occupying the K^+ site on the apical $Na^+,K^+,2Cl^-$ cotransporter (NKCC2; Figure 316-3). Some of the absorbed NH_4^+ dissociates into NH_3 and H^+ in the cytosol. The apical membrane of the cells of the TAL has the unusual property of a relatively low permeability to NH_3, whereas the basolateral membrane has a relatively high permeability. Thus NH_3, at each successive level of the TAL, accumulates in the medullary interstitium. A portion of the NH_3 also cycles back to the late proximal tubule and the descending

Table 316-2 Classifications of Renal Tubular Acidosis

PHYSIOLOGICAL	CONVENTIONAL
Reclamation type	Type 2, proximal
With Fanconi syndrome	
Primary, isolated	
Regeneration type	Type 1, distal
Nonhyperkalemic	
Hyperkalemic	Type 4
Acidification intact	
Pseudohypoaldosteronism, Ia, Ib, II	
Acidification impaired	
Medullary tubulointerstitial disease	
Hybrid	Old type 3

Ion Transport in Thick Ascending Limb of Loop of Henle

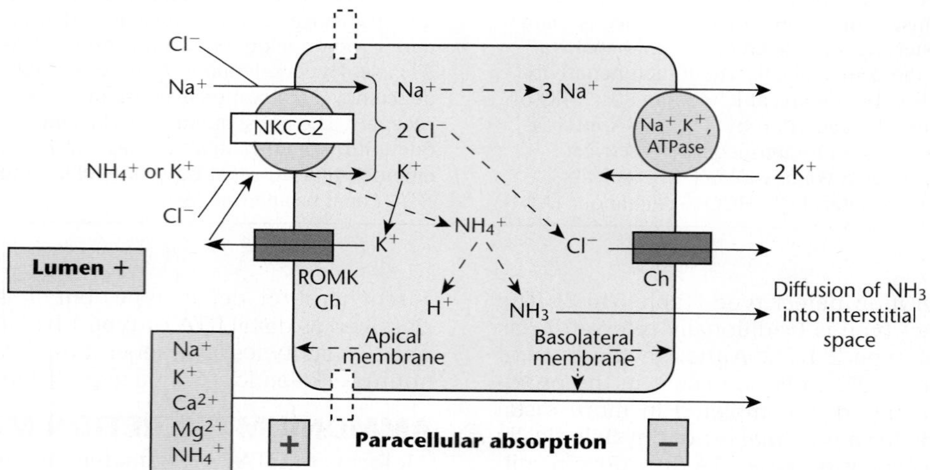

Figure 316-3 The thick ascending limb (TAL) is the site of NH_4^+ reabsorption by the apical Na^+-K^+-$2Cl^-$-cotransporter (NKCC2). The lumen-directed K^+ conductivity of the ROMK channel maintains a lumen-positive electrical gradient. NH_4^+ binds to the K^+ site of the transporter. Once inside the cell, NH_4^+ dissociates and NH_3 diffuses into the interstitium across the highly permeable basolateral membrane. The apical membrane has a low permeability to NH_3, which facilitates the medullary interstitial accumulation of NH_3. *Ch,* Basolateral chloride channel; *ROMK,* renal outer medullary (apical) K^+ channel.

thin limb of the loop of Henle. The cells of the TAL have a high outward potassium conductance via the ROMK channel, which maintains a lumen-positive potential and drives paracellular absorption of NH_4^+, adding to the accumulation in the interstitium (see Figure 316-3).

The interstitial accumulation of NH_3 constitutes the third step in the NH_4^+-excretion mechanism, which depends on an intact countercurrent system for the concentration of solute in the renal medulla. The concentration of NH_3 increases at each successively deeper stratum of the medulla, reaching the highest concentration toward the papilla.

The fourth step in the NH_4^+ excretion mechanism is the diffusion of the NH_3, which has accumulated to a relatively high concentration in the medullary interstitium, into the lumen of the collecting duct (Figure 316-4). This nephron segment has type A intercalated cells, which are solely dedicated to H^+ secretion against its concentration gradient by means of an apical proton pump (H^+-ATPase). The proton donor in these cells is H_2CO_3, which dissociates to H^+ and HCO_3^-. The HCO_3^- is extruded across the basolateral membrane of the type A intercalated cell by the Cl^-,HCO_3^--exchanger (AE1; see Figure 316-2). This fourth step of NH_4^+ excretion concludes with the titration of NH_3 diffusing into the lumen from the interstitium by H^+ secreted by the type A intercalated cell, yielding NH_4^+, which has low lipid solubility and does not readily diffuse back into the medullary interstitium. This is the process referred to as ion trapping, and as NH_3 is converted to NH_4^+ the concentration gradient for further diffusion of NH_3 from the interstitium into the lumen is maintained. The net effect is that for each NH_4^+ excreted a new HCO_3^- is returned to the extracellular pool. Thus the NH_4^+ originally produced by the proximal tubule and that then was reabsorbed in the TAL to maintain the high interstitial concentration of NH_3 is now finally out of the body.

In the context of childhood RTA, each of the four steps of NH_4^+ processing is implicated in the pathogenesis of the different forms of RTA. The initial step, proximal ammoniagenesis, is impaired by hyperkalemia occurring in mineralocorticoid deficiency or unresponsive states. The second step in the TAL, absorption of NH_4^+ by the NKCC2 cotransporter, is also impaired by hyperkalemia because K^+ more effectively competes with NH_4^+ for the same binding site on the transporter (see Figure 316-3). This impaired

The 4 Steps of Ammonium Excretion

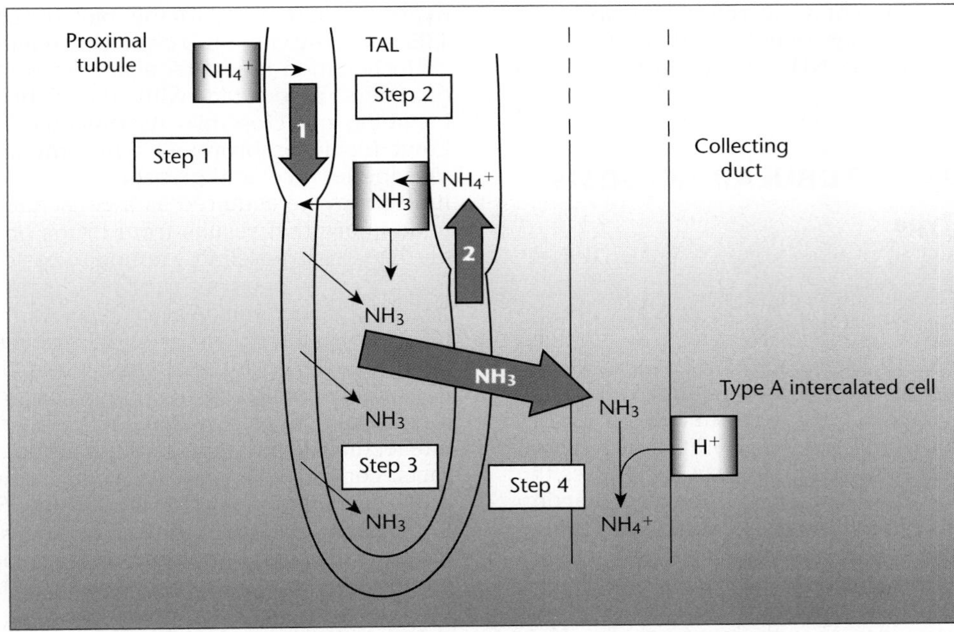

Figure 316-4 Ammonium excretion is a 4-step process. NH_4^+ is generated from glutamine within mitochondria of the proximal tubule cell and exits the cell after binding to the H^+ site of the apical Na^+-H^+-exchanger (NHE3). The broad arrow labeled "1" denotes a packet of NH_4^+ leaving the proximal tubule and entering the loop of Henle. The broad arrow labeled "2" represents a packet of NH_4^+ arriving at the TAL. NH_4^+ is reabsorbed in the TAL after binding to the K^+ site of the apical Na^+-K^+-$2Cl^-$-cotransporter (NKCC) (see Figure 316-3). After dissociation of NH_4^+, a constant input of NH_3 occurs to the medullary interstitium. The gradient between the interstitium and the lumen of the collecting duct favors diffusion of NH_3 out of the interstitium. Protonation of NH_3 in the collecting duct constitutes step 4. As a charged ion, NH_4^+ has a low lipid solubility militating against back diffusion across the cell membrane (ion trapping). As NH_4^+ is removed by excretion, a gradient for continuing diffusion of NH_3 is maintained. The shading denotes the increasing concentration of solute and NH_3 in successively deeper layers of the medulla. *TAL,* Thick ascending limb.

transport of NH_4^+ affects the third step, the accumulation of NH_3 in the medullary interstitium. Another disease process affecting this third step is inflammation and scarring of the inner medulla, distorting the architecture of the countercurrent multiplier system responsible for the increasing concentration of solutes and NH_3. Examples of disorders causing an acquired form of RTA include recurrent pyelonephritis, obstructive uropathy, and sickle cell disease. The countercurrent system is also affected by nephrocalcinosis, which occurs in regeneration-type RTA, which is typically accompanied by a low rate of citrate excretion.

The fourth and final step in NH_4^+ processing before excretion also is impaired in RTA and is the consequence of two different defects affecting the ion-trapping of NH_4^+—either a H^+ secretory defect or a voltage defect. The primary impairment of H^+ secretion is a consequence of a genetic mutation affecting either the apical H^+-ATPase transporter or the basolateral AE1 of the type A intercalated cell (see Table 316-1 and Figure 316-2). This cell type operates in the same nephron segment as the principal cell of the CCD, which, under usual physiological conditions, maintains a lumen-negative charge by means of the high inward Na^+ conductance of the ENaC. The abrogation of this lumen-negative state in mineralocorticoid deficient or unresponsive states (voltage defect) impairs both H^+ secretion by the type A intercalated cell, as well as K^+ secretion via the ROMK channel of the principal cell. This inhibition of K^+ secretion contributes to hyperkalemia and its consequent negative effects on steps one and two of the NH_4^+ excretion mechanism (see Figure 316-4).

TYPES OF RENAL TUBULAR ACIDOSIS

Reclamation Type

Reclamation-type RTA (type 2 or proximal RTA; see Table 316-2) is most commonly associated with the Fanconi syndrome (aminoaciduria, glycosuria, phosphaturia, HCO_3^- wasting, and vitamin D–dependent rickets) of cystinosis. Although the gene defect in cystinosis has been described (OMIM [Online Mendelian Inheritance in Man] 219800, a mutation of *CTNS*, encoding cystinosin, at locus 17p13), it is not known how the lysosomal accumulation of cystine causes the Fanconi syndrome and RTA. It is possible that function of the ATP-requiring basolateral Na^+,K^+-ATPase transporter system is impaired in the proximal tubule.[7] Because this system maintains a low intracellular Na^+ concentration in the face of high transcellular trafficking of Na^+, it provides the driving force for Na^+-coupled absorption of glucose, amino acids, and phosphate. Although the precise mechanism for the multiple transport abnormalities of the Fanconi syndrome has not been elucidated, the presumption is that the basic defect is a deficiency in the generation of ATP.

Urine pH in reclamation-type RTA may be appropriately acidic during acidemia, after the serum HCO_3^- has decreased to approximately 12 to 15 mEq/L. If serum HCO_3^- levels are restored to normal during treatment with alkali (sodium or potassium citrate or sodium bicarbonate), then the impaired reclamation of filtered HCO_3^- in the proximal tubule results in the flooding of the distal nephron with HCO_3^--rich fluid of alkaline pH. If luminal pH is relatively alkaline, then HPO_4^{2-} and NH_3 are not effectively protonated because the titration of HPO_4^{2-} by secreted H^+ and ion trapping of NH_4^+ depend on establishing a steep H^+ gradient between lumen and blood. After HCO_3^- replacement is stopped, the serum HCO_3^- concentration declines to a level that brings the filtered load of HCO_3^- into alignment with the tubular capacity for reclamation. The TAL and distal tubule are no longer overwhelmed by a flood of alkaline fluid. Filtered HCO_3^- is effectively reclaimed, and new HCO_3^- regeneration proceeds unimpeded by the high luminal pH that existed during HCO_3^- wasting. Under these conditions, the urine pH is in the acid range, and net acid excretion, mainly in the form of NH_4^+, matches the rate of endogenous acid production such that underexcretion of H^+ no longer occurs. However, the trade-off is a low plasma HCO_3^- and pH. Replacement of HCO_3^- restores plasma pH to normal, but massive HCO_3^- wasting ensues, requiring doses of alkali exceeding 10 mEq/kg/day.

Reclamation-type RTA is not associated with nephrocalcinosis, in contrast to the nonhyperkalemic subtype of regeneration-type RTA. However, rickets or osteomalacia may occur as a consequence of the phosphate-wasting of the Fanconi syndrome or impaired conversion by the proximal tubule cell of 25-hydroxy vitamin D_3 to the biologically active form, 1,25-dihydroy vitamin D_3, as a consequence of acidosis.

Reclamation-type RTA also occurs in other genetic disorders associated with the Fanconi syndrome, including galactosemia, tyrosinemia, Wilson disease, Lowe (oculocerebrorenal) syndrome, hereditary fructose intolerance, and glycogen storage disease type 1. It also may be acquired as a consequence of nephrotoxic injury that results from drugs or toxins such as outdated tetracycline, aminoglycosides, valproate, 6-mercaptopurine, and ifosfamide or heavy metals, such as lead, mercury, or cadmium. Reclamation-type RTA has also been reported in association with vitamin D deficiency and renal transplantation.

An autosomal-recessive inheritance of RTA without a Fanconi syndrome (OMIM 604278) associated with intellectual disability and ocular abnormalities (cataracts, corneal opacities, glaucoma, band keratopathy) is due to a loss-of-function mutation of *SLC4A4* encoding the basolateral Na^+-3HCO_3^- cotransporter (see Figure 316-1). The gene has been mapped to a locus on chromosome 4q21 (see Table 316-1). This cotransporter is also found in ocular tissues.

Isolated nonsyndromic reclamation-type RTA is rare.[8] An autosomal-dominant form may be due to a mutation of the gene encoding the NHE1 exchanger (encoded by the *SLC9A3* gene), although DNA sequencing of the putative aberrant gene has not yet been reported.

A reclamation-type RTA may also occur sporadically in infants and is believed to be due to either a transient immaturity of the basolateral NBC1 cotransporter or the apical NHE1 exchanger in the proximal tubule. This entity occurs infrequently, apparently because it is self-limited and eventually resolves in most. Affected infants are usually boys, and most no longer required alkali treatment.[9] The serum HCO_3^- concentration (or threshold) at which HCO_3^- begins to appear in urine ranges between 17.5 and 20 mEq/L whereas in healthy infants and young children the lower limit of the HCO_3^- threshold is a serum concentration of 22 mEq/L. In addition to growth retardation, infants with this transient disorder may also experience recurrent vomiting.

Treatment with sodium bicarbonate, sodium citrate, or potassium citrate requires large doses to maintain serum HCO_3^- in the reference range, and at this level, urinary excretion of HCO_3^- approaches 10% to 15% of the filtered load. The dose required to compensate for this high rate of urinary loss, coupled with impaired HCO_3^- regeneration (2-3 mEq/kg/day), may approach 10 to 20 mEq/kg/day.

Nonhyperkalemic Regeneration Type

Regeneration-type RTA refers to an impaired ability to generate new HCO_3^- and is a direct consequence of a low rate of NH_4^+ excretion. The primary defect was historically referred to as a gradient defect and was believed to be a consequence of an inability to maintain a steep transtubular pH gradient as a result of a back leak of H^+. With the advent of genomic medicine, it is now known that the basic defect is a low rate of H^+ secretion. The critical site in the distal nephron is the CCD (with one exception, PHA type 2), in which aldosterone-responsive principal cells coexist with type A intercalated cells. Unlike reclamation-type RTA, the rate of urinary loss of HCO_3^- is much lower, generally less than 5% of the filtered load (Table 316-3).

Two forms of regeneration-type RTA with autosomal-recessive inheritance are associated with mutations of genes encoding different subunits of the apical membrane proton pump of the type A intercalated cell (see Table 316-1). The proton pump, an H^+-ATPase, is a complex multimeric protein assembled from at least 13 subunits.[10] The kidney-specific isoform of H^+-ATPase has two subunits implicated in autosomal-recessive RTA; the B1 and the a4 subunits. RTA with a defect in the B1 subunit is associated with nerve deafness (see Table 316-1, OMIM 267300) and is attributed to a mutation of *ATP6V1B1* on chromosome 2. The B1 subunit is a component of the catalytic site that hydrolyzes ATP. The sensorineural hearing deficit is evident early in life and may at first present as delayed language development. The *ATP6V1B1* gene is also expressed in the cochlea, and presumably the homozygous expression of the mutant alleles accounts for the hearing impairment.[10]

Another form of autosomal-recessive distal RTA with mild or later-onset hearing impairment in some individuals (see Table 316-1, OMIM 602722) is due to a mutation of *ATP6V0A4* on chromosome 7, which encodes the a4 subunit of the apical proton pump. This gene is also expressed in the inner ear. This subunit is important for both assembly of the pump and its ATPase activity.

A rare variant with an autosomal-dominant inheritance is associated with a mutation of *SLC4A1* on chromosome 17, encoding the basolateral AE1 of the type A intercalated cell (see Table 316-1). This exchanger normally couples the extrusion of HCO_3^- across the basolateral membrane in coordination with H^+ secretion by the apical H^+-ATPase proton pump. Another rare variant is not due to a loss-of-function mutation of *SLC4A1*. Rather, nonpolarized targeting of the functional AE1 protein to the apical membrane (where it does not belong) rather than the basolateral membrane occurs because of a mutation that affects a targeting vector of the protein without impairing its transport function.[11]

These primary secretory types of RTA are classically associated with impaired growth progress, polyuria, hypercalciuria, nephrocalcinosis, nephrolithiasis, and hypokalemia. Because of impaired concentrating ability, infants are susceptible to rapid development of severe dehydration in the event of diarrheal illness or protracted vomiting. The tendency to hypovolemia stimulates aldosterone release, accounting for hypokalemia. Medullary nephrocalcinosis is apparent early in infancy and is readily detected on ultrasound examination as hyperechoic medullary regions. The further accumulation of calcium deposits may lead to chronic kidney failure in later years if acidosis is not adequately treated. Nephrocalcinosis may also interfere with the medullary recycling of NH_3 and contribute to impairment of NH_4^+ excretion. Nephrocalcinosis is attributed to hypercalciuria (calcium excretion >4 mg/kg/day), and the latter is a consequence of the release of calcium from bone under the stimulus of metabolic acidosis. Proximal tubular hyperabsorption of citrate in nonhyperkalemic regeneration-type RTA and a consequent diminished rate of citrate excretion predisposes to nephrocalcinosis. Rickets or osteomalacia is not a feature of this form of RTA unless vitamin D deficiency is present, indicated by a low serum 25-hydroxy D_3.

Some infants with primary regeneration-type RTA may also have a transient phase of impaired HCO_3^- reclamation and HCO_3^- wasting, requiring large doses of alkali. This entity was once referred to as type 3 RTA. The reclamation defect subsides during childhood and the phenotype of regeneration-type RTA emerges.

Another variant is associated with a preserved ability to lower urine pH despite a low rate of H^+ secretion, resulting in a diminished accumulation of CO_2 in urine (and a low urinary CO_2 partial pressure [P_{CO_2}]) during bicarbonate administration. The low urine-to-blood P_{CO_2} gradient has been interpreted as a rate-dependent defect because of a diminished rate of secretion of H^+.[12] However, this entity may simply be a milder expression of a primary secretory defect resulting from partial impairment of the apical H^+-ATPase.[7] Nevertheless, H^+ secretion is sufficient to establish a steep transtubular H^+ gradient with a low luminal pH. Consequently, urine pH alone cannot be relied on for the diagnosis of RTA because individuals with a rate-limited defect will not be identified.

In the context of a rate-dependent defect, the ability to acidify urine and establish a steep H^+ gradient does not demand much of the H^+ secretory mechanism. A urine of pH 4.4 has only 0.04 mEq/L of H^+. Therefore to produce 1 L of very acid urine (at a urine pH of 4.4,

Table 316-3 Comparison of Reclamation Defect Type Renal Tubular Acidosis and Regeneration Defect Type Renal Tubular Acidosis

PARAMETER	RECLAMATION DEFECT		REGENERATION DEFECT		
	DURING ACIDEMIA	AFTER TREATMENT OF ACIDEMIA	NON-HYPERKALEMIC	HYPERKALEMIC	
Urine pH	<5.5	>5.5	>5.5	>5.5	<5.5
UAG	Negative	Not reliable	Positive	Positive	Positive
NH_4^+ excretion	Normal	Decreased	Decreased	Decreased	Decreased
Plasma K^+	Normal or decreased	Normal or decreased	Normal or decreased	Increased	Increased
Fractional excretion of HCO_3^- as percentage of filtered load	<5	>10-15	<5	<5	>5-10
(U − B) Pco_2 (mm Hg)	>20	—	<20	>20	>20
Ca^{2+} excretion	Normal	Normal	Increased	Increased	Normal or decreased
Citrate excretion	Normal	Normal	Decreased	Decreased	Normal
Nephrocalcinosis, nephrolithiasis, or both present	Not present	Not present	Common	Common	Not present
Bone disease	Rickets or osteomalacia	Rickets or osteomalacia	Rarely present	Rarely present	—
Alkali dose (mEq/kg/day)	10-20	10-20	5-8 (infancy), 3-4 (children)	5-8 (infancy), 3-4 (children)	Not needed if response to fludrocortisone is adequate

B, Blood; *RTA*, renal tubular acidosis; *U*, urine; *UAG*, urinary anion gap.

the urine-to-blood H^+ gradient is 1000:1), much less than 1 mEq of H^+ is secreted. However, this hypothetical calculation does not reflect the actual capacity to secrete H^+. The task of excreting H^+ at a rate equivalent to the endogenous acid load of 3 mEq/kg/day means that a 10-kg infant must excrete 30 mEq of H^+ per day, or 750 times as much H^+ as was needed to acidify 1 L of urine to pH 4.4. Some infants with a delayed-maturation type of RTA may have a transient rate-limited defect.

An entity referred to as incomplete RTA, or compensated RTA, without overt metabolic acidosis has been described in adults with apparent idiopathic hypercalciuria, nephrocalcinosis, or nephrolithiasis. Urine pH is alkaline, but a sufficiently high rate of NH_4^+ excretion compensates for the reduced capacity to lower urine pH. It has been diagnosed after finding hypocitraturia in an individual with nephrocalcinosis, after passage of a kidney stone, or a family history of nephrolithiasis. The unexpected passage of a calcium oxalate or calcium phosphate kidney stone in a child without a known syndrome should raise consideration of incomplete RTA.

Hypocitraturia is common in patients with a primary H^+ secretory defect and contributes to the susceptibility to nephrolithiasis and nephrocalcinosis. Citrate is the predominant urinary organic anion. It acts as an inhibitor of calcium stone formation by chelating ionized calcium as a soluble complex, thereby lowering the supersaturation index of calcium oxalate. Filtered citrate, which exists as the tricarboxylate anion at physiologic pH, is preferentially absorbed as the dicarboxylate anion by an apical Na^+-dependent transporter in the proximal tubule. Urinary citrate reflects the proportion of filtered citrate that is not absorbed and is influenced by the state of acid-base balance. Absorption is enhanced by acidosis, which accounts for hypocitraturia in nonhyperkalemic regeneration-type RTA. Hyperkalemia appears to suppress the apical dicarboxylate transporter, possibly accounting for the normal-to-high urinary citrate in the hyperkalemic form of RTA. Hypokalemia enhances proximal citrate absorption and must be corrected if hypocitraturia is to be prevented or effectively treated.

Citrate is a key substrate for the ATP-generating citric acid cycle. It is transported into mitochondria, and its further metabolism ultimately yields $2H_2O$ and $2CO_2$ per molecule. The latter is converted to $2HCO_3^-$, and the consequent small increment in plasma HCO_3^- and pH inhibits proximal tubular citrate absorption, increasing urinary citrate excretion. In healthy children between 3 and 15 years of age, the random urine citrate-to-creatinine ratio ranges between 127 and 300 mg/g creatinine or 75 to 177 mcmol/mM of creatinine.[1] The lower limit of the reference range of citrate excretion in healthy boys is 130 mg/g of creatinine and in girls is 300 mg/g of creatinine.

The nonheritable occurrence of regeneration-type RTA is usually in association with medications such as lithium. The only instance of an inability to lower urine pH due to back-diffusion of H^+, a true gradient defect, is attributable to amphotericin B, which breaks down the permeability barrier of the cell membrane lipid bilayer and, in essence, creates pores in the membrane.

Hyperkalemic Regeneration Type

Two subtypes of hyperkalemic regeneration defect RTA are delineated (see Table 316-2). One subtype has an intact ability to acidify urine; the second subtype resembles the classic regeneration-type RTA in its inability to establish a steep H^+ gradient by lowering urine pH to less than 5.5. In each instance, hyperkalemia suppresses both the production of NH_4^+ in the proximal tubule and the transport of NH_4^+ from the lumen of the TAL to the medullary interstitium. The subtype with intact acidification is most closely associated with rare heredofamilial conditions, including PHA type 1. The unresponsiveness of the principal cell to aldosterone causes a voltage defect (diminished lumen negativity). As a consequence, K^+ secretion by the principal cell and H^+ secretion by the type A intercalated cell are impaired. A voltage defect can also occur in the instance of decreased delivery of Na^+ from the distal tubule to the CCD. The net effect is that the medullary accumulation of NH_3, and the ion trapping of NH_4^+ in the lumen of the medullary collecting duct are impaired. The low rate of H^+ excretion as NH_4^+ results in metabolic acidosis, but the proximate cause is the voltage defect, which causes impaired K^+ secretion and hyperkalemia. However, sufficient capacity remains for H^+ secretion in the inner medullary collecting duct to achieve a urine pH less than 5.5. Possibly the voltage defect limiting H^+ secretion by the apical proton pump in the CCD is partially offset by acidosis-induced upregulation of the apical H^+,K^+-ATPase of the type A intercalated cell in the medulla.

Most primary hyperkalemic RTA is due to PHA type 1, which has two main subtypes. The renal or classic subtype has autosomal-dominant inheritance of a mutant *MLR* gene on chromosome 4 encoding the mineralocorticoid receptor (MR) protein (see Table 316-1). Phenotypic expression is highly variable.[13] A severe salt-losing condition in neonates may result in death; adults may have normal electrolytes and have an increased plasma aldosterone as the only manifestation of the disorder. Some children have a relatively mild disorder and are readily managed with salt replacement and alkali. In some instances, treatment is not needed beyond childhood, suggesting that upregulated expression of the nonmutated gene has compensated for the haplo-insufficient state by increasing the production of the MR protein. Some individuals without a history of affected family members may have a de novo mutation. The severe neonatal phenotype with salt wasting, hyponatremia, hyperkalemia, vomiting, dehydration, and metabolic acidosis resembles salt-losing congenital adrenal hyperplasia due to an adrenal 21-hydroxylase deficiency, an autosomal-recessive disorder.

The autosomal-recessive (systemic, or PHA with multiple target organ defects) subtype of PHA type 1 (OMIM 269350) is a consequence of a mutation affecting any one of the three genes encoding separate subunits of the ENaC (see Table 316-1). ENaC is also expressed in the lung, sweat gland, salivary gland, and colon. The concentrations of Na^+ and Cl^- are increased in sweat, and because respiratory symptoms may also be present, this disorder may be confused with cystic fibrosis. The lung ENaC is active in the immediate postnatal period in clearing fluid from the lung, but well-documented instances of neonatal respiratory distress syndrome attributable to the systemic subtype of PHA type 1 have not been observed. After the electrolyte abnormalities have been treated with salt and alkali, recurrent respiratory infections may dominate the clinical course during infancy. This subtype does not have a spontaneous remission. Treatment is life long.

Some low–birth-weight infants with a PHA type 1 phenotype may not actually have a heritable disorder but rather transient unresponsiveness of the MR protein to aldosterone. One entity, referred to as early childhood hyperkalemia, may be a consequence of the delayed appearance of MRs, resulting in impaired lumen negativity.[7] However, it is not associated with the severe sodium wasting and hypovolemia seen in typical neonatal PHA type 1. Plasma renin and aldosterone may be normal or high. This variant appears to be self-limited, but though hyperkalemia persists (serum K^+ consistently >5.5 mEq/L), it can be treated with furosemide to promote urinary K^+ loss or with oral administration of a sodium polystyrene sulfonate resin that binds K^+ (Kayexalate). Infant formula can be depleted of K^+ by adding the resin and then providing the supernatant for oral ingestion.[14]

Another rare form of hyperkalemic regeneration-type RTA is familial hyperkalemic hypertension, or PHA type 2 (OMIM 145260). This autosomal-dominant condition is also referred to as Gordon syndrome or chloride shunt syndrome. Hyperabsorption of Na^+ and Cl^- in the distal tubule by the thiazide-sensitive Na^+,Cl^- cotransporter (NCCT) results in hypervolemia and low-renin hypertension. The consequent decreased delivery of Na^+ to the principal cells of the CCD limits the ability to generate a lumen-negative potential and diminishes the driving force for H^+ and K^+ secretion. The hyperabsorption is not due to a gain-of-function mutation of *SLC12A3*, encoding the NCCT cotransporter. Rather, mutations of genes (*WNK1* and *WNK4*) encoding cytosolic kinases regulating the NCCT have been identified (see Table 316-1). The nonmutated *WNK4* gene product (WNK4 kinase), in particular, downregulates the NCCT but also affects the apical ROMK channel and paracellular absorption of Cl^-.[15] PHA type 2 is the only regeneration-type RTA that does not primarily involve the CCD. Although it typically occurs in adolescents with hypertension, it may also appear in neonates with affected mothers.[16] This syndrome in younger, normotensive children is known as Spitzer-Weinstein syndrome. A low dose of a thiazide diuretic is effective treatment for the hypertension and hypervolemia. The increased delivery of Na^+ to the CCD after beginning treatment with a thiazide enables lumen negativity, promoting H^+ and K^+ secretion and correcting both the metabolic acidosis and hyperkalemia. This diagnosis should be considered in a family with early-onset hypertension and hyperkalemia.

The subtype of hyperkalemic RTA with impaired acidification is often associated with acquired renal parenchymal damage caused by recurrent pyelonephritis, obstructive uropathy, or sickle cell disease, which may interfere with aldosterone binding to its receptor, as well as the medullary recycling of NH_3. Inner medullary acidification may be impaired in these chronic tubulointerstitial nephropathies, and urine pH is generally above 5.5.

Other nonheritable causes of hyperkalemic regeneration-type RTA are due to medications, such as inhibitors of the renin-angiotensin system (angiotensin-converting enzyme [ACE] inhibitors or angiotensin-receptor blockers). In some instances, RTA is the expected consequence of the pharmacologic action of a medication. For example, amiloride, triamterene, and trimethoprim inhibit the ENaC of the principal cell. Spironolactone, an aldosterone-antagonist, binds to the MR, and indirectly causes a voltage defect by downregulation of ENaC.

Calcineurin inhibitors (cyclosporine or tacrolimus) have been implicated in causing mild metabolic acidosis and hyperkalemia after solid organ transplantation. The mechanism appears to be impaired responsiveness of the MR or acquired hypoaldosteronism that results from a hyporeninemic state, which responds to fludrocortisone.

A child with nephrotic syndrome or hepatic cirrhosis and an intensely Na^+ avid state who is not receiving diuretics may not have sufficient delivery of Na^+ to the CCD to maintain lumen negativity, although this is rare. In essence, this is an acquired form of hyperkalemic regeneration-type RTA caused by a voltage defect.

Hybrid

This rare type of RTA was once referred to as type 3 RTA. One well-characterized entity is marble bone disease, which has elements of both HCO_3^- wasting (a reclamation defect) and impaired acidification (a regeneration defect). The cytosolic enzyme, CA II, is present in both the cells of the proximal tubule and the type A intercalated cells of the CCD. CA II is also present in osteoclasts. A bi-allelic loss-of-function mutation of *CA2* at locus 8q22 has been identified in children with failure to thrive, osteopetrosis, cerebral calcifications, and mental impairment (see Table 316-1). Most reports are of children of Arabic origin, and in many instances, a history of consanguinity exists.[17] Osteoclastic resorption of bone is dependent on H^+ secretion at the osteoclast-bone mineral interface. The impairment of osteoclast activity that occurs as result of a deficiency of CA II causes low bone turnover, osteopetrosis, and an increased susceptibility to fractures. The dose of alkali required to correct the metabolic acidosis is comparable to that for reclamation-type RTA.

Medications inhibiting CA II and CA IV, such as acetazolamide, sulfonamides, or topiramate, are rare causes of a hybrid RTA.

Delayed Maturity

Some infants with failure to thrive and acidosis are suspected of having RTA and referred for further evaluation. Because the kidney is not an excretory organ during intrauterine life, glomerular filtration rate and other functions are low in the immediate newborn period. The postnatal maturation of tubular transport functions is load driven, but the capacity to augment function in response to the excretory load may lag in some infants. Some low–birth-weight infants may have a lower renal HCO_3^- threshold, maintaining a steady-state serum HCO_3^- as low as 17 to 19 mEq/L. The presumption is that this reclamation defect is a consequence of a delay in the development of a full complement of either NHE1 or NBC1 transporters in the proximal tubule. In addition to some degree of a reclamation defect, low–birth-weight infants also have an impaired ability to conserve Na^+. This impairment may represent an impaired capacity of the distal nephron to respond to aldosterone, perhaps because of a delay in the emergence of an adequate complement of MRs, analogous to the renal subtype of PHA type 1. As a consequence, activity of the basolateral Na^+,K^+-ATPase is also diminished and the number of Na^+ channels in the apical membrane is decreased, both of which are aldosterone dependent.

Reduced Na^+ absorption by the principal cell impairs the luminal electronegativity required by the type A intercalated cell for proton pump activity. In essence, this transient form of RTA is a consequence of a voltage defect. Moreover, the impaired response to aldosterone may also lead to hyperkalemia and its consequent inhibition of NH_4^+ production in the proximal tubule (early childhood hyperkalemia). The impaired response to aldosterone in infants in the first few months of life may explain the somewhat higher reference range (mean $\pm$ standard deviation) for plasma K^+, 5.2 ± 0.8 mEq/L.[18] A reasonable presumption is that, in addition to an impaired response to aldosterone, delayed maturation of either the H^+-ATPase or the AE1 transporter of the type A intercalated cell may produce a transient regeneration defect in some infants. Thus this type of RTA, a consequence of delayed maturity, is also a hybrid disorder in some infants and has elements of both reclamation and regeneration defects. The risk for RTA is further amplified in low–birth-weight infants with nephrocalcinosis as a consequence of furosemide treatment, resulting in impaired accumulation of NH_3 in the medullary interstitium.

Evaluation

The comprehensive evaluation of suspected RTA entails studies in the setting of a kidney function laboratory, and referral to a nephrologist is appropriate. However, the clinician can perform several simple tests. One pathway of decision making for a systematic evaluation is depicted in an algorithm and includes elements of history and physical examination in addition to biochemical findings (Figure 316-5).

Once it is established that the patient has a renal etiology for hyperchloremic metabolic acidosis, the principal assessment is an estimate of urinary NH_4^+ by measuring Na^+, K^+, and Cl^- concentration in a random urine specimen and calculating the urinary anion gap (UAG):

$$UAG = [Na^+] + [K^+] - [C1^-]$$

On a typical diet, Cl^- is the main anion accompanying urinary NH_4^+ and the concentration of Cl^- exceeds the sum of Na^+ and K^+. Because urinary NH_4^+ is not directly measured the UAG is a negative quantity or close to zero. In the instance of regeneration-type RTA the rate of NH_4^+ excretion is low, and the rate of Cl^- excretion is accordingly also low and its concentration is usually less than the sum, $[Na^+] + [K^+]$. In this instance the UAG is positive. This estimate is less reliable if urine pH is relatively alkaline, exceeding 6.7, at which HCO_3^- becomes a significant component of the unmeasured anions. For example, at a urine pH of 7.0 the concentration of HCO_3^- in urine is approximately 10 mEq/L; at a pH of 7.3, it is approximately 20 mEq/L. The UAG is normal in reclamation-type RTA during the acidemia that ensues after stopping alkali treatment. The UAG estimate in such patients is not reliable during alkali treatment because of massive HCO_3^- wasting.

Another surrogate measure for urinary NH_4^+ is the urine osmolal gap (UOG), estimated from urinary constituents as

$$UOG = [\text{measured urine Osm}] - (2\,[Na_u^+ + K_u^+] + urea_u)$$

The concentration of urea (mM/L) is calculated as $urea_u$ = (urea nitrogen in urine [mg/dL]/2.8). This calculation assumes that glycosuria is not present. A UOG of more than 100 mOsm/kg suggests that urinary NH_4^+ excretion is not impaired. The actual NH_4^+ is approximately one half of the UOG because the concentrations of NH_4^+ and Cl^- are approximately equal.

Although an estimate of urinary NH_4^+ is the principal assessment, a pH meter should be used to determine urine pH. A provocative test of the capacity to acidify urine entails the administration of furosemide and then later measurement of urine pH. Fludrocortisone (Florinef) should be administered approximately an hour before the infusion of furosemide. The inhibition of Na^+ reabsorption by the action of furosemide on the NKCC2 transporter of the TAL delivers more Na^+ to the CCD (see Figure 316-3). Furosemide also stimulates renin and aldosterone release, which upregulates the ENaC of the principal cell, enhancing the lumen-negative charge, if mineralocorticoid responsiveness is intact. This transepithelial voltage difference favors H^+ secretion and a lower urine pH. The failure to acidify the urine to a pH less than 5.5 suggests a defect of H^+ secretion.

The assessment of the rate of H^+ secretion in the collecting duct by measuring the urine-to-blood P_{CO_2}gradient has traditionally entailed intravenous administration of $NaHCO_3$ load in a clinical research center. However, in an ambulatory setting, a similar effect can be accomplished by aggressive treatment of regeneration-type RTA with a bicarbonate precursor (eg, oral sodium or potassium citrate). As the serum HCO_3^- approaches 28 to 30 mEq/L, the urine pH should be above 7.6, at which the urine HCO_3^- concentration will be 50 mEq/L or more, simulating HCO_3^- loading. In the setting of this large load of HCO_3^-, if the rate of H^+ secretion by the type A intercalated cell is not impaired, then the limited dissociation of H_2CO_3 in the medullary collecting duct and during passage in the urinary tract results in a urine P_{CO_2} at least 20 mm Hg greater than that of blood. If the urine-to-blood P_{CO_2} gradient is less than

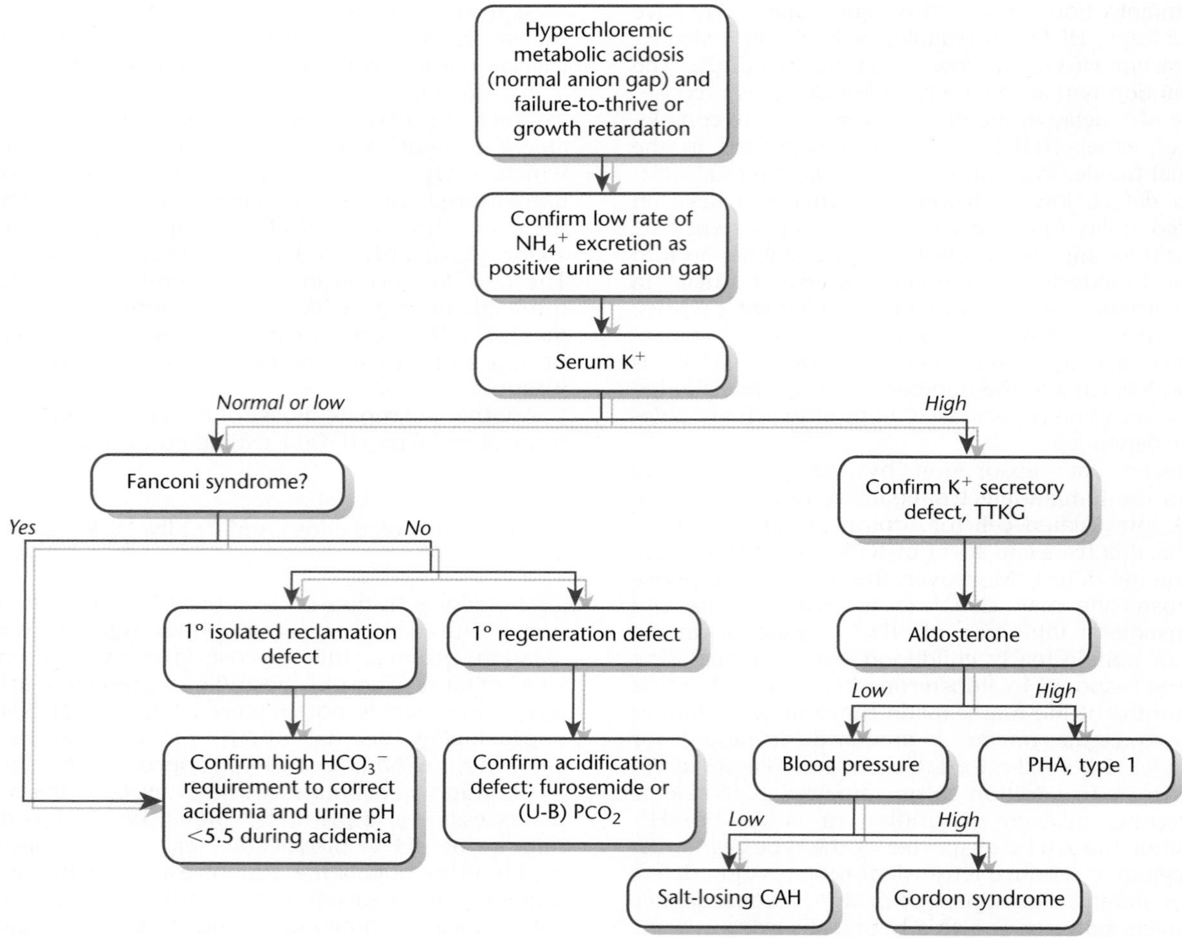

Figure 316-5 This decision tree presumes that nonrenal causes of hyperchloremic metabolic acidosis, such as viral gastroenteritis, have been ruled out. The usual presentation of RTA is either failure-to-thrive during infancy or growth retardation in early childhood. CAH, congenital adrenal hyperplasia; RTA, Renal tubular acidosis; *PHA*, Pseudohypoaldosteronism; *TTKG*, Transtubular potassium gradient; *U-B*, Urine minus blood.

20 mm Hg, then an H^+ secretory defect is likely. The voided urine specimen should be promptly aspirated into a syringe, eliminating dead space, so as to minimize the loss of CO_2. Loading the distal H^+ secretory sites with HCO_3^- can also be accomplished by administering a single dose of acetazoleamide.[4]

An estimate of the renal HCO_3^- threshold in a child suspected of having a reclamation defect may be accomplished over several days after beginning treatment with alkali. Urine pH and blood HCO_3^- are monitored. The threshold is identified as the level of blood HCO_3^-, at which a marked increase in urine pH occurs, indicating bicarbonaturia, approaching 10% to 15% of the filtered load.

If the serum K^+ is low or normal, then the diagnostic possibilities include either a reclamation defect or a nonhyperkalemic-regeneration defect RTA (see Figure 316-5). If urine glucose is positive, then further testing is performed to establish the presence of a Fanconi syndrome in association with the reclamation defect. Empiric treatment with a citrate solution may confirm the diagnosis of a reclamation defect if the dose required for correcting the serum HCO_3^- approaches 10 to 15 mEq/kg/day, well above the endogenous rate of acid production. However, an increased dose requirement may also occur in some infants with regeneration-type RTA as a transient phenomenon during the first few years of life.

The presence of medullary nephrocalcinosis on ultrasound examination confirms nonhyperkalemic regeneration-type of RTA because this type is also associated with hypercalciuria and hypocitraturia. In young infants, obtaining a reliable 24-hour urine collection for the estimation of calcium excretion is not possible without an indwelling catheter. One recourse is to collect multiple random specimens throughout the day. The norms for calcium-to-creatinine ratio of a random urine specimen vary with age (Table 316-4).

If the serum K^+ is high, suggesting the diagnosis of hyperkalemic regeneration-type RTA, then the impaired capacity to secrete K^+ may be confirmed by the measurement of K^+ and osmolality in plasma, a

Table 316-4 95th Percentiles for Urinary Calcium/Creatinine Ratios by Age

AGE RANGE (YR)	mol/mol	mg/mg
1/12-1	2.2	0.81
1-2	1.5	0.56
2-3	1.4	0.50
3-5	1.1	0.41
5-7	0.8	0.30
7-10	0.7	0.25

From Matos V, van Melle G, Boulat O, et al. Urinary phosphate/creatinine, calcium/creatinine, and magnesium/creatinine ratios in a healthy pediatric population. *J Pediatr.* 1997;131:252-257. Copyright © 1997, Elsevier, with permission.

random urine specimen, and calculation of the transtubular potassium gradient (TTKG).

$$\frac{[K^+]_u/[K^+]_p}{[Osm]_u/[Osm]_p}$$

The TTKG is a snapshot of the extent to which secretion of K^+ in the CCD has established an aldosterone-driven K^+ gradient between lumen and plasma, before the tubular fluid is further concentrated in the medulla. The actual transtubular gradient in the collecting duct, $[K^+]_u/[K^+]_p$, is obscured when urine is further concentrated, and this is accounted for by the ratio, $[Osm]_u/[Osm]_p$, in the denominator. This assessment is not reliable if urine is dilute and $[Osm]_u/[Osm]_p$ is less than 1. In the setting of hyperkalemia, the TTKG should be at least 8 if the distal tubule is responsive to mineralocorticoid. A value less than 8 suggests either insufficient production of aldosterone or a lack of responsiveness of the MR to aldosterone.

The diagnosis of PHA type 1 is suggested by an increased level of plasma aldosterone and renin (see Figure 316-5). If aldosterone and renin are suppressed and blood pressure is increased, the rare familial hyperkalemic hypertension syndrome (type 2 PHA) is a possibility. If blood pressure is normal or low and aldosterone is low in a clinical setting of salt-wasting, consideration should include congenital adrenal hyperplasia or if aldosterone is high, then the severe, potentially lethal neonatal presentation of PHA type 1 should be considered.

TREATMENT

The aims of treatment are to correct metabolic acidosis, growth impairment, mitigate osteopenia, and in the instance of a primary H^+ secretory defect, prevent chronic kidney failure caused by progression of nephrocalcinosis. Appropriate treatment with alkali restores growth to its expected trajectory, but the requirement to sustain growth was 2- to 5-fold greater than the expected rate of endogenous acid production.[19]

The mainstay of treatment in most children is a citrate solution. Because hypokalemia and K^+ depletion are characteristic of nonhyperkalemic regeneration-type RTA, a potassium citrate preparation is optimal (eg, Polycitra-K). The solution contains 2 mEq/mL of K^+ and 2 mEq/mL of HCO_3^- precursor as citrate. It also contains citric acid to make it taste better. The solution has a pH of approximately 5 before further dilution. The solution is hyperosmolar and must first be diluted 4- or 5-fold with water or formula before oral administration. Citrate is a substrate in the citric acid cycle, and its further oxidative metabolism ultimately yields HCO_3^- in a molar ratio of two HCO_3^- for each citrate transported into a mitochondrion. Potassium citrate is also available as a capsule, Urocit-K, in two dose forms, providing either 5 mEq or 10 mEq of K^+. Because it is slowly released from a wax matrix, the capsule must be swallowed whole and not opened or crushed.

Serum potassium should be monitored, especially if glomerular filtration rate is reduced or if the patient is receiving an ACE inhibitor or an angiotensin-receptor blocker.

Polycitra (not Polycitra-K) provides 1 mEq of K^+/mL and 1 mEq of Na^+/mL and also requires dilution before administration. However, K^+ containing solutions must be avoided in hyperkalemic forms of RTA.

Sodium-containing solutions, such as Bicitra, may be used for buffer repletion in the hyperkalemic subtype of regeneration defect RTA. Bicitra provides 1 mEq of Na^+/mL and thus has a lower osmolality than Polycitra K or Polycitra, but it still requires dilution to a lower strength for safety and palatability.

The total daily dose requirement should be divided into three or four doses so as to minimize the amplitude of fluctuations of the serum HCO_3^- level that may occur with less frequent administration. In view of data suggesting that metabolic acidosis inhibits growth hormone secretion, administration of a somewhat larger dose of a citrate solution at bedtime to coincide with the nocturnal peak of growth hormone release has been advocated.[4]

$NaHCO_3$ may also be used, but the rapid buildup of CO_2 in the stomach after ingesting it may cause gastric distention. However, this approach may be a preferable means of buffer repletion in infants who refuse citrate solutions. A quarter teaspoon of baking soda powder ($NaHCO_3$) provides 13 mEq each of Na^+ and HCO_3^- and should be diluted in water or infant formula. Tablets of $NaHCO_3$ are also available, which may be crushed.

Adequate treatment of nonhyperkalemic RTA with citrate should lessen hypercalciuria. However, nephrocalcinosis, once established, is not reversible. The aim of treatment is to prevent its further progression to end-stage kidney disease. In view of the risk of hypokalemia, severe K^+ depletion, muscle weakness, and even paralysis, treating hypercalciuria with a thiazide should only be done with frequent monitoring of serum K^+ and provision of an adequate dose of potassium citrate. However, adequate treatment with potassium citrate should correct the metabolic acidosis, lower urinary calcium excretion, and obviate the need for a thiazide. Correction of acidosis does not ameliorate the hearing impairment of the autosomal-recessive forms of proton pump defects of the type A intercalated cells (see Table 316-1).

Growth and serum electrolytes should be monitored periodically. The serum HCO_3^- should be maintained near the upper limit of the range between 25 and 29 mEq/L. Blood should be drawn just before the next dose of alkali.

ROLE OF THE PRIMARY CARE PHYSICIAN

The RTAs are complex disorders. A correct diagnosis must be made early in life and appropriate treatment initiated. The role of the primary care physician is to be aware of the possibility of RTA and to take some initial steps in the patient's work-up, such as calculation of the UAG or UOG. More detailed studies and explanations of this complex disorder to parents are best accomplished by a pediatric kidney disease specialist. Moreover, genetic counseling is needed for parents with a child affected with a monogenic RTA disorder, in anticipation of possible future pregnancies. Because commercially available gene testing is not yet available, the consultant-nephrologist may have access to a research laboratory capable of sequencing DNA. Once a child is established on an effective treatment regimen and is clinically stable, periodic follow-up by the primary care physician may be done in collaboration with a nephrologist.

Most children with RTA, and especially those with nephrocalcinosis, have an impairment of the urinary concentrating mechanism and a consequent obligatory polyuria. A superimposed dehydrating illness such as diarrhea or protracted vomiting can culminate in profound hypovolemia. This susceptibility warrants prompt hospitalization and fluid administration before signs of severe dehydration emerge. The susceptibility to hypokalemia in children with regeneration-type RTA calls for regular monitoring of the serum K^+ and, if it is found to be low, an increase in the dose of the potassium-containing citrate solution should be prescribed. If profound hypokalemia exists with a serum K^+ less than 2.5 mEq/L accompanied by muscle weakness, then prompt hospitalization is needed. A newborn with a salt-losing tendency, such as is common in the lethal form of type 1 PHA, should be monitored closely, and if the disorder was not recognized before discharge from the nursery, then the emergence of vomiting, feeding difficulty, listlessness, hypotonia, hyperventilation, pallor, and signs of dehydration call for urgent readmission and vigorous volume repletion. In the absence of virilization, the presence of congenital adrenal hyperplasia in a male infant may not be recognized at birth, and an infant may be discharged from the nursery only to develop profound salt wasting and hypovolemic shock 1 to 2 weeks later. Newborn screening in many states now includes congenital adrenal hyperplasia.[20]

If compliance with the medication regimen or an intercurrent illness interferes with taking medication, then hospitalization may be needed for parenteral administration of HCO_3^- for the treatment of severe metabolic acidosis.

A child with nonhyperkalemic regeneration-type RTA may experience severe pain during passage of a kidney stone and require hospitalization. If the stone is impacted in a ureter, then monitoring for the development of obstructive hydronephrosis will be needed along with urological consultation.

WHEN TO REFER

- Renal tubular acidosis is suspected

WHEN TO ADMIT

- Hypovolemia (often caused by diarrhea or vomiting illness)
- Hypokalemia with a serum K^+ less than 2.5 mEq/L accompanied by muscle weakness
- If adherence with the medication regimen or an intercurrent illness interferes with taking medication, then hospitalization may be needed for parenteral administration of HCO_3^- for the treatment of severe metabolic acidosis
- Kidney stone

REFERENCES

1. Norman ME, Feldman NI, Cohn RM, et al. Urinary citrate excretion in the diagnosis of distal renal tubular acidosis. *J Pediatr.* 1978;92(3):394-400.
2. Rodriguez-Soriano J. New insights into the pathogenesis of renal tubular acidosis—from functional to molecular studies. *Pediatr Nephrol.* 2000;14(12):1121-1136.
3. Batlle D, Ghanekar H, Jain S, et al. Hereditary distal renal tubular acidosis: new understandings. *Annu Rev Med.* 2001;52:471-484.
4. Chan JC, Scheinman JI, Roth KI. Consultation with the specialist: renal tubular acidosis. *Pediatr Rev.* 2001;22(8): 277-287.
5. Hsu SY, Tsai IJ, Tsau YK. Comparison of growth in primary Fanconi syndrome and proximal renal tubular acidosis. *Pediatr Nephrol.* 2005;20(4):460-464.
6. Carlisle EJF, Donnelly SM, Halperin ML. Renal tubular acidosis (RTA): *R*ecognize *T*he *A*mmonium defect and pH or get the urine pH. *Pediatr Nephrol.* 1991;5(2): 242-248.
7. Rodriguez-Soriano J. Renal tubular acidosis: the clinical entity. *J Am Soc Nephrol.* 2002;13(8):2160-2170.
8. Igarashi T, Sekine T, Inatomi J, et al. Unraveling the molecular pathogenesis of isolated proximal renal tubular acidosis. *J Am Soc Nephrol.* 2002;13(8):2171-2177.
9. Nash MA, Torrado AD, Greifer I, et al. Renal tubular acidosis in infants and children. Clinical course, response to treatment, and prognosis. *J Pediatr.* 1972;80(5): 738-748.
10. Karet FE. Inherited distal renal tubular acidosis. *J Am Soc Nephrol.* 2002;13(8):2178-2184.
11. Rungroj N, Devonald MAJ, Cuthbert A, et al. A novel missense mutation in AE1 causing autosomal dominant distal renal tubular acidosis retains normal transport function but is mistargeted in polarized epithelial cells. *J Biol Chem.* 2004;279:13833-13838.
12. Strife CF, Clardy CW, Varade WS, et al. Urine-to-blood carbon dioxide tension gradient and maximal depression of urine pH to distinguish rate-dependent from classic distal renal tubular acidosis in children. *J Pediatr.* 1993; 122:60-65.
13. Geller DS, Zhang J, Zennaro M-C, et al. Autosomal dominant pseudohypoaldosteronism type 1: mechanisms, evidence for neonatal lethality, and phenotypic expression in adults. *J Am Soc Nephrol.* 2006;17:1429-1436.

14. Bunchman TE, Wood EG, Schenck MH, et al. Pretreatment of formula with sodium polystyrene sulfonate to reduce dietary potassium intake. *Pediatr Nephol.* 1991; 5:29-32.
15. Bonny O, Rossier BC. Disturbances of Na/K balance: pseudohypoaldosteronism revisited. *J Am Soc Nephrol.* 2002;13:2399-2414.
16. Gereda JE, Bonilla-Felix M, Kalil B, et al. Neonatal presentation of Gordon syndrome. *J Pediatr.* 1996;129: 615-617.
17. Sly WS, Whyte MP, Sundaram V, et al. Carbonic anhydrase II deficiency in 12 families with the autosomal recessive syndrome of osteopetrosis with renal tubular acidosis and cerebral calcification. *N Engl J Med.* 1985; 313:139-145.
18. Satlin LM. Maturation of renal potassium transport. *Pediatr Nephrol.* 1991;5:260-269.
19. McSherry E, Morris RC Jr. Attainment and maintenance of normal stature with alkali therapy in infants and children with classic renal tubular acidosis. *J Clin Invest.* 1978;61:509-527.
20. Shulman DI, Palmer MR, Kemp SF. Adrenal insufficiency: still a cause of morbidity and death in childhood. *Pediatrics.* 2007;119:e485-e494.

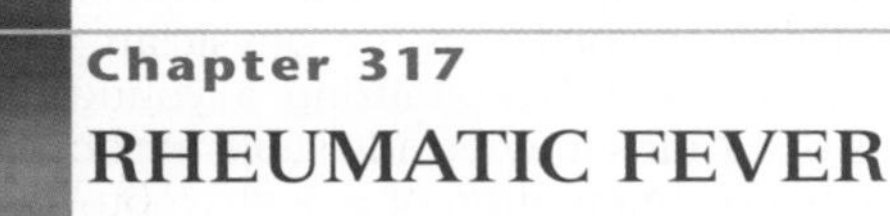

Chapter 317

RHEUMATIC FEVER

Welton M. Gersony, MD; Thomas J. Starc, MD, MPH

INTRODUCTION

Acute rheumatic fever is a systemic connective tissue disorder that is characterized by polyarthritis, carditis, and chorea, either singly or in combination. The major long-term consequence is the potential for inflammatory cardiac valvar involvement, leading to chronic heart disease. The other manifestations are self-limiting with no late sequelae. Arthritis clears without joint dysfunction or deformity, and chorea leaves no neuromuscular impediment. Therefore preventing recurrent attacks that carry the risk of recrudescent heart involvement and further cardiac damage is the most important concern.[1]

EPIDEMIOLOGIC FEATURES

Incidence

An immunologic reaction to group A beta-hemolytic streptococci infection is the established cause of rheumatic fever, and hence the incidence of the first attack of rheumatic fever can be reduced by adequate penicillin treatment of all cases of streptococcal pharyngitis. The incidence of rheumatic fever observed in epidemics of streptococcal pharyngitis is approximately 2% to 3%, whereas the attack rate after sporadic streptococcal upper respiratory tract infection is only approximately 0.2% to 0.3%.[2] In patients who have already had one or more attacks of rheumatic fever, however, the recurrence rate of carditis increases to approximately 15% after subsequent streptococcal infection.[2]

Age

Rheumatic fever is predominantly a disease of school-aged children, with most first occurrences between 5 and 15 years of age. It is uncommon in patients younger than 5 years and extremely rare in patients younger than 3 years. When occurring in infancy, acute rheumatic fever is usually associated with severe carditis and congestive heart failure. Polyarthritis caused by rheumatic fever is unusual in the preschool-aged group; rheumatoid arthritis and other inflammatory diseases of the joint are more likely diagnoses. Chorea also is uncommon in early childhood; most of the cases occur in patients older than 8 years.

Host Susceptibility

Rheumatic fever has often been called a *social status disease,* and most studies have noted its strong association with poverty. The major social risk factors that predispose patients to rheumatic fever appear to be crowding and lack of medical attention. Crowding increases the likelihood of transmission of the group A beta-hemolytic *Streptococcus* from person to person, and lack of medical care precludes timely treatment of streptococcal pharyngitis and leads to late attention to signs and symptoms of acute rheumatic fever.[3]

The tendency for rheumatic fever to occur in more than one family member has long been recognized. The observation is noted even when family members are not concurrently living in the same household, indicating that environmental influences are probably not solely responsible for the disease. No genetic factors have been clearly established.[4]

Sex predisposition does not exist in the incidence of arthritis or carditis in childhood, although chorea has been noted to be more common in girls. However, sex differences exist in the type of valvular lesions that develop with carditis, with boys having a higher incidence than girls of aortic regurgitation. In young adults, mitral stenosis is more common in women than in men.

Numerous community primary prevention programs have demonstrated the efficacy of identifying streptococcal infection by performing throat cultures on susceptible children and treating them early.[5] Furthermore, the widespread application of secondary prevention in the form of antistreptococcal prophylaxis programs for patients after their first attack has significantly reduced the recurrence rate and the additive effects of repeated bouts of carditis.[2]

The incidence of acute rheumatic fever has declined in the last 5 decades in the United States and Europe. However, in underdeveloped countries, rheumatic fever remains a common illness in childhood. Continued immigration from the Caribbean Islands, South America, and Southeast Asia is also a factor in the prevalence of the disease in the United States. An apparent resurgence of acute rheumatic fever in certain areas of the United States, both urban and suburban, was reported between 1984 and 1988[6-8] and again in 1997 and 1998,[9] but no evidence indicates that this trend has continued. Although the disease persists, the annual incidence may be so low, even at large teaching medical centers, that during 3 years of pediatric training a resident physician may not see many children who have acute rheumatic fever.

DIAGNOSIS

Jones Criteria

No pathognomonic clinical findings and specific laboratory tests are available to confirm the diagnosis of rheumatic fever, and hence the diagnosis must be somewhat arbitrary and empirical. A list of major and minor criteria for the evaluation and diagnosis of rheumatic fever and rheumatic heart disease was published more than 50 years ago by Dr T. Duckett Jones.[10] These guidelines have been accepted as diagnostic criteria throughout the world and have been modified (1955) and revised (1984) by specifically appointed committees of the American Heart Association. The most recent review of the Jones criteria was designated a 1992 update[11] and was reviewed in 2002.[12] These guidelines are given in Box 317-1. The five major manifestations in order of decreasing frequency are (1) polyarthritis, (2) carditis, (3) chorea, (4) erythema marginatum, and (5) subcutaneous nodules. The two major manifestations involving the skin, especially the nodules that were most often seen only after multiple attacks of rheumatic fever, have been extremely uncommon during the late 1900s in the United States.[10]

The category of minor manifestations includes two laboratory findings: (1) elevated acute phase reactants (erythrocyte sedimentation rate and C-reactive protein) and (2) electrocardiographic (ECG) evidence of prolongation of the PR interval. The clinical observation of fever, usually a temperature under 102°F (38.8°C), may be present early in the course of polyarthritis or carditis. Arthralgia, another minor manifestation, is nonspecific and may affect any joint without objective signs of inflammation; it should not be considered to be a minor manifestation if arthritis is counted as a major manifestation.

Under the current guidelines, laboratory confirmation of recent streptococcal infection should be part of the diagnostic evaluation. The absence of evidence of streptococcal infection should make the clinician suspicious of the diagnosis of rheumatic fever except in cases in which indolent carditis or chorea are the major manifestations. The tendency to label any low-grade febrile illness with arthralgia for which no obvious cause can be found as rheumatic fever should be avoided.

The Jones criteria should be viewed as a guide to a probable diagnosis of rheumatic fever, but the final diagnosis must remain a clinical judgment. The institution of prophylactic regimens requires prolonged administration of antistreptococcal agents, which places an important responsibility on the physician who diagnoses rheumatic fever. Hospitalizing a youngster who has arthritis or carditis may be advisable for observation, appropriate documentation of a poststreptococcal illness, and initiation of treatment. Hospitalization also emphasizes to the parents the seriousness of the disease and the importance of prophylaxis to prevent recurrence. Because of the specific association of Sydenham chorea with rheumatic fever, hospitalizing a child who has this manifestation should not be mandatory if abnormal neuromuscular activity is mild and unlikely to cause self-inflicted injury.

BOX 317-1 Jones Criteria for the Diagnosis of an Initial Episode of Rheumatic Fever

Evidence of antecedent group A streptococcal infections, two major manifestations, or one major and two minor manifestations indicates a high probability of acute rheumatic fever as the diagnosis.

MAJOR MANIFESTATIONS

Carditis
Polyarthritis
Chorea
Erythema marginatum
Subcutaneous nodules
Minor manifestations

Clinical Findings

Arthralgia
Fever

Laboratory Findings

Elevated acute-phase reactants:
  Erythrocyte sedimentation rate
  C-reactive protein
Prolonged PR interval

SUPPORTING EVIDENCE OF ANTECEDENT GROUP A STREPTOCOCCAL INFECTIONS

Positive throat culture or rapid streptococcal antigen test
Elevated or rising streptococcal antibody titer

From American Heart Association, Council of Cardiovascular Disease in the Young, Special Writing Group of the Committee on Rheumatic Fever, Endocarditis, and Kawasaki Disease. Guidelines for the diagnosis of rheumatic fever. Jones Criteria, 1992. *JAMA*. 1992;268(15):2069-2073, with permission.

Major Clinical Manifestations

The sequence of the manifestations of rheumatic fever is noteworthy: polyarthritis, when it occurs, is usually present before the onset of carditis. Although carditis may be present without preceding joint symptoms, most often the apical systolic murmur of mitral valvulitis occurs within 2 weeks of the onset of arthritis. The diastolic murmur of isolated aortic valvulitis takes longer to appear and may not be heard for 6 to 8 weeks after the joint signs and symptoms appear. Chorea may develop during the convalescent phase of carditis, although a longer latent period usually occurs. Classically, chorea appears as an independent manifestation of rheumatic fever long after the initial streptococcal infection. The majority of cases begin 2 months after streptococcal infection, with episodes still occurring up to 6 months afterward. Although chorea and carditis may coexist, chorea and polyarthritis rarely appear concurrently, presumably because of the difference in the latent periods.

Polyarthritis

Polyarthritis is the most common manifestation of rheumatic fever at the onset and usually involves the large joints of the lower extremities, particularly the ankles or knees. Polyarthritis may result in the complaint of joint pain while walking and is often initially considered to be secondary to trauma. Other large joints (for example, wrists or elbows) become involved in a migratory fashion. An affected joint characteristically is warm and reddened but minimally swollen. Involved joints are exquisitely sensitive to touch, as well as painful on motion. Arthralgias, or aching in the joints without objective signs of inflammation, are suggestive of but not specific for rheumatic fever. Fever is almost always present, but temperatures are usually below 102°F (38.8°C).

Carditis

Inflammation of cardiac tissue is characteristically expressed as valvulitis, but pancarditis involving the myocardium and pericardium may be present in severe cases. The murmurs audible in rheumatic carditis are the result of mitral or aortic valvulitis, or both, with mitral involvement by far the most common. The auscultatory diagnosis of valvulitis often includes the presence of an apical mid-diastolic murmur. Pericarditis typically is silent, but a friction rub and distant heart sounds may occasionally be noted. However, isolated pericarditis without associated auscultatory findings of mitral or aortic involvement is not consistent with the diagnosis of acute rheumatic fever. Although viral inflammation of the heart by coxsackievirus type B or Kawasaki disease may be associated with myocarditis and pericarditis, these entities do not cause valvulitis.

Carditis, clinically diagnosed by the presence of valvulitis with characteristic murmurs, may be arbitrarily designated as mild, moderate, or severe. Such a categorization is useful in the approach to management and to establishing a prognosis for developing rheumatic heart disease. Auscultation of the heart and evaluation of murmurs are influenced by fever and tachycardia; therefore the patient should be reexamined frequently after the diagnosis of acute rheumatic fever and after the temperature has normalized with aspirin therapy. A changing functional murmur in an anxious or febrile child does not indicate the presence of carditis.

MILD CARDITIS. Mild carditis is characteristically defined by the presence of a prominent, high-pitched, apical systolic murmur typical of mitral insufficiency. The heart murmur of mild carditis is usually of grade 2 to 3 (on a scale of 1 to 6) intensity and occupies all or most of systole. A mid-diastolic rumble at the apex is not present. Heart size on chest radiogram is usually normal.

MODERATE CARDITIS. Moderate carditis is defined as (1) both long systolic and prominent mid-diastolic apical murmurs, reflecting greater severity of mitral valvulitis, (2) a basilar diastolic murmur of aortic valvulitis, or (3) a combination of mitral and aortic valvulitis. An aortic diastolic murmur, which is high pitched and decrescendo in character, is usually heard best during end expiration, with the diaphragm of the stethoscope firmly held at the third left intercostal space. A chest radiograph may show mild cardiac enlargement.

SEVERE CARDITIS. Severe carditis is defined by the presence of either pericarditis or congestive heart failure in addition to mitral or aortic valvulitis. The quality of the heart sounds may be poor because of either pericardial effusion or low cardiac output. Murmurs may become more intense as cardiac compensation improves. The chest radiograph shows obvious cardiomegaly and may reveal pulmonary vascular congestion compatible with left-sided heart failure and pulmonary edema; an appearance also may be consistent with what is referred to as rheumatic pneumonia.

IMAGING. Two-dimensional echocardiography is invaluable for the documentation and quantification of pericardial effusion. However, the interpretation of valvular regurgitation by Doppler ultrasound should not constitute the basis of a diagnosis of carditis without auscultatory evidence of significant mitral or aortic involvement. Doppler studies in healthy individuals frequently show a small degree of regurgitation across the mitral valve; trivial aortic valve regurgitation also may be noted occasionally.[13]

Chorea

The clinical picture of Sydenham chorea includes that of poor neuromuscular coordination, sometimes first detected by a change or sloppiness in handwriting. A wide variety of jerky, involuntary movements may occur for 6 to 8 weeks when most cases of chorea are active. Neurologic examination may give evidence of specific deficiencies, particularly in trunk and upper extremity control of movements. A protective environment is recommended while the process is active. Occasionally, mild sedation is indicated, and agents such as clonazepam (Klonopin) or haloperidol (Haldol) may help in the treatment of more severe movement disorders.

When chorea occurs as an isolated manifestation, the patient is usually afebrile, and the sedimentation rate is normal. Because of the long interval after the initiating streptococcal infection, the antistreptolysin O (ASLO) titer is typically normal or only mildly elevated. The murmur of mild mitral insufficiency may be noted.

Erythema Marginatum

Erythema marginatum is a transient pink rash that has irregular, deeper-colored serpiginous borders that may be seen on the smooth, hairless surfaces of the inner aspect of the upper arms and thighs or trunk. This manifestation, although a specific finding for acute rheumatic fever, has been encountered infrequently in recent decades.

Subcutaneous Nodules

Subcutaneous nodules are characteristically pea-sized and are usually located on extensor surfaces of fingers, toes, elbows, and other joints and less often on the occiput. They usually reflect a longstanding or smoldering illness after severe carditis; nodules may persist for weeks or months. Subcutaneous nodules are rarely found in children with rheumatic fever in the present era.

Minor Clinical Manifestations

Among the minor criteria, fever, although almost always present, is nonspecific, as is arthralgia, which is defined as joint discomfort without objective signs of joint inflammation. An elevated acute-phase reactant, such as the erythrocyte sedimentation rate, is an invaluable though nonspecific laboratory sign of inflammation in acute rheumatic fever. Initial values usually range from 60 to 120 mm/hour. However, in chorea the sedimentation rate is normal because of the long interval beyond the antecedent streptococcal infection. Elevated C-reactive protein, although helpful in diagnosing cases with borderline findings, is also elevated in a variety of other diseases.

Prolongation of the PR interval (first-degree heart block) on ECG is considered to be a vagal effect and supports the diagnosis of rheumatic fever. It is most commonly noted when polyarthritis is apparent and is not necessarily associated with carditis. The ECG is almost always otherwise normal regardless of cardiac involvement. Although PR interval prolongation is the common manifestation, occasionally, second- or third-degree heart block occurs, indicating further heightening of vagal tone, perhaps more pronounced in the rheumatic state than in other acute illnesses. First- or second-degree heart block is not a major criterion for carditis, a harbinger of potential rheumatic heart disease, a threat to progress to complete heart block, or a cause of symptoms.

Streptococcal pharyngitis presumptively precedes an attack of rheumatic fever, even though some patients fail to report such a history. Scarlet fever will occasionally be followed by signs of polyarthritis or carditis, but suppurative streptococcal disease, such as skin infection, is not a precursor of rheumatic fever. Throat cultures may be misleading in the evaluation of patients suspected of having rheumatic fever because the streptococcal infection antedates the common manifestations of polyarthritis and carditis by periods varying from 3 to 8 weeks; only 50% or fewer of patients who have rheumatic fever continue to harbor streptococci during the course of their illness.[3]

The most reliable evidence of a preceding streptococcal infection is obtained by demonstration of an antibody response to one or more of the streptococcal antigens. The most common of these, the ASLO titer, reaches maximal levels 3 to 5 weeks after infection and gradually declines to preinfection levels 6 to 12 months later. The ASLO titer is elevated in approximately 85% of patients who have rheumatic fever; titers are never extremely low. Serologic evidence of an antecedent streptococcal infection rises to 95% if other streptococcal antibody tests (eg, antihyaluronidase, antideoxyribonuclease B, antistreptokinase) are performed.

The temporal relationship between the onset of the common manifestations of rheumatic fever and the antecedent streptococcal infection is illustrated in Figure 317-1. As shown, polyarthritis and carditis usually occur 3 to 5 weeks after infection. The streptococcal antibody titer (ASLO) peaks before the onset of the clinical symptoms and then declines gradually. Occasionally, children complain of abdominal pain after a streptococcal infection for which medical or surgical evaluation is sought, and this symptom may occasionally precede signs of joint or cardiac involvement.

MANAGEMENT

Therapeutic management of acute rheumatic fever includes the use of antistreptococcal antibiotics and antiinflammatory agents.

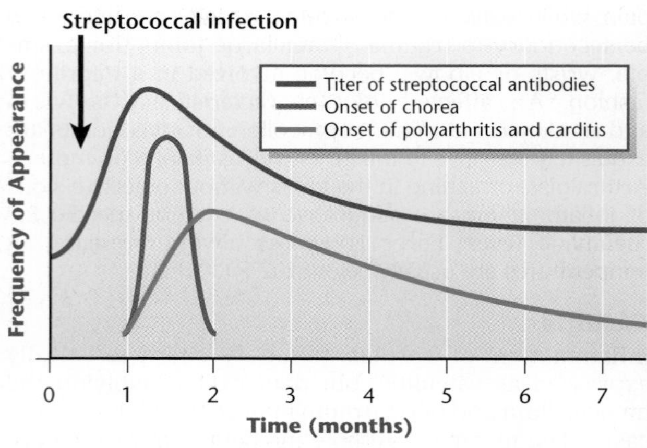

Figure 317-1 The relationship of the onset of rheumatic manifestations in relationship to antecedent streptococcal infection and streptococcal antibody titer (ASLO) is shown. *(Modified from Stollerman GH.* Rheumatic Fever and Streptococcal Infection. *New York, NY: Grune & Stratton; 1975.)*

Antistreptococcal Therapy

Eradication of group A beta-hemolytic streptococcal infection (even in the absence of a positive throat culture) by antibiotic treatment is the foremost principle in management of acute rheumatic fever. Antibiotic treatment must always be immediately followed by institution of a prophylactic program to prevent reinfection (see the discussion under Recurrence of Rheumatic Fever). Penicillin is the drug of choice prescribed initially in dose and duration to maintain therapeutic blood levels for 10 days. Several treatment schedules, which periodically are revised, are outlined by the American Heart Association.[14] The intramuscular administration of the long-acting repository benzathine penicillin G (Bicillin) is the preferred treatment method because it ensures therapeutic levels for a sufficient length of time. A single injection of 1.2 million units for children 5 to 15 years of age is recommended, to be followed by prophylactic injections of 1.2 million units every 3 to 4 weeks. An alternative method is (1) oral penicillin, 200,000 or 250,000 units (penicillin G or V), given 3 or 4 times a day for a full 10 days, followed by the same dose twice daily thereafter; or (2) a combination of oral and intramuscular penicillin (see the discussion under Recurrence of Rheumatic Fever).

For patients sensitive to penicillin, erythromycin may be used for antistreptococcal therapy. The sulfonamide drugs, which are bacteriostatic rather than bactericidal, are not effective for streptococcal eradication. They can be used in rheumatic prophylaxis programs to prevent reinfection; however, they are rarely used in the present era.

Antiinflammatory Therapy

Salicylates are indicated in the presence of acute, painful arthritis during the febrile phase of acute rheumatic fever. The duration of salicylate therapy usually ranges from 4 to 8 weeks, the average initial amount prescribed should be approximately 50 to 75 mg/kg/day given in four divided doses,[15] and extremely high doses are not required. Aspirin is used for symptomatic relief only. Aspirin administration is usually associated with a rapid and significant improvement in objective arthritis signs and symptoms and with almost immediate defervescence of fever. Specific blood levels do not need to be reached or maintained if clinical signs have disappeared. No evidence exists that salicylate administration affects the clinical course or later manifestations of cardiac involvement. The administration of steroid hormones, most commonly prednisone, is indicated for severe cardiac involvement characterized by pancarditis with congestive heart failure. When myocarditis appears to be fulminant, steroid therapy has been shown to significantly improve survival; however, as with salicylates, no evidence of long-term palliative effects on chronic rheumatic valvular disease is available.[15] The duration of steroid treatment may be extended to 1 to 3 months in severe cases, with varying schedules of tapering the dose and possibly adding salicylate therapy.

Additional, specific therapeutic measures to control congestive heart failure may be useful (ie, diuretics, digitalis). Furosemide (Lasix) is used for the management of pulmonary congestion with left-ventricular failure. Digitalis (digoxin) should be administered cautiously; the threshold for toxicity may be reduced in the presence of inflammatory myocarditis. Withholding digitalis for 1 or 2 days until steroid therapy has begun to suppress the myocarditis may be prudent. Serum potassium levels should be monitored because steroids and furosemide both decrease body potassium, predisposing the patient to digitalis intoxication. Enalapril is also sometimes used in patients with mitral valve insufficiency.

Limitation of Activity

The role of bed rest in the treatment of rheumatic fever has been deemphasized in recent years. For children with arthritis, ambulation can be permitted when pain and joint tenderness improve. Patients who have stable, mild cardiac involvement can be allowed to ambulate when they feel well enough. For patients who have more severe carditis, the length of restricted activity is individualized according to the severity of cardiac involvement.

OUTCOMES OF RHEUMATIC HEART DISEASE

In the months and years that follow an attack of rheumatic fever, the auscultatory findings frequently change from those heard during the acute episode. Apical systolic murmurs heard initially may diminish or even completely disappear. This finding is in contrast to the aortic diastolic murmur, which will almost always persist during the follow-up period. An initial diagnosis of carditis does not necessarily imply progression to permanent heart damage. When a child is labeled as having history of acute rheumatic fever, the additional appellation of rheumatic heart disease must be reevaluated continually. Even patients with severe carditis in the acute phase will show remarkable improvement in the weeks and months after the recuperative period; more than one half of murmurs of mild or moderate mitral insufficiency will disappear completely. Nevertheless, the ultimate development of rheumatic heart disease after a first attack of rheumatic fever can be correlated with the severity of the acute carditis. In the 10-year follow-up study of treatments begun in 1951, approximately 30% of patients who had mild carditis, and 50% of those who had moderate carditis developed chronic rheumatic heart disease (mitral insufficiency or stenosis or aortic regurgitation, or any combination). With severe carditis, nearly 75% of the patients will have residual heart disease.[16]

Most children who develop rheumatic heart disease after a single attack of rheumatic fever have mitral regurgitation. The others either have both mitral and aortic regurgitation or aortic regurgitation alone. Mitral stenosis evolves slowly, usually after repeated episodes of acute rheumatic fever, but it sometimes evolves unexpectedly, many years after initial mild mitral valvulitis, which was perhaps previously undiagnosed. Isolated mitral stenosis is unusual before early adulthood and has become a rare finding in developed nations.

An issue that arises in the follow-up of children who have rheumatic heart disease is the amount of physical activity permitted. In general, children who have mild mitral regurgitation with normal heart size should be allowed to engage in all athletic activities, except perhaps for the most strenuous, competitive sports. Children who have more severe mitral regurgitation or aortic insufficiency with cardiomegaly should have some restriction of their activities and a continuing appropriate regimen. If symptoms of fatigue or exercise intolerance persist despite medical management, then a full diagnostic evaluation should be performed; if appropriate, surgical intervention with valvuloplasty or valve replacement should be considered.

Recurrence of Rheumatic Fever

One of the most striking characteristics of rheumatic fever is its tendency to recur. Before the introduction of preventive measures, most patients who had an initial attack of rheumatic fever had one or more recurrences. The recurrence rate is highest during the first 3 years after an initial attack; it diminishes with time after the original episode, and recurrence is rare in adulthood.

Continuous antimicrobial prophylaxis should be performed in all children who have a history of rheumatic fever, including those who present with chorea. If by the time of high school graduation or at 18 years of age, patients who initially had cardiac involvement have no auscultatory evidence of heart disease, then prophylaxis may be discontinued. If, however, chronic mitral or aortic valvular disease exists, then prophylaxis should be maintained into adulthood. In children who had no cardiac involvement during the initial attack, prophylaxis can be discontinued after 5 years.

Prevention of Recurrence of Rheumatic Fever

The rationale for antibiotic prophylaxis in a patient with known rheumatic fever is protection against recurrence of rheumatic fever through prevention of group A streptococcal infection. The most effective method for reducing streptococcal infections and rheumatic fever recurrence is by intramuscular injections of long-acting penicillin (benzathine penicillin G, 1.2 million units).[14] This preventive regimen is most effective when given every 3 to 4 weeks; with residual cardiac involvement this approach is recommended for at least a 1- or 2-year period, before initiating oral prophylaxis. An every-3-week regimen is recommended for the first 6 to 12 months. Parenteral therapy is the most effective method of prophylaxis, given that strict adherence to a program of daily oral medication is especially difficult for children and adolescents. Some transient discomfort at the injection site (anterior thigh or buttock) may be relieved by a hot bath and aspirin on the evening of injection.

Alternative methods of prophylaxis include the oral administration of penicillin G (200,000 or 250,000 units, twice a day) or sulfisoxazole (Gantrisin, 0.5 g twice a day). For the exceptional patient who may be sensitive to both penicillin and sulfisoxazole, daily prophylaxis with another agent may be considered. Successful oral prophylaxis is hard to maintain, and if used, its value and need for compliance should be reinforced constantly by the primary care physician. Because rheumatic fever recurrence is less likely after 2 to 5 years, for patients with chronic rheumatic heart disease, an oral regimen can be substituted for intramuscular penicillin. Oral prophylaxis can be instituted immediately for patients who did not have carditis during the acute attack, because under these circumstances recurrences with carditis are extremely rare.

Bacterial Endocarditis

Individuals who have a history of rheumatic fever without evidence of significant murmurs on follow-up examination are not susceptible to bacterial endocarditis because they do not have damaged heart valves. Recent guidelines from the American Heart Association report that patients with heart disease are more likely to get infective endocarditis from frequent exposure to random bacteremic events associated with daily activities than from bacteremia following dental or surgical procedures. Therefore the latest guidelines for prevention of infective endocarditis recommend antibiotic prophylaxis for patients with prosthetic cardiac valves, previous infective endocarditis, and certain types of repaired and unrepaired congenital heart diseases. Antibiotic prophylaxis prior to dental or surgical procedures is no longer recommended for patients with mitral or aortic valve disease following rheumatic fever.[17] The recommendations for prevention of recurrent episodes of rheumatic fever have not changed.

Contraception and Pregnancy

Patients who have severe rheumatic heart disease are at high risk of cardiac complications during pregnancy and delivery. Mitral stenosis has an especially high-risk profile. However, mild rheumatic heart disease is well tolerated during pregnancy.

Adolescent girls who have rheumatic heart disease should be counseled in regard to contraceptive methods. Oral medication with a low level of estrogen can be prescribed and instructions given on the use of a diaphragm. An intrauterine device, however, should be avoided because of the risk of bacteremia.

Because of the added cardiovascular burden during pregnancy, thorough obstetrical care should be provided from the first trimester through delivery. Prophylaxis against streptococcal infection should be continued. Psychosocial support may be needed, especially for pregnant teenagers with significant rheumatic heart disease who may face medical complications during pregnancy. If early termination of a pregnancy is sought, then therapeutic abortion should be performed in the hospital.

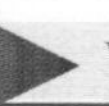

When to Refer and When to Admit

All children with acute rheumatic fever should be hospitalized and referred to a cardiologist for evaluation and management.

TOOLS FOR PRACTICE

Medical Decision Support

- *Guidelines for the Diagnosis of Rheumatic Fever* (guideline), American Heart Association (jama.ama-assn.org/cgi/content/abstract/268/15/2069).
- *Proceedings of the Jones Criteria Workshop* (other), Ferrieri P, Jones Criteria Working Group (circ.ahajournals.org/cgi/content/full/106/19/2521?ck=nck).
- Treatment of Acute Streptococcal Pharyngitis and Prevention of Rheumatic Fever: A Statement for Health Professionals, Dajani A, Taubert K, Ferrieri P, et al. *Pediatrics.* 1995:96(4):758-764 (pediatrics.aappublications.org/cgi/content/abstract/96/4/758).

REFERENCES

1. Stollerman GH. Rheumatic fever in the 21st Century. *Clin Infect Dis.* 2001;33(6):806-814.
2. Stollerman GH. *Rheumatic Fever and Streptococcal Infection.* New York, NY: Grune & Stratton; 1975.
3. Massell BF. *Rheumatic Fever and Streptococcal Infection: Unraveling the Mysteries of a Dread Disease.* Boston, MA: Harvard University Press; 1997.
4. Veasy LG, Hill HR. Immunologic and clinical correlations in rheumatic fever and rheumatic heart disease. *Pediatr Infect Dis J.* 1997;16(4):400-407.
5. Griffiths SP, Gersony WM. Acute rheumatic fever in New York City (1969 to 1998): a comparative study of two decades. *J Pediatr.* 1990;116(6):882-887.
6. Centers for Disease Control and Prevention. Acute rheumatic fever at a navy training center—San Diego, California. *MMWR Morb Mortal Wkly Rep.* 1988;37(7):101-104.
7. Kaplan EL, Hill HR. Return of rheumatic fever: consequences, implications and needs. *J Pediatr.* 1987;111(2):244-246.
8. Veasy LG, Wiedmeier SE, Orsmond GS, et al. Resurgence of acute rheumatic fever in the intermountain area of the United States. *N Engl J Med.* 1987;316(8):421-427.
9. Veasy LG, Tani LY, Daly JA, et al. Temporal association of the appearance of mucoid strains of Streptococcus pyogenes with a continuing high incidence of rheumatic fever in Utah. *Pediatrics.* 2004;113(3 pt 1):168-172.
10. Jones TD. Diagnosis of rheumatic fever. *JAMA.* 1944;126:481.

11. American Heart Association, Council of Cardiovascular Disease in the Young, Special Writing Group of the Committee on Rheumatic Fever, Endocarditis and Kawasaki Disease. Guidelines for the diagnosis of rheumatic fever. Jones criteria, 1992 update. *JAMA*. 1992;268(15): 2069-2073.
12. Ferrieri P, Jones Criteria Working Group. Proceedings of the Jones Criteria Workshop. *Circulation*. 2002;106(19): 2521-2523.
13. Vasan RS, Shrivastava S, Vijayakumar M, et al. Echocardiographic evaluation of patients with acute rheumatic fever and rheumatic carditis. *Circulation*. 1996;94(1): 73-82.
14. Dajani A, Taubert K, Ferrieri P, et al, American Heart Association, Council on Cardiovascular Disease in the Young, Committee on Rheumatic Fever, Endocarditis, and Kawasaki Disease. Treatment of acute streptococcal pharyngitis and prevention of rheumatic fever: a statement for health professionals. *Pediatrics*. 1995;96(4 pt 1): 758-764.
15. Taranta A, Markowitz M. *Rheumatic Fever*. Boston, MA: Kluwer Academic Publishers; 1989.
16. Albert DA, Harel L, Karrison T. The treatment of rheumatic carditis: a review and meta-analysis. *Medicine (Baltimore)*. 1995;74(1):1-12.
17. Wilson W, Taubert KA, Gewitz M, et al. Prevention of infective endocarditis: guidelines from the American Heart Association: a guideline from the American Heart Association Rheumatic Fever, Endocarditis and Kawasaki Disease Committee, Council on Cardiovascular Disease in the Young, and the Council on Clinical Cardiology, Council on Cardiovascular Surgery and Anesthesia, and the Quality of Care and Outcomes Research Interdisciplinary Working Group. *J Am Dent Assoc*. 2007;138(6):739-745, 747-760.

Chapter 318

ROCKY MOUNTAIN SPOTTED FEVER

Robert T. Seese, MD; Lara A. Danziger-Isakov, MD, MPH

INTRODUCTION

Rocky Mountain spotted fever (RMSF), an acute infectious disease caused by *Rickettsia,* is characterized by fever, headache, myalgia, and a distinctive exanthem. The major pathological lesion, vasculitis, makes RMSF a multisystem disease. Most important, it is a disease that requires clinical diagnosis and treatment before laboratory confirmation.

RMSF is an infectious disease that produces a vasculitis, giving rise to symptoms in multiple organ systems, including skeletal muscle, brain, lungs, kidneys, testes, adrenal glands, liver, and heart. Rickettsiae multiply in endothelial cells and may produce cellular injury by various mechanisms. These mechanisms include cell wall penetration, disturbance of intracellular metabolism, production of toxic metabolites, and use of metabolites required by the host cell. Necrosis of endothelial cell walls, an increase in vascular permeability, fibrin extravasation, and thrombosis of small blood vessels ensues because of perivascular mononuclear cell infiltration caused by the reproducing organism. Resulting cell damage in multiple locations is responsible for the clinical picture.[1]

INCIDENCE

The disease was first reported in patients from the Rocky Mountain region. Today, however, the incidence of the disease is greatest east of the Mississippi River, with most cases being reported from the southeastern and south central United States. From 1994 to 2003, 54% of the cases of RMSF reported in the United States were in North Carolina, Tennessee, Oklahoma, South Carolina, and Arkansas.[2] Although the disease occurs predominantly in the United States, it has been reported in other areas in the Western Hemisphere, specifically Canada, Central America, and South America. The reported frequency of the disease in the United States has increased slightly during the last several years from more than 500 cases per year in the 1990s to more than 1000 cases per year since 2000.[3]

EPIDEMIOLOGIC FEATURES

Ticks serve as a vector for the infectious agent *Rickettsia rickettsii*. Transmission to humans occurs when the tick takes a blood meal or when the abraded skin is contaminated by tick feces or a crushed tick, which may occur when ticks are removed. Usually, tick attachment lasting 12 to 24 hours is needed to transfer the disease to a human host.[3] Two specific ticks serve as major carriers: the wood tick, *Dermacentor andersoni,* is the more important vector in the western United States; the dog tick, *Dermacentor variabilis,* is the usual vector in the eastern United States. Ticks, in turn, acquire the rickettsiae by feeding on infected wild mammals, such as squirrels, opossums, rabbits, dogs, and mice. Infection of laboratory workers has been reported independently of exposure to ticks. The seasonal incidence of RMSF, which occurs primarily in spring, summer, and fall, is in accordance with the activity of ticks.[4] Dog ticks infected with *R rickettsii* have been found in urban areas, which suggests this tick's ubiquitous nature and places individuals at risk without travel to endemic areas.[5] Additional work has also implicated the brown dog tick, *Rhipicephalus sanguineus,* in causing an outbreak of *R rickettsii* infection in Arizona.[6]

In adults, occupational or recreational exposure to ticks increases the risk of infection; however, children are the most frequently affected, with two thirds of cases occurring in children younger than 15 years and peak ages of infection of 5 to 9 years. Fifteen percent of deaths from RMSF occur in children younger than 10 years. The illness occurs more frequently in boys than girls and more in white people than people of other races. RMSF can occur at any time of the year, but 90% of cases occur from April to September.[2,7]

A recent study by Marshall et al described positive serologic tests for RMSF in 12% of healthy children living in the southeast United States.[8] This finding seems to indicate that many infections may be subclinical.

Exposure to a tick is not elicited in every case. Only 60% of patients with RMSF can recall a specific tick exposure or encounter.[3] The tick bite is painless and leaves no local lesion or regional lymphadenopathy;

the clinician should therefore question the patient specifically about prior activities that increase the risk of exposure (eg, removal of a tick from a pet dog, camping or picnicking in a high-risk area). The overall risk to patients, even when in high-risk areas, is low, given that only approximately 1% to 3% of the tick population carries *R rickettsii* at any given time.[3]

DIFFERENTIAL DIAGNOSIS

Illnesses to be considered and differentiated from RMSF, especially after the rash appears, include rubeola (measles), meningococcemia, Henoch-Schönlein purpura, Kawasaki disease, immune thrombocytopenic purpura, leukemia, typhus, ehrlichiosis, and infectious mononucleosis. Of these illnesses, meningococcemia and ehrlichiosis require consideration, along with RMSF, because of their severe consequences with delay of diagnosis.

Meningococcemia

The petechial rash of meningococcemia differs from that of RMSF in its distribution, rapid extension, and coalescence of lesions into larger hemorrhagic, purpuric areas. Prostration develops rapidly if the patient remains untreated and is often apparent on admission to the hospital. Absence of myalgia and an extremely abrupt onset are helpful points in differentiating meningococcemia from RMSF. Although the white blood cell count may be elevated in meningococcemia, the sickest patients are frequently leukopenic. Meningitis with pleocytosis, low glucose levels, and organisms in the cerebrospinal fluid (CSF) also may be present. However, distinguishing between these entities clinically is not often possible; therefore treatment for both diseases in an ill patient is warranted.

Ehrlichiosis

Ehrlichiosis is a rickettsial disease with clinical similarity to RMSF. Although a rash occurs with less frequency, more than 60% of children with ehrlichiosis have been noted to have rash. The rash, although variable in location and appearance, may be petechial and can be confused with rickettsial exanthems. Early diagnosis and treatment of patients with ehrlichiosis with doxycycline (also the drug of choice for RMSF) reduces morbidity.

Rubeola

Rubeola (measles) is characterized by a macular rash (infrequently becoming hemorrhagic), which begins on the face and neck and is preceded by an enanthem, and Koplik spots on the buccal mucosa. The coryza and cough in the prodromal stage of illness are not consistent with RMSF. A history of adequate immunization with rubeola vaccine greatly diminishes this possibility.

Henoch-Schönlein Purpura

Henoch-Schönlein purpura may produce a petechial or purpuric rash, which is frequently concentrated on the lower extremities and buttocks. These cutaneous lesions may be multiform and occur on other parts of the body. Frequently, an arthralgia with periarticular swelling and accompanying signs and symptoms of upper respiratory tract inflammation, intense abdominal pain, or nephritis occurs. (See Chapter 272, Henoch-Schönlein Purpura.)

Kawasaki Disease

Kawasaki disease shares many of the features of RMSF: fever, puffy hands and feet, rash, and conjunctival injection. Usually, Kawasaki disease is not considered seriously until 5 days of fever, and an enlarged cervical node, pharyngeal hyperemia, dry cracked lips, strawberry tongue, and marked irritability tend to suggest the diagnosis. Although patients with Kawasaki disease also have a rash, it typically does not begin peripherally and spread centrally or become petechial in 1 to 2 days. Leukocyte and erythrocyte sedimentation rates are usually elevated significantly. In addition, Kawasaki syndrome usually occurs in the winter and spring months, in contrast to RMSF, which peaks during the summer.[2] Typically, children with Kawasaki disease do not give a history of tick exposures. An elevated platelet count begins during the second week of illness. (See Chapter 289 for a more detailed discussion of Kawasaki disease.)

Other Illnesses

Other illnesses that produce petechiae must also be mentioned, even though they lack the distinctive distribution of the rash. Immune thrombocytopenic purpura is seen as a petechial rash in an otherwise-healthy patient. Patients with leukemia who initially have fever and petechiae would be expected to be anemic and have lymphadenopathy or hepatosplenomegaly. Patients who have infectious mononucleosis, if they have a petechial eruption, usually have lymphadenopathy, hepatosplenomegaly, and a gradual onset. Typhus is a rickettsial infection to be excluded. Murine typhus produces a milder disease, with a rash that is macular and not petechial. Epidemic typhus may produce a petechial rash that typically begins proximally and extends peripherally but does not usually involve the palms or soles; a history of a tick bite is also absent.

CLINICAL FEATURES

After inoculation with the rickettsiae, the incubation period ranges from 2 to 12 days; the usual period is 5 to 7 days. In general, shorter incubation periods are associated with more serious disease.

In the typical case, the prodromal period lasts 2 to 3 days, with low-grade fever, chills, and muscle aches predominating.[9] Muscle pain is most commonly in the calf region in younger patients.[2] Headache is also an early symptom, and infants and toddlers may express pain from this or myalgias as crying or fussiness. Malaise, anorexia, vomiting, and photophobia also frequently occur. The prodrome is followed by accentuation of symptoms, especially fever, with temperatures often as high as 104°F (40°C) or more. The lowest temperatures, although still elevated, are recorded in the mornings. Lethargy and mental obtundation become prominent. Although the symptoms seen at this stage are not diagnostic, the triad of fever, headache, and myalgia, combined with a history of tick bite or removal within the previous 2 weeks, mandates treatment for RMSF until the diagnosis can be excluded.

Of RMSF symptoms and signs, rash is most distinctive. It usually appears 3 to 5 days after the onset of fever and begins peripherally on the wrists, ankles, hands, and feet. Initially, the lesions are macular, discrete, and erythematous and blanch on pressure. The rash rapidly spreads centrally, involving the arms, legs, axillae, buttocks, trunk, neck, and face. The lesions deepen in color, becoming dusky red, maculopapular, and petechial, but true petechiae may not form until day 6 of illness and 35% to 60% of patients never develop petechiae. When present, petechial lesions may coalesce and form large ecchymotic areas. In severe cases and when treatment is delayed, these ecchymotic areas may ulcerate, and distal regions (eg, fingers and toes) may become gangrenous in as many as 4% of cases. Furthermore, as many as 15% of patients do not develop rash, or they develop a fine rash that may be difficult to appreciate in patients with darker skin tones.[2] Because the rash does not occur until day 4 of the illness (and petechiae may be a much later finding) and some patients never develop a discernible exanthem, the pediatrician must not withhold treatment of a suspected case of RMSF until the rash appears. Tachycardia and an elevated pulse rate are noted early and are proportional to the degree of hyperpyrexia. A sudden increase in pulse rate or a decrease in blood pressure may indicate peripheral circulatory collapse, severe bleeding, or myocardial failure. Photophobia is associated with conjunctival ecchymosis involving both bulbar and palpebral conjunctivae. Retinal hemorrhages also may be seen.

Abdominal pain, vomiting, hepatomegaly, and splenomegaly with generalized abdominal tenderness may occur.[10] Jaundice is not usually seen except in the most critically ill patients, such as those with disseminated intravascular coagulation (DIC). Fever, poor fluid intake from nausea, and vomiting all contribute to a diminished urinary output. Mild azotemia caused by these fluid losses should respond to rehydration.

In addition to the lethargy and obtunded state of consciousness, the patient may exhibit nuchal rigidity as a result of a vasculitic reaction in the meninges. Disorientation and confusion, as well as seizures, may occur. Coma, central deafness, cortical blindness, and sixth nerve palsies are other neurovascular complications that have been reported with RMSF. Vasculitis, hemorrhage from coagulopathy, or secondary metabolic changes caused by circulatory collapse are responsible for these neurologic manifestations.[11] When these symptoms occur early in RMSF, they may mask its diagnosis.

LABORATORY EVALUATION

The diagnosis of RMSF is made clinically. Treatment should be started before laboratory diagnosis is confirmed because the disease still has a significant risk of morbidity and mortality when treatment is delayed. Available laboratory tests to confirm the presence of *R rickettsii* include a rise in antibody titer detected by immunofluorescence or latex agglutination, polymerase chain reaction testing, immunofluorescence of a skin biopsy, or isolation of the organism from a clinical specimen. Immunofluorescent staining of the skin biopsy specimen may identify *R rickettsii* and may provide early proof of RMSF, but this study is not readily available to most clinicians.[12] Appropriate antibiotic therapy started 3 days before biopsy has resulted in negative immunofluorescence. Therefore when appropriate treatment has been initiated before biopsy, clinical criteria justify a full course of antibiotic therapy. Polymerase chain reaction testing provides a specific diagnostic tool for early diagnosis but is expensive and not commonly available to most clinicians.[1]

Complement fixation and immunofluorescent antibody studies in serum will identify patients who have RMSF, but results of these tests do not become positive until 7 to 10 days after the onset of illness or later if antibiotic therapy has begun early. Thus titers should be performed during the acute illness and repeated 3 weeks later. A 4-fold increase in titer in the convalescent sera is diagnostic for infection.

The Weil-Felix reaction, agglutination of *Proteus vulgaris* by the patient's serum, is at best a nonspecific test for RMSF. Again, acute and convalescent serums must be compared, although *P agglutinins* may appear by the end of the first week of illness. Availability of the more specific and sensitive tests makes this test obsolete.

Rickettsiae can be isolated from body fluid or tissue specimens when grown in laboratory animals or chick embryos. However, the high rate of disease transmission to laboratory technicians makes such techniques feasible only in laboratories engaged in *Rickettsia*-related research in which all workers are immunized; thus culture identification of rickettsiae is not available in most clinical settings.

Blood leukocyte counts and differential counts are usually within normal limits, but neutrophils often predominate. This predominance may help distinguish RMSF from ehrlichiosis, given that most patients with ehrlichiosis have lymphopenic leukopenia. Thrombocytopenia is a complication seen in the later stages of the disease and may be the result of platelet adherence to damaged endothelium.

Up to 20% of patients may have hyponatremia, possibly caused by increased vascular permeability of the kidney to sodium. However, this finding is nonspecific and does not exclude other diagnoses, such as ehrlichiosis. The remainder of the electrolyte profile is usually normal, but hypochloremia is also seen in some patients. Up to 25% of patients will also display increased blood urea nitrogen levels and increased liver enzymes.[2] Abnormalities of prothrombin time, partial thromboplastin time, fibrinogen, and fibrin split products can occur with the development of DIC.

Patients with neurologic manifestations may have normal CSF cell counts, and most have normal CSF glucose and protein levels. However, CSF analysis might reveal neutrophilic or lymphocytic pleocytosis and elevated protein.[3] As with many of the laboratory findings, these are nonspecific and may not help distinguish RMSF from meningococcal disease or ehrlichiosis.

Neurologic complications, in addition to the lethargy, have already been discussed, but long-term morbidity from these complications, though rare, is still significant. Hematuria and anemia also may occur, but transfusion or renal dialysis is rarely required.

MANAGEMENT

Treatment

Treatment should never be withheld or delayed because of absence of rash, lack of exposure to ticks, or the desire to await confirmatory laboratory study results. Furthermore, delaying treatment is not acceptable because the patient is not from an area where RMSF is common or because the pediatrician is uncomfortable using doxycycline in a child younger than 8 years. If a pediatrician strongly suspects RMSF because of the patient's clinical history and physical findings, then therapy should be initiated immediately and can be given concurrently with treatment for meningococcemia.[2]

Pharmacotherapy

Doxycycline

The drug of choice for all ages is doxycycline, an antibiotic in the tetracycline class of antibiotics that is given and continued for at least 3 days after clinical improvement and defervescence. The usual length of therapy is 7 to 10 days.[3] Intravenous therapy should be given to all ill patients, who should then be transitioned to oral therapy when their condition has improved. Doxycycline is also effective against ehrlichiosis, which may mimic RMSF. Because doxycycline has a broad therapeutic index, levels do not need to be monitored as required with other RMSF medications, such as chloramphenicol.

Tetracycline

Tetracycline has been shown to be effective against RMSF but can lead to increased dental staining compared with doxycycline in children younger than 9 years. For this reason, and because tetracycline is no more effective than doxycycline, tetracycline is less commonly used in children.

Chloramphenicol

Chloramphenicol is no longer the drug of choice for RMSF. Data have shown doxycycline may be more effective than chloramphenicol.[13] In addition, the toxic effects of this drug (aplastic anemia) make it an undesirable treatment option. However, chloramphenicol may be given to patients who cannot tolerate doxycycline or tetracycline.

Combination Therapy

Initiating treatment for meningococcal disease, as well as RMSF and ehrlichiosis, in an ill patient may be necessary. When this situation arises, doxycycline will provide treatment for both ehrlichiosis and RMSF and can be used in conjunction with a third-generation cephalosporin to treat meningococcal infection.

Hospitalization

Hospitalization is desirable initially for most patients, both to confirm the diagnosis and to observe the effect of therapy. Therapy should be continued until the patient has improved and has been afebrile for 72 hours, which generally occurs after a total of 7 to 10 days of therapy.

Supportive Therapy

Supportive therapy includes maintenance of hydration and nutrition with appropriate intravenous fluids and oral feedings (if tolerated). Management of DIC may include therapeutic maneuvers such as administering fresh-frozen plasma, fresh platelets and packed red blood cells, and vitamin K. Seizures may require the use of anticonvulsant medications.

PROGNOSIS

RMSF now has a mortality of approximately 2% to 4% in recognized cases, but patients with RMSF who escaped clinical detection have been identified by serologic evidence, suggesting that the disease may occur in a mild or subclinical form.[14] The importance of abdominal pain mimicking an acute abdominal condition and dominating as an early symptom before the development of a rash must be emphasized. Rocky Mountain spotless fever has also been described.[9] Of great concern is a report suggesting that patients who have *spotless or almost spotless* fever have a significantly higher mortality as a result of delayed diagnosis and treatment.[15,16]

RMSF can be considered a potentially lethal illness, even though younger patients are likely to be less severely affected than older patients. Early diagnosis and prompt therapy lessen disease severity. Under such circumstances, death would be extremely unusual; in most patients, early clinical diagnosis and adequate therapy shorten the duration of illness appreciably. Normal temperatures within the first 3 to 4 days may be expected, and patients recover rapidly from other signs of illness (eg, headache, myalgia, lethargy). Extension of the rash ceases.[9] Recovery from the illness is accompanied by immunity to *R rickettsii*.

COMPLICATIONS

Vascular necrosis and thrombosis may result in local gangrene and loss of tissue. Although uncommon, DIC may develop. Patients with this complication have the greatest risk of dying. Myocardial failure may result from myocarditis and arrhythmias. Edema may be generalized as a result of an increase in capillary permeability caused by the vasculitis, of heart failure, of iatrogenic fluid overload, or any combination.

Neurologic complications in addition to the lethargy have already been discussed, but long-term morbidity from these complications, though rare, is still significant. Hematuria and anemia also may occur, but transfusions or renal dialysis are rarely required.

PREVENTION

N-N-diethyl-M-toluamide (DEET) skin repellents in conjunction with permethrin-containing repellents used on clothes have been shown to be effective against ticks and avoiding exposures. Systemic reactions to DEET are possible when the repellents contain a high concentration of the chemical.[3] The best preventive measure is avoidance of tick exposure, but when exposure is likely, daily searches for ticks should be performed. For tick-infested areas, twice-daily searches are advised. Careful inspection at bath time is an excellent way to discover the presence of ticks. They may be removed by gentle traction with forceps or tweezers, but care must be taken not to crush them. The skin should be disinfected both before and after tick exposure to clear it of tick feces that may carry *R rickettsii*. The tick should never be covered in petroleum jelly, nail polish remover, or alcohol, and no one should attempt to burn the tick to coax it to detach itself. These attempts may lead the tick to defecate or aerosolize infected body fluids.[16] Antimicrobial prophylaxis is not indicated after a tick bite. The chances of a tick carrying the disease, even in an endemic area, are low, and no demonstrable benefit of prophylaxis has been found.

WHEN TO REFER

- Uncertain of diagnosis
- Clinical suspicion of disease

WHEN TO ADMIT

- Most patients need to be hospitalized until they show clinical improvement
- Hemodynamic instability
- Dehydration
- Requires intensive monitoring
- RMSF with its complications

TOOLS FOR PRACTICE

Engaging Patient and Family

- *A Parents Guide to Insect Repellents* (brochure), American Academy of Pediatrics (patiented.aap.org).

Medical Decision Support

- *Red Book: 2006 Report of the Committee on Infectious Diseases,* American Academy of Pediatrics (www.aap.org/bookstore).
- *Rocky Mountain Spotted Fever* (Web page), Centers for Disease Control and Prevention (www.cdc.gov/ncidod/dvrd/rmsf/index.htm).

Practice Management and Care Coordination

- *Tick-borne Rickettsial Disease Case Report Form,* Centers for Disease Control and Prevention (www.cdc.gov/ncidod/dvrd/rmsf/Case_Rep_Fm.pdf).

SUGGESTED RESOURCES

Centers for Disease Control and Prevention. Rocky Mountain Spotted Fever. Available at: www.cdc.gov/ncidod/dvrd/rmsf/index.htm. Accessed July 2, 2007.

Edwards MS, Feigen RD. Rickettsial disease. In: Feigin RD, Cherry JD, eds. *Textbook of Pediatric Infectious Diseases*. 4th ed. Philadelphia, PA: WB Saunders; 1998.

Razzaq, S., Schutze, G. Rocky Mountain spotted fever: a physician's challenge. *Pediatr Rev*. 2005;26:125-130.

REFERENCES

1. Edwards MS, Feigin RD. Rickettsial disease. In: Feigin RD, Cherry JD, eds. *Textbook of Pediatric Infectious Diseases*. 4th ed. Philadelphia, PA: WB Saunders; 1998.
2. Razzaq S, Schutze GE. Rocky Mountain spotted fever: a physician's challenge. *Pediatr Rev*. 2005;26(4):125-130.
3. Chapman AS. Diagnosis and Management of Tickborne Rickettsial Diseases: Rocky Mountain Spotted Fever, Ehrlichioses, and Anaplasmosis—United States. *MMWR Morb Mortal Wkly Rep*. 2006;55(RR04);1-27. Available at: www.cdc.gov/mmwr/preview/mmwrhtml/rr5504a1.htm. Accessed July 2, 2007.
4. Lange JV, Walker DH, Wester TB. Documented Rocky Mountain spotted fever in Wintertime. *JAMA*. 1982; 247(17):2403-2404.
5. Salgo MP, Telzak EE, Currie B, et al. A focus of Rocky Mountain spotted fever within New York City. *N Engl J Med*. 1988;318(21):1345-1348.
6. Demma LJ, Traeger MS, Nicholson WL, et al. Rocky Mountain spotted fever from an unexpected tick vector in Arizona. *N Engl J Med*. 2005;353(6):587-594.
7. Abramson JS, Givner LB. Rocky Mountain spotted fever. *Pediatr Infect Dis J*. 1999;18(6):539-540.
8. Marshall GS, Stout GG, Jacobs RF, et al. Antibodies reactive to Rickettsia rickettsii among children living in the southeast and south central regions of the United States. *Arch Pediatr Adolesc Med*. 2003;157(5):443-448.
9. Haynes RE, Sanders DY, Cramblett HG. Rocky Mountain spotted fever in children. *J Pediatr*. 1970;76(5):685-693.
10. Davis AE Jr, Bradford WD. Abdominal pain resembling acute appendicitis in Rocky Mountain spotted fever. *JAMA*. 1982;247(20):2811-2812.
11. Bell WE, Lascari AD. Rocky mountain spotted fever. Neurological symptoms in the acute phase. *Neurology*. 1970;20(9):841-847.
12. Fleisher G, Lennette ET, Honig P. Diagnosis of Rocky Mountain spotted fever by immunofluorescent identification of Rickettsia rickettsii in skin biopsy tissue. *J Pediatr*. 1979;95(1):63-65.
13. American Academy of Pediatrics. Rocky Mountain spotted fever. In: Pickering LK, ed. *Red Book: 2006 Report of the Committee on Infectious Diseases*. 27th ed. Elk Grove Village, IL: American Academy of Pediatrics; 2006.
14. Marx RS, McCall CE, Abramson JS, et al. Rocky Mountain spotted fever. Serological evidence of previous subclinical infection in children. *Am J Dis Child*. 1982; 136(1): 16-18.
15. Sexton DJ, Corey GR. Rocky Mountain "spotless" and "almost spotless" fever: a wolf in sheep's clothing. *Clin Infect Dis*. 1992;15(3):439-448.
16. Westerman EL. Rocky Mountain spotless fever: a dilemma for the clinician. *Arch Intern Med*. 1982;142(6):1106-1107.

Chapter 319

SEBORRHEIC DERMATITIS

Elizabeth Alvarez Connelly, MD; Lawrence Schachner, MD

Seborrheic dermatitis (SD) is a common, usually asymptomatic, dermatosis of unknown cause that is seen primarily in infants but also in adolescents and adults. The incidence in the general population is 2% to 5%. In 50% of affected infants, symptoms begin before 5 weeks of age. Although SD is occasionally seen in infants who are infected with HIV, a true increased incidence has not been documented. No evidence suggests a genetic predisposition. Infants with SD may be at an increased risk of developing atopic dermatitis and, less often, psoriasis.

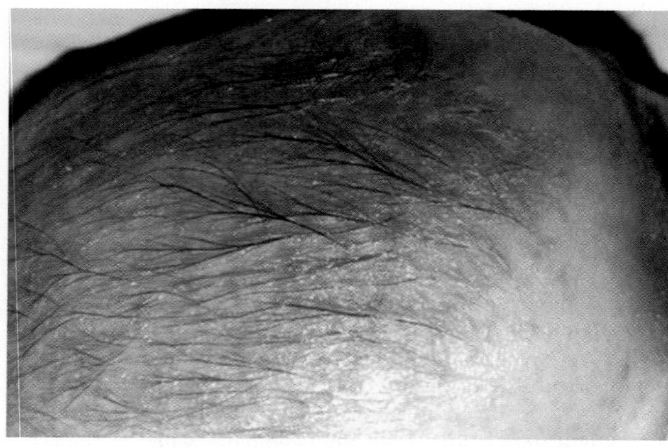

Figure 319-1 Cradle cap.

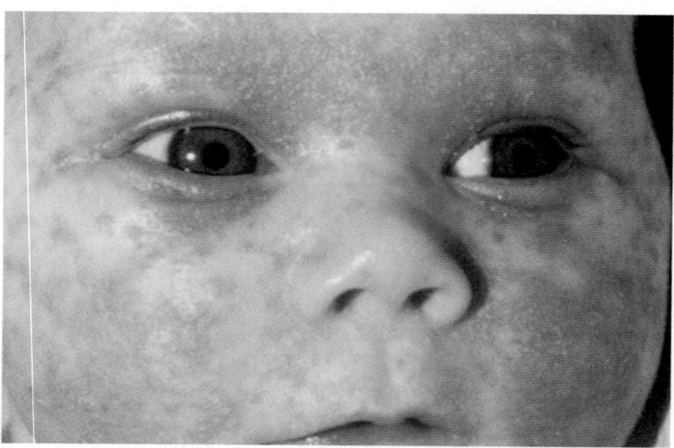

Figure 319-2 Seborrheic dermatitis in the retroauricular creases, eyebrows, and nasolabial folds.

EVALUATION

SD is most commonly characterized as a greasy, scaly dermatitis, less often as psoriasiform SD and rarely as erythrodermic SD. SD in infancy, cradle cap, is characterized by diffuse, red, crusted, and yellow scaling plaques on the vertex of the scalp (Figure 319-1). Similar lesions also may be found in the retroauricular creases, the eyebrows, and the nasolabial folds (Figure 319-2). In the axillary and inguinal folds, the neck, and the diaper area lesions appear as shiny red patches with foul-smelling scale in the folds. Posterior lymphadenopathy has been shown to be significantly associated with SD in patients with a negative fungal culture. The lesions are usually asymptomatic and distributed symmetrically. The presentation is similar in adolescents. Patients may note a greasy, scaling, pruritic eruption on the scalp. Except for lack of inguinal area involvement, the distribution of the lesions is the same as that for infants. HIV-positive children aged 2 to 5 years may exhibit SD with lesions similar to those seen in adolescents and adults. This circumstance is distinctly unusual in immunocompetent children and appears to be a manifestation of HIV infection.

Psoriasiform SD, also known as *sebopsoriasis* or *seborrhiasis*, produces features of both SD and psoriasis and may represent a bridge between the two conditions. Psoriasiform plaques—that is, annular, red-brown plaques having a silvery scale—may be present among the classic greasy, yellow, scaling lesions of SD. Patients may or may not have *pitted* nails, which are seen with classic psoriasis. Erythrodermic SD is rare and causes widespread exfoliative erythroderma. Diffuse desquamation usually begins in the flexures and then spreads.

The patient may exhibit signs and symptoms of systemic involvement—that is, fever, chills, lymphadenopathy, peripheral edema, and dehydration. This involvement also may be the presentation of Leiner disease (see Differential Diagnosis).

ETIOLOGY

The cause of SD remains unknown. In recent years, different pathogenic mechanisms have been proposed. Despite early evidence that *Pitysporum ovale* may play a role in the evolution of SD, recent data supports a causal link between *Malassezia* yeast and SD. Many studies have demonstrated clinical improvement of SD when interventions reduce *Malassezia* counts on the body. Separate research has shown that the use of antifungal agents effectively treat SD. However, no difference has been found in the *Malassezia* carriage rates in patients with and without SD. Thus authorities have proposed that the immunomodulatory factors of the host may influence the manifestation of SD rather than the actual colonization counts. *Malassezia* may serve as the primary trigger in an inflammatory reaction that ultimately results in SD. Studies have revealed an increase in both lymphocyte transformation response and leukocyte migration inhibition. This differing immunogenic host theory may explain the increase prevalence of SD in patients with AIDS. Other research postulates that lesions of SD are induced by the toxin production or lipase activity of *Malassezia*. The location of SD lesions tend to occur on the scalp, face, eyebrows, nasolabial, axillary, and inguinal folds. These locations are also areas of highest sebaceous gland concentration. Experts have proposed that an abnormality in the sebaceous gland or an increased sensitivity to circulating maternal or endogenous hormones may result in SD. However, patients with SD have normal sebaceous secretion and hormonal levels.

DIFFERENTIAL DIAGNOSIS

The differential diagnosis of SD includes atopic dermatitis, psoriasis, dermatophyte infection, diaper dermatitis, histiocytosis X, and Leiner disease. Atopic dermatitis is usually distinguished by the presence of extreme pruritus, extensoral distribution in infancy, and flexural distribution in older children (tending to spare the scalp and to involve the hands and feet), as well as a family history in 70% of persons affected. SD may also occur concomitantly with atopic dermatitis (see Chapter 240, Atopic Dermatitis). Psoriasis is a common inherited papulosquamous skin disorder characterized by well-demarcated, annular, thick, red-brown, scaling plaques usually present on the trunk,

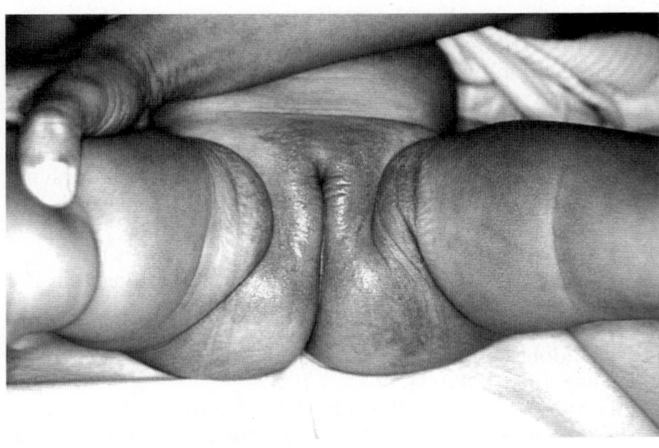

Figure 319-3 Irritant diaper dermatitis.

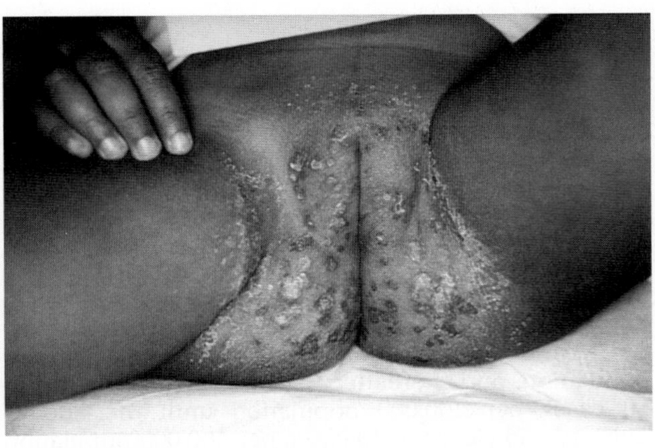

Figure 319-4 Candidal diaper dermatitis.

the extensor areas on the arms, the knees, the elbows, the diaper area, and the scalp, as well as by nail pitting. Psoriasis usually lacks the specific distribution and the greasy component of SD. However, some cases of SD may overlap with psoriasis. Extensive cases of SD become persistent; when the family history of psoriasis is positive, patients should be referred to a dermatologist for biopsy and, potentially, long term follow-up care. Symptoms of dermatophyte infection of the scalp (tinea capitis) may include scaling, pruritus, and redness of the scalp. It usually results in alopecia. In addition, performing a fungal culture by swabbing the affected area vigorously will yield a positive result. Tinea corporis appears as annular, red, scaly plaques with central clearing. Cultures from the skin may be obtained in a similar fashion to the scalp. Potassium hydroxide preparation of scales from body lesions will demonstrate septate hyphae.

Diaper dermatitis, or irritant diaper rash, is characterized by involvement primarily of the convex surfaces by red, scaling plaques; the inguinal folds are spared (Figure 319-3). In candidal diaper dermatitis, similar red, scaling plaques involve the skin folds, but satellite pustules in areas not covered by the diaper may also be found (Figure 319-4). SD in the diaper area involves the skin folds; however, no satellite lesions are found. Histiocytosis X refers to a group of Langerhans cell histiocytoses: Letterer-Siwe disease (diffuse disseminated histiocytosis), Hand-Schüller-Christian disease, and eosinophilic granuloma (chronic multifocal or focal histiocytosis). Letterer-Siwe disease may be confused with SD because its pattern of distribution is similar. However, Letterer-Siwe disease is also characterized by axillary, inguinal, and oral mucosal erosions, purpura and petechiae, and hepatosplenomegaly. A skin biopsy specimen will distinguish the two disorders easily and is recommended in cases of SD that are unresponsive to treatment. Leiner disease, sometimes referred to as *erythrodermic SD,* is an inherited immunologic disorder characterized by generalized SD, persistent diarrhea, failure to thrive, and recurrent gram-negative infections. The diagnosis is made by demonstrating deficient yeast opsonic activity in the patient's serum. In addition, other immunodeficiencies and metabolic disorders may occur in an erythrodermic SD pattern.

TREATMENT

Effective treatment for SD may involve a wide range of keratolytic agents, low-potency corticosteroids, and antifungal therapies. Choice of the medication is tailored to fit the age of the patient. A more conservative approach is suggested when treating infantile SD (cradle cap). Application of mineral oil or white petrolatum to the scalp followed by a nonmedicated shampoo is an initial therapy. If unresponsive, then second-line agents include a 1% to 2% salicylic acid in liquid or petrolatum form, followed by a keratolytic shampoo (eg, Sebulex, Neutrogena T/Sal, or P & S) and a topical low-potency corticosteroid (1% to 2.5% hydrocortisone, Synalar solution, or Derma-Smoothe). Topical antifungals, specifically the azoles, are effective as well. More recently, the use of topical macrolactam immunomodualtors have been successful in treating this inflammatory skin condition. Tacrolimus also has antifungal properties, which contributes to its therapeutic effectiveness.

Therapy for adolescent SD consists of topical corticosteroids and keratolytic shampoos applied to the scalp. In addition, topical and oral ketoconazole may be used in severe cases. Psoriasiform SD of the scalp is treated as described for cradle cap. Psoriasiform lesions on the face and trunk respond to treatment with topical corticosteroid ointments and emollients. If lesions persist into childhood, then a modified Goeckerman regimen consisting of application of a tar preparation followed by outdoor exposure to sunlight and topical corticosteroids is therapeutic. Generalized erythrodermic SD may require systemic corticosteroids and antibiotics to control superinfection in addition to the antiseborrheic therapies already mentioned. Hospitalization for intravenous antibiotic administration may be required.

In treating infantile SD, the salicylic acid solution or petrolatum should be applied for only 10 minutes and then shampooed out carefully, avoiding the face and particularly the eyes because severe contact irritation may occur. The corticosteroid solution should be applied sparingly and left on for several hours. This regimen may be repeated up to twice daily as needed and then tapered. Dramatic improvement occurs usually within a week. Lesions occurring on the face, intertriginous areas, and the diaper area may be treated with a low-potency topical corticosteroid cream (1% hydrocortisone cream) twice a day. A mid-potency corticosteroid such as 0.1% Kenalog cream may be used on the body twice a day. A mid-potency or strong halogenated corticosteroid should not be used on the face, intertriginous areas, and diaper area. Topical ketoconazole (Nizoral), which has been used to treat adult SD, has been found to be beneficial in treating infantile SD. Lesions in the diaper and intertriginous areas may become superinfected with *Candida* species and require topical antifungal creams twice a day in addition to a topical corticosteroid.

PROGNOSIS

The prognosis for infantile SD is usually excellent. Most cases resolve within the first 6 months of life. Adolescent-onset and HIV-related SD may be more persistent; however, it usually responds readily to topical therapy. Infants who have SD may be at an increased risk of developing atopic dermatitis or psoriasis later.

TOOLS FOR PRACTICE

Engaging Patient and Family

- *Diaper Rash* (brochure), American Academy of Pediatrics (patiented.aap.org).

Medical Decision Support

- *Pediatric Dermatology: A Quick Reference Guide* (book), American Academy of Pediatrics (www.aap.org/bookstore).

RELATED WEB SITE

- American Academy of Dermatology (AAD) (www.aad.org/default.htm).

REFERENCES

1. Caputo R. Papulo-squamous disease. In: Schachner LA, Hansen R, eds. *Pediatric Dermatology*. New York, NY: Churchill-Livingstone; 1988.
2. Prose N. HIV infection in children. *J Am Acad Dermatol.* 1990;22:1223-1231.
3. Menni SM, Piccinno R, Baietta S, et al. Infantile seborrheic dermatitis: seven-year follow-up and some prognostic criteria. *Pediatr Dermatol.* 1989;6:13-15.
4. Ruiz-Maldonado R, Lopez-Martinez R, Perez Chavarria EL, et al. Pityrosporum ovale in infantile seborrheic dermatitis. *Pediatr Dermatol.* 1989;6:16-20.
5. Gupta AK, Madzia SE, Batra R. Etiology and management of seborrheic dermatitis *Dermatology*. 2004;208: 89-93.
6. McGinley KJ, Leyden JJ, Marples RR, et al. Quantitative microbiology of the scalp in non-dandruff, dandruff and seborrheic dermatitis. *J Invest Dermatol.* 1975;64: 401-405.
7. Gupta AK, Nicol K, Batra R. Role of antifungal agents in the treatment of seborrheic dermatitis. *Am J Clin Dermatol.* 2004;5(6):417-422.
8. Bergbrant IM, Faergmann J. Adherence of Malassezia furfur to human stratum corneum cells in vitro: a study of health individuals and patients with seborrheic dermatitis. *Mycoses.* 1994;37:217-219.
9. Faergemann J, Bergbrandt IM, Dohse M, et al. Seborrheic dermatitis and Pitysporum (Malassezia) folliculitis: characterization of inflammatory cells and mediators in the skin by immunohistochemistry. *Br J of Dermatol.* 2001;144:549-556.
10. Parry ME, Sharpe GR. Seborrheic dermatitis is not caused by an altered immune response to Malassezia yeast. *Br J Dermatol.* 1998;139:254-263.
11. McDonald LL, Smith M. Diagnostic dilemmas in pediatric/adolescent dermatology: scaly scalp. *J Pediatr Health Care.* 1998;12:80-84.
12. Gupta AK, Nicol K, Batra R. Role of antifungal agents in the treatment of seborrheic dermatitis. *Am J Clin Dermatol.* 2004;5(6):417-422.
13. Braza TJ, Di Carlo JB, Soon SL, et al. Tacrolimus 0.1% ointment for seborrheic dermatitis: An open-label pilot study. *Br J Dermatol.* 2003;148:1242-1244.
14. Crutchfield CE III. Pimecrolimus: a new treatment for seborrheic dermatitis. *Cutis.* 2002;70:207-208.

Chapter 320

SEIZURE DISORDERS

Sarah M. Roddy, MD; Margaret C. McBride, MD

Seizures occur in approximately 1% of all children up to the age of 14 years.[1] The incidence is greatest in the first year of life, approximately 120 cases per 100,000 population, and thereafter the incidence rate is 40 to 50 cases per 100,000 population until the age of puberty and closer to 10 cases per 100,000 population in the early and mid teens.[2]

Seizures are caused by abnormal discharges of neurons and may have a wide variety of clinical manifestations. A seizure should be considered a symptom of systemic or central nervous system (CNS) dysfunction. Management consists not only of controlling seizures, but also of diagnosing any potentially treatable underlying condition. Acute conditions associated with seizures include metabolic disturbances, fever, meningitis, encephalitis, and toxic encephalopathy. The terms *seizure disorder* and *epilepsy* are synonymous and are applied to the condition in which a tendency for recurrent, unprovoked seizures exists. Care of patients who have epilepsy includes managing the psychosocial impact of epilepsy on the child and family, as well as any associated comorbidities such as learning disabilities and behavioral problems.

CLASSIFICATION

Classification of seizures has provided a means to study seizures that have similar pathophysiological features and to determine which medications are effective for which seizure types. Electroencephalographic (EEG) monitoring has aided in the current classification,[3] which is based on characterization of seizure onset and progression. Seizures are either partial or generalized. *Generalized* seizures result from

BOX 320-1 Classification of Seizures and Epilepsy Syndromes

PRIMARY GENERALIZED	PARTIAL
Seizure Types	***Seizure Types***
Absence	Simple partial
Myoclonic	Complex partial
Atonic, astatic	Partial seizures with secondary generalization
Tonic-clonic	
Epilepsy Syndromes	***Epilepsy Syndromes***
Infantile spasms (West syndrome)	Benign partial epilepsy of childhood
Lennox-Gastaut syndrome	Epilepsia partialis continua
Childhood absence epilepsy	***Unclassified***
Juvenile myoclonic epilepsy	Neonatal seizures
	Febrile seizures
	Pseudoseizures

Data from Commission of Classification and Terminology of the International League Against Epilepsy. *Epilepsia* 1985;26:268.

involvement of both cerebral hemispheres simultaneously from the onset of the seizure. Types of generalized seizures include absence, myoclonic, atonic, tonic, clonic, and tonic-clonic seizures. *Partial* seizures are caused by seizure discharges that begin in 1 hemisphere. Partial seizures are divided further into *simple partial seizures,* in which consciousness is preserved, and *complex partial seizures,* in which consciousness is impaired. Partial seizures of either type may progress to become secondarily generalized.

Epilepsy syndromes have also been defined in terms of a cluster of signs and symptoms, including age of onset, severity, diurnal or nocturnal occurrence, clinical course, associated neurologic dysfunction, inheritance, and EEG findings.[4] Generalized epilepsy syndromes include juvenile myoclonic epilepsy, Lennox-Gastaut syndrome, infantile spasms (West syndrome), and childhood absence epilepsy. A common partial epilepsy syndrome is benign partial epilepsy of childhood. Neonatal seizures have different characteristics and causes and are considered separately, as are febrile seizures. Box 320-1 outlines the classification of the various seizure types and epilepsy syndromes.

Generalized Seizures

Absence Seizures

Absence seizures are generalized, nonconvulsive seizures characterized by interruption of activity, staring, and unresponsiveness; they usually last between 5 and 15 seconds. The episode starts abruptly without warning and ends abruptly with resumption of the child's preictal activity. The child may be unaware that the episode occurred. At times, unresponsiveness is accompanied by eyelid fluttering and upward rotation of the eyes and occasionally by mild clonic movements or automatisms such as lip smacking, grimacing, or swallowing. Seizures may occur more than 100 times per day and may interfere with the child's learning ability. The age of onset is generally between 3 and 8 years; rarely does it occur before 2 years or after 15 years of age. Girls are affected more commonly than boys. The influence of genetic factors in the etiology of absence seizures is suggested by the finding that 15% to 44% of first-degree relatives have a history of absence seizures, paroxysmal EEG abnormalities, or both.[5]

The classic finding on the EEG in patients who have absence seizures is bilaterally synchronous 3-Hz spike-and-wave discharges. Hyperventilation may be used to precipitate the electrical discharge and a clinical seizure. Photic stimulation during the EEG also induces the seizure discharge in some patients. Generalized tonic-clonic seizures may occur in some children, especially those who have an onset of absence seizures after 8 years of age. The prognosis for remission is good for children with younger age of onset and in whom absence is the sole seizure type but is less favorable for those who have associated tonic-clonic seizures.

Monotherapy with ethosuximide, valproate, or lamotrigine usually controls absence seizures effectively. Valproate or lamotrigine are the drugs of choice if associated tonic-clonic seizures exist. Any two of these medications may be used together when absence seizures are not completely controlled with one.[6-8] Benzodiazepines also are effective in controlling absence seizures, but their adverse effects on behavior make them second-line therapeutic agents. Phenytoin, phenobarbital, and carbamazepine are usually ineffective for treating absence seizures and may exacerbate them.

Myoclonic Seizures

Myoclonic jerks are characterized by brief, sudden muscle contractions that may involve only part of the body or may be generalized. They may occur in clusters, especially when falling asleep or shortly after awakening, and, in most instances, no alteration in consciousness is associated with the jerks.

Atonic Seizures

Atonic, or astatic, seizures have also been termed *drop attacks.* They are characterized by a sudden decrease in muscle tone, which may result in head nodding or mild flexing of the legs. More significant decreases in muscle tone may cause the patient to slump to the floor. In most instances, no alteration in consciousness is detectable with these seizures.

Generalized Tonic-Clonic Seizures

Generalized tonic-clonic seizures are also known as *grand mal seizures* and consist of motor manifestations and loss of consciousness. The tonic phase is characterized by a sustained contraction of muscles; as a result, the patient falls to the ground, usually in opisthotonus. In most instances, extensor posturing occurs with tonic contraction of the diaphragm and intercostal muscles, which halts respirations and, in turn, produces cyanosis. The tonic phase lasts less than 1 minute and is followed by the clonic phase, which consists of bilateral rhythmic jerking. The jerks may be accompanied by expiratory grunts produced by diaphragmatic contractions against a closed glottis. The frequency of the clonic jerks decreases as the seizure progresses, although the intensity may actually increase. The tongue may be bitten, and bowel and bladder incontinence may occur. The clonic activity usually stops within several minutes. The seizure may be followed by vomiting, confusion, and lethargy, with gradual recovery of consciousness during minutes to hours.

Generalized tonic-clonic seizures may be primary or secondary. Primary generalized seizures are usually idiopathic or genetic in origin and are associated with bilaterally synchronous electrical discharges on EEG. Secondary generalized seizures begin as partial seizures but may generalize so rapidly that any suggestion of focal origin is lacking. The EEG may demonstrate a focal discharge that may spread to both hemispheres or may show only bilateral synchronous discharges. The history that is helpful in determining that a seizure is secondary generalized is the presence of an aura, head or eye deviation, or focal clonic movement at the onset of the seizure. Neurologic examination may reveal subtle focal signs such as a mild hemiparesis or visual field defect. Complete seizure control is less likely in secondary generalized epilepsy than in primary generalized epilepsy.[5]

Effective antiepileptic medications for treating primary generalized tonic-clonic seizures include valproate, lamotrigine, phenobarbital, topiramate, and zonisamide. Secondary generalized seizures may be effectively treated with these medications, as well as with carbamazepine, oxcarbazepine, and phenytoin. Evidence is growing that one of the newest anticonvulsants, levetiracetam, may be effective in both types of generalized seizures.

Infantile Spasms (West Syndrome)

Infantile spasms are a unique form of epilepsy, with onset during the first year of life. The seizures are characterized by a sudden contraction of neck, trunk, and extremity muscles. The spasms may be flexor, extensor, or mixed flexor-extensor and last only a few seconds each, but they often occur in clusters of up to 100 individual spasms. A typical episode is characterized by dropping of the head along with abduction of the shoulders and flexion of the lower extremities. The infant may cry during or after the spasm. Pallor, flushing, grimacing, laughter, and nystagmus are observed during some episodes. Episodes are common on awakening from sleep, during drowsiness, and with feedings but are rare during sleep. The peak age of infantile spasm onset is between 3 and 7 months,[5] with an estimated incidence of 0.24 to 0.60 per 1000 infants.[9] Boys are more likely to be affected than girls.

Infantile spasms are usually divided into symptomatic and cryptogenic groups based on the presence of a predisposing etiologic factor. Included among symptomatic infantile spasms are infants who have abnormal neurologic development before the onset of spasms. Causes include structural abnormalities of the brain, hypoxic-ischemic insults, CNS infections or hemorrhages, and inborn errors of metabolism. Children who have tuberous sclerosis account for up to 25% of patients who have symptomatic infantile spasms.[5] The cryptogenic group includes patients in whom no etiologic factor can be found. Infants in this group tend to be older at the onset of infantile spasms compared with infants in the symptomatic group.

The EEG pattern associated with infantile spasms is known as *hypsarrhythmia* and is characterized by high-voltage slow waves with irregularly interspersed multifocal spike-and-sharp waves. Hypsarrhythmia may precede the onset of clinical manifestations, or it may occur later or not at all. Over time, the hypsarrhythmia usually evolves into other focal or generalized abnormalities; in some cases, the EEG may normalize.

Infantile spasms are resistant to treatment with most anticonvulsants. The treatment used most commonly in the cryptogenic group is adrenocorticotropic hormone (ACTH). ACTH in a long-acting form is administered as a single daily intramuscular dose of 20 to 40 IU. Adverse effects of ACTH and steroids are significant and include Cushing syndrome, hypertension, susceptibility to infections, hyperglycemia, gastrointestinal bleeding, and electrolyte disturbance. In the symptomatic group, alternative anticonvulsants may be tried before ACTH. The benzodiazepines are also effective in controlling infantile spasms. Nitrazepam seems to be more effective than clonazepam or diazepam. Both valproic acid and topiramate are effective therapy for infantile spasms in some infants.[10] Zonisamide can be effective against infantile spasms.

The prognosis for infants who have infantile spasms remains grave. The average mortality is approximately 20%, with aspiration pneumonia related to severe developmental abnormalities being a common cause of death.[5] Approximately 80% of survivors are intellectually disabled. The spasms usually remit by a few years of age, but 55% to 60% of patients subsequently develop other forms of seizures.[5] The prognosis is more favorable for infants whose neurologic development was normal before the onset of the spasms.

Lennox-Gastaut Syndrome

Lennox-Gastaut syndrome is a severe epileptic encephalopathy characterized by a variety of generalized seizures. Tonic seizures cause sudden, sustained contraction of the muscle groups, at times causing the patient to fall. Atypical absence seizures consist of a brief period of staring and immobility. The onset and recovery of atypical absence seizures are less abrupt than those of typical absence seizures. The episodes may be associated with mild tonic motor manifestations, automatisms, or loss of postural tone. Atonic seizures occur and may be preceded by myoclonic jerks. Tonic-clonic seizures and partial seizures also may occur in patients who have Lennox-Gastaut syndrome.

Most of these patients begin to have seizures between 3 and 5 years of age[11]; boys are affected slightly more frequently than girls. Many patients have neurologic deficits before the onset of Lennox-Gastaut syndrome, including intellectual disability and cerebral palsy, which may be related to hypoxic or other insults to the brain or abnormal brain development. Patients may have a history of infantile spasms. The EEG typically shows an irregular, high-voltage, slow (2.5 Hz or slower) spike-wave pattern. The discharges are bilaterally synchronous.

Valproate has been the most successful agent used in treating different seizure types and is the drug of choice. Lamotrigine, topiramate, and felbamate have been shown to reduce significantly the frequency of atonic and generalized tonic-clonic seizures.[12,13] The benzodiazepines have also been successful in controlling atonic, myoclonic, and atypical absence seizures. Unfortunately, with increasing doses the frequency of adverse effects also increases. The development of tolerance is also is a problem associated with the use of benzodiazepines. Ethosuximide can help control the atypical absence episodes, and phenytoin can be used for tonic seizures. A ketogenic diet has also been beneficial in seizure control, but because of the nature of the diet, compliance may be a problem. Generally, the goal of treatment is to achieve reasonable seizure control with as few medications as possible to minimize adverse effects. In some instances, the seizures typical of Lennox-Gastaut syndrome occur in otherwise healthy preschool-aged children, associated with normal background and fast polyspike-and-wave changes on EEG. These children have a much better prognosis for seizure control and cognitive development.

Juvenile Myoclonic Epilepsy

Juvenile myoclonic epilepsy is a primary generalized epilepsy with an age of onset of 12 to 18 years. It represents 7% of all epilepsy and is characterized by myoclonic jerks that affect mainly the upper extremities and less commonly the lower extremities. The jerks usually occur shortly after awakening, and patients may complain of clumsiness or difficulty holding objects early in the morning. Approximately 80% of patients have generalized tonic-clonic seizures, and 25% have absence seizures in addition to myoclonic seizures.[14] Myoclonic jerks almost always precede the onset of generalized tonic-clonic seizures by months to years. A teenager who has generalized tonic-clonic seizures should be questioned carefully regarding myoclonic jerks. Both the myoclonic jerks and the tonic-clonic seizures may be precipitated by sleep deprivation, stress, alcohol, and hormonal changes. Patients remain neurologically normal. Juvenile myoclonic epilepsy is genetic; a locus on the short arm of chromosome 6 has been identified.[15] The ictal EEG typically shows generalized, symmetrical polyspike and waves at 4 to 6 Hz. Photic stimulation precipitates the electrical discharges in some patients.

Valproate will control the myoclonic jerks, absence seizures, and generalized tonic-clonic seizures in more than 80% of patients but is often avoided in women of childbearing age. Lamotrigine is also effective in most patients. Topiramate, zonisamide, and levetiracetam may be effective, but phenytoin is not, and carbamazepine may exacerbate the seizures. The rate of seizure recurrence among patients who discontinue therapy is high. Juvenile myoclonic epilepsy therefore is considered a lifelong condition that requires continuous treatment.

Partial Seizures

Simple Partial Seizures

Simple partial seizures are characterized by seizure activity with focal or limited manifestations and preserved consciousness. The symptoms may be motor, sensory, or cognitive, depending on the location of the neuronal discharge. Motor seizures may be restricted to part of the body, such as the face or a limb, or they may spread to involve the entire side. If the seizure discharge spreads to structures involved in consciousness, then the seizure will become a complex partial seizure. The seizure activity may also spread to the opposite side of the brain, causing a generalized seizure. A partial or secondary generalized seizure may be followed by Todd paralysis, a weakness of the limbs most involved in the seizure. Partial sensory seizures are most often displayed by paresthesias lasting less than 1 to 2 minutes. Seizure discharges from one occipital lobe may cause visual symptoms such as scintillating colored spots or scotomata in the visual field contralateral to the discharge. Seizures with more complex visual hallucinations often progress to complex partial seizures with diminished consciousness. Auditory seizures are manifested by hearing noises and less commonly by having elaborate but usually nonverbal auditory hallucinations such as hearing music.

Although simple partial seizures are caused by focal epileptiform discharges, a focal structural lesion may not be found in most patients. Identifiable causes associated with these seizures include prenatal and perinatal insults, CNS malformations and tumors, and, rarely, inborn errors of metabolism. Most anticonvulsants are equally effective in the treatment of simple partial seizures, but these seizures are sometimes hard to control.

Complex Partial Seizures

Complex partial seizures are seizures that originate in a limited area of one cerebral hemisphere and result in impaired consciousness. A complex partial seizure may begin as a simple partial seizure that progresses to impairment of consciousness. The initial portion of a seizure that occurs before consciousness is lost is referred to as the *aura*. The aura may consist of any of a wide variety of symptoms, depending on the location of cortical discharges. Auditory, olfactory, or visual illusions or hallucinations may occur. Affective symptoms such as fear or other unpleasant feelings can occur. Anger and rage are extremely rare as seizure manifestations but may occur during postictal confusion if the patient is restrained.

Déjà vu, the feeling that an experience has occurred before, and jamais vu, the feeling that a previously experienced sensation is unfamiliar and strange, and a *rising* epigastric sensation are common auras. Young children have difficulty describing their aura and may say only that a "funny feeling" occurred in the head or stomach. Staring and automatisms, which are involuntary coordinated motor activities, occur when clouding of consciousness occurs. Automatisms include simple phenomena such as chewing, lip smacking, swallowing, and hissing, as well as more complicated activities such as picking at clothes, searching, or ambulating. Automatisms are usually followed by postictal amnesia. The child may become tired and go to sleep.

Complex partial seizures must be distinguished from absence seizures, which are also characterized by staring and unresponsiveness. Episodes of absence seizures have an abrupt onset and termination compared with complex partial seizures, which have a more gradual onset and termination. Absence seizures last less than 30 seconds and are not associated with postictal confusion. Automatisms can occur if absence episodes are prolonged, but they are often just a continuation of motor activity present before the onset of the seizure.

The most frequent EEG finding in complex partial seizures is an anterior temporal lobe spike discharge, although some patients will have spike discharges from other areas. Interictal EEG findings are often normal. Repeating the EEG increases the likelihood of demonstrating the abnormal discharge. Nasopharyngeal or sphenoidal electrodes rarely add information that is not obtained by scalp recordings that include special temporal placements.

Causes of complex partial seizures include perinatal insults, head trauma, encephalitis, and possibly status epilepticus, all of which may be associated with scarring of the temporal lobe. Indolent tumors such as hamartomas and low-grade gliomas can also cause complex partial seizures and are found in approximately 20% of persons who have intractable partial seizures. Genetic factors play a secondary role in the etiology of complex seizures.[5]

Anticonvulsant drugs used in the treatment of complex partial seizures include carbamazepine, oxcarbazepine, and valproate. These and most of the newer anticonvulsant medications are used preferentially to phenytoin, phenobarbital, and primidone. Carbamazepine is the drug of choice in children because of its efficacy and relatively mild adverse effects. If seizures are not controlled with carbamazepine, then the addition of acetazolamide may result in improved seizure control.[16] For some patients, oxcarbazepine is less sedating. In infants and very young children, phenobarbital may be tried first. Patients who have medically intractable partial seizures should be evaluated at a comprehensive epilepsy center to determine their candidacy for surgical intervention, which results in complete seizure control in up to 90% of patients.[17]

Benign Partial Epilepsy of Childhood

Benign partial epilepsy of childhood also is known as *rolandic epilepsy, sylvian seizures,* and *centrotemporal epilepsy.* This epilepsy syndrome is a common type of partial motor epilepsy in childhood. The onset is usually between 5 and 8 years of age. Boys are more often affected than girls. Genetic factors play a role in the etiology. The seizures typically occur during sleep, although patients may occasionally have episodes during wakefulness. Episodes are characterized by the child awakening with one side of the face twitching. The oropharyngeal muscles are also often involved, causing the child to make unintelligible gurgling sounds. The ipsilateral upper extremity may be involved, but only rarely is the lower extremity involved. In rare cases, a seizure episode will become generalized. Consciousness is often retained during the seizure, although the child may not be able to speak. Most seizure episodes last less than 2 minutes. The frequency of seizures is low, with 25% of patients having a single-seizure episode and 50% having fewer than five episodes.[5] The typical EEG findings are midtemporal or centrotemporal spike discharges occurring unilaterally or independently bilaterally, often frequent in light sleep and sometimes induced by hyperventilation. Neuroradiologic studies show no abnormalities to correlate with the EEG focus. If a child has infrequent episodes, then no treatment may be needed. If the episodes frighten the child and a decision is made to initiate treatment, then carbamazepine has been the drug of choice, and most anticonvulsants are effective. Some children with rolandic epilepsy are also prone to absence seizures, and carbamazepine may exacerbate the absences. The partial seizures remit when the child is approximately 9 to 12 years of age, but no later than 17 years of age. Remission is long lasting, and no developmental or neurologic impairment is associated with these seizures other than some increased incidence of attention deficit.

Epilepsia Partialis Continua

Epilepsia partialis continua is a rare type of seizure in which twitching is continuous and limited to one side of the body. The twitching frequently involves only a few muscles and occurs most often in the hand or foot. Consciousness is preserved, but the seizure activity might weaken the extremity involved. Seizure activity may persist for hours to months. Focal encephalitis and tumor have been associated with this type of seizure. Most anticonvulsants have some efficacy, but medical control of epilepsia partialis continua is generally difficult to achieve.

Unclassified Seizures

Neonatal Seizures

Seizures are the most common manifestation of neonatal neurologic disease and occur in approximately 0.5% of all newborns.[18] For a long time, seizures have been identified only clinically, but as EEG has become more available to intensive care nurseries, it has been recognized that acute injury of the neonatal brain results in frequent subclinical electrographic seizures that can only be recognized with an EEG. In fact, particularly after initiating antiseizure medication, only 10% or less of electrographic seizures in the neonate may be recognized clinically. Additionally, the antiseizure medications that are available for newborns in parenteral forms (phenobarbital, phenytoin, and lorazepam) are not effective in stopping these electrographic seizures, which tend to last several days after the injury. Genuine debate exists about whether seizures in the neonate can further the brain damage that caused them.[19] Hence uniformity of opinion is lacking about how aggressive to be in identifying and treating neonatal seizures, particularly the larger portion of neonatal seizures that are not recognized clinically.[20]

The combination of clinical manifestations of neonatal seizures and their likelihood of being associated with simultaneous electrographic seizures has led to revised classifications of seizures in the neonate. The clinical manifestations are classified as follows:

1. Subtle seizures occur in both full-term and premature infants and are often overlooked. These seizures consist of eye deviation, blinking, sucking, swimming movements of the arms, pedaling movements of the legs, and apnea. EEG recordings do not always show correlation of electrical seizure discharges with

the clinical seizure activity. This finding has raised the possibility that, in some instances, the abnormal movements arise from regions of the brain from which abnormal electrical activity cannot be detected with surface electrodes or that they may not be seizures. Subtle seizures usually occur in infants who have severe CNS insults.

2. Clonic seizures are either focal or multifocal. Focal clonic seizures are characterized by clonic jerking that remains localized and is almost always associated with electrographic seizure discharges from the central part of the opposite hemisphere. Although focal clonic seizures can result from focal CNS lesions such as cerebral infarction, they can also occur with metabolic disturbances. Multifocal clonic seizures are characterized by clonic activity in one extremity that migrates randomly and often rapidly from side to side and place to place within the body. The EEG shows multifocal independent areas of electrical discharge.

   Clonic seizures should be differentiated from benign neonatal sleep myoclonus, which consists of small-amplitude clonic activity that may wax and wane in various parts of the body. These movements occur in healthy term neonates and infants only during sleep and are accompanied by a normal EEG throughout the jerking period. Benign neonatal sleep myoclonus is self-limited and not associated with later epilepsy.

3. Tonic seizures are focal or generalized. Focal tonic seizures are characterized by sustained posturing of a limb or asymmetrical posturing of the neck and trunk and possibly accompanying subtle seizure activity such as eye deviation. Generalized tonic seizures are characterized by tonic extension of the limbs. Less commonly, the upper extremities are flexed and the lower extremities are extended. They often have no electrographic correlate and may be some kind of brain stem phenomenon rather than seizures. They are usually associated with severe EEG background abnormalities. In premature infants, they may occur at the onset of severe intraventricular bleeding.

4. Myoclonic seizures are flexion jerks of the upper or lower extremities. They may occur singly or in a series of repetitive jerks, and they are sometimes associated with tonic spasms and multifocal seizures. Myoclonic seizures may persist into infancy and become or be followed by infantile spasms. The EEGs in infants with myoclonic seizures are usually abnormal. They may show a burst suppression pattern, although the EEG may not change during the myoclonic event. Infants with myoclonic seizures tend to have severely abnormal dysgenetic brains, or metabolic defects. Occasionally, the seizures are cryptogenic. Infants with these seizures may later develop infantile spasms. These myoclonic seizures should be differentiated from benign myoclonic jerks that occur during sleep in neonates and are accompanied by a normal EEG.

   Jitteriness is a movement in neonates that may be confused with seizure activity. The movement is a tremor that is stimulus sensitive and can be stopped by passively flexing the affected limb. Jitteriness is not associated with ocular phenomena.

Some investigators advocate the identification of neonatal seizures by EEG recording, maintaining that only electrical seizures are true seizures and require treatment. However, this theory remains controversial because identical clinical seizures in the same infant may, at times, not be associated with electrical seizures.[21] Clearly, however, electrical seizures may not have clinical correlates; hence EEG recording should be done for all infants at risk for seizures to identify these clinically silent electrical seizures.

When managing neonatal seizures, the clinician must pursue rapidly the treatable causes such as hypoglycemia, electrolyte imbalance, and infection, as well as to pursue EEG confirmation of seizure activity to help avoid the pitfall of treating coarse jitteriness or other transient abnormal movements with antiseizure medication.[22] Treating the seizures themselves is urgent if they interfere with vital functions such as maintaining good arterial oxygen saturation. An approach to the treatment of neonatal seizures is outlined in Box 320-2.

The prognosis of neonatal seizures relates to the underlying diseases that caused them. Intellectual disability and cerebral palsy are more common sequelae than seizures. Infants who have seizures related to

BOX 320-2 An Approach to the Treatment of Neonatal Seizures

- Ensure adequate ventilation and perfusion.
- Obtain blood for glucose, calcium, magnesium, and electrolyte studies. Check a Dextrostix for an immediate determination of glucose.
- Correct any associated metabolic abnormality.
- Hypoglycemia: If glucose level is low (<40 mg/dL), immediately give 10% dextrose intravenously in a dose of 2 mL/kg. Maintain blood glucose levels above 40 mg/dL by continuous intravenous infusion, and monitor the levels in both full-term and premature infants.
- Hypocalcemia: Correct by administering 5% calcium gluconate solution, 4 mL/kg, intravenously at a rate of 1 mL/min to maintain serum calcium levels above 7 mg/dL while monitoring cardiac rate and rhythm.
- Hypomagnesemia: Correct serum magnesium levels to 1 mmol/L with 50% magnesium sulfate solution, 0.2 mL/kg, intramuscularly.
- Continued seizure activity requires administration of anticonvulsants.
- Phenobarbital is given in a loading dose of 20 mg/kg intravenously over 10 minutes. Additional doses of 5 or 10 mg/kg can be given, up to a total of 40 mg/kg.
- Phenytoin or fosphenytoin is given in a loading dose of 20 mg/kg intravenously while monitoring cardiac rhythm.
- Lorazepam can be given in doses of 0.1 mg/kg intravenously for persistent seizures.* Respiratory status should be monitored.

*Maytal J, Novak GP, King KC. Lorazepam in the treatment of refractory neonatal seizures. *J Child Neurol.* 1991;6(4):319-323.

hypoxic-ischemic encephalopathy, hypoglycemia, or bacterial meningitis have a 50% chance of developing normally; those whose seizures result from late-onset hypocalcemia and primary subarachnoid hemorrhage have a greater than 90% chance of developing normally.[23] The interictal EEG is helpful in determining the prognosis. A normal background EEG pattern is usually associated with a good neurologic outcome; a markedly abnormal background pattern such as burst suppression or marked suppression of voltage is associated with a high risk of neurologic sequelae.

Febrile Seizures

Febrile seizures are seizures that occur in young children who have fever but no evidence of intracranial infection or acute neurologic illness. Simple febrile seizures are generalized tonic-clonic convulsions that last less than 15 minutes and do not recur within 24 hours. Complex febrile seizures are less common and are focal or prolonged beyond 15 minutes or recur within 24 hours. Febrile seizures occur in children between 3 months and 5 years of age; the median age of occurrence is 18 to 22 months. Approximately 2% to 5% of children will experience a febrile convulsion; boys are more susceptible than girls. Familial clustering of febrile seizures occurs[5] and mutations of the *SCN1A* gene have been found in some families.

A febrile seizure may be the first sign that a child is ill. Whether the seizure activity is triggered by the rapid rise of fever or the actual height of the temperature is unknown. Febrile seizures can be triggered by any illness that causes fever, most frequently by otitis media and upper respiratory tract infections. The rate of febrile seizures with shigellosis, salmonellosis, and roseola is high, possibly related to a direct effect the causative organism has on the CNS or to a neurotoxin they produce.

One third of children who have a febrile seizure will have another one with another febrile illness. The younger the child is at the time of the first episode, the greater the risk is of recurrence. Approximately 50% of the recurrences occur within 6 months of the initial seizure; 75% occur within 1 year.

Usually, seizure activity has stopped by the time the child is evaluated. However, if the seizure continues, then lorazepam or diazepam should be administered (see Chapter 360, Status Epilepticus). The temperature should be brought down by using rectal antipyretics, removing blankets and clothing, and sponging. Once seizure activity is controlled, evaluation is directed toward finding the cause of the fever. If the child is younger than 1 year, or if the child has not rapidly returned to normal, then a lumbar puncture should be strongly considered to evaluate for meningitis.

The EEG is generally not helpful in evaluating children who have febrile seizures. EEG tracings recorded within 1 week of the seizure often show posterior slowing. Paroxysmal activity is seen in the EEGs of 35% to 45% of patients who are followed up for several years.[5] These EEG abnormalities do not predict recurrence of febrile seizures or the development of epilepsy.

Treatment of febrile seizures includes family education that addresses the benign nature of the seizures, the use of antipyretics, and first aid for seizures. Oral diazepam (0.33 mg/kg body weight administered every 8 hours during febrile illness) reduces the risk of recurrent febrile seizures.[24] Administration of phenobarbital, however, at the onset of a febrile illness does not prevent seizure activity because therapeutic blood levels are not achieved soon enough. Prophylactic treatment with anticonvulsant agents should be considered if neurologic development is abnormal, it is a complex febrile seizure, or the child is younger than 1 year. Administration of phenobarbital in doses that achieve blood levels of 15 mcg/mL reduces the recurrence of febrile seizures. Valproate also appears to be effective in prophylaxis; phenytoin and carbamazepine do not prevent recurrences. The adverse effects of anticonvulsant therapy must be weighed against the possible benefits. No evidence has been found that prophylactic treatment reduces the risk of subsequent epilepsy.

The risk of subsequent epilepsy in children who have febrile seizures is less than 5%. Factors associated with subsequent development of afebrile partial seizures include focal seizures, prolonged seizures, and repeated episodes of seizures with the same febrile illness. Factors associated with development of afebrile, generalized seizures include more than 3 febrile seizures, a family history of afebrile seizures, and age over 3 years at the time of the first febrile seizure.[25]

Pseudoseizures

Pseudoseizures are uncommon but must be recognized if inappropriate treatment is to be prevented. They differ from epileptic seizures in several respects. The movements are usually not clonic but may be quivering or random thrashing movements. Usually, no incontinence, injury, or tongue biting is associated with pseudoseizures. Episodes may be dramatic, with screaming and shouting. Episodes also may vary greatly in the same patient. Usually, no postictal period occurs. Pseudoseizures can occur in early childhood but are more frequent in adolescence, especially in girls.[5] Pseudoseizures may occur in children who have epileptic seizures. A detailed history and observation of an episode may be all that is needed to diagnose pseudoseizures. Capturing the pseudoseizures during video EEG monitoring establishes the diagnosis in patients in whom the distinction cannot be made clinically. Treatment is directed toward the psychosocial issues involved.

ETIOLOGY

Neonatal Seizures

Neonatal seizures have multiple origins; however, only a few causes account for most cases. Determining the cause of neonatal seizures is important because specific treatment may be indicated. The cause of the seizures is also an important factor influencing prognosis. Some of the most common causes of seizure are described as follows:

1. Hypoxia-ischemia is the most common cause of seizures in both premature and full-term infants.[22] These seizures usually begin within the first 24 hours of life and may be difficult to control for several days. Metabolic disturbances in the infant also may complicate seizure control.

2. Intracranial hemorrhage is another cause of seizures in both premature and full-term infants. Intraventricular hemorrhage is seen mainly in premature infants within the first 3 days of life. Generalized tonic seizures may be associated with severe hemorrhage involving the brain parenchyma. Infants who have a primary subarachnoid hemorrhage may not have any clinical symptoms or may develop seizures on the 2nd day of life. These infants often are full term and normal neurologically except for their seizures. Subdural hemorrhage is associated with trauma and may be associated with focal seizure activity.
3. Metabolic disturbances, especially hypoglycemia and hypocalcemia, are also associated with seizures in neonates. Infants who are small for gestational age, postterm infants, or infants of diabetic mothers are at risk for hypoglycemia, and the blood glucose level should be monitored closely. Low–birth-weight infants and infants of diabetic mothers are at risk for hypocalcemic seizures, which occur when calcium levels decrease below 7 mg/dL during the first 2 to 3 days of life. In many instances, infants who have hypocalcemia also have a history of hypoxia, which contributes to the risk of seizure. Hypocalcemic seizures that occur later are usually related to a low-calcium and high-phosphate intake. Late hypocalcemic seizures are now rare as a result of the development of formula that has an appropriate ratio of calcium and phosphorus supplementation. Other metabolic disturbances less frequently associated with seizures in neonates include hyponatremia, hypernatremia, local anesthetic intoxication, pyridoxine dependence, and a variety of inborn errors of metabolism.
4. Infection, including bacterial and viral intracranial infections, is an important cause of neonatal seizures. The most common bacterial causes are group B streptococci and *Escherichia coli*. Onset of seizures with meningitis is usually after the first 3 to 4 days of life. Prenatal nonbacterial infections causing neonatal seizures include toxoplasmosis, rubella, herpes simplex virus, coxsackievirus type B, and cytomegalovirus.
5. Malformations of the brain can cause seizures at any time during the newborn period. The malformations associated most commonly with seizures are those that have cortical dysgenesis such as lissencephaly, pachygyria, and polymicrogyria.[22]

Childhood Seizures

In most children with seizures, if an underlying cause is going to be identifiable, then the child's history or physical examination will provide clues. Whereas, in most neonates, a cause is identifiable (see section on Neonatal Seizures), in older children and adolescents, a cause is identifiable in less than 20%, and if a child has no abnormalities by history or examination at the time of onset of seizures, then a cause is rarely identified. The more abnormal the neurodevelopmental status of the child is, the more likely a cause will be identified or may already have been determined before the onset of seizures. These causes include brain malformations, genetic disorders, disorders of metabolism, traumatic or previous infectious injury of the brain, and neoplasm. Children with infantile spasms and Lennox-Gastaut syndrome are more likely to have an identifiable cause. Idiopathic generalized epilepsies such as childhood absence epilepsy and juvenile myoclonic epilepsy are more likely to be related to genetic factors.

Genetic Factors in Childhood Epilepsy

Family histories and twin studies clearly show that genetic factors play a role in some children with epilepsy. Additionally, the fact that some genetic syndromes such as Angelman syndrome and Rett syndrome predispose a child to seizures raises interest in the role of different genes in the susceptibility to seizures. Several genes have been identified that govern the formation of the subunits of potassium and sodium channels and of the gamma-aminobutyric acid type A and acetylcholine receptors in nerve cell membranes. Aberrations in these genes lead to increased excitability of nerve cell membranes. Benign familial neonatal and infantile convulsions have been linked to potassium channel subunit genes *KCNQ2* and *KCNQ3* and to the *SCN2A* gene, which governs the α-2 subunit of the neuronal sodium channel. Other genes have been identified in a group of familial epilepsies called generalized epilepsy with febrile seizures plus (GEFS+). The epilepsies within these families include a range of severity from recurrent febrile seizures to febrile seizures followed by multiple seizure types including absence, myoclonic and astatic seizures, and even partial seizures of temporal lobe origin. The most commonly found genetic abnormalities in these families are mutations of the *SCN1A* gene. In several relatively rare familial focal epilepsies, mutations of other genes have been found.

Even in families with identifiable mutations of one of these genes, the severity of the epilepsy may vary, suggesting that other genes modify the expression of their primary genetic abnormality. Probably a significant number of yet-to-be-identified genes play a direct or indirect role in the excitability of the nerve cell membrane and together define each individual's seizure threshold that is then modified by environmental factors. A helpful overview of the current knowledge of genetic factors in epilepsy has been written by Scheffer and Berkovic.[26]

DIFFERENTIAL DIAGNOSIS

The first step in treating the child who has a seizure is making the correct diagnosis. Seizures must be differentiated from other paroxysmal disorders in childhood such as syncope, breath-holding spells, staring related to inattention, paroxysmal vertigo, cardiac arrhythmias, and stereotypic behaviors (see Chapter 206, Nonconvulsive Periodic Disorders). Additionally, the type of seizure should be identified to decide what diagnostic tests to pursue.

EVALUATION

Laboratory Evaluation

Laboratory tests usually performed at the time of the initial seizure include measurement of serum electrolytes, calcium, magnesium, and blood glucose. In some cases, the history or examination may indicate that a more extensive laboratory evaluation is required.

Electroencephalography

The EEG, which measures the physiological function of the brain, changes throughout childhood, reflecting brain maturation. The EEG is important in evaluating a child who has seizures because it helps define the seizure type. An epileptiform EEG may support the diagnosis of epilepsy, but a normal tracing does not exclude the diagnosis. Other abnormalities, such as slowing and background disorganization, are much less specific. Repeat tracings increase the likelihood of detecting epileptiform discharges in patients who have seizures. Procedures such as hyperventilation, photic stimulation, and sleep should be used when obtaining EEG recordings. Nasopharyngeal and sphenoidal electrodes may be used to detect mesial temporal discharges, but they rarely add information to that obtainable by special scalp electrode placements. Video EEG monitoring is useful in correlating clinical symptoms with electrical seizure activity and may be useful when clinical manifestations are atypical or pseudoseizures are in question. Although the EEG provides electrophysiological evidence to support the diagnosis of epilepsy, EEG abnormalities must be interpreted in view of the clinical symptoms. Some individuals have epileptiform discharges and other EEG abnormalities without ever having a clinical seizure; anticonvulsant treatment is not indicated for such individuals. The two most common epileptiform abnormalities seen in children who have not had a seizure are centrotemporal spikes and 3-Hz spike and wave in drowsiness or light sleep.

Neuroimaging Studies

Plain radiographs of the skull can detect calcifications that may be seen in some syndromes, but they rarely help in evaluating children who have epilepsy. Computed tomography (CT) and magnetic resonance imaging (MRI) have replaced skull radiographs in the evaluation of seizures. CT and MRI scanning detect structural abnormalities; MRI is more sensitive than CT in detecting low-grade tumors, changes in myelination, and heterotopic gray matter. Neuroimaging studies are not warranted in every child who has epilepsy; however, an MRI should be performed in children who have focal neurologic abnormalities on examination or have intractable epilepsy. Positron emission tomographic and single-photon emission computed tomographic scans are useful in localizing metabolic alterations with seizure activity and seizure foci, but their clinical relevance is only in individuals with intractable epilepsy being evaluated for epilepsy surgery.

Lumbar Puncture

The cerebrospinal fluid should be examined in patients in whom meningitis or encephalitis is suspected. In other patients, the lumbar puncture is rarely helpful and is not indicated routinely.

Screening for Associated Learning and Behavioral Problems

Children with epilepsy and without retardation tend to have more learning problems, especially reading problems[27,28] and attention deficit,[29,30] than children without epilepsy. Additionally, behavioral problems may be identified in up to 50% of children with epilepsy[22,31] and this number may increase with the added adverse effects of medication and the burden of a chronic disorder. Hence determining by history, school records, behavioral checklists, or any combination whether these comorbidities exist is essential so that they may also be addressed, thus improving the overall outcome of the child with epilepsy.

MANAGEMENT

Seizures in Neonates

After clinical seizures are controlled, electrographic seizures may continue and, if frequent or prolonged, may merit further anticonvulsant therapy. In general, seizures related to acute injuries such as asphyxia, stroke, or acute CNS infections other than herpes are self-limited and stop after several days, though they may recur months or years later. No evidence has been found that continuing treatment past the neonatal period will change the chance of recurrence later. Therefore seizures caused by acute injuries are usually treated short term, and, in many nurseries, infants are not sent home on anticonvulsants; or if they are, then anticonvulsants are continued for only a few weeks. Because phenobarbital has a long half-life, especially in asphyxiated infants, it will remain at good levels after a full loading dose for several days, and no maintenance therapy may be needed. Seizures related to brain malformations or inborn errors of metabolism may be much more persistent, and the duration of treatment will depend on the infant's clinical course.

Seizures in Children Beyond the Neonatal Period

The risk of seizure recurrence is important when deciding whether to initiate antiepileptic therapy. Some types of seizures, such as absence, myoclonic, akinetic, and infantile spasms, have a recurrence rate of virtually 100% and have usually recurred by the time the child is seen by the primary care physician. These types of seizures require treatment. However, children who have a generalized tonic-clonic or partial seizure have a recurrence risk of approximately 40%.[32,33] Factors that increase the risk of recurrence include a partial complex seizure, an abnormal neurologic examination, and focal epileptiform abnormalities on the EEG. The best prognosis is in children who have a generalized seizure, normal neurologic examination, and a nonepileptiform EEG. Many patients who have a single seizure should be observed for recurrence but should not be given antiepileptic medication. More than 50% of the recurrences occur within 6 months, up to 69% within 1 year, and 88% within 2 years.[33] If a second seizure occurs, then initiation of antiepileptic medication should be considered because approximately 80% of children who have a second seizure will have more seizures.[34]

Once the child has had recurrent seizures and antiepileptic medication is indicated, the primary care physician is faced with the decision of which medication to prescribe. Diagnosing seizure type correctly is the critical first step in treatment because some seizure disorders respond to certain medications. With the increasing understanding of gene aberrations that predispose individuals to epilepsy and the growing field of pharmacogenetics, the hope of being able to choose the best medication at the best dose for a particular individual with epilepsy may soon be realized. Meanwhile, in choosing among potentially effective antiepileptic agents for the specific individual's seizures, the drug that has the least adverse effects should be selected. The medication is given at a dose that will result in a low therapeutic blood level. The dose should be increased until seizures are controlled or adverse effects become unacceptable. If the initial medication is not fully effective, then a second medication may be added. Consideration should be given to discontinuing use of the first medication if seizures are fully controlled with the second medication. Striving for monotherapy is important, if possible, given that polytherapy often does not improve seizure control but may significantly increase toxicity. Closely monitoring for the potential cognitive and behavioral adverse effects[35] of the antiepileptic medications is essential.

When devising an optimal dosing regimen, primary care physicians should consider the pharmacokinetics of the various antiepileptic medications. The dosing frequency is determined by the *half-life,* defined as the time in which the serum level decreases to 50% of the initial value. The dosing interval should be no longer than the half-life of the medication, which means that most antiepileptic agents may be administered twice a day and some only once daily. The efficacy of an antiepileptic medication should be evaluated only after 5 half-lives have elapsed because this period is required for the medication to reach a steady state. In antiepileptic medications that induce hepatic enzymes (eg, phenobarbital, phenytoin, carbamazepine), the half-life decreases during the first weeks of treatment. If breakthrough seizures occur at times of low (trough) serum drug levels, or if toxic effects occur at times of peak serum drug levels, then the frequency of dosing should be increased. Patients requiring higher antiepileptic medication levels usually need more frequent dosing to avoid toxic effects.

Serum drug levels can guide the adjusting of doses of antiepileptic medications. A baseline level should be obtained when the patient has been taking an appropriate dose long enough to have stable levels. Other indications for obtaining levels include verification of compliance, breakthrough seizures, and toxic effects. Levels may also be checked when other medications have been added or deleted from the patient's regimen. The timing of the sample in relation to the last dose is important in the interpretation of the levels, especially in drugs with short half-lives.

Specific Antiepileptic Medications

In the last 13 years, multiple new anticonvulsant drugs have been approved for use in the United States. These drugs include felbamate (1993), gabapentin (1994), lamotrigine (1995), topiramate (1996), tiagabine (1997), levetiracetam (1999), oxcarbazepine (2000), zonisamide (2000), and pregabalin (2006). All of these drugs were originally tested and approved as add-on therapy for partial seizures. Most have undergone trials with additional seizure types and in younger children after their original approval, and some have thus received additional US Food and Drug Administration (FDA)-approved indications or evidence exists for wider use than their current FDA-approved indications. Lamotrigine, topiramate, and zonisamide have been demonstrated to have efficacy in primary generalized seizures and similar evidence is emerging for levetiracetam.[36,37] Except for gabapentin and tiagabine, which have been generally less effective than the others, these newer anticonvulsants are becoming more widely used than many of the older ones because of their better side effect profiles. The newest, pregabalin, is approved for adjunctive therapy in individuals older than 18 years; undoubtedly, trials in children will be available soon.

Table 320-1 outlines commonly used antiepileptic medications and their properties.

Phenobarbital

Phenobarbital is one of the oldest antiepileptic agents still in use. Because of its long half-life, it has the advantage of requiring dosing only once or twice a day. The dose per kilogram decreases as body weight increases. Failure to decrease the per-kilogram dose levels in older children will result in toxic levels. Because phenobarbital is a relatively safe medication in terms of serious toxic effects, monitoring of parameters other than serum levels is not necessary. The major disadvantage of phenobarbital is its effect on behavior and cognitive function, including hyperactivity, irritability, and attention deficits. Maintaining serum levels at the minimum level for seizure control may help decrease these adverse effects. Phenobarbital administration will lower the serum levels of carbamazepine and valproate. Administration of valproate will increase phenobarbital levels; therefore phenobarbital doses should be decreased by 25% to 50% to prevent toxic effects when prescribed concomitantly with valproate.

Phenytoin

Phenytoin is also an older antiepileptic medication, used widely in the past. It is used infrequently now for long-term therapy because alternatives with fewer adverse effects and more steady pharmacokinetics are available. Phenytoin has zero-order kinetics, causing blood levels to vary significantly with small changes in dose. Therefore changes in dose should be monitored via serum levels, and only small dose changes should be made when serum levels are close to or within the therapeutic range. Phenytoin is commonly used for treatment of status epilepticus because intravenous administration results in rapid penetration into the CNS. Fosphenytoin is a water-soluble prodrug of phenytoin with a more neutral pH and less tissue irritation. It can be administered intravenously or intramuscularly,[38] whereas phenytoin may not be used intramuscularly. Although phenytoin is an effective antiepileptic agent in generalized tonic-clonic and partial seizures, its adverse effects limit its use. Cosmetic

Table 320-1 Common Antiepileptic Medications

DRUG	INDICATIONS	HALF-LIFE (HOURS)	USUAL DAILY DOSE (mg/kg)	THERAPEUTIC LEVELS (mcg/mL)	ADVERSE EFFECTS
Carbamazepine	Partial, secondary generalized	18-55, initially 3-23 on chronic therapy	2-5, initially 5-25	4-12	Allergic rashes, nausea, diplopia, blurry vision, dizziness, hypersensitivity, hepatitis, aplastic anemia
Phenytoin	Partial, secondary generalized	7-42 (nonlinear kinetics)	5-7	10-20 (occasionally lower)	Rashes, hirsutism, gingival hyperplasia, coarse features, psychomotor slowing, neuropathy, folate deficiency, myelosuppression, drug-induced lupus
Valproic acid	Primary generalized, absence, myoclonic, akinetic, febrile, infantile spasms, Lennox-Gastaut syndrome, partial	6-16	10-30, monotherapy May need more in polytherapy	50-100 (150 if tolerated)	Nausea, tremor, weight gain, hair loss, thrombocytopenia, hepatic failure, pancreatitis
Phenobarbital	Neonatal, febrile, partial, secondary generalized, primary generalized, akinetic	36-120	3-5 (<25 kg) 2-3 (25-50 kg) 1-2 (>50 kg)	10-40	Sedation, inattention, hyperactivity, irritability, cognitive impairment, rare hypersensitivity reactions
Ethosuximide	Absence, myoclonic, akinetic	15-68	15-40	40-100	Nausea, abdominal discomfort, hiccups, drowsiness, behavioral problems, dystonias, myelosuppression, drug-induced lupus
Primidone	Partial, secondary generalized, primary generalized	3-20	1-2, initially 5-10	5-12	Sedation, irritability, psychomotor slowing, rare hematological and hypersensitivity reactions
Clonazepam	Absence, primary generalized, infantile spasms	20-36	0.01-0.2	0.01-0.07	Sedation, hyperactivity, inattention, aggressiveness, tolerance, ataxia, withdrawal seizures
Acetazolamide	Absence, myoclonic, akinetic, partial	10-12	10-20	10-14	Diuresis, paresthesias, sedation, carbon dioxide retention, rashes
Felbamate	Partial (in patients >12 years), Lennox-Gastaut syndrome	20 (in monotherapy)	15-45 (maximum of 3600 mg)		Anorexia, weight loss, nausea, insomnia, headache, fatigue, aplastic anemia

Table 320-1 Common Antiepileptic Medications—cont'd

DRUG	INDICATIONS	HALF-LIFE (HOURS)	USUAL DAILY DOSE (mg/kg)	THERAPEUTIC LEVELS (mcg/mL)	ADVERSE EFFECTS
Gabapentin	Partial, with or without secondary generalized seizures in patients >12 years	5-7	Total daily dose 900-1800 mg		Somnolence, dizziness, ataxia, fatigue
Lamotrigine	Partial, primary generalized, absence, atypical absence, atonic, myoclonic	7-45	5-15 without valproic acid, 1-5 with valproic acid MUST start at very low doses and titrate slowly over 2-3 months		Rash, including Stevens-Johnson syndrome, vomiting
Topiramate	Partial, primary generalized, tonic, atonic, atypical absence, infantile spasms	20-30	1-9		Somnolence, anorexia, fatigue, difficulty with concentration, nervousness, kidney stones, oligohidrosis
Tigabine	Partial	3-9	0.25-1.5 (maximum of 56 mg)		Dizziness, somnolence, headache, depression
Oxcarbazepine	Partial, secondarily generalized	4-9	10-50 mg/kg; start at 10 mg/kg up to 600 mg divided into 2 daily doses		Somnolence, nausea, dizziness, rash, hyponatremia
Zonisamide	Partial, primary generalized, infantile spasms	24-60	Start at 1-2 mg/kg and may work up to 10 mg/kg; top adult dose is 600 mg		Somnolence, dizziness, kidney stones, oligohidrosis
Levetiracetam	Partial, secondarily generalized	6-8	Start at 10-20 mg/kg/day, increase every 2 weeks; top dose 60 mg/kg or 3000 mg		Somnolence, irritability, hostility

adverse effects include gingival hypertrophy, hirsutism, and coarsening of the facial features. Also of concern are its effects on mood and cognitive function, which include depressed mood, slowed psychomotor functioning, and, in a few patients, depressed IQ scores.[35] Other adverse effects include folate-deficiency anemia, cerebellar degeneration, and allergic dermatitis including Stevens-Johnson syndrome. Valproic acid may lower total serum phenytoin levels, but the free phenytoin level transiently increases and then returns to its original level; thus no adjustment in dose is necessary. Phenytoin may decrease carbamazepine levels and increase phenobarbital levels.

Carbamazepine

Carbamazepine is widely used because it has relatively few effects on cognitive function. It may also affect behavior positively.[35] The most serious adverse effect associated with carbamazepine has been aplastic anemia. This effect is extremely rare, occurring at a rate of less than one case per 200,000 treatment years.[39] A complete blood cell count should be obtained before carbamazepine therapy is initiated and should be repeated after 2 to 3 weeks. Whether further blood cell counts are useful when the initial counts are normal is unclear, but they should be obtained more readily when the child is ill and are often repeated biannually or annually. Neutropenia as low as 3000/mm^3 may occur,[40] especially in association with a viral infection but does not predict more serious myelosuppression. The dose of carbamazepine may need to be changed during treatment because the drug tends to induce its own metabolic breakdown. Phenobarbital, phenytoin, primidone, and clonazepam decrease carbamazepine serum levels.

Valproic Acid

Valproic acid has a broad spectrum of efficacy and also has the advantage of minimal cognitive adverse effects. Tremor may occur with high serum levels. Other dose-related adverse effects include increased appetite, weight gain, reversible hair loss, nausea and vomiting, and thrombocytopenia. Rarely, fatal hepatotoxicity has been associated with valproic acid. Most cases occur during the first 3 months of treatment. Patients at greatest risk for hepatotoxicity are children younger than 2 years who receive valproic acid as part of antiepileptic polytherapy.[41] Patients younger than 2 years and those who develop hyperammonemia without liver failure are generally supplemented with L-carnitine, although this supplementation does not necessarily prevent the serious liver toxic effects.[42] Valproic acid should be administered extremely cautiously to patients who have preexisting hepatic dysfunction. Liver function should be monitored in patients taking valproic acid, especially those in the high-risk group. Valproic acid raises the level of phenobarbital; therefore the dose of phenobarbital must be decreased by 25% to 50% if valproic acid is added. Carbamazepine, phenobarbital, and phenytoin decrease valproic acid serum levels.

Ethosuximide

Ethosuximide has a limited spectrum of efficacy; it is used mainly for treating absence seizures and some forms of myoclonic seizures. Behavioral disturbances can occur in some children taking ethosuximide, and pancytopenia has been associated with long-term administration. Periodic blood cell counts therefore may be necessary. Ethosuximide does not interact significantly with other antiepileptic medications.

Primidone

Primidone is not a commonly used antiepileptic agent because it has no specific advantage over other agents, and it tends to be more sedating. Primidone is metabolized to phenobarbital and phenylethylmalonamide and has many of the same characteristics of phenobarbital, including behavioral and cognitive adverse effects. Because one third of primidone is metabolized to phenobarbital, phenobarbital levels should be monitored. Phenobarbital levels may be 1.3 to 2 times higher than primidone levels. Valproate increases primidone serum levels; phenytoin and carbamazepine increase the phenobarbital-to-primidone ratio.

Clonazepam

Clonazepam, a benzodiazepine, is not a first-line antiepileptic medication because of its adverse effects. It causes significant behavioral changes, including hyperactivity, decreased attention span, aggressiveness, and restlessness. It also causes increased secretions, which may be a problem in children with reactive airways or children with cerebral palsy and associated compromised swallowing mechanisms; it also may lead to swallowing dysfunction in higher levels. Additionally, similar to all of the other benzodiazepines, its efficacy is relatively short term because of tachyphylaxis. Because withdrawal of the drug may cause irritability, myoclonus, and increased seizures, it should be withdrawn slowly. Treatment with clonazepam is usually reserved for myoclonic seizures that are refractory to ethosuximide and valproic acid.

Other Benzodiazepines

Clorazepate is the least sedating of the benzodiazepines and is sometimes used adjunctively for resistant seizures. Diazepam and lorazepam may also be used. However, all of the benzodiazepines are associated with tachyphylaxis and some sedation and withdrawal seizures. Sometimes rotating from one to another helps this class of medications retain its efficacy. Their most significant place in epilepsy is in intermittent use, as in status epilepticus, for which intravenous lorazepam is the drug of choice. The rectal preparation of diazepam may be administered safely during a prolonged seizure outside the hospital setting. These drugs may also be used to stop flurries of seizures in patients predisposed to them or sometimes for nocturnal seizures.

Acetazolamide

Acetazolamide is an inhibitor of the enzyme carbonic anhydrase. It is an effective adjunctive therapy for treatment of several types of seizures, although its antiepileptic properties are not well understood.[42] Acetazolamide can be used in combination with valproic acid for treatment of absence, myoclonic, and akinetic seizures. Adding acetazolamide to carbamazepine may improve control of partial seizures.[35] Acetazolamide metabolism is not affected significantly by other medications.

Felbamate

Felbamate was approved by the FDA in 1993 for treatment of partial seizures in adults and for adjunctive therapy in children who have Lennox-Gastaut syndrome.[12] The most common adverse effects of felbamate are anorexia, weight loss, nausea, insomnia, headache, and fatigue. No serious cardiac effects have been reported. A year after felbamate was approved and widely used because of its lack of associated sedation, more than 20 cases of aplastic anemia among persons taking felbamate were reported. The incidence of and predisposing factors to this problem have not been fully determined. Its use decreased significantly after these reports and the associated warning. Only one additional case has been reported in the last 12 years, and no cases have been reported in children younger than 13 years. A few cases of hepatic toxicity have also been reported. Currently, felbamate should only be used in patients whose epilepsy is so severe that the benefits from its use outweigh the risk of aplastic anemia.[43] Felbamate interacts with phenytoin, carbamazepine, and valproate; therefore doses of these medications must be reduced by 25% to 50% when felbamate is added. Felbamate levels are lowered by medications that induce liver enzymes; consequently, felbamate doses may need to be increased.

Gabapentin

Gabapentin is approved as adjunctive therapy for partial seizures with and without secondary generalization in patients 3 years and older. Although gabapentin treatment has been shown to result in a significant reduction in seizure frequency among patients refractory to conventional anticonvulsants,[44] it has not proven to be as effective an anticonvulsant as most other agents and is currently used more for neuritic pain than for seizure control. One advantage of gabapentin is that it does not interact with other drugs. Additionally, it is 100% excreted renally, offering an advantage to patients with liver failure. In add-on trials, the most common adverse effects were somnolence, dizziness, ataxia, and fatigue.

Lamotrigine

Lamotrigine is approved for treatment of partial seizures in patients older than 16 years and as add-on therapy in patients 3 years and older with Lennox-Gastaut syndrome. Studies in children reveal that lamotrigine reduces the frequency of both partial and generalized seizures.[45-47] It was particularly effective in patients with absence,[48] atypical absence, and atonic seizures.[45] The most common adverse effects of lamotrigine are somnolence, rash, and vomiting. The rash is usually maculopapular or morbilliform, but a few cases of Stevens-Johnson syndrome have occurred. Comedication with valproic acid increases the incidence of rash. Starting a low dose of lamotrigine and slowly increasing the dose throughout 10 to 12 weeks helps minimize the risk of rash. Lamotrigine administration has no effect on the metabolism of other antiepileptic drugs; however, phenobarbital, phenytoin, and carbamazepine decrease the half-life of lamotrigine. Valproic acid increases the half-life of lamotrigine by 2- or 3-fold; therefore doses of lamotrigine should be lower when given in combination with valproic acid. The range of therapeutic plasma concentrations is wide (1 to ≥12 mcg/mL), making monitoring of serum levels less useful.

Topiramate

Topiramate is approved as initial monotherapy for partial seizures and primary generalized tonic-clonic seizures in patients 10 years and older and for adjunctive therapy in patients 2 years and older for partial and primary generalized tonic-clonic seizures and for Lennox-Gastaut syndrome.[13,36,37,49] Topiramate has also been effective for treating infantile spasms in some patients.[10] The most common adverse effects of topiramate are somnolence, anorexia, fatigue, difficulty with concentration and nervousness, and oligohidrosis. It also increases the chances of kidney stones and is rarely associated with open-angle glaucoma. Topiramate administration has minimal effects on the metabolism of other antiepileptic drugs. However, concomitant therapy with phenytoin or carbamazepine will lower topiramate levels. Topiramate is also now used for mood disorders and headache prevention.

Tiagabine

Tiagabine is approved for adjunctive therapy of partial seizures in adults. Studies show that tiagabine is effective as adjunctive or monotherapy for partial seizures in some children.[50,51] Its efficacy in generalized seizures is unclear. Adverse effects include dizziness, somnolence, and headache. Tiagabine does not alter the concentrations of other antiepileptic drugs except for a slight decrease in valproate levels. Enzyme inducers such as carbamazepine, phenytoin, and phenobarbital lower tiagabine levels. Therapeutic plasma concentrations for tiagabine have not been established. Tiagabine is used only infrequently for seizure control in children because other anticonvulsants are more effective.

Levetiracetam

Levetiracetam is approved as adjunctive therapy for partial seizures in patients 4 years and older. Evidence is emerging that it may be effective in treating primary generalized seizures. Its lack of significant adverse effects and significant drug interactions is leading to its increasing use. Adverse effects include somnolence, hostility, and nervousness. Its half-life of 6 to 8 hours means that it must be given at least 2 times a day.

Oxcarbazepine

Oxcarbazepine is approved for initial monotherapy and adjunctive therapy for partial seizures in patients 4 years and older. It is well tolerated with generally fewer adverse effects and especially less sedation than most other anticonvulsants. Infrequent dose-related adverse effects include somnolence, dizziness, diplopia, nausea, and vomiting. More serious but infrequent adverse events include rash and hyponatremia. An advantage over many drugs is its lack of drug interactions. Studies comparing oxcarbazepine with phenytoin and carbamazepine indicate similar efficacy but lower rates of discontinuation because of adverse effects, and a study comparing it with valproate indicated similar efficacy and rates of discontinuation because of adverse effects. Oxcarbazepine is rapidly becoming a drug of first choice for partial seizures. It has been shown to be effective as adjunctive therapy and well tolerated in infants and young children.[52]

Zonisamide

Zonisamide is approved as adjunctive therapy in adults with partial seizures. Few studies have evaluated its use in children in the United States. However, in Japan, where it has been available longer, zonisamide is used widely in children with both partial and primary generalized epilepsy and infantile spasms.[53] Adverse effects of zonisamide include somnolence, anorexia, dizziness, kidney stones, oligohidrosis, and rash. An advantage of zonisamide is its half-life of 24 to 60 hours, allowing once-a-day dosing.

Other Treatments for Seizures

Ketogenic Diet

In some children, the ketogenic diet has proved to be an effective alternative treatment, with one half of patients with intractable epilepsy showing a decrease in seizure frequency of 50% and some being seizure free at 1 year.[54] The benefits of fasting as a treatment for seizures were reported years ago, but the diet was not consistently used. Its popularity has waxed and waned since its introduction in the 1960s. A multicenter prospective study of the efficacy of the ketogenic diet in children with intractable epilepsy found that 10% of treated patients were seizure free at 1 year. A greater than 50% decrease in seizure frequency occurred in an additional 50% of the patients. Seizure type, patient age, and EEG abnormalities were not related to outcome.[54]

The exact mechanism by which the diet controls seizures is unknown, although ketone body formation is critical for the diet to be effective. To achieve ketosis, the patient is given a high-fat, low-protein, and low-carbohydrate diet, sometimes with calorie restriction. The patient is usually admitted to the hospital for initiation of the diet, which allows for monitoring for hypoglycemia and other complications. During the hospitalization, the dietitian teaches the parents about the diet, giving them sample menus and explaining how to measure foods. The initial use of 24 hours of fasting to initiate the diet is no longer adhered to. Strict adherence to the diet is needed for it to be successful. Complications of the diet include constipation, renal stones, fatigue, and metabolic acidosis.

Vagal Nerve Stimulation

A treatment for intractable epilepsy that emerged during the late 1980s and the 1990s is vagal nerve stimulation. The first vagal nerve stimulation device was implanted into a human in 1988.[55] Several studies have reported the use of vagal nerve stimulation in children, including children as young as 4 years. Most studies report an approximately 50% improvement of seizure frequency in one half of the children, with a few becoming seizure free. Patients selected for vagal nerve stimulation had seizures that were intractable to medical treatment or unacceptable adverse effects from medication. Some patients were continuing to have seizures despite having had epilepsy surgery. Positive effects seemed to be maintained over several years of follow-up.[56-58]

Vagal nerve stimulation is associated with alertness, a benefit to many children with intractable epilepsy who have often been experiencing sedation from their anticonvulsant therapy. Adverse effects associated with vagal nerve stimulation are generally uncommon and mild and include infection, hoarseness, neck pain, insomnia, and, occasionally, emergence of behavioral abnormalities, which may be related to increasing alertness. Improvements in language function have been noted in some patients.[59]

The vagal nerve stimulation device is surgically implanted subcutaneously in the anterior chest wall and stimulates the left vagus nerve. The mechanism for the antiepileptic effect of vagal nerve stimulation is not known, but changes in cerebrospinal fluid amino acids and activation of the noradrenergic system in the locus ceruleus occur with the stimulation.[40,60,61]

Psychosocial Issues

Treatment of the child with a seizure disorder must also address psychosocial issues. Parents and patients may have many fears and need reassurance. The terms *epilepsy* and *seizure disorder* must be explained, and parents need to understand that the diagnosis of epilepsy does not mean that their child is intellectually disabled or has a psychiatric disorder. Guidelines should be given on what to do when a child has a seizure, including positioning on the side and putting nothing in the mouth. Witnessing a seizure can be frightening. Parents may be afraid that the child is going to die and should be told that death from a seizure is rare. Helpful pamphlets are available from the Epilepsy Foundation of America, and some parents appreciate the information available in several books[62,63] for families of children with epilepsy. The Web sites for the Epilepsy Foundation of America (www.epilepsyfoundation.org) and the American Epilepsy Society (www.aesnet.org) are also helpful sources of information. Many larger communities have local chapters of the Epilepsy Society of America or independent epilepsy associations that provide education and support for individuals and families.

Activities of patients with seizures should be restricted as little as possible. A child with a seizure disorder should not swim alone or go bike riding without a helmet. However, these rules apply to all children, whether they have epilepsy or not. Contact sports are permissible when epilepsy is controlled. The decision about climbing up to certain heights should be based on how well the child's seizures are controlled. Older children who are not supervised when bathing should be encouraged to take showers rather than baths to minimize the risk of drowning if a seizure occurs. Parents need encouragement to treat the child normally and not be overprotective.

Discontinuation of Antiepileptic Therapy

After seizures have been controlled for a period of 2 years, consideration should be given to discontinuing the use of antiepileptic medications. Studies have shown that approximately 75% of children who were seizure free for longer than 2 years remained seizure free after the use of antiepileptic medications was discontinued.[64] The EEG can be helpful when considering discontinuing the use of antiepileptic medications. In children who have idiopathic epilepsy and a normal EEG, the prognosis for remaining seizure free after discontinuation of medications is good, except in juvenile myoclonic epilepsy (discussed earlier in this chapter). However, if the EEG demonstrates slowing, the risk of seizure recurrence is higher.[65] The risk of recurrence is not increased if medication is tapered over a period as short as 6 weeks.[66] Long-term follow-up of children after withdrawal of medication has shown that 50% of the recurrences occur within 6 months and 60% to 80% within 2 years.[65]

Intractable Seizures

When seizures continue despite anticonvulsant therapy, three possibilities should be considered before deciding that the child's seizures are intractable to anticonvulsant therapy:

1. Seizures may be occurring at times when the child has lower blood levels of medication because of incomplete compliance or because dosing intervals are too long.
2. The medication may not be appropriate to the child's type of seizures. Primary generalized seizures will often not respond and may even worsen if treated with medications that are indicated for partial or secondary generalized seizures (eg, carbamazepine, phenytoin). Any medication may worsen seizures in some individuals, sometimes because of associated drowsiness, but, in many instances, the reason is not currently understood.
3. The child's repeated events may represent one of the nonepileptiform paroxysmal disorders rather than an electrical seizure. Pseudoseizures can be especially difficult to differentiate from seizures because they tend to occur in persons who have epilepsy.

If a child is having electrographic seizures and the seizures continue despite appropriate amounts of the correct medications, then the child has intractable seizures. Approximately 15% of children who have epilepsy have intractable seizures, and approximately 50% of these may be appropriate candidates for epilepsy surgery. Therefore children who have intractable seizures should be referred to a center that has a multidisciplinary team of professionals, including epileptologists, specialized neurosurgeons, neurophysiologists, neuropsychologists, neuroradiologists, psychologists, and family therapists. These professionals can best determine the location of the epileptic zone within the child's brain and the potential morbidity from loss of function in that area or adjacent tissue, can perform the surgery, and can treat the secondary effects of the surgery on the child and the family. Although epilepsy surgery can be performed at any age, if it is performed soon after intractability of seizures has been established, then some of the secondary physiological and psychosocial effects of growing up with epilepsy may be prevented, and children are more likely to be able to live up to their potential in adult life.

Epilepsy surgery consists either of resecting the epileptic focus, such as a temporal lobectomy, a cortical resection, or a hemispherectomy, or of disconnecting the pathways that may facilitate the spread of epileptic activity within the brain, such as a corpus callosotomy.

The outcome from temporal lobectomies in appropriately chosen children is as good as in adults—at least 65% become seizure free, and another 15% are significantly improved; morbidity is minimal.[17,67] Hemispherectomies in children who have a congenital hemiparesis and resistant seizures originating in the damaged hemisphere result in control of seizures in 75% of cases and often result in improvement of function because the normal, opposite hemisphere is no longer being interrupted by seizure discharges.[7,13] A few cases of intractable infantile spasms associated with focal brain disturbances may also benefit from partial or complete hemispherectomies.[22] Corpus callosotomy is a palliative procedure for individuals who do not qualify for a local resection. It can be effective in controlling *drop* attacks and the resultant injuries in children who have multiple seizure types. Results are best in higher-functioning individuals who have localized CNS dysfunction as opposed to diffuse CNS dysfunction.

WHEN TO REFER

- Type of seizure is unclear.
- Seizures are refractory to medication.

WHEN TO ADMIT

- Seizures are uncontrolled or prolonged.
- Video EEG monitoring is needed.
- Rapidly changing anticonvulsant medication is needed.
- Ketogenic diet is initiated.

TOOLS FOR PRACTICE

Engaging Patients and Family

- *Epilepsy Foundation* (Web page), Epilepsy Foundation (www.epilepsyfoundation.org/).
- *Febrile Seizures* (fact sheet), American Academy of Pediatrics (www.aap.org/publiced/BR_FebrileSeizures.htm).
- *Seizures, Convulsions and Epilepsy* (fact sheet), American Academy of Pediatrics (www.aap.org/publiced/BK0_SeizuresConvulsions.htm).

Medical Decision Support

- *Epilepsy—Medical Home Initiative and Special Health Care Needs* (fact sheet), American Academy of Pediatrics (www.medicalhomeinfo.org/health/epilepsy.html).
- *Febrile Seizures* (book), Academic Press; edited by Tallie Z. Baram and Shlomo Shinnar (www.aap.org/bookstore).

AAP POLICY STATEMENTS

American Academy of Pediatrics, Baumann RJ. Technical report: treatment of the child with simple febrile seizures. *Pediatrics*. 1999;103(6):e86. (aappolicy.aappublications.org/cgi/content/full/pediatrics;103/6/e86).

American Academy of Pediatrics, Committee on Quality Improvement and the Subcommittee on Febrile Seizures. Practice parameter: long-term treatment of the child with simple febrile seizures. *Pediatrics*. 1999:103(6):1307-1309. (aappolicy.aappublications.org/cgi/content/full/pediatrics;103/6/1307).

REFERENCES

1. Hauser WA, Hersdorffer DC. *Epilepsy, Frequency, Causes, and Consequences*. New York, NY: Demos Publications; 1990.
2. Camfield CS, Camfield PR, Wirrell E, et al. Incidence of epilepsy in childhood and adolescents: a population based study in Nova Scotia from 1977-1985. *Epilepsia*. 1996;37:19.
3. Commission on Classification and Terminology of the International League Against Epilepsy. Proposal for revised clinical and electroencephalographic classification of epileptic seizures. *Epilepsia*. 1981;22(4):489-501.
4. Commission on Classification and Terminology of the International League Against Epilepsy. Proposal for classification of epilepsies and epileptic syndromes. *Epilepsia*. 1985;26(3):268-278.
5. Aicardi J. *Epilepsy in Children*. New York, NY: Raven Press; 1986.
6. Ferrie CD, Robinson RO, Knott C, et al. Lamotrigine as an add-on drug in typical absence seizures. *Acta Neurol Scand*. 1995;91(3):200-202.
7. Coppola G, Auricchio G, Federico R, et al. Lamotrigine versus valproic acid as firstline monotherapy in newly diagnosed typical absence seizures: an open-label, randomized, parallel-group study. *Epilepsia*. 2004;45:1049-1053.
8. Frank LM, Enlow T, Holmes GL, et al. Lamictal (lamotrigine) monotherapy for typical absence seizures in children. *Epilepsia*. 2000;41:357-359.
9. Holmes GL, Vigevano F. Infantile spasms. In: Engel J, Pedley TA, eds. *Epilepsy: A Comprehensive Textbook*. Philadelphia, PA: Lippincott-Raven; 1997.
10. Glauser TA, Clark PO, Strawsburg R. A pilot study of topiramate in the treatment of infantile spasms. *Epilepsia*. 1998;39(12):1324.
11. Genton P, Dravet C. Lennox-Gastaut syndrome and other childhood epileptic encephalopathies. In: Engel J, Pedley TA, eds: *Epilepsy: A Comprehensive Textbook*. Philadelphia, PA: Lippincott-Raven; 1997.
12. The Felbamate Study Group in Lennox-Gastaut Syndrome. Efficacy of felbamate in childhood epileptic encephalopathy (Lennox-Gastaut syndrome). *N Engl J Med*. 1993;328(1):29-33.
13. Glauser TA. Topiramate. *Semin Pediatr Neurol*. 1997; 4(1):34-42.
14. Janz D. Juvenile myoclonic epilepsy with typical absences. In: Duncan JS, Panayiotopoulos CP, eds. *Typical Absences and Related Syndromes*. London, UK: Churchill; 1994.
15. Durner M, Sander T, Greenberg DA, et al. Localization of idiopathic generalized epilepsy on chromosome 6p in families of juvenile myoclonic epilepsy patients, *Neurology*. 1991;41:1651-1655.
16. Ramsey RE, De Toledo J. Acetazolamide. In: Engel J, Pedley TA, eds. *Epilepsy: A Comprehensive Textbook*. Philadelphia, PA: Lippincott-Raven; 1997.
17. Engel J Jr, ed. *Surgical Treatment of the Epilepsies*. 2nd ed. New York, NY: Raven Press; 1993.
18. Mizrahi EM, Kellaway P. *Diagnosis and Management of Neonatal Seizures*. Philadelphia, PA: Lippincott-Raven; 1998.
19. Holmes GL. Do seizures cause brain damage? *Epilepsia*. 1991;32(5):S14-S28.
20. Lombroso CT. Neonatal seizures: historic note and present controversies. *Epilepsia*. 1996;37(3):5-13.
21. Weiner SP, Painter MJ, Geva D, et al. Neonatal seizures: electroclinical disassociation. *Pediatr Neurol*. 1991;7(5):363-368.
22. Uthman BM, Reid SA, Wilder BJ, et al. Outcome for West syndrome following surgical treatment. *Epilepsia*. 1991; 32(5):668-671.
23. Volpe JJ. *Neurology of the Newborn*. 4th ed. Philadelphia, PA: WB Saunders; 2001.
24. Rosman NP, Colton T, Labazzo J, et al. A controlled trial of diazepam administered during febrile illness to prevent recurrence of febrile seizure. *N Engl J Med*. 1993; 329(2):72-84.
25. Annegers JF, Hauser WA, Shirts SB, et al. Factors prognostic of unprovoked seizures after febrile convulsions. *N Engl J Med*. 1987;316:493-498.
26. Scheffer IE, Berkovic SF. Genetics of epilepsy. In: Swaiman KF, Ashwal S, Ferriero DM, eds. Pediatric *Neurology Principles & Practice*. 4th ed. St Louis, MO: Mosby-Elsevier; 2006.
27. Mitchell WG, Chavez JM, Lee H, et al. Academic underachievement in children with epilepsy. *J Child Neurol*. 1991;6:65-72.
28. Sturniola MG, Galletti F. Idiopathic epilepsy and school achievement. *Arch Dis Child*. 1994;70:424-428.
29. Stores G. School children with epilepsy at risk for learning and behavioral problems. *Dev Med Child Neurol*. 1978;20:502-508.
30. Kinney RO, Shaywitz BA, Shaywitz SE, et al. Epilepsy in children with attention deficit disorder: cognitive, behavioral and neuroanatomic indices. *Pediatr Neurol*. 1990;6:31-37.
31. Oostrom KJ, Smeets-Schouten A, Kruitwagen CL. et al. Not only a matter of epilepsy: early problems of cognition and behavior in children with epilepsy onlya prospective, longitudinal, controlled study starting at diagnosis. *Pediatrics*. 2003;112:1338-1344.
32. Berg AT, Shinnar S. The risk of seizure recurrence following a first unprovoked seizure: a quantitative review. *Neurology*. 1991;41(7):965-972.
33. Shinnar S, Berg AT, Moshe SL, et al. The risk of seizure recurrence after a first unprovoked afebrile seizure in childhood: an extended follow-up. *Pediatrics*. 1996;98(2:1): 216-225.
34. Camfield PR, Camfield CS. Pediatric epilepsy: an overview. In: Swaiman KF, Ashwal S, Ferriero DM, eds. *Pediatric Neurology Principles & Practice*. 4th ed. St Louis, MO: Mosby-Elsevier; 2006.
35. Trimble MR, Cull CA. Antiepileptic drugs, cognitive function, and behavior in children. *Cleve Clin J Med*. 1989;56(1): S140-S146.
36. French JA, Kanner AM, Bautista J, et al. Efficacy and tolerability of the new antiepileptic drugs I: treatment of new onset epilepsy: report of the Therapeutics and Technology Assessment Subcommittee and Quality Standards, Subcommittee of the American Academy of Neurology and the American Epilepsy Society. *Neurology*. 2004;62:1252-1260.
37. French JA, Kanner AM, Bautista J, et al. Efficacy and tolerability of the new antiepileptic drugs II: treatment of refractory epilepsy: report of the Therapeutics and Technology Assessment Subcommittee and Quality Standards, Subcommittee of the American Academy of Neurology and the American Epilepsy Society. *Neurology*. 2004;62:1261-1273.
38. Pellock JM. Fosphenytoin use in children. *Neurology*. 1996;46(6:1):S14-S16.

39. Kriel RL, Birnbaum AK, Cloyd JC. Antiepileptic drugtherapy in children. In: Swaiman K, Ashwal S, eds. *Pediatric Neurology Principles & Practice*. St Louis, MO: Mosby; 1999.
40. Ben-Menachem E, Hambergerr A, Hedner T, et al. Effects of vagus nerve stimulation on amino acids and other metabolites in the CSF of patients with partial seizures. *Epilepsy Res*. 1995;20:221-227.
41. Dreifuss FE, Santilli N, Langer DH, et al. Valproic acid hepatic fatalities: a retrospective review. *Neurology*. 1987; 37(3):379-385.
42. Ramsey RE, De Toledo J. Acetazolamide. In: Engel J, Pedley TA, eds. *Epilepsy: A Comprehensive Textbook*. Philadelphia, PA: Lippincott-Raven; 1997.
43. French J, Smith M, Faught E, et al. Practice advisory: the use of felbamate in the treatment of patients with intractable epilepsy. *Epilepsia*. 1999;40:803-808.
44. Anhut H, Ashman P, Feuerstein TJ, et al. Gabapentin (Neurontin) as add-on therapy in patients with partial seizures: a double-blind, placebo-controlled study. The International Gabapentin Study Group. *Epilepsia*. 1994; 35:795-801.
45. Besag FMC, Wallace SJ, Dulac O, et al. Lamotrigine for the treatment of epilepsy in childhood. *J Pediatr*. 1995; 127:991-997.
46. Mims J, Penovich P, Ritter F, et al. Treatment with high doses of lamotrigine in children and adolescents with refractory seizures. *J Child Neurol*. 1997:12(1):64-67.
47. Schlumberger E, Cavez F, Palacios L, et al. Lamotrigine in treatment of 120 children with epilepsy. *Epilepsia*. 1994;35:359-367.
48. Frank LM, Enlow T, Holmes GL, et al. Lamictal (lamotrigine) monotherapy for typical absence seizures in children. *Epilepsia*. 1999;40:973-979.
49. Elterman RD, Glauser TA, Wyllie E, et al. A double-blind, randomized trial of topiramate as adjunctive therapy for partial-onset seizures in children. Topiramate YP Study Group. *Neurology*. 1999;52(7):1338-1344.
50. Pellock JM. Tiagabine (Gabatril) experience in children. *Epilepsia*. 2001;42(3):49-51.
51. Uldall P, Bulteau C, Pedersen SA, et al. Tiagabine adjunctive therapy in children with refractory epilepsy: a single-blind dose escalating study. *Epilepsy Res*. 2000;42(2-3):159-168.
52. Pina-Garza JE, Espinoza R, Nordli D, et al. Oxcarbazepine adjunctive therapy in infants and young children with partial seizures. *Neurology*. 2005;65:1370-1375.
53. Glauser TA, Pellock JM. Zonisamide in pediatric epilepsy: review of the Japanese experience. *J Child Neurol*. 2002; 17:87-96.
54. Vining EP, Freeman JM, Ballaban-Gil K, et al. Multicenter study of the efficacy of the ketogenic diet. *Arch Neurol*. 1996;55(11):1433-1437.
55. Penry JK, Dean JC. Prevention of intractable partial seizures by intermittent vagal stimulation in humans: preliminary results. *Epilepsia*. 1990;31(suppl 2):40-43.
56. Murphy JV, Torkelson R, Dowler I, et al. Vagal nerve stimulation in refractory epilepsy: the first 100 patients receiving vagal nerve stimulation at a pediatric epilepsy center. *Arch Pediatr Adolesc Med*. 2003;157(6):560-564.
57. Patwardhan RV, Stong B, Bebin EM, et al. Efficacy of vagal nerve stimulation in children with medically refractory epilepsy. *Neurosurgery*. 2000;47(6):1353-1358.
58. Bremer A, Eriksson AS, Roste GK, et al. Vagal nerve stimulation in children with drug-resistant epilepsy. *Tidsskr Nor Laegeforen*. 2006;126(7):896-898.
59. Murphy JV, Wheless JW, Schmoll CM. Left vagal nerve stimulation in six patients with hypothalamic hamartomas. *Pediatr Neurol*. 2000;23(2):167-168.
60. Krahl SE. Possible mechanism of the seizure attenuating effects of vagus nerve stimulation. *Soc Neurosci Abst*. 1994;20:1453.
61. Naritoku DK, Wendy JT, Helfert RH. Regional induction of fos-like immunoreactivity in the brain by anticonvulsant stimulation of the vagus nerve. *Epilepsy Res*. 1995; 22(1):53-62.
62. Freeman JM, Vining EPG, Pillas DJ. *Seizures and Epilepsy in Childhood: A Guide for Parents*. 3rd ed. Baltimore, MD: Johns Hopkins University Press; 2002.
63. Jan JE, Ziegler RG, Erba G. *Does Your Child Have Epilepsy?* 2nd ed. Baltimore, MD: University Park Press; 1991.
64. [No authors listed]. Practice parameter: a guideline for discontinuing antiepileptic drugs in seizure-free patients—summary statement. Report of the Quality Standards Subcommittee of the American Academy of Neurology. *Neurology*. 1996;47(2):600-602.
65. Shinnar S, Berg AT, Moshe SL, et al. Discontinuing antiepileptic drugs in children with epilepsy: a prospective study. *Ann Neurol*. 1994;35(5):534-545.
66. Tennison M, Greenwood R, Lewis D, et al. Discontinuing antiepileptic drugs in children with epilepsy. A comparison of a six-week and a nine-month taper period. *N Engl J Med*. 1994;330(20):1407-1410.
67. Wyllie E, Comair YG, Kotogal P, et al. Seizure outcome after epilepsy surgery in children and adolescents. *Ann Neurol* 1998;44(5):740-748.

Chapter 321

SEPTIC ARTHRITIS

Stephanie Yee-Guardino, DO; Johanna Goldfarb, MD

DEFINITION OF TERMS

Pyogenic, or septic, arthritis refers to a bacterial infection of the joint space. Other forms of arthritis include reactive or postinfectious arthritis (an immunologically induced inflammatory response to a distant infection) and the arthritis associated with rheumatologic disorders (eg, juvenile idiopathic arthritis [JIA]). These latter forms of arthritis are aseptic in that no pathogens are found in the joint space or fluid. Pyogenic arthritis most commonly affects young children and infants, but it can occur at any age. Pyogenic arthritis constitutes a clinical emergency because complications of untreated infection include dissolution of articular cartilage, necrosis of the underlying epiphysis, destruction of the adjacent growth plate, and dislocation of the joint itself. Complications can be minimized by prompt diagnosis and by aggressive treatment. A high index of suspicion is necessary to avoid missing a case of septic arthritis.[1-6]

Hematogenous seeding of the synovial membrane is the most common cause of bacterial arthritis in children. Infection also can occur by contiguous spread from an adjoining osteomyelitis or by direct inoculation of bacteria into the joint after a penetrating wound, after intraarticular injection, or after joint surgery. (For a more complete discussion, see Chapter 303, Osteomyelitis.) Spread of bacteria from a bone infection into a joint occurs most often in infancy. Transphyseal blood vessels in the very young child allow early spread of bacteria from the metaphysis of the bone across the growth plate to the epiphysis and into the joint cavity. In infants therefore, infections that begin in the bone often spread quickly into the joint and often exhibit as joint symptoms.[7-9] This manifestation must be considered when evaluating a young child with localized pain, especially involving the femur or hip.[7]

The organism most commonly responsible for septic arthritis across all age groups is *Staphylococcus aureus*. In neonates, Gram-negative organisms, coagulase-negative staphylococci, and *Streptococcus agalactiae* (group B) also cause pyogenic arthritis.[5] In older infants and young children, *Haemophilus influenzae* type b was a common pathogen, but vaccination against this organism has made it extremely rare as a cause of bacterial infection in children in this country.[10] After *S aureus*, group A *Streptococcus* is the next most common cause of septic arthritis in children older than 5 years. In children younger than 5 years, *Kingella kingae* is an unusual cause of septic arthritis that requires special attention for successful culture. First described in Israel, this organism has been identified with increasing frequency in the United States.[11] Monoarticular gonococcal arthritis can occur after genital infection with *Neisseria gonorrheae*. In a sexually active teenager who has monoarticular arthritis of a large joint, evaluation should include gonococcus as a possible cause. Evaluation for genital gonococcal infection and other sexually transmitted infections should be part of the initial evaluation. The organism can be isolated from the joint and genital sites but requires attention to culture technique and prompt plating in the microbiology laboratory on media appropriate for its growth. This infection can follow, and is distinct from, the reactive arthritis involving multiple joints of disseminated gonococcal disease.[12] Gonococcal septic arthritis is a result of hematogenous seeding of the joint and can follow the bacteremia of untreated disseminated gonococcal disease. The bacteremic illness associated with *N gonorrheae* causes a reactive (sterile or aseptic) arthritis involving multiple joints and a vesicular rash. Similar to *N gonorrheae, N meningitides* also can cause a reactive arthritis. Multiple joints are involved; but unlike with the gonococcus, this arthritis occurs *after* recovery from the acute infection with meningococci and after treatment for meningitis or meningococcemia with antimicrobial therapy. This reactive arthritis resolves spontaneously over time and requires only symptomatic therapy.[13]

The consequences of bacterial arthritis can be severe. In addition to the direct destructive effects of the infection, the host's inflammatory response can add to the damage. By raising intraarticular pressure, intracapsular infection can obstruct blood flow, leading to necrosis of the epiphysis and the underlying growth plate. Finally, an untreated joint infection can result in joint instability through destruction of the ligamentous fibers of the capsule. These factors are of special concern for the hip joint in children.

Considering the possible consequences and, particularly in the young child, the potential for permanent deformity and disability, the need for accurate diagnosis and expeditious treatment of septic arthritis cannot be overly stressed.

DIFFERENTIAL DIAGNOSIS

The differential diagnosis of pyogenic arthritis includes the other forms of arthritis, reactive and rheumatologic or inflammatory, and, on occasion, leukemia. Reactive and inflammatory arthritis often involve multiple joints, whereas pyogenic arthritis almost always involves 1 joint. Although children with infective arthritis are often very ill from an associated bacteremia, rheumatologic disease is usually more subacute or chronic. A reactive arthritis often follows a prior obvious infection, such as the polyarthritis that can follow meningococcal infections; this history helps guide the diagnosis. The pattern of the inflammatory arthritis is sometimes helpful in making the diagnosis, such as the occurrence of multiple and alternating joint involvement in the arthritis associated with rheumatic fever. JIA is a diagnosis of exclusion, which can be confused with septic arthritis. When children with JIA have high fever and with single joint involvement, the diagnosis can be more confusing. In many instances, the diagnosis is made only with time when fevers persist, other joints become involved, or the single joint fails to have a pathogen isolated and fails to respond to therapy for a pyogenic infection. The diagnosis of JIA can remain unclear for weeks to months until the course clarifies the chronicity of the disease. At times, both JIA and a bacterial infection of the bones and joints can be confused with leukemia. Children with leukemia have fever and bone pain. The bone pain of leukemia can cause a limp or other nonspecific signs and can be confused with a septic joint, osteomyelitis, or JIA. Examining the bone marrow is often required to confirm the diagnosis. The laboratory tests that support a diagnosis of pyogenic arthritis can help point the evaluation in the proper direction. A child with leukemia may have anemia, low white blood cell count (see Chapter 291, Leukemias), or low platelet count. If not present at first, these signs will occur over time.

Some bacterial pathogens that cause arthritis are more difficult to identify, such as *Mycobacteria tuberculosis* or *Borrelia burgdorferi*. A history of exposure to tuberculosis or the occurrence of infection in the summer in an endemic area for Lyme disease will help direct the evaluation. These pathogens are identified by special testing, which may be prompted by abnormalities in the fluid aspirates. In both of these conditions, the fluid does not grow a common pathogen on routine cultures despite fluid analysis, which is suggestive of bacterial infection. For example, evaluation of a child for possible tuberculosis includes culturing the joint fluid for *Mycobacteria* on special media, placing a tuberculin skin test and ordering a chest radiograph to look for signs of primary infection. The child with possible Lyme disease will often have a history of the rash of erythema migrans; serologic testing can help confirm the diagnosis. Knowing the frequency of these unusual pathogens in the pediatrician's area of practice is crucial in guiding the evaluation of a child with presumed bacterial arthritis.

At times, septic arthritis causing decreased movement at a joint can be confused with an isolated neuropathy. Additionally, septic arthritis of the shoulder can cause a brachial plexus neuropathy, and septic arthritis of the hip can cause neuropathies of the femoral and sciatic nerves. These diagnoses, occurring without infection, should not be associated with pain or fever.[14]

EVALUATION

Clinical History

Signs of acute illness most often accompany the onset of septic arthritis. The onset of fever, malaise, poor appetite, irritability, and localized symptoms and signs is usually acute.[5,6] In septic arthritis, as in osteomyelitis, the neonate presents a unique challenge because systemic signs may be less apparent.[7] However, localized signs are usually prominent, particularly pain with motion of the involved joint. The failure of an infant to move an infected joint should suggest this diagnosis. When septic arthritis is present, passive movement of the affected extremity almost invariably elicits severe pain.

Physical Findings

Swelling, erythema, tenderness, and redness of the skin over the joint are usually present but are difficult to detect in a deep joint such as the hip. The most characteristic finding is pain with joint motion. When a lower extremity joint is involved, the child usually refuses to bear weight or limps. Manipulation of the hip joint, such as with diaper changes, causes significant pain. This pain is often the first sign to a parent or nurse caring for the child that a problem exists. Limited range of motion of an infected upper extremity joint may result in concerns about a neurologic problem, a *pseudoparalysis*. Although older children and teenagers are usually able to localize pain, the clinician should remember that pain can be referred to an unaffected joint. Joints of the lower extremities are the most common sites of septic arthritis, with the knee the most affected joint. Rarely, and usually with prolonged bacteremia, more than 1 joint can become infected.

Some characteristic signs help suggest the diagnosis. To decrease pain, the child will usually hold an infected joint very still. The joint is held immobile by muscle spasm in a position that maximizes capsular volume, thus minimizing the intraarticular pressure. For the hip, the preferred position is a combination of moderate flexion, abduction, and external rotation; for the knee, gentle flexion; and for the shoulder, adduction against the trunk. For a child to appear entirely well and in no distress is not unusual, so long as the affected joint is allowed to remain undisturbed. If a child holds a joint still and has a fever, then the diagnosis of septic joint is assumed.

Laboratory Testing

Laboratory results can be helpful in supporting the diagnosis of septic arthritis. The erythrocyte sedimentation rate is typically elevated, though it may be normal early in the course of infection. The C-reactive protein is also increased, and it is a more sensitive test during the initial illness because it rises earlier than the sedimentation rate. Blood cultures should always be obtained because the majority of pyogenic arthritis cases in children are of hematogenous origin. Blood cultures are positive in at least 40% of children with septic arthritis.[15]

Joint fluid in pyogenic arthritis is generally cloudy or purulent, with a leukocyte count of more than 50,000 cells/mcL and has a predominance of polymorphonuclear cells. Although the fluid of JIA can also contain many neutrophils, in general, levels are lower than with bacterial infection. Fluid should be sent quickly to the microbiology laboratory for Gram stain and culture of the joint fluid. If this action is not possible, then inoculating a blood culture bottle is acceptable, but this process may delay identification of pathogens. Though the culture is sometimes negative in cases that appear to be acute bacterial arthritis, the combination of clinical data and fluid characteristics help confirm the diagnosis. Positive joint fluid cultures are encountered in approximately 50% to 60% of cases caused by bacterial infection.[6] A joint effusion with a low white blood cell count and normal glucose suggests that the arthritis may be caused by a sympathetic effusion from an adjacent osteomyelitis, or possibly an aseptic arthritis caused by a reactive arthritis or JIA or other rheumatologic diseases.

Imaging

Early in the course of septic arthritis, bone changes are unlikely, but soft tissue changes may occur, including swelling and edematous infiltration into fatty tissue planes. Plain films, however, should be obtained to look for these early changes and to exclude other bone abnormalities. Ultrasonography has proven useful in detecting the capsular distention that accompanies septic arthritis of the hip.[16] An experienced radiologist can define the presence of a joint effusion by ultrasound of the joint and, if one is present, can assist the operator in accurate needle placement during diagnostic aspiration. Magnetic resonance imaging is sensitive and may be helpful in defining adjacent bony involvement and soft-tissue abscesses, especially in areas of complex anatomy such as the hip, sacroiliac joint, or pelvic bones. However, in clear cases of infection, therapy should not be delayed by waiting for this study to confirm a clinical diagnosis.

MANAGEMENT

Joint aspiration with a large-bore needle is the most important diagnostic maneuver, and an orthopedic surgeon skilled in the care of pediatric patients should be consulted to aspirate joints. Fluoroscopy or, possibly, ultrasonography, may be used to confirm entrance into the relatively inaccessible hip and shoulder joints. Failure to obtain pus from a joint that appears clinically to be infected can be caused by the thickness of pus in the joint, and open drainage of the joint may be necessary to confirm the diagnosis and to treat the infection.

Empiric therapy with antimicrobial agents that are appropriate for the likely pathogen should be started urgently after aspiration of the joint. Most infections are caused by *S aureus;* thus an effective antistaphylococcal antimicrobial is almost always part of the initial treatment. A penicillinase-resistant penicillin such as nafcillin or oxacillin or a 1st-generation cephalosporin is often sufficient initially. However, if the child is severely ill or has signs of bacteremia and sepsis, then broader coverage is appropriate, especially in areas with a high incidence of methicillin-resistant *S aureus*. In these children, vancomycin should be considered as initial therapy instead of a β-lactam.

A 1st-generation cephalosporin should not be used in a neonate as empiric therapy because of poor cerebrospinal fluid penetration and the concern for a bacteremia seeding the central nervous system. A safer approach would be to start empiric therapy with high doses of a penicillin that is effective for treating *S aureus*, such as oxacillin, combined with an antibiotic to treat Gram-negative enterics, such as ceftazidime or an aminoglycoside. Once a pathogen is identified, therapy should be narrowed to treat the specific organism.

Broad coverage is also appropriate for the child who is immunocompromised and the adolescent thought to be abusing an intravenous drug as the cause of a bacteremia. Antibiotics selected empirically for such patients should be effective against *S aureus*, enteric Gram-negative bacilli, and *Pseudomonas*. A broad-spectrum penicillin such as ceftazidime and an aminoglycoside with vancomycin might be empiric therapy in these children, pending final joint and blood cultures. The adolescent with possible gonococcal joint infection should be treated for staphylococci and gonococci until the diagnosis is clarified. In this situation, cefuroxime or ceftriaxone, perhaps with vancomycin, might be selected, depending on the specifics of the case.

Parenteral antibiotic therapy is continued at least until the child is doing well and signs of acute infection have resolved. Oral therapy can sometimes be used to finish treatment. This approach is possible when an organism has been identified by blood or joint fluid culture and when an effective oral agent is available. Oral antibiotics can be used only if the child's social situation guarantees reliably that the antibiotics will be given as directed and the antibiotic does not cause a gastrointestinal disturbance that might interfere with absorption or compliance. The organism must be susceptible to the oral antibiotic, and the antibiotic must achieve therapeutic levels in bone and joint. Laboratory tests such as the sedimentation rate and C-reactive protein should be normalizing before switching to an oral agent. Antibiotic therapy should continue for a minimum of 3 to 4 weeks, but treatment should not be discontinued until the clinical response is complete and the markers of inflammation such as the C-reactive protein level and erythrocyte sedimentation rate have returned to normal.[4] Treatment will be longer if concurrent osteomyelitis is present, and lengthening therapy is sometimes advisable if most of the course of therapy is oral.

A surgical referral is required because of the necessity to aspirate the joint and, at times, for diagnosing, surgery, and treating the infection. All children with septic arthritis of the hip should be seen emergently by an orthopedic surgeon because these patients require immediate drainage of the joint. Delay in draining a major joint, such as the hip joint, is associated with poorer outcome. Open debridement may be required. Other infected joints less often require open debridement but should also be evaluated for surgical treatment. Repeated aspirations of a joint may be necessary if fluid reaccumulates.

Septic arthritis is an urgent situation and requires consultation among the primary physician, orthopedic surgeon, and radiologist. Treatment is often coordinated by an infectious diseases specialist to aid in selecting an appropriate antibiotic, to monitor response, and to organize and coordinate follow-up after hospital discharge, which may include outpatient home intravenous therapy.

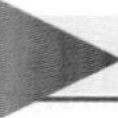

WHEN TO REFER

Children who are being evaluated for bone or joint infection should be evaluated by an orthopedic surgeon or infectious diseases specialist.

WHEN TO ADMIT

All children thought to have bacterial infection of a major joint should be hospitalized.

SUGGESTED RESOURCES

Barton LL, Dunkle LM, Habib FH. Septic arthritis in childhood. A 13-year review. *Am J Dis Child*. 1987;141(8):898-900.

Dagan R. Management of acute hematogenous osteomyelitis and septic arthritis in the pediatric patient. *Pediatr Infect Dis J*. 1993;12(1):88-92.

Fink CW, Nelson JD. Septic arthritis and osteomyelitis in children. *Clin Rheum Dis*. Aug 1986;12(2):423-435.

Green NE. Bone and joint infections in children. *Orthoped Clin North Am*. 1987;18:555-576.

Nelson JD. The bacterial etiology and antibiotic management of septic arthritis in infants and children. *Pediatrics*. 1972; 50(3):437-440.

REFERENCES

1. Dagan R. Management of acute hematogenous osteomyelitis and septic arthritis in the pediatric patient. *Pediatr Infect Dis J*. Jan 1993;12(1):88-92.
2. Green NE. Bone and joint infections in children. *Orthoped Clin North Am*. 1987;18:555-576.
3. Barton LL, Dunkle LM, Habib FH. Septic arthritis in childhood. A 13-year review. *Am J Dis Child*. Aug 1987; 141(8):898-900.
4. Nelson JD. The bacterial etiology and antibiotic management of septic arthritis in infants and children. *Pediatrics*. Sep 1972;50(3):437-440.
5. Fink CW, Nelson JD. Septic arthritis and osteomyelitis in children. *Clin Rheum Dis*. Aug 1986;12(2):423-435.
6. Nelson JD, Koontz WC. Septic arthritis in infants and children: a review of 117 cases. *Pediatrics*. Dec 1966;38(6): 966-971.
7. Morrissy R. Bone and joint infection in the neonate. *Pediatric Annals*. 1989;18:33-40.
8. Ogden JL. The pathology of neonatal osteomyelitis. *Pediatrics*. Apr 1975;55:474-478.
9. Griffin PP, Green WT Sr. Hip joint infections in infants and children. *Orthop Clin North Am*. Jan 1978;9(1):123-134.
10. Peltola H, Kallio MJ, Unkila-Kallio L. Reduced incidence of septic arthritis in children by Haemophilus influenzae type-b vaccination. Implications for treatment. *J Bone Joint Surg Br*. May 1998;80(3):471-473.
11. Morrison VA, Wagner KF. Clinical manifestations of Kingella kingae infections: case report and review. *Rev Infect Dis*. Sep-Oct 1989;11(5):776-782.
12. Masi At EB. Disseminated gonococcal infection and gonococcal arthritis: II. Clinical manifestation, diagnosis, complications, treatment and prevention. *Semin Arthritis Rheum*. Feb 1981;10:173-197.
13. Schaad UB. Arthritis in disease due to *Neisseria meningitidis*. *Rev Infect Dis*. Nov-Dec 1980;2(6):880-888.
14. Gabriel SR, Thometz JG, Jaradeh S. Septic arthritis associated with brachial plexus neuropathy. A case report. *J Bone Joint Surg Am*. Jan 1996;78(1):103-105.
15. Nade S. Acute septic arthritis in infancy and childhood. *Aust Paediatr J*. Sep 1975;11(3):145-153.
16. Chau CL, Griffith JF. Musculoskeletal infections: ultrasound appearances. *Clin Radiol*. Feb 2005;60(2):149-159.

Chapter 322

SEXUALLY TRANSMITTED INFECTIONS

Alain Joffe, MD, MPH

Fifteen to 24 year olds represent only a quarter of sexually active individuals in the United States, but almost one half of all sexually transmitted infections (STIs) occur in this age group. Several possible explanations can be given for this observation (Box 322-1). Although rates of sexual activity among adolescents decreased from 1991 to 2001 (remaining level from 2001 to 2005), approximately 47% of teenagers are sexually active and at risk for acquiring 1 or more STIs.[1,2] By virtue of their cognitive developmental level, adolescents often feel invulnerable and minimize their potential for becoming infected. They may ignore symptoms or believe that as long as they (or their sex partners) are symptom free, they are neither at risk of being infected nor capable of infecting someone else.

Much evidence indicates that consistent and correct use of condoms provides significant protection against many STIs.[3,4] Adolescents' use of condoms at last intercourse increased from 46% in 1991 to 63% in 2005, but many teenagers do not use them consistently or correctly.[1] Oral contraceptives, which are still a popular method of contraception among adolescents, may increase the risk for chlamydial infection, but they may also protect against the development of symptomatic pelvic inflammatory disease (PID).[5] Injections of the contraceptive depot medroxyprogesterone acetate (Depo-Provera) may also increase the risk for chlamydia infection.[5] No data have been collected for other forms of hormonal contraception.

Adolescents often have trouble discussing sexual matters with their partners or their parents, and they may be reluctant to reveal that they are infected or have been treated. They may postpone a visit to a physician because they are embarrassed, fear a lecture, are concerned about the physician maintaining confidentiality, or lack the money or social skills to get to a source of health care. Some physicians hesitate to provide confidential services to an adolescent with a suspected STI because they are uncertain about the adolescent's capacity to consent to treatment without parental involvement. Currently, all 50 states have laws that permit a physician to treat most minors seeking treatment for STIs without parental consent or notification.[6]

BOX 322-1 Why Adolescents Are at Risk for Sexually Transmitted Infections

- Sense of invulnerability ("It can't happen to me.")
- Lack of information ("If I don't feel sick, I can't be sick.")
- Inconsistent and improper use of condoms
- Poor communication skills with partners and physicians
- Barriers to care (legal obstacles, concerns about confidentiality)
- Inability to adhere to treatment regimens
- Sexual networks with high prevalence of infection
- Physiological changes associated with puberty

A physiological basis may be found for adolescent girls being particularly susceptible to infection with a sexually transmitted organism on exposure. The transformation zone of the pubertal cervix, which has a relatively large surface area compared with that of a mature woman, is particularly vulnerable to infection with *Chlamydia trachomatis* and human papillomavirus. Not surprisingly therefore, current data indicate that adolescent girls and young adult women have higher infection rates with these organisms than any other age group in the United States. The most recent age-specific infection rates from the Centers for Disease Control and Prevention (CDC) for *C trachomatis* and *Neisseria gonorrhoeae* are shown in Figure 322-1. Rates of infection among 10 to 19 year olds may actually be higher than indicated because the pool of truly susceptible individuals (those sexually active) is smaller in this age group than in the older ones. For example, only 47% of 9th to 12th graders have had intercourse compared with most adults.

The list of organisms that can be transmitted sexually is extensive. Box 322-2 lists the most common of these. Gonorrhea, chlamydia, herpes, human papillomavirus, and syphilis are discussed in detail in this chapter. Herpes infections are also discussed in Chapter 275, Human Herpesvirus-6 and Human Herpesvirus-7 Infections; Chapter 276, Human Immunodeficiency Virus Infection and Acquired Immunodeficiency Syndrome, reviews HIV infection and AIDS. Chapter 227, Vaginal Discharge, provides an overview of organisms causing vaginal discharge. Information about other STIs should be sought through the index.

An alternative way of conceptualizing the spectrum of health problems attributable to STIs is to focus on symptoms or diseases rather than on specific organisms. More than 1 organism can produce various symptoms, physical findings, or syndromes, and many teenagers deny or are reluctant to discuss their sexual activity. Hence, when an adolescent seeks care for symptoms and clinical findings that might be caused by an STI, the physician must proceed with appropriate diagnostic tests or therapy, even though the history may appear to exclude such a cause. Most sexually active teenagers, however, will be truthful when questioned respectfully without a parent or guardian present and when given appropriate guarantees about confidentiality. Box 322-3 lists a variety of symptoms and syndromes that are frequently caused by STIs.

Primary care physicians generally concern themselves with the short-term morbidity associated with STIs, but the complications of infection extend into adulthood. Cervical cancer, infertility, ectopic pregnancy, chronic pelvic pain, and AIDS are all long-term sequelae of infections acquired during adolescence and young adulthood. In addition, ample evidence now exists that STIs increase an individual's risk for acquiring HIV infection.[7] Additionally, HIV-positive

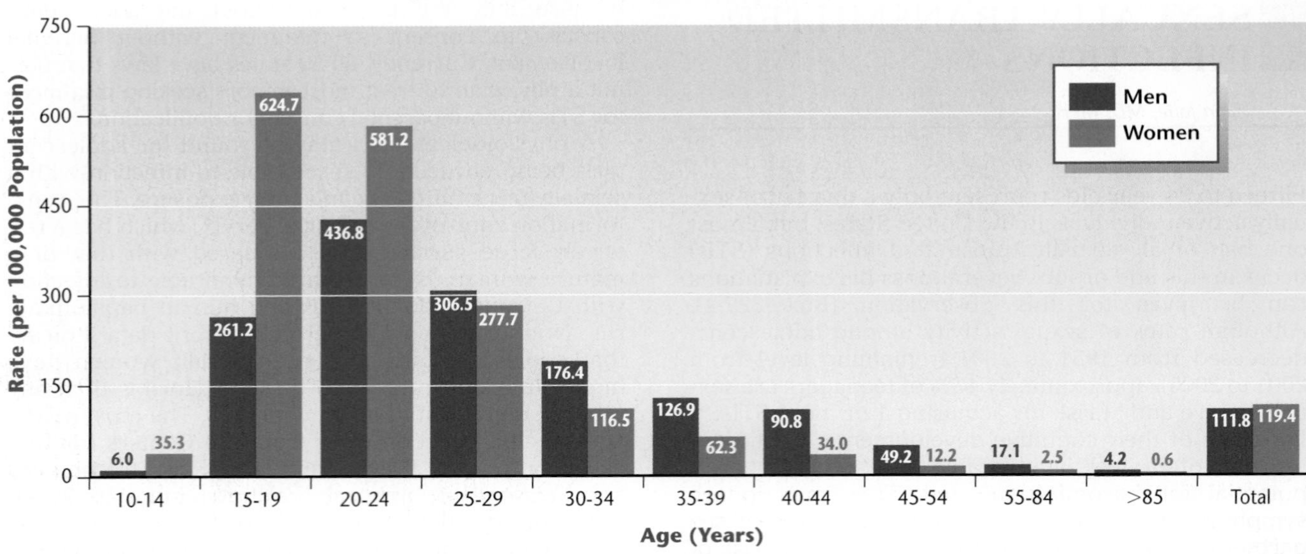

Figure 322-1 Rates of infection of *Chlamydia trachomatis* and *Neisseria gonorrhoeae* in the United States, by age and sex, 2005 data. *(Centers for Disease Control and Prevention. STD Surveillance 2005. National Profile. Available at: www.cdc.gov/std/stats05/default.htm. Accessed August 28, 2008.)*

BOX 322-2 Sexually Transmitted Organisms

Campylobacter species
Chlamydia trachomatis
Cytomegalovirus
Entamoeba histolytica
Giardia lamblia
Hepatitis A and B
Herpes simplex virus types 1 and 2
HIV
Human papillomavirus
Molluscum contagiosum (papovavirus)
Mycoplasma genitalium
Mycoplasma hominis
Neisseria gonorrhoeae
Phthirus pubis (pubic lice)
Salmonella species
Sarcoptes scabiei (mites)
Shigella species
Treponema pallidum
Trichomonas vaginalis
Ureaplasma urealyticum

individuals who contract STIs shed increased amounts of HIV in genital body fluids and therefore are more likely to transmit HIV to an uninfected partner. Aggressive control of STIs is accompanied by a reduction in the incidence of new cases of HIV infection.[8]

This perspective underscores the importance of preventing, diagnosing, and treating STIs among adolescents. Hence the increasingly widespread availability and use of nucleic acid amplification tests (NAAT) for the diagnosis of *C trachomatis* and *N gonorrhoeae* infections represent major advances in achieving this goal. These tests are more sensitive than both culture and previous generations of nonculture tests, they do not require the recovery of viable organisms, and they can be performed on urine specimens.[9] By eliminating or reducing the need for invasive testing, NAAT have the potential to expand greatly the number of at-risk youth who are screened. Self-collection of vaginal specimens will also enhance detection efforts.[10,11]

SPECIFIC AGENTS

Chlamydia trachomatis

The obligate intracellular *Chlamydia* microorganism causes a wide spectrum of disease and is the most common sexually transmitted bacterial organism in the United States.[12] Of greatest importance is its causative role in urethritis and epididymitis in men and cervicitis and PID in women.

Chlamydia appears to cause 35% to 50% of symptomatic nongonococcal urethritis among heterosexual men.[12] The organism can also be recovered from men with urethral gonorrhea. Approximately 2% to 10% of asymptomatic adolescent boys will test positive for chlamydia, depending on the population studied.[13] In a recent national study of young adult men ages 18 to 26, a total of 3.7% tested positive for chlamydia (with a range of 1% to 11%, depending on the racial or ethnic group studied). Ninety-five percent reported no symptoms in

BOX 322-3 Signs, Symptoms, and Clinical Syndromes Consistent With Sexually Transmitted Infections in Adolescents

BOYS

Dysuria, discharge, urethral itching (urethritis)
Scrotal pain, swelling (epididymitis)
Rectal discharge, tenesmus, anorectal pain (proctitis, proctocolitis, colitis)*

GIRLS

Mucopurulent cervicitis
Vaginitis (vaginal discharge)
Dysuria, urgency, frequency
Right upper quadrant abdominal pain
Pelvic inflammatory disease (low abdominal pain)
Bleeding between periods (cervicitis) or a heavier, more prolonged period (pelvic inflammatory disease)

BOTH

Dermatitis†
Genital ulcers (single or multiple)
Genital warts
Hepatitis A or B infection
Lymphadenopathy, especially inguinal or generalized (associated with HIV)
Persistent pharyngitis
Septic arthritis

*Usually seen in adolescents who practice anal receptive intercourse or oral-anal contact.
†Especially generalized papulosquamous (secondary syphilis); papular with central umbilication (molluscum contagiosum); localized pubic itching, or localized itching involving the webs of fingers and the wrists (*Phthirus pubis*, pubic lice; or *Sarcoptes scabiei*, mites); and erythematous macules turning pustular or necrotic, accompanied by tenosynovitis (disseminated gonococcal infection).

the 24 hours before urine collection.[14] When symptoms do appear, they generally develop 1 to 3 weeks after infection. Male adolescents may complain only of mild dysuria or itching at the terminal urethra, or they may have a scanty, mucoid discharge that is easily ignored and may disappear without treatment. The best time to examine an adolescent with a suggestive history, but no discharge, is 1st thing in the morning, before he has urinated that day. Alternatively, having him strip his urethra may produce some discharge. A profuse, purulent discharge should raise the possibilities of *N gonorrhoeae* co-infection or of its being the single causative agent. Adolescents also may complain of testicular pain, scrotal pain, or both, suggesting that urethral infection has spread to the epididymis.

Because the organism can infect the urethra and the cervix, dysuria can be the primary manifestation of infection. Hence *C trachomatis* infection should be considered in any adolescent girl with symptoms of a urinary tract infection. She may complain of spotting between periods as a result of cervicitis, or if the infection has spread to the upper genital tract, she may complain of low abdominal pain or right upper quadrant pain (Fitz-Hugh–Curtis syndrome). The latter is caused by organisms tracking up the abdominal cavity and causing inflammation of the liver capsule along with adhesions to the diaphragm. Unless a thorough history is obtained, the combination of dysuria and right upper quadrant or right flank pain might lead a clinician to the erroneous diagnosis of pyelonephritis. Lower abdominal pain suggests the possibility of PID. Vaginal discharge is more likely to indicate the presence of another infection (see Chapter 227; Vaginal Discharge), although chlamydia may be found incidentally. *Chlamydia* also may infect the Bartholin ducts, resulting in an exudative vaginal discharge or an abscess.

Infections in teenage girls are often asymptomatic, just as they are in teenage boys. Rates of infection vary according to region of the country and other factors.[13,14] At pelvic examination, clues to infection are the presence of mucopurulent discharge from the cervical os (known as *mucopus*; Figure 322-2), cervical erythema, and friability. Gram stain of cervical tissue will reveal the presence of 10 to 30 polymorphonuclear white blood cells (WBCs) per oil-immersion field. However, many patients lack any symptoms or signs of infection. Given the high prevalence of infection among adolescents and the serious morbidity associated with untreated disease, every sexually active teenager should be screened for chlamydia at least annually; some researchers suggest testing twice a year, especially in areas where the prevalence of infection is high.[15] Screening programs for chlamydia have been shown to reduce the incidence of PID.[16]

Culture of urethral or cervical samples was previously the gold standard for detecting infection. However, NAAT are considerably more sensitive than culture or older nonculture techniques.[9,17] For example, the sensitivity of culture for chlamydia is 54% to 85% from endocervical specimens, versus 88% to 100% by using various NAAT. NAAT are currently more expensive than other methods but have the advantage of being noninvasive (ie, specimens can be obtained without performing a pelvic examination or swabbing the urethral orifice). Older nonculture tests, such as DNA probes or enzyme-linked immunoabsorbent assays, are only 54% to 84% sensitive. Because detection of infection is critical to preventing serious morbidity, the most sensitive diagnostic test available should be used. However, chlamydia culture remains the only diagnostic test for chlamydia infection admissible in a court of law (eg, in cases of child sexual abuse). Box 322-4 lists drugs and dose information for treatment.

As with treatment for any STI, the patient's abstinence from intercourse is imperative until therapy is complete and the patient's partner is notified and treated. Reinfection rates among teenagers treated for chlamydia are lower if the patient knows for certain that her partner was treated.[18] Short-term complications of chlamydial infection include epididymitis and PID; long-term complications include reactive arthritis and the sequelae of PID. Although infection with chlamydia is not an independent risk factor for the development of cervical dysplasia, it may play some role.[19] An untreated, infected woman can pass the infection to her infant through colonization during birth.

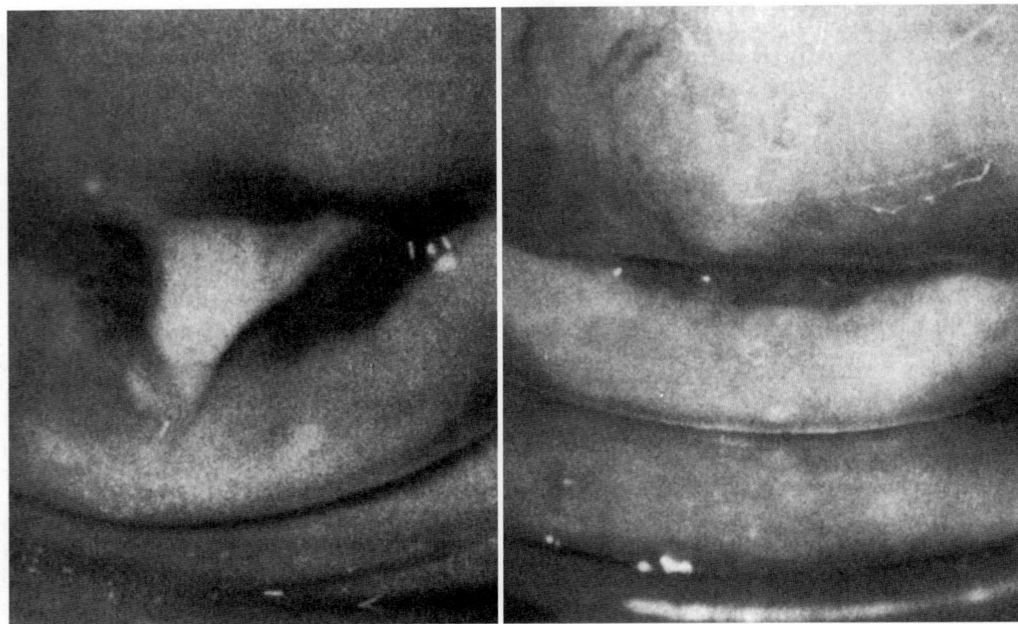

Figure 322-2 Colpophotograph showing mucopurulent cervicitis before and 2 weeks after treatment with 500 mg of tetracycline 4 times a day for 7 days. Note disappearance of endocervical exudate after therapy. *(Brunham RC, Paavonen J, Stevens CE, et al. Mucropurulent cervicitis—the ignored counterpart in women of urethritis in men.* N Engl J Med. *1984;311;1-6. Copyright © 1984 Massachusetts Medical Society. All rights reserved.)*

BOX 322-4 Treatment for Sexually Transmitted Infections

CHLAMYDIAL INFECTION IN ADOLESCENTS AND ADULTS

Treatment

Treatment of infected patients prevents transmission to sex partners, and, for infected pregnant women, treatment usually prevents transmission of *Chlamydia trachomatis* to infants during birth. Treatment of sex partners helps prevent reinfection of the index patient and infection of other partners.

Co-infection with *C trachomatis* often occurs among patients who have gonococcal infection; therefore presumptive treatment of such patients for chlamydia is appropriate (see Gonococcal Infection, Dual Therapy for Gonococcal and Chlamydial Infections). The following recommended treatment regimens and alternative regimens cure infection and usually relieve symptoms.

Recommended regimens

Azithromycin 1 g orally in a single dose OR

Doxycycline 100 mg orally twice a day for 7 days

Alternative regimens

Erythromycin base 500 mg orally 4 times a day for 7 days OR

Erythromycin ethylsuccinate 800 mg orally 4 times a day for 7 days OR

Ofloxacin 300 mg orally twice a day for 7 days OR

Levofloxacin 500 mg orally once daily for 7 days

A recent meta-analysis of 12 randomized clinical trials of azithromycin versus doxycycline demonstrated that the 2 treatments were equally efficacious, with cure rates of 97% and 98%, respectively. These investigations were conducted primarily in populations in which follow-up was encouraged, adherence to a 7-day regimen was effective, and culture or enzyme-linked immuno-absorbent assays (rather than nucleic acid amplification tests [NAAT]) were used to determine microbiological outcome. Azithromycin should always be available to treat patients for whom compliance with multiday dosing is questionable.

In populations with erratic health-care-seeking behavior, poor compliance with treatment, or unpredictable follow-up, azithromycin may be more cost effective because it offers single-dose, directly observed therapy. Doxycycline costs less than azithromycin and has no greater risk of adverse events. Erythromycin might be less efficacious than both azithromycin and doxycycline, mainly because the gastrointestinal side effects frequently discourage patients from complying with this regimen. Ofloxacin and levofloxacin are effective treatment alternatives but are more expensive and offer no advantage with regard to the dose regimen. Other quinolones either are not reliably effective against chlamydial infection or have not been adequately evaluated.

To maximize compliance with recommended therapies, medications for chlamydial infections should be dispensed on site, and the 1st dose should be directly

BOX 322-4 Treatment for Sexually Transmitted Infections—cont'd

observed. To minimize further transmission of infection, patients treated for chlamydia should be instructed to abstain from sexual intercourse for 7 days after single-dose therapy or until completion of a 7-day regimen. Patients should also be instructed to abstain from sexual intercourse until all of their sex partners are treated to minimize the risk for reinfection.

Follow-up

Except for pregnant women, patients do not need to be retested for chlamydia after completing treatment with the recommended or alternative regimens unless compliance is in question, symptoms persist, or reinfection is suspected. False-negative results might occur because of small numbers of chlamydial organisms. In addition, NAAT conducted less than 3 weeks after completion of therapy for patients who were treated successfully might yield false-positive results because of the continued presence of dead organisms.

Studies have demonstrated high rates of infection among women retested several months after treatment presumably because of reinfection by an untreated sex partner; infection from a new partner with chlamydia is also possible. Repeat infections confer an increased risk for pelvic inflammatory disease (PID) and other complications compared with the initial infection. Clinicians should consider advising all women with chlamydial infection to be retested approximately 3 months after treatment. Clinicians are strongly encouraged to retest all women treated for *C trachomatis* whenever they next seek medical care in the next 3-12 months, regardless of whether the woman believes her sex partner or partners were treated.

GONOCOCCAL INFECTION IN ADOLESCENTS AND ADULTS

Dual therapy for gonococcal and chlamydial infections

Patients infected with *Neisseria gonorrhoeae* often are co-infected with *C trachomatis;* this finding led to the recommendation that patients treated for gonococcal infection also be treated routinely with a regimen effective against uncomplicated genital *C trachomatis* infection. Because most gonococci in the United States are susceptible to doxycycline and azithromycin, routine co-treatment might hinder the development of antimicrobial-resistant *N gonorrhoeae.*

Because of the high sensitivity of NAAT for chlamydial infection, patients with a negative chlamydial NAAT result at the time of treatment for gonorrhea do not need to be treated for chlamydia as well. However, if test results for chlamydia are not available or a non-NAAT was negative for chlamydia, then patients should be treated for both chlamydia and gonorrhea.

Quinolone-resistant N gonorrhoeae

Because the prevalence of fluoroquinolone resistance among *N gonorrhoeae* isolates in the United States has increased and become widespread, the CDC "no longer recommends the use of fluoroquinolones for the treatment of gonococcal infections and associated conditions such as pelvic inflammatory disease."[21]

UNCOMPLICATED GONOCOCCAL INFECTIONS OF THE CERVIX, URETHRA, AND RECTUM

Recommended regimens

Ceftriaxone 125 mg IM in a single dose OR

Cefixime 400 mg orally in a single dose PLUS

Treatment for chlamydia if *C trachomatis* infection is not ruled out

Ceftriaxone in a single injection of 125 mg provides sustained, high bactericidal levels in the blood. Extensive clinical experience indicates that ceftriaxone is safe and effective for the treatment of uncomplicated gonorrhea at all anatomic sites, curing 98.9% of uncomplicated urogenital and anorectal infections in published clinical trials.

Cefixime has an antimicrobial spectrum similar to that of ceftriaxone, but the 400-mg oral dose does not provide as high or as sustained a bactericidal level as that provided by the 125-mg dose of ceftriaxone. In published clinical trials, the 400-mg dose cured 97.4% of uncomplicated urogenital and anorectal gonococcal infections. The advantage of cefixime is that it can be administered orally. Cefixime may not be available in many areas; the CDC or state health departments can provide updates on its availability.

Alternative regimens

Spectinomycin 2 g IM in a single dose OR

Single-dose cephalosporin regimens

Spectinomycin is expensive and must be injected; however, it has been effective in published clinical trials, curing 98.2% of uncomplicated urogenital and anorectal gonococcal infections. Spectinomycin is useful for treatment of patients who cannot tolerate cephalosporins and quinolones.

Single-dose cephalosporin regimens other than ceftriaxone 125 mg IM and cefixime 400 mg orally that are safe and highly effective against uncomplicated urogenital and anorectal gonococcal infections include (a) ceftizoxime 500 mg IM, (b) cefoxitin 2 g IM with probenecid 1 g orally, and (c) cefotaxime 500 mg IM. None of the injectable cephalosporins offer any advantage over ceftriaxone.

(Additional information on alternative oral regimens is available at www.cdc.gov/std.)

UNCOMPLICATED GONOCOCCAL INFECTIONS OF THE PHARYNX

Gonococcal infections of the pharynx are more difficult to eradicate than infections at urogenital and anorectal sites. Few antimicrobial regimens can reliably cure such infections more than 90% of the time. Although chlamydial co-infection of the pharynx is unusual, co-infection at genital sites sometimes occurs. Therefore treatment for both gonorrhea and chlamydia is suggested.

Recommended regimens

Ceftriaxone 125 mg IM in a single dose PLUS

Treatment for chlamydia if *C trachomatis* infection is not ruled out

Continued

BOX 322-4 Treatment for Sexually Transmitted Infections—cont'd

Follow-up

Test of cure is not indicated for patients with uncomplicated gonorrhea treated with any of the recommended or alternative regimens. Patients who have symptoms that persist after treatment should be evaluated with culture for *N gonorrhoeae,* and any gonococci isolated should be tested for antimicrobial susceptibility. Persistent urethritis, cervicitis, or proctitis also might be caused by *C trachomatis* or other organisms.

A high prevalence of *N gonorrhoeae* is observed in patients who have had gonorrhea in the preceding several months. The majority of these infections are due to reinfection rather than treatment failure. Repeat infection might confer an elevated risk for PID and other complications, when compared with the initial infection. Clinicians should consider advising all patients with gonorrhea to be retested in 3 months, and those not seeking retesting in 3 months should be tested when they next seek medical care in the ensuing 12 months.

DISSEMINATED GONOCOCCAL INFECTION

Disseminated gonococcal infection (DGI) results from gonococcal bacteremia. DGI often results in petechial or pustular acral skin lesions, asymmetrical arthralgia, tenosynovitis, or septic arthritis. The infection is complicated occasionally by perihepatitis, and rarely by endocarditis or meningitis. Some strains of *N gonorrhoeae* that cause DGI may cause minimal genital inflammation.

No studies on the treatment of DGI have been published since the publication of the last CDC sexually transmitted disease treatment guidelines. The following recommendations reflect the opinions of consultants; no treatment failures have been reported with these regimens.

Treatment

Hospitalization is recommended for initial therapy, especially for patients who cannot be relied on to comply with treatment, for those in whom the diagnosis is uncertain, and for those who have purulent synovial effusions or other complications. Patients should be examined for clinical evidence of endocarditis and meningitis. Patients treated for DGI should be treated presumptively for concurrent *C trachomatis* infection unless appropriate testing excludes this infection.

Recommended regimen

Ceftriaxone 1 g IM or IV every 24 hours

Alternative regimens

Cefotaxime 1 g IV every 8 hours OR

Ceftizoxime 1 g IV every 8 hours OR

Spectinomycin 2 g IM every 12 hours

All regimens should be continued for 24-48 hours after improvement begins, at which time therapy may be switched to one of the following regimens to complete at least 1 week of antimicrobial therapy:

Cefixime 400 mg orally twice a day OR

Cefixime suspension 400 mg twice daily orally (200 mg/5 mL) OR

Cefpodoxime 400 mg orally twice daily

Fluoroquinolones may be an alternative treatment option if antimicrobial susceptibility can be documented by culture.

HUMAN PAPILLOMAVIRUS INFECTION—GENITAL WARTS

Treatment

The primary goal of treating visible genital warts is the removal of the warts. In most patients, treatment can induce wart-free periods. Left untreated, visible warts may resolve, may remain unchanged, or may increase in size or number. Treatment possibly reduces, but does not eliminate, human papillomavirus (HPV) infection. Current evidence indicates that presently available treatments might reduce, but probably do not eradicate, HPV infectivity. Whether the reduction in HPV viral DNA resulting from treatment impacts future transmission remains unclear. No evidence indicates that the presence of genital warts or their treatment is associated with the development of cervical cancer.

Regimens

Treatment of genital warts should be guided by the preference of the patient, the available resources, and the experience of the primary care physician. No definitive evidence has been found to suggest that any of the available treatments is superior to other treatments, and no single treatment is ideal for all patients or all warts. Because of the uncertainty regarding the effect of treatment on future transmission of HPV and the possibility of spontaneous resolution, an acceptable alternative for some people is to forego treatment and wait for spontaneous resolution.

The available treatments for visible genital warts are patient-applied therapies (ie, podofilox, imiquimod) and physician-administered therapies (ie, cryotherapy, podophyllin resin, trichloroacetic acid [TCA], bichloroacetic acid [BCA], interferon, surgery). Most patients have fewer than 10 genital warts (with a total wart area of 0.5 to 1.0 cm^2), which are responsive to various treatment modalities. Factors that might influence selection of treatment include wart size, wart number, anatomic site of wart, wart morphology, patient preference, cost of treatment, convenience, adverse effects, and provider experience. Having a treatment plan or protocol is important because the majority of patients require a course of therapy rather than a single treatment. In general, warts located on moist surfaces and in intertriginous areas respond better to topical treatment (eg, TCA, podophyllin, podofilox, imiquimod) than do warts on drier surfaces.

The treatment modality should be changed if a patient has not improved substantially. The majority of genital warts respond within 3 months of therapy. The response to treatment and its side effects should be evaluated throughout the course of therapy.

Complications rarely occur if treatments for warts are employed properly. Patients should be warned that persistent hypo- or hyperpigmentation is common with ablative modalities. Depressed or hypertrophic scars are rare but can occur, especially if the patient has had insufficient time to heal between treatments. Treatment

BOX 322-4 Treatment for Sexually Transmitted Infections—cont'd

can result rarely in disabling chronic pain syndromes (eg, vulvodynia or analdynia, hyperesthesia of the treatment site) or, in the case of rectal warts, painful defecation or fistulas. A limited number of case reports of severe systemic effects from podophyllin resin and interferon have been documented.

Patient-applied treatments are preferred by some patients because they can be administered in the privacy of the patient's home. For these treatments to be effective, patients must be able to comply with the treatment regimen and be able to identify and reach all genital warts.

Recommended regimens for external genital warts

Patient applied

Podofilox 0.5% solution or gel. Patients should apply podofilox solution with a cotton swab, or podofilox gel with a finger, to visible genital warts twice a day for 3 days, followed by 4 days of no therapy. This cycle may be repeated as necessary for a total of 4 cycles. The total wart area treated should not exceed 10 cm^2, and a total volume of podofilox should not exceed 0.5 mL per day. If possible, the primary care physician should apply the initial treatment to demonstrate the proper application technique and identify which warts should be treated. *The safety of podofilox during pregnancy has not been established.*

OR

Imiquimod 5% cream. Patients should apply imiquimod cream once daily at bedtime, 3 times a week for up to 16 weeks. The treatment area should be washed with mild soap and water 6 to 10 hours after the application. *The safety of imiquimod during pregnancy has not been established.*

Physician administered

Cryotherapy with liquid nitrogen or cryoprobe. Repeat applications every 1 to 2 weeks.

OR

Podophyllin resin 10% to 25% in compound tincture of benzoin. A small amount should be applied to each wart and allowed to air dry. The treatment can be repeated weekly if necessary. To prevent the possibility of complications associated with systemic absorption and toxicity, 2 important guidelines should be followed: (1) Application should be limited to less than 0.5 mL of podophyllin or an area less than 10 cm^2 of warts per session, and (2) no open lesions or wounds should exist in the area to which the treatment is to be applied. Some experts suggest that the preparation should be thoroughly washed off 1 to 4 hours after application to reduce local irritation. *The safety of podophyllin during pregnancy has not been established.*

OR

TCA or BCA 80% to 90%. Apply a small amount only to warts and allow to dry, at which time a white *frosting* develops. Powder with talc, sodium bicarbonate (ie, baking soda), or liquid soap to remove unreacted acid if an excess amount is applied. Repeat weekly if necessary.

OR

Surgical removal either by tangential scissor excision, tangential shave excision, curettage, or electrosurgery.

Alternative treatments

Intralesional interferon OR

Laser surgery

Podofilox 0.5% solution or gel is relatively inexpensive, easy to use, safe, and self-applied by patients. Podofilox is an antimitotic drug that results in destruction of warts. Most patients experience mild or moderate pain or local irritation after treatment. Imiquimod is a topically active immune enhancer that stimulates production of interferon and other cytokines. Local inflammatory reactions are common; these reactions include redness and irritation and are usually mild to moderate. Traditionally, follow-up visits are not usually recommended for patients using self-administered treatments, but they may be useful several weeks into therapy to determine if the treatment is being applied correctly and to measure the response to treatment.

Cryotherapy destroys warts by thermal-induced cytolysis. Clinicians must be trained in the proper use of this treatment because overtreatment or undertreatment can result in complications or low efficacy. Pain after application of the liquid nitrogen, followed by necrosis and sometimes blistering, are not unusual. Local anesthesia (topical or injected) might facilitate treatment if warts are present in many areas or if the area of warts is large.

Podophyllin resin contains several compounds, including the podophyllin lignans that are antimitotic. The resin is most frequently compounded at 10% to 25% in tincture of benzoin. However, podophyllin resin preparations differ in the concentration of active components and contaminants. The shelf life and stability of podophyllin preparations are unknown. A thin layer of podophyllin resin should be applied to the warts and allowed to air dry before the treated area comes into contact with clothing. Overapplication or failure to air dry can result in local irritation caused by spread of the compound to adjacent areas.

Both TCA and BCA are caustic agents that destroy warts by chemical coagulation of proteins. Although these preparations are widely used, they have not been investigated thoroughly. TCA solutions have a low viscosity comparable to water and can spread rapidly if applied excessively, thus damaging adjacent normal tissue. Both TCA and BCA should be applied sparingly and allowed to dry before the patient sits or stands. If pain is intense, then the acid can be neutralized with soap or sodium bicarbonate (ie, baking soda).

Because of the shortcomings of available treatments, some clinics employ combination therapy (ie, the simultaneous use of 2 or more modalities on the same wart at the same time). No data support the use of more than 1 therapy at a time to improve the efficacy of treatment, and some specialists believe that combining modalities may increase complications.

Continued

BOX 322-4 Treatment for Sexually Transmitted Infections—cont'd

Recommended regimens for cervical warts

For women who have exophytic cervical warts, high-grade squamous intraepithelial lesions must be excluded before treatment is begun. Management of exophytic cervical warts should include consultation with an expert.

Recommended regimens for vaginal warts

Cryotherapy with liquid nitrogen. The use of a cryoprobe in the vagina is not recommended because of the risk for vaginal perforation and fistula formation.

OR

TCA or BCA 80% to 90% applied to warts. Apply a small amount only to warts and allow to dry, at which time a white *frosting* develops; powder with talc or sodium bicarbonate (ie, baking soda) or with liquid soap preparations to remove unreacted acid if an excess amount is applied. Repeat weekly if necessary.

Recommended regimens for urethral meatus warts

Cryotherapy with liquid nitrogen

OR

Podophyllin 10% to 25% in compound tincture of benzoin. The treatment area must be dry before contact with normal mucosa. Podophyllin can be applied weekly if necessary. *The safety of podophyllin during pregnancy has not been established.* Although data evaluating the use of podofilox and imiquimod for the treatment of distal meatal warts are limited, some specialists recommend their use in some patients.

Recommended regimen for anal warts

Cryotherapy with liquid nitrogen

OR

TCA or BCA 80% to 90% applied to warts. Apply a small amount only to warts and allow to dry, at which time a white *frosting* develops; powder with talc or sodium bicarbonate (ie, baking soda) or with liquid soap preparations to remove unreacted acid if an excess amount is applied. Repeat weekly if necessary.

OR

Surgical removal

Warts on the rectal mucosa should be managed in consultation with a specialist. Many individuals with anal warts also have warts on the rectal mucosa; hence these patients can benefit from inspection of the rectal mucosa by digital examination or anoscopy.

Follow-up

After visible genital warts have cleared, a follow-up evaluation may be helpful. Patients should be cautioned to watch for recurrences, which occur most frequently during the first 3 months. Because identifying external warts may be difficult, having a follow-up evaluation 3 months after treatment may be useful for patients. Earlier follow-up visits also may be useful to (a) document a wart-free state, (b) monitor for or treat complications of therapy, and (c) provide the opportunity for patient education and counseling. Women should be counseled regarding the need for regular Papanicolaou screening as recommended for women without genital warts.

Management of sex partners

Examination of sex partners is not necessary for the management of genital warts because no data indicate that reinfection plays a role in recurrences. Additionally, providing treatment solely for the purpose of preventing future transmission cannot be recommended because the value of treatment in reducing infectivity is unknown. However, sex partners of patients who have genital warts might benefit from counseling and examination to assess the presence of genital warts and other sexually transmitted infections. Female sex partners of patients who have genital warts should be reminded that cytological screening for cervical cancer is recommended for all sexually active women.

GENITAL HERPES SIMPLEX VIRUS INFECTION

Genital herpes is a chronic, life-long viral infection. The majority of cases of recurrent genital herpes are caused by herpes simplex virus type 2 (HSV-2), although HSV-1 might become more common as a cause of 1st episode genital herpes. The majority of people with HSV-2 have not been diagnosed; many of them have mild or unrecognized disease but shed virus intermittently in the genital tract. The majority of genital herpes infections are transmitted by people who do not know they are infected or who are asymptomatic at the time transmission occurs.

Up to 50% of 1st-episode cases of genital herpes are caused by HSV-1 but recurrences and subclinical shedding are much less frequent with genital HSV-1 infection than genital HSV-2 infection. Therefore identification of the type of the infecting strain has prognostic importance and may be useful for counseling purposes.

First clinical episode of genital herpes

Many patients with 1st-episode herpes have mild clinical manifestations but later develop severe or prolonged symptoms. Therefore patients with initial genital herpes should receive antiviral therapy.

Recommended regimens

Acyclovir 400 mg orally 3 times a day for 7 to 10 days OR

Acyclovir 200 mg orally 5 times a day for 7 to 10 days

OR

Famciclovir 250 mg orally 3 times a day for 7 to 10 days

OR

Valacyclovir 1 g orally twice a day for 7 to 10 days

Treatment may be extended if healing is incomplete after 10 days of therapy.

ESTABLISHED HERPES SIMPLEX VIRUS TYPE 2 INFECTION

The majority of patients with symptomatic, 1st-episode genital HSV-2 infection will have recurrent episodes of genital lesions; recurrences are less frequent after initial genital HSV-1 infection. Intermittent asymptomatic shedding occurs in persons with genital HSV-2 infection, even in those with longstanding or clinically silent infection. Antiviral therapy for recurrent disease can be administered either episodically to ameliorate or shorten the duration of lesions or continuously as suppressive therapy to reduce the frequency of recurrences. Many

BOX 322-4 Treatment for Sexually Transmitted Infections—cont'd

persons, even those with mild or infrequent outbreaks, benefit from antiviral therapy; therefore options for treatment should be discussed. Some persons may prefer suppressive therapy, which has the additional advantage of decreasing the risk of genital HSV-2 transmission to susceptible partners.

Daily suppressive therapy reduces the frequency of genital herpes recurrences by 70% to 80% in patients who have frequent recurrences (ie, 6 or more recurrences per year). Treatment is also effective in patients with less frequent recurrences. Safety and efficacy have been documented among patients receiving daily therapy with acyclovir for as long as 6 years and with valacyclovir or famciclovir for 1 year. The frequency of recurrences diminishes over time in many patients and the patient's psychological adjustment to disease might change. Therefore, periodically (eg, once a year), clinicians should discuss the need to continue suppressive therapy with the patient.

Suppressive therapy with valacyclovir 500 mg daily decreases the rate of HSV-2 transmission in discordant, heterosexual couples in which the source partner has a history of genital HSV-2 infection. Suppressive antiviral therapy probably reduces transmission when used by persons who have multiple partners (including men who have sex with men) and by those who are HSV-2 seropositive without a history of genital herpes.

Recommended regimens for daily suppressive therapy

Acyclovir 400 mg orally twice a day OR

Famciclovir 250 mg orally twice a day OR

Valacyclovir 500 mg orally once a day OR

Valacyclovir 1.0 g orally once a day

Valacyclovir 500 mg once a day may be less effective than other valacyclovir or acyclovir dosing regimens in patients who have very frequent recurrences (ie, at least 10 episodes per year). Several studies have compared valacyclovir or famciclovir with acyclovir. The results of these studies suggest that valacyclovir and famciclovir are comparable to acyclovir in clinical outcome. However, ease of administration and cost are also important considerations for prolonged treatment.

Episodic therapy for recurrent genital herpes

Effective episodic therapy of recurrent herpes requires initiation of therapy within 1 day of lesion onset or during the prodrome that precedes some outbreaks. The patient should be provided with a supply of drug or a prescription for the medication with instructions to initiate treatment as soon as symptoms begin.

Recommended regimens

Acyclovir 400 mg orally 3 times a day for 5 days OR

Acyclovir 800 mg orally twice a day for 5 days OR

Acyclovir 800 mg orally 3 times a day for 2 days OR

Famciclovir 125 mg orally twice a day for 5 days OR

Famciclovir 1.0 g orally twice daily for 1 day OR

Valacyclovir 500 mg orally twice a day for 3 days OR

Valacyclovir 1.0 g once a day for 5 days

PRIMARY AND SECONDARY SYPHILIS

Treatment

Parenteral penicillin G is the preferred drug for treatment of all stages of syphilis. The preparation or preparations used (ie, benzathine, aqueous procaine, aqueous crystalline), the dose, and the length of treatment all depend on the stage and clinical manifestations of the disease.

Recommended regimen for adults

Adults who have primary or secondary syphilis should be treated with benzathine penicillin G 2.4 million units IM in a single dose

Recommended regimen for children

After the newborn period (≥1 month), children with syphilis should have a cerebral spinal fluid (CSF) examination to detect asymptomatic neurosyphilis, and birth and maternal medical records should be reviewed to assess whether the child has congenital or acquired syphilis. Children with acquired primary or secondary syphilis should be evaluated (including consultation with child-protection services) and treated by using the following pediatric regimen:

Benzathine penicillin G 50,000 units/kg IM up to the adult dose of 2.4 million units in a single dose. (A child or adolescent weighing ≥48 kg would receive the adult dose.)

Other management considerations

All patients who have syphilis should be tested for HIV infection. In geographic areas in which the prevalence of HIV is high, patients who have primary syphilis should be retested for HIV after 3 months if the 1st HIV test result was negative.

Patients who have syphilis and symptoms or signs suggesting neurological disease (eg, meningitis) or ophthalmic disease (eg, uveitis, iritis, neuroretinitis, optic neuritis) should be evaluated fully for neurosyphilis and syphilitic eye disease; this evaluation should include CSF analysis and ocular slit-lamp examination. Such patients should be treated appropriately according to the results of this evaluation.

Invasion of CSF by *Treponema pallidum* accompanied by CSF abnormalities is common among adults who have primary or secondary syphilis. However, neurosyphilis develops in only a few patients after treatment with the regimens described here. Therefore, unless clinical signs or symptoms of neurologic or ophthalmic involvement are present, lumbar puncture is not recommended for routine evaluation of patients who have primary or secondary syphilis.

Follow-up

Treatment failure can occur with any regimen. However, assessing response to treatment is often difficult, and no definitive criteria for cure or failure have been established. Nontreponemal test titers may decline more slowly for patients who previously had syphilis. Patients should be reexamined clinically and serologically 6 and 12 months after treatment; more frequent evaluation may be prudent if follow-up is uncertain.

Continued

BOX 322-4 Treatment for Sexually Transmitted Infections—cont'd

Patients who have signs or symptoms that persist or recur or who have a sustained 4-fold increase in nontreponemal test titer (ie, compared with the maximum or baseline titer at time of treatment) probably failed treatment or were reinfected. These patients should be retreated and reevaluated for HIV infection. Because treatment failure usually cannot be reliably distinguished from reinfection with *T pallidum,* a lumbar puncture also should be performed. Clinical trial data have demonstrated that 15% of patients with early syphilis treated with recommended therapy will not achieve a 2-dilution decline in nontreponemal titer used to define response at 1 year after treatment.

Failure of nontreponemal test titers to decline 4-fold within 6 months after therapy for primary or secondary syphilis might be indicative of probable treatment failure. Persons whose titers remain serofast should be reevaluated for HIV infection. Optimal management of such patients is unclear. At a minimum, these patients should have additional clinical and serologic follow-up. HIV-infected patients should be evaluated more frequently (ie, at 3-month intervals instead of 6-month intervals). If additional follow-up cannot be ensured, retreatment is recommended. Because treatment failure might be the result of unrecognized central nervous system infection, many specialists recommend CSF examination in such situations. When patients are retreated, most experts recommend weekly injections of benzathine penicillin G 2.4 million units IM for 3 weeks, unless CSF examination indicates that neurosyphilis is present.

LATENT SYPHILIS

Latent syphilis is defined as syphilis characterized by seroreactivity without other evidence of disease. Patients who have latent syphilis and who acquired syphilis within the preceding year are classified as having early latent syphilis. Patients can be diagnosed as having early latent syphilis if, within the year preceding the evaluation, they had (a) a documented seroconversion or 4-fold or greater increase in titer of a nontreponemal test; (b) unequivocal symptoms of primary or secondary syphilis; (c) a sex partner documented to have primary, secondary, or early latent syphilis; or (d) reactive nontreponemal and treponemal tests whose only possible exposure occurred within the previous 12 months. Nontreponemal serological titers are usually higher during early latent syphilis than late latent syphilis. However, early latent syphilis cannot be reliably distinguished from late latent syphilis based solely on nontreponemal titers. All patients with latent syphilis should have thorough examination of all accessible mucosal surfaces (oral cavity, perineum in women, perianal area, and underneath the foreskin in uncircumcised men) to evaluate for internal mucosal lesions. All patients who have syphilis should be tested for HIV infection.

Treatment

Treatment of latent syphilis usually does not affect transmission and is intended to prevent late complications. Although clinical experience supports the effectiveness of penicillin in achieving this goal, limited evidence is available for guidance in choosing specific regimens.

Recommended regimens for adults

The following regimens are recommended for nonallergic patients who have normal CSF examination (if performed).

Early latent syphilis: benzathine penicillin G 2.4 million units IM in a single dose.

Late latent syphilis or latent syphilis of unknown duration: benzathine penicillin G 7.2 million units total, administered as 3 doses of 2.4 million units IM each at 1-week intervals.

Recommended regimens for children

After the newborn period, children with syphilis should have a CSF examination to exclude neurosyphilis. Birth and maternal records should be reviewed to assess whether the child has congenital or acquired syphilis. Older children with acquired latent syphilis should be evaluated as described for adults and treated using the following pediatric regimens. These regimens are for penicillin-nonallergic children with acquired syphilis who have normal CSF examination results.

Early latent syphilis: benzathine penicillin G 50,000 units/kg IM, up to the adult doe of 2.4 million units, in a single dose. (A child or adolescent who weighs ≥48 kg would receive the adult dose.)

Late latent syphilis or latent syphilis of unknown duration: benzathine penicillin G 50,000 units/kg IM, up to the adult dose of 2.4 million units, administered as 3 doses at 1-week intervals (total 150,000 units/kg up to the adult dose of 7.2 million units).

All patients who have latent syphilis should be evaluated clinically for evidence of tertiary disease (eg, aortitis, gumma) and syphilitic ocular disease (eg, iritis, uveitis). Patients with syphilis who demonstrate any of the following should have a prompt CSF examination: (a) neurologic or ophthalmic signs or symptoms, (b) evidence of active tertiary syphilis (eg, aortitis, gumma), (c) treatment failure, or (d) HIV infection with late latent syphilis or syphilis of unknown duration.

Some specialists recommend performing a CSF examination on all patients who have latent syphilis and a nontreponemal serologic test of at least 1:32 or if the patient is HIV infected with a CD4 count at or below 350 cells/mm^3. However the likelihood of neurosyphilis in this circumstance is unknown. If the CSF examination demonstrates abnormalities consistent with neurosyphilis, then the patient should be treated for neurosyphilis.

Follow-up

Quantitative nontreponemal serologic tests should be repeated at 6, 12, and 24 months. Patients with a normal CSF examination should be retreated for latent syphilis if (a) titers increase 4-fold, (b) an initially high titer (at least 1:32) fails to decline at least 4-fold (ie, 2 dilutions) within 12 to 24 months, or (c) signs or symptoms attributable to syphilis develop.

PELVIC INFLAMMATORY DISEASE

PID comprises a spectrum of inflammatory disorders of the upper female genital tract, including any combination

BOX 322-4 Treatment for Sexually Transmitted Infections—cont'd

of endometritis, salpingitis, tuboovarian abscess, and pelvic peritonitis. Sexually transmitted organisms, especially *N gonorrhoeae* and *C trachomatis,* are implicated in many cases; however, microorganisms that comprise the vaginal flora (eg, anaerobes, *Gardnerella vaginalis, Haemophilus influenzae,* enteric gram-negative rods, *Streptococcus agalactiae*) also have been associated with PID. In addition, cytomegalovirus, *Mycoplasma hominis, Ureaplasma urealyticum,* and *Mycoplasma genitalium* might be associated with some cases of PID. All women who are diagnosed with acute PID should be tested for *N gonorrhoeae* and *C trachomatis* and screened for HIV infection.

Treatment

PID treatment regimens must provide empiric, broad-spectrum coverage of likely pathogens. All regimens should be effective against *N gonorrhoeae* and *C trachomatis* because negative endocervical screening for these organisms does not preclude upper-reproductive tract infection. The need to eradicate anaerobes from women who have PID has not been demonstrated definitively. Anaerobic bacteria have been isolated from the upper-reproductive tract of women who have PID, and data from in vitro studies have revealed that anaerobes such as *Bacteroides fragilis* can cause tubal and epithelial destruction. In addition, bacterial vaginosis also is diagnosed in many women who have PID. Until treatment regimens that do not adequately cover these microbes have been shown to prevent sequelae as successfully as the regimens that are effective against these microbes, the use of regimens with anaerobic activity should be considered. Treatment should be initiated as soon as the presumptive diagnosis has been made because prevention of long-term sequelae is dependent on immediate administration of appropriate antibiotics. When selecting a treatment regimen, primary care physicians should consider availability, cost, patient acceptance, and antimicrobial susceptibility.

Parenteral treatment

For women with mild to moderate PID, parenteral therapy and oral therapy appear to have similar clinical efficacy. Many randomized trials have demonstrated the efficacy of both parenteral and oral regimens. In the majority of clinical trials, parenteral treatment for at least 48 hours has been used after the patient has demonstrated substantial clinical improvement. Clinical experience should guide decisions regarding transition to oral therapy, which usually can be initiated within 24 hours of clinical improvement. The majority of clinicians recommend at least 24 hours of direct inpatient observation for patients who have tuboovarian abscess.

Recommended parenteral regimen A

Cefotetan 2 g IV every 12 hours OR

Cefoxitin 2 g IV every 6 hours PLUS

Doxycycline 100 mg orally or IV every 12 hours

Because of pain associated with infusion, doxycycline should be administered orally when possible, even when the patient is hospitalized. Both oral and IV administration of doxycycline provide similar bioavailability. Parenteral therapy may be discontinued 24 hours after a patient improves clinically, and oral therapy with doxycycline (100 mg twice a day) should continue for a total of 14 days. When tuboovarian abscess is present, many primary care physicians use clindamycin or metronidazole with doxycycline for continued therapy, rather than doxycycline alone, because they provide more effective anaerobic coverage.

Clinical data are limited regarding the use of other 2nd- or 3rd-generation cephalosporins (eg, ceftizoxime, cefotaxime, ceftriaxone), which also might be effective therapy for PID and might replace cefotetan or cefoxitin. However, they are less active than cefotetan or cefoxitin against anaerobic bacteria.

Recommended parenteral regimen B

Clindamycin 900 mg IV every 8 hours PLUS

Gentamicin loading dose IV or IM (2 mg/kg of body weight) followed by a maintenance dose (1.5 mg/kg) every 8 hours. Single daily dosing may be substituted.

Although use of a single daily dose of gentamicin has not been evaluated for the treatment of PID, it is efficacious in analogous situations. Parenteral therapy may be discontinued 24 hours after a patient improves clinically; continuing oral therapy should consist of doxycycline 100 mg orally twice a day or clindamycin 450 mg orally 4 times a day to complete a total of 14 days of therapy. When tuboovarian abscess is present, many primary care physicians use clindamycin for continued therapy rather than doxycycline because clindamycin provides more effective anaerobic coverage.

Alternative parenteral regimens

Ampicillin/sulbactam 3 g IV every 6 hours PLUS

Doxycycline 100 mg orally or IV every 12 hours

Oral treatment

Oral therapy can be considered for women with mild-to-moderately severe acute PID, given that the clinical outcomes among women treated with oral therapy are similar to those treated with parenteral therapy. The following regimens provide coverage against the frequent etiologic agents of PID. Patients who do not respond to oral therapy within 72 hours should be reevaluated to confirm the diagnosis and should be administered parenteral therapy on either an outpatient or inpatient basis.

Recommended oral regimen

Ceftriaxone 250 mg IM in a single dose

PLUS

Doxycycline 100 mg orally twice a day for 14 days

WITH OR WITHOUT

Metronidazole 500 mg orally twice a day for 14 days

OR

Cefoxitin 2 g IM in a single dose and Probenecid, 1 g orally administered concurrently

PLUS

Doxycycline 100 mg orally twice a day for 14 days

Continued

BOX 322-4 Treatment for Sexually Transmitted Infections—cont'd

WITH OR WITHOUT

Metronidazole 500 mg orally twice a day for 14 days

OR

Other parenteral 3rd-generation cephalosporin (eg, ceftizoxime or cefotaxime)

PLUS

Doxycycline 100 mg orally twice a day for 14 days

WITH OR WITHOUT

Metronidazole 500 mg orally twice a day for 14 days

The optimal choice of a cephalosporin is unclear; although cefoxitin has better anaerobic coverage, ceftriaxone has better coverage against *N gonorrhoeae.* Clinical trials have demonstrated that a single dose of cefoxitin is effective in obtaining short-term clinical response in women who have PID; however, the theoretical limitations in its coverage of anaerobes may require the addition of metronidazole. Metronidazole also will effectively treat bacterial vaginosis, which is frequently associated with PID. No data have been published regarding the use of oral cephalosporins for the treatment of PID. Limited data suggest that the combination of oral metronidazole and doxycycline after primary parenteral therapy is safe and effective.

Alternative oral regimens

If parenteral cephalosporin therapy is not feasible, then use of fluoroquinolones (levofloxacin 500 mg orally once daily or ofloxacin 400 mg orally twice daily for 14 days) with or without metronidazole (500 mg orally twice daily for 14 days) may be considered if the community prevalence and individual risk of gonorrhea is low (see reference 21, pages 42-49). Tests for gonorrhea must be performed prior to instituting therapy and the patient managed as follows if the test is positive:

- If NAAT are positive, then parenteral cephalosporin is recommended.
- If culture for gonorrhea is positive, then treatment should be based on the results of antimicrobial susceptibility. If isolate isquinolone-resistant *N gonorrhoeae*, or if antimicrobial susceptibility cannot be assessed, then parenteral cephalosporin is recommended.

Although data are limited, amoxicillin/clavulinic acid and doxycycline or azithromycin with metronidazole has demonstrated short-term clinical cure.

EPIDIDYMITIS

Recommendation are that all patients receive ceftriaxone plus doxycycline for the initial treatment of epididymitis. Additional therapy may include a quinolone if acute epididymitis is not caused by gonorrhea (results from culture or NAAT are negative) or if the infection is most likely caused by enteric organisms.

Recommended regimens

For acute epididymitis most likely caused by gonococcal or chlamydial infection:

Ceftriaxone 250 mg IM in a single dose PLUS

Doxycycline 100 mg orally twice a day for 10 days

For acute epididymitis most likely caused by enteric organisms, or with negative culture or NAAT, or for patients allergic to cephalosporins or tetracyclines or both:

Ofloxacin 300 mg orally twice a day for 10 days OR

Levofloxacin 500 mg orally once daily for 10 days

PROCTITIS, PROCTOCOLITIS, AND ENTERITIS

Sexually transmitted gastrointestinal syndromes include proctitis, proctocolitis, and enteritis. Evaluation should include appropriate diagnostic procedures (eg, anoscopy or sigmoidoscopy, stool examination, culture).

Proctitis is inflammation of the rectum (the distal 10 to 12 cm) that may be associated with anorectal pain, tenesmus, or rectal discharge. *N gonorrhoeae, C trachomatis* (including LGV serovars), *T pallidum,* and HSV are the most common sexually transmitted pathogens involved. In patients co-infected with HIV, herpes proctitis may be especially severe. Proctitis occurs predominately among persons who participate in receptive anal intercourse.

Proctocolitis is associated with symptoms of proctitis plus diarrhea or abdominal cramps (or both) and inflammation of the colonic mucosa extending to 12 cm above the anus. Fecal leukocytes may be detected on stool examination depending on the pathogen. Pathogenic organisms include *Campylobacter* species, *Shigella* species, *Entamoeba histolytica,* and, rarely, LGV serovars of *C trachomatis.* Cytomegalovirus (CMV) or other opportunistic agents may be involved in immunosuppressed HIV-infected patients. Proctocolitis can be acquired by the oral route or by oral-anal contact, depending on the pathogen.

Enteritis usually results in diarrhea and abdominal cramping without signs of proctitis or proctocolitis; it occurs among persons whose sexual practices include oral-anal contact. In otherwise healthy patients, *Giardia lamblia* is most frequently implicated. When outbreaks of gastrointestinal illness occur among social or sexual networks of men who have sex with men, clinicians should consider sexual transmission as a mode of spread. Among HIV-infected patients, other infections that usually are not sexually transmitted may occur, including those caused by CMV, *Mycobacterium avium-intracellulare, Campylobacter* species, *Shigella* species, *Salmonella* species, *Cryptosporidium, Microsporidium,* and *Isospora.* Multiple stool examinations may be necessary to detect *Giardia,* and special stool preparations are required to diagnose cryptosporidiosis and microsporidiosis. Additionally, enteritis may be a primary effect of HIV infection.

When laboratory diagnostic capabilities are available, treatment should be based on the specific diagnosis. Diagnostic and treatment recommendations for all enteric infections are beyond the scope of these guidelines.

Treatment

Acute proctitis of recent onset among persons who have recently practiced receptive anal intercourse is most often sexually transmitted. Such patients should be examined by anoscopy and should be evaluated for infection with HSV, *N gonorrhoeae, C trachomatis,* and *T pallidum.* If an anorectal exudate is found on examination, or if

BOX 322-4 Treatment for Sexually Transmitted Infections—cont'd

polymorphonuclear leukocytes are found on a Gram-stained smear of anorectal secretions, the following therapy may be prescribed pending results of additional laboratory tests.

Recommended regimen

Ceftriaxone 125 mg IM (or another agent effective against rectal and genital gonorrhea) PLUS

Doxycycline 100 mg orally twice a day for 7 days

Patients with suspected or documented herpes proctitis should be managed in the same manner as those with genital herpes. If painful perianal ulcers are present or mucosal ulcers are detected on anoscopy, then presumptive therapy should include a regimen for treating genital herpes. In addition, LGV proctitis and proctocolitis also should be considered. Appropriate diagnostic testing for LGV should be conducted and doxycycline therapy should be administered (100 mg orally twice daily for 3 weeks).

From Centers for Disease Control and Prevention. Sexually transmitted diseases treatment guidelines, 2006. *MMWR* 2006;55(No. RR-11):1-94, and Centers for Disease Control and Prevention. Updated Recommended Treatment Regimens for Gonococcal Infections and Associated Conditions—United States, April, 2007 (www.cdc.gov/STD/treatment/2006/updated-regimens.htm.) (Most of the information contained in Box 322-4 is reproduced *verbatim* from the Treatment Guidelines or updated recommendations. In some cases, the author has edited the text to condense it.)

Neisseria gonorrhoeae

Infection with *N gonorrhoeae* produces a constellation of symptoms similar to that produced by *C trachomatis*. In general, men who are symptomatic with gonococcal infection tend to have more pronounced symptoms (more severe dysuria and a greater amount of and more purulent discharge), and they usually seek health care more quickly than those infected with *C trachomatis*. However, many patients have no symptoms at all. In a recent study of young adult men, the overall prevalence was 0.4%, with a range up to 2.4%; more than 95% were asymptomatic. Among young adult women, the overall rate of infection was 0.4%, (range up to 1.9%); almost 87% were asymptomatic.[14] The gonococcus can cause pharyngitis and proctitis; adolescent and young adult women may harbor the organism in the rectum even if they do not engage in anal intercourse.

The gonococcus can be grown from urethral or cervical discharge; from swabs of the vagina, cervix, urethra, pharynx, or rectum; and in many instances from urine sediment. In the past, the diagnosis of gonococcal infection rested on culture or on the classic findings of WBCs and gram-negative intracellular diplococci in Gram stains of discharge or material obtained from a urethral swab. Even under ideal conditions, the organism can be difficult to grow, and physicians relying on culture should be familiar with the yield from the laboratory they use. In men, a typical Gram stain from a urethral discharge is diagnostic (Figure 322-3). For samples taken from women, sorting out gram-negative organisms that truly are intracellular versus those that may be overlying or near the cells is more difficult. However, when at least 8 pairs of such diplococci are seen in at least 2 polymorphonuclear leukocytes, the culture will be positive 96% of the time.[20]

As is the case with chlamydia, diagnosis of *N gonorrhoeae* infections is now possible by NAAT. These tests are at least as sensitive as culture results but have the added advantage of eliminating the need for pelvic examination or swabbing the urethral meatus to obtain specimens; instead, a urine specimen or vaginal swab can be used.[9,17] Treatment regimens for uncomplicated gonococcal infections are listed in Box 322-4; as a result of increasing gonococcal resistance to fluoroquinolones, the CDC no longer recommends this class of antibiotics for treatment of gonococcal infection.[21] Because of the high likelihood of co-infection with chlamydia, treatment for gonorrhea must also include an effective regimen for *C trachomatis* unless a NAAT for chlamydia is known to be negative. Pharyngeal infection is more difficult to treat than infection at other sites.

Gonorrhea also may produce epididymitis and PID. In addition and in contrast to chlamydia, the gonococcal organism has the capacity to become blood borne and can lead to the so-called arthritis-dermatitis syndrome, or disseminated gonococcal infection (DGI). Approximately 1% to 3% of untreated patients develop DGI. Strains of *N gonorrhoeae* that lead to DGI characteristically tend to cause little in the way of genital symptoms. Typically, the patient develops fever (although not always) and may have anorexia, malaise, or both. Skin lesions then appear, generally distributed on the extremities (arms more often than legs). The lesions appear as erythematous macules less than 5 mm in diameter; they become pustular and occasionally hemorrhagic or necrotic (Figure 322-4). They are most often noticed near the small joints of the hands and feet. Accompanying the dermatitis is a tenosynovitis that tends to occur over the extensor and flexor tendons of the hands and feet. During this early phase of the infection, especially if evaluated within 2 to 3 days of onset of symptoms, 25% to 50% of patients will have positive blood cultures.[22]

In general, once the tenosynovitis and dermatitis clear, the patient develops polyarthralgia but usually seeks care only when an oligoarthritis develops. The knee is the joint most commonly infected, followed by the elbow, ankle, and small joints of the hands and feet. Hence, among adolescents, DGI should always be considered in the differential diagnosis of septic arthritis. Aspirates of joint fluid reveal the typical changes of septic arthritis, but joint fluid cultures are usually negative. Meningitis or endocarditis may also be present. Patients with DGI, especially those with arthritis, should be hospitalized—at least initially—for treatment (see Box 322-4).

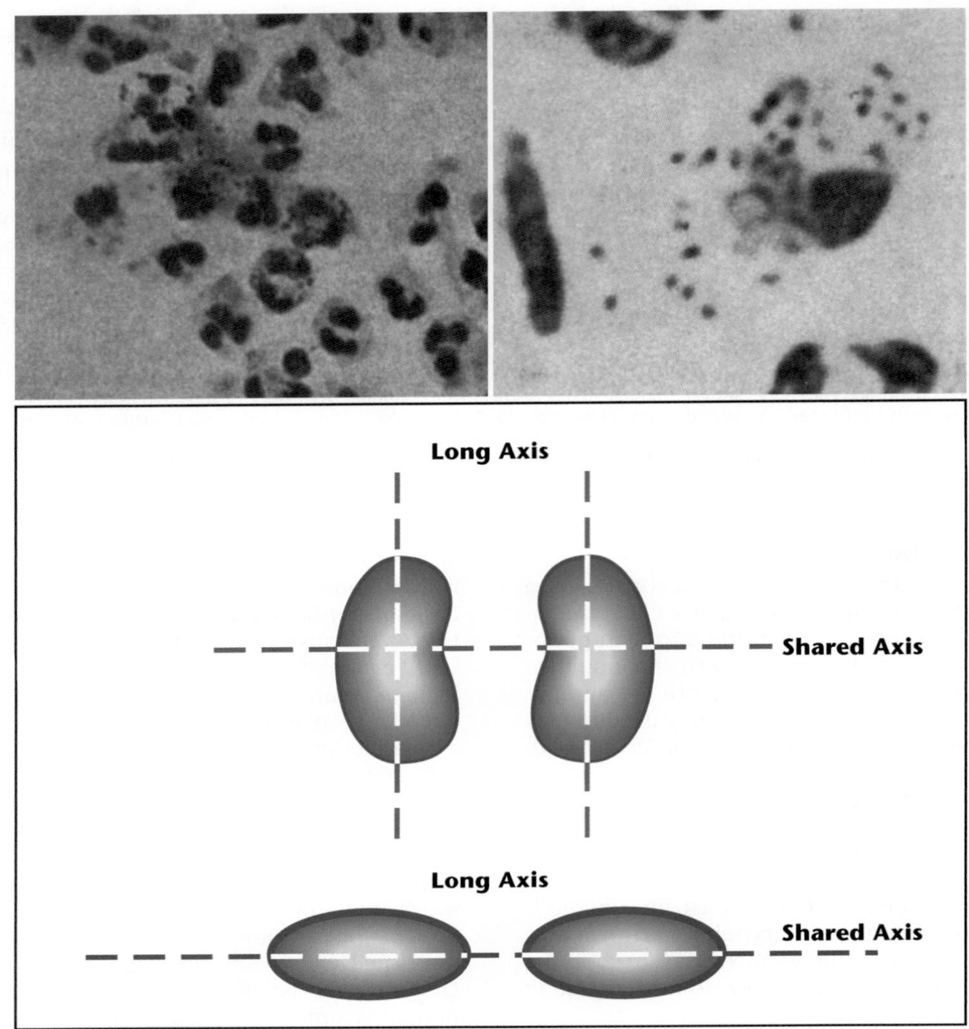

Figure 322-3 *Neisseria gonorrhoeae* on Gram stain of male urethral smears (original magnification ×1500 and ×4000) appear as tiny gram-negative diplococci within polymorphonuclear leukocytes with pink-stained nuclei *(top)*. *Neisseria* organisms are kidney bean–shaped, and their long axes are perpendicular to the shared axis *(bottom)*. *(Gilchrist MJR, Rauch JL. Office microscopy: low-cost screening for STDs.* Contemp Pediatr. *1987;4:54.)*

Human Papillomavirus (Genital Warts)

Infections with human papillomavirus (HPV) are the most prevalent STI in the United States. Such infections have always drawn attention because they cause unsightly warts (condylomata acuminatum), and because HPV infection represents the most common cause of an abnormal Papanicolaou test (Pap smear screening) among adolescent and young adult women. Concerns about HPV focus on its role in the development of cervical neoplasia. HPV infection has been associated with more than 90% of cervical dysplasia worldwide.[23]

More than 100 different types of HPV have been identified. The low-risk types 6 and 11 account for 97% of genital wart manifestations (external genital warts). Types 16, 18, 31, and 45 are responsible for approximately 80% of cervical cancers worldwide, with type 16 alone causing 40% to 60% of the disease burden.[24] An individual can be infected with more than 1 type of HPV.

As with other STIs, infection rates among adolescents and young adults are high. The prevalence of cervical HPV infection among adolescents ages 12 to 21 is approximately 51% to 64%. Longitudinal studies of adolescent girls suggest that approximately 45% to 55% become infected over a 3-year period of observation.[24]

Male adolescents constitute a significant reservoir of undetected HPV infection. Few male partners of HPV-positive women have clinical evidence of warts, but when magnification and acetic acid soaks are used to produce the acetowhite changes seen in HPV-infected skin, far more men are found to be infected (Figure 322-5).[25] Almost all data regarding HPV among men is drawn from those aged 18 and older; little information exists about younger adolescent boys.

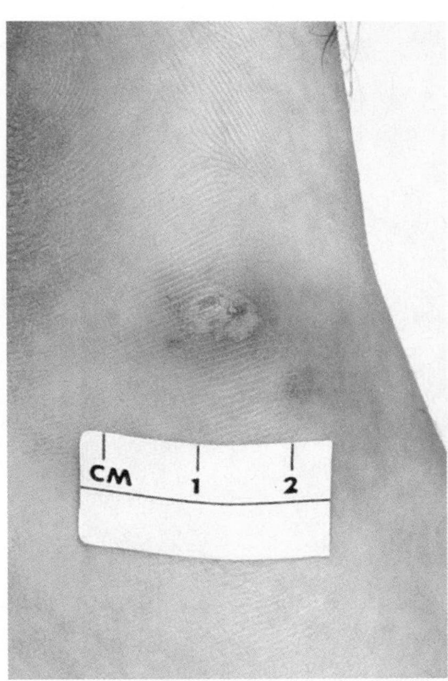

Figure 322-4 Disseminated gonococcal infection (DGI). If a gonorrhea infection is allowed to go untreated, the *N gonorrhoeae* can become disseminated throughout the body, forming lesions in extragenital locations. *(Baker CJ, ed.* Red Book Atlas of Pediatric Infectious Diseases. *Elk Grove Village, IL: American Academy of Pediatrics; 2007.)*

Visible warts usually develop within 6 weeks to 8 months after infection, but the incubation period may be even longer. The typical pedunculated wart with a keratotic and irregular surface is easy to recognize, but warts may also be flat and more difficult to detect. The use of a handheld magnifying glass or even a colposcope is extremely helpful. Among male adolescents, warts are usually seen on the penile shaft, prepuce, frenulum, corona, and glans, but they may also be present on the skin of the scrotum and the anus (Figure 322-6). The presence of anal warts is often associated with anal receptive intercourse, but warts in this location have been described in boys who deny this type of behavior. Occasionally, warts are seen at the urethral opening.

The posterior vaginal introitus, labia minora, and vestibule represent the most common sites of infection among female adolescents (Figure 322-7); again, however, warts can be seen anywhere on the external or internal genitalia. Perianal warts can be seen even in women who have not had anal intercourse. Subclinical disease is most likely to occur on the cervix; the relatively large transformation zone of the maturing adolescent cervix affords a hospitable site of infection for the virus. Extensive disease should raise the possibility of underlying HIV infection.

Evidence continues to accumulate linking the presence of HPV with the development of dysplastic and malignant changes in the cervix, making routine Pap smear screening to detect precancerous lesions extremely important. However, because most HPV infections among adolescents resolve spontaneously, Pap smear screening in adolescents may lead to additional diagnostic testing that can be psychologically upsetting, unnecessary, and expensive. In an attempt to balance the need for screening with an approach that minimizes the potential for harm, the American Cancer Society developed guidelines for initiating Pap smear screening for cervical neoplasia and cancer in young women.[26] Their guidelines recommend that Pap smear screening begin within 3 years of initiation of voluntary sexual intercourse or age 21, whichever comes first. Some experts suggest initiating earlier screening for adolescents who have a high number of sexual partners, who are immunosuppressed, or who are at risk for nonadherence to follow-up advice. These experts also recommend initial screening of teenagers who have been sexually abused (with penetration) whenever feasible by someone skilled in examining this population. Immunosuppressed women should be screened every 6 months in the 1st year and then yearly as long as the result is normal.

Use of HPV DNA typing has become an important adjunct to the management of abnormal Pap smear screening findings in adult women. However, its use may be limited in teenagers because HPV infection is so common among sexually active adolescents yet tends to be self-limited (ie, rarely progresses to cervical cancer).[27] Current guidelines from the American Society for Colposcopy and Cervical Pathology do not include the use of HPV DNA typing for the management of adolescents (aged 20 and under) with atypical squamous cells of undetermined significance or low-grade squamous intraeptithelial on Pap smear screening (Figure 322-8).[28] HPV DNA typing may be used to manage abnormal Pap smears in women who are 21 or older.

A variety of treatments for genital warts exist, including those applied by clinicians or by the patient (see Box 322-4); treatment is primarily directed toward symptomatic warts. Clinicians who choose to treat genital warts should determine which technique is most suitable to their practice and become familiar with that technique; clinicians should be knowledgeable about at least 1 physician-applied and 1 patient-applied regimen. Regardless of which approach is chosen, careful follow-up (initially at weekly intervals) is essential to monitor the results and to prevent regrowth between too widely spaced treatment intervals. The benefit of treating subclinical HPV infection in the absence of cervical dysplasia is unclear. Examination and treatment of sex partners is of uncertain benefit.

Because HPV infection is so prevalent, and because it is uncertain whether treatment reduces infectivity, current approaches to the prevention and eradication of HPV infection focus on HPV vaccines.[29] The US Food and Drug Administration recently approved a 3-dose (0, 2, and 6 months) quadrivalent HPV vaccine containing virus-like particles of types 6, 11, 16, and 18. In 1 clinical trial, the vaccine was 89% effective in preventing persistent infection with the 4 viral types contained in the vaccine; no cases of cervical intraepithelial neoplasia occurred in the vaccine group versus 3 among the placebo recipients.[30] Based on these and other data, the Advisory Committee on Immunization

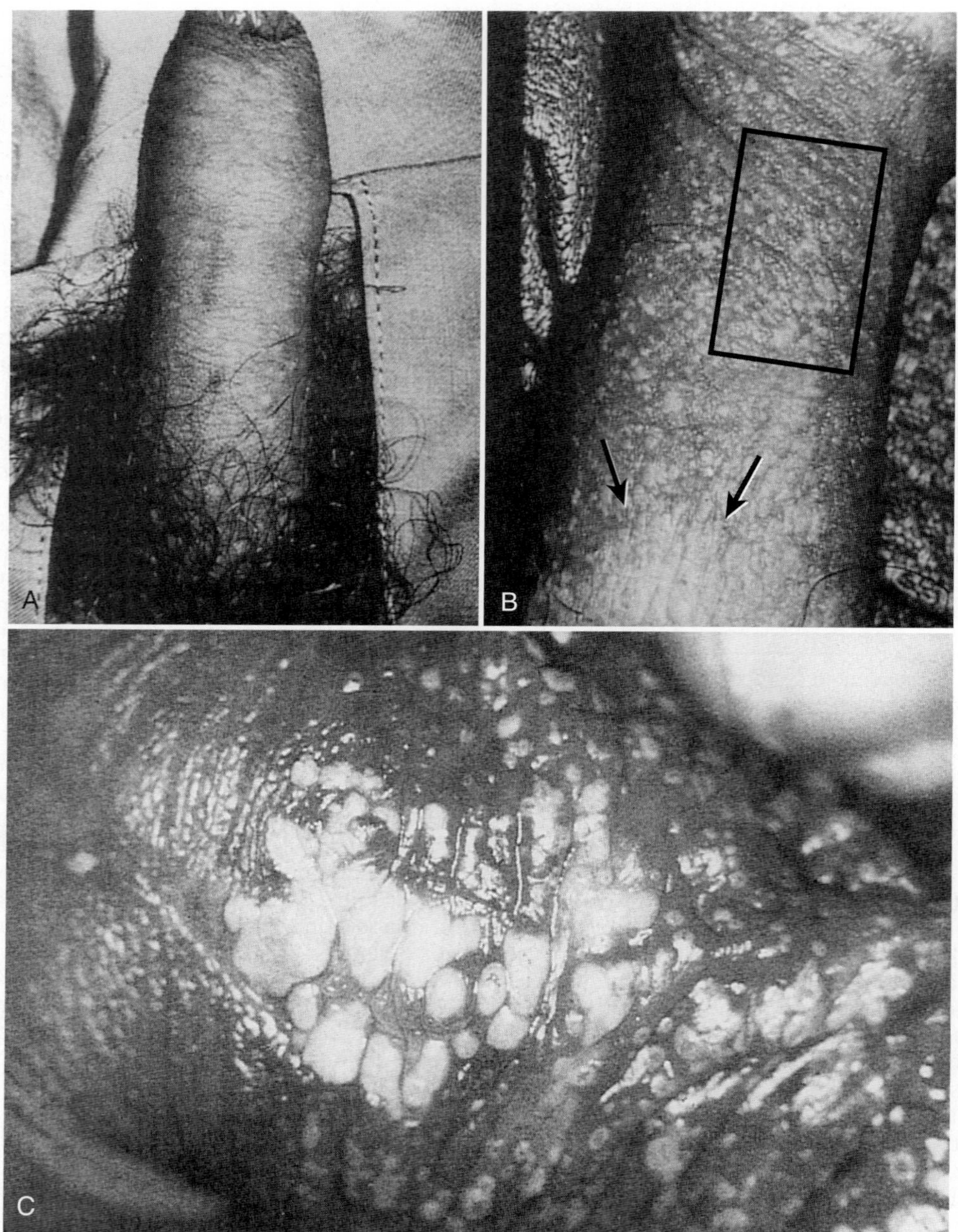

Figure 322-5 Demonstration of subclinical lesions. **A**, Appearance of penis before application of acetic acid. **B**, Penis after 5-minute application of gauze soaked in 5% acetic acid. Note coalescing sheets *(arrows)* and discrete dots of acetowhite staining *(inset)*. **C**, Magnified view of apparent subclinical human papillomavirus infection shown in panel B. *(Katelaris PM, Cossart YE, Rose BR, et al. Human papilloma virus: the untreated male reservoir.* J Urol. *1988;140:300-305. Copyright © 1988, Elsevier, with permission.)*

Practices recommends that the vaccine be administered to girls ages 11 to 12 as a priority, but the vaccine can be offered to girls as young as 9 and is also recommended for those aged 13 to 26 who have not been vaccinated or have not received all 3 doses.[31] The protective effect appears to last for 2.5 to 3.5 years; whether a booster dose will be needed is unknown at this time. A 2nd vaccine is currently under review by the US Food and Drug Administration.[29]

Herpes Genitalis

Herpes simplex viral infections of the male and female genital tract are particularly distressing to patients because of the potential for recurrence after an initial episode, especially if caused by infection with herpes simplex virus (HSV) type 2. HSV-1 and HSV-2 can cause genital tract disease; in recent years, infection with HSV-1 has accounted for an increasing proportion of genital herpes infections.[32] Although genital

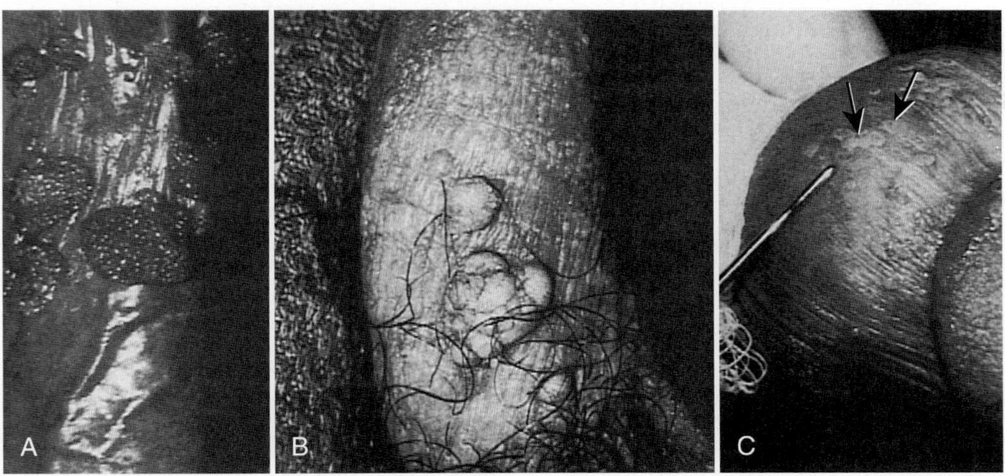

Figure 322-6 Morphology of macroscopic warts. **A**, Condylomata demonstrated by preputial retraction. **B**, Verrucous wart at penoscrotal junction. **C**, Small, flat warts *(arrows)* on distal third of penis. *(Katelaris PM, Cossart YE, Rose BR, et al. Human papilloma virus: the untreated male reservoir.* J Urol. *1988;140:300-305. Copyright © 1988, Elsevier, with permission.)*

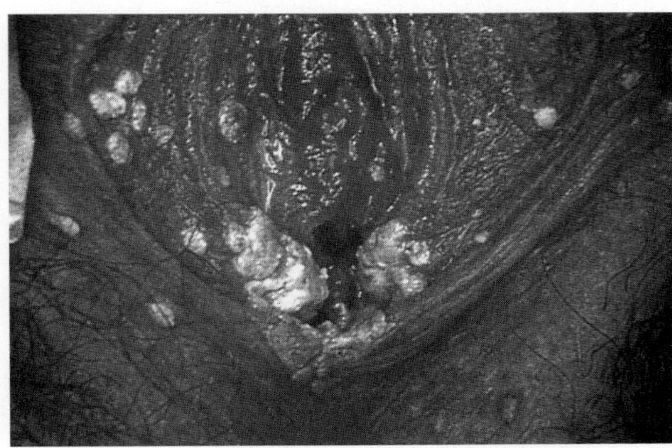

Figure 322-7 Condyloma acuminatum of the vulva appears as a polypoid mass with a keratotic fissured and irregular surface. *(Moscicki AB. HPV infections: an old STD revisited.* Contemp Pediatr. *1989;6:24. Reprinted by permission.)*

herpes infections were once believed to be associated with the development of cervical cancer, current evidence indicates that HSV more likely acts as a cofactor. Seroprevalence surveys indicate that the prevalence of HSV-2 infection among young people has decreased dramatically in the last decade (with a smaller decline for HSV-1).[33]

Infections with the virus can be classified as primary or nonprimary. Primary infection refers to infection with HSV-1 or HSV-2 in an individual without prior antibody to either virus. Nonprimary infection occurs in those with existing antibody to either HSV-1 or HSV-2 who become infected with the other strain. This type of infection, which almost always occurs in individuals who have existing antibody to HSV-1 who then become infected with HSV-2, tends to be less symptomatic. At least 10% of individuals (but probably many more) with a 1st symptomatic clinical episode of genital herpes have serologic evidence of previous HSV-2 infection.[34]

In primary infection, symptoms usually occur within 2 to 20 days after sexual exposure. The patient experiences burning or itching at the site of inoculation, followed by erythema and the development of discrete vesicles. Initially, the vesicles contain clear fluid, but they rapidly form pustules with an erythematous base. Typically, a patient may have 15 to 30 vesicles, each full of infectious viral particles. Lesions are located on the vulva, cervix, clitoris, or perineum. In male adolescents, they may occur on the penile shaft, glans, or prepuce (Figure 322-9). Infection also can involve the urethra, leading to dysuria or urinary retention. Vesicles can be seen on the thighs, buttocks, groin, or perianal region as a result of autoinoculation or anal receptive intercourse.

Because primary infection represents the 1st episode of infection with the particular virus type, systemic symptoms such as fever, malaise, and headache are common. Approximately 50% of patients have tender inguinal lymphadenopathy.

After 2 to 4 days, the pustules break open and coalesce to form wet ulcers. This event is usually when patients seek health care. New lesions still may be developing at this point (with a peak at 7-11 days), but within 20 days, all the lesions have crusted over, and the pain and other symptoms have disappeared. The lesions generally heal without scarring.

The diagnosis of herpes genitalis is made most often on clinical grounds. Cultures of intact vesicles are generally positive, as are cultures of the cervix. Because recurrence rates for genital HSV-1 and HSV-2 differ

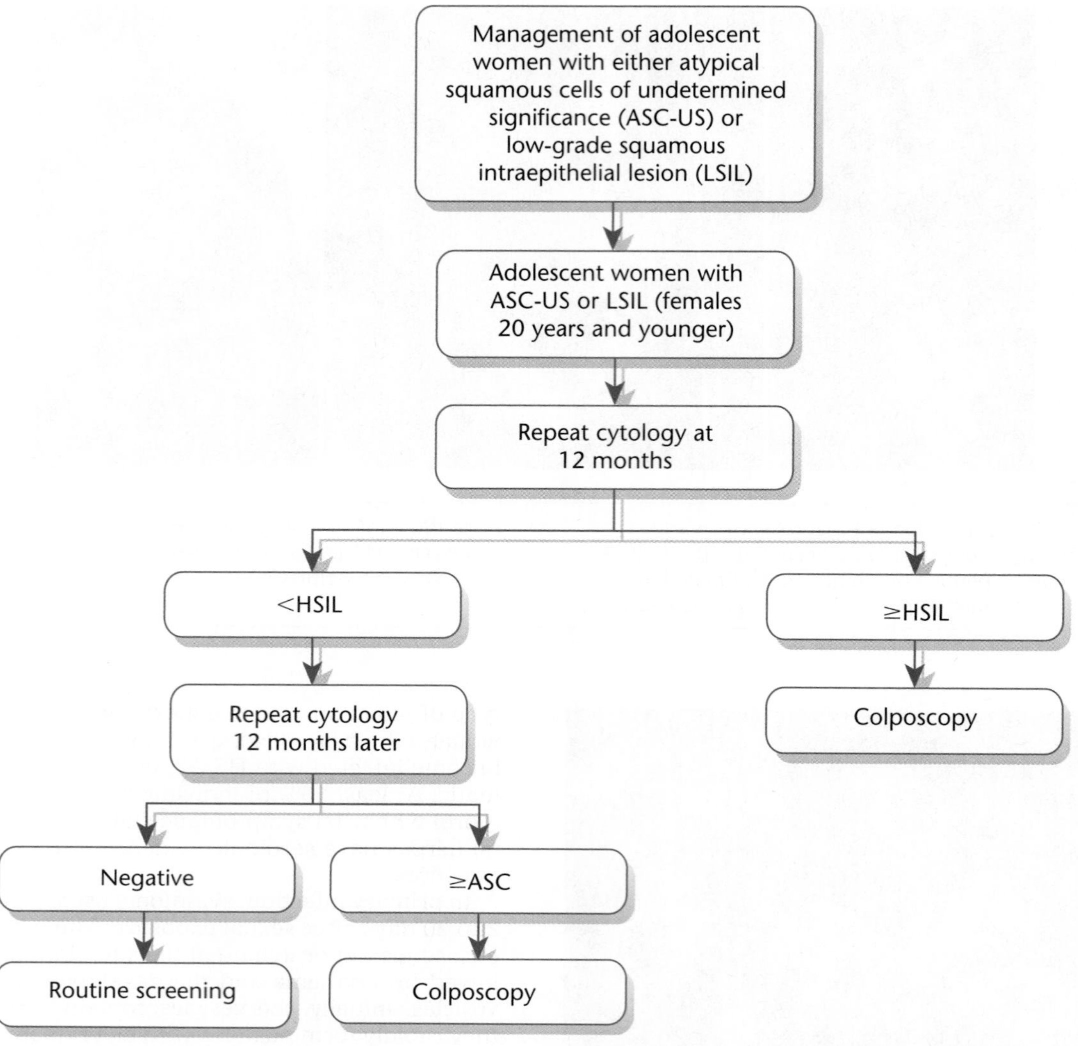

Figure 322-8 Papanicolaou test (Pap smear) guidelines. American College of Obstetricians and Gynecologists. *(American College of Obstetricians and Gynecologists, Committee on Adolescent Health Care. Evaluation and management of abnormal cervical cytology and histology in the adolescent.* Obstet Gynecol. *2006;107:963-968. Reprinted by permission.)*

significantly, culture should be obtained whenever a patient presents with new-onset genital herpes.

After the infection resolves, the virus remains latent in the sacral ganglia and may reactivate at any time. This reactivation is referred to as *recurrent disease.* Recurrences may occur in association with stress, local trauma, fever, or menstruation and tend to be shorter and less symptomatic. Vesicles usually occur near the initial infection site but tend to be fewer in number. Just before the recurrence, the patient may experience burning or itching at the site of infection. Healing takes place within 1 to 2 weeks.

Female adolescents whose only site of recurrence involves the cervix may be unaware of it, although they are shedding the virus. Approximately one third of male adolescents also may have inapparent recurrences but are still infectious. Asymptomatic reactivation is most likely to happen within 6 months after the initial infection. Hence, unless sex partners reveal their history of infection, many exposures can occur without an individual being aware that contact with the virus has been made. Many HSV-seropositive patients who deny a history of genital herpes actually have lesions that they fail to recognize as herpes. Nevertheless, they are capable of infecting their sex partners.

In the year after a 1st documented episode of genital HSV-2 infection, 90% of individuals will have at least 1 recurrence; approximately one third will have 6 or more, and one fifth will have 10 or more.[32] The risk of recurrence depends on many factors. Male adolescents are somewhat more likely to have recurrent disease, as are those whose infection was caused by HSV-2. Once a 2nd episode occurs, the patient is likely to have multiple recurrences.

Development of antiviral drugs such as acyclovir, famciclovir, or valacyclovir has dramatically altered the

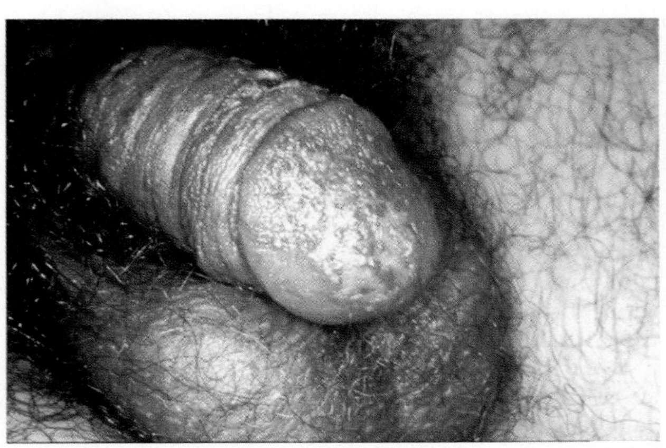

Figure 322-9 In herpes genitalis, the blisters break, leaving tender ulcers that may take 2 to 4 weeks to heal the first time they occur. *(Baker J, ed.* Red Book Atlas of Pediatric Infectious Diseases. *Elk Grove Village, IL: American Academy of Pediatrics; 2007.)*

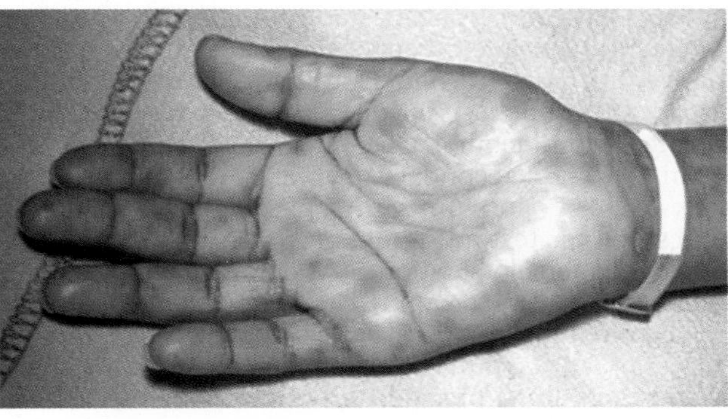

Figure 322-10 A 16-year-old girl with the rash of secondary syphilis. The signs and symptoms of secondary syphilis generally occur 6 to 8 weeks after the primary infection, when primary lesions are healed. *(Baker CJ, ed.* Red Book Atlas of Pediatric Infectious Diseases. *Elk Grove Village, IL: American Academy of Pediatrics; 2007.)*

nature of herpes therapy. These agents greatly reduce the symptoms associated with primary episodes of genital herpes and decrease the duration of virus shedding and the time to resolution of lesions (see Box 322-4). Some patients with recurrent disease may derive benefit from therapy if the medication can be initiated during the prodrome or within 1 day after onset of lesions. Those who have 6 or more recurrences per year have a 75% reduction in recurrences with daily suppressive therapy (see Box 322-4).[7] Patient-initiated administration of a single-day course of famciclovir also shortens the duration of recurrences. Valacyclovir reduces asymptomatic virus shedding and reduces the risk of infection in couples serodiscordant for HSV-2.[35] A glycoprotein vaccine for prevention of HSV-2 infection has a protective effect at 5 months but not at 1 year for persons receiving the vaccine.[36]

Syphilis

Rates of primary and secondary syphilis decreased by 90% from 1990 to 2000, then increased from 2000 to 2004. The increase was seen only among men, although for the 1st time in a decade, the rate of syphilis among women did not continue to decrease from 2003 to 2004. Syphilis remains a significant problem in the South and in some urban areas. Rates have increased since 2000 among men who have sex with men, and it often co-occurs with HIV infection.[37]

The typical chancre of syphilis develops at the site of intimate sexual contact approximately 2 to 3 weeks after exposure to an infected individual. This lesion, which varies in size from a few millimeters to a few centimeters, is clean based, painless, and has sharply demarcated, indurated borders. Multiple ulcers may be present. Lymphadenopathy is usually present, often bilaterally. Because the ulcer is painless, its appearance in the vagina or rectum or even in the mouth is likely to go unnoticed. While the ulcer is present, the exudate overlying it is highly infectious. Untreated, the chancre disappears in 3 to 6 weeks.

The rash of secondary syphilis appears 4 to 10 weeks after the chancre appears in the untreated patient. Hence the rash and the chancre may coexist. Because the spirochetes spread hematogenously from the site of initial infection, constitutional symptoms such as fever, malaise, sore throat, and generalized lymphadenopathy may be present.

The rash is typically papulosquamous but can be macular or pustular. Initially, it involves the trunk and flexor surfaces of the arms but then spreads to the entire body, including the palms, soles, and mucous membranes (Figure 322-10). Clinicians should strongly consider screening any sexually active adolescent with a generalized eruption (eg, that seen with pityriasis rosea) for syphilis. Annular papules can appear on the face, and the rash can resemble impetigo or eczema. In some cases, moist, fissured papules or raised, thickened papules (condyloma lata) are seen; both are highly infectious. Finally, loss of scalp or eyebrow hair can be associated with secondary syphilis. The rash disappears spontaneously 3 to 12 weeks after its appearance; at this point, the patient is classified as having latent syphilis.

At the time the chancre is present, a dark-field examination of the nonbloody exudate should be performed by an expert in dark-field microscopy. If performed on 3 successive days, the likelihood of obtaining a positive result from an infected individual is extremely high. If the results of all 3 examinations are negative, then the diagnosis of primary syphilis should be reconsidered. If the dark-field examination is unavailable, then a serologic test for syphilis should be obtained. If the examiner is relatively certain that the chancre is one of primary syphilis, a request for fluorescent treponemal antibody absorption test should then be made because the sensitivity of the VDRL (Venereal Disease Research Laboratory) flocculation test, the rapid plasma reagin (RPR), test, and the microhemagglutination assay for antibody to *Treponema pallidum* at this point in the disease process are relatively low. However, because all the symptoms of syphilis may not be consistently present in everyone infected, most adolescents infected with syphilis will be identified only through routine serologic screening; therefore testing at-risk youth is important.

The recommended CDC treatment guidelines for primary and secondary syphilis are outlined in Box 322-4. Follow-up with repeat clinical evaluation and serologic testing should occur at 6 and 12 months; more frequent evaluation is warranted if findings at follow-up are uncertain. Criteria for reevaluation or retreatment include persistence or recurrence of clinical signs and symptoms, a sustained 4-fold or more increase in titers, or failure of nontreponemal tests to decline 4 fold within 6 months after treatment for primary or secondary syphilis. All patients with syphilis should be screened for HIV infection.

Patients who are seroreactive but do not have any physical findings of infection are classified as having latent syphilis. Patients who are known to have seroconverted within the previous 12 months are classified as early latent syphilis, as are those who, within the previous year (1) have had unequivocal symptoms of primary or secondary syphilis; (2) have had a sex partner documented to have primary, secondary, or early latent syphilis; or (3) have reactive treponemal and nontreponemal tests with the only possible exposure occurring within the previous year. However, early and late latent syphilis cannot be distinguished from one another based on titers alone; hence all patients with latent syphilis should have a thorough physical examination with particular attention directed to examination of the oral cavity, the perineum in women, the perianal area, and beneath the foreskin in uncircumcised men. Patients with latent syphilis should be treated as indicated in Box 322-4. According to the 2006 CDC guidelines, patients with latent syphilis should undergo examination of the cerebrospinal fluid if they (1) have any neurologic or ophthalmic signs or symptoms, (2) have any evidence of tertiary syphilis, (3) do not respond to initial treatment, or (4) have HIV infection concomitant with late latent syphilis or syphilis of unknown duration.

Mycoplasma genitalium

Increasing evidence indicates that infection with *Mycoplasma genitalium* is an important cause of urethritis in men and women and of cervicitis in women.[38] The association is particularly strong in men with urethritis who test negative for gonorrhea and chlamydia.[39] A high concordance rate of infection exists among sexual partners of infected patients. Treatment is more effective with azithromycin than with the tetracyclines.

SYNDROMES ASSOCIATED WITH SEXUALLY TRANSMITTED DISEASES

Pelvic Inflammatory Disease

PID refers to infection involving the upper genital tract (uterus, fallopian tubes, ovaries, and pelvis) of women; it often occurs as a result of undetected or inadequately treated STIs of the lower genital tract (endocervix). In the short term, PID can lead to such problems as a tuboovarian abscess. In the long run, infertility, chronic pelvic pain, and increased risk for ectopic pregnancy are attributable to this condition, even when the acute episode has been managed appropriately. Among all sexually active girls and women, teenagers younger than 19 years are at greatest risk for contracting this disease; the risk is 1:8 for sexually active 15 year olds and 1:16 for 16 year olds, but only 1:80 for 24 year olds.[40] Because a major risk factor for developing PID is a prior episode, adolescent girls who experience this illness early in their reproductive life cycle are at great risk for having further significant problems.

Even though the condition is common, the diagnosis of PID is imprecise. Studies have shown that clinical diagnosis of PID has a positive predictive value for salpingitis of 65% to 90%, with the positive predictive value being higher for adolescents and in clinical settings in which the prevalence of STIs such as chlamydia or gonorrhea are high.[7] Signs and symptoms can be nonspecific, and the only sure method for diagnosis, laparoscopy, is not routinely performed for diagnostic purposes in the United States. Primary care physicians must therefore maintain a high index of suspicion, obtain an extensive history, and perform a thorough physical examination to avoid a misdiagnosis.

When eliciting a history from a patient who has lower abdominal pain, the physician should keep in mind specific factors that place an individual at risk for infection. Hence failure to use barrier methods of contraception, douching, the presence of an intrauterine device, multiple partners, a recent change in partner, or history of other STIs or PID should raise concern. The presence of a new vaginal discharge (or a change in odor, color, or amount), abnormal menstrual bleeding (increased or prolonged; occurring at the wrong time in the cycle), or dyspareunia are all suggestive of PID. Other symptoms include dysuria, dysmenorrhea (usually more severe than normal), nausea, vomiting, diarrhea, fever, and malaise. Except for dysmenorrhea, these symptoms also can be seen in patients who have diseases of the urinary tract (eg, pyelonephritis) or gastrointestinal tract (eg, appendicitis).

Depending on the extent of upper genital tract involvement, physical signs may include pain on movement of the cervix and endometrial or adnexal tenderness, or both. Fever is present in less than 50% of patients who have documented PID. If the infection has spread to involve the capsule of the liver, then right upper quadrant tenderness also may be elicited. With extensive infection, signs of peritonitis, particularly rebound tenderness, are present. The palpation of an adnexal mass raises the concern of a coexisting tuboovarian abscess. Mucopus visible in the cervical os strongly suggests the presence of infection, but its absence does not rule out the diagnosis. Acute-phase reactants lack the necessary sensitivity and specificity to be helpful in establishing the diagnosis of PID. Although 60% to 80% of patients have an increased WBC count, sedimentation rate, or C-reactive protein,[41] so do 20% to 50% of patients with abdominal pain who do not have PID. Estimates suggest that up to 60% of cases of PID are subclinical.

BOX 322-5 Diagnostic Considerations of Pelvic Inflammatory Disease

Acute pelvic inflammatory disease (PID) is difficult to diagnose because of the wide variation in the symptoms and signs. Many women with PID have subtle or mild symptoms that do not readily indicate PID. Consequently, delay in diagnosis and effective treatment probably contributes to inflammatory sequelae in the upper reproductive tract. Laparoscopy can be performed to obtain a more accurate diagnosis of salpingitis and a more complete bacteriologic diagnosis. However, in many instances, this diagnostic tool is not readily available for acute cases, and its use is not easy to justify when symptoms are mild or vague. Moreover, laparoscopy will not detect endometritis and may not detect subtle inflammation of the fallopian tubes. Consequently, a diagnosis of PID is usually based on clinical findings.

The clinical diagnosis of acute PID is imprecise. Data indicate that a clinical diagnosis of symptomatic PID has a positive predictive value of 65% to 90% for salpingitis in comparison with laparoscopy. The positive predictive value of a clinical diagnosis of acute PID differs depending on epidemiologic characteristics and the clinical setting, with higher positive predictive value among sexually active young (especially adolescent) women, among patients attending sexually transmitted disease clinics, or in settings in which rates of gonorrhea or chlamydia are high. In all settings, however, no single historical, physical, or laboratory finding is both sensitive and specific for the diagnosis of acute PID (ie, can be used both to detect all cases of PID and to exclude all women without PID). Combinations of diagnostic findings that improve either sensitivity (ie, detect more women who have PID) or specificity (ie, exclude more women who do not have PID) do so only at the expense of the other. For example, requiring 2 or more findings excludes more women who do not have PID but also reduces the number of women with PID who are identified.

Many episodes of PID go unrecognized. Although some cases are asymptomatic, others are undiagnosed because the patient or the primary care physician fails to recognize the implications of mild or nonspecific symptoms or signs (eg, abnormal bleeding, dyspareunia, vaginal discharge). Because of the difficulty of diagnosis and the potential for damage to the reproductive health of women, even by apparently mild or subclinical PID, primary care physicians should maintain a low threshold for the diagnosis of PID. The optimal treatment regimen and long-term outcome of women with asymptomatic or subclinical PID are unknown. The following suggestions for diagnosing PID are intended to help primary care physicians recognize when PID should be suspected and when they need to obtain additional information to increase diagnostic certainty. These suggestions are based partially on the fact that diagnosis and management of other common causes of lower abdominal pain (eg, ectopic pregnancy, acute appendicitis, functional pain) are unlikely to be impaired by initiating empiric antimicrobial therapy for PID.

Empiric treatment of PID should be initiated in sexually active young women and others at risk for sexually transmitted diseases if they are experiencing pelvic or lower abdominal pain, if no other cause for the illness other than PID can be identified, and if 1 or more of the following minimal criteria are present on pelvic examination: cervical motion tenderness *or* uterine tenderness *or* adnexal tenderness. Requiring that all 3 of the minimal criteria listed previously be present before initiating antibiotic treatment might result in insufficient sensitivity for diagnosing PID.

More elaborate diagnostic evaluation is frequently needed because incorrect diagnosis and management might cause unnecessary morbidity. Additional criteria that can be used to enhance the specificity of the minimal criteria and support a diagnosis of PID include the following:

- Oral temperature above 101°F (38.3°C)
- Abnormal cervical or vaginal mucopurulent discharge
- Presence of abundant numbers of white blood cells on saline microscopy of vaginal secretions
- Increased erythrocyte sedimentation rate
- Increased levels of C-reactive protein
- Laboratory documentation of cervical infection with *Neisseria gonorrhoeae* or *Chlamydia trachomatis*

From Centers for Disease Control and Prevention. Sexually transmitted diseases treatment guidelines, 2006. *MMWR.* 2006;55(RR-11):56-57. (Most of the information contained herein is reproduced verbatim from the Treatment Guidelines. In some cases, the author has edited the text to condense it.)

The CDC's 2006 sexually transmitted disease treatment guidelines recommend that treatment of PID be initiated in sexually active young women if "they are experiencing pelvic or lower abdominal pain, if no cause for the illness other than PID can be identified, and if 1 or more of the following minimum criteria are present on pelvic examination: cervical motion tenderness OR uterine tenderness OR adnexal tenderness."[7] Other supportive criteria for PID are listed in Box 322-5. The physician should take particular note that certain surgical emergency conditions can mimic PID. Hence the differential diagnosis, as outlined in Box 322-6, should be kept in mind. Because many teenagers at risk for PID are similarly at risk for pregnancy, and because ectopic pregnancy can mimic PID, a urine or serum pregnancy test should be routinely obtained at the time of evaluation. If an adnexal mass is palpated or suspected, then an ultrasound should be obtained to determine whether a tuboovarian abscess is present. Testing for *C trachomatis* and *N gonorrhoeae* should occur routinely.

In the past, hospitalization of adolescents with PID was common. However, the outcomes of teenagers with PID treated as inpatients or outpatients are similar; younger and older women respond the same to outpatient treatment. The decision to hospitalize a teenager with suspected PID should therefore be chosen based on the same criteria as used for older women (Box 322-7). If outpatient treatment is chosen, then careful follow-up is essential.

BOX 322-6 Differential Diagnosis of Acute Lower Abdominal Pain in Adolescent Girls by Organ System

URINARY TRACT
Cystitis
Pyelonephritis
Urethritis
Other

GASTROINTESTINAL TRACT
Appendicitis
Constipation
Diverticulitis
Gastroenteritis
Inflammatory bowel disease
Irritable bowel syndrome
Other

REPRODUCTIVE TRACT
Acute pelvic inflammatory disease
Cervicitis
Dysmenorrhea (primary or secondary)
Ectopic pregnancy
Endometriosis
Endometritis
Mittelschmerz
Ovarian cyst (torsion, rupture)
Pregnancy (intrauterine, ectopic)
Ruptured follicle
Septic abortion
Threatened abortion
Torsion of adnexa
Tuboovarian abscess

From Shafer M, Sweet RL. Pelvic inflammatory disease in adolescent females. *Pediatr Clin North Am.* 1989;36:513-532. Copyright © 1989, Elsevier, with permission.

BOX 322-7 Suggested Indications for Hospitalization of Patients With Pelvic Inflammatory Disease

In the past, some experts suggested that all patients who had pelvic inflammatory disease (PID) be hospitalized so that bed rest and supervised treatment with parenteral antibiotics might be initiated. However, in women with PID of mild or moderate clinical severity, outpatient therapy can provide short- and long-term clinical outcomes similar to inpatient therapy. Limited data support the use of outpatient therapy in women with more severe disease. The decision of whether hospitalization is necessary should be based on the discretion of the primary care physician.

The following criteria for hospitalization are suggested:

- Surgical emergencies such as appendicitis cannot be excluded.
- The patient is pregnant.
- The patient does not respond clinically to oral antimicrobial therapy.
- The patient is unable to follow or tolerate an outpatient oral regimen.
- The patient has severe illness, nausea and vomiting, or high fever.
- The patient has a tuboovarian abscess.

Many practitioners have preferred to hospitalize adolescents with suspected acute PID. However, no evidence exists to support this approach. Adolescents with mild to moderate acute PID have similar outcomes with either outpatient or inpatient therapy. Clinical response to outpatient therapy is similar among adolescents and older women. The decision to hospitalize an adolescent should be based on the same criteria as for older women.

Most clinicians favor at least 24 hours of direct inpatient observation for patients who have tuboovarian abscesses.

From Centers for Disease Control and Prevention. Sexually transmitted diseases treatment guidelines, 2006. *MMWR.* 2006;55(RR-11):56-57. (Most of the information contained herein is reproduced verbatim from the Treatment Guidelines. In some cases, the author has edited the text to condense it.)

Treatment is directed toward eradicating the organism responsible for the infection. Unfortunately, the exact nature of the infection is established with great difficulty. Test results obtained from cervical specimens do not necessarily reflect the nature of the tubal infection. Many organisms believed to play a role in PID are difficult to grow in culture; thus, studies that did not use state-of-the-art culture techniques may not have identified all relevant organisms. Studies that have been performed emphasize the polymicrobial nature of the infection. *N gonorrhoeae, C trachomatis,* or both are recovered from approximately 25% to 75% of adolescents and young adults with PID.[40] Facultative and anaerobic bacteria, as well as organisms associated with bacterial vaginosis, have been recovered from various points in the upper genital tract of women who have PID.

As a result of the uncertainty concerning the nature of the infecting organisms, the CDC treatment regimens outlined in Box 322-4 reflect empirical therapy based on the assumption that the infection is polymicrobial. The suggestion for doxycycline as part of therapy, with its potential to stain developing teeth, underscores the need for obtaining a pregnancy test before treatment. If outpatient therapy is to be attempted, then careful follow-up at 48 hours must be ensured, and a mechanism for hospitalizing the patient before that time if symptoms worsen must be in place.

Once therapy is initiated, the patient should improve within 48 to 72 hours. Failure to see improvement should raise concerns about the accuracy of the diagnosis or the presence of complications. The pelvic examination should be repeated to look for a tuboovarian abscess if one has not already been detected. Approximately 10% to 20% of patients who have PID develop a tuboovarian abscess; 3% to 15% of these abscesses rupture.[42] Depending on the experience of the clinician, consultation with a gynecologist should be considered if an abscess is detected or if the patient fails to improve. Consultation with a surgeon should be obtained if concern exists that the patient has appendicitis.

If hospitalized, the patient may be switched to oral therapy 24 hours after she demonstrates substantial clinical improvement. Treatment must include a total of 14 days of therapy with doxycycline (or other suitable oral regimens), and follow-up at completion of treatment is essential. The patient should be instructed not to have intercourse until her therapy is completed and her partner is notified and treated. Because an episode of PID is a major risk factor for development of a 2nd episode, the use of barrier methods of contraception must be stressed to the patient.

Even with optimal diagnosis and treatment, the long-term morbidity from a single episode of PID can be significant. Long-term complications include tubal factor infertility, increased risk for ectopic pregnancy, and chronic pelvic pain. Risk for infertility and ectopic pregnancy increases with the number of episodes of PID and with the severity of infection; women younger than 25 years at time of diagnosis are less likely to develop either complication.

Perihepatitis (Fitz-Hugh–Curtis Syndrome)

Perihepatitis associated with gonococcal salpingitis was described in 1920. Subsequently, Fitz-Hugh described a patient who had *violin string* adhesions between the liver and anterior abdominal wall, and Curtis described localized peritonitis of the liver's anterior surface in a woman who had upper abdominal pain and tenderness who was undergoing laparotomy for suspected gallbladder disease. Since then, the fact that *C trachomatis* infections can cause a similar picture has been well documented.

Onset of upper abdominal pain usually follows the onset of lower abdominal pain, but it can precede it. The pain generally occurs on the patient's right side and can radiate to the shoulder. Less than 50% of patients have mildly increased liver enzyme levels. Treatment for PID also eliminates the perihepatitis.

Epididymitis

Epididymitis is characterized by the acute or subacute onset of unilateral scrotal pain; adolescent boys may complain of testicular pain. Preceding symptoms include urethral discharge and dysuria, but these symptoms may be so mild that they are easily ignored. Fever may be present. At physical examination, tenderness may occur on palpation of the epididymis, but the testicle may also be slightly tender. A hydrocele may be present, and the spermatic cord may also be swollen and tender. Urethral discharge may or may not be present at the time of diagnosis.

Supportive laboratory evidence for the diagnosis of epididymitis includes (1) a positive leukocyte esterase test on a 1st-catch urine specimen (the first 20 mL of urine voided) or the presence of more than 10 WBCs per high-power field if the 1st-catch urine specimen is spun down and the sediment examined, or (2) Gram stain of urethral secretions showing more than 5 WBCs per oil-immersion field. If the Gram stain also shows WBCs containing intracellular gram-negative diplococci, *N gonorrhoeae* should be considered the causative agent.

In adolescents, the primary care physician must rule out testicular torsion. Depending on the presentation and laboratory evidence, additional studies (nuclear scan or Doppler flow study) or consultation with a specialist may be necessary.

Among sexually active adolescents, acute epididymitis is most frequently caused by *N gonorrhoeae* or *C trachomatis*. Sexually transmitted enteric organisms (eg, *Escherichia coli*) may be the causative agent in male adolescents who practice anal insertive intercourse. Patients with epididymitis should be tested for *N gonorrhoeae* and *C trachomatis*.

Most patients can be managed on an outpatient basis. Hospitalization should be considered if the pain is particularly severe (suggesting an alternate diagnosis such as torsion, testicular infarction, or abscess), when patients are febrile, or if noncompliance is of concern.

Treatment of epididymitis is outlined in Box 322-4. Adolescents treated as outpatients should be followed up within 48 to 72 hours of initiating treatment. Failure to improve should prompt reevaluation of the diagnosis and the treatment. The sex partners of adolescents with epididymitis suspected of being or confirmed to be caused by chlamydia or gonorrhea should be evaluated and treated if their contact with the index patient occurred fewer than 60 days before the onset of the patient's symptoms.

Enteric Infections

The syndromes of proctitis and proctocolitis are limited mostly to adolescent boys who practice anal receptive intercourse. Symptoms include anorectal pain, tenesmus, constipation, and anal discharge. Those who have proctocolitis or enteritis will have diarrhea. Patients who have proctitis (the distal 10-12 cm of the rectum) should be examined with anoscopy and evaluated for *C trachomatis* (including lymphogranuloma venereum [LGV] serovars), *N gonorrhoeae*, herpes simplex, and *Treponema pallidum* infection. Treatment should be with standard doses of ceftriaxone and doxycycline (see Box 322-4).

Patients who have symptoms suggesting proctocolitis (the symptoms of proctitis plus diarrhea or abdominal cramps) should receive more extensive evaluation. Organisms such as *Entamoeba histolytica*, *Campylobacter* species, and *Shigella* species can be sexually transmitted. HIV-infected patients may be infected with opportunistic organisms such as cytomegalovirus.

Enteritis usually occurs among patients whose sexual behaviors include oral-anal contact. Symptoms are usually limited to abdominal pain and diarrhea; the other symptoms of proctitis and proctocolitis are absent. Among immunocompetent patients, *Giardia lamblia* is the most likely organism; a variety of organisms can cause enteritis in HIV-infected patients.

Vaginitis

As discussed in Chapter 227, Vaginal Discharge, *Trichomonas vaginalis*, an important cause of vaginitis among sexually active adolescents, is a sexually transmitted infectious agent. Bacterial vaginosis, which is associated with the overgrowth of *Gardnerella vaginalis*, displays some characteristics of an STI. Bacterial vaginosis is associated with having multiple sex partners, with having a new sex partner, and with douching. Male sex partners of women who have bacterial vaginosis more often have *G vaginalis* recovered from the urethra than do controls. However, this same organism can be recovered from approximately 15% of women who have never been active sexually. Furthermore, treatment of male partners does not appear to influence recurrence risks for women who are treated for bacterial vaginosis.[7]

Vaginitis, in and of itself, can be distressing enough. However, current concerns about bacterial vaginosis center on its possible role in the pathogenesis of PID. Nongonococcal, nonchlamydial pathogens associated with PID are recovered more often from the endometrium of women who have bacterial vaginosis than from those who do not. Bacterial vaginosis has been causally related to postpartum endometritis. Hence treatment of symptomatic women who have bacterial vaginosis is warranted; asymptomatic women who are scheduled to undergo abortion or hysterectomy should also be treated.

Cervicitis

Cervicitis is characterized by a purulent or mucopurulent discharge from the endocervical os or by significant endocervical bleeding (or both) that is induced when a swab is introduced into the os. It may be detected during a routine pelvic examination even if an adolescent has no genital complaints.

Both *C trachomatis* and *N gonorrhoeae* can cause cervicitis (an association that is stronger in women younger than 25 years[43]), as can trichomonas and HSV, especially HSV-2. *M genitalium,* bacterial vaginosis, and douching also may cause cervicitis. However, in most cases of cervicitis, no etiologic agent is identified.

Women with cervicitis should be carefully evaluated for PID and for the presence of trichomonas and bacterial vaginosis; they should also be tested for chlamydia and gonorrhea. Adolescents with cervicitis should be presumptively treated for *C trachomatis* (see Box 322-4), especially if follow-up is uncertain or if the clinician does not have access to NAAT. Appropriate therapy for gonorrhea (see Box 322-4) should also be provided if the prevalence of infection in the patient population is more than 5%. Sex partners should be identified, evaluated, and treated, depending on the characteristics of the index patient.

WHEN TO REFER

If the clinician is inexperienced in the diagnosis or management of:

- Pelvic inflammatory disease
- Disseminated gonococcal arthritis
- Syphilis (or positive VDRL or RPR test)
- Anogenital warts
- Genital herpes
- Abnormal Pap smears

TOOLS FOR PRACTICE

Community Advocacy and Coordination

- *Male Latex Condoms and Sexually Transmitted Diseases* (fact sheet), Centers for Disease Control and Prevention (www.cdc.gov/nchstp/od/condoms.pdf).

Engaging Patient and Family

- *Bacterial Vaginosis* (fact sheet), Centers for Disease Control and Prevention (www.cdc.gov/std/BV/STDFact-Bacterial-Vaginosis.htm).
- *Chlamydia* (fact sheet), Centers for Disease Control and Prevention (www.cdc.gov/std/Chlamydia/STDFact-Chlamydia.htm).
- *Correct Use of Condoms* (fact sheet), American Academy of Pediatrics (www.aap.org/patiented/condoms.htm).
- *Deciding to Wait: Guidelines for Teens* (brochure), American Academy of Pediatrics (patiented.aap.org).
- *Genital Herpes* (fact sheet), Centers for Disease Control and Prevention (www.cdc.gov/std/Herpes/STDFact-Herpes.htm).
- *Genital HPV Infection* (fact sheet), Centers for Disease Control and Prevention (www.cdc.gov/std/HPV/STDFact-HPV.htm).
- *Go Ask Alice* (Web page), Columbia University (www.goaskalice.columbia.edu/).
- *Gonorrhea* (fact sheet), Centers for Disease Control and Prevention (www.cdc.gov/std/Gonorrhea/STDFact-gonorrhea.htm).
- *Hepatitis B* (fact sheet), Centers for Disease Control and Prevention (www.cdc.gov/std/hepatitis/STDFact-Hepatitis-B.htm).
- *HPV and Men* (fact sheet), Centers for Disease Control and Prevention (www.cdc.gov/std/HPV/STDFact-HPV-and-men.htm).
- *HPV Vaccine Questions and Answers* (fact sheet), Centers for Disease Control and Prevention (www.cdc.gov/std/HPV/STDFact-HPV-vaccine.htm).
- *Making Healthy Decisions About Sex* (brochure), American Academy of Pediatrics (patiented.aap.org).
- *Pelvic Inflammatory Disease (fact sheet)* Centers for Disease Control and Prevention (www.cdc.gov/std/PID/STDFact-PID.htm).
- *STDs and Pregnancy—CDC Fact Sheet,* Centers for Disease Control and Prevention (www.cdc.gov/std/STDFact-STDs&Pregnancy.htm).
- *Syphilis—CDC Fact Sheet,* Centers for Disease Control and Prevention (www.cdc.gov/std/Syphilis/STDFact-Syphilis.htm).
- *Teenwire* (Web page), Planned Parenthood (www.teenwire.com).
- *The Pelvic Exam* (brochure), American Academy of Pediatrics (patiented.aap.org).
- *The Role of STD Detection and Treatment in HIV Prevention—CDC Fact Sheet,* Centers for Disease Control and Prevention (www.cdc.gov/std/hiv/STDFact-STD&HIV.htm).
- *Trichomoniasis* (fact sheet), Centers for Disease Control and Prevention (www.cdc.gov/std/Trichomonas/STD Fact-Trichomoniasis.htm).

Medical Decision Support

- *Covering the Bases: Adolescent Sexual Health PediaLink* (online course), American Academy of Pediatrics (www.pedialink.org).
- *HPV and HPV Vaccine—Information for Healthcare Providers* (fact sheet), Centers for Disease Control and Prevention (www.cdc.gov/std/HPV/STDFact-HPV-vaccine-hcp.htm).

- *Red Book: 2006 Report of the Committee on Infectious Diseases*, 27th edition, American Academy of Pediatrics (www.aap.org/bookstore).
- *Sexually Transmitted Diseases* (Web page), Centers for Disease Control and Prevention (www.cdc.gov/std/default.htm).
- *Sexually Transmitted Diseases 2006 Treatment Guidelines*, Centers for Disease Control and Prevention (www.cdc.gov/std/treatment/).
- *Youth Risk Behavior Surveillance System (YRBSS)* (Web page), Centers for Disease Control and Prevention (www.cdc.gov/HealthyYouth/yrbs/index.htm).

RELATED WEB SITES

- American Social Health Association (www.ashastd.org/index.cfm).
- Center for Young Women's Health (CYWH) (www.youngwomenshealth.org/sexuality_menu.html).
- Guttmacher Institute (www.guttmacher.org/).

AAP POLICY STATEMENTS

American Academy of Pediatrics, Committee on Adolescence. Condom use by adolescents. *Pediatrics*. 2001;107(6):1463-1469. (aappolicy.aappublications.org/cgi/content/full/pediatrics;107/6/1463).

American Academy of Pediatrics, Committee on Adolescence. Confidentiality in adolescent health care. *AAP News*. 1989;4:151. (aapnews.aappublications.org/cgi/content/full/e2005175v1).

American Academy of Pediatrics, Committee on Pediatric AIDS and Committee on Adolescence. Adolescents and human immunodeficiency virus infection: the role of the pediatrician in prevention and intervention. *Pediatrics*. 2001;107(1):188-190. (aappolicy.aappublications.org/cgi/content/full/pediatrics;107/1/188).

American Academy of Pediatrics, Committee on Psychosocial Aspects of Child and Family Health and Committee on Adolescence. Sexuality education for children and adolescents. *Pediatrics*. 2001:108(2):498-502. (aappolicy.aappublications.org/cgi/content/full/pediatrics;108/2/498).

SUGGESTED RESOURCES

American Social Health Association. Available at: www.ashastd.org/. Accessed January 28, 2007.

Center for Young Women's Health. Children's Hospital Boston. Available at: www.youngwomenshealth.org/sexuality_menu.html. Accessed January 28, 2007.

Health Services at Columbia, Columbia University's Health Promotion Program. Go Ask Alice: Columbia University's Health Q&A Internet Service. Available at: www.goaskalice.columbia.edu/. Accessed January 28, 2007.

Planned Parenthood of America. Teenwire.com. Available at: www.teenwire.com/. Accessed January 28, 2007.

REFERENCES

1. Centers for Disease Control and Prevention. Youth risk behavior surveillance—United States, 2005. *MMWR Morb Mortal Wkly Rep*. 2006;55(SS-5):19-22.
2. Centers for Disease Control and Prevention, National Center for Disease Prevention and Health Promotion. Healthy youth! Data and Statistics. YRBSS: Youth Risk Behavior Surveillance System. Available at: www.cdc.gov/HealthyYouth/yrbs/index.htm. Accessed January 28, 2007.
3. Winer RL, Hughes JP, Feng Q, et al. Condom use and the risk of genital human papillomavirus infection in young women. *N Engl J Med*. 2006;354:45-54.
4. Warner L, Stone KM, Macaluso M, et al. Condom use and risk of gonorrhea and chlamydia: a systematic review of design and measurement factors assessed in epidemiologic studies. *Sex Transm Dis*. 2006;33:36-51.
5. Mohllajee AP, Curtis KM, Martins SL, et al. Hormonal contraceptive use and risk of sexually transmitted infections: a systematic review. *Contraception*. 2006;73:154-165.
6. Guttmacher Institute. State policies in brief as of January 1, 2007: An Overview of Minors' Consent Law. Available at: www.guttmacher.org/statecenter/spibs/spib_omcl.pdf. Accessed April 23, 2007.
7. Centers for Disease Control and Prevention. Sexually transmitted diseases treatment guidelines, 2006. *MMWR Morb Mortal Wkly Rep*. 2006;55 (RR-11):1-92.
8. Centers for Disease Control and Prevention. HIV prevention through early detection and treatment of other sexually transmitted diseases—United States. Recommendations of the Advisory Committee for HIV and STD Prevention. *MMWR Recomm Rep*. 1998;47(RR-12):1-24.
9. Cook RL, Hutchison SL, `stergaard L, et al. Systematic review: noninvasive testing for Chlamydia trachomatis and Neisseria gonorrhoeae. *Ann Intern Med*. 2005;142:914-925.
10. Serlin M, Shafer M-A, Tebb K, et al. What sexually transmitted disease screening method does the adolescent prefer? *Arch Pediatr Adolesc Med*. 2002;156:588-591.
11. Schachter J, Chernesky MA, Willis DE, et al. Vaginal swabs are the specimen of choice when screening for Chlamydia trachomatis and Neisseria gonorrhoeae: results from a multicenter evaluation of the APTIMA assays for both infections. *Sex Transm Dis*. 2005;32:725-728.
12. Peipert JF. Genital chlamydial infections. *N Engl J Med*. 2003;349:2424-2430.
13. Cohen DA, Kanouse DE, Iguchi MY, et al. Screening for sexually transmitted diseases in non-traditional settings: a personal view. *Int J STD AIDS*. 2005;16:521-527.
14. Miller WC, Ford CA, Morris M, et al. Prevalence of chlamydial and gonococcal infections among young adults in the United States. *JAMA*. 2004;291:2229-2236.
15. Burstein GR, Gaydos CA, Diener-West M, et al. Incident Chlamydia trachomatis infections among inner-city adolescent females. *JAMA*. 1998;280:521-526.
16. Scholes D, Stergachis A, Heidrich FE, et al. Prevention of pelvic inflammatory disease by screening for cervical chlamydial infection. *N Engl J Med*. 1996;334:1362-1366.
17. Blake DR, Woods ER. The future is here: noninvasive diagnosis of STDs. *Contemp Pediatr*. 2001;18:71-87.
18. Niccolai LM, Ickovics JR, Zeller K, et al. Knowledge of sex partner treatment for past bacterial STI and risk of current STI. *Sex Transm Infect*. 2005;81:271-275.
19. Samoff E, Koumans EH, Markowitz LE, et al. Association of Chlamydia trachomatis with persistence of high-risk types of human papillomavirus in a cohort of female adolescents. *Am J Epidemiol*. 2005;162:668-675.
20. Wald ER. Gonorrhea. Diagnosis by gram stain in the female adolescent. *Am J Dis Child*. 1977;131:1094-1096.
21. Centers for Disease Control and Prevention. Update to CDC's sexually transmitted diseases treatment guidelines, 2006: fluoroquinolones no longer recommended for treatment of gonococcal infections. *MMWR Morb Mortal Wkly Rep*. 2007;56(14):332-336.
22. Handsfield HH. Gonorrhea and nongonococcal urethritis. *Med Clin North Am*. 1978;62:925-943.
23. Munoz N, Bosch FX, de Sanjose S, et al. Epidemiologic classification of human papillomavirus types associated with cervical cancer. *N Engl J Med*. 2003;348:518-527.

24. Moscicki AB. Impact of HPV infection in adolescent populations. *J Adolesc Health*. 2005;37:S3-S9.
25. Barrasso R, De Brux J, Croissant O, et al. High prevalence of papillomavirus-associated penile intraepithelial neoplasia in sexual partners of women with cervical intraepithelial neoplasia. *N Eng J Med*. 1987;317:916-923.
26. Saslow D, Runowicz CD, Solomon D, et al. American Cancer Society guideline for the early detection of cervical neoplasia and cancer. *CA Cancer J Clin*. 2002;52:342-362.
27. Moscicki AB, Shiboski S, Hills NK, et al. Regression of low-grade squamous intra-epithelial lesions in young women. *Lancet*. 2004;364:1678-1683.
28. Wright TC, Massad LS, Dunton CJ, et al. 2006 American Society for Colposcopy and Cervical Pathology-sponsored Consensus Conference. 2006 consensus guidelines for the management of women with abnormal cervical cancer screening tests. *Am J Obstet Gynecol*. 2007;346-355.
29. Roden R, Wu T-C. How will HPV vaccines affect cervical cancer? *Nat Rev Cancer*. 2006;6:753-763.
30. Villa LL, Costa RLR, Petta CA, et al. Prophylactic quadrivalent human papillomavirus (types 6, 11, 16, and 18) L1 virus-like particle vaccine in young women: a randomized double-blind placebo-controlled multicentre phase II efficacy trial. *Lancet Oncol*. 2005;6:271-278.
31. Centers for Disease Control and Prevention. Quadrivalent human papillomavirus vaccine. Recommendations of the Advisory Committee on Immunization Practices (ACIP). *MMWR Morb Mortal Wkly Rep*. 2007;56(RR2):1-19.
32. Kimberlin DW, Rouse DJ. Genital herpes. *N Engl J Med*. 2004;350:1970-1977.
33. Xu F, Sternberg MR, Kottiri BJ, et al. Trends in herpes simplex virus type 1 and type 2 seroprevalence in the United States. *JAMA*. 2006;296:964-973.
34. Scoular A. Using the evidence base on genital herpes: optimizing the use of diagnostic tests and information provision. *Sex Transm Infect*. 2002;78:160-165.
35. Corey L, Wald A, Patel R, et al. Once-daily valacyclovir to reduce the risk of transmission of genital herpes. *N Engl J Med*. 2004;350:11-20.
36. Stanberry L. Clinical trials of prophylactic and therapeutic herpes simplex virus vaccines. *Herpes*. 2004;11(suppl 3):161A-169A.
37. US Department of Health and Human Services, Centers for Disease Control and Prevention. Sexually Transmitted Diseases. STD Surveillance 2005: National Profile. Syphilis. Available at: www.cdc.gov/std/stats/syphilis.htm. Accessed January 28, 2007.
38. Taylor-Robinson D. Mycoplasma genitalium—an update. *Int J STD AIDS*. 2002;13:145-151.
39. Anagrius C, Lore B, Jensen JS. Mycoplasma genitalium: clinical significance, and transmission. *Sex Transm Infect*. 2005;81:458-462.
40. Westrom L, Eschenbach O. Pelvic inflammatory disease. In: Holmes KK, Sparling PF, Mardh PA, et al, eds. *Sexually Transmitted Diseases*. 3rd ed. New York, NY: McGraw-Hill; 1999.
41. Banikarim C, Chacko MR. Pelvic inflammatory disease in the adolescent. *Adolesc Med*. 2004;15:273-285.
42. Washington AE, Sweet RL, Shafer MB. Pelvic inflammatory disease and its sequelae in adolescents. *J Adolesc Health Care*. 1985;6:298-310.
43. Marrazzo JM, Handsfield HH, Whittington WLH. Predicting chlamydial and gonococcal cervical infection: implications for management of cervicitis. *Obstet Gynecol*. 2002;100:579-584.

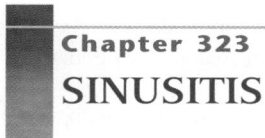

Chapter 323

SINUSITIS

Tina Q. Tan, MD

Infection of the paranasal sinuses in children occurs frequently. Estimates indicate that 5% to 13% of viral upper respiratory tract infections in children are complicated by acute bacterial sinusitis.[1,2] On average, children develop 5 to 10 upper respiratory tract infections yearly. The distinction between viral infections and acute bacterial sinusitis is based on the persistence and severity of upper respiratory symptoms.

PATHOPHYSIOLOGY

The paranasal sinuses arise during fetal development as outpouchings beneath the turbinates in the nasopharynx. Only the maxillary and ethmoid sinuses are present at the time of birth. The sinuses continue to develop and grow until adulthood (Table 323-1). Growth may be asymmetrical, and some individuals lack 1 or more sinuses altogether. Various functions have been ascribed to the sinuses, but none of these have been proved. These functions include warming and humidifying inspired air, reducing the weight of the skull, providing thermal insulation to the central nervous system and sensory organs, affecting facial form, and serving as vocal resonators. Recent theories suggest that the sinuses serve as reservoirs for the production and absorption of antigens, allowing for the tolerance of infections until effective specific immunity develops.[3]

The lining of the mucosa of the sinuses is similar to that of the nasopharynx, with pseudostratified, ciliated, columnar epithelium interspersed with goblet cells and submucosal glands. Cilia beat toward the ostium of the sinus to expel mucus and particulate matter into the nasopharynx.[4] The ostia of the maxillary sinuses are located in the upper part of the chamber where cilia must battle gravity to clear secretions. This circumstance probably contributes to the high frequency of infection in these sinuses.[5] Occlusion of the ostia, impairment of ciliary motility, and alterations in the consistency of mucus secretions alone or in combination can predispose the sinuses to infection.

Sinusitis occurs most frequently after a viral upper respiratory tract infection or as the result of nasal allergy. Inflammation and edema of the respiratory mucosa lead to obstruction of the ostium. Pressure changes in the sinus that result from occlusion or from blowing and sniffing through the nose allow bacteria to invade the normally sterile sinus cavity. Other disorders associated with sinusitis in children are listed in Box 323-1.

Respiratory viruses such as adenoviruses, influenza viruses, parainfluenza viruses, and rhinoviruses contribute to the development of sinusitis. The most common bacterial pathogens associated with acute sinusitis are *Streptococcus pneumoniae, Haemophilus influenzae,* and *Moraxella catarrhalis. Staphylococcus*

Table 323-1 Sinus Development

SINUS	FIRST APPEARANCE	SIZE (ML) BIRTH	3 YEARS	10 YEARS	14 YEARS	AGE OF CLINICAL IMPORTANCE
Maxillary	3 wk of fetal life	0.13	2.5	10.4	11.6	Birth
Ethmoid	6 mo of fetal life	0.06	0.16	2.4	4.8	Birth
Sphenoid	3 mo of fetal life	0.02	0.68	1.8	2.1	5 yr
Frontal	1 yr of life	—	0.08	1.0	3.6	10-12 yr

Modified from Schaeffer JP. *The Embryology, Development and Anatomy of the Nose, Paranasal Sinuses, Nasolacrimal Passageways and Olfactory Organ in Man.* Philadelphia, PA: Blakiston; 1920.

BOX 323-1 Disorders Associated With Paranasal Sinusitis

1. Anatomic
   a. Nasal malformations
   b. Nasal trauma
   c. Tumors and polyps
   d. Cleft palate
   e. Foreign bodies
   f. Dental infection
   g. Cyanotic congenital heart disease
2. Physiological barotrauma
3. Abnormalities of local defense mechanisms
   a. Allergy
   b. Cystic fibrosis
   c. Immotile-cilia syndrome and Kartagener syndrome
4. Abnormalities of systemic defense mechanisms
   a. Primary immunodeficiency
   b. Secondary immunodeficiency

From Shurin PA. Etiology and antimicrobial therapy of paranasal sinusitis in children. *Ann Otol Rhinol Laryngol Suppl.* 1981;90(3Pt3):72-74. Reprinted by permission of Annals Publishing Co.

aureus and anaerobes are prevalent in chronic sinusitis and *Streptococcus pyogenes* (group A *Streptococcus*) may be associated with both acute and chronic disease.[5,6]

CLINICAL PRESENTATION AND DIAGNOSIS

Sinusitis is primarily a clinical diagnosis, and differentiating upper respiratory tract infections or allergic rhinitis from acute sinusitis can be difficult in children. Most uncomplicated upper respiratory tract infections improve after 5 to 7 days. Symptoms that persist without improvement for more than 10 but fewer than 30 days suggest bacterial superinfection, and a diagnosis of acute sinusitis can be made.[7] Cough and nasal discharge are the most common clinical manifestations of acute sinusitis. The cough occurs during the day and is frequently worse at night or when the child is supine. Nasal discharge may be clear or purulent. Parents of young children may report fetid breath. Headache and facial pain are manifestations of acute sinusitis that are uncommon in children. Painless swelling of the periorbital tissues without erythema, usually in the morning, is an occasional manifestation of sinusitis that may be confused with periorbital cellulitis in its early stage.

A less common presentation of acute sinusitis is an unusually severe upper respiratory tract infection. In most cases of viral upper respiratory infection, fever precedes the onset of watery nasal discharge and is associated with constitutional symptoms. Thickening of nasal secretions occurs later in the course, before resolution. A high fever and purulent discharge that coexist for 3 or more days suggests the diagnosis of acute sinusitis.

Cough and nasal discharge persisting for more than 30 days occurs with both subacute or chronic sinusitis.[7]

On physical examination, the nasal mucosa is usually erythematous and swollen but may be pale and boggy.[2] Mucopurulent material can sometimes be seen in the nose or draining into the nasopharynx. The presence of a foreign body in the nose must be ruled out. Palpation or percussion of the sinuses may elicit tenderness.

Sinus radiographs can help confirm the diagnosis of sinusitis.[8] When clinical signs and symptoms suggest acute sinusitis and maxillary sinus roentgenograms show air-fluid levels, complete opacification, or mucosal thickening of at least 4 to 5 mm, bacteria are present in a sinus aspirate 75% of the time.[2] Routine use of radiographs to confirm the diagnosis of uncomplicated sinusitis is not recommended in young children. Sinus radiographs are more specific and therefore more helpful in children older than 6 years of age. Cysts and polyps also may be seen on sinus roentgenograms.

Computed tomography (CT) imaging of the sinuses should be reserved for patients who have frequent recurrences or persistent symptoms that are not improving, those who have complicated sinusitis accompanied by orbital or intracranial complications, and those for whom sinus surgery is being contemplated.[5,9]

Transnasal aspiration of the maxillary sinuses can be performed by an otolaryngologist for diagnostic purposes in specific situations. Nasopharyngeal culture results correlate poorly with sinus culture results. Sinus aspiration and lavage are indicated only in children who fail to respond to conventional antibiotic therapy, in immunosuppressed patients, and in those whose illness is severe or life threatening.

COMPLICATIONS

Complications of sinusitis are most often due to local extension of the disease. Orbital cellulitis is the most common serious complication of sinusitis. The ethmoid sinus is separated from the orbit by the thin lamina papyracea. Erosion of this bone leads to invasion of the orbit by bacterial pathogens. Staging of orbital cellulitis is described in Table 323-2. The eyelids appear intensely red and swollen on physical examination. Fever, malaise, and an increased white blood cell count are present. Orbital pain, proptosis, and limitation of eye movement (ophthalmoplegia) help distinguish this condition from preseptal (periorbital) cellulitis, although CT scanning may be needed to differentiate the 2 conditions. Treatment of orbital cellulitis involves parenteral antibiotics; an ophthalmologist and an otolaryngologist should be consulted to determine whether surgical drainage is indicated[7] (see Chapter 313, Preseptal and Orbital Cellulitis). This complication has been reported most frequently in male adolescents who, in many cases, lack the common symptoms of sinusitis.[10,11] However, more recent reports have shown a shift in the occurrence of orbital cellulitis toward a younger population, including infants. The reasons for this shift are unclear.[12]

Intracranial infection, most commonly subdural empyema, is the second most common complication of sinusitis. Infection can occur by direct extension through necrotic bone or by bacterial spread through the venous system. Because the frontal sinuses are involved most often, the peak age of incidence of this complication is between 10 and 20 years, although it can develop in younger children. Patients have a low-grade fever, malaise, and a frontal headache. Vomiting and a decreased level of consciousness appear as the disease progresses.

If a patient is thought to have an intracranial abscess, then a head CT scan with contrast should be obtained. Lumbar puncture should be avoided until intracranial mass effect has been ruled out. Treatment with high-dose parenteral antibiotics and neurosurgery to drain the abscess and to debride necrotic bone are required. Steroids and hypertonic agents such as mannitol or glycerol may be necessary to control intracranial hypertension.

Other less common complications of sinusitis in children include meningitis, osteomyelitis of the frontal bone *(Pott puffy tumor)*, epidural abscess, and cavernous sinus thrombosis.

TREATMENT

Treatment of sinusitis in children involves antibiotic therapy, symptomatic relief measures, and drainage, if necessary.[13] Amoxicillin is an appropriate initial choice for treating uncomplicated sinusitis in geographic areas where the prevalence of beta-lactamase–producing strains of *H influenzae* and *M catarrhalis* is low.[14] Broader coverage with amoxicillin plus clavulanate, a carbacephem, a macrolide, or a 3rd-generation cephalosporin should be considered for children who are allergic or fail to respond to amoxicillin. These alternatives should also be considered for the child who has recently been treated with amoxicillin, has frontal or sphenoid sinusitis, has complicated ethmoid sinusitis, or has very protracted symptoms.[5] Clinical improvement should be expected within 48 hours, and a minimum of 10 days of antibiotic therapy usually is adequate. If symptoms fail to resolve completely within 10 days, then patients should be treated for an additional 7 days beyond the resolution of symptoms.[7]

Decongestants, antihistamines, and saline nose drops have been recommended to help drain the sinuses, but no proof of the efficacy of these agents exists.[15] Intranasal steroids may provide some benefit, particularly in the second week of therapy, but further research is necessary to define their role in management.[5]

In unusually severe cases, hospitalization and parenteral antibiotics may be required and otolaryngologic consultation is indicated. Some experts have recommended antibiotic prophylaxis for the child who has recurrent sinusitis and no underlying disorder, although no scientific studies support this practice, and it may lead to the rapid development of antibiotic resistance.[7] Surgery may be required in cases of medically recalcitrant severe chronic sinusitis in children.[16,17]

Table 323-2 Classification of Orbital Cellulitis

STAGE	DESCRIPTION
I Inflammatory edema	Inflammatory edema beginning in medial or lateral upper eyelid; usually nontender with only minimal skin changes No induration, visual impairment, or limitation of extraocular movements
II Orbital cellulitis	Edema of orbital contents with varying degrees of proptosis, chemosis, limitation of extraocular movement, and visual loss
III Subperiosteal abscess	Proptosis down and out with signs of orbital cellulitis (usually severe) Abscess beneath the periosteum of the ethmoid, frontal, or maxillary bone (in that order of frequency)
IV Orbital abscess	Abscess within the fat or muscle cone in the posterior orbit Severe chemosis and proptosis; complete ophthalmoplegia and moderate to severe visual loss present (globe displaced forward or down and out)
V Cavernous sinus thrombosis	Proptosis, globe fixation, severe loss of visual acuity, prostration, signs of meningitis; progresses to proptosis, chemosis, and visual loss in contralateral eye

From Wald ER, et al. Sinusitis and its complications in the pediatric patient. *Pediatr Clin North Am.* 1981;28(4):777-796; modified from Chandler JR, Langenbrunner DJ, Stevens ER: The pathogenesis of orbital complications in acute sinusitis. *Laryngoscope.* 1970;80:1414-1428.

The author acknowledges the contributions of Rickey L. Williams, MD, to the preparation of this manuscript in the previous editions.

TOOLS FOR PRACTICE

Engaging Patients and Family

- *Sinusitis and Your Child* (brochure), American Academy of Pediatrics (patiented.aap.org).
- *Sinusitis* (fact sheet), American Academy of Allergy, Asthma, and Immunology (www.aaaai.org/patients/resources/easy_reader/sinusitis.pdf).
- Breathing Easy and Bringing Up Healthy Active Children (book), American Academy of Pediatrics (www.aap.org/bookstore).
- *What Is a Pediatric Allergist/Immunologist* (fact sheet), American Academy of Pediatrics (www.aap.org/family/pedspecfactsheets.htm).

Medical Decision Support

- Clinical Practice Guideline: Management of Sinusitis, American Academy of Pediatrics (http://aappolicy.aappublications.org/cgi/content/full/pediatrics;108/3/798).
- Pediatric Prescribing Update—Allergy and Asthma (on line course), American Academy of Pediatrics (www.pedialink.org/cme/_coursefinder/CMEdetail.cfm?aid=30368&area=liveCME).
- Management of Acute Bacterial Sinusitis, Cincinnati Children's Hospital Medical Center (www.cincinnatichildrens.org/NR/rdonlyres/4A6C17AD-4855-403F-A6EE-3F6D852A3FE2/0/sinusitisguideline.pdf).
- Highlights—Sinusitis Guidelines, Cincinnati Children's Hospital Medical Center (www.cincinnatichildrens.org/NR/rdonlyres/A9801F4A-E611-46A5-9226-B5F69F5CCED2/0/sinusitishighlight.pdf).
- Treatment Algorithm for Sinusitis (algorithm), Cincinnati Children's Hospital Medical Center (www.cincinnatichildrens.org/NR/rdonlyres/36FD4504-82AF-4563-AA84-4EEED1CCC745/0/sinusitisalgorithm.pdf).
- Table for Antibiotic Therapy, Cincinnati Children's Hospital Medical Center (www.cincinnatichildrens.org/NR/rdonlyres/36FD4504-82AF-4563-AA84-4EEED1CCC745/0/sinusitisalgorithm.pdf).

AAP POLICY STATEMENTS

American Academy of Pediatrics, Ioannidis JPA, Lau J. Technical report: evidence for the diagnosis and treatment of acute uncomplicated sinusitis in children: a systematic overview. *Pediatrics.* 2001;108(3):e57. (aappolicy.aappublications.org/cgi/content/full/pediatrics;108/3/e57).

American Academy of Pediatrics, Subcommittee on Management of Sinusitis and Committee on Quality Improvement. Clinical practice guideline: management of sinusitis. *Pediatrics.* 2001;108(3):808. (aappolicy.aappublications.org/cgi/content/full/pediatrics;108/3/798).

REFERENCES

1. Altemeier WA, Ward C. A pediatrician's view. Why do we have paranasal sinuses? *Pediatr Ann.* 1998;27:784-785.
2. Brook I. Bacteriologic features of chronic sinusitis in children. *JAMA.* 1981;246:967-969.
3. Fireman B. Diagnosis of sinusitis in children: emphasis on the history and physical examination. *J Allergy Clin Immunol.* 1992;90(3Pt2):433-436.
4. Giebink GS. Childhood sinusitis: pathophysiology, diagnosis and treatment. *Pediatr Infect Dis J.* 1994;13(suppl):S55-S65.
5. Johnson DL, Markle BM, Wiedermann BL, Hanahan L. Treatment of intracranial abscesses associated with sinusitis in children and adolescents. *J Pediatr.* 1988;113:15-23.
6. Kovatch AL, Wald ER, Ledesma-Medina J, et al. Maxillary sinus radiographs in children with nonrespiratory complaints. *Pediatrics.* 1984;73:306-308.
7. Lund VJ. Bacterial sinusitis: etiology and management. *Pediatr Infect Dis J.* 1994;13(suppl):S58-S63.
8. Parsons DS, Phillips SE. Functional endoscopic surgery in children: a retrospective analysis of results. *Laryngoscope.* 1993;103:899-903.
9. Rachelefsky GS, Katz RM, Siegel SC. Diseases of paranasal sinuses in children. *Curr Probl Pediatr.* 1982;12:1-57.
10. Rosenfeld EA, Rowley AH. Infectious intracranial complications of sinusitis, other than meningitis, in children: 12-year review. *Clin Infect Dis.* 1994;18:750-754.
11. Siegel JD. Diagnosis and management of acute sinusitis in children. *Pediatr Infect Dis J.* 1987;6:95-99.
12. Nageswaran S, Woods CR, Benjamin DK, et al. Orbital cellulitis in children. *Pediatr Infect Dis J.* 2006;25:695-699.
13. Wald ER. Management of sinusitis in infants and children. *Pediatr Infect Dis J.* 1988;7:449-452.
14. Wald ER. Sinusitis. *Pediatr Ann.* 1998;27:811-818.
15. Nash D, Wald E. Sinusitis. *Pediatr Rev.* 2001;22:111-117.
16. Wald ER. Sinusitis in children. *N Engl J Med.* 1992;326:319-323.
17. Yousem DM. Imaging of sinonasal inflammatory disease. *Radiology.* 1993;188:303-314.

Chapter 324
SPINA BIFIDA

Gregory S. Liptak, MD, MPH

Meningomyelocele (myelomeningocele) is a serious and complex congenital malformation, occurring at a rate of 0.4 to 0.8 cases per 1000 live births in the United States.[1] The incidence is greater among girls, among those of lower socioeconomic status, and among families of English, Irish, or Welsh extraction. The incidence of meningomyelocele (and other neural tube defects) has been declining for the last several decades. Improved nutrition, including the fortification of food with folic acid and the establishment of prenatal diagnosis with elective termination has significantly decreased the birth prevalence in the United States.[2]

ETIOLOGY

Meningomyelocele belongs to the family of neural tube defects that includes abnormalities of the head (anencephaly, cranial meningocele, encephalocele) and of the spine (spina bifida occulta, occult spinal dysraphism [OSD], meningocele, and meningomyelocele). In spina bifida occulta, which is a common, benign condition, the spinal cord and soft tissues are normal, but the vertebral arches are incomplete. In OSD, unlike spina bifida occulta, the underlying spinal cord is at risk for deterioration. In OSD the infant is born with a visible abnormality on the lower back, which may be a birthmark (eg, hemangioma), tuft of hair, dermal sinus, lipoma, or atypical dimple.[3,4] Although many healthy infants are born with a small, midline sacral dimple, if the dimple is not in the middle, is above the sacral region, is large, or does not have a visible base, then it may be associated with OSD. The spinal cord may be connected to the surface through a sinus that increases the risk for meningitis. The cord itself may be tethered to surrounding tissue, or it may be split (diastematomyelia or diplomyelia).[5] These defects can lead to subsequent neurologic damage as the child grows. Babies who have these findings on the back should have an evaluation of the underlying soft tissue and spinal cord using ultrasound or magnetic resonance imaging scan. Surgical treatment to correct the OSD should be performed early, even in asymptomatic infants, to prevent progressive neurologic damage.[6]

In meningocele, the spinal cord is normal, but the meninges protrude through abnormal vertebral arches and soft tissue. On rare occasions, the meningocele may appear as an anterior mass in the pelvis, abdomen, or thorax. In meningomyelocele the malformed spinal cord and nerve roots protrude through abnormal vertebral arches and soft tissue. Lipomas or dermoid cysts may accompany meningomyelocele or occult spinal dysraphism.

The cause of neural tube defects is unknown, although faulty closure of the neural groove by day 28 of gestation seems to be the primary mechanism. The most recent etiologic hypothesis is that neural tube defects result from the interaction of many genes (polygenic expression) that can be modified by factors in the embryonic (maternal) environment.[7] Assuming an overall incidence of 1 per 1000, the risk for a second affected child from the same parent is 2 or 3 per 100; for a third, it is 10 per 100. An adult who has meningomyelocele has a 2% to 3% chance of having a child who has a neural tube defect—the same risk that exists for the sibling of an affected child.

Maternal exposure to hyperthermia, valproic acid (Depakene, Depakote), carbamazepine (Tegretol), isotretinoin (Accutane), and ethanol increase the risk for neural tube defects. The incidence of neural tube defects is greater in mothers who have diabetes, obesity, and maternal malnutrition, especially folic acid deficiency. Meningomyelocele may be associated with certain chromosomal aberrations, including trisomy 13, trisomy 18, and cri du chat syndrome. It may be associated with malformations of multiple organ systems, including the gastrointestinal system (tracheoesophageal fistula, diaphragmatic hernia, and imperforate anus), the genitourinary system (cryptorchism, inguinal hernias and renal anomalies), craniofacial (cleft palate), and cardiovascular system (ventricular septal defect). Most cases, however, are isolated occurrences.

PATHOLOGICAL CONSIDERATIONS

Four major malformations account for the findings of meningomyelocele: (1) soft-tissue malformation, (2) brain malformation, (3) vertebral body malformation, and (4) spinal cord malformation (Figures 324-1 and 324-2).

Soft-Tissue Malformation

The failure of skin and other soft tissues to close leaves the spinal cord open to infection. The lipomas that occasionally accompany the defect may grow larger, compressing the spinal cord, and cause progressive neurologic symptoms as the child grows. The surgery to cover the cord may itself result in loss of neurologic function or may lead to scar tissue that tethers the cord and results in further neurologic deterioration as the child grows.

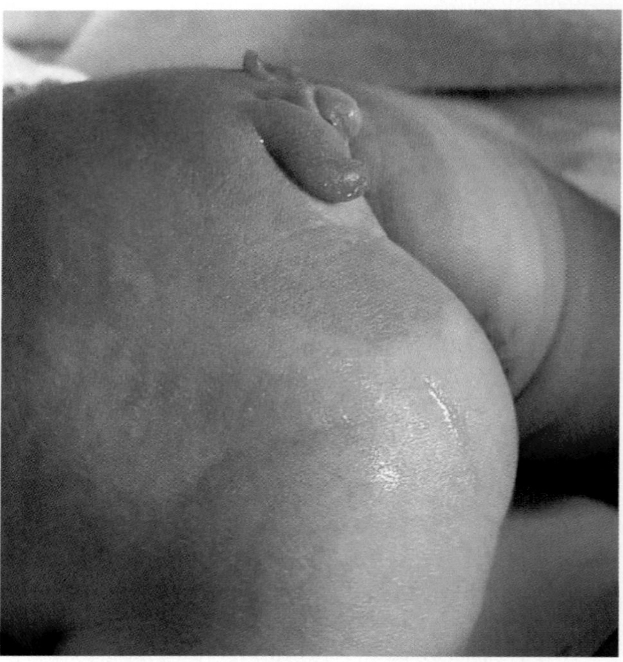

Figure 324-1 Skin tags and pigmentation associated with spinal cord tethering.

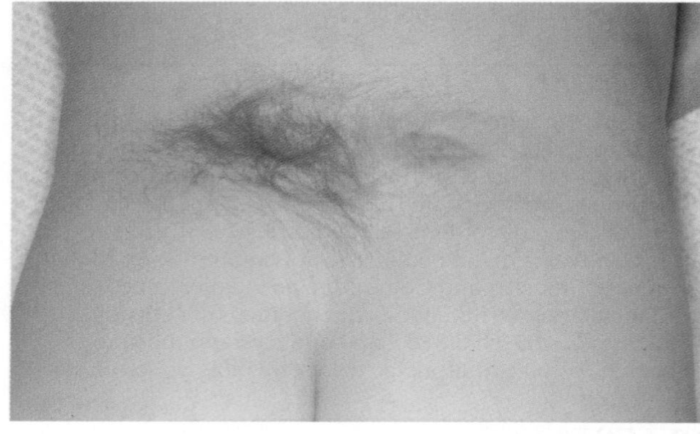

Figure 324-2 Hair tuft and pigmented lesion associated with occult spinal dysraphism (OSD).

Brain Malformation

Malformations of the brain include the Chiari type II deformity, in which the pons and medulla are distorted and elongated and the cerebellar vermis is displaced inferiorly into the spinal canal.[7] This abnormality is often associated with progressive hydrocephalus. Brainstem malformations may lead to laryngeal nerve palsy and difficulty in swallowing, as well as hypoventilation,[9] apnea, and sudden death. Subtle abnormalities of cranial nerve nuclei occur in many affected children. Seizures occur in 15% to 20% of children and adolescents who have meningomyelocele.

Approximately 25% of children who have meningomyelocele are born with evidence of hydrocephalus, with an additional 25% to 60% developing such signs within the first year of life. The higher (ie, the more cephalad) the spinal lesion is, the greater the likelihood is of developing hydrocephalus. Strabismus secondary to anomalies of the centers that control conjugate gaze occurs in approximately 50% of children who have hydrocephalus and meningomyelocele. In addition, central precocious puberty develops in many girls who have hydrocephalus.

Sudden shunt malfunction may produce life-threatening elevations of intracranial pressure, requiring emergency intervention. Signs and symptoms of acute shunt malfunction include headache, lethargy, irritability, paralysis of upward gaze, sixth cranial nerve palsy, a bulging fontanelle (in infants), and vomiting. Progression to loss of consciousness, abnormal pupillary reflexes, papilledema, deterioration of vital signs, and death may ensue rapidly.

Most children with meningomyelocele have normal overall IQ scores; yet most of these youngsters have selective cognitive disabilities, including nonverbal learning disabilities and impairment of executive functions.[10] Even children who have very low performance scores may have surprising verbal fluency, a trait sometimes referred to as the *cocktail party syndrome*. Specific cognitive testing often reveals deficiencies of selective visual attention, visual-spatial perception, tactile perception, auditory concentration, and higher-order functioning (eg, organizational skills). Children who have hydrocephalus and higher spinal lesions are more likely to have these deficits. Manifestations seen in school include short attention span, distractibility, perseveration, poor comprehension, poor handwriting, disorganization, poor memory, faulty problem-solving and decision-making skills, reduced social skills, emotional instability, impulsivity, irritability, and difficulty with subjects requiring visual-motor integration and visual-perceptual integration, such as arithmetic.

Vertebral Malformation

Vertebral malformations are caused by abnormal segmentation or formation and include absent vertebrae, fused vertebrae, hemivertebrae, and butterfly vertebrae. Occasionally, bony or ligamentous spurs lead to diastematomyelia. Of children who have thoracic lesions, 10% are born with kyphosis; by adolescence this rate increases to 33%. Children who have lumbar lesions have a 5% occurrence of kyphosis by adolescence. In addition to cosmetic deformity, severe kyphosis can lead to back pain, pulmonary and cardiac dysfunction, recurrent skin ulceration; and interference with walking.

The occurrence of scoliosis is related to the level of the lesion, with curves of 30 degrees or more appearing in 81% of adolescents who have thoracic lesions and 23% of those who have lower lumbar lesions. The consequences of scoliosis are similar to those of kyphosis. Lordosis also is much less common.

Spinal Cord Malformation

Spinal cord malformation results in both loss of sensation and motor function. Loss of sensation leaves these children vulnerable to burns and abrasions. Pathological fractures can go unnoticed. Decubitus ulcers also occur, especially among adolescents and adults who spend extensive time in wheelchairs. Skin lesions may become infected and lead to osteomyelitis.

Loss of motor function leads to decreased movement in utero, which may lead to deformities seen at birth, such as clubfoot (talipes equinovarus) and dislocated hips.

Loss of efferent nerve stimuli to the urinary bladder and sphincter results in neurogenic voiding dysfunction in virtually all children who have meningomyelocele. Bladder dysfunction may be classified as (1) failure to store urine or (2) failure to empty completely. Failure to store urine may result from a hypotonic urinary outlet or a spastic, hypertonic bladder, or both. Inability to void completely may result from spastic urinary sphincter or hypotonic bladder or both. The combination of spastic outlet and hypertonic bladder is especially serious because of reflux and hydronephrosis that occur frequently with this combination. In addition to incontinence and hydronephrosis, these children have frequent urinary tract infections.[11] These infections lead to fibrosis of the bladder and to chronic renal damage, which remains a significant source of morbidity and mortality. Repeated urinary infections in the presence of reflux lead to renal failure.[12]

Altered sexual function occurs, especially in men. Approximately 25% of men who have meningomyelocele are unable to have erections, and of those who can, most have retrograde ejaculation and decreased fertility. Although women have decreased sensation and decreased lubrication in response to sexual stimulation, most can experience orgasm and have normal fertility.

Children who have meningomyelocele usually have neurogenic bowel as a result of diminished function of the external rectal sphincter and the levator ani muscles. Most children have intact internal rectal sphincter function, and many have intact rectal sensation. Abnormal migration of neural cells in utero can lead to diminished peristalsis. Abnormal rectal function, poor peristalsis, limited mobility, and the ingestion of a low-fiber diet because of difficulty swallowing or fear of incontinence may lead to constipation or to obstipation with overflow soiling.

Loss of motor function in the lower extremities leads to loss of mobility. The degree of mobility is related closely to the level of the lesion; thus children who have intact quadriceps (L2-L4) are much more likely to be ambulatory through adolescence than are those with higher level lesions.[13] Muscle function around the joints is related directly to the level of the lesion

Table 324-1 Correlation Between Function and Level of Motor Involvement

FUNCTIONAL AREA—LEVEL OF LESION	BOWEL AND BLADDER FUNCTION	TOE INTRINSICS	FOOT	
			DORSIFLEXION—INVERSION	PLANTAR FLEXION—EVERSION
S2-3	?	?	+	?
S1-2	–	–	+	?
L5-S1	–	–	+	–
L4-5	–	–	?	–
L3-4	–	–	–	–
L2-3	–	–	–	–
L1-2	–	–	–	–

FUNCTIONAL AREA—LEVEL OF LESION	KNEE		HIP			
	EXTENSION	FLEXION	FLEXION	ADDUCTION	ABDUCTION	EXTENSION
S2-3	+	+	+	+	+	+
S1-S2	+	+	+	+	+	?
L5-S1	+	?	+	+	+	–
L4-5	+	–	+	+	–	–
L3-4	+	–	+	+	–	–
L2-3	?	–	?	?	–	–
L1-2	–	–	–	–	–	–

?, May be present; +, present; –, absent.

(Table 324-1). Joint contractures develop in children who have an imbalance of forces around a joint and in those who have no function; thus the child with a thoracic level lesion who has no hip function is at risk for developing hip flexion contractures because the child spends all day sitting in a wheelchair. Loss of mobility and innervation also increases the risk for osteoporosis and for pathological fractures in the lower extremities.

EVALUATION

History

Because meningomyelocele is inherited polygenically, affected newborns may have a family history of neural tube defects or spontaneous abortions (miscarriages). Other historical facts worth noting in the newborn period include length of gestation, type of delivery, complications with and length of labor, maternal nutrition and environmental exposures, current family functioning (including social support and stress), and parental expectations and understanding of the malformation. For the older child, information about current and past therapies for neurologic, orthopedic, urologic, ophthalmologic, dermatologic, and gastrointestinal conditions should be obtained. Educational and social functioning, the child's knowledge of the condition, and sexual function and understanding of sexuality should be ascertained. The child's growth, development, mobility, and independence in activities of daily living (personal hygiene, ability to self-feed, self-help skills) should be assessed. The onset of new neurologic symptoms, such as pain, fatigue, weakness, changes in bowel and bladder function, tripping, and clumsiness, should be determined because these symptoms usually indicate treatable conditions, such as tethered spinal cord, diastematomyelia, syringomyelia, or ventricular shunt malfunction. Up to 50% of children who have meningomyelocele have allergies to latex.[14] A history of reactions to products made of latex, such as balloons, bandages, and balls, should be sought. Contact with latex-containing products should be restricted from the first day of life in these children. All operative procedures should be performed in a latex-free environment.

Physical Examination

The backs of all children should be examined for pigmented spots, hairy patches, and sinuses that extend into the spine, because these signs may indicate occult spinal dysraphism. These children are at high risk for meningitis and for neurologic deterioration secondary to diastematomyelia, lipoma, and tethering of the spinal cord.

Children who have meningomyelocele should have a complete physical examination that emphasizes neurologic, orthopedic, and gastrointestinal function. The neurologic examination should include determination of motor function (see Table 324-1) and sensory functional levels. A rectal examination and assessment of the anal wink can assist in the evaluation of lesions at S2-S4. Upper extremity strength and function should be assessed. Palpation of the anterior fontanelle, ophthalmoscopic visualization of the *eyegrounds,* assessment of the cranial nerves (especially of extraocular movements), and palpation of the shunt valve and tubing help evaluate shunt function.

The orthopedic examination should include an assessment of posture (scoliosis, lordosis, kyphosis), as well as of joint mobility and stability. Erythema and swelling of a joint or bone in an area that lacks sensation means a fracture until proved otherwise.[9] The skin should be examined for evidence of erythema and ulcers in insensate areas.

Formal and informal developmental assessments should be part of the routine examination of these children and should include verbal, performance, sensory integration, and educational measures, as well as the more standard measures of fine-motor, gross-motor, language, and social-adaptive skills. Determining the child's learning profile before school entry is especially important to help facilitate the school in providing appropriate interventions that will optimize the child's learning. To identify the academic strengths and weaknesses of these children, formal psychoeducational testing is a critical part of their evaluation, before an individualized education plan is developed.

Laboratory Evaluation

Laboratory assessments of the newborn should include measurement of length, weight, and head circumference, with the last of these factors being measured daily. Ultrasound or computed tomography (CT) scan, or both, of the head, radiograms of the spine, and a urine culture should be performed. The kidneys should be examined by ultrasound; serum blood urea nitrogen and creatinine levels should be obtained as a baseline assessment of renal function. As the child grows, urinalysis and urine cultures should be performed as indicated, and head circumference, height, and weight should be monitored. Some clinicians recommend substituting arm span for height because growth below the waist is disproportionately slow.[15] A CT scan of the head should be performed periodically to detect asymptomatic ventricular enlargement. The condition of the spine and joints should be monitored by radiograms. Screen kidneys using routine renal ultrasound; voiding cystourethrograms, renal scans, and urodynamics are performed when indicated.

Special studies that may be indicated include (1) skinfold thickness measurements to evaluate nutritional status, (2) magnetic resonance imaging of the spine and hind brain (posterior fossa), including evaluation of cerebrospinal flow in the posterior fossa, and (3) Tc-99m dimercaptosuccinic acid renal scan to evaluate kidney structure and function, including damage from recurrent infections. A child who has signs and symptoms of ventricular shunt malfunction or other neurologic deterioration should undergo a head CT scan and a shunt series (to evaluate the integrity of the tubing).

PSYCHOSOCIAL CONSIDERATIONS

The birth of a child who has meningomyelocele is potentially devastating.[16] Most parents are shocked and begin a journey through the phases characteristic of people undergoing a loss (in this case a loss of the expected normal child). These stages include shock, denial, sadness, anger, guilt, and ultimately, acceptance and equilibrium. (Some families may go through part of the grief process several times during the child's life, particularly at significant milestones such as birthdays and the start of school.) In addition to grieving, parents must share in difficult medical decisions. Parents will require support from medical professionals and others. An evaluation of their current levels of social support and the presence of other stressors is critical. Because most children with meningomyelocele have multiple medical problems, they require the expenditure of much money,[16] time, patience, and understanding. Such demands stress parents and can lead to isolation of one parent from the other. This situation may be reinforced by a medical system that sees patients during working hours and that is content to deal exclusively with one parent only. The stresses may affect siblings, who can develop behavioral problems.

Parents may begin mourning but never reach equilibrium, and the clinician may notice telltale denial, guilt, or anger. In addition, one spouse may be able to reach equilibrium but be emotionally unavailable to the spouse still struggling with the earlier stages.

Children with meningomyelocele may have difficulty at home if parents are unable to provide affection or to set consistent limits. These children may have difficulty with peers who see them as *cripples* rather than as children who have disabilities. They may have difficulty performing academically and may lose interest in school because of frequent negative reinforcement. They may have no adult role models. Finally, they may lose self-esteem from frequent clinic visits that are often characterized by the identification of new problems without any recognition or positive reinforcement of their ongoing successes.

TREATMENT

The two overriding goals in the care of these patients are (1) to prevent dysfunctions (eg, neurologic defects) from becoming disabilities (eg, *cannot walk*) and (2) to prevent the disabilities from becoming handicaps (the social disadvantages experienced from the disabilities, (eg, difficulty in finding work). Achieving these goals requires comprehensive, coordinated care, in addition to routine care such as immunizations and anticipatory guidance. The newborn and family should be evaluated by a team, usually consisting of a pediatrician, nurse, social worker, neurosurgeon, orthopedist, physical therapist, and urologist.

Initial Concerns

Once the neonate has been examined initially and given supportive care, central nervous system infection must be prevented. For infants who have an open lesion, parenteral antibiotics that provide coverage against gram-negative bacilli and *Staphylococcus aureus* organisms should be given as soon as possible. Surgery to close the open defect typically occurs within the first 72 hours of life. Daily measurement of the head circumference and ultrasound or CT scans of the head should be used as guides for ventriculoperitoneal shunt placement to reduce hydrocephalus. No universally accepted criteria exist to determine the need for or the timing of shunt placement.

Baseline radiograms of the spine should be taken. Genetic counseling and social support should be provided to the family, and assistance with finances should be a priority. As the child grows, the primary care physician should coordinate the child's care and be the child's advocate. Another goal should be enhancing natural learning opportunities in typical routines and activities in home, school, and community settings to increase participation and optimize cognitive development. In most instances, children may benefit from formal early-intervention programs, including special education services and physical and occupational therapies. These services are mandated under the Individuals with Disabilities Education Act. Opportunities for interactions with people and objects (toys) should be provided. Similarly, the child should be encouraged to develop the best social interaction and self-help skills possible, including the development of independence in hygiene and eating. All children with meningomyelocele and hydrocephalus should have at least one visit by an ophthalmologist during infancy because of the risk of strabismus leading to amblyopia.

Long-Term Goals

According to Bronfenbrenner,[18] learning and development are facilitated by (a) the participation of the child in progressively more complex patterns of reciprocal activity with the child's parents and (b) when the balance of power gradually shifts in favor of the developing person. A child who has a disability has the same psychosocial needs as a healthy child; the clinician should help the family achieve this shifting of power. If a child has a learning disability, then the school should provide *remediation* (additional instructional time or different instructional approaches to *fix* a certain area of weakness and build strength in a particular area to facilitate potential learning) and *compensation* (alternative approaches [eg, assistive technology] to offset, or counter balance, a learning disability and produce the desired level of performance). Children, especially teens, with meningomyelocele are at increased risk for depression, anxiety, or both.[19] These conditions should be considered as causes for changes in physical functioning or problems at school.

Orthopaedic Treatment

Orthopaedic goals include optimal alignment, maximal range of motion, stability of the spine and extremities, and maximal function and comfort, while protecting the skin. Deformities such as clubfeet and joint contractures should be managed with range-of-motion exercises, splinting, and casting. Orthopedic management may include surgery for joint contractures, scoliosis, or kyphosis. One or both hips may become dislocated. However, surgical treatment may not be indicated if the dislocation is bilateral and the child has complete paraplegia. Prevention of contractures and dislocations may require regular passive range-of-motion exercises, splints, body jackets, and casts. Various exercises and orthoses (braces) may be used to enhance locomotion. The parapodium—a standing brace that allows the child to be in an upright position with hands unencumbered—and reciprocal gait orthosis can be started between 18 and 24 months of age. Crutches or walkers in conjunction with more standard bracing may be used, and early use of wheeled mobility is encouraged, especially for children who have quadriceps paralysis. Adaptive equipment such as carts and hand-pedaled tricycles also can enhance the function and self-esteem of these children.

Urologic Treatment

Urologic goals include (1) protecting the kidneys and ureters (by emptying the bladder, lowering intravesicular pressure, preventing urinary tract infections, and treating reflux) and (2) achieving continence. The urologic system should be evaluated by urine culture and renal ultrasound. In the past, urinary diversion via ileal loops was performed in most children who had meningomyelocele to achieve these goals. Clean intermittent catheterization, introduced in 1972, is safer, is more acceptable, and results in better renal function than does urinary diversion. Vesicostomy may be indicated in the infant who has vesicoureteral reflux or hydronephrosis. Most families are able to perform clean intermittent catheterization when the child is 4 to 5 years of age, and many children, even those this young, are able to perform the procedure themselves. Clean intermittent catheterization has also been used in children younger than 3 years of age and can be helpful in the management of vesicoureteral reflux with or without hydronephrosis or in those who have frequent urinary tract infections. The addition of drugs that relax the detrusor muscle or increase sphincter tone, such as imipramine hydrochloride, oxybutynin chloride, or pseudoephedrine, can enhance continence. For older children in whom catheterization does not provide continence, the use of a surgical procedure such as bladder augmentation plus the creation of a continent stoma with clean intermittent catheterization may provide continence.[20] Obtaining regular urine cultures to detect urinary tract infection and administering prophylactic antibiotics in children who have frequent infections may prevent renal damage. Trimethoprim-sulfamethoxazole, sulfisoxazole, nitrofurantoin, and cephalexin given in less than the therapeutic dose have been used for prophylaxis.

Neurosurgery

Neurosurgical goals include monitoring for signs and symptoms of ventricular shunt dysfunction and the occurrence of spinal cord problems such as tethering. Monitoring includes assessment of functioning (eg, decrease in school performance may indicate chronic shunt malfunction) and of the occurrence of signs and symptoms. Occasional cranial imaging (ultrasonography in infants and CT scans in older children) is performed. The optimal frequency of these studies has not been determined.

Continence

Bowel continence after 4 years of age and avoidance of severe constipation is often difficult to achieve. However, a high-fiber diet, stool softeners, regular toileting, regular stimulants, and biofeedback in children who have rectal sensation may be used singly or in combination to attain this goal. Regular enemas, using 20 mL/kg of normal saline, are effective in some children. Other options are suppositories and small-volume enemas (Enemeez). Several surgical procedures (antegrade colonic enema) have been developed to help children achieve fecal continence. The original surgical procedure (Malone) removes the appendix, opens its distal end, and uses it to create a channel between the colon and the abdominal wall.[21] In a related procedure (cecostomy) an opening is made in the cecum, either surgically or in the radiology suite, and a gastrostomy button is placed into the cecum.[22] In a newer antegrade colonic enema procedure, an opening is placed into the descending colon.[23] After all of these procedures, irrigation fluids are flushed into the colon, washing out stool. These procedures are used on a regular basis and show promise for a select group of children and adolescents in whom more conventional constipation-relieving techniques have failed.

Reproductive Issues

Impotence in the male patient may be managed surgically via penile implants, vacuum pumps, the injection or insertion of prostaglandin, or medications such as sildenafil (Viagra). Women with meningomyelocele have normal fertility and should use the same precautions to prevent pregnancy and sexually transmitted infections as the general population. Precocious puberty is a common occurrence in young women who have meningomyelocele with hydrocephalus because of a disorder of the hypothalamus. Precocious puberty can be treated with leuprolide (Lupron).[24] Pregnant women who have meningomyelocele may need to have their babies delivered by cesarean because of hip contractures. Their intervertebral disks also may become herniated, with neurologic sequelae; therefore they should have frequent neurologic evaluations throughout pregnancy.

Allergies

Because 50% or more of children who have meningomyelocele may have allergies to latex, including anaphylaxis during surgery, contact with products made from latex should be avoided. For example, all surgical procedures should occur in latex-free settings. Catheterization should be performed with nonlatex catheters, gloves used during care should be of nonlatex material, and toys that contain significant amounts of latex should be avoided, as should products that contact the skin, such as adhesive or Ace bandages.

Management Goals

The goal of treatment should be to optimize the child's activities and participation in society. Achieving this goal requires tremendous resources and effort and an ongoing relationship with the parents and child. However, the best efforts may still be inadequate in the absence of social changes. To prevent disabilities from becoming handicaps, society's attitudes and practices must be altered. The clinician can advocate for these children by helping remove architectural barriers in the community, which will allow people who have disabilities access to places such as banks, public buildings, transportation, and recreation areas. Altering the attitudes of people who have no disabilities may be more difficult, but the clinician can help enable the child and adult who have disabilities to serve as role models in the community—for instance, by encouraging the hiring of workers who have disabilities. Performing all the aforementioned tasks requires persistent effort and can be achieved only with a multidisciplinary team that is willing to collaborate with the family. All of these children should have healthy diets and regular physical activities to optimize health and well being; they also should have access to appropriate recreation and leisure activities.

Use of Alternative Medicine

Alternative therapies, such as cutaneous electrical field stimulation, therapeutic electrical stimulation, transrectal electrostimulation, bladder stimulation, biofeedback, and acupuncture, have been tried with varying success, and little evidence-based research exists to support their use. Because many of the conventional therapies are ineffective in treating the symptoms of spina bifida, and because no cure exists, families often turn to alternative therapies, including herbal medications. The pediatrician should inquire about the use of these treatments and be aware of their nature, possible interactions with medications, and potential for harm.

PREVENTION

Periconceptual supplementation of the diets of mothers of children who have neural tube defects has been shown to decrease the recurrence of these defects in families and to decrease the primary occurrence of such defects as well.[25] The American Academy of Pediatrics and the Centers for Disease Control and Prevention recommend that all women of child-bearing age receive 0.4 mg of folic acid daily. Women who have a first-degree relative who has a neural tube defect should receive 4.0 mg of folic acid daily.[26]

Open neural tube defects may be diagnosed prenatally by the measurement of alpha-fetoprotein levels in maternal serum between 14 and 16 weeks of gestation, coupled with confirmation of the diagnosis via high-resolution ultrasound. Amniocentesis is recommended for women who have elevated serum alpha-fetoprotein levels to confirm the diagnosis. In addition to termination, the prenatal detection of a neural tube defect allows the family to plan postnatal care, including the decision to have the delivery by cesarean section, if they elect to continue the pregnancy. Prenatal surgery to cover the open lesion on the back during the second trimester may decrease the severity of hydrocephalus and the Chiari malformation.[27] Premature delivery of the infant and maternal complications (bleeding and infection) remain major risks with this procedure. A multicenter controlled clinical trial is underway in the United States to evaluate the effects of prenatal surgery (www.spinabifidamoms.com). Social support should be offered to these families, whatever their decision.

WHEN TO REFER

- Infants born with meningomyelocele should be referred to a tertiary medical center that specializes in the care of these children, ideally before delivery.
- All infants born with meningomyelocele should be monitored during childhood by a multidisciplinary team that includes experts in child

development, neurosurgery, orthopedics, urology, orthotics, social work, nursing, physical and occupational therapies, and plastic surgery.

- Referral to an ophthalmologist, geneticist, and to an early intervention program should be accomplished early on.

WHEN TO ADMIT

- When the child is acutely ill and cannot be managed at home, and when the child requires surgical intervention

TOOLS FOR PRACTICE

Engaging Patient and Family

- *Caring for Your Baby and Young Child: Birth to Age 5* (book), American Academy of Pediatrics (www.aap.org/bookstore).

RELATED WEB SITE

- Spina Bifida Association (www.sbaa.org).

AAP POLICY STATEMENTS

American Academy of Pediatrics, Committee on Genetics. Folic acid for the prevention of neural tube defects. *Pediatrics*. 1999;104(2):325-327. (aappolicy.aappublications.org/cgi/content/full/pediatrics;104/2/325).

American Academy of Pediatrics, Cunniff C, Committee on Genetics. Prenatal screening and diagnosis for pediatricians. *Pediatrics*. 2004;114(3):889-894. (aappolicy.aappublications.org/cgi/content/full/pediatrics;114/3/889).

SUGGESTED RESOURCES

Allen PJ, Vessey JA, Carroll LH. *Primary Care of the Child with a Chronic Condition*. St Louis, MO: Mosby; 2004.

Batshaw ML, Pellegrino L, Roizen NJ. *Children with Disabilities*. 6th ed. Baltimore, MD; 2008.

Batshaw ML. *When Your Child Has a Disability: The Complete Sourcebook of Daily and Medical Care*. Revised ed. Baltimore, MD: Brooks Publishing; 1991.

Nickel RE, Desch LW. *The Physician's Guide to Caring for Children with Disabilities and Chronic Conditions*. Baltimore, MD: Paul H. Brookes; 2000.

Wilson GN, Cooley WC. Preventive management of children with congenital anomalies and syndromes. *Arch Pediatr Adolesc Med*. 2001;155:424-425.

REFERENCES

1. Williams LJ, Rasmussen SA, Flores A, et al. Decline in the prevalence of spina bifida and anencephaly by race/ethnicity: 1995-2002. *Pediatrics*. 2005;116:580-586.
2. Forrester MB, Merz RD, Yoon PW. Impact of prenatal diagnosis and elective termination on the prevalence of selected birth defects in Hawaii. *Am J Epidemiol*. 1998;148:1206-1211.
3. Tubbs RS, Wellons JC, Iskandar BJ, et al. Isolated flat capillary midline lumbosacral hemangiomas as indicators of occult spinal dysraphism. *J Neurosurg*. 2004;100:86-89.
4. Guggisberg D, Hadj-Rabia S, Viney C, et al. Skin markers of occult spinal dysraphism in children: a review of 54 cases. *Arch Dermatol*. 2004;140:1109-1115.
5. Dias MS, Pang D. Split cord malformations. *Neurosurg Clin North Am*. 1995:6:339-358.
6. Kang JK, Lee KS, Jeun SS, et al. Role of surgery for maintaining urological function and prevention of retethering in the treatment of lipomeningomyelocele: experience recorded in 75 lipomeningomyelocele patients. *Childs Nerv Syst*. 2003;1919:23-29.
7. Copp AJ, Greene ND, Murdoch JN. The genetic basis of mammalian neurulation. *Nat Rev Genet*. 2003;4:784-793.
8. Pollack IF, Kinnunen D, Albright AL. The effect of early craniocervical decompression on functional outcome in neonates and young infants with myelodysplasia and symptomatic Chiari II malformations: results from a prospective series. *Neurosurgery*. 1996;38:703-710.
9. Kirk VG, Morielli A, Brouillette RT. Sleep disordered breathing in patients with myelomeningocele: the missed diagnosis. *Dev Med Child Neurol*. 1999;41:40-43.
10. Burmeister R, Hannay HJ, Copeland K, et al. Attention problems and executive functions in children with spina bifida and hydrocephalus. *Neuropsychol Dev Cogn C Child Neuropsychol*. 2005;11:265-283.
11. Elliott SP, Villar R, Duncan B. Bacteriuria management and urological evaluation of patients with spina bifida and neurogenic bladder: a multicenter survey. *J Urol*. 2005;173:217-220.
12. Muller T, Arbeiter K, Aufricht C. Renal function in meningomyelocele: risk factors, chronic renal failure, renal replacement therapy and transplantation. *Curr Opin Urol*. 2002;12:479-484.
13. Schoenmakers MA, Uiterwaal CS, Gulmans VA, et al. Determinants of functional independence and quality of life in children with spina bifida. *Clin Rehabil*. 2005;19(6):677-685.
14. Rendeli C, Nucera E, Ausili E, et al. Latex sensitisation and allergy in children with myelomeningocele. *Childs Nerv Syst*. 2006;22(1):28-32.
15. Satin-Smith MS, Katz LL, Thornton P, et al. Arm span as measurement of response to growth hormone (GH) treatment in a group of children with meningomyelocele and GH deficiency. *J Clin Endocrinol Metab*. 1996;81(4):1654-1656.
16. McCormick MC, Charney EB, Stemmler MM. Assessing the impact of a child with spina bifida on the family. *Dev Med Child Neurol*. 1986;28(1):53-61.
17. Waitzman NJ, Romano PS, Scheffler RM. Estimates of the economic costs of birth defects. *Inquiry*. 1994;31:188-205.
18. Bronfenbrenner U. *The Ecology of Human Development*. Cambridge, MA: Harvard University Press; 1979.
19. Appleton PL, Ellis NC, Minchom PE, et al. Depressive symptoms and self-concept in young people with spina bifida. *J Pediatr Psychol*. 1997;22(5):707-722.
20. Macneily AE, Morrell J, Secord S. Lower urinary tract reconstruction for spina bifida—does it improve health related quality of life? *J Urol*. 2005;174(4 pt 2):1637-1643.
21. Curry JI, Osborne A, Malone PS. How to achieve a successful Malone antegrade continence enema. *J Pediatr Surg*. 1998;33(1):138-141.
22. King SK, Sutcliffe JR, Southwell BR, et al. The antegrade continence enema successfully treats idiopathic slow-transit constipation. *J Pediatr Surg*. 2005;40(12):1935-1940.
23. Calado AA, Macedo A Jr, Barroso U Jr, et al. The Macedo-Malone antegrade continence enema procedure: early experience. *J Urol*. 2005;173(4):1340-1344.
24. Carel JC, Lahlou N, Jaramillo O, et al. Treatment of central precocious puberty by subcutaneous injections of leuprorelin 3-month depot (11.25 mg). *J Clin Endocrinol Metab*. 2002;87:4111-4116.
25. De Villarreal LM, Perez JZ, Vasquez PA, et al. Decline of neural tube defects after a folic acid campaign in Nuevo Leon, Mexico. *Teratology*. 2002;66:249-256.

26. American Academy of Pediatrics, Committee on Genetics. Folic acid for the prevention of neural tube defects. *Pediatrics*. 1999;104:325-327.
27. Sutton LN, Adzick NS. Fetal surgery for myelomeningocele. *Clin Neurosurg*. 2004;51:155-162.

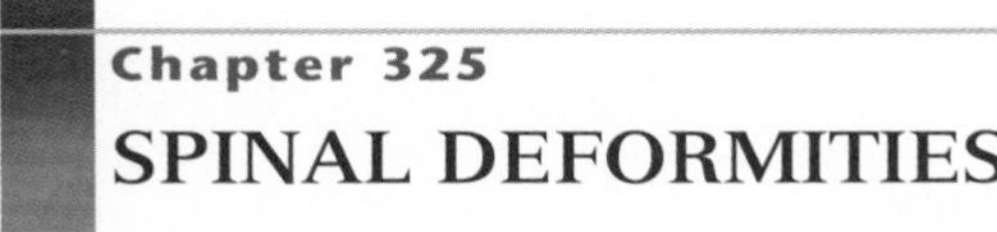

Chapter 325

SPINAL DEFORMITIES

Edward M. Sills, MD

SPINAL CORD AND VERTEBRAL EMBRYONIC DEVELOPMENT

Genetic abnormalities and teratogen exposure occurring during the embryonic period can adversely affect normal differentiation of the musculoskeletal system, resulting in malformations of the extremities or the spine. Formation of the defined spinal column occurs from the fourth through the sixth week of gestation. Somatic mesodermal tissue surrounding the notochord differentiates into a less cellular and dense upper portion and a more dense and cellular lower portion. The somites cleave together, the lower portion of the superior somite joining with the upper portion of the inferior somite. The intervertebral disk develops at the site of the cleavage. The notochord, which is contained within the newly joined primitive vertebral bodies, degenerates, and specific portions at the site of cleavage become the nucleus pulposus of the intervertebral disk. The neural arches and ribs develop from the more dense portions of the somite, and the vertebral body develops from the less dense portions.

Chondrification begins in the primitive mesodermal vertebrae during the sixth week of pregnancy. It progresses rapidly to form cartilaginous models of the vertebral body by the end of the first trimester. Ossification of the cartilaginous models begins during the second trimester. The ossification of each side of the neural arch and of the body at each level proceeds separately. In the neonate, the ossified vertebral body and neural arches at each level are clearly visible radiographically, separated by the nonossified synchondritic junctions. The ossification centers of the neural arches and body coalesce during the first 3 years of postnatal development.

The first and second cervical segments are distinct from the remainder of the spinal column. The first cervical vertebra lacks the physical form characteristic of other vertebrae, having instead only a narrow anterior arch. This arch is not ossified at birth or during the neonatal period but is most often visible by 1 year of age.

Errors in the embryologic sequence of the spine cause several congenital defects of the spinal column and spinal cord. These errors range in severity from isolated hemivertebrae to complex errors of vertebral formation and segmentation associated with defects of the neural tube or spinal cord. When such errors result in asymmetric vertebral formation or produce asymmetric vertebral growth potential, structural spinal curves such as congenital scoliosis or kyphosis develop.

Malformations of the head and neck, especially the internal and external auditory apparatuses, maxillae, and mandibles, occur frequently in patients with high thoracic and cervical curves. The association of a short neck, low posterior hairline, and restriction in neck motion caused by the congenital fusion of cervical vertebrae represents Klippel-Feil syndrome. Renal anomalies, the congenital elevation of the scapulae (ie, Sprengel deformity), impaired hearing, and congenital heart disease are common associated anomalies in affected patients. The VATER syndrome (*v*ertebral defects, imperforate *a*nus, *t*racheo*e*sophageal fistula, and *r*adial and *r*enal dysplasia) and the VACTERL complex (see later discussion), in association with limb defects, underscores the complex nature of the relationships between the rapidly evolving organ systems and the musculoskeletal system during the first trimester of pregnancy.

SPINE ABNORMALITIES

Postural

Back pain in children is often a sign of an underlying disorder. Postural abnormalities may or may not indicate an underlying spine disorder; the challenge to the physician is to determine whether the child's posture is caused by an underlying skeletal deformity or is merely a habit that has altered—exaggerates, increases, or decreases—the normal spinal curves. Abnormal curvatures and protrusions merit careful investigation. The thoracic spine normally has some kyphosis, and the lumbar spine normally has slight lordosis. If either condition is excessive, progressive, or painful, then concern is appropriate. Scoliosis, a side-to-side curve, is always abnormal (a classification of spinal deformities is provided in Box 325-1).

Congenital Malformations

When a newborn is held prone in the examiner's palm, the infant's back falls into slight flexion, allowing detection of meningomyelocele, scoliosis, kyphosis, or dorsolumbar hyperflexion. Lumbar spinal deformity may be indicated by a hair tuft, dimple, discoloration, or a palpable spina bifida lamina defect (see Chapter 324, Spina Bifida).

Congenital Scoliosis

The vertebral anomalies are present at birth, and the clinical deformity develops with spinal growth and may not become apparent until later childhood. These anomalies are due to failure of formation or failure of segmentation. They are sometimes related to cardiac or urologic abnormalities that develop during the same period (before 48 days of gestation). Vertebral developmental defects can be classified as defects of segmentation or defects of formation. This disorder shows progression in 75% of cases. Curve progression is strongly related to the type of vertebral abnormality with the poorest prognosis for unilateral unsegmented bars with contralateral hemivertebrae (up to a 10-degree/year progression), a less severe progression in cases of hemivertebrae (seen in 40% of cases) or double hemivertebrae (1-2.5 degrees/year and

BOX 325-1 Classification of Spinal Deformity

A. Idiopathic
   1. Infantile
   2. Juvenile
   3. Adolescent
B. Neuromuscular
   1. Neuropathic
      a. Upper motor neuron lesions
         (1) Cerebral palsy
         (2) Spinocerebellar degenerations
         (3) Syringomyelia
         (4) Spinal cord tumor
         (5) Spinal cord trauma
      b. Lower motor neuron lesion
         (1) Poliomyelitis
         (2) Other viral myelitis
         (3) Trauma
         (4) Spinal muscular atrophy
         (5) Meningomyelocele (paralytic)
      c. Dysautonomia (Riley-Day syndrome)
   2. Myopathic
      a. Arthrogryposis
      b. Muscular dystrophy
      c. Fiber-type disproportion
      d. Congenital hypotonia
      e. Myotonia dystrophica
C. Congenital
   1. Congenital scoliosis
      a. Failure of formation
         (1) Wedge
         (2) Hemivertebra
      b. Failure of segmentation
         (1) Unilateral bar
         (2) Bilateral bar
   2. Congenital kyphosis
      a. Failure of formation
      b. Failure of segmentation
      c. Mixed
   3. Congenital lordosis
   4. Associated with neural tissue defect
      a. Meningomyelocele
      b. Meningocele
      c. Spinal dysraphism (diastematomyelia)
D. Neurofibromatosis
E. Mesenchymal
   1. Marfan syndrome
   2. Ehlers-Danlos syndrome
F. Traumatic
   1. Fracture or dislocation
   2. After irradiation
   3. After laminectomy
G. Soft-tissue contractures
   1. After thoracoplasty
   2. Burns
H. Osteochondrodystrophies
   1. Achondroplasias
   2. Spondyloepiphyseal dysplasia
   3. Diastrophic dwarfism
   4. Mucopolysaccharidosis
I. Scheuermann disease
J. Infection
K. Tumor
L. Rheumatoid disease
M. Metabolic
   1. Rickets
   2. Juvenile osteoporosis
   3. Osteogenesis imperfecta
N. Lumbosacral anomalies
O. Hysterical
P. Functional
   1. Postural
   2. Secondary to short limb
   3. Secondary to pain

2-5 degrees/year, respectively), and a least severe progression in patients who have block and wedge vertebrae.

The management of congenital scoliosis requires frequent clinical and radiographic follow-up to detect progression. When located near the middle of the spine, the segments of the spine above and below compensate for it by curving in opposite directions. The result is a balanced spine and a straight back. Treatment is unnecessary. When, however, the asymmetrical vertebra is at the base of the spine (lumbar, sacral, or lumbosacral), the compensatory curve that develops above is insufficient, and a curvature progresses as the patient grows. This low spine congenital condition requires surgical correction before adolescence. When the deformity occurs in the cervical spine, a *wryneck* deformity results, and thoracolumbar compensatory curvature severely distorts posture. Unilateral surgical fusions are required to minimize deformity. The overall incidence of congenital anomalies of the spine is unknown, but one estimate of thoracic spine congenital deformity is 0.5 per 1000.[1]

Congenital Kyphosis

Congenital kyphosis is caused by lack of segmentation of vertebral bodies anteriorly or by lack of formation of a vertebral body. Deformities in the coronal plane produce congenital scoliosis, whereas those in the sagittal plane produce congenital kyphosis. The more severe deformities are usually recognized in the neonate, and they rapidly progress thereafter. The less obvious deformities may not appear until several years later. After progression begins, it does not cease until the end of growth. The most important factor regarding congenital kyphosis is the possibility that a progressive deformity in the thoracic spine can result in paraplegia. This potential outcome is usually associated with failure of the formation of the vertebral body. When necessary, the treatment is fusion.

Spina Bifida

Spina bifida can be mild and of no clinical significance (occulta), or it can be severe (vera), with meningeal protrusion (meningocele) or protrusion, or both, of meninges and neural elements (myelomeningocele) protruding posteriorly. When the protrusion includes bony elements, it may transfix the spinal cord. This transfixing spur is called *diastematomyelia*. Most of the lesions occur in the lower lumbar and upper sacral areas, but a few spinal defects are at a higher level. The physician should assess the level accurately because it affects prognosis. All thoracic lesions are associated with paraparesis. Lesions below L4 are associated with normal ambulation. The prognosis with lesions between L1 and L4 is mixed. Severe forms of spina bifida require prompt neurosurgical correction. Exercises to maintain the neck's functional range of motion are indicated, but surgery is contraindicated in mild cases because of the danger of injuring the cervical spinal cord. Spina bifida can be mild and of no clinical significance (occulta), or it can be severe (vera), with meningeal and neural elements protruding posteriorly. When the protrusion includes bony elements, it may transfix the spinal cord. This transfixing spur is called *diastematomyelia*. Severe forms of spina bifida require prompt neurosurgical correction.

Congenital vertebral anomalies also are seen in several syndromes in which other anomalies may be present. These anomalies are discussed in the following sections.

Larsen Syndrome

Larsen syndrome is an autosomal-dominant osteochondrodysplasia. Recently, Larsen syndrome was shown to be caused by missense mutations or small in-frame deletions in the *FLNB* gene. Larsen syndrome has a characteristic pattern of spinal deformity consisting of vertebral anomalies, spondylolysis, and scoliosis. The cervical spine is the most severely involved, and dysraphism (failure of closure of the primary neural tube), as well as hypoplasia, represents the most consistent patterns of deformity. Scoliosis is the most common deformity seen in the thoracic spine, whereas dysraphism, scoliosis, and spondylolysis are common in the lumbar spine. Dysraphism is the most common anomaly in the sacrum. Various joint, facial, and palate abnormalities are seen in some children with this syndrome. Tracheomalacia is not rare.

Goldenhar Syndrome—Ocular-Auricular-Vertebral Spectrum

Abnormalities in Goldenhar syndrome include a variety of ocular, auricular, and vertebral anomalies and was appropriately renamed the ocular-auricular-vertebral spectrum (OAVS). However, of note, the terms Goldenhar syndrome and OAVS are used interchangeably to describe this myriad of congenital anomalies.

The incidence of OAVS is rare; the prevalence is estimated to be approximately 1 in 45,000 live births. Male infants are affected more often than female infants, and the right side of the face or body (or both) is generally more commonly and severely affected than the left. OAVS has wide phenotypic variation, and, at present, no clear standard for diagnosis exists. However, authorities generally agree that the spectrum includes two or more of the following abnormalities: ear malformations (including microtia and accessory tragi), low-set ears, hemifacial microsomia (including micrognathia), coloboma, and vertebral anomalies (fused or cervical hemivertebrae). Of these abnormalities, multiple accessory tragi in a preauricular-mandibular distribution is one of the more constant findings and is an important diagnostic clue to recognizing the syndrome. Multiple malformations, including congenital heart, brain and renal disease have been seen in small numbers of patients with OAVS.

Morquio Syndrome (Mucopolysaccharidosis Type IV)—Odontoid Dysplasia With Atlantoaxial Subtuxation

Mucopolysaccharidosis type IV (MPS IV-A and -B) is also known as Morquio syndrome. This disorder consists of two forms with similar clinical findings and autosomal inheritance. MPS IV-A results from mutations in the gene-encoding galactosamine-6-sulfatase, located at *16q24.3*. MPS IV-B (a milder variant) is due to beta-galactosidase deficiency. The clinical features result from accumulation of keratan sulfate and chondroitin-6-sulfate. In both forms, mental symptoms are absent or only mildly present. Neurologic symptoms may result from compression of the spinal cord or medulla. The skeletal changes include joint laxity, short stature, pectus carinatum, shortened vertebrae, genu valgum, pes planus, and enlarged joints. Corneal clouding is present in 50% of cases. The neck is short, and the odontoid process in the cervical region is often dysplastic and fails to ossify. This circumstance can lead to atlantoaxial instability and C1-C2 subluxation. Insidious onset of cervical cord compression, beginning with fatigue and progressing to weakness, can occur but more ominously; acute cord compression and respiratory arrest may occur after minor falls. Surgery to stabilize the upper cervical spine, before the development of cervical myelopathy, usually by posterior spinal fusion, can be lifesaving.

VACTERL Complex

VACTERL complex refers to anomalies of the *vertebrae* (V), *atresias* in the gastrointestinal tract (A), congenital *cardiac* lesions (C), *tracheoesophageal* defects (TE), *renal* and distal urinary tract anomalies, and *rib* (R) and *limb* lesions (L). The categorical breakdown of anomalies in a large series were as follows: vertebral (25%), anal, esophageal (or other gastrointestinal) atresia (15%), cardiac (33%), tracheoesophageal fistula (95%), urinary (renal dysplasia, urethral valves) (17%), and skeletal (16%). The overall incidence of infants born with 3 or more components of this spectrum is estimated to be 1 in 25,000 live births.

Treatment Advances

Several groups have reported exciting advances in spinal surgery techniques to correct deformities. Research concerning the successful implementation of growing rods have revived this technique as a viable option for preserving near normal growth of the spine in both congenital and acquired disorders.[2,3]

New techniques have also been recently described, including vertebral stapling that produces asymmetric and corrective growth of the concavity of a deformity,[4] and vertical expandable prosthetic titanium rib instrumentation that indirectly corrects spine deformity and protects spine growth remaining to treat an associated thoracic insufficiency syndrome [5,6]

Acquired Abnormalities

Scoliosis

Acquired scoliosis can be nonstructural (corrects with side bending) or structural (no improvement with position change). Nonstructural scoliosis results from posture habit, splinting because of pain, muscle spasm, or hysteria. Of the structural forms of scoliosis, the congenital (eg, absent or fused spinal segments), metabolic (eg, juvenile osteoporosis), or neuromuscular (eg, poliomyelitis, cerebral palsy) types are less common than idiopathic scoliosis, which accounts for 75% of all cases.

Although most cases are idiopathic, an increased familial risk exists for scoliosis. Idiopathic scoliosis can appear clinically at any age, although the majority of cases begin in adolescence and most are girls who usually exhibit a right thoracic or right thoracolumbar pattern.

Infantile Idiopathic Scoliosis

The vast majority of these curves are self-limiting. The few that progress (usually double structural curves) can be difficult to manage. In cases in which the rib vertebral angle difference is larger than 20 degrees, progression is likely. The rib vertebral angle difference is defined as the difference in angulation of the left and right ribs on the apical vertebra as measured on an anteroposterior radiograph.

Juvenile Idiopathic Scoliosis

Juvenile idiopathic scoliosis is often progressive (estimated at approximately 70%). The potential for trunk deformity with cardiac and pulmonary compromise exists, especially in scoliosis with onset before 5 years of age. Curves of greater than 30 degrees are almost always progressive, at a rate of 1 to 3 degrees/year before 10 years of age and at a rate of 4.5 to 11 degrees/year after 10 years of age. If the scoliosis is in the thoracic region, surgery is required in more than 95% of these cases.

Adolescent Idiopathic Scoliosis

Roughly 2% of adolescents have a scoliosis (>10 degrees), but only 5% of these have a progression of the curve to greater than 30 degrees. The progression of scoliosis is dependent on the growth velocity and the magnitude of the curve at the first visit. Progression is most notable with a growth velocity of greater than 2 cm/year, between 9 and 13 years of age, at bone ages between 9 and 14 years, and between 0.5 and 2 years before menarche. The key risk factors for curve progression are the remaining spinal growth (skeletal immaturity) combined with the curve magnitude at a given time. The main progression occurs at the time of most rapid skeletal growth, occurring at 11 to 13 years of age for girls and at 13 to 15 years of age for boys. Primary thoracic curve scoliosis progresses more than primary lumbar curve scoliosis.

Scoliosis is usually painless and is discovered on routine physical examinations or at school scoliosis screening programs. The incidence of pain in children with idiopathic scoliosis is no different than in the general population in which approximately 30% report back pain at some time. Pain may arise during a phase of rapid progression of the scoliosis, or it might be related to an underlying neurologic disorder. The physician should be concerned about pain that arouses a child from sleep rather than the usually benign pain that delays falling asleep. Constant pain is also reason for concern.

When the patient bends forward, prominence of one scapula, of one side of the rib cage, or of the lumbar paraspinous muscles can indicate the site and direction of the scoliosis. When performing an Adams forward-bend test to screen for scoliosis (with the child bent forward until the spine is horizontal with the neck relaxed, knees fully extended, feet together, upper limbs dependent and palms opposed), truncal rotation (prominence) may be quantified with an inclinometer or *scoliometer*, which is centered over the apical spinous process (at the maximal degree of rotation and prominence). Seven degrees of rotation corresponds with 20 degrees of coronal deviation, which is the point at which referral to a pediatric orthopedist should be made.

Treatment is undertaken because pulmonary restriction, significant back pain, and cosmetic deformity are the sequelae of untreated severe scoliosis. Exercises are of no benefit in retarding or reversing the progress of scoliosis. A curvature in excess of 40 degrees requires surgical fusion regardless of the patient's age. Curves between 20 and 40 degrees should not require treatment if skeletal maturation is complete, but bracing is often recommended in the growing child. A curve milder than 20 degrees should be observed for possible progression but does not require treatment.

Kyphosis

An acquired dorsal hump, or kyphosis, can be secondary to a spinal tumor, radiation, infection, or surgery. The most common cause of acquired kyphosis is an osteochondrosis known as Scheuermann disease (see Chapter 302, Osteochondroses), which occurs in 5% of the population. Alternatively, glucocorticoid-induced osteoporosis, caused either by supraphysiological levels of endogenous (Cushing disease) or by exogenously administered glucocorticoids, can provoke kyphosis. Excess glucocorticoids often act to suppress bone formation and increase bone resorption, leading to trabecular bone loss, vertebral body collapse, and pathological fractures and causing an increased propensity toward kyphotic spinal malalignment. The most common site is in the lower thoracic vertebrae; but this condition can occur in any site in the vertebral column. The initial event is a bulging of the intervertebral disks in the direction of contiguous vertebral bodies, which exerts pressure against the cartilage plates covering the bodies, causing thinning of the plates. This event interferes with endochondral bone formation on the growth surface of the plates, causing gaps that are the basis for the herniation of the disk into the bodies, isolating the apophyseal ossification center from the vertebral body. The disk space narrows, more so anteriorly, causing increased pressure on the anterior portions of contiguous vertebral bodies and impeding their longitudinal growth anteriorly, resulting in attendant kyphosis.

An aching pain aggravated by physical exertion is present in the affected part of the vertebral column. The affected area is tender to palpation. Having the patient assume a stooping position often causes the pain to increase. Once the backache has been present for a year or so, the kyphosis is easily apparent as a round-back deformity. In many instances the pain is so minor that the patient first complains to the physician about pain caused by *poor posture,* and then the kyphosis is noted. Radiographs reveal a narrowing of the anterior disk space and defects on the surfaces of adjacent vertebrae at sites where the disk tissue has penetrated the bodies. The prolapsed disk tissue, in time, becomes walled off by osseous tissue, forming a bulbous mass of extruded tissue appearing as an area of lucency in the affected body (Schmorl nodule). In some children the condition can progress to cause severe deformity and dysfunction; in others, it stabilizes and the deformity may disappear. Treatment is aimed at preventing further deformity by casting or bracing. In rare instances of rapid progression or very severe pain, spinal fusion is necessary. The majority of youngsters, however, require careful observation with intervention only if progression of the deformity occurs.

Back Pain

Although scoliosis and kyphosis can be painful, they are usually painless postural deformities. The pediatrician should be aware of several painful disorders related to spinal deformity (see also Chapter 163, Back Pain).

Spondylolysis and Spondylolisthesis

Spondylolysis, a defect in the continuity of the pars interarticularis of the posterior portion of L4 or L5, may lead to forward slippage of the vertebral body, known as leading to a condition known as *spondylolisthesis.* The horizontal slippage usually involves the L5 vertebral body moving anteriorly in relationship to S1. This deformity, however, can occur anywhere in the vertebral column. Spondylolysis often causes back pain before spondylolisthesis develops. Because spondylolysis is fairly common in young athletes with low back pain, primary care physicians need to have a high index of suspicion with this group of patients. Trauma, causing disruption of the pars interarticularis, is believed to be the cause of spondylolysis in a genetically susceptible host. Gymnasts and other athletes who repeatedly hyperextend the spine have a higher incidence of spondylolysis than the general population. In adolescence and adulthood the incidence is estimated at 5%. In the absence of symptoms, it requires no treatment or activity restriction. If a child has significant low back pain, then activity modification or a brace is employed in an effort to ameliorate the symptoms. The propensity for spondylolysis to become spondylolisthesis with forward slippage is increased during growth spurts. Single photon emission computed tomography scans are important aids in diagnosis.

A flattening of the normal lumbar lordosis with posterior tilting of the pelvis is noted in spondylolysis. Spondylolisthesis is a forward slippage of one vertebra on the vertebra below. The defect in the arch dissociates the vertebra from its inferior facet and posterior ligamentous restraints. This separation may allow for a slow forward slippage of the vertebra on the vertebra below. Progression is estimated to occur in 5% to 7% of patients with spondylolisthesis. Progression and symptoms are most likely to occur during the adolescent growth spurt. Low back pain is the most common symptom. Some cases are diagnosed because the patient has an abnormal gait or postural deformity. Only 10% to 15% of patients ever develop symptoms.

An oblique radiograph roentgenogram reveals the pars interventricularis defect; a standing lateral radiograph demonstrates spondylolisthesis.

Treatment is typically aimed at the alleviation of back pain. This task can usually be accomplished with activity restrictions or a period of bracing. Activities that hyperextend the lumbar spine should be avoided. Exercises to reduce lumbar lordosis relieve the pain of spondylolysis. Once slippage occurs, surgical spinal fusion is necessary.

Infections of the Spine

Infections involving the spinal structures are exceedingly rare. Acute pyogenic osteomyelitis and tuberculosis (Pott disease) cause bone destruction, initially in the anterior portion of the vertebrae, leading to collapse. Vigorous antibiotic therapy and immobilization are indicated.

Disk space inflammation, or diskitis, can appear as a fever of unknown origin accompanied by a limp, low back pain, or refusal to walk. Narrowing of the disk space is the usual radiographic finding. In all cases, blood cultures are indicated. The majority of younger patients do not have evidence bacterial infection and require only immobilization. Children older than age 8 years occasionally have staphylococcal infections of the spine. The indications for using antibiotics include positive blood culture results, recurrences of back pain accompanied by systemic signs such as fever, leukocytosis with a *left shift* in the differential white blood cell count, erythrocyte sedimentation rate elevation, bone erosion, or clinical advancement of disease despite immobilization.

Bone scanning with technicium-99 is helpful in assessing and localizing inflammatory spine lesions.

TOOLS FOR PRACTICE

Engaging Patient and Family

- *Back Pack Safety* (fact sheet), American Academy of Pediatrics (www.aap.org/publiced/BR_Backpack.htm).
- *Spina Bifida* (fact sheet), American Academy of Pediatrics (www.aap.org/publiced/BK0_SpinaBifida.htm).

Medical Decision Support

- *Sports Shorts—Back Pain in Athletes* (fact sheet), American Academy of Pediatrics (www.aap.org/family/SportsShorts_10.pdf).

Other

- *Birth Defects* (Web page), Centers for Disease Control and Prevention (www.cdc.gov/ncbddd/bd/default.htm).

AAP POLICY STATEMENT

American Academy of Pediatrics, Committee on Psychosocial Aspects of Child and Family Health and Task Force on Pain in Infants, Children, and Adolescents. The assessment and management of acute pain in infants, children, and adolescents. *Pediatrics*. 2001;108(3):793-797. (aappolicy.aappublications.org/cgi/content/full/pediatrics;108/3/793).

SUGGESTED RESOURCES

Akbarnia BA, Marks DS, Boachie-Adjei O, et al. Dual growing rod technique for the treatment of progressive early-onset scoliosis: a multicenter study. *Spine*. 2005; 30(17 suppl):S46-S57.

Betz RR, D'Andrea LP, Mulcahey MJ, et al. Vertebral body stapling procedure for the treatment of scoliosis in the growing child. *Clin Orthop Relat Res*. 2005;434:55-60.

Bicknell LS, Farrington-Rock C, Shafeghati Y, et al. A molecular and clinical study of Larsen syndrome. *J Med Genet*. 2007;44(2):89-98.

Keckler SJ, St Peter SD, Valusek PA, et al. VACTERL anomalies in patients with esophageal atresia: an updated delineation of the spectrum and review of the literature. *Pediatr Surg Int*. 2007;23(4):309-313.

Montaño AM, Tomatsu S, Gottesman GS, et al. International Morquio A Registry: clinical manifestation and natural course of Morquio A disease. *J Inherit Metab Dis*. 2007; 30(2):165-174.

REFERENCES

1. Samadani AF, Storm PB. Other causes of pediatric deformity. *Neurosurg Clin North Am*. 2007;18:317-323.
2. Akbarnia BA, Mark DS, Boachie-Adjei O, et al. Dual growing rod technique for the treatment of progressive early-onset scoliosis: a multicenter study. *Spine*. 2005;30(17 suppl): S46-S57.
3. Takaso M, Moriya H, Kitahara H, et al. New remote-controlled growing-rod spinal instrumentation possibly applicable for scoliosis in young children. *J Orthop Sci*. 1998;3(6):336-340.
4. Betz RR, Kim J, D'Andrea LP, et al. An innovative technique of vertebral body stapling for the treatment of patients with adolescent idiopathic scoliosis: a feasibility, safety and utility study. *Spine*. 2003;28(20):5255-5265.
5. Emans JB, Caubet JF, Ordonez CL, et al. The treatment of spine and chest wall deformities with fused ribs by expansion thoracostomy and insertion of vertical expandable prosthetic titanium rib: growth of thoracic spine and improvement of lung volumes. *Spine*. 2005;30(17 suppl): S58-S68.
6. Hell AK, Campbell RM, Hefti F. The vertical expandable prosthetic titanium rib implant for the treatment of thoracic insufficiency syndrome associated with congenital and neuromuscular scoliosis in young children. *J Pediatr Orthop*. 2005;14(4):287-293.

Chapter 326
SPORTS INJURIES

Srinivasan Suresh, MD, MBA

Sport injuries result from acute trauma or repetitive stress associated with athletic activities. Increasing numbers of young athletes are involved in organized sports. Many athletes now train in sports year round and frequently play several sports at a time. Organized sports account for only approximately one third of sports injuries, with the remainder occurring in physical education classes and in recreational sports.[1] Wrestling and football have the highest significant injury rates per participant in high school, followed by softball, gymnastics, track and field, and soccer.[1] Tennis and swimming produce the fewest injuries.[1] Other sports fall somewhere in between. Frequency of injury, however, is not always the best measure of a sport's risk. The trampoline, for example, accounts for a disproportionately large number of injuries that cause paralysis.[1] Although, intuitively, younger athletes appear to be at greater risk for injury than older athletes, statistics from soccer and football demonstrate just the opposite. The risk of injury is much greater among senior high school students than among junior high and younger participants.[1]

This chapter discusses some of the medical issues regarding sports participation such as heatstroke and drug use, overuse syndromes, and acute trauma. It also discusses the common problem of anterior knee pain in young athletes. Sports medicine is a discipline in itself. This chapter can serve only as an introduction to some of the more common problems. Sports medicine texts should be consulted for more information on treatment and exercises for rehabilitation.[1] Sports medicine centers, which are located in many urban areas, provide consultation and continuing education for interested physicians.

Although many sports injuries are random events, estimates suggest that nearly two thirds of all injuries might be reduced by improvements in conditioning, equipment, compliance with rules, coaching and supervision, rehabilitation of existing injuries, and efforts to prevent reinjury.[1] Many schools now use certified athletic trainers for the prevention of and rehabilitation from sports injuries. These programs should be encouraged and supported. Inexperienced coaches with high expectations of young athletes and a poor understanding of training may contribute to injury.

Competition is often emphasized, but the greatest value of sports participation may lie in fostering lifelong habits of exercise and recreation. Especially for younger children, programs should emphasize participation by all children, not just the physically gifted.

Participation in organized sports provides an opportunity for young people to increase their physical activity and develop physical and social skills. However, when the demands and expectations of organized sports exceed the maturation and readiness of the participant, the positive aspects of participation can be negated. The nature of parental or adult involvement can also influence the degree to which participation in organized sports is a positive experience for preadolescents. The American Academy of Pediatrics (AAP) offers recommendations on how primary care physicians can help determine a child's readiness to participate, how risks can be minimized, and how child-oriented goals can be maximized.[2] The AAP also provides information for primary care physicians on sports participation for children and adolescents with medical conditions.[3]

HEAT INJURY

Heat injury is commonly divided into 3 syndromes: (1) heat cramps, (2) heat exhaustion, and (3) heatstroke. Heat is lost in 5 ways[1]: (1) convection (when heat from the body is transferred to cooler air moving across its surface); (2) conduction (heat transfer to another object by direct contact, as occurs when the skin comes in direct contact with a cooler object, such as a wet towel or shirt); (3) radiation (when heat from the body radiates into a cooler environment; this is not particularly effective when the ambient temperature is greater than the typical skin temperature, which is approximately 87°F [30.6°C]); (4) respiration (when heat is lost during exhalation and cooler air is inspired); and (5) evaporation (typically of sweat).

When the environmental temperature is warmer than the body temperature, the primary method of heat loss is evaporation of sweat, and the other 4 heat loss methods become less effective. Blood vessels close to the surface of the skin dilate to increase blood flow and heat dissipation. As the humidity increases, evaporation is less effective in producing loss of heat. Some acclimatization to high humidity occurs with training and exposure to warm temperatures.

Heat cramps, heat exhaustion, and heatstroke all appear to be increasingly common in athletes who do not drink adequate fluids, who are not acclimatized to local heat and humidity, and who are poorly conditioned. Most authorities suggest that adult-sized athletes drink 0.5 L of fluids per hour during persistent activity. Water is usually adequate. Thirst is not a reliable indicator of fluid requirements during vigorous exercise. Salt tablets should not be provided because most athletes receive abundant salt in their diets.

Heat cramps usually involve the arms, abdomen, or legs. Affected individuals usually have been sweating profusely. Treatment consists of rest in a cool environment, stretching, and fluids. Many people fail to recognize that these cramps are a symptom of dehydration and heat stress, rather than a muscle problem.

Heat exhaustion is a more severe syndrome than heat cramps and is probably caused by ineffective cardiovascular and autonomic responses to heat. Patients feel weak, faint, dizzy, and nauseous. They may vomit and appear pale. Syncope sometimes occurs. They may sweat profusely, or if severely dehydrated, the skin may feel warm and dry. Body temperature is often normal. Treatment consists of providing cool fluids and placing the athlete in a cool environment. Cool compresses and fanning also help. If the affected athlete is unable to tolerate oral fluids, then administering intravenous fluids should be considered.

Heatstroke is a medical emergency in which mechanisms for cooling are overwhelmed. The rectal temperature is high. The skin is hot and dry. Patients show signs of central nervous system dysfunction, such as irritability, combativeness, and disorientation, which may progress to obtundation. Tachycardia and hypotension are often present. Heatstroke is most often seen in long-distance runners and is the second-most common cause of death in football players, head and neck injuries being the most common.[1] To treat heatstroke, ice water–soaked towels or wet sheets with fans (if ice is not available) should be applied. The patient should be taken to an emergency room immediately. Heatstroke is most common when the temperature is greater than 95°F (35°C) and the humidity is higher than 50%.[1]

DRUG USE IN ATHLETES

Athletes frequently use drugs and nutritional supplements that they believe will give them a competitive advantage or will improve their strength or appearance. The AAP and the American College of Sports Medicine have issued policy statements condemning the use of these supplements.[4] Despite this warning, use of drugs and stimulants is exceedingly common. Anabolic steroid use, for example, has been reported to be as high as 5% to 11% among high school boys and 2.5% among high school girls.[5-7]

Anabolic steroid use is most common among football players and track participants. Clues to excessive use include jaundice, increased acne, behavioral changes (aggressiveness, irritability, marked mood swings), gynecomastia, and testicular atrophy. Hirsutism and deepening of the voice may occur in women. Liver enzymes may be elevated. Anabolic steroid withdrawal may cause side effects such as mood changes, irritability, hot flashes, nausea, myalgia, malaise, tachycardia, and hypertension.[4] Although controversy exists, anabolic steroids do appear to increase muscle mass and decrease catabolism of muscle in some situations.[8] Anabolic steroids adversely affect lipid profiles. Physicians may have overestimated and overstated short-term side effects, causing them to lose credibility with athletes, who see their peers taking these drugs without obvious problems.[8,9] Little information is available on long-term effects.

The Anabolic Steroids Control Act of 1990 made most anabolic steroids schedule-3 controlled substances. Illicit distribution is a felony. However, androstenedione, often mentioned in the media as a drug used by major league baseball player and home run king Mark McGwire, is still available without a prescription.

Creatine supplements, often advertised in bodybuilding magazines and sold at many gyms and health food stores, are also popular with adolescents. Unlike most androgen supplements, they can be obtained legally. In fact, some colleges provide them free of charge to athletes. They are not banned in professional sports or in the Olympic games. Creatine is converted to phosphocreatine in muscle with the help of the enzyme creatine kinase. Phosphocreatine is believed to serve as a reservoir for the high-energy phosphate bonds of adenosine triphosphate (ATP), which are the sources of energy for muscle contraction. The idea behind the supplements is that excess phosphocreatine will lead to a higher rate of ATP resynthesis during exertion and delay the fatigue that results from ATP depletion.[10] Some studies do show some benefit from creatine for activities requiring short bursts of high-intensity muscle contraction.[11,12] Little evidence exists that creatine is helpful in endurance sports. Some athletes argue that it helps them train more vigorously by reducing the time to recover from exertion.

Creatine supplements appear to increase serum creatinine levels, which is not an indication of any renal dysfunction but just a reflection of an increased load of creatinine. Long-term effects are unknown, and most sports medicine experts do not recommend creatine supplement use.

Over-the-counter supplements are not under government control, and being sure that these medications contain what is printed on their labels can be difficult. In addition, some supplements have been found to contain small doses of stimulants that cause athletes to test positive for banned substances.[13]

INJURIES TO BONE AND SOFT TISSUES

Injuries related to sports participation fall into the general categories of overuse syndromes that develop over time and acute traumatic injuries.

Overuse Syndromes

Overuse injuries are characterized by injury to bone, cartilage, or soft tissue caused by repetitive submaximal physical stress. In contrast to an acute fracture or soft-tissue injury, the tissue breakdown in overuse injuries occurs gradually. This phenomenon of hard- and soft-tissue breakdown is a normal, daily occurrence. The body continually remodels these tissues so that they recuperate fully.

Athletic training is a process of repetitively stimulating the musculoskeletal system and relying on remodeling and ultimately hypertrophy and strengthening to occur. Training strengthens not only the muscles, but also bones and connective tissues. When an imbalance occurs between the rate of breakdown of the connective tissues and the body's ability to remodel them, stress injuries occur. In young athletes, the frequency with which these problems occur has grown tremendously over the last several decades. Box 326-1 lists factors that contribute to overuse injuries in young athletes.

BOX 326-1 Factors Contributing to Overuse Injuries in Young Athletes

- Training errors
- Increased recreational time
- Increased intensity and duration of competition
- Increasing standards of competition
- Inadequate preseason conditioning
- Suboptimal facilities and equipment
- Overly enthusiastic coaches and parents
- Participation in multiple sports
- Lengthy seasons

More young athletes are training harder and longer than before as competition intensifies. An increasing proportion of youths also are becoming involved in competitive sports. Many athletes now train year round for participation in one sport, whereas others participate in several sports each year, even playing several sports at one time. Time off is not usually considered a priority. Inexperienced coaches may have unrealistic expectations of young athletes. All of these factors contribute to the growing number of training errors that often underlie these conditions.

Prevention of overuse syndromes involves the education of young athletes, their parents, their coaches, and the entire health care team, from trainers to physicians. Understanding these principles is crucial to returning an athlete to sports successfully after experiencing one of these overuse conditions. Failure to change the underlying problem often simply results in reinjury.

Stress Fracture

Stress fracture of bone is conceptually the simplest overuse syndrome of the musculoskeletal system. Repetitive loading of this relatively rigid tissue leads to work hardening. Unless remodeling occurs, the bone becomes brittle and eventually breaks. Along the way, the athlete begins to experience progressive discomfort with activities. Stress fracture commonly occurs with long-distance running.

Metaphyseal and Diaphyseal Stress Injuries

The athlete may experience gradual onset of symptoms of metaphyseal and diaphyseal stress injuries. Eventually, pain may preclude running. In some circumstances, the weakened bone may fail completely and result in a complete or displaced fracture. Although most of these injuries occur in later adolescence (ages 16-19 years), some do occur at younger ages. Typically, the distribution of male and female patients is equal.

Only approximately 10% of radiographs are abnormal at the onset of symptoms. A bone scan may detect an early stress fracture of the metaphysis or diaphysis (Table 326-1). The bone scan findings, however, must be correlated to the clinical symptoms. As many as 50% of adolescents with stress fractures will show multiple areas of stress response on bone scan, many of which do not correlate to areas of symptoms. Magnetic resonance imaging (MRI) may be the most sensitive study for stress fractures.

Metaphyseal and diaphyseal stress fractures in young athletes most commonly involve the fibula, metatarsals, tibia, femur, and ulna, but virtually any bone can be affected. Stress fractures of the metatarsals (typically

Table 326-1 Parts of the Growth Plate of a Long Bone

NAME	ROOT ORIGIN	DEFINITION
Physis	—	Specialized area of growth cartilage occurring at both ends of major long bones or at one end of the smaller tubular bones, such as metatarsals and phalanges
Epiphysis	Epi- (on)	Secondary ossification center interposed between the physis and joint articulation
Metaphysis	Meta- (next to)	Flared transition from the primary spongiosa of the physis to the dense tubular bone of the diaphysis
Diaphysis	Dia- (in between)	Dense cortical and tubular bone comprising the shaft
Apophysis	Apo- (arising from)	Specialized growth cartilage area to accommodate insertion of a major tendon

the second or third) and the distal fibula rarely have complications other than pain and temporary disability. Fractures of the tibia, humerus, and forearm rarely displace, but they have the potential to do so. Stress fractures of the hip are rare but have the highest potential for morbidity; displaced femoral neck fractures can disrupt the blood supply to the femoral head and lead to avascular necrosis and arthritis.

Most diaphyseal and metaphyseal stress fractures are managed by rest. Crutches are often necessary. Occasionally, casts and immobilization are needed. Healing time ranges from 4 to 12 weeks. A well-designed plan of alternative training, gradual resumption of participation in sports, and monitoring for recurrent symptoms is necessary.

Occasionally, stress fractures require surgical intervention. A suspected stress fracture of the proximal femur is probably best managed by an orthopedic surgeon. A slipped capital femoral epiphysis must be considered. Screw stabilization for either the slipped epiphysis or stress fracture may be needed. Stress fractures of the fifth metatarsal tend to be recurrent and are often best managed with an intramedullary screw.

Apophyseal Conditions

Osgood-Schlatter Disease

In 1903, Osgood and Schlatter separately described a disorder of the proximal tibial apophysis that commonly affects young athletes but may bother other active youngsters who are not involved in formal, organized sports.[14] The tubercle of the proximal tibia is the insertion site of the patellar tendon. The quadriceps is the strongest muscle group in the body, and the tensions it generates through the patellar tendon are enormous. Stresses applied at the interface between the tendon and the apophysis create a disruption of the normal transition from the ossified and unossified tubercle into the tendon.[15] Although mechanics undoubtedly play a key role, some individuals appear to be predisposed to this condition.

Patients are typically 10 to 15 years of age at the time of onset of this disorder. Boys are more commonly affected than girls; however, female gymnasts are particularly prone to this problem. Approximately 15% of teenage boys and 10% of teenage girls have complained of pain at their tibial tubercle at some point.[15] Bilaterality is high, although its reported incidence varies considerably. The average youngster with symptomatic Osgood-Schlatter disease has significant pain, tenderness, and swelling of the tubercle on the presenting side and usually has some degree of findings on the contralateral side as well. Many of these patients have a history of heel pain compatible with Sever disease (calcaneal apophysitis). As many as 20% to 30% have siblings who also have had apophysitis.[16]

The pain in Osgood-Schlatter disease is usually well localized to the tibial tubercle; it typically increases with activity. Signs and symptoms of intraarticular problems of the knee joint itself are absent. A lateral radiograph of the knee can help confirm the diagnosis by showing irregularity of the tibial tubercle and rule out a tumor or infection, which can mimic Osgood-Schlatter disease.

In most patients, Osgood-Schlatter disease will run its course with time. Symptoms can last for 1 to 4 years. In approximately 3% of patients, a persistent ossicle will form that can remain symptomatic and may ultimately require surgical excision.[14] Fracture of the tibial tubercle has been reported in patients with Osgood-Schlatter disease; its incidence is not known, but it appears to be low. As such, remaining active in sports is not an absolute contraindication.

The symptoms are often relieved with topical application of an ice pack to the area, intermittent use of oral nonsteroidal antiinflammatory drugs (NSAIDs), application of a compression band over the area, activity modifications as indicated by the symptoms, and hamstring stretching.

Casts are not routinely used because immobilization may weaken ligament insertions. However, brief periods of rigid immobilization may be necessary for acute exacerbations.

Sinding-Larsen-Johansson Disease

Sinding-Larsen-Johansson (SLJ) disease affects the inferior pole of the patella as a result of the same stresses that create the problem of Osgood-Schlatter disease.[16] Although an apophysis is not present at the inferior pole of the patella, a transition of the patellar ligament fibers occurs as they join the bone. In response to chronic repetitive stresses, the patellar periosteum can create a bony reaction, which is a classic finding of SLJ disease.

Affected youngsters are typically 10 to 13 years of age. They complain of well-localized pain at the inferior pole of the patella. As with patients with Osgood-Schlatter disease, they have no signs or symptoms of internal derangement of the knee joint itself. On physical examination, they exhibit point tenderness at the inferior edge of the patella, and they typically have no other abnormal findings. A lateral radiograph of the knee may demonstrate irregular ossification at the inferior pole of the patella. Some clinicians mistake this finding for a fracture.

Pain in the same area without radiographic change is often due to patellar tendonitis, or jumper's knee. This phase is an early stage of SLJ disease. With advanced skeletal maturity, the periosteal reaction is usually not seen.

This entity is self-limited and typically lasts 3 to 12 months. Similar to Osgood-Schlatter disease, treatment with ice, NSAIDs, and activity modification may be helpful. Immobilization and surgery are rarely necessary. Rupture of the patellar tendon or a sleeve fracture (avulsion of the inferior pole of the patella with attached cartilage) is not a well-recognized complication of this disorder. In general, athletes may participate in sports as tolerated.

Calcaneal Apophysitis

Calcaneal apophysitis, or Sever disease, occurs at the apophyseal insertion of the Achilles tendon into the calcaneus.[17] The patient is typically 9 to 14 years of age, with a substantial peak occurring at 10 and 11 years of age. Most (60% to 80%) cases are bilateral.

Patients may complain of heel, ankle, or foot pain. On physical examination, however, the discomfort is typically well localized at the region of the calcaneal apophysis. It is typically medial or posterior, although occasionally the tenderness may be on the lateral side. Rarely does the tenderness occur distal near the origin of the plantar fascia. No swelling, warmth, or limitation of motion should be present. Occasionally, because of concurrent tendonitis, some tenderness can occur along the course of the Achilles tendon itself. No classic radiographic change of calcaneal apophysitis is seen. Significant irregularity of the ossifying calcaneal apophysis is a normal finding at this age and should not be confused with evidence of a fracture.

Radiographs of the heels can be obtained to rule out other osseous processes, such as tumor or infection. In bilateral cases, radiographs are only necessary if some atypical component of the history and physical examination exists that raises concern about some other diagnosis.

Treatment focuses primarily on symptom management. This condition almost always resolves with time, and complications are extremely rare.

Shoe inserts that provide padding beneath the heel can be helpful. The material must be resilient enough so that it does not collapse. Typically, a 3/8-inch silicone or felt pad works best. Ice, NSAIDs, and activity modification are dictated by symptoms. Casts or Cam walkers (removable rigid walking splint) are occasionally necessary for severe cases. Surgery is not indicated.

Repetitive Physeal Injuries

Little League Shoulder

Little League shoulder, or physiolysis of the proximal humerus, is a widening of the proximal humeral physeal plate.[18] It occurs almost exclusively in Little League baseball players. It typically affects pitchers, but occasionally, players who do a lot of throwing from other positions can develop Little League shoulder.

Usually the patient is a 12- to 15-year-old boy who complains of pain in the shoulder related to overhead throwing. The key consideration in the differential diagnosis is rotator cuff tendonitis. Many of the signs and symptoms are the same. The patient with Little League shoulder typically has more pain in the deltoid region as opposed to the subacromial region.

Another differential diagnostic consideration is impending pathological fracture from a simple bone cyst in the upper humerus. Radiographic widening of the proximal humeral physis on the affected side confirms the diagnosis of Little League shoulder.

The essence of treatment is rest. Complications are uncommon. If the symptoms are minimal, then the young baseball player can often be allowed to bat and play in an infield position that involves minimal throwing. Clinical and radiographic resolution can take up to 6 months. A carefully planned resumption of pitching can then begin, but monitoring for recurrence of symptoms is necessary.

Physeal Widening of the Distal Radius

Physeal stress injury of the distal radius occurs almost exclusively in young female gymnasts. These injuries usually cause progressive pain in the wrists. Most often the pain is bilateral, but it may be more prominent on one side. On physical examination, point tenderness is often present, and a prominence may be noted on the dorsum of the distal radial physis.

Differential diagnoses include carpal laxity with dorsal wrist capsular impingement, posterior interosseous neuroma, and avascular necrosis of the lunate.

Anteroposterior and lateral radiographs should demonstrate the physeal widening. Comparison films of the other side are almost always obtained, although both sides may be involved. Typically, some asymmetry is noted.

Premature closure of the distal radial physis has been described, resulting in relative overgrowth of the ulna at the wrist. This closure causes asymmetrical loading of the carpal bones that can lead to chronic wrist disability. The goal of treatment is resolution of symptoms and normalization of the radiographs, which usually takes 3 months or longer. Once the athlete returns to gymnastics, clinical and radiographic monitoring are required.

Epiphyseal Overuse Conditions

Perhaps the best example of a repetitive stress-related injury of the epiphyses occurs at the capitellum (the lateral condyle of the distal humerus where it articulates with the radius). These injuries are typically classified as osteochondroses rather than stress fractures. In osteochondroses, a segment of epiphyseal bone and overlying articular cartilage becomes loose.

Panner Disease

Panner disease is a lesion of a young boy's capitellum that can be compared with Legg-Calve-Perthes disease. In patients younger than 10 years who develop irregularity of the capitellum, the course is usually benign. An avascular segment appears to exist in the center of the capitellum. It will revascularize with time. A substantial cartilaginous cap is noted around this area, and loose bodies typically do not form. Sequelae are rare, and treatment simply involves rest.

Osteochondritis Dissecans of the Capitellum

Although the term *osteochondritis dissecans* implies that an inflammatory process is present, histologic studies have failed to confirm this circumstance. Osteochondritis dissecans is clearly a repetitive stress phenomenon, and it occurs most commonly in baseball pitchers. As the ball is released during the pitching motion, a valgus movement occurs at the elbow. Tension occurs on the medial side of the elbow, and compressive forces are created across the radial capitellar articulation. The capitellum has an end arterial blood supply, which may be partially responsible for its susceptibility to developing avascular necrosis from these chronic repetitive compression forces.

Any pitching style that releases the ball lateral to the body's midsagittal plane accentuates the valgus moment at the elbow. Therefore side-arm pitches, many curve-ball techniques, and others can increase the compression loads across the lateral side of the elbow.

Patients typically experience aching pain in the lateral side of the elbow. With time, they can lose range of motion. Osteochondral fragments can displace acutely, resulting in a loose body sensation, a locked elbow, significant synovitis and pain, or any combination.

Plain-film radiographs often demonstrate a lesion of the capitellum. Either a sclerotic region or simply radiolucency may be present. Tangential views may be necessary to see the lesion. Occasionally, computed tomography scanning or MRI or both are helpful.

Unlike most overuse syndromes in young athletes, the sequelae of this condition are not always benign. Osteochondritis of the capitellum can result in permanent arthrosis of the elbow joint.

The most important lesson about this condition is the opportunity for prevention. Junior baseball programs typically have rules limiting the frequency and duration that youngsters can pitch. Typically, this limit is 3 innings per game and up to 6 innings per week. Young athletes, parents, and coaches need to be educated about this condition so that excessive pitching does not occur at other times.

Cases of osteochondritis dissecans of the capitellum occasionally heal with prolonged rest. However, surgery is often necessary to remove an unstable or displaced bone fragment.

Overuse Syndrome of Soft Tissues

Tendonoses

Overuse injuries of tendons can occur in younger patients. In adults, tendonitis is divided into 3 stages based on the progression of the disease (1) from inflammation of the paratenon (the fatty or synovial tissue between a tendon and its sheath) (2) through inflammation of the tendon itself and (3) into degenerative change of the tendon that ultimately results in rupture. Typically in young athletes, only the earliest inflammatory stage is seen.

The most common tendonitis in young athletes is that of the Achilles tendon.[17] The cause is not clear. Symptoms are typically located 2 to 6 cm above the insertion of the Achilles tendon into the calcaneus. Some lack of flexibility in the gastrocnemius muscle group may be found on physical examination.

The diagnosis typically made clinically. Radiographs and MRIs are rarely indicated. The treatment in young athletes is entirely nonoperative. If analysis of lower extremity mechanics during gait suggests a hyperpronation pattern, then custom foot orthoses to control this hyperpronation can be helpful. Ice, stretching, and NSAIDs also are used. Training modifications and heel lifts can be helpful as well. Immobilization rarely is necessary.

Occasionally a physical therapist may aid in a carefully planned program of muscle strengthening, and gradual reintroduction of sporting activities is achieved.

Rotator Cuff Tendonitis

The rotator cuff is a convergence of the tendons of the subscapularis, supraspinatus, infraspinatus, and teres minor muscles. These tendons extend laterally from the scapula over the humeral head. Together, they function to help stabilize the humeral head in the glenoid fossa of the scapula. A particularly important function of the rotator cuff is preventing the upper humerus from rubbing beneath the arch of the acromion. The supraspinatus muscle is the most important for this function.

Many factors contribute to rotator cuff tendonitis.[19] In young athletes, inherent laxity of the glenohumeral capsule (ligament complex) is likely to be a significant factor. Sporting activities that stress the shoulder joint with the arm extended overhead are particularly prone to precipitate symptoms. Some typical activities include overhead throwing in baseball, swimming, tennis serves, and gymnastics. Once a shoulder becomes irritated, a reflex arc inhibits the firing of the rotator cuff muscles. This precipitates further dysfunction of the shoulder muscle and leads to impingement of the humeral head beneath the acromion. With time, a well-established bursitis and tendonitis develop. Typically, the patient complains of pain with overhead activities. In many instances the athlete will complain of the arm becoming heavy or tired or feeling dead.

A thorough examination of the neck and shoulder should be conducted, assessing for range-of-motion limitation, muscle atrophy, and focal tenderness in the subacromion region, both anteriorly and laterally. Tenderness may occur along the course of the biceps tendon as well. Bringing the shoulder fully overhead may produce pain; this finding is referred to as a positive impingement test. The supraspinatus strength should be tested, and glenohumeral laxity should be assessed as well.

Plain-film radiographs are not diagnostic of rotator cuff tendonitis but are often obtained to rule out other

Table 326-2 Severity Grading of Sprains

GRADE	DESCRIPTION	CLINICAL PRESENTATION	TYPICAL RECUPERATION TIME
I (mild)	Stretching of the ligament with minimal microscopic injury	Mild swelling, limp	0-2 wk
II (minor)	Partial disruption of the ligament	Modest swelling, diffuse tenderness, difficulty weight bearing	1-4 wk
III (severe)	Complete disruption of the ligament	Extensive swelling and bleeding, instability, and disability	4-12 wk

bony abnormalities. An MRI can be diagnostic for rotator cuff tendonitis but is often not necessary. The diagnosis can usually be made clinically. Full-thickness rotator cuff tears are almost never seen in patients younger than 18 years.

Acute Trauma

Acute injuries include sprains, muscle tears, and fractures. Sprains are injuries to ligaments, and they typically are graded from mild to severe (Table 326-2).

The fundamental principles of treatment for many musculoskeletal injuries go by the acronym RICE (*r*est, *i*ce, *c*ompression, and *e*levation). Rest is especially important for the first 24 to 72 hours after a significant injury. For lower-extremity injuries, crutches should be used to avoid weight bearing. Randomized studies have demonstrated that athletes can return to full activity faster if cryotherapy is begun immediately after the injury.[20] Ice may be applied for 20 minutes every 2 to 4 waking hours. A wet cloth can be used between the ice and skin to decrease the chance of cold injury. Many trainers advise continuing the use of ice until the swelling disappears completely. Compression may be applied with an elastic bandage. The goal of elevation is to place the injured extremity above the level of the heart to aid in reducing edema.

Ankle Sprains

Ankle sprains are the most common musculoskeletal injury in sports.[21] Approximately 97% involve the lateral ankle ligaments.[21] The typical mechanism of injury involves inversion and external rotation of the foot, which results in a sequential tearing of the anterior talofibular ligament, calcaneal fibular ligament, and finally the posterior talofibular ligament. Occasionally the anterior talofibular ligament and the syndesmosis complex are involved. These injuries are much more severe. The deltoid ligament also may be injured.

The presence of bony tenderness should be determined, particularly over the distal fibula, the anterolateral tibia, the medial malleolus, the base of the fifth metatarsal, or the proximal fibula. In the skeletally immature athlete, the bone is usually weaker than the ligaments; thus lateral ankle injuries often result in physeal fractures of the distal fibula. Sometimes, separating focal tenderness over the physis from diffuse tenderness of the lateral ankle ligaments can initially be difficult. Percussing with the tip of the finger can often separate tenderness at the proximal physis from tenderness around the ligaments.

The decision to obtain radiographs is based on several factors, including the patient's age, history of injury, physical findings, ability to bear weight, and progress since injury. The typical fracture of the distal fibular physis has a Salter-Harris type I fracture pattern without displacement, which results in a normal radiograph of the bone, showing only soft-tissue swelling. The diagnosis is therefore made clinically. The radiograph simply excludes displacement of the fracture or other fractures being present.

As simple as the injury may sound, the treatment options for ankle sprains are complicated. Treatment modalities vary widely and are chosen based on the severity of the injury (see Table 326-2), the demands of the athlete, and the experience of the treating health care team.

If the injury does not appear severe, then the RICE principles can be applied and the ankle periodically reevaluated. Some injuries respond quickly. At reevaluation, if the pain is minimal, then the ankle should be tested for stability. The athlete should then be observed in functional tasks such as running, cutting, and twisting. If these tasks are performed well without significant pain, then the individual may return to competition. Ideally, the ankle should be taped or splinted to lessen the risk of reinjury, and a preventive physical therapy program should be considered.

For ankle sprains of moderate grade, many other options come into play. For the less-serious athlete, an expectant approach can be used, including crutches, elastic bandage wrap, and gradual progression of weight bearing, with return to sports only after resolution of symptoms. Occasionally a cast or Cam walker is helpful.

For the serious athlete with moderate-grade sprains, referral to a physical therapist is often helpful. A variety of physical therapy modalities can help reduce the swelling. Range of motion is begun early, and strengthening is emphasized. As the ankle becomes comfortable, a proprioception training phase of rehabilitation begins. Many lace-up and Velcro ankle supports are available. For some athletes, taping may be an option. In all cases, functional criteria for return to sports, prevention of reinjury, and reassessment of progress are key components.

Severe-grade sprains should be managed by someone with advanced skills in dealing with musculoskeletal problems. This person might be an experienced primary care physician or an orthopedic surgeon. A period of immobilization to reduce bleeding and swelling is often helpful. A myriad of rehabilitation protocols can be used successfully. Assessment for chronic laxity and tarsal coalitions should be made.

Persistent anterolateral ankle pain can occur after even mild ankle sprains. In many instances, this ankle pain is due to an area of fibrosis or synovial hypertrophy in the anterior lateral corner of the joint. The differential diagnosis should include chondral and osteochondral injuries at the dome of the talus, chronic laxity of the ankle or subtalar joints (or both), and tarsal coalition. Initial treatment includes NSAIDs, ankle supports, and physical therapy modalities. Occasionally, steroid injection is helpful. If symptoms persist, then referral to an orthopedist or sports medicine specialist is indicated.

Collateral Ligament Injuries of the Knee

Injuries to the ligaments do occur in skeletally immature individuals. The collateral ligaments of the knee originate from the epiphyses of the femur and insert into the epiphyses of the tibia and fibula, with one exception. The distal portion of the superficial medial collateral ligament inserts over a broad area of the proximal tibial metaphysis. As in the lateral ankle, physeal injuries should always be suspected in persons with open growth plates. Plain-film radiographs may not be diagnostic. Stress radiographs or an MRI are occasionally needed to make this diagnosis. Concurrent injury to the cruciate ligaments, menisci, and articular surfaces need to be considered as well.

Most medial collateral ligament injuries heal satisfactorily.[22] Initially, the principles of RICE are used. Depending on the severity of the injury, the knee is mobilized as the swelling and tenderness diminish. As range of motion returns, strength should be assessed. A physical therapist or athletic trainer can be helpful in designing an adequate rehabilitation program. For moderate- and severe-grade sprains, consideration should be given to using a dual, upright, hinged, functional knee orthosis.

Lateral knee and ligament injuries are uncommon in young athletes. This diagnosis should raise suspicion that another explanation can be found for the patient's signs and symptoms, and referral is wise. For true lateral collateral ligament injuries, the principles of treatment are similar to those for medial collateral ligament injuries.

Anterior Cruciate Ligament Injuries

As adolescents become skeletally mature, the incidence of anterior cruciate ligament (ACL) injuries rises rapidly. The incidence of injuries to young female athletes, particularly in soccer, basketball, and gymnastics, is rising rapidly.[23] For boys, football, soccer, and basketball are common sources of these injuries.

The ACL is a key stabilizer of the knee joint, particularly to rotational movements. As such, it is frequently injured in sports that involve cutting and twisting. Alternatively, the knee may be struck from the lateral side, first injuring the medial collateral ligament and then the ACL.

Classically, athletes describe an acute pop and pain in the knee. They often fall to the ground and experience moderate to severe pain. The knee may not swell immediately, but typically it does swell within the first few hours because of the development of a hemarthrosis. Occasionally the tenderness is not marked, and athletes will attempt to return to their sporting competition, only to discover that the knee is not stable, which may worsen the injury. A high index of suspicion should be maintained for ACL injury, and it must be ruled out before the young athlete who has a knee injury returns to practice or competition.

The physical examination will vary considerably depending on the severity, the other structures involved, the time that has elapsed, and whether the injury is truly acute or actually an exacerbation of a chronic instability.

The most sensitive physical examination component is the Lachman examination, which is performed with the patient lying supine; the knee is gently flexed to approximately 30 degrees. The patient must be able to relax the quadriceps and hamstrings enough to allow the examiner to attempt to slide the proximal tibia anteriorly. Although the amount of movement of the tibia has some importance, the key factor is the end point. If the test is negative (ie, the ligament is intact), then a distinct end point or cessation of forward movement should be felt. This end point should feel similar to holding the 2 ends of a short piece of rope and quickly pulling the ends apart until the movement suddenly stops.

Comparison with the uninjured knee can be helpful. Performing this examination competently requires experience. The size of the patient's leg, the ability of the patient to relax, and the size of the examiner's hands are factors that contribute to successful performance of the test. If doubt exists, then the knee should be reevaluated later on or the patient referred to an orthopedist. Occasionally an MRI is indicated, but in most cases, a properly performed Lachman physical examination is diagnostic.

In contrast to the collateral ligaments of the knee, the healing potential of the ACL is limited because of its susceptible vascular supply. As a result, most injuries to the ACL do not heal well, and primary surgical repairs (as opposed to reconstructive surgery) are not effective.

Left without the stability of the ACL, most knees in young, active patients eventually become symptomatically unstable, and reinjury will occur.[23] In older and less-active individuals, nonoperative management of these injuries plays a role; however, most ACL injuries in young athletes should be reconstructed. Leaving the knee unstable makes it vulnerable to injury to the other ligaments, the joint capsule, and the menisci.

Most reconstructive techniques currently in use involve drilling holes through the proximal tibia and distal femur to insert grafts along the anatomic course of the ACL. For the skeletally immature individual, this procedure raises some concerns about potential injury to the physis.

Many factors go into the decision to reconstruct the ACL. During the last year that the physes are open, very little growth of the distal femur and proximal tibia occurs, thus any disturbance to them should result in minimal problems. Most studies have not demonstrated any complications of ACL reconstruction in skeletally immature individuals, although few data exist about youngsters younger than 10 years. The risk of further damaging the knee ligaments and the menisci by not repairing the ACL must be weighed against the risk of surgical injury to the physis, which is unusual and largely correctable. For the very young patient, a brace, physical therapy, and activity modifications is probably the best approach to managing ACL injuries.

Meniscal Tears

The meniscal cartilages have several important functions within the knee joint. These functions include providing mechanical shock absorption between the weight-bearing articular cartilages of the femur and tibia, enhancing the distribution of synovial fluid, which provides nourishment to the superficial portion of the articular cartilage, and enhancing the stability of the articulation between the tibia and femur. Loss of the meniscal cartilages has little detectable effect on the knee joint initially. However, over the ensuing decades, particularly after 20 years, the rate of degenerative joint disease rises significantly. As a result, all reasonable efforts should be made to protect, preserve, and repair menisci of younger patients.[24]

For many years, investigators thought that the menisci, which are relatively avascular structures, had virtually no ability to heal. Microangiographic studies have shown, however, that even the adult meniscus is vascular in its capsular one third. Very early in life, the vascular proportion is even greater. Clearly, many meniscal tears, particularly in young patients, have the potential to heal.

In youths 10 years of age and younger, most meniscal tears are related to discoid menisci. These menisci are congenitally abnormal that are almost always on the lateral side of the joint. When viewed from the top down, the discoid meniscus does not have the usual C shape but rather has a variable degree of excessive tissue covering the tibial plateau. The complete discoid meniscus covers the plateau entirely. Discoid menisci are smaller than normal menisci, less mobile, and much more prone to tear. A discoid variant, the Wrisberg type, has thick margins and is usually not attached to the capsule posteriorly. These patients exhibit a classic finding of a snapping knee. As the knee actively extends, it suddenly shifts and pops as the thick, mobile discoid meniscus shifts between the weight-bearing surfaces of the tibia and femur.

The diagnosis of a discoid lateral meniscus can often be made clinically by the sound and shift of the cartilage itself, but MRI confirmation is often sought. Symptomatic discoid lateral menisci require surgical intervention. The principles of treatment are to preserve as much of a normal functioning rim of meniscal cartilage as possible while alleviating the mechanical snapping that ultimately leads to degenerative changes of the articular surfaces.

For patients older than 10 years, the incidence of tearing of normal menisci rises.[24] Most commonly, this tearing occurs in association with significant ligament injury, such as a tear of the ACL. Rarely do normal menisci in teenagers tear without a substantial injury. As a result, meniscal tears are not typically at the top of the list of differential diagnoses of a young person with gradual onset of nonspecific knee pain.

If a meniscal tear is suspected, then referral or MRI is appropriate. Arthrograms are now performed much less commonly than before. If a normal meniscus is torn, then the general principles of surgical treatment are preservation of meniscal tissue and reconstruction of the unstable joint. The pattern and location of the tear determine whether the meniscus may heal on its own or will require arthroscopic partial removal or repair.

Quadriceps Contusion

Minor contusions of the quadriceps muscle are common events in contact sports such as football, soccer, and lacrosse. However, significant hematomas can develop within the quadriceps, which can be quite disabling.[25] More extensive hematomas have a propensity to rebleed. Myositis ossificans traumatica (heterotopic ossification of the muscle) may develop, which can also be disabling.

The key finding for separating minor hematomas from major ones is limitation of knee flexion. Minor hematomas should not limit knee motion, whereas large ones can. Occasionally, differentiating a large quadriceps hematoma from a malignant tumor of the thigh becomes challenging, such as Ewing sarcoma and osteosarcoma, both of which have a propensity to occur in teenagers and which may bleed internally themselves.

Initial treatment of quadriceps hematoma involves RICE and crutches. As pain and swelling diminish, active knee flexion exercises are begun. Full return of motion is the minimal requirement for return to contact sports, at which time a padded guard should be used. Monitoring for reinjury is essential.

Avulsion Fractures of the Pelvis

Six major apophyses are present on each side of the pelvis. These apophyses include the iliac crest, the anterior-superior iliac spine, the anterior-inferior iliac spine, the lesser trochanter, the greater trochanter, and the ischial apophysis. Each of these areas is prone to develop an apophysitis, and, except for the greater trochanter, avulsion fractures also are fairly common.[26]

An avulsion fracture typically causes acute onset of pain during a sudden athletic motion. Examples include an explosive start for a sprint, an extreme pike maneuver (hips flexed and knees extended) in gymnastics, or a combination twisting movement and direct blow to the iliac crest. A complete history will sometimes reveal mild antecedent symptoms consistent with a preexisting apophysitis.

Findings include focal tenderness to palpation over the affected apophysis and pain with resisted strength testing of the corresponding muscle insertion or origin. The diagnosis can often be confirmed with plain-film radiographs. Special oblique views and occasionally a computed tomographic scan or an MRI are helpful.

Most of these avulsions do not displace significantly; almost all heal with time and rest. Typically, crutches and rest are suggested for the first few weeks. Stretching may inhibit healing and should be avoided until the site is pain free. Complete healing typically takes 6 weeks to several months. The athlete should be gradually returned to activity and monitored for recurrence of symptoms.

Muscle Strains

Injuries to muscle tendon units almost always occur at the musculotendinous junction. Similar to sprains, muscle tendon injuries vary in severity from mild through severe. Mild injuries heal fairly rapidly, whereas severe strains can lead to large areas of scar tissue that are prone to reinjury.

The diagnosis of muscle strain has several pitfalls. Muscle strains are not as common in young athletes as they are in older ones. The diagnosis of a strain is too often applied to a musculoskeletal malady for which the true diagnosis is not obvious to the examiner. Particularly around the hip and thigh area, the examiner should be careful not to miss a slipped capital femoral epiphysis, an avulsion fracture, an infection, or a tumor as causes of pain.

Slipped capital femoral epiphysis is the most common disorder of the hip in adolescents. Although classically exhibiting with hip pain, discomfort may be referred to the thigh or knee joint. Delay in diagnosis and treatment is a common problem and can result in the severe complication of avascular necrosis of the femoral head.

The most common muscle strain in teenaged athletes is of the hamstring. Hamstring strain causes pain at the musculotendinous junction, which is at the junction of the middle and distal thirds of the posterior thigh. More proximal hamstring tenderness should raise suspicion of an occult injury to the ischial apophysis.

The treatment principles for hamstring strain initially involve RICE and crutches. Reduction of tenderness can take days to weeks, depending on the initial severity of the injury. Once comfortable, a gradual stretching and strengthening program is initiated. The athlete is returned to activities as tolerated and monitored for recurrent symptoms. Reinjury is a problem with hamstring strains.

Dislocations

The most common dislocations of young athletes include patella, shoulder (glenohumeral joint), elbow, and fingers. With severe trauma, dislocations and fracture dislocations can occur in virtually any joint, and musculoskeletal specialists generally manage these injuries.

PATELLAR DISLOCATION. A common musculoskeletal dislocation in young athletes involves the patella. Patellar dislocation should not be labeled as knee dislocation, which denotes displacement of the articulation between the tibia and femur. The latter is a high-energy injury and has a high associated morbidity including, occasionally, loss of limb.

By contrast, patellar dislocation is often the result of a trivial injury. Many individuals are predisposed to dislocation of the patella as a result of genetic variability in their knee extensor mechanism. Variations leading to easy dislocation include a shallow sulcus in the distal femur, lateral translation of the insertion of the patellar tendon into the tibia, relative underdevelopment of the vastus medialis muscle, and tightness of the lateral retinaculum.

Almost all patellae dislocate to the lateral side. Occasionally the patient will report having seen a medial prominence, but this is typically due to the medial femoral condyle being exposed by the displaced patella.

The history of injury can vary from a minor twisting episode to a significant direct blow to the knee. The patella may spontaneously reduce or remain displaced and require manipulation.

Manipulative reduction can often be achieved relatively easily. Ideally the patient is placed in a prone position, which facilitates hip extension and thereby starts to relax the hamstrings. The knee then is gently extended, and as it extends, the patella should reduce without forced manipulation.

Unless the patellar dislocation or subluxation is a trivial event that incites little pain in the joint, radiographs should be obtained to assess for osteochondral fragments. These loose pieces typically arise from the lateral femoral condyle or the patella.

After a significant patellar dislocation, the knee is immobilized, and the principles of RICE are used. As the pain and swelling subside, a rehabilitation program is initiated that emphasizes strengthening of the quadriceps muscles, particularly the vastus medialis. The hamstrings are stretched, and a lower extremity rehabilitation program is undertaken. A patellar-stabilizing knee sleeve is used during the initial phases of return to activity.

Most patellar dislocations can be successfully managed with a single therapeutic program. Recurrent patellar instability, particularly in those with a familial history, may require reconstruction.

SHOULDER DISLOCATION. As with patellar dislocation, dislocations of the glenohumeral joint can occur from relatively minor trauma in predisposed individuals or as a result of major trauma in the average person. Reduction can occur spontaneously; however, fixed dislocations can be difficult to reduce. These dislocations may require transportation to an emergency care facility. Reduction may require expertise, local anesthesia, sedation, and occasionally, general anesthesia. Unless the episode is minor, radiographs are generally obtained to confirm reduction and rule out an associated fracture. Pathological collagen disorders, such as Marfan syndrome, need to be considered in these patients. Physical findings consistent with Marfan syndrome include tall, thin body habitus, arachnodactyly, pectus excavation, heart murmur, dislocated lens, and myopia.

Traditionally, shoulder dislocations have been treated with 3 weeks of immobilization, followed by a rigorous physical therapy program. The therapy should be directed at strengthening the rotator cuff muscles. The principle is to strengthen these dynamic stabilizers of the joint to help compensate for laxity of the shoulder joint capsule (ligaments). The patient's program is advanced, and an experienced therapist monitors progress.

Recurrent instability despite a therapy program is generally an indication for surgical stabilization. Support is growing for earlier surgical intervention, particularly with less-invasive arthroscopic techniques. The exact indications and preferred techniques currently are in a significant state of evolution.

Anterior Knee Pain

The most common knee complaint of adolescents is that of anterior knee pain. This ubiquitous symptom can arise from a wide variety of disorders. In many cases, a specific diagnosis such as Osgood-Schlatter disease, SLJ disease, patellar tendonitis, or patellar instability can be made. A complete history, physical examination, and diagnostic studies can help reach these diagnoses. However, a specific diagnosis cannot always be made. In some instances, a degree of psychological overlay to the symptoms can be found, which can make management challenging.

For patients who have anterior knee pain, diagnostic imaging, including MRI, often does not reveal its source. Occasionally, these studies are indicated to rule out other definable abnormalities. In general, consultation from a physician with appropriate expertise should be obtained before embarking on diagnostic studies beyond plain-film radiographs.

Some of the more common causes of anterior knee pain have been discussed previously, and 2 additional entities—chondromalacia patella and patellofemoral pain syndrome—are discussed here. A wide variety of less-common disorders not discussed in detail here can cause anterior knee pain. These disorders include quadriceps tendonitis, bipartite patella, osteochondritis dissecans of the femur or patella, iliotibial band tendonitis, popliteus tendonitis, inflamed plica, prepatellar bursitis, and synovial flat pin impingement syndrome. Osteomyelitis, septic arthritis, inflammatory arthritis, and tumors should always be kept in mind.

Chondromalacia Patella

The term *chondromalacia patella* refers to softening of the articular surface of the patella, which can occur in mild to severe grades, ranging from edema of the cartilage to complete ulceration of the articular surface. This term had previously been misapplied to virtually any case of anterior knee pain. The diagnosis should be reserved for specific instances of symptomatic articular change of the surface of the patella.

Particularly in mild cases, the pain from chondromalacia patella will abate with intermittent use of NSAIDs, a quadriceps-strengthening program, and judicious activity modification. Although a therapy program can be helpful, the patient must have a clear understanding that the goal is to reduce symptoms. Completely eliminating symptoms may not be possible. Occasionally, surgical intervention to alter the patella's articular surface is indicated.

Patellofemoral Pain Syndrome

Many adolescents complain of a symptom complex that shares many similar features. Although patellofemoral pain syndrome is seen in boys, the typical patient is a teenage girl older than 12 years who complains of a diffuse pain over the anterior surface of her knee.[27] The typical onset is insidious and without a specific history of trauma. Usually, no history of erythema, warmth, induration, or true effusion is noted. Occasionally, patients describe the knee having become slightly puffy. Typically, mechanical complaints of catching or locking are absent. Popping may be present, because this is a fairly ubiquitous symptom, but the popping is usually painful.

On physical examination, tenderness is often present along the medial and lateral sides of the patellofemoral articulation. Mild discomfort may be felt over the anterior portion of the joint line, but typically no tenderness occurs over the middle or posterior portion of the tibial femoral articulation. The joint has full range of motion with no crepitation. The knee is stable. Predisposing biomechanical factors, including femoral anteversion, external tibial torsion, pronating gait, and increased valgus alignment at the knees, may be present. Plain-film radiographs are usually negative. Further diagnostic evaluation is not indicated.

Although the cause of this problem is not clear, investigators believe that an abnormality of the tracking of the patella is responsible. Abnormal stresses in the patellofemoral articulation or the surrounding soft tissues are probably responsible. Better clarification is not yet available. Typically the long-term natural history of this presentation is benign, although the symptoms can be troublesome.

The most important role of the physician in this case is to rule out other more serious or more specifically treatable disorders. From this point, education, reassurance, and symptom management are the cornerstones of treatment. Psychological concerns need to be considered as well.

In some cases the syndrome may result from training errors. Sudden increase in mileage, running on hard surfaces, poor preseason conditioning, and inadequate footwear may be contributing factors. For patients with significant flexible flat feet, foot orthoses such as arch supports may reduce pronation at the foot and thereby diminish torsional stresses applied at the knee.

Stretching and strengthening the quadriceps muscles often reduces anterior knee pain. The principles are to strengthen the vastus medialis and improve patellar tracking. Occasionally, taping or supportive knee sleeves will provide relief. The intermittent and judicious use of NSAIDs may help as well. In some cases, adjustment of expectations and activities is necessary.

In refractory cases, referral to a musculoskeletal specialist may become appropriate. Surgery is occasionally performed, although the exact indications and preferred techniques are controversial.

WINTER SPORTS INJURIES

Millions of people ski, snowboard, and sled each year in the United States. These cold-weather activities result in many injuries each year. Various winter sports have distinct injury characteristics (Table 326-3).

In general, children are more likely to experience upper extremity injuries, and lower extremity injuries are more frequent in adolescents and adults.[28] Children younger than 10 years incur more fractures and catastrophic injuries (head injuries) with individual recreational activities than they do with organized sports.[28]

Table 326-3 Injuries Associated With Winter Sports

SPORT	INJURY
Downhill snow skiing	Knee contusions, anterior cruciate ligament sprains, spiral fracture of tibia
Cross-country snow skiing	Medial collateral ligament sprain, acute ankle inversion strain, acromioclavicular joint separation, skier's toe, hypothermia
Snowboarding	Wrist, ankle, and knee injuries
Snowmobiling	Multisystem trauma with head injury
Sledding	Head and face, extremity, abdominal injuries
Water skiing	Lower extremity and trunk injuries
Wakeboarding	Head and face injuries

INJURY PREVENTION

Four basic principles should be used in the development of injury-prevention measures:

1. Passive strategies will be more effective than those requiring repeated actions.
2. Specific advice is more effective than generalized information.
3. Injury control must also include postinjury care and rehabilitation.
4. Attention should be focused on common problems for which effective interventions are available.[29,30]

WHEN TO REFER

- When the diagnosis of the musculoskeletal injury is uncertain
- When the patient is not responding to initial treatment
- When injuries involve the growth plate in which future growth may be compromised
- When uncertainty exists in the safety of the young athlete to return to a competitive sports environment

WHEN TO ADMIT

- Fractures requiring open reduction
- Internal organ injuries
- Possible or definite traumatic brain injury

TOOLS FOR PRACTICE

Engaging Patient and Family

- *Steroids: Play Safe, Play Fair* (brochure), American Academy of Pediatrics (patiented.aap.org).
- *What is a Pediatric Sports Medicine Specialist?* (fact sheet), American Academy of Pediatrics (www.aap.org/sections/sportsmedicine/PedSportsMedfacts.pdf).

Medical Decision Support

- *Care of the Young Athlete* (book), American Academy of Orthopaedic Surgeons (www.aap.org/bookstore).
- *Essentials of Musculoskeletal Care, 3rd edition* (book), American Academy of Orthopaedic Surgeons (www.aap.org/bookstore).
- *Sports Medicine in the Pediatric Office* (book), Jordan Metzl (www.aap.org/bookstore).
- *Sports Shorts—facts for physicians and patients* (Web page), American Academy of Pediatrics (www.aap.org/family/sportsshort.htm).

AAP POLICY STATEMENTS

American Academy of Pediatrics, Committee on Sports Medicine and Fitness. Adolescents and anabolic steroids: a subject review. *Pediatrics*. 1997;99(6):904-908. (aappolicy.aappublications.org/cgi/content/full/pediatrics;99/6/904).

American Academy of Pediatrics, Committee on Sports Medicine and Fitness and Committee on School Health. Organized sports for children and preadolescents. *Pediatrics*. 2001;107(6):1459-1462. (aappolicy.aappublications.org/cgi/content/full/pediatrics;107/6/1459).

American Academy of Pediatrics, Committee on Sports Medicine and Fitness. Use of performance-enhancing substances. *Pediatrics*. 2005;115(4):1103-1106. (aappolicy.aappublications.org/cgi/content/full/pediatrics;115/4/1103). (doi:10.1542/peds.2005-0085).

American Academy of Pediatrics, Committee on Sports Medicine. Climatic heat stress and the exercising child and adolescent. *Pediatrics*. 2000;106(1):158-159. (aappolicy.aappublications.org/cgi/content/full/pediatrics;106/1/158).

American Academy of Pediatrics, Committee on Sports Medicine. Medical conditions affecting sports participation. *Pediatrics*. 2001;107(5):1205-1209. (aappolicy.aappublications.org/cgi/content/full/pediatrics;107/5/1205).

Brenner JS, American Academy of Pediatrics Council on Sports Medicine and Fitness. Overuse injuries, overtraining, and burnout in child and adolescent athletes. *Pediatrics*. 2007;119(6):1242-1245. (aappolicy.aappublications.org/cgi/content/full/pediatrics;119/6/1242).

SUGGESTED RESOURCE

Yang J, Peek-Asa C, Allareddy V, et al. Patient and hospital characteristics associated with length of stay and hospital charges for pediatrics sports-related injury hospitalizations in the United States 2000-2003. *Pediatrics*. 2007; 119(4):e813-e820.

REFERENCES

1. Starkey C, Johnson G, American Academy of Orthopaedic Surgeons. *Athletic Training and Sports Medicine*. 4th ed. Sudbury MA: Jones & Bartlett Publishers; 2005.
2. American Academy of Pediatrics, Committee on Sports Medicine and Fitness. Organized sports for children and preadolescents. *Pediatrics*. 2001;107(6):1459-1462.
3. American Academy of Pediatrics, Committee on Sports Medicine and Fitness. Medical conditions affecting sports participation. *Pediatrics*. 2001;107(5):1205-1209.
4. American Academy of Pediatrics. Adolescents and anabolic steroids: a subject review. *Pediatrics*. 1997;99:904-908.
5. Buckley WE, Yesalis CE, Friedl KE, et al. Estimated prevalence of anabolic steroid use among male high school seniors. *JAMA*. 1988;260(23):3441-3445.

6. Johnson MD, Jay MS, Shoup B, et al. Anabolic steroid use by male adolescents. *Pediatrics.* 1989;83(6): 921-924.
7. Windsor RE, Dumitru D. Prevalence of anabolic steroid use by male and female adolescents. *Med Sci Sports Exerc.* 1989;21(5):494-497.
8. Knopp WD, Wang TW, Bach BR Jr. Primary care of the injured athlete. Part 1. Ergogenic drugs in sports. *Clin Sports Med.* 1997;16(3):375-392.
9. Sturmi JE, Diorio JD. Sports pharmacology: anabolic agents. *Clin Sports Med.* 1998;17(2):261-282.
10. Mujika I, Padilla S. Creatine supplementation as an ergogenic acid for sports performance in highly trained athletes: a critical review. *Int J Sports Med.* 1997;18(7): 491-496.
11. Grindstaff PD, Kreider R, Bishop R, et al. Effects of creatine supplements on repetitive sprint performance and body composition in competitive swimmers. *Int J Sport Nutr.* 1997;7(4):330-346.
12. Kreider RB, Ferreira M, Wilson M. Effects of creatine supplementation on body composition, strength, and sprint performance. *Med Sci Sports Exerc.* 1998;30(1): 73-82.
13. Leach RE. Supplements. *Am J Sports Med.* 1999;27(3): 275.
14. Kujala UM, Kvist M, Heinonen O. Osgood-Schlatter's disease in adolescent athletes. *Am J Sports Med.* 1985; 13(4):236-241.
15. Ogden JA, Southwick WO. Osgood Schlatter's disease and tibial tuberosity development. *Clin Orthop Related Res.* 1976;116:180-189.
16. Medlar RC, Lyne ED. Sinding-Larsen-Johansson disease: its etiology and natural history. *J Bone Joint Surg.* 1978; 60(8):1113-1116.
17. Micheli LJ, Ireland ML. Prevention and management of calcaneal apophysitis in children: an overuse syndrome. *J Pediatr Orthop.* 1987;7(1):34-38.
18. Torg JS, Pollack H, Sweterlitsch P. The effect of competitive pitching on the shoulders and elbows of preadolescent baseball players. *Pediatrics.* 1972;49(2): 267-272.
19. Hawkins RJ, Kennedy JC. Impingement syndrome in athletes. *Am J Sports Med.* 1980;8(3):151-158.
20. Hocutt JE, Jaffe R, Rylander CR et al. Cryotherapy in ankle sprains. *Am J Sports Med.* 1982;10(5): 316-319.
21. Smith RW, Reischl SF. Treatment of ankle sprains in young athletes. *Am J Sports Med.* 1986;14(6):465-471.
22. Indelicato PA. Non operative treatment of complete tears of the medial collateral ligament of the knee. *J Bone Joint Surg.* 1983;65(3):323-329.
23. McCarroll JR, Rettig AC, Shelbourne KD. Anterior cruciate ligament injuries in the young athlete with open physes. *Am J Sports Med.* 1988;16(1):44-47.
24. Busch MT. Meniscal injuries in children and adolescents. *Clin Sports Med.* 1990;9(3):661-680.
25. Jackson DW, Feagin JA. Quadriceps contusions in young athletes. *J Bone Joint Surg.* 1973;55(1):95-105.
26. Metzmaker JN, Pappas AM. Avulsion fractures of the pelvis. *Am J Sports Med.* 1985;13(5):349-358.
27. Yates C, Grana WA. Patellofemoral pain: a prospective study. *Orthopedics.* 1986;9(5):663-667.
28. Purvis JM, Burke RG. Recreational injuries in children: incidence and prevention. *J Am Acad Orthop Surg.* 2001; 9(6):365-374.
29. National Committee for Injury Prevention Control. Injury prevention: meeting the challenge. *Am J Prev Med.* 1989; 5(suppl 3):1-278.
30. Haddon W, Suchman EA, Klein D. *Accident Research Methods and Approaches.* New York, NY: Harper and Row; 1964.

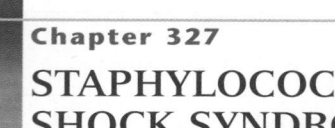

Chapter 327

STAPHYLOCOCCAL TOXIC SHOCK SYNDROME

Michael E. Pichichero, MD

Staphylococcal toxic shock syndrome (TSS) is a distinct clinical entity characterized by fever; diffuse, nonexudative mucous membrane inflammation; vomiting and profuse diarrhea; generalized myalgia; scarlatiniform erythroderma; hypotension; and shock associated with multiple organ failure—renal, myocardial, pulmonary, hepatic, hematologic, and central nervous system (CNS).

Staphylococcal TSS is an important consideration in the evaluation of toxic exanthematous diseases in children and adolescents. It must be distinguished from other serious or potentially life-threatening disease, including streptococcal TTS, staphylococcal scalded-skin syndrome, Stevens-Johnson syndrome, Kawasaki disease, streptococcal scarlet fever, measles, leptospirosis, and drug-related toxic epidermal necrolysis.

Although first described in association with menstruation and tampon use, a public health information campaign resulted in a shift to predominantly nonmenstrual cases. Currently, the incidence of nonmenstrual TSS exceeds that of menstrual TSS.[1-5] Of the nonmenstrual cases of TSS, 18.3% were reported after surgical procedures, 11.5% were postpartum or postabortion, and 23% were associated with nonsurgical cutaneous lesions.[6,7] In the United Kingdom, approximately 3% to 13% of children admitted to the burns unit develop TSS.[8,9] The incidence of postoperative cases of TSS after all types of surgery was estimated to be 3 per 100,000 population, but it was higher after ear, nose, and throat surgery (16.5 per 100,000 population).[10] A relationship between the use of nonsteroidal antiinflammatory drugs (NSAIDs) and the development of TSS caused by *Staphylococcus aureus* has been reported. NSAIDs can impair granulocyte function and enhance production of cytokines. NSAIDs may mask signs of disease progression by relieving pain, reducing swelling, and suppressing fever, thus contributing to a delay in diagnosis.[11,12] Staphylococcal TSS may occur whenever a patient becomes colonized or infected with a strain of *S aureus,* which produces a toxin, and the patient lacks protective antibody to that toxin. Clinical associations of staphylococcal TSS are shown in Table 327-1. TSS is probably underrecognized in children because of a persistent misconception that a foreign body is required for development of illness.[3] The overall annual incidence of staphylococcal TSS is 0.53 cases per 100,000 population, although wide variations exist in different geographic regions.

CAUSE AND PATHOGENESIS

Patients who develop staphylococcal TSS are colonized or infected with specific strains of *S aureus.* TSS is thought to be a superantigen-mediated disease. Superantigens are a group of proteins that can activate the

Table 327-1 Summary of Clinical and Laboratory Data Associated With Staphylococcal Toxic Shock Syndrome

CONDITION	RELATIVE FREQUENCY OF OCCURRENCE (%)
CLINICAL	
Fever	100
Temperature: ≥40°C (104°F)	70
Rash	100
Diffuse erythema	87
Desquamation	90
Myalgia	99
Hypotension (orthostatic hypotension or syncope)	95
Disorientation, irritability, or lethargy	89
Diarrhea	83
Vomiting	82
Sore throat	80
Strawberry tongue	80
Headache	78
Abdominal pain and tenderness	70
Vaginal hyperemia	67
Conjunctivitis	65
Vaginal discharge	42
Stiff neck	36
Arthralgia	15
Joint effusion	12
Adult respiratory distress syndrome	10
LABORATORY	
Hematologic	
Increased fibrinolytic split products	100
Immature neutrophils	95
Anemia	82
Leukocytosis	76
Prolonged prothrombin time	70
Decreased fibrinogen	68
Thrombocytopenia	64
Prolonged partial thromboplastin time	60
Metabolic	
Hypoproteinemia	95
Hypoalbuminemia	85
Hypocalcemia	83
Hypokalemia	75
Hypophosphatemia	62
Hyponatremia	47
Hepatic	
Elevated hepatic enzymes	67
Hyperbilirubinemia	63
Renal	
Pyuria	100
Increased creatinine	82
Increased blood urea nitrogen	75
Proteinuria	70
Microscopic hematuria	50
Musculoskeletal	
Increased creatinine phosphokinase	75
Metabolic acidosis	75
Myoglobinuria	66

immune system by bypassing certain steps in the usual antigen-mediated immune response sequence. A specific staphylococcal exotoxin known as TSS toxin type 1 (TSST-1) and staphylococcal exotoxins (SEs) A, B, C, D, E, and H are a family of superantigens and are the major toxins associated with staphylococcal TSS.[13,14] TSST-1 is responsible for 75%, SE-B for 23% and SE-C for approximately 2% of patients with TSS. TSST-1 is found in over 90% of menstrual TSS cases and approximately 50% of nonmenstrual TSS cases. Various SEs are found in the other 50% of nonmenstrual TSS.[15]

The absence of antibodies to the superantigens appears to be a major risk factor of the development of staphylococcal TSS and explains, partly, why not all patients exposed to virulent strains develop TSS. The prevalence of antibodies against TSST-1 is over 90% in adults but lower in the pediatric population.[16]

Approximately 20% of all clinical isolates of *S aureus* produce TSST-1, which is regulated by a gene known as *agr*.[17] All strains possessing the *agr* gene produce TSST-1, but the amount of toxin produced varies by strain. Physical and chemical factors are known to influence production of TSST-1. These factors include pH (toxin production increases between pH 6 and 8), oxygen concentration (toxin production increases at lower oxygen levels), concentration of carbon dioxide (toxin production increases with rising carbon dioxide levels), and concentration of divalent cations (especially magnesium).[18] The production of TSST-1 is associated with massive release of tumor necrosis factor alpha and interleukin-1.[19] These cytokines produce the fever, rash, hypotension, tissue injury, and shock associated with the syndrome.[20] The absence of antibody to TSST-1 is a major risk factor for acquisition of TSS, and failure to generate anti-TSST-1 antibody after an episode of TSS predisposes patients to recurrent episodes.[21-23] SEs also are potent mediators of cytokine production and release. They behave in a similar fashion to TSST-1 in producing clinically similar TSS disease.

CLINICAL FEATURES

Strict criteria for a case definition have been established by the Centers for Disease Control and Prevention (Box 327-1). The time sequence of the clinical manifestations of staphylococcal TSS is outlined in Figure 327-1. Patients are usually healthy before the onset of symptoms. Occasionally a prodrome consisting of low-grade fever, malaise, myalgia, or vomiting occurs in the week preceding the beginning of the acute illness. The patient abruptly develops a spiking fever of 102.2°F to 105.8°F (39°C to 41°C), chills, and severe gastrointestinal symptoms consisting of abdominal cramps, nausea, vomiting, and profuse, watery, nonbloody diarrhea. Many patients also complain of headache, myalgia, and a sore throat. At this stage of the illness, a diagnosis of acute viral gastroenteritis may well be entertained incorrectly and the youngster treated symptomatically. However, over the next 24 to 72 hours, additional clinical signs suggest the diagnosis of staphylococcal TSS. A diffuse, blanching, macular erythroderma (sunburn-like) or scarlatiniform rash appears. The rash may be faint or evanescent and is therefore sometimes missed or attributed to high fever. The rash is not pruritic but is

BOX 327-1 Case Definition of Staphylococcal Toxic Shock Syndrome

Fever: temperature: $\geq$38.9°C

Rash: diffuse macular erythroderma; desquamation of palms and soles 1 to 2 weeks after onset of illness

Hypotension: systolic blood pressure 90 mm Hg for adults or below 5th percentile by age for children under 16 years of age; orthostatic drop in diastolic blood pressure 15 mm Hg from lying to sitting, or orthostatic syncope

Multisystem involvement—3 or more of the following:

- Gastrointestinal: vomiting or diarrhea at onset of illness
- Muscular: severe myalgia or creatinine phosphokinase level at least twice the upper limit of normal for laboratory
- Mucous membrane: vaginal, oropharyngeal, or conjunctival hyperemia
- Renal: blood urea nitrogen or creatinine at least twice the upper limit of normal for laboratory or urinary sediment with pyuria (>5 white cells per high-power field) in the absence of urinary tract infection
- Hepatic: total bilirubin, serum glutamic oxaloacetic transaminase, or serum glutamic pyruvate transaminase at least twice the upper limit of normal for laboratory
- Hematologic: platelets $<100,000/mm^3$
- Central nervous system: disorientation or alterations in consciousness without focal neurologic signs when fever and hypotension are absent

Negative results on the following tests, if obtained:

- Blood, throat, cerebrospinal fluid cultures
- Antibody titer: Rocky Mountain spotted fever, leptospirosis, and rubeola

occasionally petechial. Patients demonstrate bilateral conjunctival hyperemia without discharge and may complain of photophobia. Oropharyngeal inflammation, sometimes with an associated strawberry tongue or buccal ulcerations, also occurs, as does vaginal erythema with minimal clear watery discharge in cases associated with menstruation.

Within 24 to 72 hours of onset, most patients experience orthostatic dizziness or syncope or both because of orthostatic hypotension. These symptoms can occur abruptly and may precede the development of hypovolemic shock. The peak of illness occurs on the 2nd or 3rd day and involves multiple organ systems. CNS dysfunction may consist of headache, confusion, disorientation, hallucinations, and complaints of paresthesias of the hands and feet. Some patients have a stiff, tender neck. If a lumbar puncture is performed, then normal values for cerebrospinal fluid glucose and protein are found, although patients may have up to 100 white blood cells/mm^3, 50% of which may be polymorphonuclear cells. Abdominal musculature tenderness, absent or hypoactive bowel sounds, and radiologic evidence of a nonobstructive ileus are common. Azotemia and a diminished creatinine clearance occur as evidence of renal involvement. Oliguria is typical; complete renal shutdown occurs rarely. The musculoskeletal system is nearly always affected. Exquisite muscle tenderness and severe myalgias are common. Arthralgias and joint effusions may be seen. Nonpitting edema over the wrists and ankles and synovitis of the small joints of the hands and feet have been reported to occur. Patients may experience shock lung or adult-type respiratory distress syndrome. Hematologic involvement includes a progressive normochromic normocytic anemia, thrombocytopenia, and leukocytosis. Arrhythmias or prolonged shock may lead to eventual myocardial failure.

DIFFERENTIAL DIAGNOSIS

In some aspects, staphylococcal TSS might be confused with staphylococcal scalded-skin syndrome, staphylococcal scarlet fever, Stevens-Johnson syndrome, Kawasaki disease, streptococcal scarlet fever, streptococcal TSS, measles, leptospirosis, or toxic epidermal necrolysis. The differentiating features among these diagnoses are presented in Table 327-2. The strict case definition presented in Box 327-1 is particularly useful for epidemiologic purposes and serves to exclude patients who have other diseases. However, this strict definition may also exclude patients who have milder forms of staphylococcal TSS, and this circumstance should be kept in mind when confronted with a patient who demonstrates some but not all of the clinical findings of staphylococcal TSS.

LABORATORY EVALUATION

No laboratory test is available to confirm the diagnosis of staphylococcal TSS. Initial laboratory findings often include leukocytosis, with a striking increase in the percentage of immature neutrophils, progressive anemia, and thrombocytopenia. These hematologic abnormalities are self-correcting during the convalescent stage. Thrombocytopenia may be accompanied by prolongation of prothrombin time and partial thromboplastin time and the appearance of increased fibrin split products. However, neither serious bleeding during the acute phase of illness nor thrombosis resulting from rebound thrombocytosis during recovery has been a significant clinical problem. A majority of patients have hypoproteinemia and hypoalbuminemia, probably as a consequence of increased capillary permeability caused by exotoxin-mediated vascular cell membrane change (see Cause and Pathogenesis). A significant number of patients also experience metabolic acidosis from inadequate tissue perfusion, which may be complicated by hyponatremia and hypokalemia as a result of accompanying persistent vomiting and diarrhea. Serum concentrations of calcium may appear dangerously low; however, tetany is rarely seen. The blood urea nitrogen and creatinine levels are usually elevated early in the illness. Peak abnormal values occur after 5 to 7 days and then return rapidly to normal. However, some patients have required hemodialysis or peritoneal dialysis to correct these and other metabolic imbalances. Despite abnormal renal function, hypophosphatemia is typically present in the first days of illness. The creatinine phosphokinase level

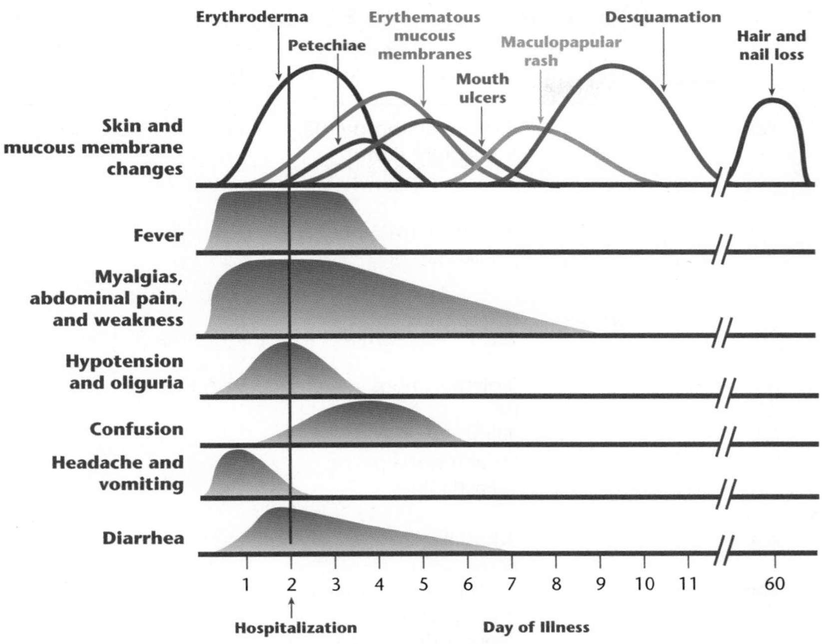

Figure 327-1 Major systemic, skin, and mucous membrane manifestations of toxic shock syndrome. *(Chesney PJ, Davis JP, Purdy WK, et al. Clinical manifestations of toxic shock syndrome.* JAMA. *1981;246(7):741-748. Reprinted by permission of the American Medical Association.)*

is often elevated, and, occasionally, patients experience myoglobinemia. These findings normalize with resolution of the myalgias, usually between the 5th and 10th day of disease. Hepatic enzyme and bilirubin levels are typically elevated initially but tend to revert to normal in convalescence. The relative frequency of these abnormal laboratory findings is presented in Table 327-1.

MANAGEMENT

The initial steps in management of staphylococcal TSS are outlined in Box 327-2. Nearly all patients should be hospitalized, although a few who have a very mild form of the illness may be managed cautiously as outpatients. The 1st and major resuscitative goal is to administer large volumes of crystalloid (lactated Ringer's) or colloid (fresh-frozen plasma or albumin) solutions to restore normal intravascular volume and correct hypotension, given that shock is the initial threat to intact survival (see Chapter 358, Shock). Patients may require enormous volumes of fluid (2 to 4 times normal daily maintenance) to maintain tissue perfusion. Adequate treatment of hypotension may also require vasopressor therapy such as dopamine or dobutamine. Much of the administered fluid is sequestered outside the intravascular space, and many patients become markedly edematous. Therefore having a central venous pressure line or a Swan-Ganz catheter in place is advisable to monitor left-ventricular end-diastolic pressure to prevent the development of congestive heart failure caused by overly vigorous fluid resuscitation. If significant hypotension exists, multiple organ system failure is likely imminent. The management outlined in Box 327-2 should be pursued while transport to a tertiary care medical facility is arranged. There, continued management largely will be supportive and dictated by the degree of organ dysfunction.

BOX 327-2 Management of Staphylococcal Toxic Shock Syndrome

1. Consider other possible diagnoses.
2. Remove potentially infected foreign bodies (eg, tampons).
3. Obtain cultures of blood, throat, vagina, nares, rectum, and other appropriate sites.
4. Drain and irrigate infected sites.
5. Give an intravenous antistaphylococcal β-lactamase-resistant antimicrobial agent at maximal dose for weight and age.
6. Consider methylprednisolone for severe cases.
7. Treat aggressively and monitor for the following:
   - Hypovolemia and inadequate tissue perfusion
   - Adult respiratory distress syndrome
   - Myocardial dysfunction
   - Acute renal failure
   - Cerebral edema
   - Hypocalcemia, hypophosphatemia
   - Metabolic acidosis
   - Disseminated intravascular coagulation
   - Fluid and electrolyte abnormalities

Table 327-2 Differential Diagnosis of Staphylococcal Toxic Shock Syndrome

DISEASE	HYPOTENSION	RASH	LIPS	ORAL CAVITY
Staphylococcal toxic shock syndrome	Yes	Diffuse erythroderma, Nikolsky sign	Red	Erythematous
Staphylococcal scalded-skin syndrome	No	Erythroderma, bullae, Nikolsky sign	—	—
Stevens-Johnson syndrome	No	Erythema multiforme	Bleeding, fissured	Bullous enanthem
Kawasaki disease	No	Polymorphous	Red, fissured	Erythematous, strawberry tongue
Scarlet fever	No	Diffuse erythroderma, circumoral pallor, Pastia lines	—	Strawberry tongue
Measles	No	Morbilliform	—	Koplik spots
Leptospirosis	Sometimes	Erythematous, macular, petechial, purpuric	—	Pharyngitis
Toxic epidermal necrolysis (drug related)	Sometimes	Painful erythroderma, bullae, Nikolsky sign	—	—
Streptococcal toxic shock syndrome	Yes	Diffuse erythroderma, maculopapular	Cracked	Erythematous

A multidisciplinary approach usually is required to manage the patient who has staphylococcal TSS. Patients who develop adult-type respiratory distress syndrome or shock lung require endotracheal intubation and ventilatory assistance with positive end-expiratory pressure and high oxygen flow rates. Renal failure, severe electrolyte and acid-base abnormalities, ventricular ectopy, refractory ventricular arrhythmias, and disseminated intravascular coagulation all can occur.

In addition to hemodynamic stabilization, a thorough search for possible sites of staphylococcal infections is mandatory to eliminate any preformed toxin and to prevent synthesis of new toxins. Vaginal examination and removal of a tampon or other foreign body are mandatory. Surgical wounds should be considered as possible reservoirs of infection, even if no superficial signs of local infection or purulent discharge are present. Infected wounds should be opened and debrided, and any packing should be removed. Abscesses need to be drained and irrigated. Culture specimens from all possible sites should be obtained.[24] Because staphylococcal TSS appears to be an exotoxin-mediated disease, the importance of antibiotics might be questioned. Nevertheless, high-dose β-lactamase-resistant antistaphylococcal antibiotics are recommended to eradicate the organism and prevent recurrences.[10,25] Nafcillin, oxacillin, and 1st-generation cephalosporins are the 1st-line agents for *S aureus*. Vancomycin should not be used routinely as initial empiric therapy because methicillin-resistant *S aureus* causes fewer than 1% of cases of staphylococcal TSS.[26] However, methicillin-resistant *S aureus* recently emerged as a community pathogen and thus raised an important issue of initial empiric antibiotic therapy in these patients.

Clindamycin, erythromycin, rifampin, and fluoroquinolones have been shown to reduce TSST-1 by 90%, whereas β-lactamase inhibitors, including nafcillin and 1st-generation cephalosporins, increase TSST-1 in culture, probably by lysis or increased cell membrane permeability.[27] Thus the use of clindamycin in combination with a β-lactamase-resistant antistaphylococcal agent results in a potentially beneficial effect by decreasing the synthesis of TSST-1. Antimicrobial therapy should be continued for at least 10 to 14 days to eradicate the organism and prevent recurrences.[28] The total duration should be based on the usual duration established for the underlying focus of infection.[29]

High levels of antibody to TSST-1 have been found in intravenous immunoglobulin (IVIg) preparations; animal model studies and small case series suggest that its administration early in the course of disease can reduce the morbidity and mortality of staphylococcal TSS.[30] IVIg may be an effective adjunctive therapy for diseases associated with superantigens. The usual dose of IVIg is 400 mg/kg over a period of 4 to 8 hours as a single dose.[30-32] Staphylococcal superantigens are not inhibited as efficiently as streptococcal superantigens by IVIg, and hence a higher dose of IVIg may be required for therapy of staphylococcal TSS to achieve protective titers and clinical efficacy.[33]

EYES	HANDS AND FEET	DESQUAMATION	OTHER FINDINGS	DIAGNOSIS
Nonpurulent conjunctivitis	Erythematous, edematous	Hands and feet; can be generalized	Diarrhea, renal, hepatic, CNS, hematologic abnormalities	Clinical, culture of *S aureus* from nasopharynx, vagina, or wound
Purulent conjunctivitis	Relatively spared or grossly involved	Gross	—	Clinical, culture of *S aureus* from nasopharynx or wound, skin biopsy
Purulent conjunctivitis	Involved	Involves only individual lesions	Respiratory and GI tract involvement	Clinical, skin biopsy
Nonpurulent conjunctivitis	Erythematous, edematous	Fingertips	Coronary aneurysms, generalized vasculitis	Clinical; no diagnostic test
—	Relatively spared	Fine, flaky	Rheumatic fever, glomerulonephritis	Clinical, culture of group A streptococci from pharynx, serology
Conjunctivitis	Involved	Fine	Respiratory tract involvement	Clinical, serology
Conjunctivitis	Relatively spared	—	CNS, renal, hepatic involvement	Clinical, serology
Conjunctivitis	Involved	Gross	—	Clinical, serology
Injected	—	—	Confusion, abdominal pain and vomiting, hyperesthesia	Clinical, culture of group A streptococci

CNS, Central nervous system; *GI,* gastrointestinal.

Use of high-dose corticosteroids has sometimes been advocated to be of possible benefit in the treatment of shock syndromes. However, such therapy should not be administered routinely to patients with TSS because it may result in a shorter time to defervescence and clinical stability while making no difference in overall risk of mortality.[34] NSAIDs are contraindicated because they actually may increase the progression to TSS by enhancing production of tumor necrosis factor.[12]

PROGNOSIS AND CONVALESCENCE

The majority of patients who have staphylococcal TSS recover within 7 to 10 days. The case fatality rate is 2% to 5%. Although most patients with TSS do not experience pulmonary compromise, mortality is increased significantly if early or prolonged adult respiratory distress syndrome becomes apparent.[35] Nongenital TSS seems to carry a worse prognosis than vaginal disease, probably because of delayed diagnosis and the more serious nature of the primary infection.[3] Refractory hypotension is associated with mortality rates of up to 50%. Convalescence is characterized by a desquamation of the palms and soles within 1 to 2 weeks after the onset of illness. Some patients also experience hair and nail loss. Fatigue and weakness for as long as 3 months may occur in the recovery phase.

The incidence of recurrent staphylococcal TSS may be as high as 28% if the patient does not receive antistaphylococcal antibiotics and does not produce antibody to toxin. The criteria for recurrent disease are less stringent than those required for defining an initial episode. Recurrent vaginal TSS occurs but much less frequently than genital vaginal disease. Persistent neuropsychological symptoms, such as fatigue, depression, and memory loss, have been described in up to 50% of patients who recover from nonvaginal TSS.[36,37]

WHEN TO REFER

All patients must be managed in consultation with infectious disease and critical care specialists. The pediatrician plays a key role in coordinating the care.

WHEN TO ADMIT

Nearly all patients with staphylococcal TSS should be hospitalized.

TOOLS FOR PRACTICE

Medical Decision Support

- *Toxic Shock Syndrome* (fact sheet) Centers for Disease Control and Prevention (www.cdc.gov/ncidod/dbmd/diseaseinfo/toxicshock_t.htm).

- *Red Book: 2006 Report of the Committee on Infectious Diseases*, 27th edition, American Academy of Pediatrics (www.aap.org/bookstore).

SELECTED RESOURCES

Bohach GA, Fast DJ, Nelson RD, et al. Staphylococcal and streptococcal pyrogenic toxins involved in toxic shock syndrome and related illnesses. *Crit Rev Microbiol.* 1989; 17:251-272.

Bonventre PF, Wechbach L, Staneck J. Production of staphylococcal enterotoxin F and pyrogenic enterotoxin C by Staphylococcus aureus isolates from toxic shock syndrome-associated sources. *Infect Immun.* 1983;40: 1023-1029.

Chow AW, Wong CK, MacFarlane AM. Toxic shock syndrome: clinical and laboratory findings in 30 patients. *Can Med Assoc J.* 1984;130:425-430.

Crass BA, Bergdoll MS. Involvement of staphylococcal enterotoxin in nonmenstrual toxic shock syndrome. *J Clin Microbiol.* 1986;23:1138-1139.

Davis JP, Chesney PJ, Wand PJ, and the Investigation and Laboratory Team. Toxic-shock syndrome: epidemiologic features, recurrence, risk factors, and prevention. *N Engl J Med.* 1980;303:1429-1435.

Graham G, O'Brien M, Hayes J, et al. Postoperative toxic shock syndrome. *Clin Infect Dis.* 1995;20:895-899.

Kreiswirth BN. Genetics and expression of toxic shock syndrome toxin 1: overview. *Rev Infect Dis.* 1989; 11(suppl 1):S97-S100.

Larkin SM, Williams DN, Osterholm MT. Toxic shock syndrome: clinical, laboratory, and pathologic findings in nine fatal cases. *Ann Intern Med.* 1982;96:858-864.

Lee VY, Chang AH, Chow AW. Detection of staphylococcal enterotoxin B among toxic shock syndrome (TSS) and non-TSS-associated Staphylococcus aureus isolates. *J Infect Dis.* 1992;166:911-915.

Manders SM. Toxin-mediated streptococcal and staphylococcal disease. *J Am Acad Dermatol.* 1998;39:383-398.

Toxic shock syndrome. In: Pickering LK, Baker CJ, Long SS, McMillan JA, eds. Red Book: 2006 Report of the Committee on Infectious Diseases. 27th ed. Elk Grove Village, IL: American Academy of Pediatrics; 2006.

Reingold AL, Broome CV, Gaventa S. Risk factors for menstrual toxic shock syndrome: results of a multistate case-control study. *Rev Infect Dis.* 1989;11(suppl 1):S35-S42.

Reingold AL, Hargrett NT, Schands KN, et al. Toxic shock syndrome surveillance in the United States, 1980 to 1981. *Ann Intern Med.* 1982;96(pt 2):875-880.

Schlievert PM. Staphylococcal enterotoxin B and toxic-shock syndrome toxin-1 are significantly associated with nonmenstrual TSS. *Lancet.* 1986;1:1149-1150.

Schlievert PM. Role of toxic shock syndrome toxin 1 in toxic shock syndrome: overview. *Rev Infect Dis.* 1989;11(supp 1): S107-S109.

Schlievert PM, Kelly JA. Clindamycin-induced suppression of toxic-shock syndrome-associated exotoxin production. *J Infect Dis.* 1981;143:471.

Schlievert PM, Bohach GA, Ohlendorf DH, et al. Molecular structure of staphylococcus and streptococcus superantigens. *J Clin Immunol.* 1995;15(suppl):S4-S10.

Shands KN, Schmid GP, Dan BB, et al. Toxic-shock syndrome in menstruating women: association with tampon use and Staphylococcus aureus and clinical features in 52 cases. *N Engl J Med.* 1980;303:1436-1442.

Stevens DL, Yan S, Bryant AE. Penicillin-binding protein expression at different growth stages determines penicillin efficacy in vitro and in vivo: an explanation for the inoculum effect. *J Infect Dis.* 1993;167:1401-1405.

Stolz S, Davis J, Vergeront J, et al. Development of serum antibody to toxic shock among individuals with toxic shock syndrome in Wisconsin. *J Infect Dis.* 1985;151: 883-889.

Todd JK, Ressman M, Caston SA, et al. Corticosteroid therapy for patients with toxic shock syndrome. *JAMA.* 1984; 252:3399-3402.

Van Langevelde P, van Dissel JT, Meurs CJ, et al. Combinations of flucloxacillin and gentamycin inhibits toxic shock syndrome toxin 1 production by Staphylococcus aureus in both logarithmic and stationary phases of growth. *Antimicrob Agents Chemother.* 1997;41:1682-1685.

REFERENCES

1. Centers for Disease Control. Reduced incidence of menstrual toxic-shock syndrome United States: 1980-1990. *MMWR.* 1990;39:421-424.
2. Chesney PJ. Clinical aspects and spectrum of illness of toxic shock syndrome: overview. *Rev Infect Dis.* 1989; 11(suppl):S1-S7.
3. Parsonnet J. Nonmenstrual toxic shock syndrome: new insights into diagnosis, pathogenesis, and treatment. *Curr Clin Top Infect Dis.* 1996;16:1-20.
4. Reingold AL, Dan BB, Shands KN, et al. Toxic-shock syndrome not associated with menstruation. *Lancet.* 1982; 1:1-4.
5. Strausbaugh LJ. Toxic shock syndrome: are you recognizing its changing presentations? *Postgrad Med.* 1993; 94:107-118.
6. Gaventa S, Reingold AL, Hightower AW, et al. Active surveillance for toxic shock syndrome in the United States: 1986. *Rev Infect Dis.* 1989;11(suppl 1):S28-S34.
7. Hajjeh RA, Reingold A, Weil A, et al. Toxic shock syndrome in the United States: surveillance update, 1979-1996. *Emerg Infect Dis.* 1999;6(5):807-810.
8. Childs C, Jones V, Dawson M, et al. Toxic shock syndrome toxin-1 (TSST-1) antibody level in burned children. *Burns.* 1999;25:473-476.
9. Edwards-Jones V, Dawson M, Childs C. A survey into toxic shock syndrome (TSS) in UK burn units. *Burns.* 2000;26:323-333.
10. Chesney J, Davis J. Toxic shock syndrome. In: Feigin R, Cherry J, eds. *Textbook of Pediatric Infectious Diseases.* 4th ed. Philadelphia, PA: WB Saunders; 1998.
11. Huang Y, Hsueh P, Lin T, et al. A family cluster of streptococcal toxic shock syndrome in children: clinical implication and epidemiological investigation. *Pediatrics.* 2001; 107:1181-1183.
12. Stevens DL. Could nonsteroidal antiinflammatory drugs (NSAIDs) enhance the progression of bacterial infections to toxic shock syndrome? *Clin Infect Dis.* 1995;21:977-980.
13. Schlievert PM, Shands KN, Dan BB, et al. Identification and characterization of an exotoxin from Staphylococcus aureus associated with toxic-shock syndrome. *J Infect Dis.* 1981;143:509-516.
14. Dinges M, Orwin P, Schlievert P. Exotoxins of Staphylococcus aureus. *Clin Microbiol Rev.* 2000;13:16-34.
15. Garbe PL, Arko RJ, Reingold AL, et al. Staphylococcus aureus isolates from patients with nonmenstrual toxic shock syndrome: evidence for additional toxins. *JAMA.* 1985;253:2538-2542.
16. Crass BA, Bergdoll MS. Toxin involvement in toxic shock syndrome. *J Infect Dis.* 1986;153:918-926.
17. Kreiswirth BN. Genetics and expression of toxic shock syndrome toxin 1: overview. *Rev Infect Dis.* 1989;11(1): S97.
18. Kass EJ, Parsonnet J. On the pathogenesis of toxic shock syndrome. *Rev Infect Dis.* 1987;9:382-385.

19. Parsonnet J, Hickman RK, Eardley DD, et al. Induction of human interleukin-1 by toxic-shock-syndrome toxin-1. *J Infect Dis.* 1985;151:514-522.
20. Ikejima T, Okusawa S, van der Meer JW, et al. Induction by toxic-shock-syndrome toxin-1 of a circulating tumor necrosis factor-like substance in rabbits and of immunoreactive tumor necrosis factor and interleukin-1 from human mononuclear cells. *J Infect Dis.* 1998;158:1017-1025.
21. Bonventre PF, Linnemann C, Weckbach LS, et al. Antibody responses to toxic-shock syndrome (TSS) toxin by patients with TSS and by healthy staphylococcal carriers. *J Infect Dis.* 1984;150:662-666.
22. Leung DYM, Travers JB, Norris DA. The role of superantigens in skin disease. *J Invest Dermatol.* 1995;105(suppl):37s-42s.
23. Rosten PM, Bartlett KH, Chow AW. Serologic responses to toxic shock syndrome (TSS) toxin-1 in menstrual and nonmenstrual TSS. *Clin Invest Med.* 1988;11:187-192.
24. Chuang Y, Huang Y, Lin T. Toxic shock syndrome in children. *Pediatr Drugs.* 2005;7(1):11-25.
25. Kain K, Schulzer M, Chow A. Clinical spectrum of nonmenstrual toxic shock syndrome (TSS): comparison with menstrual TSS by multivariate discriminant analyses. *Clin Infect Dis.* 1993;16:100-106.
26. Kum W, Laupland K, Chow A. Defining a novel domain of staphylococcal toxic shock syndrome toxin-1 critical for major histocompatibility complex class II binding, superantigenic activity, and lethality. *Can J Microbiol.* 2000;46:171-179.
27. Parsonnet J, Modern P, Giacobbe K. Effect of subinhibitory concentrations of antibiotics on production of toxic shock syndrome toxin-1 (TSST-1) [abstract]. Presented at the 32nd Meeting of the Infectious Disease Society of America, Orlando, FL, 1994.
28. Andrews M, Parent E, Barry M, et al. Recurrent nonmenstrual toxic shock syndrome: clinical manifestations, diagnosis and treatment. *Clin Infect Dis.* 2001;32:1470-1479.
29. American Academy of Pediatrics. Toxic shock syndrome. In: Pickering LK, Baker CJ, Long SS, et al, eds. *Red Book: 2006 Report of the Committee on Infectious Diseases.* 27th ed. Elk Grove Village, IL: American Academy of Pediatrics; 2006.
30. Barry W, Hudgins L, Donta ST, et al. Intravenous immunoglobulin therapy for toxic shock syndrome. *JAMA.* 1992;267:3315-3316.
31. Lamothe F, D'Amico P, Ghosn P, et al. Clinical usefulness of intravenous human immunoglobulins in invasive group A streptococcal infections: case report and review. *Clin Infect Dis.* 1995;21:1469-1470.
32. Melish ME, Frogner K, Hirata S, et al. Use of IVIg for therapy in the rabbit model of TSS. *Clin Res.* 1987;35:220A.
33. Darenberg J, Soderquist B, Normark B, et al. Differences in potency of intravenous polyspecific immunoglobulin G against streptococcal and staphylococcal superantigens: implications for therapy of toxic shock syndrome. *Clin Infect Dis.* 2004;38:836-842.
34. Todd J, Fishaut M. Toxic shock syndrome associated with phage-group-I staphylococci. *Lancet.* 1978;2:1116-1118.
35. Davis D, Gash-Ki TL, Heffernan EJ. Toxic shock syndrome: case report of a postpartum female and a literature review. *J Emerg Med.* 1998;16:607-614.
36. Chesney PJ, Crass BA, Polyak MB, et al. Toxic-shock syndrome: management of long-term sequelae. *Ann Intern Med.* 1982;96:847-851.
37. Rosene KA, Copass MK, Kastner LS, et al. Persistent neuropsychological sequelae of toxic shock syndrome. *Ann Intern Med.* 1982;96:865-870.

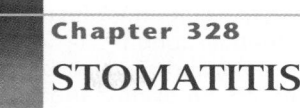

Chapter 328

STOMATITIS

Linda S. Nield, MD

Stomatitis, or inflammation of the oral mucosa, is characterized by multiple ulcerations inside the mouth. Frequently painful, this condition may lead to decreased oral intake and dehydration.

ETIOLOGY

Stomatitis can be a disease entity unto itself, such as recurrent aphthous stomatitis (RAS), or it may be a symptom of an underlying condition. Infection, trauma, irritant exposure, medical interventions, and systemic disorders are the major causes of oral inflammation.

Recurrent Aphthous Stomatitis

RAS is a benign condition characterized by painful oral ulcers that recur at irregular intervals. In otherwise healthy individuals, most cases are idiopathic. Although the exact cause of RAS is not known, stress, genetics, hormonal and immunologic influences, trauma, and smoking are suggested triggers for this common condition.[1,2]

Infection

Viruses, bacteria, and fungi can inflame the oral mucosa. Some viral causes include herpes simplex, varicella-zoster, various subtypes of coxsackie, rubeola, Epstein-Barr virus, and HIV. Several coxsackieviruses cause an acute febrile illness associated with the development of lesions in the posterior oropharynx known as herpangina. Coxsackie A16 is the most common cause of hand-foot-mouth disease (HFMD), but other enteroviral subtypes have been implicated as causative agents.

Borrelia vincentii and *Fusobacterium dentium* are bacterial causes of oral inflammation known as necrotizing ulcerative gingivitis. Syphilis, gonorrhea, and tuberculosis can also lead to oral inflammation.

Fungal infections rarely occur in the immunocompetent child except for *Candida* mucositis in the first several months of life. Histoplasmosis can develop in otherwise healthy children and produce mucosal ulceration along with other systemic manifestations.

Irritants

Exposure to a large array of external irritants can lead to stomatitis.[3] The irritant may directly traumatize the mucosal surface (irritant contact stomatitis) or incite an allergic delayed-type hypersensitivity reaction (allergic contact stomatitis).[3]

Trauma secondary to biting one's own mucosa or exposure to friction from dental appliances will cause irritant contact stomatitis. A rare condition known as Riga-Fede syndrome is characterized by the formation of ulcerative lesions of the lower lip, lingual frenulum, and ventral tongue secondary to repeated rubbing of the teeth against these mucosal surfaces.[4] The age of onset of Riga-Fede syndrome is 6 to 8 months and coincides with the age of primary tooth eruption.

Exposure to excessive heat, cold, and acidic or basic substances can irritate the mouth. Smokeless tobacco is another mucosal irritant that has been found to lead to oral lesions in older school-age children.[5,6]

The most common causes of allergic contact stomatitis include preservatives and oral flavorings such as cinnamon, menthol, and peppermint. Metals, such as nickel found in dental instruments, may also elicit an oral allergic reaction.[3]

Iatrogenic Causes

Stomatitis may arise from medical interventions. Chemotherapy agents and radiation are the most notorious iatrogenic causes of mucosal breakdown. These treatments disrupt the mucosal barrier of the mouth, allowing ulceration, desquamation, and secondary infection by both acquired and endogenous flora.[1] Infrequently, medications such as cyclooxygenase-2 inhibitors, nonsteroidal antiinflammatory agents, and sertraline (an antidepressant) lead to oral dryness and the development of aphthous stomatitis.[2] The misuse of commercial mouthwash with high alcohol content can also cause oral mucosal ulceration.[7]

SYSTEMIC DISORDERS

Although typically a benign, self-limiting process, stomatitis may be one of the presenting symptoms of a serious, systemic illness such as Behçet syndrome, inflammatory bowel disease, gluten-sensitive enteropathy, diabetes mellitus, systemic lupus erythematosus, scleroderma, dermatomyositis, and Wegener granulomatosis. Stomatitis is also caused by periodic fever accompanied by aphthous stomatitis, pharyngitis, and (cervical) adenopathy (PFAPA syndrome),[8,9] as well as cyclic neutropenia. Nutritional deficiencies of iron, vitamins B12 and B6, folate, and zinc can also cause oral mucosal breakdown. Some dermatologic disorders associated with oral lesions include pemphigus, erythema multiforme, Stevens-Johnson syndrome, erosive lichen planus, and epidermolysis bullosa.

EPIDEMIOLOGIC FACTORS

Because of the many diverse causes of stomatitis, a large number of children suffer from stomatitis at some time in childhood. RAS is the most common form of painful oral ulcers, and Kleinman and colleagues found that 37% of surveyed school-age children reported a history of suffering from RAS.[5] The peak age of onset of RAS is in the second decade of life,[10] and bouts may recur throughout adulthood.

Viruses are the most common infectious cause of stomatitis. In the Kleinman study, 33% of the 5- to 17-year-old participants reported a history of recurrent herpes labialis.[5] Herpangina and HFMD are also quite frequently experienced by young children. Outbreaks of acute stomatitis caused by herpangina are most likely to occur in the summer and early fall; HFMD is most likely to occur in the spring and summer. Bacteria and fungi infrequently cause stomatitis in otherwise healthy children, except for *Candida* infection in the first several months of life. The presence of syphilis and gonorrhea pharyngitis in a young child is rare and suggests sexual abuse and warrants a thorough child abuse investigation.

The number of children who suffer from stomatitis caused by irritants is not known; however, the use of orthodontic devices is quite prevalent, and oral flavorings and preservatives are ubiquitous in many commercial products.[3] Oral inflammation secondary to medications is likely to occur only in the select group of children who use the offending agents.

Stomatitis as the only presenting feature of one of the systemic disorders does occur, but it is rare. Approximately 15% of patients with aphthous ulcers and other symptoms will have a systemic disorder.[1] PFAPA syndrome is a relatively newly described entity, with multiple case series reported in the medical literature.[8,9]

DIFFERENTIAL DIAGNOSIS

The differential diagnosis of stomatitis in children consists of the entities listed in Box 328-1.

CLINICAL MANIFESTATIONS

Each of the conditions that are associated with stomatitis will display unique clinical features. The history of presentation of the oral lesions will provide the clues

BOX 328-1 Differential Diagnosis of Stomatitis

RAS: Infection

- Viruses: herpes simplex type 1, varicella-zoster, coxsackie and other enteroviruses, rubeola, Epstein-Barr virus, HIV
- Bacteria: *Borrelia vincentii, Fusobacterium dentium*, syphilis, gonorrhea, tuberculosis
- Fungi: *Candida, Histoplasmosis*

Irritant contact stomatitis

Allergic contact stomatitis

Iatrogenically induced stomatitis

Systemic disorders:

- Behçet syndrome
- Inflammatory bowel disease
- Celiac disease
- Diabetes mellitus
- Systemic lupus erythematosus
- Scleroderma
- Dermatomyositis
- Wegener granulomatosis
- PFAPA syndrome
- Cyclic neutropenia
- Nutritional deficiencies
- Dermatologic disorders

PFAPA, Periodic fever accompanied by aphthous stomatitis, pharyngitis, and (cervical) adenopathy; *RAS*, recurrent aphthous stomatitis.

for the possible diagnosis. The time of year, the presence of local outbreaks, and the accompanying systemic symptoms should be noted. The physical examination will determine the location of the lesions and the presence of failure to thrive, fever, lymphadenopathy, organomegaly, and dermatologic and joint abnormalities.

The recurrence of 1 or more painful ulcers on the buccal, labial, and lingual surfaces, as well as on the floor of the mouth, characterizes RAS. The oral lesions will be the only physical examination finding. Three clinically distinct types of RAS have been described.[10] Small, round craters, smaller than 5 mm in diameter and surrounded by an erythematous halo, typify the minor variety that heals in 1 to 2 weeks. The major variety may last 6 weeks and is characterized by lesions larger than 5 mm that often scar. The herpetiform variety is named as such not because herpesvirus is the etiologic agent but because of its herpes-like appearance of multiple, small clusters of pinpoint lesions that resolve in 1 week to 10 days. The child with RAS is otherwise healthy.

The primary infection with herpes simplex virus type 1 is associated with systemic signs and symptoms of fever, malaise, sore throat, and cervical adenopathy. Vesicles can develop anywhere on the oral mucosa but most typically in the anterior oropharynx on the lips, tongue, and buccal mucosa (Figure 328-1). The gingiva may be swollen and erythematous. The perioral area may also display vesicles and small ulcers that coalesce and continue to appear for the next week. Anorexia as a result of the oral pain may produce dehydration that is severe enough to warrant hospitalization. Children in the first few years of life are most likely to experience a primary infection, and recurrences vary in number. The recurrences are less severe than the initial bouts and are not usually associated with systemic symptoms. Spontaneous resolution occurs in a week to 10 days.

Herpangina is characterized by ulcers surrounded by erythematous halos located in the posterior oropharynx (Figure 328-2). Spontaneous resolution occurs in 3 to 5 days. In HFMD, along with lesions of the posterior oropharynx, blanching red macules or vesicles appear on the palms, soles, and buttocks. Erythematous halos may also surround the macules. Spontaneous resolution occurs within a week. Systemic symptoms of fever, malaise, dysphagia, and anorexia accompany these coxsackie infections, which can lead to dehydration in children with either herpangina or HFMD.

The bacterial condition necrotizing ulcerative gingivitis is characterized by painful, erythematous, and friable gingiva. Foul breath accompanies the necrotic tissue that accumulates as a pseudomembrane over the gingival surface. Fever, malaise, anorexia, and dehydration may be part of its clinical presentation as well.

Candidal mucositis produces white, curdlike patches on many of the surfaces of the oral mucosa. If scraped, then a white patch can be removed, unveiling ulceration at the base. Diaper dermatitis may also be present.

Contact stomatitis can present in 4 general ways: (1) red lesions with general mouth erythema, (2) white lesions and leukoplakia, (3) erosions and ulcerations, or (4) no obvious lesions accompanied by mouth pain and burning.[3] Location of the lesions in close proximity to dental appliances, for example, will provide the clue that the etiology may be irritant contact stomatitis. The manifestation of stomatitis in the multitude of potential underlying multisystem diseases will vary depending on the diagnosis. Immunocompromised patients may experience more frequent and severe episodes of oral ulceration that take longer to resolve. The appearance of the individual aphthae in stomatitis secondary to a benign or self-limiting condition may be indistinguishable from those associated with a serious underlying

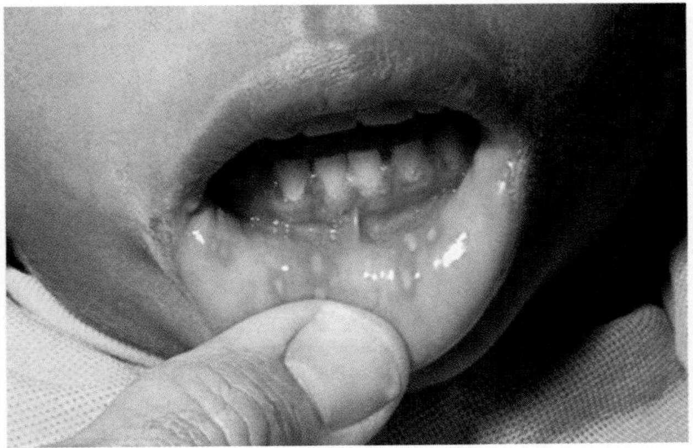

Figure 328-1 Herpes simplex stomatitis is a primary infection of the anterior oral mucous membranes. Tongue lesions also are common with primary herpes simplex virus infections.

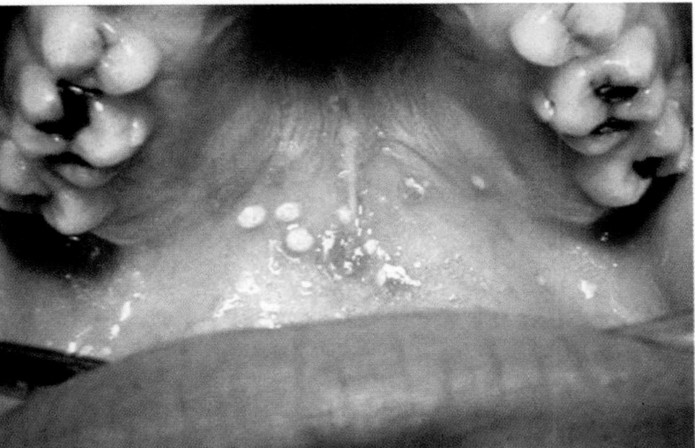

Figure 328-2 Herpangina (coxsackievirus) lesions on the posterior palate of a young male adult. Coxsackievirus lesions are usually found in the posterior aspect of the oropharynx and may progress rapidly to painful ulceration.

systemic disease.[11] Therefore the search for other symptoms and physical examination findings are important to help determine the appropriate etiology.

Ulcerations may occur in other body parts also, such as in the genitals and gastrointestinal tract in Behçet syndrome. Gastrointestinal symptoms, fever, weight loss, joint and ocular abnormalities, and rash are sample constitutional complaints that the child with an underlying disease may experience.

PFAPA syndrome is characterized by recurrent fevers every 4 to 6 weeks with onset in the first 6 years of life.[12] Along with the symptoms described in its name, PFAPA syndrome may also cause general malaise, anorexia, headache, abdominal pain, and arthralgias[12] that typically resolve within 1 week. The child has complete resolution of symptoms between the recurrences.

LABORATORY EVALUATION

In most of the cases of stomatitis, laboratory evaluation is not helpful in the diagnosis or management of the patients. Monitoring serum electrolytes in patients with severe dehydration is prudent during the rehydration process. In the case of a child with stomatitis of uncertain etiology or oral lesions that persist for longer than 2 weeks, a further evaluation should be undertaken while the pain-relieving and hydrating measures continue. If frequently recurring or persistent oral aphthae are present, along with genital lesions or other systemic findings, an initial evaluation for an underlying cause may then include laboratory studies of complete blood count, erythrocyte sedimentation rate, and serum levels of iron, folate, vitamin B12, and zinc.[11] Depending on the history, screening for antinuclear antibodies, HIV, and celiac disease may be necessary. Establishing the definitive diagnosis and appropriate treatment may require the expertise of an allergist-immunologist, rheumatologist, dermatologist, gastroenterologist, ophthalmologist, oral surgeon, or otolaryngologist, depending on the clinical scenario. A biopsy of an oral lesion may be needed, especially if the child chews tobacco and has a persistent, nonhealing ulcer.

MANAGEMENT

Uncomplicated Case

Relieving pain and preventing dehydration are the goals of treatment for the child with RAS or stomatitis caused by an acute infectious process or for a child with contact stomatitis. By maximizing pain relief, the child will be able to remain hydrated and consume a soft diet. Systemic ibuprofen, acetaminophen, or opiates may help with the pain, but more relief may be obtained from the application of soothing, topical substances. In a cooperative child, the topical substances may be administered by allowing the child to swish and then spit or, alternatively, by painting the substance on the sores with a cotton-tip swab. The many topical agents that have been studied minimally for safety and efficacy include the following: saline rinses, diphenhydramine–aluminum hydroxide with magnesium hydroxide–viscous lidocaine compounded in various combinations, benzocaine, kaolin, and pectin.[13] Most of these agents, if used too aggressively, can lead to overdose and adverse side effects. The topical anesthetic preparations, in particular, must be used cautiously because of the risk of aspiration, loss of protective airway reflexes, and systemic toxicity caused by absorption through the inflamed oral mucosa.

Antimicrobials are of limited value, except in the instance of necrotizing ulcerative gingivitis, in which case chlorhexidine mouth rinses and systemic antibiotics, such as penicillin may be required. Oral acyclovir is of limited therapeutic benefit in the otherwise healthy child with herpes stomatitis, and topical acyclovir is ineffective.[14]

Complicated Cases

An immunocompromised child or one with stomatitis secondary to cancer treatment should receive topical and systemic analgesics and be monitored for secondary infection. Topical sucralfate and capsaicin[15] have been found to relieve the pain of chemotherapy or radiation-induced mucositis and are not routinely used for children with benign, self-limiting conditions.[13] However, these agents may be an option for an otherwise healthy child with persistent pain despite aggressive use of the standard medications. On a case-by-case basis, topical corticosteroids, local anesthetics, topical tacrolimus, and systemic medications (colchicines, dapsone, thalidomide) may be used to treat the oral symptoms in these complicated patients[11]; but these medications are not typically prescribed in general pediatric practice. PFAPA syndrome typically responds well to a short course of oral steroids (1 to 2 mg/kg/day for 5 days) if prescribed at the onset of symptoms.

PREVENTION

Most causes of stomatitis cannot be prevented. In general, along with avoidance of tobacco products and any possible irritants, good oral hygiene should be promoted to reduce the risk of dental caries and gingivitis. Exposure to the proposed triggers for RAS should be lessened. Based on adult studies, continuous oral acyclovir is a therapeutic option for preventing recurrences in a child with frequent herpetic flares.[14] Children with cancer may benefit from a preventive protocol that includes frequent plaque biofilm removal and teeth brushing, chlorhexidine or saline rinses, and nystatin.[16,17]

WHEN TO REFER

If the underlying cause of the stomatitis is uncertain, or if oral lesions persist for greater than 2 weeks, then referral to an oral surgeon or otolaryngologist should be considered for definitive diagnosis. Biopsy of a lesion may be necessary, especially for a child who uses smokeless tobacco.

A child with stomatitis plus multiple symptoms and abnormal physical examination findings may require the expertise of an allergist-immunologist, rheumatologist, dermatologist, gastroenterologist, or ophthalmologist to establish the definitive diagnosis and administer appropriate treatment.

SUGGESTED RESOURCES

Bruce AJ, Rogers RS. Acute oral ulcers. *Dermatol Clin*. 2003;21:1-15.

Padeh S. Periodic fever syndromes. *Pediatr Clin North Am*. 2005;52(2):577-609.

Patel NJ, Sciubba J. Oral lesions in young children. *Pediatr Clin North Am*. 2003;50(2):469-486.

Zunt SL. Recurrent aphthous stomatitis. *Dermatol Clin*. 2003;21(1):33-39.

REFERENCES

1. Bruce AJ, Rogers RS 3rd. Acute oral ulcers. *Dermatol Clin*. 2003;21:1-15.
2. Zunt SL. Recurrent aphthous stomatitis. *Dermatol Clin*. 2003;21(1):33-39.
3. LeSueur BW, Yiannias JA. Contact stomatitis. *Dermatol Clin*. 2003;21(1):105-114, vii.
4. Patel NJ, Sciubba J. Oral lesions in young children. *Pediatr Clin North Am*. 2003;50:469-486.
5. Kleinman DV, Swango PA, Pindborg JJ. Epidemiology of oral mucosal lesions in the United States schoolchildren: 1986-87. *Community Dent Oral Epidemiol*. 1994;22:243-253.
6. Tomar SL, Winn DM, Swango PA, et al. Oral mucosal smokeless tobacco lesions among adolescents in the United States. *J Dent Res*. 1997;76:1277-1286.
7. Moghadam BK, Gier R, Thurlow T. Extensive oral mucosal ulcerations caused by misuse of a commercial mouthwash. *Cutis*. 1999;64:131-134.
8. Padeh S, Brezniak N, Zemer D, et al. Periodic fever, aphthous stomatitis, pharyngitis, and adenopathy syndrome: clinical characteristics and outcome. *J Pediatr*. 1999;135:98-101.
9. Miller LC, Sisson BA, Tucker LB, et al. Prolonged fevers of unknown origin in children: patterns of presentation and outcome. *J Pediatr*. 1996;129:419-423.
10. Ship JA. Recurrent aphthous stomatitis. An update. *Oral Surg Oral Med Oral Pathol Oral Radiol Endod*. 1996;81:141-147.
11. Lestinger JA, McCarty MA, Jorizzo JL. Complex aphthosis: a large case series with evaluation algorithm and therapeutic ladder from topicals to thalidomide. *J Am Acad Dermatol*. 2005;52(3 pt 1):500-508.
12. Padeh S. Periodic fever syndromes. *Pediatr Clin North Am*. 2005;52:577-609.
13. Zempsky WT, Schechter NL. Office-based pain management. The 15-minute consultation. *Pediatr Clin North Am*. 2000;47(3):601-615.
14. American Academy of Pediatrics. Herpes simplex. In: Pickering LK, ed. *Red Book: 2003 Report of the Committee on Infectious Diseases*. 26th ed. Elk Grove Village, IL: American Academy of Pediatrics; 2003.
15. Berger A, Henderson M, Nadoolman W, et al. Oral capsaicin provides temporary relief for oral mucositis pain secondary to chemotherapy/radiation therapy. [Erratum in: *J Pain Symptom Manage*. 1996;11(5):331] *J Pain Symptom Manage*. 1995;10(3):243-248.
16. Levy-Polack MP, Sebelli P, Polack NL. Incidence of oral complications and application of a preventive protocol in children with leukemia. *Spec Care Dentist*. 1998;18:189-193.
17. Cheng KK, Molassiotis A, Chang AM, et al. Evaluation of an oral care protocol intervention in the prevention of chemotherapy-induced oral mucositis in pediatric cancer patients. *Eur J Cancer*. 2001;37:2056-2063.

Chapter 329

STREPTOCOCCAL TOXIC SHOCK SYNDROME

Chokechai Rongkavilit, MD

Streptococcus pyogenes, also known as group A β-hemolytic *Streptococcus* (GAS), is the cause of purulent pharyngitis, impetigo, and scarlet fever and is occasionally complicated by rheumatic fever and glomerulonephritis. Less frequently, GAS causes severe invasive diseases including necrotizing fasciitis, necrotizing myositis, bacteremia, and sepsis with vascular collapse, hypotension, and multiorgan failure, a syndrome known as the streptococcal toxic shock syndrome (STSS).[1]

Beginning in the 1980s, reports began to appear of a shift in the epidemiology of GAS disease toward the occurrence of more severe clinical illness.[2-6] Subsequent reports indicated the emergence of a toxic shock–like syndrome caused by GAS.[7-9] Patients with STSS have epidemiologic features that distinguish them from patients with other invasive GAS infections, including younger age, alcohol abuse, and fewer underlying illnesses.[9,10] Published incidence rates of severe invasive GAS infections have ranged from 1.5 to 7.0 cases per 100,000 population annually.[9,11,12] Outbreaks of severe invasive GAS infections have occurred in some closed environments, such as military bases, nursing homes, and hospitals.[13,14] A population-based surveillance study in the United States indicated a high fatality rate associated with invasive GAS infections, with rates of 22% for necrotizing fasciitis and 45% for STSS.[15] The case-fatality rate among patients with neither STSS nor necrotizing fasciitis was 10%. Although the overall fatality rate of invasive GAS diseases is lower in children (5%-10%) than in adults (30%-80%),[11,16,17] the case fatality rate associated with STSS remains high in both pediatric and adult populations.[10,11,16]

ETIOLOGY AND PATHOGENESIS

The pathogenic mechanisms responsible for invasive GAS infections have yet to be completely defined. Skin and mucous membrane, frequently at the site of minimal or inapparent local trauma, is a common portal of entry of GAS. The opened lesion of chickenpox has been identified as a risk factor for acquiring invasive GAS diseases, including STSS, in otherwise healthy children.[11,16,18,19] However, severe invasive GAS infections rarely occur after an episode of acute GAS pharyngitis.[20,21]

The major human host defense against invasive GAS infection is that of phagocytosis and killing by polymorphonuclear leucocytes. Thus a critical somatic GAS virulence factor is an antiphagocytic surface constituent known as M protein. M protein exerts its antiphagocytic effect by interfering with opsonization via alternate complement pathway. Strains of GAS isolated from patients with STSS are not of a single

M type,[7,22] but M1 and M3 infections have been commonly associated with invasive diseases and STSS.[10,15]

Most cases of STSS are caused by GAS strains that produce bacterial superantigens known as the streptococcal pyrogenic exotoxins (Spe).[7,8,22] This group of exotoxins includes the bacteriophage-encoded SpeA and SpeC, as well as SpeB, SpeF (mitogenic factor), SpeG, SpeH, SpeJ, SpeK, SpeL, Streptococcal superantigen (SSA), streptococcal mitogenic exotoxin Z (SMEZ), and SMEZ-2.[23] Their structures are similar to each other and to the structures of staphylococcal superantigens.[24] Superantigens are potent immunostimulators that are able to simultaneously bind to the major histocompatibility complex class 2 molecules and the T-cell receptor. This binding results in activation of a large number of T cells that express specific V-β subsets of T-cell repertoire and leads to increased secretion of large quantities of specific cytokines such as tumor necrosis factor α and interleukin 1β and T-cell mediators such as interleukin 2 and interferon γ. The probable direct importance of streptococcal pyrogenic exotoxins, particularly exotoxin A (SpeA), for the development of STSS is emphasized by the total inability of STSS sera to neutralize the lymphocyte mitogenic properties of SpeA, the known biologic property of SpeA as a superantigen.[25] Among the streptococcal pyrogenic exotoxins, SpeA is the most potent inducer of massive T-cell proliferation and interferon γ and tumor necrosis factor β production.[26] Unrestrained release of these immunomodulators may activate the complement, coagulation, and fibrinolytic cascades, resulting in the hypotension, tissue injury, and multiorgan failure characteristic of STSS.

BOX 329-1 Case Definition for Streptococcal Toxic Shock Syndrome*

I. Isolation of group A β-hemolytic streptococci
  A. From a normally sterile site (eg, blood, cerebrospinal fluid, peritoneal fluid, tissue biopsy specimen)
  B. From a nonsterile site (eg, throat, sputum, vagina)

II. Clinical signs of severity
  A. Hypotension (systolic blood pressure ≤90 mm Hg in adults or less than the 5th percentile for age in children)
  B. Two or more of the following signs:
    - Renal impairment, creatinine ≥2 mg/dL for adults or twice the upper limit or more of normal for age
    - Coagulopathy (platelets ≤100,000/mcL or disseminated intravascular coagulation)
    - Hepatic involvement (alanine aminotransferase, aspartate aminotransferase, or total bilirubin levels twice the upper limit of normal or more for age)
    - Acute respiratory distress syndrome
    - Generalized erythematous macular rash that may desquamate
    - Soft-tissue necrosis, including necrotizing fasciitis, myositis, or gangrene

*An illness fulfilling criteria IA and IIA and IIB can be defined as a definite case. An illness fulfilling criteria IB and IIA and IIB can be defined as a probable case if no other cause of the illness is identified.

EVALUATION

Clinical Presentation

STSS is characterized by fever, rapid-onset hypotension, rapidly accelerated renal failure, and multisystem organ involvement. Pharyngitis and local soft-tissue infection (eg, cellulitis, abscess, myositis, necrotizing fasciitis) associated with sudden severe pain is common with STSS.[27] The pain, the most common initial symptoms of STSS, usually involves an extremity, but it may also mimic peritonitis, pelvic inflammatory disease, or acute chest syndrome. Twenty percent of patients may have preceding influenza-like syndrome, characterized by fever, chills, myalgia, nausea, vomiting, and diarrhea.[21] Fever is the most common early sign, although hypothermia may be present in patients with shock. A diffuse scarlatina-like erythema occurs in only 10% of patients.[20] Confusion is present in 55% of patients, and in some, coma or combativeness may occur.[21] The case definition for STSS was developed by the Centers for Disease Control and Prevention in 1993 (Box 329-1).[1]

Soft-tissue swelling and erythema is present in 80% of patients, and up to 70% can progress to necrotizing fasciitis or myositis and will require surgical debridement, fasciotomy, or amputation.[20] Necrotizing fasciitis is a life-threatening soft-tissue infection primarily involving the superficial fascia with relative sparing of the skin and muscles, both of which may be infected secondarily.[28,29] The patient may have a history of soft-tissue injury from an animal or insect bite, blunt or penetrating trauma, surgical wounds, or subcutaneous injections of insulin or illicit drugs. It may occur after varicella infection; 15% to 30% of invasive GAS diseases were reported as associated with varicella.[16,17,30] In some instances, an inconsequential scratch or abrasion may be implicated.[29] Most patients have an erythematous, tender, swollen area that resembles cellulitis with disproportionately severe pain at the site of involvement.[31,32] Other less-common presenting complaints include fever, chills, weakness, confusion, and rash. An ominous sign of necrotizing fasciitis is the progression of soft-tissue swelling to the formation of vesicles, then bullae, which appear violaceous or hemorrhagic. The line of demarcation becomes sharply defined, and the dead skin begins to separate at the margins or breaks in the center, revealing an extensive necrosis of the subcutaneous tissue. The presence of crepitus on physical examination or soft-tissue air by plain-film radiograph, which is pathognomonic for necrotizing soft-tissue infections, is seen in only one third and one half of cases, respectively.[33]

Severe pain, swelling, erythema, and fever may be the early signs of myositis. Pain is often out of proportion to the clinical findings, possibly related to muscle compartment syndrome, which may develop rapidly.[34] Both necrotizing fasciitis and myositis are difficult to diagnose; therefore clinical acumen and suspicion are important. Some patients with STSS may have both necrotizing fasciitis and myositis. Emergent surgical exploration should be performed to establish and distinguish GAS infection from other soft-tissue infections. Nearly one half of patients with STSS may have normal blood pressure at the time of admission but soon develop hypotension.[20] The presence of hypotension is a significant risk factor for death.[10]

Renal dysfunction, which may occur before or after hypotension, progresses or persists in all patients for 48 to 72 hours in spite of treatment, and many patients require dialysis.[21] In patients who survive, serum creatinine values return to normal within 4 to 6 weeks. Acute respiratory distress syndrome occurs in one half of the cases and generally develops after the onset of hypotension. Profuse watery diarrhea, vomiting, abdominal pain, generalized erythroderma, conjunctival injection, and severe myalgias commonly present with *Staphylococcus aureus*–mediated toxic shock syndrome are present but less common with STSS (see Chapter 327, Staphylococcal Toxic Shock Syndrome). STSS also may be associated with invasive GAS infections, such as pneumonia, meningitis, peritonitis, osteomyelitis, bacteremia, or septic arthritis. However, STSS may occur without a readily identifiable focus of infection in 21% of cases.[10] Recurrent episodes have not been reported for STSS.

Laboratory Evaluation

Renal involvement is indicated by the presence of hemoglobinuria and by rising serum creatinine values. Renal impairment precedes hypotension in 40% to 50% of patients.[20] Hypoalbuminemia, hypocalcemia, lactic acidosis, hyperglycemia, thrombocytopenia, and altered coagulation profiles may be observed. The serum creatinine kinase level is useful in detecting deeper soft-tissue infections; when the level is increased, a good correlation exists with necrotizing fasciitis or myositis. Mild leucocytosis may be seen initially, but the mean percentage of immature neutrophils can reach 40% to 50%. Blood cultures are positive for GAS in 60% of cases.[20]

Subcutaneous fluid may be aspirated from the affected limb for Gram stain and culture. All tissues obtained at the time of initial surgical debridement should be subjected to Gram staining and to culturing for aerobic and anaerobic microorganisms. Rapid antigen detection tests for GAS have not been approved for any specimen besides pharyngeal swab specimens; however, GAS may be identified from necrotic tissue with a rapid antigen test.[35] In necrotizing soft-tissue infections in children, GAS is identified as a single organism in only 25% of cases; the remaining cases are polymicrobial.[36]

Imaging Studies

The presence of soft-tissue air at the affected area may be observed in plain films.[33,37,38] Computed tomography and magnetic resonance imaging play an important role in the diagnosis of necrotizing fasciitis and myositis and in the delineation of the extent of infection. Features that indicate necrotizing fasciitis by computed tomography or magnetic resonance imaging include deep fascial thickening and enhancement and the presence of fluid and gas in the fascial planes.[39,40] The typical radiologic findings of myositis are of a general homogenous enlargement of the muscle, with low attenuation values and edema or the presence of intramuscular gas.[34,39,41]

Imaging studies are only adjuncts in the evaluations of patients with STSS and necrotizing soft-tissue infections, and they should not be relied on to exclude the diagnosis. The diagnosis of invasive GAS infection, including STSS, is still based primarily on clinical grounds.

TREATMENT

Treatment of a child with severe invasive GAS infection includes hemodynamic stabilization and specific antibiotic therapy. Prompt and aggressive surgical exploration, fasciotomy, and debridement of suspected deep-seated infection are mandatory. Surgical exploration and incisional biopsy provide both definitive diagnosis and treatment. Survival is possible with early surgical debridement, reexploration at 24 to 36 hours, and intensive supportive care. The extent of debridement is determined not only by the radiographic findings, but also by physical findings at the time of surgery.

Patients suspected of having STSS, regardless of the presence of necrotizing soft-tissue infections, should receive empiric broad-spectrum antibiotic therapy with drugs that cover gram-positive, gram-negative, and anaerobic organisms. The most frequently advocated antibiotic regimens include (a) the combination of ampicillin, penicillin, aminoglycosides, and clindamycin or (b) the combination of expanded-spectrum penicillin or cephalosporins, clindamycin, and aminoglycosides.* Patients who are allergic to penicillin may receive vancomycin in place of ampicillin or penicillin. The antibiotic regimen can be changed once the causative organism is identified.

Penicillin is less efficacious in overwhelming GAS infections when large numbers of organisms are present (the so-called *Eagle* effect).[43,44] Penicillin fails to halt this type of infection because of the physiologic state of the organism. Large inocula of GAS reach the stationary growth phase quickly both in vitro and in vivo, and penicillin is less efficacious against slowly growing organisms. Certain penicillin-binding proteins are not expressed by GAS during the stationary phase.[45] The loss of penicillin-binding proteins may be responsible for the inocula effects observed both in vivo and in vitro and may account for the failure of penicillin to control severe GAS infection.

Conversely, the greater efficacy of clindamycin in experimental models of fulminant GAS infection is probably related to its mechanism of action—the inhibition of protein synthesis, which is independent of the size of the inoculum or the stage of bacterial growth.[43,45] In addition, clindamycin suppresses the synthesis of bacterial toxins, facilitates phagocytosis of GAS by inhibiting M protein synthesis, has a postantimicrobial effect, and suppresses the synthesis of penicillin-binding proteins that, in addition to being targets for penicillin, are also enzymes involved in cell-wall synthesis and

*References: 29, 31-33, 37, 38, 42.

degradation.[46,47] Research has shown that clindamycin suppresses lipopolysaccharide-induced monocyte synthesis of tumor necrosis factor α.[48] The efficacy of the drug may thus also be related to its ability to modulate the immune response. Although no clinical evidence has determined that clindamycin improves outcome, administering clindamycin in addition to penicillin seems advisable in patients with overwhelming invasive GAS infection. Clindamycin should not be used alone because strains of GAS with clindamycin resistance have been reported.[49]

Previous studies have shown that protective humoral immunity to both cell-associated and soluble GAS virulence factors is important in preventing invasive disease.[22,50-52] Patients with invasive GAS disease have significantly lower serum levels of protective antibodies against M protein and superantigens compared with serum samples from noninvasive cases.[22,50,52] These findings provide evidence that lack of protective humoral immunity against GAS virulence factors contributes to susceptibility to invasive infection. Intravenous immunoglobulin (IVIg) therapy in patients with STSS results in decreased mortality rates.[53,54] Patients who received IVIg had significant improvement of organ dysfunction after therapy, as well as a significant increase in plasma-neutralizing activity against superantigens. Considering the high mortality rates associated with STSS, IVIg may be provided as adjunctive therapy for patients with STSS.

Hyperbaric oxygen, a form of medical treatment in which the patient is enclosed in a chamber and breathes 100% oxygen at a pressure greater than 1 atmosphere absolute, has gained acceptance for treatment of a variety of medical conditions. Although a physiologic rationale can be found for the use of hyperbaric oxygen therapy in the treatment of necrotizing fasciitis, the results of clinical studies have been inconsistent. Some studies have shown that such therapy can improve patent survival and decrease the number of debridements required to achieve wound control,[55-57] whereas others have shown no benefit.[58-60]

PREVENTION

Opportunities for preventing STSS are few. Because of the association between invasive GAS infections, including STSS and varicella infection, in healthy children,[16,61,62] routine childhood immunization against varicella is suggested. Children who receive the varicella vaccine are less likely to be hospitalized for varicella-related invasive GAS infections.[63] A relationship between the use of nonsteroidal antiinflammatory drugs (NSAIDs) and necrotizing fasciitis has been reported.[64,65] Evidence suggests that NSAIDs can impair granulocytic function and enhance production of cytokines.[66] Although some physicians have suggested that NSAIDs should not be used to treat children with varicella, a causal relationship between NSAID use and severe invasive GAS infections has not been established. Nosocomial GAS infections should be prevented by improving infection-control practices for surgical and obstetric procedures and for placement and care of intravascular devices.

GAS can easily spread through the household.[67] In many of these clusters, additional family members, usually children, are identified with pharyngitis or with carriage of the same strain of GAS that caused the invasive disease.[11,13,14] The relative risks of invasive GAS infections among household contacts of patients with invasive GAS infections are 19 to 200 times the baseline risk in general population.[11,68] Secondary cases of invasive GAS infections, including STSS within the same household, have been reported.[13,14,69,70] Although the risk of subsequent invasive GAS disease among household contacts is higher than the risk among the general population, such infections are rare. No studies have evaluated the effectiveness of chemoprophylaxis in preventing invasive GAS disease among household contacts of patients with invasive GAS infections; thus routine chemoprophylaxis among household contacts is not warranted. Health care providers should inform members of the household about the clinical manifestations of pharyngeal and invasive GAS infections and emphasize the importance of seeking immediate medical attention if they develop such symptoms, particularly within 30 days after the diagnosis is made in the index case.[71] Routine use of cultures to identify household contacts who are colonized with GAS is not suggested.

Because of the high mortality of invasive GAS infections among persons older than 65 years, or those with underlying illnesses or other host factors, chemoprophylaxis to prevent secondary cases may be offered to household members aged 65 years or older and those with HIV infection, concurrent varicella infection, diabetes mellitus, cancer, chronic cardiac or pulmonary diseases, injection drug use, alcoholism, known immunodeficiency disorder, and corticosteroid use.[71] Because the source of GAS in households is not necessarily the person with invasive infection, physicians who elect to prescribe chemoprophylaxis for an elderly or high-risk household member should prescribe chemoprophylaxis for all members in that household. If available, then antibiotic susceptibility data should be used to select the most appropriate chemoprophylactic agent. Everyone who receives chemoprophylaxis should watch for sign and symptoms of invasive GAS disease for 30 days after the diagnosis of invasive disease in the index case. The chemoprophylactic regimens are as follows:[71]

a. A single dose of benzathine penicillin G (600,000 units intramuscularly for persons weighing <27 kg or 1,200,000 units intramuscularly for persons weighing ≥ 27 kg) and oral rifampin 20 mg/kg/day (maximum daily dose, 600 mg) in 2 divided doses for 4 days
b. Clindamycin 20 mg/kg/day (maximum daily dose, 900 mg) in 3 divided doses for 10 days
c. Azithromycin 12 mg/kg/day (maximum daily dose, 500 mg) once a day for 5 days

There is limited evidence that first- and second-generation cephalosporins are effective in eradicating pharyngeal colonization of GAS and these agents could be considered for patients allergic to penicillin whose allergic reactions are not anaphylactic. Rifampin is not recommended for pregnant women due to its teratogenic effect.

Enhanced surveillance by the infection control personnel should be implemented after identification of a case of postpartum or postsurgical invasive GAS infections.[71] All GAS isolates from suspected cases should be stored and compared by serotyping or molecular techniques. The occurrence of $\geq$2 cases of invasive GAS infection by the same GAS type within 6-month period suggests that a healthcare worker might be the source of the cluster; therefore screening of healthcare workers who are epidemiologically linked to the case patients by obtaining cultures from throat, anus, vagina and skin lesions is strongly recommended. One of the three prophylactic regimens mentioned above can be prescribed to healthcare workers who are colonized with GAS. Follow-up culture should be done at 7-10 days after the completion of therapy.

WHEN TO REFER

- All patients with STSS should be managed in consultation with infectious diseases specialists.

WHEN TO ADMIT

- All patients with STSS need to be admitted.

TOOLS FOR PRACTICE

Medical Decision Support

- *Red Book: 2006 Report of the Committee on Infectious Diseases*, 27th edition, American Academy of Pediatrics (www.aap.org/bookstore).

REFERENCES

1. The Working Group on Severe Streptococcal Infections. Defining the group A streptococcal toxic shock syndrome. Rationale and consensus definition. *JAMA.* 1993; 269:390-391.
2. Chiobotaru P, Yagupsky P, Fraser D, et al. Changing epidemiology of invasive Streptococcus pyogenes infections in southern Israel: differences between 2 ethnic population groups. *Pediatr Infect Dis J.* 1997;16:195-199.
3. Cone LA, Woodard DR, Schlievert PM, et al. Clinical and bacteriologic observations of a toxic shock-like syndrome due to Streptococcus pyogenes. *N Engl J Med.* 1987;317:146-149.
4. Martin PR, Hoiby EA. Streptococcal serogroup A epidemic in Norway 1987-1988. *Scand J Infect Dis.* 1990;22: 421-429.
5. Stromberg A, Romanus V, Burman LG. Outbreak of group A streptococcal bacteremia in Sweden: an epidemiologic and clinical study. *J Infect Dis.* 1991;164:595-598.
6. Bartter T, Dascal A, Carroll K, et al. "Toxic strep syndrome." A manifestation of group A streptococcal infection. *Arch Intern Med.* 1988;148:1421-1424.
7. Stevens DL, Tanner MH, Winship J, et al. Severe group A streptococcal infections associated with a toxic shock-like syndrome and scarlet fever toxin A. *N Engl J Med.* 1989;321:1-7.
8. Wheeler MC, Roe MH, Kaplan EL, et al. Outbreak of group A streptococcus septicemia in children. Clinical, epidemiologic, and microbiological correlates. *JAMA.* 1991;266:533-537.
9. Hoge CW, Schwartz B, Talkington DF, et al. The changing epidemiology of invasive group A streptococcal infections and the emergence of streptococcal toxic shock-like syndrome. A retrospective population-based study. *JAMA.* 1993;269:384-389.
10. Eriksson BK, Andersson J, Holm SE, et al. Epidemiological and clinical aspects of invasive group A streptococcal infections and the streptococcal toxic shock syndrome. *Clin Infect Dis.* 1998;27:1428-1436.
11. Davies HD, McGeer A, Schwartz B, et al. Invasive group A streptococcal infections in Ontario, Canada. Ontario Group A Streptococcal Study Group. *N Engl J Med.* 1996;335:547-554.
12. Centers for Disease Control and Prevention. Group A beta-hemolytic streptococcal bacteremia—Colorado, 1989. *MMWR Morb Mortal Wkly Rep.* 1990;39:3-6, 11.
13. Schwartz B, Elliott JA, Butler JC, et al. Clusters of invasive group A streptococcal infections in family, hospital, and nursing home settings. *Clin Infect Dis.* 1992;15:277-284.
14. DiPersio JR, File TM Jr, Stevens DL, et al. Spread of serious disease-producing M3 clones of group A streptococcus among family members and health care workers. *Clin Infect Dis.* 1996;22:490-495.
15. O'Brien KL, Beall B, Barrett NL, et al. Epidemiology of invasive group A streptococcus disease in the United States, 1995-1999. *Clin Infect Dis.* 2002;35:268-276.
16. Laupland KB, Davies HD, Low DE, et al. Invasive group A streptococcal disease in children and association with varicella-zoster virus infection. Ontario Group A Streptococcal Study Group. *Pediatrics.* 2000;105:E60.
17. Davies HD, Matlow A, Scriver SR, et al. Apparent lower rates of streptococcal toxic shock syndrome and lower mortality in children with invasive group A streptococcal infections compared with adults. *Pediatr Infect Dis J.* 1994;13:49-56.
18. Begovac J, Marton E, Lisic M, et al. Group A beta-hemolytic streptococcal toxic shock-like syndrome. *Pediatr Infect Dis J.* 1990;9:369-370.
19. Cowan MR, Primm PA, Scott SM, et al. Serious group A beta-hemolytic streptococcal infections complicating varicella. *Ann Emerg Med.* 1994;23:818-822.
20. Stevens DL. Streptococcal toxic-shock syndrome: spectrum of disease, pathogenesis, and new concepts in treatment. *Emerg Infect Dis.* 1995;1:69-78.
21. Stevens DL. Invasive group A streptococcus infections. *Clin Infect Dis.* 1992;14:2-11.
22. Eriksson BK, Andersson J, Holm SE, et al. Invasive group A streptococcal infections: T1M1 isolates expressing pyrogenic exotoxins A and B in combination with selective lack of toxin-neutralizing antibodies are associated with increased risk of streptococcal toxic shock syndrome. *J Infect Dis.* 1999;180:410-418.
23. Bisno AL, Brito MO, Collins CM. Molecular basis of group A streptococcal virulence. *Lancet Infect Dis.* 2003; 3:191-200.
24. Papageorgiou AC, Acharya KR. Microbial superantigens: from structure to function. *Trends Microbiol.* 2000; 8:369-375.
25. Schlievert PM. Role of superantigens in human disease. *J Infect Dis.* 1993;167:997-1002.
26. Norrby-Teglund A, Norgren M, Holm SE, et al. Similar cytokine induction profiles of a novel streptococcal exotoxin, MF, and pyrogenic exotoxins A and B. *Infect Immun.* 1994;62:3731-3738.
27. Chiang MC, Jaing TH, Wu CT, et al. Streptococcal toxic shock syndrome in children without skin and soft tissue infection: report of 4 cases. *Acta Paediatr.* 2005;94: 763-765.
28. Wilson B. Necrotizing fasciitis. *Am Surg.* 1952;18: 416-431.

29. Cunningham JD, Silver L, Rudikoff D. Necrotizing fasciitis: a plea for early diagnosis and treatment. *Mt Sinai J Med.* 2001;68:253-261.
30. Givner LB. Invasive disease due to group A beta-hemolytic streptococci: continued occurrence in children in North Carolina. *South Med J.* 1998;91:333-337.
31. Majeski JA, Alexander JW. Early diagnosis, nutritional support, and immediate extensive debridement improve survival in necrotizing fasciitis. *Am J Surg.* 1983;145: 784-787.
32. Sudarsky LA, Laschinger JC, Coppa GF, et al. Improved results from a standardized approach in treating patients with necrotizing fasciitis. *Ann Surg.* 1987;206:661-665.
33. Elliott DC, Kufera JA, Myers RA. Necrotizing soft tissue infections. Risk factors for mortality and strategies for management. *Ann Surg.* 1996;224:672-683.
34. Dalal M, Sterne G, Murray DS. Streptococcal myositis: a lesson. *Br J Plast Surg.* 2002;55:682-684.
35. Ault MJ, Geiderman J, Sokolov R. Rapid identification of group A streptococcus as the cause of necrotizing fasciitis. *Ann Emerg Med.* 1996;28:227-230.
36. Brook I. Aerobic and anaerobic microbiology of necrotizing fasciitis in children. *Pediatr Dermatol.* 1996;13: 281-284.
37. Rubinstein E, Dehertogh D, Brettman L. Severe necrotizing soft-tissue infections: report of 22 cases. *Conn Med.* 1995;59:67-72.
38. McHenry CR, Piotrowski JJ, Petrinic D, et al. Determinants of mortality for necrotizing soft-tissue infections. *Ann Surg.* 1995;221:558-563.
39. Wong CH, Wang YS. The diagnosis of necrotizing fasciitis. *Curr Opin Infect Dis.* 2005;18:101-106.
40. Wysoki MG, Santora TA, Shah RM, et al. Necrotizing fasciitis: CT characteristics. *Radiology.* 1997;203:859-863.
41. Tang WM, Wong JW, Wong LL, et al. Streptococcal necrotizing myositis: the role of magnetic resonance imaging. A case report. *J Bone Joint Surg Am.* 2001; 83-A:1723-1726.
42. Bisno AL, Stevens DL. Streptococcal infections of skin and soft tissues. *N Engl J Med.* 1996;334:240-245.
43. Stevens DL, Gibbons AE, Bergstrom R, et al. The Eagle effect revisited: efficacy of clindamycin, erythromycin, and penicillin in the treatment of streptococcal myositis. *J Infect Dis.* 1988;158:23-28.
44. Eagle H. Experimental approach to the problem of treatment failure with penicillin. I. Group A streptococcal infection in mice. *Am J Med.* 1952;13:389-399.
45. Stevens DL, Yan S, Bryant AE. Penicillin-binding protein expression at different growth stages determines penicillin efficacy in vitro and in vivo: an explanation for the inoculum effect. *J Infect Dis.* 1993;167:1401-1405.
46. Stevens DL, Maier KA, Mitten JE. Effect of antibiotics on toxin production and viability of Clostridium perfringens. *Antimicrob Agents Chemother.* 1987;31:213-218.
47. Gemmell CG, Peterson PK, Schmeling D, et al. Potentiation of opsonization and phagocytosis of Streptococcus pyogenes following growth in the presence of clindamycin. *J Clin Invest.* 1981;67:1249-1256.
48. Stevens DL, Bryant AE, Hackett SP. Antibiotic effects on bacterial viability, toxin production, and host response. *Clin Infect Dis.* 1995;20(suppl 2):S154-S157.
49. Tanz RR, Shulman ST, Shortridge VD, et al. Community-based surveillance in the united states of macrolide-resistant pediatric pharyngeal group A streptococci during 3 respiratory disease seasons. *Clin Infect Dis.* 2004; 39:1794-1801.
50. Norrby-Teglund A, Pauksens K, Holm SE, et al. Relation between low capacity of human sera to inhibit streptococcal mitogens and serious manifestation of disease. *J Infect Dis.* 1994;170:585-591.
51. Basma H, Norrby-Teglund A, Guedez Y, et al. Risk factors in the pathogenesis of invasive group A streptococcal infections: role of protective humoral immunity. *Infect Immun.* 1999;67:1871-1877.
52. Basma H, Norrby-Teglund A, McGeer A, et al. Opsonic antibodies to the surface M protein of group A streptococci in pooled normal immunoglobulins (IVIG): potential impact on the clinical efficacy of IVIG therapy for severe invasive group A streptococcal infections. *Infect Immun.* 1998;66:2279-2283.
53. Kaul R, McGeer A, Norrby-Teglund A, et al. Intravenous immunoglobulin therapy for streptococcal toxic shock syndrome—a comparative observational study. The Canadian Streptococcal Study Group. *Clin Infect Dis.* 1999;28:800-807.
54. Darenberg J, Ihendyane N, Sjolin J, et al. Intravenous immunoglobulin G therapy in streptococcal toxic shock syndrome: a European randomized, double-blind, placebo-controlled trial. *Clin Infect Dis.* 2003;37:333-340.
55. Eltorai IM, Hart GB, Strauss MB, et al. The role of hyperbaric oxygen in the management of Fournier's gangrene. *Int Surg.* 1986;71:53-58.
56. Riseman JA, Zamboni WA, Curtis A, et al. Hyperbaric oxygen therapy for necrotizing fasciitis reduces mortality and the need for debridements. *Surgery.* 1990;108: 847-850.
57. Korhonen K, Hirn M, Niinikoski J. Hyperbaric oxygen in the treatment of Fournier's gangrene. *Eur J Surg.* 1998; 164:251-255.
58. Tehrani MA, Ledingham IM. Necrotizing fasciitis. *Postgrad Med J.* 1977;53:237-242.
59. Brown DR, Davis NL, Lepawsky M, et al. A multicenter review of the treatment of major truncal necrotizing infections with and without hyperbaric oxygen therapy. *Am J Surg.* 1994;167:485-489.
60. Shupak A, Shoshani O, Goldenberg I, et al. Necrotizing fasciitis: an indication for hyperbaric oxygenation therapy? *Surgery.* 1995;118:873-878.
61. Vugia DJ, Peterson CL, Meyers HB, et al. Invasive group A streptococcal infections in children with varicella in Southern California. *Pediatr Infect Dis J.* 1996;15:146-150.
62. Doctor A, Harper MB, Fleisher GR. Group A beta-hemolytic streptococcal bacteremia: historical overview, changing incidence, and recent association with varicella. *Pediatrics.* 1995;96(3 pt 1):428-433.
63. Patel RA, Binns HJ, Shulman ST. Reduction in pediatric hospitalizations for varicella-related invasive group A streptococcal infections in the varicella vaccine era. *J Pediatr.* 2004;144:68-74.
64. Brogan TV, Nizet V, Waldhausen JH, et al. Group A streptococcal necrotizing fasciitis complicating primary varicella: a series of fourteen patients. *Pediatr Infect Dis J.* 1995;14:588-594.
65. Rimailho A, Riou B, Richard C, et al. Fulminant necrotizing fasciitis and nonsteroidal anti-inflammatory drugs. *J Infect Dis.* 1987;155:143-146.
66. Stevens DL. Could nonsteroidal antiinflammatory drugs (NSAIDs) enhance the progression of bacterial infections to toxic shock syndrome? *Clin Infect Dis.* 1995;21:977-980.
67. Falck G, Holm SE, Kjellander J, et al. The role of household contacts in the transmission of group A streptococci. *Scand J Infect Dis.* 1997;29:239-244.
68. Robinson KA, Rothrock G, Phan Q, et al. Risk for severe group A streptococcal disease among patients' household contacts. *Emerg Infect Dis.* 2003;9:443-447.
69. Ichiyama S, Nakashima K, Shimokata K, et al. Transmission of *Streptococcus pyogenes* causing toxic shock-like syndrome among family members and confirmation by DNA macrorestriction analysis. *J Infect Dis.* 1997;175: 723-726.

70. Huang YC, Hsueh PR, Lin TY, et al. A family cluster of streptococcal toxic shock syndrome in children: clinical implication and epidemiological investigation. *Pediatrics.* 2001;107:1181-1183.
71. [No author listed]. Prevention of invasive group A streptococcal disease among household contacts of case patients and among postpartum and postsurgical patients: recommendations from the Centers for Disease Control and Prevention. *Clin Infect Dis.* 2002;35:950-959.

Chapter 330

SUDDEN INFANT DEATH SYNDROME

Rachel Y. Moon, MD; John Kattwinkel, MD

DEFINITION AND DIAGNOSIS

Sudden infant death syndrome (SIDS) is a disease of unknown cause. Despite a recent decrease in the incidence, SIDS continues to be the leading cause of death of infants between 1 month and 1 year of age. It currently accounts for approximately 2200 deaths per year in the United States. SIDS is defined as "the sudden death of an infant under 1 year of age, which remains unexplained after a thorough case investigation, including performance of a complete autopsy, examination of the death scene, and review of the clinical history."[1]

INCIDENCE

In 1992 the American Academy of Pediatrics (AAP) recommended that infants be placed in a nonprone position for sleep as a strategy to reduce the risk of SIDS,[2] and the *Back to Sleep* campaign was launched in the United States in 1994. Since 1992 the rate of prone sleeping has decreased from 70% to 13% in 2004,[3] and the rate of SIDS has decreased from 1.2 deaths per 1000 live births to 0.57 deaths per 1000 live births in 2002.[4] Similar decreases in SIDS have been experienced in other countries that have initiated similar educational campaigns.

However, a racial disparity exists in both prone sleeping and SIDS. The rate of SIDS in black infants was 2.5-fold that of white infants in 2001,[5] and this disparity may be partially attributed to the increased prevalence of prone positioning in black infants (21%, as opposed to 11% in 2001).[3]

The occurrence of SIDS is rare in the first month of life, peaks between 2 and 3 months of age, and then decreases thereafter. Approximately 90% of SIDS deaths occur in the first 6 months of life.

ETIOLOGY

SIDS likely represents a variety of causes of death. However, the leading hypothesis regarding the etiology of SIDS is that certain infants, for reasons yet unknown, have a maldevelopment or delay in maturation of the brainstem neural network that is responsible for arousal and the physiological responses to life-threatening challenges during sleep. Postmortem examination of the brainstems of a series of infants dying of SIDS, using quantitative techniques, have demonstrated deficits in serotonin receptors throughout the ventral medulla, when compared with age-matched control infants who had died from some other well-defined cause. Authorities believe that these brainstem regions are involved with arousal, chemosensitivity, respiratory drive, thermoregulation, and blood pressure responses.[6] In addition, polymorphisms in the promoter region of serotonin transporter protein genes (5-HTT) have been associated with SIDS in several studies.[7,8] When the physiological stability of such infants becomes compromised during sleep, they may not arouse sufficiently to avoid the fatal noxious insult or condition. One theory proposes that rebreathing and associated hypoxia and hypercarbia provide the noxious stimulus, whereas another proposes hyperthermia, perhaps in combination with asphyxia, as the stimulus. Investigators have argued that prone sleep position, soft sleeping surfaces, and covering of the head increase the likelihood of rebreathing, hyperthermia, or both.[9-16]

DIFFERENTIAL DIAGNOSIS

Because SIDS is a diagnosis of exclusion, other conditions must be ruled out by autopsy, death scene investigation, and review of the clinical history.[1] Illnesses that should be considered in the differential diagnosis include sepsis, pneumonia, myocarditis, cardiomyopathy, congenital heart defect, arrhythmia, prolonged QT syndrome, trauma (accidental or nonaccidental), suffocation, adrenal hypoplasia, and inherited metabolic disorders, such as fatty acid oxidation disorders.

The large majority of SIDS cases have no evidence suggesting parental psychiatric disease or neglect of the infant. However, much media attention has been given to a few cases of Münchausen-by-proxy causing apparent life-threatening events[17] and of multiple cases of SIDS within a family later determined to be multiple homicides.[18,19] The proportion of SIDS deaths attributable to homicide is probably less than 10%.[20] A family in which an infant has previously died of SIDS has a 2% to 6% risk of a second SIDS death.[21]

Suffocation, either accidental or nonaccidental, is difficult to distinguish on autopsy from SIDS. Indeed, since 1999, some deaths that would previously have been classified as SIDS are now being classified as suffocation.[22]

EPIDEMIOLOGIC CONSIDERATIONS

The following characteristics have consistently been identified as independent risk factors for SIDS: prone or side sleep position, sleeping on a soft surface, maternal smoking during pregnancy, overheating, late or no prenatal care, young maternal age, preterm birth or low birth weight (or both), and male gender.[15,23-30] Blacks and American Indian/Alaska Native infants consistently have SIDS rates that are 2 to 3 times the national average.[31,32]

The AAP, in its 1992 recommendations on sleeping position, recommended side or supine to reduce SIDS risk.[2] However, with the large decrease in the proportion of infants placed to sleep prone since the initiation of Back to Sleep campaigns internationally, the contribution of side sleep position to SIDS risk has increased.[24,33-36] The side sleep position is unstable, and a large proportion of infants placed on the side will roll to prone,[37,38] which confers an exceptionally high risk for SIDS.[34,36,39] Secondary caregivers (grandparents, babysitters, child care providers, relatives) are more likely to place infants prone, which also increases the risk for SIDS, particularly if the infant is unaccustomed to the prone position.[34,36,39]

Soft surfaces, such as pillows, quilts, comforters, sheepskins, and porous mattresses, have been identified as a significant risk factor.[11,15,40-44] A strong interaction has been found between prone sleep position and soft bedding surface, indicating that these 2 factors together are very hazardous.[44] Soft surfaces have also been implicated in infant deaths occurring on adult beds.[45-47]

Maternal smoking during pregnancy has been shown to be a major risk factor in almost every epidemiologic study of SIDS.[28,29,48] Postnatal exposure to tobacco smoke has emerged as a separate risk factor in a few studies,[28,49] although separating this variable from maternal smoking prenatally is difficult.

An increased risk of SIDS has been associated with increased layers of clothing or blankets on the infant and warmer room temperatures.[10,15,50] The increased risk of overheating is particularly evident when infants sleep prone[15] but is less clear when they sleep supine. Also unclear is whether overheating is an independent factor or merely a reflection of the use of more clothing, quilts, and other potentially asphyxiating objects in the sleeping environment during cold weather.

Infants born preterm or who are low birth weight are at increased risk for SIDS, and the risk increases with decreasing gestational age or birth weight.[26,30] The increased risk cannot be explained by a greater likelihood of apnea of prematurity among preterm SIDS victims while they are in the hospital after birth.[26] Whether other complications of prematurity can explain the increased risk is unclear. The association of sleep position and SIDS is equally strong for infants born preterm as for those born at term.[51] Strategies designed to reduce risk in full-term infants should also be applied to infants born preterm after they are no longer in an intensive care setting.

Physiologic and behavioral studies demonstrate that bed sharing between an infant and adult facilitates breastfeeding and enhances maternal-infant bonding.[52,53] However, epidemiologic studies of bed sharing have shown that it can be hazardous. The risk of sudden unexpected death with bed sharing seems to be particularly high when multiple people share the bed,[44] when the infant is younger than 11 weeks,[54,55] when bed sharing occurs on a couch,[44,55-57] and when bed sharing occurs for the whole night.[58,59] Bed sharing may be increased when the bed sharer has consumed alcohol or is overtired.[54,59] Bed sharing is particularly hazardous with mothers who smoke,[58,59] but bed sharing with nonsmoking mothers is a risk factor among infants younger than 11 weeks.[54,55] Evidence is growing that room sharing without bed sharing is associated with a reduced risk of SIDS.[54,55,58] Notably, breastfeeding in bed has not been shown to carry a risk if the baby is returned to the crib after the feeding. Because breastfeeding has many benefits, parents should be encouraged to bring the infant into bed for breastfeeding and for bonding. However, the baby should be returned to the crib or bassinet when the parent is ready for sleep.

Pacifiers, by a yet unidentified mechanism, appear to reduce the risk of SIDS when used at sleep time.[44,54,57,60-64] Two recent meta-analyses demonstrate a strong protective effect.[65,66] However, several studies have shown a negative correlation between pacifier use and breastfeeding duration; apparently the biggest factor is early pacifier use that may interfere with establishment of good breastfeeding practices.[67] Thus, in breastfed infants, pacifiers should not be offered for the first month of life until breastfeeding has been well established and while the incidence of SIDS is low. In addition, practices that encourage breastfeeding (rooming in, skin-to-skin holding) should be encouraged in delivery hospitals, and continued breastfeeding support for the parents should be offered.

RISK REDUCTION

For many years, apnea was thought to be the predecessor of SIDS, and home apnea monitors were used in an effort to prevent SIDS.[18] However, although they may be useful in some infants who have had an apparent life-threatening event, no evidence has been found that home monitors are effective in reducing the risk of SIDS when no event has occurred in a particular infant.[68-71]

SIDS risk reduction has centered on eliminating risk factors that have been shown epidemiologically to be associated with SIDS. The AAP has made the following recommendations for SIDS risk reduction[72]:

- Infants should be placed for sleep in a supine position for every sleep. Side sleeping is not as safe as supine sleeping and is not advised.
- A firm sleep surface should be used, such as a firm crib mattress covered by a well-fitted sheet.
- Soft materials or objects such as pillows, quilts, comforters, sheepskins, stuffed toys, and other soft objects should be kept out of an infant sleeping environment. Loose bedding, such as blankets and sheets, should be avoided.
- Smoking during pregnancy or in the infant's environment is strongly discouraged.
- A separate but proximate sleeping environment is recommended; the infant should sleep in the same room, in a crib or bassinet, next to the parent's bed.
- Offering a pacifier at nap time and bedtime should be considered; it does not need to be reinserted once the infant falls asleep and should not be forced if the infant refuses it. Introduction of the pacifier should be delayed in breastfeeding infants until 1 month of age to ensure that breastfeeding is fully established.
- Overheating should be avoided.
- Commercial devices marketed to reduce the risk of SIDS should be avoided.
- Home monitors should not be used as a strategy to reduce the risk of SIDS.

Supine Sleeping and Plagiocephaly

With the increased rate of supine sleeping, the incidence of plagiocephaly without synostosis has increased.[73-75]

Infants with plagiocephaly are more likely not to have had the head position altered when put down to sleep, more likely to spend little awake time in the prone position (tummy time), and less likely to have been held in the upright position while awake.[76] Development of positional plagiocephaly can be avoided by altering the supine head position during sleep; encouraging upright cuddle time; avoiding excessive time in car seats, infant carriers, and bouncers, all of which place pressure on the occiput; and encouraging tummy time when the infant is awake and observed.[72] Awake tummy time will also enhance upper body motor development. For more information on plagiocephaly, see Chapter 311, Plagiocephaly.

Supine Sleeping and Gastroesophageal Reflux

A perception exists that sleeping supine may increase the risk of gastroesophageal reflux, choking, and aspiration. However, evidence indicates that infants who vomit are at greater risk of choking when they are prone.[77,78] Indeed, the incidence of aspiration or complaints of vomiting has not increased with increased supine sleeping.[77]

MANAGEMENT AND SUPPORT

The loss of an infant to SIDS is devastating for the family, friends, and health care providers. The lack of certainty as to how the infant died adds an additional and difficult element to the grief process. The physician can play an active role by ensuring that an autopsy is performed in all cases of sudden unexpected death, discussing the results of the autopsy with the parents, and providing emotional support to the entire family, including age-appropriate support for surviving siblings. The family should be directed to local counseling and support groups.

TOOLS FOR PRACTICE

Community Advocacy and Coordination

- *Reducing the Risk of Sudden Infant Death Syndrome* (booklet), American Academy of Pediatrics (www.aap.org/bookstore).

Engaging Patient and Family

- *SIDS: Important Information for Parents* (fact sheet), American Academy of Pediatrics (www.aap.org/bookstore).

RELATED WEB SITE

- First Candle (firstcandle.org).

AAP POLICY STATEMENTS

American Academy of Pediatrics, Committee on Fetus and Newborn. Apnea, sudden infant death syndrome, and home monitoring. *Pediatrics.* 2003;111:914-917. (aappolicy.aappublications.org/cgi/content/full/pediatrics;111/4/914).

American Academy of Pediatrics, Task Force on Infant Sleep Position and Sudden Infant Death Syndrome. Changing concepts of sudden infant death syndrome: implications for infant sleeping environment and sleep position. *Pediatrics.* 2000;105: 650-656. (aappolicy.aappublications.org/cgi/content/full/pediatrics;105/3/650).

American Academy of Pediatrics, Task Force on Sudden Infant Death Syndrome. The changing concept of sudden infant death syndrome: diagnostic coding shifts, controversies regarding the sleeping environment, and new variables to consider in reducing risk. *Pediatrics.* 2005;116: 1245-1255. (aappolicy.aappublications.org/cgi/content/full/pediatrics;116/5/1245).

REFERENCES

1. Willinger M, James LS, Catz C. Defining the sudden infant death syndrome (SIDS): deliberations of an expert panel convened by the National Institute of Child Health and Human Development. *Pediatr Pathol.* 1991;11:677-684.
2. Kattwinkel J, Brooks J, Myerberg D, American Academy of Pediatrics, Task Force on Infant Positioning and SIDS. Positioning and SIDS [Erratum in: *Pediatrics.* 1992;90(2 pt 1):264]. *Pediatrics.* 1992;89(6):1120-1126.
3. National Infant Sleep Position. Back to Sleep. Available at: dccwww.bumc.bu.edu/ChimeNisp/Main_Nisp.asp. Accessed November 2, 2004.
4. Kochanek KD, Murphy SL, Anderson RN, et al. Deaths: final data for 2002. *Natl Vital Stat Rep.* 2004;53(5):1-115.
5. Mathews TJ, Menacker F, MacDorman MF. Infant mortality statistics from the 2002 period: linked birth/infant death data set. *Natl Vital Stat Rep.* 2004;53(10):1-29.
6. Panigraphy A, Filiano J, Sleeper LA, et al. Decreased serotonergic receptor binding in rhombic lip-derived regions of the medulla oblongata in the sudden infant death syndrome. *J Neuropathol Exp Neurol.* 2000;59(5):377-384.
7. Narita N, Narita M, Takashima S, et al. Serotonin transporter gene variation is a risk factor for sudden infant death syndrome in the Japanese population. *Pediatrics.* 2001;107(4):690-692.
8. Weese-Mayer DE, Berry-Kravis EM, Maher BS, et al. Sudden infant death syndrome: association with a promoter polymorphism of the serotonin transporter gene. *Am J Med Genet.* 2003;117A(3):268-274.
9. Dwyer T, Ponsonby A-L, Blizzard L, et al. The contribution of changes in the prevalence of prone sleeping position to the decline in sudden infant death syndrome in Tasmania. *JAMA.* 1995;273(10):783-789.
10. Fleming P, Gilbert R, Azaz Y, et al. Interaction between bedding and sleeping position in the sudden infant death syndrome: a population based case-control study. *BMJ.* 1990;301:85-89.
11. Kemp JS, Kowalski RM, Burch PM, et al. Unintentional suffocation by rebreathing: a death scene and physiologic investigation of a possible cause of sudden infant death. *J Pediatr.* 1993;122:874-880.
12. Kemp Js, Thach BT. Sudden death in infants sleeping on polystyrene-filled cushions. *N Engl J Med.* 1991;324: 1858-1864.
13. Markestad T, Skadberg B, Hordvik E, et al. Sleeping position and sudden infant death syndrome (SIDS): effect of an intervention programme to avoid prone sleeping. *Acta Paediatr.* 1995;84:375-378.
14. Nelson EAS, Taylor BJ, Weatherall IL. Sleeping position and infant bedding may predispose to hyperthermia and the sudden infant death syndrome. *Lancet.* 1989;1(8631): 199-200.
15. Ponsonby A-L, Dwyer T, Gibbons LE, et al. Factors potentiating the risk of sudden infant death syndrome associated with the prone position. *N Engl J Med.* 1993; 329:377-382.
16. Skadberg BT, Markestad T. Consequences of getting the head covered during sleep in infancy. *Pediatrics.* 1997; 100(2):E6.
17. Southall DP, Plunkett MCB, Banks M, et al. Covert video recordings of life-threatening child abuse: lessons for child protection. *Pediatrics.* 1997;100(5):735-760.

18. Steinschneider A. Prolonged apnea and the sudden infant death syndrome: clinical and laboratory observations. *Pediatrics*. 1972;50:646-654.
19. Firstman R, Talan J. *The Death of Innocents: A True Story of Murder, Medicine, and High-Stakes Science*. New York, NY: Bantam Books; 1997.
20. Levene S, Bacon CJ. Sudden unexpected death and covert homicide in infancy. *Arch Dis Child*. 2004;89(5): 443-447.
21. Oyen N, Skjaerven R, Irgens LM. Population-based recurrence risk of sudden infant death syndrome compared with other infant and fetal deaths. *Am J Epidemiol*. 1996;144(3):300-305.
22. Malloy MH, MacDorman M. Changes in the classification of sudden unexpected infant deaths: United States, 1992-2001. *Pediatrics*. 2005;115(5):1247-1253.
23. Choidini BA, Thach BT. Impaired ventilation in infants sleeping facedown: potential significance for sudden infant death syndrome. *J Pediatr*. 1993;123:686-692.
24. Fleming PJ, Blair PS, Bacon C, et al. Environment of infants during sleep and risk of the sudden infant death syndrome: results of 1993-1995 case-control study for confidential inquiry into stillbirths and deaths in infancy. Confidential Enquiry into Stillbirths and Deaths Regional Coordinators and Researchers. *BMJ*. 1996;313(7051): 191-195.
25. Hoffman HJ, Damus K, Hillman L, et al. Risk factors for SIDS. Results of the National Institute of Child Health and Human Development SIDS Cooperative Epidemiological Study. *Ann N Y Acad Sci*. 1988;533:13-30.
26. Hoffman HJ, Hillman LS. Epidemiology of the sudden infant death syndrome: maternal, neonatal, and postneonatal risk factors. *Clin Perinatol*. 1992;19(4):717-737.
27. Kemp JS, Nelson VE, Thach BT. Physical properties of bedding that may increase risk of sudden infant death syndrome in prone-sleeping infants. *Pediatr Res*. 1994; 36(1):7-11.
28. Schoendorf KC, Kiely JL. Relationship of sudden infant death syndrome to maternal smoking during and after pregnancy. *Pediatrics*. 1992;90(6):905-908.
29. MacDorman MF, Cnattingius S, Hoffman HJ, et al. Sudden infant death syndrome and smoking in the United States and Sweden. *Am J Epidemiol*. 1997;146(3):249-257.
30. Malloy MH, Hoffman HJ. Prematurity, sudden infant death syndrome, and age of death. *Pediatrics*. 1995;96 (3 pt 1):464-471.
31. Hoyert DL, Arias E, Smith BL, et al. Deaths: final data for 1999. *Natl Vital Stat Rep*. 2001;49(8):1-113.
32. Mathews TJ, MacDorman MF, Menacker F. Infant mortality statistics from the 1999 period linked birth/infant death data set. *Natl Vital Stat Rep*. 2002;50(12):1-28.
33. Hauck FR, Moore CM, Herman SM, et al. The contribution of prone sleeping position to the racial disparity in sudden infant death syndrome: the Chicago Infant Mortality Study. *Pediatrics*. 2002;110(4):772-780.
34. Li DK, Petitti DB, Willinger M, et al. Infant sleeping position and the risk of sudden infant death syndrome in California, 1997-2000. *Am J Epidemiol*. 2003;157(5): 446-455.
35. Mitchell EA, Tuohy PG, Brunt JM, et al. Risk factors for sudden infant death syndrome following the prevention campaign in New Zealand: a prospective study. *Pediatrics*. 1997;100(5):835-840.
36. Oyen N, Markestad T, Skjaerven R, et al. Combined effects of sleeping position and prenatal risk factors in sudden infant death syndrome: the Nordic epidemiological SIDS study. *Pediatrics*. 1997;100(4):613-621.
37. Waters KA, Gonzalez A, Jean C, et al. Face-straight-down and face-near-straight-down positions in healthy, prone-sleeping infants. *J Pediatr*. 1996;128:616-625.
38. Willinger M, Hoffman HJ, Wu K-T, et al. Factors associated with the transition to nonprone sleep positions of infants in the United States: the National Infant Sleep Position Study. *JAMA*. 1998;280:329-335.
39. Mitchell EA, Thach BT, Thompson JMD, et al. Changing infants' sleep position increases risk of sudden infant death syndrome. *Arch Pediatr Adolesc Med*. 1999;153: 1136-1141.
40. Brooke H, Gibson A, Tappin D, et al. Case-control study of sudden infant death syndrome in Scotland, 1992-1995. *BMJ*. 1997;314(7093):1516-1520.
41. Mitchell EA, Thompson JMD, Ford RPK, et al. Sheepskin bedding and the sudden infant death syndrome. New Zealand Cot Death Study Group. *J Pediatr*. 1998;133:701-704.
42. Ponsonby A-L, Dwyer T, Couper D, et al. Association between use of a quilt and sudden infant death syndrome: case-control study. *BMJ*. 1998;316:195-196.
43. Scheers NJ, Dayton CM, Kemp JS. Sudden infant death with external airways covered: case-comparison study of 206 deaths in the United States. *Arch Pediatr Adolesc Med*. 1998;152:540-547.
44. Hauck FR, Herman SM, Donovan M, et al. Sleep environment and the risk of sudden infant death syndrome in an urban population: the Chicago Infant Mortality Study. *Pediatrics*. 2003;111(5 pt 2):1207-1214.
45. Flick L, White DK, Vemulapalli C, et al. Sleep position and the use of soft bedding during bed sharing among African American infants at increased risk for sudden infant death syndrome. *J Pediatr*. 2001;138:338-343.
46. Kemp JS, Livne M, White DK, et al. Softness and potential to cause rebreathing: differences in bedding used by infants at high and low risk for sudden infant death syndrome. *J Pediatr*. 1998;132:234-239.
47. Scheers NJ, Rutherford GW, Kemp JS. Where should infants sleep? A comparison of risk for suffocation of infants sleeping in cribs, adult beds, and other sleeping locations. *Pediatrics*. 2003;112(4):883-889.
48. Haglund B. Cigarette smoking and sudden infant death syndrome: some salient points in the debate. *Acta Paediatr Suppl*. 1993;82(suppl 389):37-39.
49. Mitchell EA, Milerad J. Smoking and Sudden Infant Death Syndrome. WFO/TFI Reports 1999. Available at: tobacco.who.int/en/health/background-papers-ets.html. Accessed July 12, 2007.
50. Ponsonby A-L, Dwyer T, Gibbons LE, et al. Thermal environment and sudden infant death syndrome: case-control study. *BMJ*. 1992;304:277-282.
51. Blair PS, Ward Platt M, Smith IJ, et al. Sudden infant death syndrome and sleeping position in pre-term and low birthweight infants: an opportunity for targeted intervention. *Arch Dis Child*. 2006;91:101-106.
52. McKenna JJ, Mosko S, Richard CA. Bedsharing promotes breastfeeding. *Pediatrics*. 1997;100(2):214-219.
53. Mosko S, Richard C, McKenna J. Infant arousals during mother-infant bed sharing: implications for infant sleep and sudden infant death syndrome research. *Pediatrics*. 1997;100(5):841-849.
54. Carpenter RG, Irgens LM, Blair PS, et al. Sudden unexplained infant death in 20 regions in Europe: case control study. *Lancet*. 2004;363:185-191.
55. Tappin D, Ecob R, Brooke H. Bedsharing and sudden infant death syndrome in Scotland: a case control study. *J Pediatr*. 2005;147(9413):32-37.
56. Carpenter RG, Waite A, Coombs RC, et al. Repeat sudden unexpected and unexplained infant deaths: natural or unnatural? *Lancet*. 2005;365(9453):29-35.
57. McGarvey C, McDonnell M, Chong A, et al. Factors relating to the infant's last sleep environment in sudden infant death syndrome in the Republic of Ireland. *Arch Dis Child*. 2003;88(12):1058-1064.

58. Blair PS, Fleming PJ, Smith IJ, et al. Babies sleeping with parents: case-control study of factors influencing the risk of the sudden infant death syndrome. CESDI SUDI research group. *BMJ*. 1999;319(7223):1457-1462.
59. Scragg R, Mitchell EA, Taylor BJ, et al. Bed sharing, smoking, and alcohol in the sudden infant death syndrome. New Zealand Cot Death Study Group. *BMJ*. 1993;307(6915):1312-1318.
60. Arnestad M, Andersen M, Rognum TO. Is the use of dummy or carry-cot of importance for sudden infant death? *Eur J Pediatr*. 1997;156:968-970.
61. Fleming PJ, Blair PS, Pollard K, et al. Pacifier use and sudden infant death syndrome: results from the CESDI/SUDI case control study. CESDI SUDI Research Team. *Arch Dis Child*. 1999;81:112-116.
62. L'Hoir MP, Engleberts AC, van Well GTJ, et al. Dummy use, thumb sucking, mouth breathing and cot death. *Eur J Pediatr*. 1999;158:896-901.
63. Mitchell EA, Taylor BJ, Ford RPK, et al. Dummies and the sudden infant death syndrome. *Arch Dis Child*. 1993;68:501-504.
64. Tappin D, Brooke H, Ecob R, et al. Used infant mattresses and sudden infant death syndrome in Scotland: case-control study. *BMJ*. 2002;325:1007-1012.
65. Hauck FR, Omojokun OO, Siadaty MS. Do pacifiers reduce the risk of sudden infant death syndrome? A meta-analysis. *Pediatrics*. 2005;116(5):e716-723.
66. Mitchell EA, Blair PS, L'Hoir MP. Should pacifiers be recommended to prevent SIDS? *Pediatrics*. 2006;117(5):1755-1758.
67. Howard CR, Howard FM, Lanphear B, et al. Randomized clinical trial of pacifier use and bottle-feeding or cupfeeding and their effect on breastfeeding. *Pediatrics*. 2003;111:511-518.
68. Ward SL, Keens TG, Chan LS, et al. Sudden infant death syndrome in infants evaluated by apnea programs in California. *Pediatrics*. 1986;77(4):451-458.
69. Ramanathan R, Corwin MJ, Hunt CE, et al. Cardiorespiratory events recorded on home monitors: comparison of healthy infants with those at increased risk for SIDS. *JAMA*. 2001;285(17):2199-2207.
70. Hodgman JE, Hoppenbrouwers T. Home monitoring for the sudden infant death syndrome. The case against. *Ann N Y Acad Sci*. 1988;533:164-175.
71. Monod N, Plouin P, Sternberg B, et al. Are polygraphic and cardiopneumographic respiratory patterns useful tools for predicting the risk for sudden infant death syndrome? A 10-year study. *Biol Neonate*. 1986;50(3):147-153.
72. Kattwinkel J, Hauck FR, Keenan ME, et al, American Academy of Pediatrics, Task Force on Sudden Infant Death Syndrome. The changing concept of sudden infant death syndrome: diagnostic coding shifts, controversies regarding the sleeping environment, and new variables to consider in reducing risk. *Pediatrics*. 2005;116(5):1245-1255.
73. Argenta LC, David LR, Wilson JA, et al. An increase in infant cranial deformity with supine sleeping position. *J Craniofacial Surg*. 1996;7(1):5-11.
74. Kane AA, Mitchell LE, Craven KP, et al. Observations on a recent increase in plagiocephaly without synostosis. *Pediatrics*. 1996;97(6):877-885.
75. Persing J, James H, Swanson J, et al. Prevention and management of positional skull deformities in infants. *Pediatrics*. 2003;112(1 pt 1):199-202.
76. Hutchison BL, Thompson JM, Mitchell EA. Determinants of nonsynostotic plagiocephaly: a case-control study. *Pediatrics*. 2003;112(4):e316.
77. Hunt L, Fleming P, Golding J. Does the supine sleeping position have any adverse effects on the child? I. Health in the first six months. The ALSPAC Study Team. *Pediatrics*. 1997;100(1):E11.
78. Pickens DL, Schefft GL, Thach BT. Pharyngeal fluid clearance and aspiration preventive mechanisms in sleeping infants. *J Appl Physiol* 1989;66(3):1164-1171.

Chapter 331

TONSILLECTOMY AND ADENOIDECTOMY

Louis G. Petcu, MD, MS; Ian Scott Goodman, MD; James J. Burns, MD

Tonsillectomy and adenoidectomy are 2 of the most common surgical procedures performed on children worldwide over the last several decades. From the 1st century to modern times, the use of medical and surgical treatments for adenotonsillar disease has varied significantly.[1] Improvement in diagnostic techniques and medical therapy of adenotonsillar disease, along with questions about proper indications for surgery, has led to a gradual de-emphasis of tonsillectomy and adenoidectomy as primary therapy.

A consensus is just beginning to emerge regarding the proper indications for these procedures.

DIAGNOSIS AND INDICATIONS

Obstructive Sleep Apnea

In his book, *The Pickwick Papers*, published in 1836, author Charles Dickens introduced a character with a collection of symptoms that included the uncanny ability to fall asleep in any situation (indeed, the inability to remain awake unless in constant motion), obesity, snoring, and unexplained behavioral changes. Over 100 years later, Burwell et al first used the term *pickwickian* to describe an alveolar hypoventilation syndrome associated with obesity.[2] However, only a minority of persons with physical features consistent with this description have waking hypoxia or hypercapnia, or both; the remainder have symptoms that likely result from disrupted sleep patterns.

Clinical practice guidelines published by the American Academy of Pediatrics in 2002 define obstructive sleep apnea syndrome (OSAS) as "a disorder of breathing during sleep characterized by prolonged partial upper airway obstruction and/or intermittent complete obstruction (obstructive apnea) that disrupts normal ventilation and sleep patterns."[3] Patients with this problem demonstrate nighttime snoring, respiratory pauses, snorts, or gasps. The quality of sleep is thought to lead to emotional problems and increased school difficulties, including deficits in memory, vocabulary, and learning.[4] Severe and untreated airway obstruction may contribute to growth failure and the development of cor pulmonale.[5]

Enlargement of adenoids and tonsils are a common cause of obstructive sleep apnea. Additionally OSAS can also be found in children who have obesity, genetic syndromes, neuromuscular disorders, and abnormalities of the oropharynx.

The guidelines recommend obtaining a history of snoring in the routine clinical assessment of all children at each visit. Although the history and physical examination are useful screening tools, they are not reliable for diagnosis or for recommending intervention.[6] Approximately 10% of the population has benign primary snoring, whereas only approximately 2% of children have true obstructive sleep apnea. Thus additional diagnostic testing is needed in the habitually snoring child before proceeding with surgical intervention. However, referring all children who have snoring as the only symptom for further testing is impractical. Approximately 40% of children who display a combination of snoring and other symptoms (mouth breathing, adenoid facies, hyponasal speech, tonsillar enlargement) have OSAS[4,7,8] and should be referred for further testing (Box 331-1). Additionally, further testing should be strongly considered in snoring children who are struggling academically or are being evaluated for hyperactivity.

The gold standard of tests used to diagnose OSAS accurately is the nocturnal polysomnogram (Figure 331-1). Polysomnography is useful to identify patients who are at risk for adverse outcomes, to avoid unnecessary intervention in patients who are not at risk for adverse outcomes, and to evaluate which patients are at risk of complications resulting from adenotonsillectomy so that appropriate precautions can be taken. Overnight pulse oximetry, unsupervised home study, and nap studies are diagnostic if positive results are obtained, but they are not sensitive enough to rule out OSAS. Thus, when these test results are negative, the patient should be referred for polysomnography. If positive, then the patient should be referred for surgery (Figure 331-2). Reviewing home audiotaping or videotaping has insufficient specificity to be useful diagnostic tools. Studies looking at the cost effectiveness of using abbreviated testing modalities are lacking.

BOX 331-1 Evaluation of Patients With Snoring and Obstructive Symptoms

High-risk patient:
- Cardiac disease
- Peritonsillar abscess
- Craniofacial anomalies (including mandibular hypoplasia or macroglossia)
- Trisomy 21 syndrome
- Cerebral palsy
- Neuromuscular disease
- Chronic lung disease
- Sickle cell disease
- Central hypoventilation syndromes
- Genetic, metabolic, or storage diseases

From American Academy of Pediatrics, Section on Pediatric Pulmonology, Subcommittee on Obstructive Sleep Apnea Syndrome. Clinical practice guideline: diagnosis and management of childhood obstructive sleep apnea syndrome. *Pediatrics*. 2002;109(4):704-712.

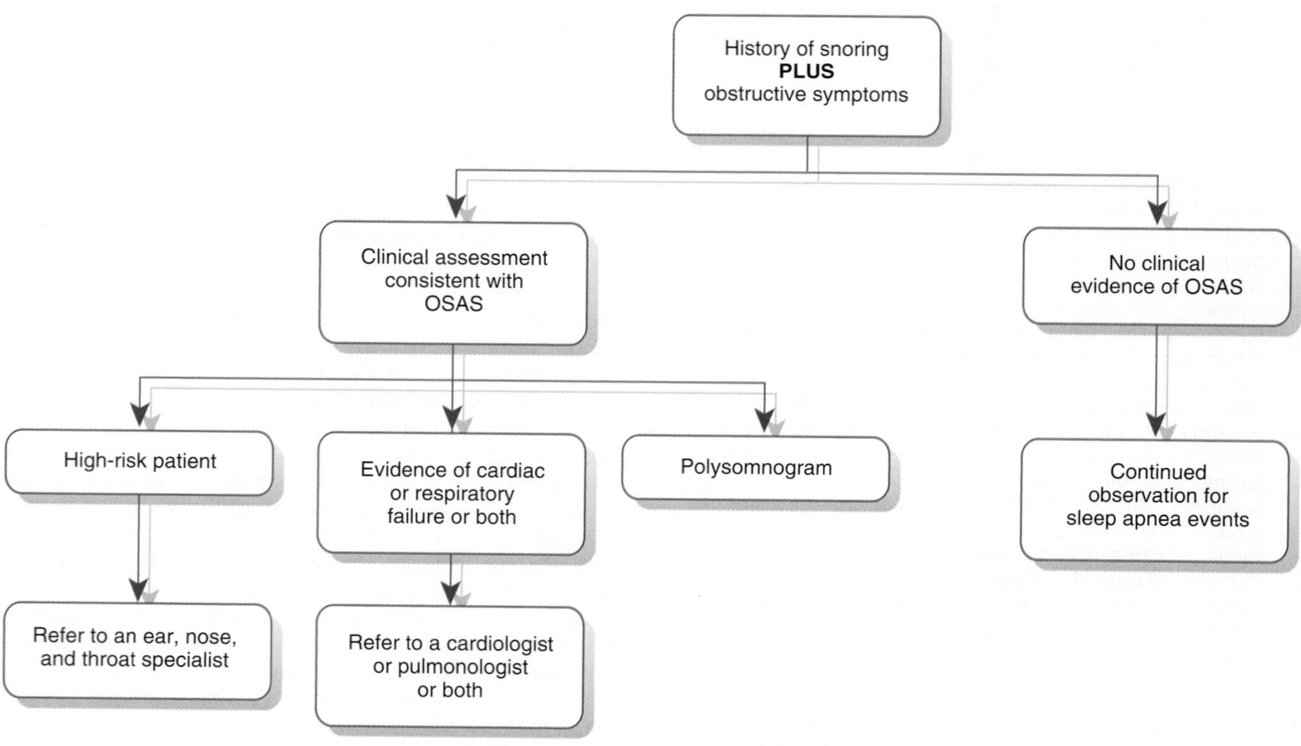

Figure 331-1 Logical approach for the evaluation and management of OSAS.

The vast majority of patients with OSAS will have clinical resolution of symptoms and normalization of polysomnography after a adenotonsillectomy. Obese children and those with neuromuscular weakness, craniofacial anomalies, and severe OSAS are less likely to have complete resolution of sleep abnormalities after an adenotonsillectomy and warrant restudies postoperatively. Some patients have significant improvement after adenotonsillectomy despite negative polysomnograms.[9] These patients may respond to treatment with montelukast or nasal steroids[10] More controlled trials are needed to delineate adequate criteria for recommending surgery in patients with negative polysomnograms.

Tonsillitis

Many children with recurrent tonsillitis are referred for tonsillectomy (Figure 331-3). The criteria for recommending this surgery have been the subject of significant controversy in the medical literature. The *Cochrane Database of Systematic Reviews* states that the "effectiveness of tonsillectomy has not been formally evaluated" and that "further trials addressing relevant outcome measures are required."[11] The American Academy of Otolaryngology supports surgery in patients with 3 or more infections of tonsils or adenoids per year.[12]

Paradise studied children severely affected by recurrent pharyngitis. The inclusion criteria for this study are now known as the Pittsburgh criteria (Box 331-2). The children who had tonsillectomy had consistently lower throat infection rates than the observation group, especially in relation to episodes rated moderate or severe. After 1 year, the surgical group had a 14-fold reduction in throat infections episodes rated as moderate or severe; after 2 years, a 6-fold reduction occurred. In addition, sore throat days and sore throat–associated school absences were reported more often for individuals who were treated nonsurgically. Despite the better outcomes in the surgical group, rates of having more than 1 moderate or severe infection in the control group in the subsequent follow-up years were relatively low (year 1: 26%; year 2: 24%; and year 3: 5%). Therefore the conclusion might be made that this

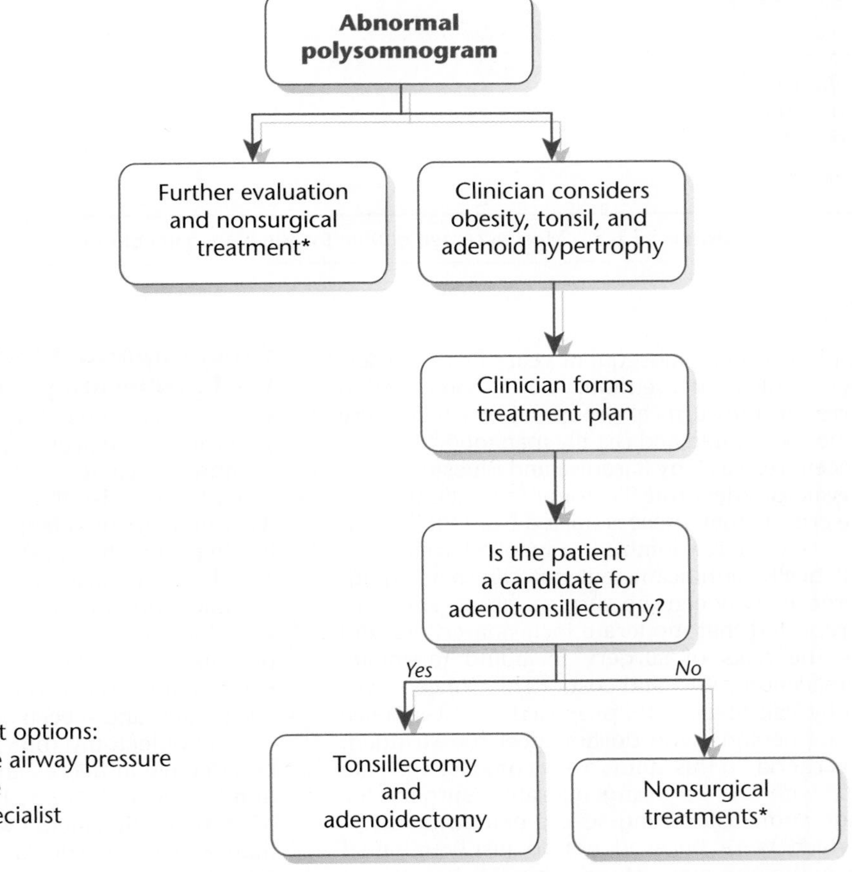

Figure 331-2 Management of patients after abnormal polysomnography. *(American Academy of Pediatrics, Section on Pediatric Pulmonology, Subcommittee on Obstructive Sleep Apnea Syndrome. Technical report: diagnosis and management of childhood obstructive sleep apnea syndrome.* Pediatrics. *2002;109(4):e69.*

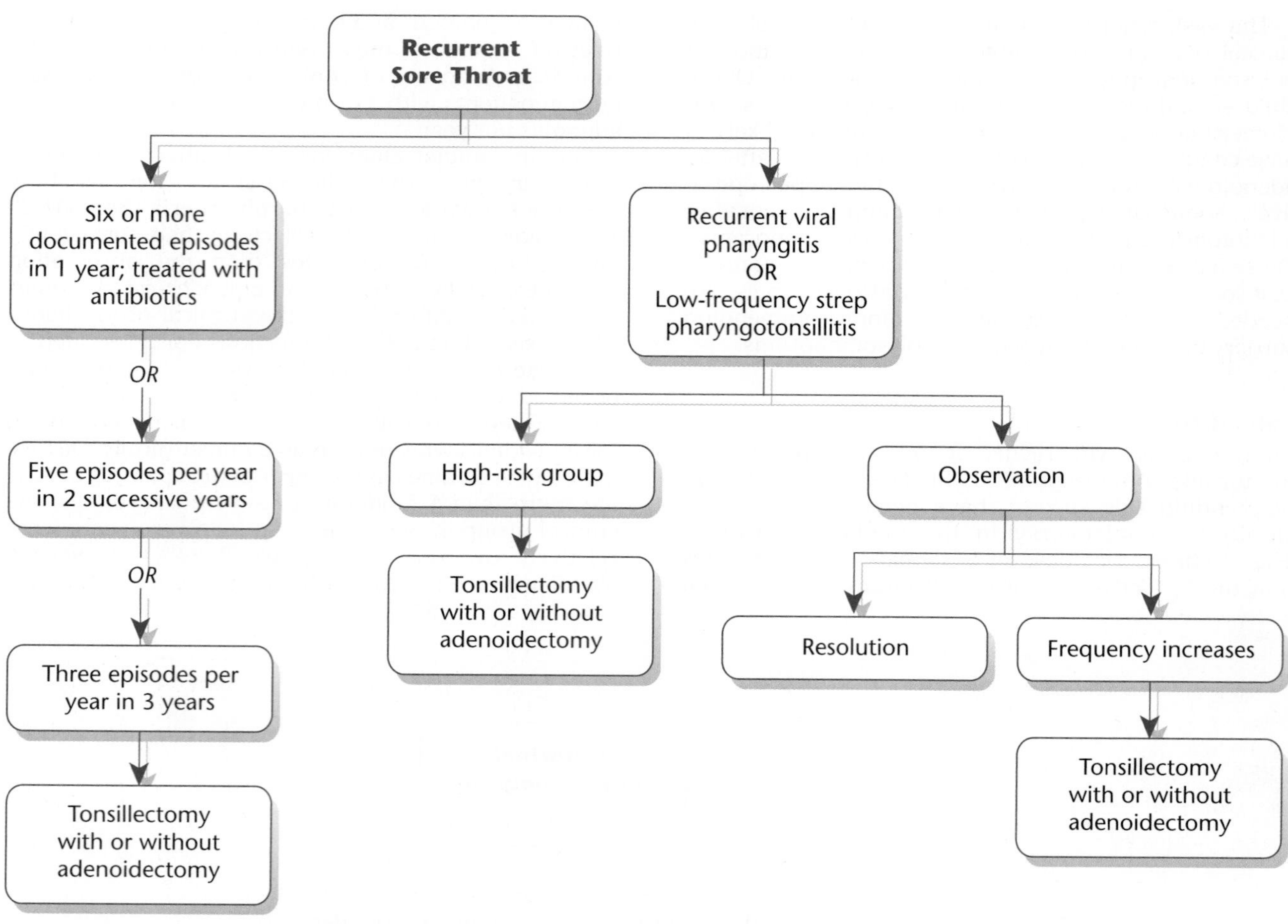

Figure 331-3 Most accepted outline for the management of recurrent sore throat.

low rate of infection in subsequent years favors observation over surgical intervention. A 14% complication rate occurred in the surgical group, all of which were judged to be self-limited and readily managed.[5]

More recent research by Paradise and Bluestone analyzes the issue of adenotonsillectomy for patients with less severe criteria than those reported from their original study. Using a randomized controlled trial, they found statistically significant, but *not clinically* significant, differences between the surgical group and controls and reported that moderate inclusion criteria did not justify the risks of surgery including morbidity (7.9% complication rates) and cost.[13] This concept was supported by Van Staaij, who proposed a wait-and-see approach for persons who do not meet the stringent Pittsburgh criteria. In this study, a 4% complication rate was noted, with 1% requiring operative surgery for hemorrhage and 2.6% having severe nausea or dehydration, which were believed not to justify minimal reductions in the frequency of tonsillitis.[14,15] Because of the cost and complications associated with surgery, most experts recommend surgery only for patients with recurrent pharyngitis who meet the stringent Pittsburgh criteria.[13-15]

Other Important Indications for Tonsillectomy and Adenoidectomy

Clear indications for tonsillectomy are recurrent peritonsillar abscess, infectious mononucleosis with immunodeficiency, malignancy—which should be thought to exist if lymphadenopathy is larger than 3 centimeters or splenomegaly with asymmetric tonsillar hypertrophy—and hemorrhagic tonsillitis. These conditions are also uncommon.[1,16]

Indications for adenoidectomy are not well studied and include chronic otitis media with effusion if pressure-equalization (PE) tubes have to be reinserted,[17] significant nasal obstruction, recurrent sinusitis, chronic adenoiditis, and speech or orthognathic issues.

Adenoidectomy (but not tonsillectomy) appears to be effective in decreasing the rate of PE tube reinsertion.[18] Adenoidectomy has a limited role in treatment of chronic otitis media with effusion for children older than 4 years, particularly if nasal obstruction, recurrent sinusitis, or chronic sinusitis are present.[19-24] Finally, adenoidectomy does not reduce the incidence of recurrent acute otitis media when performed in conjunction with insertion of PE tubes for children younger than 4 years.[24]

BOX 331-2 Selection of Recurrent Tonsillitis Patients for Tonsillectomy With or Without Adenoidectomy (Pittsburgh Criteria)

Requires documenting 1 of the following clinical features:
- Temperature more than 38.3° C (101° F)
- Tender cervical lymphadenopathy (>2 cm)
- Tonsillar exudate
- Positive cultures

PLUS antibiotics for proven or possible streptococcal infection

High-risk patient:
- Cardiac disease
- Peritonsillar abscess
- Craniofacial anomalies
- Trisomy 21 syndrome
- Cerebral palsy
- Neuromuscular disease
- Chronic lung disease
- Sickle cell disease
- Central hypoventilation syndromes
- Genetic, metabolic, or storage diseases

From Paradise JL, Bluestone CD, Bachman RZ, et al. Efficacy of tonsillectomy for recurrent throat infection in severely affected children. Results of parallel randomized and nonrandomized clinical trials. *N Engl J Med.* Mar 1984;15;310(11):674-683.

PROCEDURES

Although the technique for adenoidectomy remains blunt curettage with a ring curette or vaporization using an electrocautery device, various techniques for tonsillectomy have evolved over the last several years. The objective in developing new techniques is to devise a surgical approach that can be performed with fewer complications in an ambulatory surgery setting and with less postoperative pain.

Dissection and snare tonsillectomy is the traditional technique, as practiced by otolaryngologists for the last 75 years. The procedure involves blunt dissection of the tonsillar capsule from the adherent pharyngeal constrictor muscle, working from the superior to the inferior pole of the tonsil. Blunt dissection causes stretching and avulsion of the small tonsillar arteries, causing arterial spasm and subsequent hemostasis. Although the procedure has been proven as safe, it has been virtually abandoned by otolaryngologists because of the relatively large amount of intraoperative blood loss that this technique produces.

Electrocautery is currently the most common and popular technique for tonsillectomy. It is safe and rapid, and it has the potential for little or no blood loss. Dissection is conducted in a manner similar to the dissection and snare technique (Figure 331-4 and Figure 331-5). Minimal additional safety precautions are required to prevent inadvertent injury to the patient. The equipment is relatively inexpensive and widely available. It has the disadvantage of higher postoperative pain because of thermal injury to the underlying constrictor muscle and a delayed return to normal diet.

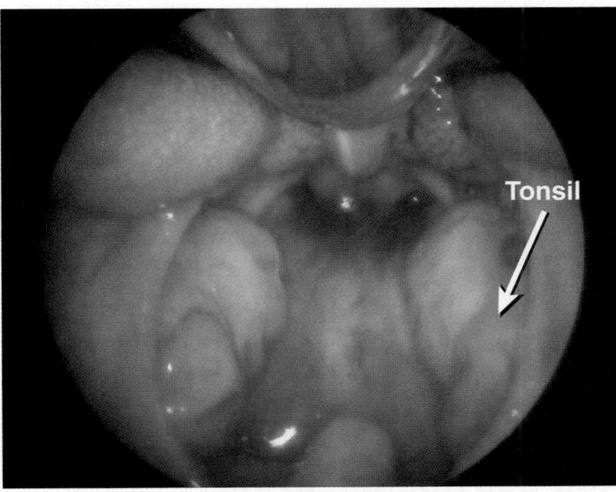

Figure 331-4 Operative field prepared for electrocautery tonsillectomy.

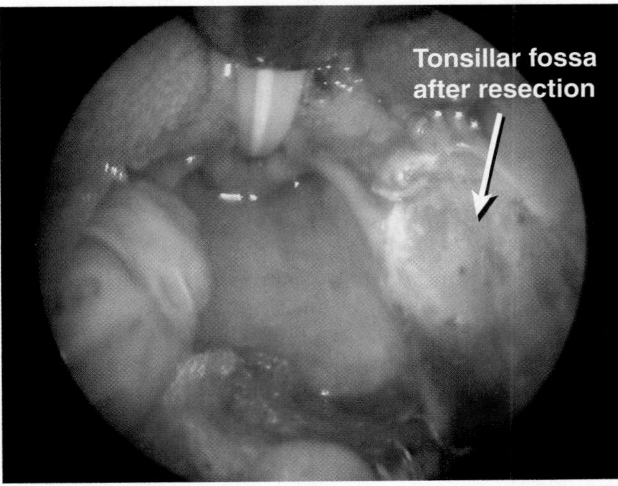

Figure 331-5 Tonsil completely removed from the pharyngeal constrictor.

Surgical lasers have been used in tonsillectomy for the last 2 decades. The oropharynx and tonsils are easily accessible with laser handpieces used in either illumination (thermocoagulation) or contact (vaporization) modes. The advantages to using lasers include less superior pharyngeal constrictor muscle injury, better hemostasis, and less pain when compared with the more popular electrocautery technique. Lasers have the distinct disadvantage of requiring special and extensive precautions to avoid injury to the patient or operating room staff by reflected or misdirected laser light.

Extracapsular tonsillectomy involves using traditional or powered instrumentation to remove 90% to

95% of the tonsil tissue medial to the tonsillar capsule. The rationale is that decreased injury to the pharyngeal constrictor muscle will yield decreased postoperative pain. This technique is frequently accomplished with the use of a microdebrider. Harmonic scalpel tonsillectomy involves using ultrasound to disrupt and coagulate tissues at a lower temperature than that encountered with laser or electrocautery.

In radio-frequency tonsillectomy, radio-frequency energy is applied directly to tissues to generate heat, vaporizing tonsillar tissue. This technique was associated with less postoperative pain and a faster return to normal diet when compared with electrocautery[25] or dissection tonsillectomy.[26]

COMPLICATIONS AND CONTRAINDICATIONS

Complications

Life-threatening complications in tonsillectomy and adenoidectomy are rare and generally produce a catastrophic hemorrhagic and respiratory complication (Table 331-1). Mortality rates after tonsillectomy have been difficult to estimate because death is a very rare outcome of this procedure. Postmortem examinations have indicated that death generally occurs from aspiration of blood into the lungs and not from exsanguination. Therefore, during an acute and catastrophic bleeding event, if the patient can be intubated and the airway protected, then the mortality decreases dramatically. The estimated mortality rate in England was 1:10,000 (1945 to 1965),[27] 1:10,000 (1957 to 1961),[28] 1:16,000 (1961 to 1969), and 1:35,000 (1970s).[29] This improvement in mortality is probably attributed to improved anesthesia, monitoring equipment, medications, and preparation for hemorrhagic consequences. As anesthetic and surgical techniques and medications continue to evolve and improve, this mortality rate will likely be further reduced.

A relatively common complication of tonsillectomy and adenoidectomy is minor postoperative bleeding, which is thought to occur at a frequency of 1% to 2% of all cases in the United States.[30] Postoperative hemorrhage can be divided into 2 groups. The immediate postoperative hemorrhage occurs within 24 hours of the tonsillectomy or adenoidectomy and is generally thought to be related to surgical technique. The 2nd form of posttonsillectomy bleeding occurs without identifiable cause and is delayed; it occurs approximately 1 to 2 weeks after surgery. Postoperative airway obstruction occurs mainly in the child younger than 3 years. In most cases, this complication is caused by edema of the palate, tongue, or lateral pharynx. High-risk patients with preexisting craniofacial deformities, obesity, and neuromuscular disorders should be identified preoperatively and observed closely in the postoperative period. Occasionally, patients with severe OSAS will exhibit postoperative, postobstructive pulmonary edema or central apnea. Other rare complications of tonsillectomy include Grisel syndrome (atlantoaxial subluxation—more common in trisomy 21 syndrome),[31] Lemierre syndrome (parapharyngeal infection with internal jugular vein thrombosis),[32] and posttonsillectomy taste distortion.[33]

Patients at high risk for complications postoperatively who require special attention in maintaining airway include infants and patients with craniofacial disorders, trisomy 21 syndrome, cerebral palsy, neuromuscular disorders, chronic lung disease, sickle cell disease, central hypoventilation syndromes, obesity, and genetic or metabolic storage diseases.[4]

Contraindications

The relative contraindications for tonsillectomy and adenoidectomy include cleft palate or submucous cleft palate because these patients are at risk for velopharyngeal insufficiency. Clinicians should evaluate for the presence of a bifid uvula or a notched hard palate as clues to making this diagnosis preoperatively. In

Table 331-1 Posttonsillectomy and Adenoidectomy Complications

COMPLICATION	ONSET	PRESENTATION	TREATMENT
Immediate hemorrhage	<24 hr	Oral bleeding Hemoptysis Hematemesis	Exploration and ligation of blood vessel
Delayed hemorrhage	5-14 days	Oral bleeding Hemoptysis Hematemesis	Ice pack to neck and iced liquids Elevation of head and neck $AgNO_3$ cautery Blood vessel ligation Coagulopathy work-up
Immediate airway compromise	Extubation—2 hr	Cyanosis Stridor	Rule out pulmonary edema Rule out aspiration Rule out laryngospasm
Delayed airway compromise	2-24 hr	Shortness of breath Stridor	Intravenous or oral steroid Nasopharyngeal airway
Dehydration	1-6 days	Lethargy Tachycardia Anuria	Intravenous rehydration Pain control Parent education

$AgNO_3$, Silver nitrate.

addition, severe bleeding disorders should be given special consideration (see Chapter 271, Hemophilia and Other Hereditary Bleeding Disorders).

IMPACT OF ADENOTONSILLAR DISEASE ON QUALITY OF LIFE

Objective review of the literature demonstrates a relative lack of randomized, blinded studies evaluating the effectiveness of adenoidectomy and tonsillectomy for OSAS and recurrent tonsillitis. Attention has therefore been recently directed at quality-of-life measurements. Using the Child Health Questionnaire to measure the quality of life for children with adenotonsillar disease, scores shows similar quality-of-life indices for children with adenotonsillar disease and children with juvenile rheumatoid arthritis.[34] This finding suggests a significant effect of adenotonsillar disease on quality of life. Additionally, upper airway obstruction and sleep disorders have been postulated to contribute to behavioral problems and diminution of intellectual skills.[35]

Polysomnography and parental questionnaires assessing sleep disturbance, growth, breathing problems, emotional problems, hyperactivity, aggression, swallowing disorders, speech problems, parental anxiety or concerns, activity limitations, somatization behaviors show significant resolution of these symptoms after adenotonsillectomy.[36,37]

TOOLS FOR PRACTICE

Engaging Patients and Family

- *Sleep Apnea and Your Child* (brochure), American Academy of Pediatrics (patiented.aap.org).
- *Tonsils and the Adenoids* (fact sheet), American Academy of Pediatrics (www.aap.org/pubed/ZZZFVOR0R7C.htm?&sub_cat=107).
- *What is a Pediatric Otolaryngologist* (fact sheet), American Academy of Pediatrics (www.aap.org/sections/sap/he3008.pdf).

Medical Decision Support

- *Clinical Practice Guideline: Diagnosis and Management of Childhood Obstructive Sleep Apnea Syndrome* (guideline), American Academy of Pediatrics (aappolicy.aappublications.org/cgi/content/abstract/pediatrics;109/4/704).

AAP POLICY STATEMENT

American Academy of Pediatrics. Technical report: diagnosis and management of childhood obstructive sleep apnea syndrome. *Pediatrics* 2002;109(4):e69. (aappolicy.aappublications.org/cgi/content/full/pediatrics;109/4/e69).

SUGGESTED RESOURCE

The American Academy of Otolaryngology—Head and Neck Surgery (AAO-HNS). Working for the Best Ear, Nose, and Throat Care. Available at: www.entnet.org.

REFERENCES

1. Discolo CM, Darrow DH, Koltai PJ. Infectious indications for tonsillectomy. *Pediatr Clin North Am.* 2003;50(2):445-458.
2. Burwell CS, Robin ED, Whaley RD. Extreme obesity associated with alveolar hypoventilation: a Pickwickian syndrome. *Am J Med.* 1956;21:811-818.
3. American Academy of Pediatrics, Section on Pediatric Pulmonology, Subcommittee on Obstructive Sleep Apnea Syndrome. Clinical practice guideline: diagnosis and management of childhood obstructive sleep apnea syndrome. *Pediatrics.* 2002;109(4):704-712.
4. Sterni LM, Tunkel DE. Obstructive sleep apnea in children: an update. *Pediatr Clin North Am.* 2003;50:427-443.
5. Paradise JL, Bluestone CD, Bachman RZ, et al. Efficacy of tonsillectomy for recurrent throat infection in severely affected children. Results of parallel randomized and nonrandomized clinical trials. *N Engl J Med.* 1984;310(11):674-683.
6. Suen JS, Arnold JE, Brooks LJ. Adenotonsillectomy for treatment of obstructive sleep apnea in children. *Arch Otolaryngol Head Neck Surg.* 1995;121(4):525-530.
7. Nieminen P, Lopponen T, Tolonen U, et al. Growth and biochemical markers of growth in children with snoring and obstructive sleep apnea. *Pediatrics.* 2002;109(4):e55.
8. Zucconi M, Strambi LF, Pestalozza G, et al. Habitual snoring and obstructive sleep apnea syndrome in children: effects of early tonsil surgery. *Int J Pediatr Otorhinolaryngol.* 1993;26(4):235-243.
9. Goldstein NA, Pugazhendhi V, Rao SM, et al. Clinical assessment of pediatric obstructive sleep apnea. *Pediatrics.* 2004;114(1):33-43.
10. Kheirandish L, Goldbart AD, Gozal D. Intranasal steroids and oral leukotriene modifier therapy in residual sleep-disordered breathing after tonsillectomy and adenoidectomy in children. *Pediatrics.* 2006;117(1):e61-e66.
11. Burton MJ, Towler B, Glasziou P. Tonsillectomy versus nonsurgical treatment for chronic/recurrent acute tonsillitis. *Cochrane Database System Rev.* 2000;2:CD001802.
12. American Academy of Otolaryngology. Head and neck surgery. *Clin Indic Compend.* 2000;19:6.
13. Paradise JL, Bluestone CD, Colborn DK, et al. Tonsillectomy and adenotonsillectomy for recurrent throat infection in moderately affected children. *Pediatrics.* 2002;110(1):7-15.
14. van Staaij BK, van den Akker EH, Rovers MM, et al. Effectiveness of adenotonsillectomy in children with mild symptoms of throat infections or adenotonsillar hypertrophy: open, randomized controlled trial. *BMJ.* 2004;329:651-656.
15. Little PL. Watchful waiting is useful for children with recurrent throat infections. *BMJ.* 2004;329:654.
16. Gigante JG. Tonsillectomy and adenoidectomy. *Pediatr Rev.* 2005;26(6):199-203.
17. American Academy of Family Physicians, American Academy of Otolaryngology—Head and Neck Surgery, American Academy of Pediatrics Subcommittee on Otitis Media With Effusion. Otitis media with effusion. *Pediatrics.* 2004;113(5):1412-1429.
18. Gates GA, Avery CA, Prihoda TJ, et al. Effectiveness of adenoidectomy and tympanostomy tubes in the treatment of chronic otitis media with effusion. *N Engl J Med.* 1987;317:1444-1451.
19. Gates GA, Avery CA, Prihoda TJ. Effect of adenoidectomy on children with chronic otitis media with effusion. *Laryngoscope.* 1988;95:58-63.
20. Paradise JL, Bluestone CD, Rogers KD. Efficacy of adenoidectomy for recurrent otitis media in children previously treated with tympanostomy-tube placement: results of parallel randomized and nonrandomized trials. *JAMA.* 1990;263:2066-2073.
21. Coyte PC, Croxford R, McIsaac W, et al. The role of adjuvant adenoidectomy and tonsillectomy in the outcome of the insertion of tympanostomy tubes. *N Engl J Med.* 2001;344:1188-1195.

22. Paradise JL, Bluestone CD, Colborn DK. Adenoidectomy and adenotonsillectomy for recurrent acute otitis media: parallel, randomized, clinical trials in children not previously treated with tympanostomy tubes. *JAMA*. 1999; 282:945-953.
23. Darrow DH, Siemens C. Indications for tonsillectomy and adenoidectomy. *Laryngoscope*. 2002;112(8 pt 2, suppl 100):6-10.
24. Hammaren-Malmi S, Saxen H, Tarkanen J, et al. Adenoidectomy does not significantly reduce the incidence of otitis media in conjunction with the insertion of tympanostomy tubes in children who are younger than 4 years: a randomized trial. *Pediatrics*. 2005;116(1):185-189.
25. Walner DL. Pediatric tonsillectomy: coblation versus electrocautery. *Otolaryngol Head Neck Surg*. 1999;121: 277-282.
26. Belloso A, Chidambaram A, Morar P. Coblation tonsillectomy versus dissection tonsillectomy. *Laryngoscope*.2003;113:2010-2013.
27. Williams RC. Hemorrhage following tonsillectomy and adenoidectomy in a review of 18,184 operations. *J Laryngol Otol*. 1967;81:805-808.
28. Tate N. Deaths from tonsillectomy. *Lancet*.1963;2:1090-1091.
29. Maw AR. Tonsillectomy today: annotations. *Arch Dis Child*. 1986;61:421-423.
30. Windfuhr JP, Chen YS, Remmert S. Hemorrhage following tonsillectomy and adenoidectomy in 15,218 patients. *Otolaryngol Head Neck Surg*. 2005;132(2):281-286.
31. Hirth K, Welkoborsky HJ. Grisel's syndrome following ENT-surgery: report of two cases. *Laryngothinootolgie*. 2003;82:794-798.
32. Sagowski C, Koch U. Lemierre syndrome; thrombosis of the internal jugular vein after tonsillectomy. *HNO*. 2004; 52:251-254.
33. Goins MR, Pitovski DZ. Posttonsillectomy taste distortion: a significant complication. *Laryngoscope*. 2004;114: 1206-1213.
34. Georgalas C, Tolley N, Kanagalingam J. Measuring quality of life in children with adenotonsillar disease with the child health questionnaire: a first UK study. *Laryngoscope*. 2004;114:1849-1855.
35. Ali N, Pitson D, Stradling J. Snoring, sleep disturbance and behavior in 4-5 year olds. *Arch Dis Child*. 1993;68: 360-366.
36. Lim J, McKean M. Adenotonsillectomy for obstructive sleep apnea in children. *Cochrane Database System Rev*. 2003;1:CD003136.
37. Helfaer MA, McColley SA, Pyzik PL, et al. Polysomnography after adenotonsillectomy in mild pediatric obstructive sleep apnea. *Crit Care Med*. 1996;24(8):1323-1327.

Chapter 332

TUBERCULOSIS AND LATENT TUBERCULOSIS INFECTION

Ann M. Loeffler, MD; Mark N. Lobato, MD

Tuberculosis (TB) is a serious disease caused by *Mycobacterium tuberculosis*. TB disproportionately affects young children as a result of their increased risk of progression to disease once infected by *M tuberculosis* and the increased likelihood of disseminated disease. In the United States, children who are at the highest risk for TB are children of color, children born in countries with a high prevalence of TB or into families from these countries, children who live with or in contact with adults who are at risk for TB, and children younger than 4 years.

DEFINITIONS

Tuberculosis

TB disease is caused by a member of the *M tuberculosis* complex, which includes *M tuberculosis* and *M bovis*, and is distinguished from latent TB infection (LTBI). Common clinical presentations of TB include pneumonia, intrathoracic or peripheral lymphadenopathy, meningitis, disseminated TB, and bone and joint disease. In the United States, children diagnosed with TB disease are often asymptomatic but have radiographic evidence of disease such as an infiltrate or intrathoracic adenopathy. Asymptomatic presentations of TB disease are treated with multidrug therapy because they will progress in most children if not treated. Table 332-1 provides epidemiologic data for TB in children. Among U.S. children with TB in 2006, 485 were <5 years of age, 322 were ages 5-14; 48% were Hispanic (most from Mexico), and 31% were black. A total of 25% of TB cases in children occurred in the foreign born: 15% of children were <5 years of age and 40% of children were 5-14 yrs of age. Thirty-six percent of the cases were reported from California, Texas, and New York. A total of 73% had pulmonary TB (with or without extrapulmonary TB).

Latent Tuberculosis Infection

Infection with *M tuberculosis* occurs when the organism is in a metabolically dormant state and replicating slowly within granulomata in the lung and other tissues. The patient usually has a positive tuberculin skin test (TST) result but no clinical or radiographic evidence

Table 332-1 Tuberculosis (TB) Among Children, United States, 2006

GROUP	TB CASE RATE PER 100,000 CHILDREN
Children ages 0-14 yrs	1.3
Children <5 yrs	2.4
Foreign born	21.9
US born	2.1
Hispanic or Latino	5.5
Asian	5.2
Black or African American	4.5
White	0.2

From Centers for Disease Control and Prevention, Division of Tuberculosis Elimination. *Reported Tuberculosis in the United States, 2006*. Atlanta, Ga: US Department of Health and Human Services, Centers for Disease Control and Prevention; September 2007. Available at: www.cdc.gov/tb/surv/surv2006/default.htm. Rates were computed using population denominator data from the Community Population Survey; available at: www.census.gov/cps.

of TB disease. Until new diagnostic tests become better studied in children and are more readily available, a positive TST result is used to define LTBI. An interferon-gamma release assay such as the QuantiFERON-TB test may also diagnose LTBI in children. Patients should be treated with isoniazid (isonicotinyl hydrazine [INH]) monotherapy daily for 9 months, unless they have a medical contraindication (including infection with a known INH-resistant strain). Because LTBI is not a reportable condition in most states, the number of children who have LTBI is unknown.

Tuberculosis Exposure

A person exposed to TB is one who has spent time in close proximity to a potentially contagious patient with TB disease. The exposed individual may or may not be infected. Young children can progress rapidly to TB once infected; thus they should be quickly evaluated and treated prophylactically while awaiting completion of the evaluation if they are exposed to TB.

DIFFERENTIAL DIAGNOSIS

TB symptoms mimic many different diseases. Because TB is uncommon in the United States among most populations, the clinician must maintain a high index of suspicion for TB, especially among children who fit the epidemiologic profile and who have risk factors for infection and disease. The differential diagnosis for TST results is outlined in Box 332-1. The differential diagnosis for forms of TB disease is provided in Box 332-2.

Tuberculin Skin Testing

Universal skin testing for TB is not recommended. Annual assessment for TB risk factors and testing of children with defined risk factors are the standard of care.[1] Testing asymptomatic children without known risk factors for TB is no longer performed. The TST is used to diagnose LTBI and support the diagnosis of TB disease. Because of the poor sensitivity and specificity of the TST in low-incidence populations, it is given only to children identified as having increased risks of TB exposure or disease. TSTs should be undertaken only for children who have clinical disease that raises concern for TB, children at high risk for progression to TB disease, or children who have new risk factors for TB exposure since their last TST. Most children with US-born parents never require a TST.

In the United States, the only recommended TST is intradermal instillation of 5 TU (0.1 mL) purified protein derivative (PPD) by the Mantoux method. The skin test should be placed and interpreted by a trained health care professional. The definition of a positive TST result depends on risk factors for infection and the likelihood of TB disease. Box 332-3 lists the breakpoints used to interpret TB skin test results in children.

In areas with low TB rates, most positive TST reactions are in fact falsely positive.[2] (See Box 332-1, Differential Diagnosis for Tuberculin Skin Test Results for details.) If a child is found to have a positive TST result, the evaluation includes a chest radiograph, focused history, and physical examination. A two-view chest radiograph (frontal and lateral views) is particularly helpful in differentiating intrathoracic lymphadenopathy from other hilar structures. National guidelines suggest obtaining two-view radiographs on all children when resources permit. If resources are limited, children over 6 years of age should be screened with one-view chest radiographs.[3]

Targeted testing is the strategy of skin testing only for children who are at high risk of contracting TB infection of developing TB disease if infected. This strategy results in fewer unnecessary skin tests and avoids evaluation

BOX 332-1 Differential Diagnosis for Tuberculin Skin Test Results

TRULY POSITIVE

- Caused by infection with *M tuberculosis* complex

FALSELY POSITIVE

- Cross-reaction with nontuberculous mycobacteria, such as *M avium* complex and *M scrofulaceum*. These reactions are frequently, but not always, smaller than those caused by *M tuberculosis*.
- Cross-reaction with a recent or multiple vaccinations with BCG. In general, the public health strategy in the United States is to discount the history of BCG vaccination when deciding to administer or interpreting the TST. If a patient has received only a single BCG vaccination in the newborn period and several months have elapsed since the last BCG, then a positive TST reaction due to BCG is unlikely.*
- Allergic-type reactions. These reactions peak within 24 hours of TST placement and should be gone within 48-72 hours. Induration that peaks >24 hours after TST placement is due to a delayed-type hypersensitivity, the mechanism of a true positive TST reaction.
- Irritation from a circular Band-Aid or tape
- Injection with a substance other than PPD

FALSELY NEGATIVE

- Recent infection with *M tuberculosis* (delayed-type hypersensitivity reaction takes 2-8 weeks after infection to develop)
- Infancy
- Improper storage of the PPD skin test material (eg, not refrigerated, prolonged storage in syringe)
- Improper placement (eg, subcutaneous placement, pressure by gauze or a Band-Aid leading to the absorption of PPD solution)
- Vaccination with a live virus vaccine within the previous 6 weeks
- Generalized or specific anergy associated with extensive or disseminated TB or as seen in immunocompromised patients, especially those infected with HIV

BCG, Bacille Calmette-Guérin; *PPD*, purified protein derivative; *TB*, tuberculosis; *TST*, tuberculin skin test.

*From Centers for Disease Control and Prevention. Guidelines for the investigation of contacts of persons with infectious tuberculosis: recommendations from the National Tuberculosis Controllers Association and CDC. *MMWR Morb Mortal Wkly Rep.* 2005;54(RR-:1- American Academy of Pediatrics. Tuberculosis. In: Pickering LK, Baker CJ, Long SS, et al, eds. *2006 Red Book: 2006 Report of the Committee on Infectious Diseases.* 27th ed. Elk Grove Village, IL: American Academy of Pediatrics; 2006.?

BOX 332-2 Differential Diagnosis for Forms of Tuberculosis Disease

PULMONARY INFILTRATE

- Community acquired pneumonia (ie, bacterial pneumonia, including lung abscess and necrotizing pneumonia; viral pneumonia)
- Atelectasis caused by reactive airways disease or other processes
- Other granulomatous diseases (eg, coccidiomycosis, histoplasmosis)

INTRATHORACIC LYMPHADENOPATHY

- Infections caused by fungus, virus, or bacteria
- Nontuberculous mycobacterial infections
- Malignancies
- Round pneumonia
- Other granulomatous diseases (eg, coccidiomycosis, histoplasmosis)

SUBACUTE PERIPHERAL ADENOPATHY

- Scrofula caused by nontuberculous mycobacteria
- Cat-scratch disease
- Toxoplasmosis
- Partially treated pyogenic infection

MENINGITIS

- Viral, bacterial, fungal, and chemical meningitis

and treatment of children with false positive TST results. At each well-child visit, the child should be screened with a risk-factor questionnaire. The child should undergo skin testing only if a new risk factor has been identified since the last TST. Foreign birth, foreign travel, and close contact with individuals with a positive TST result or TB disease predict increased risk of LTBI. Individual questionnaires should be modified based on local risks.[1] A sample questionnaire is provided in Box 332-4, and the general strategy for targeted TB testing is outlined in Figure 332-1.

Prior bacille Calmette-Guérin (BCG) vaccination sometimes causes a small, transient TST reaction as a result of cross-reactivity among antigens. The effect of BCG vaccination on TST reaction is an ongoing challenge for clinicians. The Centers for Disease Control and Prevention and the American Academy of Pediatrics advise clinicians to discount the history of BCG vaccination when interpreting the TST.[1,4,5] The following factors decrease the likelihood that the skin test reaction is caused by BCG:

- TST reaction (induration) >10 mm
- Previous receipt of a single rather than multiple BCG vaccines
- BCG given in the first month of life
- A long period since the BCG dose
- Receipt of no other recent TST[6,7]

New blood tests may further clarify the impact of BCG on TST reactions and allow for more accurate TST cutoff points in individuals who have received BCG.[8]

BOX 332-3 Breakpoints for Interpretation of Tuberculin Skin Test Results

A ≥5-mm induration is interpreted as positive in the following circumstances:

- Child is immunosuppressed (receiving immunosuppressive therapy) or immunocompromised, including HIV infection.
- Child is a recent contact of a person with TB or suspected TB disease.
- Radiograph or clinical evidence suggests TB disease.
- Fibrotic changes on chest x-ray are consistent with prior TB infection.

A ≥10 mm induration is interpreted as positive in the following circumstances:

- Child is <4 years of age.
- Child has medical conditions (lymphoma, Hodgkin disease, diabetes mellitus, chronic renal failure, malnutrition).
- Child or parent was born in a country with a high prevalence of TB.
- Child has frequent exposure to high-risk adults (HIV infected, homeless, residents of nursing homes, institutionalized, incarcerated, users of illicit drugs, migrant farm workers).
- Child has traveled to a high-prevalence country.
- Child is a resident of California.

A ≥15-mm induration is interpreted as positive in the following circumstance:

- Child is ≥4 years of age and has no risk factors

TB, Tuberculosis.
From California Tuberculosis Controllers Association (CTCA). CDHS/CTCA Joint Guidelines. Targeted Testing and Treatment of Latent Tuberculosis Infection in Adults and Children. Available at: ctca.org/guidelines/IIA2targetedskintesting.pdf. Accessed June 25, 2007.

MANAGEMENT

Tuberculosis Exposure

A child exposed to an adult or adolescent with potentially contagious TB requires prompt and thorough evaluation to determine whether the child already has evidence of LTBI or TB disease. All exposed individuals should undergo a symptom review, TST, and a focused history and physical examination. These evaluations should be coordinated with the local health department. Children younger than 5 years and all immunocompromised individuals with significant exposure should receive *window prophylaxis* after TB disease has been ruled out by a normal chest radiograph and negative physical examination. Window prophylaxis is the practice of treatment with INH until a repeat TST given 8 to 10 weeks after their last exposure (Figure 332-2) is performed and is negative.[9]

Latent Tuberculosis Infection

Management of LTBI is reasonably easy once TB disease is eliminated as a possibility. INH monotherapy should be initiated[1] unless strong evidence exists of INH drug resistance in the source case (not merely LTBI acquisition in an area with a high level of INH

BOX 332-4 Tuberculosis Risk Assessment Questionnaire

Name: ______________________ DOB: ____________________

Last tuberculin skin test (TST) date: ________ Results: __________ mm induration OR _____ not read by health care professional

If positive TST result in the past: Chest radiograph date and result: ______________

1. Was your child born outside the United States? ______Yes ______No

   Country: ______________________________

2. Since the last TB skin test, has your child traveled outside the United States? ______Yes ______No

   Country or countries visited: ___________________________________

   Dates of travel and how long did they travel? ___________________________________

   Where did they stay (hotel, family, resort)? ___________________________

3. Since the last TB skin test, has your child been exposed to anyone with TB disease? ______Yes ______No

   Name of their disease? ___________________________

   Positive TST result with normal chest radiograph taking one medicine or no treatment OR TB disease taking many pills and different kinds of medicine?

   Name of person: ____________________________ DOB: ___________________

   Where is the person being treated? ____

4. Since the child's last skin test, has your child had close contact with a person who has a positive TST result? ______Yes ______No

   Nature of their disease? ____

   Positive TST result with normal chest radiograph taking medicine or no treatment OR TB disease taking many pills and different kinds of medicine?

   Name of person: _________________________ DOB: ____________________

   Where is the person being treated? ____

   Optional questions depending on local epidemiology:

   Since the last skin test, has your child consumed unpasteurized milk or cheese (from Mexico or Central America)? ______Yes ______No

   Since the last skin test, has your child been around people in jail, homeless or in shelters, people who have HIV, or use illegal drugs? ______Yes ______No

   Since the last skin test, has your child lived with a new person who was born or traveled outside the US? ______Yes ______No

   INSTRUCTIONS FOR PROVIDERS: Test only children who have a new risk factor since their last TST.

   If the child has previously had a positive TST result, then do not administer another TST.

   Significant travel is considered travel to a country with a high prevalence of TB (eg, in Africa, Asia, Latin American, and Eastern Europe) for >1 week AND had a substantial contact with indigenous people from such countries (did not stay in a resort).

From Pediatric Tuberculosis Collaborative Group. Targeted tuberculin skin testing and treatment of latent tuberculosis infection in children and adolescents. *Pediatrics.* 2004;114:1175-1201.

resistance). Dosing is 270 daily doses (or twice a week administered by directly observed therapy [DOT]) within a 12 month period. Table 332-2 lists INH doses by weight. When a prolonged break occurs after a short initial treatment period, then therapy should be restarted, but short lapses are tolerated, especially if the regimen is well underway. If interruption of therapy is greater than 2 months, then the child should be reevaluated for possible TB disease before restarting INH. Vitamin-B6 (pyridoxine) supplementation is indicated only for exclusively breastfed infants, children and adolescents on milk- and meat-deficient diets, children who experience paresthesias while receiving isoniazid therapy, and those with HIV infection.[3]

INH is available as 100-mg and 300-mg scored tablets and as a liquid suspended in sorbitol. The liquid formulation causes cramping and diarrhea in more

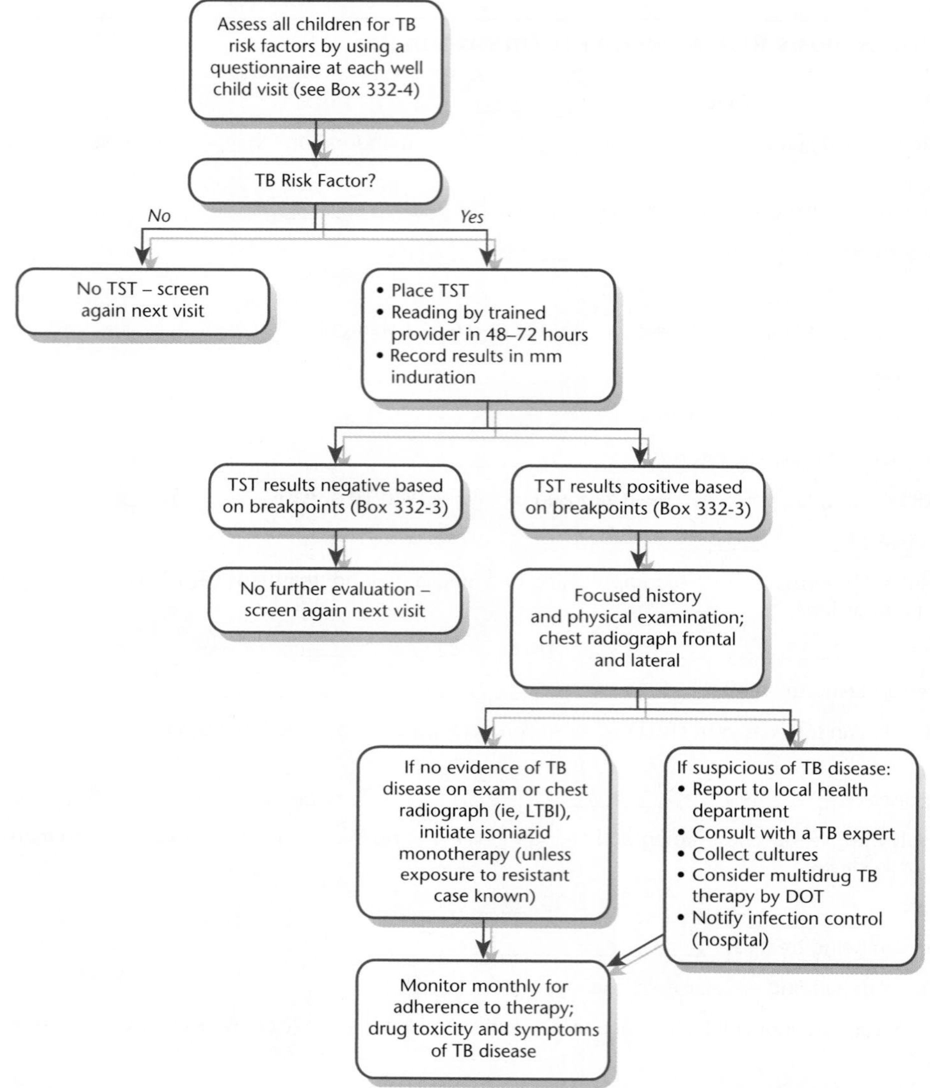

Figure 332-1 General strategy for targeted tuberculosis testing. *LTBI,* Latent tuberculosis infection; *TST,* tuberculin skin test; *DOT,* directly observed therapy.

than one half of children because of its osmotic load. The tablet can be crushed and mixed with or layered into a strong-flavored semisoft food in a spoon. Children should be examined monthly and questioned about symptoms of toxicity. INH-related transient increase of transaminases has been noted in children, with the effects increasing with increasing age; however, INH rarely causes clinical hepatotoxicity in children.[10] Routine monitoring of liver transaminases is not indicated for asymptomatic children who do not have underlying liver disease and who are not receiving other hepatotoxic drugs.[1] Families should be thoroughly educated about and instructed on recognizing symptoms of hepatotoxicity (eg, anorexia, malaise, abdominal pain, vomiting) and to stop the therapy and return to the clinic if these symptoms arise. Lack of association with other viral symptoms and lack of improvement after a few days should suggest the possibility of hepatotoxicity rather than an intercurrent illness. Patients receiving antiepileptic drugs (particularly phenytoin and carbamazepine) should have these drug levels monitored.

Parents should be asked about the child's adherence to therapy and results of skin testing of family members and other contacts. Figure 332-3 shows an example of a flow sheet for monitoring LTBI treatment. Every effort should be made to promote and facilitate adherence through enablers such as walk-in visits for refills (nurse visits) or school-based dosing or monthly monitoring. Incentives such as stickers and calendars, prizes, and end-of-treatment rewards can also be used to promote adherence (for an example, see www.maine.gov/dhhs/boh/ddc/treasure_chest_program_tb.htm). Children receiving antiepileptic drugs should be

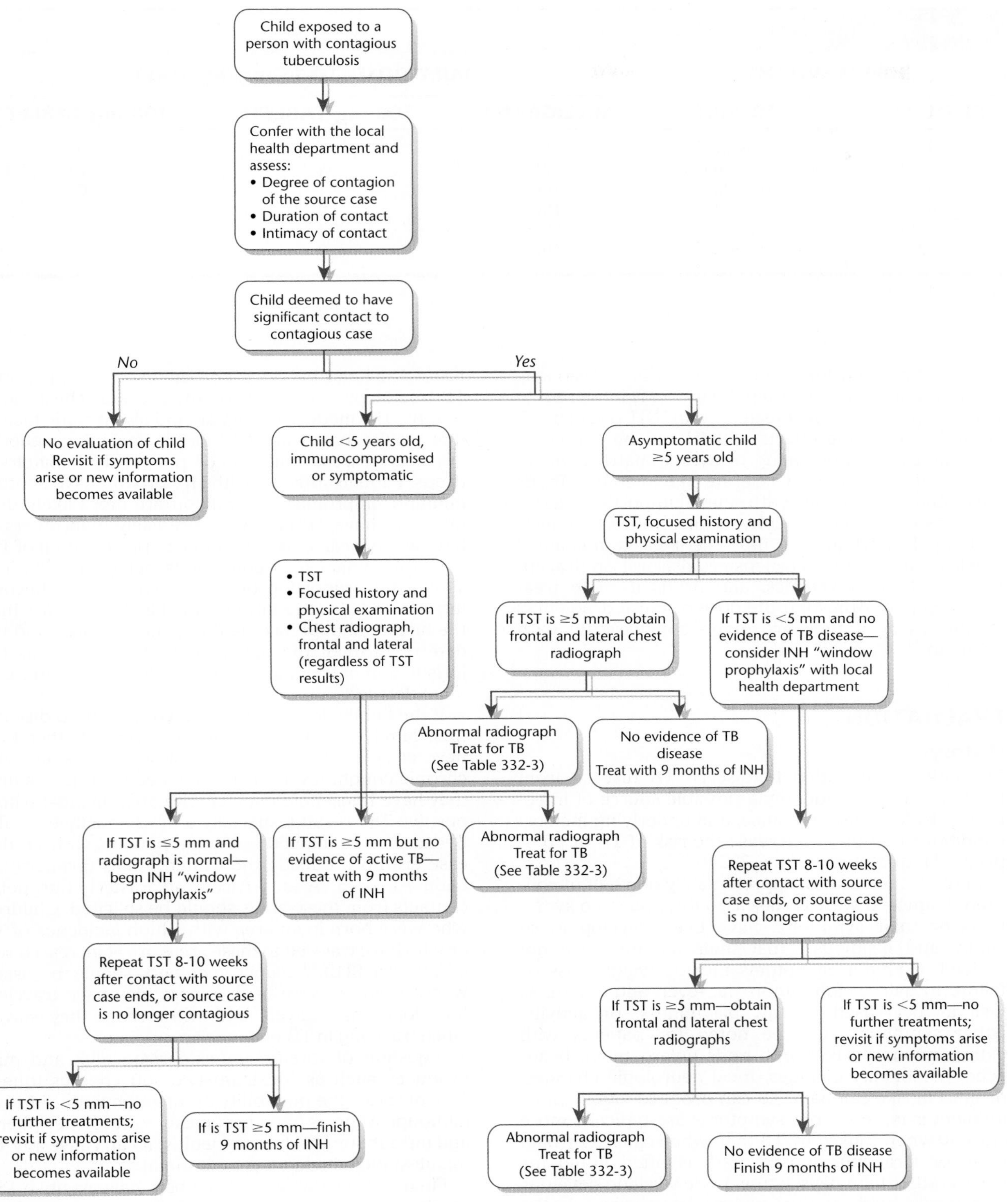

Figure 332-2 Evaluation of a child exposed to a person with contagious tuberculosis. *INH,* Isoniazid; *TST,* tuberculin skin test.

monitored closely because INH affects the drug levels of some of these medications.

After completing the 270 doses of INH for LTBI, the family should be provided with a card or letter documenting completion of therapy and reminded that the child should not undergo tuberculin testing in the future. An end-of-completion radiograph is not necessary.[1]

Table 332-2 Isoniazid Daily Dosing

CHILD'S WEIGHT		DAILY DOSE (10-15 mg/kg/DAY)*		
KILOGRAMS	POUNDS	MILLIGRAMS	100-mg TABLETS	300-mg TABLETS
3-5	6.6-11	50	1/2	0
5-7.5	11-16.4	75	3/4	OR 1/4
7.5-10	16.5-22	100	1	0
10-15	22-33	150	0	1/2
15-20	33-44	200	2	0
>20	>44	300	0	1

*Maximal dose, 300 mg.

Rifampin given for 180 daily doses is occasionally used as an alternative for a patient who is intolerant to INH or is known to be infected by an INH-resistant TB strain.[1,3] Most side effects of INH can be overcome with adjustments of timing or symptomatic management. Rifampin may accelerate the metabolism or have other interactions with several important classes of drugs, including anticonvulsants, antiarrhythmics, antifungals, barbiturates, β-blockers, calcium channel blockers, antibiotics, corticosteroids, oral contraceptives, oral hypoglycemics, and drugs used to treat HIV infection. Adjusting the dose of these drugs may be necessary if they are given concurrently with rifampin.[11]

EVALUATION

History

Evaluation is intended to discern TB disease from LTBI, as well as to identify a possible source of infection, risks for drug resistance, and underlying medical conditions that might increase the risk of TB or complicate TB treatment (Figure 332-4).

In the United States, approximately one half of children diagnosed with TB disease either have no symptoms or their symptoms have been developing so subtly and insidiously that their parents have not noticed. Common symptoms include weight loss or failure to gain weight, anorexia, fever, and cough, as well as decreased energy, playfulness, or activity. Other symptoms may be noted for patients with extrapulmonary TB: lymph node enlargement, headache, personality changes, focal neurologic changes, or musculoskeletal pain. TB can produce fulminant or indolent symptoms, but symptoms are typically more chronic when caused by TB than when caused by bacterial or viral infections. Cough is often noted for weeks rather than days; lymph node swelling develops over weeks, with gradual and modest changes in the overlying skin. Occasionally, symptoms such as cough and fever are actually improving at the time of diagnosis.

The history should include information that would suggest an alternative diagnosis, such as reactive airways disease, bacterial or viral pneumonia, pyogenic lymphadenitis, or viral meningitis. Pertinent medical history includes previous TB skin test results, previous TB treatment, and results of any previous chest radiographs. The medical history should also include factors that would complicate TB therapy, including underlying liver disease and use of potentially hepatotoxic drugs. Patients infected with HIV or who have another immunocompromising condition are more likely than others to have TB and are more likely than others to have an atypical or extrapulmonary presentation of TB.

Close contact to a contagious person results in a significant proportion of household contacts becoming infected. If the family knows of a TB exposure, then the history should include the name, address, and the date of birth of the patient with TB, as well as the jurisdiction of treatment, susceptibility data, and treatment details.[9]

If the family does not know anyone with TB disease, then family members should be asked whether they have close contact with an adolescent or adult with chronic cough, fever, or unexplained weight loss or if they have household contact with an individual with a positive TST result (especially a newly positive result). Because more than 50% of adult patients with TB disease are born outside the United States (primarily in Latin America, Asia, Africa, and Eastern Europe),[12] contacts from these areas should be solicited. Children who were born in an area with a high incidence of TB or who have traveled to these areas are at increased risk of TB and LTBI.[13] Family members should be asked where children were born, where they have traveled, how long they stayed, and with whom they stayed when traveling in TB-endemic areas.

Ingestion of foreign unpasteurized milk and milk products, such as Mexican-style soft cheeses (queso fresco) raises the possibility of infection with *M bovis*. (although *M bovis* has a propensity to cause peripheral and intraabdominal lymphadenitis, it can cause any TB manifestation, including pneumonia).[14]

Finally, if several family members have positive TST results, then the likelihood that the patient's disease is TB increases. The primary care physician should immediately perform a TST on any family member who has not recently undergone such a test (and has never had a positive result in the past). To prevent possible continued transmission of TB, chest radiographs of adults with a previous or newly positive TST result or suspicious TB-like symptoms should be obtained.

TUBERCULOSIS MANAGEMENT RECORD

Name: ____________________ Parent name: ____________________

DOB: ____________________ Parent telephone: (____) ____________________

Language spoken by parent: ____________________

VISIT DATE:											
PATIENT WEIGHT:											

Prescribe 1 bottle of 30 doses each visit. When 9 bottles (270 doses) are consumed, therapy is complete.

MEDICATION:

Isoniazid (IHN) dose in milligrams:											
Bottle number:											
Date on current bottle:											
Number of pills in bottle:											

Recalculate dose if weight increases significantly (10-15 mg/kg/dose)

DRUG SCREEN (yes or no answers):

Taking medications regularly?											
Fatigue?											
Loss of appetite?											
Rash or itching?											
Nausea or vomiting?											
Tingling of fingers or toes?											
Color change in skin or eyes?											
Tender abdomen?											
See progress note?											

Remind the family during each visit to stop medication and call if concerning side effects (3 days of anorexia or malaise that does not improve)

FOLLOW-UP:

Tuberculois education:											
Return appointment:											
Provider's initials:											

Phramacy name: ____________________ Pharmacy telephone: (____) ____________________

Prescription number: ____________________

Figure 332-3 Tuberculosis medication flow sheet.

Physical Examination

The focused physical examination should emphasize vital signs, growth parameters, conjunctival examination, neck flexion, lymph node palpation, auscultation of heart and lungs, abdomen and flank palpation, spine and bone palpation, brief skin examination, and neurologic examination (depending on concerns for TB of the central nervous system). Children diagnosed as having LTBI will have no examination abnormalities that suggest TB disease.[1,3] Even children with pulmonary TB may have no findings at physical examination. The findings on chest radiograph are frequently more useful than those found by physical examination or history.

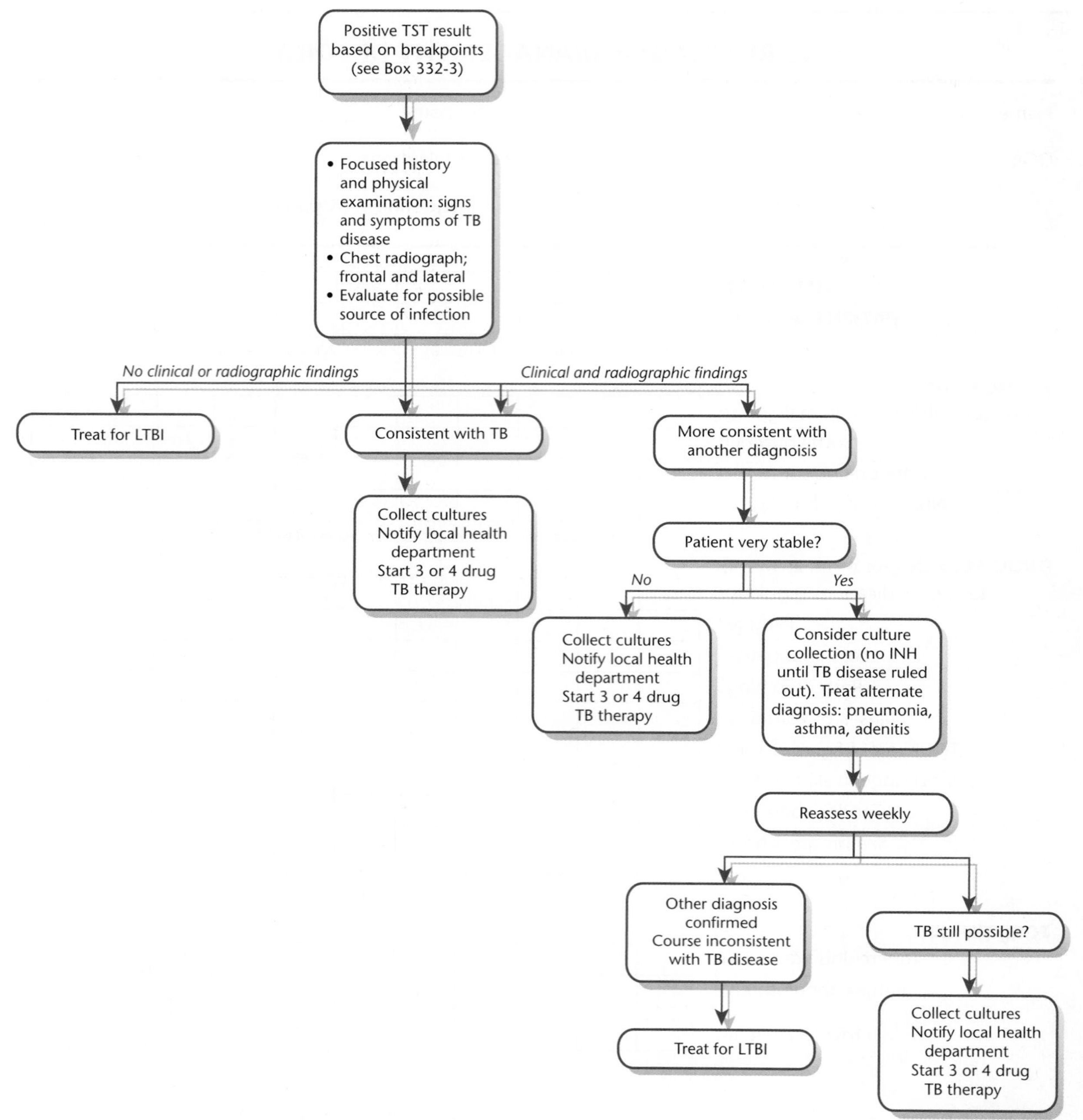

Figure 332-4 Evaluation of a child with a positive TST result. *LTBI,* Latent tuberculosis infection; *TST,* tuberculin skin test.

Laboratory Evaluation

Routine testing for children suspected of having TB includes HIV serologic testing and mycobacterial cultures. Sputum specimens are challenging to collect from young children, but they can be collected by gastric aspiration (Box 332-5),[15] induction, or bronchoalveolar lavage. Gastric aspirates are typically collected on three consecutive mornings after an overnight fast.[16] Historically, yields are between 30% and 50%, with the highest yields being in the youngest infants and from the initial sample collected. If the patient is not otherwise ill enough to require inpatient management, then gastric aspirates can be collected in the outpatient setting.[17]

In older children, sputum induction with hypertonic saline can be attempted; inducing sputum in infants is difficult.[18] Bronchoalveolar lavage is used primarily when diagnostic possibilities other than TB are being strongly considered. Yield for bronchoalveolar lavage in culturing *M tuberculosis* in children is between 10% and 21%, and yields are less than that for gastric lavage in children.[15]

BOX 332-5 Gastric Aspirate Procedure for Culture of *Mycobacterium tuberculosis*

- For health care workers present during gastric aspirate procedures of a patient with suspected or confirmed infectious TB disease, at least N-95 disposable respirators should be worn.
- Collect all supplies and have everything ready: N-95 respirators, papoose board or sheet, No. 10 or larger French nasogastric or suction tube, 30-mL syringe with appropriate connector for tube; pen; sterile water; specimen cup or laboratory-preprepared tube containing bicarbonate for bedside neutralization; requisition and label; helper.
- Child should not take anything by mouth for at least 6 hours before the procedure.
- Immobilize the child with a sheet with or without a papoose board.
- Measure the distance from the nose to the stomach.
- Insert a No. 10 French nasogastric tube through the nose into the stomach.
- Puff in the child's face as the tube enters the throat to elicit a swallow reflex.
- Gently aspirate the tube with an appropriately fitted 30- to 60-mL syringe.
- If no significant yield, then advance and withdraw the tube slightly while aspirating.
- If yield is still less than 5 to 10 mL, then place any collected mucus into a container.
- Check tube position by auscultating the stomach while pushing air from the syringe into tube.
- Instill 20 mL of sterile water into the stomach and quickly aspirate again.
- If yield is less than 5 to 10 mL, then roll the child on the side, advance the tube, aspirating continuously to find the pool of mucus in the stomach.
- As tube is withdrawn, continuously aspirate the syringe.
- Place any yield, including any spontaneously vomited emesis, in the specimen container.
- Label the specimen and order AFB smear and culture.
- Promptly transport the specimen to the laboratory for processing (tell the laboratory if the specimen has already been neutralized).

AFB, Acid-fast bacillus; *TB*, tuberculosis.
From Francis J. Curry National Tuberculosis Center. Pediatric Tuberculosis: A Guide to the Gastric Aspirate Procedure. 2006. www.nationaltbcenter.ucsf.edu/catalogue/epub/index.cfm?uniqueID=13&tableName=GAP. Accessed March 7, 2007. Reprinted by permission.

Guided by the physical examination and clinical scenario, other specimens may be collected, including cerebrospinal fluid (CSF). CSF culture has a 50% to 75% yield in diagnosis of TB meningitis. Acid-fast bacillus (AFB) smear has an even lower yield, but it can be improved by centrifugation of large volumes of CSF.[19] The use of the polymerase chain reaction technique has been disappointing, but it may play a role as an adjunct diagnostic method.[19] AFB smear and culture of other tissues should be undertaken as indicated for lymph node tissue, abscess drainage, bone or synovial fluid, urine, blood, bone marrow, or other tissue. Specimens for AFB smear and culture should be submitted in a sterile cup (rather than on a swab) and without formalin preservative.

Regardless of the culture-collection method or specimen being collected, culture for *M tuberculosis* in children has suboptimal yields. Families should understand that AFB smears are not usually positive from specimens from children, that cultures must be incubated for several weeks before any results are available, and that cultures have less than 50% yield in most situations.[15] Specimens are collected so that if cultures are positive and yield susceptibility data, then the treatment regimen can be optimized. In most cases, the diagnosis of TB in a child is a clinical diagnosis, influenced by the probability of exposure to a person with infectious TB, TST results, clinical symptoms and signs, and results of imaging tests. Although none of these elements is diagnostic for TB disease, the experienced TB clinician weighs all these factors along with the risk to the child of not treating TB when considering whether to begin treatment. Unless an alternative diagnosis is established, most often, once TB therapy is begun, the course should be completed.

Other laboratory evaluations should be considered based on individual circumstances. Patients who have TB-HIV coinfection, severe TB disease, symptoms or signs of hepatitis, or known underlying liver disease or those who are receiving other hepatotoxic medications should have liver transaminase levels measured.

The QuantiFERON-TB Gold test is an in vitro diagnostic test for detecting interferon gamma (IFN-γ) when a patient's whole blood is incubated with specific TB proteins and controls. The detection of IFN-γ indicates a T-cell response by the patient's lymphocytes and probable infection with *M tuberculosis*.[8] Few data support its applicability to children, although studies are underway.[20]

Imaging Studies

Any child whose TST result is positive or who is suspected of having pulmonary or extrapulmonary TB should have a chest radiograph performed. For the best-quality radiograph, the child should be in full inspiration and should not be rotated. Guidelines suggest obtaining 2-view radiographs on all children when resources permit. If resources are limited, children older than 6 years can be screened with 1-view chest radiographs.[1] The lateral view is particularly helpful in distinguishing other central shadows from intrathoracic lymph nodes, which are spherical and can frequently be seen on both views.[15] Ideally the films should be interpreted by a clinician or radiologist experienced in pediatric TB. Computed tomography is not indicated in the evaluation of an asymptomatic child with a normal chest radiograph and a positive TST result. A computed tomography scan can be helpful when the radiograph is equivocal and when looking for other causes of lung disease is necessary.[22]

Findings on chest radiographs of children with TB are variable. Enlarged intrathoracic lymph nodes and infiltrate are the most common abnormalities. Intrathoracic adenopathy is frequently seen in children and is reported to be present in up to 85% of children under 3 years of age.[21,23] Hilar, mediastinal, paratracheal, and subcarinal nodes may be seen and are most often found on the right side. Isolated adenopathy should be treated as TB disease.[3] Figure 332-5 shows the radiograph of a child with typical intrathoracic adenopathy caused by TB.

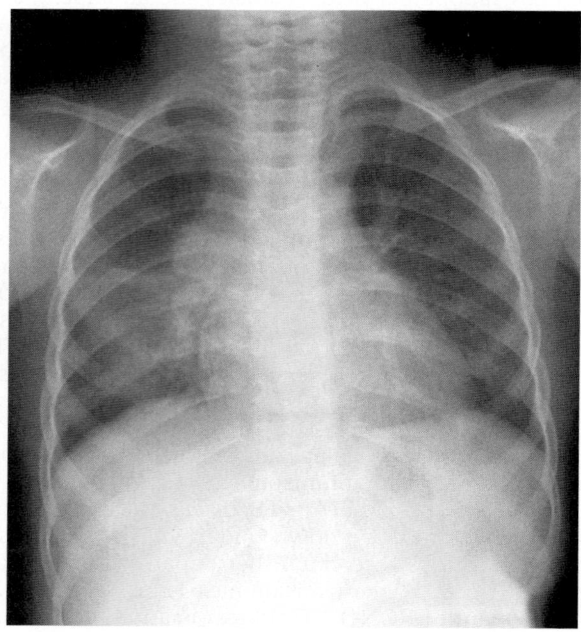

Figure 332-5 Chest radiograph of a child with enlarged intrathoracic lymph nodes.

An infiltrate may be seen in any lung field and is seen in multiple lobes in one quarter of children. Parenchymal disease may be caused by several processes. A larger consolidation may be associated with advancement of the infection—the so-called progressive primary process—or it may be due to atelectasis or collapse-consolidation that results from lymph node obstruction. Lymph node obstruction can also cause air trapping behind the node with resultant wheezing and hyperinflation. Older children, especially adolescents, may have radiographic findings that are consistent with adult reactivation (postprimary) TB, including upper lobe disease with fibronodular infiltrates, volume loss, hilar retraction, and cavities.

Infection is sometimes spread to other parenchymal locations after erosion of a lymph node with spilling of infectious material (bronchogenic spread). This situation can cause a segmental lesion when the material is limited to one bronchus, or it may result in diffuse bronchopneumonia when the organism spreads throughout the lung.

Distribution of *M tuberculosis* via hematogenous dissemination that causes disease to the lung and other organs is termed *disseminated disease,* although the term *miliary disease* was formerly used because of the small, round, millet-like appearance of the diffuse lesions. Figure 332-6 shows the radiograph of an infant with disseminated TB. Primary bacillemia occurs during the initial process of the proximal lymph nodes draining into the thoracic duct. The infection may also be disseminated secondarily if a necrotizing lymph node or airspace focus erodes into a blood vessel. These disseminated processes do not always appear radiographically in the classic disseminated pattern. Larger, patchy, reticulonodular lesions may

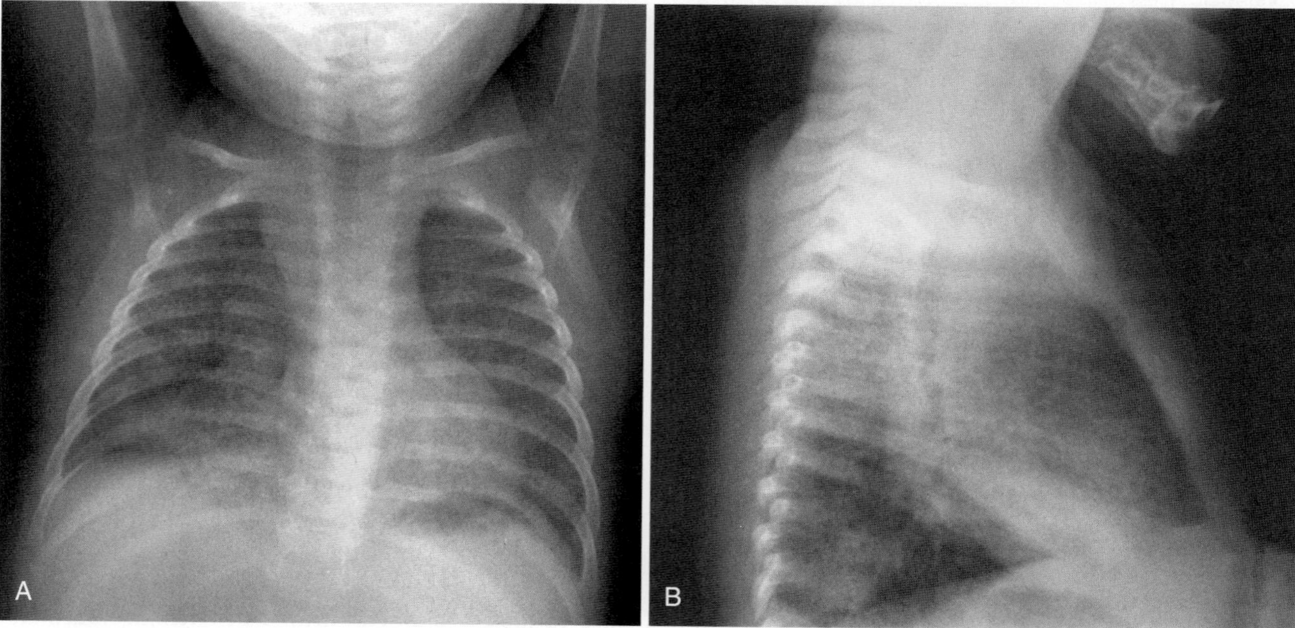

Figure 332-6 Chest radiograph of infant with disseminated tuberculosis.

Table 332-3 Treatment Regimens for Tuberculosis in Children*

TB MANIFESTATION	MINIMAL DURATION OF THERAPY	INITIAL REGIMEN	FOLLOW-UP REGIMEN	COMMENTS
Pulmonary TB	6 mo	Isoniazid, rifampin, pyrazinamide, and ethambutol daily for 2 wk to 2 mo (three-drug therapy only if no risk of resistance)	Stop ethambutol as soon as the patient or reliable source case isolate is found to be drug susceptible. Document a follow-up chest radiograph 2 mo into therapy. If the isolate is sensitive and the patient is clinically well and radiographically improving or stable, then change to isoniazid and rifampin at 2 mo to complete a 6-mo course; twice-weekly therapy can be provided by directly observed therapy. Document chest radiograph at end of treatment—frequently not quite normal.	Four-drug initial therapy is provided if any risks exists of drug resistance, including previous TB treatment or exposure to a person with known drug-resistant TB.If a cavitary lesion was present on the chest radiograph and sputum culture is positive after 2 mo of treatment, then the total treatment should be extended to 9 rather than 6 mo.
Extrapulmonary (meningitis, bone or joint, disseminated)	9-12 mo	Same as pulmonary disease	7-10 mo of isoniazid and rifampin, either daily or twice a week by directly observed therapy.	Some clinicians use an injectable drug (eg, amikacin, kanamycin) for initial treatment of disseminated or meningeal disease. Strongly consider corticosteroid therapy for some types of extrapulmonary disease (eg, meningitis, pericarditis).
Other extrapulmonary (cervical adenopathy)	Same as pulmonary disease	Same as pulmonary disease	Same as pulmonary disease except no need to follow chest radiographs if initially normal	Same as pulmonary disease

TB, Tuberculosis.
*Directly observed therapy by a trained health care worker is the standard of care for all children with TB.

be present and difficult to distinguish from other diffuse lung infections.

Pleural effusion and empyema are less common in children with TB compared with adults. Isolated, dense nodules with calcification, nonenlarged calcified lymph nodes, and isolated pleural thickening are considered signs of healed *M tuberculosis* infection and are not considered to be TB disease. Peribronchial cuffing or thickening is commonly associated with reactive airway disease and viral infection and, in isolation, is not consistent with TB.

The clinician should obtain a chest radiograph 2 months after therapy for TB disease has begun and again when therapy has ended. Radiographic abnormalities in children with TB resolve slowly, and enlargement of lymph nodes may persist for a long period. The chest radiograph is not normal in more than one half of children at the end of therapy. However, they continue to improve gradually. The radiograph at the completion of therapy should be greatly improved compared with the original radiograph, which will serve as a baseline for monitoring future changes. The chest radiograph need not be repeated for children receiving or completing LTBI treatment unless they develop symptoms compatible with TB disease.

Treatment of Tuberculosis Disease

In all states, Puerto Rico, and US territories, providers are legally mandated to report persons suspected of having or confirmed to have TB to the local health department. Reporting is an important public health function because the health department assumes responsibility for collaboration in case management, provides DOT, and tests exposed contacts.

Children with TB disease should be managed in a dedicated TB clinic or by the most experienced pediatric TB clinician available. In areas where this treatment is not feasible, close and ongoing consultation with an experienced clinician should be sought.

Children with clinical or radiographic evidence of active TB, regardless of the TST result, should be evaluated immediately, as outlined in Figure 332-4. Specimens for AFB smear and culture should be collected.[3] TB disease is hard to diagnose definitively in children because culture confirmation is frequently lacking or can be delayed for several weeks. Children who have a positive TST result, who have known exposure to TB or risk factors for TB exposure, who have radiographic changes consistent with TB, or who have relatively few symptoms compared with their radiographic changes are more likely to have TB as opposed to alternative diagnoses such as community-acquired pneumonia or reactive airways disease.

Table 332-3 shows recommended treatment regimens for TB disease in children. A four-drug empiric regimen (INH, rifampin, pyrazinamide, and ethambutol) is recommended for individuals who are at higher risk for having INH-resistant TB, including exposure to an individual from an area of high prevalence of drug-resistant TB, with known drug-resistant TB, or previous treatment for TB.[24] DOT by a health care professional (not parents) is recommended for treatment of TB in children and adolescents.[24] After 2 months of treatment, a repeat chest radiograph should be performed. For children from whom sputum can be obtained, follow-up sputum should be obtained to document culture conversion. If the patient has been adherent to therapy, is clinically well, has an improving or at least stable radiograph, and no reason exists to suspect drug resistance, the regimen can then be changed to two drugs (INH and rifampin) after completing 2 months of pyrazinamide so as to complete a 6-month course. Twice-weekly dosing by DOT can be used after the induction phase of daily treatment if the child is tolerating the regimen well and has shown considerable clinical improvement. The number of doses actually observed should be counted when considering whether a patient has completed therapy. Patients receiving daily doses for the first 2 months will typically receive 40 observed doses (Monday through Friday for approximately 8 weeks) followed by 36 twice-weekly doses in the following 18 weeks.[24]

Treatment of INH-monoresistant TB disease requires at least 6 months of rifampin, pyrazinamide, and ethambutol. Treatment of drug-resistant TB should be performed in consultation with an expert in this area.

The most important element of TB therapy is the actual ingestion of the drugs. Children are difficult to dose with TB drugs, given that the formulations are not particularly child friendly. See dosing suggestions in the previous section on Latent Tuberculosis Infection.[25] The parents and public health staff should be warned that they might have to endure a several-week period of trial and error. Patients should be monitored monthly during therapy. Routine laboratory evaluation need not be performed unless the patient has symptoms of toxicity or underlying liver disease or unless the patient is taking other medications, which might interfere with the TB drugs or cause similar toxicities.

An end-of-therapy chest radiograph should be obtained. Most children do not have a normal radiograph at the end of therapy, but significant improvement is expected.

Corticosteroids have been shown to be beneficial in central nervous system disease, particularly stage 2 and 3 (altered mental status).[19,24] Some clinicians would use steroids for any child with symptomatic TB meningitis. Steroids are also frequently used for TB pericarditis.[24] Two reports support the use of steroids in children with symptomatic airways compression caused by lymphatic disease.[15] Prednisone is generally used at a dose of 1 to 2 mg/kg/day given for 4 to 8 weeks and then tapered over several weeks.

CONCLUSION

TB is a focal problem in the United States, disproportionately affecting immigrant, Hispanic, and black populations. TB risk assessments at well-child and other visits have replaced universal screening of children by TST.[26] Only children who have a new risk for TB exposure since the last TST or who have features suggestive of TB disease should undergo the TST. All children diagnosed as having LTBI should be treated and closely monitored for adherence and toxicity. Clinics should develop or modify systems to remove barriers to completion of therapy, including walk-in nurse visits, minimal paperwork, easy chart forms, and incentives. Many children with TB in the United States are asymptomatic at the time of diagnosis. TB disease in children is diagnosed clinically and radiographically, often without culture confirmation. Experienced TB clinicians are best qualified to manage TB disease, but ongoing consultation should be sought when local resources are limited.

Prevention of TB includes identification of children at risk for exposure to TB, aggressive evaluation and treatment of children exposed to potentially contagious adolescents and adults with TB (young children are generally not contagious), treatment of LTBI, and prompt treatment of contagious TB patients.

The authors thank Phil LoBue, MD, Ann Lanner, and Michael Iademarco, MD, Centers for Disease Control and Prevention, for their input on this chapter.

The findings and conclusions in this report are those of the authors and do not necessarily represent the views of the Centers for Disease Control and Prevention, Agency for Toxic Substances and Disease Registry.

WHEN TO REFER

- All patients suspected of having active TB should be reported to the local health department according to state statute (eg, within 1 working day).
- In many jurisdictions, young children with LTBI should be reported to the local health department, according to local regulations.
- Ideally, an experienced pediatric TB clinician should manage children with TB disease. If local resources are not available, then close and ongoing consultation with a pediatric TB expert should be established.

WHEN TO ADMIT

- Children should be admitted to the hospital for culture collection if local resources are not available for outpatient culture collection.
- Few children require admission to the hospital based on clinical severity of TB disease. Patients with increased work of breathing, meningitis, or complicating simultaneous conditions or patients who require diagnostic evaluation should be admitted.

TOOLS FOR PRACTICE

Engaging Patient and Family

- *Tuberculosis* (fact sheet), American Academy of Pediatrics (www.aap.org/publiced/BK0Tuberculosis.htm).
- *Tuberculosis: General Information* (fact sheet), Centers for Disease Control and Prevention (www.cdc.gov/tb/pubs/tbfactsheets/tb.htm).
- *Pediatric Tuberculosis: An Online Presentation* (www.nationaltbcenter.ucsf.edu/pediatric_tb/resources.cfm).

Medical Decision Support

- *Division of Tuberculosis Elimination* (Web page), Centers for Disease Control and Prevention (www.cdc.gov/tb/default.htm).
- *Interactive Core Curriculum on Tuberculosis* (other), Centers for Disease Control and Prevention (www.cdc.gov/tb/webcourses/CoreCurr/index.htm).
- *Red Book: 2006 Report of the Committee on Infectious Diseases*, 27th edition, American Academy of Pediatrics (www.aap.org/bookstore).
- *TB Education and Training Resources* (interactive tool), Centers for Disease Control and Prevention and the National Prevention Information Network (www.findtbresources.org/scripts/index.cfm).
- *TB Guidelines* (Web page), Centers for Disease Control and Prevention (www.cdc.gov/tb/pubs/mmwr/Maj_guide/List_date.htm).

AAP POLICY STATEMENT

American Academy of Pediatrics, Committee on Community Health Services. Providing care for the immigrant, homeless, and migrant children. *Pediatrics*. 2005;115(4):1095-1100. (aappolicy.aappublications.org/cgi/content/full/pediatrics;115/4/1095)

REFERENCES

1. Pediatric Tuberculosis Collaborative Group. Targeted tuberculin skin testing and treatment of latent tuberculosis infection in children and adolescents. *Pediatrics*. 2004; 114:1175-1201.
2. Huebner RE, Schein MF, Bass JB Jr. The tuberculin skin test. *Clin Infect Dis*. 1993;17:968-975.
3. American Academy of Pediatrics. Tuberculosis. In: Pickering LK, Baker CJ, Long SS, et al, eds. *2006 Red Book: 2006 Report of the Committee on Infectious Diseases*. 27th ed. Elk Grove Village, IL: American Academy of Pediatrics; 2006.
4. Centers for Disease Control and Prevention. Targeted tuberculin testing and treatment of latent tuberculosis infection. *MMWR Morb Mortal Wkly Rep*. 2000;49 (RR-6): 1-51.
5. Farhat M, Greenaway C, Pai M, et al. False-positive tuberculin skin tests: what is the absolute effect of BCG and non-tuberculous mycobacteria? *Int J Tuberc Lung Dis*. 2006;10:1192-1204.
6. Menzies D. What does tuberculin reactivity after bacille Calmette-Guérin vaccination tell us? *Clin Infect Dis*. 2000; 31:S71-S74.
7. Bozaykut A, Ozahi Ipek I, Ozkars MY, et al. Effect of BCG vaccine on tuberculin skin tests in 1-6-year-old children. *Acta Paediatr*. 2002;91:235-238.
8. Mazurek GH, Jereb J, Lobue P, et al. Guidelines for using the QuantiFERON-TB Gold Test for detecting Mycobacterium tuberculosis infection, United States. *MMWR Recomm Rep*. 2005;54(RR-15):49-55. Erratum in *MMWR Morb Mortal Wkly Rep*. 2005;54:1288.
9. Centers for Disease Control and Prevention. Guidelines for the investigation of contacts of persons with infectious tuberculosis: recommendations from the National Tuberculosis Controllers Association and CDC. *MMWR Morb Mortal Wkly Rep*. 2005;54(RR-15):1-37.
10. Palusci VJ, O'Hare D, Lawrence RM. Hepatotoxicity and transaminase measurement during isoniazid chemoprophylaxis in children. *Pediatr Infect Dis J*. 1995;14:144-148.
11. Centers for Disease Control and Prevention, Division of Tuberculosis Elimination. TB/HIV drug interactions. Updated Guidelines for the Use of Rifamycins for the Treatment of Tuberculosis Among HIV-Infected Patients Taking Protease Inhibitors or Nonnucleoside Reverse Transcriptase Inhibitors. Updated January 20, 2004. Available at: www.cdc.gov/tb/TB_HIV_Drugs/default.htm. Accessed June 25, 2007.

12. Centers for Disease Control and Prevention. Trends in tuberculosis—United States, 2005. *MMWR Morb Mortal Wkly Rep.* 2006;55:305-308.
13. Lobato MN, Hopewell PC. Mycobacterium tuberculosis infection after travel to or contact with visitors from countries with a high prevalence of tuberculosis. *Am Rev Respir Dis Crit Care Med.* 1998;158:1871-1875.
14. LoBue PA, Betacourt W, Peter C, et al. Epidemiology of Mycobacterium bovis disease in San Diego County, 1994-2000. *Int J Tuberc Lung Dis.* 2003;7:180-185.
15. Loeffler AM. Pediatric tuberculosis. *Semin Respir Infect.* 2003;18:272-291.
16. Francis J. Curry National Tuberculosis Center. Pediatric Tuberculosis: A Guide to the Gastric Aspirate Procedure, 2006. Available at: www.nationaltbcenter.ucsf.edu/catalogue/epub/index.cfm?uniqueID=13&tableName=GAP. Accessed June 25, 2007.
17. Lobato MN, Loeffler AM, Furst K, et al. Detection of Mycobacterium tuberculosis in gastric aspirates collected from children: hospitalization is not necessary. *Pediatrics.* 1998;102:e40.
18. Zar HJ, Hanslo D, Apolles P, et al. Induced sputum versus gastric lavage for microbiological confirmation of pulmonary tuberculosis in infants and young children: a prospective study. *Lancet.* 2005;365:130-134.
19. Starke JR. Tuberculosis of the central nervous system in children. *Semin Pediatr Neurol.* 1999;6:318-331.
20. Starke JR. Interferon-gamma release assays for diagnosis of tuberculosis infection in children. *Pediatr Infect Dis J.* 2006;25(10):941-942.
21. Smuts NA, Beyers N, Gie RP, et al. Value of the lateral chest radiograph in tuberculosis in children. *Pediatr Radiol.* 1994;24:478-480.
22. Neu N, Saiman L, San Gabriel P, et al. Diagnosis of pediatric tuberculosis in the modern era. *Pediatr Infect Dis J.* 1999;18:122-126.
23. Cremin BJ, Jamieson DH. Childhood tuberculosis. In: *Modern Imaging and Clinical Concepts.* London, UK: Springer-Verlag; 1995.
24. American Thoracic Society, Centers for Disease Control and Prevention, Infectious Diseases Society of America. Treatment of tuberculosis. *MMWR Recomm Rep.* 2003; 52(RR-11):1-77.
25. Francis J. Curry National Tuberculosis Center. Pediatric Tuberculosis, 2007. Available at: www.nationaltbcenter.ucsf.edu/pediatric_tb. Accessed May 22, 2007.
26. Bright Futures at Georgetown University. Appendices. In: *Bright Futures: Guidelines for Health Supervision of Infants, Children, and Adolescents.* 2nd rev ed.Washington, DC: National Center for Education in Maternal and Child Health; 2002. Available at: www.brightfutures.org/bf2/pdf/pdf/Appendices.pdf. Accessed June 26, 2007.

Chapter 333

UMBILICAL ANOMALIES

Robert W. Marion, MD

"It [the umbilicus] is all that remains of the stem that bound us to the parental stalk. It is a reminder that we have been plucked and must sooner or later die. It might be said that when the stem is severed, we cease to live in any true sense. We may be ornamental like roses or useful like cabbages but only for a little while. Our dissolution has begun."[1]

Despite its essential role in the survival of the fetus during prenatal life, the umbilicus, the external vestige of the umbilical cord, is frequently ignored or overlooked by the pediatric primary care physician. However, aberrations in either the formation or the position of this structure can offer helpful clues to underlying disease in the young child. Major congenital anomalies of the ventral abdominal wall, such as omphalocele, gastroschisis, and exstrophies of the bladder and cloaca, are described in detail elsewhere. This chapter deals with minor anomalies in configuration, placement, and formation of the umbilicus. In addition to the conditions described here, the umbilicus can be the site of both tumors (either vascular or teratomatous neoplasms) and infections (omphalitis).[2]

To understand the causes and significance of anomalies of the umbilicus, a review of some basic fundamentals of the embryologic development of the umbilical cord is necessary.

EMBRYOLOGIC DEVELOPMENT OF THE UMBILICAL CORD

Appearing within the first 6 weeks of gestation, the umbilical cord is derived from the fusion of 3 separate embryonic structures: (1) the primitive or primary yolk sac, which contains the allantois and a portion of the vitelline duct, transient structures that ultimately form the central portion of the embryonic gut, the urinary bladder, the urachus, and the umbilical blood vessels (usually 2 arteries and 1 vein); (2) the secondary yolk sac, composed of the remainder of the vitelline duct; and (3) the mesenchyme of the connecting body stalk of the embryo, the tissue that produces Wharton jelly, which is the packing substance that holds the cord together. After fusion is complete, these unified structures become covered by the amnion and are ultimately surrounded by amniotic fluid.[3]

Many of these embryonic structures that form the umbilical cord are present for only brief periods during embryogenesis. After the 7th week of gestation, the vitelline duct regresses and is ultimately completely resorbed. Similarly the allantois, which is contiguous with the urinary bladder, degenerates, forming a fibrous cord called the *urachus,* which connects the apex of the bladder with the umbilicus. Anomalies may result when these structures fail to undergo normal regression, causing them to persist into postnatal life.

ANOMALIES

Abnormalities of Position and Morphology

Anatomically, the level of the umbilicus is usually at the top of the iliac crest ventral to the 3rd or 4th lumbar vertebra.[4] Variations in the position of the umbilicus can result from abnormalities in the way in which the abdominal wall itself has formed and, as such, may be a clue to the diagnosis of specific dysmorphic syndromes. For example, as described in Table 333-1, the umbilicus has been noted to be low set in achondroplasia (in which disproportionate growth of the trunk accounts for the aberration in position), in bladder and

Table 333-1 Conditions Associated With Abnormalities in Position or Morphology of the Umbilicus

DISORDER	ABNORMALITY IN POSITION	ABNORMALITY IN MORPHOLOGY
Aarskog-Scott syndrome	X	Prominent, protruding, pouting
Achondroplasia	Low placement	X
Bladder exstrophy	Low placement	X
Cloacal exstrophy	Low placement	X
Cornelia de Lange syndrome	X	Hypoplasia
Rieger syndrome	X	Prominent, broad, redundant periumbilical skin
Robinow syndrome	High placement	Broad, scar is poorly epithelialized

From Curry CJR, Honore L, Boyd E: The ventral wall of the trunk. In: Stevenson RE, Hall JG, Goodman RM, eds: *Human Malformations and Related Anomalies.* Vol 2. New York, NY: Oxford University Press; 1993.

cloacal exstrophy,[5] and in association with various anomalies of the urinary tract.[6] Higher-than-normal placement of the umbilicus occurs in Robinow syndrome, a condition also known as *fetal face syndrome* because of the striking ocular hypertelorism and macrocephaly that occurs in affected individuals.[5]

Variations in the appearance of the umbilicus, as well as abnormal location, can suggest the presence of a syndrome. In Aarskog-Scott syndrome, also known as *faciogenital dysplasia,* a disorder that combines abnormalities of the face (ocular hypertelorism, small nose with anteversion of the nares, minor anomalies of the ears), digits (mild soft-tissue webbing with clinobrachydactyly of the 5th fingers), and genitalia (*shawl* scrotum, cryptorchidism), the umbilicus is prominent and appears pouting and protuberant. In Robinow syndrome, previously described, the umbilical scar is broad and poorly epithelized.[5] Hypoplasia of the umbilicus occurs in Cornelia de Lange syndrome, a disorder combining growth and developmental retardation with a characteristic facial appearance and multiple congenital anomalies. Finally, in Rieger syndrome, which combines iris dysplasia and other ophthalmologic malformations with hypodontia (absence of the upper incisors), failure of involution of the periumbilical skin occurs, leading to a protruding umbilicus.[7]

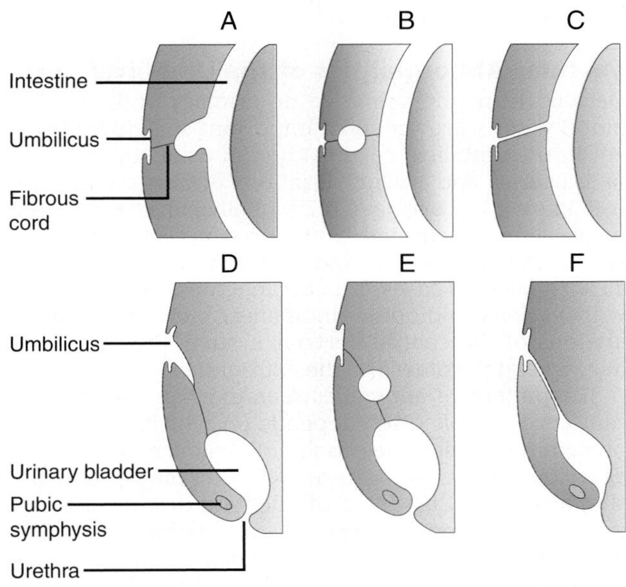

Figure 333-1 Embryonic umbilical remnants. **A**, Meckel diverticulum. **B**, Enterocystoma. **C**, Enteric (vitelline) fistula. **D**, Urachal sinus. **E**, Urachal cyst. **F**, Urachal fistula.

Embryonic Umbilical Remnants

As previously noted, the umbilical cord is formed of the vitelline duct, which connects the yolk sac to the midgut, the allantois, which ultimately degenerates into the urachus, a structure that forms a connection between the apex of the urinary bladder and the umbilicus, and the umbilical blood vessels. Persistence of these structures can lead to the presence of anomalies within the newborn.

Failure of the closure and total regression of the vitelline duct by the 7th week of gestation may lead to the presence of Meckel diverticulum (an outpouching of the gut without attachment to the anterior abdominal wall), a vitelline cyst or enterocystoma (a connection between the midgut and umbilicus without communication with either structure), an enteric or vitelline fistula (formed from a communicating connection between the midgut and the umbilicus), or a urachal sinus, cyst, or fistula (resulting from a connection between the bladder and the urachus)[3] (Figure 333-1). In a child, the presence of these anomalies may be signaled by the presence of signs of infection and of a lower midline abdominal mass (caused by infection of a vitelline cyst); the discharge of feces and urine, which can lead to an erosive dermatitis (from enteric and urachal fistulas); and urinary tract infections (also resulting from urachal fistulas). Furthermore, the persistence of a fibrous band of tissue attached to the gut, the result of incomplete involution, may serve as the lead point for a volvulus or the cause of intestinal obstruction.

Of all these anomalies, Meckel diverticula clearly are the most common. Present in 2.5% of newborns in the United States,[3] they are a well-known cause of clandestine lower intestinal bleeding in children and adults. The bleeding results from the presence of ectopic gastric mucosa within the diverticulum, which is prone to ulceration and hemorrhage. Additionally, given that these diverticula, which can occur anywhere from the ileocecal valve to a point 3 feet or more proximal to the valve, resemble a supernumerary vermiform appendix, their presence may be signaled by symptoms and signs of acute appendicitis.

Embryonic umbilical remnants that are lined with gastric mucosa can be detected by gastrointestinal radionuclide scans using ^{99m}Tc pertechnetate. Sonography or computed tomography is helpful in delineating vitelline cysts that, after onset of infection, exhibits as abdominal masses. The presence of a urachal fistula can best be documented by noting the presence of methylene blue dye in the urine after the dye has been instilled at the umbilicus. The treatment of all internal umbilical cord remnants that are symptomatic is surgical excision and repair.

Vascular Abnormalities of the Umbilical Cord

Derived from the primitive or primary yolk sac, the blood vessels are the most important structures present in the umbilical cord. Although usually consisting of 2 arteries and 1 vein, variations on this pattern are well known, occurring in 0.7% of all births.[3] By far, the most common variation is the presence of only 2 vessels in the cord, consisting of 1 vein and 1 artery. In 25% to 50% of cases, this arrangement is associated with various additional anomalies, including malformations of the central nervous system, the genitourinary tract, the spine, and the extremities.

The pattern of anomalies seen in infants with aberrant cord vessels often depends on which vessels are present and which are missing. Blackburn and Cooley describe 3 separate patterns.[3] In the 1st pattern, the single umbilical artery is of allantoic origin; this pattern is associated with growth retardation, anomalies of the central nervous system such as anencephaly and spina bifida, and abnormalities of the lower genitourinary tract. In the 2nd pattern, the single artery is of vitelline origin; associated anomalies include sirenomelia, sacral agenesis, reduction defects of the lower extremities, anal atresia (features of the VACTERL [vertebral, anal atresia, cardiac, trachea, esophageal, renal, and limb defects] association), and trisomy 18. Infants with the 3rd pattern have cords that have 3 vessels, including a single umbilical artery (of either allantoic or vitelline origin), a left umbilical vein, and a persistent and aberrant right umbilical vein; such a pattern has been described in some children with Noonan syndrome and *47,XXY* karyotype.

Umbilical Hernia

The predisposition to develop an umbilical hernia occurs during the 2nd trimester, after the midgut, which has until then been developing extraabdominally, returns to the abdominal cavity. Failure to form the normal fascial reinforcements that keep the midgut in place leads to a weakness in the abdominal wall.[4]

Umbilical hernias are so common that they should be considered as a variation of normal. The incidence varies with race and age. Evans found that at 6 weeks of age, 32% of black infants had umbilical hernias, whereas only 4% of white babies did. At 1 year, the prevalence decreased to 12% and 2%, respectively.[8] Low–birth-weight babies are also at markedly increased risk.[8] No gender predilection has been noted; boys and girls are equally affected.

In the vast majority of affected individuals, umbilical hernias are associated with no medical sequelae. One study revealed that incarceration, strangulation, rupture, or skin breakdown occurred in less than 5% of 590 children.[8] Other studies have revealed even lower rates of complication. Furthermore, in most cases, the hernia will close spontaneously without any medical intervention.[9] Thus the major indication for surgical treatment of the condition is cosmetic. As such, surgery should only be considered in carefully selected individuals.

Although most umbilical hernias occur as isolated findings in otherwise healthy children, they can also be associated with a variety of known conditions, many of which feature increased abdominal girth or hypotonia. As shown in Table 333-2, these conditions include the common autosomal trisomies, the mucopolysaccharidoses and other inborn errors of metabolism that are associated with organomegaly, and various dysmorphic syndromes, such as Beckwith-Wiedemann syndrome.

Umbilical Granulomas

At birth, the normal umbilical cord contains only the umbilical vessels surrounded by the protective

Table 333-2 Some Conditions Associated With Umbilical Hernias

CHROMOSOMAL ANOMALIES	METABOLIC DISORDERS	DYSMORPHIC SYNDROMES
Trisomy 21	Hypothyroidism	Aarskog syndrome
Trisomy 18	Mucolipidosis III (pseudo-Hurler syndrome)	Beckwith-Wiedemann syndrome
Trisomy 21	Mucopolysaccharidoses	Fetal hydantoin syndrome
Deletion 9p	Type 1 (Hurler syndrome)	Marfan syndrome
Duplication 3q	Type 2 (Hunter syndrome)	Opitz syndrome
	Type 4 (Morquio syndrome)	Weaver syndrome
	Type 6 (Maroteaux-Lamy syndrome)	

From Curry CJR, Honore L, Boyd E: The ventral wall of the trunk. In: Stevenson RE, Hall JG, Goodman RM, eds. *Human Malformations and Related Anomalies.* Vol 2. New York, NY: Oxford University Press; 1993.

Wharton jelly. Within the first 2 weeks after birth, the umbilical stump normally dries and separates from the abdomen; the region is completely covered by skin in 3 to 4 weeks. Delayed healing with the accumulation of excessive amounts of granulation tissue produces an umbilical granuloma, a small, reddened mass. The lesion may be associated with infection at its base or with a foreign body such as talcum, but it recedes rapidly after repeated topical applications of silver nitrate. Persistence of a granulomatous-appearing lesion after treatment, the presence of erosive dermatitis at the site, or the egression of gas, feces, or urine from it should suggest the persistence of one of the embryonic remnants described previously.[10]

Umbilical Polyps

Although polyps may superficially resemble umbilical granulomas, those at the umbilicus actually represent external remnants of the umbilical cord. They may be sinuses of the vitelline duct or the urachus. Often larger in size than granulomas, umbilical polyps are bright red and do not respond to treatment with silver nitrate. Diagnosis depends on histologic examination, and treatment is surgical excision.

SUGGESTED RESOURCES

Blackburn W, Cooley NR. The umbilical cord. In: Stevenson RE, Hall JG, Goodman RM, eds. *Human Malformations and Related Anomalies*. New York, NY: Oxford University Press; 1993.

Curry CJR, Honore L, Boyd E. The ventral wall of the trunk. In: Stevenson RE, Hall JG, Goodman RM, eds. *Human Malformations and Related Anomalies*. New York, NY: Oxford University Press; 1993.

Minkes RK, Chen LE, Mazziotta MV, et al. Disorders of the Umbilicus. eMedicine. Available at: www.emedicine.com/ped/topic2948.htm. Accessed March 7, 2007.

REFERENCES

1. Cullen TS. *Embryology Anatomy and Disease of the Umbilicus Together With Disease of the Urachus*. Philadelphia, PA: WB Saunders; 1916.
2. Campbell J, Beasley SW, McMullin N, et al. Clinical diagnosis of umbilical swellings and discharges in children. *Med J Aust*. 1986; 145:450-453.
3. Blackburn W, Cooley NR. The umbilical cord. In: Stevenson RE, Hall JG, Goodman RM, eds. *Human Malformations and Related Anomalies*. Vol 2. New York, NY: Oxford University Press; 1993.
4. Curry CJR, Honore L, Boyd E. The ventral wall of the trunk. In: Stevenson RE, Hall JG, Goodman RM, eds: *Human Malformations and Related Anomalies*. Vol 2. New York, NY: Oxford University Press; 1993.
5. Friedman JM. Umbilical dysmorphology. *Clin Genet*. 1985;28:343-347.
6. Aase JM. Caudal displacement of the umbilicus: implications for diagnosis of genitourinary anomalies. *Proc Greenwood Genet Center*. 1991;10:120.
7. Jones KL. *Smith's Recognizable Patterns of Human Behavior*. 5th ed. Philadelphia, PA: WB Saunders; 1997.
8. Evans AG. Comparative incidence of umbilical hernias in colored and white infants. *J Natl Med Assoc*. 1944;33:158.
9. Walker SH. The natural history of umbilical hernia. *Clin Pediatr*. 1967;6:29-32.
10. Cresson SL, Pilling GP. Lesions about the umbilicus in infants and children. *Pediatr Clin North Am*. 1959;6:1085.

Chapter 334

URINARY TRACT INFECTIONS

Timo J. Jahnukainen, MD, PhD; Abhay N. Vats, MD

INCIDENCE

Urinary tract infection (UTI) is a common childhood infectious disease. Approximately 2% to 8% of children experience at least one UTI episode by 10 years of age.[1] The susceptibility to UTI depends on age and gender, with the highest incidence in children younger than 1 year. Boys constitute the majority of infants 6 months of age or younger with UTI, and UTIs occurring beyond 6 months are most commonly seen in girls.[2] Approximately 30% of the children younger than 12 months are affected by recurrent infections after the first UTI.[3] A majority (85%) of the recurrences occur within 6 months after the primary episode of UTI.[3] Recurrence rates of UTI do not differ significantly between boys and girls. In school-aged children, symptomatic UTI is 5 times more common in girls than boys. Febrile UTI (pyelonephritis) is more common in children younger than 12 months, whereas cystitis mostly occurs in older children. Table 334-1 shows the common organisms and incidence of UTI for various age groups. The symptoms of cystitis in infants can be nonspecific and therefore difficult to recognize, which may partly explain the higher incidence of more severe UTIs in younger age groups.[1-3]

ETIOLOGY

Community-Acquired Infections

Escherichia coli, occurring naturally in the feces, is responsible for more than 75% cases of community acquired UTI (see Table 334-1). Other commonly occurring pathogens are *Enterococcus*, *Klebsiella*, coagulase-negative *Staphylococcus*, and *Proteus*, with each accounting for approximately 3% to 5% of cases. Genotypic analysis of pathogens causing second-time UTIs has shown that 65% of the recurrences are caused by the same pathogen as the first episode of UTI. The same bacteria were also found in the feces of the patients, suggesting that the colon is a reservoir of uropathogenic bacteria. The prevalence of anatomic abnormalities of the urinary tract is significantly higher among patients with non–*E coli* UTI or infections caused by the nonvirulent *E coli* strains. Researchers have speculated that anatomic or functional abnormality can enhance the invasion of bacteria with low virulence into urinary tract.[4]

Non–Community Acquired and Unusual Infections

Non–*E coli* organisms such as *Neisseria gonorrhoeae* and *Chlamydia trachomatis* should be considered as possible causes of UTI in sexually active adolescents. Multidrug-resistant *E coli* strains and non–*E coli* pathogens, including *Candida*, are the most common pathogens causing nosocomial infections. The vast

Table 334-1 Common Pathogens and Incidence of Urinary Tract Infection in Different Age Groups

AGE	GENDER	INCIDENCE (%)	COMMON ORGANISM	SYSTEMIC/ PYELONEPHRITIS/ CYSTITIS/ ASYMPTOMATIC BACTERIURIA (%)
0-1 yr	Female Male	0.4-1 0.2-0.7	*E coli* *Proteus mirabilis* *Klebsiella* *Enterococcus* *Staphylococcus*	4-9/70/30/2.5
1-5 yr	Female Male	0.9-1.4 0.1-0.2	*E coli* *Proteus mirabilis* *Staphylococcus*	1-5/60/40/1.5
>6 yr	Female Male	0.7-2.3 0.04-0.2	*E coli* *Staphylococcus* *Sexually transmitted organisms in adolescents*	0-4/40/60/0.5-1.0
Cumulative incidence, 0-6 yr	Female Male	6.6 1.8	—	—
SPECIAL SCENARIOS				
Myelomeningocele, Spina bifida	—	100%	*E coli* *Pseudomonas aeruginosa*	Asymptomatic Bacteriuria 90%
Obstructive uropathy	—	—	*Klebsiella* *Staphylococcus* *Enterococcus* *E coli*	—
Immunocompromised patients and those in intensive care units	—	10-20/1%	*E coli* *Candida albicans* *Pseudomonas aeruginosa* *Enterococcus* *Staphylococcus* *Klebsiella*	—

majority of these infections are associated with urinary tract instrumentation or catheterization, which makes critically ill children especially prone to UTI. Fungal infections are significant in immunocompromised or diabetic patients. Fungal overgrowth, however, may complicate antibiotic treatment of immunologically normal children with abnormal urinary tract emptying or those with indwelling urinary catheters.

Viral uropathogens are relatively uncommon except for the adenovirus infections in patients with acute hemorrhagic cystitis. Several viruses, including adenovirus, polyomavirus, and cytomegalovirus, can also cause UTI and hemorrhagic cystitis in immunocompromised patients, especially those undergoing solid organ or bone marrow transplantation. Although protozoan infections of the urinary tract are important in many parts of the world, they remain uncommon in the United States. Urinary infections with *Mycobacterium tuberculosis* occur rarely in secondary tuberculosis but should be considered when sterile pyuria is found in a suspect clinical setting, particularly because the prevalence of tuberculosis currently is increasing in the United States.

Pathogenesis

Generally, UTI occurs when bacteria adhere to the uroepithelium and induce an inflammatory response. Asymptomatic bacteriuria (ABU) is a condition with bacterial growth in urine culture but with no symptoms or signs typical for UTI. UTI is, in most cases, considered to be of the ascending type. The invasion of uropathogens may be restricted to the distal part of the urinary tract, causing urethritis or cystitis (ie, lower infection), or they may reach upper urinary tract, causing ureteritis and pyelitis or pyelonephritis (or both) (ie, upper infection). The probability and level of UTI depends on virulence factors of the bacteria and on the defense mechanisms of the host.[5]

Bacterial Virulence Factors

Uropathogenicity of the bacteria depends on the presence of virulence genes, which determine their adhesive capacity, resistance to host defense mechanisms, and ability to cause tissue damage by toxin production. Expression of these genes varies among different strains. Some of the virulence genes are located on segments of genome called mobile pathogenity islands, allowing them to be spread among different bacterial strains.

Bacterial adhesion depends on the presence of the fimbriae or pili on the surface of the pathogen. Adhesins, which are situated at the tips of the bacterial fimbriae, recognize specific receptors on uroepithelial cells and enable adhesion to these cells. Bacteria may also use fimbriae to invade bladder epithelial cells and thus avoid the wash effect of urine flow.

Bacterial toxins also have an important role in induction of inflammation and tissue damage in the host. These factors influence the severity of symptoms, such as fever or dysuria, and long-term effects of UTI (renal cell damage and scarring). Several *E coli*–derived toxins, such as lipopolysaccharide, α-hemolysin, cytotoxic necrotizing factor type 1, and secreted autotransporter toxin, have been recognized, but their exact role in UTI is still unclear. Some of these toxins have been postulated to use the toll-like receptor-dependent pathway, which finally initiates nuclear translocation of nuclear factor-κB and transcription of inflammatory response genes. Researchers have speculated that toll-like receptor gene polymorphisms may influence a patient's susceptibility to UTI.

Host Defense

Local and systemic host defense mechanisms are relatively effective in preventing UTI. Uroepithelium forms a physical barrier against microorganisms. In addition to providing a passive shield, uroepithelium produces antimicrobial proteins and responds to bacterial invasion by activation of immune cascade.

Under physiologic conditions, overgrowth of uropathogenic bacteria at the periurethral area is controlled by colonization of low-virulence bacterial strains that are considered to be normal flora. Disturbances in normal periurethral flora can allow enrichment of pathogenic bacteria, leading to their spread into urinary tract. The vast majority of bacteria entering the urinary tract are eliminated by the wash effect of urine flow. Adherence of remaining bacteria is decreased by antibodies (immunoglobulin A) and Tamm-Horsfall protein. Pathogens that survive this first line of defense can later adhere to the urothelium. These organisms then face the next level of defense mechanism, which is a set of proteins called *defensins*. Defensins are a family of cysteine-rich peptides with antimicrobial properties and have an important role in eradicating bacteria at the epithelial level. The urinary concentration of one of the defensins, β-defensin-1, is increased up to threefold during acute pyelonephritis. However, the exact mechanism by which defensins kill the microorganisms is unclear.

Once the pathogens cross the mucosal barrier, they may be cleared by the systemic immune defense mechanisms. Local production of inflammatory chemokines and cytokines represents an important defense mechanism of the uroepithelium during acute infection. Adhesion molecules, such as murine intercellular adhesion molecule-1 and E-selectin, and chemokine receptors–mediate recruitment of inflammatory cells and clearance of pathogens. Abnormalities in any of the defense layers can predispose a person to develop UTI.

Bladder dysfunction (detrusor instability) is known to be a significant risk factor for UTI and recurrent infections. Constipation can cause incomplete bladder emptying, leading to retention of residual urine, which disturbs hydrokinetic defense mechanisms.[6] Constipation has therefore been suggested to lessen innate host defense mechanisms and to predispose the individual to UTI. The role of circumcision in prevention of UTI has also been debated. According to some reports, circumcision reduces the risk for UTI, especially in early infancy.[7,8] The possible benefits of circumcision can be explained partly by better penile hygiene when compared with uncircumcised boys.

EVALUATION

History

The clinical presentation of UTI depends on the age of the child, virulence of underlying pathogen, and on the inflammatory response of the host. Dysuria, frequency, urgency, and lower back pain are the symptoms most often associated with UTI. However, in young children, especially in infants, the symptoms of UTI are variable and nonspecific. Even bacteremic UTI can be clinically indistinguishable from other types of infection in very young children. This ambiguity may sometimes lead clinicians to think of alternate possibilities, causing a delay in diagnosis and appropriate treatment.

Small children are not usually able to localize pain or report their precise symptoms. By the age of 4 years, their capability to report more specific symptoms such as abdominal pain or pain at micturition improves. UTI should always be considered as a possible cause of unexplained fever and should be included in the sepsis work-up of seriously ill infants and younger children.

Fever is the most prominent and often the only clearly recognized sign of UTI in children. With some caveats, fever can be used as a rough estimate of the level of UTI. Body temperature less than 38°C suggests cystitis, whereas fever of 38.5°C or more most often is associated with upper UTI. In newborn infants, however, normal body temperature does not exclude the possibility of upper UTI, and they might often be hypothermic. Fever can, however, be an inconsistent finding and exists in only approximately 10% to 40% of UTI cases in children younger than 2 years. In these cases, other symptoms such as vomiting, irritability, abnormal crying, lethargy, failure to thrive, and feeding problems should be considered as indications for urine screening.

Physical Examination

The physical findings of UTI vary depending on the severity of the infection. Especially in infants, the findings are nonspecific and are rarely suggestive of a definitive diagnosis. In addition to fever, other findings suggestive of septicaemia, including irritability, abnormal crying, peripheral cyanosis or hypothermia, and long capillary filling time, can be seen in young infants. Tenderness on palpation of the abdomen in the suprapubic region can be found with cystitis, whereas costovertebral angle tenderness is elicited with pyelonephritis in older children. However, absence of these findings does not rule out the possibility of UTI.

Examination of the urethral meatus should be included in the physical examination of every child with suspected UTI. In some cases, dysuria can be caused by local inflammation or irritation of external genitalia. The external genitalia in girls should be examined carefully, given that labial adhesions are often associated with UTI.

Laboratory Testing

Correct diagnosis is crucial for successful treatment and follow-up of childhood UTI. An incorrect diagnosis of UTI may lead either to missing a potentially harmful urinary tract abnormality or to unnecessary studies, costs, and stress. UTI must be always confirmed by adequate urine collection and culture.

Urine Collection

Adequate urine collection is essential for correct diagnosis. All samples should be collected, stored, and analyzed carefully to prevent contamination. Sample collection at home is discouraged because of the high risk of contamination. The urine samples should be kept at 4°C until cultured.

Before micturation, the periurethral area and surrounding skin should be washed and dried properly. In incontinent children, a urine bag or absorbent pad may be suitable for urine collection, but such methods can have a high risk of contamination. Urine contamination rates are similar for bag and pad (75% of positive cultures) and significantly higher than for clean-catch urine, a catheterization, or suprapubic aspiration. Positive culture results from urine bag or urine pad sample should always be verified by catheterization or suprapubic aspiration (Box 334-1). A negative culture result from urine collected by bag or pad does exclude UTI. For toilet-trained children and adolescents, the midstream urine sample is preferred for culture. If the child is critically ill, then subrapubic aspiration or catheterization is preferred in all age groups.

Urine Culture

The diagnosis of UTI is confirmed by the growth of a single pathogen on urinary culture. The bacteria level that is considered significant depends on the method used for urine collection. For voided samples (clean-catch urine, urine bag, and absorbent pad) bacterial count of 100,000 or more colony forming units (CFU)/mL is considered significant. The contamination risk for catheterization and suprapubic aspirate is considerably lower, and therefore any bacterial growth in suprapubic aspirate or a bacterial count of 50,000/mL or more in a catheter sample is indicative of UTI[9]; signs and symptoms strongly suggest UTI, and even lower numbers of bacteria (≥10,000/mL), particularly in the presence of pyuria, may be considered diagnostic. Urine cultures showing growth of more than 1 pathogen should be considered as contamination, and a repeat sample is required before starting any treatment.

BOX 334-1 Guidelines for Suprapubic Percutaneous Aspiration of Urine

1. Indications
   - Verification of UTI in newborns and infants
   - Sepsis work-up in critically ill children
2. Equipment
   - 21- to 25-gauge needle
   - 5- to 10-mL syringe
   - EMLA cream
   - Sterile gloves
   - Portable ultrasonography equipment
3. Technique
   - Put small amount of EMLA cream on a circle area (approx 3 cm) approximately 2-3 cm above symphysis midline; wait about 30 minutes.
   - Set child in a supine position.
   - Clean the patient's skin with antiseptic solution.
   - Insert needle percutaneously at approximately 1 fingerbreadth above the symphysis pubis.
   - Advance slowly with continuous suction, usually urine is obtained at the depth of 2-3 cm
4. Complications
   - Generally safe and reliable
   - Occasionally transient hematuria (2-3%)
   - Intestinal puncture not harmful

Urinalysis

The results of urine culture are not generally available on the same day that the sample is collected, which may cause a delay in diagnosis. Urinalysis can help in suggesting the presence of UTI, but a normal urine analysis does not rule out UTI. Therefore, if UTI is suspected, then urine culture should always be sent in spite of normal urine analysis. Urinalysis showing leukocytouria can support the diagnosis of UTI. However, urinalysis is not sufficient by itself to diagnose UTI because leukocytes may be present in urine (pyuria) for several reasons besides UTI.

Pyuria is defined as 10 or more leukocytes/mcL in an uncentrifuged urinary specimen. A count of less than 10 leukocytes/mcL is almost invariably associated with a sterile urine culture, whereas a count of 10 or more leukocytes/mcL is found in 90% of patients with bacterial growth of 50,000 or more CFU/mL. UTI can also be an important cause of microscopic hematuria. However, the presence of red blood cells in urine does not have diagnostic or prognostic value. The dipstick leukocyte esterase test can be used for detecting urinary leukocytes, but this method has a low sensitivity of approximately 53% and 67% in detecting 10 or more leukocytes/mcL and 20 or more leukocytes/mcL, respectively. A combination of cell count and Gram stain can be a more sensitive (87.7%) and specific

(99.2%) method to assess the risk for UTI.[9] The combination of leukocyte esterase test and nitrite can also improve sensitivity (78.7%) and specificity (98.3%).[9] Nitrite test is usually positive if the bacterial counts are high enough (>10^5 CFU/mL). However, this chemical reaction requires that urine be present in the bladder for some time. A positive nitrite test usually requires bladder time of at least 4 hours.

Determining the Location of Urinary Tract Infection

Reliable differentiation of upper UTI from lower UTI can be difficult. Several investigations or findings can, however, help in making this distinction. Only 55% to 85% of children with febrile UTI have changes on radionuclide studies, such as 99m technetium dimercaptosuccinic acid (DMSA) scan, which has been suggested as a gold standard for diagnosing pyelonephritis.[10] In addition, infants may have afebrile bacteremic UTI. However, fever of 38.5° C or higher, increased levels of C-reactive protein (≥40 mg/L), and leukocytosis should suggest pyelonephritis. Several biomarkers are currently being evaluated as possible indicators for upper UTI. Procalcitonin is one such marker and has recently been proposed as a possible indicator for pyelonephritis. Increased serum procalcitonin levels have been shown to correlate significantly with renal parenchymal involvement in children with febrile UTI. This method, however, is not currently routinely available or used in the diagnostic testing of UTI in the clinics.

No correlation between the level of UTI and serum electrolyte, creatinine, and blood urea nitrogen concentrations has been reported. However, these parameters should be measured in children younger than 12 months and in patients with febrile UTI or with associated symptoms such as vomiting or diarrhea to assess level of hydration or other attendant complications.

IMAGING STUDIES

The association of anatomic abnormalities in the kidneys or in the urinary tract is increased in children with UTI. The risk is higher in children with non–*E coli* UTI versus those with *E coli*–associated UTI.[11] Imaging studies of the urinary tract are recommended for children with first-time UTI[12,13] to exclude obstructive disorders, vesicoureteral reflux (VUR), severe loss of renal parenchyma, and significant bladder abnormalities. All of these abnormalities are considered as risk factors for renal scarring and for eventual development of hypertension and renal failure. The imaging studies used in UTI include renal ultrasonography (RUS), voiding cystourethrography (VCUG), and DMSA scan. Most of the recommendations have suggested imaging studies for children younger than 2 years in both boys and girls. However, in the last few years, the importance of imaging in routine management of uncomplicated UTI in older children is being reconsidered.

RUS is the least invasive and most widely available imaging modality that can be performed during the acute phase of UTI. It can detect dilated collecting system, thinning of kidney parenchyma, and the size of the kidneys, as well as the thickness and size of urinary bladder. However, ultrasonography may not be able to detect VUR or smaller renal scars. The reliability of ultrasonography is highly dependent on the experience of the radiologist. Recent studies have suggested that ultrasonography results may have little or no influence on the treatment of children with UTI because of routine prenatal ultrasonography.[14] Therefore the need for ultrasonography after UTI has been questioned. The widespread use of maternal-fetal ultrasonography in industrialized countries has possibly lessened the need for ultrasonography later in childhood. However, several studies have shown that a significant kidney or urinary tract abnormality may be missed in spite of prenatal RUS in 5% to 6% of the children with first-time febrile UTI.[15,16] These findings suggest that RUS will probably continue to play a major role as a primary imaging study after the first-time febrile UTI in children.[15,16]

BOX 334-2 International Classification of Vesicoureteral Reflux

Grade I: involves only ureters

Grade II: involves ureters and intrarenal collecting systems

Grade III: mild ureteral and pelvic dilatation; no or slight obliteration of caliceal fornices

Grade IV: moderate ureteral and pelvic dilatation; clear obliteration of caliceal fornices

Grade V: gross dilatation of ureters and renal pelvis and calyces

From Medical versus surgical treatment of primary vesicoureteral reflux: report of the International Reflux Study Committee. *Pediatrics.* 1981;67(3):392-400.

VCUG is traditionally used to diagnose VUR, which predisposes patients to pyelonephritis and recurrent infections and may be associated with renal scarring. The incidence of VUR is highest in children younger than 2 years. VCUG can be performed using either radiocontrast medium or radiolabeled nuclides. Contrast voiding cystography is usually preferred in boys because it is more reliable than other methods in detecting urethral valves, and it allows more exact grading of reflux (Box 334-2); it is recommended as a base-line study in all children with first-time UTI.[14] On the contrary, isotope voiding cystography is recommended for follow-up studies. Cystography requires catheterization, which is relatively invasive and stressful, especially in older children. Spontaneous resolution of VUR occurs in a high proportion of children; hence isotope voiding cystography is recommended every 1 to 3 years until resolution of VUR is documented.

One of the most reliable methods to differentiate pyelonephritis from lower UTI is a DMSA scan. DMSA is a radionuclide that is taken up by renal tubular cells and provides information on functional anatomy, as well as scarring of renal parenchyma. It is more often abnormal in patients with documented reflux than in children without VUR. Based on these results, some authors have suggested that VCUG be performed only on select patients with abnormalities on the DMSA scan.[17] This approach would reduce the number of

BOX 334-3 Indications for Imaging Studies in Children

ULTRASONOGRAPHY

First-time UTI and age younger than 2 years

Febrile UTI, all ages

Non–*E coli* UTI, all ages

Second episode of afebrile cystitis, age older than 2 years

VOIDING CYSTOURETHROGRAM

First-time UTI and age younger than 2 years

All ages if ultrasound or DMSA (or both) is abnormal and suggestive of VUR

Consider if family history of VUR

Consider if recurrent pyelonephritis

DMSA SCAN

Abnormal ultrasound (parenchymal thinning, suggestive of renal dysplasia or hypoplasia)

High grade VUR

Consider before VCUG if febrile UTI and age older than 2 years

Consider if recurrent UTIs

DMSA, Dimercaptosuccinic acid; *UTI,* urinary tract infection; *VUR,* vesicoureteral reflux.

VCUGs performed by approximately 50% without adding any major risk for the patient. VCUG should be performed only if a positive family history of VUR exists or if urinary tract dilation is detected prenatally or a history is found of recurrent pyelonephritis.[17] Box 334-3 summarizes indications for various imaging studies in children. The American Academy of Pediatrics[12] recommends that children younger than 2 years with first-time UTI should be studied by means of ultrasonography in the acute phase and cystography or renal cortical scan thereafter as soon as possible (Box 334-4). The optimal time for VCUG is approximately 2 to 6 weeks after the infection. The recommendations about imaging studies after UTI in older children are more variable and are dependent on clinical presentation. Because the probability to have factors predisposing the patient to renal damage is relatively low in children older than 2 years, imaging studies are therefore recommended in this age group in the following scenarios: recurrent UTI, non–*E coli* infection, or positive family history (see Box 334-3).

TREATMENT

The cornerstones of successful treatment of UTI are early recognition and early, appropriate treatment. Before initiating treatment, adequate samples of urine should be collected for culture and antibiotic sensitivities of organisms. If the patient is septic or dehydrated, then adequate rehydration should coincide with antibiotic therapy. The route of antibiotic administration (oral or parenteral) depends on the age and clinical condition of the patient.

BOX 334-4 Diagnosis, Treatment, and Evaluation of the Initial Urinary Tract (UTI) Infection in Febrile Infants and Young Children

DIAGNOSIS

- The presence of UTI should be suspected in infants and young children with unexplained fever.
- The degree of toxicity, dehydration, and ability to retain oral intake should be thoroughly assessed.
- If the child is critically ill, then a urine specimen should be obtained by catheterization or suprapubic percutaneous aspiration.
- If the child is assessed as not being too ill to require antibiotics, then the options are (1) obtain and culture a urine specimen by catheterization or suprapubic aspiration, or (2) obtain urine by the most convenient method and repeat the urine collection by catheterization or suprapubic aspiration if the urinalysis suggests a UTI.
- Diagnosis of UTI requires a culture of the urine.

TREATMENT

- If the child with suspected UTI is septic or dehydrated or is unable to retain oral intake, then initial antibiotics should be administered parenterally.
- In a child who may not appear ill but who has a urine culture confirming the presence of UTI, antibiotic therapy should be initiated parenterally or orally.
- Infants and children who do not demonstrate the expected clinical response within 2 days of antimicrobial therapy should be reevaluated.
- Infants and young children should complete a 7- to 14-day antimicrobial course.
- After a 7- to 14-day course of antimicrobial therapy and sterilization of the urine, infants and young children should receive prophylactic antimicrobial doses until the imaging studies are completed.

IMAGING

- Infants and children who do not demonstrate the expected clinical response within 2 days of antimicrobial therapy should undergo ultrasonography promptly and either voiding cystourethrography (VCUG) or radionuclide scan should be performed at the earliest convenient time.
- Infants and young children who have the expected response to antimicrobials should have a sonogram and either VCUG or radionuclide scan performed at the earliest convenient time.

From American Academy of Pediatrics, Committee on Quality Improvement, Subcommittee on Urinary Tract Infection. Practice parameter: the diagnosis, treatment, and evaluation of the initial urinary tract infection in febrile infants and young children. *Pediatrics.* 1999;103(4 pt 1):843-852.

Pyelonephritis

Infants younger than 1 year are usually hospitalized and treated with parenteral antibiotics for at least 3 days followed by oral antibiotic therapy for 11 days (a total of 14 days). However, research has shown that oral antibiotics are as effective as parenteral antibiotics

Table 334-2 Antibiotics for Treatment and Prophylaxis in Children With Urinary Tract Infection

DRUG	TREATMENT REGIMEN	PROPHYLAXIS REGIMEN
PARENTERAL THERAPY		
Ampicillin	100 mg/kg/day divided every 6 hr	—
Amikacin	15-22.5 mg/kg/day divided every 8 hr	—
Ampicillin-sulbactam	100-200 mg/kg/day ampicillin divided every 6 hr	—
Cefepime	100-150 mg/kg/day divided every 8 hr	—
Cefotaxime	100-150 mg/kg/day divided every 8 hr	—
Ceftazidime	100-150 mg/kg/day divided every 8 hr	—
Gentamicin	5-7.5 mg/kg/day divided every 8 hr	—
TMP-SMX	6-12 mg/kg/day TMP with 30-60 mg/kg/day SMX divided every 12 hr	—
ENTERAL THERAPY		
Amoxicillin	30-40 mg/kg/day divided every 12 hr	10-15 mg/kg once daily at bedtime
Amoxicillin-clavulanate	30 mg/kg/day divided every 12 hr	25 mg/kg once daily at bedtime
Cefixime	8-16 mg/kg/day once daily or divided every 12 hr	—
Cephalexin	40-50 mg/kg/day divided every 6 to 8 hr	12-15 mg/kg once daily at bedtime
Cefpodoxime	10 mg/kg/day divided every 12 hr	—
Methenamine mandelate	40-50 mg/kg/day divided every 8 to 12 hr	—
Nitrofurantoin	5-7 mg/kg/day divided every 6 hr	1-2 mg/kg once daily at bedtime
Sulfisoxazole	150 mg/kg/day divided every 6 hr	50 mg/kg once daily at bedtime
TMP-SMX	6-12 mg/kg/day TMP with 30-60 mg/kg SMX divided every 8 to 12 hr	2 mg/kg TMP with 10 mg/kg/day SMX once every night

TMP-SMX, Trimethoprim-sulfamethoxazole.
From American Academy of Pediatrics, Committee on Quality Improvement, Subcommittee on Urinary Tract Infection. Practice parameter: the diagnosis, treatment, and evaluation of the initial urinary tract infection in febrile infants and young children. *Pediatrics.* 1999;103(4 pt 1):843-852.

even in young children with febrile UTI.[18] Hence, if the child with UTI does not appear septic and is able to tolerate oral medications, then initial treatment with an oral antibiotic might possibly be appropriate. However, follow-up is essential to ensure complete recovery.

Cystitis

Oral therapy alone is usually adequate to treat cystitis. The first-line therapy for outpatient treatment of UTI is usually trimethoprim-sulfamethoxazole (TMP-SMX) or amoxicillin. Other choices include amoxicillin-clavulanate or first-generation cephalosporins such as cephalexin. The suggested dosing is shown in Table 334-2; 5 days of treatment with appropriate antibiotics is adequate.[18]

Asymptomatic Bacteriuria

Studies on infants and schoolgirls have shown that untreated ABU does not increase the risk for pyelonephritis or renal damage. In fact, children treated with antibiotics for ABU can have a higher incidence of pyelonephritis than untreated children.[12] Researchers have suggested that pathogens causing ABU have low virulence, which may protect against overgrowth of uropathogenic bacteria. Current recommendations for ABU are that it should not be treated with antibiotics,[19] in children who use intermittent catheterization, or in those with neurologic bladder dysfunction. These children frequently have ABU but are asymptomatic and often do not have leukocyturia.

Prophylaxis

Prophylactic antibiotics are recommended for all children after their first UTI until imaging studies are performed.[12] Thereafter, prophylaxis should be considered for children with an increased risk of UTI, that is, children with higher grades of VUR (higher than grade II) or obstructive uropathy and previous history of UTI or children with recurrent UTIs (more than two a year). The most common prophylactic regimen is of co-trimoxazole (TMP-SMX [2 mg of TMP and 10 mg of SMX/kg/day]) or nitrofurantoin (1 to 2 mg/kg/day) as a single daily bedtime dose. The duration of prophylaxis depends on the indication. In children with VUR, the prophylaxis is usually continued until reflux has resolved spontaneously or has been surgically corrected and the child has been free of symptoms and bacteriuria for at least 1 year.

Supplemental Therapy

Constipation and encopresis are known to be risk factors for UTI and should be especially anticipated in children with recurrent UTI. Treatment of these problems by dietary modification or medication is important to prevent recurrent UTI.[6] Besides constipation, the role of circumcision in preventing UTI has also been studied. Although the relative risk of UTI in uncircumcised male infants compared with circumcised male infants is increased from 4- to as much as 10-fold during the first year of life, the absolute risk of developing a UTI in an uncircumcised male infant is low (at most, approximately 1%). Currently, the data are not sufficient to recommend routine neonatal circumcision.[20]

COMPLICATIONS—RENAL SCARRING

Isotope uptake studies (DMSA scans) have shown that the renal parenchyma is affected in approximately 55% to 75% of children with febrile UTI. Approximately 20% to 40% of these children will develop permanent renal parenchymal damage, that is, renal scarring. In some cases, renal disease may be congenital rather than acquired and therefore is not dependent on UTI. In an analysis of 1221 children with first-time UTI, the incidence of permanent renal damage was 86% in boys and 30% in girls. The mean age of boys at the time of UTI was significantly lower compared with girls, and VUR was present in 67% of the boys and in only 19% of the girls.[21] These data suggest that boys have a higher incidence of congenital renal disease and damage to the kidney parenchyma, whereas in girls, the renal damage is acquired and results from UTI. Infants (mean age 4 months) with high-grade VUR without UTI have been shown to have fewer scars than patients with VUR with a history of UTI. In children with high-grade VUR, UTI, and renal damage, determining the exact contribution of congenital factors, reflux, and infection to renal dysfunction may be difficult. The risk factors for renal parenchymal damage include gross VUR, young age at the time of first infection, delayed initiation of treatment, and recurrent infections. Thorough radiologic investigation of young children with UTI and appropriate treatment and follow-up can dramatically reduce the incidence of complications after UTI.

LONG-TERM EFFECTS OF URINARY TRACT INFECTION

UTI is supposed to be an infectious disease with good prognosis. However, several sequelae can be associated with UTI. A risk exists of permanent renal damage, which may increase risk of hypertension and ultimately cause varying degrees of renal failure. UTI may also increase the risk of pre-eclampsia during pregnancy. The risk for end-stage kidney disease, however, is relatively small in children with UTI. According to the North American Pediatric Renal Transplant Cooperative Study (NAPRTCS) (www.naprtcs.org), which collects data on all pediatric patients with renal failure in the United States, pyelonephritis or interstitial nephritis accounts for renal failure in only 1.8% of all patients who require renal transplantation. The respective numbers for obstructive uropathy, renal hypoplasia or dysplasia, and reflux nephropathy are 16.1%, 16%, and 5.2%, indicating that anatomic abnormality with or without UTI is a more important threat for kidney function than UTI itself.

Hypertension has been shown to be a significant long-term complication of childhood febrile UTI associated with renal scarring. The exact risk for developing this complication ranges from 6% to 23%.[22,23] Lower incidences of hypertension may be the result of increased awareness of risk factors related to childhood UTI. Hypertension remains an important long-term complication of childhood UTI, but its incidence may be lowered by careful attention to risk factors and early treatment.

Bacteriuria and symptomatic UTI are significantly more frequent in pregnant women with history of childhood UTI.[22] UTI may also contribute to increased risk to pre-eclampsia (hypertension and proteinuria) and may be harmful for the fetus and cause premature labor.[24]

WHEN TO REFER

- Abnormal findings on imaging
- Frequently relapsing UTI
- Suspicion of voiding dysfunction

WHEN TO ADMIT

- Suspected urosepsis
- Infant younger than 3 months with UTI
- Suspected UTI in dehydrated patient or patient unable to retain oral fluids
- Patient whose symptoms worsen or do not improve despite oral treatment

TOOLS FOR PRACTICE

Medical Decision Support

- *North American Pediatric Renal Transplant Cooperative Study* (Web page), North American Pediatric Renal Transplant Cooperative Study (web.emmes.com/study/ped/index.htm).

AAP POLICY STATEMENTS

American Academy of Pediatrics, Committee on Quality Improvement, Subcommittee on Urinary Tract Infection. The diagnosis, treatment, and evaluation of the initial urinary tract infection in febrile infants and young children. *Pediatrics.* 1999;103(4):843-852. (aappolicy.aappublications.org/cgi/content/full/pediatrics;103/4/843).

American Academy of Pediatrics, Task Force on Circumcision. Circumcision policy statement. *Pediatrics.* 1999; 103(3):686-693. (aappolicy.aappublications.org/cgi/content/full/pediatrics;103/3/686).

Downs S, American Academy of Pediatrics. Urinary tract infections in febrile infants and young children. *Pediatrics.* 1999;103(4):e54. (aappolicy.aappublications.org/cgi/content/full/pediatrics;103/4/e54).

REFERENCES

1. Hellstrom A, Hanson E, Hansson S, et al. Association between urinary symptoms at 7 years old and previous urinary tract infection. *Arch Dia Child.* 1991;66:232-234.
2. Winberg J, Andersen HJ, Bergstrom T, et al. Epidemiology of symptomatic urinary tract infection in childhood. *Acta Paediatr Scand Suppl.* 1974;252:1-20.
3. Nuutinen M, Uhari M. Recurrence and follow-up after urinary tract infection under the age of 1 year. *Pediatr Nephrol.* 2001;16:69-72.
4. Jantunen M, Siitonen A, Koskimies O, et al. Predominance of class II papG allele of Escherichia coli in pyelonephritis in infants with normal urinary tract anatomy. *J Infect Dis.* 2000;181:1822-1824.

5. Jahnukainen T, Chen M, Celsi G. Mechanisms of renal damage owing to infection. *Pediatr Nephrol.* 2005;20: 1043-1053.
6. Hellerstein S, Linebarker JS. Voiding dysfunction in pediatric patients. *Clin Pediatr (Phila).* 2003;42:43-49.
7. Singh-Grewal D, Macdessi J, Craig J. Circumcision for the prevention of urinary tract infection in boys: a systematic review of randomised trials and observational studies. *Arch Dis Child.* 2005;90:853-858.
8. Zorc JJ, Levine DA, Platt SL, et al. Multicenter RSV-SBI Study Group of the Pediatric Emergency Medicine Collaborative Research Committee of the American Academy of Pediatrics. Clinical and demographic factors associated with urinary tract infection in young febrile infants. *Pediatrics.* 2005;116:644-648.
9. Hoberman A, Wald ER. Urinary tract infections in young febrile children. *Pediatr Infect Dis J.* 1997;16:11-17.
10. Majd M, Rushton HG. Renal cortical scintigraphy in the diagnosis of acute pyelonephritis. *Semin Nucl Med.* 1992; 22:98-111.
11. Honkinen O, Lehtonen OP, Ruuskanen O, et al. Cohort study of bacterial species causing urinary tract infection and urinary tract abnormalities in children. *BMJ.* 1999; 318:770-771.
12. American Academy of Pediatrics, Committee on Quality Improvement, Subcommittee on Urinary Tract Infection. Practice parameter: the diagnosis, treatment, and evaluation of the initial urinary tract infection in febrile infants and young children. *Pediatrics.* 1999;103:843-852.
13. Jodal U, Lindberg U. Guidelines for management of children with urinary tract infection and vesico-ureteric reflux. Recommendations from a Swedish state-of-the-art conference. *Acta Paediatr.* 1999;431:87-89.
14. Hoberman A, Charron M, Hickey RW, et al. Imaging studies after a first febrile urinary tract infection in young children. *N Engl J Med.* 2003; 348:195-202.
15. Giorgi LJ Jr, Bratslavsky G, Kogan BA. Febrile urinary tract infections in infants: renal ultrasound remains necessary. *J Urol.* 2005;173:568-570.
16. Jahnukainen T, Honkinen O, Ruuskanen O, et al. Ultrasonography after the first febrile urinary tract infection in children. *Eur J Pediatr.* 2006;165:556-559.
17. Hansson S, Dhamey M, Sigström O, et al. Dimercapto-succinic acid scintigraphy instead of voiding cystourethrography for infants with urinary tract infection. *J Urol.* 2004;172:1071-1073
18. Hoberman A, Wald ER, Hickey RW, et al. Oral versus initial intravenous therapy for urinary tract infections in young febrile children. *Pediatrics.* 1999;104:79-86.
19. Hansson S, Martinell J, Stokland E, et al. The natural history of bacteriuria in childhood. *Infect Dis Clin North Am.* 1997;11:499-512.
20. American Academy of Pediatrics, Task Force on Circumcision. Circumcision policy statement. *Pediatrics.* 1999; 103;686-693.
21. Marra G, Oppezzo C, Ardissino G, et al; ItalKid Project. Severe vesicoureteral reflux and chronic renal failure: a condition peculiar to male gender? Data from the ItalKid Project. *J Pediatr.* 2004;144:677-681.
22. Jacobson SH, Eklöf O, Eriksson CG, et al. Development of hypertension and uraemia after pyelonephritis in childhood: 27 year follow up. *BMJ.* 1989;299:703-706.
23. Wennerström M, Hansson S, Hedner T, et al. Ambulatory blood pressure 16-26 years after the first urinary tract infection in childhood. *J Hypertens.* 2000;18:485-491.
24. Martinell J, Jodal U, Lidin-Janson G. Pregnancies in women with and without renal scarring after urinary infections in childhood. *BMJ.* 1990;300:840-844.

Chapter 335

VERRUCAE (WARTS) AND MOLLUSCUM CONTAGIOSUM

Catherine Chen, MD; Judith V. Williams, MD

VERRUCAE (WARTS)

Verrucae (warts) are virally induced tumors of the skin.[1-3] They are a frequent cause of physician office visits. Cutaneous warts affect up to 10% of children between 2 and 12 years of age and rank among the top three dermatoses in this age group, with no gender predilection.[4] Genital warts are uncommon in children before puberty but represent one of the most common sexually transmitted infections in adolescents and adults.

Etiology

The wart virus is a human papillomavirus[1,5] (HPV) that infects epidermal cells and causes focal epidermal proliferation, expressed clinically as a verrucous papule.

More than 100 types of HPV have been characterized, and the number continues to grow. Specific types have been associated with specific warts. For example, HPV types 1 (HPV-1), 2, and 4 are found in plantar warts; HPV-2 and HPV-7 in common warts; HPV-3 and HPV-10 in flat warts; HPV types 1, 6, and 11 in benign genital warts; HPV types 6, 7, 11, 16, and 32 in laryngeal papillomas; and HPV types 16, 18, 31, 33, 35, 39, 45, 51, 52, 56, 58, 59, and 68 in genital warts that have malignant potential (eg, cervical carcinoma). Thus HPV typing holds promise in helping identify premalignant warts, as well as sources of the transmission of warts.[3,6] Gardasil, a vaccine for HPV types 6, 11, 16, and 18, which together cause 70% of cervical cancers and 90% of genital warts, was approved by the US Food and Drug Administration (FDA) in June 2006 for use in female patients 9 to 26 years of age.[7] It is administered 3 times over a 6-month period. The question about whether it should become mandatory or remain voluntary is currently being addressed at the state level.

Physical Findings

The clinical appearance of warts varies, depending on the type and location. The common wart, or verruca vulgaris, is easily recognized as a superficial, light-colored papule that has a coarse, roughened surface. Warts are often studded with black specks, which many patients call *seeds,* but which are actually small, superficial dermal capillaries. Warts are sometimes found in linear array, presumably as a result of auto-inoculation through scratching. Not all warts appear as verrucous papules. Variants include flat (planar) warts, plantar warts, periungual warts, and anogenital warts.

Laboratory Findings

Warts are almost always diagnosed clinically. If doubt exists, then a skin biopsy can provide histologic confirmation.

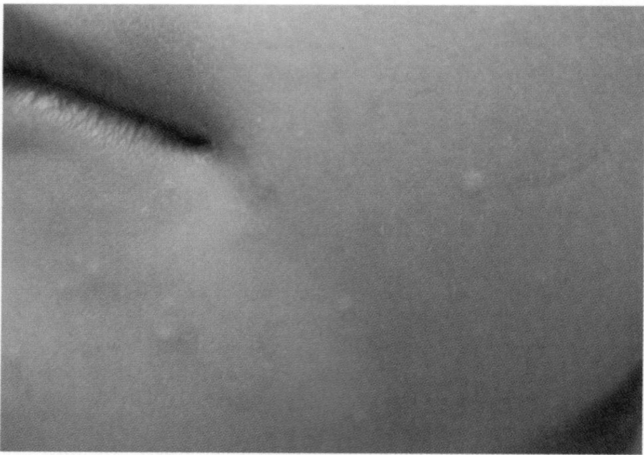

Figure 335-1 Flat warts. Flat warts may be confused with comedones.

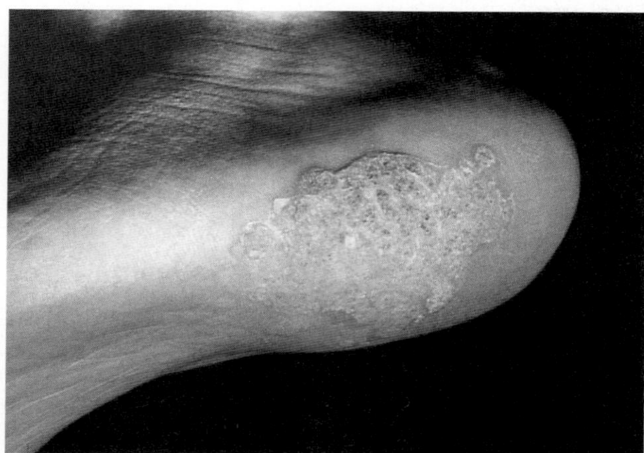

Figure 335-2 A mosaic plantar wart with a roughened surface punctuated with black specks.

Differential Diagnosis

The distinctive clinical appearance of the common wart usually presents no problem in diagnosis. Although epidermal nevi, which are hamartomas, may be confused with warts, they are usually softer, more pigmented, more persistent, and much less common. Flat (planar) warts appear as small, flesh-colored papules (Figure 335-1). When located on the face, epidermal nevi are often confused with the closed comedones (whiteheads) seen in acne. On very close inspection, however, flat warts are seen to have sharp borders and a finely verrucous surface, whereas closed comedones are smooth, dome-shaped lesions.

Plantar warts are so named because they appear on the plantar surface of the foot (Figure 335-2). They are often confused with calluses and corns, although corns are much less common in children than are warts. Large plantar warts are often composed of confluent smaller warts, which form a mosaic wart surrounded by satellite lesions. Additionally, plantar warts differ from corns by having a verrucous surface that interrupts skin markings and are often punctuated with black specks. In some cases, the 2 entities can only be distinguished by paring down the surface; wart tissue still has a roughened texture, whereas a corn is smooth. A corn also becomes smaller in diameter as it is pared; a wart does not.

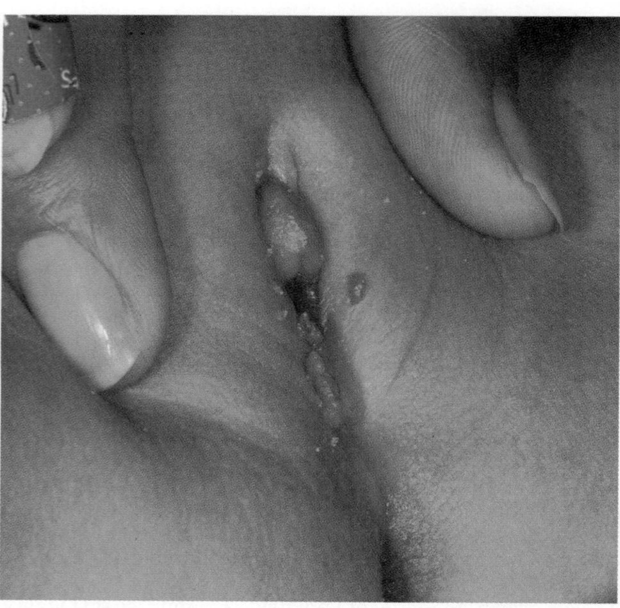

Figure 335-3 Condylomata acuminate appear as skin-colored papules and plaques.

Periungual warts that occur around the nail fold should not pose diagnostic difficulty. Warts under the free edge of the nail, however, can cause the nail plate to separate from the nail bed and may be confused with a fungal infection. On close inspection, the verrucous nature of the wart usually can be appreciated.

Anogenital warts (condylomata acuminata) are sometimes, but not always, acquired by sexual contact.[6,8,9] They can usually be easily identified as verrucous papules (Figure 335-3), but they are sometimes small or flat and therefore more difficult to see. In this situation the acetowhitening technique can aid in the diagnosis. A compress containing 5% acetic acid is applied for several minutes to the suspected area, which is then reexamined, ideally under magnification. With this technique, warty tissue turns white and thus is visualized more easily.

Genital warts may be confused with the less common condylomata lata, skin lesions found in secondary syphilis. In general, condylomata acuminata are drier and usually more verrucous than condylomata lata, which are flat and moist. If doubt exists, then a serologic test for syphilis should settle the issue.

Epidemiologic Features

The wart virus is presumably inoculated into the skin from some external source, but usually neither the source nor event of inoculation is elicitable. Frogs and toads have been unfairly incriminated as carriers.[10] However, asking about and searching for warts on other areas of the body is reasonable; for example, patients who have warts on their lips often have them on their fingers. Given that warts are transmissible, other family members may also have them.

In young infants, warts (including those in laryngeal and genital locations) are assumed to have been acquired from the mother's vaginal tract during delivery. Genital warts in children can raise the question of sexual abuse.[5,9] No clear age exists below which sexual abuse is not a concern; however, several recent studies of anogenital warts in children found no evidence of sexual abuse in most of the subjects under the age of 3 years.[6,8] Based on HPV typing, anogenital HPV infection in most infants appears to be acquired either by nonsexual transmission or perinatally. In fact, a study demonstrating a high incidence of HPV-2 in anogenital warts in prepubertal children suggested that innocent auto- or heteroinoculation from cutaneous warts may be a common means of acquisition.[11] Evidence also exists pointing to the possibility of in utero transmission of HPV, although the exact mechanism (hematogenous, infected semen at fertilization, ascending maternal infection) is unclear.[12] A complete social history and thorough physical examination may be helpful in determining the need for evaluation for possible sexual abuse.

Patients who have systemic defects in cell-mediated immunity are more susceptible to warts, which are often recalcitrant to treatment.[13] In addition, because cellular immune responses in the skin are impaired with atopic dermatitis, these patients, too, have more difficulty with warts and other viral infections of the skin.

Psychosocial Considerations

Among schoolchildren, warts are often a focus for teasing and insensitive remarks. Consequently, when children ask that their warts be treated, they usually do so because of social pressure. Successful therapy gives patients the opportunity to feel better about themselves and their appearance.

Management

Over the years, a wide variety of treatments has been recommended, including some interesting unscientific approaches, such as applying banana peels or slices of raw potato, which probably worked because most warts eventually regress spontaneously. One prospective study of untreated common warts in children showed that two thirds of the warts underwent spontaneous regression within 2 years.[3] This finding must be kept in mind when physicians credit their treatment for a successful result. Nonetheless, when a patient requests treatment of a wart, practitioners are usually inclined to oblige. However, because a specific antiviral medication for warts has not yet been developed, clinicians still rely on nonspecific destructive techniques as therapy; the following techniques are used most often.

Cryotherapy

Tissue is frozen by applying liquid nitrogen (–195°C) to the wart either with a swab or through a canister delivery system. The freeze should extend beyond the wart to include a 1- to 2-mm rim of normal skin. To destroy affected tissue more effectively, the wart may be refrozen after the initial thaw. The patient must be advised that (1) the frozen area will be sore for several days, (2) a blister may form, and (3) several weeks are usually needed for the wart to turn dark and drop off. Cryotherapy is a favorite office therapy for common warts. For small warts, a single treatment is often successful, but large warts frequently need to be refrozen approximately every 3 weeks. Scars may result but are uncommon. The skin may also become hypopigmented. In freezing warts on the fingers, care must be taken to avoid freezing too deeply because underlying structures such as digital nerves can be damaged. Over-the-counter freezing treatments are now available, but these products may not be as effective as liquid nitrogen.

Keratolytic (Acid) Therapy

Acid therapy is slower and involves more patient participation than freezing, but it is less immediately painful and is least likely to cause scarring. A variety of acids are available for treating warts. A convenient outpatient medication incorporates 17% salicylic acid in a polyacrylic or flexible collodion vehicle (Occlusal-HP, Duofilm). The vehicle dries rapidly to prevent spread of the acid onto surrounding skin. The patient is instructed to apply the medication to the wart at bedtime and to cover the area with thick tape. Superficial necrotic tissue should be pared daily, with either a pumice stone or, for thick palmar or plantar warts, a callus grater. The latter warts often require a stronger acid, such as a 40% salicylic acid plaster. These products can be bought over the counter (Mediplast and Duofilm patches), but patients need instruction in application. A piece of plaster is cut to match the size of the wart, and its adhesive, medicated side is applied to the wart and held in place with tape. The plaster is changed every 24 hours and the macerated wart pared daily, as previously described.

Flat warts are often treated successfully with topical adapalene (Differin), tretinoin (Retin-A), or imiquimod (Aldara; see later discussion), applied nightly to the entire affected area. In this situation, these products probably act as *peeling* agents. Painful irritation may occur, necessitating less frequent use.

These home acid therapies usually require at least 1 month of continuous use to be effective. If no progress has been made after several months, then other treatments should be considered. For deeply seeded warts, paring followed by a combination of acid and cryotherapy usually provides successful treatment. Caustic acids such as trichloroacetic acid at concentrations of 30% to 100% are reserved for office treatment of palmar or plantar warts. These acids must be carefully applied because they can cause destruction of normal tissue as well. Cantharidin is a protein phosphatase inhibitor produced by the Spanish fly, *Lytta vesicatoria*. It penetrates the epidermis and causes acantholysis, resulting in vesiculation and destruction of infected keratinocytes. Cantharidin can be used for almost all nongenital warts.[14] Reapplication may be required at 1 to 3 week intervals. It has the advantage of being painless when initially applied and causes little risk of scarring. Occasionally, a ring wart will develop at the edge of the treated site.

All of these treatments are nonspecific, and none of them are foolproof. In some instances, different modalities are used in sequence. Although warts commonly regress spontaneously, the time required for this varies considerably. In some patients, therapy may only serve to appease the patient while nature takes its course. In other patients the destructive techniques may initiate an inflammatory reaction, exposing the wart viral antigen to the body's immune system, which finally rejects the wart. This reaction may explain the occasionally observed phenomenon that by treating the mother wart, the baby goes away. In any event, whenever warts are treated, the physician must guard against doing harm by being overzealous. Accordingly, surgical excision is usually discouraged, and radiotherapy is contraindicated.

Imiquimod

Imiquimod (Aldara) 5% cream is an immunomodulator that augments cellular immunity by inducing a variety of cytokines.[15] It can be self-administered daily or every other day and should be left on overnight. Controlled, multicenter trials have evaluated its role in treating genital warts, but trials will soon be underway for common warts as well. In addition, some smaller studies and case reports are already suggesting its potential as an alternative treatment, either alone or in combination with other modalities such as cryotherapy and salicylic acid.[16,17] Imiquimod's mechanism of action may also make it especially useful in treating nongenital warts in immunosuppressed patients.[18]

Electrodesiccation and Laser Therapy

Electrodesiccation of a wart can be preceded or followed by curettage. One advantage of this technique is that the patient leaves the office without visible evidence of the wart, although the cure rate is probably no higher than with cryotherapy. The disadvantages are that (1) the procedure requires local anesthesia, and (2) scarring is more likely. The carbon dioxide laser can be used to destroy large or refractory warts, but the risk of scarring is significant. The pulsed dye laser, which destroys the vascular component of the wart, may become another alternative, with less risk of scarring. It is used for some recalcitrant warts, particularly in palmar, plantar, periungual, and anogenital areas.[14,19]

Other Treatments

A recent study showed that duct tape occlusion therapy was significantly more effective than cryotherapy in treating nongenital warts.[20]

The efficacy of oral cimetidine in the treatment of warts is still controversial.[21-25] It may be useful in the treatment of flat warts.[23] Use of oral cimetidine in other types of warts is under investigation.

Immunotherapy, which involves sensitization to antigens, such as *Candida,* mumps, or *Trichophyton,* is another technique used by dermatologists when topical therapies fail. Studies have demonstrated response rates ranging from 54% to 74% in treated warts and 34% to 78% in untreated, distant warts.[26,27]

Treatment of Genital Warts

Although condylomata in children are usually asymptomatic, they may be treated to curtail their spread and allay parental concerns. Some forms of therapy may be painful, and recurrence rates may be as high as 50%. Weighing the risks versus the benefits is wise before treating genital warts in children.

Two therapeutic options for condyloma have been approved by the FDA in adults, and case reports with children have shown promise: imiquimod[28] (described previously) and podophyllotoxin.[29,30] Podophyllin is derived from the May apple plant and is available in 10% to 25% solutions in alcohol or benzoin. It is exclusively for office use. Podophyllin is painless when applied but can be toxic if used over large areas. It must be washed off within 6 to 8 hours of application. Podophyllin is also marketed as purified 0.5% podophyllotoxin (Condylox) solution or gel. Podophyllotoxin has also been shown to be effective in case reports involving children and infants. It is available for home use but can be very irritating for some patients. Other options for treatment of condylomata include cryotherapy, lasers, caustic acids, and cimetidine.

Complications

The major complications of warts are those caused by overzealous therapy, resulting in short-term discomfort or scarring. The annoyance of the presence of a wart, which is usually temporary, must be balanced against the inconvenience of a scar, which is usually lifelong, may be unsightly and is sometimes tender, particularly if present on a pressure-bearing surface such as the sole of the foot.

Prognosis

Most warts eventually involute spontaneously, probably through immunologic rejection.[13] Because the time required for involution varies greatly, predicting when it might occur for an individual patient is impossible. The goal of therapy, then, is to shorten the time required for the wart to disappear. The therapies outlined in this chapter result in clearing in most cases; but patients who have resistant, persistent warts will continue to be plagued by them. More specific therapy is needed for these patients especially, and these patients may benefit from an evaluation by a dermatologist.

MOLLUSCUM CONTAGIOSUM

Since the eradication of smallpox, molluscum contagiosum is the only poxvirus infection that specifically affects humans.[31] Similar to warts, molluscum lesions are virally induced tumors of the skin. In children, molluscum contagiosum is a common, benign, self-limited process.

Etiology

Molluscum contagiosum is caused by molluscum contagiosum virus (MCV), a large double-stranded DNA virus of the *Molluscipoxvirus* genus.[32] Four subtypes of the virus have been identified. Although most cases of infection are caused by the first subtype, MCV-1, the subtypes are clinically indistinguishable.[33]

Epidemiologic Features

In the United States, fewer than 5% of children demonstrate MCV infection, with approximately 80% of cases occurring in children younger than 8 years.[32] Gender distribution is equal. It is spread by contact, through skin-to-skin contact (eg, certain sports, sexual activity), fomites (eg, sponges, towels, beauty parlors, heated public pools and baths), or autoinoculation.[34-36] Of note, patients with impaired cell-mediated immunity have increased incidence and severity. Examples include HIV-positive patients (though incidence has been somewhat controlled with the success of highly active antiretroviral therapy),[37,38] patients with atopic dermatitis,[39,40] and patients receiving immunosuppressants.[11,41]

Physical Findings

The lesions of molluscum contagiosum are discrete, dome-shaped, umbilicated, waxy papules, and their color can be skin colored, pink, or white.[42] Their translucence may cause them to resemble vesicles. The lesions may also resemble milia or skin tags. Their diameter usually does not exceed 5 mm, although they can sometimes be as wide as 15 mm (ie, giant molluscum). Lesions may occur anywhere on the body, although the most common locations are the axilla, sides of the trunk, lower abdomen, thighs, and face. Although genital molluscum contagiosum in young children do not necessarily indicate sexual abuse, it should be considered.[43]

Laboratory Findings

Molluscum contagiosum is usually diagnosed clinically. If the diagnosis is unclear, then a skin biopsy can confirm it.

Differential Diagnosis

The diagnosis of molluscum contagiosum is generally straightforward. However, it may occasionally be mistaken for verrucae, varicella, folliculitis, furunculitis, milia, juvenile xanthogranuloma, spitz nevi, and skin tags.[42]

Management

Active Nonintervention

Some lesions resolve spontaneously within a few weeks, though the average lesion takes 2 to 3 years to clear, with some lesions taking up to 5 years. For most active children, avoiding situations that promote spread and proliferation is sufficient,[44] Behaviors to avoid include excoriating lesions, walking barefoot in public places, and sharing personal items such as towels and sponges. However, if lesions are numerous or persistent, or if new lesions continue to appear, then therapeutic intervention can be helpful. In the case of periocular molluscum contagiosum, the risk of iatrogenic injury justifies active nonintervention unless symptomatic conjunctivitis is present, when surgical removal under general anesthesia is merited.[45]

Tretinoin

The ability of topical tretinoin to induce local inflammation has also been helpful in treating molluscum contagiosum, though controlled trials are needed to confirm its efficacy. It can be applied daily for 2 to 3 months, and it can be used safely on the face and other sensitive areas. Side effects are usually mild and include site irritation, dryness, and photosensitivity; thus patients should be advised to wear sunscreen and limit sun exposure while using tretinoin.

Duct Tape

Duct tape can be used for recalcitrant molluscum contagiosum.[46] It can be cut to the size of each lesion and applied (and reapplied if needed) until all lesions have cleared. Duct tape is an attractive treatment option because it is affordable, available over the counter, nondestructive, and painless (or minimally painful), and it can be used at home, reducing the need for office visits. Controlled studies comparing it with conventional treatments are needed to further establish its efficacy.

Cantharidin

Cantharidin, a vesiculating agent derived from the Spanish fly, is a helpful in-office treatment for molluscum contagiosum lesions. Although it has not been approved by the FDA, cantharidin has been recommended by the FDA's Pharmacy Compounding Advisory Committee for inclusion as a compounded medication to be used in physicians' offices since 1998. Local pharmacies may compound the 0.7% solution, or it can be obtained in compounded form by several American and Canadian manufacturers. Cantharidin is administered in the office using the blunt wooden end of a cotton-tipped swab and applied sparingly to the lesions. It should be rinsed off with liberal amounts of water in 4 to 6 hours, or sooner if the patient complains of pain or if vesiculation occurs. Cantharidin may be reapplied in 2 to 4 weeks. In a recent study involving 300 children with molluscum contagiosum treated with catharidin, 90% had clearance of their lesions after an average of 2 treatment visits, and an additional 8% had improvement of their lesions.[47] The most common side effects were related to site irritation. Experts have suggested that occlusion with translucent tape 5 minutes after cantharidin application can enhance clearance of persistent lesions; the tape can be removed when blistering or soreness develops.[48] On rare occasions, patients may have an exaggerated response with large blister formation. Some experts recommend that every patient have a test dose of the agent to a few lesions and wait up to a week to assess the response before proceeding to treat extensive areas. Some patients never get blisters—just irritation and erythema.

Cryotherapy

A light freeze with liquid nitrogen can be helpful in treating older children with a small number of large lesions. Treatment may need to be repeated in 2 to 4 weeks.

Curettage or Needle Extraction

Curettage or needle extraction done with local anesthesia is an older technique that may be used for larger lesions that do not respond to topical treatments but are best reserved for older children who can better tolerate these procedures.

Cimetidine

Cimetidine is an H_2-antihistamine that is thought to stimulate the cell-mediated immune response and remains an adjunctive therapy.[49] Controlled studies are needed to verify its efficacy.

Podophyllin

Podophyllin 25% solution acts as a keratolytic. It is applied in the office sparingly to lesions, and should be washed off within the first 6 hours of treatment to minimize site irritation.[49] Podophyllin can be reapplied weekly up to 4 weeks. Controlled studies are needed to establish its efficacy in comparison to other treatment modalities.

Pulsed Dye Laser

Although very effective and generally well-tolerated, the use of pulsed dye laser is limited by its high cost, the need for special equipment, and the risk of transient hyperpigmentation.[50,51] Pulsed dye laser remains a third-line treatment for recalcitrant lesions.

Complications

MCV infection is considered a benign condition. During resolution, mild erythema and irritation can occur as part of the local cellular immune response. These signs should not be confused with those of bacterial superinfection, which can occur secondary to excoriation and resulting impetiginization. If significant tenderness, crusting, or purulent drainage occurs, then treatment with topical or oral antibiotics would be warranted.[51]

Atopic individuals frequently develop patches of eczema (molluscum dermatitis) in the area of the lesions, presumed to be a result of their immune response to the virus or repeated excoriation of the lesions.

Prognosis

Although most healthy children do not experience recurrences of MCV infection, extensive molluscum infections can occur in immunocompromised individuals, especially patients with HIV or AIDS.

WHEN TO REFER

- A child with warts or molluscum contagiosum in the perineal or perianal area
- Unresponsive/persistent or extensive warts or molluscum contagiosum

TOOLS FOR PRACTICE

Engaging Patient and Family

- *What is a Pediatric Dermatologist?* (fact sheet), American Academy of Pediatrics (www.aap.org/family/PedDermatologistfacts.pdf).

Medical Decision Support

- *Pediatric Dermatology: A Quick Reference Guide* (book), American Academy of Pediatrics (www.aap.org/bookstore).
- *Red Book: 2006 Report of the Committee on Infectious Diseases,* 27th edition, American Academy of Pediatrics (www.aap.org/bookstore).

REFERENCES

1. Androphy EJ. Human papillomavirus: current concepts. *Arch Dermatol.* 1989;125:683-685.
2. Birkett DA. Warts and their management. *Practitioner.* 1982;226:1251-1254.
3. Cobb MW. Human papillomavirus infection. *J Am Acad Dermatol.* 1990;22:547-566.
4. Kirnbauer, Lenz P, Okun MM. Human papillomavirus. In: Bolognia JL, Jorizzo JL, Rapini RP, eds. *Dermatology.* Philadelphia, PA: Mosby; 2003.
5. Bender ME. New concepts of condylomata acuminata in children. *Arch Dermatol.* 1986;122:1121-1124.
6. Obalek S, Jablonska S, Favre M, et al. Condylomata acuminata in children: frequent association with human papillomaviruses responsible for cutaneous warts. *J Am Acad Dermatol.* 1990;23:205-213.
7. Centers for Disease Control and Prevention, Division of STD Prevention. STD Facts—HPV Vaccine. August 2006. Available at: www.cdc.gov/std/hpv/STDFact-HPV-vaccine.htm. Accessed June 25, 2007.
8. Cohen BA, Honig P, Androphy E. Anogenital warts in children: clinical and virologic evaluation for sexual abuse. *Arch Dermatol.* 1990;126:1575-1580.
9. Rock B, Naghashfar Z, Barnett N, et al. Genital tract papillomavirus infection in children. *Arch Dermatol.* 1986; 122:1129-1132.
10. Ross MS. Warts in the medical folklore of Europe. *Int J Dermatol.* 1979;18:505-509.
11. Handley J, Hanks E, Armstrong K, et al. Common association of HPV 2 with anogenital warts in prepubertal children. *Pediatr Dermatol.* 1997;14:339-343.
12. Syrjanen S, Puranen M. Human papillomavirus infections in children: the potential role of maternal transmission. *Crit Rev Oral Biol Med.* 2000;11:259-274.
13. Adler A, Safai B. Immunity in wart resolution. *J Am Acad Dermatol.* 1979;1:305-309.
14. Goldfarb MT, Gupta AK, Gupta MA, et al. Office therapy for human papillomavirus infection in nongenital sites. *Dermatol Clin.* 1991;9:287-296.
15. Rivera A, Tyring SK. Therapy of cutaneous human papillomavirus infections. *Dermatol Ther.* 2004;17:441-448.
16. Hengge UR, Esser S, Schultewolter T, et al. Self-administered topical 5% imiquimod for the treatment of common warts and molluscum contagiosum. *Br J Dermatol.* 2000;143:1026-1031.
17. Housman TS, Jorizzo JL. Anecdotal reports of 3 cases illustrating a spectrum of resistant common warts treated with cryotherapy followed by topical imiquimod and salicylic acid. *J Am Acad Dermatol.* 2002;47: S217-S220.
18. Harwood CA, Perrett CM, Brown VL, et al. Imiquimod 5% cream for recalcitrant cutaneous warts in immunosuppressed individuals. *Br J Dermatol.* 2005;152:122-129.
19. Webster GF, Satur N, Goldman MP, et al. Treatment of recalcitrant warts using the pulsed dye laser. *Cutis.* 1995; 56:230-232.
20. Focht DR III, Spicer C, Fairchok MP. The efficacy of duct tape vs cryotherapy in the treatment of verruca vulgaris (the common wart). *Arch Pediatr Adolesc Med.* 2002;156: 971-974.
21. Bauman C, Francis JS, Vanderhooft S, et al. Cimetidine therapy for multiple viral warts in children. *J Am Acad Dermatol.* 1996;35:271-272.
22. Glass AT, Solomon BA. Cimetidine therapy for recalcitrant warts in adults. *Arch Dermatol.* 1996;132:680-682.
23. Karablut AA, Sahin S, Eksioglu M. Is cimetidine effective for nongenital warts? A double-blind, placebo-controlled study. *Arch Dermatol.* 1997;133:533.
24. Orlow SJ, Paller A. Cimetidine therapy for multiple viral warts in children. *J Am Acad Dermatol.* 1993;28:794-796.

25. Yilmaz E, Alpsoy E, Bajaran E. Cimetidine therapy for warts: a placebo-controlled, double-blind study. *J Am Acad Dermatol.* 1996;34:1005-1007.
26. Clifton MM, Johnson SM, Roberson PK, et al. Immunotherapy for recalcitrant warts in children using intralesional mumps or Candida antigens. *Pediatr Dermatol.* 2003;20:268-271.
27. Johnson SM, Roberson PK, Horn TD. Intralesional injection of mumps or Candida skin test antigens. *Arch Dermatol.* 2001;137:451-455.
28. Bayerl C, Feller G, Goerdt S. Experience in treating molluscum contagiosum in children with imiquimod 5% cream. *Br J Dermatol.* 2003;149:S25-S29.
29. Beutner KR, Spruance SL, Hougham AJ, et al. Treatment of genital warts with an immune-response modifier (imiquimod). *J Am Acad Dermatol.* 1998;38:230-239.
30. Moresi JM, Herbert CR, Cohen BA. Treatment of anogenital warts in children with topical 0.5% podofilox gel and 5% imiquimod cream. *Pediatr Dermatol.* 2001;18: 448-450.
31. Mancini AJ, Shani-Adir A. Other viral diseases. In: Bolognia JL, Jorizzo JL, Rapini RP, eds. *Dermatology.* Philadelphia, PA: Mosby; 2003.
32. Dohil MA, Lin P, Lee J, et al. The epidemiology of molluscum contagiosum in children. *J Am Acad Dermatol.* 2006; 54:47-54.
33. Diven DG. An overview of poxviruses. *J Am Acad Dermatol.* 2001;44:1-14.
34. Becker TM, Blount JH, Judson DJ. Trends in molluscum contagiosum in the United States, 1933-1983. *Sex Transm Dis.* 1986;13:88-92.
35. Choong KY, Roberts LJ. Molluscum contagiosum, swimming and bathing: a clinical analysis. *Australas J Dermatol.* 1999;40:89-92.
36. Niizeki K, Kano O, Kondo Y. An epidemic study of molluscum contagiosum. Relationship to swimming. *Dermatologica.* 1984;169:197-198.
37. Calista D, Boschini A, Landi G. Resolution of disseminated molluscum contagiosum with highly active antiretroviral therapy (HAART) in patients with AIDS. *Eur J Dermatol.* 1999;9:211-213.
38. Schwarz JJ, Myskowski PL. Molluscum contagiosum in patients with human immunodeficiency virus infection. *J Am Acad Dermatol.* 1992;27:583-588.
39. Leung D, Soter N. Cellular and immunologic mechanisms in atopic dermatitis. *J Am Acad Dermatol.* 2001; 44:S1-S12.
40. Pauly C, Artis W, Jones H. Atopic dermatitis, impaired cellular immunity, and molluscum contagiosum. *Arch Dermatol.* 1978;114:391-393.
41. Hellier F. Profuse mollusca contagiosa of the face induced by corticosteroids. *Br J Dermatol.* 1971;85:398.
42. Mancini AJ, Bodemer C. Viral infections. In: Schachner LA, Hansen RC, eds. *Pediatric Dermatology.* New York, NY: Mosby; 2003.
43. Bargman H. Is genital molluscum contagiosum a cutaneous manifestation of sexual abuse in children? *J Am Acad Dermatol.* 1986;14:847-849.
44. Weston WL, Lane AT. Should molluscum be treated? *Pediatrics.* 1980;65:865.
45. Margo C, Katz NNK. Management of periocular molluscum contagiosum in children. *J Pediatr Ophthalmol Strabismus.* 1983;20:19-21.
46. Lindau MS, Munar MY. Use of duct tape occlusion in the treatment of recurrent molluscum contagiosum. *Pediatr Dermatol.* 2004;21:609.
47. Silverberg NB, Sidbury R, Mancini AJ. Childhood molluscum contagiosum: experience with cantharidin therapy in 300 patients. *J Am Acad Dermatol.* 2000;43: 503-507.
48. Epstein E. Cantharidin therapy for molluscum contagiosum in children. *J Am Acad Dermatol.* 2001;45: 638.
49. Smolinski KN, Yan AC. How and when to treat molluscum contagiosum and warts in children. *Pediatr Ann.* 2005;34:211-221.
50. Hindson C, Cotterill J. Treatment of molluscum contagiosum with the pulsed tuneable dye laser. *Clin Exp Dermatol.* 1997;22:255.
51. Michel JL. Treatment of molluscum contagiosum with 585 nm collagen remodeling pulsed dye laser. *Eur J Dermatol.* 2004;14:103-106.

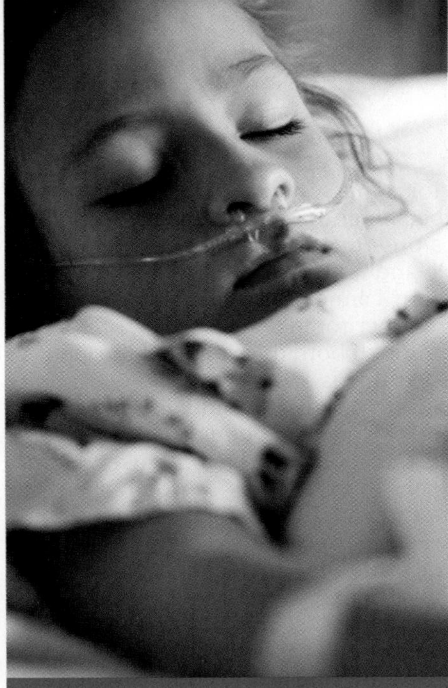

PART 10

Critical Situations

336 Acute Surgical Abdomen
337 Airways Obstruction
338 Altered Mental Status
339 Anaphylaxis
340 Croup (Acute Laryngotracheobronchitis)
341 Dehydration
342 Diabetic Ketoacidosis
343 Disseminated Intravascular Coagulation
344 Drowning and Near Drowning
345 Drug Overdose
346 Envenomations
347 Esophageal Caustic Injury
348 Head Injuries
349 Heart Failure
350 Hypertensive Emergencies
351 Hypoglycemia
352 Increased Intracranial Pressure
353 Meningococcemia
354 Pneumothorax and Pneumomediastinum
355 Poisoning
356 Rape
357 Acute Renal Failure
358 Shock
359 Status Asthmaticus
360 Status Epilepticus
361 Thermal Injuries

Chapter 336

ACUTE SURGICAL ABDOMEN

Michael D. Klein, MD

Some abdominal pain can be evaluated in a measured way, but the acute surgical abdomen may require immediate surgical intervention. Three major diagnoses must be considered that are the most common and the most likely to cause complications if treatment is delayed. These diagnoses are (1) malrotation and midgut volvulus, which usually presents in the newborn period, (2) intussusception, which occurs most often in children between the ages of 2 months and 2 years, and (3) appendicitis, which is most common in children older than 5 years. Other causes of abdominal pain, some requiring immediate surgical intervention, are highlighted in Box 336-1.

APPROACH TO THE CHILD WITH ACUTE ABDOMINAL PAIN

History

A complete history is important in evaluating all patients with abdominal pain. Emphasis should be placed on eliciting the nature, location, radiation, and timing of the pain and whether it is associated with physical activity or eating. Most patients with an acute surgical problem will have anorexia and will usually have nausea and vomiting. Generally, their bowel habits are unchanged, or they will have constipation. Diarrhea is unusual in diseases requiring urgent operation. The pain usually precedes vomiting. Systemic symptoms such as headache and myalgia are seldom present. Pharyngitis, however, does not rule out a surgical problem. The clinician must certainly ask specifically about genitourinary tract symptoms, other illnesses, and prior operations.

Physical Examination

The physical examination of the abdomen is crucial. Inspection can reveal distension or a mass. Palpation should begin by gently stroking all abdominal quadrants while looking at the patient's face. With peritonitis, cutaneous hyperesthesia is often present, which can be determined by narrowing of the outer canthus of the eye (wincing). The clinician should next gently percuss the entire abdomen; pain on percussion is termed rebound and indicates peritonitis, which can be localized or general. Other tests for rebound, such as pushing in on the abdomen and then suddenly letting go, are very painful and unnecessary. Gentle palpation and percussion will provide sufficient information. Percussion can also indicate gaseous distension of the intestine by the resonant note of tympany. The next step in the abdominal examination is to palpate the abdomen quadrant by quadrant, again while looking at the patient's face. The clinician should make several passes of each quadrant, with each one being deeper, looking for a mass, tenderness, and guarding. Guarding is a specific and important sign. When the examiner pushes on a quadrant of the abdomen over the rectus muscle and it pushes back, this is known as *guarding*. Guarding cannot occur voluntarily, and it indicates localized peritonitis and, most often, the need for an operation. If both the right and the left rectus push back, then this is known as *rigidity*. Rigidity indicates generalized peritonitis, and in contrast to guarding, it can be performed voluntarily.

Auscultation of the abdomen offers no useful information. Possibly no bowel sounds can be heard with an ileus or high-pitched hyperactive bowel sounds heard with obstruction, but no data support this distinction. The rectal examination is useful if the clinician suspects a pelvic abscess or if stool is needed for guaiac to screen for intussusception, but these events are unusual. The clinician should assess structures or organs superior and inferior to the abdomen because pneumonia, inguinal hernia, and testicular torsion can cause abdominal pain.

Evaluation

Laboratory Tests

Laboratory tests are helpful when the history and physical examination are not conclusive. Patients with anemia can have one of many medical conditions such as sickle cell anemia, Henoch-Schönlein purpura, and lead toxicity. An elevated white blood cell (WBC) count is revealing. In acute appendicitis without perforation, the count is elevated from 9000 to 14,000/mm^3. If the bowel is perforated or gangrenous, or if an intra-abdominal abscess exists, then the WBC count will exceed 12,000/mm^3. The urinalysis can also be revealing. A high specific gravity indicates hypovolemia. Ketones in the urine indicate significant anorexia and emesis. WBCs and bacteria indicate a urinary tract infection. Red blood cells indicate trauma or stone. Casts may indicate glomerulonephritis that can be associated with primary peritonitis. Most patients with intussusception will have a positive stool guaiac test result.[1]

Imaging

Imaging studies can also aid in diagnosis. Plain-film radiographs of the abdomen can show bowel obstruction (distended loops of bowel, air-fluid levels, absence of colonic gas), localized ileus, free air in the abdomen, scoliosis, or the impression of a mass. The chest radiograph may show free air under the diaphragm or pneumonia. Ultrasound is especially useful in locating ovarian disease; it can also suggest appendicitis, intussusception, and even malrotation with midgut volvulus (reversal of the normal superior mesenteric artery and superior mesenteric vein relationship). Computed tomography (CT) scan is useful in diagnosing appendicitis in patients with sickle cell anemia or who are immunocompromised (transplant patients and those being treated for malignancy).

Observation

In most cases of acute surgical abdomen an operation is emergent. When considering malrotation and midgut volvulus or intussusception, immediate surgical

BOX 336-1 Causes of Abdominal Pain in Children

I. Peritoneum—inflammatory
- Bacterial
- Primary
- Secondary
- Perforated viscus*
- Stomach, duodenum*
- Appendix*
- Foreign body*

II. Hollow intestinal organs—inflammatory
- Appendicitis (C)*
- Cholecystitis*
- Gastroenteritis (C)
- Regional enteritis (C)
- Meckel diverticulitis*
- Colitis—ulcerative, Crohn, bacterial, amebic (C)
- Typhlitis

III. Hollow-intestinal organs—noninflammatory
- Intussusception*
- Malrotation and midgut volvulus*
- Intestinal obstruction (C)*
- Inguinal hernia*
- Biliary colic*
- Peptic ulcer
- Constipation (C)
- Cystic fibrosis

IV. Enteric infections (gastroenteritis)
- *Shigella*
- *Salmonella*
- *Campylobacter*
- *Clostridium difficile*
- Viral gastroenteritis (C)

V. Unusual infections
- Malaria
- Tuberculosis of the spine
- Osteomyelitis
- Psoas abscess
- Helminthic infestation

VI. Solid viscera
- Acute hepatosplenomegaly
- Abscess of spleen or liver
- Pancreatitis
- Hepatitis
- Fitzhugh-Curtis syndrome
- Mesenteric lymphadenitis
- Torsion of:
  - Testicle*
  - Scrotal appendages*
  - Omentum*
  - Spleen*
- Appendix epiploica*

VII. Gynecologic (C)
- Salpingitis
- Mittelschmerz
- Ovarian cyst (usually ruptured)
- Menstrual pain
- Threatened abortion
- Ectopic gestation*
- Ovarian torsion*
- Pelvic inflammatory disease
- Endometritis
- Endometriosis

VIII. Urinary tract (C)
- Pyelonephritis
- Hydronephrosis
- Calculi*
- Cystitis

IX. Trauma (C)
- Rectus muscle tear
- Hematoma
- Solid-organ injury*
- Hollow-organ injury*

X. Trauma to a previously unsuspected mass
- Hydronephrosis*
- Wilms tumor*

XI. Medical diseases
- Pneumonia
- Sickle cell anemia (C)
- Henoch-Schönlein purpura
- Streptococcal pharyngitis
- Lead poisoning
- Green-apple bellyache
- Hemolytic-uremic syndrome
- Diabetic ketoacidosis (C)
- Porphyria
- Hyperlipidemia
- Rheumatic fever
- Epilepsy
- Migraine
- Hemophilia
- Herpes zoster
- Lupus erythematosus

XII. Immunosuppressed
- Ischemic colitis
- Typhlitis
- Primary peritonitis

XIII. Nonorganic—chronic
- Recurrent
- Psychogenic
- Functional
- Psychophysiological

C, indicates most common causes of abdominal pain.
*Diagnoses considered acute surgical problems.

intervention can prevent intestinal necrosis. When considering appendicitis, however, observation is a useful diagnostic aid. If a diagnosis of appendicitis cannot be made with history, physical examination, complete blood count, urinalysis, and plain films, then a period of 6 to 12 hours of observation with serial examination and a repeat WBC count may be diagnostic. Patients with appendicitis generally worsen; those without appendicitis usually improve. If observation for 6 to 12 hours does not clarify the diagnosis, then a CT scan is indicated. In performing the CT scan, the patient should have a good enteric preparation with contrast, or the contrast should be instilled rectally so that it can reach the cecum. Intravenous contrast is also important because it makes the presence of inflammation much clearer.

THREE COMMON CAUSES OF ACUTE ABDOMINAL PAIN IN CHILDREN REQUIRING URGENT INTERVENTION

Malrotation and Midgut Volvulus

At 5 to 6 weeks of gestation the elongating midgut pushes out into the umbilical coelom. When it returns to the abdominal cavity at 10 to 12 weeks' gestation, it rotates and fixes to the posterior abdominal wall. The duodenum returns first and is mainly retroperitoneal. It courses behind the mesenteric vessels and enters the peritoneal cavity at the duodenojejunal junction, just to the left of L2, the ligament of Treitz. The colon enters the abdomen last and rotates so that the ileocecal region is in the right lower quadrant. The right and left colon are fixed to the posterior abdominal wall by avascular attachments. Thus the small bowel mesentery is normally fixed along a line from the ligament of Treitz in the left upper quadrant just to the left of L2 to the right lower quadrant at the right sacroiliac joint (Figure 336-1). This long fixation prevents the lengthy mass of small bowel from rotating with the superior mesenteric artery and vein as a center. This rotation, twisting, or volvulus would obstruct blood flow to the intestine and cause gangrene (Figure 336-2). If an anomaly of rotation is present, or if this long fixation does not occur, then volvulus can occur. In such anomalies of rotation and fixation (usually termed malrotation or nonrotation) the avascular adhesion of the cecum still appears to occur, although in this case the cecum is usually in the midabdomen and the adhesive bands (now called Ladd's bands) cross the duodenum to the right upper quadrant (Figure 336-3). This obstruction of the duodenum in malrotation causes bilious emesis. The possibility of volvulus in malrotation requires urgent intervention.

Malrotation and midgut volvulus usually develops in the newborn period but can occur at any age. The characteristic symptom is bilious emesis. The occurrence of this symptom should provoke urgent gastrointestinal contrast studies. Approximately one third of all children who have bilious emesis will require operative intervention (although not always for malrotation and midgut volvulus).[2] Any child with bilious emesis who has abdominal pain or tenderness should have either an operation or a contrast examination. An upper gastrointestinal (GI) series to assess for the position of the ligament of Treitz is the surest way to determine malrotation. Normally the ligament of Treitz should be at the level of the pylorus and just to the left of the midline, with the second portion of the duodenum coursing posteriorly on a lateral view. If the imager is not experienced, then a barium enema can help find the position of the cecum, which is normally below the iliac crest and to the right of the midline (although it can occasionally be in this position in malrotation).[3] Once the diagnosis has been made in a patient with symptoms, an operation is urgently required to untwist the bowel and to perform a Ladd procedure. If the diagnosis of malrotation is serendipitous and symptoms are not present, then a Ladd procedure should be performed to decrease the likelihood of volvulus. In this procedure the Ladd's bands are lysed, and the duodenum and colon are separated in an attempt to create a broad mesentery. The appendix is removed because it will not usually be in the right

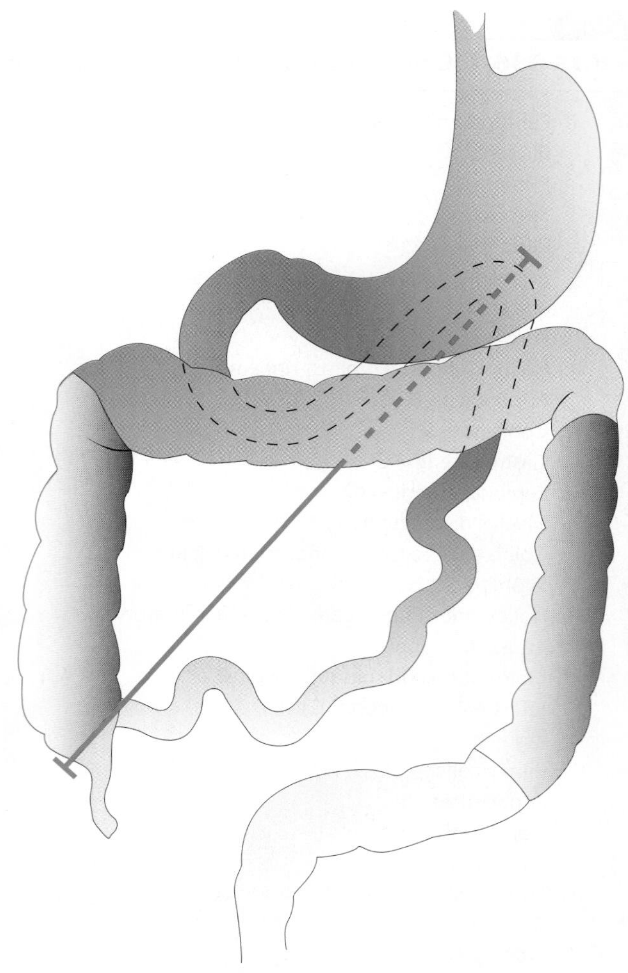

Figure 336-1 Normal rotation and fixation of the intestine. The small bowel mesentery is fixed to the duodenojejunal junction just to the left of L2 to the ileocecal junction at the sacroiliac joint. This arrangement prevents twisting or volvulus.

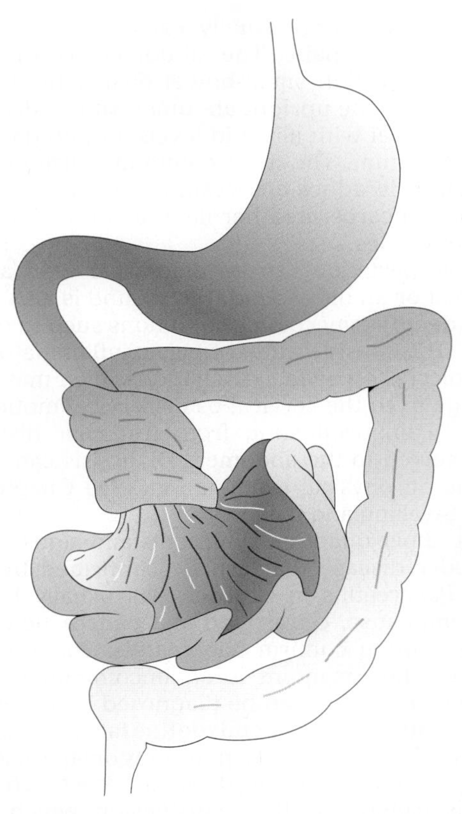

Figure 336-2 Malrotation with midgut volvulus. The small-bowel mesentery has no attachment, and, with the peristaltic motion of the intestine, the entire small bowel can twist around the axis of the superior mesenteric artery.

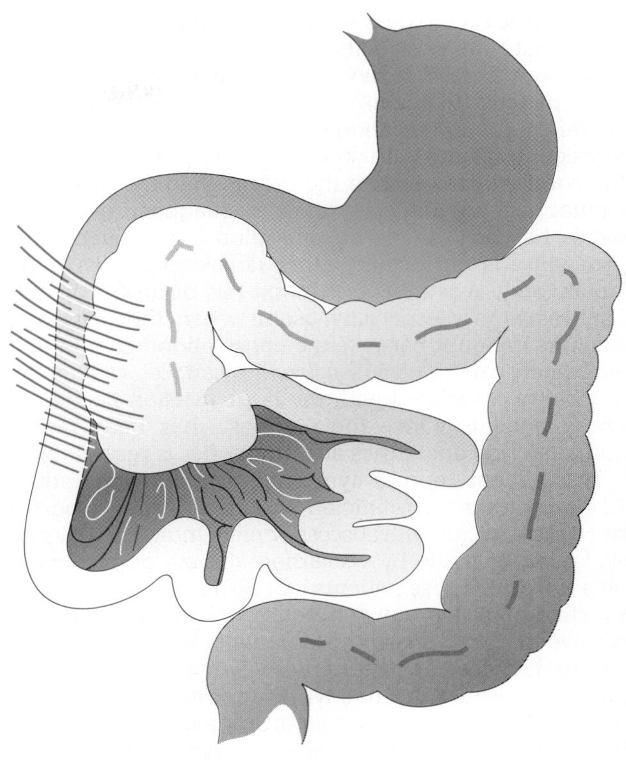

Figure 336-3 Malrotation with Ladd's bands. No attachment of the small-bowel mesentery to the posterior abdominal wall is seen. The avascular adhesions that would normally perform this task instead extend across the duodenum, causing an obstruction.

lower quadrant and thus will complicate any future diagnosis of appendicitis. Hopefully some adhesions will be created to help decrease the chance of volvulus postoperatively.

Intussusception

Intussusception occurs when the terminal ileum telescopes into the right colon. This circumstance causes not only bowel obstruction, but also ischemia because the mesenteric vessels are dragged along with the ileum. Intussusception is most likely due to hypertrophic ileal lymphatic tissue, which acts as a food bolus that can be *swallowed* by the more distal bowel. Most children exhibit intermittent colicky abdominal pain, although some children will be lethargic. They appear well between bouts of pain (approximately 20 minutes). Physical examination reveals a mass in the epigastrium and a feeling of emptiness in the right lower quadrant (signe de Dance). Tenderness and guarding are present as ischemia progresses. Stool is usually guaiac positive, and a *currant jelly* bloody stool may be passed. Diagnosis is made most rapidly by ultrasound or contrast enema. Reduction of the intussusception often can be made by contrast enema using barium, nonionic contrast, or air. When contrast enema reduction fails, an operation is necessary. During the operation the clinician can usually reduce the intussusception, or a resection and anastomosis can be performed. The appendix is also removed. Recurrence occurs in 15% of cases, usually within 72 hours of the original disease. Treatment is the same as that in the initial occurrence.

Appendicitis

Appendicitis is probably caused by obstruction of the lumen by feces or hypertrophic lymphatic tissue that allows stasis and bacterial multiplication to occur in the closed space. Early symptoms of appendicitis are diffuse or periumbilical abdominal pain followed by anorexia, nausea, vomiting, and localization of the pain to the right lower quadrant. Physical examination reveals a fever to 38.6°C, right lower quadrant tenderness, and guarding. The WBC count is usually elevated to 9000 to 14,000/mm^3. Symptoms usually progress over 36 hours until perforation occurs; usually diffuse peritonitis follows. After perforation the tenderness is no longer localized and the guarding becomes rigidity. The temperature rises above 38.6°C, and the WBC count exceeds 14,000/mm^3. Abdominal radiographs may reveal scoliosis to the right, an ileus pattern, and a fecalith early on. In perforated appendicitis the impression of a right lower quadrant soft-tissue mass may be present, as well as a gas pattern of bowel obstruction, with multiple loops of bowel with air-fluid levels. In female patients an ultrasound can be helpful to evaluate the possibility of ovarian or tubal disease, and some experts believe this evaluation is helpful in male patients to identify appendicitis. Most surgeons currently prefer an abdominal CT scan with intravenous contrast and with contrast of the GI tract in which the contrast has reached the colon when the diagnosis cannot be made clinically. Once the diagnosis of appendicitis has been made an operation is indicated. This procedure is performed either laparoscopically or by laparotomy, whether perforation has occurred or not. Laparoscopy is especially useful when the diagnosis remains in doubt because the entire abdomen and pelvis usually can be well visualized; it can also reduce the morbidity associated with the large incision needed in obese patients. Once the diagnosis has been made, administering analgesics and antibiotics is reasonable.

If a patient reports symptoms lasting longer than 72 hours, then the clinician should consider a perforated appendicitis with abscess or phlegmon. This diagnosis is usually made by visualizing abscess or phlegmon on a CT scan. These patients can be treated with broad-spectrum intravenous antibiotics.[4,5] If their symptoms resolve in 2 to 3 days, these patients can then be discharged home on antibiotics. Some clinicians ask patients to return in 6 to 8 weeks for interval appendectomy, which can be done laparoscopically. Little morbidity exists to an elective laparoscopic appendectomy, even after perforation. Most patients will eat the evening of the operation and be discharged the next day. Immediate operation for a delayed presentation of perforated appendicitis can result in a very large incision and a long, complicated hospital course.

DIFFERENTIAL DIAGNOSIS

Secondary bacterial peritonitis is usually caused by appendicitis, but it can be the result of any hollow-organ perforation. Other organs that can rupture and lead to peritonitis are the spleen and kidney, although the peritonitis and pain from these ruptured organs are likely caused by the irritation from blood and urine in the peritoneal cavity.

The second-most common organ to perforate is the jejunum as a result of blunt abdominal trauma. A radiograph of the patient's upright abdomen may not show free air, and a CT scan may show only a small amount of fluid. Persistent abdominal tenderness after blunt abdominal trauma may be the only sign of a perforated jejunum. In children, a history of trauma causing such a rupture may not be obvious (a fall or wrestling match) and may be difficult to elicit, particularly if the child is injured while playing in an unsafe area and is reluctant to admit this activity to the parents. Injury to the spleen or kidney may be related to a previously undiagnosed enlarged kidney (hydronephrosis, Wilms tumor) or spleen (mononucleosis). A perforated ulcer is rare in children and is characterized by free air on abdominal and chest radiographs. Meckel diverticulitis is less common than bleeding from a Meckel diverticulum. The signs, symptoms, and other findings are not especially different from those of appendicitis. Most foreign bodies, including open safety pins, will pass through a child's GI tract without event, but perforation can occur.

Bowel obstruction usually causes bilious emesis and abdominal pain. The abdomen is distended (unless it is a high small-bowel obstruction), and a radiograph of the upright abdomen shows distended loops of bowel with air-fluid levels and no gas in the colon or rectum. The most common cause of bowel obstruction is adhesions resulting from a previous operation; incarcerated hernia and congenital bands are other causes.

Ectopic gestation can be diagnosed with a pregnancy test or an ultrasound. Ultrasound is also important to identify gynecologic conditions such as ovarian torsion. The consideration of pelvic inflammatory disease indicates a pelvic examination which may reveal discharge from the cervical os or cervical motion tenderness. Pain originating from testicular disease is often referred to the abdomen. Diagnosis can usually be made on physical examination. (See Chapter 216, Scrotal Swelling and Pain.)

Right upper quadrant symptoms and signs suggest gallbladder disease that can be confirmed by ultrasound. Pancreatitis in children will usually have an underlying cause. Ultrasound and pancreatic enzyme levels will often confirm pancreatitis. Torsion of the spleen or the omentum is an uncommon cause of abdominal pain that can be diagnosed by ultrasound. Torsion of an epiploic appendage (the fat hanging off the colon) is only diagnosed at laparotomy or laparoscopy.

Although the GI mucosa does not have touch sensation, it is acutely sensitive to distension, which is why constipation can cause abdominal pain. When cystic fibrosis is responsible for abdominal pain, it is usually because of the meconium ileus equivalent even in older children, which is constipation, although intussusception also occurs more frequently in patients with cystic fibrosis.

In immunocompromised patients, right lower quadrant pain and tenderness usually indicates typhlitis and not appendicitis. The inflammatory mass can be seen on CT scan and can be monitored with ultrasound. Treatment is generally nonoperative with broad-spectrum antibiotics.

Most medical diagnoses of abdominal pain can be ruled out by their lack of tenderness or guarding on physical examination. Patients with sickle cell anemia frequently have abdominal pain. They also usually have WBC counts of approximately 14,000 to 16,000/mm^3, so this test is not helpful. If the clinician is not sure of the diagnosis, then treatment for sickle cell crisis, even including transfusion, is best. If the pain resolves, then the diagnosis was not appendicitis. If the pain does not resolve, then the patient needs to go to the operating room.

ROLE OF THE PRIMARY CARE PHYSICIAN

The primary care physician must be able to recognize which patients with abdominal pain have an acute surgical abdomen. In brief, indicators of an acute surgical abdomen include the following:

- Pain lasting more than 1 hour that is severe enough to require analgesics
- Bilious emesis

Table 336-1 Most Common Diagnoses in Boys with a Chief Complaint of Abdominal Pain by Age

<2 YR (n = 56)		2-5 YR (n = 128)		5-12 YR (n = 230)		>12 YR (n = 86)	
DIAGNOSIS	FREQUENCY (%)	DIAGNOSIS	FREQUENCY (%)	DIAGNOSIS	FREQUENCY (%)	DIAGNOSIS	FREQUENCY (%)
Abdominal pain	30 (60)	Abdominal pain	59 (46)	Abdominal pain	117 (51)	Abdominal pain	33 (38)
Constipation	9 (18)	Constipation	21 (16)	Constipation	27 (12)	Appendicitis	14 (16)
Infection	4 (8)	Infection	13 (10)	Appendicitis	24 (10)	Constipation	7 (8)
Bowel obstruction	2 (4)	Gastroenteritis	13 (10)	Gastroenteritis	14 (6)	Gastritis, esophagitis	5 (6)
Dental	1 (2)	Hematologic	4 (3)	Gastritis, esophagitis	14 (6)	Infection	4 (5)
Gastritis, esophagitis	1 (2)	Gastritis, esophagitis	4 (3)	Infection	10 (4)	Diabetes	2 (2)
Crohn disease	1 (2)	Bowel obstruction	4 (3)	Hematologic	5 (2)	Hematologic	2 (2)
Abdominal trauma	1 (2)	Appendicitis	3 (2)	Cancer	2 (1)	Cancer	2 (2)

Reprinted from Klein MD, Rabbani AB, Rood KD, et al. Three quantitative approaches to the diagnosis of abdominal pain in children; practical applications of decision theory. *J Pediatr Surg.* 2001;36(9):1375-1380.

Table 336-2 Most Common Diagnoses in Girls with a Chief Complaint of Abdominal Pain by Age

<2 YR (n = 25)		2-5 YR (n = 94)		5-12 YR (n = 248)		>12 YR (n = 150)	
DIAGNOSIS	FREQUENCY (%)	DIAGNOSIS	FREQUENCY (%)	DIAGNOSIS	FREQUENCY (%)	DIAGNOSIS	FREQUENCY (%)
Abdominal pain	11 (44)	Abdominal pain	53 (56)	Abdominal pain	126 (51)	Abdominal pain	59 (39)
Constipation	6 (24)	Gastroenteritis	9 (10)	Constipation	42 (17)	Genital, pregnancy	14 (10)
Gastroenteritis	2 (8)	Infection	6 (6)	Gastritis, esophagitis	17 (7)	Pelvic inflammatory disease	14 (10)
Infection	1 (4)	Constipation	6 (6)	Gastroenteritis	17 (7)	Urinary	10 (7)
Hematologic	1 (4)	Urinary	5 (5)	Appendicitis	12 (5)	Constipation	10 (7)
Malabsorption	1 (4)	Bowel obstruction	4 (4)	Urinary	8 (3)	Gastritis, esophagitis	9 (6)
		Gastritis, esophagitis	3 (3)	Infection	5 (2)	Appendicitis	6 (4)
		Appendicitis	3 (3)	Hematologic	4 (2)	Gastroenteritis	5 (3)

Reprinted from Klein MD, Rabbani AB, Rood KD, et al. Three quantitative approaches to the diagnosis of abdominal pain in children; practical applications of decision theory. *J Pediatr Surg.* 2001;36(9):1375-1380.

- Abdominal pain of any sort lasting more than 6 hours
- Obstipation
- Localized abdominal tenderness
- Guarding
- Rebound
- Guaiac positive stools, melena, or hematochezia

Indicators of nonsurgical problems include the following:

- Diarrhea
- Symptoms of systemic illness: headache, sore throat, and myalgia
- Emesis precedes pain
- High fever very early in the illness
- No abdominal tenderness

Ordering a complete blood count with differential and urinalysis is reasonable for the primary care practitioner when abdominal pain is the chief complaint. Examination by a (pediatric) surgeon before any other tests, including imaging studies, are ordered is in the patient's best interest. Certainly, when appendicitis is suspected the diagnosis can often be made without resorting to imaging studies. When malrotation is in question, an upper GI series is the best test. However, if the patient already has signs of peritonitis and abnormal signs on plain-film radiograph, then prompt operation might be a better course. When intussusception is being considered, a contrast enema is indicated unless signs of obstruction or necrotic bowel are present, which should prompt immediate operation. When appendicitis is a possibility the first imaging studies should be radiographs of the chest and abdomen. If the diagnosis is not clear, then an ultrasound is the next step in girls and a CT scan in boys. The subtleties of the individual case might alter these judgments; involving the surgeon early will allow a more prompt and accurate diagnosis.

All patients with an acute surgical abdomen have volume depletion. Administering intravenous hydration at one-and-one-half times the maintenance requirement with appropriate solutions is reasonable. Broad-spectrum antibiotics (ampicillin, gentamicin, and metronidazole) and analgesics (morphine) are also of benefit but should probably be started only after consultation with the surgeon. If a patient is vomiting or has marked abdominal distension, then a nasogastric tube should be placed. Certainly, any patient with abdominal pain as any part of their chief complaint should not have any food or drink until a diagnosis and disposition are decided.

IMPROVING DIAGNOSTIC ABILITY

Making a diagnosis is certainly the most difficult task in medicine. Knowledge of the prevalence of a disease can aid the differential diagnosis (Tables 336-1 and 336-2).

This information allows emergency room personnel or primary care physician to approach the child with abdominal pain in an efficient and accurate manner. The clinician should consider common conditions first while evaluating a child with abdominal pain. Once these possibilities are exhausted, which will be infrequently, the clinician can look for more esoteric diseases.

TOOLS FOR PRACTICE

Medical Decision Support

- *Acute Abdominal Pain Clinical Guideline* (guideline), Royal Children's Hospital Melbourne (www.rch.org.au/clinicalguide/cpg.cfm?doc_id=5036).
- *Children and Infants with Acute Abdominal Pain—Acute Management* (guideline), New South Whales Health (www.health.nsw.gov.au/policies/PD/2005/PD2005_384.html).

RELATED WEB SITE

University of Leeds and Media Innovations Ltd: AAPHelp (www.media-innovations.ltd.uk/AAP.htm).

REFERENCES

1. Losek JD, Fiete RL. Intussusception and the diagnostic value of testing stool for occult blood. *Am J Emerg Med.* 1991;9:1-3.
2. Godbole P, Stringer D. Bilious vomiting in the newborn: How often is it pathologic? *J Pediatr Surg.* 2002;37:909-911.
3. Slovis TL, Klein MD, Watts FB. Incomplete rotation of the intestine with a normal cecal position. *Surgery.* 1980;87:325-330.
4. Yamini D, Vargas H, Bongard F, et al. Perforated appendicitis: is it truly a surgical urgency? *Am Surg.* 1998;64:970-975.
5. Vane DW, Fernandez N. Role of interval appendectomy in the management of complicated appendicitis in children. *World J Surg.* 2006;30:51-54.

Chapter 337 AIRWAYS OBSTRUCTION

Carol K. Conrad, MD; David N. Cornfield, MD

Respiratory distress is common in children. Airways obstruction is an event that can be precipitated acutely by infections, trauma, inhalational injury, a mass lesion, or foreign-body aspiration. Alternatively, an acute illness can significantly worsen an obstruction caused by either a chronic process or an anatomic abnormality. Acute upper airways obstruction presents an immediate threat to life. If the airways obstruction is relieved quickly, then rapid clinical improvement can be effected. Acute obstruction of the airways can occur throughout the respiratory tract. Knowledge of developmental respiratory physiology and anatomy, combined with historical information, can help determine the anatomic site of the obstruction. In the event of airways obstruction, definitive treatment and relief of the obstruction is of critical importance to prevent hypoxic-ischemic injury.

Airways obstruction results either from blockage of the airway from aspiration of a foreign object or can occur when the inner diameter of the airway is reduced, such as occurs with mucosal edema in the case of acute laryngotracheobronchitis, or with constriction of the peribronchiolar muscles, as occurs with status asthmaticus. Alternatively, the airway can be compressed from an external mass, such as a mediastinal tumor; the onset can seem to occur quite rapidly, even with a slowly growing tumor. A patient with chronic airways obstruction, such as a prematurely born infant, can experience acute airways obstruction caused by an acute viral infection, such as respiratory syncytial virus bronchiolitis.[1]

Infants have a greater incidence of respiratory compromise compared with older children because they have a smaller airway diameter and exponentially increased airway resistance. Second, the connective tissue in infants has incompletely hardened cartilaginous structures (malacia). Such is the case for the cartilaginous structures such as the larynx (epiglottis, aryepiglottic folds, arytenoid cartilage, tracheal cartilage), the trachea, bronchi, bronchioles, and the chest wall itself. As a result, any increase in airways obstruction results in relatively higher airflows, thereby increasing the dynamic obstruction caused by relatively flexible airway structures. In infants younger than 1 year, collateral lower airway circulation in the alveoli and the bronchioles, the pores of Kohn, and the canals of Lambert are absent, predisposing the infant to atelectasis. The narrowest portion of the airways in the infant and child is the cricoid ring, unless an infant is born with congenital airways anomalies such as tracheal stenosis or bronchomalacia. In the older child and adolescent the narrowest portion of the airway is the vocal cord aperture.[2]

CLINICAL APPROACH

Initial Assessment

To determine whether a child requires emergent intervention, consideration should focus on upper airway patency, the degree of respiratory effort, and the effectiveness of respiratory function. Complete upper airway obstruction or respiratory failure mandates immediate intervention. The child should be kept calm and comfortable. Anxiety and crying can substantially increase dynamic airway obstruction and the work of breathing in young children. Simple observation of the child, without an examination, is an invaluable tool. By determining the respiratory rate, whether the child is using accessory muscles, has retractions, recognizes parents, can speak, or suck on a bottle or pacifier, an examiner can match the appropriate level of support to the condition of the patient.

HISTORY

Contingent on the degree of acuity, historical information can be obtained before initiating therapy. Historical information can establish a cause for the respiratory disease. Acute onset, particularly in the absence of fever, prompts concern about an aspirated foreign body. Conversely, if a child has had respiratory problems before the acute process, then dynamic obstruction caused by underlying laryngomalacia, subglottic stenosis, or malacia of the trachea or bronchus may be worsened by superimposed infection or reactive airways disease.

The pulmonary history should elicit information regarding the duration of the problem and factors that either worsen or improve the signs or symptoms. Historical information regarding the prenatal and neonatal periods can guide diagnosis and treatment. A history of decreased fetal motion may indicate a neuromuscular disorder that would lead to alveolar hypoventilation and restrictive chest wall disease. A history of oligohydramnios can indicate the presence of pulmonary hypoplasia. Knowledge of whether resuscitation efforts were required in the perinatal period and for what reason is helpful. The gestational age at birth and whether the infant required intubation, mechanical ventilation, or supplemental oxygen can provide information regarding the presence of either upper or lower respiratory tract disease. The quality of a child's cry can provide information regarding vocal cord function and tracheal patency. A history of cyanosis in the absence of cardiac anomalies may prompt concern over respiratory disease.

PHYSICAL EXAMINATION

Initial evaluation should include careful observation. Observation of the child and of the quality and timing of the respiratory pattern is important. Close attention to the child's work of breathing, level of consciousness, and degree of interaction can be particularly instructive. Attention to whether accessory muscles are being used, the relative ratio of inspiration to expiration, and movement of the head and neck with respirations provide important clinical information. By approaching the child from a distance and observing the child in the relative comfort of parental arms, an assessment can be made without biasing the examination by introducing fear and anxiety. Careful attention to the facial expressions of the child can provide further insight into the clinical presentation. The child with incipient respiratory collapse may demonstrate furrowed eyebrows, may be unable to regard and to focus on the examiner, and may appear fatigued and anxious. The child may demonstrate nasal flaring and may be diaphoretic.[3]

Abnormal breath sounds and physical examination findings are either more prominent on the inspiratory or the expiratory phase of breathing depending on the site of disease.[4] In the presence of complete upper airways obstruction, no effective air movement is present. In such an emergency situation, the child would be unable to cough audibly, speak, or produce any sound. Audible phonation or breath sounds indicate airway patency, though partial obstruction may be present. Partial extrathoracic upper airways obstruction results in stridulous respirations with increased obstruction to airflow on inspiration relative to expiration. Retractions and nasal flaring with diminished air movement or worsening hypoxemia (poor color and decreased mental status) portend impending respiratory failure.

Children with respiratory failure have inadequate oxygenation, ventilation, or both. Children in extremis appear ashen, obtunded, lethargic, or extremely anxious. Central cyanosis may be present. Chest wall movement may be diminished because of weak or inefficient breaths, thereby decreasing any signs of respiratory distress. Extreme tachypnea can precede hypopnea. Given that respiratory insufficiency leads to respiratory failure, the pattern of respirations becomes irregular. In the presence of a tenuous airway, avoiding components of the examination that will increase the child's anxiety is prudent. Comprehensive airway evaluation ought to be deferred pending the presence of critical personnel and access to equipment that will allow for definitive airway management if necessary.

For the chest examination, the physician should observe the breathing pattern and the respiratory effort. Removing the child's shirt allows observation of how accessory muscles of respiration are used. Patients with obstructive disease (cystic fibrosis and asthma) may have a prolonged expiratory phase and a hyperinflated thorax that may be clinically evident as an increase in anteroposterior diameter. A normal inspiratory/expiratory ratio is 1:2. In the presence of small airways obstruction the ratio will appreciably increase. Children with restrictive lung disease breathe rapidly and with smaller tidal volumes. The examiner should inspect the chest wall for symmetry, pectus deformity, and the size of the thorax. Retractions are more clinically apparent in younger children compared with adolescents and adults, owing to the relatively high compliance of the chest wall. Retractions are evident in the lower part of the thorax as the rib cage is pulled inward with diaphragmatic contraction on inspiration. Head bobbing is a result of the use of the suprasternal accessory muscles of respiration and is a sign of increased airway resistance. For any rate of airflow, the degree of respiratory effort is directly proportional to the degree of obstruction. Percussion of the thorax can reveal localized air trapping, hyperresonance, or lobar consolidation or dullness.[5]

When auscultating breath sounds, the examiner should listen for crackles, wheezing, or stridor. The examiner should also determine whether the sounds occur on inspiration, on expiration, or throughout the respiratory cycle. The distribution, pitch, and quality of sounds can differentiate between upper and lower airway pathology. Table 337-1 describes the types of sounds that can be appreciated in various forms of disease as described by the American Thoracic Society and the American College of Chest Physicians.[6] Causes of intra- and extrathoracic obstructing lesions of the upper airway are detailed in Table 337-2. A lesion in the extrathoracic trachea increases airflow resistance primarily during inspiration and is characterized by stridor. Obstruction in the intrathoracic trachea results in an increase in airflow resistance during expiration and is clinically characterized by wheezing. A lesion may be a *fixed* or a *variable* form. If airflow limitation does not vary during the respiratory cycle, then the lesion is fixed. Noise that occurs on both

Table 337-1 Sounds Produced From Lower Airways

SOUND (ATS)	FREQUENTLY USED SYNONYM	ACOUSTIC CHARACTERISTICS	LIKELY LOCATION OF FLUID, MUCUS, OR OBSTRUCTION
Crackle:	—	Usually inspiratory sound	—
Coarse	Rhonchi	Loud, low in pitch	Larger to medium-size bronchi
Fine	Rale	Softer and shorter in duration, higher in pitch	Alveoli or small bronchioles
Wheeze:	—	Usually expiratory sound	—
High pitched		Long, musical	Small airways, typical of asthma
Low pitched		Loud, long, sonorous	Large airways, such as bronchi or trachea, such as in tracheo- or broncho-malacia

ATS, American Thoracic Society.
From Pasterkamp H, Kraman S, Wodicka G, et al. Respiratory sounds: advances beyond the stethoscope. A state of the art review. *Am J Respir Crit Care Med.* 1997;156:974-987. Reprinted by permission of the American Thoracic Society.

Table 337-2 Localize the Source of the Noise

LESION	NOISE: INTRATHORACIC LOCATION	NOISE: EXTRATHORACIC LOCATION
Fixed: Tracheal stenosis Double aortic arch anomaly Cricoid ring	Noise occurs on inspiration and expiration	Noise occurs on inspiration and expiration
Variable: Foreign body aspiration Laryngomalacia	Wheeze predominates on expiration	Stridor dominates on inspiration

inspiration and expiration suggests a fixed stenosis of the airway.[5]

In a child or infant, the dynamics of the lesion can be assessed for the change in character of the stridor by making the child breathe more forcefully. By making the child inspire with high inspiratory flow, a dynamic compression (an acute airway narrowing) will develop below an extrathoracic lesion and above an intrathoracic lesion. Variable lesions are those that can be distended or compressed during the phases of respiration. An extrathoracic variable obstruction (laryngomalacia) worsens on *inspiration* and improves during expiration, given that positive intraluminal pressures will distend this portion of the airway during exhalation but will compress the airway during a forceful inhalation. A variable intrathoracic obstruction is appreciated on *expiration* primarily, given that the airway is dilated on inspiration by the negative intrathoracic pressure but compressed during forceful exhalation.

DIFFERENTIAL DIAGNOSIS

Causes of airways obstruction differ at various developmental stages. A summary of the causes of stridor in children is found in Table 337-3. Determining the correct pathological cause of the obstruction entails consideration of the patient's age.

EARLY INFANCY

Laryngomalacia

Infants have more compliant chest walls and soft tissue, breathe faster, and have smaller caliber airways than older children. These factors combine to increase the likelihood that infants will have respiratory difficulty. The most common cause of stridor in an infant is laryngomalacia.[7] The onset is typically within the first 2 weeks of life. The stridor is positional, with greater severity with the infant lying supine and diminished severity with prone positioning. Stimuli that increase the rate of airflow on inspiration such as crying, feeding, or an upper respiratory tract infection worsen the dynamic inspiratory obstruction associated with laryngomalacia. The symptoms come from immature cartilaginous structures of the larynx. The condition can aggravate underlying gastroesophageal reflux.[8] Moreover, the relatively more negative intrathoracic pressure that is necessary to bypass the dynamic and intermittently obstructive upper airway can result in microaspiration. Generally, laryngomalacia worsens in the first several months of life and resolves by the end of the first year of life.[7]

In severe cases of laryngomalacia with constitutional symptoms of failure to thrive or an evolving chest wall deformity, epiglottoplasty with or without tracheostomy may be necessary. Respiratory distress, thoracic deformities (caused by severe and chronic retractions), failure to thrive, and hypoxia may occur in severe cases.[9] Generally, diagnosis can be achieved with a complete history and physical examination. Definitive diagnosis, often unnecessary, can be made with flexible laryngoscopy. Endoscopically, the epiglottis folds over the larynx on inspiration as the arytenoid cartilages move to the midline on inspiration. Such infants often have feeding problems as their first symptom. Stridor often worsens with minor respiratory tract infections. Through continuous noninvasive monitoring, studies have demonstrated that infants who have laryngomalacia are more likely than age-matched controls to have transient, albeit non-life-threatening, episodes of hypoxemia and hypercapnia. As their disorder improves over time, these infants rarely require an artificial airway.

Table 337-3 Causes of Stridor and Guide for Diagnostic Evaluation

CONDITION	DIAGNOSTIC STUDIES
STRIDOR—ACUTE	
Laryngotracheobronchitis	Anteroposterior neck radiograph
Epiglottis	Lateral neck or direct visualization in an operating room with a qualified surgeon
Spasmodic croup	History diagnostic
Foreign-body aspiration	Inspiratory and expiratory films, right and left lateral decubitus films, fluoroscopy, barium esophogram, rigid bronchoscopy
Retropharyngeal abscess	Lateral neck radiograph
Trauma	History
Allergic reactions	History
Peritonsillar abscess	History and physical examination of oropharynx, lateral neck radiograph
Angioneurotic edema	History, C1 esterase level
STRIDOR—CHRONIC	
Choanal atresia	Inability to pass a nasogastric tube
Laryngomalacia	History, fluoroscopy, flexible bronchoscopy
Subglottic stenosis	History, pulmonary function test, flexible bronchoscopy
Laryngeal cysts, webs, hemangiomas	Flexible bronchoscopy
Vocal cord dysfunction	Flexible bronchoscopy, history
Laryngotrachealesophageal clefts	Suspension laryngoscopy
Retained foreign body	Rigid bronchoscopy
Epiglottic cysts	Flexible bronchoscopy
Laryngeal papilloma	Flexible bronchoscopy

Vocal Cord Paralysis

Unilateral or bilateral vocal cord paralysis may occur in otherwise healthy newborns and has been associated with birth trauma. A neonate with a shoulder dystocia, forceps delivery, or vacuum extraction is more likely to have unilateral vocal cord paralysis than a neonate experiencing an atraumatic delivery. Trauma associated with airway instrumentation can cause vocal cord paralysis as well. Infants intubated in the delivery room or those who have undergone mechanical ventilation may also have injury to the vocal cords as a result of airway instrumentation. Diagnosis is best made by flexible laryngoscopy while the baby is breathing spontaneously. If the endoscopic evaluation is performed during positive pressure ventilation, then discerning vocal cord paralysis is difficult. In the spontaneously breathing patient with vocal cord paralysis, the true cord or cords move passively to the midline with inspiration. Unilateral cord paralysis often requires no specific therapy and resolves over time. However, bilateral cord paralysis is associated with chronic aspiration and hypoxemia. In the presence of bilateral paralysis, a tracheotomy may be necessary.[10]

To determine the feasibility of feeding the infant, a video swallowing study is essential. In some cases, infants can protect the airway if highly textured, thickened food is consumed, but they are unable to do so if thin food is consumed.

Vocal cord paralysis may also result from elevated intracranial pressure, a congenital Arnold-Chiari malformation, or from an intracranial mass. In the presence of bilateral cord paralysis, determining the underlying cause is particularly important.[11] In an otherwise healthy child whose vocal cord paralysis is thought to be caused by birth trauma, improvement over time is the rule.

Data indicate that vocal cord paralysis, either unilateral or bilateral, is a relatively frequent complication of congenital heart disease surgery. In the presence of a patent ductus arteriosus the recurrent laryngeal nerve can be compressed, resulting in unilateral vocal cord paralysis.[12] In the course of repairing congenital heart disease, injury to the recurrent laryngeal nerve frequently occurs, leading to vocal cord paralysis. Contingent on the lesion, the incidence may be approximately 10%.[13,14]

Extrinsic Compression of the Trachea

Compression of the trachea can lead to stridor. The potential causes of airway compression include thyroglossal duct cyst, ectopic thyroid tissue, esophageal duplication cyst, lymphoma, cardiac anomaly, or vascular anomaly. The optimal diagnostic and therapeutic approach depends on the condition of the child and the rate of progression of the symptoms. Clearly a relatively asymptomatic patient with gradual onset can be evaluated at a less urgent pace than an acutely ill child with rapidly progressive illness.[15]

Craniofacial Anomalies

Congenital craniofacial anomalies can place newborns and older children at risk for chronic and severe obstruction of the upper airway. Obstruction of the upper airway can occur because of micrognathia (Pierre Robin sequence and Treacher Collins syndrome), macroglossia (Beckwith-Wiedemann syndrome), small mid-face or small oropharyngeal space (achondroplasia), and adenotonsillar hypertrophy (Down syndrome). Macroglossia can develop in children with lipid or glycogen storage disorders; this anomaly is rarely present at birth and develops slowly.[16] Apnea studies that monitor nasal and oral airflow, chest wall movement, and pulse oximetry or a full polysomnogram can grade the level of severity of hypoventilation and hypoxemia in these children. Some infants require treatment with noninvasive or invasive (via tracheostomy) mechanical ventilation before reconstructive surgery can be performed.

Tracheomalacia

Tracheomalacia is a congenital disorder of the trachea characterized by respiratory distress and wheezing. Typically symptoms appear before the infant is 2 months of age. The predisposing risk factors include a previous history of intubation, prematurity, and gastroesophageal reflux.[17] Tracheomalacia results from incompletely formed cartilaginous rings. Normally the cartilaginous component of the trachea comprises approximately two thirds of the airway circumference, with the membranous trachea comprising the remainder of the tracheal circumference. In tracheomalacia the proportion of membranous to cartilaginous trachea is increased, resulting in less well-supported tracheal structures. Depending on the position of the diminished cartilaginous structure in the airway, the dynamic obstruction to airflow may be more apparent in inspiration or expiration. If the tracheomalacia is particularly severe, then both phases of respiration may be affected. Tracheomalacia can be either primary or secondary.[18] The primary form is characterized by relatively decreased cartilage in the tracheal rings. Secondary tracheomalacia results from extrinsic compression of the trachea. Causes of extrinsic compression might include an anomalous vascular structure, mediastinal tumor, lymphadenopathy, or enlargement of the left atrium.[7]

The child with moderate or severe tracheomalacia will exhibit chronic wheezing that is frequently diagnosed as asthma. Many premature infants have some component of tracheo- and bronchomalacia. In children with tracheomalacia, treatment with beta-agonists may relax the tracheal smooth muscle in the membranous trachea, thereby worsening airflow obstruction.[19] Use of medications that increase tracheal airway smooth-muscle cell tone can improve airflow.

CHILDREN BEYOND THE NEWBORN PERIOD

Acquired Infectious Causes of Airways Obstruction

Croup (laryngotracheobronchitis) is the most common upper respiratory obstruction in childhood, with peak incidence in the second year of life (range 6 months to 3 years). (See Chapter 340 for more information on croup.) Admission rates for croup in children seen in outpatient settings range from 1.5% to 31% of cases seen; these figures vary widely, depending on hospital admission practices and the severity of the disease in the population being assessed. Croup occurs most commonly in late fall and early winter. Croup is caused by inflammation and edema of the mucosal and submucosal tissues of the subglottic space. The swollen mucosa expands into the airway lumen and narrows the trachea.[20]

Most children with croup have an uncomplicated course and are managed without formal medical care. Only a small percentage of children who require urgent care require hospitalization. Croup is diagnosed clinically and causes a barky cough, hoarse voice, high-pitched inspiratory stridor, and fever. The clinical presentation follows a prodrome of mild fever and upper respiratory tract infection symptoms lasting several days. Croup severity is generally worse at night compared with daytime. Mild croup is characterized by intermittent barky cough, stridor only with agitation, mild tachypnea, and tachycardia. A child with mild croup is minimally distressed, well hydrated, and has a normal mental status. Moderate croup produces audible stridor at rest, worsening stridor with agitation, barky cough, and increased work of breathing (retractions, tachypnea, tachycardia). A patient with moderate croup may be fussy but is alert, interactive, and comforted by parents. Hypoxia is atypical in mild or moderate croup. Laboratory tests are nondiagnostic. Radiographic studies of the neck are confirmatory but do not alter management. Classically the trachea appears narrowed in the subglottic space in a characteristic *steeple-like* appearance.

Peritonsillar Abscess and Retropharyngeal Abscess

Peritonsillar and retropharyngeal abscesses are frequent infections that occur in childhood and can be life threatening. Retropharyngeal abscess occurs most commonly in children between the ages of 2 and 4 years. A retropharyngeal abscess may extrinsically compress structures in the upper airway. Prominent presenting complaints are usually neck pain, fever, and sore throat rather than acute, severe airways obstruction. The symptoms caused by a retropharyngeal abscess relate to pressure and inflammation produced by the abscess on either the airway or the upper digestive tract and pharynx. The patient may have intense dysphagia, drooling, and odynophagia, or some element of respiratory distress from edema and inflammation of the airway (stridor, tachypnea, or both) may be present. Unwillingness to move the neck because of discomfort is often a prominent presenting feature and should lead to consideration of retropharyngeal abscess if the child is febrile and irritable. Usually, extension of the neck is affected more than flexion. This circumstance causes the patient to hold the neck stiffly or have torticollis.[21]

Peritonsillar abscess is the most common deep neck infection in children and adolescents, accounting for at least 50% of cases. Peritonsillar abscess generally occurs in later childhood and adolescence, although it can occur at any age. (See details in Chapter 308, Pharyngitis and Tonsillitis). The sudden onset of severe respiratory distress is rare. The infection is usually in the superior pole of the tonsil, where a defined collection of pus is located between the tonsillar capsule, the superior constrictor, and the palatopharyngeus muscle. The typical clinical presentation of peritonsillar abscess is a severe sore throat, fever, and a *hot potato* muffled voice. Drooling may be present. Trismus is common; patients will often have swelling of the neck and complain of neck pain. The discomfort associated with the peritonsillar abscess creates fatigue and irritability in the patient.[22,23]

Bacterial Tracheitis

Bacterial tracheitis has been termed membranous croup, bacterial croup, and pseudomembranous croup. Although the incidence is low, bacterial tracheitis is a serious illness. It generally affects children between 4 and 8 years of age. The pathogenesis of bacterial tracheitis remains controversial. Bacterial tracheitis often occurs as a secondary bacterial infection complicating a preexisting viral infection, including adenovirus, influenza A, and influenza B. Bacteria gain access to the trachea epithelium after a viral infection that compromises epithelial integrity. The tracheal epithelial inflammation occurs, and thick mucopurulent secretions accrue. Although *Staphylococcus aureus* used to be the primary causative organism, more recently the predominant organisms are *Moraxella catarrhalis*, Streptococcal species, and oral anaerobes.[24] The incidence of bacterial tracheitis caused by *Haemophilus influenzae* is decreasing because of the routine practice of childhood vaccinations in most areas of the United States.

Bacterial tracheitis can be distinguished from croup by patient age and the degree of toxicity[25] (Table 337-4). Patients commonly experience a viral prodrome of fever, barky cough, and stridor. In contrast to croup, in bacterial tracheitis, symptoms worsen over time. To evaluate the patient, lateral and anteroposterior radiographs of neck and chest may be helpful. Findings on plain-film radiographs include subglottic narrowing, a ragged edge to the usually smooth tracheal air column, and a hazy density within the tracheal lumen. The epiglottis and supraglottic structures appear normal on neck films. In the event of respiratory collapse or an inability to mobilize secretions effectively, then mechanical ventilation will be necessary. Careful attention to the suctioning and mobilization of secretions is essential. Occlusion of the endotracheal tube has been reported as a frequent cause of death in intubated and mechanically ventilated children with bacterial tracheitis. For this reason, some otolaryngologists have advocated for expectant placement of tracheotomy tubes in children with bacterial tracheitis. Antibiotics and supportive care are essential for full recovery. Complications associated with bacterial tracheitis include toxic shock syndrome, septic shock, postintubation pulmonary edema, acute respiratory distress syndrome, and subglottic stenosis.[26]

Laryngeal Papillomatosis

Respiratory papillomatosis is a disease caused by infection of the airway by human papilloma virus (HPV). The lesion is benign but can transform to a malignant lesion particularly in the lung parenchyma.

Table 337-4 Comparison of Epiglottitis, Laryngotracheobronchitis, Spasmodic Croup, and Bacterial Tracheitis

FACTOR	EPIGLOTTITIS	VIRAL CROUP	SPASMODIC CROUP	BACTERIAL TRACHEITIS
Age (yr)	2-6	0.6-2	0.5-3	4-8
Organism	*Haemophilus influenzae* type b	Parainfluenza 1,2,3	Gastroesophageal reflux	*Staphylococcus aureus, Haemophilus influenzae* type b
Season	All year	Late spring, late fall	All year	All year
Clinical presentation	Child sitting Toxic Drooling Dysphagia Muffled voice	Child lying down Nontoxic Barking cough Hoarseness	Nontoxic Barking cough Hoarseness	Toxic Barking cough
Onset prodrome	Rapid over a few hours	Variable; few hours to 4 days	Sudden	Variable; few hours to 5 days
Stridor	Less common	Common	Very common	Common
Fever	High	Low-grade	Afebrile	High
Chest retractions	Less common	Common	Common	Common
Lateral neck film	Swollen epiglottis	Subglottic narrowing	None	Pseudomembrane
Progression	Rapid	Usually slow	Rapid	Usually slow
Recurrence	Rare	Common	Very common	Rare

More commonly, HPV is life threatening if aggressive growth and rapid proliferation of the papilloma lesions in the airway cause airway obstruction. HPV infection in children is most commonly acquired as the neonate passes through the birth canal. HPV-6 and -11 are the most common subtypes in this population, as is true for genital HPV infection in women.[27,28]

In most instances, children with HPV infection of the larynx exhibit hoarseness, though advanced cases can have stridor and respiratory distress. Most commonly, it occurs on the vocal cords but can infect the trachea and even the bronchi. In children, HPV infection of the larynx is diagnosed most commonly at age 2 to 4 years. The earlier it occurs, the more aggressive the growth of the papilloma will be.[29] Treatment is generally focused on removing the obstructing lesions with laser ablation of the root of the papilloma to prevent regrowth. Frequently, recurrent ablations are necessary as lesions regrow at sites of ablation. Adjuvant therapies using antivirals injected into the lesion such as alpha-interferon[30] and vaccine trials are being evaluated as therapeutic alternatives. Should a clinical need to instrument the airway exist, then great care must be taken to avoid introducing infection by inoculating the more distal components of the airway with viral particles.[27]

Vascular Anomalies

Stridor or dysphagia can be a manifestation of extrinsic compression of the airway or esophagus by an anomalous vascular structure. The anomalies result from abnormal persistence or regression of embryonic structures. The most common anomaly—aberrant right subclavian artery—produces minimal symptoms. In many cases the only clinical manifestation is dysphagia caused by compression on the esophagus. A barium swallow can yield diagnostic information.[31] In the presence of a severe obstruction, infants can be quite ill. Poor feeding may lead to failure to thrive. Wheezing and stridor may be consistently present and exacerbated by feeding. In the most profound cases, cyanosis and apnea may occur.

In the presence of a right-sided aortic arch, a child may experience vascular impingement on the airway as a result of a double aortic arch, wherein the aortic arches encircle the esophagus and trachea. The disease results when resorption of the fourth embryonic aortic arch is incomplete. The problem may cause stridor or wheezing.[32] The right and left arches compress the right and left sides of the trachea and the esophagus. The right arch indents the esophagus posteriorly. Division of one of the arches, usually the smaller posterior one, opens the constricting ring and is curative.[15]

In the context of right-sided arches, a residual patent ductus arteriosus or ligamentum arteriosum can form a complete ring around the airway. Division of the ductus or ligamentum is curative. Occasionally a carotid or innominate artery compresses the anterior margin of the trachea. This compression may show on radiographs of the tracheal air column or on a tracheogram, but the esophagram is normal. If needed, the compressing artery can be displaced anteriorly at surgery.[33]

Although not a vascular ring, the anomalous left pulmonary artery also causes airways obstruction. The left pulmonary artery arises from the right pulmonary artery and passes between the esophagus and trachea, compressing the trachea and the right main bronchus. This lesion causes compression on the anterior edge of the esophagus. Collapse or hyperinflation of part of the right lung may occur. Diagnosis is made by a combination of esophagrams, bronchoscopy, computed tomographic angiography, or magnetic resonance imaging. Surgical reattachment of the left pulmonary artery to the main pulmonary artery relieves the obstruction, but residual tracheomalacia may be present.

ACQUIRED, NONINFECTIOUS CAUSES OF AIRWAYS OBSTRUCTION

Vocal Cord Dysfunction

Vocal cord dysfunction (VCD) is characterized by the inappropriate adduction of the vocal cords during inspiration. Typically, vocal cord dysfunction causes a sudden onset of labored breathing with inspiratory stridor. The sound is often erroneously characterized as wheezing. For some patients the symptoms are precipitated by physical activity. The inappropriate adduction during inspiration may result in severe airflow limitation that is characterized by profound high-pitched stridor and dyspnea. The acute onset and severity of symptoms in some patients with VCD have resulted in intervention with endotracheal intubation or tracheotomy for severe upper airways obstruction. Diagnosis entails flexible laryngoscopy during an acute exacerbation.[34] Subsequent to the definitive diagnosis, patient education, speech therapy, and biofeedback have produced favorable results. Techniques taught by a speech therapist who is familiar with this disorder results in the ability of patients to control the vocal cord movement in the event that symptoms recur. Techniques focus on training the extrinsic laryngeal muscles. In the short term, high rates of success associated with this treatment course exist.

The diagnosis of VCD is often complicated by an initial diagnosis of asthma. Current data indicate that VCD is often a self-limiting disorder. Most patients have no long-term sequelae once the diagnosis has been established. For some patients, only high-level exercise can precipitate the VCD.[35] For such patients, insight-driven biofeedback is difficult to use. Data suggest that the use of ipratropium bromide may be a safe and effective measure for treating exercise-induced VCD.[36]

Anaphylaxis

Anaphylaxis and anaphylactoid reactions may be severe and life threatening when edema involves the retropharynx or larynx. The increasing incidence of food allergies correlates with more anaphylactic reactions. Onset of symptoms is usually sudden. Presenting signs and symptoms can include urticaria and facial edema. Treatment needs to be initiated immediately. Initial therapy should include intramuscular injection of epinephrine. Patients at risk for anaphylactic reaction should always have immediate access to portable epinephrine devices that can be used in an ambulatory setting (home or school) when the first signs of anaphylaxis are noted.[37] Even if the device is effective, the patient should be transported to a local emergency room for monitoring as the effects of initial treatment wane and to ensure that the late phase of the allergic response does not compromise the child. After the initial treatment with epinephrine, systemic corticosteroids should be provided to mitigate any biphasic or prolonged effect of the allergic response.[38]

Foreign-Body Aspiration

Foreign-body aspiration (FBA) is a common and potentially life-threatening event. The number of emergency room visits for FBA in 2001 exceeded 17,000. Ten percent of these events resulted in death.[39] The vast majority of these events occur in children younger than 3 years, and the peak incidence occurs between 1 and 2 years of age. The most commonly aspirated objects are peanuts and other types of nuts and seeds, food particles, hardware, and pieces of toys. Balloons are the most common object involved in fatal FBA, but aspiration of small marbles and balls results in considerable morbidity and mortality. The majority of foreign bodies are found in the major bronchi; laryngeal and tracheal foreign bodies are less common. The right lung was involved in 60% of the cases, the left lung in 23% of cases, the trachea or carina in 13%, the larynx in 3%, and bilateral FBA occurred in 2%.[40]

The presentation of FBA depends on whether the event was witnessed, the age of the child, the type of object aspirated, the amount of time that has elapsed since the event, and the anatomic location of the object. Presentation and diagnosis within 24 hours of aspiration occurs in approximately 50% to 75% of cases. Children who have signs of severe respiratory distress, such as cyanosis, stridor, or wheeze, and altered mental status have to be evaluated and treated immediately with rigid bronchoscopic removal of the foreign body. More commonly, the situation is less emergent. The examination may reveal localized wheezing, cough, and diminished breath sounds, but this is not universally present.[39] A history of choking or a sudden onset of coughing, dyspnea, or cyanosis may be present in a previously healthy child. The choking phase occurs immediately after the episodes but tends to resolve quickly because of tachyphylaxis of cough receptors in the lower airways. The lack of ongoing symptoms should not be construed as a sign of resolution, given that a delay in diagnosis may result in chronic infection of the lung parenchyma distal to the foreign body. Children may have fever and other signs of pneumonia.[40]

Plain-film radiographs may or may not be helpful to establish the diagnosis of FBA. If the child is able to cooperate, then chest radiographs obtained in the exhalation phase can demonstrate asymmetric gas trapping. Given that most inhaled objects are not radiopaque, direct radiographic evidence of their presence will be absent. Other radiographic signs can include focal segmental or entire lung hyperinflation, atelectasis, mediastinal shift, and pneumonia.

The most sensitive and specific method is that of direct visualization by bronchoscopy. If the index of suspicion is high, then an otorhinolaryngologist or general surgeon should be consulted. In children, rigid bronchoscopy is the preferred mode of visualization and airway instrumentation, as the rigid bronchoscopy provides control of the airway throughout the removal process.[41]

REFERENCES

1. Tuffaha A, Gern JE, Lemanske RFJ. The role of respiratory viruses in acute and chronic asthma. *Clin Chest Med.* 2000;21(2):289-300.

2. Pohunek P. Abstract. Development, structure and function of the upper airways. *Paediatr Respir Rev.* 2004; 5(1):2-8.
3. Sigillito RJ, DeBlieux PM. Abstract. Evaluation and initial management of the patient in respiratory distress. *Emerg Med Clin North Am.* 2003;21(2):239-258.
4. Kelly HW. The assessment of childhood asthma. *Pediatr Clin North Am.* 2003;50(3):593-608.
5. Margolis P, Gadomski A. The rational clinical examination. Does this infant have pneumonia? *JAMA.* 1998; 279(4):308-313.
6. Pasterkamp H, Kraman S, Wodicka G. Respiratory sounds: advances beyond the stethoscope. A state of the art review. *Am J Respir Crit Care Med.* 1997;156:974-987.
7. Bobin S, Attal P. Laryngotracheal manifestations of gastroesophageal reflux in children. *Pediatr Pulmonol Suppl.* 1999;18:73-75.
8. Masters IB, Chang AB, Patterson L, et al. Series of laryngomalacia, tracheomalacia, and bronchomalacia disorders and their associations with other conditions in children. *Pediatr Pulmonol.* 2002;34:189-195.
9. McCray PBJ, Crockett DM, Wagener JS, et al. Hypoxia and hypercapnia in infants with mild laryngomalacia. *Am J Dis Child.* 1988;142(8):896-899.
10. Greenberg SJ, Kandt RS, D'Souza BJ. Birth injury-induced glossolaryngeal paresis. *Neurology.* 1987;37(3): 533-535.
11. Hillel AD, Benninger M, Blitzer A, et al. Evaluation and management of bilateral vocal cord immobility. *Otolaryngol Head Neck Surg.* 1999;121(6):760-765.
12. Fan LL, Campbell DN, Clarke DR, et al. Paralyzed left vocal cord associated with ligation of patent ductus arteriosus. *J Thorac Cardiovasc Surg.* 1989;98(4):611-613.
13. Skinner ML, Halstead LA, Rubinstein CS, et al. Laryngopharyngeal dysfunction after the Norwood procedure. *J Thorac Cardiovasc Surg.* 2005;130(5):1293-1301.
14. Khariwala SS, Lee WT, Koltai PJ. Laryngotracheal consequences of pediatric cardiac surgery. *Arch Otolaryngol Head Neck Surg.* 2005;131(4):336-339.
15. McElhinney DB, Reddy VM, Pian MS, et al. Compression of the central airways by a dilated aorta in infants and children with congenital heart disease. *Ann Thorac Surg.* 1999;67(4):67.
16. Daniel SJ. The upper airway: congenital malformations. *Paediatr Respir Rev.* 2006;7(suppl 1):S260-S263.
17. Sheikh S, Allen E, Shell R, et al. Chronic aspiration without gastroesophageal reflux as a cause of chronic respiratory symptoms in neurologically normal infants. *Chest.* 2001;120(4):1190-1195.
18. Boogaard R, Huijsmans SH, Pijnenburg MW, et al. Tracheomalacia and bronchomalacia in children: incidence and patient characteristics. *Chest.* 2005;128(5):3391-3397.
19. Panitch HB, Keklikian EN, Motley RA, et al. Effect of altering smooth muscle tone on maximal expiratory flows in patients with tracheomalacia. *Pediatr Pulmonol.* 1990;9(3):170-176.
20. Marx A, Torok TJ, Holman RC, et al. Pediatric hospitalizations for croup (laryngotracheitis): biennial increases associated with human parainfluenza virus 1 epidemics. *J Infect Dis.* 1997;176:1423-1427.
21. Craig FW, Schunk JE. Retropharyngeal abscess in children: clinical presentation, utility of imaging, and current management. *Pediatrics.* 2003;111:1394-1398.
22. Schraff S, McGinn JD, Derkay CS. Peritonsillar abscess in children: a 10-year review of diagnosis and management. *Int J Pediatri Otorhinolaryngol.* 2001;57:213-218.
23. Johnson RF, Stewart MG, Wright CC. An evidence-based review of the treatment of peritonsillar abscess. *Otolaryngol Head Neck Surg.* 2003;128(3):332-343.
24. Brook I. Aerobic and anaerobic microbiology of bacterial tracheitis in children. *Pediatr Emerg Care.* 1997;113:16-18.
25. Bernstein T, Brilli R, Jacobs B. Is bacterial tracheitis changing? A 14-month experience in a pediatric intensive care unit. *Clin Infect Dis.* 1998;27(3):458-462.
26. Burns JA, Brown J, Ogle JW. Group A streptococcal tracheitis associated with toxic shock syndrome. *Pediatr Infect Dis J.* 1998;17(10):933-935.
27. Andrus JG, Shapshay SM. Contemporary management of laryngeal papilloma in adults and children. *Otolaryngol Clin North Am.* 2006;39(1):135-158.
28. Wiatrak BJ, Wiatrak DW, Broker TR, et al. Recurrent respiratory papillomatosis: a longitudinal study comparing severity associated with human papilloma viral types 6 and 11 and other risk factors in a large pediatric population. *Laryngoscope.* 2004;114(11 pt 2, suppl 104):1-23.
29. Derkay CS. Recurrent respiratory papillomatosis. *Laryngoscope.* 2001;111:57-69.
30. Gerein V, Rastorguev E, Gerein J, et al. Use of interferon-alpha in recurrent respiratory papillomatosis: 20-year follow-up. *Ann Otol Rhinol Laryngol.* 2005;114(6):463-471.
31. Kussman BD, Geva T, McGowan FX. Cardiovascular causes of airway compression. *Paediatr Anaesth.* 2004; 14(1):60-74.
32. Sladek KC, Byrd RPJ, Roy TM. A right-sided aortic arch misdiagnosed as asthma since childhood. *J Asthma.* 2004; 41(5):527-531.
33. Bove T, Demanet H, Casimir G, et al. Tracheobronchial compression of vascular origin. Review of experience in infants and children. *J Cardiovasc Surg (Torino).* 2001; 42(5):663-666.
34. Newman KB, Mason UG 3rd, Schmaling KB. Clinical features of vocal cord dysfunction. *Am J Respir Crit Care Med.* 1995;152(4):1382-1386.
35. Wilson JJ, Wilson EM. Practical management: vocal cord dysfunction in athletes. *Clin J Sport Med.* 2006;16(4):357-360.
36. Doshi DR, Weinberger MM. Long-term outcome of vocal cord dysfunction. *Ann Allergy Asthma Immunol.* 2006; 96(6):794-799.
37. McIntyre CL, Sheetz AH, Carroll CR, et al. Administration of epinephrine for life-threatening allergic reactions in school settings. *Pediatrics.* 2005;116(5):1134-1140.
38. Brown SG. Clinical features and severity grading of anaphylaxis. *J Allergy Clin Immunol.* 2004;114(2):371-376.
39. Nonfatal choking-related episodes among children—United States, 2001. *MMWR Morb Mortal Wkly Rep.* 2002;51:945-948.
40. Eren S, Balci AE, Dikici B, et al. Foreign body aspiration in children: experience of 1160 cases. *Ann Trop Paediatr.* 2003;23:31-37.
41. Tan HK, Brown K, McGill T, et al. Airway foreign bodies: a 10-year review. *Int J Pediatr Otorhinolaryngol.* 2000;56:91-99.

Chapter 338

ALTERED MENTAL STATUS

Rene J. Forti, MD; Jeffrey R. Avner, MD

Many disease processes act directly or indirectly on the central nervous system to cause an alteration in the level of consciousness. Although in severe cases the child appears unresponsive, the initial changes in mental status are often subtle. These changes are recognized by assessing the child's actions and responses to external and internal stimuli in what is collectively known as *behavior*. Behavior is a combination of a variety of observations, including appearance, level of alertness, speech, affect, mood, thought, and judgment. These actions are child and age specific. For example, apprehension, avoidance, and crankiness may be normal responses of a toddler to a physician's physical examination, whereas a similar response by an adolescent may be abnormal. Although major changes in behavior are readily apparent, subtle changes are often best appreciated by parents and caretakers.

DEFINITION OF TERMS

Consciousness is the awareness of self and the environment. Alteration of the level of consciousness usually begins with becoming unaware of self, followed by reduced awareness of the environment, and finally an inability to be aroused. A child who is in a coma is unresponsive to all stimuli, including pain. Although consciousness and coma represent the extremes of mental status, many intermediate levels of consciousness exist. Although specific definitions are given to each stage of consciousness, a progression of symptoms is not an all-or-nothing phenomenon. Rather, a continuum of the levels of consciousness may exist.

Confusion is a state in which a person's responses are slowed and cognitive abilities are impaired, usually accompanied by some disorientation. Infants and toddlers may exhibit irritability as a sign of confusion. Delirium is a succession of confused and unconnected ideas. Children with delirium are often aggressive, agitated, and combative, with episodes of somnolence and withdrawal. Lethargy is a state of profound slumber in which the child has limited movement and speech. The lethargic child can be awakened with moderate stimuli but then returns to a state of slumber. In stupor, the child appears unresponsive and can be aroused only by repeated, vigorous stimuli. In the vegetative state, the child has lost all cognitive neurologic function, communication, and awareness but may retain some noncognitive functions (eg, eye opening) and a sleep-wake cycle. In coma, the child is totally unresponsive, and the eyes remain closed.

ETIOLOGY

An altered level of consciousness in children has many causes. The mnemonic AEIOU TIPS is helpful when considering the major categories of illness or injury (Table 338-1). Although these disorders can occur at any age, certain conditions are more prevalent at certain ages (Box 338-1). Nontraumatic coma has a bimodal distribution and is most common in infants and toddlers, with a smaller peak in adolescence.[1] Infection of the brain, meninges, or both is the most common cause of altered level of consciousness, accounting for more than one third of nontraumatic cases.[1] Exposure to or ingestion of toxic substances is the next most common cause.[1] Many medications are brightly colored and taste similar to candy, resulting in accidental ingestion, especially in toddlers. Ingestion by adolescents is often intentional and typically involves over-the-counter medication or psychotropic drugs such as antidepressants.[2] Commonly ingested agents that cause an altered level of consciousness are listed in Box 338-2. Congenital heart and brain malformations typically present in the first few months after birth, but complications from surgical correction of such problems—for example, ventriculoperitoneal shunt obstruction—may occur at any age.

Inborn errors of metabolism, including urea cycle defects, organic acidemias, and specific disorders of amino acid metabolism, typically occur in infancy. Diabetic ketoacidosis is the most common metabolic disorder that can present with an alteration of consciousness. It can occur at any age but is more common in adolescence. Prolonged seizures, anticonvulsive therapy, and the postictal state can alter the level of consciousness at any age.

Although the overall incidence of traumatic and nontraumatic coma is similar, the rate of traumatic injury tends to increase throughout childhood. Head trauma can cause intracerebral, epidural, or subdural bleeding, as well as contusions and diffuse axonal injury. These conditions can lead to cerebral

Table 338-1 Mnemonic for Altered Mental Status (AEIOU TIPS)

A	Alcohol, abuse
E	Epilepsy, encephalopathy, electrolyte abnormalities, endocrine
I	Insulin, intussusception, inadequate fluid
O	Overdose, oxygen deficiency, occult trauma, obstructed ventriculoperitoneal shunt
U	Uremia
T	Trauma, temperature abnormality, tumor
I	Infection
P	Poisonings, psychiatric, postictal
S	Shock, stroke, space-occupying lesion (intracranial)

BOX 338-1 Common Causes of Altered Mental Status by Age

INFANT
- Infection
- Complication of congenital malformation (cardiac or central nervous system)
- Metabolic
- Inborn error of metabolism
- Seizure
- Abuse

CHILD
- Infection
- Seizure
- Toxin
- Trauma
- Metabolic
- Abuse
- Intussusception

ADOLESCENT
- Toxin
- Trauma
- Infection
- Psychiatric
- Seizure

BOX 338-2 Commonly Ingested Agents That Cause Altered Mental Status

Amphetamines	Ethanol
Anticholinergics	Haloperidol
Anticonvulsants	Narcotics
Barbiturates	Phenothiazines
Benzodiazepines	Salicylates
Clonidine	Selective serotonin reuptake inhibitors
Cocaine	Tricyclic antidepressants
Dextromethorphan	

dysfunction, either by primary neuronal damage or the effects of cerebral herniation with brainstem compression. Child abuse should always be considered in any infant with an altered level of consciousness.

DIFFERENTIAL DIAGNOSIS

The differential diagnosis of a child with altered mental status can be divided into structural (anatomic) causes and medical (toxic, infectious, metabolic) causes (Box 338-3). This framework is useful in the context of the pathophysiological factors of maintaining a state of consciousness. Normal mental status requires the combination of thought content (ie, cognition, affect) and a state of arousal. The content is controlled by the cerebral hemispheres, whereas the state of arousal is controlled by the ascending reticular activating system (ARAS). The ARAS, also known as the sleep center, is a core brainstem structure that courses from the medulla to the thalamus. As part of the normal cycling of behavior, consciousness moves from the awake state to drowsiness to sleep. At any time during this transition, sensory impulses may reach the ARAS, leading to an increased awareness and a more awake state. These sensory impulses may be external, such as noise, touch, or smell, or they may be internal, such as headache or abdominal pain.

To maintain a normal level of consciousness, functioning cerebral hemispheres and a functioning ARAS must be present. Defects in either of these components will cause an alteration in mental status. Thus altered mental status can result from depression of both cerebral hemispheres, a localized abnormality of the sleep center, or a global central nervous dysfunction in which both the cerebral cortex and the ARAS are affected. In general, structural causes, such as an epidural hematoma, a cerebral vascular accident, or an intracranial tumor, produce dysfunction in the region of the ARAS. Medical causes, such as meningitis, hypoglycemia, or ingestion of a toxic substance, cause dysfunction of both cerebral hemispheres.

The differentiation of structural and medical causes therefore rests on the ability to assess the function of the ARAS. The ARAS is located in the vicinity of several brainstem reflexes, the most important of which is the pupillary light reflex. Pupil size is a balance of parasympathetic and sympathetic inputs. For example, lesions in the midbrain affect the parasympathetic and sympathetic fibers equally, resulting in pupils that are fixed at midsize. Lesions of the pons preferentially affect the descending sympathetic fibers and result in fixed, pinpoint pupils. Importantly, the pupillary reflex is relatively resistant to metabolic insult. Thus preservation of the pupillary response to light, even if sluggish, is one of the most important ways to differentiate structural from medical cause of altered mental status. The cranial nerves that control reflex eye movements and maintain conjugate gaze are also located in the vicinity of the ARAS. Therefore asymmetric eye movements, such as a fixed gaze or an inability to abduct an eye, suggest dysfunction in the region of the ARAS, which is often caused by structural problems.

BOX 338-3 Differential Diagnosis of Altered Level of Consciousness

STRUCTURAL CAUSES
- Cerebral vascular accident
- Cerebral vein thrombosis
- Hydrocephalus
- Intracerebral tumor
- Subdural empyema
- Trauma (intracranial bleeding, diffuse cerebral swelling, shaken baby syndrome)

MEDICAL CAUSES (TOXIC-INFECTIOUS-METABOLIC)
- Anoxia
- Diabetic ketoacidosis
- Electrolyte abnormality
- Encephalopathy
- Hypoglycemia
- Hypothermia or hyperthermia
- Infection (sepsis)
- Inborn errors of metabolism
- Intussusception
- Meningitis and encephalitis
- Psychogenic
- Postictal state
- Toxin
- Uremia (hemolytic uremic syndrome)

Structural lesions compress or destroy areas of the brainstem and are often characterized by unequal or unreactive pupils, as well as focal neurologic findings. Medical causes produce dysfunction in both cerebral hemispheres but result in preserved pupillary reflexes and nonfocal neurologic findings. Structural causes sometimes occur without focality, such as acute bilateral cerebrovascular disease or early acute hydrocephalus. Similarly, some medical causes, such as hypoglycemia, hypercalcemia, uremia, and a postictal state with Todd paralysis, may be accompanied by focal neurologic findings.

EVALUATION

Regardless of the underlying cause, patients with an acute change in mental status may exhibit a reduced awareness of self, may have a reduced awareness of the environment, may be agitated with periods of heightened mental activity, or may be unable to be aroused. A complete history and thorough physical examination are crucial in identifying the underlying cause and managing these patients appropriately.

HISTORY

The history of the manifesting event is often the part of the clinical evaluation with the greatest diagnostic value. Specific detail should be obtained concerning the circumstances of the onset of the neurologic symptoms, including events and actions directly preceding the change in mental status. Associated symptoms may include weakness, headache, vomiting, dizziness, diplopia, and seizure-like activity. If the alteration in consciousness occurred abruptly, then the clinician should consider intracranial hemorrhage, seizure, sudden cardiac arrhythmia, trauma, or ingestion of a toxic substance. A more gradual change in mental status may suggest infection, metabolic abnormality, or a slowly growing intracranial mass. If the altered mental status is preceded by headache (especially on wakening), double vision, or nausea and vomiting, then increased intracranial pressure should be suspected. Vomiting and decreased oral intake, especially if accompanied by bloody stool, is seen with intussusception.

A history of trauma is important because it directs the differential diagnosis toward a structural lesion such as an epidural hematoma or cerebral contusion. However, the possibility of nonaccidental trauma, especially if the caregiver's history is inconsistent with the clinical findings, should not be excluded.

Ingestion of toxic substances is a common cause of altered mental status in toddlers and adolescents.[1] In the young child, the history of an accidental exposure is often obtained from the child's caretaker. However, sometimes the ingestion is not witnessed; thus a detailed list of potential poisons to which the child may have access, including prescription and nonprescription medications, should be obtained. The adolescent may admit to an intentional overdose, but the history is often obscure or unobtainable. In these cases, interviews with accompanying friends and family members are essential.

The medical history may include an underlying disorder that predisposes the child to a condition that results in altered mental status. A child with diabetes may have ketoacidosis or hypoglycemia. Children with a metabolic disorder or with hepatic or renal failure may develop encephalopathy.

PHYSICAL EXAMINATION

A thorough physical examination may not only lead to a probable diagnosis, but may also provide a baseline with which future examinations can be compared so as to assess the improvement or deterioration of the child's clinical status. The level of consciousness can be determined by the child's appearance, interactiveness, consolability, speech, cry, and gaze. Care must be taken, especially for young children and those with chronic illness, to ascertain the child's baseline state of functioning and responsiveness.

Vital signs are particularly important. Hyperthermia may be present with infection, heatstroke, or certain toxins (eg, cocaine, anticholinergics, phencyclidine). Hypothermia occurs with exposure to cold or with alcohol overdose. Hypertension, bradycardia, and irregular respirations (the Cushing triad) are signs of impending cerebral herniation but only appear late in the course of increasing intracranial pressure. Abnormalities in heart rate and blood pressure can also occur with fever, pain, arrhythmias, hypovolemia, myocardial injury, and status epilepticus. Abnormal respirations can be seen with pain, hypoxia, acidosis, intoxication, and brainstem lesions. In some cases, the respiratory pattern may be a clue to the level of neurologic dysfunction. Posthyperventilation apnea—a short apnea after deep breathing—occurs with lesions in the cerebral hemispheres. As dysfunction moves rostrally from the midbrain to the medulla, the respiratory pattern progresses from Cheyne-Stokes breathing (crescendo-decrescendo hyperpnea followed by apnea) to central neurogenic hyperventilation (sustained, rapid, deep breathing). Finally, irregular, sporadic, apneustic respiration occurs with low brainstem dysfunction.

The mouth and throat should be examined for signs of airway obstruction causing hypoxia. A budging fontanel and nuchal rigidity are signs of meningitis or meningeal irritation from an intracranial mass. The skin examination can be helpful in identifying hypoxia, anemia, jaundice, carbon monoxide and other poisonings, trauma, and certain infections. Adolescents who are pretending to be unresponsive usually resist opening their eyes, and they avoid hitting themselves when their hand is raised and then allowed to drop to their face. Furthermore, when feigning coma, the eyes close quickly and deliberately after being held open by the examiner, as opposed to true coma, during which the eyes close slowly.

The neurologic examination should be directed at determining whether the underlying diagnosis is of structural or medical origin. The pupillary reflex and extraocular movements may provide essential clues. In pathological states confined to the cerebral hemispheres, the pupils function normally, unless this state results in herniation. At the level of the diencephalon (thalamus and hypothalamus), pupils are miotic but react to light. With midbrain involvement, pupils may be midposition, irregular, or widely dilated; light reflexes may be absent if oculomotor nerves are involved. Bilateral fixed and dilated pupils indicate massive central nervous system dysfunction. A unilateral dilated pupil is a common early sign of uncal herniation. Extraocular muscle positions should be noted at rest (deviation may mean seizure activity or structural lesions); spontaneous abnormal eye movements should be identified, and ocular responses to vestibular stimulation should be tested. As with pupillary response, extraocular movements will vary with the level of the lesion. In general, asymmetry is seen with midbrain and upper pons involvement, and lack of extraocular movements is present with lower pons and medullary involvement. Negative doll's eyes—a condition in which the eyes appear painted on the face because the eyes remain stationary with respect to head movement—is seen in comatose patients with a low brainstem lesion.

Not all abnormal pupillary response is due to increased intracranial pressure. Mydriasis can be seen in Horner syndrome and in exposure to certain toxic substances, including anticholinergics, amphetamines, cocaine, and tricyclic antidepressants. Miosis may be caused by cold exposure, opiates, ethanol, barbiturates, cholinergic agents such as organophosphates, and clonidine.

When assessing motor function in patients with an altered mental status, spontaneous movements should be evaluated for signs of hemiparesis that may suggest a structural lesion or uncal herniation. Tone should be assessed for flaccidity and responses to painful stimuli. Patients who are unresponsive may have depressed brainstem function, and those who have increased tone may have diffuse cortical injury. Posturing is a bad sign, and the type of posturing aids in determining the extent of the injury. Decorticate posturing occurs when the patient flexes the arms, wrists, and hands, and adducts the upper extremities while internally rotating and plantar flexing the lower extremities. This form of posturing occurs as a result of diffuse damage to the cerebral cortex, white matter, and basal ganglia. Decerebrate posturing is when the patient exhibits marked opisthotonus with extended arms and hands, which is usually the result of extensive damage involving the midbrain.

LABORATORY EVALUATION

In the setting of altered mental status, laboratory testing should focus first on determining life-threatening metabolic derangements and then determination of the underlying cause. Rapid bedside glucose determination can identify hypoglycemia within minutes of clinical evaluation. In addition to being a common cause of altered mental status, hypoglycemia also accompanies many other underlying causes, such as diabetes, metabolic disorders, and sepsis. Calcium and sodium abnormalities can be identified on a serum chemistry panel. Serum bicarbonate and arterial blood gas levels may show acidemia, either as a direct result of an underlying metabolic disorder or as a result of abnormal respiratory effort. Hemoglobin levels can help determine whether anemia is present, and the white blood cell count may be high if the altered mental status is due to an infection. Serum ammonia is an important screening test for many inborn errors of metabolism, although mild hyperammonemia can be a nonspecific finding in children.

If ingestion of a toxic substance is considered, then directed drug levels (eg, phenytoin, salicylates) might pinpoint a diagnosis. A qualitative urine toxicology screening can identify a variety of commonly ingested agents, but its usefulness is limited because of the delay until the results become available. Measurement of serum osmolarity may be helpful if poisoning with methanol, ethylene glycol, or isopropanol is suspected. Serum cooximetry is needed for determining carbon monoxide level. If the child is febrile, then a blood culture should be obtained.

Abnormalities on an electrocardiogram (ECG) may be seen in cardiac causes such as myocarditis or dysrhythmias. However, a normal ECG finding does not rule out these disorders. In addition, many serious drug overdoses have ECG findings. Tricyclic antidepressants cause sodium-channel blockage, resulting in primary conduction delays and prolongation of the QRS interval. Ischemic changes on the ECG are seen with cocaine overdose. Neuroleptic overdose (phenothiazines, thioridazine, haloperidol, chlorpromazine) causes QT prolongation.

Imaging Studies

Although the history and physical examination may provide clues to the underlying diagnosis, neuroimaging of the brain is the fastest, most reliable test to differentiate structural from medical causes of altered mental status. The decision whether to obtain a computed tomographic (CT) scan or a magnetic resonance imaging (MRI) study depends on a variety of factors, including the clinical situation, the stability of the patient, and the availability of the test. MRI uses no ionizing radiation and therefore poses reduced risk to the developing brain of the child. In addition, MRI provides more detail of the soft tissues and better imaging of the brain parenchyma, cerebellum, and brainstem than CT. However, in the setting of an acute change in mental status, a CT scan is usually a readily available, rapid screening test that can identify acute intracranial bleeding, masses, or contusions in emergency situations.

MANAGEMENT

Management of a child with altered mental status is similar to any emergency condition. The primary objective is to stabilize the child's clinical status and correct any acute life-threatening conditions. Once stabilized, the child should be transported to an acute care facility for additional evaluation and management.

Initial management begins with the ABCs—airway, breathing, and circulation. If the airway is obstructed, which is usually identified by the presence of stridor or an abnormal breathing pattern, then immediate maneuvers to open the airway either by manual positioning or artificial methods (oral airway or endotracheal intubation) should be performed. Oxygen should be routinely administered. Because many of the causes of an altered mental status require intravenous (IV) fluid or medication, a peripheral IV catheter should be placed. Immediate bedside blood glucose levels should be determined because hypoglycemia is readily identified and easily corrected with administration of IV dextrose. Additional blood tests to help determine the underlying cause should be performed. Empiric administration of naloxone should be considered if the underlying cause is unknown. Naloxone can reverse the depressive cardiorespiratory effects of narcotic ingestion, but it may also be helpful in ingestions of clonidine, dextromethorphan, valproic acid, and captopril. A fluid bolus with normal saline should be administered if signs exist of poor perfusion or hypotension. Acid-base and electrolyte abnormalities, if present, should be corrected.

If the patient has a history of trauma, or if the suspected cause is structural, then intracranial pressure may be high. To control the intracranial pressure, the head should be elevated to 30 degrees and placed in a midline position. Hyperventilation can be a temporizing measure to reduce intracranial pressure. Every effort should be made to stabilize the child as soon as possible and obtain an emergent CT scan, as well as a consultation with a neurosurgeon. Obstructive hydrocephalus resulting from an intracranial mass lesion or obstructed ventriculoperitoneal shunt may need to be relieved emergently with a ventriculoperitoneal shunt tap or ventriculostomy.

If a medical cause is suspected, then additional laboratory and radiologic testing may help determine whether the cause is infectious, metabolic, or toxicologic. Fever may indicate an infectious origin, and the child should be provided with IV antibiotics after a blood culture is obtained. If meningitis is suspected, then a lumbar puncture can be performed to help confirm this diagnosis. It should be performed if the patient is stable and does not have focal neurologic signs. However, if the child is clinically unstable, then the lumbar puncture should be deferred but without delay in administration of empiric IV antibiotics. If herpes encephalitis is a concern, then empiric acyclovir should be provided. A positive stool guaiac test raises the concern of intussusception, which can be diagnosed by plain-film radiography or ultrasonography and reduced by an air-contrast enema. ECG can identify cardiac dysrhythmias or conduction abnormalities. If unexplained bruising exists, then child abuse should be considered.

When a clear cause cannot be identified, ingestion of a toxic substance should be suspected. Family members should be questioned about the availability of any medication. If possible, the bottle of the medication should be checked and the remaining pills counted to estimate the maximal amount ingested. For some ingestions, antidotes are available. Specialists at the local poison control center can assist in the management of a suspected overdose. Many children will require a dose of activated charcoal, which binds the toxin and limits intestinal absorption.

After stabilization and initial management, the patient should be observed in a monitored setting until mental status improves.

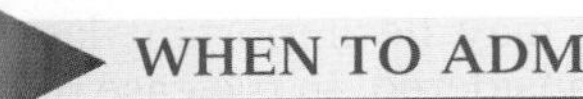

WHEN TO ADMIT

Any child with altered mental status

SUGGESTED RESOURCES

Avner JR. Altered states of consciousness. *Pediatr Rev.* 2006;72:331-337.

Burton B. Inborn errors of metabolism in infancy: a guide to diagnosis. *Pediatrics.* 1998;102:e69. Available at: http://pediatrics.aappublications.org/cgi/content/full/102/6/e69. Accessed May 28, 2007.

Kanich W, Brady WJ, Huff S, et al. Altered mental status: evaluation and etiology in the ED. *Am J Emerg Med.* 2002;20:613-617.

Key CB, Roghrock SG, Falk JL. Cerebrospinal fluid shunt complications: an emergency medicine perspective. *Pediatr Emerg Care.* 1995;11:265-273.

King D, Avner JR. Altered mental status. *Clin Pediatr Emerg Med.* 2003;4:171-178.

Kirkham FJ. Non-traumatic coma in children. *Arch Dis Child.* 2001;85:303-312.

Meyer PG, Ducrocq S, Carli P. Pediatric neurologic emergencies. *Curr Opin Crit Care.* 2001;7:81-87.

Pattisapu JV. Etiology and clinical course of hydrocephalus. *Neurosurg Clin North Am.* 2001;36:651-659.

Plum F, Posner J. *The Diagnosis of Stupor and Coma.* Philadelphia, PA: FA Davis; 1980.

REFERENCES

1. Wong CP, Forsyth RJ, Kelly TP, et al. Incidence, aetiology, and outcome of non-traumatic coma: a population based study. *Arch Dis Child.* 2001;84:193-199.
2. Lai M, Klein-Schwartz W, Rodgers GC, et al. 2005 Annual report of the American Association of Poison Control Centers' National Poisoning and Exposure Database. *Clin Toxicol.* 2006;44:803-932.

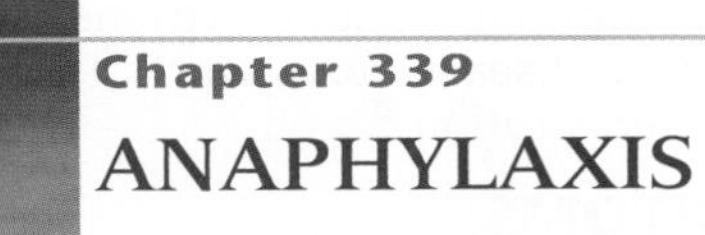

Chapter 339

ANAPHYLAXIS

Elizabeth Secord, MD; Michael R. Simon, MD

DEFINITION OF TERMS

Severe allergic reactions mediated by immunoglobulin E (IgE) and involving 2 or more organ systems are classically referred to as anaphylaxis. Clinically similar events that are not attributable to IgE are historically referred to as anaphylactoid. The terms are often used interchangeably because the clinical syndromes are often indistinguishable, and the treatment recommendations are the same regardless of the cause.

ETIOLOGY

Classical anaphylactic reactions are mediated through antigen-induced, IgE-mediated mast cell and basophil degranulation.[1] The majority of these reactions are induced by foods or medications.[2] Anaphylactoid reactions are often the result of direct mast cell degranulation; some causes of direct mast cell degranulation are radiocontrast media or opioids.[3] Some cases of exercise-induced anaphylaxis also are thought to be caused by direct mast cell degranulation. In anaphylactic and anaphylactoid reactions to nonsteroidal anti-inflammatory agents, the majority of cases appear to be due to an inhibition of the cyclooxygenase pathway.[4]

The final common step in the pathway for all of these reactions is mast cell and, usually, basophil degranulation. Histamine may account for the majority of symptoms.[5] Nevertheless, antihistamines alone cannot prevent or reverse all anaphylactic symptoms. Other mediators such as leukotrienes may contribute to some symptoms in anaphylactic and anaphylactoid reactions. Although reproducing the symptoms of anaphylaxis is possible by infusion of histamine, animal studies suggest that nitric oxide production may contribute to the cardiovascular manifestations of this syndrome.[6-8] Nitric oxide increases the activity of guanylyl cyclase, which produces cyclic guanosine monophosphate, which causes vasodilation.[9,10] Methylene blue is an inhibitor of guanylyl cyclase and nitric oxide synthase.[11]

EPIDEMIOLOGIC MECHANISM

The estimates of the incidence of anaphylaxis and anaphylactoid reactions vary, but it is generally reported as less than 1% and can be from 0.04% to 0.4%.[2,12,13] Theories suggest that the incidence is higher than reported because of underreporting and underrecognition of the syndrome.[14,15] No racial predisposition is present. In childhood, boys are more likely to experience anaphylaxis than girls, and in adult life, women are more likely than men.[13,16,17] Atopy is a predisposing factor for food-induced anaphylaxis.[18] Reactions to injected agents tend to be more severe and more rapid than for ingested agents.[19,20] Risk factors associated with death from anaphylaxis include extremes of age, concomitant cardiac disease, asthma,[21,22] and delay of epinephrine administration.[20]

SIGNS AND SYMPTOMS

Ninety percent or more of patients experiencing anaphylactic and anaphylactoid reactions will report skin manifestations of urticaria, facial swelling (angioedema), pruritus, or flushing.[2,23,24] Difficulty breathing (shortness of breath, chest tightness, or wheezing) is the second most common complaint. Lightheadedness or weakness and palpitations are often reported. Gastrointestinal symptoms, such as diarrhea and vomiting, may occur. Headache may also be present. Some patients report a sense of impending doom accompanying the onset of anaphylaxis.

DIFFERENTIAL DIAGNOSIS

Vasodepressor reactions: Hypotension, pallor, weakness, nausea, and bradycardia, which are common features of vasodepressor reactions and often occur after an emotional stressor. Loss of consciousness may also occur. Lack of skin and airway manifestations, which are usually seen in anaphylactic reactions, and prompt recovery after assuming a recumbent position help differentiate the syndromes. Given that bradycardia occurs in 5% of patients with anaphylaxis, even in the absence of the use of beta-adrenergic blockers,[25] it alone does not differentiate anaphylaxis from vasovagal reactions. An important point to remember, however, is that anaphylaxis may produce only cardiovascular and no cutaneous signs or symptoms.[26]

Panic attacks: Palpitations, flushing, shortness of breath, and gastrointestinal symptoms are frequent with panic attacks. If they are accompanied by vocal cord dysfunction and stridor, then they may mimic anaphylaxis. Even if these latter symptoms are not accompanied by upper airway involvement, such as stridor, anaphylaxis must be excluded.

Mastocytosis: Idiopathic and antigen-induced anaphylaxis may occur in patients with systemic mastocytosis because these mast cells bind IgE and release histamine and other mast cell mediators. Urticaria pigmentosa, the most typical skin lesions of mastocytosis, may suggest the diagnosis. If the lesions are primarily internal, then a higher level of suspicion will be necessary to make the diagnosis.[27] Tests that include total serum tryptase, urinary histamine metabolites, and genetic testing for mastocytosis may be necessary to differentiate mastocytosis from anaphylaxis. Serum concentrations of total tryptase are acutely elevated in patients with anaphylaxis, whereas total tryptase is increased in patients with mastocytosis even when they are not acutely ill. These tests are, however, not useful for managing acute episodes, which are indistinguishable from anaphylaxis.[28]

Hypoglycemia: Flushing can occur with hypoglycemia, mimicking an early allergic skin reaction. In hypoglycemia, flushing may be associated with tachycardia, anxiety, diaphoresis, and lightheadedness.

EVALUATION

Relevant History

A history of recent food ingestion should always be sought. Food-induced anaphylaxis is more common in children than in adults.[29] Most anaphylactic reactions to foods occur in the first 2 hours after eating, with the vast majority occurring within the first 30 minutes. Cases of reactions beginning up to several hours later have been reported. Peanuts, tree nuts, fish, and shellfish account for the vast majority of anaphylactic reactions to foods, with peanut being the most frequent (up to 62% of cases). These foods are usually responsible for lifelong allergies in affected persons, and children are not likely to outgrow these reactions.[30] Milk, soy, and eggs are also responsible for severe allergic reactions in infants and toddlers; but unlike children who are allergic to peanuts, nuts, fish, and shellfish, most children will become tolerant to milk and soy with time, and some will become tolerant to eggs.[29,30] In some patients with severe food allergy, inhalation of the offending antigen is sufficient to lead to a reaction in a sensitized individual. Some with apparent idiopathic anaphylaxis may actually be reacting to inhalation of pollen to which they are exquisitely sensitive.[31] Injected venoms from a *Hymenoptera* insect sting (ie, bees, yellow jackets, hornets, wasps, fire ants) can cause anaphylaxis in sensitized individuals. From 0.5% to 3.0% of the population experiences a systemic reaction after *Hymenoptera* stings.[32,33] A history of exposure to particular insects may be important later if immunotherapy is to be considered. In the case of bee sting, removing the stinger early is important to avoid further venom injection. Identification of the wound or stinger helps identify the species. Bees (and very rarely yellow jackets) leave a stinger, whereas other *Hymenoptera* do not.

Ingestion of medications is another common cause of anaphylactic reactions. Penicillin does so most commonly. Aspirin and other nonsteroidal anti-inflammatory agents may also induce anaphylactoid reactions. Drugs that are administered intravenously or intramuscularly are absorbed more rapidly and are associated with more frequent and more severe reactions.[19,20] Anaphylactic and anaphylactoid reactions occurring in hospitalized patients are most frequently caused by allergy to antibiotics, radiocontrast media reactions, and latex allergy, although latex allergy is becoming less common.[34]

Exercise-induced anaphylaxis usually occurs in teenagers and young adults. A prodrome of flushing and abdominal pain may occur followed by collapse during exercise. Some cases of exercise-induced anaphylaxis occur only after ingesting foods that cross-react with pollens (eg, melons that cross-react with ragweed, apples that cross-react with birch). The combination of exercise with food ingestion appears to be necessary for the event in these persons.[35,36] Some individuals also have exercised-induced anaphylaxis after nonspecific food ingestion combined with exercise. Exercise-induced anaphylaxis may follow episodes of exercise-induced urticaria.

Physical Examination[2]

Respiratory

Bronchospasm with wheezing is frequent. Edema of the airway may cause stridor or hoarseness. Cyanosis may occur. Upper respiratory findings include nasal congestion, rhinorrhea, sneezing, and lingual and pharyngeal edema.

Skin

Urticaria, angioedema, or flushing are evident in approximately 90% of cases.

Cardiovascular

Tachycardia is a frequent finding resulting from the adrenergic response to decreased intravascular volume or histamine activity through the H2 receptor. Hypotension may then occur and be followed by anaphylactic shock.

Ocular

Tearing, conjunctival erythema, and edema (chemosis) may be present.

Laboratory Testing

The history and clinical assessment are far more important in the initial evaluation of anaphylaxis than laboratory testing. Plasma concentration of histamine, which mediates many of the symptoms in anaphylaxis, has a very short half-life (peaks within 5 minutes to an hour after an anaphylactic event). Histamine plasma concentration is not a reliable or useful marker in most instances. However, histamine metabolites in the urine may be clinically useful in the diagnosis of systemic mastocytosis.[28] Identifying specific IgE (skin prick tests for specific allergens or serum antigen–specific IgE tests such as radioallergosorbent assay, and the enzyme-linked immunosorbent assay) may be useful to help determine the cause of the reactions. However, at the time of presentation these tests will not be valid because the specific IgE may no longer be in the skin or serum. It has been consumed in the reaction, and testing for specific IgE may not reliably be done for up to 6 weeks after the incident. In any case, the acute management is not altered by specific identification of the agent.

If uncertainty exists as to whether the reaction is anaphylaxis and the incident has occurred within the last 1 to 2 hours, then serum tryptase may be useful in establishing the diagnosis. It may remain elevated in the blood for up to 6 hours after the event[37,38] and is measurable for up to several days later in serum samples that have been refrigerated. This time frame allows its determination after the fact from samples that were obtained for other laboratory studies.

Pulse oximetry and arterial blood gas determinations may be appropriate in patients with cyanosis or respiratory compromise. Imaging is not important in evaluating anaphylaxis.

Management

The airway should be secured; the respiratory rate, blood pressure, and pulse should be obtained; and patient should be placed in supine position with feet elevated if blood pressure is decreased. If the child is wheezing, then a compromise may have to be made regarding the recumbent position to allow adequate air exchange. Oxygen should be administered. A tourniquet applied on an extremity proximal to a *Hymenoptera* sting or medication injection will slow systemic absorption of antigen and anaphylactic mediators.[39]

Epinephrine is the most important initial treatment for anaphylaxis. Epinephrine should be administered intramuscularly, preferably in the outer thigh, while the assessment is being made. The dose may be repeated as needed every 10 to 15 minutes. Administering epinephrine as a 1:10,000 solution intravenously may be necessary in the event of severe hypotension with peripheral vasoconstriction resulting from severely decreased intravascular volume.[39]

Fluid replacement may be necessary if hypotension from increased vascular permeability is present. Children should receive up to 30 mL/kg of crystalloid solution in the first hour to treat hypotension. Adults often require 1 to 2 liters over the first hour.

Intravenous Vasopressors

In severe refractory hypotension, continuous intravenous infusions of dopamine, norepinephrine, or epinephrine may be required.

Nebulized β2 Agonists

Inhaled albuterol may be used for wheezing that is not responsive to parenteral epinephrine.

Antihistamines

H1 antihistamines are often given to relieve symptoms and are highly effective for relieving skin manifestations and oropharyngeal angioedema. These drugs are not effective for treating life-threatening symptoms that do not involve the upper airway, and they do not replace the need for epinephrine. First-generation H1 antihistamines commonly cause drowsiness and may impair the patient's ability to relate the progress or resolution of their symptoms.

The intravenous administration of the combination of an H1 antihistamine (eg, diphenhydramine) with the H2-blocker cimetidine (intravenously by piggyback infusion) has been demonstrated to block both the cardiac and peripheral vascular effects of histamine.[40,41]

The use of adrenal corticosteroids is recommended based on their efficacy in asthma and their beneficial effect in decreasing vascular permeability. The data, however, do not indicate that use of corticosteroids prevents biphasic reactions.[42]

In cases in which the patient is prescribed a beta blocker (more frequent in adults than children), resistance to standard therapy may occur, causing refractory hypotension, bradycardia, and relapsing symptoms.[43,44] These patients are at increased risk of death from anaphylaxis. Glucagon (1 mg) is recommended when the patient has been taking a beta blocker and should be considered in cases of anaphylaxis with refractory hypotension even without a clear history of beta blockade.[45] Methylene blue (1-2 mg/kg), which is used to treat methemoglobinemia, has been successfully used to treat patients with severe anaphylactic hypotension.[46-48]

Anaphylaxis may be uniphasic, biphasic, or protracted. Biphasic reactions occur in from 4% to 20% of patients with anaphylaxis.[42,49] Patients with biphasic reactions often experience the recurrence of their initial signs and symptoms several hours after their apparent resolution.

Patients who have an anaphylactic episode should be discharged with epinephrine in an autoinjection device for self-administration.[39] The patient must be able to use the device and must understand that it should be available at home, school, work, or anywhere the patient travels. The patient also needs to understand that the devices have expiration dates and should be renewed periodically.

A reasonable work-up should be undertaken to identify the cause of the reaction, and education on avoidance should be provided. This assessment is particularly important for foods, insect stings, and medications. A medic alert bracelet should be advised. Venom immunotherapy is indicated for treatment of insect sting reactions. In cases of exercise-induced anaphylaxis, patients should be advised to avoid exercising alone.

WHEN TO REFER

All patients with anaphylaxis and anaphylactoid reactions should be referred to an allergist for identification of the responsible agent and for patient education and management.

WHEN TO ADMIT

Observation for up to 24 hours is recommended because biphasic reactions cannot reliably be prevented with corticosteroids and cannot be predicted.[42] When hypotension or airway compromise is present, hospital admission is warranted.

TOOLS FOR PRACTICE

Engaging Patients and Family

- *What is Anaphylaxis?* (fact sheet), American Academy of Allergy, Asthma, and Immunology (www.aaaai.org/patients/resources/easy_reader/anaphylaxis.pdf).
- *Students with Chronic Health Conditions* (brochure), American Academy of Pediatrics (patiented.aap.org).
- *Common Childhood Allergies* (fact sheet), American Academy of Pediatrics (www.aap.org/topics.html).
- Food Allergy (Web site), American Academy of Allergy, Asthma, and Immunology (www.aaaai.org/patients/gallery/foodallergy.asp).
- *What You Should Know About Food Allergy* (fact sheet), American Academy of Allergy, Asthma, and Immunology, AAP endorsed (www.aaaai.org/members/allied_health/tool_kit/educational/food.pdf).
- *Food Allergies and Reactions—Kids* (fact sheet), American Academy of Allergy, Asthma, and Immunology, AAP endorsed (www.aaaai.org/patients/resources/easy_reader/food.pdf).

Medical Decision Support

- *Pediatric Nutrition Handbook* (policy manual), American Academy of Pediatrics (www.aap.org/bookstore).

Community Coordination and Advocacy

- Food Allergy Action Plan (form), Food Allergy Organization (www.foodallergy.org/actionplan.pdf).

REFERENCES

1. Martin KC, Janis KS, Andrew FW. Mast cell-derived mediators. In: Adkinson FNJ, Yunginger JW, Busse WW, et al, eds. *Middleton's Allergy Principles and Practice*. Philadelphia, PA: Mosby; 2003:189-212.
2. Yocum MW, Butterfield JH, Klein JS. et al. Epidemiology of anaphylaxis in Olmstead County, a population-based study. *J Allergy Clin Immunol*. 1999;104:452-456.
3. Lieberman P. Anaphylaxis and anaphylactoid reactions. In: Adkinson FNJ, Yunginger JW, Busse WW, et al, eds. *Middleton's Allergy Principles and Practice*. Philadelphia, PA: Mosby; 2003:1497-1522.
4. Lee TH, Smith CM, Arm JP, et al. Mediator release in aspirin-induced reactions. *J Allergy Clin Immunol*. 1991; 88:827-829.
5. Winbery SL, Lieberman PL. Histamine and antihistamines in anaphylaxis. *Clin Allergy Immunol*. 2002;17: 287-317.
6. Thiemermann C, Wu CC, Szabo C, et al. Role of tumor necrosis factor in the induction of nitric oxide synthase in a rat model of endotoxin shock. *Br J Pharmacol*. 1993; 110(1):177-182.
7. Amir S. An inhibitor of nitric oxide production, NG nitro L arginine methyl ester, improves survival in anaphylactic shock. *Eur J Pharmacol*. 1991;203(1):125-127.
8. Mitsuhata HSJ, Takeuchi H, Hasome N, et al. Production of nitric oxide in anaphylaxis in rabbits. *Shock*. 1994;2(5): 381-384.
9. Friebe A, Koesling D. Regulation of nitric oxide-sensitive guanylyl cyclase. *Circ Res*. 2003;93(2):96-105.
10. Kawada T, Ishibash T, Sasage H, et al. Modification by LY83583 and methylene blue of relaxation induced by nitric oxide, glyceryl trinitrate, sodium nitroprusside and atriopeptin in aorta of the rat, guinea-pig and rabbit. *Gen Pharmacol*. 1994;25:1361-1371.
11. Mayer B, Brunner F, Schmidt K. Novel actions of methylene blue. *Eur Heart J*. 1993;14(suppl):22-26.
12. van der Klauw MM, Wilson JH, Stricker BH. Drug-associated anaphylaxis: 20 years of reporting in the Netherlands (1974-1994) and review of the literature. *Clin Exp Allergy*. 1996;26:1355-1363.
13. Pastorello E, Rivolta F, Bianchi M, et al. Incidence of anaphylaxis in the emergency department of a general hospital in Milan. *J Chromatogr B Biomed Sci Appl*. 2001; 756(1-2):11-17.
14. Barclay WR. Adverse drug reactions. *JAMA*. 1979;242: 656.
15. Pumphrey RSH, Davis D. Under-reporting of antibiotic anaphylaxis may put patients at risk. *Lancet*. 1999;3:1157-1158.

16. Simons FE, Peterson S, Black CD. Epinephrine dispensing for the out-of-hospital treatment of anaphylaxis in infants and children: a population-based study. *Ann Allergy Asthma Immunol.* 2001;86:622-626.
17. Kaufman D. An epidemiologic study of severe anaphylactic and anaphylactoid reactions among hospital patients: methods and overall risks: abstract from report from the International Collaborative Study of severe anaphylaxis. *Epidemiology.* 1998;9:141-146.
18. Salvaggio JE, Cavanaugh JJ, Lowell FC. A comparison of the immunologic responses of normal and atopic individuals to intranasally administered antigens. *J Allergy Clin Immunol.* 1964;35:62-69.
19. Lieberman P. Difficult allergic drug reactions. *Immunol Allergy Clin North Am.* 1991;11:213-231.
20. Pumphrey R. Lessons for management of anaphylaxis from a study of fatal reactions. *Clin Exp Allergy.* 2000;30:1144-1150.
21. Lang DM, Alpern MB, Visintainer PF, et al. Elevated risk of anaphylactoid reaction from radiographic contrast media is associated with both beta-blocker exposure and cardiovascular disorders. *Arch Intern Med.* 1993;153(17):2033-2040.
22. Lang DM, Alpern MB, Visintainer PF, et al. Increased risk for anaphylactoid reaction from contrast media in patients on beta-adrenergic blockers or with asthma. *Ann Intern Med.* 1991;115(4):270-276.
23. DeShazo RD, Kemp SF. Allergic reactions to drugs and biologic agents. *JAMA.* 1997;278:1895-1905.
24. Yocum MW, Khan DA. Assessment of patients who have experienced anaphylaxis: a 3-year survey. *Mayo Clin Proc.* 1994;69(1):16-23.
25. Fisher MM. Clinical observations on the pathophysiology and treatment of anaphylactic cardiovascular collapse. *Anaesth Intensive Care.* 1986;14(1):17-21.
26. Viner NA, Rhamy RK. Anaphylaxis manifested by hypotension alone. *J Urol.* 1975;113(1):108-110.
27. Florian S, Krauth MT, Simonitsch-Klupp I, et al. Indolent systemic mastocytosis with elevated serum tryptase, absence of skin lesions, and recurrent severe anaphylactoid episodes. *Int Arch Allergy Immunol.* 2005;136(3);273-280.
28. Metcalfe D. Mastocytosis Syndromes. In: Adkinson FNJ, Yunginger JW, Busse WW, et al, eds. *Middleton's Allergy Principles and Practice.* Philadelphia, PA: Mosby; 2003: 1523-1535.
29. Bock SA, Munoz-Furlong A, Sampson HA. Fatalities due to anaphylactic reactions to foods. *J Allergy Clin Immunol.* 2001;107:191-193.
30. Sampson H. Adverse Reactions to Foods. In: Adkinson FNJ, Yunginger JW, Busse WW, et al, eds. *Middleton's Allergy Principles and Practice.* Philadelphia, PA: Mosby; 2003:1619-1644.
31. Broom BC, Fitzharris P. Life-threatening inhalant allergy: typical anaphylaxis induced by inhalational allergen challenge in patients with idiopathic recurrent anaphylaxis. *Clin Allergy.* 1983;13(2):169-179.
32. Golden DB, Marsh DG, Freidhoff LR, et al. Natural history of Hymenoptera venom sensitivity in adults. *J Allergy Clin Immunol.* 1997;100(6pt1):760-766.
33. Golden DB, Addison BI, Gadde J, et al. Prospective observations on stopping prolonged venom immunotherapy. *J Allergy Clin Immunol.* 1989;84(2):162-167.
34. Neugut AJ, Ghatak AT, Miller RL. Anaphylaxis in the United States: an investigation into its epidemiology. *Arch Intern Med.* 2001;161:15-21.
35. Stratbucker WB, Summit PH, Stratbucker WB. Exercise-induced anaphylaxis. Park CL, Windle ML, Georgitis JW et al eds. Available at: www.emedicine.com/ped/topic724.htm.
36. Kaplan A. Urticaria and angioedema. In: Adkinson FNJ, Yunginger JW, Busse WW, et al, eds. *Middleton's Allergy Principles and Practice.* Philadelphia. PA: Mosby; 2003: 1537-1558.
37. Schwartz LB, Metcalfe DD, Miller JS, et al. Tryptase levels as an indicator of mast-cell activation in systemic anaphylaxis and mastocytosis. *N Engl J Med.* 1987;316(26): 1622-1626.
38. Schwartz LB, Yunginger JW, Miller J, et al. Time course of appearance and disappearance of human mast cell tryptase in the circulation after anaphylaxis. *J Clin Invest.* 1989;83(5):1551-1555.
39. Joint Task Force on Practice Parameters, American Academy of Allergy, Asthma and Immunology. The diagnosis and management of anaphylaxis. *J Allergy Clin Immunol.* 1998;101(6 pt 2):S465-S528.
40. Kaliner M, Sigler R, Summers JH. Effects of infused histamine: analysis of the effects of H-1 and H-2 histamine receptor antagonists on cardiovascular and pulmonary responses. *J Allergy Clin Immunol.* 1981;68:365-371.
41. Dachman WD, Bedarida G, Blaschke TF, et al. Histamine-induced venodilation in human beings involves both H1 and H2 receptor subtypes. *J Allergy Clin Immunol.* 1994; 83:606-614.
42. Stark BJ, Sullivan TJ. Biphasic and protracted anaphylaxis. *J Allergy Clin Immunol.* 1986;78(1pt1):76-83.
43. Toogood JH. Beta-blocker therapy and the risk of anaphylaxis. *CMAJ.* 1987;137(7):587-588, 590-591.
44. Hart LL, Sue D. Potentiated anaphylaxis during chronic beta-blocker therapy. *Drug Intell Clin Pharm.* 1988;22: 720-721.
45. Zaloga GP, Delacey W, Holmboe E, et al. Glucagon reversal of hypotension in a case of anaphylactic shock. *Ann Int Med.* 1986;105:65-66.
46. Evora PR, Roselino CH, Schiavetto PM. Methylene blue in anaphylactic shock. *Ann Emerg Med.* 1997;30:240.
47. Evora PR, Oliveira Neto AM, Duarte NM, et al. Methylene blue as treatment for contrast medium-induced anaphylaxis. *J Postgrad Med.* 2002;48:327.
48. Oliveira Neto AM, Duarte NM, Vicente WV, et al. Methylene blue: an effective treatment for contrast medium-induced anaphylaxis. *Med Sci Monit.* 2003;9(11):102-106.
49. Lee JM, Greenes DS. Biphasic anaphylactic reactions in pediatrics. *Pediatrics.* 2000;106(4);762-766.

Chapter 340

CROUP (ACUTE LARYNGOTRACHEOBRONCHITIS)

Caroline Breese Hall, MD; William J. Hall, MD

DEFINITION

Viral croup (acute laryngotracheobronchitis) is an age-specific viral syndrome characterized by acute laryngeal and subglottic swelling, resulting in hoarseness, cough, respiratory distress, and inspiratory stridor. Inflammation at the subglottic area is apt to cause marked airflow obstruction because the anatomy of the cricoid and thyroid cartilage make this area the narrowest and the least distensible part of the larynx. Inflammation, however, commonly affects the conducting airways at all levels.

This syndrome, recognized and respected by physicians for centuries, inherited its name, croup, from the

Anglo-Saxon word *kropan*,[1] or from an old Scottish word *roup*, which meant to cry out in a hoarse voice. *Spasmodic croup* is a term sometimes used to denote afebrile episodes of croup that may be recurrent.[2,3] Airway hyperreactivity resulting from allergens may play a role in predisposing these children to repetitive bouts of croup. In the past, *membranous croup was* commonly referred to as diphtheria, which, until the 20th century, was considered the cause of most croup cases. Occasionally, *membranous croup* is still used for crouplike cases caused by bacteria.

ETIOLOGY AND EPIDEMIOLOGY

Viral Agents

A variety of agents may be associated with croup (Table 340-1). The parainfluenza viruses are identified most frequently as causing this disease, with parainfluenza virus type 1 as the major single agent.[4-7] In an 11-year study of croup in a private practice in Chapel Hill, North Carolina, the parainfluenza viruses constituted 75% of viral isolates obtained from children who had croup; 65% of the parainfluenza viral isolates were parainfluenza virus type 1.[8] Influenza viruses A and B and respiratory syncytial virus (RSV) are usually the next most frequently identified agents. Influenza virus, especially influenza A virus, has been associated with more severe croup than the more commonly occurring cases caused by the parainfluenza viruses.[4,9] More recently, human metapneumovirus (hMPV) has been identified as causing lower respiratory tract illness, including croup in young children. The presentation and epidemiologic features of hMPV infections appear to be similar to those caused by RSV.[10,11] Human coronaviruses (HCoV) are increasingly being recognized as potentially important causes of croup.[12] In Germany, a large prospective study of lower respiratory tract disease in children younger than 3 years identified a novel human coronavirus (HCoV-NL63) in 5% of the children, and HCoV infection was strongly associated with croup. This agent was more frequently identified in the winter than it was during other times of the year and in ambulatory rather than hospitalized children.[12] In the United States, measles was once a major cause of croup cases, which were often severe. Measles should still be considered in inadequately immunized populations.[13,14]

Croup occurs primarily in children between 3 months and 3 years of age and accounts for approximately 10% to 15% of respiratory tract disease in children.[5,6,15] The peak incidence of croup occurs between 6 and 24 months.[6,8,16,17] A study of croup requiring hospitalization in Canada over 14 years showed the rates of hospitalization for croup among children up to and including 4 years of age was highest in the first year of life.[6]

In a prepaid group practice in Seattle, the annual incidence of croup was 7 per 1000 children under 6 years of age.[16] However, between 1 and 2 years of age, this incidence approximately doubled. In the Chapel Hill practice, the attack rate during the second year of life was 4.7 per 100 children per year, and the yearly incidence per 100 children for all ages was 1.82 for boys and 1.27 for girls.[8] Boys appear more susceptible to croup than girls. Among both hospitalized and ambulatory croup cases, the ratio of boys to girls is approximately 2:1.[8,16-18]

The number of hospital admissions from croup in the United States has been declining since the 1990s, despite the concurrent increase in the population of young children.[7] This decline is most likely explained by the improved and more widely used therapeutic modalities of corticosteroids and nebulized epinephrine.[6]

Seasonal Occurrence

The singular seasonal patterns of croup cases correlate closely with activity of the major viral agents causing the syndrome, predominately the parainfluenza viruses (Figure 340-1; see also Table 340-1). Parainfluenza virus type 1, the most common cause of croup (Figure 340-2),

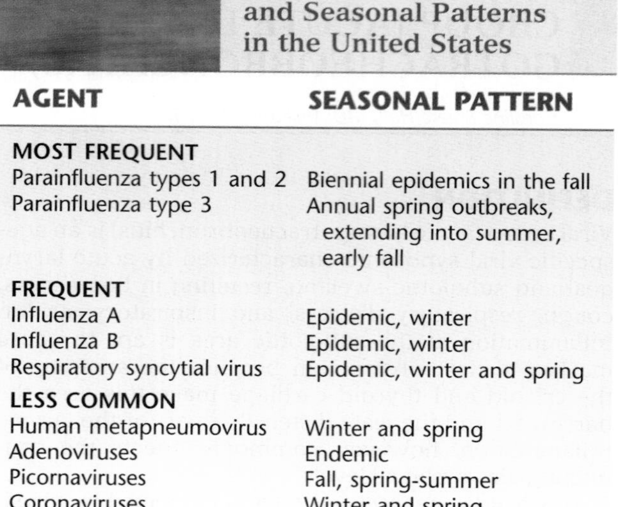

Table 340-1 Agents of Viral Croup and Seasonal Patterns in the United States

AGENT	SEASONAL PATTERN
MOST FREQUENT	
Parainfluenza types 1 and 2	Biennial epidemics in the fall
Parainfluenza type 3	Annual spring outbreaks, extending into summer, early fall
FREQUENT	
Influenza A	Epidemic, winter
Influenza B	Epidemic, winter
Respiratory syncytial virus	Epidemic, winter and spring
LESS COMMON	
Human metapneumovirus	Winter and spring
Adenoviruses	Endemic
Picornaviruses	Fall, spring-summer
Coronaviruses	Winter and spring

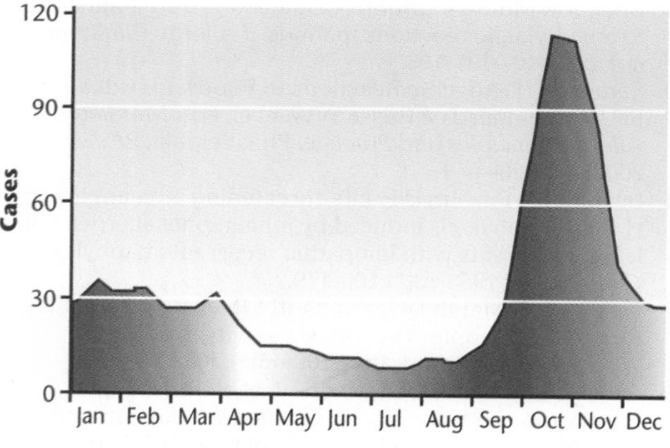

Figure 340-1 Seasonal occurrence of croup in patients in pediatric practices participating in an ongoing community surveillance program initiated in 1975 in Monroe County, New York. Most cases observed in the fall resulted from outbreaks for parainfluenza virus type 1 occurring during odd-numbered years.

has the distinctive pattern of producing epidemics of croup and other associated respiratory illnesses every other year in the autumn.[4,6,18,19] In a continuing surveillance program conducted in Monroe County, New York, the parainfluenza viruses constituted approximately 17% of all the viral isolates obtained from outpatients in private practices and for 67% of the isolates from children who had croup.[19] Smaller peaks of croup are associated with outbreaks of influenza, RSV, and parainfluenza virus types 2 and 3.[4,8,19,20] Although the proportion of RSV infections that are exhibited as croup is relatively small (approximately 5%), RSV is associated with up to 11% of all croup cases. Cases of croup that occur in the fall are most likely related to the parainfluenza viruses, especially type 1 and to a lesser extent type 2. Winter cases are associated most frequently with influenza and RSV. In the warmer months of spring and summer, parainfluenza type 3 is the agent isolated most often.

Host Factors Affecting Croup

RSV tends to cause croup in younger children, primarily in the first year of life, and often results in prolonged symptoms and hospitalization. The parainfluenza viruses cause croup predominately in toddlers, but these viruses may infect younger and, sometimes, school-aged children.

The age predilection of viral croup can be partly explained by the anatomic features of the airway. Smaller airways are prone to greater degrees of obstruction from any inflammation of the lining membranes, as illustrated by the fact that resistance to airflow is inversely related to the fourth power of the radius of the airway. The subglottic trachea of a young child is relatively smaller and also more pliable than that of an older individual. The narrowing that occurs with inspiratory effort may therefore be exaggerated in a young child with croup. In addition, obstruction above the subglottic area, such as may occur with nasal congestion, increases the collapsing force, and an increased respiratory rate associated with crying or anxiety may compromise the child's ventilation further.

Other host factors (eg, genetic and immunologic mechanisms), as yet poorly defined, are likely to contribute to the development and severity of croup.[2,3,15,21] Atopy or hyperreactivity of the airways has been suggested as playing a role in spasmodic or recurrent croup by the higher incidence of a family history of allergy and positive skin tests for allergens in such children.[22,23] The role in croup of genetic and anatomic host factors is further supported by the Tucson, Arizona, studies of lower respiratory tract disease, in which children enrolled at birth were prospectively monitored from birth through 13 years of age with periodic pulmonary function tests and markers of atopy.[15] Children with croup were divided into 2 major groups according to associated and without associated wheezing. The group with wheezing had significantly lower levels of indices of intrapulmonary airway function as infants, before any lower respiratory tract illness, and an increased risk of persistent wheezing in later life. In contrast, premorbid inspiratory resistance was significantly higher among children who subsequently developed croup without wheezing compared with those who developed croup with wheezing or who never developed croup.

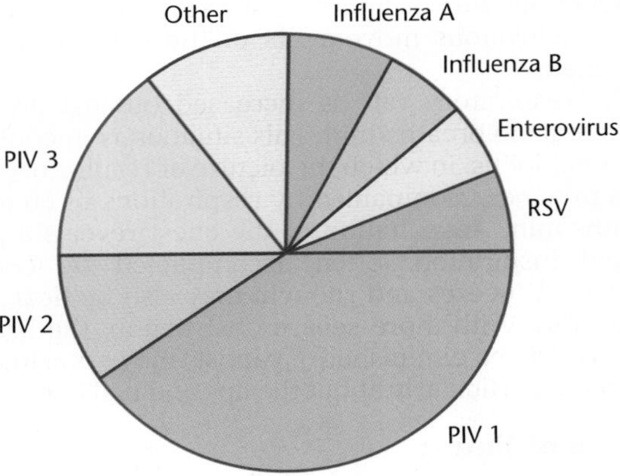

Figure 340-2 Viral cause of croup in patients in pediatric practices participating in a community surveillance program in Monroe County, New York. *PIV,* Parainfluenza virus; *RSV,* respirtory syncytial virus.

DIFFERENTIAL DIAGNOSIS

Viral croup must be differentiated from the 2 bacterial causes of stridor: (1) bacterial tracheitis and (2) epiglottitis, which may be fatal without immediate therapy (Box 340-1). Since the conjugated *Haemophilus influenzae* type b vaccines were licensed and incorporated into the routine immunization schedule of young children, epiglottitis has become rare in the United States. The differentiating features of epiglottitis are

BOX 340-1 Differential Diagnosis of Acute Viral Laryngotracheobronchitis

INFECTIOUS CAUSES OF STRIDOR

Epiglottitis
Bacterial tracheitis
Human papillomavirus (acquired perinatally)
Retropharyngeal and parapharyngeal abscess

NONINFECTIOUS CAUSES OF STRIDOR

Foreign body aspiration
Vocal cord paralysis
Angioneurotic edema of upper airway
Hypocalcemic tetany
Congenital malformations of upper airway
Laryngotracheal malacia, web, cleft
Vascular ring
Tracheal stenosis
Hemangioma, cyst of larynx or trachea
Cystic hygroma
Trauma

the rapidly progressive and unrelenting course, the drooling, and the toxic appearance. In most instances, the coryza and barking cough characteristic of viral croup are not present with epiglottitis.[24]

Bacterial tracheitis is the second emergent entity that needs to be differentiated from viral croup.[25] Bacterial tracheitis is a relatively uncommon infection that may affect children of any age and sometimes occurs after an episode of viral croup. The onset is acute with respiratory stridor, high fever, and, often, copious, purulent secretions. As with epiglottitis, the child appears toxic, and the respiratory obstruction rapidly progresses, often necessitating tracheal intubation. The pathogens most often involved are *Staphylococcus aureus,* and group A β-hemolytic streptococci. The diagnosis may be confirmed by direct laryngoscopy, which shows the purulent secretions and inflammation in the subglottic area and sometimes by a lateral neck radiograph, which may reveal an area of subglottic narrowing with a shaggy membrane.

A retropharyngeal abscess may occasionally have features similar to those of croup and should be especially considered in a child with a history of a penetrating pharyngeal injury, such as that caused by a fishbone. A retropharyngeal abscess is usually preceded by a mild pharyngitis and is more gradual in onset than croup. The child may be febrile with complaints of a sore throat and have difficulty in swallowing. Stridor is not usually present until the disease has markedly progressed. Important differential findings include a muffled voice, rather than a hoarse voice, the head held in a position allowing extension of the neck, the child resisting oropharyngeal examination, and progressive drooling and visible asymmetry to the wall of the posterior oropharynx.

Fortunately, other infectious agents that may mimic croup are now rare.

Diphtheria may be excluded by a history of adequate immunizations and by the absence of the characteristic gray pharyngeal or laryngeal diphtheritic membrane. However, several noninfectious entities cause stridor, most of which (eg, congenital malformations, trauma) can be differentiated by obtaining a thorough history (see Box 340-1).[26,27] An aspirated foreign body may produce stridor. Abrupt onset of the stridor, respiratory distress, and the lack of preceding respiratory symptoms, fever, and a history of previous choking on food or foreign body suggest this diagnosis. Acute edema of the upper respiratory tract caused by an allergic reaction may cause abrupt swelling and severe respiratory distress with stridor. The history of the circumstances of the abrupt onset, the lack of previous respiratory signs, and the concurrent onset of other manifestations of an allergic reaction, such as swollen lips and tongue and urticaria, are helpful in differentiation from viral croup.

EVALUATION

History

The history is integral in both making the diagnosis of viral croup, as noted previously, and in assessing the severity of the illness on which the management depends. The child's prodromal signs, the characteristics of the onset of the illness, and the course of the development of the respiratory signs should be carefully obtained. A child with an atypical onset, with a rapidly progressive illness, with a history of recurrent episodes of illness with respiratory distress, or with an underlying condition may be at an increased risk for developing severe disease.

The typical history of a child with viral croup includes the child having had signs of an upper respiratory tract infection for 1 to 2 days. This period is then followed by a characteristic cough, indicating the progression of the infection. The cough may be spasmodic, with a deep *brassy* or harsh *barking* quality. This cough has been likened to a *seal's bark* and a *brass bell.* In 1836, Ley[28] described the stridor as "the crowing of a cock, the yelping of a fox, the barking of a dog, the braying of an ass, or a ringing sound, as if the voice came from a brazen tube." Laryngitis with a raspy-sounding voice may also develop. Fever is commonly present, particularly with influenza and parainfluenza viral infections; fever in this age group often reaches 103°F and 104°F. Patients with higher temperatures and more toxic appearance should be suspected of having bacterial tracheitis.

In addition, the child may then awaken at night with spasms of the cough and the acute onset of respiratory distress and inspiratory stridor.

Physical Examination

The stridor results from obstruction to airflow during both inspiration and expiration but is most marked during inspiration. Because the subglottic region is outside the pleural cavity, the negative pressures generated on inspiration tend to narrow the passage further, similar to sucking on an occluded straw.

On physical examination, therefore, the child's distress is most evident during inspiration. Each inspiratory effort is marked audibly by the stridulous sound and is accentuated visibly by the retractions of the accessory muscles of the chest wall. The suprasternal, supraclavicular, and particularly the substernal retractions are characteristic of the inspiratory obstruction. Furthermore, distress may be marked by asynchronous movements of the chest wall and abdomen.

The respiratory rate is increased but usually not more than 50 breaths/min. This situation is in contrast to bronchiolitis, in which the picture of respiratory distress may be accompanied by respirations of 80 to 90 breaths/min. Auscultation of the chest reveals a prolonged inspiration, often accompanied by coarse crackles. Wheezes and rhonchi may also be heard on expiration. With more severe obstruction, the breath sounds may be diminished. Cyanosis may occasionally be noted, particularly about the lips and nail beds.

Course of Illness

A varying intensity of the respiratory distress is characteristic of croup. The child may appear severely compromised and an hour later appear improved, only to worsen over the next hour. In some children, the symptoms appear to abate on waking in the morning but may worsen again as the day progresses. For most

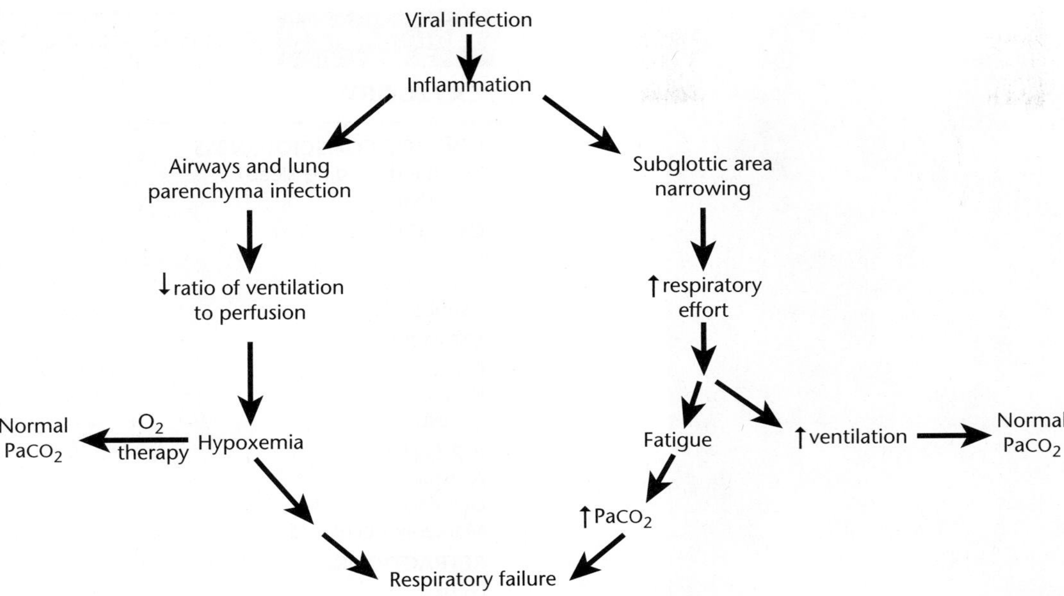

Figure 340-3 Physiological abnormalities in viral croup. Viral infection of the subglottic area produces inflammation and obstruction, resulting in an initial decrease in the child's tidal volume. To maintain an adequate alveolar ventilation, the child increases the respiratory rate. With greater degrees of obstruction, however, the work of breathing may increase such that the child can no longer compensate by the increased respiratory effort. The ensuing decrease in tidal volume and respiratory rate may then result in hypercapnia and secondary hypoxemia.

children, the signs of croup extend over 3 or 4 days, but the upper respiratory tract signs and cough may last longer.

In a few children, the respiratory distress may be unremitting or associated with significant pneumonitis and hypoxemia. As the child tires, respirations may become increasingly rapid but also shallow, indicating the need for ventilatory assistance (Figure 340-3).

Laboratory Testing

Croup is usually diagnosed based on the characteristic clinical findings and a compatible history. Laboratory testing is usually not necessary for most outpatients and may upset the child, causing an increased respiratory effort, which will augment the subglottic narrowing and obstruction to airflow. In severe cases, measurement of the oxygen saturation level may detect hypoxemia (see Figure 340-3). If the child's appearance or history suggests dehydration, then serum chemistries may be warranted. The white blood cell count and differential are not usually helpful. The total white blood cell count may be normal or low from the viral infection. However, a shift to the left with an increased number of neutrophils and band forms may also occur in more distressed and hypoxemic children or, infrequently, may suggest a bacterial infection.

Multiple laboratory assays are available to determine the specific viral agent, including viral isolation, rapid antigen detection techniques, such as immunofluorescence assays and enzyme immunoassays, and methods to detect viral RNA, as by reverse transcriptase polymerase chain reaction.[5,29] In most cases, however, specific diagnosis of the viral agent is not necessary. In some instances, determination of the specific viral cause may be helpful in determining infection control procedures or when antiviral therapy, such as for influenza or RSV, is being considered.

Imaging

Imaging is not usually necessary in diagnosing or managing children with viral croup. In some cases that are atypical or apt to be confused with other syndromes characterized by stridor, the diagnosis of croup may be aided by a lateral inspiratory and expiratory radiograph or by a posteroanterior radiograph of the neck (Figure 340-4).[30-32] The air shadow of the larynx is seen to narrow, resembling an hourglass or a steeple, in the subglottic region as a result of the characteristic inflammation in this area. An inspiratory lateral view may also show distension of the hypopharynx (see Figure 340-4). However, the sensitivity and specificity of diagnosing viral croup by use of neck radiographs has been variable.[31,33-35] In some instances, the radiograph is not interpretable, or the classic signs may not be evident.

MANAGEMENT

The first phase of management is to evaluate which children may be managed at home and which require hospitalization. Severity is often difficult to determine in this fluctuating disease, and no clinical signs are consistently prognostic of a complicated course. Clinical scoring

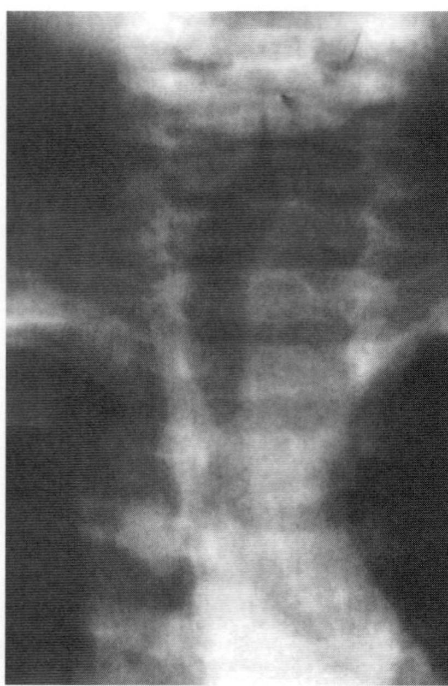

Figure 340-4 Radiograph of the posteroanterior neck of a child with viral croup, showing narrowing in the subglottic area.

Table 340-2 Clinical Scoring System

CATEGORY	SCORE
LEVEL OF CONSCIOUSNESS	
Normal (including sleep)	0
Disoriented	5
CYANOSIS	
None	0
Cyanosis with agitation	1
Cyanosis at rest	2
STRIDOR	
None	0
When agitated	1
At rest	2
AIR ENTRY	
Normal	0
Decreased	1
Markedly decreased	2
RETRACTIONS	
None	0
Mild	1
Moderate	2
Severe	3

Reprinted with permission from Westley CR, Cotton EK, Brooks JG. Nebulized racemic epinephrine by IPPB for the treatment of croup: a double-blind study. *Am J Dis Child.* 1975;132:484-487. Copyright American Medical Association.

systems, such as the Westley croup score,[36] have been used to aid in the decision as to which children should be hospitalized (Table 340-2). Toxic appearance, dehydration, and fatigue are indications for hospitalization.

Supportive Care

Supportive care is of prime importance for children with croup, whether they are outpatients or hospitalized. The child should be made comfortable to avoid unnecessary anxiety and fatigue. Crying and anxiety tend to make the young child take rapid, short breaths, which aggravate the narrowing of the airway and the metabolic need for gas exchange. Fluids should be encouraged, and antipyretics may be given for fever and to diminish the associated increased respiratory rate and fluid requirements. Despite a cornucopia of cures passed down from generation to generation, few other home therapies have proved beneficial. Because of croup's fluctuating nature, several unverified therapeutic modalities may appear to work.

Humidified Air

Vaporizers and home-devised mist tents, from showers to teakettles, have commonly been tried. The water particles that these devices produce, nevertheless, are generally too large to reach the lower respiratory tract, and they humidify primarily the anterior nares and oropharynx. Furthermore, devices that use hot water and steam pose the potential hazard of accidental burns. A cool mist may help cool the airway and may be beneficial to some children who have croup. This method may also explain the improvement that some children experience when taken out in the cold night air. In a dog model of croup, cold-dry, cold-moist, and warm-dry air, all of which contain little moisture compared with warm-moist air, were found to be more effective than warm-moist air in decreasing airway resistance.[37] Studies in children, evaluating the efficacy of humidified air in treating croup are few and involve small numbers of patients. Nevertheless, no significant benefit has been shown.[38-41]

Nebulized Epinephrine

Nebulized epinephrine has been shown to be beneficial for children with more severe croup.[17,40,42-45] Clinical improvement occurs in most cases by reducing the degree of stridor and retractions. Epinephrine causes diminished subglottic swelling via its stimulus of α- and β-adrenergic receptors, resulting in decreased blood flow and swelling in the upper respiratory tract. Racemic epinephrine, which contains both D and L isomers, has been preferably used because it was believed to have fewer adverse effects. However, controlled evaluation of the 2 isomers indicated no difference in effect or in adverse reactions.[45,46]

Nebulized epinephrine should be used with the understanding that (1) amelioration of the clinical signs is transient, and the child again may worsen within 2 to 3 hours; (2) the arterial oxygen saturation is not affected[42,47,48]; and (3) nebulized epinephrine should be used only for children with moderately severe or severe croup, and these children should usually be concurrently treated with corticosteroids.

Corticosteroid Therapy

The major advance and mainstay in the management of both ambulatory and hospitalized children with viral croup is the use of systemic or nebulized corticosteroids.[49] Multiple well-designed trials have shown both systemic and nebulized corticosteroid therapy has resulted in significant clinical improvement, decreased hospitalization, and fewer follow-up visits.[40,42,49-52]

A recent Cochrane[49] systematic review of 31 studies involving 3736 children found significant clinical improvement in the Westley score at 6 to 12 hours. By 24 hours, the benefit was no longer significant. The clinical efficacy did not differ significantly according to the agent or route of administration. The review concluded that (1) dexamethasone and budesonide show clinical benefit as early as 6 hours after administration; (2) treatment was associated with fewer and shorter hospital stays, return visits, and need for other therapies; and (3) dexamethasone was also effective for mild cases of croup.

Antibiotic Therapy

Because croup is of viral etiology, antibiotics are rarely indicated. Secondary or concurrent bacterial infection is unusual, and antibiotics should be reserved for such documented cases.[40,42,53]

WHEN TO REFER

- When the child has wheezing condition predisposing to more severe croup
- When child has history of recurrent episodes of croup
- When the episode of croup occurs during the neonatal period
- When symptoms progress despite supportive care at home

WHEN TO ADMIT

- When child appears toxic, lethargic, in respiratory distress, or dehydrated
- When the onset of illness was sudden with rapid progression of symptoms
- When signs of respiratory distress are unresponsive to outpatient drug therapy

TOOLS FOR PRACTICE

Engaging Patients and Family

- *Common Childhood Infections* (brochure), American Academy of Pediatrics (patiented.aap.org).
- *Croup and Your Young Child* (brochure), American Academy of Pediatrics (patiented.aap.org).
- *What is Croup?* (fact sheet), American Academy of Pediatrics (www.aap.org/topics.html).

Medical Decision Support

- *Human Parainfluenza Viruses (Common Cold and Croup)* (fact sheet), Centers for Disease Control and Prevention (www.cdc.gov/ncidod/dvrd/revb/respiratory/hpivfeat.htm).
- *National Respiratory and Enteric Virus Surveillance System (NREVSS)* (database), Centers for Disease Control and Prevention (www.cdc.gov/ncidod/dvrd/revb/nrevss/index.htm).
- *Westley Croup Score* (form), CR Westley, EK Cotton, and JG Brooks (practice.aap.org/content.aspx?aid=2001).

AAP POLICY STATEMENT

American Academy of Pediatrics, Committee on Drugs. Drugs for pediatric emergencies. *Pediatrics.* 1998;101:e13. (aappolicy.aappublications.org/cgi/content/full/pediatrics;101/1/e13).

SUGGESTED RESOURCES

Castro-Rodriguez J, Holberg C, Morgan W, et al. Relation of two different subtypes of croup before age three to wheezing, atopy, and pulmonary function during childhood: a prospective study. *Pediatrics.* 2001;170:512-518.

Klassen T. Croup. A current perspective. *Pediatr Clin North Am.* 1999;46:1167-1178.

Knott A, Long C, Hall C. Parainfluenza viral infections in pediatric outpatients: seasonal patterns and clinical characteristics. *Pediatr Infect Dis J.* 1994;13:269-273.

Segal A, Crighton E, Moineddin R, et al. Croup hospitalizations in Ontario: a 14-year time-series analysis. *Pediatrics.* 2005;116:51-55.

Wright R, Pomerantz W, Luria J. New approaches to respiratory infections in children: bronchiolitis and croup. *Emerg Med Clin North Am.* 2002;20:93-114.

REFERENCES

1. Cherry JD. Croup. In: Kiple K. *Cambridge History and Geography of Human Disease Project.* Bowling Green, OH: University of Cambridge Press; 1990.
2. Leung AK, Cho H. Diagnosis of stridor in children. *Am Fam Physician.* 1999;60:2289-2296.
3. van Bever HP, Wieringa MH, Weyler JJ, et al. Croup and recurrent croup: their association with asthma and allergy. An epidemiological study on 5-8-year-old children. *Eur J Pediatr.* 1999;158:253-257.
4. Peltola V, Heikkinen T, Ruuskanen O. Clinical courses of croup caused by influenza and parainfluenza viruses. *Pediatr Infect Dis J.* 2002;21:76-78.
5. Henrickson KJ, Hoover S, Kehl KS, et al. National disease burden of respiratory viruses detected in children by polymerase chain reaction. *Pediatr Infect Dis J.* 2004; 23:S11-S18.
6. Segal AO, Crighton EJ, Moineddin R, et al. Croup hospitalizations in Ontario: a 14-year time-series analysis. *Pediatr.* 2005;116:51-55.
7. Counihan ME, Shay DK, Holman RC, et al. Human parainfluenza virus-associated hospitalizations among children less than five years of age in the United States. *Pediatr Infect Dis J.* 2001;20:646-653.
8. Denny FW, Murphy TF, Clyde WA Jr. Croup: an 11-year study in a pediatric practice. *Pediatrics.* 1983;71:871-876.
9. Howard JB, McCracken GH Jr, Luby JP. Influenza A 2 virus as a cause of croup requiring tracheotomy. *J Pediatr.* 1972;81:1148-1150.
10. McIntosh K, McAdam AJ. Human metapneumovirus—an important new respiratory virus. *N Engl J Med.* 2004;350:431-433.
11. Konig B, Konig W, Arnold R, et al. Prospective study of human metapneumovirus infection in children less than 3 years of age. *J Clin Microbiol.* 2004;42:4632-4635.

12. van der Hoek L, Sure K, Ihorst G, et al. Croup is associated with the novel coronavirus NL63. *PLoS Med.* 2005; 2:e240.
13. Fortenberry JD, Mariscalco MM, Louis PT, et al. Severe laryngotracheobronchitis complicating measles. *Am J Dis Child.* 1992;146:1040-1043.
14. Ross LA, Mason WH, Lanson J, et al. Severe laryngotracheobronchitis as a complication of measles during an urban epidemic. *J Pediatr.* 1992;121:511-515.
15. Castro-Rodriguez JA, Holberg CJ, Morgan WJ, et al. Relation of two different subtypes of croup before age three to wheezing, atopy, and pulmonary function during childhood: a prospective study. *Pediatrics.* 2001;170:512-518.
16. Foy HM, Cooney MK, Maletzky AJ, et al. Incidence and etiology of pneumonia, croup, and bronchiolitis in preschool children belonging to a prepaid medical care group over a four-year period. *Am J Epidemiol.* 1973;97:80-92.
17. Ewig JM. Croup. *Pediatr Ann.* 2002;31:125-130.
18. Leung AK, Kellner JD, Johnson DW. Viral croup: a current perspective. *J Pediatr Health Care.* 2004;18:297-301.
19. Knott AM, Long CE, Hall CB. Parainfluenza viral infections in pediatric outpatients: seasonal patterns and clinical characteristics. *Pediatr Infect Dis J.* 1994;13:269-273.
20. Glezen WP, Denny FW. Epidemiology of acute lower respiratory disease in children. *N Engl J Med.* 1973;288: 498-505.
21. Welliver RC, Sun M, Rinaldo D. Defective regulation of immune responses in croup due to parainfluenza virus. *Pediatr Res.* 1985;19:716-720.
22. Litmanovitch M, Kivity S, Soferman R, et al. Relationship between recurrent croup and airway hyperreactivity. *Ann Allergy.* 1990;65:239-241.
23. Welliver RC, Wong DT, Middleton E Jr, et al. Role of parainfluenza virus-specific IgE in pathogenesis of croup and wheezing subsequent to infection. *J Pediatr.* 1982; 101:889-896.
24. Mauro RD, Poole SR, Lockhart CH. Differentiation of epiglottitis from laryngotracheitis in the child with stridor. *AJDC.* 1988;142:679-682.
25. Bernstein T, Brill R, Jacobs B. Is bacterial tracheitis changing? A 14-month experience in a pediatric intensive care unit. *Clin Infect Dis.* 1998;27:458-462.
26. Hammer J. Acquired upper airway obstruction. *Paediatr Respir Rev.* 2004;5:25-33.
27. Tan HKK, Holinger LD. Tachypnea is often the first sign of respiratory distress. How to evaluate and manage stridor in children. *J Respirat Dis.* 1994;15:245-260.
28. Ley H. *An Essay on the Laryngismus Stridulus or Croup-like Inspiration of Infants.* London, UK: Churchill; 1836.
29. Storch GA, ed. *Essentials of Diagnostic Virology.* New York, NY: Churchill Livingstone; 2000.
30. Currarino G, Williams B. Lateral inspiration and expiration radiographs of the neck in children with laryngotracheobronchitis (croup). *Radiology.* 1982;195:365-366.
31. Rapkin RH. The diagnosis of epiglottitis: simplicity and reliability of radiographs of the neck in the differential diagnosis of the croup syndrome. *J Pediatr.* 1972;80: 96-98.
32. Mills JL, Spackman TJ, Borns P, et al. The usefulness of lateral neck roentgenograms in laryngotracheobronchitis. *Am J Dis Child.* 1979;133:1140-1142.
33. Jones JL. False positives in lateral neck radiographs used to diagnose epiglottitis. *Ann Emerg Med.* 1983;12:797.
34. Shackelford GD, Siegel MJ, McAlister WH. Subglottic edema in acute epiglottitis in children. *AJR.* 1978;131:603-605.
35. Stankiewicz JA, Bowes AK. Croup and epiglottitis: a radiologic study. *Laryngoscope.* 1985;95:1159-1160.
36. Westley CR, Cotton EK, Brooks JG. Nebulized racemic epinephrine by IPPB for the treatment of croup: a double-blind study. *Am J Dis Child.* 1978;132:484-487.
37. Wolfsdorf J, Swift DL. An animal model simulating acute infective upper airway obstruction of childhood and its use in the investigation of croup therapy. *Pediatr Res.* 1978;12:1062-1065.
38. Bourchier D, Dawson KP, Fergusson DM. Humidification in viral croup: a controlled trial. *Aust Paediatr J.* 1984;20: 289-291.
39. Lenney W, Milner AD. Treatment of acute viral croup. *Arch Dis Child.* 1978;53:704-706.
40. Skolnik NS. Treatment of croup. *Am J Dis Child.* 1989; 143:1045-1049.
41. Neto GM, Kentab O, Klassen TP, et al. A randomized controlled trial of mist in the acute treatment of moderate croup. *Acad Emerg Med.* 2002;9:873-879.
42. Klassen TP. Croup. A current perspective. *Pediatr Clin North Am.* 1999;46:1167-1178.
43. Kaditis AG, Wald ER. Viral croup: current diagnosis and treatment. *Pediatr Infect Dis J.* 1998;17:827-834.
44. Wright RB, Pomerantz WJ, Luria JW. New approaches to respiratory infections in children: bronchiolitis and croup. *Emerg Med Clin North Am.* 2002;20:93-114.
45. Osmond M. Croup. *Clin Evid.* 2002;June:297-306.
46. Waisman Y, Klein BL, Boenning DA, et al. Prospective randomized double-blind study comparing L-epinephrine and racemic epinephrine aerosols in the treatment of laryngotracheitis (croup). *Pediatrics.* 1992;89:302-306.
47. Geelhoed GC. Croup. *Pediatr Pulmonol.* 1997;23:370-374.
48. Tunnessen WW, Feinstein AR. The steroid-croup controversy: an analytic review of methodologic problems. *J Pediatr.* 1980;96:751-756.
49. Russell K, Wiebe N, Saenz A, et al. Glucocorticoids for croup. *Cochrane Database Syst Rev.* 2004:1-40.
50. Johnson DW, Jacobson S, Edney PC, et al. A comparison of nebulized budesonide, intramuscular dexamethasone, and placebo for moderately severe croup. *N Engl J Med.* 1998;339:498-503.
51. Kairys SW, Olmstead EM, O'Connor GT. Steroid treatment of laryngotracheitis: a meta-analysis of the evidence from randomized trials. *Pediatrics.* 1989;83:683-693.
52. Ausejo-Segura M, Saenz A, Pham B, et al. Glucocorticoids for croup. *The Cochrane Library,* Issue 2, 2003.
53. Pianosi P, Feldman W, Robson MG, et al. Inappropriate use of antibiotics in croup at three types of hospital. *Can Med Assoc J.* 1986;134:357-359.

Chapter 341
DEHYDRATION

Prashant V. Mahajan, MD, MPH, MBA

The terms *volume depletion* or *hypovolemia* (a condition in which extracellular fluid is lost) and *dehydration* (a condition in which pure water loss occurs) are used interchangeably. The most common cause of dehydration is diarrheal illness, which results in 2.5 million deaths annually.[1-4] Gastroenteritis causes over 200,000 hospital admissions and over 1.5 million outpatient visits every year in the United States. Although not a leading cause of death in the United States, gastroenteritis and related disorders result in a substantial amount of morbidity and generate significant health care costs.

Table 341-1 Causes of Pediatric Gastroenteritis

TYPE OF ORGANISM	COMMON	UNCOMMON
Viral	Rotavirus Norwalk Enteric adenovirus	*Calicivirus* *Astrovirus*
Bacterial	*Salmonella* *Shigella* *Campylobacter jejuni*	*Yersinia enterocolitica* *Vibrio cholerae* *Escherichia coli* *Clostridium difficile*
Parasitic	*Giardia lamblia*	*Entamoeba histolytica* *Cryptosporidium*

BOX 341-1 Nondiarrheal Causes of Dehydration

Water deficit	Nephrogenic diabetes insipidus Central diabetes insipidus
Increased insensible losses	Premature infants Radiant warmers Phototherapy Tracheostomy, tachypnea
Inadequate intake of water	Ineffective breastfeeding Child abuse
Water and sodium deficits	Burns Excessive sweating
Renal losses	Diuretic use or abuse Diabetes mellitus Chronic renal disease, obstructive uropathy
Miscellaneous	Surgical drains and third spacing

ETIOLOGY

Dehydration in infants and children is overwhelmingly the result of infectious processes. Of these processes, viral agents are of primary importance in the industrialized countries. Rotavirus and the Norwalk agent account for most cases of viral gastroenteritis in children. Some other causes of gastroenteritis are given in Table 341-1.

Noninfectious causes of dehydration in children include agents that produce osmotic diarrhea, such as laxatives or cathartics that contain high concentrations of sugars; obstructive processes in the gastrointestinal tract; and, occasionally, vomiting as a sign of elevated intracranial pressure. Although each of these conditions occurs only rarely, they should be borne in mind when evaluating the child who is dehydrated and has a history that is not typical for infectious gastroenteritis. Finally, nondiarrheal causes of water and electrolyte loss can also result in severe dehydration. Losses can occur through the skin, respiratory system (ie, increase in insensible losses), or renal conditions. Losses that occur through the skin because of fever are usually in the range of a 10% to 15% rise in insensible losses for each 1°C rise in temperature above 38°C. A few common causes of nondiarrheal dehydration are given in Box 341-1.

PATHOPHYSIOLOGIC MECHANISM OF DEHYDRATION IN GASTROENTERITIS

Children are at an increased risk for hypovolemia and dehydration because of the following[5]:

1. The frequency of gastroenteritis is higher in children as compared with adults.
2. Very young children have higher surface area-to-volume ratios than adults; thus they have a proportionally higher rate of insensible losses, which can be accentuated in disease states.
3. Young children are often unable to communicate or actively seek fluids to replenish their losses.

To make the best informed decisions about appropriate treatment of dehydration, primary care physicians should understand the basic principles underlying dehydrating diarrhea and the mechanisms by which rehydration occurs.

Regardless of which pathogen is involved, diarrhea and fluid loss ultimately result when intestinal fluid secretion exceeds the rate of absorption. In the case of viral agents and cytopathic bacteria such as *Shigella, Salmonella, Campylobacter,* and enteropathogenic strains of *Escherichia coli,* fluid absorption is diminished because absorptive cells at the intestinal villus tip are destroyed, whereas secretory processes that occur at the level of intestinal crypt cells remain unimpaired. On the other hand, toxin-producing bacterial pathogens such as *Vibrio cholerae,* toxigenic *E coli,* and some strains of *Shigella* cause significant increases in fluid secretion from crypt cells by deranging modulation of ion channels in the crypt cell membranes. Intestinal absorptive function is normal in such cases but does not keep pace with secretion, and diarrhea results.

Substantial fluid loss from the intestines or other sites depletes intravascular volume, resulting in end-organ hypoperfusion and poor nutrient and oxygen delivery; ultimately, tissue acidosis develops. Elevated aldosterone levels resulting from hypovolemia lead to renal potassium loss. Eventually, circulatory collapse and shock occur; irreversible organ damage and death may follow. The chain of events can be interrupted by very rapid repletion of fluids to restore circulating volume, reverse acidosis, and improve perfusion and end-organ function.[6]

EVALUATION

All children with dehydration should be systematically evaluated with the following 5-point assessment[7]:

1. What is the magnitude of volume deficit?
2. Is osmolar imbalance present?
3. Is acid-base disturbance present?
4. Is abnormality in potassium metabolism present?

5. Is the renal function impaired?

The 5-point assessment can be evaluated by a combination of clinical and laboratory techniques as detailed in Table 341-2.

Physical Examination

During the initial evaluation of a child with dehydration, primary care physicians must determine and document the degree of dehydration. Volume depletion is most objectively measured as a change in weight from baseline. Ideally, the preillness weight should be used to determine the exact proportion of weight loss that is attributable to the fluid deficit. Given that the preillness weight is often unavailable, primary care physicians should use pulse rate, blood pressure, urine output, skin turgor, and other signs (Table 341-3) to categorize the child as having mild (3% to 5% volume loss), moderate (6% to 9% volume loss), or severe dehydration (≥10% volume loss).

Table 341-2 Five-Point Assessment of Dehydration

POINT OF ASSESSMENT	METHOD
Volume deficit	History and physical examination
Osmolar disturbance	Serum sodium and serum osmolality measurement
Acid-base disturbance	Blood pH, Pco_2, and serum bicarbonate measurement
Potassium	Serum potassium
Renal function	Blood urea nitrogen, creatinine, urine specific gravity

PCO_2, Partial pressure of carbon dioxide.

Laboratory Evaluation

Laboratory testing is used to determine the clinical condition of the child and the origin of dehydration. Many children with mild or moderate dehydration do not need any laboratory tests. The minimal amount of testing in the patients with moderate to severe dehydration is measurement of serum electrolytes, including sodium, potassium, chlorides, and bicarbonates, along with blood urea nitrogen, serum creatinine, urine specific gravity, and serum glucose (by the finger-prick method at the bedside). Laboratory testing is less useful in assessing the degree of volume depletion. A review of the literature and a prospective study found that only serum bicarbonate (<17 mEq/L) differentiated a child with moderate or severe hypovolemia from those with mild hypovolemia.[8,9] Serum sodium measurements are useful in categorizing the child as having isonatremic, hyponatremic (<130 mEq/L), or hypernatremic (>150 mEq/L) dehydration. The signs of dehydration (see Table 341-3) will be delayed if the patient has hypernatremic dehydration (ie, higher relative loss of free water as compared with loss of sodium) because the increased serum sodium causes an osmotically driven fluid shift from the intracellular compartment to the extracellular compartment. Similarly, the signs of dehydration are present earlier if the child has hyponatremic dehydration. Serum potassium levels may be falsely elevated (acidosis causes a shift from the intracellular compartment) or low (caused by losses in the gastrointestinal tract). Urine osmolality and specific gravity will be high (often exceeding 450 mOsm/kg) but may be low if the patient has lost renal concentrating ability (in patients with osmotic diuresis or diabetes insipidus). Stool diagnostic studies should similarly be used sparingly. Bacterial cultures should certainly be obtained in ill-appearing children, those with fever (≥38°C in infants younger than 3 months and 39°C in children older than 3 months), those who have bloody or mucoid stools, or those in whom a travel

Table 341-3 Degree of Dehydration

	DEGREE OF DEHYDRATION		
PARAMETER	MILD	MODERATE	SEVERE
Weight loss (%)—infants	5	10	15
Weight loss (%)—children	3	6	>9
Skin color	Pale	Gray	Mottled
Skin turgor	May be normal	Decreased	Tenting
Mucous membranes	Slightly dry	Dry	Dry, parched, collapse of sublingual veins
Eyes	Normal	Decreased tears	Sunken, absence of tears
Central nervous system	Alert but thirsty	Irritable	Lethargic, grunting, coma
Pulse	Normal and strong	Rapid and slightly weak	Significantly tachycardic and very weak to not palpable
Capillary refill	Normal (<2 sec)	2-4 sec	>4 sec
Blood pressure	No change	Orthostatic decrease	Shock
Urine	Normal to mildly reduced	Significantly reduced	Anuria
Volume of deficit—infants	50 mL/kg	60 mL/kg	150 mL/kg
Volume of deficit—children	30 mL/kg	100 mL/kg	>90 mL/kg

or exposure history is suggestive of enteric pathogens. Most children will not meet these criteria, and routine stool cultures should be discouraged. Similarly, little additional diagnostic or therapeutic guidance is provided by detection of the rotavirus antigen in stool samples, and such studies should rarely be obtained.

TREATMENT

Principles of Fluid Therapy

In children, dividing fluid therapy into replacement therapy (corrects deficit) and maintenance therapy (replaces ongoing losses, including insensible losses) is useful. Details of maintenance therapy are provided in Chapter 58, Body Fluids, Electrolyte Concentration, and Acid-Base Composition. Replacement therapy is based on 2 steps:

1. First-fluid (emergent) phase: This phase restores moderately or severely compromised effective circulating volume and prevents tissue damage. This phase is typically begun with a 20-mL/kg fluid bolus with isotonic saline (0.9 normal saline) or lactated Ringer solution over 1 to 2 hours. Fluid boluses should be repeated until signs of shock begin to disappear. Although some advantages can be found for using colloid solutions (albumin or hetastarch, namely that the colloid solutions remain for a longer time in the intravascular space and have a lower risk of developing pulmonary edema caused by dilutional hypoalbuminemia), many clinical trials have failed to demonstrate these theoretical benefits.[10-13]
2. Second-fluid phase: This phase essentially replaces the body's fluid and electrolyte loss and can be in the form of parenteral intravenous fluids or oral replacement as oral rehydration therapy (ORT). Primary care physicians should recognize that in mild to moderate cases of dehydration, this phase will often suffice and the clinician may not have to resort to the first fluid or emergent phase. Administration of ORT is discussed later in this chapter. Intravenous fluids are often indicated if the child is unable to undergo ORT because of altered mental status or persistent vomiting, or has severe electrolyte abnormalities. The type of intravenous fluids depends on the serum sodium levels (ie, whether the child has isonatremia, hyponatremia, or hypernatremia). Most cases of dehydration in children are associated with isonatremia and can be managed over a few hours in an ambulatory setting (either the primary care provider's office or the observation unit in an emergency department).

Table 341-4 provides details about the estimated water and electrolyte deficits associated with moderate-to-severe dehydration.

Controversies Regarding Optimal Fluid Management in Dehydration

Although rapid reexpansion of the extracellular fluid volume with 0.9% saline followed by ORT has become the gold standard therapy in infants with moderate-to-severe dehydration, few physicians are actually using this therapeutic regimen.[14-16] Tables 341-5, 341-6, and 341-7 provide examples of a child who is 10% dehydrated with isonatremic, hyponatremic, and hypernatremic dehydration.[17]

Oral Rehydration

Fluid absorption can be promoted by the enteral administration of properly designed fluids, even in the face of ongoing losses. In healthy adults, over 6500 mL per day of fluids, including both ingested liquids and intestinal secretions, are introduced into the intestinal tract and reduced to form a stool output of less than 100 mL per day. Oral rehydration exploits a normal cellular process known as co-transport, in which absorption of a molecule of an organic substrate promotes the absorption of an ion of sodium from the small intestine. With enhanced absorption of sodium, water, in turn, is absorbed rapidly into the circulation. Intravascular fluid volume can be restored in this fashion rapidly and reliably.[18,19]

A fluid that is designed to promote water and electrolyte absorption through the co-transport system in the gut is referred to as an oral rehydration solution (ORS). A physiologically appropriate ORS contains 70 to 90 mEq/L sodium and not more than 25 g/L of glucose. In addition, an ORS typically contains 20 mEq/L of potassium and 30 mEq/L of base in the form of citrate. Almost all juices, soft drinks, and punches contain much higher concentrations of sugars and almost no sodium, making them inappropriate for use as ORSs. In fact, the higher sugar concentrations in these fluids may exacerbate diarrhea by presenting a large osmotic load within the intestinal lumen.

An ORS can be used to restore both fluid and electrolyte balance in children who have a wide range of initial serum sodium values. By the end of the rehydration period, both hypernatremia and hyponatremia generally have resolved.

Table 341-4 Estimated Fluid and Electrolyte Deficits in Moderate-to-Severe Dehydration

TYPE OF DEHYDRATION	WATER (mL/kg)	SODIUM (mEq/kg)	POTASSIUM (mEq/kg)	CHLORIDE AND BICARBONATE (mEq/kg)
Isonatremic	100-150	8-10	8-10	16-20
Hyponatremic	50-100	10-14	10-14	20-28
Hypernatremic	120-180	2-5	2-5	4-10

Table 341-5 Intravenous Fluids for a 5-kg Child With 10% Dehydration and Normal Serum Sodium

	WATER	SODIUM	POTASSIUM
Maintenance*	5 kg × 100 cc/kg/d = 500 mL	3 mEq/100 mL = 15 mEq	2 mEq/100 mL = 10 mEq
Deficit†	Weight × % dehydration	Sodium in ECF × proportion of fluid loss from ECF × deficit (cc)	Potassium in ICF × proportion of fluid loss from ECF × deficit (cc)
	5 kg × 0.1 = 0.5 g (500 mL)	135 mEq/L × 0.6 × 500 mL = 40 mEq	150 mEq/L × 0.4 × 500 mL = 30 mEq
Ongoing losses	Replace cc-for-cc	Add sodium in proportion to expected fluid loss (stool, gastric contents, etc.)	Add potassium in proportion to expected fluid loss (stool, gastric contents, etc.)
Total	1000 mL	55 mEq	40 mEq

*After the initial bolus, maintenance fluids are administered over 24 hours, and one half the deficit is given over 8 hours and the remainder over 24 hours.
†The water and sodium content in the initial bolus of normal saline does not count toward either maintenance or replacement of ongoing losses or deficit therapy.
ECF, Extracellular fluid; *ICF*, intracellular fluid.

Table 341-6 Intravenous Fluids for a 5-kg Child With 10% Dehydration and Hyponatremia (Serum Sodium = 128 mEq/L)

	WATER	SODIUM	POTASSIUM
Maintenance*	5 kg × 100 cc/kg/d = 500 mL	3 mEq/100 mL = 15 mEq	2 mEq/100 mL = 10 mEq
Deficit†	Weight × % dehydration	Sodium in ECF × proportion of fluid loss from ECF × deficit (cc) PLUS (desired sodium – observed sodium) × weight × sodium in ECF	Potassium in ICF × proportion of fluid loss from ECF × deficit (cc)
	5 kg × 0.1 = 0.5 g (500 mL)	135 mEq/L × 0.6 × 500 mL = 40 mEq PLUS (135 mEq/L – 128 mEq/L) × 5 × 0.6 = 21 mEq	150 mEq/L × 0.4 × 500 mL = 30 mEq
Ongoing losses	Replace mL-for-mL	Add sodium in proportion to expected fluid loss (stool, gastric contents, etc.)	Add potassium in proportion to expected fluid loss (stool, gastric contents, etc.)
Total	1000 mL	76 mEq	40 mEq

*After the initial bolus, maintenance fluids are administered over 24 hours, and one half the deficit is given over 8 hours and the remainder over 24 hours.
ECF, Extracellular fluid; *ICF*, intracellular fluid.
†The water and sodium content in the initial bolus of normal saline does not count toward either maintenance or replacement of ongoing losses or deficit therapy.

MANAGEMENT

Most dehydrated children can be rehydrated successfully without resorting to parenteral (intravenous or intraosseous) therapy. The combined use of an ORS and an appropriate regimen of refeeding is referred to as ORT. The number of deaths attributable to diarrhea in children younger than 5 years fell from 4.6 million to 1.5 million per year from 1980 to 2000 concomitant with the increased use of ORT.[1] In addition, ORT has been found to have a low failure rate (4%), reduced hospital stays, and fewer adverse events and was less expensive when compared with intravenous therapy.[20]

Intravenous Rehydration

Patients who have severe dehydration (shock) should receive initial rehydration fluids parenterally via either the intravenous or, when line placement proves difficult, the intraosseous route. Patients treated parenterally should be given rapid boluses of 0.9% sodium chloride in initial volumes of 20 mL/kg for not more than 20 minutes. In especially severe cases, for patients to require 60 to 100 mL/kg before the restoration of circulating volume is apparent, is not unusual. Enteral fluid therapy may begin immediately by either the mouth or a nasogastric tube, provided the patient is conscious and airway protective reflexes are intact.

Oral Rehydration

In the conscious child who has mild or moderate dehydration, fluid replacement should always be initiated orally. Successful ORT depends on proper fluid selection and skilled administration.[21] Simply instructing parents

Table 341-7 Intravenous Fluids for a 5-kg Child With 10% Dehydration and Hypernatremic Dehydration (Serum Sodium = 16 mEq/L)

	WATER	SODIUM	POTASSIUM
Maintenance	5 kg × 100 mL/kg/d = 500 mL	3 mEq/100 mL = 15 mEq	2 mEq/100 mL = 10 mEq
Deficit	Weight × % dehydration	Free water deficit = ([observed sodium –desired sodium] weight × 4 mL/kg), thus: Free water deficit = (160 – 145) × 5 kg × 4 mL/kg = 300 mL	Potassium in ICF × proportion of fluid loss from ECF × deficit (cc), thus: Free water deficit = (160 – 145) × 5 kg × 4 mL/kg = 300 mL
	5 kg × 0.1 = 0.5 g (500 mL)	Sodium in ECF × proportion of fluid loss from ECF × (total deficit – free water deficit) 135 eq/1000 mL × 0.6 × (500 – 300 mL) = 16 mEq/L	150 mEq/L × 0.4 × (500 – 300 mL) = 12 mEq
Ongoing losses	Replace mL-for-mL	Add sodium in proportion to expected fluid loss (stool, gastric contents. etc.)	Add potassium in proportion to expected fluid loss (stool, gastric contents. etc.)
Total	1000 mL	31 mEq	22 mEq

Table 341-8 Solutions Commonly Used in Children Who Have Diarrhea

SOLUTION	GLUCOSE/ PHENOL (g/L)	SODIUM (mEq/L)	BASE (mEq/L; CITRATE OR BICARBONATE)	POTASSIUM (mEq/L)	OSMOLALITY (mMol/L)
PHYSIOLOGICALLY APPROPRIATE SOLUTIONS					
Pedialyte	25	45	30	20	270
Ricelyte	30*	50	30	25	200
Rehydralyte	25	75	30	20	310
WHO and UNICEF oral replacement solution	20	90	30	20	310
PHYSIOLOGICALLY INAPPROPRIATE SOLUTIONS					
Cola	700	2	13	0.1	750
Apple juice	690	3	0	32	730
Gatorade	255	20	3	3	330

*Rice syrup solids.
UNICEF, United Nations Children's Fund; *WHO*, World Health Organization.

to purchase and feed a child an ORS is unlikely to result in success and satisfaction.[22]

Types of Oral Rehydration Solutions

ORSs are most widely available commercially in the industrialized world as premixed liquids. These solutions contain sodium levels varying from 50 to 70 mEq/L. For the mildly dehydrated child, any of these solutions is appropriate. For more significantly dehydrated infants and children, a solution containing 70 to 90 mEq/L of sodium should be chosen. Packets of oral rehydration salts for preparation of a solution containing 90 mEq/L of sodium are available for mixing with 1 L of water to provide an inexpensive and reliable alternative. These packets always should be distributed with a 1-L bottle to promote proper mixing. Juices, punches, and other soft drinks are inappropriate solutions for children who have diarrhea because of the high osmotic load they introduce into the intestines. Table 341-8 lists the most commonly available solutions and their compositions. Information on juices and soft drinks is provided for comparison. The World Health Organization formula (2002) contains 13.5 g/L of carbohydrates, 75 mEq/L of sodium, 20 mEq/L of potassium, and 30 mEq/L of bicarbonate base and has an osmolarity of 245 mOsm/kg of water. The desired properties for an ORS as recommended by the World Health Organization and the United Nations Children's Fund for global use include the following[23]:

1. Total osmolality between 200 and 310 mmol/L
2. Equimolar concentrations of glucose and sodium

3. Glucose concentration not in excess of 20 g/L (111 mmol/L)
4. Sodium concentration between 60 and 90 mEq/L
5. Potassium concentration between 15 and 25 mEq/L
6. Citrate concentration between 8 and 12 mmol/L
7. Chloride concentration between 50 and 80 mEq/L

Although homemade sugar-salt solutions can be prepared to produce an appropriate ORS, the risk of incorrect mixing is high. Such homemade solutions should not be used when commercial solutions are available.

Administration of Oral Replacement Therapy

In general, ORT can be started in the office or emergency department immediately after assessment excludes acute abdominal processes (eg, appendicitis, volvulus, intussusception, pyloric stenosis) and extra-intestinal causes of fluid losses (eg, intracranial hypertension caused by tumor, meningitis, or hydrocephalus, all of which may induce volume loss as a result of vomiting). Ideally, the goal is to replace the entire fluid deficit in the first 4 to 6 hours (Table 341-9).

Rehydration Phase

Fluids are best administered initially by a parent who is instructed to place the fluids into the child's mouth (via a needleless syringe) 1 teaspoon (5 mL) per minute for infants, 10 mL per minute for toddlers, and 15 mL per minute for older children. This amount, at a steady rate of administration, provides 300, 600, and 900 mL/hr, respectively, which generally replaces the calculated deficit within a 4- to 6-hour period. Frequent reassessment of the child and encouragement of the parent are crucial during this rehydration period. The rehydration phase should be completed in the office, clinic, or emergency department before the child is sent home. In general, vomiting is not a contraindication to ORT. Even when vomiting occurs, steady fluid replacement is continued orally. Children usually do not discharge their entire stomach contents when they vomit. As dehydration and tissue acidosis are corrected, the frequency and severity of vomiting are generally reduced. However, children who only have vomiting (without diarrhea) warrant especially careful evaluation for conditions other than gastroenteritis, such as appendicitis, intussusception, volvulus, or pyloric stenosis, depending on age.

Maintenance Phase

At the end of 4 hours, the state of hydration should be reassessed by using the original clinical criteria. If detectable dehydration remains, then the rehydration phase should be repeated based on the remaining calculated volume deficit. If rehydration has been completed, then the maintenance phase is begun. In this phase, the parent is instructed to continue to administer an ORS in ad libitum quantities but to alternate this fluid intake with human milk, formula, or other appropriate feedings.

Table 341-9 Fluid Therapy for Dehydration

DEGREE OF DEHYDRATION*	SIGNS	REHYDRATION PHASE (FIRST 4 HR; REPEAT UNTIL NO SIGNS OF DEHYDRATION REMAIN)	MAINTENANCE PHASE‡ (UNTIL ILLNESS RESOLVES)
Mild (3-5%)	Slightly dry mucous membranes, increased thirst	ORS 60 mL/kg†	Breastfeeding, undiluted lactose-free formula, half-strength cow milk, or lactose-containing formula
Moderate (6-9%)	Sunken eyes, sunken fontanelle, loss of skin turgor, dry mucous membranes, decreased urine output	ORS 80 mL/kg	Same as above
Severe (>10%)	Signs of moderate dehydration plus 1 or more of the following: rapid thready pulse, hypotension, cyanosis, rapid breathing, delayed capillary refill, markedly reduced or absent urine output, lethargy, coma	Intravenous or intraosseous isotonic fluids (0.9% saline or lactated Ringer solution), 20 mL/kg over 1 hr; repeat until pulse and state of consciousness return to normal, then 50-100 mL/kg of ORS based on remaining degree of dehydration§	Same as above

ORS, Oral rehydration solution.
*Percent of total body weight lost.
†If no signs of dehydration are present, the rehydration phase may be omitted. Proceed with maintenance therapy and replacement of ongoing losses.
‡In addition to the rehydration amounts shown, replace ongoing stool losses and vomitus with ORS, 10 mL/kg for each diarrheal stool and 5 mL/kg for each episode of vomitus.
§While parenteral access is being sought, nasogastric infusion of ORS may be administered at 30 mL/kg/hr, provided airway protective reflexes remain intact.

Regular feedings should not be withheld once rehydration is complete. Strong evidence suggests that both the volume and the duration of diarrhea are reduced when children are fed immediately following rehydration.[24,25]

Children Treated in Emergency Departments

The subpopulation of children who seek treatment at emergency departments may represent a distinct group of patients. These children have often seen a primary care physician earlier in the illness, and the physicians may have attempted to rehydrate the children orally. Although use of ORT in the emergency department should be strongly encouraged and should always be attempted in the mild and moderately dehydrated child, primary care physicians should realize that ORT in these children will likely fail, and therefore intravenous treatment will probably be required, especially in the older (school-age) child in whom vomiting is the most prominent feature. Such children are often simply too exhausted to continue with efforts to drink. A brief trial of ORT followed, if necessary, by a brief course of intravenous fluids and subsequent reintroduction of liquids and solids is a reasonable approach in such children.[26]

COMPLICATIONS

Complications of inadequately treated dehydration may be severe, ultimately including full-blown shock and multiorgan dysfunction syndrome, with end-organ damage to the kidneys, liver, and brain, culminating in death. In practice, such extreme consequences may be prevented readily by early and aggressive fluid therapy, using the oral or occasionally the intravenous or intraosseous routes. As a rule, risking overhydration is far better than being exceptionally cautious with fluid administration. On rare occasions, aggressive oral hydration has resulted in mild overhydration, with some transient periorbital puffiness and a 2% to 3% weight gain.[22] These findings are generally self-limited and of no clinical consequence.

Hypokalemia, which results from the losses of total body potassium as a consequence of the increased aldosterone activity in the kidney, is a common occurrence in severe dehydration. As sodium is avidly retained, potassium is lost in the urine. Hypokalemia can result in ileus, which may impair fluid and electrolyte absorption from the intestines. An ORS generally contains 20 mEq/L potassium chloride; such a solution is capable of restoring potassium balance.

PROGNOSIS

Although diarrheal dehydration is the leading cause of death among children globally, when appropriately treated, it carries an excellent prognosis. Rapid restoration of circulating volume coupled with proper dietary management results in maintenance of hydration and earlier resolution of diarrheal symptoms. Parents should be warned, however, that even with ideal therapy, typical episodes of gastroenteritis last 3 to 7 days. Parents and primary care providers should be reassured about the child's state of good hydration. The physician should reinforce the idea that the diarrheal illness itself is of little consequence as long as hydration is maintained and feeding reintroduced in a timely fashion.

SUMMARY

Dehydration resulting from gastroenteritis is a common condition generally managed by ORT on an outpatient basis. Little laboratory evaluation is necessary. Parenteral therapy is reserved for severe or unusual cases. Regardless of the route of delivery, fluid should be administered rapidly and with the intent to restore the entire fluid deficit in 4 to 6 hours. Proper dietary management is essential to minimize the severity and duration of symptoms.

WHEN TO ADMIT

- The child has a persistently abnormal mental status, persistently abnormal electrolyte levels, or chronic diarrhea (>14 days' duration).
- The child has other medical problems, such as short-gut and inflammatory bowel disease.
- The child's hydration status cannot be restored or maintained after a 6-hour outpatient treatment period.

TOOLS FOR PRACTICE

Engaging Patients and Family

- *Diarrhea and Dehydration* (brochure), American Academy of Pediatrics (patiented.aap.org).
- *Rotavirus* (brochure), American Academy of Pediatrics (patiented.aap.org).
- *Sports Shorts—Exertional Heat Related Illness* (fact sheet), American Academy of Pediatrics (www.aap.org/family/SportsShorts_02.pdf).
- *Sports Shorts—Nutrition in Sports* (fact sheet), American Academy of Pediatrics (www.aap.org/family/SportsShorts_06.pdf).
- *Treating Diarrhea and Dehydration* (fact sheet), American Academy of Pediatrics (www.aap.org/topics.html).
- *Treatment of Vomiting* (fact sheet), American Academy of Pediatrics (www.aap.org/topics.html).

Medical Decision Support

- *Managing Acute Gastroenteritis Among Children* (guideline), Centers for Disease Control and Prevention (www.cdc.gov/mmwr/PDF/RR/RR5216.pdf).
- *Sports Shorts—Exertional Heat Related Illness* (fact sheet), American Academy of Pediatrics (www.aap.org/family/SportsShorts_02.pdf).
- *Sports Shorts—Nutrition in Sports* (fact sheet), American Academy of Pediatrics (www.aap.org/family/Sports Shorts_06.pdf).

AAP POLICY STATEMENTS

American Academy of Pediatrics, Committee on Sports Medicine and Fitness. Climatic heat stress and the exercising child and adolescent. *Pediatrics.* 2000;106(1):158-159. (aappolicy.aappublications.org/cgi/content/full/pediatrics;106/1/158).

Centers for Disease Control and Prevention. Managing acute gastroenteritis among children: oral rehydration, maintenance, and nutritional therapy. *MMWR Recomm Rep*. 2003;52(RR-16):1-16. (Endorsed by the American Academy of Pediatrics April 29, 2004.) Available at: www.cdc.gov/mmwr/PDF/RR/RR5216.pdf.

REFERENCES

1. Batra B, Stanton B. Oral Rehydration Therapy. Available at: www.uptodate.com. Accessed March 14, 2006.
2. Kosek M, Bern C, Guerrant RL. The global burden of diarrhoeal disease, as estimated from studies published between 1992 and 2000. *Bull World Health Organ*. 2003;81:197-204.
3. Parashar UD, Bresee JS, Glass RI. The global burden of diarrhoeal disease in children. *Bull World Health Organ*. 2003;81:236.
4. Bryce J, Boschi-Pinto C, Shibuya K, et al. WHO estimates of the causes of death in children. *Lancet*. 2005;365:1147-1152.
5. Endom EE, Kim MS. Clinical Assessment and Diagnosis of Hypovolemia (Dehydration) in Children. Available at: www.uptodate.com. Accessed March 13, 2006.
6. Goepp J. Oral rehydration. In: Henretig FJ, King C, eds. *Textbook of Pediatric Emergency Procedures*, Baltimore, MD: Williams & Wilkins; 1994.
7. Kallen RJ. The management of diarrheal dehydration in infants using parenteral fluids. *Pediatr Clin North Am*. 1990;37(2):265-287.
8. Steiner MJ, Dewalt DA, Byerley JS. Is this child dehydrated? *JAMA*. 2004;291:2746-2754.
9. Vega RM, Avner JR. A prospective study of usefulness of clinical and laboratory parameters for predicting percentage of dehydration in children. *Pediatr Emerg Care*. 1997;13:179-182.
10. Endom EE, Kim MS. Treatment of Hypovolemia (Dehydration) in Children. Available at: www.uptodate.com. Accessed March 13, 2006.
11. Alderson, P, Schierhout, G, Roberts, I, et al. Colloids versus crystalloids for fluid resuscitation in critically ill patients. *Cochrane Database Syst Rev*. 2000;(2): CD000567.
12. Wilkes MM, Navickis RJ. Patient survival after human albumin administration. A meta-analysis of randomized, controlled trials. *Ann Intern Med*. 2001;135:149-164.
13. Finfer S, Bellomo R, Boyce N, et al. A comparison of albumin and saline for fluid resuscitation in the intensive care unit. *N Engl J Med*. 2004;350:2247-2256.
14. Hirschhorn N, Greenough WB. Progress in oral rehydration therapy. *Sci Am*. 1991;264:50-56.
15. American Academy of Pediatrics, Provisional Committee on Quality Improvement, Subcommittee on Acute Gastroenteritis. Practice parameter on management of acute gastroenteritis in young children. *Pediatrics*. 1996;97:427-430.
16. Holliday M. The evolution of therapy for dehydration: should deficit therapy still be taught? *Pediatrics*. 1996;98:171-172.
17. Cronan KM, Kost SI. Renal and electrolyte emergencies. In: Fleisher GR, Ludwig S, Henretig FM, eds. *Textbook of Pediatric Emergency Medicine*. 5th ed. Philadelphia, PA: Lippincott, Williams and Wilkins; 2005.
18. Goepp J. Dehydration. In: Hoekelman RA, Adam HM, Nelson NM, et al, eds. *Primary Pediatric Care*. 4th ed. St Louis, MO: Mosby; 2001.
19. Hirschhorn N. The treatment of acute diarrhea in children: an historical and physiological perspective. *Am J Clin Nutr*. 1980;33:637-663.
20. Fonseca BK, Holdgate A, Craig JC. Enteral vs intravenous rehydration therapy for children with gastroenteritis: a meta-analysis of randomized controlled trials. *Arch Pediatr Adolesc Med*. 2004;158(5):483-490.
21. Goepp J. Oral rehydration. In: Henretig FJ, King C, eds. *Textbook of Pediatric Emergency Procedures*. Baltimore, MD: Williams & Wilkins; 1994.
22. Goepp J, Katz S. Oral rehydration therapy: a practice-oriented approach. *Am Fam Phys*. 1993;47:843-851.
23. World Health Organization. *Reduced Osmolarity Oral Rehydration Salts (ORS) Formulation*. New York, NY: UNICEF House; 2001. Available at: www.who.int/child-adolescent-health/New_Publications/NEWS/Expert_consultation.htm. Accessed June 15, 2006.
24. Santosham M, Foster S, Reid R, et al: Role of soy-based, lactose-free formula during treatment of acute diarrhea. *Pediatrics*. 1985;76:292-298.
25. Santosham M, Goepp J, Bums B, et al. Role of a soy-based, lactose-free formula in the outpatient management of diarrhea in infants. *Pediatrics*. 1991;87:619-622.
26. Conners GP, Goepp J. Emergency department oral rehydration of children: the best solution? *Clin Pediatr Emerg Med*. 1999;1:27.

Chapter 342

DIABETIC KETOACIDOSIS

Peter J. Tebben, MD; W. Frederick Schwenk II, MD

Diabetic ketoacidosis (DKA) is the metabolic consequence of insulin deficiency. The biochemical hallmarks of this disorder are hyperglycemia and acidosis. Historically, DKA has been associated with type 1 diabetes (T1D); however, clearly, many patients with type 2 diabetes (T2D) may have DKA.[1-4] Hispanic and African-American youth with T2D appear to be more prone to developing DKA than other populations. With the increasing incidence of both T1D and T2D, early recognition and appropriate intervention are imperative to prevent significant morbidity and mortality associated with DKA.[5-8] This condition represents a medical emergency and requires meticulous attention to optimize outcomes.

DKA is present at the time of initial diagnosis in many patients with T1D. The risk of developing DKA at the onset of diabetes has been associated with factors such as younger age and lower socioeconomic status.[9-11] Most children with newly diagnosed TID who have DKA will have symptoms consistent with the diagnosis, including polyuria, fatigue, weight loss, or any combination.[12]

Despite improvement in the understanding of diabetes and methods for treatment, recurrent DKA remains a significant problem for patients with previously diagnosed diabetes. Box 342-1 lists several factors associated with an increased risk of DKA in patients with established diabetes. Girls 13 to 19 years of age, patients with high HbA_{1C} values, and patients with high reported daily insulin doses have been reported to have an increased incidence of DKA.[13] A high risk of DKA has also been reported in children who were underinsured or were diagnosed as having a

BOX 342-1 Risk Factors for Diabetic Ketoacidosis in Patients with Established Type 1 Diabetes

Poor glycemic control (higher HbA_{1C})
Previous episode of diabetic ketoacidosis
Coexisting psychiatric disorders
Lower socioeconomic status (underinsured)
Adolescent age (especially girls)

coexisting psychiatric disorder.[13,14] The presence of previous episodes of DKA may also predict which patients are at particularly high risk of recurrence. Several investigators have reported that only a few patients account for a significant proportion of DKA cases.[13,15]

DEFINITION

DKA results from a lack of insulin, which leads to decreased peripheral glucose utilization despite continued hepatic glucose production. Counter-regulatory hormones including glucagon, catecholamines, and cortisol may have elevated levels and contribute to the hyperglycemia.[16-18] Fat stores are broken down in the absence of adequate insulin action, which leads to ketone body formation and subsequent metabolic acidosis. Criteria for the biochemical diagnosis of DKA were proposed in a consensus statement from the European Society for Pediatric Endocrinology and the Lawson Wilkins Pediatric Endocrine Society (ESPE/LWPES). The 2 biochemical requirements include a blood glucose level more than 200 mg/dL and metabolic acidosis with a venous pH less than 7.3 or bicarbonate level less than 15 mmol/L.[19] Although these criteria will identify most patients, a glucose concentration of less than 200 mg/dL does not always rule out the possibility of DKA.

DIFFERENTIAL DIAGNOSIS

When these criteria are applied to define DKA, the diagnosis is usually straightforward. During the initial assessment of a patient with DKA, the precipitating factors associated with the episode should be identified. Many factors have been described to precipitate an episode of DKA (Box 342-2). In adults with diabetes, myocardial infarction and stroke should also be considered. The omission of insulin is the most common cause of DKA in children and young adults with established diabetes mellitus.[1,20,21] Insulin doses are sometimes not given during illness, especially if the patient is not eating. Failure to recognize the ongoing need for insulin (and sometimes increased requirements) during illness is a common mistake that can be prevented by providing adequate education to the patient and family. In addition to missed or inadequate insulin dosing, illness and trauma may contribute to the occurrence of DKA. Primary care physicians should also consider the relative contribution of other illnesses to the metabolic acidosis. Lactic acidosis as a result of sepsis or poor perfusion may coexist with DKA, and its cause should be treated concurrently.

BOX 342-2 Factors Associated with Diabetic Ketoacidosis in Children and Adolescents

Omission of insulin	Alcohol
Illness	Medications
Trauma	Pancreatitis

EVALUATION

Relevant History

Most patients with T2D will have a family history of diabetes. However, a relatively small percentage of patients with T1D will have another family member with the disease. The symptoms a patient with DKA reports will vary and are consistent with the degree of metabolic disturbance. As insulin deficiency progresses and blood glucose levels rise, the renal threshold for glucose reabsorption in the proximal tubule is surpassed ($\approx$ 180 mg/dL). An osmotic diuresis ensues, leading to symptoms of polyuria and polydipsia. With excess renal water loss, obligate losses of sodium, potassium, and phosphorus also occur. The osmotic diuresis can lead to enuresis in previously continent children. Weight loss caused by dehydration and loss of calories in the urine is often reported but difficult to quantify unless a recent accurate weight is available. If the child has limited access to fluids or is vomiting, dehydration can be severe. Fatigue is a common symptom reported that may be evident even before significant dehydration and acidosis. Polyphagia may be evident early in the disease but is typically replaced with a loss of appetite as ketosis and metabolic acidosis worsens. Patients who develop moderate to severe ketoacidosis often experience abdominal pain and vomiting, which will contribute to the dehydration, thereby reducing glomerular filtration rate and thus impairing the clearance of glucose and ketones.

Early recognition of DKA in infants and young children can be particularly challenging. Infants and young children are not able to verbalize their symptoms. In addition, an infant's inability to access fluids freely may mask the polyuria. Increased urine production may also be difficult to judge based on how wet infants' diapers are or how frequently the diapers need to be changed. Parents are less likely to recognize symptoms of hyperglycemia and DKA in children younger than 2 years.[22] This circumstance may lead to a delay in the diagnosis of diabetes and partially explain why more children in this age group have DKA at the time of initial diagnosis compared with older children.

Physical Examination

Similar to historical clues that should prompt consideration of the diagnosis of DKA, physical findings are commensurate with the degree of metabolic disturbance. Despite many patients having moderate to severe dehydration at the time of diagnosis, few become hypotensive. If a patient is in shock, a coexisting illness should be considered.

Dehydration

Clinically assessing the degree of dehydration can be difficult, but tachycardia and weight loss may be useful findings. Most patients with moderate to severe DKA are considered to be at least 5% to 10% dehydrated. True dehydration (intracellular and extracellular fluid loss) rather than simple hypovolemia (intravascular fluid loss) is the rule. As the intravascular osmolality increases resulting from hyperglycemia, water shifts from the intracellular space into the vascular space. This process results in an osmotic diuresis, leading to profound water and electrolyte loss if the cycle remains uninterrupted.

Acid Load

As would be expected in a patient with metabolic acidosis, compensatory respiratory mechanisms attempt to correct the excess acid load. This correction is accomplished by increasing the minute ventilation, which may be evident as rapid, deep respirations (Kussmaul breathing). Beta-hydroxybutyrate, acetoacetic acid, and acetone are produced in excess in patients with DKA. Although acetone does not contribute to the acid load, as it is exhaled, a *fruity* breath may be detected.

Neurologic Signs

When DKA goes untreated and becomes severe, neurologic signs may become prominent. Confusion and an altered sensorium may be observed. Seizures and coma may also occur as a complication of DKA. Although cerebral edema has typically been reported after the initiation of therapy, cases have been described where edema has been present before therapeutic intervention.[23] Cerebral edema should be considered in all patients with DKA who exhibit signs or symptoms of neurologic compromise regardless of whether treatment has been initiated.

Laboratory Findings

As previously mentioned, hyperglycemia (glucose >200 mg/dL) and acidosis (pH <7.3 or bicarbonate <15 mmol/L) are the defining biochemical characteristics of DKA. In addition to these findings, several other biochemical features of DKA are consistent with the diagnosis. Electrolyte depletion is a prominent feature of DKA that requires close attention (Table 342-1).[24]

Sodium

Sodium concentrations are commonly low at initial evaluation. Hyponatremia during DKA is the result of the combined effect of renal sodium losses and dilutional effects. As dehydration from the osmotic diuresis ensues, sodium is lost in excess through the kidney. In addition, hyperglycemia and the elevation of other osmotically active solutes (blood urea nitrogen [BUN] and ketone bodies) provide a gradient between the intracellular and extracellular spaces such that water is drawn into the extracellular space, resulting in a dilutional effect and exhibiting as a low serum or plasma sodium concentration. A commonly used correction factor for hyponatremia has been to add 1.6 mEq/L to the measured sodium concentration for every 100 mg/dL the glucose is over the normal range. Other researchers have suggested that a correction factor of 2.4 mEq/L is more appropriate than 1.6 mEq/L.[25]

Alternatively, pseudohyponatremia may also be seen in patients with significant elevations in plasma lipid concentrations. Insulin is a stimulator of lipoprotein lipase, which is necessary for clearance of triglyceride from the blood. DKA is a state of inadequate insulin, and hyperlipidemia is not an uncommon finding. Sodium is primarily a part of the aqueous fraction of blood, and when the lipid fraction is significantly elevated, the result is apparent hyponatremia (pseudohyponatremia). Because some laboratory methods take this into account when measuring sodium, such as direct potentiometry using an ion selective electrode, primary care physicians need to know the method being used by the laboratory to determine if pseudohyponatremia is contributing to this biochemical abnormality.[26] Accurate assessment of the sodium concentration is necessary to determine appropriate fluid management. A slower rate of rise in sodium concentration during treatment of DKA has been associated with a higher risk of cerebral edema.[27,28]

Potassium

Potassium is primarily an intracellular electrolyte that becomes depleted in DKA. In a state of metabolic acidosis, excess hydrogen ion is exchanged for intracellular potassium, which is then excreted through the kidney. Additional potassium may be lost through the gastrointestinal tract if vomiting occurs. Because of the multiple factors influencing potassium in a patient with DKA, the serum potassium concentration can be variable before therapeutic intervention. However, even if the initial serum potassium concentration is elevated, DKA represents a state of total body potassium depletion as intracellular stores are reduced. At initial evaluation, potassium levels are typically normal or elevated. When treatment with insulin is begun, potassium shifts to the intracellular compartment, resulting in a decrease in the measured potassium concentration. Profound hyperkalemia or hypokalemia may lead to cardiac arrhythmias, and this

Table 342-1 Estimate of Fluid and Electrolyte Deficits in Children with Diabetic Ketoacidosis

FLUID OR ELECTROLYTE	EXTENT OF LOSS PER kg BODY WEIGHT
Water	60-100 mL/kg
Sodium	6 mEq/kg (range 5-13)
Potassium	5 mEq/kg (range 4-6)
Chloride	4 mEq/kg (range 3-9)
Phosphate	3 mEq/kg (range 2-5)

Modified from Schwenk WF 2nd, Haymond MW. Treatment of diabetic ketoacidosis in children and young adults. *Prim Care.* 1983;10(4):663-676.

electrolyte must be monitored closely and replaced appropriately.

Phosphorus

Phosphorus is another predominantly intracellular electrolyte that becomes depleted during DKA. The mechanism is similar to that of potassium with the primary loss occurring through the kidney. Patients with DKA may have profound hypophosphatemia that may only become apparent during therapy.

Other Laboratory Components

Assessment of renal function and dehydration should be performed, including measurement of BUN and creatinine. These values are typically elevated in a pattern consistent with a prerenal state. Insulin and C-peptide concentrations are generally low in patients with newly diagnosed T1D. Although antibody levels against islet cell antigens and insulin are frequently elevated at the time of diagnosis, they are not useful in the diagnosis or management of DKA. The principles of managing DKA are the same whether the underlying diagnosis is T1D or T2D.

MANAGEMENT

The management of DKA should be focused on correction of the metabolic disturbances while preventing potential complications. The major complications that arise during treatment of DKA include cerebral edema and hypoglycemia. An increased risk of venous thrombosis has also been associated with DKA, especially in children with a central venous catheter.[29,30] Effective treatment of DKA includes insulin administration and fluid and electrolyte replacement. Many algorithms have been proposed to assist the clinician in the management of DKA. The following principles have been used successfully in the authors' institution. However, the fact that no single protocol will be appropriate for all patients must be stressed. Specific therapy must be designed according to the clinical circumstances and coexisting diseases, such as infection, which should be treated concomitantly.

ASSESSMENT AND DISPOSITION

Initial assessment of a child with DKA should include an estimation of the severity of disease (Table 342-2). The patient's cardiovascular and respiratory status should be evaluated and addressed immediately if compromise is present. Signs of neurologic dysfunction should prompt evaluation for cerebral edema, which can be present before any therapeutic intervention.[23] Laboratory assessment should include measurement of the patient's blood glucose, pH, bicarbonate, ketone (β-hydroxybutyrate), and electrolyte (sodium, potassium, chloride, phosphorus, and calcium) levels. Coexisting illness often contributes to the precipitation of DKA and additional studies including cultures (blood, urine, and cerebral spinal fluid) should be obtained when clinically indicated. Urine should also be assessed for glucose and ketones.

Patients with mild DKA may not exhibit any clinical findings of dehydration. In many instances, in patients with established diabetes, mild DKA can be managed in the outpatient setting for patients who are able to maintain oral intake. As a part of chronic diabetes care, patients and families should be educated on treatment strategies for mild ketosis. Written education materials and access to a primary care provider experienced in the care of patients with diabetes may prevent some emergency department visits and hospitalizations. For patients with moderate to severe DKA, admission to a pediatric intensive care unit or general pediatric ward is indicated. Familiarity with the level of care available within a particular institution is essential for proper placement of the child. Most patients with severe DKA will require a level of care only offered in an intensive care setting. However, some hospitals are equipped to manage moderate ketoacidosis on a general pediatric ward.

FLUID REPLACEMENT

Patients with moderate to severe DKA are generally considered to be between 5% and 10% dehydrated. Ten to 20 mL/kg intravenous fluids are suggested for initial fluid replacement. The ESPE/LWPES recommends isotonic solutions such as lactated Ringer's solution or 0.9% saline,[19] which are commonly used for the treatment of dehydration or hypovolemia from any cause. Additional fluid resuscitation may be required in some patients but caution must be used, especially for patients with signs or symptoms suggestive of cerebral edema. Aggressive fluid resuscitation caused by hemodynamic instability is rarely required even for patients with severe DKA. In this setting, other causes of hypotension such as sepsis should be considered. The goal of initial fluid resuscitation is not to replace the entire fluid deficit. Rehydration should take place over the subsequent 36 to 48 hours. In adults and children with DKA, less aggressive rates of fluid replacement have been associated with more rapid correction of the

Table 342-2 Assessment of the Severity of Diabetic Ketoacidosis

	MILD	MODERATE	SEVERE
Sensorium	Alert	Drowsy, lethargic	Obtundation, coma
Hyperpnea	Absent	Mild	Severe
Hydration	No dehydration	Mild to moderate (3-5%)	Severe (>5%)
Plasma bicarbonate	>16-18 mEq/L	>10 mEq/L	<10 mEq/L
Anion gap	18-20 mEq/L	<20-25 mEq/L	>25 mEq/L

Modified from Schwenk WF 2nd, Haymond MW. Treatment of diabetic ketoacidosis in children and young adults. *Prim Care.* 1983;10(4):663-676. Copyright © 1983, Elsevier, with permission.

acidosis.[31,32] A gradual rehydration strategy may reduce the risk of cerebral edema compared with more aggressive fluid administration.[27] Fluid therapy (even before insulin) will result in a reduction of the blood glucose concentration.[33,34] This reduction is partially the result of a dilutional effect, as well as improved glomerular filtration rate and increased renal clearance of glucose.

After the initial fluid bolus, the content of the intravenous fluid should be changed to address additional electrolyte abnormalities present and to prevent hyperchloremic metabolic acidosis that may occur if isotonic saline solutions are continued. The ESPE/LWPES guidelines suggest that rehydration should take place over at least 48 hours and that the rate of fluid administration should rarely exceed 1.5 to 2 times the maintenance fluids. The ESPE/LWPES also recommends that urinary losses not be added to the calculated fluid requirement. Because total body stores of potassium are invariably depleted, potassium should be added to the intravenous solution when the potassium concentration is normal or low and urine flow has been established. When the patient transitions to oral intake, after correction of the acidosis, intravenous fluids should be reduced or discontinued accordingly.

INSULIN THERAPY

Delivery

Insulin is essential to correct the metabolic disturbances present in patients with DKA. Intravenous regular insulin is the preferred route of administration.[19] Subcutaneous and intramuscular insulin have been used successfully in the treatment of DKA.[35-39] These modes of insulin delivery should only be used when intravenous access in not possible, especially in severely dehydrated patients in whom insulin absorption may be impaired because of poor circulatory status. Intravenous insulin can be titrated frequently if necessary because of its relatively short half-life.

Dosing

An initial infusion rate of 0.1 unit/kg/hour of intravenous regular insulin is generally an effective dose. The insulin infusion will act to decrease gluconeogenesis, decrease lipolysis and ketogenesis, and increase peripheral glucose utilization. The blood glucose concentration should not be used alone to determine when to discontinue or decrease the rate of insulin infusion. Ketosis and metabolic acidosis will not correct without adequate insulin administration. The metabolic acidosis often corrects many hours after euglycemia has been restored. For this reason, a constant insulin infusion rate should be used, and glucose should be added to the intravenous fluids when the blood glucose level falls below 250 to 300 mg/dL. An infusion of 5% dextrose may be sufficient for many patients. However, higher rates of dextrose infusion may be required to prevent hypoglycemia while the ketoacidosis is resolving. The rate of insulin infusion may need to be increased in some children if the ketoacidosis does not improve or worsens. In this circumstance, additional causes of acidosis or coexisting illnesses should be considered and treated appropriately.

Monitoring

Monitoring the patient's response to therapy frequently is imperative to assess when a change in treatment is required. Such monitoring should include hourly glucose determinations. Electrolytes, bicarbonate, ketones, and pH should be measured every 2 to 4 hours to ensure correction of the metabolic disturbances. More frequent monitoring is suggested (every 2 hours) with severe DKA and less frequent monitoring (every 4 hours) when improvement in the ketoacidosis has been established.

ELECTROLYTES

Sodium

Sodium concentrations are frequently low because of the reasons previously mentioned. The isotonic solutions suggested for initial fluid management are intended to increase the intravascular volume and improve the glomerular filtration rate. Sodium depletion is also addressed with this therapy. After the initial fluid administration, 0.45% saline is often used to prevent excessive sodium and chloride delivery. Excessive isotonic sodium chloride should not be given because hyperchloremic metabolic acidosis may result. Electrolytes such as potassium and phosphorus that have been depleted can be easily added to 0.45% saline. Sodium concentrations should be monitored closely. Some authors have suggested that failure of an increase in the sodium concentration with therapy for DKA may be associated with a higher risk of developing cerebral edema.[28,40]

Potassium

Potassium concentrations may be elevated, normal, or low before the initiation of therapy in patients with DKA. The concentration likely depends on several factors, including the severity and duration of DKA and the presence of gastrointestinal losses caused by vomiting. In patients with significantly elevated potassium concentrations, an electrocardiogram should be obtained to determine if cardiac abnormalities are present. With the initiation of insulin therapy, potassium concentrations invariably decline and may become normal or low. Insulin facilitates intracellular transport of potassium and the correction of acidosis also results in the exchange of intracellular hydrogen for extracellular potassium leading to further reductions in potassium concentrations. Adding 20 mEq/L potassium acetate and 20 mEq/L potassium phosphate to 0.45% saline works well in most patients. This combination of salts prevents excess chloride while replacing not only potassium, but also phosphorus, which is frequently depleted. This solution is a safe and effective means to prevent profound hypokalemia. Potassium should be replaced after the initial isotonic fluid bolus has been given, the serum potassium concentration becomes normal or low, and urine output is established. Potassium levels should be monitored closely and therapy adjusted according to individual patient needs.

Phosphorus

Phosphate depletion occurs as a result of many of the same mechanisms as potassium depletion. Phosphate concentrations may also be variable before initiation of therapy. Hypophosphatemia may become profound as intracellular phosphate transport from the extracellular space is facilitated by insulin. Phosphate replacement in the treatment of patients with DKA has not been shown to provide clinically important improvements in outcome or to eliminate significant complications.[41-43] However, the possibility of a decrease in oxygen delivery to tissues caused by a shift of the oxyhemoglobin dissociation curve to the left is present.[44,45] The addition of potassium phosphate to the rehydration solution is safe and effective at maintaining a normal or near-normal phosphate concentration. If phosphate therapy is used, then serum calcium concentrations should be monitored because hypocalcemia may occur.

Bicarbonate

Bicarbonate therapy for patients with mild to moderate DKA lacks data to support its use.[46-50] Even for patients with severe DKA, bicarbonate therapy has not been proven to be beneficial.[49,51] Use of bicarbonate in patients with DKA may not be appropriate for several reasons. The ketoacidosis can be completely corrected by the administration of intravenous fluids and insulin. Treatment with bicarbonate will result in additional sodium administration that may not be required. Paradoxical central nervous system acidosis that may occur as a result of bicarbonate treatment is a potential concern. Bicarbonate therapy has also been associated with an increased risk of cerebral edema.[46] Despite these concerns, some patients with cardiovascular dysfunction caused by severe acidosis or hyperkalemia (or both) may benefit from cautious alkali administration.[19]

CONVERTING TO SUBCUTANEOUS INSULIN

Converting to subcutaneous insulin should be considered when the serum bicarbonate level is more than 16 to 18 mmol/L (or pH more than 7.3) and the patient is able to begin oral intake. If DKA has occurred in a child with a previous diagnosis of diabetes, then the home insulin regimen may serve as a guide in choosing initial subcutaneous insulin doses and the type of program to use (split-mixed versus multiple daily injection). For patients with newly diagnosed diabetes, 0.5 to 1.0 units/kg/day in divided doses is appropriate. Frequently, adjustments to the initial doses are necessary depending on the child's meal plan, level of activity, and pubertal status. Children with and children without diabetes have an increased insulin requirement to maintain euglycemia during puberty compared with prepubertal children.[52,53] Additional details regarding subcutaneous insulin therapy are discussed in Chapter 256, Diabetes Mellitus.

COMPLICATIONS

The incidence of clinically apparent cerebral edema in children has been estimated to be approximately 1%.[15,23,46] Some, but not all, studies suggest that the incidence of subclinical cerebral edema is higher when using imaging criteria to diagnose the condition.[54-56] The reported mortality rate in children with DKA is low (<0.5%).[57,58] However, most of these deaths have been in those who developed clinically apparent cerebral edema.[46,58] In adults, coexisting conditions such as myocardial infarction contribute to a larger percentage of the mortality associated with DKA.[59]

Although cerebral edema is a rare complication of DKA, the consequences are severe. Several studies in children have reported a mortality rate of approximately 20% to 25% for those who developed cerebral edema.[15,23,46] A significant proportion of those who survive will have permanent neurologic consequences. Symptoms of cerebral edema attributed to increased intracranial pressure include a decreased level of consciousness, elevated blood pressure, and bradycardia. Nonspecific symptoms such as headache may also be present, and a high index of suspicion should be maintained to identify this potentially fatal condition early. If these clinical findings are encountered at any time during the treatment of DKA, prompt assessment including imaging of the head should be undertaken.

The precise etiology of cerebral edema is not clear; however, several potential risk factors have been identified (Box 342-3). Few data are available to establish optimal therapy for cerebral edema associated with DKA. If cerebral edema occurs, the EPES/LWPES consensus statement recommends that the rate of fluid administration be reduced.[19] Intravenous mannitol may be given and repeated after 2 hours if clinically indicated. Case reports of improvement in cerebral edema with this therapy have been published, but not all studies suggest a clear benefit.[60,61] Hypertonic saline has also been suggested as an alternative to the use of mannitol in the treatment of children with cerebral edema.[19,62] If intubation is required, then hyperventilation should be avoided because this has been associated with worse outcomes.[60] Frequent neurologic examinations should be performed in children with DKA in an attempt to identify and intervene early. Because cerebral edema can be present before therapy for DKA, prevention of DKA may be the only effective strategy to prevent this potentially devastating complication.

BOX 342-3 Potential Risk Factors for Cerebral Edema

- Lower partial pressure of arterial carbon dioxide at presentation
- Severity of dehydration (higher initial BUN)
- Smaller rise in serum sodium during treatment
- New-onset diabetes
- Treatment with bicarbonate
- Younger age
- Longer duration of symptoms before presentation

BUN, Blood urea nitrogen.

PREVENTION

In patients with established T1D, ketoacidosis is largely preventable with proper attention to glycemic control, especially during times of illness. Most children develop DKA because of the omission of insulin, which may occur for a variety of reasons, including financial constraints or a lack of knowledge regarding proper management during illness.[21] This finding emphasizes the importance of ongoing diabetes education for the patients and their families to help them understand the factors that lead to DKA in an effort to prevent its occurrence.

Few prospective studies have been performed with the goal of preventing DKA in patients with newly diagnosed diabetes. An Italian study investigated the impact of raising public awareness regarding diabetes and found significantly fewer episodes of DKA at the time of diagnosis in this region compared with surrounding communities.[63] Raising public awareness of the symptoms of diabetes may be a cost-effective way to prevent this potentially fatal illness.

In patients with established diabetes, the most often cited cause of DKA is the omission of insulin, which is a preventable problem. Effective education should be a part of any comprehensive diabetes program and has the potential to decrease the rates of recurrent DKA. Clinical experience and review of the literature would indicate that a small percentage of patients with diabetes account for a disproportionate number of episodes of DKA.[13,15] Interventions targeted at this high-risk population would seem appropriate.

WHEN TO REFER

- When facilities to provide frequent patient assessment (clinical and laboratory) are not available
- When a physician experienced in the diagnosis and treatment of DKA is not available

WHEN TO ADMIT

- Patients with moderate to severe DKA
- Patients with dehydration or those who are unable to maintain adequate oral intake
- All patients with newly diagnosed diabetes regardless of the severity of ketoacidosis

SUGGESTED RESOURCE

European Society for Pediatric Endocrinology/Lawson Wilkins Pediatric Endocrine Society consensus statement on diabetic ketoacidosis in children and adolescents. Dunger DB, Sperling MA, Acerini CL, et al. European Society for Paediatric Endocrinology/Lawson Wilkins Pediatric Endocrine Society consensus statement on diabetic ketoacidosis in children and adolescents. *Pediatrics*. 2004;113(2): e133-e140.

REFERENCES

1. Newton CA, Raskin P. Diabetic ketoacidosis in type 1 and type 2 diabetes mellitus: clinical and biochemical differences. *Arch Int Med*. 2004;164(17):1925-1931.
2. Valabhji J, Watson M, Cox J, et al. Type 2 diabetes presenting as diabetic ketoacidosis in adolescence. *Diabet Med*. 2003;20(5):416-417.
3. Pinhas-Hamiel O, Dolan LM, Zeitler PS. Diabetic ketoacidosis among obese African-American adolescents with NIDDM. *Diabetes Care*. 1997;20(4):484-486.
4. Sellers EA, Dean HJ. Diabetic ketoacidosis: a complication of type 2 diabetes in Canadian aboriginal youth. *Diabetes Care*. 2000;23(8):1202-1204.
5. Cooper GS, Stroehla BC. The epidemiology of autoimmune diseases. *Autoimmun Rev*. 2003;2(3):119-125.
6. Gale EA. The rise of childhood type 1 diabetes in the 20th century. *Diabetes*. 2002;51(12):3353-3361.
7. Fagot-Campagna A, Pettitt DJ, Engelgau MM, et al. Type 2 diabetes among North American children and adolescents: an epidemiologic review and a public health perspective. *Pediatrics*. 2000;136(5):664-672.
8. Pinhas-Hamiel O, Dolan LM, Daniels SR, et al. Increased incidence of non-insulin-dependent diabetes mellitus among adolescents. *Pediatrics*. 1996;128(5 pt 1):608-615.
9. Neu A, Willasch A, Ehehalt S, et al. Ketoacidosis at onset of type 1 diabetes mellitus in children—frequency and clinical presentation. *Pediatr Diabetes*. 2003;4(2):77-81.
10. Mallare JT, Cordice CC, Ryan BA, et al. Identifying risk factors for the development of diabetic ketoacidosis in new onset type 1 diabetes mellitus. *Clin Pediatr*. 2003; 42(7):591-597.
11. Komulainen J, Lounamaa R, Knip M, et al. Ketoacidosis at the diagnosis of type 1 (insulin dependent) diabetes mellitus is related to poor residual beta cell function. Childhood Diabetes in Finland Study Group. *Arch Dis Child*. 1996;75(5):410-415.
12. Rosenbauer J, Icks A, Giani G. Clinical characteristics and predictors of severe ketoacidosis at onset of type 1 diabetes mellitus in children in a North Rhine-Westphalian region, Germany. *J Ped Endocrinol*. 2002;15(8):1137-1145.
13. Rewers A, Chase HP, Mackenzie T, et al. Predictors of acute complications in children with type 1 diabetes. *JAMA*. 2002;287(19):2511-2518.
14. Maniatis AK, Goehrig SH, Gao D, et al. Increased incidence and severity of diabetic ketoacidosis among uninsured children with newly diagnosed type 1 diabetes mellitus. *Pediatr Diabetes*. 2005;6(2):79-83.
15. Edge JA, Hawkins MM, Winter DL, et al. The risk and outcome of cerebral oedema developing during diabetic ketoacidosis. *Arch Dis Child*. 2001;85(1):16-22.
16. Alberti KG. Role of glucagon and other hormones in development of diabetic ketoacidosis. *Lancet*. 1975;1(7920):1307-1311.
17. Bolli G, Compagnucci P, Cartechini MG, et al. Urinary excretion and plasma levels of norepinephrine and epinephrine during diabetic ketoacidosis. *Acta Diabetologica Latina*. 1979;16(2):157-167.
18. Gerich JE, Lorenzi M, Bier DM, et al. Prevention of human diabetic ketoacidosis by somatostatin. Evidence for an essential role of glucagon. *N Engl J Med*. 1975; 292(19):985-989.
19. Dunger DB, Sperling MA, Acerini CL, et al. European Society for Paediatric Endocrinology/Lawson Wilkins Pediatric Endocrine Society consensus statement on diabetic ketoacidosis in children and adolescents. *Pediatrics*. 2004;113(2):e133-e140.
20. Thompson CJ, Cummings F, Chalmers J, et al. Abnormal insulin treatment behaviour: a major cause of ketoacidosis in the young adult. *Diabet Med*. 1995;12(5):429-432.
21. Musey VC, Lee JK, Crawford R, et al. Diabetes in urban African-Americans. I. Cessation of insulin therapy is the major precipitating cause of diabetic ketoacidosis. *Diabetes Care*. 1995;18(4):483-489.

22. Quinn M, Fleischman A, Rosner B, et al. Characteristics at diagnosis of type 1 diabetes in children younger than 6 years. *Pediatrics*. 2006;148(3):366-371.
23. Lawrence SE, Cummings EA, Gaboury I, et al. Population-based study of incidence and risk factors for cerebral edema in pediatric diabetic ketoacidosis. *Pediatrics*. 2005; 146(5):688-692.
24. Schwenk WF 2nd, Haymond MW. Treatment of diabetic ketoacidosis in children and young adults. *Prim Care*. 1983;10(4):663-676.
25. Hillier TA, Abbott RD, Barrett EJ. Hyponatremia: evaluating the correction factor for hyperglycemia. *AJM*. 1999;106(4):399-403.
26. Weisberg LS. Pseudohyponatremia: a reappraisal. *AJM*. 1989;86(3):315-318.
27. Duck SC, Weldon VV, Pagliara AS, et al. Cerebral edema complicating therapy for diabetic ketoacidosis. *Diabetes*. 1976;25(2):111-115.
28. Harris GD, Fiordalisi I, Harris WL, et al. Minimizing the risk of brain herniation during treatment of diabetic ketoacidemia: a retrospective and prospective study. *Pediatrics*. 1990;117(1 pt 1):22-31.
29. Worly JM, Fortenberry JD, Hansen I, et al. Deep venous thrombosis in children with diabetic ketoacidosis and femoral central venous catheters. *Pediatrics*. 2004; 113(1 pt 1):e57-e60.
30. Gutierrez JA, Bagatell R, Samson MP, et al. Femoral central venous catheter-associated deep venous thrombosis in children with diabetic ketoacidosis. *Crit Care Med*. 2003;31(1):80-83.
31. Adrogue HJ, Barrero J, Eknoyan G. Salutary effects of modest fluid replacement in the treatment of adults with diabetic ketoacidosis. Use in patients without extreme volume deficit. *JAMA*. 1989;262(15):2108-2113.
32. Felner EI, White PC. Improving management of diabetic ketoacidosis in children. *Pediatrics*. 2001;108(3): 735-740.
33. Owen OE, Licht JH, Sapir DG. Renal function and effects of partial rehydration during diabetic ketoacidosis. *Diabetes*. 1981;30(6):510-518.
34. Waldhausl W, Kleinberger G, Korn A, et al. Severe hyperglycemia: effects of rehydration on endocrine derangements and blood glucose concentration. *Diabetes*. 1979;28(6):577-584.
35. Della Manna T, Steinmetz L, Campos PR, et al. Subcutaneous use of a fast-acting insulin analog: an alternative treatment for pediatric patients with diabetic ketoacidosis. *Diabetes Care*. 2005;28(8):1856-1861.
36. Umpierrez GE, Latif K, Stoever J, et al. Efficacy of subcutaneous insulin lispro versus continuous intravenous regular insulin for the treatment of patients with diabetic ketoacidosis. *AJM*. 2004;117(5):291-296.
37. Umpierrez GE, Cuervo R, Karabell A, et al. Treatment of diabetic ketoacidosis with subcutaneous insulin aspart. *Diabetes Care*. 2004;27(8):1873-1878.
38. Drop SL, Duval-Arnould JM, Gober AE, et al. Low-dose intravenous insulin infusion versus subcutaneous insulin injection: a controlled comparative study of diabetic ketoacidosis. *Pediatrics*. 1977;59(5):733-738.
39. Sacks HS, Shahshahani M, Kitabchi AE, et al. Similar responsiveness of diabetic ketoacidosis to low-dose insulin by intramuscular injection and albumin-free infusion. *Ann Intern Med*. 1979;90(1):36-42.
40. Hale PM, Rezvani I, Braunstein AW, et al. Factors predicting cerebral edema in young children with diabetic ketoacidosis and new onset type I diabetes. *Acta Paediatrica*. 1997;86(6):626-631.
41. Fisher JN, Kitabchi AE. A randomized study of phosphate therapy in the treatment of diabetic ketoacidosis. *J Clin Endocrinol Metab*. 1983;57(1):177-180.
42. Wilson HK, Keuer SP, Lea AS, et al. Phosphate therapy in diabetic ketoacidosis. *Arch Intern Med*. 1982;142(3):517-520.
43. Gibby OM, Veale KE, Hayes TM, et al. Oxygen availability from the blood and the effect of phosphate replacement on erythrocyte 2,3-diphosphoglycerate and haemoglobin-oxygen affinity in diabetic ketoacidosis. *Diabetologia*. 1978;15(5):381-385.
44. Clerbaux T, Reynaert M, Willems E, et al. Effect of phosphate on oxygen-hemoglobin affinity, diphosphoglycerate and blood gases during recovery from diabetic ketoacidosis. *Int Care Med*. 1989;15(8):495-498.
45. Clerbaux T, Detry B, Reynaert M, et al. Reestimation of the effects of inorganic phosphates on the equilibrium between oxygen and hemoglobin. *Int Care Med*. 1992; 18(4):222-225.
46. Glaser N, Barnett P, McCaslin I, et al. Risk factors for cerebral edema in children with diabetic ketoacidosis. The Pediatric Emergency Medicine Collaborative Research Committee of the American Academy of Pediatrics. *N Engl J Med*. 2001;344(4):264-269.
47. Hale PJ, Crase J, Nattrass M. Metabolic effects of bicarbonate in the treatment of diabetic ketoacidosis. *Br Med J (Clin Res Ed)*. 1984;289(6451):1035-1038.
48. Okuda Y, Adrogue HJ, Field JB, et al. Counterproductive effects of sodium bicarbonate in diabetic ketoacidosis. *J Clin Endocrinol Metab*. 1996;81(1):314-320.
49. Green SM, Rothrock SG, Ho JD, et al. Failure of adjunctive bicarbonate to improve outcome in severe pediatric diabetic ketoacidosis. *Ann Emerg Med*. 1998;31(1):41-48.
50. Kaye R. Diabetic ketoacidosis—the bicarbonate controversy. *Pediatrics*. 1975;87(1):156-159.
51. Morris LR, Murphy MB, Kitabchi AE. Bicarbonate therapy in severe diabetic ketoacidosis. *Ann Intern Med*. 1986;105(6):836-840.
52. Bloch CA, Clemons P, Sperling MA. Puberty decreases insulin sensitivity. *Pediatrics*. 1987;110(3):481-487.
53. Kerouz N, el-Hayek R, Langhough R, et al. Insulin doses in children using conventional therapy for insulin dependent diabetes. *Diabetes Res Clin Pract*. 1995;29(2): 113-120.
54. Hoffman WH, Steinhart CM, el Gammal T, et al. Cranial CT in children and adolescents with diabetic ketoacidosis. *AJNR*. 1988;9(4):733-739.
55. Krane EJ, Rockoff MA, Wallman JK, et al. Subclinical brain swelling in children during treatment of diabetic ketoacidosis. *N Engl J Med*. 1985;312(18):1147-1151.
56. Smedman L, Escobar R, Hesser U, et al. Sub-clinical cerebral oedema does not occur regularly during treatment for diabetic ketoacidosis. *Acta Paediatrica*. 1997;86(11): 1172-1176.
57. Curtis JR, To T, Muirhead S, et al. Recent trends in hospitalization for diabetic ketoacidosis in Ontario children. *Diabetes Care*. 2002;25(9):1591-1596.
58. Edge JA, Ford-Adams ME, Dunger DB. Causes of death in children with insulin dependent diabetes 1990-96. *Arch Dis Child*. 1999;81(4):318-323.
59. Basu A, Close CF, Jenkins D, et al. Persisting mortality in diabetic ketoacidosis. *Diabet Med*. 1993;10(3):282-284.
60. Marcin JP, Glaser N, Barnett P, et al. Factors associated with adverse outcomes in children with diabetic ketoacidosis-related cerebral edema. *Pediatrics*. 2002; 141(6):793-797.
61. Franklin B, Liu J, Ginsberg-Fellner F. Cerebral edema and ophthalmoplegia reversed by mannitol in a new case of insulin-dependent diabetes mellitus. *Pediatrics*. 1982;69(1):87-90.
62. Kamat P, Vats A, Gross M, Checchia PA. Use of hypertonic saline for the treatment of altered mental status associated with diabetic ketoacidosis. *Pediatr Crit Care Med*. 2003;4(2):239-242.

63. Vanelli M, Chiari G, Ghizzoni L, et al. Effectiveness of a prevention program for diabetic ketoacidosis in children. An 8-year study in schools and private practices. *Diabetes Care*. 1999;22(1):7-9.

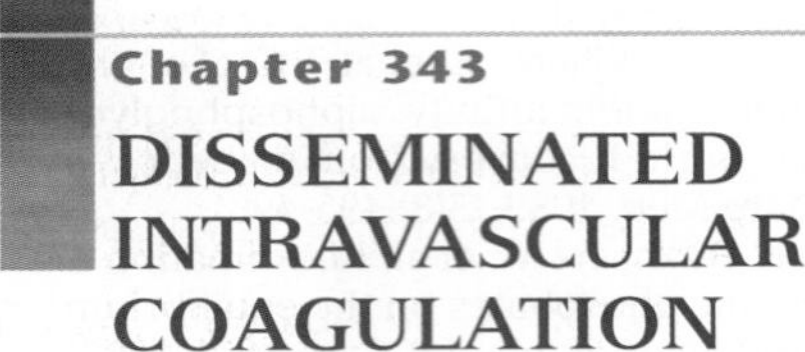

Chapter 343

DISSEMINATED INTRAVASCULAR COAGULATION

Steven W. Pipe, MD; Anjali A. Sharathkumar, MD

DEFINITION

Disseminated intravascular coagulation (DIC) is a pathological syndrome that arises from a heterogeneous group of medical disorders. It is characterized by *simultaneous* activation of both *clotting* and *fibrinolysis*. This action leads to widespread intravascular deposition of fibrin with resultant thrombotic end-organ complications and consumption of platelets and coagulation proteins, resulting in severe bleeding. DIC is always a secondary phenomenon and not a disease entity in its own right. The clinical expression of DIC varies and may be displayed by laboratory abnormalities alone or in combination with hemorrhagic and thrombotic complications. Because of the variable clinical manifestations and heterogeneity of primary disorders associated with the development of DIC, this entity has been recognized under various different names, including consumptive coagulopathy,[1] hemorrhagic syndrome,[2] defibrination syndrome,[3] or consumptive thrombohemorrhagic disorder.[4]

INCIDENCE

Given that DIC frequently occurs in combination with sepsis, trauma, and systemic inflammatory syndrome, the precise incidence of this condition is difficult to assess.[5,6] The frequency of DIC in hospitalized children is approximately 0.4% to 1%.[7,8] The incidence of DIC according to the underlying disease process is not known. Infection is the most common etiologic factor, contributing to DIC in almost 95% of children, and multiorgan dysfunction occurs in almost 85% of children.[7] Associated comorbidities, such as the underlying disease, multiorgan dysfunction, and respiratory failure, determine the outcome of DIC.[7]

PATHOGENESIS

Physiological Features of Hemostasis

Improved understanding of molecular mechanisms involved in the physiological features of hemostasis has led to better understanding of the pathogenesis of DIC. In healthy individuals, physiological hemostasis is tightly controlled as a balance of forces promoting and impeding coagulation and fibrinolysis. Normally, in response to injury, coagulation is limited to the site of vascular injury. After such injury, platelets adhere to the exposed collagen mediated by the von Willebrand factor, which activates platelets. A signaling cascade within activated platelets causes release of platelet granule contents and facilitates thrombin generation on their surface. As a result of platelet activation and thrombin formation, platelets aggregate, leading to a primary hemostatic plug. Simultaneously, the extrinsic pathway of coagulation is activated. Tissue factor (TF), up-regulated on endothelial cells adjacent to the vascular injury and present on monocytes, forms a complex with circulating factor VII, resulting in the activation of factor VII and the formation of a TF–factor VII/VIIa complex.[9] This complex then activates factors IX and X on the negatively charged phospholipid surface of platelets. Factor Xa, in turn, converts prothrombin to thrombin, the major procoagulant. Thrombin generation is greatly amplified through activation of a feedback loop (intrinsic pathway) through activation of factor XI, which, in turn, activates more factor IX. Thrombin also activates the coagulation cofactors, factor VIII and factor V. Activated factors VIII (VIIIa) and V (Va) increase the efficiency of factor Xa and thrombin generation, respectively, by several orders of magnitude. Once thrombin is generated, it converts soluble fibrinogen to insoluble fibrin. Fibrin monomers polymerize, and adjacent fibrin monomers are cross-linked between their respective D domains by factor XIIIa. The insoluble, cross-linked fibrin enmeshes the platelet plug, forming a secondary hemostatic plug.

This process is kept in check by anticoagulant and fibrinolytic pathways. TF pathway inhibitor is an endogenous anticoagulant protein that binds to and inactivates the TF–factor VIIa complex and factor Xa. Thrombin is quickly inactivated by antithrombin (AT) by forming thrombin-AT (TAT) complexes that are rapidly cleared from plasma. Thrombin also binds to thrombomodulin (TM) on the endothelial surface, abrogating its procoagulant activity. Thrombin-TM complexes, in turn, activate protein C, which, in the presence of its cofactor, protein S, proteolytically inactivates factors VIIIa and Va, dampening further thrombin generation. Fibrinolysis is promoted by thrombin-induced tissue-type plasminogen activator release from endothelial cells, generating plasmin. Plasmin will degrade both soluble fibrinogen and insoluble fibrin. The resultant fragments can be measured as fibrinogen-fibrin degradation products. When plasmin cleaves cross-linked fibrin, it liberates a soluble D-D dimer. Plasmin generation is also regulated through inhibition by plasminogen activator inhibitor type 1. As shown in Figure 343-1, thrombin generation plays a crucial role in interconnecting all of these pathways.[10]

Primary Events of Disseminated Intravascular Coagulation

In DIC, the normal physiological feature of coagulation is disturbed by the simultaneous action of 4 mechanisms: (1) increased thrombin generation, (2) suppressed physiological anticoagulant pathways, (3) activation and subsequent impairment of fibrinolysis, and (4) activation of the inflammatory pathway.[11] Figure 343-2 illustrates the primary events involved in DIC. During an inciting event such as sepsis, monocytes and endothelial cells are injured by toxic

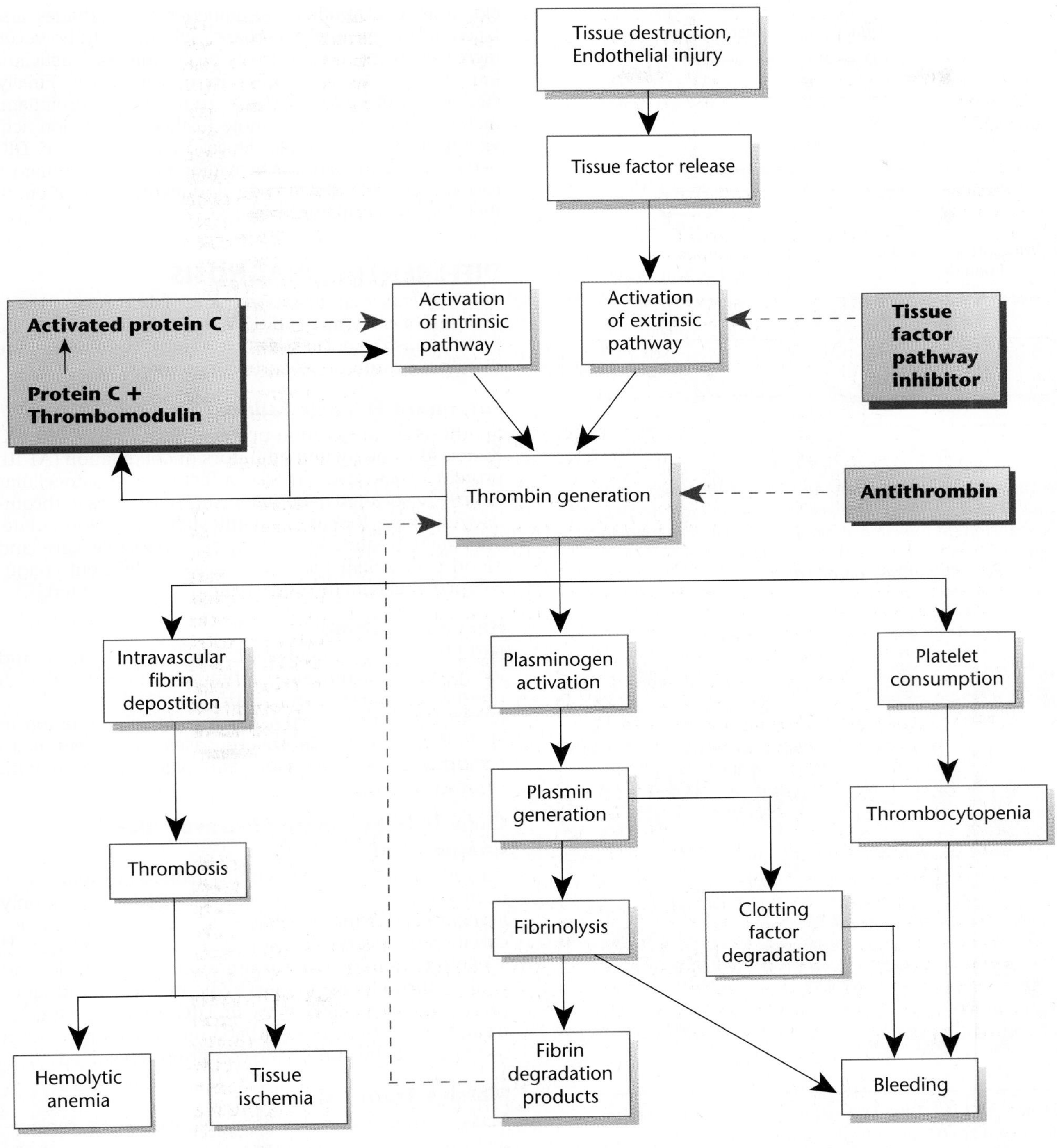

Figure 343-1 Pathophysiological mechanism of disseminated intravascular coagulation.

substances that are elaborated during the disease process. They generate TF, which activates the coagulation cascade (see Figure 343-1). Continuous activation of coagulation leads to an unregulated and explosive generation of thrombin, which, in turn, depletes clotting factors and platelets and activates the fibrinolytic system. Activation of clotting leads to generalized fibrin deposition and microthrombi formation. These microthrombi deposit in various organs, leading to tissue ischemia and multiorgan failure.

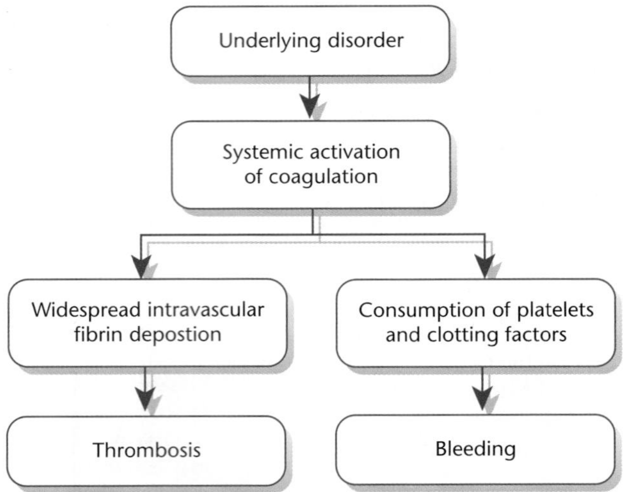

Figure 343-2 Primary events in disseminated intravascular coagulation. *(Levi J, de Jonge E, van der Poll T, et al. Advances in the understanding of the pathogenetic pathways of disseminated intravascular coagulation result in more insight in the clinical picture and better management stategies. Semin Thromb Hemost. 2001;27(6):569-575. Reprinted with permission of Thieme.)*

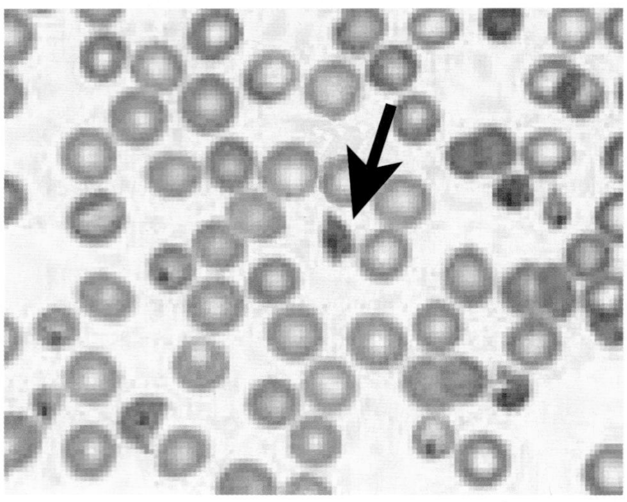

Figure 343-3 Blood smear of a patient with disseminated intravascular coagulation showing schistocytes *(arrow)*.

Deposition of fibrin in microvasculature also leads to mechanical fragmentation of erythrocytes, causing microangiopathic hemolytic anemia (Figure 343-3; see also Figure 343-1). Impaired function of the physiological anticoagulant pathways can amplify thrombin generation and contribute to fibrin formation. Plasma levels of AT are reduced in septic patients, and significant depression of the activated protein C system may occur through consumption and down-regulation of TM expression on the endothelium. An initial hyperfibrinolytic response causes clot lysis, contributing to cutaneous hemorrhages and bleeding into the internal organs. Subsequently, however, increases in the plasma levels of plasminogen activator inhibitor type 1 can suppress fibrinolytic activity. Finally, stimulation of endothelial cells to synthesize proinflammatory cytokines can promote further coagulation activation. Thus the overall clinical manifestation of DIC depends on simultaneous activation of the inflammatory cascade, coagulation cascade, and involvement of endothelial microvasculature.[12,13]

DIFFERENTIAL DIAGNOSIS

The clinical manifestations and laboratory abnormalities of several conditions may mimic or may be indistinguishable from DIC yet may require unique diagnostic evaluations and management.

Fulminant Hepatic Failure

Synthesis of coagulation proteins (factors II, V, VII, IX, X, and fibrinogen) and inhibitors of coagulation (AT III, protein C, and protein S) is affected in hepatocellular failure. Associated hypersplenism contributes to thrombocytopenia. Bleeding manifestations predominate. The main treatment strategy is supportive care and blood component therapy to provide deficient coagulant proteins until the underlying disease is treated.

HELLP Syndrome

HELLP (hemolysis, elevated liver function tests, and low platelets) syndrome is commonly associated with pregnancy. Clinical and laboratory features are similar to DIC, but hypertension is relatively common in HELLP syndrome. In severe cases, treatment is to promptly deliver the fetus and placenta along with supportive care.

Chronic Disseminated Intravascular Coagulation

Chronic DIC, also known as Trousseau syndrome, occurs rarely in children. Chronic DIC is commonly associated with malignancies such as mucinous adenocarcinomas, ovarian cancer, and pancreatic tumors.[14] It exhibits as migratory thrombophlebitis, arterial and venous thrombosis, hemorrhagic diathesis, and laboratory values consistent with DIC. The mainstay of treatment is long-term anticoagulation with heparin therapy until the underlying condition is resolved.

Massive Transfusion

Massive transfusion has been defined as the replacement of more than 1 blood volume in 24 hours or the replacement of 50% of the total blood volume within 3 hours.[15] For example, considering the blood volume of a 30-kg child to be roughly 2400 mL, such a transfusion would require approximately 8 units of blood products over 24 hours or 4 units over 3 hours. Hemostatic failure can result from dilution of clotting factors or acquired platelet dysfunction. Hemostatic tests typically show prolongation of the prothrombin time (PT) and activated partial thromboplastin time (PTT), reduced fibrinogen, and thrombocytopenia. Clinical bleeding associated with hemostatic failure can be managed first with prompt transfusion with cryoprecipitate and fresh-frozen plasma (FFP), although platelet transfusion may be required if bleeding persists. Recent randomized, placebo-controlled, double-blind trials have suggested a benefit of recombinant factor VIIa in the management of excessive perioperative bleeding.[16,17]

Thrombotic Thrombocytopenic Purpura

Thrombotic thrombocytopenic purpura (TTP) is considered a primary disorder in which platelet-rich thrombi form within the microvasculature, leading to tissue ischemia. TTP is caused by congenital (Upshaw-Schulman syndrome) or acquired deficiency of a von Willebrand factor–cleaving protease (ADAMTS13).[18] Patients can exhibit fever, thrombocytopenia, microangiopathic hemolytic anemia, renal failure, and neurologic signs. Screening coagulation tests (PT) and fibrin degradation products are usually normal. Treatment is plasmapheresis and supplementation of ADAMTS13 protease through FFP infusion.

Hemolytic Uremic Syndrome

Hemolytic-uremic syndrome (HUS), the triad of microangiopathic hemolytic anemia, thrombocytopenia, and renal insufficiency, is clinically similar to TTP and is often confused with DIC. HUS occurs in children younger than 3 years. Most cases are caused by Shiga toxin–producing strains of *Escherichia coli*, most often the O157:H7 subtype.[19] Acute mortality in HUS is 3% to 5%, mostly from central nervous system involvement, cardiac failure, or multiorgan failure. Laboratory findings in HUS include microangiopathic hemolytic anemia, with a hemoglobin level of less than 10 g/dL and a negative direct antiglobulin (Coombs) test. HUS is a clinical diagnosis; the presence of schistocytes and helmet cells on the blood smear suggests mechanical trauma. Typical findings accompanying hemolysis include increased indirect bilirubin, decreased haptoglobin, and increased lactate dehydrogenase values. Thrombocytopenia usually is approximately 40×10^3/mcL (40×10^9/L). PT and PTT are normal. Urinalysis shows hematuria and proteinuria. Blood urea nitrogen and creatinine concentrations are elevated, and the albumin concentration may be decreased from protein loss in the gastrointestinal tract. Management is primarily supportive, which includes renal replacement therapy.[20]

EVALUATION

DIC is a clinical diagnosis[21] based on the evaluation of laboratory results in a patient with a clinical condition known to be associated with DIC (Box 343-1).[22] A practical approach to categorize and understand many clinical presentations of DIC is by (1) rate of progression (acute or chronic), (2) extent (localized or systemic), and (3) chief clinical manifestations (thrombotic or hemorrhagic, with or without progressive organ dysfunction).

Relevant History and Physical Examination Findings

Clinical manifestations of DIC include bleeding, thrombosis, or both. However, in general, bleeding manifestations predominate. Bleeding is typically acute and occurs from multiple sites. Bleeding from venipuncture sites and intravascular access sites, such as intra-arterial lines or surgical wounds, is an important early indication of DIC. Mucocutaneous bleeding, such as petechiae, purpura, epistaxis, gum bleeding, bleeding after tracheal suctioning, gastrointestinal bleeding, and hematuria, is commonly observed. In more advanced cases, internal bleeding in vital organs such as brain, lung, heart, and gastrointestinal system may constitute a medical emergency, with patients experiencing raised intracranial pressure, brain herniation, respiratory compromise, or shock. Generalized microvascular thrombosis may produce purpura fulminans, peripheral acrocyanosis, and pregangrenous changes in

BOX 343-1 Causes of Disseminated Intravascular Coagulation in Children

SEPSIS OR SEVERE INFECTION
Any microorganism
(eg, HIV, cytomegalovirus, varicella, hepatitis)
Fungal (eg, *Histoplasma*)
Parasitic (eg, malaria)

TRAUMA
Polytrauma
Neurotrauma
Fat embolism

ORGAN FAILURE
Severe pancreatitis
Liver cell failure

MALIGNANCY
Acute promyelocytic leukemia
Lymphoproliferative disorders
Hemophagocytic lymphohistiocytosis
Solid tumors

OBSTETRICAL CALAMITIES
Dead fetus syndrome
Abruptio placentae
Amniotic fluid embolism

VASCULAR ABNORMALITIES
Kasabach-Merritt syndrome
Large vascular aneurysms

IMMUNOLOGIC CONDITIONS
Systemic lupus erythematosus
Autoimmune hemolytic anemia
Crohn disease
Ulcerative colitis
Transfusion reactions
Transplant rejection

MISCELLANEOUS
Snake bites
Recreational drugs
Poisoning
Burns
Massive transfusions

digits, genitalia, and nose. Microvascular thrombosis in various organs further contributes to multiorgan failure and hemodynamic instability.

Laboratory Testing

The role of laboratory tests in DIC is to show evidence of a consumptive coagulopathy with activation of the fibrinolytic cascade. A complete blood cell count may show moderate to severe thrombocytopenia with or without anemia. Thrombocytopenia is present in approximately 50% of patients and suggests consumption of platelets, whereas anemia might be caused by bleeding or mechanical destruction of red blood cells. Presence of fragmented red blood cells (schistocytes) on blood smear confirms the diagnosis of microvascular angiopathy (see Figure 343-3). Screening tests for the extrinsic and intrinsic coagulation cascade such as the PT and PTT, respectively, are prolonged in 50% to 60% of patients, reflecting consumption of many coagulation proteins, including prothrombin; factors V, VII, and VIII; and fibrinogen. Fibrinogen-fibrin degradation products or D-dimers are both increased in concentration in most patients with DIC, suggesting activation of the fibrinolytic process.

The most sensitive tests for diagnosis of DIC are markers of endogenous thrombin generation: prothrombin fragment 1.2 and TAT complexes. Prothrombin fragment 1.2 is released when thrombin is generated from prothrombin. TAT complexes are generated by binding of thrombin with its inhibitor AT.

In practice, although the standard assays are relatively rapid and simple to perform, changes in these test results do not always occur at the same time, and laboratory values change rapidly based on the patient's clinical status, which may create confusion in patient management. These changes also make the diagnosis of DIC at an early stage particularly difficult. A scoring system based on clinical and laboratory criteria to diagnose DIC has been established and is still being validated.[22,23] The International Society for Thrombosis and Hemostasis Scientific Standardization, Subcommittee on DIC, proposed a scoring system developed from a previously described set of diagnostic criteria.[24] The 5-step algorithm assigns a score based on the severity of abnormality for each of the following: platelet count ($>100 \times 10^9$/L = 0; $<100 \times 10^9$/L = 1; $<50 \times 10^9$/L = 2), elevated fibrin-related markers (no increase = 0; moderate increase = 2; strong increase = 3), prolonged PT (<3 seconds = 0; >3 seconds but <6 seconds = 1; >6 seconds = 2), and fibrinogen level (>1 g/L = 0; <1 g/L = 1). A total score of 5 or more is considered compatible with DIC. The sensitivity and specificity of this scoring system are more than 90%. However, the algorithm should only be applied in the presence of an underlying disorder known to be associated with DIC. Recent observations have suggested that scoring for rates of change in the PT, platelet count, and D-dimer levels can help identify non-overt DIC in the early stages.[25]

MANAGEMENT

Most children with DIC will either already be in the intensive care unit because of their underlying disease or require admission because of the disease complications that can occur. The fundamental principal of DIC treatment is the specific and vigorous treatment of the underlying disorder. In some cases, DIC will completely resolve within hours after resolution of the underlying condition (for example, in cases of DIC induced by placental abruption or intrauterine fetal demise). However, in other cases, supportive measures are required to control the DIC until the underlying condition is resolved (for example, the use of all-trans-retinoic acid and chemotherapy for the treatment of acute promyelocytic leukemia and DIC).[26] Recent insights[27] into mechanisms that contribute to DIC have been helpful in developing new preventive, supportive, and therapeutic management strategies, although therapeutic decisions remain controversial and need to be individualized according to the underlying basis for the DIC and severity of the clinical symptoms. Box 343-2 lists the key components of management of DIC.

Clinical Monitoring

The underlying condition, the DIC itself, and response to therapy can rapidly change the clinical manifestations of the disease in the children. Therefore frequent clinical monitoring along with monitoring of PT, PTT, fibrinogen, and platelet counts may be needed several times per day. Monitoring of D-dimer levels once every day is usually enough.

Treatment Modalities

Blood Component Therapy

Low levels of platelets and coagulation factors may increase the risk of bleeding. Hence treatment with

BOX 343-2 Treatment of Disseminated Intravascular Coagulation

- Aggressive treatment of the underlying cause
- Obtaining reliable venous access and considering central venous access
- Possible multiorgan support required:
  - Ventilatory support
  - Circulatory resuscitation or inotropic agents
  - Hemodialysis
- Blood product support if evidence of active bleeding:
  - Platelets if less than 50×10^9/L
  - Fresh frozen plasma if clotting times prolonged (dose: 15 mL/kg)
  - Cryoprecipitate to keep fibrinogen more than 100 mg/dL (dose: 1-1.5 bags/10 kg)
  - Packed red blood cell transfusion (dose: 10 mL/kg)
  - Recombinant VIIa for intractable bleeding or volume overload (dose: 75 mcg/kg every 2 hours)
  - Recombinant human activated protein C in desperate situations with severe sepsis and multiple organ failure, provided platelet count is not less than 50×10^9/L (dose: 24 mcg/kg per hour for 24-72 hours)

FFP, fibrinogen, cryoprecipitate, or platelets appears to be a rational therapy in bleeding patients or patients who are at risk for bleeding with a significant depletion of these hemostatic factors. However, blood component therapy should not be instituted based on laboratory results alone; it is indicated only in patients with active bleeding, those who require an invasive procedure, or those who are otherwise at risk for bleeding complications.[28] Using large volumes of plasma may be necessary to correct the coagulation defect.

Anticoagulants

Use of heparin or other anticoagulants appears reasonable to inhibit thrombin generation, considering the central role played by thrombin in DIC. Experimental studies and case reports have shown that heparin can at least partly inhibit the activation of coagulation in sepsis and other causes of DIC.[29] However, a beneficial effect of heparin on clinically important outcome events in patients with DIC has never been demonstrated in controlled clinical trials. In addition, the safety of heparin treatment is debatable in patients who have DIC and who are prone to bleeding. Hence using heparin is not a standard of care in overt cases of DIC. However, therapeutic doses of heparin are indicated in patients with clinically overt thromboembolism, chronic DIC, or extensive fibrin deposition such as seen in purpura fulminans or acral ischemia.

Restoration of Natural Anticoagulant Pathways

Another therapeutic option that seems appealing is to restore natural coagulation inhibitors to physiological levels. Use of FFP as a source of AT, protein C, and protein S is not practical because of the short plasma half-life of these proteins. Hence AT concentrates and protein C concentrates were extensively evaluated in patients with DIC.[30-32] Although trials of AT[33] were not so successful, the double-blind, placebo-controlled, phase III trial of recombinant human activated PA **w**orldwide **e**valuation in **s**evere **s**epsis (known as the PROWESS trial) was successful, creating a significant decrease in mortality when compared with the placebo group.[24] Hence recombinant activated protein C has been used in patients with sepsis. Bleeding is the only recognized adverse effect with this therapy. Maintaining platelets above 30×10^9/L is prudent during this therapy. The dose of recombinant activated protein C is 24 mcg/kg/hour.[34] Newer anticoagulants against the TF–factor VIIa complex, such as recombinant nematode anticoagulant protein c2, are currently being evaluated in phase II/III clinical studies.[35-38]

Other Agents

Recently, recombinant factor VIIa (rVIIa) has become an attractive strategy to control bleeding in various scenarios. In situations in which volume overload is an issue or bleeding persists despite adequate blood component support, use of rVIIa (75 mcg/kg every 2 hours) has been shown to be effective.[39,40] High doses of rVIIa (250 mcg/kg every 2-4 hours) have been shown to inhibit fibrinolysis in patients with severe hemophilia A with inhibitors.[41]

CONCLUSION

DIC has been associated with unacceptably high mortality. New information about the pathophysiological features and treatment of DIC promises new hope of an improved prognosis for this disorder. Understanding the relationship between inflammation and coagulation has led to a conceptual shift in the treatment strategy for DIC. Coordinated clinical efforts are required to study the safety and efficacy of newer agents in the treatment of DIC.

REFERENCES

1. Bick RL. Disseminated intravascular coagulation and related syndromes: a clinical review. *Semin Thromb Hemost*. 1988;14:299-338.
2. Rodriguez-Erdmann F. Bleeding due to increased intravascular blood coagulation. Hemorrhagic syndromes caused by consumption of blood-clotting factors (consumption-coagulopathies). *N Engl J Med*. 1965;273:1370-1378.
3. Merckey C, Johnson AJ, Kleiner GJ, et al. The defibrination syndrome: clinical features and laboratory diagnosis. *Br J Haematol*. 2006;13:528.
4. Pateiuk VG. Thrombohemorrhagic syndrome in patients with meningococcal infection. *Klin Med (Mosk)*. 1975;53:60-65.
5. Gando S, Kameue T, Nanzaki S, et al. Disseminated intravascular coagulation is a frequent complication of systemic inflammatory response syndrome. *Thromb Haemost*. 1996;75:224-228.
6. Gando S, Kameue T, Nanzaki S, et al. Cytokines, soluble thrombomodulin and disseminated intravascular coagulation in patients with systemic inflammatory response syndrome. *Thromb Res*. 1995;80:519-526.
7. Oren H, Cingoz I, Duman M, et al. Disseminated intravascular coagulation in pediatric patients: clinical and laboratory features and prognostic factors influencing the survival. *Pediatr Hematol Oncol*. 2005;22:679-688.
8. Manco-Johnson MJ. Disseminated intravascular coagulation. In: Hoekelman RA, ed. *Primary Pediatric Care*. 3rd ed. St Louis, MO: Mosby Elsevier; 1997.
9. Lwaleed BA, Bass PS. Tissue factor pathway inhibitor: structure, biology and involvement in disease. *J Pathol*. 2006;208:327-339.
10. Levi M. Disseminated intravascular coagulation: what's new? *Crit Care Clin*. 2005;21:449-467.
11. van der Poll T, Buller HR, ten Cate H, et al. Activation of coagulation after administration of tumor necrosis factor to normal subjects. *N Engl J Med*. 1990;322:1622-1627.
12. Levi M, Keller TT, van Gorp E, et al. Infection and inflammation and the coagulation system. *Cardiovasc Res*. 2003;60:26-39.
13. van der Poll T, de Jonge E, Levi M. Regulatory role of cytokines in disseminated intravascular coagulation. *Semin Thromb Hemost*. 2001;27:639-651.
14. Rak J, Milsom C, May L, et al. Tissue factor in cancer and angiogenesis: the molecular link between genetic tumor progression, tumor neovascularization, and cancer coagulopathy. *Semin Thromb Hemost*. 2006;32:54-70.
15. Hardy JF, de Moerloose P, Samama CM. The coagulopathy of massive transfusion. *Vox Sang*. 2005;89:123-127.
16. Boffard KD, Riou B, Warren B, et al. Recombinant factor VIIa as adjunctive therapy for bleeding control in severely injured trauma patients: two parallel randomized, placebo-controlled, double-blind clinical trials. *J Trauma*. 2005;59:8-15.

17. Friederich PW, Geerdink MG, Spataro M, et al. The effect of the administration of recombinant activated factor VII (NovoSeven) on perioperative blood loss in patients undergoing transabdominal retropubic prostatectomy: the PROSE study. *Blood Coagul Fibrinolysis.* 2000;11(1);S129-S132.
18. Murrin RJ, Murray JA. Thrombotic thrombocytopenic purpura: aetiology, pathophysiology and treatment. *Blood Rev.* 2006;20:51-60.
19. Karmali MA, Steele BT, Petric M, et al. Sporadic cases of haemolytic-uraemic syndrome associated with faecal cytotoxin and cytotoxin-producing Escherichia coli in stools. *Lancet.* 1983;1:619-620.
20. Tarr PI, Gordon CA, Chandler WL. Shiga-toxin-producing Escherichia coli and haemolytic uraemic syndrome. *Lancet.* 2005;365:1073-1086.
21. Mant MJ, King EG. Severe, acute disseminated intravascular coagulation. A reappraisal of its pathophysiology, clinical significance and therapy based on 47 patients. *Am J Med. October.* 1979;67(4):557-563.
22. Taylor FB, Toh CH, Hoots WK, et al. Towards definition, clinical and laboratory criteria, and a scoring system for disseminated intravascular coagulation. *Thromb Haemost.* 2001;86:1327-1330.
23. Gando S, Wada H, Asakura H, et al. Evaluation of new Japanese diagnostic criteria for disseminated intravascular coagulation in critically ill patients. *Clin Appl Thromb Hemost.* 2005;11:71-76.
24. Taylor FB, Toh CH, Hoots WK, et al. Towards definition, clinical and laboratory criteria, and a scoring system for disseminated intravascular coagulation. *Thromb Haemost.* 2001;86:1327-1330.
25. Bakhtiari K, Meijers JC, de Jonge E, et al. Prospective validation of the International Society of Thrombosis and Haemostasis scoring system for disseminated intravascular coagulation. *Crit Care Med. December.* 2004;32(12); 2416-2421.
26. Falanga A, Rickles FR. Pathogenesis and management of the bleeding diathesis in acute promyelocytic leukaemia. *Best Pract Res Clin Haematol.* 2003;16:463-482.
27. Levi M, de Jonge E, van der Poll T. New treatment strategies for disseminated intravascular coagulation based on current understanding of the pathophysiology. *Ann Med.* 2004;36(1);41-49.
28. Levi M, de Jonge E, van der Poll T. Plasma and plasma components in the management of disseminated intravascular coagulation. *Best Pract Res Clin Haematol.* 2006;19:127-142.
29. Pernerstorfer T, Hollenstein U, Hansen J, et al. Heparin blunts endotoxin-induced coagulation activation. *Circulation.* 1999;100:2485-2490.
30. Hoffmann JN, Muhlbayer D, Jochum M, et al. Effect of long-term and high-dose antithrombin supplementation on coagulation and fibrinolysis in patients with severe sepsis. *Crit Care Med.* 2004;32:1851-1859.
31. Dhainaut JF, Yan SB, Joyce DE, et al. Treatment effects of drotrecogin alfa (activated) in patients with severe sepsis with or without overt disseminated intravascular coagulation. *J Thromb Haemost.* 2004;2:1924-1933.
32. Fourrier F, Chopin C, Huart JJ, et al. Double-blind, placebo-controlled trial of antithrombin III concentrates in septic shock with disseminated intravascular coagulation. *Chest.* 1993;104:882-888.
33. Wiedermann CJ, Hoffmann JN, Juers M, et al. High-dose antithrombin III in the treatment of severe sepsis in patients with a high risk of death: efficacy and safety. *Crit Care Med.* 2006;34:285-292.
34. Sajan I, Da-Silva SS, Dellinger RP. Drotrecogin alfa (activated) in an infant with gram-negative septic shock. *J Intensive Care Med.* 2004;19:51-55.
35. Lee AY, Vlasuk GP. Recombinant nematode anticoagulant protein c2 and other inhibitors targeting blood coagulation factor VIIa/tissue factor. *J Intern Med.* 2003;254:313-321.
36. Moons AH, Peters RJ, Bijsterveld NR, et al. Recombinant nematode anticoagulant protein c2, an inhibitor of the tissue factor/factor VIIa complex, in patients undergoing elective coronary angioplasty. *J Am Coll Cardiol.* 2003;41:2147-2153.
37. Barton P, Kalil AC, Nadel S, et al. Safety, pharmacokinetics, and pharmacodynamics of drotrecogin alfa (activated) in children with severe sepsis. *Pediatrics.* 2004;113:7-17.
38. Abraham E, Reinhart K, Svoboda P, et al. Assessment of the safety of recombinant tissue factor pathway inhibitor in patients with severe sepsis: a multicenter, randomized, placebo-controlled, single-blind, dose escalation study. *Crit Care Med.* 2001;29:2081-2089.
39. Bielanow T, Sidor M, Maciejewski M, et al. Effectiveness of recombinant activated factor VIIA (NovoSeven) in case of severe obstetric complication with coagulopathy. *Ginekol Pol.* 2003;74:1055-1059.
40. Franchini M, Zaffanello M, Veneri D. Recombinant factor VIIa. An update on its clinical use. *Thromb Haemost.* 2005;93:1027-1035.
41. Lisman T, Mosnier LO, Lambert T, et al. Inhibition of fibrinolysis by recombinant factor VIIa in plasma from patients with severe hemophilia A. *Blood.* 2002;99: 175-179.

Chapter 344

DROWNING AND NEAR DROWNING

Lorry R. Frankel, MD

Drowning and *near drowning* refer to submersion accidents. *Drowning* is defined as death caused by suffocation within 24 hours after submersion in a liquid medium. *Near drowning* refers to an event whereby a person has survived this initial time period through resuscitative efforts. *Submersion injury* is now the term more commonly used for *drowning* and *near drowning.*[1] Drowning remains an important cause of accidental death among children and adolescents, ranking second to motor vehicles as the leading cause of accidental death in this age group.[2]

Submersion injuries are among the most tragic and catastrophic accidents that can occur to children. Within a matter of minutes, a perfectly healthy child may die from submersion or may be left with severe neurologic injury. Although the mortality rates for submersion injuries have declined, survival may result in neurologic injuries ranging from a permanent vegetative state to motor and cognitive disabilities.[3,4]

The most important determinant in the patient's outcome is the success of resuscitative measures at the scene of submersion. Patients who are conscious at arrival at a hospital have an excellent chance of intact survival. Pulmonary injury can be managed successfully with newer innovative approaches to mechanical ventilation. Persons with the worst prognosis are those who continue to require resuscitation in the emergency department (ED).[5] This remains true despite the age of the patient, duration of submersion, pH at the time of care, or body temperature. The best predictor of outcome is return of normal neurologic function within 24 to 72 hours. The fact that people who do not have a return of cognitive function within 72 hours of the hypoxic episode either do not survive or do so in a persistent vegetative state has been well documented. Other poor prognostic findings include continuation of cardiopulmonary resuscitation (CPR) beyond 25 minutes; fixed, dilated pupils; seizures; flaccidity; a Glasgow coma score of less than 5; and decreased cerebral blood flow.[6,7] Cold-water submersions that produce severe hypothermia may influence the outcome, but not all victims of hypothermic submersion escape serious neurologic sequelae.

EPIDEMIOLOGIC CONSIDERATIONS

In the United States, approximately 1400 drowning deaths occur each year in patients younger than 19 years. The groups most at risk include children younger than 5 and boys between ages 5 and 19.[2-4] The drowning rate is higher for white children than for black children younger than 5.[8] The overall outcome for submersion injuries appears to be bimodal, with children either dying or being discharged home. A few children are either discharged home with skilled nursing care or discharged to a long-term or chronic care facility.

The circumstances that surround submersion injuries vary by age and geographic region. Bathtub submersion injuries are more common in children younger than 1 year of age who are left in the care of an older sibling or who are without adult supervision. Child abuse should be suspected when bathtub submersion events occur. Bathtub submersion injuries may be associated with scald burns from hot water.[3-5,9] Toddlers are more likely than older children to experience submersion injuries in family swimming pools, hot tubs, or on top of pools by falling into a puddle of water on top of the pool cover. Older children and adolescents may experience submersion injuries during a diving accident. Adolescent and adult drowning incidents are often associated with drinking alcohol or using drugs, which may impair judgment and increase risk-taking behaviors.

Not all submersion injuries are fatal. However, the morbidity may not be inconsequential. For every submersion injury that results in a death within 24 hours, approximately 4 hospital admissions and 14 ED visits occur. Despite efforts to educate children about pool safety, submersion injuries continue to plague the pediatric community. Community education and mandatory barriers around private pools have resulted in a reduction in the number of submersion injuries.[2,4,10]

PATHOPHYSIOLOGICAL FEATURES OF SUBMERSION INJURIES

Asphyxia, anoxia, hypothermia, and reperfusion injuries are the hallmarks of submersion injuries. The child initially panics, then holds his/her breath and loses consciousness.[3,5,7,10,11] During this period, the child may lose cough and gag reflexes, then aspirate large amounts of water. This action produces anoxia, resulting in decreased oxygen delivery to the tissues. The child's heart rhythm becomes abnormal, with evidence of fibrillation and finally asystole. In addition, the child's core temperature begins to drop. Theoretically the type of fluid aspirated will affect the circulatory volume and electrolyte balance. Fresh water is hypotonic and is rapidly absorbed across the alveoli, which may result in increased blood volume, hemodilution, a reduction in serum electrolytes, and hemolysis. On the other hand, a submersion injury in salt water may result in hemoconcentration, decreased blood volume, and an elevation in serum electrolytes.

For blood volume to be seriously altered, the patient must aspirate at least 11 mL of fluid per kilogram of body weight; at least twice this amount must be aspirated to result in marked electrolyte changes. However, most children aspirate less than 4 mL/kg of fluid, which means that, practically speaking, little clinical relevance exists to the type of water in which the child is submerged. Most patients who experience near drowning are intravascularly hypovolemic as a result of capillary leak from asphyxia. The effects on the body may be on a single system or may be multisystem. In addition to hypovolemia, patients who experience near drowning may experience serious injury to other organ systems, including the following: (1) pulmonary injury with surfactant washout and aspiration of gastric contents or contaminated water contents, (2) central nervous system (CNS) injury resulting from anoxic or ischemic events, (3) myocardial injury, (4) renal impairment, (5) injury to the gut mucosa, and (6) liver function abnormalities.[3,5,7,10]

Pulmonary Effects

Usually the lungs are the most seriously affected organs. The decrease in the functional residual capacity of the lungs results in hypoxia and hypercarbia. The lung injury may progress from either aspiration pneumonia or simple pulmonary edema with alterations in surfactant to the acute lung injury commonly referred to as *acute respiratory distress syndrome*. The child may have apnea or agonal respirations or may have difficulty with airway protection. Understanding these changes will enable the astute clinician to act appropriately to prevent further hypoxic or anoxic injury.

If spontaneous respirations are present, then the clinician should first administer oxygen to the child. If the child does not possess the capability to protect the airway, then the airway must be intubated with the endotracheal tube of appropriate size. Initial ventilatory settings will require enough tidal volume (6-10 mL/kg) or inspiratory pressure to allow for adequate rising of the chest wall. Higher tidal volumes may be associated with ventilator-induced lung injury. Positive end-expiratory pressure (4-8 cm H_2O) must be used to help alveolar distension.[3,12] An age-appropriate respiratory rate and a fraction of inspired oxygen of 1.0 should be provided. The child should undergo a chest radiograph examination so the degree of lung injury can be evaluated and to make certain that the endotracheal tube is correctly placed.[10]

Hemodynamic Effects

The cardiovascular system may be seriously affected as a result of the period of anoxia. Myocardial contractility may be greatly reduced, and the patient may require inotropic support in the form of dopamine, epinephrine, or dobutamine. The goal will be to hydrate the child adequately with 20 to 40 mL/kg of isotonic crystalloid or colloid. If the hemodynamic response is suboptimal, then inotropes should be added. To accomplish this task safely and effectively, a central venous catheter and an arterial line should be inserted. A double-lumen catheter should be used for the central venous access. The distal port should be used to transduce the central venous pressure (CVP) and the proximal port used to infuse inotropes. The line may be inserted into any one of several vessels (subclavian, internal jugular, external jugular, femoral).

The child will require continuous monitoring of vital signs as well as CVP. CVP monitoring enables the clinician to understand better the child's volume status, which helps guide fluid administration. An arterial line will enable continuous monitoring of the mean arterial pressure, which should be kept in the correct range for age. If the patient continues to struggle with high CVPs and poor cardiac output, then the clinician should consider placing a pulmonary artery catheter to measure the wedge pressure, which is a reflection of a true CVP. Cardiovascular instability, hypotensive shock and metabolic acidosis may persist. Therefore the clinician must understand that hypovolemia and decreased myocardial function may result from the asphyxial component of submersion injuries. The cardiogenic component may be related to hypoxic injury, dysrhythmia, or metabolic acidosis. In addition, pulmonary vascular resistance may be increased as a result of pulmonary vasoconstriction and the release of various inflammatory mediators. This increased resistance will affect right-sided heart function and further decrease left-sided heart performance. This additive effect will result in decreased left-sided filling pressures and a further decrease in oxygen delivery to an already compromised periphery, which will further potentiate the metabolic acidosis seen with submersion injuries. If cardiovascular instability continues, then the clinician must consider sepsis or further myocardial dysfunction.[3,13]

Effects on the Central Nervous System

Profound CNS dysfunction is the ultimate complication of submersion injuries. The duration of hypoxia and hypotension determine the severity of the neurologic injury seen after serious submersion events. As the neurons are deprived of oxygen, the patient loses consciousness. After this stage, blood flow to the CNS may be increased, resulting in a reperfusion injury, followed by a marked decrease in cerebral blood flow. Thus the clinician may see severe CNS injury even after the restoration of cardiac output, normalization of blood pressure, and adequate oxygenation.

Given that intensive care unit techniques have advanced to improve cardiac output and innovations in mechanical ventilation have resulted in restoration of a favorable acid-base status and oxygenation, the degree of CNS injury remains the major determinant of survival and neurologic morbidity in patients with asystole who are resuscitated and then transferred to a pediatric intensive care unit (PICU).[7,11] The exact mechanism of CNS injury is complex and includes increased intracranial pressure, vasogenic changes in autoregulation and cytotoxic cerebral edema, and the accumulation of various metabolites and oxygen free radicals. Although hypothermia may have some protective effects on the CNS, the child's outcome after submersion injuries will be determined within the first 24 to 72 hours.[11]

Multisystem Organ Effects

In addition to the pulmonary, hemodynamic, and CNS effects, the other organ systems in the body may also be adversely affected. These organ systems include the gastrointestinal system, the liver, kidney, and hematopoietic systems with disseminated intravascular coagulation. One of the other ominous signs is discharge from the rectum of material sloughed from the intestinal mucosa mixed with blood. This discharge is commonly associated with severe hypoxic-ischemic injury after the perfusion to the gastrointestinal tract becomes severely reduced, followed by gut necrosis. In addition, severe hypoxic-ischemic injuries may result in coagulopathy, renal failure, and predisposition to infection.[2,3]

Other Effects

One of the most commonly associated physiological changes that occur in submersion injuries is hypothermia. Children submerged in cold water (<5°C [41°F]) have had astonishing outcomes. The period of submersion hypothermia may protect the CNS. Severe hypothermia results in a decrease in energy use and thus decreases the metabolic rate of the brain. For each 1°C reduction in core temperature, the cerebral blood flow is reduced by 6% to 7%. Severe hypothermia may result in cardiac dysrhythmia, loss of consciousness, and a predisposition to infection.[3,4,11]

During a submersion incident, the diving reflex may provide some form of protection. This well-known reflex, which is present in diving mammals such as seals, allows oxygen to be conserved. The diving reflex enables these animals to be submerged for 15 or 20 minutes. The reflex results in a marked reduction of blood flow to tissues that are more resistant to hypoxia while preserving blood flow to more sensitive organs such as the brain and heart. However, the role of the diving reflex in submersion in children is uncertain.

In addition to hypothermia and the diving reflex, other preexisting associated conditions may be relevant in submersion injuries. Children with underlying seizure disorders, occult cardiomyopathy, or alterations in the conduction system may be predisposed to submersion injuries.[14,15]

APPROACH TO SUBMERSION INJURY

The approach to a child who has experienced significant submersion injury has been standardized and involves a minimum of 4 phases: (1) initial lay person rescue at the scene, (2) emergency medical team or paramedic response, (3) stabilization in the ED, and (4) care in the PICU.

Initial Lay Person Rescue

The initial lay person rescue at the scene consists of identifying the problem, calling 911, removing the child from the water, and clearing the airway and performing CPR until the emergency medical team arrives. Effective CPR at the scene is one of the major determinants of success in submersion injuries. The lay rescuer should note the time that CPR was initiated. If possible, an estimation of length of time of submersion should be noted, as should the temperature of the water.

Emergency Medical Team or Paramedic Response

At the scene, determining the extent of the CNS injury is initially often difficult. Therefore every effort is made to resuscitate the child to restore cardiac output, oxygenation, and acid-base status. The best approach is to ignore the down time that the child may have had during this initial resuscitative phase. Assessing the patency of the airway is critical, as is clearing the airway of any debris before attempting to ventilate the patient with either a bag-mask device or through intubation in the field. Efforts should be made to protect the airway from the aspiration of stomach contents and the lungs from aggressive positive pressure ventilation, which may produce overdistention of the lungs and possibly barotrauma.

Once a heart rate has been established and adequate chest wall rise is observed, the child should be transported to the closest ED that can deal with children. The child's vital signs, including temperature, should be assessed, and the child's cardiorespiratory status should be monitored, which includes continuous electrocardiographic monitoring, recording of oxygen saturation, and, if possible, intermittent recording of blood pressure.[16]

Stabilization in the Emergency Department

On arrival in the ED, for further stabilization and evaluation in the ED, the child should be placed in a room large enough to provide enough space for the many interventions that will be required: a careful examination, which includes a survey to ascertain whether any other traumatic injuries exist that are associated with the submersion event (eg, head injury, thoracoabdominal injury); further stabilization of the patient, which will include the use of equipment needed for vascular access, gastric decompression, and bladder catheterization; and provision of appropriate respiratory support.

For children who are spontaneously moving and breathing, close observation and monitoring are required to ensure that response to the submersion injury is not delayed. Children who are well saturated in room air and who have age-appropriate responses and a normal Glasgow coma score may be discharged after 4 to 8 hours; however, those who require significant amounts of oxygen or who have abnormal sensorium need to be admitted to the hospital. They may also require imaging studies while in the ED to make certain that the internal organs are not adversely affected.[3,5,6]

Patients who were intubated in the field will require thorough evaluation in the ED before being extubated. At most institutions, these children will probably remain intubated and mechanically ventilated, then they will be transferred to the closest PICU. The stomach must be decompressed with a nasogastric tube, a bladder catheter must be placed to measure urine output, and appropriate vascular access lines must be inserted. If the patient was not intubated in the field but now has poor oxygenation, displays signs that indicate increased work of breathing, or has a high oxygen requirement, then positive pressure ventilation is indicated. The child should then be intubated with an appropriately sized endotracheal tube. The patient should be placed on the appropriate ventilator setting for the patient's underlying condition.

To facilitate intubation, the physicians may administer a muscle relaxant and an analgesic-amnesic agent. Before the patient is transferred to the PICU, the child's neurologic condition must be carefully determined. In addition, if indicated, the physician may wish to order a head computed tomographic scan to evaluate the brain and to determine whether an associated traumatic head injury has occurred.[3-5] The cervical spine must be cleared.[17] All lines and tubes must be stabilized to make certain that the patient cannot dislodge any of the lines or the endotracheal tube.

Efforts should be made to restore vascular volume with an isotonic solution (10-20 mL/kg). The patient should be warmed to prevent hypothermia, which is associated with abnormal cardiac rhythms.[18] Antibiotic treatment may be initiated if the patient aspirated contaminated water or if pulmonary infection is suspected. Before transfer to the PICU, radiographic studies must be performed to confirm the placement of the endotracheal tube, vascular access catheters, and contour of the lungs. Patients should also be assessed to ensure that no pneumothorax or other evidence of air leak exists.[12]

Care in the Pediatric Intensive Care Unit

On arrival into the PICU, the clinician will closely monitor all aspects of the patient's vital signs, including oxygen saturation and, if intubated, end-tidal carbon dioxide. All PICU efforts are aimed at minimizing any injury that resulted from the submersion event itself because the primary injury—the hypoxic-ischemic event—cannot currently be treated.

If the patient is intubated, an arterial line should be placed, and if the child requires cardiovascular support with inotropes, then a central venous catheter should be placed. Further management is aimed at restoring cardiac output, minimizing injury to the brain, and preventing catastrophic complications. Neurointensive care support is often required; however, aggressive management of intracranial hypertension with osmotic agents, hypothermia, hyperventilation, steroids, or barbiturate-induced coma has not proven to be of much benefit. In fact, these interventions may increase the risk for nosocomial infections, pulmonary insufficiency, and cardiac dysfunction.[3-5]

The approach taken in the PICU varies from institution to institution, but the major goal is always to restore the child, if possible, to the previous state of health by preventing further injury to the brain. Efforts should be made to assess the degree of neurologic injury over the first 24 to 48 hours. Electroencephalographic monitoring may help recognize electrical seizures. Seizure activity should be treated quickly and aggressively. Monitoring intracranial pressure has not proven to be of benefit for these patients.[19] Patients should only receive sedation if it is clinically indicated. The severity of the encephalopathy is the main determinant of outcome.

When possible, nutritional support is provided either in the form of parenteral nutrition or enteral nutrition if the intestinal tract can tolerate feeds. Normalization of blood gases by various ventilatory strategies (to ensure adequate oxygenation and acid-base status) is preferred to hyperventilation.[3-5] Appropriate support of the cardiovascular system with inotropes as needed to maintain an adequate blood pressure is required to maintain blood flow to vital organs.[13] Minimizing the development of stress ulcers in the gastric mucosa is vitally important; thus agents may be used to maintain a gastric pH of more than 5. Appropriate use of antibiotics to treat suspected or proven infections is often necessary because submersion victims are susceptible to bacterial infections that result from aspiration of water. Bacterial infections may also result from complications of mechanical ventilation or vascular access attempts. Therefore initiating empiric antibiotic treatment may be reasonable.

A periodic review of blood tests for changes in hematocrit level, coagulation profile, or white blood cell count is also important. A review of liver and renal function studies helps the clinician ascertain whether other organs have been injured. Unusual forms of ventilatory support may include the use of high-frequency ventilation for acute pulmonary injury, inhaled nitric oxide for severe hypoxia-induced respiratory failure, and extracorporeal oxygenation. Extracorporeal oxygenation, which may be used for rewarming, theoretically allows the lungs to rest and prevent barotraumas associated with high airway pressures.[20-22]

When Neurologic Function Is Likely to Be Impaired

When a child has experienced a serious submersion injury and is still comatose after 72 hours after the incident despite interventions, the child will not likely recover neurologic function. This fact must be explained to the child's parents within 12 to 24 hours after the child's admission to the PICU. A multidisciplinary meeting (neurologists, primary care physician, PICU nurses, and a social worker assigned to the case) should be held with the family to explain in great detail the potential outcomes of children who have experienced a serious submersion injury and who are still comatose.

At this initial meeting, depending on the child's clinical condition, the full spectrum of outcome should be presented in an open and forthright manner: the child may regain much, but not all, of previous neurologic function; the child may experience less severe neurologic sequelae; or the child may remain in a vegetative state or may experience brain death.

During the next 48 to 72 hours, if the patient does not return to appropriate neurologic functioning, then the family is presented with this information again so that the difficult process of deciding what to do next can begin. The parents need to make informed decisions about aggressive approaches to care. Once the determination has been made that the child's chances for meaningful survival are remote, the family may be presented with information about the potential need for technology-based ongoing support; long-term mechanical ventilation, tracheostomy, gastrostomy feeds, and fundoplication should all be discussed. In addition, the parents may consider placing the child in a long-term or chronic care facility or nursing the child at home.

A pediatric palliative care consultation will help the parents make these complex decisions.[23] Family members must participate in decisions about further aggressive care or decisions to limit or withdraw care based on the potential for poor outcome. This participation empowers the parents to decide to limit aggressive interventions that will not change the ultimate outcome. A natural death may result from withdrawing life support. If the parents choose this route, then they must be prepared to deal with an extubation that results in the child's death. In such instances, if possible, a *do-not-resuscitate* order should be obtained.

Some parents may wish to attempt extubation with the idea that if the child does not succeed with breathing without mechanical ventilation, then the child will be reintubated, thereby providing the parents with more time to come to a consensus about what to do next. Nonetheless, once the medical team has established that the most likely neurologic outcome for the child is the potential for severe encephalopathy or a persistent vegetative state, some parents request that the child be extubated, not reintubated, and permitted to die naturally. A do-not-resuscitate order on record ensures that no further heroic efforts will be undertaken to save the child.

An open, honest policy enables parents to participate in decisions that will profoundly affect them for years to come.[24,25] The health care team should provide resources to the family as needed: support for sustaining the child in a long-term care facility should be provided to the family or after a child's death, the palliative care team or another specialist may provide bereavement support for the family. (See Chapter 69, Palliative, End-of-Life, and Bereavement Care.)

PREVENTION

The overall effect of submersion injury prevention and pool safety cannot be overstated. The efforts of the American Academy of Pediatrics and community efforts have resulted in a reduction in serious submersion injuries by advocating standards for pool safety. Primary care physicians need to educate families during routine office visits about pool safety.

A swimming pool in the yard can be dangerous for children. If possible, swimming pools should not be built until the children in the household are older than 5 years. If a pool is already in place, then safety measures should be undertaken to prevent drowning. Box 344-1 provides tips on how to protect children from drowning.

BOX 344-1 How to Protect Children From Drowning

- Never leave your children alone in or near the pool, even for a moment.
- Put up a fence to separate your house from the pool. Most young children who drown in pools wander out of the house and fall into the pool. Install a fence at least 4 feet high around all 4 sides of the pool. This fence will completely separate the pool from the house and play area of the yard. Use gates that auto-close and auto-latch, with latches higher than your children's reach.
- Consider the use of a safety cover. A power safety cover that meets the standards of the American Society for Testing and Materials adds to the protection of your children but should not be used in place of the fence between your house and the pool. Even fencing around your pool and using a power safety cover will not prevent all drownings.
- Keep rescue equipment (eg, a shepherd's hook, life preserver) and a telephone by the pool.
- Do not let your child use air-filled swimming aids because they are not a substitute for approved life vests and can be dangerous.
- Know CPR. Anyone watching young children around a pool should learn CPR and be able to rescue a child if needed. Stay within an arm's length of your child.
- Remove all toys from the pool after use so children are not tempted to reach for them.
- After the children are finished swimming, secure the pool so they cannot get back into it.
- Teaching your child how to swim does not mean that your child is safe in water.

From American Academy of Pediatrics, The Injury Prevention Program (TIPP). *Pediatrics.* 2000 Apr;105(4 Pt 1):868-870.

TOOLS FOR PRACTICE

Engaging Patient and Family

- *Home Water Hazards for Young Children* (fact sheet), American Academy of Pediatrics (www.aap.org/bookstore).
- *Pool Safety for Children* (fact sheet), American Academy of Pediatrics (www.aap.org/bookstore).
- *Water-Related Injuries* (fact sheet), Centers for Disease Control and Prevention (www.cdc.gov/ncipc/factsheets/drown.htm).
- *Water Safety for Your School-aged Child* (fact sheet), American Academy of Pediatrics (www.aap.org/bookstore).

Medical Decision Support

- *The Pediatric Emergency Medicine Resource* (book), American Academy of Pediatrics and American College of Emergency Physicians (ACEP) (www.aap.org/bookstore).

AAP POLICY STATEMENTS

American Academy of Pediatrics Committee on Injury, Violence and Poison Prevention. Prevention of Drowning in Infants, Children, and Adolescents. *Pediatrics.* 2003;112(2):437-439. (aappolicy.aappublications.org/cgi/content/full/pediatrics;112/2/437).

American Academy of Pediatrics Committee on Injury, Violence and Poison Prevention. Prevention of Drowning in Infants, Children, and Adolescents. *Pediatrics.* 2003;112(2):440-445. (aappolicy.aappublications.org/cgi/content/full/pediatrics;112/2/440).

REFERENCES

1. Falk JL, Escowitz HE. Submersion injuries in children and adults. *Semin Respir Crit Care Med.* 2002;23:47-55.
2. Lee LK, Mao C, Thompson KM. Demographic factors and their association with outcomes in pediatric submersion injury. *Acad Emerg Med.* 2006;13:308-313.
3. Sarnaik AP, Lieh-Lai MW. Near-Drowning. In: Furhman BP, Zimmerman JJ, eds. *Pediatric Critical Care.* 3rd ed. Philadelphia, PA: Mosby; 2006.
4. Kallas HJ. Drowning and near-drowning. In: Behrman RE, Kliegman RM, Jenson HB, eds. *Nelson Textbook of Pediatrics.* 17th ed. Philadelphia, PA: WB Saunders; 2004.
5. Hodge D. Submersion injury. In: Gausche-Hill M, Fuchs S, Yamamoto L, eds. *The Pediatric Emergency Medicine Resource.* 4th ed. Sudbury, MA: Jones and Bartlett; 2004.
6. Donoghue AJ, Nakkarni V, Berg RA, et al. Out-of-hospital pediatric cardiac arrest: an epidemiologic review and assessment of current knowledge. *Ann Emerg Med.* 2005;46:512-522.
7. Orlowski JP, Szpilman D. Drowning: rescue, resuscitation, and reanimation. *Pediatr Clin North Am.* 2001;48:627-646.
8. Nagaraja J, Menkedick J, Phelan KJ, et al. Deaths from residential injuries in US children and adolescents, 1985-1997. *Pediatrics.* 2005;116:454-461.
9. Allasio D, Fischer H. Immersion scald burns and the ability of young children to climb into a bathtub. *Pediatrics.* 2005;115:1419-1421.
10. Salomez F, Vincent JL. Drowning: a review of epidemiology, pathophysiology, treatment and prevention. *Resuscitation.* 2004;63:261-268.
11. Modell JH, Idris AH, Pineda JA, et al. Survival after prolonged submersion in freshwater in Florida. *Chest.* 2004;125:1948-1951.
12. Acute Respiratory Distress Syndrome Network. Ventilation with lower tidal volumes as compared with traditional tidal volumes for acute lung injury and the acute respiratory distress syndrome. *N Engl J Med.* 2000;342:1301-1308.
13. Carcillo JA, Fields AI, American College of Critical Care Medicine, Task Force Committee Members. Clinical practice parameters for hemodynamic support of pediatric and neonatal patients in septic shock. *Crit Care Med.* 2002;30:1365-1378.
14. Ackerman MJ, Tester DJ, Porter CJ. Swimming, a gene-specific arrhythmogenic trigger for inherited long QT syndrome. *Mayo Clin Proc.* 1999;74:1088-1094.
15. Yoshinaga M, Kamimura J, Fukushige T, et al. Face immersion in cold water induces prolongation of the QT syndrome. *Am J Cardiol.* 1999;83:1494-1497.
16. Habib DM, Tecklenburg FW, Webb SA, et al. Prediction of childhood drowning and near-drowning morbidity and mortality. *Pediatr Emerg Care.* 1996;12:255-258.
17. Watson RS, Cummings P, Quan L, et al. Cervical spine injuries among submersion victims. *J Trauma.* 2001;51:658-662.
18. Steele MT, Nelson MJ, Sessler DI, et al. Forced air speeds rewarming in accidental hypothermia. *Ann Emerg Med.* 1996;27:479-484.
19. Bratton SL, Jardine DS, Morray JP. Serial neurologic examinations after near-drowning and outcome. *Arch Pediatr Adolesc Med.* 1994;148:167-170.

20. Vitali SH, Arnold JH. Bench-to-bedside review: ventilator strategies to reduce lung injury—lessons from pediatric and neonatal intensive care. *Crit Care.* 2005;9:177-183.
21. Dobyns EL, Anas NG, Fortenberry JD, et al. Interactive effects of high-frequency oscillatory ventilation and inhaled nitric oxide in acute hypoxemic respiratory failure in pediatrics. *Crit Care Med.* 2002;30:2425.
22. Thalmann M, Trampitsch E, Haberfellner N, et al. Resuscitation in near drowning with extracorporeal membrane oxygenation. *Ann Thorac Surg.* 2001;72:607-608.
23. Sourkes B, Frankel LR, Brown M, et al. Food, toys and love: pediatric palliative care. *Curr Prob Pediatr Adolesc Health Care.* 2005;35:349-387.
24. Mathers LH. Letting go: a study in pediatric life-and-death decision making. In: Frankel LR, Goldworth A, Rorty MV, Silverman WA, eds. *Ethical Dilemmas in Pediatrics: Cases and Commentaries.* Cambridge, MA: Cambridge University Press; 2005.
25. Whitney SN. Near-drowning, futility, and the limits of shared decision making. In: Frankel LR, Goldworth A, Rorty MV, et al, eds. *Ethical Dilemmas in Pediatrics: Cases and Commentaries.* Cambridge, MA: Cambridge University Press; 2005.

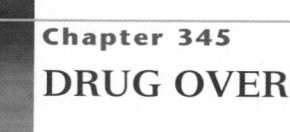

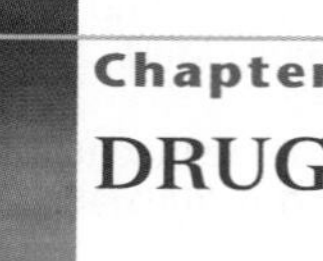

Chapter 345

DRUG OVERDOSE

Ian M. Paul, MD, MSc

Drug overdose, whether from unintentional ingestion, a therapeutic mistake, or a suicide attempt, is a major problem in pediatric practice. In 2004 the American Association of Poison Control Centers, Toxic Exposure Surveillance System, tabulated 2,473,570 case reports of human exposure to potentially toxic substances.[1] The participating poison control centers serve 292.2 million people. Children younger than 6 years accounted for 51.6% of case reports, and 39.1% occurred in children 2 years or younger.[2] Annually, 1.4 million children aged 12 or younger are exposed to drugs that are potentially able to cause toxicity, and in 2002 these exposures resulted in 29 deaths.[2]

DEFINITION

Drug overdose occurs when a child ingests or is given an amount of a substance that exceeds the recommended dose.

EPIDEMIOLOGY AND ETIOLOGY

The incidence of drug overdose varies by patient age (Table 345-1). The bimodal frequency of deaths peaks at 5 years or younger and again at 15 to 19 years. The former peak reflects unintentional ingestions, the latter usually suicidal events. For some compounds, acetaminophen being a prime example, therapeutic mistakes may play a significant role. Many acetaminophen poisonings are drug overdosing caused by errors in one of the following: inappropriate dosing, unintentional multiple overdosing, ingestion of acetaminophen along with another hepatotoxic drug, administration of adult rather than pediatric preparations, concurrent administration of an over-the-counter fixed-dose combination product that also contains acetaminophen, or supervision of medication administration by another child.[3] Preventive measures, such as child-resistant bottle tops, are effective in eliminating acute, single-dose, unintentional exposures. The most common drug overdoses causing death are analgesics, antidepressants, and over-the-counter cough and cold preparations. Chapter 355, Poisoning, provides detailed information on the management of the most common drug ingestions in children.

Table 345-1 Substances Causing Toxic Exposure (by Patient Age)*

SUBSTANCE	AGE <6 YR	AGE 6-19 YR
Pharmaceutical agents	504,725	168,053
Nonpharmaceutical agents (chemicals, plants, gases)	725,941	188,002

DEATHS	AGE <6 YR	AGE 6-12 YR	AGE 13-19 YR
Number	25	4	48

*Occurrence in 1 year or per year.
Modified from Litovitz TL, Holm KC, Clancy C, et al. 1992 annual report of the American Association of Poison Control Centers Toxic Exposure Surveillance System. *Am J Emerg Med.* 1993;11(5):494-555. Copyright © 1993, Elsevier, with permission.

IMMEDIATE ASSESSMENT

Immediately on encountering the overdosed patient, as much information as possible should be gathered. The person or persons who brought the child to the hospital or office should be detained. If initial contact is made by telephone, then the caller's name and telephone number should be obtained, and then the caller should be instructed to proceed immediately with the child to the hospital. Obtaining the precise description of the ingested drug is important, including, if known, the name, dose, pharmacy of origin, and prescription number. The parents should be instructed to bring the actual container when they come with the patient. An attempt should be made to determine the amount of drug ingested. This determination is frequently impossible, and such information, even if obtained, is occasionally misleading. Maximal exposure is assumed unless a precise tablet count or liquid amount is available.

Initial Procedures for Stabilization and Life Support

As always with an acute, life-threatening event, the patient's airway, breathing, and circulation, the ABCs, should be promptly assessed. The vital signs (temperature, pulse, respirations, blood pressure) should be determined and pulse oximetry and continuous electrocardiography instituted. The sensorium should be monitored frequently—that is, every 15 minutes—until the patient's condition is stable. Changes in frequency and duration of monitoring will depend on the drug, dose, and clinical course.

Adequacy of the airway must be closely assessed. Most drug overdoses do not affect the upper airway (larynx, trachea) but interfere with air exchange by either depressing the central nervous system or paralyzing neuromuscular transmission. An intravenous line should be established. An arterial line should be considered if danger exists of respiratory depression or ingestion of drugs that alter cardiovascular status. Some toxic substances, such as insecticides, have significant dermal absorption, especially if the skin is inflamed or abraded, and in such instances, the skin should be cleansed.

Gastric Decontamination

Gastric decontamination procedures have undergone recent changes in recommendations. Before 2003 the American Academy of Pediatrics recommended that a 1-ounce bottle of ipecac syrup be kept in the home so that it might be administered to children on the direction of a physician or poison control center after an ingestion. The Academy reversed this recommendation in a 2003 policy statement because research has shown that ipecac does not completely remove an ingested substance from the stomach, has side effects of its own (including lethargy), may be given inappropriately by caregivers, and, importantly, does not improve health outcomes or reduce utilization of emergency services.[4] Another form of gastric emptying—gastric lavage—may still be used on occasion in an emergency setting but is reserved for patients who have ingested a near-lethal or lethal amount of a toxic agent within the prior 1 to 2 hours. Activated charcoal is now considered the best method of gastrointestinal decontamination.[5] It is given at a dose of 1 g/kg usually via nasogastric tube; most children refuse to drink the slurry. Use of a cathartic remains controversial, with no firm evidence supporting its use.[5,6] Only a very small number of compounds appear not to be adsorbed by the charcoal (acids, alkali, iron salts). For substances that are poorly adsorbed by charcoal, the use of whole-bowel irrigation (with a polyethylene glycol–electrolyte solution [Colyte or Golytely]) at a dose of 25 to 40 mL/kg/hour may be used. This technique may be especially helpful in treating for overdoses of the increasing numbers of delayed-release drugs.[7] Gastrointestinal fluid obtained by any of the aforementioned methods should be saved for drug analysis.

DIFFERENTIAL DIAGNOSIS

Other conditions can mimic the signs and symptoms of drug overdose. Head trauma is a prime consideration in patients who have alterations in sensorium. Additionally, adolescents who have head trauma may have ingested ethanol. Near-drowning victims also may have ingested ethanol. Use of illicit drugs can also alter mental status and should be considered in a differential diagnosis. General urine toxicologic screens ordered in an emergency department will test for tetrahydrocannabinol (marijuana), cocaine, opioids, benzodiazepines, barbiturates, and phencyclidine.

Spontaneous intracranial hemorrhages in the pediatric age group are rare; they usually produce focal neurologic signs rather than global depression of consciousness.

Metabolic conditions such as diabetes mellitus, hypoglycemia, and addisonian crisis may cause clinical states that resemble drug ingestion. Awareness of these possibilities will help narrow the diagnostic considerations. Head injury with drug overdose in a child may indicate child abuse. Infections of the central nervous system, particularly viral encephalitis, should also be considered.

The most difficult situation of all is presented by the patient who has a psychiatric illness and who may develop tremors, hallucinations, or hysterical paralysis. In these patients, precise and rapid laboratory analyses are most important in ruling out drug ingestion. If the patient has been receiving psychoactive medications and is having an untoward reaction, then management is identical to that presented previously, with special attention directed to the emotional needs of the patient.

MANAGEMENT

The 2 factors to consider in managing the patient are (1) expertise of the physician in the management of drug overdose and (2) available hospital support facilities. The latter point is of most concern because even the best-trained physician cannot provide care properly in an institution that is inadequately equipped with support staff, equipment, and laboratory facilities. The well-trained pediatrician will not always be able to predict the clinical course of a patient who has overdosed. Will the patient require charcoal perfusion, renal or peritoneal dialysis, or an exchange transfusion? Is the hospital able to offer pediatric intensive care unit monitoring? Can the hospital provide prolonged ventilation and airway management? Can the nursing staff monitor intracranial or intra-arterial

BOX 345-1 Steps to Treat the Patient with a Drug Overdose

1. Stabilize the patient.
2. Identify the drug ingested and determine the amount ingested.
3. Contact the local poison control center for toxicology data and information regarding the signs and symptoms and clinical course. The toll-free telephone number for poison control centers across the United States has become uniform: 800-222-1222.
4. Use gastrointestinal decontamination (see text).
5. If a specific antidote exists, then administer it. A table of specific antidotes (Table 345-2) and their location in the hospital should be available; the best location is the emergency department. All staff members must know the precise location.
6. Provide supportive care in an intensive or intermediate care unit as appropriate.
7. Meet social service needs as indicated (eg, drug ingestion by a toddler as a symptom of chaotic family structure or by an adolescent as a symptom of depression or as a suicidal gesture).
8. Provide counseling concerning the institution of poison-control measures in the home.

pressure properly? Deciding early in the clinical course whether special facilities will be needed is best. The preferable course of action would be to transfer a stable patient earlier than a critically ill child requiring mobile life support later.

Frequent and open communication with the patient's family should be maintained. Regardless of the cause of their child's poisoning, these parents are in constant need of counseling, especially with regard to any guilt feelings they may be experiencing. Adolescents with intentional drug overdoses often have complex psychosocial problems that typically require psychiatric consultation. Box 345-1 highlights the steps to take in treating a drug overdose.

General Homeostatic Support

Thermal monitoring is an important aspect of management in drug overdose. Centrally and peripherally induced hypothermia is a common problem—for example, the hypothermia that occurs with phenothiazine ingestion. Hyperthermia can occur with salicylate, atropine, or selective serotonin reuptake inhibitor poisoning.

Monitoring fluid and electrolyte homeostasis is important. Deficits must be replaced, and the amount of maintenance fluids required depends on changes in the vital and physical signs. For example, hyperventilation and increased body temperature require higher volume of maintenance fluids. Continuing losses through vomiting and diarrhea should be replaced as they occur.

Central venous pressure and arterial pressure should be monitored to assess vascular volume and tone. Respiratory function and oxygenation (with pulse oximetry) also require monitoring. Intracranial pressure may need to be assessed to determine the need for treatment of cerebral edema. The need for peritoneal dialysis, hemodialysis, charcoal perfusion, or exchange transfusion to remove the ingested drug must be considered.

Diagnostic Procedures

Assays of blood, urine, and gastric contents for barbiturates, antidepressants, phenytoin, iron, digoxin, salicylate, acetaminophen, narcotics, alcohol, cocaine, and propoxyphene must be available. Rapid drug screens should be available; quantitative analyses should follow as quickly as possible.

A flat plate radiographic examination of the abdomen may be required to identify radiopaque tablets (eg, iron) or foreign bodies. A computed tomography scan of the head should be performed if intracranial hemorrhage is suspected after amphetamine or cocaine ingestion. A chest radiograph is needed if narcotic-induced pulmonary edema or aspiration is suspected.

The clinician should remember that trauma may have occurred in any poisoned patient, especially in adolescents. One half of adolescent drownings are associated with alcohol use. Because near-drownings often follow diving, in which the head and neck may be injured, immobilization of the cervical spine should be accomplished immediately on site.

Definitive Therapy

Specific antidotes exist for some drugs but unfortunately not for most (Table 345-2). Thus definitive therapy consists of intensive supportive care and treatment of signs and symptoms as they develop (eg, hypotension and hypertension, thermal instability, cardiac arrhythmias).

Complications

Possible complications of drug overdose are many and varied. Therapy itself can have side effects, such as overzealous treatment of seizures that may cause apnea. Many poisoned patients require ventilator therapy. Such therapy, especially if prolonged, may lead to complications such as pneumothorax, oxygen toxicity, and airway infections. Nosocomial infections are not uncommon, especially hypostatic pneumonia, urinary tract infection

Table 345-2 Common Antidotes

DRUG	DIAGNOSTIC FINDINGS REQUIRING TREATMENT	ANTIDOTE	DOSAGE
Acetaminophen	History of ingestion and toxic serum level	N-acetylcysteine	140 mg/kg/dose PO, then 70 mg/kg/dose every 4 hr PO × 17
Anticholinergics Antihistamines Atropine Phenothiazines Tricyclic antidepressants	Supraventricular tachycardia (hemodynamic compromise); unresponsive ventricular dysrhythmia, seizures, pronounced hallucinations or agitation	Physostigmine	Child: 0.5 mg IV slowly (over 3 min) every 10 min as needed
Benzodiazepines	Drowsiness, ataxia, hallucinations, confusion, agitation, respiratory depression, hypotension	Flumazenil	0.01 mg/kg IV every min × 1-5 doses; max 0.2 mg/dose
Cholinergics Insecticides	Cholinergic crisis: salivation, lacrimation, urination, defecation, convulsions, fasciculations	Atropine sulfate Physostigmine	0.05 mg/kg/dose (usual dose 1-5 mg; test dose for child 0.01 mg/kg) every 4-6 hr IV or more frequently as needed
Carbon monoxide	Headache, seizure, coma, dysrhythmias	Oxygen, hyperbaric oxygen	100% oxygen (half-life 40 min); consider hyperbaric chamber

Table 345-2 Common Antidotes—cont'd

DRUG	DIAGNOSTIC FINDINGS REQUIRING TREATMENT	ANTIDOTE	DOSAGE
Cyanide	Cyanosis, seizures, cardiopulmonary arrest, coma	Amyl nitrite	Inhale pearl every 60-120 sec
		Sodium nitrite (3%)	0.27 mL (8.7 mg)/kg (adult: 10mL [300 mg]) IV slowly (Hb ≥10 g/dL)
		Sodium thiosulfate (25%)	1.35 mL (325 mg)/kg (adult: 12.5 g) IV slowly (Hb ≥10g/dL)
		Also consider hyperbaric chamber	15 mg/kg IV over 30 min
Ethylene glycol	Metabolic acidosis, urine Ca^{++} oxalate crystals	Fomepizole	
		Ethanol (100% absolute, 1 mL-790 mg)	1 mL/kg in 5% dextrose in water IV over 15 min, then 0.16 mL (125 mg/kg/hr) IV; maintain ethanol level of 100 mg/dL
Iron	Hypotension, shock, coma, serum iron >350 mg/dL (or greater than iron-binding capacity)	Deferoxamine	Shock or coma: 15 mg/kg/hr IV for 8 hr No shock or coma: 90 mg/kg/dose IM every 8 hr
Phenothiazines Chlorpromazine Thioridazine	Extrapyramidal dyskinesis, oculogyric crisis	Diphenhydramine (Benadryl)	1-2 mg/kg/dose (max: 50 mg/dose) every 6 hr IV, PO
Methanol	Metabolic acidosis, blurred vision; level >20 mg/dL	Fomepizole	15 mg/kg IV over 30 min
		Ethanol (100% absolute)	1 mL/kg in 5% dextrose in water over 15 min, then 0.16 mL (125 mg)/kg/hr IV
Methemoglobin Nitrate Nitrites Sulfonamide	Cyanosis, methemoglobin level 30%, dyspnea	Methylene blue (1% solution)	1-2 mg (0.1-0.2 mL)/kg/dose IV; repeat in 4 hr if necessary
Narcotics Heroin Codeine Propoxyphene	Respiratory depression, hypotension, coma	Naloxone (Narcan)	0.1 mg/kg up to 0.8 mg initially IV, if no response give 2 mg IV
Organophosphates Malathion Parathion	Cholinergic crisis: salivation, lacrimation, urination, defecation, convulsions, fasciculations	Atropine sulfate	0.05 mg/kg/dose (usual dose 1-5 mg; test dose for child 0.01 mg/kg) every 4-6 hr IV or more frequently as needed
		Pralidoxime	After atropine, 20-50 mg/kg/dose (max: 2000 mg) IV slowly (<50 mg/min) every 8 hr IV as needed × 3

Hb, Hemoglobin; *IV*, intravenously; *PO*, orally.
From Barkin RM. Toxicologic emergencies. *Pediatr Ann.* 1990;19(11):629-633. Reprinted by permission of Slack Inc.

(secondary to catheter placement), or septicemia from vascular catheters. Thrombotic and embolic episodes also can result from vascular catheters.

Permanent central nervous system damage sometimes follows periods of hypoxia or hypoglycemia, usually before therapy is instituted. Skin, mucous membrane, and deeper-tissue injuries often result from acids, substances containing lye, or corrosives. Specific compounds can cause permanent organ damage (eg, to the lungs from hydrocarbons, the kidneys from ethylene glycol, the liver from acetaminophen, the retina from methanol).

Hazards of treatment for drug overdose include overtreatment, the wrong treatment, an insufficient period of observation, and failure to appreciate drug ingestion as an indication of child neglect or abuse. Child abuse or neglect should be particularly suspected in a child younger than 12 months who is admitted with accidental ingestion or the child who has a history of repeated drug ingestions. Overtreatment occurs when errors are made in assessing the amount of drug ingested. A nontoxic ingestion may be vigorously but inappropriately treated with potentially toxic antidotes, for example, using sodium nitrate-sodium thiosulfate for the treatment of cyanide ingestion.

The wrong treatment can occur when a mistake is made in identifying the drug ingested, for example, from a mislabeled prescription vial. An insufficient period of observation can worsen the situation. For example, hepatic necrosis may not occur until day 3 after acetaminophen ingestion, and renal disease may not occur until day 7 to 10.

WHEN TO REFER

- Ingestion of any substance unfamiliar to the primary care physician
- Any patient who potentially may require a therapy unfamiliar to the primary care physician

WHEN TO ADMIT

- Any patient strongly suspected of ingesting a toxic or lethal dose of any substance
- An unstable patient
- Any patient requiring gastrointestinal decontamination, intravenous therapy, hemoperfusion, or charcoal perfusion, even if clinically well
- A patient in an environment suggesting child abuse

TOOLS FOR PRACTICE

Medical Decision Support

- *2004 Poison Center Survey Results* (report), American Association of Poison Control Centers (www.aapcc.org/2004_poison_center_survey_results.htm).

RELATED WEB SITE

- American Association of Poison Control Centers (www.1-800-222-1222.info/poisonhelp.asp).

AAP POLICY STATEMENTS

American Academy of Pediatrics Committee on Drugs. Acetaminophen Toxicity in Children. *Pediatrics*. 2001;108(4):1020-1024. (aappolicy.aappublications.org/cgi/content/full/pediatrics;108/4/1020).

American Academy of Pediatrics Committee on Injury, Violence, and Poison Prevention. Poison Treatment in the Home. *Pediatrics*. 2003;112(5):1182-1185. (aappolicy.aappublications.org/cgi/content/full/pediatrics;112/5/1182).

REFERENCES

1. American Association of Poison Control Centers. 2004 Poison Center Survey. Available at: www.aapcc.org/2004_poison_center_survey_results.htm. Accessed June 28, 2007.
2. Watson WA, Litovitz TL, Rodgers GC Jr, et al. 2002 annual report of the American Association of Poison Control Centers Toxic Exposure Surveillance System. *Am J Emerg Med*. 2003;21:353-421.
3. American Academy of Pediatrics, Committee on Drugs. Acetaminophen toxicity in children. *Pediatrics*. 2001;108:1020-1024.
4. American Academy of Pediatrics, Committee on Injury, Violence, and Poison Prevention. Poison treatment in the home. *Pediatrics*. 2003;112:1182-1185.
5. Perry H, Shannon M. Emergency department gastrointestinal decontamination. *Pediatr Ann*. 1996;25:19-26.
6. Rivera-Penera T, Gugig R, Davis J, et al. Outcome of acetaminophen overdose in pediatric patients and factors contributing to hepatotoxicity. *J Pediatr*. 1997;130:300-304.
7. Snodgrass WR. Clinical toxicity. In: Klaasen CD, ed. *Casarett and Doull's Toxicology*. 5th ed. New York, NY: McGraw-Hill; 1996.

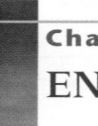

Chapter 346

ENVENOMATIONS

Shireen Banerji, PharmD; Alvin C. Bronstein, MD

Venoms are complex chemical mixtures designed either for defending or for hunting. Animal venoms used for immobilizing prey may also have predigestive effects to aid the hunter.[1] Envenomations present unique problems in the pediatric population. Although the amount of venom injected may not be enough to cause morbidity in an adult, an equal amount of venom may be disastrous for a child.

Various venom delivery systems exist. Most systems of clinical relevance consist of specially evolved exocrine gland mechanisms to make and store venom and a sophisticated delivery apparatus. Snake fangs resemble hypodermic needles, and the Hymenoptera sting device is similar to a blood sampling stylet. *Envenomation* is the injection of venom through the bite or sting of venomous creatures. *Bites* refer to the injection through structures associated with the mouth and are primarily evolved for handling prey, whereas *stings* are delivered through a posterior structure (stinger) and are primarily defensive.[2] Primary care and emergency medicine physicians often receive complaints of envenomation. Concerns about allergic reactions, mostly from insects, result in referrals to allergy and immunology specialists.

EPIDEMIOLOGIC FEATURES

In 2005 the American Association of Poison Control Centers (AAPCC) National Poison Database reported 2,547,394 exposures, with 82,151 (3.2%) as a result of a

Table 346-1 American Association of Poison Control Centers 2005 Envenomation Exposures in the United States

ANIMAL	TOTAL	CHILDREN AGES <6 YEARS (%)
Ants, fire ants	2101	812 (39%)
Hymenoptera	10,972	2051 (19%)
Scorpions	14,521	1243 (9%)
Snakes	2971	117 (4%)
Crotalines	2913	116 (4%)
Coral	58	1 (2%)
Spiders	22,961	2446 (11%)

From Lai MW, Klein-Schwartz W, Rodgers GC, et al. 2005 annual report of the American Association of Poison Control Centers' National Poisoning and Exposure Database. *Clin Toxicol*. 2006;44:803-932. Reprinted by permission of Taylor & Francis.

bite or sting (Table 346-1). Of the 1460 deaths reported, 7 (0.5%) were from bites and stings, and none involved children.[3] Although bites and envenomations ranked number 10 in all age groups in the National Poison Database, they did not make the top 20 in children younger than 6 years.[3]

Although most cases are minor, serious local and systemic injury can result. Consequently the primary care clinician must be aware of local venomous species and be able to recognize and treat the injuries caused by them. In North America, venomous species include arthropods, specifically Hymenoptera (bees, wasps, hornets, ants), arachnids (spiders, scorpions), and snakes (pit vipers and coral snakes).

HYMENOPTERA

In the United States, Hymenoptera are responsible for most insect stings. These creatures include the family Apidae (honeybees), family Bombidae (bumblebees), superfamily Vespidae (paper wasps, white-faced hornets, yellow hornets, and yellow jackets), and superfamily Formicidae (harvester ants and native and imported fire ants).[1,4,5] All Hymenoptera possess a stinger located posteriorly.

Hymenoptera stings can cause local or systemic reactions. Reactions may be a direct effect of the venom, or they may occur through an IgE-mediated allergic reaction. Systemic reactions occur in less than 5% of patients.[6] Their prevalence in the general population ranges from 0.15% to 3.9%.[7] Large local cutaneous reactions to stings occur in approximately 2.3% to 18.6% of the general population.[8,9] Biphasic anaphylactic reactions, characterized by return of symptoms 6 to 10 hours after initial symptom resolution, may occur in up to 20% of patients.[10] Death by honeybee or wasp envenomation is rare. IgE-mediated type-1 anaphylaxis, although uncommon, is usually responsible for related deaths. Massive envenomation involving hundreds of stings may also result in death.

Winged Hymenoptera

Characteristics and Distribution

Winged Hymenoptera are found in most areas of the United States. Honeybees usually nest in hollow trees and crevices, whereas bumblebees prefer nesting underground. Wasp nests can often be found under roofs and eaves, hornets prefer to nest in the branches of trees, and yellow jackets tend to build their nests in the ground.

Most social bees and wasps sting primarily in defense of their nest or while in search of food. Yellow jacket wasps are common near exposed food and garbage, resulting in stings not associated with nest protection. Yellow jackets have also been implicated in frequent stings in late summer and early fall associated with *yellow jacket delirium,* a poorly understood seasonal behavior characterized by aggressiveness toward objects that are not threatening or provocative.[11] If disturbed, any wasp or bee will sting in self-defense. Mass envenomations occur when a human is perceived to be intruding or threatening the colony. Honeybee colonies consist of approximately 40,000 workers, with Africanized honeybees having slightly smaller colonies. In contrast, yellow jackets and hornets maintain colonies of several hundred to a few thousand insects.[12]

The sting apparatus, or *aculeus,* of wasps (vespids) and honeybees resembles a stylet with 2 shafts. The shafts, propelled by muscular attachments, alternatively slide back and forth, pulling the sting deep into the flesh. Barbs located in the tips of the stylet help anchor the aculeus.[13] Venom is then pumped down a central channel into the wound. Unlike the aculeus of the honeybee, the vespid sting stylet is wider than the stylet shaft barbs, and the dorsal stylet surface is smooth, decreasing the likelihood that the sting will remain in the victim. The insect dies after stinging because stinging eviscerates the insect, the result of the morphology of the honeybee aculeus. However, because vespids can withdraw their stingers, they are able to sting multiple times.[2,5]

Much attention has been garnered by Africanized honeybees, commonly referred to as *killer bees,* which are now found in southern Texas, Arizona, and California.[14] The original colonies of these bees were imported to South America to breed with European varieties in an attempt to increase honey production. However, the ensuing generations of bees retained the ferocity of the African bees. The bees are not more individually dangerous than European bees. Their venom is similarly potent, and similar amounts are delivered per sting. However, their aggressive nature results in massive envenomation because of the sheer number of stings delivered in an attack.[10]

Venoms of the winged Hymenoptera contain many protein components that account for the reactions that have been observed. Phospholipids A_2, hyaluronidase, histamine, apamin, melittin, mast cell degranulating peptide, acid phosphatase, norepinephrine, dopamine, and allergen C are the main constituents of honeybee venom. Mast cell degranulating protein causes cell breakdown and histamine release. Bumblebee venom contains acid phosphatase, tryptic amidase, and melittin. Melittin is the main pain-inducing compound, and it causes membrane integrity alteration.[12] The major vespid allergens are antigen 5 and hyaluronidase, but they also contain histamine, kinins, serotonin, phospholipase A_1 and B, and mastoparans.[4,5] Cross-reactivity between the apid and the vespid venoms is limited, but a marked cross-reactivity exists between the different vespid venoms.[8,15]

The most common areas to be stung are the head, neck, feet, and hands. Stinging is most common during the summer months, and children are often affected.[5] Most patients cannot reliably identify the insect that stung them. Bees and wasps are strongly attracted to dark colors. Therefore eyes, mouth, and nostrils may be selectively targeted. Although stings to the eye are uncommon, when they occur, the cornea is the most common site.[16]

Physical Examination

LOCAL. Both nonallergic and allergic local reactions may occur after a sting. The nonallergic reaction is a direct result of envenomation through mast cell degranulation and the production of a wheal-and-flare response. This response produces erythema, swelling, pain, and itching. These signs and symptoms usually subside in a few hours.

Allergic local reactions occur in approximately 17% of people stung by winged Hymenoptera. They consist of erythema and local edema more than 10 cm in diameter; they often persist for 48 to 72 hours, and they may become indurated for a period of up to 5 days.[5,9] Some patients may experience headache, nausea, or malaise with these reactions.

As mentioned previously, a stinger may sometimes be found at the sting site, which usually indicates a honeybee sting or, in some cases, a yellow jacket sting. Skin and soft-tissue necrosis in the weeks after a Hymenoptera sting have also been reported.[17,18]

Corneal stings may result in local damage through toxic and immunologic reactions.[19] Stingers retained in the eye may cause corneal edema with striate and toxic keratopathy.[20] Immunologic reactions can result in extensive inflammation and uveitis. Inflammatory glaucoma may occur as a result of severe uveitis. Severe neuroophthalmic complications such as optic neuritis, loss of vision, and cataracts have also been reported.[19,20]

SYSTEMIC. The more common systemic manifestations of an allergic reaction to Hymenoptera stings include urticaria, angioedema, wheezing, shortness of breath, stridor, nausea, vomiting, diarrhea, abdominal pain, malaise, dizziness, and anaphylaxis. Dysphagia, dysarthria, hoarseness, weakness, and confusion also have been described. Effects on the hematologic system include hemolysis with associated hematoglobinuria and hematoglobinemia, thrombocytopenia, and disseminated intravascular coagulation.[12] Respiratory and cardiovascular complications are observed in adults more often than in children.[9] Fatal anaphylaxis is rare, especially in children.[8,14] However, the sheer number of exposures makes Hymenoptera envenomation the second-leading cause of anaphylactic reactions after penicillin exposure, and it accounts for more deaths in the United states than any other envenomation.[21-23]

The risk of developing a systemic reaction appears to be increased in the patient with a history of multiple stings or after being stung within a few weeks after a previous sting. The risk is also increased in patients who have a history of anaphylaxis. Their risk of anaphylaxis with subsequent stings is 35% to 60%.[9,15] However, the pattern of reaction is difficult to predict.[8] Atopic patients do not appear to be at greater risk of developing systemic complications, but the severity of their symptoms may be greater than in nonatopic individuals.[9] A history of a large local reaction does not reliably predict progression to systemic complications. The risk of subsequent anaphylaxis after a large local reaction is approximately 5% to 10%.[8,24]

Systemic reactions may also be caused by direct action of bee venom. In rare cases, serum sickness, vasculitis, encephalopathy, neuritis, and renal disease with or without rhabdomyolysis have been observed.[25] Renal failure or death may occur when 20 to 200 wasp stings and 150 to 1000 or more honeybee stings have been inflicted.[12,26,27] The human 50% lethal dose for honeybee stings has been estimated to be between 500 and 1200 stings.[12] However, recovery has been reported in children involving incidents of 200 to 1000 or more honeybee stings. Children are considered to be at high risk because of their failure to perceive the risk, and they are less apt to be able to escape while being stung. The presence of Africanized bees may result in multiple stings resulting in high doses of venom, in turn resulting in hemolysis, thrombocytopenia, rhabdomyolysis (skeletal and myocardial), and acute tubular necrosis.[28-31] Systemic damage may develop within 24 hours, although delayed onset (2 to 6 days) has been reported.[12]

Differential Diagnosis

Differential diagnosis of the local reaction includes other arthropod envenomations, puncture wounds with reactive erythema or cellulitis, or simple cellulitis.[24] Differential diagnosis of systemic reactions includes any other cause of allergic reaction, reactive airway disease, or infectious processes. Other causes of stridor, wheezing, and allergic reaction should be considered if a sting site cannot be identified.

Laboratory Studies

No specific laboratory test is useful in the acute management of Hymenoptera stings.

Management

Insect sting sites should be inspected for the presence of a stinger. Honeybee stingers remain present and will further embed themselves and continue to pump venom after separation from the bee. The venom sac is emptied within 2 minutes of entering the skin[2,32]; therefore quick removal of the stinger is imperative.[33-35] Traditional teaching advocates the removal of the stinger by scraping it with a hard-edged object, such as a credit card, to prevent pressure on the venom sac. Such pressure would theoretically result in an increase in envenomation.[6] However, experimental data show that removal of the stinger with the fingers does not increase envenomation.[35] Rapid removal of the stinger by any means is most effective in minimizing envenomation. Removal of bee stingers that have been embedded for more than 1 minute will not reduce envenomation because most of the venom empties from detached honeybee stings within 10 to 20 seconds.[32]

Nonallergic local reactions require symptomatic treatment, including cool compresses (ice should not be placed directly on the skin), elevation, and local wound care. No further evaluation is necessary. If local itching is bothersome, then an oral histamine-1 (H_1) antagonist such as diphenhydramine may help. Local allergic reactions require similar care as nonallergic reactions. For very large cutaneous reactions, prednisone (0.5 to 2 mg/kg/day given in 1 to 4 doses for 3 to 5 days) may be useful.[6,14]

Acute management of corneal bee sting is aimed at preventing secondary infection with broad-spectrum topical antibiotics, reducing inflammation with topical corticosteroids, treating anterior uveitis, early detection and treatment of inflammatory glaucoma, and providing pain relief.[19] Surgical removal of the embedded stinger is controversial. Pulse corticosteroids may prevent permanent loss of vision.[19]

Mild systemic allergic reactions may be treated with diphenhydramine or another H_1 antihistamine, supportive care, and observation. Epinephrine is the mainstay of therapy for severe systemic allergic reactions, along with H_1 antagonists, corticosteroids, and intensive supportive care.[10] A 0.01-mL/kg dose of 1:1000

BOX 346-1 How to Avoid Insect Stings

- Do not disturb nests or hives—have someone else remove them.
- Do not wear perfume, cologne, scented sunscreens, or hairspray when outdoors.
- Use footwear when outside.
- Avoid picnic areas, garbage sites, orchards, fields of clover, and flowerbeds.
- Be extra careful when gardening, and cover the hands and body.
- Avoid trips outdoors if medical help is not readily available or until maintenance immunotherapy is established.
- Do not wear brightly colored clothes or jewelry.
- Install screens on windows and doors to prevent insects from entering the home.

aqueous epinephrine solution is injected subcutaneously. The original dose should not exceed 0.3 mL, but it may be repeated in 15 minutes. Susceptible individuals should carry epinephrine self-administered kits when they go outdoors. After such a kit is used, medical help should be sought because the effect of the drug is short lasting. Severe systemic reactions from direct toxic effects of massive envenomation require intensive supportive care, therapy similar to that for anaphylactic reactions and careful monitoring for rhabdomyolysis, thrombocytopenia, cardiac arrhythmias, and renal failure. Dialysis may be required.[10,30,31]

Patients with systemic reactions who respond completely to therapy in the emergency department should be observed for 6 to 8 hours after the sting because of the possibility of a delayed anaphylactic episode. The mechanism of this delayed complication is not well understood.[15] Patients with severe symptoms, including airway, cardiovascular, or pulmonary compromise, or persistent symptoms should receive a short course of corticosteriods.[6]

At the time of discharge after a systemic reaction, all patients should be given a prescription for a self-administered epinephrine kit. The patient or caretaker should be instructed in its proper use before discharge from the emergency department. They also should be encouraged to wear a Medic Alert bracelet identifying them as being allergic to insect stings. Patients should be taught how to prevent further stings (Box 346-1).

The perception that children generally outgrow Hymenoptera sting allergies is not always true. Research has found that the long-term risk of a systemic allergic reaction to a sting among patients who do not receive venom immunotherapy is far higher in those with a history of moderate to severe reactions than in those with strictly mild (cutaneous) systemic reactions.[36]

Children who experience extracutaneous systemic reactions should be referred to an allergist for risk analysis and possible venom immunotherapy.[5,37,38] Various immunotherapy regimens exist; consequently, susceptible patients may be effectively protected within hours to days, although typical regimens take weeks to months.[39] Immediate access to aqueous epinephrine and a thorough understanding of its administration remain important aspects of care for children undergoing immunotherapy until maintenance doses are reached.[37,38]

Fire Ants

Characteristics

Approximately 20 species of ants comprise the genus *Solenopsis* (commonly known as fire ants) in the United States. Of these, 2 imported species have the most clinical importance: *Solenopsis invicta* and *Solenopsis richteri*. Three common species of native fire ant, *Solenopsis xyloni, Solenopsis geminata,* and *Solenopsis aurea,* are less aggressive, have limited geographic range, and have largely been displaced by the imported species.[40]

S invicta is red, 3 to 4 mm in length, and native to northern Argentina, Paraguay, and western Brazil. It arrived in Mobile, Alabama, in the late 1930s and has spread aggressively throughout the Southeast from Texas to Virginia, as well as into California. *S invicta* is expected to spread north along the West Coast and may reach the Canadian border by the end of 2010, displacing native species as it spreads.[41] In infested areas, imported fire ants can make up 90% of the ant population.[42]

S richteri is black, slightly larger than *S invicta,* and is native to Argentina and Uruguay. *S richteri*'s importation to southern Alabama preceded *S invicta* by approximately 20 years, and *S invicta* has largely displaced *S richteri*.[41] Currently, *S richteri* is found only in northeastern Mississippi and northwestern Alabama.

Significant changes in the characteristics of imported fire ants have occurred in the United States. *S invicta* and *S richteri* have formed hybrid species with a greater tolerance to cold, which will likely increase their geographic distribution.[43] Spread of fire ants is largely passive, commonly through soil or plant matter.[43]

Imported fire ants are extremely aggressive, which results in a high frequency of envenomation among humans in endemic areas. The literature suggests a 20% to 30% annual attack rate in endemic areas, although rates as high as 58% have been reported.[43,44] Children are especially vulnerable. The highest sting rate (close to 50%) occurs in persons younger than 20 years.[45,46] Trespassing into the fire ants' territory or disturbing a nest will incite aggressive, swarming behavior, often resulting in multiple stings. Cases of ants attacking victims indoors are not uncommon.[47-49] Heavy rains appear to increase this occurrence, although increasingly the ants are noted to nest in human-made structures.[44]

Fire ants bite the skin of their victims with their mandibles, then they arch their bodies to inject venom through a lancet-shaped stinger located at the distal end of their abdomen. If undisturbed, they will continue to sting the victim repeatedly in a circular pattern, using their mandibles as a pivot; venom is injected with each sting.[50,51,53]

Fire ant venom differs from bee and wasp venom in that it is mostly composed of alkaloid piperidine hemolytic factors and contains very little protein. However, this protein moiety is responsible for the IgE-mediated allergic reactions sometimes encountered with fire ant stings. Antigenic similarity exists between these proteins and bee and wasp venoms.[54] The alkaloid portion is believed to be responsible for releasing histamine, leading to the common local dermal reactions; it also has some neurotoxic properties.[40,45,49,50,52,54]

Fire ant envenomations are becoming an increasingly important public health concern in the United States, resulting in fatalities caused by fire ant-induced anaphylaxis.[54]

Physical Examination: Signs and Symptoms

LOCAL. Stings from imported fire ants frequently occur on children's ankles and feet in the summer. Stings tend to be multiple and cause immediate local burning and itching. Soon after, the area becomes erythematous and raised. This reaction usually subsides after 30 to 60 minutes. The classic pathognomonic finding of small, sterile pustules develops between 4 and 24 hours after the sting and is more common with stings of imported fire ants.[6,43] Pustules may occur in rings or lines consistent with fire and stinging behavior. Pustules usually resolve over 3 to 10 days. Some patients develop a large local reaction similar to that of other Hymenoptera stings. An initial wheal-and-flare reaction evolves into an erythematous, pruritic, warm, indurated area around the sting site. Large local reactions may progress for 48 hours and may not subside for 7 days. The pathophysiological mechanism of large local reactions is not clear, and they may be confused with cellulites.

Secondary bacterial infections from excoriation and open erosions are not uncommon after fire ant stings.[54] These infections are usually minor and localized. However, sepsis may result from superinfected lesions.[48]

SYSTEMIC. Systemic allergic reactions occur in up to 16% of patients treated for fire ant stings, with serious reactions, including anaphylaxis, occurring in up to 2%.[41,43] Systemic allergic reactions are similar to those associated with other insects and include bronchospasm, angioedema, urticaria, pruritus, laryngeal edema, hypotension, and anaphylaxis. Seizures, mononeuritis, Guillain-Barré syndrome, serum sickness, nephritic syndrome, and worsening of preexisting cardiopulmonary disease have also occurred.[41,43,54] The venoms of native and imported fire ants are highly cross-reactive, and phospholipase components of fire ant venom have been shown to be cross-reactive with vespid venom phospholipases.[4,40] Direct systemic toxic effects of fire ant venom are not well understood. No deaths have been attributed to date to fire ant venom toxicity.

Laboratory Studies

The diagnosis of fire ant sting is a clinical one; no confirmatory laboratory test has been developed.

Management

Mild local reactions are treated conservatively with cool compresses, oral antihistamines, and wound care. Large local reactions may require oral antihistamines and systemic corticosteroids,[10,41] and they must be carefully examined to differentiate them from cellulitis. The absence of lymphadenopathy and lymphangitis supports the diagnosis of large localized reaction.[10] Systemic allergic reactions are treated similarly to those from any cause. Epinephrine is the mainstay of therapy, coupled with H_1 antagonists, systemic corticosteroids, and vigorous supportive care as appropriate.[10,41] Patients who have experienced severe allergic reactions to stings should be referred to an allergist or immunologist for venom immunotherapy assessment.[14,55]

Harvester Ants

Harvester ants (genus *Pogonomyrmex*) belong to the Hymenoptera order, subfamily Myrmicinae, which includes the genus *Solenopsis* (fire ants). More than 20 native species inhabit the United States, but only 3 have been associated with anaphylaxis: *Pogonomyrmex barbatus, Pogonomyrmex rugosus,* and *Pogonomyrmex maricopa*.[53] Harvester ants occupy a wide geographic area and are found in the southern and western United States and in Mexico.

Similar to fire ants, harvester ants attach to the skin with their mandibles and envenomate their victim through a sting. Their venom differs from fire ant venom in that it contains a much larger fraction of protein constituents; in this regard, it is more similar to other Hymenoptera venoms.

Unlike imported fire ants, harvester ants do not leave characteristic skin lesions. Their sting resembles that of other insects and may be associated with allergic reactions. Treatment of *Pogonomyrmex* stings is the same as that for other Hymenoptera stings.

ARACHNIDS

The class Arachnida, which includes spiders, belongs to the phylum Arthropoda. In addition to spiders, other members of Arthropoda include Crustacea (shrimp and crab), Myriapoda (centipedes and millipedes), Chelicerata (a subphylum of Arachnida; spiders and scorpions), and Uniramia (Insecta; bees and flies). Members of Arachnida are distinguished from Insecta by the fact that they have 2 main body regions (cephalothorax and trunk) and Insecta have 3 (head, thorax, and abdomen). Arachnids have 4 pairs of legs to insects' 3, and arachnids are always wingless and lack antennae.

Two arachnid orders that will be discussed here are Araneae (spiders) and Scorpionidae (scorpions). Although creatures from both of these orders can inflict envenomations that result in significant morbidity, fatalities are rare. The 2005 AAPCC National Poison Database reports no fatalities as a result of spider envenomations.[3]

Spiders

The order Araneae, which includes all spiders, covers a diverse group numbering 105 families with approximately 40,000 species worldwide.[56] In North America the spiders most commonly involved in human exposures are *Loxosceles* species (brown recluse spider, also known as the violin spider or fiddleback spider), *Latrodectus* species (black widow spider), and tarantulas. All tarantulas are in the family Theraphosidae. Tarantulas are composed of 13 subfamilies, with multiple genera and species.

Approximately 50 spider species are of medical importance. Most are venomous and can sometimes cause serious injury. The differential diagnosis includes other arthropod bites, skin infections, and injury caused by chemical and physical agents.[57]

Eradicating brown recluse spiders, black widow spiders, and tarantulas is not possible. Most spiders are not aggressive and only bite in self-defense when humans invade their territory or when the spider becomes lost in items such as bedclothes. Tarantulas, which are sometimes kept as pets, pose a risk to the unsuspecting child. Prevention is therefore mostly focused on caution in areas inhabited by spiders. A clean house greatly decreases the risk of spider bite. Wearing long-sleeved shirts and gloves when outside gardening or wearing long pants tucked into socks when hiking are good preventive measures.[57] Insect repellants that contain meta-N,N-diethyltoluamide (DEET) or picaridin may offer some protection.

Loxosceles (Brown Recluse Spider)

CHARACTERISTICS AND DISTRIBUTION. Eleven *Loxosceles* species have been identified in the United States.[58] *Loxosceles* are usually found in the Southeast and Southwest United States. Although they have been suspected of traveling in baggage or cargo to other areas,[59,60] the spider has only rarely been verified outside its normal habitat.[58] In the United States, the brown recluse spider, *Loxosceles reclusa,* is usually responsible for most envenomations. Its natural habitat includes the states of southeastern Nebraska, Kansas, Oklahoma, Texas, Louisiana, Arkansas, Missouri, Kentucky, Tennessee, Mississippi, Alabama, northern Georgia, and southern areas of Ohio, Indiana, Illinois, and Iowa. *Loxosceles* species are not found in Canada.[61] Other *Loxosceles* species include *arizonica, deserta, devia,* and *rufescens.*[58] They are hearty and live in dry areas such as woodpiles, rodent burrows, vacant buildings, attics, or closets. They are reclusive and nonaggressive unless disturbed. Their web is irregular and common in appearance.

The body of the brown recluse spider is oval (10 to 15 mm long, 4 mm wide) and light fawn to dark chocolate in color. The leg span is approximately 25 mm. The eye pattern easily distinguishes them from other spiders. *Loxosceles* differ from other US spiders in that they have 6 eyes arranged in pairs—one anterior and 2 lateral—instead of 8 eyes.[58] The other often-quoted physical feature, which gives rise to the names *violin spider* or *fiddleback spider,* is a violin-shaped marking on the dorsal side of its cephalothorax, with the violin's neck pointing toward the abdomen. Although this pigmented area is seen on adult spiders, it is not always found on some species in the West and on young spiders.[58]

Bites are usually the result of accidental contact, such as looking through boxes or woodpiles, or contact with linens or clothing in which the spider has become trapped.[60]

PHYSICAL EXAMINATION: SIGNS AND SYMPTOMS

Local. The bite itself does not cause much discomfort and may go unnoticed. Sometimes a minor stinging or burning sensation may be felt at the site. Erythema, pruritus, pain, and edema typically develop within 2 to 8 hours. These symptoms may be followed in the next 24 to 48 hours by the appearance of a blue-gray halo surrounding the erythematous center. Vesicles or bullae containing serous or hemorrhagic fluid soon follow.[56]

Local ischemia and necrosis result in the formation of a black eschar within 7 to 10 days of the bite. This necrotic area may expand slowly in diameter for weeks, especially in fatty areas that have delicate blood supplies such as the abdomen, buttocks, and thighs.[62] The eschar is shed after 2 to 5 weeks and an ulcer remains that may take weeks to months to heal.

Systemic. Systemic manifestations of the bite are less common than cutaneous ones. The most common symptoms are fever, chills, and malaise. Symptoms usually occur within 24 hours of the bite and also may include nausea, vomiting, diarrhea, arthralgia, urticaria or maculopapular rash, hemolytic anemia, disseminated intravascular coagulation, jaundice, renal failure, transverse myelitis, seizures, and shock.[63,64]

DIFFERENTIAL DIAGNOSIS. In the absence of a definitive history of spider bites, other diagnostic possibilities must be considered, such as emboli, thrombi, focal vasculitis, envenomation by other insects or reptiles, fat herniation with infarction, pressure sore, pyoderma gangrenosum, poison oak or ivy, cutaneous manifestation of gonorrhea or herpes simplex, diabetic ulcer, purpura fulminans, erythema nodosum, erythema multiforme, Stevens-Johnson syndrome, or abusive or self-inflicted trauma.[58] Cutaneous anthrax has also been misdiagnosed as *Loxosceles* envenomation.[58]

Other species of spiders have been implicated in the cause of necrotic skin lesions similar to *Loxosceles.* These are *Argiope* (orb weaver spider), *Chiracanthium* (sac spider), *Lycosa* (wolf spider), *Phidippus* (jumping spider), and *Tegenaria agrestis.*[63,65] Although other spiders can produce a necrotizing skin lesion, the temptation to diagnose all necrotizing skin lesions as *Loxosceles* bites should be avoided. Positive identification of the spider is important not only for the correct diagnosis, but also to understand better the true clinical course of *Loxosceles* envenomation.

LABORATORY STUDIES. No current clinical laboratory study can confirm the presence of arachnid venom–related necrosis. Several research tests, including enzyme-linked immunosorbent assay and passive hemagglutination inhibition test, have been studied; but no such test is in clinical use.[66,67] Complete blood counts, coagulation profiles, electrolytes, and renal function should be monitored in systemic illness.

MANAGEMENT. Management is controversial because the unpredictable natural course of the wounds makes prospective trials difficult.[58] Serial observations, cleansing, cool compresses, splinting of the affected extremity, and tetanus prophylaxis are often-suggested measures. Symptomatic relief with antipruritics and analgesics may be useful in some cases.

Different therapies have been proposed, including systemic corticosteroids, antibiotics, antihistamines, colchicine, dapsone, electric shock, hyperbaric oxygen, metronidazole, and surgical excision and skin graft.[58,68,69] None of these therapies is of proven efficacy for *Loxosceles* envenomation. Although the most suitable therapy in children is unclear, general agreement exists on delaying any surgical repair of skin defects until the necrotic demarcation is discrete and no further spread occurs. This period is approximately 8 weeks.

Latrodectus (Black Widow Spider)

CHARACTERISTICS. Although both male and female black widow spiders have venom, only the female spider has fangs that are powerful enough to bite through skin and envenomate humans. Black widow spiders are among the largest spiders in the world, with a leg span of 40 mm and a body of 1.5 cm. The mature female spider is black, with a red or orange hourglass-shaped marking on the ventral surface. The immature female spider may be red, brown, or cream in color, and the hourglass marking may be cream colored or even incomplete.[63]

The web, usually built close to the ground in dimly lit, moist areas, is distinguishable by its irregular pattern. It may be found in barns, outhouses, lumber piles, and sheds where insects are plentiful. Bites are usually a result of the spider being disturbed and acting in self-defense.[70]

DISTRIBUTION. *Latrodectus* spiders are found in both temperate and tropical climates throughout the world. Five species are found in the United States; Alaska is the only state that does not have this genus. The most common spiders implicated in bites are *Latrodectus mactans, Latrodectus variolus,* and *Latrodectus hesperus.* Envenomations by any of these species result in the same clinical syndrome.

PHYSICAL EXAMINATION: SIGNS AND SYMPTOMS

Local. A bite may go unnoticed or may be experienced as a pinprick or burning sensation. Two small puncture lesions may be visible. Within 30 minutes, pain develops at the site and in the regional lymph nodes. Central pallor at the bite site with surrounding erythema has been described. Unlike the bite of *Loxosceles,* the black widow bite does not usually induce an impressive inflammatory response. An unusual reaction may include compartment syndrome, which may improve after antivenin administration.[71]

Systemic. The onset of systemic symptoms is frequently sudden, with crampy, skeletal muscle pains in the legs, abdomen, back, and chest and associated autonomic dysfunction. The most frequent systemic signs and symptoms are generalized abdominal pain or back pain, local or extremity pain, hypertension, diaphoresis, and isolated abdominal or chest pains. Nausea and vomiting and tachycardia may also be present.[72] Restlessness, salivation, bronchorrhea, priapism, urinary retention, periorbital edema, tremor, and convulsions may also be seen.[5,59] Abdominal rigidity may mimic peritoneal irritation. Respiratory paralysis, heart failure, and myocarditis have been reported.[73] In children, symptoms include abdominal pain, hypertension, muscle complaints, target-shaped skin lesions, and irritability or agitation.[74] Treatment may alleviate symptoms.

Patients who do not receive antivenin may experience protracted symptoms that may last for several days to a week.[70,75] Symptoms can include fatigue, weakness, paresthesias, generalized aches, diaphoresis, headache, sleeplessness, excessive sweating, impotence, mental status changes, and transient hemiparesis.[55]

The primary protein component of *Latrodectus* venom is α-lactrotoxin. This protein binds to motor end plate receptors, causing increased synaptic concentration of catecholamines. This excess catecholamine results in characteristic muscle cramps, hypertension, nausea, vomiting, weakness, tremors, and malaise.[75]

LABORATORY STUDIES. No specific laboratory test helps establish a diagnosis. Leukocytosis and hyperglycemia are common. Creatine phosphokinase may be increased as a result of increased muscle activity. Serum calcium levels are normal.

DIFFERENTIAL DIAGNOSIS. The causes of acute abdominal pain should be part of the differential diagnosis. Of interest is the close resemblance of the autonomic hyperactivity seen after black widow spider bites and those seen in organophosphate poisoning.

MANAGEMENT. Most black widow spider bites require only cool compresses, elevation of the affected extremity, tetanus update (if needed), and analgesics. In more severe cases, administration of oxygen, cardiac monitoring, and intravenous access are suggested.

Muscle cramps may be relieved with opiates and muscle relaxants. Diazepam, methocarbamol, and calcium gluconate have been used with varying results. The efficacy of 10% calcium gluconate has been questioned.[72] Patients who do not receive antivenin will gradually improve over the next 12 to 48 hours, and some patients may experience protracted symptoms.

Latrodectus antivenin of equine origin is available and neutralizes venom from all related species.[76] Patients should be tested for horse serum hypersensitivity before it is administered because death from anaphylaxis may result.[72] It should be considered in cases of severe envenomation when the patient shows evidence of respiratory distress, marked hypertension, and cardiovascular compromise. *Latrodectus* antivenin should also be considered in pregnant women and for protracted symptoms that do not respond to analgesics and muscle relaxants. Response is usually dramatic after antivenin infusion. The administration of antivenin may decrease the length of hospital stay and prevent lingering neurologic complications.[56,76]

Tarantulas (Mygalomorphs)

CHARACTERISTICS. Tarantulas, more appropriately called *mygalomorphs,* are considered primitive forms of true spiders. In the United States, the species spends most of the daytime hours in burrows, emerging to hunt at night.[56,60] They are docile, and bites are unusual. Body size varies; they can reach up to 10 cm in diameter. These spiders possess large fangs that point straight down and require them to lean back on their hind legs to bite—a characteristic defensive posture. More than 30 species of tarantulas are found in the tropical and subtropical desert areas of the southwestern United States. Some North American and foreign species are kept as pets.

PHYSICAL EXAMINATION: SIGNS AND SYMPTOMS. Most bites are no more severe than a bee sting and occasionally result in local erythema, swelling, and pain. Nausea and vomiting may occur from the bite. Some genera (*Lasiodora, Grammostola, Acanthoscurria,* and *Brachypelma*) are capable of releasing urticaria-producing hairs from their abdomen by rubbing their hind legs on the area. This event can result in local histamine release with mild pruritus. However, the itching can last for weeks.[56,60,63] The hairs may cause itching in eyes or airways and cause considerable discomfort.[56]

MANAGEMENT. Local wound care and a tetanus update are all that is needed in most cases; antihistamines and oral analgesics may be helpful. Adhesive tape or irrigation with saline solution may be used to remove the urticaria-producing hairs from the skin.

Scorpions

Characteristics

Centruroides exilicauda, formerly *Centruroides sculpturatus,* or the bark scorpion, is the only medically relevant species of scorpion in the United States.[77] Envenomation may be life threatening in children. The bark scorpion's habitat is Arizona and adjacent states in the southwestern United States.[77] Scorpions are found in Arizona and parts of southern California, Nevada, New Mexico, and Texas. *C exilicauda,* which is considered a climbing scorpion, can be sighted on trees, fence posts, and rocks and in cracks and trash piles. It measures 1.3 to 7.5 cm in length and envenomates its victim with a stinger located at the tip of its tail. The venom is a potent neurotoxin that activates neuronal sodium channels and results in excessive firing of the affected neurons, including both adrenergic and parasympathetic systems.[78,79] Patients may exhibit both adrenergic and cholinergic symptoms.

Stings usually result from accidental contact with a scorpion trapped in linen or clothing or during outdoor play. Not all stings result in clinical evidence of envenomation. Although most stings take place in scorpion-endemic areas, scorpions can be accidentally transported to other areas by travelers.

Physical Examination: Signs and Symptoms

LOCAL. Pain at the sting site with or without paresthesias is common, especially with species other than *Centruroides.*[80] In mild envenomations, pain may be the only symptom. Infants may exhibit this symptom as unexplained crying.[78] Local erythema and swelling may surround a small puncture wound, but the sting site is often unidentifiable. Paresthesias and pruritus are also frequent.[80]

SYSTEMIC. Systemic manifestations of scorpion envenomation can be dramatic and usually develop within 60 minutes of the sting. They tend to be more common in children younger than 10 years.[77,79] Cardiovascular findings include tachycardia or bradycardia.[81] Children may experience central nervous system dysfunction, a finding that is rare in adults. Severe hypertension may be present in one-third to two-thirds of the victims. Hypertension is sometimes associated with acute hypertensive encephalopathy. Heart failure and acute lung injury may also be seen. An ischemic electrocardiographic pattern may be present. Hypertension may not respond to medical management.[81]

Echocardiographic, scintigraphic, and hemodynamic evaluations reveal hypodynamic ventricular motion with decreased systolic performance.[81,82] Pulmonary edema is a common feature and is likely due to decreased ventricular performance in the setting of increased venous return, arterial hypertension, kinin-induced increased permeability of the pulmonary vasculature, and impaired left-ventricular filling caused by tachycardia.[81-83] Electrocardiographic changes are common and include nonspecific ST-T changes or ST elevation or depression consistent with myocardial infarction.[81,82]

Pathological cardiac specimens show evidence of ischemia and direct toxicity.[81,82] The primary mechanism of cardiovascular toxicity is thought to be the result of excessive stimulation of the autonomic nervous system, with the sympathetic influence generally being greater than the parasympathetic. Cardiac effects may also be mediated by electrolyte changes, in particular a relative hyperkalemia.[82]

Neurologic toxicity includes excessive cholinergic stimulation resulting in salivation, sweating, and vomiting.[81] Profound sialorrhea may be evident.[80,84]

Skeletal muscle findings include twitching or jerking of the extremities, which, in some cases, may be severe enough to be mistaken for seizure activity. Rhabdomyolysis may result from this event.[78] Nystagmus may be present.[80] Seizures and agitation may also occur.

Differential Diagnosis

Two factors make establishing the correct diagnosis difficult. The first is that the sting site may not be identifiable; the second is that the child may not be able to communicate the history of a sting clearly. Seizure disorders, intra-abdominal catastrophes, phenothiazine or cholinergic poisoning, and allergic reactions are some of the differential diagnostic possibilities. Some children have been misdiagnosed as having asthma in the presence of wheezing and respiratory distress.[79]

Progression of symptoms is not predictable; progression to serious symptoms usually occurs in less than 5 hours, if at all. Numbness, tingling, and pain may persist for 2 weeks.[85] The duration of symptoms has been found to be inversely related to the age of the patient.[79]

Laboratory Studies

Scorpion envenomation is a clinical determination; no confirmatory laboratory test exists. Leukocytosis, cerebrospinal fluid pleocytosis, and increased creatine phosphokinase have been reported.[78,81]

Management

The treatment of scorpion envenomation is primarily supportive, with the use of cold compresses and analgesics. Severe cases require aggressive supportive therapy. Although various therapies have been tried, no clear standard therapy has been developed.[81,82] Antihypertensives, including calcium-channel blockers, hydralazine, prazosin, and captopril, have all been used. At present, afterload reducers such as angiotensin-converting enzyme inhibitors, calcium-channel blockers, or prazosin are front-line therapeutic agents for hypertension.[81,82] Concern about reflex tachycardia has led some clinicians to favor prazosin and captopril.[81,82] The use of diuretics for pulmonary edema is controversial.[81,82] Atropine may be used with caution if cholinergic symptoms become severe.[81,82,84] Atropine may improve hypersecretion, obviating the need for more aggressive therapy. Treatment should be guided by thorough hemodynamic monitoring. Benzodiazepines are generally administered for the treatment of seizures and agitation.[82] Corticosteroid therapy has been shown to be of no benefit.[86]

Currently, no scorpion antivenin is approved in the United States by the US Food and Drug Administration. Clinical trials at the University of Arizona are ongoing with an equine-derived antigen-binding fragment (Fab_2) antivenin.[87] In the future, antivenin therapy may decrease the need for hospitalization, the length of stay, and the number of intensive care procedures required.

SNAKES

In 2005 the AAPCC National Poison Database recorded almost 3000 coral and Crotalinae snake envenomations.[3] The venomous snakes of North America can be divided into 2 families: Viperidae (subfamily Crotalinae) and Elapidae. The Crotalinae includes genera *Crotalus* (rattlesnakes), *Agkistrodon* (water moccasins or cottonmouths and copperheads), and *Sistrurus* (pygmy rattlesnakes and Massasauga rattlesnakes). As a group, these snakes are known as *pit vipers* because of a heat-sensitive pit found behind and below their nostrils. Snakes use this organ to locate the victim of a strike. The Elapidae family includes coral snakes, as well as the nonindigenous cobras and mambas.

Epidemiologic Features

Type of Snake

Envenomations by snakes in North America are overwhelmingly caused by indigenous Crotalinae; Elapidae constitute less than 1% of envenomations.[88] Nonindigenous snakes in North American zoos or kept as exotic house pets are responsible for only a small percentage of envenomations.[89] All sea snakes are venomous, but fortunately, none inhabit the coastal waters of North America.[90]

Host Factors

The typical snakebite victim is a young adult white male who is bitten while handling or playing with a snake. Many of those bitten have a blood alcohol level of more than 0.1%. Less than one-half of rattlesnake bites occur before an encounter with a snake was recognized or while the person was attempting to move away from the snake.[91] Most bites in the United States occur in the southwestern states (Figure 346-1).

Body Area

Most bites are inflicted on the upper extremity, including fingers, hand, and arm. Other, less commonly affected sites are leg or foot, and torso.[92] Given the high percentage of bites experienced while the snake was intentionally being handled, these sites are less surprising than reports of snakebites to the tongue[93] and the glans penis.[94]

Mortality

The number of deaths from snakebite in the United States ranges from 0 to 14 per year.[3,88,95] Most snakebite deaths are associated with the absence of medical care, errors in medical management, or the presence of an underlying medical condition. Children are at increased risk for serious sequelae because of their lower body mass and the relatively high venom dose per kilogram of body weight compared with adults.

Prevention

Historically, Native Americans used numerous plants, animal tissues, oils, and excrement to prevent snakebites.[95] Box 346-2 provides current practical

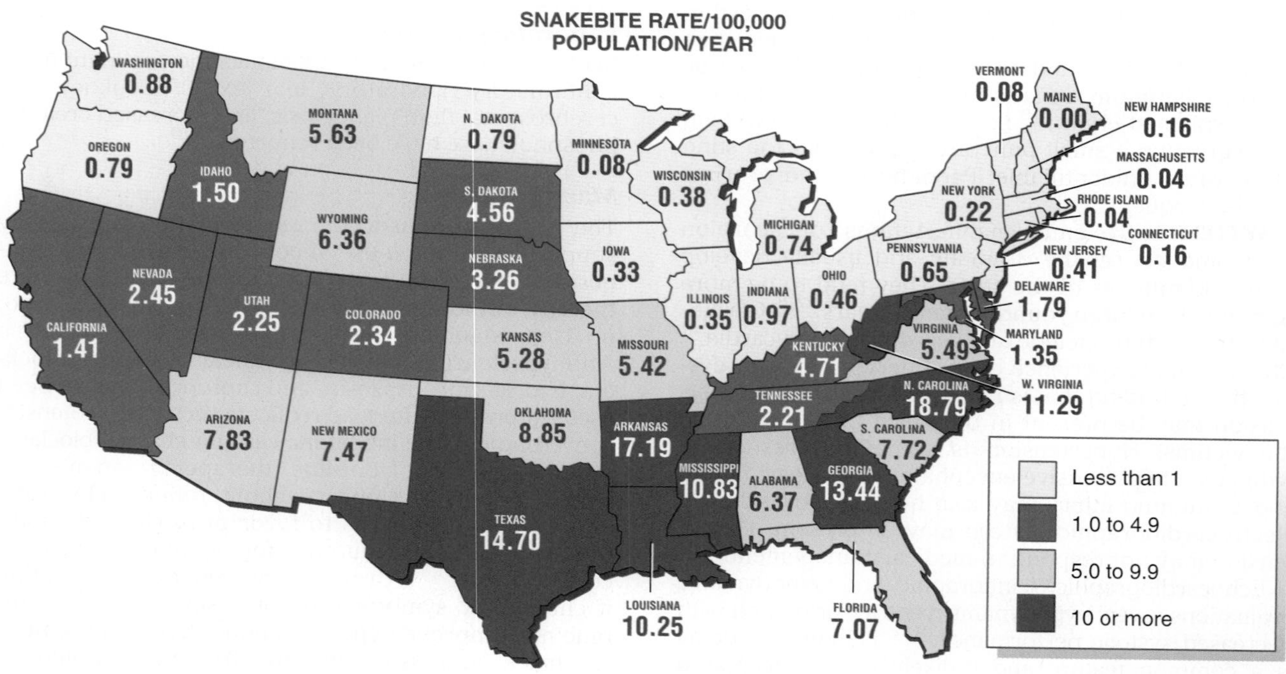

Figure 346-1 Incidence of snake venom poisoning by state. (*Russell FEL.* Snake Venom Poisoning. *New York, NY: Scholium International; 1983. Reprinted by permission.*)

suggestions for preventing snakebites that are based on the epidemiologic mechanism of these injuries and the medical community's understanding of snake behavior.

BOX 346-2 Snakebite Prevention

1. Differentiating poisonous from nonpoisonous snakes is impossible without years of experience. Therefore children should not approach, disturb, play with, capture, or kill any snake. These practices are dangerous for both the human and the snake.
2. Children should not put their hands or feet in places they cannot see. Children should not put their hands or feet anywhere without first looking.
3. Snakes frequently can be found under rocks, boulders, fallen trees, fences, rubbish piles, and boats that have been left on shore for several hours; in tall grass and heavy underbrush; or sunning themselves on logs, boulders, trees, walls, or cliffs. Extra caution should be used in these areas.
4. The striking distance of a snake is roughly half its length. Children should be taught to keep a safe distance from snakes.
5. The striking reflex remains intact for up to an hour after the snake has died. Therefore, even if certainty exists that the snake is dead, it must be examined or transported at the opposite end of a long stick.
6. Rattlesnakes are nocturnal feeders and therefore are active after dark. Never gather firewood after dark. Camp should be set up on open ground, never near wood, rubbish piles, swampy areas, or the entrance of a cave.
7. Children should wear boots when walking in areas endemic for snakes.
8. Children should not be allowed to walk alone in an area endemic for snakes.
9. Children should not be allowed to swim in waters known to be infested with snakes.
10. Once bitten, everyone present should get away from the snake as quickly as possible. The benefit of identifying the snake is small in comparison to the risk of additional bites.

Characteristics

Some key characteristics can help distinguish between venomous and nonvenomous snakes; however, overlap and exceptions create difficulty in distinguishing the difference (Table 346-2).[96,97] Crotalinae are characterized by a heat-sensing pit on either side of the head between the eye and the nostril. This apparatus is used to locate and estimate the size of prey and predators. The snake can estimate a venom dose in accordance with the size of the prey that is to be immobilized, killed, and digested.[7]

Crotaline snakes have highly mobile and retractable, hollow fangs that function similarly to a hypodermic needle. They usually penetrate to subcutaneous tissue, but large snakes can reach a depth of 8 to 19 mm.[79] The speed of a pit viper's strike has been clocked at 8 feet per second, and the animal can reach distances of approximately one-half of its body length.[96] Consequently, larger snakes may penetrate dermal or subcutaneous structures and deposit venom into the muscle. Venom is generally absorbed through the lymphatic system, although rare cases of intra-arterial and intravenous deposition of venom have been reported. For an envenomation to take place, the pit viper must be venomous at the time of the strike, penetrate the skin, and inject venom during penetration. Approximately 20% to 25% of pit viper bites are *dry*, meaning they do not result in envenomation.[97]

Crotaline venom is a complex mixture of biologically active proteins and peptides capable of damaging vascular endothelial cells, leading to increased permeability to plasma and erythrocytes into the extravascular space, which can ultimately result in hypotension and shock.[96,98,99] This process may also occur in the lungs, myocardium, kidneys, peritoneum, and central nervous system.[98] Other enzymes specific to pit viper venom include proteolytic enzymes, hyaluronidase, thrombin-like enzymes, phospholipase-A_2, L–amino acid oxidase, collagenase, RNase, DNAse, and arginine ester hydrolase.[96,98] Venom is spread throughout the body as a result of the action of hyaluronidase and its integrity-reducing effect on connective tissue.

Pit viper venoms, which are derived from the salivary glands, are designed to immobilize and digest prey. Prominent effects include direct tissue injury resulting from enzymatic degradation. Local inflammatory responses are exaggerated by metalloproteinases, which cleave pro–tumor necrosis factor alpha (TNF-α),

Table 346-2 Characteristics of Venomous Versus Nonvenomous Snakes*

CHARACTERISTIC	VENOMOUS SNAKE	NONVENOMOUS SNAKE
Triangular head shape	+	+/–
Elliptical pupils	+	+/–†
Single row of subcaudal scales	+/–‡	+/–
Presence of fangs	+	+/–
Pit sensor	+	–
Rattle	+/–	–

*+ indicates present; –, absent.
†Some North American boas have cat's-eye pupils.
‡Coral snakes have a double row of scales.

releasing activated TNF-α.[88,98,100] Myotoxin-α acts to increase intracellular calcium in skeletal muscle, resulting in prolonged contraction and necrosis.[88] The presence of systemic myotoxin-α and phospholipase-A_2 is thought to be the cause of myonecrosis and rhabdomyolysis.[88] Phospholipids A_2 also increase permeability of red blood cell membranes, changing their morphology and potentially causing hemolysis. One of the byproducts of the enzymatic action of phospholipase-A_2 is lysolecithin, which can damage mast cell membranes and cause histamine release.[96]

Coagulopathy caused by fibrinolysis and thrombin-like peptide actions may result in isolated defibrination.[88] Thrombocytopenia occurs as a result of platelet aggregation at sites of tissue injury, as well as from a direct effect of venom on individual platelets, particularly rattlesnake venom.[88,101] Given that thrombocytopenia and defibrination both occur independently, the clinician must distinguish between these processes occurring simultaneously and true disseminated intravascular coagulation, which may also occur. Neurotoxins are also present in varying degrees, notably in the Mojave and timber rattlesnakes, and can produce weakness and paralysis, as well as myokymia, which appears as involuntary wormlike muscle movements under the skin.[102] The cause of crotaline-induced neurotoxicity remains under study.[88,102]

The notion that juvenile rattlesnakes are more dangerous than adult snakes is a misconception. The venom of some juvenile rattlesnakes may be slightly more toxic, but larger rattlesnakes are capable of delivering more venom in a single bite.[103] Additionally, venom composition appears to change as the rattlesnake matures. Specifically, phospholipase-A_2 activity decreases with the snake's age, but proteolytic activity increases.[103] The clinical relevance of these differences is uncertain.

Distribution

Box 346-3 lists the indigenous locations for North American pit vipers.[104]

First Aid

Commonly accepted guidelines for snakebite first aid are summarized in Box 346-4.[91] Other forms of first aid are controversial and are discussed here because the physician may see patients who are less damaged by the snake than by the field treatment of well-meaning but untrained (and possibly inebriated) attendants.

Identification

The helpfulness of identifying the type of snake is controversial. Snake parts should never be handled directly because the bite reflex in recently killed or decapitated snakes can remain intact, rendering them capable of biting even when they are dead.[92] Snakebite victims should be rushed to medical attention, and the rescue party should not expose themselves to risk while trying to find and identify the snake. If medically necessary, a herpetologist from a zoo or aquarium may be able to help with positive identification.

BOX 346-3 Indigenous Locations for North American Pit Vipers

SOUTHEAST
- Cottonmouths and copperheads*
- Eastern diamondback *(Crotalus adamanteus)*
- Timber *(Crotalus horridus)*
- Southeastern pygmy rattlesnakes *(Sistrurus miliarius barbouri)*

MIDWEST
- Cottonmouths and copperheads*
- Eastern diamondback *(Crotalus adamanteus)*
- Timber *(Crotalus horridus)*
- Prairie *(Crotalus viridis)*

NORTHEAST
- Cottonmouths and copperheads*
- Eastern diamondback *(Crotalus adamanteus)*
- Timber *(Crotalus horridus)*
- Eastern Massasauga rattlesnakes *(Sistrurus catenadus)*

NORTHWEST
- Great Basin *(Crotalus viridis lutosus)*
- Northern Pacific *(Crotalus viridis oreganus)*

SOUTHWEST
- Western diamondback *(Crotalus atrox)*
- Sidewinder *(Crotalus cerastes)*
- Rock *(Crotalus lepidus)*
- Speckled *(Crotalus mitchelli)*
- Black-tailed *(Crotalus molossus)*
- Twin-spotted *(Crotalus pricei)*
- Red diamond *(Crotalus ruber)*
- Mojave *(Crotalus scutulatus)*
- Tiger *(Crotalus tigris)*
- Prairie *(Crotalus viridis)*
- Grand Canyon *(Crotalus viridis abyssus)*
- Southern Pacific *(Crotalus viridis helleri)*
- Great Basin *(Crotalus viridis lutosus)*
- Ridge-nosed *(Crotalus willardi)*

**Agkistrodon* species.
From Banner W. Bites and stings in the pediatric patient. *Curr Probl Pediatr.* 1988;18:1-69.

Cryotherapy

Cryotherapy is a form of snakebite treatment that is theorized to constrict blood flow, thus diminishing systemic venom absorption and inactivating the venom enzymes and proteins. Freezing does not inactivate snake venom. Cases of limb ischemia have been reported from cryotherapy. Cryotherapy should not be used to treat snake envenomation.

Incision and Suction

Incision at the bite site and suction has shown mixed results in clinical and laboratory trials.[24,88,105,106] Complications of incision and suction include damage to

BOX 346-4 First Aid for Snakebites

1. Observe the approximate size and characteristics of the snake if this can be done without danger of remaining within the snake's striking range.
2. Move the patient as little as possible.
3. Mark the victim's skin with a pen to indicate the area of swelling and the time. Repeat this every 15 minutes.
4. Remove rings, watches, and constrictive clothing.
5. Immobilize the affected limb by splinting as if for a fracture, and keep the limb below the level of the heart.
6. Regardless of early symptoms, transport the victim to the nearest medical facility at a safe speed.
7. Avoid the use of ice (tissue damage), aspirin (anticoagulation), alcohol or sedative drugs (vasodilation), or stimulants such as caffeine (acceleration of venom absorption).
8. As soon as possible, start basic life support, including volume expansion and Trendelenburg position for patients with hypotension.

underlying neurovascular structures, increased rate of wound infection, and further tissue damage.[88,106] Given that no clear benefit has been demonstrated, incision and suction should not be performed.

Constricting Bands

Constricting bands that impede blood flow should not be used. Only loose-fitting bands placed in an effort to reduce lymphatic flow have been advocated, but these have not been shown to be of clear benefit.[88,106] Thus constricting bands of either type should not be used.[88,106] Although the routine use of an extractor device for care in the field is not advocated, patients who have an extractor or suction device in place should not remove it until they arrive at a health care facility.[107]

Immobilization

Splinting of the affected extremity and placing it in a position below the level of the heart should be performed without delaying transport to a medical facility. Patients should be kept as calm as possible during transport because agitation hastens venom distribution.

In-Hospital Care

Information elicited in the medical history of known envenomations include the size and species of the snake, the circumstances of the bite (eg, through clothing, alcohol related), the number of bites and body area affected, first-aid methods used, time of bite and transport time, previous snakebite history, allergy to horse- or sheep-derived products (eg, drugs, food, animal products), and tetanus immunization status.[92] The patient's coexisting medical conditions, with special attention paid to the cardiovascular, pulmonary, and neurologic systems, should be factored into the clinical management of the exposure. Snakebites from exotic (nonindigenous) species, which usually occur in zoo employees or in those illegally keeping the snake as a house pet, also occur, and clinicians must address this issue as part of the history-gathering process. The clinical presentation and medical management of an exotic bite may differ from bites of North American poisonous snakes.

Physical Examination: Signs and Symptoms

Local

Local signs and symptoms usually include the presence of one or more fang marks, as well as pain, edema, ecchymosis, and erythema from 15 minutes to 4 hours after the bite. The notion that copperhead envenomations are generally benign as compared with other pit viper envenomations is not true. Although ecchymosis and swelling are considered to be less common after copperhead bites, significant local injury after copperhead envenomation has been reported.[99,108,109] Pain is present in more than 90% of envenomations, although an exception is the Mojave rattlesnake, the bites of which inflict little or no pain.[99] Fang marks typically have ragged edges, but these edges may be obscured as a result of trauma experienced during the flight from the snake or trauma resulting from first-aid attempts. Because of the presence of hemorrhagic toxins in pit viper venom, blood may ooze from the puncture sites, and hemorrhagic bullae may develop. Muscle necrosis also may become apparent. Lymphangitis and lymphadenopathy with tender regional lymph nodes and warmth in the injured body part may occur as a result of lymphatic spread of venom components.[98,99]

Systemic

Typical systemic findings may include malaise, weakness, lightheadedness, diaphoresis, visual disturbances, nausea, vomiting, syncope, myokymia, perioral paresthesias, and a metallic or minty taste.[99,110] More severe systemic effects include altered sensorium, acute respiratory distress syndrome, respiratory depression, hemodynamic instability leading to circulatory collapse, and renal failure. A consumptive coagulopathy is frequently present in serious envenomations characterized by hemolysis, unmeasurable international normalized ratio (INR) and activated partial thromboplastin time, hypofibrinogenemia, the presence of fibrin degradation products, thrombocytopenia (<20,000/mm^3), and generalized hemorrhage.[99] When combined with defibrination, venom-induced thrombocytopenia may appear as disseminated intravascular coagulation; it may also be a contributing factor to disseminated intravascular coagulation.[98] The Mojave rattlesnake may cause more neurotoxicity, specifically myokymia, than other rattlesnakes.

Laboratory Studies

Laboratory studies have been found to be of only minor assistance when severity of rattlesnake envenomation is being assessed.[81] However, they may be useful in determining whether envenomation has actually occurred early in the course of treatment.[88] Studies should include a complete blood count with differential, red blood cells morphology (to assess for spherocytosis), INR and prothrombin time, plasma thromboplastin time, fibrinogen levels, fibrin-split products, and platelet count. If these studies reveal any abnormalities, or if the patient has clinical symptoms, then envenomation must be assumed, and analysis of electrolytes, blood urea nitrogen, and blood type and cross-match should be performed, as well as a urinalysis. Patients may require further testing as the clinical situation dictates.

Disposition

After pit viper envenomation, all patients should be observed in the emergency department for a minimum of 8 hours.[99] Patients who remain asymptomatic and whose coagulation study results are normal may then be discharged with instructions to return if symptoms develop. Symptomatic patients and all patients treated with antivenin should be admitted to intensive care.

Local Therapy

Local wound care includes gentle irrigation, non-constrictive immobilization, elevation of the bitten extremity, and close observation. Circumferential measurements at several points along the affected limb should be performed at baseline and regularly repeated to monitor the progression of swelling. Intercompartmental pressures should only be measured in cases when the patient's symptoms are consistent with compartment syndrome. The snakebite extremity may appear nearly identical to an extremity with a compartment syndrome.[98] In cases of suspected compartment syndrome, clinical diagnosis requires objective evidence of increases in compartment pressure to more than 30 mm Hg.[99] Fasciotomy has not been shown to be of benefit and may lengthen the hospitalization and cause significant long-term morbidity.[88,111,112] No evidence exists for the use of excisional therapy, and its use is discouraged.[88,98,111,112] Digital dermotomy may be indicated on clinical grounds.[88]

Shock

Patients may have marked decrease in intravascular volume as a result of hemorrhage, third-space fluid loss, vomiting, and diaphoresis. Crystalloid replacement should begin immediately in envenomated patients. In the case of hypotension caused by extravascular fluid shifts or hemorrhage, antivenin therapy should be considered.

Fluid and Electrolyte Abnormalities

Extensive third-space fluid loss may cause fluid and electrolyte imbalances. Electrolyte and urine output monitoring with fluid and electrolyte replacement with crystalloid is essential.

Hematologic Complications

Treatment of thrombocytopenia and anemia (caused by hemolysis) may require multiple transfusions. Transfusions of fresh-frozen plasma and cryoprecipitate may be required in severely envenomated patients. Therapy with blood products is rarely effective, however, in the absence of antivenin therapy. Treatment with coagulation factors may actually worsen the coagulopathy by adding more substrate for unneutralized venom, thus increasing the levels of degradation products, which are also anticoagulants.[99] Thrombocytopenia often corrects with antivenin therapy alone, and clotting factor levels rarely improve when blood products are provided without antivenin.[88] Disseminated intravascular coagulopathy caused by snakebite does not respond to heparin; antivenin is the treatment of choice.

Use of Antivenom

The sole antivenin used from 1954 to 2000 in the United States to treat pit viper envenomations was antivenin (Crotalidae) polyvalent (ACP). It was produced by injecting horses with venom from *Crotalus adamanteus, Crotalus atrox, Crotalus durissus teriffi-cus,* and *Bothrops atrox.* A high incidence of serum sickness and serious allergic reaction was associated with its use. Skin testing was necessary before administration of antivenin. After December 2000, crotaline polyvalent immune Fab (ovine) antivenin (CroFab, Savage Laboratories, a division of Altana Inc, Melville, NY) was released. CroFab has replaced the horse serum-based antivenin ACP as the drug of choice for crotaline envenomations, and ACP is no longer manufactured. CroFab is a purified ovine polyvalent Fab immunoglobulin fragment product produced by immunizing sheep with venoms of 4 crotaline snakes: *C adamanteus* (eastern diamondback), *C atrox* (western diamondback), *Crotalus scutulatus* (Mojave rattlesnake), and *Agkistrodon piscivorus* (cottonmouth).[99,113,114]

Indications for CroFab therapy are for the treatment of patients with minimal or moderate North American crotaline envenomation (Table 346-3). Administration of CroFab within 6 hours is advised to prevent clinical deterioration and the occurrence of systemic coagulation abnormalities.[114] However, delayed use of CroFab has been reported with successful correction of significant toxicity incurred after crotaline envenomation.[115]

Antivenin use should proceed simultaneously with supportive therapy (Box 346-5). CroFab is administered with the goal of achieving *initial control,* which is defined as the reversal or marked attenuation of all effects of venom.[99] This process encompasses 3 general areas: (1) coagulation abnormalities, (2) systemic effects, and (3) local effects (progression of swelling). Box 346-5 outlines the dosing. If *initial control* is not achieved, then the loading dose of 4 to 6 vials should be repeated until the envenomation syndrome is halted. Once initial control has been established, maintenance doses of 2 vials every 6 hours for 3 doses is recommended. Epinephrine, corticosteroids, antihistamines, and airway maintenance equipment should be provided at the bedside. Volume depletion should be aggressively treated before initiating antivenin therapy because of the risk of rapid vasodilatation and third-space fluid loss associated with anaphylaxis. Anaphylaxis associated with antivenin therapy should be treated in the standard fashion.[88]

Recurrence Phenomena

Recurrence phenomena are described as worsening status caused by return of venom effect after it has been successfully abated with antivenin. *Local recurrence* indicates return of swelling after initial control achieved, and *coagulopathic recurrence* describes the return of thrombocytopenia or hypofibrinogenemia

Table 346-3 Envenomation Categories and Definitions

ENVENOMATION CATEGORY	DEFINITION
Minimal	Swelling, pain, and ecchymosis are limited to the immediate bite site. Systemic signs and symptoms are absent. Coagulation parameters are normal, with no clinical evidence of bleeding.
Moderate	Swelling, pain, and ecchymosis involves less than a full extremity, or, if bite was inflicted on the trunk, head, or neck, extends less than 50 cm. Systemic signs and symptoms may be present but not life threatening, including but not limited to nausea, vomiting, oral paresthesia or unusual tastes, mild hypotension (systolic blood pressure >90 mm Hg), mild tachycardia (heart rate <150 beats/min), and tachypnea. Coagulation parameters may be abnormal, but no clinical evidence of bleeding present. Minor hematuria, gum bleeding, and nosebleeds are allowed if they are not considered severe in the investigator's judgment.
Severe	Swelling, pain, and ecchymosis involves more than an entire extremity or threatens the airway. Systemic signs and symptoms are markedly abnormal, including several alteration of mental status, severe hypotension, severe tachycardia, tachypnea, or respiratory insufficiency. Coagulation parameters are abnormal, with serious bleeding or severe threat of bleeding.

From CroFab [package insert]. Melville, NY: Savage Laboratories, a division of Altana, Inc; 2006.

after initial control is achieved. Recurrent coagulopathy has been reported after the use of both ACP and CroFab.[116] With CroFab, the cause of recurrence is probably due to the clearance of unbound antivenin being faster than the absorption and clearance of some venom components.[117,118] Such may not be the case with coagulopathic recurrence. All CroFab recipients should be reevaluated at least once during the 5 days after antivenin treatment.[119] The decision to administer additional antivenin in patients who develop delayed coagulopathy must be made on a case-by-case basis.

An isolated hematologic abnormality after envenomation poses a low risk for significant bleeding, whereas *multicompartment coagulopathies* (critically abnormal INR, activated partial thromboplastin time, fibrinogen, platelets) may represent a risk for bleeding and may warrant additional antivenin consideration.[120] Conservative management for this scenario may be adequate; however, clinicians should consult with someone experienced in treating crotaline envenomations or with a regional poison control center.[121]

Antivenin Use in Copperhead Bites

Envenomations by copperheads are not considered to be as serious as rattlesnake or cottonmouth bites.[99,109] However, clinically significant local effects may occur, suggesting that these bites should be cautiously managed.[108] Victims of copperhead envenomation treated with CroFab had a marked improvement in local tissue effects, but clinical failures and recurrence of local effects also occurred.[122] The use of CroFab in copperhead bites has been shown to halt local tissue effect; however, more data are needed to define the role of CroFab for treatment of copperhead envenomation.[109,122,123] Suggested dosing of CroFab in copperhead envenomation is a single loading dose. Additional maintenance doses after initial control did not reduce the incidence of recurrent swelling in one study.[122] After administering the loading dose, the patient should be monitored for progressive swelling, coagulopathy development, and systemic effects. The need for additional antivenin should be evaluated on a case-by-case basis, and poison control center consultation is advised.

Antivenin Use in Children

The use of CroFab in pediatrics is loosely defined. Children with crotaline envenomation may be more likely to experience serious effects as a result of the larger ratio of venom to serum volume. Any child with a crotaline envenomation that meets the criteria for antivenin therapy should receive the same dosing regimen as adults. Weight-based (ie, per-kilogram) dosing is not appropriate for antivenin neutralization because the dose should reflect venom load, not patient size.[113,124] CroFab use in children ages 14 months to 13 years has been found to be safe and effective.[123-125]

Prevention and Treatment of Serum Sickness

Delayed reactions to antivenin are thought to be the result of serum sickness-like reactions attributable to immune complexes as a result of an immune response against antivenin proteins.[126] *Serum sickness* is a type-3 hypersensitivity reaction that may occur 7 to 21 days after completion of treatment.[99] Many patients develop serum sickness sometime within 4 weeks after being treated with antivenin, but only a few require hospitalization for this complication. Oral corticosteroids (prednisone) should be prescribed at the first signs (usually urticaria and pruritus) and should be continued for 24 hours after all symptoms have subsided. The corticosteroid should then be tapered over 72 hours. If necessary, diphenhydramine or hydroxyzine may be added to control pruritus.

BOX 346-5 Steps in Using Antivenin

1. Prepare to manage anaphylaxis. An anaphylactic reaction to CroFab is uncommon but has been reported.[a-c] All patients receiving antivenin should be monitored and 2 sites for intravenous access should be considered—1 for the antivenin and 1 for emergency drugs and fluids. Intravenous epinephrine, diphenhydramine, and plasma expanders, as well as cardiorespiratory support, must be readily available.
2. Test for sensitivity. Unlike the previous horse serum-based antivenin, skin testing is not needed for the administration of CroFab. Pretreatment with epinephrine, H_1- and H_2-receptor antagonists, or corticosteroids are not routinely recommended unless the patient has a history of hypersensitivity.
3. Start the infusion.[d] The dosing is based on estimated venom injected; no dosing adjustment is required for children. Each vial of CroFab is reconstituted with 10 mL sterile water for injection. After reconstitution, the entire dose (4 to 6 vials) is diluted in 250 mL of 0.9% sodium chloride and mixed by swirling gently. Use reconstituted and diluted product within 4 hours. This dose should be infused intravenously over 60 minutes with careful observation for allergic or anaphylactoid reactions.
4. Repeat infusion.[d] If initial control is not achieved, the loading dose of 4 to 6 vials of CroFab should be repeated until initial control of the envenomation syndrome has been achieved. After initial control has been achieved, additional 2-vial doses of CroFab every 6 hours for 3 doses is recommended. Additional doses may be necessary, as guided by the patient's clinical status and consultation with a clinician experienced in treating snakebite envenomations or a regional poison control center.

[a]Holstege CP, Wu J, Baer AB. Immediate hypersensitivity reaction associated with the rapid infusion of Crotalidae polyvalent immune Fab (ovine). *Ann Emerg Med.* 2002;39:677-679.
[b]Dart RC, McNally J. Efficacy, safety, and use of snake antivenoms in the United States. *Ann Emerg Med.* 2001;37:181-188.
[c]Dart RC, Seifert SA, Carroll L, et al. Affinity-purified, mixed monospecific crotalid antivenom ovine Fab for the treatment of cortalid venom poisoning. *Ann Emerg Med.* 1997;30:33-39.
[d]CroFab [package insert]. Melville, NY: Savage Laboratories, a division of Altana, Inc; 2006.

Additional Therapeutic Measures

Pain Control

Analgesics should not be overlooked in the management of snakebites. Adequate pain control allows rehabilitation to begin as early as possible to prevent contractures. However, opioid analgesics should be used cautiously if the venom is known to have neurotoxicity (eg, Mojave rattlesnake). Nonsteroidal anti-inflammatory agents should also be used with caution, especially in patients with evidence of coagulopathy.[101]

Infection Control

Although snakes have been found to carry a wide variety of bacteria in their mouth (histotoxic *Clostridia, Bacteroides,* and many gram-positive and gram-negative aerobes), infection is rare in the absence of severe necrosis, and good wound care is usually sufficient to prevent secondary infection. Systemic and local changes produced by envenomation and the subsequent vascular damage may be difficult to differentiate from infection. If infection is suspected by clinical and microbiological evidence, then antibiotic therapy should be instituted. Antibiotic prophylaxis is not currently suggested.[98,99,127]

Corticosteroids

Corticosteroids should not be used to reduce inflammation caused by pit viper envenomation. They are not considered a standard of care,[98] and they should not be routinely administered to snakebite victims. However, their use is efficacious in patients who develop serum sickness after antivenin administration.

Tetanus Prophylaxis

Clostridium tetani are not part of the mouth flora of snakes. Updating the patient's tetanus immunization is the only necessary intervention.

Follow-Up Care

Preservation of joint mobility and muscle strength is a goal after pit viper envenomation. Patients who experience full-thickness tissue damage may require referral to a surgeon. Pain control may be needed in the weeks after discharge. If the patient received antivenin therapy, then serum sickness should be discussed and the patient taught how to monitor for this syndrome. Physical or occupational therapy may also be needed to encourage joint mobilization of the affected extremity.

CORAL SNAKES

Coral snakes are the members of the Elapidae family that are indigenous to North America. Although their venom can cause a life-threatening paralysis, coral snakes tend to be small, secretive, and mild-mannered unless provoked. Few bites are reported, and death is rare.

Characteristics

The Eastern coral snake is often mistaken for the nonvenomous scarlet king snake because of similar colorful bands encircling the body. The mnemonic *red to yellow, kill a fellow; red to black, venom lack; head of black, step back, Jack!* refers to the color patterns of these snakes. The poisonous black-snouted snake has broad red and black bands separated by narrow yellow ones; the nonpoisonous variety's snout is red, and its broad red bands are separated by narrow yellow ones bounded on each side by black. Despite these distinctions, many people bitten by coral snakes thought they were handling a harmless scarlet king snake.[47]

Unlike pit vipers, coral snakes lack facial pits, are diurnal, and have fixed fangs and nearly round pupils. Their bites may produce superficial scratches or definite fang marks. Their retroverted teeth gnaw or chew on their prey, which makes coral snakes difficult to shake off. Because they must stay attached long enough for their venom to be deposited around their teeth, 50% of coral snake bites are dry. Elapidae venom is primarily neurotoxic; systemic neurologic symptoms are the rule, and local tissue injury is uncommon. Elapidae venom causes paresthesias and paralysis by inhibiting acetylcholine receptors at the neuronal synapse.

Distribution

Three types of coral snakes are found in the United States: (1) the Eastern coral snake *(Micrurus fulvius)*, (2) the Texas coral snake *(Micrurus fulvius tenere)*, and (3) the Arizona or Sonoran coral snake *(Micruroides euryxanthus)*. Their distribution is shown in Figure 346-2. The bite of the Sonoran coral snake produces no more than local pain and a small amount of nausea.

Venom Characteristics

Micrurus and *Micruroides* venoms have minimal proteolytic activity but contain hyaluronidase and some phospholipase-A_2.[96] The venom contains a neurotoxic compound that blocks acetylcholine binding sites at the neuromuscular junction.[96] Despite the relatively simple composition of coral snake venom, its potency should not be underestimated.

First Aid

Cryotherapy, incision and suction (including the Sawyer extractor), and constricting bands should not be used in any snakebites, including coral snake bites. The Australian pressure mobilization technique has been used, which involves wrapping the entire bitten extremity with a crepe bandage, elastic bandage, or article of clothing as tightly as possible, then splinting it.[128] This approach is different than first aid for pit viper envenomations because, in this setting, differences in venom characteristics mean that local necrosis is not expected.

Physical Examination: Signs and Symptoms

Local

Erythema and local pain from a coral snake bite are transient or absent.[99] Although most patients have evident fang marks, envenomations have been reported that were not associated with apparent fang marks on close examination.[129]

Systemic

Systemic manifestations may be delayed for 12 hours and may appear suddenly. They may include bulbar paralysis with ptosis, dysphagia, dysarthria, excessive salivation, paresthesias, euphoria or apprehension, drowsiness, dizziness, weakness, confusion, nausea, vomiting, diaphoresis, muscle tenderness or fasciculations, tremors, altered sensorium, drowsiness, and ophthalmoplegias that cause visual disturbances. These manifestations may be followed by seizures, respiratory paralysis, and pulmonary hemorrhage. Often unclear is which findings are the result of the venom itself and which are the result of hypoxia.

Laboratory Studies

Coral snake bites do not mandate routine laboratory screening. Transcutaneous pulse oximetry, arterial blood gases, or both should be assessed if respiratory insufficiency is suspected.

Supportive Therapy

Elective intubation before impending respiratory paralysis tends to prevent aspiration pneumonia. Elective intubation should be performed if any signs of bulbar paralysis develop.[130] The patient should receive cardiac and pulse oximetry monitoring (if not intubated), and intravenous access should be established.

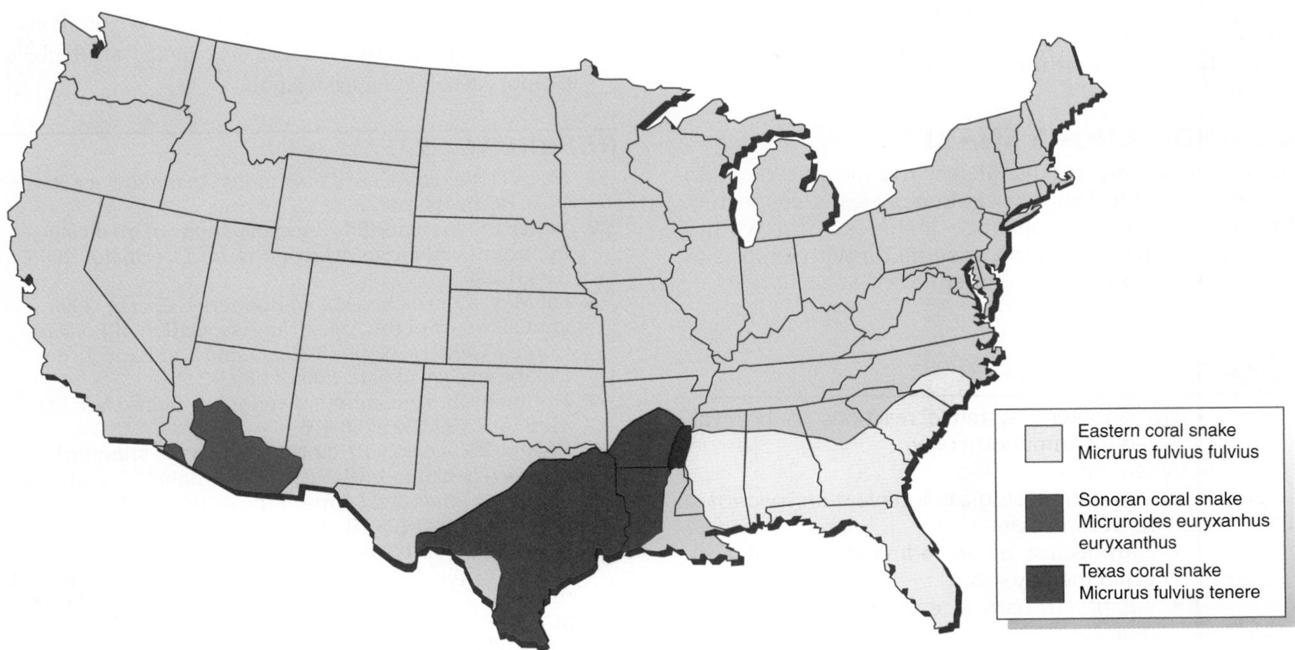

Figure 346-2 Distribution of coral snakes by type in the United States. *(Russell FEL. Snake Venom Poisoning. New York, NY: Scholium International; 1983. Reprinted by permission.)*

All victims of potential coral snake envenomation should be admitted to an intensive care unit for close monitoring for a minimum of 12 hours because the effects of envenomation may develop precipitously hours after a bite and are not easily reversed once they occur.[96,99]

Use of Antivenin

Antivenin effective against Eastern and Texas coral snake venom *(M fulvius)*, produced by Wyeth Ayerst, is used if a patient has definitely been bitten or if any signs or symptoms develop.[95] These guidelines are based on the judgment that the risks of intravenous hyperimmune horse serum are offset by the potential prevention of respiratory paralysis, which may occur if therapy is not immediately administered. If the snake cannot be found, then victims of bites suspected to be from coral snakes should be admitted to the hospital for 12 hours of observation.[99]

Skin testing may be performed, but skin testing yields many false-negative findings and is of little benefit in making therapeutic decisions. Three to 5 vials of antivenin are mixed in 250 to 500 mL of normal saline, and 1 to 2 mL is given intravenously over 3 to 5 minutes. The medical team must be prepared for anaphylaxis and have necessary drugs and equipment at bedside. If the patient does not exhibit any signs of an allergic reaction, then the remainder of the solution is infused slowly as tolerated. An additional 3 to 5 vials of antivenin-saline mixture may need to be infused if the patient's signs and symptoms do not abate or worsen. Rarely are more than 10 vials of antivenin required for victims of coral snake envenomations.[96]

Additional Therapeutic Measures

Prophylaxis for infection and tetanus are the same as for pit viper bites. Additional measures may become necessary if aspiration pneumonia develops. Patients should be aware that muscular weakness may persist for 3 to 6 weeks.

NONINDIGENOUS SNAKES

The variety of imported snakes is too great to detail in this text. If a bite from an exotic species is suspected, then the suggested approach includes local wound care, supportive care, and consultation with experts at a regional poison control center.

WHEN TO REFER

- Hymenoptera: systemic reactions to be evaluated for immunotherapy
- Arachnids
  - *Loxosceles:* surgical intervention necessary for wound care
  - *Latrodectus:* before administration of antivenin therapy
  - *Tarantulas:* hairs in eyes that are not easily removed
  - *Scorpions:* considered use of antivenin
- Snakes
  - *Pit vipers*
    - Considered use of antivenin
    - Surgical intervention necessary for wound care
  - *Coral snakes:* anticipated need for airway control or intensive care unit monitoring

WHEN TO ADMIT

- Hymenoptera: severe systemic allergic reactions or severe systemic reactions caused by massive envenomation
- Arachnids
  - *Loxosceles*
    - Secondary infection requiring intravenous antibiotics
    - Inability to provide adequate wound care at home
    - Severe systemic symptoms
  - *Latrodectus*
    - Severe systemic symptoms
    - After use of antivenin
  - *Tarantulas*
    - Significant comorbidity
    - Inability to tolerate oral fluids
  - *Scorpions*
    - Cardiac or neurological toxicity
    - Severe systemic signs or symptoms
- Snakes
  - *Pit vipers:* chance of envenomation
  - *Coral snakes:* chance of envenomation

TOOLS FOR PRACTICE

Medical Decision Support

- *2005 Annual Report of the American Association of Poison Control Centers' National Poisoning and Exposure Database* (other), American Association of Poison Control Centers (www.aapcc.org/Annual%20Reports/05report/2005%20Publsihed.pdf).

REFERENCES

1. Mebs D. *Venomous and Poisonous Animals.* Boca Raton, FL: CRC Press; 2002.
2. Vetter RS, Visscher PK. Bites and stings of medically important venomous arthropods. *Int J Dermatol.* 1998; 37:481-496.
3. Lai MW, Klein-Schwartz W, Rodgers GC, et al. 2005 annual report of the American Association of Poison Control Centers' National Poisoning and Exposure Database. *Clin Toxicol.* 2006;44:803-932.
4. Hoffman DR. Hymenoptera venom proteins. *Adv Exp Med Biol.* 1996;391:169-186.
5. Wright DN, Lockey RF. Local reactions to stinging insects (Hymenoptera). *Allerg Proc.* 1990;11:23-28.
6. Kemp ED. Bites and stings of the arthropod kind. *Postgrad Med.* 1998;103:88-90.
7. Charpin D, Birnbaum J, Lanteaume A, et al. Prevalence of allergy to Hymenoptera stings in different samples of the general population. *J Allerg Clin Immunol.* 1992;90: 331-334.
8. Golden DB. Diagnosis and prevalence of stinging insect allergy. *Clin Rev Allergy.* 1987;5:119-136.
9. Muller UR. Epidemiology of insect sting allergy: epidemiology of clinical allergy. *Monogr Allergy.* 1993;31: 131-146.

10. Jerrard DA. Management of insect stings. *Am J Emerg Med.* 1996;14:429-433.
11. Bischof RO. Seasonal incidence of insect stings: autumn "yellow jacket delirium." *J Fam Pract.* 1996;43:271-273.
12. Vetter RS, Visscher PK, Camazine S. Mass envenomations by honey bees and wasps. *West J Med.* 1999;170: 223-227.
13. Mulfinger L, Yunginger J, Styer W, et al. Sting morphology and frequency of sting autotomy among medically important vespids (Hymenoptera: Vespidae) and the honey bee (Hymenoptera: Apidae). *J Med Entomol.* 1992;29:325-328.
14. Reisman RE. Insect stings. *N Engl J Med.* 1994;331:523-527.
15. Li JT, Yunginger JW. Management of insect sting hypersensitivity. *Mayo Clin Proc.* 1992;67:188-194.
16. Greene A, Breisch NL. Avoidance of bee and wasp stings: an entomological perspective. *Curr Opin Allergy Clin Immonol.* 2005;5:337-341.
17. Koçer U, Tiftikcioglu YO, Aksoy HM. Skin and soft tissue necrosis following Hymenoptera sting. *J Cutan Med Surg.* 2003;7:133-135.
18. Keskin M, Duymaz A, Tosun Z, et al. Tissue necrosis following a honey bee sting. *Ann Plast Surg.* 2005;55: 114-115.
19. Teoh SCB, Lee JJ, Fam HB. Corneal honeybee sting. *Can J Ophthalmol.* 2005;40:469-471.
20. Arcieri ES, Franca ET, de Oliveria HB, et al. Ocular lesions arising after stings by Hymenopteran insects. *Cornea.* 2002;21:328-330.
21. Valentine M. Insect sting anaphylaxis. *Ann Intern Med.* 1993;118:225-226.
22. Tome R, Somri M, Teszler CB, et al. Bee stings of children: when to perform endotracheal intubation? *Am J Otolaryngol.* 2005;26:272-274.
23. Smoley BA. Oropharyngeal Hymenoptera stings: a special concern for airway obstruction. *Mil Med.* 2002;167:161-163.
24. Zuckerberg AL, Schweich PJ. An arm red and hot: infection or not? *Pediatr Emerg Care.* 1990;6:275-277.
25. Maguire JF, Geha RS. Bee, wasp, and hornet stings. *Pediatr Rev.* 1986;8:5-11.
26. Gabriel DP, Rodrigues AG Jr, Barsante RC, et al. Severe acute renal failure after massive attack of Africanized bees. *Nephrol Dial Transplant.* 2004;19:2680-2682.
27. Bresolin NL, Carvalho LC, Goes EC, et al. Acute renal failure following massive attack by Africanized bee stings. *Pediatr Nephrol.* 2002;17:625-627.
28. Ariue B. Multiple Africanized bee stings in a child. *Pediatrics.* 1994;94:115-117.
29. dos Reis MA, Costa RS, Coimbra TM, et al. Acute renal failure in experimental envenomation with Africanized bee venom. *Renal Failure.* 1998;20:39-51.
30. Mejia G, Arbelaez M, Henao JE, et al. Acute renal failure due to multiple stings by Africanized bees. *Ann Intern Med.* 1986;104:210-211.
31. Schumacher MJ, Egen NB. Significance of Africanized bees for public health. *Arch Intern Med.* 1995;155: 2038-2043.
32. Schumacher MJ, Tveten MS, Egen NB. Rate and quantity of delivery of venom from honeybee stings. *J Allergy Clin Immunol.* 1994;93:831-835.
33. Bansal AS. Bee stings. *Lancet.* 1996;348:900.
34. Simini B. Bee stings. *Lancet.* 1996;348:900.
35. Visscher PK, Vetter RS, Camazine S. Removing bee stings. *Lancet.* 1996;348:301-302.
36. Golden DBK, Kagey-Sobotka A, Norman PS, et al. Outcomes of allergy to insect stings in children, with and without venom immunotherapy. *N Engl J Med.* 2004; 351:668-674.
37. Lockey RF. Immunotherapy for allergy to insect stings. *N Engl J Med.* 1990;323:1627-1628.
38. Valentine MD, Schuberth KC, Kagey-Sobotka A, et al. The value of immunotherapy with venom in children with allergy to insect stings. *N Engl J Med.* 1990;323: 1601-1603.
39. Mosbech H. Hymenoptera immunotherapy. *Allergy.* 1997;52:1-3.
40. Hoffman DR. Reactions to less common species of fire ants. *J Allergy Clin Immunol.* 1997;100:679-683.
41. Stafford CT. Hypersensitivity to fire ant venom. *Ann Allergy Asthma Immunol.* 1996;77:87-95.
42. Rhoades RB, Stafford CT, James FK. Survey of fatal anaphylactic reactions to imported fire ant stings. *J Allerg Clin Immunol.* 1989;84:159-162.
43. Hoffman DR. Fire ant venom allergy. *Allergy.* 1995;50: 535-544.
44. deShazo RD. The continuing saga of imported fire ants: evolution before our eyes. *Ann Allergy Asthma Immunol.* 1996;77:85-86.
45. Adams CT, Lofgren CS. Red imported fire ants (Hymenoptera: Formicidae): frequency of sting attacks on residents of Sumter County, Georgia. *J Med Entomol.* 1981; 18:378-382.
46. Adams CT, Lofgren CS. Incidence of stings or bites of the red imported fire ant (Hymenoptera: Formicidae) and other arthropods among patients at Ft Stewart, Georgia, USA. *J Med Entomol.* 1982;19:366-370.
47. deShazo RD, Banks WA. Medical consequences of multiple fire ant stings occurring indoors. *J Allergy Clin Immunol.* 1994;93:847-850.
48. deShazo RD, Butcher BT, Banks WA. Reactions to the stings of the imported fire ant. *N Engl J Med.* 1990; 323:462-466.
49. Hardwick WE, Royall JA, Petitt BA, et al. Near-fatal fire ant envenomation of a newborn. *Pediatrics.* 1992;90:622-624.
50. Cohen PR. Imported fire ant stings: clinical manifestations and treatment. *Pediatr Dermatol.* 1992;9:44-48.
51. Fox RW, Lockey RF, Bukantz SC. Neurologic sequelae following the imported fire ant sting. *J Allerg Clin Immunol.* 1982;70:120-124.
52. Ginsburg CM. Fire ant envenomation in children. *Pediatrics.* 1984;73:689-692.
53. Stablein JJ, Lockey RF. Adverse reactions to ant stings. *Clin Rev Allergy.* 1987;5:161-175.
54. Ralston JP, Rapini RP. Fire Ant Bites. eMedicine. January 2006. Available at: www.emedicine.com/derm/topic607.htm. Accessed April 2, 2006.
55. Freeman TM, Hylander R, Ortiz A, et al. Imported fire ant immunotherapy: effectiveness of whole body extracts. *J Allerg Clin Immunol.* 1992;90:210-215.
56. Saucier JR. Arachnid envenomation. *Emerg Med Clin North Am.* 2004;22:405-422.
57. Diaz JH. The global epidemiology, syndromic classification, management, and prevention of spider bites. *Am J Trop Med Hyg.* 2005;72:361-364.
58. Swanson DL, Vetter RS. Bites of brown recluse spiders and suspected necrotic arachnidism. *N Engl J Med.* 2005;352:700-707.
59. Anderson PC. Spider bites in the United States. *Dermatol Clin.* 1997;15:307-311.
60. Bennett RG, Vetter RS. An approach to spider bites: erroneous attribution of dermonecrotic lesions to brown recluse or hobo spider bites in Canada. *Can Fam Physician.* 2004;50:1098-1101.
61. Wong RC, Hughes SE, Voorhees JJ. Spider bites. *Arch Dermatol.* 1987;123:98-104.
62. Wasserman GS, Anderson PC. Loxoscelism and necrotic arachnidism. *J Toxicol Clin Toxicol.* 1983-1984; 21:451-472.

63. Allen C. Arachnid envenomations. *Emerg Med Clin North Am.* 1992;20:269-298.
64. Ingber A, Trattner A, Cleper R, et al. Morbidity of brown recluse spider bites: clinical picture, treatment and prognosis. *Acta Dermatol Venereol.* 1991;71:337-340.
65. Willis GA. Loxoscelism in Canada. *CMAJ.* 1988;139:11-12.
66. Krywko DM, Gomez HF. Detection of *Loxosceles* species venom in dermal lesions: a comparison of 4 venom recovery methods. *Ann Emerg Med.* 2002;39:475-480.
67. Barrett SM, Romine-Jenkins M, Blick KE. Passive hemagglutination inhibition test for diagnosis of brown recluse spider. *Clin Chem.* 1993;39:2104-2107.
68. Phillips S, Kohn M, Baker D, et al. Therapy of brown spider envenomation: a controlled trial of hyperbaric oxygen, dapsone, and cyproheptadine. *Ann Med.* 1995;25:363-68.
69. Wasserman GS. Wound care of spider and snake envenomations. *Ann Emerg Med.* 1988;1331-1335.
70. Stack LB. Images in clinical medicine. Latrodectus mactans. *N Engl J Med.* 1997;336:1649.
71. Cohen J, Bush S. Case report: compartment syndrome after a suspected black widow spider bite. *Ann Emerg Med.* 2005;45:414-416.
72. Clark RF, Wethern-Kestner S, Vance MV, et al. Clinical presentation and treatment of black widow spider envenomation: a review of 163 cases. *Ann Emerg Med.* 1992;21:782-787.
73. Pneumatikos IA, Galiatsou E, Goe D, et al. Acute fatal toxic myocarditis after black widow spider envenomation [letter]. *Ann Emerg Med.* 2003;41:158.
74. Woestman R, Perkin R, Van Stralen D. The black widow: is she deadly to children? *Pediatr Emerg Care.* 1996;12:360-364.
75. O'Malley GF, Dart RC, Kuffner EF. Successful treatment of latrodectism with antivenin after 90 hours. *N Engl J Med.* 1999;340:657.
76. Isbister GK, Graudins A, White J, et al. Antivenom treatment in arachnidism. *J Toxicol Clin Toxicol.* 2003;41:291-300.
77. LoVecchio F, McBride C. Scorpion envenomations in young children in central Arizona. *J Toxicol Clin Toxicol.* 2003;41:937-940.
78. Berg RA, Tarantino MD. Envenomation by the scorpion Centruroides exilicauda (C sculpturatus): severe and unusual manifestations. *Pediatrics.* 1991;87:930-933.
79. Rimsza ME, Zimmerman DR, Bergeson PS. Scorpion envenomation. *Pediatrics.* 1980;66:298-302.
80. Diaz P, Chowell G, Ceja G, et al. Pediatric electrocardiograph abnormalities following Centruroides limpidus tecomanus scorpion envenomation. *Toxicon.* 2005;45:27-31.
81. Gueron M, Ilia R, Sofer S. The cardiovascular system after scorpion envenomation: a review. *J Toxicol Clin Toxicol.* 1992;30:245-258.
82. Ismail M. The scorpion envenoming syndrome [review]. *Toxicon.* 1995;33:825-858.
83. Karnad DR. Haemodynamic patterns in patients with scorpion envenomation. *Heart.* 1998;79:485-489.
84. Curry SC, Vance MV, Ryan PJ, et al. Envenomation by the scorpion Centruroides sculpturatus. *J Toxicol Clin Toxicol.* 1983-1984;21:417-449.
85. Suchard JR, Hilder R. Atropine use in Centruroides scorpion envenomation. *J Toxicol Clin Toxicol.* 2001;39:595-598, discussion 599.
86. Abroug F, Nouira S, Haguiga H, et al. High-dose hydrocortisone hemisuccinate in scorpion envenomation. *Ann Emerg Med.* 1997;30:23-27.
87. McNally J. Personal Communication.
88. Holstege CP, Miller MB, Wermuth M, et al. Crotalid snake envenomation. *Med Toxicol.* 1997;13:889-921.
89. Gold BS. Neostigmine for the treatment of neurotoxicity following envenomation by the Asiatic cobra. *Ann Emerg Med.* 1996;28:87-89.
90. Tu AT. Biotoxicology of sea snake venoms. *Ann Emerg Med.* 1987;16:1023-1028.
91. Clark RF, Williams SR, Nordt SP, et al. Successful treatment of crotalid-induced neurotoxicity with a new polyspecific crotalid Fab antivenom. *Ann Emerg Med.* 1997;30:54-57.
92. Wingert WA, Chan L. Rattlesnake bites in southern California and rationale for recommended treatment. *West J Med.* 1988;148:37-44.
93. Danzl DF, Carter GL. "Kiss and yell": a rattlesnake bite to the tongue [letter]. *Ann Emerg Med.* 1988;17:549.
94. Crane DB, Irwin JS. Rattlesnake bite of glans penis. *Urology.* 1985;26:50-52.
95. Russell FEL. *Snake Venom Poisoning.* Philadelphia, PA: JB Lippincott; 1980.
96. Norris RL Jr, Bush SP. North American venomous reptile bites. In: Auerbach PS, ed. *Wilderness Medicine.* 4th ed. St Louis, MO: Mosby; 2001.
97. Kunkel DB, Curry SC, Vance MV, et al. Reptile envenomations. *J Toxicol Clin Toxicol.* 1983-1984;21:503-526.
98. Singletary EM, Rochman AS, Bodmer JCA, et al. Envenomations. *Med Clin North Am.* 2005;89:1195-1224.
99. Gold BS, Dart RC, Barish RA. Bites of venomous snakes. *N Engl J Med.* 2002;347:347-356.
100. Teixeira Cde F, Fernandes CM, Zuliani JP, et al. Inflammatory effects of snake venom metalloproteinases. *Mem Inst Oswaldo Cruz.* 2005;100(suppl 1):181-184.
101. Bond GR, Burkhart KK. Thrombocytopenia following timber rattlesnake envenomation. *Ann Emerg Med.* 1997;30:40-44.
102. Clark RF, Williams SR, Nordt SP, et al. Successful treatment of crotalid-induced neurotoxicity with a new polyspecific crotalid fab antivenom. *Ann Emerg Med.* 1997;30:54-57.
103. Wagner CW, Colladay ES. Crotalid envenomation in children: selective conservative management. *J Pediatr Surg.* 1989;24:128-131.
104. Banner W. Bites and stings in the pediatric patient. *Curr Probl Pediatr.* 1988;18:1-69.
105. Bronstein AC, Russell FE, Sullivan JB, et al. Negative pressure suction in field treatment of rattlesnake bite. *Vet Hum Toxicol.* 1985;27:297.
106. Lawrence WT, Giannopoulos A, Hansen A. Pit viper bites: rational management in locales in which copperheads and cottonmouths predominate. *Ann Plast Surg.* 1996;36:276-285.
107. McKinney PE. Out-of-hospital and interhospital management of crotaline snakebite. *Ann Emerg Med.* 2001;37:168-174.
108. Scharman EJ, Noffsinger VD. Copperhead snakebites: clinical severity of local effects. *Ann Emerg Med.* 2001;38:55-61.
109. Thorson A, Lavonas EJ, Rouse AM, et al. Copperhead envenomations in the Carolinas. *J Toxicol Clin Toxicol.* 2003;29-35.
110. Burch JM, Agarwal R, Mattox KL, et al. The treatment of crotalid envenomation without antivenin. *J Trauma.* 1988;28:35-43.
111. Hall EL. Role of surgical intervention in the management of crotaline envenomation. *Ann Emerg Med.* 2001;37:175-180.
112. Lawrence WT, Giannopoulos A, Hansen A. Pit viper bites: rational management in locales in which copperheads and cottonmouths predominate. *Ann Plast Surg.* 1996;36:276-285.
113. Schmidt JM. Antivenom therapy for snakebites in children: is there evidence? *Curr Opin Pediatr.* 2005;17:234-238.

114. CroFab [package insert]. Melville, NY: Savage Laboratories, a division of Altana, Inc; 2006.
115. Bebarta V, Dart RC. Effectiveness of delayed use of Crotalidae polyvalent immune Fab (ovine) antivenom. *J Toxicol Clin Toxicol.* 2004;42:321-324.
116. Bogdan GM, Dart RC, Falbo SC, et al. Recurrent coagulopathy after antivenom treatment of crotalid snakebite. *South Med J.* 2000;93:562-566.
117. Seifert SA, Boyer LV. Recurrence phenomena after immunoglobulin therapy for snake envenomations: part 1. Pharmacokinetics and pharmacodynamics of immunoglobulin antivenoms and related antibodies. *Ann Emerg Med.* 2001;37:189-195.
118. Ruha AM, Curry SC, Beuhler M, et al. Initial postmarketing experience with Crotalidae polyvalent immune Fab for treatment of rattlesnake envenomation. *Ann Emerg Med.* 2002;39:609-615.
119. Boyer LV, Seifert SA, Cain JS. Recurrence phenomena after immunoglobulin therapy for snake envenomations: part 2. Guidelines for clinical management with crotaline fab antivenom. *Ann Emerg Med.* 2001;37:196-201.
120. Yip L. Rational use of Crotalidae polyvalent immune Fab (ovine) in the management of crotaline bite. *Ann Emerg Med.* 2002;39:648-650.
121. Camilleri C, Offerman S, Gosselin R, et al. Conservative management of delayed, multicomponent coagulopathy following rattlesnake envenomation. *Clin Toxicol (Phila).* 2005;43:201-206.
122. Lavonas EJ, Gerardo CJ, O'Malley G, et al. Initial experience with Crotalidae polyvalent immune Fab (ovine) antivenom in the treatment of copperhead snakebite. *Ann Emerg Med.* 2004;43:200-206.
123. Trinh HH, Hack JB. Use of CroFab antivenin in the management of a very young pediatric copperhead envenomation. *J Emerg Med.* 2005;29:159-162.
124. Offerman SR, Bush SP, Moynihan JA, et al. Crotaline Fab antivenom for the treatment of children with rattlesnake envenomation. *Pediatrics.* 2002;110:968-971.
125. Richardson WH III, Barry JD, Tong TC, et al. Rattlesnake envenomation to the face of an infant. *Pediatr Emerg Care.* 2005;21:173-176.
126. Lalloo DG, Theakston RDG. Snake antivenoms. *J Toxicol Clin Toxicol.* 2003;41:277-290.
127. Kerrigan KR, Mertz BL, Nelson SJ, et al. Antibiotic prophylaxis for pit viper envenomation: prospective, controlled trial. *World J Surg.* 1997;21:369-372.
128. Norris RL Jr, Minton SA. Non-North American venomous reptile bites. In: Auerbach PS, ed. *Wilderness Medicine.* 4th ed. St Louis, MO: Mosby; 2001.
129. Norris RL, Dart RC. Apparent coral snake envenomation in a patient without visible fang marks. *Am J Emerg Med.* 1989;7:402-405.
130. Kitchens CS, Van Mierop LHS. Envenomation by the Eastern coral snake (Micrurus fulvius). *JAMA.* 1987; 258:1615-1618.

Chapter 347

ESOPHAGEAL CAUSTIC INJURY

Jill M. Cholette, MD; George T. Drugas, MD

Caustic injury of the esophagus is a major, though preventable, pediatric health concern. Corrosive esophageal injuries continue to occur despite federal legislation mandating preventive packaging and labeling, injury-prevention programs designed for children and parents, and laws restricting the potency and availability of caustic substances. In fact, the number of toxic exposures to cleaning substances (acid and alkaline) rose between 2000 and 2003.[1] Cleaning substances were the second-most frequent substance involved in pediatric exposures in 2003, comprising 9.7% of the total.[1] Thirty-nine percent of exposures occur in children younger than 3 years, and 52% occur in those younger than 6 years.[1] Of victims younger than 13 years, most caustic injuries occur in boys; this gender association is reversed during adolescence when intentional suicide attempts are more prevalent.[1] Twenty percent of caustic ingestions result in some form of esophageal injury, and although death from caustic ingestion is rare, the morbidity can be devastating. Medical treatment for corrosive esophageal injury is reasonably well established, but surgical management remains controversial.

PATHOPHYSIOLOGICAL FEATURES

The extent of injury after a caustic ingestion depends on the type of agent (acid versus alkaline), whether the substance was liquid or solid, the concentration, the volume ingested, and the duration of contact between the substance and the gut mucosa. Agents with a pH under 2 or over 12 are extremely corrosive. Solid or powder substances adhere to the oropharynx, maximally burning focally with sparing of the esophagus. Liquids rapidly reach the esophagus and stomach, causing greatest damage to these more distal sites. Alkaline substances are more available than acidic substances in Western countries and are involved in the majority of corrosive ingestions.[1] Household bleaches, drain cleaners, automatic dishwasher detergents, anhydrous Benedict's reagent tablets, and denture cleaning tablets are common alkaline household products. Common household acids are toilet bowl cleaners, rust removers, battery fluids, and swimming pool cleaners (Table 347-1).

Ingestion of liquid laundry detergents and dishwasher solutions found in the home usually results in mild esophageal injury that heals without complication. Household bleaches have rarely been associated with severe esophageal injury because of their low concentration of sodium hypochlorite. Strong alkalis cause liquefaction necrosis that allows penetration of the corrosive agent transmurally through the esophagus and into adjacent mediastinal tissues. Heat production and small-vessel thrombosis resulting from the reaction compound the initial damage. The ensuing inflammatory reaction can result in gangrene, perforation, mediastinitis, fibrosis, or severe contracture of the esophagus. Lye is the lay term for the alkaline agent found in most cleaning substances. Liquid lye is the most common cause of esophageal caustic injury and is associated with the greatest morbidity.[2] Lye is odorless, tasteless, and viscous, which allow it to be easily ingested by children and in massive volumes by suicidal teens and adults. Lye's high viscosity retards transit through the esophagus, making it particularly injurious; tissue injury is rapid in the first few minutes but can persist for hours. Solid alkalis, such as anhydrous Benedict's reagent tablets and batteries, tend to

Table 347-1 Household Agents Causing Caustic Exposures

CHEMICAL	PRODUCT
ACIDIC	
Hydrochloric acid	Swimming pool cleaners, toilet bowl cleaner, metal cleaner
Hydrofluoric acid	Rust remover
Sulfuric acid	Automotive batteries, drain cleaners
ALKALINE	
Ammonia	Toilet bowl cleaners, hair dyes, floor strippers, glass cleaners
Sodium hydroxide	Anhydrous Benedict's reagent tablets, detergents, laundry powders, paint removers, drain cleaners, button batteries, oven cleaner
Sodium borates, carbonates, phosphates	Detergents, electric dishwasher detergents, water softeners
Sodium hypochlorite	Bleaches, household cleaners, mildew remover

lodge during transit, resulting in focal burns and perforations at their point of impaction.

Lesions caused by lye injury occur in 3 phases. The acute *necrotic* phase usually lasts 24 to 96 hours after ingestion. An intense inflammatory reaction surrounds nonviable tissue. During the second *ulceration and granulation* phase 3 to 5 days after injury, superficial necrotic tissue sloughs and is replaced by an ulcerated and inflamed granulation bed. The healing tissue lacks collagen deposition and has very little tensile strength. Although perforation can occur at any point during the first 2 weeks after injury, during this phase (lasting 10 to 12 days) the esophagus is most vulnerable. The third phase of *scarring and cicatrization* begins during the third week after injury. In this period, contracture of the wound may lead to stricture formation and alteration of lower esophageal sphincter pressure, leading to gastroesophageal reflux.

Strong acids, unlike alkalis, have an offensive odor and bitter taste that usually results in rapid expectoration after accidental ingestion. Because acids exhibit rapid esophageal transit, they were previously thought to cause more damage to the stomach or intestine; however, recent studies have revealed that acids also cause extensive esophageal injury as well.[2] Acids cause coagulation necrosis, resulting in superficial eschar formation, which may, in part, limit penetration into deeper tissues. Acids and alkalis alike can induce pylorospasm, resulting in pooling of the caustic agent in the gastric antrum, with extensive damage to this area.

DIAGNOSIS AND INITIAL MANAGEMENT

After caustic ingestion, symptoms can consist of searing or burning pain of the mouth and lips, drooling or hypersalivation, and difficulty with swallowing. An important point to recognize is that the absence of pain does not exclude significant injury. Epiglottic or vocal cord edema may result in stridor, dysphonia, or aphonia. Substernal or back pain usually results from esophageal disruption and mediastinitis. Acute epigastric pain may indicate gastric perforation. The presence of fever is strongly correlated with significant esophageal injury. The primary care physician must recognize that the absence of oral burns does not exclude an esophageal burn injury and that 20% to 45% of patients with esophageal burns have no evidence of oral burns.[3] Oropharyngeal damage, however, does not reliably indicate esophageal involvement; 70% of persons with oropharyngeal injuries do not have esophageal lesions.[4] Bleeding can occur and results from mucosal sloughing, with persistent ooze from the exposed submucosa or muscularis. Life-threatening hematemesis from the development of an aortoesophageal fistula is, however, a rare event. No single symptom, sign, or combination has been found to predict accurately the degree of esophageal injury after corrosive ingestion.

Every attempt should be made to identify the agent ingested. In the case of young children, parents are usually aware of the offending agent and often bring the container to the emergency department. With suicidal intent, the caustic agent may be unknown. Stridor or aphonia indicate laryngoepiglottic injury and may require urgent orotracheal intubation for airway protection. Occasionally, severe laryngeal destruction necessitates emergency cricothyroidotomy or tracheostomy. Adequate vascular access should be obtained to allow for correction of hypovolemia or hypotension. A chest roentgenogram may identify concomitant aspiration, subcutaneous cervical emphysema, or pneumomediastinum corroborating perforation. Gastric lavage and emetics should be avoided because of the risk of reexposing the esophagus to the ingested corrosive agent and because of the threat of aspiration. Any attempt to neutralize an ingested caustic agent poses an additional danger because the resultant exothermic reaction frequently exacerbates the primary burn injury. Activated charcoal is not recommended, is ineffective, and obscures visualization with endoscopy. Gastric lavage is contraindicated because it may result in propagation of injury beyond the level of the pylorus. Placement of a nasogastric tube should be deferred because of risk of esophageal perforation.

Only after the patient is stabilized should the airway and gastrointestinal tract be inspected. The initial examination should include laryngoscopy. Evidence of a supraglottic or epiglottic burn indicates a risk for airway obstruction and requires endotracheal intubation. Presence of a third-degree burn to the hypopharynx precludes advancement of the endoscope beyond that level. Once the upper airway integrity is confirmed, endoscopy should be performed, even in the absence of oropharyngeal burns, to establish extent of injury.[5] More than 50% of victims of caustic ingestion will have no evidence of damage to the gastrointestinal tract,[6] and many will have extensive esophageal damage in the absence of oropharyngeal lesions. Flexible, rather than rigid, esophagoscopy is preferred to minimize the risk of iatrogenic perforation. Most endoscopists, fearing perforation, will advance the scope only to the level at which maximal injury is

BOX 347-1 Grading of Caustic Esophageal Burns

Grade 0: normal
Grade I: mucosal hyperemia and edema
Grade IIa: mucosal hemorrhage, exudate, superficial ulceration, sloughing, and pseudomembrane formation
Grade IIb: IIa plus deep discrete or circumferential ulcerations
Grade IIIa: deep ulcerations and necrosis, massive hemorrhage, obliteration of the lumen, charring, and perforation
Grade IIIb: extensive necrosis

Modified from Zargar SA, Kochhar R, Mehta S, et al. *Gastrointest Endosc.* 1991;37(2):165-169. Copyright © 1991, Elsevier, with permission.

encountered; others advocate full examination of the stomach and, if possible, the duodenum. The degree of injury can be graded similarly to that of thermal skin burns and holds similar prognostic implications[7] (Box 347-1). Endoscopy only allows examination of superficial mucosa, which makes differentiating between grade-IIb and -III lesions difficult. Circumferential burns limit full visualization with endoscopy, and contrast radiography may be required for identification of grade-III injuries. Contrast radiography uses water-soluble contrast followed by thin barium (Figure 347-1).

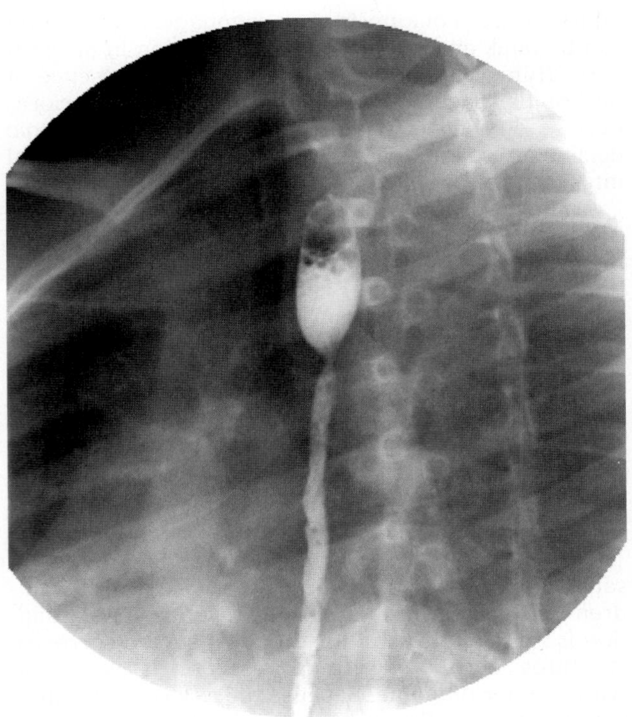

Figure 347-1 Esophagram demonstrating long-segment esophageal stricture after lye ingestion in a 2-year-old girl.

MEDICAL MANAGEMENT

Therapy for a caustic injury to the esophagus depends on the grade assigned at endoscopy. Children with no injury or grade-I injuries are usually admitted and observed for 24 to 48 hours. Children with more severe injuries are admitted to the pediatric intensive care unit for monitoring and management. As with any patient, close attention to the ABCs (airway, breathing, and circulation) is of paramount importance. A nasogastric tube placement is not recommended routinely because it may be associated with subsequent stricture formation.[8]

Initially, these patients may have nothing orally and require proper fluid resuscitation, nutritional support through total parenteral nutrition, and pain management. After disruption of the mucosal barrier by caustic ingestion, bacterial translocation and secondary bacterial invasion are likely events. This rationale is offered for early institution of prophylactic antibiotic therapy; however, controlled trials do not support antibiotic use, and therefore most experts no longer advocate empirical therapy.[9] Vigilance for mediastinitis or systemic infection must be maintained and appropriate antimicrobials reserved for any evidence of local or systemic infection. For grade-II and -III injuries, parenteral nutrition is begun, and oral feedings are withheld until the dysphagia of the initial phase has regressed and no evidence exists of clinical or radiographic deterioration.

Proton pump inhibitors should be prescribed because loss of lower esophageal sphincter tone occurs secondary to corrosive esophageal injury, and acid reflux can exacerbate the underlying injury and accelerate stricture formation.[10] The use of steroids to limit fibrosis after caustic injury has debatable efficacy in humans. Most studies demonstrate a lack of proven benefit, and the potential side effects of steroids argue against routine use.[11] Strictures after grade-I and -IIa injuries are rare, and follow-up contrast esophagography is unnecessary. After grade-IIb and -III injuries, a barium esophagram for the early detection of stricture development is performed 2 to 4 weeks later. Early stricture detection is important because the less-mature stricture is more responsive to dilation. Esophageal dilation to prevent adhesion formation in the injured segment, intraluminal stenting, and prolonged esophageal rest (maintenance of nothing-by-mouth status; total parenteral nutrition) have all been proposed for prophylaxis against stricture formation, but none have demonstrated a proven benefit.[12,13] Multiple animal studies with a variety of agents (heparin, epidermal growth factor, caffeic acid phenethyl ester) have demonstrated varying degrees of success in ameliorating stricture formation, but none of these agents have been studied in humans.[14,15]

SURGICAL INTERVENTIONS

Early surgical intervention is vital and can be life saving. Full and immediate resection of devitalized tissue is necessary to prevent expansion of the corrosive injury. Delay in diagnosis of an esophageal perforation can be fatal, and a high index of suspicion in grade-II and -III injuries must be maintained. The presence of peritonitis, pneumoperitoneum, or clinical deterioration, as evidenced by refractory acidosis, neurologic decline, or coagulopathy, requires immediate surgical intervention.

Complete surgical exposure of the foregut—esophagus, stomach, and duodenum—is necessary to assess the extent of the damage and allow for possible resection. Full-thickness injury to the stomach or duodenum invariably predicts severe esophageal injury and is an indication for complete esophagogastrectomy.[16] Full-thickness circumferential injury to the esophagus carries 20% mortality, mandating surgical resection.[16] Conservative management, including later esophageal dilation, may be considered for short segments of full-thickness esophageal mucosal damage. If any question persists after the initial exploration, then a second-look operation (often within 24 hours) is required.

Primary treatment with esophageal dilation offers a satisfactory outcome for most otherwise-healthy children with grade-IIa injuries. However, repeated dilation is rarely successful for the most severe corrosive strictures, and early surgical resection is associated with a better outcome. Because the risk of perforation is highest in the first weeks after injury, most experts advocate waiting 6 weeks before initiating dilation therapy. Dilation can be accomplished by 2 methods: (1) passing graded bougies over endoscopically or radiographically placed guide wires (pulsion dilation) or (2) using endoscopically or radiographically controlled balloon dilation (radial dilation). Dilation with bougies passed endoscopically is difficult with tortuous or complicated strictures and warrants fluoroscopic guidance. Dilation is typically performed every other week with the goal to dilate the stricture to 18 mm, which is the required diameter for normal swallowing. Typically, 3 or more dilations are required to achieve this goal.

Esophageal rupture is a potentially fatal complication of dilation and warrants immediate surgical repair; the incidence ranges from 17% to 32%.[17,18] In addition to the risk of perforation, serial dilations are also complicated by dysphagia between treatments, which may precipitate pulmonary aspiration. An adequate lumen is usually attained within 6 months to 1 year, with progressively longer intervals between dilations. Consider esophageal replacement if dilation is ineffective beyond 1 year.

Surgical management is required for the most severe corrosive injuries and for intractable esophageal strictures. The surgical options include bypass with placement of an esophageal substitute or resection, or both, or esophagoplasty (Figure 347-2). Bypass with complete esophageal resection is the preferred approach because retained proximal esophagus may distend forming a mucocele or abscess; distal esophagus may develop reflux esophagitis, ulceration, and hemorrhage; and retained esophagus carries increased risk for malignant transformation.[19] Resection, however, is not without risk; the extensive dissection necessary to remove the damaged esophagus can result in significant morbidity. Colonic interposition, gastric advancement, gastric tube esophagoplasty, and jejunal interposition are accepted procedures to replace the injured esophagus.[20] Esophagoplasty with a colonic patch over less-extensive but persistent strictures has also been used in the management of focal strictures.[21] Decisions regarding surgical management are based on patient age, general health, severity and extent of stricture, and risk of long-term complications.

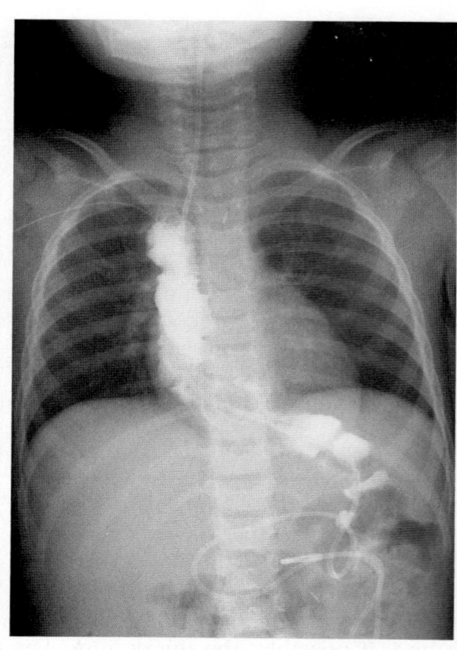

Figure 347-2 Colonic interposition in a child 6 months after esophageal injury. This is the same child in Figure 347-1.

DELAYED COMPLICATIONS

Long-term complications of corrosive ingestions include stricture formation (see Medical Management), gastric outlet obstruction, and esophageal carcinoma. Not surprisingly, the long-term morbidity after corrosive esophageal ingestion correlates with the grade of injury.

Gastric outlet obstruction occurs in approximately 9% of corrosive ingestions[22] and is characterized by early satiety and weight loss. The obstruction can occur years after the initial injury and follows acid or alkaline ingestions with equal frequency. The treatment of gastric outlet obstruction is surgical, and balloon dilation of the pylorus, pyloroplasty, and Billroth I reconstruction are each effective. The type of operation performed depends on findings at laparotomy and surgeon preference.

For victims in which the native esophagus is retained, the risk of postcorrosive esophageal carcinoma is estimated to be 1000- to 3000-fold higher than the incidence for esophageal cancer in the general population, and up to 3% of patients with esophageal carcinoma have a history of corrosive ingestion.[23] These squamous cell carcinomas usually originate in the mid-esophagus. Local dissemination occurs infrequently so that the potential for curative resection is slightly improved over primary esophageal malignancies. The interval between burn injury and the development of carcinoma ranges from 10 to 70 years, with a mean of 50 years.[24] Long-term follow-up of children who have grade-II and -III burns is warranted, regardless of their symptoms. Esophagography and surveillance esophagoscopy should be performed annually or biannually.

TOOLS FOR PRACTICE

Engaging Patient and Family

- *Protect Your Child From Poison* (brochure), American Academy of Pediatrics (patiented.aap.org).

REFERENCES

1. Watson WA, Litovitz TL, Klein-Schwartz W, et al. 2003 annual report of the American Association of Poison Control Centers Toxic Exposure Surveillance System. *Am J Emerg Med.* 2004;22(5):335-404.
2. Zargar SA, Kochhar R, Nagi B, et al. Ingestion of corrosive acid. Spectrum of injury to upper gastrointestinal tract and natural history. *Gastroenterology.* 1989;97: 702-707.
3. Lovejoy FH Jr, Woolf AD. Corrosive ingestions. *Pediatr Rev.* 1995;16:473-474.
4. Haller JA Jr, Andrews HG, White JJ, et al. Pathophysiology and management of acute corrosive burns of the esophagus: results of treatment in 285 children. *J Pediatr Surg.* 1971;6:578-584.
5. Ferguson MK, Migliore M, Staszak VM, et al. Early evaluation and therapy for caustic esophageal injury. *Am J Surg.* 1989;157:116-120.
6. Gumaste VV, Dave PB. Ingestion of corrosive substances by adults. *Am J Gastroenterol.* 1992;87:1-5.
7. Zargar SA, Kochhar R, Mehta S, et al. The role of fiberoptic endoscopy in the management of corrosive ingestion and modified endoscopic classification of burns. *Gastrointest Endosc.* 1991;37:165-169.
8. Ramasamy K, Gumaste VV. Corrosive ingestion in adults. *J Clin Gastroenterol.* 2003;37:119-124.
9. Rao RB, Hoffman RS. Caustics and batteries. In: Goldfrank LR, ed. *Goldfrank's Toxicologic Emergencies.* Norwalk, CT: Appleton & Lange; 1998.
10. Mutaf O, Genc A, Herek O, et al. Gastroesophageal reflux: a determinant in the outcome of caustic esophageal burns. *J Pediatr Surg.* 1996;31:1494-1495.
11. Anderson KD, Rouse TM, Randolph JG. A controlled trial of corticosteroids in children with corrosive injury of the esophagus. *N Engl J Med.* 1990;323:637-640.
12. Berkovits RN, Bos CE, Wijburg FA, et al. Caustic injury of the oesophagus. Sixteen years experience, and introduction of a new model of esophageal stent. *J Larnygol Otol.* 1996;110:1041-1045.
13. Lahoti D, Broor SL, Basu PP, et al. Corrosive esophageal strictures: predictors of response to endoscopic dilation. *Gastrointest Endosc.* 1995;41:196-200.
14. Bingol-Kologlu M, Tanyel FC, Muftuoglu S, et al. The preventive effect of heparin on stricture formation after caustic esophageal burns. *J Pediatr Surg.* 1999;34: 291-294.
15. Koltuksuz U, Mutus HM, Kutlu R, et al. Effects of caffeic acid phenethyl ester and epidermal growth factor on the development of caustic esophageal stricture in rats. *J Pediatr Surg.* 2001;36:1504-1509.
16. Kirsh MM, Peterson A, Brown JW, et al. Treatment of caustic injuries of the esophagus: a ten year experience. *Ann Surg.* 1978;188:675-678.
17. Cox JGC, Winter RK, Maslin SC, et al. Balloon or bougie for dilatation of benign esophageal stricture? *Dig Dis Sci.* 1994;39:184:373-378.
18. Broor SL, Raju GS, Bose PP, et al. Long term results of endoscopic dilatation for corrosive esophageal strictures. *Gut.* 1993;34:1498-1501.
19. Song HY, Han YM, Kim HN, et al. Corrosive esophageal stricture: safety and effectiveness of balloon dilation. *Radiology.* 1992;184:373-378.
20. Watson TJ, DeMeester TR, Kauer WK, et al. Esophageal replacement for end-stage benign esophageal disease. *J Thorac Cardiovasc Surg.* 1998;115:1241-1247.
21. Othersen HB Jr, Parker EF, Chandler J, et al. Save the child's esophagus. Part II: colic patch repair. *J Pediatr Surg.* 1997;32:328-333.
22. Gumaste VV, Dave PB. Ingestion of corrosive substances by adults. *Am J Gastroenterol.* 1992;87:1-5.
23. Tekant G, Eroglu E, Erdogan E, et al. Corrosive injury-induced gastric outlet obstruction: a changing spectrum of agents and treatment. *J Pediatr Surg.* 2001;36:1004-1007.
24. Ribeiro U Jr, Posner MC, Safatle-Ribeiro AV, et al. Risk factors for squamous cell carcinoma of the esophagus. *Br J Surg.* 1996; 83(9):1174-1185.

Chapter 348

HEAD INJURIES

Prashant V. Mahajan, MD, MPH, MBA

Traumatic brain injury (TBI) is the leading cause of death and disability in the United States. An estimated 1.6 million head injuries occur every year, with more than 250,000 requiring hospitalization.[1-3] Overall, 60,000 deaths caused by head injuries occur every year, and an estimated 70,000 to 90,000 patients are left with permanent neurologic sequelae.[1,4,5] The financial burden in terms of medical costs and lost productivity has been estimated at $100 billion per year.[1,4,5] Among children ages 0 to 14 years, TBI results in an estimated 2685 deaths, 37,000 hospitalizations, and 435,000 emergency department (ED) visits annually.[6] Approximately 50% of patients hospitalized with head injury are younger than 20 years.[7] Boys are injured at least twice as often as girls. More than 75% of trauma deaths in children are due to brain injury.[8] In 2000 the injuries that children and adolescents ages 14 and younger experienced will have lasting impacts, including total lifetime economic costs of more than $50 billion in medical expenses and lost productivity.[9]

The causes of severe head injury vary with age. In infants, falls and child abuse predominate; in preschool- and school-aged children, vehicular accidents are most common; and during the adolescent years, sports injuries and assault are seen most frequently. For all ages combined, falls are the most common cause of head trauma, but vehicular accidents are the leading cause of serious injury. In most vehicular accidents, the child is a pedestrian. Most children hit by a vehicle are not supervised by an adult at the time of the accident.[10] Education regarding prevention of head injury is an essential role for the primary care physician. Anticipatory guidance regarding appropriate supervision of children, high-risk activities, and advice regarding protective equipment such as car seats for infants and bicycle helmets for older children can dramatically reduce the morbidity and mortality that result from head injury.[11,12]

PATHOPHYSIOLOGICAL FEATURES

The brain is covered by 3 layers of meningeal tissue (pia mater, arachnoid mater, and dura mater) followed by the skull bones (calvarium) and scalp, which has a strong layer of tissue (galea aponeurotica). The brain does not adhere to the skull but is able to move freely within it, cushioned to some extent by the cerebrospinal fluid in which it bathes. *Primary brain injury* refers to the neural injury caused by the traumatic insult itself and exhibits in the form of contusions, intracranial bleeding, fractures, or diffuse axonal injuries. *Secondary brain injury* refers to the subsequent injury to the neural tissue after a trauma has occurred. It results from numerous causes, including hypoxia, hypoperfusion, excitotoxic damage, free radical damage, or metabolic derangements. Sometimes the damage caused by secondary brain injury is more devastating than that from the primary insult itself. The most important cause for secondary brain injury is brain ischemia resulting from inadequate cerebral blood flow. Adequate cerebral blood flow depends on the cerebral perfusion pressure, which is the difference between mean arterial pressure and intracranial pressure (ICP). Normally the cerebral perfusion pressure fluctuates inside a narrow range, the result of cerebral autoregulation. However, when this control mechanism is lost because of brain injury and secondary brain tissue damage, an increase in intracranial volume (mainly the result of intracranial hemorrhage or cerebral edema) will lead to a disproportionate increase in ICP. This increase further accentuates neuronal damage by reducing cerebral blood flow. An increase in ICP leads to cerebral herniation syndromes.[13] These syndromes are characterized by worsening of sensorium, pupillary changes, bradycardia, irregular respirations, and hypertension (the Cushing triad).

INITIAL CARE

The improved prognosis for survival and neurologic recovery of the child after a severe head injury compared with an adult,[14,15] plus the potential for organ donation in patients who are brain dead, dictate that the physician providing emergency care make every effort to resuscitate the child who has a severe head injury. The basic ABCs of resuscitation (airway, breathing, and circulation) should be addressed first. Maintaining normal oxygenation is imperative, as was aptly stated by Haldane in 1919: "Anoxia not only stops the machine but wrecks the machinery."[16] In addition, ischemia, increased ICP, and uncontrolled seizures may cause further brain injury. The correction of anoxia and poor cerebral perfusion is more important than detection of an intracranial hematoma.

In patients with severe head injury, a coexisting cervical spine injury should be assumed until proved otherwise. The neck should not be moved until cervical spine films can rule out a fracture or dislocation, which may result in spine trauma if movement occurs. The preferred initial radiographs are cross-table lateral, anteroposterior, and odontoid views. In the severely injured patient the airway requires intubation to ensure adequate ventilation to reduce the chance of developing increased ICP. When possible an anesthesiologist should perform the intubation. Rapid sequence intubation is indicated for most patients with head injuries to ensure that they are comfortable and that intubation can be safely achieved. This task is usually accomplished with a combination of a sedative to induce anesthesia (thiopental, etomidate, fentanyl, or midazolam are commonly used sedatives), atropine to reduce secretions and prevent vagal reflexes, and a neuromuscular blocking agent to produce paralysis (rocuronium or succinylcholine). Close attention to blood pressure is necessary because sedatives may cause hypotension. Cricoid pressure may be applied to reduce the risk of aspiration. In the past, prolonged hyperventilation was suggested for patients with acute severe head injury. Such is no longer the case.[17] Although hyperventilation constricts intracranial blood vessels and lowers ICP, concerns exist that hyperventilation may decrease cerebral perfusion.[18] Meticulous attention to pressure of carbon dioxide in the arterial blood is required to prevent hypercapnia at all costs. The optimal level of carbon dioxide pressure is unknown and may vary from patient to patient. Acute hyperventilation may be useful, however, in an emergency situation in which the patient's condition deteriorates acutely because of increased ICP.

Secondary Brain Damage

Once TBI has been detected and the patient resuscitated, the subsequent management is directed at preventing secondary insults. The most important causes of secondary brain damage are hypoxia, systemic hypotension, and raised ICP (intracranial hypertension). These situations must be prevented. Vital signs should be frequently assessed to ensure adequacy of circulation. Shock leads to further brain injury despite adequate airway management and oxygenation. Vigorous fluid therapy to restore adequate circulating blood volume and sufficient cerebral perfusion is essential. Isotonic solutions or blood products should be administered because hypotonic solutions may promote movement of free water into damaged brain tissue, increasing the potential for cerebral edema. Some authorities have even argued for the use of hypertonic solutions in acute severe brain trauma,[19] although this approach has not achieved widespread use. If the patient is in shock, then a source of bleeding should be sought. Patients rarely sequester sufficient blood volume in the head to produce shock (notable exceptions include the infant with an expansible skull and the presence of a large subgaleal hematoma). Additional measures directed at reducing secondary brain injury include elevating the patient's head 30 degrees and keeping it in a midline position to maximize venous outflow from the cranial vault.

ICP should be monitored and lowered if necessary. Placement of an intracranial ventricular catheter is the

Table 348-1 Glasgow Coma Scale*

EYE-OPENING RESPONSE

SCORE	>1 YEAR	<1 YEAR
4	Spontaneous	Spontaneous
3	To verbal command	To shout
2	To pain	To pain
1	None	None

MOTOR RESPONSE

SCORE	>1 YEAR	<1 YEAR
6	Obeys commands	Spontaneous response
5	Localizes pain	Localizes pain
4	Withdraws from pain	Withdraws from pain
3	Displays abnormal flexion to pain (decorticate rigidity)	Displays abnormal flexion to pain (decorticate rigidity)
2	Displays abnormal extension to pain (decerebrate rigidity)	Displays abnormal extension to pain (decerebrate rigidity)
1	None	None

VERBAL RESPONSE

SCORE	>5 YEARS	2 TO 5 YEARS	0-23 MONTHS
5	Is oriented and converses	Uses appropriate words and phrases	Babbles, coos appropriately
4	Conversation is confused	Use inappropriate words	Cries but is consolable
3	Words are inappropriate	Cries or screams persistently to pain	Cries or screams persistently to pain
2	Sounds are incomprehensible	Grunts or moans to pain	Grunts or moans to pain
1	None	None	None

*The Glasgow Coma Scale score is the sum of best eye-opening, motor, and verbal responses. Scores range from 3 to 15. Severe indicates a score of <9; moderate, 9-12; and mild, 13-15.
Modified from Teasdale G, Jennett B. Assessment of coma and impaired consciousness: a practical scale. *Lancet.* 1974;2:81-84. Copyright © 1974, Elsevier, with permission.

most accurate and reliable method for monitoring ICP.[13] Intracranial hypertension is defined as an ICP of more than 20 mm of Hg. The Cushing response (hypertension and bradycardia) is an ominous sign that implies increased ICP. This response and unilateral pupillary dilation (a sign of impending catastrophic temporal lobe herniation) should prompt the administration of mannitol. Reduction of cerebral metabolism by initiating barbiturate coma may improve outcomes and should be considered when pediatric neurosurgeons and pediatric intensive care units are available.[20] The role of therapeutic hypothermia in the treatment of children with severe TBI is still unclear. Corticosteroids do not improve outcome when used in the acute-phase management of TBI.[17,21]

Antipyretics should be administered if fever exists. Hyperthermia may increase cerebral metabolic demands, further taxing delivery of nutrients to the injured brain. Similarly, seizures greatly increase the metabolic demands of the brain and should be treated promptly with intravenous diazepam or lorazepam, followed by intravenous phenytoin. The latter should be provided if the patient is pharmacologically paralyzed because it results in an inability to detect seizure activity. Intravenous phenytoin is also advisable before transfer to another medical center.

Glasgow Coma Scale

A more detailed neurologic evaluation should be performed only when adequacy of the airway, breathing, and circulation are ensured. The Glasgow Coma Scale (GCS) (Table 348-1), or a modified GCS for children and infants, can be used to evaluate mental status and is valuable in assessing prognosis and in following the patient's progress. The scale is based on the patient's response in 3 areas: (1) motor response, (2) verbal response, and (3) eye-opening response. Severe head injury may be defined as that resulting in a GCS score of less than 9, whereas moderate head injury is associated with a score of 9 to 12. A score of 13 to 15 indicates a mild head injury.

Motor response is evaluated by noting symmetry of tone, movement, and reflexes. Cranial nerve examination may reveal signs of focal injury to the brainstem. Pupil size, symmetry, and reactivity should be noted carefully, and the fundus should be examined for signs of papilledema. Retinal hemorrhages suggest child abuse from shaken-baby syndrome. Pontine and midbrain function may be assessed by examining oculovestibular reflexes. In the unconscious patient, the head should be rotated briskly from side to side after making certain that the cervical spine has not been injured. Normally, when the head moves to the right, the eyes move to the left, and vice versa. Loss of these reflex eye movements in a comatose patient suggests an injury to the midbrain or pons. Alternatively, if the tympanic membranes are intact, then ice water caloric responses should be elicited. With the patient's head elevated to 30 degrees, 120 mL of ice water is infused alternately into each ear canal. The eyes should turn toward the irrigated ear. If they do not, then a brainstem injury is likely. To assess pontine function further, the quality and symmetry of the grimace evoked by painful stimulation of the face should be observed. In patients who do not respond to this stimulation, or in those who do so minimally, the corneal reflex should be tested. Failure to react by blinking is consistent with pontine injury or deep coma.

Medullary function is evaluated by assessing the patient's gag reflex and tongue movement. Examination of the patient's craniospinal axis should be performed in concert with the neurologic assessment, assessing for signs of trauma. Swelling and bony depression of the skull suggest an underlying fracture. Ecchymoses behind the ear (the Battle sign) or around the orbits (raccoon sign), cerebrospinal fluid rhinorrhea, otorrhea, or hemotympanum suggest a basilar skull fracture. Basilar fractures or scalp lacerations overlying fractures are important to detect because they serve as portals of entry for bacteria into the subarachnoid space and may cause meningitis. This neurologic evaluation is the baseline for serial assessments of neurologic function while neuroimaging studies are being obtained and for transferring the patient to the care of pediatric neurosurgeons and intensivists.

Neuroimaging studies for the severely injured patient typically consist of cervical spine films to rule out fracture or subluxation and a noncontrast computed tomographic (CT) scan of the brain with bone windows. The bone windows identify skull fractures and obviate the need for a skull roentgenogram. CT scan is the imaging study of choice in acute trauma. It is easier to obtain than a magnetic resonance image (MRI) and may not require sedation. CT identifies the relationship between bone fragments and intracranial contents, and it reveals extraaxial fluid collections such as epidural and subdural hematomas, as well as injury to brain parenchyma. The MRI may be useful later on because it is more sensitive than CT at detecting intrinsic brain injuries.[22]

Types of Traumatic Brain Injury

Concussion

Concussion is defined as any head injury associated with alteration in mental status. Most clinicians use this term to refer to mild head injuries with a GCS score of 13 to 15 and no focal neurologic findings. CT scans are often normal in children with transient loss of consciousness, amnesia, confusion, headache, nausea, vomiting, or dizziness. Many patients with concussion have subtle findings that suggest diffuse axonal injury on MRI scans in spite of a normal CT scan. Most patients can be discharged home after a period of evaluation and observation. Thorough evaluation is important, and the physician should advise parents regarding the child's return to sports. Table 348-2 gives details about grades of concussion and management guidelines after sports injuries, as suggested by the American Academy of Neurology.[23]

Skull Fractures

Skull fractures occur in approximately 2 per 1000 infants and 0.5 to 1 per 1000 older children and adolescents.[13]

Table 348-2 Classification of Concussion*

GRADE	DEFINITION	MANAGEMENT
1	Transient confusion No loss of consciousness, mental status abnormalities for <15 min	Return to sports activities same day only if all symptoms resolve within 15 min. If a second grade-1 concussion occurs, no sports activity until asymptomatic for 1 week.
2	Transient confusion No loss of consciousness, mental status abnormalities for >15 min	No sports activity until asymptomatic for 1 week. If a grade-2 concussion occurs on the same day as a previous grade-1 concussion, no sports activity for 2 weeks.
3	Concussion involving any loss of consciousness	No sports activity until asymptomatic for 1 week if loss of consciousness was brief (seconds). No sports activity until asymptomatic for 2 weeks if loss of consciousness was prolonged (minutes or longer). Second grade-3 concussion. No sports activity until asymptomatic for 1 month. Any abnormality on CT or MRI. No sports activity for remainder of season. Patient should be discouraged from any future return to contact sports.

*Concussion symptoms: early (minutes and hours)—headache, dizziness or vertigo, lack of awareness of surroundings, nausea or vomiting. Late (days to weeks)—persistent low-grade headache, light-headedness, poor attention and concentration, memory dysfunction, easy fatigability, irritability and low frustration tolerance, intolerance to bright lights or difficulty focusing vision, intolerance of loud noises, sometimes ringing in the ears, anxiety or depressed mood, sleep disturbance.
CT, Computed tomography; *MRI,* magnetic resonance imaging.
Modified from McQueen JK, Blackwood DHR, Harris P, et al. Low risk of late posttraumatic seizures following severe head injury: implications for clinical trials of prophylaxis. *J Neurol Neurosurg Psychiatry*. 1983;46:899-904. Reprinted by permission of BMJ Publishing Group Ltd.

The most common bone to fracture is the parietal bone. Most fractures can be diagnosed by plain-film radiographs or CT with bone windows. Linear skull fractures often require no intervention, although most clinicians would admit these children for a period of observation. Depressed skull fractures are often associated with underlying brain abnormalities and may require surgical interventions. Basilar skull fractures are often associated with cerebrospinal fluid leakage and cranial nerve damage. These fractures require pediatric neurosurgical intervention and should ideally be managed at tertiary-care pediatric trauma centers.

Parenchymal Injuries

Cerebral contusions are bruises of the cerebral cortex that can occur as a result of direct injury (coup injury) or at the opposite point where the relatively mobile brain strikes the bone on the other side (contrecoup injury). Clinical manifestations vary, but patients often exhibit some alteration in consciousness, focal seizures, or focal neurologic findings (eg, cortical blindness in cases of occipital lobe injury). Most cases are diagnosed by CT scan, and management depends on the extent of injury. Patients may thus need to be observed with ICP monitoring, and some may require craniotomies for drainage of intracerebral hematomas.

Diffuse Axonal Injury

Diffuse axonal injury is often seen after an acceleration-deceleration mechanism (whiplash injury); the damage is at the gray-white matter junction. Most children will experience changes in sensorium, and some studies have reported that 82% will develop coma.[13] Although some changes with diffuse axonal injury may be seen on CT scan, MRI is often diagnostic. Most patients with diffuse axonal injury will need hospitalization along with monitoring of ICP in the intensive care unit.

Intracranial Hematoma

Although hematomas can occur anywhere in the intracranial space, the 2 most common types—epidural and subdural—are described in Table 348-3.

CARE OF THE LESS SEVERELY INJURED PATIENT

Most physicians have little trouble identifying patients who require intensive care at a regional medical center. More difficult is deciding whether to admit the less severely injured child to the hospital for observation. Information from published studies concerning the indications for such action is scant because most head trauma studies have focused just on hospitalized patients.[24] Decisions regarding the hospitalization of less severely injured patients must be made individually.

History

When taking the history, the possibility of abuse must be kept in mind. Children rarely experience a serious injury when they fall out of bed; therefore such a history,

Table 348-3 Differences Between Epidural and Subdural Hematomas

CHARACTERISTIC	EPIDURAL HEMATOMA	SUBDURAL HEMATOMA
Mechanism	Direct trauma that leads to bleeding from middle meningeal artery or shearing of epidural veins	Shaking (acceleration-deceleration) injury leading to tearing of bridging veins in the subdural space. In young children, this may result from child abuse.
Clinical manifestations	Lucid interval—symptom-free interval between time of injury and time of manifestation can be seen. Patients run the gamut from asymptomatic to those who exhibit focal seizures and coma	Lucid interval unlikely. Many children exhibit coma, seizures, or evidence of chronic changes (tense anterior fontanel, macrocephaly).
Investigations	CT scan is diagnostic for a lenticular lesion with an overlying fracture	CT scans reveal blood collection as a hyperdense crescentic collection along the cerebral hemisphere. In cases of child abuse, hemorrhage of different ages can be seen with changes suggestive of hydrocephalus.
Management	Craniotomy with drainage of hematoma and repair of the ruptured blood vessel	Management will vary depending on extent of bleeding, and in some cases, ICP monitoring with expectant observation may be the only therapy; intracranial evacuation of blood clot may be the therapy of choice for some cases.
Prognosis	Excellent after initial insult is adequately treated	Poor with high mortality and high morbidity (sequelae).

CT, Computed tomography; *ICP,* intracranial pressure.

when given as the cause of severe injury, may be an indication of child abuse. Loss of consciousness, seizures, amnesia for the circumstances surrounding the injury, and focal neurologic deficits are indicators of more severe head trauma. Vomiting and headache are common symptoms after head trauma, and their presence, if not persistent or severe, is not particularly ominous or suggestive of any specific pathological finding.[25] Persistent clouding of consciousness is the most reliable sign of a significant brain injury. In addition, the duration of posttraumatic amnesia, defined as an inability to generate new memories after head injury, correlates positively with the severity of the injury.[27]

Physical Examination

Examination of the patient should begin with assessment of mental status and assignment of a GCS score. Neurologic examination should proceed with assessment of the cranial nerves. Particular attention needs to be given to pupillary responses and symmetry, funduscopic examination (to rule out papilledema or hemorrhage), eye movements (to assess for dysconjugate gaze), asymmetries of facial sensation or movement, tongue movement, and gag reflex. As a sensory screening examination, symmetrical responses to pain in all 4 limbs should be determined. Symmetry of muscle tone and movement and of the deep-tendon reflexes and plantar responses needs to be determined, as should the alert, cooperative child's ability to manipulate small objects. The child's gait and station also need to be assessed. The general physical examination should focus on the presence of injury to other body systems and on seeking evidence of physical neglect or abuse.

Imaging Studies

The decision to perform neuroimaging studies is difficult and must be individualized. As a general rule, if the clinician is sufficiently worried about a child's clinical status to desire radiographic studies, then a noncontrast CT with bone windows is the preferred imaging study and has supplanted the use of skull roentgenograms.[28] In addition, CT scan often detects parenchymal brain injury.

TREATMENT

Similar to the performance of neuroimaging studies, the decision to admit a child with mild to moderate head trauma must be individualized. Much controversy exists in the literature regarding the ability of the physician to use clinical signs and symptoms to identify children at risk for TBI after blunt trauma. Guidelines have been proposed in the approach of children with blunt injury. These children have been traditionally divided into 2 groups: (1) those ages 2 years and younger or (2) those between 2 and 20 years of age.[20,29]

In children younger than 2 years, a multidisciplinary panel suggested stratifying patients into risk categories based on clinical features (eg, history and physical examination, mechanism of injury, presence or absence of skull fracture).[29]

Patient Characteristics

High-risk patients have any of the following characteristics: depressed mental status, focal neurologic findings, signs of depressed or basilar skull fracture, seizure, irritability, acute skull fracture, bulging fontanel, more than 5 episodes of vomiting or vomiting for more than 6 hours, and loss of consciousness that lasts more than a minute. All high-risk patients require a cranial CT scan.

Intermediate-risk patients have any of the following characteristics: vomiting 3 to 4 times; loss of consciousness that lasts for less than a minute; history of lethargy or irritability now resolved; caretakers concerned about current behavior; higher force mechanism, hematoma (especially large or nonfrontal in location), unwitnessed trauma; fall onto a hard surface, vague or no history of trauma with evidence of trauma; and nonacute skull fracture older than 24 to 48 hours. Patients in this category might be managed in 1 of 2 ways: a 4- to 5-hour period of observation and reevaluation or a head CT scan.

Low-risk patients are defined as having low-energy mechanism (eg, a fall of less than 3 feet), no signs or symptoms, and more than 2 hours since the injury; in addition, as the patient's age increases, the risk decreases. These patients may be observed in the ED or at home with reliable caretakers.[29]

Management of Closed Head Trauma

In 1999 the American Academy of Pediatrics published guidelines for the management of closed head trauma in previously healthy children 2 to 20 years of age.[30] This consensus statement used the historical features of loss of consciousness and the presence of symptoms as an indication for obtaining a CT scan of the head. For children without a loss of consciousness, a complete history should be taken and a physical examination should be performed, and a competent caregiver should observe the patient for any deterioration in mental status. For patients who have a history of a brief loss of consciousness, along with amnesia, headache, or vomiting at the time of evaluation, the prevalence of intracranial injury may be as high as 7%.[31-33] Although many of these brain injuries may have little clinical consequence, a minority of these children may require neurosurgical intervention.[32-34] Therefore, in this group of symptomatic children with a brief loss of consciousness, CT scans of the head may be useful. However, with a brief loss of consciousness alone in an otherwise asymptomatic patient, observation of the patient for neurologic deterioration may be an acceptable alternative to obtaining a CT scan of the head.[30]

The following 5 clinical findings have been found to identify 99% of all children with TBI at CT scan and 100% of those who required neurosurgery: (1) abnormal mental status, (2) clinical signs of skull fracture, (3) scalp hematoma, (4) history of headache, and (5) vomiting. A clinical decision rule excludes TBI in need of neurosurgical intervention (negative predictive value of 100%) when none of these 5 clinical variables is present.[35] Use of this rule will reduce unnecessary exposure to the radiation of the CT scan by 25%. Although CT is the diagnostic test of choice for evaluating children with head trauma, this procedure has disadvantages, including exposure to radiation,[36] transport of the child away from supervision in the ED, the frequent need for pharmacologic sedation, additional health care costs, and increased time for completing the ED evaluation. In fact, the lifetime attributable cancer mortality risk for a child after a typical head CT scan is estimated at 1 per 5000.[37] Therefore cranial CT scans should be used selectively in the ED evaluation of children with minor blunt head trauma.

Whenever a head injury occurs, the question of a coexisting cervical spine injury always exists. Most ED physicians do not obtain cervical spine radiographs if mental status and neurologic examinations are normal, if no tenderness of the spine is present, and if the child moves the head around without difficulty, especially if the child is older than 5 years. The younger the child is, the lower the threshold will be for obtaining cervical spine films.[38]

Discharge Home

Patients with mild head injury who promptly recover their neurologic function, who are not suspected of being abused, and who have reliable caregivers can be discharged home with appropriate instructions. Children with normal neurologic examinations and negative CT scans rarely have neurologic deterioration after discharge from the ED.[39,40] Parents are often instructed to observe the child carefully for at least 24 hours, periodically awakening the child during periods of sleep. Caregivers should return immediately to the ED if their child (1) cannot be awakened; (2) demonstrates decreasing mental status while awake; or (3) develops seizures, focal weakness, increasing headache, progressive instability, or vomiting to the point of dehydration. Linear skull fractures do not require admission to the hospital if the child is asymptomatic, but they do require close observation because the force required to fracture a child's skull is significant. A reliable observer at home is required.

After hospital or emergency room discharge, office follow-up is suggested at 2 weeks. The child's recovery can be reviewed and further anticipatory guidance provided to the family regarding relevant neurologic sequelae of the child's head injury. Children younger than 2 years who have diastatic fractures (fractures that involve normal suture lines) should be evaluated again in 6 to 8 weeks to check for a *growing fracture*. These enlarging fractures occur as a result of leptomeningeal cyst formation, and they frequently require neurosurgical closure.

PROGNOSIS

Children who experienced mild head trauma (GCS score of 13 to 15) are indistinguishable from their peers 1 year after their injuries.[40] Despite this fact, significant neurologic dysfunction may be seen in the period immediately after the child's injury and may persist for as long as 8 weeks. Symptoms include irritability, sleep disturbance, clinging behavior, hyperactivity, and headache.[18,41] Providing anticipatory guidance to parents regarding the transient nature of these symptoms in mild head injuries is important.

Children who have moderate head injury (GCS score of 9 to 12) and severe head injury (a score of 3 to 8) may suffer from multiple physical, cognitive, and psychological disabilities. However, prognosis is generally more favorable for head-injured children than adults.[42] For example, children with an initial GCS score of 6 or more have an 80% chance of achieving functional independence.[14] Intellectual recovery continues for as long as 2 years after head injury in children[43]; thus long-term rehabilitative services are needed. Formal psychological assessment for staging school reentry and for ongoing adjustment of the child's academic curriculum should be obtained.[44,45]

Five percent of patients will experience seizures within the first week after their head injury. The occurrence of these early-onset seizures does not accurately predict the development of later posttraumatic epilepsy.[46] The risk of subsequently developing epilepsy is significantly increased if seizures are present beyond the first week after head injury, particularly when severe head trauma, intraparenchymal hematoma, or depressed skull fracture occurs. With these risk factors, approximately one third of patients will develop posttraumatic epilepsy.[46] Electroencephalographic studies do not accurately predict its subsequent development,[10,47] and the use of prophylactic anticonvulsant medications does not appear to reduce the risk of its occurrence. These medications are generally not used in mild brain injury.[48-50] They are indicated for children who have had severe brain injury to prevent increased ICP caused by the seizures per se.

WHEN TO REFER

- Deteriorating mental status
- Coma or persistent alteration in mental status
- A GCS score of less than 9
- Subdural, epidural, or intraparenchymal hematoma
- Focal abnormalities on neurologic examination
- Seizures after the first week or recurrent seizures
- Shock
- Signs of Cushing response (bradycardia and hypertension)
- Suspicion of child abuse (refer to appropriate local governmental agency)
- Cervical spine injury
- Basilar skull fracture
- Depressed skull fracture
- Increasingly severe headaches
- Facial laceration or suspicion of significant trauma at other locations

WHEN TO ADMIT

- Persistent alteration in mental state
- Focal neurologic deficits
- Seizures
- Persistent vomiting that precludes adequate hydration
- Severe headache
- Suspicion of abuse
- Unreliable caregivers or observers at home
- Any injury requiring neurosurgical intervention
- CT scan indicating intracranial bleeding or brain injury

TOOLS FOR PRACTICE

Community Advocacy and Coordination

- *Heads Up: Concussion in Youth Sports* (tool kit), Centers for Disease Control and Prevention (www.cdc.gov/ConcussionInYouthSports/).

Engaging Patient and Family

- *About Bicycle Helmets* (fact sheet), American Academy of Pediatrics (www.aap.org/family/thelmabt.htm).
- *Minor Head Injuries in Children* (tool kit), American Academy of Pediatrics (www.aap.org/bookstore).
- *Tips for Getting Your Kid to Wear a Bicycle Helmet* (fact sheet), American Academy of Pediatrics (www.aap.org/family/thelmabt2.htm).
- *What is a Pediatric Neurologist?* (fact sheet), American Academy of Pediatrics (www.aap.org/family/WhatisChildNeurologist.pdf).

Medical Decision Support

- *Head Injuries Sports Shorts* (fact sheet), American Academy of Pediatrics (www.aap.org/family/SportsShorts_01.pdf).
- *Heads Up: Brain Injury in Your Practice—A Tool Kit for Physicians* (tool kit), Centers for Disease Control and Prevention (www.cdc.gov/ncipc/tbi/Physicians_Tool_Kit/).

RELATED WEB SITE

- American Academy of Pediatrics: Car Safety Seats and Transportation Safety—Health Topic Page (www.aap.org/healthtopics/carseatsafety.cfm).

AAP POLICY STATEMENTS

American Academy of Pediatrics, Committee on Injury and Poison Prevention. Bicycle helmets. *Pediatrics*. 2001; 108(4):1030-1032. (aappolicy.aappublications.org/cgi/content/full/pediatrics;108/4/1030).

American Academy of Pediatrics, Committee on Injury and Poison Prevention. Selecting and using the most appropriate car safety seats for growing children: guidelines for counseling parents. *Pediatrics*. 2002;109(3):550-553. (aappolicy.aappublications.org/cgi/content/full/pediatrics;109/3/550).

American Academy of Pediatrics, Committee on Quality Improvement, and American Academy of Family Physicians, Commission on Clinical Policies and Research. The management of minor closed head injury in children. *Pediatrics*. 1999;104(6):1407-1415. (aappolicy.aappublications.org/cgi/content/full/pediatrics;104/6/1407).

Homer CJ and Kleinman L. Technical report: minor head injury in children. *Pediatrics*. 1999;104(6):e78. (aappolicy.aappublications.org/cgi/content/full/pediatrics;104/6/e78).

REFERENCES

1. Thurman D, Guerrero J. Trends in hospitalization associated with traumatic brain injury. *JAMA*. 1999;282: 954-957.
2. Guerrero JL, Thurman DJ, Sniezek JE. Emergency department visits associated with traumatic brain injury, United States, 1995-1996. *Brain Inj*. 2000;14:181-186.
3. Marik PE, Varon J, Trask T. Management of head trauma. *Chest* 2002;122:699-711.
4. Kraus JF. Epidemiology of head injury. In: Cooper PR, ed. *Head Injury*. Baltimore, MD: Williams and Wilkins; 1993.
5. Sosin DM, Sniezek JE, Waxweiler RJ. Trends in death associated with traumatic brain injury, 1979 through 1992; success and failure. *JAMA*. 1995;273:1778-1780.
6. Langlois JA, Rutland-Brown W, Thomas KE. Traumatic brain injury in the United States: emergency department visits, hospitalizations, and deaths. Atlanta, GA: Centers for Disease Control and Prevention, National Center for Injury Prevention and Control; 2004.
7. Field JH. *Epidemiology of Head Injuries in England and Wales*. London, UK: Her Majesty's Stationery Office; 1976.
8. Mayer T, Walker ML, Johnson DG, et al. Causes of morbidity and mortality in severe pediatric trauma. *JAMA*. 1981;245:719-721.
9. Finkelstein EA, Corso PS, Miller TR. *Incidence and Economic Burden of Injuries in the United States*. New York, NY: Oxford University Press; 2006.
10. Jennett B. *Epilepsy After Non-Missile Head Injuries*. 2nd ed. London, UK: William Heinemann; 1975.
11. Johnston C, Rivara FP, Soderberg R. Children in car crashes: analysis of data for injury and use of restraints. *Pediatrics*. 1994;2:960-965.
12. Thompson RS, Rivara FP, Thompson DC. A case-control study of the effectiveness of bicycle safety helmets. *N Engl J Med*. 1989;320:1361-1367.
13. Greenes DS. Neurotrauma. In: Fliesher GR, Ludwig, Henretig FM, eds. *Textbook of Pediatric Emergency Medicine*. 5th ed. Baltimore, MD: Lippincott Williams & Wilkins.
14. Bruce DA. Outcome: does it work? In: Harris BH, ed. *Progress in Pediatric Trauma*. Boston, MA: Nobb Hill Press; 1985.
15. Luersson T, Klauber M, Marshall L. Outcome from head injury related to patient's age: a longitudinal prospective study of adult and pediatric head injury. *J Neurosurg*. 1988;68:409-416.
16. Kalbag RM. Management of head injuries. In: Cartilidge NEF, Shaw DA, eds. *Head Injury*. London, UK: WB Saunders; 1981.
17. Allen E, et al. Head and spinal cord injury. In: Rogers MC, Helfaer M, eds. *Handbook of Pediatric Intensive Care*. Baltimore, MD: Williams and Wilkins; 1999.
18. Chesnut R. Hyperventilation in traumatic brain injury: friend or foe? *Crit Care Med*. 1997;25:1275-1278.
19. Simma B. A prospective, randomized, and controlled study of fluid management in children with severe head injury: lactated Ringer's solution versus hypertonic saline. *Crit Care Med*. 1998;26:1265-1270.
20. Bechtel K. 2004. Pediatric Controversies: Diagnosis and Management of Traumatic Brain Injuries. Trauma Report. Supplement to Emergency Medicine Reports, Pediatric Emergency Medicine Reports, ED Management, and Emergency Medicine Alert. Volume 5, Number 3. Thompson American Health Consultants.
21. Gudeman SK, Miller JD, Becker DP. Failure of high-dose steroid therapy to influence intracranial pressure in patients with severe head injury. *J Neurosurg*. 1979;51: 301-306.
22. Mansfield RT. Common issues in pediatric and adult clinical care. *Crit Care Clin*. 1997;13:611-628.
23. American Academy of Neurology. Report of the Quality Standards Committee: practice parameter: the management of concussion in sports [summary statement]. *Neurology*. 1997;48:581-585.
24. Casey R, Ludwig S, McCormick MC. Morbidity following minor head trauma in children. *Pediatrics*. 1986;78: 497-502.

25. Cheung D, Kharasch M. Evaluation of the patient with closed head trauma: an evidence based approach. *Emerg Med Clin North Am.* 1999;17:9-23.
26. Hall DE, Goldstein EM. *Hoekelman's Primary Pediatric Care.* 4th ed. St Louis, MO: Mosby; 2001.
27. Rutter M, Chadwick O, Shaffer D, et al. A prospective study of children with head injuries. *Psychol Med.* 1980;10:633-645.
28. Frush D, O'Hara, SM, Kliewer M. Pediatric imaging perspective: acute head trauma—is skull radiography useful? *J Pediatr.* 1998;132:553-554.
29. Schutzman SA, Barnes P, Duhaime AC, et al. Evaluation and management of children younger than 2 years old with apparently minor head trauma: proposed guidelines. *Pediatrics.* 2001;107:983-993.
30. American Academy of Pediatrics. The management of minor closed head trauma in children. *Pediatrics.* 1999; 104:1407-1415.
31. Dietrich AM, Bowman MJ, Ginn-Pease ME, et al. Pediatric head injuries: can clinical factors reliably predict an abnormality on computed tomography? *Ann Emerg Med.* 1993;22:1535-1540.
32. Dacey RG, Alves WM, Rimel RW, et al. Neurosurgical complications after apparently minor head injury: assessment of risk in a series of 610 patients. *J Neruosurg.* 1986; 65:203-210.
33. Hahn YS, McLone DG. Risk factors in the outcome of children with minor head injury. *Pediatr Neurosurg.* 1993;19:135-142.
34. Rosenthal BW, Bergman I. Intracranial injury after moderate head trauma in children. *J Pediatr.* 1989;115: 346-350.
35. Palchak MJ, Holmes JF, Vance CW, et al. A decision rule for identifying children at low risk for brain injuries after blunt head trauma. *Ann Emerg Med.* 2003;42:492-506.
36. Paterson A, Frush DP, Donnelly LF. Helical CT of the body: are settings adjusted for pediatric patients? *AJR Am J Roentgenol.* 2001;176:297-301.
37. Brenner DJ, Elliston C, Hall E, et al. Estimated risks of radiation-induced fatal cancer from pediatric CT. *AJR Am J Roentgenol.* 2001;176:289-296.
38. Hall D, Boydston W. Pediatric neck injuries. *Pediatr Rev.* 1999;20:13-19.
39. Davis RL, Hughes M, Gubler KD, et al. The use of cranial CT scans in the triage of pediatric patients with mild head injury. *Pediatrics.* 1995;95:345-349.
40. Roddy S, Cohn S, Moller B, et al. Minimal head trauma in children revisited: is routine hospitalization required? *Pediatrics.* 1998;101:575-577.
41. Farmer MY, Singer HS, Melleits ED, et al. Neurobehavioral sequelae of minor head injuries in children. *Pediatr Neurosci.* 1987;13:304-308.
42. Bacco E, et al. Early outcome prediction in severe head injury: comparison between children and adults. *Childs Nerv Syst.* 1986;2:67-71.
43. Chadwick O, Rutter M, Shaffer D, et al. A prospective study of children with head injuries. II. Cognitive sequelae. *Psychol Med.* 1981;11:49-61.
44. Chadwick O, Rutter M, Thompson J, et al. Intellectual performance and reading skills after localized head injury in childhood. *J Child Psychol Psychiatry.* 1981; 22:117-139.
45. Levine HS, Bento AL, Grossman RG. *Neurobehavioral Consequences of Closed Head Injury.* New York, NY: Oxford University Press; 1982.
46. Jennett WB, Lewin W. Traumatic epilepsy after closed head injuries. *J Neurol Neurosurg Psychiatry.* 1960;23: 295-301.
47. Raimondi AJ, Hirschauer J. Head injury in the infant and toddler. *Childs Brain.* 1984;11:12-35.
48. McQueen JK, Blackwood DHR, Harris P, et al. Low risk of late posttraumatic seizures following severe head injury: implications for clinical trials of prophylaxis. *J Neurol Neurosurg Psychiatry.* 1983;46:899-904.
49. Yablon S. Posttraumatic seizures. *Arch Phys Med Rehabil.* 1993;74:983-1001.
50. Young B, Rapp RP, Norton JA, et al. Failure of prophylactically administered phenytoin to prevent late posttraumatic seizures. *J Neurosurg.* 1983;58:236-241.

Chapter 349

HEART FAILURE

Tanvi S. Sharma, MD; Liana Perez Loughlin, Esq; Tracie L. Miller, MD, MS; Steven E. Lipshultz, MD

Congestive heart failure (CHF) is defined in the broadest sense as an inability to perfuse the body tissues adequately. CHF can occur in infants or children of any age, but up to 90% of cases occur during the 1st year of life, and most of these occur during the neonatal period.[1] This chapter reviews the pathophysiological mechanism of CHF, especially as it relates to differences in age at presentation. Then the signs and symptoms of CHF are discussed, after which the specific causes and associated findings in children with CHF at different ages are explored—an important topic because, in many children, CHF takes a chronic, smoldering course and may not be recognized early. Finally, the chapter presents the various medical and surgical treatment options for these children. Understanding the causes and associations for pediatric CHF and being able to recognize its signs and symptoms will help with early identification, which may, in turn, reduce morbidity and mortality.

PATHOPHYSIOLOGICAL FEATURES

The heart's generation of left-ventricular force differs at each developmental stage.[2] The inotropic forces of myocardial contractions are higher in neonates than in fetuses, and higher in adults than in neonates. Thus, for a particular left-ventricular preload, cardiac output or stroke volume rises progressively from the fetal to neonatal to adult stages of life. Although the mechanisms are not entirely clear, the properties of contractile proteins, ion channels, and cell surface receptors are expressed differently at each developmental stage. These changes in protein expression affect the contractility of the left-ventricular myocardium at different developmental stages. Animal studies suggest that neonates operate closer to their maximal inotropic potential than adults, and neonates may have less reserve to handle excess ventricular preload, making them more likely than adults to experience episodes of CHF. Several human clinical examples support this likelihood. For example, during the 3rd trimester of pregnancy, intravascular volume in pregnant women is approximately 50% greater than baseline. Nonetheless, only 1 in 4000 pregnant women develops peripartum cardiomyopathy. In contrast, in a normal 3-kg neonate, intravascular volume may be 240 mL, and a 50% increase of 120 mL would likely result in CHF. Although this simplified example does not consider the difference between acute and longer-lasting increases in intravascular volume, it implies that results of animal studies may apply to humans. Table 349-1 summarizes the major differences between neonatal and mature hearts.[3]

SIGNS AND SYMPTOMS OF CONGESTIVE HEART FAILURE

CHF in children occurs most frequently in the very young. A thoroughly obtained clinical history often provides clues to the cause of CHF. For example, in a 6-week-old infant who develops CHF as a result of a ventricular septal defect, the child's history is critical to appropriate management.

Feeding

Feeding history helps quantify nutritional intake and allows this data to be compared with weight gain. The average 6-week-old child takes roughly 3 to 4 oz of formula per feeding and nutritively sucks no longer than 20 minutes per feeding. Much lower intake or much longer feeding times may be a basis for concern. Most healthy, full-term, 6-week-old infants gain 10 to 30 g a day and consume more than 90 kcal/kg a day. Children who have CHF often have greater nutritional needs because of increased metabolic demands, and they often require 150 kcal/kg a day or more to gain adequate weight. Frequently, infants with CHF do not feed vigorously and may feed only in short, interrupted periods. Mothers will report that the infant feeds all day long, yet the child may have a nutritional intake of only 65 kcal/kg a day or less, and the child may gain little or no weight. For older children, CHF over long intervals results in malnutrition. Weight is usually the initial anthropometric measurement to be affected, followed by height and then head circumference. Evaluating growth velocity is critical to understanding the true nutritional impact of CHF.

Activity Level

Children with CHF usually change their activity level. In some cases, they become less active, and, in other situations, they become more irritable and anxious.

Tachycardia

Infants and children are expected to have a low resting heart rate. Children who have CHF may have persistent sinus tachycardia, with heart rates far higher than the normal range for their age.

Tachypnea

Healthy infants and children typically have low sleeping respiratory rates. Higher rates are often found in children with CHF.

Rales

Clinically evident rales are less likely to be found in infants and young children who have CHF than in older patients. In a young child, rales may suggest active pulmonary disease.

Jugular Venous Distention

Although jugular venous distention is found in many older patients who have heart failure, it is not seen as frequently in infants and children, largely because observing their jugular veins is difficult.

Hepatomegaly

The liver is frequently enlarged in infants and children who have CHF. Measuring the total liver span by

Table 349-1 Summary of Major Differences Between Neonatal and Mature Hearts

CHARACTERISTIC	NEONATAL	MATURE
PHYSIOLOGIC FEATURES		
Contractility	Limited	Normal
Heart rate dependence	High	Low
Contractile reserve	Low	High
Afterload tolerance	Low	Higher
Preload tolerance	Limited	Better
Ventricular interdependence	Significant	Less
CA^{2+} CYCLING		
Predominant site of Ca^{2+} flux	Sarcolemma	SR
Dependence on normal ionized Ca^{2+}	High	Lower
Circulating catecholamines	High	Lower
Adrenergic receptors	Downregulation, insensitive β_2, α_1 predominant	Normal, β_1
Predominant innervation	Parasympathetic predominates; sympathetic incomplete	Complete
Cytoskeleton	Higher water content	Lower water content
Cellular elements	Incomplete SR, disorganized myofibrils	Mature SR, organized myofibrils

Ca^{2+}, Calcium ion; *SR*, sarcoplasmic reticulum.

From Altman C, Kung G. Clinical recognition of heart failure in children. In: Chang AC, Towbin JA, eds. *Heart Failure in Children and Young Adults: From Molecular Mechanisms to Medical and Surgical Strategies.* Philadelphia, PA: Saunders Elsevier; 2006.

percussion is more useful than determining how far the liver edge extends below the right costal margin. The left lobe of the liver is frequently enlarged in infants and young children who have CHF, and thus a palpable liver edge that crosses the midline is suggestive of CHF.

Third Heart Sound Gallop

A 3rd heart sound (S_3) gallop is frequently observed in children of all ages who have CHF. However, during the neonatal period, an S_3 gallop may not indicate CHF. For example, a child with a patent ductus arteriosus with a left-to-right shunt will experience increased left-ventricular preload, which may result in an S_3 gallop.

Pulses and Perfusion

Because CHF is the inability to adequately perfuse the tissues, diminished strength of the peripheral pulses and perfusion are common signs. Simultaneously palpating the upper and lower extremity pulses may reveal differences in intensity or timing of the pulses, indicating a coarctation of the aorta, an interrupted aortic arch, or another lesion interfering with arterial blood flow.

Arrhythmias and Sudden Death

Arrhythmias can occur as both a cause and a result of heart failure in children and young adults. Ventricular dysfunction resulting from dilated cardiomyopathy may be associated with high-grade ectopy, which may increase the risk of death associated with heart failure. Unexplained syncope or palpitations in children with heart failure or cardiomyopathy should prompt an evaluation for arrhythmias. Syncope, in particular, may be an important predictor of sudden death in these children.

Scoring Systems

In 2004 the International Society for Heart and Lung Transplantation published practice guidelines for managing heart failure in children—guidelines that differ from those for adults with heart failure.[4] In adults, the New York Heart Association (NYHA) classification is used to provide a practical assessment of functional limitation as a result of heart failure (Table 349-2).[3] This classification system is not particularly useful in infants and children because of the variation in normal respiratory rates, different developmental stages reflecting different exercise capabilities, and different causes for heart failure across age groups. The Ross classification grading system for pediatric heart failure has been validated to address some of these issues (Tables 349-3, 349-4, 349-5).[3] The Ross classification system and the NYHA classification system both denote only current symptoms. Therefore the American College of Cardiology (ACC) and the American Heart Association (AHA) have also supported the use of a staging system to complement the NYHA classification system. The International Society for Heart and Lung Transplantation's practice guidelines describe a proposed heart failure staging system for infants and children that is modified from the ACC-AHA guidelines and that complements the Ross classification system (Table 349-6).[4]

Table 349-2 New York Heart Association Classification

CLASS	DESCRIPTION
I	No limitations to normal exertion
II	Symptoms on ordinary exertion
III	Symptoms with less than ordinary exertion
IV	Symptoms at rest

From Altman C, Kung G. Clinical recognition of heart failure in children. In: Chang AC, Towbin JA, eds. *Heart Failure in Children and Young Adults: From Molecular Mechanisms to Medical and Surgical Strategies.* Philadelphia, PA: Saunders Elsevier; 2006.

Table 349-3 Ross Scoring System of Heart Failure in Infants

CHARACTERISTIC	0 POINTS	1 POINT	2 POINTS
Volume per feed (oz)	>3.5	2.5-3.5	<2.5
Time per feed (min)	<40	>40	—
Respiratory rate (breaths/min)	<50	50-60	>60
Respiratory pattern	Normal	Abnormal	—
Peripheral perfusion	Normal	Decreased	—
S_3 or diastolic rumble	Absent	Present	—
Liver edge from costal margin, cm	<2	2-3	>3
Totals			
No CHF	0-2 points	—	—
Mild CHF	3-6 points	—	—
Moderate CHF	7-9 points	—	—
Severe CHF	10-12 points	—	—

CHF, Congestive heart failure; *S_3,* 3rd heart sound.
From Ross RD. Grading the severity of congestive heart failure in infants. *Pediatr Cardiol.* 1992;13:72-75. Reprinted with kind permission from Springer Science and Business Media.

LEADING CAUSES OF CONGESTIVE HEART FAILURE AT DIFFERENT AGES

The age at onset of heart failure in children, especially in infants, is important in determining its cause. The transition from fetal circulation to postnatal circulation requires precise steps, any of which may be compromised and lead to heart failure.[3]

Prenatal Period

Fetuses can develop CHF from a variety of causes. Infections, such as those caused by parvovirus, can lead to CHF with or without myocarditis. Abnormalities of heart rhythm can lead to CHF as well. Prolonged supraventricular tachycardia is not well tolerated by fetuses, and the mother must often be treated with antiarrhythmic medications to control the condition in the fetus. Fetuses with chronic or severe CHF have a greater likelihood of developing hydrops fetalis and dying.

Table 349-4 Ross Classification of Heart Failure in Infants

CLASS	DESCRIPTION
I	No limitations or symptoms
II	Mild tachypnea or diaphoresis with feeding in infants Dyspnea on exertion in older children No growth failure
III	Marked tachypnea or diaphoresis with feeds or exertion Prolonged feeding times Growth failure from CHF
IV	Symptoms at rest with tachypnea, retractions, grunting, or diaphoresis

CHF, Congestive heart failure.
From Ross RD. Grading the severity of congestive heart failure in infants. *Pediatr Cardiol.* 1992;13:72-75. Reprinted with kind permission from Springer Science and Business Media.

Table 349-6 Proposed Heart Failure Staging for Infants and Children

STAGE	INTERPRETATION
A	Patients with increased risk of developing HF but who have normal cardiac function and no evidence of cardiac chamber volume overload. Examples: previous exposure to cardiotoxic agents, family history of heritable cardiomyopathy, univentricular heart, congenitally corrected transposition of the great arteries.
B	Patients with abnormal cardiac morphology or cardiac function, with no symptoms of HF, past or present. Examples: aortic insufficiency with LV enlargement, history of anthracycline with decreased LV systolic function.
C	Patients with underlying structural or functional heart diseases and past or current symptoms of HF.
D	Patients with end-stage HF requiring continuous infusion of inotropic agents, mechanical circulatory support, cardiac transplantation, or hospice care.

HF, Heart failure; *LV,* left-ventricular.
Adapted from Rosenthal D, Chrisant MR, Edens E, et al. International Society for Heart and Lung Transplantation: practice guidelines for the management of heart failure in children. *J Heart Lung Transplant.* 2004;23:1313-1333. Copyright © 2004, Elsevier, with permission.

Table 349-5 Pediatric Clinical Heart Failure Score

CHARACTERISTIC	0 POINTS	1 POINT	2 POINTS
HISTORY			
Diaphoresis	Head only	Head and body during exercise	Head and body at rest
Tachypnea	Rare	Several times	Frequent
PHYSICAL EXAMINATION			
Breathing	Normal	Retractions	Dyspnea
RESPIRATORY RATE (BREATHS/MIN)			
Age 0-1 yr	<50	50-60	>60
Age 1-6 yr	<35	35-45	>45
Age 7-10 yr	<25	25-35	>35
Age 11-14 yr	<18	18-28	>28
HEART RATE (BEATS/MIN)			
Age 0-1 yr	<160	160-170	>170
Age 1-6 yr	<105	105-115	>115
Age 7-10 yr	<90	90-100	>100
Age 11-14 yr	<80	80-90	>90
Liver edge from costal margin, cm	<2	2-3	>3

From Reithmann C, Reber D, Kozlik-Feldman R, et al. A post-receptor defect of adenylyl cyclase in severely failing myocardium from children with congenital heart disease. *Eur J Pharmacol.* 1997;330:79-86. Copyright © 1997, Elsevier, with permission.

First Day of Life

Persistent fetal circulation or persistent pulmonary hypertension is the leading cause of CHF in the 1st day of life. This disorder is associated with meconium aspiration and neonatal acidosis. Newborns who have persistent pulmonary hypertension often have CHF that may not be clinically apparent. Many of the therapies for neonates with persistent pulmonary hypertension are directed to CHF. When the condition is recognized early, careful use of fluids, inotropes, and oxygen can be beneficial.

Neonatal sepsis is another leading cause of CHF in the 1st day of life. Prolonged rupture of membranes, maternal infection, and associated findings are risk factors. CHF is usually accompanied by the classic signs or symptoms outlined previously. Treating the sepsis with antibiotics and judicious use of fluids in conjunction with anticongestive therapy is often effective.

Hematologic or metabolic disorders should be considered in the differential diagnosis of CHF in the 1st day of life. Children who have hematocrit levels that are too high or too low are at risk for heart failure. Polycythemia resulting in sludging and hyperviscosity can lead to CHF, most commonly in infants of mothers with diabetes. A partial exchange transfusion will often lead to a rapid improvement in signs of heart failure.

Severe anemia in the 1st day of life can also cause CHF. Determining if the reduced red blood cell numbers have an acute or a chronic cause is important. An acute blood loss, such as occurs from abruptio placentae, can be managed with blood transfusion and by otherwise increasing intravascular fluid volume. On the other hand, a chronic anemia, such as that caused by Rh sensitization, may also produce a low red blood cell count and a low hematocrit level. However, in these cases, the intravascular volume may actually be high, and transfusion may worsen the heart failure. Such patients may benefit from double-volume exchange transfusion.

Metabolic causes of cardiomyopathy in the 1st day of life include hypoglycemia and hypocalcemia. The neonatal myocardium uses glucose for energy metabolism, by which fat reserves are diminished. A newborn who has low blood sugar and signs or symptoms of CHF will often improve when blood sugar levels are normalized. Hypocalcemia is another metabolic cause of CHF in the 1st day of life. Normalization of calcium, a potent inotrope, can reduce signs or symptoms of CHF. Hypoglycemia and hypocalcemia are often seen together in infants of mothers with diabetes.

Rare congenital heart defects such as absent pulmonary valve syndrome, free tricuspid orifice, or severe anomaly of the tricuspid valve associated with severe pulmonary stenosis can cause CHF in the 1st day of life.

Heart rate abnormalities may also lead to CHF in the 1st day of life. A newborn can tolerate supraventricular tachycardia of 250 to 300 beats per minute for only 12 to 36 hours before developing signs and symptoms of CHF. Sinus rhythm should be established immediately in symptomatic neonates who have supraventricular tachycardia and CHF. If vagal maneuvers or intravenous administration of adenosine do not result in normal sinus rhythm, and if a pacemaker is unavailable, then cardioversion should be attempted, followed by treatment with drugs. Slow heart rates may also lead to CHF; heart rates less than 60 beats per minute result in symptomatic CHF. For example, bradycardia can occur in infants with congenital complete heart block. When congenital complete heart block is diagnosed in a child, the mother should be screened for rheumatologic and connective tissue disorders.

Days 1 to 2 of Life

Between 1 and 2 days of age, CHF should be considered in an infant who has persistent or progressive tachypnea and hypoxia and whose chest radiographs show a *snowman* or *snowball* pattern with vessels radiating from a small cardiac silhouette. This scenario is typical for an infant who has obstructed total anomalous pulmonary venous return. Early identification is essential because surgery is the only effective intervention. Echocardiography can confirm the diagnosis.

Days 2 to 3 of Life

The leading cause of CHF at days 2 and 3 of life is ductus arteriosus-dependent lesions. These abnormalities include the following: (1) right-sided obstructive lesions such as pulmonary atresia, maximal tetralogy of Fallot, or tricuspid atresia; (2) transposition of the great arteries (the most common type of cyanotic heart disease); and (3) left-sided obstructive lesions such as hypoplastic left heart syndrome, critical aortic stenosis, or complex coarctation of the aorta. CHF is less likely when any of these conditions is accompanied by a patent ductus arteriosus but may develop at 2 to 3 days of age after the ductus arteriosus has closed, especially in cases of left-sided obstructive lesions. If diagnosed in time, these patients can often be stabilized by infusions of prostaglandin E_1, which maintains patency of the ductus arteriosus.

Days 3 to 7 of Life

Later in the 1st week of life, CHF can follow from endocrine disorders, including congenital adrenal hypoplasia, hyperthyroidism, or renal disorders, such as renal vein thrombus, renal artery stenosis, and hypertension or oliguria of any cause.

Weeks 1 to 2 of Life

Complex coarctation of the aorta is a leading cause of CHF between 1 and 2 weeks of age. Other similar lesions such as an interrupted aortic arch also may be present at this age. Typically, the ductus arteriosus closes by 3 days of life in children who do not have these conditions. However, in infants with complex coarctation of the aorta, the ductus remains open for up to 1 or 2 weeks. A child who has coarctation of the aorta and who has CHF at 1 to 2 weeks of age may have no pulse differential between the upper and lower extremities if cardiac output is low; thus any suspected complex coarctation or interrupted aortic arch should be investigated by echocardiography. When diagnosed early, the child can often be stabilized quickly with anticongestive therapy and prostaglandin E_1.

Months 1 to 2 of Life

Left-to-right shunt lesions are most common at 1 to 2 months of age. A typical example is a child who has a ventricular septal defect in whom pulmonary artery resistance has fallen over the 1st few postnatal weeks, resulting in increased left-to-right shunting. Other examples include atrial level shunts (eg, atrial septal defect), common atria, ventricular-level left-to-right shunts (eg, complete atrioventricular canal defects, ventricular septal defects, single ventricle), and great vessel-level shunts such as patent ductus arteriosus. The timing of presentation often suggests the existence of a left-to-right shunt. Whether CHF in this circumstance is easily treated is unclear. In the past, hypertransfusion therapy to reduce shunting was found to be useful, but this therapy is not commonly used at this time.

Months 6 to 12 of Life

Metabolic, genetic, infectious, and inflammatory cardiomyopathies often present between 6 and 12 months of age.[5] Children with metabolic or genetic cardiomyopathy would be asymptomatic for the first 6 months of life, according to the family. However, when the child contracts a viral illness, CHF results. The child may also exhibit growth failure and hypotonia. Disorders such as glycogen storage diseases would also present in this way. Infectious and inflammatory diseases such as HIV, enteroviral infections, and Kawasaki disease can cause myocarditis at this age.[6,7]

Years 1 to 18 of Life

CHF in children older than 1 year occurs most commonly in children with comorbid severe or chronic illnesses. For example, a child treated for cancer is at risk for CHF during active treatment with anthracycline chemotherapy[8,9] or radiation[10] to the chest. This child continues to be at risk for CHF for many years thereafter because of long-term cardiotoxicity from these agents. Nevertheless, during childhood, beyond the 1st year of life, CHF is unusual. Older children with congenital heart disease, other than those who have had corrective surgery, rarely develop CHF. In fact, the leading indications for pediatric heart transplantations, which indicate a failure of the medical management of CHF, are congenital heart disease during the 1st year of life and cardiomyopathies thereafter.[11]

THERAPY FOR CONGESTIVE HEART FAILURE IN CHILDREN

Pharmacotherapy

The 4 classes of drugs used most frequently in the management of CHF in children include diuretics, inotropes, agents to reduce afterload, and β-adrenergic antagonists.[12,13] Each class targets a different aspect of the pathophysiological features of CHF, and they are often used in combination. A pediatric cardiologist should direct the treatment of CHF in children.

Symptomatic left-ventricular dysfunction or CHF in children can be caused by many different pathophysiological mechanisms. Increased preload is one common mechanism. In this situation, although the left-ventricular myocytes are healthy and have normal contractility, the overall systolic performance of the ventricle is reduced.[14] Preload reduction with diuretic therapy is often beneficial.[15]

CHF can also result from depressed contractility of unhealthy left-ventricular myocytes. In this case, inotropic support frequently brings early symptomatic relief.[16] However, determining the cause of heart failure in a child becomes critical because many children with unexplained heart failure may have mitochondrial defects that impair their ability to respond to inotropic support. Aggressive use of inotropic support in such patients may hasten their deaths.

Digoxin, an inotrope that can be administered orally or intravenously, will raise a child to a higher inotropic state and, in the process, lead to a reduction in preload. Frequently, digoxin is used in combination with a diuretic. Some studies suggest a synergy between digoxin and diuretics that potentiates primary ventricular function and reduces preload[17] more than either agent alone.[15] Combination therapy can also reduce the chance of individual agent toxicity. β-Adrenergic agonists such as dopamine and dobutamine are also inotropic and are useful for treating children with heart failure, especially children in a decompensated state. Newer inotropic agents are being investigated in children. Calcium-sensitizing agents, in particular, improve cardiac output with minimal increases in heart rate, a common side effect of β-adrenergic agonists.

Agents that reduce afterload constitute the 3rd major class of pharmacotherapy for the management of heart failure. Left-ventricular afterload reduction in a child with symptomatic left-ventricular dysfunction will improve function and reduce symptoms of CHF. Several classes of afterload reducers are available. The angiotensin-converting enzyme (ACE) inhibitors, such as captopril and enalapril, are used most frequently.[18] These agents are vasodilators, but they also affect neurohormonal mechanisms. In adults with asymptomatic left-ventricular dysfunction or CHF, the use of ACE inhibitors has been associated with slowing the progression from asymptomatic left-ventricular dysfunction to CHF and reducing mortality from heart failure. These beneficial effects are believed to be caused by the combination of vasodilatory and neurohormonal activation. The vasodilatory effects of ACE inhibitors will often move a child to a more favorable preload state and reduce afterload, thus improving left-ventricular contractility.

A 4th class of therapy for left-ventricular dysfunction in children is the β-adrenergic antagonists, such as atenolol and carvedilol.[19] β-adrenergic antagonists reverse adrenergically mediated intrinsic myocardial dysfunction and remodeling. In adults who have CHF, β-antagonists improve symptoms, ventricular function, and survival. Results of small studies suggest that β-antagonists improve ventricular function in children who have CHF,[20] but these agents have not been used extensively, and further evaluation of this class of drugs is underway.

Newer agents for the management of CHF include angiotensin-receptor blockers, endothelin-receptor antagonists, phosphodiesterase inhibitors, aldosterone antagonists, calcium-sensitizing agents, tumor necrosis factor α inhibitors, neural endopeptidase inhibitors, and vasopressin antagonists.[3]

Few large, controlled clinical trials have been conducted on the indications, dosages, and optimal use of existing therapy for CHF. The basis for using these agents is therefore extrapolated from adults, and, generally, they are used for the palliative relief of symptoms in children. Figure 349-1 demonstrates some of the therapies used for adults with heart failure.[21] Treatments directed at prevention or cure of CHF in children have not been evaluated.

Arrhythmias

In addition to pharmacotherapy aimed at the specific symptoms of heart failure in children, management of arrhythmias is also critical. Arrhythmias are a major cause of morbidity and mortality in children with heart failure, especially in the later stages of disease.[4] Acute treatment with intravenous antiarrhythmic agents and cardioversion or defibrillation should be considered for all children with hemodynamic instability. Chronic suppressive therapy or radio-frequency surgical ablation therapy may be required for long-term management of recurring arrhythmias. In adults with heart failure and arrhythmias, implantable cardiac defibrillators have greatly improved survival.[4] These devices have not been used extensively in young children, and only a few small studies have assessed their use. However, technologic advances in the development of these devices suggest the potential for decreased complications and infections, and they thus hold promise for use in younger children.

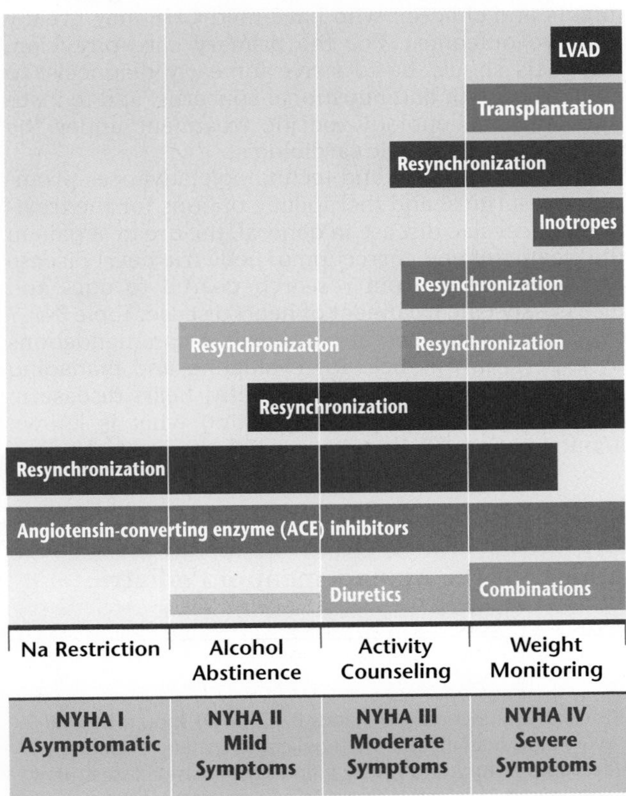

Figure 349-1 Management of systolic heart failure in adults. Because very few large, controlled studies have been conducted regarding treatment of CHF in children, management strategies have been extrapolated from adults. This figure describes the therapies used for adults with heart failure, and many of the same principles of treatment are used in children as well. *LVAD,* Left ventricular assist devices; *NYHA,* New York Heart Association. *(Massie BM. Management of the patient with chronic heart failure. In: Crawford MH, DiMarco JP, Paulus WJ, eds.* Cardiology. *Philadelphia: Mosby; 2004: 893. Copyright © 2004, Elsevier, with permission.)*

Nutritional Management

A classic symptom—failure to thrive—can impede even the most cutting-edge medical advancements in children with heart failure. Children with congenital heart disease often exhibit a range of delays in weight gain and linear growth. The danger of growth and development disturbances is not limited to the threat of permanent effects on these outcomes; they can also lead to worse clinical outcomes after corrective surgery.[22] A systematic approach to overcoming failure to thrive has been suggested, starting with dietary intervention: counseling and educating the patient and parents to optimize feeding to increase mean caloric intake and weight.[23] Nutritional education and counseling alone will not work for all children or infants with congenital heart disease because the high energy cost of eating might actually prevent a child from consuming larger quantities of food. In these cases, fortified formula and breast milk have improved weight gain.[22] However, this approach should be closely monitored because high-energy formula can induce thermogenesis and increase metabolic inefficiency. Breastfeeding is less stressful than bottle feeding for infants with congenital heart disease. The decision to breastfeed or bottle feed should be made on an individual basis with the cooperation of the parents, primary care physician, and other health care professionals familiar with the particular needs of the infant. Gastrostomy placement and parenteral feeding may also be important considerations in severely malnourished infants, in part, because they do not incur the energy costs of feeding.

Most children with congenital heart disease require surgical correction, which is usually performed as soon as the child reaches an ideal weight.[22] Mortality and morbidity associated with cardiac surgery increase in underweight infants. Conversely, some findings show that energy expenditures decrease and return to normal after surgery.[24,25] Therefore, if an infant fails to thrive after all aggressive feeding and nutrition measures have been tried, then surgery may be advisable even if the infant is not at an ideal weight.

Other nutritional considerations include managing electrolyte abnormalities that may occur from diuretic use and balancing fluid intake with fluid overload in children with heart failure.[26]

Surgery

Surgical correction of congenital cardiac defects is crucial in managing heart failure in children. However, heart failure occurring after surgery may be a complicating factor. Children with cardiomyopathy or heart failure after repair of a congenital cardiac defect may be candidates for a heart transplant. Aggressive pretransplantation evaluation is required, given the potential for long-term complications after transplantation.

Newer surgical techniques for congenital cardiac defects include techniques to correct failed procedures or revise older, less effective surgical procedures. As children with congenital heart disease live longer as a result of improved medical and surgical care, revision procedures in young adulthood may become a key component of long-term management.

For children at risk of sudden death from arrhythmias, implantable cardioverter defibrillators may be considered, although these devices have not been well studied or used extensively in children. Children present a unique challenge to the use of these devices because of the large size of the device and leads, difficult surgical access resulting from previous cardiac surgeries, and difficulties with programming the devices as a result of inconsistent rate patterns.[3]

SUMMARY

CHF can occur at any age in infants and children. It is most common in the neonatal period and the 1st year of life. Although it can be acute and fulminant, CHF is most often a chronic, smoldering process, and it is associated with substantial morbidity and mortality. Recognizing the signs and symptoms of CHF in infants and children as soon as possible is important because prompt therapy can reduce morbidity and improve the quality of life. Some therapies may even prevent mortality.

The causes of CHF vary with the age of the infant or child. Prenatally, infectious and heart rate abnormalities are most common. In the 1st day of life, persistent fetal circulation and neonatal sepsis resulting in CHF are common, as are metabolic and hematologic causes of CHF. Days 2 and 3 of life are associated with ductus arteriosus-dependent cardiovascular lesions. At age 1 to 2 weeks, complex coarctation and other aortic obstructions are associated with CHF. One to 2 months of age finds CHF onset most commonly associated with left-to-right cardiovascular shunts. The 2nd half of the 1st year of life is most commonly associated with metabolic genetic cardiomyopathies, as well as infectious and inflammatory conditions. Later on, the onset of CHF is most commonly associated with chronic illnesses, including toxic exposures and infectious and inflammatory conditions.

The early recognition and effective management of infants and children who have mild CHF may greatly improve outcomes. For the primary care physician, the goals should be to strive for early diagnosis, to address growth and nutritional concerns, and to institute effective, etiology-specific treatment under the direction of a pediatric cardiologist.

Although medical and technologic advances promise new surgical and therapeutic options for the treatment of cardiac disease in general, the greatest gain in the treatment and correction of pediatric heart disease will likely result from research geared to age- and disease-specific treatment of heart disease. Table 349-7 summarizes the current consensus recommendations by experts in this field for evaluating and managing heart failure in children.[4] Currently, heart disease in children is treated by extrapolating what is known about treating adults with cardiac disease.[27] Lack of

Table 349-7 Current Consensus Recommendations for the Management of Pediatric Heart Failure*

RECOMMENDATION	DESCRIPTION
Recommendation 1	The underlying cause of new-onset ventricular dysfunction (HF stages B, C, or D) should be evaluated thoroughly in all patients. The evaluation may include metabolic and genetic evaluation in selected cases, as indicated by the available history and physical findings. Invasive assessment, including myocardial biopsy, may be considered in selected cases. In infants, particular care should be paid to the exclusion of coronary artery anomalies and other anatomic causes.
Recommendation 2	Screening of 1st-degree relatives should be considered in patients with new-onset ventricular dysfunction caused by dilated cardiomyopathy (HF stages B, C, or D).
Recommendation 3	Patients with fluid retention associated with ventricular dysfunction (HF stage C) should be treated with diuretics to achieve a euvolemic state using clinical criteria of fluid status and cardiac output.
Recommendation 4	Digoxin should be used in patients with ventricular dysfunction and symptoms of HF (HF stage C) to relieve symptoms. Lower doses of digoxin are preferred for this purpose.
Recommendation 5	For the treatment of moderate or severe degrees of left-ventricular dysfunction with or without symptoms (HF stages B and C), ACE inhibitors should be routinely used unless a specific contraindication exists. These medications should be started at low doses and titrated up to a maximal tolerated safe dose. Uptitration may require a reduction in the dose of diuretics.

Table 349-7 Current Consensus Recommendations for the Management of Pediatric Heart Failure*—cont'd

RECOMMENDATION	DESCRIPTION
Recommendation 6	In all cases of HF associated with structural heart disease (HF stages B, C, or D), consideration should be given to surgical repair of significant lesions because the long-term outlook may be more favorable than with medical management alone.
Recommendation 7	Clinical management of diastolic dysfunction should address symptoms and attempt to address the underlying cause of the diastolic dysfunction, if known. This management should include a careful evaluation for pericardial disease, and coronary insufficiency with attendant myocardial ischemia. Systemic hypertension, if present, should be aggressively controlled.
Recommendation 8	Fluid management to control symptoms remains a cornerstone in the management of symptomatic diastolic dysfunction (HF stage C). Diuretics can help control symptoms but must be used cautiously because cardiac output depends on increased filling pressures. Renal function should be followed closely, with care taken not to administer too much. Finally, sodium and fluid restriction may be helpful in controlling symptoms.
Recommendation 9	Atrial arrhythmias are not infrequent in patients with diastolic dysfunction caused by atrial enlargement. However, atrial contribution to ventricular filling is particularly important for this group of patients (HF stages B and C). Therefore efforts should be made to maintain sinus rhythm by use of antiarrhythmic therapy and pacemakers.
Recommendation 10	Patients with diastolic dysfunction refractory to optimal medical or surgical management should be evaluated for heart transplantation because such patients are at high risk for developing pulmonary hypertension and of dying suddenly (HF stage C).
Recommendation 11	Institution of mechanical cardiac support should be considered in patients without structural congenital heart disease, who present with acute low cardiac output, or who have intractable arrhythmias during a presumably temporary condition that is refractory to medical therapy (HF stage D), such as myocarditis, septic shock, or acute rejection after receiving a heart transplant.
Recommendation 12	Institution of mechanical cardiac support should be considered in patients with or without structural congenital heart disease and who have acute decompensation of end-stage HF, primarily as a bridge to heart transplantation (HF stage D).
Recommendation 13	In patients with significant arrhythmias in the setting of HF associated with structural heart disease (HF stages B, C, or D), consideration should be given to surgical repair of important uncorrected or residual defects because this is likely to be essential in achieving adequate rhythm control.
Recommendation 14	In patients with significant arrhythmias in the setting of HF associated with structural heart disease (HF stages B, C, or D), consideration should be given to improving or optimizing the medical treatment for HF and correcting aggravating factors such as electrolyte abnormalities because this is likely to be a key determinant of the successful control of arrhythmias.
Recommendation 15	In patients with significant arrhythmias in the setting of HF associated with structural heart disease (HF stages B, C, or D), maintenance of atrioventricular synchrony is of great importance in optimizing hemodynamics, and management of intraatrial arrhythmias should be oriented toward restoration of sinus rhythm rather than on ventricular rate control alone.

*All recommendations presented are class I (conditions for which general agreement exists that a given therapy is useful and effective) (American College of Cardiology and American Heart Association evidence grade).
ACE, Angiotensin-converting enzyme; *HF,* heart failure.
Adapted from Rosenthal D, Chrisant MR, Edens E, et al. International Society for Heart and Lung Transplantation: practice guidelines for the management of heart failure in children. *J Heart Lung Transplant.* 2004;23:1313-1333. Copyright © 2004, Elsevier, with permission.

resources and difficulty in undertaking pediatric trials are important issues. Therapies can work differently and cause idiosyncratic reactions in children. Therefore, although innovation and cooperation will be required, the greatest potential for advancement will be found in evidence-based medicine geared specifically to treating and correcting cardiac disease in children.

AAP POLICY STATEMENTS

American Academy of Pediatrics, Section on Cardiology and Cardiac Surgery. Guidelines for pediatric cardiovascular centers. *Pediatrics.* 2002;109(3):544-549. (aappolicy.aappublications.org/cgi/content/full/pediatrics;109/3/544).

American College of Cardiology, American Heart Association, American Academy of Pediatrics. ACC/AHA/AAP recommendations for training in pediatric cardiology. *Pediatrics.* 2005;116(6):1574-1575. (aappolicy.aappublications.org/cgi/content/full/pediatrics;116/6/1574).

SUGGESTED RESOURCES

Chang AC, Towbin JA, eds. *Heart Failure in Children and Young Adults: From Molecular Mechanisms to Medical and Surgical Strategies.* Philadelphia, PA: Saunders Elsevier; 2006.

Shaddy RE, Wernovsky G, eds. *Pediatric Heart Failure.* Boca Raton, FL: Taylor and Francis; 2005.

REFERENCES

1. Towbin JA, Lipshultz SE. Genetics of neonatal cardiomyopathy. *Curr Opin Cardiol.* 1999;14:250-262.
2. Auslender M. Pathophysiology of heart failure. *Prog Pediatr Cardiol.* 2000;11:175-184.
3. Altman C, Kung G. Clinical recognition of heart failure in children. In: Chang AC, Towbin JA, eds. *Heart Failure in Children and Young Adults: From Molecular Mechanisms to Medical and Surgical Strategies.* Philadelphia, PA: Saunders Elsevier; 2006.
4. Rosenthal D, Chrisant MR, Edens E, et al. International Society for Heart and Lung Transplantation: practice guidelines for the management of heart failure in children. *J Heart Lung Transplant.* 2004;23:1313-1333.
5. Schwartz ML, Cox GF, Lin AE, et al. Clinical approach to genetic cardiomyopathy in children. *Circulation.* 1996; 94:2021-2038.
6. Bowles NE, Kearney DL, Ni J, et al. The detection of viral genomes by polymerase chain reaction in the myocardium of pediatric patients with advanced HIV disease. *J Am Coll Cardiol.* 1999;34:857-865.
7. Lipshultz SE, Easley KA, Orav EJ, et al for the Pediatric Pulmonary and Cardiovascular Complications of Vertically Transmitted HIV Infection Study Group. Left ventricular structure and function in children infected with human immunodeficiency virus: the prospective P2C2 HIV Multicenter Study. *Circulation.* 1998;97: 1246-1256.
8. Krischer JP, Epstein S, Cuthbertson DD, et al. Clinical cardiotoxicity following anthracycline treatment for childhood cancer: the pediatric oncology group experience. *J Clin Oncol.* 1997;15:1544-1552.
9. Lipshultz SE, Lipsitz SR, Mone SM, et al. Female sex and higher drug dose as risk factors for late cardiotoxic effects of doxorubicin therapy for childhood cancer. *N Engl J Med.* 1995;332:1738-1743.
10. Cameron EH, Lipshultz SE, Tarbell NJ, Mauch PM. Cardiovascular disease in long-term survivors of pediatric Hodgkin's disease. *Prog Pediatr Cardiol.* 1998;8:139-144.
11. Grenier MA, Osganian SK, Cox GF, et al. Design and implementation of a North American pediatric cardiomyopathy registry. *Am Heart J.* 2000;139(2:3):S86-S95.
12. Auslender M, Artman M. Overview of the management of heart failure. *Prog Pediatr Cardiol.* 2000;11:231-241.
13. Giantris A, Lipshultz SE. Cardiac therapeutics in HIV-infected patients. In: Lipshultz SE, ed. *Cardiology in AIDS.* New York, NY: Chapman and Hall; 1998.
14. Lipshultz SE, Orav EJ, Sanders SP, et al. Limitations of fractional shortening as an index of contractility in HIV-infected children. *J Pediatr.* 1995;125:563-570.
15. Lowrie L. Diuretic therapy of heart failure in infants and children. *Prog Pediatr Cardiol.* 2000;12:45-55.
16. Latifi S, Lidsky K, Blumer JL. Pharmacology of inotropic agents in infants and children. *Prog Pediatr Cardiol.* 2000;12:57-79.
17. Hougen TJ. Digitalis use in children: an uncertain future. *Progr Pediatr Cardiol.* 2000;12:37-43.
18. Grenier MA, Fioravanti J, Truesdell SC, et al. Angiotensin converting enzyme inhibitor therapy for ventricular dysfunction in infants, children, and adolescents. *Prog Pediatr Cardiol.* 2000;12:91-111.
19. Shaddy RE, Tani LY, Gidding SS, et al. Beta-blocker treatment of dilated cardiomyopathy with congestive heart failure in children: a multiinstitutional experience. *J Heart Lung Transplant.* 1999;18:269-274.
20. Rusconi P, Gomez-Marin O, Rossique-Gonzalez M, et al. Carvedilol in children with cardiomyopathy: 3-year experience at a single institution. *J Heart Lung Transplant.* 2004;23:832-838.
21. Massie BM. Management of the patient with chronic heart failure. In: Crawford MH, DiMarco JP, Paulus WJ, eds. *Cardiology.* Philadelphia, PA: Mosby; 2004.
22. Wheat JC. Nutritional management of children with congenital heart disease. *Nutr Bytes.* 2002;8:1.
23. Unger R, DeKleermaeker M, Gidding SS, et al. Calorie count: improved weight gain with dietary intervention in congenital heart disease. *Am J Dis Child.* 1992;146:1078-1084.
24. Mitchell IM, Davies PS, Day JM, et al. Energy expenditure in children with congenital heart disease, before and after cardiac surgery. *J Thoracic Cardiovasc Surg.* 1994; 107:374-385.
25. Leitch CA, Karn CA, Ensing GJ, et al. Energy expenditure after surgical repair in children with cyanotic congenital heart disease. *J Pediatr.* 2000;137:381-385.
26. Leitch CA. Nutritional aspects of pediatric heart failure. In: Shaddy RE, Wernovsky G, eds. *Pediatric Heart Failure.* Boca Raton, FL: Taylor and Francis; 2005.
27. Burch M. Heart failure in the young. *Heart.* 2002;88:198-202.

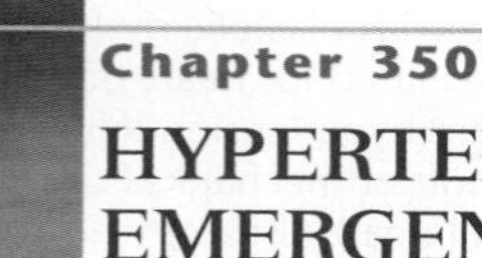

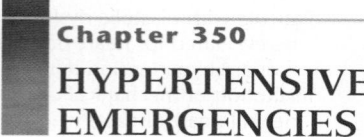

Chapter 350 HYPERTENSIVE EMERGENCIES

Srinivasan Suresh, MD, MBA

Hypertension, defined as the systolic or diastolic blood pressure (BP) above the 95th percentile for sex, age, and height, is a significant health issue in children. The risk of hypertension increases with the child's body mass index (BMI); approximately 30% of children with BMI that exceeds the 95th percentile have hypertension.[1] This increase in prevalence has led to more children being evaluated in various settings, including clinics, offices, and emergency departments (EDs). Acute hypertensive emergencies are relatively infrequent in the pediatric population. However, their full clinical manifestations represent potential life-threatening events, demanding prompt identification and carefully implemented therapeutic intervention. The increasing array of potent oral and parenteral antihypertensive agents, as well as the widespread availability of dialysis, has resulted in marked reductions of morbidity and mortality associated with hypertensive crises.

Hypertensive emergency is distinguished from *hypertensive urgency* by the presence of acute end-organ dysfunction discovered in the history, physical examination, or laboratory studies, and not from the child's BP (Figure 350-1). The division into these 2 categories determines where treatment should be administered: in the ED, intensive care unit (ICU), or routine hospital unit. Classifying the hypertensive episode as *urgent* or *emergent* governs the approach to treatment.

Malignant hypertension is characterized by marked increases in systolic BP, diastolic BP, or both (eg, ≥160 mm Hg systolic and ≥105 mm Hg diastolic for children younger than 10 years; ≥170 mm Hg systolic and ≥110 mm Hg diastolic for children older than 10 years) and is often associated with spasm and

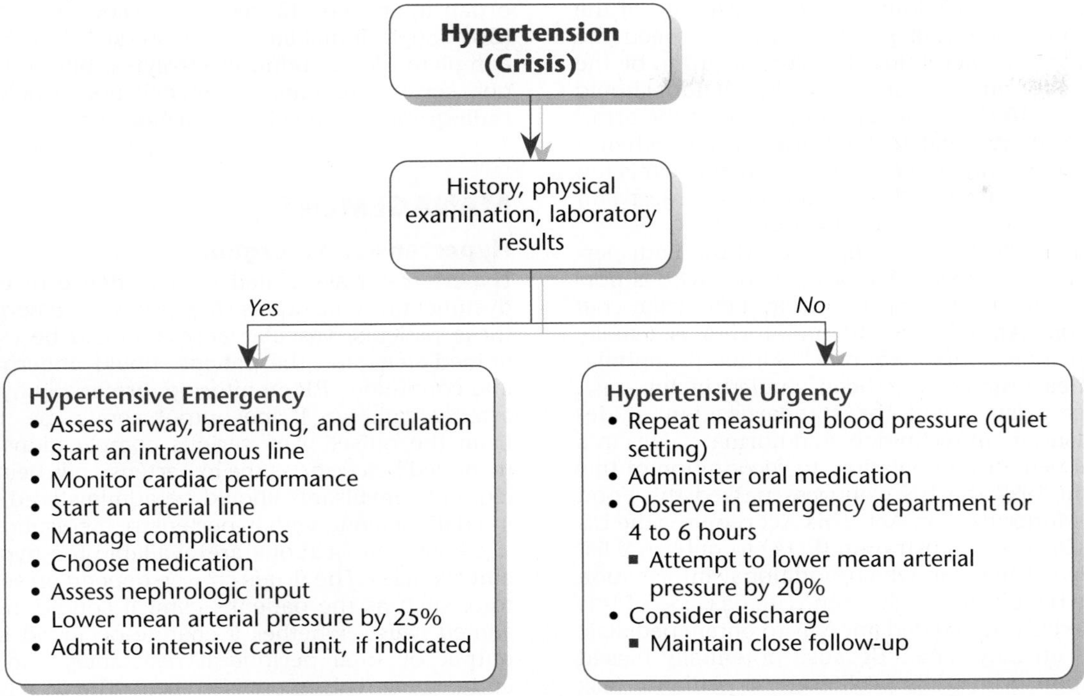

Figure 350-1 Diagnostic approach for management of acute hypertension. *(Fleisher G, Ludwig S.* Textbook of Pediatric Emergency Medicine. *5th ed. Baltimore, MD: Lippincott Williams & Wilkins; 2006. Reprinted by permission.)*

tortuosity of the retinal arteries, papilledema, and hemorrhages and exudates on funduscopic examination. Hypertensive encephalopathy (an example of hypertensive emergency) is often seen in malignant hypertension and consists of a combination of signs and symptoms that vary from patient to patient and that include nausea, vomiting, headaches, altered mental status, visual disturbances, seizures, and stroke. This condition describes the transient migratory neurologic symptoms associated with a malignant hypertensive state.

EVALUATION

As part of the initial physical assessment, all children evaluated for hypertension must have their BP measured in both upper extremities and in at least 1 lower extremity. When confronted with newly diagnosed hypertension in the child, the physician should ask 3 important questions: (1) Is the hypertension primary or secondary? (2) Does evidence exist of target organ injury? (3) Do associated risk factors exist that would worsen the prognosis if the hypertension is not treated or is treated unsuccessfully?

History

A brief but thorough history and physical examination should be performed with the goal of classifying the severity of the hypertension. Some key features in the history would be the duration and onset of hypertension, degree of compliance with any drug therapy, and possibility of renal disease. Therefore clinicians should be alert to any history of urinary tract infections, failure to thrive, hematuria, edema, or umbilical artery catheterization. Clinicians should also inquire about any history of joint pain, palpitations, weight loss, flushing, weakness, drug ingestion, headaches (including characterization), nausea, and vomiting and should ask about a family history of renal disease or hypertension.

Physical Examination

With severe hypertension, this evaluation should progress only after the ABCs (airway, breathing, and circulation) of resuscitation have been accomplished. After BP has been taken several times, a focused physical examination should immediately be performed, with a focus on checking for any evidence of neurologic dysfunction and congestive heart failure. Funduscopy should be performed to assess for hemorrhage, papilledema, or infarcts. Any discrepancy in the upper and lower extremity BP measurements should be noted. Presence of an abdominal bruit suggests a renovascular cause of hypertension.

Improper cuff size can affect the diagnosis; thus taking BP with the proper-size cuff is important. By convention, an appropriate cuff size is a cuff with an inflatable bladder width that is at least 40% of the arm circumference at a point midway between the olecranon and the acromion. For such a cuff to be the optimal size for an arm, the cuff bladder length should cover 80% to 100% of the circumference of the arm.[2] BP measurements tend to be overestimated when a cuff is too small and underestimated when a cuff is too big. If a cuff is too small, then the next largest cuff should be used, even if it appears large.

A patient with BP levels that exceed the 95th percentile in a physician's office or clinic but who is normotensive outside a clinical setting has *white-coat hypertension*. Ambulatory BP monitoring is usually required to make this diagnosis.[3] Although ambulatory BP measurement has been studied in the past, uncertainty exists about the standardization of devices, measurement technique, and normal values in a multiracial pediatric population. In recognition of this problem, in 1997 the US Congress passed the Food and Drug Modernization Act. This Act requires the US Food and Drug Administration (FDA) to publish a list of approved drugs for which additional information may prove beneficial for children. The passage of this act provided a long-needed impetus to obtain pediatric safety and efficacy data.[4] Because potentially biased industry-sponsored trials proliferate, a pediatric task force has suggested guidelines for antihypertensive trials in children.[5] The task force concluded that the use of children in antihypertensive trials is highly complex, partly related to a low incidence and prevalence, the lability of BP values, and technical problems in measurement of BP.

Laboratory Evaluation

The laboratory and radiologic workup can then be divided into 3 categories: (1) tests for diagnosis of primary or secondary hypertension, (2) tests for target organ injury, and (3) tests for associated risk factors (Box 350-1). Initial laboratory studies should include a complete blood count, electrolytes, blood urea nitrogen, serum creatinine, serum calcium, urinalysis, chest radiograph, and an electrocardiogram.

MANAGEMENT

Hypertensive Emergency

Hypertension associated with evidence of end-organ dysfunction constitutes *hypertensive emergency*. In these patients, vascular access should be established immediately, and the patient should undergo cardiac and continuous BP monitoring, preferably by an intra-arterial catheter. Urine output should be monitored from the outset. Any serious complications must be managed before or as the hypertension is being treated (eg, anticonvulsants should be administered to a seizing patient along with hypertensive medications).

Several medications are available for hypertensive emergencies. The drugs chosen depend on several factors, such as the patient's clinical condition, the presumed cause, whether a change occurred in cardiac output or total peripheral resistance, and whether end-organ involvement is present. The goal is to lower the BP promptly but gradually because a sudden decrease in BP can lead to neurologic complications, such as intracranial bleeding. Hypertensive emergencies should be treated by an intravenous antihypertensive drug that produces a controlled reduction in the BP, with the aim of decreasing the pressure by 25% or less over the first 8 hours, then gradually normalizing the BP over 26 to 48 hours.[6,7] Each of the most commonly used medications has advantages and disadvantages (Table 350-1), and each clinical situation requires its own mode of management. However, some helpful general guidelines exist.

BOX 350-1 Laboratory Tests for Hypertension

TESTS FOR DIAGNOSIS OF PRIMARY OR SECONDARY HYPERTENSION

Laboratory

Urinalysis
Urine culture
Urinary catecholamines
Complete blood count with platelet count and blood smear
Serum electrolytes, calcium, phosphorus
Serum blood urea nitrogen, creatinine
Serum C3 complement, antistreptolysin O titer, antinuclear antibody
Plasma renin

Radiology

Chest radiograph
Intravenous pyelogram
Voiding cystourethrogram
Cardiac catheterization
Renal ultrasound
Renal scan
Renal arteriogram

Other

Electrocardiogram

TESTS FOR TARGET ORGAN INJURY

Urinalysis
Chest radiograph
Electrocardiogram

TESTS FOR ASSOCIATED RISK FACTORS

Serum lipid profile (eg, lipoprotein electrophoresis)
Serum uric acid

From Fleisher G, Ludwig S. *Textbook of Pediatric Emergency Medicine*. 5th ed. Baltimore, MD: Lippincott Williams & Wilkins; 2006. Reprinted by permission.

Table 350-1 Drugs Used in Cases of Hypertensive Emergency

DRUG CHARACTERISTIC	NITROPRUSSIDE	DIAZOXIDE	HYDRALAZINE	LABETALOL	NIFEDIPINE	PHENTOLAMINE
Initial dose	0.5 mcg/kg/min	3-5 mg/kg (max 150 mg/dose)	0.1-0.5 mg/kg (max 20 mg)	0.25 mg/kg (max 3-4 mg/kg)	0.25-0.5 mg/kg (max 20 mg)	0.1 mg/kg/dose
Administration	IV infusion	Rapid IV push	IV infusion over 15-30 min	IV infusion while supine	Bite and swallow or sublingual	IV
Onset of action	Instantaneous	Minutes	30 min	5 min	15-30 min	Instantaneous
Interval to repeat or increase dose	30-60 min	15-30 min	10 min	10 min	30-60 min	30 min
Duration of action	Only during infusion	4-12 hr	4-12 hr	To 24 hr	6 hr	30-60 min
Side effects	Headache; chest and abdominal pain	Hyperglycemia, hyperuricemia	Tachycardia, headache, flushing, vomiting	GI upset, scalp tingling, headache, sedation	Dizziness, facial flushing, nausea	Tachycardia, abdominal pain

GI, Gastrointestinal; *IV*, intravenous.
Modified from Fleisher G, Ludwig S. *Textbook of Pediatric Emergency Medicine.* 5th ed. Baltimore, MD: Lippincott Williams & Wilkins; 2006. Reprinted by permission.

Therapy with sodium nitroprusside, an arteriolar and venous vasodilator, is always effective. BP decreases with little change in cardiac output, and reflex tachycardia does not occur. Sodium nitroprusside is administered by constant infusion. Its effect is immediate, and it lasts only as long as the infusion is continued. Use requires close observation, and therefore sodium nitroprusside may be inappropriate in the ED. Other disadvantages are that the drug requires 10 minutes to prepare and is photosensitive, and a potential exists for cyanide accumulation.

Diazoxide is an arteriolar vasodilator, has little effect on capacitance vessels, and has no direct cardiac effect. It is potent and has a rapid onset, resulting in sometimes dramatic effects. Providing a long duration of BP control (8 to 12 hours), diazoxide causes marked salt and water retention and in patients with edema should be followed with a diuretic agent. Diazoxide also causes reflex tachycardia and hyperglycemia.

Hydralazine is an arteriolar vasodilator that is not as potent as diazoxide or nitroprusside. However, it has an excellent safety profile. The half-life is short (3 to 7 hours); thus frequent dosing is required. Reflex tachycardia often occurs, which may require the introduction of a β-blocker.

Labetalol is an α1- and nonselective β-adrenergic blocker. Dosing is independent of renal function. It has been reported to be effective in the management of severe hypertension that results from pheochromocytoma and coarctation of the aorta, and it is a reasonable alternative in the treatment of hypertensive crises in patients with end-stage renal disease.

Nifedipine, a calcium channel blocker, reduces peripheral vascular resistance and does not affect cardiac output. It can be administered sublingually, but biting the capsule and swallowing its contents achieves measurable blood levels more rapidly than administration by the sublingual route. Use depends on the patient's state of consciousness. Nifedipine is contraindicated in the presence of intracerebral bleeding.

Nicardipine, another calcium channel blocker, is an excellent drug for use in emergencies because it can be administered as an easily prepared and titrated infusion.

Phentolamine is a pure α-adrenergic blocker used almost exclusively for the treatment of catecholamine crisis, as seen in patients with pheochromocytoma or in patients who ingested sympathomimetic agents such as cocaine. The effect is immediate. Phentolamine carries a high risk of hypotension after the primary lesion (eg, pheochromocytoma) is excised, and care should be exercised and surgeons alerted to this possibility.

Hypertensive Urgency

Hypertensive urgency is defined as severe hypertension without evidence of end-organ involvement. Patients with known hypertension who experience an urgent hypertensive crisis may not require hospitalization if the therapy in the ED is successful and if follow-up is adequate. In many instances, oral antihypertensive agents (Table 350-2) are sufficient, although parenteral therapy is sometimes indicated. Theories suggest that one third of the total planned BP reduction should be done during the first 6 hours, another third during the next 24 to 36 hours, and the final third during the next 24 to 96 hours or even longer.[8] A 4- to 6-hour period of observation should follow the administration of the antihypertensive agent in the ED to identify any untoward effects of the medication, such as orthostasis. Patients should be discharged with the same medications that were used in the ED to treat the hypertension.

Results of pediatric studies of amlodipine, felodipine, isradipine, intravenous nicardipine, and nitrendipine have been published.[9] Enalapril, an angiotensin-converting enzyme inhibitor, is commonly used as an antihypertensive agent in children. The maximum serum

Table 350-2 Drugs Used in Cases of Hypertensive Urgency

DRUG CHARACTERISTIC	DOSE	ADMINISTRATION	ONSET	DURATION
Nifedipine	0.25-0.5 mg/kg	Bite and swallow or sublingual	15-30 min	6 hr
Captopril	Age <6 mo: 0.05-0.5 mg/kg Age >6 mo: 0.3-2.0 mg/kg	By mouth	15-30 min	8-12 hr
Minoxidil	2.5-5.0 mg	By mouth	2 hr	12 hr

From Fleisher G, Ludwig S. *Textbook of Pediatric Emergency Medicine*. 5th ed. Baltimore, MD: Lippincott Williams & Wilkins; 2006. Reprinted by permission.

concentration occurs approximately 1 hour after administration, and that of its metabolite, enalaprilat, peaks 4 to 6 hours after the 1st dose and 3 to 4 hours after multiple doses.[10] Amlodipine is a safe and effective antihypertensive drug in children with chronic renal disease.[11] When administered in the ICU, intravenous nicardipine is safe and effective in lowering the BP in children with severe hypertension.[12]

The 4th report on the diagnosis, evaluation, and treatment of high BP in children and adolescents sponsored by the National Heart, Lung and Blood Institute (NHLBI) was published in August 2004.[3] It defines the 50th, 90th, 95th, and 99th percentiles of BP separately for boys and girls, depending on age and height. In the absence of established outcome measures for the treatment of hypertension in children, the goal of treatment is to reduce the BP to a level below the 95th percentile. A more aggressive reduction of BP to below the 90th percentile has been suggested for children with associated conditions such as diabetes mellitus.[13] When hypertension is discovered by accident and is not the reason for the patient's visit, medical follow-up for repeated BP measurements is indicated before therapy is initiated, especially if the increase is mild (no more than 5 mm Hg above the 99th percentile, as defined in the NHLBI report).

If the BP is moderately increased (>5 mm Hg above the 99th percentile, as defined in the NHLBI report) but the patient is asymptomatic, 2 options exist. Arrangements can be made for a future outpatient workup, and a low-dose thiazide diuretic or a β-blocker may be initiated. Alternatively, the patient may be admitted to begin evaluation and therapy while under hospital observation.

Malignant Hypertension

The urgency of prompt treatment of malignant hypertension is attested to by the fact that one third of severely hypertensive children develop neurologic abnormalities that may be sudden in onset and leave permanent neurologic deficits. These abnormalities include cortical blindness, infarction of the optic nerve, and hemiplegias. Patients with malignant hypertension are usually admitted to an ICU for continuous cardiac monitoring and frequent assessment of neurologic status and urine output. An intravenous line is placed to permit administration of fluids and medications. Patients typically have altered BP autoregulation, and overzealous reduction of BP to reference range levels may result in organ hypoperfusion.

The initial goal of therapy is to reduce the mean arterial pressure by approximately 25% over the first 24 hours. An intra-arterial line is helpful for continuous titration of BP. Sodium and volume depletion may be severe, and volume expansion with isotonic sodium chloride must be considered. No trials have been performed that compare the efficacy of various agents in the treatment of malignant hypertension in children. Drugs are chosen based on their rapidity of action, ease of use, special situations, and convention.

PROGNOSIS

The immediate prognosis of the child who has symptoms resulting from a hypertensive emergency depends on the rapidity of recognition of the problem and achievement of appropriate BP reduction thereafter. Although the initial neurologic and visual disturbances may improve or resolve with time, risks remain for residual abnormalities such as seizure disorders, cranial nerve palsies, hemiplegia, and blindness. Renal function often deteriorates acutely in patients who have chronic renal diseases after a hypertensive emergency or urgency. With sustained BP control, renal function may improve over a period of weeks or longer. The long-term prognosis also depends, to some extent, on the underlying cause, as well as the success in managing the malignant hypertension. Some causes, such as acute poststreptococcal glomerulonephritis, may resolve on their own. Others, such as isolated vascular abnormalities, are amenable to correction. In other settings, such as hypertension associated with chronic glomerulonephritis, the condition may be controlled by continued antihypertensive therapy, although failure to comply with medication regimens remains a problem. Regardless, the longevity of the patient and the subsequent development of end-organ damage (eg, hypertensive cardiomyopathy, stroke) are directly related to the adequacy of long-term BP control.

CONCLUSIONS

With the increase in the prevalence of obesity in children, the incidence of hypertension among children is also on the rise. Not infrequently, these children seek care at an ED with hypertension with or without symptoms related to hypertension. Hypertensive emergencies in symptomatic children should be treated without delay to avoid further damage to vital organs. When treating children with hypertensive emergencies, BP should be brought down by no more than 25% within the first 2 hours.[14] A pathogenesis for hypertension may be evident in individual cases, and management decisions must be made based on the cause of the hypertension. With the development of databases and the FDA modernization act in place (including endeavors such as the Best Pharmaceuticals for Children Act[15]), studies for the evaluation and management of hypertension in children will be forthcoming.[16]

WHEN TO REFER

Consultation with a pediatric nephrologist
- Diagnostic evaluation of cause of hypertension
- Short- and long-term management suggestions

Consultation with a pediatric cardiologist or pediatric neurologist
- If end-organ cardiac or central nervous system injury is suspected
- If a question exists of the relationship between end-organ dysfunction and hypertension

WHEN TO ADMIT

- All hypertensive emergencies
- Most cases of hypertensive urgencies

TOOLS FOR PRACTICE

Engaging Patient and Family

- *Children's Health: Cardiovascular Health* (Web page), American Academy of Pediatrics (www.aap.org/healthtopics/cardiology.cfm).

AAP POLICY STATEMENT

National High Blood Pressure Education Program Working Group on High Blood Pressure in Children and Adolescents. The fourth report on the diagnosis, evaluation, and treatment of high blood pressure in children and adolescents. *Pediatrics*. 2004;114(2/S2):555-576. AAP endorsed.

REFERENCES

1. Sorof J, Daniels S. Obesity hypertension in children: a problem of epidemic proportions. *Hypertension*. 2002; 40:441-447.
2. Gomez-Marin O, Prineas RJ, Rastam L. Cuff bladder width and blood pressure measurement in children and adolescents. *J Hypertens*. 1992;10:1235-1241.
3. National High Blood Pressure Education Working Group on High Blood Pressure in Children and Adolescents. The fourth report on the diagnosis, evaluation, and treatment of high blood pressure in children and adolescents. *Pediatrics*. 2004;114:555-576.
4. Wells TG. Trials of antihypertensive therapies in children. *Blood Press Monit*. 1999;4:189-192.
5. Chesney RW, Adamson P, Wells T, et al. The testing of antihypertensive medications in children. Report of the Antihypertensive Agent Guidelines Subcommittee of the Pediatric Pharmacology Research Units. *Pediatrics*. 2001; 107:558-561.
6. Adelman RD, Coppo R, Dillon MJ. The emergency management of severe hypertension. *Pediatr Nephrol*. 2000; 14:422-427.
7. Vaughan CJ, Delanty N. Hypertensive emergencies. *Lancet*. 2000;356:411-417.
8. Farine M, Arbus GS. Management of hypertensive emergencies in children. *Pediatr Emerg Care*. 1989;3:51-55.
9. Flynn JT, Pasko DA. Calcium channel blockers: pharmacology and place of therapy in pediatric hypertension. *Pediatr Nephrol*. 2002;15:302-316.
10. Rocchini AP. Pediatric hypertension. *Curr Opin Cardiol*. 2002;17:385-389.
11. Blaszak RT, Savage JA, Ellis EN. The use of short-acting nifedipine for the treatment of severe hypertension in childhood. *J Pediatr*. 2001;139:34-37.
12. Flynn JT, Mottes TA, Brophy PD, et al. Intravenous nicardipine for treatment of severe hypertension in children. *J Pediatr*. 2001;139:7-9.
13. Blowey DL. Safety of the newer antihypertensive agents in children. *Expert Opin Drug Saf*. 2002;1:39-43.
14. Porto I. Hypertensive emergencies in children. *J Pediatr Health Care*. 2000;14:312-319.
15. US Food and Drug Administration. Best Pharmaceuticals for Children Act. Available at: www.fda.gov/opacom/laws/pharmkids/contents.html. Accessed July 5, 2006.
16. Nehal US, Ingelfinger JR. Pediatric hypertension: recent literature. *Curr Opin Pediatr*. 2002;14:189-196.

Chapter 351

HYPOGLYCEMIA

Srinivasan Suresh, MD, MBA

INTRODUCTION

Any acutely ill child should be evaluated for hypoglycemia, especially when the history reveals diminished oral intake. Diagnosing hypoglycemia promptly is essential because low blood glucose levels that persist or recur may have catastrophic effects on the brain, particularly in infants. Accordingly, the primary care physician must recognize the clinical symptoms associated with hypoglycemia, document the low blood glucose level, and treat appropriately with glucose. Delineating the cause of the hypoglycemia is necessary to initiate effective continuing treatment.

DEFINITIONS

A child who has a serum or plasma glucose concentration less than 40 mg/dL or a whole blood glucose concentration less than 35 mg/dL should be investigated and treated for hypoglycemia; those who have plasma glucose concentrations between 40 and 50 mg/dL should be followed up carefully.[1] If hypoglycemia is suspected, then the blood glucose level may be approximated quickly at the bedside using a visual test strip or glucose meter and later confirmed by an appropriate chemical laboratory test. Although these thresholds have been commonly quoted and used, the level of plasma glucose that is safe is uncertain, and some authorities advocate a therapeutic goal of maintaining a plasma glucose level above 60 mg/dL in both neonates and older children to prevent permanent brain damage.[2]

CLINICAL MANIFESTATIONS

The clinical findings in hypoglycemia are those caused mainly by cerebral dysfunction and adrenergic discharge. Incoordination of eye movements, strabismus, excessive irritability, motor incoordination, and convulsions may occur after 1 month of age. In the older child, pallor, tachycardia, sweating, limpness, inattention, staring, listlessness, hunger, abdominal pain, ataxia, stupor, coma, and convulsions are frequent findings. Episodes of hypoglycemia may be present at any age without obvious clinical manifestations.

ETIOLOGY

The blood glucose level is the final balance between the sum of hepatic glucose production and dietary intake minus peripheral glucose use. An adequate fasting blood glucose concentration depends on sufficient amounts of endogenous nonglucose precursors (eg, alanine, lactate, glycerol), effective hepatic enzyme pathways for gluconeogenesis and glycogenolysis, and normal hormonal activities (insulin, growth hormone [GH], cortisol, glucagon, and epinephrine) for the mobilization of substrates and the regulation of these processes.

INCIDENCE

The overall incidence of symptomatic hypoglycemia in newborns varies from 1.3 to 3 per 1000 live births. Early feeding decreases the incidence of hypoglycemia. Prematurity, hypothermia, hypoxia, maternal diabetes, maternal glucose infusion in labor, and intrauterine growth retardation increase the incidence of hypoglycemia.

DIFFERENTIAL DIAGNOSIS

Metabolic acidosis, ketonemia, or hepatomegaly in association with hypoglycemia strongly suggests the presence of an inborn error of metabolism of carbohydrate, amino acid, or organic acid.[3] Hypotonia and hyperammonemia may also be present in infants who have defects in organic acid and amino acid metabolism. The presence of non–glucose-reducing substances in the urine may indicate galactosemia or hereditary fructose intolerance (HFI). Nonketotic hypoglycemia in patients who have hepatomegaly, with or without metabolic acidosis, suggests 3-hydroxy-3-methylglutaric aciduria,[4] glutaric aciduria type II,[5] systemic carnitine deficiency,[6] carnitine palmityl transferase deficiency,[7] or long- and medium-chain acyl-coenzyme A dehydrogenase (MCAD) deficiencies.[1] In contrast, hepatomegaly, ketonuria, and metabolic acidosis are usually absent in patients with hypoglycemia accompanied by hyperinsulinism.[8] The findings of ketonuria and hypoglycemia without hepatomegaly among small and underweight boys older than 1 year suggest ketotic hypoglycemia,[3,9] although ketosis may be present in some hypoglycemic patients who have hypopituitarism[10] and adrenocorticotropic hormone (ACTH) unresponsiveness.[11]

Hyperinsulinism

Hyperinsulinism may be caused by any of several abnormalities of the β-cell (Box 351-1) and is the most common cause of persistent or recurrent hypoglycemia in the first year of life.[12] In Beckwith-Wiedemann syndrome (omphalocele, macroglossia, and gigantism), hypoglycemia occurs in many of the affected infants and resolves at several months of age.[13] Some of these infants also have hemihypertrophy. An increased incidence of adrenal, liver, and kidney (Wilms) tumors occurs in these patients. More commonly, hyperinsulinism is transient and associated with infants of diabetic mothers.[2]

Most children who have hypoglycemia caused by persistent hyperinsulinism (previously called *nesidioblastosis, islet cell dysplasia,*[1] or *congenital hyperinsulinism*[14]) have symptoms beginning during the first year of life. The understanding of the genetic basis of this condition has advanced enormously in the last several years. Pancreatic β-cell insulin secretion is regulated through a multistep signaling pathway. Glucose, amino acids, and other fuels are metabolized in the β-cells, raising the ratio of adenosine triphosphatase to adenosine diphosphate. This action, in turn, activates a plasma protein, the sulfonylurea receptor (SUR), to close a potassium channel (K_{ATP}), depolarizing the membrane and leading to an influx of calcium and release of insulin. The rate-limiting step in glucose metabolism is the enzyme glucokinase. The most severe form of congenital hyperinsulinism has been found to be caused by a recessive mutation in the K_{ATP}. Other forms of congenital hyperinsulinism are caused by mutations in the SUR, potassium pore, glucokinase, and other steps of the signaling path. Congenital hyperinsulinism appears to occur associated with either focal or diffuse abnormalities of the β-cells.

Pancreatic islet cell adenomas are uncommon in children. Although hypoglycemia caused by varying histologic types of insulinoma may have its onset in the newborn period, symptoms begin after the age of 4 years in 85% of patients.[9]

Inborn Errors of Metabolism

Carbohydrate Enzyme Defects

Several enzymatic defects of carbohydrate metabolism result in deficiencies of hepatic glucose formation and release. Glucose-6-phosphatase deficiency is the most common deficiency, and the symptoms are more severe than those in other glycogen storage disease (GSD) types (see Box 351-1).[3] Patients who have GSD types Ia and Ib have growth retardation, cherubic facies, a protuberant abdomen, a large smooth liver, enlarged kidneys, normal intelligence, fasting hypoglycemia of only a few hours' duration, ketosis, lacticacidemia, hyperlipidemia, hyperuricemia, and bleeding diathesis. In type Ib the patients also have neutropenia and an increased frequency of infections. Among infants and young children, poor food intake during an illness may result in severe lactic acidosis and hypoglycemia. Death

BOX 351-1 Causes of Hypoglycemia in Childhood

HYPERINSULINISM
- Islet cell dysplasia (functional β-cell secretory disorder)
- Islet cell adenoma
- Adenomatosis
- Beckwith-Wiedemann syndrome

HEREDITARY DEFECTS IN CARBOHYDRATE METABOLISM
- Glycogen storage diseases
- Glucose-6-phosphatase deficiency types Ia and Ib
- Amylo-1,6-glucosidase deficiency type III
- Defects of liver phosphorylase enzyme system

ENZYME DEFICIENCIES OF GLUCONEOGENESIS
- Fructose-1,6-diphosphatase
- Phosphoenolpyruvate carboxykinase
- Pyruvate carboxylase

OTHER ENZYME DEFECTS
- Galactose-1-phosphate uridyltransferase (galactosemia)
- Fructose-1-phosphate aldolase (hereditary fructose intolerance)
- Glycogen synthetase

HEREDITARY DEFECTS IN AMINO ACID AND ORGANIC ACID METABOLISM
- Maple syrup urine disease
- Propionic acidemia
- Methylmalonic aciduria
- Tyrosinosis
- 3-Hydroxy-3-methylglutaric aciduria
- Glutaric aciduria type II

HEREDITARY DEFECTS IN FAT METABOLISM
- Systemic carnitine deficiency
- Carnitine palmitoyl transferase deficiency
- Long- and medium-chain acyl-coenzyme A dehydrogenase deficiencies

HORMONE DEFICIENCIES
- Congenital hypopituitarism or hypothalamic abnormality
- Growth hormone
- Cortisol
- Adrenocorticotropic hormone (ACTH)
- ACTH unresponsiveness
- Glucagon
- Thyroid hormone
- Catecholamine

KETOTIC HYPOGLYCEMIA
- Nonpancreatic tumors
- Mesenchymal tumors
- Epithelial tumors
- Hepatoma
- Adrenocortical carcinoma
- Wilms tumor
- Neuroblastoma

POISONING OR TOXINS
- Salicylate
- Alcohol
- Propranolol
- Oral hypoglycemic agents (eg, sulfonylureas)
- Insulin
- Unripe ackees (hypoglycin) (Jamaican vomiting sickness)
- Pentamidine

LIVER DISEASE
- Hepatitis, cirrhosis
- Reye syndrome

OTHER CAUSES
- Malnutrition
- Malabsorption
- Chronic diarrhea
- Cyanotic congenital heart disease
- Postsurgery

Data from Cornblath MD, Schwartz R. *Disorders of Carbohydrate Metabolism in Infancy.* 2nd ed. Philadelphia, PA: WB Saunders; 1976; Kogut MD. Hypoglycemia: pathogenesis, diagnosis, and treatment. In: Gluck L, ed. *Current Problems in Pediatrics.* Chicago, IL: Mosby; 1974; Kogut MD. Neonatal hypoglycemia: a new look. In: Moss AJ, ed. *Pediatrics Update: Review for Physicians.* New York, NY: Elsevier; 1980.

may result if hypoglycemia and lactic acidemia are not treated adequately and promptly with intravenous glucose and sodium bicarbonate.

Reye Syndrome

Because children who have an inborn error of metabolism may exhibit a Reye syndrome-like illness, the primary care physician must be alert to the possibility of an underlying metabolic defect, particularly in young children or in a child who has a recurrence of Reye syndrome-like symptoms.[1,15]

Galactosemia

Galactosemia in a lactose-fed infant is characterized by failure to thrive, jaundice, vomiting, susceptibility to infection, hepatomegaly, edema, ascites, a tendency to bleed, cataracts, proteinuria, aminoaciduria, and galactosuria.[3] Intellectual disability, progressive liver failure, and death may occur unless galactose-containing feedings are eliminated. Symptomatic hypoglycemia is not a common finding and is reversed quickly by intravenous glucose.

Hereditary Fructose Intolerance

Clinical manifestations of HFI develop only after fructose ingestion and include vomiting, profound hypoglycemia, and convulsions. Continued ingestion of fructose is associated with failure to thrive, prolonged vomiting, jaundice, hepatosplenomegaly, hemorrhage, abnormal liver function, fructosuria, defects in proximal renal tubular function (including proteinuria, glucosuria, and aminoaciduria), and, in some cases, hepatic failure and death.

Fructose-1,6-Diphosphatase Deficiency

Patients who have fructose-1,6-diphosphatase (FDPase) deficiency may have episodic hyperventilation, fasting hypoglycemia, lactic acidosis, ketosis, hyperuricemia, and hepatomegaly. Refusal to eat and vomiting, often associated with febrile illness, precipitate the attacks. The disorder is life threatening in neonates and in young children. In contrast to those who have HFI, these patients do not vomit after fructose intake and do not develop an aversion to sweets.

Amino Acid and Organic Acid Metabolic Defects

Hypoglycemia has been noted in a variety of inborn errors of amino acid and organic acid metabolism (see Box 351-1).[3] Although symptoms usually begin in the neonatal period, they may occur later. The infants tend to improve when protein feedings are discontinued and glucose is administered intravenously. Occasionally, peritoneal dialysis or exchange transfusion may be lifesaving. Amino acid analysis and gas chromatography of blood and urine are often helpful in detecting these inborn errors (Table 351-1). Diagnosis and treatment of a specific disorder depend on detection of its characteristic metabolites in blood and urine and on assays of specific enzyme activities in skin fibroblasts or white blood cells.

MCAD deficiency is the most common defect of fatty acid oxidation. This condition may exhibit as nonketotic hypoglycemia (similar to Reye syndrome), an acute life-threatening event, or even sudden death. In fact, an association has been made between infants with known MCAD deficiency and a history of a sibling dying of sudden infant death syndrome. Initial screening for defects of fatty acid oxidation is best performed with analysis of urine organic acids, plasma acylcarnitine profile, and measurement of serum carnitine.[16]

Hormonal Deficiencies

GH deficiency, cortisol deficiency, or combined hormonal deficiencies may cause hypoglycemia.

Hypopituitarism

Congenital hypopituitarism, caused by either a hypothalamic abnormality or aplasia of the anterior pituitary gland, is associated with severe hypoglycemia during the first few days of life.[8,9,17] Occasionally, however, hypoglycemia may appear first later in infancy or childhood. A few patients may have midline deformities, including hypotelorism, abnormality of the frontonasal process, and cleft lip or palate. Septo-optic dysplasia

Table 351-1 Hypoglycemia in Infancy and Childhood

	INBORN METABOLIC ERRORS OF CARBOHYDRATE AND AMINO ACIDS	HORMONE DEFICIENCY	HYPERINSULINISM
Family history	+	Variable	Variable
Hypoglycemia			
Fasting	GSD, fructose-1,6-diphosphatase deficiency	+	+
After lactose	Galactosemia	–	–
After sucrose	Hereditary fructose intolerance	–	–
After protein	Amino acids, organic acids	–	Variable
Hepatomegaly	+	Variable	–
Ketosis	+	Variable	–
Acidosis	+	–	–
Tests	Glucose, glucagon, galactose, fructose tolerance tests; amino acids, gas chromatography	Blood growth hormone, cortisol; stimulation tests	Random blood glucose and immunoreactive insulin; leucine tolerance test
Liver biopsy (enzymes)	Diagnostic for carbohydrate errors (not for galactosemia; use red blood cells)	Not indicated	Not indicated
White blood cells, fibroblasts (enzymes)	Amino acids, organic acids	—	—
Treatment	Specific	Specific	Diazoxide; somatostatin analog; partial excision of the pancreas

+, Present; –, absent.
GSD, Glycogen storage diseases, types I, III, and defects of liver phosphorylase enzyme system.
Data from Cornblath MD, Schwartz R. *Disorders of Carbohydrate Metabolism in Infancy.* 2nd ed. Philadelphia, PA: WB Saunders; 1976; Kogut MD. Hypoglycemia: pathogenesis, diagnosis and treatment. In: Gluck L, ed. *Current Problems in Pediatrics.* Chicago, IL: Mosby; 1974; Kogut MD. Neonatal hypoglycemia: a new look. In: Moss AJ, ed. *Pediatrics Update: Review for Physicians.* New York, NY: Elsevier; 1980.

(optic nerve hypoplasia and absence of the septum pellucidum) is present in some patients and may be accompanied by nystagmus. Some male patients who have congenital hypopituitarism may have a small penis (microphallus) or genitalia, and children with hypopituitarism are often overweight. Measurement of height and weight is essential for the evaluation of a child in whom GH deficiency is suspected because these children have significant growth retardation, which may begin within the first 1 to 2 years of life.

Cortisol Deficiency

Deficient cortisol production may be caused by Addison disease, congenital adrenal hyperplasia, ACTH deficiency, or ACTH unresponsiveness.[8,9,11,17] Patients who have ACTH unresponsiveness and Addison disease may have abnormal pigmentation.

Ketotic Hypoglycemia

Although the pathogenesis of hypoglycemia in ketotic hypoglycemia has not been defined, the evidence suggests that it represents an exaggeration of the starvation state.[9] During hypoglycemia, blood insulin levels are appropriately low; blood alanine levels also may be low; GH, glucagon, cortisol, β-hydroxybutyrate, and free fatty acid levels in the blood are elevated; urinary ketones are present; and blood glucose levels fail to rise after the administration of glucagon.

Ketotic hypoglycemia is the most common cause of hypoglycemia after 1 year of age.[3,9] Symptoms mimicking those noted in ketotic hypoglycemia have occurred in children who have GH deficiency, ACTH unresponsiveness, FDPase deficiency, glycogen synthetase deficiency, and Reye syndrome. Before a child is classified as having ketotic hypoglycemia, therefore, a thorough laboratory investigation must be conducted to consider these and other diseases.

The combination of ketonuria, hypoglycemia, and central nervous system symptoms, which may vary from unresponsiveness, pallor, and vomiting to coma and convulsions and which often occur in the early morning hours in association with an upper respiratory tract infection or prolonged fast, is typical of ketotic hypoglycemia for which no cause is known.[3] The onset is between 9 months and 5.5 years of age, with a peak incidence at 2 years. Hypoglycemic episodes occur at intervals of a few months to a year or more; they then decrease in frequency and tend to disappear, usually by 7 to 8 years of age.

EVALUATION

Hypoglycemia reflects the failure of one or more factors that regulate the concentration of glucose in the blood (see Box 351-1). Clinical clues enable the physician to plan a logical approach to the diagnostic evaluation of a patient who has hypoglycemia. The age at onset of hypoglycemia is important. The inborn errors of carbohydrate, amino acid, organic acid metabolism, and hormonal deficiencies become apparent during the first 2 years of life.[9] Hyperinsulinism has 2 peak times of onset: (1) during the first year of life and (2) after the age of 3 years.[3,9] Ketotic hypoglycemia is the most likely cause of hypoglycemia with onset after 1 year of age.[9] In toddlers, hypoglycemia may result from ingestion of alcohol, aspirin, and other drugs (see Box 351-1). Hypoglycemia is rare after the age of 5 years.[18]

History

A history of other affected family members or the occurrence of unexplained infant deaths among close relatives suggests the possibility of one of the inherited metabolic disorders. Some disorders associated with hormonal deficiencies[19] and hyperinsulinism[14] also may be familial. The physician should inquire about the frequency of hypoglycemic episodes, the possibility of drug ingestion, and the malicious administration of drugs.[17,18] The temporal relationship of symptoms to food intake is important in assessing for hypoglycemia. In hereditary defects of amino acid and organic acid metabolism, hypoglycemic symptoms may occur shortly after the ingestion of protein. Symptoms that occur after the ingestion of lactose suggest galactosemia; those that occur after sucrose ingestion suggest HFI.[3] In contrast, fasting hypoglycemia is characteristic of ketotic hypoglycemia, hormonal deficiencies, hyperinsulinism, GSD, and FDPase deficiency[20] (see Table 351-1).

Laboratory Evaluation

At the time hypoglycemia is suspected in a child, a diagnostic blood sample for glucose, insulin, GH, cortisol, ketone bodies, lactic acid, and amino acids must be obtained, generally before the low blood glucose level has been corrected.[17,18] These measurements provide important information concerning cause. Unnecessary blood sampling can be minimized by using a bedside glucose meter to decide if the patient is truly hypoglycemic during a symptomatic episode. If available blood volume is a limiting factor, then judgment must be used in ranking the importance of these tests, with measurement of the blood glucose and insulin levels receiving priority. Urinary ketones, as well as specific tests for urinary glucose and non–glucose-reducing substances, should also be determined. If ketones are present, then the urine should be tested further for presence of amino acids and organic acids. For diagnostic purposes, the administration of glucagon can be useful; a robust glycemic response to glucagon strongly suggests hyperinsulinism.[18]

Diagnostic Evaluation for Specific Disorders

Hyperinsulinism

Hyperinsulinism in infants and older children is usually characterized by fasting hypoglycemia, even if of only a few hours' duration, and low fasting plasma levels of β-hydroxybutyrate and free fatty acids.[21] Frequent random simultaneous measurements of blood glucose and insulin levels, particularly before feeding and as hypoglycemia occurs, help identify patients who have hyperinsulinism (see Table 351-1). The diagnosis depends on detecting inappropriate insulin secretion by demonstrating insulin levels disproportionately high relative to blood glucose values, particularly during hypoglycemia. A high rate of glucose infusion (greater than 12 mg/kg/min) is often necessary to maintain euglycemia. Leucine or tolbutamide challenges are not helpful in delineating the specific cause of hyperinsulinism.[3,12]

In any child who has intermittent attacks of nonketotic hypoglycemia, the physician should always investigate the possibility of malicious or self-administration of insulin or oral sulfonylurea drugs.[19,22,23] Measurement of C-peptide, insulin, and insulin antibodies in blood may identify the patient who has an exogenous source of insulin. In contrast to patients who have endogenous hyperinsulinism, C-peptide levels are suppressed; insulin antibodies may be present in patients to whom insulin has been administered.[19,23] In children who have received oral hypoglycemic agents, plasma insulin and C-peptide levels may be misleading; however, the drug may be detected in the child's blood or urine.

Inborn Errors of Metabolism

A suggested outline for the investigation of hypoglycemia caused by inborn errors of carbohydrate metabolism is provided in Table 351-1 and Table 351-2. These studies should be performed in a pediatric metabolic center but only when the child's condition is stable and the blood glucose level is normal. Judgment must be exercised in choosing the proper diagnostic test to delineate the underlying abnormality. The presence of specific hepatic enzyme deficiencies may be determined by the use of other tolerance tests (see Table 351-2). The tolerance tests are performed after a variable period of fasting and only with a primary care physician in attendance, who must be prepared to interrupt the test by administering intravenous glucose should symptoms and signs of hypoglycemia occur or should a low blood glucose level be detected. Definitive diagnosis of any of the inherited disorders of carbohydrate metabolism (see Box 351-1) except galactosemia depends on assay of specific hepatic enzyme activities (see Table 351-2). Galactosemia, on the other hand, may be detected by the absence of galactose-1-phosphate uridyltransferase activity in red blood cells; thus liver biopsy is unnecessary for its definitive diagnosis.

Hormone Deficiencies

Laboratory studies should include determination of GH and cortisol in the blood, particularly when the child has hypoglycemia (see Table 351-1). Hypoglycemia is an excellent stimulus for GH and cortisol secretions; therefore low values of either hormone in the presence of hypoglycemia raise suspicion of deficiencies of these hormones and the need for further studies. In patients who have suspected hypopituitarism or GH deficiency, magnetic resonance imaging and computed tomography of the brain may be of diagnostic help. Correction of hypoglycemia by intravenous administration of glucose makes up the treatment of acute episodes. Specific treatment depends on identifying the underlying hormonal deficiency. However, if GH or cortisol deficiency is suspected on clinical grounds, then empiric replacement therapy should be started while awaiting test results. Patients should be encouraged to avoid prolonged fasting.

MANAGEMENT

Healthy, full-term infants are functionally and metabolically programmed to make the transition from their intrauterine-dependent environment to their extrauterine existence without the need for metabolic

Table 351-2 Differential Diagnosis of Hepatic Enzyme Defects

BLOOD VALUES	GSD-I	GSD-III	GSD, PHOSPHORYLASE ENZYME SYSTEM	FDPase	HFI
FASTING					
Glucose	↓	↓ or N	↓ or N	↓	N
Lactic acid	↑	N	N	↑	N
AFTER GLUCOSE*					
Glucose	↑	↑	↑	↑	↑
Lactic acid	↓	↑	↑	↓	↔
AFTER GLUCAGON*					
Glucose	↔	↑†	↑ or ↔	↑ or ↔‡	↑§
Lactic acid	↑	↔	↔	↓ or ↑	↔
AFTER GALACTOSE*					
Glucose	↔	↑	↑	↑	↑
Lactic acid	↑	↑	↑	↔	↔
AFTER FRUCTOSE*					
Glucose	↔	↑	↑	↓	↓
Lactic acid	↑	↑	↑	↑	↑

*Tolerance tests done after variable fasting period.
†Two hours after feeding.
‡Variable; dependent on duration of fast.
§No increase in glucose at time of fructose-induced hypoglycemia.
FDPase, Fructose-1,6-diphosphatase; *GSD*, glycogen storage diseases; *HFI*, hereditary fructose intolerance.
↑, increased; ↓, decreased; ↔, no change; *N*, normal.

monitoring. Full-term infants are equipped with homeostatic mechanisms that preserve adequate energy substrate to the brain and other vital organs. Thus routine newborn screening for blood glucose concentration is not necessary.[24] Glucose water supplement should not be given to breastfeeding newborn infants unless a medical indication exists.[25] However, many healthy infants and young children, in contrast to adults, cannot maintain normoglycemia during a 24-hour fast.[26] The glycogen stores of healthy infants are sufficient only to meet glucose requirements for 8 to 12 hours in the absence of caloric intake[27]; therefore after 24 to 36 hours of fasting the young child depends totally on gluconeogenesis for glucose production.[28] Because of relatively lower protein and fat stores, fasting infants and young children may not be able to supply sufficient substrates for adequate glucose production. Hence the primary care physician caring for a child requiring surgery or other procedures accompanied by fasting must prevent hypoglycemia by ensuring that extended fasting is avoided, by administering parenteral glucose before and after surgery, and by monitoring the patient's blood glucose level.

Immediate Management

Once appropriate laboratory tests are sent, hypoglycemia should be corrected by administering 2 to 4 mL/kg of 10% to 25% glucose intravenously. Intravenous fluids containing appropriate electrolytes and glucose should be given at a rate sufficient to maintain plasma or serum glucose levels above 50 to 60 mg/dL. A common mistake is to believe that the hypoglycemia resolved after the initial bolus and failing to follow up with sufficiently frequent blood glucose monitoring to determine the adequacy of the continuous glucose infusion. The blood glucose level should be monitored initially every 30 to 60 minutes at the bedside until stable then every 2 to 4 hours, and the rate of glucose administered should be adjusted accordingly. Overcorrection with subsequent hyperglycemia may complicate fluid management by causing an osmotic diuresis.

Significant hypoglycemia should be evaluated on an inpatient basis to allow for close monitoring. During transport to the hospital, personnel experienced in intravenous techniques and rapid bedside blood glucose determinations must ensure that adequate amounts of glucose are infused continuously. The previously obtained diagnostic blood samples should be sent with the patient to the hospital, preferably on ice. The patient who has hypoglycemia should be under the combined care of a pediatric specialist and the child's primary care physician.

Hyperinsulinism

Patients with hyperinsulinism require higher rate of glucose infusion (more than 12 to 14 mg/kg/min) to maintain normal blood glucose level as compared with other conditions causing hypoglycemia. The further management depends on the age of the onset of the condition.

Diazoxide

An infant's response to diazoxide is of great diagnostic and therapeutic value in hyperinsulinism. Diazoxide raises blood glucose levels primarily by suppressing pancreatic insulin secretion.[29] In patients in whom diazoxide results in restoration of normal glucose levels, use of the drug is continued and the patients are assessed periodically until approximately 5 to 7 years of age. Some patients remain euglycemic without medication by this age. The knowledge that many of these patients harbor genetic defects supports the concept that although clinical improvement may occur with increasing age, abnormalities of glucose regulation remain. Because hyperglycemia, ketosis, and hyperosmolar nonketotic coma can occur with diazoxide therapy, the parents should be instructed to monitor urinary glucose and ketones.[3]

Diazoxide acts by inhibiting the β-cell SUR. Although it is effective in many children, hyperinsulinism caused by SUR mutations may not respond to this drug. If hypoglycemia associated with hyperinsulinism persists or recurs despite diazoxide therapy, then octreotide, a long-acting analog of somatostatin, may be used. Tachyphylaxis has prevented its long-term use in all but a small number of severely affected children.[13]

Surgery

Surgery is needed if medical therapy fails. Although the traditional approach has favored controlling hyperinsulinism with removal of 95% of the pancreas, resulting in a significant risk of subsequent diabetes, new insights may change this approach. Preoperative catheterization and intraoperative histologic studies may allow partial pancreatectomy in approximately 40% of infants with focal abnormalities, thus reducing the postoperative incidence of diabetes.[20]

Carbohydrate Enzyme Defects

In treating carbohydrate enzyme defects, a significant advance has been the introduction of continuous nocturnal glucose-containing gastric feedings.[30] To maintain normal blood glucose levels during the day, frequent feedings, at least every 3 to 4 hours, are essential. Foods rich in fructose and galactose should be avoided. The daily oral administration of an uncooked cornstarch suspension has been beneficial in older children but not as effective in infants in maintaining normoglycemia and attaining adequate metabolic control.[31]

Galactosemia

When the diagnosis of galactosemia is suspected, the patient should be given a galactose-free diet immediately. This diet should be maintained carefully while the primary care physician awaits the results of erythrocyte enzyme studies and should be continued if the diagnosis is confirmed. Long-term management consists of avoidance of lactose- and galactose-containing foods.

Hereditary Fructose Intolerance

The acute episodes of hypoglycemia are reversed promptly by the intravenous administration of glucose. Long-term treatment consists of strict elimination of dietary fructose and of fructose in cough syrups and other drugs.

Fructose-1,6-Diphosphatase Deficiency

Treatment of acute attacks of FDPase deficiency consists of correcting the hypoglycemia and acidosis by intravenous infusion of glucose and sodium bicarbonate. Long-term management should emphasize the avoidance of fasting and the provision of a fructose-free, high-carbohydrate diet.

Ketotic Hypoglycemia

In patients with ketotic hypoglycemia, the primary care physician should document hypoglycemic blood glucose levels at the time of symptoms by obtaining a diagnostic blood sample. After the child has had several days to recover from the acute episode and is eating well, the administration of a provocative low-calorie, high-fat ketogenic diet has been useful in establishing the diagnosis if a blood sample is unobtainable.[3,9] The child must be observed carefully for hypoglycemia during the test period.

The acute hypoglycemic attacks are reversed by the intravenous administration of glucose; glucagon usually has no effect. Because the attacks occur infrequently, long-term drug therapy is not indicated. A liberal carbohydrate diet, including a bedtime snack, should be followed. Prolonged overnight fasting, particularly during weekends or holidays and periods of illness, should be avoided. The parents should be encouraged to test their child's urine for ketones during illness or periods of fasting. Carbohydrate-containing foods, given promptly when acetonuria develops, are usually successful in aborting attacks.

WHEN TO ADMIT

- Any child with documented hypoglycemia not caused by insulin therapy should be hospitalized for careful monitoring and diagnostic testing. These patients need to be referred to an endocrinologist.
- If hypoglycemia is diagnosed in an infant younger than 3 months, then surgical intervention may be necessary. Surgical exploration is usually performed in severely affected neonates who are unresponsive to glucose and somatostatin therapy.

REFERENCES

1. Haymond MW. Hypoglycemia in infants and children. *Endocrinol Metab Clin North Am.* 1989;18(1):211-252.
2. Stanley CA, Baker L. The causes of neonatal hypoglycemia. *N Engl J Med.* 1999;340(15):1200-1201.
3. Aynsley-Green A. Hypoglycemia in infants and children. *Clin Endocrinol Metab.* 1982;11(1):159-194.
4. Cornblath M. Hypoglycemia in infancy and childhood. *Pediatr Ann.* 1981;10:356.
5. Eidelman AI. Hypoglycemia and the breastfed neonate. *Pediatr Clin North Am.* 2001;48(2):377-387.
6. American Academy of Pediatrics, Section on Breastfeeding. Policy statement: breastfeeding and the use of human milk. *Pediatrics.* 2005;115(2):496-506.
7. Chaussain JL. Glycemic response to 24 hour fast in normal children and children with ketotic hypoglycemia. *J Pediatr.* 1973;82(3):438-443.
8. Shelly HJ, Neligan GA. Neonatal hypoglycemia. *Br Med Bull.* 1966;22(1):34-39.
9. Pagliara AS, Karl IE, Haymond M, et al. Hypoglycemia in infancy and childhood, part 1. *J Pediatr.* 1973;82(3):365-379.
10. Cornblath M, Schwartz R. *Disorders of Carbohydrate Metabolism in Infancy.* 2nd ed. Philadelphia, PA: WB Saunders; 1976.
11. Kogut MD. Hypoglycemia: pathogenesis, diagnosis and treatment. In: Gluck L, ed. *Current Problems in Pediatrics.* Vol 4. Chicago, IL: Mosby; 1974.
12. Mayefsky JH, Sarnaik AP, Postellon DC. Factitious hypoglycemia. *Pediatrics.* 1982;69(6):804-805.
13. Thornton PS, Summer AE, Ruchelli ED, et al. Familial and sporadic hyperinsulinism: histopathologic findings and segregation analysis support a single autosomal recessive disorder. *J Pediatr.* 1991;119(5):721-724.
14. de Lonlay-Debeney P, Poqqi-Travert F, Fournet JC, et al. Clinical features of 52 neonate with hyperinsulinism. *N Engl J Med.* 1999;340(15):1169-1175.
15. Schutgens RB, Heymans H, Ketel A, et al. Lethal hypoglycemia in a child with a deficiency of 3-hydroxy-3-methylglutaryl coenzyme A lyase. *J Pediatr.* 1979;94(1):89-91.
16. Dusheiko G, Kew MC, Joffe BI, et al. Recurrent hypoglycemia associated with glutaric aciduria type II in an adult. *N Engl J Med.* 1979;301(26):1405-1409.
17. Ware AJ, Burton WC, McGarry JD, et al. Systemic carnitine deficiency: report of a fatal case with multisystemic manifestations. *J Pediatr.* 1978;93(6):959-964.
18. Bougneres PF, Saudubray JM, Marsac C, et al. Fasting hypoglycemia resulting from hepatic carnitine palmitoyl transferase deficiency. *J Pediatr.* 1981;998(5):742-746.
19. Kogut MD. Neonatal hypoglycemia: a new look. In: Moss AJ, ed. *Pediatrics Update: Review for Physicians.* New York, NY: Elsevier; 1980.
20. Roe TF, Kogut MD. Hypopituitarism and ketotic hypoglycemia. *Am J Dis Child.* 1971;121(4):296-299.
21. Kershnar AK, Roe TF, Kogut MD. Adrenocorticotropic hormone unresponsiveness: report of a girl with excessive growth and review of 16 reported cases. *J Pediatr.* 1972;80(4):610-619.
22. Greene CL, Blitzer MG, Shapira E. Inborn errors of metabolism and Reye syndrome: differential diagnoses. *J Pediatr.* 1988;113(1 pt 1):156-159.
23. Stanley CA, Baker L. Hyperinsulinism in infants and children: diagnosis and therapy. *Adv Pediatr.* 1976;23:315-355.
24. Stanley CA. Hyperinsulinism is infants and children. *Pediatr Clin North Am.* 1997;44(2):363-374.
25. Stanley CA, Baker L. Hyperinsulinism in infancy: diagnosis by demonstration of abnormal response to fasting hypoglycemia. *Pediatrics.* 1976;57(5):702-711.
26. Dershewitz R, Vestal B, Maclaren NK, et al. Transient hepatomegaly and hypoglycemia: a consequence of malicious insulin administration. *Am J Dis Child.* 1976;130(9):998-999.
27. Scarlett JA, Mako ME, Rubenstein AH, et al. Factitious hypoglycemia: diagnosis by measurement of serum C-peptide immunoreactivity and insulin-binding antibodies. *N Engl J Med.* 1977;297(19):1029-1032.
28. Roe TF, Kogut MD. Idiopathic leucine-sensitive hypoglycemia syndrome: insulin and glucagon responses and effects of diazoxide. *Pediatr Res.* 1982;16(1):1-4.
29. Greene HL, Slonim AE, Burr IM, et al. Type I glycogen storage disease: five years of management with nocturnal intragastric feeding. *J Pediatr.* 1980;96(3 pt 2):590-595.
30. Chen YT, Cornblath M, Sidbury JB. Cornstarch therapy in type I glycogen-storage disease. *N Engl J Med.* 1984;310(3):171-175.
31. Burton BK. Inborn errors of metabolism in infancy: a guide to diagnosis. *Pediatrics.* 1998;102(6):E69.

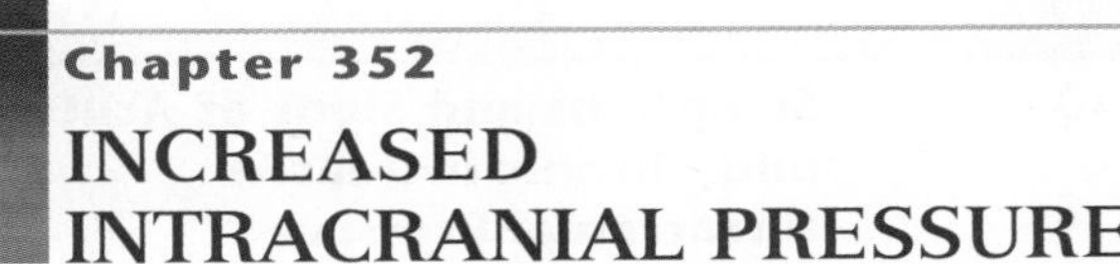

Chapter 352

INCREASED INTRACRANIAL PRESSURE

M. Mohsin Shah, MD; Matthew D. Smyth, MD

Elevated intracranial pressure (ICP) is a potentially life-threatening neurologic or neurosurgical emergency. Rapidly identifying and managing the cause can prevent serious morbidity and possible mortality. Elevated ICP has many causes, and symptoms can be acute, subacute, or chronic.

PATHOPHYSIOLOGICAL CONSIDERATIONS

The skull in older children and adults is closed and rigid and is filled with 3 compartments: (1) the brain (80% to 90% of the volume), (2) circulating cerebrospinal fluid (CSF; 5% to 10% of the volume), and (3) circulating blood (remainder of the volume).[1,2] The Monro-Kellie doctrine dictates the pathophysiological relationship of these compartments when altered. Based on this dictum that the relative volume is fixed, small increases in any one of these compartments will result in a compensatory decrease in the other 2. ICP rises if the increase exceeds normal compensatory mechanisms. Also affecting this variable is the brain's compliance (stiffness), which is altered in various disease states. Changes in brain compliance dampen compensatory mechanisms because the brain accounts for most of the intracranial volume.[2]

Normal ICP in older children and adults is usually 10 to 15 mm Hg in the recumbent position and is less in young children.[1] ICP is pulsatile and varies around a baseline; variation results from cardiac and respiratory activity.[2,3] Transient increases of up to 50 mm Hg or higher normally occur with actions that increase intrathoracic pressure or that impede venous return, such as coughing, sneezing, and straining. However, ICP returns rapidly to baseline when these maneuvers are discontinued.

Under normal conditions, blood flow to the brain is autoregulated, maintaining a constant perfusion level over a range of blood pressures.[2,3] A disruption in autoregulation makes blood flow pressure passive, which, in turn, can lead to significant changes in cerebral perfusion with any change in blood pressure. The cerebral perfusion pressure (CPP) is the mean arterial pressure minus the ICP.[2] CPP falls when ICP increases, leading to further cerebral compromise, ischemia, and swelling and further increases in ICP. This cycle may persist and ultimately cause death if not treated.

ETIOLOGY

Many factors can cause increased ICP in children, which can be classified as shown in Box 352-1. Depending on the cause, intracranial hypertension can be chronic (as with pseudotumor cerebri) or acute (as with head trauma resulting in cerebral edema or intracerebral hemorrhage). Common causes of increased ICP in children include head trauma, infection, hydrocephalus, and mass lesions.

BOX 352-1 Causes of Increased Intracranial Pressure in Children

HEAD TRAUMA
Cerebral edema
Intracerebral hemorrhage
Extracerebral hemorrhage (subdural, epidural)

VASCULAR CAUSES
Arterial or venous infarctions
Intracerebral hemorrhage
Dural sinus thrombosis
Subarachnoid hemorrhage
Vascular anomalies (vein of Galen malformation, arteriovenous malformations)

NEOPLASTIC CAUSES
Primary brain tumors
Metastatic (intracerebral, meningeal infiltration)
Hydrocephalus (congenital or acquired, communicating or noncommunicating)
Pseudotumor cerebri (benign intracranial hypertension)
Central nervous system infections
Meningitis (bacterial, fungal, mycobacterial)
Encephalitis (focal or diffuse)
Abscess

METABOLIC CAUSES
Inborn errors of metabolism (hyperammonemia)
Hepatic encephalopathy
Diabetic ketoacidosis
Renal failure
Reye syndrome
Hypoxic-ischemic encephalopathy
Fluid-electrolyte abnormalities (hyponatremia, hypernatremia)

STRUCTURAL CAUSES
Craniosynostosis
Status epilepticus

Modified from Pickard JD, Czosnyka M. Management of raised intracranial pressure. *J Neurol Neurosurg Psychiatry.* 1993;56(8):845-858. Reprinted by permission of BMJ Publishing Group Ltd.

In idiopathic intracranial hypertension (pseudotumor cerebri), the mechanism is less clear but based on experimental data is thought to be derived from 2 primary mechanisms[4]: (1) vasogenic extracellular brain edema and (2) delayed reabsorption through the arachnoid villa. Idiopathic intracranial hypertension may be compounded by secondary exacerbation of intracranial venous sinus compression that results in further reduction of flow across the arachnoid villi. This condition predominantly affects young obese women of childbearing age. In the young, risk factors include:

1. Medications (vitamin A in infants, isotretinoin [Accutane], corticosteroids, all-trans-retinoic acid for treatment of promyelocytic leukemia, levothyroxine, tetracycline, trimethoprim-sulfamethoxazole,

cimetidine, nalidixic acid, nitrofurantoin, recombinant growth hormone)
2. Endocrinopathies (recent weight gain, menstrual irregularity, adrenal insufficiency, Cushing disease, hypoparathyroidism, hypothyroidism, and excessive thyroxine replacement)
3. Chronic renal failure
4. Systemic lupus erythematosus

SIGNS AND SYMPTOMS

Signs and symptoms of both acute and chronic increased ICP are presented in Box 352-2. Many of these signs and symptoms are the same, demonstrating their somewhat nonspecific nature. The temporal pace of development differs between the 2 forms. Acute signs of rapidly increasing ICP result from displaced neuronal tissue through the several dural openings, with subsequent compression and ischemic changes to the cerebral structures. For example, with uncal herniation in association with supratentorial masses the uncus is displaced through the tentorial opening, leading to compression of the ipsilateral third nerve and displacement of the peduncles and brainstem laterally[5] (Figure 352-1). Clinically the patient is comatose and has an ipsilateral pupillary dilation (third nerve palsy) and ipsilateral hemiparesis, which suggests a falsely localizing lesion in the contralateral hemisphere. The pupil reliably localizes the side of the lesion. Downward herniation of the cerebellar tonsils through the foramen magnum leads to compression and vascular compromise of the lower brainstem structures (medulla) (see Figure 352-1). Patients are comatose and exhibit decorticate or decerebrate rigidity and autonomic (respiratory and circulatory) changes. The symptoms of a widened pulse pressure, bradycardia, and deep, slow respiration are classically referred to as the *Cushing triad*. Clinically, this triad is rarely seen.[3]

BOX 352-2 Symptoms and Signs of Acute and Chronic Increased Intracranial Pressure in Children

INFANTS

Acute

Irritability
Poor feeding or emesis
Split sutures (especially lambdoidal)
Bulging fontanelle
Altered mental status
Seizures
Parinaud sign (upgaze paresis)

Chronic

Irritability
Poor feeding or emesis
Increased head circumference
Bulging fontanelle
Split sutures (especially lambdoidal)
Apparent developmental arrest or regression
Parinaud sign (upgaze paresis)

CHILDREN

Acute

Severe, acute headache
Seizures
Emesis
Rapidly deteriorating mental status
Decerebrate or decorticate posture
Focal neurologic deficits
Papilledema
Pupillary abnormalities
Autonomic dysfunction (Cushing triad)

Chronic

Chronic, progressive headache
Seizures
Early morning emesis
Change in school performance
Altered mental status
Cranial neuropathy (eg, sixth cranial nerve palsy)
Focal neurologic deficits
Papilledema
Visual changes

DIAGNOSIS

Key to managing increased ICP is rapidly recognizing intracranial hypertension in a patient. As with any individual with neurologic complaints, the history and physical *and* neurologic examinations are the most important aspects of the initial diagnostic evaluation. These examinations provide the physician with information on the pace of the illness, which allows the clinician to discern the need for urgent versus emergent management. If a rapidly evolving process (eg, impending herniation) is evident, then stabilizing the patient is essential before proceeding to definitive diagnosis and therapy.

Performing a lumbar puncture (LP) provides an opportunity to evaluate the ICP by inserting a spinal needle into the thecal sac, attaching a manometer, and measuring the CSF column height while the patient is in the lateral decubitus position with legs extended. Between 12 and 18 cm is normal. However, if a mass lesion is suspected, then withdrawing lumbar CSF may create a pressure gradient intracranially and precipitate a herniation syndrome; therefore neuroimaging is generally recommended before an LP. The one exception is in children suspected of having meningitis, in which case, neuroimaging before an LP may unnecessarily delay antibiotic treatment.[6] If meningitis is a serious consideration and a computed tomography (CT) scan is still desired, then antibiotic therapy should not be delayed pending completion of the CT scan and, in turn, the LP. A spinal fluid analysis should always include glucose and protein measurement and a total and differential cell count. Depending on the clinical situation, other studies can be obtained, including microbial cultures (bacterial, fungal, viral, mycobacterial), special stains, and cytology.

CT or magnetic resonance imaging (MRI) can provide essential information in diagnosing and managing

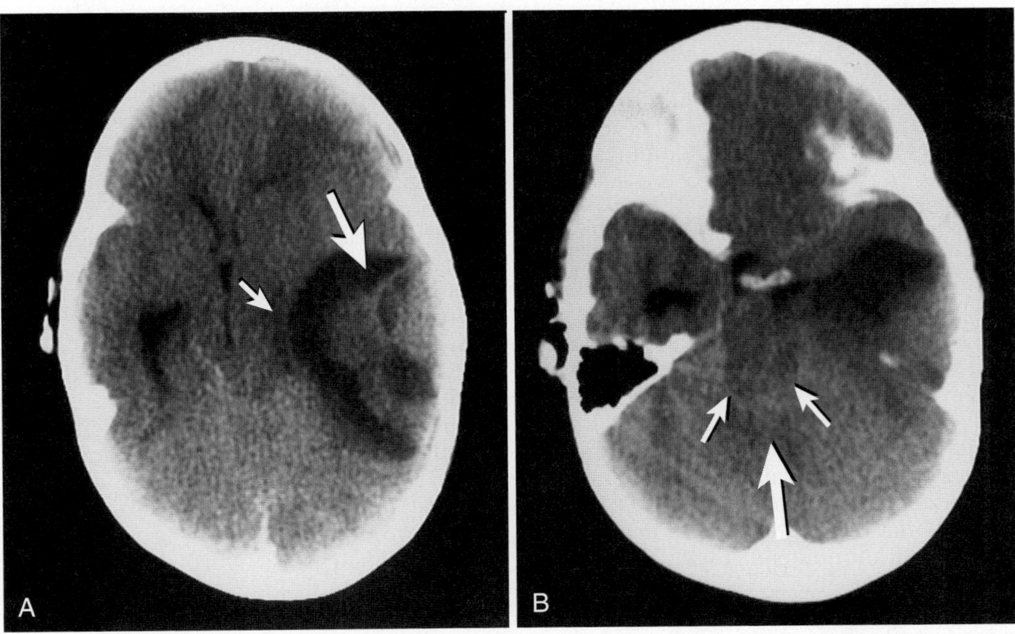

Figure 352-1 Two sections from a computed tomography scan of a 5-year-old girl who is comatose and has increased intracranial pressure. **A,** Large, cystic left temporal lobe mass *(large arrow)* causing left uncal herniation *(small arrow)* with loss of perimesencephalic cistern and midline shift. **B,** A lower cut demonstrating loss of the fourth ventricle (large arrow) and a quadrigeminal cistern *(small arrows),* suggesting downward (tonsillar) herniation.

patients with increased ICP. Although MRI provides better anatomic differentiation than CT, it is frequently unavailable in the emergency setting; therefore CT is performed more often than MRI. If a mass lesion is suspected, then neuroimaging (regardless of modality) should include contrast enhancement. Both modalities are effective in evaluating the cause of intracranial hypertension and are performed primarily to determine the presence of a mass lesion. The one exception is in the patient suspected of having a subarachnoid hemorrhage, when CT followed by LP remains the mainstay of initial diagnosis. Finally, ultrasonography is a reasonable alternative to CT or MRI in infants suspected of having aqueductal stenosis (Figure 352-2). Other neuroimaging studies, such as angiography, rarely play a role in the initial diagnostic management of intracranial hypertension.

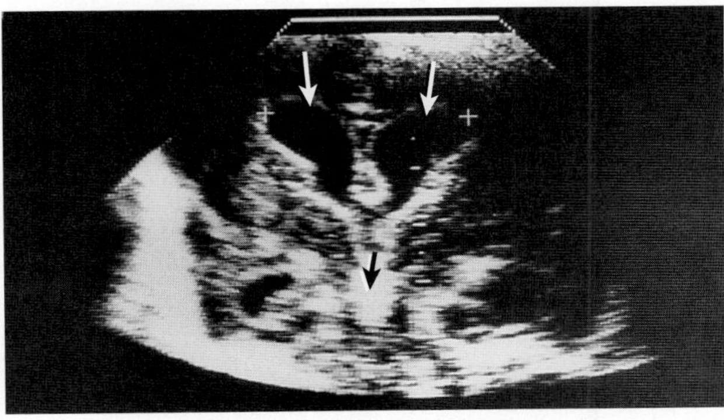

Figure 352-2 A coronal head ultrasound of a baby born at 30 weeks' gestation with a history of an intraventricular hemorrhage with increasing head circumference. Prominent dilated lateral ventricles *(white arrows)* and a clot-filled third ventricle *(black arrow)* are demonstrated.

MANAGEMENT

Rapidly recognizing and stabilizing the patient suspected of having acutely increased ICP is essential in preventing greater morbidity and mortality. The goal of early management is to lower ICP without compromising cerebral perfusion and to identify the cause so that definitive therapy can be provided, whether medical or neurosurgical. Management is usually directed toward definitive therapy for patients with chronically elevated ICP.

As in any emergency, the first step in management is to assess the airway, breathing, and circulation (the ABCs). Also useful is to obtain a urine dextrostick and, in the case trauma, to expose the patient completely so as to identify injuries. The following initial steps should be taken when acute increased ICP is suspected:

1. Stabilize the airway. In most instances this step requires rapid, controlled intubation, taking care to minimize any patient Valsalva maneuvers, which increase ICP further, albeit transiently.

2. Obtain intravenous (IV) access. Use only isotonic solutions, minimizing fluids initially unless circulatory compromise is evident.
3. Measure the vital signs, and assess the neurologic state rapidly and frequently.
4. Position the head at 30 degrees, and maintain a midline position in the event an injury to the cervical spine exists or is suspected.
5. Maintain adequate intravascular volume and blood pressure.
6. Maintain adequate oxygenation.

Following these initial maneuvers, further interventions should be attempted based on the patient's clinical situation. The pediatric section of the Society of Critical Care Medicine and the World Federation of Pediatric Intensive and Critical Care issued evidence-based practice guidelines for the acute medical management of severe traumatic brain injury in infants, children and adolescents that provide specific recommendations as they relate to acute intracranial hypertension treatment. These guidelines were adapted from previously published guidelines for adult traumatic brain injury treatment. Based on these guidelines, further interventions to consider for treating intracranial hypertension are discussed in the following sections.

Monitoring Intracranial Pressure and Removing Cerebrospinal Fluid

Recent studies indicate the benefit of monitoring ICP, especially in traumatic brain injury.[7-9] Maintaining normal ICP allows for the maintenance of adequate cerebral perfusion pressure, oxygenation, and metabolic substrate delivery while preventing cerebral herniation. ICP-targeted protocols and therapies have clearly improved outcomes.[9,10] The guidelines recommend treatment goals to keep ICP under 20 mm Hg and maintain CPP above 40 mm Hg.

Numerous invasive devices are available to assess ICP, including intraventricular catheters that allow CSF drainage, therefore reducing ICP. The disadvantage is the higher risk of infection, seizures, and hemorrhage compared with other available devices. A fiberoptic catheter tip pressure transducer or strain gauge device (Camino catheter or Codman catheter) placed within the brain parenchyma provides an effective way to continuously monitor ICP with minimal morbidity. Intraparenchymal catheters that measure brain tissue oxygenation (Pbo_2) and oxygen delivery (Do_2) (Licox catheter, Integra Neurosciences) and microdialysis catheters that allow for measurement of substrates, such as pyruvate and lactate, enable monitoring for brain ischemia and can be used in conjunction with ICP monitoring. Jugular bulb indwelling catheters enable measurement of cerebral venous oxygenation. Transcutaneous, transcranial near infrared spectroscopy can assess ICP and cerebral perfusion indirectly and noninvasively.[3,11,12]

In severe traumatic brain injury, standard ICP and CPP monitoring often do not reflect true Do_2. The combination of ICP and Pbo_2 monitoring (Licox) using Pbo_2-directed critical care are associated with improved outcomes.[7,8] High ICP correlates with decreased cerebral Do_2. Monitoring ICP and Pbo_2 allows early recognition of low oxygen delivery states, hence enabling appropriate therapeutic interventions.

Hyperventilation

Cerebral blood flow is exquisitely sensitive to carbon dioxide levels. Low carbon dioxide levels lead to cerebral vasoconstriction, whereas elevated levels lead to dilation. Early hyperventilation (HV) of the patient with increased ICP leads to a decrease in cerebral blood volume and a decrease in ICP. This method is the most rapid, effective way to lower ICP acutely. This effect is transient; therefore other methods must be employed to maintain normal or near-normal ICP. In general, carbon dioxide should be lowered to the low thirties (mm Hg). Further decreases can lead to a significant decrease in cerebral blood flow, producing ischemia and further increasing ICP. Failure to respond to HV is often a poor prognostic sign.[12] Evidence suggests that the alkalizing effect of HV—and therefore lowered ICP—can be minimized through IV buffers, such as tris hydroxymethyl aminomethane.[12]

HV, although long a mainstay in the treatment of increased ICP, was recently called into question as possibly causing more harm than good.[1,9,13] HV induces a more pronounced change in cerebral blood flow than in cerebral blood volume, which can lead to a reduction in oxygen pressure despite the beneficial affect on CPP and ICP.[14] One study found that aggressive HV had worse outcomes for patients with early, severe head trauma than those who were normocapnic.[15] Although HV is the most rapid method to lower ICP acutely, aggressive HV is not beneficial for the chronic treatment of increased ICP.[1] The recent guidelines suggest considering aggressive HV (carbon dioxide pressure <30 mm Hg) for short periods and mild HV (carbon dioxide pressure 30-35 mm Hg) for longer periods for intracranial hypertension refractory to other maneuvers. HV should be used judiciously with cerebral oxygenation monitoring if at all possible.

Osmotic Agents and Diuretics

Intravenous osmotic agents (mannitol and glycerol) do not permeate the blood-brain barrier and therefore draw fluid from the intracellular brain compartment to the vascular space, thereby reducing ICP and allowing increased cerebral perfusion.[16] Traditionally, mannitol is favored over glycerol; however, one study found that although mannitol decreased ICP, it did not improve cerebral oxygen pressure.[17] Mannitol is given rapidly in an initial IV bolus of 0.5 to 1 g/kg. Following this administration, additional boluses ranging from 0.25 to 0.5 g/kg should be given every 2 to 5 hours, depending on the patient's status. Response to IV mannitol is rapid and usually occurs within 10 to 20 minutes. Serum osmolarity should be maintained in the 295- to 320-mOsm/L range. Mannitol is excreted renally; thus it cannot be given in the setting of renal failure because it can provoke potentially life-threatening pulmonary edema.

Glycerol acts in a similar fashion to mannitol but is used less often.[16] It has the advantage of being a physiological agent with caloric value, which can be beneficial for nutritional support. Glycerol has less diuretic effects such that, unlike mannitol, it does not depend solely on renal function and can be given to patients with renal insufficiency. The main side effect is intravascular hemolysis, which can be prevented by giving a low concentration (<20%) at a slow infusion rate (>1 hour). Glycerol is most effective via enteroduodenal administration. Direct oral intake or gastric tube administration is less effective. Unlike mannitol, which is most effective when given as intermittent boluses, glycerol is usually given as a continuous drip. In summary, mannitol and glycerol are probably equally effective and may be complementary because of their different properties.

Loop diuretics, such as furosemide, reduce ICP by provoking a diuresis of water and electrolytes, thereby establishing a gradient between the intravascular compartment and the brain. Diuretics must be used cautiously in patients with traumatic brain injury and subarachnoid hemorrhage because volume depletion can worsen the outcome. Diuretics are frequently used in combination with osmotic diuretics but are infrequently used alone. Care must be given when using any of the aforementioned agents to maintain intravascular volume and adequate blood pressure. Electrolytes must be monitored carefully.

Hypertonic Saline

A more recent treatment for increased ICP is administering 3% to 23.4% hypertonic saline via IV.[18-20] IV boluses can reduce ICP and augment CPP for several hours.[2,5,21] It creates an osmotic gradient and draws water from the intracellular and extracellular spaces into the intravascular compartment.[3,5] Hypertonic saline can be given quickly and requires lower fluid volumes than osmotic agents. No immediate concern exists for volume depletion, as can occur with mannitol. The potential side effects include hyperosmolar central pontine myelosis, congestive heart failure, subdural hematomas, and, rarely, coagulopathy. As an option, the trauma guidelines recommend the continuous infusion of 3% saline between 0.1 and 1.0 mL/kg/hour administered on a sliding scale with the minimal dose needed to maintain ICP under 20 mm Hg. Serum osmolarity should be maintained below 360 mOsm/L when using hypertonic saline as the only hyperosmolar therapy to control brain edema.

Neuromuscular Blockade

Using agents such as pancuronium and vecuronium can effectively decrease ICP by preventing maneuvers that increase intrathoracic pressure, such as coughing, straining, or *bucking* the ventilator. The physician must remember that these agents do not provide analgesia or sedation; therefore they should be used in conjunction with analgesic agents and short-acting sedatives.

Temperature Control

Hyperthermia leads to greater cerebral metabolism; therefore measures should be taken to prevent body temperature elevation. This process generally includes judicious use of antipyretics, cooling blankets, and antibiotics if infection is suspected. Conversely, hypothermia decreases cerebral metabolism and may be advantageous in managing elevated ICP, as long as shivering is prevented and efforts are made to maintain full cardiorespiratory function. Body temperature should be maintained between 96.8°F and 98.6°F (36°C and 37°C).[3,22]

Seizure Control

Seizure activity, whether clinical or subclinical, places excessive metabolic demand on already-compromised brain tissue. Treatment with antiepileptic drugs is necessary for any patient who is having or is suspected of having seizures, especially if neuromuscular blocking agents are to be used. In general, diazepam (0.1 mg/kg/dose IV) or lorazepam (0.05 to 0.1 mg/kg/dose IV) is to be used in treating acute seizures. For more prolonged therapy, phenytoin, fosphenytoin (a water-soluble prodrug of phenytoin), or phenobarbital can be used. Phenytoin and fosphenytoin have the distinct advantage of not depressing mental status. Phenytoin needs to be given slowly (50 mg/min). Although fosphenytoin can be given more rapidly (150 mg/min), it is water soluble, therefore it can also be given intramuscularly. If possible, the cause of seizure activity (eg, fever, drug toxicity, hypoglycemia, electrolyte abnormalities) should be identified and treated.

Corticosteroids

The use of corticosteroids remains controversial in managing acutely elevated ICP associated with head trauma, intracerebral hemorrhage, and ischemic stroke.[12] Several controlled studies involving the use of glucocorticoids in head injury did not find any change in outcome or benefit for controlling increased ICP.[23] Thus steroids are rarely used to treat increased ICP in patients with head injury; however, they do have clear utility in managing edema associated with brain tumors and refractory pseudotumor cerebri. Their mechanism of action is unknown, but hypotheses include stabilizing the blood-brain barrier, enhancing brain energy supplies, decreasing tumor growth, reducing CSF production, and stabilizing cellular membranes.[3,22] Dexamethasone is generally used.

Glycemic Control

Hyperglycemia after head injury is associated with a poorer outcome than that for patients who are normoglycemic.[23] Many centers now remove glucose from intravenous fluids and aggressively treat hyperglycemia.

High-Dose Barbiturates

Treating refractory increased ICP with high doses of barbiturates can sometimes be effective. These agents act to decrease cerebral blood flow and metabolism. Pentobarbital is given for prolonged therapy; in general, an IV loading dose of 3 to 10 mg/kg is given followed by a maintenance infusion of 1 to 2 mg/kg/hour. The dose should be titrated on the electroencephalogram with a goal of obtaining a burst-suppression pattern. This therapy should be maintained for 24 hours or more and then tapered. Side effects are frequent and include myocardial suppression and hypotension, often requiring pressors. Which groups of refractory increased ICP patients benefit from this therapy has

Table 352-1 Glasgow Coma Scale*

EYE-OPENING RESPONSE

SCORE	>1 YEAR	<1 YEAR
4	Spontaneous	Spontaneous
3	To verbal command	To shout
2	To pain	To pain
1	None	None

MOTOR RESPONSE

SCORE	>1 YEAR	<1 YEAR
6	Obeys commands	Displays spontaneous response
5	Localizes pain	Localizes pain
4	Withdraws from pain	Withdraws from pain
3	Displays abnormal flexion to pain (decorticate rigidity)	Displays abnormal flexion to pain (decorticate rigidity)
2	Displays abnormal extension to pain (decerebrate rigidity)	Displays abnormal extension to pain (decerebrate rigidity)
1	None	None

VERBAL RESPONSE

SCORE	>5 YEARS	2 TO 5 YEARS	0-23 MONTHS
5	Is oriented and converses	Uses appropriate words and phrases	Babbles, coos appropriately
4	Conversation is confused	Uses inappropriate words	Cries, but is consolable
3	Words are inappropriate	Cries or screams persistently to pain	Cries or screams persistently to pain
2	Sounds are incomprehensible	Grunts or moans to pain	Grunts or moans to pain
1	None	None	None

*Glasgow coma scale score equals sum of best eye opening, motor, and verbal responses. Range is 3 to 15. Usual definitions of severity of head injury: severe = <9; moderate = 9 to 12; mild = 13 to 15.

From Teasdale G, Jennett B. Assessment of coma and impaired consciousness: a practical scale. Lancet. 1974;2:81-84.

not yet been determined.[3,12] Pentobarbital should be used only when all other medical and surgical therapies have failed.

Surgical Decompression

Obviously, removing large intracranial masses causing acutely increased ICP can be life saving. Surgery may also play a role in decreasing ICP in select patients with large intracerebral hemorrhages by removing the clot and in trauma patients with massive edema and contusion or in patients who have a large cerebral infarction through craniectomy or decompression of the edematous mass. In the latter 2 instances, surgery is performed after all other measures have failed and increased ICP becomes refractory, but it should be considered before the ICP critically impairs the CPP.[1,3,24]

The trauma guidelines recommend considering decompressive craniectomy to treat severe traumatic brain injury and medically refractory intracranial hypertension, particularly when a potentially recoverable brain injury occurs. Although mortality in children with severe traumatic brain injury remains high, craniotomy has shown to be effective in reducing ICP and can be associated with favorable outcomes in surviving patients.[15]

In pseudotumor cerebri, management is based on symptoms (intractable headache) or when signs of papilledema or visual loss are detected. Imaging studies are recommended to screen for mass lesions or hydrocephalus although the vast majority have normal scans. CT of the head may show small, slit ventricles. MRI of the brain with gadolinium enhancement is the preferred modality for its sensitivity in screening other conditions. Magnetic resonance venography is recommended for patients with suspected dural venous sinus thrombosis and may show extraluminal narrowing of the transverse sinus that may be a typical feature of pseudotumor cerebri.[25] LP is recommended to document opening CSF pressure and may be used therapeutically to decrease ICP by draining CSF. Medical management includes the use of carbonic anhydrase inhibitors (acetazolamide) to decrease CSF production. Digoxin has also been suggested as a comparable alternative with the same effect but lesser side effects. Patients with severe symptoms, visual loss, or failing standard medical therapy may also benefit from a short course of high-dose corticosteroids (prednisone).

Patients with pseudotumor cerebri failing medical therapy or those experiencing progressive visual loss may be considered for surgical treatment that includes CSF shunting procedures (ventriculoperitoneal, ventriculoatrial, or lumboperitoneal shunt) or optic nerve sheath fenestration.

Future Trends

In the future, cerebral protectants, such as free radical scavengers, excitotoxic amino acid antagonists, lazeroids, and *N*-methyl-d-aspartate–receptor antagonists, may be part of the *cocktail* in the initial emergent management of acutely increased ICP.[3,12]

With respect to neurologically stable patients who exhibit evidence of chronically increased ICP, management is directed toward definitive therapy, that is, evacuating the chronic subdural hematoma, appropriate tumor management (corticosteroids, surgery or radiation plus chemotherapy or both), and treatment with acetazolamide, loop diuretics, steroids, or a lumbar drain in patients who have more benign causes of intracranial hypertension.

OUTCOME

Increased ICP is a major complication that affects morbidity and, possibly, ultimate outcome in at least 50% of children who have severe head injuries and in children who are comatose from other cerebral insults (hypoxia, infections, metabolic disorders).[14,26,27] Determining which variables—ICP, CPP, or initial Glasgow coma scale score (Table 352-1)—are helpful in predicting prognosis remains uncertain.[14,26] Regardless, significant morbidity remains for children with increased ICP. Clearly, in select children with mass lesions or treatable metabolic disorders, early identification and treatment before a catastrophic increase in ICP occurs will improve outcome.

WHEN TO REFER

- Macrocephaly or accelerating head growth *(crossing percentiles)*
- Chronic unremitting headache or new onset of severe headache
- Mild papilledema
- Visual abnormalities (field cuts, diplopia)
- Developmental arrest or regression

WHEN TO ADMIT

- Bulging fontanel
- Altered mental status
- Prolonged seizures
- New focal neurologic deficits
- Moderate to severe papilledema
- Cushing triad (widened pulse pressure; bradycardia; and deep, slow respirations)

TOOLS FOR PRACTICE

Medical Decision Support

- *Glasgow Coma Scale* (scale), Graham Teasdale and Bryan J. Jennett.

REFERENCES

1. Allen CH, Ward JD. An evidence-based approach to management of increased intracranial pressure. *Crit Care Clin*. 1998;14(3):485-495.
2. Ropper AH, Rockoff MA. Physiology and clinical aspects of raised intracranial pressure. In: Ropper AH, ed. *Neurological and Neurosurgical Intensive Care*. 2nd ed. New York, NY: Raven Press; 1993.
3. Pickard JD, Czosnyka M. Management of raised intracranial pressure. *J Neurol Neurosurg Psychiatry*. 1993; 56:845-858.
4. Radhakrishnan K, Ahlskog JE. Garrity JA, et al. Idiopathic intracranial hypertension. *Mayo Clinic Prod*. 1994;69(2):169-180.
5. Plum F, Posner JB. *The Diagnosis of Stupor and Coma*. 3rd ed. Philadelphia, PA: FA Davis; 1982.
6. Haslam RHA. Role of computed tomography in the early management of bacterial meningitis. *J Pediatr*. 1991; 119(1 pt 1):157-159.
7. Narotam PK, Burjonrappa SC, Raynor SC, et al. Cerebral oxygenation in major pediatric trauma: its relevance to trauma severity and outcome. *J Pediatr Surg*. 2006; 41(3):505-513.
8. Stiefel MF, Udoetuk JD, Storm PB, et al. Brain tissue oxygen monitoring in pediatric patients with severe traumatic brain injury. *J Neurosurg*. 2006;105(4 suppl):281-286.
9. Wahlström MR, Olivecrona M, Koskinen LO, et al. Severe traumatic brain injury in pediatric patients: treatment and outcome using an intracranial pressure targeted therapy—the Lund concept. *Intensive Care Med*. 2005; 31(6):832-839.
10. Tilford, JM, Aitken ME, Anand KJ, et al. Hospitalizations for critically ill children with traumatic brain injuries: a longitudinal analysis. *Crit Care Med*. 2005;33(9):2074-2081.
11. McKinley BA, Parmley CL, Tonneson AS. Standardized management of intracranial pressure: a preliminary clinical trial. *J Trauma*. 1999;46(2):271-279.
12. Ropper AH. Treatment of intracranial hypertension. In: Ropper AH, ed. *Neurological and Neurosurgical Intensive Care*. 2nd ed. New York, NY: Raven Press; 1993.
13. Schneider GH, Sarrafzadeh AS, Kiening KL, et al. Influence of hyperventilation on brain tissue—PO2, PCO2, and pH in patients with intracranial hypertension. *Acta Neurochir Suppl*. 1998;71:62-65.
14. Barzilay Z, Augarten A, Sagy M, et al. Variables affecting outcome from severe brain injury in children. *Inten Care Med*. 1998;14(4):417-421.
15. Jagannathan J, Okonkwo DO, Dumont AS, et al. Outcome following decompressive craniectomy in children with severe traumatic brain injury: a 10-year single-center experience with long-term follow up. *J Neurosurg*. 2007;106(4 suppl):268-275.
16. Biestro A, Alberti R, Galli R, et al. Osmotherapy for increased intracranial pressure: comparison between mannitol and glycerol. *Acta Neurochir (Wein)*. 1997; 139(8):725-732.

17. Härtl R, Bardt TF, Kiening KL, et al. Mannitol decreases ICP but does not improve brain-tissue pO2 in severely head-injured patients with intracranial hypertension. *Acta Neurochir (Wein)*. 1997;70:40-42.
18. Prough DS, Zornow MH. Hypertonic maintenance fluids for patients with cerebral edema: does the evidence support a "phase II" trial? *Crit Care Med*. 1998;26(3):421-422.
19. Prough DS, Zornow MH. Mannitol: an old friend on the skids? *Crit Care Med*. 1998;26(6):997-998.
20. Suarez JI, Qureshi AI, Bhardwaj A, et al. Treatment of refractory intracranial hypertension with 23.4% saline. *Crit Care Med*. 1998;26(6):1118-1122.
21. Khanna S, Davis D, Peterson B, et al. Use of hypertonic saline in the treatment of severe refractory posttraumatic intracranial hypertension in pediatric traumatic brain injury. *Crit Care Med*. 2000;28(4):1144-1151.
22. Shapiro K, Morris WJ, Teo C. Intracranial hypertension: mechanisms and management. In: Cheek WR, ed. *Pediatric Neurosurgery*. 3rd ed. Philadelphia, PA: WB Saunders; 1994.
23. Giannotta SL, Weiss MH, Apuzzo ML, et al. High dose glucocorticoids in the management of severe head injury. *Neurosurgery*. 1984;15(4):497-501.
24. Rutigliano D, Egnor MR, Priebe CJ, et al. Decompressive craniectomy in pediatric patients with traumatic brain injury with intractable elevated intracranial pressure. *J Pediatr Surg*. 2006;41(1):83-87.
25. Farb RI, Vanek I, Scott JN, et al. Idiopathic intracranial hypertension: the prevalence and morphology of sinovenous stenosis. *Neurology*. 2003;60(9):1418-1424.
26. Lieh-Lai MW, Theodorou AA, Sarnaik AP, et al. Limitations of the Glasgow coma scale in predicting outcome in children with traumatic brain injury. *J Pediatr*. 1992; 120(2 pt 1):193-199.
27. Young A, Willatts S. Controversies in management of acute brain trauma. *Lancet*. 1998;352(9123):164-166.

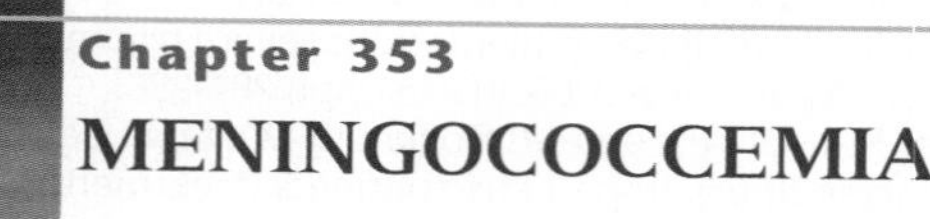

Chapter 353

MENINGOCOCCEMIA

Mary T. Caserta, MD

DEFINITION OF TERMS

Meningococcemia is a classic example of fulminant bacterial sepsis and is the most dreaded consequence of infection with *Neisseria meningitidis*. Although occult or chronic meningococcemia is occasionally detected, children who have the severe form of the disease can progress from a state of good health to death in hours, regardless of whether meningitis is present.

EPIDEMIOLOGY AND ETIOLOGY

N meningitidis is an aerobic gram-negative coccus that appears typically in pairs (diplococci) with the adjacent sides flattened. The organism is enclosed by a cell envelope containing outer membrane proteins and lipopolysaccharide (endotoxin) and by a polysaccharide capsule. Thirteen serogroups have been identified based on the antigenic structure of the capsular polysaccharide. Five of these serogroups are responsible for the majority of human disease, serogroups A, B, C, Y, and W-135. Additional methods of typing outer membrane proteins and lipooligosaccharides have led to classifications of serosubtypes, serotypes, and immunotypes that are useful in epidemiologic investigations.[1]

N meningitidis is found only in the human nasopharynx and is spread from person to person via respiratory droplets or direct contact with secretions. Invasive meningococcal disease is a relatively uncommon event, with most individuals colonized only intermittently with the organism. Approximately 5% to 30% of adolescents and adults in nonepidemic conditions are colonized. Subgroups, such as military recruits, can have rates as high as 80%, and carriage rates are even higher in household contacts of infected patients.[2] Colonization with both pathogenic and nonpathogenic *Neisseria*, in addition to other gram-negative organisms that have similar capsular polysaccharides, induces the development of natural immunity to *N meningitidis*. Nonetheless, *N meningitidis* causes both epidemic and endemic disease worldwide. Since the introduction of an effective vaccine against *Haemophilus influenzae* type b, meningococcal infection is the leading cause of meningitis and sepsis in children and young adults in the United States, with approximately 2600 cases reported annually.[3] Data from the Centers for Disease Control and Prevention show that between 1992 and 1996, the overall incidence of meningococcal disease was 1.1 cases per 100,000 people.[4] The highest incidence of disease is consistently found in infants, with a peak attack rate of 15.9 cases per 100,000 population.[4] From 20% to 25% of all cases of meningococcal disease occur in children younger than 2 years, when passively acquired maternal antibody concentrations have reached their nadir and a substantial number of children have not yet acquired protective antibodies after colonization. A second smaller peak of disease is found in adolescents and young adults[5] (Figure 353-1).

Historically, the majority of cases of invasive meningococcal disease in the United States have been caused by serogroup B meningococcus. However, in the mid-1990s, organisms of serogroup B and C were each identified in approximately 35% of cases of meningococcal disease, with serogroup Y accounting for 26% of isolates.[4] Despite the relative equality in the overall number of cases caused by each of these 3 serogroups, 57% of disease caused by serogroup C occurred in persons between 2 and 30 years of age, whereas 40% of disease caused by group B occurred in children younger than 2 years, making serogroup B meningococci more of a threat to the younger age groups. Serogroup Y disease has been found to be associated with older age groups and the clinical syndrome of pneumonia.[6] The occurrence of meningococcal infection also varies with the seasons. Winter and spring constitute the peak time of disease in the United States. Several studies have shown an association between meningococcal disease and influenza and other viral respiratory infections, although the exact nature of the interaction is not clear.[7]

Fifty percent of cases of invasive meningococcal disease are associated with meningitis; approximately 35% are classified as sepsis without central nervous system involvement. The overall mortality for meningococcal

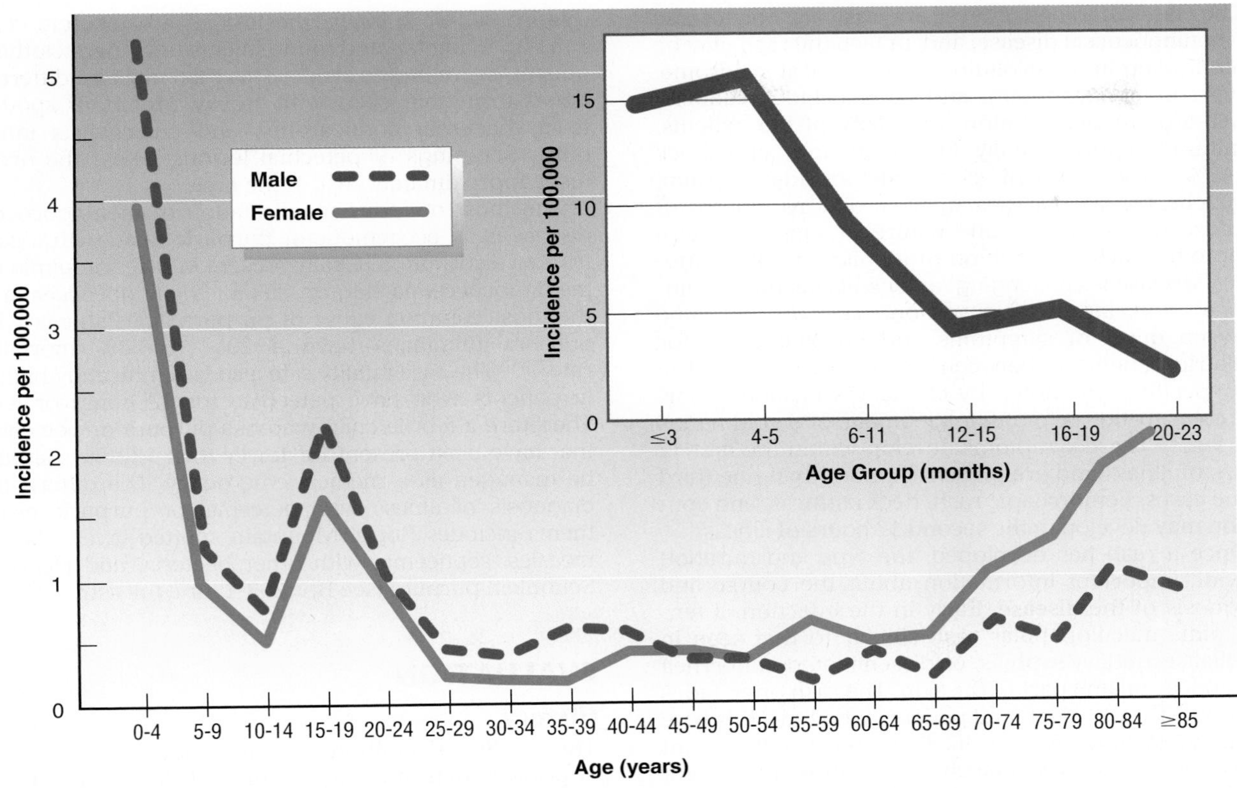

Figure 353-1 Race-adjusted rates of meningococcal disease by age group and sex in California, Georgia, Maryland, Tennessee, Connecticut, Minnesota, and Oregon, 1992-1996. (*Rosenstein NE, Perkins BA, Stephens DS, et al. The changing epidemiology of meningococcal disease in the United States, 1992-1996.* J Infect Dis. *1999;180:1894-1901. Reprinted by permission of the University of Chicago Press.*)

disease is 5% to 15%.[8] Subgroups of patients, such as those who have fulminant meningococcemia, can have fatality rates as high as 50% to 80% despite aggressive intensive care therapy.

CLINICAL MANIFESTATIONS AND DIFFERENTIAL DIAGNOSIS

The classic signs of invasive meningococcal disease are hemorrhagic rash, meningism, and impaired consciousness[9] (Figure 353-2). Fever and rash are consistent findings noted in approximately 70% of patients.[9] Unfortunately, fever and rash are not specific to meningococcemia and have been described in many other infectious and noninfectious diseases (Box 353-1). In a study of more than 200 children in an emergency department with a nonblanching rash, 11% were found to have meningococcal disease.[10] Children with meningococcemia were more likely to be judged ill by the investigators, have fever >38.5°C, a purpuric rash, and a capillary refill time of >2 seconds. In a similar study by Nielson and colleagues, 15% of children with fever and hemorrhagic rash had documented invasive meningococcal disease. After a full evaluation 45% of the children did not have a specific diagnosis identified, and presumably most of these children had self-limited viral illnesses. Poor general condition, the presence of nuchal rigidity, >2-mm maximal diameter of skin hemorrhages, and a generalized distribution of the rash were highly associated with a diagnosis of invasive meningococcal disease.[11] These 2 studies also confirmed the absence of meningococcal disease in children with petechial rashes confined to the area of distribution of the superior vena cava (above the nipple line).[10,11]

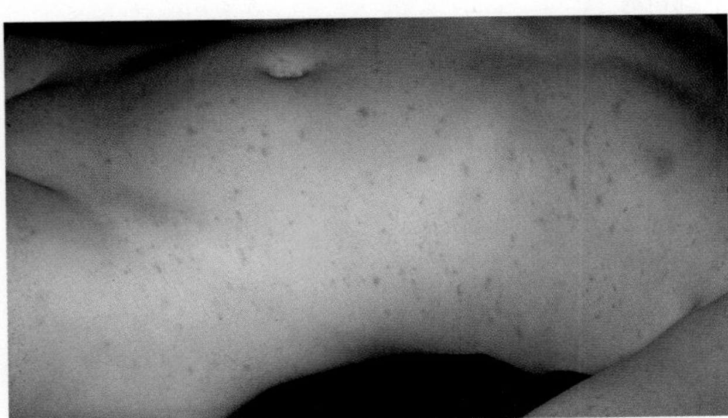

Figure 353-2 A 4-year-old white girl with acute meningococcemia without meningitis with a near uniform distribution of petechiae over the trunk and extremities.

The classic findings of fever and rash are not specific for meningococcal disease, and, in fact, the rash may be a late finding in the evolution of the clinical syndrome. Other common symptoms and signs include irritability or lethargy in slightly more than 50% of the patients, vomiting in approximately 35% of children, and shock in 42%. Less frequent symptoms include delirium, headache, coryza, diarrhea, myalgia, and hypothermia.[9] Because of the nonspecific nature of many of these symptoms, early recognition of a child with meningococcal disease is challenging, and clinicians must maintain a high index of suspicion. The median time between onset of symptoms and hospitalization for pediatric patients is between 13 and 22 hours.[12] The first specific signs noted by caretakers include abnormal color (pallor or mottling), leg pain, and cold hands and feet.[12] These symptoms develop within the first 12 hours of illness and are present in more than one third of the cases; hemorrhagic rash, neck stiffness, and confusion may develop in the second 12 hours of illness.

Once a rash has developed, the type and duration provide important information about the course and prognosis of the disease. Early in the infection, a tender, pink, maculopapular rash similar to that seen in rubella, secondary syphilis, or disseminated gonorrhea can appear on any part of the skin. The rash often fades rapidly with treatment, and patients who have this type of manifestation are less likely to have a fulminant course. A generalized petechial rash most prominent on the distal extremities, including the palms and soles, is usually associated with meningococcal disease (Figure 353-3). Initially, the lesions are discrete, 1 to 2 mm in diameter, and found in clusters where clothing puts pressure on the skin.[13] This rash must be differentiated from that seen with Rocky Mountain spotted fever, bacterial endocarditis, and enterovirus infections. Scrapings of petechial lesions reveal the organism approximately 70% of the time.

The most ominous manifestation of meningococcal disease is an ecchymotic or purpuric rash, with a centrifugal distribution usually present in cases of fulminant meningococcemia (Figure 353-4). Meningococcemia is the most common cause of purpura.[14,15] Patients with purpura fulminans have a 20% to 50% mortality rate.[14,15] The case fatality rate also is significantly higher in patients who have petechiae for 12 hours or less. Therefore a febrile child who has purpura or petechiae that have been present for fewer than 12 hours should be managed as a medical emergency. The differential diagnosis of illness with petechial or purpuric exanthems includes Rocky Mountain spotted fever, plague, measles, septicemia with other bacteria, and Henoch-Schönlein purpura (see Box 353-1 for a full list).

EVALUATION

History

The early recognition of meningococcemia is an important determinant of survival. The majority of children with invasive meningococcal disease have an illness with symptoms and signs lasting only a few

BOX 353-1 Causal Agents and Illnesses in Which Petechiae or Purpura Occurs

- Viruses
  - Varicella-zoster virus
  - Cytomegalovirus (congenital infection)
  - Variola virus
  - Coxsackie viruses
- Echoviruses
  - Colorado tick fever virus
  - Rubella virus
  - Measles virus
  - Alpha viruses (ie, Ross River fever)
  - Lassa virus
  - Marburg viruses
- Nonviral Agents
  - *Rickettsia typhi* (murine typhus)
  - *Rickettsia prowazekii* (epidemic typhus)
  - *Rickettsia rickettsii* (Rocky Mountain spotted fever)
  - *Ehrlichia canis*
  - *Mycoplasma pneumoniae*
  - *Streptococcus pyogenes* (scarlet fever)
  - *Streptococcus pneumonia*
  - Enterococcal and viridans group streptococci (endocarditis)
  - *Neisseria gonorrhoeae*
  - *Neisseria meningitides*
  - *Moraxella catarrhalis*
  - *Haemophilus influenzae*
  - *Streptobacillus moniliformis* (rat bite fever)
  - *Pseudomonas aeruginosa* (erythema gangrenosa)
  - *Yersinia pestis* (plague)
  - *Bartonella henselae* (cat-scratch disease)
  - *Treponema pallidum* (congenital syphilis)
  - *Borrelia* species (relapsing fever)
  - *Trichinella spiralis* (trichinosis)
  - *Toxoplasma gondii* (congenital toxoplasmosis)
- Miscellaneous
  - Henoch-Schönlein purpura
  - Immune thrombocytopenic purpura
  - Kawasaki disease
  - Serum sickness
  - Poisons
  - Erythema multiforme
  - Erythema nodosum
  - Systemic lupus erythematosus

Modified and reprinted from: Cherry JD. Cutaneous manifestations of systemic infections. In: Feigen RD, Cherry JD, eds. *Textbook of Pediatric Infectious Diseases.* 4th ed. Philadelphia, PA: WB Saunders; 1998:713-737, with permission from Elsevier, and Ferguson LE, Hormann MD, Parks DK, et al. *Neisseria* meningitides: presentation, treatment, and prevention. *J Pediatr Health Care.* 2002;16:119-124, with permission from The National Association of Nurse Practitioners.

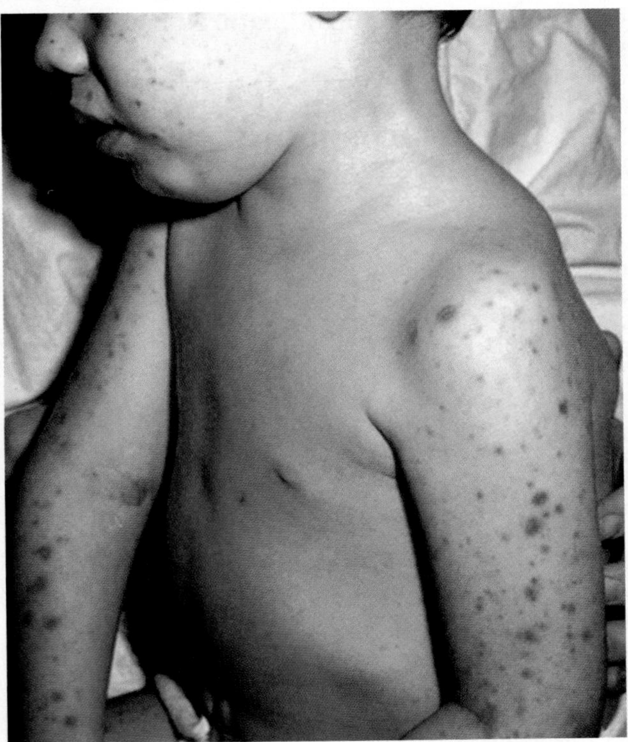

Figure 353-3 Meningococcemia showing striking involvement of the extremities with relative sparing of the skin of the child's body surface.

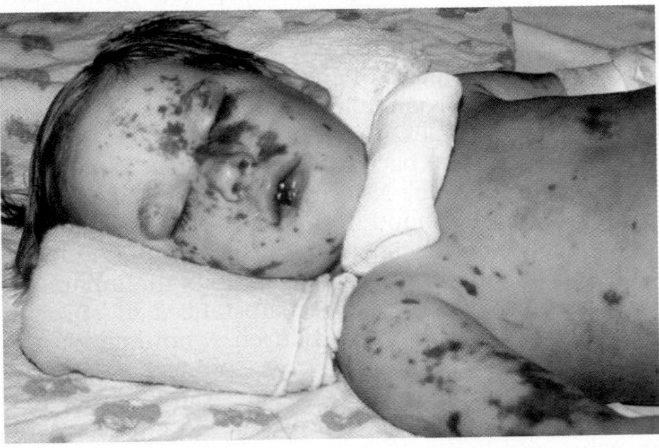

Figure 353-4 Ecchymotic or purpuric rash is the most significant manifestation of meningococcal disease, showing a centrifugal distribution present in the child with fulminant meningococcemia.

hours to a day. Approximately 25% may report a recent respiratory illness, but, in general, the children have no significant medical history.[12] Patients often describe the acute onset of fever, nausea, vomiting, irritability or lethargy, and rash. Other symptoms include myalgia, leg pain, cold hands and feet, neck pain or stiffness, sore throat, diarrhea, headache, and abnormal skin color[9,12] (Table 353-1).

Physical Examination

The physical examination of a child or adolescent with suspected meningococcemia should be performed expeditiously and with close attention to the vital signs and skin findings. A maculopapular rash may precede the more classic generalized petechiae. Petechiae are often clustered, 1 to 2 mm in size, and more prominent on the distal extremities including the palms and soles. Purpura may also be present with the petechiae. In addition to the skin findings, the adequacy of respiration, the central and peripheral circulation, and mental status need to be evaluated to determine the presence of shock.[16] Because of the rapid evolution of meningococcemia, frequent reassessments are warranted.

Laboratory Testing

An infant or child with signs and symptoms of invasive meningococcal disease should be evaluated immediately with aggressive monitoring and treatment as soon as the diagnosis is reasonably thought to be present. If the patient must be transported to a pediatric intensive care unit, then blood should be drawn, antibiotics given, and intravenous access secured beforehand. The patient should be attended during transport by a physician prepared to treat shock and respiratory failure because the disease may worsen when endotoxin is liberated after antibiotic therapy. Initial laboratory tests should include a blood culture, a complete blood count and differential, a partial thromboplastin time, a prothrombin time, measurement of fibrin breakdown products, and serum chemistries. If the patient is stable when first evaluated, then a lumbar puncture should be performed to examine the cerebral spinal fluid for organisms, obtain cultures, and assess the prognosis more accurately. If the patient is not stable on initial assessment, then the lumbar puncture should be deferred until a later time. Antibiotic therapy should never be withheld while waiting to obtain cerebrospinal fluid.

Management

The recommended antibiotic regimen for treatment of meningococcemia is aqueous penicillin G 250,000 units/kg of body weight/day in 4 to 6 divided doses.[17] Although a small number of meningococcal isolates with intermediate susceptibility to penicillin have been identified in the United States, no resistance to penicillin has been reported.[18] Ceftriaxone, cefotaxime, and chloramphenicol are alternative antibiotics recommended for patients who are allergic to penicillin. Antibiotic therapy generally is continued for 5 afebrile days or 7 days total. Rifampin (10 mg/kg per dose given twice a day for 2 days) is prescribed at the end of the course of penicillin to eliminate carriage of the organism from the nasopharynx.[19] Rifampin is not necessary if the patient has been treated with a third-generation cephalosporin because these agents are effective in eliminating carriage.[20]

In addition to antibiotic therapy, children who have meningococcemia often require aggressive supportive therapy in a pediatric intensive care setting, with invasive monitoring of hemodynamic, neurologic, and respiratory function. Mechanical ventilation often is necessary to treat respiratory failure. Maintenance of

Table 353-1 Cumulative Proportion of Children Developing Clinical Features During the Course of Meningococcal Disease

	FATAL CASES (*N*=103)	NONFATAL CASES (*N*=345)	OVERALL (95% CONFIDENCE INTERVAL [CI])	MEDIAN HOUR OF ONSET
EARLY SYMPTOMS				
Leg pain	22.3%	38%	36.7% (28-47)	7
Thirst	41.7%	40.6%	40.7% (31-50)	8
Diarrhea	54.4%	44.6%	45.2% (36-56)	9
Abnormal skin color	73.8%	53.9%	55.1% (45-65)	10
Breathing difficulty	75.7%	58.0%	59.1% (50-69)	11
Cold hands and feet	81.6%	75.7%	76.1% (67-85)	12
CLASSIC SYMPTOMS				
Hemorrhagic rash	94.2%	88.4%	88.8% (82-95)	13
Neck pain or stiffness	94.2%	91.6%	91.8% (86-97)	13
Photophobia	94.2%	92.5%	92.6% (87-97)	15
Bulging fontanel	94.2%	93.0%	93.1% (88-98)	15
LATE SYMPTOMS				
Confusion or delirium	94.2%	95.1%	95.0% (90-99)	16
Seizure	96.1%	95.4%	95.4% (91-99)	17
Unconsciousness	97.1%	95.9%	96.0% (92-99)	22

Reprinted from Thompson MJ, Ninis N, Mayon-White R, et al. Clinical recognition of meningococcal disease in children and adolescents. *Lancet.* 2006;367:402-403, with permission from Elsevier.

optimal plasma expansion with intravenous fluids is the first step in stabilizing the circulatory system. Large amounts of fluid may be needed because of the capillary leak associated with endotoxic shock. In addition, multiple transfusions with platelets and fresh-frozen plasma may be necessary to correct the coagulopathy associated with meningococcemia. Several studies have demonstrated that myocardial dysfunction precedes shock in adult and pediatric patients who have meningococcal sepsis.[21] This phenomenon is believed to be caused by endotoxemia. The use of inotropic agents aimed at reversing myocardial depression and improving tissue perfusion is recommended based on these observations.

Supportive measures for severe purpura include treatments aimed at relieving the ischemic complications associated with vasculitis. Continuous epidural anesthesia may help in improving perfusion of the lower extremities and preventing gangrenous necrosis.[22] The mechanism of action is thought to be vasodilatation of partially occluded vessels via sympathetic blockade. If no evidence of coagulopathy exists, then an anesthesiologist can perform this type of regional block with an indwelling catheter in the caudal space. Systemic thrombolytic therapy with recombinant tissue plasminogen activator (r-TPA) has been used in a limited number of patients in an attempt to dissolve microthrombi and restore organ and tissue perfusion.[23] However, the risks of bleeding complications caused by this intervention have not been fully evaluated, and it is not recommended for use outside of a research setting. The topical administration of nitroglycerin has also been reported to be useful in restoring blood flow to limited areas of skin and superficial tissues without notable adverse effects although this has not been systematically studied.[24,25]

Other ancillary treatments evaluated experimentally are aimed at interrupting the disease process pathophysiology via interference with both endotoxin and the secondary mediators of inflammation induced by endotoxin.[26] These treatments include plasmapheresis, whole blood exchange, extracorporeal membrane oxygenation, and continuous venovenous hemodiafiltration.[27,28] Several studies have shown a correlation between plasma levels of endotoxin or tumor necrosis factor and multiorgan failure or disease severity, making these strategies theoretically attractive.[29,30] Recombinant human bactericidal-permeability-increasing protein ($rBPI_{21}$) is the N-terminal fragment of a human protein naturally found in the azurophilic granules of polymorphonuclear leukocytes. This compound binds to bacteria and endotoxin and inhibits the inflammatory response caused by these substances. In a preliminary trial of $rBPI_{21}$ in children who had severe meningococcemia, mortality was reduced compared with historical controls.[31] A large, randomized, placebo-controlled trial of this product in children with invasive meningococcal disease did demonstrate a lower incidence of multiple and severe amputations, improved functional outcome, and less need for blood product support but failed to show a substantial benefit in mortality.[32] Based on this study, the product remains in clinical development and is not available for general use. Reports have associated purpura fulminans induced by sepsis with acquired deficiencies of the natural anticoagulation factor proteins C and S and deficiency in the activation pathway for protein C.[33,34] Drotrecogin alfa (activated) is an activated protein C compound licensed for use in adults with severe sepsis and organ dysfunction. Although efficacy has been demonstrated in adult populations, a recent pediatric trial of this compound was halted because of

Table 353-2 Glasgow Meningococcal Septicemia Prognostic Score

POINTS	SCORE
Blood pressure <75 mm Hg systolic, age <4 yr and <85 mm Hg systolic, age >4 yr	3
Skin to rectal temperature difference >3°C	3
Modified Glasgow Coma Scale score less than 8 or deterioration of at least 3 points in 1 hr	3
Clinical deterioration in hour before scoring	2
Absence of meningitis	2
Extending purpuric rash or widespread ecchymoses	1
Base deficit (capillary or arterial) >8.0	1
Maximum score	15

A score of at least 9 has a sensitivity of 100%, a specificity of 95%, a positive predictive value of 73.7%, and a negative predictive value of 100% in predicting mortality.
Reprinted from Thomson AJ, Sills JA, Hart A. Validation of the Glasgow Meningococcal Septicemia Prognostic Score: a 10-year retrospective survey. *Crit Care Med* 1991;19:26-30, with permission from Lippincott Williams & Wilkins.

concerns over lack of benefit and an increased number of intracranial hemorrhages in patients receiving the product.[35] The use of high-dose steroids in children who have meningococcal disease remains controversial.

Numerous investigators have attempted to predict the outcome for individual patients who have meningococcal disease based on laboratory and clinical data. In 1966, Stiehm and Damrosch[36] developed a prognostic score whereby patients who had 3 or more symptoms (the presence of petechiae for fewer than 12 hours before admission, shock, the absence of meningitis, normal or low white blood cell counts, or normal or low erythrocyte sedimentation rates) had fatality rates of 85% or greater when the score was validated. The Glasgow Meningococcal Septicemia Prognostic Score was developed in 1987 (Table 353-2) and is designed for rapid bedside assessment without the need for multiple laboratory tests.[37] Points are assigned for shock, a skin-to-rectal temperature differential of greater than 3°C, a pediatric-modified coma scale score of less than 8, absence of meningismus, an extending purpuric rash, deterioration in the hour before scoring, and a base deficit greater than 8. The scale was tested retrospectively on a group of 123 children who had meningococcemia. A score of 10 or greater had a positive predictive value of 87.5% and a negative predictive value of 100%. Although multiple scoring systems have been developed for invasive meningococcal disease the Glasgow Meningococcal Septicemia Prognostic Score continues to perform well in clinical studies compared to other methods.[38,39] In general, these scoring systems are used to determine which patients might benefit from more aggressive or experimental therapies and to help evaluate the usefulness of newer treatments.

COMPLICATIONS

The majority of children who survive meningococcal disease recover completely; 15% to 40% of patients, however, develop a complication of infection that may be categorized broadly as suppurative, neurologic, ischemic, or allergic. The suppurative complications include subdural effusions, subdural empyema, and acute suppurative arthritis.[40] Suppurative complications occur in approximately 9% of children.[40] Deafness is the most common neurologic sequelae (2% to 6%). The percentage of survivors who have ischemic complications such as gangrenous necrosis of the skin or extremities requiring skin grafting or amputation varies from 3% to 20%.[9,41] Arthritis and pericarditis are the most common sequelae of meningococcal infection and are reported in 4% to 10% of pediatric cases.[9,40] These complications are thought to be caused by an allergic phenomenon with immune complex deposition rather than a direct invasion of the heart or joints by the organism. Allergic arthritis and pericarditis are late in onset and more common in adults than in children. The symptoms are usually self-limited. Specific therapy is generally not required; however, drainage of pericardial or joint fluid occasionally is necessary.

Although not a true complication, complement deficiency has been reported in approximately 15% of adolescents and children who have meningococcal disease.[42] These patients are at high risk for recurrent episodes of invasive infection. Based on this information, screening for complement deficiencies with a total hemolytic complement assay should be considered in any pediatric patient who has meningococcemia.

DISEASE CONTROL AND PREVENTION

Antimicrobial chemoprophylaxis is an integral component in the control of invasive meningococcal disease. Several studies have demonstrated that household, child care, and preschool contacts of patients who have invasive disease have a rate of infection approximately 100 to 800 times that of the general population.[8,43] In addition, 50% of secondary cases occur within 5 days of the index case and 70% within 1 week.[43] Rifampin is highly effective in eliminating carriage of the meningococcus from the nasopharynx.[20] The American Academy of Pediatrics recommends that all household, child care, or preschool contacts or anyone directly exposed to a patient's secretions be given rifampin within 24 hours of recognizing the primary case.[17] The dose is 10 mg/kg per dose (maximal adult dose is 600 mg) every 12 hours for 2 days for children older than 1 month of age and 5 mg/kg per dose every 12 hours for 2 days for infants younger than 1 month of age (Table 353-3).

Table 353-3 Recommended Chemoprophylaxis Regimens for High-Risk Contacts and People With Invasive Meningococcal Disease

AGE OF INFANTS, CHILDREN, AND ADULTS	DOSE	DURATION	EFFICACY (%)	CAUTIONS
RIFAMPIN*				
<1 mo	5 mg/kg, orally, every 12 h	2 days		
≥1 mo	10 mg/kg (maximum 600 mg), orally, every 12 hr	2 days	90-95	May interfere with efficacy of oral contraceptives and some seizure prevention and anticoagulant medications; may stain soft contact lenses
CEFTRIAXONE				
<15 yr	125 mg, intramuscularly	Single dose	90-95	To decrease pain at injection site, dilute with 1% lidocaine
≥15 yr	250 mg, intramuscularly	Single dose		
CIPROFLOXACIN*				
≥18 yr	500 mg, orally	Single dose	90-95	Not recommended for people younger than 18 years of age

*Not recommended for use in pregnant women.
American Academy of Pediatrics. Meningococcal infections. In: Pickering LK, Baker CJ, Long SS, et al., eds. *Red Book: 2006 Report of the Committee on Infectious Diseases*. 27th ed. Elk Grove Village, IL; American Academy of Pediatrics; 2006:452-460.

Alternative agents proven to be effective in chemoprophylactic regimens include ceftriaxone and ciprofloxacin.[20] Although ceftriaxone is not recommended for widespread chemoprophylactic use, a single 250-mg intramuscular dose has the advantage of being safe for pregnant women. Ciprofloxacin is not approved for children or pregnant women, but it can be used in older adolescents and young adults and has the advantage of being administered as a single oral 500-mg dose.

Vaccination is another important aspect of disease control and prevention. A new tetravalent meningococcal polysaccharide-protein conjugate vaccine was licensed for use in January 2005 among individuals from 11 to 55 years of age.[44] In May 2005 the Centers for Disease Control and Prevention's Advisory Committee on Immunization Practices recommended adding meningococcal conjugate vaccine to the routine immunization schedule for all children at age 11 to 12 years.[44] The vaccine contains purified capsular polysaccharide of serogroups A, C, Y, and W-135 conjugated to diphtheria toxoid. The conjugated protein elicits a T cell–dependent antibody response and induces immunologic memory. In a trial comparing meningococcal polysaccharide vaccine with the new conjugate meningococcal vaccine among more than 800 children age 11 to 18 years who received conjugate vaccine, 82% to 97% of children achieved 4-fold or greater rises in serum bactericidal antibody titers, and 98.6% to 99.8% achieved protective levels to all 4 serogroups.[44] Adverse reactions are mild and infrequent and are usually limited to local reactions and fever.

Unfortunately, no vaccine is available for protection from group B meningococcal disease. The group B capsule is not strongly immunogenic in humans and has been found to share cross-reacting antigens with human neural tissue. Attempts to create vaccine by using outer membrane proteins are ongoing. In addition, studies aimed at evaluating the immunogenicity and safety of the new meningococcal conjugate vaccine in younger age groups are underway.

TOOLS FOR PRACTICE

Engaging Patients and Family

- *Vaccine Information Statement: Meningococcal Vaccine* (fact sheet), Centers for Disease Control and Prevention and American Academy of Pediatrics (www.aap.org/bst/showdetl.cfm?&DID=15&Product_ID=2239).
- *Meningococcal Disease—Information for Teens and College Students* (brochure), American Academy of Pediatrics (patiented.aap.org).
- *Meningococcal Disease* (fact sheet), Centers for Disease Control and Prevention (www.cdc.gov/ncidod/dbmd/diseaseinfo/meningococcal_g.htm).
- *Meningitis on Campus: Don't Wait, Vaccinate* (brochure), National Meningitis Association (www.cdc.gov/nip/vaccine/mening/meni_NMA_brochure.pdf).
- *Meningococcus Vaccine—FAQ* (fact sheet), Vaccine Education Center Children's Hospital of Philadelphia (www.chop.edu/consumer/jsp/division/generic.jsp?id=75734).

Medical Decision Support

- PediaLink Hot Topics 2006—Meningococcal Vaccines (on-line course), American Academy of Pediatrics (www.pedialink.org)
- *Vaccine Delivery Tip Sheet* (fact sheet), National Foundation for Infectious Diseases (66.11.193.178/materials/vaccinedeliverytipsheet.pdf)

AAP POLICY STATEMENTS

American Academy of Pediatrics, Committee on Infectious Diseases. Prevention and control of meningococcal disease: recommendations for use of meningococcal vaccines in pediatric patients. *Pediatrics*. 2005;116(2):496-505. (aappolicy.aappublications.org/cgi/content/full/pediatrics;116/2/496).

American Academy of Pediatrics, Committee on Infectious Diseases. Prevention and control strategies for practice-based physicians (Addendum: recommendations for college students). *Pediatrics*. 2000;106(6):1500-1504. (aappolicy.aappublications.org/cgi/content/full/pediatrics;106/6/1500).

American Academy of Pediatrics, Committee on Infectious Diseases. Recommended childhood and adolescent immunization schedule—United States, 2006. *Pediatrics*. 2006, 117(1):239-240. (aappolicy.aappublications.org/cgi/content/full/pediatrics;115/1/182).

REFERENCES

1. Rosenstein NE, Perkins BA, Stephens DS, et al. Meningococcal disease. *N Engl J Med*. 2001;344(18):1378-1388.
2. Cartwright KA, Stuart JM, Robinson PM. Meningococcal carriage in close contacts of cases. *Epidemiol Infect*. 1991;106(1):133-141.
3. Control and prevention of meningococcal disease: recommendations of the Advisory Committee on Immunization Practices (ACIP). *MMWR Recomm Rep*. 1997;46(RR-5):1-10.
4. Rosenstein NE, Perkins BA, Stephens DS, et al. The changing epidemiology of meningococcal disease in the United States, 1992-1996. *J Infect Dis*. 1999;180(6):1894-1901.
5. Schaffner W, Harrison, Lee H, et al. Reducing the impact of meningococcal disease in adolescents and young adults. National Foundation for Infectious Diseases. Available at: www.nfid.org/publications/meningococcalepid.pdf. Accessed July 2005 and July 2007.
6. Winstead JM, McKinsey DS, Tasker S, et al. Meningococcal pneumonia: characterization and review of cases seen over the past 25 years. *Clin Infect Dis*. 2000;30(1):87-94.
7. Cartwright KA, Jones DM, Smith AJ, et al. Influenza A and meningococcal disease. *Lancet*. 1991;338(8766):554-557.
8. Barquet N, Domingo P, Cayla JA, et al. Meningococcal disease in a large urban population (Barcelona, 1987-1992): predictors of dismal prognosis. Barcelona Meningococcal Disease Surveillance Group. *Arch Intern Med*. 1999;159(19):2329-2340.
9. Wong VK, Hitchcock W, Mason WH. Meningococcal infections in children: a review of 100 cases. *Pediatr Infect Dis J*. 1989;8(4):224-227.
10. Wells LC, Smith JC, Weston VC, et al. The child with a non-blanching rash: how likely is meningococcal disease? *Arch Dis Child*. 2001. 2001;85(3):218-222.
11. Nielsen HE, Andersen EA, Andersen J, et al. Diagnostic assessment of haemorrhagic rash and fever. *Arch Dis Child*. 2001;85(2):160-165.
12. Thompson MJ, Ninis N, Perera R, et al. Clinical recognition of meningococcal disease in children and adolescents. *Lancet*. 2006;367(9508):397-403.
13. Baxter P, Priestley B. Meningococcal rash. *Lancet*. 1988; 1(8595):1166-1167.
14. Toews WH, Bass JW. Skin manifestations of meningococcal infection; an immediate indicator of prognosis. *Am J Dis Child*. 1974;127(2):173-176.
15. Tesoro LJ, Selbst SM. Factors affecting outcome in meningococcal infections. *Am J Dis Child*. 1991;145(2):218-220.
16. Hazelzet JA. Diagnosing meningococcemia as a cause of sepsis. *Pediatr Crit Care Med*. 2005;6(3 Suppl):S50-54.
17. Pickering LK, Baker CJ, Long SS, et al. *The Red Book: Report of the Committee on Infectious Diseases*. 27th ed. Elk Grove Village, IL: American Academy of Pediatrics; 2006.
18. Rosenstein NE, Stocker SA, Popovic T, et al. Antimicrobial resistance of *Neisseria* meningitidis in the United States, 1997. The Active Bacterial Core Surveillance (ABCs) Team. *Clin Infect Dis*. 2000;30(1):212-213.
19. Alvez F, Aguilera A, Garcia-Zabarte A, et al. Effect of chemoprophylaxis on the meningococcal carrier state after systemic infection. *Pediatr Infect Dis J*. 1991;10(9):700.
20. Cochrane Database of Systematic Reviews 2006, Issue 4. Art. No. DOI: 10.1002/14651858.CD004785.pub.3.
21. Monsalve F, Rucabado L, Salvador A, et al. Myocardial depression in septic shock caused by meningococcal infection. *Crit Care Med*. 1984;12(12):1021-1023.
22. Tobias JD, Haun SE, Helfaer M, et al. Use of continuous caudal block to relieve lower-extremity ischemia caused by vasculitis in a child with meningococcemia. *J Pediatr*. 1989;115(6):1019-1021.
23. Zenz W, Zoehrer B, Levin M, et al. Use of recombinant tissue plasminogen activator in children with meningococcal purpura fulminans: a retrospective study. *Crit Care Med*. 2004;32(8):1777-1780.
24. Irazuzta J, Jarrell J, Portillo A, et al. Compared contralateral application of topical nitroglycerin on purpura fulminans. *W V Med J*. 1998;94(1):29-30.
25. Meyer MT, Irazuzta JE, Tozibikian H. Topical nitroglycerin and pain in purpura fulminans. *J Pediatr*. 1999; 134(5):639-641.
26. Cohen J. Meningococcal disease as a model to evaluate novel anti-sepsis strategies. *Crit Care Med*. 2000;28(9 Suppl):S64-S67.
27. Goldman AP, Kerr SJ, Butt W, et al. Extracorporeal support for intractable cardiorespiratory failure due to meningococcal disease. *Lancet*. 1997;349(9050):466-469.
28. Best C, Walsh J, Sinclair J, et al. Early haemo-diafiltration in meningococcal septicaemia. *Lancet*. 1996;347(8995):202.
29. Brandtzaeg P, Kierulf P, Gaustad P, et al. Plasma endotoxin as a predictor of multiple organ failure and death in systemic meningococcal disease. *J Infect Dis*. 1989;159(2):195-204.
30. Waage A, Halstensen A, Espevik T. Association between tumour necrosis factor in serum and fatal outcome in patients with meningococcal disease. *Lancet*. 1987; 1(8529):355-357.
31. Giroir BP, Quint PA, Barton P, et al. Preliminary evaluation of recombinant amino-terminal fragment of human bactericidal/permeability-increasing protein in children with severe meningococcal sepsis. *Lancet*. 1997; 350(9089):1439-1443.
32. Levin M, Quint PA, Goldstein B, et al. Recombinant bactericidal/permeability-increasing protein (rBPI21) as adjunctive treatment for children with severe meningococcal sepsis: a randomised trial. rBPI21 Meningococcal Sepsis Study Group. *Lancet*. 2000; 356(9234);961-967.

33. Powars DR, Rogers ZR, Patch MJ, et al. Purpura fulminans in meningococcemia: association with acquired deficiencies of proteins C and S. *N Engl J Med.* 1987;317(9):571-572.
34. Faust SN, Levin M, Harrison OB, et al. Dysfunction of endothelial protein C activation in severe meningococcal sepsis. *N Engl J Med.* 2001;345(6):408-416.
35. Eli Lilly and Co., *Dear Doctor* [letter].
36. Stiehm ER, Damrosch DS. Factors in the prognosis of meningococcal infection. Review of 63 cases with emphasis on recognition and management of the severely ill patient. *J Pediatr.* 1966;68(3):457-467.
37. Thomson AP, Sills JA, Hart CA. Validation of the Glasgow Meningococcal Septicemia Prognostic Score: a 10-year retrospective survey. *Crit Care Med.* 1991;19(1):26-30.
38. Riordan FA, Marzouk O, Thomson AP, et al. Prospective validation of the Glasgow Meningococcal Septicaemia Prognostic Score. Comparison with other scoring methods. *Eur J Pediatr.* 2002;161(10):531-537.
39. Derkx HH, van den Hoek J, Redekop WK, et al. Meningococcal disease: a comparison of eight severity scores in 125 children. *Intensive Care Med.* 1996;22(12):1433-1441.
40. Edwards MS, Baker CJ. Complications and sequelae of meningococcal infections in children. *J Pediatr.* 1981; 99(4):540-545.
41. Kirsch EA, Barton RP, Kitchen L, et al. Pathophysiology, treatment and outcome of meningococcemia: a review and recent experience. *Pediatr Infect Dis J.* 1996;15(11): 967-978, quiz 979.
42. Leggiadro RJ. Systemic meningococcal infection and complement deficiency. *Pediatr Infect Dis J.* 2003;22(8): 760-761.
43. De Wals P, Hertoghe L, Borlee-Grimee I, et al. Meningococcal disease in Belgium. Secondary attack rate among household, day-care nursery and pre-elementary school contacts. *J Infect.* 1981;3(1 Suppl):53-61.
44. Prevention and Control of Meningococcal Disease. Recommendations of the Advisory Committee on Immunization Practices (ACIP). *MMWR Recomm Rep.* 2005;54(RR-7):1-23.

Chapter 354

PNEUMOTHORAX AND PNEUMOMEDIASTINUM

Michelle Zebrack, MD; Susan L. Bratton, MD, MPH

Pneumothorax and pneumomediastinum are uncommon events in healthy children. A pneumothorax is a collection of air in the potential space between the parietal and visceral layers of the pleura. Pneumothoraces are typically classified as spontaneous, traumatic, or iatrogenic.[1,2] Pneumomediastinum is a condition in which air is present in the mediastinum. The 3 main causes of pneumomediastinum are (1) alveolar rupture; (2) perforation or rupture of the esophagus, trachea, or main bronchi; and (3) dissection of air from the neck or the abdomen.[3,4] Failure to recognize and properly manage pneumothorax or pneumomediastinum can have serious consequences.

PNEUMOTHORAX

Spontaneous Pneumothorax

Spontaneous pneumothoraces occur in the absence of antecedent thoracic trauma and are further subdivided into primary or secondary spontaneous pneumothorax. Primary spontaneous pneumothorax affects patients who do not have *clinically apparent* lung abnormality or an underlying condition known to promote pneumothorax. Secondary spontaneous pneumothorax occurs in the setting of underlying pulmonary disease such as pneumonia, asthma, or cystic fibrosis.[1,2]

Little is known about the true incidence of spontaneous pneumothorax in children; however, it is infrequent and usually related to underlying lung disease.[5,6]

Primary Spontaneous Pneumothorax

Although primary spontaneous pneumothorax is said to occur without a precipitating event or underlying lung disease, patients initially diagnosed with primary spontaneous pneumothorax frequently (76%-100%) have unrecognized lung disease, usually subpleural bullae.[1,7,8] The incidence of primary spontaneous pneumothorax in children is not reported, but 1 study documents only 58 children with primary spontaneous pneumothorax in a 20-year period.[9] In adults the estimated incidence is between 7.4 and 18 cases per 100,000 population per year among men and between 1.2 and 6 cases per 100,000 population per year among women.[1,10-12] The typical patient is a tall, thin, male patient between the ages of 10 and 30 years. Smoking increases the risk of primary spontaneous pneumothorax 9-fold among women and 22-fold among men.[11]

Secondary Spontaneous Pneumothorax

Secondary spontaneous pneumothorax occurs in patients with lung disease. Pediatric incidence related specifically to secondary spontaneous pneumothorax has not been reported, but the adult estimated incidence is 6.3 cases per 100,000 population per year among men and 2 cases per 100,000 population per year among women[1,10,11] Pneumothorax is a known complication of asthma, and, by some estimates, tension pneumothorax is present in almost 30% of patients who die suddenly from asthma.[13] Nearly 3.5% of all patients with cystic fibrosis will experience a pneumothorax, and subsequent pneumothoraces are common.[14] The risk of spontaneous pneumothorax is also increased in various inherited disorders, such as α_1-antitrypsin deficiency, Marfan syndrome, and Ehlers-Danlos syndrome. Some familial cases without evidence of connective tissue disease do occur. Spontaneous pneumothorax is a well-recognized complication of AIDS in pediatric patients and is associated with *Pneumocystis carinii* pneumonia. Catamenial pneumothorax, a condition related to endometriosis with diaphragmatic hernia, should be considered in female patients with spontaneous pneumothorax temporally related to menstruation.

Other Precipitating Factors

Foreign body ingestion must be considered in any child with an unexplained pneumothorax, particularly children ages 6 months to 6 years. Exposure to loud music has been reported as a precipitating factor in patients with spontaneous pneumothorax.[15] Spontaneous pneumothorax is associated with illicit drug use and may result from attempted jugular or subclavian vessel injection (mainlining), cavitating septic thromboemboli, forceful exhalation of crack smoke into another individual's respiratory tract (shotgunning), or from deep inhalation and Valsalva maneuvers while smoking marijuana.[16] Emesis and coughing, both Valsalva maneuvers, can also cause spontaneous pneumothorax.

Traumatic Pneumothorax

When a child has a traumatic pneumothorax, the clinician must recognize that chest trauma is often an indicator of multisystem injury (eg, life-threatening head injury, abdominal injury).[17] Trauma to the chest is classified as blunt or penetrating. The leading causes of blunt thoracic trauma are vehicle-pedestrian injuries and motor-vehicle crashes.[18] Falls and child abuse are also causes of blunt traumatic pneumothorax.[19] The leading causes of penetrating thoracic trauma are gunshot and stab wounds. In 1 report of children with blunt trauma, 38% had an associated pneumothorax, hemothorax, or both. In children with penetrating thoracic trauma, 64% had an associated pneumothorax, hemothorax, or both.[20]

Iatrogenic Pneumothorax

Iatrogenic pneumothoraces are caused by diagnostic or therapeutic interventions, including transthoracic-needle aspiration, central venous catheter insertion, thoracocentesis, and barotrauma or volutrauma related to mechanical ventilation. Rates of pneumothorax caused by mechanical ventilation have fallen in all age groups because of improved modes of mechanical ventilation with better patient synchrony and lower tidal-volume strategies that limit delivered airway pressure.[2,21-24] Use of surfactant has also been credited with substantial decreases in pneumothorax rates for preterm neonates (30%-65%).[25] The observed rate of iatrogenic pneumothorax in the hospitalized pediatric population was recently reported as 0.06 per 1000 discharges.[22] Some reports note an incidence of iatrogenic pneumothorax that exceeds that of spontaneous pneumothorax.[26,27]

Neonatal Pneumothorax

The incidence of neonatal pneumothorax depends on gestational age, birth weight, and the presence of lung disease. Spontaneous pneumothorax is present in 1% to 2% of live births, and most are term infants. Of affected infants, approximately one half of them have symptoms. A history of delivery-room resuscitation efforts or infant aspiration of meconium or blood often exists.[28-30] Pneumothoraces are very common in critically ill ventilated neonates, and the incidence increases with prematurity. Pneumothorax in an infant with the neonatal respiratory distress syndrome is associated with mortalities exceeding 60% in some studies.[31] Familial cases of spontaneous pneumothorax in neonates have also been described.[32,33]

PNEUMOMEDIASTINUM

Pneumomediastinum is uncommon in the pediatric population and is usually self-limited. Although no apparent consensus exists regarding classification of pneumomediastinum, the term *spontaneous pneumomediastinum* is used frequently in the medical literature and is applied to younger patients who have no obvious precipitating event.[34] The incidence of spontaneous pneumomediastinum detected by screening symptomatic infants was 25 of 10,000 live births.[35] The incidence of spontaneous pneumomediastinum in the noninfant pediatric population is not known. The most common etiology of spontaneous pneumomediastinum in pediatric patients is bronchospasm related to respiratory tract infection.[36] Because healthy young people do not often have severe symptoms or physical examination findings, spontaneous pneumomediastinum may go undetected, and the actual incidence is thus difficult to ascertain.

Pneumomediastinum is seen in a variety of clinical circumstances; it is often associated with exaggerated Valsalva maneuvers during cough, emesis, hiccupping, heavy lifting, straining at stool, illicit drug inhalation, and sports activities.[37,38] Pneumomediastinum has been noted in situations in which external pressure changes occur, such as scuba diving and air travel. Marked decreases in interstitial pressure such as that seen with hyperpnea from diabetic ketoacidosis can also cause pneumomediastinum.[39] Asthma is a well-recognized risk factor.[40,41] Pneumomediastinum is associated with barotrauma or volutrauma secondary to mechanical ventilation or manual resuscitative ventilation. The clinician must consider the possibility of foreign body as a cause of pneumomediastinum, especially in children younger than 6 years. Spontaneous esophageal perforation (Boerhaave syndrome) and mediastinitis must be considered in the differential diagnosis.

Pneumomediastinum can be secondary to trauma and has been reported in child abuse and other blunt thoracic trauma such as motor-vehicle crashes. Isolated facial trauma has also been reported as a cause.[42] Tracheobronchial and esophageal rupture can also cause pneumomediastinum. Care must be taken to evaluate for penetrating injury because air can enter the mediastinum from penetrating neck or chest wall injury.

EVALUATION OF PNEUMOTHORAX

History

Patients often note abrupt ipsilateral pleuritic chest pain with or without acute dyspnea. Pleuritic pain may be more prevalent in primary than in secondary spontaneous pneumothorax. Dyspnea is typically quite severe in patients with secondary spontaneous pneumothorax because they have decreased cardiopulmonary reserve at baseline. Symptoms associated with primary spontaneous pneumothorax often resolve within 24 hours, even if untreated. This feature contrasts with the progressive course of secondary spontaneous pneumothorax.[1] Respiratory symptoms might be vague in young children, and parents may note sudden dyspnea and irritability.

Physical Examination

The physical examination findings in primary spontaneous pneumothorax are variable and depend on the pneumothorax size and patient age. A patient with a pneumothorax occupying less than 15% of the hemithorax may have a normal physical examination.[1] Most commonly, vital signs demonstrate tachycardia and tachypnea. Hypoxemia caused by a small primary spontaneous pneumothorax is uncommon in older children because most will have adequate alveolar reserve to preserve oxygenation. However, smaller children are often hypoxemic.[5] Because the underlying lung function is normal, hypercarbia does not typically develop in patients with primary spontaneous pneumothorax. In contrast, patients with secondary spontaneous pneumothorax often have hypoxemia and hypercarbia, and as the size of the pneumothorax increases, characteristic signs such as diminished or absent breath sounds, hyper-resonance to percussion on the involved side, and chest asymmetry may be noted.

Neonates may have severe respiratory distress with marked tachypnea, grunting, retractions, and cyanosis.[29] In infants with respiratory distress syndrome or other underlying lung disease, pneumothorax can be rapidly life threatening. Such infants may demonstrate cardiorespiratory instability and progress to cardiac arrest.[43] Detection of pneumothorax by physical examination in infants can be difficult because of the small thorax size; however, a shift of the apical heart impulse away from the side of the pneumothorax has been reported to be a reliable sign.[29]

Iatrogenic pneumothorax should be suspected in any patient who becomes more dyspneic after a medical or surgical procedure known to be associated with the development of a pneumothorax. Iatrogenic pneumothorax should also be suspected in any patient treated with positive pressure ventilation who experiences a sudden clinical deterioration or demonstrates an unexplained increase in peak and plateau pressures or decreased tidal volume.

No matter the pneumothorax classification, hypotension, profound hypoxemia, or tracheal deviation in the setting of diminished breath sounds herald *tension* pneumothorax, which is life threatening and requires immediate attention. Intervention for tension pneumothorax should not be delayed for radiologic imaging to confirm the diagnosis.

Laboratory Testing

Pneumothorax diagnosis is routinely made by chest radiograph, preferably with the patient in an upright position. The main radiologic feature of a pneumothorax is a white visceral pleural line, separated from the parietal pleura by an avascular collection of gas (Figure 354-1). In many instances, no pulmonary vessels are visible beyond the visceral pleural edge. In films in which the patient is upright, the accumulation of gas occurs primarily in an apicolateral location. In supine views, more pleural gas is needed for definitive diagnosis of a pneumothorax. The pleural gas accumulates in a subpulmonic location, outlining the anterior pleural reflection, the costophrenic sulcus (the so-called *deep sulcus sign*), and the anterolateral border of the mediastinum.[44]

A computed tomographic (CT) scan can detect pneumothoraces that do not appear on radiograph (occult pneumothoraces) but is often not practical in the initial work-up. Portable ultrasound devices may play a role in the future, but application of thoracic ultrasound for pneumothorax in children has yet to be established. In young infants, neonatal pneumothorax must be differentiated from congenital lobar emphysema, which can appear as an expanded radiolucent pulmonary segment. A CT scan may be required to make this differentiation, which is important because the treatment for congenital lobar emphysema is lobectomy. Aspiration or chest tube placement in a patient with congenital lobar emphysema is associated with substantial risk of mortality.

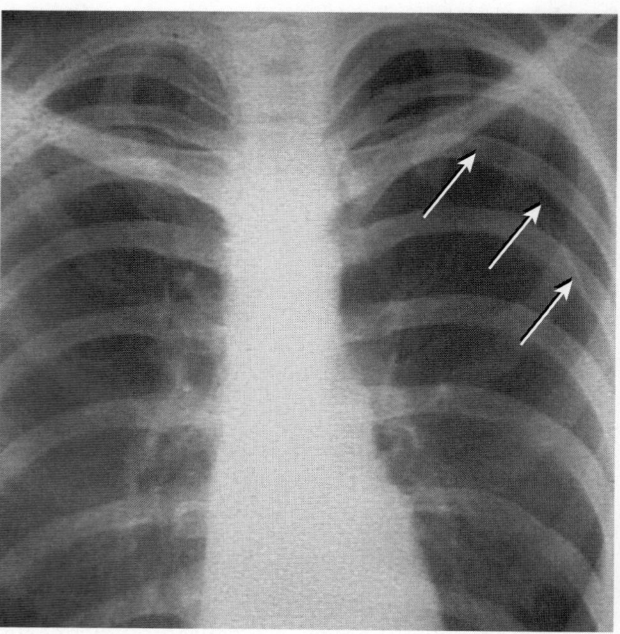

Figure 354-1 Pneumothorax: a white visceral pleural line, separated from the parietal pleura by radiolucent air. *(Used with permission by Richard Wiggins, MD.)*

In trauma patients, the presence of a large pneumothorax with persistent air leak into the pleural space despite tube thoracostomy is an indication for fiberoptic bronchoscopy to assess the possibility of a bronchial tear. Clinicians must also rule out traumatic rupture of the esophagus because the mortality approaches 100% if surgical treatment is not prompt.[45]

EVALUATION OF PNEUMOMEDIASTINUM

History and Physical Findings

Patients with pneumomediastinum may complain of chest pain, cough, and dyspnea, as well as dysphonia, dysphagia, or neck pain. The examination will often reveal subcutaneous cervical emphysema with crepitance. Less commonly, Hamman sign (a mediastinal crunching sound synchronized with systole) may be heard.

Laboratory Testing

Pneumomediastinum is recognized by air outlining mediastinal structures such as the thymus (sail sign) or the superior surface of the diaphragm (continuous-diaphragm sign). Pneumomediastinum is usually bilateral and does not move with decubitus positioning, which helps differentiate it from anteromedial

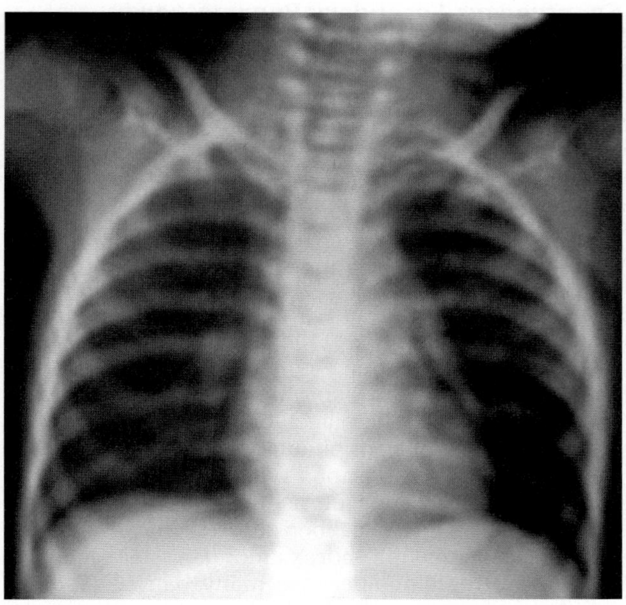

Figure 354-2 Pneumomediastinum. The mediastinal structures, usually invisible, are outlined, particularly the medial side of the descending aorta. (*Reprinted from Shaw,* Semin Pediatr Surg. *2003:12(1):55-61, with permission from Elsevier.)*

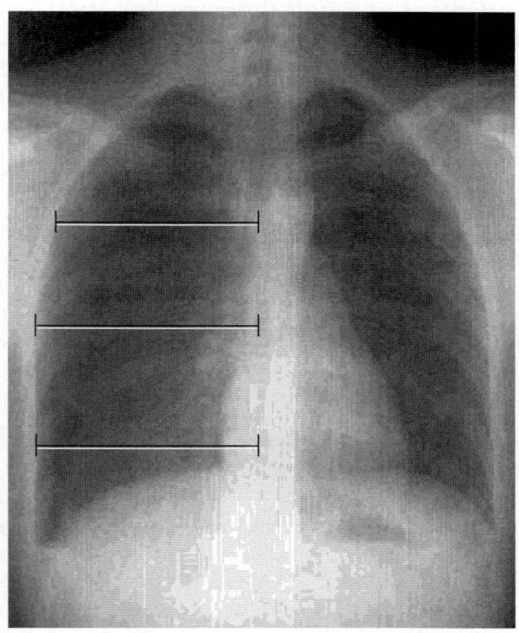

Figure 354-3 Measurements estimating volume of pneumothorax.

pneumothorax (Figure 354-2). However, pneumothorax may also be present.

MANAGEMENT OF PNEUMOTHORAX

Primary Spontaneous Pneumothorax

Management of Small Primary Spontaneous Pneumothorax in Adolescents and Young Adults

Although guidelines for the management of spontaneous pneumothorax in adult patients have been published by both the British Thoracic Society[27] and the American College of Chest Physicians,[2] no similar guidelines exist for treatment of infants and small children. The British and American adult guidelines distinguish between small and large primary spontaneous pneumothorax in the recommended treatment pathways. Small pneumothoraces are defined as less than 15% to 20% of the chest volume.

These guidelines estimate loss of lung volume by the distance from the lung apex to the ipsilateral thoracic cupola at the parietal surface on a standard upright radiograph.[2] This method is, however, a poor way of quantifying pneumothorax volume, usually underestimating it. The British Thoracic Society defines *small* as a rim less than 2 cm, whereas the American College of Chest Physicians define *small* as a rim less than 3 cm. This simple linear measurement is of little use for infants and small children but can be applied in adolescents and young adults. Another way to estimate the size of a pneumothorax is to realize that the volume of the lung approximates the ratio of the lung diameter to the hemithorax cubed. The clinician can measure the ratio of length of the lung to the hemithorax at several rib levels and apply the following formula:

$$\text{Estimated size of pneumothorax (\%)} = (1 - L^3/H^3) \times 100,$$

where H = diameter of the hemithorax, and L = diameter of the *collapsed* lung[45,46] (Figure 354-3).

Using this formula, a pneumothorax smaller than 15% would be considered small. If the pneumothorax size is small, and if the severity of acute symptoms is mild with unlabored breathing, and if room air saturations are greater than 90%, then supplemental oxygen and observation in the emergency department for 3 to 6 hours, followed by a repeat chest radiograph to exclude progression of the pneumothorax, is recommended for adolescents and young adults. Patients must have careful instructions to return for worsening shortness of breath and have follow-up in 12 hours to 2 days with a planned chest radiograph to document improvement.[2,27] Breathless patients should undergo intervention, regardless of pneumothorax size.[27] All patients should be referred to a lung specialist for follow-up care because they have recurrent risk of spontaneous pneumothorax. Smoking is a risk factor for primary spontaneous pneumothorax recurrence, and smoking cessation should be encouraged.[11] Supplemental oxygen is administered to all pneumothorax patients because it increases the pleural air reabsorption rate 3- to 4-fold above the baseline of 1.25% per day and is recommended to hasten resolution.[47] A 15% pneumothorax is expected to resolve in approximately 12 days without oxygen therapy.

Management of Small Primary Spontaneous Pneumothorax in Children

Children with small primary spontaneous pneumothorax are typically admitted for observation.[6,9,46] However, based on the adult guidelines, older children and adolescents with asymptomatic small primary spontaneous pneumothorax who have been observed in the emergency department for 3 to 6 hours can be discharged to home with close follow-up as recommended for adult patients. Any patient with breathlessness should be admitted and should undergo intervention to remove the air. Although simple needle aspiration has been advocated by experts in the United Kingdom, such is not standard practice in the United States.

Management of Moderate to Large Primary Spontaneous Pneumothorax in Adolescents and Young Adults

The British Guidelines recommend simple aspiration as the first-line treatment for all symptomatic primary spontaneous pneumothoraces and for all with greater than 2 cm rim of air on chest radiograph (large); however, the United States guidelines do not generally endorse attempts at simple aspiration over placement of a chest drain. Recent publications regarding primary spontaneous pneumothorax in adults show that aspiration is successful in more than 50% of cases but is more likely to fail if the pneumothorax is greater in size than 40%.[48] A randomized study of 50 adult participants showed that aspiration was immediately successful in 59% of adults compared with immediate resolution of the pneumothorax in 64% of patients treated with a chest drain. Of note, 48% of the patients who had simple aspiration were discharged from the emergency department compared with none of the patients treated with chest tube placement.[49] Success at 1 week did not differ between groups (93% vs 85%), and recurrence of spontaneous pneumothorax within 1 year was also similar (26% vs 27%). A meta-analysis of 3 randomized studies showed significantly shorter length of hospital stay with simple aspiration and equivalent success at 1 week compared with chest tube drainage.[50] No difference in recurrence of pneumothorax was noted for a year after the initial spontaneous pneumothorax between treatment groups.

In the British Guidelines, patients who have successful aspiration of a primary pneumothorax may be observed in the emergency department for similar follow-up.[27] The American College of Chest Physicians recommends placement of a chest drain for symptomatic or any large (>3 cm rim) primary spontaneous pneumothorax.[2] Patients are then managed with either a Heimlich value (one-way valve) or a chest tube to water seal or suction.

Management of Large Primary Spontaneous Pneumothorax in Children

Simple aspiration versus chest tube placement for children with large pneumothorax is based on experience of the treating physician. However, published pediatric series suggest that hospital admission with placement of a pleural catheter or chest tube is usual practice.[6,9,46]

Spontaneous Secondary Pneumothorax in Young Adults and Children

Guidelines recommend hospital admission for patients with spontaneous secondary pneumothorax for treatment of the underlying condition and symptomatic treatment of the pneumothorax, if needed. Small pneumothoraces can be treated with oxygen therapy and observed, whereas large pneumothoraces are drained either by aspiration[27] or by chest tube placement.[2,27]

Traumatic Pneumothorax

If a tension pneumothorax is suspected, then emergency needle aspiration of the second intercosal space in the midclavicular line is required. If the patient improves with needle aspiration, then a chest drain should immediately be placed on that side.[2] However, a substantial number of pneumothoraces are not seen on initial chest radiographs but are found on subsequent imaging (CT or ultrasound) of the chest.[51,52] Placement of a larger-caliber chest drain for symptomatic or large pneumothorax among trauma victims is customary treatment because many patients require positive pressure ventilation and may have an accompanying hemothorax. Small asymptomatic pneumothorax may be observed if the patient is not receiving positive pressure and radiographic evaluation does not reveal chest multitrauma.

Iatrogenic Pneumothorax

Treatment of iatrogenic pneumothorax should be tailored to the patient's clinical circumstance. Patients receiving positive pressure ventilation are at risk of extension of the pneumothorax and generally require chest tube placement. Patients who are not on mechanical support who have a small pneumothorax and limited symptoms can receive supportive care with close observation.

Chest Tube Insertion and Management

Planning

Before inserting a chest tube, a predrainage risk assessment is appropriate. Risk of hemorrhage should be corrected when possible; however, routine platelet count and bleeding times are recommended only for patients with known risk factors.[53] When possible, the clinician should obtain informed consent and provide sedation with standard monitoring.[54] Risks include bleeding, infection, failure of pneumothorax resolution, laceration of the lung, and extrathoracic placement with potential injury of abdominal organs. In 1 report, 3% of tubes were placed in an extrathoracic position, and 6% were placed in the lung parenchyma.[55]

Positioning

The preferred position for chest drain insertion is supine with the ipsilateral arm above the patient's head to expose the axilla. Alternative positions are for the patient to sit upright leaning over an adjacent table with a pillow or in a lateral decubitus position. The triangle in Figure 354-4 illustrates the safe area that is bordered by the lateral margin of pectoralis major muscle, the anterior margin of the latissimus dorsi muscle, the line superior to the horizontal level of the nipple, and an apex below the axilla. This supine

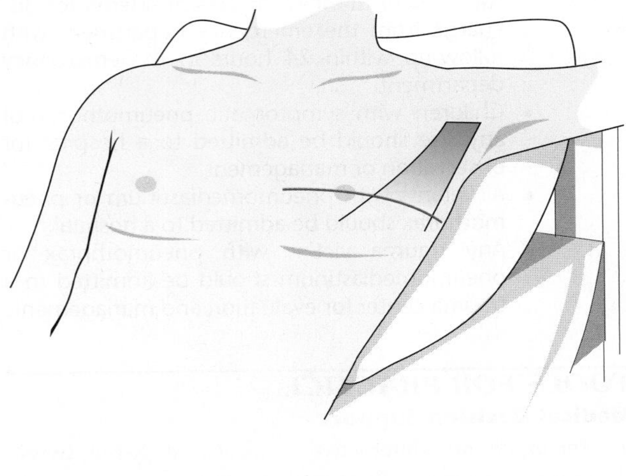

Figure 354-4 Diagram to illustrate the safe triangle. *(Laws D, Neville E, Duffy J, et al. BTS guidelines for the insertion of a chest drain.* Thorax. *2003;58(suppl 2):ii53-ii59. Reproduced with permission from the BMJ Publishing Group.)*

position minimizes risk to underlying structures such as the internal mammary arteries, breast tissue, and solid organs. A more posterior position is chosen if the pneumothorax is loculated and posterior. However, loculated collections are most safely approached under fluoroscopic guidance.[56] Although a more posterior position is safe, it is uncomfortable for the patient on which to lie after insertion and is at risk for kinking. The second intercostal space in the midclavicular line may be chosen for apical pneumothorax; however, this position is uncomfortable and may leave a visible scar. A survey of house officers showed that approximately one half did not know the recommended anatomic landmarks for safe chest tube insertion.[57]

Thoracostomy Tube Size Selection

Smaller tubes are recommended for aspirating air and are more comfortable compared with larger tubes, which are recommended for draining blood or a large air leak. Age-based sizes for thoracostomy tubes recommended for trauma victims by the American Heart Association[58] are shown in Table 354-1. These tubes are relatively large based on the patient size and are intended to drain blood if needed. The Adult Guidelines for pneumothorax management recommend relatively smaller tubes for draining air. The British Guidelines[27] recommend a No. 10 to 14 French tube for the management of pneumothorax in adults, whereas the American College of Chest Physicians recommends initial management with a No. 16 to 22 French tube in patients not at risk for large air leaks.[2] Roberts et al reported use of No. 7 and No. 8.5 French percutaneous pigtail catheters (polyurethane) in children, with resolution of pneumothorax in 75% of cases. In that study, the pigtail catheters drained serous fluid well (96% success) but were less effective for draining blood (81%) and

Table 354-1 Age-Based Sizes for Tracheostomy Tubes

AGE (WEIGHT IN KG)	CHEST TUBE SIZE (FRENCH)
Newborns (2-5 kg)	8-12
<1 yr (5-11 kg)	14-20
Children 1-8 yr (12-30 kg)	20-28
Children >8 yr (>30 kg)	29-36

ineffective for draining pus (0%).[59] The catheters are much more pliant and can be kinked by the chest wall in obese patients; the tubing connection also can be kinked.

Insertion Techniques

Small-bore chest tubes are usually inserted with the aid of a needle and guidewire using a modified Seldinger technique. Blunt dissection is not needed because a dilator is used. Blunt dissection of the subcutaneous tissue and muscle into the pleural cavity is performed for insertion of medium and large chest drains. A finger-sized opening allows exploration to ensure that no underlying organs will be damaged by tube insertion; creation of the track prevents excessive force. Once the tube is past the chest wall, it is directed apically to drain air and basally to drain fluid. The chest tube is then sutured in place. If an incision has been made, then 1 stitch is placed to assist with wound closure after tube removal, and 1 stitch is placed to secure the drain. A chest radiograph is obtained after insertion to check placement and resolution of the pneumothorax.

Management of Chest Drain

The chest tube is connected to a closed system with a water seal device. If the lung fails to expand quickly, then continuous suction delivered through a measured column of water is applied and remains until the lung has completely reexpanded.[2,27] The closed system allows detection of air bubbles through the water chamber, suggesting continued visceral pleural air leak. However, an air leak may be caused by a leak in the system; the chest tube air holes are outside the chest or the chest tubing connections are not airtight.

The chest tube should remain in place as long as persistent air leak is present. Surgical referral is recommended if air leak persists for longer than 4 to 7 days in patients without preexisting lung disease, and earlier referral is recommended if the lung fails to expand or in patients with a large air leak and underlying lung disease.[2,27] Chest tubes are removed in a staged manner after a pneumothorax is resolved. Suction is discontinued and the chest tube is placed on water seal. Opinions differ regarding the appropriate length of time for a water seal trial, ranging from 3 to 24 hours. After a trial on water seal, a chest radiograph is obtained to rule out recurrence.[2,60] The chest tube may then be removed. Clamping of a chest tube should never be done unless the clinician is expert in chest tube management and the patient has constant nursing supervision.[2,27]

Risk of Recurrence

Children with primary spontaneous pneumothorax have a 17% to 54% risk of recurrence,[6,61] with a greatest risk of recurrence within a year. Some experts recommend CT imaging to detect pleural blebs after initial pneumothorax to help determine risk of recurrence. However, at this point, surgical treatment is generally limited to children with recurrent pneumothorax.[61] Surgery usually involves repair of the air leak and adhering the visceral pleura to the parietal pleura (pleurodesis). Surgical approach via a mini thoracotomy or video-assisted thoracoscopic surgery (VATS) is based on surgeon's preference; however, VATS is associated with less postoperative pain and shorter hospital length of stay.[62]

MANAGEMENT OF PNEUMOMEDIASTINUM

Initial therapy for pneumomediastinum is directed at the underlying disease process. Because mediastinal air decompresses into the cervical fascia and rarely causes tamponade, observation is standard management. Efforts to lower intrathoracic pressures or tidal volume among patients receiving mechanical ventilation may decrease continued air leakage. If signs of tamponade occur, then placement of a mediastinal tube via echocardiographic guidance should be done by a specialist with skills in this procedure. Because of the high prevalence of asthma-related pneumomediastinum, children for whom the underlying cause of pneumomediastinum is unknown should undergo diagnostic pulmonary function tests after the acute episode.

WHEN TO REFER

- Infants and children with primary or secondary spontaneous pneumothorax or spontaneous pneumomediastinum should be referred to either a hospital or an emergency department for evaluation and management. All children with spontaneous pneumothorax should be referred to a lung specialist for follow-up because of the risk of recurrent pneumothorax.
- Infants and children with traumatic pneumothorax should be referred to a trauma center for evaluation and management.
- Infants and children with iatrogenic pneumothorax should be cared for by physicians with expertise in chest drain insertion and management.
- Infants and children with pneumomediastinum and signs of cardiac tamponade should be evaluated by a cardiologist or surgeon able to place a mediastinal drain.

WHEN TO ADMIT

- Children with asymptomatic small primary spontaneous pneumothorax who have been observed for 6 hours in the emergency department and who have reliable transportation and social circumstances can be considered for discharge from the emergency department with follow-up within 24 hours in the emergency department.
- Children with symptomatic pneumothorax of any size should be admitted to a hospital for observation or management.
- All infants with pneumomediastinum or pneumothorax should be admitted to a hospital.
- Any trauma victim with pneumothorax or pneumomediastinum should be admitted to a trauma center for evaluation and management.

TOOLS FOR PRACTICE

Medical Decision Support

- *Pneumothorax* (interactive tool), Chest X-ray (www.chestx-ray.com/calculator/PTX.html).

SUGGESTED RESOURCES

Baumann MH, Strange C, Heffner JE, et al. Management of spontaneous pneumothorax: an American College of Chest Physicians Delphi consensus statement. *Chest.* 2001;119(2):590-602.

Henry M, Arnold T, Harvey J. BTS guidelines for the management of spontaneous pneumothorax. *Thorax.* 2003;58(suppl 2):ii39-ii52.

Laws D, Neville E, Duffy J. BTS guidelines for the insertion of a chest drain. *Thorax.* 2003;58(suppl 2):ii53-ii59.

REFERENCES

1. Sahn SA, Heffner JE. Spontaneous pneumothorax. *N Engl J Med.* 2000;342(12):868-874.
2. Baumann MH, Strange C, Heffner JE, et al. Management of spontaneous pneumothorax: an American College of Chest Physicians Delphi consensus statement. *Chest.* 2001;119(2):590-602.
3. Macklin C. Transport of air along sheaths of pulmonic blood vessels from alveoli to mediastinum: clinical implications. *Arch Intern Med.* 1939;64:913-926.
4. Light RW. Disorders of the pleura, mediastinum, and diaphragm. In: Isselbacher KJ, ed. *Harrison's Principles of Internal Medicine.* 13th ed. New York, NY: McGraw-Hill; 1994.
5. Alter SJ. Spontaneous pneumothorax in infants: a 10-year review. *Pediatr Emerg Care.* 1997;13(6):401-403.
6. Wilcox DT, Glick PL, Karamanoukian HL, et al. Spontaneous pneumothorax: a single-institution, 12-year experience in patients under 16 years of age. *J Pediatr Surg.* 1995;30(10):1452-1454.
7. Lesur O, Delorme N, Fromaget JM, et al. Computed tomography in the etiologic assessment of idiopathic spontaneous pneumothorax. *Chest.* 1990;98(2):341-347.
8. Bense L, Lewander R, Eklund G, et al. Nonsmoking, non-alpha 1-antitrypsin deficiency-induced emphysema in nonsmokers with healed spontaneous pneumothorax, identified by computed tomography of the lungs. *Chest.* 1993;103(2):433-438.
9. Poenaru D, Yazbeck S, Murphy S. Primary spontaneous pneumothorax in children. *J Pediatr Surg.* 1994;29(9):1183-1185.
10. Melton LJ, Hepper NG, Offord KP. Incidence of spontaneous pneumothorax in Olmsted County, Minnesota: 1950 to 1974. *Am Rev Respir Dis.* 1979;120(6):1379-1382.

11. Bense L, Eklund G, Wiman LG. Smoking and the increased risk of contracting spontaneous pneumothorax. *Chest*. 1987;92(6):1009-1012.
12. Gupta D, Hansell A, Nichols T, et al. Epidemiology of pneumothorax in England. *Thorax*. 2000;55(8): 666-671.
13. Afessa B,. Morales I, Cury JD. Clinical course and outcome of patients admitted to an ICU for status asthmaticus. *Chest*. 2001;120(5):1616-1621.
14. Flume PA, Strange C, Ye X, et al. Pneumothorax in cystic fibrosis. *Chest*. 2005;128(2):720-728.
15. Noppen M, Verbanck S, Harvey J, et al. Music: a new cause of primary spontaneous pneumothorax. *Thorax*. 2004;59(8):722-724.
16. Wilson KC, Saukkonen JJ. Acute respiratory failure from abused substances. *J Intensive Care Med*. 2004;19(4): 183-193.
17. Crankson SJ, Fischer JD, Al-Rabeeah AA, et al. Pediatric thoracic trauma. *Saudi Med J*. 2001;22(2):117-120.
18. Peclet MH, Newman KD, Eichelberger MR, et al. Thoracic trauma in children: an indicator of increased mortality. *J Pediatr Surg*. 1990;25(9):961-965; discussion 965-966.
19. Ruddy RM. Trauma and the paediatric lung. *Paediatr Respir Rev*. 2005;6(1):61-67.
20. Cooper A, Barlow B, DiScala C, et al. Mortality and truncal injury: the pediatric perspective. *J Pediatr Surg*. 1994;29(1):33-38.
21. Horbar JD, Badger GJ, Carpenter JH, et al. Trends in mortality and morbidity for very low birth weight infants, 1991-1999. *Pediatrics*. 2002;110(1 pt 1):143-151.
22. Sedman A, Harris JM, Schulz K, et al. Relevance of the Agency for Healthcare Research and Quality Patient Safety Indicators for children's hospitals. *Pediatrics*. 2005;115(1):135-145.
23. McCallion N, Davis PG, Morley CJ. Volume-targeted versus pressure-limited ventilation in the neonate. *Cochrane Database Syst Rev*. 2005(3):CD003666.
24. Greenough A, Milner AD, Dimitriou G. Synchronized mechanical ventilation for respiratory support in newborn infants. *Cochrane Database Syst Rev*. 2004(4): CD000456.
25. Suresh GK, Soll RF. Overview of surfactant replacement trials. *J Perinatol*. 2005;25(suppl 2):S40-S44.
26. Despars JA, Sassoon CS, Light RW. Significance of iatrogenic pneumothoraces. *Chest*. 1994;105(4): 1147-1150.
27. Henry M, Arnold T, Harvey J. BTS guidelines for the management of spontaneous pneumothorax. *Thorax*. 2003;58(suppl 2):ii39-ii52.
28. Norton LE, DiMaio VJ, Zumwalt RE. Spontaneous pneumothorax in the newborn: a report of two fatalities. *J Forensic Sci*. 1978;23(3):508-510.
29. Chernick V, Avery ME. Spontaneous alveolar rupture at birth. *Pediatrics*. 1963;32:816-824.
30. Steele RW, Metz JR, Bass JW, et al. Pneumothorax and pneumomediastinum in the newborn. *Radiology*. 1971;98(3):629-632.
31. Walker MW, Shoemaker M, Riddle K, et al. Clinical process improvement: reduction of pneumothorax and mortality in high-risk preterm infants. *J Perinatol*. 2002; 22(8):641-645.
32. Bagchi I, Nycyk JA. Familial spontaneous pneumothorax. *Arch Dis Child Fetal Neonatal Ed*. 2002;87(1):F70.
33. Kugelman A, Riskin A, Weinger-Abend M, et al. Familial neonatal pneumothorax associated with transient tachypnea of the newborn. *Pediatr Pulmonol*. 2003; 36(1):69-72.
34. Newcomb AE, Clarke CP. Spontaneous pneumomediastinum: a benign curiosity or a significant problem? *Chest*. 2005;128(5):3298-3302.
35. Morrow G, Hope JW, Boggs TR, Jr. Pneumomediastinum, a silent lesion in the newborn. *J Pediatr*. 1967; 70(4):554-560.
36. Chapdelaine J, Beaunoyer M, Daigneault P, et al. Spontaneous pneumomediastinum: are we overinvestigating? *J Pediatr Surg*. 2004;39(5):681-684.
37. Abolnik I, Lossos IS, Breuer R. Spontaneous pneumomediastinum. A report of 25 cases. *Chest*. 1991;100(1): 93-95.
38. Morgan EJ, Henderson DA. Pneumomediastinum as a complication of athletic competition. *Thorax*. 1981; 36(2):155-156.
39. Bratton SL, O'Rourke PP. Spontaneous pneumomediastinum. *J Emerg Med*. 1993;11(5):525-529.
40. Eggleston PA, Ward BH, Pierson WE, et al. Radiographic abnormalities in acute asthma in children. *Pediatrics*. 1974;54(4):442-449.
41. Stack AM, Caputo GL. Pneumomediastinum in childhood asthma. *Pediatr Emerg Care*. 1996;12(2):98-101.
42. Monksfield P, Whiteside O, Jaffe S, et al. Pneumomediastinum, an unusual complication of facial trauma. *Ear Nose Throat J*. 2005;84(5):298-301.
43. Ogata ES, Gregory GA, Kitterman JA, et al. Pneumothorax in the respiratory distress syndrome: incidence and effect on vital signs, blood gases, and pH. *Pediatrics*. 1976;58(2):177-183.
44. Stark P. The Pleura. In: Taveras JM, Ferrucci JT, eds. Radiology: Diagnosis/imaging/intervention. Philadelphia, Pa: Lippincott-Raven; 2000:1-29.
45. Light R. Pneumothorax, chylothorax, hemothorax, and fibrothorax. In: Mason RJ, ed. *Murray & Nadel's Textbook of Respiratory Medicine*. 4th ed. Philadelphia, PA: Saunders Elsevier; 2005.
46. Shaw KS, Prasil P, Nguyen LT, et al. Pediatric spontaneous pneumothorax. *Semin Pediatr Surg*. 2003;12(1):55-61.
47. Northfield TC. Oxygen therapy for spontaneous pneumothorax. *BMJ*. 1971;4(779):86-88.
48. Chan SS, Lam PK. Simple aspiration as initial treatment for primary spontaneous pneumothorax: results of 91 consecutive cases. *J Emerg Med*. 2005;28(2):133-138.
49. Noppen M, Alexander P, Driesen P, et al. Manual aspiration versus chest tube drainage in first episodes of primary spontaneous pneumothorax: a multicenter, prospective, randomized pilot study. *Am J Respir Crit Care Med*. 2002;165(9):1240-1244.
50. Devanand A, Koh MS, Ong TH, et al. Simple aspiration versus chest-tube insertion in the management of primary spontaneous pneumothorax: a systematic review. *Respir Med*. 2004;98(7):579-590.
51. Jaffer U, McAuley D. Best evidence topic report. Transthoracic ultrasonography to diagnose pneumothorax in trauma. *Emerg Med J*. 2005;22(7):504-505.
52. Trupka A, Waydhas C, Hallfeldt KK, et al. Value of thoracic computed tomography in the first assessment of severely injured patients with blunt chest trauma: results of a prospective study. *J Trauma*. 1997;43(3):405-411.
53. Laws D, Neville E, Duffy J, et al. BTS guidelines for the insertion of a chest drain. *Thorax*. 2003;58(suppl 2): ii53-ii59.
54. Hoffman GM, Nowakowski R, Troshynski TJ, et al. Risk reduction in pediatric procedural sedation by application of an American Academy of Pediatrics/American Society of Anesthesiologists process model. *Pediatrics*. 2002;109(2):236-243.
55. Baldt MM, Bankier AA, Germann PS, et al. Complications after emergency tube thoracostomy: assessment with CT. *Radiology*. 1995;195(2):539-543.
56. O'Connor AR, Morgan WE. Radiological review of pneumothorax. *BMJ*. 2005;330(7506):1493-1497.

57. Griffiths JR, Roberts N. Do junior doctors know where to insert chest drains safely? *Postgrad Med J.* 2005; 81(957):456-458.
58. Chameides L, Hazinski MF, American Academy of Pediatrics, American Heart Association, Subcommittee on Pediatric Resuscitation. *Pediatric Advanced Life Support.* 1998 ed. Dallas, TX: American Heart Association; 1997.
59. Roberts JS, Bratton SL, Brogan TV. Efficacy and complications of percutaneous pigtail catheters for thoracostomy in pediatric patients. *Chest.* 1998;114(4): 1116-1121.
60. Schulman CI, Cohn SM, Blackbourne L, et al. How long should you wait for a chest radiograph after placing a chest tube on water seal? A prospective study. *J Trauma.* 2005;59(1):92-95.
61. Qureshi FG, Sandulache VC, Richards, et al. Primary vs delayed surgery for spontaneous pneumothorax in children: which is better? *J Pediatr Surg.* 2005;40(1): 166-169.
62. Sawada S, Watanabe Y, Moriyama S. Video-assisted thoracoscopic surgery for primary spontaneous pneumothorax: evaluation of indications and long-term outcome compared with conservative treatment and open thoracotomy. *Chest.* 2005;127(6):2226-2230.

Chapter 355
POISONING

Jeffrey S. Fine, MD; Marc A. Auerbach, MD; Kevin Y. Ching, MD; Katherine T. Fullerton, MD; Eric R. Weinberg, MD

Injuries are a leading cause of pediatric morbidity and mortality, and poisoning is one important mechanism of injury. As a result, physicians who provide primary care to children have been at the forefront in promoting the field of medical toxicology, particularly in the area of poison prevention. This chapter reviews the epidemiologic considerations of pediatric poisoning and provides more specific information on some important poisonings.

EPIDEMIOLOGIC FEATURES

Ingestion of potentially toxic substances is a common pediatric problem. More than 2 million exposures are reported each year to the American Association of Poison Control Centers (AAPCC); 65% are exposures that involve children and adolescents up to 19 years of age. Children under the age of 6 account for approximately 80% of these pediatric exposures. Boys account for 55% of childhood exposures and 45% of the adolescent reports.[1]

Childhood exposures peak in children between 1 and 3 years of age. In young children, ingestions result from the natural curiosity, increasing mobility and dexterity, and typical oral exploration displayed by toddlers.[2] The toxicity, if it occurs, is unintentional.

Several characteristics differentiate childhood exposures from adolescent and adult exposures: (1) they are unintentional; (2) only one agent is involved; (3) the agents are frequently nontoxic; (4) the amount ingested is small; and (5) toddlers are brought in for evaluation soon after the ingestion is discovered.

Certain behavioral characteristics increase the risk of ingestion, such as hyperactivity, impulsive risk-taking behavior, rebelliousness, and negativistic attitude.[3] In addition, social isolation, poor parenting skills, and maternal depression have been identified as family variables that predispose young children to unintentional poisonings.[4] Unintentional exposures occur at times of family disorganization, with deviations from normal routines (eg, household moving, spring cleaning, vacation, holidays), and during times of family stress (eg, sickness, death, divorce).[5] Repeat exposures may occur in 10% to 40% of childhood poisoning victims.[6,7]

Most childhood exposures occur in the child's own home.[8,9] One common site of exposure within the home is the kitchen, where cleaning and polishing products are often stored underneath the sink or on easily accessible lower cabinet shelves. Improper storage of solvents and cleaning agents in drinking glasses, cups, and beverage bottles contributes to the risk of unintentional exposures.[10] Medications are sometimes stored in the refrigerator or left out on the kitchen table. In the bedroom, medications are left out on the dresser or on the bedside table. Medications and cosmetics are also kept in the bathroom, another common site for an unintentional exposure. The grandparents' home is another setting where unintentional exposures may occur.[11] Grandparents often have cardiovascular or psychotropic medications at home and may not be as vigilant as parents in child-proofing their home.[8] Grandparents' medications may not be in child-resistant containers.

Poisoning is unusual in children younger than 6 months. It may result from a medication error,[12] intentional administration of a drug by a parent or sibling,[13,14] or passive exposure to a psychoactive substance—for example, exposure to the smoke of crack cocaine.[15-20] Child abuse and neglect should be part of the differential diagnosis of all cases of childhood poisoning, particularly when the child is younger than 1 year.[13] Children who ingest poisons may also be at risk for other types of injuries.[21,22]

Unintentional ingestion is unusual after age 5 years. For school-aged children, poisoning may be a reflection of intrafamilial stress or suicidal intent. For older children and adolescents, exposure is intentional, the result of either a suicidal gesture or the use of psychoactive substances; the resulting toxicity may be unintentional. Adolescents are also at risk for repeat exposures.[23]

Table 355-1 lists the AAPCC categories of agents to which children and adolescents are frequently exposed. Most pediatric exposures are to common plants and products found around the house, as well as to pharmaceutical products. Pharmaceutical agents account for the majority of fatalities. Table 355-2 lists the categories of agents responsible for poisoning fatalities. A comparison with Table 355-1 demonstrates that many exposures do not cause significant toxicity. Most childhood poisoning fatalities are caused by analgesic agents, carbon monoxide, hydrocarbons, and cold preparations. In contrast, most adolescent fatalities are caused by analgesic agents, drugs of abuse, psychiatric medications, and hydrocarbons. In adolescents, hydrocarbon fatalities are related to inhalant abuse.

Poison-related mortality is low overall; poisoning deaths represent 2.5% of annual childhood and adolescent

Table 355-1 Top Poison Exposure Categories*

CATEGORY	PERCENTAGE OF ALL REPORTED EXPOSURES
AGE <6 YR	
Cosmetics and personal care products	13
Cleaning substances	10
Analgesics	7
Topical agents	6
Plants	6
Cough and cold preparations	5
Insecticides, pesticides, rodenticides	4
Vitamins	3
Gastrointestinal preparations	3
Antimicrobial drugs	3
Other	40
AGE 6-19 YR	
Analgesics	14
Cough and cold preparations	6
Antidepressants	5
Cleaning substances	5
Cosmetics and personal care products	5
Stimulants and street drugs	4
Sedative-hypnotic drugs	4
Antihistamines	3
Art and craft supplies	3
Plants	3
Other	44

*Does not include envenomations or foreign bodies. Data from Fine J. Pediatric principles. In: Goldfrank LR, Flomenbaum NE, Lewin NA, et al, eds. *Goldfrank's Toxicologic Emergencies.* 8th ed. New York, NY: McGraw-Hill; 2006. Reprinted by permission of The McGraw-Hill Companies.

Table 355-2 Top Fatal Poisoning Categories

CATEGORY	PERCENTAGE OF ALL REPORTED FATALITIES
AGE <6 YR	
Analgesic agents	24
Carbon monoxide	14
Hydrocarbons	11
Cough, cold, antihistamine preparations	10
Insecticides, pesticides, rodenticides	5
Envenomations	4
Cardiovascular agents	4
Anticonvulsants	3
Antidepressants and antipsychotics	3
Drugs of abuse	3
AGE 6-19 YR	
Analgesic agents	26
Drugs of abuse	26
Antidepressants, antipsychotics	12
Hydrocarbons	10
Cough, cold, antihistamine preparations	4
Alcohols	3
Carbon monoxide	3
Cleaning agents and chemicals	3
Cardiovascular agents	2
Sedative hypnotic agents	2

Adapted from Fine J. Pediatric principles. In: Goldfrank LR, Flomenbaum NE, Lewin NA, et al, eds. *Goldfrank's Toxicologic Emergencies.* 8th ed. New York, NY: McGraw-Hill; 2006. Reprinted by permission of The McGraw-Hill Companies.

deaths from unintentional injury.[24] For children younger than 6 years, the AAPCC reports an average of 24 deaths per year from 1983 to 2004. These deaths represent almost 4% of the poisoning fatalities for all age groups and a 94% decrease from a high of 456 in 1959.[25] Factors contributing to this decline include parental anticipatory guidance, preventive measures that include child-resistant closures and unit-dose packaging, and improved medical care.

Childhood exposures have changed in recent years. Aspirin overdoses, once a leading cause of death in children, are now rare.[26,27] This change may be related to packaging changes and to the decreased antipyretic and analgesic use of aspirin at home because of its association with Reye syndrome.[28-31] Some agents, such as kerosene or lye, which remain a significant risk in other countries, are rare causes of poison-related mortality in the United States.

Iron poisoning was also formerly a leading cause of poison-related mortality; but now, childhood iron poisoning is rare. This reduction is the result of changes in packaging. In 1997 the US Food and Drug Administration (FDA) issued a regulation to package products with 30 mg or more of elemental iron per tablet in unit-dose packages such as blister packs.[32] In 2003 this rule was overturned when the determination was made that the FDA did not have the statutory authority to regulate a drug for the purpose of poison prevention.[33]

PREVENTION

Every child is at risk for a potentially toxic exposure; thus effective prevention strategies are directed toward the environment of all children and require parental cooperation. Primary care physicians must educate parents and caregivers in the importance of safe storage practices for household products and prescription drugs, as well as the use of child-resistant closures, the only preventive measure of proven efficacy.[34] The American Academy of Pediatrics (AAP) recommends anticipatory guidance about poisoning prevention beginning with the 6-month well-child visit. Educational materials are available from the AAP as part of the Injury Prevention Program. All parents should be given the telephone number of the local or regional poison control center and should be advised to keep the number posted by the telephone for immediate use if necessary.

With respect to prevention, a caretaker's primary responsibilities include selecting appropriate products for storage within the home, selecting an appropriate place to store these products, and practicing prompt disposal of old, unused, and unnecessary medications and potentially toxic materials. Toxic substances (medications, psychoactive substances, alcohol, household chemicals and products) must be inaccessible to children

BOX 355-1 Agents With Significant Toxicity in Toddlers After a Small Dose

AntihistaminesBenzocaine
β-Adrenergic antagonists (sustained release)
Calcium-channel antagonists (sustained release)
Camphor
Clonidine
Diphenoxylate-atropine (Lomotil)
Ethylene glycol
Methanol
Methylsalicylate (oil of wintergreen)
Opioids (methadone, codeine, OxyContin)
Phenothiazine
Quinine, chloroquine
Sulfonylurea antidiabetic agents
Theophylline
Tricyclic antidepressants

and stored in locked cabinets or boxes. These agents should be kept in their original containers so that they are not mistaken for food, beverages, or nontoxic products. If toxic substances are no longer being used, then they should be safely discarded in a manner that prevents access by the child, such as flushing unused medications down the toilet.

Parents should be advised to exercise particular care with agents that can be fatal to a toddler in small doses (Box 355-1).[35,36] They should also be cautioned about a few agents to which children are infrequently exposed but which cause severe toxicity, such as acetonitrile (artificial fingernail remover), ammonium fluoride (wheel cleaner, rust-removal agent), selenious acid (gun bluing compound), and brodifacoum (superwarfarin rat poison).[37]

PRINCIPLES OF MANAGEMENT

General Considerations

Primary care physicians should be familiar with the signs, symptoms, and management of common acute ingestions. Specific, recent toxicology textbooks are an important part of an office library.[38-40] Poisindex, a commercial poison information software package available as part of Micro Medex, is generally available in emergency treatment facilities and in many medical libraries.[41]

Primary care physicians should be familiar with community resources that can provide information or practical help with acute poisonings. Pharmacists can provide information about medications when the name of the medication or the amount dispensed does not appear on the label. Manufacturers can help identify the chemicals in a commercial product. An emergency care facility should be readily available for the transfer of patients who are in need of immediate evaluation.

Poison control centers provide comprehensive information on poison management and can usually help organize referral to an appropriate treatment facility. A list of regional poison centers can be found at the Web site of the AAPCC (www.aapcc.org/). The AAPCC toll-free telephone number is 800-222-1222.

Telephone Calls

Telephone triage is an important first step in managing potentially toxic exposures. Many exposures can be managed over the telephone, although home therapy of serious poisonings is limited. The practitioner should determine the name and type of agent, the quantity involved, the weight of the child, and the presence or absence of symptoms. The relative risk of toxicity can then be estimated. Alternatively, symptoms alone may indicate toxicity, despite the fact that, by history, neither the agent nor the dose would have predicted it. In the case of nontoxic exposures, reassurance is appropriate.

Prompt decontamination may reduce subsequent symptoms and the need for further treatment. Skin and eyes may be washed in the home or office, if appropriate. Activated charcoal is available in some areas for home administration, but its use has not gained widespread acceptance.

When the history of the exposure or the reported signs and symptoms suggest likely acute toxicity, the patient will be expeditiously transferred to an emergency care facility, preferably one with pediatric and toxicologic expertise and experience.

Although many of these initial calls can be managed by primary care practitioners, especially in the case of nontoxic exposures, all calls regarding potentially toxic exposures should be referred to trained poison information specialists at local and regional poison control centers.

Poisoning and injury prevention should be discussed with parents within a few days of a poison exposure call. Experience suggests that addressing prevention at the time of the initial call is less effective than doing so later. The recent exposure focuses the mind of the parents, providing a valuable opportunity to impart advice on poison prevention.

Approach to the Symptomatic Patient

When no specific history of a toxic exposure can be found, the diagnosis of poisoning can be challenging. The signs and symptoms of poisoning can mimic those of many acute illnesses; therefore the possibility of toxic exposure should be considered in the differential diagnosis. The rapid onset of central nervous system (CNS), gastrointestinal (GI), or respiratory symptoms should alert the physician to ask about possible exposure to medications, gases or fumes (eg, carbon monoxide), or to other potentially harmful substances around the home. The physician should always consider the possibility of poisoning when faced with a puzzling situation in which the diagnosis is unclear. Any patient with a possible or confirmed exposure to a toxic substance should be managed in consultation with poison specialists available through a local or regional poison control center.

Some toxins such as opioids or anticholinergic agents produce a typical constellation of signs and symptoms known as a *toxidrome*, or toxic syndrome

Table 355-3 Toxidromes

Sympathomimetic	*Opioid*
Agitation	Respiratory depression
Diaphoresis	Miosis
Fever	Coma
Mydriasis	Bradycardia
Tachycardia	
Anticholinergic	*Cholinergic*
Blind as a bat—mydriasis	D-efecation
Dry as a bone—dry skin	U-rination
Hot as Hades—fever	M-iosis, muscle fasciculations, muscle weakness
Red as a beet—red	B-ronchorrhea, bradycardia, bronchospasm
Mad as a hatter—central nervous system stimulation	E-mesis
Decreased gastrointestinal motility—decreased bowel sounds	L-acrimation
Urinary retention—full bladder	S-alivation

(Table 355-3). When present, these toxidromes may suggest a likely toxin.

This chapter focuses on the medical management of acute poisonings. For many patients, this part represents only the first phase of a complete evaluation. The term *medically clear* is used to describe the status of a patient once the risk of toxic effects is past or actual toxic manifestations are resolved. At that point, many patients will require appropriate consultation with mental health services for evaluation of acute suicidal thoughts and assessment for psychiatric admission.

THERAPEUTIC MODALITIES

The important principles of management of acute poisonings are (1) resuscitation—attention to the ABCs (airway, breathing, and circulation) and D (disability—altered mental status and seizures), (2) decontamination, (3) administration of specific antidotes, (4) enhanced elimination, and (5) supportive care. Although management will typically follow this sequence, in certain cases, priorities will differ. For example, in a chemical terrorism event, decontamination may need to precede any medical intervention, even resuscitation. After an opioid overdose with respiratory arrest, administration of naloxone, an opioid antidote, is part of resuscitation.

Resuscitation

Some poisons cause toxicity that requires immediate attention. Such effects include airway obstruction, difficulty breathing, dysrhythmias, hypotension, and seizures. Specific details of the resuscitation of the poisoned patient are beyond the scope of this chapter; however, resuscitation generally proceeds according to the recommendations of pediatric advanced life support (PALS) and advanced cardiac life support (ACLS).

Patients with airway obstruction or respiratory failure require urgent airway management and may require assisted ventilation or endotracheal intubation. Patients with respiratory depression should receive an empiric trial of naloxone. This agent will be both diagnostic and therapeutic for opioid (or clonidine) intoxication and may preclude the need for intubation. An escalating dosing scheme allows administration of sufficient naloxone to reverse respiratory depression without precipitating withdrawal in a chronic user (Table 355-4).[42,43] For patients with a prolonged opioid effect that outlasts the effect of a single dose of naloxone, it can be administered as a continuous infusion. Although naloxone administration may precipitate seizures as part of the withdrawal syndrome in newborns born to opioid-dependent mothers, seizures are not a typical part of the withdrawal syndrome in chronic users.

Hypotension should be treated with a saline bolus and infusion. Hypotension unresponsive to fluid alone may require the use of a vasopressor. Although use of dopamine is common, it acts indirectly by releasing epinephrine and norepinephrine, which are stored within the nerve terminal. When these stores are depleted, a direct-acting agent such as norepinephrine may be useful.

Patients experiencing cardiovascular toxicity from certain agents such as clonidine, β-blockers, calcium-channel blockers, tricyclic antidepressant agents, cocaine, and type 1 antidysrhythmic agents (eg, quinidine) may benefit from antidotal therapy (see Table 355-4).

Many toxins cause altered mental status, and several antidotes may be appropriately administered during the resuscitation phase. Although the primary reason for administering naloxone is to reverse respiratory depression, patients who have coma related to opioid intoxication may wake up after administration of naloxone.

All patients with altered mental status should be evaluated for hypoglycemia at the bedside by a glucose oxidase test strip. Hypoglycemia should be promptly treated with dextrose (see Table 355-4). However, there is little risk associated with empirically administering a large dose of glucose to a child or adolescent with altered mental status, and many clinicians opt to administer glucose without specific bedside testing. If a patient is intoxicated with an antidiabetic agent that has a long half-life (eg, glipizide), then a continuous intravenous dextrose infusion or the administration of octreotide may be required (see Table 355-4).

Table 355-4 Antidote Table*

SUBSTANCE	ANTIDOTE	DOSE	COMMENTS
Acetaminophen	N-acetylcysteine	IV: 150 mg/kg over 15 min, then 50 mg/kg over 4 hr, then 100 mg/kg over 16 hr PO: 140 mg/kg load, then 70 mg/kg/dose every 4 hr for 17 doses	AE: vomiting (PO); anaphylactoid reaction (IV). IV protocol requires large volumes of free water, which may cause hyponatremia and seizures in children.
Anticholinergic agents (eg, atropine)	Physostigmine	P: 0.5 mg IV slowly A: 2 mg IV slowly	May repeat dose after 15 min. AE: cholinergic symptoms occur with excessive dosing.
Benzodiazepines	Flumazenil	P: 0.01 mg/kg IV slowly every min (max 1 mg) A: 0.1-0.2 mg IV slowly every min (max 1 mg)	Titrate to effect or maximal dose. May not reverse respiratory depression. If positive response is of short duration, may be administered as a continuous infusion. AE: withdrawal symptoms in dependent or chronic use; seizures or dysrhythmias in cyclic antidepressant overdose.
β-Adrenergic antagonists (BB)	Glucagon	P: 0.1 mg/kg IV slowly A: 3-5 mg IV slowly	If positive response is of short duration, may be administered as a continuous infusion. AE: vomiting, hyperglycemia, hypocalcemia.
	Insulin and dextrose	Insulin 0.5 U/kg/hr IV with Dextrose 1 g/kg/hr	AE: hypo- or hyperglycemia, hypokalemia.
	Amrinone	750 mcg/kg over 3-5 min slowly (max 3 mg/kg)	May use other phosphodiesterase inhibitors with equal efficacy (eg, milrinone). AE: hypotension.
Carbon monoxide	Oxygen (100%)	100% Oxygen by nonrebreather	Treat until normal CO level or until hyperbaric oxygen initiated.
	Oxygen (hyperbaric)	100% Oxygen at 2-3 atmosphere for 20 min	AE: pneumothorax, perforated tympanic membrane.
Calcium-channel blockers (CCB)	Calcium chloride (10%)	P: 20 mg/kg (0.2 mL/kg) IV slowly, via central line A: 1-2 g (10-20 mL) IV slowly	May use glucagon, insulin, and dextrose as adjunctive treatment in CCB as in BB toxicity.
	Calcium gluconate (10%)	P: 60 mg/kg (0.6 mL/kg) A: 3-6 g (30-60 mL) IV	AE: hypercalcemia, phlebitis, nausea, vomiting, flushing, confusion, angina.
Cyanide	Amyl nitrate	One ampule by inhalation for 30 seconds every 3 min until IV access	AE: methemoglobinemia (see caution for sodium nitrite below).
	Sodium nitrite (3%)	P: 0.33 mL (10 mg) IV (for Hb at 12) A: 10 mL IV over 10 min	Dose varies according to weight and Hb level. See package insert. AE: methemoglobinemia. Use with caution in unconfirmed or unlikely cyanide poisoning (eg, in the setting of smoke inhalation), because induced methemoglobinemia may exacerbate hypoxemia from other causes.
	Sodium thiosulfate (25%)	P: 1.6 mL/kg IV (for Hb at 12) A: 50 mL IV over 3 min	Dose varies according to weight and Hb count. See package insert. AE: hypotension, CNS toxicity.
Digoxin	Digoxin-specific antibody fragments (Digibind)	For known ingested dose: number of vials = mg ingested × 1.5 For known serum digoxin concentration (SDC, ng/mL): number of vials = SDC × weight (kg)/100 For unknown SDC or dose acute overdose: 10-20 vials For chronic overdose: P: 2 vials; A: 5 vials	Each 40-mg vial binds 0.6 mg digoxin. AE: hypokalemia, worsening CHF.

Table 355-4 Antidote Table*—cont'd

SUBSTANCE	ANTIDOTE	DOSE	COMMENTS
Ethylene glycol and methanol	Ethanol (10%)	800 mg/kg (8 mL/kg) IV over 20-60 min, then 80-130 mg/kg/hr (0.8-1.3 mL/kg/hr) IV	Titrate to serum ethanol 100 mg/dL. Increase dose during dialysis and in chronic alcoholics. Oral dosing may be used in select cases.
	Fomepizole (4-methylpyrazole)	15 mg/kg over 30 min IV, then 10 mg/kg/dose every 12 hr × 4 doses, then 15 mg/kg/dose every 12 hr	Continue therapy until serum methanol or ethylene glycol level <20 mg/dL. Increase dose during dialysis. AE: headache, nausea, dizziness bradycardia, eosinophilia, transient increase of liver enzyme levels
Heparin	Protamine sulfate	Use 1 mg protamine for every 100 units of heparin to be neutralized.	AE: hypotension, bradycardia, hemorrhage. Use with caution with known fish allergy.
Iron	Deferoxamine	5-15 mg/kg/hr IV (max 6 g/24 hr)	Titrate dose slowly to avoid hypotension. Continue therapy until *vin rose* urine color clears, symptoms clinically resolve, or maximal dose attained. Deferoxamine challenge no longer suggested. AE: flushing, hypotension, acute respiratory distress syndrome.
Isoniazid (INH)	Pyridoxine (vitamin B_6)	Known INH dose: 1g per g of INH ingested IV slowly Unknown INH dose: 5 g IV over 10 min	Administer 1 g every 2-3 min. AE: CNS toxicity—headache, seizure, peripheral neurotoxicity.
Lead	Succimer (DMSA)	10 mg/kg/dose PO every 8 hr × 5 days, then 10 mg/kg/dose twice daily × 14 days	AE: rash, neutropenia, increased LFTs, GI upset.
	Dimercaprol (BAL)	75 mg/m^2/dose IM every 4 hr. Max: 450 mg/m^2/dose/24 hr	Pretreatment with diphenhydramine suggested. Contraindicated with peanut allergy, hepatic insufficiency. AE: G6PD hemolytic crisis, nausea, vomiting, histamine release.
	$CaNa_2EDTA$	1-1.5 g/m^2/day continuous IV infusion × 5 days	In cases of encephalopathy, administer after dimercaprol to prevent increased CNS lead levels. AE: phlebitis.
Methanol	*See* Ethylene glycol		
Methemoglobinemia	Methylene blue (1%)	1-2 mg/kg IV over 5 min	Repeat doses as needed. AE: dyspnea, chest pain, and hemolysis.
Opioids	Naloxone	0.5-2 mg IV/IM/SC/ET (max 10 mg)	Higher dose may be required for certain agents. Can repeat dose every 2-3 min until response or max dose. If no response to total 10-mg dose, unlikely opioid intoxication. If positive response is of short duration, may be administered as a continuous infusion. In setting of possible opioid dependence, consider initial dose of 0.05 mg to avoid withdrawal. AE: opioid withdrawal (piloerection, agitation, vomiting).

*Pediatric (P) and adult (A) doses are the same unless specifically noted.
AE, Adverse effects; *BB,* β-adrenergic blocker; *CCB,* calcium-channel blocker; *CHF,* congestive heart failure; *CNS,* central nervous system; *CO,* carbon monoxide; *D10W,* 10% dextrose and water; *ET,* endotracheally; *G6PD,* glucose-6-phosphate dehydrogenase; *GI,* gastrointestinal; *Hb,* hemoglobin; *IM,* intramuscular; *INR,* international normalized ratio of prothrombin time; *IV,* intravenous; *LFT,* liver function tests; *max,* maximum; *PO,* oral; *PRN,* as needed; *SC,* subcutaneous; *SDC,* serum digoxin concentration.

Continued

Table 355-4 Antidote Table*—cont'd

SUBSTANCE	ANTIDOTE	DOSE	COMMENTS
Cholinergic agents (eg, malathion)	Atropine	P: 0.02 mg/kg IV initial dose (minimum 0.1 mg) A: 0.5-1 mg IV initial dose	Double dose every 3-5 min. Titrate to reduced bronchorrhea or improved oxygen saturation. May require total doses 5 or 10 times the initial dose or higher. AE: anticholinergic toxicity.
	Pralidoxime	P: 25-50 mg/kg over 30-60 min, then 20 mg/kg/hr A: 1-2 g IV over 15-30 min, then 0.5 g/hr	Pralidoxime should be administered in addition to atropine. Continue therapy for 24-72 hr.
Oral antidiabetic agents	Octreotide	P: 1-2 mcg/kg SC/IV every 6-12 hr A: 50-100 mcg SC/IV, then 50 mcg every 12 hr	Continue therapy until euglycemic. May require several days of therapy. AE: bradycardia, dysrhythmias, GI upset, hyperglycemia.
	Dextrose	Neonatal: 0.2 g/kg IV (use D10W, 2 mL/kg) P: 0.5-1 g/kg IV (use D25W, 2-4 mL/kg) A: 25 to 50 g IV (use D50W)	AE: hyperglycemia, extravasation may cause local tissue reaction.
Tricyclic antidepressants	Sodium bicarbonate	1-2 mEq/kg IV bolus, then titrate to pH ~7.5 with additional doses or with continuous infusion	AE: volume overload, hypernatremia, metabolic alkalosis.
Warfarin	Vitamin K	P: 1-5 mg SC/IM/IV/PO, every 6-8 hr PRN A: 10 mg SC/IM/IV/PO, every 6-8 hr PRN	Much larger doses may be required. Continue therapy until INR within normal limits.

*Pediatric (P) and adult (A) doses are the same unless specifically noted.
AE, Adverse effects; *BB,* β-adrenergic blocker; *CCB,* calcium-channel blocker; *CHF,* congestive heart failure; *CNS,* central nervous system; *CO,* carbon monoxide; *D10W,* 10% dextrose and water; *ET,* endotracheally; *G6PD,* glucose-6-phosphate dehydrogenase; *GI,* gastrointestinal; *Hb,* hemoglobin; *IM,* intramuscular; *INR,* international normalized ratio of prothrombin time; *IV,* intravenous; *LFT,* liver function tests; *max,* maximum; *PO,* oral; *PRN,* as needed; *SC,* subcutaneous; *SDC,* serum digoxin concentration.

The empiric use of the benzodiazepine antagonist flumazenil to treat CNS depression after an overdose of an unknown agent is controversial.[44] Flumazenil administration is appropriate in the setting of a known acute benzodiazepine exposure associated with significant CNS or respiratory depression. Flumazenil may precipitate withdrawal seizures in the patient with benzodiazepine dependence, and it may induce dysrhythmias or seizures in patients exposed to tricyclic antidepressant agents. If the duration of flumazenil effect is shorter than that of the toxin, then repeat doses or a continuous intravenous infusion of flumazenil may be required (see Table 355-4).

Intoxication or poisoning is only one cause of altered mental status. Other important causes are trauma and CNS infection. Trauma is especially important to consider because intoxication is common before trauma. When the cause of altered mental status is unclear, cranial computed tomographic imaging should be considered. A lumbar puncture may also be performed in cases of altered mental status, especially in the presence of fever.

Seizures require urgent intervention. Many of the toxins that cause seizures are listed in Box 355-2. Benzodiazepines, specifically lorazepam or diazepam, are the preferred agents for the initial treatment of most toxin-induced seizures. However, seizures related to isoniazid or the *Gyromitra* species of mushrooms (false morel) should be treated with pyridoxine (vitamin B_6); seizures related to hypoglycemia should be treated with dextrose (see Table 355-4).

BOX 355-2 Agents That Cause Seizures

P—phenothiazine, phencyclidine, pesticides, propranolol
L—lithium, lidocaine, lindane
A—anticholinergics, alcohol withdrawal, amphetamine
S—salicylate, sedative-hypnotic withdrawal, sympathomimetics, strychnine
T—theophylline
I—insulin, isoniazid
C—carbon monoxide, camphor, cocaine

Agitation is a common manifestation of altered mental status and places the patient at risk of injury, hyperthermia, and rhabdomyolysis. Evaluating a highly agitated patient is difficult. Benzodiazepines are the preferred sedative agents, and the dose should be titrated to effect. Extremely agitated patients may require high doses.

Decontamination

Decontamination is considered in 2 large categories: (1) surface decontamination of the skin and eyes and

(2) GI decontamination. Because most exposures in children are ingestions, GI decontamination must be discussed. However, in an era when chemical terrorism is a serious concern, the issues related to surface decontamination take on added importance.

Skin exposures require thorough washing with soap followed by copious rinsing. Eye exposures also require copious irrigation with water or saline. For certain agents such as organophosphate (OP) pesticides or nerve agents, in which significant dermal absorption occurs, decontamination must occur before other interventions, even resuscitation, can proceed. Clothing must be removed and secured. Health care workers involved in the decontamination process must be appropriately protected with gowns and gloves; some exposures require using complete personal protective equipment. If the patient is not appropriately decontaminated, then health care workers are at risk of toxicity from secondary exposure. The prehospital approach to managing chemical incidents includes decontamination at the site of the incident, although decontamination facilities are being built at many health care facilities. Detailed information on decontamination techniques can be found at the Web site of the Centers for Disease Control and Prevention (www.bt.cdc.gov/planning/personalcleaningfacts.asp).

GI decontamination refers to any procedure that removes toxin or reduces absorption from the GI tract and includes the use of emetic agents, lavage, activated charcoal, and cathartic agents.

Until recently, gastric emptying with syrup of ipecac (SOI) has occupied a central place in the management of poisonings. However, both the AAP and the American Academy of Clinical Toxicology currently recommend against the use of SOI for poison management, even at home.[45,46] In fact, the overall use of SOI has greatly declined, from 13% of cases in 1983 to only 0.2% in 2004.[1] Several reasons can be cited for the change in approach. (1) SOI does not provide additional benefit after a patient has vomited spontaneously. (2) Although the evidence is strong that SOI causes vomiting and that some ingested substance can be recovered in the vomitus, the evidence that SOI prevents toxicity after poison ingestion is weak. (3) SOI is contraindicated for use after ingesting agents such as acids, alkalis, and hydrocarbons. (4) SOI is contraindicated for use after ingesting any agent that causes or is likely to cause dysrhythmia, hypotension, heart failure, respiratory depression or failure, altered mental status, CNS depression, or seizures because of the serious risk of protracted vomiting and aspiration of stomach contents. As such, SOI is contraindicated for almost all serious poisonings—the ones leading to significant cardiac, respiratory, or CNS symptoms. (5) SOI, which is available over the counter, is frequently abused by adolescents and adults with eating disorders.

Gastric lavage describes the procedure of irrigating the stomach with a large volume of fluid through a large-bore tube passed through the mouth into the stomach. Gastric lavage should be performed when the risk of toxicity is great, when the likelihood of recovering the toxin is high, or when other treatment modalities are unavailable.[47] Limited data show a benefit of this procedure, at least when used within an hour after ingestion.[48] Certain agents such as anticholinergic agents or opioid agents may delay gastric emptying and slow GI transit time. These agents may remain in the stomach for more than an hour and may be available for removal by lavage. Gastric lavage is contraindicated after the ingestion of hydrocarbons, acids, or alkaline agents.

The most likely complication of gastric lavage is vomiting with the aspiration of stomach contents. The risk is highest in a patient with a depressed level of consciousness and a diminished gag reflex. This risk can be reduced by intubating the patient with a cuffed endotracheal tube. Other unusual complications related to gastric lavage include esophageal or gastric perforation, dysrhythmias, hypothermia, and fluid and electrolyte abnormalities.

Activated charcoal is a mainstay in poison management.[49] Activated charcoal adsorbs toxins in the GI tract to prevent absorption into the blood stream and can interrupt the enterohepatic circulation of some drugs, such as salicylate. Activated charcoal effectively binds most large molecules such as acetaminophen, aspirin, and phenobarbital but does not adsorb small molecules such as lithium or iron. Activated charcoal can be administered in single or multiple doses.[50]

The most common side effect related to activated charcoal administration is vomiting. Again, if the patient has a depressed level of consciousness, then the airway must be protected. The only real contraindication to using activated charcoal is GI tract obstruction or perforation. Activated charcoal should not be provided after acid or alkali exposures, especially when endoscopy is planned, because the charcoal will obscure the endoscopist's view of the esophagus and stomach.

Cathartic agents are used to enhance elimination from the GI tract; however, evidence supporting this therapy is not strong.[51] Agents such as magnesium citrate and magnesium sulfate are rarely used because of associated fluid and electrolyte abnormalities. Sorbitol is the most frequently used cathartic agent and is typically administered along with activated charcoal. Fluid and electrolyte abnormalities are uncommon unless multiple doses of sorbitol are administered; therefore only 1 combination dose of sorbitol and charcoal is suggested, even for cases in which multiple doses of activated charcoal are planned.

Whole-bowel irrigation (WBI) describes a procedure of flushing the entire GI tract with an isoosmotic electrolyte solution, polyethylene glycol, a procedure frequently used to prepare the bowel for surgery.[52] In this procedure, large volumes (liters) of polyethylene glycol are infused until the effluent turns clear, at which point the GI tract is presumed to be empty. WBI is not associated with fluid and electrolyte abnormalities, but patients sometimes experience GI discomfort and bloating. WBI may be particularly helpful for agents that cannot be adsorbed to activated charcoal, such as iron or lithium, and for extended-release medications.

Antidotes are available for many different agents (see Table 355-4). Some of these antidotes are administered empirically during resuscitation or when the history or a toxidrome points strongly to a particular agent. Other antidotes are administered later when a specific toxin has been identified.

Enhanced Elimination

Ion trapping, particularly urinary alkalinization, is a method to enhance drug clearance and is most often used for salicylate poisoning.[53] At physiological pH levels, salicylate is a weak acid; but in acidosis, salicylate exists mostly in the un-ionized state and can freely traverse cell membranes. When sodium bicarbonate is administered, the bicarbonate ion is excreted in the urine. In alkaline urine, salicylate exists in the ionized state and cannot be reabsorbed across the renal tubule; the salicylate ion has been trapped in the urine. The net effect is to create a concentration gradient that moves salicylate from the CNS into the urine.

Ion trapping may also enhance the elimination of phenobarbital, chlorpropamide, and myoglobin. Theoretically, the elimination of weak bases such as phencyclidine and amphetamines should be enhanced in acidic urine. However, urinary acidification has greater risk than benefit and is not used therapeutically.

Hemodialysis provides definitive therapy for a limited number of agents, including ethylene glycol, lithium, methanol, and salicylate. Charcoal hemoperfusion is generally suggested for theophylline and sometimes for carbamazepine poisonings. However, specialized charcoal cartridges have been difficult to obtain recently, and these poisonings are being treated with new high-efficiency, high-flux hemodialysis techniques.

Supportive Care

Supportive care continues the management outlined in the previous section on Resuscitation, with ongoing attention paid to cardiorespiratory and neurologic status.

Laboratory testing should be directed to the diagnosis of particular toxins or to medical management. However, a few screening tests have been developed that are generally appropriate, especially for adolescent patients. An electrocardiogram (ECG) can be a useful screening test for agents such as tricyclic antidepressants that have characteristic ECG findings. Pregnancy testing should be part of the evaluation of adolescent girls because suicidal adolescents often have an acute stressor (such as pregnancy) that precipitates toxin ingestion. Because acetaminophen is widely available, because most patients are asymptomatic after acetaminophen ingestion, and because a window exists for antidotal therapy, acetaminophen levels should be assessed after a suicidal ingestion.

SPECIFIC AGENTS

Analgesics

Acetaminophen

Acetaminophen is one of the most commonly used antipyretic and analgesic agents in the United States. It is available in many formulations and dose forms and is often formulated in combination with other medicines such as opioids, diphenhydramine, dextromethorphan, and pseudoephedrine. Acetaminophen-containing products lead to 7% of all childhood exposures, 4% of all adolescent exposures, and 12% of all childhood and adolescent poisoning fatalities.[1] At therapeutic doses, acetaminophen is remarkably safe. Toxicity occurs after overdose or therapeutic error. Therapeutic dosing errors result from confusion related to the multitude of formulations and strengths and account for many of the childhood fatalities.[54]

More than 90% of a therapeutic dose of acetaminophen is metabolized by the liver to nontoxic sulfate and glucuronide conjugates. The remainder is metabolized by cytochrome P-450 CYP2E1 and CYP3A4 to a toxic intermediate, N-acetyl-p-benzoquinoneimine (NAPQI), which is conjugated with glutathione to form a nontoxic metabolite. In overdose, metabolic pathways are saturated, more acetaminophen is shunted through the P-450 system, larger quantities of NAPQI are generated, and glutathione stores are depleted. Unconjugated NAPQI causes hepatic necrosis. Young children have relatively greater stores of glutathione, which may explain the apparent lower incidence of serious acetaminophen toxicity in children.

After an overdose, patients are usually asymptomatic for the first 24 hours, although they may have some mild GI distress. Clinical hepatitis develops over the next 2 days and may progress to fulminant hepatic failure. Although patients may recover spontaneously, liver transplantation may be necessary in severe cases.

Poison control centers will refer children for evaluation after an ingestion of 150 mg/kg[55]; toxicity in an adult is expected after an ingestion of 15 g.[56] GI decontamination with activated charcoal is appropriate. When an otherwise healthy patient takes an overdose of immediate-release acetaminophen, the only test necessary is an acetaminophen level test performed on samples drawn 4 hours after the exposure. Levels drawn before this time will not reliably predict the need for antidotal therapy. Additional laboratory testing may be appropriate when an overdose of an extended-release preparation or a mixed overdose occurs, if the patient seeks care late, if an underlying chronic disease is present, or when otherwise medically indicated.

N-acetylcysteine (NAC), the specific antidote for acetaminophen overdose, replenishes glutathione in the P-450 pathway (see Table 355-4).[57] The decision to initiate NAC therapy requires using the Rumack-Matthew nomogram (Figure 355-1). If a level on samples drawn 4 hours or later is above the *possible toxicity* line (eg, 150 mcg/mL at 4 hours), then the patient should receive NAC. Although this treatment approach was developed in the context of a single acute exposure to an immediate-release preparation, it is also applicable to patients who overdose with an extended-release preparation of acetaminophen.[58]

Before intravenous NAC was approved for use in the United States in 2004, only the oral formulation was available. The oral formulation may still be available for use in some locations. The sulfurous smell and foul taste of oral NAC frequently lead to nausea and vomiting. The incidence of adverse reactions to intravenous NAC administration, primarily anaphylactoid reactions, may be as high as 20%.[59-61] These side effects are not completely mitigated by lowering the

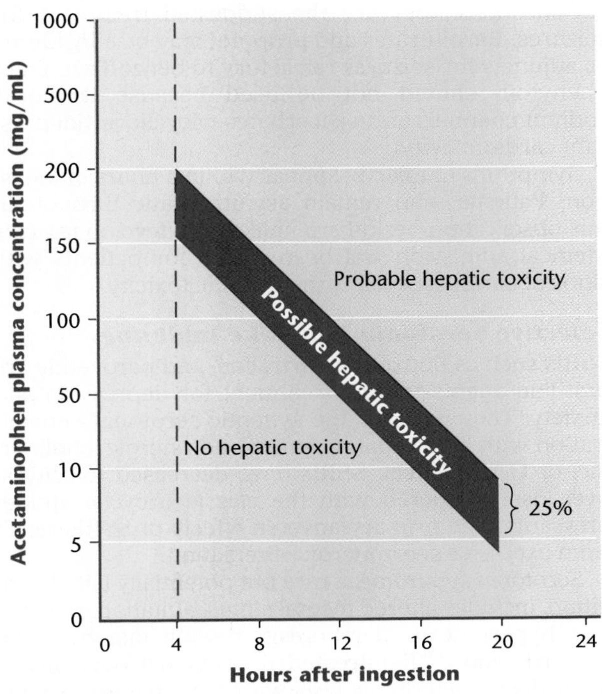

Figure 355-1 Rumack-Matthew nomogram for deciding whether to use N-acetylcysteine (NAC) as an antidote in treating acetaminophen overdose.

infusion rate,[62] but they are usually amenable to therapy, after which treatment can be restarted.[58]

Intravenous NAC is reconstituted in 5% dextrose in water and administered according to a complex regimen that delivers a large volume of free water to the patient. As a result, reports have been issued of children developing hyponatremia and seizures.[63] Intravenous NAC should be administered in consultation with a toxicologist familiar with its use.

Sick patients show altered mental status and hypovolemic shock. Hepatotoxicity is unlikely if NAC is administered within 8 to 10 hours of the time of ingestion. After this time, efficacy may be reduced, especially when patients wait a long time before seeking care. Therefore, if a patient arrives 4 hours or more after the ingestion and a level will not be available within the 8-hour window, then NAC should be administered pending the results. Although the efficacy of NAC is reduced after 8 hours, it should still be administered, even to patients who seek care very late after the time of ingestion.

If patients progress to fulminant hepatic failure, then they may require liver transplantation. This process should be initiated early in the hospital course if a possibility of liver failure exists. Spontaneous recovery is not associated with long-term clinical or pathological sequelae.

If a patient's acetaminophen levels are assessed on samples drawn 4 hours or more after an ingestion and the level is below the *possible toxicity* line of the nomogram, then the patient is medically clear. If the level is above the line and the patient begins NAC therapy within 8 to 10 hours, then the patient is medically clear at the end of treatment.

Salicylates

Salicylate formulations comprise one of the oldest and most commonly used classes of analgesic and antipyretic medicines and are available in many formulations, including standard, enteric-coated, extended-release, and chewable tablets. Salicylates are formulated together with opioids and over-the-counter cold remedies, and they can be found in antidiarrheal agents, herbal medications, and analgesic ointments.

Patients ingesting more than 150 mg/kg are at risk of toxicity and generally require direct evaluation. Methyl-salicylate is a liquid formulation used as a topical analgesic (oil of wintergreen); a 100% solution contains 1.5 g/mL, and even a single teaspoon of this formulation presents a significant risk for toxicity in a toddler.

Salicylates stimulate the chemoreceptor trigger zone to cause nausea and vomiting and the respiratory center of the medulla to cause hyperpnea and respiratory alkalosis. Salicylates are weak acids that uncouple oxidative phosphorylation and cause a positive anion gap metabolic acidosis. Thus patients may have a respiratory alkalosis, a metabolic acidosis, or a mixed acid-base disturbance. Children usually exhibit acidosis.

Sick patients demonstrate altered mental status and hypovolemic shock. Other acute effects include seizures, coma, hyperthermia, hypoglycemia, hypokalemia, and sometimes noncardiogenic pulmonary edema. Laboratory evaluation requires assessment of electrolytes, blood gas, and salicylate level. With acute intoxication, symptoms are typically seen with salicylate levels more than 30 mg/dL, although severe toxicity is typically found with levels of 80 to 100 mg/dL.

Ferric chloride can be used as a quick bedside test to confirm exposure to salicylates. Urine that contains salicylate turns purple or brown when 1 or 2 drops of 1% ferric chloride are added to 1 mL of urine. This qualitative test is positive after taking even 1 aspirin tablet; thus proof of salicylism still requires a salicylate level.

The Done nomogram was formerly used to assess the risk of clinical toxicity based on the salicylate level, but its use has fallen out of favor as a clinical tool. Salicylate toxicity is likely with elevated salicylate levels, but toxicity does not specifically correlate with salicylate levels; hence decisions regarding therapy are based on clinical evidence of toxicity.

Although patients can be quite sick, the need for intubation is unusual, and hypoventilation after intubation may worsen acidosis. Fluid resuscitation is critical, and patients may require treatment for hypoglycemia. Several doses of activated charcoal are useful to prevent the absorption of ingested salicylate and may interrupt salicylate's enterohepatic circulation. Rarely, salicylate tablets form a conglomeration in the stomach that requires surgical removal. In the case of methyl-salicylate, patients may require skin decontamination to prevent ongoing dermal absorption.

The first intervention to enhance salicylate elimination is to alkalinize the urine as described in the previous section on Enhanced Elimination. Optimal elimination occurs at urine pHs of more than 8. Any patient with clinical evidence of salicylate toxicity is a candidate for alkalinization unless administering large volumes of fluid is contraindicated.

Hemodialysis is used to eliminate salicylate and to correct acidosis. Indications for hemodialysis include persistent CNS toxicity; severe, worsening, or intractable acidosis; extremely high salicylate levels (usually >100 mg/dL); or any condition that precludes the administration of a high-volume bicarbonate infusion, such as pulmonary edema, renal insufficiency, or congestive heart failure.

Any patient with evidence of significant toxicity requires hospital admission for further evaluation and management. If no evidence of toxicity is found after 4 to 6 hours of observation, then the patient is medically clear.

Antidepressants

Tricyclic Antidepressants

The classic tricyclic antidepressants such as imipramine or amitriptyline have largely been replaced by selective serotonin reuptake inhibitors (SSRIs) as first-line agents in the treatment of depression. Nonetheless, tricyclic antidepressants are still used to augment SSRIs and to treat conditions such as insomnia or neuropathic pain. Tricyclic antidepressant overdose is a leading cause of poisoning morbidity and mortality, and ingestion of only 1 or 2 pills may be toxic in a toddler.

Tricyclic antidepressants affect many neurotransmitters and have a myriad of effects. They inhibit norepinephrine and serotonin reuptake from the nerve synapse. α1-Adrenergic blockade leads to hypotension. Sodium-channel blockade impairs depolarization throughout the myocardium, leading to prolonged QRS and QT intervals on ECG, right bundle branch block, and wide, complex dysrhythmias. γ-Aminobutyric acid (GABA) receptor inhibition lowers the seizure threshold; brief generalized seizures occur 1 to 2 hours after ingestion. Anticholinergic effects also contribute to delirium, coma, and seizures. The risk of seizures and ventricular dysrhythmias is increased with a QRS duration of more than 100 ms, R wave amplitude in aVR more than 3 mm, and R/S ratio in aVR more than 0.7.[64,65]

Because of the high risk of coma, seizures, and dysrhythmias in tricyclic antidepressant overdose, gastric lavage should only be performed when adequate airway protection is ensured. Reversal agents such as flumazenil and physostigmine are contraindicated in the setting of known or possible tricyclic antidepressant overdose.

The initial management of patients with significant cardiovascular or CNS toxicity follows the principles outlined in the previous section on Resuscitation. The specific therapy for tricyclic antidepressant–related wide complex ventricular dysrhythmias and hypotension is hypertonic sodium bicarbonate administration to raise the serum pH to approximately 7.5. A more alkaline pH lowers the concentration of free drug by stimulating protein binding; the increased serum sodium overcomes the sodium-channel blockade. Adverse effects of bicarbonate infusion include volume overload, hypernatremia, and severe metabolic alkalosis. For persistent wide-complex tachycardias or Torsades de pointes, limited evidence supports the use of magnesium.[66,67]

Benzodiazepines are the suggested treatment for seizures. Barbiturates and propofol may be considered as adjuncts for seizures refractory to benzodiazepines. Phenytoin should not be used because it blocks sodium channels and exacerbates tricyclic antidepressant cardiotoxicity.

Symptoms of toxicity appear within 6 hours of ingestion. Patients who remain asymptomatic throughout this observation period are unlikely to develop toxicity. Medical admission will be required for patients with signs of cardiovascular or neurologic toxicity.

Selective Serotonin Reuptake Inhibitors

SSRIs such as fluoxetine, sertraline, and paroxetine are first-line agents for the treatment for depression and anxiety. They increase the synaptic serotonin concentration with little sodium channel, adrenergic, cholinergic, or GABA effect. SSRIs have decreased toxicity in overdose compared with the classic tricyclic antidepressants. The primary adverse effects of SSRIs result from excessive serotonergic stimulation.

Serotonin syndrome, a rare but potentially lethal condition, includes altered mental status, agitation, myoclonus, hyperreflexia, diaphoresis, tremor, diarrhea, and incoordination.[68] If untreated, patients may develop lactic acidosis, rhabdomyolysis with renal failure, hepatic dysfunction, disseminated intravascular coagulation, and acute respiratory distress syndrome. Serotonin syndrome most commonly results from therapy with a combination of serotonergic agents or the combination of a SSRI with a monoamine oxidase inhibitor.

The main focus of therapy is to decrease muscle rigidity and its sequelae, myoglobinuria and renal failure. Initial therapy for muscle relaxation is with benzodiazepines. Adjunctive therapy may be provided with cyproheptadine, a histamine and serotonin antagonist.[69] Severe hyperthermia should be treated with aggressive cooling. If muscle rigidity is severe and unresponsive to conventional measures, then neuromuscular blockade can be used after the patient is intubated.

Asymptomatic patients do not require medical admission. Patients with symptoms of serotonin syndrome should be admitted to the hospital for further evaluation and management.

Antihistamines

Antihistamines are commonly available prescription and over-the-counter allergy medications, antinausea medications, and sleep aids. They are available in both short- and long-acting formulations and are found in combination with other medications such as acetaminophen.

Antihistamines are broadly categorized as H_1-receptor and H_2-receptor antagonists. First-generation H_1 antagonists (eg, diphenhydramine) typically cause sedation and CNS depression. Second-generation H_1 antagonists (eg, loratadine) generally have less sedation than the first-generation agents; however, several agents in this class (eg, terfenadine) were withdrawn from the US market because of the high risk of Torsades de pointes. H_2-receptor antagonists such as ranitidine and cimetidine primarily act in the GI tract.

Antihistamine toxicity is marked by either CNS depression with somnolence or coma or by CNS excitation with tremor, hyperactivity, hallucinations, or seizures. Peripherally, antihistamines cause an anticholinergic toxidrome (see Table 355-3). The association of fever and altered mental status may be confused with meningitis or encephalitis.

Most patients with antihistamine toxicity do well with supportive care alone.[70] For large ingestions or for ingestions of sustained-release formulations, gastric lavage or WBI may be useful. Administration of activated charcoal is appropriate. Significant agitation or seizures should be treated with benzodiazepines, as described in the previous section on Resuscitation.

Physostigmine, a carbamate with cholinergic properties, is an antidote for patients with anticholinergic toxicity and is appropriate for use in a pure antihistamine overdose with moderate to severe symptoms (see Table 355-4).[71,72] Adverse effects of physostigmine include seizures and ventricular dysrhythmias. Therefore physostigmine is contraindicated for patients with evidence of cardiotoxicity or for treatment of overdoses of cardiotoxic agents such as tricyclic antidepressants, which may also exhibit anticholinergic effects. Physostigmine therapy should not be administered as nonspecific therapy for unknown coma or agitation.

Patients who remain asymptomatic after 4 to 6 hours may be medically cleared. However, symptoms may sometimes be delayed after a large ingestion, and patients may require a longer period of observation.

Carbon Monoxide

Carbon monoxide (CO), an odorless, colorless, tasteless, and nonirritating gas, is a by-product of hydrocarbon combustion and is the leading cause of poisoning deaths in the United States. Vehicular exhaust is one of the most common sources of exposure, and children have even been exposed in the back of pickup trucks.[73] House fires are another significant source of unintentional exposure to CO and, in some cases, cyanide. CO exposure also occurs with the use of poorly vented kerosene space heaters, charcoal grills, camping stoves, and gas generators. The paint-stripping agent methylene chloride is converted to CO in vivo and may occasionally cause toxicity. Prevention of CO poisoning involves educating people about the safe use of space heaters and other small CO-generating devices in closed spaces and encouraging the use of CO detectors and smoke detectors in the home and workplace.

The toxic effects of CO poisoning are the result of a variety of mechanisms. CO binds to hemoglobin with a much greater affinity than oxygen and blocks the binding of oxygen. The binding of CO also leads to structural changes in the hemoglobin molecule that decrease the oxygen-carrying capacity and the tissue delivery of oxygen and that shift the hemoglobin-oxygen dissociation curve to the left. CO also binds to myoglobin and impairs oxygen delivery to the heart. The binding of CO to cytochrome oxidase may impair the utilization of energy that is generated from oxidative phosphorylation. Finally, CO leads to increased nitric oxide production and free radical formation, which causes lipid peroxidation, damage to myelin, and neurotoxicity.

Symptoms of mild CO poisoning can be nonspecific. Headache is the most common symptom. Malaise, nausea, and dizziness may accompany the headache and mimic a nonspecific viral syndrome. Severe disease produces CNS (altered mental status, seizure, syncope, and coma) and cardiac toxicity (dysrhythmias and myocardial ischemia).[74,75] Significant toxicity is often associated with metabolic acidosis and increased lactate levels. Cherry-red skin, although frequently mentioned, is rarely seen. Higher carboxyhemoglobin (CO-Hb) levels are associated with more severe disease, but no correlation exists between a particular symptom and a particular level. Children develop symptoms at lower CO-Hb levels than adults.[75]

CO causes lesions in the deep white matter and damage to the thalamus, basal ganglia, hippocampus, and globus pallidus.[76,77] Neurocognitive deficits, personality changes, focal neurologic symptoms, and movement disorders may be delayed for 2 weeks after exposure. Although children can experience delayed effects, adults have a higher risk, particularly if loss of consciousness occurs during the early phase of the exposure. Again, these delayed symptoms do not correlate well with the presenting level of CO.

When a pregnant woman is exposed to CO, the fetus is at particular risk. In animal models, peak fetal CO-Hb levels are approximately 10% to 15% higher and peak later than maternal levels.[78,79] Brain damage and fetal death have been reported, generally after severe maternal exposures.[80-82]

The best measure of CO exposure is the CO-Hb level. Normal CO-Hb levels are 1% to 2%; smokers may have levels of 5% to 10%. Fetal hemoglobin may be assayed as CO-Hb, and infants may have a CO-Hb of approximately 3%.[83] Standard pulse oximeters cannot differentiate CO-Hb from oxyhemoglobin. Blood gas CO oximetry is necessary to obtain accurate measurements of CO-Hb and methemoglobin. Although levels do not specifically correlate with symptoms, high levels indicate significant exposure.

Seriously poisoned patients will have impaired CNS and cardiovascular function. Standard PALS and ACLS protocols should be initiated. All exposed patients should initially receive 100% oxygen until an accurate estimate of exposure can be determined or a CO-Hb level can be measured, or both. A pH and blood lactate should be obtained concurrently because lactate seems to correlate to some extent with severity of disease.[84]

Hyperbaric oxygen therapy is the preferred treatment for serious CO poisoning. The half-life of CO-Hb in a patient breathing room air is 4 to 8 hours but decreases to 1 hour while breathing 100% oxygen and to 15 to 30 minutes when hyperbaric oxygen is administered. Thus hyperbaric oxygen therapy increases the concentration of dissolved oxygen to displace CO from binding sites on hemoglobin, myoglobin, and cytochrome oxidase; improves the delivery of oxygen to tissues; and reduces lipid peroxidation. Limited data suggest that hyperbaric oxygen therapy reduces the incidence of delayed neurologic and neuropsychiatric effects, particularly if administered within 6 hours, although data are conflicting.[85,86] Hyperbaric therapy seems to be safe for pregnant women and may benefit the fetus.[80,81,87] Hyperbaric chambers can be located through the Undersea and Hyperbaric Medicine Web site (www.uhms.org/).

Potential candidates for hyperbaric oxygen therapy include patients with (1) significant CNS, cardiovascular, or neuropsychiatric symptoms; (2) persistent metabolic acidosis or other symptoms that do not respond to standard 100% oxygen therapy; (3) CO-Hb levels exceeding 25%; or (4) pregnant women or children with a CO-Hb levels exceeding 15%.

In general, symptomatic patients will require hospitalization for further evaluation and management. Patients with relatively low CO-Hb levels and mild symptoms, especially when symptoms resolve after a short course of oxygen therapy, do not require hospitalization. Identifying and ameliorating the source of CO is imperative; contacting other potentially exposed persons who may require evaluation is also important.

Cardiovascular Medications

Although childhood poisoning with cardiovascular agents is unusual, even small doses may cause serious toxicity. Cardiovascular agents may be divided into 4 important classes: (1) cardiac glycosides, (2) calcium-channel blockers (CCBs), (3) β-adrenergic blockers (BBs), and (4) α2-adrenergic agonists.

Cardiac Glycosides

Cardiac glycosides include digoxin, digitalis, and related compounds found in plants such as oleander and foxglove, as well as in some toad venoms (bufotoxin). Bufotoxins have become popular as hallucinogens and aphrodisiacs, and their use has resulted in death.[88]

The cardiac glycosides inhibit myocyte sodium-potassium-adenosine triphosphatase pumps and increase the concentration of intracellular sodium and calcium during systole. Cardiac glycosides increase inotropy and automaticity, shorten repolarization intervals, and decrease conduction through the sinoatrial and atrioventricular (AV) nodes. The result is to increase the force and velocity of myocardial contractions.

Symptoms associated with acute overdose are typically nausea, vomiting, headache, weakness, confusion, changes in vision, palpitations, and dizziness. Severe acute overdose will lead to hyperkalemia, bradycardia, hypotension, and dysrhythmia. Hypercalcemia, hypokalemia, hyperkalemia, or hypomagnesemia can exacerbate cardiac toxicity. Chronic overdose is often characterized by nausea and vomiting, psychiatric disturbances, drowsiness, headache, and hallucinations.

A serum digoxin level will help in management. Levels above the therapeutic range may be associated with toxicity; higher levels are generally associated with a higher risk of and more serious toxicity. Children may tolerate high digoxin levels with less clinical toxicity.[89] The laboratory assays used to measure digoxin cross-react incompletely with plant- and toad-derived digoxin-like substances; thus an increased digoxin level may at least indicate exposure to one of these substances. Specific digitoxin levels are sometimes available.

Activated charcoal and steroid binding resins such as cholestyramine will adsorb cardiac glycosides in the GI tract and may interrupt their enterohepatic circulation.[90] Hyperkalemia should be aggressively treated with bicarbonate, insulin, and glucose. Calcium administration is contraindicated for the treatment of hyperkalemia in this setting because it can exacerbate glycoside toxicity, but magnesium sulfate should be used in patients with hypomagnesemia.[91,92] Kayexalate can also be administered.

Significant toxicity is treated with digoxin-specific antibody antigen-binding fragments (Fab) (Digibind; see Table 355-4). In the acute setting, Digibind therapy is used to treat significant dysrhythmia, serum digoxin levels of more than 15 ng/mL at any time or more than 10 ng/mL 6 hours after ingestion, serum potassium level of more than 5 mEq/L, hypotension, second- or third-degree heart block, or a digoxin dose of more than 10 mg in a teenager or adult or more than 4 mg in a child.[93] Because administration of Digibind causes a marked increase in the measured serum digoxin level, posttreatment levels do not reliably indicate a response to therapy.

Adjunctive therapy includes atropine for bradycardia and phenytoin and lidocaine for ventricular dysrhythmias. Cardioversion should be avoided because the ensuing sympathetic discharge can be fatal.[94] Classes Ia, Ic, II, and IV antidysrhythmics are contraindicated because they decrease AV conduction and worsen bradycardia and other dysrhythmias.

β1-Adrenergic Antagonists and Calcium-Channel Antagonists

BBs such as propranolol, atenolol, and metoprolol are commonly prescribed for treatment of hypertension, angina, dysrhythmias, and headache. β1-Receptor blockade results in decreased myocardial contractility and conduction; β2-receptor blockade increases smooth muscle tone (bronchospasm) and peripheral vascular tone (hypertension).

After an oral overdose of BBs, symptoms begin within 2 hours; sustained-release formulations may result in delayed onset. Cardiovascular manifestations include hypotension, bradycardia, wide QRS and PR intervals on ECG, bundle branch block, and ventricular dysrhythmias such as ventricular tachycardia and Torsades de pointes. CNS depression ranging from drowsiness to coma and seizures can also occur. Bronchospasm may occur in patients with a history of asthma. Metabolic effects include hyperkalemia and hypoglycemia.

CCBs such as verapamil, diltiazem, and nifedipine are used to treat hypertension, angina, and cardiac arrhythmias and are available in both immediate-release and long-acting formulations.

Calcium channels are found in the sinoatrial and AV nodes, the myocardium, and vascular smooth muscle. CCBs block the influx of calcium into myocytes and reduce contractility and conduction; smooth muscle relaxation also occurs. CCBs cause sinus bradycardia, hypotension, AV block, CNS depression, hyperglycemia, and lactic acidosis. CCB overdoses are clinically similar to BB toxic ingestions.

For both BB and CCB ingestions, activated charcoal can be administered. WBI should be considered for ingestions of sustained-release preparations. Glucagon is considered the specific antidote for significant cardiovascular symptoms related to BB overdose, but it may also be useful for CCB ingestions.[95,96] Glucagon increases cyclic adenosine monophosphate (cAMP) activity, leading to positive inotropy.[97] High-dose insulin and glucose is another therapeutic option; insulin may increase myocardial glucose utilization or alter myocardial calcium handling.[98-100] Calcium chloride may be useful after CCB or BB overdose.[101,102] Amrinone, a phosphodiesterase inhibitor, may be useful for refractory hypotension.[103] By inhibiting the breakdown of cAMP, amrinone, as with glucagon, increases inotropy. Table 355-4 provides additional information on glucagon, insulin, amrinone, and calcium.

In both CCB and BB overdose, adjunctive therapy for severe refractory bradycardia includes atropine, epinephrine, isoproterenol, and cardiac pacing. Patients may require therapy for hyperglycemia, hyperkalemia, or seizures.

All symptomatic patients with a history of a BB or CCB overdose should be admitted to an intensive care unit. Patients who are asymptomatic 6 hours after ingestion may be discharged unless they ingested a sustained-release formulation.

α2-Adrenergic Agonists (Clonidine)

Clonidine is used to treat hypertension and other disorders such as attention-deficit/hyperactivity disorder and nicotine withdrawal. Oral and patch formulations are both available. Even 1 or 2 clonidine pills may cause toxicity in a toddler.[104] The patches contain high doses of clonidine to ensure transdermal delivery, and they are a particular problem when ingested by children.[105-108]

Clonidine stimulates central α2-adrenergic receptors and can modulate opiate receptors. At therapeutic doses, clonidine primarily affects α2 receptors, but at high doses, both α1 and α2 receptors can be stimulated.

Toxic symptoms begin within an hour of ingestion and can last up to 24 hours.[109] Clonidine toxicity mimics opioid toxicity, with altered mental status, coma, respiratory depression, and miosis. Hypotension and bradycardia may develop, and dysrhythmias such as first- and second-degree AV block may also occur.

Naloxone should be administered in cases of respiratory depression; high doses may be required (see Table 355-4). Naloxone may also be useful in cases of CNS depression or hypotension.[110] When naloxone is effective but clonidine toxicity outlasts naloxone's effect, a continuous infusion of naloxone is indicated. Decontamination with activated charcoal is appropriate, and WBI may be indicated for children who have ingested clonidine patches.[107] Atropine may have modest effects on bradycardia, and fluids and pressors are indicated for hypotension.[111]

Patients may be discharged if they are asymptomatic 4 hours after ingestion. All symptomatic patients should be admitted to the hospital.

Caustic Ingestions

Caustic agents are broadly categorized as *acids* and *alkalis*. Common sources of acid in the home include toilet bowl cleaners, rust removal products, and automotive battery liquids. Common alkaline-containing products include drain cleaners, bleaches, ammonia-containing cleaners, oven cleaners, dishwasher detergents, and hair relaxers. Serious caustic exposures are unusual in childhood, but these agents have the potential to cause significant injury.

Acids injure tissue by coagulation necrosis.[112] Even though the resulting eschar may limit the initial depth of injury, esophageal, gastric, or intestinal injuries frequently occur. Significant exposures may cause metabolic acidosis or acute renal failure.

Alkali ingestions injure tissue rapidly by liquefactive necrosis.[112] Within minutes, tissue edema develops in the oropharynx and esophagus, potentially leading to airway obstruction. Scar tissue from full-thickness burns in the esophagus may progress to strictures over several weeks.[113]

Caustic ingestions produce dysphagia, odynophagia, drooling, stridor, hoarseness, abdominal pain, nausea, and vomiting.[114] GI hemorrhage and perforation may occur. Tissue eschar may sometimes mask findings despite a significant acid ingestion.

Gastric lavage is contraindicated after caustic ingestions because of the risk of esophageal or gastric perforation. Activated charcoal absorbs caustic chemicals poorly and may interfere with endoscopy. Plain-film radiographs of the chest and abdomen are helpful to rule out pneumomediastinum, pneumoperitoneum, and aspiration pneumonitis.[115] Esophagoscopy defines the extent of injury and should be performed in symptomatic patients.[116]

If any suspicion of perforation exists, then a surgical consultation should be obtained, and broad-spectrum antibiotics should be administered. In the case of large-volume acid ingestions, nasogastric suction performed within 30 minutes of exposure may prevent the passage of acid into the small intestine.[117] Neutralization of acids and bases should be avoided because of the excessive heat it generates and the risk of emesis.[118] A repeat esophagram will be required 3 to 4 weeks after caustic ingestion to check for strictures.

Hydrocarbons

Hydrocarbons are organic compounds that have significant toxicity. They are categorized into 3 classes: (1) aliphatics (kerosene, gasoline, mineral seal oil, solvent, paint thinners), (2) aromatics (industrial solvents such as benzene and toluene), and (3) terpenes (turpentine and pine oils). Hydrocarbon aspiration after unintentional exposure to such household products is a leading cause of poison-related death in young children.

Pulmonary toxicity results from chemical pneumonitis after aspiration. Local or diffuse infiltrates, pleural effusions, and pneumatoceles may develop.[119] Lipoid pneumonitis may result from ingesting hydrocarbons with high viscosity, such as petroleum jelly.

Most patients will experience some coughing after hydrocarbon exposure, but cough does not by itself indicate pulmonary toxicity. Significant exposures cause gasping, choking, gagging, and vomiting that begins within 30 minutes, and patients may develop cough, tachypnea, rales, rhonchi, wheeze, and diminished breath sounds. In the most severe cases, acute lung injury, hemorrhagic pulmonary edema, and respiratory failure may occur with long-term respiratory dysfunction. Respiratory effects may progress over the first 24 hours and resolve over the next 2 to 5 days. Associated acute symptoms may include CNS depression and fever.

Contaminated clothing should be disposed of properly, and the skin should be washed with soap and water to limit continuing exposure to hydrocarbon vapors. GI decontamination plays only a limited role; toxicity is related more to pulmonary exposure than to GI absorption. Most patients experience nausea and vomiting after hydrocarbon exposure and do not require further gastric emptying. Gastric emptying is contraindicated after most hydrocarbon ingestions because the risk of aspiration increases with any gastric-emptying procedure.

Gastric emptying is controversial, but it may be considered in 2 cases. The first is when the patient has swallowed a large volume of hydrocarbon but has not already vomited. The second is when the swallowed hydrocarbon can have systemic toxicity or is the carrier for another toxin. These particular hydrocarbons and additives are characterized by the mnemonic CHAMP (camphor, halogenated hydrocarbons, aromatic hydrocarbons, heavy metals, and pesticides).

Symptomatic patients have radiographic evidence of aspiration as early as 30 minutes after exposure. Asymptomatic patients occasionally develop radiographic changes, but the importance of these changes is unclear.

Management of pulmonary toxicity includes supplemental oxygen, humidified air, and intravenous fluids. Nebulized β2 agonists may be useful. Severely ill patients may require continuous positive airway pressure, mechanical ventilation with positive end-expiratory pressure, or extracorporeal membrane oxygenation. Corticosteroids are not beneficial in hydrocarbon ingestions.[120] Leukocytosis and fever are associated with hydrocarbon aspiration, and at least early in the course, do not signify infection.

Patients with persistent respiratory symptoms should be hospitalized. Patients who are asymptomatic or whose initial symptoms have resolved and whose radiographic findings are normal should be observed for 6 hours. If they are asymptomatic at the end of the observation period, then they may be medically cleared.

Insect Repellants

Diethyltoluamide

Insect repellents are used worldwide in the prevention of infectious disease transmission. N,N-diethyl-3-methylbenzamide (known as DEET) provides broad protection against many insects and is available in a variety of formulations.

Toxicity may occur after an acute ingestion or with dermal exposures. Systemic toxicity causes confusion, ataxia, generalized seizures, and encephalopathy. Hypotension and bradycardia have been reported in severe exposures. Encephalopathy may result from oral ingestions or chronic cutaneous exposures at high doses. Chronic exposures can also lead to insomnia, muscle cramps, mood changes, and rash.[121,122]

Lindane

Lindane (γ-hexachlorocyclohexane) is an organochlorine insecticide used topically to treat scabies and pediculosis. The organochlorines are absorbed from the skin and are distributed into fat. The elimination half-life is between 20 hours and 10 to 20 days.[123] A prodrome of headache, dizziness, ataxia, and tremors may be followed within 1 to 2 hours by self-limited seizures. Other complications include disseminated intravascular coagulation, anemia, and myoglobinuria. Repeat and chronic exposures may be associated with elevated transaminase levels, leukopenia, leukocytosis, thrombocytopenia, pancytopenia, and aplastic anemia.[124,125] Treatment entails avoidance of the medication and decontamination with soap and water.

Iron

In spite of consumer product safety improvements, iron poisoning remains a problem for toddlers. Prenatal vitamins typically contain 62 mg of elemental iron per tablet and can resemble candies such as M&Ms or Good'n'Plenty, making them appealing to children. Most significant toxicity is related to ingestion of adult iron tablets, not children's liquid or chewable vitamin preparations.

Iron is a GI irritant that causes abdominal pain, nausea, vomiting, and diarrhea.[40,126,127] Severe poisoning causes mucosal ulceration and hemorrhagic necrosis, leading to hematemesis, melena, or hematochezia.[127] GI fluid losses lead to hypovolemic shock and contribute to positive anion gap metabolic acidosis.[128,129] Absorbed iron leads to the production of free radicals, with adverse effects on cellular metabolism, which exacerbate the acidosis. The combination of the shock state in addition to iron's direct toxic effects contribute to progressive myocardial dysfunction and acute hepatic injury.[1,128,130] As hepatocellular damage progresses, coagulation is disrupted, further exacerbating the GI hemorrhage.[131] In rare cases, corrosive injury to the GI tract leads to gastric outlet obstruction weeks after the ingestion.

In general, the higher the dose of iron ingested, the greater the likelihood is of toxicity (Table 355-5). Poison control center specialists use this formula to predict toxicity and to refer patients for evaluation if the ingested dose of elemental iron is more than 20 mg/kg.[132] Similarly, the higher the serum iron level, the greater the likelihood is of resultant toxicity (see Table 355-5).[133] A peak serum iron level is best measured 4 to 6 hours after ingestion.[40]

Table 355-5 Iron Toxicity Based on Dose and Serum Iron Level

INGESTED DOSE*	EXPECTED TOXICITY
<20	None or minor
20-40	Mild-moderate
40-60	Moderate-severe
>60	Severe
Serum iron level (mg/dL)	Expected toxicity
<300	None or minor
300-500	Mild-moderate
<500	Severe

*Ingested dose of elemental iron (mg/kg).

GI symptoms alone do not necessarily predict severe toxicity but do confirm exposure. Because GI distress is a marker of exposure, asymptomatic patients do not require gastric emptying. Patients experiencing toxicity vomit spontaneously, and, in these cases, no additional benefit exists to gastric emptying.

Nonetheless, a limited role for gastric lavage exists after a significant ingestion or when pills are radiologically evident in the stomach. Gastric lavage is often unsuccessful at removing pills from the stomach, and lavage cannot remove pills that have passed into the lower GI tract. WBI may be more effective than other treatments at removing these residual pills.[134] In rare cases, surgery may be necessary to remove the iron pills.

Radiographs detect residual iron pills in less than 3% of all ingestions.[135] However, the absence of pills on radiographs does not exclude a toxic overdose. In particular, chewable and liquid iron formulations do not appear on abdominal radiographs, but they do not account for most toxic exposures either.

Although significant iron poisoning is associated with both an increased serum glucose and an increased white blood cell count, normal values do not rule out significant exposure. A total iron-binding capacity greater than the serum iron level was once thought to be protective in poisoning; however, the total iron-binding capacity is factitiously increased in the setting of iron poisoning. Deferoxamine also interferes with the accurate measurement of total iron-binding capacity.

In addition to the initial GI symptoms, patients with significant poisoning are in shock with a positive anion gap metabolic acidosis. These patients are very ill and need immediate and vigorous resuscitation. Although a serum iron level might be useful, because the optimal time to draw the level is 4 to 6 hours, and because these levels are often not rapidly available, decisions regarding treatment will usually have to be made on clinical grounds alone.

Chelation therapy with deferoxamine should be considered for any symptomatic child who is in shock, has an altered mental status, or is experiencing protracted vomiting or GI bleeding[136] (see Table 355-4). Serum iron levels exceeding 500 mcg/dL or abdominal radiographs suggesting a serious ingestion may also be an indication for chelation. Desferrioxamine, the deferoxamine-iron chelate, is excreted in the urine and imparts a dark brown or *vin rose* color to the urine. This color change is only a qualitative measure of desferrioxamine and is an unreliable marker of iron elimination.[137,138] Chelation therapy should continue until the child is clinically improved and the metabolic acidosis is resolved but duration of therapy greater than 24 hours may present an increased risk of toxicity.[139]

Patients who remain asymptomatic without treatment for 6 hours after ingestion are medically clear.

Isoniazid

Isoniazid (isonicotinyl hydrazine [INH]) is a medication primarily used for the prophylaxis and treatment of tuberculosis. It can cause hepatic toxicity, peripheral neuropathy, and optic neuritis even at therapeutic doses. INH doses of more than 30 mg/kg are likely to cause acute toxicity. Effects occur within 2 hours of ingestion. Patients initially experience nausea, vomiting, slurred speech, dizziness, tachycardia, urinary retention, and hyper- or hyporeflexia. Significant toxicity causes a anion gap metabolic acidosis, coma, and refractory seizures. INH inhibits the effects of vitamin B_6 (pyridoxine), an essential cofactor for the synthesis of GABA, an inhibitory neurotransmitter. Seizures occur as a result of decreased GABA activity.

If an asymptomatic patient seeks care soon after a significant exposure, then gastric lavage is appropriate. Activated charcoal may be provided.[140] To prevent seizures, prophylactic pyridoxine should be administered to patients who seek care within 2 hours of ingestion.[141]

Seizure therapy can begin with typical anticonvulsants such as the benzodiazepines or phenobarbital; phenytoin is not useful in treating INH-related seizures.[142] Definitive therapy requires administration of pyridoxine, the specific antidote for INH toxicity (see Table 355-4). If intravenous pyridoxine is unavailable, then crushed tablets can be given by nasogastric tube.[143] Hemodialysis may be considered for patients with massive toxic ingestions.[144]

Patients who remain asymptomatic for 6 hours can be medically cleared.

Lead Poisoning

Public health efforts over the last 2 decades have dramatically reduced environmental lead exposure by limiting its concentration in automotive gasoline and paints; the decline in lead poisoning parallels this change. Today the principal childhood source of lead is from deteriorating paint in pre-1970s-era houses. Although pica may result in oral lead exposure, more children are exposed to aerosolized lead paint flakes or contaminated dust inside the home or in the soil.[145] Other sources of lead include lead-based plumbing, ceramics, or imported goods in lead-soldered cans.[146,147] Folk remedies for colic advocated by some Chinese, South Asian, and Hispanic cultures may also result in lead exposure.[148-150]

Ingestion of lead-containing material is the predominant mode of exposure in children. GI absorption is facilitated by deficiencies in essential trace elements such as iron, calcium, and zinc, which compete for the same absorption sites. Absorbed lead is bound to erythrocytes and distributed into relatively labile soft-tissue storage sites such as the liver and brain and into more stable reservoirs such as bone. Although inhalation of lead fumes occurs in occupational exposures among adults, in children, aerosolized lead particles are inhaled, coughed up, and swallowed.[151]

Lead inhibits heme biosynthetic enzymes to produce a hypochromic, microcytic anemia. It also interferes with vitamin D biosynthesis, impairing calcium metabolism. Chronic lead poisoning can produce a reversible but progressive lead nephropathy with a Fanconi-like syndrome of glycosuria, aminoaciduria, and phosphaturia. As lead accumulates in the CNS, it compromises the capillary endothelium, causing cerebral edema and increased intracranial pressure. Irreversible neuronal damage and alterations in neurotransmitter function can also cause more subtle neurocognitive disabilities.

The initial clinical manifestations of chronic lead poisoning are subtle; most children with a long history of lead exposure and absorption are asymptomatic. A threshold *no effect* level for lead has not been defined, and decreased IQ has been observed among children with whole blood lead (BPb) levels less than 10 mcg/dL.[145]

Pallor, hearing impairment, constipation, and behavioral disturbances may be the first signs of chronic lead poisoning, but loss of developmental milestones and declines in school performance are sometimes seen. BPb levels as low as 15 to 20 mcg/dL have been associated with learning disabilities and mild decrements in IQ.[152]

Encephalopathy is the most significant clinical manifestation of lead toxicity. Children with BPb levels that exceed 70 mcg/dL may experience coma, intractable seizures, or even death.[153,154] Patients with BPb less than 70 mcg/dL may exhibit ataxia, incoordination, lethargy, or irritability. Subacute encephalopathy may cause anorexia, intermittent abdominal pain, nausea, vomiting, or constipation.[155] Peripheral neuropathy is uncommon in children, but wrist and foot drops may occasionally occur with sickle cell disease.[156]

In all cases of suspected lead poisoning, any sources of lead exposure should be identified and abated, and parents should be counseled regarding optimal nutrition. Symptomatic children are typically hospitalized to remove them from the source of lead and to administer chelation therapy. Oral intake should be restricted and intravenous fluid resuscitation should be started if the use of EDTA is anticipated. If abdominal radiography finds radiopaque material, then WBI with polyethylene glycol should be initiated.

Blood lead levels less than 45 mcg/dL represent excessive exposure to lead but do not require chelation therapy, which is reserved for symptomatic children or those with modest to severe lead burdens.[145,157] Three lead chelating agents are available in the United States: (1) dimercaprol (also known as British anti-lewisite [BAL]), (2) $CaNa_2EDTA$, and (3) succimer (dimercaptosuccinic acid [DMSA]) (see Table 355-4). A fourth agent, D-penicillamine, is not approved by the FDA, but its use may be necessary in the unusual event of adverse reactions to both DMSA and $CaNa_2EDTA$.[145,158] Asymptomatic children with BPb between 45 and 70 mcg/dL are chelated with oral succimer; intravenous $CaNa_2$ EDTA is also an option. Children with BPb more than 70 mcg/dL are chelated in the hospital with intramuscular BAL and intravenous $CaNa_2EDTA$. Encephalopathy is treated with the same two-drug regimen but for a longer course. After initial chelation therapy, the decision to repeat treatment depends on symptoms and follow-up BPb levels.

Organophosphates

Pesticides

OP agents such as parathion or malathion are highly toxic compounds that are found in a variety of pesticides. Ingestion of the agent directly or of contaminated fruit is the most common route of exposure in children, although these agents are highly lipophilic and are well absorbed through the skin, eyes, and lungs.[159] Assistance in identifying individual agents can be obtained from the US National Pesticide Telecommunications Network at 800-858-7378 or http://npic.orst.edu.

OPs bind to and inactivate acetylcholinesterase; acetylcholine accumulates in nerve terminals of the autonomic nervous system and CNS and at the neuromuscular junction. This bond, which is initially reversible, becomes permanent after a 24- to 48-hour period. Once inactivation is permanent, new acetylcholinesterase must be synthesized.[159]

Acute OP poisoning causes cholinergic symptoms (see Table 355-3). CNS symptoms are often the presenting symptoms in younger children. The diagnosis of OP poisoning is made when a patient has a confirmed exposure or a history of a suspected exposure and consistent physical findings. The hydrocarbon carrier may produce an odor of garlic. Symptoms occur within several hours but may be delayed for several days with the more fat-soluble compounds.

The poisoned patient has pinpoint pupils, vomiting, changes in mental status, and copious secretions. Untreated, the combination of bronchial hypersecretion, bronchial constriction, and failure of respiratory musculature leads to respiratory failure, which may be complicated by coma and convulsions. Atypical presentations can occur in children. For example, a child might have only mydriasis and tachycardia.[160] Other clinical sequelae that have been reported in children include hyperglycemia, metabolic acidosis, and prolongation of the QT interval with subsequent Torsades de pointes.[161]

The *intermediate syndrome*, uncommon in children, describes delayed toxicity that occurs after the resolution of initial cholinergic symptoms. Symptoms include proximal muscle weakness, cranial nerve deficits, and hyporeflexia. These symptoms are present 1 to 3 days after the cholinergic crisis, are not responsive to atropine, and require supportive care for several weeks. An increased risk of the intermediate syndrome appears to exist with the more lipophilic agents, which may not have been accessible to antidote and which are released from fat-storage sites into the circulation.[159,162] Delayed polyneuropathy, ataxia, neuropsychiatric symptoms, peripheral neuropathy, and spasticity have also been reported up to 3 weeks after exposure. Most of these cases improve with time and do not cause permanent disability.[163]

Although serum levels of both butyrylcholinesterase (pseudocholinesterase) and red blood cell cholinesterase (true cholinesterase) can be measured, red blood cell cholinesterase is a more sensitive measure of OP toxicity. However, red blood cell cholinesterase testing is not available in most hospital laboratories. Treating a patient for suspected poisoning should not wait for laboratory confirmation.

When a patient seeks care for a suspected or confirmed OP exposure, decontamination should follow the principles outlined previously. Rescuers and health care workers are at risk of exposure if a patient has not been appropriately decontaminated. Contaminated clothing must be safely discarded. After ingestions, gastric lavage may be appropriate, and activated charcoal can be administered. Lavage fluid is contaminated and must be safely discarded. For ocular exposures, the eyes should be copiously irrigated.

The immediate life-threatening problem is bronchorrhea (copious airway secretions). A patient in severe respiratory distress should be intubated, and atropine should be administered (see Table 355-4). Succinylcholine should not be used for rapid-sequence intubation because it requires the inactivated cholinesterase for its metabolism. The goal of therapy is to dry the airway secretions with atropine. High-dose, continuous infusions of atropine may be required.[164,165] Tachycardia, which may be related to atropine administration but which may also be related to hypoxia, is not a contraindication to use of higher doses of atropine.

The OP-acetylcholinesterase enzyme complex ages over time, leading to irreversible inactivation of the enzyme. 2-Pralidoxime, also known as 2-PAM, can hydrolyze the bond and reactivate the cholinesterase when administered before complete aging. Because this agent does not cross the blood-brain barrier, the reversal of neurologic symptoms requires atropine. Pralidoxime's efficacy varies with the different OP compounds, but it should be administered in all cases of severe toxicity.[165]

All patients with OP toxicity require admission. Time to full recovery depends on the agent and can range from a few hours to several weeks.

Nerve Agents

OP compounds that were too toxic to be used as pesticides were developed as nerve agents in the 1940s. Sarin, soma, tabun, and VX are all agents with very rapid rates of permanent cholinesterase inactivation, leading to the rapid onset of severe cholinergic symptoms. These agents can be dispersed through a blast or can be aerosolized. Sarin, soma, and tabun are volatile liquids with easily inhaled fumes. VX is less volatile than the others and is more likely to be absorbed through the skin. The volatile fumes of sarin, soma, and tabun are quickly dispersed in the air and degrade within several hours. Patients exposed to these agents are not at further risk once they are removed from the site of exposure. VX is more persistent in the environment and may present a risk for ongoing exposure. Overall, these agents are more dense than air and are concentrated near the ground; thus children may have an increased exposure risk.[166] More information on OPs and other chemical agents with potential for use as chemical weapons can be found at www.bt.cdc.gov/chemical.

Treatment for these agents is the same as that outlined for OP insecticides above. In June 2003, the FDA approved an atropine autoinjector for children that is available for prehospital use.

Plants

Plant exposures are common in children because they are easy to reach in the home and environment. More than 750 toxins have been identified in more than 100 plant species.[167] Plants do not require labeling for potential toxins, as is done for pharmaceuticals and household products, and no federal regulations exist on sales of plants or herbs.

Exposure to plants occurs by contact with the skin or eyes or by ingestion. Although plant exposures are common, only a very few patients seek medical attention, and even fewer require intervention.[168] For example, common plants such as the dandelion pose little hazard. The most common plants that result in clinical sequelae are peace lilly, holly, philodendron, poinsettia, pokeweed, poison ivy, rubber tree, and nightshade (Table 355-6).

Prevention of plant exposures occurs through education. Parents must learn the names of the plants they purchase, be familiar with plants that are toxic, and keep them safely away from children.

Substance Abuse

The high prevalence of substance use among adolescents despite educational efforts makes it an important issue for parents and physicians alike. Marijuana is the illicit drug most commonly used by children and adolescents in the United States, with 40% of students reporting use at some point in their life.[169] Marijuana is considered a gateway to other substance use. Adolescents use other drugs in addition to marijuana, such as ethanol, cocaine, methamphetamine, hallucinogens, inhalants, and prescription medications. In 2003, 9% of students reported having used cocaine in their lifetime, representing an increase over previous years, although the overall use of cocaine appears to be slightly decreasing. Methamphetamine use is rising dramatically throughout the United States, especially in the western and southwestern states. Inhalant abuse is also becoming more prevalent, with 12% of students reporting inhalant use at some point in their lifetime.[169] The illicit use of prescription medications such as Vicodin and OxyContin represent an advanced stage of drug abuse. The recognition of drug abuse is a challenging but necessary skill of any pediatric care physician.[170] The primary outpatient management of substance use and abuse per se is beyond the scope of this chapter.[171-174]

Marijuana

Marijuana is made from the dried leaves from the plant *Cannabis septiva*. Extracts of the *Cannabis* plant are available as hashish (dried resin) and hash oil (liquid extract). These various forms can be smoked or eaten. Medical marijuana is available in pill form (Dronabinol).

The active component in marijuana is tetrahydrocannabinol (THC), a psychoactive compound. THC is lipophilic and easily crosses the blood-brain barrier; when inhaled, the onset of action is 10 to 30 seconds, and the effects last from 1 to 4 hours.[175] Ingestion results in slower onset of action (30-60 minutes) and more prolonged effects. THC stimulates cannabinoid receptors, activates the mesolimbic dopaminergic pathway (the *reward* pathway), and increases turnover in the GABA pathway. THC metabolites accumulate in adipose tissue and can be detected by urine toxicologic screens up to 1 month after use.

The clinical effects of marijuana include euphoria, impaired motor coordination and speech, impaired short-term memory, paranoia, and agitation. In rare circumstances, patients may experience hallucinations, delusions, and psychosis. Other effects include dry mouth, conjunctival injection, tachycardia, and

Table 355-6 Toxic Plants

PLANT	TOXIN OR TOXIC PART	TOXICITY AND TREATMENT
HOUSEPLANTS AND CULTIVATED FLOWERS		
Aloe	Latex contains anthraquinones	Oral irritation, nausea, vomiting, diarrhea
Anemone	Protoanemonin aglycone	Irritation of mucous membranes and GI
Autumn crocus, glory lily	Colchicine	GI, respiratory, renal, CNS toxicity
Christmas pepper	Capsicum	Strong irritant, stinging or burning of mucous membranes
Chrysanthemum	Sesquiterpene, lactones, pyrethrins	Skin reactions
Iris	Resin-like podophyllotoxin	Gastroenteritis
Jerusalem cherry	Solanine alkaloids	GI, CNS depression
Lily-of-the-valley, foxglove, oleander	Cardiac glycosides	Irritation of mucous membranes, CV toxicity
Monkshood, larkspur	Alkaloid aconitine	Restlessness, salivation, irregular heartbeat Rx: gastric decontamination
Narcissus, amaryllis, daffodil	Alkaloid lycorine	Vomiting and diarrhea
Philodendron, caladium, dumb cane, elephant ear, peace lily, pothos	Oxalates	Irritation of buccal mucosa, edema, gastroenteritis, hypocalcemia Rx: rinse mouth with milk; administer calcium
Snow-on-the-mountain	Unknown acrid principle in milky sap	Irritation of mucous membranes and GI
WILDFLOWERS AND WEEDS		
Buttercup, morning glory	Protoanemonin; seeds contain lysergic acid monoethylamide	GI irritation, CNS stimulation, hallucinations
Deadly or black or climbing nightshade, jimson weed, henbane	Atropine, solanine, and related glycoalkaloids	Anticholinergic Rx: physostigmine
Death camus	Veratrum alkaloids	Nausea, vomiting, hypotension, bradycardia, syncope, paresthesia, weakness Rx: Atropine
Green or false hellebore	Veratrum alkaloids	GI irritation, respiratory, CV depression Rx: Atropine
Horse nettle	Solanine alkaloid	GI, CNS depression
Jack-in-the-pulpit, wild calla, skunk cabbage	Calcium oxalate crystals	Irritation and burning of mouth Rx: rinse with milk and magnesium hydroxide
May apple	Podophylloresin	May produce peripheral neuropathy, vomiting, colic, diarrhea, drowsiness, impaired vision
Poison hemlock	Alkaloid coniine	Salivation, nausea, vomiting, diarrhea, sensory disturbances, seizure, coma; death from respiratory paralysis
Poison ivy, oak, sumac, wood	Urushiol	Rhus dermatitis—red, itchy, and clear blisters that exude serum; if ingested, causes severe mucosal irritation Rx: topical or oral corticosteroids
Pokeweed	Podophyllotoxins	Vomiting, sweating, colic, diarrhea, CNS depression
Rosary pea	Abrin	Burning sensation of mouth and throat, delayed GI, depression of vasomotor center, CV collapse
Spurges	Unknown acid principle	Severe mucosal irritation
Water hemlock	Cicutoxin	Generalized seizures Rx: symptomatic to prevent/control seizures
White snakeroot	Tremetol, may be in milk of poisoned cow	Weakness, vomiting, tremor, and death
CULTIVATED FLOWERS AND CROPS		
Castor bean	Ricin, must be chewed to release	Burning sensation of mouth and throat, delayed GI, depression of vasomotor center, hepatic, hemolysis, convulsions, and death

Table 355-6 Toxic Plants—cont'd

PLANT	TOXIN OR TOXIC PART	TOXICITY AND TREATMENT
Potato, tomato	Foliage and sprouts contain solanine alkaloids	GI irritation, headache, CNS depression, dermatitis
Rhubarb	Leaves contain oxalate crystals and soluble oxalates	Irritation of mucosa, hypocalcemia with seizures Rx: rinse mouth with milk, replace calcium
Tobacco	Nicotine	Salivation, gastroenteritis, seizures
TREES AND WOODY SHRUBS		
Black locust	Toxalbumin	Anorexia, weakness, GI, dilated pupils, irregular and weak pulse
Cherry, apple, peach, apricot, choke cherry	Leaves, pits, or seeds contain glycosides hydrolyzed to hydrocyanic acid upon chewing	Dyspnea, paralysis, convulsions, coma, and death Rx: cyanide antidote kit
Daphne	Glycoside in which the aglycone is dihydroxycoumarin	Burning and irritation to the skin and GI tract, bloody diarrhea, stupor, weakness, and convulsions
English holly	Ilexanthin and ilex acid	Vomiting and diarrhea
Mistletoe	Berries contain lectins, phoratoxin, viscotoxin, polysaccharides	Gastroenteritis and CV collapse
Mountain laurel, rhododendrons	Grayanotoxin	Local and GI irritation, respiratory and CV depression Rx: atropine
Yew	Alkaloid taxine	Vomiting, colic, hypotension, respiratory depression

CNS, Central nervous system; *CV*, cardiovascular; *GI*, gastrointestinal; *Rx*, treatment; and *Sx*, symptoms.
Adapted from Rodgers GC, Matyunas NJ. *Handbook of Common Poisonings in Children.* 3rd ed. Elk Grove, IL: American Academy of Pediatrics; 1994.

urinary retention.[176] Compared with other hallucinogens, the effects of marijuana are usually mild and self-limited and require minimal medical intervention.

Hallucinogens

Hallucinogens are substances that principally alter perception, thought, and mood. This section examines 3 common hallucinogens: (2) lysergic acid diethylamide (LSD), (2) phencyclidine (or phenylcyclohexylpiperidine, [PCP]), and (3) ketamine.

LYSERGIC ACID DIETHYLAMIDE. LSD was first synthesized in 1938 from ergot alkaloids extracted from the plant *Claviceps purpurea*. In the 1950s, LSD was used to facilitate psychotherapy, and by the 1960s, it had became a popular recreational drug. LSD is available in several forms, including liquid-impregnated blotter paper, microdots, tiny tablets, windowpane gelatin squares, liquid, powder, and tablets.[177] LSD is usually ingested and has rapid GI absorption.

LSD's psychedelic effects include existential experiences, intensified perceptions, hallucinations, and paranoia. Clinical signs of LSD intoxication include tachycardia, palpitations, blurred vision, tremors, incoordination, and mydriasis.[178] These effects are most intense in the early part of the intoxication. LSD users may experience flashbacks during which an individual reexperiences aspects of the acute intoxication. These episodes are short-lived and self-limited but may provoke anxiety.

PHENCYCLIDINE AND KETAMINE. PCP was commercially available in the 1950s as an anesthetic and reemerged as a recreational drug in the 1960s. PCP can be used orally, intravenously, smoked, or inhaled. Ketamine is a derivative of PCP and is used medically as a dissociative anesthetic. Ketamine is also a popular recreational agent because of its short duration, low cost, and hallucinatory effects. Recreational ketamine is not manufactured by drug users but is diverted from medical, dental, and veterinary sources and is administered orally, intramuscularly, and intravenously.

PCP blocks the N-methyl-D-aspartic acid receptor to produce its dissociative and psychotic effects. PCP also produces sympathomimetic effects by blocking the reuptake of dopamine and norepinephrine. The clinical effects of PCP can last up to 48 hours after a large dose is ingested.[179] Ketamine is pharmacologically similar to PCP but differs with respect to pharmacokinetics. Intoxication will typically last for approximately 8 hours after oral exposure and 90 to 120 minutes after intramuscular or nasal exposure.

PCP and ketamine cause a dissociative psychotic reaction manifesting as changes in body image and feelings of spiritual separation from the body. Users may have difficulty seeing themselves as separate from their environment. PCP users may experience dangerous or violent behavior, and the emotional state created by PCP is frequently unpleasant. Physical signs of PCP and ketamine intoxication include nystagmus, ataxia, sensory impairment, catatonia, tachycardia, hypertension, and increased secretions.[179] Ketamine intoxication is usually less severe and more short-lived than PCP intoxication. Both ketamine and PCP also have sympathomimetic effects.

Supportive care in a quiet environment with minimal loud or noxious stimuli is usually all that is needed, although verbal and physical contact with friends or family members may be helpful. When agitated, patients should be sedated with appropriate doses of benzodiazepines. Prolonged or severe psychosis will require psychiatric evaluation.

Stimulants

Cocaine, amphetamine, and related compounds are the most commonly used stimulants. All the stimulants have sympathomimetic effects.

Cocaine is a short-acting stimulant with local anesthetic properties. It is extracted from the leaves of the *Erythroxylum* coca plant. Cocaine can be insufflated (snorted), smoked, or injected. Crack is a purified alkaloid form of cocaine that vaporizes instead of burning, allowing it to be smoked. *Freebasing* describes a technique of heating a cocaine solution until it vaporizes and then inhaling the fumes.

When smoked or used intravenously, cocaine effects begin almost immediately and peak within several minutes. With nasal use, effects begin in a few minutes and peak after 30 minutes. Cocaine is rapidly metabolized to benzoylecgonine and ecgonine methylester.[180] These inactive metabolites have a half-life of 4 to 6 hours and can be detected in a urine drug screen up to 48 hours after single use and longer after chronic use. Cocaine interferes with the reuptake of adrenergic neurotransmitters and causes CNS stimulation, vasoconstriction, and blockade of fast sodium channels in axons and in myocardial tissue.

α-Methylphenylethylamine and its derivatives are generically referred to as *amphetamines*. Although amphetamines have been used to treat narcolepsy, asthma, and obesity, their primary current medical indication is for treatment of attention-deficit/hyperactivity disorder (eg, methylphenidate). Methylenedioxymethamphetamine (MDMA) is an amphetamine derivative commonly known as *ecstasy*, a popular club drug that is used at raves and rock concerts.[181,182] MDMA stimulates feelings of enhanced emotion and arousal, and hallucinations can occur at high doses.

Amphetamines stimulate the release of dopamine and norepinephrine to cause altered perception, stereotypical and psychotic behaviors, and locomotor stimulation. MDMA stimulates serotonin release and inhibits serotonin synthesis and reuptake. Acute ingestion causes a functional increase in the serotonin concentration; with chronic use, however, serotonin stores are depleted.[183]

The clinical effects associated with these agents are related to stimulation of the CNS and cardiovascular system. Severe effects include seizures and intracranial hemorrhage. Cardiac toxicity of stimulants can cause tachycardia, hypertension, myocardial ischemia, and dysrhythmias.[184] Specific sequelae of cocaine use include endocarditis, pneumothorax, and tactile hallucinations. Amphetamines have been reported to cause choreoathetoid movements and compulsive behaviors. MDMA can cause hyponatremia resulting from the intake of large volumes of water combined with the release of alcohol dehydrogenase.[185]

Treatment of stimulant intoxication requires good supportive care. Benzodiazepine sedation is the most effective treatment for agitation, chest pain, hypertension, hyperthermia, and seizures. Rhabdomyolysis is a common complication of stimulant use and may require aggressive intravenous hydration, urinary alkalinization, and rarely hemodialysis. Hyperthermia requires aggressive cooling.

Patients who respond appropriately to sedation and remain asymptomatic for a 4- to 6-hour period of observation are medically clear.

Cocaine associated chest pain is an issue of concern. Although most cocaine-related chest pain is short-lived and benign, approximately 6% of patients will have an acute myocardial infarction.[186] Most cases occur in the absence of underlying heart disease and can occur in adolescence.[187] The management of myocardial ischemia and dysrhythmias may require the use of benzodiazepines, nitroglycerin, phentolamine, aspirin, morphine, and CCBs.[186] Wide-complex tachycardias associated with cocaine may respond to the use of bicarbonate.[188]

If patients display any persistent signs of cardiac involvement (eg, chest pain, ECG changes, abnormal cardiac enzymes), then they should be admitted to a chest pain observation unit. Patients are medically clear if they have normal levels of troponin I, no new ischemic ECG changes, and no cardiovascular complications during a 12-hour observation period.[189]

Inhalants

Inhalation of volatile hydrocarbons such as glue, spray paint, or gasoline is a common form of adolescent substance abuse.[190-192] Typically, patients will *sniff* (inhale directly), *huff* (soak a rag and inhale from it), or *bag* (squirt or spray hydrocarbon in a bag and inhale from the bag or place the bag over the head). The acute presentation and management of inhalant intoxication differs from the hydrocarbon aspiration syndrome described previously. The primary acute effect of hydrocarbon inhalation is altered mental status. At high doses, inhalation may cause significant CNS depression, coma, and respiratory depression. Alternatively, when a person covers the head with a bag, the individual may pass out and become asphyxiated.

Halogenated hydrocarbons such as typewriter correction fluid (trichloromethane) or Freon are cardiotoxic; these agents sensitize the heart to catecholamines and can cause malignant dysrhythmias. *Sudden sniffing death* occurs when a patient has been using these agents, experiences a catecholamine surge (eg, when running away from police), and develops sudden ventricular fibrillation.[193]

Sedative-Hypnotic Agents

Sedative-hypnotic agents encompass a diverse group of agents, including benzodiazepines, barbiturates, ethanol, and γ-hydroxybutyrate (GHB).

Benzodiazepines such as diazepam or alprazolam are commonly prescribed anxiolytic agents. Flunitrazepam (Rohypnol, or *roofies*) is an illicit benzodiazepine common in drug-facilitated sexual assault (date rape); its anxiolytic effects are also used to soften the coming-down phase after cocaine or heroin use.

Barbiturates such as phenobarbital, thiopental, or pentobarbital are commonly used sedative, anesthetic, or anticonvulsant agents.

Benzodiazepine and barbiturate effects are mediated by GABA, the predominant inhibitory neurotransmitter in the brain. Enhanced GABA activity leads to increased sedation. Subtle variations in the GABA receptor allow for the variable physiologic effects of these agents (sedation, hypnosis, anxiolysis, amnesia, and muscle relaxation), and at least 2 types of benzodiazepine receptors have been identified.

Ethanol (ethyl alcohol) is commonly used by teens and preteens and is a contributing factor to injuries related to motor-vehicle collisions, homicide, fire, drowning, and suicide attempts. At high doses, ethanol intoxication progresses to CNS depression, with coma and death resulting from respiratory suppression. Ethanol is frequently ingested with other drugs. Ethanol's inhibitory effects are the result of enhanced GABA transmission and inhibition of NMDA glutamate receptors.

GHB was introduced as an anesthetic agent and gained popularity with body builders as a reputed facilitator of growth hormone release. In the late 1980s, its illicit use as a sedative agent and for drug-facilitated sexual assault became more common. It is currently a schedule-3 drug prescribed for narcolepsy and other sleep disorders.

GHB is available in either pill or powder form. It crosses the blood-brain barrier and acts on GHB-specific receptors, the function of which is poorly understood but which may involve dopaminergic pathways. GHB receptor activation may cause agitation or sedation, vomiting, bradycardia, hypotension, coma, and seizures.[194]

Sedative hypnotic agents are usually identified on urine drug screens. Barbiturates may be detected up to 4 days after ingestion, although phenobarbital may be detected in urine up to 4 weeks later. Benzodiazepines can be detected from 1 to 30 days after ingestion, depending on the individual agent. Blood alcohol concentrations are routinely available. Standard urine drug assays do not screen for GHB.

The hallmark of sedative-hypnotic intoxication is CNS depression with or without respiratory depression. Respiratory depression can be seen with barbiturate intoxication but is unusual after benzodiazepine intoxication alone. Any combination of agents, including ethanol, increases the risk of respiratory depression. Most sedated patients do well with supportive care. Significant CNS and respiratory depression may require urgent endotracheal intubation to ventilate the patient and to protect the patient from aspiration. Medical interventions should be focused on drug-specific side effects.

Administration of flumazenil, a specific benzodiazepine antagonist (see Table 355-4), is appropriate in the setting of a known benzodiazepine exposure associated with significant CNS depression, respiratory depression, or both. Empiric use of flumazenil to treat respiratory or CNS depression after overdose of an unknown agent is not suggested.[44] Flumazenil should not be administered to patients with possible chronic benzodiazepine use because of the high risk of inducing withdrawal.

Patients with suspected sedative-hypnotic intoxication should be admitted for monitoring of respiratory and neurologic status. Barbiturate and benzodiazepines may require prolonged hospitalization as a result of prolonged duration of effect. Patients with uncomplicated ethanol ingestion can usually be observed and discharged after observation in an emergency department setting. GHB and Rohypnol usually have short durations of action and can typically be managed in the emergency department.

Opioids

Opioid medications such as morphine, meperidine, codeine, hydrocodone, oxycodone, and propoxyphene are commonly used analgesic agents. Heroin is primarily used for its psychoactive effects; methadone is prescribed to treat heroin addiction. Different formulations of these agents are available for oral, intravenous, intramuscular, and subcutaneous administration. These agents can also be insufflated or smoked. Intravenous administration (morphine, meperidine, and heroin) leads to rapid onset of effect and carries the highest risk for adverse effects.[195] All opioids bind to specific opioid receptors; mu (OP_3) receptors mediate analgesia, euphoria, and respiratory function.

Management of intoxication is based on the history of exposure and the presence of clinical symptoms. The classic opioid toxidrome includes respiratory depression, CNS depression, and miosis (see Table 355-3). Patients with respiratory or CNS depression related to known or presumed opioid intoxication should receive naloxone as described in the previous section on Resuscitation (see Table 355-4). Opioid metabolites are excreted in the urine and can be detected on a urine drug screen up to 4 days after acute use and longer after chronic use.

Patients who are awake and alert after opioid use do not require further medical evaluation. Patients whose status is reversed by a single dose of naloxone should be observed for at least several hours in case of recurrence of symptoms. Patients with significant opioid symptoms who have received high doses or a continuous infusion of naloxone require hospitalization.

Toxic Alcohols

Methanol and Ethylene Glycol

Methanol is found in many commercial products, including antifreeze, windshield washing fluid or de-icer, and picnic stove fuel. Ethylene glycol has a sweet taste and is found in antifreeze, inks, pesticides, adhesives, cosmetics, and paints. The metabolites of methanol and ethylene glycol are toxic. Methanol is initially metabolized to formaldehyde via alcohol dehydrogenase and then to formic acid by aldehyde dehydrogenase. Although absorption of methanol after ingestion is rapid, metabolism and symptoms can sometimes be delayed up to 24 hours.[196] Ethylene glycol is metabolized to glycoaldehyde and then to glycolic acid, glyoxylate, and oxalic acid. Oxalic acid can chelate calcium and calcium oxalate crystals can precipitate within renal tubules.

Methanol intoxication causes nausea, headache, decreased vision with mydriasis, and weakness. These symptoms may progress to blindness, coma, and death without treatment. Ethylene glycol intoxication produces neurologic symptoms ranging from drunkenness to coma followed by tachypnea and pulmonary edema. Ethylene glycol toxicity may cause acute renal failure with precipitated oxalate crystals. Both methanol and ethylene glycol cause a positive anion gap acidosis and an increase in serum osmolality; ethylene glycol may cause hypocalcemia. Methanol and ethylene glycol do not cause lactic acidosis or ketonuria. Antifreeze often contains fluorescein as an additive to help mechanics locate radiator leaks; thus a Wood lamp examination of the urine for fluorescence is sometimes suggested to help identify ethylene glycol. However, this test lacks sensitivity.[197]

Because these agents have rapid absorption from the GI tract, gastric lavage and activated charcoal have limited utility but may be useful for patients who seek care soon after large-volume ingestions. Maintaining the pH near normal with sodium bicarbonate will reduce the availability of and enhance the elimination of some of the toxic metabolites.

Fomepizole is available for the treatment of methanol and ethylene glycol intoxication.[198] Both fomepizole and ethanol competitively inhibit alcohol dehydrogenase and prevent the formation of toxic metabolites (see Table 355-4).[199-201] Therefore, if the patient ingested ethanol along with methanol or ethylene glycol, the onset of toxicity may be delayed. Folate enhances the metabolism of formic acid and is adjunctive therapy for methanol poisoning. Thiamine and pyridoxine shunt ethylene glycol metabolism toward less toxic metabolites and are adjunctive therapy for ethylene glycol poisoning.

Definitive therapy requires hemodialysis to remove both the toxic alcohols and their metabolites. Indications for hemodialysis are severe acidosis, visual or mental status changes, or high serum concentrations (methanol or ethylene glycol >25 mg/dL).[202-204]

Isopropyl Alcohol (Isopropanol)

Isopropanol is found in common household products such as rubbing alcohol. In some instances, isopropanol is ingested intentionally as a substitute for ethanol. Unmetabolized isopropanol causes clinical toxicity; as little as 20 mL can cause symptoms.[205] It is metabolized to acetone, which is nontoxic and is excreted by the kidneys and the lungs.

GI toxicity causes nausea and vomiting and can progress to hemorrhagic gastritis. CNS findings include ataxia, muscle weakness, areflexia, lethargy, and coma. Patients with isopropanol ingestion can develop myocardial depression with tachycardia and hypotension, renal tubular acidosis, and tracheobronchitis. Patients with isopropanol intoxication have increased serum osmolality and ketonuria but do not have metabolic acidosis.

The clinical presentation of patients with isopropanol ingestion is not usually severe and is rarely fatal. These patients require supportive care and symptomatic therapy. In severe cases, hemodialysis may be necessary for persistent hypotension, plasma levels exceeding 400 mg/dL, prolonged coma, or underlying renal or hepatic disease that limits the metabolism and excretion of isopropanol.[202]

Any patient with suspected or confirmed significant toxic alcohol ingestion and any symptomatic patient should be hospitalized. Patients who have no symptoms and who are treated early have an excellent prognosis. However, patients with seizures, coma, or pH less than 7.20 have a poor prognosis.[206] Asymptomatic patients who ingested small volumes of isopropanol can be medically cleared after several hours of observation.

Warfarin-Like Rodenticides

The most common rodenticides (rat poisons) are coumarin anticoagulants that cause the rodent to bleed to death. When rodents became resistant to the short-acting warfarins, long-acting *superwarfarins* such as brodifacoum were developed in response.

Warfarins inhibit vitamin K epoxide reductase, block the conversion of vitamin K to its active form, and prevent carboxylation of the vitamin K–dependent factors 2, 7, 9, and 10 and proteins C and S. Signs of coagulopathy become apparent when the active factor levels fall below 30% and may not occur until days after ingestion. Superwarfarins are more lipophilic and occupy hepatic binding sites with a higher affinity. Whereas warfarin ingestion may produce symptoms for approximately a week, the superwarfarins may cause effects that persist for months.[207-209]

Single toddler exposures to standard warfarin or superwarfarin rodenticides do not typically lead to toxicity. Toxicity has been reported in children who repeatedly ingest superwarfarins or in large suicidal ingestions by adolescents or adults. The prothrombin time will remain normal for 1 to 2 days until factor levels have decreased; therefore testing immediately after exposure is not very helpful.

Ingestions exceeding 0.0125 mg/kg of brodifacoum should be treated with charcoal and decontamination.[210,211] Blood products (fresh-frozen plasma, packed red blood cells, whole blood) should be administered for significant bleeding such as intracranial hemorrhage. Symptomatic patients should receive vitamin K (see Table 355-4); oral administration of vitamin K is preferred to intravenous administration, which has been associated with anaphylactoid reactions.[210-212]

An asymptomatic patient whose samples have abnormal laboratory values should be monitored and provided oral vitamin K. Asymptomatic patients with an international normalized ratio of prothrombin time less than 3.0 should not receive vitamin K and may be monitored as outpatients.

Drs Teresa M. Herbert and Michael L. Weitzman contributed to this chapter in a previous edition.

TOOLS FOR PRACTICE

Engaging Patient and Family

- *Poison Help Line* 1-800-222-1222 (hotline), American Association of Poison Control Centers (www.aapcc.org).
- *TIPP: Children Can Get Very Sick if They Are Poisoned. Children Ages 1 to 3 Are at Highest Risk* (fact sheet), American Academy of Pediatrics (www.aap.org/family/poistipp.htm).
- *What do I do if my child has been poisoned?* (fact sheet), American Academy of Pediatrics (www.aap.org/publiced/BR_Poison.htm).

Medical Decision Support

- *Chemical Agents: Facts About Personal Cleaning and Disposal of Contaminated Clothing* (fact sheet), Centers for Disease Control and Prevention (www.bt.cdc.gov/planning/personalcleaningfacts.asp).
- *Medical Management Guidelines for Chemical Agents*, Centers for Disease Control and Prevention (www.bt.cdc.gov/chemical/mmg.asp).

AAP POLICY STATEMENTS

American Academy of Pediatrics Committee on Drugs. Acetaminophen Toxicity in Children. *Pediatrics*. 2001; 108(4):1020-1024. (aappolicy.aappublications.org/cgi/content/full/pediatrics;108/4/1020).

American Academy of Pediatrics Committee on Environmental Health. Lead Exposure in Children: Prevention, Detection, and Management. *Pediatrics*. 2005;116(4):1036-1046. (aappolicy.aappublications.org/cgi/content/full/pediatrics;116/4/1036) (doi:10.1542/peds.2005-1947).

American Academy of Pediatrics Committee on Injury, Violence, and Poison Prevention. Poison Treatment in the Home. *Pediatrics*. 2003;112(5):1182-1185. (aappolicy.aappublications.org/cgi/content/full/pediatrics;112/5/1182).

OTHER RESOURCES

American Association of Poison Control Centers (Web page), American Association of Poison Control Centers (www.aapcc.org).

Carbon Monoxide Poisoning (Web page), Centers for Disease Control and Prevention (www.cdc.gov.co/).

Chemical Emergencies (Web page), Centers for Disease Control and Prevention (www.bt.cdc.gov/chemical).

Childhood Lead Poisoning Prevention Program (Web page), Centers for Disease Control and Prevention (www.cdc.gov/nceh/lead).

Poisoning (Web page), Centers for Disease Control and Prevention (www.cdc.gov/health/poisoning.html).

The Agency for Toxic Substances and Disease Registry (ATSDR) (Web page), The Agency for Toxic Substances and Disease Registry (ATSDR) (www.atsdr.cdc.gov).

REFERENCES

1. Watson WA, Litovitz TL, Rodgers GC Jr, et al. 2004 Annual report of the American Association of Poison Control Centers Toxic Exposure Surveillance System. *Am J Emerg Med*. 2005;23:589-666.
2. Zuckerman BS, Duby JC. Developmental approach to injury prevention. *Pediatr Clin North Am*. 1985;32:17-29.
3. Sobel R. The psychiatric implications of accidental poisoning in childhood. *Pediatr Clin North Am*. 1970;17:653-685.
4. Bithoney WG, Snyder J, Michalek J, et al. Childhood ingestions as symptoms of family distress. *Am J Dis Child*. 1985;139:456-459.
5. Sibert R. Stress in families of children who have ingested poisons. *Br Med J*. 1975;3:87-89.
6. Flagler SL, Wright L. Recurrent poisoning in children: a review. *J Pediatr Psychol*. 1987;12:631-641.
7. Jones JG. The child accident repeater: a review. *Clin Pediatr*. 1980;19:284-288.
8. Jacobson BJ, Rock AR, Cohn MS, et al. Accidental ingestions of oral prescription drugs: a multicenter survey. *Am J Public Health*. 1989;79:853-856.
9. Wiseman HM, Guest K, Murray VS, et al. Accidental poisoning in childhood: a multicentre survey. 2. The role of packaging in accidents involving medications. *Hum Toxicol*. 1987;6:303-314.
10. Thompson JN. Corrosive esophageal injuries. I. A study of nine cases of concurrent accidental caustic ingestion. *Laryngoscope*. 1987;97:1060-1068.
11. Litovitz T, Klein-Schwartz W, Veltri J, et al. Prescription drug ingestions in children: whose drug? *Vet Hum Toxicol*. 1986;28:14-15.
12. Gaudreault P, McCormick MA, Lacouture PG, et al. Poison exposures and use of ipecac in children less than 1 year old. *Ann Emerg Med*. 1986;15:808-810.
13. Bays J, Feldman KW. Child abuse by poisoning. In: Reece RM, Ludwig S, eds. *Child Abuse: Medical Diagnosis and Management*. Philadelphia, PA: Lippincott Williams & Wilkins; 2001.
14. Densen-Gerber J. The forensic pathology of drug-related child abuse. *Leg Med Annu*. 1978:135-147.
15. Bateman DA, Heagarty MC. Passive freebase cocaine ("crack") inhalation by infants and toddlers. *Am J Dis Child*. 1989;143:25-27.
16. Heidemann SM, Goetting MG. Passive inhalation of cocaine by infants. *Henry Ford Hosp Med J*. 1990;38:252-254.
17. Mirchandani HG, Mirchandani IH, Hellman F, et al. Passive inhalation of free-base cocaine ("crack") smoke by infants. *Arch Pathol Lab Med*. 1991;115:494-498.
18. Schwartz RH, Einhorn A. PCP intoxication in seven young children. *Pediatr Emerg Care*. 1986;2:238-241.
19. Schwartz RH, Peary P, Mistretta D. Intoxication of young children with marijuana: a form of amusement for "pot"-smoking teenage girls. *Am J Dis Child*. 1986; 140:326.
20. Welch MJ, Correa GA. PCP intoxication in young children and infants. *Clin Pediatr*. 1980;19:510-514.
21. Baraff LJ, Guterman JJ, Bayer MJ. The relationship of poison center contact and injury in children 2 to 6 years old. *Ann Emerg Med*. 1992;21:153-157.
22. Eriksson M, Larsson G, Winbladh B, et al. Accidental poisoning in pre-school children in the Stockholm area. Medical, psychosocial and preventive aspects. *Acta Paediatr Scand Suppl*. 1979;275:96-101.
23. Gauvin F, Bailey B, Bratton SL. Hospitalizations for pediatric intoxication in Washington State, 1987-1997. *Arch Pediatr Adolesc Med*. 2001;155:1105-1110.
24. National Safety Council. *Injury Facts*. Itasca, IL: National Safety Council; 2003.
25. Centers for Disease Control and Prevention. Update: childhood poisonings—United States. *MMWR Morb Mortal Wkly Rep*. 1985;34:117-118.
26. Craft AW. Circumstances surrounding deaths from accidental poisoning. 1974-80. *Arch Dis Child*. 1983;58: 544-546.
27. Deeths TM, Breeden JT. Poisoning in children—a statistical study of 1,057 cases. *J Pediatr*. 1971;78:299-305.
28. Belay ED, Bresee JS, Holman RC, et al. Reye's syndrome in the United States from 1981 through 1997. *N Engl J Med*. 1999;340:1377-1382.
29. Hurwitz ES. Reye's syndrome. *Epidemiol Rev*. 1989;11: 249-253.
30. Monto AS. The disappearance of Reye's syndrome—a public health triumph. *N Engl J Med*. 1999;340:1423-1424.
31. Rodgers GB. The effectiveness of child-resistant packaging for aspirin. *Arch Pediatr Adolesc Med*. 2002;156: 929-933.
32. US Department of Health and Human Services, US Food and Drug Administration. Code of Federal Regulations. Section 111.50: Packaging of Iron-Containing Dietary Supplements, 1997-2003. In: Title 21, Part III: *Good Manufacturing Practice for Dietary Supplements*. Washington DC: US Government Printing Office; 2001.
33. Nutritional Health Alliance v. FDA. 318 F.3d. 2d Cir, 2003:92.

34. Rodgers GB. The safety effects of child-resistant packaging for oral prescription drugs. Two decades of experience. *JAMA*. 1996;275:1661-1665.
35. Koren G. Medications which can kill a toddler with one tablet or teaspoonful. *J Toxicol Clin Toxicol*. 1993;31: 407-413.
36. Liebelt EL, Shannon MW. Small doses, big problems: a selected review of highly toxic common medications. *Pediatr Emerg Care*. 1993;9:292-297.
37. Litovitz T, Manoguerra A. Comparison of pediatric poisoning hazards: an analysis of 3.8 million exposure incidents. A report from the American Association of Poison Control Centers. *Pediatrics*. 1992;89:999-1006.
38. Dart RC. *Medical Toxicology*. Philadelphia, PA: Lippincott, Williams & Wilkins; 2004.
39. Goldfrank LR, Flomenbaum NE, Lewin NA, et al, eds. *Goldfrank's Toxicologic Emergencies*. 8th ed. New York, NY: McGraw-Hill; 2006.
40. Ling LJ, Hornfeldt CS, Winter JP. Absorption of iron after experimental overdose of chewable vitamins. *Am J Emerg Med*. 1991;9:24-26.
41. Thompson Healthcare, Inc. Toxicology Information. Available at: www.micromedex.com/products/health care/toxicology/. Accessed July 12, 2007.
42. Chamberlain JM, Klein BL. A comprehensive review of naloxone for the emergency physician. *Am J Emerg Med*. 1994;12:650-660.
43. Howland MA. Antidotes in depth: naloxone. In: Goldfrank LR, Flomenbaum NE, Lewin NA, et al, eds. *Goldfrank's Toxicologic Emergencies*. 8th ed. New York, NY: McGraw-Hill; 2006.
44. Weinbroum AA, Flaishon R, Sorkine P, et al. A risk-benefit assessment of flumazenil in the management of benzodiazepine overdose. *Drug Saf*. 1997;17:181-196.
45. American Academy of Clinical Toxicology, European Association of Poisons Centres and Clinical Toxicologists. Position paper: ipecac syrup. *J Toxicol Clin Toxicol*. 2004;42:133-143. Available at: www.clintox.org/pos_statements/ipecacsyrup.pdf. Accessed July 12, 2007.
46. American Academy of Pediatrics. Poison treatment in the home. *Pediatrics*. 2003;112:1182-1185.
47. Vale JA, Kulig K. Position paper: gastric lavage. *J Toxicol Clin Toxicol*. 2004;42:933-943. Available at: www.clintox.org/pos_statements/gastriclavage.pdf. Accessed July 12, 2007.
48. Kulig K, Bar-Or D, Cantrill SV, et al. Management of acutely poisoned patients without gastric emptying. *Ann Emerg Med*. 1985;14:562-567.
49. Chyka PA, Seger D, Krenzelok EP, et al. Position paper: single-dose activated charcoal. *Clin Toxicol*. 2005;43: 61-87. Available at: www.clintox.org/pos_statements/singledoseactivatedcharcoal.pdf. Accessed July 12, 2007.
50. American Academy of Clinical Toxicology, European Association of Poisons Centres and Clinical Toxicologists. Position statement and practice guidelines on the use of multi-dose activated charcoal in the treatment of acute poisoning. *J Toxicol Clin Toxicol*. 1999;37:731-751. Available at: www.clintox.org/pos_statements/multiple-doseactivatedcharcoal.pdf. Accessed July 12, 2007.
51. American Academy of Clinical Toxicology, European Association of Poisons Centres and Clinical Toxicologists. Position paper: cathartics. *J Toxicol Clin Toxicol*. 2004;42:243-253. Available at: www.clintox.org/pos_statements/cathartics.pdf. Accessed July 12, 2007.
52. American Academy of Clinical Toxicology, European Association of Poisons Centres and Clinical Toxicologists. Position paper: whole bowel irrigation. *J Toxicol Clin Toxicol*. 2004;42:843-854. Available at: www.clintox.org/pos_statements/wholebowelirrigation.pdf. Accessed July 12, 2007.
53. Proudfoot AT, Krenzelok EP, Vale JA. Position paper on urine alkalinization. *J Toxicol Clin Toxicol*. 2004;42:1-26.
54. American Academy of Pediatrics. Acetaminophen toxicity in children. *Pediatrics*. 2001;108:1020-1024.
55. Prescott LF. Paracetamol overdosage. Pharmacological considerations and clinical management. *Drugs*. 1983; 25:290-314.
56. Mitchell JR, Thorgeirsson SS, Potter WZ, et al. Acetaminophen-induced hepatic injury: protective role of glutathione in man and rationale for therapy. *Clin Pharmacol Ther*. 1974;16:676-684.
57. Marzullo L. An update of N-acetylcysteine treatment for acute acetaminophen toxicity in children. *Curr Opin Pediatr*. 2005;17:239-245.
58. Hendrickson RG, Bizovi KE. Acetaminophen. In: Goldfrank LR, Flomenbaum NE, Lewin NA, et al, eds. *Goldfrank's Toxicologic Emergencies*. 8th ed. New York, NY: McGraw-Hill; 2006.
59. Mant TG, Tempowski JH, Volans GN, et al. Adverse reactions to acetylcysteine and effects of overdose. *Br Med J (Clin Res Ed)*. 1984;289:217-219.
60. Perry HE, Shannon MW. Efficacy of oral versus intravenous N-acetylcysteine in acetaminophen overdose: results of an open-label, clinical trial. *J Pediatr*. 1998;132: 149-152.
61. Vale JA, Proudfoot AT. Paracetamol (acetaminophen) poisoning. *Lancet*. 1995;346:547-552.
62. Yip L, Dart RC, Hurlbut KM. Intravenous administration of oral N-acetylcysteine. *Crit Care Med*. 1998;26:40-43.
63. Sung L, Simons JA, Dayneka NL. Dilution of intravenous N-acetylcysteine as a cause of hyponatremia. *Pediatrics*. 1997;100:389-391.
64. Boehnert MT, Lovejoy FH Jr. Value of the QRS duration versus the serum drug level in predicting seizures and ventricular arrhythmias after an acute overdose of tricyclic antidepressants. *N Engl J Med*. 1985;313:474-479.
65. Liebelt EL, Francis PD, Woolf AD. ECG lead aVR versus QRS interval in predicting seizures and arrhythmias in acute tricyclic antidepressant toxicity. *Ann Emerg Med*. 1995;26:195-201.
66. Citak A, Soysal DD, Ucsel R, et al. Efficacy of long duration resuscitation and magnesium sulphate treatment in amitriptyline poisoning. *Eur J Emerg Med*. 2002;9:63-66.
67. Knudsen K, Abrahamsson J. Magnesium sulphate in the treatment of ventricular fibrillation in amitriptyline poisoning. *Eur Heart J*. 1997;18:881-882.
68. Boyer EW, Shannon M. The serotonin syndrome. *N Engl J Med*. 2005;352:1112-1120.
69. Graudins A, Stearman A, Chan B. Treatment of the serotonin syndrome with cyproheptadine. *J Emerg Med*. 1998;16:615-619.
70. Ten Eick AP, Blumer JL, Reed MD. Safety of antihistamines in children. *Drug Saf*. 2001;24:119-147.
71. Burns MJ, Linden CH, Graudins A, et al. A comparison of physostigmine and benzodiazepines for the treatment of anticholinergic poisoning. *Ann Emerg Med*. 2000; 35:374-381.
72. Padilla RB, Pollack ML. The use of physostigmine in diphenhydramine overdose. *Am J Emerg Med*. 2002; 20:569-570.
73. Hampson NB, Norkool DM. Carbon monoxide poisoning in children riding in the back of pickup trucks. *JAMA*. 1992;267:538-540.
74. Herman LY. Carbon monoxide poisoning presenting as an isolated seizure. *J Emerg Med*. 1998;16:429-432.
75. Klasner AE, Smith SR, Thompson MW, et al. Carbon monoxide mass exposure in a pediatric population. *Acad Emerg Med*. 1998;5:992-996.

76. Mandal NG, White N, Wee MY. Carbon monoxide poisoning in a parturient and the use of hyperbaric oxygen for treatment. *Int J Obstet Anesth*. 2001;10:71-74.
77. Silver DA, Cross M, Fox B, et al. Computed tomography of the brain in acute carbon monoxide poisoning. *Clin Radiol*. 1996;51:480-483.
78. Hill EP, Hill JR, Power GG, et al. Carbon monoxide exchanges between the human fetus and mother: a mathematical model. *Am J Physiol*. 1977;232: H311-H323.
79. Longo LD, Hill EP. Carbon monoxide uptake and elimination in fetal and maternal sheep. *Am J Physiol*. 1977; 232:H324-H330.
80. Greingor JL, Tosi JM, Ruhlmann S, et al. Acute carbon monoxide intoxication during pregnancy. One case report and review of the literature. *Emerg Med J*. 2001; 18:399-401.
81. Koren G, Sharav T, Pastuszak A, et al. A multicenter, prospective study of fetal outcome following accidental carbon monoxide poisoning in pregnancy. *Reprod Toxicol*. 1991;5:397-403.
82. Longo LD. The biological effects of carbon monoxide on the pregnant woman, fetus, and newborn infant. *Am J Obstet Gynecol*. 1977;129:69-103.
83. Perrone J, Hoffman RS. Falsely elevated carboxyhemoglobin levels secondary to fetal hemoglobin. *Acad Emerg Med*. 1996;3:287-289.
84. Sokal JA, Kralkowska E. The relationship between exposure duration, carboxyhemoglobin, blood glucose, pyruvate and lactate and the severity of intoxication in 39 cases of acute carbon monoxide poisoning in man. *Arch Toxicol*. 1985;57:196-199.
85. Silverman RK, Montano J. Hyperbaric oxygen treatment during pregnancy in acute carbon monoxide poisoning. A case report. *J Reprod Med*. 1997;42:309-311.
86. Waisman D, Shupak A, Weisz G, et al. Hyperbaric oxygen therapy in the pediatric patient: the experience of the Israel Naval Medical Institute. *Pediatrics*. 1998; 102:E53.
87. Van Hoesen KB, Camporesi EM, Moon RE, et al. Should hyperbaric oxygen be used to treat the pregnant patient for acute carbon monoxide poisoning? A case report and literature review. *JAMA*. 1989;261:1039-1043.
88. Centers for Disease Control and Prevention. Deaths associated with a purported aphrodisiac—New York City, February 1993-May 1995. *MMWR Morb Mortal Wkly Rep*. 1995;44:853-855, 861.
89. Lewander WJ, Gaudreault P, Einhorn A, et al. Acute pediatric digoxin ingestion. A ten-year experience. *Am J Dis Child*. 1986;140:770-773.
90. Lalonde RL, Deshpande R, Hamilton PP, et al. Acceleration of digoxin clearance by activated charcoal. *Clin Pharmacol Ther*. 1985;37:367-371.
91. Nola GT, Pope S, Harrison DC. Assessment of the synergistic relationship between serum calcium and digitalis. *Am Heart J*. 1970;79:499-507.
92. Reisdorff EJ, Clark MR, Walters BL. Acute digitalis poisoning: the role of intravenous magnesium sulfate. *J Emerg Med*. 1986;4:463-469.
93. Hack JB, Lewin NA. Cardioactive steroids. In: Goldfrank LR, Flomenbaum NE, Lewin NA, et al, eds. *Goldfrank's Toxicologic Emergencies*. 8th ed. New York, NY: McGraw-Hill; 2006.
94. Taboulet P, Baud FJ, Bismuth C, et al. Acute digitalis intoxication—is pacing still appropriate? *J Toxicol Clin Toxicol*. 1993;31:261-273.
95. Bailey B. Glucagon in beta-blocker and calcium channel blocker overdoses: a systematic review. *J Toxicol Clin Toxicol*. 2003;41:595-602.
96. Taboulet P, Cariou A, Berdeaux A, et al. Pathophysiology and management of self-poisoning with beta-blockers. *J Toxicol Clin Toxicol*. 1993;31:531-551.
97. Mery PF, Brechler V, Pavoine C, et al. Glucagon stimulates the cardiac Ca2+ current by activation of adenylyl cyclase and inhibition of phosphodiesterase. *Nature*. 1990;345:158-161.
98. Kerns W, Schroeder D, Williams C, et al. Insulin improves survival in a canine model of acute beta-blocker toxicity. *Ann Emerg Med*. 1997;29: 748-757.
99. Shepherd G, Klein-Schwartz W. High-dose insulin therapy for calcium-channel blocker overdose. *Ann Pharmacother*. 2005;39:923-930.
100. Yuan TH, Kerns WP 2nd, Tomaszewski CA, et al. Insulin-glucose as adjunctive therapy for severe calcium channel antagonist poisoning. *J Toxicol Clin Toxicol*. 1999;37:463-474.
101. Brimacombe JR, Scully M, Swainston R. Propranolol overdose—a dramatic response to calcium chloride. *Med J Aust*. 1991;155:267-268.
102. Henry M, Kay MM, Viccellio P. Cardiogenic shock associated with calcium-channel and beta blockers: reversal with intravenous calcium chloride. *Am J Emerg Med*. 1985;3:334-336.
103. Kollef MH. Labetalol overdose successfully treated with amrinone and alpha-adrenergic receptor agonists. *Chest*. 1994;105:626-627.
104. Eddy O, Howell JM. Are one or two dangerous? Clonidine and topical imidazolines exposure in toddlers. *J Emerg Med*. 2003;25:297-302.
105. Broderick-Cantwell JJ. Case study: accidental clonidine patch overdose in attention-deficit/hyperactivity disorder patients. *J Am Acad Child Adolesc Psychiatry*. 1999; 38:95-98.
106. Hamblin JE, Martin CA. Transdermal patch poisoning. *Pediatrics*. 1987;79:161.
107. Horowitz R, Mazor SS, Aks SE, et al. Accidental clonidine patch ingestion in a child. *Am J Ther*. 2005;12: 272-274.
108. Killian CA, Roberge RJ, Krenzelok EP, et al. "Cloniderm" toxicity: another manifestation of clonidine overdose. *Pediatr Emerg Care*. 1997;13:340-341.
109. Seger DL. Clonidine toxicity revisited. *J Toxicol Clin Toxicol*. 2002;40:145-155.
110. Kulig K, Duffy J, Rumack BH, et al. Naloxone for treatment of clonidine overdose. *JAMA*. 1982;247:1697.
111. Anderson RJ, Hart GR, Crumpler CP, et al. Clonidine overdose: report of six cases and review of the literature. *Ann Emerg Med*. 1981;10:107-112.
112. Ashcraft KW, Padula RT. The effect of dilute corrosives on the esophagus. *Pediatrics*. 1974;53:226-232.
113. Gorman RL, Khin-Maung-Gyi MT, Klein-Schwartz W, et al. Initial symptoms as predictors of esophageal injury in alkaline corrosive ingestions. *Am J Emerg Med*. 1992;10:189-194.
114. Gaudreault P, Parent M, McGuigan MA, et al. Predictability of esophageal injury from signs and symptoms: a study of caustic ingestion in 378 children. *Pediatrics*. 1983;71:767-770.
115. Woodring JH, Heiser MJ. Detection of pneumoperitoneum on chest radiographs: comparison of upright lateral and posteroanterior projections. *AJR*. 1995;165: 45-47.
116. Poley JW, Steyerberg EW, Kuipers EJ, et al. Ingestion of acid and alkaline agents: outcome and prognostic value of early upper endoscopy. *Gastrointest Endosc*. 2004; 60:372-377.
117. Penner GE. Acid ingestion: toxicology and treatment. *Ann Emerg Med*. 1980;9:374-379.

118. Homan CS, Maitra SR, Lane BP, et al. Effective treatment for acute alkali injury to the esophagus using weak-acid neutralization therapy: an ex-vivo study. *Acad Emerg Med*. 1995;2:952-958.
119. Lifshitz M, Sofer S, Gorodischer R. Hydrocarbon poisoning in children: a 5-year retrospective study. *Wilderness Environ Med*. 2003;14:78-82.
120. Marks MI, Chicoine L, Legere G, et al. Adrenocorticosteroid treatment of hydrocarbon pneumonia in children—a cooperative study. *J Pediatr*. 1972;81: 366-369.
121. Fradin MS. Mosquitoes and mosquito repellents: a clinician's guide. *Ann Intern Med*. 1998;128:931-940.
122. Sudakin DL, Trevathan WR. DEET: a review and update of safety and risk in the general population. *J Toxicol Clin Toxicol*. 2003;41:831-839.
123. Ginsburg CM, Lowry W, Reisch JS. Absorption of lindane (gamma benzene hexachloride) in infants and children. *J Pediatr*. 1977;91:998-1000.
124. Rugman FP, Cosstick R. Aplastic anaemia associated with organochlorine pesticide: case reports and review of evidence. *J Clin Pathol*. 1990;43:98-101.
125. Sunder Ram Rao CV, Shreenivas R, Singh V, et al. Disseminated intravascular coagulation in a case of fatal lindane poisoning. *Vet Hum Toxicol*. 1988;30:132-134.
126. Linakis JG, Lacouture PG, Woolf A. Iron absorption from chewable vitamins with iron versus iron tablets: implications for toxicity. *Pediatr Emerg Care*. 1992;8: 321-324.
127. Tenenbein M, Littman C, Stimpson RE. Gastrointestinal pathology in adult iron overdose. *J Toxicol Clin Toxicol*. 1990;28:311-320.
128. Vernon DD, Banner W Jr, Dean JM. Hemodynamic effects of experimental iron poisoning. *Ann Emerg Med*. 1989;18:863-866.
129. Whitten CF, Chen YC, Gibson GW. Studies in acute iron poisoning. 3. The hemodynamic alterations in acute experimental iron poisoning. *Pediatr Res*. 1968;2: 479-485.
130. Gleason WA Jr, deMello DE, deCastro FJ, et al. Acute hepatic failure in severe iron poisoning. *J Pediatr*. 1979; 95:138-140.
131. Tenenbein M, Israels SJ. Early coagulopathy in severe iron poisoning. *J Pediatr*. 1988;113:695-697.
132. Klein-Schwartz W, Oderda GM, Gorman RL, et al. Assessment of management guidelines. Acute iron ingestion. *Clin Pediatr*. 1990;29:316-321.
133. Bosse GM. Conservative management of patients with moderately elevated serum iron levels. *J Toxicol Clin Toxicol*. 1995;33:135-140.
134. Everson GW, Bertaccini EJ, O'Leary J. Use of whole bowel irrigation in an infant following iron overdose. *Am J Emerg Med*. 1991;9:366-369.
135. Everson GW, Oudjhane K, Young LW, et al. Effectiveness of abdominal radiographs in visualizing chewable iron supplements following overdose. *Am J Emerg Med*. 1989;7:459-463.
136. Fine JS. Iron poisoning. *Curr Probl Pediatr*. 2000;30: 71-90.
137. Eisen TF, Lacouture PG, Woolf A. Visual detection of ferrioxamine color changes in urine. *Vet Hum Toxicol*. 1988;30:369-370.
138. Villalobos D. Reliability of urine color changes after deferoxamine challenge. *Vet Hum Toxicol*. 1992; 34:330.
139. Tenenbein M. Benefits of parenteral deferoxamine for acute iron poisoning. *J Toxicol Clin Toxicol*. 1996;34: 485-489.
140. Siefkin AD, Albertson TE, Corbett MG. Isoniazid overdose: pharmacokinetics and effects of oral charcoal in treatment. *Hum Toxicol*. 1987;6:497-501.
141. Boyer E. Antituberculous agents. In: Goldfrank LR, Flomenbaum NE, Lewin NA, et al, eds. *Goldfrank's Toxicologic Emergencies*. 8th ed. New York, NY: McGraw-Hill; 2006.
142. Holdiness MR. Neurological manifestations and toxicities of the antituberculosis drugs. A review. *Med Toxicol*. 1987;2:33-51.
143. Santucci KA, Shah BR, Linakis JG. Acute isoniazid exposures and antidote availability. *Pediatr Emerg Care*. 1999;15:99-101.
144. Cash JM, Zawada ET Jr. Isoniazid overdose. Successful treatment with pyridoxine and hemodialysis. *West J Med*. 1991;155:644-646.
145. American Academy of Pediatrics. Lead exposure in children: prevention, detection, and management. *Pediatrics*. 2005;116:1036-1046.
146. Browder AA. Lead poisoning from glazes. *Ann Intern Med*. 1972;76:665.
147. Centers for Disease Control and Prevention. Lead poisoning following ingestion of homemade beverage stored in a ceramic jug—New York. *MMWR Morb Mortal Wkly Rep*. 1989;38:379-380.
148. Centers for Disease Control and Prevention. Lead poisoning from Mexican folk remedies—California. *MMWR Morb Mortal Wkly Rep*. 1983;32:554-555.
149. Centers for Disease Control and Prevention. Lead poisoning-associated death from Asian Indian folk remedies—Florida. *MMWR Morb Mortal Wkly Rep*. 1984; 33:638, 643-645.
150. Centers for Disease Control and Prevention. Childhood lead poisoning associated with tamarind candy and folk remedies—California, 1999-2000. *MMWR Morb Mortal Wkly Rep*. 2002;51:684-686.
151. Schneitzer L, Osborn HH, Bierman A, et al. Lead poisoning in adults from renovation of an older home. *Ann Emerg Med*. 1990;19:415-420.
152. National Research Council. *Measuring Lead Exposure in Infants, Children, and Other Sensitive Populations*. Washington, DC: National Academy Press; 1993.
153. Centers for Disease Control and Prevention. Fatal pediatric lead poisoning—New Hamphshire, 2000. *MMWR Morb Mortal Wkly Rep*. 2001;50:457-459.
154. Wiley JF, Henretig F, Foster R. Status epilepticus and severe neurologic impairment from lead encephalopathy. *J Toxicol Clin Toxicol*. 1995;33:529-530.
155. Piomelli S, Rosen JF, Chisolm JJ Jr, et al. Management of childhood lead poisoning. *J Pediatr*. 1984;105: 523-532.
156. Erenberg G, Rinsler SS, Fish BG. Lead neuropathy and sickle cell disease. *Pediatrics*. 1974;54:438-441.
157. Henretig FM. Lead. In: Goldfrank LR, Flomenbaum NE, Lewin NA, et al, eds. *Goldfrank's Toxicologic Emergencies*. 8th ed. New York, NY: McGraw-Hill; 2006.
158. American Academy of Pediatrics. Treatment guidelines for lead exposure in children. *Pediatrics*. 1995;96:155-160.
159. Kwong TC. Organophosphate pesticides: biochemistry and clinical toxicology. *Ther Drug Monit*. 2002;24: 144-149.
160. Lifshitz M, Shahak E, Sofer S. Carbamate and organophosphate poisoning in young children. *Pediatr Emerg Care*. 1999;15:102-103.
161. Nel L, Hatherill M, Davies J, et al. Organophosphate poisoning complicated by a tachyarrhythmia and acute respiratory distress syndrome in a child. *J Paediatr Child* Health. 2002;38:530-532.
162. Mattingly JE, Sullivan JE, Spiller HA, et al. Intermediate syndrome after exposure to chlorpyrifos in a 16-month-old girl. *J Emerg Med*. 2003;25:379-381.

163. Hsieh BH, Deng JF, Ger J, et al. Acetylcholinesterase inhibition and the extrapyramidal syndrome: a review of the neurotoxicity of organophosphate. *Neurotoxicology.* 2001;22:423-427.
164. Goswamy R, Chaudhuri A, Mahashur AA. Study of respiratory failure in organophosphate and carbamate poisoning. *Heart Lung.* 1994;23:466-472.
165. Rotenberg JS, Newmark J. Nerve agent attacks on children: diagnosis and management. *Pediatrics.* 2003; 112:648-658.
166. Buckley NA, Roberts D, Eddleston M. Overcoming apathy in research on organophosphate poisoning. *BMJ.* 2004;329:1231-1233.
167. Dyer S. Plant exposures: wilderness medicine. *Emerg Med Clin North Am.* 2004;22:299-313, vii.
168. Ogzewalla CD, Bonfiglio JF, Sigell LT. Common plants and their toxicity. *Pediatr Clin North Am.* 1987;34: 1557-1598.
169. Grunbaum JA, Kann L, Kinchen S, et al. Youth risk behavior surveillance—United States, 2003. *MMWR Morb Mortal Wkly Rep Surveill Summ.* 2004;53:1-96.
170. Kaye DL. Office recognition and management of adolescent substance abuse. *Curr Opin Pediatr.* 2004;16: 532-541.
171. Dias PJ. Adolescent substance abuse. Assessment in the office. *Pediatr Clin North Am.* 2002;49:269-300.
172. Greydanus DE, Patel DR. Substance abuse in adolescents: a complex conundrum for the clinician. *Pediatr Clin North Am.* 2003;50:1179-1223.
173. Levy S, Vaughan BL, Knight JR. Office-based intervention for adolescent substance abuse. *Pediatr Clin North Am.* 2002;49:329-343.
174. Simkin DR. Adolescent substance use disorders and comorbidity. *Pediatr Clin North Am.* 2002;49:463-477.
175. Chait LD, Burke KA. Preference for high- versus low-potency marijuana. *Pharmacol Biochem Behav.* 1994; 49:643-647.
176. Ashton CH. Pharmacology and effects of cannabis: a brief review. *Br J Psychiatry.* 2001;178:101-106.
177. Schwartz RH. LSD: its rise, fall, and renewed popularity among high school students. *Pediatr Clin North Am.* 1995;42:403-413.
178. Leikin JB, Krantz AJ, Zell-Kanter M, et al. Clinical features and management of intoxication due to hallucinogenic drugs. *Med Toxicol Adverse Drug Exp.* 1989;4:324-350.
179. Young T, Lawson GW, Gacono CB. Clinical aspects of phencyclidine (PCP). *Int J Addict.* 1987;22:1-15.
180. Benowitz NL. Clinical pharmacology and toxicology of cocaine. *Pharmacol Toxicol.* 1993;72:3-12.
181. Koesters SC, Rogers PD, Rajasingham CR. MDMA ("ecstasy") and other "club drugs." The new epidemic. *Pediatr Clin North Am.* 2002;49:415-433.
182. Maxwell JC. Party drugs: properties, prevalence, patterns, and problems. *Subst Use Misuse.* 2005;40:1203-1240.
183. Rattray M. Ecstasy: towards an understanding of the biochemical basis of the actions of MDMA. *Essays Biochem.* 1991;26:77-87.
184. Wilkerson RD. Cardiovascular toxicity of cocaine. *NIDA Res Monogr.* 1988;88:304-324.
185. Henry JA, Jeffreys KJ, Dawling S. Toxicity and deaths from 3,4-methylenedioxymethamphetamine ("ecstasy"). *Lancet.* 1992;340:384-387.
186. Levis JT, Garmel GM. Cocaine-associated chest pain. *Emerg Med Clin North Am.* 2005;23:1083-1103.
187. Cregler LL, Mark H. Relation of acute myocardial infarction to cocaine abuse. *Am J Cardiol.* 1985;56:794.
188. Winecoff AP, Hariman RJ, Grawe JJ, et al. Reversal of the electrocardiographic effects of cocaine by lidocaine. Part 1. Comparison with sodium bicarbonate and quinidine. *Pharmacotherapy.* 1994;14:698-703.
189. Weber JE, Shofer FS, Larkin GL, et al. Validation of a brief observation period for patients with cocaine-associated chest pain. *N Engl J Med.* 2003;348:510-517.
190. Brouette T, Anton R. Clinical review of inhalants. *Am J Addict.* 2001;10:79-94.
191. Kurtzman TL, Otsuka KN, Wahl RA. Inhalant abuse by adolescents. *J Adolesc Health.* 2001;28:170-180.
192. Spiller HA, Krenzelok EP. Epidemiology of inhalant abuse reported to two regional poison centers. *J Toxicol Clin Toxicol.* 1997;35:167-173.
193. Bass M. Sudden sniffing death. *JAMA.* 1970;212: 2075-2079.
194. Shannon M, Quang LS. Gamma-hydroxybutyrate, gamma-butyrolactone, and 1,4-butanediol: a case report and review of the literature. *Pediatr Emerg Care.* 2000;16:435-440.
195. Schwartz RH. Adolescent heroin use: a review. *Pediatrics.* 1998;102:1461-1466.
196. Palatnick W, Redman LW, Sitar DS, et al. Methanol half-life during ethanol administration: implications for management of methanol poisoning. *Ann Emerg Med.* 1995;26:202-207.
197. Wallace KL, Suchard JR, Curry SC, et al. Diagnostic use of physicians' detection of urine fluorescence in a simulated ingestion of sodium fluorescein-containing antifreeze. *Ann Emerg Med.* 2001;38:49-54.
198. Brent J, McMartin K, Phillips S, et al. Fomepizole for the treatment of methanol poisoning. *N Engl J Med.* 2001;344: 424-429.
199. Barceloux DG, Krenzelok EP, Olson K, et al. American Academy of Clinical Toxicology Practice Guidelines on the treatment of ethylene glycol poisoning. *J Toxicol Clin Toxicol.* 1999;37:537-560.
200. Baud FJ, Bismuth C, Garnier R, et al. 4-Methylpyrazole may be an alternative to ethanol therapy for ethylene glycol intoxication in man. *J Toxicol Clin Toxicol.* 1986; 24:463-483.
201. Baud FJ, Galliot M, Astier A, et al. Treatment of ethylene glycol poisoning with intravenous 4-methylpyrazole. *N Engl J Med.* 1988;319:97-100.
202. Garella S. Extracorporeal techniques in the treatment of exogenous intoxications. *Kidney Int.* 1988;33:735-754.
203. Gonda A, Gault H, Churchill D, et al. Hemodialysis for methanol intoxication. *Am J Med.* 1978;64:749-758.
204. Peterson CD, Collins AJ, Himes JM, et al. Ethylene glycol poisoning: pharmacokinetics during therapy with ethanol and hemodialysis. *N Engl J Med.* 1981;304:21-23.
205. Lacouture PG, Wason S, Abrams A, et al. Acute isopropyl alcohol intoxication. Diagnosis and management. *Am J Med.* 1983;75:680-686.
206. Liu JJ, Daya MR, Carrasquillo O, et al. Prognostic factors in patients with methanol poisoning. *J Toxicol Clin Toxicol.* 1998;36:175-181.
207. Babcock J, Hartman K, Pedersen A, et al. Rodenticide-induced coagulopathy in a young child. A case of Munchausen syndrome by proxy. *Am J Pediatr Hematol Oncol.* 1993;15:126-130.
208. Chong LL, Chau WK, Ho CH. A case of "superwarfarin" poisoning. *Scand J Haematol.* 1986;36:314-315.
209. Hoffman RS, Smilkstein MJ, Goldfrank LR. Evaluation of coagulation factor abnormalities in long-acting anticoagulant overdose. *J Toxicol Clin Toxicol.* 1988;26:233-248.
210. Jones EC, Growe GH, Naiman SC. Prolonged anticoagulation in rat poisoning. *JAMA.* 1984;252:3005-3007.
211. Smolinske SC, Scherger DL, Kearns PS, et al. Superwarfarin poisoning in children: a prospective study. *Pediatrics.* 1989;84:490-494.
212. Watts RG, Castleberry RP, Sadowski JA. Accidental poisoning with a superwarfarin compound (brodifacoum) in a child. *Pediatrics.* 1990;86:883-887.

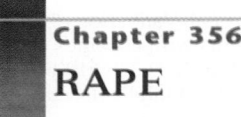

Chapter 356

RAPE

Marianne E. Felice, MD; Christine E. Barron, MD

Rape is a legal definition, not a medical diagnosis; every state has statutory definitions of sexual assault and rape. Clinicians should be familiar with the statutes in their local jurisdictions. In general, *rape* refers to sexual intercourse with force or the threat of force or without a person's consent. Sexual intercourse may include penile-oral, penile-vaginal, or penile-anal penetration. The threat may be an overt physical threat, verbal threat, or an implicit threat as a result of age and power differentials between sexual partners. Rape can occur at all ages; however, this chapter focuses on adolescent victims of rape. Rape entails an assault acted out sexually, rather than a sexual act per se. Not only is rape an unchosen act for the victim, but it also causes health risks unchosen by the victim. In this chapter, information is provided on rape, not chronic sexual abuse, such as incest.

INCIDENCE

Exact statistics on the incidence and prevalence of adolescent rape are not available because many victims never report the crime. Estimates of unreported rape range from 40% to 90%.[1] Between 40% and 60% of all rape victims are younger than 18 years, and most are adolescents.[2,3]

Female adolescents aged 16 to 19 are 4 times more likely to be sexually assaulted than women in all other age groups.[4] Worldwide, estimates indicate that between one third and two thirds of rape victims are 15 years and younger.[5] Although most rape victims are women, 5% to 10% are men.[2,6] Ninety percent of adolescent rape victims are assaulted by someone they know, and more than 50% of these cases occur on a date.[7] Survivors of prior sexual abuse are at particular risk of revictimization.[8] Adolescents who engage in high-risk behaviors, such as running away and using drugs and alcohol, are at an increased risk for rape.[9] Approximately one half of all reported rapes in the United States eventually lead to arrests; approximately two thirds of those arrested are prosecuted, and approximately one half of those prosecuted are found guilty. In other words, for every 100 reported rapes, only 16 of the perpetrators are convicted.[1]

TYPES OF RAPES

Types of rape vary considerably based on the relationship of the victim to the assailant. The various types of rapes raise different issues that are crucial to consider when providing care for the pediatric survivor. Psychosocial sequelae of rape often vary according to the type of rape involved.

Known Assailant

In most reported pediatric rape cases the victim knows the assailant, who may be a parent, a stepparent, an adult relative or friend of the family, a neighbor, an acquaintance, or a classmate. The victim-assailant relationship may cause conflicting family or social loyalties. In these cases, victims are less likely to report the rape. Furthermore, rape victims who know their assailants are prone to self-doubt and self-blame, and when they do report the rape, their reports may be received with skepticism and disbelief, even by the professionals to whom they turn for help.[10]

Stranger Rape

An estimated 15% to 55% of reported rapes are committed by individuals who are not known by the victim.[11] Stranger rape is more likely to entail threats or use of violence and fear of immediate danger, and it is associated with a higher incidence of reporting the rape and of subsequent conviction of the assailant. Stranger rape is most likely to occur in areas of poverty and in high-crime districts where walking and playing pose risks of danger.

Date Rape

Estimates of the incidence of date rape are unclear. However, in 1 survey of middle and high school students, nearly 20% of the girls and more than 10% of the boys reported a history of unwanted sexual activity on dates.[12] Surveys of college students indicate that approximately 25% of female students and 6% of male students report a history of sexual assault that meets the definition of rape while on a date.[6,12] Almost none of the college students in these surveys reported the sexual assault to authorities. Particularly in cases of young female adolescents (ages 10 to 15) and older men, questions of statutory rape arise, along with questions of consent, refusal skills, and exploitation.[13]

Of the various types of rape, date rape is the least likely to be reported. The fact that the incidence of date rape appears highly correlated with 1 or both parties having been drinking or using other drugs before the rape is of particular concern to adolescents. As would be expected, date rapes are more likely to occur on weekends between 10 PM and 1 AM, in automobiles or at the home of the assailant.[11]

Date rape may not be reported if the rape was facilitated by the administration of pharmaceuticals, including gamma hydroxybutyric acid, flunitrazepam (Rohypnol), and ketamine hydrochloride (Ketamine), known as *date rape drugs,* given that these medications cause anterograde amnesia.

Long-term issues of trust, self-blame, and vulnerability are important issues for victims of date rape, as in any other form of rape. The female date rape victim may not trust her judgment concerning men, and she may blame herself for the rape, erroneously believing that she did not resist clearly or did not resist convincingly enough. She may be ashamed that she ended up in a situation that resulted in rape. These thoughts of guilt may be reinforced by the response and degree of support provided by parents, guardians, and friends. Parents' and friends' understanding and support of the victim is a significant prognostic factor for recovery. The tendency for victims to have reservations about reporting date rape is easy to understand.

Unfortunately, such secrecy also applies to discussing the incident in general, making catharsis, as well as verbal and emotional support from others, difficult to obtain.

Gang Rape

Gang rape typically involves a group of young men raping a solitary female victim. This type of rape may be associated with ritualistic behavior, as well as displaced rage on the part of the assailants. Issues of sexualized rites of passage apply both to stereotypical adolescent gangs and to college fraternities. Victims of college campus gang rapes are more likely to drop out of college after the rape than to pursue legal recourse,[11] avoiding confrontation with the perpetrators at the long-term expense of the victims.

Male Rape

In this discussion, *male rape* refers to same-sex rape. Although sporadic reports have surfaced of male rape by women, data are limited.[10] The area of male rape remains understudied and is far less understood than female rape. Specific subgroups of young men are at particular risk for sexual abuse: those in institutionalized settings (such as the criminal justice system), street youth (who may engage in prostitution), young male homosexuals (who may be runaways), and youth who have a parental history of physical or sexual abuse (parents who were abused themselves may become abusers as adults).[14] The occurrence of male rape in institutionalized settings is often attributed to displaced heterosexual behavior or undifferentiated sexual orientation, along with aggressive dominance of a weaker partner.[15,16] Male rape outside institutions often occurs through coercion by an individual perceived as an authority figure to the victim.[1]

Although male rape victims are more likely than their female counterparts to sustain physical trauma,[17,18] the treatment of male victims should parallel that described for women. Issues of loss of control are particularly relevant for the male rape victim, along with subsequent symptoms of depression, anxiety, sleep disturbances, and suicidal ideation. Conflicted sexual identity is common among all male rape victims, whether they are homosexual or not. Male rape victims are often controlled by entrapment, intimidation, physical force, or any combination. The intimidation is accomplished by threats of physical harm, by brandishing a weapon, or both. Male rape victims frequently perceive the rape as a life-threatening event[18] (a perception that may result in long-term psychological problems).[16] Because of the pervasive reluctance of boys and men to report rape, the preclusion of social support and intervention is a particularly challenging issue.

MALE PERPETRATORS

Just as female adolescents constitute a large proportion of reported rape victims, male adolescents make up a large proportion of convicted rape assailants; 40% of convicted rapists are 16 to 20 years of age, and another 25% are between 20 and 24 years of age.[1]

Perpetrators tend to fall into 1 of 3 clusters: (1) those for whom anger is the primary dynamic; (2) those for whom power or conquest is the central issue; and (3) the sadistic person, for whom anger and control are, in and of themselves, erotic.[19] For the anger-driven rapist, the act tends to be impulsive, with the intent of hurting, humiliating, and degrading the victim. Physical brutality is common. Rape functions as the outlet for anger, essentially by using sex as a weapon. The power-oriented rapist is more likely to engage in premeditated, obsessive, or stalking behavior, in which the rape essentially compensates for social and sexual incompetence or inadequacy. Aggression for the power-oriented rapist is less likely to be violent than a means of dominating his prey. Both anger- and power-driven rapists have serious deficits in social skills and the inability to interpret and respond to social cues from others. For the sadistic rapist, eroticism and violence are enmeshed; victims are typically subjected to premeditated, deliberate acts of cruelty and dehumanization. The sadistic perpetrator finds gratification in his victim's pain and powerlessness.

Although some rapists are dysfunctional sexually at the time of the rape, most rapists are sexually active with available, consensual partners outside the rape.[19] Perpetrators usually appear ordinary by most standards; most do not have symptoms of major psychiatric illnesses such as psychoses, nor does a preponderance exist of intellectual disability. However, other conditions such as antisocial, schizoid, paranoid, and narcissistic personality disorders are noted more commonly among convicted rapists than in the general population.[3,14]

Alcohol and drug use have been associated with the occurrence of rape. Ironically, alcohol intoxication sometimes seems to have the effect of both diminishing a perpetrator's sense of responsibility and increasing a victim's culpability. Specifically, the perpetrator's act of rape is *excused* because he was drinking and not responsible for his actions. Whereas, victim intoxication is consistently coupled with the process of *unfounding,* or disproving, rape charges. For date rape victims, having been seen drinking with the perpetrator before the attack has serious implications in relation to public, social, and legal responses to the charges.

RESPONSE TO RAPE

Immediate Response to Rape By the Victim

Immediate responses to rape vary considerably, ranging from distraught histrionics to near-mute withdrawal. Most victims have intense levels of fear and anxiety. Varying levels of cognitive disorganization, *shock,* and disbelief also characterize this postrape acute phase.[19] As occurs in any crisis, many adolescents regress to previous stages of development. An adolescent rape victim who was previously self-assured and appropriately independent may become clinging and dependent on the parent or health professional.

Immediate Response By the Family

Unlike other crime victims, the victim of rape rarely contacts the police immediately. Typically, the victim contacts an intermediary (a friend or family member) first. This individual's response is crucial in the ensuing medical and legal processes; but most family and friends need guidance to know how best to be supportive to the victim. The disclosure of rape is usually traumatic for the family, as well as the victim. Parents may blame themselves inappropriately for the rape. In other instances, parental activities (eg, neglect) may have contributed to the rape. In either scenario, the issues are highly sensitive and need to be addressed with skill and compassion.

Familial responses to a child's rape range from denial and disbelief to shame and outrage. No guarantee exists that a family is prepared to respond appropriately to a raped child's needs at this time. In some cases, a victim's mother's financial dependence on a perpetrator may confound reactions. During the initial evaluation session, health care professionals must therefore spend some time with the family members and friends of the victim to determine their own psychological response and their ability to be supportive of the victim.

LEGAL ISSUES

All states have laws that require physicians to report cases involving violent assault, including rape. To report statutory rape, the clinician should be familiar with state's laws regarding reporting sexual abuse and the legal age of consent. Statutory rape is defined as sexual activity of an adult with an adolescent under the age of legal consent. Reporting concerns include the possibility that reporting statutory rape can cause barriers for adolescents to obtain appropriate medical care. Clinicians have expressed the desire to use their clinical judgment in reporting cases of sexual activity that fall within the definition of statutory rape.[20] Some states require parental notification of a minor's sexual assault, and in those states, this statute overrides issues of confidentiality.

Most states permit a minor to receive treatment for sexual assault without parental consent. All clinicians must be familiar with local statutes.[21,22] Health care providers should seek additional guidance from their legal counsel or from their state attorney general's office.

Consent for treatment of rape is different than consent for collection of evidence. An adolescent patient above the legal age of consent has the ability to consent to a medical evaluation and treatment and may refuse collection of forensic evidence, or the patient may consent to both. Many victims are reluctant to give permission because they fear social isolation and possible retribution by the perpetrator. Adolescent victims who decide not to report the rape to law enforcement should be informed that if the victim wanted to pursue possible prosecution in the future, then the evidence must be collected at this time. Therefore the physician must ask the adolescent patient for permission to complete a full evidentiary examination and to release the evidence to the police. The exceptions are cases identified by state law to be child sexual abuse that requires mandatory reporting to a child welfare agency, law enforcement, or both, which does not require consent from patient or family to report.

From a medical-legal perspective, physicians must realize that their responsibility is limited to the documentation of evidence. Determining whether a rape really occurred is not the physician's role; this determination is a court decision. The physician will be of most help to the victim and the authorities by presuming that the victim is telling the truth, being thorough in the evaluation, and keeping accurate medical records.

MEDICAL EVALUATION

Rape is a serious medical and psychological emergency for both the victim and the family. The purpose of the initial evaluation is 4 fold: (1) treatment of injury and infection, (2) prevention of pregnancy, (3) collection of evidence, and (4) psychological assessment with referral for follow-up counseling.

General Concepts

Many metropolitan areas have treatment centers with trained interdisciplinary teams available for adolescent and child victims of rape; these treatment centers are ideal sites for an initial evaluation[23] and are usually staffed with an interdisciplinary care team, most frequently consisting of a physician, nurse, and social worker. An interdisciplinary approach is beneficial for several reasons, including the ability to provide support to the child and family simultaneously and to serve as a resource for future services. For various reasons, most pediatric rape victims do not use such specialized facilities, and they may receive medical evaluations at emergency departments or private medical offices. To minimize the physical and psychological trauma of the evaluation, eliminate the need for repeat evaluations, and maximize the probability of collecting forensic evidence, the most skilled professional available should perform the initial evaluation. The gender of the examiner is less important than the individual's comfort with adolescents and children, skill at conducting the examination, and level of compassion.

The rape evaluation can be long and tedious, but it should never be rushed. Although the youngster is coping with personal outrage and physical and psychological pain, the patient is expected to tolerate and cooperate with uncomfortable procedures that may feel similar to the acts of intrusion and aggression experienced previously. The approach to the evaluation should be calm, gentle, and private. Rape protocols, if available, are helpful and will serve to minimize the chance for error or omission in the evidence-collection process. Most jurisdictions have printed standardized forms for the evidence-procurement process[5]; these forms are available in each state's *forensic evidence kit*. Before examining a victim, the clinician should become familiar with these forms.

The clinician should avoid making inappropriate assumptions about the victim based on the patient's psychological state. Many victims are in a state of shock or denial immediately after the event. How a patient responds in the emergency room varies and depends on numerous factors, including developmental maturity. Appearing physically mature but functioning cognitively at the level of a preadolescent is not uncommon for a 13-year-old child. Therefore the patient's psychological state should not alter the physician's approach to care. Furthermore, the clinician should not attempt to minimize the victim's sense of personal guilt, shame, and anxiety by offering reassurance immediately. Taking a few minutes to empathize with the patient and acknowledge the patient's feelings before proceeding with the evaluation helps both the patient and the physician. Particularly in cases in which acute trauma may compromise a pediatric patient's existing coping skills, the establishment of the patient's safety is crucial. The clinician should never leave the patient alone, if at all possible.

Taking whatever time is necessary at the beginning of the evaluation to explain the process of the examination and allow for questions is always prudent, particularly for rape victims who never had previous sexual relationships or a prior gynecologic examination; such is also the case for more experienced patients who understandably may still be anxious and fearful of anticipated pain and discomfort. Whenever possible, the clinician should allow the patient some control over the proceedings; the patient should set the pace of the examination. The clinician should be careful to inform the patient in advance of what tasks must be accomplished. The patient should be the one who signals when to begin the procedure. If the victim becomes visibly agitated with the proceedings, then the clinician should stop and allow the patient to regain composure before continuing with the examination. At no point should a physician continue to examine a child or adolescent against the patient's will.

Whenever applicable, making reference to prior experience with other similar-aged rape survivors may help establish that the patient is not the only child or adolescent to whom this ordeal has happened; it also establishes that the physician is not shocked at such circumstances and has some practical knowledge with which to anticipate concerns.

After obtaining consent from the patient, the physician should obtain a detailed and relevant history, followed by a thorough general physical examination and a gentle but complete pelvic examination. A female nurse or assistant must be present during this process; for some young adolescents, having a parent present during the examination is usually helpful if the parent is reassuring, rather than openly distraught during the procedure. Some aspects of the evaluation will change depending on the temporal proximity of the evaluation to the alleged event. The following guidelines are recommended for evaluations conducted within 72 hours of the assault. Modifications are necessary if the evaluation is conducted after this time. In some centers the interdisciplinary team obtains the history simultaneously and together so that the victim does not have to repeat the history unnecessarily.

History

History taking necessarily entails asking some very personal and potentially awkward questions. The patient should be assured of privacy and offered respectful compassion. The history should include the time, date, and location of both the event and the examination. Recalling the event may be emotionally traumatic for the patient; thus beginning with a relevant, but relatively neutral, medical history is sometimes useful. Such information as medical history, physical and behavioral symptoms, and a thorough menstrual history—including the age of menarche; the date of the last menstrual period; the frequency of menses; sexual activity if relevant; previous pregnancies, miscarriages, and abortions; and the use of contraceptives and feminine hygiene products—is important. Additional history should include parental response to disclosure, fear of parental reaction and risk of running away, and fully exploring past and current suicidal ideation.

Next, the event itself should be the focus. Questions should be asked calmly and with sensitivity and patience. The victim's own words should be recorded whenever possible. The medical chart is a legal document and will be subjected to the same scrutiny as any other form of evidence. Only the historical facts, without embellishment or interpretation, should be recorded.

The patient should be asked about the use of intoxicating substances before or during the event, as well as whether any loss of consciousness that may have occurred. The clinician needs to ask whether weapons or restraints were used during the assault. The patient should be asked to describe in detail the location of the event, the appearance of the perpetrator, the type of sexual contact and the positions used, the use of force (by both the perpetrator and the victim), the removal of clothing and the manner in which it was removed, and what measures, if any, the patient took to cleanse or relieve himself or herself (eg, bathing, douching, changing clothes, urinating, defecating). Whether the assailant used a condom or any other means of contraception should be determined. Finally, the physician should ask about the presence of clinical symptoms in the musculoskeletal, gastrointestinal, and genitourinary system.

Physical Examination

A detailed history and physical examination, as well as specimens for forensic and laboratory evaluation, should be obtained for all rape victims. Particular focus should be placed on the evaluation of the oral cavity, the genitals, and the anus.

Although a complete physical examination from head to toe is warranted, 40% to 60% of sexual assault victims will have no visible physical injuries.[17,18] Inspection of the entire body may provide the corroborative evidence necessary to convict the perpetrator, and follow-up examinations may reveal emerging bruising or injuries in areas initially noted to have tenderness or swelling but no visible bruising on the initial examination.

The patient's physical appearance and emotional state and the condition of the patient's clothing should be noted. If the patient is wearing the same clothing worn at the time of the event, then its condition should be noted and each piece saved in a separate, labeled bag. Applying a fluorescent lamp to the clothing and skin may illuminate the presence of dried semen. Semen fluoresces best at wavelengths of 420 and 450 nm, when viewed through orange goggles. A Wood lamp emits light at only 360-nm wavelength. Therefore specialized alternate light sources that emit wavelengths at 420 and 450 nm, such as a Bluemaxx, should be used. Although this type of lamp will improve the detection of dried semen, many other substances will fluoresce as well; thus confirmation of semen cannot be made with this method.[24] These specimens should be marked for later analysis for the presence of seminal vesicle–specific antigen. Next, a topical survey of the body, documenting any evidence of recent trauma or bruising, should be done. The use of photographs may be useful during subsequent litigation. Use of a diagram to indicate locations of visible injuries can be helpful. The clinician should use the fluorescent lamp to identify any fluorescent areas on the skin and obtain swabs of these areas.

Particular attention should be given to the examination of the head and neck. Compression injuries of the neck are fairly common if force is used. This type of injury may lead to obstruction of venous return from the head, causing the development of neck bruising or petechial hemorrhages in the eyelids and conjunctiva. The inner surface of the lips may have tiny abrasions resulting from forced pressure applied to the mouth by the perpetrator to prevent the victim from screaming. Common injuries to the mouth include torn frenulums and palate petechiae.

The breasts may show bite marks or bruises. The clinician should swab all bite marks to collect genetic markers (ABO group) and photo-document these injuries because the bite impression may be matched to a potential perpetrator. Tanner staging to determine the victim's level of sexual maturation (breasts and pubic hair in female patients, genitalia and pubic hair in male patients) should also be performed.

Genital Examination

Female Patient

After the initial physical examination, the patient can be draped and placed in the lithotomy position. If the patient seems too anxious and a speculum examination is not required to investigate for a source of undiagnosed internal bleeding, then the supine frog-leg position may be a suitable alternative. A speculum examination is not necessary for younger adolescents or children, unless active vaginal bleeding is present, which is a rare occurrence. In these rare instances of active vaginal bleeding, performing the pelvic examination with the patient under sedation or under general anesthesia may be necessary.

The pelvic examination should begin with inspection of the thighs and perineum for evidence of trauma, bruising, semen, or blood. Appropriate forensic evidence should be taken at this time (Box 356-1). General inspection of the external genitalia should be performed, with documentation of any erythema, edema, ecchymosis, or abrasions noted.

In some cultures, an intact hymen is important as an indicator of virginity, and the patient and parents will be concerned with its structural integrity. An intact hymen does not rule out the diagnosis of rape. Acute injuries to the hymen such as bruising, petechiae, or acute transactions should be documented by describing any active bleeding and the location, as though a face of a clock were superimposed over the hymen (eg, acute swelling and transaction of hymen with active bleeding at 8 o'clock position). The entire rim of the hymen must be visualized; proper labial traction along with saline-moistened cotton swab rolled around the edges of the hymen is necessary.[25] The use of a light source or the application of aqueous toluidine blue (1%) to the posterior fourchette may help locate and identify acute tears.[26] Many experts use colposcopy, which provides a light source, magnification, and photo-documentation of the examination. Colposcopy or photo-documentation with a camera is essential in providing documentation of the examination, and images can later be evaluated by expert review.[27,28]

Older female adolescents should be able to undergo a speculum examination of the internal genitals, which will allow a clear view of the vaginal walls, fornices, and cervix. Appropriate specimens for culture and forensics should be obtained (see Box 356-1).

BOX 356-1 Recommended Procedures for Collecting Forensic Data

Forensic evidence kit: Complete forms for authorization and release of evidence, history, and physical examination. Individual envelopes will be completed if indicated by the history provided.

Additional tests:

- Pregnancy test
- Syphilis screening
- HIV test
- Cultures for gonorrhea (oral, urethral, vaginal, and anal)
- Cultures for *Chlamydia* (urethral, vaginal, and anal)
- Wet mount for detection of *Trichomonas* and spermatozoa

Male Patient

The testes, epididymis, vas deferens, penile shaft, foreskin, and glans penis should be examined thoroughly for the presence of infection or trauma.

Anal Examination

A history of sodomy in both male and female victims indicates the need to conduct a thorough anal inspection. The clinician should document any erythema, ecchymosis, abrasions, or rectal bleeding noted. Aqueous toluidine blue (1%) may be applied to help visualize acute microtrauma to the perianal area.[25]

Summarizing the Examination

When the physical examination is complete, the patient should be given ample time to dress and regain composure before discussing any findings. Most patients will benefit from knowing that their genital anatomy is normal. Several studies have demonstrated that over 90% of anogenital examination are normal.[29-31] Discussing physical findings, treatment options, and plans for follow-up is also important.

Forensic and Laboratory Information

The recovery of laboratory and forensic data is probably the most controversial aspect of the evaluation,[32] especially when recovery of semen and sperm is involved; nonetheless, the finding of male ejaculate is neither predictive nor essential for criminal conviction. In one study, physical evidence of rape was found in only 23% of all of the cases that resulted in felony convictions.[33] Forensic evidence identified in younger victims is more often obtained from the child's clothing, bed linens, or both.[34] The newest developments in forensic science have occurred in the laboratory analysis of semen and include the demonstration of quantifiable levels of acid phosphatase and a positive monoclonal antibody test, the MH5 enzyme-linked immunosorbent assay (specific for seminal vesicle antigen) in vaginal fluids.

Sexually Transmitted Infection

Most patients are concerned about the risk of acquiring a sexually transmitted infection (STI) as a result of the rape. This risk is related directly to the health status of the assailant and the victim, the site of the assault, and the infectivity of the disease in question. Overall, the risk of contracting an STI from a single encounter is small.[35,36] Repeat assaults or assaults by more than one assailant increase the risk of infection.[36] Many adolescent victims of rape, however, also engage in high-risk behaviors that put them at increased risk of having a preexisting STI. Additionally, as many as 50% of sexual assault survivors do not return for follow-up appointments.[37] The Centers for Disease Control and Prevention recommends using prophylactic antibiotics for treating potential sexually acquired infections (see Chapter 322, Sexually Transmitted Infections).[38,39] A prophylactic hepatitis B vaccination against possible exposure is recommended.

Regardless of the antibiotics given, the clinician must emphasize to the patient that the incubation period for STIs varies and that a high possibility exists that an infection may not be detected or may be missed or treated inadequately at the time of the evaluation examination. Therefore, although baseline studies should be obtained at the initial evaluation, medical follow-up is absolutely crucial. After 2 weeks the patient should be reexamined for the presence of an STI. Serial testing for syphilis, human papillomavirus, and HIV infection should be performed after the assault in most cases.

Pregnancy

The occurrence of pregnancy after rape is strongly influenced by whether a female patient is in the fertile interval of her menstrual cycle, as well as the possible sexual dysfunction of the assailant (eg, failure to maintain an erection or to ejaculate).[3,14,40] Many adolescents, however, have irregular menstrual cycles; therefore the occurrence of ovulation for any particular cycle may be in question. If the assault occurred within 5 days of the evaluation, then emergency contraception (see the discussion of postcoital *morning after* contraception in Chapter 156, Contraception and Abortion) should be offered to the patient after a negative pregnancy test has ruled out the presence of an already existing pregnancy.[41] Two types of emergency contraceptive medications are available. The 1st type contains only progestin. Plan B is a progestin-only emergency contraceptive that reduces the risk of pregnancy by 89%.[41] Because Plan B contains only progestin, it has less side effects of nausea or vomiting. The 2nd type contains both progestin and estrogen. Most brands of the daily oral contraception pill contain both progestin and estrogen that reduces the risk of pregnancy by 75%.[42] When medication containing both progestin and estrogen is used, antiemetics should be offered because of the frequent side effects of nausea and vomiting. The occurrence of pregnancy after unprotected exposure should be strongly suspected when menses does not occur within 4 weeks of the rape, at which point the patient should return for a repeat evaluation.[42]

PSYCHOLOGICAL ASSESSMENT

The psychosocial and emotional implications of rape in children and adolescents are complex. This circumstance is tempered further by the young person's stage of development and the family's response to the rape. For example, young adolescents who are just beginning to grapple with their own sexuality may believe that they deserved to be raped because of having begun to experience sexual urges. A female child who sees her mother respond with tearful distress to the news that her child was raped may feel guilt not just because of the rape but also because of the emotional trauma inflicted on the mother.

How the youngster copes with the rape is also related to how society responds to victims of rape. Unlike most crimes, the crime of rape is often blamed on the victim rather than on the perpetrator, particularly in adolescents. Following no other crime are the victim's prior reputation, appearance, and behavior subject to such scrutiny as in rape. Running away, sexual activity, and even hitchhiking are used as justification for the rape, placing further blame on an already-troubled young victim. Providers of care must avoid compounding such punitive dynamics.

Follow-Up Care

After the initial evaluation is complete, arrangements should be made for follow-up care, not only for the medical issues discussed previously, but also to assess the victim's ability to cope with the rape and to accept counseling concerning the rape. All rape victims and their families should be seen as soon as possible after the rape by a mental health professional who is trained to work with adolescents and who is knowledgeable about the emotional sequelae to rape.

Short- and Long-Term Psychological Sequelae

Multiple factors will determine how a child or adolescent responds to the rape, such as level of social support, coping styles and strengths, and developmental variables and cognitive functions. How any given individual will respond to rape cannot be predicted. However, children and adolescents who have been rape victims consistently have lower levels of self-esteem after rape than the general population.[5] In addition, sexually traumatized children have been noted to have higher levels of precocious sexualization than nontraumatized children.[2,43] Confusion may exist about what is normal adult sexual behavior, sometimes leading to inappropriate sexual, acting-out behaviors. Some children experience developmental arrests at the time of the trauma; such arrests are not necessarily readily apparent. Although child and adolescent studies are still too scarce to be considered definitive, apparently the earlier and more traumatic the rape is, the greater the chance is of developmental and functional impairment.[15]

Behavioral concerns frequently associated with adolescent rape sequelae include school phobias, generalized fearfulness and withdrawal, and, especially in adolescents, the onset of truancy. Suicidal ideations are not uncommon, with increased lifetime risks of major depression and suicide attempts being associated with women in the aftermath of rape.[15] For male rape victims the existing research is less clear; however, male sexual trauma in childhood may be associated with sexually abusive behavior toward other boys during adolescence.[14,16] Obviously, though not all children and adolescents who have been raped will have psychiatric sequelae, all of those who have been raped should be assessed and monitored for serious sequelae. Particularly in cases in which sexual *acting out* follows a rape, careful clinical attention to issues such as posttraumatic stress disorder and depression is required. Self-medication with various substances is an ongoing clinical hazard after rape and deserves consideration as a *red flag* for health care providers working with at-risk patients.

SUMMARY

Rape is an act of violence that involves a disparity of power between the perpetrator and the victim. Because of its sexual context, rape is easily misinterpreted as erotic or sexual behavior, which it is not.

Adolescents who have been raped should have sensitive and thorough evaluations and follow-up assessments. From the time of initial disclosure through eventual legal outcome, many developmental, familial, and social variables can shape the experience for young survivors and their families. Long-term adjustment following rape varies considerably, with both developmental and familial factors having considerable impact.

TOOLS FOR PRACTICE

Community Advocacy and Coordination

- *Center for Adolescent Health & Law* (Web page), Center for Adolescent Health & Law (cahl.org/).
- *State Laws on Reporting Child Abuse and Neglect*, US Department of Health & Human Services (www.childwelfare.gov/responding/reporting.cfm).

Medical Decision Support

- *2006 Guidelines for the Treatment of Sexually Transmitted Disease*, Centers for Disease Control and Prevention (www.cdc.gov/std/treatment/).
- *Management of Possible Sexual, Injecting-Drug-Use, or Other Nonoccupational Exposure to HIV, Including Considerations Related to Antiretroviral Therapy Public Health Service Statement* (guideline), Centers for Disease Control and Prevention (www.cdc.gov/mmwr/preview/mmwrhtml/00054952.htm).
- *Strategies for the Treatment and Prevention of Sexual Assault* (guideline), American Medical Association (www.ama-assn.org/ama1/pub/upload/mm/386/sexualassault.pdf).
- *Visual Diagnosis of Child Abuse on CD-ROM, 2nd edition* (CD-ROM), American Academy of Pediatrics (www.aap.org/bookstore).

AAP POLICY STATEMENTS

American Academy of Pediatrics, Committee on Adolescence. Care of the adolescent sexual assault victim. *Pediatrics*. 2001;107(6):1476-1479. (aappolicy.aappublications.org/cgi/content/full/pediatrics;107/6/1476).

American Academy of Pediatrics, Committee on Adolescence. Emergency contraception. *Pediatrics*. 2005;116(4):1026-1035. (aappolicy.aappublications.org/cgi/content/full/pediatrics;116/4/1026).

American Academy of Pediatrics, Committee on Adolescence. Sexual assault and the adolescent. *Pediatrics*. 1994;94(5):761-765. (aappolicy.aappublications.org/cgi/content/full/pediatrics;94/5/761).

Havens PL, American Academy of Pediatrics, Committee on Pediatric AIDS. Clinical report: postexposure prophylaxis in children and adolescents for nonoccupational exposure to human immunodeficiency virus. *Pediatrics*. 2003;111(6):1475-1489. (aappolicy.aappublications.org/cgi/content/full/pediatrics;111/6/1475).

Kellogg N, American Academy of Pediatrics, Committee on Child Abuse and Neglect. Clinical report: the evaluation of sexual abuse in children. *Pediatrics*. 2005;116(2):506-512. (aappolicy.aappublications.org/cgi/content/full/pediatrics;116/2/506).

REFERENCES

1. Neinstein LS, ed. *Adolescent Health Care: A Practical Guide*. 3rd ed. Baltimore, MD: Urban & Schwarzenberg; 1996.
2. American Academy of Pediatrics, Committee on Adolescence. Sexual assault and the adolescent. *Pediatrics*. 1994;94:761-765.
3. Raine A. *The Psychopathology of Crime*. San Diego, CA: Academic Press; 1993.
4. Rickert VI, Wiemann CM. Date rape among adolescents and young adults. *J Pediatr Adolesc Gynecol*. 1998;11:167-175.
5. Koss MP, Heise L, Russo NF. The global health burden of rape. *Psychol Women Q*. 1994;18:509-537.
6. Greenfield L. *Sex Offenses and Offenders: An Analysis of Data on Rape and Sexual Assault*. Publication No NCJ-163392. Washington, DC: US Department of Justice, Bureau of Justice Statistics; 1997.
7. Heger A, Emans SJ. *Evaluation of the Sexually Abused Child: A Medical Textbook and Photographic Atlas*. New York, NY: Oxford University Press; 1992.
8. Wyatt GE, Guthrie D, Notgrass C. Differential effects of women's child sexual abuse and subsequent sexual revictimization. *J Consult Clin Psychol*. 1992;60:167-173.
9. Nagy S, Adcock AG, Nagy MC. A comparison of risky health behaviors of sexually active, sexually abused, and abstaining adolescents. *Pediatrics*. 1994;93:570-575.
10. Petrak JA. Current trends in the psychological assessment and treatment of victims of sexual violence. *Sex Marital Ther*. 1996;11:37-45.

11. Allison J, Wrightsman LS. *Rape: The Misunderstood Crime.* Newbury Park, CA: Sage Publications; 1993.
12. Erickson PI, Rapkin AJ. Unwanted sexual experiences among middle and high school youth. *J Adolesc Health.* 1991;12:319-325.
13. Elstein S, Davis N. *Sexual Relationships Between Adult Males and Young Teen Girls: Exploring the Legal and Social Responses.* Chicago, IL: American Bar Association; 1997.
14. Knight R, Rosenberg R, Schneider B. Classification of sex offenders: perspectives, methods, and validation. In: Burgess AW, ed. *Rape and Sexual Assault: A Research Handbook.* New York, NY: Garland Press; 1985.
15. Calhoun K, Atkeson B. *Treatment of Rape Victims: Facilitating Psychosocial Adjustment.* New York, NY: Pergamon; 1991.
16. Lacey HB, Roberts R. Sexual assault of men. *Int J STD AIDS.* 1991;2:258-260.
17. American Medical Association. Strategies for the Treatment and Prevention of Sexual Assault. 1995. Available at: www.ama-assn.org/ama1/pub/upload/mm/386/sexualassault.pdf. Accessed May 8, 2007.
18. Botash AS, Braen R, Gilchrist VJ. Acute care for sexual assault victims. *Patient Care.* 1994;Aug:112-137.
19. Groth N, Burges AW. Male rape: offenders and victims. *Am J Psychiatry.* 1980:137:806-810.
20. Burgess A, Holstrom L. *Rape Crisis and Recovery.* Bowie, MD: Prentice-Hall; 1979.
21. American Academy of Family Physicians, American Academy of Pediatrics, American College of Obstetricians and Gynecologist, and Society for Adolescent Medicine. Position paper. Protecting adolescents: ensuring access to care and reporting sexual activity and abuse. *J Adolesc Health.* 2004;35:420-423.
22. US Department of Health and Human Services. State Laws on Reporting Child Abuse and Neglect. Available at: www.childwelfare.gov/responding/reporting.cfm. Accessed May 8, 2007.
23. English A, Kenney KE. *State Minor Consent Laws: A Summary.* 2nd ed. Chapel Hill, NC: Center for Adolescent Health & Law; 2003. Available at: www.cahl.org. Accessed May 8, 2007.
24. Nelson DG, Santucci KA. An alternate light source to detect semen. *ACAD Emerg Med.* Oct 2002;9(10):1045-1048.
25. Jenny C, Lowen D. *The Visual Diagnosis of Child Sexual Abuse.* Elk Grove Village, IL: American Academy of Pediatrics; 1998.
26. McCauley J, Gorman RL, Guzinski G. Toluidine blue in the detection of perineal lacerations in pediatric and adolescent sexual abuse victims. *Pediatrics.* 1986;78(6):1039-1043.
27. Jones JG, Lawson L, Rickert CP. Use of optical glass binocular magnifiers in the examination of sexually abused children. *Adolesc Pediatr Gynecol.* 1990;3:146-148.
28. Bays J, Chadwick D. Medical diagnosis of the sexually abused child. *Child Abuse Negl.* 1993;17:91-110.
29. Adams JA, Harper K, Knudson S, et al. Examination findings in legally confirmed child sexual abuse: it's normal to be normal. *Pediatrics.* 1994;94(3):310-317.
30. Berenson AB, Chacko MR, Wiemann CM, et al. A case-control study of anatomic changes resulting from sexual abuse. *Am J Obstet Gynecol.* 2000;182:820-834.
31. Kellogg ND, Menard SW, Santos A. Genital anatomy in pregnant adolescents: "normal" does not mean "nothing happened". *Pediatrics.* 2004;113(4):e67-e69.
32. Young WW, Bracken AC, Goddard MA, et al. Sexual assault: review of a national model protocol for forensic and medical evaluations. *Obstet Gynecol.* 1992;80:878-883.
33. De Jong AR, Rose M. Legal proof of child sexual abuse in the absence of physical evidence. *Pediatrics.* 1991;88:506-511.
34. Christian C, Lavalle J, Dejong A, et al. Forensic evidence findings in prepubertal victims of sexual assault. *Pediatrics.* 2000;106:100-104.
35. Centers for Disease Control and Prevention. Management of possible sexual, injecting-drug-use, or other nonoccupational exposure to HIB, including considerations related to antiretroviral therapy. Public Health Service statement. *MMWR.* 47(RR17):1-14, 1198. Available at: www.cdc.gov/mmwr/preview/mmwrhtml/00054952.htm. Accessed May 8, 2007.
36. Fong C. Post-exposure prophylaxis for HIV infection after sexual assault: when is it indicated? *Emer Med J.* 2001;18:242-245.
37. Holmes MM, Resnick HS, Frampton D. Follow-up of sexual assault victims. *Am J Obstet Gynecol.* 1998;179:336-342.
38. Centers for Disease Control and Prevention. 2006 guidelines for treatment of sexually transmitted disease. *MMWR.* 2006;55(RR-36):997. Available at: www.cdc.gov/std/treatment/. Accessed May 8, 2007.
39. Centers for Disease Control and Prevention. 1993 Sexually transmitted diseases treatment guidelines. *MMWR.* 1993;42(RR-14):1-102.
40. Wilcos AJ, Weinberg CR, Baird DD. Timing of sexual intercourse in relation to ovulation. *N Engl J Med.* 1995;333:1517-1527.
41. Hatcher R, Trussell J, Stewart F, et al. Emergency contraception. In: Hatcher R, Trussell J, Stewart F, et al, eds. *Contraceptive Technology.* 17th ed. New York, NY: Ardent Media; 1998.
42. Gold MA. Emergency contraception. *Adv Pediatr.* 2000;47:309-334.
43. Friedrich W. Behavior problems in sexually abused children. In: Wyatt GE, Powell GJ, eds. *Lasting Effects of Child Sexual Abuse.* Newbury Park, CA: Sage Publications; 1998.

Chapter 357

ACUTE RENAL FAILURE

Stuart L. Goldstein, MD; Horacio Esteban Adrogué, MD

DEFINITION OF TERMS

Acute renal failure is a syndrome of sudden diminution or cessation of kidney function. Despite the significant morbidity and mortality associated with acute renal failure, over 30 definitions exist in the published literature.[1] Definitions vary according to specific patient populations and the outcome measure (eg, rise in creatinine versus need for renal replacement therapy). Given that most acute renal failure definitions are based on a serum creatinine rise, lack of a uniform definition may result in lack of recognition of significant kidney injury and delay in treatment. In addition, creatinine-based acute renal failure definitions are problematic for infants and small children because their normal serum creatinine level is 0.2 to 0.4 mg/dL. As a result, a serum creatinine change of 0.1 mg/dL represents a 25% to 50% change for small children.

A graded acute renal failure classification system, which identifies patients at risk for developing significant kidney insult and metabolic disturbance, is needed to assess best the state of kidney injury in patients with a renal insult. One such system uses the RIFLE criteria (*r*isk, *i*njury, *f*ailure, *l*oss and *e*nd-stage renal disease) to classify the degree of kidney insult by changes in serum creatinine and the duration of decreased urine output.[1] Furthermore, a change in terminology from acute renal failure to acute kidney injury (AKI) focuses attention on early recognition of kidney insult and interventions to prevent or mitigate the effects of significant renal failure.

Until RIFLE or other AKI classification systems undergo systematic validation, clinicians still rely on historical definitions based on urine output to characterize the degree of acute renal failure. For the purposes of this chapter the following definitions are used for decreased urine output:

Anuria: less than 100 mL/m^2/day

Oliguria: less than 300 mL/m^2/day

Nonoliguric state: sufficient urine volume to allow for administration of necessary fluids, nutrition, blood products, and medication without resulting volume overload

Oligoanuric state: insufficient urine volume to allow for administration of necessary fluids, nutrition, blood products, and medication without resulting volume overload

EPIDEMIOLOGIC FEATURES

The causes of AKI in children have changed from primary kidney diseases[2-4] to secondary effects of other systemic illnesses or their treatment. In studies of acutely ill hospitalized patients, the most common causes of AKI in children are congenital heart disease, sepsis, and nephrotoxic medicines.[5,6]

The 3- to 5-year patient survival of an AKI episode is 57%; approximately 60% of patients demonstrate evidence of chronic kidney injury.[7,8] Routine evaluation of all pediatric AKI survivors for evidence of chronic kidney disease, hypertension, and microalbuminuria may help prevent the long-term sequelae of AKI.

ETIOLOGY

The classification of AKI should focus on determining the cause and site of kidney insult (Table 357-1). Factors leading to diminished kidney function are often grouped according to prerenal, renal (parenchymal), postrenal, or a combination of these mechanisms. Prerenal causes are those that diminish kidney perfusion without producing actual parenchymal injury. In children, hypovolemia is the most common clinical situation in which diminished kidney function occurs and it usually results from dehydration associated with acute gastrointestinal losses. Hypovolemia may also occur in shock as the result of hemorrhage, burns, sepsis, and trauma. Less-common causes of prerenal AKI are those that diminish renal blood flow in the absence of hypovolemia, such as congestive heart failure, kidney vascular obstruction from thrombosis or embolism, liver failure, and increased kidney vascular resistance occasionally after anesthesia or surgery. Although oliguria or AKI (or both) occur in the prerenal syndrome, normal compensatory kidney tubular function usually persists, characterized by high urinary osmolality and low urinary sodium concentrations as the result of kidney water and sodium conservation.

AKI from intrinsic parenchymal injury may result from glomerular, tubular, or interstitial disorders. AKI from glomerular injury results most commonly from any of the glomerulonephritides or the microangiopathy of the hemolytic-uremic syndrome. (See Chapter 269, Hemolytic-Uremic Syndrome.) Tubular injury is frequently the result of prolonged ischemia or exposure to a variety of nephrotoxins. Renal ischemia may be seen in hypotensive episodes, severe dehydration, sudden hemorrhage, or sepsis. Tubular toxins may be endogenous (eg, hemoglobin, myoglobin) or exogenous (eg, medications such as aminoglycoside antibiotics), and various chemicals (eg, carbon tetrachloride, diethylene glycol, heavy metals) may cause acute parenchymal kidney failure. Drugs can also produce acute kidney failure by inducing a hypersensitivity reaction (drug-induced interstitial nephritis). Diffuse pyelonephritis also may result in AKI, particularly in infants. Kidney cortical necrosis associated with

Table 357-1 Clinical Tests to Differentiate Functional from Parenchymal Oliguric Acute Kidney Injury (AKI)

TEST	FUNCTIONAL AKI	PARENCHYMAL AKI	DISCRIMINATION
SODIUM CONSERVATION			
Urine sodium concentration (U_{Na})	<20 mEq/L	>40 mEq/L	Poor
Fractional excretion of sodium (FE_{Na})*; $FE_{Na} = (U_{Na} \times S_{Cr})/(S_{Na} \times U_{Cr}) \times 100$	<1	>1	Good
WATER CONSERVATION			
Urine osmolality (Uosm)	>500 mOsm/L	>350 mOsm/L	Poor
Urine-serum osmolality ratio (Uosm/Sosm)	>2	<1.1	Fair
Response to diagnostic challenge with intravenous mannitol and furosemide	Urine flow increase	No change	Good

AKI, acute kidney injury *U,* Urine; *Na,* sodium; *Cr,* creatinine; *S,* serum.

*Children with nonoliguric acute tubular necrosis (ATN) can have fractional excretion of sodium less than 1%. The FE_{Na} test is only helpful for oliguric ATN. The threshold for FE_{Na} in neonates is 3% and not 1%.

infection, hemorrhage, or dehydration can produce significant irreversible injury to both glomeruli and tubules.

EVALUATION

Relevant History

The processes contributing to kidney functional impairment can frequently be identified from the patient's history. Reduction in urine production is not included in the definition of AKI because kidney failure occurs not only in anuric states, but also in patients with oliguric or nonoliguric states. Some kidney insults, such as various glomerulonephritides and hemolytic-uremic syndrome, are frequently associated with oligoanuric AKI; others, such as aminoglycoside toxicity, will more often cause nonoliguric kidney failure. Determining the type of insult provides the clinician with insights into the possible manifestations of kidney failure, the probable duration of AKI, and the overall prognosis. The history often helps distinguish between an episode of AKI in an otherwise healthy child and the acute deterioration of kidney function in a child who has preexisting, undiagnosed, chronic kidney disease. History of urinary abnormalities, fatigue, pallor, slowed linear growth, poor school performance, and anorexia extending over a period would lead the practitioner to suspect the latter.

AKI may be heralded by seizures. Seizures can be precipitated by hypocalcemia, hypertensive encephalopathy, uremia, and water intoxication. To first have a sudden onset of seizures and other signs of central nervous system dysfunction, only to be found to have AKI is not unusual for a child.

Physical Findings

Many children with AKI will have markedly diminished urine output. Complete anuria is unusual and leads to consideration of a catastrophic renovascular event or urinary obstruction. In the child who has anuria or oliguria, fluid retention can produce edema, water intoxication, vascular overload with congestive heart failure, pulmonary edema, hypertension, or any combination. In many instances, the fluid overload is iatrogenic, resulting from attempts to increase urinary output by increasing fluid intake. Early detection of fluid retention is determined best by short-term weight gain on serial measurements and carefully recorded intakes and outputs, with appropriate allowances for insensible fluid losses. In contrast, nonoliguric AKI may be clinically covert; it is usually suspected only after laboratory tests reveal an elevation in serum creatinine or electrolyte imbalance.

Laboratory Findings

The biochemical disturbances that contribute to clinical findings in AKI are complex and interrelated. Inherent to the diagnosis of acute renal failure is the accumulation of nitrogenous waste products characterized by a rise in blood urea nitrogen and creatinine. If hypotonic fluids have been used in excess to hydrate the patient, then dilutional hyponatremia and anemia may affect central nervous system and cardiac function adversely.

Hyperkalemia (Table 357-2) is often the result of injudicious potassium administration or inadequate renal potassium excretion (Table 357-2 lists treatment options). Hyperkalemia is a potentially life-threatening complication of AKI and can be especially severe in disease states associated with cellular damage and the consequent release of intracellular potassium (hemolysis, burns, trauma, and infections). Hyperkalemia produces a state of increased neuromuscular excitability, including a vulnerability to cardiac arrhythmias. Unfortunately, hyperkalemia produces no consistent physical signs; diagnosis depends on the measurement of serum potassium and, if indicated, assessment of the electrocardiogram for evidence of altered cardiac electrical activity.

In AKI, metabolic acidosis develops as the result of the kidney's failure to excrete hydrogen ions and reabsorb bicarbonate. Furthermore, any state associated with increased catabolism, such as shock, fever, poor caloric intake, or extensive tissue damage, may accentuate the degree of acidosis as a result of increased production of organic and inorganic acid radicals. The acidosis promotes further hyperkalemia resulting from movement of intracellular potassium into the extracellular space as the body attempts to accommodate the higher hydrogen ion concentration. Respiratory compensation for an underlying metabolic acidosis may cause low carbon dioxide pressure resulting from tachypnea or Kussmaul breathing.

Failure of phosphate excretion can lead to hyperphosphatemia. The hypocalcemia associated with hyperphosphatemia may exhibit clinically as tremors, tetany, or seizures.

MANAGEMENT

Acute kidney injury management should begin before consulting with a nephrologist and before initiating renal replacement therapy. Maintenance of adequate urine volumes and prevention and treatment of metabolic derangements comprise the goals of therapy in children with acute renal failure. Preservation or restoration of renal perfusion with appropriate fluid resuscitation and inotropic agents is essential and is the first measure to maintain urine output in critically ill patients.

Goal-directed fluid therapy is a term that represents the use of physiological endpoints such as heart rate, central venous pressure, and mean arterial pressure to guide initiation and termination of fluid resuscitation of patients in shock. Goal-directed fluid therapy leads to better survival in adults with shock.[9] Adult patients who receive early goal-directed fluid therapy in the emergency center received more fluid in the emergency center but received less fluid and have better survival in the intensive care unit compared with patients who receive standard therapy. Although fluid resuscitation in critically ill children is essential to treat acute hypovolemic and septic shock state,[10] the concept that worsening fluid overload is associated with worse outcomes in critically ill pediatric patients who require renal replacement therapy has been the focus of recent pediatric study. Both single-center data[11-14] and a multicenter effort, the Prospective Pediatric Continuous Renal Replacement Therapy Registry

Table 357-2 Treatment of Hyperkalemia in Pediatric Patients

AGENT	DOSE	EFFECT	REMARKS
Calcium gluconate (10%)	0.5 mL/kg IV over 2-4 min	Rapid but transient	Monitor electrocardiogram for bradycardia during injection; may be repeated but *not likely* to be effective.
Sodium bicarbonate (7.5%)	2.5 mEq/kg (approximately 3 mL/kg) IV by slow push	Rapid but transient	Repetition *not* recommended.
Glucose (50%)	1 mL/kg IV by slow push	Within 1-2 hr	Attempt to increase blood glucose to 250 mg/dL; may be maintained by infusion of 30% glucose at rate equal to insensible fluid loss.
Insulin (regular)	0.1 U/kg IV	Rapid	Give *only* with hypertonic glucose infusion (30%).
Sodium polystyrene sulfonate (Kayexalate)	1 g/kg PO or PR	3-6 hr	Side effects: gastric irritation (nausea and vomiting), diarrhea, *or* fecal impaction; PO more effective than PR; enemas should be retained >60 min—removed by cleansing enema; may cause *hypokalemia:* use cautiously in patients who tolerate sodium loads poorly; also chelates Ca^+ and Mg^+.

Ca+, Calcium ion; *IV,* intravenous; *Mg+,* magnesium ion; *PO,* orally; *PR,* rectally.

Group (known as the ppCRRT Registry)[15,16] demonstrate that worsening fluid overload is an independent risk factor for mortality, irrespective of severity of illness by the *pediatric risk of mortality* score, in patients who receive continuous renal replacement therapy (CRRT). These data, coupled with the predilection for early multiorgan system failure and death in critically ill children,[17,18] argue for early and aggressive initiation of renal replacement therapy. Earlier initiation at lesser fluid overload degrees may allow for (1) more expeditious optimal nutrition and blood product provision without further fluid or waste product accumulation and (2) preventing the worsening volume overload and, in particular, pulmonary edema. Given that most pediatric drug dosing is based on intensive care unit admission weight, worsening fluid overload might increase the volume of distribution of inotropes, antimicrobials, and chemotherapeutic agents, thereby resulting in underdosing.

Medication dosing should be altered for specific drugs that are primarily eliminated by the kidneys; drug dose or interval (or both) may need to be altered based on the level of kidney dysfunction. In addition, drug concentrations can be wholly or partially reduced by dialysis in patients who receive either intermittent or continuous renal replacement therapy. Factors associated with enhanced dialytic elimination include low volume of distribution and low protein binding.

Well-designed prospective randomized studies of adult patients at risk for acute tubular necrosis have called into question the utility of intravenous furosemide or *renal-dose* dopamine in preventing oliguria.[19,20] Other recent studies support the use of fenoldopam, a dopamine α1-agonist, to prevent AKI in certain critically ill adult populations.[21,22] To date, no published pediatric study has been conducted with respect to the optimal pharmacologic management of pediatric AKI.

In the last decade, survival rates stratified by the renal replacement therapy modality have been stable; survival rates for patients receiving hemodialysis (73% to 89%) are higher than those receiving peritoneal dialysis (49% to 64%) or CRRT (34% to 42%).[5,12,23] Better survival in patients who receive hemodialysis likely results from improved hemodynamic stability, but no prospective pediatric study that controls for patients illness severity has compared survival across modalities. Improvements in pediatric specific technology[24] and CRRT techniques[25,26] have led to preferential use of CRRT in pediatric patients with AKI and has decreased morbidity in patients who require CRRT.[27]

WHEN TO REFER

- For guidance on diagnostic evaluation
- Management of complex fluid, mineral, electrolyte, and blood pressure abnormalities
- Evaluation of dialysis options and preparation for and implementation of dialysis or CRRT treatment
- Disease-specific management

WHEN TO ADMIT

- When AKI is unexplained, rapidly progressive, or oliguric or anuric
- In the presence of severe or potentially dangerous fluid or metabolic abnormalities (eg, hyperkalemia, hypocalcemia, acidosis, clinical fluid overload, dehydration)
- For renal biopsy

TOOLS FOR PRACTICE

Engaging Patient and Family

- *What is a Pediatric Nephrologist?* (fact sheet), American Academy of Pediatrics (www.aap.org/family/WhatisPedNephrologist.pdf).

REFERENCES

1. Bellomo R, Ronco C, Kellum JA, et al. Acute renal failure—definition, outcome measures, animal models, fluid therapy and information technology needs: the Second International Consensus Conference of the Acute Dialysis Quality Initiative (ADQI) Group. *Crit Care.* 2004;8:R204-R212.
2. Andreoli SP. Acute renal failure. *Curr Opin Pediatr.* 2002;14:183-188.
3. Counahan R, Cameron JS, Ogg CS, et al. Presentation, management, complications, and outcome of acute renal failure in childhood: five years' experience. *BMJ.* 1977;1:599-602.
4. Williams DM, Sreedhar SS, Mickell JJ, et al. Acute kidney failure: a pediatric experience over 20 years. *Arch Pediatr Adolesc Med.* 2002;156:893-900.
5. Bunchman TE, McBryde KD, Mottes TE, et al. Pediatric acute renal failure: outcome by modality and disease. *Pediatr Nephrol.* 2001;16:1067-1071.
6. Hui-Stickle S, Brewer ED, Goldstein SL. Pediatric ARF epidemiology at a tertiary care center from 1999 to 2001. *Am J Kidney Dis.* 2005;45:96-101.
7. Askenazi DJ, Feig DI, Graham NM, et al. 3-5 year longitudinal follow-up of pediatric patients after acute renal failure. *Kidney Int.* 2006;69:184-189.
8. Georgaki-Angelaki HN, Steed DB, Chantler C, et al. Renal function following acute renal failure in childhood: a long-term follow-up study. *Kid Int.* 1989;35(1):84-98.
9. Lassnigg A, Donner E, Grubhofer G, et al. Lack of renoprotective effects of dopamine and furosemide during cardiac surgery. *J Am Soc Nephrol.* 2000;11:97-104.
10. Baldwin L, Henderson A, Hickman P. Effect of postoperative low-dose dopamine on renal function after elective major vascular surgery. *Ann Intern Med.* 1994;120:744-747.
11. Samuels J, Finkel K, Gubert M, et al. Effect of fenoldopam mesylate in critically ill patients at risk for acute renal failure is dose dependent. *Ren Fail.* 2005;27:101-105.
12. Tumlin JA, Finkel KW, Murray PT, et al. Fenoldopam mesylate in early acute tubular necrosis: a randomized, double-blind, placebo-controlled clinical trial. *Am J Kidney Dis.* 2005;46:26-34.
13. Rivers E, Nguyen B, Havstad S, et al. Early goal-directed therapy in the treatment of severe sepsis and septic shock. *N Engl J Med.* 2001;345:1368-1377.
14. Carcillo JA, Fields AI. Clinical practice parameters for hemodynamic support of pediatric and neonatal patients in septic shock. *Crit Care Med.* 2002;30:1365-1378.
15. Gillespie RS, Seidel K, Symons JM. Effect of fluid overload and dose of replacement fluid on survival in hemofiltration. *Pediatr Nephrol.* 2004;19(12):1394-1399.
16. Goldstein SL, Currier H, Graf C, et al. Outcome in children receiving continuous venovenous hemofiltration. *Pediatrics.* 2001;107:1309-1312.
17. Michael M, Kuehnle I, Goldstein SL. Fluid overload and acute renal failure in pediatric stem cell transplant patients. *Pediatr Nephrol.* 2004;19:91-95.
18. Foland JA, Fortenberry JD, Warshaw BL, et al. Fluid overload before continuous hemofiltration and survival in critically ill children: a retrospective analysis. *Crit Care Med.* 2004;32:1771-1776.
19. Goldstein SL, Somers MJ, Brophy PD, et al. The Prospective Pediatric Continuous Renal Replacement Therapy (ppCRRT) Registry: design, development and data assessed. *Int J Artif Organs.* 2004;27:9-14.
20. Goldstein SL, Somers MJ, Baum MA, et al. Pediatric patients with multi-organ dysfunction syndrome receiving continuous renal replacement therapy. *Kidney Int.* 2005;67:653-658.
21. Proulx F, Fayon M, Farrell CA, et al. Epidemiology of sepsis and multiple organ dysfunction syndrome in children. *Chest.* 1996;109:1033-1037.
22. Proulx F, Gauthier M, Nadeau D, et al. Timing and predictors of death in pediatric patients with multiple organ system failure. *Crit Care Med.* 1994;22:1025-1031.
23. Flynn JT. Choice of dialysis modality for management of pediatric acute renal failure. *Pediatr Nephrol.* 2002;17:61-69.
24. Bunchman TE, Maxvold NJ, Kershaw DB, et al. Continuous venovenous hemodiafiltration in infants and children. *Am J Kidney Dis.* 1995;25:17-21.
25. Brophy PD, Somers MJ, Baum MA, et al. Multi-centre evaluation of anticoagulation in patients receiving continuous renal replacement therapy (CRRT). *Nephrol Dial Transplant.* 2005;20:1416-1421.
26. Bunchman TE, Maxvold NJ, Barnett J, et al. Pediatric hemofiltration: Normocarb dialysate solution with citrate anticoagulation. *Pediatr Nephrol.* 2002;17:150-154.
27. Warady BA, Bunchman T. Dialysis therapy for children with acute renal failure: survey results. *Pediatr Nephrol.* 2000;15:11-13.

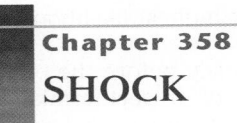

Chapter 358

SHOCK

Monika Gupta, MD; Joseph R. Custer, MD

The primary care physician can have a dramatic effect on the outcome of a patient with shock. Recognizing and treating shock early in the community setting, following consensus guidelines and algorithms, can dramatically reduce mortality and morbidity.[1]

Early treatment for shock remains the same regardless of the cause of shock. Prompt recognition and management of shock minimizes mortality and morbidity, even if transfer to a tertiary care facility is eventually required. Simple principles of fluid and pressor therapy are effective despite the cause. The clinician should be confident in treating the hemodynamic abnormalities first and establishing the cause later.[2]

EPIDEMIOLOGIC FACTORS

Shock, especially septic shock and hypovolemic shock caused by diarrhea or blood loss remains a common cause of pediatric morbidity and mortality. Severe sepsis is one of the most common causes of death in infants and children in the world.[3]

In 1995, severe sepsis was the 4th leading cause of death in infants. In children ages 1 to 14 years, it was the 2nd leading cause of death.[4] Diarrhea leading to dehydration severe enough to produce shock is no longer a common cause of death in the United States but remains a world health problem.

The presence of shock increases morbidity and mortality when it complicates other childhood diseases. Investigators at the University of Pittsburgh evaluated 1766 children with respiratory disease who required transport to a tertiary facility. Shock complicated the respiratory failure presentation in 25% (440) of the children, and this group had a mortality rate of 38%. In the group of children transferred for respiratory failure only, without shock present, the mortality rate was only 3%.[5]

The cost to treat shock is substantial. In an analysis of data from 1997 hospitalizations, children with severe sepsis had an average hospital stay of 31 days at a cost of $40,600 per case. In a 2005 report, the national annual cost of caring for children with severe sepsis alone is estimated at $2.3 billion.[3]

CLINICAL DIAGNOSIS

A high index of suspicion and prompt recognition can affect dramatically the outcome for pediatric patients in shock.[1,2] Shock can be defined by clinical signs and symptoms, by hemodynamic variables, or by parameters of oxygen delivery. In the primary care setting, the diagnosis is based on clinical signs and symptoms.

Shock can be considered a progressive process of compensated, decompensated, and irreversible states. The diagnosis may be made in the early, compensated state by easily detectable clinical signs: tachycardia, decreased capillary refill, and altered mental status. Intervention in this state has the highest likelihood of success.

Shock can be diagnosed clinically before the onset of hypotension. The presence of hyperthermia or hypothermia, altered mental status, and altered perfusion (brisk in warm shock [vasodilated] or delayed in cold shock [vasoconstricted]) confirms the diagnosis of shock. Poor perfusion is diagnosed by capillary refill (>2 seconds) before the onset of hypotension.

Mental status is a remarkably sensitive indicator of degree of illness and response to therapy. Shock must be ruled out in children who demonstrate changes in mental status, such as agitation, lethargy, confusion, and coma. The presence of coma or neurologic compromise implies significant brain hypoperfusion. Restoration of neurologic well being is the goal of therapy.[6]

Urine output is usually an accurate indicator of blood volume and perfusion to the kidneys. Oliguria is defined as urine output of less than 0.5 mL/kg/hr. However, several caveats are important. Many children have multiple caretakers during a typical day; thus the frequency and volume of urination may not be accurately recounted. Patients who have high-output renal failure, hyperglycemia (diabetes mellitus), patients on diuretics, and children who have received mannitol will have high obligatory urine losses.

An unexplained metabolic acidosis (defined as a base deficit of >3.0 mEq/L) or an increased arterial lactate (2 times upper limits of normal) in a patient with cardiovascular symptoms confirms inadequate perfusion. In the decompensated phase of shock, hypotension occurs as the child's compensatory mechanisms are exhausted. Hypotension and tachycardia are the hallmarks of severe shock in a decompensating patient. Restoration of blood pressure and reduction of heart rate are indicators of therapeutic success.[7,8] Ranges of heart rate and blood pressure by age group are seen in Table 358-1. Hypotension represents a decompensated state in the patient and is confirmatory of the severity of shock. The diagnosis of shock is based on clinical findings.[7] If organ failure develops, then the child can enter a phase of refractory shock, with increased morbidity and mortality. These children are not responsive to aggressive volume resuscitation, catecholamines, steroids, vasopressin, and inotropic agents.

In practice, the diagnosis of septic shock in children is confirmed with the use of simple physical assessments: mental status, pulse rate and quality, capillary refill, blood pressure, and urine output. The phase of shock is defined by the response to treatment (Table 358-2 highlights decision points for increasing therapeutic interventions).[9]

DIAGNOSIS OF SHOCK: HISTORY

After the patient is stabilized, an accurate history may help choose appropriate treatments and guide referral. Infants younger than 6 weeks who are in shock merit special attention, and a broader differential diagnosis should be considered than that in older children. Early discharge of newborns shortly after birth requires attention to both acquired and congenital or

Table 358-1 Vital Signs and White Blood Counts by Age

AGE GROUP	HEART RATE—TACHYCARDIA	HEART RATE—BRADYCARDIA	RESPIRATORY RATE	SYSTOLIC BLOOD PRESSURE	LEUKOCYTE COUNT × 10/mm
0 days to 1 wk	>180	<100	>50	<65	>34
1 wk to 1 mo	>180	<100	>40	<75	>19.5 or <5
1 mo to 1 yr	>180	<90	>34	<100	>17.5 or <5
2-5 yr	>140	NA	>22	<94	>15.5 or <6
6-12 yr	>130	NA	>18	<105	>13.5 or <4.5
13-<18 yr	>110	NA	>14	<117	>11 or <4.5

From Goldstein B, Giroir B, Randolph A, et al. International pediatric sepsis consensus conference: Definitions for sepsis and organ dysfunction in pediatrics. *Pediatr Crit Care Med.* 2005; 6:2-8. Reprinted with permission from Lippincott Williams & Wilkins.

Table 358-2 Definitions of Shock Classified by Physical Examination and Response to Therapy

TYPE	RESPONSE
Cold shock	Altered mental status, capillary refill >2 sec, cool extremities, diminished pulses, and urine output of <1 mL/kg/hr
Warm shock	As above, but with flash capillary refill and bounding pulses
Fluid refractory—dopamine-resistant shock	Persistence of symptoms with >60 mL/kg/in the 1st hour of fluid therapy and dopamine infusion of 10 mcg/kg/min
Catecholamine-resistant shock	Shock persists despite addition of epinephrine or norepinephrine or both
Refractory shock	Shock persists despite use of pressor, fluid, maintenance of glucose and calcium, thyroid and adrenal status

Septic shock is classified by perfusion status and is further defined by lack of response to treatment. The order also indicates progressive severity of the patient's illness, and decision points in treatment algorithms.
From Carcillo JA, Fields AI, task force committee members. Clinical practice parameters for hemodynamic support of pediatric and neonatal patients in septic shock. *Crit Care Med.* 2002;30:1365-1378. Reprinted with permission from Lippincott Williams & Wilkins.

BOX 358-1 Causes of Shock in Infants

Cardiac
Hypoplastic left heart syndrome
Coarctation of the aorta
Myocarditis
Arrhythmia
Infectious
Bacterial meningitis
Urinary tract sepsis
Herpes (meningitis and sepsis)
Streptococcal sepsis
Metabolic
Hypoglycemia
Inborn errors of metabolism
Traumatic
Child abuse
Occult central nervous system hemorrhage
Surgical
Bowel obstruction
Occult blood loss

Infants in shock present unique diagnostic challenges. Algorithmic approaches to shock diagnosis developed for children and adults may not be appropriate.
From Perkin RM, Levin DL. Shock in the pediatric patient. I. Therapy, *J Pediatr.* 1982;101:319-327; Perkin RM, Levin DL. Shock in the pediatric patient II. Therapy, *J Pediatr.* 1982;101:613-621.

inherited conditions in infants who subsequently exhibit in extremis. Several of these conditions are listed in Box 358-1.

Shock in toddlers usually has a determinable, apparent cause. The clinician should be aware of the propensities that are unique to this age group, especially poisonings, ingestions of medications, inhaling and swallowing of foreign bodies, trauma resulting from falls, playground and household accidents, and child abuse.

The adolescent may not be forthright in volunteering an accurate history. The risk-taking behavior of the teen years should be taken into consideration when considering the differential diagnosis in this age group. Poisoning after attempted suicide or experimentation with drugs and alcohol may not be reported by persons who are available to give a history. Antipsychotic medications can cause cardiovascular collapse and arrhythmias. Ingestion of antihypertensive agents and opiates in the home should also be considered in the differential diagnosis of an adolescent in shock.

In all age groups, history of travel may lead to further clues. In a child with recent exposure to pets and who has diarrhea, the possibility of *Salmonella* infection must be considered. Recent ingestion of meat and early onset of central nervous system symptoms with bloody diarrhea imply hemolytic uremic syndrome. Exposure to organophosphates should be sought if weakness is part of the presentation.[10]

Finally, family history is important. In a study of Danish families, the risk of death was increased 5-fold in children whose parent had died with a severe infection before the age of 50.[11]

CLINICAL PHYSIOLOGICAL MECHANISM OF SHOCK

In all shock states, oxygen delivery and blood flow to vital organs is decreased or cellular oxygen needs are increased, and metabolic demands are not met, resulting in multiple organ failure.

The signs, symptoms, and sequelae of shock are the result of inadequate perfusion of oxygen and nutrients (eg, glucose) to vital organs. Perfusion is a clinical representation of the combined effects of cardiac output and systemic vascular resistance. Shock can be defined in terms of oxygen delivery and consumption parameters. Delivery of oxygen to tissue is the product of content of oxygen in blood and the cardiac output.

In young children, pulse rate is a reasonable proxy of cardiac output, and capillary refill is a reliable indicator of perfusion. Cardiac output is the product of heart rate and stroke volume, which is expressed in liters of blood flow per minute. Hypotension (loss of peripheral vascular tone) is sensed by baroreceptors, which act through mediators to increase both the heart rate and the stroke volume. In older children and adults, stroke volume is dependent on contractility (inotropy) and preload (venous return to the right heart). Contractility of the myocardium is depressed by acidosis, hypoglycemia, and hypocalcemia. Epinephrine and other catecholamines act as inotropic agents, increasing contractility.

Preload is the vascular volume presented to the heart during diastole, which stretches cardiac muscle, to enable optimal contraction during systole. Clinically, the central venous pressure or a pulmonary capillary wedge pressure and left atrial pressure represent preload to right and left ventricles, respectively. A patient with hypovolemia is said to have a low preload, and if blood volume is restored, then preload increases and stroke volume is increased (Figure 358-1 [point a]). In hypovolemic shock caused by trauma or diarrhea, pulses would be thready, heart rate would be high, and the capillary refill is over 2 seconds. Physiologically, the patient has a low vascular volume, heart rate is high in an effort to restore blood flow, and the systemic vascular resistance is elevated; thus the skin is cool and poorly perfused.

In cardiogenic shock, high volumes may stretch the heart muscle, and either or both diastolic and systolic function may be altered. Preload is high, but contractility (inotropy) is greatly diminished (see Figure 358-1 [point b]). This circumstance requires invasive monitoring in a sophisticated tertiary intensive care unit.

Children with sepsis may exhibit symptoms of hyperdynamic, vasodilated shock (see Figure 358-1 [point c]). Physiologically, cardiac output is high, peripheral vasculature is vasodilated, venous return (preload) to the heart is diminished, and systemic vascular resistance is low. On physical examination, the patient has brisk capillary refill, is warm to the touch, and has bounding pulses, tachycardia, and a hyperdynamic precordium. Symptoms result not from low cardiac output, but rather from maldistribution of blood flow.

Peripheral vascular resistance can be estimated clinically. A patient who is cold to the touch with capillary refill of over 2 seconds has an increase in peripheral vascular resistance and is said to be in *cold shock*. A patient who is warm to the touch, has a rapid blush of capillary refill, and has a vasodilated, low peripheral resistance shock and is in *warm shock*.[1]

Heart rate is a valuable clinical sign both for diagnosis and treatment in children. Infants cannot increase stroke volume as readily as adults can and rely on an increase in heart rate as a compensatory mechanism to increase blood flow to vital organs.[12] Thus an infant in shock whose heart rate is 2 standard deviations above normal is attempting to increase cardiac output. The return of pulse rate and blood pressure to normal values is a valuable indicator of therapeutic success.[7,13,14]

CLASSIFICATION OF SHOCK

Shock can be classified by cause and mechanism: hypovolemic, cardiogenic, and distributive. Again, the primary clinician should recall that despite complexities of cause, the early stages of shock are easy to recognize, and the treatments are straightforward.[13]

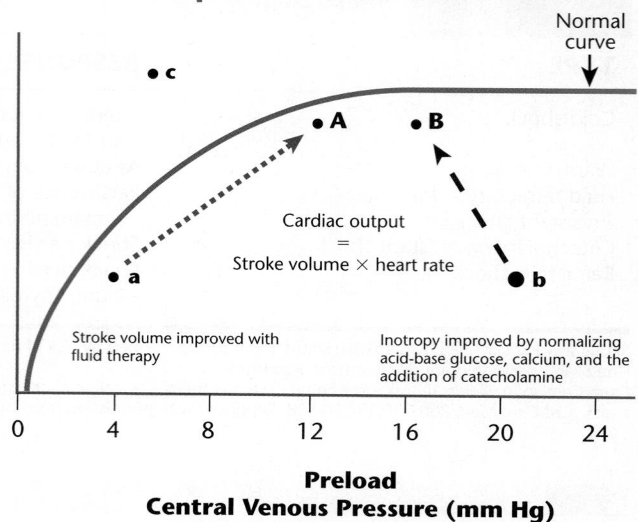

Figure 358-1 The figure demonstrates the interaction of adequate volume status (Preload or CVP) and contractility (cardiac output). Note the plateau in cardiac output relative to central venous filling pressure. As cardiac out reaches its maximum (in this example at a central venous pressure of 10-12), further increase in central venous pressure does not improve cardiac output.

Point a represents the situation in hypovolemic shock. Here cardiac output is low, as is the Central Venous Pressure. The arrow demonstrates that as fluid administration increases preload, there is an improvement in cardiac output to **Point A.**

Point b is a patient with a high preload (venous congestion) who would most likely have congestive signs on exam: rales, hepatomegaly, edema, distended neck veins, with low cardiac output causing poor perfusion. This could be secondary to primary cardiogenic shock, as in myocarditis or after an ischemic event, or with myocardial dysfunction in late stages of septic shock. Evidence of poor perfusion would be obvious on examination: cold clammy skin, prolonged capillary refill, and thready rapid peripheral pulses.

The restoration of acid base balance, glucose, calcium and magnesium levels to normal, and the addition of inotropic agents can dramatically improve function. The line from point **b** to point **B**, demonstrates an improvement in output and with a reduction in filling pressure. (It should be noted that in infants, resting cardiac output is near maximum, and infants rely on increasing heart rate whereas adults increase cardiac output by mechanisms intended to increase stroke volume.)

Point c represents a patient who is vasodilated, with hyperdynamic cardiac output and relatively low cardiac preload. This would occur in distributive forms of shock: anaphylaxis and septic shock. This state would be reflected in the physical exam by presence of rapid capillary refill, bounding cardiac pulses, and a hyperdynamic precordium with tachycardia. (See text.)

Hypovolemic Shock

Shock from loss of blood volume caused by trauma, diarrhea, burns, and 3rd spacing (as in peritonitis) is the most common form of shock in children. Loss of fluid leads to low intravascular volume and preload to the heart is decreased. If such losses (up to 30% of circulating blood volume) occur over days, then patients can compensate by increasing thirst, heart rate, and retention of fluid by concentrating urine. Large volumes of fluid loss that occur acutely lead to decompensation represented by diminished mental status, tachycardia, poorly perfused skin with prolonged capillary refill, oliguria, and, eventually, hypotension.

Nonhemorrhagic shock is seen in diarrhea, vomiting, urinary losses, evaporative losses, 3rd spacing of fluid (peritonitis, edema), and burns. The causes of hypovolemic shock are seen in Box 358-2.

Physical signs in hypovolemic shock occur as a result of decreased venous return to the heart, which leads to diminished cardiac output. Catecholamines are released, which produces the hallmark vasoconstriction in skin, muscle, and splanchnic blood vessels. The renin-angiotensin system is activated, promoting the retention of salt and water. Fluid resuscitation restores preload, and cardiac output is increased with resolution of symptoms. Physical signs in dehydration reliably indicate the percentage of body fluid compartment losses (Table 358-3). In hemorrhagic shock, physical findings correlate to the amount of blood loss[15] (Table 358-4).

Cardiogenic Shock

Cardiac shock can be caused by mechanical obstruction or muscle (pump) failure. In obstructive cardiogenic shock, air and fluid in the pericardium or pleural spaces (rarely) can impede venous return to the heart and decrease systolic ejection. Common causes are listed in Box 358-3. These patients usually exhibit distended neck veins because of increased jugular venous pressure and hypotension. Massive pulmonary embolus, rare in children, can obstruct flow from the right to the left side of the heart. In coarctation of the aorta, hypoplastic left heart syndrome, and left ventricular outflow tract stenosis, cardiac output is compromised.

The heart can fail as a mechanical pump from a variety of causes (Box 358-4). Patients with cardiac failure have low cardiac output resulting in the clinical signs of altered mental status, tachycardia, decreased capillary refill, and evidence of venous congestion (hepatomegaly, rales). Children with pericardial effusion may have muffled heart tones.

BOX 358-2 Causes of Hypovolemic Shock

- Gastrointestinal losses
- Excess urine output, diuretic agent administration
- Mannitol administration
- Hypoalbuminemia
- Burns
- 3rd space fluid losses (peritonitis, edema)
- Traumatic blood loss

Table 358-3 Physical Signs in Dehydration

PERCENTAGE OF DEHYDRATION	PHYSICAL SIGNS
5% (mild)	Dry skin, mild tachycardia, concentrated urine
10% (moderate)	Lethargy, poor perfusion
15% (severe)	Obtundation, tachycardia, hypotension, very poor perfusion to skin

Table 358-4 Physical and Vital Signs in Hemorrhagic Shock

BLOOD VOLUME LOST (%)	SIGNS
<15%	Minimal tachycardia, normal respiratory rate, blood pressure, and capillary refill
15-30%	Tachycardia, tachypnea, decreased pulse pressure, normal systolic pressure, prolonged capillary refill, anxiety
30-40%	Hypotension, decreased urine output, mental status changes
>40%	Hypotension, loss of consciousness

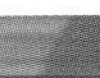

BOX 358-3 Causes of Obstructive Cardiogenic Shock

- Tamponade (air, blood, or effusion)
- Coarctation of the aorta
- Aortic valve stenosis or atresia

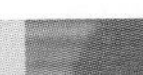

BOX 358-4 Pump Failure

- Arrhythmia
- Hypoplastic left heart syndrome
- Decreased contractility acquired in sepsis syndrome or shock of any cause
- Myocardiopathy
- Myocarditis
- Anomalous coronary artery
- Cardiac contusion
- Storage disease—glycogen storage disease

Septic Shock

Septic shock is the most common and certainly best-studied cause of cardiovascular collapse the primary caregiver will encounter.[9] The causes of bacterial septic shock have changed since vaccination against *Haemophilus influenzae* type b was instituted in 1988. If sepsis in the (increasingly common) immunocompromised patient is excluded, meningococci and streptococci are then the most frequently encountered bacterial causes of sepsis.

Patients with infections caused by *Staphylococcus aureus, Pseudomonas aeruginosa,* Candida species, and *Streptococcus pyogenes* have higher mortality rates compared with patients with infections caused by coagulase-negative *Staphylococcus* and *Acinetobacter* species.[16]

Studies of children who have meningococcemia highlight important issues in the care of children in septic shock (see Chapter 353, Meningococcemia). Mortality remains high despite modern advances in critical care.[17] An unfortunate characteristic of meningococcal disease is its rapid progression in fatal cases. Characteristics of cases rapidly progressing to death include young age, absence of meningitis, thrombocytopenia, leukopenia, multiorgan failure, and severity of petechiae.[17] Invasive meningococcal disease is most common in children younger than 4 years. Meningitis and sepsis occurs in 1.3:100,000 in the United States, but incidence in Ireland is 15:100,000.[17] Clinicians who encounter these clinical stigmata in primary care settings should recognize the importance of early stabilization, the need for referral for definitive therapy, and the high mortality despite aggressive intervention.

Children and adults exhibit developmental differences in the hemodynamic response to sepsis. In adults, mortality is caused by a pressor and volume resistant state characterized as vasomotor paralysis. Myocardial dysfunction is common in adults, but cardiac output is maintained by tachycardia and ventricular dilatation.[7,18]

In pediatric septic shock, low cardiac output, not vasodilatation, is associated with mortality.[19] In children, oxygen delivery is the major determinant of oxygen consumption, whereas in adults, oxygen used by tissues (oxygen extraction) is more important. Survival correlates to the restoration of cardiac output and oxygen delivery.[8,20]

Some patients with severe septic shock may develop a hypoadrenal response to shock. This scenario is clinically characterized as patients who are in refractory shock (see Table 358-2) who are, by definition, unresponsive to volume resuscitation, the addition of 2 catecholamine drugs, and normalization of acid base, glucose, and calcium homeostasis. Infants and children at risk include those with septic shock and purpura, those with known or suggested adrenal abnormalities, and children who have received a therapeutic course of steroids in the 6 months before the onset of sepsis.[21]

In patients whose shock state is refractory to volume, dopamine or dobutamine, and the addition of epinephrine or norepinephrine (catechol resistant shock), empirically initiating stress-dose steroids (hydrocortisone at stress doses of 50 to 100 mg/m^2/day would be reasonable. If time and condition allow it, a baseline serum cortisol level is drawn, followed by a 250 microgram dose of corticotropin, and a repeat cortisol level is drawn at 30 minutes. The response (or absence of) will determine the presence of a hypoadrenal state and the need for continued steroid administration. A baseline serum cortisol of less than 18 mcg/dL and a poststimulation increment of less than 9 mcg/dL indicate a hypoadrenal state.[9,21] If a stimulation test cannot be done, then continued steroid therapy for 3 to 5 days should be based on clinical response.

Distributive Shock

In distributive shock disorders, global disorder in vasomotor control is present, resulting in maldistribution of blood flow and oxygen to tissue. Anaphylaxis and spinal cord injury are the 2 types most likely to be encountered in primary care. Cardiac output may be normal or increased. These patients lose sympathetic control of the vascular system, which reduces peripheral vascular tone. This circumstance produces pooling of blood in the periphery, which, in turn, leads to decreased venous return to the heart.

In anaphylactic shock, the inciting agent should be removed if possible. These patients uniformly respond well to volume administration, epinephrine infusion, antihistamines that include an H_2-receptor blocker, and steroid therapy.

TREATMENT

Three basic principles that should guide the therapy of a patient in shock are (1) prompt recognition of a patient in shock, (2) rapid restoration of systemic and regional perfusion to prevent ongoing shock and cellular injury, and (3) preventing the development of end-organ failure.

Primary caregivers can make an enormous difference in the morbidity and mortality of shock. The most important predictor of outcome is appropriate resuscitation and reversal of shock within 75 minutes of recognition. Han and his co-investigators at Pittsburgh documented increased survival and decreased morbidity in a group of infants and children in shock treated by community physicians.[1] Children who were treated following the American College of Critical Care Medicine *Pediatric Advanced Life Support* (ACCM-PALS) practice parameters for hemodynamic support of pediatric patients were compared with children who were treated by physicians who did not adhere to these algorithms.[22] Figure 358-2 graphically portrays the results.

In a 9-year study, community physicians successfully achieved shock reversal within 75 minutes of recognition in 24 of 91 children. In these patients, survival increased to 96% and more than 9-fold increase in the odds of survival. Each additional hour of persistent shock was associated with more than 2-fold increase in the odds of mortality. Shock resuscitation was consistent with ACCM-PALS guidelines in 30% of patients. When practice was consistent with these guidelines, mortality was only 8% compared with 38% in the children treated without following the guidelines. These data parallel and corroborate a study in adults of early and aggressive

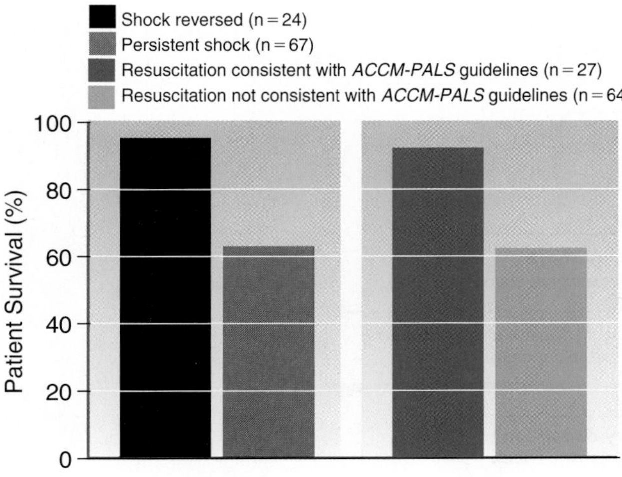

Figure 358-2 When community physicians implemented therapy and followed ACCM-PALS guidelines, almost all patients survived. Odds of mortality doubled with each hour of persistent shock. *(Han Y, Carcillo JA, Dragotta MA, et al. Early reversal of pediatric and neonatal septic shock by community physicians is associated with improved outcome. Pediatrics. 2003;112:793-799.)*

intervention that documented the importance of early goal-directed therapy.[23]

The guidelines for diagnosis, care, and treatment of infants and children are simple to understand and follow (Figure 358-3). The importance of timely recognition and treatment are highlighted. Review articles detail evidence-based development of the protocols.[9,21] Features of the guidelines are worth emphasis for the primary caregiver.

American College of Critical Care Medicine Clinical Practice Parameters for Hemodynamic Support of Pediatric and Neonatal Shock

Five minutes:

- First, secure airway and ventilation. Children have low lung volumes and are at risk for hypoxemia. Establish venous access within 5 minutes of recognition of shock. An intraosseous device or peripheral intravenous device suffices for this purpose. (Central access is not part of the 1st response.)
- Begin monitoring the child (see monitoring guidance in Box 358-5).

Fifteen minutes: In the first 15 minutes, administer intravenous fluids. Fluid needs can exceed 60 mL/kg of body weight. The volume of each fluid bolus should be 20 mL/kg.

Thirty minutes (15 minutes after fluid therapy begins):

- For children who do not immediately respond to fluid administration (15 minutes from beginning of fluid therapy), begin infusion of dopamine, catecholamine agent of 1st choice, at a dose of 5 to 20 mcg/kg/min. Infants younger than 6 months may not respond as well to dopamine.[9]
- Children who do not respond to dopamine infusion up to 20 mcg/kg/min and fluid resuscitation have dopamine-fluid refractory shock. Institute epinephrine (for cold shock) or norepinephrine (for warm shock) infusions. Glucose, serum hemoglobin or hematocrit, acid-base homeostasis, and ionized calcium should be monitored and restored to normal values.

Sixty minutes:

- Children who do not respond to fluid and an infusion of 2 catecholamine agents within 60 minutes have catecholamine resistant shock, and adrenal insufficiency should be considered.
- Refer to a tertiary care pediatric intensive care unit if children do not respond to fluid administration and to dopamine and epinephrine or norepinephrine infusions. These children require diagnostic evaluation for cardiac function and will require central venous access, echocardiography, and mixed venous oxygen saturation monitoring.

Treatment of shock, especially in primary care settings, is based on principles of restoring adequate circulating blood volume, thereby achieving adequate delivery of glucose and oxygen to all tissues. Drugs and fluids for the treatment of shock are listed in Table 358-5. Monitoring and documenting the patient's response to each intervention is essential. Patients who develop organ failure have a markedly worse prognosis in shock. Specific definitions of organ failure are listed in Box 358-6.

Early volume resuscitation and vasopressor therapy are always indicated in the treatment of shock. Hepatomegaly is a reliable clinical indicator of volume overload. In children who develop hepatomegaly but remain hemodynamically unstable, cardiac or renal failure must be considered. Clinicians should bear in mind that fluid requirements in shock may exceed 60 mL/kg, and a more common error is to give too little fluid too slowly. Rather than fearing fluid overload and thus undertreating the vast majority of patients, the clinician should gauge the patient's response to fluid administration. Patients who remain tachycardic with poor capillary refill and have inadequate urine output (<0.5 mL/kg/hr) after 60 mL/kg of fluid and the addition of 2 vasopressors are critically ill and in catecholamine-resistant shock. Placement of a central venous catheter is recommended at this point. Patients in this decompensated state will require referral to a tertiary pediatric intensive care unit for further diagnosis and treatment.

No conclusive data are found in the literature proving superiority of one fluid over another.[19,24,25] Commonly used solutions are normal saline, lactated Ringer solution, or 5% albumin. The volume of the bolus should be 20 mL/kg of body weight.

Children consume glucose at a faster rate than adolescents and adults. In infants and toddlers, glucose levels should be considered a vital sign, and blood glucose needs to be added to maintain adequate blood glucose levels. Glucose replacement is crucial, especially in very young patients. Glucose should be maintained at over 60 mg/dL.

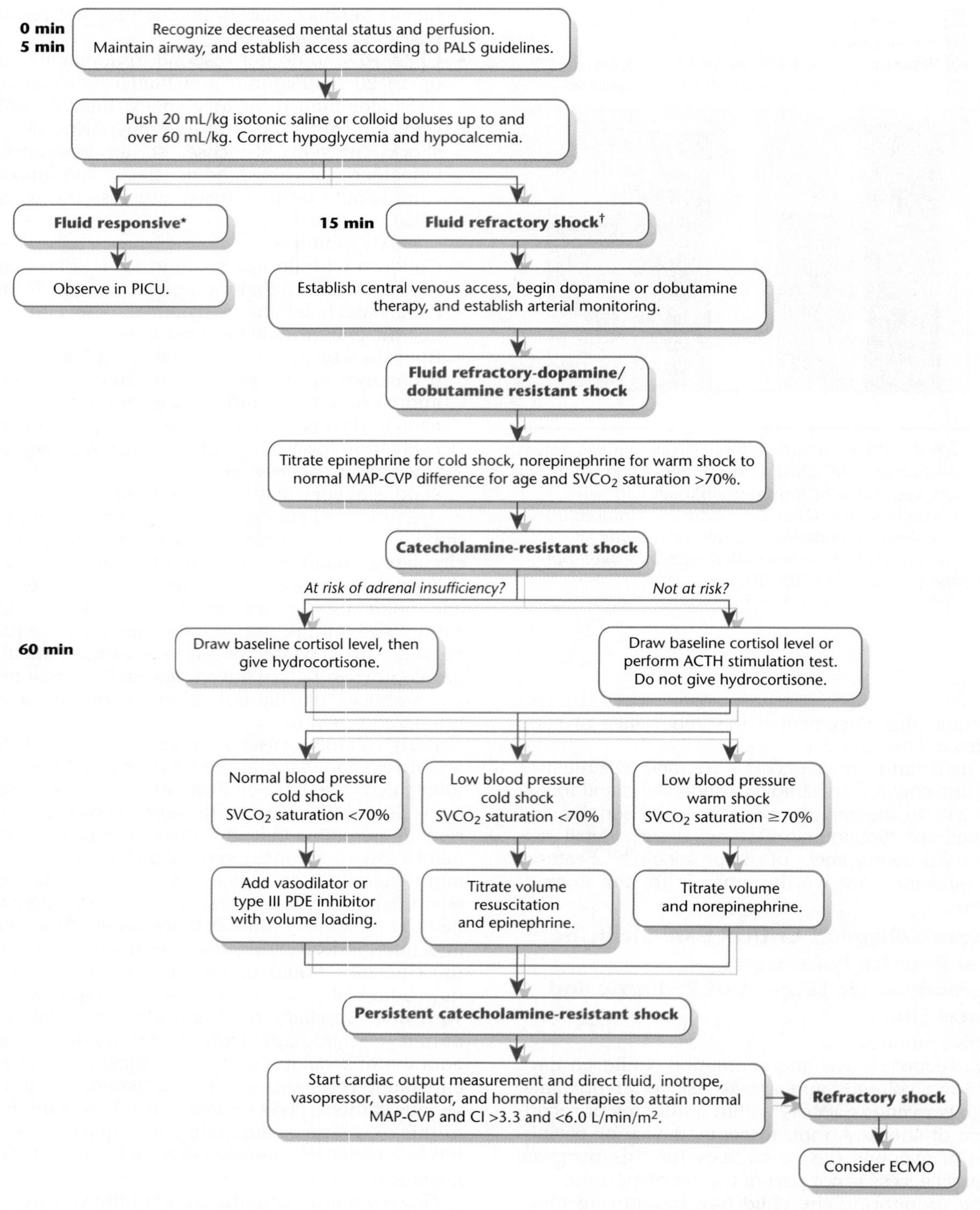

Figure 358-3 American College of Critical Care Medicine *Pediatric Advanced Life Support* (ACCM-PALS) guidelines for children in septic shock. The 1st hour of care can be crucial to outcome and is easily accomplished in the primary care setting. Recommendations are presented for stepwise management of hemodynamic support in infants and children with goals of normal perfusion and perfusion pressure (MAP-CVP). Proceed to next step if shock persists.

ACTH, adrenocorticotropic hormone; *CI,* cardiac index; *ECMO,* extracorporeal membrane oxygenation; MAP-CVP, mean arterial pressure minus central venous pressure; *PALS,* pediatric advanced life support: *PDE,* phosphodiesterase; *PICU,* pediatric intensive care unit; *$SVCO_2$,* superior vena cava oxygen; *(Carcillo JA, Fields AI (task force committee members). Clinical practice parameters for hemodynamic support of pediatric and neonatal patients in septic shock.* Crit Care Med. *2002;30:1365-1378. Reprinted by permission from Lippincott Williams & Wilkins.)*

BOX 358-5 Monitoring the Child in Shock in the Primary Care Setting

Capillary refill
Documentation of mental status
Pulse oximetry
Continuous electrocardiogram
Blood pressure (cuff)
Temperature
Urine output
Glucose and ionized calcium level
Serum hemoglobin or hematocrit

Hepatomegaly is a reliable indicator of volume overload and cardiac compromise. Successful resuscitation is recognized by:

- Return of pulse rate to normal
- Improvement in mental status
- Return of capillary refill
- Improvement in acid-base status

Table 358-5 Drugs and Fluids Used in the Treatment of Shock in Children and Infants

MEDICATIONS AND FLUIDS FOR TREATMENT OF SHOCK	DOSES
FLUIDS	
Normal saline	20-80 mL/kg
Albumin 5%	20-80 mL/kg
MEDICATIONS	
Dopamine	5-20 mcg/kg/min
Epinephrine	0.01-0.2 mcg/kg/min
Norepinephrine	0.01-0.2 mcg/kg/min
Dobutamine	5-20 mcg/kg/min
Milrinone	0.3-0.7 mcg/kg/min
Hydrocortisone (vasopressor resistant)	2 mg/kg/dose
Vasopressin	0.0003 units/kg/min to 0.01 units/kg/min
Calcium chloride (10%)	20 mg/kg

All patients in shock should immediately be given 100% oxygen; oxygenation should be monitored continuously with a pulse oximeter and the values documented in the patient's record. Because normal oxygen saturation does not reflect adequate oxygen content, the hemoglobin (the carrying vehicle for oxygen) should be maintained at a normal level. In hypovolemic shock, occult blood loss is in the differential diagnosis. In septic shock, the outcome in children may depend on adequate oxygen delivery. Clinicians need to appreciate that normal oxygen saturation on a pulse oximeter does not imply adequate tissue delivery.[20,26,27]

Blood transfusions may be necessary to ensure adequate oxygen delivery. If the circulation is compromised and cardiac output falls, then oxygen delivery to tissues will be compromised. In septic shock, adequate oxygen delivery is associated with improved survival.[10]

Oxygen delivery is the product of oxygen content and cardiac output. Oxygen content = 1.36 × the percentage of saturation × hemoglobin (in grams) and is expressed as milliliters of oxygen per 100 mL of blood. In healthy children, oxygen consumption is 25% of oxygen delivery. In shock states, oxygen consumption may increase simultaneously with inadequate cardiac output, leading to inadequate tissue oxygenation. If lung disease is present or hypoventilation occurs, then hemoglobin is desaturated, and oxygen delivery is compromised further. Despite concerns over the adverse effect of transfusion, the hemoglobin or hematocrit must be monitored, and maintaining the hemoglobin at least 10-g percentage is reasonable.[23]

Arterial lactic acidosis (normal is <2 mmol/L) or an increasing base deficit (>3 mEq) document inadequate perfusion. The effects of restoring the pH to over 7.25 are important: Myocardial contractility is enhanced, sensitivity to catecholamines is improved, and potassium is returned to the intracellular space.

Sodium bicarbonate may be required to improve blood pH to over 7.25 and serum bicarbonate levels to more than 15 mEq/dL. Any remaining base deficit may be corrected by using the following guide: 0.3 × body weight in kilograms × base deficit = milliequivalents of sodium bicarbonate.[28]

Hypocalcemia is common. Total calcium measurements do not correlate with measurements of the biologically important ionized calcium.[29] Restoring ionized calcium to normal levels improves myocardial contractility.[24]

In general, unless bleeding is evident, platelet counts of 20,000 to 50,000 cells/mm^3 are tolerated well. Prothrombin time and partial thromboplastin time should be maintained at approximately 1.3 times the normal values. Fresh frozen plasma, administered at 10 mL/kg, is a reasonable method of both repairing volume deficit and replenishing coagulation factors. Rapid infusion of fresh frozen plasma can contribute to hypotension resulting from the presence of vasoactive kinins.[2]

Vasopressor Drugs

Catecholamines do not replace adequate, aggressive, and early fluid administration as the initial treatment of shock. Dopamine, norepinephrine, epinephrine, and dobutamine are the drugs of choice in the early treatment of shock. In the majority of cases of shock encountered in primary care, dopamine with adequate fluid replacement saves the day. A vasoactive drug should be infused continuously with a calibrated

BOX 358-6 Definitions of Organ Failure for Pediatric Patients in Septic Shock*

CARDIOVASCULAR DYSFUNCTION

Despite administration of isotonic intravenous fluid bolus ≥40 mL/kg in 1 hr:

- Decrease in blood pressure (BP) levels (hypotension): <5th percentile for age; or systolic BP >2 standard deviation below normal for age

OR

- Need for vasoactive drug to maintain BP in normal range (dopamine >5 mcg/kg/min or dobutamine, epinephrine, or norepinephrine at any dose)

OR

- Two of the following:
  Unexplained metabolic acidosis: Base deficit >5.0 mEq/L
  Increased arterial lactate: >2 times upper limit of normal
  Oliguria: Urine output <0.5 ml/kg/hr
  Prolonged capillary refill: >5 sec
  Core to peripheral temperature gap: >3°C

RESPIRATORY

- PaO_2/FiO_2: <300 in absence of cyanotic heart disease or preexisting lung disease

OR

- $PaCO_2$: >65 torr or 20 mm Hg over baseline $PaCO_2$

OR

- Proven need or >50% FiO_2 to maintain saturation ≥92%

OR

- Need for nonelective invasive or noninvasive mechanical ventilation

NEUROLOGIC

- Glasgow coma score: ≤11 (57)

OR

- Acute change in mental status with a decrease in Glasgow coma score of ≥3 points from abnormal baseline

HEMATOLOGIC

- Platelet count: <80,000/mm^3 or a decline of 50% in platelet count from highest value recorded over the last 3 days (for patients with chronic hematologic disease or cancer)

OR

- International normalized ratio: >2

RENAL

- Serum creatinine: ≥2 times upper limit of normal for age, or 2-fold increase in baseline creatinine level

HEPATIC

- Total bilirubin: ≥4 mg/dL (not applicable for newborn)

OR

- Alanine aminotransferase (ALT): 2 times upper limit of normal for age

*Each additional organ failure increases the risk of death.
From Goldstein B, Giroir B, Randolph A, et al. International pediatric sepsis consensus conference: Definitions for sepsis and organ dysfunction in pediatrics. *Pediatr Crit Care Med.* 2005; 6:2-8. Reprinted with permission from Lippincott Williams & Wilkins.

infusion pump, and continuous heart rate and blood pressure monitoring is required.

Catecholamines are classified by their relative effects on the α or β receptor. The α receptor produces vasoconstriction, which accounts for its salutary effect in raising blood pressure. Beta agonists have 2 receptor sites. Beta-1 receptors stimulate heart rate and cardiac muscle contractility; thus toxicity is reflected in cardiac tachyarrhythmias and ischemia. Beta-2 agonist receptors are present in bronchial and arteriole smooth muscles, and these muscles relax when stimulated. These agents stimulate adenyl cyclase activity, and one of the effects is increased entry of potassium into cells.

Dopamine is the drug of choice and is administered at doses of 5 to 20 mcg/kg/min and titrated to effect. The α-adrenergic effects predominate with vasoconstriction and reduced peripheral perfusion. Patients who do not respond to fluid resuscitation of 60 mL/kg

Sample Case Report

A 3-year-old child exhibits a lung contusion and splenic hematoma. The hemoglobin is 10, heart rate is 180 beats per minute, systolic blood pressure is 80 mm Hg, and arterial saturation of oxygen by pulse oximetry is 90%. On examination, the patient is difficult to rouse, tachycardic, and has capillary refill >4 seconds. Evidence is ample that the patient's cardiac output is compromised because heart rate is elevated, perfusion is inadequate, and mental status is depressed.

The patient's oxygen content is (1.36 × serum hemoglobin × arterial saturation) or 1.36 × 10 × 0.90 = 12.3 mL of oxygen/100 mL blood, whereas normal oxygen content is 1.36 × 13 × 100 = 17.68 mL oxygen/100 mL blood. Transfusion of red blood cells to reach a hemoglobin count of 13 thus increases oxygen content of the patient's arterial blood nearly 50% (from 12.3 to 17.8 mL/100 mL blood)!

and 20 mcg/kg/min of dopamine are in a state defined as *dopamine fluid resistant shock* and require addition of epinephrine (cold shock) or norepinephrine (warm shock).[9] Infants younger than 6 months may not respond well to dopamine and epinephrine may be more effective.

Children who are thought to have low cardiac output may benefit from dobutamine. Dobutamine differs from dopamine because of its enhanced inotropic effect with less chronotropic effect than dopamine; it also has less effect on systemic vascular resistance. In some circumstances, especially shock after hypoxemic-ischemic injury, epinephrine or dobutamine may be preferred because dopamine may precipitate tachyarrhythmias and increase myocardial oxygen consumption.[28]

Hydrocortisone is indicated in limited circumstances. Children with anaphylaxis, those with known or suggested adrenal abnormalities, and children who have received a therapeutic course of steroids for chronic illness in the 6 months before the onset of shock will require stress-dose steroids at 1 to 2 mg/kg hydrocortisone.[21] Children in *refractory septic shock* (see Table 358-2) are, by definition, unresponsive to volume resuscitation, the addition of 2 catecholamine drugs, and normalization of acid base, glucose, and calcium homeostasis; they may respond to hydrocortisone.[2,21]

In selected situations, and in tertiary care settings only, the use of vasodilator drugs (nitroprusside, milrinone, nitroglycerin) may be beneficial in reducing afterload when high peripheral vascular resistance and low cardiac output is encountered. This therapy optimizes myocardial contractility and improves cardiac output but requires sophisticated monitoring, including pulmonary arterial oximetry, cardiac output measurement, and pulmonary vascular pressure catheters.[6]

Trials of several novel therapies that include activated protein C, granulocyte macrophage colony stimulating factor have been unsuccessful or have not affected outcomes for pediatric patients.[21] Extracorporeal membrane oxygenation has not been explored adequately in children in shock and should be performed only at the few centers that are capable of supporting this technology.[25] Trials of ibuprofen, antibody to endotoxin, and antibody to tumor necrosis factor-α did not improve survival in cases of septic shock.[30]

Therapeutic endpoints are capillary refill of under 2 seconds, normal peripheral pulses, warm limbs, a urine output of more than 1 mL/kg/hr, a decreasing lactic acid or improved base deficit, and normalization of mental status.[21]

SEQUELAE OF SHOCK

Several organ systems may be affected by shock (see Table 358-5). A common form of hypoxemic respiratory failure known as acute respiratory distress syndrome occurs 24 to 48 hours after presentation in shock. The child becomes dyspneic and hypoxemic, with a P/F ratio of less than 200 (partial pressure of oxygen/Fraction of inspired oxygen). Physical examination reveals rales and tachypnea; a chest radiograph reveals diffuse infiltrates. These changes may be delayed for 24 hours or more. The interstitial edema that develops appears to be caused by a capillary leak syndrome. This complication is life threatening, and the patient should be referred to a tertiary intensive care unit. Mechanical ventilation and positive end-expiratory pressure, right heart catheters, high-frequency oscillatory ventilation, or extracorporeal membrane support may be required.

Myocardial depression is commonly encountered in septic shock. Inadequate perfusion, increased work, and distension in the presence of inflammatory mediators affect contractility and may lead to a decrease in cardiac output.

Renal failure, especially acute tubular necrosis, is common. A serum creatinine more than twice normal for age is diagnostic. Renal failure is suggested when the urine output is under 0.5 mL/kg/hr, despite adequate restoration of blood volume. Aggressive use of dialysis and hemofiltration has minimized the morbidity resulting from this complication. Unrecognized renal failure will increase the mortality resulting from shock. Serum levels of drugs in the blood become uncertain. Doses of antibiotics, sedatives, and analgesics must be monitored carefully, following blood levels in serum whenever possible. Fluid therapy must be titrated carefully to insensible fluid loss replacement; otherwise congestive heart failure will result. Anuria or oliguria complicating shock requires referral or consultation with a nephrologist or intensivist. Diuretics may increase mortality in acute renal failure.[31]

The central nervous system is most susceptible to hypoxemia and ischemia. A child may suffer significant neurologic impairment, although other organs are spared. Early central nervous system signs of shock include delirium, irritability, confusion, and coma. Signs of increased intracranial pressure are usually delayed 24 to 72 hours after a hypoxemic-ischemic insult. The presence of increased intracranial pressure accompanying the acute presentation of shock implies a traumatic or metabolic etiology.[6] A Glasgow coma score of under 11, or a decrease of 3 points from baseline, are diagnostic of central nervous system compromise.

Liver function may become impaired as a result of inadequate perfusion. Bilirubin levels of more than 4 mg/dL and alanine aminotransferase levels greater than twice normal are diagnostic of hepatic failure. Clotting factors may be diminished. In septic shock, liver perfusion may be adequate, but bacteria or toxins may damage hepatic cells. Liver failure is usually transient.

SUMMARY

Shock in the pediatric setting is a relatively common emergency. Community caregivers can make a significant difference in the outcome of children in shock. The diagnosis of shock is clinical, based on mental status, tachycardia, and peripheral perfusion. Early treatment does not require sophisticated monitors, central venous catheters, or invasive monitoring.

SUGGESTED RESOURCES

Carcillo JA. Fluid resuscitation of hypovolemic shock in children. *Pediatr Crit Care Med.* 2001;2(suppl):s10-s13.

Finfer S, Bellomo R, Boyce N, et al, (SAFE Investigators Committee). A comparison of albumin and saline for fluid resuscitation in the intensive care unit. *N Engl J Med.* 2004;350:2247-2256.

REFERENCES

1. Han Y, Carcillo JA, Dragotta MA, et al. Early reversal of pediatric and neonatal septic shock by community physicians is associated with improved outcome. *Pediatrics.* 2003;112:793-799.
2. Carcillo JA, Davis AL, Zaritsky A. Role of early fluid resuscitation in pediatric septic shock. *JAMA.* 1991;266: 1242-1249.
3. Watson RS, Carcillo JA. Scope and epidemiology of pediatric sepsis. *Ped Crit Care Med.* 2005;6(suppl): S3-S5.
4. Watson RS, Carcillo JA, Linde-Zwirble WT, et al. The epidemiology of severe sepsis is children in the United States. *Am J Respir Crit Care Med.* 2003;167: 695-701.
5. Orr RA, Kuch B, Carcillo J, et al. Shock is under-reported in children transported for respiratory distress: a multicenter study. *Crit Care Med.* 2003;31(Suppl):A18.
6. Tobin JR, Wetzel RC: Shock. In: Rogers M, ed. *Textbook of Pediatric Intensive Care.* 3rd ed. Baltimore, MD: Williams & Wilkins; 1996.
7. Parker MM, Shelhamer JH, Natanson C, et al. Serial cardiovascular variables in survivors and nonsurvivors of human septic shock; heart rate as an early predictor of prognosis. *Crit Care Med.* 1987;15: 923-929.
8. Pollack MM, Fields AI, Ruttiman UE. Distributions of cardiopulmonary variables in pediatric survivors and nonsurvivors of septic shock. *Crit Care Med.* 1985;13: 454-459.
9. Carcillo JA, Fields AI (task force committee members). ACCM clinical practice parameters for hemodynamic support of pediatric and neonatal patients in septic shock. *Crit Care Med.* 2002;30:1365-1378.
10. Perkin RM: Shock states. In: Fuhrman BH, Zimmerman JR, eds. *Pediatric Critical Care.* St Louis, MO: Mosby; 1992.
11. Sorenson IA, Nielson GG, Andersen PK, et al. Genetic and environmental influences on premature death in adult adoptees. *N Engl J Med.* 1988;328: 727-732.
12. Friedman WF, George BL. Treatment of congestive heart failure by altering loading conditions of the heart. *J Pediatr.* 1985;106:697-705.
13. Carcillo JA, Pollack MM, Ruttiman U. Sequential physiologic interactions in pediatric cardiogenic and septic shock. *Crit Care Med.* 1989;17:12-16.
14. Bangur AR, Meliones JN. Cardiogenic shock. *New Horiz.* 1998;6:139-149.
15. Thomas NJ, Carcillo J. Hypovolemic shock in pediatric patients. *New Horiz.* 1998;6:120-129.
16. Opal SM. Concept of Piro as a new conceptual framework to understand sepsis. *Pediatr Crit Care Med.* 2005; 6(suppl):s55-s60.
17. Hazelzet JA. Diagnosing meningococcemia as a cause of sepsis. *Pediatr Crit Care Med.* 2005;6(suppl): s50-s54.
18. Landry DW, Oliver JA. The pathogenesis of vasodilatory shock. *N Engl J Med.* 2001;345:588-595.
19. Ceneviva G, Paschall JA, Maffei F, et al. Hemodynamic support in fluid refractory pediatric septic shock. *Pediatrics.* 1998;102:e19.
20. Pollack MM, Fields AI, Ruttiman UE. Distributions of cardiopulmonary variables of infants and children in septic shock. *Crit Care Med.* 1984;12:554-559.
21. Parker MM, Hazelzet JA, Carcillo, JA. Pediatric considerations. *Crit Care Med.* 2004;32(suppl): S591-S594.
22. Zaritsky AL, Nadkarni VM, Hickey RW, et al. *Pediatric Advanced Life Support Manual.* Dallas, TX: American Heart Association; 2002.
23. Rivers E, Nguyen B, Havstad S, et al. Early goal-directed therapy in the treatment of severe sepsis and septic shock. *New Eng J Med.* 2001;345:1368-1377.
24. Cardenas-Rivero N, Chernow B, Stoiko MA, et al. Hypocalcemia in critically ill children. *J Pediatr.* 1989;114: 946-951.
25. Goldman AP, Kerr SJ, Butt W, et al. Extracorporeal support for intractable cardiorespiratory failure due to meningococcal disease. *Lancet.* 1997;349:466-469.
26. Rodriguez LR, Koten N, Lowenthal D. A study of pediatric house staffs' knowledge of pulse oximetry. *Pediatrics.* 1994;93:810-813.
27. Mink RB, Pollack M. Effect of blood transfusion on oxygen consumption in pediatric septic shock. *Crit Care Med.* 1987;18:1087-1091.
28. Zaritsky A. Recent advances in pediatric cardiopulmonary resuscitation and advanced life support. *New Horiz.* 1998;6:201-211.
29. Meliones JM, Moler FW, Custer JR. Hemodynamic instability after the initiation of extracorporeal membrane oxygenation: role of ionized calcium. *Crit Care Med.*1987; 19:1247-1251.
30. Saez-Llorens X, McCracken GH Jr: Sepsis syndrome and septic shock in pediatrics: current concepts of terminology, pathophysiology, and management, *J Pediatr.* 1994; 123:497-507.
31. Uchino S, Doig GS, Bellomo R, et al. Diuretics and mortality in acute renal failure. *Crit Care Med.* 2004;32: 1669-1677.

Chapter 359

STATUS ASTHMATICUS

Alan R. Schroeder, MD

Asthma is a major cause of morbidity and mortality in children. Asthma exacerbations impose a significant strain on health care systems and can compromise the quality of life of patients and their families.[1,2] Asthma death rates in US children increased progressively between 1980 and 1999, with the highest mortality rates in blacks.[3] The term *status asthmaticus* generally refers to an acute exacerbation that does not respond to initial doses of nebulized bronchodilating agents,[4] thereby placing the asthmatic patient at risk for respiratory failure.[5]

Risk factors for near-fatal and fatal asthma differ across studies and between pediatric and adult populations. The risk of fatal or near-fatal asthma is greater in patients with more longstanding disease[6] and in patients with more severe disease.[6-10] Signs of increased asthma severity include multiple hospitalizations, prior intubations, and previous attacks with severe, unexpected, and rapid deterioration. Many studies have demonstrated associations between β-agonist use and death or near death.[7,8,11-13]

A putative link exists between the use of long-acting β-agonists and significant adverse events. The association between significant adverse events and β-agonist exposure underscores the importance of familiarity with a patient's medical regimen when treating an asthma exacerbation. Abrupt cessation of inhaled corticosteroids may further increase risk of death.[7]

Overall, most asthma deaths (80%-85%) occur in patients with severe and poorly controlled asthma with progressive deterioration characterized by histologic evidence of extensive mucus plugging and eosinophilic inflammation.[5] These patients tend to respond slowly to treatment. More optimal chronic antiinflammatory therapy may assist in preventing the death of these patients. A smaller proportion of deaths occurs in patients who have acute deterioration (eg, sudden asphyxic asthma), in whom mucus plugging is substantially reduced and the inflammatory cells are neutrophils. These attacks are less preventable given their acute onset; however, if appropriately treated, they usually demonstrate faster response to treatment.[5]

CLINICAL MANIFESTATIONS

Asthma exacerbations are most frequently triggered by viral infections in children. Other common triggers include aeroallergens (animal dander, dust mites, cockroaches, molds, and pollens), tobacco smoke, pollutants, cold or dry air, gastroesophageal reflux disease, exercise, and laughter.[14]

The hallmark of asthma is cough and wheezing, although wheezing may not be evident if air entry is limited. Patients in status asthmaticus may complain of shortness of breath or chest tightness and demonstrate signs of increased work of breathing, including tachypnea, accessory muscle use, nasal flaring, head bobbing, and grunting. Patients may have difficulty speaking or completing short sentences in 1 breath. Patients are often anxious and, in severe cases, may have altered mental status or lethargy. Signs of impending respiratory failure include cyanosis, decreased breath sounds, altered level of consciousness, diaphoresis, and inability to speak.[4]

Physical examination should include a complete set of vital signs, including pulse oximetry. Patients in status asthmaticus often have tachycardia, tachypnea, hypoxemia, and pulsus paradoxus, defined as a drop in systolic blood pressure of 10 mm Hg or more during inspiration. Close attention should be paid to the neurologic examination, hydration status, and peripheral perfusion. The eyes, ears, nose, and throat should be examined to assess for a possible source of infection that may have triggered the asthma. The nares should be inspected for polyps and signs of allergic rhinitis. A heart examination is necessary to rule out a cardiac cause of wheezing. During the abdominal examination, hepatomegaly may be noted if the lungs are hyperinflated.

The chest should be directly inspected to assess the work of breathing, to gauge the anterior-posterior diameter, to assess for the presence of chest wall deformities, and to observe whether chest movement is bilaterally symmetric. Auscultation should be performed to evaluate air entry (depth and symmetry), inspiration-to-expiration ratio, and to detect wheezing or rales. Spirometry is helpful in older children and should be performed serially to follow the disease trajectory but is of little value in the context of an acute exacerbation. Comparison of peak expiratory flow rates to baseline values or to normal values based on age and height can be helpful in assessing the severity of an acute exacerbation.[15]

Chest radiographs are often ordered but rarely add meaningfully to the diagnosis and management of severe asthma exacerbations.[16] Findings may include hyperinflation, an area of opacification, and, rarely, pneumothorax or pneumomediastinum. The history and physical examination should guide the decision to obtain a radiograph. Indications include asymmetry or focal abnormality on auscultation, endotracheal intubation, and a suspicion of foreign body aspiration, in which case unilateral hyperinflation may be present or the lung distal to the obstructed airway may be hyperinflated as demonstrated on lateral decubitus films.

Arterial or venous blood gas analysis can provide additional assessment of the adequacy of ventilation and oxygenation, although venipuncture or arterial puncture may increase anxiety and distress in a borderline patient. Hypoxemia and respiratory alkalosis are present initially,[4,5] but the pressure of carbon dioxide in the blood will slowly start to increase as airway obstruction increases. Historically, a finding of carbon dioxide retention has been considered as an indication for endotracheal intubation and mechanical ventilation,[17] However, more recent reviews advocate basing intubation decisions on clinical parameters such as altered mental status or hemodynamic instability rather than blood gas results alone.[4,5]

Patients in status asthmaticus may have some degree of metabolic acidosis caused by either compensatory renal bicarbonate loss (as compensation for respiratory alkalosis if the exacerbation has been longstanding) or lactate accumulation.[5] The source of lactic acidosis is unclear, but it may be the result of a combination of high-dose parenteral β-agonist use, anaerobic metabolism from overused respiratory muscles, or tissue hypoxia.[17] The presence of lactic acidosis is an ominous sign but is rare in children with status asthmaticus.[18]

PATHOPHYSIOLOGICAL CONSIDERATIONS

Asthma is an inflammatory condition characterized by widespread, variable obstruction of the lower airways. The airflow limitation results from inflammation of the lower airways, mucosal edema, epithelial sloughing, mucus plugs, and bronchospasm. The inflammation is a complex response that includes eosinophils, mast cells, T lymphocytes, macrophages, neutrophils, and epithelial cells.[19] The primary event is generally activation of mast cells in response to local irritation, which leads to mast-cell degranulation and promotes activation of T lymphocytes (Figure 359-1). Multiple proinflammatory mediators are released, including histamine, leukotrienes, platelet-activating factor, and several T2 helper cell cytokines (interleukin [IL]-4, IL-5, IL-8, and IL-13).[4,20] These cytokines augment immunoglobulin E production by B lymphocytes, thereby augmenting leukotriene release from mast cells. Ultimately, this inflammatory environment is rich in leukotrienes, prostaglandins, nitric oxide, adhesion molecules, and platelet-activating factor, causing overproduction of mucus and epithelial cell destruction. The loss of epithelial cells exposes nerve endings, rendering the airway even more hyperirritable in response to environmental triggers.[20] Epithelial damage is correlated with the severity of airway reactivity.[21]

Airway caliber and mucus secretion are regulated by the autonomic nervous system. Bronchial nerve ganglia receive direct vagal innervation, but they are also modulated by circulating catecholamines. Vagal parasympathetic stimulation leads to the release of postganglionic acetylcholine, causing bronchoconstriction, and mucus secretion.[22,23] β-Receptors are found on airway smooth muscle, epithelium, and mucous glands, as well as on various inflammatory cells.[4] Stimulation of β-receptors causes cyclic adenosine monophosphate activation of protein kinase A, which in smooth muscle leads to muscle relaxation and bronchodilation. Polymorphisms in the β2-adrenergic receptor have been described in children and may explain some ethnic differences in asthma severity and response to bronchodilators.[24,25]

Airway obstruction compromises inspiratory and expiratory gas flow, leading to ventilation and perfusion mismatch. Distal lung segments become hyperinflated as alveoli empty incompletely. In the respiratory cycle, inspiration begins before exhalation is complete. This process of dynamic hyperinflation creates large end-expiratory lung volumes, which may be evident on clinical or chest x-ray examination. Hyperinflation worsens ventilation as large residual volumes creates difficulty in generating effective tidal volumes. As obstruction worsens, hyperinflation can lead to

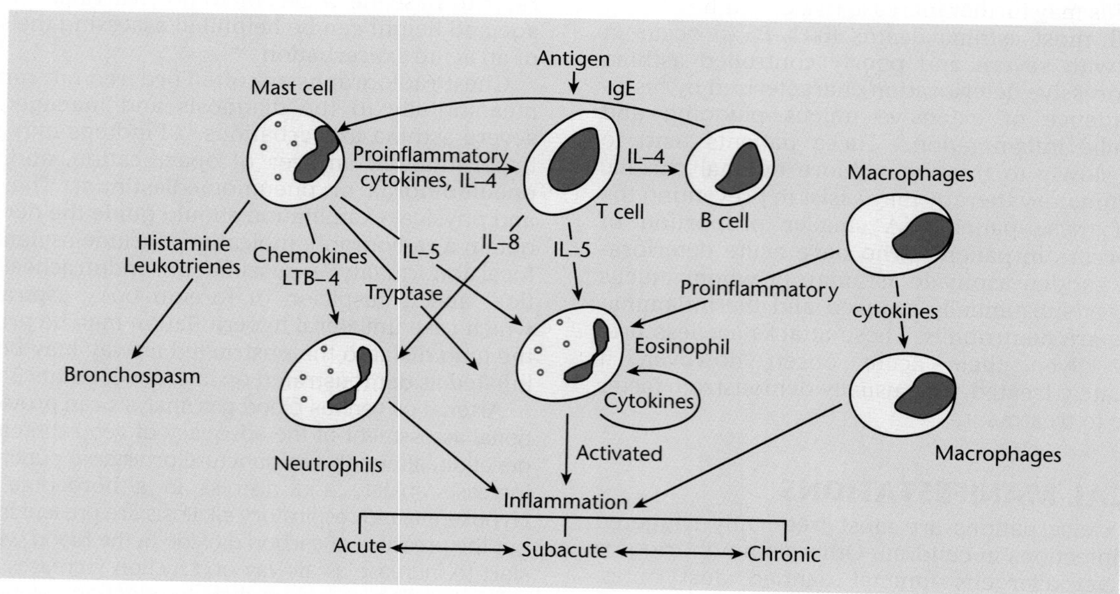

Figure 359-1 Cellular mechanisms involved in airway inflammation. (*National Asthma Education and Prevention Program.* Guidelines for the Diagnosis and Management of Asthma, Expert Panel Report 2. *Bethesda, MD: National Heart, Lung, and Blood Institute, National Institutes of Health, US Department of Health and Human Services; 1997. NIH Publication 97-4051.*)

ventilation and perfusion mismatch and hypoxemia. If airway obstruction is not relieved, then muscle fatigue can further compromise ventilation, resulting in hypercarbia and ultimately respiratory failure.

The severe obstruction that characterizes status asthmaticus leads to complex cardiopulmonary interactions. With severe obstruction, the increased residual volume in the lungs can diminish venous return to the right atrium, thereby decreasing cardiac output. Pulmonary vascular resistance can be increased by hypoxia, acidosis, and hyperinflation, further increasing the workload of the right ventricle. Spontaneously breathing patients in status asthmaticus generate large negative intrapleural pressures, with inspiratory pressures as low as −35 cm water.[4] Negative pleural pressure increases left-ventricular oxygen demand and work by increasing left-ventricular transmural pressure. Furthermore, the generous degree to negative intrapleural pressure creates a gradient for fluid movement from capillaries to alveoli, leading to a decrease in cardiac output and a potential for pulmonary edema.[26] Pulsus paradoxus occurs when systemic cardiac output drops markedly during inspiration, resulting primarily from increased capacitance of the pulmonary vasculature and resulting in decreased left-ventricular preload.[27]

MANAGEMENT

Supportive Care

Any child in status asthmaticus should be hospitalized on a monitored bed. Indications for pediatric intensive care unit (PICU) admission vary across hospitals and may depend on hospital policies and staffing issues. Any child requiring positive pressure ventilation, sedation, or continuous intravenous bronchodilator infusions should be monitored in a PICU.

In the context of status asthmaticus, administration of supplemental oxygen can address hypoxemia. Supplemental oxygen is often required to improve oxygen saturation and ease the work of breathing. Oxygen can be delivered via nasal canula, but in cases of significant hypoxemia, it is better given by mask. According to National Institutes of Health guidelines, the target oxygen saturation should be more than 90% in most patients and more than 95% in infants, children with acyanotic heart disease, and pregnant women.[19]

Most asthma exacerbations are caused by viral infections or noninfectious triggers. Antibiotics should therefore not be provided for acute asthma exacerbations except as needed for comorbid conditions and in cases in which a strong suspicion of pneumonia exists (eg, fever and purulent sputum, chest radiograph demonstrating focal infiltrate).[28]

Patients are often dehydrated as a result of poor oral intake and increased insensible losses from the respiratory tract. Rehydration is necessary to maintain euvolemia and cardiac output, but overhydration can lead to pulmonary edema.[4] Urine output and electrolytes should be monitored closely, given that the syndrome of inappropriate antidiuretic hormone may occur in severe asthma.[29]

Patients with respiratory failure or impending failure should be intubated and mechanically ventilated. However, patients with severe asthma should receive prompt and aggressive therapy as soon as possible to avoid endotracheal intubation because manipulation of the airway may exacerbate bronchospasm. Furthermore, positive pressure ventilation, even noninvasive ventilation, increases the risk of pneumothorax and may result in untoward hemodynamic sequelae.[4] Noninvasive positive pressure ventilation prevents the risks inherent in intubation and may be considered as an alternative to intubation and mechanical ventilation.[30,31]

In the event of a clinical decision that respiratory failure is imminent and intubation is necessary, great care must be exercised in the course of induction and intubation. Induction medications that minimize the effects on the patient's cardiovascular status should be chosen. Intravenous access should be established before intubation because administration of analgesic and sedative agents can cause vasodilation, leading to profound hypotension. If a patient is intubated and mechanically ventilated, then sedation should be used.

Neuromuscular blockade may be necessary to minimize peak inspiratory pressures on the ventilator. However, neuromuscular blocking agents metabolized via Hoffman degradation pathways should be used because agents such as pancuronium or vecuronium can lead to prolonged paralysis, the result of the half-life of its active metabolites being prolonged by corticosteroids.[32,33] In nonintubated patients, sedation may be used if patient agitation is contributing to respiratory distress. However, because sedation confounds the neurologic examination and may contribute to diminished respiratory effort, judicious use of sedative-hypnotic agents is indicated. If sedation is used, then objective criteria to assess respiratory status, such as blood gases, should be monitored even more closely than usual. Because of its bronchodilatory effects, ketamine is the sedative agent of choice, and it has been used successfully in nonintubated[34] and intubated[35-37] children.

Bronchodilators

β2-agonists are the mainstay of status asthmaticus pharmacotherapy, and they are most often provided in the inhaled form. These drugs stimulate β2-receptors in airway smooth muscle, leading to smooth-muscle relaxation and subsequent bronchodilation. Inhaled albuterol can be given via a metered dose inhaler with a spacer chamber or via nebulization. Studies comparing the efficacy of the 2 methods of delivery for acute asthma show no significant difference,[38-40] although patients receiving albuterol via metered dose inhaler or spacer appear to have a shorter length of stay in the emergency department than patients using nebulization.[39] For severe exacerbations, however, nebulization is generally the preferred route,[4] and continuous nebulization appears to be better than intermittent doses, even when the same cumulative dose is used.[41] The standard dose of continuous albuterol is 5 to 20 mg/hr, although doses as high as 40 to 150 mg/hr have been reported.[4]

The standard formulation of albuterol is a 50/50 mixture of the (R)- and (S)-enantiomer forms of the drug. (R)-albuterol (levalbuterol) is the active form of the drug that leads to bronchodilation, whereas (S)-albuterol has a longer half-life and may contribute to side effects. In 1999 the US Food and Drug Administration approved the use of levalbuterol for asthma.[42] Studies comparing levalbuterol with the racemic form have yielded inconsistent results, with some studies showing no differences in efficacy,[43,44] some showing no differences in efficacy but a better side-effect profile for levalbuterol,[45] and some showing increased efficacy with levalbuterol.[46,47] These studies generally evaluate acute asthma with either hospitalization rates or forced expiratory volume in 1 second measures as the primary outcome. Because definitive data are absent and the significantly increased cost of levalbuterol,[48] routine use is not recommended at this time.[4,20] However, levalbuterol may be considered for patients who are experiencing significant side effects from albuterol, such as tachycardia and agitation.

Other β-agonists include epinephrine and terbutaline, which can be given via aerosolized, subcutaneous, or intravenous routes. Epinephrine is rarely used because of its lack of β2 selectivity and the resulting dangerous side-effect profile. Terbutaline is often provided subcutaneously during a severe exacerbation when intravenous access is not readily available. The usual dose is 0.01 mg/kg given subcutaneously every 20 minutes in 3 doses, as necessary.[20] In the PICU, terbutaline can be administered as a continuous infusion,[49-51] with a dose range of 0.4 to 10 mcg/kg/min. It is generally well tolerated, although it may cause a decrease in diastolic blood pressure.[50] Given in a protocol-based fashion as an adjunct to aerosolized bronchodilators, terbutaline has been shown to reduce length of stay in both the PICU and the hospital.[49]

Anticholinergics are often used as adjuncts to β-agonists in managing status asthmaticus. These agents produce bronchodilation by blocking the effects of acetylcholine-induced bronchoconstriction. The prototypical anticholinergic drug is ipratropium bromide, which is similar to atropine but has the advantage of not inhibiting ciliary beating and mucociliary clearance.[52] When given as an adjunct to albuterol and corticosteroids, ipratropium has been demonstrated to reduce hospitalization rates of asthmatic children[53] and adults[54] seen in the emergency department for asthma exacerbations. In the inpatient setting, ipratropium is generally given at a dose of 250 to 500 mcg inhaled or nebulized every 6 to 8 hours. Ipratropium produces minimal systemic side effects, although inadvertent spread of the aerosolized drug to the eyes may cause unilateral or bilateral mydriasis,[55-57] which can be alarming in the intensive care unit setting.

Whether magnesium sulfate plays a meaningful role in the management of the patient with severe asthma remains unclear. Magnesium exerts its bronchodilatory effects through inhibition of calcium uptake. A recent meta-analysis demonstrated that intravenous magnesium sulfate improves pulmonary function and modestly decreases the rate of hospitalization in children seeking emergency care, although in adults with asthma, a meta-analysis of intravenous magnesium sulfate use demonstrated a reduction in hospitalization rates occurred only with severe asthma.[58,60] Intravenous magnesium sulfate is usually given over 20 to 30 minutes at reported doses of 25, 40, and 75 mg/kg.[58] A dose of 75 mg/kg does not produce any added benefit, and therefore the 40-mg/kg dose is recommended.[61] Adverse effects include flushing, nausea, and hypotension. Serious toxicities such as cardiac arrhythmias, muscle weakness, and respiratory depression are rare.

Corticosteroids

Corticosteroids are indicated for any moderate to severe asthma attack. The anti-inflammatory properties of corticosteroids include reduction in the number and activation of inflammatory cells, inhibition of the vascular leak induced by proinflammatory mediators, restoration of disrupted epithelium, normalization of ciliated cell/goblet cell ratio, a decrease in mucus secretion, and the downregulation of proinflammatory cytokine production and release.[4,20] Corticosteroids also increase β-adrenergic receptors density on bronchial smooth-muscle cells, thereby increasing β-agonist efficacy.[19]

Corticosteroids can be administered by inhaled, oral, intravenous, or intramuscular routes. Although the bioavailability of oral and intravenous corticosteroids is similar, intravenous administration is preferred in status asthmaticus to decrease the risk of aspiration in case the child needs to be intubated and requires administration of sedative agents and medications delivered via the oral route.[4,20,62] Inhaled corticosteroids, which are a mainstay of chronic asthma therapy, reduce hospitalizations in acute asthma when compared with placebo, but they are probably less efficacious than intravenous corticosteroids.[63] Common oral corticosteroids include prednisone and prednisolone. Intravenous corticosteroids include methylprednisolone, hydrocortisone, and dexamethasone. For status asthmaticus, methylprednisolone is administered most often. Adverse effects of corticosteroid therapy usually occur only after prolonged administration (ie, >3 weeks). In the short term, hyperglycemia, hypertension, leukocytosis, and mood and appetite changes may be encountered. A varicella vaccination should be administered, and a complete exposure history should be taken before corticosteroid therapy is initiated because of the rare but serious risk of disseminated varicella.[64-66]

Methylxanthines

Methylxanthines used in asthma include theophylline and its water-soluble salt analog, aminophylline. The primary effect of theophylline lies in phosphodiesterase inhibition, which reduces the degradation of cyclic adenosine monophosphate, resulting in dilation of airway smooth muscle.[67,68] Theophylline also strengthens diaphragmatic contractility and increases respiratory drive.[69,70] The addition of intravenous aminophylline to β2-agonists and corticosteroids in children with severe asthma improves lung function within 6 hours of treatment; however, it does not lead to any apparent reduction in symptoms or length of hospital stay and is associated with a significantly increased risk of vomiting.[71] Because of the narrow therapeutic window of theophylline (5-15 mcg/dL), use of this agent should be reserved for patients with severe asthma whose disease is not responding to maximal conventional therapy.[4,20]

Helium-Oxygen Mixtures

Helium-oxygen (heliox) mixture was used for treating upper and lower airway obstruction as early as 1935, and its use in asthma increased in the 1980s when asthma deaths began to rise.[72] Helium gas is less dense than air and therefore facilitates laminar gas flow and decreases turbulent flow and thereby reduces work, leading to easier breathing in patients with high airway resistance.[4,20,72] Heliox is used most frequently in children with upper airway obstruction,[73-78] but a recent randomized trial demonstrated that heliox decreased work of breathing, diminished pulsus paradoxus, and may have prevented intubation in children hospitalized with status asthmaticus because it decreases the work of breathing and diminishes pulsus paradoxus.[79] Data supporting the use of heliox in pediatric asthma are not compelling; studies conflict regarding whether children experienced improvement in pulmonary index scores and were discharged home earlier when provided with albuterol nebulized with heliox as opposed to albuterol with oxygen alone.[80] However, a similar study done in the emergency department setting found no significant improvement in work of breathing in patients using heliox.[81] Data supporting the use of heliox in pediatric asthma remain less than compelling. Although heliox possesses a favorable toxicity profile, the theoretical benefit of heliox is lost if less than 60% helium is in the mixture. Thus heliox may not be tolerated in patients with significant hypoxemia.[20]

Other Therapeutic Strategies

In severe, refractory cases of status asthmaticus, inhalational anesthetics have been used. The mechanism of action remains unknown but may involve inhibition of baseline vagal tone.[82] In children, halothane[83-86] and isoflurane[87-91] have been described most extensively, and ventilation improved in most patients. Bronchoscopy with lavage and instillation of mucolytic agents is another treatment modality in severe cases in which extensive mucus plugging or bronchial casts (or both) are suspected.[20] Finally, extracorporal life support has been used in both adults and children,[90,92-96] and it may be lifesaving in its ability to ameliorate severe hypoxemia, hypercarbia, or cardiovascular collapse.

TOOLS FOR PRACTICE

Medical Decision Support

- *Guidelines for the Diagnosis and Management of Asthma* National Heart, Lung, and Blood Institute (www.nhlbi.nih.gov/guidelines/asthma/asthgdln.htm).

REFERENCES

1. Lane S, Molina J, Plusa T. An international observational prospective study to determine the cost of asthma exacerbations (COAX). *Respir Med.* 2006;100:434-450.
2. Skrepnek GH, Skrepnek SV. Epidemiology, clinical and economic burden, and natural history of chronic obstructive pulmonary disease and asthma. *Am J Manag Care.* 2004;10(5 suppl):S129-S138.
3. Mannino D, Homa D, Akinbami L, et al. Surveillance for asthma—United States, 1980-1999. *MMWR Morb Mortal Wkly Rep.* 2002;51(SS01):1-13.
4. Werner HA. Status asthmaticus in children: a review. *Chest.* 2001;119:1913-1929.
5. Papiris S, Kotanidou A, Malagari K, et al. Clinical review: severe asthma. *Crit Care.* 2002;6:30-44.
6. Belessis Y, Dixon S, Thomsen A, et al. Risk factors for an intensive care unit admission in children with asthma. *Pediatr Pulmonol.* 2004;37:201-209.
7. Alvarez GG, Schulzer M, Jung D, et al. A systematic review of risk factors associated with near-fatal and fatal asthma. *Can Respir J.* 2005;12:265-270.
8. Ernst P, Habbick B, Suissa S, et al. Is the association between inhaled beta-agonist use and life-threatening asthma because of confounding by severity? *Am Rev Respir Dis.* 1993;148:75-79.
9. Fletcher HJ, Ibrahim SA, Speight N. Survey of asthma deaths in the Northern region, 1970-85. *Arch Dis Child.* 1990;65:163-167.
10. Mountain RD, Sahn SA. Clinical features and outcome in patients with acute asthma presenting with hypercapnia. *Am Rev Respir Dis.* 1988;138:535-539.
11. Ernst P, Spitzer WO, Suissa S, et al. Risk of fatal and near-fatal asthma in relation to inhaled corticosteroid use. *JAMA.* 1992;268:3462-3464.
12. Spitzer WO, Suissa S, Ernst P, et al. The use of beta-agonists and the risk of death and near death from asthma. *N Engl J Med.* 1992;326:501-506.
13. Suissa S, Ernst P, Boivin JF, et al. A cohort analysis of excess mortality in asthma and the use of inhaled beta-agonists. *Am J Respir Crit Care Med.* 1994;149(3 pt 1):604-610.
14. Liu A, Spahn J, Leung D. Childhood asthma. In: Behrman RE, ed. *Nelson Textbook of Pediatrics.* 17th ed. Philadelphia, PA: Elsevier; 2004.
15. Pollack CV Jr, Pollack ES, Baren JM, et al. A prospective multicenter study of patient factors associated with hospital admission from the emergency department among children with acute asthma. *Arch Pediatr Adolesc Med.* 2002;156:934-940.
16. Brooks LJ, Cloutier MM, Afshani E. Significance of roentgenographic abnormalities in children hospitalized for asthma. *Chest.* 1982;82:315-318.
17. Corbridge TC, Hall JB. The assessment and management of adults with status asthmaticus. *Am J Respir Crit Care Med.* 1995;151:1296-1316.
18. Yousef E, McGeady SJ. Lactic acidosis and status asthmaticus: how common in pediatrics? *Ann Allergy Asthma Immunol.* 2002;89:585-588.
19. National Heart, Lung, and Blood Institute. *Guidelines for the Diagnosis and Management of Asthma, Expert Panel Report 2.* Publication 97-4051. Bethesda, MD: National Institutes of Health; 1997.
20. Furhman BP, Zimmerman J. *Pediatric Critical Care.* St Louis, MO: Mosby; 2006.
21. Laitinen LA, Heino M, Laitinen A, et al. Damage of the airway epithelium and bronchial reactivity in patients with asthma. *Am Rev Respir Dis.* 1985;131:599-606.
22. Joos GF. The role of neuroeffector mechanisms in the pathogenesis of asthma. *Curr Allergy Asthma Rep.* 2001;1:134-143.
23. Joos GF, Germonpre PR, Pauwels RA. Neural mechanisms in asthma. *Clin Exp Allergy.* 2000;30(suppl 1):60-65.
24. Binaei S, Christensen M, Murphy C, et al. Beta2-adrenergic receptor polymorphisms in children with status asthmaticus. *Chest.* 2003;123(3 suppl):375S.
25. Elbahlawan L, Binaei S, Christensen ML, et al. Beta2-adrenergic receptor polymorphisms in African American children with status asthmaticus. *Pediatr Crit Care Med.* 2006;7:15-18.
26. Stalcup SA, Mellins RB. Mechanical forces producing pulmonary edema in acute asthma. *N Engl J Med.* 1977;297:592-596.

27. Blaustein AS, Risser TA, Weiss JW, et al. Mechanisms of pulsus paradoxus during resistive respiratory loading and asthma. *J Am Coll Cardiol.* 1986;8:529-536.
28. National Heart, Lung, and Blood Institute. *Expert Panel Report: Guidelines for the Diagnosis and Management of Asthma. Update on Selected Topics 2002.* Publication 02-5074. Bethesda, MD: National Institutes of Health; 2003.
29. Baker JW, Yerger S, Segar WE. Elevated plasma antidiuretic hormone levels in status asthmaticus. *Mayo Clin Proc.* 1976;51:31-34.
30. Carroll CL, Schramm CM. Noninvasive positive pressure ventilation for the treatment of status asthmaticus in children. *Ann Allergy Asthma Immunol.* 2006;96:454-459.
31. Meduri GU, Cook TR, Turner RE, et al. Noninvasive positive pressure ventilation in status asthmaticus. *Chest.* 1996;110:767-774.
32. Road J, Mackie G, Jiang TX, et al. Reversible paralysis with status asthmaticus, steroids, and pancuronium: clinical electrophysiological correlates. *Muscle Nerve.* 1997; 20:1587-1590.
33. Leatherman JW, Fluegel WL, David WS, et al. Muscle weakness in mechanically ventilated patients with severe asthma. *Am J Respir Crit Care Med.* 1996;153:1686-1690.
34. Denmark TK, Crane HA, Brown L. Ketamine to avoid mechanical ventilation in severe pediatric asthma. *J Emerg Med.* 2006;30:163-166.
35. Nehama J, Pass R, Bechtler-Karsch A, et al. Continuous ketamine infusion for the treatment of refractory asthma in a mechanically ventilated infant: case report and review of the pediatric literature. *Pediatr Emerg Care.* 1996;12:294-297.
36. Youssef-Ahmed MZ, Silver P, Nimkoff L, et al. Continuous infusion of ketamine in mechanically ventilated children with refractory bronchospasm. *Intensive Care Med.* 1996;22:972-976.
37. Rock MJ, Reyes de la Rocha S, L'Hommedieu CS, et al. Use of ketamine in asthmatic children to treat respiratory failure refractory to conventional therapy. *Crit Care Med.* 1986;14:514-516.
38. Amirav I, Newhouse MT. Metered-dose inhaler accessory devices in acute asthma: efficacy and comparison with nebulizers: a literature review. *Arch Pediatr Adolesc Med.* 1997;151:876-882.
39. Cates CJ, Crilly JA, Rowe BH. Holding chambers (spacers) versus nebulisers for beta-agonist treatment of acute asthma. *Cochrane Database Syst Rev.* 2006; CD000052.
40. Kerem E, Levison H, Schuh S, et al. Efficacy of albuterol administered by nebulizer versus spacer device in children with acute asthma. *J Pediatr.* 1993;123:313-317.
41. Papo MC, Frank J, Thompson AE. A prospective, randomized study of continuous versus intermittent nebulized albuterol for severe status asthmaticus in children. *Crit Care Med.* 1993;21:1479-1486.
42. [No author listed]. Levalbuterol for asthma. *Med Lett Drugs Ther.* 1999;41(1054):51-53.
43. Hardasmalani MD, DeBari V, Bithoney WG, et al. Levalbuterol versus racemic albuterol in the treatment of acute exacerbation of asthma in children. *Pediatr Emerg Care.* 2005;21:415-419.
44. Qureshi F, Zaritsky A, Welch C, et al. Clinical efficacy of racemic albuterol versus levalbuterol for the treatment of acute pediatric asthma. *Ann Emerg Med.* 2005;46:29-36.
45. Milgrom H, Skoner DP, Bensch G, et al. Low-dose levalbuterol in children with asthma: safety and efficacy in comparison with placebo and racemic albuterol. *J Allergy Clin Immunol.* 2001;108:938-945.
46. Carl JC, Myers TR, Kirchner HL, et al. Comparison of racemic albuterol and levalbuterol for treatment of acute asthma. *J Pediatr.* 2003;143:731-736.
47. Gawchik SM, Saccar CL, Noonan M, et al. The safety and efficacy of nebulized levalbuterol compared with racemic albuterol and placebo in the treatment of asthma in pediatric patients. *J Allergy Clin Immunol.* 1999;103:615-621.
48. Asmus MJ, Hendeles L. Levalbuterol nebulizer solution: is it worth five times the cost of albuterol? *Pharmacotherapy.* 2000;20:123-129.
49. Carroll CL, Schramm CM. Protocol-based titration of intravenous terbutaline decreases length of stay in pediatric status asthmaticus. *Pediatr Pulmonol.* 2006;41:350-356.
50. Stephanopoulos DE, Monge R, Schell KH, et al. Continuous intravenous terbutaline for pediatric status asthmaticus. *Crit Care Med.* 1998;26:1744-1748.
51. Wheeler DS, Jacobs BR, Kenreigh CA, et al. Theophylline versus terbutaline in treating critically ill children with status asthmaticus: a prospective, randomized, controlled trial. *Pediatr Crit Care Med.* 2005;6:142-147.
52. Gross NJ. Ipratropium bromide. *N Engl J Med.* 1988;319:486-494.
53. Qureshi F, Pestian J, Davis P, et al. Effect of nebulized ipratropium on the hospitalization rates of children with asthma. *N Engl J Med.* 1998;339:1030-1035.
54. Lanes SF, Garrett JE, Wentworth CE, et al. The effect of adding ipratropium bromide to salbutamol in the treatment of acute asthma: a pooled analysis of three trials. *Chest.* 1998;114:365-372.
55. Bond DW, Vyas H, Venning HE. Mydriasis due to self-administered inhaled ipratropium bromide. *Eur J Pediatr.* 2002;161:178.
56. Openshaw H. Unilateral mydriasis from ipratropium in transplant patients. *Neurology.* 2006;67:914.
57. Ryan CA. Ipratropium bromide induced unilateral mydriasis. *Ir Med J.* 1997;90:76.
58. Cheuk DK, Chau TC, Lee SL. A meta-analysis on intravenous magnesium sulphate for treating acute asthma. *Arch Dis Child.* 2005;90:74-77.
59. Rowe BH, Bretzlaff JA, Bourdon C, et al. Magnesium sulfate for treating exacerbations of acute asthma in the emergency department. *Cochrane Database Syst Rev.* 2000;CD001490.
60. Blitz M, Blitz S, Beasely R, et al. Inhaled magnesium sulfate in the treatment of acute asthma. *Cochrane Database Syst Rev.* 2005;CD003898.
61. Scarfone RJ, Loiselle JM, Joffe MD, et al. A randomized trial of magnesium in the emergency department treatment of children with asthma. *Ann Emerg Med.* 2000; 36:572-578.
62. Warner JO, Naspitz CK. Third International Pediatric Consensus statement on the management of childhood asthma. International Pediatric Asthma Consensus Group. *Pediatr Pulmonol.* 1998;25:1-17.
63. Edmonds ML, Camargo CA Jr, Pollack CV Jr, et al. Early use of inhaled corticosteroids in the emergency department treatment of acute asthma. *Cochrane Database Syst Rev.* 2003;CD002308.
64. Dowell SF, Bresee JS. Severe varicella associated with steroid use. *Pediatrics.* 1993;92:223-228.
65. Silk HJ, Guay-Woodford L, Perez-Atayde AR, et al. Fatal varicella in steroid-dependent asthma. *J Allergy Clin Immunol.* 1988;81:47-51.
66. Kasper WJ, Howe PM. Fatal varicella after a single course of corticosteroids. *Pediatr Infect Dis J.* 1990;9: 729-732.
67. Miech RP, Niedzwicki JG, Smith TR. Effect of theophylline on the binding of cAMP to soluble protein from tracheal smooth muscle. *Biochem Pharmacol.* 1979;28: 3687-3688.
68. Nicholson CD, Shahid M. Inhibitors of cyclic nucleotide phosphodiesterase isoenzymes—their potential utility in the therapy of asthma. *Pulm Pharmacol.* 1994;7:1-17.

69. Aubier M, De Troyer A, Sampson M, et al. Aminophylline improves diaphragmatic contractility. *N Engl J Med.* 1981;305:249-252.
70. Mayock DE, Standaert TA, Watchko JF, et al. Effect of aminophylline on diaphragmatic contractility in the piglet. *Pediatr Res.* 1990;28:196-198.
71. Mitra A, Bassler D, Goodman K, et al. Intravenous aminophylline for acute severe asthma in children over two years receiving inhaled bronchodilators. *Cochrane Database Syst Rev.* 2005;CD001276.
72. Rodrigo GJ, Rodrigo C, Pollack CV, et al. Use of helium-oxygen mixtures in the treatment of acute asthma: a systematic review. *Chest.* 2003;123:891-896.
73. Beckmann KR, Brueggemann WM Jr. Heliox treatment of severe croup. *Am J Emerg Med.* 2000;18:735-736.
74. Connolly KM, McGuirt WF Jr. Avoiding intubation in the injured subglottis: the role of heliox therapy. *Ann Otol Rhinol Laryngol.* 2001;110:713-717.
75. Kemper KJ, Izenberg S, Marvin JA, et al. Treatment of postextubation stridor in a pediatric patient with burns: the role of heliox. *J Burn Care Rehabil.* 1990;11:337-339.
76. Myers TR. Use of heliox in children. *Respir Care.* 2006;51:619-631.
77. Terregino CA, Nairn SJ, Chansky ME, et al. The effect of heliox on croup: a pilot study. *Acad Emerg Med.* 1998;5:1130-1133.
78. Weber JE, Chudnofsky CR, Younger JG, et al. A randomized comparison of helium-oxygen mixture (heliox) and racemic epinephrine for the treatment of moderate to severe croup. *Pediatrics.* 2001;107:E96.
79. Kudukis TM, Manthous CA, Schmidt GA, et al. Inhaled helium-oxygen revisited: effect of inhaled helium-oxygen during the treatment of status asthmaticus in children. *J Pediatr.* 1997;130:217-224.
80. Kim IK, Phrampus E, Venkataraman S, et al. Helium/oxygen-driven albuterol nebulization in the treatment of children with moderate to severe asthma exacerbations: a randomized, controlled trial. *Pediatrics.* 2005;116:1127-1133.
81. Rivera ML, Kim TY, Stewart GM, et al. Albuterol nebulized in heliox in the initial ED treatment of pediatric asthma: a blinded, randomized controlled trial. *Am J Emerg Med.* 2006;24:38-42.
82. Brown RH, Mitzner W, Zerhouni E, et al. Direct in vivo visualization of bronchodilation induced by inhalational anesthesia using high-resolution computed tomography. *Anesthesiology.* 1993;78:295-300.
83. Habre W, Matsumoto I, Sly PD. Propofol or halothane anaesthesia for children with asthma: effects on respiratory mechanics. *Br J Anaesth.* 1996;77:739-743.
84. Jeudy C, Granry JC, Chassevent JL, et al. [Use of halothane in the treatment of severe asthmatic crisis in children. A propos of 2 cases]. *Cah Anesthesiol.* 1985;33:421-422.
85. Restrepo RD, Pettignano R, DeMeuse P. Halothane, an effective infrequently used drug, in the treatment of pediatric status asthmaticus: a case report. *J Asthma.* 2005;42:649-651.
86. O'Rourke PP, Crone RK. Halothane in status asthmaticus. *Crit Care Med.* 1982;10:341-343.
87. Johnston RG, Noseworthy TW, Friesen EG, et al. Isoflurane therapy for status asthmaticus in children and adults. *Chest.* 1990;97:698-701.
88. Otte RW, Fireman P. Isoflurane anesthesia for the treatment of refractory status asthmaticus. *Ann Allergy.* 1991;66:305-309.
89. Rice M, Hatherill M, Murdoch IA. Rapid response to isoflurane in refractory status asthmaticus. *Arch Dis Child.* 1998;78:395-396.
90. Shankar V, Churchwell KB, Deshpande JK. Isoflurane therapy for severe refractory status asthmaticus in children. *Intensive Care Med.* 2006;32:927-933.
91. Wheeler DS, Clapp CR, Ponaman ML, et al. Isoflurane therapy for status asthmaticus in children: a case series and protocol. *Pediatr Crit Care Med.* 2000;1:55-59.
92. Cooper DJ, Tuxen DV, Fisher MM. Extracorporeal life support for status asthmaticus. *Chest.* 1994;106:978-979.
93. Kukita I, Okamoto K, Sato T, et al. Emergency extracorporeal life support for patients with near-fatal status asthmaticus. *Am J Emerg Med.* 1997;15:566-569.
94. Leiba A, Bar-Yosef S, Bar-Dayan Y, et al. Early administration of extracorporeal life support for near fatal asthma. *Isr Med Assoc J.* 2003;5:600-602.
95. Sakai M, Ohteki H, Doi K, et al. Clinical use of extracorporeal lung assist for a patient in status asthmaticus. *Ann Thorac Surg.* 1996;62:885-887.
96. Tobias JD, Garrett JS. Therapeutic options for severe, refractory status asthmaticus: inhalational anesthetic agents, extracorporeal membrane oxygenation and helium/oxygen ventilation. *Paediatr Anaesth.* 1997;7:47-57.

Chapter 360

STATUS EPILEPTICUS

Sarah M. Roddy, MD; Margaret C. McBride, MD

Status epilepticus is defined by the World Health Organization as "a condition characterized by an epileptic seizure that is sufficiently prolonged or repeated at sufficiently brief intervals as to produce an unvarying and enduring epileptic condition."[1] Much variability exists in the interpretation of what constitutes an "unvarying and enduring epileptic condition." The most widely accepted criterion for diagnosis of status epilepticus is any seizure that continues for 30 minutes or intermittent seizures lasting for 30 minutes or longer in which the person does not regain consciousness between the episodes.

Status epilepticus can be classified in terms of the type of seizure. *Generalized convulsive status epilepticus* is the most common and easily recognized type in children. The seizure activity usually is tonic-clonic or clonic and is less often tonic or myoclonic. In *simple partial status epilepticus,* also known as *epilepsia partialis continua,* focal seizure activity is prolonged and restricted to 1 side of the body without loss of consciousness. *Nonconvulsive status epilepticus* exhibits as a confused, drowsy state in which the patient seems to move in slow motion. This condition results from continuing or repetitive absence seizures or partial complex seizures (see Chapter 320, Seizure Disorders).

INCIDENCE

The incidence of status epilepticus in patients who have epilepsy ranges from 4% to 16%.[2] Its frequency is highest in the younger age groups.[3,4] Infants and children also are far more likely than adults to have status epilepticus as the manifestation of their 1st seizure.[4] Up to 70% of children with epilepsy beginning before the age of 1 year experience status epilepticus.[3]

BOX 360-1 Treatment of Status Epilepticus

- Assess cardiopulmonary function by making sure the airway is clear, the patient is breathing, and circulation is adequate. Provide oxygen or respiratory support and cardiac stimulation (cardiopulmonary resuscitation) as necessary.
- Establish an intravenous line, and obtain blood samples for electrolytes, blood urea nitrogen, calcium, complete blood count, and anticonvulsant medication levels. A blood Dextrostix test should be performed immediately; and, if the glucose is under 60 mg/dL, then 1 to 2 mL/kg of D25W should be administered.
- One member of the emergency team should obtain a history while another does a brief physical examination.
- Administer anticonvulsant drugs in the following order until seizure activity is controlled:
  - Lorazepam should be the initial anticonvulsant administered intravenously at a dose of 0.1 mg/kg (maximum 4 mg) over 2 minutes; a dose of 0.05 to 0.1 mg/kg may be repeated every 5 minutes if necessary up to a maximum of 0.5 mg/kg, but not over 10 mg in total. Lorazepam has a 6- to 8-hour duration of effect. Therefore, unlike diazepam, another anticonvulsant need not be administered right away if the status epilepticus has stopped.
  - If lorazepam is not available, then diazepam should be administered intravenously at a dose of 0.1 to 0.2 mg/kg (maximum 10 mg) by pushing one half the dose over 1 minute and the remainder at 1 mg/min. A dose of 0.1 mg/kg may be repeated in 5 minutes if necessary. Because of diazepam's short duration of anticonvulsant effect, another anticonvulsant such as phenytoin must be administered immediately, even if the status epilepticus has stopped.
  - If the patient is known to be receiving phenytoin on a chronic basis, then it should be administered as the initial anticonvulsant.
  - If status epilepticus continues, then administer phenytoin or fosphenytoin, which is a water-soluble prodrug of phenytoin with a more neutral pH value. The dose for both drugs is 15 to 20 mg/kg up to a total dose of 1000 mg. Phenytoin must be administered intravenously, but fosphenytoin can be administered intramuscularly if intravenous access is not available. A quarter of the dose may be administered during the first 2 minutes, then at a rate of 1 to 2 mg/kg/min (maximal rate of 50 mg/min) for phenytoin and 3 mg/kg/min (maximal rate of 150 mg/min) for fosphenytoin. If the patient is known to be receiving phenytoin chronically, then 5 to 8 mg/kg of phenytoin may be administered as the initial anticonvulsant. Monitor the heart rate, and slow the rate of phenytoin infusion if bradycardia occurs. If seizure activity continues despite a full loading dose of phenytoin, then correction of underlying acidosis with sodium bicarbonate (0.25 to 0.5 mEq/kg) is indicated.
  - If status epilepticus continues, then phenobarbital is usually the next drug given in a dose of 15 to 20 mg/kg intravenously up to a total of 800 mg. Administer this amount over 15 minutes, monitoring respirations and blood pressure, especially if the patient has been treated with a benzodiazepine. An alternative or additional medication for status epilepticus is intravenous valproate, which has the advantage of not depressing respirations but is less well understood than phenobarbital. It is administered as 25 mg/kg over 8 to 10 minutes.[6] Valproate is not a good choice in a patient with liver dysfunction.
- If seizure activity still persists, then consult a neurologist to determine the need for other anticonvulsants, general anesthesia, or induction of pentobarbital, diazepam, midazolam, or propofol coma. If a child cannot be aroused for hours after the end of status epilepticus, then electroencephalogram monitoring to look for subclinical status should be considered.[7]

ETIOLOGY

In approximately 25% of cases, status epilepticus is idiopathic. In another 20% to 25%, it is provoked solely by fever.[5] Acute symptomatic status epilepticus accounts for another 25% of cases and is an expression of an acute encephalopathy or brain injury. Causes in this group include meningitis, electrolyte disturbance, drug ingestion, and poor compliance with antiepileptic medication. Remote symptomatic status epilepticus occurs in patients with a history of central nervous system insult known to be associated with increased risk of seizure. This group accounts for another 20% of the cases of status epilepticus in children; most of the affected patients have cerebral palsy or intellectual disability. The cause of status epilepticus in a small percentage of cases is a progressive encephalopathy. This category includes neurodegenerative diseases and neurocutaneous syndromes (phakomatoses).

History

A history should be obtained from an accompanying family member and should include any history of previous seizures, chronic and recent medication use, intercurrent illness, head trauma, and details of the onset of status epilepticus.

Physical Examination

At physical examination, fever, any evidence of head trauma, increased intracranial pressure, or infection should be noted. A urine toxicologic screen is helpful in determining whether drug ingestion precipitated the seizures.

Laboratory Evaluation

Blood samples should be drawn to assess levels of electrolytes, blood urea nitrogen, calcium, complete blood count, and anticonvulsant medication. A blood

Dextrostix test should be performed immediately, and if the glucose is under 60 mg/dL, then 1 to 2 mL/kg of 25% dextrose in water (D25W) should be administered.

Imaging Studies

Computed tomographic scanning may be required to rule out an intracranial lesion if the cause of status epilepticus remains unclear.

TREATMENT

The objectives of treating convulsive status epilepticus are to maintain vital functions, identify and correct any precipitating factors, and control seizure activity. Box 360-1 outlines a plan for treatment. Most episodes of status epilepticus are controlled by 1 or more of the drugs named in Box 360-1.

Nonconvulsive status epilepticus and epilepsia partialis continua require prompt treatment, but less urgency exists because these seizures do not alter the body's homeostatic mechanisms to the degree that convulsive status epilepticus does. Convulsive status epilepticus is considered a medical emergency because it is life threatening and is sometimes followed by severe neurologic sequelae. The longer convulsive status epilepticus continues, the more resistant it is to therapy and the greater the incidence is of mortality and morbidity. Studies have shown that continued seizure activity for more than 60 minutes results in permanent cell damage, even in ventilated animals whose metabolic parameters are kept in the normal range. Neurologic sequelae from status epilepticus include intellectual impairment and motor dysfunction.

If the history or physical examination suggest a central nervous system infection, then antibiotics should be administered immediately and a lumbar puncture performed as soon as seizure activity has been controlled. Because neurologic sequelae of status epilepticus can result from precipitating factors such as hypoxia, hypotension, and acidosis, immediate attention should be given to the respiratory and cardiovascular status of the child. If the patient is febrile, then the clinician's priority is reducing body temperature because of the synergy between fever and status epilepticus in producing brain damage.[8-10]

Over the last 25 years, morbidity and mortality from status epilepticus have declined, probably because of better access to medical care, more aggressive treatment, and the availability of benzodiazepines. In children with idiopathic or febrile status epilepticus, less than 5% develop new neurologic dysfunction.[11] Mortality in children attributable to status epilepticus currently does not exceed 6%,[12] with most deaths caused by the illness that precipitated the seizure.[11]

Once seizure activity is controlled, management should be directed toward preventing recurrence of seizures, including maintenance anticonvulsant therapy. The appropriate duration of therapy after an initial episode of idiopathic status epilepticus is not clear. Recurrence of seizures in this situation may be as low as 25%,[12] and recurrence of status epilepticus only 4%.[13] For a child prone to generalized convulsive status epilepticus, consideration should be given to prescribing rectal diazepam gel to be administered by caregivers for seizures lasting longer than 5 minutes.

WHEN TO REFER

- When seizure activity cannot be controlled
- After seizure activity is controlled, if a history of previous afebrile seizures is present and a physician with experience in prescribing maintenance anticonvulsant medication is not available

WHEN TO ADMIT

- Always for a child with status epilepticus
- Virtually always for a child who is unresponsive after status epilepticus

REFERENCES

1. Gastaut H, ed. *Dictionary of Epilepsy, I. Definitions.* Geneva, Switzerland: World Health Organization; 1973.
2. Hauser WA. Status epilepticus: epidemiologic considerations. *Neurology.* 1990;40(2):9-13.
3. Hesdorffer DC, Logroscino G, Cascino G, et al. Incidence of status epilepticus in Rochester, Minnesota, 1965-1984. *Neurology.* 1998;50:735-741.
4. Shinnar S, Pellock JM, Moshe SL, et al. In whom does status epilepticus occur: age-related differences in children. *Epilepsia.* 1997;38:907-914.
5. Shinnar S, Berg AT, Moshe SL, et al. The risk of seizure recurrence after a first unprovoked afebrile seizure in childhood: an extended follow-up. *Pediatrics.* 1996;98:216-225.
6. Yu KT, Mills S, Thompson N, et al. Safety and efficacy of intravenous valproate in pediatric status epilepticus and acute repetitive seizures. *Epilepsia.* 2003;44:724-726.
7. Scheuer ML. Continuous EEG monitoring in the intensive care unit. *Epilepsia.* 2002;43:114-127.
8. Lundgren J, Smith ML, Blennow G, et al. Hyperthermia aggravates and hypothermia ameliorates epileptic brain damage. *Exp Brain Res.* 1994;99:43-55.
9. van Esch A, Ramlal IR, van Steensel-Moll HA, et al. Outcome after febrile status epilepticus. *Dev Med Child Neurol.* 1996;38:19-24.
10. Shinnar S, Pellock JM, Berg AT, et al. Short-term outcomes of children with status epilepticus. *Epilepsia.* 2001;42:47-53.
11. Gross-Tsur V, Shinnar S. Convulsive status epilepticus in children. *Epilepsia.* 1993;34(1):S12-S20.
12. Maytal J, Shinnar S, Moshe SL, et al. Low morbidity and mortality of status epilepticus in children. *Pediatrics.* 1989;83:323-331.
13. Shinnar S, Maytal J, Krasnoff L, et al. Recurrent status epilepticus in children. *Ann Neurol.* 1992;31:598-604.

Chapter 361
THERMAL INJURIES

Robert L. Sheridan, MD

Burns are common injuries. Most practitioners caring for children will be required to deal with thermal injuries periodically. Public expectations for the quality of burn care and outcomes are high. In recent years, survival has improved significantly for children with serious burns.[1,2] Even if their burns are severe, the quality of their long-term outcomes is generally good if children participate in a burn aftercare program.[3] Coincident with increasing survival and improving outcome quality has been the evolution of the burn center paradigm, in which all aspects of necessary care are coordinated in one program.[4]

EPIDEMIOLOGIC FEATURES

Approximately 70% of pediatric burns are caused by hot liquid. In older children and young working adults, flame injuries are more common than other kinds.[5] Approximately 20% of burns in young children involve abuse or neglect.[6] Organized burn-prevention efforts have met with mixed success when based on public education, but legislation has been more effective than these efforts. Examples include factory settings of hot water heaters, fire-safe cigarettes, and flammability standards for children's bedclothes.

CLINICAL PRESENTATION AND EVALUATION

Despite a broad spectrum of burn injury severity, from a practical perspective, the number of burn-injured children can be divided into 2 categories: (1) those reasonably managed in the outpatient setting and (2) those requiring inpatient or burn center care. This decision is based on an evaluation of the child and of the wound.

Evaluating the Burn Patient

An evaluation of the child should precede an evaluation of the wound, especially if the burn is large or physiologically threatening. Patient evaluation is organized into a primary and a secondary survey, following the guidelines of the American College of Surgeons Committee on Trauma and the Advanced Burn Life Support Course of the American Burn Association.

As in trauma, the primary survey begins with an assessment and control, if necessary, of the airway. Deep burns of the face and neck can result in progressive airway edema. Occasionally, a child will aspirate hot liquids, resulting in very severe upper airway edema and mandating urgent intubation.

A burn-specific secondary survey evaluates issues uniquely associated with burn injury (Box 361-1). This process may take just a few seconds in a child with a small burn, but it can be much more time consuming if the injury is large. In children with small injuries, essentials include a detailed determination of the mechanism of injury, a screen for associated trauma, consideration of the possibility of abuse, and a detailed assessment of the burn wound. Delayed presentation for care, confusing and conflicting stories, sharply demarcated margins, immersion patterns, and contact injuries are physical findings worrisome for abuse or neglect. All such children should be admitted for evaluation (Figure 361-1).[7]

Evaluating the Burn Wound

After the patient has been evaluated, the burn wound should be examined for size, extent, depth, and circumferential components.[8] Decisions regarding outpatient care, hospitalization, or transfer will generally be made based on this information.

Burn extent is best estimated using a chart based on the Lund-Browder diagram that compensates for the changes in body proportions with age (Figure 361-2). An alternative is a modified *rule of nines,* in which the head and neck area is given 18% (instead of the adult 9%), each lower extremity is given 15% (instead of the adult 18%), each upper extremity is given 10% (instead of the adult 9%), and the anterior and posterior torso are each given 16% (instead of the adult 18%). For scattered or irregular burns, the entire palmar surface of the patient's hand represents approximately 1% of the body surface over all ages.

Burn depth is classified as 1st, 2nd, 3rd, or 4th degree. First-degree burns are red, dry, and painful and are often deeper than they appear, sloughing the next day. Second-degree burns are red, wet, and very painful (Figure 361-3, *A*). Enormous variability exists in their depth, ability to heal, and propensity to hypertrophic scar formation. Third-degree burns are leathery, dry, insensate, and waxy (Figure 361-3, *B*). Fourth-degree burns involve underlying subcutaneous tissue, tendon, or bone (Figure 361-3, *C*).

Near or completely circumferential burns should be identified for special monitoring and possible escharotomy. If across the torso, such wounds will interfere with ventilation. When they involve an extremity, limb-threatening ischemia may occur during resuscitation. This complication usually becomes an issue 12 to 24 hours after injury. These procedures can be performed with coagulating electrocautery. They can be frightening and painful, and anesthesia or sedation is generally required in children. The physician should avoid damaging uninjured skin or superficial neurovascular structures.

Selection for Outpatient Versus Inpatient Care

The majority of burns can be successfully managed in the outpatient setting.[9] However, poorly provided outpatient burn care can be frustrating and painful for patients and providers. The key is careful patient selection and a detailed care plan. Several issues should be considered when making this decision (Box 361-2).

MANAGEMENT

Outpatient Burns

Many correct answers exist to the question, "How should outpatient burn wounds be treated?" However, certain characteristics are universal. The wound should be kept clean and inspected regularly for infection. Accumulated exudate and topical medications should be periodically cleansed. The small superficial burns managed in this setting present a low risk of infection; therefore clean rather than sterile technique is reasonable. If topical agents rather than membrane dressings are used, then wounds may be cleansed with lukewarm tap water and a bland soap. Soaking adherent dressings before removal will decrease the pain associated with daily wound care. The wound is gently cleansed with a gauze or clean washcloth, inspected

BOX 361-1 Burn-Specific Secondary Survey

HISTORY

Mechanism of injury

Closed space exposure and extrication time

Delay in seeking attention

Fluid and pain medication given during transport

Prior illnesses and allergies

Prior child protective services involvement

HEAD, EARS, EYES, NOSE, AND THROAT

Early examination of the globes for corneal burns

Clinical assessment for intraocular hypertension if deep facial burns

Perioral and intraoral burns and carbonaceous material

Check for intraocular hypertension if extreme periorbital swelling or very deep periorbital burns are noted. Patient may need lateral canthotomy orbital decompression.

Progressive hoarseness

Consider hot liquid aspiration.

Continuously assess endotracheal tube security.

NECK

Radiographic evaluation if indicated by injury mechanism

Rare need for neck escharotomies

CARDIAC SYSTEM

Cardiac monitoring after significant electrical injury

PULMONARY SYSTEM

Chest escharotomies indicated if near circumferential torso burn and difficulty with ventilation

Inhalation injury associated with airway obstruction and bronchospasm initially

VASCULAR SYSTEM

Perfusion of burned extremities should be closely monitored.

Escharotomy indicated for decreasing perfusion.

Fasciotomy indicated after electrical or deep thermal injury when flow compromised.

Compartment pressures can followed in equivocal extremities.

Worrisome extremities should be decompressed based on serial examination.

ABDOMEN

Nasogastric tubes are often indicated, especially before air transport.

Inappropriate volume requirement may be a sign of an occult intra-abdominal injury.

Torso escharotomies may be required to facilitate ventilation.

Ulcer prophylaxis indicated in all with serious burns.

Consider abdominal compartment syndrome in very large burns or delayed resuscitation.

GENITOURINARY SYSTEM

Catheterization is appropriate in those who require a fluid resuscitation.

Ensure that the foreskin is reduced over the bladder catheter.

NEUROLOGIC SYSTEM

Level of consciousness often reduced during the hours after injury.

Computed tomographic scanning useful to exclude head injury if mechanism appropriate.

EXTREMITIES

Monitor perfusion if near circumferential burns or electrical injury is present.

Limbs at risk should be dressed so they can be easily reexamined.

WOUNDS

Evaluate wounds for size, depth, and circumferential components.

Wounds are often underestimated in depth and size initially.

ELECTRICAL FACTORS

Monitor cardiac rhythm for high (>1000) or intermediate (>220) volt exposures.

Neurologic and ocular examination is important.

Extremities should be serially evaluated for intracompartmental edema.

Bladder catheters useful in high-voltage exposures to document clearing of pigment.

CHEMICAL FACTORS

Irrigate wounds with tap water for at least 30 minutes.

Irrigate eyes with isotonic crystalloid solution.

Blepharospasm may require ocular anesthetic.

Hydrofluoric acid may be complicated by life-threatening hypocalcemia.

TAR

Cool with tap water irrigation and remove later with a lipophilic solvent.

LABORATORY AND RADIOGRAPHY DATA

Evaluate blood gas when inhalation injury present.

Normal carboxyhemoglobin does not eliminate significant exposure.

Baseline hemoglobin and electrolytes can be helpful later.

Perform a urinalysis for occult blood in patients with deep thermal or electrical injuries.

Perform radiographic evaluation as needed for mechanism of injury.

for any sign of infection, patted dry with a clean towel, and redressed. Teaching the patient and family to return promptly if they notice erythema, swelling, increased tenderness, lymphangitis, odor, or drainage is important so that infectious complications can be addressed early. The frequency of wound cleansing and dressing change is debated, but most small burns are adequately managed with a daily cleansing and dressing change. In some cases, a membrane dressing, designed not to be changed daily, is applied once early surgery is clearly not needed and early infection has not occurred. Pain and anxiety can be an issue for many children. Some of these children will benefit from an oral narcotic given 30 to 60 minutes before a planned dressing change. Especially if dressings are occlusive, pain in between dressing changes tends to be modest for most children.

Increasing pain and anxiety associated with dressing changes, inability to keep scheduled follow-up appointments, delayed healing, signs of infection, or a wound that appears deeper than appreciated at the time of the initial examination should prompt early return and specialty evaluation. Wounds selected for outpatient management are usually fairly superficial and heal within 2 weeks. Patients with mid and deep dermal injuries may have a deeper component, with resulting scarring that may benefit from specialty evaluation. Finally, wounds of the face, ears, hands, genitals, and feet have a functional and cosmetic importance out of proportion to their wound size. In some cases, early specialty evaluation may be prudent because initial care can have an impact on long-term outcome.

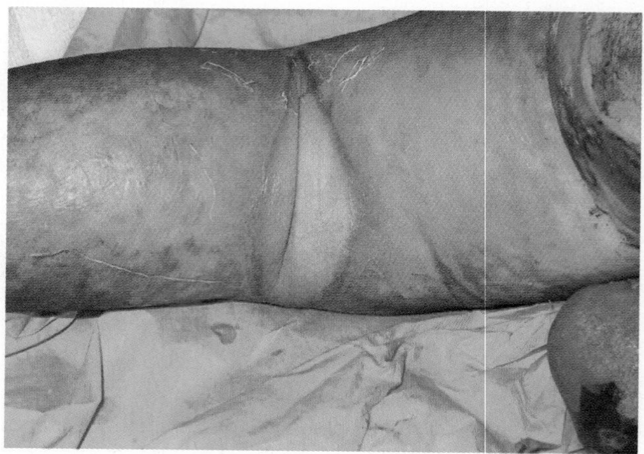

Figure 361-1 Some burn patterns are worrisome for abuse or neglect. This photograph illustrates popliteal flexor sparing, which may indicate abuse or neglect.

Wound Medications and Membranes

The proliferation of wound medications and membranes is increasingly confusing.[10] Thankfully, most superficial wounds heal well under any of these products. Wound medications and membranes provide 3 benefits: (1) pain control, (2) prevention of wound desiccation, and (3) reduction of wound colonization.

A wide variety of topical wound medications are available, ranging from aqueous solutions to antibiotic containing ointments and debriding enzymes. Most topical agents in outpatient use have a viscous carrier that prevents wound desiccation and a more or less broad antibacterial spectrum that reduces wound colonization. A gauze wrap minimizes soiling of clothing and protects the wound from trauma. Silver sulfadiazine is commonly used because it is painless on application and has a broad spectrum of antibacterial activity. Superficial burns are commonly treated with a clear, viscous, antibacterial ointment containing low concentrations of various antibiotics. Wounds around the eyes can be treated with topical ophthalmic antibiotic

Burn Estimate: Age Versus Area

	Birth-1 yr	1-4 yr	5-9 yr	10-14 yr	15 yr	2°	3°	Total
Head	19	17	13	11	9			
Neck	2	2	2	2	2			
Anterior trunk	13	13	13	13	13			
Posterior trunk	13	13	13	13	13			
Right buttock	2½	2½	2½	2½	2½			
Left buttock	2½	2½	2½	2½	2½			
Genitalia	1	1	1	1	1			
Right upper arm	4	4	4	4	4			
Left upper arm	4	4	4	4	4			
Right lower arm	3	3	3	3	3			
Left lower arm	3	3	3	3	3			
Right hand	2½	2½	2½	2½	2½			
Left hand	2½	2½	2½	2½	2½			
Right thigh	5½	6½	8	8½	9			
Left thigh	5½	6½	8	8½	9			
Right Leg	5	5	5½	6	6½			
Left Leg	5	5	5½	6	6½			
Right foot	3½	3½	3½	3½	3½			
Left foot	3½	3½	3½	3½	3½			
					Total			

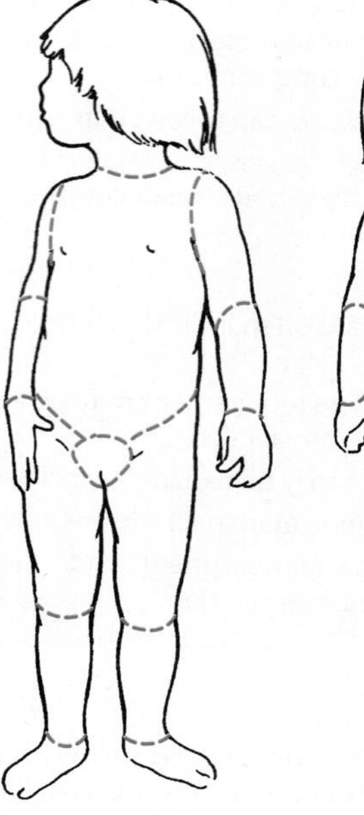

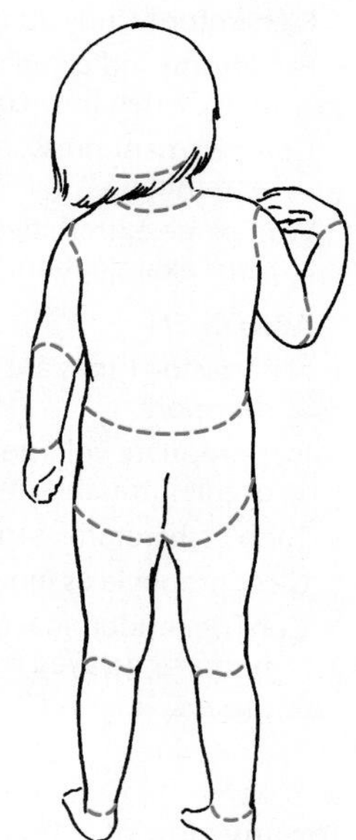

Figure 361-2 Burn chart for estimating the extent of injury. Numbers equal the percentage of total body surface.

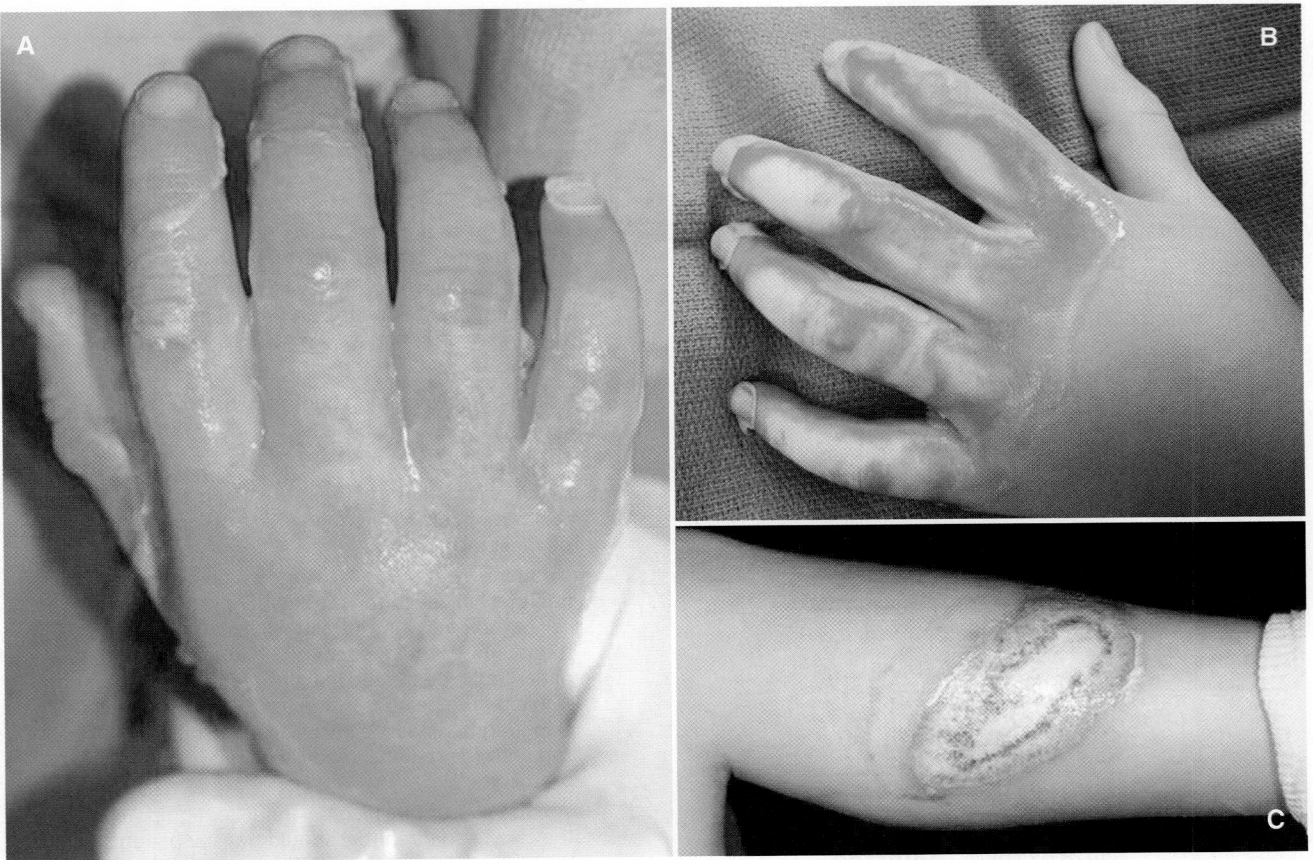

Figure 361-3 **A,** Second-degree burns are red, wet, and very painful. Enormous variability exists in their depth, ability to heal, and propensity to hypertrophic scar formation. **B,** Third-degree burns are leathery, dry, insensate, and waxy. This wound demonstrates peripheral 2nd-degree component with central 3rd-degree areas. **C,** Fourth-degree burns involve underlying subcutaneous tissue, tendon, or bone.

ointments. Significant ear burns should be treated with mafenide acetate because it is the only agent that will penetrate the relatively avascular cartilage.

Wound membranes provide transient physiological wound closure while the underlying wound heals (Box 361-3). Physiological closure implies a degree of protection from mechanical trauma, vapor transmission characteristics similar to skin, and a physical barrier to bacteria. The major benefit of wound membranes is that when successful, they minimize wound manipulations. These membranes help create a moist wound environment with a low bacterial density and are generally intended for use on selected clean superficial wounds and donor sites. Occlusive synthetic membranes must be used with caution if wounds are not completely clean and superficial because submembrane infection can occur, deepening underlying wounds and causing systemic infection and toxicity. When used, these products are often applied after a period of care with a topical medication that allows the wound to be inspected and a clear determination made that the wound is superficial and will likely heal.

Inpatient Burns

Inpatient burn care is resource intensive.[11] A system of burn center verification has evolved to ensure that children requiring such care receive coordinated efforts by experienced providers. An increasing body of data supports the efficacy of this approach.[12] Transfer to a burn center should be considered for patients meeting American Burn Association transfer criteria (Box 361-4). Care of severe burns can be divided into 4 phases: (1) initial evaluation and resuscitation, (2) initial excision and biological closure, (3) definitive wound closure, and (4) rehabilitation and reconstruction. Significant critical care needs often exist during the first 3 phases of care.

Priorities during the initial evaluation and resuscitation phase are to document the entire extent of the injury, including nonburn trauma, and to address the physiological changes that accompany burns. This phase occupies the first 24 to 72 hours after injury. These needs will vary with the mechanism of injury, extent of burn, and the child's social and medical history. If burns involve more than approximately 15% of the body surface, then a poorly understood syndrome

BOX 361-2 Requirements for Outpatient Burn Management

Clear airway—has no need for airway monitoring.

Wound size should be generally less than 10% (fluid resuscitation not needed).

Child must be able to take in adequate fluid by mouth.

No significant burns occur to the face, ears, hands, genitals, or feet.

Family must have the resources to support an outpatient care plan.

Adult caregiver should be able to stay at home with the child.

Adult who is able to perform wound cleansing, inspection, and dressing changes should be available.

Child must have transportation and access to clinic follow-up.

Family must have transportation for clinic and emergency visits.

No suspicion of abuse or neglect is noted.

No clearly full-thickness areas that will require surgery are found.

BOX 361-3 Partial Listing of Some Commonly Used Wound Membranes—Selected Characteristics

Porcine Xenograft[a]: adheres to coagulum, excellent pain control

Biobrane[b]: bilaminate, fibrovascular in growth into inner layer

Acticoat[c]: nonadherent dressing that delivers silver

Aquacel-Ag[d]: absorptive hydrofiber that delivers silver

Various semipermeable membranes: provide vapor and bacterial barrier

Various hydrocolloid dressings: provide vapor and bacterial barrier; absorb exudate

Various impregnated gauzes: provide barrier while allowing drainage

[a]Brennan Medical, St. Paul, MN.
[b]Dow-Hickham, Sugar Land, TX.
[c]Westhaim Biomedical, Saskatchewan, Can.
[d]Convatec, Princeton, NJ.

of reduced capillary integrity is seen, necessitating a fluid resuscitation. This complication typically abates after approximately 24 hours. Any one of several burn formulas may be used to initiate resuscitation, but all should be carefully titrated to individual patient needs. One commonly cited formula is listed in Box 361-5.

In the initial excision and biological closure phase, large full-thickness injuries are identified and excised, ideally within the first few days of injury, to avoid otherwise inevitable local and systemic sepsis, before systemic inflammation develops. Resulting wounds are

BOX 361-4 American Burn Association Burn Center Transfer Criteria

2nd- and 3rd-degree burns over more than 10% of total body surface area (TBSA) in patients younger than 10 years or older than 50 years

2nd- and 3rd-degree burns over more than 20% over TBSA in patients aged 10 to 50 years

2nd- and 3rd-degree burns that involve the face, hands, feet, genitalia, perineum, and major joints

3rd-degree burns over more than 5% of TBSA in any age group

Electrical burns, including lightning injury

Chemical burns

Inhalation injury

Burn injury in patients with preexisting medical disorders that might complicate management, prolong recovery, or affect mortality

Any patients with burns and concomitant trauma (eg, fractures) in which the burn injury poses the greatest risk of morbidity or mortality. (In such cases, if the trauma poses the greater immediate risk, then the patient may be treated initially in a trauma center until stable before being transferred to a burn center. Physician judgment will be necessary and should be in concert with the regional medical control plan and triage protocols.)

Hospitals without qualified personnel or equipment for the care of children that should transfer patients with burns to a burn center with these capabilities

Burn injury in patients who will require special social or emotional or long-term rehabilitative support, including cases involving suspected child abuse or substance abuse

closed with autograft or, in some circumstances, temporary wound membranes. This strategy changes the natural history of the injury from inevitable sepsis and inflammation to a more controlled wound-closure situation.

In the definitive wound-closure phase, which varies in duration with wound size and complexity, temporary wound membranes are replaced with autologous tissue, and small complex wounds, such as those on the hands and face, are addressed. In very large burns, this process may take many weeks. Intensive care is often a prominent part of the first 3 phases of care. Proper attention to pain and anxiety management is essential in all phases of care.[13]

The final phase of care, rehabilitation and reconstruction, is of the longest duration.[14] This phase begins as soon as the child is able to participate and lasts well past discharge, again depending on wound size and complexity. This process requires initially ranging and splinting and progresses through strength and endurance training. Long-term scar management and emotional support must be a part of this plan.[15,16] As children grow and scars contract, burn reconstruction procedures become important.[17] A long-term follow-up plan is an essential part of discharge.

BOX 361-5 Consensus Resuscitation Formula

FIRST 24 HOURS

Adults and Children Over 20 kg

Ringer's lactate: 2-4 mL/kg per percentage of total body surface area (TBSA) burned per 24 hours (first half in first 8 hours)

Colloid: in most circumstances, none

Children Less Than 20 kg

Ringers lactate: 2-3 mL/kg per percentage of TBSA burned per 24 hours (first half in first 8 hours)

Ringers lactate with 5% dextrose: maintenance rate (approximately 4 mL/kg/hr for the first 10 kg, 2 mL/kg/hr for the next 10 kg, and 1 mL/kg/hr for weight over 20 kg)

Colloid: in most circumstances, none; however, many clinicians initiate colloid infusions in children with large burns.

SECOND 24 HOURS—ALL PATIENTS

Crystalloid: to maintain urine output. If silver nitrate is used, then sodium leeching will mandate continued isotonic crystalloid. If other topical is used, then free-water requirement is significant. Serum sodium should be monitored closely. Nutritional support should begin, ideally by the enteral route.

Colloid (5% albumin in Ringer's lactate solution):

- 0-30% burn: none
- 30-50% burn: 0.3 mL/kg per percentage of TBSA burned per 24 hours
- 50-70% burn: 0.4 mL/kg per percentage of TBSA burned per 24 hours
- 70-100% burn: 0.5 mL/kg per percentage of TBSA burned per 24 hours
- Colloid, generally as 5% albumin solution, is increasingly used early in resuscitation of children with large burn injuries.

From Sheridan RL. Comprehensive management of burns. *Curr Probl Surg.* 2001;38 (9):641-756. Copyright © 2001, Elsevier, with permission.

Complications

In the outpatient setting, patient selection should ensure that major complications are few. The most common issues that arise are wound sepsis, excessive pain and anxiety, and underestimation of burn depth. The most common wound infection in this setting is streptococcal cellulitis, which initially produces surrounding erythema that progresses to lymphangitis and systemic toxicity (Figure 361-4). Children with cellulitis often need admission for antibiotics, observation, and, sometimes, surgery. In some situations, adequate pain and anxiety management is difficult in the outpatient setting, especially around dressing changes. This problem can be addressed with judicious medication and, in some instances, carefully monitored membrane dressings. Some children will require admission. For burn depth to be underestimated initially is common, with areas of full-thickness injury not appreciated for several days. These children may require admission for surgery.

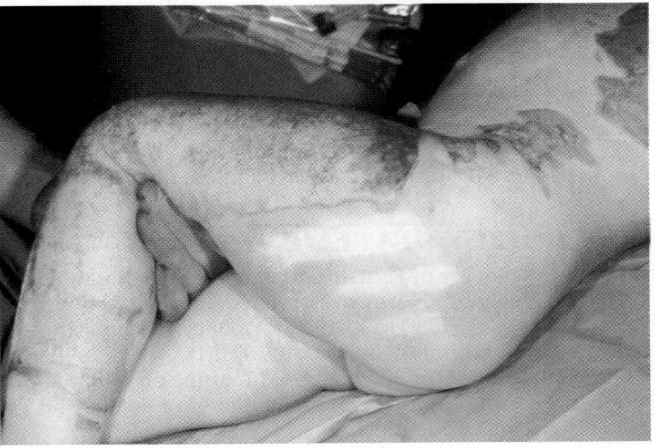

Figure 361-4 The most common infectious complication in the outpatient setting is streptococcal cellulitis, as demonstrated here. Note blanching by examiner's fingers, suggesting surrounding erythema.

As burn severity increases, the local injury is accompanied by an increasing degree of systemic derangement. An initial phase of reduced perfusion and metabolic rate, which lasts 24 to 48 hours, is followed by a phase of protein catabolism and a hyperdynamic circulation, lasting until well after wound closure. Management of this physiological process is an essential part of inpatient burn care. Children with large burns are susceptible to a host of other complications related to sepsis and organ failures. Careful monitoring and early intervention are essential to successful outcomes.[18]

LONG-TERM CARE

Burn wounds and grafts typically develop some degree of hypertrophy. This process involves a gradual increase in vascularity and collagen deposition in the months after healing.[19] Some wounds will demonstrate significant contracture formation, with important functional and aesthetic consequences. Many children will have bothersome pruritus. A long-term follow-up plan consisting of scar management strategies, rehabilitation, reconstructive surgery, and emotional support will facilitate optimal outcomes. This care is best provided in a multidisciplinary burn clinic, ideally part of a comprehensive burn program. With such supports in place, the long-term outcome for children is surprisingly good.[20] When managed in a comprehensive follow-up program, even patients who have suffered devastating burns may become happy and productive adults.

TOOLS FOR PRACTICE

Engaging Patients and Family

- *Fire Safety* (Web page), American Academy of Pediatrics (www.aap.org/healthopics/safety.cfm).
- *Keep Your Family Safe: Fire Safety and Burn Prevention at Home* (brochure), American Academy of Pediatrics (patiented.aap.org).

Medical Decision Support

- *TIPP The Injury Prevention Program* (fact sheet), American Academy of Pediatrics (www.aap.org/family/tippmain.htm).
- *The Burn-Specific Secondary Survey* (checklist), Robert Sheridan, MD (practice.aap.org/content.aspx?aid=2001).

AAP POLICY STATEMENTS

American Academy of Pediatrics, Committee on Injury and Poison Prevention. Fireworks-related injuries to children. *Pediatrics.* 2001;108(1):190-191. (aappolicy.aappublications.org/cgi/content/full/pediatrics;108/1/191).

American Academy of Pediatrics, Committee on Injury and Poison Prevention. Reducing the number of deaths and injuries from residential fires. 2000; 105(6):1355-1357. (aappolicy.aappublications.org/cgi/content/full/pediatrics;105/5/1355).

REFERENCES

1. Sheridan RL, Remensnyder JP, Schnitzer JJ, et al. Current expectations for survival in pediatric burns. *Arch Pediatr Adolesc Med.* 2000;154:245-249.
2. Sheridan RL, Schnitzer JJ, Weber JM, et al. Young age is not a predictor of mortality in burns. *Pediatr Crit Care Med.* 2001;2(3):223-224.
3. Sheridan RL, Hinson MM, Liang MM, et al. Long-term outcome of children surviving massive burns. *JAMA.* 2000;283(1):69-73.
4. Sheridan RL. Burn care: results of technical and organizational progress. *JAMA* 2003;290(6):719-722.
5. Pereira CT, Barrow RE, Sterns AM, et al. Age-dependent differences in survival after severe burns: a unicentric review of 1,674 patients and 179 autopsies over 15 years. *J Am Coll Surg.* 2006;202(3):536-548.
6. Sheridan RL, Ryan CM, Petras LM, et al. Burns in children younger than two years of age: an experience with 200 consecutive admissions. *Pediatrics.* 1997;100(4):721-723.
7. Greenbaum AR, Donne J, Wilson D, et al. Intentional burn injury: an evidence-based, clinical and forensic review. *Burns.* 2004;30(7);628-642.
8. Sheridan RL. Evaluating and managing burn wounds. *Dermatol Nurs.* 2000;12(1);17-31.
9. Sheridan R. Outpatient burn care in the emergency department. *Pediatr Emerg Care.* 2005;21(7):449-456.
10. Sheridan RL, Tompkins RG. Skin substitutes: current state of the art. *Burns.* 1999;25:97-103.
11. Sheridan RL. Comprehensive management of burns. *Curr Probl Surg.* 2001;38(9):641-756.
12. Sheridan RL, Weber JM, Prelack K, et al. Early burn center transfer shortens the length of hospitalization and reduces complications in children with serious burns [lead article]. *J Burn Care Rehabil.* 1999;20(5):347-350.
13. Stoddard FJ, Sheridan RL, Saxe GN, et al. Treatment of pain in acutely burned children. *J Burn Care Rehabil.* 2002;23(2):135-156.
14. Esselman PC, Thombs BD, Magyar-Russell G, et al. Burn rehabilitation: state of the science. *Am J Phys Med Rehabil.* 2006;85(4);383-413.
15. Simons M, King S, Edgar D, ANZBA. Occupational therapy and physiotherapy for the patient with burns: principles and management guidelines. *J Burn Care Rehabil.* 2003;24(5):323-335.
16. Stoddard FJ, Saxe G, Ronfeldt H, et al. Acute stress symptoms in young children with burns. *J Am Acad Child Adolesc Psychiatry.* 2006;45(1):87-93.
17. Rea SM, Goodwin-Walters A, Wood FM. Surgeons and scars: differences between patients and surgeons in the perceived requirement for reconstructive surgery following burn injury. *Burns.* 2006;32(3):276-283.
18. Sheridan RL. Sepsis in pediatric burn patients. *Pediatr Crit Care Med.* 2005;6(3):S112-S119.
19. Greenhalgh DG. Models of wound healing. *J Burn Care Rehabil.* 2005;26(4):293-305.
20. Patterson DR, Ptacek JT, Cromes F, et al. The 2000 Clinical Research Award. Describing and predicting distress and satisfaction with life for burn survivors. *J Burn Care Rehabil.* 2000;21(6):490-498.

Index

A

AAIDD. *See* American Association on Intellectual and Developmental Disabilities
Aarskog-Scott syndrome, 2605, 2605t
Abatacept, 2216b, 2217
Abdomen. *See also* Abdominal pain
  circular burns on, 67t
  distention of. *See* Abdominal distention
  of infants, 132–133
  of newborns, 132–133
  percussion of, 133
  physical examination of, 132–134
  tenderness of, 133
  trauma to, 1097
  tumors of, 1373–1375
  tympanitic, 1370, 1372–1373
Abdominal distention
  causes of, 1370b
  diagnosis of, 1370, 1370t, 1374f
  family history and, 1369
  physical examination for, 1369–1370
  radiographic diagnosis of, 1375, 1375f
  secondary torsion, 1371f
  symptoms of, 1369
Abdominal masses, 1373–1374
Abdominal migraine, 1783
Abdominal pain
  acute, 1372, 1376, 1378, 1378b
  appendicitis in, 2627–2728
  causes of, 1379b, 2625b, 2626–2628
  characteristics of, 1376, 1379–1383, 1380f
  conversion reaction causing, 1226
  diagnosis of, 1377b, 1377–1379, 1378b
  differential diagnosis, 2530b, 2628, 2629t
  evaluation of, 1379–1382, 1380f, 2624, 2626
  history-taking, 2624
  imaging studies for, 1281–1282
  intussusception, 2627
  malrotation and midgut volvulus, 2626f–2627f, 2626–2627
  physical examination for, 1380–1381, 2624
  recurrent, 1376–1377, 1379–1380, 1381
  surgery for, 2628, 2630
  treatment for, 1382
Abdominal sepsis, 506t
Abdominal wall defects
  newborn assessment, 767–768
  ultrasound detection of, 610
Abdominal wall hypotonia, 1375
Abduction, 1529b
ABO incompatibility in newborn, 942
Abortion
  description of, 1348, 1356–1357
  minor consent to, 76
Abrasion, corneal, 2346–2347, 2347f
Abruption of the placenta, 632
Abscess
  brain, 506t
  characteristics of, 1856–1857
  dental, 125
  peritonsillar, 126, 2635
  retropharyngeal, 2635, 2650
Absence seizures, 2489, 2489b
Absenteeism, 1145b, 1145–1146
Abstinence syndromes, 1249
Abuse
  child. *See* Child abuse and neglect
  dissociative disorders and, 1745
  drug. *See* Drug abuse
  ocular trauma caused by, 2349–2350, 2350f
  sexual. *See* Sexual abuse
  substance. *See* Substance abuse
Abuse Assessment Screen, 369
Academic difficulties, 1558–1559, 1559t
Academic underachievement, 1215
Access to health care. *See* Health care, access to
Accessory tarsonavicular, 1535, 1536
Accessory tragi, 783
Accommodative esotropia, 1735–1736, 1736f
Accreditation, 1019
Accreditation Committee in Acupuncture and Oriental Medicine, 460
Acculturation, 182
ACE inhibitors. *See* Angiotensin-converting enzyme inhibitors
Acellular pertussis vaccines, 2423b
Acetaminophen
  antidote for, 2684t, 2766t
  chronic pain managed using, 440, 441t
  mild-to-moderate acute pain managed using, 426
  overdose of, 2682, 2770–2771, 2771f
Acetazolamide, 2498t, 2500–2501
Acetylcholine, 1603
Acetylcholinesterase, 605
Acetyl-CoA, 981
Acetylsalicylic acid
  acute pain managed using, 428t
  adverse effects of, 427
Achalasia, 2057
Achondroplasia
  description of, 2604–2605, 2605t
  megalencephaly and, 1648
  ultrasound detection of, 612
Acid excretion, 2460–2463, 2461f, 2463f
Acid load, in diabetic ketoacidosis, 2664
Acid (poison)
  in caustic esophageal injuries, 2705–2706, 2706b
  poisoning by, 2775
Acid therapy, for warts, 2617–2618
Acid-base system
  balance of, 2460–2463, 2461f, 2463f
  composition of, 467–471
Acidemias, 984–985
Acid-fast bacillus smear, 2599
Acidosis
  medical-legal issues and, 746
  metabolic
    in acute renal failure, 2799
    in diabetic ketoacidosis, 2662–2664
    in status asthmaticus, 2814
  in neonates, 665
  renal tubular
    ammonium excretion mechanism and, 2463–2466, 2464f–2465f, 2464t
    causes of, 2460
    classifications of, 2463, 2464t
    clinical presentations of, 2459–2460
    definition of, 2459–2460, 2460t
    delayed maturity caused by, 2470–2471
    diagnosis of, 2459
    disorders of, 2459, 2460t
    evaluation of, 2471–2473, 2472f, 2473t
    failure to thrive and, 2459–2460
    heredofamilial, 2459, 2460t
    hybrid, 2470
    primary care physician's role in, 2474
    reclamation-type, 2466–2467, 2468t
    regeneration-type
      hyperkalemic, 2468t, 2469–2470
      nonhyperkalemic, 2467–2469, 2468t

Page numbers followed by "f" denote figures; "t" denote tables; "b" *denote* boxes.

Acidosis—cont'd
  renal tubular—cont'd
    renal mechanisms for acid excretion and, 2460–2463, 2461f, 2463f
    treatment of, 2473–2474
    types of, 2466–2471, 2468t
Acne
  bacterial causes of, 1802
  blackheads/whiteheads (open/closed comedones), 1803
  clinical findings, 1802–1803
  complications of, 1807
  cystic, 1802–1805, 1807
  description of, 1690, 1690f
  differential diagnosis of, 1803–1804, 1804f
  etiology of, 1802, 1802f
  follicular obstruction and, 1802, 1802f
  hirsutism and, 1590, 1595
  hormonal causes of, 1802
  inflammatory, 1802–1805
  instruction sheet, 1806b
  management of
    antibiotics, 1805
    cleanliness, 1806
    comedolytics, 1804–1805
    cosmetics, 1806
    diet, 1806
    female patients, 1805
    hormonal therapy, 1805–1806
    isotretinoin. *See* Isotretinoin
    patient compliance, 1806
    picking, 1806–1807
    systemic retinoids, 1805
    topical retinoids, 1805
    tretinoin preparations, 1805t
  pathogenesis of, 1802
  in prepubertal children, 1803
  prognosis, 1807
  Propionibacterium acnes, 1802, 1805
  psychosocial considerations, 1804, 1807
  referral for, 1807
  scarring caused by, 1807
  steroid, 1804
Acne conglobata, 1804
Acne fulminans, 1804
Acne rosacea, 1803, 1804f
ACP Journal Club, 39t
Acquired autoimmune myasthenia gravis, 1607
Acquired hemolysis, 942
Acquired hypothyroidism, 1728
Acquired torticollis, 1764–1765
Acrocephaly, 117
Acrocyanosis, 114
Acrodermatitis enteropathica, 1389, 1451, 1691f
Acropustulosis of infancy, 784
Actinomycin D, 1875
Activities of daily living devices, 579
Acupoint stimulation, 459–460
Acupuncture, 440, 459–460
Acute abdomen
  appendicitis in, 2627–2628
  description of, 1611
  differential diagnosis of, 2628, 2629t
  evaluation of, 2526, 2624
  history-taking, 2624
  indicators of, 2628, 2630
  intussusception, 2627
  malrotation and midgut volvulus, 2626–2627, 2627f
  pain in, 2625b, 2626–2628
  physical examination for, 2624
Acute bowel wall trauma, 2080
Acute diarrhea
  description of, 1443, 1443b, 1445b
  evaluation of, 1444–1445, 1445b
  treatment of, 1445–1447
Acute fetal hypoxia, 656–658
Acute glomerulonephritis
  characteristics of, 2287, 2287f
  with no or mild renal failure, 2287b, 2287–2290, 2289b
  with rapidly progress renal failure, 2289–2290, 2289b
Acute hemolytic transfusion reaction, 487
Acute hemorrhagic conjunctivitis, 2036
Acute lung injury, 489
Acute lymphoblastic leukemia
  classification of, 2235f, 2235t, 2236
  clinical features of, 2239t
  clinical manifestations of, 2333t
  cytogenetic and molecular markers in, 2237–2238, 2237t, 2239t
  frequency of, 2235, 2235f
  immunophenotype of, 2235t, 2236
  in infants, 2240
  laboratory findings in, 2233t
  relapsed, 2242
  treatment of, 2238–2244, 2239t
Acute mastoiditis, 122
Acute myelogenous leukemia
  classification of, 2236, 2236t
  clinical features of, 2235f, 2239t
  clinical manifestations of, 2333t
  cytogenetic and molecular markers in, 2238, 2239t
  laboratory findings in, 2233t
  prevalence of, 2236
  relapsed, 2242
  treatment of, 2240
Acute osteomyelitis, 2355–2356
Acute otitis media
  complications of, 2363
  description of, 2360
  diagnosis of, 2361
  epidemiologic features of, 2360
  follow-up for, 2362
  management of, 2361–2362
  pathogenesis of, 2360–2361
  tympanic membrane findings in, 122
Acute pain
  analgesic ladder for, 424, 424b
  description of, 423
  measurement of, 423–424
  mild-to-moderate, 424–427, 425t
  moderate-to-severe, 427–428, 427f, 428t
  pharmacologic management of
    administration mode, 430–431
    hydromorphone, 429
    intravenous administration, 430
    meperidine, 429
    methadone, 429–430
    morphine, 429, 429b
    nonintravenous administration, 430–431
    opioids
      adverse effects of, 431–432, 431b, 431t
      strong, 428–433, 428t, 429b, 431b, 431t
      weak, 426–427
    prostaglandin synthesis inhibitors, 424–426, 425t
    regional anesthetic techniques, 432–433
Acute poststreptococcal glomerulonephritis
  causes of, 2287
  clinical presentation of, 2288
  course of, 2288
  description of, 2287
  laboratory findings in, 2288
  pathological features of, 2287
  prognosis of, 2289
  treatment of, 2288–2889
Acute promyelocytic leukemia, 2240
Acute renal failure, 1825–1826, 2797–2800. *See also* Anuria; Oliguria
Acute respiratory distress syndrome
  in drowning injuries, 2677
  in shock, 2811
Acute tubular necrosis, 1826, 1827
Acute upper respiratory infection, 323t
Acyclovir
  chickenpox treated with, 1916
  genital herpes treated with, 2516b, 2517b
  indications for, 510t
ADA. *See* American Diabetes Association
Adapalene, 1804
Addison, Thomas, 1811
Addison disease, 1511, 1811–1813
Adduction
  definition of, 1529b
  of forefoot, 1532
Adefovir, 510t, 2124
Adenoid hypertrophy, 1820
Adenoidectomy
  complications, 2588, 2588t
  contraindications, 2588–2589

Page numbers followed by "f" denote figures; "t" denote tables; "b" *denote* boxes.

Adenoidectomy—cont'd
indications for, 2583–2586, 2585f–2586f, 2587b
Pittsburgh criteria for, 2587b
procedures, 2587
quality of life after, 2589
with tonsillectomy, 2585, 2586
Adenoma sebaceum, 1803, 2310–2311, 2310f
Adenomatous polyps, 1545
Adenopathy, intrathoracic, 2599, 2600f
Adenosine, 1414
Adenotonsillar hypertrophy, 525
Adenovirus
description of, 1981
pertussis vs., 2420
pharyngitis caused by, 2425b, 2426
ADHD. *See* Attention deficit/ hyperactivity disorder
Adherence
communication effects, 163
definition of, 161, 196
determinants of, 162, 196
difficulties with, 161–162
family factors that affect, 163
to healthy lifestyle, 196–197
patient-family knowledge effects on, 163
patient-physician interaction effects on, 164
reward systems for, 196
strategies for improving, 163t, 163–164
treatment regimen effects on, 163–164
Adipose tissue, fetal, 113
Adjustment disorders, 1258b
Adolescence
behaviors established during, 56
dating violence, 1076–1078
definition of, 1745
developmental tasks, 211
early, 211
foster care and, 1064, 1068–1069
health outcomes for NICU infants in, 856–861
homelessness and, 1090
late, 211
media exposure effects on, 1114–1120
middle, 211
psychological development during, 1009–1010
self-care effects in, 1104
sexual abuse and, 1112–1113
stages of, 211
Adolescent(s). *See also* Late childhood; Parent-adolescent relationship
abdomen of, 133–134
abdominal pain in, 2530b
abortions in, 76
acne. *See* Acne
amenorrhea in, 1390–1394
autonomy of, 1322–1323, 1331
back pain in, 1405, 1407–1410
blood pressure in, 108t, 110t, 1584–1585

Adolescent(s)—cont'd
cardiac arrhythmias in, 1412–1413, 1416–1417
cardiovascular screening in, 338–340
chest of, 129–130
coercive feelings by, 204
cognition by, 1322
confidential discussions with, 77
contraception for, 75–76
conversion reactions of, 1226–1232
death of, leading causes of, 239, 240t–241t
depression, 1313–1315, 1342
development of, 1331
diet for, 219
Down syndrome, 2022b, 2022–2023
drug testing of, 76–77
dysuria in, 1476f
empowerment of, 1132
essential hypertension in, 132
fatigue in, 1511
gastrointestinal bleeding in, 1545–1546
genitalia of, 136–137
heart of, 131–132
heart rate in, 106t
hoarseness in, 1599b, 1599–1600
homosexuality in, 1341–1342. *See also* Gay, lesbian, and bisexual youth; Transgender youth
hospitalization preparations for, 172b
hypertension in, 1584b
identity of, 1323
interviewing of, 1331–1338
leading causes of death in, 239, 240t–241t
lean body mass growth spurt in, 221
lungs of, 129–130
mortality, 1323, 1342
cardiac arrhythmias and, 1418
encopresis and, 1256
substance abuse and, 1245
suicide and, 1312–1313
as mothers, 184. *See also* Adolescent pregnancy
musculoskeletal system examination in, 140
neck of, 127–128
nervous system of, 145
nose of, 123
parent and, relationship between
assessment of, 1329–1330
communication and, 1328–1329, 1329b
conflict management and, 1328, 1330
goals of, 1328
sexuality and, 1343–1344, 1364
pelvic examination in, 137
pneumothorax and, 1423
privacy issues, 31
protein requirements, 223t
psychopathological conditions, 1166

Adolescent(s)—cont'd
puberty in, 1322, 1339–1340
rashes in, 1694b–1695b
respiratory rate in, 106
risk avoidance discussions with, 15
scoliosis in, 2548
sexuality, 1339–1343
sexually transmitted infections in, 2509, 2509b, 2510f
skin examination, 116
specialty care for, 9
strange behavior in, 1745–1746
substance abuse in
definition of, 398–404
effects of, 398
epidemiologic features of, 398, 398f
prevalence of, 398, 398f, 399
smoking and, 398
suicide, 1312–1315, 1314b, 1342
transgender youth and, 1240
transitional planning for, 53
uterus palpation in, 137
vaccinations for, 246f
violence prevention in, 274–275
vision screening in, 344–345
Adolescent pregnancy
demographic data regarding, 235–236, 236t
discussions about, 75–76
prevalence of, 75
statistics regarding, 235–236
Adoption. *See also* Foster care
countries with highest rates of, 1043
culture and diversity issues, 1048–1051
demographics of, 1042–1043
description of, 1348
Down syndrome patients, 2020, 2023
ethical issues, 80–81
etiquette guidelines, 1050
first-year home issues, 1046–1048
ICD-9 diagnoses in newly adopted children, 1049
language guidelines, 1050
long-term issues, 1048
medical issues, 1045–1046
new-arrival issues, 1044–1048
physician services billing and payment, 1048–1049
preadoption care, pediatrician's role in, 1043–1044
social and emotional issues, 1044–1045
Adoption studies, 998–1000
Adrenal carcinomas, 1815
Adrenal glands
anatomy of, 1808
atrophy of, 1811
congenital deficiency, 982–983
description of, 1808
dysfunction of. *See* Adrenal insufficiency; Adrenocortical hyperfunction
hyperandrogenism, 1593–1594

Adrenal glands—cont'd
physiology of, 1808
sex hormones, 1804, 1808, 1814
Adrenal hyperplasia, 1594
Adrenal hypoplasia congenita, 1812
Adrenal insufficiency
acute
chronic replacement therapy, 1813–1814
stress dosing, 1814
age of onset, 1811
causes of, 1809–1812, 1810b
congenital adrenal hyperplasia. *See* Congenital adrenal hyperplasia
description of, 1811–1812
glucocorticoids for, 1812–1813
history-taking for, 1808–1809
hyperpigmentation, 1808–1809, 1811–1812, 1814
imaging studies, 1812
in intensive care unit patients, 1813
laboratory evaluation of, 1812
management of, 1812
pathological, 1809
physical examination for, 1808–1809
secondary, 1809, 1812–1813
signs and symptoms of, 1808, 1812
tuberculosis as cause of, 1811
Adrenal medulla
description of, 1808
diseases involving, 1816
Adrenarche, 1593–1594, 1686, 1814–1815
Adrenergic agonists
alpha, 2775
beta
anaphylaxis treated with, 2645
heart failure treated with, 2722
shock treated with, 2810–2811
status asthmaticus treated with, 2815–2816
Adrenergic antagonists
beta. *See* Beta-blockers
heart failure treated with, 2722
Adrenocortical hyperfunction
adrenal medullary diseases, 1816
causes of, 1814b
Cushing syndrome, 1815–1816
premature adrenarche, 1814–1815
Adrenocorticotropic hormone, 1808–1815
Adrenoleukodystrophy, 1812
Adventitious breath sounds, 129
Advice
delivery and timing of, 202
rejection of, 203–204
Aerobic exercise, 190, 191b
Affective education, 1131–1132
African folk illnesses, 64t, 66t
African trypanosomiasis, 2370
After-hours programs, 7
After-school care programs, 1104–1105
Age. *See also* Gestational age
bacterial meningitis and, 2252
Age—cont'd
childhood death by, 593, 593t
cysticercosis and, 2395
hypertension and, 1579, 1580f, 1581t–1582t
obesity and, 2321
pertussis and, 2419, 2420f
pneumonia and, 2437
rheumatic fever and, 2475
Agency for Healthcare Research and Quality, 365
Ages and Stages Questionnaire, 315
Ages and Stages Social-Emotional screening tool, 186
Aggressiveness
description of, 1220
media exposure and, 1114–1120
Agitation, 1656–1657
β_2-agonists, 1844, 1845t, 1847t, 1848
Agoraphobia, 1281, 1283
AIDS. *See also* HIV
description of, 2138–2139
in hemophilia patients, 2110
meningoencephalitis caused by, 2269
Air conduction, 122
Air flights, supplemental oxygen for infants in, 714
Airborne allergens, 1850
Airways
compression of, 1796f
fluoroscopy of, 1793f
in general anesthesia, 521–524, 521b, 523f–524f
management of, in neonatal stabilization, 675–678
Airways, breathing, and circulation
acute fetal hypoxia and asphyxia, 657–658
in altered mental status, 2642
in drug overdose, 2682
neonatal transitional cardiorespiratory physiology, 654–655
postnatal evaluation and intervention, 659–661
premature infant neonatal resuscitation, 663–664
seizure management, 746–747
Airways obstruction
assessment of, 2631
breath sounds in, 2631, 2632, 2632t
clearing of, 2048
differential diagnosis, 2633, 2633t
in early infancy, 2631, 2633–2634
history, 2631
infectious causes, 2634–2636
in neonates, 656
noninfectious causes, 2637
physical examination for, 2631–2633
in status asthmaticus, 2814–2815
stridor and, 1747–1748
vascular anomalies, 2636–2637
wheezing and, 1790–1991, 1792f
Alabama Parenting Questionnaire, 1170
Albendazole
ascariasis treated with, 2390
description of, 70
giardiasis treated with, 2086
hookworm infections treated with, 2388–2389
pinworm treated with, 2389, 2433
trichinellosis treated with, 2386
Albumin, 487
Albumin-globulin ratio, 1527
Albuterol
anaphylaxis treated with, 2645
anticholinergic agents in combination with, 1844
asthma treated with, 1844
status asthmaticus treated with, 2815–2816
Alcohol
abuse of, 1131, 2791
adolescents use of, 1337
breastfeeding and, 813
education about, 1131
ethyl, 2783
isopropyl, 2784
media images, 1115–1120
neonatal drug withdrawal syndrome, 949
Alcoholism, 1378, 1511
Aldosterone deficiencies, 1808
Alfentanil, 425t
Aliases, 32
Alignment, ocular, 1776, 1780
Alkaline substances
esophageal injuries caused by, 2705–2706, 2706b
poisoning by, 2775
ALL. *See* Acute lymphoblastic leukemia
Allergic contact stomatitis, 2569–2570
Allergic rhinitis
anatomic abnormalities and, 1820
clinical features of, 1819
complications of, 1819
description of, 123
differential diagnosis of, 1820
etiology of, 1819
laboratory evaluation of, 1819–1820
prognosis for, 1821
referral for, 1821
treatment, 1820–1821
Allergies
bee sting, 2688–2689
breastfeeding effects on prevention of, 810
complementary and alternative medicine and, 461–462
conjunctivitis caused by, 1715
constipation caused by, 1427
cow milk protein, 1932, 2057, 2065b, 2065–2067
diarrhea caused by, 1450–1452
early education and child care programs, 1020
fatigue caused by, 1510
food, 1614

Page numbers followed by "f" denote figures; "t" denote tables; "b" *denote* boxes.

Allergies—cont'd
gastrointestinal. *See* Gastrointestinal allergy
history-taking about, 92b, 93
prevalence of, 242
in spina bifida patients, 2543
transfusion-related, 488
Allodynia, 1554
Alloimmune hemolysis
anemia with, 941–942
perinatal morbidity and mortality and, 634
Aloe, 458t
Alopecia
alopecia areata, 1386–1387
androgenetic, 1387
definition of, 1384, 1385t
diagnosis of, 1385–1389, 1387f
management of, 1389t
prognosis for, 1385
referrals for, 1389–1390
traumatic, 1388
Alpha-2-adrenergic agonists, 2775
Alpha-agonists
in chronic pain management, 444
description of, 1313t
Alpha-blockers, 1587t–1588t
Alphanumeric organisms, 1823
Alpha-thalassemia, 1396–1398
Alport syndrome, 2291–2292
Alprazolam, 2782
Alternative medical systems, 459–460
Alternative medicine. *See* Complementary and alternative medicine
Alveoli, 128
Amantadine, 510t
Ambient potassium levels, 1808
Ambiguous genitalia
congenital anomalies, 794
ultrasound detection of, 611
Ambivalence, 202–203
Amblyopia. *See also* Vision screening
causes of, 120, 1777
classification of, 1778b
definition of, 343, 1776–1777
description of, 1736f
early identification of, 343–344
infantile esotropia and, 1734b, 1734–1735
ocular trauma and, 2343
pathological feature of, 1778f
prevalence of, 343
strabismus and, 1776–1778
treatment of, 1736
vision test for, 1736f
Ambulatory blood pressure monitoring, 1585
Ambulatory patients, 479–480
Amebiasis, 2372–2373
Amendments to the Education of the Handicapped Act, 346
Amenorrhea
causes of, 1391b
Amenorrhea—cont'd
description of, 1390–1392
evaluation of, 1392f, 1392–1394, 1393t
laboratory testing for, 1394
management of, 1394
physical examination for, 1392–1393
referrals for, 1394
secondary sex characteristics, 1393
stress and, 1391
American Association on Intellectual and Developmental Disabilities, 2184
American trypanosomiasis, 2368–2369. *See also* Chagas disease
Amikacin
dosage, peak serum concentrations, and MIC_{95} for, 493t
urinary tract infections treated with, 2613t
uses of, 500
Amino acids
description of, 222
metabolic defects of, 2733b, 2734, 2734t
Aminoglycosides
bacterial resistance to, 499
description of, 825
mechanism of action of, 499
pharmacologic properties of, 499
side effects of, 499–500
uses of, 500
Aminophylline
apnea, bradycardia and desaturation in neonates, 686–688
status asthmaticus treated with, 2816
Amitriptyline
dosing strategies for, 445t
headaches and, 1554
AML. *See* Acute myelogenous leukemia
Amlodipine, 2730
Ammoniacal dermatitis, 136
Ammonium excretion
mechanism for, 2463–2466, 2464f–2465f, 2464t
steps in, 2465, 2465f
Amniocentesis
fetal assessment, 644
Rh sensitization testing, 619
Amniotic fluid, 643
Amniotocele, 1707, 1708f–1709f
Amoebic meningoencephalitis
clinical manifestations of, 2374
description of, 2373–2374
diagnosis of, 2374–2375
epidemiologic features of, 2374
prevention of, 2375
treatment of, 2375
Amoxicillin
acute otitis media treated with, 2362
dosage, 493t
Lyme disease treated with, 2250–2251, 2251t
MIC_{95} for, 493t
peak serum concentrations, 493t
sinusitis treated with, 2536
Amoxicillin—cont'd
urinary tract infections treated with, 2613, 2613t
Amoxicillin-clavulanate, 2613t
Amphetamines
abuse of, 2782
neonatal drug withdrawal syndrome, 950–951
tics caused by, 1759
Amphotericin B
dosage of, 512t
leishmaniasis treated with, 2368
Ampicillin
dosage, peak serum concentrations, and MIC_{95} for, 493t
urinary tract infections treated with, 2613t
uses of, 495
Ampicillin-sulbactam
pelvic inflammatory disease treated with, 2519b
urinary tract infections treated with, 2613t
Anabolic steroids, 2551
Anaerobic infections, 560–561
Anal development stage, 1006
Anal warts, 2516b, 2523
Analgesics
adjuvant, 443–444, 445t
nonopioid, 440, 441t
opioid. *See* Opioids
overdose of, 2700–2772
rebound headaches, 1554
for snakebites, 2700
Anaphylactic allergy, 248
Anaphylactoid reactions, 2643. *See also* Anaphylaxis
Anaphylaxis. *See also* Allergies
airways obstruction in, 2637
definition, 2643
differential diagnosis, 2644
epidemiology, 2644
etiology, 2643
evaluation, 2644–2645
hospitalization for, 2646
insect stings, 2644, 2688–2689
management of, 2645–2646
referrals for, 2646
shock in, 2806
signs and symptoms, 2644
Ancestry-specific genetic disease, 604
Ancylostoma sp.
A braziliense, 2389
A duodenale, 2388–2389
Androgen
biosynthesis defects, 2196
body hair and, 1590–1591
defects in action of, 2196
excess of, 1591, 2195, 2195t
production of, 1809, 1811
Androstenedione, 1808, 1811
Anemia
of chronic disease and inflammation, 2205

Anemia—cont'd
classification of, 1395–1403, 1400t
definition of, 1395
differential diagnosis of, 342–343
evaluation of, 1401–1404
family history of, 1403
fatigue caused by, 1510
fetal, 619
hematologic causes of, 1401
hemolytic, 941–942
iron-deficiency. *See* Iron-deficiency anemia
laboratory findings for, 1404
management of, 1481
microcytic, 1395–1396, 1398f
neonatal
in congestive heart failure, 2721
management of, 683–685, 940–944
normocytic, 1401–1402
physical examination for, 1403–1404
prevalence of, 342
referrals and, 1404
risk factors for, 342, 342b
screening for, 342b, 342–343
sickle cell. *See* Sickle cell anemia
sideroblastic, 1401
treatment of, 343, 1404
Anesthesia/anesthetics. *See also specific indications*
adverse reactions to, 376
American Society of Anesthesiologists Physical Status Classification, 517–518, 517t
asthma and, 522
bronchopulmonary dysplasia and, 524–525
cardiovascular disease and, 526–529, 527t–528t
cerebral palsy and, 538
congenital adrenal hyperplasia and, 532
connective tissue disorders and, 540
cystic fibrosis and, 526
diabetes mellitus
considerations for, 529–532, 530t, 531f, 533f
insulin regimen in preoperative period, 530–531, 530t, 531f, 533f
Down syndrome and, 538–539, 539f
endocrine diseases and, 529–534, 530t, 531f, 533f, 534b, 534t
general
airways function in, 521–524, 521b, 523f–524f
early postoperative surgical problems related to, 558t–559t, 558–560
effects of, 516
emergence phenomena after, 556–557
intubation-related complications from, 557
Anesthesia/anesthetics—cont'd
general—cont'd
postintubation croup, 557
pulmonary function in, 521–524, 521b, 523f–524f
succinylcholine-induced myalgia, 557–558
genetic diseases and, 538
heart murmur and, 526–527, 527t
hematologic diseases and, 534–538, 537b
hemophilias and, 537–538
hyperthyroidism and, 534
hypothyroidism and, 532, 534
inherited coagulopathies and, 537–538
malignant hyperthermia and, 539b–540b, 539–540
medications and, 541, 542t
morbidity and mortality rates with, 517, 518f
obstructive sleep apnea syndrome and, 525–526
oncologic diseases and, 538
in outpatient surgical procedures, 545
Pediatric Anesthesia Malpractice Closed Claims Registry on, 519
Pediatric Perioperative Cardiac Arrest Registry on, 518–519, 518t, 519f
platelet abnormalities, 538
post-delivery breastfeeding and, 801
postoperative events
apnea, 522, 524, 524f
nausea and vomiting, 552–556, 553f, 554t–555t
preanesthetic history and physical examination, 519–521, 520f, 521b
prematurity and, 524
preoperative fasting, 543–544, 544t
prolonged QT syndrome and, 527–529, 528t
regional, 432–433
risks associated with, 517t–518t, 517–521, 518f–520f, 521b
secondary adrenal insufficiency and, 532, 534b, 534t
sickle cell disease and, 535–537, 537b
skin diseases and, 540
subacute bacterial endocarditis prophylaxis and, 529, 529b
thyroid diseases and, 532, 534, 534b
transfusions and, 545–546
upper respiratory tract infections and, 521–522, 521b
von Willebrand disease and, 537
Williams syndrome and, 527
Aneuploidy
cystic hygroma, 607
pregnancy-associated plasma protein A, 604
Anger, 734–735
Angiofibromas, 2310–2311, 2310f
Angiography, computed tomography
renal, 147, 151, 151f
Angiomatosis, encephalotrigeminal, 2312–2314, 2313f. *See also* Sturge-Weber syndrome
Angiotensin-converting enzyme inhibitors
dilated cardiomyopathy treated with, 1961
heart failure treated with, 2722
hemolytic-uremic syndrome treated with, 2096
hypertension treated with, 1587t–1588t, 2114
nephrotic syndrome treated with, 2301, 2301b
Angiotensin-receptor blockers, 1587t
Angle classification system for malocclusion, 1650–1652
Animal bites. *See also* Bite(s)
anticipatory guidance, 1824
bacteria associated with, 1823
cats, 1822–1824
dogs, 1822–1824
evaluation, 1823
infection risk factors, 1822t
management of, 1823–1824
rabies vaccination guidelines, 1824t
referral for, 1825
wild, 1824
wound care, 1823–1824
Animal dander, 1819
Ankle sprains, 2556t, 2556–2557
Ankyloglossia, 124, 766
Ankylosing spondylitis, 1626
Annulus, 1692f
Anomalous left coronary artery, 1612
Anomalous pulmonary venous return, 1946–1947
Anorectal disorders, 1427
Anorexia
end-of-life care, 598
Anorexia nervosa. *See also* Eating disorders
causes of, 1638b
description of, 1745–1746, 1788
differential diagnosis of, 1637–1638
evaluation for, 1638–1639
manifestations of, 1188
pathophysiological features, 1637
physical examination for, 1189–1190
prognosis for, 1193
referral for, 1639
sports participation with, 322t
treatment of, 1639
Antacids, 2061
Antalgic gait, 1630
Antenatal hydronephrosis, 775–776
Antenatal period
maternal medical history, 752–753
newborn assessment, 775–777
Anterior cruciate ligament injuries, 2557–2558

Anterior horn cell disease, 1606
Anterior saccular cyst, 1751f
Anterior segment trauma
chemical injuries, 2345–2346
conjunctival foreign bodies, 2347–2348, 2347f
cornea
abrasion, 2346–2347, 2347f
foreign bodies, 2347–2348, 2347f
hyphema, 2348, 2348f
iritis, 2348
mydriasis, 2348
subconjunctival hemorrhages, 2346, 2346f
Anteversion, 1529b
Anthralin, 2452t, 2453
Antibacterial agents, 492–508
Antibiotics
acne treated with, 1805
acute otitis media treated with, 2361–2362
during breastfeeding, 825
cellulitis treated with, 1858
Chlamydia treated with, 2512b–2513b
croup treated with, 2653
gonococcal infections treated with, 2513b–2514b
health outcomes affected by, 11–12
impetigo treated with, 1854–1855
macrolide, 501–503
bacterial resistance to, 501
Lyme disease treated with, 2251, 2251t
mechanism of action of, 501
neonatal meningitis treated with, 2262–2263
osteomyelitis treated with, 2358
pelvic inflammatory disease treated with, 2519b–2520b
pertussis treated with, 2422, 2422t
pneumonia treated with, 2439
proctitis treated with, 2521b
prophylactic, 1823–1824
rheumatic fever treated with, 2478
septic arthritis treated with, 2507–2508
sinusitis treated with, 2536
staphylococcal TSS treated with, 2566
streptococcal TSS treated with, 2575, 2576
syphilis treated with, 2517b–2518b
urinary tract infections treated with, 2612–2613, 2613t
Anticholinergics
antidote for, 2684t, 2766t
asthma treated with, 1844, 1847t
postoperative nausea and vomiting managed using, 555t
status asthmaticus treated with, 2816
Anticipatory grief, 594
Anticipatory guidance
adolescence, 211
behavioral, 1165–1166
breastfeeding guidelines, 816–817
Anticipatory guidance—cont'd
conduct disorders and, 1221
description of, 49
end-of-the-day crying and, 1158
feeding and visual stimuli and, 1158–1159
goals achieved through, 207
infants, 209–210
information gathering before, 207–208, 208b
literature resources about, 211
newborns, 209
parent education, 208
phobias and, 1284
prenatal visits, 209
preschool-age child, 210–211
school-age child, 211
scope of, 208
sexuality and, 1344
sick and dying infant management, 733–735
sleep disturbance and, 1159
substance abuse and, 1246–1247
temper tantrums and, 1316–1317
therapeutic alliance, 207–208
toilet training and, 1159–1160
topics for, 208–211, 209b
Anticoagulants
in disseminated intravascular coagulation, 2675
as plasma product, 487
Anticonvulsants, 443–444, 2820b
Antidepressants
atypical, 1313t
chronic pain managed using, 444
neonatal drug withdrawal syndrome, 951
selective serotonin reuptake inhibitors, 2772
neonatal drug withdrawal syndrome, 951
overdose of, 2772
treatment for insomnia, 1309
tricyclic, 1313t
antidote for, 2684t, 2768t
in chronic pain management, 444
headaches and, 1554
overdose of, 2772
Antidiabetic agents, 2768t
Antidotes, 2684t–2685t, 2766t–2768t
Antiemetics
pharmacology of, 556
postoperative nausea and vomiting managed using, 555–556, 555t
vomiting and, 1785
Antiepileptics
acetazolamide, 2498t, 2500–2501
carbamazepine, 2498t, 2500
clonazepam, 2498t, 2500
clorazepate, 2500
diazepam, 2500
discontinuation of, 2503
ethosuximide, 2498t, 2500
Antiepileptics—cont'd
felbamate, 2498t, 2501
gabapentin, 2499t, 2501
headaches and, 1554
ketogenic diet, 2502
lamotrigine, 2499t, 2501
levetiracetam, 2499t, 2501
lorazepam, 2500
oxcarbazepine, 2499t, 2501–2502
phenobarbital, 2497, 2498t
phenytoin, 2497, 2498t, 2500
primidone, 2498t, 2500
seizures treated with, 2743
tiagabine, 2499t, 2501
topiramate, 2499t, 2501
valproic acid, 2498t, 2500
zonisamide, 2499t, 2502
Antifolate metabolism, 2243
Antifungal drugs, 512t–513t
Antihistamines
allergic rhinitis treated with, 1820–1821
anaphylaxis treated with, 2645
antidote for, 2684t
atopic dermatitis treated with, 1852
cough treated with, 1435
overdose of, 2772–2773
postoperative nausea and vomiting treated with, 555t
pruritus and, 1682
Anti-inflammatories
bacterial meningitis treated with, 2259
neonatal meningitis treated with, 2263
nonsteroidal
adverse effects of, 427b
asthma treated with, 1844, 1845t
description of, 2215–2216, 2216b
dysmenorrhea treated with, 1461–1462
headaches and, 1553
hives and, 2028
moderate-to-severe acute pain treated with, 427, 427b
staphylococcal TSS and, 2562, 2567
Stevens-Johnson syndrome treated with, 2030
streptococcal TSS and, 2576
toxic epidermal necrolysis treated with, 2030
rheumatic fever treated with, 2478–2479
Antimicrobial agents, 489–515. *See also* Antibiotics
aminoglycosides, 499–500
approach to, 490
azalides, 501–503
azithromycin, 502
bactericidal titers and, 491
bacteriostatic vs. bactericidal agents, 491
cephalosporins, 496–498, 496b
chloramphenicol, 503
clarithromycin, 502

Antimicrobial agents—cont'd
  classes of, 492–508
  clindamycin, 502–503
  culture in, 491–492, 495f
  efficacy of, 490
  endocarditis prophylaxis using, 508–509, 508t, 509t
  erythromycin, 501–502
  fungal infections treated with, 512t–513t
  HIV prophylaxis using, 2143
  laboratory's role in, 491–492, 495f
  ß-lactam, 498–499
  macrolides, 501–503
  maternal health and risk of, 630
  metronidazole, 505
  minimal bactericidal concentrations of, 491
  minimal inhibitory concentrations of, 491
  parasitic infections treated with, 514
  penicillins, 492, 493t, 494–496
  pharmacokinetics and pharmacodynamics of, 490–492
  postantibiotic effect, 490
  preoperative, 507t
  prophylactic uses, 508t–509t, 508–509
  rifampin, 505–506, 508
  serum inhibitory titers and, 491
  sulfonamides, 500–501
  susceptibility testing in, 491–492, 495f
  tetracycline, 503–504
  tolerance to, 491
  trimethoprim, 500–501
  vancomycin, 504–505
  viral infections treated with, 509–514, 510t–512t
Antimonials, 2367–2368
Antiretroviral therapy, 2143–2144
Anti-Rho, 2173
Antiserotonin(s), 555t
Antistreptococcal therapy, 2478
Antithrombin concentrates, 2675
Antithyroid medications, 2156
Antitrypsin deficiency, 387–388
Antivenin
  in copperhead bites, 2699
  in coral snakebites, 2702
  recurrence phenomenon with, 2698–2699
  serum sickness due to, 2699
  steps in using, 2700b
  use in children, 2699
Ants
  fire, 2689–2690
  harvester, 2690
Anuria
  in acute renal failure, 2799
  causes of, 1826t
  comorbid conditions of, 1826
  definition of, 2798
  etiology of, 1825–1826
  evaluation of, 1826–1827
Anuria—cont'd
  incidence of, 1825
  management of, 1827–1829, 1828f
  referral for, 1829
Anus
  examination of, in rape, 2794
  newborn assessment, 768–769
  sexual abuse signs in, 1107–1113
Anxiety/anxiety disorders
  attention deficit/hyperactivity disorder and, 1204, 1212
  description of, 1171, 1281–1282, 1656–1657
  in end-of-life care, 598
  medication for, 1181b
  in palliative care, 598
  self-hypnosis for, 452
  tics and, 1762
Aorta, coarctation of the
  evaluation, 1952
  in infants, 1951f
  management of
    prognosis after surgery, 1953–1954
    surgical, 1952–1953, 1953f
  pressure overload, 925
Aortic arch
  interrupted, 2721
  right-sided, 2636
Aortic stenosis
  characteristics of, 1949–1952, 1951f
  syncope and, 1755
Apgar score
  acute fetal hypoxia and asphyxia, 657–658
  description of, 114, 128, 129t
Apheresis, 486
Aphthous stomatitis, 2569–2571
Apical impulse, 130
Aplasia cutis congenita, 782–783
Apnea
  American Academy of Pediatrics recommendations, 1835
  aminophylline for, 686–688
  cyanotic heart disease and, 1966
  definition, 1830t
  gastroesophageal reflux and, 2055b, 2058b
  gastroesophageal reflux disease and, 2056b, 2059–2060
  home monitoring in NICU-discharged infants, 716
  laryngopharyngeal reflux and, 2059
  neonatal
    causes of, 656
    description of, 910–912
    management of, 685–688
  NICU-discharged infants, 715
  obstructive sleep, 525–526, 2583–2585
  postoperative, 522, 524, 524f
  pulse oximetry for, 1832
Apneic spells, 129
Apocrine glands, 113
Apophyseal overuse conditions, 2553–2554
Apophysis, 2553t
Apophysitis, calcaneal, 2554
Apparent life-threatening events
  breathing patterns and concepts related to, 1830t
  cardiorespiratory monitor tracing, 1832f
  differential diagnosis of, 1830
  evaluation of, 1830–1832
  gastroesophageal reflux disease and, 1830, 1832, 2059–2060
  history-taking, 1831b
  management of, 1832–1835
  neurologic disorders, 1830
  polysomnographic tracing, 1833f. 1834f
  prevalence of, 1829
  referral for, 1836
  respiratory disorders, 1830
  SIDS and, 1829–1830
Appendicitis
  computed tomography of, 150, 150f
  definitions, 1836
  description of, 2627–2628
  diagnosis of, 149–150, 2626, 2630
  differential diagnosis, 1837–1838, 1838b
  etiology of, 1836
  evaluation of, 1836–1837
  imaging modalities for, 149–150
  in infants, 1838
  irritability and, 1611
  management of, 1838
  pathophysiology of, 1836
  prognosis, 1838
  referral for, 1838
  signs and symptoms of, 134
Appendicolith, 149f
Appendix testis torsion, 1720
Appetite
  loss of. *See* Anorexia
  pain and, 1639
  pathophysiological features of, 1637
Apprehension, 1656–1657
Apraxia, 356
Apt-Downey test, 1544
Aqueductal stenosis, 2151–2152
Arachidonic acid pathway, 1840
Arachnids
  scorpions, 2693–2694
  spiders, 2690–2692
  tarantulas, 2692–2693
Arboviruses, 2268
Arcanobacterium hemolyticum, 2425b, 2426–2427
Arguments, 204
Arnold-Chiari malformation, 1748
Aromatase deficiency, 2195
Arrhythmias
  approach to, 1411
  atrial fibrillation, 1415f, 1416–1417
  atrial flutter, 1416, 1416f
  cardiovascular defects, 918–921
  conduction abnormalities, 1417–1418
  in heart failure, 2719, 2723
  normal rhythm variations, 1412

Page numbers followed by "f" denote figures; "t" denote tables; "b" *denote* boxes.

Arrhythmias—cont'd
premature beats, 1412–1413
primary disease and, 1413
referrals for, 1419
sudden cardiac death, 1418–1419
supraventricular tachycardia, 1413–1416
ultrasound detection of, 610
ventricular tachycardia, 1417
Arrhythmogenic right-ventricular dysplasia, 1963
Artemisinin derivatives, 2382t, 2383
Arterial blood gas
neonatal stabilization, 679
respiratory failure in newborns, 905
Arteriovenous malformation, 1942–1943
Arthralgia
definition of, 1625–1626
in rheumatic fever, 2477
Arthritis, 1625
enthesitis-related, 2214
juvenile idiopathic, 1626, 2211–2220
causes of, 2211
clinical manifestation of, 2212
course of, 2218
differential diagnosis of, 2214–2215, 2215b
oligoarticular, 2213
ophthalmologic examination in, 2214t
pharmacologic management of
abatacept, 2216b, 2217
corticosteroids, 2216b, 2217
COX-2 inhibitors, 2216, 2216b
leflunomide, 2216, 2216b
methotrexate, 2216, 2216b
nonsteroidal anti-inflammatory drugs, 2215–2216, 2216b
rituximab, 2216b, 2217
sulfasalazine, 2216, 2216b
polyarticular, 2212–2214, 2213t
prevalence of, 2211
prognosis of, 2218
systemic-onset, 2212
limp and, 1635
psoriatic, 2214, 2449–2450
pyogenic, 506t
rheumatoid disorders with, 2211–2212
septic
causes of, 2505–2506
definition of, 2505
differential diagnosis of, 2506
empirical therapy for, 506t
evaluation of, 2507
hospitalization in, 2508
limp and, 1635
management of, 2507–2508
referrals for, 2508
Arthritis-dermatitis syndrome, 2514b, 2521, 2523f
Arthrogryposis, 613
Artificial insemination with donor sperm, 620–621
Arytenoid dislocation, 1602
Ascariasis, 2390–2391
Ascaris lumbricoides, 2071, 2390–2391
Ascending reticular activating system, 2640
Aseptic meningitis
causes of, 2256t
clinical manifestations of, 2263–2264
description of, 2036, 2252, 2263
diagnosis of, 2264
incidence of, 2254
management of, 2264
outcome of, 2264
viruses causing, 2268f–2269f, 2268–2270, 2270t
Asia
cultural healing practices confused with child abuse, 69t
folk illnesses in, 65t, 68t
Asperger disorder, 1197, 1742
Asphyxia
birth injury and, 745–746
hemoptysis and, 1573
in large-for-gestational-age infants, 890
neonatal, 656–658, 746
neurological impairment, 862–863
Aspiration
pneumothorax treated with, 2758
suprapubic, 2610, 2610b
Aspirin. *See also* Salicylates
Kawasaki disease managed using, 2226
mild-to-moderate acute pain managed using, 426
rheumatic fever managed using, 2479
Assisted reproductive technologies
adoption rate decreases secondary to, 80
congenital malformations and chromosomal anomalies, 623
description of, 620–621
growth and development issues, 624
maternal medical history, 752–753
multiple birth risk, 623–624
neonatal issues, 622–625
overview, 621
perinatal outcomes, 622–625
psychosocial effect and family functioning, 624–625
Assistive technology
description of, 579
in rehabilitation process, 579
Associations, 789, 1496–1497
Asthma
anesthesia effects on, 522
child care programs for, 1020
in children under 5 years, 1848–1849
classification of, 1843
diagnosis of, 1841–1842
differential diagnosis, 1842
difficult-to-manage, 1849
early education about, 1020
epidemiologic features, 1839–1840
factors that exacerbate, 1840b
Asthma—cont'd
FEV_1, 1842b
gastroesophageal reflux disease and, 1840, 2059
in infants, 1848–1849
management of
description of, 1843–1844, 1849
drugs. *See* Asthma, pharmacologic therapy
therapy assessment questionnaire, 1843
pathophysiological features of, 1840–1841
pharmacologic therapy
β_2-agonists, 1844, 1845t, 1847t, 1848
albuterol, 1844
anticholinergics, 1844, 1847t
appropriate, selecting, 1848t
compliance with, 1843b
controller, 1844
cromolyn sodium and nedocromil sodium, 1848
inhaled corticosteroids, 1844, 1845–1846t, 1847–1848
leukotriene modifiers, 1846t, 1848
levalbuterol, 1844
long-term control, 1845–1846t
methylxanthines, 1846t, 1848
nonsteroidal antiinflammatory agents, 1844, 1845t
omalizumab, 1848
oral corticosteroids, 1844, 1846t–1847t
quick relief of symptoms using, 1844, 1847t
racemates, 1844
Rules of Two when considering maintenance therapy, 1849
prevalence of, 242, 242t
referrals for, 1849
risk factors for, 1839, 1842
severity of, 1842b, 1842–1843, 1843t
signs and symptoms of, 1841b
sleep-related, 1309
sports participation with, 323t
status asthmaticus, 2813–2817
wheezing and, 1790–1791
Asthma control questionnaire, 1843
Asthma control score, 1843
Asthma control test, 1843
Astragalus, 458t
Asymmetric lid fissures, 1780f
At risk for overweight, 2320–2321
Ataxia-telangiectasia
description of, 1699, 2317
differential diagnosis of, 2317, 2318t
evaluation of, 2318
management of, 2318
prevalence of, 2317
Atherosclerosis
cardiac disease risks and, 279t–281t, 280–288, 281b, 282f, 283t, 284f, 285b–286b, 287f, 288b

Atherosclerosis—cont'd
clinical manifestations of, 280
description of, 189, 230
environment and, 280
hypercholesterolemia prevention and, 280–281, 280t
mortality related to, 280
prevention of, 280–281, 280t
risk factors for, 280
treatment of, 281b, 283, 285–288, 286b, 287f, 288b, 289f
Athletes
back pain and, 1406, 1497
cardiovascular screening in, 340
drug use in, 2551–2552
extremity pain and, 1491–1492
hypertrophic obstructive cardiomyopathy in, 81
sports injuries in, 2550–2561
Atlantoaxial instability, 322t, 2021
Atonic seizures, 2489, 2489b
Atopic conjunctivitis, 1716
Atopic dermatitis
clinical manifestations of, 1851
definition of, 1850
diagnostic criteria for, 1851, 1851b
differential diagnosis of, 1851
epidemiology of, 1850–1851
etiology of, 1850
laboratory evaluation for, 1851–1852
management of, 1852
prevention of, 1852–1853
pruritus and, 1681–1682
referrals for, 1853
Atresia
duodenal
description of, 2076, 2079f
postnatal evaluation, 777
ultrasound detection of, 610–611
esophageal, 777, 915, 2076, 2078f
ileal, with meconium peritonitis, 2077–2078, 2079f
newborns and, 1371f, 1375
pulmonary
with intact ventricular septum, 1946
tetralogy of Fallot management, 1944–1946
tricuspid, 1957
Atrial fibrillation, 1415f, 1416–1417
Atrial flutter
description of, 1416, 1416f
in newborn, 920, 922
Atrial premature contractions
description of, 1412f, 1412–1413
in newborn, 921, 923–924
Atrial septal defect
clinical manifestations of, 1939–1940
evaluation of, 1940–1941, 1941f–1942f
management of, 1941
prognosis of, 1941–1942
ultrasound detection of, 608–610
Atrial trigeminy, 921, 924
Atrioventricular block, 1417–1418, 1418f, 1755
Atrioventricular canal defects, 608–609
Atrioventricular septal defects, 1942, 1943f
Atropine, 2684t
Attachment
benefits of, 179
definition of, 179
description of, 210
disorders, interventions for, 186
insecure, 179, 210
pregnancy and precursors of, 1004–1005
temperament and, 1001
Attention deficit/hyperactivity disorder, 242, 1744
case report of, 1201–1202, 1215–1216
coexisting conditions and, 1204, 1204b, 1208, 1221
definition of, 1202, 1207t
diagnosis of, 1202–1204, 1205t, 1207–1209
criteria for, 1203b, 1205–1209, 1207t
failure to meet, 1207t, 1207–1208
tools for, 1205–1208
evaluation of, 1204–1209
flowchart for, 1206f
imaging studies for, 1205
irritability and, 1614
laboratory studies for, 1205
management of, 1208–1215, 1214t
manifestations of, 1207
prevalence of, 1202
resources for, 1203
tics and, 1759, 1760, 1762
treatments for
description of, 1171, 1215
medications, 1181b, 1209–1211, 1210t, 1212t–1213t
Attention disorders, 452
Attunement, 183
Atypical measles, 1980
Audiologic Assessment Panel's Guidelines for Audiologic Screening, 329, 330, 356
Auditory hallucinations, 1744
Auditory neuropathy/dyssynchrony, 1558
Auditory screening. *See also* Hearing loss
goals of, 326
in infants, 326–328, 327b, 328f, 330b
justification for, 326
in newborns, 121, 326–328, 327b, 328f, 330b
permanent hearing loss and, 1557, 1559
in preschool-age children, 328–329, 329b
primary care physician's role in, 332
in school-age children, 330
in toddlers, 328–329, 329b
Aura, 1551–1553, 1552b
Auscultation
cardiac, 1562f, 1562–1563
chest, 129
heart, 130
lungs, 129
Autism
in children, 1196–1197
diagnosis of, 1197–1198, 1199t
irritability and, 1614
laboratory evaluations for, 1197–1198
management of, 1198–11991
measles-mumps-rubella vaccine and, 79
medication for, 1181b
megalencephaly and, 1648
physical examination for, 1197
prognosis for, 1199
treatment of, 1198–1199
Autism Diagnostic Interview Revised, 1198
Autoimmune adrenal insufficiency, 1812
Autoimmune adrenalitis, 1811
Autoimmune diseases
fever caused by, 1517, 1525, 1526b
hemoptysis and, 1571
Autoimmune enteropathy, 1452
Autoimmune hepatitis, 2124–2126
Autoimmune hypoparathyroidism, 1811
Autoimmune polyendocrine syndrome type 1/type 2, 1811
Autoinflammatory diseases, 1628
Autonomy, 74, 210
Autosomal-recessive chromosomal fragility disorders of Bloom syndrome, 2232
Autosomal-recessive disease, 604
Avulsion fracture, of pelvis, 2558–2559
Axillary apocrine bromhidrosis, 1661
Axillary hyperhidrosis, 1603–1604
Axillary odor, 1661
Azalides, 501–503
Azithromycin
Chlamydia treated with, 2512b
description of, 502
pertussis treated with, 2422, 2422t
streptococcal TSS treated with, 2576
Aztreonam, 499

B

Babesiosis
clinical manifestations of, 2385
description of, 2384
diagnosis of, 2385
epidemiologic features of, 2384
life cycle of, 2384–2385
pathogenesis of, 2384–2385
prevention of, 2385
treatment of, 2385
Babinski reflex, 143
Bacille Calmette-Guérin vaccine, 2592
Back pain
chronic causes of, 1406, 1407
definition of, 1305
diagnosis of, 1405–1406, 1406t
epidemiology of, 1405
evaluation of, 1407–1409
management of, 1409–1410
postural abnormalities and, 2545
psychosocial considerations of, 1407

Page numbers followed by "f" denote figures; "t" denote tables; "b" *denote* boxes.

Back pain—cont'd
referrals for, 1410
spinal abnormalities and, 2549
Back to Sleep campaign, 2434, 2579
Bacterial infections
endocarditis
rheumatic fever and, 2480
subacute, 529, 529b
fever caused by, 1517–1518, 1521–1522, 1525, 1526b
hematuria and, 1566, 1567f, 1568
hemoptysis caused by, 1571
joint pain and, 1627, 2505–2508
lymphadenopathy caused by, 1643
meningitis. *See* Bacterial meningitis
neonatal skin conditions, 785
ophthalmia neonatorum and, 801–802
pharyngitis caused by, 2425b, 2426
pneumonia, 2420
recurrent, 1696
skin
cellulitis, 1857–1859
folliculitis, 1856
furuncles and abscesses, 1856–1857
impetigo. *See* Impetigo
pyoderma, 1855f, 1855–1856
referrals for, 1859
after snakebites, 2700
in spine, 2549
splenomegaly and, 1731–1732
stomatitis caused by, 2569, 2570
tracheitis, 2635, 2636t, 2649–2650
in urinary tract, 406–407, 2607–2608, 2613
vaginosis, 491, 2531
Bacterial meningitis
age and, 2252
anti-inflammatory therapy for, 2259
antimicrobial agents for, 2259–2261, 2260t
causes of, 2253–2254, 2255t
cerebrospinal fluid in, 2257–2258
characteristics of, 2267
clinical manifestations of, 2255–2257, 2257f
complications of, 2261
description of, 2252, 2254–2255
differential diagnosis of, 2255
distribution of, 2254f
fluid therapy for, 2259
glucocorticoids for, 2259
incidence of, 2253, 2254f
laboratory testing and findings in, 2257–2258
lumbar puncture in, 2257–2258
management of, 2258–2261
prevention of, 2261–2262
sequelae of, 2261
syndrome of inappropriate antidiuretic hormone caused by, 2258
Bacterial sepsis, 2746–2752
Bactericidal titers, 491
Bactericidal-permeability-increasing protein, recombinant human, 2750
Bacteriuria, 406–407, 2608, 2613
Bad breath, 1661–1662
Balanitis, 136, 1477, 2431
Balanitis xerotica obliterans, 2430
Balanoposthitis, 1477, 2431
Ballard score, 757–759
Bamboo spine, 1626
Banana sign, 605, 618
Banti syndrome, 1732
Barbiturates
abuse of, 2783
increased intracranial pressure treated with, 2743–2744
neonatal drug withdrawal syndrome, 948–949
Barium esophagogram, 148f, 337
Barky cough, 1748
Barlow test, 771
Barrel chest, 128
Barrett esophagus, 2054, 2058
Barriers to health care, 847, 849–850
Bartonella henselae, 1823
Basilar skull fracture, 122
Bathing
of healthy newborn, 844
postponement in neonatal period, 778–779
Bayley Scales, 349, 1742
Baylor University, 35t
BCR-ABL gene, 2237–2238
Beck Depression Inventory, 366
Becker dystrophy
complications of, 2278t
symptoms, genetics and diagnostic tests for, 2274t
treatment of, 2278t
Beckwith-Wiedemann syndrome, 888, 976–977, 2634, 2732
Bed sharing, with infants, 2580
Bedbugs, 2179, 2179f
Bedtime fears, 1301
Bedwetting. *See* Enuresis
Bee stings, 2644, 2687–2689, 2689b
Behavior
cultural expectations regarding, 159
definition, 2639
modification techniques for, 1211–1214, 1214t
self-stimulating, 1724–1726
strange. *See* Strange behavior
Behavioral change, 49
Behavioral development
behavioral genetics perspective, 998–1000
decreasing undesirable behavior, 1032–1033
discipline and, 1029–1035
encouragement of desirable behavior, 1032
homelessness and, 1089–1090
media exposure and, 1114–1120
Behavioral development
in neonatal intensive care infants, 879
sexual abuse and, 1107–1113
Behavioral disabilities
early identification and intervention for, 350
prevalence of, 349
Behavioral disorders. *See also* Mental health
considerations of, 1165–1168
consultation referrals and, 1163–1164
in Down syndrome patients, 2020, 2023
hearing loss and, 1558–1559, 1559t
prevalence of, 200
referrals, 1164–1165
seizure-related, 2496
self-hypnosis for, 452
Behavioral genetics, 998–1000
Behavioral screening
benefits of, 349–350
description of, 69–70
office process in, 350, 353
tools for, 350, 351t, 352t
Behavioral specialists, 1167–1168
Behavioral style, 1746
Behçet syndrome, 2570, 2572
Benchmarking, 47
Benign cardiac murmurs, 916–917
Benign familial hematuria, 2291
Benign familial megalencephaly, 758, 760
Benign neonatal sleep myoclonus, 1658
Benign paroxysmal positional vertigo, 1458
Benign paroxysmal torticollis, 1764
Benign paroxysmal vertigo, 1658
Benign partial epilepsy of childhood, 2489b, 2492
Benign positional molding, 2433–2437. *See also* Plagiocephaly
Benzamide, 555t
Benzathine penicillin
dosage, peak serum concentrations, and MIC_{95} for, 493t
syphilis treated with, 2518b
Benzodiazepines
abuse of, 2782–2783
antidote for, 2684t, 2766t, 2768
neonatal drug withdrawal syndrome, 949
seizures managed using, 2498t, 2500
Benzoyl peroxide, for acne, 1804–1805
Bereavement
care, 593–602
definition of, 594
perinatal care, 736–738
Beriberi, 627–629
Best interest of the child standard, 74
Beta thalassemia, 943
Beta-adrenergic agonists
anaphylaxis treated with, 2645
heart failure treated with, 2722
shock treated with, 2810–2811
status asthmaticus treated with, 2815–2816

Beta-blockers
  adjuvant, for hyperthyroidism, 2156
  anaphylaxis treated with, 2645–2646
  antidote for, 2766t
  headaches and, 1554
  heart failure treated with, 2722
  hypertension and, 1587t, 1588t
  overdose of, 2774–2775
  syncope and, 1757
Beta-lactamase inhibitors, 495–496
Beta-thalassemia, 1396
Bezoars, 1375
Bhutani curve, 893
Bicarbonate, 2667
Bichloracetic acid, for warts, 2515b, 2516b
Bier block, 445
Bifid uvula, 126, 126f
Bilateral vestibular schwannomas, 2308, 2308b, 2308f
Bilharziasis, 2393–2395. *See also* Schistosomiasis
Biliary obstruction
  hepatomegaly and, 1577
  jaundice and, 1620
Biliary tree, 148f
Bilious emesis, 2626
Bilirubin
  breastfeeding and, 821–822
  chemicals for displacement of, 895
  conjugation of, 1617–1618
  increased production of, 1616–1617
  jaundice and, 893–895, 899–900, 1616
  laboratory evaluation of, 895–896
  metabolism, 1616
Bill coding, 24
Binocular fusion, 1776
Biobehavioral therapy, 1554–1555
Biofeedback, 448–449, 449f, 448b, 1555
Biologically based therapies, 457
Biopsy
  liver, 1622
  lymphadenopathy and, 1643–1646
  renal, 1567
Biopsychosocial approaches
  abdominal pain and, 1382
  behavioral and emotional problems, 1164
  school refusal and, 1147
Biotin, 228t
Biotinidase deficiency
  diagnosis and management, 984
  newborn screening for, 386
Biphenotypic leukemia, 2236–2237, 2237t
Bipolar disorder, 1745
  diagnosis of, 1259b
  medication for, 1181b
  treatment of, 1261–1262
Birth(s). *See also* Childbirth
  demographic data regarding, 235–238
  multiple. *See* Multiple births
  to teenagers, 235–236
  to unmarried mothers, 236, 237t
Birth control. *See* Contraception
Birth defects, 774–775
Birth families, 1066
Birth history, 91b
Birth injuries
  in large-for-gestational-age infants, 890
  medical-legal issues in, 745–746
Birth weight
  infant mortality and, correlation between, 238
  newborn assessment and, 758–760
  statistics regarding, 236–237
Birthmarks, 779–781
Bisexuality. *See* Gay, lesbian, and bisexual youth
Bite(s). *See also* Animal bites; Envenomations
  ant, 2689–2690
  cat, 1822–1824
  child abuse and, 1095
  definition, 2686
  dog, 1822–1824
  insect, 2179–2181
  scorpion, 2693–2694
  snake. *See* Snakebites
  spider, 2690–2692
  tarantula, 2692–2693
  tick. *See* Tick bites
Black widow spider, 2692
Blackheads, 1803
Bladder
  dysfunction of, 2609
  exstrophy of, 2605t
Bleeding. *See also* Hemophilia; Hemorrhage
  in disseminated intravascular coagulation, 2673
  gastrointestinal
    adolescents with, 1545–1546, 1546b
    causes of, 1544–1546, 1546b
    diagnostic testing of, 1544, 1547–1549
    differential diagnosis of, 1544–1546
    history-taking, 1546–1547
    infants and young children with, 1544–1545, 1546b
    lower, 1544
    management of, 1547–1549
    newborns with, 1544, 1546b
    physical examination for, 1547
    treatment of, 1544–1546
  immune thrombocytopenic purpura and, 2172
  postoperative, 559
  vaginal
    causes of, 1768b
    diagnostic testing for, 1769
    evaluation of, 1767–1768
    history-taking, 1768–1769
    management of, 1769–1770
    physical examination for, 1769
    in prepubertal girls, 1767
    in pubertal girls, 1767–1770
Blended payments, 22t
Blepharitis, 1702, 1713f–1714f, 1713–1714
Blood
  coughing or spitting up. *See* Hemoptysis
  in diaper or underwear, 1569
  loss of, 482
  in urine, 1568f
Blood count
  description of, 1401
  dyspnea and, 1470
  epistaxis and, 1484–1485
  neonatal stabilization, 679–680
Blood donors, 481
Blood glucose. *See also* Glucose, metabolism of
  in infants of diabetic mothers, 889
  intrauterine growth restriction and, 885
  in large-for-gestational-age infants, 889
  neonatal stabilization, 679
Blood pressure. *See also* Hypertension; Hypertensive emergencies
  in adolescents, 108t, 110t
  by age, 2802t
  ambulatory monitoring of, 1585
  auscultation of, 106, 108
  in boys, 107t–108t, 1580f, 1581t–1582t
  cardiovascular health promotion and, 279t
  definition of, 1585
  factors influencing, 1579–1580
  in girls, 109t–110t, 1580f, 1583t–1584t
  measurement of
    cuff size for, 2727–2728
    techniques for, 106–108, 107t–110t, 1584–1585
  neonatal stabilization, 678–679
  regulation, 1585
  screening of, 339
Blood pressure cuffs, 108, 2727–2728
Blood products
  albumin, 487
  anticoagulants, 487
  exchange transfusion, 486, 486f
  granulocyte transfusions, 485–486
  handling of, 481
  immune globulin, 487
  plasma products, 487
  platelet transfusions, 484–485, 485b, 486t
  red blood cell transfusions, 482–484, 482t, 483b
  therapeutic apheresis, 486
  uses of, 481–489
Blood transfusion. *See also* Red blood cell transfusions
  complications of, 487–488
  in disseminated intravascular coagulation, 2674–2675
  indications for, 481
  massive, 2672–2673
Blood urea nitrogen, 1827
Bloodletting, 56
Bloody vomitus, 1543

Page numbers followed by "f" denote figures; "t" denote tables; "b" *denote* boxes.

Bloom syndrome, 2232
Blount disease, 139
Blueberry muffin lesions, 786
Blurred image, 1778b
Board certification, 4
Body composition, 193
Body fat, 222f
Body fluid(s), 467–471. *See also* Fluid(s)
Body fluid compartments, 467, 467f
Body hair
  definition of, 1590
  early growth of. *See* Precocious sexual hair growth
  excessive growth of. *See* Hirsutism
Body mass index
  for boys, 114f
  calculation of, 111, 112t, 279t, 288–289, 289f
  classification of children by, 299b
  for girls, 112f
  pre-exercise measurement of, 193
  recommendations for, 297, 299b
Body odor
  causes of, 1661–1665, 1662t–1665t
  differential diagnosis of, 1660
  physical examination of, 1661
Body temperature. *See also* Hyperthermia; Hypothermia
  circadian rhythm of, 104, 106f
  in increased intracranial pressure, 2743
  measurement of, 104, 105f–106f
  normal, 1516
  oral, 104
  rectal, 104, 105f
  regulation of, in NICU-discharged infants, 712–713
Body twirling, 1726
Body-based therapy, 457–459
Bogalusa Heart Study, 280
Bohn nodules, 123
Bonding. *See* Maternal-infant bonding
Bone
  growth of, 137
  growth plate in, 2553t
  imaging of, 151, 151f
  overuse injuries to, 2552–2555
  stress fractures in, 2552–2553
Bone marrow failure, 1668
Bone scans, 2357
Bone scintigraphy, 1635
Bordetella sp., 2419–2420
Bornholm disease, 2036
Borrelia burgdorferi
  joint pain and, 1627
  in Lyme disease, 2249
Bottle feeding
  breastfeeding vs., 213, 215
  formulas. *See* Formula
  schedule for, 215–216
  weaning from, 218
Botulism
  in infants, 1607, 1611
  in neonates, 991–992
Bourneville disease, 2309–2312, 2310b, 2310f–2311f. *See also* Tuberous sclerosis
Bowed legs, 1537f, 1537–1538, 1542
Bowel. *See also* Intestine(s)
  echogenic
    postnatal evaluation, 776–777
    ultrasound detection of, 611
  irrigation of
    for drug overdose, 2683
    for poisoning, 2769
  obstruction of, 2628
Boys. *See also* Male(s)
  blood pressure levels, 107t–108t, 1580f, 1581t–1582t
  body mass index for, 114f
  calorie recommendations for, 194t
  growth patterns in, 1727
  head circumference of, 113f
  length for age measurements, 113f–114f
  puberty in, 1683–1687
Brace, 579–580
Brachial cleft cysts, 766, 782, 1996
Brachial plexus injury
  medical-legal issues, 747
  neurological evaluation, 992
  newborn assessment, 770–771
Brachycephaly, 763
Bradyarrhythmias, 918–919, 1755
Bradycardia
  by age, 2802t
  description of, 1412, 1412t
  folk illness remedies associated with, 68t
  management of, in neonates, 685–688
  neonatal hypocalcemia and, 966
  NICU-discharged infants, 715
Brain
  abscess of, 506t
  computed tomography of, 152
  development of
    dysmorphic features associated with, 2190t
    experience-dependent learning for, 181
    parent-baby environment effects on, 181
    stimulation for, 181
  growth of
    head circumference and, 117
    during infancy, 116
    parental effects on, 181
  injuries to, 1609
  magnetic resonance imaging of, 152
  malformation of, 2539
  traumatic injury to, 2709–2715
  ultrasound of, 151–152
Brain tumors
  classification of, 1861
  definition of, 1860
  diagnostic delays, 1861
  differential diagnosis of, 1861, 1861b
  evaluation of, 1861–1863, 1862b
  incidence, 1860
Brain tumors—cont'd
  management of, 1863
  referrals for, 1863–1864
  risk factors, 1860b, 1860–1861
  treatment guidelines, 1863
Branchio-oto-renal syndrome, 792
Breast(s)
  development of
    in boys, 1683–1684
    in girls
      delayed, 1684–1685, 1687
      early, 1685–1687
      normal, 1683
    pubertal, 128
    transgender youth and, 1238–1239
  review of systems for, 92b
Breast pumping, 817
Breast surgery, 811
Breastfeeding. *See also* Lactation
  American Academy of Pediatrics recommendations, 213, 218
  artificial feeding vs., 213, 215
  benefits of
    infant protective benefits, 809–811
    maternal benefits, 811
  complementary feeding, 822
  complications of
    hypoglycemia, 819
    inadequate milk intake, 819–820
    insufficient milk syndrome, 820–821
    jaundice, 821–822, 897–899
    mastitis, 819
    nipple pain, 818–819
    plugged ducts (milk stasis), 819
  contraindications to, 811–813
  decisions regarding, 215
  declines in, 230
  discontinuation of, 218
  drug administration and, 824–825
  duration of, 822
  electric pumps for, 215
  elimination patterns in newborn and, 818
  energy requirements, 221
  engorgement, 819
  environmental toxins and, 827–828
  evaluation of, 816
  extremely low–birth-weight infants, 855
  failure of, 811–813
  family counseling and, 841–842
  feeding patterns and frequency, 816–817
  first week of, 817, 820
  growth patterns in infants, 822
  guidelines for, 814
  herbal medicines and, 825–827
  hunger cues, 816–817
  infant assessment, 817–818
  initiation of, 814
  latch-on guidelines, 815–816
  maternal complications, 818–819
  mother-infant relationship building through, 215

Breastfeeding—cont'd
neonatal drug withdrawal syndrome, 956
of neonatal intensive care infants, 710–712, 871–872
pacifier use and, 2580
perinatal, 801, 813–817
positioning at breast, 814–815
premature infants, 695–696, 835
prevalence of, 809
primary insufficient milk syndrome, 812
promotion of
description of, 701, 799–800, 813
in neonatal intensive care infants, 872
office visit guidelines, 820
protein requirements, 223t, 224
psychological benefits for infant, 215
schedule for, 215–216
second-hand smoke exposure during, 723–724
sleep and, 843, 1300, 1302
transition to, 702
weaning from, 218
weight loss in infants and, 1786
Breath sounds
adventitious, 129
in airways obstruction, 2631–2632, 2632t
auscultation of, 129
Breath-holding spells
description of, 1318–1319, 1657
syncope and, 1753, 1754–1755
Breathing. *See* Airways, breathing, and circulation
Breathing disorders
apnea. *See* Apnea
blood gas studies, 905
cardiac tests, 906
dyspnea, 1467–1473
imaging studies for, 906
laboratory tests for, 906
lung development disorders, 912–915
meconium aspiration syndrome, 908–910
newborn assessment, 903–905
overview of, 902–903
pathophysiology of, 907–908
pneumomediastinum, 911–912
pneumothorax, 911–912
pulmonary air leak syndrome, 911–912
pulse oximetry, 905
sleep related, 1303, 1309–1310
transient tachypnea of newborn, 906–907
Brigance Screens-II, 315
Bright Futures, 1203
Bright Futures in Practice: Mental Health, 364
Bright Futures Practice Guidelines, 50, 197, 359, 364, 369, 404–408
Bromhidrosis, 1604, 1660
Bronchiectasis
folk illness remedies associated with, 67t–68t
hemoptysis and, 1572–1573, 1574
Bronchiolitis
definition of, 1865–1866
differential diagnosis of, 1866–1867
epidemiology of, 1866
evaluation of, 1867–1868
management of, 1868–1869
prognosis for, 1869
referrals for, 1869
respiratory syncytial virus, 1865, 1865f
seasonal occurrence of, 1866f
Bronchitis, 1790
Bronchodilators
cystic fibrosis treated with, 1989
status asthmaticus treated with, 2815–2816
Bronchopulmonary dysplasia
anesthesia and, 524–525
management of, 688–690
in neonatal intensive care infants
follow-up care protocols, 877–878
incidence of, 853–858
nutrition management, 696
Bronchopulmonary sequestration, 607, 915
Bronchoscopy
hemoptysis and, 1574
wheezing and, 1795f, 1796f
Brown recluse spider, 2691
Brown syndrome, 1741, 1741f
Bruckner test, 1780, 1781
Brudzinski sign, 127
Bruising, 1094–1095
Bruits, auscultation for, 118
Brushfield spots, 118, 764
Bruxism, 1306–1307
Budesonide, 1847–1848
Bulbar conjunctiva, 2343
Bulimia nervosa. *See also* Eating disorders
definition of, 1186
description of, 1745–1746, 1788
diagnosis of, 1187b
manifestations of, 1188
physical examination for, 1190–1191
sports participation with, 322t
Bullae, 1690, 1691f
Bullous disease, 1691f
Bullous impetigo, 785, 1854f
Bullous myringitis, 122
Bullying, 274
Bunionette, 1532
Bunyavirus sp., 2268
Bureau of Primary Health Care, 7
Burn(s)
abuse or neglect as cause of, 1095, 2822, 2824f
burn center transfer criteria, 2826b
caustic esophageal, 2705–2709
circular, on abdomen, 67t
Burn(s)—cont'd
clinical presentation of, 2822
complications, 2827, 2827f
depth classifications, 2822, 2825f
epidemiology of, 2822
estimating extent of, 2822, 2824f
evaluation of, 2822, 2823b, 2824f
fluid therapy for, 479, 2826, 2827b
inpatient, 2822, 2825–2826
long-term care for, 2827
management of, 2822–2827
outpatient, 2822–2824, 2826b
wound medications and membranes for, 2824–2825, 2826b
Burn centers, 2825, 2826b
Butorphanol, 425t
Butyrophenone(s), 555t
BXO. *See* Balanitis xerotica obliterans

C

Cadmium, 828
Café-au-lait macules, 780, 1689f, 2305, 2305f, 2306t
Caffeine
apnea, bradycardia and desaturation in neonates, 686–688
breastfeeding and intake of, 825–826
Caffey disease, 1628
CAH. *See* Congenital adrenal hyperplasia
Calcaneal apophysitis, 2554
Calcaneocavus, 1536
Calcaneonavicular coalition, 1535
Calcaneovalgus, 139, 1532, 1533f, 1538
Calcaneus, 1529b, 1531f
Calcineurin inhibitors
atopic dermatitis treated with, 1848
orthotopic heart transplantation uses of, 1965
psoriasis treated with, 2452t, 2453
Calcipotriol, 2451, 2452t
Calcium
description of, 227t
disorders involving
fetal metabolism and birth adaptation, 966–967
maternal nutritional status and, 627–629
Calcium channel blockers
antidote for, 2766t
headaches and, 1554
hypertension treated with, 1587t–1588t, 1816
overdose of, 2774–2775
Calcium salts, 967
Calendula, 458t
Calories
from carbohydrates, 193–194
from fats, 224
in infant formulas, 216
low-birth-weight neonate requirements, 221
maintenance requirements for, 472
total daily amount of, 194t

Page numbers followed by "f" denote figures; "t" denote tables; "b" *denote* boxes.

CAM. *See* Complementary and alternative medicine
Cancer. *See also* Malignancies; Sarcoma
  breastfeeding during therapy for, 813
  Ewing tumors
    clinical manifestations, 1886
    differential diagnosis of, 1886t
    etiology, 1885–1886
    evaluation, 1886
    follow-up, 1887
    management of, 1887
    prognosis, 1887
  germ cell tumors and teratomas
    clinical manifestations, 1884
    etiology, 1883–1884
    evaluation, 1884–1885
    follow-up, 1885
    management of, 1885
    prognosis, 1885
  Hodgkin disease
    chemotherapy for, 1892–1894, 1995
    clinical manifestations of, 1892–1893
    etiology of, 1892
    evaluation of, 1893
    follow-up, 1894–1895
    management of, 1893–1894
    prognosis of, 1894
  incidence of, 2231, 2231f
  neuroblastoma, 1876–1879
  non-Hodgkin lymphoma
    clinical manifestations, 1890–1891
    etiology, 1890
    evaluation, 1891
    follow-up, 1892
    management of, 1891
    prognosis, 1892
  oncologic care, general, 1895
  osteosarcoma
    clinical manifestations, 1888–1889
    etiology, 1887–1888
    evaluation, 1889
    follow-up, 1890
    management of, 1889
    prognosis, 1889–1890
    radiation side effects, 1888t
  retinoblastoma
    case study of, 77
    clinical manifestations, 1880
    etiology, 1879–1880
    evaluation, 1880
    follow-up, 1881
    management of, 1880–1881
    prognosis, 1881
  rhabdomyosarcoma
    chemotherapy-related side effects, 1883t
    clinical manifestations, 1881–1882
    etiology, 1881
    follow-up, 1883
    management of, 1882
    prognosis, 1882–1883
  Wilms tumor, 1873–1876
Candida albicans
  breastfeeding and, 818–819
  diaper rash/dermatitis, 2013–2014, 2487, 2487f
  neonatal conditions caused by
    sepsis, 936
    skin conditions, 786
  stomatitis, 124, 2569–2571
Cantharidin, 2619
Capitation, 22, 22t
Capitellum, 2554–2555
CAP-RAST tests, 2066, 2068
Captopril, 2730t
Caput succedaneum
  description of, 117
  neurological evaluation, 992
  newborn head assessment, 761–762
Car safety seats
  for healthy newborn, 845
  injury prevention uses of, 269–270, 270t
  positioning for NICU-discharged infants, 717
  premature infants, 838
Carbamazepine, 1262, 2498t, 2500
Carbohydrate(s)
  calories from, 193–194
  characteristics of, 225
Carbohydrate enzyme defects
  diagnostic evaluation, 2736
  differential diagnosis, 2732–2733, 2733b, 2734t
  hypoglycemia in, 2732–2733, 2733b, 2734t, 2736–2737
  management of, 2737
Carbon monoxide
  poisoning caused by
    antidote for, 2684t, 2766t
    description of, 2773–2774
    irritability and, 1612
  sources of, 845
Cardiac arrhythmias
  approach to, 1411
  atrial fibrillation, 1415f, 1416–1417
  atrial flutter, 1416, 1416f
  cardiovascular defects, 918–921
  conduction abnormalities, 1417–1418
  in heart failure, 2719, 2723
  normal rhythm variations, 1412
  premature beats, 1412–1413
  primary disease and, 1413
  referrals for, 1419
  sudden cardiac death, 1418–1419
  supraventricular tachycardia, 1413–1416
  ultrasound detection of, 610
  ventricular tachycardia, 1417
Cardiac catheterization, 1757
Cardiac cycle, 1561, 1561f
Cardiac pacing, 1757
Cardiac transplantation, 1963–1965
Cardiogenic shock, 2804f, 2805, 2805b
Cardioinhibitory syncope, 1753
Cardiomyopathy
  arrhythmogenic right-ventricular dysplasia, 1963
  in congestive heart failure, 2721, 2722
  description of, 1960
  dilated, 1960–1962, 1961f
  hypertrophic, 1962–1963
  in infants of diabetic mothers, 891
  left-ventricular noncompaction, 1963
  restrictive, 1963
Cardiopulmonary resuscitation, 723
Cardiorespiratory endurance, 190–191, 191t
Cardiorespiratory monitoring
  home monitoring in NICU-discharged infants, 716–717
  monitor tracing, 1832f
  neonatal drug withdrawal syndrome, 953
  in neonatal intensive care infants, 877–878
Cardiovascular disease and disorders
  anesthesia considerations, 526–529, 527t–528t
  arrhythmias. *See* Arrhythmias
  atherosclerosis. *See* Atherosclerosis
  congestive heart failure, 921–926
  cyanosis, 926–927
  fetal assessment, 646–647
  health outcomes for, 861–862
  in infants of diabetic mothers, 891
  maternal health and risk of, 630–631
  murmurs. *See* Heart murmurs
  newborn assessment, 670, 766
  nutrition management for infants with, 696
  post-delivery screening for, 803–804
  premature, 280t
  prevalence, 916
  prolonged QT syndrome, 527–529, 528t
  respiratory failure in newborns, 905
  ultrasound detection of, 608–610
  Williams syndrome, 527
Cardiovascular screening, 334–341
  in athletes, 340
  blood pressure screening, 339
  description of, 335–336, 335b
  of fetus, 336
  medical history in, 339
  in neonates and infants, 336–338
  obesity-related, 339–340
Cardiovascular system
  anatomy, 1561, 1562f
  auscultation, 1562f
  in drowning injuries, 2678
  evaluation of, 335b, 336, 1562–1563, 1586–1587
  examination of, 319t, 320
  irritability and, 1612
  obesity effects on, 2323
  review of systems for, 92b
  screening of, 334–341. *See also* Cardiovascular screening
  syncope, 1755

Carditis
in rheumatic fever, 2477
sports participation with, 322t
Care coordination of hospitalized children, 175
Care Model for Child Health, 45–46, 46f
Caregiver
Caregiver Strain Questionnaire, 1170
primary care physician's questions for, 179, 180t–181t
CARES Foundation, 1812
Caries
in adulthood, 230
causes of, 293–294
definition of, 293
description of, 63, 293
diet in, 296, 296f
fluoride products for
dentifrice, 295
description of, 294–295, 295t
rinses, 295
supplements, 294, 295t
varnish, 295
oral hygiene in, 295
pediatrician's role in, 296
prevention of, 293–297
sealants in, 296
water fluoridation in, 294
Caroli disease, 1577
Carpal semilunar end plate, 2353b, 2354
Carrier screening
ancestry-specific genetic disease, 604
new techniques in, 388
Cascara, 458t
Case control study, 40t
Case management
description of, 173b
foster care, 1063
of NICU-discharged infants, 722
Casein, 213
Casein hydrolysate infant formula, 2067
Caspofungin, 512t
Cast, 579
Cat bites, 1822, 1823, 1824
Cataplexy, 1659
Cataracts, 764
Catch-up growth, in premature infants, 857
follow-up monitoring of, 876
toddler and early childhood years, 870–871
Catecholamines, 1808, 2810–2811
Cathartic agents, 2769
Catheterization
cardiac, 1757
thromboembolic disease in neonates and, 945
Cat-scratch disease, 1823
Caustics
esophageal injury, 2705–2709
poisoning by, 2775
Cavernous hemangiomas, 123, 1997
Cavovarus, 1536
Cavus, 1529b, 1536, 1536f
Cayenne, 458t
Cefaclor, 497–498
Cefadroxil, 497
Cefazolin, 493t, 497
Cefepime, 498, 2613t
Cefixime
gonococcal infections treated with, 2513b, 2514b
urinary tract infections treated with, 2613t
uses of, 498
Cefmetazole, 497
Cefotaxime
dosage, peak serum concentrations, and MIC_{95} for, 493t
gonococcal infections treated with, 2514b
meningococcemia treated with, 2749
urinary tract infections treated with, 2613t
uses of, 498
Cefotetan, 497, 2519b
Cefoxitin
dosage, peak serum concentrations, and MIC_{95} for, 493t
pelvic inflammatory disease treated with, 2519b, 2520b
uses of, 497
Cefpodoxime, 498, 2514b
Ceftazidime
dosage, peak serum concentrations, and MIC_{95} for, 493t
urinary tract infections treated with, 2613t
uses of, 498
Ceftibuten, 498
Ceftriaxone
dosage, peak serum concentrations, and MIC_{95} for, 493t
epididymitis treated with, 2520b
gonococcal infections treated with, 2513b, 2514b
meningococcemia treated with, 2749, 2752, 2752t
pelvic inflammatory disease treated with, 2519b, 2520b
proctitis treated with, 2520b
uses of, 498
Cefuroxime, 497
Celiac crisis, 2090
Celiac disease, 1427, 1728
Celiac sprue. *See* Gluten-sensitive enteropathy
Cellular immunity defects, 1697–1699
Cellular rejection after organ transplantation, 1964
Cellulitis
description of, 1823, 1857–1859
folk illness remedies associated with, 66t
orbital
description of, 120, 2536, 2536t
empirical therapy for, 506t
infectious causes of, 2441–2442, 2441b
Cellulitis—cont'd
pathogenesis of, 2440–2442, 2441b, 2441f
periorbital, 2442–2443, 2443f
preseptal, 2440–2445
infectious causes of, 2441–2442, 2441b
inflammatory edema of sinusitis and, 2443–2445, 2443f
trauma-related, 2442
streptococcal, 2827, 2827f
Central alpha-agonist, 1587t, 1588t
Central diabetes insipidus, 1671
Central medical record, 53
Central nervous system. *See also* Nervous system
abnormalities of, 1604
child abuse-related injuries of, 1096
defects of
antenatal identification of, 776
fetal assessment for, 645–646
neurological evaluation, 991–992
respiratory failure in newborns, 905
ultrasound second- and third-trimester testing for, 605–606
drowning and, 2678
hemangioblastomas of, 2315, 2315t
hypotonia, 1606–1607
neonatal drug withdrawal syndrome, 952–953
sensation of dyspnea and, 1468
in shock, 2811
tuberous sclerosis-related manifestations in, 2309–2310
tumors of, 1860–1861, 1863. *See also* Brain tumors
Central precocious puberty, 1592, 1685
Central syncope, 1753
Central venous catheter, 1265
Central venous pressure, 2678
Cephalexin
dosage, peak serum concentrations, and MIC_{95} for, 493t
urinary tract infections treated with, 2613t
uses of, 497
Cephalocele, 783
Cephalohematoma
neurological evaluation, 992
newborn head assessment, 761–762
Cephalosporins. *See also specific drug*
bacterial resistance to, 496
classification of, 496–497, 496b
first-generation, 497
fourth-generation, 498
gonococcal infections treated with, 2513b
mechanism of action of, 496
meningococcemia treated with, 2749
pelvic inflammatory disease treated with, 2519b, 2520b
pharmacologic properties of, 497
second-generation, 497–498
septic arthritis treated with, 2507–2508

Page numbers followed by "f" denote figures; "t" denote tables; "b" *denote* boxes.

Cephalosporins—cont'd
side effects of, 497
staphylococcal TSS treated with, 2566
streptococcal TSS treated with, 2576
third-generation, 498
types of, 496b
urinary tract infections treated with, 2613, 2613t
uses of, 497–498
Cerebral contusions, 2713
Cerebral edema, 2664, 2667, 2667b
Cerebral malaria, 2381
Cerebral palsy
anesthesia and, 538
birth injury and, 745–746
classification of, 1904, 1904b
diagnosis of, 1904b, 1904–1905
differential diagnosis of, 1904–1905
disorders associated with, 1905, 1906t
epidemiologic features, 1903
etiology of, 1903–1904
evaluation of, 1905
hypotonia and, 1604
in infants of diabetic mothers, 891
interventions for, 1906t, 1906–1907
in neonatal intensive care infants, 854–858
prognosis for, 1907–1908
referrals for, 1908
sports participation with, 322t
Cerebral perfusion pressure, 2739
Cerebrospinal fluid, 2146–2147. *See also* Hydrocephalus
leakage of, 123
meningitis findings
bacterial, 2257–2258
description of, 2252, 2253t
neonatal, 2262, 2262t
meningoencephalitis findings, 2270, 2270t
shunting of
aqueductal stenosis, 2151–2152
Dandy Walker syndrome, 2151
description of, 2149, 2152b
distal catheter, 2150–2151
endoscopic third ventriculostomy, 2151
hydrocephalus treatment in specific clinical contexts, 2151
intraventricular hemorrhage of prematurity, 2151
multiloculated hydrocephalus, 2151
myelomeningocele, 2151
posterior fossa tumors, 2151
postinfectious hydrocephalus, 2151
valve, 2150
ventricular catheter, 2149–2150
Certification
electronic health record systems, 33
practitioner, 3–4
Certification Commission for Health Information Technology, 33
Cervical adenitis, 118
Cervical ectopy, 1342
Cervical lymph nodes, 127
Cervical warts, 2516b, 2523
Cervicitis
in *Chlamydia* infection, 2511, 2512f
description of, 2532
in *Mycoplasma genitalium* infection, 2528
Cervix
development of, 134
gonococcal infection of, 2513b
CF Foundation Patient Registry Annual Data Report, 1988
CFS. *See* Chronic fatigue syndrome
CGD. *See* Constitutional growth delay
Chagas disease
clinical manifestations of, 2368–2369
description of, 2368
diagnosis of, 2369
epidemiologic features of, 2368
life cycle of, 2368
treatment of, 2369
Chalazion, 1714, 1715f
Chamomile, 458t
Change
behavioral, 49
implementation of, 46–47
Charcoal, activated
for drug overdose, 2683
for poisoning, 2769
CHARGE dysmorphologies
neonatal assessment, 671
newborn eye assessment, 764
Cheilosis, 125
Chelation therapy, 2777
Chemotherapy
adjuvant, 1889–1890
antiretroviral, 2139
indications for
central nervous system tumors, 1863
Ewing tumors, 1886, 1887
germ cell tumors, 1885
Hodgkin disease, 1892–1894, 1995
malaria, 2382–2383, 2382t
neuroblastoma, 1877, 1879
non-Hodgkin lymphoma, 1891, 1892
osteosarcoma, 1889–1890
posttransplant lymphoproliferative disease, 1965
retinoblastoma, 1880–1881
rhabdomyosarcoma, 1881–1882
Wilms tumor, 1875–1876
long-term side effects/toxicities of, 1883t
MOPP regimen, 1894–1895
myelosuppression secondary to, 1896
varicella treatment withheld during, 1896, 1917
Chest
auscultation of, 129
circumference of, 112
fetal development of, 128
imaging of, 148, 148f
of newborns, 128–129, 760, 792
physical examination of, 128–130
Chest pain. *See also* Arrhythmias
causes of, 1421–1424, 1422t
diagnosis of, 1420, 1428b
evaluation of, 1421
history and, 1421
idiopathic causes of, 1423
laboratory evaluation and, 1421
pathophysiological features of, 1420–1421
psychogenic, 1423–1444
symptoms of, 1421b, 1422t
Chest physiotherapy, 1989
Chest radiograph
achalasia evaluations, 2057
aortic stenosis evaluations, 1950
apparent life-threatening events evaluations, 1831–1832
atrial septal defect evaluations, 1940
bronchiolitis evaluations, 1868
cardiovascular screening uses of, 337
coarctation of the aorta evaluations, 1952
common cold evaluations, 1936
cystic fibrosis evaluations, 1988–1989
dilated cardiomyopathy evaluations, 1961
Ebstein anomaly evaluations, 1946, 1947f
esophageal atresia indications, 2076, 2078f
esophageal foreign body evaluations, 2048, 2049
Hodgkin disease evaluations, 1893–1894
hypoplastic left heart syndrome evaluations, 1954
lymphadenopathy evaluations, 1643
lymphoid interstitial pneumonitis evaluations, 2140
Mycoplasma pneumonia evaluations, 1980
myocarditis evaluations, 1958, 1959f
non-Hodgkin lymphoma evaluations, 1891–1892
osteosarcoma evaluations, 1890
pediatric cardiologist consultations, 1967–1968
pericarditis evaluations, 1960
Pneumocystis jirovecii pneumonia evaluations, 2140
right-to-left shunting lesions evaluations, 1944, 1944f
roseola evaluations, 2137
status asthmaticus evaluations, 2813
Stevens-Johnson syndrome evaluations, 2030
toxic epidermal necrolysis evaluations, 2030
transposition of the great arteries evaluations, 1948
tuberculosis evaluations, 2591, 2599–2600, 2600f, 2602
varicella pneumonia evaluations, 1914
ventricular septal defect evaluations, 1940

Chest radiograph—cont'd
wheezing evaluations, 1793f–1794f
Wilms tumor evaluations, 1875–1876
Chest tubes
insertion and management of, 2758–2759
position of, 2758–2759, 2759f
Chest wall injuries, 1422, 1422t
Chiari type II deformity, 618
Chickenpox. *See also* Varicella zoster
in adults, 1912
breakthrough, in previously immunized children, 1912
clinical manifestations of, 1912–1913
complications of
hematologic, 1914
hepatitis, 1914
neurologic, 1913–1914
Reye syndrome, 1913
secondary bacterial infection, 1913
varicella pneumonia, 1914
zoster, 1914
congenital, 1913
conjunctivitis and, 1713
diagnosis of, 1914–1915
differential diagnosis of, 1915
epidemiology of, 1911–1912
etiology of, 1911
in healthy children, 1912
in HIV-infected children, 2142
immunization for, 1911, 1916–1917
in immunocompromised children, 1912–1913
neonatal, 1913
in older children, 1912
pathogenesis, 1912
prevention of, 1916
referrals for, 1917
transmission of, 1911
treatment of, 1915–1916
varicella vaccine, 1916–1917
Chief complaint, 90, 91b
Child abuse and neglect
advocacy for, 1100
apparent life-threatening events, 1830
burns as sign of, 1095, 2822, 2824f
cultural healing practices that can be confused with, 69t
definitions, 1091–1092
description of, 184, 1263–1264
dislocations, 2053
domestic violence and, 1075
evaluation of, 1093–1098
fractures, 2053
health outcomes of, 1098
incidence, 1092–1093
legal issues, 1098–1099
Münchausen syndrome. *See* Münchausen syndrome
parent education, 1093
prevention, 1093, 1100
protective factors, 1093
risk factors, 1093
Child abuse and neglect—cont'd
screening, 1093
sexual
assessment of, 1109–1111
clinical manifestations of, 1107–1109
definition of, 1092, 1106–1107
diagnosis of, 1109–1111
differential diagnosis of, 1111
dissociative disorders and, 1745
epidemiology of, 1106–1107
etiology of, 1107
management and treatment of, 1112
prevention of, 1113
psychosocial consequences, 1112–1113
vaginal bleeding and, 1767
suspicion of, 139–140
treatment, 1099–1100
Child advocacy, 1063
Child Behavior Checklist, 1233
Child care services and programs. *See also* After-school care programs
child health professionals and, 1022–1025
enrollment rates, 1019
family arrangements for, 1018–1019
health risks and promotion opportunities, 1020–1022
parents as advisors and consultants, 1024
prevalence of, 184
psychosocial outcomes, 1019–1020
regulation, accreditation and quality control, 1019
subsidized, 24
Child custody
arrangements, 1053–1054
divorce and, 1057–1059
history, 1053
pediatrician's role in, 1054–1055
Child Find system, 724
Child Health and Illness Profile Adolescent and Child Editions, 1169–1170
Child health supervision
effectiveness of, 49–50
preventive services visit, 48–49
visit for, 50
Child life services, 175
Child life specialists, 173b
Child mortality
age-related, 593, 593t
cardiac arrhythmias and, 1418
causes of, 593, 593t
encopresis and, 1256
Münchausen syndrome and, 1264–1268
prevalence of, 593, 593t
Child neglect. *See* Child abuse and neglect
Childbirth
at-home, 82–83
psychological development and, 1005
skull changes during, 117
vaginal birth after cesarean, 82
Childhood. *See* Early childhood; Late childhood; Middle childhood
Childhood disintegrative disorder, 1197
Childhood traumatic grief, 1288
Childless families, 1040–1041
Children's Cancer Study Group, 2242
Children's Oncology Group, 1863, 1895–1896
Chiropractic, 457–459
Chlamydia, 1342
Chlamydia trachomatis
conjunctivitis caused by, 1705, 1706f
description of, 2510–2511
detection of, 2511
in infants, 120
infection rates, 2510f
newborn eye assessment for, 764
ocular manifestations of, 120
ophthalmia neonatorum, 801–802
in perinatal period, 935
pertussis vs., 2420
sexual abuse and, 1109
symptoms of, 2511, 2512f
treatment of, 2511, 2512b–2513b
in urinary tract infection, 2607
Chloramphenicol
bacterial resistance to, 503
dosage, peak serum concentrations, and MIC_{95} for, 494t
mechanism of action of, 503
meningococcemia treated with, 2749
pharmacologic properties of, 503
Rocky Mountain spotted fever treated with, 2484
side effects of, 503
use of, 503
Chlordiazepoxide, 949
Chlorhexidine, 779
Chloromas, 2234
Chlorpromazine, 555t, 2685t
Choanal atresia, 122
C-hold, for breastfeeding, 815
Cholelithiasis, 1620
Cholera, 1442
Cholestasis, 699, 873, 1622
Cholestatic jaundice, 1618
Cholestatic liver disease, 2118
Cholesteatoma, 122
Cholesterol. *See also* Hypercholesterolemia
cardiovascular health promotion and, 279t
exercise effects on, 190
health effects of, 194–195
high serum levels of, 189, 194–195
low-density lipoprotein, 195
metabolic roles of, 224

Page numbers followed by "f" denote figures; "t" denote tables; "b" *denote* boxes.

Cholesterol—cont'd
screening for
American Academy of Pediatrics on, 281
American Heart Association on, 281
description of, 195
recommendations for, 281b, 281t, 282–283, 282f, 283t, 284f
United States Preventive Services Task Force on, 281
studies of, 194–195
Choline magnesium trisalicylate
acute pain managed using, 428t
chronic pain managed using, 440, 441t
Cholinergic drugs, 2684t, 2768t
Chondrodystrophies, 766–767
Chondromalacia patella, 1628, 2560
Chorea
in rheumatic fever, 2477
tics and, 1760
Chorionic gonadotropin-secreting tumors, 1593
Chorionic villus sampling
fetal assessment, 644–645
first- and second-trimester testing, 604–605
prenatal diagnoses, 604
Choroid plexus cysts
antenatal identification of, 776
ultrasound detection of, 606
Chromosomal anomalies, 623–624
Chromosome analysis
congenital anomaly diagnosis, 794
dysmorphism diagnosis and, 1500
Chronic care model, 45–46
Chronic cough, 2058, 2059t
Chronic disease and illness. *See also* Ongoing health conditions; *specific disease*
activity limitations secondary to, 242, 242t
in adolescents, 1326–1327
anemia and, 1400–1401
breastfeeding effects on prevention of, 810
child care programs, 1022
constipation, 1454
demographic data regarding, 239, 241, 242t
description of, 1137, 1145–1146
early education about, 1022
electronic health record benefits for management of, 32
epidemiologic trends for, 239, 241
in extremely low–birth-weight infants, 856–857
follow-up care checklist, 870
prevalence of, 241, 242t
short stature caused by, 1728
Chronic fatigue syndrome
chronic fatigue vs., 1512
clinical manifestations of, 1920
Chronic fatigue syndrome—cont'd
criteria for, 1512
description of, 1511
differential diagnosis, 1920b
Epstein-Barr virus and, 2178
laboratory evaluations for, 1921
pathogenesis of, 1921, 1921f
prognosis for, 1922
psychological factors, 1920
referrals for, 1922
treatment of, 1921–1922, 1922b
Chronic glomerulonephritis
Alport syndrome, 2291–2292
benign familial hematuria, 2291
description of, 2290
IgA nephropathy, 2290–2291
membranoproliferative glomerulonephritis, 2293–2294
systemic lupus erythematosus, 2292–2293
Chronic immune thrombocytopenic purpura, 2173
Chronic inflammation, 1400–1401
Chronic irritability, 1613–1614
Chronic liver disease, 2110
Chronic lung disease
cerebral palsy with, 855
follow-up care protocols, 877–878
in neonatal intensive care infants, 853, 856–857
Chronic meningoencephalitis, 2037
Chronic myelogenous leukemia, 2240–2241
Chronic osteomyelitis, 2355–2356
Chronic pain
consultation for, 438
definition of, 435
effects on patient and family, 436–437
evaluation of, 437–438
history-taking for, 437
laboratory tests for, 438
management of
acupuncture, 440
algorithm for, 439f
bier block, 445
cognitive-behavioral interventions, 438
description of, 438
discontinuation, 446
implanted devices, 446
interventional therapy, 444–446
intravenous regional block, 445
nonpharmacologic, 438
palliative care, 446
patient care, 443
pharmacologic. *See* Chronic pain, pharmacotherapy for
sympathetic blocks in, 445–446
transcutaneous electrical nerve stimulation in, 439–440
pain specialist referral for, 446
pathophysiologic mechanisms of, 435
Chronic pain—cont'd
pharmacotherapy for, 441t–442t
adjuvant analgesics, 443–444, 445t
alpha agonists, 444
anticonvulsants, 443–444
antidepressants, 444
controlled substances, 443
membrane stabilizers, 444
nonopioid analgesics, 440
opioids, 440–443, 442t
physical examination of, 438–439
prevalence of, 436
referral for, 446
types of, 435–436
Chronic tic disorder, 1760
Churg-Strauss syndrome, 1848
Chvostek sign, 118
Cidofovir, 510t
Cigarette smoking. *See* Smoking
Ciliary body destructive procedures, 1710
Cimetidine
molluscum contagiosum treated with, 2619–2620
warts treated with, 2618
Ciprofloxacin, 2752, 2752t
Circadian rhythms
description of, 1295
sleep disorder involving, 1303–1304
Circulation. *See* Airways, breathing, and circulation
Circulatory transition in newborn, 656
Circumcision
cancer risk and, 829
complications, 829
hygiene issues, 829
in NICU-discharged infants, 722
pain management during, 829
penile cancer and, 829
procedures, 829
rates of, 828
recommendations for, 828–829
sexually transmitted disease and, 830
urinary tract infection and, 829, 2609, 2613
Circumduction gait, 1630
Citrate solution, for renal tubular acidosis, 2473–2474
Civil Rights Act of 1964, 62
Clarithromycin, 502
Classical conditioning, 1004
Claudication, 1490
Clavicle, fractured, 2052
Claw toe, 1530–1531, 1531f
Clawfoot, 1536
Cleanliness, 1806
Cleft lip and palate. *See also* Orofacial cleft
bifid uvula with, 126, 126f
definition of, 1923
embryology
incomplete and complete, 1923, 1924f
normal palatal anatomy, 1923f, 1924f

Cleft lip and palate—cont'd
fetal assessment for, 649–650
genetics of, 1924–1925, 1925t
incidence of, 1924
management of
auditory dysfunction, 1926–1927
cleft palate speech, 1927
feeding, 1925–1926
fetal surgery, 1925
Latham appliance, 1927f
lip and nose revisions, 1927, 1928f–1929f
orthodontics/cleft alveolus, 1929
orthognathic surgery, 1929, 1930f
Pierre Robin sequence, 1929–1930
presurgical orthopedics, 1927
repair, 1927
newborn assessments, 765–766, 792
prenatal evaluation, 1925
referrals for, 1930–1931
risk factors for, 1924–1925, 1925t
ultrasound detection of, 606
Clindamycin
dosage, peak serum concentrations, and MIC_{95} for, 494t
mechanism of action of, 502
pelvic inflammatory disease treated with, 2519b
pharmacologic properties of, 502
resistance to, 502
side effects of, 502–503
staphylococcal TSS treated with, 2566
streptococcal TSS treated with, 2575–2576
use of, 502–503
Clinical Evidence, 39t
Clinical interview, 401
Clinical Practice Guidelines, 39
Clinodactyly, 769–771
Clitoromegaly, 794
Cloacal exstrophy, 2605t
Clonazepam, 2498t, 2500
Clonidine, 2775
Clorazepate, 2500
Clotrimazole, 512t
Clove oil, 458t
Clubfoot
characteristics of, 139, 1531f–1533f, 1532–1534, 1541
newborn assessment, 771
physical examination, 793
ultrasound detection of, 613
Cluster headaches, 1550b
Clutton joints, 1627
Coach Care Center, Inc., 572
Coagulation disorders
description of, 2111
disseminated intravascular coagulation
causes of, 2673b
chronic, 2672
definition of, 2670
description of, 944
differential diagnosis, 2672–2673
Coagulation disorders—cont'd
disseminated intravascular coagulation —cont'd
evaluation of, 2673–2674
incidence of, 2670
management of, 2674b, 2674–2675
pathogenesis of, 2670–2672, 2671f–2672f
hemophilia. *See* Hemophilia
hereditary, 944
von Willebrand disease
anesthesia and, 537
description of, 944, 1484, 2110–2111
petechiae and purpura caused by, 1668
Coagulopathies, 537–538
Coal tar preparations, 2451, 2452t
Coarctation of the aorta
evaluation of, 1952
in infants, 1951f
pressure overload, 925
prognosis for, 1953–1954
surgical management of, 1952–1953, 1953f
Cobalamin, 228t
Cobalamin disease, 987
Cobb syndrome, 781
Cocaine
neonatal drug withdrawal syndrome, 949–950
neonatal health and, 630
overdose of, 2782
Cochlear implants, 332, 332b, 1559
Cochrane Database of Systematic Reviews, 39, 39t
Cockroaches, 1819
Co-coordinator, 52
Codeine, 442t, 2685t
Coding, 24
Coercion, 204
Coffee, 458t
Cognitive behavioral treatment
abdominal pain and, 1382
behavioral and emotional problems, 1171–1172
eating disorders and, 1193
phobias and, 1283
psychostimulants and, 1209–1211
Cognitive development
from 1 to 2 years, 210
concrete operational stage, 1009
formal operational period, 1011
Piaget's theory of, 1002
preoperational period, 1007–1008
sensorimotor period, 1006
Cognitive impairment
definition of, 2184
irritability and, 1614
Cognitive-developmental theory, 1746–1747
Cohort study, 40t
Coin rubbing, 69t
Cold. *See* Common cold
Cold sores, 125
Colic
definitions, 1931–1932
differential diagnosis, 1932
evaluation, 1932
irritability and, 1611
management of, 1932–1933
referrals for, 1933
Collaborative care, 52–53
Collaborative decision-making
bereavement, 738
for neonatal drug withdrawal syndrome, 956
sick and dying infant care, 729–735
Collaborative learning, 47
Collaborative management, 167
Collateral ligament injuries, 2557
Collection of payments, 17
Collodion baby, 13
Coloboma, 764
Colon
contrast enema of, 150
obstruction of, 2082
Colorado intrauterine growth charts, 639–641
Coma. *See also* Mental status alterations
definition, 2639
in drowning injuries, 2680
Glasgow Coma Scale, 2711t, 2711–2712, 2744t
Comedolytics, 1804–1805
Comedonal lesions, 1803, 1803f
Coming out, 1240, 1363
Common cold
causative agents of, 1934t
clinical presentation, 1935
complications of, 1936
differential diagnosis, 1935
epidemiologic features, 1934
etiology, 1934
management of, 1935–1936
pathophysiological features, 1934–1935
Communication
adherence affected by, 163
barriers to, 165–166
clarification during, 95
concerns of patients, 201–202
confrontation during, 95
empathy during, 95
facilitation of, 94–95, 165–166
with family, 52, 2185
follow-up care, 846–847
hindrances to, 95
between hospitalist and primary care physician, 168–170
interpretation during, 95
in interview, 94–95
malpractice avoidance through, 12b
medical-legal issues in, 750
methods of, 169
parent-child arguments, 205
patient safety through, 169
recapitulation of, 95
reflection during, 95
in rehabilitation process, 577

Page numbers followed by "f" denote figures; "t" denote tables; "b" *denote* boxes.

Communication—cont'd
sick and dying infant care and role of, 730
Community health centers, 7
Community pediatrics
accessible medical services, 56
definition of, 55
disease, 55–56
health, 55–57
history of, 55
practical activities to promote, 57–58
sudden infant death syndrome prevention, 56
Community support personnel, 50
Community-based care, 53–54
Community-based organizations, 57–58
Complement system, 1699–1700
Complementary and alternative medicine
abdominal pain managed using, 1382
acupuncture, 459–460
allergies, 461
alternative medical systems, 459–460
attention deficit/hyperactivity disorder managed using, 1215
biologically based therapies, 457
body-based methods, 457–459
categories of, 456–460
chiropractic, 457–459
communication with patients about, 460–462, 461b–462b
counseling of families about, 462–463, 462b
current and past medication assessments, 461
definition of, 456
description of, 455–460
energy therapies, 460
homeopathy, 459–460
manipulative methods, 457–459
massage, 457–459
medical history, 461–462
mind-body medicine, 456–457
osteopathy, 457–459
pediatricians' knowledge about, 456
practitioners of, 463
social history, 460–461, 461b
spina bifida managed using, 2543
spirituality, 461b, 463
Complete heart block, 919–920
Complex carbohydrates, 193–194
Complex partial seizures, 2489b, 2491–2492
Complex vocal tics, 1758
Compliance. *See* Adherence
Complicated grief, 594
Comprehensive Addiction Severity Index, 401
Comprehensive care model, 1017
Comprehensive school health education, 1132
Computed tomography
adrenal hemorrhage evaluations, 1812
altered mental status evaluations, 2642
appendicitis evaluations, 150, 150f, 1837
Computed tomography—cont'd
atlantoaxial instability evaluations, 2021
brain
description of, 152
tumors of, 1862–1863
central nervous system disease evaluations, 2141
cerebral palsy evaluations, 1905
chest evaluations, 148, 148f
cleft palate evaluations, 1929
cystic fibrosis evaluations, 1982
description of, 147
gastrointestinal obstruction evaluations, 2079
growth plate injury evaluations, 2051
head injury evaluations, 2714–2715
helical, 147
hydrocephalus evaluations, 2149
increased intracranial pressure evaluations, 2740–2741, 2741f
limitations of, 147
limp and, 1635
multidetector, 147
musculoskeletal system evaluations, 151
neurofibromatosis type 1 evaluations, 2307
pericarditis evaluations, 1960
pneumothorax evaluations, 2756
retropharyngeal abscess evaluations, 2049
sinus abnormality evaluations, 1935
soft-tissue bleeding evaluations, 2107
solid mass evaluations, 1996
streptococcal toxic shock syndrome evaluations, 2575
tuberculosis evaluations, 2599
Wilms tumors evaluations, 1875
Computed tomography renal angiography, 147, 151, 151f
Computed tomography urography, 147
Computers
description of, 27
diagnostic decision support uses of, 34, 36
Concrete operational stage of cognitive development, 1009
Concussion
description of, 2712, 2712t
irritability and, 1609
preparticipation physical evaluation, 324–325
Condoms
adolescent use of, 2509
female, 1356
male, 1355
Conduct disorder
assessment of, 1221–1224
attention deficit/hyperactivity disorder and, 1204, 1221
description of, 1744
diagnostic criteria of, 1222b–1223b, 1224–1225
etiology of, 1221
Conduct disorder—cont'd
medication for, 1181b
prevalence of, 1221
prevention of, 1224
severity of, 1222–1223, 1223
Conduction abnormalities, 1417–1418, 1418f
Condylomata acuminatum. *See* Genital warts
Confetti lesions, 2311
Confidentiality, 77, 100
Confusion, 2639
Confusional arousals, 1304
Congenital adrenal hyperplasia
anesthesia and, 532
description of, 2195, 2195t
genetic factors, 1809–1811
glucocorticoids for, 1809, 1811, 1813
laboratory evaluation of, 1809
long-term follow-up for, 1811
management of, 1811
newborn screening for, 386
Congenital aganglionosis of the colon, 2079–2080, 2080f
Congenital atrioventricular block, 1418f
Congenital cystic adenomatoid malformation
description of, 914
fetal intervention for, 617
ultrasound detection of, 607–608
Congenital cysts, 1995–1997
Congenital diaphragmatic hernia
description of, 912–914
fetal intervention for, 616–617
ultrasound detection of, 608
Congenital disorders
assisted reproductive technologies and risk of, 623–624
cardiovascular. *See* Congenital heart defects
cataracts, 764
chromosome analysis for, 794
definitions, 788–789
diagnosis of, 790–795
fluorescent in situ hybridization for, 794–795
Goldenhar syndrome, 2547
high-risk delivery management, 654
hyperinsulinism, 974–976
hypoplastic anemia, 943–944
imaging studies for, 795
in infants of diabetic mothers, 890–891
intrauterine growth restriction and, 885
kyphosis, 2546–2547
Larsen syndrome, 2547
lobar emphysema, 914
medical history for, 790–791
melanocytic nevi, 780
metabolic tests for, 794–795
Morquio syndrome, 2547
neonatal care procedures, 789–790
physical examination for, 791–794
respiratory failure in newborns, 905

Congenital disorders—cont'd
rubella syndrome, 786
scoliosis, 2545–2546
spina bifida, 2537–2544
spinal, 2547–2548
Congenital fibrosis syndrome, 1741–1742
Congenital heart defects
aortic stenosis, 1949–1952, 1951f
arrhythmias, 918–921
arteriovenous malformation, 1942–1943
atrial septal defect
clinical manifestations of, 1940
evaluation of, 1940–1941, 1941f–1942f
management of, 1941
prognosis of, 1941–1942
ultrasound detection of, 608–610
atrioventricular septal defects, 1942, 1943f
cardiac transplantation, 1963–1965
cardiomyopathies
arrhythmogenic right-ventricular dysplasia, 1963
dilated, 1960–1962, 1961f
hypertrophic, 1962–1963
left-ventricular noncompaction, 1963
restrictive, 1963
classification of, 130
coarctation of the aorta
evaluation, 1952
in infants, 1951f
pressure overload, 925
prognosis for, 1953–1954
surgical management of, 1952–1953, 1953f
complete mixing lesions or the single-ventricle heart, 1954
congestive heart failure, 921–926
cyanosis, 926–927
Ebstein anomaly, 1946, 1947f
Eisenmenger syndrome, 1943, 1946
embryology, 1937–1938, 1937–1939f
endocarditis, 1957–1958
health outcomes for, 861–862
hemoptysis and, 1570, 1573
hypoplastic left heart syndrome
evaluation of, 1954f–1955f, 1954–1955
management of, 1955–1956
pressure overload, 925–926
prognosis, 1956–1957
ultrasound detection, 906
in infants of diabetic mothers, 891
maternal health and risk of, 630–631
murmurs, 916–918
myocarditis, 1958–1959, 1959f
nutrition management for infants with, 696
partial anomalous pulmonary venous return, 1947
patent ductus arteriosus, 1942
pediatric cardiologist consultation for, 1965–1968

Congenital heart defects—cont'd
pericarditis, 1959–1960
post-delivery screening for, 803–804
prevalence, 916
pulmonary atresia with intact ventricular septum, 1946
pulmonary hypertension, 1943
shunting lesions
intracardiac, 1938–1939
left-to-right, 1939–1943
right-to-left, 1943–1946
sports participation with, 322t
tetralogy of Fallot
cyanosis and, 927
description of, 1943, 1944f
management of, 1944–1946
with pulmonary atresia, 1945–1946
surgical management of, 1945f
syncope and, 1756
ultrasound detection of, 609
without pulmonary atresia, 1944–1945
total anomalous pulmonary venous return, 1946–1947
transposition of the great arteries, 1947–1949, 1949f
tricuspid atresia, 1957
ventricular septal defect
clinical manifestations of, 1940
evaluation of, 1940–1941, 1941f–1942f
management of, 1941
murmur with, 917–918
prognosis of, 1941–1942
ultrasound detection of, 608–610
volume overload, 926
Congenital hepatic fibrosis, 1577
Congenital infections
cytomegalovirus, 929–930
parvovirus B19, 932
rubella virus, 931
syphilis, 931–932
Toxoplasma gondii, 930–931
Congestive heart failure
arrhythmias in, 2723
causes of, 925, 2720–2722
definition of, 2717
nutritional management, 2723–2724
orthopnea in, 129
pathophysiological features, 2717–2718
pharmacotherapy for, 2722–2723, 2723f
recommendations for, 2724t–2725t
scoring systems for, 2719, 2719t–2720t
signs and symptoms of, 132, 2718–2719
surgery for, 2724
tachycardia caused by, 105
Congestive splenomegaly, 1732
Conjugated bilirubin, 1616, 1621
Conjugated hyperbilirubinemia, 1618

Conjunctiva
foreign bodies in, 2347–2348, 2347f
nevi of, 1717, 1717f
pseudomembrane, 1706f
Conjunctivitis
allergic, 1715–1716
bacterial, 1710, 1710f, 1711b
causes of, 1702b, 1704t, 1705–1710
definition of, 1702
evaluation of, 1702–1705, 1703b
features of, 1703t
inflammatory, 1715–1716
in Kawasaki disease, 120, 2220, 2220f
neonatal
causes of, 1703, 1704t, 1705–1710
definition of, 1703
evaluation and treatment of, 1703–1705, 1704b, 1704f
referral for, 1717
systemic disease and, 1716–1717
treatment of, 1702–1705, 1703b
viral, 1711–1715
Connective tissue disorders, 540
Consciousness
altered, 2639–2643
definition, 2639
loss of, 2714
Consent, for abortion, 76
Consortium of Academic Health Centers for Integrative Medicine, 456
Constipation. *See also* Encopresis
abdominal pain in, 2628
causes of, 1426–1427
chronic, 1454
definition of, 1424b, 1424–1425
diagnosis of, 1426b, 1426–1427
in end-of-life care, 598
evaluation of, 1428–1429, 1429b
functional, 1425–1426, 1427t, 1428–1431
Hirschsprung disease comparison, 1427t
idiopathic, 1372–1373
irritability and, 1613–1614
in neonatal intensive care infants, 875–876
in newborn, 842–843
in palliative care, 598
referrals for, 1431
studies and, 1427b
treatment of, 1429–1431, 1431b
Constitutional growth delay, 1727
Constricting bands, for snakebites, 2697
Consultations
chronic pain, 438
collaborative management secondary to, 167
purpose of, 166, 166b
requesting of, 166–167
Consumer Assessment of Health Plan Survey, 44
Consumer-driven health plans, 20–21
Contact dermatitis
allergic, 1974
clinical manifestations, 1975
differential diagnosis, 1974–1975

Contact dermatitis—cont'd
epidemiologic considerations, 1974
illustration of, 1691f
irritant, 1973–1974, 1974f
management of, 1975
prevention, 1975–1976
pruritus and, 1682
referrals for, 1976
Contact stomatitis, 2569–2572
Continence, in spina bifida, 2542–2543
Continuing medical education, 35t, 36
Continuous positive airway pressure
apnea treated with, 687–688
bradycardia treated with, 687–688
bronchopulmonary dysplasia treated with, 688–689
desaturation treated with, 687–688
neonatal infant stabilization, 675–678
Continuous professional development, 36
Contraception/contraceptives
access to, 1351–1352
in acne patients, 1806
adolescent use of, 2509
barrier method, 1355–1356
breastfeeding, 811
condoms. *See* Condoms
description of, 1346–1347
diaphragm, 1355–1356
dysmenorrhea and, 1462
emergency, 1355
hormonal, 1352–1355, 1353t
information sources about, 1117–1120
management of, 1353–1354
rheumatic fever and, 2480
Contraction stress test, 643
Controller therapy, for asthma, 1844
Contusions
cerebral, 2713
quadriceps, 2558
Convergence insufficiency, 1738f
Conversion reactions. *See also* Stress
case reports for, 1227b–1229b
diagnosis of, 1227–1229, 1229–1230
management of, 1230–1231
referrals and, 1231–1232, 1232b
symptoms and, 1226–1227, 1229
Conversions, 34
Convulsive disorder, 323t
Coping
dissociative disorders as mechanisms for, 1745
posttraumatic stress disorder and, 1286–1287
Copper, 227t
Coprolalia, 1758
Copropraxia, 1758
Coral snakes, 2700–2702
Cordocentesis. *See* Percutaneous umbilical blood sampling
Core muscles, 192
Core-binding factor, 2238
Cornea
abrasion of, 120, 2346–2347, 2347f
bee sting to, 2688
Cornea—cont'd
description of, 2343
foreign bodies in, 2347–2348, 2347f
postnatal increases in, 118
subepithelial infiltrates of, 1712f
ulcer of, 1706f
Corneal light reflex test, 1780–1781, 1781f
Cornelia de Lange syndrome, 763, 1726, 2605, 2605t
Coronary arteries, 1756
Coronary artery disease, 2226–2227, 2227b, 2227t
Coronary heart disease
physical inactivity and, 189
screenings for, 195
Coronaviruses, 2648
Corporal punishment, 81–82, 273–274, 1033
Cortical collecting duct, 2462, 2463f
Corticosteroids
acne treated with, 1804
allergic rhinitis treated with, 1821
anaphylaxis treated with, 2645
asthma treated with, 1844, 1845t–1847t, 1847–1848
atopic dermatitis treated with, 1852
croup treated with, 2653
immune thrombocytopenic purpura treated with, 2172
increased intracranial pressure treated with, 2743
infectious mononucleosis treated with, 2175–2177, 2176f, 2177t
inhaled, 1844, 1845t–1846t, 1847–1848
juvenile idiopathic arthritis treated with, 2216b, 2217
Kawasaki disease treated with, 2226
nasal, 1821
nephrotic syndrome treated with, 2300–2301, 2301b
oral, 1844, 1846t–1847t
psoriasis treated with, 2451, 2452t
seborrheic dermatitis treated with, 2487–2488
snakebites treated with, 2700
status asthmaticus treated with, 2816
topical, 2451, 2452t, 2487–2488
toxoplasmosis treated with, 2380
tuberculosis treated with, 2602
Cortisol
deficiency of
diagnosis of, 2736
hyperandrogenism and, 1594
hypoglycemia in, 2735
description of, 1808
Co-sleeping, mother-child, 843
Cosmetics, 1806
Cough
classification of, 1432
in croup, 2635, 2650
diagnosis of, 1433
evaluation of, 1433–1435
family and personal history, 1433
laboratory evaluation of, 1434–1435
Cough—cont'd
neonatal history, 1433–1434
pathophysiological features of, 1432–1433
physical examination for, 1434
referrals for, 1436
treatment of, 1435–1436
whooping, 2419–2425. *See also* Pertussis
Cough suppressants, 1435
Counseling
for at-risk adolescents for violence, 275
gay, lesbian, and bisexual youth and, 1362
learning disabilities and, 1154
substance abuse and, 1247–1248
for teenage drivers, 270
transgender youth and, 1239
Cover test, 1781–1782, 1782f
Cow milk
bacterial contamination of, 226, 229
dietary recommendations, 194
digestibility issues for, 229
human milk vs., 213, 214t, 226, 229
pasteurization of, 229
protein allergy, 1932, 2057, 2065b, 2065–2067
protein content of, 229
supplements added to, 229
COX. *See* Cyclooxygenase
COX-2 inhibitors, 2216, 2216b
Coxa vara, 1529
Coxsackievirus, 2036, 2268, 2268f
Crack, 2782
Crackles, 2632
Cradle cap, 2486, 2486f
Cradle hold for breastfeeding, 814–815
CRAFFT screening tool, 401, 1246b, 1246–1247, 1337b
Cramps, heat, 2551
Cranial nerves, 144
Cranial ultrasonography
neurologic evaluation in NICU-discharged infants, 720–721
newborn screening, 702–703
Craniofacial defects
description of, 2634
ultrasound detection of, 606
Cranioscoliosis, 117
Craniosynostosis, 117, 762–763, 1652
Craniotabes, 117, 762
C-reactive protein, 1527
Creatine supplements, 2551–2552
Creatinine, 2797
Cremasteric reflex, 141f
Cromolyn sodium for asthma, 1848
Cross-cradle/transitional hold for breastfeeding, 815
Crossed extensor reflex, 141f
Crotamiton 10%, 2183
Croup
airways obstruction in, 2634–2635
bacterial, 2635

Croup—cont'd
definition of, 2647–2648
differential diagnosis, 2636t, 2649b, 2649f, 2649–2650
epidemiology of, 2648–2649
etiology of, 2648–2649
evaluation of, 2650–2651, 2651f–2652f, 2652t
hospitalization for, 2653
management of, 2651–2653
membranous, 2635, 2648
postintubation, 557
referral for, 2653
scoring system for, 2652t
seasonal occurrence, 2648f, 2648t, 2648–2649
spasmodic, 2636t, 2648–2649
viral, 2636t, 2647–2653
Crying
end-of-the-day, 1158
in newborn
congenital anomalies and, 792
description of, 758
mouth defects, 765–766
Cryotherapy
description of, 1710
genital warts treated with, 2515b, 2516b
leishmaniasis treated with, 2368
molluscum contagiosum treated with, 2619
snakebites treated with, 2696
warts treated with, 2515b–2516b, 2617
Cryptorchidism, 768–769, 794, 2157–2161
Cryptosporidiosis
causes of, 2375
clinical manifestations of, 2376
description of, 2375
diagnosis of, 2376
epidemiologic features of, 2375
life cycle of, 2375–2376
pathogenesis of, 2375–2376
prevalence of, 2375
prevention of, 2377
transmission of, 2375
treatment of, 2376–2377
Cryptosporidium, 2086, 2142
CT. *See* Computed tomography
Cultural assessment, 157–159
Cultural competence/competency, 63, 70b, 157, 1016
Cultural norms, 157, 159
Culturally effective pediatric health care, 160
Culture
adoption processes and, 1048–1051
behavioral expectations based on, 159
cross-cultural situations, 156b–157b
definition of, 157
dietary practices affected by, 159
ethical issues, 160
family's role based on, 159, 182
folk illnesses, 63, 64t–65t
Culture—cont'd
gender and, 1235–1236
health beliefs and practices based on, 158
health care affected by, 62–63
language barriers, 158
learning disorders and, 1151
media exposure and, 1114–1120
mental health issues, 1016
nonverbal communication, 158
parenting styles based on, 159
perceptual differences among, 159–160
racial background, 158
religious influences, 158
rituals, 158
stereotypical assumptions, 158
Culture, urine, 2610
Cupping, 69t
CureSearch, 1895
Curettage, 2619
Curfew, 1329–1330
Curly toe, 1531f, 1531–1532
Currant jelly stools, 2075
Cushing disease, 1815
Cushing syndrome, 1728, 1815–1816
Cushing triad, 2740
Cutaneous larva migrans, 2389
Cutaneous leishmaniasis, 2366–2367
Cuticle biting, 1725
Cyanide poisoning, 2685t, 2766t
Cyanosis, 904, 926–927
Cyanotic breath-holding spells, 1657
Cyanotic heart disease, 1948, 1966
Cyberphysiology, 448
Cyclic vomiting, 1783, 2057
Cyclooxygenase
chronic pain managed using, 440, 441t
moderate-to-severe acute pain managed using, 427–428
Cyclospora cayetanensis, 2377–2378
Cyclosporiasis, 2377–2378
Cyclosporine, 2453–2454, 2453t
Cyclothymic disorders, 1259b
Cyproheptadine, 1554
Cyst(s)
brachial cleft, 766, 782, 1996
cavernous hemangiomas, 1997
choroid plexus
antenatal identification of, 776
ultrasound detection of, 606
cystic hygromas, 1996–1997
definitions, 1995
description of, 1690, 1995
differential diagnosis, 1995
enteric (vitelline), 2605–2606
epidermoid, 1997
epithelial, 1373
evaluation, 1995–1996
management of, 1997
neck masses, solid, 1997
ovarian, 777
preauricular, 1997
referrals for, 1997–1998
Cyst(s)—cont'd
sites of, 1995f
thyroglossal duct, 1996
urachal, 2605
Cystic acne, 1802–1805, 1807
Cystic adenomatoid malformation
description of, 914
fetal intervention for, 617
ultrasound detection of, 607–608
Cystic fibrosis
abdominal pain in, 2628
anesthesia and, 526
BMI percentile, 1983f
clinical manifestations
body fluids, 1984
gastrointestinal tract, 1982–1984
infection, 1982
lower respiratory tract, 1982
pancreas, 1984
puberty, 1984–1985
skeletal complications, 1984
upper respiratory tract, 1982
description of, 1427
diabetes mellitus secondary to, 1984
differential diagnosis, 1985
evaluation of
abdomen, 1986
chest, 1985–1986
diabetes patients, 1987f
extremities, 1986
genitourinary tract, 1986
growth parameters, 1985
head and neck, 1985
heart, 1986
imaging, 1988–1989
lungs, 1985–1986
microbiological assessment, 1988, 1988f
newborn screening, 1986
patients with established diagnosis of cystic fibrosis, 1987–1988
relevant history, 1985
spirometry, 1988, 1988f
sweat testing and genotype analysis, 1986
vital signs, 1985
evolution of, 1983f
hemoptysis and, 1570, 1572
incidence of, 1982
liver disease caused by, 1984, 1991
management of
gastrointestinal therapy, 1990–1991
pulmonary therapy, 1989–1990
vitamin supplementation, 1990–1991, 1991t
pathophysiological features, 1982
referrals for, 1991
screening for, 386, 702
summary, 1991
weight loss and, 1787
Cystic Fibrosis Foundation, 1988
Cystic hygroma, 606–607, 1996–1997
Cysticercal encephalitis, 2396

Page numbers followed by "f" denote figures; "t" denote tables; "b" *denote* boxes.

Cysticercosis
clinical manifestations of, 2396
description of, 2396
diagnosis of, 2396–2397
epidemiologic features of, 2395
extraneural, 2396
life cycle of, 2395–2396
seizures and, 2397
treatment of, 2397
Cystitis, 2607, 2613
Cytogenetic markers, 2237–2238, 2237t
Cytomegalic inclusion disease, 635–636
Cytomegalovirus
breastfeeding and, 812–813
congenital infection, 929–930
maternal-fetal infection, 635–636

D

Dacryocystitis, 1703
Dacryocystocele, 1707
Dance sign, 2075
Dancing eyes-dancing feet (opsoclonus-myoclonus) syndrome, 2037
Dandelion, 458t
Dandy Walker syndrome, 618, 2151
Data norms, 29t, 31
Data sets, 14
Database of Abstracts of Reviews of Effects, 39t
Date rape, 2782, 2790–2791
Dating violence, 1076–1077, 1079
Daydreaming, 1745
Day-night reversal, 1299
Daytime enuresis, 2040–2043
DDH. *See* Developmental dysplasia of the hip
De Lange syndrome, 1653
Death. *See also* Mortality
childhood
age-related, 593, 593t
causes of, 593, 593t
leading causes, 239, 240t
prevalence of, 593, 593t
due to poisoning, 2762–2763, 2763t
in heart failure, 2719
of infant, management protocols for, 733
leading causes of
in adolescents, 239, 240t–241t
in children, 239, 240t
in infants, 238
statistics regarding, 238–239
sudden infant death syndrome, 2579–2581
Debranching-enzyme deficiency, 979
DEC, 2392–2393
Decision making
by child, 75
ethical guidelines, 74–75
by family, 171–172
sexual, 1240, 1364
shared, 49
Decision support
diagnostic systems, 34, 36
electronic health record used for, 30t, 32
Decongestants
allergic rhinitis treated with, 1821
cough treated with, 1435
Decontamination, after poisoning, 2768–2770
DEET. *See* Diethyltoluamide
Defensins, 2609
Defensive medicine, 11
Deferasirox, 2100–2101
Deformation
defined, 789
definition of, 1496
Dehydration
complications of, 2661
degree of, 2656t
in diabetic ketoacidosis, 2664
etiology of, 2654–2655, 2655b, 2655t
evaluation of, 2655–2657, 2656t
fluid and electrolyte deficits in, 2657t
fluid therapy for, 2657–2661, 2658t–2660t
folk illness remedies associated with, 67t
in gastroenteritis, 2654–2655
hospitalization for, 2661
in infants, 1786
management of, 479t, 480, 2658–2661, 2659t–2660t
prognosis, 2661
signs and symptoms of, 473–474, 473t, 2805t
vomiting secondary to, 1785
Dehydroepiandrosterone, 1808, 1814–1815
Dehydroepiandrosterone sulfate, 1803, 1815
Delayed hemolytic transfusion reaction, 487
Delayed maturity, 2470–2471
Delayed puberty
causes of, 1685b
description of, 1684–1685
diagnostic testing for, 1686b
referral for, 1687
Delayed settling, 1299–1300
Delayed-onset hearing loss, 719
Delirium, 556, 2639
Delivery room management. *See also* Childbirth
intrauterine growth restriction, 884–885
large-for-gestational-age infants, 889
medical-legal considerations, 743–744
perinatal stabilization and health, 653–666, 800–807
acute fetal hypoxia/asphyxia, 656–658
airways obstruction, 656
apnea/hypopnea causes, 656
Delivery room management—cont'd
perinatal stabilization and health—cont'd
assessment protocol, 665
breastfeeding, 801
congenital heart defect screening, 803–804
delivery room resuscitation, 658–659
developmental dysplasia screening, 805
disposition, 665
eye care, 801–802
glucose screening, 803
hearing screening, 805
hepatitis B virus vaccine and screening, 806–807
high-risk deliveries, 654
HIV transmission prevention, 804–805
inadequate circulatory transition, 656
initial postnatal evaluation and intervention, 659–663
neonatal resuscitation, 655, 665–666
newborn blood-spot screening, 804
physical examinations, 803–807
postresuscitation assessment and stabilization, 663–664
transitional cardiorespiratory physiology, 654–656
umbilical cord, 664–665, 805
vitamin-K prophylaxis, 802
physical assessment of newborn, 757–773
risk minimization strategies, 743
Demographic profiles
births, 235–238
chronic illness, 239, 241–242, 242t
deaths, 238–239
dependency ratio, 233
disability, 239, 241
diversity, 234
family, 234
future population projections, 235
life expectancy, 239
minorities, 234, 234f
multiple births, 236
poverty, 234–235
prenatal care, 236
preterm births, 238
race, 234f
socioeconomic status, 234–235
teenage pregnancies, 235–236, 236t
in United States, 233–235
vital statistics, 235t
Dental abscess, 125
Dental caries. *See* Caries
Dental fluorosis, 294–295
Dental health
maternal health and, 630
natal teeth, newborn assessment, 765–766
in premature infants, 857

Dental stains
coloration, 1438–1439t
extrinsic stains, 1437
intrinsic stains, 1147–1148
management of, 1438
Dentistry
antimicrobial prophylaxis for procedures in, 508t–509t, 508–509
description of, 6
Dentition. *See* Teeth
Dependency ratio
definition of, 233
elderly, 235
future projections for, 235
Depigmentation disorders, 779
Depo-medroxyprogesterone acetate, 1354–1355
Depression. *See also* Mood disorders
adolescents and, 1313–1315
attention deficit/hyperactivity disorder and, 1204
children and, 1260, 1308–1309
description of, 1745
family history and, 1260
insomnia caused by, 1308
maternal
attachment issues secondary to, 181
caregiver questioning about, 180t
causes of, 365, 365b
definition of, 365
effects on children, 365–366, 366b
prevalence of, 365
risk factors for, 184, 185t
screening for
questions in, 367b–368b
rationale for, 365
strategies in, 366
tools in, 366–369, 367b–368b
signs and symptoms of, 365, 365b
medication for, 1181b
postpartum
attachment issues secondary to, 181
caregiver questioning about, 180t
clinical features of, 185t
description of, 1172
incidence of, 184, 185t
onset of, 184–185
risk factors for, 184, 185t
tics and, 1762
in women, 365
Depressive disorders, 1256–1261
Depth perception, 1776
Dermabrasion, 1807
Dermatitis
atopic
clinical manifestations of, 1851
definition, 1850
diagnostic criteria for, 1851, 1851b
differential diagnosis, 1851
Dermatitis—cont'd
atopic—cont'd
epidemiology of, 1850–1851
etiology, 1850
laboratory evaluations, 1851–1852
management of, 1852
prevention of, 1852–1853
pruritus and, 1681–1682
referrals for, 1853
contact
allergic, 1974
clinical manifestations of, 1975
differential diagnosis, 1974–1975
epidemiology of, 1974
illustration of, 1691f
irritant, 1973–1974, 1974f
management of, 1975
prevention, 1975–1976
pruritus and, 1682
referrals for, 1976
diaper, 2487, 2487f
seborrheic
causes of, 2486
description of, 2485
differential diagnosis of, 2486–2487, 2487f
evaluation of, 2486, 2486f
incidence of, 2485
prognosis of, 2488
treatment of, 2487–2488
Dermatogenic torticollis, 1765
Dermatoglyphics, 116
Dermatomal distribution, 1692f
Dermatophytes, 1663
Dermoid cysts, 783
Desaturation syndromes
neonatal management of, 685–688
NICU-discharged infants, 715
Desferrioxamine, 2777
Desmopressin, 2043
Development. *See* Growth and development
Developmental delays
children and, 1143
definition of, 2184
early intervention for, 346–349, 347b
follow-up for, 347, 347b
identification of, 346–349
management of, barriers to, 347–348
overidentification concerns, 347–348
primary care physician's role in, 346–348
sleep-related problems, 1309
Developmental disabilities
early identification and intervention for, 350
prevalence of, 349
screening for, 349–354
Developmental disorders
early recognition of, 184
parental support, 184
prevalence of, 184
strange behavior and, 1742
Developmental dysplasia of the hip
characteristics of, 2052–2053
limp and, 1632–1633, 1633f, 1635–1636
metatarsus adductus and, 1534
newborn assessment, 771
Ortolani maneuver, 138, 138f
screening for, 805
Developmental surveillance, 315
Developmentally supportive care, 705–706
Dexamethasone, 1813
Diabetes mellitus
anesthesia
considerations for, 529–532, 530t, 531f, 533f
insulin regimen in preoperative period, 530–531, 530t, 531f, 533f
breastfeeding and, 810
complications of
celiac disease, 2007
diabetic nephropathy, 2006
diabetic retinopathy, 2006
hyperlipidemia, 2006–2007
hypoglycemia, 2006
thyroid disease, 2007
Diabetes Control and Complications Trial, 2001, 2005–2006
differential diagnosis of, 2000
evaluation of, 2000–2001
fatigue caused by, 1510
glycemic control guidelines, 2002
hyperglycemia in, 2000b
incidence of, 1998
infants of mothers with, 888–892
insulin
continuous subcutaneous insulin injection program, 2004
exercise, 2005
illness, 2005
meal plan, 2004–2005
monitoring and adjusting, 2004
multiple daily injection program, 2003–2004
onset of, 2003t
split-mixed program, 2003
insulin-dependent, 1998–1999, 2001–2002
management of, 2001–2002. *See also* American Diabetes Association
maternal, 631, 888–892
maturity-onset diabetes of the young, 1999–2000
referrals for, 2007
self-hypnosis for, 453
sports participation with, 322t
type 1, 1998–2002
complications of,
diabetic ketoacidosis, 2662-2663, 2663b
hyperlipidemia, 2006,2007
thyroid diseases, 2007

Diabetes mellitus—cont'd
type 1—cont'd
diagnosis of, 2000, 2000b
incidence of, 2000, 2003t
insulin
bolus, 2003, 2003t
duration of action, 2003t
insulin-dependent, 1998-1999, 2001-2002
weight loss and, 1788
type 2, 1999-2002
diabetic ketoacidosis, 2662-2663
screening, 1999
Diabetes Prevention Program, 2002
Diabetic ketoacidosis
assessment of, 2665, 2665t
complications of, 2667, 2667b
definition of, 2663
description of, 1837, 1984, 2001
differential diagnosis of, 2663
electrolyte therapy in, 2666–2667
evaluation of, 2663–2665
factors associated with, 2663b
fluid and electrolyte deficits in, 2664t
fluid replacement in, 2665–2666
hospitalization for, 2668
insulin therapy in, 2666–2667
management of, 2665
prevention of, 2668
referrals for, 2668
risk factors for, 2662–2663, 2663b
Diagnosis. *See also specific diagnosis*
disclosure to parents and patients, 153–156
inconclusive determination, 1274
validity of, 1202, 1273b
Diagnosis-related groups, 2
Diagnostic and Statistical Manual for Primary Care, 1163–1164, 1207
Diagnostic and Statistical Manual of Mental Disorders
on maternal depression, 365
Primary Care Version (DSM-IV-PC), 358–359
on psychosocial dysfunction, 358
shortcomings of, 186
on substance abuse and dependence, 399–400
Diagnostic Classification of Mental Health and Developmental Disorders of Infancy and Early Childhood, 186
Diagnostic decision support systems, 34, 36
Diagnostic test study, 40t
Diamond-Black anemia, 943–944
Diaper dermatitis, 2487, 2487f
candidal, 2487, 2487f
Diaper rash
differential diagnosis of, 2013
etiology of, 2010
Diaper rash—cont'd
history-taking, 2011
laboratory evaluation for, 2013
less common conditions associated with, 2013t
management of, 2013–2014
pathologic studies, 2011, 2011f
physical examination for, 2011–2013, 2012f
prevention of, 2014–2015
referrals for, 2015
Diaphragm, 1355–1356
Diaphyseal stress injuries, 2552–2553
Diaphysis, 2553t
Diarrhea
acute
description of, 1443, 1443b, 1445b
evaluation of, 1444–1445, 1445b
treatment of, 1445–1447
adrenal insufficiency and, 1808, 1813, 1837
anuria and, 1826–1827
appendicitis and, 1837
celiac disease and, 2020, 2090, 2092–2093
chronic, 144–1454, 1448b
in common cold, 1935
definition of, 1440
dehydration in, 2654–2655
diaper rash and, 2011, 2011f
enteroviral illness and, 2034, 2036
eosinophilic gastrointestinal disorders and, 2067–2068
exudative, 1443
factitious, 1451
gastrointestinal obstruction and, 2075
Giardia intestinalis, 2084–2086
hemolytic-uremic syndrome and, 2094–2096
HIV-infected children with, 2140–2142
hormone-related, 1452
medication for, 1446b
milk protein intolerance and, 1932, 2057, 2065
motility, 1443
neuroblastoma and, 1877
oliguria and, 1826, 1827
osmotic, 1441–1442
oxybutynin-related, 2043
pathophysiological factors of, 1441–1443
protracted, 1448–1449
referrals for, 1454
scarlet fever and, 1981
secretory, 1442–1443
sports participation with, 322t
toxic epidermal necrolysis and, 2031
transplantation rejection and, 1968
Diastematomyelia, 2547
Diastole, 1561
Diastolic blood pressure, 1585
Diastolic murmurs, 1563t, 1564, 1564f
Diazepam
abuse of, 2782
seizures treated with, 2500, 2743
status epilepticus treated with, 2820b
Diazoxide
hyperinsulinism treated with, 2737
hypertensive emergency treated with, 2729, 2729t
Dicloxacillin, 493t
Diencephalic syndrome, 1862
Diet
acne and, 1806
adolescent, 219
American Heart Association recommendations, 219, 281t
atopic dermatitis managed using, 1852
calories, 193–194, 194t
carbohydrates, 193–194
cardiovascular health promotion and, 279t
cultural variations in, 159
dental caries and, 293–294, 296, 296f
fats, 194
genetic-metabolic diseases screening uses of, 376
gluten-free, 2090, 2092–2093
healthy, 193–195
hypertension and, 1588
insulin meal plan, 2004–2005
ketogenic, 2502
obesity prevention through modifications in, 2327b, 2328
protein, 194, 222–223
for school-aged child, 219
USDA recommendations, 193
well-balanced, 231
yo-yo, 193
Dietary Supplement Health and Education Act of 1994, 457
Dietary supplements, 825–827
Diethyltoluamide, 2180–2181, 2776
Difficult temperament, 1746
Diffuse axonal injury, 2713
Diffuse mesangial sclerosis, 2300
Diffuse pulmonary hemorrhage, 1571
Digibind, 2774
Digit abnormalities
newborn assessment, 769–771
physical examination, 793
supernumerary digits, 783
Digoxin
antidote for, 2766t
heart failure treated with, 2722
overdose of, 2774
Dihydroergotamine, 1553
Diisopropyl iminodiacetic acid, 147
Dilated cardiomyopathy, 1960–1962, 1961f
Dilated pouch in esophageal atresia, 2076, 2078f
Dill, 458t
Diphenhydramine, 555t

Diphtheria, tetanus, and pertussis
in adolescents, 246f
adverse reactions to, 252
catch-up schedule for, 250t
characteristics of, 252
contraindications, 252
description of, 2650
guidelines for, 245f
Diphtheria toxoids, 2423b
Diphyllobothriasis, 2399–2400
Diphyllobothrium latum, 2399–2400
Diplopia, 1733–1734
Dipstick test, for urine screening, 1676
Direct bilirubin, 1616, 1621. *See also* Conjugated bilirubin
Direct current synchronized cardioversion, 1414
Direct fluorescent antibody testing, 2421
Direct questions, 94
Directional distortion, 1150
Directory of State Title V CSHCN Programs, 584
Disability
cultural differences in beliefs and perceptions about, 158
definition of, 574
developmental. *See* Developmental disabilities
intellectual. *See* Intellectual disability
Disaccharides, 224
Discharge instructions, 174b
Discharge planning
attention to, 173–174
considerations for, 174b
family involvement in, 174–175
follow-up appointments, 174, 174b
healthy newborns, 840–847, 849–850
neonatal intensive care patients, 709–726, 868
Child Find and early intervention, 724
circumcision, 722
feeding and nutrition, 709–712
follow-up care, 721–722, 726
hearing screening, 718–720
immunizations, 717–718
insurance coverage, 722–723
laboratory studies, 722
neurologic evaluation, 720–721
parent education, 723
prescriptions and medication administration, 724
respiratory management, 713–717
retinopathy of prematurity screening, 720–721
safety issues, 723–724
screening procedures, 720–721
social services and case management, 722
summary and checklist, 724–726
temperature regulation, 712–713
patient education, 174
primary care physician's role in, 173–175
Discharge planning—cont'd
roles and resources necessary for, 173, 173b
Discharge summaries, 174b
Discharge teaching, 174b
Discipline
corporal punishment for, 81–82
description of, 10–11
history-taking about, 92b
principles of, 1029–1035
time-outs vs. spanking, 82
Discomfort, 14t, 15
Disease. *See also specific disease*
chronic. *See* Chronic disease
community dimensions of, 55–56
detection of, 49
health care focus on, 12, 14
Disease prevention, 49
Disimpaction, 1430, 1430t
Disk space inflammation, 2549
Diskitis, 1407, 1409, 1627, 2549
Dislocation
patellar, 2559
shoulder, 2559–2560
Disruption, 789
Disseminated gonococcal infection, 2514b, 2521, 2523f
Disseminated intravascular coagulation
causes of, 2673b
chronic, 2672
definition of, 2670
description of, 944
differential diagnosis, 2672–2673
evaluation of, 2673–2674
incidence of, 2670
management of, 2674b, 2674–2675
pathogenesis of, 2670–2672, 2671f–2672f
Dissociative disorders, 1744–1745
Distal airways obstruction, 1790
Distal catheter, 2150–2151
Distribution system (of lacrimal system), 1707f
Distributive shock, 2804f, 2806
Diuretics
heart failure treated with, 2722
hypertension and, 1587t
increased intracranial pressure treated with, 2743
Diurnal enuresis, 2040–2043
Divalproex, 1261–1262
Diving reflex, 2678
Divorce
custody issues, 1058
family changes, 1056
pediatrician's role, 1059
preventive intervention, 1059
psychological impact on children, 1056–1057
remarriage after, 1058–1059
stages of, 1055
stepfamilies, 1058–1059
tasks for parents and children, 1057–1058
Dizziness
attention deficit/hyperactivity disorder and, 1212t
causes of, 1457
conversion reactions and, 1226
definition of, 1457
diagnosis of, 1458f, 1460t
evaluation of, 1459
management of, 1459–1460
referrals for, 1460
DMSA scan, 2611–2612
DNA analysis, 1500
DNA testing, 1606
Dobutamine
heart failure treated with, 2722
shock treated with, 2811
Documentation
child abuse and neglect, 1098–1099
delivery room, 743–744
malpractice avoidance through, 12b
medicolegal issues, 750–751
neonatal assessment and stabilization, 665
sexual abuse, 1111
Dog bites, 1822, 1823, 1824
Domestic violence. *See also* Child abuse and neglect; Sexual abuse
assessment of, 1077–1078
breaking cycle of, 1080
child abuse and, 1075
dating violence, 1076–1077
definition of, 1074–1075
detection of, 1079
health care system and, 1075–1076
statistics regarding, 1074–1075
treatment of, 1079–1080
victims
assistance for, 1078–1079
identification of, 1076
witnessing of, 272
Do-not-resuscitate orders, 2680
Dopamine
heart failure treated with, 2722
shock treated with, 2807, 2810–2811
Dopamine antagonists, 1553
Dopamine receptor agonists, 1588t
Dopaminergic drugs, 1759
Dornase alfa, 1989–1990
Double aortic arch, 148f
Double bubble sign, 777
Double duodenal bulb appearance, 2078
Double elevator palsy, 1741
Down syndrome
adolescents with, 2022b, 2022–2023
anesthesia and, 538–539, 539f
cystic hygroma, 607
diagnosis of, 792, 2017
facial characteristics associated with, 118
features of, 2017f, 2189t
ß-human chorionic gonadotropin, 604
hypotonia and, 1604
incidence, 2016
infants with, 2019b, 2019–2020

Page numbers followed by "f" denote figures; "t" denote tables; "b" *denote* boxes.

Down syndrome—cont'd
leukemia and, 2232
management of, 2018, 2020–2023
microcephaly and, 1653
newborns with
description of, 2018, 2018b
eye assessments, 764
screening for, 389
preschool-age child with, 2020b, 2020–2021
referrals for, 2024–2025
school-age child with, 2020–2021, 2022b
simian line associated with, 116
trisomy 21 defect in
free, origin of, 2016
molecular pathological features of, 2016–2017
translocation, origin of, 2016–2017
young adults with, 2023–2024, 2024b
Doxepin, 445t
Doxycycline
acne treated with, 1805
Chlamydia treated with, 2512b
epididymitis treated with, 2520b
Lyme disease treated with, 2250–2251, 2251t
pelvic inflammatory disease treated with, 2519b–2520b
proctitis treated with, 2520b
Rocky Mountain spotted fever treated with, 2484
Drainage, postoperative, 559
Drawings, 100
Drop attacks, 2489, 2489b
Droperidol, 555t
Drowning
central nervous system effects of, 2678, 2680
clinical features of, 2677–2678
definition of, 2676
epidemiology of, 2677
family consultations in, 2680
fluid aspiration in, 2677
hemodynamic effects of, 2678
management of, 2678–2680
multisystem organ effects of, 2678
near, 2676
prevention of, 2680, 2681b
prognosis of, 2676–2677, 2680
pulmonary effects of, 2677
Drug(s). *See also* Psychopharmacology therapy; *specific drug*
abdominal pain managed using, 1382
abortion, 1356–1357
adherence issues, 164
administration of
apnea, 686–688
bradycardia, 686–688
breastfeeding and, 813, 824–825
bronchopulmonary dysplasia, 689–690
desaturation, 686–688
maternal-fetal transport, 629–630
Drug(s)—cont'd
administration of—cont'd
neonatal resuscitation, 662
in NICU-discharged infants, 724
in adolescents, 1335t, 1337
anaphylactic reactions to, 2643, 2644
anesthesia and, 541, 542t
chronic pain managed using, 440–444, 441t–442t
concentration of, 490
date rape, 2782, 2790
description of, 1177
electronic health record used for prescribing of, 29t, 31
family involvement with, 1182
financial resources and, 1177–1179
hepatitis induced by, 2117
history-taking about, 92b
illicit. *See* Substance abuse
irritability and, 1612–1613
laxatives, 1253
mental status alterations and, 2640b
misuse of, 14
nonadherence to, 164
postoperative nausea and vomiting effects on, 556
prescribing of, 29t, 31
psychoactive, 1181b
safety concerns, 1180, 1209–1211, 1213t
in schools, 1130, 1178–1179
side effects of, 1180, 1209–1211, 1213t
skin eruptions caused by
allergic skin reactions, 2027t
drug rash with eosinophilia and systemic symptoms, 2029
erythema multiforme, 2029–2030
management of, 2028
morbilliform (measles-like) eruptions, 2027–2028
referrals for, 2031
Stevens-Johnson syndrome, 2030–2031, 2031t
toxic epidermal necrolysis, 2030–2031, 2031t
urticaria (drug-induced hives), 2028
sleep affected by, 1309
stimulants, 1209–1211
training and, 1177
trial periods for, 1180
washout period and, 1180–1182
weight-based dosages, 31
Drug abuse. *See also* Substance abuse
in athletes, 2551–2552
breastfeeding and, 813
in Down syndrome patients, 2022
dyspnea caused by, 1472
fatigue caused by, 1511
foster care for children from, 1061–1062
hallucinogens, 2781–2782
inhalants, 2782
marijuana, 2779, 2781
maternal health and, 629–630
Drug abuse—cont'd
media images and, 1115–1120
neonatal drug withdrawal. *See* Drug withdrawal in neonates
opioids, 2783
sedative-hypnotics, 2782–2783
stimulants, 2782
Drug overdose
antidotes for, 2684t–2685t, 2766t–2768t
assessment of, 2682–2683
complications, 2684–2686
definition of, 2682
differential diagnosis, 2683
epidemiology of, 2682
etiology of, 2682, 2682t
gastric decontamination in, 2683
hallucinogens, 2781–2782
hospitalization for, 2686
inhalants, 2782
life support procedures, 2682–2683
management of, 2683b, 2683–2686
marijuana, 2779, 2781
opioids, 2783
referrals for, 2686
sedative-hypnotics, 2782–2783
stabilization procedures, 2682–2683
stimulants, 2782
Drug rash, 2029
Drug testing, 76–77
Drug withdrawal in neonates
assessment of, 672
breastfeeding, 956
cardiorespiratory signs, 953
caregiver decision making regarding, 956
central nervous system effects, 952–953
complications of, 956
cutaneous signs, 953
diagnosis of, 953
differential diagnosis of, 953
duration of, 951–952
gastrointestinal signs, 953
hypnosedatives, 948–949
incidence of, 947
narcotics, 947–948
nonnarcotic drugs, 953
onset of, 951–952
pathophysiology, 947
severity of, 954
social/protective service referral and follow-up, 957
stimulants, 949–951
supportive treatment, 954–956
Dry bed training, 2043
DS. *See* Down syndrome
DSM-IV-TR, 1282
Duane syndrome, 1739f–1740f, 1739–1740, 1740b
DUB. *See* Dysfunctional uterine bleeding
Dubin-Johnson syndrome, 1621
Duchenne muscular dystrophy
characteristics of, 2274t
clinical presentation of, 2273, 2274t, 2276, 2276f–2277f, 2278t, 2280

Duchenne muscular dystrophy—cont'd
complications of, 2278t
definition of, 2273
diagnostic tests for, 2274t, 2277f
differential diagnosis of, 2273, 2274t, 2276, 2276f–2277f, 2278t, 2280
evaluation of, 2280
genetics of, 2273, 2274t
hypotonia and, 1607
incidence of, 2274t
prednisone for, 2281
supportive care for, 2280–2281
symptoms of, 2274t
treatment of, 2278t, 2280–2281
Duct tape, 2619
Ductus arteriosus
in airways obstruction, 2636
in congestive heart failure, 2721
Duodenal atresia
description of, 2076, 2079f
postnatal evaluation, 777
ultrasound detection of, 610–611
Duodenal obstructions, 2081
Duplication cysts, 2078
Durable medical equipment
description of, 579
discharge planning of, 174b
in rehabilitation process, 579–580
Dust mites, 1819
Dxplain, 35t
Dysfunctional uterine bleeding, 1768, 1769
Dysfunctional voiding, 1477
Dysmenorrhea
primary, 1461–1462
referrals for, 1463
secondary, 1462
Dysmorphism, facial
body, 1499–1500
causes of, 1498t
craniofacial features, 1498–1499
definition of, 1496
description of, 1727
diagnosis of, 1497b, 1500–1501
growth, 1498
history-taking, 1497–1498
laboratory evaluation for, 1500
physical examination for, 1498–1500
proportions, 1498
Dysphagia
causes of, 1463–1464, 1464b
clinical manifestation of, 1464–1465
diagnostic studies of, 1465–1466
evaluation of, 1465–1466
imaging studies for, 1465
laboratory studies for, 1465
management of, 1466–1467
physical examination for, 1465
referrals for, 1467
symptoms of, 1465b
Dysphoric mood, 1212t
Dysplasia
bronchopulmonary
anesthesia and, 524–525
management of, 688–690
Dysplasia—cont'd
bronchopulmonary—cont'd
neonatal intensive care infants with follow-up care protocols, 877–878
incidence of, 853–858
nutrition management for, 696
hip. *See* Developmental dysplasia of the hip; Hip dysplasia
Dyspnea
clinical evaluation of, 1468–1469, 1469b
clinical presentation of, 1469–1472
definition of, 1466–1467
in end-of-life care, 598
etiology of, 1469–1472
history-taking, 1468
management of, 598, 1472–1473
in palliative care, 598
pathophysiological features of, 1468
psychogenetic causes of, 1472
referrals for, 1473
Dysrhythmia, 322t
Dysthymic disorders, 1258b
Dystonic torticollis, 1765
Dystrophica myotonia, 2281–2283, 2282t
Dystrophy. *See* Muscular dystrophy
Dysuria
adolescents with, 1476f
associated symptoms, 1474–1475
causes of, 1474b, 1477–1478
folk illness remedies associated with, 66t
physical examination for, 1464–1467
prepubertal children with, 1475f

E

E2A/PBX gene, 2237
Ear(s)
congenital anomalies, 792
ear pits, 783
of infants, 121–122
infection of. *See* Otitis media
newborn assessment, 764–765
of newborns, 120–121
physical examination of, 120–122
review of systems for, 92b
swimmer's, 2364
Early adolescence, 211
Early and Periodic Screening, Diagnosis, and Treatment program
description of, 23–24, 50
in home health care funding, 572
Early childhood. *See also* Infant(s); Neonate(s); Newborn(s)
abdomen examination in, 133–134
blood pressure in, 107t, 109t
chest examination, 129–130
developmental tasks, 210–211
ear examination, 121–122
eye examination, 120
genitalia examination in, 136
heart examination in, 131–132
heart rate in, 106t
Early childhood—cont'd
lung examination, 129–130
neonatal intensive care unit infants, follow-up care, 870–871
nervous system examination in, 145
nose examination, 123
respiratory rate in, 106
Early education programs. *See also* After-school care programs
child health professionals and, 1022–1025
enrollment rates, 1019
family arrangements for, 1018–1019
health risks and promotion opportunities, 1020–1022
parents as advisors and consultants, 1024
psychosocial outcomes, 1019–1020
regulation, accreditation and quality control, 1019
East African cultural practices, 159
Eating disorders, 1788. *See also* Anorexia nervosa; Bulimia nervosa
in adolescents, 1745–1746
collaborative care, 1191
complications of, 1189b
definition of, 1186, 1187
diagnosis of, 1187b, 1188–1191
dietary plan for, 1191–1192
etiology of, 1187
fitness concerns in patients with, 193
high-risk groups for, 193
in infants, 1743
laboratory evaluations and, 1190
manifestations of, 1188
media images and, 1118
monitoring of, 193
multimodal therapy, 1191
prevention of, 1194
prognosis for, 1193–1194
rehabilitation for, 1191
sports participation with, 322t
in young children, 1743
Ebstein anomaly, 921, 1946, 1947f
EBV. *See* Epstein-Barr virus
Eccrine bromhidrosis, 1662–1663
ECG. *See* Electrocardiogram
Echinacea
preoperative discontinuation of, 542t
uses of, 458t
Echinococcal disease
causes of, 2397–2398
clinical manifestations of, 2398–2399
description of, 2397
diagnosis of, 2399
epidemiologic features of, 2397–2398
life cycle of, 2398
treatment of, 2399
Echinococcus sp.
E granulosus, 2398–2399
E multilocularis, 2399
E oligarthrus, 2399
E vugeli, 2399
hydatid disease caused by, 2397

Page numbers followed by "f" denote figures; "t" denote tables; "b" *denote* boxes.

Echocardiogram
aortic stenosis evaluations, 1950, 1952
apparent life-threatening events evaluations, 1832
arrhythmogenic right-ventricular dysplasia evaluations, 1963
atrial septal defect evaluations, 1940
atypical Kawasaki disease evaluated using, 2224b
cardiovascular screening using, 338–340
coarctation of the aorta evaluations, 1952
congenital anomalies evaluated using, 795, 804
dilated cardiomyopathy evaluations, 1961
heart transplantation rejection evaluations, 1964
hypoplastic left heart syndrome evaluations, 1955
Kawasaki disease evaluations, 1967
myocarditis evaluations, 1960
partial anomalous pulmonary venous return evaluations, 1947
pericarditis evaluations, 1960
restrictive cardiomyopathy evaluations, 1963
right-to-left shunting lesions evaluations, 1944
syncope evaluations, 1757
tetralogy of Fallot evaluations, 1967
total anomalous pulmonary venous return evaluations, 1947
transposition of the great arteries evaluations, 1947
ventricular septal defect evaluations, 1940
Echogenic bowel
postnatal evaluation, 776–777
ultrasound detection of, 611
Echokinesis, 1758
Eclampsia, 634–635
Economics
adoption physician billing and payment, 1048–1049
early education and child care programs, payment for, 1024
foster care, 1065–1066
homelessness and, 1088–1090
insurance coverage, for NICU-discharged infants, 722–723
newborn length of stay and, 840–841
prenatal care fees, 800
Ecstasy, 2782
Ectopic pregnancy, 2628
Ectopic ureter, 2335
Edema. *See also* Inflammation
causes of, 1479b, 1479–1480
cerebral, 2664, 2667, 2667b
evaluation of, 1480
laboratory evaluation of, 1480
management of, 1481
pathophysiology of, 1479
Edema—cont'd
physical examination for, 1480
preseptal cellulitis caused by, 2443–2445, 2443f
referrals for, 1481
test interpretation and, 1480
Edginess, 1656–1657
Edinburgh Postpartum Depression Scale, 366, 367b–368b
Education
parent
adoption, 1046–1050
American Academy of Pediatrics materials for, 207
bereavement for sick and dying infant, 736–738
breastfeeding, 813–817
child abuse prevention, 1093
child health professionals, 1024
discipline guidelines, 1029–1035
divorce, 1057–1058
domestic violence, 1078–1079
early education and child care programs and, 1020–1024
electronic health records used for, 32
foster care and, 1066
healthy newborn follow-up care, 840–847, 849–850
hospital rounds and, 733
on media effects on children, 1114–1120
medical-legal issues in, 750–751
mental health diagnosis and treatment, 1016–1017
neonatal intensive care infants, 723, 869–880
newborn screening, 78
prenatal visit procedures, 797–800
self-care by children and, 1103–1105
sick and dying infants, 730
patient
during discharge planning, 174
electronic health records used for, 32
primary care physician–hospitalist partnership in, 169
Education for All Handicapped Children Act. *See* Individuals with Disabilities Education Act
Effective care, 42
Effective circulating volume, 467
Effective Early Hearing Detection and Intervention Systems, 327b
Efficient care, 43
Egg freezing, 625
EGIDS. *See* Eosinophilic gastrointestinal disorders
Egocentrism, 210
Ehlers-Danlos syndromes, 1605
Ehrlichiosis, 2482
Eikenella corrodens, 1823
Eisenmenger syndrome, 1943, 1946
Ejection murmurs, 1563–1564, 1564f
Elbow pain, 2555
Electrocardiogram
aortic stenosis evaluations, 1950
apparent life-threatening events evaluations, 1831–1833
arrhythmia evaluations, 1411–1412, 1414
atrial septal defect evaluations, 1940
bradyarrhythmia evaluations, 918–919
cardiovascular screening uses of, 337–340
chest pain evaluations, 1421
coarctation of the aorta evaluations, 1952
dyspnea evaluations, 1470
heart murmur evaluations, 918
hypoplastic left heart syndrome evaluations, 1954
pressure overload, 925–926
right-to-left shunting lesions evaluations, 1944
syncope evaluations, 1756–1757
transposition of the great arteries evaluations, 1948
ventricular septal defect evaluations, 1940
Electrodessication, 2618
Electroencephalograms, 1318, 2496
Electrolysis, 1242
Electrolytes
abnormalities of
hyperkalemia, 477–478, 478t
hypernatremia, 475–477, 476t
hypokalemia, 477, 477t
hyponatremia, 474–475, 475t
potassium-related, 477t–478t, 477–478
in preoperative laboratory evaluation, 544
sodium-related, 474–477, 475t–476t
absorption of, 1442, 1453
in clinical practice, 471–481
composition of, 468, 468t
concentration of, 467–471
deficits in
estimation and correction of, 473–474, 473t
shock due to, 474
dehydration and, 2656, 2657t
diabetic ketoacidosis and, 2664t, 2664–2667
imbalance of, 1785
maintenance requirements for, 472
in snakebites, 2698
Electronic health records
aliases stored in, 32
benefits of, 27, 33–34
certification of, 33
chronically ill children managed using, 32
data norms use of, 29t, 31
decision support uses of, 30t, 32
definition of, 28

Electronic health records—cont'd
electronic medical record vs., 28
functions of, 28–32, 29t–30t
granularity, 30t, 32
growth monitoring uses of, 28, 29t, 30–31
illustration of, 30f
immunization management uses of, 29t, 31
implementation of, 32–36
increased use of, 28
information-gathering uses of, 36
integration abilities of, 32
medical prescribing uses of, 29t, 31
paper chart transition to, 33
parental access to, 53
patient and parent education uses of, 32
privacy issues, 29t, 31
systems
cost of, 33
selection of, 32–33
support for physicians, 33
terminology systems, 29t–30t, 31–32
Web-based resources, 34
Electronic medical record. *See* Electronic health records
Electrophysiological testing, 1757
Elicit-provide-elicit model, 202
Elimination patterns
breastfeeding, 818, 820
family counseling regarding, 842–843
Ellis van Creveld syndrome, 792
Embryonic umbilical remnants, 2605f, 2605–2606
Emedicine.com, 35t
Emergence delirium, 556
Emergency contraception, 1355
Emery-Dreifuss muscular dystrophy
complications and treatment of, 2279t
prevalence of, 2283
symptoms, genetics and diagnostic tests for, 2275t
Emesis. *See* Vomiting
Emollients, for psoriasis, 2451, 2452t
Emotional disorders. *See also* Depression; Mood disorders
barriers to referral, 1164–1165
considerations of, 1165–1168
consultation referrals and, 1163–1164
fatigue caused by, 1511
interventions for, 186
prevalence of, 186, 200
risk factors for, 185–186
Emotional well-being, 179
Empathy, 95
Employee Retirement Income Security Act of 1974, 19
Employer-based health insurance, 17, 18f
Enalapril, 2729–2730
Enamel hypoplasia, 126f
Enanthem disease, 2036
Encephalitis
cysticercal, 2396
description of, 2037
in HIV-infected children, 2142
Encephalocele, 123
Encephalopathy
hypertensive, 2727
vaccination-related, 248
Encephalotrigeminal angiomatosis, 2312–2314, 2313f. *See also* Sturge-Weber syndrome
Encopresis
definition of, 1251
diagnosis of, 1251
disimpaction, 1253
evaluation of, 1251–1252
hospitalization for, 1255b
incidence of, 1251
laboratory evaluations for, 1252
management of, 1252–1253, 1255
nonretentive, 1251, 1255
physical examination for, 1252
prognosis for, 1255–1256
radiographic finding and, 1252
referrals for, 1255b
retentive, 1252t
treatment of, 1255b
Endocardial cushion defect. *See* Atrioventricular canal defect
Endocarditis
bacterial, 2480
description of, 1957–1958
infective, 506t
prophylaxis, for dental procedures, 508t–509t, 508–509
Endocrine disorders, 529–534, 530t, 531f, 533f, 534b, 534t
adrenal insufficiency. *See* Adrenal insufficiency
congenital adrenal hyperplasia. *See* Congenital adrenal hyperplasia
diabetes mellitus. *See* Diabetes mellitus
fatigue caused by, 1510
short stature caused by, 1728
Endocrine system
leukemia treatment effects on, 2243–2244
review of systems for, 93b
End-of-life care
components of, 594–595, 595b
definition of, 594
ethical issues related to, 595–596
pain management in, 597–598, 597b
patient and family conversations about, 596–597
planning of, 587
psychosocial support in, 598–599, 599b
spiritual support in, 598–599, 599b
symptom management in, 597–598, 597b
End-of-the-day crying, 1158
Endophthalmitis, 1702
Endoscopy
Barrett esophagus, incidence of, 2054
description of, 1544–1545, 1547–1549
diarrhea in HIV-infected children evaluations, 2142
esophageal foreign objects removed using, 2049
gastrointestinal obstruction evaluations, 2078
gluten-sensitive enteropathy evaluations, 2088, 2091–2092, 2092f
third ventriculostomy, 2151
Endotracheal tube
neonatal airway stabilization, 676–677
neonatal resuscitation, 662–663
Endurance
cardiorespiratory, 190–191, 191t
large-muscle, 191–192
Energy
conditions resulting in deficiency, 1504b
daily requirements, 221f
expenditure of, 221, 221t
during lactation, 221
metabolism of, 220–222
needs in children, 1503b
physical activity requirements for, 220–221
during pregnancy, 221
Energy therapies, 460
Engorgement of breasts, 819, 826
Enmeshment, 1183
Entamoeba histolytica, 2142, 2372–2373
Enteral nutrition, 692–693
Enteric fistula, 2605
Enteric infections, 2531
Enteritis, 2520b–2521b, 2531
Enterobius vermicularis, 2389–2390
Enterocolitis, 1545
Enterocystoma, 2605
Enterohemorrhagic *Escherichia coli,* 2094
Enteroviral disease, 2037
Enteroviral exanthems, 1977
Enterovirus infections
acute hemorrhagic conjunctivitis, 2036
aseptic meningitis. *See* Aseptic meningitis
classification of, 2032, 2033t
clinical syndromes, 2034, 2036t, 2036–2037
encephalitis, 2037
enteroviral disease, 2037
epidemiology of, 2032–2033
exanthem diseases, 2036
gastrointestinal diseases, 2036
laboratory procedures for, 2037–2038
meningoencephalitis caused by, 2037, 2268, 2268f
molecular genetic analysis for, 2038
myocarditis, 2037
nonspecific febrile illness, 2034

Page numbers followed by "f" denote figures; "t" denote tables; "b" *denote* boxes.

Enterovirus infections—cont'd
orchitis, 2037
paralytic disease, 2036–2037
parechovirus infections, 2037
parotitis, 2037
pathogenesis of, 2033–2034
pericarditis, 2037
perinatal period, 934–935
pharyngitis caused by, 2425b, 2426
prevention of, 2039
rapid virus identification for, 2038
referrals for, 2039
respiratory tract disease, 2034, 2036
serological diagnosis of, 2038
treatment of, 2038–2039
virus isolation, 2038
Enthesitis-related arthritis, 2214
Enuresis
definition of, 2040
differential diagnosis, 2041
diurnal, 2040–2043
epidemiology of, 2040–2041
etiology of, 2041
evaluation of, 2041–2042, 2042b
management of, 2043–2044
medical conditions associated with, 2041b
referrals for, 2044
self-hypnosis for, 451–452
treatment of, 2043–2044
Envenomations
Arachnid, 2690–2694
definition, 2686
epidemiology, 2686t, 2686–2687
hospitalization for, 2702
Hymenoptera, 2687–2690, 2689b
referrals for, 2702
snake, 2694–2702
Environment
atherosclerosis and, 280
conduct disorders and, 1221
conversion reactions and, 1228
eating disorders and, 1188
gay, lesbian, and bisexual youth and, 1359
heredity vs., 998
hypercholesterolemia and, 280
intrauterine growth restriction and, 884
learning disorders and, 1151
leukemia and, 2231b, 2232–2233
maternal nutritional status and, 629
neonatal health and, 630
obesity and, 299–300, 301t, 2322, 2322t, 2323f
school health and, 1124–1125, 1126
school readiness and, 1142
school refusal and, 1146, 1147
sexuality and, 1339–1340
Environmental tobacco smoke, 369
Environmental toxins
breastfeeding and, 827–828
in home environment, 845–846
Enzymatic defects of steroidogenesis, 1594
Enzyme disorders, 942–943
Eosinophil(s)
chronic inflammation of asthma and, 1840–1841
nasal smear for, 1819–1820
Eosinophilic esophagitis, 2055–2057
Eosinophilic gastrointestinal disorders
clinical manifestations of, 2068
differential diagnosis of, 2068–2069
etiology of, 2068
features of, 2068b
incidence of, 2068
management of, 2069
pathological considerations, 2068–2069
prognosis of, 2069
Eosinophilic pustular folliculitis, 784
Ephedra, 458t, 542t
Epicanthal fold, 764
Epidemic keratoconjunctivitis, 1711f–1712f, 1711–1712
Epidemic pleurodynia, 2036
Epidemiologic transition, 56
Epidemiologic triangle, 56
Epidemiology of Diabetes Interventions and Complications trial, 2001, 2006
Epidermal nevus, 781–782
Epidermoid cysts, 1997
Epidermolytic hyperkeratosis, 781–782
Epididymal cysts, 1723
Epididymitis, 1720, 2520b, 2531
Epidural hematoma, 2713t
Epiglottis, 127
Epiglottitis
differential diagnosis, 2636t, 2649–2650
empirical therapy for, 506t
Epilepsia partialis continua, 2489b, 2492, 2819
Epilepsy, 2488–2505. *See also* Seizure(s); Seizure disorders
causes of, 2495
classification of, 2489, 2489b
electroencephalograms and, 1318
false diagnosis of, 1273b
genetics in, 2495
in infants of diabetic mothers, 891
myoclonic, 2489b, 2491
neonatal epileptic syndromes, 990–992
sleep-related, 1309
status epilepticus, 2819–2821
Epilepsy Foundation of America, 2502
Epinephrine
anaphylaxis treated with, 2645, 2646
bee stings treated with, 2688–2689
croup treated with, 2652
description of, 1808
shock treated with, 2807
status asthmaticus treated with, 2816
Epiphyseal overuse conditions, 2554–2555
Epiphysis, 2553t
Episcleral hemorrhages, 118
Epispadias, 135, 2158
Epistaxis
cause of, 1484
definitions of, 1482
diagnosis of, 1483–1484
epidemiologic factors of, 1482
evaluation of, 1484–1485, 1485t
management of, 1485–1488, 1486f, 1487b
referrals for, 1488
treatment of, 1486f
Epstein pearls, 123
Epstein-Barr virus
chronic fatigue syndrome and, 2178
description of, 1511, 1965
malignancy and, 2178–2179
negative infectious mononucleosis, 2178
pharyngitis caused by, 2425b, 2426
prevalence of, 2175
serologic findings in, 2175–2177, 2176f, 2177t
Equinovarus, 1532, 1532f–1533f, 1538
Equinus, 1529b, 1531f, 1532
Equity in health care, 44
Erb palsy, 137
Erectile dysfunction, 1343
Ergot alkaloids, 1553
Erikson, Erik
description of, 98
theory of psychosocial development, 1003
Erogenous zones, 1002–1003
Erosions, 1690, 1691f
Erysipelas, 1858
Erythema infectiosum (fifth disease), 1977
Erythema marginatum, 2477
Erythema migrans, 1627
Erythema multiforme, 1716, 2029–2030
Erythema toxicum, 760, 783–785
Erythematous papules, 1690f
Erythematous patch, 1689f
Erythrocytapheresis, 486
Erythrocyte sedimentation rate, 1526–1527
Erythroderma, 2220, 2220f
Erythrodermic psoriasis, 2448t, 2449, 2450f
Erythromycin
acne treated with, 1805
Chlamydia treated with, 2512b
description of, 501–502
feeding intolerance in neonates and, 695
pharmacologic properties of, 501
side effects of, 501–502
staphylococcal TSS treated with, 2566
use of, 502
Erythromycin estolate, 494t
Erythromycin ethylsuccinate, 494t

Escherichia coli
neonatal sepsis, 936
in urinary tract infections, 2607
Esophageal manometry, 1466
Esophageal pH monitoring for gastroesophageal reflux disease, 2057
Esophageal pH probe study, 1466
Esophagogastroduodenoscopy, 1466
Esophagram, 1793f
Esophagus
atresia of, 777, 915, 2076, 2078f
caustic injury of
causes, 2705, 2706t
delayed complications, 2708–2709
diagnosis, 2706
grading, 2707b
initial management, 2706–2707
medical management, 2707
pathophysiological features, 2705–2706
surgical interventions, 2707–2708, 2708f
Esotropia
characteristics of, 1734b, 1734f–1736f, 1734–1737, 1781f
definition of, 1733
Espundia, 2367
ESR. *See* Erythrocyte sedimentation rate
Essential amino acids, 222
Essential fatty acids, 224
Essential hypertension, 132
Estriol, 604
Estrogen, 1354
Etanercept, 2453t, 2454
Ethambutol, 2602
Ethanol. *See* Alcohol
Ethical issues
adolescents
drug testing of, 76–77
sexual activity in, 75–76
adoption, 80–81
assisted reproductive technologies and, 625
barriers to follow-up care for newborns, 847, 849–850
case studies of, 74–85
child abuse and neglect and, 1098–1100
corporal punishment, 81–82
cross-cultural medicine, 160
description of, 74
end-of-life care-related, 595–596
genetic testing, 795–796
hypertrophic obstructive cardiomyopathy, 81
immunizations, 79–80
maternal-fetal interventions, 615
newborn screening and, 78–79, 389
palliative care-related, 595–596
right to know genetic inheritance, 80–81
Ethinyl estradiol, 1354
Ethnicity, 1580
Ethosuximide, 2498t, 2500
Ethyl alcohol. *See* Alcohol
Ethylene glycol
antidote for, 2685t, 2767t
poisoning by, 2783–2784
Etonogestrel, 1355
Euglycemia, 978
European Group for Immunological Characterization of Leukemias, 2236–2237, 2237t
Evening primrose oil, 458t
Event monitors, 1757
Eversion, 1529b
Evidence-Based Clinical Practice Guidelines, 39t
Evidence-based medicine
acquisition step of, 38–39
application step of, 40–41
appraisal step of, 39–40
definition of, 38
getting started, 41
information acquisition, 38–39
questions, 38, 38b
steps involved in, 38–41
terminology in, 40t
time efficiency of, 41
Ewing tumors
clinical manifestations, 1886
differential diagnosis of, 1886t
etiology, 1885–1886
evaluation, 1886
follow-up, 1887
management of, 1887
prognosis, 1887
Exanthematous diseases. *See also* Measles
adenovirus, 1981
differentiating common childhood exanthems, 1978–1979t
enteroviral exanthems, 1977
erythema infectiosum (fifth disease), 1977
exanthem subitum (roseola), 1977
infectious mononucleosis, 1980
influenza A and B, 1981
parainfluenza virus, 1981
respiratory syncytial virus, 1981
rubella (German measles), 1977, 1979–1980
viruses associated with, 2269, 2269f
Exchange transfusion, 486, 486f
Excretory system (of lacrimal system), 1707f
Exercise. *See also* Physical activity
activities for, 191t
adherence to, 196–197
aerobic, 190, 191b
anaphylaxis caused by, 2644–2645
barriers to, 196–197
body mass index measurements before beginning, 193
cholesterol levels reduced through, 190
dyspnea secondary to, 1470
Exercise—cont'd
in eating disorder patients, 193
frequency of, 191
heart rate during, 190–191, 191t
hypertension and, 1588
muscle strength increases through, 192, 192f
opportunities for talking about, 197
overuse syndromes secondary to, 191
variations in, 196
weight training, 192
Exhaustion, heat, 2551
Exotropia, 1733, 1734b, 1737, 1737f, 1781f
Expectorants, 1435
Experience-dependent learning, for brain development, 181
Extended oligoarthritis, 2213–2214
External tibial torsion, 1540–1541
Extracellular fluid, 467
Extracorporeal membrane oxygenation, 862
Extra-family learning, 1009, 1012
Extramedullary hematopoiesis, 1732
Extraocular movements, 2641
Extrauterine growth restriction, 690–691
Extreme temperament, 1746
Extremely low–birth-weight infants. *See also* Low-birth-weight infants; Very low–birth-weight infants
chronic conditions, functional limitations, and special health needs, 856–857
growth outcomes in, 857
health and developmental outcomes, 852–863
neurodevelopmental outcomes in, 856
pain sensitivity in, 857–858
retinopathy of prematurity in, 757
transition to adulthood for, 858–861
Extremities. *See also* Foot; Leg
defects in
newborn assessment, 769
ultrasound detection of, 613
pain in
diagnosis of, 1491–1495, 1492–1493b
evaluation of, 1489–1491
history and, 1489–1490
laboratory examination and, 1490–1491
physical examination for, 1490
unexplained, 1490
Eye(s). *See also* Cellulitis
alignment of, 1776
anatomy of, 2343–2344
assessment of
congenital anomalies, 791–792
fetal development, 649–650
newborn, 763–764
post-delivery, 801–802
cataracts, 764
congenital anomalies of, 791–792
cornea. *See* Cornea
fetal development of, 649–650

Page numbers followed by "f" denote figures; "t" denote tables; "b" *denote* boxes.

Eye(s)—cont'd
inspection, 1780f
iris of. *See* Iris
newborn assessment of, 763–764
ophthalmologic evaluation
congenital anomaly diagnosis, 795
in neonatal intensive care infants, 879
paranasal sinuses relationship to, 2441, 2441f
physical examination of, 118–120
retina. *See* Retina
retinopathy of prematurity. *See* Retinopathy of prematurity
review of systems for, 92b
sports participation despite disorders of, 322t
swollen, 2440–2445
toxoplasmosis effects on, 2379
trauma to. *See* Ocular trauma
tuberous sclerosis complex effects on, 2311
Eyelids
description of, 2343
injuries of, 2345, 2345f

F

Face
abnormalities of, 2605
congenital anomalies, 791–792
development of, 116
Down syndrome characteristics, 118
dysmorphic, 1498–1499
examination of, 118
newborn assessment, 763
Face, legs, activity, cry, and consolability scoring system, 424
Facial angiofibromas, 2310–2311, 2310f
Facial dysmorphism
body, 1499–1500
causes of, 1498t
craniofacial features, 1498–1499
definition of, 1496
diagnosis of, 1497b, 1500–1501
growth, 1498
history-taking, 1497–1498
laboratory evaluation for, 1500
physical examination for, 1498–1500
proportions, 1498
Facial hair, 1238–1239
Facial palsy, 117
Facilitative responses, 1333, 1334
Faciogenital dysplasia, 2605
Facioscapulohumeral dystrophy
complications and treatment of, 2279t
diagnostic tests for, 2275t
hypotonia and, 1608
prevalence of, 2282–2283
symptoms of, 2275t
Factitious fever, 1522
Factitious hemoptysis, 1573
Factor H inhibitors, 2095
Factor replacement, 2108–2109, 2111
Factor VIIa, recombinant, 2675
Fad diets, 231
Failure to thrive
in congestive heart failure, 2723
definition of, 1501–1502
description of, 1743
evaluation of, 1504–1506
family dynamics and, 1504
follow-up for, 1506–1507
history-taking, 1505
laboratory evaluation of, 1506
pathogenesis of, 1503–1504
physical examination for, 1505–1506
prognosis for, 1507
renal tubular acidosis and, 2459–2460
treatment of, 1506–1507
Famciclovir
genital herpes treated with, 2516b, 2517b
indications for, 511t
Familial dysautonomia, 1754
Familial gonadotropin-independent puberty, 1593, 1728–1729
Familial short stature, 1727, 1729
Family. *See also* Parents
abuse in. *See* Child abuse and neglect; Domestic violence
adherence affected by, 163
adopted children
first year home, 1046–1048
long-term issues, 1048
unique issues, 1049
alternative, 1036–1037
American patterns in, 1037–1041
assessment of, 364–373. *See also* Family, screening of; Maternal depression
intimate partner violence, 369
parental smoking in, 369
rationale for, 364–365
attachment, 179, 181
behavioral genetics, 998–1000
changing demographics and definitions, 1027
changing structures in, 1027
child abuse. *See* Child abuse and neglect
child care, 1018–1019
child custody, 1053–1055
chronic pain effects on, 436–437
communication with, 52
complementary and alternative medicine counseling of, 462–463, 462b
cultural differences in, 159, 182
decision-making role of, 171–172
demographics of, 234, 1038–1039
dietary habits influenced by, 219
in discharge planning, 174–175
divorce effects, 1056–1059
domestic violence. *See* Domestic violence
dysfunctional, 1039
early education programs, 1018–1019
Family—cont'd
education of, about health insurance plans, 25
electronic health records used to support, 36
end-of-life care discussions with, 596–597
failure to thrive and, 1504
foster care effects on, 1062–1072
future issues in, 1041
gay- and lesbian-parented, 1082–1085
genetic disease screening, 604
grandparents, 182
health outcomes affected by, 13t, 15
healthy newborn discharge and, 841
homeless, 1087–1090
during hospitalization, 171–172
hypoglycemia, 970
of intellectually disabled children, 2185
marital strain effects on, 182
marriage patterns and trends and, 1037
maternal health and, 754–756
mental health diagnosis and treatment, 1015–1016
mood disorders and, 1260
origins of, 1036–1037
palliative care discussions with, 596–597
partnerships with, 567, 583–588
primary care physician's role in supporting, 179
psychosocial development and, 1036–1041
psychosocial support to, 580–581
resiliency in, 179
screening of
environmental tobacco smoke screening, 369
intimate partner violence, 369
maternal depression, 365–369. *See also* Maternal depression
parental smoking, 369
rationale for, 364–365
self-care by children and, 1103–1105
siblings, 182–183
of sick and dying infants
bereavement, 736–738
coping strategies, 738
core principles of, 731–732
death, 733
management of, 730–735
psychosocial issues in, 733–735
rounds and, 733
social learning and, 1008
support for, 179–188
transgender youth and, 1234
unexplained physical symptoms, 1183–1185
US Census data on, 1038
Family advisory council, 26–27
Family history
in adopted children, 80
cardiovascular health promotion and, 279t

Family history—cont'd
construction of, 93, 93f
in genetic-metabolic diseases screening, 376
in prenatal interview, 89–90
purpose of, 92b, 93
Family Voices, Inc., 584
Family-centered care
assisted reproductive technologies and, 624–625
description of, 53, 171
discipline principles, 1029–1035
fetal-maternal health and, 650
healthy newborn discharge and, 841–846
key elements of, 1027–1028
maternal medical history and, 753–754
neonatal intensive care infants, 879–880
pediatric medical home planning, 1028
pediatrician as ally, 1028–1029
prenatal visit procedures, 797–800
principles of, 569–570, 570b
Family-directed home health care, 570–571
Fasting
in genetic-metabolic diseases screening, 376
metabolic interrelationships, 973
preoperative, 543–544, 544t
Fat excretion, 1440–1441
Fatigue. *See also* Chronic fatigue syndrome
in adolescents, 1511
definition and etiology of, 1509
description of, 1509–1511
diagnostic testing of, 1513–1514
differential diagnosis of, 1509–1512, 1510b
end-of-life care and, 598
in infants, 1509
management of, 598, 1514
palliative care and, 598
patient history and, 1512
physical examination of, 1512–1513
pronation as cause of, 1535
weakness vs., 1509, 1510
Fats
calories from, 224
daily consumption of, 194
definition of, 224
dietary, 224–225
digestion of, 224
formation of, 224
in human vs. cow milk, 213
polyunsaturated, 224
recommendations for, 195–196
saturated, 224
Fatty acid oxidation disorders
hypothermia and, 833
pathophysiology, 981
rare defects, 982
Fatty acids, 224
Fatty liver, 2121
FDA. *See* US Food and Drug Administration
Febrile seizures
description of, 1516–1517, 2489b, 2494
management of, 420–421
Febrile transfusion reaction, 487–488
Feces
energy excretions in, 220
impaction of, 1372f
water loss in, 225
Fee for service, 21, 22t, 24
Feeding
abnormalities, 1504
artificial (bottle)
breastfeeding vs., 213, 215
formulas
breastfeeding vs., 816
description of, 213
family counseling for use of, 842
iron supplementation in, 217
in neonatal intensive care infants, 710–712, 871–872
nutrients in, 214t
premature infants, 695–698
preparation of, 216, 217b
vitamin supplementation of, 229
schedule for, 215–216
weaning from, 218
breastfeeding. *See* Breastfeeding
diarrhea and, 1448
dietary recommendations, 212
disorders involving, 1743
dysphagia caused by, 1464–1465
equipment, 1466
failure to thrive and, 1504–1505
fluoride supplements, 217
history-taking, 91b
iron supplements, 217
overview of, 212–213
sleep and, 1300–1302
solid foods, 213, 218–219
thermic effect of, 220
vitamin D supplements, 217
vitamin K supplements, 216–217
water-soluble vitamins, 217
Feeding center, 1637
Feeding intolerance
infants of diabetic mothers with, 890
neonates with
assessments, 840–841
description of, 694–695
neonatal intensive care infants, 874–876
neurological evaluation, 992
in premature infants, 835
Feeding therapy, 577–579
Felbamate, 2498t, 2501
Female genitalia
in newborn, 769, 845
sexual abuse signs, 1107–1113
Femoral anteversion, 1530, 1541–1542
Femoral head osteochondroses, 2353, 2353b
Femoral torsion deformities, 1541–1542
Fennel seed, 826
Fentanyl
chronic pain managed using, 442t
half-life of, 425t
oral transmucosal, 442t
potency of, 425t
Fenugreek, 826
Ferritin, 2208
Fertilization. *See* In vitro fertilization
Fetal alcohol syndrome
diagnosis, 792
features of, 2189t
microcephaly and, 1654
Fetal face syndrome, 2605
Fetal hemoglobin, 648
Fetal surgery
for cleft lip and cleft palate, 1925
fetal assessment for, 644
for gastrointestinal obstruction, 2082–2083
Fetal-to-maternal hemorrhage, 941
Fetus
adipose tissue of, 113
anemia in, 619
assessment of, 637–651
amniocentesis, 644
biophysical profile, 643
cardiovascular system, 646–647
central nervous system, 645–646
checklist for, 642
chorionic villus sampling, 644–645
gastrointestinal system, 647
hematopoietic system, 648
immune system, 648–649
intrauterine growth and nutrition, 638–639
life span conceptual and menstrual dating, 637–638
musculoskeletal system, 646–647
nonstress and contraction stress tests, 642–643
percutaneous umbilical blood sampling, 645
preconception care inventory and recommendations, 641
pre-labor assessment, 641–643
respiratory system, 648
risk assessment and diagnostic testing, 644
risk identification and management, 639–642
system formation and malformation, 645–650
ultrasound techniques, 643–644
urogenital system, 649
uterine size, 643
cardiovascular screening of, 336
disorders involving
categories of, 615–616
congenital cystic adenomatoid malformation, 617
congenital diaphragmatic hernia, 616–617

Page numbers followed by "f" denote figures; "t" denote tables; "b" *denote* boxes.

Fetus—cont'd
disorders involving—cont'd
delivery room medical-legal considerations and, 743–744
ethical considerations, 615
fetal anemia, 619
future techniques, 619
gastroschisis and omphalocele, 617
hydrocephalus, 618
neural tube defects, 617–618
obstructive uropathy, 615–616
sacrococcygeal teratoma, 617
twin reversed arterial perfusion syndrome, 618–619
twin-twin transfusion syndrome, 618
growth and development of
abnormalities
description of, 633–634
infants of diabetic mothers, 888–892
intrauterine growth restriction, 883–885
large-for-gestational-age infants, 888–892
pathophysiology and management, 885–887
assisted reproductive technologies and, 624
intrauterine growth and nutrition, 638–639
maternal nutritional status and, 628–629
stages, 638–639
growth chart, 694
heart rate of, 642
lung masses, 776
pre-labor assessment of activity, 641–642
skin development, 113
Fever. *See also specific types*
bacterial infections as cause of, 1517–1518, 1521–1522
in Bornholm disease, 2036
in bronchiolitis, 1867
in cellulitis, 1858
in chickenpox, 1912
clinical presentation of, 1516–1517
in compromised child, 420
in cystic fibrosis, 1985
definition of, 418–419
diagnostic testing of, 1518, 1519f–1520f, 1521–1522
dysuria and, 1476
empirical therapy for, 506t
evaluation of, 1516–1517
factitious, 1522
in genetic-metabolic diseases screening, 376
in hepatitis, 2116t
in hives, 2028
in human herpesvirus 6 and 7, 2135t
hyperthermia-related, 420
joint pain and, 1626
Fever—cont'd
in Kawasaki disease, 2221
management of, 418–422, 1515–1516, 1519f–1520f
pain relief-related, 420
patient history and, 1521
in PFAPA syndrome, 2572
postoperative, 558, 558t
rheumatic. *See* Rheumatic fever
Rochester criteria, 1521, 1521t
in rubella, 1979
scarlet
description of, 1981
differential diagnosis, 2566t–2567t
staphylococcal, 2222t
streptococcal, 2222t
seizure-related, 420–421, 1516–1517
signs and symptoms of, 1516
sports participation with, 322t
thermoregulation and, 418–419
of unknown origin. *See* Fever of unknown origin
in urinary tract infections, 2607, 2609
viral infections as cause of, 1517, 1522
weight loss and, 1787
Fever of unknown origin
autoimmune diseases as cause of, 1525, 1526b
definition of, 1524–1525
diagnostic testing of, 1527
differential diagnosis of, 1525–1526, 1526b
infectious diseases as cause of, 1525, 1526b
malignancies as cause of, 1525–1526, 1526b
patient history and, 1526–1527
periodic fever syndromes as cause of, 1526, 1526b
physical examination of, 1527
pseudo-fever of unknown origin vs., 1524–1525, 1525b
rate of incidence of causes of, 1527t
Fever phobia, 419
Feverfew, 458t
Fiber, 1431
Fiberoptic endoscopic evaluation of swallowing, 1466
Fighting, 275, 275b
Filariasis, 2392–2393
Fingernails, 116
Finger-sucking, 1651
Fire ants, 2689–2690
Firearm injuries, 270–271
First aid, 2696, 2697b, 2701
First heart sound, 131
Fistula
enteric (vitelline), 2605
urachal, 2605, 2606
Fitness. *See also* Exercise; Physical activity
description of, 189
opportunities for discussing, 197
Fitz-Hugh-Curtis syndrome, 2511, 2531
5-Lipoxygenase inhibitors for asthma, 1848
FLACC scoring system. *See* Face, legs, activity, cry, and consolability scoring system
Flat villus lesion, 2090–2091, 2091b
Flat warts, 1803, 1803f
Flatfoot, 1530, 1534, 1536
Flea bites, 2179, 2180f
Flexibility, 192
Flexible flatfoot, 1536
Flexible foot, 1534
Flexible laryngoscopy, 1750f
Flexner Report, 459
Floppiness. *See* Hypotonia
Fluconazole
dosage of, 512t–513t
leishmaniasis treated with, 2368
Flucytosine, 513t
Fluid(s)
in clinical practice, 471–481
maintenance
inadequate, 471f, 472–473
for parenteral use, 472
requirements for, 471–472, 471f, 472t
polyuria, 1671–1672
Fluid compartments, 471, 471f
Fluid deficits
in diabetic ketoacidosis, 2664t
estimation and correction of, 473–474, 473t
shock due to, 474
in snakebites, 2698
Fluid therapy
ambulatory patient treated with, 479–480
bacterial meningitis after neonatal period treated with, 2259
burns treated with, 479, 2826, 2827b
controversies regarding, 2657
dehydration treated with, 2657–2661
diabetic ketoacidosis treated with, 2665–2666
goal-directed, 2799
intravenous rehydration, 2658
neonatal meningitis treated with, 2263
in neonates, 478–480, 479t
oral rehydration, 2657–2661
principles of, 2657
renal failure treated with, 2799–2800
situations requiring, 478–480, 479t
Fluid volumes, 226f
Flumazenil, 2768, 2783
Flunitrazepam (Rohypnol), 2782, 2790
Fluorescent in situ hybridization
congenital anomaly diagnosis, 794–795
dysmorphism diagnosis and, 1500
Fluoride
characteristics of, 227t
in dental caries prevention, 294–295, 295t
dentifrices, 295
description of, 63

Fluoride—cont'd
rinses, 295
supplements, 217, 294, 295t
varnish, 295
Fluoroquinolones
gonococcal infections treated with, 2513b, 2514b
pelvic inflammatory disease treated with, 2520b
staphylococcal TSS treated with, 2566
Fluoroscopy, 146–147
Fluorosis, dental, 294–295
Focal fat necrosis, 1721
Focal segmental glomerulosclerosis, 2296, 2299
Folacin, 228t
Folic acid
deficiency of, 605
supplementation of, 226
Folk illnesses
characteristics of, 63, 64t–65t
child abuse confused with healing practices for, 69t
Folliculitis, 1691f, 1804, 1856
Follow-up appointments, 174, 174b
Follow-up care
growth-restricted infants, 885–887
healthy newborn, 846–847, 849–850
in infants of diabetic mothers, 891
jaundice, 899–900
neonatal drug withdrawal syndrome, 957
NICU-discharged infants, 721–722, 726
Fomivirsen, 511t
Fontanelles
assessment of, 760–762
description of, 116–117, 117f
percussion of, 117–118
Food
abdominal pain correction and, 1382
anaphylactic reactions to, 2643, 2644
anemia and, 1396
constipation and, 1426, 1431
diarrhea and, 1444b
dysphagia and, 1466
for eating disorder patients, 1191–1192
failure to thrive correction and, 1506b
refusal of, 1503–1504. *See also* Eating disorders
in schools, 1124
supplementation programs for, 24
Food allergy
American Academy of Pediatrics recommendations for prevention of, 2066b
clinical manifestations, 2065
cow's milk protein allergy, 2065, 2065b, 2066–2067
gastroesophageal reflux disease and, 2057
human milk allergy, 2065–2066
infant formulas, nonstandard, 2066t
laboratory abnormalities in, 2066
Food allergy—cont'd
management of, 2066
partial vs. extensive hydrolysates, 2067t
soy protein, 2065–2067
Food and Agricultural Organization, 230
Food and Drug Administration
acyclovir not approved by, 1916
adefovir dipivoxil approved by, 2124
deferasirox approved by, 2100–2101
H_2RA therapy approved by, 2061
inhaled corticosteroids approved by, 1847
α-interferon and oral ribavirin combination approved by, 2124
isotretinoin guidelines, 1805
in Lyme disease, 2251
on supplements, 457
tacrolimus ointment and pimecrolimus cream warnings, 1852
varicella vaccine licensed by, 1916
Food and Nutrition Board, 230
Food assistance programs, 229–230
Food groups, 231
Food Guide Pyramid, 193
Foot disorders. *See also* Limp
clubfoot, 1532–1533, 1541
femoral torsion deformities, 1541–1542
forefoot, 1533–1534, 1541
pes cavus, 1542
positional deformities, 1530, 1531f
pronation, 1534–1536, 1542
referral for, 1541–1542
shoes and, 1529–1530
terminology, 1529b
tibial torsion, 1540–1542
toe deformities, 1530–1532, 1531f, 1541
toeing-in and toeing-out, 1538–1540, 1542
toe-walking, 1536–1537, 1542
Foot odor, 1662–1663
Football position for breastfeeding, 814–815
Forced expiratory volume in 1 second, 1840, 1988
Forefoot, 1533f–1534f, 1533–1534
Foreground question, 38, 38b
Foreign bodies
in airway, 2047–2048
aspiration of
description of, 2637, 2650
hemoptysis caused by, 1571, 1574
stridor caused by, 1749t
wheezing and, 1793f
in conjunctiva, 2347–2348, 2347f
in cornea, 2347–2348, 2347f
in ear, 1613, 2045–2046
in esophagus, 2048–2049
in eye, 1613
gastrointestinal bleeding caused by, 1544
in nose, 1613, 2046–2047
Foreign bodies—cont'd
referrals for, 2049
retention of, 1663
vaginal bleeding caused by, 1767
Forensic evidence kit, 2792, 2794b
Foreskin of penis, 135
Formal operational period of cognitive development, 1011
Formula
breastfeeding vs., 816
description of, 212, 2066t, 2066–2067
family counseling for use of, 842
iron supplementation in, 217
in neonatal intensive care infants, 710–712, 871–872
nutrients in, 214t
premature infants, 695–698
preparation of, 216, 217b
vitamin supplementation of, 229
46,XX/XY disorders of sexual development, 2194–2195
Foscarnet, 511t
Fosphenytoin
seizures treated with, 2743
status epilepticus treated with, 2820b
Foster care. *See also* Adoption; Kinship care
adolescents in, 1065
caseworkers' role in, 1063
child advocates and, 1063
foster family structure, 1065–1066
history of, 1060–1062
honeymoon period, 1063–1064
parental rights termination, 1063
parents, 182
psychological issues in, 1063–1064
psychotropic medicines and, 1072–1073
risk factors for placement in, 1062
Fourth nerve palsy, 1737–1738
Fractional excretion of sodium, 1827
Fractures
avulsion, of pelvis, 2558–2559
child abuse, 2053
classification, 2051f, 2051–2052
clavicle, fractured, 2052
definition, 2051
developmental dysplasia of the hip, 2052–2053
evaluation of, 2051
management of, 2052
nursemaid's elbow, 2053, 2053f
referral for, 2053
skull, 2712–2713
stress, 2552–2553
toddler's, 2053
Fragile X syndrome, 2189t
Freckling, 2305, 2306f
Free ß-human chorionic gonadotropin, 604
Frenulum, 124
Fresh-frozen plasma, 482
Freudian psychoanalysis, 1002–1003, 1006–1010

Frog-leg position, 1512
Frontal sinus, 122
Fructose intolerance, hereditary
  hypoglycemia in, 2733–2734, 2736t
  management, 2737
Fructose-1,6-diphosphatase deficiency
  description of, 980
  hypoglycemia in, 2734, 2736t
  management, 2738
Fructosemia, 984
Fukuyama-type congenital muscular dystrophy, 2275t, 2279t
Fulminant hepatic failure, 2122, 2126
Functional activity training, 576–577
Funduscopic examination, 119
Fungal infections
  antimicrobial therapy for, 512t–513t
  lymphadenopathy caused by, 1642t, 1643
  in stomatitis, 2569, 2570
  in urinary tract, 2608
Fungi
  meningoencephalitis caused by, 2270, 2270t
  pharyngitis caused by, 2427
  splenomegaly and, 1731–1732
Fungistatic agents, 1388–1389
FUO. *See* Fever of unknown origin
Furazolidone, 2086, 2372
Furosemide, 2743
Furuncles, 1856–1857

G

Gabapentin
  in chronic pain management, 443–444
  dosing strategies for, 445t
  in seizure management, 2499t, 2501
GABHS. *See* Group A beta-hemolytic streptococcal infection
Gag reflex, 125, 144
Gait. *See also* Limp
  assessment of, 139
  examination, 1632
Galactagogues, 826
Galactose, 213
Galactosemia
  diagnosis and management, 983–984
  hypoglycemia in, 2733
  management, 2737
  newborn screening for, 385
Galeazzi sign, 771, 2052
Galeazzi test, 1633f
Gallbladder disease, 2628
Gallop sounds, 2719
Gallstones, 148, 873
Gamma globulin, 897
Gamma-hydroxybutyrate, 2783
Ganciclovir, 511t
Gang rape, 2791
Gardnerella vaginalis, 2531
Garlic
  preoperative discontinuation of, 542t
  uses of, 458t
Gas exchange, 129–130
Gastric antral web, 2078
Gastric aspirates, 2598, 2599b
Gastric lavage
  for drug overdose, 2683
  for poisoning, 2769
Gastric obstructions, 2081
Gastroduodenoscopy, 1548
Gastroenteritis
  dehydration in, 2654–2655
  description of, 1447
Gastroesophageal reflux
  complications of, 2058b
  description of, 1599–1601, 1785, 2054, 2054f
  irritability and, 1613
  neonatal management of, 696, 699
  prevalence, 2054f
  and supine sleeping, 2581
  symptoms, 2055b
Gastroesophageal reflux disease
  apparent life-threatening events and, 1830, 1832, 2059–2060
  clinical manifestations of, 2055
  complications of, 2058, 2060
  definitions, 2054
  diagnostic methods
    endoscopy and biopsy, 2058
    esophageal pH monitoring, 2057
    multiple intraluminal electrical impedance measurement, 2057–2058
    scintigraphy, 2058
    upper gastrointestinal radiography (barium swallow), 2058
  differential diagnosis
    achalasia, 2057
    cyclic vomiting syndrome, 2057
    eosinophilic esophagitis, 2055–2057
    food allergy, 2057
    infectious esophagitis, 2057
    pill esophagitis, 2057
    rumination syndrome, 2057
    vomiting, 2056b
  history-taking, 2055, 2056b
  lifestyle changes, 2060–2061
  in neonates, 696, 699
  pathophysiology of, 2055
  pharmacologic therapy for
    antacids, 2061
    H_2-receptor antagonists, 2061, 2061t
    prokinetic agents, 2062
    proton pump inhibitors, 2058, 2061–2062, 2062t
  physical examination for, 2055, 2056b
  prevalence of, 2054
  respiratory complications
    apnea or apparent life-threatening event, 2059–2060
    asthma, 1840, 2059
    chronic cough, stridor, hoarseness, 2058, 2059t
Gastroesophageal reflux disease—cont'd
  respiratory complications—cont'd
    laryngeal edema, 2058, 2059t
    laryngopharyngeal reflux, 2058, 2059b
    recurrent pneumonia, 2058–2059
    Sandifer syndrome, 2060
  sleep-related affects, 1310–1311
  summary of, 2062
  surgery for, 2062
Gastroesophageal varices, 1544–1545
Gastrointestinal allergy. *See also* Eosinophilic gastrointestinal disorders; Food allergy
  conclusion, 2069
  introduction to, 2064–2065
  referrals for, 2069
Gastrointestinal bleeding
  adolescents with, 1545–1546, 1546b
  causes of, 1544–1546, 1546b
  diagnostic testing of, 1544, 1547–1549
  differential diagnosis of, 1544–1546
  history-taking, 1546–1547
  infants and young children with, 1544–1545, 1546b
  lower, 1544
  management of, 1547–1549
  newborns with, 1544, 1546b
  physical examination for, 1547
  treatment of, 1544–1546
Gastrointestinal decontamination, 2769
Gastrointestinal obstructions
  bowel wall trauma, 2080
  causes of, 1371
  clinical findings for, 2073t, 2074f
  colonic and rectal obstruction, 2082
  diagnostic work-up, 2077f
  double duodenal bulb appearance, 2078
  duodenal atresia, 2076, 2079f
  duodenal obstructions, 2081
  duplication cysts, 2078
  effects of, 1373
  esophageal atresia, 2076, 2078f
  esophageal obstruction, 2081
  fetal surgery, 2082–2083
  gastric obstructions, 2081
  ground-glass or soap-bubble appearance, 2078, 2080f
  Hirschsprung disease, 2080, 2080f
  hypertrophic pyloric stenosis, 2078
  ileal atresia with meconium peritonitis, 2077–2078, 2079f
  ileal obstructions, 2081–2082
  imaging studies for, 2075–2080
  intussusception, 2079–2080
  jejunal obstructions, 2081–2082
  management of
    medical, 2080–2081
    surgical, 2072t, 2081–2082
  meconium ileus, 2079
  meconium peritonitis, 2079
  meconium plug syndrome, 2079

Gastrointestinal obstructions—cont'd
minimally invasive surgery, 2082
partial gastric antral web, 2078
physical examination, 2075
referrals for, 2083
roentgenographic findings, 2076, 2076t
signs and symptoms of
abdominal pain, 2074
stool, 2074–2075
vomiting, 2071, 2074
small left colon syndrome, 2080
string of beads sign, 2079
surgical management of, 2072t
volvulus, 2076–2077
Gastrointestinal system
bleeding. *See* Gastrointestinal bleeding
imaging of, 147–150
obstructions. *See* Gastrointestinal obstructions
review of systems for, 92b
ultrasound of, 147–150
Gastrointestinal tract
cystic fibrosis and, 1982–1984
defects
fetal assessment, 647
in neonatal intensive care infants, 873–874
postnatal evaluation, 777
ultrasound detection of, 610–611
function of, 1441f
glucose absorption, 972–976
illness risks, early education and child care programs and, 1020–1022
neonatal drug withdrawal syndrome, 953
Gastroschisis
fetal intervention, 617
ultrasound detection of, 610
Gateway hypothesis, 399
Gay, lesbian, and bisexual youth
advocacy for, 1364–1365
clinical reports and, 1358
definitions and, 1359
development and, 1359
environmental effects and, 1359–1360
laboratory evaluation of, 1362
management of, 1362–1363
optimism and, 1364
physical examination of, 1361–1362
sexual decision making of, 1364
well-being of, 1362–1363
Gay-parented families, 1082–1085
Gender. *See also* Boys; Girls; Transgender youth
culture and, 1235–1236
nephrotic syndrome and, 2296
pectus excavatum and, 2416
psoriasis and, 2447
pyloric stenosis and, 2455
Gender dysphoria, 1233
Gender identity disorder, 1743
Gender reassignment, 794
Gene therapy
for brain tumors, 1863
for hemophilia, 2110
for unstable hemoglobins, 2103
General anesthesia
airway function in, 521–524, 521b, 523f, 524f
early postoperative surgical problems related to, 558t–559t, 558–560
effects of, 516
emergence phenomena after, 556–557
intubation-related complications from, 557
postintubation croup, 557
pulmonary function in, 521–524, 521b, 523f–524f
succinylcholine-induced myalgia, 557–558
Generalized seizures
absence seizures, 2489, 2489b
atonic seizures, 2489, 2489b
grand mal seizures, 2489–2490, 2489b
infantile spasms, 2489b, 2490
juvenile myoclonic epilepsy, 2489b, 2491
Lennox-Gastaut syndrome, 2489t, 2490–2491
myoclonic seizures, 2489, 2489b
tonic-clonic seizures, 2489–2490, 2489b
Genetic counseling, 790, 795–796
Genetic diseases. *See also* Genetic-metabolic diseases; *specific disease*
anesthesia and, 538
assisted reproductive technologies and, 622–625
ethical issues in testing of, 795–796
familial disease screening, 604
intrauterine growth restriction, 884
prenatal diagnoses, 604–613
thromboembolic disease, 945
Genetic factors
abdominal distention and, 1369
attention deficit/hyperactivity disorder and, 1202
childhood epilepsy and, 2495
conduct disorders and, 1221
Duchenne muscular dystrophy, 2273
environment and, 998, 1001
epistaxis and, 1483–1484
hearing loss and, 1558
hepatomegaly and, 1577
hypercholesterolemia and, 280
hypertension and, 1580
hypotonia and, 1604–1605
intrauterine growth restriction, 884
leukemia and, 2231–2232, 2231b
microcephaly and, 1653b, 1653–1654
migraine headache and, 1552
in nephrotic syndrome, 2299–2300
obesity and, 298
stuttering and, 1291–1292
tics and, 1759
Genetic imprinting disorders, 622–625
Genetic inheritance, 80–81
Genetic screenings
congenital anomalies, 790, 795–796
prenatal diagnoses, 604–613
Genetic-metabolic diseases
case examples, 379–382
chronic, 376
classification of, 373, 374t
clinical presentation of, 373, 375
evaluation of
anesthesia and surgery reactions in, 376
dietary history in, 376
family history in, 376
laboratory tests in, 377, 378t
physical examination in, 376–377
response to infection, fever, and fasting in, 376
late-onset presentation of, 375–376
neonatal presentation of, 375, 375t
neuropsychological regression with, 376
newborn screening for
availability of tests in, 389
biotinidase deficiency, 386
congenital adrenal hyperplasia, 386
congenital hypothyroidism, 384–385
cystic fibrosis, 386
description of, 383–384
ethical issues in, 389
galactosemia, 385
genetic susceptibilities, 387
glucose-6-phosphate dehydrogenase deficiency, 387
homocystinuria, 387
legal issues in, 389
maple syrup urine disease, 385–386
medium-chain Acyl-CoA dehydrogenase deficiency, 387
new techniques in
α_1-antitrypsin deficiency, 387–388
carrier screening-related, 388
Down syndrome, 389
glucose-6-phosphate dehydrogenase deficiency, 387
neural tube defects, 388
prenatal screening-related, 388
phenylketonuria, 384
sickle cell anemia, 385
tandem mass spectrometry in, 387
screening for, 373–393
false-negative findings in, 382–383
false-positive findings in, 382–383
future of, 389–390
in newborns. *See* Genetic-metabolic diseases, newborn screening for
treatment of, 377, 379–381
Genetic-plus-environment parents, 998–1000
Genital stage of psychosexual development, 1010

Page numbers followed by "f" denote figures; "t" denote tables; "b" *denote* boxes.

Genital warts
  description of, 2522–2524
  morphology of, 2525f, 2616, 2626f
  subclinical lesions, 2524f
  treatment of, 2514b–2516b, 2523, 2618
Genitalia
  abnormalities of, 2158
  adolescents, 136–137
  ambiguous
    congenital anomalies, 794
    description of, 134
    ultrasound detection of, 611
  congenital anomalies, 794
  embryologic development of, 134–135
  examination of, in rape, 2794
  female
    description of, 135f
    in newborn, 769, 845
    sexual abuse signs, 1107–1113
  herpes simplex virus of, 2516b–2517b, 2524–2527
  of infants, 136
  irritation of, 1726
  male
    anatomy of, 134f
    newborn, 768–769, 845
    sexual abuse signs in, 1107–1113
  maturity ratings for, 134f–135f
  of newborn, 135–136, 768–769, 845
  sexual abuse signs, 1107–1113
Genitourinary system
  defects of, 611–612
  female, 93b
  male, 92b
  review of systems for, 92b–93b
Genitourinary tract
  imaging of, 150f, 150–151
  malformation of, 1370
Genograms, 1039–1040
Genotype-environment correlation/ interaction, 998
Gentamicin
  dosage, peak serum concentrations, and MIC_{95} for, 494t
  pelvic inflammatory disease treated with, 2519b
  urinary tract infections treated with, 2613t
  uses of, 500
Genu valgum. *See* Knock-knees
Genu varum. *See* Bowed legs
Geographic tongue, 126
GER. *See* Gastroesophageal reflux
GERD. *See* Gastroesophageal reflux disease
Germ cell tumors and teratomas
  clinical manifestations, 1884
  etiology, 1883–1884
  evaluation, 1884–1885
  follow-up, 1885
  management of, 1885
  prognosis, 1885
Germinal matrix
  intraventricular hemorrhage, 992
  newborn cranial ultrasonography screening, 702–703
Gesell's categories for infant assessment, 1742
Gestational age
  Ballard score for, 757–759
  eye examination based on, 721
  growth and development and, 857
  health outcomes for moderate- to late-preterm infants, 858
  high-risk delivery management, 654
Gestational hypertension, 634–635
GI bleeding. *See* Gastrointestinal bleeding
Giant papillary conjunctivitis, 1716
Giant vascular malformations, 1669
Giardia sp.
  description of, 2142
  G duodenalis, 2086
  G intestinalis, 2084–2086, 2370–2371. *See also* Giardiasis
  screening for, 70
Giardiasis
  clinical manifestations of, 2086, 2371
  description of, 2370–2371
  diagnosis of, 2372
  epidemiology of, 2085, 2371
  etiology, 2084–2085, 2085f
  laboratory evaluation, 2086
  life cycle of, 2371
  pathogenesis of, 2085, 2371
  prevalence of, 2371
  prevention of, 2087, 2372
  in travelers, 2371
  treatment of, 2086–2087, 2372
GID. *See* Gender identity disorder
Gilbert syndrome, 1618, 1619
Ginger, 458t
Gingiva
  in children, 125
  in infants, 125
  in newborns, 123–124
Gingivitis, necrotizing ulcerative, 2569, 2571
Ginkgo biloba, 458t, 542t
Ginseng, 458t, 542t
GIO. *See* Gastrointestinal obstruction
Girls. *See also* Female(s)
  adolescent, 2530b
  blood pressure levels, 109t–110t, 1580f, 1583t–1584t
  body mass index for, 112f
  calorie recommendations for, 194t
  puberty in, 1683–1687
  short stature in, 1729
Glabella tap reflex, 141f
Glasgow Coma Scale, 2711t, 2711–2712, 2744t
Glasgow Meningococcal Septicemia Prognostic Score, 2751, 2751t
Glaucoma, 118, 1703, 1707–1710, 1710f
GLB. *See* Gay, lesbian, and bisexual Youth
Global Appraisal of Individual Needs, 401
Global developmental delay
  definition of, 2184
  hypotonia and, 1604
Globe
  description of, 2343
  ruptured, 2348–2349
α-Globin chain, 2100, 2101f
Globin Gene Server, 342
Glomerular disease, 1566–1567, 1567f
Glomerular hematuria, 1567, 1569
Glomerular lesions, 1826
Glomerular proteinuria, 1677
Glomerulonephritides, 2286, 2286b
Glomerulonephritis. *See also* Nephritis
  acute
    characteristics of, 2287, 2287f
    with no or mild renal failure, 2287b, 2287–2290, 2289b
    with rapidly progress renal failure, 2289–2290, 2289b
  acute poststreptococcal
    causes of, 2287
    clinical presentation of, 2288
    course of, 2288
    description of, 2287
    laboratory findings in, 2288
    pathological features of, 2287
    prognosis of, 2289
    treatment of, 2288–2889
  chronic
    Alport syndrome, 2291–2292
    benign familial hematuria, 2291
    description of, 2290
    IgA nephropathy, 2290–2291
    membranoproliferative glomerulonephritis, 2293–2294
    nephritis of SLE, 2292–2293
  membranoproliferative, 2293–2294, 2296–2297
  postinfectious, 2289, 2289b
  rapidly progressive, 2289–2290, 2289b
Glottic web, 1751f
Glottis, 1750f, 1751f
Glucocorticoids
  Addison disease treated with, 1813
  adrenal insufficiency treated with, 1812–1813
  bacterial meningitis after neonatal period treated with, 2259
  congenital adrenal hyperplasia treated with, 1809, 1811, 1813
  inflammatory and neoplastic diseases treated with, 1815
  leukemia treated with, 1812
  potencies, 1811t
  regulation of, 1808
  replacement therapy, 1815
  short stature secondary to, 1728
  stress doses of, 1814
Gluconeogenesis, 973, 980–981

Glucose. *See also* Hyperglycemia; Hypoglycemia
  blood levels of. *See* Blood glucose
  in hypoglycemia, 2731–2732
  infusion of, 976
  metabolism of
    fetal metabolism and perinatal metabolic adaptation, 960
    gastrointestinal absorption, 972–976
    potassium-ATP channels, 974
  screening of, 679, 803
Glucose-6-phosphatase dehydrogenase deficiency
  description of, 2732
  hemolytic anemia, 942–943
  medical-legal issues in management of, 747–748
  newborn screening for, 387
Glucosuria, 406
Gluten-free diet, 2090, 2092, 2093
Gluten-sensitive enteropathy
  clinical manifestations of, 2090, 2090b
  differential diagnosis, 2090–2091, 2091b
  genetic markers, 2091
  incidence of, 2088
  intestinal biopsy, 2091–2092, 2092f
  laboratory evaluation, 2091, 2092f
  management of, 2092–2093
  pathogenesis of, 2089–2090
  pathological features, 2088, 2089f
  profile of patient with, 2090f
  referrals for, 2093
  serologic markers, 2091
  short stature caused by, 1728
Glycerol, 2742–2743
Glycogen storage diseases
  differential diagnosis, 2732–2733, 2736t
  hypotonia and, 1608
  type I, 978–979
  type III, 979
Glycogen synthase deficiency, 979
Glycogenolysis, 973, 976–979
Glycosuria, 1672
Glycosylation, 1453
Goiter, 607
Goldenhar syndrome, 2547
Gomco clamp, 829
Gonadal androgen production
  by ovaries, 1591–1592
  by testes, 1592–1593
Gonadal differentiation disorders, 2196–2197
Gonadal dysgenesis, 2197
Gonadarche, 1591
Gonadotropin-releasing hormone analogue, 1242
Gonads radiation exposure and infertility, 1896
Goniotomy, 1709
Gonococcal infection, 2521
  cervix, 2513b
  conjunctivitis caused by, 66t, 1705, 1705f
  diagnosis of, 2521, 2522f
  disseminated, 2514b, 2521, 2523f
  pharynx, 2513b–2514b
  rectum, 2513b
  in septic arthritis, 2506
  treatment of, 2513b–2514b, 2521
  urethra, 2513b
  in young children, 2570
Gonorrhea. *See Neisseria gonorrhoeae*
Good Manufacturing Practice regulations, 457
Goodpasture syndrome, 1571, 1827
Goose flesh, 1851
Gowers sign, 2273, 2276f
Graft-versus-host disease, 1717
Gram stain, 1823, 1854, 1857, 1858
Gram-negative aerobes, 1823
Gram-negative bacteria, 1823
Gram-negative folliculitis, 1804
Gram-positive bacteria, 1663
Gram-positive infections, 560
Grand mal seizures, 2489–2490, 2489b
Grandparents, 90, 182, 734
Granularity, 30t, 32
Granulocyte transfusions, 485–486
Granuloma, umbilical, 2606–2607
Granulomatous diseases, 1813
Graves disease
  management of, 2156
  signs and symptoms of, 2154t
  thyrotoxicosis caused by, 2154
Grief, 594
Griseofulvin, 513t
Gross hematuria. *See* Macroscopic hematuria
Ground glass appearance, 2078, 2080f
Group A beta-hemolytic streptococcal infection
  maternal-fetal infection, 637
  neonatal blood count/blood culture, 679–680
  neonatal sepsis, 935–936
  pharyngitis caused by, 2425
  placental health and, 632
  in rheumatic fever management, 2478
  in streptococcal TSS, 2573–2574
Group practice, 6t, 6–7
Growing pains, 1491, 1628
Growth and development
  abnormalities in, 63
  aggressiveness and, 1220
  anomalies. *See also* Congenital disorders
    in low–birth-weight infants, 856
    skin conditions, 782–783
  behavioral
    behavioral genetics perspective, 998–1000
    decreasing undesirable behavior, 1032–1033
Growth and development—cont'd
  behavioral—cont'd
    discipline and, 1029–1035
    encouragement of desirable behavior, 1032
    homelessness and, 1089–1090
    media exposure and, 1114–1120
    in neonatal intensive care infants, 879
    sexual abuse and, 1107–1113
  behavioral genetics, 998–1000
  breastfed infants, 822
  child abuse and neglect effects, 1098
  cognitive
    from 1 to 2 years, 210
    concrete operational stage, 1009
    formal operational period, 1011
    Piaget's theory of, 1002
    preoperational period, 1007–1008
    sensorimotor period, 1006
  conduct disorders and, 1220–1221
  congenital heart disease and, 861–862
  disorders, 1197, 1200
  early childhood development, in NICU patients, 870–871
  energy requirements for, 220
  Erikson's stages of, 98
  family role in, 999–1000
  fetal
    abnormalities
      description of, 633–634
      infants of diabetic mothers, 888–892
      intrauterine growth restriction, 883–885
      large-for-gestational-age infants, 888–892
      pathophysiology and management, 885–887
    assisted reproductive technologies and, 624
    in fetal stage, 638–639
    intrauterine growth and nutrition, 638–639
    maternal nutritional status and, 628–629
  foster care and, 1066–1072
  gay- and lesbian-parented children, 1082–1085
  health care assessments of, 13t, 15
  heredity-environment interaction, 998, 1001
  high-risk infants
    chronic lung disease infants, 696
    congenital heart disease, 696
    enteral nutrition, 693–694
    feeding intolerance, 694–695
    growth and maturity assessment and classification, 667–668
    human milk and preterm infant formula use, 695–696
    maternal health, abnormal growth and gestation, 633–634

Growth and development—cont'd
high-risk infants
osteopenia, 700
parenteral nutrition, 691–693
post-NICU care protocols, 690–698
history-taking about, 91b, 93
homelessness and, 1089–1090
language and, 1150
media impact on, 1114–1120
milestones in, history-taking about, 91b
neonatal intensive care infants, 853–858, 870–876
neurodevelopment. *See* Neurodevelopment
peer group and, 1000
phobias and, 1281
physical examination of, 108, 110–112
physiological-psychological factors in, 1004–1012
premature infants
brain maturation and neurodevelopment, 836–837
description of, 857
fetal-infant growth chart, 694, 836
growth and nutrition in, 690–696, 835–836
psychological
adolescence and young adulthood, 1009–1010
birthing process and, 1005
cognitive-intellectual theory, 1003
Erikson's psychosocial development theory, 1003
infancy, 1005–1006
intermediate postpartum period, 1004
learning theory, 1004
middle childhood, 1008–1009
physiological development and, 1004–1012
pregnancy precursors, 1004–1005
stages of, 1012
theoretical background, 1001–1004
toddlerhood and preschool age, 1007
psychosexual
genital stage, 1010
latency stage, 1008
oral and anal stages, 1006
phallic stage, 1007
psychosocial development
identity vs. role confusion and intimacy vs. isolation, 1010–1011
industry vs. inferiority, 1009
initiative vs. guilt, 1007–1008
trust vs. mistrust, autonomy vs. shame and guilt, 1006
school environment and, 1000
screenings, 349–354, 351t–352t
shared/nonshared environment, 998
sleep and, 1295t

Growth and development—cont'd
social learning development, 1007–1008, 1012
surveillance for, 49
temper tantrums and, 1316
temperament and attachment, 1001
theories and concepts, 997
timeframe for, 1147–1148
transgender youth and, 1238–1239
Growth charts, 110, 111f–114f
Growth curves
breastfed infants, 822
NICU discharge feeding plan and, 710–712
postnatal infants, 690–691
short stature and, 1728–1729
Growth delay, 1727
Growth hormone
deficiency of
diagnosis, 2736
hypoglycemia in, 2734, 2735
short stature and, 1728
description of, 1808, 1809, 1813
Growth monitoring
description of, 13t, 14–15
electronic health record used for, 28, 29t, 30–31
Growth patterns, 1727
GSE. *See* Gluten-sensitive enteropathy
Guarded alliance model, 733–735
Guarding, 2624
Guide to Community Preventive Services, 308
Guidelines for Adolescent Preventative Services, 1351
Guidelines for Health Supervision, 359
Guilt, 210
Guthrie card, 78
Guttate psoriasis, 2447, 2448f, 2449f
Gynecomastia, 1683–1684

H

Habilitation
definition of, 574
disorders treated with, 574b
Habit disorders, 451
Haddon's matrix of strategies in injury prevention, 267, 268t
Haemophilus influenzae type b
breastfeeding and, 810
description of, 1518, 1988
ophthalmia neonatorum and, 801–802
pharyngitis caused by, 2425b, 2426
prevention of, 810
vaccine
adverse effects of, 254
catch-up schedule for, 251t
characteristics of, 253–254
contraindications, 254
description of, 1857
guidelines for, 245f
intervals between doses, 248t

Haemophilus influenzae type b—cont'd
vaccine—cont'd
minimum age for, 248t
schedule for, 254t
Haggerty, Robert J., 55
Hair
growth of, 763, 1384
lanugo, 116
loss, 1384–1385. *See also* Alopecia
pulling and twisting of, 1726
shaft anomalies, 1386
Hair follicles, 113
Hair tourniquet, 1613
Hairball, 1726
Halitosis, 1660, 1661–1662
Hallucinogens, 2781–2782
Hallux valgus, 1530, 1531f
Haloperidol, 555t
Hamartomas, 781–782
Hammer toe, 1530, 1531f
Hand coordination, 144, 145f
Hand flapping, 1726
Hand-foot-mouth disease, 2569–2571
Handicap, 574
Happiness, 15
Hard palate
growth of, 123
in infants, 126
petechiae on, 126
Harvester ants, 2690
Hawthorn, 458t
Head
asymmetry of, 117
circumference of
brain growth and, 117
measurement of, 111f, 111–112, 113f
neonatal growth and development, 690–692
newborn assessment, 758–762
of infant, 117–118
of newborn, 116–117
percussion of, 117–118
physical examination of, 116–118
review of systems for, 92b
transillumination of, 117
tumors of, 1877t
Head banging, 1724–1725, 1726
Head injuries
causes, 2709–2710
child abuse evaluation, 1096–1097
concussion in, 2712, 2712t
diffuse axonal injuries in, 2713
hospitalization for, 2715
incidence, 2709
initial care in, 2710–2713
intracranial hematomas in, 2713, 2713t
irritability and, 1609
less severe, care of, 2713–2714
neonatal, 992
neurologic evaluation, 2711t, 2711–2712
parenchymal injuries in, 2713
pathophysiology of, 2710

Head injuries—cont'd
 prognosis, 2715
 referrals for, 2715
 secondary brain damage in, 2710–2711
 skull fracture in, 2712–2713
 sports participation with, 323t
 syncope and, 1756
 treatment of, 2714–2715
Head lice, 2181, 2181f
Head Start, 24, 1142
Headaches
 allodynia and, 1554
 analgesic rebound, 1554
 evaluation of, 1550–1551
 migraine
  characteristics of, 1550b, 1550–1555, 1552b
  irritability and, 1609
  self-hypnosis for, 453b
  syncope and, 1756
  vertigo caused by, 1457–1458
 pathophysiological features of, 1552–1553
 primary
  cluster, 1550b
  migraine, 1550b, 1550–1555, 1552b
  tension-type, 1550, 1550b, 1551, 1553
 referral for, 1555
 secondary
  causes of, 1551b
  definition of, 1550
  primary vs., 1550–1551
 sleep-related, 1309
 treatment of, 1553–1555
Healing touch, 460
Health
 community dimensions of, 55–56
 cultural differences on, 158
 maternal. *See* Maternal health
 World Health Organization definition of, 48
Health and developmental outcomes
 assisted reproductive technologies and, 622–625
 child abuse and neglect and, 1098
 foster care affected by, 1066–1072
 growth-restricted infants, 885–887
 health care barriers and, 847, 849–850
 homelessness and, 1088–1090
 in infants of diabetic mothers, 891
 jaundice, 899–900
 in neonatal intensive care unit infants, 852–863
  adolescence and adulthood, 858–861
  chronic conditions, functional limitations and special health care needs, 856–857
  congenital heart disease, 861–862
  early intervention in, 860
  growth problems, 857
  infancy and childhood health-related outcomes, 853
Health and developmental outcomes—cont'd
 in neonatal intensive care unit infants—cont'd
  moderate- to late-preterm infants, 858
  neurodevelopment and school-aged outcomes, 855–856
  pain sensitivity, 857–858
  post-hypoxic-ischemic encephalopathy, 862–863
  premature infants, 853–858
  respiratory failure, neurodevelopment and, 862
  visual function and retinopathy of prematurity, 857
 in premature infants, 837–838, 869
Health care
 access to
  community pediatrics, 56
  description of, 3
  financial barriers, 6
  for immigrants, 60–61
  language barriers, 61–62, 158
  for Latinos, 60–61
  outpatient care facilities, 6
 equity in, 44
 financial barriers to, 6
 financing of
  acronyms associated with, 19b
  adolescents and, 1326
  collection of payments, 17
  complexity of, 24
  consumer-driven health plans, 20–21
  description of, 17
  employer-based, 17, 18f
  family education about, 25
  health savings accounts, 20–21
  indemnity insurance plans, 17–18, 20t
  managed care, 17–19, 19b, 20t
  Medicaid, 23–24
  preferred provider organizations, 19b, 20t
  provider payment methods, 21–22, 22t
  self-funded or self-insured plans, 19–20
  State Children's Health Insurance Plan, 23–24
  summary of, 24–25
 metrics, 44
 processes of, 8–11
 purpose of, 11
Health care delivery systems. *See also* Mental Health services
 accessing of, 3, 410–416, 411f, 412t–413t, 415f
 challenges for, 3, 1322–1327
 collaborative care, 1138, 1186
  conversion reactions and, 1230–1231
  eating disorders and, 1191
Health care delivery systems—cont'd
  mood disorders and, 1260
  Münchausen syndrome by proxy and, 1276
  suicide and, 1314
 confidentiality and, 1322, 1326
 context of, 1324–1325
 ill children, 410–416, 411f, 412t–413t, 415f
 interactions in, 46
 outcomes of
  data sets, 14
  description of, 11
  disease, 12–14, 13t
  family, 13t, 15
  framework for assessing, 11, 13t–14t
  functioning and development, 13t, 15
  growth, 13t, 14–15
  injury, 12–14, 13t
  risk behaviors, 13t, 15
  survival, 11–12
  symptoms and comfort, 14t, 15
  well-being, 14t, 15
 overview of, 2
 pediatric workforce
  certification of, 3–4
  international medical graduates, 3
  licensure of, 3–4
  medical training of, 3–4
  nonphysician clinicians, 5
  nurse practitioners, 5
  physician assistants, 5
  statistics regarding, 2–3
 in schools, 1123
 sites for
  inpatient care facilities, 5–6
  outpatient care facilities. *See* Outpatient care
 structure of, 2–7
Health care professionals
 domestic violence and role of, 1075–1076
 in early education and child care programs, 1022–1025
 fetal-maternal health and role of, 650–651
 as parents, 1024
Health care spending, 416–417, 416f
Health education
 adolescents and, 1323
 pediatricians and, 1131–1133
 in schools, 1123, 1132
 substance abuse and, 1131
 trends in, 1131–1132
Health employer and data information set, 43
Health insurance
 adolescents and, 1326
 early-onset disorder diagnosis effects on, 77
 employer-based, 17, 18f

Health insurance—cont'd
- family education about, 25
- indemnity plans, 17–18, 20t
- lack of, 23
- Latinos, 61
- managed care, 17–19, 19b, 20t
- self-funded or self-insured, 19–20

Health maintenance organizations, 18–19, 19b

Health problems
- commonly referred types of, 9, 10t
- recognition of, 12

Health promotion
- activities for, 49
- early education and child care programs and risk of, 1022–1023
- focus of, 51
- for immigrants, 61

Health reimbursement account, 21

Health savings accounts, 20–21

Health screening
- for CRAFFT tool, 1246b, 1246–1247
- of immigrants and refugees, 69–70
- for phobias, 1283
- for posttraumatic stress disorder, 1287–1288, 1288f
- for school readiness, 1141, 1141b, 1143
- in schools, 1137
- for sleep complaints, 1296–1297t, 1297–1298
- for substance abuse, 1246–1247

Health supervision
- effectiveness of, 49–51
- preventive services visit, 48–49
- visit for, 50

Health-promoting school
- community involvement, 1126
- components of, 1122f
- health education and, 1123
- health services, 1123–1124
- nutrition services, 1124
- physical education, 1123
- physical environment of, 1124–1125
- social environment of, 1126
- staff health promotion and, 1126

Health-related quality of life outcomes, 853

Healthy lifestyle
- adherence to, 196–197
- components of
  - body composition, 193
  - cardiorespiratory endurance, 190–191, 191t
  - flexibility, 192
  - healthy diet, 193–195
  - large-muscle strength and endurance, 191–192
  - overview of, 190b
  - smoking cessation, 196
  - stress management, 195, 195b
- diseases prevented through, 189–190

Healthy lifestyle—cont'd
- learning of, 189
- programs for promoting, 190

Healthy People 2010
- on lead poisoning screening, 395
- on maternal depression, 365

Hearing. *See also* Hearing loss.
- assessment of, 356–357
- language development and, correlation between, 122
- loss of, 1458
- screening of, 122, 718–719

Hearing aids, 1559, 1560

Hearing loss
- adaptive equipment for, 1559, 1560
- cochlear implants for, 332, 332b
- consequences of, 326
- follow-up care for children with, 330–332, 331f, 332b
- identification of, 1559
- in neonatal intensive care infants, 879
- normal hearing vs., 1557f–1558f
- parental concerns and, 1559t
- permanent, 1557–1560
- post-delivery screening for, 805
- prevalence of, 326
- risk factors and indicators for, 719
- screening for, 326–334, 879. *See also* Auditory screening
- signs and symptoms of, 1558
- speech development affected by, 1558–1559, 1559t
- treatment of, 330–332, 331f, 332b

Heart
- of adolescents, 131–132
- auscultation of, 130
- of children, 131–132
- congenital defects of. *See* Congenital heart defects
- of infants, 130–131
- leukemia treatment effects on, 2243
- of newborns, 130–131
- physical examination of, 130–132
- point of maximal impulse, 130
- tuberous sclerosis complex effects on, 2311

Heart beat. *See also* Cardiac Arrhythmias
- normal rhythm variation, 1412
- premature, 1412–1413

Heart block, 105

Heart disease
- burden of, 335
- dyspnea caused by, 1470
- heart sounds and, 1561
- hepatomegaly and, 1577
- management of, 1481
- National Cholesterol Education Program guidelines for, 281
- obesity effects on, 288–290, 289f
- prevalence of, 335
- prevention of, 278–293. *See also* Preventive cardiology
- risk factors for, 56, 279t, 280

Heart disease—cont'd
- screening for, 334–341. *See also* Cardiovascular screening
- serum markers of, 338
- signs of, 1562b, 1562–1563
- smoking and, 290–291

Heart failure, congestive
- arrhythmias in, 2723
- causes of, 925, 2720–2722
- definition of, 2717
- nutritional management, 2723–2724
- orthopnea in, 129
- pathophysiological features, 2717–2718
- pharmacotherapy for, 2722–2723, 2723f
- recommendations for, 2719, 2720t, 2724t–2725t
- scoring systems for, 2719, 2719t–2720t
- signs and symptoms of, 132, 2718–2719
- surgery for, 2724
- tachycardia caused by, 105

Heart murmurs
- anesthesia and, 526–527, 527t
- atrioventricular valve regurgitant, 131
- cardiac evaluation and, 1562–1563
- continuous, 132
- definition of, 1563
- description of, 916–918
- diastolic, 132
- diastolic flow, 132
- evaluation of, 1563t, 1563–1565
- hemoptysis and, 1574
- information suggestive of, 130
- innocent, 131, 131f, 1564–1566
- localization of, 131
- middiastolic, 132
- patient evaluation for, 1561–1562
- protodiastolic, 132
- referral for, 1566
- sports participation with, 322t
- systolic, 131

Heart rate
- abnormalities of
  - by age, 2802t
  - in congestive heart failure, 2721
- circadian rhythm of, 105
- during exercise, 190, 191t
- measurement of, 104–105, 106t
- during physical activity, 190, 191t
- during sleep, 105

Heart sounds
- abnormalities of, 131
- cardiac cycle and, 1561
- in congestive heart failure, 2719
- in infants, 130–131

Heat cramps, 2551

Heat exhaustion, 2551

Heat illness, 322t

Heatstroke, 2551

HEEADSS interview, 1334, 1335–1336t

Height
- of girls, 112f
- hypertension and, 1579, 1580f, 1581t–1582t
- measurement of, 110–111, 112f, 115f
- short stature, 1727–1730

Heimlich maneuver, 2048
Heiner syndrome, 1571
Helical computed tomography, 147
Helium-oxygen mixtures, for status asthmaticus, 2817
HELLP syndrome, 981, 2672
Hemangioblastomas, 2315, 2315t
Hemangiomas
- gastrointestinal bleeding caused by, 1546
- stridor and, 1748–1749
- stridor caused by, 1749t
- vascular birthmarks, 780–781

Hemarthrosis, 2107
Hematemesis, 1543, 1573t
Hematochezia, 1543, 2075
Hematologic diseases and disorders
- alloimmune hemolysis, 941–942
- anemia. *See* Anemia
- anesthesia and, 534–538, 537b
- in congestive heart failure, 2721
- dyspnea caused by, 1471
- edema caused by, 1480
- hemostatic disorders, 944–945
- hereditary hemolytic anemia, 942–943
- hypoplastic anemia, 943–944
- inherited coagulopathies, 537–538
- maternal health and, 631
- neonatal assessment, 671, 941–945
- platelet disorders, 538, 945–946
- sickle cell disease, 535–537, 537b
- in snakebites, 2698
- splenomegaly and, 1732
- thromboembolic disease, 945

Hematoma
- epidural, 2713t
- intracranial, 2713, 2713t
- septal, 123
- subdural, 66t, 2713t
- subgaleal, 762, 992

Hematuria
- benign familial, 2291
- causes of, 1566
- description of, 2107
- macroscopic, 1566–1568, 1567f
- microscopic, 1567b, 1568–1569, 1569f
- referral for, 1569–1570
- screening for, 405–406
- urine color change and, 1568f

Hemodialysis, 2770
Hemoglobin
- $A1_c$, 162
- C, 2104
- concentration of, in iron-deficiency anemia evaluation, 2205
- D, 2104
- determination of, 544

Hemoglobin—cont'd
- E, 943, 2104
- with high/low oxygen affinity, 2103
- H, disease
  - description of, 2099–2100
  - iron-deficiency anemia vs., 2204–2205
- M, 2103–2104
- production of, 1396–1401
- reticulocyte, 2208
- structure of, 2098
- synthesis of, 2098
- unstable, 2103

Hemoglobin Bart disease, 2100
Hemoglobinopathies, 943, 2098. *See also* Sickling disorders; Thalassemia
- genetic diagnosis of, 2098
- red blood cell transfusions and, 484
- referrals for, 2104
- reproductive options for carriers of, 2104
- screening of, 2098
- stem cell transplantation, 2104
- structural, 2102–2104, 2103t
- transfusion safety, 2104

Hemoglobinuria, 1567
Hemolysis, 1617
Hemolytic anemia, 941–942
Hemolytic-uremic syndrome
- in acute renal failure, 1826
- clinical entities, 2095t
- clinical presentation of, 2095
- description of, 1669, 2094
- diarrhea associated with, 2094–2096
- differential diagnosis of, 2095–2096, 2673
- epidemiology of, 2095
- gene mutations, 2095
- kidney transplant after, 2096–2097
- prognosis of, 2097
- referrals for, 2097
- sequelae of, 2097
- shigatoxin, 2094
- treatment of, 2096, 2096t

Hemophilia
- A, 2105, 2107
- anesthesia and, 537–538
- B, 2105, 2107
- bleeding associated with, 2107, 2109t
- classification, 944
- coagulation cascade, 2106f
- diagnosis, 2107
- hemarthrosis, 2107
- hematuria, 2107
- mild, 2109–2110
- mouth bleeding, 2107
- referrals for, 2111
- soft-tissue bleeding, 2107
- sports participation considerations, 322t
- treatment of
  - for AIDS and other viral infections, 2110

Hemophilia—cont'd
- treatment of—cont'd
  - factor replacement, 2109–2111
  - gene therapy, 2110
  - health care maintenance, 2109
  - home management, 2109
  - inhibitors, 2105, 2108, 2110
  - principles of, 2107–2108
  - products for, 2108t
  - prophylaxis, 2110
- von Willebrand disease, 2110–2111

Hemoptysis
- description of, 1990
- diagnostic testing for, 1574–1575
- differential diagnosis of, 1573, 1573t
- etiology of, 1571–1573, 1572t
- history-taking for, 1573–1574
- pathogenesis of, 1570–1571
- physical examination for, 1573–1574
- referral for, 1575

Hemorrhage. *See also* Bleeding
- gastrointestinal. *See* Gastrointestinal bleeding
- intracranial, 2172
- intraventricular
  - in extremely low–birth-weight infants, 854–855
  - neurological evaluation, 992
  - of prematurity, 2151
  - school-aged outcomes and, 855–856
  - in very low–birth-weight infants, 855
- posttonsillectomy, 559–560
- subconjunctival, 2346, 2346f

Hemorrhagic conjunctivitis, 1711f–1712f, 1712
Hemorrhagic disease of newborn
- acquired disorders, 944–945
- anemia and, 941
- description of, 1544
- hemophilia, 944
- inherited diseases, 944
- vitamin-K prophylaxis, 802

Hemosiderosis. *See* diffuse pulmonary hemorrhage
Hemostasis
- in disseminated intravascular coagulation, 2670–2672, 2671f–2672f
- newborn assessment, 944–945
- physiology of, 2670

Henoch-Schönlein purpura
- appendicitis vs., 1838
- clinical presentation of, 2112–2113
- description of, 1658, 1668
- differential diagnosis of, 2113
- epidemiology of, 2112
- evaluation of, 2113
- joint pain, 1627–1628
- nephritis, 2289, 2289b
- prognosis for, 2113–2114
- referrals for, 2114
- Rocky Mountain spotted fever vs., 2482

Page numbers followed by "f" denote figures; "t" denote tables; "b" *denote* boxes.

Henoch-Schönlein purpura—cont'd
  scrotal swelling and, 1720–1721
  treatment of, 2113–2114
  vascular lesions in, 1826
Heparin
  antidote for, 2767t
  in disseminated intravascular coagulation, 2675
Hepatic failure, 2672
Hepatic fibrosis, congenital, 1577
Hepatic veno-occlusive disease, 66t
Hepatitis. *See also* Metabolic liver disease
  acute, clinical features of, 2116t
  autoimmune, 2117, 2124–2126
  in chickenpox, 1914
  description of, 1362
  differential diagnosis of, 2116t
  drug-induced, 2117, 2126
  fulminant hepatic failure, 2126
  in human herpesvirus 6 and 7, 2136
  immunizations, 2109, 2115, 2120t, 2122–2123, 2124b
  jaundice and, 1620
  liver transplantation, 2126
  metabolic liver disease, 2126
  referrals for, 2126
  therapy and prevention, 2115–2117, 2120t
  TT-virus, 2117
Hepatitis A
  description of, 2115
  therapy and prevention, 2122b, 2122–2123, 2123t
  vaccine for
    in adolescents, 246f
    characteristics of, 252
    contraindications, 252
    guidelines for, 245f
    in immigrants and refugees, 71
Hepatitis B
  breastfeeding and, 813
  description of, 2115–2117, 2120t
  high-risk groups for, 253
  immune globulin, 250
  maternal screening for, 806–807
  perinatal infection, 932–933
  during pregnancy, 253
  therapy and prevention, 2123–2124, 2124b, 2125t
  vaccine
    in adolescents, 246f
    catch-up schedule for, 250t–251t
    characteristics of, 252t–253t
    combinations, 253
    contraindications, 253
    guidelines for, 245f
    for healthy infants, 806
    intervals between doses, 248t
    in low-birth-weight infants, 253
    minimum age for, 248t
    for NICU-discharged infants, 718
    in premature infants, 704, 838
Hepatitis C
  breastfeeding and, 813
  description of, 2117
  perinatal infection, 932–934
  therapy and prevention, 2124
Hepatitis D, 2117
Hepatitis E
  description of, 2117
  therapy and prevention, 2124
Hepatitis G, 2117
Hepatoblastoma, 1374
Hepatomegaly
  congestive heart failure and, 2718–2719
  definition of, 1575
  diagnostic testing for, 1578
  differential diagnosis of, 1576b, 1576–1577
  history-taking for, 1577–1578
  management of, 1578
  palpable liver and, 1576b, 1577
  physical examination for, 1577–1578
Heptavalent pneumococcal vaccine, 1518
Herbal therapies. *See also* Complementary and alternative medicine
  during breastfeeding, 825–827
  commonly used, 458t
  preoperative discontinuation of, 542t
  uses of, 457, 458t
Hereditary elliptocytosis, 942
Hereditary hemolytic anemia, 942–943
Hereditary hemorrhagic telangiectasia, 1574
Hereditary sensorimotor neuropathies, 1606
Hereditary spherocytosis, 942
Heredofamilial renal tubular acidosis syndromes, 2459, 2460t
Hernia
  characteristics of, 1721f, 1721–1722
  congenital diaphragmatic
    fetal intervention for, 616–617
    ultrasound detection of, 608
  umbilical, 133, 767, 2606
Heroin, 2685t
Herpangina, 2034, 2569–2571, 2571f
Herpes keratitis, 1713, 1713f
Herpes simplex virus
  breastfeeding and, 812–813
  conjunctivitis caused by, 1705
  definitions, 2129–2130
  description of, 1692f
  epidemiologic factors, 2130
  genital, 2516b–2517b, 2524–2527, 2527f
  maternal-fetal infection, 636
  meningoencephalitis caused by, 2268
  neonatal, 785–786, 2131–2132
  ocular herpes, 2130
  perinatal period, 934, 2132
  pharyngitis caused by, 2425b, 2426
  referrals for, 2133
  stomatitis, 125, 2571, 2571f
Herpes simplex virus—cont'd
  treatment of, 2132–2133, 2133b
  type 1, 2130–2131
  type 2, 2131
Herpes zoster
  conjunctivitis and, 1713
  in HIV-infected children, 2142
  lesions, 1692f
Heterosexual precocious puberty, 1685, 1686b, 1687
High blood pressure. *See* hypertension
High-risk infants. *See also* Low-birth-weight infants; Neonatal resuscitation; Premature infants; Sick and dying infants
  clinical signs of, 875
  delivery management, 654
  diagnostic categories for, 672–673
  discharge planning from intensive care, 709–726
  growth and maturity assessment and classification, 667–668
  health and developmental outcomes
    adolescence and adulthood, 858–861
    chronic conditions, 856–857
    congenital heart disease, 861–862
    early intervention and, 860
    growth problems, 857
    moderate- to late-preterm infants, 858
    neurodevelopmental and school-aged outcomes, 855–856
    pain sensitivity, 857–858
    post-hypoxic-ischemic encephalopathy, 862–863
    premature infants, 853–858
    severe respiratory failure, 862
    very low–birth-weight, extremely preterm infants, 853–855
    visual function and retinopathy of prematurity, 857
  levels of care guidelines, 683
  maternal health and, 627–637
    abnormal growth and gestation, 633–634
    alloimmunization, 634
    cytomegalovirus infection, 636
    dental health, 630
    drug/other substance abuse, 629–630
    gestational hypertension, 634–635
    herpes simplex virus infection, 636
    human immunodeficiency virus, 635
    intrauterine infection, 635–637
    maternal-fetal unit, 632
    multiple gestation, 633
    nutritional status, 627–629
    obstetric complications, 633
    pharmacologic intervention, 633
    placenta and membrane disorders, 631–632

High-risk infants—cont'd
maternal health and—cont'd
premature birth, 632–633
reproductive capability, 630–631
rubella exposure, 635–636
toxoplasmosis, 636–637
medical-legal considerations in care of, 744–745
metabolic derangements, 670–672
neonatal intensive care unit
needs assessment and referral, 667
post-NICU care protocols
anemia, 683–685
apnea, bradycardia, and desaturation, 685–688
bronchopulmonary dysplasia, 688–690
Child Find and early intervention, 724
cholestasis, 699
circumcision, 722
developmentally supportive care, 705–706
feeding and nutrition, 709–712
follow-up care, 721–722, 726
gastroesophageal reflux/ gastroesophageal reflux disease, 696, 699
health maintenance guidelines, 700–705
hearing screening, 718–720
immunizations, 717–718
insurance coverage, 722–723
laboratory studies, 722
neurologic evaluation, 720–721
nutrition and growth issues, 690–698
osteopenia, 700
pain assessment and management, 705
parent education, 723
prescriptions and medication administration, 724
respiratory management, 713–717
retinopathy of prematurity screening, 720–721
safety issues, 723–724
screening procedures, 720–721
social services and case management, 722
summary and checklist, 724–726
temperature regulation, 712–713
transition to oral feeding, 700
neonatal return transfer to community setting, 684–685
pre-transport care of, 673–680
primary care physician's responsibilities for, 729–730
respiratory distress signs, 668
sepsis syndrome, 668–670
warning signs of, 875
Hip dysplasia
developmental. *See* Developmental dysplasia of the hip
limp and, 1632–1633, 1633f, 1635–1636
metatarsus adductus and, 1534
newborn assessment, 771
screening for, 805
Hip rotation test, 1633f
Hirschberg test, 120, 1780–1781
Hirschenual diagnosis, 1426
Hirschsprung disease
description of, 1428, 2080, 2080f
diarrhea caused by, 1450
postnatal evaluation, 777
Hirsutism
causes of, 1591b, 1595t
definition of, 1590
diagnostic testing for, 1595t
evaluation for, 1595
hyperandrogenism and, 1591–1594
hypertrichosis and, 1590, 1591b
idiopathic, 1595
treatment of, 1595–1596
Histoplasmosis, 1731–1732
History-taking
definition of, 88
information gathering through, 207
interviews and interviewing
with child, 95–96
direct questions, 94
facilitation of communication during, 94–95
pediatric history, 90–94, 91b–92b
prenatal, 89–90
techniques for, 94–96
present illness, 90, 91b, 96
questionnaires, 96
questions asked in, 88
recording of information, 96
reflexive self-concept, 88
review of systems, 92b–93b, 94
setting for, 88–89
HITS questions, 369
HIV
adolescents with, 2145
age-specific immunologic categories, 2141t
antimicrobial prophylaxis, 2143
antiretroviral therapy, 2143–2144
breastfeeding and, 812
categories of, 2141t
child care considerations, 2145
clinical manifestations of, 2140–2141
clinical problems caused by, 2141–2142
description of, 1342
diagnosis of, 2140
diarrhea associated with, 2142
disseminated varicella associated with, 2142
growth failure secondary to, 2142
in hemophilia patients, 2110
herpes zoster in, 2142
HIV—cont'd
immunizations, 2139–2140, 2142–2143, 2145
maternal-infant transmission of, 2142
needlestick injuries, 2144–2145
neurocognitive effects of, 2142
pathophysiological features of, 2139–2140
perinatal infection
diagnosis and management, 932
morbidity and mortality, 635
transmission prevention, 804–805
pneumonia in, 2142
postexposure prophylaxis for, 2144–2145
schooling considerations, 2145
secondary infection and, 1696–1697
sports participation with, 322t
transmission of, 2139
HIV encephalitis, 2142
HIV meningitis, 2142
Hives, 1682, 2028
HLA-DQ2 allele combination, 2089–2090
HLA-DQ8 allele combination, 2090
HLHS. *See* Hypoplastic left heart syndrome
HMOs. *See* Health maintenance organizations
Hoarseness
causes of, 1598
definition of, 1598
diagnostic testing for, 1600–1601
differential diagnosis of, 1598b–1599b, 1598–1599
gastroesophageal reflux disease and, 2058, 2059t
history-taking, 1600
management of, 1601–1602
physical examination for, 1600
Hodgkin disease
chemotherapy for, 1892–1894, 1995
clinical manifestations of, 1892–1893
etiology of, 1892
evaluation of, 1893
follow-up, 1894–1895
management of, 1893–1894
prognosis of, 1894
Holosystolic murmurs, 1564f
Holter monitors, 1757
Home births, 82–83
Home care
diagnoses that commonly receive, 569
Early and Periodic Screening, Diagnosis, and Treatment program in, 572
family-centered care, 569–570, 570b
family-directed, 570–571
ill child, 409–410, 410t
Medicaid, 571–572
medical day treatment programs, 572
oxygen therapy
discharge criteria for, 713–717
equipment requirements, 714

Home care—cont'd
pediatric home health care providers, 571
public funding of, 571–572
reimbursement for, 571–572
supplemental security income in, 572
ventilation therapy, in NICU-discharged infants, 714–715
Home health visits, 723
Home monitoring, in neonatal intensive care infants, 716–717, 877–878
Home nursing, 174b
Homelessness
behavioral effects of, 1089–1090
causes of, 1088
health effects of, 1088–1089
statistics regarding, 1087–1088
trends in, 1087–1088
Homeopathy, 459–460
Homeostasis
potassium, 470
sodium, 469–470
Homicide
of children, 1265–1266
statistics regarding, 239
Homocystinuria, 387, 987
Homosexual behavior, 1341
Honesty, 155
Hookworm infections
clinical manifestations of, 2388
diagnosis of, 2388
epidemiologic features of, 2388
prevalence of, 2388
prevention of, 2389
treatment of, 2388–2389
Hops, 458t
Hormonal regulation disorders
counterregulatory hormone deficiency, 982–983
fasting metabolic systems, 983
Hormonal therapy, for acne, 1805–1806
Hormone(s)
birth control uses of, 1352
deficiencies of
in cortisol deficiency, 2735
diagnostic evaluation, 2736
hypoglycemia in, 2733b, 2734t, 2734–2736
in hypopituitarism, 2734–2735
sexuality and, 1339
transgender youth and, 1238, 1241–1242
Horner syndrome, 119
Hornet stings, 2687–2689
Hospice, 594
Hospital(s)
admission to, 171–173, 172b
emergent admission to, 171, 172b
family's role in decision making, 171–172
health care delivery in, 5–6
infections in
neonatal sepsis against, 936
prophylaxis, 705
nonprofit status, 5–6
Hospital(s)—cont'd
primary care physician's role in, 172b, 173
selection of, 171
socioeconomic status influences, 5
statistics regarding, 5
teaching, 6
Hospitalists
benefits of, 170
communication with patient and family by, 168–170
description of, 4–5
primary care physicians and, 168–169, 169b
Hospitalization
abdominal distention, 1375–1376
abdominal pain, 1383
adolescents and, 1324–1325
anemia, 1404
back pain, 1410
cardiac arrhythmias, 1419
chest pain, 1421b, 1424
constipation, 1431
cough, 1436
description of, 171–173, 172b
diarrhea, 1454
dizziness, 1460
dysmenorrhea, 1463
dysphagia, 1467
dyspnea, 1474
dysuria, 1478
eating disorders, 1192
edema, 1481–1482
encopresis, 1253, 1255b
epistaxis, 1488
failure to thrive, 1506, 1507
history-taking about, 92b
of ill child, 414–415, 415f
of patient with indemnity insurance, 17–18
recurrent, 171
statistics regarding, 5
stress associated with, 171, 173, 175
suicidal adolescents, 1314
variations in rates of, 14
vertigo, 1460
Hot tub folliculitis, 1856
HPO axis. *See* Hypothalamic-pituitary-ovarian axis
H_2-receptor antagonists for gastroesophageal reflux disease, 2061, 2061t
Huffman vaginoscope, 136, 136f
Human chorionic gonadotropin, 604
Human herpesvirus-6 and -7
classification, 2134
clinical characteristics of, 2135, 2135t
diagnosis, 2137
differential diagnosis, 2137
epidemiologic features, 2134–2135
hepatitis, 2136
in immunocompromised patients, 2136–2137
Human herpesvirus-6 and -7—cont'd
management of, 2137
meningoencephalitis, 2136
mononucleosis-like disease, 2136
nonspecific viral illness, 2135
referrals for, 2137–2138
roseola, 2135–2136
seizures, 2136
Human milk. *See also* Breastfeeding
allergy to, 2065–2066
breast milk jaundice, 822
cow milk vs., 213, 214t, 226, 229
expression of, 817
for extremely low–birth-weight infants, 855
medications in, 813, 824–825
NICU discharge feeding plan including, 710–712
for preterm infants, 695–696
protein in, 213, 222
Human papillomavirus
atopic dermatitis and, 1852
description of, 1342
in laryngeal papillomatosis, 2635–2636
morphology, 2525f
sexual abuse and risk of, 1109
subclinical lesions of, 2524f
treatment of, 2514b–2516b
vaccine for
in adolescents, 246f
description of, 2523–2524
interval between doses, 249t
minimum age for, 249t
Human rabies immunoglobulin, 1824
Human T-cell lymphotropic virus, 812
Humerus, proximal, 2554
Humidified air, for croup, 2652
Humoral immunodeficiencies, 1697–1699, 1698t
HUS. *See* Hemolytic-uremic syndrome
Hydatid disease, 2397–2399. *See also* Echinococcal disease
Hydralazine, 2729, 2729t
Hydrocarbon poisoning, 2775–2776
Hydrocele, 134, 1721f–1722f, 1721–1722
Hydrocephalus. *See also* Cerebrospinal fluid, shunting of
cerebrospinal fluid and, 2146–2147
classification of, 2147, 2148t
clinical manifestations of, 2149
complications of
infection, 2152
intracerebral hemorrhage, 2152
mechanical failure, 2152
overdrainage, 2152–2153
shunt obstruction, 2152
definition of, 2147
description of, 1646–1647, 1647b
epidemiologic features of, 2147
etiology of, 2147–2149
evaluation of, 2149
fetal intervention, 618
follow-up, 2153

Hydrocephalus—cont'd
obstructive, 2147–2148
outcome of, 2153
pathophysiological features, 2147
plagiocephaly caused by, 2434
prognosis of, 2153
radiological findings in, 2150t
signs and symptoms of, 2148t–2149t
stridor and, 1748
treatments of, 2149, 2152–2153
ultrasound detection of, 605–606
Hydrocortisone
adrenal insufficiency treated with, 1813
shock treated with, 2811
Hydrolysates, 2067t
Hydrolyzed casein hydrolysate infant formula, 2066–2067
Hydrometrocolpos, 1373
Hydromorphone
acute pain managed using, 429
chronic pain managed using, 442t
potency and half-life of, 425t
Hydronephrosis
antenatal hydronephrosis, 775–776
differential diagnosis of, 2333, 2333b
prenatal, 2334, 2334t
ultrasound detection of, 611
17-Hydroxylase deficiency, 2196
11ß-hydroxylase enzyme deficiency, 1594
17-Hydroxyprogesterone
NICU-discharged infant screening, 719
premature infant screening, 702
3ß-Hydroxysteroid deficiency, 1594
Hymenolepiasis, 2400–2401
Hymenolepis nana, 2400–2401
Hymenoptera
anaphylactic reaction to, 2644, 2687–2690
fire ants, 2689–2690
harvester ants, 2690
winged, 2687–2689
Hyperactivity in Down syndrome patients, 2022
Hyperacute rejection, 1963–1964
Hyperandrogenism
adrenal, 1593–1594
gonadal androgen production and, 1591–1593
Hyperbaric oxygen
carbon monoxide poisoning treated with, 2773–2774
streptococcal TSS treated with, 2576
Hyperbilirubinemia
conjugated, 1615–1616, 1617b, 1618, 1620b, 1620–1621
definition of, 1615
follow-up care, 897–899
in infants of diabetic mothers, 890
management guidelines, 893
medical history, 893–895
medical-legal issues in management of, 747–748
Hyperbilirubinemia—cont'd
neonatal assessment, 671
in premature infants, 836–837
risk factors for, 748, 895
severity definitions, 893
unconjugated, 1616–1619, 1617b, 1620b, 1621
Hypercalcemia, 966–967
Hypercalciuria
dysuria caused by, 1477
microhematuria caused by, 1569
Hypercholesterolemia. *See also* Cholesterol
breastfeeding and incidence of, 810
cholesterol levels in children and adolescents from families with, 280t
environment in, 280
genetics in, 280
prevention of, 280–281, 280t
Hyperextension test, 1408f
Hyperglycemia
causes of, 2000b. *See also* Diabetes mellitus
in diabetic ketoacidosis, 2662–2664
in increased intracranial pressure, 2743
neonatal, 965
prevention and management, 966
Hyperhidrosis, 1603–1604
Hyperimmunoglobulin E, 745–746
Hyperinsulinism
congenital, 974–976
diagnostic evaluation, 2735–2736
differential diagnosis, 2732, 2733b, 2734t
in infants of diabetic mothers, 889–890
management, 2737
neonatal, 973
Hyperinsulinism-hyperammonemia syndrome, 975
Hyperkalemia
in acute renal failure, 2799, 2800t
characteristics of, 477–478, 478t
in diabetic ketoacidosis, 2664–2665
regeneration-type renal tubular acidosis, 2468t, 2469–2470
Hyperlipidemia, 2006–2007, 2298
Hypermagnesemia, 969
Hypermobility syndrome, 1628
Hypernatremia, 475–477, 476t, 2657, 2659t
Hyperphosphatemia, 2799
Hyperpigmentation, 1808–1809, 1811–1812, 1814
Hyperpigmented lesions
description of, 779–780
incontinentia pigmenti, 784–785
Hypertelorism, 791–792
Hypertension. *See also* Gestational hypertension
ACE inhibitors for, 2114
antihypertensive drugs and, 1587t–1588t, 1588
Hypertension—cont'd
blood pressure regulation and, 1585
body size and, 1579, 1580f, 1581t–1582t, 1588
calcium channel blockers for, 1816
causes of, 1580–1584, 1584b
definition of, 1579, 2726
diagnostic evaluation for, 1585–1587, 1586f
essential, 132
factors influencing, 1579–1580
gestational, 634–635
idiopathic intracranial, 2739
laboratory tests for, 2728, 2728b
malignant, 2726–2727, 2730
persistent pulmonary, 2721
prevalence of, 188
primary, 1580, 1582
pulmonary, 1943
referral for, 1589
renal causes of, 132
sports participation with, 322t
treatment of, 1588–1589
in urinary tract infections, 2614
white coat, 2728
Hypertensive emergencies
definition of, 2726–2727
description of, 1588–1589
drugs used in, 2729t–2730t, 2729–2730
evaluation, 2727–2728
hospitalization for, 2731
hypertensive urgency, 2726, 2727f, 2729–2730
laboratory tests for, 2728, 2728b
malignant hypertension, 2726–2727, 2730
management of, 2727f, 2728–2730
prognosis, 2729
referral for, 2731
Hyperthermia
definition of, 418
fever vs., 1516
increased intracranial pressure and, 2743
malignant, anesthesia and, 539b–540b, 539–540
management of, 420
Hyperthyroidism
anesthesia and, 534
complications of, 2157
definition of, 2154
differential diagnosis of, 2154
evaluation of, 2154–2156, 2155f
history-taking for, 2154–2155, 2154t
laboratory tests for, 2155–2156
management of
adjuvant ß-adrenergic blockers, 2156
antithyroid medications, 2156
definitive therapy in, 2156–2157
iodide, 2156
side effects of, 2156
thioamides, 2156
neonatal thyrotoxicosis caused by, 2157

Page numbers followed by "f" denote figures; "t" denote tables; "b" *denote* boxes.

Hyperthyroidism—cont'd
physical examination for, 2154–2155, 2154t, 2155f
thyrotoxic crisis caused by, 2157
Hypertonia, 991–992, 1738
Hypertrichosis, 1590
Hypertrophic cardiomyopathy
definition of, 340
description of, 81, 1962–1963
syncope and, 1755
Hypertrophic pyloric stenosis, 1611, 2078
Hypertropia, 1738, 1738f
Hyperventilation
description of, 1226, 1424
increased intracranial pressure treated with, 2742
syncope and, 1755
Hyphema, 2348, 2348f
Hypnagogic hallucinations, 1659
Hypnosis
definition of, 448
research in, 454
self-hypnosis, 449–454
Hypnotherapy, 448
Hypocalcemia
in congestive heart failure, 2721
in infants of diabetic mothers, 889
in large-for-gestational-age infants, 889
neonatal, 966–967
Hypochondriasis, 1282
Hypoglycemia
Beckwith-Wiedemann syndrome, 976
blood-urine sampling, 975
breastfeeding and, 819
clinical manifestations, 2732
congenital hyperinsulinism, 974–976
congestive heart failure and, 2721
definition of, 2731–2732
description of, 2006
differential diagnosis of, 2644, 2732–2735
etiology of, 971, 2732, 2733b
evaluation of, 2735–2736
fatty acid oxidation and ketogenesis, 981–982
fructose-1,6-diphosphatase deficiency, 980
glucose screening, 803
glycogen storage diseases, 978–979
glycogen synthase deficiency, 979
in hormonal deficiencies, 2733b, 2734t, 2734–2735, 2736
hormonal regulation disorders, 982–987
hospitalization for, 2738
hyperinsulinism and, 2732, 2733b, 2734t, 2735–2737
incidence of, 2732
in infants of diabetic mothers, 889
intrauterine growth restriction and, 884
irritability and, 1612
ketotic, 2733b, 2735, 2738
Hypoglycemia—cont'd
in large-for-gestational-age infants, 889
management, 2736–2738
medical-legal issues in management of, 745
medium-chain acyl-CoA dehydrogenase deficiency, 981–982
in metabolic disorders, 2732–2734, 2733b, 2734t, 2736–2737
mitochondrial respiratory-chain disorders, 979
neonatal
clinical signs, 962
counterregulatory hormone deficiency, 982–987
diagnosis of, 961–965
differential diagnosis of, 962
etiologic factors, 972
evaluation of, 970–971
family history, 970
fatty acid oxidation and ketogenesis, 981–982
gastrointestinal glucose absorption, 972–976
gluconeogenesis, 980–981
glycogenolysis, 976–979
incidence, 962
infant of diabetic mother, 974
management of, 961–965
persistent hypoglycemia, 972–987
physical examination for, 970–971
signs and symptoms, 971
stabilization, 674
persistent, 972–987
phosphoenolpyruvate-carboxylase deficiency, 980
pituitary deficiency, 983
in premature infants, 834, 965
pyloric stenosis and, 2457
pyruvate carboxylase deficiency, 980–981
signs and symptoms, 971
Hypokalemia, 477, 477t, 2664–2665
Hypomagnesemia, 968
Hypomelanotic macules, 779
Hypomyelinating neuropathy, 1606
Hyponatremia
in dehydration, 2657, 2658t
description of, 474–475, 475t
in diabetic ketoacidosis, 2664
polyuria and, 1674
Hypophosphatemia, 2665
Hypopigmentation, 779
Hypopituitarism, congenital, 2734–2735
Hypoplasia, 1499
Hypoplastic anemia, 943–944
Hypoplastic left and right ventricles
pressure overload, 925–926
ultrasound detection of, 609
Hypoplastic left heart syndrome
evaluation of, 1954–1955
illustration of, 1954f–1955f
Hypoplastic left heart syndrome—cont'd
management of, 1955–1956
pressure overload, 925–926
prognosis, 1956–1957
ultrasound detection, 906
Hypopnea, 656
Hypoprothrombinemia, 216
Hypospadias
description of, 135, 2158, 2159f
newborn assessment, 768–769
physical examination, 794
Hypotelorism, 791–792
Hypotension
differential diagnosis, 2566t
neonatal blood pressure assessment, 678–679
syncope and, 1753
Hypotensive crisis, 1809, 1816
Hypothalamic corticotrophin-releasing hormone, 1808
Hypothalamic-pituitary-ovarian axis, 1767–1768
Hypothalamus tumors, 1862
Hypothermia
in drowning injuries, 2678
increased intracranial pressure and, 2743
neonatal infant stabilization, 674–676
in premature infants, 833
Hypothyroidism
acquired, 2165
anesthesia and, 532, 534
causes of, 2161–2162, 2162b
clinical manifestations of, 2161
congenital
causes of, 2162b
management of, 2165, 2165t
newborn screening for, 384–385
definition of, 2161
description of, 1375, 2161–2167
differential diagnosis of, 2162, 2163b
evaluation of, 2162–2164, 2163b–2164b
fatigue caused by, 1510
history-taking, 2162–2163
hypotonia and, 1605
incidence of, 2162
juvenile, 2162b
laboratory tests for, 2163–2164
management of, 2164t–2165t, 2164–2165
physical examination for, 2163, 2164f
prognosis of, 2165
radioisotopic studies for, 2164
short stature and, 1728
thyroid function tests for, 2163–2164
L-thyroxine for, 2164t–2165t, 2164–2165
Hypotonia. *See also* Weakness
causes of, 1605–1608
definition of, 1604
diagnostic testing for, 1605–1606
history-taking, 1605
neonatal, 990–992
physical examination for, 1605
referral for, 1608

Hypovolemia. *See* Dehydration
Hypovolemic shock
  description of, 2804f, 2804–2805, 2805b
  neonatal stabilization, 678–679
Hypoxia
  acute fetal, 656–658
  neurological evaluation, 991–992
  neurological impairment, 862–863
Hypoxic ischemic encephalopathy, 669–670
Hysterical personality, 1227

I

Iatrogenic disease
  case report, 2167–2168
  causes of, 2168, 2169t
  database for, 2168
  description of, 2167
  differential diagnosis of, 2168, 2170t
  management of, 2169–2170
  prevention of, 2168–2169
Ibuprofen
  acute pain managed using, 428t
  chronic pain managed using, 440, 441t
Identity, 1010–1011
Idiopathic hypersomnia, 1308
Idiopathic short stature, 1728
Ileal atresia with meconium peritonitis, 2077–2078, 2079f
Ileal obstructions, 2081–2082
Ill children
  accessing health care system for, 410–416, 411f, 412t–413t, 415f
  description of, 409, 409f
  disposition in, 415–416
  home care of, 409–410, 410t
  hospitalized, 414–415, 415f
  levels of care in, 409, 409f
  office emergency, 412, 412t–413t
  practitioner-patient encounter in, 412t–413t, 412–414
  special needs children, 416–417, 416f
  substance overdose, 410, 410t
  telephone care flow chart in, 411–412, 411f
Illness fabrication, 1269–1276
Image blur, 1777
IMAGe syndrome, 1812
Imaginary companions, 1744
Imaging
  acute abdomen evaluations, 2624
  bone, 151
  chest, 148, 148f
  computed tomography. *See* Computed tomography
  congenital anomaly diagnosis, 795
  croup evaluations, 2651, 2652f
  fluoroscopy, 146–147
  genitourinary tract, 150f, 150–151
  head injuries evaluations, 2714
Imaging—cont'd
  increased intracranial pressure evaluations, 2740–2741, 2741f
  magnetic resonance imaging. *See* Magnetic resonance imaging
  mental status alteration evaluations, 2642
  nervous system evaluations, 151–152
  nuclear scintigraphy, 147–148
  pneumothorax evaluations, 2756, 2756f
  respiratory failure in newborns, 906
  septic arthritis evaluations, 2507
  skeletal system, 151
  status asthmaticus evaluations, 2813
  status epilepticus evaluations, 2821
  streptococcal TSS evaluations, 2575
  tuberculosis evaluations, 2591, 2599–2600, 2602
  ultrasound. *See* Ultrasound
  urinary tract infection evaluations, 2611–2612, 2612b
Imipenem, 498–499
Imiquimod
  genital warts treated with, 2515b
  warts treated with, 2618
Imitative learning, 1004
Immigrants
  behavioral health screening of, 69–70
  blood lead level testing in, 63
  countries of origin, 60f
  cultural issues, 62–63
  demographics of, 60
  functional health screening of, 69–70
  growth abnormalities in, 63
  health care access for, 60–61
  health promotion for, 61
  immunizations for, 71
  lack of insurance, 60
  language barriers, 61–62
  limited English proficiency among, 61–62
  malaria screening in, 70
  nutritional disorders in, 63
  oral health among, 63, 69
  parasitic infection screening in, 70
  screening tests for, 70–71
  serologic testing in, 71
  statistics regarding, 59–60
  tuberculosis screening in, 70–71
Immobilization, for snakebites, 2697
Immune globulin, 487
Immune system, 648–649
Immune thrombocytopenic purpura
  chronic, 2173
  clinical presentation of, 2170–2171
  complications of, 2173
  description of, 2170
  differential diagnosis of, 2171
  evaluation of, 2171
  incidence of, 2170
  intracranial hemorrhage in, 2172
Immune thrombocytopenic purpura—cont'd
  management of
    anti-Rho, 2173
    bleeding-related, 2172
    corticosteroids, 2172
    follow-up care, 2173
    general advice in, 2172
    intravenous immunoglobulin, 2172–2173
    outcomes after, 2173
    splenectomy, 2173–2174
  in neonates, 2173
Immunizations. *See also* Vaccinations
  acellular pertussis, 2423b
  adolescents, 246f
  anaphylactic allergy caused by, 248
  animal bites and, 1823
  autoimmune disorders and, 1999
  benefits of, 244
  childhood, 245f
  conjugate, 2254, 2255t
  contagious exanthematous diseases treated with, 1976
  contraindications, 247–250
  diphtheria, tetanus, and pertussis
    in adolescents, 246f
    adverse reactions to, 252
    catch-up schedule for, 250t
    characteristics of, 252
    contraindications, 252
    guidelines for, 245f
  in Down syndrome patients, 2019b, 2022b, 2024
  electronic health record used for management of, 29t, 31
  in foreign countries, 247
  4-week separation rule for, 244
  Haemophilus influenza type b vaccine
    adverse effects of, 254
    catch-up schedule for, 251t
    characteristics of, 253–254
    contraindications, 254
    guidelines for, 245f
    intervals between doses, 248t
    minimum age for, 248t
    schedule for, 254t
  hemophilia patients, 2109
  hepatitis A vaccine
    in adolescents, 246f
    characteristics of, 252
    contraindications, 252
    guidelines for, 245f
    in immigrants and refugees, 71
  hepatitis B vaccine
    in adolescents, 246f
    catch-up schedule for, 250t–251t
    characteristics of, 252t–253t
    combinations, 253
    contraindications, 253
    guidelines for, 245f
    for healthy infants, 806

Page numbers followed by "f" denote figures; "t" denote tables; "b" *denote* boxes.

Immunizations—cont'd
hepatitis B vaccine—cont'd
intervals between doses, 248t
in low–birth-weight infants, 253
minimum age for, 248t
for NICU-discharged infants, 718
in premature infants, 704, 838
history-taking about, 92b
in HIV-infected child, 2139–2140, 2142–2143, 2145
human papillomavirus vaccine
in adolescents, 246f
interval between doses, 249t
minimum age for, 249t
in ill children, 248–249
in immigrants, 71
in immunocompromised children, 249–250
inactivated polio virus
in adolescents, 246f
catch-up schedule for, 250t
characteristics of, 257
intervals between doses, 248t
minimum age for, 248t
inactivated vaccines, 244
influenza vaccine
administration of, 254–255
in adolescents, 246f
adverse effects of, 255
characteristics of, 254–255
contraindications, 255
guidelines for, 245f
interval between doses, 248t
minimum age for, 248t
intervals between, 247, 248t
live injected, 247
live vaccines
contraindications, 250
description of, 244
Lyme disease, 2251
malignancies and, 1896
measles, mumps, rubella vaccine
administration of, 255
in adolescents, 246f
adverse reactions to, 255
catch-up schedule for, 250t–251t
characteristics of, 255–256
contraindications, 255–256
guidelines for, 245f
in HIV-infected children, 2143
before immune globulin-containing products, 247
in immunocompromised patients, 250
intervals between doses, 248t
minimum age for, 248t
meningococcal polysaccharide vaccine
in adolescents, 246f
guidelines for, 245f
interval between doses, 248t
minimum age for, 248t
in NICU-discharged infants, 717–718
Immunizations—cont'd
in orthotopic heart transplantation patients, 1964
parental refusal for, 79
pneumococcal vaccine
in adolescents, 246f
catch-up schedule for, 251t
characteristics of, 256
conjugated, 256
guidelines for, 245f
intervals between doses, 248t
minimum age for, 248t
polysaccharide, 256–257, 257t
schedule for, 251t, 256t
for poliovirus, 2034, 2039
precautions for, 247–250
during pregnancy, 250
in preterm/premature infants, 250, 704–705
principles of, 244–252
recommended, 244, 245f–246f
in refugees, 71
religious exemption for, 79
rotavirus vaccine
adverse reactions to, 257–258
characteristics of, 257–258
contraindications, 257
guidelines for, 245f
interval between doses, 249t
minimum age for, 248t
safety concerns, 250, 252
schedule for
catch-up, 250t–251t
recommended, 244, 245f–246f, 247
simultaneous administration of, 244, 247
stress dosing, 1814
underimmunization risk factors, 79
varicella vaccine
in adolescents, 246f
catch-up schedule for, 250t
description of, 1911, 1916–1917
guidelines for, 245f
before immune globulin-containing products, 247
in immunocompromised patients, 250
Immunocompromised patients, 249–250
Immunodeficiencies. *See also* AIDS; HIV
combined, 1698–1699, 1699t
diagnostic testing for, 1700, 1700t
history-taking, 1700
physical examination for, 1700
primary, 1697–1701
recurrent infections and, 1696
secondary, 1696–1697, 1697t
signs and symptoms of, 1701b
treatment of, 1700
Immunoglobulin, intravenous
immune thrombocytopenic purpura treated with, 2172–2173
in staphylococcal TSS, 2566
in streptococcal TSS, 2566
Immunoglobulin A nephropathy, 1568, 2290–2291
Immunoglobulin E
allergic rhinitis and, 1819–1820
asthma and, 1839–1841, 1848
atopic dermatitis and, 1850, 1852
eosinophilic gastrointestinal disorders and, 2067–2068
gastrointestinal allergy and, 2064–2066
hives and, 2028
Immunoglobulin M, 2030, 2090, 2115, 2119
Immunophenotype, 2235–2237, 2235t
Immunoreactive trypsinogen
cystic fibrosis screening in neonates, 702
NICU-discharged infant screening for, 719
Immunotherapy, for warts, 2618
Impaired attachment, 1157
Impairment
cognitive
definition of, 2184
irritability and, 1614
definition of, 574
Impetigo
bullous, 1854f
complications of, 1855
differential diagnosis of, 1854
etiology of, 1853
exclusion from school, 1854
history-taking, 1853–1854
laboratory evaluation of, 1854
management of, 1854–1855
physical findings of, 1854
prognosis of, 1855
Implanted devices, for chronic pain, 446
Impulse control disorders, 1726
In vitro fertilization
assisted reproductive technologies and, 623
ethical issues, 625
fetal/neonatal growth and development issues with, 624
legal issues, 625
overview, 621
perinatal outcomes and neonatal issues, 622–625
pregnancy rates after, 621
Inactivated polio virus
in adolescents, 246f
catch-up schedule for, 250t
characteristics of, 257
intervals between doses, 248t
minimum age for, 248t
Inborn errors of metabolism. *See also* Metabolic disorders
breastfeeding and, 813
neonatal assessment, 671–672
Incontinence, 66t
Incontinentia pigmenti, 784–785
Indemnity insurance plans, 17–18, 20t

Independent living issues, 590
Independent practice organization, 19b, 20t
Indirect bilirubin, 1616–1617. *See also* Unconjugated bilirubin
Indirect laryngoscopy, 1600
Indirect questions, 94
Individual educational program, 589, 2021
Individuals with Disabilities Education Act
  amendments to, 346
  description of, 24, 53, 184, 346, 588–589, 1127
  reauthorization of, 153–154
Indoor air pollution, 845
Industry, 210, 1009
Infant(s). *See also* Early childhood; Newborn
  abdomen of, 132–133
  acute lymphoblastic leukemia in, 2240
  anorexia in, 1638b
  apical impulse in, 130
  arrhythmias in, 1415–1416
  assessment of, 1742
  auditory behaviors commonly seen in, 122
  auditory screening in, 326–328, 327b, 328f, 330b
  back pain in, 1405–1407, 1409–1410
  blood pressure in, 107t, 109t, 1584–1585
  botulism in, 1607, 1611
  brain growth in
    description of, 116
    parental effects on, 181
  breastfed. *See* Breastfeeding
  caloric intake in, 1786
  cardiovascular screening in, 336–338
  caregiver questioning about, 180t
  chest of, 128–130
  conjunctivitis in
    causes of, 1703, 1704t, 1705–1710
    definition of, 1703
    differential diagnosis of, 1703
    evaluation and treatment of, 1703–1705, 1704b, 1704f
  constipation in, 1428–1429
  corneal abrasions in, 120
  crying evaluations, 124, 144
  death of
    description of, 2579–2581
    leading causes, 238, 240t
  development of
    communication and, 1226
    feeding, 1157–1159
    night feeding, 1302–1303, 1305t
    sleep, 59, 1294
    timeframe for, 1156–1161
  developmental tasks for, 209–210
  of diabetic mother
    diagnosis and management of, 888–892
    hypoglycemia in, 974
Infant(s)—cont'd
  diarrhea in
    acute, 1440–1441, 1444
    chronic, 1447–1454
    description of, 1787
  dietary recommendations for, 213
  diffuse pulmonary hemorrhage in, 1575
  dying. *See* Sick and dying infants
  dysphagia and, 1465
  ears of, 121–122
  eating disorders in, 1743
  emotional range of, 183
  esotropia in, 1734f, 1734–1735
  extremely low-birth-weight. *See* Extremely low-birth-weight infants
  eyes of, 119–120
  fatigue in, 1509
  feeding of. *See* Feeding
  feet of, 139
  fever in, 1517–1518, 1519f–1520f, 1522
  gastrointestinal bleeding in, 1544–1545, 1546b
  genitalia of, 136
  growth chart, 694
  hand coordination monitoring, 144, 145f
  head of
    circumference measurements, 111f, 111–112
    physical examination of, 117–118
  hearing in
    loss of, 1558–1560
    screening of, 122
  heart of, 130–131
  heart rate in, 106t
  hepatitis in, 1618
  high-risk. *See* High-risk infants
  hoarseness in, 1598–1599, 1599b
  hospitalization preparations for, 172b
  hypertension in, 1584b
  hypotonia in, 1512, 1607
  irritability and, 1609, 1613–1614
  jaundice in, 1616–1621
  leading causes of death in, 238, 240t
  length measurements, 111, 111f, 113f, 115f
  liver of, 133
  low-birth-weight. *See* Low-birth-weight infants
  lower extremities of, 139
  lungs of, 129–130
  lymph nodes in, 127
  maternal bonding with
    breastfeeding and, 801, 810–811
    in neonatal intensive care unit, 734
  maturation of, 183–184
  morbidity and mortality of, 729
  mother's responses to, 183, 183t
  neck of, 127–128
  nervous system of, 142–144
  nose of, 123
  otoscopic examination in, 121
Infant(s)—cont'd
  pharynx of, 124–125, 125f
  physical examination of, 102–103
    chest circumference, 112
    description of, 102–103
    eyes, 119–120
    head circumference, 111f, 111–112, 113f
    length of, 111, 111f, 113f, 115t
    nervous system of, 142–144
    skin, 116
    weight, 111
  premature. *See* Premature infants
  progressive spinal muscular atrophy, 1606, 1606t
  protein requirements, 223t
  rashes in, 1693b–1695b
  reactive attachment disorder in, 1743
  rectal examination in, 133
  regurgitation and, 1783
  reorganization periods for, 183–184
  respiratory rate in, 106
  salivation in, 125
  sick. *See* Sick and dying infants
  SIDS. *See* SIDS
  skin of, 116
  sleep myoclonus in, 1658–1659
  social behaviors by, 184
  spasms in, 2489b, 2490
  spleen of, 133
  strange behavior in, 1742–1743
  stress in, 181
  syncope in, 1657
  teeth in, 125
  temperament of, 183
  tongue in, 125–126
  vaginal discharge in, 1771
  very low-birth-weight. *See* Very low-birth-weight infants
  vision screening in, 344
  vomiting and, 1783, 1787
  vulva of, 135f
  weight gain, 1502–1503
  weight loss, 1787
Infant CPR Anytime program, 723
Infant mortality rate
  birth weight and, 238
  declines in, 233, 238, 238f
  international, 238–239, 239t
  low-birth-weight neonates, 238
  statistics, 238
  in United States, 238, 239t
Infantile cortical hyperostosis, 1628
Infection. *See also specific infection*
  acquired hemolysis, 942
  bacterial. *See* Bacterial infections
  breastfeeding and, 809–810
  community-acquired methicillin-resistant *Staphylococcus aureus*, 937
  conjunctivitis. *See* conjunctivitis
  diarrhea caused by, 1450
  early education and child care programs and, 1020–1022

Infection—cont'd
empirical therapy for, 506t
fatigue caused by, 1510, 1511
fever caused by, 1517–1518, 1521–1522, 1525, 1526b
fungal. *See* Fungal infections
hematuria caused by, 1566–1568, 1567f
hemoptysis caused by, 1571
hoarseness caused by, 1599, 1601–1602
homelessness and, 1088–1090
incidence in newborns, 928–929
irritability caused by, 1611
joint pain caused by, 1627
limp caused by, 1635
lymphadenopathy caused by, 1641t–1642t, 1642–1643
maternal, 635–636, 755, 928–929
neonatal skin, 785–786
nephrotic syndrome, 2298
newborn assessment for, 928–937
normal pattern of, 1696
odor caused by, 1664t
orbital, 2245–2446, 2444f–2445f
perinatal, 932–935
petechiae and purpura caused by, 1667
in premature infants, 834–835
prevention of, 809–810
recurrent
diagnostic testing for, 1700–1701
immune disorders and, 1696
immunodeficiency and, 1701b
patient history and examination for, 1700
primary immunodeficiencies and, 1697t, 1697–1701
referrals for, 1701b
secondary immunodeficiencies and, 1696–1697, 1697t
susceptibility to, 1696
treatment of, 1701
response to, 376
splenomegaly and, 1731–1732
transfusion-transmitted, 488
urinary tract. *See* Urinary tract infections
vaginal bleeding caused by, 1768–1769
vaginal discharge caused by. *See* Vaginal discharge
viral. *See* Viral infections
weight loss and, 1788
wound, 558, 559t, 561
Infectious cellulitis, 2440–2445, 2441b, 2441f
Infectious esophagitis, 2057
Infectious mononucleosis
clinical presentation of, 2175
complications of, 2177, 2177t
deaths caused by, 2177
description of, 1980
diagnosis of, 2175–2177, 2176f, 2177t
epidemiology of, 2175
Epstein-Barr virus–negative, 2178
management of, 2177–2178
Infectious mononucleosis—cont'd
prevalence of, 2175
serologic findings in, 2175–2177, 2176f, 2177t
tonsillar signs of, 126
Infective endocarditis, 506t
Inferiority, 211
Infertility, 620–622
Infiltrative disorders
hepatomegaly and, 1577
splenomegaly and, 1732
Inflammation. *See also* Edema
chronic, 1400–1401
conjunctival. *See* Conjunctivitis
hoarseness and, 1601–1602
limp and, 1635
Inflammatory acne, 1802–1805
Inflammatory bowel disease
diarrhea caused by, 1453–1454
fatigue caused by, 1511
gastrointestinal bleeding caused by, 1546
joint pain and, 1627
short stature caused by, 1728–1729
Inflammatory diseases
fatigue caused by, 1510
hepatomegaly and, 1577
lymphadenopathy and, 1643
splenomegaly and, 1732
Inflammatory edema of sinusitis, 2443–2445, 2443f
Influenza
in croup, 2648, 2649f
description of, 1981
vaccine
administration of, 254–255
in adolescents, 246f
adverse effects of, 255
characteristics of, 254–255
contraindications, 255
guidelines for, 245f
interval between doses, 248t
minimum age for, 248t
for NICU-discharged infants, 718
in premature infants, 704
InfoPOEMs/InfoRetriever, 39t
Information gathering
before anticipatory guidance, 207–208, 208b
electronic health records used for, 36
in evidence-based medicine, 38–39
methods of, 207–208
Informed consent
cultural differences in, 160
management of sick and dying infants and, 730
Inguinal hernia
description of, 1721f, 1721–1722
irritability and, 1611–1612
palpation of, 135
Inhalant abuse, 951, 2782
Inherited coagulopathies, 537–538
Inhibin, 604
Initiative, 210, 1007
Injuries. *See also* Trauma
child abuse, 1093–1098
comorbidity associated with, 267
domestic violence and, 1075
early education and child care programs and risk of, 1022
firearm-related, 270–271
head. *See* Head injuries
history-taking about, 92b
intentional vs. unintentional, 268
sports, 2550–2561
unintentional deaths caused by, 266–267, 267t
in violence history, 275, 275b
Injury control
description of, 266
principles of, 267–268, 268t
Injury prevention, 266–272
active strategies, 267–268
anticipatory guidance, 268–271, 269b, 270t
car safety seats, 269–270, 270t
counseling teen drivers, 270
education in, 268
enforcement in, 268
engineering in, 268
firearms-related, 270–271
Haddon's matrix of strategies in, 267, 268t
passive strategies in, 267–268
pediatricians' role in, 268
principles of, 267–268, 268t
topics for office-based counseling, 269, 269b
traffic safety in, 269–270, 270t
Injury Prevention Program, 269
Innocent murmurs, 1563, 1565, 1565t
Inotropes, 2722
Inpatient care
facilities for, 5–6
hospitalist effects on, 168
Insect bites and stings
anaphylactic reaction to, 2644, 2688
avoiding of, 2689b
bedbugs, 2179, 2179f
body sites of, 2179–2180, 2180f
DEET for, 2180–2181
flea, 2179, 2180f
Hymenoptera, 2687–2690
mites, 2179, 2180f
papular urticaria caused by, 2180–2181
prevention of, 2180–2181
ticks, 2179
treatment of, 2181–2182
Insect repellents, 2776
Insecticides, 2684t
Insecure attachments, 179
Insensible water loss, 225
Insomnia
attention deficit/hyperactivity disorder and, 1212t
primary, 1301–1302
Institute of Medicine, 42, 297
Instrumental conditioning, 1004

Insufficient milk syndrome, 820–821
Insulin
adjustments in, 2004
bolus, 2003, 2003f
continuous subcutaneous injection, 2004
diabetic ketoacidosis treated with, 2666, 2667
duration of action for, 2003t
exercise, 2005
illness, 2005
meal plan considerations, 2004–2005
monitoring of, 2004
multiple daily injections, 2003–2004
omission of doses, 2663, 2668
onset of, 2003t
during preoperative period, 530–531, 530t, 531f, 533f
sensitivity, in preterm infants, 692
split-mixed program, 2003
Insulin-like growth factor 1, 1729
Integrative medicine, 456. *See also* Complementary and alternative medicine
Intellectual development, 15
Intellectual disability
case studies, 2186–2190, 2188t–2191t
classification of, 2185, 2185t
communicating with families about, 2185
definitions of, 2184–2185
diagnosis of, 2185b
differential diagnosis of, 2186–2190, 2188t–2191t
evaluation of, 2188t, 2190–2192, 2191t
functioning with, 2188t
levels of, 2185t
management of, 2186–2190, 2188t–2191t
neurocutaneous findings with, 2190t
syndromes associated with, 2189t
terminology use, 2184
Intelligence quotient, 2184–2185
Interdisciplinary team, 574–575, 574b
α-Interferon and oral ribavirin combination, 2124
Intermediate syndrome, 2778
Intermittent esotropia, 1737
Internal tibial torsion, 1540–1541
International Association for the Study of Pain, 435
International Children's Continence Society, 2041
International Classification of Diseases, 1207
International Classification of Headache Disorders II, 1550, 1550b
International medical graduates, 3
Internet
continuing medical education using, 35t, 36
parenting materials from, 1170
resources on, 34
Interpreter, 62b
Interpretive conference, 154–156
Intersex. *See also* Sexual development disorders
causes of, 2193
definitions associated with, 2194
epidemiology of, 2193
evaluation of, 2197–2200, 2198f–2199f
history-taking, 2198–2199
imaging of, 2200
laboratory tests for, 2200
management of, 2200–2201
physical examination for, 2199–2200
Interstitial disease, 1567f
Interstitial fluid, 467
Interstitial hydrostatic pressure, 1480
Interstitial nephritis, 2293
Interviews/interviewing
adolescent developmental level and, 1331
child
behavioral assessment, 98
closure, 99–100
confidentiality issues, 100
data collection, 98–99
nonverbal behavior, 98
overview of, 95–96
parent-child interactions assessed during, 95–96
parents' role in, 100
psychodiagnostic techniques, 100–101
psychological functioning assessments, 99
rapport, 97–98
structure of, 97–100
third-person techniques, 98
typical day technique for, 96
clinical, 401
communication during, 94–95
direct questions, 94
gay, lesbian and bisexual youth and, 1361
indirect questions, 94
motivational, 402
open-ended questions, 94
parent role in, 1332
pediatric history, 90–94, 91b–92b
posttraumatic stress disorder and, 1287b
prenatal, 89–90
privacy of, 1287
in psychosocial dysfunction recognition, 359–361
rapport and, 1331–1332
sensitive issues and, 1334–1337
techniques, 1226, 1332–1334
Intestinal Lymphangiectasia, 1451
Intestine(s). *See also* Bowel
disorders of, 1787
failure of, 873–874
malrotation of
irritability and, 1611
upper gastrointestinal series for, 148
obstruction of, 1371–1372
Intimacy, 1010–1011
Intimate partner violence, 369
Intraabdominal fetal echogenic lesions, 776–777
Intracellular fluid, 467
Intracranial hematomas, 2713, 2713t
Intracranial hemorrhage, 2172
Intracranial pressure, increased
brain tumors, 1861–1862, 1863
diagnosis, 2740–2741, 2741f
etiology, 2739b, 2739–2740
hospitalization for, 2745
hydrocephalus, 2147, 2150, 2152
irritability and, 1609
lateral rectus muscle palsy and, 120
management of
barbiturates, 2743–2744
cerebrospinal fluid removal for, 2742
corticosteroids, 2743
diuretics, 2743
future trends in, 2745
glycemic control, 2743
hypertonic saline, 2743
hyperventilation, 2742
neuromuscular blockade, 2743
osmotic agents, 2742–2743
seizure control, 2743
surgical decompression, 2744–2745
temperature control, 2743
monitoring of, 2742
outcomes of, 2745
pathology of, 2739
referral for, 2745
signs and symptoms of, 2740, 2740b
Intractable seizures, 2503
Intracytoplasmic sperm injection
assisted reproductive technologies and risk of, 623
ethical and legal issues, 625
fetal/neonatal growth and development issues with, 624
overview, 621
perinatal outcomes and neonatal issues, 622–625
Intrathoracic airways obstruction, 1791
Intrauterine device, 1356
Intrauterine growth restriction
definition and etiology, 883–885
management of, 885–887
maternal factors
health, 630–631
nutritional status, 627–629
pathophysiology of, 885–887
symmetric vs. asymmetric, 884
ultrasound detection of, 613
Intrauterine infections, 635–637
Intrauterine insemination, 620–621
Intravenous immunoglobulin
immune thrombocytopenic purpura treated with, 2172–2173
staphylococcal TSS treated with, 2566
streptococcal TSS treated with, 2566
Intravenous regional block, 445

Page numbers followed by "f" denote figures; "t" denote tables; "b" *denote* boxes.

Intraventricular hemorrhage
in extremely low–birth-weight infants, 854–855
neurological evaluation, 992
of prematurity, 2151
school-aged outcomes and, 855–856
in very low–birth-weight infants, 855
Intrinsic renal disease, 1827, 2107
Intubation
difficult
anatomic abnormalities causing, 541, 543t
Mallampati signs in, 541, 543f
general anesthesia, 557
in status asthmaticus, 2815
Intussusception
description of, 2079–2080, 2627, 2630
gastrointestinal bleeding caused by, 1545
imaging assessments, 149
irritability and, 1611
ultrasound evaluations, 149
Inverse psoriasis, 2447, 2448t, 2449f
Inversion, 1529b
Iodide, 2156
Iodine, 227t
Ion transport, 2464, 2464f
Ion trapping, 2770
IPA, 19b, 20t
Ipecac syrup, 2683, 2769
IPEX syndrome, 1452
Ipratropium bromide, 2816
Iris
defects in, 118–119
pigmentation of, 118
Iritis, traumatic, 2348
Iron
antidote for, 2685t, 2767t
characteristics of, 227t
iron-deficiency anemia treated with, 2208
poisoning, 2763, 2776t, 2776–2777
supplementation of, 217, 685
Iron deficiency
anemia and. *See* Iron-deficiency anemia
breath-holding spells and, 1318
causes of, 2202–2203, 2202t
differential diagnosis of, 2203–2204, 2206f, 2207t
incidence of, 2202
prevention of, 2209b, 2210, 2210b
sleep disturbance and, 1307
stages of, 2203, 2205t
treatment of, 2208–2210, 2209b–2210b, 2209t
Iron-deficiency anemia
anemia of chronic disease and inflammation vs., 2205
causes of, 2202–2203, 2202t
evaluation of, 2205–2208, 2207t, 2208f, 2209t
Hb H disease vs., 2204–2205
hemoglobin concentration in, 2205
Iron deficiency—cont'd
history-taking, 2205
incidence of, 2202
iron therapy for, 2208–2209, 2209t
laboratory tests for, 2205
lead poisoning and, 2205
management of, 2208–2210, 2209b–2210b, 2209t
pathophysiology of, 2202–2203, 2202t
peripheral blood smear for, 2208, 2208f
physical examination for, 2205
prevalence of, 2201–2202
prevention of, 2209b, 2210, 2210b
red blood cell indices in, 2206–2207, 2207t
reticulocyte hemoglobin in, 2208
screening of, 2205–2208, 2207t, 2208f, 2209t
serum ferritin in, 2208
serum iron and transferrin saturation in, 2205–2206, 2207t
serum transferrin receptor in, 2207t, 2208
tests for, 2208
thalassemia trait vs., 2203–2204
zinc protoporphyrin in, 2207, 2207t
Irregular cardiac rhythms, 920–921
Irritability
acute, 1609–1613, 1610f
causes of, 1609, 1613
chronic, 1610f, 1613–1614
Irritable bowel syndrome, 1453
Irritant diaper dermatitis. *See* Diaper rash
Irritants
dysuria caused by, 1477
stomatitis and, 2569–2570
Isabel, 35t
Islet cell dysplasia, 2732
Isolation
psychosocial development and, 1010–1011
transgender youth and, 1240, 1363
Isometric exercises, 1757
Isoniazid
antidote for, 2767t
dosing for, 2596t
overdose of, 2777
toxicity to, 2594
tuberculosis treated with, 2591–2595
Isopropanol, 2784
Isopropyl alcohol poisoning, 2784
Isosexual precocious puberty, 1685–1687, 1686b
Isospora belli, 2377
Isosporiasis, 2377
Isotretinoin
acne conglobata treated with, 1804
acne fulminans treated with, 1804
dermabrasion, 1807
FDA guidelines for, 1805
fetal malformations caused by, 1805, 1925
therapeutic effect of, 1805
Isovaleric acidemia, 984–985
ISS. *See* Idiopathic short stature
Itch, 1681–1682
Itraconazole, 513t
Ivermectin
ascariasis treated with, 2390
description of, 70
lice treated with, 2182
onchocerciasis treated with, 2393
strongyloidiasis treated with, 2388
Ixodes scapularis, 2249

J

Jacobi, Abraham, 55
Jaundice
bilirubin metabolism and, 1616
breastfeeding and, 821–822
definition of, 892, 1615
description of, 2119–2121
diagnosis of
algorithm for, 894
testing for, 1621–1622
differential diagnosis of, 892, 1616, 1617b
follow-up for, 899–900
history-taking for, 1621
hyperbilirubinemia and. *See* Hyperbilirubinemia
incidence, 892
in infants, 115, 2118–2119
of diabetic mothers, 890
laboratory testing, 895–896
long-term outcomes for, 899–900
management of, 896–897, 1622–1623
medical history, 893–895
in newborns, 115, 841, 2118–2119
physical examination for, 895, 1621
prevention of, 897–899
treatment of, 894
Jejunoileal atresia, 777
Jejunum
injury to, 2628
mucosa of, in gluten-sensitive enteropathy, 2088, 2089f
obstruction of, 2081–2082
Jervell and Lange-Nielsen syndrome, 1418
Jeune asphyxiating thoracic dystrophy, 792
Joint(s)
bacterial infection in, 2505–2508
examination of, 1632–1633
injured or symptomatic, 320b, 321
Joint Committee on Infant Hearing
description of, 326, 356
high-risk register screening, 315
permanent hearing loss and, 1558–1560
Joint pain
definition of, 1625–1626
differential diagnosis of, 1626–1628
etiology of, 1626
evaluation for, 1628
referral for, 1629
treatment of, 1628–1629

Joint sepsis, 1633
Jones criteria, for rheumatic fever, 2476, 2476b
Joule, 220
Jugular venous distention, 2718
Junk food, 231
Juvenile glaucoma, 1709, 1710f
Juvenile idiopathic arthritis
  causes of, 2211
  clinical manifestation of, 2212
  course of, 2218
  description of, 1626
  differential diagnosis of, 2214–2216, 2215b
  fatigue caused by, 1510
  oligoarticular, 2213
  ophthalmologic examination in, 2214t
  pharmacologic management of
    abatacept, 2216b, 2217
    corticosteroids, 2216b, 2217
    COX-2 inhibitors, 2216, 2216b
    leflunomide, 2216, 2216b
    methotrexate, 2216, 2216b
    nonsteroidal anti-inflammatory drugs, 2215–2216, 2216b
    rituximab, 2216b, 2217
    sulfasalazine, 2216, 2216b
  polyarticular, 2212–2214, 2213t
  prevalence of, 2211
  prognosis of, 2218
  systemic-onset, 2212
Juvenile myelomonocytic leukemia, 2241
Juvenile myoclonic epilepsy, 2489b, 2491
Juvenile plantar dermatosis, 1851
Juvenile rheumatoid arthritis. *See* Juvenile idiopathic arthritis

K

Kala-azar, 2367
Kasabach-Merritt syndrome, 1669
Kava kava, 458t, 542t
Kawasaki disease
  atypical, 2224–2226, 2224b, 2225f, 2226b
  causes of, 2221
  clinical manifestations of, 2221–2224, 2222t, 2223b, 2223f
  complications of, 2226–2227, 2227b, 2227t
  conjunctivitis associated with, 120, 1716–1717, 2220, 2220f
  course of, 2221
  definition of, 2220
  description of, 1967, 2011
  diagnostic criteria for, 2223b
  differential diagnosis of, 2221, 2566t–2567t
  echocardiogram for, 2224b
  epidemiologic features of, 2220–2221
  erythroderma of, 2220, 2220f
  features of, 2220, 2220f, 2222t
  fever in, 2221
  incidence of, 2220–2221
  irritability and, 1611
Kawasaki disease
  laboratory findings in, 2224, 2224b
  lymph node manifestations of, 127
  management of
    coronary artery disease secondary to, 2226–2227, 2227b, 2227t
    description of, 2226
  ocular manifestations of, 120
  oral manifestations of, 125
  pathogenesis of, 2221
  pharyngitis caused by, 2427
  prognosis of, 2227
  psychosocial aspects of, 2227
  rash in, 2220, 2220f
  Rocky Mountain spotted fever vs., 2482
Kenalog cream, 2488
Keratitis, 1705, 1706f
Keratoconjunctivitis, 1705
Keratolytic therapy
  seborrheic dermatitis treated with, 2487–2488
  warts treated with, 2617–2618
Keratosis pilaris, 1851
Kernicterus, 127, 747–748, 899–900
Kernig sign, 127
Ketamine, 2781–2782, 2790
Ketoacidosis, diabetic
  assessment of, 2665, 2665t
  complications of, 2667, 2667b
  definition of, 2663
  description of, 1837, 1984, 2001
  differential diagnosis of, 2663
  electrolyte therapy in, 2666–2667
  evaluation of, 2663–2665
  factors associated with, 2663b
  fluid and electrolyte deficits in, 2664t
  fluid replacement in, 2665–2666
  hospitalization for, 2668
  insulin therapy in, 2666–2667
  management of, 2665
  prevention of, 2668
  referrals for, 2668
  risk factors for, 2662–2663, 2663b
Ketoconazole, 513t
Ketogenesis, 981
Ketogenic diet, 2502
Ketorolac, 427
Ketotic hypoglycemia, 2733b, 2735, 2738
Kidney(s)
  acid-base balance and, 2460–2463, 2461f, 2463f
  acute injury of
    definition, 2798
    etiology, 2798t, 2798–2799
    evaluation, 2799
    hospitalization for, 2800
    hyperkalemia in, 2799, 2800t
    management, 2799–2800, 2800t
    referral for, 2800
  congenital anomalies of, 133
  failure of. *See* Renal failure
  multicystic, 1373
  physical examination of, 133
Kidney(s)—cont'd
  rupture of, 2628
  singular, sports participation with, 322t
  tuberous sclerosis complex effects on, 2311
Kidney stones, 1477
KidsHealth, 35t
Kienbock disease, 2353b, 2354
Kiesselbach plexus, 123, 1482
Kilocalorie, 220
Kindergarten, 1140. *See also* School readiness
Kinship care, 182, 1066, 1068–1069. *See also* Foster care
Kleine-Levin syndrome, 1309
Klinefelter syndrome, 2196–2197
Klippel Feil syndrome, 127, 2545
Klippel-Trénaunay syndrome, 781
Knee
  anterior cruciate ligament injuries, 2557–2558
  collateral ligament injuries in, 2557
  meniscal tears in, 2558
  pain in, 2560
Knock-knees, 1537–1538, 1538f, 1542
Koebner response, 2013
Komoto syndrome, 119
Koplik spots, 125
Korotkoff sounds, 1585
Kwashiorkor, 158
Kyphosis
  acquired, 2548–2549
  congenital, 2546–2547

L

Labetalol, 2729, 2729t
Labial adhesions
  case examples, 2229–2230, 2230f
  causes of, 2228–2229
  clinical manifestations of, 2229
  definition of, 2228
  description of, 2228
  differential diagnosis of, 2229, 2229f
  dysuria caused by, 1477
  epidemiologic mechanisms in, 2229
  management of, 2229–2230, 2230f
  prevention of, 2230
Labial agglutination, 2228–2230
Lacrimal injury, 2345, 2345f
Lacrimal system, 1707f
ß-lactam antibiotics, 498–499
Lactation. *See also* Breastfeeding
  energy requirements during, 221
  protein requirements, 223t, 224
Lactose, 213
Laminectomy, 1877
Lamivudine, 511t
Lamotrigine
  chronic pain managed using, 444
  description of, 1262
  seizures managed using, 2499t, 2501
Language
  adopted children, 1049–1050
  assessment of, 354–358

Page numbers followed by "f" denote figures; "t" denote tables; "b" *denote* boxes.

Language—cont'd
barriers to health care caused by, 61–62, 158
development of. *See also* Speech, development of
from 2 to 5 years of age, 210–211
description of, 355, 1150
hearing and, correlation between, 122
in preschool-age children, 355–356
disorders of, 357, 1197
learning of, 160
in preschool-age children, 355–356
Lanugo hair, 116
Laparoscopy, for gastrointestinal obstruction, 2079
Large-for-gestational-age infants, 888–892
Large-muscle strength and endurance, 191–192
Larsen syndrome, 2547
Larva migrans, 2389
Laryngeal clefts, 1599, 1601
Laryngeal edema, 2058, 2059t
Laryngeal papilloma, 1751f
Laryngeal papillomatosis, 1749t, 2635–2636
Laryngeal saccular cysts, 1599, 1601
Laryngeal trauma, 1602
Laryngeal webs
hoarseness and, 1599
stridor caused by, 1749t
Laryngitis, 1601–1602
Laryngomalacia, 1748, 1749t, 1751f, 2633
Laryngopharyngeal reflux, 1599–1601, 2058, 2059b
Laryngoscopy, 1601, 1750f
Laryngotracheobronchitis, 1601–1602. *See also* Croup
Larynx, 1750f, 1751f
Laser surgery, 1710
Laser therapy, 2618
Latch-on technique in breastfeeding, 815–816
Late childhood. *See also* Adolescent(s); School-age child
abdomen examination in, 133–134
blood pressure in, 107t, 109t
chest examination, 129–130
description of, 211
developmental tasks, 211
ear examination, 121–122
eye examination, 120
genitalia examination in, 136
heart examination in, 131–132
heart rate in, 106t
lung examination, 129–130
musculoskeletal system examination in, 140
nervous system examination in, 145
nose examination, 123
respiratory rate in, 106
testes examination in, 136
Late talkers, 355
Latency stage of psychosexual development, 1008
Latent tuberculosis
definition, 2590–2591
management, 2592–2596
physical examination for, 2597
Latham appliance, 1927f
Latin America
cultural healing practices confused with child abuse, 69t
folk illnesses in, 64t, 66t
Latino(s)
health care access for, 60–61
health insurance status of, 61
language barriers, 61
limited English proficiency among, 61
Laudanum, 955
Lavender, 458t
Law(s), 1127–1128
Law of Dilutions, 459
Law of Similars, 459
Laxatives, 1429–1430, 1430t
L-carnitine deficiency
medium-chain acyl-CoA dehydrogenase deficiency, 981–982
non-hypoglycemic neonatal onset metabolic disease, 983
Lead
adverse health effects associated with, 394
blood levels of, 394–396, 395b–396b, 395t
exposure to
breastfeeding and, 827–828
home environment, 845
sources of, 393–394
Lead poisoning
adverse health effects associated with, 394
anemia and, 2205
antidote for, 2767t
description of, 1400, 2777–2778
epidemiologic features of, 393
folk illness remedies associated with, 66t–68t
in immigrant children, 63
lead sources, 393–394
screening for, 393–397, 395b–396b, 395t
Lean body mass, 221
Learning
collaborative, 47
focus on, 15
Learning disabilities
description of, 1149–1150, 1152b
in low-birth-weight infants, 856
prevalence of, 242
Learning problems
in Down syndrome patients, 2021
evaluation of, 1151–1154, 1152t
interventions for, 1154
laboratory studies for, 1153
physical examination for, 1152–1153
Learning problems—cont'd
reasons for, 1149, 1150t, 1150–1151
seizure-related, 2496
sleep-related symptoms of, 1309
Learning theory, 1004
Leflunomide, 2216, 2216b
Left-ventricular noncompaction cardiomyopathy, 1963
Leg disorders. *See also* Limp
bowed legs, 1537f, 1537–1538, 1542
femoral torsion deformities, 1541–1542
knock-knees, 1537–1538, 1538f, 1542
positional deformities, 1530, 1531f
pronation, 1534–1536, 1542
referral for, 1541–1542
terminology, 1529b
tibial torsion, 1540–1542
Legal issues. *See also* Malpractice
adoption process, 1042–1051
assisted reproductive technologies, 625
case studies of, 74–85
child abuse and neglect, 1098–1099
child custody, 1053–1055
conduct disorders, 1224
description of, 74
gay- and lesbian-parented children, 1083–1085
hyperbilirubinemia, 899–900
Münchausen syndrome by proxy, 1277–1278
in newborn screening for genetic-metabolic diseases, 389
newborn-related
birth injury, 745–746
brachial plexus injuries, 747
communication issues, 750
delivery room, 743–744
healthy newborn nursery, 744
hyperbilirubinemia, 747–748
hypoglycemia management, 745
liability risk minimization, 750–751
medical malpractice, 742–743
office care procedures, 749–750
procedure risk-benefit analysis, 748–749
safety issues, 750
seizure management, 746–747
sick newborn care, 744–745
transport and referral procedures, 749
umbilical cord blood gases, 746
umbilical line complications, 749
of rape, 2792
Legg-Calve-Perthes disease, 140
Leg-length discrepancy, 1633f
Leishmania sp., 2368
Leishmaniasis
causes of, 2368
clinical manifestations of, 2366–2367
cutaneous, 2366–2367
diagnosis of, 2367
epidemiologic features of, 2366
life cycle of, 2368

Leishmaniasis—cont'd
- mucosal, 2367
- Old World vs. New World disease, 2368
- pathogenesis of, 2368
- prevention of, 2368
- transmission of, 2368
- treatment of, 2367–2368
- visceral, 2367

Lemon sign, 605, 618
Lennox-Gastaut syndrome, 2489t, 2490–2491
Lens
- description of, 2344
- postnatal increases in, 118

Leptospirosis
- clinical features of, 2222t
- differential diagnosis, 2566t–2567t

Lesbian youth. *See* Gay, lesbian, and bisexual youth
Lesbian-parented families, 1082–1085
Lesch-Nyhan syndrome, 1628, 1726
Let-down reflex, 1786
Lethargy, 2639
Leukemia, 2231–2249
- acute lymphoblastic
  - classification of, 2235f, 2235t, 2236
  - clinical features of, 2239t
  - clinical manifestations of, 2333t
  - cytogenetic and molecular markers in, 2237–2238, 2237t, 2239t
  - frequency of, 2235, 2235f
  - immunophenotype of, 2235t, 2236
  - in infants, 2240
  - laboratory findings in, 2233t
  - relapsed, stem cell transplantation for, 2242
  - treatment of, 2238–2240, 2239t
- acute myelogenous
  - classification of, 2236, 2236t
  - clinical features of, 2239t
  - clinical manifestations of, 2333t
  - cytogenetic and molecular markers in, 2238, 2239t
  - laboratory findings in, 2233t
  - prevalence of, 2236
  - relapsed, 2242
  - treatment of, 2240
- acute myeloid, 2235f, 2236, 2236t
- acute promyelocytic, 2240
- antifolate metabolism in, 2243
- autosomal-recessive chromosomal fragility disorders of Bloom syndrome and, 2232
- biphenotypic, 2236–2237, 2237t
- causes of, 2231–2233, 2231b
- chloromas and, 2234
- chronic myelogenous, 2240–2241
- classification of, 2235–2238, 2235f, 2235t–2237t
- clinical manifestations of, 2233–2234, 2233t
- cytogenetic and molecular markers, 2237–2238, 2237t

Leukemia—cont'd
- differential diagnosis of, 2234–2235, 2234b
- Down syndrome and, 2232
- environmental factors in, 2231b, 2232–2233
- epidemiologic features of, 2231, 2231f
- extramedullary, 2234
- frequency of, 2235, 2235f
- genetic predisposition to, 2231–2232, 2231b
- immunophenotype classification of, 2235–2237, 2235t
- incidence of, 2231, 2231f
- laboratory findings in, 2232–2233, 2232t
- leukemogenesis, 2231–2233, 2231b
- mixed-lineage, 2237
- in monozygotic twins, 2232
- myelodysplasia and, 2241
- myelomonocytic, 2241
- pharmacogenetics in, 2242–2243
- prognostic features of, 2238, 2239t
- relapsed, 2242
- signs and symptoms of, 2232, 2232t
- TPMT metabolism in, 2242
- treatment of
  - cardiac effects of, 2243
  - cognitive function effects of, 2243
  - endocrine effects of, 2243–2244
  - late effects of, 2243–2244
  - second malignant neoplasm resulting from, 2244

Leukemogenesis, 2231–2233, 2231b
Leukocoria, 119
Leukocytapheresis, 486
Leukocytes
- counts, by age, 2802t
- in urine, 2610–2611

Leukocytosis, 1858
Leukotriene modifiers, 1846t, 1848
Levalbuterol
- asthma treated with, 1844
- status asthmaticus treated with, 2815–2816

Levamisole, 2301, 2301b
Levetiracetam, 2499t, 2501
Levofloxacin
- *Chlamydia* treated with, 2512b
- epididymitis treated with, 2520b

Levonorgestrel, 1354
Liability, 10–11. *See also* Malpractice
Lice
- head, 2181, 2181f
- pubic, 2181
- treatment of, 2181–2182

Licensing, 1167
Licensure, 4
Lichen spinulosus, 1851
Licorice, 458t
Life course model of health, 11
Life expectancy
- description of, 239
- health care spending vs., 416–417, 416f

Lifestyle
- foster care and, 1070–1072
- neonatal health and, 630

Ligament injuries, 2557–2558
Ligamentum arteriosum, 2636
Limb abnormalities
- newborn assessment, 769–771
- physical examination, 793

Limb girdle muscular dystrophy, 2282t
Limb pain. *See* Extremities, pain in
Limited English proficiency, 61–62
Limit-setting disorder, 1300–1301
Limp
- causes of, 1632t, 1635–1636
- diagnostic testing for, 1633–1635
- differential diagnosis of, 1630, 1631t, 1635–1636
- management of, 1635–1636
- patient history for, 1630–1631
- physical examination for, 1631–1633

Lindane, 2776
Linoleic acid, 213
Lipid Research Clinics Prevalence Study, 285
Lipoid nephrosis, 2298–2299
Lipoid pneumonia, 67t–68t
Lipolysis, 973
Listening skills, 1333b, 1333–1334
Listeria monocytogenes
- maternal-fetal infection, 637
- neonatal sepsis, 936

Lithium, 1261
"Little League" shoulder, 2554
Liver
- bilirubin transport defects, 1620
- biopsy of, 1622
- enlarged
  - in congestive heart failure, 2718–2719
  - sports participation with, 323t
- fatty, 2121
- fulminant failure, 2672
- function of, 2811
- in infants, 133
- in newborns, 133
- palpation of, 133, 1575
- span, 1575–1576
- transplantation of, 1622

Liver disease. *See also* Hepatitis
- acute viral hepatitis progressing to, 2115
- cholestatic, 2118
- chronic, 2110
- in cystic fibrosis, 1984, 1991
- diagnosis of, 2119t
- edema caused by, 1481
- factor replacement and, 2109–2111
- in HIV infection, 2141
- jaundice and, 1620
- metabolic
  - abnormal liver enzyme levels, 2121–2122
  - diagnostic investigations for, 2119t

Page numbers followed by "f" denote figures; "t" denote tables; "b" *denote* boxes.

Liver disease—cont'd
metabolic—cont'd
fulminant hepatic failure, 2122
jaundice
in children, 2119–2121
in newborns and infants, 2118–2119
therapy and prevention, 2126
metformin contraindications in, 2002
neonatal coagulopathies, 945
theophylline affected by, 1848
Loa loa, 70
Long QT syndrome, 1418–1419
Loop of Henle, 2464, 2464f
Loose anagen syndrome, 1386
Loracarbef, 497–498
Lorazepam
neonatal drug withdrawal syndrome treated with, 949
seizures treated with, 2500, 2743
status epilepticus treated with, 2820b
Loss of appetite. *See* Anorexia
Louis Bar syndrome, 2317–2319, 2318t. *See also* Ataxia-telangiectasia
Low-birth-weight infants. *See also* Extremely low–birth-weight infants; Very low–birth-weight infants
adulthood transition of, 858–861
anemia in, 940–944
caloric requirements, 221
early intervention for, 860
growth outcomes in, 857
health outcomes in, 852–863
hepatitis B vaccine in, 253
mortality rates, 238
prevalence of, 236
protein requirements, 224
statistics regarding, 236, 729
sudden infant death syndrome and, 2580
Low-density lipoprotein cholesterol, 195
Lower esophageal sphincter, 2055
Lower extremities. *See also* Foot; Leg
of infants, 139
of newborns, 137–138, 138f
Lower gastrointestinal bleeding, 1544–1545, 1546b, 1547, 1549
Lower thoracic vertebrae osteochondroses, 2353b, 2354
Lower urinary tract obstructions, 2335, 2335f
LSD. *See* Lysergic acid diethylamide
Lumbar puncture
bacterial meningitis evaluations, 2257–2258
cellulitis evaluations, 1858
in hemophilia patients, 2108
in HIV-infected children, 2142
hydrocephalus evaluations, 2149, 2151
increased intracranial pressure evaluations, 2740
non-Hodgkin lymphomas evaluations, 1891
Lumbar puncture—cont'd
nonspecific febrile illness evaluations, 2034
seizure evaluations, 2496
Lung(s)
Apgar score evaluations, 128, 129t
auscultation of, 129
developmental disorders, 912–915
in drowning injuries, 2677
fetal development of, 128
fetal lung masses, postnatal evaluation, 776
gas exchange evaluations, 129–130
newborn, 128–129, 766–767
physical examination of, 128–130
transplantation of, 1990
Lung density evaluation, 906
Lung parenchymal type 1 airway disorders, 905
Lupus erythematosus
description of, 1389
drug-induced, 2026, 2029
systemic
in anuria, 1827
cervical lymphadenopathy caused by, 1997
herpes simplex virus type 1 and, 2130
in oliguria, 1827
proteinuria present in, 2113
Luteinizing hormone–receptor defects, 2195–2196
Lye, 2705
Lyell syndrome, 2030–2031
Lyme disease
causes of, 2249
clinical manifestations of, 2249–2250
coinfections, 2250
congenital infection, 2250
description of, 105
differential diagnosis of, 2250
early disseminated phase in, 2249–2250
early localized phase in, 2249
epidemiology of, 2249
joint pain and, 1627, 1633
late-stage of, 2250
management of, 2250–2251, 2251t
pathogenesis of, 2249
pharmacotherapy for, 2250–2251, 2251t
prophylaxis after tick bite in, 2251
serologic testing, 2250
vaccine for, 2251
LYMErix, 2251
Lymph nodes
cervical, 127
disease origin in, 1640t
enlarged. *See* Lymphadenopathy
of head and neck, 1640f
in infants, 127
intrathoracic, 2599, 2600f
in newborns, 127
Lymphadenopathy
age-based incidence of, 1641t
definition of, 1639
diagnostic testing for, 1643–1645
differential diagnosis of, 1642–1643
etiology of, 1640t–1642t
evaluation of, 1644t
history-taking for, 1643–1644
infectious, 1644–1645
physical examination for, 1643–1644
referral for, 1646
treatment of, 1645–1646
Lymphatic dysplasia syndrome, 912
Lymphatic filariasis, 2392–2393
Lymphatic system, 1639–1640
Lymphoid interstitial pneumonitis, 2140
Lymphoma, non-Hodgkin, 1890–1892
Lymphonodular hyperplasia, 1545
Lymphoproliferative disease, 1574
Lysergic acid diethylamide, 2781
Lysosomal storage disorders, 376

M

Macrocephaly
causes of, 1647b
definition of, 1646
diagnostic testing for, 1649
differential diagnosis of, 1646–1648
management of, 1649
patient history and examination for, 1648–1649
referral for, 1649
Macrocytic anemia, 1402
Macroglossia, 766, 2634
Macrolides
description of, 501–503
Lyme disease treated with, 2251, 2251t
mechanism of action of, 501
Macronutrients, 692
Macroscopic hematuria, 1566–1570
Macrosomia, 888–890
Macules
café-au-lait, 1689f
definition of, 1689
Magical thinking, 210
Magnesium, 967–968
Magnesium sulfate, 2816
Magnetic resonance imaging
brain, 152, 1861
central nervous system defect evaluations, 606, 1863
cerebral palsy evaluations, 1904–1905, 1907
congenital anomaly diagnosis, 795
Cushing syndrome evaluations, 1815
description of, 147
Ewing family of tumors evaluated using, 1886
hydrocephalus evaluations, 2149–2151, 2153
increased intracranial pressure evaluations, 2740–2741
limp evaluations, 1635
mental status alteration evaluations, 2642

Magnetic resonance imaging—cont'd
neuroblastoma evaluations, 1816
neurofibromatosis type 1 evaluations, 2306–2307
neurofibromatosis type 2 evaluations, 2309
neurologic evaluation in NICU-discharged infants, 719–721
osteomyelitis evaluations, 2357
osteosarcoma evaluations, 1889
paravertebral lesions evaluations, 1878
pituitary stalk abnormality evaluations, 1812
retinoblastoma evaluations, 1880
rhabdomyosarcoma evaluations, 1882–1883
streptococcal TSS evaluations, 2575
Wilms tumors evaluations, 1875
Magnetic resonance urography, 151
Major depressive disorder, 1745. *See also* Depression
Mal ojo, 64t
Malabsorption
diarrhea and, 1442, 1447
syndromes, 1441–1442, 1449–1450
weight loss caused by, 1787
Malaria
cerebral, 2381
chemotherapy for, 2382–2383, 2382t
clinical manifestations of, 2381
diagnosis of, 2381–2382
epidemiologic features of, 2380
life cycle of, 2380–2381
pathogenesis of, 2381
Plasmodium sp., 2380–2384, 2382t–2383t
prevention of, 2383–2384, 2383t
screening for, 70
treatment of, 2382t, 2382–2383
Malathion
antidote for, 2685t, 2768t
head and pubic lice treated with, 2181
Male(s)
blood pressure levels, 1580f, 1581t–1582t
genitalia of
newborns, 768–769, 845
sexual abuse signs in, 1107–1113
growth patterns in, 1727
puberty in, 1683–1687
Malformations. *See also* Congenital disorders
defined, 788–789
definition of, 1496–1497
Pierre Robin sequence of, 1496
sequence, 789
Malignancies. *See also* Cancer; Sarcoma
Epstein-Barr virus and, 2178–2179
fatigue caused by, 1510–1511
petechiae and purpura caused by, 1668
sports participation with, 323t
weight loss and, 1788
Malignant hypertension, 2726–2727, 2730
Malignant hyperthermia, 539b–540b, 539–540
Malignant otitis externa, 2364
Malingering, 1229–1230
Mallampati signs, 541, 543f
Mallet toe, 1530, 1531f
Mallory-Weiss tear, 1544
Malnutrition. *See also* Nutrition
in adopted children, 1045–1046, 1048
diarrhea as cause of, 1448
failure to thrive and, 1505–1506
homelessness and, 1090
intrauterine growth restriction and, 884
prevalence of, 230
secondary immunodeficiency and, 1697
Malocclusion
assessment, 1651–1652
classification of, 1650
description of, 125
etiology of, 1650–1651
referral for, 1652
thumb sucking and, 1725
treatment of, 1651
Malpractice
avoidance of, 11, 12b
birth injury, 745–746
hyperbilirubinemia follow-up and outcomes, 899–900
newborn-related issues
brachial plexus injuries, 747
communication issues, 750
delivery room, 743–744
healthy newborn nursery, 744
hyperbilirubinemia, 747–748
hypoglycemia management, 745
liability risk minimization, 750–751
medical malpractice, 742–743
minimization of risk for, 750–751
office care procedures, 749–750
procedure risk-benefit analysis, 748–749
safety issues, 750
seizure management, 746–747
sick newborn care, 744–745
transport and referral procedures, 749
umbilical cord blood gases, 746
umbilical line complications, 749
statistics regarding, 10–11
Malrotation
intestinal, 2626–2627, 2627f, 2630
newborns and, 1371
postnatal evaluation, 777
with secondary midgut volvulus, 1783
Managed care
description of, 17–19, 19b, 20t
Medicaid, 24
Manic depression, 1745
Manipulative methods, 457–459
Mannitol, 2742–2743
Maple syrup urine disease
diagnosis and management, 986–987
newborn screening for, 385–386
Marfan syndrome, 112, 1409, 1498
Marijuana, 950, 2779, 2781
Marital strain, 182
Marriage
divorce and, 1055–1059
family structure and, 1037
Masculinization, 1590–1591
Massage, 457–459
Mastitis, 819
Mastocytosis, 2644
Masturbation, 1340–1341, 1725–1726
Maternal and Child Health Block Grant, 24
Maternal and Child Health Bureau, 53, 564
Maternal depression
attachment issues secondary to, 181
caregiver questioning about, 180t
causes of, 365, 365b
definition of, 365
effects of, on children, 365–366, 366b
prevalence of, 365
risk factors for, 184, 185t
screening for, 366–369, 367b–368b
signs and symptoms of, 365, 365b
Maternal health
breastfeeding. *See* Breastfeeding
high-risk infant care and
abnormal growth and gestation, 633–634
alloimmunization, 634
cytomegalovirus infection, 636
dental health, 630
drug/other substance abuse, 629–630
gestational hypertension, 634–635
herpes simplex virus infection, 636
human immunodeficiency virus, 635
intrauterine infection, 635–637
maternal-fetal unit, 632
multiple gestation, 633
nutritional status, 627–629
obstetric complications, 633
pharmacologic intervention, 633
placenta and membrane disorders, 631–632
premature birth, 632–633
reproductive capability, 630–631
rubella exposure, 635–636
toxoplasmosis, 636–637
homelessness effects on, 1090
newborn affected by, 755
placenta/membrane disorders and, 631–632
preconception care inventory and recommendations, 641
prenatal visit procedures, 797–800
risk identification and management, 639–641
uterine size, 643
Maternal medical history
family history, 754–756
intrapartum course, 755

Maternal medical history—cont'd
  preconception and antenatal history, 752–753
  pregnancy duration, 756
  prenatal testing and diagnosis, 753–754
Maternal morbidity, 624
Maternal sensitive period, 1005
Maternal serum alpha-fetoprotein
  neural tube defect detection, 605
  prenatal serum testing, 604
Maternal-fetal interventions
  delivery room medical-legal considerations and, 743–744
  ethical issues, 615
Maternal-fetal transport patterns, 629
Maternal-infant bonding
  breastfeeding and, 801, 810–811
  in neonatal intensive care unit, 734
Maturity, delayed, 2470–2471
Maturity-onset diabetes of the young, 1999–2000
Maxillary sinus, 122
MCAD deficiency, 2734
McBurney point, 1837
MCHAT. *See* Modified Checklist for Autism in Toddlers
MC2R, 1812
MD Consult, 35t
MDMA, 1248
Measles
  atypical, 1980
  description of, 1980–1981, 2566t–2567t
  Mycoplasma pneumonia, 1980
  scarlet fever, 1981
  vaccine for. *See* Measles, mumps, rubella vaccine
Measles, mumps, rubella vaccine
  administration of, 255
  in adolescents, 246f
  adverse reactions to, 255
  autism and, 79
  catch-up schedule for, 250t–251t
  characteristics of, 255–256
  concerns about, 79
  contraindications, 255–256
  guidelines for, 245f
  in immunocompromised patients, 250
  before immunoglobulin-containing products, 247
  intervals between doses, 248t
  minimum age for, 248t
Meatal stenosis, 1477
Mebendazole
  ascariasis treated with, 2390
  hookworm infections treated with, 2388–2389
  pinworms treated with, 2389, 2433
  trichinellosis treated with, 2386
  trichuriasis treated with, 2387
Meckel diverticulum
  description of, 133, 2605–2606
  gastrointestinal bleeding caused by, 1545
  nuclear scintigraphy evaluations, 149
Meconium aspiration syndrome, 908–909
Meconium ileus, 777, 1372f, 2079
Meconium peritonitis, 1879, 2079
Meconium plug syndrome, 777, 2079
Media
  adolescents and, 1114–1120
  children and, 1114–1120, 1142
  content analyses of, 1115–1116
Mediastinal masses, 1643b
Mediastinal tumors, 1878t
Medicaid
  Early and Periodic Screening, Diagnostic, and Treatment program, 23–24
  fee-for-service, 24
  history of, 23–24
  in home health care funding, 571–572, 572
  managed care, 24
  NICU-discharged infant coverage, 722
  in schools, 1138
Medical day treatment programs, 572
Medical history
  adoption process and importance of, 1045–1046
  breastfeeding assessment, 817
  child abuse evaluation, 1096–1098
  congenital anomaly diagnosis, 790–791
  description of, 90, 91b
  jaundice evaluation, 893–895
  maternal
    family history, 754–756
    intrapartum course, 755
    preconception and antenatal history, 752–753
    pregnancy duration, 756
    prenatal testing and diagnosis, 753–754
  questions on preparticipation physical evaluation, 318t, 319–320
  sexual abuse assessment and diagnosis, 1110
Medical home
  description of, 7
  first contact in, 52–53
  preventive service visits in, 50
  role of, 52–53
Medical home physician, 52
Medical liability, 10–11
Medical literature
  acquisition of, 38–39
  application of, 40–41
  appraisal of, 39–40
  validity of, 39, 41b
Medical reference materials, 34, 35t
Medications. *See also* Drug(s); Psychopharmacology therapy; *specific medications*
  abdominal pain managed using, 1382
  abortion, 1356–1357
  adherence issues, 164
  administration of
    apnea, 686–688
    bradycardia, 686–688
Medications—cont'd
  administration of—cont'd
    breastfeeding and, 813, 824–825
    bronchopulmonary dysplasia, 689–690
    desaturation, 686–688
    maternal-fetal transport, 629–630
    neonatal resuscitation, 662
    in NICU-discharged infants, 724
  adolescent use of, 1335t, 1337
  anaphylactic reactions to, 2643, 2644
  anesthesia and, 541, 542t
  chronic pain managed using, 440–444, 441t–442t
  concentration of, 490
  date rape, 2782, 2790
  description of, 1177
  electronic health record for, 29t, 31
  family involvement with, 1182
  financial resources and, 1177–1179
  hepatitis induced by, 2117
  history-taking about, 92b
  irritability and, 1612–1613
  laxatives, 1253
  mental status alterations and, 2640b
  misuse of, 14
  nonadherence to, 164
  postoperative nausea and vomiting effects on, 556
  prescribing of
    electronic health record used for, 29t, 31
    weight-based dosages, 31
  psychoactive, 1181b
  safety concerns and side effects of, 1180, 1209–1211, 1213t
  in schools, 1130, 1178–1179
  skin eruptions caused by
    allergic skin reactions, 2027t
    drug rash with eosinophilia and systemic symptoms, 2029
    erythema multiforme, 2029–2030
    management of, 2028
    morbilliform (measles-like) eruptions, 2027–2028
    referrals for, 2031
    Stevens-Johnson syndrome, 2030–2031, 2031t
    toxic epidermal necrolysis, 2030–2031, 2031t
    urticaria (drug-induced hives), 2028
  sleep affected by, 1309
  stimulants, 1209–1211
  training and, 1177
  trial periods for, 1180
  washout period and, 1180–1182
  weight-based dosages, 31
Medium-chain acyl-CoA dehydrogenase deficiency, 387, 981–982
  A985G mutation frequency, 982t
Medline Plus, 35t
Medroxyprogesterone acetate, 1355
Medscape, 35t
Medullary vomiting center, 1783

Megalencephaly, 1646, 1647b, 1648
Megaureter, obstructed, 2334
Megestrol acetate, 1639
Meglumine antimonite, 2368
Meibomian gland dysfunction, 1714–1715, 1715f
Melanin, 115
Melanoblasts, 113
Melena, 1543
Membrane defects, 942–943
Membrane stabilizers, 444
Membranoproliferative glomerulonephritis
- description of, 2293–2294
- in nephrotic syndrome, 2296–2297, 2299

Membranous nephropathy, 2299
Menarche, 1399, 1767–1768
Meninges, 2252
Meningitis
- aseptic
  - causes of, 2256t
  - clinical manifestations of, 2263–2264
  - description of, 2036, 2252, 2263
  - diagnosis of, 2264
  - incidence of, 2254
  - management of, 2264
  - outcome of, 2264
  - viruses causing, 2268f–2269f, 2268–2270, 2270t
- bacterial
  - age and, 2252
  - anti-inflammatory therapy for, 2259
  - antimicrobial agents for, 2259–2261, 2260t
  - causes of, 2253–2254, 2255t
  - cerebrospinal fluid in, 2257–2258
  - characteristics of, 2267
  - clinical manifestations of, 2255–2257, 2257f
  - complications of, 2261
  - description of, 2252, 2254–2255
  - differential diagnosis of, 2255
  - distribution of, 2254f
  - fluid therapy for, 2259
  - glucocorticoids for, 2259
  - incidence of, 2253, 2254f
  - laboratory testing and findings in, 2257–2258
  - lumbar puncture in, 2257–2258
  - management of, 2258–2261
  - prevention of, 2261–2262
  - sequelae of, 2261
  - syndrome of inappropriate antidiuretic hormone caused by, 2258
- breastfeeding and prevention of, 810
- causes of, 2252
- cerebrospinal fluid findings in, 2252, 2253t
- definition of, 2252
- empirical therapy for, 506t

Meningitis—cont'd
- epidemiology of, 2253f–2254f, 2253–2254, 2255t
- febrile seizures and, 1517
- in HIV-infected children, 2142
- in meningococcemia, 2746
- neonatal
  - anti-inflammatory therapy for, 2263
  - antimicrobial agents for, 2262–2263
  - cause of, 2262
  - cerebrospinal fluid findings in, 2262, 2262t
  - clinical signs of, 2262
  - description of, 2262
  - fluid therapy for, 2263
  - incidence of, 2262
  - management of, 2262–2263
  - prognosis of, 2263
  - supportive care for, 2263
- partially treated, 2252, 2263
- pyogenic. *See* Bacterial meningitis
- recurrent, 1696

Meningococcemia
- clinical manifestations of, 2747–2748, 2748f–2749f
- complications of, 2751
- definition of, 2746
- differential diagnosis, 2747–2748, 2748b
- disease control for, 2751–2752, 2752t
- epidemiology of, 2746–2747, 2747f
- etiology of, 2746–2747
- evaluation of, 2748–2749, 2750t
- management of, 2749–2751
- prevention of, 2751–2752, 2752t
- prognosis of, 2751, 2751t
- Rocky Mountain spotted fever vs., 2482
- septic shock in, 2806
- vaccine for, 245f–246t, 248t, 2752

Meningoencephalitis
- amoebic
  - clinical manifestations of, 2374
  - description of, 2373–2374
  - diagnosis of, 2374–2375
  - epidemiologic features of, 2374
  - prevention of, 2375
  - treatment of, 2375
- cerebrospinal fluid findings in, 2270, 2270t
- clinical features of, 2270
- description of, 2136, 2267
- differential diagnosis of, 2270–2271
- incidence of, 2270
- laboratory evaluation of, 2271
- prevention of, 2271
- prognosis of, 2271
- treatment of, 2271
- viral causes of
  - AIDS, 2269
  - arboviruses, 2268
  - childhood exanthems-related, 2269, 2269f

Meningoencephalitis—cont'd
- viral causes of—cont'd
  - enteroviruses, 2268, 2268f
  - fungi, 2270, 2270t
  - herpesviruses, 2268
  - parasites, 2270, 2270t
  - prions, 2270
  - rabies, 2268–2269
  - spirochetes, 2270, 2270t
  - varicella zoster virus, 2269, 2269f

Meningomyelocele. *See* Spina bifida
Meniscal tears, 2558
Menstrual cycle, 1767
Menstrual dating, 637–638
Menstrual pain. *See* Dysmenorrhea
Menstruation. *See also* Amenorrhea
- restoration and eating disorders, 1192
- tracking of, 1347

Mental developmental index
- in congenital heart disease patients, 862
- health and development outcomes, in neonatal intensive care infants, 854–858

Mental health
- children's services role in, 1014–1015
- comprehensive care and, 1017
- cultural competence, 1016
- cultural differences in, 160
- diagnosis and treatment, 1014
- divorce and, 1056–1059
- foster care and, 1063–1072
- health outcomes for NICU infants, 858–861
- models of, 1015–1016
- obesity effects on, 2324–2325
- overview, 1014
- parent education and communications, 1016–1017
- primary care physician's role, 1017
- psychological development and, 1017
- sexual abuse of children, 1106–1113

Mental health disorders
- assessment measures and, 1169t, 1172
- collaborative care, 1171–1174, 1173t
- detection of, 200
- encopresis and, 1255b
- intervention resources and, 1163–1165, 1170–1172
- prevalence of, 186
- problems in schools, 1137
- psychoeducation and, 1172
- referrals for, 200
- risk factors for, 185–186
- services in schools, 1123–1124
- transgender youth and, 1236
- trauma-related, 1285–1289
- treatment, 1172–1174. *See also specific disorders*

Mental health services
- children and, 1164–1165, 1167–1168
- conversion behavior and, 1231
- posttraumatic stress disorder and, 1289

Page numbers followed by "f" denote figures; "t" denote tables; "b" *denote* boxes.

Mental health specialists, 1167
Mental retardation, 1196–1197, 2184. *See also* Intellectual disability.
Mental status alterations
  commonly ingested agents in, 2640b
  definition of, 2639
  differential diagnosis, 2640, 2640b
  etiology of, 2639b, 2639t, 2639–2640
  evaluation of, 2640–2641
  history-taking, 2641
  hospitalization for, 2643
  laboratory evaluation of, 2642
  management of, 2642–2643
  physical examination for, 2641–2642
  in poisonings, 2765, 2768
Meperidine, 425t, 429
Merck Medicus, 35t
Mercury exposure
  breastfeeding and, 827–828
  maternal nutritional status and, 629
Meropenem, 499
Mesmerism, 448
Mesoblastic nephroma, 1373
Meta-analysis, 40t
Metabolic acidosis
  in acute renal failure, 2799
  in diabetic ketoacidosis, 2662–2664
  in status asthmaticus, 2814
Metabolic disorders
  calcium metabolism, 965–966
  congenital, 2732–2734, 2733b, 2734t, 2736
  in congestive heart failure, 2721
  description of, 1427, 1471, 1662t, 1663
  diagnosis and screening of, 373–393
  fetal glucose metabolism, 960
  fetal magnesium metabolism and adaptation, 966–967
  high-risk scenarios for, 375t
  hypercalcemia, 966–967
  hyperglycemia, 965
  hypermagnesemia, 969
  hypocalcemia, 966
  hypoglycemia, 961–965, 970–987
  hypomagnesemia, 967–968
  hypotonia and, 1605
  inherited. *See* Genetic-metabolic diseases
  maternal health and, 631
  newborn/neonatal assessment, 670–672, 970
  non-hypoglycemic neonatal onset disease, 983–987
  phosphorus metabolism, 965–966
  physical findings, 971
  respiratory failure in newborns, 905
  suspicion of, 373–376, 374t–375t
Metabolic liver disease
  abnormal liver enzyme levels, 2121–2122
  diagnostic investigations for, 2119t
  fulminant hepatic failure, 2122
Metabolic liver disease—cont'd
  jaundice
    in children, 2119–2121
    in newborns and infants, 2118–2119
  therapy and prevention, 2126
Metabolic syndrome
  hypertension and, 1579–1580
  obesity and, 2323b, 2323–2324. *See also* Obesity
  polycystic ovary syndrome and, 1592
  waist circumference measurements, 112
Metabolism
  antifolate, 2243
  bilirubin, 1616
  cholesterol's role in, 224
  energy, 220–222
  glucose. *See* Glucose, metabolism of
  inborn errors of. *See* Inborn errors of metabolism
  after meal, 220
  phosphorus, 966–967
  thiopurine methyltransferase, 2242
Metacognitive skills, 1150
Metaiodobenzylguanidine, 147–148, 1816
Metals, 827–828
Metaphyseal osteomyelitis, 151
Metaphyseal stress injuries, 2552–2553
Metaphysis, 2553t
Metapneumovirus, 2648
Metatarsal heads, 2353b, 2354
Metatarsus adductus, 771, 1533–1534, 1534f
Metatarsus varus, 1533–1534, 1534f, 1538
Metformin, 2002
Methadone
  acute pain managed using, 429–430
  chronic pain managed using, 442t
  neonatal drug withdrawal syndrome management, 955
  potency and half-life of, 425t
Methanol
  antidote for, 2685t, 2767t
  poisoning by, 2783–2784
Methemoglobin, 2685t, 2767t
Methemoglobinemia, 1612
Methenamine mandelate, 2613t
Methicillin, 493t
Methicillin-resistant *Staphylococcus aureus*, 937, 1854–1855, 1859
Methotrexate
  during breastfeeding, 825
  juvenile idiopathic arthritis treated with, 2216, 2216b
  psoriasis treated with, 2452t, 2453
Methylenedioxymethamphetamine, 2782
Methylmalonic acidemia, 984
Methylxanthines
  asthma treated with, 1846t, 1848
  status asthmaticus treated with, 2816
Metoclopramide, 555t
Metrics, 44
Metronidazole
  bacterial resistance to, 505
  during breastfeeding, 825
  description of, 505
  dosage, peak serum concentrations, and MIC_{95} for, 494t
  giardiasis treated with, 2086, 2372
  mechanism of action, 505
  pelvic inflammatory disease treated with, 2519b, 2520b
  properties of, 505
  side effects of, 505
  use of, 505
Mezlocillin, 493t, 496
Micafungin, 513t
Microangiopathic hemolysis, 942
Microarray comparative genomic hybridization, 1500
Microcephaly
  causes of, 1653b
  definition of, 1652–1653
  description of, 117, 1652, 1654
  differential diagnosis of, 1653–1654
  evaluation of, 1654–1655
  management of, 1655
Microcytic anemia, 1395–1396, 1398f
Microenvironment, 731–732
Microphthalmia, 119
Microscopic hematuria
  causes of, 1567b
  description of, 1566, 1568–1569
  evaluation of, 1569f
Microvillus inclusion disease, 1452–1453
MIDAS. *See* Migraine Disability Assessment
Middle adolescence, 211
Middle childhood
  definition of, 1744
  psychological development during, 1008
  strange behavior in, 1744–1745
Middle Eastern folk illness remedies, 68t
Midgut volvulus, 777, 2626–2627
Mifepristone, 1356
Migraine Disability Assessment, 1551–1552
Migraine headaches
  characteristics of, 1550b, 1550–1555, 1552b
  irritability and, 1609
  self-hypnosis for, 453b
  syncope and, 1756
  vertigo caused by, 1457–1458
Milia, 1803
Miliaria, 116, 784
Milk
  cow. *See* Cow milk
  human. *See* Human milk
Milk thistle
  breastfeeding and intake of, 826
  uses of, 458t
Millennial morbidity, 52
Miller-Dieker syndrome, 1653

Miltefosine, 2368
Mind-body medicine, 456–457
Mineral(s)
  characteristics of, 226t
  deficiency of, 628–629
  description of, 224–225
Mineralocorticoids, 1808
Minimal bactericidal concentration, 491
Minimal change nephrotic syndrome, 2296, 2298–2299
Minimal inhibitory concentration, 491
Minocycline, 1805
Minor blood group incompatibility, 942
Minorities
  demographic profile of, 234, 234f
  urban, 273
Minoxidil, 2730t
Mite bites, 2179, 2180f
Mitochondrial encephalomyopathies, 1608
Mitochondrial respiratory-chain disorders, 979
Mitral valve prolapse, 322t, 1423
Mobility devices, 579
Möbius syndrome, 1740
Model for improvement, 47
Modified Checklist for Autism in Toddlers, 360, 1198
Mogan clamp, 829
Mold, 1570, 1819
Molding, 761–762
Molecular genetic analysis, 2032, 2038
Molluscum contagiosum, 1715, 1715f, 2618–2620
Mongolian spots, 115, 779
Monilethrix, 1386
Monoamine oxidase inhibitors for giardiasis, 2086
Mononucleosis, infectious
  clinical presentation of, 2175
  complications of, 2177, 2177t
  deaths caused by, 2177
  description of, 1980
  diagnosis of, 2175–2177, 2176f, 2177t
  epidemiology of, 2175
  Epstein-Barr virus–negative, 2178
  fatigue caused by, 1511
  management of, 2177–2178
  prevalence of, 2175
  serologic findings in, 2175–2177, 2176f, 2177t
  splenomegaly and, 1731–1732
  tonsillar signs of, 126
Mononucleosis-like disease, 2136
Monosaccharides, 225
Monosymptomatic nocturnal enuresis, 2041–2043
Monozygotic twins, 2232
Montelukast, 1821
Mood and Feelings Questionnaire, 1170
Mood disorders
  bipolar disorder, 1261–1262
  classification of, 1256
Mood disorders—cont'd
  clinical picture of, 1257–1258
  depression. *See* Depression
  diagnosis of, 1257b–1259b, 1258–1260
  epidemiological description of, 1256
  prognosis for, 1260
  risk factors for, 1256–1257
MOPP chemotherapy, 1894, 1895
Morbidity and mortality. *See also* Death
  infant. *See* Infant mortality rate
  in infants of diabetic mothers, 891
  perinatal period, 637–638, 729, 736–737
  preeclampsia, 634–635
  premature infants, 632, 831–833, 854–855
  rubella virus and, 635–636
Morbilliform (measles-like) eruptions, 2027–2028
Moro reflex
  asymmetrical, 137
  description of, 102
  development of, 141f
  evaluation of, 143, 144f
Morphine
  acute pain managed using, 429, 429b
  chronic pain managed using, 442t
  potency and half-life of, 425t
Morquio syndrome, 2547
Mortality. *See also* Death
  age-related, 593, 593t
  cardiac arrhythmias and, 1418
  causes of, 593, 593t
  encopresis and, 1256
  infant mortality rate
    birth weight and, 238
    declines in, 233, 238, 238f
    international, 238–239, 239t
    low-birth-weight neonates, 238
    statistics, 238
    in United States, 238, 239t
  Münchausen syndrome and, 1264–1268
  prevalence of, 593, 593t
Mother
  "blues" in. *See* Postpartum blues
  breastfeeding discontinuation by, 218
  depression in. *See* Maternal depression; Postpartum depression
  health of. *See* Maternal health
  Münchausen syndrome by proxy in, 1268–1269
  responses to infant, 183, 183t
  unmarried, 236, 237t
  working, 184
Motility assessment (ocular), 1780
Motivational interviewing, 402
Motor disability, 575, 575t
Motor function, 2539–2540
Motor system impairments, 1226
Motor tics, 1758
Motor unit disorders, 1605–1608
Mourning, 594
Mouth
  congenital anomalies, 792
  gingiva. *See* Gingiva
  of infants, 124–125
  newborn assessment, 765–766
  of newborns, 123–124
  physical examination of, 123–127
  review of systems for, 92b
  stomatitis in, 2569–2573
  teeth. *See* Teeth
Mouth odor, 1661
Moxibustion, 69t
MPGN. *See* Membranoproliferative glomerulonephritis
MRI. *See* Magnetic resonance imaging
MSBP. *See* Münchausen syndrome by proxy
Mucocele, 766
Mucocutaneous candidiasis, 1811
Mucolytic agents, 1435
Mucopolysaccharidosis
  diagnosis, 792
  type IV, 2547
Mucopus, 2511, 2512f
Mucosal leishmaniasis, 2366–2367
Mucus-retention cysts, 123
Multicystic dysplastic kidney, 611–612
Multifetal pregnancy, 624
Multiloculated hydrocephalus, 2151
Multiple births
  assisted reproductive technologies and risk of, 623–624
  fetal risk with, 633
  percentage of, 729
  statistics regarding, 236
Multiple daily injection program, 2003–2004
Multiple intraluminal electrical impedance measurement, 2057–2058
Multiple personality disorder, 1745
Multiple suture craniosynostosis, 1654
Mumps, 1980–1981
Mumps orchitis, 1721
MUMs National Parent-to-Parent Network, 584
Münchausen syndrome by proxy
  alternatives, 1270
  clinical findings for, 1265–1268, 1266t–1267t
  definition of, 1263–1264
  demographics and, 1264–1265
  diagnosis of, 1269–1275, 1272t–1273t, 1273b–1275b
  gastrointestinal bleeding and, 1544
  hemoptysis and, 1573
  intervention and, 1275–1277
  laboratory findings and, 1265–1268
  legal considerations, 1278
  symptoms of, 1272–1273t
Mupirocin, 1854

Page numbers followed by "f" denote figures; "t" denote tables; "b" *denote* boxes.

Murmurs
anesthesia and, 526–527, 527t
atrioventricular valve regurgitant, 131
cardiac evaluation and, 1562–1563
continuous, 132, 1564–1565, 1565f
definition of, 1563
description of, 916–918
diastolic, 132
diastolic flow, 132
evaluation of, 1563t, 1563–1565
hemoptysis and, 1574
information suggestive of, 130
innocent, 131, 131f, 1564–1566
localization of, 131
middiastolic, 132
patient evaluation for, 1561–1562
protodiastolic, 132
referral for, 1566
sports participation with, 322t
systolic, 131
Muscle biopsies, 1606
Muscle growth, 137
Muscle strains, 2559
Muscle strength
core muscles, 192
exercises for increasing, 192, 192f
healthy lifestyle and, 191–192
Muscular dystrophy
Becker
complications of, 2278t
symptoms, genetics and diagnostic tests for, 2274t
treatment of, 2278t
complications of, 2278t–2279t
description of, 2273
diagnostic tests for, 2274t–2275t
Duchenne
characteristics of, 2274t
clinical presentation of, 2273, 2274t, 2276, 2276f–2277f, 2278t, 2280
complications of, 2278t
definition of, 2273
diagnostic tests for, 2274t, 2277f
differential diagnosis of, 2273, 2274t, 2276, 2276f–2277f, 2278t, 2280
evaluation of, 2280
genetics of, 2273, 2274t
hypotonia and, 1607
incidence of, 2274t
prednisone for, 2281
supportive care for, 2280–2281
symptoms of, 2274t
treatment of, 2278t, 2280–2281
Emery-Dreifuss
complications and treatment of, 2279t
prevalence of, 2283
symptoms, genetics and diagnostic tests for, 2275t
facioscapulohumeral
complications and treatment of, 2279t
Muscular dystrophy—cont'd
facioscapulohumeral—cont'd
hypotonia and, 1608
prevalence of, 2282–2283
symptoms, genetics and diagnostic tests for, 2275t
Fukuyama-type, 2275t, 2279t
genetics of, 2274t–2275t
Gowers sign in, 2273, 2276f
hypotonia and, 1607–1608
symptoms of, 2274t–2275t
treatment of, 2278t–2279t
Muscular Dystrophy Association, 2280
Muscular dystrophy type 1, 2281–2283, 2282t
Muscular dystrophy type 2, 2282
Muscular torticollis, 1764, 1766
Musculoskeletal injuries
anterior knee pain, 2560
avulsion fractures of the pelvis, 2558–2559
description of, 1422, 1422t
dislocations, 2559–2560
knee ligaments, 2557–2558
meniscal tears, 2558
muscle strains, 2559
quadriceps contusion, 2558
sprains, 2556t, 2556–2557
in winter sports, 2560–2561
Musculoskeletal system
adolescents, 140
computed tomography of, 151
deformities of, 137–138
examination of, 137–140, 320–321, 320b, 1632–1633
fetal assessment, 646–647
imaging of, 151, 151f
newborns, 137–139, 769–771
review of systems for, 93b
Music therapy, 457
Mutation analysis, 719, 794
Mutational voice disorder, 1600
Mutual influence, 997
MVP. *See* Mitral valve prolapse
Myasthenia gravis, 1607
Myasthenic syndromes, 990–992
Mycobacterium bovis, 2590, 2596
Mycobacterium tuberculosis, 2590, 2599, 2608
Mycoplasma genitalium, 2528
Mycoplasma pneumonia
description of, 1980, 2030
fatigue caused by, 1511
pharyngitis caused by, 2425b, 2427
Mydriasis, traumatic, 2348
Myelodysplasia, 2241
Myelomeningocele, 618, 2151
Myeloproliferative diseases, 2241–2242
Myelosuppression, 1896
Myelocardial depression, 2811
Myocarditis
description of, 1423, 1958–1959, 1959f
heart failure secondary to, 132
irritability and, 1612
Myoclonic jerks, 2489, 2489b
Myoclonic seizures, 2489, 2489b
Myoclonus, 1658–1659
Myoglobinuria, 1567
Myoneural junction disorders, 1607
Myopathies, 1607–1608
Myositis, 2574–2575
Myotonic dystrophy
complications of, 2278t
hypotonia and, 1607
symptoms, genetics and diagnostic tests for, 2274t
treatment of, 2278t
Myxedema, 1481

N

N-acetylcysteine, 2770–2771, 2771f
Nafcillin
dosage, peak serum concentrations, and MIC_{95} for, 493t
staphylococcal TSS treated with, 2566
uses of, 496
Nail biting, 1725
Nail care, 844
Nalbuphine, 425t
Naloxone, 2765, 2775
Naproxen
acute pain managed using, 428t
chronic pain managed using, 440, 441t
Narcolepsy, 1307–1308, 1659
Narcotics
antidote for, 2685t
neonatal drug withdrawal syndrome, 947–948
Nasal gliomas, 783
Nasal polyps, 123
Nasal septum, 123
Nasogastric feedings, 872–873
Nasogastric tubes
curling, 2076, 2078f
description of, 1548
Nasolacrimal duct
description of, 119
obstruction of, 1704f, 1706–1707, 1707f
probing of, 1707
Nasolacrimal sac, 1707
Nasolacrimal stent, 1708f
Nasolacrimal system, 1707f
Natal history, 91b
National Academy of Sciences, 364
National Adolescent Health Information Center, 1325
National Adrenal Diseases Foundation, 1812
National Association of School Nurses, 1136
National Cancer Institute, 1895
National Cholesterol Education Program
Expert Panel on Blood Cholesterol Levels in Children and Adolescents, 285
heart disease prevention, 281–283

National Committee on Quality Assurance, 43–44
National Down Syndrome Congress, 2018
National Educational Goals Panel, 1141
National Health and Nutrition Examination, 285–286, 1390, 2323
National Health Examination Survey, 1390
National Health Interview Survey, 349
National Heart, Lung, and Blood Institute Guidelines for Asthma Severity, 1842b
National Institute of Drug Abuse, 398
National Institutes of Health
  Consensus Conference on Early Identification of Hearing Impairment, 356
  Consensus Statement on Screening, 312
  hearing loss, 326
  in pertussis prevention, 2423
National Kidney Foundation, 2041
National Notifiable Diseases Surveillance System, 2419
National Safety Council, 2045
Natural family planning, 1356
Nausea and vomiting
  management of, 598
  postoperative, 552–556, 553f, 554t–555t
    anesthetic technique as factor in, 554
    concomitant medications affected by, 556
    description of, 552–554
    postoperative oral intake and, 554–555
    prolonged, 556
    treatment of, 555–556, 555t
Necator americanus, 2388–2389
Neck
  of adolescents, 127–128
  of children, 127–128
  of newborns, 127
  physical examination of, 116–118, 127–128
  prenatal defects
    newborn assessment, 766
    ultrasound detection of, 606–607
  range of motion evaluations, 128
  review of systems for, 92b
  short, 127
  tumors of, 1877t
Necrotizing enterocolitis
  breastfeeding and, 810
  description of, 1371f
  in extremely low–birth-weight infants, 854–855
  feeding intolerance in, 694–695
  gastrointestinal bleeding and, 1544
  in infants of diabetic mothers, 890
  irritability and, 1611
  prevention of, 810
Necrotizing fasciitis, 2574–2575
Necrotizing ulcerative gingivitis, 2569, 2571
Nedocromil sodium for asthma, 1848
Needle extraction, for molluscum contagiosum, 2619
Neglect. *See* Child abuse and neglect
Neisseria gonorrhoeae
  joint pain and, 1627
  ophthalmia neonatorum and, 801–802
  pharyngitis caused by, 2425b, 2426
  sexual abuse and, 1109
  sexually transmitted, 2521, 2522f–2523f
  in urinary tract infections, 2607
Neisseria meningitidis
  joint pain and, 1627
  in meningococcemia, 2746
Nematode infections
  ascariasis, 2390–2391
  cutaneous larva migrans, 2389
  hookworm infections, 2388–2389
  lymphatic filariasis, 2392–2393
  onchocerciasis, 2393
  pinworm, 2389–2390
  strongyloidiasis, 2387–2388
  toxocariasis, 2391
  trichinellosis, 2385–2386
  trichuriasis, 2386–2387
Neonatal behavioral assessment scale, 102, 1157
Neonatal drug abstinence syndrome, 1453
Neonatal history, 91b
Neonatal intensive care unit
  discharge criteria
    Child Find and early intervention, 724
    circumcision, 722
    description of, 868
    feeding and nutrition, 709–712
    follow-up care, 721–722, 726
    hearing screening, 718–720
    immunizations, 717–718
    insurance coverage, 722–723
    laboratory studies, 722
    neurologic evaluation, 720–721
    parent education, 723
    prescriptions and medication administration, 724
    respiratory management, 713–717
    retinopathy of prematurity screening, 720–721
    safety issues, 723–724
    screening procedures, 720–721
    social services and case management, 722
    summary and checklist, 724–726
    temperature regulation, 712–713
  family adjustment to, 733–734
  follow-up care
    chronic lung disease management, 877–878
    family adjustment, 879–880
    growth and nutrition management, 871–876
Neonatal intensive care unit—cont'd
  follow-up care—cont'd
    health and development surveillance protocols, 869
    home monitoring discharge criteria, 877–878
    home transition, 869–870
    management issues, 868–880
    neurodevelopment and behavior, 879
    outpatient screening, 879
    risk categories, 867–868
    toddler and early childhood years, 870–871
  full-term newborn admissions to, 729
  health and developmental outcomes
    adolescence and adulthood, 858–861
    chronic conditions, functional limitations and special health care needs, 856–857
    congenital heart disease, 861–862
    early intervention in, 860
    growth problems, 857
    infancy and childhood health-related outcomes, 853
    moderate- to late-preterm infants, 858
    neurodevelopment and school-aged outcomes, 855–856
    pain sensitivity, 857–858
    post-hypoxic-ischemic encephalopathy, 862–863
    premature infants, 853–858
    respiratory failure, neurodevelopment and, 862
    visual function and retinopathy of prematurity, 857
  hospital-induced infection, 936
  intrauterine growth restriction infants, 884
  needs assessment for, 667
  prenatal conditions and need for, 671
  referral protocols, 667
  sick and dying infant management, 731–732
Neonatal resuscitation
  assessment after, 663–664
  delivery room, 658–659, 662
  endotracheal tube size and depth, 662
  ethical principles, 732
  evaluation, 665–666
  extensive or complicated, 662–663
  initial postnatal evaluation and intervention, 659–664
  needs assessment guidelines, 661
  oxygen delivery and monitoring equipment, 661
  premature newborns, 663–664
  preparation for, 658–659
  quality improvement, 665–666
  risk factors for, 655
  stabilization after, 663–664
  unresponsive newborns, 663

Neonatal resuscitation—cont'd
ventilation assistance and monitoring equipment, 661
withholding, limiting, and withdrawing of, 658
Neonate. *See also* Early childhood; Newborn
acne in, 784
alloimmune thrombocytopenia in, 946
assessment of. *See* Newborn assessment
auditory screening in, 326–328, 327b, 328f
botulism in, 1607, 1611
breastfed. *See* Breastfeeding
cardiovascular screening in, 336–338
conjunctivitis in
causes of, 1703, 1704t, 1705–1710
definition of, 1703
differential diagnosis of, 1703
evaluation and treatment of, 1703–1705, 1704b, 1704f
prophylaxis, 1705–1706
diffuse pulmonary hemorrhage in, 1575
drug withdrawal in
assessment of, 672
breastfeeding, 956
cardiorespiratory signs, 953
caregiver decision making regarding, 956
central nervous system effects, 952–953
complications of, 956
cutaneous signs, 953
diagnosis of, 953
differential diagnosis of, 953
duration of, 951–952
gastrointestinal signs, 953
hypnosedatives, 948–949
incidence of, 947
narcotics, 947–948
nonnarcotic drugs, 953
onset of, 951–952
pathophysiology, 947
severity of, 954
social/protective service referral and follow-up, 957
stimulants, 949–951
supportive treatment, 954–956
fever in, 1518, 1522
fluid therapy for, 478–480, 479t
gastroesophageal reflux disease in, 696, 699
gastrointestinal bleeding in, 1544, 1546b
genetic-metabolic diseases in
presentation of, 375
screening for, 383–387. *See also* Genetic-metabolic diseases, newborn screening for
growth and maturity
assessment and classification, 667–668
premature infants, 690–696
Neonate—cont'd
growth and maturity—cont'd
psychological development, 1005–1006
hemoptysis in, 1575
herpes infection in, 2131–2132
hoarseness in, 1598–1599, 1599b
hypertension in, 1584b
hypoglycemia in
clinical signs, 962
counterregulatory hormone deficiency, 982–987
diagnosis of, 961–965
differential diagnosis of, 962
etiologic factors, 972
evaluation of, 970–971
family history, 970
fatty acid oxidation and ketogenesis, 981–982
gastrointestinal glucose absorption, 972–976
gluconeogenesis, 980–981
glycogenolysis, 976–979
incidence, 962
infant of diabetic mother, 974
management of, 961–965
persistent hypoglycemia, 972–987
physical examination for, 970–971
signs and symptoms, 971
stabilization, 674
hypotonia in, 1512, 1607
immune thrombocytopenia in, 2173
irritability in, 1609, 1614
jaundice in, 1616–1619
measuring blood pressure of, 1584–1585
meningitis in
anti-inflammatory therapy for, 2263
antimicrobial agents for, 2262–2263
cause of, 2262
cerebrospinal fluid findings in, 2262, 2262t
clinical signs of, 2262
description of, 2262
fluid therapy for, 2263
incidence of, 2262
management of, 2262–2263
prognosis of, 2263
supportive care for, 2263
rashes in, 1693b
regurgitation and, 1783
screenings. *See* Newborn screening
seizures in, 2489b, 2493b
causes of, 2494–2495
treatment of, 2493b, 2496
types of, 2492–2493
sleep myoclonus in, 1658–1659
testicular torsion in, 1720
thyrotoxicosis, 2157
vaginal discharge in, 1771
vomiting and, 1783
Neoplasia
glucocorticoids for, 1815
hoarseness and, 1601
Neoplasia—cont'd
limp and, 1636
lymphadenopathy and, 1643, 1646
Neoplasms
extremity pain caused by, 1495
torticollis and, 1765
Nephritis. *See also* Glomerulonephritis
clinical manifestation of, 2286
definition of, 2286
Henoch-Schönlein purpura, 2289, 2289b
incidence of, 2286
interstitial, 2293
suspected, 2286–2287, 2286b
systemic lupus erythematosus, 2292–2293
Nephrogenic diabetes insipidus, 1671–1672, 1675
Nephrolithiasis, 1567
Nephropathy
IgA, 2290–2291
membranous, 2299
reflux, 2338
Nephrotic syndrome
causes of, 2296, 2296b, 2299–2300
clinical presentation of, 2297, 2297f
complications of, 2298
definition of, 2296
epidemiologic features of, 2296–2297
evaluation of, 2297–2298, 2297f
focal segmental glomulerosclerosis in, 2296, 2299
gender predilection for, 2296
genetic causes of, 2299–2300
hyperlipidemia in, 2298
incidence of, 2296
infection in, 2298
laboratory evaluation of, 2297–2298
management of, 2300–2302, 2301b
membranoproliferative glomerulonephritis in, 2299
membranous nephropathy in, 2299
minimal change, 2296, 2298–2299
pathophysiological features of, 2298
primary
causes of, 2296, 2296b
histopathological entities associated with, 2298–2300
secondary, 2296, 2296b
thromboembolism in, 2298
Nerve agents, 2779
Nerve stimulation, vagal, 2502
Nervous system
of adolescents, 145
central. *See* Central nervous system
of children, 145
growth of, 140
hand coordination monitoring, 144, 145f
imaging of, 151–152
of infants, 142–144
Moro reflex assessments, 143, 144f
of newborns, 142–144
physical examination of, 140–145
sleep-wake cycle changes, 142
Nervousness, 1656–1657

Nesidioblastosis, 974–976, 2732
Neural tube defects
causes, 2538
cranial, 605
fetal intervention, 617–618
newborn screening for, 388
prevention, 2543
second- and third-trimester testing for, 605
spina bifida, 2537–2544
spine, 792–793
ultrasound testing for, 605
Neurobiologic development disorder, 1196. *See also* Autism
Neurobiologic process, 1156, 1158, 1196
Neuroblastoma
clinical manifestations of, 1877
description of, 1816
differential diagnosis of, 1877t–1878t
etiology of, 1876–1877
evaluation of, 1878–1879
follow-up of, 1879
head and neck tumors vs., 1877t
management of, 1879
mediastinal tumors vs., 1878t
meta-iodobenzylguanidine scanning of, 147–148
prognosis of, 1879
Neurocardiogenic syncope, 1318, 1753
Neurocutaneous syndromes
ataxia-telangiectasia, 2317–2319, 2318t
characteristics of, 2304, 2304t
description of, 2303
megalencephaly and, 1648
neurofibromatosis, 2304–2309, 2304f–2306f, 2304t, 2305b, 2306t, 2308b, 2308f
Sturge-Weber syndrome, 2312–2314, 2313f
tuberous sclerosis, 2309–2312, 2310b, 2310f–2311f
von Hippel-Lindau disease, 2314–2317, 2315t–2316t
Neurocysticercosis, 2396
Neurodevelopment
assessment of, 1153
assisted reproductive technologies and, 624
brain development, 989
hyperbilirubinemia, 899–900
in infants of diabetic mothers, 891
in neonatal intensive care infants, 879
premature infants
description of, 836–837
health and developmental outcomes, 853–858
morbidity factors, 854–855
neurologic disability rates in extremely premature infants, 732
surveillance checklist for, 869
school-aged outcomes in NICU infants, 855–856
severe respiratory failure and, 862
Neurofibromas, 1690f, 2304f, 2304–2305
Neurofibromatosis
classification of, 2304t
definition of, 2304
description of, 1689f, 1690f
intellectual disability and, 2190t
type 1
description of, 2304–2305, 2305f, 2304t
diagnosis of, 2305, 2305b, 2306t
evaluation of, 2305–2307, 2306f
management of, 2307–2308
type 2
bilateral vestibular schwannomas in, 2308, 2308b, 2308f
description of, 2308
evaluation of, 2308–2309
management of, 2309
Neurogenic diabetes insipidus, 1671
Neuroimaging, 2496
Neurologic disorders. *See also specific disorder*
in diabetic ketoacidosis, 2664
irritability and, 1614
sleep-related symptoms of, 1309
Neurologic examination
components of, 142b
goals of, 989
head and skull injuries, 911
indications for, 142
muscle tone and movement disorders, 990–991
newborn assessment, 670–671, 771–773, 988–989
NICU-discharged infants, 720–721, 879
post-hypoxic-ischemic encephalopathy, 862–863
premature and full-term newborn, 988–989
respiratory failure in newborn, 904
seizures, 989–992
Neurologic system, 93b
Neuromuscular blockade, 2743
Neuropathic pain, 435
Neuropsychological regression, 376
Neurosurgery, for spina bifida, 2542
Neurotransmitters, 1783
Nevoid hypermelanosis, 780
Nevus
depigmentosus, 779
epidermal, 781–782
flammeus, 115, 781
hyperpigmented lesions, 779–780
of Ito, 779
of Ota, 779
sebaceous, 782
simplex, 781
New Ballard Score, 654
New York Heart Association heart failure classification, 2719, 2719t
Newborn. *See also* Early childhood; Neonate
abdomen of, 132–133, 767–768
anemia and, 1402–1403
Newborn—cont'd
anus of, 768–769
atresia and, 1371
auditory screening of, 121
blood pressure in, 107t, 109t
body measurements, 758–760
body temperature of, 104, 105f
cardiac arrhythmias and, 1412–1413, 1417
cardiovascular system, 766
caregiver questioning about, 180t
chest of, 128–129, 766–767
congenital anomalies, 789–790
cry assessment, 758
developmental tasks for, 209
diarrhea in, 1444, 1453
Down syndrome
description of, 2018, 2018b
eye assessments, 764
screening for, 389
dysmorphism and, 1497–1500
ears of, 120–121, 764–765
eyes of, 118–119, 763–764
face of, 763
feet of, 139
fingernails of, 116
fontanelles of, 116–118, 117f
funduscopic examination in, 119
genitalia of, 135–136, 768–769
gingiva in, 123–124
hair of, 116
head of
anatomy of, 116–117
measurements, 758–762
healthy
discharge procedures, 840–847
family counseling for, 841–846
follow-up care for, 846–847, 849–850
nursery management, medical-legal considerations, 744
post-delivery care of, 801–802
postnatal evaluation, 775–777
signs of illness in, 846
heart of, 130–131
hemorrhagic disease of
acquired disorders, 944–945
anemia and, 941
description of, 1544
hemophilia, 944
inherited diseases, 944
vitamin-K prophylaxis, 802
hernia in, 1372f
liver of, 133
lower extremities of, 137–138, 138f
lungs of, 128–129, 766–767
malrotation and, 1371
mouth of, 123–124, 765–766
musculoskeletal system of, 137–139
neck of, 127, 766
nervous system of, 142–144
neurologic examination, 670–671, 771–773
nose of, 122–123, 765
penis of, 135

Page numbers followed by "f" denote figures; "t" denote tables; "b" *denote* boxes.

Newborn—cont'd
- pharynx of, 124
- physical examination of, 757–773
- respiratory distress in, 128–129
- respiratory rate in, 106, 128–129
- scalp, 762–763
- scrotum of, 135, 768–769
- skin of, 114–115, 760
- skull of, 116–117, 117f
- strabismus in, 119
- testes of, 135
- tympanitic abdomen and, 1370–1372
- umbilical cord, 767–768
- visual acuity in, 119
- vulva of, 135

Newborn assessment
- blood spot testing, 718–719, 804
- cardiac murmurs, 918
- hemostatic disorders, 944–945
- hypoglycemia, 970–971
- infants of diabetic mothers, 889
- intrauterine growth restriction, 885
- large-for-gestational-age infants, 889
- medical-legal issues
  - birth injury, 745–746
  - brachial plexus injuries, 747
  - communication issues, 750
  - delivery room, 743–744
  - healthy newborn nursery, 744
  - hyperbilirubinemia, 747–748
  - hypoglycemia management, 745
  - liability risk minimization, 750–751
  - medical malpractice, 742–743
  - office care procedures, 749–750
  - procedure risk-benefit analysis, 748–749
  - safety issues, 750
  - seizure management, 746–747
  - sick newborn care, 744–745
  - transport and referral procedures, 749
  - umbilical cord blood gases, 746
  - umbilical line complications, 749
- physical examination, 757–773
  - abdomen, 767–768
  - body measurements, 758–760
  - cardiovascular system, 766
  - chest and lungs, 766–767
  - congenital anomalies, 789–790
  - cry assessment, 758
  - ears, 764–765
  - eyes, 763–764
  - face, 763
  - genitalia and anus, 768–769
  - head measurements, 758–762
  - mouth, 765–766
  - neck, 766
  - neurologic examination, 670–671, 771–773
  - nose, 765
  - scalp, 762–763
  - skin, 760
  - umbilical cord, 767–768
- premature infants, 838

Newborn screening
- α_1-antitrypsin deficiency, 387–388
- availability of tests in, 389
- biotinidase deficiency, 386
- carrier screening-related, 388
- congenital adrenal hyperplasia, 386
- congenital hypothyroidism, 384–385
- cystic fibrosis, 386
- description of, 383–384
- Down syndrome, 389
- ethical issues in, 389
- galactosemia, 385
- genetic susceptibilities, 387
- glucose-6-phosphate dehydrogenase deficiency, 387
- homocystinuria, 387
- legal issues in, 389
- maple syrup urine disease, 385–386
- medium-chain Acyl-CoA dehydrogenase deficiency, 387
- neural tube defects, 388
- new techniques in, 387–388
- parental education about, 78
- phenylketonuria, 384
- prenatal screening-related, 388
- refusal of, 78
- sickle cell anemia, 385
- state-mandated programs for, 78
- tandem mass spectrometry in, 387
- World Health Organization criteria for, 78

NHL. *See* Non-Hodgkin lymphoma
Niacin, 228t–229t
Nicardipine, 2729, 2730t
Nicotine, 950
Nifedipine, 2729, 2729t
Night terrors, 1614, 1659
Night waking, 210
Night walking, 1303
Nightmare disorder, 1305–1307
Nightmares
- irritability and, 1614
- night terrors vs., 1659

Nighttime pruritus, 1767
Nil disease, 2298–2299
Nipple pain, 818–819
Nissen fundoplications, 1265
Nitazoxanide, 2086
Nitrate, 2685t
Nitrites, 2685t
Nitrofurantoin, 2613, 2613t
"No Fears No Tears," 451
Nodding spasms, 1765
Nodules, 1689, 2477
Nonadherence
- consequences of, 162
- determinants of, 162f, 162–163
- extent of, 162
- history of, 161–162

Nonalcoholic steatohepatitis, 2324
Nonallergic rhinitis with eosinophilia, 1820
Noncommunicative children's pain checklist, 424
Nonconvulsive periodic disorders, 1657–1659
Nonexudative pharyngitis, 2034
Non-Hodgkin lymphoma, 1890–1892
Non-hypoglycemic neonatal onset disease
- biotinidase deficiency, 984
- cobalamin disease, 987
- fructosemia, 984
- galactosemia, 983–984
- homocystinuria, 987
- L-carnitine deficiency, 983
- maple syrup urine disease, 986
- organic acidemias, 984–985
- phenylketonuria, 986
- pyruvate-dehydrogenase complex deficiency, 987
- tyrosemia type I, 986
- urea-cycle defects, 985–986

Nonoliguric state
- in acute renal failure, 2799
- definition, 2798

Nonopioid analgesics, 440, 441t
Nonpathological proteinuria, 1677
Nonphysician health professionals, 167–168
Nonspecific febrile illness, 2034
Nonsteroidal anti-inflammatory drugs
- asthma treated with, 1844, 1845t
- dysmenorrhea treated with, 1461–1462
- headaches treated with, 1553
- hives and, 2028
- moderate-to-severe acute pain treated with, 427, 427b
- staphylococcal TSS treated with, 2562, 2567
- Stevens-Johnson syndrome treated with, 2030
- streptococcal TSS and, 2576

Nonstress test, 642–643
Nonsynostotic plagiocephaly, 763
Nonverbal communication, 98, 158, 1334
Noonan syndrome
- congenital anomalies with, 792
- short stature and, 1727

Norepinephrine, 2807
Norepinephrine reuptake inhibitors, 1313t
North American Society of Homeopaths, 460
Nortriptyline, 445t, 1554
Norwegian scabies, 2182
Nose
- of adolescents, 123
- bleeding. *See* Epistaxis
- blood supply, 1483f
- of children, 123
- of infants, 123
- of newborns, 122–123, 765
- physical examination of, 122–123
- review of systems for, 92b

Nothing by mouth, 543–544, 544t
NSAIDs. *See* Nonsteroidal antiinflammatory drugs

Nuchal rigidity, 127
Nuchal translucency, 604–605
Nuclear scintigraphy
  description of, 147–148
  Meckel diverticulum evaluations, 149
Nucleoside reverse transcriptase inhibitors, 2144
Number needed to treat, 39–40
Nurse. *See also* School nurses
  as pediatric home health care providers, 571
  qualifications for, 1136
  in school health, 1135–1139
Nurse practitioners
  description of, 5
  discharge planning role of, 173b
Nursemaid's elbow, 2053, 2053f
Nurse-to-student ratio, 1137–1138
Nutrition. *See also* Malnutrition
  adoption assessments, 1045–1046
  adult health affected by, 230–231
  allowances, 230
  breastfeeding and, 819–820
  carbohydrates, 193–194, 225
  changes over last two decades, 2322, 2322b
  in chronic lung disease infants, 696
  congenital heart disease effects, 696
  in congestive heart failure, 2718, 2723–2724
  cystic fibrosis treated with, 1990–1991
  disorders of
    in immigrants, 63
    short stature caused by, 1728
  energy requirements, 220–222
  enteral, 692–693
  in extremely low–birth-weight infants, 854–855
  fats. *See* Fats
  feeding intolerance effects, 694–695
  food groups, 231
  growth-restricted infants, 885–887
  intrauterine growth and, 638–639, 884
  maternal health and, 627–629
  minerals, 225–226
  in neonatal intensive care infants, 709–712, 871–876
  osteopenia and, 700
  overview of, 219–220
  parenteral, 691–693
  preterm infants, 693–696
  protein. *See* Protein
  suggestions for, 194b
  supplements, 24, 324–325, 2551–2552
  in United States, 226, 229–230
  vitamins, 226
Nystatin, 513t

O

Oats, 458t
Obesity
  adults with, 230
  age and, 2321
  assessment of, 300b, 302
Obesity—cont'd
  breastfeeding and, 810
  cardiovascular health promotion and, 279t
  causes of, 2320, 2322, 2322t, 2323f
  comorbidities and complications of, 297, 2320, 2323–2324, 2323b, 2324t
  costs associated with, 2320, 2325
  definitions, 288, 2320–2321
  description of, 297
  differential diagnosis of, 2325, 2325t
  in Down syndrome, 2021, 2022
  dyspnea caused by, 1472
  environment and, 299–300, 301t, 2322, 2322t, 2323f
  epidemiology of, 2321
  factors associated with, 298–300, 301t, 2322, 2322t, 2323f
  genetics of, 298
  heart disease effects of, 288–290, 289f
  hypertension and, 1579, 1588
  incidence of, 297, 298f–299f
  in infants of diabetic mothers, 891
  knock-knees and, 1537
  laboratory evaluation of, 2325–2326, 2326b, 2326t
  maternal health and, 627–629
  media images and, 1118
  mental health comorbidities, 2324–2325
  metabolic syndrome and, 1579–1580, 2323b, 2323–2324
  nonalcoholic steatohepatitis caused by, 2324
  pathophysiological features of, 2321–2322
  polycystic ovarian syndrome caused by, 2324
  premature adrenarche in, 1814–1815
  preparticipation physical evaluation, 324
  prevalence of, 189, 2320–2321, 2321f
  prevention of
    age-appropriate guidance for, 301t
    description of, 44, 302, 810
    dietary modifications, 2327b, 2328
    parent's role in, 2327b, 2328
    physical activity in, 2328, 2328b
    physician's role in, 1999, 2327–2328, 2327b
    primary, 2326–2327
    secondary, 2327b–2328b, 2327–2328, 2328f
  pronation and, 1535
  screening for, 300b, 339–340
  sports participation with, 323t
  television viewing and, 2322, 2323f
  treatment of, 196, 300b, 302–303
Object permanence, 183, 210
Observational learning, 1004
Obsessive-compulsive behaviors, 1725, 1726
Obsessive-compulsive disorder, 1282, 1759–1760
Obstetric complications
  fetal/perinatal morbidity and mortality and, 633
  respiratory failure in newborn, 903
Obstetric pharmacology, 630
Obstipation, 2074
Obstructed megaureter, 2334
Obstruction
  airways. *See* Airways obstruction
  biliary
    hepatomegaly and, 1577
    jaundice and, 1620
  bowel, 2628
  colon, 2082
  distal airways, 1790
  duodenal, 2081
  gastrointestinal. *See* Gastrointestinal obstruction
  ileal, 2081–2082
  intrathoracic airways, 1791
  jejunal, 2081–2082
  nasolacrimal duct, 1704f, 1706–1707, 1707f
Obstructive hydrocephalus, 2147–2148
Obstructive pulmonary disease, 1469–1470
Obstructive sleep apnea, 525–526, 2583–2585
Obstructive uropathy
  causes of, 2333–2335, 2334f, 2335f
  differential diagnosis of, 2333–2335, 2334f–2335f, 2333b, 2334t
  fetal intervention for, 615–616
  management of, 2336–2338
  radiologic evaluation of, 2335–2336, 2336f
  urinary tract infections and, 2333
  voiding cystourethrogram in, 2336
Occipital plagiocephaly, 2433–2437. *See also* Plagiocephaly
Occipital-frontal circumference, 758–760
Occlusion
  assessment of, 1651
  description of, 125
  malocclusion. *See* Malocclusion
Occult spinal dysraphism, 2537–2538
Occupational therapists, 571
Occupational therapy
  discharge planning role of, 173b
  in rehabilitation process, 576–577, 578t
OCD. *See* Obsessive-compulsive disorder
Octreotide, 975–976
Ocular alignment, 1776
Ocular diseases and disorders
  herpes simplex virus, 1712f, 1712–1713, 2130
  sports participation with, 322t
  vision testing for, 1779–1782
Ocular inspection, 1780b, 1780f
Ocular misalignment. *See* Strabismus
Ocular toxoplasmosis, 2379
Ocular trauma
  abusive, 2349–2350, 2350f
  accidental, 2343

Page numbers followed by "f" denote figures; "t" denote tables; "b" *denote* boxes.

Ocular trauma—cont'd
amblyopia caused by, 2343
anatomic considerations in, 2343–2344
anterior segment
chemical injuries, 2345–2346
conjunctival foreign bodies, 2347–2348, 2347f
cornea
abrasion, 2346–2347, 2347f
foreign bodies, 2347–2348, 2347f
hyphema, 2348, 2348f
iritis, 2348
mydriasis, 2348
subconjunctival hemorrhages, 2346, 2346f
evaluation of
fundus in, 2345
history-taking, 2344
ocular motility in, 2344
physical examination, 2344–2345
pupils in, 2344–2345
vision testing, 2344
eyelids, 2345, 2345f
lacrimal injury, 2345, 2345f
orbit, 2349
ruptured globe, 2348–2349
shaken baby syndrome, 2350
Ocular-auricular-vertebral spectrum, 2547
ODD. *See* Oppositional defiant disorder
Odontoid dysplasia, 2547
Odor, 1664t–1665t, 1664–1665
Office setting, 53
Ofloxacin
Chlamydia treated with, 2512b
epididymitis treated with, 2520b
Oligoanuric state, 2798
Oligoarthritis
extended, 2213–2214
persistent, 2213
Oligoarticular juvenile idiopathic arthritis, 2213
Oligohydramnios, 1369
Oliguria
in acute renal failure, 2799
causes of, 1826t
comorbid conditions, 1826
definition of, 2798
etiology of, 1825–1826
evaluation of, 1826–1827
incidence of, 1825
management of, 1827–1829, 1828f
referrals for, 1829
Omalizumab, 1848
Omentum, torsion of, 2628
Omphalocele
fetal intervention, 617
ultrasound detection of, 610
Onchocerca volvulus, 2393
Onchocerciasis, 2393
Oncologic care, 1895–1897. *See also* Cancer
Ondansetron, 555t
Ongoing health conditions. *See also* Chronic disease and illness
coordination of care, 568
definition of, 564
developing and promoting partnerships with families, 567
diagnosis of, 566–567
effects of, 565
goals of care for, 567–568
involving and preparing child in care, 568
periodic reassessment of, 568
prevalence of, 564–565
special care considerations for, 565–566, 566b
Online Mendelian Inheritance in Man, 35t, 1809
Open-ended questions, 94, 201
Ophthalmia neonatorum, 801–802
Opiate toxicity, 68t
Opioids
abuse of, 2783
acute pain managed using, 431–432, 431b, 431t
antidote for, 2767t
chronic pain managed using, 440–443, 442t
half-life of, 425t
potency of, 425t
strong, 428–433, 428t, 429b, 431b, 431t
weak, 426–427
Opisthotonos, 127
Opportunistic infections, 1696
Oppositional behavior, 1220–1221, 1221b, 1223. *See also* Conduct disorder
Oppositional defiant disorder, 1223b, 1744
Oral contraception, 1352–1354
Oral development state, 1006
Oral health, 63, 69
Oral hygiene
in dental caries prevention, 295
description of, 1661–1662
promotion of, 63, 69
Oral lesions, 2569–2573
Oral motor therapy, 1466
Oral rehydration therapy, 2657–2661, 2659t
Oral-motor therapy, 577–579
Orbit
description of, 2343
infections of, 2245–2446, 2444f–2445f
trauma to, 2349
valveless venous system of, 2441f
Orbital cellulitis
description of, 120
empirical therapy for, 506t
infectious causes of, 2441–2442, 2441b
in sinusitis, 2536, 2536t
Orchitis, 1720, 2037
Organ transplantation
kidney, 2096–2097
liver, 2126
Organ transplantation—cont'd
lung, 1990
orthotopic heart, 1963–1965
rejection, 1963–1965
Organic acids, 2733b, 2734
Organochlorine compounds, 827
Organogenesis, 629–630
Organophosphates, 2685t, 2778–2779
Ornithine transcarbamoylase deficiency, 985–986
Orofacial cleft. *See also* Cleft lip and palate
fetal assessment for, 649–650
newborn assessment, 765–766, 792
ultrasound detection of, 606
Orofacial injuries, 1097
Orthodontic treatment, 1651–1652
Orthognathic surgery, 1929, 1930f
Orthopedic treatment, 2542
Orthopedics
definition of, 1528–1529
foot and leg problems. *See* Foot disorders; Leg disorders
terminology, 1529, 1529b
Orthopnea, 129
Orthoses, 579
Orthostatic hypotension, 1753, 1808
Orthostatic proteinuria, 1677
Orthotopic heart transplantation, 1963–1965
Orthotropias, 1781f
Ortolani test/maneuver, 138, 138f, 771, 805, 2052
Oseltamivir, 511t
Osgood-Schlatter disease, 140, 1636, 2553
Osmidrosis axillae, 1661
Osmolality, 468–469
Osmole, 225
Osmotic agents, 2742–2743
Osmotic diuresis, 1672
Osmotic pressure, 468
Osteochondritis dissecans, 2555
Osteochondrodysplasia, 2547
Osteochondroses
carpal semilunar end plate, 2353b, 2354
clinically significant sites of, 2353b
description of, 2352–2353, 2352b
extremity pain caused by, 1494
femoral head, 2353, 2353b
lower thoracic vertebrae, 2353b, 2354
metatarsal heads, 2353b, 2354
tarsal navicular, 2353b, 2354
tibia, 2353, 2353b
tibial shaft, 2353–2354, 2353b
Osteogenesis imperfecta
newborn eye assessment, 764
ultrasound detection of, 612–613
Osteomalacia, 700
Osteomyelitis
acute, 2355–2356
bone scan and scintigraphy evaluations, 151, 2357

Osteomyelitis—cont'd
causes of, 2355–2356
chronic, 2355–2356
definitions of, 2355–2356
description of, 2355
differential diagnosis of, 2356
empirical therapy for, 506t
evaluation of, 2356–2357
extremity pain caused by, 1494–1495
frontal bone bossing and, 117
joint pain and, 1627
limp and, 1635
magnetic resonance imaging of, 151, 152f, 2357
management of, 2357–2358
metaphyseal, 151
ultrasound of, 2357
Osteopathy, 457–459
Osteopenia, 700
Osteosarcoma
clinical manifestations, 1888–1889
etiology, 1887–1888
evaluation, 1889
follow-up, 1890
management of, 1889
prognosis, 1889–1890
radiation side effects, 1888t
Otitis externa, 2364
Otitis media
breastfeeding and, 810
classification of, 2360
complications of, 2363
costs of, 2360
definition of, 2360
description of, 2360
diagnosis of, 2361
early education and child care programs for, 1010–1022
with effusion
description of, 2360
management of, 2362–2363
epidemiologic features of, 2360
follow-up for, 2362
irritability and, 1613
management of, 2361–2362
pathogenesis of, 2360–2361
permanent hearing loss and, 1560
prevalence of, 2360
prevention of, 810
recurrent, 1696, 2360, 2363
referrals for, 9, 10t
treatment for, 162
tympanic membrane findings in, 122
Otoacoustic emissions, 327
Otorrhea, 2363
Otoscopic examination, 121
Outcomes
data sets, 14
description of, 11
disease, 12–14, 13t
family, 13t, 15
framework for assessing, 11, 13t–14t
functioning and development, 13t, 15
growth, 13t, 14–15
Outcomes—cont'd
injury, 12–14, 13t
risk behaviors, 13t, 15
survival, 11–12
symptoms and comfort, 14t, 15
well-being, 14t, 15
Outcomes assessment, 14
Outpatient care
access to, 6
of adolescents, 1324
after-hours coverage, 6–07
description of, 6
for eating disorders, 1192
medical home, 7
patient-call centers, 7
physician organizations, 6–7
surgical procedures, 515b
anesthesia in, 545
patient selection for, 552
postoperative anesthetic problems, 552–556, 553f, 554t–555t
postoperative care for, 552–563. *See also* Postoperative care
by specialty, 552b
visits to, 6, 9
Ovaries
absence of, 323t
androgen production, 1591–1592
cysts of, 777
Overbite, 125
Overdose, drug
antidotes for, 2684t–2685t, 2766t–2768t
assessment of, 2682–2683
complications, 2684–2686
definition of, 2682
differential diagnosis, 2683
epidemiology of, 2682
etiology of, 2682, 2682t
gastric decontamination in, 2683
hallucinogens, 2781–2782
hospitalization for, 2686
inhalants, 2782
life support procedures, 2682–2683
management of, 2683b, 2683–2686
marijuana, 2779, 2781
opioids, 2783
referrals for, 2686
sedative-hypnotics, 2782–2783
stabilization procedures, 2682–2683
stimulants, 2782
Overeating, 2322
Overheating, 2580
Overnight sleep study, 1298
Overnutrition, 231
Overprotectiveness, 1183–1184
Overuse syndromes
apophyseal conditions, 2553–2554
description of, 191
epiphyseal conditions, 2554–2555
extremity pain caused by, 1491–1492
factors contributing to, 2552, 2552b
physeal conditions, 2554
soft tissue, 2555–2556
stress fractures, 2552–2553
Overweight. *See also* Obesity
definition of, 2320
prevalence of, 14
Ovotesticular disorders of sexual development, 2197
Ovulation, 621
Oxacillin, 2566
Oxcarbazepine, 2499t, 2501–2502
Oxybutynin, 2043
Oxycodone, 442t
Oxygen saturation, 689
Oxygen therapy
bronchopulmonary dysplasia in neonates, 688–689
discharge criteria for home therapy, 713–717
hyperbaric
carbon monoxide poisoning treated with, 2773–2774
streptococcal TSS treated with, 2576
neonatal infant stabilization, 674–676
neonatal resuscitation, 661
in status asthmaticus, 2815
supplemental oxygen in air flights, 714
Oxymorphone, 425t

P

Pacemaker malfunction, 1755
Pacific Islands
cultural healing practices confused with child abuse, 69t
folk illnesses in, 65t, 68t
Pacifiers
breastfeeding effects, 817
malocclusion and, 1651
sudden infant death syndrome and, 2580
Packed red blood cells, 482
Pain
abdominal
acute, 1372, 1376, 1378, 1378b
appendicitis in, 2627–2728
causes of, 1379b, 2625b, 2626–2628
children and, 1376, 1379–1383, 1380f
conversion reaction causing, 1226
diagnosis of, 1377b, 1377–1379, 1378b
differential diagnosis, 2530b, 2628, 2629t
evaluation of, 1379–1382, 1380f, 2624, 2626
history, 2624
imaging studies for, 1281–1282
intussusception, 2627
malrotation and midgut volvulus, 2626f–2627f, 2626–2627
physical examination for, 1380–1381, 2624
recurrent, 1376–1377, 1379–1381
surgery in, 2628, 2630
treatment for, 1382
acute. *See* Acute pain

Page numbers followed by "f" denote figures; "t" denote tables; "b" *denote* boxes.

Pain—cont'd
back
chronic causes of, 1406, 1407
definition of, 1305
diagnosis of, 1405–1406, 1406t
epidemiology of, 1405
evaluation of, 1407–1409
management of, 1409–1410
postural abnormalities and, 2545
psychosocial considerations of, 1407
referrals for, 1410
spinal abnormalities and, 2549
chest. *See also* Arrhythmias
causes of in children, 1421–1424, 1422t
diagnosis of, 1420, 1428b
evaluation of, 1421
history and, 1421
idiopathic causes of, 1423
laboratory evaluation and, 1421
pathophysiological features of, 1420–1421
psychogenic, 1423–1444
symptoms of, 1421b, 1422t
circumcision and, 829
definition of, 435
extremities
diagnosis of, 1491–1495, 1492b–1493b
evaluation of, 1489–1491
history and, 1489–1490
laboratory examination and, 1490–1491
physical examination for, 1490
unexplained, 1490
fever-related, 420
joint
definition of, 1625–1626
differential diagnosis of, 1626–1628
etiology of, 1626
evaluation for, 1628
referral for, 1629
treatment of, 1628–1629
management of, 597–598, 597b
neuropathic, 435
postoperative, 556
premature infant, 705, 857–858
self-hypnosis for, 451, 451b
in snakebites, 2700
somatic, 435
types of, 435–436
Palate, cleft. *See* Cleft lip and palate
Palilalia, 1758
Palivizumab, 705
Palliative care, 593–602
chronic pain management, 446
components of, 594–595, 595b
definition of, 594
ethical issues related to, 595–596
indications for, 593–594
pain management in, 597–598, 597b
psychosocial support in, 598–599, 599b
for sick and dying infant, 737–738
Palliative care—cont'd
spiritual support in, 598–599, 599b
symptom management in, 597–598, 597b
talking with patient and families, 596–597
Pallid breath-holding spells, 1657
Pallor, 1395, 1403
Palmar grasp reflex, 141f, 143f
Palmoplantar hyperhidrosis, 1603
Palpation, 1562
Palpebral fissures, 119
Pamelor, 1313t
Pancreas, 1984
Pancreatic enzyme supplements, 1991
Pancreatitis, 1378–1379, 2628
Pancuronium, 2743
Panhypopituitarism, 1812
Panic attacks, 2644
Panner disease, 2555
Pansystolic murmurs, 1564f
Pantothenic acid, 229t
Pap smear, 2523, 2526f
Papilledema, 119
Papillomatosis, laryngeal, 2635–2636
Papular urticaria, 2180–2181
Papules, 1689, 1691f
Papulopustules, 1690f
Paradoxical vocal fold dysfunction, 1600
Parainfluenza viruses, 1981, 2648–2649
Paralysis of vocal cords, 2634
Paralytic disease, 2036–2037
Paraphimosis, 2431
Parasites, 2366–2416
antimicrobial therapy for, 514
diarrhea caused by, 1450
immigrant screening for, 70
meningoencephalitis caused by, 2270, 2270t
nematodes, 2385–2393
protozoa, 2366–2385
refugee screening for, 70
trematodes, 2393–2401
Parathion, 2685t
Parechovirus infections, 2037
Paregoric, 955
Parent(s). *See also* Family; Parent-adolescent relationship; Parent-child relationship
adolescent interviews and, 1332
amenorrhea diagnosis and, 1391
behavioral concerns of, 1221b
behavioral consultations and, 1165–1166
brain development of infant, 181
breath-holding spells, 1318–1319
child mental illness, 1170–1171, 1172
of children with special health care needs, 53
concerns of, 179
conduct disorders and, 1221b, 1221–1222
conflict among, 76–77
consanguinity of, 93–94
Parent(s)—cont'd
constipation and, 1425, 1429–1430
conversion reactions and, 1228
counseling of, 1328–1330
decision making by, 75
diagnosis disclosure with, 153–156
dysmorphism and, 1501
family history of. *See* Family history
foster, 182. *See also* Foster care
gay, lesbian, and bisexual youth and, 1364
goals of, 1328
grandparents as, 182
immunization refusal by, 79
interpretive conference with, 154–156
learning disabilities and, 1154
marital strain among, 182
medications and, 1177–1179
Münchausen syndrome by proxy, 1268–1269
newborn screening refusal by, 78–79
physician and, relationship between, 101
posttraumatic stress disorder and, 1283
prenatal interview with, 89–90
preparticipation physical evaluation questions, 317b, 318–319
primary care physician's questions for, 179, 180t–181t
questionnaires for, 360
resources for, 1170–1171, 1242
responsibilities of, 179
restraint of child by, 103
school health and, 1126, 1137
school readiness and, 1140–1141
school refusal and, 1146–1148
sleep disturbance and, 1297
stress assessments, 186
styles of, 1328
support for, 182
teenage
challenges for, 184
imaging studies, 1348
laboratory evaluation of, 1347–1348
management of, 1348, 1348b
physical examination for, 1347
temper tantrums and, 1316–1317
termination of rights
foster care and, 1063, 1067
substance abuse issues, 956
transgender youth and, 1237, 1242–1243, 1243b
unexplained physical symptoms and, 1183–1185
Parent education
adoption, 1046–1050
American Academy of Pediatrics materials for, 208
bereavement for sick and dying infant, 736–738
breastfeeding, 813–817
child abuse prevention, 1093
child health professionals, 1024

Parent education—cont'd
discipline guidelines, 1029–1035
divorce, 1057–1058
domestic violence, 1078–1079
early education and child care programs and, 1020–1024
electronic health records used for, 32
foster care and, 1066
healthy newborn follow-up care, 840–847, 849–850
hospital rounds and, 733
on media effects on children, 1114–1120
medical-legal issues in, 750–751
mental health diagnosis and treatment, 1016–1017
neonatal intensive care infants, 723, 869–880
newborn screening, 78
prenatal visit procedures, 797–800
self-care by children and, 1103–1105
sick and dying infants, 730
Parent Stress Index Short Form, 186
Parent-adolescent relationship
assessment of, 1329–1330
communication and, 1328–1329, 1329b
conflict management and, 1328, 1330
goals of, 1328
sexuality and, 1343–1344, 1364
Parental conflict, 1184
Parent-child relationship, 1156–1157, 1161, 1242–1243, 1243b
Parenteral drugs, 512t–513t
Parenteral fluid, 472, 479–480
Parenteral nutrition
in neonatal intensive care infants, 872–873
preterm infants, 691–693
Parenthetical statements, 1333–1334
Parent–infant relationship
goodness of fit, 179, 180t–181t, 183
temperament effects, 183
Parenting
overintellectualizing of, 211
stress in, 181
styles of, 159
violence-free, 273–274
without corporal punishment, 273–274
Parents' Evaluation of Developmental Status, 184, 315, 360
Parinaud syndrome, 1862
Parkes-Weber syndrome, 781
Paromomycin, 2368
Parotid gland, 118
Parotitis, 125, 2037
Paroxysmal nonepileptic disorders, 1657–1659
Partial anomalous pulmonary venous return, 1947
Partial exchange transfusion, 486
Partial seizures, 2489b, 2491–2492. *See also* Seizure(s), partial
Partially hydrolyzed infant formula, 2067
Partially treated meningitis, 2252, 2263
Participatory Management theory, 1171
Parvovirus B19, 932
Passive activism, 57
Pasteurella multocida, 1823
Patches, 1689, 1689f
Patella
chondromalacia, 1628, 2560
dislocation of, 2559
Patellofemoral arthralgia, 1636
Patellofemoral pain syndrome, 1628, 2560
Patent ductus arteriosus, 917, 1942
Pathobiological Determinants of Atherosclerosis in Youth, 280
Pathological cardiac murmurs, 917–918
Pathological proteinuria, 1677, 1678t
Patient(s)
communicating the concerns of, 201–202
diagnosis disclosure with, 153–156
education of
during discharge planning, 174
electronic health records used for, 32
primary care physician–hospitalist partnership in, 169
questionnaires, 360
Patient call centers, 7
Patient centeredness, 43
Patient Health Questionnaire, 366, 1170
Patient-physician relationship
adolescents and, 1331–1332
communication and, 1333
sexuality and, 1343–1344
Pay-for-performance programs, 22–23
PCOS. *See* Polycystic ovary syndrome
PCP. *See* Phencyclidine
PDD. *See* Pervasive developmental disorder
Peak flow monitoring, 1841–1842
Pectus carinatum, 128, 2418
Pectus excavatum
clinical features of, 2416–2417, 2417b
description of, 128, 2416
disorders associated with, 2417b
evaluation of, 2417
gender as factor in, 2416
prevalence of, 2416
prognosis of, 2418
treatment of, 2417–2418
PediaLink, 35t
Pediatric Advanced Life Support, 2806–2807, 2808f, 2809–2810
Pediatric Anesthesia Malpractice Closed Claims Registry, 519
Pediatric Brain Tumor Consortium, 1863
Pediatric history interview, 90–94, 91b–92b
Pediatric Migraine Disability Assessment, 1551–1552, 1554
Pediatric nurse practitioners, 5
Pediatric Perioperative Cardiac Arrest Registry, 518–519, 518t, 519f
Pediatric Quality of Life Measurement Model, 1170
Pediatric subspecialists
description of, 2, 4, 4t
referrals to, 9
Pediatric workforce
certification of, 3–4
international medical graduates, 3
licensure of, 3–4
medical training of, 3–4
nonphysician clinicians, 5
nurse practitioners, 5
physician assistants, 5
statistics regarding, 2–3
Pediatricians
appearance of, 89
children and, ratio between, 3
clothing worn by, 89
community activities to promote, 57–58
in community health centers, 7
cultural education of, 160
disciplining of, 10–11
gender of, 3
in group practice, 6t, 6–7
international medical graduates as, 3
medical liability of, 10–11
part-time, 9
payment methods for, 21–22, 22t
practice settings for, 6t, 6–7
recruitment and retention of, 26
reimbursement issues for, 17–18
residency programs for, 3
rural practice, 3
scope of practice for, 8b, 8–9
in solo practice, 6, 6t
specialization by, 2, 4, 4t
statistics regarding, 2–3
time management by, 9, 9f
visits to, 6, 9, 11t
women as, 3
Pediculosis, 2181–2182, 2181f
PedMIDAS. *See* Pediatric Migraine Disability Assessment
PEDS. *See* Parents Evaluation of Developmental Status
PedsCORI project, 2054
Peer groups
behavioral development and, 1000
media exposure and, 1116–1120
Peer violence, 272
PEG, 1430–1431
Pelvic examination
in adolescents, 137
description of, 1392, 1461–1462
in rape, 2794
Pelvic fractures, 2558–2559
Pelvic inflammatory disease
description of, 1462
diagnosis, 2528, 2529b
differential diagnosis, 2530b
dysuria caused by, 1477
hospitalization in, 2530b
treatment of, 2518b–2520b, 2529–2530
Penicillin
acute unilateral cervical adenitis treated with, 1997

Page numbers followed by "f" denote figures; "t" denote tables; "b" *denote* boxes.

Penicillin—cont'd
allergic interstitial nephritis caused by, 2028
allergic skin reactions, 2027t
animal bite wound uses of, 1824
bacterial resistance to, 492
bacterial skin infections treated with, 1855–1856
benzathine
dosage, peak serum concentrations, and MIC_{95} for, 493t
syphilis treated with, 2518b
classification of, 492
desensitization to, 495
G, 493t, 495
infectious mononucleosis treated with, 1980
mechanism of action of, 492
meningococcemia treated with, 2749
pharmacologic properties of, 492, 495
septic arthritis treated with, 2507–2508
sickling disorders treated with, 2103
side effects of, 495
streptococcal infections treated with
description of, 1981
toxic shock syndrome, 2575–2576
syphilis treated with, 2517b–2518b
uses of, 495–496
V, 493t
Penis
circumcision. *See* Circumcision
genital warts on, 2523, 2524f–2525f
herpes lesions on, 2525, 2527f
hygiene, 829
newborn assessment, 768–769
in newborns, 135
physical examination of, 135
Pentamidine isethionate, 2368
Pentazocine, 425t
Pentobarbital, 2743–2744
Peptic ulcer disease, 1545–1546
Percutaneous umbilical blood sampling, 645
Perfusion, in congestive heart failure, 2719
Perianal dermatitis, 1858
Pericarditis, 1423, 1959–1960
Periderm, 13
Perihepatitis, 2531
Perinatal asphyxia, 1654
Perinatal care. *See also* Neonatal intensive care unit; Sick and dying infants
assistive reproductive technologies, 622–625
bereavement issues, 736–738
birth injuries, 745–746
breastfeeding, 801, 813–817
circumcision, 828–830
congenital anomalies, 791
delivery room procedures
acute fetal hypoxia/asphyxia, 656–658
airways obstruction, 656
Perinatal care—cont'd
delivery room procedures—cont'd
apnea, 656
assessment protocol, 665
blood-spot screening, 804
breastfeeding, 801
congenital heart defect screening, 803–804
delivery room resuscitation, 658–659
developmental dysplasia screening, 805
disposition, 665
eye care, 801–802
glucose screening, 803
hearing screening, 805
hepatitis B virus vaccine and screening, 806–807
high-risk deliveries, 654
HIV transmission prevention, 804–805
hypopnea, 656
inadequate circulatory transition, 656
initial postnatal evaluation and intervention, 659–663
neonatal resuscitation, 655, 665–666
physical examinations, 803–807
postresuscitation assessment and stabilization, 663–664
transitional cardiorespiratory physiology, 654–656
umbilical cord, 664–665, 805
vitamin-K prophylaxis, 802
healthy newborn, 801–807
hemorrhage, 941
high-risk infant care
fetal assessment, 637–651
maternal conditions, 627–637
post-delivery care procedures, 801
sepsis prevention, 805
infectious disease, 932–935
medical-legal issues in, 742–751
metabolic derangements, 670–672
morbidity and mortality statistics, 634–636, 729, 736–737
neonatal growth and maturity indicators, 667–668
neonatal intensive care unit
needs assessment and screening, 667
referral protocol, 667
post-NICU continuing care protocols, 682–706
prenatal diagnosis, 604–619
respiratory distress symptoms, 668
sepsis syndrome, 668–670
sick and dying infants, collaborative decision making, 729–735
well-appearing infant assessment, 672–673
Periodic breathing, 129
Periodic fever, aphthous stomatitis, pharyngitis and cervical adenopathy, 1526, 2570, 2572
Periodic limb movements, 1307
Periodicity Schedule, 50
Periods (menstrual), 1767
Periorbital cellulitis, 120, 2442–2443, 2443f
Peripheral alpha-agonists, 1587t
Peripheral blood smear, 2208, 2208f
Peripheral nerve disorders, 1606–1607
Peripheral precocious puberty, 1592, 1595
Peripheral pulmonary stenosis murmur, 916–917
Peristalsis, 132
Peritonitis, 2624, 2628
Peritonsillar abscess, 126, 2635
Periventricular leukomalacia, 855
Permanent teeth, 123
Permethrin
lice treated with, 2181
scabies treated with, 2182–2183
Persistent oligoarthritis, 2213
Persistent pulmonary hypertension, 677–678
Personal Experience Inventory, 401
Personality
history-taking about, 92b
traits, 997
Pertussis
age as factor in, 2419, 2420f
characteristics of, 2419
clinical features of, 2420–2421
complications of, 2421–2422
definition of, 2419
diagnosis of, 2421
differential diagnosis of, 2420
epidemiologic features of, 2419f–2420f, 2419–2420
evaluation of, 2420–2422
management of
antibiotics, 2422, 2422t
close contact care, 2422
household care, 2422
supportive care, 2422
prevalence of, 2419, 2419f–2420f
prevention of, 2422–2423
Pervasive Development Disorder Behavior Inventory, 1198
Pervasive developmental disorder, 1197, 1742
Pes, 1529b
Pes cavus, 1536, 1536f, 1542
Pes planovalgus, 1535, 1536, 1538
Pes planus, 1530, 1534, 1536
Pesticides, 845–846, 2778–2779
Petechiae
causes, 2748b
description of, 1667–1669
in meningococcemia, 2747f, 2749
PFAPA. *See* Periodic fever, aphthous stomatitis, pharyngitis and cervical adenopathy
Phagocytic immunodeficiencies, 1699, 1699t
Phallic stage of psychosexual development, 1007

Pharmacodynamics
definition of, 490
description of, 490–492
efficacy related to, 490
Pharmacogenetics, 2242–2243
Pharmacokinetics
apnea, bradycardia and desaturation in neonates, 686–688
bronchopulmonary dysplasia in neonates, 689–690
definition of, 490
description of, 490–492
efficacy related to, 490
maternal-fetal transport and, 629–630
neonatal considerations
drug withdrawal syndrome, 954–956
resuscitation, 662
Pharyngitis
causes of
adenoviruses, 2425b, 2426
bacteria, 2425b, 2426–2427
cigarette smoke exposure, 2427
enteroviruses, 2425b, 2426
Epstein-Barr virus, 2425b, 2426
fungi, 2427
herpes simplex virus, 2425b, 2426
Kawasaki disease, 2427
Mycoplasma pneumoniae, 2425b, 2427
viruses, 2425–2426, 2425b
complications of, 2428–2429
definition of, 2425
description of, 2425
differential diagnosis of, 2427
evaluation of, 2427–2428
rheumatic fever caused by, 2429
streptococcal, 2478–2479
treatment of, 2428
Pharyngoconjunctival fever, 1711
Pharyngotonsillitis, 2425
Pharynx
gonococcal infection of, 2513b–2514b
of infants, 124–125, 125f
of newborns, 124
physical examination of, 123–127
recurrent infections of, 2585–2589
Phencyclidine, 950, 2781–2872
Phenobarbital
seizures treated with, 2497, 2498t, 2743
status epilepticus treated with, 2820b
Phenothiazines
antidote for, 2684t–2685t
postoperative nausea and vomiting managed using, 555t
Phentolamine, 2729, 2729t
Phenylketonuria
diagnosis and management, 986
newborn screening for, 384
Phenytoin
seizures treated with, 2497, 2498t, 2500, 2743
status epilepticus treated with, 2820b
Pheochromocytoma, 1816, 2315–2316, 2315t
Phimosis, 2430f, 2430–2432
Phlyctenular conjunctivitis, 1714
PHO, 19b
Phobia
agoraphobia, 1281
definition of, 1280
development and, 1281
diagnosis of, 1282
etiology of, 1281
evaluation of, 1282–1283
fever, 419
management of, 1283–1284
prevalence of, 1281
referrals for, 1284
relevant history and, 1282–1283
school, 1146–1147
social, 1281
specific, 1281
Phonemes, 159–160
Phonocardiogram, 131f
Phonotrauma, 1599–1600, 1602
Phosphoenolpyruvate-carboxykinase deficiency, 980
Phosphorus
in diabetic ketoacidosis, 2665, 2667
metabolism of, 966–967
Phototherapy
jaundice treated with, 821–822, 896–897
psoriasis treated with, 2452t, 2453
Physeal injuries, repetitive, 2554
Physiatrists, 575
Physical abuse
defined, 1092
joint pain and, 1628
Physical activity. *See also* Exercise
activities for, 191b
adherence to, 196–197
American College of Sports Medicine daily recommendations, 190
barriers to, 196–197
benefits of, 189–190
body mass index measurements before starting, 193
cardiorespiratory endurance through, 190–191, 191t
cardiovascular health promotion and, 279t
changes over last two decades, 2322, 2322b, 2323f
congestive heart failure and, 2718
in eating disorder patients, 193
energy requirements, 220–221
frequency of, 191
in heart disease prevention, 288–290, 289f, 291b
heart rate levels, 190–191, 191t
obesity prevention through, 2328, 2328b
opportunities for talking about, 197
poverty effects on, 241f, 242
Physical education, 1123
Physical examination
abdomen, 132–134
adolescents, 105, 116
blood pressure, 106–108, 107t–110t
body temperature, 104, 105f–106f
breastfeeding, 818
cardiac murmurs, 918
chest, 112, 128–130
early childhood, 103, 116, 120
ears, 120–122
epiglottis, 127
eyes, 118–120
face development, 116
feet, 139
genitalia. *See* Genitalia
hand coordination monitoring, 144, 145f
head, 116–118
heart, 130–132
heart rate, 104–105, 106t
height, 110–111, 112f, 115f
infants
chest circumference, 112
description of, 102–103
of diabetic mothers, 889
eyes, 119–120
head circumference, 111f, 111–112, 113f
length of, 111, 111f, 113f, 115t
nervous system of, 142–144
skin, 116
weight, 111
jaundice evaluation, 895
kidneys, 133
large-for-gestational-age infants, 889
late childhood, 104, 116, 120
length of infants, 111, 111f, 113f, 115f
liver, 133
lower extremities, 138–139
lungs, 128–130
mouth, 123–127
musculoskeletal system, 137–140
neck, 116–118, 127–128
nervous system, 140–145
newborn, 757–773
abdomen, 767–768
body measurements, 758–760
cardiovascular system, 766
chest and lungs, 766–767
chest circumference, 112
congenital anomalies, 789–790
cry assessment, 758
description of, 101–102
ears, 764–765
eyes, 118–119, 763–764
face, 763
genitalia and anus, 768–769
head, 111f, 111–112, 113f, 758–762
metabolic disorders, 970–971
mouth, 765–766
musculoskeletal system, 137–139
neck, 766

Physical examination—cont'd
newborn—cont'd
nervous system of, 142–144
neurologic examination, 670–671, 771–773
nose, 765
scalp, 762–763
skin, 114–115, 760
skull, 116–118
umbilical cord, 767–768
nose, 122–123
overview of, 101
pharynx, 123–127
post-delivery, 803–807
preanesthetic, 541, 543, 543f, 543t
pulse, 104–105, 106t
reflexes, 141f, 142–143
respirations, 106
respiratory failure in newborn, 903–904
screening uses of, 316–317
sexual abuse, 1110
skin, 113–116
skull, 116–118
somatic growth, 108, 110–112
spleen, 133
tongue, 124
tonsils, 126
vital signs, 104–108
weight, 111
Physical inactivity, 189–190
Physical therapists, 571
Physical therapy
discharge planning role of, 173b
in rehabilitation process, 576–577, 578t
Physician(s)
collaborative management by, 167
cultural education of, 160
disciplining of, 10–11
hospitalists, 4–5
licensed, 2
medical home, 52
medical liability of, 10–11
med-peds, 3
parents and, relationship between, 101
pay-for-performance programs, 22–23
payment methods for, 21–22, 22t
as pediatric home health care providers, 571
practice settings for, 6t, 6–7
recruitment and retention of, 26
refusal to participate in home births, 82–83
Physician assistants, 5
Physician hospital organization, 19b
Physician organizations, 6–7
Physician-patient relationship
adolescents and, 1326
therapeutic effects for parents, 1160–1161
Physis, 2553t
Physostigmine, 2766t, 2773
Piaget's cognitive development theory, 1002, 1015
Pica, 1743
PICOTT format, 38
PID. *See* Pelvic inflammatory disease
Piebaldism, 113, 779
Pierre Robin sequence/syndrome, 525, 1929–1930
Pigeon toe, 1538–1540
Pigmentary birthmarks, 779–780
Pili Torti, 1386
Pill esophagitis, 2057
Pimecrolimus cream, 1852
Pine bark extract, 458t
Pineal tumors, 1862
Ping-pong skull fracture, 992
Pinhole test, 1780
Pink eye. *See* Conjunctivitis
Pinworms
causes of, 2432
clinical manifestations of, 2432–2433
description of, 2389–2390
dysuria caused by, 1477
laboratory evaluation of, 2433
prevalence of, 2432
prevention of, 2433
treatment of, 2433
vaginal bleeding caused by, 1767
Pitted keratolysis, 1662–1663
Pittsburgh criteria, 2585, 2587b
Pituitary deficiency, 982
Pituitary hormone deficiencies, 1812
Placenta disorders
fetal/neonatal care and, 631–632
placenta previa, 632
Plagiocephaly
definition of, 2433
description of, 117, 2433, 2580–2581
differential diagnosis of, 2434
epidemiologic features of, 2434
newborn assessment, 763
pathogenesis of, 2433–2434
positional, 2434
posterior deformational
diagnosis of, 2434–2435, 2435f
prevention of, 2436
sequelae of, 2436
treatment of, 2435–2436
prevention of, 2435
risk factors for, 2434
sequelae of, 2436
treatment of, 2435–2436
Plan-do-study-act cycle, 47
Planned visits, 46
Plantar flexion, 1532
Plantar grasp reflex, 143f
Plantar hyperhidrosis, 1603
Plants, toxic, 2779, 2780t–2781t
Planus, 1529b
Plaque
description of, 1689
psoriasis, 2447–2448, 2448f, 2448t
scaling, 1690f
Plasma products, 487
Plasma volume, 1480
Plasma water, 467
Plasmodium sp.
malaria caused by, 2380–2384, 2382t–2383t
P falciparum, 70
PlastiBell, 829
Platelet disorders
anesthesia and, 538
in neonates, 945–946
petechiae and purpura, 1667–1669
Platelet transfusions, 484–485, 485b, 486t
Plexiform neurofibroma, 2305
Ploidy, 2237
Plugged milk ducts (milk stasis), 819
PMI. *See* point of maximal impulse
PML/RAR gene, 2238
Pneumococcal disease, 1518
Pneumococcal vaccine
in adolescents, 246f
catch-up schedule for, 251t
characteristics of, 256
conjugated, 256
description of, 1518
guidelines for, 245f
intervals between doses, 248t
minimum age for, 248t
polysaccharide, 256–257, 257t
schedule for, 251t, 256t
Pneumocystis jirovecii pneumonia, 2140
Pneumomediastinum
causes of, 2754–2755
definition of, 2754
diagnosis of, 911–912
evaluation of, 2756–2757, 2757f
hospitalization for, 2760
management of, 2760
pathophysiology of, 911–912
referral for, 2760
spontaneous, 2755
Pneumonia
acute, 2437
age as factor in, 2437
bacterial, 2420
causes of, 2438
definition of, 2437
description of, 2437–2438
empirical therapy for, 506t
evaluation of, 2438–2439
in HIV-infected children, 2142
management of, 2439
Mycoplasma
description of, 1980, 2030
fatigue caused by, 1511
pharyngitis caused by, 2425b, 2427
Pneumocystis jirovecii, 2140
recurrent, 1696, 2058–2059
varicella, 1914
Pneumoperitoneum, 1372
Pneumothorax
in adolescents, 2757–2758
causes of, 2754–2755

Pneumothorax—cont'd
- chest tube insertion and management, 2758–2759, 2759f
- definition of, 2754
- description of, 1990, 2758
- diagnosis of, 911–912
- evaluation of, 2755–2756, 2756f
- hospitalization for, 2760
- iatrogenic, 2755–2756, 2758
- management of, 2757–2760
- neonatal, 678, 2755
- pathophysiology of, 911–912
- recurrence of, 2760
- referral for, 2760
- size estimations, 2757, 2757f
- spontaneous, 2754–2755, 2757–2758
- tension, 2756, 2758
- traumatic, 2755, 2758
- in young adults, 2757–2758

Podofilox, 2515b
Podophyllin
- molluscum contagiosum treated with, 2620
- warts treated with, 2618

Point of maximal impulse, 130, 1562
Point-of-service plans, 18, 19b, 20t
Poison control centers, 2764
Poison ivy, 1691f
Poisoning
- acetaminophen, 2766t, 2770–2771, 2771f
- acid, 2775
- α_2-adrenergic agonists, 2775
- β_1-adrenergic antagonists, 2766t, 2774–2775
- alcohols, 2767t, 2783–2784
- alkali, 2775
- antidepressants, 2768t, 2772
- antidotes for, 2766t–2768t
- antihistamines, 2772–2773
- calcium-channel blockers, 2766t, 2774–2775
- carbon monoxide
  - antidote for, 2684t, 2766t
  - description of, 2773–2774
  - irritability and, 1612
- cardiac glycosides, 2766t, 2774
- decontamination in, 2768–2770
- description of, 1265–1266
- enhanced elimination in, 2770
- epidemiology, 2762–2763, 2763t
- fatalities caused by, 2762–2763, 2763t
- general management of, 2764–2765
- hallucinogens, 2781–2782
- hydrocarbons, 2775–2776
- inhalants, 2782
- insect repellents, 2776
- iron, 2766t–2767t, 2776–2777
- isoniazid, 2767t, 2777
- lead
  - adverse health effects associated with, 394
  - anemia and, 2205
  - antidote for, 2767t

Poisoning—cont'd
- lead
  - description of, 1400, 2777–2778
  - epidemiologic features of, 393
  - folk illness remedies associated with, 66t–68t
  - in immigrant children, 63
  - lead sources, 393–394
  - screening for, 393–397, 395b–396b, 395t
- marijuana, 2779, 2781
- mental status alterations in, 2640b, 2641–2643
- nerve agents, 2779
- opioids, 2767t, 2783
- pesticides, 2778–2779
- plants, 2779, 2780t–2781t
- prevention, 2763–2764
- resuscitation in, 2765, 2768
- rodenticides, 2784
- salicylates, 2771–2772
- sedative-hypnotics, 2782–2783
- seizures caused by, 2768, 2768b
- selective serotonin reuptake inhibitors, 2772
- stimulants, 2782
- supportive care in, 2770
- in toddlers, 2764b
- toxidromes, 2764t, 2764–2765

Pollens, 1819
Polyarthritis, 2476–2477
Polyarticular juvenile idiopathic arthritis, 2212–2214, 2213t
Polycystic ovary syndrome, 19b, 20t, 1590, 1592, 1809, 1815, 2324
Polycythemia, 890
Polydactyly
- description of, 1531f, 1532
- newborn assessment, 769–771
- physical examination, 793
- supernumerary digits, 783

Polydipsia, 1670, 1672–1674
Polyhydramnios
- description of, 1369
- fetal goiter, 607
- tracheoesophageal fistula, 777

Polymerase chain reaction
- description of, 2038, 2140
- meningitis diagnosis using, 2264
- neonatal blood viruses, 929–930
- pertussis diagnosis using, 2421

Polypharmacy, 1180
Polyps
- description of, 1545
- gastrointestinal bleeding caused by, 1545
- umbilical, 2607

Polysaccharides, 225
Polysomnographic tracing, 1833f–1834f
Polysomnography
- description of, 1832, 1834, 1985, 2584–2585
- predischarge monitoring of NICU infants, 715–716

Polyunsaturated fats, 224

Polyuria
- definition of, 1670
- diagnostic testing for, 1672–1674, 1673t
- differential diagnosis of, 1670–1672, 1671b
- management of, 1674–1675
- pathophysiological features of, 1670, 1670f
- patient history and examination for, 1672
- referral for, 1673, 1675

Pool safety, 2680, 2681b
Population projections, 235
Port wine stain, 781, 1689f
Positional plagiocephaly, 705, 2434
Positive D test, 495f
Positive pressure ventilation, 657–658
Postanesthetic apnea, 522, 524, 524f
Postantibiotic effect, 490
Posterior fontanelle, 116, 117f
Posterior fossa tumors, 2151
Posterior plagiocephaly, 2433–2437
Post-hypoxic-ischemic encephalopathy, 862–863
Postinfectious glomerulonephritis, 2289, 2289b
Postinfectious hydrocephalus, 2151
Postintubation croup, 557
Postnatal assessment
- breastfeeding, 819–822
- health and development outcomes, in neonatal intensive care infants, 854–858
- sonographic findings, 774–777

Postoperative care
- anesthesia-related problems, 552–556, 553f, 554t–555t
- bleeding, 559
- complications in, 552
- description of, 552
- drainage, 559
- early problems, 558t–559t, 558–560
- fever, 558, 558t
- pain management, 556
- posttonsillectomy hemorrhage, 559–560
- scar formation, 562
- scrotal swelling, 560
- surgical problems, 560–561
- urinary retention, 560
- venous thromboembolism, 561, 561b
- wound healing, 561–562
- for wound infections, 558, 559t, 561

Postoperative nausea and vomiting, 554t–555t
- anesthetic technique as factor in, 554
- concomitant medications affected by, 556
- description of, 552–554
- postoperative oral intake and, 554–555
- prolonged, 556
- treatment of, 555–556, 555t

Primary care physician—cont'd
  hospitalists and, 168–169, 169b
  illnesses commonly treated by, 8
  learning problems and, 1149, 1151–1154
  legal considerations of, 1278
  media effects on children, 1119–1120
  mental health services
    assessment tools, 1168–1170
    collaborative care, 1171–1174, 1173t
    description of, 1164–1165, 1168
    implementation of, 1171
    treatment, 1014–1017
  Münchausen syndrome by proxy, 1275–1278
  neutrality of, 1332
  nurse and, collaboration between, 1138
  parent-adolescent relationship and, 1329–1330
  parental distress, 1172
  physical education, 1123
  posttraumatic stress disorder, 1289
  preadoption care role of, 1043–1044
  prenatal visit procedures, 797–800
  referral to specialty care, 9
  responsibilities of, 8
  role of, 165
  school outreach by
    description of, 1122, 1124, 1126–1130, 1128t, 1129b
    health education and, 1131–1133
  school readiness and, 1143–1144
  self-care by children, 1105
  sexual abuse assessment and diagnosis, 1107–1113
  sick and dying infant care responsibilities, 729–730, 732
  substance abuse and, 1246
  therapists and, collaboration between, 1186
  transgender youth and, 1236–1237, 1238–1244
  unexplained physical symptoms and, 1185–1186
Primary insufficient milk syndrome, 812
Primary prevention, 12
Primary teeth, 123, 124f
Primidone, 2498t, 2500
Primitive neuroectodermal tumors, 1860–1861, 1885, 1887
Prions, 2270
Priorities, 43–45
Privacy
  adolescents, 31
  electronic health record and, 29t, 31
Problem Oriented Screening Instrument for Teenagers, 401
Procaine penicillin, 493t
Procedure notes and protocols, 748–749
Processus vaginalis, 1721
Prochlorperazine, 555t
Proctitis, 2520b–2521b, 2531
Proctocolitis, 2520b–2521b, 2531
Progesterone-only injection, 1354–1355
Progestin, 1354
Program for Renewal of Certification in Pediatrics, 4
Progressive hearing loss, 719
Prokinetic agents for gastroesophageal reflux disease, 2062
Prolapsed urethra, 1767
Prolonged QT syndrome, 527–529, 528t
Promethazine, 555t
Pronation
  description of, 1534–1536, 1535f, 1542
  knock-knees and, 1537
  toeing-in and, 1538
Propionibacterium acnes, 1802, 1805
Propionic acidemia, 984
Propoxyphene, 2685t
Prostaglandin synthesis inhibitors, 424–426, 425t
Protease inhibitors, 2139–2140, 2144
Protein
  amino acids, 222
  biological quality of, 222–223, 223t
  daily consumption of, 194
  daily requirements, 223f, 223–224
  essential amino acids, 222
  functions of, 222
  in human vs. cow milk, 213, 222, 229
  hydrolysis of, 222
  inadequate supply of, 222
  low-birth-weight newborn requirements for, 224
  pregnancy requirements, 224
  sources of, 223–224
  vegetable, 222–223
Protein C
  deficiency of, 2750–2751
  in disseminated intravascular coagulation, 2675
Protein S deficiency, 2750
Proteinuria
  description of, 2113
  diagnostic testing for, 1676, 1678, 1679f
  etiology of, 1677–1678
  history-taking for, 1678
  management of, 1679–1680
  pathophysiology of, 1676
  physical examination for, 1678
  prevalence of, 1677
  renal biopsy and, 1680b
  screening for, 405
  warning sings of, 1678b
Proton pump inhibitor, 2058, 2061–2062, 2062t
Protozoal infections, 2366–2385. *See also specific types, eg, Leishmaniasis*
  African trypanosomiasis, 2370
  amebiasis, 2372–2373
  amoebic meningoencephalitis, 2373–2375
  babesiosis, 2384–2385
Protozoal infections—cont'd
  Chagas disease, 2368–2369
  cryptosporidiosis, 2375–2377
  cyclosporiasis, 2377–2378
  giardiasis, 2370–2372
  isosporiasis, 2377
  leishmaniasis, 2366–2368
  malaria, 2380–2384, 2382t–2383t
  toxoplasmosis, 2378–2380
Provider payment, 21–22, 22t
Provitamin A, 228t
Proximal tubule cell, 2461, 2461f
Pruritus, 1681–1682, 1851–1852
Pseudoesotropia, 1735, 1735f
Pseudo-fever of unknown origin, 1524–1525, 1525b
Pseudohermaphrodite, 2194
Pseudomonas aeruginosa, 1856, 1989–1990
Pseudomonas multocida, 1823–1824
Pseudoseizures, 2489b, 2494
Pseudotumor cerebri, 2739, 2744–2745
Psoriasis, 1690f
  in adults, 2447
  causes of, 2447
  clinical variants of, 2447–2449, 2448f–2450f, 2448t
  description of, 2447
  diagnosis of, 2450, 2451t
  differential diagnosis of, 2450, 2451b, 2451t
  erythrodermic, 2448t, 2449, 2450f
  evaluation of, 2450, 2451b
  gender and, 2447
  guttate, 2447, 2448f, 2449f
  incidence of, 2447
  inverse, 2447, 2448t, 2449f
  joint pain and, 1626
  laboratory testing for, 2450, 2451t
  management of
    anthralin, 2452t, 2453
    calcineurin inhibitors, 2452t, 2453
    calcipotriol, 2451, 2452t
    corticosteroids, 2451, 2452t
    cyclosporine, 2453–2454, 2453t
    emollients, 2451, 2452t
    etanercept, 2453t, 2454
    methotrexate, 2452t, 2453
    phototherapy, 2452t, 2453
    retinoids, 2451, 2452t–2453t, 2453
    systemic agents, 2452t–2453t, 2453–2454
    tar preparations, 2451, 2452t
    topical therapies, 2451, 2452t, 2453
  plaque-type, 2447–2448, 2448f, 2448t
  pustular, 2448–2449, 2448t
  types of, 2447–2449, 2448f–2450f, 2448t
Psoriatic arthritis, 2214, 2449–2450
Psychiatric syncope, 1755
Psychoeducation
  for learning disorders, 1153
  for mental illness, 1172
  for mood disorders, 1260

Psychological development. *See also* Mental health
- adolescence, 1009–1010
- adoption and, 1044–1045
- birthing process and, 1005
- child abuse and, 1092
- cognitive-intellectual theory, 1003
- discipline principles, 1029–1035
- divorce effects on, 1056–1059
- Erikson's psychosocial development theory, 1003
- infancy, 1005–1006
- intermediate postpartum period, 1004
- learning theory, 1004
- media impact on, 1114–1120
- mental health issues and, 1017
- middle childhood, 1008–1009
- physiological development and, 1004–1012
- pregnancy precursors, 1004–1005
- preschool-age child, 1007
- stages of, 1012
- theoretical background, 1001–1004
- toddlers, 1007
- young adulthood, 1009–1010

Psychologists, 1167

Psychopharmacology therapy. *See also* Drug(s); Medications
- autism and, 1198
- eating disorders and, 1193
- phobias and, 1283

Psychosexual development
- Freudian analysis and, 1002–1003
- gay- and lesbian-parented families, children in, 1082–1085
- genital stage, 1010
- latency stage, 1008
- media images and, 1115–1120
- oral and anal stages, 1006
- phallic stage, 1007

Psychosis
- in children, 1166
- definition of, 1745
- postpartum, 365

Psychosocial development
- adoption and, 1044–1045
- autonomy vs. shame and guilt, 1006
- discipline principles, 1029–1035
- divorce effects on, 1056–1059
- early education and child care programs, 1019–1020
- family genogram techniques, 1039–1040
- family structure and environment and, 1036–1041
- gay- and lesbian-parented children, 1082–1085
- identity vs. role confusion, 1010–1011
- industry vs. inferiority, 1009
- initiative vs. guilt, 1007–1008
- intimacy vs. isolation, 1010–1011
- self-care by children and, 1103–1104
- sexual abuse and, 1112–1113
- socialization norms, 1040
- trust vs. mistrust, 1006

Psychosocial dysfunction
- causes of, 361, 361t
- detection of, 359
- evaluation of, 361–362
- management of, 362
- prevalence of, 358–359
- recognition of, 359–361
- screening for, 359
- secondary consequences of, 359
- severity of, 360–361

Psychosocial health, 361, 361t

Psychosocial history, 92b, 94

Psychosocial issues
- assisted reproductive technologies, 624–625
- behavioral and emotional outcomes, very low–birth-weight infants, 856
- breastfeeding and, 810–811
- fetal influences on mother and family, 650
- healthy newborn discharge, 846
- infants of diabetic mothers, 891
- Kawasaki disease, 2227
- maternal health and, 631
- neonatal intensive care infants
  - family adjustment to, 879–880
  - health outcomes, 858–861
  - parents, 733–735
- pre-transfer neonatal stabilization, 680
- psychosocial development
  - autonomy vs. shame and guilt, 1006
  - Erikson's theory, 1003
  - identity vs. role confusion, 1010–1011
  - industry vs. inferiority, 1009
  - initiative vs. guilt, 1007–1008
  - intimacy vs. isolation, 1010–1011
  - trust vs. mistrust, 1006
- in seizure management, 2502

Psychosocial screening
- changing pediatric practice environment in, 362
- description of, 349
- future directions in, 362
- goals of, 359
- interviewing in, 359–361
- need for, 358–359
- parent questionnaires in, 360
- patient questionnaires in, 360
- in psychosocial dysfunction severity, 360–361
- reasons for, 359
- in special areas, 360
- strategies in, 359–361
- tools in, 360–361

Psychosocial stress, 189

Psychosocial support
- adolescents and, 1334–1337, 1335t, 1337t
- autism, 1198–1199
- in end-of-life care, 598–599, 599b
- family and patient, 580–581
- in palliative care, 598–599, 599b

Psychostimulants, 1209–1211

Psychotherapy
- for behavioral and emotional problems, 1177, 1179
- for eating disorders, 1193
- for mood disorders, 1261–1262

Psychotic disorders, 1745

Psychotropic medications, 1072–1073

Pterygium colli, 1764

PTSD. *See* Posttraumatic stress disorder

Puberty
- breast development during, 128
- cystic fibrosis and, 1984–1985
- delayed
  - causes of, 1685b
  - description of, 1684–1685
  - diagnostic testing for, 1686b
  - referral for, 1687
- delayed tooth eruption and, 123
- description of, 1339–1340, 1595
- gynecomastia, 1683–1684
- normal, 1663
- onset of, 1684t
- precocious
  - causes of, 1686b
  - diagnostic testing for, 1687b
  - referral for, 1687
  - sexual hair growth and, 1591–1593, 1595
- short stature and, 1729
- Tanner stages of
  - in boys, 134f
  - in girls, 135f

Pubic hair. *See also* Puberty
- definition of, 1590
- precocious, 1596

Pubic lice, 2181

Public funding, for home health care, 571–572

Public health nurse visits, 723

Public Law 94-142, 588

Public speaking, 58

Pulmonary air leak syndrome, 911–912

Pulmonary artery, anomalous left
- in airways obstruction, 2636–2637
- in congestive heart failure, 2721

Pulmonary atresia
- with intact ventricular septum, 1946
- tetralogy of Fallot management, 1944–1946

Pulmonary diseases and disorders
- description of, 1422t, 1422–1423
- dyspnea caused by, 1469–1470
- fatigue caused by, 1510

Pulmonary function
- in general anesthesia, 521–524, 521b, 523f–524f
- in neonatal intensive care infants, 853

Pulmonary function tests
- cough and, 1434–1435
- preoperative evaluation uses of, 545
- wheezing and, 1792f

Pulmonary hemosiderosis, 1571

Page numbers followed by "f" denote figures; "t" denote tables; "b" *denote* boxes.

Pulmonary hypertension
description of, 1943
hemoptysis and, 1574
syncope and, 1756
Pulmonary neoplasms, 1572
Pulmonary system
in drowning injuries, 2677
tuberous sclerosis complex effects on, 2311
Pulse
in congestive heart failure, 2719
measurement of, 104–105, 106t
Pulse oximetry
for apnea, 1832
for bronchiolitis, 1868
congenital heart defect screening, 803–804
for cystic fibrosis, 1985
in NICU-discharged infants, 713–714
Pulsed dye laser, 2620
Punishment
corporal, 81–82
guidelines for, 1033–1034
Pupillary light reflex, 118, 141f, 2640–2641
Purpura
causes, 2748b
description of, 1667–1669
Henoch-Schönlein
appendicitis vs., 1838
clinical presentation of, 2112–2113
description of, 1658, 1668
differential diagnosis of, 2113
epidemiology of, 2112
evaluation of, 2113
joint pain, 1627–1628
nephritis, 2289, 2289b
prognosis for, 2113–2114
referrals for, 2114
Rocky Mountain spotted fever vs., 2482
scrotal swelling and, 1720–1721
treatment of, 2113–2114
vascular lesions in, 1826
immune thrombocytopenic
chronic, 2173
clinical presentation of, 2170–2171
complications of, 2173
description of, 2170
differential diagnosis of, 2171
evaluation of, 2171
incidence of, 2170
intracranial hemorrhage in, 2172
management of, 2171–2173
anti-Rho, 2173
bleeding-related, 2172
corticosteroids, 2172
follow-up care, 2173
general advice in, 2172
intravenous immunoglobulin, 2172–2173
outcomes after, 2173
splenectomy, 2173–2174
in neonates, 2173
in meningococcemia, 2748–2749, 2749f
Pustules, 1690, 1691f
Pyelectasis, 775–776
Pyelonephritis, 2611, 2612–2613
Pyloric stenosis
abdominal findings, 132
causes of, 2455
characteristics of, 2454–2455
complications of, 2457
description of, 2454–2455
diagnosis of, 2455–2456, 2456f
differential diagnosis of, 2456
discharge criteria, 2457
epidemiologic features of, 2455
gender as factor in, 2455
history-taking findings, 2455
imaging studies for, 2456, 2456f
incidence of, 2455
laboratory studies for, 2455–2456
management of, 2456–2457
mortality rate in, 2457
physical examination of, 2455
surgical management of, 2457
ultrasound evaluations, 147–148, 148f
Pyoderma, 1855f, 1855–1856
Pyogenic arthritis. *See* Septic arthritis
Pyogenic meningitis. *See* Bacterial meningitis
Pyrantel pamoate
hookworm infections treated with, 2388–2389
pinworms treated with, 2389, 2433
Pyrazinamide, 2602
Pyrethrin(s), 2181
Pyrexia, 560
Pyridoxine, 228t
Pyrimethamine-sulfadiazine, 2380
Pyruvate carboxylase deficiency, 980–981
Pyruvate-dehydrogenase complex deficiency, 987
Pyuria, 2610

Q

QRS morphology, 1412–1414, 1417
QT interval, 1418–1419
Quadriceps contusion, 2558
Quadruple births, 604–605
Quality control, 1019, 1025
Quality improvement
definitions, 42–45
description of, 26, 42
focus of, 43
goals of, 45
model for improvement, 47
performance measures, 45
preventive care, 44
priorities, 43–45
undertaking a project in, 45–47
QuantiFERON-TB test, 2591, 2599
Questionnaires
description of, 96
mental health and, 1170
parent, 360
patient, 360
prescreening, 315
screening-related, 315
Questions
in evidence-based medicine, 38, 38b
foreground, 38, 38b
Quinacrine, 2086, 2372
Quinidine gluconate, 2382–2383, 2382t

R

Rabies, 1824, 1824t, 2268–2269
Race
demographic profile based on, 234f
hypertension and, 1580
prenatal care use by, 236
preterm births and, 238
Racemics, 1844
Racial background, 158
Radiation
brain tumors treated with, 1860, 1863
embryonal histology and residual disease treated with, 1882
Ewing tumors treated with, 1887
exposure to, 1989, 2075
gonadal, 1896
Hodgkin disease treated with, 1893, 1894, 1895
neuroblastomas treated with, 1877, 1879
non-Hodgkin lymphomas treated with, 1891
retinoblastoma treated with, 1880–1881
rhabdomyosarcoma treated with, 1882–1883
side effects of, 1888t
thyroid, 1896
toxicities of, 1888t
Wilms tumors treated with, 1875–1876
Radiographs
abdominal distention and, 1375
abdominal pain and, 1381–1382
amenorrhea and, 1394
back pain and, 1407–1408
chest. *See* Chest radiograph
chest pain and, 1421
dizziness and, vertigo and, 1459
dysmorphism and, 1500
dysphagia and, 1465
dyspnea and, 1470
epistaxis and, 1485
extremity pain and, 1491
facial dysmorphism and, 1500
limp and, 1634, 1634f
wheezing and, 1793f–1794f
Radius, distal, 2554
Rales, 129, 2718
Randomized controlled trial, 40t
Rape
anal examination in, 2794
date, 2782, 2790–2791
definition, 2790
forensic and lab information in, 2794–2795
gang, 2791
genital examination in, 2794
history in, 2793

Rape—cont'd
incidence, 2790
by known assailant, 2790
legal issues in, 2792
male, 2791
male perpetrators of, 2791
medical evaluation in, 2792–2795
physical examination in, 2793–2794
pregnancy and, 2795
psychological assessment in, 2795–2796
response to, 2791–2792
sexually transmitted infections and, 2795
statutory, 2792
stranger, 2790
Rapid virus identification, 2036, 2038
Rapidly progressive glomerulonephritis, 2289–2290, 2289b
Rapport, 97–98, 196
Rash
appearance of, 1689–1692
causes of, 2748b
diaper. *See* Diaper rash
differential diagnosis of, 1692–1695, 1693b–1695b, 2566t
examples of, 1689f–1692f
extremity pain and, 1490
in Kawasaki disease, 2220, 2220f
in meningococcemia, 2747f, 2747–2749, 2749f
patient history and, 1688–1689
physical examination of, 1689–1692
in Rocky Mountain spotted fever, 2481–2483
secondary changes in, 1692
in staphylococcal TSS, 2563–2564, 2566t
in syphilis, 2527, 2527f
types of, 1689–1692
Rat-bite fever, 1824
Reactive airway disease, 1696
Reactive arthritis, 1626
Reactive attachment disorder, 1743
Reading disability, 1150
Rebound
attention deficit/hyperactivity disorder and, 1212t
definition, 2624
Reciprocity, 209
Reclamation-type renal tubular acidosis, 2466–2467, 2468t
Recombinant factor VIIa (Novoseven), 2111
Recombinant human erythropoietin, 684–685
Rectal examination
in children, 136
in infants, 133, 136
Rectum
body temperature measurements, 104, 105f
gonococcal infection of, 2513b
newborn assessment, 769
obstruction of, 2082
Recurrence phenomenon, 2698–2699
Recurrent aphthous stomatitis, 2569–2571
Recurrent otitis media, 2360, 2363
Recurrent respiratory papillomatosis, 1600–1601
Red blood cell(s), 1395, 1399–1400b, 1400–1404. *See also* Anemia
Red blood cell indices, 2206–2207, 2207t
Red blood cell preparations, 482, 482t
Red blood cell transfusions
acute blood loss treated with, 482
chronic, 483
complications of, 487–488
description of, 482–484, 482t, 483b
fresh-frozen plasma in, 482
hemoglobinopathy and, 484
in immunosuppressed patients, 484
in infants younger than 4 months, 483b, 484
in oxygen-carrying capacity restoration, 482–483, 483b
packed red blood cells in, 482
in potential stem cell transplant recipients, 484
in surgery, 483–484
Red Book, 1824
Red eye. *See* Conjunctivitis
Red reflex, 119–120, 764, 1780, 1781t
5α-Reductase-2 deficiency, 2196
Referrals
abdominal pain, 1383
acne, 1807
adolescents, 1326–1327
allergic rhinitis, 1821
alopecia, 1389–1390
amenorrhea, 1394
anemia, 1404
animal bites, 1825
anuria, 1829
apparent life-threatening events, 1836
appendicitis, 1838
asthma, 1849
atopic dermatitis, 1853
at-risk adolescents for violence, 275
attention deficit/hyperactivity disorder and, 1216–1217
back pain, 1410
bacterial skin infections, 1859
behavioral problems, 1164–1165
brain tumors, 1863–1864
bronchiolitis, 1869
cardiac arrhythmias, 1419
cerebral palsy, 1908
chest pain, 1424
chickenpox, 1917
chronic fatigue syndrome, 1922
chronic pain, 446
cleft lip and palate, 1930–1931
colic, 1933
complementary and alternative medicine, 463
conjunctivitis, 1702, 1711, 1716–1717
constipation, 1431
Referrals—cont'd
contact dermatitis, 1976
conversion reactions, 1231–1232
cough, 1436
cystic fibrosis, 1991
cysts, 1997–1998
description of, 9, 19t, 167
diabetes mellitus, 2007
diaper rash, 2015
diarrhea, 1454
dislocations, 2053
dizziness, 1460
Down syndrome, 2024–2025
drug eruptions, 2031
dysmenorrhea, 1463
dysphagia, 1467
dyspnea, 1473
dysuria, 1478
eating disorders, 1194
edema, 1481
encopresis, 1255b
enterovirus infections, 2039
enuresis, 2044
epistaxis, 1488
extremity pain, 1495
failure to thrive, 1507
foreign bodies, 2049
fractures, 2053
gastrointestinal allergy, 2069
gastrointestinal obstruction, 2083
gay, lesbian, and bisexual youth, for, 1365
gluten-sensitive enteropathy, 2093
hemoglobinopathies, 2104
hemolytic-uremic syndrome, 2097
hemophilia, 2111
Henoch-Schönlein purpura, 2114
hepatitis, 2126
herpes simplex virus, 2133
human herpesvirus-6 and -7, 2137–2138
medical-legal issues, 749
mental health, 199, 1147b, 1163–1165, 1167–1168
nosebleeds, 1488
oliguria, 1829
oncologist, 1895–1896
phobias, 1284
posttraumatic stress disorder, 1289
pregnancy, 1348
reasons for, 167
scrotal swelling and pain, 1723
self-stimulating behaviors, 1725, 1726
short stature, 1729, 1730
sleep disturbances, 1311
splenomegaly, 1742
staphylococcal toxic shock syndrome, 2567
stuttering, 1293
substance abuse, 398–404
transgender youth, 1243
urinary tract infections, 2614
vertigo, 1460
vision screening, 345

Page numbers followed by "f" denote figures; "t" denote tables; "b" *denote* boxes.

Referred pain
abdomen and, 1379
extremities and, 1489, 1490
Reflection, 95
Reflex
Babinski, 143
corneal light, 1780–1781, 1781f
cremasteric, 141f
crossed extensor, 141f
development of, 141f
diving, 2678
gag, 125, 144
glabella tap, 141f
let-down, 1786
Moro. *See* Moro reflex
palmar grasp, 141f, 143f
plantar grasp reflex, 143f
pupillary light, 118, 141f, 2640–2641
rooting, 141f, 143f, 815–816
stretch, 141
sucking, 123, 816
tonic myotactic, 141
types of, 141f, 143f
vesicoureteral. *See* Vesicoureteral reflex
Reflex syncope, 1753
Reflexive self-concept, 88
Reflux
gastroesophageal. *See* Gastroesophageal reflux
hoarseness and, 1599
laryngopharyngeal, 1599–1601, 2058, 2059b
testing, 1600–1601
Reflux nephropathy, 2338
Refugees
behavioral health screening of, 69–70
blood lead level testing in, 63
demographics of, 60
functional health screening of, 69–70
growth abnormalities in, 63
immunizations in, 71
malaria screening in, 70
nutritional disorders in, 63
oral health among, 63, 69
parasitic infection screening in, 70
screening tests for, 70–71
serologic testing in, 71
tuberculosis screening in, 70–71
Regional anesthesia, 432–433
Regions
chest, 1423
pelvic, 1462, 1477
scalp, 1388, 1388f
spinal, 1427
Regression
developmental, 1156–1157
procedures, 1170–1171
Regurgitation
in neonatal intensive care infants, 874–875
vomiting vs., 1783
Rehabilitation
ADL devices in, 579
assistive technology in, 579
barriers to effective care coordination in, 581–582
braces in, 579–580
casts in, 579
communication therapy in, 577
definitions related to, 573–574
description of, 573
disorders treated with, 574b
durable medical equipment for, 579–580
educational planning in, 581
feeding therapy in, 577–579
functional activity training in, 576–577
functional impaired areas for, 575, 575t
goals of, 576
interdisciplinary team in, 574–575, 574b
interventional plan for, 575–576
medical management in, 576
mobility devices in, 579
occupational therapy in, 576–577, 578t
oral-motor therapy in, 577–579
orthopedic management in, 576
orthoses in, 579
pain management in, 576
physical therapy, 576–577, 578t
psychosocial support to family and patient in, 580–581
spasticity management in, 576
speech therapy in, 577
splints in, 579
sports and recreation programs in, 580
therapeutic management in, 576–579, 578t
transfer aids in, 579
vocational planning in, 581
wheelchair in, 579
Rehabilitation Act, 589, 1128
Rehydration
diarrhea management and, 1445–1447
intravenous, 2658
oral, 2657–2661
Reiki, 460
Reimbursement, 17–18
Reiter syndrome, 1626
Rejection after heart transplantation, 1963–1965
Relative value unit, 21
Relaxed foot, 1534
Remarriage, 1058–1059
Remifentanil, 425t
Renal agenesis, 612
Renal ARF, 1825, 1826
Renal arteries, 151, 151f
Renal biopsy, 1567
Renal disease
edema caused by, 1480–1481
maternal health and, 631
proteinuria and, 1677
short stature caused by, 1728
Renal failure
acute, 1825–1826, 2797–2800. *See also* Anuria; Oliguria
in acute glomerulonephritis, 2287–2290, 2287b, 2289b
definition, 2797–2798
epidemiology, 2798
etiology, 2798t, 2798–2799
evaluation, 2799
hospitalization for, 2800
hyperkalemia in, 2799, 2800t
management, 2799–2800, 2800t
referral for, 2800
in shock, 2811
after urinary tract infection, 2614
Renal masses, 150, 1373
Renal scarring, 2614
Renal tubular acidosis
ammonium excretion mechanism and, 2463–2466, 2464f–2465f, 2464t
causes of, 2460
classifications of, 2463, 2464t
clinical presentations of, 2459–2460
definition of, 2459–2460, 2460t
delayed maturity caused by, 2470–2471
description of, 2459, 2460t
diagnosis of, 2459
evaluation of, 2471–2473, 2472f, 2473t
failure to thrive and, 2459–2460
heredofamilial, 2459, 2460t
hybrid, 2470
primary care physician's role in, 2474
reclamation-type, 2466–2467, 2468t
regeneration-type
hyperkalemic, 2468t, 2469–2470
nonhyperkalemic, 2467–2469, 2468t
renal mechanisms for acid excretion and, 2460–2463, 2461f, 2463f
treatment of, 2473–2474
types of, 2466–2471, 2468t
Renal ultrasonography, 2611, 2612b
Renal vein thrombosis
in infants of diabetic mothers, 891
neonatal disease, 945
Renin-angiotensin axis, 1808
Renovascular hypertension, 150–151
Reperfusion syndrome, 991–992
Repetitive stereotypic behavior, 1742
Repetitive stress-related injuries. *See* Overuse syndromes
Representative assessment tools, 1169t, 1169–1170
Residency programs, 3
Residential treatments, 402–403
Resiliency, 179
Resource-based relative value scale, 19, 21
Respirations, 106
Respiratory compromise, 323t
Respiratory cycle, 1747, 1790, 1791f
Respiratory disease and disorders
apnea, 910–911
cardiac tests for, 906
in cystic fibrosis, 1982

Respiratory disease and disorders—cont'd
differential diagnosis, 905
early education and child care programs and risk of, 1020–1022
in gastroesophageal reflux disease
apnea or apparent life-threatening event, 2059–2060
asthma, 2059
chronic cough, stridor, hoarseness, 2058, 2059t
laryngeal edema, 2058, 2059t
laryngopharyngeal reflux, 2058, 2059b
recurrent pneumonia, 2058–2059
Sandifer syndrome, 2060
imaging studies of, 906
laboratory testing, 906
lung development disorders and, 912–915
meconium aspiration syndrome and, 908–910
neonatal drug withdrawal syndrome, 953
neurodevelopmental issues, 862
in NICU-discharged infants
apnea, bradycardia, and desaturations, 715
apnea monitoring, 716–717
cardiorespiratory monitoring, 716
home oxygen therapy and pulse oximetry, 713–714
home ventilation, 714–715
predischarge polysomnography, 715–716
sleep position, 717
supplemental oxygen requirements, air-flight, 714
vehicle seat safety, 717
overview, 902–903
pathophysiology, 907–908
pneumomediastinum, 911–912
pneumonia, 909–910
pneumothorax, 911–912
pulmonary air leak syndrome, 911–912
pulse oximetry and blood gas studies, 905
transient tachypnea of newborn, 906–907
Respiratory distress syndrome
in airways obstruction, 2630–2637
breastfeeding and prevention of, 810
in infants of diabetic mothers, 890
in neonatal intensive care infants, 853
in newborns, 128–129, 903–905
postnatal evaluation, 776
in premature infants, 833–834
signs of, 129, 668
Respiratory infections
description of, 2534–2535
upper
acute, 323t
allergic rhinitis confused with, 1820
general anesthesia and, 521–522, 521b, 523f
Respiratory rates
by age, 2802t
assessment of, 106
in newborns, 128
postnatal changes in, 128
Respiratory syncytial virus
in croup, 2648, 2649
description of, 1865, 1865f, 1981
in-hospital prophylaxis, 705
neonatal sepsis, 936–937
pertussis vs., 2420
prophylaxis in NICU-discharged infants, 718
Respiratory system
in drowning injuries, 2677
fetal assessment, 648
review of systems for, 92b
Respiratory tract infections, 520b, 521–522, 523f
Respite House, Inc., 572
Resting metabolic rate, 220
Restless leg syndrome, 1307
Restraints, during physical examination, 103
Restrictive cardiomyopathy, 1963
Restrictive pulmonary disease, 1470, 1471b
Resuscitation
cardiopulmonary, 723
neonatal
assessment and stabilization after, 663–664
delivery room, 658–659, 662
endotracheal tube size and depth, 662
ethical principles, 732
evaluation, 665–666
extensive or complicated, 662–663
initial postnatal evaluation and intervention, 659–664
needs assessment guidelines, 661
oxygen delivery and monitoring equipment, 661
premature newborns, 663–664
preparation for, 658–659
quality improvement, 665–666
risk factors for, 655
unresponsive newborns, 663
ventilation assistance and monitoring equipment, 661
withholding, limiting, and withdrawing of, 658
after poisoning, 2765, 2768
Retapamulin, 1854–1855
Retching, 1783
Reticulocyte hemoglobin, 2208
Retina
development of, 118
examination of, 119
hemangioblastomas, 2315, 2315t
Retinal image, blurred, 1777
Retinoblastoma, 1879–1881
case study of, 77
clinical manifestations, 1880
Retinoblastoma—cont'd
etiology, 1879–1880
evaluation, 1880
follow-up, 1881
management of, 1880–1881
prognosis, 1881
Retinoids
acne treated with, 1805
psoriasis treated with, 2452t–2453t, 2453
Retinol, 228t
Retinopathy of prematurity
description of, 703–704
in NICU infants
health outcomes, 857
ophthalmologic evaluation, 879
screening for, 719–721
in very low–birth-weight infants, 855
Retropharyngeal abscess, 1749t, 2049, 2635, 2650
Retroversion, 1529b
Rett syndrome, 1197, 1654, 2189t
Review of systems, 92b–93b, 94
Reward systems for adherence, 196
Reye syndrome, 1913, 2733
Rh sensitization
alloimmunization, 634
fetal intervention, 619
hemolytic disease, 941–942
Rhabdomyosarcoma
clinical manifestations, 1881–1882
etiology, 1881
follow-up, 1883
long-term side effects of chemotherapy, 1883t
management of, 1882
prognosis, 1882–1883
Rheumatic fever
activity limitations for, 2479
acute, 2475
age as factor in, 2475
anti-inflammatory therapies for, 2478–2479
antistreptococcal therapies for, 2478
aspirin for, 2479
bacterial endocarditis and, 2480
cardiac effects of, 2479–2480
clinical manifestations of
arthralgia, 2477
carditis, 2477
chorea, 2477
erythema marginatum, 2477
polyarthritis, 2476–2477
streptococcal infection, 2478, 2478f
streptococcal pharyngitis, 2478
subcutaneous nodules, 2477
contraception and, 2480
diagnosis of, 2476, 2476b
epidemiologic features of, 2475
group A beta-hemolytic streptococcal infection eradication in, 2478
host susceptibility for, 2475
incidence of, 2475
joint pain and, 1626
management of, 2478–2479

Page numbers followed by "f" denote figures; "t" denote tables; "b" *denote* boxes.

Rheumatic fever—cont'd
manifestations of, 2475
pharyngitis and, 2429
pregnancy and, 2480
recurrence of, 2479–2480
salicylates for, 2478–2479
Rheumatic heart disease, 2479–2480
Rhinitis, allergic
anatomic abnormalities and, 1820
clinical features of, 1819
complications of, 1819
description of, 123
differential diagnosis of, 1820
etiology of, 1819
laboratory evaluation of, 1819–1820
prognosis for, 1821
referral for, 1821
treatment, 1820–1821
Rhinolith, 2047
RhoGAM testing
alloimmunization, 634
fetal intervention, 619
Rhonchi, 129
Rhubarb root, 458t
Ribavirin, 511t
Rickets
craniotabes and, 117
vitamin D insufficiency and, 217
Rickettsia sp., 2481
Rieger syndrome, 2605, 2605t
Rifampin
bacterial resistance to, 505
description of, 505–506, 508
dosage, peak serum concentrations, and MIC_{95} for, 494t
mechanism of action of, 505
meningococcemia treated with, 2749, 2751, 2752t
pharmacologic properties of, 506
side effects of, 506, 508
staphylococcal TSS treated with, 2566
streptococcal TSS treated with, 2576
tuberculosis treated with, 2576, 2602
use of, 508
RIFLE criteria, 2798
Riga-Fede syndrome, 2569–2570
Rigidity, 1184, 2624
Rimantadine, 511t
Rinne test, 122
Risk avoidance, 15
Risk behaviors
description of, 13t, 15
health outcomes affected by, 13t, 15
Rituals, 158
Rituximab, 2216b, 2217
Robinow syndrome, 2605, 2605t
Rochester criteria, 1521, 1521t
Rocking, 1724–1726
Rocky Mountain spotted fever
appendicitis vs., 1838
cause of, 2481
clinical features of, 2482–2483
complications of, 2484
description of, 2481
Rocky Mountain spotted fever—cont'd
differential diagnosis of, 2482
epidemiologic features of, 2481–2482
geographic distribution of, 2481
incidence of, 2481
laboratory evaluation of, 2483–2484
management of, 2484
petechiae in, 2481–2482
prevention of, 2484–2485
prognosis of, 2484
rash in, 2481–2483
Rickettsia sp. and, 2481
ticks and, 2481–2482
Rodenticides, 2784
Rohypnol, 2782, 2790
Role confusion, 1010–1011
Rome I, II, & III for abdominal pain, 1376
"Roofies," 2782
Rooting reflex, 141f, 143f, 815–816
Roseola, 1977, 2135–2136, 2137
Ross heart failure grading system, 2719, 2719t–2720t
Rotator cuff tendonitis, 2555–2556
Rotavirus vaccine
adverse reactions to, 257–258
characteristics of, 257–258
contraindications, 257
guidelines for, 245f
interval between doses, 249t
minimum age for, 248t
for NICU-discharged infants, 718
in premature infants, 704–705
RRP. *See* recurrent respiratory papillomatosis
RTA. *See* Renal tubular acidosis
Rubella
congenital infection, 931
description of, 1977, 1979–1980
neonatal skin infections, 786
perinatal morbidity and mortality and, 635–636
Rubeola, 2482
Rubinstein-Taybi syndrome, 1653
Rules of Two when considering maintenance therapy, 1849
Rumination, 1743
Rumination syndrome, 2057
Rural practices, 3
Russell-Silver syndrome, 1727
Rutgers Alcohol Problem Index, 401

S

S4 gallop, 1561
Sacrococcygeal teratoma, 617
Safety
communication benefits for, 169
Institute of Medicine definition of, 42
medical-legal issues in, 750
medication use during breastfeeding, 813, 824–825
newborn, 845
for NICU-discharged infants, 723–724
transgender youth and, 1240, 1362
vaccinations, 250, 252
Safety-net provider systems, 7
Salaam spasms, 1765
Salary, 22t
Salicylates. *See also* Aspirin
chronic pain managed using, 440, 441t
overdose of, 2763, 2770–2772
rheumatic fever treated with, 2478–2479
Salicylic acids, for seborrheic dermatitis, 2487–2488
Saline, hypertonic, 2743
Saliva, 293–294
Salivation, 125
Salmon patches, 781
Salmonella Arizona infection, 66t
Salter-Harris fracture, 2052
Salt-wasting, 1594
Sandfly, 2368
Sandifer syndrome, 1765, 2060
Sarcoma
osteosarcoma
clinical manifestations, 1888–1889
etiology, 1887–1888
evaluation, 1889
follow-up, 1890
management of, 1889
prognosis, 1889–1890
radiation side effects, 1888t
rhabdomyosarcoma
clinical manifestations, 1881–1882
etiology, 1881
follow-up, 1883
long-term side effects of chemotherapy, 1883t
management of, 1882
prognosis, 1882–1883
Sarcoptes scabiei hominis, 2182
Sarin, 2779
SASSI. *See* Substance Abuse Subtle Screening Inventory
Satellite offices, 6
Satiety center, 1637
Saturated fats, 224
SBS. *See* Shaken baby syndrome
Scabies, 2182–2183
Scale for Anxiety and Related Emotional Disorders, 1170
Scalp, 762–763
Scaphocephaly, 117, 763
Scar formation, 562
Scarlet fever
description of, 1981
differential diagnosis, 2566t–2567t
staphylococcal, 2222t
streptococcal, 2222t
SCFE. *See* Slipped capital femoral epiphysis
Scheuermann disease, 1409, 1410
Schistosoma sp., 2393–2395
Schistosomiasis
causes of, 2394
clinical manifestations of, 2394–2395
description of, 70, 2393–2394
diagnosis of, 2395

Schistosomiasis—cont'd
epidemiologic features of, 2394
life cycle of, 2394
pathogenesis of, 2394
prevention of, 2395
treatment of, 2395
Schizophrenia, 1745
medication, 1181b
medications for, 1181
Schmidt syndrome, 1811
School health. *See also* School health programs
cardiac arrhythmias and, 1419
collaborative care and, 1153–1154
cooperative approach, 1122, 1126–1127, 1129–1133, 1138
education programs, 1131–1134
laws and, 1128
medication policies and, 1178–1179
nurses and, 1135–1139
parents and, 1137
pediatricians and, 1122, 1124, 1126–1130, 1128t, 1129b, 1131–1133
quality of care, 1138–1139
timeline, 1125f
School health programs. *See also* Health education; School health
attention deficit/hyperactivity disorder and, 1214–1215
change implementation, 1134
coordinated
components of, 1122–1124, 1123f, 1126, 1132
school nurses and, 1136
evaluation of, 1126, 1127t
goals of, 1122, 1127f, 1132–1133
government policy, 1129b
planning committees, 1133–1134
primary health physician involvement, 1127–1130
quality of, 1139–1140
School nurses
collaboration with physicians, 1138
health programming and, 1136–1138
models of service and, 1138
preparations and qualifications for, 1136
School outcomes
behavioral development and, 1000
homelessness and, 1089
impact of foster care on, 1066
moderate- to late-preterm infants, 858
neonatal intensive care infants, 855–856
self-care by children and, 1104
School phobia, 1146, 1147
School physicians, 1127
School readiness
age and, 1141
definition of, 1140–1141
health considerations, 1141–1142
health risk factors and, 1141b
parent and teacher expectations of, 1140–1141
School readiness—cont'd
pediatricians role, 1143–1144
success factors of, 1140b–1141b, 1141–1142, 1143b
unpreparedness and, 1142–1143
School refusal
child related factors of, 1146
definition of, 1145
environmental factors of, 1146, 1147
family related factors of, 1146
management of, 1147
parents and, 1146, 1147, 1148
prevalence of, 1146
prevention of, 1147–1148
School-age child. *See also* Late childhood
anticipatory guidance for, 211
auditory screening in, 330
diet for, 219
Down syndrome, 2020–2021, 2022b
hospitalization preparations for, 172b
protein requirements, 223t
violence among, 274
vision screening in, 344–345
Schooling
children with special health care needs
child-specific guidance, 589, 590b
collaboration of school staff and health professionals, 590–591
independent living issues, 590
job achievement issues, 590
medical issues, 589, 589b, 590b
school achievement issues, 589–590
history-taking about, 92b
Schwannoma, bilateral vestibular, 2308, 2308b, 2308f
SCID. *See* Severe combined immunodeficiency
Scintigraphy, 147–148, 1466, 2058
Sclera, 2344
Sclerosis
diffuse mesangial, 2300
tuberous. *See* Tuberous sclerosis
Scoliosis
acquired, 2548
congenital, 2545–2546
description of, 1407
examination for, 140, 140f
idiopathic, 2548
Scope of practice, 8b, 8–9
Scopolamine, 555t
Scorecards, 43
Scorpions, 2693–2694
Screenings, 312–408
alternative approaches, 315
anemia, 342–343
auditory. *See also* Hearing loss
goals of, 326
in infants, 326–328, 327b, 328f, 330b
justification for, 326
in newborns, 121, 326–328, 327b, 328f, 330b
permanent hearing loss and, 1557, 1559
Screenings—cont'd
auditory—cont'd
in preschool-age children, 328–329, 329b
primary care physician's role in, 332
in school-age children, 330
in toddlers, 328–329, 329b
behavioral
benefits of, 349–350
office process in, 350, 353
tools for, 350, 351t, 352t
cardiovascular
in athletes, 340
blood pressure screening, 339
description of, 335–336, 335b
of fetus, 336
medical history in, 339
in neonates and infants, 336–338
obesity-related, 339–340
Centers for Disease Control and Prevention on, 312
cholesterol
American Academy of Pediatrics on, 281
American Heart Association on, 281
recommendations for, 281b, 281t, 282–283, 282f, 283t, 284f
United States Preventive Services Task Force on, 281
conditions appropriate for
criteria for, 312–313
evidence-based recommendations in, 314–315
coronary heart disease, 195
CRAFFT tool, 1246b, 1246–1247
cystic fibrosis, 386, 702
definition of, 312
description of, 312
developmental
benefits of, 349–350
office process in, 350, 353
tools for, 350, 351t, 352t
developmental delays, 346–349
environmental tobacco smoke, 369
family
environmental tobacco smoke screening, 369
intimate partner violence, 369
maternal depression, 365–369. *See also* Maternal depression
parental smoking, 369
rationale for, 364–365
general considerations in, 312–316
genetic-metabolic diseases, 373–393
hearing, 122, 356–357, 718–719
high serum cholesterol, 195
high-risk register, 315
history-taking about, 92b
immigrants, 69–70
intimate partner violence, 369
in language assessment, 354–358
lead poisoning, 393–397
maternal depression, 366–369, 367b–368b

Page numbers followed by "f" denote figures; "t" denote tables; "b" *denote* boxes.

Screenings—cont'd
National Institutes of Health Consensus Statement on, 312
parental refusal, 78–79
phobias, 1283
physical examination in, 316–317
posttraumatic stress disorder, 1287–1288, 1288f
preparticipation physical evaluation in, 317–326
proteinuria, 405
psychosocial, 349, 358–364
public health service, 314
questionnaires in, 315
refugees, 69–70
school readiness, 1141, 1141b, 1143
selective vs. high-risk, 315
sleep complaints, 1296–1297t, 1297–1298
speech, 354–358
substance abuse, 398–404, 1246–1247
surveillance in, 315
tests for, 313–314
United State Congress Office of Technology Assessment on, 312
United States Department of Health and Human Services on, 312
urinalysis in, 404–408
urine culture in, 404–408
violence-related, 275, 275b, 276f
vision
in adolescents, 344–345
benefits of, 343–344
description of, 1779f, 1779–1782
equipment for, 345
goals of, 344
improvements in, 345
in infants, 344
ocular trauma evaluations using, 2344
personnel for, 345
in preschoolers, 344
referral for, 345
in school-age children, 344–345
in toddlers, 344
tools for, 344
World Health Organization criteria for, 78
Scrotal skin disease, 1721
Scrotum
anatomy of, 1719f
of newborns, 135, 768–769
palpation of, 136
swelling of
causes of, 1718b
diagnostic testing for, 1718, 1719
pain and, 1718–1721
patient history and examination for, 1718–1720, 1722
postoperative, 560
referral for, 1723
treatment of, 1719–1721
without pain, 1721–1723
Sealants, 296
Seal-like cough, 1748
Sebaceous glands, 113
Seborrheic dermatitis
causes of, 2486
description of, 2485
differential diagnosis of, 2486–2487, 2487f
evaluation of, 2486, 2486f
incidence of, 2485
prognosis of, 2488
treatment of, 2487–2488
Seckel syndrome, 1653
Second diagnosis, 88
Second heart sound, 131
Second impact syndrome, 1609
Second opinions, 167
Secondary prevention, 12
Second-hand smoke exposure
in home environment, 845
NICU-discharged infants and, 723–724
Secretory system (of lacrimal system), 1707f
Sedative-hypnotic agents, 2782–2783
Seizure(s)
absence, 2489, 2489b
antiepileptic agents for
acetazolamide, 2498t, 2500–2501
carbamazepine, 2498t, 2500
clonazepam, 2498t, 2500
clorazepate, 2500
diazepam, 2500
ethosuximide, 2498t, 2500
felbamate, 2498t, 2501
gabapentin, 2499t, 2501
ketogenic diet, 2502
lamotrigine, 2499t, 2501
levetiracetam, 2499t, 2501
lorazepam, 2500
after neonatal period, 2496–2497
oxcarbazepine, 2499t, 2501–2502
phenobarbital, 2497, 2498t
phenytoin, 2497, 2498t, 2500
primidone, 2498t, 2500
psychosocial issues in, 2502
tiagabine, 2499t, 2501
topiramate, 2499t, 2501
vagal nerve stimulation, 2502
valproic acid, 2498t, 2500
zonisamide, 2499t, 2502
atonic, 2489, 2489b
behavioral problems associated with, 2496
benign neonatal sleep myoclonus vs., 1658–1659
causes of, 2494–2495, 2495
classification of, 2488–2494, 2489b, 2493b
complex partial, 2489, 2489b
cysticercosis and, 2397
description of, 2488
differential diagnosis of, 2495
electroencephalography of, 2496
evaluation of, 2495–2496
Seizure(s)—cont'd
febrile
description of, 1516–1517, 2489b, 2494
management of, 420–421
generalized. *See* Generalized seizures
grand mal, 2489–2490, 2489b
after head injury, 2715
human herpesvirus 6 and 7 and, 2136
hypertension and, 1588–1589
increased intracranial pressure and, 2743
intractable, 2503
irritability and, 1609, 1611
laboratory tests for, 2495–2496
learning problems associated with, 2496
lumbar puncture evaluations, 2496
meningitis and, 1517
myoclonic, 2489, 2489b
neonatal. *See* Neonate(s), seizures in
neuroimaging studies for, 2496
night terrors vs., 1659
paroxysmal nonepileptic disorders vs., 1657–1659
partial
benign partial epilepsy of childhood, 2489b, 2492
complex, 2489b, 2491–2492
epilepsia partialis continua, 2489b, 2492
simple, 2489b, 2491
prevalence of, 2488
simple partial, 2489, 2489b
in status epilepticus, 2819
syncope and, 1756
tonic-clonic, 2489–2490, 2489b
toxic agents causing, 2768, 2768b
unclassified
febrile seizures, 2489b, 2494
neonatal seizures, 2489b, 2492–2494, 2493b
pseudoseizures, 2489b, 2494
Seizure disorders
benign partial epilepsy of childhood, 2489b, 2492
causes of, 2488, 2494–2495
differential diagnosis of, 2495
electroencephalography in, 2496
epilepsia partialis continua, 2489b, 2492
evaluation of, 2495–2496
incidence of, 2488
infantile spasms, 2489b, 2490
juvenile myoclonic epilepsy, 2489b, 2491
laboratory tests in, 2495–2496
Lennox-Gastaut syndrome, 2489t, 2490–2491
lumbar puncture in, 2496
management of, 2496–2503, 2498t–2499t. *See also* Seizure(s), management of
maternal health and, 631

Seizure disorders—cont'd
medical-legal issues, 746–747
neonatal assessment for, 670–671
neuroimaging studies for, 2496
neurological evaluation, 989–992
screening for associated learning and behavioral problems in, 2496
Selective mutism, 1282
Selective serotonin reuptake inhibitors
description of, 1261, 1554
neonatal drug withdrawal syndrome, 951
overdose of, 2772
Self-acceptance, 1239, 1362–1363
Self-biting, 1726
Self-care
adolescents, effect on, 1104
after-school care programs, 1104–1105
pediatrician's role in, 1105
school outcomes and, 1104
trends in, 1103–1104
Self-defense, 275, 275b
Self-discovery, 1235
Self-esteem, 1729
Self-funded/self-insured plans, 19–20
Self-hypnosis
in anxiety, 452
in behavioral and attention disorders, 452
clinical applications of, 450–451, 450b
in diabetes, 453
in enuresis, 451–452
in habit disorders, 451
learning of, 449–450, 449b, 450b
in medical problems, 452–453, 453b
in medical procedures, 453
in migraine headache, 453b
in pain management, 451, 451b
research in, 454
in routine office visit, 453–454
in stress management, 452
teaching of, 449–450, 449b, 450b
in wart eradication, 453b
Self-management support, 46
Self-mastery, 210
Self-mutilation, 1726
Self-regulation, 1008
Self-regulation therapies
commonalities in, 449
definitions of, 448–449, 448b
history of, 448–449, 449f
self-hypnosis. *See* Self-hypnosis
terminology related to, 448–449, 448b
Self-report
adolescents and, 1336–1337
children and, 1287–1288, 1288f
Self-stimulating behaviors
hair pulling and twisting, 1726
head banging and rocking, 1724
masturbation, 1725–1726
referral for, 1724–1726
thumb sucking and nail biting, 1725
tics vs., 1760
Sensorimotor cognitive development, 1006
Sensory, motor, reflex grid, 1407f
Sensory abnormalities, 1425
Sensory esotropia, 1736–1737
Sensory impairment, 1151
Sentence completion tasks, 100
Separation, 1271
Separation anxiety, 210, 1282, 1743
Sepsis
abdominal, 506t
bacterial
in congestive heart failure, 2721
in meningococcemia, 2746–2752
breastfeeding and, 810
empirical therapy for, 506t
neonatal infection, 935–937
prevention of, 810
risk factors in infants, 805
Septal hematoma, 123
Septic arthritis
causes of, 2505–2506
definition of, 2505
differential diagnosis of, 2506
empirical therapy for, 506t
evaluation of, 2507
hospitalization in, 2508
limp and, 1635
management of, 2507–2508
referrals for, 2508
Septic shock, 2804f, 2806
Serologic tests
description of, 71
pertussis diagnosis using, 2421
pharyngitis diagnosis using, 2428
Serological diagnosis, 1979, 2038
Serotonin syndrome, 2772
Serum bilirubin, 1616
Serum ferritin, 2208
Serum glucose management, 674–675
Serum inhibitory titers, 491
Serum iron saturation, 2205–2206, 2207t
Serum sickness, 2699
Serum transferrin receptor, 2207t, 2208
Serum transferrin saturation, 2205–2206, 2207t
Setting-sun sign, 119
17-hydroxyprogesterone, 1803, 1809, 1811
Sever disease, 2554
Severe combined immunodeficiency, 1698
Sex chromosome disorders of sexual development, 2196–2197
Sex steroids, 1808
Sexual abuse
assessment of, 1109–1111
clinical manifestations of, 1107–1109
definition of, 1092, 1106–1107
diagnosis of, 1109–1111
differential diagnosis of, 1111
dissociative disorders and, 1745
epidemiology of, 1106–1107
Sexual abuse—cont'd
etiology of, 1107
prevention of, 1113
psychosocial consequences, 1112–1113
treatment of, 1112
vaginal bleeding and, 1767
Sexual activity
among adolescents, 75–76
consent statutes regarding, 76
Sexual behavior
definition of, 1340
homosexual, 1341
masturbation and, 1340–1341
noncoital, 1340
prevalence of, 1340, 1341t
Sexual development disorders. *See also* Intersex
androgen-related, 2195–2196
aromatase deficiency, 2195
congenital adrenal hyperplasia, 2195, 2195t
defects in androgen action, 2196
evaluation of
diagnostic algorithms in, 2198f, 2199f
history-taking, 2198–2199
imaging, 2200
laboratory tests, 2200
physical examination, 2199–2200
fetal sources of androgen excess, 2195, 2195t
46,XX, 2194–2195
46,XY, 2195–2196
gonadal differentiation disorders, 2196–2197
17-hydroxylase deficiency, 2196
Klinefelter syndrome, 2196–2197
luteinizing hormone-receptor defects, 2195–2196
management of, 2200–2201
ovotesticular, 2197
5α-reductase-2 deficiency, 2196
sex chromosome, 2196–2197
Turner syndrome, 2197
types of, 2194–2197, 2195t
Sexual differentiation, 2194
Sexual dysfunction, 1343
Sexual orientation, 1358–1365
Sexual victimization, 1342–1344
Sexual violence, 275, 275b
Sexuality. *See also* Sexual behavior
adolescent, 1336t, 1337
communication and, 1343–1344
in Down syndrome patients, 2023
history-taking about, 92b
practitioner-parent-adolescent relationship and, 1343–1344
Sexually transmitted diseases
in adolescents, 2509
Chlamydia trachomatis, 2510f, 2510–2511, 2512b–2513b, 2512f
circumcision and, 830
complications, 2509–2510
description of, 1341–1342

Sexually transmitted diseases—cont'd
genital herpes simplex virus, 2516b–2517b, 2524–2527, 2527f
gonococcal, 2510f, 2513f–2514f, 2521, 2522f–2523f
human papillomavirus (genital warts), 2514b–2516b, 2522–2524, 2525f
Mycoplasma genitalium, 2528
Neisseria gonorrhoeae. *See Neisseria gonorrhoeae*
organisms in, 2510b
prevention, 1355
after rape, 2795
referrals for, 2532
sexual abuse and risk of, 1108–1109
signs and symptoms, 2511b
syndromes associated with
cervicitis, 2532
enteritis, 2520b–2521b, 2531
epididymitis, 2520b, 2531
pelvic inflammatory disease, 2518b–2520b, 2528–2531, 2529b–2530b
perihepatitis, 2531
proctitis, 2520b–2521b, 2531
proctocolitis, 2520b–2521b, 2531
vaginitis, 2531–2532
syphilis. *See* Syphilis
treatment of, 2512b–2521b
Shaken baby syndrome, 2350
Shared decision making, 49
Shared environment, 999
Shargreen patches, 2311, 2311f
Shewhart cycle, 47
Shigatoxin related to hemolytic-uremic syndrome, 2094
Shingles. *See* Herpes zoster
Shivering episodes, 1658
Shock
anaphylactic, 2804f, 2806
cardiogenic, 2804f, 2805, 2805b
catecholamine-resistant, 2803t, 2806–2807, 2808f
classification of, 2804–2806
cold, 2803t, 2804
definitions, 2803t
diagnosis, 2802t, 2802–2803
distributive, 2804f, 2806
drugs and fluids used in, 2809t
empirical therapy for, 506t
epidemiology, 2801–2802
fluid refractory-dopamine-resistant, 2803t, 2807, 2808f, 2811
hemorrhagic, 2805, 2805t
history in, 2802–2803
hypovolemic, 2804f, 2804–2805, 2805b
in infants, 2803b
management of, 474
monitoring of, 2809b
organ failure in, 2810b
Shock—cont'd
physiological mechanism, 2803–2804, 2804f
refractory, 2803t, 2806, 2808f, 2811
septic, 2804f, 2806, 2808f
sequelae of, 2810b, 2811–2812
in snakebites, 2698
treatment, 2806–2807, 2807f–2809f, 2809–2811
warm, 2803t, 2804
Shoes
anatomy of, 1530b
fitting of, 1529–1530
foot problems and, 1529
function of, 1529
leg problems and, 1529–1530
Short bowel syndrome, 873–874
Short stature
diagnostic testing for, 1729
differential diagnosis of, 1727–1728
history-taking, 1728–1729
management of, 1729–1730
physical examination for, 1728–1729
Short-bowel syndrome, 1451
Shoulder
dislocation of, 2559–2560
"Little League," 2554
Shuddering attacks, 1658
Shuffle gaits, 1630
Shy temperament, 1746
SIADH. *See* Syndrome of inappropriate antidiuretic hormone
Siblings, 182–183, 734
Sick and dying infants
bereavement issues, 736–738
collaborative decision making and family support, 729–735
congenital anomalies, 789–790
medical-legal considerations, 744–745
palliative care, 737–738
Sick sinus syndrome, 1755
Sickle cell anemia
abdominal pain in, 2628
irritability and, 1612
newborn screening for, 385
penicillin prophylaxis, 162
splenomegaly and, 1732
Sickle cell disease
anesthesia and, 535–537, 537b
complications of, 535–536
description of, 535, 943
hospitalization for, 536–537
physiologic features of, 535
preoperative preparation for, 537, 537b
sports participation with, 323t
stroke caused by, 536
surgical procedures in, 536–537
vasoocclusion in, 535
Sickle cell trait, 323t, 2102–2103
Sickling disorders, 2102–2103. *See also* Hemoglobinopathies
Side-lying position for breastfeeding, 814
SIDS
as apparent life-threatening event, 1829–1830
community campaigns to prevent, 56
description of, 1268, 2579–2581
sleeping patterns and positioning, 723, 843–844, 1834–1835, 2060
Silicon, 828
Silicone stent, 1708f
Simian line, 116
Simple partial seizures, 2489b, 2491
Simple vocal tics, 1758
Sinding-Larsen-Johansson disease, 2553–2554
Single umbilical artery, 767–768
Single-photon emission computed tomography, 1408
Sinus(es)
development of, 2535t
physical examination of, 122–123
review of systems for, 92b
transillumination of, 123
Sinus arrhythmia, 920–921
Sinus bradycardia, 918–919
Sinus tachycardia, 920
Sinusitis
clinical presentation of, 2535
complications of, 2536
diagnosis of, 2535
disorders associated with, 2535b
pathophysiology of, 2534–2535
preseptal cellulitis caused by inflammatory edema of, 2443–2445, 2443f
signs and symptoms of, 123
treatment of, 2536
Situational syncope, 1753
Sixth nerve palsy, 1739, 1739f
SJS. *See* Stevens-Johnson syndrome
Skeletal defects
chest measurements, 792
fetal assessment, 646–647
ultrasound detection of, 612–613
Skeletal trauma, 1095–1096
Skill development methods, 1132
Skin
care of, 778–779, 844
child abuse signs, 1094–1095
decontamination of, 2769
drug-related eruptions
allergic skin reactions, 2027t
drug rash with eosinophilia, 2029
erythema multiforme, 2029–2030
morbilliform (measles-like) eruptions, 2027–2028
urticaria, 2028
embryologic development of, 113
infant, 116
melanin variations, 115
neonatal drug withdrawal syndrome signs, 953
newborn, 114–115
physical examination of, 113–116

Skin—cont'd
review of systems for, 92b
Skin disorders
acne. *See* Acne
anesthesia and, 540
developmental anomalies, 782–783
hamartomas and lesions, 781–782
infectious lesions of newborn, 785–786
lesions. *See* Rash
newborn assessment, 760
pigmentary birthmarks, 779–780
rashes. *See* Rash
sports participation with, 323t
vascular birthmarks, 780–781
vascular malformations, 781
vesiculopustular diseases, 783–785
Skin gouging, 1726
Skin picking, 1726
Skin tags, 116, 2538f
Skinner, B. F., 1015
Skull
abnormalities of, 1646, 1647b, 1648
childbirth effects on, 117
congenital anomalies, 791
fracture of, 2712–2713
injuries to, 992
newborn, 116–117, 117f, 760–762
physical examination of, 116–118
sutures of, 116, 117f
Skullcap, 458t
Sleep
average hours, 1295t, 1298t
developmental milestones and, 1159, 1295t
evaluation of, 1295–1298
excessive, 1307t
heart rate decreases during, 105
history-taking about, 91b
hygiene principles and, 1300b
inadequate, 1301b
in newborn, 843–844
position during
in infants, 2579–2581
in newborn, 843–844
NICU-discharged infants, 717, 723
stabilization of, 1306f
violence during, 1306
Sleep apnea, obstructive, 525–526, 2583–2585
Sleep center, 2640
Sleep disorders
apnea. *See* Apnea
behavioral disorder associations, 1308t, 1308–1309
benign neonatal sleep myoclonus, 1658–1659
causes of, 1301t, 1302t
classification of, 1296t–1297t, 1299
developmental disorder associations, 1305f, 1309
maturational issues and, 1299–1307
medical problem associations, 1309–1311, 1310t
narcolepsy, 1659
Sleep disorders—cont'd
night terrors, 1659
referrals and, 1311
Sleep myoclonus, 1658–1659
Sleep paralysis, 1659
Sleep terrors, 1304, 1659
Sleep walking, 1304–1305
Sleep-onset association disorder, 1300, 1302–1303, 1307–1308
Sleep-wake cycle, 142
Sleep-wake transition disorder, 1307
Slew foot. *See* Toeing-in and toeing-out
Slipped capital femoral epiphysis, 1493, 1636
Slippery elm bark, 458t
Slow transit, 1426
Slow-to-warm-up temperament, 1746
Slump test, 1409f
Small intestine polyps, 149
Small left colon, 891, 2080
Small-for-gestational-age infants
definition and etiology, 883–885
description of, 1727
follow-up care of, 876
growth and development in, 857
management of, 885–887
pathophysiology of, 885–887
Smoking
breastfeeding and, 723–724, 813
cardiovascular health promotion and, 279t
cessation of, 196
dangers from, 305–306
description of, 305
in Down syndrome patients, 2023
health outcomes affected by, 15
heart disease caused by, 290–291
hemoptysis and, 1570
in home environment, 845
life cycle effects on health, 306, 306f
morbidity and mortality associated with, 305–306
neonatal drug withdrawal syndrome, 950
parental, 369
pharyngitis caused by, 2427
prevalence of, 189
prevention of
barriers to implementation of standard recommendations in, 307–308
community-level tobacco control in, 308
counseling parents in, 307
evidence-based guidelines for, 308
failure in, 307–308
pediatricians' role in, 306–308, 306f
second-hand smoke exposure, 723–724
SIDS and, 2580
substance abuse and, 398
Smooth-muscle hamartoma, 782
Snakebites
antivenom use for, 2698–2699, 2700b
categories, 2699t
Snakebites—cont'd
characteristics of, 2695t, 2695–2696
constricting bands for, 2697
copperhead snakes, 2699
coral snakes, 2700–2702, 2701f
disposition of, 2698
electrolyte abnormalities in, 2698
epidemiology, 2694f, 2694–2695
first aid for, 2696, 2697b
fluid abnormalities in, 2698
hematologic complications in, 2698
immobilization for, 2697
indigenous locations for, 2696b
laboratory studies, 2697–2698
nonindigenous snakes, 2702
physical exam, 2697
pit vipers, 2694–2700, 2696b
prevention, 2694–2695, 2695b
recurrence phenomena in, 2698–2699
serum sickness in, 2699
shock in, 2698
treatment, 2696–2698, 2697b, 2700
venomous vs. nonvenomous, 2695t
Snellen E chart, 120
Snellen illiterate E chart, 120
Snoring, 2583–2584
Soap bubble appearance, 2078, 2080f
Social anxiety, 1282
Social development, 91b–92b
Social difficulties, 1558–1559
Social influences approach, 1132
Social issues. *See also* Psychosocial development
adoption. *See* Adoption
child abuse. *See* Child abuse
fetal-maternal health and, 650–651
foster care, 1063
gay- and lesbian-parented children, 1083–1085
homelessness, 1087–1090
media impact, 1114–1120
self-care, 1103–1105
sexual abuse, 1106–1113
Social learning method, 1132
Social learning theory
basic principles, 1004
rudimentary behavior phase, 1007
Social modeling theory, 1116–1120
Social phobia, 1281
Social Security Administration, 572
Social self, 157
Social services
description of, 173b, 1224
mental health diagnosis and treatment, 1014–1015
neonatal drug withdrawal syndrome referral and follow-up, 957
NICU-discharged infants, 722
sexual abuse assessment and diagnosis, 1109–1113
Social stigma
homosexuality and, 1342
transgender youth and, 1235–1236
Social support, 1170, 1501

Page numbers followed by "f" denote figures; "t" denote tables; "b" *denote* boxes.

Social workers, 571, 1167
Socialization norms, 1040
Socioeconomic status, 5
Sodium
- in dehydration, 2656, 2657t–2658t
- in diabetic ketoacidosis, 2664, 2664t, 2666
- electrolyte abnormalities effects on, 474–477, 475t–476t
- homeostasis of, 469–470

Sodium nitroprusside, 2729, 2729t
Sodium stibogluconate, 2367–2368
Sodium sulfacetamide, 1805
Soft tissues
- malformation of, 2538
- overuse injuries to, 2555–2556

Solid foods, 213, 218–219, 876
Solo practice, 6, 6t
Solution-focused therapy, 204
Soma, 2779
Somatic delusions, 1230
Somatic growth assessments, 108, 110–112
Somatic pain, 435
Somatization, 69–70
Somnambulism, 1304–1305
Sonography
- abdominal distention evaluations, 1369
- fatty liver evaluations, 2121
- meconium peritonitis evaluations, 1879
- soft-tissue bleeding evaluations, 2107
- testicular adrenal rests evaluations, 1811

Sotos syndrome, 1648
Southeast Asian cultural practices, 159
Soy protein allergy, 2065–2067
Space-occupying lesions, 1646, 1647b, 1648
Spanking, 82
Spasms, infantile, 2489b, 2490
Spasmus nutans, 1765
Spastic flatfoot, 1535–1536
Spasticity, 576
Special needs children, 564–592
- demographic data regarding, 241
- description of, 184
- end-of-life planning, 587
- financial considerations, 586–587
- home health care, 569–573
- ongoing health conditions, 564–569
- parenting of, 583–588
- partnering with families in hospital and community settings, 583–588
- physician's first contact with parent, 583–584
- prevalence of, 241
- rehabilitation, 573–582
- school-aged, 588
- school-related issues, 588–592
- treatment of, 416–417, 416f

Special Olympics, 2021
Special Supplemental Nutrition Program for Women, Infants, and Children, 63
- on lead poisoning, 396

Specialists. *See* Pediatric subspecialists
Specific phobia, 1281
Spectinomycin, 2513b, 2514b
Speech
- apraxia of, 356
- assessment of, 354–358
- development of, 355–356
- disorders of, 357, 1291–1293
- history-taking about, 92b
- intelligibility of, 356
- late talkers, 355
- preschool, 355–356
- prespeech assessment, 355

Speech language pathologists, 1291, 1293
Speech therapists, 571
Speech therapy
- discharge planning role of, 173b
- in rehabilitation process, 577

Sperm, intracytoplasmic injection of
- assisted reproductive technologies and risk of, 623
- ethical and legal issues, 625
- fetal/neonatal growth and development issues with, 624
- overview, 621
- perinatal outcomes and neonatal issues, 622–625

Spermatoceles, 1723
Spermicides, 1156
Spiders, 2690–2692
Spina bifida
- allergies and, 2543
- alternative medicine in, 2543
- brain malformation in, 2539
- continence in, 2542–2543
- etiology, 2537–2538, 2547
- evaluation, 2540–2541
- hospitalization in, 2544
- motor function in, 2539–2540, 2540t
- with myelomeningocele and hydrocephalus, 2149
- neurosurgery in, 2542
- orthopaedic management of, 2542
- pathology of, 2538f, 2538–2540
- prevention of, 2543
- psychosocial considerations in, 2541
- referrals for, 2543–2544
- reproductive issues in, 2543
- soft tissue malformation in, 2538
- spinal cord malformation in, 2539–2540
- treatment, 2541–2543
- urologic management of, 2542
- vertebral malformation in, 2539

Spinal cord
- growth of, 140
- malformation of, 2539–2540

Spinal muscular atrophy, 991–992
Spine
- congenital anomalies, 792–793
- deformities of
  - acquired, 2548–2549
  - classification of, 2546b
  - congenital, 2545–2548
  - postural, 2545
- embryonic development of, 2545
- infections of, 2549
- newborn assessment of, 769
- trauma to, 323t

Spinning behavior, 1726
Spirituality
- complementary and alternative medicine, 461b, 463
- in palliative and end-of-life care, 598–599, 599b

Spirochetes, 2270, 2270t
Spirometry
- for asthma, 1841
- for cystic fibrosis, 1988, 1988f

Spleen
- disorders of, 1732
- dysfunction of, 1696
- enlargement of. *See* Splenomegaly
- function of, 1731
- in infants, 133
- in newborns, 133
- palpation of, 133, 1730
- rupture of, 2628
- torsion of, 2628

Splenectomy, 2173–2174
Splenic cysts, 1732
Splenomegaly
- definition of, 1730
- differential diagnosis of, 1731b, 1731–1732
- imaging for, 1732–1733
- laboratory testing for, 1732
- patient history and, 1732
- physical examination for, 1732
- referral for, 1733
- referrals for, 1742
- sports participation with, 323t
- treatment of, 1733

Splenoptosis, 1732
Splints, 579
Split-mixed program, 2003
Spondyloarthropathy, 1626
Spondylolisthesis, 1408, 2549
Spondylolysis, 1406, 1408, 1410, 2549
Spontaneous pneumothorax, 1423
Spoon scratching, 69t
Sports
- contact-based classification of, 320b, 321, 321t
- intensity-based classification of, 321t
- participation in, 2550–2551

Sports injuries
- ankle sprains, 2556t, 2556–2557
- anterior cruciate ligament injuries, 2557–2558
- anterior knee pain, 2560

Sports injuries—cont'd
avulsion fractures of the pelvis, 2558–2559
causes, 2550–2551
collateral ligament injuries of the knee, 2557
dislocations, 2559–2560
and drug use, 2551–2552
heat injury, 2551
hospitalization in, 2562
meniscal tears, 2558
muscle strains, 2559
overuse syndromes
apophyseal conditions, 2553–2554
epiphyseal conditions, 2554–2555
factors contributing to, 2552, 2552b
physeal conditions, 2554
of soft tissues, 2555–2556
stress fractures, 2552–2553
prevention, 2562
quadriceps contusion, 2558
referrals for, 2562
winter, 2561t, 2561–2562
Sprains
ankle, 2556t, 2556–2557
extremity pain caused by, 1491
Sputum collection, 2598
St. John's wort, 458t, 542t
Stabilization protocols, for sick and dying infants, 674–680, 732
Staphylococcal infection, 1409–1410
Staphylococcal scalded skin syndrome, 2566t–2567t
Staphylococcal scarlet fever, 2222t
Staphylococcal toxic shock syndrome
case definition, 2564b
cause of, 2562–2563
clinical features of, 2222t, 2562–2564, 2563t, 2565f
convalescence for, 2567
description of, 2562–2563
differential diagnosis, 2564, 2566f–2567f
hospitalization for, 2567
incidence of, 2562
laboratory evaluation of, 2564–2565
management of, 2565b, 2565–2567
nonsteroidal anti-inflammatory drugs for, 2562
pathogenesis of, 2562–2563
prognosis of, 2567
referrals for, 2567
Staphylococcus aureus
description of, 1852–1853, 1856–1857
joint pain and, 1627
methicillin-resistant, 937, 1854–1855, 1859
neonatal skin conditions, 785
Startle response, 102
State Children's Health Insurance Plan, 23–24
Static stretching, 192
Status asthmaticus
clinical manifestations, 2813–2814
deaths caused by, 2813
definition, 2813
management, 2815–2817
pathophysiology, 2814f, 2814–2815
Status epilepticus
classification, 2819
convulsive, 2819, 2821
etiology, 2820–2821
hospitalization for, 2821
incidence, 2819
nonconvulsive, 2819, 2821
partial, 2819
referral for, 2821
treatment, 2820b, 2821
Steatohepatitis, nonalcoholic, 2324
Steatorrhea, 1440
Steinert disease, 2281–2283, 2282t
Stem cell transplantation
hemoglobinopathies treated with, 2104
red blood cell transfusions in, 484
relapsed leukemias treated with, 2242
Stent, nasolacrimal, 1708f
Stepfamilies, 1058–1059
Steppage gait, 1630
Stereopsis, 1776
Stereotypies, 1724, 1759, 1760
Steroid acne, 1804
Steroid creams, 2430–2431
Steroid hormones, 1808
Steroids. *See* Corticosteroids; Glucocorticoids
Stevens-Johnson syndrome
clinical features of, 2222t
description of, 1716, 2030–2031, 2031t
differential diagnosis, 2566t–2567t
Still disease, 1626
Still heart murmur, 917
Stimulants
abuse of, 2782
neonatal drug withdrawal syndrome, 949–951
short stature caused by, 1728, 1730
treatment for insomnia, 1309
Stings
anaphylactic reaction to, 2644
definition, 2686
by winged Hymenoptera, 2687–2689, 2689b
Stomach
age-related capacity increases, 132
distended, 1372f
Stomatitis
Candida albicans, 124
clinical manifestations of, 2569–2572, 2571f
differential diagnosis of, 2570, 2570b
epidemiologic factors of, 2570
Stomatitis—cont'd
etiology of, 2569–2570
herpes simplex, 125
laboratory evaluation of, 2572
management of, 2572
prevention of, 2572
recurrent aphthous, 2569–2571
referrals for, 2572–2573
systemic disorders, 2570
Stool. *See also* diarrhea
blood in, 1444, 1445
failure to thrive diagnosis and, 1505
withholding of, 1425
Stool guaiac test, 1544
Stooped gaits, 1630
Storage disorders, 1577
Storytelling, 100–101
Strabismus
alternating, 1776, 1777f
amblyopia and, 1776–1778, 1778b
causes of, 1734b
characteristics of, 1734b
in children, 120
concomitant, 1734–1737
definition of, 119, 1733–1734
esotropias, 1733–1737, 1734b, 1734f–1736f
exotropias, 1733, 1734b, 1737, 1737f
Hirschberg test for, 120
incomitant, 1737–1742
in newborns, 119
referral for, 1742
during visual development, 1776
Strains, muscle, 2559
Strange behaviors
in adolescents, 1745–1746
in infants, 1742–1744
in medically ill child, 1746–1747
in middle-aged children, 1744–1745
referral for, 1747
temperament and, 1746
in young children, 1742–1744
Stranger rape, 2790
Strawberry tongue, 126
Streptococcal infections
cellulitis, 2827, 2827f
rheumatic fever after, 2478, 2478f
Streptococcal pharyngitis, 2478–2479
Streptococcal scarlet fever, 2222t
Streptococcal toxic shock syndrome
case definition, 2574b
differential diagnosis, 2566t–2567t
etiology and pathogenesis, 2573–2574
evaluation, 2574–2575
hospitalization for, 2577
prevention, 2576–2577
referrals for, 2577
treatment, 2575–2576
Streptococcus sp.
S pneumoniae, 1857
description of, 256
joint pain and, 1627

Page numbers followed by "f" denote figures; "t" denote tables; "b" *denote* boxes.

Streptococcus sp.—cont'd
S pneumoniae—cont'd
vaccine for
in adolescents, 246f
catch-up schedule for, 251t
characteristics of, 256
conjugated, 256
guidelines for, 245f
intervals between doses, 248t
minimum age for, 248t
polysaccharide, 256–257
schedule for, 251t, 256t
S pyogenes
description of, 1855
neonatal skin conditions, 785
pharyngitis caused by, 2425b, 2426
in streptococcal TSS, 2573–2574
Streptomycin, 500
Stress. *See also* Conversion reactions; Posttraumatic stress disorder
hospitalization-related, 171, 173, 175
in parents, 181, 186
psychosocial, 189
Stress dosing, 1814
Stress fractures, 2552–2553
Stress management
family activities for, 195b
self-hypnosis for, 452
techniques for, 195
Stretch reflexes, 141
Stretching, 192
Stridor
in airways obstruction, 2632–2633, 2633t
causes, 2633t, 2649b, 2649–2650
definition of, 1747–1748
diagnostic testing for, 1751–1752
differential diagnosis of, 1748, 1749t
gastroesophageal reflux disease and, 2058, 2059t
history-taking for, 1748–1749
hoarseness and, 1600
management of, 1752–1753
physical examination for, 1749–1751
spirometry findings for, 1749f
String of beads sign, 2079
Stroke
neonatal, 945
sickle cell disease and, 536
Strongyloidiasis, 70, 2387–2388
Stupor, 2639
Sturge-Weber syndrome
clinical manifestations of, 2313, 2313f
description of, 2312–2313
differential diagnosis of, 2314
evaluation of, 2314
features of, 2313
intellectual disability and, 2190t
leptomeningeal involvement in, 2312–2313
management of, 2314
Stuttering
affects of, 1292–1293
amenorrhea and, 1391
characteristics of, 1291, 1292b
diagnosis of, 1292
etiology of, 1291–1292
referrals and, 1293
Stye, 1714, 1715f
Subacute bacterial endocarditis, 529, 529b
Subclavian artery, 2636
Subconjunctival hemorrhage, 118, 1712, 2346, 2346f
Subcutaneous nodules, 2477
Subdermal rod implant, 1355
Subdural hematoma, 66t, 2713t
Subgaleal hematoma, 762, 992
Subglottic hemangiomas, 1599, 1601
Subglottic lesions, 1752f
Subglottic obstruction, 1750f
Subglottic stenosis, 1749t
Subluxation, radial head, 1493
Submentobregmatic diameter, 760–762
Submersion injuries. *See* Drowning
Subspecialists. *See* Pediatric subspecialists
Substance abuse. *See also* Alcohol, abuse of
in adolescents
definition of, 398–404
effects of, 398
epidemiologic features of, 398f, 398–399
gateway hypothesis related to, 399
prevalence of, 398f, 398–399
smoking and, 398
in athletes, 2551–2552
clinical interview for, 401
clinical presentation of, 400
commonly abused substances, 1247–1248
counseling for, 1247–1248
diagnosis of, 1249
differential diagnosis of, 399–400, 400b
in Down syndrome patients, 2022
DSM-IV-TR criteria for, 399–400, 400b
dyspnea caused by, 1472
early identification of, 398–404
evaluation of, 400–402
fatigue caused by, 1511
hallucinogens, 2781–2782
inhalants, 2782
laboratory testing and, 1249
management of, 402–403, 1249–1250
marijuana, 2779, 2781
medical history and, 1246–1247
opioids, 2783
physical examination for, 1248b, 1248–1249
prevalence of, 398f, 398–399, 1245–1246
referrals for, 398–404
Substance abuse—cont'
school health education and, 1131–1132
sedative-hypnotics, 2782–2783
stimulants, 2782
urine drug screens for, 401–402
Substance Abuse Subtle Screening Inventory, 401
Substance dependence, 399–400, 400b
Succinylcholine, 557–558
Sucking reflex, 123, 816
Sudden cardiac death, 340, 1418–1419
Sudden infant death syndrome. *See* SIDS
Sufentanil, 425t
Suffocation death, 1268
Suicide, 239, 1312
Sulfasalazine, 2216, 2216b
Sulfisoxazole
dosage, peak serum concentrations, and MIC_{95} for, 494t
urinary tract infections treated with, 2613t
uses of, 501
Sulfonamide
antidote for, 2685t
bacterial resistance to, 500
mechanisms of action of, 500
pharmacologic properties of, 500–501
side effects of, 501
uses of, 501
Superior oblique palsy, 1737–1739, 1739f
Supernumerary digits, 783
Supernumerary nipple, 766–767, 783
Supplement(s)
Dietary Supplement Health and Education Act of 1994 on, 457
fluoride, 217
iron, 217
nutritional, 2551–2552
vitamin D, 217
vitamin K, 216–217
water-soluble vitamins, 217
Supplemental nutrition program
breastfeeding and interference from, 817, 825–827
neonatal eligibility for, 711–712
Supplemental security income, 23, 572, 722–723
Support groups, 1240
Suppression
of appetite. *See* Anorexia
strabismus and, 1733–1734
Suprapubic aspiration, 2610b
Supratentorial tumors, 1862
Supraventricular tachycardia
definition of, 1413–1414, 1415f
diagnosis of, 1413–1414, 1415f
irritability and, 1612
management of, 1414–1416
in newborn, 920–921
presentation of, 1414
syncope and, 1755

Surfactant protein deficiency, 907–908
Surgery
abdominal, 2624–2630
abdominal pain treated with, 1377–1378, 1378b
adenoidectomy, 2583–2589
back pain treated with, 1410
caustic esophageal injuries treated with, 2707–2708
congestive heart failure treated with, 2724
dysmenorrhea treated with, 1462
extremity pain treated with, 1493
fetal
assessment for, 644
cleft lip and cleft palate treated with, 1925
gastrointestinal obstruction treated with, 2082–2083
gastroesophageal reflux disease treated with, 2062
hyperinsulinism treated with, 2737
increased intracranial pressure treated with, 2744–2745
outpatient, 515b, 545
tonsillectomy, 2583–2589
Surveillance, 49, 315
Survival outcomes, 11–12
SVT. *See* Supraventricular tachycardia
Swallowing
development and phases of, 1463
disorders of. *See* Dysphagia
Sweat glands, 113
Sweating, excessive, 1603–1604
Swimmer's ear, 2364
Swimming pool safety, 2680, 2681b
Swollen eye, 2440–2445, 2445f
SWOT analysis, 27
Sympathetic blocks, 445–446
Symptomatic proteinuria, 1678
Syncope
causes of, 1753–1756, 1754b
characteristics of, 1657–1658
definition of, 1657, 1753
diagnostic testing for, 1756–1757
management of, 1757
patient history and examination for, 1756
Syndactyly, 793, 1531f, 1532
Syndrome of gonadal dysgenesis, 2197
Syndrome of inappropriate antidiuretic hormone, 475, 2258
Syndrome X, 2323, 2323b
Synechia vulvae, 2228–2230. *See also* Labial adhesions
Synophrys, 763
Syphilis
congenital, 931–932, 1627
joint pain and, 1627
maternal-fetal transmission, 636–637
neonatal skin infections, 785
primary, 2527–2528
secondary, 2527f, 2527–2528
sexual abuse and, 1109
Syphilis—cont'f
treatment, 2517b–2518b
in young children, 2570
Syrup of ipecac, 2683, 2769
Systemic lupus erythematosus
in anuria, 1827
cervical lymphadenopathy caused by, 1997
drug-induced, 2026, 2029
herpes simplex virus and, 2130
joint pain and, 1626–1627
nephritis of, 2292–2293
in oliguria, 1827
proteinuria present in, 2113
Systemic retinoids, 2453, 2453t
Systemic-onset disease, 1626
Systems theory, 1156
Systole, 1561
Systolic blood pressure, 1585
Systolic murmurs, 1563, 1563t, 1564f

T

T cells, 1698
Tabun, 2779
Tachyarrhythmias, 610, 920, 1755
Tachycardia
by age, 2802t
in congestive heart failure, 2718, 2719
pulse associated with, 105
supraventricular
definition of, 1413–1414, 1415f
diagnosis of, 1413–1414, 1415f
irritability and, 1612
management of, 1414–1416
in newborn, 920–921
presentation of, 1414
syncope and, 1755
ventricular
description of, 1417, 1417f
in newborn, 920, 923
syncope and, 1755
Tachypnea, 2718, 2721
Tacrolimus ointment, 1852
Taenia sp., 2395–2397
Taeniasis
clinical manifestations of, 2396
description of, 2395–2396
diagnosis of, 2396–2397
epidemiologic features of, 2395
life cycle of, 2395–2396
treatment of, 2397
Tai chi, 195
Tailor bunion, 1532
Talipes, 1529b, 1531f
Talipes calcaneovalgus, 1532, 1533f, 1538
Talipes equinovarus
description of, 139, 1532, 1532f–1533f, 1538
newborn assessment, 771
physical examination, 793
ultrasound detection of, 613
Talipes varus, 1533f, 1533–1534
Talocalcaneal coalition, 1535–1536
Tandem mass spectrometry, 387
Tar preparations, 2451, 2452t
Tarantulas, 2692–2693
Tarsal coalition, 1535–1536
Tarsal navicular bone, 2353b, 2354
Task Force on Community Preventive Services, 308
Tazarotene for acne, 1804–1805
TBMN. *See* thin basement membrane nephropathy
^{99m}Tc dimercaptosuccinic acid renal scan, 2339–2340, 2340f
Tea treeoil, 458t
Teaching hospitals, 6
Tear duct obstruction, 1706
Tear secreting glands, 1714f
Teenage drivers, 270
Teenage parents
challenges for, 181
imaging studies, 1348
laboratory evaluation and, 1347–1348
management of, 1348, 1348b
physical examination for, 1347
Teenage pregnancy
demographic data regarding, 235–236, 236t
discussions about, 75–76
prevalence of, 75
statistics regarding, 235–236
Teenagers. *See* Adolescent(s)
Teeth
delayed eruption of, 123, 125
growth of, 123, 124f
in infants, 125
intrauterine growth of, 123
newborn assessment, 765–766
in newborns, 123
permanent, 123
primary, 123, 124f
tetracycline staining of, 125
tuberous sclerosis complex effects on, 2311
Teeth stains
coloration, 1438–1439t
extrinsic stains, 1437
intrinsic stains, 1147–1148
management of, 1438
tetracycline, 125
Teething, 1613
TEL/AML1 gene, 2238
Telemedicine, 1138
Telephone care flow chart, 411–412, 411f
Television viewing, 190
Television violence, 272–273
Telogen effluvium, 1384
Temper tantrums, 1316–1319
Temperament, 1746
attachment and, 1001
infant, 183
Temperament and Behavior Scale, 186
Temporal-sequential deficits, 1150
Temporomandibular joint dysfunction, 1651
TEN. *See* Toxic epidermal necrolysis
Tendon injuries, 2555–2556, 2559

Page numbers followed by "f" denote figures; "t" denote tables; "b" *denote* boxes.

Tendonitis, 2555–2556
Tenex, 1313t
TENS. *See* Transcutaneous electrical nerve stimulation
Tension-type headaches, 1550b, 1550–1551, 1553
Teratogenic agent, 1496
Teratomas. *See* Germ cell tumors and teratomas
Terbinafine, 513t
Terbutaline, 2816
Terminal hair, 1590
Terminology systems, 29t–30t, 31–32
Terrible twos, 210
Testes
- absent, 323t
- androgen production, 1592–1593
- development. *See* Puberty
- fetal, 134
- of newborns, 135
- nonsalvageable, 1719f
- undescended
  - in cryptorchism, 2158–2159
  - description of, 134–136
  - sports participation with, 323t

Testicular adrenal rests, 1811
Testicular torsion, 1718–1720
Testicular tumors, 1592–1593, 1723
Testosterone
- in acne, 1802, 1803
- in cancer survivors, 1896
- in cystic fibrosis patients, 1984
- dosing in acne management, 1811
- free, 1806, 1814

Tetanus
- prophylaxis against, in snakebites, 2700
- toxoids, in pertussis prevention, 2423b

Tetracycline
- acne treated with, 1805, 1806b
- bacterial resistance to, 504
- dosage, peak serum concentrations, and MIC_{95} for, 494t
- mechanism of action of, 503
- pharmacologic properties of, 504
- Rocky Mountain spotted fever treated with, 2484
- side effects of, 504
- teeth staining caused by, 125
- use of, 504

Tetralogy of Fallot, 1943, 1944f
- cyanosis and, 927
- management of, 1944–1946
- with pulmonary atresia, 1945–1946
- surgical repair, 1945f
- syncope and, 1756
- ultrasound detection of, 609
- without pulmonary atresia, 1944–1945

Thalassemia
- α-
  - definitions and clinical manifestations, 2099
  - Hb Bart disease, 2100
  - Hb H disease, 2099–2100

Thalassemia—cont'd
- ß-
  - clinical forms, 2100
  - definitions and clinical manifestations, 2100
  - α-globin chain production, 2100, 2101f
  - management of, 2100–2102
  - thalassemia major, 2100
- description of, 943
- iron-deficiency anemia vs., 2203–2204
- major, 1396, 2100

Thelarche, 1686
Theobromine, 825–826
Theophylline
- apnea, bradycardia and desaturation in neonates, 686–688
- asthma treated with, 1848
- status asthmaticus treated with, 2816

Therapeutic alliance, 207–208
Therapeutic apheresis, 486
Therapeutic relationships, 1160–1161
Therapeutic touch, 460
Therapists
- collaboration with pediatricians, 1186
- medication for, 1178, 1179

Thermal injuries. *See* Burn(s)
Thermic effect of feeding, 220
Thermometer, rectal, 104, 105f
Thermoregulation
- fever and, 418–419, 1516
- infant stabilization, 674–676
- in neonates
  - NICU-discharged infants, 712–713
  - resuscitation, 658–659
  - transition, 656
- in premature infants, 833

Thermotherapy, 2368
Thin basement membrane nephropathy, 1567f, 1568–1569
Thioamides, 2156
Thiopurine methyltransferase metabolism, 2242
Third heart sound, 131, 2719
Third nerve palsy, 1740–1741, 1741f
Thioridazine, 2685t
Thoracic defects
- physical examination, 793
- ultrasound detection of, 607

Thoracic index, 112
Thoracic vertebrae, 2353b, 2354
Thoracostomy, 2759, 2759t
Three-dimensional airway reconstruction, 1795f
Throat. *See* Pharynx
Thrombocytopenia
- description of, 945–946
- epistaxis caused by, 1483
- immune. *See* Immune thrombocytopenic purpura
- intrauterine infection and, 946
- neonatal assessment, 671, 946
- petechiae and purpura and, 1667–1969

Thromboembolism
- neonatal, 945
- in nephrotic syndrome, 2298
- venous, 561, 561b

Thrombotic thrombocytopenic purpura, 1669, 2673
Thrush, 124, 1696
Thumb-sucking, 1651, 1725
Thyme, 458t
Thyroglossal duct cysts, 1996
Thyroid disease
- anesthesia and, 532, 534, 534b
- description of, 2007
- maternal health and, 631

Thyroid function tests, 2163–2164
Thyroid gland
- enlargement of, 128
- palpation of, 127–128
- ultrasonography of, 1996

Thyrotoxic crisis, 2157
Thyrotoxicosis
- definition of, 2154
- fatigue caused by, 1510
- Graves disease and, 2154
- neonatal, 2157

L-Thyroxine, 2164t–2165t, 2164–2165
Tiagabine, 2499t, 2501
Tibial osteochondroses, 2353–2354, 2353b
Tibial torsion, 1540–1541, 1542
Tick bites
- description of, 2179
- joint pain and, 1627
- Lyme disease prevention after, 2251
- prevention of, 2251
- Rocky Mountain spotted fever caused by, 2481–2482

Tics
- attention deficit/hyperactivity disorder and, 1212t
- clinical manifestations of, 1758
- comorbid disorders, 1760
- definition of, 1758
- differential diagnosis of, 1760
- etiology of, 1758–1760
- incidence of, 1758
- management of, 1762
- pharmacotherapy for, 1761
- treatment of, 1760–1762

Tide mark dermatitis, 2013
Tilt-table testing, 1757
Time efficiency, 41
Timed urine sample, 1676
Timeliness, 43
Time-outs, 82, 1033–1034
Tinea capitis, 1388–1389
Tinea corporis, 1692f
TMJ. *See* Temporomandibular joint dysfunction
To-and-fro murmurs, 1564–1565, 1565f
Tobacco smoking. *See* Smoking
Tobramycin
- dosage, peak serum concentrations, and MIC_{95} for, 494t
- uses of, 500

Tocolytic therapy, 633
Toddlers
auditory screening in, 328–329, 329b
neonatal intensive care unit infants as, 870–871
psychological development in, 1007
vision screening in, 344
Toddler's fracture, 2053
Toe deformities, 1530–1532, 1531f, 1541
Toeing-in and toeing-out, 1538–1540, 1542
Toe-walking, 1536–1537, 1542, 1630
Toilet habits
encopresis and, 1253
Tolerance, 491
Tolmetin, 428t
Tongue
abnormalities of, 124
geographic, 126
in infants, 125–126
physical examination of, 124
strawberry, 126
Tongue tie, 124
Tonic myotactic reflexes, 141
Tonic neck position, 142
Tonsillectomy
with adenoidectomy, 2585, 2586
complications of, 2588, 2588t
contraindications of, 2588–2589
indications for, 2583–2586, 2585f–2586f, 2587b
Pittsburgh criteria for, 2585, 2587b
procedures for, 2587f, 2587–2588
quality of life after, 2589
Tonsillitis, 2425–2430, 2585–2586, 2587b
Tonsillopharyngitis, 2425
Tonsils, 126
Tooth stains
coloration, 1438–1439t
extrinsic stains, 1437
intrinsic stains, 1147–1148
management of, 1438
Topical calcineurin inhibitors, 2452t, 2453
Topical corticosteroids
psoriasis treated with, 2451, 2452t
seborrheic dermatitis treated with, 2487–2488
Topical retinoids, 2452t, 2453
Topiramate
dosing strategies for, 445t
seizures managed using, 2499t, 2501
TORCH, 152, 635–636, 928–932
Torsades de pointes, 527, 528t
Torsion, 1529b
Torticollis
clinical manifestations of, 1764
congenital, 2434
definition of, 1764
description of, 127–128
differential diagnosis of, 1764–1765, 1765b
evaluation of, 1765–1766
management of, 1766
Total anomalous pulmonary venous return, 1946–1947
Total body water, 467–470
Tourette syndrome, 1181b, 1758–1759, 1760
Toxic epidermal necrolysis, 2030–2031, 2031t, 2566t–2567t
Toxic shock syndrome
staphylococcal
case definition, 2564b
cause and pathogenesis, 2562–2563
clinical features of, 2222t, 2562–2564, 2563t, 2565f
differential diagnosis, 2564, 2566f–2567f
hospitalization for, 2567
incidence, 2562
laboratory evaluation, 2564–2565
management, 2565b, 2565–2567
NSAIDs and, 2562
prognosis and convalescence, 2567
referrals for, 2567
streptococcal, 2573–2577
Toxic substances. *See* Poisoning
Toxic synovitis, 1493–1494
Toxicology, 1265–1266
Toxidromes, 2764–2765, 2765t
Toxins
body odor and, 1663
irritability and, 1612–1613
Toxocariasis, 2391
Toxoplasma gondii, 930–931, 2378–2380
Toxoplasmosis
acquired, 2379
causes of, 2378
clinical manifestations of, 2378–2379
congenital, 2378–2379
description of, 2378
diagnosis of, 2379–2380
epidemiologic features of, 2378
in immunodeficient patients, 2379
life cycle of, 2378
maternal-fetal infection, 635–636
ocular, 2379
pathogenesis of, 2378
prevention of, 2380
treatment of, 2380
TPMT metabolism. *See* Thiopurine methyltransferase metabolism
Trabeculectomy, 1709
Trabeculotomy ab externum, 1709
Trachea
compression of, 2634
obstruction of, 2634
stenosis of, 1796f
Tracheitis, bacterial, 2635, 2636t, 2649–2650
Tracheoesophageal fistula, 777, 915
Tracheomalacia, 2634
Traction response test, 141f, 143, 144f
Tramadol, 426–427
Transcutaneous electrical nerve stimulation, 439–440
Transdermal patch, 1354
Transfer aids, 579
Transfer protocols for high-risk neonates, 683–685, 749
Transfusions
anesthesia and, 545–546
blood
complications of, 487–488
in disseminated intravascular coagulation, 2674–2675
indications for, 481
massive, 2672–2673
complications of, 487–488
acute hemolytic transfusion reaction, 487
acute lung injury, 489
allergic reactions, 488
delayed hemolytic transfusion reaction, 487
febrile transfusion reaction, 487–488
infections, 488
in disseminated intravascular coagulation, 2674–2675
exchange, 486, 486f
granulocyte, 485–486
massive, 2672–2673
neonatal anemia, 684–685
partial exchange, 486
platelet, 484–485, 485t
red blood cell
acute blood loss treated with, 482
chronic, 483
complications of, 487–488
description of, 482–484, 482t, 483b
fresh-frozen plasma in, 482
hemoglobinopathy and, 484
in immunosuppressed patients, 484
in infants younger than 4 months, 483b, 484
in oxygen-carrying capacity restoration, 482–483, 483b
packed red blood cells in, 482
in potential stem cell transplant recipients, 484
in surgery, 483–484
safety in, 2104
Transgender youth
adverse effects of, 1235–1236
advocacy for, 1243
definition of, 1233–1234
etiology of, 1234–1235
evaluation of, 1236–1239
laboratory evaluation of, 1239
management of, 1239–1241
parents and, 1237, 1242–1243
physical examination of, 1238–1239
referrals for, 1243
transitional care and, 1241–1242
Transient lower esophageal sphincter relaxation, 699
Transient neonatal pustular melanosis, 784

Transient proteinuria, 1677
Transient synovitis of hip, 1635
Transient tachypnea of newborn
pathophysiology and diagnosis, 906–907
in premature infants, 833–834
signs of, 668
Transient tic disorder, 1760
Transient tricuspid regurgitation, 918
Transitional cardiorespiratory physiology
acute fetal hypoxia and asphyxia, 656–658
delivery management and, 654–656
Transitional objects, 1744
Transitional planning, 53
Translocation, 2016–2017
Transplantation
kidney, 2096–2097
liver, 2126
lung, 1990
orthotopic heart, 1963–1965
rejection, 1963–1965
stem cell
hemoglobinopathies treated with, 2104
red blood cell transfusions in, 484
relapsed leukemias treated with, 2242
Transposition of the great arteries, 609, 927
Trauma. *See also* Injuries
abdominal, 1097
description of, 1285–1286
dissociative disorders and, 1745
dysuria caused by, 1477
extremity pain caused by, 1489
head
description of, 2709–2715
sports participation with, 323t
syncope and, 1756
hoarseness and, 1599–1600, 1602
irritability and, 1609, 1611
limp and, 1635
musculoskeletal injuries, 2556–2561
ocular. *See* Ocular trauma
preseptal cellulitis after, 2442
scrotal pain and swelling caused by, 1721
spinal, 323t
Traumatic brain injury, 2709. *See also* Head injuries
Trazodone, 445t
Treacher Collins syndrome, 792
Treatment adherence, 163–164
Trematode infections
cysticercosis, 2395–2397
diphyllobothriasis, 2399–2400
echinococcal disease, 2397–2399
hydatid disease, 2397–2399
hymenolepiasis, 2400–2401
schistosomiasis, 2393–2395
taeniasis, 2395–2397
Trendelenburg gait, 1630
Trendelenburg sign, 139f
Treponema pallidum, 931–932
Tretinoin
acne treated with, 1805t
molluscum contagiosum treated with, 2619
Trichinella spiralis, 2385–2386
Trichinellosis
causes of, 2385
clinical manifestations of, 2386
diagnosis of, 2386
epidemiologic features of, 2385
life cycle of, 2385–2386
pathogenesis of, 2385–2386
prevention of, 2386
treatment of, 2386
Trichloroacetic acid, 2515b, 2516b
Trichobezoar, 1374f, 1726
Trichomonas vaginalis, 2531
Trichorrhexis nodosa, 1386
Trichotillomania, 1387–1388, 1388f, 1726
Trichuriasis
causes of, 2386
clinical features of, 2386–2387
diagnosis of, 2387
epidemiologic features of, 2386
prevention of, 2387
treatment of, 2387
Trichuris trichiura, 2386–2387
Tricuspid atresia, 1957
Tricyclic antidepressants
antidote for, 2684t, 2768t
chronic pain managed using, 444
headaches and, 1554
overdose of, 2772
Triglycerides, 224
Trigonocephaly, 763
Trimethoprim-sulfamethoxazole
dosage, peak serum concentrations, and MIC_{95} for, 494t
urinary tract infections treated with, 2613, 2613t
uses of, 501
Triple A syndrome, 1812
Triptans, 1553
Trisomy 13
cystic hygroma, 607
neonatal assessment, 671
talipes equinovarus with, 793
Trisomy 18
chest measurements, 792
cystic hygroma, 607
neonatal assessment, 671
talipes equinovarus with, 793
Trisomy 21. *See also* Down syndrome
free, origin of, 2016
molecular pathological features of, 2016–2017
neonatal assessment, 671
translocation, 2016–2017
Trousseau syndrome, 2672
Truancy, 1145, 1148
True precocious puberty, 1591–1593
Truncus arteriosus, 609
Trust, 209
of parents of NICU infants, 733–734
primary care physician and, 729–730
Trypanosoma sp.
T brucei, 2370
T cruzi. See Chagas disease
Trypanosomiasis
African, 2370
American, 2368–2369
Tube feedings, 872–873
Tuberculin skin test, 2590, 2591–2592
Tuberculosis
adrenal insufficiency caused by, 1811
breastfeeding and, 812
definition of, 2590–2591
differential diagnosis of, 2591b–2592b, 2591–2592
directly observed therapy for, 2593, 2602
disseminated disease, 2600, 2602
evaluation of, 2595f, 2596–2600, 2598f, 2599b, 2600f, 2602
exposure to, 2591, 2592
gastrointestinal obstruction caused by, 2071
hospitalization for, 2603
isoniazid for, 2591, 2592–2595, 2596t
latent
definition, 2590–2591
management, 2592–2596
physical examination for, 2597
management of, 2592–2596
medication flow sheet, 2597f
perinatal infection, 935
rates of, 2590t
referrals for, 2603
risk assessment questionnaire, 2592, 2593b
treatment of, 2592–2596, 2597f, 2601t, 2602
tuberculin skin testing, 2591–2592, 2592b, 2594f
Tuberous sclerosis
cardiac manifestations of, 2311
central nervous system manifestations of, 2309–2310
cutaneous manifestations of, 2310f–2311f, 2310–2311
definition of, 2309
dental manifestations of, 2311
diagnostic criteria for, 2310b
differential diagnosis of, 2311–2312
evaluation of, 2312
features of, 2309
hypomelanotic macules, 779
intellectual disability and, 2190t
management of, 2312
ocular manifestations of, 2311
prevalence of, 2309
pulmonary manifestations of, 2311
renal manifestations of, 2311
vascular manifestations of, 2311

Tubular disease, 1567f
Tufting enteropathy, 1453
Tumor(s)
abdominal, 1373–1375
adrenal, 1593, 1595
brain
classification, 1861
definitions, 1860
diagnostic delays, 1861
differential diagnosis, 1861, 1861b
evaluation of, 1861–1863, 1862b
incidence, 1860
management of, 1863
referrals for, 1863–1864
risk factors, 1860b, 1860–1861
central nervous system, 1860–1861, 1863
chorionic gonadotropin-secreting, 1593
Ewing
clinical manifestations, 1886
differential diagnosis of, 1886t
etiology, 1885–1886
evaluation, 1886
follow-up, 1887
management of, 1887
prognosis, 1887
germ cell
clinical manifestations, 1884
etiology, 1883–1884
evaluation, 1884–1885
follow-up, 1885
management of, 1885
prognosis, 1885
hoarseness caused by, 1600
ovarian, 1592
testicular, 1592–1593, 1723
Wilms
abdominal and pelvic tumors, differential diagnosis of, 1874t
clinical manifestations, 1874
description of, 1374f
etiology, 1873–1874
evaluation of, 1874–1875
follow-up, 1876
management of, 1875–1876
prognosis, 1876
staging, 1875b
Turner syndrome, 2197
congenital anomalies with, 792
cystic hygroma, ultrasound detection of, 607
neck findings in, 127
short stature in girls and, 1727
21-hydroxylase deficiency, 1594
Twins
monozygotic, 2232
reversed arterial perfusion syndrome, 618–619
ultrasound detection of, 613
Twin-to-twin transfusion syndrome, 114, 618
2-Nitro 4-trifluoromethylbenzoyl-1-1, 3-cyclohexanedione inhibitor, 2126
Tympanic membrane
in acute otitis media, 122
anatomy of, 121–122
Tympanitic abdomen
children and, 1372–1373
newborns and, 1370–1372
Tympanostomy tubes, 2363
Type 1 diabetes. *See* Diabetes mellitus
Type 2 diabetes. *See* Diabetes mellitus
Typhlitis, 2628
Tyrosinase, 113
Tyrosinemia type 1, 986

U

Ulcers
inside mouth, 2569–2573
perforated, 2628
skin, 1690
Ultrasound/ultrasonography
adrenal hemorrhage evaluations, 1812
appendicitis evaluations, 149–150, 1837
brain imaging using, 151–152
cerebral palsy evaluations, 1904, 1905
congenital anomaly diagnosis, 795
description of, 147
fetal assessment with, 643–644
gallstone evaluations, 148
gastrointestinal system evaluations, 147–150
intussusception evaluations, 149
jaundice and, 1622
limp and, 1635
neonatal screening, 702–703
osteomyelitis evaluations, 2357
prenatal diagnoses
first-trimester ultrasound, 604–605
postnatal assessment, 774–777
pyloric stenosis evaluations, 147–148, 148f, 2456, 2456f
renal, 1826–1827, 1875, 2096, 2611, 2612b
renal mass evaluations, 150
retinoblastoma evaluations, 1880
second- and third-trimester
abdominal wall defects, 610
cardiovascular defects, 608–610
central nervous system defects, 605–606
clubfoot, 613
craniofacial defects, 606
extremities anomalies, 613
gastrointestinal defects, 610–611
genitourinary defects, 611–612
intrauterine growth restriction, 613
neck defects, 606–607
skeletal defects, 612–613
thoracic defects, 607–608
twins diagnosis, 613
umbilical cord anomalies, 612
thyroid gland evaluations, 1996
vesicoureteral reflux evaluations, 2338–2339, 2339f
Umbilical anomalies
embryonic umbilical remnants, 2506f, 2605–2606
granulomas, 2606–2607
hernia, 2606, 2606t
polyps, 2607
of position and morphology, 2604–2605, 2605t
vascular, 2606
Umbilical cord
blood gas analysis
medical-legal issues and, 746
neonatal assessment, 664–665
care of
home care, in healthy newborn, 844
post-delivery procedures, 805
defects
placental health and, 632
ultrasound detection of, 612
description of, 2604
newborn assessment, 767–768
Umbilical hernia, 133, 767
Umbilical line complications, 749
Umbilical stump, 132–133
Umbilicus, 133
Umbo, 121, 121f
Unclassified seizures, 2489b, 2492–2494, 2493b
Unconjugated bilirubin, 1616, 1617
Underbite, 125
Underinsurance, 6
Unexplained adrenal insufficiency, 1812
Uninsured children, 23
Unintended pregnancy, 1342, 1351
Unintentional injuries, 239
United States Congress Office of Technology Assessment, 312
United States Department of Health and Human Services, 312
United States Preventive Services Task Force, 281
Universal Newborn Hearing, Screening, Diagnosis, and Intervention, 326, 328f
Unmarried mothers, 236, 237t
Unsaturated fatty acids, 225
Up to Date, 35t, 39t
Upper airway hemorrhage, 1573t
Upper gastrointestinal tract
barium study of, 1465
bleeding in, 1544, 1546b, 1547–1548
radiography of, 2058
Upper respiratory infections
acute, 323t
allergic rhinitis confused with, 1820
general anesthesia and, 521–522, 521b, 523f
Upper-body strength, 192
Urachal cyst, 2605
Urachal fistula, 2605, 2606
Urachal sinus, 2605
Urban minority communities, 273
Urea-cycle defects, 985–986
Ureaplasma infection, 935

Page numbers followed by "f" denote figures; "t" denote tables; "b" *denote* boxes.

Ureterocele, 2335, 2335f
Ureteropelvic junction obstruction, 2334, 2334f
Ureterovesical junction obstruction, 2334, 2334f
Urethral gonococcal infection, 2513b
Urethral meatus warts, 2516b
Urethral prolapse, 1477
Urethral strictures, 1477
Urethritis
- in *Chlamydia* infection, 2510
- dysuria caused by, 1477
- in *Mycoplasma genitalium* infection, 2528

Urinalysis, 404–408, 2610–2611. *See also* Urine screening
Urinary tract
- description of, 1373
- obstructions, 1375
- pain, 1474. *See also* Dysuria
- review of systems for, 92b

Urinary tract infections
- breastfeeding and, 810
- circumcision and, 829, 2609, 2613
- complications of, 2614
- diagnosis of, 2612b
- dysuria caused by, 1477
- empirical therapy for, 506t
- etiology of, 2607–2609
- evaluation of, 2609–2611, 2610b, 2612b
- folk illness remedies associated with, 66t
- hematuria and, 1566, 1568f, 1569
- hospitalization for, 2614
- imaging studies in, 2611–2612, 2612b
- incidence of, 2607, 2608t
- long-term effects of, 2614
- macroscopic hematuria and, 1567f
- obstructive uropathy and, 2333
- pathogens in, 2607–2609, 2608t
- prevention of, 810
- recurrent, 1696
- referrals for, 2614
- treatment of, 2612b, 2612–2613, 2613t

Urine
- alkalinization of, 2770
- blood or color change in. *See* Hematuria
- collection of, 2610
- culture of, 2610
- drug screening, for substance use disorders evaluation, 401–402
- leukocytes in, 2610–2611
- nitrogen excretion in, 220
- normal output, 1670t
- odor of. *See also* Polyuria
  - causes of, 1661–1665, 1662t–1665t
  - differential diagnosis of, 1660
  - physical examination of, 1661
- postoperative retention of, 560
- protein excretion and. *See* Proteinuria
- protein-creatinine ratio, 1676–1677
- retention of, 66t, 560
- testing of, 2610–2611

Urine—cont'd
- water loss in, 225

Urine output, in acute renal failure, 2798–2799
Urine screening
- bacteriuria evaluations, 406–407
- glucosuria evaluations, 406
- hematuria evaluations, 405–406
- proteinuria evaluations, 405

Urogenital system
- fetal assessment, 649
- in infants of diabetic mothers, 891

Uropathies, obstructive, 2333–2338
Urticaria
- description of, 1690f, 2028
- papular, 2180–2181
- pruritus and, 1682

US Food and Drug Administration, 1177
Users' Guides to the Medical Literature, 41
Utah Growth Study, 1727, 1728
Uterine bleeding, 1768b
Uterine contractility, 811
Uterine size, 643
Uterocele, 611
Uterus
- in adolescents, 137
- palpation of, 136–137

Utilization review, 17
UTIs. *See* Urinary tract infections
Uvula, bifid, 126, 126f

V

Vaccinations
- acellular pertussis, 2423b
- adolescents, 246f
- anaphylactic allergy caused by, 248
- benefits of, 244
- childhood, 245f
- conjugate, 2254, 2255t
- contraindications, 247–250
- diphtheria, tetanus, and pertussis
  - in adolescents, 246f
  - adverse reactions to, 252
  - catch-up schedule for, 250t
  - characteristics of, 252
  - contraindications, 252
  - guidelines for, 245f
- in foreign countries, 247
- 4-week separation rule for, 244
- *Haemophilus influenza* type b
  - adverse effects of, 254
  - catch-up schedule for, 251t
  - characteristics of, 253–254
  - contraindications, 254
  - guidelines for, 245f
  - intervals between doses, 248t
  - minimum age for, 248t
  - schedule for, 254t
- hepatitis A
  - in adolescents, 246f
  - characteristics of, 252
  - contraindications, 252
  - guidelines for, 245f

Vaccinations—cont'd
- hepatitis B
  - in adolescents, 246f
  - catch-up schedule for, 250t–251t
  - characteristics of, 252t–253t
  - combinations, 253
  - contraindications, 253
  - guidelines for, 245f
  - health infants, 806
  - intervals between doses, 248t
  - in low-birth-weight infants, 253
  - minimum age for, 248t
  - NICU-discharged infants, 718
  - in perinatal period, 806–807
  - premature infants, 704, 838
- human papillomavirus
  - in adolescents, 246f
  - interval between doses, 249t
  - minimum age for, 249t
- in ill children, 248–249
- in immunocompromised children, 249–250
- inactivated polio virus
  - in adolescents, 246f
  - catch-up schedule for, 250t
  - characteristics of, 257
  - intervals between doses, 248t
  - minimum age for, 248t
- inactivated vaccines, 244
- influenza vaccine
  - administration of, 254–255
  - in adolescents, 246f
  - adverse effects of, 255
  - characteristics of, 254–255
  - contraindications, 255
  - guidelines for, 245f
  - interval between doses, 248t
  - minimum age for, 248t
  - NICU-discharged infants, 718
  - premature infants, 704
- intervals between, 247, 248t
- irritability and, 1613
- live injected, 247
- live vaccines
  - contraindications, 250
  - description of, 244
- Lyme disease, 2251
- measles, mumps, rubella
  - administration of, 255
  - in adolescents, 246f
  - adverse reactions to, 255
  - catch-up schedule for, 250t–251t
  - characteristics of, 255–256
  - contraindications, 255–256
  - guidelines for, 245f
  - before immune globulin-containing products, 247
  - in immunocompromised patients, 250
  - intervals between doses, 248t
  - minimum age for, 248t
- meningococcal polysaccharide
  - in adolescents, 246f
  - description of, 2752

Vaccinations—cont'd
meningococcal polysaccharide—cont'd
guidelines for, 245f
interval between doses, 248t
minimum age for, 248t
pneumococcal
in adolescents, 246f
catch-up schedule for, 251t
characteristics of, 256
conjugated, 256
guidelines for, 245f
intervals between doses, 248t
minimum age for, 248t
polysaccharide, 256–257, 257t
schedule for, 251t, 256t
precautions for, 247–250
during pregnancy, 250
in preterm infants, 250
principles of, 244–252
recommended, 244, 245f–246f
rotavirus vaccine
adverse reactions to, 257–258
characteristics of, 257–258
contraindications, 257
guidelines for, 245f
interval between doses, 249t
minimum age for, 248t
NICU-discharged infants, 718
premature infants, 704–705
safety concerns, 250, 252
schedule for
catch-up, 250t–251t
recommended, 244, 245f–246f, 247
simultaneous administration of, 244, 247
varicella
in adolescents, 246f
in HIV-infected children, 2143
catch-up schedule for, 250t
guidelines for, 245f
before immune globulin-containing products, 247
in immunocompromised patients, 250
VACTERL complex, 671, 2545, 2547–2548
Vagal nerve stimulation, 2502
Vagina
digital examination of, 136
embryologic development of, 134
inspection of, 136, 136f
odor of, 1661
Vaginal birth after cesarean
American College of Obstetrics and Gynecology recommendations, 82
risks associated with, 82
Vaginal bleeding
causes of, 1768b
diagnostic testing for, 1769
evaluation of, 1767–1768
history-taking, 1768–1769
management of, 1769–1770
physical examination for, 1769
in prepubertal girls, 1767
in pubertal girls, 1767–1770
Vaginal contraceptive ring, 1354
Vaginal discharge
causes of, 1771b, 1772t–1773t
evaluation of, 1771–1773
management of, 1773–1775
in newborns, 1771
in prepubertal girls, 1771, 1771b
in pubertal and postpubertal girls, 1772t–1773t, 1774–1775
Vaginal warts, 2516b, 2523
Vaginitis
description of, 2531–2532
vaginal bleeding and, 1767, 1769
vaginal discharge and, 1772, 1774
Vaginoscope, 136, 136f
Vaginosis, bacterial, 2531
Valacyclovir
genital herpes simplex treated with, 2516b, 2517b
indications for, 512t
Valerian
preoperative discontinuation of, 542t
uses of, 458t
Valgus, 1529b, 1531f
Validity, 39, 41b
Valproic acid, 2498t, 2500
Valve, 2150
Vancomycin
bacterial resistance to, 504
dosage, peak serum concentrations, and MIC_{95} for, 494t
mechanism of action of, 504
pharmacologic properties of, 504
septic arthritis treated with, 2507–2508
side effects of, 504–505
use of, 505
Vanderbilt ADHD Diagnostic Parent Rating Scale, 1168
Varicella pneumonia, 1914
Varicella zoster. *See also* Chickenpox
breastfeeding and, 812
conjunctivitis and, 1713
immunoglobulin, 1916, 2142
meningoencephalitis caused by, 2269, 2269f
neonatal skin infections, 786
perinatal infection, 934
rash, 1691f
recurrent infections and, 1696
streptococcal TSS and, 2573, 2576
vaccine for
in adolescents, 246f
in HIV-infected children, 2143
catch-up schedule for, 250t
guidelines for, 245f
before immune globulin-containing products, 247
in immunocompromised patients, 250
Varicocele, 1723
Varus, 1529b, 1531f
Vascular abnormalities
in airways obstruction, 2636–2637
imaging of, 1793f
of umbilical cord, 2626
Vascular birthmarks, 780–781
Vascular congestion, 1577
Vascular disease
hemoptysis and, 1573
macroscopic hematuria and, 1567f
Vascular lesions, 1546, 1826
Vascular malformations, 781
Vascular pulmonary disease, 1470
Vascular system, 2311
Vasculitis. *See also* Henoch-Schönlein purpura
in Churg-Strauss syndrome, 1848
drug eruptions, 1827
gastrointestinal bleeding caused by, 1545
in oliguria patients, 1827
Vasodepressor reactions, 2644
Vasodepressor syncope, 1753
Vasodilators, 1587t, 1588t
Vasomotor function, 953
Vasomotor rhinitis, 1820
Vasoocclusion, 535
Vasopressin, 1670–1671, 1673t, 2043
Vasopressors
anaphylaxis treated with, 2645
shock treated with, 2810–2811
Vasovagal syncope, 1753
VATER syndrome, 2545
Vaulting gait, 1630
VCUG. *See* Voiding cystourethrogram
Vecuronium, 2743
Vegetable proteins, 222–223
Vegetative state, 2639
Vellus hair, 1590
Velocardiofacial syndrome, 2189t
Velocity growth curves, 110, 115f
Venn diagram, 41f
Venom, 2686
Venous hum, 131
Venous hypertension, 1480
Venous thromboembolism
description of, 1353
edema caused by, 1481
postoperative, 561, 561b
Ventilator therapy
home ventilation, NICU-discharged infants, 714–715
neonatal airway stabilization, 676–677
positive pressure ventilation, 657–658
Ventricular catheter, 2149–2150
Ventricular septal defect
clinical manifestations of, 1940
evaluation of, 1940–1941, 1941f, 1942f
management of, 1941
murmur with, 917–918
prognosis of, 1941–1942
ultrasound detection of, 608–610
volume overload, 926
Ventricular tachycardia
description of, 1417, 1417f
in newborn, 920, 923
syncope and, 1755
Ventriculomegaly
antenatal identification of, 776
ultrasound detection of, 605–606

Page numbers followed by "f" denote figures; "t" denote tables; "b" *denote* boxes.

Vermiform, 1836
Vernal conjunctivitis, 1716, 1716f
Vernix caseosa, 114
Verrucae. *See* Warts
Version, 1529b
Vertebrae
embryonic development of, 2545
thoracic, 2353b, 2354
Vertebral malformations
in Goldenhar syndrome, 2547
in kyphosis, 2546–2549
in Larsen syndrome, 2547
in Morquio syndrome, 2547
newborn assessment, 769–771
in scoliosis, 2545–2546, 2548
in spina bifida, 2539, 2547
in VACTERL complex, 2547–2548
Vertical strabismus, 1733, 1738
Vertical talus, 1535
Vertigo
benign paroxysmal, 1658
causes of, 1457
definition of, 1457
diagnosis of, 1460t
evaluation of, 1459
management of, 1459–1460
referrals and, 1460
Very low–birth-weight infants
early intervention for, 860
growth outcomes in, 857
health outcomes in
description of, 852–863
neurodevelopmental outcomes in, 856
school-aged outcomes, 855–856
infection risk in, 928–929
longitudinal growth in, 690–691
retinopathy of prematurity in, 757
transition to adulthood for, 858–861
Vesicles, 1689–1690, 1691f–1692f
Vesicoureteral reflex
definition of, 2338
description of, 150, 2611, 2611b
differential diagnosis of, 2338
epidemiological features of, 2338
evaluation of, 2338–2340, 2339f–2340f, 2339t
incidence of, 2338
management of, 2340–2341, 2341t
on nuclear cystogram, 2339, 2340f
prevalence of, 2338
on ^{99m}Tc dimercaptosuccinic acid renal scan, 2339–2340, 2340f
ultrasound in, 2338–2339, 2339f
voiding cystourethrogram in, 2338–2339, 2339f
Vesiculopustular diseases, 783–785
Video games, 190
Videofluorographic swallowing study, 1465–1466
Videostroboscopy, 1600
Videotaping, 1270, 1298, 1465–1466
Vincristine, 1875
Vineland Adaptive Behavior Scales, 2185
Violence
in adolescents, 274–275
dating, 1076–1077, 1079
domestic
assessment of, 1077–1078
breaking cycle of, 1080
child abuse and, 1075
dating violence, 1076–1077
definition of, 1074–1075
detection of, 1079
health care system and, 1075–1076
statistics regarding, 1074–1075
treatment of, 1079–1080
victims
assistance for, 1078–1079
identification of, 1076
witnessing of, 272
experiences with, 275, 275b
gay, lesbian, and bisexual youth and, 1363
history of, 275, 275b
intimate partner, 369
as learned behavior, 272
media exposure to, 1115
parenting free of, 273
peer, 272
prevention of, 272–278
advocacy in, 276–277
anticipatory guidance in, 273
bullying prevention in, 274
after a fight, 276
violence-free parenting in, 273
in school-age children, 274
in schools, 1126
screening for, 275, 276f
sexual, 275, 275b
television, 272–273
transgender youth and, 1235, 1236
understanding of, 272
in urban minority communities, 273
witnessing of
domestic violence, 272
television violence, 272–273
Viral croup, 1748, 1749t
Viral hepatitis. *See* Hepatitis
Viral infections
antimicrobial therapy for, 509–514, 510t–512t
croup, 2636t, 2647–2653
fever caused by, 1517, 1522, 1525, 1526b
gastroenteritis, 2655
hematuria and, 1567f, 1568
hemoptysis caused by, 1571
joint pain and, 1627
lymphadenopathy caused by, 1641t
neonatal skin infections, 785–786
splenomegaly and, 1731
in stomatitis, 2569, 2570
in urinary tract, 2608
Viral laryngitis, 1601–1602
Virilization, 1590–1591, 1803
Virus(es)
adenovirus
description of, 1981
Virus(es)—cont'd
adenovirus—cont'd
pertussis vs., 2420
pharyngitis caused by, 2425b, 2426
arboviruses, 2268
coronavirus, 2648
coxsackievirus, 2036, 2268, 2268f
cytomegalovirus
breastfeeding and, 812–813
congenital infection, 929–930
maternal-fetal infection, 635–636
enterovirus
acute hemorrhagic conjunctivitis, 2036
aseptic meningitis. *See* Aseptic meningitis
classification of, 2032, 2033t
clinical syndromes, 2034, 2036t, 2036–2037
encephalitis, 2037
enteroviral disease, 2037
epidemiology of, 2032–2033
exanthem diseases, 2036
gastrointestinal diseases, 2036
laboratory procedures for, 2037–2038
meningoencephalitis caused by, 2037, 2268, 2268f
molecular genetic analysis for, 2038
myocarditis, 2037
nonspecific febrile illness, 2034
orchitis, 2037
paralytic disease, 2036–2037
parechovirus infections, 2037
parotitis, 2037
pathogenesis of, 2033–2034
pericarditis, 2037
perinatal period, 934–935
pharyngitis caused by, 2425b, 2426
prevention of, 2039
rapid virus identification for, 2038
referrals for, 2039
respiratory tract disease, 2034, 2036
serological diagnosis of, 2038
treatment of, 2038–2039
virus isolation, 2038
Epstein-Barr
chronic fatigue syndrome and, 2178
description of, 1511, 1965
malignancy and, 2178–2179
negative infectious mononucleosis, 2178
pharyngitis caused by, 2425b, 2426
prevalence of, 2175
serologic findings in, 2175–2177, 2176f, 2177t
herpes simplex
breastfeeding and, 812–813
conjunctivitis caused by, 1705
definitions, 2129–2130
description of, 1692f
epidemiologic factors, 2130
genital, 2516b–2517b, 2524–2527, 2527f
maternal-fetal infection, 636

Virus(es)—cont'd
herpes simplex—cont'd
meningoencephalitis caused by, 2268
neonatal, 785–786, 2131–2132
ocular herpes, 2130
perinatal period, 934
pharyngitis caused by, 2425b, 2426
referrals for, 2133
stomatitis, 125, 2571, 2571f
treatment of, 2132–2133, 2133b
type 1, 2130–2131
type 2, 2131
human papillomavirus. *See* Human papillomavirus
parainfluenza, 1981, 2648–2649
parechovirus, 2037
parvovirus B19, 932
respiratory syncytial
in croup, 2648, 2649
description of, 1865, 1865f, 1981
in-hospital prophylaxis, 705
neonatal sepsis, 936–937
pertussis vs., 2420
prophylaxis in NICU-discharged infants, 718
rotavirus, vaccine for
adverse reactions to, 257–258
characteristics of, 257–258
contraindications, 257
guidelines for, 245f
interval between doses, 249t
minimum age for, 248t
for NICU-discharged infants, 718
in premature infants, 704–705
West Nile
meningoencephalitis caused by, 2268
neonatal infection, 937
Virus isolation, 2038
Visceral leishmaniasis, 2367
Vision disorders, 1560
Vision loss, 1777
Vision screening
in adolescents, 344–345
benefits of, 343–344
description of, 1779f, 1779–1782
equipment for, 345
goals of, 344
improvements in, 345
in infants, 344
ocular trauma evaluations using, 2344
personnel for, 345
in preschoolers, 344
referral for, 345
in school-age children, 344–345
in toddlers, 344
tools for, 344
Visitation rights in foster care, 1064
Visits
advice given during, 202
agenda discussed during, 201–202
concerns discussed during, 201–202
health supervision, 50
parent-child arguments during, 205
planned, 46
Visits—cont'd
preventive services, 48–49
statistics regarding, 6, 9, 11t
topics discussed during, 201–202
Visual acuity
in children, 120
development of, 1776, 1776f, 1776t
in newborns, 119
referral criteria, 1780, 1782
testing for, 1779–1782
Visual development
amblyopia in, 1776–1779, 1779b
fixation in, 1776t
milestones in, 1776, 1776f
normal, 1775
referral for, 1782
visual acuity in, 1776t, 1777f
Visual fixation, 1776
Visual function
breastfeeding and enhancement of, 811
in premature infants, 857
Visual testing
preverbal children and, 1779, 1779f
verbal children and, 1779f
Vital signs
by age, 2802t
blood pressure. *See* Blood pressure
physical examination of, 104–108
pulse, 104–105, 106t, 2719
Vital statistics, 235t
Vitamin(s)
A, 228t
B_6, 229t
B_{12}
deficiency of, 217
vegetarian supplementation with, 231
characteristics of, 228t–229t
D, 217, 226
deficiencies of
description of, 226
maternal health and, 627–629
vitamin K deficiency, 944
in human milk, 214t
in infant formulas, 214t
K
deficiency, 944
deficiency of, 216
hemostatic disorders, 944–945
prophylaxis, in post-delivery period, 802
supplementation of, 216–217
purpose of, 226
Vitelline cyst, 2605, 2606
Vitelline fistula, 2605
Vocal cords
cyst of, 1749t
dysfunction of, 2637
paralysis of
description of, 2634
hoarseness and, 1599, 1601
stridor caused by, 1749t
Vocal tics, 1758
Vocational training, 2020, 2023
Voiding cystourethrogram
description of, 150f, 2611, 2612b
obstructive uropathy evaluations, 2336
vesicoureteral reflux evaluations, 2338–2339, 2339f
Volume depletion. *See* Dehydration
Volume expansion, 1757
Volume overload, 926
Volvulus, 2076–2077, 2626–2627, 2627f
Vomiting
in appendicitis, 1837
in brain tumors, 1861, 1862b
causes of, 1783–1784, 1784b
complications with, 1785
in cow's milk protein allergy, 2065b
cyclic vomiting syndrome, 2057
definition of, 1783
differential diagnosis of, 1783–1784
evaluation of, 1784–1785
failure to thrive diagnosis and, 1505
in gastroesophageal reflux disease, 2054f, 2055b–2056b
in gastrointestinal obstruction, 2071, 2074
in giardiasis, 2086
in gluten-sensitive enteropathy, 2090b
in hydrocephalus, 2148t
management of, 598
nausea and. *See* Postoperative nausea and vomiting
referral for, 1785
treatment of, 1785
weight loss and, 1787
von Hippel-Lindau disease
central nervous system hemangioblastomas in, 2315
classification of, 2315, 2315t
description of, 1816
differential diagnosis of, 2316, 2316t
evaluation of, 2316
management of, 2316–2317
pheochromocytomas in, 2315–2316, 2315t
prevalence of, 2314–2315
retinal hemangioblastomas in, 2315, 2315t
von Recklinghausen disease, 2304–2308. *See also* Neurofibromatosis, type 1
von Willebrand disease
anesthesia and, 537
description of, 944, 1484, 2110–2111
petechiae and purpura caused by, 1668
Voriconazole, 513t
Vulnerable child syndrome
assisted reproductive technologies and, 625
description of, 77, 1148
in neonatal intensive care infants, 853
Vulva
genital warts on, 2523, 2525f
of infant, 135f

Page numbers followed by "f" denote figures; "t" denote tables; "b" *denote* boxes.

Vulvar vestibule, 136
Vulvitis, 1767
Vulvovaginal infections, 1767
Vulvovaginitis, 1477
VX (nerve agent), 2779

W

Waardenburg syndrome, 763
Waddell test, 1407
Waddling gaits, 1630
Warfarin, 2768t
Warfarin-like rodenticides, 2784
Warts
  complications, 2618
  differential diagnosis, 2616
  epidemiology, 2616–2617
  eradication of, 453b
  etiology, 2615
  flat, 2616, 2626f
  genital
    description of, 2522–2524
    morphology of, 2525f, 2616, 2616f
    subclinical lesions, 2524f
    treatment of, 2514b–2516b, 2523, 2618
  laboratory findings, 2615
  periungual, 2616
  physical findings, 2615
  plantar, 2616, 2626f
  prognosis, 2618
  psychosocial considerations, 2617
  treatment, 2617–2618
Wasp stings, 2687–2689
Water
  daily loss of, 225
  fluoridation of, 294
  insensible loss of, 225
  maintenance requirements for, 471–472, 471f, 472t
  urinary loss of, 225
Water intoxication, 1672
Water-soluble vitamins, 217
WBC count. *See* White blood cell count
Weakness, 1512. *See also* Fatigue; Hypotonia
  definition and etiology of, 1509
  diagnostic testing for, 1514
  differential diagnosis of, 1510b
Weaning, 218
Web-based resources, 34, 35t
Weber test, 122
Wegener granulomatosis, 1571, 1574, 1827
Weight
  birth
    infant mortality and, correlation between, 238
    newborn assessment and, 758–760
    statistics regarding, [illegible]
  control of, 124[illegible]
  goals for, 23[illegible]
  hypertension [illegible]
    1581[illegible]
Weight gain. *See also* Failure to thrive
  breastfeeding and, 810–811, 817–818
  causes of, 2321
  follow-up care for healthy newborn and, 850
  healthy, 1501–1503
  large-for-gestational-age infants, 888
  premature infant growth and development, 690–696
Weight loss. *See also* Eating disorders
  admission for, 1789
  in adolescents, 1788, 1789
  attention deficit/hyperactivity disorder and, 1212t
  diagnostic testing for, 1788, 1789t
  differential diagnosis of, 1787b
  in infants, 1786–1787
  initial evaluation of, 1788–1789
  maternal, breastfeeding and, 811
  in newborns, 1786–1789
  parenting skills in, 2327b, 2328
  psychiatric causes for, 1188
  referral for, 1789
Weight measurements, 111
Weight training, 192
Well-balanced diet, 231
Well-being, 15
Well-child visits
  4 month, 1157–1159
  6 month, 1159, 1316
  12 month, 1159–1160, 1316
Well-seeming infants
  neonatal assessment, 672–673
  neonatal intensive care, 667
  underlying disorders in, 670
  warning signs, 672
Werdnig-Hoffman disease, 126
West Nile virus
  meningoencephalitis caused by, 2268
  neonatal infection, 937
West syndrome, 2489b, 2490
Wheals, 1689, 1690f
Wheelchair, 579
Wheezing
  causes of, 1792t
  definition of, 1790
  description of, 129, 2632
  diagnostic testing for, 1792f–1796f, 1793–1796
  differential diagnosis of, 1791
  management of, 1796–1797
  patient history for, 1791–1793
  physical examination for, 1793
Whiplash injury, 2713
White blood cell count
  by age, 2802t
  pharyngitis diagnosis using, 2428
Whiteheads, 1803
White's classification of diabetes during pregnancy, 888
[illegible]HO. *See* World Health Organization
[illegible]hole-bowel irrigation
  [illegible]for drug overdose, 2683
  [illegible]or poisoning, 2769
Whooping cough, 2419–2425. *See also* Pertussis
Williams syndrome
  anesthesia and, 527
  features of, 2189t
Wilms tumor
  abdominal tumors vs., 1874t
  clinical manifestations, 1874
  description of, 1374f
  differential diagnosis of, 1874t
  etiology, 1873–1874
  evaluation of, 1874–1875
  follow-up, 1876
  management of, 1875–1876
  pelvic tumors vs., 1874t
  prognosis, 1876
  staging, 1875b
Wilson disease, 1620
Wiskott-Aldrich syndrome, 1698, 2011, 2013
Witch hazel, 458t
Witch's milk, 128
Withdrawal reflex, 141f
Wolff-Parkinson-White syndrome, 918–919
Wolman disease, 1812
Woman Abuse Screening Tool, 369
Women, Infants, and Children, 230–231, 711–712
Woodruff plexus, 1482
World Health Organization
  classification of tumors, 1861
  health as defined by, 48
  Healthy Schools initiative, 1122
  polio eradication efforts, 2038
Wound
  animal bites, 1823–1824
  medications for, 2824–2825
  postsurgical, 561–562
Wound healing, 561–562
Wound infection, 66t, 558, 559t, 561
Wound membranes, 2824–2825, 2826b
Wrist, 2554

X

X-linked adrenoleukodystrophy, 1812

Y

Yeast infections, 786
Yellow jacket stings, 2687–2689
Yoga, 192, 195
Youth empowerment, 1132
Youth Risk Behavior Survey, 1340

Z

Zanamivir, 512t
Zellweger syndrome, 1812
Zinc protoporphyrin, 2207, 2207t
Zonisamide, 2499t, 2502